# CONTENTS

# Illustrated CHURCHILL'S MEDICAL DICTIONARY

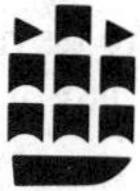

CHURCHILL LIVINGSTONE
New York, Edinburgh, London, Melbourne, Tokyo

**Library of Congress Cataloging-in-Publication Data**

Churchill's illustrated medical dictionary.

1. Medicine—Dictionaries. I. Title: Churchill's medical dictionary. [DNLM: 1. Dictionaries, Medical. W 13 C5632]
R121.I58 1989 610′.3′21 89-801

0-443-08691-5


Distributed in the United Kingdom by Churchill Livingstone, Robert Stevenson House, 1–3 Baxter's Place, Leith Walk, Edinburgh EH1 3AF, and by associated companies, branches, and representatives throughout the world.



*Cover design by Paul Moran*
*Production Assistant:* Christina Hippeli

Printed in the United States of America

First published in 1989

Third printing in 1991

# EDITOR'S PREFACE

*Churchill's Medical Dictionary* is the first entirely new, one-volume medical dictionary to be published in the United States since the early 1900's. There are about 100,000 entries in *CMD*, extracted from a database that was compiled over a ten-year period, using original definitions supplied by a distinguished group of medical authorities. The terms included represent over 63 subjects in the clinical specialties and in basic sciences related to medicine, with extensive coverage given to the vocabulary that has emerged from medical research, advanced diagnostic technology, and innovations in health care.

Our computerized database, consisting in its entirety of over 151,000 entries, also formed the basis of the three-volume *International Dictionary of Medicine and Biology* (*IDMB*), published in 1986. Among the features being introduced for this volume are pronunciations (over 32,000 of them) and original illustrations by Neil O. Hardy, especially commissioned for *CMD*. Those features of *IDMB* that were recognized as outstanding, such as its coverage of international usage, have been retained. These are described in *A Guide to the Use of This Dictionary* (p. xix).

In the three years since publication of *IDMB*, new advances in medicine have been reflected in the continuous updating of definitions and the addition of new terms. Many improvements were made during that time, some suggested by *IDMB* readers and some whose usefulness became apparent to the dictionary staff as we worked our way through the database.

*Churchill's Medical Dictionary* is intended for the use of all who are involved in the health professions, be they physicians, nurses, allied health professionals, medical students, researchers, science writers, or support staff, as well as for the educated lay public. The editors have been ever mindful of the ways in which a dictionary should serve those readers. The primary consideration, of course, has been the preciseness, scope, and currency of its definitions.

In a sense, much of the vocabulary of medicine is intended to be self-defining. Given an inventory of combining forms and affixes based on Greek roots (*cardio-*, *dys-*, *-itis*, *-opia*, etc.), any number of general concepts can be named. When preceded by strings of carefully defined modifiers, such as *chronic*, *progressive*, or *idiopathic*, the opportunities for coinage are limitless. Various nomenclature committees within the world medical community regularly review such terms, discouraging the use of any component that might be misleading. Often, however, custom prevails over scientific logic; a fact that at least makes dictionaries more interesting.

Furthermore, for many medical definitions the traditional scheme of "genus and differentia" is inadequate. The "meaning" of something as complex as *acquired immune deficiency syndrome* (*AIDS*) cannot be explicated in such a concise fashion. (This is among 1260 entries to be found under the heading *syndrome*, and at that heading the reader will find a brief discussion of the way a particular entity comes to be called a syndrome.) The task of any dictionary, medical or otherwise, is to provide all manner of information about language: spelling, notation conventions, synonyms, pronunciation, word origins (including biograph-

ical data for eponymous terms), and the like, and in those areas we have made a special effort to be helpful.

One common use of a dictionary is to resolve uncertainties of usage. A reader wishing to know, for example, whether to use a capital or lower-case *G* in the term "Gram-positive," will, in consulting most medical dictionaries, find one or the other and may conclude that the one not found is wrong. But it can be even more valuable for the reader to be assured that he or she is not necessarily wrong; that a particular usage is in dispute among experts or may be favored in a particular country, discipline, or context. *CMD* contains over 750 usage notes, many of which provide just such clarification.

Much welcome assistance has been provided in putting together this volume. We would like to express our special gratitude to Dr. H. B. F. Dixon of the University of Cambridge Department of Biochemistry for preparing the diagrams of the tricarboxylic acid cycle and the Embden-Meyerhof pathway; to Dr. Virgil F. Fairbanks of the Mayo Clinic for his diagram of the coagulation cascade, and for supplying data for blood, serum, and plasma for the Table of Normal Ranges; to Dr. Jane T. Gaede of the Durham Veterans Administration Medical Center and Duke University Medical Center for supplying urinalysis data for the Table of Normal Ranges; and to Dr. Reed E. Pyeritz of The Johns Hopkins University School of Medicine for his diagram illustrating mendelian inheritance.

Space does not permit a listing of all those contributors who assisted our Advisory Editors in the preparation of definitions, nor of the many individuals who devoted so much time and care to developing the database or adapting it for producing *CMD*. Certain contributions, however, have been so central to the success of this undertaking that they cannot go unacknowledged. Our most lasting debt is to Sidney I. Landau, Editor-in-Chief of *IDMB*, who conceived the plan for the abridgement. His support and encouragement made the entire project less daunting, and his expertise as a highly regarded lexicographer has continued to inform our editorial judgment.

Special recognition is also due to my colleague, Mark Cowell, who wrote a new, expanded introductory section on etymologies, and whose scholarship and uncompromising dedication to accuracy has greatly enhanced the quality of this dictionary.

It is the hope of all of those involved in the preparation of *CMD* that it will become an essential tool for everyone who needs to consult a comprehensive and authoritative reference for medical terminology.

RUTH KOENIGSBERG
*Managing Editor*

# EDITORIAL BOARD, PANEL ON INTERNATIONAL USAGE, AND EDITORIAL STAFF

## EDITORIAL BOARD



## PANEL ON INTERNATIONAL USAGE



† Deceased

## EDITORIAL STAFF

# ADVISORY EDITORS AND CO-ADVISORY EDITORS BY SUBJECT

*Advisory Editors* have primary responsibility for the vocabulary and definitions within their specialties. A few subjects have two or more equivalent Advisory Editors who share equally the responsibility for their subject. Some Advisory Editors have been assisted by other experts who have made very substantial contributions to the body of definitions in their field. The latter are designated *Co-Advisory Editors*.

## ANATOMY

*Advisory Editor*
**Ronald Singer, MB, ChB, DSc**
The Robert R. Bensley Professor in Biology and Medical Sciences
Professor of Anatomy and Anthropology
University of Chicago
Chicago, Illinois

## ANESTHESIOLOGY

*Advisory Editor*
**Leroy D. Vandam, PhB, MD**
Professor of Anaesthesia, Emeritus
Harvard Medical School
Anaesthesiologist
Brigham and Women's Hospital
Boston, Massachusetts

## ANTHROPOLOGY

*Advisory Editor*
**Michael H. Day, MB, BS, DSc, PhD, LRCP, MRCS**
Professor of Anatomy
United Medical and Dental Schools of Guy's and St. Thomas's Hospitals
University of London
London, England

## BIOCHEMISTRY

*Advisory Editor*
**Sir Hans Kornberg, MA, DSc, ScD, PhD, FRS**
Sir William Dunn Professor of Biochemistry
Head of Biochemistry Department
University of Cambridge
Master, Christ's College
Cambridge, England

*Advisory Editor*
**H. B. F. Dixon, ScD**
Department of Biochemistry
University of Cambridge
Cambridge, England

## BIOMEDICAL ENGINEERING

*Advisory Editor*
**John G. Webster, PhD**
Professor of Electrical and Computer Engineering
University of Wisconsin-Madison
Madison, Wisconsin

## CARDIOTHORACIC SURGERY

*Advisory Editor*
**Paul A. Ebert, MD**
Director
American College of Surgeons
Chicago, Illinois

## CARDIOVASCULAR DISEASE

*Advisory Editor*
**Desmond G. Julian, MD, FRCP**
Medical Director
British Heart Foundation
London, England

## CELL BIOLOGY

*Advisory Editor*
**Lawrence D. Koehler, PhD**
Professor of Biology
Chairman, Department of Biology
Central Michigan University
Mt. Pleasant, Michigan

## DENTISTRY

*Advisory Editor*
**R. D. Emslie, MS (Ill.), BDS (Lond.), FDS, RCS (Eng.), DRDRCS (Edin.)**
Professor Emeritus of Periodontology and Preventive Dentistry
University of London
(Formerly) Dean of Dental Studies
Guy's Hospital Dental School
London, England

*Co-Advisory Editor*
**D. W. Macfarlane, LDS, RCS (Eng.)**
(Formerly) Lecturer
Department of Periodontology and Preventive Dentistry
Guy's Hospital Medical and Dental Schools
London, England

## DERMATOLOGY

*Advisory Editor*
**Arthur Rook, MA, MD, FRCP**
Honorary Consultant Dermatologist
Addenbrooke's Hospital
Cambridge, England

## ELECTRON MICROSCOPY

*Advisory Editor*
**David R. Turner, MB, PhD, FRCPath**
Professor of Pathology
Nottingham University Medical School
Nottingham, England

## EMBRYOLOGY

*Advisory Editor*
**Sir Richard Harrison, FRS, MD, DSc**
Emeritus Professor of Anatomy
University of Cambridge
Honorary Fellow, Downing College
Cambridge, England

*Co-Advisory Editor*
**M. H. Kaufman, MB, ChB, PhD, MA, DSc**
Professor of Anatomy
Universal Medical School
University of Edinburgh
Edinburgh, Scotland

## ENDOCRINOLOGY

*Advisory Editor*
**Nicholas P. Christy, MD**
Professor Emeritus
The Health Science Center at Brooklyn, SUNY
Senior Lecturer in Medicine
College of Physicians and Surgeons
Columbia University
Writer in Residence
Attending Physician, Medicine
The Presbyterian Hospital
New York, New York

## ENTOMOLOGY

*Advisory Editor*
**Donald Heyneman, PhD**
Professor of Parasitology
Department of Epidemiology and International Health
University of California at San Francisco
San Francisco, California

## ENVIRONMENTAL HEALTH

*Advisory Editor*
**Alec E. Martin, MD, DPH**
(Formerly) Principal Medical Officer
Department of Health and Social Security
Medical Advisor, Department of the Environment
London, England

## FORENSIC MEDICINE

*Advisory Editor*
**Bert F. Morton, MD**
Senior Attending Pathologist
St. Agnes Hospital
Baltimore, Maryland

## GASTROENTEROLOGY

*Advisory Editor*
**Marvin H. Sleisenger, MD, MACP**
Professor and Vice-Chairman for Academic Affairs
Department of Medicine
University of California at San Francisco
San Francisco, California

*Advisory Editor*
**David F. Altman, MD**
Associate Clinical Professor of Medicine
Director, GI Clinic
School of Medicine
Associate Dean, Office of Student and Curricular Affairs
University of California at San Francisco
San Francisco, California

## GENETICS

*Advisory Editor*
**Victor A. McKusick, MD, ScD, FACP, FRCP (Lond.)**
University Professor of Medical Genetics
The Johns Hopkins University School of Medicine
Baltimore, Maryland

*Advisory Editor*
**Reed Edwin Pyeritz, MD, PhD, FACP, FABMG**
Associate Professor of Medicine and Pediatrics
The Johns Hopkins University School of Medicine
Director of Clinical Services, Division of Medical Genetics
Department of Medicine
The Johns Hopkins Hospital
Baltimore, Maryland

## GERIATRIC MEDICINE

*Advisory Editor*
**J. C. Brocklehurst, MD, FRCP**
Professor of Geriatric Medicine
University of Manchester
Manchester, England

## GYNECOLOGY

*Advisory Editor*
**Harold Schulman, MD**
Professor of Obstetrics and Gynecology
State University of New York at Stony Brook
Stony Brook, New York
Chairman, Department of Obstetrics and Gynecology
Winthrop University Hospital
Mineola, New York

## HEALTH SERVICES

*Advisory Editor*
**Stephen J. Williams, ScD**
Professor and Head
Division of Health Services Administration
Graduate School of Public Health
San Diego State University
San Diego, California

## HEMATOLOGY

*Advisory Editor*
**Virgil F. Fairbanks, MD, FACP**
Professor of Medicine and Laboratory Medicine
Mayo Medical School
Department of Laboratory Medicine and Pathology
Department of Internal Medicine
Mayo Clinic
Rochester, Minnesota

*Co-Advisory Editor*
**Robert M. Petitt, MD**
Division of Hematology
Mayo Clinic
Rochester, Minnesota

## HISTOLOGY

*Advisory Editor*
**David R. Turner, MB, PhD, FRCPath**
Professor of Pathology
Nottingham University Medical School
Nottingham, England

## IMMUNOLOGY

*Advisory Editor*
**Peter Lachmann, ScD, FRS**
Sheila Joan Smith Professor of Tumour Immunology
Honorary Director
MRC Unit on Mechanisms in Tumour Immunity
University of Cambridge
Cambridge, England

*Advisory Editor*
**John B. Zabriskie, MD**
Associate Professor
Laboratory of Bacteriology and Immunology
The Rockefeller University
New York, New York

## INFECTIOUS DISEASE

*Advisory Editor*
**Edward W. Hook, MD**
Henry B. Mulholland Professor and Chairman
Department of Medicine
University of Virginia School of Medicine
Physician-in-Chief
University of Virginia Hospital
Charlottesville, Virginia

*Co-Advisory Editor*
**Marcia Day Finney, MA**
Medical Editor
Department of Medicine
University of Virginia School of Medicine
Charlottesville, Virginia

## LABORATORY MEDICINE

*Advisory Editor*
**Frances K. Widmann, MD**
Associate Professor of Pathology
Duke University School of Medicine
Assistant Chief, Laboratory Service
Durham Veterans Administration Medical Center
Durham, North Carolina

## MEASURES

*Advisory Editor*
**†Edward Pyatt, BSc (Eng.), CEng, MIEE**

*Advisory Editor*
**Basil Swindells, MA, BSc, CEng, MIMechE**

† Deceased

## MICROBIOLOGY

*Advisory Editor*
**Bernard D. Davis, MD**
Adele Lehman Professor of Bacterial Physiology, Emeritus
Harvard Medical School
Boston, Massachusetts

## NEPHROLOGY

*Advisory Editor*
**David P. Earle, MD, MACP**
Otho S. A. Sprague Emeritus Professor of Medicine
Northwestern University Medical School
Chicago, Illinois

## NEUROANATOMY AND NEUROPHYSIOLOGY

*Advisory Editor*
**Carmine D. Clemente, PhD**
Professor of Anatomy
Member, Brain Research Institute
UCLA School of Medicine
Professor of Surgery (Anatomy)
Charles R. Drew Postgraduate Medical School
Center for Health Sciences
Los Angeles, California

*Advisory Editor*
**Anthony M. Adinolfi, PhD**
Associate Professor of Anatomy
UCLA School of Medicine
Center for the Health Sciences
Los Angeles, California

*Advisory Editor*
**Earl Eldred, MD**
Professor of Anatomy
Member, Brain Research Institute
UCLA School of Medicine
Center for the Health Sciences
Los Angeles, California

*Advisory Editor*
**Lawrence Kruger, PhD**
Professor of Anatomy and Anesthesiology
Member, Brain Research Institute
UCLA School of Medicine
Center for the Health Sciences
Los Angeles, California

*Advisory Editor*
**Arnold B. Scheibel, MD**
Professor of Anatomy and Psychiatry
Acting Director, Brain Research Institute
UCLA School of Medicine
Center for the Health Sciences
Los Angeles, California

## NEUROLOGY

*Advisory Editor*
**Sir John Walton, TD, MA, MD, DSc, FRCP**
Warden, Green College
University of Oxford
Oxford, England
(Formerly) Professor of Neurology
University of Newcastle upon Tyne
Newcastle upon Tyne, England

## NEUROPHYSIOLOGY
(See NEUROANATOMY)

## NEUROSURGERY

*Advisory Editor*
**Bronson S. Ray, MD**
Professor of Surgery (Neurosurgery) Emeritus
Cornell University Medical College
Honorary Surgeon
The New York Hospital
New York, New York

## NUCLEAR MEDICINE

*Advisory Editor*
**Frank H. DeLand, MD, MS (Path.)**
Chief of Staff
Veterans Administration Medical Center
Associate Dean
Health Sciences
State University of New York
Syracuse, New York

*Co-Advisory Editor*
**Douglas A. Ross, PhD, MD**
(Formerly) Research Staff Member
Medical Instrumentation Group
Oak Ridge National Laboratory
Oak Ridge, Tennessee

## NUTRITION

*Advisory Editor*
**Myron Winick, MD**
R. R. Williams Professor of Nutrition
Professor of Pediatrics
Director, Institute for Human Nutrition
Director, Center for Nutrition, Genetics and Human Development
Columbia University College of Physicians and Surgeons
New York, New York

*Co-Advisory Editor*
**Brian L. G. Morgan, PhD**
Assistant Professor of Nutrition
Columbia University College of Physicians and Surgeons
New York, New York

## OBSTETRICS AND HUMAN REPRODUCTION

*Advisory Editor*
**Ronald T. Burkman, MD**
Chairman
Department of Obstetrics and Gynecology
Henry Ford Hospital
Detroit, Michigan

## OCCUPATIONAL MEDICINE

*Advisory Editor*
**Richard Schilling, CBE, MD, DSc, FRCP, FFOM, FFCM**
Emeritus Professor of Occupational Health
University of London
Honorary Fellow
London School of Hygiene and Tropical Medicine
London, England

## ONCOLOGY

*Advisory Editor*
**Leslie H. Sobin, MD**
Department of Gastrointestinal Pathology
Armed Forces Institute of Pathology
Washington, D.C.
(Formerly) Pathologist, Cancer Unit
World Health Organization
Geneva, Switzerland

## OPHTHALMOLOGY

*Advisory Editor*
**William H. Havener, MD**
Professor and Chairman
Department of Ophthalmology
The Ohio State University
Columbus, Ohio

## ORTHOPEDICS

*Advisory Editor*
**Robert B. Duthie, CBE, MA, ChM, FRCS**
Nuffield Professor of Orthopaedic Surgery
University of Oxford
Honorary Consultant Orthopaedic Surgeon
Nuffield Orthopaedic Centre and John Radcliffe Hospital
Oxford, England

## OTORHINOLARYNGOLOGY

*Advisory Editor*
**L. F. W. Salmon, MBE, MS, FRCS**
Consultant Surgeon Emeritus
Ear, Nose and Throat Department
Guy's Hospital
London, England

*Co-Advisory Editor (Speech and Hearing)*
**J. A. M. Martin, MB, BS, FRCS, DLO**
Director
Nuffield Hearing and Speech Centre
Royal National Throat, Nose and Ear Hospital
London, England

## PARASITOLOGY

*Advisory Editor*
**Donald Heyneman, PhD**
Professor of Parasitology
Department of Epidemiology and International Health
University of California at San Francisco
San Francisco, California

## PATHOLOGY

*Advisory Editor*
**Daniel R. Alonso, MD**
Professor of Pathology
Senior Associate Dean
Cornell University Medical College
Attending Pathologist
The New York Hospital
New York, New York

## PEDIATRICS

*Advisory Editor*
**Douglas Gairdner, DM, FRCP**
(Formerly) Consultant Paediatrician
Addenbrooke's Hospital
Cambridge, England

*Advisory Editor*
**†Dermod MacCarthy, MD, FRCP**
Consultant Paediatrician
Stoke Mandeville Hospital
Aylesbury, England

## PEDIATRIC SURGERY

*Advisory Editor*
**S. Frank Redo, MD**
Professor of Surgery
Cornell University Medical College
Attending Surgeon-in-Charge of Pediatric Surgery
The New York Hospital
New York, New York

## PERIPHERAL VASCULAR SURGERY

*Advisory Editor*
**Kaj Johansen, MD, PhD**
Professor of Surgery
University of Washington School of Medicine
Harborview Medical Center
Seattle, Washington

## PHARMACOLOGY

*Advisory Editor*
**Bert N. La Du, MD, PhD**
Professor, Department of Pharmacology
University of Michigan Medical School
Ann Arbor, Michigan

*Advisory Editor*
**James J. Lipsky, MD**
Associate Professor of Medicine, Pharmacology, and Molecular Sciences
The Johns Hopkins University School of Medicine
Baltimore, Maryland

† Deceased

## PHYSICAL MEDICINE AND REHABILITATION

*Advisory Editor*
**James T. Demopoulos, MD**
Chairman
Temple University Hospital
Philadelphia, Pennsylvania

*Advisory Editor*
**Asa P. Ruskin, MD, FACP**
Associate Clinical Professor of Rehabilitation Medicine
Albert Einstein College of Medicine
New York, New York
Director of Rehabilitation Medicine
Kingsbrook Jewish Medical Center
New York, New York

## PHYSIOLOGY

*Advisory Editor*
**Eric Lewis Blair, MD, FRCP**
Professor of Physiology
Academic Sub-Dean
The Medical School
University of Newcastle upon Tyne
Newcastle upon Tyne, England

## PLASTIC AND RECONSTRUCTIVE SURGERY

*Advisory Editor*
**Robert E. Shanahan, MD**
Clinical Associate Professor of Surgery
Division of Plastic Surgery
The Medical College of Ohio
Toledo, Ohio
(Formerly) Attending Surgeon
The Burns Clinic Medical Center
Petoskey, Michigan

*Advisory Editor*
**†Frank McDowell, MD, ScD**
Professor of Surgery
University of Hawaii
Honolulu, Hawaii

## PSYCHIATRY

*Advisory Editor*
**Robert Jean Campbell, MD**
Clinical Professor of Psychiatry
New York University School of Medicine
Director, Gracie Square Hospital
New York, New York

## PSYCHOLOGY

*Advisory Editor*
**H. E. King, PhD**
Professor of Psychology
Washington and Lee University
Lexington, Virginia
Adjunct Professor of Psychiatry
University of Pittsburgh School of Medicine
Pittsburgh, Pennsylvania

## PUBLIC HEALTH

*Advisory Editor*
**G. Wynne Griffith, MD, FFCM, FSS, DPH**
(Formerly) Principal Medical Officer
Department of Health and Social Security
London, England

## PULMONARY MEDICINE

*Advisory Editor*
**John E. Stark, MA, MD, FRCP**
Consultant Physician
Addenbrooke's and Papworth Hospitals
Cambridge, England

† Deceased

## RADIOLOGY

*Advisory Editor*
**Milton Elkin, MD**
Professor and Chairman
Department of Radiology
Albert Einstein College of Medicine
Director of Radiology
Bronx Municipal Hospital Center and Hospital of the Albert Einstein College of Medicine
New York, New York

## RHEUMATOLOGY

*Advisory Editor*
**Michael D. Lockshin, MD, FACP**
Professor of Medicine
Cornell University Medical College
Attending Physician
The New York Hospital and The Hospital for Special Surgery
New York, New York

## SURGERY

*Advisory Editor*
**George E. Wantz, MD**
Associate Professor of Clinical Surgery
Cornell University Medical College
Attending Surgeon
The New York Hospital
New York, New York

*Co-Advisory Editor*
**Jeffrey P. Gold, MD**
Assistant Professor of Surgery
Cornell University Medical College
Attending Surgeon in Cardiothoracic Surgery
The New York Hospital
New York, New York

## TERATOLOGY

*Advisory Editor*
**†James G. Wilson, MA, PhD**
Professor of Research Pediatrics and Anatomy
University of Cincinnati College of Medicine
Children's Hospital Research Foundation
Cincinnati, Ohio

† Deceased

## TOXICOLOGY

*Advisory Editor*
**Harry W. Hays, PhD**
Toxicologist (Retired)
Arlington, Virginia

*Co-Advisory Editor*
**Florence M. Carleton**
(Formerly) Medical Librarian
Washington, D.C.

## TRAUMA AND BURNS

*Advisory Editor*
**David M. Heimbach, MD**
Professor of Surgery
University of Washington
Director, Burn Center
Harborview Medical Center
Seattle, Washington

## TROPICAL MEDICINE

*Advisory Editor*
**Gordon C. Cook, MD, DSc (London), FRCP, FRACP**
London School of Hygiene and Tropical Medicine
Honorary Consultant Physician
University College Hospital and
Hospital for Tropical Diseases
London, England

## ULTRASOUND

*Advisory Editor*
**Frederick W. Kremkau, PhD**
Associate Professor
Department of Diagnostic Radiology
Yale University School of Medicine
New Haven, Connecticut

## UROLOGY

*Advisory Editor*
**Jay Y. Gillenwater, MD**
Professor and Chairman
Department of Urology
University of Virginia Medical Center
Charlottesville, Virginia

## VIROLOGY

*Advisory Editor*
**R. Gordon Douglas, Jr., MD**
Chairman, Department of Medicine
Cornell University Medical College
Physician-in-Chief
The New York Hospital
New York, New York

# A GUIDE TO THE USE OF THIS DICTIONARY



## 1. FORM OF ENTRIES

### 1.1 Main entries and subentries

This dictionary groups entries according to whether they are main entries (printed in bold letters flush with the left-hand margin of each column) or subentries (printed in bold letters and run into the text following a main entry). Within the subentry term, the component that is identical to the main-entry term is represented by its initial letter only. Thus **dazzle reflex** is to be found as a subentry under the main entry **reflex**, and appears as **dazzle r.; arteria radialis** is found under the main entry **arteria**, and appears as **a. radialis**. Subentries whose main-entry components are in the plural are fully spelled out unless the plural is formed simply by adding *-s* or *-es*, in which case the component will appear as the initial followed by **.'s** or **.'es**. Thus, under the main entry **bone** there will appear **b.'s of cranium**; under the main entry **os**[2] there will appear **ossa cranii**. If the first term on a page is a subentry, the abbreviated portion will correspond to the running head at the top of the left-hand column.

## 1.2 Homographs

Main entries derived from different etymological roots are listed separately as homographs and are distinguished by superior figures, for example, **mole¹** (skin lesion), **mole²** (uterine mass), and **mole³** (unit of amount of substance), with their respective subentries, if any, appearing under the appropriate main entry.

## 1.3 Eponyms

Use of the possessive form in eponymous terms has been a subject of considerable debate among medical writers. As a style convention for this dictionary, terms for entities named after a person (eponym) are given in a form consistent with that recommended in McKusick's *Mendelian Inheritance in Man* (seventh ed., 1986), p. xxiv. Briefly stated, the conventions governing eponyms are as follows: The possessive case of a name is not used if the word following begins with a sibilant sound, for example, *Marfan syndrome*, not *Marfan's syndrome*, or if the name itself ends in a sibilant sound, for example, *Graves disease*. Compound eponyms are not made possessive. The possessive case may be used in those eponymous terms not falling into these categories, for example, *Parkinson's disease*, if usage so warrants.

# 2. VOCABULARY

## 2.1 Subjects covered

A list of the subject specialties comprehended by this dictionary can be found under *Advisory Editors and Co-Advisory Editors by Subject*, beginning on p. ix. In addition to these subjects, contributed by specialists in each discipline, the following subjects included were mainly or entirely staff-written: abbreviations, combining forms, general medical terms, and general terms. The more fundamental general medical terms (e.g., *disease, syndrome*) were submitted to Advisory Editors for review and correction, but most such terms (e.g., *high-risk, target, infirmity, Hippocrates*) were staff-written, as were virtually all those general terms (e.g., *feature, relationship*), which though not essentially medical are included because subentries are appended to them. Some main entries of a general character are included without definition.

Qualifying subject labels are not used, and as a rule no introductory phrase specifies the particular subject to which each definition applies. The branches of medicine and biology are so interconnected that such specification is often arbitrary or unduly narrow, and in most cases the definition is sufficient to indicate its range of application. However, in some cases involving multiple meanings (polysemy) or ambiguous context, an introductory phase is used to distinguish the relevant subject area.

Biographical entries are main entries consisting of an individual's name (eponym) after whom a term has been named and including usually a listing of the complete name, nationality, an indication of the individual's discipline or occupation, birth and death dates (if known), and cross-references to the eponymous term or terms. (See also *Biographical entries*, ¶ 4.3.)

## 2.2 Nomenclatures

*CMD* has made use of a number of widely used systems of nomenclature in certain subject areas. Anatomy terms generally follow the recommendations of *Nomina Anatomica* (fifth ed., Mexico City, 1980), and such terms are identified by the abbreviation NA within square brackets immediately preceding the definition. Tumor terminology is based on the classification of the International Histological Classification of Tumours of the World Health Organization. Enzymes are represented in accordance with the recommendations of *Enzyme Nomenclature*, formerly *Enzyme Commission* (International Union of Biochemistry), and are identified within parentheses by numerical code following the abbreviation EC.

## 2.3 Preferred terms

A special effort has been made to determine the preferred term in those cases where several or many variant terms are used to describe the same entity. Every Advisory Editor was asked to select the preferred term based primarily on the prevailing common usage. Due weight, however, was also given to the recommendations of official bodies charged with determining preferred nomenclature, and whenever it was reasonable to adopt such recommendations, they were incorporated into this work. Nonetheless, Advisory Editors were not bound to observe any group's official recommendations if they felt that those recommendations were in particular cases clearly contradicted by the weight of prevailing usage. To adopt little-known alternative forms over others long-established and understood worldwide would only breed confusion in the international scientific community. There are instances, therefore, although rare, in which an official term is deliberately not preferred. In some cases it was impossible to determine which of several terms was most commonly used. In such cases, therefore, the first or second variant listed may well be the preferred usage for many. In other cases, usage varied geographically or by discipline; *CMD* attempts to record such variations in usage in special linguistic notes appended to the pertinent entries. (See *Notes*, ¶ 5.3.)

### 2.4 Variants

Variants (or synonyms) of preferred terms are listed in *italic type (in which this is printed)* at the end of the definition to which they apply. They are introduced by *Also*. If a variant is appended to the last definition of a polysemous entry, it applies to the last definition only unless otherwise noted. Variants that apply to more than one definition in an entry are introduced by a phrase that indicates the definitions to which they apply. Usage information is frequently appended to variants. (See *Usage labels*, ¶ 5.1.)

Variants in *CMD* are listed both under the term of which they are variants and as cross-references to the preferred term in their respective alphabetic places. A variant may or may not be listed in its own place if it falls immediately before or after the preferred term. Thus, at **conductive deafness** a variant **conduction deafness** is not entered separately. English names of anatomical branches are given as variants under **ramus** but are not entered at **branch**. These are the only exceptions to a reciprocal listing of variants. We believe the inclusion of variants will be of immense help to those involved in biomedical research from earlier periods or from non-English traditions, where older or more obscure variants (such as those based on translations from other languages) may have been used.

## 3. ALPHABETIZATION

### 3.1 Main entries and subentries

Main entries are alphabetized in letter-by-letter sequence (except as qualified in ¶ 3.2) rather than in word-by-word sequence. Hyphens or spaces between words are ignored. Thus *bloodstream* precedes *blood type*. The main entry, usually a noun, always corresponds to a portion of each subentry. Thus, the subentry *primary spermatocyte* is alphabetized under *spermatocyte*, and *spina scapulae* under *spina*. Plural subentries such as *spinae palatinae* or *ossa cranii* appear under the corresponding singular main-entry forms, that is, *spina* and *os*², respectively. (See *Main entries and subentries*, ¶ 1.1.) Cross-references to singular forms are provided at the main-entry plural forms (as at *venae* and *ossa*) that do not follow the standard rules of pluralization in English. Irregular plural forms in English are also given within preferred singular entries following the italic label *pl.* (See ¶ 6.) Although the preferred form of almost all main entries is singular, in those cases where a plural form is preferred, a cross-reference is given from the singular to the plural form.

Letter-by-letter alphabetization within subentries is strictly observed and unless understood can cause confusion, since it sometimes results in plural forms preceding singular forms owing to changes in Latin spellings. For example, the following terms appear in this order under the main entry *nervus*:

**nervi digitales**
**nervi digitales palmares**
**n. digitalis communis**

After being primarily alphabetized under *nervus*, the last two subentries are secondarily alphabetized under DIGITALESPALMARES and DIGITALISCOMMUNIS, respectively.

Apart from chemical terms (¶ 3.3), *CMD* has relatively few exceptions to its rule of listing main entries under single words rather than phrases. When an exception must be made (as, for example, at *blood group*, a main entry), a cross-reference is included under the element (i.e., *group*) where the reader might expect to find the term.

### 3.2 Qualifications to letter-by-letter alphabetization

The following words, word elements, or symbols are ignored in alphabetization:

**3.2.1** a, an, and, as, at, between, for, from, of, on, the, to, with, without. Thus, *plane of inlet of pelvis* which appears under the main entry *plane*, is alphabetized under that heading as if it were spelled INLETPELVIS.

**3.2.2** The grammatical suffix *'s* indicating the possessive case, as in *Bell's palsy*.

**3.2.3** Chemical prefixes appearing in italic type or small capitals, as *p*-aminobenzoic acid, alphabetized as a main entry at AMINOBENZOICACID. (¶ 3.3 explains the alphabetic treatment of chemical terms.)

**3.2.4** Numerals, for example, 5-methyluracil is alphabetized at METHYLURACIL.

**3.2.5** Greek letters, for example, ε-*N*-methyllysine is alphabetized at METHYLLYSINE.

## 3.3 Chemical terms

Chemical terms are treated as main entries regardless of whether they are written in solid or hyphenated form or as several words. For example, *ammonium chloride* and *alcohol dehydrogenase* are alphabetized as main entries as if each term were written in solid form. A term that consists of an ordinary modifier, however, and a generic name (e.g., *wood alcohol*) is usually treated as a subentry under the governing noun (*alcohol*). Similarly, a chemical name modifying an ordinary word (as in *dyclonine hydrochloride solution*) is treated as a subentry under the governing noun (*solution*). In cases where the distinction may not be clear (e.g., *benzene ring*, alphabetized at *benzene*), a cross-reference is provided to direct the reader to the appropriate alphabetic position.

# 4. CROSS-REFERENCES

Cross-references are distinguished by appearing in SMALL CAPITAL LETTERS (IN WHICH THIS IS PRINTED). Cross-references occur in a variety of contexts, but they are always identified by this type.

## 4.1 Variants

By far the most common cross-reference is that of a variant to a preferred term:

> **Fabry's disease** ANGIOKERATOMA CORPORIS DIFFUSUM.

The reader seeking a definition for *Fabry's disease* is directed to *angiokeratoma corporis diffusum* (alphabetized under the governing noun, *angiokeratoma*), where a definition for this condition will be found. Moreover, the list of variants appearing at the end of the entry for *angiokeratoma corporis diffusum* includes *Fabry's disease*. This is useful for two reasons: first, because it provides information about the usage (including international usage) and history of the term; and secondly, because in cases of polysemy (i.e., should the preferred term have several different definitions), the reader will be able to determine unequivocally to which sense or senses the variant applies.

## 4.2 *See under*

Cross-references beginning with this phrase direct the reader to a different alphabetic position where the term is being sought may be found. For example, under the main entry *group*, one finds:

> **blood group** See under BLOOD GROUP.

This directs the reader to the alphabetic position BLOODGROUP. Under the main entry *ring*, one finds:

> **benzene ring** See under BENZENE.

This directs the reader to find *benzene ring* under the main entry *benzene*.

## 4.3 Biographical entries

Most other sources simply list in one grouping all the eponymous terms in which a particular name appears, regardless of whether those terms are preferred or variants of other terms. We seek to list all eponymous terms and to refer the reader in every case to the corresponding preferred term, whether or not it is eponymous. Therefore, our system is necessarily more complex than that used elsewhere, but we believe it will provide greater assistance to the reader.

Biographical entries make special use of the phrase *See under*. In order to avoid referring the reader to a variant term (a "blind" cross-reference), all the variant terms that include the eponym are listed first, followed by a *See under* reference to the preferred term where a definition can be found. For example, rather than referring the reader from the entry *Fabry* to *Fabry's disease* (found under *disease*), which is a variant of another term, we list the eponyms in order to provide this information and then direct the reader to the preferred term:

> **Fabry** [Johannes *Fabry*, German physician, 1860–1930] Fabry's disease, Fabry syndrome. See under ANGIOKERATOMA CORPORIS DIFFUSUM.

This entry informs the reader that Fabry's name is used in two terms, *Fabry's disease* and *Fabry syndrome*, both of which are variants of *angiokeratoma corporis diffusum*.

If the reference is unambiguously to a preferred term, *See under* directs the reader to the correct main entry under which the term may be found:

**Graves** [Robert James *Graves*, Irish physician, 1795–1863] See under DISEASE.

This entry directs the reader to find the term *Graves disease* under the main entry *disease*.

If more than one unambiguous eponymous terms are preferred terms, the references are listed in a single definition. *This is the only case in which references to more than one preferred term are combined in a single definition.*

**Kienböck** [Robert *Kienböck*, Austrian physician, 1871–1953] See under DISEASE, DISLOCATION.

This entry directs the reader to *Kienböck's disease* (under *disease*) and *Kienböck's dislocation* (under *dislocation*).

Whenever the main entry under which a preferred term may be found is ambiguous, the preferred term is listed followed by a *See under* reference to the main-entry word.

**Hess** [Alfred Fabian *Hess*, U.S. physician, 1875–1933] Hess capillary test. See under TEST.

**Cohnheim** [Julius Friedrich *Cohnheim*, German pathologist, 1839–1884] Cohnheim's areas. See under AREA.

Although the many variations in cross-referencing (often involving multiple names) are too complex to be described in detail here, two basic rules can be stated.

**4.3.1** *See under* always refers the reader either to a preferred term or to a main entry heading under which the preferred subentry term can be found.

**4.3.2** With the single exception noted above (¶ 4.3), every definition in biographical entries refers to one and only one preferred term. If the reader keeps this in mind, some features of our cross-referencing system that might otherwise appear puzzling or duplicative will be understood and provide more complete and accurate access to eponymous terms than that given by other sources.

### 4.4 *See also*

*See also* is used at the end of certain definitions to cross-refer to other terms where additional or fuller information that relates directly to the originating term may be found. In most instances the originating term is specifically mentioned under the term referred to. *See also* is not used in *CMD* merely to link together related terms, since that would necessitate the inclusion of many thousands of such cross-references, and the usefulness of the device would be so vitiated as to be negligible. It is used chiefly to avoid the repetition of a lengthy definition, as of a complex process, by referring the reader from each of the several steps of such a process to the term providing a full description.

### 4.5 *Compare*

*Compare* is used only to link pairs of contrasting words, such as *afferent* and *efferent*, when such contrast is likely to help the reader appreciate the significance of the distinction between them. Indeed, some words practically self-evident in meaning are included because they are used in opposition to other more important words that are not self-evident.

## 5. USAGE INFORMATION

This dictionary contains a variety of usage information, including both labels and more extensive usage and linguistic notes.

### 5.1 Usage labels

Labels conveying usage information are appended to the end of definitions of preferred terms and are also used to introduce cross-references. A preferred term that is outmoded includes the label *Outmoded*. If the term has more than one definition and only one definition is outmoded, the phrase *An outmoded usage* appears after the appropriate definition. If all of its definitions are outmoded, *Outmoded* appears after the last definition only; it should be understood as applying to the entire term. Obsolete variants of other terms are introduced by the abbreviated label *Obs.*, with the preferred term appearing in small capital letters. In the corresponding listing at the preferred term (following *Also*), the variant is also identified by the pertinent usage classification in parentheses. For example:

**incus** [NA] The middle of the three auditory ossicles of the middle ear. Also *anvil, stithe* (outmoded).

*Anvil* is a current variant, *stithe* an outmoded one.

Usage labels based on the following criteria are used:

**5.1.1** Temporal criteria, classified as *older, outmoded,* or *obsolete*. *Older* is equivalent to old-fashioned or obsolescent; it is applied to terms or senses that are still in use but would appear dated to most informed observers. Such terms include those in the process of being replaced by a newer terminology competing with the older one. *Outmoded* is equivalent to archaic; it is applied to terms or senses that are not used today except in special contexts or that have been replaced in recent years with other terms, although they may be of considerable historic importance. *Obsolete* means no longer in use; terms or senses so labeled are retained because they are of historic interest.

**5.1.2** Currency (frequency) criteria, classified as *seldom used* or *rare*. *Seldom used* means infrequently used in scientific literature; *rare* means hardly ever encountered. (An idiosyncratic usage by a world-renowned scientist can be of importance in spite of its rarity). Although there is a tendency to associate seldom used and rare terms with out-of-date terms, no such relationship is necessary: a term can be uncommon yet current.

**5.1.3** Prescriptive criteria, classified as *ambiguous, imprecise,* or *incorrect*. *Ambiguous* describes those terms having two or more meanings that can be confused in certain contexts and are thus apt to sow confusion. Not every term having multiple meanings is ambiguous. *Imprecise* is usually applied to older terms based on outmoded concepts; modern theory may have no place for such a term within its framework, yet the term may at one time have been of great importance in the development of the science. The term itself may or may not be outmoded, but it no longer has the specific referent it was once thought to have. *Incorrect*, a label sparingly applied in this dictionary, is based on an Advisory Editor's judgment that the continued use of a particular term in a given sense is seriously misleading and improper or has on good grounds been specifically rejected by an official organization.

**5.1.4** Style criteria, including the classifying label *popular*, equivalent to nontechnical and including some informal usages. It is applied to terms or definitions that are commonly used by the general public and sometimes by scientific writers in nontechnical contexts, but that are not used in the scientific literature.

**5.1.5** Although these are the standard expressions employed in this work for giving usage information, the Advisory Editors have not been constrained from using other expressions if they deemed them more suitable. One will therefore find many other phrases, including combinations of labels (such as *obsolete and misleading*) as well as those listed above.

## 5.2 British and American Spellings

This dictionary gives preference to American spellings over British in cases where the two differ. However, special attention has been given to British spelling and usage to insure that preferred British forms are fully represented and that British users will have no difficulty in finding the preferred entry. Whenever a British spelling (e.g., *oedema*) would place a term alphabetically remote from the American spelling (*edema*), a cross-reference has been provided from the British spelling. Systematic cross-references are also given at a number of strategic places (as at *oe-*) to alert the British reader that American spellings are used. Differences relating to the meaning and usage of terms in Britain and the United States are fully treated in usage notes. (See ¶ 5.3 and 5.4.)

## 5.3 Notes

Notes, which are always set off within the text by the boldface symbol **•**, are used to convey information about the entry term, especially about its current or past uses, when such information is too extensive to be compressed into a brief phrase. (See, for example, the note at *filterable virus*.) Notes may also deal with linguistic information such as etymology, spelling, or regional differences in usage.

## 5.4 Panel on International Usage

In order to determine possible differences in usage in different parts of the world where the English language is spoken as a native language or widely used as the language of scientific communication, a panel of leading medical educators was established.

(See p. vii.) Areas represented are Australia, Canada, India, Japan, New Zealand, South Africa, the United Kingdom, and the United States. Whenever an entry was suspected of having divergent regional meanings or uses, copies of the entry and its definitions were sent to all members of the panel for comment. With the information supplied by these eight panel members, a number of usage notes have been composed. (See, for example, the note at *mister*.) It is our hope that such information will be useful in clarifying terminology that often causes confusion in international scientific communication, both in personal contacts and in written papers.

## 5.5 Illustrative quotations

Our editorial staff has regularly read certain professional periodicals and books to enlarge its store of possible dictionary entries, and by this means collected a large number of citations (quotations of actual usage) to demonstrate the existence of new terms and to exemplify new meanings, uses, and spellings of older terms. Such citations were routinely forwarded to the Advisory Editor responsible for the subject most closely associated with the subject of each citation; the editor was asked to decide whether the term or sense merited inclusion and, if so, to provide a definition for it. Many terms and meanings were added by such means. In selected cases, moreover, it was deemed worthwhile to print a brief quotation in the text to illustrate actual usage. (See, for example, the quotation at *high-risk*.) Such illustrative quotations are set off from the rest of the text by angled brackets and contain full bibliographic data. Illustrative quotations are intended to augment definitions by showing specific but more or less typical contexts which often elucidate meaning better than a formal definition can.

## 5.6 Bibliographic references

Bibliographic references are cited sparingly and are usually given only when a particular source is widely regarded as the basis of the essential theory or knowledge underlying a given treatment of definition. Such references are set off from the rest of the text by angled brackets and contain full bibliographic data.

## 5.7 Associated adjectives

Adjectives associated with a particular noun may be listed without a definition after the definition of the noun and following the abbreviation *Adj*. This does not preclude the separate listing of such adjectives as entries with full definitions, but in many cases the definitions of such words conform to the formula "of or relating to" (the noun under which the particular adjective appears), and no separate definition is necessary. Some rarely used adjectives can be economically treated in this way, whereas more common adjectives always have a separate listing.

# 6. PLURALS

For entry words that have irregular or non-English plural forms, the plural is generally given in parentheses immediately before the definition. Thus, for *iris* we have (*pl*. irides); for *corpus*, (*pl*. corpora). If the preferred entry word itself is plural, an irregular singular is shown in the same way: *meninges*, (*sing*. meninx).

Some Latin and Greek plural patterns occur so regularly that they need not be shown explicitly for every term they apply to, although we do in fact show them in many instances. The plural can be deduced from the ending of the singular:

| SINGULAR | PLURAL | EXAMPLE |
|---|---|---|
| -sis | -ses | **diagnosis** (*pl*. diagnoses) |
| -itis | -itides | **meningitis** (*pl*. meningitides) |
| -um | -a | **flagellum** (*pl*. flagella) |
| -oma | -omata *or* -omas | **chondroma** (*pl*. chondromas, chondromata) |

Other plural patterns are also common but less predictable than the above:

| SINGULAR | PLURAL | EXAMPLE AND COUNTEREXAMPLE |
|---|---|---|
| -a | -ae | **vertebra** (*pl*. vertebrae), but **cornea** (*pl*. corneas) |
| -us | -i | **gyrus** (*pl*. gyri), but **plexus** (*pl*. plexus, plexuses) |
| -on | -a | **ganglion** (*pl*. ganglia), but **neuron** (*pl*. neurons) |

In these cases a Latin or Greek plural, if used, is always explicitly shown, sometimes in addition to a regular English plural. If a regular English plural is the only one ordinarily used, no plural is shown.

There are pitfalls for readers unacquainted with Latin grammar. For example, in Latin phrases the endings *-ae* and *-i* do not necessarily indicate a plural; they may be genitive (possessive) singular. Thus *arcus vertebrae* means the arch of a vertebra (vertebral arch) and *septum nasi* means the septum of the nose (nasal septum).

## 7. ETYMOLOGIES

Etymologies, or word derivations, are given in square brackets immediately after the pronunciation or, if no pronunciation is shown, immediately after the entry word.

### 7.1 Analytical etymologies

For a word coined in modern times, the etymology usually shows only its constituent parts:

**leukocyte** [LEUKO- + -CYTE]

Further information can be found at the entries for these separate constituents: *leuko-* (from Greek *leukos*) means "white," and *-cyte* (from Greek *kytos* vessel, container) means "cell." Constituents that are not themselves entered in the dictionary are identified and glossed wherever they occur in an etymology:

**spodography** [Gk *spodo(s)* ashes + -GRAPHY]

### 7.2 Historical etymologies

For a word adopted from another language, or inherited from an earlier stage of the same language, the etymology identifies the source language and shows the form and meaning of the source word:

**gout** [French *goutte* a drop, dripping, gout . . .]

Often, however, the word can be traced farther back: French *goutte* is a modern development of Latin *gutta* a drop. In some cases, when it is not obvious how the modern medical meaning developed from the original meaning, an explanation is provided. The full etymology in this case is:

[French *goutte* (from L *gutta* a drop) a drop, dripping, gout; the disease was attributed to a defluxion or dripping of morbid humors into a joint]

If the source word does not differ in spelling from the entry word, it is usually not repeated in the etymology:

**gluten** [L, glue]

This means that the Latin source word, which originally meant "glue," is *gluten*, the same as the entry word itself.

Many etymologies are both historical and analytical, as when a source word is shown to be derived from a more basic word in the same language, or broken down into its constituents in that language:

**syndrome** [Gk *syndromē* (from *syn-* together + *dromos* course, race) a concourse, concurrence, combination of symptoms]

### 7.3 Three kinds of derivation

In an etymological formula the word "from" (short for "derived from") can have any of three very different meanings, depending on context.

**7.3.1** ***Formation:*** To say that Greek *syndromē* is from *syn-* + *dromos* means it was generated from these underlying elements by the word-formative apparatus of the Greek language. This is the kind of derivation dealt with in analytical etymologies and the analytical parts of historical etymologies.

**7.3.2** ***Inheritance:*** To say that French *goutte* is from Latin *gutta* means that the French word was inherited from Latin; in the course of history Latin *gutta* became, or evolved into, French *goutte*. This evolutionary type of derivation can occur only between ancestral and descendant languages, or between earlier and later stages of the same language.

**7.3.3** ***Adoption:*** To say that English *gout* is derived from French *goutte* means that English speakers adopted, or "borrowed," this French word. Words are adopted from other languages for a variety of reasons. Sometimes an imported word accompanies an imported concept. Other times, people find a foreign word somehow more appropriate, or more fashionable, than its native counterpart.

Most of the medical and scientific vocabulary of English was either adopted from Latin or Greek or else formed out of constituents that were adopted from these languages. In many cases a Greek word was originally adopted into Latin, and the resulting Latin word later adopted into English and other modern languages. For example, Greek ἡπατικός (*hēpatikós*) was latinized as *hepaticus*, and the latter was eventually anglicized as *hepatic*.

Many medical and scientific words in French and the other Romance languages were adopted, rather than inherited, from Latin. While Latin in its popular, or "Vulgar," form was ancestral to these languages, Latin in its literary or academic form coexisted with them as the medium of scholarly discourse throughout medieval and early modern times, and was therefore a rich source of adopted vocabulary for them as well as for non-Romance languages like English.

## 7.4 New Latin

Besides providing word-building materials for modern languages, Latin is also still utilized in its own right, especially in international nomenclatures such as Nomina Anatomica and the names of species and higher taxa used in biology. Modern Latin coinages and usages, often labeled "New L" in the etymologies, include borrowings from present-day vernaculars as well as more conventional adaptations of classical Latin and Greek. They range, for example, from the prosaic *Musca domestica* (housefly) to the more exuberant sort of New Latin seen in *Lutzomyia flaviscutellata* (the yellow-scutellated sandfly), where the genus name combines Brazilian bacteriologist Adolfo *Lutz* with Greek *myia* a fly.

## 7.5 Mixtures and influences

Some derivations are complicated by "cross fertilization" of associated terms. Reanalysis (false analysis) may alter a word's original form (see ZOONOSIS) or its original meaning (see PUSTULE). In some cases a word's form comes from one source and its meaning from another, as when an adopted word undergoes assimilation to a native word (see SCURVY). Without being adopted, foreign terms wield considerable influence through translation, often causing native words to take on new meanings (see CLAVICULA) or to combine idiomatically in novel ways (see PIA MATER).

## 7.6 Collateral connections

Some etymologies show relationships in which one word is not derived from another, but two or more words are derived from an inferred common source that is not historically recorded. These collaterally related words are introduced by the phrase "akin to":

> **cutis** [L (akin to Gk *kytos* container and Old English *hȳd* skin, hide) skin]

Having in common the Indo-European stem reconstructed as "kut-," the three related words, Latin *cutis*, Greek *kytos*, and Old English *hȳd*, were inherited from the prehistoric ancestral language independently of each other. The Greek word in this case is fairly similar to the Latin in form but widely divergent in meaning. The English word, while close to the Latin in meaning, differs markedly in form, primarily because of sound shifts (*k-* to *h-* and *-t-* to *-d-*) that affected the Germanic sector of the Indo-European speech community.

## 7.7 Citation forms

Certain inflectional forms are conventionally used for citing words, such as the nominative singular for Latin and Greek nouns, the nominative singular masculine for adjectives, and the infinitive for verbs. Sometimes, however, these forms fail to show the word-stem that appears in derivatives, and need to be supplemented by another form. The supplementary citation forms most commonly used are the genitive singular for Latin and Greek nouns, and the past participle for Latin verbs:

> **galacto-** [Gk *gala*, gen. *galaktos* milk]
> **fossa** [L (from *fossus*, past part. of *fodere* to dig) a ditch, trench]

## 7.8 Alphabets and transliteration

Greek words in the etymologies are transliterated into the Roman alphabet according to the following table:

| Capital | Lowercase | Name | Transliteration |
|---|---|---|---|
| Α | α | alpha | *a* |
| Β | β | bēta | *b* |
| Γ | γ | gamma | *g*, *n*[1] |
| Δ | δ | delta | *d* |
| Ε | ε | epsilon | *e* |
| Ζ | ζ | zēta | *z* |
| Η | η | ēta | *ē* |
| Θ | θ | thēta | *th* |
| Ι | ι | iōta | *i* |
| Κ | κ | kappa | *k* |
| Λ | λ | lambda | *l* |
| Μ | μ | mu | *m* |
| Ν | ν | nu | *n* |
| Ξ | ξ | xi | *x* |
| Ο | ο | omicron | *o* |
| Π | π | pi | *p* |
| Ρ | ρ | rhō | *r* |
| Σ | σ, ς | sigma | *s* |
| Τ | τ | tau | *t* |
| Υ | υ | upsilon | *y*, *u*[2] |
| Φ | φ | phi | *ph* |
| Χ | χ | chi | *ch* |
| Ψ | ψ | psi | *ps* |
| Ω | ω | ōmega | *ō* |
| | ʽ "rough breathing" | | *h* |

[1] Gamma (γ) is transliterated *n* before a velar consonant. Thus γγ = *ng*, γκ = *nk*, γξ = *nx*, and γχ = *nch*. Otherwise, *g*.
[2] Upsilon (υ) is transliterated *u* after another vowel in the same syllable. Thus αυ = *au*, ευ = *eu*, ου = *ou*, etc. Otherwise, *y*.

The Greek accents (´,`,˜) and the "smooth breathing" ( ᾿ ) are not shown in the transliterations. Long vowels are shown only in the case of η (= ē) and ω (= ō), which are differentiated in Greek spelling from the corresponding short vowels (ε and ο, respectively).

Latin spellings in the etymologies follow the modern convention that distinguishes *v* (consonant) from *u* (vowel), and *j* (consonant) from *i* (vowel). Long vowels are not marked.

## 7.9 Abbreviations used in etymologies

| | |
|---|---|
| accus. | accusative |
| adj. | adjective |
| adv. | adverb |
| alter. | alteration |
| *a-* priv., *an-* priv. | alpha privative (Gk negative prefix) |
| contr. | contraction |
| dim. | diminutive |
| esp. | especially |
| fem. | feminine |
| fut. | future |
| gen. | genitive (possessive) |
| Gk | Greek (classical) |
| inf. | infinitive |
| irreg. | irregular |
| L | Latin (classical) |
| Late L | Late Latin (3rd–6th centuries A.D.) |
| lit. | literally |
| masc. | masculine |
| Med L | Medieval Latin (7th–15th centuries A.D.) |
| neut. | neuter |
| New L | New Latin (16th century–present) |
| nom. | nominative |
| obsol. | obsolete |
| orig. | originally |
| part. | participle |
| perf. | perfect |
| perh. | perhaps |
| pl. | plural |
| pref. | preferably |
| pres. | present |
| priv. | privative (see *a-* priv.) |
| prob. | probably |
| sing. | singular |
| superl. | superlative |
| transl. | translation |
| usu. | usually |

# 8. PRONUNCIATIONS

## 8.1 General principles

This dictionary employs a simple but clear system for rendering pronunciations. Except for foreign sounds, it employs only one symbol, the schwa (ə), that is not a common English letter, plus diacritics used in ways familiar to most readers and two stress marks following the stressed syllable: primary, or heavier, stress (**′**) and secondary, or lighter, stress (′).

In the pronunciation key given in ¶ 8.2, the schwa represents the neutral sound found in the first syllable of *abrasive* \əbrā**′**siv\. In a few instances a consonant can stand alone as a syllable and no ə is given:

**operable** \äp**′**ərəbl\
**spasm** \spaz**′**m\

Unlike other dictionaries, *CMD* gives pronunciations for combining forms. They are pronounced and given stress (usually secondary) as they would be when combined into words. Terms beginning with such a combining form will have truncated pronunciations unless the stress is changed. Thus:

**neo-** \nē′ō-\
**neonatal** \-nā**′**təl\ (to be understood as \nē′ōnā**′**təl\)
but **neonate** \nē**′**ōnāt′\

Where two vowels come together and do not represent a diphthong, a center dot (·) is used to indicate that they form separate syllables.

**arterial** \ärtir**′**ē·əl\

Occasionally the center dot is needed between two consonants that would otherwise represent a single sound.

**dyshidrosis** \dis·hīdrō**′**sis\

Since the quality of the vowels in our pronunciation system does not depend on whether a syllable is open or closed, aside from the stress marks and use of the center dot as explained above the syllables are not otherwise demarcated.

**vesicular** \vesik**′**yələr\

There are two optional sounds given: $^{h}$ and $^{y}$.

Thus, **whitlow** \\$^{h}$wit′lō\ can be pronounced either \hwit′lō\ or \wit′lō\, and **neuroma** \n$^{y}$ʊrō′mə\ can be pronounced either \nyʊrō′mə\ or \nʊrō′mə\.

When a term is pronounced differently for different meanings, the pronunciations are keyed to the definition numbers.

**colic** \(1) kō′lik; (2) käl′ik\ **1** Relating to the colon. **2** Any of various conditions characterized by abdominal pain.

## 8.2 Pronunciation key

*Vowels*

| | |
|---|---|
| \a\ | hat (carry \kar′ē\) |
| \ä\ | father, hospital (part \pärt\) |
| \ā\ | fate |
| \e\ | flesh (air \er\, ferry \fer′ē\) |
| \ē\ | she |
| \i\ | sit (ear \ir\) |
| \ī\ | eye |
| \ō\ | nose |
| \ô\ | saw |
| \oi\ | boy |
| \oo\ | move (future \fyoo′chər\) |
| \ʊ\ | book |
| \ou\ | out |
| \u\ | cup, love (first \furst\) |
| \ə\ | (about\əbout\, doctor \däk′tər\) |

*Consonants*

| | |
|---|---|
| \b\ | book |
| \ch\ | chew |
| \d\ | day |
| \f\ | fast |
| \g\ | good |
| \h\ | happy |
| \j\ | gem, join |
| \k\ | keep |
| \l\ | late |
| \m\ | make |
| \n\ | no |
| \ng\ | sing, sink (sanguineous \sang·gwin′ē·əs\) |
| \p\ | pair |
| \r\ | ring |
| \s\ | set |
| \sh\ | shoe, lotion |
| \t\ | tone |
| \th\ | thin |
| \TH\ | than |
| \v\ | very |
| \w\ | work |
| \y\ | yes (union \yoo′nyən\) |
| \z\ | zeal |
| \zh\ | azure, vision |

*Foreign sounds*

| | |
|---|---|
| \œ\ | feu, schön |
| \Y\ | tu, Walküre |
| \kh\ | loch, Bach |
| \SH\ | ich, Reich |
| \N\ | means that the preceding vowel is nasal: bon \bôN\ en face \äNfäs′\ |

# 9. ABBREVIATIONS

## 9.1 Abbreviations used in this dictionary

Exclusive of etymologies (¶ 7.9), this dictionary employs very few abbreviations. These are:

| | |
|---|---|
| Abbr. | Abbreviation |
| Adj. | Adjective |
| *Brit.* | British (spelling) |
| def(s). | definition(s) |
| EC | Enzyme Commission number |
| NA | *Nomina Anatomica* (fifth ed.) |
| *Obs.* | Obsolete |
| *pl.* | plural |
| *sing.* | singular |

The abbreviation *def.* is used only to refer to a definition number in an entry having two or more definitions.

## 9.2 Abbreviations as entries

Abbreviations abound in scientific papers, but in most cases they are explained when first introduced. Subsequently the abbreviations are routinely employed to save space. Many such abbreviations seldom if ever appear apart from an initial explanation, and it is unnecessary and unwise to encumber dictionaries with great numbers of such abbreviations, many of which are short-lived. On the other hand, there are many abbreviations in current use that are considered so commonplace or so important that they are usually given without explanation. It is these that we have sought to enter and explain in this dictionary. The expression from which the abbreviation is formed is given in full in all abbreviation entries. If the abbreviation is of a word or phrase in another language (such as Latin), the language is identified and a translation is given. Often the context in which the expression is used (as in prescription writing) is indicated. In many cases, the term abbreviated is also an entry appearing in its own alphabetic position with a definition. In other cases, the full expression of the abbreviation is sufficient to define it.

## 9.3 Abbreviations and symbols of lexical entries

Abbreviations and symbols for lexical entries are given at the end of the definition treatment following *Abbr.* or *Symbol.* If an abbreviation commonly appears without periods, no periods are given.

# A

**A** 1 Symbol for the unit, ampere. 2 Symbol for alanine. 3 Symbol for adenosine. 4 absorbance.

**$A_2$** aortic second sound.

**Å** Symbol for the unit, ångström.

**Å$^{-1}$** Symbol for the unit, reciprocal ångström.

**Ã** antinuclear antibody.

**a** 1 Symbol for atto-: used with SI units. 2 Symbol for the unit, year.

**a-$^1$** [Gk alpha privative *a-* (sometimes *an-* before vowels) not] A prefix meaning not, without, absence of. Also *an-*.

**a-$^2$** AB-$^1$.

**ā** *ante* (L, before).

***A*** 1 Symbol for mass number or nucleon number. 2 Symbol for work, expressed in joules.

*α* 1 The first letter of the Greek alphabet, alpha. 2 A symbol used in chemistry to start enumerating atoms from the atom next to a reference atom. Thus the *α*-carbon of a carboxylic acid is C-2, since the carboxyl group contains C-1.

**AA** 1 Alcoholics Anonymous. 2 achievement age (educational age).

**aa.** arteriae.

**āā** *ana* (Greek, of each, i.e., the stated amount of each of the following substances is to be taken: used in prescription writing).

**AAAS** American Association for the Advancement of Science.

**Aaron** [Charles Dettie *Aaron*, U.S. physician, 1866–1951] See under SIGN.

**AAV** adeno-associated virus.

**ab** antibody.

**ab-$^1$** \ab-, əb-\ [L *ab* (*ab-* before vowels, *h*, and sometimes consonants; *a-* before consonants except *h*; *abs-* sometimes before *c*, *q*, *t*) from] A prefix meaning from, away from, outside of. Also *a-*, *abs-*.

**ab-$^2$** \ab-\ [from ABSOLUTE] A prefix denoting a unit in the CGS electromagnetic system of units.

**Abadie** [Jean Marie Charles *Abadie*, French ophthalmologist, 1842–1932] See under SIGN.

**abandonment** In medical malpractice, negligent termination of the physician-patient relationship by the physician without consent of the patient or without giving the patient adequate time and notice to obtain the services of another physician and under circumstances where continuing medical care is required. Any denial of the patient's full benefit of the physician-patient relationship, such as not seeing a hospitalized patient as frequently as due care in treatment requires, constitutes abandonment.

**abapical** \abap′əkl\ Opposite the apex of a structure.

**abarognosia** BARAGNOSIA.

**abarthrosis** \ab′ärthrō′sis\ [AB-$^1$ + Gk *(ap)arthr(oun)* to dismember, dissect + *-ōsis* -OSIS] 1 ARTICULATIO SYNOVIALIS. 2 ABARTICULATION.

**abarticulation** \ab′ärtik′yəlā′shən\ A joint dislocation. Also *abarthrosis*.

**abasia** \əbā′zhə\ [New L, from Gk *a-* priv. + *basis* a step + -IA] Inability to walk because of motor incoordination, but without paralysis. Abasia is sometimes accompanied by astasia. Adj. abasic, abatic.

**abasia-astasia** \əbā′zhə-əstā′zhə\ ASTASIA-ABASIA.

**abaxial** \abak′sē·əl\ Located outside the axis of a part, organ, or body.

**Abbe** [Ernst Karl *Abbe*, German physicist and industrialist, 1840–1905] Abbe-Zeiss counting chamber, Abbe-Zeiss counting cell. See under THOMA-ZEISS COUNTING CHAMBER.

**Abbe** [Robert *Abbe*, U.S. surgeon, 1851–1928] 1 Abbe lip flap. See under ABBE FLAP. 2 See under OPERATION. 3 Abbe-Estlander operation. See under OPERATION.

**Abbott** [Edville Gerhardt *Abbott*, U.S. surgeon, 1870–1938] See under METHOD.

**Abbott** [William Osler *Abbott*, U.S. physician, 1902–1943] 1 Abbott-Miller tube. See under MILLER-ABBOTT TUBE. 2 Abbott-Rawson tube. See under TUBE.

**ABC** antigen binding capacity.

**abdomen** \ab′dəmən, abdō′mən\ [L (gen. *abdominis*), the belly] The region of the trunk below the diaphragm, containing the largest cavity in the body. The upper, cranial part is the abdomen proper, and the lower, caudal part is the lesser pelvis, the boundary between them being the superior aperture of the latter. The upper boundary is the diaphragm, which arches upward, so that part of the abdomen is protected by the lower bony thoracic wall. The lower boundary is formed by the pelvic and urogenital diaphragms. The abdomen proper is bounded in front by the rectus abdominis and pyramidalis muscles and the aponeuroses of the flat abdominal muscles, the fleshy parts of which form the side walls, supplemented by the iliacus muscles and iliac bones. Behind are the lumbar part of the vertebral column with the crura of the diaphragm and the psoas and quadratus lumborum muscles. The front wall and cavity are arbitrarily divided in clinical usage, for the purpose of locating the viscera contained within, into nine regions by two horizontal and two vertical imaginary planes. The abdominal contents include numerous viscera, blood and lymph vessels, lymph nodes, and nerves. The organs and the interior of the walls are lined by peritoneum. The abdomen varies in capacity and shape according to respiratory phases, the tone of the muscles of the walls, the condition of the viscera, and with age and sex. Also *venter, belly* (popular), *stomach* (incorrect). **acute a.** An acute, intra-abdominal, inflammatory process usually requiring surgical intervention, as an intestinal obstruction or ruptured appendix. *Imprecise.* Also *surgical abdomen.* **carinate a.** An abdomen that has a keel-like anterior prominence along the midline, with depression of the abdominal walls on each side. Compare SCAPHOID ABDOMEN. **navicular a.** SCAPHOID ABDOMEN. **scaphoid a.** An abdomen with a depressed anterior wall; an anterior abdominal contour that is concave rather than convex. Also *navicular abdomen.* Compare CARINATE ABDOMEN. **surgical a.** ACUTE ABDOMEN.

**abdomin-** \abdäm′ən-, ab′dəmən-\ ABDOMINO-.

**abdominal** \abdäm′ənəl\ Pertaining to the abdomen.

**abdominalgia / periodic a.** Diffuse abdominal pain, not due to specific visceral disease or infection. It occurs at specified recurrent time intervals as part of the symptom complex of periodic disease.

**abdomino-** \abdäm′ənō-\ A combining form denoting the abdomen. Also *abdomin-*.

**abdominoanterior** \-antir′ē·ər\ Having the abdomen facing forward: used especially of an intrauterine position of the fetus in which the fetal abdomen faces forward towards the mother's abdominal wall. Compare ABDOMINOPOSTERIOR.

**abdominocentesis** \-sentē′sis\ [ABDOMINO- + -CENTESIS] A procedure whereby a needle is introduced into the abdominal cavity for aspirating fluid. The procedure may be used for diagnostic or therapeutic purposes. Also *abdominal paracentesis, paracentesis abdominis, celioparacentesis, celiocentesis, peritoneocentesis.*

**abdominocystic** \-sis′tik\ **1** Pertaining to the abdomen and the gallbladder. **2** ABDOMINOVESICAL.

**abdominoperineal** \-per′inē′əl\ Relating to the abdomen and the perineum: used especially of surgical procedures involving exploration of these regions, such as total proctocolectomy or resection of the entire rectum.

**abdominoplasty** \abdäm′ənōplas′tē\ [ABDOMINO- + -PLASTY] **1** Rhytidectomy of the skin and subcutaneous tissue of the abdomen performed for cosmetic reasons. **2** Any plastic operation on the abdomen.

**abdominoposterior** \-pästir′ē·ər\ Having the abdomen facing towards the rear: used especially of an intrauterine position of the fetus in which the fetal abdomen faces towards the mother's spine. Compare ABDOMINOANTERIOR.

**abdominothoracic** \-thôras′ik\ Relating to or involving the abdomen and the thorax.

**abdominovesical** \-ves′ikəl\ Pertaining to the abdomen and the urinary bladder. Also *abdominocystic.*

**abducens** \abdoo′səns\ [L, pres. part. of *abducere* to lead or take away, relieve] NERVUS ABDUCENS.

**abducent** \abdoo′sənt\ Causing abduction.

**abduct** \abdukt′\ [L *abduct(us),* past part. of *abducere (from ab-* away + *ducere* to lead) to take or lead away] To move away from the median plane, as the hand, foot, or eye.

**abduction** \abduk′shən\ [ABDUCT + -ION] Movement of a part of the body away from the median plane of the body; or of the hand, from the median plane of the middle digit; or of the foot, from the median plane of the second digit. Abduction of the eye refers to a lateral (distal) movement away from the median plane. Compare ADDUCTION.

**abductor** \abduk′tər\ [ABDUCT + -OR] Any muscle that produces sideways movement of a limb or part away from either the median plane of the body or, in the case of the digits, the middle of the middle finger or of the second toe. Compare ADDUCTOR.

**abembryonic** \ab′embrē·än′ik\ Pertaining to a region opposite to the position of an embryo. In an implanting human blastocyst, the thicker formative mass at the region of deepest penetration is at the embryonic pole, whereas the thinner region most recently embedded is the abembryonic pole.

**abequose** \ab′əkwōs\ 3,6-Dideoxy-D-galactose. It is characteristic of the O antigen (group B) of *Salmonella typhimurium.*

**aberrant** \əber′ənt, ab′ərənt\ [L *aberrans,* gen. *aberrantis* (pres. part. of *aberrare,* from *ab-* away + *errare* to wander) wandering, divergent] Differing substantially in structure, function, or location from the norm of its kind, as a part or organism, especially when due to developmental origin; abnormal.

**aberration** \ab′ərā′shən\ [L *aberratio* (from *aberrare* to go astray, from *ab-* away + *errare* to wander) diversion, deviation] Abnormality; deviation; abnormal variant. **chromatic a.** Aberration due to the refractive differences between the various wavelengths of light, typically manifested by a fringe of color around the image. **chromosomal a.** Any abnormality in the number of chromosomes or the structure of a chromosome that is detectable by microscopy. Small changes in nucleotide sequence such as point mutations, while clearly producing an abnormal chromosome in the functional sense, usually do not result in a change in light-microscopic appearance. Also *chromosomal anomaly.* **heterosomal a.** An alteration of the structure of more than one chromosome, usually by translocation. **homosomal a.** An alteration of the structure of a single chromosome. Genetic loci or nucleotide sequences may be deleted, duplicated, inverted, or in other ways rearranged without apparent change to any other chromosome in the complement. Also *intrachromosomal aberration, intrachange.* **intrachromosomal a.** HOMOSOMAL ABERRATION. **monochromatic a.** Aberration occurring in the transmission of only a single wavelength of light. **optical a.** Failure of the light rays from a point source to form a perfect image after passing through an optical system. **penta-X chromosomal a.** The rare occurrence of five X chromosomes in a human. The subject is usually female, in which case the karyotype is designated 49,XXXXX. The clinical consequences are moderate to severe mental retardation, postnatal growth retardation, small hands, and patent ductus arteriosus. Also *penta-X syndrome.* **spherical a.** A monochromatic aberration occurring in lens refraction in which the central portion of the lens and the peripheral portion focus at different axial points. **tetra-X chromosomal a.** The rare occurrence of four X chromosomes in a human. The subject is usually female, in which case the karyotype is designated 48,XXXX. The clinical consequences are moderate mental retardation, variable facial and limb abnormalities, and menstrual problems. Males who have four X chromosomes express a different phenotype. Also *XXXX syndrome, tetra-X syndrome.* **triple-X chromosomal a.** The occurrence of three X chromosomes in a human. The subject is usually female, in which case the karyotype is designated 47,XXX. The incidence of this most common of the X-chromosomal aberrations approaches one in every 800 live female births. Affected females show no characteristic phenotype and are usually fertile. The frequency of mild mental retardation is slightly greater than it is in the general population. Also *triple-X syndrome, XXX sex chromosome constitution.*

**abetalipoproteinemia** \əbā′təlī′pōprō′tinē′mē·ə\ [A-[1] + *β-lipoprotein* + -EMIA] A rare disorder of autosomal recessive inheritance that results in retinitis pigmentosa, cerebellar ataxia, peripheral neuropathy, steatorrhea, and acanthocytosis of erythrocytes, associated with reduced serum phospholipids and the absence of β-lipoprotein. It occurs predominantly in Ashkenazi Jews, and may be due to homozygosity for the allele that causes familial hypobetalipoproteinemia. Also *Bassen-Kornzweig syndrome, Bassen-Kornzweig disease, abetalipoproteinemic neuropathy.*

**abeyance** \əbā′əns\ A state of inaction capable of reversal.

**ability** / **general a.** G FACTOR OF SPEARMAN. **impaired urinary concentrating a.** Inability to concentrate urine, as measured by specific gravity or osmolality, in response to 18 to 24 hours of fluid deprivation or in response to injection of vasopressin. Concentrating ability may be impaired by any tubular lesion, either isolated, or as a part of any nephritis. **template a.** The capacity of the DNA molecule to code information, which may be replicated or transcribed. **primary mental abilities** The hypothesized basic abilities which combine to make up the intelligence, according to group-factor theory. They include several separable factors of approximately equal importance: verbal comprehension, word fluency, number concepts, space-handling skills, perceptual speed, rote memory, and reasoning. **verbal a.** A demonstrable level of facility in the use of words, whether spoken or written, including the rapid and precise comprehension of verbally expressed concepts.

**-ability** \-əbil′itē\ [*-abl(e)* + -ITY] A combining form meaning capacity, power to do (something specified) or act (in a specified way).

**abiogenesis** \ab′ē·ōjen′əsis\ [Gk *a-* priv. + BIO- + GENESIS] SPONTANEOUS GENERATION. Adj. abiogenetic, abiogenic.

**abiotic** \ab′ē·ät′ik\ Characterized by the absence of life, as an environment that will not support life.

**abiotrophic** \ab′ē·ətrăf′ik\ **1** Pertaining to abiotrophy. **2** Describing disease processes presumed to be due to abiotrophy.

**abiotrophy** \ab′ē·ät′rəfē\ [Gk *a-* priv. + BIO- + TROPH- + -Y] Any of various processes of degeneration of unknown cause affecting nerve cells in the central nervous system. • This is an imprecise term, being used sometimes to describe aging processes and on other occasions to identify the types of neuronal degeneration occurring in such diseases as motor neuron disease and Huntington's disease.

**abirritant** \abir′ətənt\ An agent that relieves irritation.

**ablate** \ablāt′\ To remove, especially by surgery; to subject to ablation.

**ablatio** \ablā′shō\ ABLATION. **a. retinae** RETINAL DETACHMENT.

**ablation** \ablā′shən\ [Late L *ablatio* (from L *ablatus* past part. of *auferre* to carry away, remove, from *au-, ab-* away + *ferre* to carry) removal] The detachment or removal, as of an organ or part, especially by surgery. Also *ablatio.*

**-able** \-əbl\ [Old French, from L *-abilis* (from stem vowel *a* + *-bilis* adj. suffix denoting ability) able, capable] A combining form meaning (1) tending to; (2) capable of, fit to.

**ablephary** \āblef′ərē\ [Gk *a-* priv. + BLEPHAR- + -Y] A congenital deficiency of the eyelids. It can be partial or complete, unilateral or bilateral. Disorganized eye tissue is usually found beneath the skin in the region where the lids are missing. It is often associated with digital or urogenital malformations, or other facial malformations. Also *ablepharon.*

**abluent** \ab′loo·ənt\ **1** Used as or having the properties of a cleansing agent. **2** A substance or agent for cleansing or washing; a detergent.

**ablution** \abloo′shən\ [L *ablutio* (from *ablutus,* past part. of *abluere* to wash away) a washing away] The act or process of washing, especially that of washing the body. *Older term.*

**abmortal** \abmôr′tl\ [AB-[1] + MORTAL] Moving away from damaged tissue: said of an electric current. Compare ADMORTAL.

**abnormal** Describing or pertaining to any state, structure, or function that differs substantially from the norm of its kind; exhibiting abnormality; aberrant.

**abnormality** \ab′nôrmal′itē\ A departure from the normal with respect to some attribute. Where the variation involves a discontinuity, as in the case of polydactyly, the distinction between normality and abnormality is clear, but if the variation is continuous the limits of normality have to be agreed upon. The relative character of this type of abnormality must be recognized, and indeed what may be abnormal in one population may be normal in another. The essential feature of such relative abnormality is not its absolute value but its frequency in a given population. **figure-of-eight a.** An appearance of the heart and the great vessels as seen on an anteroposterior or posteroanterior chest roentgenogram, and considered characteristic for the diagnosis of total anomalous venous return.

**abort** \əbôrt\ [See ABORTION.] To expel the products of conception prematurely before viability of the fetus is reached.

**abortifacient** \əbôr′təfā′shənt\ [L *abort(us)* abortion + *i* + *faciens,* gen. *facientis,* pres. part. of *facere* to do, make] **1** Producing or bringing about an abortion. Also *abortive, abortigenic.* **2** Any agent, usually a drug or other chemical, that produces abortion.

**abortigenic** \əbôr′təjen′ik\ ABORTIFACIENT.

**abortin** \əbôr′tin\ An extract of *Brucella abortus,* formerly used in diagnostic testing for brucellosis. Like tuberculin, abortin is injected subcutaneously, and a positive reaction, marked by erythema and infiltration, indicates active brucellosis or recovery from the disease.

**abortion** [L *abortio* (from *aboriri* to abort or be aborted, from *ab-* away, off, + *oriri* to appear, emerge, be born) miscarriage] The termination of pregnancy or premature expulsion of the products of conception by any means, usually before fetal viability. Although the definition of viability varies, a human pregnancy of over 20 weeks' duration from the first day of the last menstrual period or a fetal weight of more than 500 grams is usually termed viable. **ampullar a.** A tubal abortion where the implantation site is located at the ampulla of the oviduct. **complete a.** An abortion in which the fetus and placenta have been completely expelled from the uterus. **criminal a.** An abortion that has been produced illegally. Also *illegal abortion.* **elective a.** An induced abortion that is performed voluntarily at the request of the mother for reasons other than maternal health or likely fetal disease. **habitual a.** The occurrence in the same woman of three or more consecutive spontaneous abortions. Also *recurrent abortion.* **idiopathic a.** The occurrence of a spontaneous abortion for which no cause can be readily determined. **illegal a.** CRIMINAL ABORTION. **incomplete a.** An abortion in which some but not all of the products of conception have passed from the uterine cavity. Also *partial abortion.* **induced a.** An abortion which is brought about intentionally by the use of instruments, medications, or other devices, as contrasted with a spontaneous abortion. **infected a.** An abortion in which there is evidence of uterine infection such as fever, purulent cervical discharge, or an elevated white blood cell count. **late a.** An abortion which occurs in the latter half of the second trimester. *Imprecise.* **legal a.** A legally sanctioned abortion, performed on an elective basis in the first trimester of pregnancy, or occasionally later when the cause for the abortion is therapeutic. **missed a.** Prolonged retention, usually a minimum of four weeks, of the products of conception after death of the fetus. The diagnosis is made by noting absence of expected growth in uterine size or loss of fetal heart tones which previously had been noted. **natural a.** SPONTANEOUS ABORTION. **partial a.** INCOMPLETE ABORTION. **psychiatric a.** A therapeutic abortion performed on the grounds that continuation of pregnancy would severely impair the mother's mental health. **recurrent a.** HABITUAL ABORTION. **repeat a.** The performance of more than one abortion, especially elective abortions, at the request of the patient. *Imprecise.* **septic a.** An infected abortion in which there is a serious uterine infection and, sometimes, shock. The condition may threaten the life of the mother. It is often associated with criminally induced abortion. **spontaneous a.** An abortion which has not been induced. Also *natural abortion, miscarriage* (popular). **therapeutic a.** An induced abortion performed because continuation of pregnancy might threaten the patient's life or severely affect her health, when pregnancy is a result of rape or incest, or when continuation of pregnancy is likely to result in the birth of a child with mental retardation or severe physical deformities. **threatened a.** The occurrence of vaginal bleeding or bloody discharge, felt to be of uterine origin, during the first half of pregnancy. **tubal a.** The rupture or extrusion of the products of conception into the peritoneal cavity from an ectopic pregnancy located in the oviduct.

**abortive** \əbôr′tiv\ [L *abortivus* (from *aboriri* to abort or be aborted) born prematurely; causing abortion] **1** Following a course that is unusually short or incomplete: said especially of a disease. **2** Acting to cut short the progress of a disease, as a treatment. **3** Not fully developed or formed; rudimentary. **4** ABORTIFACIENT. **5** Of or relating to an infection of a cell by bacteriophage or virus that fails to lead to the production of additional infectious vectors. **6** Characterized by a transfer of DNA to a cell, as by transformation, conjugation, or transduction, in which the foreign DNA fails to be integrated into the host genome.

**abortus** \əbôr′təs\ [L, untimely birth. See also ABORTION.] The fetal products following an abortion. In usual usage, the human abortus must weigh less than 500 g.

**abouchement** \ä′booshmäɴ′\ [French (from *aboucher* to join mouth to mouth, end to end, from *bouche* mouth) anastomosis] The junction of a small vessel terminating in a larger one.

**ABP** arterial blood pressure.

**abrachia** \əbrā′kē·ə\ [Gk *a-* priv. + BRACH- + -IA] The congenital unilateral or bilateral absence of the arms, a condition associated with high neonatal mortality. The pectoral girdle may be normal or reduced. Also *brachial amelia.*

**abrachiocephaly** \əbrā′kē·əsef′əlē\ [Gk *a-* priv. + BRACHIO- + CEPHAL- + -Y] Congenital absence of the arms and head. Also *acephalobrachia.*

**Abrahams** [Robert *Abrahams,* U.S. physician, 1861–1935] See under SIGN.

**Abrams** [Albert *Abrams,* U.S. physician, 1863–1924] Abrams heart reflex. See under REFLEX.

**abrasio** \əbrā′zhō\ ABRASION.

**abrasion** \əbrā′zhən\ [L *abrasio* (from AB-[1] + L *rasus,* past part. of *radere* to shave, scrape) a shaving off] **1** A minor wound resulting from the scraping or rubbing away of a usually small area of skin or mucous membrane. **2** The removal by mechanical friction of the epidermis and the upper part of the dermis, either accidentally or as a controlled procedure in plastic surgery. **3** The lesion created by such action. For defs. 1, 2, and 3 also *abrasio.* **4** See under DERMABRASION. **5** BRUSH BURN. **dental a.** The wearing away of tooth surface, most often buccal or labial, usually by the polishing agent in a dentifrice. It commonly occurs on that part of the root which has been exposed by recession of the gingiva, in which case the affected tissues are cementum and dentine. It sometimes occurs at the crown, where its progress is much slower because the enamel is more resistant. It may also occur proximally, where it is caused by the relative buccolingual movement of adjacent teeth during mastication. In this case dentifrice abrasive plays no part. **dicing a.'s** The angular, small, superficial lacerations on the face, upper arms, or upper torso of a driver and/or passenger who are victims of vehicular trauma. The lacerations are caused by the explosion and disintegration of the tempered safety glass of the side windows into small, angular, often cubical fragments which strike the victim. Also *dicing lacerations, dicing pattern.* • Although a misnomer, the term *abrasion* is widely used. **a. of the gingiva** Abrasion, usually of the buccal or labial gingiva, caused by the use of stiff sharp toothbrush filaments. Small circular ulcers, 0.5 to 1.0 mm in diameter, are found on the attached gingiva. When chronic, it may present as gingival recession. **marginal a.** ABRASION COLLAR.

**abrasive** \əbrā′ziv\ **1** A substance used for polishing teeth or restorations, usually as an ingredient of a paste or dentrifice. **2** Tending to abrade.

**abrasor** \əbrā′zər\ Any device or material used for abrading.

**abreaction** \ab′rē·ak′shən\ [AB-[1] + REACTION] The act of bringing repressed material into consciousness with an appropriate discharge of the affect that originally accompanied the event.

**Abrikosov** [Aleksei Ivanovich *Abrikosov,* Russian pathologist, 1875–1955] Abrikosov's tumor. See under GRANULAR CELL TUMOR.

**abrin** \ā′brin\ A protein phytotoxin produced by *Abrus* species, especially *A. precatorius.* Its ingestion causes stomach pain, nausea, diarrhea, coma, circulatory collapse, and coagulation of erythrocytes. It is a severe irritant of mucous membranes, including the conjunctivae.

**abrotanum** \ab′rətā′nəm\ [alteration of L *abrotonum* (from Gk *abrotonon* an aromatic plant) an aromatic herb] An aromatic herb, *Artemisia abrotanum,* used variously as an anthelmintic, moth repellent, detergent, astringent, and antisomnolent. It is known to be aeroallergenic. Abrotanum is a source of the alkaloid abrotine, $C_{21}H_{22}ON_2$. Also *southernwood.*

**abruptio** \abrup′shō\ [L (from *abruptus,* past part. of *abrumpere* to break off), a tearing away] A tearing or violent separation, as of the placenta from the uterus. Also *abruption.* **a. placentae** Premature separation of the placenta from the uterine wall occurring prior to the delivery of the fetus. Also *abruption of placenta, uterine apoplexy, accidental antepartum hemorrhage.*

**abruption** \əbrup′shən\ ABRUPTIO. **a. of placenta** ABRUPTIO PLACENTAE.

**abrus** \ā′brəs\ [New L (irreg. from Gk *(h)abros* delicate, dainty)] The seeds of the plant *Abrus precatorius,* known as Indian licorice, jequirity, or rosary pea. They are extremely toxic, being the source of the phytotoxin abrin.

**abs** absolute.

**abs-** \abs-, əbs-\ AB-[1].

# abscess

**abscess** \ab′səs\ [L *abscessus* (from *abscedere* to go away, slough off, suppurate, from *abs-, ab-* away, off + *cedere* to withdraw, cede) withdrawal, abscess] A focal collection of pus resulting from liquefactive necrosis of a tissue, usually caused by a pyogenic microorganism. When fully developed, it is characterized by a spherical shape and consists of a central collection of dead and dying polymorphonuclear neutrophilic leukocytes contained in a wall, or capsule, composed of granulation tissue and proliferating myofibroblasts. Also *apostema* (obs.), *abscessus* (obs.). **acute periappendicular a.** An abscess resulting from an acute inflammatory process in the region of the vermiform appendix, generally related to a perforation of the appendix but occasionally to Crohn's disease of the terminal ileum and cecum. It may become chronic if untreated, but it generally requires surgical drainage and appendectomy. Also *periappendiceal abscess.* **alveolar a.** An abscess starting adjacent to the apical foramen of a nonvital tooth, caused by infection from the root canal, and spreading through the overlying bone and soft tissues. The subsequent facial swelling may occasionally be a true pus-containing abscess, extending from the original abscess, but usually it is caused by inflammatory exudate only. The abscess may be acute or become chronic with a draining tract to the oral cavity or occasionally to the skin. The facial swelling is popularly known as a dental abscess, and in the mouth as a gumboil. Also *apical abscess, periapical abscess, apical periodontal abscess, parulis, dentoalveolar abscess, apical pericementitis.* **amebic a.** A circumscribed area of necrosis, usually involving the right lobe of the liver, caused by *Entamoeba histolytica*. Unlike most abscesses, the inflammatory response consists of mononuclear cells rather than neutrophils. **apical a.** ALVEOLAR ABSCESS. **apical periodontal a.** ALVEOLAR ABSCESS. **appendiceal a.** An abscess in the region of the vermiform appendix, generally following perforation of the appendix. Also *appendicular abscess.* See also ACUTE PERIAPPENDICULAR ABSCESS. **appendicular a.** APPENDICEAL ABSCESS. **bartholinian a.** An abscess in Bartholin's glands or their ducts. It is frequently but not exclusively the result of gonorrheal infection. **Bezold's a.** An abscess in the digastric fossa caused by rupture through the mastoid cortex of an abscess within the mastoid process of the temporal bone. The latter in turn is often a complication of suppurative otitis media. **bile duct a.** CHOLANGITIC ABSCESS. **bone a.** OSTEOMYELITIS. **brain a.** An abscess occurring in the brain, either as the result of direct extension from an adjacent focus of infection, for example in the ear, or by blood-borne metastasis from a distant site of infection, for example in the lungs or endocardium. Also *pyencephalus, pyocephalus, internal pyocephalus.* **Brodie's a.** A form of chronic osteomyelitis characterized by a localized abscess composed of inflamed, jellylike granulation tissue which is surrounded by dense, sclerotic bone. **canalicular a.** A form of breast abscess that communicates with one or more of the milk ducts, causing a purulent discharge from the nipple. **cerebellar a.** An abscess of the cerebellum, with etiology and symptoms similar to those of a cerebral abscess. One characteristic sign is spontaneous phasic nystagmus. This is usually horizontal, rarely rotatory. Vertical nystagmus is exceptional. In most cases, the quick phase of the nystagmus occurs predominantly or entirely on looking towards the side of the lesion. It is seldom affected by change in the position of the head. Conjugate deviation of the eyes to the side opposite the lesion, usually a late symptom, paralysis of gaze to that side, and ataxia in the ipsilateral limbs are other important manifestations. **cerebral a.** Any abscess within the substance of the brain. The condition may present acutely or subacutely. A chronic abscess may develop due to localization after a prior phase of suppurative encephalitis. Cerebral abscesses are sometimes loculated, occasionally multiple. They often develop as a complication of otitis media or paranasal sinusitis but may be the consequence of septic embolism in bacterial endocarditis, or can result from metastatic spread of infection from septic foci in the lungs, skin, or any part of the body. Cerebral abscess is an important complication of congenital heart disease. Clinical manifestations are firstly those of infection (mild fever and leukocytosis), secondly of raised intracranial pressure (headache, vomiting and papilledema), and thirdly those of a focal cerebral lesion, depending upon location. Also *intracerebral abscess.* **cholangitic a.** An abscess resulting from extrahepatic biliary obstruction and ascending cholangitis. Also *bile duct abscess.* **circumscribed a.** WALLED ABSCESS. **cold a.** A focal collection of caseous material devoid of any significant acute inflammatory reaction. It is usually of tuberculous origin. Also *strumous abscess.* **crypt a.** A microscopic abscess of a crypt of Lieberkühn, constituting the earliest and most characteristic histopathologic lesion of ulcerative colitis. **dental a.** The sudden painful facial swelling arising from any type of abscess associated with a tooth, most commonly an alveolar abscess. *Popular.* Also *tooth abscess.* **dentoalveolar a.** ALVEOLAR ABSCESS. **diffuse a.** An abscess that lacks a capsule and often infiltrates the adjacent tissues. **Douglas a.** A collection of pus filling the pouch of Douglas. It represents a complication of pelvic or diffuse peritonitis. **dry a.** An abscess that has been drained or has resorbed spontaneously as a result of antibiotic therapy. **Dubois a.** A lesion of the thymus characterized by multiple small cysts lined by squamous epithelium and containing keratin and necrotic debris. The condition was originally regarded as an indication of congenital syphilis, but it most likely represents enlarged Hassall's corpuscles and is probably of a hamartomatous nature. Also *thymic abscess.* **embolic a.** An abscess developing at the site of impaction of a septic embolus. Usually multiple and involving several organs, these abscesses are frequent in septicemia. **encapsulated a.** WALLED ABSCESS. **encysted a.** An abscess formed within a serous cavity and circumscribed by inflammatory adhesions. **epidural a.** EXTRADURAL ABSCESS. **extradural a.** An abscess situated between the dura mater and the skull, or outside the dura mater of the spinal cord. It occurs most frequently as a consequence of cranial or vertebral osteomyelitis, or of infection of the middle ear or frontal sinus. Intracranial extradural abscess may also result from compound fracture of the skull. Spinal extradural abscess may be tuberculous, complicating tuberculous caries of the spine, or pyogenic when it is almost always staphylococcal, due either to osteomyelitis or to metastatic spread of infection to the extradural space. It causes spinal tenderness, fever, and spinal cord compression and is a neurosurgical emergency. Also *epidural abscess, purulent pachymeningitis, pyogenic pachymeningitis, extradural empyema.* **fecal a.** An abscess which contains a mixture of fecal material and pus. It is often located in or around the colon and results from fistulas or perforations of the bowel such as acute diverticulitis or cancer. Also *stercoraceous abscess, stercoral abscess.* **gingival a.** An acute abscess near the gingival margin, chiefly associated with a suprabony pocket. It is locally painful but the tooth itself is not tender. **gravitation a.** HYPOSTATIC ABSCESS. **gummatous a.** An abscess resulting from liquefaction of a syphilitic gumma. Also *syphilitic abscess.* **helminthic a.** An abscess caused by an intestinal worm such as ancylostoma or ascaris. **hematogenous a.** An abscess, usually multiple, resulting from dissemination of a blood-borne infection. **hemorrhagic a.** An abscess in which blood is admixed with pus. **hepatic a.** LIVER ABSCESS. **hot a.** An abscess that displays signs of acute inflammation. **hypostatic a.** An abscess that migrates from its site of origin to an adjacent, dependent area of the body as a result of the force of gravity. Also *gravitation abscess, migrating abscess, wandering abscess.* **intracerebral a.** CEREBRAL ABSCESS. **intracranial a.** An abscess inside the cranium, especially in the brain but also in any of the intracranial fluid spaces, such as the epidural, subdural, subarachnoid, and ventricular spaces. **intradural a.** An abscess arising between the layers of the dura, but not in the subdural space. **intramammary a.** An abscess in the parenchyma of the breast. **intramedullary spinal a.** 1 Abscess formation within the substance of the spinal cord; a very rare manifestation of metastatic infection. 2 METASTATIC MYELITIS. **intraspinal a.** An abscess within the spinal canal, usually in the epidural or subdural space but occasionally within the spinal cord. **intratonsillar a.** An abscess located within the substance of the palatine tonsil. **kidney a.** RENAL ABSCESS. **lacunar a.** An abscess that develops in a urethral lacuna. **lateral alveolar a.** PERIODONTAL ABSCESS. **lateral root a.** PERIODONTAL ABSCESS. **liver a.** An abscess of the liver. Frequently multiple, it arises as a complication of infection of the biliary tree, pylephlebitis, septicemia, or amebiasis. Also *hepatic abscess.* **lung a.** An abscess of the pulmonary parenchyma, frequently caused by aspiration of infected material from the upper respiratory passages or as a complication of unresolved pneumonia. **lymphatic a.** An abscess of a lymph node, usually cold and of tuberculous origin. **mammary a.** An abscess located in the breast that usually affects lactating women. It is commonly caused by a staphylococcus. Also *broken breast, gathered breast.* **mastoid a.** An abscess occurring in a case of mastoiditis. It may locate within the mastoid process (intramastoid abscess), beneath the mastoid periosteum behind the ear (subperiosteal abscess), deep to the upper fibers of the sternomastoid muscle (Bezold's abscess), or between the mastoid bone and the dura mater (extradural abscess). **metastatic a.** A secondary abscess arising from the hematogenous spread of microbes from a distinct primary site. **migrating a.** HYPOSTATIC ABSCESS. **miliary a.** One of multiple small abscesses, the size of millet seeds (1–2 mm), resulting from the spread of a blood-borne infection. **milk a.** A mammary gland abscess occurring during the period of lactation. **mother a.** The oldest abscess of a group of abscesses of which the more recent ones originated by local spread of the infection. **Munro's a.'es** MUNRO'S MICROABSCESSES. **mural a.** An abscess of the wall of the abdomen. **nasal septum a.** An abscess located beneath the mucoperichondrium of the nasal septum, usually the result of infection of a traumatic nasal septum hematoma. Destruction of the septal cartilage with collapse of the nasal dorsum and the development of a characteristic deformity is usually the end result. **orbital a.** An abscess occurring in the cellular tissues of the orbit usually as the result of direct spread from an infected frontal sinus. **ossifluent a.** *Seldom used* OSTEOMYELITIS. **otic cerebral a.** An abscess in the cerebrum originating from infection in the ear. It usually occurs by direct extension, but can be blood-borne. Also *otogenic abscess.* **otogenic a.** OTIC CEREBRAL ABSCESS. **palatal a.** An abscess pointing in the palate, usually from an alveolar abscess related to an upper lateral incisor tooth or to the palatal root of a molar tooth. **pancreatic a.** An abscess located in the pancreatic parenchyma which develops as a complication of pancreatitis or trauma and is frequently associated with enzymatic fat necrosis. **paranephric a.** An abscess located in the adipose tissue surrounding the kidney. It results from extension of a renal cortical abscess or hematogenous or lymphatic spread of infection. **parapharyngeal a.** An abscess located between the superior constrictor muscle of the pharynx and the investing layer of the deep cervical fascia. In rare cases, it complicates tonsillitis, and peritonsillar abscess or, more rarely, tonsillectomy or accidental trauma to the pharynx. Parapharyngeal abscess is a dangerous condition with a risk of mediastinitis, jugular-vein thrombosis, or even massive hemorrhage with death from exsanguination. Such a condition demands prompt external surgical drainage. **parotid a.** An abscess occurring within the parotid gland in the course of acute suppurative parotitis. Predisposing factors are obstruction to the parotid duct from calculus or stricture and oral sepsis in dehydrated patients. Rupture may occur into the external auditory meatus. **Pautrier's a.'es** PAUTRIER'S MICROABSCESSES. **pelvirectal a.** An abscess of the deep tissues of the perirectal region extending into the pelvis. **periapical a.** ALVEOLAR ABSCESS. **periappendiceal a.** ACUTE PERIAPPENDICULAR ABSCESS. **periarticular a.** An abscess occurring in structures outside of, but next to, the joint space, as in a bursa or tendon sheath. **pericemental a.** PERIODONTAL ABSCESS. **pericoronal a.** An abscess affecting the dental follicle or the space between an unerupted or partially erupted tooth and the overlying gum. **peridental a.** PERIODONTAL ABSCESS. **periesophageal a.** An abscess occurring alongside the esophagus, such as may form at the site of a perforation or an erosion caused by an impacted foreign body. **perinephric a.** An abscess of the perirenal fat, usually associated with an infection of the renal pelvis (by *Escherichia coli, Proteus, Klebsiella, Enterobacter,* tuberculosis, or fungi), but sometimes hematogenous in origin *(Streptococcus* or *Staphylococcus).* Flank pain, fever and a palpable flank mass are common features. The condition usually is unilateral. Pyuria may or may not be present. **periodontal a.** An acute, inflammatory, usually painful destructive process in the periodontium, resulting in a localized collection of pus. It originates laterally to the root, usually emanating from a preexisting pocket. It may become chronic with a draining tract. Also *lateral alveolar abscess, lateral root abscess, pericemental abscess, peridental abscess.* **periproctic a.** PERIRECTAL ABSCESS. **perirectal a.** An abscess in the tissue planes around the rectum, often extending to the perianal region or into the pelvis. Also *periproctic abscess.* **peritoneal a.** A walled abscess within the peritoneal cavity, commonly seen in bacterial peritonitis resulting from perforation of a hollow viscus such as the vermiform appendix. **peritonsillar a.** An abscess located between the connective tissue capsule of the palatine tonsil and the muscular tonsillar bed. It occurs as a complication of tonsillitis. The abscess can be drained surgically or it may rupture spontaneously. Also *retrotonsillar abscess, supratonsillar abscess, quinsy.* **periureteral a.** An abscess in close approximation to a ureter, usually secondary to calculous or other conditions that cause ureteral obstruction or infection. The signs and symptoms are similar to those of perinephric abscess, but pyuria is usually present. **periurethral a.** A pyogenic infection of the glands and lacunae of the urethra following urethritis of gonorrheal or nonspecific origin. **perivesical a.** An abscess in urinary bladder tissues. **pilonidal a.** An abscess developing within a pilonidal sinus that may represent its first clinical manifestation. **Pott's a.** A cold abscess associated with tuberculosis of the spine. **premammary a.** An abscess located in the skin and subcutaneous tissue of the breast. **preperitoneal a.** An abscess located in the tissues between the parietal peritoneum and the anterior abdominal wall. Also *subperitoneal abscess.* **psoas a.** An abscess that develops as a complication of osteomyelitis of the spine in the lower thoracic or the lumbar region. It is usually of tuberculous origin. The pus or caseous exudate originates in the infected vertebrae, descends along the sheath of the psoas muscle, and may point in the inguinal region. **pulp a.** An abscess within the dental pulp; a stage of a slowly progressing closed pulpitis. **pyemic a.** SEPTICEMIC ABSCESS. **pylephlebitic a.** A hepatic abscess resulting from the spread to the liver of infected emboli that originated in portal vein tributaries, usually as a result of acute appendicitis or acute colonic diverticulitis. **renal a.** Single or multiple abscesses of the renal cortex, usually unilateral. The onset is sudden, characterized by chills and fever and costovertebral angle tenderness. Pyuria may occur. Also *kidney abscess, renal carbuncle, acute suppurative nephritis.* **residual a.** An abscess that reappears at the same site following apparent healing. **retrocecal a.** An abscess located behind the cecum, usually resulting from perforation of a retrocecal appendix. **retromammary a.** An abscess in the soft tissues behind the breast, usually having no connection with the breast parenchyma. **retropharyngeal a.** An abscess located deep to the posterior pharyngeal wall, in most cases due to suppuration in retropharyngeal lymph nodes. In such cases the swelling appears to one side of the midline of the pharyngeal wall although it may spread across it. In the past such abscesses were often due to caries tuberculosa of the cervical spine, in which case the swelling would originate in the midline. This cause is still encountered in areas where tuberculosis is uncontrolled. Also *hippocratic angina* (outmoded). **retrotonsillar a.** PERITONSILLAR ABSCESS. **secondary a.** An abscess complicating another disease process. **septal a.** A periodontal abscess occurring between the teeth. **septicemic a.** An abscess, usually multiple, affecting several organs as a result of hematogenous spread of an infectious process. Also *pyemic abscess.* **shirt-stud a.** An abscess composed of two interconnected cavities, one superficial and one deep. **spinal subdural a.** An abscess developing between the dura mater and arachnoid investing the spinal cord or cauda equina. **spirillar a.** An abscess caused by spirilla, often developing at the site of a rat or mouse bite and accompanied by lymphangitis and fever. **stellate a.** An irregular or star-shaped, coalescent, centrally necrotic, epithelioid granuloma rather than a proper abscess. It is the characteristic lymph node lesion of lymphogranuloma venereum but may also be seen in cat-scratch disease and infection with *Pasteurella septica.* **stercoraceous a.** FECAL ABSCESS. **stercoral a.** FECAL ABSCESS. **sterile a.** An abscess from which organisms cannot be demonstrated. **stitch a.** An abscess forming around a surgical suture. It is a manifestation of wound infection. **strumous a.** *Obs.* COLD ABSCESS. **subacute a.** An abscess that heals slowly, usually over a period of weeks. **subaponeurotic a.** An abscess that develops beneath a fascial layer or aponeurosis. Also *subfascial abscess.* **subarachnoid a.** An abscess situated in the subarachnoid space between the arachnoid and pia mater. A localized subarachnoid collection of pus is a very rare complication of pyogenic meningitis. **subareolar a.** A breast abscess located beneath the areola of the nipple. It often results from infection of one of the sebaceous glands of the areola. When chronic, it may lead to a milk fistula. **subdiaphragmatic a.** SUBPHRENIC ABSCESS. **subdural a.** An abscess situated in the subdural space between the arachnoid and dural membranes. It is very rare in the spinal cord, less rare intracranially when it most often results from frontal sinusitis, less often from otitis media. The usual manifestations are increasing drowsiness, convulsions, progressive hemiplegia, and fever. Also *subdural empyema, pachymeningitis intralamellaris, purulent pachymeningitis, pyogenic pachymeningitis.* **subepidermal a.** An abscess situated beneath the epidermis. **subfascial a.** SUBAPONEUROTIC ABSCESS. **subgaleal a.** An abscess beneath the epicranial aponeurosis. **submammary a.** An abscess whose location is underneath the mammary gland. Also *submammary mastitis.* **subperiosteal a.** An abscess forming deep to the periosteum and thereby raising the periosteum away from the subjacent bone, as in cases when an abscess presents behind the ear in mastoiditis. **subperiosteal orbital a.** A subperiosteal abscess located beneath the roof of the orbit as the result of direct spread of infection from an infected frontal sinus, thus causing a displacement of the eye downwards and outwards. **subperitoneal a.** PREPERITONEAL ABSCESS. **subphrenic a.** A walled peritoneal abscess beneath the diaphragm, most often on the right side, in a compartment bounded by the liver and the falciform ligament. It is frequently a complication of abdominal surgery or diffuse peritonitis. Also *subdiaphragmatic abscess, suprahepatic abscess.* **subscapular a.** An abscess between the chest wall and the scapula, usually beneath the serratus anterior. **subungual a.** A collection of pus beneath a nail. **sudoriparous a.** An abscess developing in a sweat gland. **superficial a.** An abscess located near a surface such as the skin, a serosal membrane, or a mucosa. **suprahepatic a.** SUBPHRENIC ABSCESS. **supralevator a.** An abscess developing in association with an anal fistula between the levator ani muscles and the reflection of the peritoneum. **supratonsillar a.** PERITONSILLAR ABSCESS. **sympathetic a.** A secondary or satellite abscess arising near but separate from a primary infectious focus. **syphilitic a.** GUMMATOUS ABSCESS. **temporal lobe a.** An abscess located within the temporal lobe of the brain, attributable, in the majority of cases, to direct spread from a focus of infection in the middle ear. Both incidence and mortality have been greatly reduced over a number of decades as a result of improved diagnosis and management of otitis media as well as modern neurosurgical techniques. **thymic a.** DUBOIS ABSCESS. **tooth a.** DENTAL ABSCESS. **tubo-ovarian a.** An abscess involving both the uterine tube and the ovary. This condition generally is a complication of either acute or chronic salpingitis. **urinary a.** An abscess due to infection by extravasated urine. **urinous a.** An abscess containing pus and urine, the latter originating from a communication with the urinary tract, usually a fistula. **verminous a.** An abscess containing worms of any kind. Also *worm abscess.* **walled a.** A chronic abscess surrounded by a thick fibrous capsule. Also *circumscribed abscess, encapsulated abscess.* **wandering a.** HYPOSTATIC ABSCESS. **worm a.** VERMINOUS ABSCESS.

**abscessus** \abses′əs\ *Obs.* ABSCESS.

**abscission** \absizh′ən\ [L *abscissio* (from *abscissus,* past part. of *abscindere* to tear or cut off) a tearing or cutting off] The removal of tissue by cutting.

**absconsio** \abskän′sē·ō\ [Late L, noun from L *abscondere* to conceal] A recess, cavity, depression, or fossa, usually one in bone hiding the head of an adjacent bone.

**abscopal** \ab′skəpəl\ [AB-[1] + Gk *skop(os)* target, objective + -AL] Referring to the effects induced by ionizing radiation on tissues remote from those directly irradiated.

**absence** [French, absence, absent-mindedness, abstraction, loss of awareness] **1** Abrupt, transient loss of consciousness without loss of postural tone or autonomic function and usually without convulsive movements. This is the most typical form of petit mal. Also *absentia epileptica.* ● *Absence* is commonly used in French for a variety of minor epileptic seizures, including those covered in English by the term *petit mal.* **2** The failure of any structure to develop; agenesis, as *congenital absence of arms..* Also *absentia.* ● The term in this sense is rarely applied to the failure of functional or chemical entities to develop. **atypical a.** A type of absence which may be simple or complex and which is differentiated, by definition, on the basis of its electroencephalographic characteristics which are not the same as those of a typical absence or petit mal attack. Atypical absences may be accompanied by at least three types of electroencephalographic pattern, a very rapid generalized epileptic discharge of low amplitude occurring at about 20 Hz, a generalized epileptiform rhythm which is slower (about 10 Hz) but of greater amplitude and a slow, bilateral spike-wave pattern, which is more or less synchronous and symmetrical and which is repeated more or less rhythmically at about 2 Hz. Atypical absence is easy to distinguish electroencephalographically from typical petit mal because it is never accompanied by bilaterally synchronous, symmetrical spike-wave patterns repeated rhythmically at 3 Hz. Moreover, unlike the latter, it is difficult to induce by hyperventilation or intermittent photic stimulation. Clinically, it is not of the group of common benign idiopathic varieties of epilepsy, but the attacks are variable in content and duration and are often associated with intellectual impairment (Lennox-Gastaut syndrome). **complex a.** COMPLEX PARTIAL SEIZURE. **congenital ossicular a.** Congenital absence of part of the ossicular chain, a common cause of congenital conductive deafness. The lesion most often found at exploratory tympanotomy is absence of the superstructure of the stapes. **enuretic a.** An attack of minor epilepsy in which urinary incontinence occurs. **myoclonic a.** A minor attack of epilepsy accompanied by one or two bilateral rhythmic myoclonic jerks, especially in the head and arms. This is most often seen in true petit mal, with a 3 Hz spike-wave pattern in the EEG. The myoclonic jerks occur in time with the EEG spike. **retrocursive a.** An attack of transient impairment of consciousness in which the patient may involuntarily walk backwards a few paces and the body may arch backwards due to a transient increase in extensor tone. **retropulsive a.** A transient episode of increased extensor tone with backward arching of the head, neck, and trunk. In extreme cases the patient may fall backwards. This may occur in postencephalitic parkinsonism. Despite the term *absence*, there is considerable doubt as to whether such attacks are epileptic. **subclinical a.** SUBCLINICAL EPILEPSY.

**absentia** \absen′shə\ [L, absence] ABSENCE. **a. epileptica** ABSENCE.

**abs. feb.** *absente febre* (L, in the absence of fever).

**absinthe** \ab′sinth\ [French, from L *absinthium,* from Gk *apsinthion* wormwood] A green liqueur consisting of a 60% alcohol extract of absinthium, anise, and other aromatic bitter herbs.

**absinthin** $C_{30}H_{40}O_6$. The chief bitter principle of wormwood (*Artemisia absinthium*), used as a flavoring in alcoholic beverages and formerly used as an anthelmintic and as a gastric tonic.

**absinthism** \ab′sinthizm\ A pathologic condition resulting from chronic use of absinthe, characterized by gastrointestinal symptoms, nervousness, visual disturbances, convulsions, and hallucinations. Prolonged use may be fatal.

**absinthium** \absin′thē·əm\ The dried leaves and flowering tops of *Artemesia absinthium.* It has been used as a tonic, an anthelmintic, and as a flavoring agent in alcoholic beverages. Also *wormwood.*

**absinthol** THUJONE.

**absorbance** \absôr′bəns\ [*absorb* + -ANCE] In spectrophotometry, the logarithm of the ratio of the incident intensity to the emerging intensity. If Beer's law holds, which it is likely to do if the light is monochromatic, this quantity is proportional to the concentration of the absorbing substance and the path length. Also *absorbency, optical density.*

**absorbefacient** 1 Promoting absorption. 2 An absorbefacient agent.

**absorbency** \absôr′bənsē\ ABSORBANCE.

**absorbent** \absôr′bənt\ 1 Having the property of absorbing. Also *absorptive.* 2 Any agent possessing the ability to absorb.

**absorber** \absôr′bər\ Any substance that absorbs, as radiation or sound. **carbon dioxide a.** A substance used to absorb carbon dioxide when anesthetic gases are rebreathed in an anesthesia breathing circuit. It may be either sodium hydroxide or a combination of barium hydroxide and sodium hydroxide (baralyme).

**absorptiometer** \absôrp′shē·äm′ətər\ [*absorptio(n)* + -METER] A device for determining the solubility of a gas or the amount of gas absorbed.

**absorptiometry** \absôrp′shē·äm′ətrē\ [*absorptio(n)* + -METRY] Any technique for measuring absorption of waves or particles. Each material or element has the property of absorbing light or electromagnetic waves of characteristic lengths, and analyzing absorption patterns permits analysis of constituents in complex mixtures or structures. **dual photon a.** Determination of the density of an object by measuring the relative absorption of two x-ray or gamma ray beams having different energies. **photon a.** Determination of the density of an object by measuring the absorption of a beam of x rays or gamma rays passed through the object.

**absorption** \absôrp′shən\ [Late L *absorptio* (from L *absorbere* to swallow up, absorb, from *ab-*, completive prefix, + *sorbere* to drink or suck in) absorption, swallowing up] 1 The uptake of energy from radiation in a medium traversed by such radiation. 2 The uptake of a substance by a tissue, or other phase separate from that in which the substance was originally located. **bone a.** The surface removal of bone by osteoclastic activity. **broad-beam a.** In radiation measurements, the absorption of energy as measured under conditions where the radiation beam impinges on a large area, so that some scattered radiation is included in the measurement. **cross a.** The absorption of a given antiserum with antigens which share antigenic determinants with the specific immunogen to obtain a specific antiserum. An example of cross absorption is the absorption of a group A streptococcal antiserum with other hemolytic streptococci to remove antibodies cross-reactive with hemolytic streptococci. **cutaneous a.** Absorption into the body through the skin. **intestinal a.** Absorption through the wall of the intestine. Also *enteral absorption.* **net a.** The excess of absorption over excretion. **parenteral a.** Absorption from a site other than the digestive tract. **wall a.** The absorption of an x ray or gamma radiation in the wall of an ionization chamber used for radiation measurement. **x-ray a.** The deposition of energy in a material irradiated by a beam of x rays.

**absorptive** \absôrp′tiv\ ABSORBENT.

**abst** abstract.

**abstinence** \ab′stinəns\ 1 The act or practice of voluntarily denying oneself the indulgence of a craving or desire, particularly, in alcoholism and other types of drug dependency the act of refraining from the use of the substance. Abstinence may lead to the development of withdrawal syndromes, such as delirium tremens or barbiturate withdrawal. 2 The voluntary forgoing of sexual activity and, particularly in psychoanalysis, the giving up of interests and pleasures that might permit substitute expression for the symptoms that are under analytic investigation. **periodic a.** RHYTHM METHOD.

**abstr** abstract.

**abstraction** \abstrak′shən\ [Late L *abstractio* (from L *abstractus,* past part. of *abstrahere* to drag away, exclude) abduction, exclusion] Teeth or other structures below the normal occlusal plane.

**abtorsion** \abtôr′shən\ Rotation of the eye on its anteroposterior axis so that its upper portion turns away from the nose.

**abtropfung** \ab′träpfəng, äp′trôp′fung\ [German *abtropf(en)* to drip, trickle down + *-ung* -ING] A maturation process of pigmented nevi in which those nevus cells in contact with the basal layer of the epidermis enter the dermal layer.

**abundance** / **isotopic a.** The relative number of atoms having a particular mass number, compared to the total atoms of that element. **relative isotopic a.** The amount of a particular isotope of an element compared to the total of all isotopes of the element.

**abuse** 1 Habitual and excessive misuse, as of drugs. 2 Mistreatment, as *child abuse.* **child a.** Physical or emotional damage of a child of severity greater than that generally felt to be appropriate as punishment for a child of that age. Such parents often have themselves been abused as children. The ill treatment of the child includes emotional abuse (hostility, rejection, coldness), abuse by neglect (allowing a child to incur accidents, failure of nurturing leading to malnutrition and dwarfism), sexual abuse, and physical abuse. Child abuse in any form, and sexual abuse in particular, predisposes to behavior disorders and other long-range personality disturbances. Also *child battering, baby battering* (British usage). See also BATTERED CHILD SYNDROME. **drug a.** The use of a drug for gratification, producing effects not required for therapy.

**abutment** \əbut′mənt\ [French *aboutement* (from Old French *abouter* to place end to end, from *bout* end) abutment] A tooth or root used to support a fixed or removable prosthesis. **a. of implant** The projection of an implant into the mouth to support an appliance. Also *abutment of implant substructure.*

**AC** 1 adrenal cortex. 2 air conduction.

**Ac** Symbol for the element, actinium.

**Ac-** Symbol for the acetyl group, $CH_3$—CO—.

**aC** Symbol for the unit, abcoulomb.

**ac** alternating current.

**a.c.** *ante cibum* (L, before food, i.e., before meals).

**ac-** \ak-, ək-\ AD-.

**acacia** The dried gummy exudate from the stem and branches of *Acacia senegal* and other *A.* species. It consists mainly of calcium, potassium, and magnesium salts of arabic acid, and it is used as an emollient and as a thickening agent in many food products. Also *gum arabic, acacia gum, Kordofan gum, gum senegal.*

**acalculia** \ā′kalkoo′lyə\ [A-[1] + *calcul(ate)* + -IA] Impairment in the ability to perform arithmetic operations. It may occur in a child as a specific developmental disorder, but is less common than a developmental reading disorder. When it occurs in subjects whose arithmetic skills are known to be consonant with their intellectual level, chronologic age, and schooling, it constitutes a type of aphasia, associated most often with parietal lobe lesions.

**acampsia** \əkamp′sē·ə\ [Gk *akampsia* (from *a-* priv. + *kamps(is)* a bending + -IA) inflexibility] A stiffening or rigidity of a joint irrespective of cause.

**acanth-** \əkanth-\ ACANTHO-.

**-acanth** \-əkanth\ [Gk *akantha* thorn] A combining form meaning spine, thorn.

**acantha** \əkan′thə\ A spine or spinous process.

***Acanthamoeba*** \əkan′thəmē′bə\ A genus of free-living amebas in the family Acanthamoebidae commonly found in fresh water and soil. Some species can become facultative parasites of humans and other primates, causing in some instances an extremely severe form of meningoencephalitis. See also PRIMARY AMEBIC MENINGOENCEPHALITIS. ***A. culbertsoni*** A species of variable shape and size (10–45 μm), with a wrinkled, spherical 20-μm ectocyst and polyhedral endocyst. It is the species most frequently implicated in human acanthamoebiasis.

**acanthamoebiasis** \əkan′thəmēbī′əsis\ [*Acanthamoeb(a)* + -IASIS] Infection by amebas of the genus *Acanthamoeba,* sometimes manifested as primary amebic meningoencephalitis.

**acanthesthesia** \əkan′thesthē′zhə\ An abnormality of cutaneous sensory perception in which a simple touch stimulus may give the impression that the skin is being pricked with a sharp object.

**acantho-** \əkan′thə-\ [Gk *akantha* thorn, spine] A combining form meaning (1) spine, thorn; (2) prickle cell. Also *acanth-.*

***Acanthocheilonema*** \-kī′lōnē′mə\ [ACANTHO- + CHEILO- + Gk *nēma* a thread] A genus of filarial nematodes, the adults of which are found chiefly in the body cavities, skin, or subcutaneous tissues, of their hosts. It is now considered by some to be part of the genus *Mansonella..* ***A. perstans*** MANSONELLA PERSTANS ***A. streptocerca*** MANSONELLA STREPTOCERCA.

**acanthocyte** \əkan′thəsīt\ An abnormally shaped erythrocyte, often appearing contracted, that has a small number (usually 1–5) of spurlike projections. Acanthocytes are observed in blood films taken from some persons with hemolytic disorders, or following splenectomy, and in hereditary abetalipoproteinemia. Also *spur cell.*

**acanthocytosis** \-sītō′sis\ The presence of numerous acanthocytes in blood.

**acantholysis** \ak′ənthäl′isis\ The separation of the cells of the prickle-cell layer from each other, resulting in the formation of clefts. **a. bullosa** *Obs.* EPIDERMOLYSIS BULLOSA.

**acanthoma** \ak′ənthō′mə\ [ACANTH- + -OMA] A tumor with a squamous cell component, such as adenoacanthoma. **basal cell a.** A benign tumor arising from cells of the basal layer of the epidermis.

***Acanthophis antarctica*** A deadly, oviparous species of snake widespread in tropical and warm temperate regions of Australia and New Guinea; the death adder. It is viperlike, with a stout body and a tail tipped with spine. Along with the tiger snake (*Neotechis*), it is the most feared snake of the Australian region.

**acanthosis** \ak′ənthō′sis\ A thickening of the prickle-cell layer of the skin. **congenital a.** ACANTHOSIS NIGRICANS. **a. nigricans** Hyperkeratosis of gray to black hue associated with melanosis in the larger flexures of the skin. It is a manifestation of systemic malignancy in the adult. Also *keratosis nigricans, congenital acanthosis.* **a. seborrheica** SEBORRHEIC KERATOSIS.

**a capite ad calcem** \a kap′ətē ad kal′səm\ [L *a* from + *capite,* ablative of *caput* head + *ad* to + *calcem,* accus. sing. of *calx* heel] From head to heel, specifying the sequence in which symptoms were once traditionally listed.

**acapnia** \əkap′nē·ə\ [Gk *a-* priv. + Gk *kapn(os)* smoke, vapor + -IA] The total absence of carbon dioxide in the blood. Such an absolute absence does not occur in living organisms. Also *acarbia.* Adj. acapnic. • The term has been imprecisely used, however, with the meaning of *hypocapnia.*

**acar-** \ak′ər-, əkar′-\ ACARO-.

**acarbia** \əkär′bē·ə\ ACAPNIA.

**acardiacus** \ā′kärdī′əkəs\ ACARDIUS.

**acardius** \əkär′dē·əs\ [New L, from Gk *a-* priv. + *kardia* heart] A twin lacking a heart, usually the smaller of monozygotic twins or the parasitic member of conjoined twins. Circulation in the acardiac member is sustained through major vascular anastomoses in the placenta or elsewhere. The condition is often associated with disorganization or agenesis in other regions of the affected fetus. Also *acardiacus, acardiac twin.* **a. acephalus** ACEPHALOCARDIA. **a. amorphus** A twin characterized by the congenital absence of a heart, associated with generalized disorganization or reduction of the body as a whole.

**acari-** \ak′ərē-, əkar′ē-\ ACARO-.

**acariasis** \ak′ərī′əsis\ [New L *acar(us)* a mite + -IASIS] A disease or condition induced by infection with mites, skin-inhabiting members of the family Acaridae. Also *acariosis, acaridiasis.*

**acaricide** \əkar′isīd\ An agent that is destructive to mites of the family Acaridae or to mites in general; a miticide.

**acarid** \ak′ərid\ **1** Of or belonging to the family Acaridae. **2** A member of the family Acaridae.

**Acaridae** \əkar′idē\ [*acar(o)-* + -IDAE] A family of mites (order Acarina) some members of which cause allergic skin rash in humans, such as grocers' itch, copra itch, and vanillism.

**acaridiasis** \əkar′idī′əsis\ ACARIASIS.

**acarine** \ak′ərin\ **1** Of or belonging to the Acarina or Acariformes, an order of mites. **2** A mite of the order Acarina or Acariformes.

**acariosis** \əkar′ē·ō′sis\ ACARIASIS.

**acaro-** \ak′ərō-\ [New L *acarus* (from Gk *akari* mite) mite, tick] A combining form meaning mite, tick.

**acarodermatitis** \-dur′mətī′tis\ Dermatitis secondary to infestation with mites, as *Sarcoptes scabiei.*

**acarophobia** \-fō′bē·ə\ [ACARO- + -PHOBIA] Fear of infestation with bugs or worms and of the itching they might cause.

***Acarus*** \ak′ərəs\ [New L, from Gk *akari* (from *akarēs* tiny) a mite] A genus of mites in the family Acaridae, some species of which include agents of dermatitis, allergic itch, mange, and other skin diseases in man and domestic animals. ***A. folliculorum*** *DEMODEX FOLLICULORUM.* ***A. hordei*** A barley mite that burrows under the skin of barley handlers and may induce severe allergic reactions. Multiplication is extraordinarily rapid, resulting in great numbers of mites in a stored product in a few days. ***A. scabiei*** *SARCOPTES SCABIEI.* ***A. siro*** A mite commonly infesting vanilla beans that may induce an allergic dermatitis, vanillism. Also *Tyroglyphus farinae, Tyroglyphus siro, Tyrophagus siro.*

**acaryote** \ākar′ē·ōt\ AKARYOCYTE.

**acatalasia** \əkat′əlā′zhə\ A deficiency of the enzyme catalase. About one half of persons homozygous for the deficiency develop recurrent oral infections. This autosomal recessive condition occurs predominantly among Japanese. Also *Takahara's disease.*

**acatalepsy** \əkat′əlepsē\ The ancient doctrine that nothing can be known with certitude. Thus medical diagnostic or prognostic judgments are inherently uncertain.

**acatamathesia** \əkat′əməthē′zhə\ [Gk *a-* priv. + *katamathēs(is)* knowledge, understanding + -IA] Impairment of perception or understanding, as in sensory aphasia. *Obs.*

**acathexis** \ak′əthek′sis\ [Gk *a-* priv. + CATHEXIS] An absence of psychic energy with which the ego ordinarily invests the intrapsychic representations of external objects or parts of the self. An idea or memory seems to be of no consequence or significance to the subject, even though the subject's developmental history suggests that the idea in question may in fact contain the very essence of the conflict or symptom.

**acathisia** \ak′əthē′zhə\ AKATHISIA.

**ACC** **1** alveolar cell carcinoma. **2** anodal closure contraction.

**acc** accommodation.

**accelerant** \aksel′ərənt\ ACCELERATOR.

**acceleration** [L *acceleratio* (from *accelerare* to speed up, from *ad-*, intensifying prefix, + *celerare* to hurry, from *celer* fast, quick) a speeding up] **1** An increase in speed. **2** The rate of change of velocity per unit time. **developmental a.** Precocious growth in children in some or all areas, such as motor, perceptual, language, or social functioning, most commonly appearing as part of an uneven growth pattern in which some functions are delayed, others accelerated, and still others distorted. Such a growth pattern may be a manifestation of a pervasive developmental disorder. **negative a.** DECELERATION. **standard a. of free fall** A conventional reference value of acceleration used in the reduction to a common basis of measurements made at some point on the earth's surface, defined as 9.806 65 meters per second squared. The equivalent value is 32.1740 feet per second squared approximately. Also *standard gravity.* Symbol: $g_n$

**accelerator** A substance used to accelerate or activate a chemical reaction, as in dental technology. Also *accelerant.* **electron a.** A device to accelerate electrons to high velocities, thus giving them high kinetic energy, usually in the multi-MeV region. In radiation therapy, the accelerated electrons can be used to produce x-radiation or used directly for treatment. **linear a. 1** A device which accelerates charged particles, such as electrons or protons, in a straight line. **2** In radiotherapy, a device which accelerates electrons to high energies, usually for the production of x-radiation, although in some cases electron beams may also be used directly for radiation therapy. **serum prothrombin conversion a.** *Outmoded* FACTOR VII. **serum thrombotic a.** A serum factor that, when injected intravenously, induces a clot in a subsequently ligated segment of vein. **thromboplastin generation a.** A plasma clotting activity that is often increased in patients with thrombophilia. Abbr. TGA **Van de Graaff a.** An apparatus for the rapid production of monoenergetic electron or ion beams with great precision of energy and current in the range of 1 MeV–15 MeV. It is used in bacteriology for the sterilization of materials such as nutrient media, and has been used for superficial radiotherapy of dermatologic lesions.

**accelerin** \aksel′ərin\ The activated form of plasma coagulation factor V, designated factor Va. *Outmoded.*

**accentuation** \aksen′choo·ā′shən\ Increased intensity, particularly applied to heart sounds and murmurs. **presystolic a.** Increased intensity of a diastolic murmur in the presystolic period, particularly associated with mitral stenosis.

**accentuator** \aksen′choo·ā′tər\ A substance that increases the intensity of staining of biological structures but is neither a dye nor a mordant.

**acceptor** \aksep′tər\ **hydrogen a.** A compound that acts as an oxidant by accepting hydrogen atoms or a hydride ion from a reductant.

**accessorius** \ak′sesôr′ē·əs\ [Med L (from L *access(us)*, past part. of *accedere* to assent to, be added to + *-orius* -ORY), accessory] Either supplemental, auxiliary, or additional to similar but major structures; supernumerary.

**accident** [French (from L *accidens*, gen. *accidentis*, pres. part. of *accidere* to fall down, from AC- + *cadere*, past perf. *cecidi*, to fall, happen), accident] An unintended or unexpected event or occurrence that results in bodily injury or death of the involved individual. In forensic pathology, an accident is considered immediately unpreventable and is one of the four recognized manners of death, the others being natural death, suicide, and homicide. **cerebrovascular a.** A disorder of cerebral function of vascular origin, often of abrupt onset. Among the commoner manifestations are weakness, paralysis, sensory loss, and speech disturbance. Cerebral vascular accidents are due to cerebral infarction or ischemia resulting from arterial thrombosis or embolism, much less often from venous thrombosis, or to spontaneous cerebral hemorrhage in the cerebrum, cerebellum, brainstem, or subarachnoid space. Also *stroke*. Abbr. CVA **compensation a.** An accident for which money, services, or goods are given to an injured person or his/her dependents or relatives in consequence of the injury, usually in the form of money. Compensation may be provided through a no-fault scheme or through the tort system under common law where the employer has been negligent or in breach of statutory duty.

**accidentalism** \ak′siden′təlizm\ The theory that the study of symptoms of diseases are sufficient to account for them, without considering their etiology or pathology.

**accident-proneness** \ak′sidənt-prōn′nis\ A predisposition to having accidents found to exist in certain individuals exhibiting a set of enduring and stable personality characteristics. These characteristics are said to include aggressiveness, impulsiveness, maladjustment, and antagonism toward authority.

**ACCl** anodal closure clonus.

**acclimatization** \əklī′mətīzā′shən\ [French *acclimat(er)* to accustom to a new climate + *-iz(e)* + -ATION] The physiologic differences that appear in an organism after a change in its natural environment. Also *acclimation, acclimatation*. **altitude a.** A gradual physiologic adaptation to reduced atmospheric pressure which occurs in people living at high altitudes, conventionally altitudes above 10 000 m. It also occurs in pilots who regularly fly aircraft with unpressurized cabins.

**accommodation** [L *accommodatio* (from *accommodare* to fit, apply, adapt, from *ad-* to, for + *commodus* suitable, agreeable) a fitting, adaptation] **1** The dioptric focusing of the eye, achieved by changing strength of the crystalline lens, to achieve sharp focusing of the visual image upon the retina. **2** SOCIAL ADAPTATION. **histologic a.** An adjustment of the arrangement of cells and connective tissues in response to various stimuli. **negative a.** Change in dioptric focusing of the eye to a more remote focal point. **nerve a.** The property of axons of readjusting their excitability after being electrically excited by returning the membrane potential to its equilibrium level. **obstetric a.** The adjustment of the fetus to the shape of the maternal pelvis during the last trimester of pregnancy. **positive a.** Change in dioptric focusing of the eye to a closer focal point. **reflex a.** The adjustment of the tension of the lens, and thus its radius of curvature, in order to focus light on the retina, elicited by light or accompanying autonomic reflex acts altering the pupillary aperture. **relative a.** Change in dioptric focusing of the eye without any change in convergence.

**accommodative** \əkäm′ədā′tiv\ Pertaining to the ability of the eye to change its dioptric strength by varying the tension of the zonular fibers.

**accouchement** \ä′kooshmäɴ′\ [French (from *accoucher* to give birth, from *coucher* to lay, put to bed, lie, from L *collocare* to place, set, lay) lying-in, parturition] *Older term* PARTURITION. **a. forcé** The manual dilatation of the uterine cervix during labor to forcibly bring about delivery of the infant. This practice is condemned in modern obstetrics.

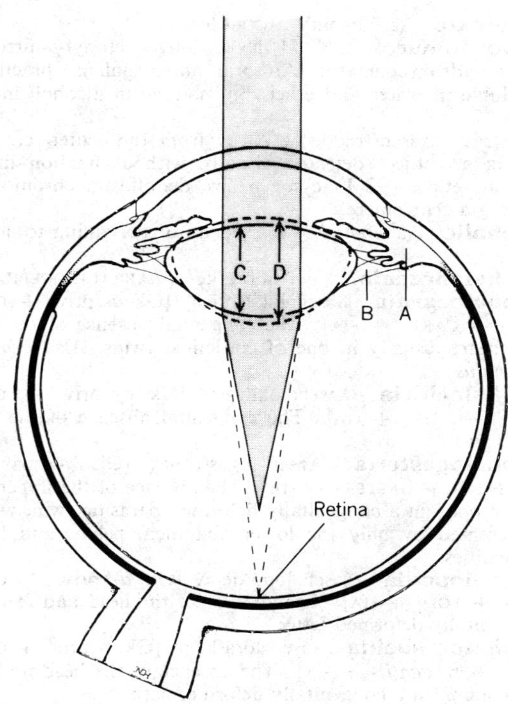


**Accommodation** (A) Ciliary muscle. (B) Suspensory ligaments. (C) Lens focuses image in front of retina; image is blurred. (D) Lens accommodates to focus on retina; image is sharp.

**accoucheur** \ä′kooshœr′\ [French, from *accouch(er)* to give birth + *-eur* -OR] OBSTETRICIAN.

**accrementition** \ak′rəmentish′ən\ [L *accre(scere)* to increase, accrue (from *ad-* to + *crescere* to grow) + *-ment(um)*, noun-forming suffix + English *-ition* (for -ATION)] The growth of a tissue by simple cell fission or budding.

**accretio** \əkrē′shō\ [L (from AC- + L *cretus*, past part. of *crescere* to grow), an increasing] Adhesion between normally separate structures such as serosal layers, resulting from a pathologic process. *Seldom used.*

**accrochage** \ä′krôshäzh′\ [French (from *accrocher* to hook, hang, fasten, from *croc* a hook) attachment, linkage, synchronization] Transient synchronization of the two pacemakers in atrioventricular dissociation.

**accuracy** **1** In a measurement, the ratio of the error of the indicated value to the true value. **2** Freedom from error. **registration a.** The accuracy with which objects are positioned on an image display.

**ACE** adrenocortical extract.

**-acea** \-ā′sē·ə\ [L, neut. pl. of *-aceus* -aceous] A suffix denoting animals characterized by (a specified property).

**-aceae** \-ā′si·ē\ [L, fem. pl. of *-aceus* -aceous] A suffix denoting plants characterized by (a specified property).

**acedapsone** $C_{16}H_{16}N_2O_4S$. Bis-(4-Acetamidophenyl)-sulfone. A compound given intramuscularly to release diaminodiphenylsulfone slowly upon hydrolysis. It is used against malaria and leprosy. Also *diacetyldapsone*. Abbr. DADDS

**acelomate** \āsē′ləmāt\ ACOELOMATE.
**acenocoumarol** $C_{19}H_{15}NO_6$. 3-(α-Acetonyl-*p*-nitrobenzyl)-4-hydroxycoumarin. An oral anticoagulant, practically insoluble in water and ether, but soluble in alcohol and alkali.
**acentric** \āsen′trik\ **1** Away from the center, e.g., denoting an object detected visually without fixation in the central retina. **2** In cytogenetics, denoting a chromosome lacking a centromere.
**acephalic** \ā′sefal′ik\ Marked by or pertaining to acephaly.
**acephalobrachia** \əsef′əlōbrā′kē·ə\ ABRACHIOCEPHALY.
**acephalocardia** \əsef′əlōkär′dē·ə\ [Gk *a-* priv. + CEPHALO- + CARD- + -IA] The congenital absence of the head and heart, usually in one of conjoined twins. Also *acardius acephalus.*
**acephalochiria** \əsef′əlōkī′rē·ə\ [Gk *a-* priv. + CEPHALO- + CHIR- + -IA] The congenital absence of the head and hands.
**acephalogasteria** \əsef′əlōgas′trē·ə\ [Gk *a-* priv. + CEPHALO- + GASTER- + -IA] The absence of the upper half of the body in a congenitally deformed parasitic twin, who is represented by only the lower abdomen, pelvis, and lower extremities.
**acephalopodia** \əsef′əlōpō′dē·ə\ [Gk *a-* priv. + CEPHALO- + POD- + -IA] The absence of the head and feet in a congenitally deformed fetus.
**acephalorrhachia** \əsef′əlôrā′kē·ə\ [Gk *a-* priv. + CEPHALO- + *rrhach(i)-* + -IA] The absence of the head and spinal column in a congenitally deformed fetus.
**acephalostomia** \əsef′əlōstō′mē·ə\ [Gk *a-* priv. + CEPHALO- + STOM- + -IA] The congenital absence of the head but the presence of a mouthlike orifice in the neck region.
**acephalus** \əsef′ələs\ [Gk *akephalos* (from *a-* priv. + *kephalē* head) headless] An infant or fetus whose head has failed to develop. • Sometimes this term is used with other terms to denote various associated conditions, either normal or abnormal, such as *acephalus dipus,* meaning without a head but with two feet, or *acephalus monopus,* meaning without a head but with only one foot. **a. athorus** PSEUDOHEMIACARDIUS.
**acephaly** \əsef′əlē\ [*acephal(us)* + -Y] The congenital absence of the head.
**acepromazine maleate** ACETYLPROMAZINE MALEATE.
**acerebral** \āser′əbrəl\ DECEREBRATE.
**acervuline** \əsur′vyəlīn\ Aggregated in small clumps, usually with reference to groups of glands.
**acervuloma** \əsur′vyəlō′mə\ [L *acervul(us)* a small heap + -OMA] PSAMMOMA.
**acervulus** \əsur′vyələs\ [New L, dim. of L *acervus* a heap] A calcareous concretion formed in later life in the pineal body and its vicinity. Also *brain sand, sabulum.*
**acesodyne** \əses′ədīn\ ANODYNE.
**acetabular** \as′ətab′yələr\ Pertaining or belonging to the acetabulum.
**acetabuloplasty** \as′ətab′yəlōplas′tē\ [*acetabul(um)* + *o* + -PLASTY] The surgical reorientation of the acetabulum. It is often performed in response to a congenital dislocation of the hip.
**acetabulum** \as′ətab′yələm\ [L (from *acet(um)* vinegar + *-bulum,* instrumental suffix) a vinegar cup, socket of hip joint] (*pl.* acetabula) [NA] The deep, cup-shaped articular socket situated near the middle of the outer surface of the hip bone at the junction of the ilium, ischium, and pubis, which are fused in the adult. The head of the femur fits and moves in this cavity, forming the hip joint. Also *cotyloid cavity, cotyle.* **sunken a.** PROTRUSIO ACETABULI.
**acetal** \as′ətəl\ The compound formed between a carbonyl compound, RR′C═O, and two molecules of an alcohol, R″—OH, to give R′C(—OR″)$_2$. Acetal formation protects the carbonyl group during transformations elsewhere in the molecule.
**acetaldehyde** $CH_3$—CHO. Ethanal.
**acetamide** $CH_3$—CO—$NH_2$. The amide of acetic acid.
**acetamido-** [*acet(ic)* + AMIDO-] A combining form denoting the group $CH_3$—CO—NH—.
**acetaminophen** $C_8H_9NO_2$. 4-Hydroxyacetanilide. A metabolite of both acetanilide and phenacetin, used as an analgesic and antipyretic. Also *paracetamol.*
**acetanilide** $C_8H_9NO$. *N*-Phenylacetamide. A white, crystalline solid, soluble in water and alcohol. It was the first of the coal-tar analgesic, antipyretic drugs. Its excessive toxicity limited its use and encouraged the search for less toxic analogues, such as phenacetin. Also *acetylaniline, acetylaminobenzine.*
**acetanisidine** $C_9H_{11}NO_2$. *p*-Methoxyacetanilide. A crystalline powder, slightly soluble in water, soluble in alcohol and organic solvents. It is a congener of phenacetin with antipyretic and analgesic properties. Also *methacetin, methoxy acetanilide.*
**acetannin** A grayish powder, very slightly soluble in water and alcohol, soluble in ethyl acetate. It is used in chronic diarrhea as an intestinal astringent. Also *acetyltannic acid, acetyltannin, diacetyltannic acid.*
**acetarsol** $C_8H_{10}AsNO_5$. *N*-Acetyl-4-hydroxy-*m*-arsanilic acid. A white, crystalline solid, almost insoluble in water and alcohol, soluble in alkali. Formerly used in the treatment of amebiasis and syphilis, it has been superseded by more effective agents. It is used locally for Vincent's angina, and leukorrhea due to *Trichomonas vaginalis.*. Also *acetarsone, acetphenarsine, Fourneau 190.*
**acetate** A salt or ester of acetic acid; the ion $CH_3$—$COO^-$
**acetate kinase** An enzyme (EC 2.4.2.1) found in yeasts and bacteria that transfers a phosphate group from ATP to acetate to form acetyl phosphate, $CH_3$—CO—O—PO(OH)$_2$, and ADP. Also *acetokinase.*
**acetazolamide** $C_4H_6N_4O_3S_2$. 5-Acetamido 1,3,4-thiadiazole-2-sulfonamide. A white, crystalline powder, slightly soluble in water. It is a carbonic anhydrase type of diuretic, useful in treating glaucoma.
**acetcarbromal** ACETYLCARBROMAL.
**acetdiamersulfonamide** A mixture containing equal amounts of sulfacetamide, sulfadiazine, and sulfamerazine. The mixture is safer than giving an equivalent amount of one drug alone because of the greater solubility of the three drugs and their metabolites in the urine, and reduced risk of renal toxicity.
**Acetest** A reagent tablet used to detect ketone bodies in body fluids, primarily urine. The tablet, containing sodium nitroprusside, disodium phosphate, glycine, and lactose, produces a purple color when acetoacetic acid or acetone is present. A proprietary name.
**acetic** \asē′tik\ [L *acet(um)* vinegar + -IC] Having the nature of vinegar.
**acetic acid** $CH_3$—COOH. Ethanoic acid. A substance of p*K* 4.7 found in vinegar. Its melting point is 16°C and its boiling point is 118°C.
**aceto-** \as′ətō-\ ACETYL-. • *Aceto-* is used now only in the common names of certain ketones, such as acetophenone and acetoacetic acid.
**acetoacetate** A salt, anion, or ester derived from acetoacetic acid.
**acetoacetate decarboxylase** An enzyme (EC

4.1.1.4) that catalyzes the conversion of acetoacetate into acetone and carbon dioxide.

**acetoacetic acid** $CH_3—CO—CH_2—COOH$. An acid found in blood in mild starvation and in diabetes. It is derived from the breakdown of fat. Its ethyl ester is a useful intermediate in chemical syntheses.

**acetocarmine** \as′ətōkär′min\ A stain consisting of carmine in 45% acetic acid that is used to stain chromatin. Also *Schneider's carmine.*

**acetoform** METHENAMINE.

**acetohexamide** $C_{15}H_{20}N_2O_4S$. 4-Acetyl-*N*-[(cyclohexylamino)-carbonyl] benzenesulfonamide. A white, crystalline powder. It is one of the sulfonylurea compounds, used as an oral hypoglycemic agent.

**acetoin** $CH_3—CO—CHOH—CH_3$. A substance which can be formed by bacteria from the hydroxyethyl derivative of thiamine pyrophosphate, an intermediate in the decarboxylation of pyruvate.

**acetokinase** ACETATE KINASE.

**acetolactic acid** $CH_3—CO—C(OH)(CH_3)—COOH$. A compound formed from two molecules of pyruvate with loss of one molecule of carbon dioxide in the pathway of biosynthesis of valine in plants and bacteria.

**acetomorphine** HEROIN.

**acetone** \as′ətōn\ [*acet(o)-* + -ONE] $CH_3—CO—CH_3$. Propanone. The simplest ketone, formed by decarboxylation of acetoacetic acid and occurring in the blood and breath of persons with high concentrations of this acid in their blood. Industrially, it is used as a solvent for paints, and is obtained from petroleum as well as by bacterial fermentation. Also *dimethylketone* (outmoded). **a. powder** The residue of a tissue after it has been extracted with acetone and dried. The acetone extracts water and lipids and prevents enzymatic autolysis. Acetone powders are conveniently stored without deteriorating, and are used as the starting point for isolating certain proteins and peptides.

**acetone diethylsulfone** SULFONMETHANE.

**acetonemia** \as′ətōnē′mē·ə\ [*aceton(e)* + -EMIA] An increased concentration of acetone in the blood, seen in uncontrolled diabetes mellitus and in starvation. Also *ketonemia.*

**acetonitrile** $CH_3—CN$. A clear, colorless liquid, used as a fairly polar, aprotic solvent for chemical reactions. On hydrolysis it yields ammonium acetate. Also *methyl cyanide.*

**acetonuria** \as′ətōnoo′rē·ə\ *Seldom used* KETONURIA.

**acetophenazine maleate** $C_{31}H_{37}N_3O_{10}S$. 1-[10-[3-[4-(2-Hydroxyethyl)-1-piperazinyl]propyl]-10H-phenothiazin-2-yl]ethanone dimaleate. A major phenothiazine tranquilizer.

**acetophenetidin** PHENACETIN.

**acetopyrine** ACOPYRINE.

**acetosal** ASPIRIN.

**acetosulfone sodium** $C_{14}H_{14}N_3NaO_3S_2$. An orally effective derivative of dapsone with similar antibacterial properties against leprosy. It is also used in the treatment of dermatitis herpetiformis.

**acetphenarsine** ACETARSOL.

**acetphenetidin** PHENACETIN.

**acetrizoate sodium** $C_9H_5I_3NNaO_3$. 3-(Acetylamino)-2,4,6-triiodobenzoic acid sodium salt, an iodine-containing x-ray contrast medium.

**acetyl** \as′ətil\ The group $CH_3—CO—$ corresponding to acetic acid. Also *ethanoyl.*

**acetyl-** \as′ətil-\ [L *acetum* vinegar + -YL] A combining form denoting the presence in a molecule of the group $CH_3CO—$. Also *aceto-.*

**acetylaminobenzine** ACETANILIDE.

**acetylaminofluorene** $C_{15}H_{13}NO$. *N*-2-Fluorenylacetamide. A very potent carcinogenic compound. Abbr. AAF

**acetylaniline** ACETANILIDE.

**acetylation** In organic chemistry, the introduction into a molecule of an acetyl group in replacement of a hydrogen atom.

**acetylcarbromal** $C_9H_{15}BrN_2O_3$. *N*-Acetyl-*N*-(α-bromo-α-ethylbutyryl)-urea. A white, crystalline powder, slightly soluble in water, soluble in alcohol, chloroform, and ether. It is a sedative. Also *acetcarbromal.*

**acetylcholine** $CH_3—CO—O—CH_2—CH_2—N^+(CH_3)_3$. An important neurotransmitter. It is produced by the vagus nerve. Also *vagusstoff* (obs.).

**acetylcholinesterase** The enzyme (EC 3.1.1.7) responsible for the hydrolysis of acetylcholine at cholinergic synapses. Its inhibition can lead to repeated stimulation of the postsynaptic nerve. Characteristic symptoms of acetylcholinesterase inhibition, as by certain organophosphorus insecticides, are headache, giddiness, nausea, sweating, blurred vision, chest tightness, abdominal cramps, vomiting, and diarrhea. In more severe cases collapse, pulmonary edema, and respiratory failure follow. Also *true cholinesterase.*

**acetyl-CoA** Acetylcoenzyme A. The *S*-acetylated form of coenzyme A. It is the form in which 2-carbon units from fat and from carbohydrate enter the citric acid cycle, and it is also an acetylating agent in many biologic reactions.

**acetyl-CoA acetyltransferase** An enzyme (EC 2.3.1.9) that transfers an acetyl group between coenzyme A and another substance. Also *3-ketoacyl-CoA thiolase* (outmoded).

**acetyl-CoA acyltransferase** The enzyme (EC 2.3.1.16) responsible for the reaction: acyl-CoA + acetyl-CoA ⇌ CoA + 3-oxoacyl-CoA, in which the acyl group is transferred from the thiol group of coenzyme A to acylate an acetyl group. This acetyl group is activated for proton loss by being itself in thioester combination. When acting from right to left the enzyme catalyzes the removal of the 2-carbon unit in the pathway by which fatty acids are broken down. Also *β-ketothiolase* (outmoded).

**acetyl-CoA carboxylase** A biotin-containing enzyme (EC 6.4.1.2) that catalyzes the carboxylation of acetyl-CoA to malonyl-CoA, which is needed for fatty acid synthesis, with concomitant cleavage of ATP to ADP and inorganic phosphate. Its control largely determines the rate of fat synthesis.

**acetyl-CoA synthetase** An enzyme (EC 6.2.1.1) that catalyzes the reaction: ATP + acetate + CoA ⇌ AMP + pyrophosphate + acetyl-CoA. It enables acetate to enter metabolic pathways.

**acetylcoenzyme A** See under ACETYL-COA.

**acetylcysteine** $C_5H_9NO_3S$. *N*-Acetyl-L-cysteine. A compound with mucolytic properties that is used in the treatment of bronchopulmonary disorders to reduce the viscocity of mucous secretions.

**acetyldigitoxin** A derivative of lanatoside C, obtained by the removal of a glucose molecule. The α and β isomers have cardiotonic activity much like that of digoxin.

**acetylene tetrachloride** TETRACHLORETHANE.

***N*-acetylgalactosamine** 2-Acetamido-2-deoxygalactose, a sugar derivative whose residues are commonly found in the oligosaccharide chains of glycoproteins.

***N*-acetylglucosamine** 2-Acetamido-2-deoxyglucose, a sugar derivative whose residues are found in the oligosaccharide chains of glycoproteins. Chitin, the material of insect cuticle, is a polymer of *N*-acetylglucosamine.

**acetylmethadol** $C_{23}H_{31}NO_2$. A derivative of methadone with analgesic properties. It has been used like methadone to

treat morphine and heroin addiction. Also *methadyl acetate.*
**acetyl-β-methylcholine** METHACHOLINE.
**acetyl-β-methylcholine chloride** METHACHOLINE CHLORIDE.
***N*-acetylmuramic acid** Muramic acid carrying an acetyl substituent on its amino group. This is the form in which its residues occur, alternating with residues of *N*-acetylglucosamine, in the peptidoglycan of bacterial cell walls.
***N*-acetylneuraminic acid** Neuraminic acid acetylated on its amino group. This is one of the commonest sialic acids, whose residues occur in glycoproteins.
**acetylphenylhydrazine** $C_8H_{10}N_2O$. A derivative of phenylhydrazine that has also been used in the treatment of polycythemia vera. It is toxic and causes hemolysis in patients with certain types of glucose-6-phosphate dehydrogenase deficiencies. Also *hydracetin.*
**acetyl phosphate** $CH_3—CO—O—PO_3H_2$. A compound formed in bacterial metabolism, either by interaction of acetate and ATP, or by interaction of acetyl-CoA and inorganic phosphate. It can act as an acetylating or a phosphorylating agent, and it can be reduced to acetaldehyde.
**acetylpromazine maleate** $C_{19}H_{22}N_2OS$, $C_4H_4O_4$. 2-Acetyl-10-(3-dimethylaminopropyl)phenothiazine hydrogen maleate. A yellow, odorless, crystalline powder, soluble in water and alcohol, and slightly soluble in ether. It has tranquilizing properties like those of chlorpromazine hydrochloride, and is used in association with etorphine hydrochloride to immobilize large animals. Also *acepromazine maleate.*
**acetylsalicylamide** $C_9H_9NO_3$. A derivative of aspirin, with analgesic, antipyretic, and antirheumatic properties. Also *salacetamide.*
**acetylsalicylic acid** ASPIRIN.
**acetylstrophanthidin** A semisynthetic, cardiotonic aglycone. It is used in experiments requiring a digitalislike compound that produces effects of rapid onset and short duration.
**acetyl sulfisoxazole** A metabolite of sulfisoxazole excreted in the urine.
**acetyltannic acid** ACETANNIN.
**acetyltannin** ACETANNIN.
**acetyltransferase** Any enzyme that catalyzes the transfer of an acetyl group. Also *transacetylase.*
**ACG** **1** angiocardiography. **2** apexcardiogram.
**AcG** accelerator globulin (factor V).
**ACh** acetylcholine.
**achalasia** \ak′əlā′zhə\ [Gk *a-* priv. + *chalas(is)* a letting loose + -IA] The inability to relax of any of various sphincters or smooth muscles at junctional areas, especially in the gastrointestinal tract. **a. of the cardia** An abnormality of the motility of the esophagus characterized by elevated resting pressure of the lower esophageal sphincter, failure of the sphincter to completely relax, and nonperistaltic contractions of the esophageal smooth muscle. The etiology is unknown. Long-term complications include recurrent pulmonary aspiration, inanition, and carcinoma of the esophagus. Also *cardiospasm, proventriculosis.* **a. of the pharyngoesophageal sphincter** Incomplete relaxation of the pharyngoesophageal sphincter. It may be a primary neuromuscular disorder, or secondary to distal esophageal disease, most commonly gastroesophageal reflux.
**Achard** [Emile Charles *Achard,* French physician, 1860–1944] Achard-Thiers syndrome. See under SYNDROME.
***Achatina fulica*** The sugar snail, a serious pest of cane sugar in Hawaii and other regions. It is also one of the intermediate hosts of the rat lungworm *Angiostrongylus cantonensis,* which can cause eosinophilic meningoencephalitis in humans.
**AChE** acetylcholinesterase.
**acheilia** \əkī′lyə\ The congenital absence of one or both lips.
**acheiria** \əkī′rē·ə\ [Gk *acheir* (from *a-* priv. + *cheir* the hand) without hands + -IA] The congenital absence of one or both hands. Also *achiria, ectrocheiry, ectrochiry.*
**acheiropodia** \əkī′rəpō′dē·ə\ The congenital absence of one or both hands and feet.
**achillobursitis** \əkil′ōbursī′tis\ ACHILLES BURSITIS.
**achillodynia** \ak′ilədin′ē·ə\ Pain about the insertion of the Achilles tendon at the heel.
**achillogram** \əkil′əgram\ [*Achill(es tendon)* + -GRAM] A reflexogram of the Achilles tendon reflex.
**achillorrhaphy** \ak′ilôr′əfē\ A surgical suturing of the Achilles tendon.
**achillotenotomy** \əkil′ōtenät′əmē\ An incision of the Achilles tendon.
**achiria** \əkī′rē·ə\ ACHEIRIA.
**achlorhydria** \ā′klôrhī′drē·ə\ Absence of hydrochloric acid from gastric secretions. Also *gastric anacidity.*
***Acholeplasma*** \ākäl′əplaz′mə\ [GK *a-* priv. + *cholē* gall, bile + PLASM] A genus of the mycoplasmas that differs from the genus *Mycoplasma* in not having a growth requirement for a sterol.
**acholic** \ākō′lik\ [Gk *a-* priv. + CHOLIC] Not containing bile or bile pigments.
**achondrogenesis** \əkän′drəjen′əsis\ [Gk *a-* priv. + CHONDRO- + GENESIS] **1** Dwarfism characterized by extreme shortening of the extremities, rudimentary digits, normal or increased head size, and autosomal recessive inheritance. **2** A lethal variant of osteogenesis imperfecta characterized by lack of ossification in long bones, ribs, and lower vertebrae. • Cartilage is formed in both conditions and therefore the term is incorrect.
**achondroplasia** \əkän′drəplā′zhə\ [Gk *a-* priv. + CHONDRO- + -PLASIA] An autosomal dominant osteochondrodysplasia that is apparent at birth and is characterized by slowed growth of those bones that are derived from cartilage and nearly normal formation of periosteal bone. The primary abnormality is deficient conversion of cartilage to bone at the epiphyses of the long bones. This abnormal skeletal development results in a form of disproportionate dwarfism with short extremities, midfacial hypoplasia, small foramen magnum, and narrow spinal canal. It is thought to arise frequently by mutation. Also *fetal rickets, achondroplasty, osteosclerosis congenita, Parrot's disease, chondrodystrophia fetalis* (outmoded), *hypoplastic fetal chondrodystrophy* (inexact and outmoded).
**achroacytosis** \əkrō′əsītō′sis\ Blood or tissue lymphocytosis. *Obs.*
**achroma** \əkrō′mə\ [Gk *a-* priv. + *chrōma* color] The absence of pigmentation, especially absence of normal pigmentation.
**achromat** \ak′rəmat′\ ACHROMATIC LENS.
**achromate** \ak′rəmāt′\ [Gk *a-* priv. + CHROM- + -ATE] An individual unable to distinguish any colors.
**achromatic** \ak′rəmat′ik\ [Gk *achrōmat(os)* (from *a-* priv. + *chrōma,* gen. *chrōmatos* color) colorless + -IC] **1** Being without color. **2** Incapable of combining with a stain or dye. **3** Designating an optical lens designed to eliminate chromatic aberration.
**achromatin** \əkrō′mətin\ The parts of the cell nucleus which stain very weakly with basic dyes.
**achromatism** \əkrō′mətizm\ [Gk *a-* priv. + CHROMAT- + -ISM] **1** COMPLETE COLOR BLINDNESS. **2** Freedom of an optical system from chromatic aberration.
**achromatocytosis** \əkrō′mətōsītō′sis\ The presence of erythrocyte ghosts.

**achromatognosia** \əkrō′mətägnō′zhə\ [Gk *a-* priv. + CHROMATO- + Gk *gnōs(is)* knowledge + -IA] COMPLETE COLOR BLINDNESS.
**achromatophil** \ā′krōmat′əfil\ [Gk *a-* priv. + CHROMATO- + -PHIL] A cell that has little or no affinity for cytoplasmic stains. Also *achromophil.*
**achromatopia** \əkrō′mətō′pē·ə\ COMPLETE COLOR BLINDNESS.
**achromatopsia** \əkrō′mətäp′sē·ə\ [Gk *a-* priv. + CHROMATOPSIA ] COMPLETE COLOR BLINDNESS.
**achromatosis** \əkrō′mətō′sis\ ACHROMODERMA.
**achromatous** \əkrō′mətəs\ Being without color; colorless.
**achromaturia** \əkrō′mətoo′rē·ə\ Excretion of colorless urine as a consequence of diuresis or chronic renal failure.
**achromia** \əkrō′mē·ə\ [Gk *a-* priv. + CHROM- + -IA] A congenital deficiency of natural pigment. See also ALBINISM. **central a.** The normal lack of color in the center of a stained erythrocyte. **consecutive a.** The secondary loss of pigment from the skin, such as that resulting from an inflammatory disease. **cortical a.** Abnormal pallor of a localized area of cerebral cortex. It is usually associated with loss of neurons in the affected area.
**achromoderma** \əkrō′mədur′mə\ [Gk *a-* priv. + CHROMO- + -DERMA] An absence of skin pigment. Also *achromatosis, achromodermia.*
**achromodermia** \əkrō′mədur′mē·ə\ ACHROMODERMA.
**achromophil** \əkrō′məfil\ ACHROMATOPHIL.
**achromophilous** \ā′krōmäf′ələs\ Characterized by achromatophilia.
**achylia** \əkī′lyə\ [New L, from GK *a-* priv. + *chyl(o)-* + -IA] **1** Absence of chyle. **2** Absence of gastric acid and pepsin secretion. Also *achylosis.*
**aciculate** \əsik′yəlit\ [Late L *acicul(a)*, dim. of L *acus* needle + -ATE] Shaped like a needle.
**acid** \as′id\ [French *acide* (from L *acidus* sour, from *acere* to be sour) acid] A substance that can donate a proton. • Such a substance may be called a *Brønsted acid* to distinquish it from the less common meaning of the word, a *Lewis acid*, which is a substance that can accept an electron pair. **bile a.** A $C_{24}$ steroid, formed from cholesterol by breaking the side chain after C-24 and leaving this atom as a carboxyl group. See also BILE SALTS. **Brønsted a.** A substance that can donate the ion $H^+$. **conjugate a.** The acid derived from a particular base by addition of a proton. **dibasic a.** A substance with two acidic groups in its molecule, so that two moles of base are required to titrate each mole of the substance. **fatty a.** See under FATTY ACID. **Lewis a.** A substance that can combine with other substances (Lewis bases) by accepting the electrons that form the bond between them. **mineral a.** An inorganic acid, usually a strong acid, such as hydrochloric or sulfuric acid. **titratable a.** Acid present in a body fluid that can be restored to physiologic neutrality by addition of measured amounts of a base, usually 0.1 N sodium hydroxide.
**acidaemia** *Brit.* ACIDEMIA.
**acid anhydride** Any of the substances that form two acid groups by reaction with water. These include carboxylic acids, in which the acid anhydride contains the —CO—O—CO— grouping. The anhydrides of phosphoric acid [—O—PO(O$^-$)—O—PO(O$^-$)—], such as ATP and ADP, are of particular metabolic importance.
**acid chloride** Any substance derived from an acid by replacing an acidic hydroxyl group with a chlorine atom. The acid is usually a carboxylic acid, so that the acid chloride contains the chloroformyl group Cl—CO— and is a powerful acylating agent.
**acidemia** \as′idē′mē·ə\ An abnormally low pH of whole blood. Mean normal arterial blood pH is 7.42 ± 0.016 at 38°C. **glutaric a. type I** GLUTARIC ACIDURIA TYPE I. **glutaric a. type IIA** GLUTARIC ACIDURIA TYPE IIA. **glutaric a. type IIB** GLUTARIC ACIDURIA TYPE IIB. **isovaleric a.** A condition in which serum isovaleric acid increases due to a block in its oxidation to $\beta$-methyl crotonic acid. The result is chronic metabolic acidosis and ketosis, with coma and death in severe cases, and mental retardation in those that survive. Some patients have a fetid breath, like that of sweaty feet, due to short-chain keto acids. **methylmalonic a.** A rare, inborn disorder of branched chain amino acid metabolism, in which there is a blockage in the conversion of methylmalonic acid to succinic acid due to a deficiency of the enzyme methyl malonyl CoA isomerase. The activity of this enzyme is partly dependent on vitamin $B^{12}$ and hence some forms of this acidemia are responsive to treatment with $B^{12}$. The clinical effects in some cases are acute severe ketoacidosis, coma, and death in the first month of life. In more chronic forms there is mental retardation, growth failure, neutropenia, and epileptic seizures. **propionic a.** A disorder of amino acid metabolism in which the major catabolic pathway of degradation of proprionic acid to methylmalonic acid is blocked by a defect of the enzyme proprionyl CoA carboxylase. The result is severe ketoacidosis, often fatal in the early weeks of life. Some cases are responsive to biotin.
**acid-fast** **1** See under ACID-FAST STAIN. **2** Distinguished by the acid-fast stain: used especially of the mycobacteria.
**acid-forming** Of or relating to substances that give rise to the production of acid in the body, such as protein. Also *acidogenic.*
**acidic** \asid′ik\ **1** Of, relating to, or being an acid. **2** Having a high concentration of $H^+$ions: used of a solution.
**acidification** \asid′ifikā′shən\ **1** The conversion of a substance into the acid state or its acquisition of certain properties of acids. **2** The addition of acid to a medium.
**acidify** \asid′ifī\ To lower the pH of (a medium).
**acidity** \asid′itē\ [French *acidité.* See ACID.] The ability of a substance to release protons and its tendency to do so. **urinary titratable a.** The amount of acid, expressed in milliequivalents, excreted in a timed collection of urine and measured by titration to the pH of the patient's blood.
**acidocyte** \as′idōsīt′\ EOSINOPHIL.
**acidogenic** \as′idōjen′ik\ ACID-FORMING.
**acidophil** \əsid′ōfil\ EOSINOPHIL.
**acidophilia** \as′idōfil′yə\ Affinity for acid stains.
**acidophilic** \as′idōfil′ik\ Having an affinity for acid dyes. Also *acidophilous, oxyphilic, oxyphilous, oxyphil.*
**acidosis** \as′idō′sis\ A disturbance of the acid-base state of the body towards the acid. Acidosis may be metabolic, respiratory, or both. Adj. acidotic. **bicarbonate wastage renal tubular a.** PROXIMAL RENAL TUBULAR ACIDOSIS. **carbon dioxide a.** RESPIRATORY ACIDOSIS. **classic renal tubular a.** DISTAL RENAL TUBULAR ACIDOSIS. **compensated a.** A condition in which the arterial blood pH is within the normal range despite the existence of a stress that causes acidosis, such as diabetes, renal disfunction, or faulty metabolism. **diabetic a.** DIABETIC KETOACIDOSIS. **distal renal tubular a.** Defective secretion of hydrogen ions by the distal tubule cells, leading to a hyperchloremic metabolic acidosis with an inappropriately high urine pH. Renal function may be otherwise normal but hypokalemia and hypercalciuria with atten-

dant bone disease, nephrocalcinosis, and nephrolithiasis may result. If symptoms begin in infancy, lethargy, anorexia, and stunted growth may be the presenting symptoms. When interstitial fibrosis develops as a complication, glomerular filtration may decrease secondarily. The condition may be of hereditary origin or secondary to excess vitamin D, dysproteinuria, or amphotericin B toxicity. Treatment involves oral administration of sodium bicarbonate or Shohl solution. Also *classic renal tubular acidosis, distal acidosis, type I renal tubular acidosis.* **hypercapnic a.** RESPIRATORY ACIDOSIS. **hyperchloremic a.** An abnormal physiologic state consisting of blood pH less than 7.40 and serum chloride ion concentration greater than 110 mEq/ml, often due to renal disease. **infantile renal tubular a.** TRANSIENT PRIMARY RENAL TUBULAR ACIDOSIS. **lactic a.** A metabolic acidosis in which the excess hydrogen ion results from increased circulating lactic acid, due either to tissue hypoxia and decreased conversion of lactate to pyruvate, or to endogenous or exogenous metabolic defects. Characterized by an increased anion gap, lactic acidosis occurs when blood lactate rises above the normal 1 to 2 mEq/l. **metabolic a.** Acidosis that arises from a disorder of metabolism in which acid (excluding carbonic acid) accumulates in, or bicarbonate is lost from, extracellular fluid. It is distinguished from respiratory acidosis, in which the primary defect is retention of carbon dioxide. **mixed renal tubular a.** A condition in which both tubular excretion of acid and reabsorption of bicarbonate are impaired out of proportion to any decrease in glomerular filtration rate. **primary renal tubular a.** Renal tubular acidosis associated with intrinsic disease of the kidney, such as inherited renal tubular acidosis, or many instances of the Fanconi syndrome. **proximal renal tubular a.** A condition characterized by defective reabsorption of bicarbonate by the proximal renal tubules. Excess bicarbonate overwhelms the distal hydrogen ion secretory mechanism resulting in impaired acidification of the urine. This disorder may develop as an isolated defect of the proximal tubule or as a feature of various syndromes, such as the Fanconi syndrome. Retarded growth is the main feature in children. In contrast to distal renal tubular acidosis, hypercalciuria is absent or slight, while bone disease and nephrocalcinosis do not develop. Correction often requires large amounts of bicarbonate or citrates. Also *bicarbonate wastage renal acidosis, proximal acidosis, type II renal tubular acidosis.* **renal a.** Acidosis secondary to renal disorders. This may occur with a normal anion gap in renal tubular acidosis or with accumulation of nonvolatile metabolic acids, and impaired ability of the kidneys to form ammonia to neutralize inorganic anions in renal failure. **renal hyperchloremic a.** Acidosis characterized by hyperchloremia and a normal anion gap, secondary to renal disease such as renal tubular acidosis. It may also result from ingestion or intravenous administration of ammonium chloride, lysine or arginine chloride, or acetazolamide, loss of bicarbonate in upper intestinal contents, diarrheal stools, or from a ureterosigmoidostomy. **renal tubular a.** Any defect in kidney function that produces systemic metabolic acidosis. The defects can be primary or acquired. At least three distinct heritable primary forms of renal tubular acidosis (RTA) occur. RTA I is a dominant condition with defective distal tubule function caused by a gradient defect and variable clinical manifestations which include nephrocalcinosis, osteomalacia, hypocalcemia, hyperchloremia, and a urinary pH greater than 6.0. RTA II is an autosomal recessive defect in proximal tubule function characterized by bicarbonate wasting. RTA III is an autosomal recessive disorder with onset in childhood and gradual improvement with age. **respiratory a.** Acidosis resulting from carbon dioxide accumulation due to insufficient alveolar ventilation. Also *carbon dioxide acidosis, hypercapnic acidosis.* **secondary renal tubular a.** Renal tubular acidosis secondary to some disease extrinsic to the kidney such as dysproteinemia or hyperparathyroidism, or to some toxic agent such as cadmium or mercury. **starvation a.** A metabolic acidosis associated with the accumulation of ketone bodies arising from a calorie deficiency. **transient primary renal tubular a.** A rare form of distal tubular acidosis that affects males 12–18 months of age. Nephrocalcinosis is rare. Familial or genetic relationships have not been demonstrated. Alkali therapy is effective and complete recovery is usual. Also *infantile renal tubular acidosis.* **type I renal tubular a.** DISTAL RENAL TUBULAR ACIDOSIS. **type II renal tubular a.** PROXIMAL RENAL TUBULAR ACIDOSIS. **uremic a.** Acidosis associated with the uremic state. It results from impaired ability of the kidneys to form ammonia to neutralize inorganic anions, thus causing loss of bicarbonate, and to retention of nonvolatile metabolic acids with an anion gap.

**acidotic** \as′idät′ik\ Characterized by or involving acidosis.

**acid phosphatase** The enzyme (EC 3.1.3.2) that catalyzes the hydrolysis of monoesters of phosphoric acid at acid pH. It is present in high concentration in the prostate, and the prostatic enzyme, which is characterized by its inhibition by tartrate and insensitivity to formaldehyde, may be raised in concentration in the blood of patients with prostatic carcinoma.

**acid sulfate** A salt of sulfuric acid containing the ion $HSO_4^-$. Also *hydrogen sulfate, bisulfate* (obs.).

**aciduria** \as′idoo′rē·ə\ A state of acidity in the urine. It may be due to any of a great variety of agents, normal and abnormal. Adj. aciduric. **β-aminoisobutyric a.** An excessive excretion of β-aminoisobutyric acid in the urine occurring in a small proportion of the population and in patients with illnesses in which there is tissue destruction and excessive catabolism of DNA. The amino acidemia and aciduria cause no symptoms. **argininosuccinic a.** An inborn error of urea-cycle metabolism resulting in elevated serum argininosuccinic acid and copious excretion in the urine. The basic defect is in the enzyme argininosuccinase. Three autosomal recessive phenotypes are differentiated by age of onset and clinical severity. The neonatal form is characterized by convulsions, coma, and death within two weeks. The subacute and late-onset forms are associated with mental retardation, hepatomegaly, and brittle hair. **glutamic a.** A disturbance of glutathione biosynthesis due to γ-glutamyl cysteine synthetase deficiency. The glutathione deficiency which results is associated with generalized neuropathies, hemolytic anemia, and amino aciduria. **glutaric a. type I** An autosomal recessive inborn error of organic acid metabolism characterized by infantile onset of opisthotonus, dystonia, and athetoid posturing. Excessive plasma and urinary levels of glutaric acid result from an inability to metabolize glutaryl-CoA, probably due to a deficiency of glutaryl-CoA dehydrogenase. Also *glutaric acidemia type I.* Symbol: GA I **glutaric a. type IIA** A severe, X-linked inborn error of organic acid metabolism characterized by neonatal onset of metabolic acidosis, hypoglycemia, hyperammonemia, and early death. Excessive urinary excretion of glutaric, lactic, ethylmalonic, butyric, isobutyric, 2-methylbutyric, and isovaleric acids results from multiple acyl-CoA dehydrogenase deficiencies. Also *glutaric acidemia type IIA.* Symbol: GA IIA **glutaric a. type IIB** An autosomal recessive, inborn error of organic acid metabolism characterized by hypoglycemia, vomiting, metabolic acidosis, coma, hepatomegaly due to fatty infiltration, and sudden death. Age of onset of clinical symptoms is variable, from infancy to adolescence, and is often precipitated by an intercurrent febrile illness. Elevations in plasma and urine of multiple organic acids is associated with deficiency of multiple acyl-CoA dehydrogenases. Also *glutaric acidemia type IIB, ethylmalonyl-adipicaciduria.* Symbol: GA IIB **glyceric a.** OXALOSIS II. **L-glyceric a.** A disturbance in the degradation of D-glyceric acid, probably due to absence of D-glyceric dehydrogenase, causing hypotonia, tonic fits with ocular crises and hyperkinetic movements. Hyperglycinemia and hyperglycinuria are present but without ketosis. The glycine in the cerebrospinal fluid is raised. **glycolic a.** OXALOSIS I. **methylmalonic a.** Any of a group of hereditary disorders in the synthesis of succinic acid from methylmalonic acid and methionine from homocysteine. Common features are metabolic ketoacidosis, recurrent infections, convulsions, developmental retardation, neutropenia, thrombocytopenia, and excretion in the urine of large quantities of methylmalonic acid, homocystine, and cystathionine. Few have megaloblastic anemia. **orotic a.** A rare heritable disorder of pyrimidine metabolism resulting in markedly increased urinary excretion of orotic acid. Two genetic forms occur. One is due to deficient activity of the enzymes orotidine-5′-pyrophosphorylase and orotidine-5′-phosphate decarboxylase. The second is due to deficiency of only the latter enzyme. The clinical syndrome is autosomal recessive and is characterized by growth and mental retardation, megaloblastic anemia, leukopenia, and crystalluria. Administration of uridine and cytidine corrects the anemia and reduces orotic acid excretion. Also *oroticaciduria.* **paradoxical a.** A condition in which a urine with pH less than 7 is excreted in patients with sustained alkalosis and an increased plasma bicarbonate, reflecting increased reabsorption of bicarbonate by the renal tubules. **pyroglutamic a.** An inborn error of glutathione biosynthesis due to an inability to convert 5-oxoproline to glutamic acid and resulting in elevated levels in the blood and cerebrospinal fluid of 5-oxoproline, as well as massive excretion of it in the urine. Subjects have a severe metabolic acidosis requiring treatment with sodium bicarbonate, and they may suffer from mental retardation. **xanthurenic a.** A disturbance in the pathway of tryptophan-nicotinamide metabolism due to an inability to convert 3-hydroxykynurenine to 3-hydroxyanthranilic acid. It may be found in cases of pyridoxine deficiency and also in pyridoxine dependency.

**acies** \ā′si·ēz\ [L, a sharp edge or point] A margin, border, or edge. **a. thalami optici** *Obs.* STRIA MEDULLARIS THALAMI.

**acinaciform** [L *acinac(es)* a scimitar, short crooked sword + *i* + -FORM] Shaped like a short, curved sword: used especially of certain fungal spores.

**acinar** \as′inər\ Pertaining to or associated with an acinus. Also *acinal, acinic.*

**acinesia** \as′inē′zhə\ AKINESIA.

**acinetic** \as′inet′ik\ AKINETIC.

***Acinetobacter*** \as′ənētōbak′tər\ [New L (from Gk *a-* priv. + CINETO- + *bacter(ium)*) a nonmotile bacterium] A genus of Gram-negative or short diplobacilli, found widely in the environment and also on mucous membranes, rarely as pathogens. They are easily mistaken for species of *Neisseria.* They are aerobic and fermentation-negative, but also oxidase-negative. *Acinetobacter lwoffi* (previously *Mima polymorpha* and *Achromobacter lwoffi*) cannot metabolize carbohydrates, but *Acinetobacter anitratum* (formerly *Herellea vaginicola* and *Achromobacter anitratum*) can.

**acinic** \əsin′ik\ ACINAR.

**aciniform** \əsin′əfôrm\ Grape-shaped, usually referring to glands. Also *acinous, acinose.*

**acinose** \as′inōs\ **1** Having acini. **2** ACINIFORM.

**acinotubular** \as′inōt$^y$oob′yələr\ Made up of tubular acini or of tubules terminating as acini. Also *tubuloacinar, tubuloacinous.*

**acinous** \as′inəs\ ACINIFORM.

**acinus** \as′inəs\ [L, seed, grape, berry] (*pl.* acini) A rounded sac, opening into a small excretory duct, in the terminal secretory portion of an exocrine gland. A number of these combine in a cluster to form a lobule. An acinus is similar to an alveolus, except for its shape. Adj. acinar, acinal, acinic. **liver a.** The glandular unit of liver parenchyma in which branches of the bile duct are central, associated with branches of the portal vein and the hepatic artery. Thus, each unit forms part of two adjacent hepatic lobules. Its function is part of the exocrine activity of the liver. **pulmonary a.** One of numerous thin-walled air sacs pouching from alveolar ducts, atria, and alveolar sacs at the termination of a respiratory bronchiole in the lung. **a. renalis malpighii** *Outmoded* CORPUSCULUM RENALE. **a. renis malpighii** *Outmoded* CORPUSCULUM RENALE.

**ackee** \akē′\ [Jamaican name of the plant, prob. from the Kru language of Liberia] The seeds and arils of *Blighia sapida.* If ingested raw, they can cause vomiting sickness, with mortality of 40 to 80 percent. The toxic principles, hypoglycine A and B, are hypoglycemic and act as antimetabolites capable of blocking oxidation of fatty acids. Also *akee.*

**aclasis** \ak′ləsis\ [Gk *a-* priv. + *klasis* a breaking] Lack of modeling or deformation in the shape of a structure during embryonic development and growth. *Obs.* Adj. aclastic. **diaphyseal a.** The abnormal deposition of bone at the metaphysis of a growing long bone, particularly one about the knee, resulting from an irregular remodeling process. Also *metaphyseal aclasis.* **metaphyseal a.** DIAPHYSEAL ACLASIS.

**acleistocardia** \əklī′stōkär′dē·ə\ [Gk *akleisto(s)* (from *a-* priv. + *kleistos* shut) not shut + -CARDIA] PATENT FORAMEN OVALE.

**acme** \ak′mē\ [Gk *akmē* a point, the highest point, bloom] The stage in the course of a disease marked by the most intense symptoms; crisis. Adj. acmic. **a. of contraction** The time of highest intrauterine pressure during a uterine contraction.

**acmesthesia** \ak′mesthē′zhə\ [Gk *akm(ē)* a point + -ESTHESIA] Sensation produced by touching with the point of a needle. *Seldom used.*

**acne** \ak′nē\ [erroneous for Gk *akmē* a point, the highest point, bloom, eruption] **1** ACNE VULGARIS. **2** Any chronic inflammatory disease of the pilosebaceous follicles characterized by keratinous obstruction of the upper part of the pilosebaceous gland. **adolescent a.** Acne vulgaris occurring in adolescence as a result of androgenic stimulation of the pilosebaceous follicles in genetically predisposed subjects. In some races it is present in about 100 percent of subjects in at least a mild degree. Emotional stress as a secondary effect of the disfigurement is common. **a. aestivalis** A seldom seen form of acne that is characterized by lesions with a uniform, papular appearance and few comedones. It is found almost exclusively among females and is believed to be provoked by sunbathing. **a. agminata** An uncommon skin eruption that affects particularly the central area of the face and consists of firm yellow-brown papules. It was once regarded as a tuberculid. Also *lupus miliaris disseminatus faciei, acne telangiectodes, acnitis, disseminated fol-*

*licular lupus.* **apocrine a.** HIDRADENITIS SUPPURATIVA. **colloid a.** COLLOID MILIUM. **common a.** ACNE VULGARIS. **a. conglobata** An extreme form of acne vulgaris that is characterized by abscesses, cysts, sinuses, and severe scarring. **a. frontalis** *Outmoded* ACNE NECROTICA. **a. fulminans** A rare, severe acne in which suppurative and ulcerating skin lesions are associated with malaise, fever, and arthralgia. Also *systemic acne.* **keloid a.** A chronic inflammatory disease of the pilosebaceous follicles that produces keloidal scarring. Also *dermatitis papillaris capillitii, keloidal folliculitis.* **a. mechanica** Acne that is provoked or aggravated by mechanical forces, such as friction or pressure. **a. medicamentosa** Acne vulgaris or an acneform rash caused by a drug or chemical. **a. necrotica** Chronic folliculitis marked by papules or pustules on the scalp that become necrotic and leave varioliform scars. Also *acne frontalis* (outmoded), *acne varioliformis.* **a. necrotica miliaris** Acne necrotica marked by pruritus and crusted excoriations. **a. neonatorum** Acne occurring in newborn infants as a result of stimulation of the pilosebaceous follicles *in utero* by maternal androgens. The lesions are superficial and are seen on the face, neck, axillae, and occasionally the chest and back. The condition clears spontaneously but commonly recurs with some severity at puberty. **oil a.** An acneform eruption which occurs on the skin, usually of the thighs and arms, of workers continuously exposed to cutting oils. It is caused by oil plugging the sebaceous follicles. Also *petroleum acne, oil folliculitis, industrial folliculitis.* **petroleum a.** OIL ACNE. **a. rosacea** *Outmoded* ROSACEA. **a. scorbutica** The acneform rash of scurvy. **steroid a.** An acneform eruption due to the use of topical or systemic glucocorticoids. **a. syphilitica** A pustular syphilid that resembles acne vulgaris. Also *syphilitic acne.* **systemic a.** ACNE FULMINANS. **a. tarsi** Meibomian gland inflammation. **a. telangiectodes** ACNE AGMINATA. **tropical a.** A severe form of acne vulgaris caused by exposure to a tropical climate. Also *acne tropicalis.* **a. varioliformis** ACNE NECROTICA. **a. vulgaris** A chronic inflammatory disease of the sebaceous follicles, characterized by the formation of comedones, papules, pustules, and scars. Lesions occur most frequently on the face, chest, and back. The condition is common in young adults. Also *acne, common acne.*

**acneform** \ak′nəfôrm\ Resembling acne in appearance. Also *acneiform.*

**acnegen** \ak′nəjən\ A substance capable of causing acne.

**acnegenic** [ACNE + -GENIC] Capable of causing acne.

**acneiform** \aknē′əfôrm\ ACNEFORM.

**acnitis** \aknī′tis\ [*acn(e)* + -ITIS] ACNE AGMINATA.

**acoasma** \ā′kō·as′mə\ ACOUSMA.

**acocantherin** OUABAIN.

**acoelomate** \āsē′ləmāt\ [Gk *a-* priv. + COELOM + -ATE] **1** Having no body cavity. **2** An animal in which there is no body cavity, the entire space between the ectoderm and the endoderm being of solid mesoderm. Most prominent in this group are the flatworms (Platyhelminthes) and proboscis worms (Nemertini). Also *acelomate.*

**acognosia** \ak′ägnō′zhə\ [Gk *ako(s)* cure, remedy + *gnōs(is)* knowledge + -IA] The study of or a knowledge of remedies. Also *acognosy.*

**acognosy** \əkäg′nəsē\ ACOGNOSIA.

**acokantherin** OUABAIN.

**acology** \akäl′əjē\ [Gk *ako(s)* cure, remedy + -LOGY] The science or study of cures and remedies.

**acolous** \ak′ələs\ [Gk *a-* priv. + *kōl(on)* a limb + -OUS] Having no limbs.

**acomplementemia** \əkäm′pləmentē′mē·ə \ HYPOCOMPLEMENTEMIA.

**aconitase** An iron-containing enzyme (EC 4.2.1.3) catalyzing the interconversion of citrate and isocitrate, via enzyme-bound aconitate, which slowly equilibrates with free aconitate. It is an enzyme of the citric acid cycle. At equilibrium under physiologic conditions, citrate forms over 90% of the mixture. Its inhibition by fluorocitrate is responsible for the toxicity of fluoroacetate.

**aconite** \ak′ənīt\ A poisonous compound derived from the tuberous root of *Aconitum napellus.* It contains several closely related alkaloids, the principal one being aconitine. It was formerly used as an antihypertensive, diaphoretic, antipyretic, and diuretic. Also *wolfsbane.*

**aconitic acid** HOOC—CH=C(—COOH)—$CH_2$—COOH. Prop-1-ene-1,2,3-carboxylic acid, whose *Z*-isomer, commonly known as *cis*-aconitic acid, is an intermediate in the interconversion of citric and isocitric acids in the tricarboxylic acid cycle. In this reaction it largely remains bound to the enzyme aconitase. It may be formed by heating citric acid.

**aconitine** \əkän′ətin\ $C_{34}H_{47}NO_{11}$. The active principle of aconite. It is an extemely poisonous alkaloid.

**aconuresis** \ak′ənoorē′sis\ [Gk *akōn* involuntary + -URESIS] Involuntary voiding of urine.

**acopyrine** A combination of antipyrine and aspirin that has antirheumatic and analgesic properties. Antipyrine, however, causes agranulocytosis in susceptible individuals. It is soluble in hot water and in alcohol. Also *acetopyrine.*

**acor** [L, sourness, acidity] Acidity; bitterness.

**acorea** \ā′kôrē′ə\ [Gk *a-* priv. + CORE- + *-(i)a*] The congenital absence of the pupil in one or both eyes.

**acormia** \əkôr′mē·ə\ [Gk *a-* priv. + Gk *korm(os)* the trunk of a tree with branches lopped off + -IA] The congenital absence of all or most of the trunk.

**acortan** \akôr′tən\ A term seldom used in the U.S. for ADRENOCORTICOTROPIC HORMONE.

**Acosta** [José de *Acosta,* Spanish missionary, 1539–1600] Acosta's disease. See under MOUNTAIN SICKNESS.

**acostate** \əkäs′tāt\ Lacking ribs; characterized by apleuria.

**acou-** \əkoo-\ [Gk *akouein* to hear] A combining form meaning hearing. Also *acu-.*

**acouasm** \əkoo′azm\ ACOUSMA.

**acoumeter** \əkoo′mətər\ [ACOU- + -METER] An instrument once used for measuring the acuity of hearing before the introduction of audiometers. The sound stimulus was generated by mechanical means. Also *acumeter.*

**-acousia** \-əkoo′zhə\ [Gk *akous(is)* hearing + -IA] -ACUSIS.

**acousma** \əkoos′mə\ [Gk *akousma* (from *akouein* to hear) a thing heard, sound, rumor] The hearing of imaginary sounds, usually indeterminate. *Obs.* Also *acoasma, acouasm.*

**acousmatagnosia** \əkoos′matagnō′zhə\ [ACOUSMA + *t* + AGNOSIA ] *Outmoded* AUDITORY AGNOSIA.

**acousmatamnesia** \əkoos′matamnē′zhə\ The inability to remember certain sounds. *Seldom used.*

**acoustic** \əkoos′tik\ [Gk *akoustikos* (from *akouein* to hear) pertaining to the sense of hearing] **1** Pertaining to the physical aspects or characteristics of sounds. **2** Referring to particular aspects of hearing, as in *acoustic nerve. Incorrect.*

**acousticofacial** \əkoos′tikōfā′shəl\ Relating to both the eighth (auditory) and seventh (facial) cranial nerves.

**acousticomotor** \əkoos′tikōmō′tər\ Pertaining to a motor response to sound.

**acoustics** \əkoos′tiks\ [See ACOUSTIC.] The science of the physical aspects or characteristics of sound. Compare AU-

DIOLOGY. **geometrical a.** That part of acoustics in which sound can be regarded as traveling in straight-line paths except when reflected or refracted, and thus limited to treating obstacles with dimensions much larger than the wavelength and to the ignoring of edge effects.

**acoustigram** ACOUSTOGRAM.

**acoustogram** \əkoos′təgram\ [*acoust(ic)* + -GRAM] A graphic representation of sounds produced during movement of a joint. Also *acoustigram.*

**ACP** American College of Physicians.

**acquired** Developed and manifested after birth; not congenital. Also *acquisitus.*

**acquisitus** ACQUIRED.

**acragnosis** \ak′ragnō′sis\ ACROAGNOSIA.

**acral** \ak′rəl\ Pertaining to or affecting the extremities, such as the limbs, fingers, and toes.

**acrania** \əkrā′nē·ə\ [Gk *a-* priv. + *cran(i)-* + -IA] The absence of the calvaria and variably other bones comprising the braincase. The condition always exists to some degree in anencephaly and exencephaly.

**acraturesis** \əkrat′yərē′sis\ [Gk *akrat(ēs)* powerless + -URESIS] Difficulty in urinating or inability to do so, due to lack of muscular contraction in the bladder.

**acrid** \ak′rid\ Sharp and biting in taste or smell.

**acridine** The ring system formed by fusion of benzene rings to the 2,3 and 5,6 bonds of pyridine. Its derivatives are dyes, which intercalate into the DNA helix and cause insertion or deletion mutations by affecting DNA replication. Acridine and its derivatives are much used in microbial genetics for eliminating plasmids from bacteria.

**acridine orange** Tetramethyl acridine. A fluorescent basic dye used for identification of DNA (green) and RNA (orange-red) under ultraviolet illumination. It is also used to identify activated macrophages.

**acrimony** \ak′rəmō′nē\ The quality of being acrid. *Outmoded.*

**acrisia** \əkrī′zhə\ **1** Absence of crisis of a disease. **2** Uncertainty about the course of a disease. *Rare.*

**acrisorcin** A compound of 4-hexylresorcinol and 9-aminoacridine, used in a topical cream for the treatment of tinea versicolor.

**acritical** \ākrit′ikəl\ Lacking a crisis, as an illness.

**acro-** \ak′rō-, ak′rə-\ [Gk *akros* outermost, at the top, extreme] A combining form meaning (1) tip, end or extremity, as of the body; (2) highest point, top.

**acroagnosia** \-agnō′zhə\ [ACRO- + AGNOSIA] Inability to appreciate or recognize the position in space of an extremity of the body, such as a hand or foot. Severe cases may involve lack of recognition of the extremity's existence. Also *acroagnosis, acragnosis.*

**acroanesthesia** \-anesthē′zhə\ [ACRO- + ANESTHESIA] Anesthesia in one or more of the extremities.

**acroarthritis** Arthritis of distal peripheral joints.

**acroblast** \ak′rəblast\ One of the granules, probably derived from the Golgi apparatus in a spermatid, giving rise to the acrosome.

**acrobrachycephaly** \-brak′əsef′əlē\ [ACRO- + BRACHYCEPHALY] A form of craniostenosis in which premature fusion at the coronal suture results in abnormal shortness of the anteroposterior diameter of the braincase.

**acrobystia** \-bis′tē·ə\ [Gk *akrobystia* prepuce] PREPUTIUM PENIS.

**acrobystiolith** \-bis′tē·əlith\ [*acrobysti(a)* + -LITH] PREPUTIAL CONCRETION.

**acrocentric** \-sen′trik\ Having the centromere close to one end of the chromosome such that one arm is much longer than the other. The short arm is often associated with satellites. Also *subtelocentric.*

**acrocephalopolysyndactyly** \-sef′əlōpälēsindak′təlē\ [*acrocephal(y)* + *poly(dactyly)* + SYNDACTYLY] Any of four heritable malformation syndromes recognizable at birth and characterized by premature craniosynostosis, syndactyly, and polydactyly. A variety of other features occur in specific syndromes. In type I, the Noack syndrome, the features and autosomal dominant inheritance are the same as in acrocephalosyndactyly type V (Pfeiffer syndrome), suggesting these are the same disorder. In type II, the Carpenter syndrome, additional features are peculiar facies, brachydactyly, and mild mental retardation, all inherited as an autosomal recessive trait. In type III, the Sakati-Nyhan syndrome, tibial hypoplasia and aural and facial anomalies occur while inheritance is unclear. In type IV, the Goodman syndrome, congenital heart disease, clinodactyly, and normal intelligence are heritable as an autosomal recessive syndrome.

**acrocephalosyndactyly** \-sef′əlōsindak′təlē\ [*acrocephal(y)* + SYNDACTYLY] A congenital syndrome that combines a peaked cranium, due to premature closure of skull sutures, and syndactyly. Four autosomal dominant variations have been identified, each recognizable at birth and designated types I through IV. Also *acrodysplasia, acrosphenosyndactalia.* **a. type I** Acrocephalosyndactyly characterized by the fusion of the second through fourth digits, which share a common nail. Also *Apert syndrome, Apert's disease.* **a. type II** Acrocephalosyndactyly in which the second through fourth digits are fused and bear a common nail and in which the mandible is hypoplastic, as is seen in the Crouzon syndrome. Also *Apert-Crouzon syndrome.* **a. type III** Acrocephalosyndactyly that is characterized by mild syndactyly and skull asymmetry. Also *Saethre-Chotzen syndrome, Chotzen syndrome.* **a. type IV** Acrocephalosyndactyly in which the preaxial digits are broad and short and the thumbs often deviate radially. Also *Pfeiffer syndrome.*

**acrocephaly** \-sef′əlē\ [ACRO- + CEPHAL- + -Y] OXYCEPHALY.

**acrocinesia** \-sinē′zhə\ The property of exhibiting excessive motility. Also *acrokinesia, acrocinesis.* Adj. acrocinetic.

**acrocyanosis** \-sī′ənō′sis\ An uncommon vasospastic disorder characterized by persistent coldness with cyanosis of the hands and fingers, feet, and toes, usually associated with excessive perspiration.

**acrodermatitis** \-dur′mətī′tis\ Dermatitis that affects primarily the extremities. **a. chronica enteropathica** A rare disease of infancy and childhood, appearing as a triad of dermatitis, diarrhea, and alopecia. Vesicobullous eruptions occur around the eyes, body orifices, and extremities. Death may ensue after a prolonged course of relapses and remissions, depression, infantilism, and malnutrition. Treatment with diiodohydroxy quinolone is effective. The cause is thought to be a disorder of tryptophan metabolism, inherited as an autosomal recessive defect. **a. continua** A form of acral pustulosis in which a sterile, pustular eruption affects primarily the skin of the distal phalanges and usually runs a chronic relapsing course. It may extend proximally, and generalized pustular psoriasis may occur. It resembles psoriasis and is sometimes associated with it. Also *acrodermatitis perstans, Hallopeau's acrodermatitis, pustular acrodermatitis.* **a. enteropathica** A periorificial erythematous eruption with bullae that arises when an infant is weaned. It is caused by a deficiency of zinc resulting from a genetically determined defect in zinc absorption. Also *Danbolt-Closs syndrome.* **Hallopeau's a.** ACRODERMATITIS CONTINUA. **infantile papular a.** An infective disease of childhood, possibly caused by the hepatitis B virus, and characterized by an acral eruption of dull red, sometimes lichenoid papules, fever, and lymphadenopathy. Also *Gianotti-Crosti syndrome, acrodermatitis papulosa infantum, infantile lichenoid acrodermatitis.* **a. perstans** ACRODERMATITIS CONTINUA. **pustular a.** ACRODERMATITIS CONTINUA. **a. vesiculosa tropica** A vesicular eruption of the fingers occurring in tropical climates.

**acrodermatoses** \-dur′mətō′sēz\ Plural of ACRODERMATOSIS.

**acrodermatosis** \-dur′mətō′sis\ [ACRO- + DERMATOSIS] Any skin disease involving the extremities.

**acrodolichomelia** \-däl′əkōmē′lyə\ [ACRO- + DOLICHO- + MEL-[1] + -IA] Abnormal largeness of hands or feet owing to disproportionate or continued growth beyond the usual time of physical maturation.

**acrodynia** \-din′ē·ə\ [*acr(o)-* + -ODYNIA] PINK DISEASE.

**acrodysesthesia** \-dis′esthē′zhə\ Dysesthesia in the extremities.

**acrodysplasia** \-displā′zhə\ [ACRO- + DYSPLASIA] ACROCEPHALOSYNDACTYLY.

**acrogeria** \-jir′ē·ə\ [ACRO- + *ger(o)-* + -IA] A genetically determined syndrome in which premature aging of the skin predominantly affects the extremities.

**acrognosia** \ak′rägnō′zhə\ [ACRO- + Gk *gnōs(is)* knowledge + -IA] Sensory recognition of the limbs and of the different portions of each limb in relation to each other. *Seldom used.* Also *acrognosis.*

**acrohypothermy** \-hī′pōthur′mē\ An abnormally low temperature of the hands and feet.

**acrokeratoelastoidosis** \-ker′ətō·ilas′toidō′sis\ [*acrokerato(sis)* + ELASTOIDOSIS] **1** A syndrome characterized by the development in middle or old age of a line of warty papules at the junction of palmar and dorsal skin, from the tip of the thumb to the radial side of the index finger. It is associated with solar elastosis. **2** A hereditary syndrome, probably determined by an autosomal dominant gene, in which warty papules develop during childhood in the same distribution as those associated with solar elastosis in later years. There appears to be no dermal abnormality.

**acrokeratosis** \-ker′ətō′sis\ [ACRO- + KERATOSIS] Any hyperkeratotic condition of the extremities.

**acrokinesia** \-kīnē′zhə\ ACROCINESIA.

**acromacria** \-mak′rē·ə\ ARACHNODACTYLY.

**acromastitis** \-mastī′tis\ [ACRO- + MASTITIS] Inflammation of the nipple.

**acromegalogigantism** \-meg′əlōjī′gantizm\ ACROMEGALIC GIGANTISM.

**acromegaly** \-meg′əlē\ [ACRO- + -MEGALY] A disease caused by oversecretion of pituitary growth hormone and characterized by an eosinophilic (acidophilic) cell adenoma of the anterior pituitary gland, enlargement of acral parts (ears, nose, jaw, hands, feet), bony overgrowth, and multiple metabolic derangements. Acromegaly occurs, rarely, as one feature of the familial syndrome, multiple endocrine neoplasia Type I (MEN I). Also *Marie syndrome* (outmoded), *pituitary syndrome, hypersomatotropism.*

**acromelia** \-mē′lyə\ [ACRO- + MEL-[1] + -IA ] **1** A relative shortening of the distal segment of the limbs. **2** ACROMELIC DWARFISM.

**acromelic** \-mē′lik\ Relating to or involving the end of a limb.

**acromial** \əkrō′mē·əl\ Pertaining to the acromion.

**acromiale os** OS ACROMIALE. **a. secundarium** OS ACROMIALE SECUNDARIUM.

**acromioclavicular** \əkrō′mē·ōkləvik′yələr\ Pertaining to the acromion and the clavicle, usually with reference to the articulation and ligaments between them. Also *scapuloclavicular.*

**acromion** \əkrō′mē·än\ [Gk *akrōmion* (from *akr(os)* at the top, extreme + *ōmos* shoulder) the upper arm, shoulder] [NA] The flattened, squarish lateral projection of the spine of the scapula, providing attachment for fibers of the deltoid and trapezius muscles. Medially it articulates with the lateral end of the clavicle at an oval facet, just in front of which is the attachment of the coracoacromial ligament. The latter, with the acromion and coracoid process, forms an arch over the glenohumeral joint, preventing upward dislocation of the humerus and limiting its upward rotation. The thick lateral border of the acromion is a palpable subcutaneous bony landmark. Also *acromial process, acromial bone.*

**acromionectomy** \əkrō′mē·ənek′təmē\ A surgical excision of the acromion.

**acromioscapular** \əkrō′mē·ōskap′yələr\ Pertaining to the acromion and the body of the scapula.

**acroneuropathy** \-n[y]Uräp′əthē\ Any neuropathy giving clinical manifestations which affect predominantly the extremities, as is the case in many varieties of polyneuropathy.

**acroneurosis** \-nyUrō′sis\ A condition giving rise to symptoms of emotional origin which involve the extremities. *Obs.*

**acronine** $C_{20}H_{19}NO_3$. 3,12-Dihydro-6-methoxy-3,3,12-trimethyl-7*H*-pyrano[2,3-*c*]acridin-7-one. An antineoplastic compound.

**acro-osteolysis** \-äs′tē·äl′isis\ The loss of terminal digits, with bone resorption, caused by diseases such as scleroderma, Raynaud's disease, hyperparathyroidism, or vinyl chloride poisoning.

**acropachy** \ak′rəpak′ē\ [ACRO- + Gk *pachy(s)* thick, large, curdled] A thickening of the fingers and toes as a consequence of a pathologic condition that affects the periosteum and subcutaneous tissues, as in hyperthyroidism or hypertrophic pulmonary osteoarthropathy.

**acroparalysis** \-pəral′isis\ Paralysis of one or more extremities. *Seldom used.*

**acroparesthesia** \-par′esthē′zhə\ **1** Paresthesia of the hands and feet. **2** Troublesome nocturnal paresthesia involving the hands, usually due to a carpal tunnel syndrome but occasionally to other causes. **Nothnagel type a.** Acroparesthesia due to ischemia of the extremities, as in Raynaud's disease. **Schultze type a.** Acroparesthesia with acrocyanosis.

**acropathy** \əkräp′əthē\ [ACRO- + -PATHY] A disease or injury of the extremities. **amyotrophic a.** Any disease characterized by muscular atrophy in the extremities, of neurogenic as distinct from myopathic origin, and caused by damage to or disease of peripheral nerves, the motor nerve roots, or the anterior horn cells of the spinal cord. *Seldom used.* Also *neural amyotrophy.* **ulcerative mutilating a.** A syndrome of multiple etiology, characterized by sensory loss, involving particularly pain and temperature sensation in the distal parts of the limbs, associated with perforating ulcers, often painless, in the feet, and frequently with progressive loss of soft tissue, bone destruction, and resorption in the phalanges and metatarsals, and consequent deformity. The commonest cause is hereditary sensory neuropathy. When destruction and resorption of bone is severe, the condition is often called the Morvan syndrome. The forms of polyneuropathy giving rise to this syndrome are often collectively entitled the acrodystrophic neuropathies.

**acropetal** \əkräp′ətəl\ Tending or preceeding toward an apex or summit.

**acrophobia** \-fō′bē·ə\ [ACRO- + -PHOBIA] Fear of heights.

**acropigmentatio reticularis** A hereditary syndrome

of autosomal dominant origin that is characterized by the development during childhood of a network of pigmentation that begins on the backs of the hands and subsequently appears elsewhere.

**acropurpura** \-pur′pərə\ Purpura of the extremities.

**acropustulosis** \-pus′tyəlō′sis\ ACRAL PUSTULOSIS.

**acrosclerosis** \-sklerō′sis\ Scleroderma involving the extremities. Also *acroscleroderma.*

**acrosome** \ak′rəsōm\ [ACRO- + -SOME] The anterior tip of a spermatozoon contained within the head cap. The acrosome is probably derived from part of the Golgi apparatus of the spermatocytes. Also *acrosomal cap, apical body.* Adj. acrosomal.

**acrospiroma** / **eccrine a.** A benign sweat gland tumor that mimics the structure of the eccrine duct. Also *clear cell hidradenoma, eccrine poroma.*

**acrostealgia** \-stē·al′jə\ [*acr(o)-* + OSTEALGIA] A painful inflammation of the bones of the hands or feet.

**acroteric** \-ter′ik\ [Gk *akrōtēr(ion)* tip, end (from *akros* topmost, outermost) + -IC] Of or relating to the extremes of the body, such as the ears, the tip of the nose, the tips of the toes, and the fingertips.

**acrotic**[1] \əkrät′ik\ [Gk *a-* priv. + *krot(os)* the sound of striking + -IC] Pertaining to or characterized by an absent pulse.

**acrotic**[2] \əkrät′ik\ [Gk *akrot(ēs)* (from *akros* outermost) an extreme + -IC] Pertaining to an external surface. *Outmoded.*

**acrotrophodynia** \-träf′ədin′ē·ə\ [ACRO- + TROPH- + -ODYNIA] Neuritic pain in the extremities occurring as a result of continued exposure to damp and cold, as in trench foot.

**acrylate** 1 A salt or ester of acrylic acid. 2 A plastic based on polymerization of a derivative of acrylic acid.

**acrylic acid** $CH_2{=}CH{-}COOH$. Propenoic acid. Its derivatives are used in the manufacture of plastics.

**acrylonitrile** \ak′rilōnī′trīl\ $CH_2{=}CH{-}CN$. A chemical compound used in the manufacture of synthetic fibers and styrene plastics. It can act as a chemical asphyxiant and irritant to mucous membranes. It is carcinogenic to rats and is suspected of causing lung cancer in exposed workers. Also *vinyl cyanide* (seldom used).

**ACS** antireticular cytotoxic serum.

**act** / **compulsive a.** COMPULSION. **forced a.** COMPULSION. **imperious a.** COMPULSION. **impulsive a.** An action performed without deliberation or reflection. The action itself is ego-syntonic, contains a pleasurable component as well as some degree of irresistibility, and expresses itself directly rather than in some disguised or distorted form. **reflex a.** A relatively constant, automatic motor response triggered by a specific afferent stimulus in the absence of, or independent of, suprasegmental control.

**ACTe** anodal closure tetanus.

**ACTH** adrenocorticotropic hormone.

**actin** \ak′tin\ [*act* + -IN; so called for its *act*ivation of, or inter*act*ion with, myosin] A protein constituent of the muscle fibril existing in two forms, globular (G-actin), with a molecular mass of 46 kilodaltons, and fibrous (F-actin), a polymer of G-actin. The interaction of F-actin, the thin filament of muscle fibril, with the thick myosin filament is responsible for muscular contraction. Many other cells also contain actin fibers as structural or motile elements.

**actin-** \ak′tən-\ ACTINO-.

**acting out** A type of displacement in which behavior that appears to be in response to the current situation is, in fact, an expression of unconscious feelings or conflicts.

**actinic** \aktin′ik\ Concerning electromagnetic radiation capable of detection by a photographic plate, usually visible radiation and radiation of shorter wavelengths.

**actinide** Any of the elements of atomic number from 90 to 103, containing filled 6s, 6p, and 7s orbitals, whereas the 5f orbitals fill as the atomic number increases. The actinides follow actinium in the periodic table, and include uranium and plutonium. Many actinides are radioactive.

**actiniform** \aktin′əfôrm\ Displaying raylike or radiate form.

**actinin** A muscle protein found in the Z-lines of striated muscle, i.e. at the midpoints of the actin filaments.

**actinium** A radioactive element having atomic number 89. Isotopes of mass numbers 221 to 231 have been identified, all having short half-lives ranging down to a fraction of a second. Most of these are synthetic. The longest lived, actinium 227 (half-life, 21.6 years) is found in association with uranium 235, of which it is a decay product. Actinium 228 (half-life, 6.13 hours) is a decay product of uranium 238. Actinium in equilibrium with its decay products is a powerful emitter of alpha radiation. Chemically, actinium resembles lanthanum. See also RADIOACTIVE SERIES. Symbol: Ac

**actino-** \ak′tənō-\ [Gk *aktis* (gen. *aktinos*) ray] A combining form meaning (1) having rays, radial; (2) light, sunlight; (3) any electromagnetic radiation of visible or shorter wavelengths. Also *actin-*.

***Actinobacillus*** \-basil′əs\ A genus of Gram-negative, facultatively anaerobic coccobacilli that cause granulomatous lesions or septicemia in various domestic animals and occasionally in man. This genus is related to *Pasteurella.* ***A. mallei*** *PSEUDOMONAS MALLEI.* ***A. pseudomallei*** *PSEUDOMONAS PSEUDOMALLEI.*

**actinocongestin** \-kənjes′tin\ CONGESTIN.

**actinodermatitis** \-dur′mətī′tis\ 1 ACTINIC DERMATITIS. 2 RADIATION DERMATITIS. 3 Any dermatitis provoked by exposure to radiation. Also *actinocutitis.*

***Actinomadura*** \-mədoo′rə\ [ACTINO- + *Madura* (India)] A genus incertae sedis of funguslike branching bacteria, presently considered to be part of the genus *Nocardia.*

***Actinomyces*** \ak′tinōmī′sēz\ A genus of actinomycetes of which the type species is *A. bovis.* ***A. bovis*** The actinomycete usually responsible for actinomycosis in cattle. It is differentiated from *A. israelii* by colonial structure and by metabolic reactions. ***A. israelii*** An anaerobic actinomycete that grows as highly pleomorphic Gram-positive rods with little branching. Longer filaments forming rays and masses of organisms (sulfur granules) are seen in lesions. The organism is very widespread in the human oral cavity and only rarely initiates lesions, which are then chronic and deep. ***A. muris*** *Obs. STREPTOBACILLUS MONILIFORMIS.* • This species causes acute disease quite different from actinomycosis. ***A. naeslundii*** A facultative actinomycete often found in the human oral cavity and occasionally in lesions.

**actinomycete** \-mī′sēt\ [ACTINO- + -MYCETE] A broad group of bacteria that grow slowly as branched filaments. Together with the mycobacteria they make up the Actinomycetales. In medicine the families of main interest are the Actinomycetaceae, which are often anaerobes, the Nocardiaceae, which are aerobes, and the Streptomycetaceae, which are the source of most antibiotics. Because of their branching growth and the fact that they cause chronic granulomatous lesions, the actinomycetes were long considered fungi, but in their fundamental properties they are typical prokaryotes. Also *ray fungus* (outmoded).

**actinomycetin** A lytic substance produced by *Streptomyces albus* with the ability to dissolve dead Gram-negative organisms and, to a lesser degree, dead Gram-positive organisms.

**actinomycin** Any of a number of antimicrobial substances with antitumor activity, produced by *Streptomyces antibioticus* and *S. chrysomallus.*. **a. $C_1$** ACTINOMYCIN D. **a. D** An antibiotic produced by the actinomycete *Streptomyces chrysomallus.* It binds to DNA, obstructing the minor groove of the double helix, thereby displacing RNA polymerase and preventing transcription. Chemically it is a heterocyclic base in combination with a cyclic peptide, the peptide containing residues modified from those of common amino acids in various ways, including methylation. It is of use experimentally in the study of nucleic acid synthesis and clinically in the treatment of rhabdomyosarcoma and Wilms tumor in children, and for choriocarcinoma. It has also been employed to inhibit immunologic responses, such as the rejection of renal transplants. Also *dactinomycin, actinomycin $C_1$, meractinomycin.*

**actinomycoma** \-mīkō′mə\ [*actinomyc(ete)* + -OMA] A reactive swelling due to actimomycetes.

**actinomycosis** \-mīkō′sis\ [*Actinomyc(es)* + -OSIS] A chronic suppurative bacterial infection caused by *Actinomyces israelii* in man, *A. bovis* in cattle, and other *Actinomyces* species in other animals. It is characterized by indolent inflammatory lesions of the cervicofacial area, lungs, or abdomen, and often formation of abscesses and external draining sinuses. Drainage from a suppurative lesion sometimes contains yellow sulfur granules, distinct conglomerate masses of Gram-positive, branching, filamentous organisms. In man the cervicofacial form is the most common, infection gaining entrance through a wound or a broken-down tooth. Typically it presents as a dark red discoloration of the skin, with boardlike induration and multiple sinuses. Prolonged antibiotic therapy, surgical drainage of abscesses, and excision of sinus tracts are curative. Also *ray-fungus disease.* **cervicofacial a.** Actinomycosis involving the cervicofacial region. Characteristically a painful indurated swelling appears over the lower jaw and tends to spread slowly into the face and neck. The overlying skin assumes a swollen bluish appearance and sinuses appear from which sulfur granules, containing colonies of *Actinomyces israelii,* may sometimes be discharged.

**actinomycotin** A preparation of cultures of *Actinomyces* that has been used in the treatment of actinomycosis.

**actinon** \ak′tinän\ An isotope of radon having a half-life of approximately four seconds. It is a member of the actinium series, (i.e., an actinide) the daughter of radium 223 by alpha decay. Also *radon 219, actinium emanation.* Symbol: An ● See note at EMANATION.

**actinorhodine** $C_{32}H_{26}O_{14}$. An antibiotic pigment produced by *Streptomyces coelicolor,* a species found in woods near Göttingen, Germany.

**actinospectacin** SPECTINOMYCIN.

**actinotherapy** \-ther′əpē\ The use of rays of light, particularly ultraviolet, for the treatment of diseases that are at or near the surface of the body. Also *actinotherapeutics.*

**action** **1** The performance of a function, as in *the action of the heart.* **2** The production of an effect, as in *chemical action.* **3** The application of a force. **4** A behavioral event, as in *a compulsive action.* **adipokinetic a.** The mobilization of fat from adipocytes, usually with liberation of free fatty acids into the blood plasma, a property of a number of several hormones, such as the growth hormone, adrenocorticotropin, thyrotropin, and the anterior pituitary lipotropins. Also *adipokinesis.* **automatic a.** AUTOMATISM. **ball-valve a.** The intermittent obstruction of the outlet from a cavity by a mobile object within the cavity that is itself too large to pass through the outlet. **capillary a.** The movement of fluid in small-bore tubes as a result of surface or interfacial forces. **compulsive a.** COMPULSION. **cumulative a.** Increased intensity of drug action due to an accumulation of a drug in the body after several doses have been given. **electrocapillary a.** ELECTROCAPILLARITY. **nicotinic a.** The paralyzing effect of acetylcholine on autonomic ganglia and skeletal muscle. **reflex a.** The response of an effector, activated by a reflex. **sparing a.** The property of a food substance that serves to safeguard the body's supply of another nutrient which is in short supply. During starvation a carbohydrate supplement is said to have a protein sparing effect, as it is used for energy production in preference to protein that would be used in its absence. **specific a.** The predominant, beneficial activity of a drug representing the basis for its use, such as an antibiotic effect against microorganisms, or the specific metabolic effects of one of the vitamins. **specific dynamic a.** The stimulation of metabolic activity and heat production associated with absorption of food. The action is believed to be partly due to the secretion of gastric juice, which has $10^6$ times more hydrogen ions than does plasma, and partly to protein synthesis. The heat produced by this action may be involved in the maintenance of body temperature. Also *specific dynamic effect.* **synergistic a.** **1** The action of muscles serving in a capacity subsidiary to prime movers in order to prevent unwanted movement and, by fixing joints, to provide a stable base for the action of the prime movers. **2** The interaction of agents resulting in a combined effect that is greater than the sum of the effects of the agents acting alone. **trigger a.** An action in which a stimulus initiates an energy-releasing process with a result unrelated to the action of the stimulus. Also *trigger reaction.*

**actithiazic acid** $C_9H_{15}NO_3S$. An antibiotic substance produced by *Streptomyces lavendulae, S. viginiae,* and several other *Streptomyces* species. Also *mycobacidin.*

**activated** \ak′tivā′tid\ Characterized by increased reactivity: said of a substance, a molecule, or an atom. Also *active.*

**activation** **1** The act or process of making active. **2** In embryology, the normal or artificial stimulation of development, usually in the egg. The two essentially independent aspects to fertilization of an ovum are activation, which initiates a series of rapid changes, and amphimixis, which involves the intermingling of the hereditary characters. Activation is marked by a number of interrelated physicochemical changes, such as increased metabolic rate and protein synthesis. Fertilizins may play a part in triggering activation, as may also genetic mechanisms resulting in activation of amino acids. Chemical treatment (butyric acid, certain ions) and temperature changes (cold shock) can activate unfertilized eggs to develop parthenogenetically. **3** In chemistry, the process of making a substance or group more reactive by chemical reaction or by altering its environment, e.g., on binding to an enzyme. **epileptic a.** Any of the many techniques which have been used for diagnostic purposes in order to induce either clinical attacks of epilepsy or, more often, subclinical epileptic discharges in the EEG. Techniques in common use include hyperventilation, flickering light (photic stimulation), recording during natural or drug-induced sleep or after sleep deprivation and the intravenous injection of graded doses of convulsive drugs such as leptazol or bemegride. The latter technique must be used with caution, as attacks of major epilepsy can sometimes be induced even in normal individuals. **macrophage a.** An enhanced bactericidal activity of macrophages due to an increase in the number of lysosomes and in the secretion of microbicidal products. It is induced, in association with specific delayed hypersensitivity, by various intracellular parasites, such as *Listeria* and *Salmonella*. **spore a.** The first stage in spore germination, in which the spore coat is made permeable to water by mechanical damage or by activation by certain ions or metabolites. **stretch a.** The excitation of contraction in a muscle fiber by abrupt stretch of the fiber, as seen in the flight muscles of some insects and in $bag_1$ intrafusal fibers of the mammalian muscle spindle. **thermal neutron a.** Induction of radioactivity in a target material by thermal neutron bombardment.

**activator** \ak′tivā′tər\ 1 A substance necessary or favorable for enzyme action. 2 CATALYST. 3 A removable orthodontic appliance acting as a passive transmitter of force produced by the function of muscles and applied to the teeth and alveolar processes in contact with it. Also *functional appliance*. **polyclonal a.** A substance that induces the physiologic function or activity of more than one clone of cells. **tissue plasminogen a.** An enzyme having a double chain configuration and a molecular weight of 72 000 that catalyzes the cleavage of plasminogen to plasmin, thus initiating fibrinolysis. It is found in endothelial and other cells. A double and single chain mixture of human forms of this enzyme, produced by genetic engineering techniques, is used as a drug in the treatment of acute myocardial infarction. It may also be useful in pulmonary embolism. It is administered intravenously, and bleeding may be a complication of its use. Also *alteplase, tissue plasminogen factor, lysokinase, vascular tissue factor*. Abbr. t-PA

**active** 1 Especially capable of reaction, as finely divided carbon which is particularly capable of absorption or adsorption. 2 ACTIVATED. 3 Endowed with rotatory power: said of a substance. For example, D- and L-tartaric acids are optically active, the racemic acid and mesotartaric acid are inactive. 4 Capable of action under defined conditions, as the *active* form of an enzyme. 5 Efficacious: said of a medicament.

**activity** [French *activité* (from Med L *activitas* activity) activity] 1 The concentration that a substance dissolved in a solvent behaves as having, which, because of departures from ideal behavior, may differ from its actual concentration. Its activity is equal to its partial molar Gibbs energy. 2 Any of the numerous waveforms recorded in the electroencephalogram or electromyogram. **asynchronous a.** Cerebral electrical activity, as recorded in the EEG, irregular and of low amplitude, arising relatively randomly from neuronal activity. Compare SYNCHRONOUS ACTIVITY. **background a.** 1 BACKGROUND RADIATION. 2 That level of spiking discharge or other recordable excitatory activity shown by neurons, axons, muscle cells, etc., before some stimulus likely to change the activity is imposed. **blocking a.** Interference with the transmission of electrical activity in nerve fibers or synapses whether produced by drugs or by nonphysiologic electrical activity. **catalytic a.** ENZYME ACTIVITY. **continuous muscle fiber a.** A syndrome in which the subject experiences muscle pain and spasms in the extremities and the affected muscles show coarse fasciculations. After voluntary contraction there is often slow relaxation, as in myotonia. The electromyogram shows continuous muscle fiber activity even with the muscles apparently at rest. Also *neuromyotonia, Isaacs syndrome*. **cumulated a.** The product of the amount of radioactivity present (in an organ, for example) and the time during which it is there. It is usually measured in microcurie-hours. **elevation activities** Activities that involve climbing and descending stairs, curbs, and other types of steps. **enzyme a.** The rate of conversion which an enzyme can catalyze, expressed as (amount of substance)/time. Also *catalytic activity*. **insulinlike a.** See under NONSUPPRESSIBLE INSULINLIKE ACTIVITY. **nonsuppressible insulinlike a.** That portion (90%) of bioassayable insulinlike activity which cannot be neutralized by antibodies against insulin. It consists of a group of peptides, some precipitable by acid-ethanol, some soluble. It is often found in excess in plasma and tumors of patients having severe hypoglycemia associated with large mesenchymal tumors, hepatocellular carcinoma, and miscellaneous neoplasms. Abbr. NSILA **optical a.** The ability of a substance to rotate the plane of vibration of polarized light either counterclockwise or clockwise. See also OPTICAL ROTATION. **plasma renin a.** The capacity of renin in a plasma sample to catalyze conversion of angiotensinogen. It is increased in hypertension secondary to renal disease, in untreated Addison's disease, and in the presence of renin-secreting tumors. It is decreased in primary aldosteronism. **specific a.** 1 Activity per unit mass of solid or teletherapy sources, measured in curies per gram, kilocuries per gram, microcuries per gram, etc. 2 Activity per unit volume of radioactive solutions, measured in microcuries per milliliter, millicuries per milliliter, etc. **spontaneous a.** A discharge arising in a sensory receptor or brain structure in the apparent absence of all afferent stimuli. **sudomotor a.** Activity of the sympathetic cholinergic fibers which innervate the sweat glands, giving rise to sweating. **surface a.** The property, possessed by soaps and other detergents, of lowering surface tension. **synchronous a.** 1 Electrical rhythms or discharges recorded in the electroencephalogram which occur simultaneously and in synchrony on the two sides of the brain. Compare ASYNCHRONOUS ACTIVITY. 2 In the electromyogram, the simultaneous appearance of electrical potentials of similar shape and amplitude when recording with two separate electrodes inserted at different points within the same muscle.

**acu-**[1] \ak′yoo-\ [L *acus* needle] A combining form meaning needle.

**acu-**[2] \əkoo-\ ACOU-.

**acuclosure** \ak′yooklō′zhər\ [ACU-[1] + *closure*] Hemostasis achieved by the placement of needles.

**acufilopressure** \ak′yoofi′lōpresh′ər\ [ACU-[1] + *fil(um)* + *o* + PRESSURE] The combined use of acupression and ligation to control bleeding.

**acuity** \əkyoo′itē\ [French *acuité* (from Med L *acuitas*, from L *acutus*, past part. of *acuere* to sharpen) sharpness] Sharpness; distinctness; acuteness. **auditory a.** The degree of sensitivity of the auditory system in the reception of sounds. **Vernier a.** DISPLACEMENT THRESHOLD. **visual a.** The clarity of eyesight, the most important clinical measurement of ocular function, expressed as a ratio. For example, in the expression 6/12 vision, the numerator signifies the distance in meters at which measurement is made, and the denominator signifies the distance in meters at which the test line subtends one minute of arc. 6/12 measured in meters corresponds to 20/40 measured in feet. 6/6 or 20/20 represents normal vision. 6/12 visual acuity indicates that the subject could recognize letters at 6 inches which would normally be recognized at 12 inches. Abbr. VA

**aculalia** \ak′oolā′lyə\ [ACU-[2] + -LALIA] SYNTACTICAL APHASIA.

**acumeter** \əkoo′mətər\ ACOUMETER.

**acuminate** \əkyoo′mənit\ [L *acuminat(us)*, past part. of *acuminare* (from *acumen* sharp point, from *acuere* to sharpen, from *acus* needle) to make sharp or pointed] Tapering or sharply pointed.

**acupression** \ak′yoopresh′ən\ [ACU-[1] + *(com)pression*] The compression of bleeding vessels by the insertion of needles into adjacent tissue. Also *acupressure.*

**acupressure** \ak′yoopresh′ər\ **1** ACUPRESSION. **2** SHIATSU.

**acupuncture** \ak′yoopungk′chər\ [ACU-[1] + PUNCTURE] An oriental method of treating pain and disease, and of producing surgical anesthesia, by means of the insertion of special needles at specific points on the body surface. As adapted in Western medicine, the needles may be twirled or weak electrical current applied. Also *stylostixis.*

**acusection** \ak′yoosek′shən\ [ACU-[1] + SECTION] The cutting of tissues by electrosurgery.

**acusector** \ak′yoosek′tər\ [ACU-[1] + SECTOR] A needle that uses an electric current to cut through tissues.

**-acusis** \-əkoo′sis\ [Gk *akousis* hearing] A combining form designating a (specified) kind or condition of hearing, as in *presbyacusis, hypoacusis.* Also *-acousia.*

**acute** \əkyoot′\ [L *acut(us),* past part. of *acuere* to sharpen, incite, stimulate] **1** Of or characterized by sudden onset, marked symptoms, and a short course: said especially of a disease. Compare CHRONIC. **2** Sharp or severe, as pain. **3** Sharply pointed; needlelike; acuate.

**acutorsion** \ak′yootôr′shən\ [ACU-[1] + TORSION] The control of hemorrhaging from a bleeding vessel by passing a needle across the open lumen and twisting it in such a way as to arrest flow through the vessel.

**acyanotic** \əsī′ənät′ik\ Not cyanotic.

**acyclic** \āsik′lik, āsī′klik\ [Gk *a-* priv. + CYCLIC] Composed of molecules containing no rings, but only open (straight or branched) chains: said of a chemical compound.

**acyclovir** \əsī′klōvir\ An acyclic nucleoside analogue of guanosine that is selectively phosphorylated by the herpescoded thymidine kinase to the triphosphate derivative of the drug. The latter is the active antiviral compound. The drug is active *in vitro* and clinically against herpes simplex virus and varicella-zoster virus infections, and herpes genitalis. The bioavailability by oral administration is variable and difficult to predict. The drug is given intravenously or, less frequently, orally, and is used in topical ointments for herpes simplex infections. However, most strains of cytomegalovirus appear to be relatively resistant.

**acyesis** \ā′sī·ē′sis\ [Gk *a-* priv. + *kyēsis* (from *kyein* to hold, be pregnant) pregnancy] **1** Female sterility. **2** The absence of pregnancy.

**acyl** \as′il\ [*ac(id)* + -YL] A univalent chemical group R—CO—, resulting from removal of a hydroxyl group from a carboxylic acid.

**acylase** An enzyme that hydrolyzes an acyl compound to form a carboxylic acid in the reaction: R—CO—X + $H_2O$ ⇌ R—COOH + HX.

**acylation** The replacement of a hydrogen atom by the group R—CO—.

**acyl carrier protein** A bacterial protein of low molecular mass that carries fatty acyl groups, attached as a thioester to a pantetheine group, during chain elongation in fatty acid biosynthesis.

**acyl-CoA dehydrogenase** An enzyme (EC 1.3.99.3) that catalyzes the oxidation of an acyl-CoA to form a 2,3-dehydroacyl-CoA with concomitant reduction of the coenzyme flavin adenine dinucleotide (FAD). It is of metabolic importance in the pathway of fatty acid oxidation.

**acyl-CoA synthetase** An enzyme (EC 6.2.1.3) catalyzing the reaction: ATP + fatty acid + CoA ⇌ acyl-CoA + AMP + pyrophosphate. This is the first reaction in the breakdown of free fatty acids, which are subsequently oxidized in the form of their thioesters with coenzyme A.

**acyl coenzyme A** Coenzyme A acylated on its thiol group.

**acyl enzyme** An intermediate in the enzymatic hydrolysis of ester or amide bonds, in which the acyl group of the substrate has been transferred onto the enzyme with release of the substance it was bound to. The catalysis is completed by hydrolysis of the acyl enzyme. Trypsin, for example, forms such an intermediate.

**acyltransferase** Any enzyme of group EC 2.3, which catalyzes the transfer of an acyl group. Also *transacylase.*

**ad** [L, to, near] To; i.e., up to a specified amount: used in prescription order writing to indicate that a substance, usually a diluent, is to be added to bring the volume up to a specified amount.

**a.d.** *auris dextra* (L, right ear).

**ad-** \ad-, əd-\ [L *ad* (as prefix, assimilated as *ac-, af-, ag-, ap-, as-, at-*) to, near] A prefix meaning (1) to, toward; (2) near, adjoining. Also *ac-, af-, ag-, ap-, as-, at-.* ● In the sense of near, the form is invariably *ad-.*

**-ad** \-ad, -əd\ [L *ad* to, near] A suffix meaning toward.

**ADA** American Dental Association.

**adactyly** \ādak′təlē\ ECTRODACTYLY.

**Adair Dighton** [Charles Allen *Adair Dighton,* English otologist, born 1885] Adair-Dighton syndrome, Dighton-Adair syndrome. See under VAN DER HOEVE-DE KLEYN SYNDROME.

**Adamantiades** [B. *Adamantiades,* French physician, flourished 20th century] Adamantiades-Behçet syndrome. See under BEHÇET SYNDROME.

**adamantinoblastoma** \ad′əman′tənōblastō′mə \ [Gk *adamantino(s)* hard as adamant + BLASTOMA] *Obs.* AMELOBLASTOMA.

**adamantinocarcinoma** \ad′əman′tənōkär′sinō′mə\ [Gk *adamantino(s)* hard as adamant + CARCINOMA] MALIGNANT AMELOBLASTOMA.

**adamantinoma** \ad′əman′tinō′mə\ [Gk *adamantinos* (from *a-* priv. + *damas,* gen. *damantos,* the hardest metal, from *daman* to conquer) hard as adamant + -OMA] AMELOBLASTOMA. **a. of long bones** A rare bone tumor, almost invariably of the tibia (tibial adamantinoma), which histologically resembles the ameloblastoma of the jaw. It is malignant, or at least locally malignant. **pituitary a.** CRANIOPHARYNGIOMA. **tibial a.** See under ADAMANTINOMA OF LONG BONES.

**adamantoblast** \ad′əman′təblast\ AMELOBLAST.

**Adamkiewicz** [Albert *Adamkiewicz,* Polish-born Austrian pathologist, 1850–1921] Artery of Adamkiewicz. See under ARTERIA RADICULARIS MAGNA.

**Adams** [Robert *Adams,* Irish physician, 1791–1875] **1** Adams disease, Adams-Stokes disease, Stokes-Adams disease, Stokes-Adams syndrome, Morgagni-Adams-Stokes syndrome. See under ADAMS-STOKES SYNDROME. **2** Adams-Stokes syncope. See under SYNCOPE.

**Adams** [William *Adams,* English surgeon, 1820–1900] See under FORCEPS.

**adamsite** DIPHENYLAMINEARSINE CHLORIDE.

**adaptability** A flexibility in behavior which assists the effective interaction between an individual and his or her environment. Adaptability is demonstrated by appropriate responses made to altered social or environmental circumstances.

**adaptation** [French (from Med L *adaptatio,* from L *adaptatus,* past part. of *adaptare* to fit + *-atio* -ATION), adaptation] **1** The change of sensitivity of the retina to light resulting from photochemical metabolism. **2** The advantageous change or changes of behavior, physiology, or structure by which an organism modifies itself to fit into a particular environment. **3** A nongenetic change in a organism that takes place in response to an environmental stimulus. 4 A progressive reduction in the sensitivity of a sense organ following prolonged exposure to the same sensory stimulus, often noted in temperature awareness, smell, or taste. 5 The fitting of a denture. 6 The degree of molding of the approximating surfaces of a restorative material to a cavity preparation in a tooth. 7 The adjustment of bands to teeth. **abnormal auditory a.** Impairment of auditory acuity during the course of sustained acoustic stimulation, demonstrated clinically by comparing the thresholds for continuous and interrupted tones on the Bekesy audiometer, and by the tone decay test. Cochlear disorders may show adaptation in excess of normal but the more extreme degrees of impairment are seen in retrocochlear pathology. Abbr. AAA **auditory a.** The ability to adapt to auditory changes, demonstrated by sensitivity to alterations in the auditory threshold on exposure to sound. **color a.** The ability of the retina to change its sensitivity to spectral discrimination. **dark a.** The ability of the retina to increase its sensitivity to light by utilizing the rods, enabling the eye to see in very dim light. Colors cannot be recognized. This function is impaired in certain conditions such as vitamin-A deficiency and retinitis pigmentosa. Also *scotopic adaptation.* **genetic a.** Improved survival or growth in a particular environment achieved by undirected genetic change and natural selection, in contrast to a reversible, environmentally induced phenotypic (physiologic) adaptation. **light a.** The ability of the retina to reduce its sensitivity to light by utilizing the cones, enabling the eye to see in daylight intensities of light. Also *photopic adaptation.* **phenotypic a.** Any changes in the properties of an organism that occur in response to environmental stress and are not associated with a change in the genotype, such as the induction of enzyme synthesis or a change in the rate of cell division. Also *physiologic adaptation.* **photopic a.** LIGHT ADAPTATION. **physiologic a.** PHENOTYPIC ADAPTATION. **retinal a.** The ability of the retina to change its sensitivity to visual stimuli. **scotopic a.** DARK ADAPTATION. **sensory a.** 1 A loss of sensitivity resulting from the prolonged stimulation of a sensory end-organ. 2 Any change in the sensitivity of a sensory end-organ, whether an increase, decrease or shift in the quality of stimulus resolution. **social a.** The adjusting of one's behavior to conform with the customs and conditions of the society in which one lives to enhance harmony in social interaction. Also *accommodation.*

**adapter** \ədap′tər\ A device for connecting two incompatible instruments that differ in size, voltage, frequency, etc. Also *connector.* Also *adaptor.*

**adaptometer** \ad′aptäm′ətər\ [*adapt(ation)* + -METER] A device to measure the rate and amount of increased sensitivity of the retina to light, as occurs when the light-adapted eye is placed in darkness.

**adaptor** \ədap′tər\ ADAPTER.

**adarticulation** \ad′ärtik′yəlā′shən\ ARTICULATIO PLANA.

**ad aur.** *ad aurem* (L, to the ear).

**adaxial** \adak′sē·əl\ To the side of, or directed toward, the axis of a structure.

**ADC** analog-to-digital converter.

**adde** [L, pres. imperative of *addere* to add] Add: used in prescription writing to indicate a substance should be added.

**ad def. an.** *ad defectionem animi* (L, to the point of fainting).

**ad deliq.** *ad deliquium* (L, to the point of weakness, or faintness).

**adder** [formerly, with article, *a nadder*; from Old English *nædre,* akin to L *natrix* a water snake] 1 A snake belonging to any of numerous poisonous genera in the serpentine subfamily Viperinae. 2 A member of any of several genera of North American snakes including the harmless hognose snake (*Heterodon*) and milk snake (*Lampropeltis*) as well as the venomous northern copperhead (*Agkistrodon*). A popular and imprecise term. **death a.** A snake of the species *Acanthophis antarctica.* **puff a.** 1 A highly poisonous snake of the genus *Bitis.* 2 A harmless snake of the genus *Heterodon.*

**addict** [L *addictus* (past part. of *addicere* to assign, give over, surrender, from AD- + *dicere* to say, declare) bound, addicted] A person with a psychological or physiologic compulsive need to take certain drugs, alcohol, or other substances.

**addiction** [L *addictio* assignment, surrender. See also ADDICT.] Physiologic dependence upon a substance as manifested by tolerance and/or an abstinence or withdrawal syndrome when intake is reduced or stopped. The most commonly abused substances that may be associated with addiction are alcohol, barbiturates and related sedatives or hypnotics, opioids, amphetamines, and caffeine. • Although *addiction* and *habituation* are often used interchangeably, *habituation* usually indicates only a psychological dependence without the physiologic dependence and increasing tolerance of addiction. **alcohol a.** ALCOHOLISM. **drug a.** Physiologic, and almost always psychological, dependency on a chemical substance, characterized by the appearance of a withdrawal reaction or abstinence syndrome when the drug is discontinued. **polysurgical a.** A chronic factitious disorder in which physical symptoms are presented so convincingly that surgical intervention is considered necessary and the patient eagerly submits to multiple operations. It is a form of Münchausen syndrome in which the relief sought is an invasive surgical procedure rather than drugs or mere hospitalization.

**Addis** [Thomas *Addis,* U.S. physician, 1881–1949] See under COUNT.

**Addison** [Christopher *Addison,* English anatomist, 1869–1951] 1 Addison's planes. See under PLANE. 2 See under POINT.

**Addison** [Thomas *Addison,* English physician, 1793–1860] 1 Addisonian crisis. See under CRISIS. 2 Addisonian dermal pigmentation. See under PIGMENTATION. 3 Addison's keloid. See under MORPHEA. 4 See under DISEASE. 5 Schilder-Addison complex. See under ADRENOLEUKODYSTROPHY. 6 Addison's anemia, addisonian anemia, Addison-Biermer anemia. See under PERNICIOUS ANEMIA.

**addisonian** \ad′isō′nē·ən\ [after Thomas *Addison,* English physician, 1793–1860 + *-ian,* adjectival suffix] Having the characteristics of a patient with Addison's disease; pertaining to Addison's disease.

**addition** A chemical reaction of two compounds to form a single product, usually by combination of one across a double bond in the other. Also *coupling.*

**additive** \ad′itiv\ [Late L *additivus* (from L *addit(us),* past part. of *addere* to add, + *-ivus* -IVE) to be added] 1 A substance added to another. 2 Characterized by addition, as in *additive effect.* **color a.'s** Substances added to foods in order to replace the natural color which has been lost in processing. They fall into three groups: natural pigments (from biological sources), inorganic pigments and lakes, and synthetic coal-tar colors. Many compounds found in the first two groups are permitted by law throughout the world; however, only a few from the coal-tar colors group are permitted in each country. **food a.** Any substance deliberately added to food during processing to ensure that it reaches the consumer in a nutritious, palatable, or appealing state. Such substances include emulsifiers, flavors, colors, vitamins, minerals, thickeners, curing agents, antioxidants, yeast, bacterial inhibitors, chelating agents, and mold.

**adducent** \ədoo′sənt\ [L *adducens*, gen. *adducentis*, pres. part. of *adducere* to bring, conduct, draw to oneself] Bringing about or promoting adduction.

**adduct** \ədukt′\ [L *adduct(us)*, past part. of *adducere* (from *ad-* to + *ducere* to lead) to lead or bring to] **1** To draw (a limb or other part) toward the median axis of the body. **2** To rotate medially, as the eye. **3** A product of a reaction of association between molecules such that they or their residues have their major axes parallel.

**adduction** \əduk′shən\ [ADDUCT + -ION] Movement of a part of the body toward the median plane of the body; or of the hand, toward the median plane of the middle digit; or of the foot, toward the median plane of the second digit. Adduction of the eye refers to a medial (proximal) movement toward the median plane. Compare ABDUCTION.

**adductor** \əduk′tər\ [ADDUCT + -OR] [NA] Any muscle that produces sideways movement of a limb or part toward either the median plane of the body or, in the case of the digits, the middle of the middle finger or of the second toe. Compare ABDUCTOR.

**Ade** Symbol for adenine.

**Adelmann** [Georg Franz Blasius *Adelmann*, German surgeon, 1811–1888] See under OPERATION.

**aden-** \ad′ən-\ ADENO-.

**adenalgia** \-al′jə\ Pain originating in a gland. Also *adenodynia.*

**adenase** \ad′ənās\ An enzyme which deaminates adenine to hypoxanthine. It is produced by the liver, kidney, and spleen.

**adendritic** \ā′dendrit′ik\ Describing neurons without dendrites.

**adenectomy** \-ek′təmē\ [ADEN- + -ECTOMY] The surgical excision of a gland.

**adenic** \ədē′nik\ Resembling or pertaining to a gland. Also *adenous.*

**adeniform** \əden′əfôrm\ Having the shape of a gland.

**adenine** \ad′ənīn\ $C_5H_5N_5$. A 6-amino purine base which is widely distributed in plant and animal cells. It is present in ATP, ADP, and AMP, and is one of the two main purines found in nucleotide coenzymes and in nucleic acids.

**adenine arabinoside** VIDARABINE.

**adenine deaminase** An enzyme (EC 3.5.4.2) responsible for the hydrolysis of adenine to form hypoxanthine and ammonia.

**adenine deoxyriboside** A nucleoside composed of the purine base adenine and the pentose deoxyribose. One of the four nucleosides present in DNA, it base-pairs with thymidine.

**adenine hypoxanthine** HYPOXANTHINE.

**adenine nucleotide** A nucleotide containing a pentose sugar linked to phosphate through one carbon and to the nitrogen atom at position 9 of adenine through another (C-1′). The main adenine nucleotides are ATP, ADP, and AMP, and the term often applies only to them.

**adenitis** \ad′ənī′tis\ [ADEN- + -ITIS] Inflammation of a gland or lymph node. **acute infectious a.** INFECTIOUS MONONUCLEOSIS. **mesenteric a.** Inflammation of the lymph nodes of the mesentery. The acute form in young children, sometimes complicated by intussusception, is usually due to an adenovirus. Suppuration of the glands may occur. The main symptom is colicky abdominal pain. The condition is difficult to distinguish from appendicitis. Also *mesenteric lymphadenitis.* **phlegmonous a.** Adenitis with inflammation of the neighboring connective tissues. Also *adenophlegmon.* **syphilitic inguinal a.** Persistent adenitis that affects the groin area as a result of primary syphilis of the genitalia. **a. tropicalis** *Obs.* LYMPHOGRANULOMA VENEREUM. **tuberculous a.** Infection of the lymph nodes by the tubercle bacillus. There is chronic swelling, then caseation and rupture of the glands, according to their situation, onto the skin, as of the neck, into the bronchial tubes, or into the peritoneum, causing tuberculous peritonitis.

**adeno-** \ad′ənō-\ [Gk *adēn* (genitive *adenos*) gland] A combining form denoting gland. Also *aden-.*

**adenoacanthoma** \-ak′anthō′mə\ [ADENO- + ACANTHOMA] An adenocarcinoma containing areas of squamous differentiation, encountered at a variety of sites but most often seen in the body of the uterus.

**adenoameloblastoma** \-am′əlōblastō′mə\ ADENOMATOID ODONTOGENIC TUMOR.

**adenoamygdalectomy** \-əmig′dəlek′təmē\ *Seldom used* ADENOTONSILLECTOMY.

**adenoblast** \ad′ənōblast′\ [ADENO- + -BLAST] Any embryonic cell from which a glandular cell is derived.

**adenocarcinoma** \-kär′sinō′mə\ [ADENO- + CARCINOMA] A malignant epithelial tumor of glandular structure. Tubular, acinar, cystic, papillary, and trabecular growth patterns occur. The cells may show evidence of glandular function, such as the production of mucus, hormones, or bile. Also *glandular epithelioma* (obs.), *glandular cancer, carcinoma adenomatosum, glandular carcinoma.* **acinar a.** An adenocarcinoma composed of small glandlike structures (acini). Also *acinous adenocarcinoma, acinar carcinoma, acinar cell carcinoma, acinous carcinoma.* **clear cell a.** An adenocarcinoma with cells having clear or very pale cytoplasm, typically found in the kidney and ovary. Also *clear cell carcinoma..* **follicular a.** An adenocarcinoma composed of cells arranged as follicles, typically found in the thyroid. **a. of kidney** RENAL CELL CARCINOMA. **mammary a.** A malignant gland-forming tumor of the breast. **mucinous a.** MUCINOUS CARCINOMA. **mucoid a.** MUCINOUS CARCINOMA. **papillary a.** An adenocarcinoma characterized microscopically by its papillary structure, that is, by glandular tumor cells covering branching stromal stalks, more commonly encountered at certain sites, such as the thyroid and stomach, than at others. **polypoid a.** An adenocarcinoma with a macroscopic appearance of a polyp; an exophytic adenocarcinoma. Such tumors grow from surfaces into lumens, as in the stomach, colon, or bladder. **renal a.** RENAL CELL CARCINOMA. **scirrhous a.** SCIRRHOUS CARCINOMA. **sebaceous a.** A malignant tumor of sebaceous cells, most frequently occurring in the eyelid. **testicular a. of infancy** YOLK SAC TUMOR.

**adenocele** \ad′ənōsēl′\ [ADENO- + -CELE[1]] CYSTADENOMA.

**adenocellulitis** \-sel′yəlī′tis\ Acute inflammation of interstitial tissues in and surrounding a gland.

**adenochondrosarcoma** \-kän′drəsärkō′mə\ [ADENO- + CHONDRO + SARCOMA] Any malignant tumor composed of glandular and cartilagelike tissue, such as a malignant mixed tumor of the salivary glands, mesodermal mixed tumor of the uterus, and nephroblastoma. *Obs.*

**adenocystic** \-sis′tik\ Denoting a tumor composed of glandular and cystic elements.

**adenocystoma** \-sistō′mə\ CYSTADENOMA. **papillary a. lymphomatosum** ADENOLYMPHOMA.

**adenocyte** \ad′ənōsīt′\ [ADENO- + -CYTE] A secretory cell of a gland.

**adenodynia** \-din′ē·ə\ ADENALGIA.

**adenoepithelioma** \-ep′ithē′lē·ō′mə\ ADENOSQUAMOUS CARCINOMA.

**adenofibroma** \-fībrō′mə\ [ADENO- + FIBROMA] A benign tumor, typically found in the ovary, composed of glandular and fibrous elements. **a. of the ovary** A benign tumor with epithelial and stromal components, the latter predominating. The epithelium may be serous (serous adenofibroma), mucinous, or endometrioid in type. The stroma is derived from ovarian stroma. **pseudomucinous a.** An adenofibroma with mucinous epithelium. **serous a.** An adenofibroma with serous epithelium.

**adenofibromyoma** \-fī′brōmī·ō′mə\ A benign tumor composed of glandular, fibrous, and smooth muscular tissues, such as an adenomatoid tumor or a hyperplastic lesion of the prostate and gallbladder. *Obs.*

**adenogenesis** \-jen′əsis\ The process of development of a gland.

**adenogenous** \ad′ənäj′ənəs\ Having a glandular origin. *Seldom used.*

**adenography** \ad′ənäg′rəfē\ Roentgenography of glands, usually after the opacification of their parenchyma or ducts by contrast medium. Adj. adenographic.

**adenohypophyseal** \-hīpäf′isē′əl\ ADENOHYPOPHYSIAL.

**adenohypophysectomy** \-hīpäf′isek′təmē\ Excision of the adenohypophysis.

**adenohypophysial** \-hī′pōfiz′ē·əl\ Pertaining to the adenohypophysis, or anterior pituitary. Also *adenohypophyseal.*

**adenohypophysis** \-hīpäf′isis\ [ADENO- + HYPOPHYSIS] [NA] The anterior lobe of the pituitary gland (hypophysis), which develops in the embryo from the buccal epithelium. Also *lobus anterior hypophyseos, anterior lobe of pituitary gland, anterior lobe of hypophysis, lobus glandularis of hypophysis, pars glandularis* (outmoded), *pars pharyngea lobi anterioris hypophyseos, pharyngeal pituitary, pituitarium anterius, prehypophysis* (rare). See also PITUITARY GLAND.

**adenoid** \ad′ənoid\ [Gk *adenoeidēs* (from *adēn* gland, gen. *adeno(s)* + *-eidēs* -like, -OID) glandular, glandlike] **1** Glandlike in form or substance. **2** LYMPHOID. **3** TONSILLA PHARYNGEALIS. **4** Pertaining to the tonsilla pharyngealis or to its enlarged state. See also ADENOIDS.

**adenoidectomy** \ad′ənoidek′təmē\ Surgical removal of the adenoids.

**adenoidism** \ad′ənoidizm\ The symptom complex attributed to gross hyperplasia of the adenoids. Among the ascribed features are adenoid facies, high-arched palate, and mental dullness which may be a consequence of hearing impairment from middle-ear effusion.

**adenoiditis** \ad′ənoidī′tis\ Inflammation of the adenoids.

**adenoids** \ad′ənoids\ Hypertrophy of the tonsilla pharyngealis. Also *adenoid vegetation.*

**adenolipoma** \-lipō′mə\ LIPOADENOMA.

**adenolipomatosis** \-lip′ōmətō′sis\ [ADENO- + *lipomat(a)*, pl. of LIPOMA + -OSIS] The presence of multiple adenolipomas (lipoadenomas).

**adenolymphitis** \-limfī′tis\ LYMPHADENITIS.

**adenolymphocele** \-lim′fəsēl\ The presence of lymph-filled cystic spaces in a lymph node, often as a result of obstruction of afferent lymphatic channels.

**adenolymphoma** \-limfō′mə\ [ADENO- + LYMPHOMA] A benign parotid tumor composed of glandular and often cystic structures, sometimes with papillary cystic arrangement, lined by characteristic eosinophilic epithelium. The stroma contains a variable amount of lymphoid tissue with follicles. In rare cases, this tumor may be found in the submaxillary gland. Also *Warthin's tumor, papillary cystadenoma lymphomatosum, papillary adenocystoma lymphomatosum.*

**adenolysis** \ad′ənäl′isis\ A decrease in glandular size resulting from destruction of tissue.

# adenoma

**adenoma** \ad′ənō′mə\ [ADEN- + -OMA] A benign epithelial tumor of glandular structure. Tubular, acinar, cystic, papillary, and trabecular growth patterns occur. The cells may show evidence of glandular function, such as the production of mucus and hormones. Also *adenoid tumor.* ● The expression *malignant adenoma* should not be used, as it is contradictory. **acidophil a.** A benign tumor, usually of the pituitary gland, composed of acidophil cells with or without an admixture of chromophobe cells. Many produce excessive growth hormone with consequent acromegaly or gigantism. Other acidophil adenomas may secrete prolactin, resulting in galactorrhea. Also *eosinophil adenoma, acidophilic adenoma, eosinophilic tumor of the pituitary.* **acinar a.** An adenoma in which the tumor cells are arranged in the form of glandular acini. **adnexal a.** A benign glandular tumor arising from skin appendages. **adrenocortical a.** A benign tumor of the adrenal cortex. It may be single or multiple, unilateral or bilateral. It may be hormonally inert or active, secreting excessive aldosterone, cortisol, or androgen. Also *adenoma substantiae corticalis suprarenalis.* **adrenocorticoid a. of the ovary** ADRENAL REST TUMOR. **apocrine a.** PAPILLARY HIDRADENOMA. **basophil a.** A pituitary adenoma composed of basophil cells possibly admixed with chromophobe cells. Cushing syndrome with hypersecretion of ACTH and consequent hyperplasia of the adrenal cortex may be associated with these adenomas. Also *mucoid cell adenoma, pituitary basophilism, pituitary basophilia.* **bronchial a.** A benign glandular tumor of the bronchus. ● Certain malignant tumors, such as adenoid cystic carcinoma, carcinoid tumor, and mucoepidermoid carcinoma, have been inappropriately referred to as bronchial adenomas. **ceruminous a.** A benign tumor of the ceruminous glands. **chief cell a. of the parathyroid** An adenoma composed predominantly of cells with slightly granular, occasionally vacuolated, cytoplasm, commonly associated with hyperfunction. A variety of growth patterns may occur, such as follicular, tubular, or trabecular. **chromophobe a.** An adenoma of the pituitary consisting only of chromophobe cells. No neoplastic acidophil or basophil cells are present. The most frequent hormonal effects are hypopituitarism due to compression of the normal glandular tissue and excessive secretion of prolactin. Some chromophobe adenomas secrete other hormones and may be associated with acromegaly, Cushing syndrome, thyrotoxicosis, etc. **clear cell a.** An adenoma composed of cells with cytoplasm which is unstained, appearing clear. It is usually found in tumors of the parathyroid, kidney, and adrenal. **colloid a.** A form of follicular adenoma, usually of the thyroid gland, with large glandular spaces containing colloid. Also *macrofollicular adenoma.* **cystic a.** An adenoma characterized by large cavities often filled with secretions. *Rare.* **duct a.** INTRADUCTAL PAPILLOMA. **embryonal a.** An adenoma whose cells resemble the embryonal appearance of the organ: used especially for thyroid tumors. **endometrioid a.** A benign ovarian tumor having microscopic features of an endometrial tumor. Also *adenoma endometrioides ovarii.* **a. endometrioides ovarii** OVARIAN ENDOMETRIOSIS.

**eosinophil a.** ACIDOPHIL ADENOMA. **fetal a.** A form of thyroid adenoma with very small follicles containing little or no colloid. The cells and their arrangement resemble the fetal appearance of the gland: used especially of the microfollicular form of thyroid adenoma. Also *microfollicular adenoma.* **a. fibrosum** FIBROADENOMA. **follicular a.** An adenoma with growth patterns and cells resembling those seen in mature or developing thyroid glands. It is characteristically solitary with a well-defined capsule. Follicles of various sizes, tubules, or trabeculae may be present. Growth patterns may be trabecular (embryonal), tubular, microfollicular (fetal), normofollicular (simple), or macrofollicular (colloid). Oxyphilic (Hürthle) cells or clear cells may occur. **a. gelatinosum** COLLOID GOITER. **Getsowa's a.** *Obs.* ONCOCYTIC ADENOMA. **hepatocellular a.** LIVER CELL ADENOMA. **a. hidradenoides** HIDRADENOMA. **Hürthle cell a.** ONCOCYTIC ADENOMA. **intrahepatic bile duct a.** An intrahepatic benign tumor composed of small bile ducts lined by normal-appearing epithelium set in a fibrous stroma. Also *benign cholangioma, cholangioadenoma, cholangioma.* **islet cell a.** A benign tumor of the cells of the islets of Langerhans. The tumor can be subdivided into alpha cell adenomas, which may be associated with hyperglycemia (glucagonoma), and beta cell adenomas, which may cause hypoglycemia (insulinoma). Islet cell tumors may be multiple, in which case they are usually associated with multiple endocrine neoplasia type 1. **a. of the kidney** A benign tumor of renal epithelium. A variety of growth patterns, such as tubular or papillary, and of cell types, such as eosinophil or clear cell, may occur. It is usually small, often multiple in a subcapsular position, and rarely the cause of symptoms. It is the most common benign renal tumor. Also *renal adenoma.* **liver cell a.** A benign tumor composed of cells resembling normal hepatocytes. The cells are arranged in thin trabeculae (two to three cells thick) separated by sinusoids lined by endothelium. Portal tracts and bile ducts are absent, but bile canaliculi are present. Large vessels are commonly found. Also *hepatocellular adenoma.* • This term should not be used for the parenchymal nodules of cirrhosis. **macrofollicular a.** COLLOID ADENOMA. **malignant a.** A well-differentiated adenocarcinoma. *Obs.* **mesonephric a.** WOLFFIAN ADENOMA. **microfollicular a.** FETAL ADENOMA. **mucinous a.** An adenoma composed of cells containing abundant amounts of mucin, typically found in the ovary as a cystic tumor (mucinous cystadenoma). Also *pseudomucinous adenoma.* **mucoid cell a.** BASOPHIL ADENOMA. **multiple endocrine a.'s** MULTIPLE ENDOCRINE NEOPLASIA. **a. of the nipple** An adenoma of the ducts of the nipple. **oncocytic a.** An adenoma composed of oncocytes. These tumors have been described in the thyroid (Hürthle cell tumors), pituitary, parathyroid, and salivary glands. They are not associated with any known function. Also *oxyphilic adenoma, oxyphilic granular cell adenoma, oncocytoma, salivary gland oncocytoma, Hürthle cell adenoma, Getsowa's adenoma* (obs.). **a. ovarii testiculare** ARRHENOBLASTOMA. **oxyphilic a.** ONCOCYTIC ADENOMA. **oxyphilic granular cell a.** ONCOCYTIC ADENOMA. **papillary a.** An adenoma which is characterized microscopically by its papillary structure, i.e., glandular tumor cells covering branching stromal stalks. **papillary cystic a.** An adenoma in which papillary processes grow into a cystic space. **pleomorphic a.** A benign tumor composed of epithelial structures showing a variety of growth patterns intermingled with stroma of mucoid, myxoid, or chondroid appearance, typically found in the salivary glands. Also *benign mixed tumor, mixed tumor of salivary glands.* **pseudomucinous a.** MUCINOUS ADENOMA. **renal a.** ADENOMA OF THE KIDNEY. **renal cortical a.** An adenoma of renal tubular epithelium. Also *adenoma of the renal cortex.* **sebaceous a.** A benign tumor of the skin resembling sebaceous glands. It is most frequently found on the face. Also *steatadenoma.* **a. simplex** An adenoma with an orderly arrangement of glandular or ductal elements. *Obs.* **a. of the stomach** A benign tumor of gastric epithelium typically growing as a polyp. It may be tubular, villous, or tubulovillous. It is considered to be a precancerous lesion. **a. substantiae corticalis suprarenalis** ADRENOCORTICAL ADENOMA. **testicular a.** **1** An adenoma of the testicular collecting ducts or rete testis. **2** TUBULAR ANDROBLASTOMA. **a. of the thyroid** A benign neoplasm of thyroid gland tissue. Virtually all thyroid adenomas are follicular in type. The histologic distinction between an adenoma and a hyperplastic nodule in an adenomatous goiter can be difficult. The existence of a true papillary adenoma of the thyroid is in question. **toxic thyroid a.** A thyroid adenoma associated with hyperthyroidism. **trabecular a.** An adenoma with a microscopic growth pattern of anastomosing epithelial cords of variable thickness. **tubular a.** An adenoma composed of cells arranged as tubules. The tubules are typically embedded in a variable amount of stroma. The most common example is the adenomatous polyp of the colon. **a. tubulare testiculare ovarii** TUBULAR ANDROBLASTOMA. **tubular a. of Pick** TUBULAR ANDROBLASTOMA. **tubulovillous a.** An adenoma with a mixture of tubular and villous structures, usually seen in the colon and rectum. **villous a.** An adenoma with fingerlike processes of stroma covered by epithelium, most frequently seen in the colon and rectum. Also *villous papilloma.* **villous a. of the colon** An adenoma of the colon characterized by fingerlike structures with epithelial cells covering delicate cores of lamina propria. It is usually sessile, and is a precancerous lesion. It may be associated with excessive mucous secretion. **water-clear cell a.** An adenoma of the parathyroid gland, composed predominantly of cells with clear cytoplasm. **wolffian a.** A benign tumor of wolffian duct origin. Also *mesonephric adenoma.*

**adenomatoid** \ad′ənō′mətoid\ [ADENOMA + *t* + -OID] Resembling an adenoma.

**adenomatosis** \-mətō′sis\ [ADENOMA + *t* + -OSIS] The presence of multiple adenomas. **endocrine a.** MULTIPLE ENDOCRINE NEOPLASIA. **familial polyendocrine a.** MULTIPLE ENDOCRINE NEOPLASIA. **fibrosing a.** SCLEROSING ADENOSIS. **multiple endocrine a.** MULTIPLE ENDOCRINE NEOPLASIA. Abbr. MEA **a. oris** Hyperplasia of the mucous glands of the lips. It is a symptomless condition seen as numerous, small, pale, circumscribed patches beneath the epithelium of the everted lip. **pancreatic-islet a.** Multiple benign tumors of the pancreatic islets, in which $\beta$-cell tumors are associated with hypoglycemia (hyperinsulinism), non-$\beta$-cell tumors with hypergastrinemia (Zollinger-Ellison syndrome). Some tumors are nonsecretory, some are the sites of ectopic hormone secretion. **pluriglandular a.** MULTIPLE ENDOCRINE NEOPLASIA. **polyendocrine a.** MULTIPLE ENDOCRINE NEOPLASIA.

**adenomatous** \ad′ənäm′ətəs\ **1** Pertaining to an adenoma. **2** Resembling an adenoma, as in *adenomatous hyperplasia.* An ambiguous term.

**adenomyohyperplasia** \-mī′əhī′pərplā′zhə \ ADENOMYOSIS.

**adenomyoma** \-mī·ō′mə\ [ADENO- + MYOMA] **1** A

benign tumor composed of smooth muscle and glandular tissue. 2 *Incorrect* FOCAL ADENOMYOMATOUS HYPERPLASIA OF THE GALLBLADDER. 3 ADENOMYOSIS.

**adenomyomatosis** \-mī′ōmətō′sis\ 1 The presence of many adenomyomas. 2 *Obs.* SALPINGITIS ISTHMICA NODOSA. **a. of the gallbladder** Hyperplasia of the gallbladder wall characterized by cystic spaces (Rokitansky-Aschoff sinuses) and histologically similar to an adenomyoma. It may produce symptoms of chronic cholecystitis, but the condition is commonly asymptomatic. Also *cholecystitis cystica, cholecystitis glandularis proliferans, diverticulosis of the gallbladder.*

**adenomyosis** \-mī·ō′sis\ [ADENO- + MY- + -OSIS] A benign condition in which there are endometrial glands and stroma in the myometrium causing a symmetrical enlargement of the uterus; endometriosis of the myometrium. Also *endometriosis interna, adenomyoma, stromal adenomyosis, adenomyosis uteri, adenomyohyperplasia, adenomyometritis, endometriosis uterina.* **a. externa** ENDOMETRIOSIS. **a. of fallopian tube** ENDOMETRIOSIS. **stromal a.** ADENOMYOSIS. **a. tubae** TUBAL ENDOMETRIOSIS. **a. uteri** ADENOMYOSIS.

**adenopathy** \ad′ənäp′əthē\ LYMPHADENOPATHY. **hilar a.** An enlargement of the lymph nodes at the pulmonary hilum, most commonly caused by sarcoidosis, pulmonary granulomatous infection, lymphoma, or pulmonary malignancy. **tracheobronchial a.** Disease of lymph nodes of the tracheobronchial group.

**adenophlegmon** \-fleg′mən\ PHLEGMONOUS ADENITIS.

**adenosalpingitis** \-sal′pinji′tis\ [ADENO- + SALPINGITIS] Inflamed endometriosis of the fallopian tube.

**adenosarcoma** \-särkō′mə\ [ADENO- + SARCOMA] A tumor containing connective tissue and glandular elements both of which are malignant. **embryonal a.** *Obs.* NEPHROBLASTOMA

**adenose** \ad′ənōs\ 1 Like a gland. 2 Having or full of glands.

**adenosine** \əden′əsin\ A nucleoside composed of one molecule of adenine and one molecule of D-ribose, a product of hydrolysis of adenylic acid. Also *ribofuranosyladenine.*

**adenosine 3′,5′-cyclic phosphate** A nucleotide formed from ATP with loss of pyrophosphate so that its phosphate group is esterified with both 3′ and 5′ hydroxyl groups. (The primes on the numerals signify that the numbering is that of the ribose, not of the adenine.) In higher organisms it is formed in response to the action of several hormones, including epinephrine and glucagon, and it stimulates various protein kinases, with resulting acceleration of glycolysis. In some bacteria, adenosine 3′,5′-cyclic phosphate stimulates synthesis of the messenger RNA required to synthesize the proteins that are needed for metabolizing other foods when glucose levels fall. Also *cyclic adenosine monophosphate, cyclic AMP.* Abbr. cAMP

**adenosine deaminase** An enzyme (EC 3.5.4.2) that catalyzes the hydrolysis of the amino group of adenosine to form inosine and ammonia.

**adenosine diphosphate** The ester formed between diphosphoric acid and the 5′-hydroxyl group of adenosine. It is formed by transfer of a phospho group from ATP to some appropriate acceptor, which could be water. Symbol: ADP

**adenosine kinase** An enzyme (EC 2.7.1.20) that catalyzes the reaction: adenosine + ATP ⇌ ADP + AMP.

**adenosine monophosphate** The ester formed between orthophosphoric acid and the 5′-hydroxyl of adenosine. Several enzymes are inhibited or activated by it. At high concentration ratios of ATP to ADP, its concentration, which is held in equilibrium with them, changes by a larger factor than the concentration of either of them does, and so provides cells with a sensitive indicator of the need for ATP synthesis. Symbol: AMP

**adenosine 5′-phosphosulfate** The anhydride formed between the phospho group of adenosine 5′-phosphate and sulfate. It can be formed from ATP and sulfate with release of diphosphate (pyrophosphate), and is phosphorylated on O-3′ to form adenosine 3′-phosphate 5′-phosphosulfate, which is the normal biologic donor of the sulfo group $—SO_3^-$. It is also an intermediate in the oxidative metabolism of inorganic sulfur compounds in microbes.

**adenosine triphosphatase** See under ATPASE.

**adenosine triphosphate** The most commonly occurring phosphate donor in biochemical systems. It functions as an energy store and is used up in muscular work, ion pumping, and many other energy-requiring reactions. It is built up again from adenosine diphosphate and orthophosphate. Green plants do this in the course of photosynthesis. Other organisms do it largely through glycolysis (which does not require oxygen) and through respiration (oxidative phosphorylation). Its concentration in muscle is about 5 mM. Abbr. ATP

**adenosis** \ad′ənō′sis\ [ADEN- + -OSIS] 1 Adenopathy or lymphadenopathy. 2 Proliferation of glandular tissue. 3 SALPINGITIS ISTHMICA NODOSA. **sclerosing a.** A form of mammary dysplasia, occurring most often in young women, characterized by firm, tender nodules and small cysts in the breast, increased fibrous tissue, and mastodynia. Microscopically, it is sometimes difficult to distinguish from carcinoma. Also *sclerosing adenomatosis, fibrosing adenomatosis, fibrosing adenosis.* **a. vaginae** The presence of columnar epithelium in the vagina. See also DES SYNDROME.

**adenosquamous** \-skwā′məs\ Both glandular and squamous, as a tumor.

***S*-adenosylhomocysteine** A thioether formed between adenosine and homocysteine by loss of the 5′-hydroxyl group of adenosine and the thiol-hydrogen of homocysteine. It remains after *S*-adenosylmethionine has donated its methyl group.

***S*-adenosylmethionine** The sulfonium compound formed by alkylation of the sulfur atom of methionine by ATP with loss of phosphate and diphosphate. It is an important biologic methylating agent, since its methyl group can be transferred to nucleophiles from the good leaving group on which it is placed. Also *active methionine* (outmoded).

**adenotome** \ad′ənōtōm′\ [ADENO- + -TOME] Any one of several instruments designed for the excision of adenoids. **La Force a.** An adenotome in which a box adjacent to the blade is so arranged as to trap the excised tissue and ensure against its accidental retention in the nasopharynx or elsewhere.

**adenotomy** \ad′ənät′əmē\ [ADENO- + -TOMY] The incision of a gland.

**adenotonsillectomy** \-tän′səlek′təmē\ The surgical removal of the palatine tonsils and the adenoids. Also *tonsilloadenoidectomy, adenoamygdalectomy* (seldom used).

**adenous** \ad′ənəs\ ADENIC.

**adenovarix** \-ver′iks\ LYMPHADENOVARIX.

**adenovirus** \-vī′rəs\ [*adeno(id)* (the tissue from which it was first isolated) + VIRUS] Any of a group of DNA viruses belonging to either of the two genera of the Adenoviridae family, *Mastadenovirus* and *Aviadenovirus.* There are human, simian, bovine, porcine, canine, murine, ovine, equine, and avian adenoviruses.

**adenyl** \ad′ənil\ ADENYLYL.

**adenylate** An anion formed from adenylic acid.

**adenylate cyclase** An enzyme (EC 4.6.1.1) that forms

adenosine 3′,5′-cyclic phosphate and inorganic pyrophosphate from ATP. In many eukaryotic cells it does this in response to the interaction of hormones with receptors on the cell envelopes. Also *adenyl cyclase, 3′,5′-cyclic AMP synthetase.*

**adenylate kinase** A widespread enzyme catalyzing the reaction: ATP + AMP ⇌ 2ADP. It enables AMP, formed in many biosynthetic reactions, to be converted into a form in which it can be phosphorylated to ATP. This enzyme is also important in the regulation of many enzymic processes through alterations in the concentrations of adenine nucleotides, especially AMP. Also *myokinase* (older term).

**adenyl cyclase** ADENYLATE CYCLASE.

**adenylosuccinate** 6-*N*-(1,2-Dicarboxyethyl)-adenosine 5′-phosphate. It is an intermediate in the biosynthesis of AMP, being formed from inosine 5′-phosphate, aspartic acid, and GTP in the reaction that introduces the 6-amino group.

**adenylyl** \ad′ənil′il\ The residue formed from AMP (adenylic acid) by removing a hydroxyl group from its phosphate group. Also *adenyl.*

**adephagia** \ad′əfā′jə\ [Gk *adēphagia* gluttony] *Obs.* BULIMIA.

**adeps** [L (gen. *adipis*), animal fat, grease] LARD. **a. anserinus** Goose grease. **a. benzoinatus** An ointment base prepared by heating lard with 1–3% benzoin. Also *benzoinated lard.* **a. lanae** ANHYDROUS LANOLIN. **a. lanae hydrosus** A preparation composed of seven parts anhydrous lanolin and three parts distilled water. **a. praeparatus** LARD.

**adequal** \adē′kwəl\ Almost equal.

**adermia** \ədur′mē·ə\ [Gk *a-* priv. + DERM- + -IA] A congenital absence of skin or a specified area of skin.

**adermine** PYRIDOXINE.

**adermogenesis** \ədur′məjen′əsis\ [Gk *a-* priv. + DERMO- + GENESIS] Imperfect development of the skin in fetuses or neonates.

**ADH** 1 antidiuretic hormone (vasopressin). 2 alcohol dehydrogenase.

**adherence** \adhir′əns\ [French *adhérence* (from Med L *adhaerentia* adherence, from AD- + L *haerens*, pres. part. of *haerere* to hold, stick) adherence] The fact or condition of sticking to something; the binding of one thing to another. **bacterial a.** 1 The attachment of bacteria either to specific antibody-forming cells or to particles coated with the antibody. 2 The adherence of bacteria to surfaces for which they carry receptors. The phenomenon is important in pathogenesis, determining the sites of colonization and persistence (e.g. buccal, respiratory, gastrointestinal epithelium), and also in the distribution of bacteria in nature. **graft a.** The fibrin seal that maintains apposition of a skin graft to the recipient bed for the first three days after grafting, until the skin graft begins to vascularize. **immune a.** Adherence of primate erythrocytes to antibody-coated and complement-coated particulate antigens or antigen-antibody-complement complexes. The receptor on the primate erythrocyte is the complement receptor CR1. This binds to C4b, C3b, and iC3b (less strongly) on the complement-coated material.

**adhesiectomy** \adhē′zē·ek′təmē\ [*adhesi(on)* + -ECTOMY] The surgical removal of adhesive tissues.

**adhesin** \adhē′zin, -sin\ A surface feature of a microbe that causes it to adhere to host cells or tissues. Most adhesins are organelles such as fimbriae or binding proteins such as lectins.

**adhesio** \adhē′zē·ō\ [L *adhaesio* an adhesive, adhesiveness] A band of tissue connecting two separated structures. **a. interthalamica** [NA] A bridge of tissue between the lateral walls of the third ventricle formed by the meeting of the thalami on the two sides during their growth and subsequent fusion. It has no known function and frequently is absent. Also *interthalamic adhesion, interthalamic commissure, conexus interthalamicus, massa intermedia, intermediate mass, massa mollis* (obs.), *middle commissure of cerebrum* (obs.).

**adhesion** \adhē′zhən\ [L *adhaesio* (from AD- + L *haesus*, past part. of *haerere* to hold, stick) an adhesive, adhesiveness] 1 The act or state of sticking together or becoming joined, as adjacent structures. 2 The abnormal union of adjoining surfaces, as may occur in association with an inflammatory process. Also *syncretio* (obs.). 3 One of the fibrous bands uniting adjoining surfaces in association with an inflammatory process. 4 The attraction between molecules of different substances in contact. **amniotic a.'s** Abnormal junction of the amnion with itself or with other structures, including the fetus. **anomalous mesenteric a.'s** The abnormal disposition and fusion of the dorsal mesentery of the embryonic midgut to the abdominal wall or to organs, due to malrotation of the intestines during development. The mesentery that forms the greater omentum is often involved in such adhesions. **fibrinous a.** The abnormal attachment of serous surfaces to one another by intervening fibrous tissue. **interthalamic a.** ADHESIO INTERTHALAMICA. **preputial a.** Abnormal union between the glans penis and the inner surface of the prepuce. **primary a.** 1 A fibrous band abnormally attaching two surfaces, resulting from natural causes rather than from previous surgical trauma. 2 HEALING BY FIRST INTENTION. **secondary a.** 1 A fibrous band abnormally connecting two surfaces as a consequence of previous surgical trauma. 2 HEALING BY SECOND INTENTION. **serologic a.** Adherence of a nonspecific particulate substance to a specific particulate antigen in the presence of antibody and complement. **traumatic uterine a.'s** ASHERMAN SYNDROME.

**adhesiotomy** \adhē′zē·ät′əmē\ [*adhesio(n)* + -TOMY] The surgical division of adhesions. Also *colliotomy.*

**adhesive** \adhē′siv\ [French *adhésive* (fem. of *adhésif* adhesive; from AD- + L *haesus*, past part. of *haerere* to hold, stick) adhesive] 1 Tending to stick fast to a surface or substance. 2 An adhesive substance; a substance used to bind together two surfaces. **cyanoacrylate a.** Any of the liquid glues derived from the methacrylate group of chemicals, which adhere tenaciously to tissues and organs, wet or dry, and harden rapidly creating a bond of great strength. In surgery, it has been applied on the cut and bleeding surfaces of such organs as the liver, spleen, and kidney to produce hemostasis, or to glue such cuts together. It has also been used as a dressing on full-thickness burns, and to repair nerves, blood vessels, and other tissues. It is also used in dentistry in cases where attachment to oral soft and hard tissues is required. **denture a.** A paste or powder which, when placed on the fitting surface of a denture, improves the adhesion of the denture to the edentulous ridge and palate. It is used chiefly with full upper dentures. Also *denture fixative.* **tissue a.** Any substance that is suitable for gluing together living tissues, such as a cyanoacrylic adhesive.

**adhib.** *adhibendus* (L, to be administered).

**adiactinic** \ədī′əktin′ik\ Resistant to the passage of ultraviolet light.

**adiadochokinesia** \ədī′ədō′kəkīnē′zhə\ [Gk *a-* priv. + *diadocho(s)* in succession + KINESIA] Inability to carry out or clumsiness in performing rapid alternating movements, such as repetitive pronation and supination of both forearms with the hands outstretched. This is a sign of cerebellar dysfunction. Also *adiadochokinesis, adiadokokinesia, adiadokokinesis.*

**adiaspiromycosis** \ədī′əspī′rəmīkō′sis\ A pulmonary disease of humans and animals caused by inhalation of spores of several species of the genus *Chrysosporium.* Also *haplomycosis, adiaspirosis.*

**adiathermance** \ədī′əthur′məns\ [Gk *a-* priv. + *dia* through + *therman(sis)* a heating, from *thermainein* to heat, from *thermos* hot] The characteristic of being impervious to heat radiation. Also *adiathermancy.*

**adicillin** CEPHALOSPORIN N.

**Adie** [William John *Adie,* English neurologist, 1886–1935] Adie's pupil, Weill-Reys-Adie syndrome, Holmes-Adie syndrome, Kehrer-Adie syndrome. See under ADIE SYNDROME.

**adietetic** \ədī′ətet′ik\ [Gk *a-* priv. + DIETETIC] Having no nutritive value.

**adipectomy** \ad′əpek′təmē\ [*adip(o)-* + -ECTOMY] LIPECTOMY.

**adiphenine hydrochloride** $C_{20}H_{26}ClNO_2$. α-Phenylbenzeneacetic acid 2-(diethylamino)ethyl ester, an anticholinergic agent that is used to treat spasms of the biliary tract, ureter, gastrointestinal tract, or uterus.

**adipic** \ədip′ik\ ADIPOSE.

**adipic acid** HOOC—$[CH_2]_4$—COOH. Hexanedioic acid. It was originally obtained by oxidation of fats.

**adipo-** \ad′əpō-\ [L *adeps,* gen. *adipis* fat] A combining form denoting fat.

**adipocele** \ad′əpōsēl′\ LIPOCELE.

**adipocellular** \-sel′yələr\ Consisting of fat and connective tissue.

**adipocere** \ad′əpōsir′\ [ADIPO- + L *cer(a)* wax] A gray-white substance with a cheesy or waxy consistency, formed by slow decomposition of the soft tissue of bodies that have been buried in moist environments or immersed in water. The substance consists principally of fatty acid salts formed from putrefactive hydrolysis of adipose tissues. The fatty acids infiltrate other tissues and inhibit putrefactive bacteria, thereby retarding complete decomposition.

**adipocyte** \ad′əpōsīt′\ [ADIPO- + -CYTE] FAT CELL.

**adipogenic** \-jen′ik\ LIPOGENIC.

**adipogenous** \ad′əpäj′ənəs\ LIPOGENIC.

**adipokinesis** \-kīnē′sis\ ADIPOKINETIC ACTION.

**adipolysis** \ad′ipäl′isis\ LIPOLYSIS.

**adipolytic** \-lit′ik\ LIPOLYTIC.

**adipoma** \ad′əpō′mə\ *Obs.* LIPOMA.

**adiponecrosis** \-nekrō′sis\ FAT NECROSIS. **subcutaneous a. in infants** SUBCUTANEOUS FAT NECROSIS.

**adipopexis** \-pek′sis\ [ADIPO- + Gk *pēxis* (from *pēgnynai* to fix in) a fixing] The storage or fixation of fats. Also *adipopexia.*

**adiposalgia** \ad′əpäsal′jə\ *Seldom used* PANNICULALGIA.

**adipose** \ad′əpōs\ [*adip(o)-* + -OSE[1]] Of or relating to fat. Also *adipic.*

**adiposis** \ad′ipō′sis\ [*adip(o)-* + -OSIS] OBESITY. **a. cerebralis** CEREBRAL ADIPOSITY. **a. dolorosa** NEUROLIPOMATOSIS DOLOROSA. **a. orchica** FRÖHLICH SYNDROME. **a. tuberosa simplex** A disease marked by painful circumscribed subcutaneous lipomas. Also *Anders disease.*

**adipositas** \ad′ipäs′itas\ [New L, fatness] ADIPOSITY. **a. cerebralis** CEREBRAL ADIPOSITY. **a. cordis** FATTY HEART. **a. ex vacuo** FATTY ATROPHY.

**adipositis** \-sī′tis\ [*adipos(e)* + -ITIS] PANNICULITIS.

**adiposity** \ad′əpäs′itē\ [*adipos(e)* + -ITY] The state of excessive deposition of fat. Also *adipositas.* **cerebral a.** Morbid obesity caused by pathologic overeating owing to disease of the brain, especially of the appetite-controlling centers of the hypothalamus. Also *adiposis cerebralis, adipositas cerebralis.*

**adipsia** \ədip′sē·ə\ [Gk *a-* priv. + DIPSIA] **1** The absence of thirst. **2** An abstention from drinking. *Outmoded.* Also *adipsy, aposia.*

**aditus** \ad′ətəs\ [L (from AD- + L *itus,* past part. of *ire* to go), approach, entry] An opening or inlet into a cavity, part, or organ. **a. ad antrum** [NA] A large irregular opening extending posteriorly from the epitympanic recess into the upper part of the mastoid or tympanic antrum. On its medial wall is the prominence of the facial canal, above which is the prominence of the lateral semicircular canal. **a. glottidis superior** The narrow part of the vestibulum laryngis just above the rima vestibuli. *Outmoded.* Also *superior entrance to glottis.* **a. laryngis** [NA] The aperture through which the pharynx communicates with the laryngeal cavity, bounded anteriorly by the upper edge of the epiglottis, laterally by the free edges of the aryepiglottic folds, and posteriorly by the mucous membrane between the two arytenoid cartilages. Also *aperture of larynx, aditus of larynx.* **a. orbitae** [NA] The roughly quadrangular base of the pyramidal shaped orbital cavity that opens on the face on each side of the nose. It is bounded above and below by the supraorbital margin and infraorbital margin, respectively; laterally by the frontal process of the zygomatic bone, and medially by the frontal bone and frontal process of the maxilla. Also *orbital aperture, orbital opening, anterior opening of orbital cavity.* **a. pelvis** *Outmoded* APERTURA PELVIS SUPERIOR.

**adjunction** The use of a combination of remedies in treatment.

**adjust** To subject to or undergo adjustment.

**adjuster** / **Negus ligature a.** An instrument resembling a long-handled, blunt, two-pronged fork, designed for use in tonsillectomy. It is used to facilitate tying ligatures around bleeding points in the tonsil bed.

**adjustment** [French *ajustement* (from AD- + L *just(us)* just, regular + *-mentum* -MENT) a making right] **1** Those changes or variations in behavior actively made by an organism to meet either physical or social demands imposed by environmental circumstances. **2** Modification of a completed denture. **3** In orthopedics, a rearrangement of apparatus, splint parts, or orthotic materials. **4** STANDARDIZATION. **coarse a.** A preliminary focusing control on either a light or electron microscope. **fine a.** A precision focusing control on either a light or electron microscope. **occlusal a.** Modification of the biting surfaces of the teeth by grinding. Also *occlusal contouring.*

**adjuvant** \ad′joovənt\ [L *adjuvans* (gen. *adjuvantis;* pres. part. of *adjuvare* to aid), aiding] **1** Assisting; auxiliary, as *adjuvant therapy.* **2** Any substance which, when mixed with an antigen, increases the immune response to that antigen. Also *immunologic adjuvant, antigen adjuvant.* **a. 65** A water-in-oil emulsion of antigen solution in peanut oil, stabilized with aluminum monostearate and Arlacel A. This adjuvant is recognized as safe for use in man because peanut oil is biologically degradable. **antigen a.** ADJUVANT. **centrally acting a.** A substance which elicits an immune response independently of time or site of antigen injection. It is thought to directly stimulate cells of the immune system. **depot-forming a.** A substance which adsorbs antigen and holds it at one site, or depot, after injection. It is thought to enhance antigenicity by slow release of antigen over a long period of time and by enhanced macrophage action at the depot site. **double emulsion a.** WATER-IN-OIL-IN-WATER EMULSION ADJUVANT. **Freund's a.** A water-in-oil emulsion administered with aqueous antigen to enhance the immune response to that antigen. The complete adjuvant contains, in addition to mineral oil, lanolin, and water, killed mycobacteria which provide immunopotentiating capacity well above that of the emulsion without organisms. **Freund's complete a.** A water-in-oil emulsion that contains killed mycobacteria, administered along with an antigen to enhance immunogenicity of the antigen. The mechanism of action is not clear, but it appears to potentiate macrophage activity and may slow the disappearance of soluble antigen from immunologically active tissue sites. Also *mycobacterial adjuvant.* **Freund's incomplete a.** A water-in-oil emulsion that lacks the mycobacteria present in Freund's complete adjuvant but nonetheless has moderate capacity to potentiate immunogenicity when administered with a soluble antigen. **immunologic a.** ADJUVANT. **multiple emulsion a.** WATER-IN-OIL-IN-WATER EMULSION ADJUVANT. **mycobacterial a.** FREUND'S COMPLETE ADJUVANT. **oil emulsion a.** WATER-IN-OIL EMULSION ADJUVANT. **pertussis a.** A mixture in which antigen is injected mixed with a saline suspension of killed *Bordetella pertussis.* **solubilized water-in-oil a.** A low-viscosity, water-in-oil adjuvant in which the antigen is contained in an aqueous phase of small volume compared with the oil phase and is dissolved in a mixture of emulsifiers. **water-in-oil emulsion a.** An adjuvant in which the antigen, dissolved or suspended in water, is dispersed as tiny droplets in a continuous phase of mineral oil in the presence of a stabilizer such as Arlacel. **water-in-oil-in-water emulsion a.** A water-in-oil emulsion adjuvant which has been redispersed in a continuous saline phase and the addition of emulsifier in order to form a free-flowing liquid. It forms three phases, namely a continuous saline phase, the primary disperse phase of oil, and a second disperse phase of antigen. Also *double emulsion adjuvant, multiple emulsion adjuvant.*

**adjuvanticity** \aj'əvantis'itē\ The ability to enhance immunogenicity.

**Adler** [Alfred *Adler,* Austrian psychiatrist, 1870–1937] Adlerian psychoanalysis, Adler's theory. See under ADLERIAN PSYCHOLOGY.

**ad lib.** *ad libitum* (L, as desired, freely).

**admaxillary** \admak'siler'ē\ Adjacent to the maxilla.

**admedian** \admē'dē·ən\ Situated near or toward the median plane of the body. Also *admedial.*

**adminiculum** \ad'minik'yələm\ [L (from *ad-* AD- + *min(ae)* pinnacle of a wall + *i* + *-culus,* diminishing suffix), a support, prop] (*pl.* adminicula) A supporting or strengthening structure. Also *adminicle, auxiliary.* **a. lineae albae** [NA] The deeper fibers of the lower end of the linea alba, which form a triangular sheet and are attached to the posterior aspect of the crest of the pubis behind the rectus abdominis muscles. Also *stay of white line* (outmoded).

**admission** The formal acceptance of a patient by an inpatient health care facility which intends to provide room, board, and nursing or other health care, as needed, usually for at least one night's stay. **voluntary a.** Admission to an inpatient facility with the free consent of the patient, who is considered capable of making such a decision. Compare COMMITMENT.

**admixture** MIXTURE.

**admortal** \admôr'tl\ [AD- + MORTAL] Moving toward damaged tissue: said of an electric current. Compare ABMORTAL.

**admov.** **1** *admove* (L, apply). **2** *admoveatur* (L, let there be applied).

**adnasal** \adnā'səl\ Adjacent to the nose.

**adnate** \ad'nāt\ [L *adnat(us),* past part. of *adnasci,* alteration of *agnasci* to be engendered or born to] Congenitally joined or attached: usually said of unlike parts.

**ad nauseam** [L *ad* to + *nauseam,* accus. of NAUSEA] To the extent of producing nausea.

**adnexa** \adnek'sə\ [L (substantive from neut. pl. of *adnexus,* past part. of *adnectere* to bind to), things bound to] Appendages or accessory parts adjoining an organ or structure. **fetal a.** The structures adjoining the fetus; the fetal membranes, including the amnion, chorion, and allantois. Also *appendages of the fetus.* **a. mastoidea** [NA] The accessory structures of the middle ear, including the paries mastoideus, membrana tympani, ossicula auditus, and tunica mucosa cavitatis tympani. **a. uteri** *Outmoded* UTERINE APPENDAGES.

**adnexal** \adnek'səl\ Pertaining to adnexa, especially those of the uterus (uterine appendages).

**adnexectomy** \ad'neksek'təmē\ The surgical removal of adnexa. Also *annexectomy.*

**adnexitis** \ad'neksī'tis\ Inflammation of adnexa.

**Ado** Symbol for adenosine.

**adolescence** \ad'əles'əns\ [L *adulescentia* (from *adulescens* a youth) youth. See ADOLESCENT.] The time of life between childhood and adulthood, during which the bodily changes of puberty take place and reproductive capacity in both sexes is achieved and emotional maturity gradually becomes adequate for child-rearing, at about age 10 to 18 years in girls and 13 to 19 years in boys. Onset is influenced by genetic, climatic, and nutritional factors. **delayed a.** DELAYED PUBERTY.

**adolescent** \ad'əles'ənt\ [L *adolescens* (also *adulescens*), gen. *adolescentis,* pres. part. of *adolescere* to grow up (past part. *adultus*), from AD- + *al(ere)* to nourish, raise, bring up + *-escere,* inchoative verb suffix] **1** An individual going through adolescence. **2** Pertaining to or characteristic of adolescence or, in a disease or abnormality, tending to occur in adolescence, as *adolescent goiter.*

**adoption** [L *adoptio* (from *ad-* to, at + *optio* liberty to choose) adoption, a looking at] The nurturing or care of a child by an adult who is not the natural parent but who may be related, by assuming the role and the rights of the child's parent. The safeguards necessary for ensuring the best interests of the child under all circumstances are laid down by statute in many countries.

**adoral** \adôr'əl\ Adjacent to or directed toward the mouth.

**ADP** **1** adenosine diphosphate. **2** automatic data processing.

**ADPglucose** The glucoside formed between glucose and ADP by glucosylation of the terminal phospho group. It is formed in plants and microorganisms by transfer of an adenylyl group from ATP onto glucose 1-phosphate, with release of diphosphate. It is the donor of glucosyl groups for starch synthesis in plants, and thus plays a role similar to that of UDPglucose in glycogen synthesis in animals.

**ad pond. om.** *ad pondus omnium* (L, to the weight of the whole).

**ADP-ribosylation** \-rī'bōsilā'shən\ A reaction, catalyzed by the enzymatically active moiety of diphtheria toxin and several other toxins, that transfers ADP-ribose from NAD to a protein.

**adren-** \adrēn-\ ADRENO-.

**adrenal** \adrē'nəl\ **1** Pertaining to or produced by the adrenal gland. **2** Situated near or on the kidney. Also *suprarenal.*

**adrenalectomize** \adrē'nəlek'təmīz\ [ADRENAL + *-ectom(y)* + -IZE] To remove surgically one or both adrenal glands; in man and most mammals, to remove simulta-

neously the adrenal cortex and adrenal medulla, which are inseparable.
**adrenalectomy** \adrē′nəlek′təmē\ Surgical excision of one or both adrenal glands. Also *epinephrectomy, suprarenalectomy* (seldom used) .
**Adrenalin** A proprietary name for epinephrine.
**adrenaline** The British term for EPINEPHRINE.
**adrenalotropic** \adren′əlōtrō′pik\ ADRENOTROPIC.
**adrenergic** \ad′renur′jik\ [ADREN- + *erg(o)-* + -IC] **1** Denoting the autonomic sympathetic neurons activated by or secreting epinephrine or norepinephrine (adrenaline). **2** Denoting neural action, endogenous chemical agents, or drugs that simulate the action of sympathetic postganglionic nerves or their transmitters. Also *sympathicomimetic, sympathomimetic, sympatheticomimetic.*
**adreno-** \adrē′nō-\ [L *ad* to, near + *ren* kidney] A combining form denoting the adrenal gland.
**adrenoceptive** \-sep′tiv\ Referring to receptors usually on the surface of effector cells with which epinephrine unites to produce a response, or to which inhibitors of adrenergic chemicals bind to block the cell's response.
**adrenoceptor** \-sep′tər\ Any of the sites on cells of effector organs that react with epinephrine ($\beta$-adrenergic receptors) or norepinephrine ($\alpha$-adrenergic receptors) and to various related blocking or stimulating agents. Usually associated with effectors innervated by postganglionic fibers of the sympathetic nervous system. Also *adrenoreceptor.* Compare ADRENERGIC RECEPTOR.
**adrenochrome** A quinone formed by the oxidation of epinephrine. Oxidation of its *o*-quinol system to the quinone makes the ring electrophilic, so that it reacts with the amino group to form a second ring. Further oxidation to regenerate the *o*-quinone forms adrenochrome.
**adrenocortical** \-kôr′tikəl\ Pertaining to, arising from, or having the characteristics of the adrenal cortex.
**adrenocorticoid** \-kôr′təkoid\ A steroid hormone arising from the adrenal cortex. *Seldom used.*
**adrenocorticosteroid** \-kôr′təkōstir′oid\ CORTICOSTEROID.
**adrenocorticotrophic** \-kôr′təkōträf′ik\ ADRENOCORTICOTROPIC.
**adrenocorticotrophin** \-kôr′təkōträf′in\ ADRENOCORTICOTROPIC HORMONE.
**adrenocorticotropic** \-kôr′təkōträp′ik\ [ADRENO- + CORTICO- + -TROPIC[1]] Exerting specific or nonspecific effects upon the structure or function of the adrenal cortex, such as stimulation of the adrenal cortex. Also *adrenocorticotrophic, corticotropic, corticotrophic.*
**adrenocorticotropin** \-kôr′təkōträp′in\ ADRENOCORTICOTROPIC HORMONE.
**adrenodoxin** A nonheme iron protein that contains two iron atoms, bridged together by two $S^{2-}$ ions, and is held by four cysteinate residues of the protein. It reduces heme-thiolate proteins that are involved in hydroxylations by dioxygen, and is recycled by reduction by NADPH. It is therefore an essential component of many biologic hydroxylations, as of steroids in hormone biosynthesis.
**adrenogenital** \-jen′ətəl\ Pertaining to the adrenal glands and the genitalia.
**adrenoglomerulotropin** \-glōmer′yŭlōträp′in\ ANGIOTENSIN.
**adrenoleukodystrophy** \-loo′kədis′trəfē\ Progressive demyelination of cerebral white matter, associated with Addison's disease. It is an X-linked recessive disorder and a variant of Schilder's disease. Also *melanodermic leukodystrophy, cerebral leukodystrophy, Schilder-Addison complex.*
**adrenolytic** \ad′renəlit′ik\ [ADRENO- + LYTIC] **1** Blunting the activity of epinephrine or norepinephrine. **2** Inhibiting the action of adrenergic nerves.
**adrenomedullary** \-med′yəler′ē\ Pertaining to or having the characteristics of the adrenal medulla.
**adrenoreceptor** \-risep′tər\ ADRENOCEPTOR.
**adrenosympathetic** \-sim′pəthet′ik\ Referring to the physiologic effects of the secretions (epinephrine, norepinephrine) of the adrenal medulla which mimic those of transmitters identified with the sympathetic nervous system.
**adrenotrophic** \-träf′ik\ ADRENOTROPIC.
**adrenotrophin** \-träf′in\ ADRENOCORTICOTROPIC HORMONE.
**adrenotropic** \-träp′ik\ [ADRENO- + -TROPIC[1]] Having a specific predilection for and stimulatory action upon the adrenal gland, especially on the adrenal cortex (adrenocorticotropic). Also *adrenotrophic, adrenalotropic, suprarenotropic.*
**adrenotropin** \-träp′in\ ADRENOCORTICOTROPIC HORMONE.
**Adriamycin** A proprietary name for doxorubicin hydrochloride.
**Adrian** [Edgar Douglas *Adrian,* English biologist, 1889–1977] Adrian-Bronk law. See under ALL-OR-NONE LAW.
**Adson** [Alfred Washington *Adson,* U.S. surgeon, 1887–1951] **1** Adson syndrome. See under SCALENUS ANTERIOR SYNDROME. **2** See under TEST.
**adsorb** \adsôrb′\ [AD- + *-sorb* as in *absorb*] To bind to a surface, usually noncovalently.
**adsorbent** **1** Capable of adsorbing other substances. **2** An adsorbent agent.
**adsorption** \adsôrp′shən\ [AD- + *-sorption* as in ABSORPTION] The adherence of a gas, a liquid, or dissolved matter to the surface of a solid.
**adsorption-hemagglutination** The agglutination of red cells on which soluble antigens have been adsorbed.
**adsternal** \adstur′nəl\ Adjacent to or toward the sternum.
**adst. feb.** *adstante febre* (L, while fever is present).
**ADTe** anodal duration tetanus.
**adtorsion** \adtôr′shən\ [AD- + TORSION] Movement of both eyes medially and inward rotation of the upper poles of their vertical meridians.
**adult** [L *adultus,* past part. of *adolescere* to grow, grow up] **1** The sexually mature stage of the life cycle of an individual; the stage of the life cycle of an animal after reproductive capacity has been attained. **2** An individual that has achieved full growth or maturity.
**adulterant** A substance added to a pharmaceutical preparation or food substance, cheapening or diluting it.
**adulteration** [L *adulteratio* (from *adulterare* to corrupt, from AD- + *alter* other) corruption, adulteration] The addition of a cheap, impure, or unnecessary substance to cheapen or dilute a preparation below the standard expected or specified on the label.
**adv.** *adversum* (L, against).
**advance** To perform a surgical advancement on (e.g. a tendon insertion).
**advancement** **1** A surgical repositioning (as of a tendon insertion) to a more forward or distal position. **2** The operation of moving the insertion of an extraocular muscle forward upon the sclera. This mechanically rotates the eye in the direction of the advanced muscle and thus may be useful in the correction of strabismus. Compare RECESSION.
**capsular a.** The surgical movement of a part of the muscle sheath to a more anterior position upon the eye.
**maxillary a.** An operation wherein a retruded maxilla is completely separated from its bony attachments, moved for-

ward into normal position, and held in place by wiring it to various points on the facial skeleton and by wiring the teeth of the maxilla to those of the mandible. **tendon a.** Surgical detachment of a tendon and reattachment at a point further back from the detached end of the tendon, having the effect of shortening the tendon.

**advehent** \ad′vēhənt\ AFFERENT.

**adventitia** \ad′ventish′ə\ [New L *(tunica) adventitia* an adventitious or outer coat. See ADVENTITIOUS.] The outermost layer of organs or structures that are not covered by a serous coat, such as the outermost layer of the three layers of an artery. It is derived from adjacent areolar connective tissue.

**adventitial** \ad′ventish′əl\ Pertaining to an adventitia, or outer coat, of a vessel or organ.

**adventitious** \ad′ventish′əs\ [Med L *adventitius,* alter. of L *adventicius* (from *adventus,* past part. of *advenire* to come to, arrive) coming from without, foreign] **1** Arising from an external source; extrinsic. **2** Accidental; unplanned.

**adversive** \advur′siv\ [L *advers(us)* against, opposite to + -IVE] Characterized by turning, usually of the head and eyes, away from the side of a cerebral lesion as in the attacks resulting from an irritative process involving the eye field (area 8) of the frontal lobe of the brain.

**ad 2 vic.** *ad duas vices* (L, for two times; for two doses).

**advocate** \ad′vəkət\ **health a.** PATIENT ADVOCATE. **patient a.** An individual who represents the patient's interests in the use of health care services by facilitating access to and use of the system to the extent and in the manner needed. Duties can vary widely, ranging from follow-up with patients to translation and social service assistance. There is usually little or no formal training and preparation for the role of patient advocate, but the duties are learned through on-the-job instruction. Also *health advocate.*

**adynamia** \ad′ənā′mē·ə\ [Gk *a-* priv. + *dynam(o)-* + -IA] Extreme muscular weakness due to physical disease. **a. episodica hereditaria** *Imprecise* PERIODIC PARALYSIS II.

**ae-** \ē-\ For words beginning *ae-,* see also under E-.

**Aeby** [Christoph Theodor *Aeby,* Swiss anatomist, 1835–1885] **1** See under MUSCLE, PLANE. **2** Aeby's muscle. See under MUSCULUS DEPRESSOR LABII INFERIORIS.

***Aedes*** \ā·ē′dēz\ [New L, from Gk *aēdēs* unpleasant, from *a-* priv. + *ēdos* pleasure] A genus of culicine mosquitoes found in tropical and subtropical regions, characterized by black and white markings on body and legs. ***A. aegypti*** The tiger mosquito, with black and white markings, and a lyre-shaped pattern on the thorax. It breeds near houses, in small pools of water, as in cans and auto tires, and transmits yellow fever, dengue, filarial worms, and encephalitis-producing arboviruses. Historically, this is the mosquito responsible for epidemic outbreaks of yellow fever that were finally controlled in Cuba and the Panama Canal Zone by General William C. Gorgas. ***A. albopictus*** An important vector mosquito of dengue, yellow fever, and equine encephalomyelitis viruses in the Pacific basin. ***A. leucocelaenus*** An important treetop-breeding mosquito in tropical South America that transmits jungle yellow fever. ***A. polynesiensis*** The vector of Bancroft's filariasis and dengue in many islands of the Pacific basin. ***A. sollicitans*** An abundant salt-marsh pest mosquito of the Atlantic and Gulf coasts of North America. It is a vector of eastern equine encephalomyelitis. ***A. taeniorhynchus*** A common salt-marsh mosquito of the southeastern United States. It is a vector of dengue in Florida. ***A. togoi*** A species found in Japan and southeast Asia, where it is a vector of Malayan filariasis. ***A. triseriatus*** A species lacking white rings on the tarsal segments. It is an important vector of viruses of the California encephalitis complex, and breeds in tree holes in the upper midwestern United States east of the Rocky Mountains.

**aeg.** *aeger* or *aegra* (L, the patient).

**-aemia** \-ē′mē·ə\ *Brit.* -EMIA.

**aequorin** \ēkwôr′in\ A protein extracted from the jellyfish *Aequorea aequorea* which exhibits luminescence in the presence of calcium ions. When aequorin is injected into cells, the degree of luminescence indicates the amount of available calcium.

**aer-** \er-\ AERO-.

**aerated** \er′ātid\ Supplied with air, especially by bubbling air through a solution.

**aeration** \erā′shən\ [French *aération* (from AERO- + *-ation* -ATION) aeration] **1** The process of exposure to air. **2** The charging of a liquid with air or other gas, as the oxygenation of blood in the bronchial alveoli.

**aeremia** \erē′mē·ə\ [AER- + -EMIA] AIR EMBOLISM.

**aero-** \er′ō-\ [Gk *aēr* (genitive *aeros*) the lower air, the atmosphere] A combining form meaning (1) air; (2) gas. Also *aer-.*

**aeroallergen** \er′ō·al′ərjən\ An air-borne allergen; specifically, any of various allergenic chemicals found in wind-borne pollen, fungal spores, and certain algae.

***Aerobacter*** \er′ōbak′tər\ An obsolete genus that has been replaced by genera *Enterobacter* and *Klebsiella.* ***A. aerogenes*** *Outmoded* ENTEROBACTER AEROGENES.

**aerobe** \er′ōb\ [AERO- + Gk *bios* life, manner of living] An organism that can grow in the presence of air. Obligate aerobes require air, facultative aerobes can grow either with or without air. Also *aerophil.* Compare ANAEROBE. **obligate a.** An organism that depends on respiration to provide energy and hence can grow only aerobically.

**aerobic** \erō′bik\ [AERO- + Gk *b(ios)* life, manner of living + -IC] **1** Using or requiring oxygen: said of an organism. Also *aerophilic, aerophilous.* **2** Denoting an environment in which free oxygen is present.

**aerobiology** \er′ōbī·äl′əjē\ [AERO- + BIOLOGY] The study of microorganisms in the atmosphere. Intramural aerobiology is concerned with aerial hygiene, while extramural aerobiology is mostly concerned with plant pathology and allergies.

**aerobullosis** \er′ōbəlō′sis\ DECOMPRESSION SICKNESS.

**aerocele** \er′ōsēl\ [AERO- + -CELE[1]] A swelling caused by air trapped in the adventitial covering of an organ, usually the trachea (tracheocele) or larynx(laryngocele), but also found in the gastrointestinal tract. Also *pneumatocele, pneumocele.* **epidural a.** A collection of air in the epidural (extradural) space. It is an occasional sequel of head injury with skull fracture. **intracranial a.** A collection of air in the cranial cavity. It may be a sequel of penetrating head injury or of communication between the middle ear or the paranasal sinuses and the intracranial cavity.

***Aerococcus*** \er′ōkäk′əs\ A genus of Gram-positive microaerophilic cocci, intermediate in properties between streptococci and staphylococci, found primarily on vegetables.

**aerocolpos** \er′ōkäl′pəs\ [AERO- + Gk *kolpos* bosom, womb, fold] The presence of gas in the vagina, usually in the submucosa.

**aerocystography** \er′ōsistäg′rəfē\ PNEUMOCYSTOGRAPHY.

**aerocystoscope** \er′ōsis′təskōp\ [AERO- + CYSTOSCOPE] An instrument for examination of the interior of the urinary bladder after the bladder has been distended with air.

**aerodontalgia** \er′ōdäntal′jə\ [AER- + ODONTALGIA] Toothache associated with the reduction in atmospheric pressure in high-altitude flying. The difference in pressure exacerbates existing pulpitis, particularly in connection with caries and restorations. Also *barodontalgia, aero-odontalgia, aero-odontodynia, odontalgia barotrauma.*

**aerodontics** \er′ōdän′tiks\ A branch of dentistry concerned with the prevention and treatment of aerodontalgia. Also *aerodontia.*

**aeroembolism** \er′ō·em′bəlizm\ AIR EMBOLISM.

**aeroemphysema** \er′ō·em′fizē′mə\ DECOMPRESSION SICKNESS.

**aerogenesis** \er′ōjen′əsis\ Production of gas, as with certain bacteria.

**aerogenic** \er′ōjen′ik\ [AERO- + -GENIC] Gas-producing: said of certain bacteria, such as *Enterobacter aerogenes.* Also *aerogenous* (outmoded).

**aeromammography** \er′ōmanäg′rəfē\ [AERO- + MAMMOGRAPHY] Radiography of the breast after the injection of gas into the retromammary space.

**aeromedicine** \er′ōmed′əsin\ AVIATION MEDICINE.

**aeromonad** \er′ōmō′nad\ Any of a group of microorganisms that includes *Aeromonas* and *Plesiomonas.*

***Aeromonas*** \er′ōmō′nas\ A genus of Gram-negative rods (family Vibrionaceae) that resemble *Escherichia coli* or *Enterobacter* species metabolically but have a single polar flagellum. They excrete several toxins. They are found in natural waters and are often pathogens in marine and freshwater animals. They occasionally cause human disease.

**aero-odontalgia** \er′ō-ō′däntal′jə\ AERODONTALGIA.

**aero-odontodynia** \er′ō-ō′däntədin′ē·ə\ AERODONTALGIA.

**aeropathy** \eräp′əthē\ Any morbid condition induced by a pronounced change in atmospheric pressure such as decompression sickness or mountain sickness.

**aerophagia** \er′ōfā′jə\ [AERO- + -PHAGIA] The swallowing of air, most commonly done while eating and usually accompanied by belching. It can result in distention of the stomach. Also *aerophagy, pneumophagia, air swallowing, sialoaerophagy, sialoaerophagia.* Adj. aerophagic.

**aerophagy** \eräf′əjē\ AEROPHAGIA.

**aerophil** \er′ōfil\ AEROBE.

**aerophilic** \er′ōfil′ik\ AEROBIC.

**aerophilous** \eräf′ələs\ AEROBIC.

**aeroplethysmograph** \er′ōplethiz′məgraf\ BODY PLETHYSMOGRAPH.

**aerosinusitis** \er′ōsīnəsī′tis\ Sinus barotrauma affecting the occupants of aircraft during flight, particularly during descent, or soon after descent.

**aerosis** \erō′sis\ [AER- + -OSIS] The formation of gas in organs or tissues of the body.

**aerosol** \er′ōsôl\ [AERO- + *sol(ution)*] **1** A suspension in the air or other gaseous medium of minute solid and/or liquid particles having a negligible falling velocity. **2** A fine mist or spray released from a pressurized container. The size of the particles frequently exceeds the normal colloidal limits of 1 nm to 1 μm. Such mists or sprays may be used for household, industrial, or pharmaceutical purposes. **mainstream a.** An aerosol produced by passing a gas through the chamber of a nebulizer. **sidestream a.** An aerosol discharged from a nebulizer into a stream of gas passing to a patient.

**aerosolization** \er′ōsäl′īzā′shən\ The dispersion of a liquid in the form of a fine mist.

**aerotaxis** \er′ōtak′sis\ [AERO- + Gk *taxis* an arranging, order] The positive or negative effect of air or oxygen on living organisms as expressed by their movement toward or away from the source of the air or oxygen.

**aerotherapy** \er′ōther′əpē\ Any treatment of disease processes utilizing air, as, for example, the use of pressurized air to treat decubitus ulcers.

**aerotitis** \er′ōtī′tis\ [AER- + OTITIS] Otitic barotrauma caused by abrupt atmospheric pressure changes such as may affect the crew and passengers of aircraft during flight, particularly during descent. Also *aviation otitis, altitude dysbarism.*

**aerotolerant** \er′ōtäl′ərənt\ Able to grow in the presence of air but deriving energy by fermentation rather than by respiration.

**aerotropism** \erō′trəpizm\ The growth or movement of an organism toward an air supply, such as an air bubble in a bacterial culture chamber.

**Aesculapius** \es′kyəlā′pē·əs\ [L, from Gk *Asklēpios,* the god of medicine] See under STAFF.

**aesthesio-** \esthē′sē·ō-\ *Brit.* ESTHESIO-.

**aesthetic** \esthet′ik\ ESTHETIC.

**aestus** \es′təs\ [L, burning heat] An increase of heat to a region of the body, as a facial flush.

**aet** *aetas* (L, age).

**aetio-** \ē′tē·ō-\ *Brit.* ETIO-.

**aetiology** \ē′tē·äl′əjē\ *Brit.* ETIOLOGY.

**aetionymous** \ē′tē·än′əməs\ Of, pertaining to, or being the cause of a disease from which the name of the disease is derived, such as *varicella pneumonia.*

**af-** \af-, əf-\ AD-.

**AFB** acid-fast bacillus.

**afebrile** \əfeb′ril\ [Gk *a-* priv. + FEBRILE] Of or characterized by the absence of fever. Also *apyrexial, athermic, apyretic.*

**affect** \af′ekt\ [L *affect(us)* (past part. of *afficere* to affect, influence) condition of mind, emotion] The feeling tone accompaniment of an idea or reaction to a stimulus, including feelings, emotions, and mood. Affect is sometimes used to refer to external manifestations in addition to internal feelings.

**affective** \əfek′tiv\ Pertaining to emotion or affect.

**affectomotor** \əfek′tōmō′tər\ [AFFECT + *o* + MOTOR] Of or pertaining to an emotional and associated muscular activity.

**affenspalte** \af′ənspal′tə, äf′ənshpäl′tə\ [German *Affe* ape, monkey + *Spalte* a cleft, fissure] SULCUS LUNATUS.

**afferent** \af′ərənt\ [L *afferens,* gen. *afferentis,* pres. part. of *afferre* (from *ad-* to + *ferre* to carry, bring) to carry, bring to, deliver] Conveying inward or toward a center, as sensory nerve impulses, fluid such as blood or lymph, or information. Also *adhevent, esodic, eisodic, inferent.* Compare EFFERENT. ● As commonly used in neurophysiology, *afferent* and *sensory* are often used interchangeably, as in *sensory* (or *afferent*) *nerve.* However, since not all afferent activity is consciously perceived, some afferent activity is not sensory, i.e., it does not give rise to sensation, and the two words are not synonymous in all contexts. **Ib a.** GROUP IB FIBER. **flexor reflex a.'s** Fibers from a variety of sensory receptors in skin, muscle, joints, and viscera, that have small caliber axons (groups II and III) and elicit flexor reflexes when excited. **pressoreceptor a.** A sensory neuron, including its receptor terminal, that is sensitive specifically to changes in blood pressure. Such endings are located in the carotid sinus and in the walls of the aorta and other large vessels. **primary a.** **1** The very large axon leading from the primary ending of a muscle spindle. The axon makes monosynaptic connections with homonymous motoneurons, and contributes to the phasic and tonic components of the stretch reflex. Also *group Ia fiber, group Ia axon, Ia fiber.* **2** The primary afferent, together with its primary ending. **somatic a.** **1** Denoting nerve fibers that transmit impulses centralward from the skin, muscles, bones, and joints (i.e., somatic structures as distinguished from viscera). 2 A somatic afferent fiber. **special somatic a.** 1 Denoting sensory fibers from the special sensory organs (i.e., the eye, cochlea, and vestibular apparatus). 2 A special somatic afferent fiber. **special visceral a.** 1 Denoting sensory fibers from the visceral sensory organs (i.e., receptors of taste and olfaction). 2 A special visceral afferent fiber. **tendon organ a.** GROUP IB FIBER. **visceral a.** 1 Denoting sensory fibers leading from the internal organs. 2 A visceral afferent fiber.

**afferentation** \af'ərentā'shən\ The sum total of sensory inflow from a body part, e.g., a limb. *Seldom used.*

**affinity** \əfin'itē\ [L *affinitas* (from AF- + *finis* boundary) vicinity, relationship by marriage] 1 The tendency to combine or interact; attraction. 2 The property of a substance that makes it more readily combine with or take up some substances, as a stain or dye, than others. **genetic a.** 1 In sexual reproduction, the preferential attraction for genetically distinct gametes. 2 The nonrandom assortment of unlinked and nonsyntenic loci brought about by the preferential migration of nonhomologous chromosomes to the same pole of the mitotic apparatus. 3 The occurrence of disparate phenotypes due to the same genotype.

**affinous** \af'ənəs\ [L *affin(is)* neighboring, related by marriage + -OUS] Denoting a marriage, usually nonconsanguineous, between individuals already related through prior marriages of their relatives.

**afibrinogenemia** \afī'brinojenē'mē·ə\ The absence of plasma fibrinogen.

**aflatoxin** \af'lātäk'sin\ [*A(spergillus)* + *fla(vus)* + TOXIN] Any of a group of chemically related fungal metabolites produced by some strains of *Aspergillus flavus* and *Aspergillus parasiticus.* They are most commonly found in various nuts and grains. Aflatoxins have been implicated in the causation of liver cell carcinomas.

**AFP** $\alpha$-fetoprotein.

**afteraction** The response occurring after stimulus cessation.

**afterbirth** The placenta, umbilical cord, and membranes that are delivered from the mother following the birth of a fetus.

**afterbrain** METENCEPHALON.

**aftercare** Medical and social surveillance of a patient after treatment.

**aftercataract** \af'tərkat'ərakt\ The opacity remaining subsequent to incomplete removal of the crystalline lens of the eye.

**aftercontraction** \af'tərkəntrak'shən\ The continuing muscular contraction that persists after a brief, strong stimulus.

**aftercurrent** An electrical current that passes through muscle and nerve following the cessation of a constant current which was applied to the tissue. Also *after current.*

**afterdamp** [*after* + *damp* as in FIREDAMP] A poisonous mixture of gases found in mines after an explosion of methane or coal dust. It consists of primarily carbon monoxide, carbon dioxide, and nitrogen. Carbon monoxide is responsible for most deaths resulting from such an explosion.

**afterdischarge** In electromyography, the electrical activity of a muscle affected by myotonia, which may continue for some time after the cessation of voluntary activity. • In electroencephalography this term has been used incorrectly to refer to a polysynaptic reflex discharge.

**aftereffect** A response to a stimulus that follows a primary response, either immediately or after an interval, such as the visual image of a complementary color that is seen after the original stimulus has been removed.

**aftergilding** \af'tərgil'ding\ GOLD TONING.

**afterglow** An emission of light from a fluorescent substance after the exciting radiation has stopped.

**afterhearing** A persistence of sound sensation after the stimulus that produced it has ceased. Also *aftersound.*

**afterhyperpolarization** \af'tərhī'pərpō'lərīzā'shən\ [*after* + HYPER- + POLARIZATION] POSITIVE AFTERPOTENTIAL.

**afterimage** A visual sensation which occurs when observing a uniform background subsequent to visual stimulation. Because of continuing retinal photochemical activity, a positive, or negative, or complementary image of the previously observed detail will appear upon the neutral background. Also *accidental image, photogene, aftervision, incidental image.* **negative a.** A persisting visual sensation subsequent to visual stimulation in which the light and dark areas of the original visual impression are reversed. **positive a.** A persisting visual sensation subsequent to visual stimulation in which light and dark remain to the original visual impression. **Purkinje a.** The second positive visual aftersensation. The hue is complementary to that of the primary sensation.

**afterimpression** AFTERSENSATION.

**afterload** / **ventricular a.** The tension, force or stress in the ventricular wall after the onset of contraction. It is largely determined by impedance to ejection.

**aftermovement** An involuntary continuing muscular contraction following strong exertion against resistance: usually referring to abduction of the arm.

**afterpains** The uterine contractions, often painful, that occur after the birth of an infant.

**afterperception** \af'tərpərsep'shən\ The image that is perceived after a sensory stimulus has terminated.

**afterpotential** The electrical potential recorded from a nerve axon following the spike potential and consisting of a negative phase (negative afterpotential) followed by a positive phase (positive afterpotential). **negative a.** The prolonged depolarization phase of an action potential before the membrane potential returns through its resting level. **positive a.** 1 The small, prolonged late hyperpolarization phase of an action potential before the membrane potential returns to its resting level. Also *afterhyperpolarization.* 2 The early, rapid repolarization or falling phase of the spike potential that "undershoots" the resting potential. This phase is absent if the resting potential is high. Also *early hyperpolarization.*

**afterpressure** A sensation of pressure that persists briefly after removal of the pressure stimulus.

**aftersensation** The sensory impression that persists after the external stimulation giving rise to it has ceased, as the result of continuing activity in the peripheral sensory receptor. Also *afterimpression.*

**aftersound** AFTERHEARING.

**afterstain** COUNTERSTAIN.

**aftertaste** The perception of a gustatory, or taste, sensation following the removal of the substance that induced the initial taste sensation.

**aftertreatment** Treatment following a surgical operation or the acute phase of an illness.

**aftervision** AFTERIMAGE.

**Ag** 1 Symbol for the element, silver. 2 antigen.

**ag-** \ag-, əg-\ AD-.

**agalactia** \ā'gəlak'shə\ [Gk *agalakt(os)* (from *a-* priv. + *gala,* gen. *galaktos,* milk) without milk + -IA] Absence of breast milk during the lactational period. *Seldom used.*

**agametic** \ā'gəmet'ik\ Reproducing asexually or without production of gametes. Also *agamic.*

**agammaglobulinemia** \əgam′əgläb′yəlinē′mē·ə\ [Gk *a-* priv. + GAMMA GLOBULIN + -EMIA] HYPOGAMMAGLOBULINEMIA. **Bruton type a.** INFANTILE SEX-LINKED HYPOGAMMAGLOBULINEMIA. **lymphopenic a.** SEVERE COMBINED IMMUNODEFICIENCY. **Swiss type a.** SEVERE COMBINED IMMUNODEFICIENCY.

**agamocytogeny** \əgam′əsītäj′ənē\ [Gk *a-* priv. + GAMO- + CYTO- + -GEN + -Y] SCHIZOGONY.

***Agamofilaria*** \əgam′əfīler′ē·ə\ [New L (from Gk *agamo(s)* unmarried + FILARIA)] A taxonomically invalid name for immature filarial worms that cannot be assigned to a known genus or species. ***A. streptocerca*** *MANSONELLA STREPTOCERCA.*

**agamogenesis** \ag′əmōjen′əsis\ [Gk *a-* priv. + GAMO- + GENESIS] SCHIZOGONY.

**agamogenetic** \ag′əmōjənet′ik\ Characterized by or relating to asexual reproduction.

**agamogony** \ag′əmäg′ənē\ [Gk *a-* priv. + GAMO- + GON-[2] + -Y] SCHIZOGONY.

**agamont** \ag′əmänt\ [Gk *a-* priv. + GAM- + *-ont,* combining form from the stem of *ōn,* pres. part. of *einai* to be] SCHIZONT.

**agamous** \ag′əməs\ [Gk *agam(os)* unmarried + -OUS] Reproducing by fission, budding, or other asexual means.

**aganglionic** \əgang′glē·än′ik\ Lacking autonomic ganglion cells as, for example, in segments of intestine in congenital megacolon (Hirschsprung's disease).

**aganglionosis** \əgang′glē·ənō′sis\ The congenital absence of autonomic ganglia.

**agar** \ä′gär, ag′ər\ [Malay, a seaweed from which gelatin is made; *agar-agar* jelly, gelatin] **1** A hydrophylic mucilagenous carbohydrate complex that is derived from several species of red algae. It is used as a laxative, a component of media for growing microorganisms, and as an emulsion in food preparation and certain laboratory procedures. Also *agar-agar.* **2** A preparation for cultivating microorganisms in which various materials are added to agar. It is usually employed in plate or tube form. Also *agar culture medium.* See also CULTURE MEDIUM, BROTH, MEDIUM. **bacteriostasis a.** A culture medium used to grow stock cultures of test organisms and in tests for antibacterial activity. It contains peptone, beef extract, sodium chloride, and agar. **bismuth sulfite a.** A selective medium for isolating *Salmonella typhi* and *Salmonella paratyphi* from clinical or environmental specimens. The medium inhibits Gram-positive organisms, coliforms, and many *Shigella* species. *Salmonella* colonies appear black because the hydrogen sulfide evolved interacts with metallic salts in the medium. Also *Wilson-Blair culture medium.* **blood a.** A general-purpose nonselective medium incorporating mammalian, usually sheep, blood. It supports both pathogenic and nonpathogenic bacteria, but does not support pathogenic *Neisseria* or *Haemophilus.* It is especially useful for demonstrating the hemolytic properties of colony growth. **Bordet-Gengou a.** A solid medium containing potato infusion, peptone, glycerol, and fresh sheep blood. It is used for detection and isolation of *Bordetella pertussis.* Also *potato-blood agar.* **brain-heart infusion a.** An agar medium incorporating peptone, dextrose, and an infusion of calf brain and beef heart, used to cultivate fastidious pathogenic bacteria. It can be used as a selective medium to isolate pathogenic fungi when blood and antibiotics are added. Also *brain-heart infusion medium.* ***Brucella* a.** A medium containing a digest of casein and animal tissue, used to isolate *Brucella* from clinical specimens and as a basal medium. ***Campylobacter* selective a.** A selective medium used to isolate *Campylobacter* species from clinical specimens. It is a *Brucella* basal medium with 5% sheep erythrocytes and the antimicrobials vancomycin, trimethoprim, polymyxin B, amphotericin B, and cephalothin. **cetrimide a.** A selective agar medium containing the quaternary ammonium compound cetrimide. It is used to isolate and grow *Pseudomonas aeruginosa.* Also *Pseudomonas-selective agar.* **charcoal yeast extract a.** A selective medium used to isolate *Legionella* species, containing supplemental iron and cysteine, which meet the specific growth requirements of these organisms. **chocolate a.** A peptone culture medium made by adding hemoglobin solution and vitamins. It contains NAD (factor V) and hemin (factor X), necessary for growing various *Haemophilus* species and suitable for growing *Neisseria.* It was originally prepared by adding sheep blood to hot agar so that the lysis of red cells imparted the characteristic chocolate brown appearance of denatured hemoglobin. **clostrisel a.** A highly selective peptone and dextrose medium used to isolate *Clostridium* from clinical and environmental specimens containing mixed flora. A combination of neomycin and sodium azide inhibits the growth of Gram-positive organisms, facultative anaerobes (coliforms), and *Pseudomonas,* thus facilitating isolation of *Clostridium.* **Czapek-Dox a.** A medium containing prescribed sources and quantities of inorganic nitrogen and of carbon, used to isolate fungi and bacteria capable of metabolizing inorganic nitrogen. It is the standard medium on which fungi are grown for morphologic studies leading to taxonomic classification. Also *Czapek-Dox solution.* **deoxycholate-citrate a.** A selective medium that inhibits growth of most Gram-positive and coliform organisms and supports *Salmonella* and *Shigella.* Lactose-fermenting organisms produce red colonies, nonlactose fermenters have colorless colonies, and colonies of *Salmonella* species that produce hydrogen sulfide have a central black spot. Also *deoxycholate-citrate medium.* **dextrose a.** A nonselective growth medium containing peptone and dextrose, to which pH indicators are sometimes added to identify various microorganisms. **egg-yolk a.** A medium containing egg yolk, in which the hydrolysis of lecithin by excreted phospholipase causes turbidity around colonies, especially of *Clostridium perfringens.* **EMB a.** EOSIN-METHYLENE BLUE AGAR. **Endo a.** A selective and differential medium originally developed for isolation of typhoid bacillus. The peptone base medium contains lactose and basic fuchsin, and allows differentiation between lactose-fermenting and nonfermenting Gram-negative bacilli. The growth of Gram-positive organisms is inhibited. **eosin-methylene blue a.** A selective and differential medium that inhibits the growth of Gram-positive organisms and allows differentiation between lactose-fermenting and nonfermenting Gram-negative bacilli by the detection of acid as a fermentation product. The peptone base medium contains lactose and the color indicators eosin-Y and methylene blue. Also *Levine's eosin-methylene blue agar, eosin-methylthionine chloride culture medium, EMB agar, Levine's EMB agar.* **GC a.** An agar base containing starch, dextrose, and peptone. It is used in the production of media used to isolate pathogenic species of *Neisseria,* especially *N. gonorrheae.* **gelatin a.** An agar medium containing gelatin, used to detect the excretion of proteolytic enzymes by growing bacterial colonies. This test for gelatinolysis is one of the biochemical tests used to differentiate nonlactose fermenting Gram-negative bacilli. **heart infusion a.** HEART INFUSION BROTH. **Kligler iron a.** A differential medium prepared in slanted tubes and containing a peptone base, phenol red as a pH indicator, and lactose and glucose in a 10:1 ratio. Various Gram-negative bacilli produce characteristic patterns of color change that reflect different carbohydrate utilization patterns, and the presence of ferrous sulfate and sodium thiosulfate in the medium allows detection of hydrogen sulfide production. **Krumwiede triple sugar a.** A differential medium similar to triple sugar iron agar except that it lacks iron and hence does not detect hydrogen sulfide production. **Levine's EMB a.** EOSIN-METHYLENE BLUE AGAR. **Levine's eosin-methylene blue a.** EOSIN-METHYLENE BLUE AGAR. **Löffler serum a.** LÖFFLER'S BLOOD CULTURE MEDIUM. **Löwenstein-Jensen a.** A culture medium of eggs, potato starch, and glycerol that is designed to isolate and grow *Mycobacterium* species. Also *Löwenstein-Jensen medium.* **MacConkey a.** A differential and selective medium used to isolate and characterize Gram-negative bacilli. The peptone base medium contains bile salts and crystal violet, which inhibit the growth of Gram-positive organisms, and lactose and a colored pH indicator, which allow differentiation of lactose-fermenting and nonfermenting organisms. **modified TM a.** A selective agar medium that is similar in purpose and composition to Thayer-Martin agar but with the antibiotic trimethoprim added. **Mueller-Hinton a.** A starch and beef-infusion medium developed originally for the isolation and growth of pathogenic *Neisseria* species, and now widely used as the standard medium for performance of antimicrobial susceptibility tests. ***Mycoplasma* a.** A culture medium containing horse serum, yeast extract, and glucose that supports the growth of *Mycoplasma* species and such antimicrobial agents as penicillin and thallium acetate to prevent overgrowth of unwanted bacteria. **neomycin assay a.** An assay medium to determine the neomycin content of pharmaceutical preparations, as specified by FDA and USP requirements. It contains beef extract, yeast extract, peptone, casein hydrolysate, and dextrose. **nystatin assay a.** An assay medium used to determine the mycostatic activity of pharmaceutical preparations, as specified by FDA and USP requirements. It contains beef extract, yeast extract, peptone, and dextrose. **phenylalanine a.** A culture medium that detects the ability of Gram-negative bacilli to produce phenylpyruvic acid from phenylalanine. **polymyxin test a.'s** Culture media used to determine polymixin in accord with FDA and USP standards. They contain peptones and dextrose in base agar (antibiotic medium 9); and polysorbate 80 in seed agar (antibiotic culture medium 10). **potato-blood a.** BORDET-GENGOU AGAR. **potato dextrose a.** A culture medium composed of potatoes and dextrose that is used to cultivate and isolate fungi. ***Pseudomonas*-selective a.** CETRIMIDE AGAR. **Russell's double sugar a.** A culture medium, prepared in slanted tubes, that contains lactose, glucose, and a colored pH indicator. It is used to differentiate lactose-fermenting from nonfermenting Gram-negative bacilli. **Sabouraud a.** A culture medium of peptone and dextrose that is used to isolate and cultivate fungi. With added antibiotics it can be used to isolate yeasts or molds from specimens contaminated with bacteria. **saccharose-mannitol a.** A differential medium, prepared in slanted tubes, that contains mannitol, saccharose, and phenol red as a pH indicator. Gram-negative bacilli with different patterns of carbohydrate usage produce different patterns of color change, reflecting the presence or absence of acid as a fermentation product. ***Salmonella-Shigella* a.** A highly selective medium that inhibits the growth of Gram-positive and many Gram-negative organisms but supports the growth of *Salmonella* and *Shigella.* The peptone base medium contains lactose and neutral red to allow differentiation of lactose-fermenting from nonfermenting organisms. The presence of sodium thiosulfate and ferric citrate permit the demonstration of hydrogen sulfide production, but only in large amounts. **seed a.** A culture medium used in antibiotic assays as specified by FDA and USP standards. It contains peptone, casein hydrolysate, yeast extract, beef extract, and dextrose. **standard methods a.** A culture medium of yeast extract, digest of casein, and glucose that is used in plate counts for bacterial growth in food, dairy products, and other nonclinical materials. Also *standard plate count agar.* **streptomycin assay a. with yeast extract** A culture medium used for the assay of streptomycin as specified by FDA and USP requirements. It contains beef extract, yeast extract, and peptone. **sulfite a.** A culture medium of peptone and sulfite used for detection and growth of thermophilic sulfide-producing anaerobes in foods and dairy products. **tellurite a.** A selective and differential medium containing cystine and tellurite in a blood agar base that is used to isolate *Corynebacterium diphtheriae* from specimens with mixed bacterial flora. *C. diphtheriae* colonies are black in color on this medium. **tellurite glycine a.** An inhibitory medium used for the detection and isolation of coagulase-positive staphylococci from food, environmental sources, or human specimens. The growth of coagulase-negative cocci, coliform bacteria, and other bacteria is inhibited. **Thayer-Martin a.** A selective medium composed of a GC agar base, hemoglobin, and the antibiotics vancomycin, colistin, and nystatin. It is used to isolate pathogenic species of *Neisseria.* **triple sugar iron a.** A differential medium containing a colored pH indicator and lactose, sucrose, and glucose in a ratio of 10:10:1. It is prepared in slanted tubes and used to characterize the fermentation patterns of Gram-negative bacilli and to detect the production of hydrogen sulfide. It is used especially in differentiating *Salmonella* and *Shigella* from other enteric organisms. Also *TSI agar.* **urea a.** A differential medium that detects urea-splitting activity in Gram-negative bacilli by demonstrating the pH change that accompanies ammonia production when urea is enzymatically attacked. **zein a.** A medium containing corn protein that is used to demonstrate chlamydospore production by *Candida albicans.*

**agar-agar** \ag′ər-ag′ər\ AGAR.

**agaric** / **fly a.** A poisonous mushroom of the species *Amanita muscaria.* A watery decoction of the fruiting body was once used to attract and kill flies.

***Agaricus muscarius*** \əgar′ikəs muskar′ē·əs\ *Incorrect* *AMANITA MUSCARIA.*

**agarose** A polysaccharide present in agar and responsible for its gelling. It consists of residues of 3,6-anhydro-L-galactose (an ether oxygen links C-3 and C-6) and D-galactose. It is used as a medium for gel chromatography.

**agastric** \əgas′trik\ [A-[1] + GASTRIC] Having no stomach.

**AGC** automatic gain control.

**age** [Middle English, from Old French *aage,* ultimately from L *aetas* age, contraction of *aevitas* age, from *aevum* time, eternity, age, life] **1** The time elapsed since an individual's birth. The age of adults is customarily expressed in solar years at the last birthday. **2** The degree or stage of development of an individual with respect to a given characteristic, expressed as the average chronological age at which the measure of development normally occurs. Examples are physiological age, skeletal age, and emotional age. **anatomic a.** The age of an individual expressed in terms of the average chronologic age of normal individuals with the same degree of anatomic development. **Binet a.** *Outmoded* MENTAL AGE. **bone a.** SKELETAL AGE. **childbearing a.** The period in a woman's life occurring between the menarche and the menopause when childbearing is possible. In statistical usage the age span is conventionally taken to be from ages 15 to 44 years. Also *reproductive age*. **chronologic a.** Age as measured in time elapsed since birth. **coital a.** The age of an embryo or fetus estimated from the date of coitus. In the human subject, it is anything up to four days more than the fertilization age. **a. of consent** In legal medicine, the chronologic age of a minor at which he or she is considered legally able to assent to sexual intercourse or marriage. The age varies among different jurisdictions, but is usually from 14 to 18 years. **developmental a.** The age of a fetus based on the degree or extent of development of various fetal parts. **fertilization a.** The age of an embryo or fetus estimated from the date of fertilization of the egg. The average fertilization age of human fetuses at term is usually given as 266 days, about 14 days less than the average menstrual age at term. **fetal a.** The estimated age of a fetus calculated from the date of such events in human reproduction as the first day of the last menstrual period, the probable date of ovulation, coitus, or fertilization of the ovum from which the fetus arose. The fetal period of human development is usually considered to start at the beginning of the third month of pregnancy by which time the embryo, although by no means exhibiting its final external form, possesses the rudiments of most of the major organs and systems and already manifests obvious human features. **functional a.** The age of an individual expressed in terms of the average chronologic age of normal individuals with the same degree of emotional, mental, and physiologic development. **gestational a.** A duration of a pregnancy. In standard obstetric practice, gestational age is timed in weeks starting with the first day of the last menstrual period. **menstrual a.** The age of an embryo or fetus estimated from the date of the first day of the last menstrual period before conception. The average menstrual age of human fetuses at term is usually given as 280 days. Two thirds of all deliveries occur between menstrual ages of 269 and 291 days. **mental a.** A unit expressing a child's intellectual level by comparing it with the performance of the average child of any given age. One whose mental age exceeds his or her chronological age is judged to be advanced in mental development, while one whose mental age falls below is correspondingly retarded. Also *Binet age* (outmoded). **ovulational a.** The age of an embryo or fetus estimated from the date of ovulation. **physiologic a.** The age of an individual expressed in terms of the average chronologic age of normal individuals with the same degree of physiologic development. **reproductive a.** CHILDBEARING AGE. **skeletal a.** The stage of development of the skeleton of an individual in terms of the average chronologic age of normal individuals with the same degree of skeletal development. In the living this is determined for all practical purposes by radiologic evidence of the closure of the fontanelles in infants and small children, and by the extent of ossification of the cartilages of the wrist and hand in older children and adolescents. In adults the estimate depends mostly on the extent of synostoses of the cranial sutures. Skeletal age does not always correspond with dental or chronologic age, and the disparity may have diagnostic and prognostic value in certain growth disorders. Also *bone age*.

**-age** \-ij\ [French, from L *-aticum*, a suffix forming nouns from verbs or other nouns] A combining form meaning (1) a collection of; (2) a process, result, or degree of.

**agency** / **home health a.** An agency, either public or private, which provides health care services to clients in their homes, usually to help them maintain themselves outside of institutional care. See also HOME HEALTH CARE.

**agenesis** \əjen′əsis\ [Gk *a-* priv. + GENESIS] A failure of development of an organ or part in the absolute sense, implying absence of a primordial or rudimentary form. Compare APLASIA, DYSPLASIA, HYPOPLASIA. **anorectal a.** The failure of development of the terminal parts of the digestive tract, particularly the rectum and anus. The distal part of the sigmoidal colon also may be involved. It is thought to result from the aberrant development of the embryonic urorectal septum. **gonadal a.** A failure of the gonads of either sex, testes or ovaries, to develop. The resulting genitalia are of the female type regardless of the chromosomal sex. **nuclear a.** MÖBIUS SYNDROME. **ovarian a.** A rare condition in which there is a total absence of recognizable ovarian tissue in individuals with feminine phenotype. Most patients so diagnosed, as in the Turner syndrome, actually have hypoplastic or streak ovaries attached to the broad ligament. The latter ovaries are typically small and are lacking in germinal tissue. **renal a.** Failure of one or both kidneys to develop or to develop grossly recognizable metanephric structure. **sacral a.** Congenital absence of the caudal spine below the fifth lumbar vertebra. Varying syndromes result, according to whether the first sacral arch is preserved, with normal separation of the iliac bones, or whether the whole sacrum is missing, the iliac bones therefore being in apposition. Involvement of sacral nerve roots may cause muscular atrophy of the legs, fecal and urinary incontinence, and dislocation of the hips.

**agenitalism** \əjen′ətəlizm\ The absence of genitalia, a rare condition except in a sirenomelus and in certain parasitic twins in which the lower half of the body is absent or aplastic. ● The term is sometimes applied to hypoplastic or infantile genitalia resulting from inadequate sex hormonal stimulation, but this usage is discouraged.

**agent** [L *agens* (gen. *agentis*; pres. part. of *agere* to do, act) doing, acting] Anything having the power to effect a change, as a substance or principle, whether chemical, biological, or physical. **activating a.** **1** One of two factors present in adult tissues which, when both factors are administered to an embryo, interact with the embryonic tissue at the site of exposure to induce localized development. When administered alone, this agent induces only archencephalic development, whereas the other agent induces only mesodermal development. Also *dorsalizing agent, neuralizing agent*. **2** Physical or chemical factors or conditions which induce unfertilized eggs to initiate parthenogenetic development. **adrenergic blocking a.** Any drug that blocks transmission at adrenergic nerve endings. Such agents are of two types, alpha-blockers and beta-blockers, depending upon whether synaptic function at alpha or beta endings is selectively blocked. **alkylating a.** A reagent capable of transferring an alkyl group onto a nucleophile. Alkylating agents contain an alkyl group on a leaving group, such as iodomethane ($CH_3$-I), triethyloxonium ($Et_3O^+$). They react with nucleic acids, and often have mutagenic and carcinogenic properties. *S*-adenosylmethionine is an important metabolic alkylating agent. Many, especially nitrogen mustards, are used in antitumor chemotherapy. **antibacterial a.** Any compound that prevents bacterial growth. Usually antibiotic or synthetic inhibitors of specific species, rather than disinfectants, are considered antibacterial agents. **antifoaming a.** Any substance that reduces foam formation, usually by lowering surface tension. It is added to laboratory materials that will be subjected to heat, or to pulmonary inhalants in order to reduce symptoms of pulmonary edema. **blocking a.** A chemical or drug which prevents the response of an effector organ to a stimulus by any of several means. It may occlude the receptors for the stimulatory chemical; interfere with the storage, synthesis, or liberation of the transmitter; or inactivate the transmitter enzymes. **caudalizing a.** One of two factors present in adult tissues which, when both factors are administered to an embryo, interact with the embryonic tissue at the site of exposure to induce localized development. When administered alone, this agent induces only mesodermal development, whereas the other agent induces only archencephalic development. Also *mesodermalizing agent.* **chelating a.** A substance that binds metal ions by chelation, i.e. by more than one group. The chelating agent often has great affinity for the metal ion, because bond formation after the first bond is formed involves little loss of translation entropy. Thus penicillamine and triethylenetetramine are chelating agents for cupric ions and are used as such in the treatment of Wilson's disease. Also *sequestering agent.* **chemotherapeutic a.** A chemical of natural or synthetic origin that can selectively inhibit or kill a parasitic microbe at drug concentrations tolerated by the host. **chimpanzee coryza a.** *Outmoded* RESPIRATORY SYNCYTIAL VIRUS. **clearing a.** A liquid used to remove a fixing or dehydrating agent from tissue in preparation for microscopy. Since many of these liquids have a similar refractive index to that of the tissue, the latter appears transparent. The essential feature of a clearing agent is that it should be miscible both with the dehydrating agent used and with the embedding medium. Xylene is the most widely used clearing agent. Also *clearer.* **delta a.** A viruslike particle consisting of an antigenic protein constituent and an RNA genome contained within a particle coated with hepatitis B surface antigen (HBsAg). It is transmissible person-to-person, but its replication in the host depends upon the presence of HBsAg. At first thought to be an immunologic marker in chronic hepatitis B, it was subsequently shown to be the cause of delta agent hepatitis. **desensitizing a.** A solution, gel, or varnish for topical application to sensitive areas of exposed dentin on the tooth surface. **disclosing a.** A solution, gel, or soluble tablet for topical application to the teeth to stain plaque and surface deposits. **dorsalizing a.** ACTIVATING AGENT. **Eaton a.** An organism of the species *Mycoplasma pneumoniae.* **embedding a.** Any of various substances within which tissues can be placed to make a structure sufficiently rigid to be cut with a knife and yet sufficiently plastic to allow deformation of the section as it is cut without fragmentation. The most satisfactory material for routine use is paraffin wax. **F a.** F FACTOR. **fixing a.** Any substance that preserves tissues in a form as close as possible to that which existed in life by preventing autolysis and bacterial decomposition and minimizing changes in shape and volume. It also facilitates subsequent staining of tissue sections. **ganglionic blocking a.** An agent which acts upon the ganglia of the autonomic nerves, retarding or preventing the passage of an impulse. See also BLOCKING AGENT. **inducing a.** EVOCATOR. **lissive a.** A medication that reduces spasticity without causing flaccidity. **luting a.** A nonadhesive substance used to hold dental inlays and crowns in place by virtue of its ability to fill microscopic irregularities of the adjacent surfaces. **mesodermalizing a.** CAUDALIZING AGENT. **mouse mammary tumor a.** MOUSE MAMMARY TUMOR VIRUS. **myoneural blocking a.** A drug that prevents the transmission of nervous impulses across the myoneural junction, causing the relaxation and paralysis of the muscles. These agents may be competitive with acetylcholine, such as curare; or depolarizing blocking agents, such as succinylcholine. **Norwalk a.** A 27-nm viruslike particle, originally found in the stools of patients in Norwalk, Ohio. It is an important cause of epidemic gastroenteritis in adults and older children. Also *Norwalk virus.* **oncotic a.** A colloid that contributes to an oncotic pressure effect. **oxidizing a.** A substance capable of acting as an oxidant in a chemical reaction. **progestational a.** Any substance that induces a secretory endometrium in mammals, i.e., which exerts the hormonal effects of progesterone, a normal secretory product of the corpus luteum, placenta, and adrenal cortex. Most synthetic antiovulatory agents (birth control drugs) exhibit progestational actions. **sequestering a.** CHELATING AGENT. **uncoupling a.** A compound capable of destroying the coupling between electron transport and ATP biosynthesis. Such compounds often act by making membranes, such as those of mitochondria or of bacteria, permeable to hydrogen ions. **virus-inactivating a.** An agent of any type which, when mixed with a virus, disrupts the virus morphologically or renders it incapable of infecting cells. **wetting a.** DETERGENT.

**Agent Orange** A mixture of 2,4-dichlorophenoxyacetic acid and 2,4,5-trichlorophenoxyacetic acid, used by the U.S. armed forces in Vietnam to defoliate enemy cover. Its principal health effect is due to the highly toxic contaminant, 2,3,7,8-tetrachlorodibenzo-*p*-dioxin.

**agerasia** \āʹjərāʹzhə\ A youthful appearance and behavior in old age.

**ageusia** \əgyooʹsē·ə\ [Gk *a-* priv. + *geus(is)* taste + -IA] Complete absence of the sense of taste. Also *ageustia, gustatory anesthesia.* **central a.** Ageusia due to a lesion of that part of the cerebral cortex (the uncinate gyrus) where taste sensation is recorded and appreciated. **conduction a.** Ageusia due to a lesion of the pathways conveying taste sensation from the peripheral receptors to the cerebral cortex. **peripheral a.** Ageusia due to a lesion of the taste receptors in the tongue.

**ageusic** \əgooʹsik\ **1** Pertaining to ageusia. **2** A person with ageusia.

**ageustia** \əgoosʹtē·ə\ AGEUSIA.

**ag. feb.** *aggrediente febre* (L, while the fever is coming on).

**agger** \agʹər, ajʹər\ [L, heap, mound, rampart] A prominence or projection. **a. nasi** [NA] A slight bony ridge curving anteroinferiorly from the upper end of the anterior margin of the middle concha and situated above the atrium of the middle meatus on the lateral wall of the nasal cavity. It is better developed in infants than in adults and is also prominent in lower mammals. Also *nasoturbinal concha, agger of the nose.* **a. valvae venae** A swelling of the wall of a vein at the site of a valve.

**aggeres** \ajʹərēz\ Plural of AGGER.

**agglutinant** \əglooʹtənənt\ AGGLUTININ.

**agglutinate** \əglooʹtənāt\ To aggregate or form into clumps, or cause to form into clumps, as *antibodies agglutinate antigen-coated cells.*

**agglutination** \əglooʹtināʹshən\ [L *agglutin(are)* (from *ad-* to, together + *glutinare* to glue, from *gluten* glue) to glue together + -ATION] The formation of clumps of cells or other particles, usually as a result of the formation of antibody bridges between cells that have the corresponding antigens on their surfaces. **cold a.** Agglutination of antigens occurring only at low temperatures. **group a.** Agglutination of all of a set of related bacterial species or corpuscles by an agglutinin specific for one member of that set. Also *cross agglutination, paragglutination, group reaction.* **H a.** The agglutination of bacteria by antibody to heat-labile flagellar antigens. **heterophil a.** Any agglutination test for the heterophil antibody characteristic of infectious mononucleosis. Also *heterophil antibody reaction.* **macroscopic a.** Agglutination in which the agglutinate can be seen with the naked eye. **microscopic a.** Agglutination in which the aggregating microorganisms can be seen only in the microscope. **O a.** Agglutination of bacteria by antibodies to the heat-stable O antigens. This property is widely used in the classification of *Salmonella.* **passive a.** Any procedure in which a soluble immune reactant is adsorbed to the surface of an inert particle so that agglutination will be the visible end point of the antigen-antibody reaction. Either antigen or antibody may be adsorbed. **spontaneous a.** Agglutination of various cell types (bacteria, tissue cells) in normal salt solutions, due to surface charge characteristics of the cells and the ionic constitution of the solution.

**agglutinin** \əgloo′tinin\ An adhesive material that holds parts together. Antibodies to particulate antigens can act as agglutinins. Also *agglutinating substance, agglutinant.* **anti-A a.** ANTI-A ANTIBODY. **anti-B a.** ANTI-B ANTIBODY. **anti-M a.** ANTI-M ANTIBODY. **anti-N a.** Antibody capable of clumping red cells bearing the N antigen. **anti-P a.** ANTI-P ANTIBODY. **anti-Rh a.** ANTI-RH ANTIBODY. **anti-S a.** ANTI-S ANTIBODY. **cold a.** An antibody that binds antigen sufficiently strongly to produce agglutination only at temperatures below 37°C. **cross a.** An agglutinin that is capable of agglutinating related microorganisms or cells by virtue of the presence of shared antigens in the cells. **flagellar a.** An antibody that agglutinates the flagella of some bacteria. **group a.** An antibody which may agglutinate different bacteria or cells by virtue of antigens common to all the cells within a given group. **H a.** An agglutinating antibody directed against the H antigen (flagellar antigen). **natural a.** An agglutinating antibody found normally in the blood of animal or man that occurs without intentional immunization to that antigen. **O a.** An antibody directed against the somatic antigens of Gram-negative bacteria. **plant a.** Agglutinin extracted from the seeds of various plants that reacts specifically with carbohydrate groups on cells and mimics the activity of antibodies, as for example with blood-group specificity. **platelet a.** Antibody capable of inducing clumping *in vitro* of platelets bearing the corresponding antigen. **saline a.** Antibody which induces clumping of red blood cells that are suspended in a medium containing a 0.85 gm/dl solution of sodium chloride in water. **serum a.** A substance in serum capable of specifically clumping red blood cells bearing the corresponding antigens. **somatic a.** An agglutinin specific for the somatic (as opposed to capsular) antigens of a microorganism. **T a.** T ANTIBODY. **warm a.** An antibody, usually IgG, that reacts best at 37°C in the agglutination reaction. It is usually applied to antierythrocyte autoantibodies that cause hemolytic anemias in patients who have not been subjected to low temperatures.

**agglutometer** \ag′lootäm′ətər\ An apparatus used to demonstrate without the aid of a microscope the agglutination of bacteria with dilutions of serum.

**aggregate** [See AGGREGATION.] **1** To form into a group or cluster. **2** A coherent assembly of different solid particles. **tubular a.** A collection of tubular structures, giving a honeycomb appearance in sections of skeletal muscle examined with the electron microscope. This is a nonspecific appearance seen in many types of metabolic myopathy.

**aggregation** \ag′rəgā′shən\ [L *aggregat(us)* (from AG- + L *grex,* gen. *gregis,* flock) gathered + *-io* -ION] A collection or mass of things; a close grouping of discrete objects or entities. **cell a.** The process by which suspensions of trypsin-dissociated embryonic cells form multicellular masses. Initial clustering is attributable to random collisions between cells, to active cell movements, and to contraction of protoplasmic filaments between cells. **platelet a.** The adherence of platelets to one another.

**aggregometer** \ag′rəgäm′ətər\ A photoelectric device to quantify and record platelet aggregation in platelet-rich plasma.

**aggressin** \əgres′in\ *Obs.* VIRULENCE FACTOR.

**aggression** \əgresh′ən\ [L *aggressio* (from *aggredi* to walk toward, accost, assault, from *ad-* toward + *-gradi* to walk) an attack] An attack on another; an attempt to injure another person. The hostility expressed is either caused by or is much increased by what is perceived to be frustration or opposition in the attainment of a goal. In psychoanalytic theory, aggression is one of the two basic drives or instincts. **displaced a.** An attack made on a substitute person instead of on the actual source of frustration either because the latter is considered too dangerous to be directly assaulted or because he is unavailable.

**aging** The process of growing old or older. **demographic a.** The aging of a population as recorded in statistical data and illustrated in tables and graphs. **placental a.** Histologic changes which occur in conjunction with an increase in placental size during the course of a pregnancy.

**agitation** \aj′itā′shən\ [L *agitatio* (from *agitatus,* past part. of *agitare,* to move to and fro, agitate, from *agere* to move, drive) a stirring, agitation] A marked increase in motor activity, generally associated with mental disturbance. There are many causes, including especially delirium and mania.

**agitophasia** \aj′ətōfā′zhə\ [L *agit(are)* to agitate, hurry + Gk *phasis* speech + -IA] Hasty speech, with involuntary omission of words or syllables. *Seldom used.* Also *agitolalia.*

**agit. vas.** *agitato vase* (L, the vial being shaken).

***Agkistrodon*** \agkis′trədän\ [New L (from Gk *ankistr(on)* fishhook + Ionic Gk *odōn* tooth)] A genus of venomous snakes of the family Viperidae, subfamily Crotilinae, inhabiting North America, Central America, Asia, Malaysia, and extreme southeastern Europe. The North American snakes include the copperheads or highland moccasins *A. contortrix* and the cottonmouths or water moccasins (*A. piscivorous*). Also *Ancistrodon.*

**aglandular** \əglan′dyələr\ Lacking glands.

**aglomerular** \ā′glōmer′ʸələr\ Lacking glomeruli.

**aglossia** \əgläs′ē·ə\ [Gk *a-* priv. + GLOSS- + -IA] The congenital absence of all or a major part of the tongue, a condition of exceptional rarity.

**aglycone** The alcohol with which a sugar is combined in a glycoside.

**agminated** \ag′minā′tid\ Clumped or massed together; aggregated.

**agmination** \agminā′shən\ The formation of groups or clusters.

**agnathia** \agnā′thē·ə\ [Gk *a-* priv. + GNATH- + -IA] The congenital absence of all or a major portion of the lower jaw. See also OTOCEPHALY.

**agnathous** \agnā′thəs\ Having or pertaining to agnathia.

**agnogenic** \ag′nōjen′ik\ Of unknown cause or origin.

**agnosia** \agnō′zhə\ [Gk *agnōsia* (from *a-* priv. + *gnōsis* knowledge) ignorance] Inability to recognize and interpret the meaning and significance of sensory information, whether visual, auditory, or tactile even though ability to perceive and record the primary sensory modality is intact. Adj. agnosic, agnostic. **acoustic a.** AUDITORY AGNOSIA.

**apraxic a.** APRACTOGNOSIA. **auditory a.** Inability to recognize the meaning and significance of sounds. Also *acousmatagnosia* (outmoded), *acoustic agnosia.* **body-image a.** AUTOTOPAGNOSIA. **chromatic a.** Disturbance of color vision in which the patient is able to see the colors but cannot differentiate between them, name them, or describe them. **developmental a.** A failure of either development or acquisition of those skills concerned with the recognition and interpretation of sensory information. It is one cause of the clumsy child syndrome. **digital a.** FINGER AGNOSIA. **a. for faces** PROSOPAGNOSIA. **finger a.** Inability to distinguish between the different fingers or to identify a specific finger in the patient or the examiner. This is one feature of the Gerstmann syndrome. Also *digital agnosia, finger aphasia.* **geometrical a.** Faulty spatial portrayal of objects and of topography, preventing the individual from copying geometrical patterns, maps, or diagrams. Also *geometric-optic agnosia.* **ideational a.** Inability to appreciate and interrelate ideas or concepts. **localization a.** Inability to localize accurately visual stimuli in space or tactile stimuli upon one's own body. **nonsymbolic visual a.** Visual agnosia not involving the recognition of printed or written symbols, such as letters or numbers. **position a.** A defect of the body image causing failure to recognize the position of parts of the body. This is similar to but not identical with autotopagnosia. **spatial a.** VISUOSPATIAL AGNOSIA. **spatial geometrical a.** GEOMETRICAL AGNOSIA. **symbolic visual a.** Inability to recognize and to understand the meaning of visual symbols, such as printed or written letters and numbers. **tactile a.** Inability to recognize objects or to assess their shape, size, and texture by touching or feeling them, although fine touch, tactile discrimination, and position and joint sense are unimpaired in the affected hand. Also *astereognosis, stereoagnosis, tactile asymbolia, anesthesognosia* (seldom used), *tactile amnesia, astereocognosy.* **time a.** Inability to recognize and appreciate time and temporal relationships. **topographical a.** Inability to find one's way, even in a familiar environment. **visual a.** Inability to recognize visually objects which are well known, although the primary visual pathways are intact. There are many forms of this condition, including inability to recognize the parts of the body on a diagram (autotopagnosia), spatial visual agnosia, visual agnosia for objects and shapes, visual agnosia for letter, word, or mathematical symbols (alexia or acalculia), and agnosia for colors, for pictures of objects, and for written music. Also *mind blindness* (obs.), *apperceptive blindness, psychic blindness, cortical psychic blindness.* **visuospatial a.** A form of visual agnosia characterized by the inability to comprehend the position of the body or of objects, in space, or the relative positions of different parts of the body or of different objects. This is often accompanied by inability to distinguish between right and left, as well as by loss of stereoscopic vision and of memory with regard to topography of the environment. Other common associations are constructional apraxia, agraphia, acalculia and visual inattention. Also *spatial agnosia.*

**agnosic** \agnō′sik\ Characteristic of, related to, or suffering from agnosia. Also *agnostic.*

**-agogue** \-əgäg\ [Gk *agōgos* (from *agein* to lead) inducing, leading] A combining form meaning leading, promoting, inducing or a substance that leads, induces, or promotes.

**agonadal** Characterized by or pertaining to a lack of gonads.

**agonal** Of or relating to the process of dying, especially to the events just prior to or at the time of death.

**agonist** \ag′ənist\ [Gk *agōnist(ēs)* (from *agōnizesthai* to contend) a combatant] **1** A muscle acting on its own or in combination with other muscles in such a way that its contraction causes movement. The contraction of an agonist is associated with relaxation of an antagonist and contraction of fixation muscle. Also *agonistic muscle.* **2** An agent capable of stimulating a biological response by occupying cell receptors.

**agonistic** \ag′ənis′tik\ Denoting or functioning as an agonist.

**agoraphobia** \ag′ərəfō′bē·ə\ [Gk *agora* the place of assembly, marketplace + -PHOBIA] Fear of public places where help might not be readily available or from which escape might be difficult. It may be accompanied by panic attacks and then extended to anticipatory fear of a recurrence of such attacks, leading to severe constriction of daily activities and avoidance of being alone. Also *agyiophobia, street phobia.*

**-agra** \-ag′rə\ [Gk *agra* seizure] A combining form meaning painful seizure, especially of acute onset.

**agrammaphasia** \əgram′əfā′zhə\ [Gk *a-* priv. + *gramm(a)* a thing drawn or written + APHASIA ] *Seldom used* SYNTACTICAL APHASIA.

**agrammatism** \əgram′ətizm\ [A-[1] + *grammat(ical)* + -ISM] A speech defect involving incorrect phrase construction, leading to infantile speech or a telegraphic style; an aphasic disorder which impairs syntax rather than vocabulary. It may take the form of paragrammatism or telegrammatism. Also *dysgrammatism, agrammatica, agrammatologia.*

**agranular** \āgran′yələr\ Without grains or granules: said of cytoplasm.

**agranulocytosis** \əgran′yooləsitō′sis\ Absence of granulocytes in the blood. Also *agranulosis, Schultz disease, Werner Schultz disease, Schultz syndrome, malignant neutropenia, malignant pernicious leukopenia.* **infantile genetic a.** CONGENITAL NEUTROPENIA. **infantile lethal a.** CONGENITAL NEUTROPENIA.

**agranulosis** \əgran′yəlō′sis\ AGRANULOCYTOSIS.

**agraphesthesia** \əgraf′esthē′zhə\ Inability to recognize letters or numbers written on the skin of a subject whose eyes are closed.

**agraphia** \əgraf′ē·ə\ [New L. from Gk *a-* priv. + *graph(ein)* to write + -IA] Inability to express oneself in writing; a form of apraxia for written letter or word symbols. Also *graphic motor aphasia, graphomotor aphasia.* Adj. agraphic. **absolute a.** LITERAL AGRAPHIA. **acoustic a.** Inability to write to dictation. *Seldom used.* **a. amnemonica** *Seldom used* JARGON AGRAPHIA. **a. atactica** LITERAL AGRAPHIA. **jargon a.** A type of dysgraphia marked by incoherent and unintelligible writing, although the affected individual is able to understand spoken or written speech and to speak normally. Also *jargonagraphia.* **literal a.** Total inability to write even single letters of the alphabet. Also *absolute agraphia, agraphia atactica.* **mental a.** Inability to express ideas or concepts in writing. **musical a.** Loss of ability to write musical notes. **sensory a.** Inability to write because of impaired understanding and recognition of language. **verbal a.** Agraphia characterized by the inability to write words, although the ability to write single letters is retained.

**agraphic** \əgraf′ik\ Related to, or resembling, agraphia.

**agravic** \əgrav′ik\ Denoting a lack of gravity (zero G), such as that produced in a spacecraft orbiting the earth.

**agremia** \əgrē′mē·ə\ *Older term* HYPERURICEMIA.

***Agrobacterium tumefaciens*** \ag′rəbaktir′rē·əm too′məfā′shē·əns\ A Gram-negative, aerobic rod of the Rhizobiaceae family, found in soil. It is not pathogenic to animals. Most strains can initiate tumors, or galls, in susceptible plants. This process is of considerable interest because it involves transfer of a plasmid, called Ti, from the bacterium to plant cells.

**agrypnia** \əgrip′nē·ə\ [Gk *agrypnia* sleeplessness] *Seldom used* INSOMNIA.

**agrypnotic** \ā′gripnät′ik\ Of or relating to wakefulness; sleepless.

**ague** \ā′gyoo\ [Med French, from Med L *acuta*, short for *febris acuta* an acute fever] **1** Malarial fever or other recurrent symptoms of malaria. **2** A chill. **3** Localized pain. *Older term.* **brass-founders' a.** METAL-FUME FEVER. **shaking a.** An acute febrile state with chills. **spelter-workers' a.** METAL-FUME FEVER. **welders' a.** METAL-FUME FEVER. **zinc-smelters' a.** METAL-FUME FEVER.

**agyiophobia** \aj′ī·ōfō′bē·ə\ AGORAPHOBIA.

**agyria** \əjī′rē·ə\ [Gk *a-* priv. + GYR- + -IA] The congenital absence or great reduction in the number of surface convolutions on the cerebral cortex. The total mass of cortical tissue is markedly reduced and as a result affected individuals are severely mentally retarded. Also *lissencephaly.*

**ah** Symbol for hyperopic astigmatism.

**AHA** **1** American Heart Association. **2** autoimmune hemolytic anemia.

**Ahlfeld** [Johann Friedrich *Ahlfeld*, German obstetrician, 1843–1929] See under SIGN.

**Ahumada** [Juan Carlos *Ahumada*, Argentinian physician, flourished 20th century] Ahumada-del Castillo syndrome. See under SYNDROME.

**AI** **1** aortic insufficiency (aortic regurgitation). **2** apical impulse (apex beat).

**AID** artificial insemination–donor (heterologous insemination).

**aid** [Old French *aïde*, *aiude* (from Late L *adjuta*, noun from L *adjutare*, variant of *adjuvare* to help, assist, relieve) help, assistance] **1** Help; assistance. **2** A device used to help or assist, especially one designed to compensate for a disability. **air conduction hearing a.** A hearing aid which conveys amplified sound to the external ear canal of the listener. **binaural hearing a.'s** Hearing aids, usually postaural, fitted one to each ear so that amplified sound may be conveyed to both ears simultaneously. **body-worn hearing a.** A hearing aid placed in a pocket or special harness, or attached to the clothing of the upper part of the body. The output is conveyed to the individual via a fine lead connected to a receiver connected to an ear mold. **bone conduction hearing a.** A hearing aid in which the output activates a vibratory electromechanical transducer held in position on the bone behind the ear. See also BONE CONDUCTION VIBRATOR. **CROS a.** A hearing aid designed to incorporate the contralateral routing of signals. **electric hearing a.** A hearing aid in which the amplification and other acoustic processing circuits are battery-powered. **first a.** The initial emergency treatment of injured or ill persons prior to the arrival of trained medical personnel. **hearing a.** An instrument which amplifies sound, especially speech, worn or used by the hearing-impaired. The majority are now electrical and may incorporate a number of other facilities, for example the gain may be limited above certain input levels or the frequency response may be altered to suit the individual's loss. Usually such aids are postaural in type and amplify air-conducted sound. They may, however, be located in the ear, or incorporated in a spectacle frame, but there are also body-worn aids and aids that work by bone conduction. **in-the-ear hearing a.** A hearing aid of such small size that the component parts are incorporated in the ear mold. **mechanical hearing a.** A hearing aid of the horn or speaking-tube variety which does not incorporate electric circuitry. **pharmaceutic a.** PHARMACEUTIC NECESSITY. **speech a.** Any device used to increase the volume or intelligibility of speech when it is impaired as a consequence of trauma or surgery to the larynx. It may be a hand-held or prosthetic aid. **ultrasonic mobility a.** An aid, usually a cane, that emits ultrasonic vibration to assist the blind in walking and other activities.

**aide** \ād\ [French (from *aider* to help, assist) assistance, an assistant] An assistant, as a paraprofessional helper. **nurse's a.** An individual who assists nurses in performing the routine tasks of patient care in an institutional setting such as a hospital. Also *nurse aide.*

**AIDS** acquired immune deficiency syndrome.

**AIH** artificial insemination–husband (homologous insemination).

**ailment** [Middle English *eilen* to ail, from Old English *eglan, eglian* to cause fear, from *egle* hurtful + -MENT] Any sickness or disorder, especially a minor one.

**AIM** acute intermittent porphyria.

**ainhum** \īnyooN′\ [Portuguese, from Yoruba *eyun*] A tropical disease characterized by the development of a fibrous band encircling digits of the foot. Continued constriction by the band leads to spontaneous amputation of the toes. This condition most often afflicts African men. Also *dactylolysis spontanea.*

**Ainu** \ī′noo\ An aboriginal people of northern Japan thought to represent the remnant of an early Caucasoid population and characterized by abundant wavy black hair, brown eyes, abundant body and facial hair, and thickset body form.

**air** [L *aer* (from Gk *aēr* the lower air, the atmosphere, akin to *aētēs* the wind) the air] The mixture of gases forming the terrestrial atmosphere, composed mainly of nitrogen (78% by volume, 76% by weight), oxygen (21% by volume, 23% by weight), and, in much smaller proportions, carbon dioxide, water vapor, ammonia, rare gases (helium, argon, krypton, neon, xenon, and radon), powders, and suspended organic particles. **alveolar a.** ALVEOLAR GAS. **ambient a.** The outdoor air breathed by the general public, in contrast to that in localized situations such as workshops, domestic rooms, or near specific appliances. **complemental a.** Air in the inspiratory reserve volume. *Obs.* **dead-space a.** The component of inspired air which takes no part in gaseous exchange with pulmonary blood. **functional residual a.** *Obs.* FUNCTIONAL RESIDUAL CAPACITY. **stationary a.** *Obs.* FUNCTIONAL RESIDUAL CAPACITY. **tidal a.** The air contained in the tidal volume. **vitiated a.** Air that has a less-than-normal amount of oxygen or has been contaminated.

**air-borne** Transported or carried by the air: commonly used in reference to pathogenic organisms and other disease-producing agents.

**airway** Part or all of the air-conducting system by which the air reaches the lungs from the external environment. **anatomical a.** ANATOMICAL DEAD SPACE. **artificial a.** A cylindrical device inserted into the nose, mouth, or trachea, through which spontaneous or artificial respiration may be attained or improved. **conducting a.** The tracheobronchial tree through which air must pass to reach the alveoli. **endotracheal a.** ENDOTRACHEAL TUBE. **esophageal a.** A cuffed tube, sealed distally and with proximal perforations which can be passed through the mouth into the esophagus. When the cuff is inflated air can be blown down the tube in an effort to ventilate the lungs.

This method of artificial ventilation has been advocated for use by paramedical personnel in emergency situations. **oropharyngeal a.** A device placed in the mouth and pharynx to correct respiratory obstruction caused by the tongue, usually during unconsciousness. **respiratory a.** 1 An anatomical air passage where gases are exchanged. 2 A tubular device used as a gas conduit in anesthesia or respiratory assistance. Also *air tube, breathing tube.*

***Ajellomyces*** \əjel′ōmī′sēz\ A genus of fungi, the ascomycetous, perfect (sexual reproductive) state of *Blastomyces dermatitidis.*

**akaryocyte** \ākar′ē·əsīt\ A cell without a nucleus, such as an erythrocyte. Also *akaryote, acaryote.*

**akatama** \ak′ətam′ə\ [A West African word] A form of chronic peripheral neuropathy endemic in West Africa, presumed to be of metabolic or toxic origin. It is characterized by sensations of burning, prickling, and numbness, erythema, and in some cases by excessive sweating.

**akatanoesis** \əkat′ənō′əsis\ [Gk *a-* priv. + *katanoēsis* observation, introspection, from *noēsis* thought, intelligence] Lack of ability to understand one's own utterances or thoughts.

**akathisia** \ak′əthē′zhə\ [Gk *a-* priv. + *kathis(is)* a sitting down + -IA] The inability to sit down or remain seated because of motor restlessness and a sensation of muscular quivering which occurs as a side effect of neuroleptic drugs, especially phenothiazine. It is also an uncommon manifestation of Parkinson's disease. Akathisia was originally described as a type of anxiety disorder in which the mere thought of sitting down provoked severe anxiety, panic, or hysterical convulsions. Also *cathisophobia.* Also *acathisia, akithisia.* **psychic a.** Akathisia associated with irrational terror at the idea of sitting down.

**akee** \akē′\ ACKEE.

**akembe** \əkem′bē\ ONYALAI.

**Akerlund** [Ake *Akerlund,* Swedish roentgenologist, 1885–1958] See under DIAPHRAGM.

**A/kg** Symbol for the unit, ampere per kilogram.

**A·kg$^{-1}$** Symbol for the unit, ampere per kilogram.

**akinesia** \āk′inē′zhə\ [Gk *a-* priv. + KINESIA] The inability to initiate movement. This is seen particularly in Parkinson's disease as, for instance, in inability to rise from a chair or to begin to walk, even though walking, once begun, can be continued. Also *akinesis, acinesia.* **a. algera** A condition in which pain, with no evident organic cause, is evoked by voluntary movement. **cerebral a.** Inability to initiate movement, as the result of a cerebral lesion. **spinal a.** Paralysis due to a spinal cord lesion. *Seldom used.*

**akinesic** \ak′inē′sik\ AKINETIC.

**akinesis** \ak′inē′sis\ AKINESIA.

**akinetic** \ā′kinet′ik\ 1 Related to akinesia. 2 Accompanied by lack of movement, as *akinetic mutism.* Also *akinesic, acinetic.*

**akithisia** \ak′ithē′zhə\ AKATHISIA.

**akiyami** \ā′kēyä′mē\ [Japanese *aki* autumn + *yami* epidemic] NANUKAYAMI.

**aklomide** $C_7H_5ClN_2O_3$. 2-Chloro-4-nitrobenzamide. An anticoccidiomycotic agent used in veterinary medicine.

**Al** Symbol for the element, aluminum.

**-al** \-əl, -al\ [L *-alis* suffix in adjectives formed from nouns, or in nouns formed from adjectives formerly used as nouns, or in nouns of action formed from verbs] 1 A suffix meaning (1) of or relating to, characterized by (in adjectives); (2) the act or process of (in nouns). 2 In chemistry, a suffix denoting an aldehyde.

**ALA** δ-aminolevulinic acid.

**Ala** Symbol for alanine.

**ala** \ā′lə\ [L (from earlier *axla,* akin to Old English *eaxl* shoulder) a wing, wing joint, shoulder joint, armpit. See also AXILLA.] (*pl.* alae) A wing or winglike structure. **a. alba medialis** *Obs.* AREA VESTIBULARIS. **a. auris** AURICULA. **a. cinerea** TRIGONUM NERVI VAGI. **a. cristae galli** [NA] The alar process that projects sideways on each side from the anterior border of the crista galli and articulates with the frontal bone, thereby completing the foramen cecum. Also *frontal hamulus.* **a. lobuli centralis cerebelli** [NA] The lateral hemispheric expansions continuous with the central lobule of the cerebellar vermis. Also *prolatio aliformis* (obs.). **a. major ossis sphenoidalis** [NA] The greater wing, or alisphenoid, that projects laterally and upward on each side of the body of the sphenoid bone in the base of the skull. Also *ala temporalis ossis sphenoidalis, alisphenoid bone, alisphenoid, greater wing of sphenoid bone, major wing of sphenoid bone, temporal wing of sphenoid bone.* **a. minor ossis sphenoidalis** [NA] The lesser wing, or orbitosphenoid, that projects sideways on each side from the superior and anterior parts of the body of the sphenoid bone. Also *alisphenoid bone, minor wing of sphenoid bone, apophysis of Ingrassia.* **alae nasi** [NA] The convex expansions of the lower posterior parts of the sides of the nose, the inferior margin of each bounding the related naris laterally. A sulcus separates the upper part of each expansion from the remaining part of the lateral surface of the nose. Also *wings of nose, flare of the nostrils.* **a. ossis ilii** [NA] The upper, flattened plate of the ilium, a portion of the innominate, or hip bone. Also *wing of ilium, blade of ilium.* **a. parva ossis sphenoidalis** ALA MINOR OSSIS SPHENOIDALIS. **a. pontis** PROPONS. **a. of sacrum** PARS LATERALIS OSSIS SACRI. **a. temporalis ossis sphenoidalis** ALA MAJOR OSSIS SPHENOIDALIS. **a. vomeris** [NA] A small horizontal projection on each side of a deep furrow at the anterior end of the superior border of the vomer. The furrow lodges the rostrum of the sphenoid bone. Also *ala of vomer, wing of vomer.*

**alactasia** \ā′laktā′zhə\ LACTASE DEFICIENCY.

**alae** \ā′lē\ Plural of ALA.

**Alajouanine** [Théophile *Alajouanine,* French neurologist, born 1890] Foix-Alajouanine syndrome, Foix-Alajouanine disease. See under SUBACUTE NECROTIC MYELITIS.

**alalia** \əlā′lyə\ [New L, from Gk *a-* priv. + *lalia* a talking, from *lalein* to speak, chatter] Inability to speak because of organic or functional disturbance. *Obs.* Adj. alalic. **developmental a.** Severe stammering or stuttering in childhood. **a. organica** Alalia attributable to an organic disease. *Obs.*

**alanine** $CH_3$—CH(—$NH_2$)—COOH. 2-Aminopropionic acid. It is one of the 20 amino acids normally found as components of proteins. It is not essential in the diet as it is easily made by transamination from pyruvate. It occupies a central position in amino-acid metabolism.

***β*-alanine** $NH_2$—$CH_2$—$CH_2$—COOH. 3-Aminopropionic acid. It occurs bound in several substances of importance, such as coenzyme A, and is an intermediate in a pathway for the catabolism of uracil.

**alanine aminotransferase** An enzyme (EC 2.6.1.2) that catalyzes the reaction: alanine + 2-oxoglutarate ⇌ glutamate + pyruvate. It contains pyridoxal phosphate and is important for the use and formation of alanine. Also *glutamate pyruvate transaminase.*

**alanine racemase** An enzyme (EC 5.1.1.1) that interconverts L-alanine and D-alanine. It occurs in bacteria, many of which require D-alanine for wall synthesis. In most species the enzyme contains pyridoxal phosphate, whose imine with the substrate can lose H-2 as a hydrogen ion to form a carbanion that is intermediate between L-alanine and D-alanine.

**alar** \ā′lär\ **1** Pertaining to or having an ala, or wing; winglike. **2** Pertaining to the axilla or the shoulder.

**alastrim** \əlas′trim\ [Portuguese (from *alastrar* to scatter, from *lastro* ballast), milk pox] A mild form of smallpox with a low mortality rate, caused by a virus less virulent than that which causes ordinary smallpox. Also *variola minor, amaas, bexia, milkpox, whitepox, glasspox, parasmallpox, pseudosmallpox, Kaffir pox, mild smallpox*. Adj. alastrimic, alastrinic.

**alastrimic** \al′əstrim′ik\ Having to do with alastrim. Also *alastrinic*.

**alate** \ā′lāt\ Possessing wings or winglike attachments; winged.

**alatus** \əlā′təs\ Having wings; winged.

**alba** \al′bə\ [L, fem. of *albus* white] White; used to describe pertinent morphologic tissues, such as substantia alba, the white matter of the brain and spinal cord.

**Albarrán** [Joaquín *Albarrán* y Domínguez, Cuban urologist, 1860–1912] Albarrán's glands. See under SUBCERVICAL GLANDS OF ALBARRÁN.

**albedo** \albē′dō\ [Late L (from L *albus* white), whiteness] The ability of a surface to reflect light. **a. retinae** The whitish reflections characteristic of retinal edema.

**Albee** [Fred Houdlett *Albee*, U.S. orthopedic surgeon, 1876–1945] **1** See under SAW, OPERATION. **2** Albee fracture table. See under TABLE.

**Albers-Schönberg** [Heinrich Ernst *Albers-Schönberg*, German roentgenologist, 1865–1921] Albers-Schönberg disease. See under OSTEOPETROSIS.

**Albert** [Eduard *Albert*, Austrian surgeon, 1841–1900] Albert's disease. See under ACHILLES BURSITIS.

**albicans** \al′bikənz\ [L, pres. part. of *albicare* (from *albus* white) to whiten, be white] White, whitish; used to describe pertinent morphologic tissues.

**albidus** \al′bidəs\ [L (from *albus* white), whitish] White; whitish.

**Albini** [Giuseppe *Albini*, Italian physiologist, 1830–1911] Albini's nodules. See under NODULE.

**albinism** \al′binizm\ [*albin(o)* + -ISM] A group of hereditary syndromes characterized by congenital hypopigmentation of the skin, hair, and eyes, caused by a lack of the enzymes responsible for the oxidation of tyrosine via dopa to dopaquinone in the pathway of melanin formation. It is usually transmitted as an autosomal recessive characteristic. Also *albinismus, albinoism, congenital leukopathia*. **acquired a.** VITILIGO. **cutaneous a.** Albinism in which the absence of pigment is confined to the skin, as distinguished from oculocutaneous albinism. **localized a.** The presence of achromic nevi on the skin. **oculocutaneous a.** A heterogenous group of hereditary disorders characterized by hypomelanosis of the skin, eyes, and hair. Also *total albinism*. **partial a.** PIEBALDISM. **piebald a.** PIEBALDISM. **rufous a.** XANTHISM. **total a.** OCULOCUTANEOUS ALBINISM.

**albinismus** \al′biniz′məs\ [German, albinism. See ALBINISM.] ALBINISM.

**albino** \albī′nō\ [Portuguese (from L *albus* white) an albino] An animal or plant affected with albinism, especially with respect to the type and/or distribution of pigment characteristic of its species.

**albinoidism** \albī′noidizm\ An inherited state of incomplete albinism.

**albinoism** \albī′nō·izm\ ALBINISM.

**Albinus** [Bernhard Siegfried *Albinus*, German anatomist and surgeon, 1697–1770] **1** Albinus muscle. See under MUSCULUS RISORIUS. **2** Albinus muscle. See under MUSCULUS SCALENUS MINIMUS. **3** See under MUSCLE.

**Albright** [Fuller *Albright*, U.S. physician, 1900–1969] **1** Albright syndrome, Albright-McCune-Sternberg syndrome, McCune-Albright syndrome. See under ALBRIGHT'S DISEASE. **2** Forbes-Albright syndrome. See under SYNDROME. **3** Albright's dystrophy, Albright syndrome. See under ALBRIGHT'S HEREDITARY OSTEODYSTROPHY.

**albuginea** \al′byoojin′ē·ə\ [New L, from *tunica albuginea* a white coat. See ALBUGINEOUS.] Denoting a white, opaque layer of fibrous tissue surrounding an organ or part, for example, the tunica albuginea of the testis, ovary, and cavernous bodies of the penis. **a. oculi** *Outmoded* SCLERA. **a. ovarii** *Outmoded* TUNICA ALBUGINEA OVARII. **a. testis** TUNICA ALBUGINEA TESTIS.

**albugineotomy** \al′bəjin′ē·ät′əmē\ [*(tunica) albugine(a)* + *o* + -TOMY] Incision into a tunica albuginea, especially that of the testis to relieve pressure due to orchitis.

**albugineous** \al′bəjin′ē·əs\ [New L *albugineus* (from L *albugo*, gen. *albuginis* a white spot) whitish. See ALBUGO.] **1** Whitish; resembling the white of the sclera. **2** Pertaining to a tunica albuginea.

**albugo** \alboo′gō\ [L (from *alb(us)* white + *-ugo*, noun-forming suffix) a white spot in the eye] A white opacity of the cornea.

**albumen** \albyoo′mən\ ALBUMIN.

**albumimetry** \al′byoomim′ətrē\ ALBUMINIMETRY.

**albumin** \albyoo′mən\ [L *albumen* (gen. *albuminis*; from *albus* white) the white of an egg] Any protein of the class that dissolves in water without the addition of salt and that, unlike a globulin, stays in solution on half saturation with ammonium sulfate. Usually serum albumin is meant. Also *albumen*. **iodine 131 human serum a.** A serum albumin labeled with iodine 131. It is used for blood-flow studies, blood and plasma determinations, and imaging of brain tumors. **iodine 125 human serum a.** Human serum albumin labeled with radioactive iodine 125. It is often preferable to $^{131}$I-labeled albumin because there is less radiation hazard and more stable shelf life of labeled material. It is largely used in measuring blood and plasma volume. **macroaggregated a.** Human serum albumin aggregated by a denaturation process. The particle size is 10–75 μm. Radiolabeled macroaggregated albumin is used in lung imaging, revealing particles lodged in pulmonary capillaries following intravenous administration. **normal human serum a.** A commercially prepared solution of fractionated pooled plasma used to provide colloid oncotic pressure as an intravenous infusion. The fractionation decreases the risk of transmitting serum hepatitis. **radioiodinated serum a.** Serum albumin that has been chemically combined with radioiodine so that the movement or behavior of the albumin in the body can be monitored externally. It is used in vascular circulation studies and in the detection of brain tumors. Abbr. RISA **serum a. 1** The albumin that is present in serum or plasma. **2** A quantification of the albumin concentration in serum or plasma. **technetium 99m human serum a.** Human serum albumin labeled with technetium 99m, used mainly for intravascular blood-pool and kinetic studies, and certain kinetic studies of cerebrospinal fluid.

**albuminimetry** \albyoo′mənim′ətrē\ The measurement of albumin in fluid, usually a body fluid like urine, plasma, or cerebrospinal fluid. Also *albumimetry*.

**albuminoid** \albyoo′mənoid\ Resembling albumin.

**albuminuria** \al′byoomənoo′rē·ə\ [ALBUMIN + -URIA] **1** Excretion of abnormal amounts of albumin in urine. **2** *Incorrect* PROTEINURIA. Adj. albuminuric.

**Albustix** Reagent-impregnated strips used for semiquantitative determination of albumin in body fluids. A proprietary name.

***Alcaligenes faecalis*** \al′kəlij′ənēz fēkā′lis\ A Gram-negative, motile, oxidase-positive, fermentation-negative rod that cannot attack sugars. The oxidation of organic acids and amino acids makes the medium alkaline. It is found in feces, and occasionally in infections.

**alcapton** *Obs.* HOMOGENTISIC ACID.

**alcaptonuria** \alkap′tōnoo′rē·ə\ ALKAPTONURIA.

**Alcian blue** \al′sē·ən\ A water-soluble cationic dye that is derived from copper phthalocyanin and is used to stain acid mucopolysaccharides in tissue sections.

**Alcock** [Benjamin *Alcock*, Irish anatomist, born 1801] Alcock's canal. See under CANALIS PUDENDALIS.

**alcohol** [Med L (from Arabic *al-* the + *kuḥl* kohl, an eye cosmetic, a fine powder) powder produced by sublimation or liquid produced by distillation; sublimate, distillate, spirit] **1** Any of a group of organic substances containing an —OH group with limited tendency to ionize (p*K* near 14) and not joined to an aromatic nucleus (in distinction from phenols, p*K* near 10) or to a —CO— group (in distinction from acids, p*K* near 5). **2** ETHANOL. **absolute a.** Ethanol not containing more than 1% by weight of water. **acid a.** 70% ethyl alcohol containing 1% hydrochloric acid. **fatty a.** An alcohol of formula $CH_3$—$[CH_2]_n$—OH, where *n* is fairly large, usually over 8. **primary a.** An alcohol containing the —$CH_2OH$ group. **rubbing a.** A solution containing not less than 68.5% and not more than 71.5% by volume of absolute alcohol, the rest consisting of water, denaturing agents, and perfume oils. It is used as a rubefacient. Its composition must meet the requirements of the United States Treasury Department. **secondary a.** An alcohol containing the —CH(OH)— group where neither of the two attached groups is hydrogen. **sugar a.** A polyhydroxylic alcohol, H—$[CHOH]_n$—H, which can be derived by reducing a sugar. **tertiary a.** Methanol bearing three substituents on its carbon atom. **wood a.** METHANOL. **wool a.** The yellow-brown solid, alcoholic fraction of the products from saponification of wool fat. It contains not less than 30% cholesterol and 500 to 1000 ppm of BHA or BHT as an antioxidant, and is used in ointments as an emulsifying agent for water-in-oil emulsions.

**alcoholate** ALKOXIDE.

**alcohol dehydrogenase** An enzyme (EC 1.1.1.71) that catalyzes the dehydrogenation of an alcohol to an aldehyde (or ketone, if the alcohol is secondary), with concomitant reduction of an electron acceptor such as nicotinamide adenine dinucleotide ($NAD^+$). Also *retinal reductase* (outmoded). Symbol: $NAD(P)^+$

**alcoholemia** \al′kəhōlē′mē·ə\ The presence of ethanol in the blood. Also *hyperalcoholemia*.

**alcohol-ether** A mixture of equal parts of 96% ethanol and diethyl ether, used as a solvent or as a fixative in bacteriology.

**alcoholic** **1** Pertaining to, caused by, or containing alcohol, particularly ethanol. **2** A person suffering from alcoholism.

**alcoholica** Designating pharmaceutical preparations containing alcohol.

**Alcoholics Anonymous** A self-help group serving to foster the rehabilitation of alcoholics. It has become an international movement with total abstinence as its cornerstone and methods which are primarily inspirational and supportive.

**alcoholism** \al′kəhôlizm\ Physiologic dependence on alcohol, characterized by a pattern of pathologic use, impaired social or occupational functioning, the development of tolerance to alcohol, and the appearance of withdrawal symptoms when alcohol intake is reduced or eliminated. Withdrawal is typically manifested in coarse tremor of the hands and tongue, nausea, weakness, autonomic hyperactivity, and anxiety or depression. Delirium tremens or alcoholic hallucinosis may result if withdrawal is prolonged. Also *alcohol addiction, alcoholic addiction, dipsomania*. **acute a.** Drunkenness due to the ingestion of excessive amounts of alcoholic beverages, characterized by muscular incoordination and mental confusion. **chronic a.** A morbid condition resulting from excessive or prolonged use of alcoholic beverages. Symptoms include anorexia, diarrhea, weight loss, liver degeneration, and severe disturbances of the nervous system. **epsilon a.** PERIODIC DRINKING BOUTS. **paroxysmal a.** PERIODIC DRINKING BOUTS.

**aldehyde** [German *Aldehyd*, from abbreviation (*Al. dehyd.*) of New L *alcohol dehydrogenatum* dehydrogenated alcohol] Any of the organic compounds containing the group —CH=O. The compounds may be prepared by oxidation (dehydrogenation) of a primary alcohol. They are named from the corresponding hydrocarbon with the suffix *-al*, as *ethanal*, or from the carboxylic acid with the same number of carbon atoms, as *acetaldehyde*.

**aldehyde dehydrogenase** An enzyme that catalyzes the dehydrogenation of an aldehyde, usually to a carboxylic acid. In the important instance of glyceraldehyde-3-phosphate dehydrogenase, however, orthophosphate is a reactant and an acyl phosphate is the product.

**aldehyde fuchsin** \al′dəhīd fook′sin\ A histologic stain that is prepared from basic fuchsin by dissolving it in a solution of hydrochloric acid and paraldehyde in isopropanol. It is used for staining elastic fibers and oxytalan fibers.

**Alder** [Albert von *Alder*, German physician, born 1888] Alder's anomaly, Alder's constitutional granulation anomaly. See under ALDER-REILLY ANOMALY.

**aldimine** The imine formed between an aldehyde and an amine, as between enzyme-bound pyridoxal phosphate and an amino acid in an aminotransferase. Compare KETIMINE.

**aldo-** \al′də-\ [*ald(ehyde)* + *o*] A combining form indicating relation to an aldose.

**aldol** $CH_3$—CHOH—$CH_2$—CHO. 3-Hydroxybutanal. **a. condensation** The reversible combination of two molecules, each containing a carbonyl group, in which one of them loses a proton from the carbon atom next to the carbonyl group, so that it becomes nucleophilic and attacks the carbonyl group of the other molecule. Such a condensation between two molecules of acetaldeyhyde produces aldol. The reverse of this condensation is involved in the dissociation of fructose 1,6-bisphosphate into triose phosphates in the glycolytic pathway.

**aldolase** **1** An enzyme that catalyzes the aldol condensation. **2** FRUCTOSE-BISPHOSPHATE ALDOLASE.

**aldonic acid** A sugar derivative formed by oxidizing an aldose and having the structure $CH_2OH$—$[CHOH]_n$—COOH.

**aldose** Any sugar whose carbonyl group is terminal; a substance of formula H—$[CHOH]_n$—CHO.

**aldosterone** 11*β*,21-Dihydroxy-3,20-dioxo-4-pregnen-18-al. The steroid secreted by the outer layer of the adrenal cortex, enabling sodium to be retained by the body and potassium excreted. Its lack is the cause of death on removal or destruction of the adrenal glands. It exists largely as the hemiacetal formed by reaction of the 11-hydroxyl group with the aldehyde group. Also *electrocortin* (outmoded).

**aldosteronism** \-ster′ōnizm\ The clinical state caused by excessive adrenocortical secretion of aldosterone. Symptoms include muscular weakness, hypertension, hypokalemic alkalosis, polyuria, and polydipsia. Also *hyperaldosteronism.* **idiopathic a.** Excessive secretion of aldosterone due to unknown cause. **primary a.** Aldosteronism due to intrinsic disease of the adrenal cortex, such as adenoma or hyperplasia of the adrenal cortex. Also *Conn syndrome.* **secondary a.** Aldosteronism resulting from elevated renin production with an excess of angiotensin II, as in hepatic cirrhosis, nephrotic syndrome, or accelerated hypertension.

**aldosteronopenia** \-ster′ənōpē′nē·ə\ HYPOALDOSTERONISM.

**Aldrich** [Robert Anderson *Aldrich,* U.S. pediatrician, born 1917] Aldrich syndrome. See under WISKOTT-ALDRICH SYNDROME.

**Aldridge** [Albert Herman *Aldridge,* U.S. gynecologist, born 1893] See under OPERATION.

**aldrin** $C_{12}H_8CL_6$. A polycyclic chlorinated hydrocarbon, largely saturated but containing two double bonds. It is used as an insecticide but it is also toxic to mammals.

**alecithal** \əles′ithal\ MIOLECITHAL.

**alembic** \əlem′bik\ [Old French *alambic* alembic, from Med L *alambicus* alembic, from Arabic *al-anbīq* the still, from *al* the + *anbīq* still, from Gk *ambix* a cup, beaker, cap of a still] An apparatus formerly used for distillation.

**aleukia** \əloo′kē·ə\ [Gk *a-* priv. + LEUK- + -IA] The absence, or near-absence, of leukocytes in the blood. Also *aleukocytosis, aleucia.* **alimentary toxic a.** A disease characterized by leukopenia and associated with the consumption of food made from grain which has remained unharvested under snow and has become moldy from contamination with a variety of microorganisms. The causative agent is believed to be a trichothecene, or T2 toxin, derived from certain species of *Fusarium, Cladosporium, Alternaria, Penicillium, Mucor, Piptocephalis, Trichoderma, Rhizopus, Trichothecium, Thammidium, Verticillium,* and *Actinomyces.* The toxin affects both humans and animals and produces vomiting, diarrhea, multiple hemorrhage, and exhaustion of bone marrow. The disease was noted in particular in the U.S.S.R. during World War II. **congenital a.** CONGENITAL NEUTROPENIA. **a. hemorrhagica** MALIGNANT THROMBOCYTOPENIA.

**aleukocytosis** \əloo′kəsītō′sis\ ALEUKIA.

***Aleurobius farinae*** \əloorō′bē·əs ferē′nē\ *ACARUS SIRO.*

**Alexander** [W. Stewart *Alexander,* English neurologist and pathologist, flourished 20th century] See under DISEASE.

**alexia** \əlek′sē·ə\ [Gk *a-* priv. + *lex(is)* (from *legein* to speak) a word + -IA] Inability to read, in the absence of any defect of visual acuity. Alexia can be regarded as a form of visual agnosia or receptive aphasia specifically impairing the ability to recognize and interpret letters and words. It can result from an acquired lesion of the dominant parietal lobe, generally involving the region of the angular and/or supramarginal gyri. It may also be developmental (congenital word blindness), and is then often familial and sometimes of dominant inheritance, though there is a marked preponderance of affected males. Acquired alexia due to cerebral lesions may sometimes be associated with agraphia, acalculia, various features of the Gerstmann syndrome, or with hemianopia, or spatial or visual object agnosia. Also *visual aphasia, text blindness, word blindness.* Adj. alexic. **a. with agraphia** Inability to decipher, understand, and use verbal symbols coupled with the inability to write them. While comprehension of the meaning of written or printed words is lost, the ability to identify letters is unimpaired. Also *cortical alexia, parietal alexia, Dejerine's alexia.* **a. without aphasia** PURE WORD BLINDNESS. **aphasic a.** Alexia in which words and letters are recognized but not the meaning which they convey. **cortical a.** ALEXIA WITH AGRAPHIA. **Dejerine's a.** ALEXIA WITH AGRAPHIA. **developmental a.** DEVELOPMENTAL DYSLEXIA. **geometric a.** PURE WORD BLINDNESS. **isolated a.** PURE WORD BLINDNESS. **motor a.** Inability to read a written text aloud although it is understood. **musical a.** MUSICAL BLINDNESS. **occipital a.** PURE WORD BLINDNESS. **optic a.** PURE WORD BLINDNESS. **parietal a.** ALEXIA WITH AGRAPHIA. **pure a.** PURE WORD BLINDNESS. **semantic a.** Alexia in which the patient can read aloud correctly but without understanding. **sensory a.** PURE WORD BLINDNESS. **subcortical a.** Alexia caused by a lesion interrupting the nervous connections between the angular gyrus and Wernicke's area. **symbolic a.** PURE WORD BLINDNESS. **tactile a.** Inability of a blind person to read Braille. **verbal a.** PURE WORD BLINDNESS.

**alexic** \əlek′sik\ Characteristic of, or resembling, alexia.

**alexin** \əlek′sin\ *Obs.* COMPLEMENT.

**aleydigism** \əlī′digizm\ Absence of androgen (testosterone) secretion by the interstitial (Leydig) cells of the testis; eunuchism.

**Alezzandrini** [Arturo Alberto *Alezzandrini,* Argentinian ophthalmologist, born 1932] See under SYNDROME.

**ALG** antilymphocyte globulin.

**alga** \al′gə\ Singular of ALGAE.

**algae** \al′jē\ [L, pl. of *alga* seaweed] (*sing.* alga) Photosynthetic eukaryotic organisms lacking a vascular system, true leaves, stems, and roots. Algae range in size from the microscopic to the macroscopic, and include many seaweeds found in freshwater and marine habitats. **blue-green a.** See under CYANOBACTERIA.

**alganesthesia** \algan′esthē′zhə\ [*alg(o)-* + ANESTHESIA] ANALGESIA.

**alge-** \al′jə-\ ALGO-.

**algesi-** \aljē′sē-\ ALGO-.

**algesia** \aljē′zē·ə\ [Gk *algēsis* sense of pain + -IA] Pain sensitivity, often to an abnormal degree.

**algesic** \aljē′sik\ Pertaining to or producing pain; painful. Also *algetic.*

**algesimeter** \al′jēsim′ətər\ [ALGESI- + -METER] An instrument designed to measure the threshold of perception and the intensity of painful stimuli. Also *algesiometer, algometer.* **Boas a.** An algesimeter designed to test the sensitivity to pain of the skin of the epigastrium.

**algesimetry** \al′jēsim′ətrē\ [ALGESI- + -METRY] The measurement of the reaction (sensitivity) to painful stimuli using an algesimeter. Also *algometry.*

**algesiogenic** \aljē′zē·əjen′ik\ Productive of pain. Also *algogenic.*

**algesiometer** \aljē′zē·äm′ətər\ ALGESIMETER.

**algesthesia** \al′jesthē′zhə\ [*alg(e)-* + ESTHESIA] Pain sensation; the ability to perceive pain. Also *algesthesis.*

**algetic** \aljet′ik\ ALGESIC.

**-algia** \-al′jə\ [Gk *alg(os)* pain + -IA] A combining form meaning a painful condition.

**algid** \al′jid\ [L *algidus* (from *algere* to be cold, chilled) cold, chilly] **1** Cold; severely chilled or chilling. **2** Characterized by hypothermia, clammy skin and prostration: used in reference to certain severe conditions or stages of disease, as *algid malaria.*

**algin** A polysaccharide extracted from seaweed. It is a cream or yellow powder which forms a viscous, colloidal emulsion in water. It is used as a stabilizing colloid in ice cream and in pharmaceuticals as a suspending agent. Also *sodium alginate, alginic acid sodium salt.*

**alginate** A 1-4$\beta$ linked polymer of mannuronic acid; the 2-epimer of glucuronic acid, obtained from seaweeds. Its sodium salt is used as a thickening agent for foods such as ice cream, and in dentistry is used mixed with water as an elastic impression material.

**alginic acid** A polymer of 1,4-linked D-mannuronic acid and L-guluronic acid that forms a mucoid capsule on strains of *Pseudomonas aeruginosa* found in the lungs of cystic fibrosis patients. It is also extracted from marine algae and used as a binder in pharmaceutical tablets and a thickening and emulsifying agent in a number of food products.

**alginic acid sodium salt** ALGIN.

**alginuresis** \al′jinoorē′sis\ [Gk *algin(oeis)* painful + -URESIS] Pain upon urinating.

**algio-** \al′jō-\ ALGO-.

**algioglandular** \al′jē·əglan′dyələr\ Of or relating to glandular activity arising from painful stimulation.

**algiometabolic** \al′jē·əmet′əbäl′ik\ Of or relating to metabolic activity brought on by painful stimulation.

**algiovascular** \al′jē·əvas′kyələr\ Pertaining to the reaction of cardiovascular structures stemming from a painful stimulation. Also *algovascular.*

**algo-** \al′gō-\ [Gk *algos* pain] A combining form meaning pain. Also *alge-, algesi-, algio-.*

**algoceptor** \al′gōsep′tər\ NOCICEPTOR.

**algogenesis** \al′gōjen′əsis\ The production or induction of pain.

**algogenic** \al′gōjen′ik\ ALGESIOGENIC.

**algolagnia** \al′gōlag′nē·ə\ [ALGO- + Gk *lagneia* lust, desire] A psychosexual disorder in which arousal depends upon pain, suffering, or humiliation being inflicted on one or more of the participants in sexual activity, as in masochism and sadism. **active a.** SADISM. **passive a.** MASOCHISM.

**algomenorrhea** \al′gōmənôrē′ə\ [ALGO- + MENORRHEA] DYSMENORRHEA.

**algometer** \algäm′ətər\ ALGESIMETER.

**algometry** \algäm′ətrē\ ALGESIMETRY.

**algophilia** \al′gōfil′yə\ [ALGO- + -PHILIA] *Obs.* MASOCHISM.

**algorithm** \al′gəriTHm\ [alteration, because of *arithmetic,* of *algorism,* from Med L *algorismus,* from Arabic *al-khuwārizmi* system of numerals, after *al-Khuwarizmi,* ninth-century Persian mathematician] A set of rules for approaching solution of a complex problem by setting down individual steps and delineating how each step follows from the preceding one. It can be expressed in algebraic notation, in computer programs, or in graphic form as a tree with branches representing alternative decisions.

**algovascular** \al′gōvas′kyələr\ ALGIOVASCULAR.

**Alibert** [Jean Louis *Alibert,* French physician, 1768–1837] See under KELOID.

**alicyclic** [*ali(phatic)* + CYCLIC] Having a ring composed only of carbon atoms: used of a cyclic, nonaromatic, organic compound. Inositol, steroids, and shikimic acid are important natural alicyclic compounds.

**alienation** \āl′yənā′shən\ [L *alienatio* (from *alienatus,* past part. of *alienare* to make a thing another or another's) an alienating] A feeling of being isolated, lonely, or out of touch either with one's own feelings or with one's environment and culture; estrangement. Alienation may progress to feelings of depersonalization or derealization, or to an identity crisis. Also *anomie.*

**aliesterase** *Obs.* CARBOXYLESTERASE.

**align** \əlīn\ **1** To adjust an optical system so that all components have the same or parallel optical axes. **2** To adjust a multistage amplifier so that resonant circuits all pass the same frequency. **3** To adjust delays in digital circuits to make them synchronous.

**alignment** \əlīn′mənt\ **1** The process of bringing into line. **2** The normal arrangement of the teeth in the dental arches. For defs. 1 and 2 also *alinement.*

**aliment** \al′əmənt\ [L *alimentum* (from *alere* to nourish) nourishment] Any substance that has nutritional value.

**alimentary** \al′əmen′terē\ [L *aliment(um)* food + -ARY ] Relating to food or to the digestive system.

**alimentation** \al′əmentā′shən\ [Med L *alimentatio* (from Late L *alimentare* to nourish, from L *alimentum nourishment) a nourishing*] The process of feeding or of receiving nutrition. **artificial a.** The supplying of nutrients to people who cannot take food orally, such as the procedure used in parenteral nutrition. **forced a.** The act of forcing a person to eat more than he would under his own volition, a procedure adopted as therapy for patients with extreme forms of anorexia nervosa. It is also used in instances of self-starvation.

**alinasal** \al′ənā′səl\ Pertaining to the alae nasi.

**alinement** \əlīn′mənt\ ALIGNMENT.

**aliphatic** [Gk *aleiphar,* gen. *aleiphat(os)* (from *aleiphein* to anoint, akin to *lipos* fat) unguent, oil + -IC] Related to paraffins and devoid of benzenoid (aromatic) character.

**aliptic** **1** Pertaining to inunction, or the administration of a drug in an ointment applied by rubbing to promote absorption of the active ingredient. **2** OINTMENT.

**aliquot** \al′əkwət\ [L indeclinable pl. adj. (from *ali(us)* other, another + *quot* how many, as many as ), some, several] **1** Divisible into a given whole without remainder. Thus 3 is an aliquot part of 15 but 2 is not. **2** Constituting a representative sample of a whole, such as an aliquot portion of a solution. **3** An aliquot part.

**alisphenoid** \al′əsfē′noid\ ALA MAJOR OSSIS SPHENOIDALIS.

**alive** Electrically connected to a source of voltage or electrically charged to a voltage different from ground. Also *live.*

**alizarin No. 6** PURPURIN.

**alizarinopurpurin** PURPURIN.

**alkalaemia** *Brit.* ALKALEMIA. See under ALKALOSIS.

**alkalemia** \al′kəlē′mē·ə\ ALKALOSIS.

**alkalescens-dispar** \al′kəles′əns-dis′pär\ See under ALKALESCENS-DISPAR GROUP.

**alkali** \al′kəlī\ [Arabic *al* the + *qalī* kali, the plant from which soda ash was obtained] A substance whose solution contains $OH^-$ ions.

**alkaline** \al′kəlīn\ [*alkal(i)* + -INE] **1** Reacting as an alkali. **2** Containing an alkali. **3** Having a high concentration of $OH^-$ ions: said of a solution. **4** Describing the six metals (lithium, sodium, potassium, rubidium, cesium, and francium) which combine with oxygen to produce alkalies.

**alkaline phosphatase** A phosphatase (EC 3.1.3.1) having an alkaline optimum (pH often close to 10). Such enzymes are widely distributed in animals and bacteria.

**alkalinity** The property of being an alkali or an alkaline solution.

**alkalitherapy** Treatment with alkali salts, as in the treatment of peptic ulcer. Also *alkalotherapy, alkali therapy.*

**alkaloid** \al′kəloid\ [*alkal(i)* + -OID] Any of a group of nitrogenous substances of vegetable origin, often of complex structure and high molecular mass. They are often heterocycles, and may be primary, secondary, or tertiary bases or may contain quaternary ammonium groups. Alkaloids are only slightly soluble in water but soluble in ethanol, benzene, ether, and chloroform. They exhibit some general characteristics which are revealed by coloration or precipitation by alkaloid reagents. They show intense physiologic action and are widely used medicinally. They may be highly toxic, even in very small doses.

**alkalometry** The administration of alkaloids in doses calculated according to scientific, quantitative rules.

**alkalosis** \al′kəlō′sis\ [*alkal(i)* + -OSIS] A disturbance of the acid-base state of the body in which arterial pH is higher than 7.45. Also *alkalemia, baseosis.* **acapnial a.** RESPIRATORY ALKALOSIS. **altitude a.** Respiratory alkalosis by hyperventilation during acclimatization to high altitudes. It follows excessive elimination of $CO_2$ from the lungs. **carbon-dioxide a.** RESPIRATORY ALKALOSIS. **compensated a.** A condition in which the pH of the arterial blood is within the normal range despite the presence of an alkalosis. **compensated metabolic a.** A condition in which the pH of the arterial blood is within the normal range despite the presence of metabolic alkalosis. **compensated nonrespiratory a.** A condition in which the pH of the arterial blood is within the normal range despite the presence of nonrespiratory alkalosis. **compensated respiratory a.** A condition in which the pH of the arterial blood is within the normal range despite the presence of respiratory alkalosis. **congenital gastrointestinal a.** A rare congenital intestinal disorder in which there is loss of chloride in abnormal amounts in watery stools. A similar alkalosis results from the vomiting of infants with congenital hypertrophic pyloric stenosis, by loss of chlorine and hydrogen ions in gastric secretions. **hypokalemic a.** A nonrespiratory alkalosis in which the plasma concentration of potassium is less than normal. **metabolic a.** A nonrespiratory alkalosis that stems from a metabolic disorder. **respiratory a.** Alkalosis resulting from reduced arterial and tissue carbon dioxide tension due to hyperventilation. Also *carbon-dioxide alkalosis, acapnial alkalosis.*

**alkalotherapy** ALKALITHERAPY.

**alkalotic** \al′kəlät′ik\ Of or relating to alkalosis.

**alkane** \al′kān\ Any hydrocarbon containing no double bonds. Also *paraffin.*

**alkapton** [German (from *al(kali)* + Gk *kaptōn* gulping down, from *kaptein* to gulp down) lit., an alkali-devouring substance] *Obs.* HOMOGENTISIC ACID.

**alkaptonuria** \al′kaptənoo′rē·ə\ [ALKAPTON + -URIA] An inborn error of tyrosine metabolism in which homogentisic acid (HGA), a metabolite of tyrosine, accumulates because of deficient activity of HGA oxidase. Oxidation and polymerization of the HGA produces a black pigment. The urine turns dark on standing or on the addition of alkali. Black pigment is deposited in cartilage and other connective tissue (ochronosis). Arthritis of the spine and large joints is often manifest in the third or fourth decade, as well as aortic valve stenosis. The trait is of autosomal recessive inheritance. Also *alcaptonuria.*

**alkene** \al′kēn\ Any unsaturated hydrocarbon with a double bond.

**alkoxide** The anion formed by removing the proton from the OH group of an alcohol, or a salt of this anion. Alkoxides are important synthetic reagents, especially for xanthogenates and ethers. Also *alcoholate.*

**alkoxy** The group $H—[CH_2]_n—O—$, possibly substituted.

**alkoxyl** The group R—O—, where R equals alkyl.

**alkyl** \al′kil\ Any univalent group obtained by loss of a hydroxyl group from an alcohol, equally by loss of a hydrogen atom from a hydrocarbon.

**alkylation** \al′kilā′shən\ The chemical process of replacing a hydrogen atom with an alkyl group.

**alkyne** Any unsaturated hydrocarbon with a triple bond.

**ALL** **1** acute lymphoblastic leukemia. **2** acute lymphocytic leukemia.

**allachesthesia** \al′əkesthē′zhə\ ALLESTHESIA. **optical a.** VISUAL ALLESTHESIA.

**allantiasis** \al′antī′əsis\ [*allant(o)-* + -IASIS] Poisoning due to consumption of sausages containing *Clostridium botulinum* toxin. Also *sausage poisoning.* See also BOTULISM.

**allanto-** \əlan′tō-, al′əntō-\ [Gk *allas* (gen. *allantos*) sausage] A combining form denoting (1) the allantois; (2) sausage.

**allantoamnion** \-am′nē·än\ The condition in which the allantois completely surrounds the amnion.

**allantochorion** \-kôr′ē·än\ A type of embryonic membrane formed by apposition of the side of the allantois with the chorionic mesoderm.

**allantoenteric** \-enter′ik\ [ALLANTO- + ENTERIC] Relating to the allantois and the intestine.

**allantogenesis** \-jen′əsis\ [ALLANTO- + GENESIS] The formation and development of the allantois.

**allantoic** \al′antō′ik\ Relating to the allantois, as *allantoic fluid.*

**allantoic acid** $(NH_2—CO—NH—)_2CH—COOH$. A product of purine catabolism in fish. Some species excrete this, but most hydrolyze it to urea and glyoxylate.

**allantoicase** An enzyme that hydrolyzes allantoic acid to urea and ureidoglycolic acid ($NH_2$—CO—NH—CHOH—COOH), which is normally further hydrolyzed to glyoxylate and more urea.

**allantoid** \əlan′toid\ [Gk *allantoeidēs* sausagelike. See ALLANTOIS.] **1** Resembling a sausage, as *allantoid membrane.* **2** Pertaining to or resembling the allantois.

**allantoin** 5-Ureidoimidazolidine-2,4-dione. Although man and most primates excrete uric acid as the major end product of purine catabolism, most animals oxidatively decarboxylate it to allantoin. This in turn is excreted by most mammals but is further broken down to allantoic acid in lower organisms.

**allantois** \əlan′tō·is\ [New L, irreg. from French *allantoïde,* from Gk *(ho) allantoiedēs (hymēn)* the sausagelike membrane, allantois, from *allas,* gen. *allantos* sausage] One of the true extraembryonic membranes of vertebrates, providing respiratory exchange. It is formed as a ventral diverticulum from the posterior part of the primitive intestinal tube. It is covered by a conjoined vascular layer containing umbilical or allantoic vessels which are the vascular connections with the placenta. In reptiles and birds the allantoic sac evolved primarily as a temporary store for urine but also became a structure vital for embryonic respiratory exchange. In some mammals, such as the horse and goat, it is very large and acts as an excretory reservoir. In others it is vestigial, but in all its vessels are essential in the establishment of the extraembryonic circulation between embryo and placenta. Also *allantoid membrane.*

**Allarton** [George *Allarton,* English surgeon, flourished late 19th century] Allarton's operation. See under MEDIAN LITHOTOMY.

**allele** \əlēl′\ [Gk *allēlōn* (from *allos* another) of one another] Any one of two or more variants of a gene that occurs at a given locus. Two alleles always differ in nucleotide sequence but may or may not produce discernibly different effects. Also *allelomorph* (obs.), *allelic gene, isomorph* (outmoded). Also *allel.* **dominant a.** DOMINANT GENE. **leaky a.** HYPOMORPH. **lethal a.** **1** An allele that directly causes the death or reproductive failure of an organism when present in one copy if the resulting phenotype is dominant or in two copies if recessive. 2 An allele that results in a total failure of reproduction of an organism. 3 An allele, particularly in microorganisms, that permits survival only under a restricted environment. For defs. 1, 2, and 3 also *lethal factor, lethal gene.* **modification a.** MODIFYING GENE. **recessive a.** RECESSIVE GENE. **silent a.** An allele that produces no detectable product or effect. Also *silent gene.* **sublethal a.** 1 An allele that reduces but does not eliminate genetic fitness. 2 An allele that impairs without killing an organism. For defs. 1 and 2 also *sublethal gene.*

**allelism** \al′ēlizm\ The existence of multiple variants of the gene that occupies a given locus.

**allelo-** \əlē′lō-\ [Gk *allēlōn* (from *allos* another) of one another] A combining form meaning from one to another; reciprocally; in mutual relation.

**allelomorph** \əlē′lōmôrf\ *Obs.* ALLELE.

**allelotaxy** \əlē′lōtak′sē\ The formation, during development, of one organ from more than one embryologic structure. Also *allelotaxis.*

**allelotype** \əlē′lōtīp′\ The frequency distribution of a given set of alleles in a population.

**Allen** [Edgar *Allen,* U.S. scientist, 1892–1943] Allen-Doisy unit. See under MOUSE UNIT.

**Allen** [Willard Myron *Allen,* U.S. gynecologist, born 1904] Corner-Allen test. See under TEST.

**allergen** \al′ərjən\ [*aller(gy)* + -GEN] A substance known to be an agent contributing to immediate hypersensitivity in man, such as pollen, animal dander, or house dust proteins. Also *allergic antigen* (outmoded), *anaphylactogen* (obs.), *sensibiligen* (obs.), *sensibilisinogen* (obs.), *sensitizin* (obs.). ● The term was formerly used synonymously with *antigen,* but is now used almost exclusively with reference to proteins or carbohydrates which induce specific IgE antibodies in humans.

**allergenic** \al′ərjen′ik\ [*aller(gy)* + -GENIC] Capable of inducing allergy.

**allergic** Pertaining to, caused by, or having an allergy.

**allergid** \əlur′jid\ [*allerg(y)* + -ID[2]] A disseminated skin eruption attributed, sometimes on inadequate evidence, to allergic sensitization to an infective organism.

**allergist** \al′ərjist\ [*allerg(y)* + -IST] A physician who specializes in the treatment of allergic disorders.

**allergologist** \al′ərgäl′əjist\ One who specializes in allergology.

**allergology** \al′ərgäl′əjē\ [*allerg(y)* + *o* + -LOGY] A medical subspecialty devoted to the study of allergy and its treatment. Adj. allergologic.

**allergy** [German *Allergie,* from Gk *all(o)-* other (altered) + Gk *erg-* work, action (reaction) + *-ie* -Y] A state of hypersensitivity, especially of the immediate or acute type with the implication of immunologically induced tissue damage. ● The term was originally introduced by Clemens Freiherr von Pirquet in 1906 to mean altered host reactivity to an antigen. **atopic a.** ATOPY. **bacterial a.** A state of altered reactivity in which the body reacts to the product or products of bacteria. It is no longer generally recognized as a form of immediate hypersensitivity. *Outmoded.* **bronchial a.** Allergy affecting the bronchi, usually resulting in asthma. **cold a.** A tendency to develop skin lesions, usually urticaria, upon exposure to cold, which can be transferred to unaffected individuals by serum. It is often seen in several autoimmune states. **contact a.** An allergic reaction of delayed type following contact of the skin with chemical substances acting as allergens or haptens. The catechols of poison ivy and poison oak and nickel ions are common causes of contact allergy. Contact allergy to dinitrocholorbenze is used as a test of immune competence. **delayed a.** An allergic reaction developing between 24 and 28 hours after contact with a substance to which cell-mediated hypersensitivity has developed. See also DELAYED HYPERSENSITIVITY. **drug a.** An allergic reaction induced by hypersensitivity to a drug. **food a.** An allergy initiated by the ingestion of a specific food, such as peanuts, shellfish, or certain berries. In children, cow's milk is a common antigen. Symptoms may include diarrhea and vomiting but are more often manifested by skin rashes (urticaria or eczema) that may appear shortly after the food has been ingested or after a delay of several hours. **gastrointestinal a.** A food allergy in which the dominant symptoms are gastrointestinal, as colic, vomiting, or diarrhea. **house dust a.** An allergic reaction to the constituents of house dusts. The principal allergen in house dust is the house dust mite (*Dermatophagoides pteronyssinus*). Other allergens which may be present include bacteria, fungi, and dander. **humoral a.** An allergic reaction mediated by antibodies to the antigen involved. IgE-mediated immediate allergy (hypersensitivity) and IgG-mediated Arthus reactions are both examples of humoral allergy. **immediate a.** IMMEDIATE HYPERSENSITIVITY. **intrinsic a.** ATOPY. **latent a.** Allergy whose presence in a subject can be demonstrated by tests although the subject is free of symptoms. **nasal a.** ALLERGIC RHINITIS. **physical a.** An allergy activated by a physical factor, such as cold, heat, or light. **pollen a.** An allergy to a variety of pollen antigens affecting the respiratory tract and eyes as in hay fever and in some cases of asthma. Also *pollinosis, pollenosis.* **seasonal nasal a.** HAY FEVER.

**allesthesia** \al′esthē′zhə\ [Gk *all(os)* other, another + -ESTHESIA] A change in the sensation experienced from a given sensory stimulus when background input from other sensory receptors is concurrently altered, as for example the dependence of thermal sensation both on sensory cues from the skin and on core temperature of the body. Also *allachesthesia.* **visual a.** A disorder of vision in which the images are transposed to the opposite half of the visual field. Also *optical allachesthesia.*

**alleviant** \əlē′vē·ənt\ A drug or other substance that alleviates pain or other symptoms of disease; anodyne or palliative.

**allicin** \al′isin\ $C_6H_{10}OS_2$. Allylthiosulfinic allyl ester, a broad-spectrum antifungal and antibacterial substance obtained from garlic, *Allium sativum.*

**alligation** [L *alligatio* (from *alligare* to bind or tie to, unite) a tying, binding] 1 In pharmacy, a method of determining the proportions of various solutions necessary to produce a final mixture of a given strength. 2 A method of determining the cost of a mixture or solution when the proportions and prices of the individual ingredients are known.

**Allingham** [William A. *Allingham,* English surgeon, 1830–1908] Allingham's ulcer. See under ANAL FISSURE.

**Allis** [Oscar Huntington *Allis,* U.S. surgeon, 1836–1921] See under FORCEPS.

**alliteration** \əlit′ərā′shən\ [AD- + L *litera* a pen stroke, letter of the alphabet + -ATION] A form of aphasia in which the patient uses consecutively words which may be inappropriate but begin with the same sound.

**allo-** \al′ō-\ [Gk *allos* (adjective) other, another] 1 A combining form meaning other, extraneous, different from, opposed to. 2 A prefix signifying that the compound referred to has a stereochemical configuration at one center opposite to that of the compound without such a prefix. Thus L-allothreonine is (2*S*,3*S*)-2-amino-3-hydroxybutyric acid, whereas L-threonine is (2*S*,3*R*)-2-amino 3-hydroxybutyric acid.

**alloantibody** \al′ə·an′tēbäd′ē\ An antibody produced in response to an alloantigen; antibody reacting with an antigen produced by a genetically different member of the same species. Also *isoimmune antibody, isoantibody* (outmoded), *isobody* (outmoded).

**alloantigen** \al′ə·an′təjən\ An antigen which can be recognized and to which a response is made by the immune system of other members of the same species. Alloantigens exist in more than one allelic form, and there are allelic differences in the molecule concerned between the individual stimulating the response and the individual responding. Also *allogeneic antigen, homologous antigen, isoantigen* (outmoded), *isophile antigen* (outmoded).

**alloarthroplasty** \al′ə·ärth′rəplas′tē\ ALLOGRAFT ARTHROPLASTY.

**allobarbital** $C_{10}H_{12}N_2O_3$. 5,5-Diallylbarbituric acid, a barbiturate with sedative and hypnotic properties.

**allocheiria** \al′əkī′rē·ə\ [ALLO- + CHEIR- + -IA] ALLOESTHESIA.

**allochesthesia** \al′əkesthē′zhə\ ALLOESTHESIA.

**allochezia** \al′əkē′zhə\ [ALLO- + Gk *chez(ein)* to defecate + -IA] **1** The discharge of nonfecal material via the anus. **2** The discharge of feces through an abnormal opening such as a fistula.

**allochiria** \al′əkī′rē·ə\ [Gk *allo(s)* other + *cheir* hand + -IA] ALLOESTHESIA.

**allocortex** \al′əkôr′teks\ The portions of cerebral cortex medial to the rhinal fissure during embryonic development that fail to differentiate into a six-layered isocortex. There are two main components of the allocortex, the archicortex and the paleocortex.

***Allodermanyssus*** \al′ədur′mənis′əs\ *LIPONYSSOIDES.*

**allodiploid** \al′ədip′loid\ [ALLO- + DIPLOID] **1** A hybrid organism that has at least one, and usually all, of its chromosomes composed of a haploid set of genes from a parent of one species and a haploid set from a parent or donor of a different species. **2** Having parents of two different species, each of whom contributes a haploid gene complement to the organism.

**alloeroticism** \al′ə·irät′isizm\ The mature stage of object relationships in which fusion and integration of drives lead to predominance of the love of the object rather than of being loved by the object. Also *alloerotism.*

**alloesthesia** \al′ə·esthē′zhə\ [ALLO- + -ESTHESIA] A disorder of the localization of tactile stimuli, in which the patient feels the sensation at a corresponding point on the opposite side of the body to that to which the stimulus is applied. Also *allocheiria, allochiria, allochesthesia, Bamberger sign.* Adj. alloesthesic.

**allogamy** \əläg′əmē\ The usual mechanism of fertilization in which the ovum of one individual combines with the spermatozoon of another individual, as distinguished from autogamy.

**allogeneic** \al′əjənē′ik\ **1** In immunology, describing material coming from a genetically distinct member of the same species, as serum, tissue, or cells. Compare SYNGENEIC. **2** Genetically distinct within the same species. Also *allogenic.*

**allogenic** \al′əjen′ik\ ALLOGENEIC.

**allogotrophia** \al′əgətrō′fē·ə\ [ALLO- + TROPH- + -IA] The growth or nourishment of one part of the body at the expense of another, as in certain neoplasms.

**allograft** \al′əgraft\ [ALLO- + GRAFT] A graft from a donor of one species to a recipient of the same species, where the two individuals are not genetically identical. Also *homograft, allogeneic graft, homogenous graft, homoplastic graft* (older term), *homologous graft* (older term), *homeograft, homeotransplant, homotransplant.* **nerve a.** A surgical graft inserted into a peripheral nerve where the donor portion of nerve comes from another individual.

**alloisoleucine** See under ISOLEUCINE.

**allokeratoplasty** \al′əker′ətōplas′tē\ [ALLO- + KERATOPLASTY] A corneal transplant composed of a different substance than corneal tissue, such as a synthetic plastic.

**allokinesis** \al′əkīnē′sis\ The involuntary copying in one limb of a voluntary movement in the opposite limb. Also *mirror movement, allokinesia.*

**allokinetic** \al′əkīnet′ik\ [ALLO- + KINETIC] Pertaining to passive or reflex movement.

**allometry** \əläm′ətrē\ [ALLO- + -METRY] The measurement of the changing shape of an organism in relation to its growth or evolution.

**allopath** \al′əpath\ A practitioner of allopathy.

**allopathic** \al′əpath′ik\ Of or relating to allopathy.

**allopathy** \əläp′əthē\ [Gk *allo(s)* other, another + -PATHY] A system of medicine in which disease is treated by producing effects opposed to or incompatible with the effects of the disease process. Compare HOMEOPATHY.

**allophene** \al′əfēn\ [ALLO- + Gk *phain(ein)* to bring to light, appear] A character that is not produced solely by the action of the genes of the cell or tissue expressing the phenotype. It may result from interaction with genetically distinct cells or tissues. Hence transplantation or transfer of the original cells or tissue to a different genetic milieu may cause disappearance or alteration of the allophenic character. Compare AUTOPHENE.

**allophenic** \al′əfen′ik\ Of or relating to an animal who bears cellular phenotypes from more than one conceptus. It is a result of the fusion of blastomeres from different genotypes *in vitro.*

**allophore** \al′əfôr\ ERYTHROPHORE.

**alloplasia** \al′əplā′zhə\ HETEROPLASIA.

**alloplast** \al′əplast\ A presumably inert inorganic material, such as plastic, used as an implant in humans or animals.

**alloplasty** \al′əplas′tē\ **1** Any plastic operation which utilizes alloplastic materials. **2** The process of adapting by changing the environment rather than by changing the self.

**alloploid** \al′əploid\ [ALLO- + -PLOID] A cell or organism having two or more sets of chromosomes derived from parents of different species or genera. Also *allopolyploid.*

**allopregnane** Pregnane in the 5α configuration, i.e., with *trans* fusion of rings A and B to give a flat molecule. *Outmoded.*

**allopurinol** \al′əpyoo′rinôl\ 5-Hydroxypyrazolopyrimidine, a pharmacologic agent used to lower serum uric acid by blocking the action of the enzyme xanthine oxidase.

**all-or-none** Characterized by effects or responses that are either maximal or absent; nongradient. See also ALL-OR-NONE LAW.

**allorphine hydrochloride** NALORPHINE HYDROCHLORIDE.

**allosome** \al′əsōm\ [ALLO- + *-some* as in *chromosome*] Any chromosome that differs in appearance or behavior from the normal chromosome complement. Also *heterochromosome, heteromorphic chromosome, heterotypical chromosome.* **paired a.** DIPLOSOME. **unpaired a.** An accessory chromosome that differs in appearance or behavior from the chromosomes of the normal complement.

**allosteric** **1** Relating to another position: said of enzyme effector molecules (activators or inhibitors) that have a binding site separate from that of the substrate-binding site. The binding of such effectors often causes a conformational change in the enzyme. 2 Having another position where an effector molecule can bind: said of a protein, usually an enzyme.

**allosynapsis** \al′əsinap′sis\ The complete or partial pairing at meiosis of chromosomes derived from genotypically distinct parents, as in parents of different species. It occurs only in polyploid or aneuploid organisms. Also *allosyndesis.*

**allosyndesis** \al′əsin′dəsis\ ALLOSYNAPSIS.

**allotetraploid** \al′ətet′rəploid\ A cell or organism that contains four chromosome sets, two each from different ancestral species. Also *amphidiploid.*

**allothreonine** The 3-epimer of threonine.

**allotransplantation** \al′ətrans′plantā′shən\ The replacement of lost or damaged tissue with an allograft. Also *homotransplantation, homeotransplantation.*

**allotrio-** \əlät′rē·ō-\ [Gk *allotrios* of another, foreign] A combining form meaning strange, foreign.

**allotriogeustia** \-goo′stē·ə\ [ALLOTRIO- + Gk *geust(os)* verbal of *geuein* to taste + -IA] A strange or perverted taste sensation in which one substance tastes like another. It is similar to but not identical with parageusia.

**allotriophagy** \əlät′rē·äf′əjē\ [ALLOTRIO- + -PHAGY] PICA.

**allotype** \al′ətip\ [ALLO- + TYPE] **1** Any of the genetic variants of a plasma protein or other molecule occurring among members of a single species. Allotypes may vary in electrophoretic charge, in antigenicity, and in molecular weight. Changes in amino acid sequence (for proteins) or sugar distribution (for carbohydrates) underlie these variations. **2** Any of the discernible phenotypes produced by a set of alleles at a given genetic locus. Seldom used in this sense. **Gm a.** Any of the genetic markers found in IgG molecules in man. They were recognized by the use of antibodies (found in the serum of rheumatoid arthritis patients and sometimes of normal multiparous women) which agglutinate antibody-coated erythrocytes only when the antierythrocyte antibody was taken from genetically defined donors.

**allotypic** \al′ətip′ik\ Of or characteristic of an allotype.

**allotypy** \əlät′ipē\ [*allotyp(e)* + -Y] Genetic variation occurring in plasma proteins and other molecules among members of the same species.

**allowance** / **recommended daily a.** The amount of a nutrient thought necessary to be ingested each day in order to maintain health. Abbr. RDA

**alloxan** 5-Oxobarbituric acid, a bright yellow compound. It is usually found as its stable, colorless monohydrate, in which the water molecule is present in combination with the carbonyl group at the 5-position in the form of a geminal diol, making 5,5-dihydroxybarbituric acid. Alloxan is readily formed chemically by oxidizing uric acid. It reacts with amino acids similarly to ninhydrin. Since it is particularly toxic to the insulin-producing cells of the pancreas, it is used to make animals diabetic for experimental purposes. Also *mesoxalyl urea.*

**alloxazine** A heterocyclic substance, $C_8H_6N_4O_2$, obtained by condensation of *o*-phenylenediamine with alloxan. Its molecules possess fused benzene, pyrazine and pyrimidine rings with oxygen substituents on the pyrimidine ring. Riboflavin, which is a vitamin and constituent of the flavoprotein enzymes, is a substituted derivative of alloxazine.

**alloxuremia** \al′äksoorē′mē·ə\ The presence of excess purine bases in the blood and associated signs of toxicity.

**alloxuria** \al′äksoo′rē·ə\ The excretion of purine bases in the urine.

**alloxuric** \al′äksoo′rik\ Related to, or characteristic of alloxuria.

**alloy** \al′oi\ [French *aloi* (from L *alligare* to bind to, unite) a combining] A metal consisting of a mixture of two or more metallic elements. **amalgam a.** An alloy for mixing with mercury to form a silver amalgam used in dentistry. Also *silver tin alloy, dental alloy.* **chrome-cobalt a.** A strong, corrosion-resistant alloy used for making dentures, particularly bases, bars, and clasps. Also *cobalt-chromium alloy.* **dental a.** AMALGAM ALLOY. **Newton's a.** MELOTTE'S METAL. **silver tin a.** AMALGAM ALLOY.

**allozygote** \al′əzī′gōt\ GENETIC COMPOUND.

**allozyme** \al′əzīm\ Any of a class of functionally identical or similar enzymes that are separable on the basis of genetically determined properties between species.

**allyl** The univalent group $CH_2{=}CH{-}CH_2{-}$. 2-Propenyl.

**allysine** $HCO{-}[CH_2]_3{-}CH(NH_3^+){-}COO^-$. The aldehydic amino acid formed by oxidation of C-6 of lysine. This process occurs to some lysine residues in collagen and elastin, and is important for the cross-linking of these proteins.

**Almeida** [Floriano Paulo de *Almeida,* Brazilian physician, born 1898] Almeida's disease, Lutz-Splendore-Almeida disease. See under SOUTH AMERICAN BLASTOMYCOSIS.

**Almén** [August Theodor Andersson *Almén,* Swedish physiologist, 1833–1903] Almén's test. See under GUAIAC TEST.

***Aloe*** \al′ō\ A large genus of shrubby or arborescent xerophytes of the family Liliaceae. The juice from the fleshy leaves of *A. vera* is widely used for treating burns of all types, including sunburn and radiation burn. Chrysophanic acid is the constituent of the juice that is believed to be most active in healing burned skin. The plant has also been used as a laxative. Cultivated varieties of *A. vera* are known as *A. barbadensis, A. chinensis,* and *A. perryi.*

**aloe** [L *aloë* (from Gk *aloē* the aloe) the aloe, bitterness] The dried juice obtained from the leaves of various species of *Aloe.* It contains aloe-emodin, a potent anthraquinone purgative that acts upon the large intestine, but it has been largely superseded by less toxic cathartics.

**aloe-emodin** 1,8-Dihydroxy 3-(hydroxymethyl)anthraquinone. A compound found in rhubarb and in various species of *Aloe,* occuring both as the free anthraquinone and as the glycoside derivative. It is used as a laxative.

**aloetic** Pertaining to or containing aloe.

**alogognosia** \al′əgägnō′zhə\ LOGAGNOSIA.

**alopecia** \al′ōpē′shə\ [L (from Gk *alōpekia* mange of foxes, from *alōpēx* fox), a falling off of the hair by the roots, morbid baldness] A loss of hair occurring at any site and from any cause. **a. acquisita** A loss of hair that results from any but hereditary or congenital causes. **androgenetic a.** CALVITIES. **a. areata** A loss of hair in clearly defined circumscribed patches, which may coalesce to give rise to alopecia totalis or alopecia universalis. It is a distinct clinicopathological entity, probably mediated by an immunologic mechanism. Also *Cazenave's vitiligo, vitiligo capitis.* **a. capitis totalis** Alopecia areata involving loss of all scalp hairs. **cicatricial a.** A loss of hair that results from the destruction of follicles by an inflammatory or neoplastic process, with the subsequent replacement by scar tissue. **a. circumscripta** A loss of hair confined to a small area. **congenital sutural a.** The absence of hair on the skin overlying the sutures of the skull, as in the Hallermann-Streiff syndrome. **congenital triangular a.** A developmental defect characterized by the appearance in early childhood of unilateral or bilateral triangular areas partially or completely deficient in follicles of normal size. The base of the triangle is at the frontal hair line in the frontotemporal region. **favic a.** Alopecia, usually with scarring, that is caused by chronic infection with one of the favus fungi. **a. leprotica** A loss of hair due to leprosy, as in the thinning or loss of eyebrows and/or eyelashes characteristic of lepromatous leprosy or the absence of hairs in skin lesions of tuberculoid leprosy. Although scalp alopecia due to leprosy has been described in Japan, such a relationship has not been established elsewhere. **a. liminaris** MARGINAL TRAUMATIC ALOPECIA. **male pattern a.** CALVITIES. **marginal a.** OPHIASIC ALOPECIA AREATA. **marginal traumatic a.** The loss of hair along the frontal hair line as a result of prolonged traction on the hair, leading to folliculitis and scarring. Also *alopecia liminaris, traction alopecia.* **mechanical a.** TRAUMATIC ALOPECIA. **ophiasic a. areata** Alopecia areata involving part or all of the scalp margin in linear distribution. Also *marginal alopecia, ophiasis.* **pityriasic a.** Common baldness associated with pityriasis capitis, which was formerly believed to be the cause of the hair loss. **postoperative pressure a.** See under PRESSURE ALOPECIA. **postpartum a.** POSTPARTUM DEFLUVIUM. **a. prematura** Common baldness developing at an age earlier than customary in the population concerned. **pressure a.** A usually temporary loss of hair from a circumscribed area of the scalp that results from ischemia induced by prolonged pressure, as during a surgical operation. **radiation a.** The loss of hair that is induced by exposure to ionizing radiation. It can either be a temporary loss following exposure to an epilatory dose or a permanent loss after exposure to a dose of sufficient intensity to cause atrophy and destruction of the hair follicles. **a. seborrheica** A loss of hair associated with seborrhea but not caused by it. Both are androgenic changes. **senile a.** A loss of hair attributed to old age. • The term is often misapplied to symptomatic hair loss in the elderly. **symptomatic a.** A loss of hair that occurs as a manifestation of systemic disease such as hypothyroidism or a high fever. **syphilitic a.** A loss of hair, most often in irregular small patches, that occurs during the secondary stage of syphilis. **a. totalis** ALOPECIA UNIVERSALIS. **traumatic a.** A loss of hair resulting from physical trauma, usually traction or friction, as from excessive brushing, massage, or scratching. Also *mechanical alopecia.* **traumatic marginal a.** See under MARGINAL TRAUMATIC ALOPECIA. **a. universalis** The loss of all hair by the universal extension of alopecia areata. Also *alopecia totalis.* **x-ray a.** Alopecia resulting from exposure to x rays.

**Alpers** [Bernard Jacob *Alpers,* U.S. neurologist, born 1900] Alpers disease, Alpers polioencephalopathy. See under SYNDROME.

**alpha** \al′fə\ The name of the first letter of the Greek alphabet. Symbol: $\alpha$

**alphabet** / **genetic a.** GENETIC CODE.

**alphalytic** \al′fəlit′ik\ **1** Effective in blocking $\alpha$-adrenergic receptors: used especially of drugs. **2** Describing the action of blocking such receptors.

**alphamimetic** \al′fəmimet′ik\ **1** Mimicking the effect of stimulation of $\alpha$-adrenergic receptors. **2** An agent that stimulates or mimics the stimulation of such receptors.

**alphanumeric** \al′fən^y^oomer′ik\ Consisting of letters, numbers, and usually punctuation marks and mathematical symbols.

**alphaprodine hydrochloride** $C_{16}H_{23}NO_2 \cdot HCl$. *cis*-1,3-Dimethyl-4-phenyl-4-piperidyl-propionate hydrochloride, an analogue of meperidine with narcotic and analgesic properties. Chronic use of the substance may lead to addiction and psychic dependence.

**alphavirus** \al′fəvī′rəs\ [Gk *alpha* first letter of Greek alphabet + VIRUS; formerly known as group A arboviruses] Any virus belonging to the *Alphavirus* genus of the Togaviridae, including eastern, western, and Venezuelan encephalitis viruses, chikungunya virus, Sindbis virus, and others.

**Alport** [Arthur Cecil *Alport,* South African physician, 1880–1959] See under SYNDROME.

**alprenolol hydrochloride** $C_{15}H_{23}NO_2 \cdot HCl$. 1(*o*-Allylphenoxy)-3-(isopropylamino)-2-propanol hydrochloride, a drug that blocks $\beta$-adrenergic receptors.

**ALS** amyotrophic lateral sclerosis.

**A.L.S.** advanced life support (designating any of a number of training programs designed to teach emergency resuscitation of the ill or injured).

**Alsberg** [Albert A. *Alsberg,* German physician, born 1856] See under ANGLE.

**alseroxylon** An alkaloid-rich extract of *Rauwolfia serpentina* that contains reserpine. It acts as a sedative and tranquilizer.

**Alsever** [John Bellows *Alsever,* U.S. Public Health Service, born 1908] See under SOLUTION.

**alstonine** $C_{21}H_{20}N_2O_3$. An alkaloid from *Alstonia constricta* with antiseptic and antipyretic properties. It has been used in the East to treat diarrhea and malaria.

**ALT** alanine aminotransferase.

**alt. dieb.** *alternis diebus* (L, every other day).

**alteplase** TISSUE PLASMINOGEN ACTIVATOR.

**alterative** Any medicine that favorably changes the functioning of an organ or system of the body.

**alternans** \ôltur′nəns\ [L, (pres. part. of *alternare* to alternate) alternating] Pulsus alternans. See under PULSUS. **auditory a.** AUSCULTATORY ALTERNANS. **auscultatory a.** Alternately soft and loud heart sounds or murmurs, in spite of a regular heart rhythm. Also *auditory alternans.* **electrical a.** Alternating high and low voltages of the P wave or QRS complex of the electrocardiogram in the absence of an arrhythmia. Also *electrical alternation of the heart.* **mechanical a.** Alternating strong and weak cardiac contractions in regular cardiac rhythm.

***Alternaria*** \ôl′tərner′ē·ə\ [L *altern(us)* acting by turns, alternate + -ARIA] A genus of fungus that has been implicated as the causal agent of human dermatitis and of lesions in the respiratory tract.

**alternation** \ôl′tərnā′shən\ [L *alternatio* (from *alternare* to do by turns, from L *alter* the other of two) a doing by turns] In neurology, the response of a nerve fiber only to each alternate stimulus when a high-frequency pattern of stimulation (900–1000 Hz or above) is employed. This phenomenon is due to the refractory period of a nerve fiber. **cardiac a.** PULSUS ALTERNANS. **electrical a. of the heart** ELECTRICAL ALTERNANS. **a. of generations** The alternate production of asexual (diploid) and sexual (haploid) individuals in the life cycle of an organism, as occurs in coelenterates, platyhelminths, and plants.

**alternobaric** \ôl′tərnōber′ik\ Having to do with or resulting from a persisting difference of gaseous pressure between the environment and air-containing compartments within the body.

**alt. hor.** *alternis horis* (L, every other hour).

**altitude** / **high a.** An altitude above 10 000 meters.

**Altmann** [Richard *Altmann,* German histologist, 1852–1900] **1** Altmann's granule. See under MITOCHONDRION. **2** Altmann's liquid. See under FLUID. **3** Altmann-Gersh method. See under METHOD.

**alum** [L *alumen* alum] **1** $KAl(SO_4)_2 \cdot 12H_2O$. The double sulfate of potassium and aluminum. **2** Any of the double sulfates of one univalent and one tervalent cation, many of which form mixed crystals with each other.

**alum hematoxylin** A hematoxylin that incorporates an aluminum salt as a mordant. Also *hemalum, ammonia hematе.*

**alumina** $Al_2O_3$. Aluminum oxide. It is amphoteric, dissolving in acids to give salts of the $Al^{3+}$cation and in alkalies to give aluminates containing the $AlO_2^-$anion. **a. gel** Alumina precipitated in a form suitable for adsorbing proteins as a step in their purification. It is made by adding ammonia to an aluminum salt under defined conditions.

**alumina and magnesia** A combination of aluminum hydroxide and magnesium hydroxide. It is used in the form of tablets as an antacid.

**aluminium** \al′oomin′ē·əm\ ALUMINUM. • This form of the word is used widely throughout the world, and was used in the United States before 1927.

**Aluminoid** A proprietary name for aluminum hydroxide gel.

**aluminosis** \əloo′mənō′sis\ Fibrosis of the lung due to inhalation of dust of metallic aluminum or aluminum-containing ores.

**aluminum** \əloo′minəm\ [New L, from L *alumen,* gen. *alumin(is)* alum] Element number 13, having atomic weight 26.9815. Aluminum is the most abundant metal in the lithosphere. It is never found free but is generally combined with oxygen. The pure metal is silvery white and light, having specific gravity of 2.7. One stable isotope (aluminum 47) occurs naturally, and six unstable isotopes are known. Also *aluminium.* Symbol: Al

**aluminum acetate** $C_6H_9AlO_6$. A compound used in a 5% solution (Burow solution) as an astringent and antiseptic.

**aluminum aminoacetate** DIHYDROXYALUMINUM AMINOACETATE.

**aluminum carbonate** $Al_2(CO_3)_3$. A chalklike compound with mild antiseptic and styptic properties. **basic a.** A complex mixture of aluminum hydroxide and aluminum carbonate. The gel is used as an antacid and in a low phosphate diet to prevent the formation of phosphate urinary stones.

**aluminum chloride** $AlCl_3{\cdot}6H_2O$. A white, crystalline, hygroscopic powder used as an astringent, antiseptic, and antiperspirant. It occurs in a trivalent form (Burow solution), widely used as an antiseptic and astringent, and in a hexavalent form, as in Shelley's formulation, which is particularly effective as an antiperspirant.

**aluminum glycinate** DIHYDROXYALUMINUM AMINOACETATE.

**aluminum hydroxide** A slightly astringent, tasteless powder used externally as a drying powder and internally as an antacid in the form of a gel. **a. gel** A suspension containing $Al_2O_3$, primarily as the hydroxide, used as an antacid.

**aluminum monostearate** A combination of aluminum with variable proportions of stearic acid and palmitic acid. It is used in preparation of a suspension of procaine penicillin G.

**aluminum penicillin** An aluminum salt of penicillin that has been used as an oral form of the antibiotic.

**aluminum subacetate** A yellow liquid prepared by combining aluminum sulfate, acetic acid, and calcium carbonate. In dilute aqueous solution it is used as an astringent wash.

**alundum** \əlun′dəm\ An extremely hard form of alumina prepared by fusion in an electric furnace. It is used as an abrasive and in laboratory apparatus that must withstand great heat.

**alveated** \al′vē·ātid\ **1** Honeycombed. **2** Canalized.

**alvei** \al′vē·ī\ Plural of ALVEUS.

**alveolar** \alvē′ələr\ Pertaining to or resembling an alveolus.

**alveolare** \al′vē·əler′ə\ PROSTHION.

**alveolate** \alvē′əlāt\ [*alveol(a)* + -ATE] Having cavities or pits like a honeycomb.

**alveolectomy** \al′vē·əlek′təmē\ [*alveol(o)*- + -ECTOMY] The removal of bone of the alveolar process, usually in preparation for the fitting of a denture. **transeptal a.** An alveolectomy in which the interdental septa are removed and the buccal bone is compressed into the resulting space. Also *interradicular alveoloplasty, intraseptal alveoloplasty.*

**alveoli** \alvē′əlī\ Plural of ALVEOLUS.

**alveolitis** \al′vē·ōlī′tis\ [*alveol(o)*- + -ITIS] **1** Inflammation of one of the dental alveoli, particularly following the extraction of a tooth. Also *dry socket, septic socket, infected socket.* **2** Inflammation of any alveoli, especially those of the lung. **allergic a.** Inflammatory damage to alveoli resulting from an allergic reaction to an inhaled substance. **extrinsic allergic a.** A hypersensitivity reaction of the lung to repeated inspiration of organic dusts. **fibrosing a.** Inflammation of lung alveoli proceeding to, or with a tendency to, fibrosis. **a. with honeycombing** Inflammation of lung alveoli with fibrosis resulting in greatly enlarged air spaces.

**alveolo-** \alvē′əlō-\ [L *alveolus* (dim. of *alveus* a hollow) a little hollow] A combining form denoting alveolus.

**alveolobasal** \-bā′səl\ Pertaining to the thicker, basal portion of the processus alveolaris that transmits pressure in the jaws.

**alveolocapillary** \-kap′iler′ē\ Relating to lung alveoli and capillaries, or the interface between them.

**alveololingual** \-ling′gwəl\ Involving or pertaining to both the alveolar process or part and the tongue.

**alveolonasal** \-nā′səl\ In craniometry, pertaining to the alveolar point and nasion.

**alveolopalatal** \-pal′ətəl\ Relating to both the alveolar process of the maxilla and the hard palate.

**alveoloplasty** \alvē′əlōplas′tē\ [ALVEOLO- + -PLASTY] Surgical recontouring of alveolar bone prior to providing a denture. **interradicular a.** TRANSEPTAL ALVEOLECTOMY. **intraseptal a.** TRANSEPTAL ALVEOLECTOMY.

**alveolus** \alvē′ələs\ [L, dim. of ALVEUS] (*pl.* alveoli) **1** A small cavity, hollow, or cell. Also *foveola, faveolus.* **2** One of the alveoli dentales. **3** A terminal rounded secretory unit of an alveolar or acinar gland. **4** One of the numerous thin-walled, polyhedral formations that line the walls of the alveolar sacs that open into the alveolar ducts at the termination of a respiratory bronchiole in the lung. Some authorities consider the term to refer to the space within the partially open polyhedral formation. Also *air cell.* **5** One of the foveolae gastricae. Adj. alveolar. **dental alveoli** Alveoli dentales mandibulae and alveoli dentales maxillae. Also *tooth sockets.* **alveoli dentales mandibulae** [NA] Conical bony sockets in the alveolar part of the body of the mandible for the roots of the teeth of which there are sixteen in the adult. They are separated from each other by the interalveolar septa. **alveoli dentales maxillae** [NA] Conical bony sockets in the alveolar process of the maxilla for the roots of the teeth of which there are sixteen in the adult. They are separated from each other by the interalveolar septa. **pulmonary alveoli** ALVEOLI PULMONIS. **alveoli pulmonis** [NA] Small pouches in the walls of the alveolar ducts, atria, and alveolar saccules or sacs at the terminal end of the respiratory bronchioles of the lungs. Their walls comprise a thin epithelial lining that rests on a layer of connective tissue which contains blood capillar-

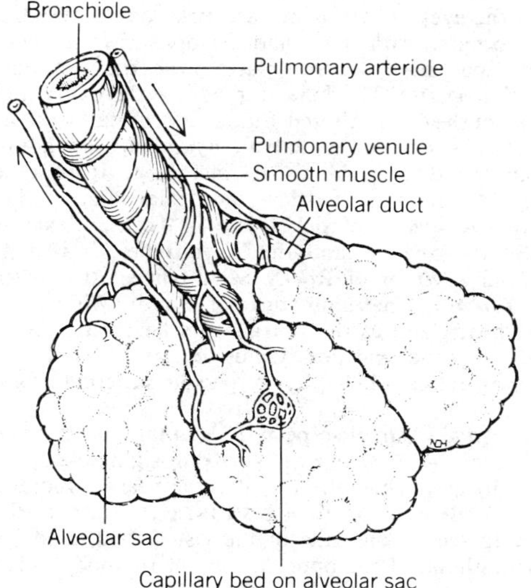


**Pulmonary alveoli**

ies. They are separated from each other by interalveolar septa. They provide an enlarged surface area for the exchange of gases between the atmospheric air and the blood capillaries. Also *pulmonary alveoli, alveoli pulmonum, Malpighi's vesicles, pulmonary vesicles, air vesicles, bronchic cells, lung vesicles.* **alveoli pulmonum** ALVEOLI PULMONIS.

**alveus** \al′vē·əs\ [L, a hollow] (*pl.* alvei) A trough, canal, or groove. **a. communis** *Outmoded* UTRICULUS. **a. hippocampi** [NA] The layer of fibers covering the ventricular surface of the hippocampus. It contains axons both leaving and entering the deeper layers.

**alvus** \al′vəs\ [L, belly, womb, hold of a ship, beehive] The abdomen and its viscera. Adj. alvine.

**alymphocytosis** \əlim′fōsītō′sis\ The absence of lymphocytes.

**alymphoplasia** \əlim′fōplā′zhə\ [Gk *a-* priv. + LYMPHO- + -PLASIA] A markedly meager or hypoplastic development of lymphoid tissue. **thymic a.** Lymphoid hypoplasia, occurring particularly in the thymus but to some degree in the lymph nodes and spleen as well. Associated peripheral lymphopenia and hypogammaglobulinemia predispose to infection in infancy.

**Alzheimer** [Alois *Alzheimer,* German neurologist, 1864–1915] **1** See under STAIN. **2** Alzheimer's dementia, Alzheimer sclerosis. See under DISEASE. **3** Alzheimer neurofibrillary change. See under CHANGE. **4** Alzheimer cells. See under CELL. **5** Alzheimer fibril. See under INTRANEURAL FIBRILLARY TANGLE.

**Am** Symbol for the element, americum.

**am** **1** ametropia. **2** Symbol for myopic astigmatism.

**am-** \am-\ ANA-.

**AMA** **1** American Medical Association. **2** against medical advice.

**amaas** \ä′mäs\ [Afrikaans, sour milk] ALASTRIM.

**amacrine** \am′əkrīn\ [Gk *a-* priv. + MACR- + Gk *is,* gen. *inos,* nerve, fiber] AMACRINE CELL.

**Amadori** [Mario *Amadori,* Italian chemist, born 1886] See under REARRANGEMENT.

**amalgam** \əmal′gəm\ [Med L *amalgama* (from Arabic *al-malgham* soft substance, from Gk *malagma* a soft mass, from *malassein* to soften) a soft mass] Any alloy of mercury with another metal or metals. **copper a.** A dental amalgam consisting of mercury and copper. Unlike a silver and tin alloy, it is prepared a moment before use by heating the required quantity over a flame. The alloy then melts and remains plastic for a time, even at room temperature. It sets after insertion in the tooth cavity. Copper amalgam has bactericidal properties. **dental a.** An amalgam for filling teeth. There are two main types, silver amalgam, which is the one chiefly used, and copper amalgam. **retrograde a.** POSTRESECTION FILLING. **silver a.** A dental amalgam containing principally mercury, silver, and tin. It is prepared a moment before use by mixing mercury and amalgam alloy in a mortar or in an amalgamator. The resultant amalgam is plastic and sets in the tooth cavity in a short time.

**amalgamator** \əmal′gəmā′tər\ A machine for mixing mercury and an alloy to make a dental amalgam. Measured quantities of mercury and alloy are placed in a capsule, which is rapidly vibrated for a few seconds by means of an electric motor.

***Amanita*** \am′ənē′tə\ [New L (from Gk *amanitai* a kind of fungus)] A genus of mushrooms generally recognized as highly toxic. ***A. muscaria*** One of the most cosmopolitan poisonous species of fungus. It is easily recognized by the yellow, orange, or red caps having white or cream flakes on the upper surface. This mushroom is commonly known as the fly agaric since during ancient times it was believed to act as an insecticide. Also *Agaricus muscarius* (incorrect). ***A. phalloides*** A deadly poisonous species of mushroom which produces phallotoxic cyclopeptides known as phalloidins. Although fairly rare in North America, the fruiting body is recognized by the olive-green cap and stem. ***A. virosa*** A species of mushroom, the destroying angel, considered to be the most poisonous known.

**amanitin** Any of a group of poisons (α-amanitin, β-amanitin, etc.) occurring in mushrooms of the genus *Amanita.* They are cyclic peptides with cross-linking between cysteine and tryptophan side chains, and they contain unusual amino acids, such as 2-amino-4,5-dihydroxy-3-methylvaleric acid. Also *amanitotoxin.*

**amanitotoxin** AMANITIN.

**amantadine** \əman′tədīn\ [*amantad-,* anagram of *adamant-* (from Gk *adamant(inos)* hard as adamant) + -INE] An antiviral agent which specifically inhibits influenza A virus *in vitro* and exerts prophylactic and therapeutic effects in experimental influenza A infections in animals and in natural infections in humans.

**amara** \əmer′ə\ BITTERS.

**amastia** \əmas′tē·ə\ [Gk *a-* priv. + MAST- + -IA] A congenital absence of the breasts.

**amastigote** \əmas′tigōt\ [irreg. from Gk *a-* priv. + *mastix,* gen. *mastigos,* a whip, flagellum] The intracellular phase of certain flagellate protozoan parasites such as *Leishmania* species or *Trypanosoma cruzi,* characterized by a round or ovoid form 2–6 μ in diameter, withdrawn flagellum, and large kinetoplast. Also *Leishman-Donovan body* (older term), *leishmania* (older term).

**amaurosis** \am′ôrō′sis\ [Gk *amaurōsis* (from *amauros* dark) darkening, dimming of vision] Loss of sight; blindness; a disease characterized by loss of sight. Adj. amaurotic. **cat's eye a.** Loss of vision associated with an abnormal reflection of light from the ocular fundus, resembling the appearance of a cat's eye glowing in the dark. This is due to reflection from neoplastic, inflammatory, or traumatic opacities within the vitreous cavity. **cerebral a.** Loss of sight due to damage to the visual pathways in the brain or the visual cortex. Also *central amaurosis, amaurosis centralis.* **compression a.** Loss of sight due to mechanical damage to the eye, visual pathways, or their blood supply. **a. congenita of Leber** A genetically heterogeneous, autosomal recessive syndrome limited to the eye, in which infantile visual loss and keratoconus are associated with choreoretinal degeneration and cataract formation. Also *congenital amaurosis.* **diabetic a.** Loss of sight due to vascular or intraocular damage caused by diabetes mellitus. **a. fugax** A fleeting or temporary loss of sight, usually implying transient retinal ischemia. **a. partialis fugax** Temporary and partial loss of sight attributable to transient ischemia of the retina, visual pathways, or visual cortex, as that associated with the aura of migraine or caused by microembolism. **saburral a.** Loss of sight associated with a gastric upset, such as might be caused by acute angle-closure glaucoma.

**amaurotic** \am′ôrät′ik\ Pertaining to amaurosis; unable to see.

**amb-** \amb-\ AMBI-.

**ambenonium chloride** $C_{28}H_{42}Cl_4N_4O_2$. N,N′-[(1,2-Dioxo-1,2-ethanediyl)bis-(imino-2,1-ethanediyl)]bis[2-chloro-N,N-diethylbenzenemethanaminium] dichloride, a cholinergic drug that acts as a cholinesterase inhibitor. Its action resembles that of neostigmine and is used in the treatment of myasthenia gravis and, to a limited extent, of intestinal and urinary tract atony.

**Amberg** [Emil *Amberg,* U.S. otologist, 1868–1948] See under LINE.

**Amberlite** Various ion-exchange resins, both cation exchangers and anion exchangers. A proprietary name.

**ambi-** \am′bi-\ [L, prefix denoting on both sides, around] A prefix meaning both. Also *amb-.*

**ambidexterity** \-dekster′itē\ The ability to perform motor acts with equal skill with either the left or right hand. Also *ambidextrality, ambidextrism.*

**ambidextrous** \-dek′strəs\ Possessing the faculty of ambidexterity.

**ambiguity** \-gyoo′itē\ The capacity of being understood in different ways. **ribosomal a.** Imperfect fidelity in translation, in which a codon is translated not into the cognate amino acid but into one with a closely related codon. The very low background rate can be increased by ribosomal ambiguity mutations and by certain antibiotics such as streptomycin.

**ambilateral** \-lat′ərəl\ Pertaining to or affecting both sides.

**ambiocularity** \-äk′yəler′itē\ [AMBI- + OCULAR + -ITY] The ability to use either eye alone with equal facility.

**ambisexual** \-sek′shoo·əl\ [AMBI- + SEXUAL] **1** Having sexual characteristics common to both sexes, as axillary hair. Also *ambosexual.* **2** BISEXUAL.

**ambisexuality** \-sek′shoo·al′itē\ [AMBI- + SEXUALITY] **1** The capacity for being associated with either or both sexes. **2** BISEXUALITY.

**ambivalence** \ambiv′ələns\ The coexistence of an emotion, wish, impulse, or the like, with its antithesis, such as the simultaneous love and hate for the same person. Also *bipolarity.*

**ambly-** \am′blē-\ [Gk *amblys* dull] A combining form meaning (1) dull, blunt; (2) dim, dimmed.

**amblyacusis** \-əkʸoo′sis\ [AMBLY- + ACU-² + -SIS] HEARING LOSS.

**amblyaphia** \-ā′fē·ə\ [AMBLY- + Gk *(h)aph(ē)* a touching, sense of touch + -IA ] TACTILE HYPOESTHESIA.

***Amblyomma*** \am′blē·äm′ə\ [New L, from AMBLY- + Gk *omma* the eye] A genus of hard ticks (family Ixodidae) generally ornate, with eyes and festoons. Males lack adanal shields, but have ventral plates near the festoons. ***A. americanum*** The lone star tick, a three-host tick found in the southeastern United States and as far west as Texas, that attacks man in its larval, nymphal, and adult stages, though the dog is the usual final host. It is a vector of Rocky Mountain spotted fever and tularemia. ***A. cajennense*** A species of tick found in Texas, Mexico, Central and South America, and the West Indies. It is a notorious biter and a vector of Rocky Mountain spotted fever. ***A. hebraeum*** The bont tick of South Africa, found on sheep, goats, and cattle. It transmits heartwater, a rickettsial disease of cattle, and tick typhus to man.

**amblyope** \am′blē·ōp′\ A person suffering from amblyopia.

**amblyopia** \am′blē·ō′pē·ə\ [Gk *amblyōpia* (from *ambly(s)* blunt, dim + *ōp(s)* eye + -IA) dim-sightedness] Reduced ability to see, while the eye itself appears structurally normal. **color a.** COLOR BLINDNESS. **crossed a.** Inability to see on one side of the visual field, associated with hemianesthesia of the opposite side of the body. Also *amblyopia cruciata.* **a. cruciata** CROSSED AMBLYOPIA. **eclipse a.** Reduced vision attributable to macular damage resulting from an ultraviolet burn to the retina caused by viewing an eclipse of the sun without adequate protection of the eyes. **a. ex anopsia** SUPPRESSION AMBLYOPIA. **nocturnal a.** NYCTALOPIA. **receptor a.** Reduced vision attributable to faulty function of the retinal cones or rods. **strabismic a.** Suppression amblyopia due to long-standing strabismus. **suppression a.** A relatively irreversible cortical inhibition of the central vision of one eye, a cerebral extinction of a competing visual image, as may occur in strabismus or anisometropia, and persisting when the affected eye is used by itself. Also *lazy eye, amblyopia ex anopsia.* **tobacco-alcohol a.** Progressive visual deterioration in smokers of thick, dark, pipe tobacco, who often also drink alcohol in excess. It may be due to conditioned deficiency of vitamin $B_{12}$. **toxic a.** Defective vision attributable to a poison. **West Indian a.** Progressive bilateral visual impairment with optic atrophy occurring in the West Indies. The cause is uncertain, but thought to be toxic (dietary cyanide intake) or nutritional (vitamin $B_{12}$ deficiency) or both.

**amblyoscope** \am′blē·əskōp′\ [AMBLY- + *o* + -SCOPE] An orthoptic instrument that can present visual objects at different angles of convergence and divergence, useful in evaluation of patients with ocular muscle imbalance.

**ambo** \am′bō\ AMBON.

**ambo-** \am′bō-\ [L *ambo* (adjective) both, two] A prefix meaning both.

**amboceptor** \-sep′tər\ [AMBO- + *(re)ceptor* (from L *captus,* past part. of *capere* to take) a receiver] Any hemolysin that binds complement. *Seldom used.* Also *desmon.*

**Ambodryl** A proprietary name for bromodiphenhydramine hydrochloride

**ambomycin** An antibiotic obtained from *Streptomyces ambofaciens.* Also *duazomycin C* (outmoded).

**ambon** \am′bän\ [Gk *ambōn* a rising, edge of a dish, raised bottom as in a bottle, round hilltop, akin to L *umbo* boss of a shield] The annular fibrocartilaginous rim attached to the edge of articular sockets in which the heads of long bones fit. Examples are the labrum acetabulare and the labrum glenoidale. Also *ambo.*

**ambosexual** \-sek′shoo·əl\ AMBISEXUAL.

**ambulance** [French (from *ambul(ant)* without fixed residence, esp. as in *hôpital ambulant* field hospital; from L *am-*

*bulans,* gen. *ambulantis,* pres. part. of *ambulare* to walk; + *-ance* -ANCE), ambulance, provisional hospital] A motor vehicle or other means of transportation designed for rapid and medically assisted transfer of a patient to a hospital or other health treatment facility.

**ambulanceman** \am′byələnsman′\ (*pl.* ambulancemen) A medical technician trained to respond to medical emergencies. • The term is used in this sense in Britain and Australia and can refer to either the driver or the driver's associate. It is used also in India, where, however, it does not imply any training in meeting medical emergencies. In New Zealand, the term corresponding to the British sense is *ambulance officer* and in South Africa, *ambulance attendant,* a term sometimes also used in the United States, where such personnel within the medical community are more often called paramedics or, more formally, emergency medical technicians.

**ambulatory** \am′byələtôr′ē\ [L *ambulatorius* (from *ambulare* to walk) mobile, pertaining to walking] **1** Able to walk: used especially to distinguish patients who are not bed-ridden from those who are. Also *ambulant.* **2** Pertaining to ambulatory patients or to the process of walking.

**ambuphylline** $C_{11}H_{19}N_5O_3$. A theophylline compound with 2-amino-2-methyl-1-propanol, it is a drug with smooth muscle relaxant properties. It is used as a diuretic and as a bronchodilator. Also *bufylline, theophylline aminoisobutanol.*

**ameba** \əmē′bə\ [variant of *amoeba.* See AMOEBA.] (*pl.* amebas, amebae) A protozoan of the superclass Rhizopoda, characterized by a flexible membrane covering the body and movement and feeding by formation of pseudopodia. The typical amebas, members of the the order Amoebida, have a single nucleus and no flagellate stage or test. Also *amoeba.*

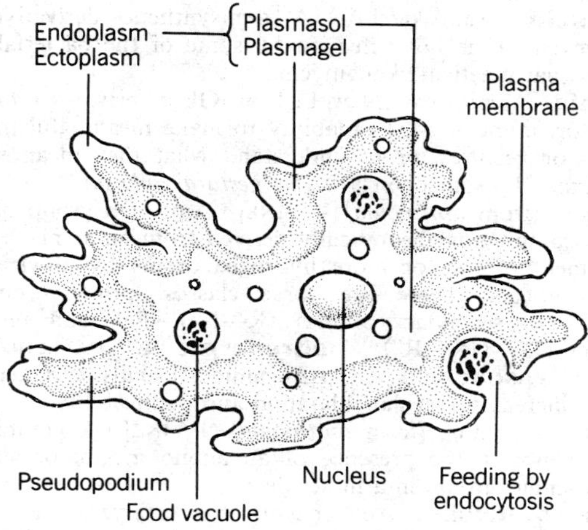


**Ameba**

**amebacidal** \əmē′bəsī′dəl\ AMEBICIDAL.

**amebacide** \əmē′bəsīd\ AMEBICIDE.

**amebaism** \əmē′bə·izm\ AMEBISM.

**amebiasis** \am′ēbī′əsis\ [*ameb(a)* + -IASIS] Infection with amebas, especially *Entamoeba histolytica,* presenting in man as an asymptomatic carrier state, as a moderate to severe colitis, or as extraintestinal amebic infection. Also *amebiosis, amebosis, amoebiasis.* **a. cutis** Amebiasis with penetration of the skin, usually an extension of an underlying infection, though it can occur at a site of direct contact. **hepatic a.** Amebiasis of the liver caused by *Entamoeba histolytica.* It usually, but not always, occurs with antecedent amebic dysentery. Hematogenous spread to the liver follows an intestinal infection and penetration of the mucosa. **intestinal a.** Infection of the intestine with a pathogenic ameba, usually *Entamoeba histolytica.* See also AMEBIC DYSENTERY. **pulmonary a.** Amebiasis involving principally the lung.

**amebic** \əmē′bik\ Relating to or caused by amebas. Also *amoebic.*

**amebicidal** \əmē′bisī′dəl\ Lethal to amebas. Also *amebacidal, amoebicidal.*

**amebicide** \əmē′bisīd\ [*ameb(a)* + *i* + -CIDE] A substance or agent that kills amebas. Also *amebacide, amoebicide.*

**amebiform** \əmē′bifôrm\ Like an ameba in shape. Also *amoebiform.*

**amebiosis** \am′ēbī-ō′sis\ AMEBIASIS.

**amebism** \am′ēbizm\ [*ameb(a)* + -ISM] Infection by amebas; amebiasis. Also *amebaism, amoebism.*

**amebocyte** \əmē′bōsīt\ [*ameb(a)* + *o* + -CYTE ] **1** An ameboid white blood cell found primarily in invertebrates. Also *amoebocyte.* **2** *Rare* LEUKOCYTE.

**ameboflagellate** \əmē′bōflaj′əlāt\ **1** Having ameboid and flagellated stages in the life cycle. **2** An ameba that has a flagellated stage in its life cycle.

**ameboid** \əmē′boid\ [*ameb(a)* + -OID] Resembling an ameba in shape or movement. Also *amoeboid.*

**ameboma** \am′ēbō′mə\ [*ameb(a)* + -OMA] A tumorlike mass of the colon caused by a chronic inflammatory reaction to intestinal amebiasis. Also *amoeboma.*

**amebosis** \am′ēbō′sis\ AMEBIASIS.

**ameiosis** \am′ī-ō′sis\ [Gk *a-* priv. + MEIOSIS] A cell division resulting in gametes without a reduction in the chromosome number.

**amelanotic** \ā′melənät′ik\ Without melanin.

**amelia** \əmē′lyə\ [Gk *a-* priv. + MEL-[1] + -IA] The congenital absence of one or more limbs. The normally associated pectoral or pelvic girdle is usually present but may be reduced. A fleshy tab is sometimes seen at the site of the missing limb. Also *ectromelia.* **brachial a.** ABRACHIA. **complete a.** TETRA-AMELIA. **unilateral brachial a.** MONOBRACHIA.

**amelification** \əmēl′ifikā′shən\ AMELOGENESIS.

**amelo-** \am′əlō-, əmel′ō-\ [obsol. English *amel* (from Old French *asmal, esmal;* see ENAMEL) enamel] A combining form denoting enamel.

**ameloblast** \əmel′ōblast\ [AMELO- + -BLAST] A tall, columnar epithelial cell of ectodermal origin located at the inner layer of the cup of the enamel organ. Each cell is responsible for the production of one enamel prism. Also *adamantoblast, ganoblast, enameloblast, enamel cell, emailloblast.*

**ameloblastoma** \əmel′ōblastō′mə\ [AMELOBLAST + -OMA] A benign but locally invasive neoplasm consisting of proliferating odontogenic epithelium in a fibrous stroma. It usually occurs in the mandible, sometimes in the maxilla. Typically, these are intraosseous tumors, but they may arise outside of the bone. A variety of histologic patterns have been described, such as follicular, plexiform, acanthomatous, basal cell, and granular cell. Most characteristic are islands of tumor cells with a peripheral layer of columnar cells resembling internal dental epithelium. Cyst formation is frequent. Also *adamantinoma, adamantinoblastoma* (obs.) . **malignant a.** An ameloblastoma in which metastases occur. This very rarely happens. Also *adamantinocarcinoma, ameloblastosarcoma.* **melanotic a.** MELANOTIC NEURO-

ECTODERMAL TUMOR. **pituitary a.** CRANIOPHARYNGIOMA.

**ameloblastosarcoma** \-blas′tōsärkō′mə\ MALIGNANT AMELOBLASTOMA.

**amelogenesis** \-jen′əsis\ [AMELO- + GENESIS] The formation of enamel. It is carried out by the ameloblasts of the enamel organ, which is part of the tooth germ. Initially a matrix is laid down which is partially calcified in a short time. Complete calcification takes place over a much longer period by the process of maturation. Also *amelification, enamelogenesis.* **a. imperfecta** Hereditary defective mineralization of enamel, quickly worn away by mastication. Also *hereditary brown enamel, hereditary brown hypoplasia of enamel, enamel dysplasia.*

**amenia** \əmē′nē·ə\ [Gk *a-* priv. + *mēn* month + -IA] AMENORRHEA.

**amenorrhea** \əmen′ôrē′ə\ [New L, from Gk *a-* priv. + MENO- + -RRHEA] Absence of menstrual bleeding. Also *amenia, menostaxis.* Adj. amenorrheal. **functional a.** Amenorrhea related to a physiologic condition, such as pregnancy. **hypothalamic a.** Absence of menses stemming from a hypothalamic disorder associated with failure of luteinizing hormone-releasing hormone. **lactation a.** Absence of menses associated with the secretion of milk. **ovarian a.** Absence of menses due to primary failure or disease of the ovaries, as in menopause, gonadal dysgenesis, or polycystic ovarian disease. **physiologic a.** Absence of menses not caused by a disease, as during pregnancy or lactation. **pituitary a.** Absence of menses caused by failure of anterior pituitary secretion or release of follicle stimulating hormone and/or luteinizing hormone. **premenopausal a.** Skipping of menstrual cycles, which may precede the menopause. **primary a.** Failure of menstruation to occur by the age of 16–18. **secondary a.** Cessation of menses for at least three months in a woman who has previously had her menarche. **traumatic a.** Cessation of menses by blockage of the cervical canal or by intrauterine adhesions.

**amenorrhoea** \əmen′ôrē′ə\ *Brit.* AMENORRHEA.

**amentia** \əmen′shə\ [L *amens,* gen. *amentis,* insane + -IA] Intellectual subnormality present since birth or very early in an individual's life; mental retardation. **nevoid a.** STURGE-WEBER SYNDROME. **phenylpyruvic a.** A severe form of mental retardation which results from a genetically transmitted metabolic disorder, namely the lack of an enzyme needed for the normal oxidation of phenylalanine, an amino acid found in most ordinary diets.

**americium** A transuranic element of atomic number 95, produced by neutron bombardment of uranium and plutonium. Symbol: Am

**Amerindian** \am′ərin′dē·ən\ Pertaining to, or a member of, the indigenous peoples of the Americas (excluding the Eskimos), characterized by reddish brown to yellowish brown skin color, straight black hair, sometimes epicanthic folds, and a variety of Mongoloid skeletal features.

**ameristic** \am′əris′tik\ Characterized by lack of segmentation.

**ametabolous** \am′ətab′ōləs\ Developing without undergoing metamorphosis: said chiefly of certain insects.

**amethopterin** METHOTREXATE.

**ametria** \əmē′trē·ə\ [Gk *a-* priv. + METR- + -IA] Agenesis of the uterus.

**ametrometer** \am′əträm′ətər\ [Gk *ametro(s)* (from *a-* priv. + *metron* measure) disproportionate, unequal + -METER] A device for measurement of the refractive error of the eye.

**ametropia** \am′ətrō′pē·ə\ [Gk *ametr(os)* (from *a-* priv. + *metron* measure) disproportionate, unequal + -OPIA] The failure to focus light accurately upon the retina without the aid of accommodation or optical aids. This condition includes hyperopia, myopia, and astigmatism. Adj. ametropic. **axial a.** A refractive error attributable to the anteroposterior length of the eye. **curvature a.** A refractive error attributable to the radius of curvature of a refractive surface of the eye. **index a.** A refractive error attributable to the index of refraction of the transparent ocular media.

**ametropic** \am′əträp′ik\ Marked by or pertaining to ametropia or refractive error.

**Amh** Mixed astigmatism with a larger myopic error than hyperopic.

**amicroscopic** \əmī′krəskäp′ik\ ULTRAMICROSCOPIC.

**amide** A substance formed by acylation of ammonia or of a primary or secondary amine. Usually the acyl group is derived from a carboxylic acid, but the name is sometimes used for derivatives of other acids. The peptide link in proteins is an amide bond.

**amidino** The group $NH_2$—C(=NH)—. Also *guanyl* (obs.).

**amidinotransferase** Any enzyme that transfers the amidino group —C(=NH)—$NH_2$. The most important such enzyme is glycine amidinotransferase, which is responsible for a step in the biosynthesis of creatine. Also *transamidinase.*

**amido-** [from *am(monia)* + *-id(e)* + *o*] A combining form indicating the presence of an amide group in a molecule. • *Amido-* has sometimes been used incorrectly in the past in place of *amino-*.

**amidoazotoluene** $C_{14}H_{15}N_3$. *o*-Amino-azo-toluene. A carcinogenic red dye derived from scarlet red, formerly used to promote regeneration of epithelium.

**amidopyrine** AMINOPYRINE.

**amikacin** \am′əkā′sin\ A semisynthetic derivative of kanamycin. It is not acted on by some of the bacterial enzymes that inactivate kanamycin.

**amimia** \əmim′yə\ [New L, from Gk *a-* priv. + *mim(os)* imitator, mime + -IA] Inability to make meaningful movements or gestures, or to understand what they mean when performed by someone else. Also *gestural aphasia.*

**amine** [from *am(monia)* + -INE] Any of a group of organic compounds theoretically derived from ammonia by replacement of one or more hydrogen atoms by alkyl, aryl, etc., radicals. There are three classes: primary amines (R—$NA_2$), secondary amines (R—NH—R′), and tertiary amines (R′—NR—R″). **adrenergic a.** CATECHOLAMINE. **vasoactive a.** Any amine, usually endogenous, which increases vascular dilatation and permeability.

**-amine** \-əmin\ [from *am(monia)* + -INE] A combining form denoting the presence of an amino group, or substituted amino group, in a molecule.

**amine oxidase** Any enzyme that catalyzes the oxidation of amines. Such enzymes include those responsible for the inactivation of catecholamine neurotransmitters. There are two main types: the flavin-containing one (EC 1.4.3.4), traditionally known as monoamine oxidase, which acts on primary amines, and also on secondary and tertiary amines with small substituents; and the copper-containing one (EC 1.4.3.6), which acts on primary amines, including diamines. The former is associated with the outer mitochondrial membrane and is often used as a marker for the outer membrane in mitochondrial fraction studies.

**amino** \əmē′nō\ The chemical group —$NH_2$.

**amino-** \əmē′nō\ [from AMINE] A combining form denoting the presence of the group —$NH_2$ in a molecule, which is therefore an amine.

**aminoacetic acid** See under GLYCINE.

**amino acid** Any acid containing an amino group; usually, in biologic contexts, an α-amino carboxylic acid, R—CH(—$NH_2$)—COOH, unless otherwise specified. Especially important are the 20 different amino acids that can be incorporated into proteins. **aromatic a.** **1** Those amino acids that contain an aromatic ring and are incorporated into proteins, namely phenylalanine, tyrosine, tryptophan, and histidine. **2** Any amino acid containing an aromatic ring. **basic a.'s** Amino acids that carry a positive charge at neutral pH, and whose isoelectric forms contain basic groups. Of the 20 common amino acids, arginine, lysine, and histidine are the basic ones. **essential a.** Any of the amino acids that must be supplied in the diet to maintain health or nitrogen balance when all other amino acids of the 20 incorporated in proteins are present in excess. **ketogenic a.** Any amino acid that increases the excretion of ketone bodies when administered to animals, usually dogs, whose kidneys have been damaged by phloridzin treatment. Amino acids were classed as ketogenic or glucogenic to obtain indications about their routes of catabolism. The ketogenic ones are those that form acetyl-CoA. **a. residue** The residue that remains of an amino-acid molecule when it is in peptide combination. In a protein the residue derived from an amino acid of formula $NH_3^+$—CHR—$COO^-$ will have the formula —NH—CHR—CO— if it is internal, and $NH_3^+$—CHR—CO— or —NH—CHR—$COO^-$ if it is terminal. **a. sequence** The linear order of amino acids in a peptide or protein, usually specified beginning with the N-terminus. Determination of this sequence defines the covalent structure of a protein, which in turn is believed to specify its folding. **sulfur-containing a.'s** Usually, the amino acids cysteine and methionine, which are incorporated into proteins, and cystine, the oxidation product of the former, which is found especially in extracellular proteins. **uncoded a.** An amino acid other than one of the twenty that can be incorporated into proteins because they are coded for by mRNA.

**D-amino acids** Amino acids of dextral configuration. They are not found in proteins but are found in simpler bacterial polypeptides, such as some antibiotics and the peptidoglycan.

**amino acid decarboxylase** An enzyme catalyzing the reaction: R—CH($NH_2$)COOH $\rightleftharpoons$ R—$CH_2$—$NH_2$ + $CO_2$. Such enzymes often contain pyridoxal phosphate and are involved in the biosynthesis of histamine, epinephrine, spermine, and many other derivatives of the amino acids.

**aminoacidemia** \-as′idē′mē·ə\ An abnormal increase in concentration of amino acids in the plasma or serum.

**aminoacidopathy** \-as′idäp′əthē\ [AMINO ACID + *o* + -PATHY] A disease state in which amino acids are excreted in abnormal amounts in the urine. It is due to a defective enzymatic step in the metabolism of the amino acid or acids involved, or a defect in a mediator necessary for cellular transport of the amino acid or acids involved.

**L-amino acid oxidase** An enzyme (EC 1.4.3.2) that oxidizes an L-amino acid by dioxygen to form a 2-oxoacid, ammonia, and hydrogen peroxide. It is a flavoprotein and occurs in, for example, snake venom.

**aminoaciduria** \-as′idoo′rē·ə\ [AMINO ACID + -URIA] An excessive amount of amino acids excreted in the urine. This may involve increased excretion of a single amino acid, a group of :elated amino acids, or amino acids in general, as in the Fanconi syndrome or in tubular lesions. **imidazole a.** The urinary excretion of imidazole dipeptides, especially anserine and carnosine. Small amounts are normally excreted, but increased levels of excretion are characteristic of individuals on high protein diets and those with certain disorders of renal transport and amino acid metabolism. **overflow a.** An enzymatic deficiency in renal tubule cells which reduces the tubular secretion of one or more amino acids, and which leads to an accumulation of the amino acids in blood. This, in turn, results in increased amounts filtered by the glomeruli, and therefore, increased urinary excretion. **renal a.** The excessive urinary excretion of one or more amino acids due to decreased tubular reabsorption. The concentration of the pertinent amino acids in blood may be normal or decreased. Also *transport aminoaciduria*. **transport a.** RENAL AMINOACIDURIA.

**aminoacyl** Usually 2-aminoacyl, the group R—CH($NH_2$)—CO—. Amino acids are incorporated into proteins by reacting initially with ATP to form an enzyme-bound aminoacyl-AMP (the aminoacyl group is on the phosphate group of the AMP) and this group is then passed onto transfer RNA. Elongation of the growing protein chain occurs by acylation of the aminoacyl-tRNA by the peptidyl group from peptidyl-tRNA.

**aminoacyl adenylate** Adenosine 5′-phosphate carrying an aminoacyl group on its phosphate group. It is in nature an acid anhydride. Such compounds are enzyme-bound intermediates in the synthesis of aminoacyl-tRNA by amino-acid-tRNA ligases (aminoacyl-tRNA synthetases). They are formed by the action of an amino acid with ATP by release of diphosphate (pyrophosphate), and they can transfer the aminoacyl group onto O-2′ or O-3′ of the terminal adenosine group of tRNA.

**aminoacyl-tRNA** A transfer RNA carrying an aminoacyl group on adenosine of its terminal adenylate residue. Such groups pass freely between atoms O-2′ and O-3′. In protein biosynthesis a peptidyl group on one molecule of tRNA is transferred onto the amino group of an aminoacyl-tRNA to lengthen the chain by one residue.

**aminoacyl-tRNA synthetase** Any enzyme that catalyzes the formation of aminoacyl-tRNA, AMP, and diphosphate (pyrophosphate) from an amino acid, ATP, and tRNA. There is at least one such enzyme for each of the twenty amino acids incorporated into proteins. The fidelity of protein synthesis depends on their specificity, since the mRNA specifies the amino acid by recognizing a trinucleotide sequence in the tRNA. Such enzymes are classed as EC 6.1.1.

***p*-aminobenzoic acid** 4-Aminobenzoic acid, a constituent of folic acid. It antagonizes the action of the sulfonamide drugs because these compete with it in the reactions by which bacteria make folic acid. It is an essential growth factor for those bacteria unable to synthesize it for the production of folic acid. Deficiency has never been described in humans, but it causes graying of the hair in rats. Abbr. PABA

**γ-aminobutyric acid** $NH_3^+$—$[CH_2]_3$—$COO^-$. A neurotransmitter in arthropods and possibly in mammals. It is present in mammalian brain tissue and is also formed by plants. Formed from glutamate by glutemate decarboxylase, it can donate its amino group by transamination, forming 4-oxobutyrate (succinic semialdehyde), which can in turn be metabolized by being oxidized to succinate. Abbr. GABA

**ε-aminocaproic acid** $NH_2(CH_2)_5COOH$. 6-Aminohexanoic acid. A water-soluble substance that inhibits plasmin and plasminogen activators, and thus may be used to prevent or retard fibrinolysis.

**aminocyclitol** **1** A hydroaromatic ring, with free or substituted amino groups, present in aminoglycoside antibiotics and in spectinomycin. **2** The group of antibiotics containing this ring.

**2-aminoethanol** $NH_2$—$CH_2$—$CH_2OH$. A constituent of phospholipids and the decarboxylation product of serine. It is formed by decarboxylation of serine and is a component of phospholipids and a precursor of choline. Also *glycinol, ethanolamine* (trivial name).

**aminoglutaric acid** GLUTAMIC ACID.

**aminoglycoside** 1 A glycoside of an aminosugar. 2 A major group of bactericidal antibiotics, containing an aminocyclitol (with two amino or guanidino groups) and one or more aminosugars. They are effective against various Gram-positive and Gram-negative bacteria and also *Mycobacterium tuberculosis.* They act by causing misreading and blockade of protein synthesis on bacterial ribosomes. Examples include streptomycin, kanamycin, paromomycin, gentamicin, and neomycin.

***p*-aminohippuric acid** $C_9H_{10}N_2O_3$. A compound, usually given intravenously in the form of its sodium salt, used to measure the effectiveness of renal plasma flow and the functional capacity of renal tubular excretion. Abbr. PAH, PAHA

***p*-aminohippuric acid synthethase** A liver enzyme that catalyzes the formation of *p*-aminohippuric acid from *p*-aminobenzoic acid and glycine.

**aminohydroxybenzoic acid** AMINOSALICYLIC ACID.

**$\beta$-aminoisobutyricaciduria** \əmē′nō-i′sōbyootir′ik-as′idoo′rē-ə\ The excessive urinary excretion of the non-protein amino acid $\beta$-aminoisobutyrate. Inherited as an autosomal recessive trait, the condition by itself is clinically benign. Increased excretion may also be associated with certain leukemias and in hyperbetaalaninemia, in which specific interference with renal tubular transport occurs.

**aminoisocaproic acid** *Obs.* LEUCINE.

**$\delta$-aminolevulinic acid** $NH_2$—$CH_2$—CO—$CH_2$—$CH_2$—COOH. 5-Amino-4-oxovaleric acid. It is made from succinyl-CoA and glycine by an enzyme that contains pyridoxal phosphate, and is an intermediate in the biosynthesis of porphyrins and related compounds.

**2-amino-6-mercaptopurine** THIOGUANINE.

**aminometradine** $C_9H_{13}N_3O_2$. 6-Amino-3-ethyl-1-(2-propenyl)-2,4-(1*H*,3*H*)-pyrimidinedione, a uracil derviative that is given orally to treat edema from congestive heart failure and other causes through its effective diuretic properties.

**6-aminopenicillanic acid** A precursor of penicillin. It accumulates instead of penicillin in media deficient in sources for side chain, or it may be formed by treating penicillin with an amidase. Semisynthetic penicillins are made by acylating the amino group of this compound. Symbol: 6-APA

**aminopeptidase** An enzyme that hydrolyzes the peptide bond between the amino-acid residue that bears a free amino group and the rest of the molecule of a peptide or protein substrate.

**aminophenylstibinic acid** $C_6H_9NO_3Sb$. 4-Aminobenzenestibonic acid. An organic antimony compound that has been used in the treatment of kala-azar.

**aminophylline** THEOPHYLLINE ETHYLENEDIAMINE.

**aminopterin** An analogue of pteroylglutamic acid. It has an amino group on C-4 of the pterin ring in place of the (potential) hydroxyl group of the natural compound. It inhibits dihydrofolate reductase and is used in the chemotherapy of leukemia.

**aminopyrine** $C_{13}H_{17}N_3O$. 4-(Dimethylamino)-1,2-dihydro-1,5-dimethyl-2-phenyl-3*H*-pyrazol-3-one, an effective analgesic and antipyretic agent. Although it is commonly used in Europe, it has not been approved for use in the U.S. because it occasionally causes agranulocytosis. Also *amidopyrine.*

**aminoquinoline** The 4-aminoquinolines and 8-aminoquinolines that represent two major classes of important antimalarial drugs. Examples are chloroquine, pentaquine, and primaquine.

**aminosalicylic acid** $C_7H_7NO_3$. *p*-Aminosalicylic acid, used as a bacteriostatic agent in the treatment of tuberculosis. Also *aminohydroxybenzoic acid.*

**aminosis** \am′inō′sis\ [*amin(o)* + -OSIS] The excessive production of amino acid by the body.

**aminosugar** A monosaccharide in which one of the hydroxyl groups, usually the one on C-2 of an aldose, is replaced by an amino group, e.g. glucosamine.

**amino-terminal** N-TERMINAL.

**aminotransferase** Any enzyme that transfers amino groups. It is usually one catalyzing the reaction R—CH($NH_2$)COOH + R′—CO—COOH ⇌ R—CO—COOH + R′—CH($NH_2$)COOH. Such enzymes normally contain pyridoxal phosphate and are important in protein catabolism. Also *transaminase.*

**amisometradine** $C_9H_{13}N_3O_2$. 6-Amino-3-methyl-1-(2-methyl-2-propenyl)-2,4(1*H*,3*H*)-pyrimidinedione, an orally active diuretic agent that is closely related chemically to aminometradine.

**amitosis** \am′itō′sis\ [A-[1] + MITOSIS] Cell division in which the nuclear material is divided by direct division. The events associated with chromosome formation and movement are not observed. Also *Remak's nuclear division, holoschisis.* Adj. amitotic.

**ammeter** \am′ətər\ [*am(pere)* + -METER] An instrument calibrated to measure the magnitude of electric current in amperes.

**ammine** \am′īn\ Ammonia as a neutral ligand in a complex, such as hexamminecobalt (3+) for $Co(NH_3)_6^{3+}$.

**Ammon** [Friedrich August von *Ammon,* German ophthalmologist and pathologist, 1799–1861] Ammon's operation. See under DACRYOCYSTOTOMY.

**ammonemia** \am′ōnē′mē-ə\ HYPERAMMONEMIA.

**ammonia** \amō′nē-ə\ [*(sal) ammonia(c),* so named from being obtainable from camel dung near temple of Jupiter *Ammon*] $NH_3$. An easily liquefied gas, of boiling point −33°C. The liquid is an ionizing solvent like water. In water ammonia is a weak base, of p*K* 9.3. Many biologic reactions involve it, one of the most important being the reaction of glutamate dehydrogenase: $H^+$ + $NH_3$ + NAD(P)H + 2-oxoglutarate ⇌ glutamate + $NAD(P)^+$. This reaction allows the synthesis and probably the breakdown of glutamate. Ammonia can be converted in the liver into carbamoyl phosphate for incorporation into urea. In the blood it is highly toxic.

**ammonia hemate** ALUM HEMATOXYLIN.

**ammonia-lyase** An enzyme that catalyzes the dissociation of a substrate into ammonia and another product. It usually acts on an amino acid of structure R—$CH_2$—CH($NH_2$)COOH, such as histidine or phenylalanine, to produce $NH_3$ and R—CH=CH—COOH.

**ammonification** \əmō′nifikā′shən\ The formation or release of ammonia by the decomposition of proteins.

**ammonio-** \amō′nē-ō-\ [from *ammonium*] A combining form signifying the group $NH_3^+$—.

**ammonium** [*ammoni(a)* + New L *-ium,* noun suffix] The ion $NH_4^+$ or its substituted derivatives.

**ammonium carbonate** A solid of variable composition, comprising not only the carbonate of ammonia, $(NH_4)_2CO_3$, but also the carbamate, $NH_4^+NH_2$—$CO_2^-$. It is obtained from solutions of ammonia and carbon dioxide containing an excess of ammonia. As it picks up moisture from the air it gives off ammonia. It has been used to give controlled sniffs of ammonia to revive someone who had fainted. Also *sal volatile, smelling salts.*

**ammonium chloride** $NH_4Cl$. A colorless or white crystalline salt, given orally to produce acidification of the urine. Also *sal ammoniac* (obs.).

**ammonium ichthyosulfonate** ICHTHAMMOL.

**ammonium oxalate crystal violet** A metachromatic stain used for the demonstration of amyloid. The addition of ammonium oxalate is said to enhance the metachromatic effect of the crystal violet.

**ammonium sulfate** $(NH_4)_2SO_4$. It is a highly soluble salt (2.1 M) often used in protein purification. Most proteins change solubility very rapidly with increasing ammonium sulfate concentration, so that much of each protein precipitates over a narrow range of increasing salt concentration. Since this range differs for different proteins, such precipitation can achieve good separation.

**ammotherapy** \am′ōther′əpē\ PSAMMOTHERAPY.

**amnesia** \amnē′zhə\ [Gk *amnēsia* (from *a-* priv. + root of *mnēsasthai* to remember) forgetfulness] Partial or complete loss of memory. This may occur as a result of brain injury, of focal cerebral lesions, and of many forms of organic cerebral dysfunction, but it may also be hysterical. Adj. amnesic, amnestic. **affective a.** ELECTIVE AMNESIA. **anterograde a.** Loss of memory for events occurring after the head injury or incident which caused the condition. Also *post-traumatic amnesia.* **auditory a.** Inability to recall or understand the meaning of spoken words; a form of word deafness. **Broca's a.** Inability to remember spoken words. *Seldom used.* **circumscribed a.** Amnesia in which the boundaries of the time for which memory is lost are precisely delineated. **elective a.** Forgetfulness with regard to certain specific facts, brought about by subconscious repression of memory; a form of hysterical amnesia. Also *affective amnesia.* **graphokinetic a.** Loss of memory of writing movements, leading to agraphia. **hysterical a.** Amnesia resulting not from organic brain disease or dysfunction but from hysteria, and consequent upon a subconscious desire to escape from a stressful situation. The patient usually loses all sense of time, place, and personal identity but may seem outwardly normal. **immunologic a.** Loss of a previously established immune response. **incomplete a.** LACUNAR AMNESIA. **lacunar a.** Inability to recall events occurring in certain isolated episodes. Also *incomplete amnesia, patchy amnesia.* **localized a.** Amnesia for events connected with a certain place, time or incident. **mimokinetic a.** Loss of memory for gestures, leading to amimia. **olfactory a.** Inability to recall or recognize smells. **organic a.** Any amnesia due to organic brain disease. **patchy a.** LACUNAR AMNESIA. **posthypnotic a.** The inability of a hypnotic subject to recall, after being awakened from the hypnotic state, the suggestions or commands given during the hypnotic trance. **post-traumatic a.** ANTEROGRADE AMNESIA. **retroactive a.** RETROGRADE AMNESIA. **retrograde a.** Loss of memory for events occurring prior to the injury or incident which caused the condition. Also *retroactive amnesia.* **systematic a.** Inability to remember a specific group of ideas. **tactile a.** TACTILE AGNOSIA. **transient global a.** A stereotyped clinical syndrome of abrupt onset in middle-aged or elderly subjects, believed to be due to temporal lobe ischemia. There is total loss of memory with inability to record new impressions but with retention of the sense of personal identity, usually lasting for about 24 hours and usually followed by complete recovery. **traumatic a.** Loss of memory due to a head injury. **verbal a.** Inability to remember or recognize written or printed words. It is a form of visual agnosia. **visual a.** **1** Inability to recognize an object or person previously seen. **2** Inability to identify a written word.

**amnesiac** \amnē′sē·ak\ A person suffering from amnesia.

**amnesic** \amnē′sik\ Causing or suffering from amnesia. Also *amnestic, letheral.*

**amnestic** \amnes′tik\ AMNESIC.

**amnio-** \am′nē·ō-\ [Gk *amnion* (dim. of *amnos* lamb) bowl in which blood of victims was caught] A combining form denoting the amnion.

**amniocardiac** \-kär′dē·ak\ [AMNIO- + CARDIAC] Concerning the embryonic heart and coelom.

**amniocele** \am′nē·əsēl′\ [AMNIO- + -CELE[1]] Failure of closure of the anterior abdominal wall during intrauterine development. The intestines protrude into the amniotic cavity covered only by a thin peritoneal membrane. After birth, the condition in the neonate is called omphalocele.

**amniocentesis** \-sentē′sis\ [AMNIO- + -CENTESIS] A procedure in which a needle is placed transabdominally into the amniotic cavity in order to remove fluid for analysis, instill solutions that will induce abortion, or infuse dyes for radiographic studies.

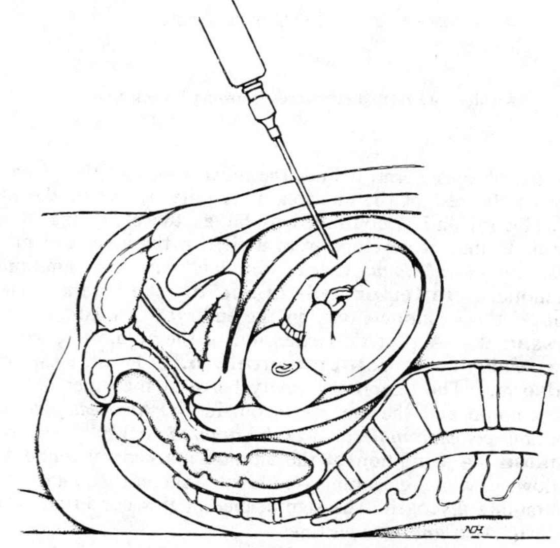

**Amniocentesis** (performed at 15 weeks)

**amnioclepsis** \-klep′sis\ [AMNIO- + Gk *klep(sō),* fut. of *kleptein* to steal, + -SIS] Leakage of amniotic fluid, usually gradual and often unnoticed.

**amniogenesis** \-jen′əsis\ [AMNIO- + GENESIS] The process of formation of the amnion.

**amniography** \am′nē·äg′rəfē\ [AMNIO- + -GRAPHY] A radiologic method for the examination of the amniotic cavity by making radiographs after the injection of a radiopaque agent into the amniotic sac.

**amnioma** \am′nē·ō′mə\ [*amni(on)* + -OMA] A tumor of the amnion.

**amnion** \am′nē·än\ [Gk (dim. of *amnos* lamb), a bowl in which blood of victims was caught, the membrane around a fetus] The thin, transparent, tough membrane lining the fluid-filled cavity which contains the embryo of reptiles, birds, and mammals (amniotes). Made of ectoderm and

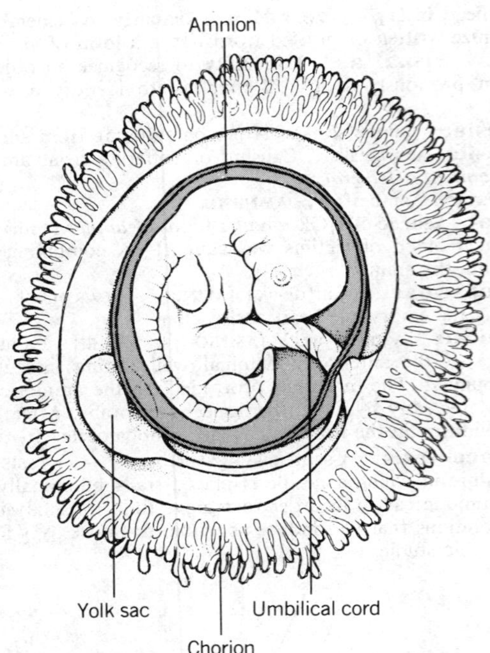


**Amnion and related structures** (showing 5-week embryo)

backed by mesoderm, it lines the inner aspect of the placenta and of the rest of the chorion. It is reflected on to the umbilical cord and is continued as far as the epidermis of the navel. In man it develops from a cleft in the inner cell mass. Also *amnioembryonic vesicle, amniotic sac.* Adj. amnionic, amniotic. **anterior cul-de-sac a.** An anterior extension of the amniotic cavity in the embryo. **caudal cul-de-sac a.** A posterior extension of the amniotic cavity in the embryo. **ectoplacental a.** FALSE AMNION. **false a.** The temporary cavity between the inner layer of the amnion and the mesoderm outside it. Also *ectoplacental amnion, ectoplacental cavity, false amniotic cavity.* **a. nodosum** A condition of the amnion marked by numerous, yellowish white elevations made of adherent squames and containing glycogen. The significance of this condition is unknown. Also *amniotic pustules.*

**amnionitis** \-nī′tis\ [AMNION + -ITIS] Infection or inflammation involving the amnion.

**Amnioplastin** \-plas′tin\ A prepared amniotic membrane used particularly in neurosurgery to minimize adhesions. A proprietary name.

**amnioscope** \am′nē·əskōp′\ [AMNIO- + -SCOPE] An instrument, usually cone-shaped, which is passed transcervically to lie against the fetal membranes in order to note the character and color of the underlying ammniotic fluid.

**amnioscopy** \am′nē·äs′kəpē\ Observation of the character and color of the amniotic fluid through the use of an amnioscope.

**amniotic** \am′nē·ät′ik\ Pertaining to or developing on or from the amnion, as *amniotic fluid.*.

**Amniotin** A preparation of estrogens obtained from the urine of pregnant mares.

**amniotomy** \am′nē·ät′əmē\ [AMNIO- + -TOMY] The process of puncturing the fetal membranes.

**amobarbital** $C_{11}H_{18}N_2O_3$. 5-Ethyl-5-isopentylbarbituric acid. A barbiturate used as a sedative and hypnotic. Also *amylobarbitone, isoamylethylbarbituric acid.*

**amodiaquin dihydrochloride dihydrate** $C_{20}H_{24}Cl_3N_3O$. 7-Chloro-4-(3-diethyl-aminomethyl-4-hydroxyanilino)quinoline dihydrochloride dihydrate, an antimalarial agent with properties that are similar to those of chloroquine.

***Amoeba*** \əmē′bə\ [New L, from Gk *amoibē*, a change, exchange] A genus of amebas in the order Amoebida, suborder Tubulina. Various medically significant species were originally grouped together in this genus but have been reclassified and assigned to a number of different genera. ***A. buccalis*** *ENTAMOEBA GINGIVALIS.* ***A. coli*** *ENTAMOEBA COLI.* ***A. dentalis*** *ENTAMOEBA GINGIVALIS.* ***A. dysenteriae*** *ENTAMOEBA HISTOLYTICA* ***A. histolytica*** *ENTAMOEBA HISTOLYTICA* ***A. proteus*** An abundant free-living species found in fresh water, noted for the number and variety of shapes of its pseudopodia. It is often used in laboratory studies.

**amoeba** \əmē′bə\ [New L. See *AMOEBA*. (*pl.* amoebae, amoebas) AMEBA.

**amoebiasis** \am′ēbī′əsis\ [*amoeb(a)* + -IASIS] AMEBIASIS.

**amoebic** \əmē′bik\ AMEBIC.

**Amoebida** \əmē′bidə\ [*Amoeb(a)* + *-ida*, suffix designating a taxonomic order] An order of protozoa (superclass Rhizopoda, class Lobosea) including free-living amebas in soil and water and those found as commensals and parasites of animals and man.

**amoebiform** \əmē′bifôrm′\ AMEBIFORM.

**amoebism** \am′ēbizm\ AMEBISM.

**amoebocyte** \əmē′bəsīt\ **1** AMEBOCYTE. **2** *Rare* LEUKOCYTE.

**amoeboid** \əmē′boid\ AMEBOID.

**amoeboma** \am′ēbō′mə\ AMEBOMA.

**amorph** \əmôrf′\ AMORPHIC GENE.

**amorphagnosis** \əmôr′fagnō′sis\ AMORPHOGNOSIA.

**amorphic** \əmôr′fik\ Of or relating to a gene that produces either no product or a nonfunctional one.

**amorphinism** \əmôr′finizm\ [Gk *a-* priv. + MORPHINISM] The state produced by morphine deprivation in a morphine addict.

**amorphognosia** \əmôr′fägnō′zhə\ [Gk *a-* priv. + MORPHO- + *(a)gnosia*] A form of agnosia marked by difficulty in recognizing the shape of objects. Also *amorphosynthesis, amorphagnosis.*

**amorphosynthesis** \əmôr′fōsin′thəsis\ [Gk *a-* priv. + MORPHOSYNTHESIS] AMORPHOGNOSIA.

**amorphous** \əmôr′fəs\ [Gk *amorphos* without form, from *a-* priv. + *morphē* form] Without definite form: used especially of solid substances that lack crystalline structure.

**amorphus** \əmôr′fəs\ [New L (from Gk *amorphos* shapeless)] An embryo or fetus which lacks the external features characteristic of its species. The heart is usually absent.

**amotio** \amō′shō\ [L (from *amotus*, past part. of *amovere* to remove from a place), a removing] A removal or detachment. **a. retinae** RETINAL DETACHMENT.

**amount** / **catalytic a.** The amount of substance used in a chemical reaction for catalytic purposes, expressed in katals or moles per second. Symbol: *z* **a. of substance** The physical quantity proportional to the number of specified elementary entities of a substance. These entities may be atoms, molecules, ions, electrons, photons, etc., or any specified group of such particles. The SI base unit of amount of substance is the mole, and its symbol is *n*.. **a. of substance concentration** The amount of substance of a solute divided by the volume of the solution, often expressed as mol/l though the preferred SI usage is mol/m$^3$. Symbol: $C_B$

**amoxacillin** \əmäk′səsil′in\ A semisynthetic penicillin, with *p*-hydroxyphenylglycine substituted on the 6-aminopenicillanic acid nucleus. It is active against many Gram-negative bacteria.

**AMP** 1 adenosine monophosphate. 2 average mean pressure.

**ampere** \am′pir\ [after André Maria *Ampère*, French physicist and writer, 1775–1836] The SI base unit of electric current. That constant current which, if maintained in two straight parallel conductors of infinite length, of negligible circular cross-section, and placed one meter apart in vacuum, would produce between these conductors a force equal to $2 \times 10^{-7}$ newton per meter of length. Symbol: A • The symbol *amp* is often but incorrectly used. **a. per kilogram** An alternative SI derived unit of radiation exposure rate, identical with coulomb per kilogram second. Symbol: A/kg, A·kg$^{-1}$

**ampere-second** \am′pir\ COULOMB. Symbol: A·s

**amperometry** \am′piräm′ətrē\ A titration method of determining solute concentration by measuring electric current generated in the medium.

**amphetamine** $C_9H_{13}N$. (+)-α-Methylbenzeneethanamine, a racemic mixture of dextroamphetamine and levamphetamine. The mixture of isomers has the capability of strong central nervous system stimulation, but chronic use may lead to tolerance and physical dependence.

**amphetamine sulfate** $(C_9H_{13}N)_2{\cdot}H_2SO_4$. A white, crystalline powder with a slightly bitter taste, used as a central nervous system stimulant. Because of its potential for abuse and dependency, it is a Schedule II drug under the Controlled Substances Act of 1970.

**amphi-** \am′fē-, am′fə-\ [Gk *amphi* on both sides, around] A prefix meaning both, on both sides, around. For words beginning *amphi-*, see also under AMPHO-.

**amphiarthrodial** \-ärthrō′dē·əl\ Pertaining to a cartilaginous joint.

**amphiarthrosis** \-ärthrō′sis\ [AMPHI- + Gk *arthrōsis* jointing, articulation] *Outmoded* ARTICULATIO CARTILAGINEA.

**amphiaster** \-as′tər\ A figure formed by two asters and the connecting spindle, observed during mitosis or meiosis. Also *diaster, dyaster.*

**amphibolic** \-bäl′ik\ 1 Ambiguous; uncertain. Also *amphibolous.* 2 Referring to a metabolic intermediate, or a pathway, that can act in either anabolic or catabolic processes.

**amphidesmous** \-dez′məs\ Possessing a double ligament. Also *amphidesmic.*

**amphidiarthrosis** \-dī′ärthrō′sis\ [*amphi(arthrosis)* + DIARTHROSIS] The temporomandibular joint, previously conceived as combining the movements of a ginglymus joint and an arthrodial joint. Also *amphidiarthrodial joint.*

**amphidiploid** \-dip′loid\ ALLOTETRAPLOID.

**amphigastrula** \-gas′troolə\ [AMPHI- + GASTRULA] A gastrula in which the upper and lower halves are composed of cells of unequal size.

**amphigenesis** \-jen′əsis\ [*amph(o)-* + *i* + GENESIS] The ability to have heterosexual relations when one's preference is predominantly homosexual.

**amphigony** \amfig′ənē\ [AMPHI- + -GONY] SEXUAL REPRODUCTION.

**amphikaryon** \-kar′ē·än\ [AMPHI- + Gk *karyon* a nut, nucleus] A diploid nucleus; nucleus containing two sets of chromosomes.

**amphimixis** \-mik′sis\ [AMPHI- + Gk *mixis* a mixing, mingling, sexual intercourse] Fusion of the female and male pronucleifollowing fertilization of an egg.

**amphimorula** \-môr′yələ\ [AMPHI- + MORULA] A morula in which the two halves are composed of cells of unequal size.

**amphinucleus** \-n$^y$oo′klē·əs\ A single-bodied nucleus containing a centrosome and spindle fibers surrounded by masses of chromatin. It is characteristic of the nucleus of many protozoans. Also *centronucleus.*

**amphistome** \am′fistōm\ [AMPHI- + English *-stome*, suffix denoting mouth, from Gk *stoma* mouth] A fluke with the acetabulum located at the posterior end, where it is usually enlarged. This morphological feature typifies members of the family Paramphistomatidae, formerly placed in the now obsolete genus *Amphistomum.*.

**amphitene** \am′fitēn\ [French *amphitène* (from Gk *amphi-* on both sides, around + *tain(ia)* a band, fillet) a pairing of chromosomes in meiosis] A stage of meiosis during which synapsis or chromosome pairing occurs. Homologous chromosomes pair and become twisted around one another. Pairing is initiated at one, or more, contact points and proceeds from these points along the chromosome.

**amphitheater** \-thē′ətər\ An operating room with a gallery of tiered seats for observers.

**amphitypy** \amfit′ipē\ The condition of being characteristic of two discrete types.

**ampho-** \am′fō-\ [Gk *amphō* (noun) both] A prefix meaning both.

**ampholyte** [AMPHO- + Gk *lyt(os)* (verbal of *lyein* to loose) that may be loosed] A substance whose molecules bear both positive and negative charges.

**amphomycin** An antimicrobial substance from *Streptomyces canus.* It has activity against Gram-positive bacteria and was used in ointments with neomycin and hydrocortisone to treat skin infections.

**amphophilic** \-fil′ik\ [AMPHO- + -PHILIC] Characterized by a similar tintorial affinity to basic and acid dyes. If hematoxylin and eosin are used, a structure so stained will appear neither blue nor pink but of a hue reflecting a variable combination of the two colors. Also *amphophile.* **a. -basophil** Readily stained by acid and basic dyes but preferring basic dyes. **a. -oxyphil** Readily stained by acid and basic dyes but preferring acid dyes.

**amphoric** \amfôr′ik\ [L *amphor(a)* (from Gk *amphoreus* a jar) a jar, vessel with handles, flask] Characterizing a sound likened to that produced by blowing air over the opening of a large bottle or jar. It is heard, for example, on auscultation over a lung cavity.

**amphoteric** \-ter′ik\ [Gk *amphoter(os)* either, both + -IC] 1 Having divergent or even opposite properties, such as the capacity of reacting in the presence of either acids or bases, or of behaving as either an acid or a base. 2 Reacting as an acid with bases and as a base with acids, as glycine, $NH_3^+{-}CH_2{-}CO_2^-$, which can donate $H^+$ from its $-NH_3^+$group and combine with $H^+$on its $-CO_2^-$ group.

**amphotericin** A mixture of antifungal compounds from certain strains of *Streptomyces nodosus.* It is used for the treatment of several types of fungal infections having either a cutaneous or general, systemic distribution. **a. B** A USP designated form of amphotericin, including a preparation suitable for administration by injection.

**ampicillin** A semisynthetic penicillin for oral and parenteral use, having the same antibiotic spectrum of activity as penicillin G. It is active against Gram-positive organisms, and even more effective against Gram-negative bacteria.

**amplification** \am′pləfəkā′shən\ An increasing of magnitude, as of voltage, power, acoustic intensity, or light intensity. **compression a.** Nonlinear amplification of acoustical input particularly at higher sound-pressure levels, so that a given increase does not result in the same increase of output but rather less. This is a common feature of modern hearing aids. **gene a.** Any process by which a gene is duplicated once or, more typically, many times in specific cells in response to defined developmental signals or environmental stresses. The functional consequence is an increased ability to transcribe RNA from the gene. For example, gene amplification occurs in the oocyte, producing multiple copies of the gene for ribosomal RNA, which is associated with the nucleolar organizer center. In *Xenopus* oocytes the nucleolar organizer gene may be amplified about 1000 times. **image a.** In radiology, the increase of the brightness of a fluoroscopic image by electronic means.

**amplitude** \am′plitood\ [L *amplitudo* (from *amplus* large) size, extent] **a. of accommodation** The range between the relaxed state of accommodation and the maximum amount of accommodation of which the eye is capable. It is equal to the refracting power of a thin lens which when placed at the first principal point of the eye would produce by itself an image of the far point at the near point. **a. of convergence** The range between the maximum convergence and the maximum divergence of which the eyes are capable.

**ampoule** \am′pool\ AMPULE.

**amprotropine phosphate** $C_{18}H_{32}NO_7P$. α-(Hydroxymethyl)-benzeneacetate-3-(diethylamino)-2,2-dimethylpropyl ester phosphate, an anticholinergic agent that is used as an antispasmodic drug. Its properties resemble those of atropine.

**ampule** \am′pyool\ [French *ampoule* (from L *ampulla* a bottle, flask; see AMPULLA) a phial] A small glass vial that can be sterilized and sealed. It is used primarily to store solutions that are to be administered by injection. Also *ampoule.*

**ampulla** \ampyoo′lə, ampul′ə\ [L (dim. of *amphora* a jar, from Gk *amphoreus* a jar with handles, from *amphi* on both sides + *pherein* to carry), a flask] (*pl.* ampullae) **1** A small saclike dilatation in a tube, duct, or canal, usually at or near its beginning or termination. **2** Any membranous vesicle. **a. canaliculi lacrimalis** [NA] A dilatation of each of the lacrimal canaliculi, situated at their angles about midway along their length. Also *ampulla of lacrimal canaliculus, ampulla of lacrimal duct.* **a. chyli** CISTERNA CHYLI. **a. ductus deferentis** [NA] A dilatation of the ductus deferens behind the urinary bladder beyond which its lumen narrows again to terminate in the duct of the seminal vesicle. Also *Henle's ampulla, ampulla of vas deferens.* **a. duodeni** [NA] The portion of the superior part of the duodenum that is adjacent to the pylorus and is usually seen prominently in roentgenograms. Also *duodenal cap, duodenal bulb, duodenal antrum, bishop's cap.* **a. of the gallbladder** HARTMANN'S POUCH. **Henle's a.** AMPULLA DUCTUS DEFERENTIS. **a. hepatopancreatica** [NA] The dilatation at the junction of the common bile duct and the pancreatic duct, usually situated in the wall of the left side of the descending part of the duodenum. Distally it constricts before opening on the summit of the duodenal papilla. Also *ampulla of Vater.* **a. of lacrimal canaliculus** AMPULLA CANALICULI LACRIMALIS. **a. of lacrimal duct** AMPULLA CANALICULI LACRIMALIS. **a. of Mascagni** AMPULLA OF THORACIC DUCT. **a. membranacea** A dilatation of the membranous labyrinth at one end of either the anterior (ampulla membranacea anterior or superior), the lateral (ampulla membranacea lateralis), or the posterior (ampulla membranacea posterior) semicircular canal just before it opens into the utricle. The internal wall of each is thickened to form the prominent ampullary crest that receives the nerve endings of the vestibular division of the vestibulocochlear nerve. **a. ossea anterior** [NA] A rounded dilatation of the anterolateral end of the bony anterior semicircular canal just before it enters the vestibule. It contains the membranous ampulla and perilymph. **a. ossea lateralis** [NA] A rounded dilatation of the anterior end of the bony lateral semicircular canal just before it opens into the vestibule below the ampulla of the anterior canal. It contains the membranous ampulla and perilymph. **a. ossea posterior** [NA] A rounded dilatation of the anterior end of the bony posterior semicircular canal just before it opens into the lower part of the vestibule where the macula cribrosa inferior provides passage for the nerves to the ampulla. It contains the membranous ampulla and perilymph. **phrenic a.** An abnormal dilatation or diverticulum in the wall of the esophagus immediately above the diaphragm. Also *supradiaphragmatic esophageal dilatation.* **a. recti** [NA] The dilatation at the lower end of the rectum just proximal to the anorectal junction. Also *rectal ampulla.* **a. of Thoma** A dilatation claimed to be in a terminal arterial capillary beyond a sheathed arteriole in the red pulp of the spleen. **a. of thoracic duct** A small dilatation at the terminal end of the thoracic duct which is observed in about 50% of cases. Also *ampulla of Mascagni.* **a. tubae uterinae** [NA] The thin-walled, broad, tortuous portion of the uterine tube, occupying about one half of its total length between the isthmus medially and the infundibulum laterally. Also *ampulla of uterine tube.* **a. of vas deferens** AMPULLA DUCTUS DEFERENTIS. **a. of Vater** AMPULLA HEPATOPANCREATICA.

**ampullae** \ampyoo′lē\ Plural of AMPULLA.

**ampullar** \ampyoo′lər\ Pertaining to or resembling an ampulla. Also *ampullary.*

**ampullate** \ampul′āt\ Having or shaped like an ampulla.

**ampullifugal** \ampul′əfyoo′gəl, am′pulif′yəgəl\ Away from an ampulla: used especially of endolymph movement in the semicircular canals of the inner ear.

**ampullipetal** \ampul′əpet′əl, am′pulip′itəl\ Toward an ampulla: used especially of endolymph movement in the semicircular canals of the inner ear.

**ampullitis** \am′pulī′tis\ [*ampull(a)* + -ITIS] Inflammation of an ampulla, especially the ampulla ductus deferentis.

**ampullula** \ampul′yələ\ [Late L, dim. of L *ampulla* flask, cruet] A small ampulla, such as those found in minute blood, lymphatic, and lacteal vessels.

**amputate** [See AMPUTATION.] To excise a limb, part of a limb, or other body appendage.

## amputation

**amputation** [L *amputatio* (from *am(b)-* + L *putatus,* past part. of *putare* to cut, lop off) amputation] The removal of a limb, part of a limb, or other body appendage. Also *apocope* (outmoded). **Alanson's a.** A circular amputation that leaves a cone-shaped stump. **amniotic a.** CON-

GENITAL AMPUTATION. **Anderson's a.** ANDERSON'S OPERATION. **aperiosteal a.** An amputation that includes removal of all of the periosteum from the remaining stump of bone. Also *Bunge's amputation.* **Berger's a.** BERGER'S OPERATION. **bloodless a.** An amputation performed after blood flow to the limb has been cut off by application of tourniquet or another technique. **Bunge's a.** APERIOSTEAL AMPUTATION. **Carden's a.** An amputation at the level of the femoral condyles, using a single flap for closure. **cervix a.** Excision of the cervix, usually by a vaginal operation. **chop a.** GUILLOTINE AMPUTATION. **Chopart's a.** A midtarsal amputation through the foot. Also *Chopart's operation.* **circular a.** The sequential division of skin, muscle, and bone, each excision performed at a higher level. It is followed by a single flap closure. **closed a.** An amputation that uses primary closure of the flaps to cover the stump wound. Also *flap amputation.* **coat-sleeve a.** An amputation in which the wound is closed with a single long flap that is usually secured with tape. **complete a.** The removal of an entire limb or limb segment. **congenital a.** The loss during intrauterine development of a limb or other appendage. It was formerly attributed to constricting bands from or adhesions to the amnion, but is now generally thought to be of genetic, vascular, or other intrinsic origin. Also *intrauterine amputation, natural amputation, amniotic amputation.* **definitive a.** An amputation that results in a viable limb segment. **eccentric a.** An amputation that leaves a scar at a location away from the center of the stump. **elliptic a.** An amputation that uses an elliptic incision with respect to the axis of the limb. **end-bearing a.** An amputation in which the weight of the remaining limb segment is borne on the end of the stump. **flap a.** CLOSED AMPUTATION. **Forbes a.** A foot amputation that preserves the calcaneus, astragalus, scaphoid, and a portion of the cuboid bones. **forequarter a.** The surgical removal of the upper extremity, including the scapula and distal clavicle. Also *interscapulothoracic amputation.* **Gritti's a.** An amputation through the knee that uses the patella as an osteoplastic flap to cover the femur. Also *Gritti's operation.* **Gritti-Stokes a.** A modification of the Gritti amputation that uses an anterior flap which is oval in shape. Also *Stokes operation, Stokes amputation.* **guillotine a.** An amputation that uses a direct cut through the limb tissues without the formation of flaps or skin closure. It is used when ongoing suppuration makes primary closure unwise. Also *chop amputation.* **Guyon's a.** An amputation of an extremity above the level of the malleoli. Also *Guyon's operation.* **hindquarter a.** The amputation of the lower limb with all or part of the ilium of the pelvis. Also *interilioabdominal amputation, interinnominoabdominal amputation, hemipelvisectomy.* **intermediary a.** An amputation performed during the period of inflammation, before suppuration sets in. Also *mediate amputation, intermediate amputation, intrapyretic amputation.* **interpelviabdominal a.** An amputation of the thigh with resection of the lateral aspect of the pelvis. Also *Jaboulay's amputation, Jaboulay's operation.* **interscapulothoracic a.** FOREQUARTER AMPUTATION. **intrapyretic a.** INTERMEDIARY AMPUTATION. **intrauterine a.** CONGENITAL AMPUTATION. **Jaboulay's a.** INTERPELVIABDOMINAL AMPUTATION. **kineplastic a.** An amputation with preservation of the tissues within the stump in order to preserve motor function. **Kirk's a.** An amputation above the femoral condyles with coverage of the divided end with the quadriceps tendon. **Lisfranc's a.** An amputation of the foot through the tarsometatarsal joint. Also *Lisfranc's operation.* **MacKenzie's a.** An amputation at the level of the ankle joint, with a flap originating from the medial aspect of the ankle. **major a.** An amputation above the ankle or above the wrist. **mediate a.** INTERMEDIARY AMPUTATION. **mediotarsal a.** An amputation of the foot that preserves the calcaneus, talus, and parts of the tarsus. It uses the soft tissues of the foot to close the wound. Also *Chopart's operation.* **metacarpal a.** An amputation of the toe or metacarpal bone. **minor a.** The amputation of a finger or a toe. **multiple a.** The simultaneous amputation of more than one part. **natural a.** CONGENITAL AMPUTATION. **open a.** An amputation in which the incision is not closed primarily. **osteoplastic a.** An amputation in which the cut ends of the bone are brought into apposition, as in Syme's amputation. **partial a.** The amputation of less than a full segment of a limb. **pathological a.** An amputation necessitated by a diseased condition of the part. **periosteoplastic a.** SUBPERIOSTEAL AMPUTATION. **primary a.** An amputation performed prior to the development of inflammatory changes. **provisional a.** An amputation that is unlikely to be the only one required because of the questionable viability of the remaining tissues. **pulp a.** PULPOTOMY. **racket a.** An amputation that uses two spiral incisions connected with a single longitudinal incision. **ray a.** The amputation of a single digital bony unit including its metacarpal, if in the hand, or its metatarsal, if in the foot. **rectangular a.** An amputation that uses long and short rectangularly shaped flaps. **root a.** Surgical removal of part or the whole of a tooth root. Complete removal of a root from a multirooted tooth is a treatment for chronic periodontitis. It is usually preceded by devitalization and filling of the remaining roots to prevent infection. See also APICOECTOMY. **secondary a.** An amputation that is performed during a period of healing. **semicircular-flap a.** An amputation in which closure is obtained with a semicircular flap. **spontaneous a.** The loss of a portion of an extremity, usually a toe or a finger, without surgical intervention. Although this condition is rare, it may be seen in diabetics with gangrene resulting from vascular disease and in patients with leprosy. **Stokes a.** GRITTI-STOKES AMPUTATION. **submalleolar a.** An amputation immediately distal to the malleoli. **subperiosteal a.** Amputation whereby a sleeve of periosteum covers the cut end of the bone. Also *periosteoplastic amputation.* **supracondylar a.** An amputation immediately above the femoral condyles. **Syme a.** An amputation of the foot at the ankle joint in which the malleoli are removed and the distal os calcis is approximated to the distal sawed end of the tibia. Also *Syme's operation.* **Teale's a.** A limb amputation that utilizes a long myocutaneous flap on one side of the limb and a short rectangular flap on the other side. Also *Teale's operation.* **tertiary a.** An amputation that is performed after the resolution of inflammation or the reestablishment of an adequate blood supply. **through-knee a.** An amputation of the lower limb through the knee joint, thus dividing no bone. Rarely it is performed as a definitive amputation. More often it is employed in the the rapid removal of an irreversibly damaged or infected leg. Also *knee disarticulation.* **transmetatarsal a.** An amputation through the distal foot that divides one or more of the metatarsals immediately distal to the metatarsal head. **transverse a.** An amputation in the transverse plane of the extremity. **traumatic a.** Severance of a part through injury.

**Amsler** [Marc *Amsler,* Swiss ophthalmologist, 1891–1968] **1** Amsler's charts. See under CHART. **2** See under GRID.

**amu** atomic mass unit

**amusia** \əmyoo′sē·ə\ [Gk *amousia* (from *amous(os)* unmusical, without the Muses) a lack of musicality or refinement] The inability to distinguish between different musical notes, making it impossible to sing in tune or to play a musical instrument properly. This may occur as a developmental disorder or, more often, as the consequence of a cerebral lesion. Also *tonal amusia, musical deafness, tone deafness, musical aphasia, asonia.* **amnesic a.** Inability to name a piece of music that the affected individual is familiar with. *Seldom used.* **motor a.** Loss of the ability to sing or play an instrument. **receptive a.** 1 MUSICAL BLINDNESS. 2 SENSORY AMUSIA. **sensory a.** Inability to differentiate between musical sounds. Also *receptive amusia.* **tonal a.** AMUSIA. **vocal motor a.** Inability to sing in tune.

**Amussat** [Jean Zulema *Amussat,* French surgeon, 1796–1856] 1 See under VALVULA. 2 Amussat's valvula. See under PLICA SPIRALIS.

**amyctic** \əmik′tik\ [Gk *amyktik(os)* (from *amyssein* to mangle, scratch) scratching] Abrasive, caustic, or irritating.

**amydriasis** \am′idrī′əsis\ [Gk *a-* priv. + MYDRIASIS] The absence of pupillary dilatation.

**amydricaine** $C_{16}H_{26}N_2O_2$. 1-(Dimethylamino)-2-[(dimethylamino)-methyl]-2-butanol benzoate, a compound whose hydrochloride salt is used as a topical anesthetic agent.

**amyelencephaly** \əmī′əlensef′əlē\ [Gk *a-* priv. + MYEL- + ENCEPHAL- + -Y] The absence of the brain and spinal cord. Such a malformation is rare if not improbable, except in an amorphous fetus.

**amyelia** \am′ī-ē′lyə\ [Gk *a-* priv. + MYEL- + -IA] The congenital absence of the spinal cord. This condition is probably not a primary developmental defect but is more likely a secondary result of the erosion of exposed spinal cord tissue in rachischisis totalis.

**amyelinated** \əmī′əlinā′tid\ Lacking a myelin sheath, either as a result of failure to develop or secondary to disease process or to injury: said of nerve fibers. Also *amyelinic.*

**amyelination** \əmī′əlinā′shən\ [Gk *a-* priv. + MYELINATION] Failure to form a myelin sheath, or loss of the myelin after it has formed as a result of disease or injury, the latter usually being referred to as demyelination.

**amyelinic** \əmī′əlin′ik\ AMYELINATED.

**amygdala** \əmig′dələ\ [Med L (from Gk *amygdalē* almond) tonsil] 1 CORPUS AMYGDALOIDEUM. 2 TONSIL. **a. accessoria** *Outmoded* TONSILLA LINGUALIS. **accessory a.** *Outmoded* TONSILLA LINGUALIS. **a. of cerebellum** *Seldom used* TONSILLA CEREBELLI.

**amygdaline** \əmig′dəlīn\ TONSILLAR.

**amygdalo-** \əmig′dəlō-\ [Med L *amygdala* tonsil, from Gk *amygdalē* almond] A combining form denoting (1) almonds; (2) tonsil; (3) corpus amygdaloideum.

**amygdaloid** \əmig′dəloid\ [Gk *amygdaloeidēs* (from *amygdal(ē)* almond + *-eidēs* -like, -OID) like an almond] 1 Shaped like or suggestive of an almond. 2 Pertaining to the corpus amygdaloideum. 3 Pertaining to the tonsilla palatina.

**amygdaloidectomy** \əmig′dəloidek′təmē\ [AMYGDALOID + -ECTOMY] The excision of the amygdaloid nucleus.

**amygdalotomy** \əmig′dəlät′əmē\ An incision into the amygdaloid nucleus.

**amyl-** \am′əl-\ AMYLO-.

**amylase** An enzyme that hydrolyzes starch. Two main types occur, α-amylase and β-amylase. α-Amylase hydrolyzes 1,4-α-D-glucosidic bonds within molecules, whereas β-amylase hydrolyzes this bond only when it is the second such bond from the nonreducing end of a chain, so that it releases maltose and leaves a chain shortened by two glucose residues. The salivary amylase is an α-amylase. **serum a.** The concentration in serum of any form of amylase. **urinary a.** Amylase present in urine, an abnormal finding that accompanies or follows elevation of serum amylase levels.

**amylasuria** \am′iləsoo′rē·ə\ [*amylas(e)* + -URIA] The excretion of an increased amount of amylase in the urine, especially in acute pancreatitis. Excretion of more than 300 Somogyi units of amylase per hour is abnormal, while more than 1000 units per hour is common in acute pancreatitis.

**amylemia** \am′ilē′mē·ə\ [AMYL- + -EMIA] The presence of starch in the blood plasma or serum.

**amyl nitrite** $C_5H_{11}$—O—N═O. An ester of pentanol. It has been used for the relief of asthma and angina, since breathing the vapor dilates blood vessels and relaxes muscles. Also *isoamyl nitrite.*

**amylo-** \am′əlō-\ [Gk *amylon* (from *amylos* not ground at the mill, from *a-* priv. + *mylē* mill) the finest meal, starch] A combining form denoting starch. Also *amyl-.*

**amylobarbitone** AMOBARBITAL.

**amylo-1,6-glucosidase** An enzyme (EC 3.2.1.33), which is one of those responsible for the hydrolysis of starch. It breaks α1-6 glucoside bonds between chains of 1,4-linked α-glucose residues.

**amyloid** \am′iloid\ [AMYL- + -OID] 1 Starchlike. 2 Any of various starchlike substances occurring in nature or in certain manufacturing processes. 3 Any of several complex proteins characteristically deposited in tissues in amyloidosis. They have a hyaline gross structure, a unique type of fibrillar ultrastructure, high refractility, and an affinity for Congo red dye. The amino acid sequences vary greatly, depending in part on the disease processes involved. 4 Pertaining to amyloids or amyloidosis.

**amyloidemia** \am′iloidē′mē·ə\ The presence of amyloid fibrils in the circulating blood.

**amyloidosis** \am′iloidō′sis\ An incurable, multisystemic disease process of uncertain etiology characterized by the interstitial accumulation of amyloid fibrils. The affected tissues have a firm, waxy texture. Diagnosis is made by microscopic examination which shows extracellular, hyalinelike deposits of Congo red-positive material that have a green birefringence under polarized light. Organs principally affected include the liver, kidney, spleen, heart, and gastrointestinal tract. This condition occurs in disorders of B lymphocytes, such as multiple myeloma and monoclonal gammopathies, following chronic infections or inflammatory conditions such as rheumatoid arthritis, regional enteritis, and tuberculosis. Amyloidosis may also affect the hearts of elderly individuals, causing a form of restrictive cardiomyopathy and heart failure. Also *amyloid disease, amyloid thesaurismosis.* **Andrade type a.** PORTUGUESE TYPE AMYLOIDOSIS. **cutaneous a.** Amyloidosis affecting the skin, most commonly lichen amyloidosus, and marked by the eruption of pigmented papules and by itching. Also *amyloidosis cutis.* **familial renal a.** A form of renal amyloidosis transmitted as an autosomal dominant, probably is a variant of familial Mediterranean fever. Progressive decline in hearing begins in the first decade, while episodic fever, pain in extremities, and painful red papules begin in adolescence, with progressive renal failure beginning in the third to fifth decade. **Indiana type a.** A dominantly inherited amyloid neuropathy which usually appears clinically as a bilateral carpal tunnel syndrome due to deposition of amyloid beneath the carpal ligaments. Also *Indiana type amyloid neuropathy.* **Iowa type of a.** A dominantly inherited progressive polyneuropathy due to primary amyloidosis in which the affected individual usually also develops nephropathy and peptic ulcer. Also *Iowa type amyloid neuropathy.* **kidney a.** RENAL AMYLOIDOSIS. **a. of the larynx** The occurrence in the larynx of either diffuse or localized deposits of amyloid material. If the deposits are diffuse they may be part of a widespread condition with amyloid involvement of other parts. If they are localized they may present as a primary localized amyloid tumor of the larynx. **lichenoid a.** LICHEN AMYLOIDOSUS. **macular a.** A clinical form of cutaneous amyloidosis marked by lesions that arise as closely grouped macules. **a. of multiple myeloma** A form of systemic amyloidosis occurring in 10–15% of patients with multiple myeloma. The tumor cells synthesize immunoglobulin light chains (Bence-Jones protein), which are excreted in the urine. **nodular a.** A clinical form of cutaneous amyloidosis that is marked by lesions occurring almost exclusively on the lower legs. **Portuguese type a.** Primary amyloidosis of autosomal dominant inheritance giving rise to severe, progressive, sensorimotor polyneuropathy. It is seen especially in individuals of Portuguese descent. Also *Andrade type amyloidosis, Portuguese type amyloid neuropathy, Andrade type amyloid neuropathy.* **renal a.** A renal disease resulting from extracellular deposition of amyloid, a proteinaceous material that has affinity for certain stains, such as Congo red, and which electron microscopy shows to consist of characteristic fine fibrils 75 to 100 Å wide. Amyloid is deposited in arterial walls, along glomerular capillaries and later in the interstitium. The disease may be primary, a part of the aging process, familial, or secondary to chronic inflammation or multiple myeloma. Renal amyloidosis often occurs as part of a process that involves other organs as well. Clinically the disease may be asymptomatic, but proteinuria usually and the nephrotic syndrome sometimes are present. Uremia develops within two to ten years. Also *kidney amyloidosis, amyloid kidney, lardaceous kidney, waxy kidney.* **secondary a.** A common systemic form of amyloidosis that usually occurs in a context of a chronic infection or chronic inflammatory condition. Among diseases associated with this form of amyloidosis today are rheumatoid arthritis, regional enteritis, ulcerative colitis, scleroderma, dermatomyositis, and bronchiectasis. The amyloid protein is principally deposited in the kidney, where it causes the nephrotic syndrome. **senile a.** A form of amyloidosis affecting elderly individuals, in which amyloid deposits are found in the brain, heart, and spleen, as well as in blood vessels of most organs. Though usually asymptomatic, this form of amyloidosis may seriously affect cardiac function, causing restrictive cardiomyopathy. A special type of amyloid protein, chemically related to prealbumin, is deposited in the tissues.

**amylopectin** A constituent of starch that has considerable 1,6-branching of 1,4-linked chains of $\alpha$-glucose residues.

**amylopectinosis** \-pek′tinō′sis\ GLYCOGEN STORAGE DISEASE IV.

**amylophagia** \-fā′jə\ [AMYLO- + -PHAGIA] The ingestion of starch in forms not normally used for food; a kind of pica.

**amyloplast** \am′ilōplast′\ A leucoplast that produces and stores starch.

**amylose** The constituent of starch that consists of straight chains of 1,4-linked $\alpha$-glucopyranose residues. Amylose with water forms hydrated micelles, which give a blue color with iodine. This reaction is the basic of a test for starch that is much used.

**amylosuria** \-soo′rē·ə\ [*amylos(e)* + -URIA] The excretion of amylose or other starches in the urine.

**amylpenicillin sodium** $C_{14}H_{21}NaN_2O_4S$. A penicillin antibiotic that is derived from *Aspergillus flavus* as well as from *Penicillium notatum.* Also *flavicin, flavacidin, penicillin dihydro F sodium, sodium n-amylpenicillinate.*

**amylum** \am′iləm\ [L (from Gk *amylon*; see AMYLO-) fine meal, starch] STARCH.

**amyoesthesia** \əmī′ō·esthē′zhə\ [Gk *a-* priv. + MYOESTHESIA] An impaired muscle sense that leads to a diminished position sense and muscle movement sense. *Seldom used.* Also *amyoaesthesia, amyoesthesis.*

**amyoplasia** \əmī′ōplā′zhə\ [Gk *a-* priv. + MYO- + -PLASIA] A state in which there is absent or deficient muscle development. **a. congenita** CONGENITAL MULTIPLE ARTHROGRYPOSIS.

**amyosthenia** \əmī′ästhē′nē·ə\ MYASTHENIA.

**amyosthenic** \əmī′ästhen′ik\ MYASTHENIC.

**amyotaxia** \əmī′ōtak′sē·ə\ ATAXIA.

**amyotonia** \əmī′ōtō′nē·ə\ [Gk *a-* priv. + MYO- + *ton(o)-* + -IA] MYATONIA. **a. congenita** MYATONIA CONGENITA. **Oppenheim's a.** MYATONIA CONGENITA.

**amyotrophia** \əmī′ōtrō′fē·ə\ AMYOTROPHY.

**amyotrophic** \əmī′ōträf′ik\ Relating to amyotrophy.

**amyotrophy** \am′ī·ät′rəfē\ [Gk *a-* priv. + MYO- + *(a)-trophy*] Muscular atrophy of neurogenic origin. Also *myoatrophy, amyotrophia, myatrophy.* • By common usage, the term *amyotrophy* is not applied to wasting of skeletal muscle due to primary disease of the muscles. **Aran-Duchenne a.** PROGRESSIVE MUSCULAR ATROPHY. **diabetic a.** Asymmetrical weakness and wasting of the musculature of the pelvic girdle and thighs with hyporeflexia and diffuse pain, associated with uncontrolled diabetes mellitus. The role of diabetic neuropathy is not ruled out, but atrophy of single muscle fibers from biopsied muscle suggests a primary myopathy. In some cases the condition is due to an ischemic mononeuropathy of one or both femoral nerves. **neural a.** AMYOTROPHIC ACROPATHY. **neuralgic a.** SHOULDER GIRDLE SYNDROME. **neuritic a.** HEREDITARY HYPERTROPHIC INTERSTITIAL NEUROPATHY. **primary progressive a.** MUSCULAR DYSTROPHY. **progressive nuclear a.** PROGRESSIVE NUCLEAR MUSCULAR ATROPHY. **syphilitic a.** Muscular atrophy and weakness secondary to syphilitic arachnoiditis or meningomyelitis.

**Amytal** Barbituric acid substituted in position 5 with ethyl and 3-methylbutyl (i.e., isoamyl) groups. It is a hypnotic, and it is used in biochemistry to inhibit the respiratory chain by blocking electron transfer from NADH to the cytochrome system. A proprietary name.

**amyxorrhea** \əmik′sôrē′ə\ [Gk *a-* priv. + MYXO- + -RRHEA] The condition of lacking secretion of mucus.

**An** **1** Symbol for the element, actinon. **2** anode.

**an-** \an-, ən-\ **1** A-[1]. **2** ANA-.

**-an** \-an\ [shortening of -ANE] A suffix usually indicating an unsaturated hydrocarbon or an anhydride of a carbohydrate.

**ANA** antinuclear antibody.

**ana** [Gk] Of each: used in prescription writing to indicate that the stated amount of each ingredient specified is to be taken. Symbol: $\overline{aa}$

**ana-** \an′ə-\ [Gk *ana* (sometimes *am-, an-*) up, upward, back again] A prefix meaning (1) up, upward; (2) back, backward; (3) again. Also *am-, an-.*

**anabasine** \ənab′əsin\ $C_{10}H_{14}N_2$. A pyridine alkaloid obtained from the leaves of *Anabasis aphylla* of the family Chemopodiaceae. It resembles nicotine in action and has been used as an insecticide.

**anabatic** \an′əbat′ik\ [Gk *anabatik(os)* (from *anabainein* to go up) skilled in ascending] **1** Increasing in intensity. **2** Moving upward.

**anabiotic** \an′əbī·ät′ik\ **1** Seemingly lifeless but capable of revival. **2** Any agent used to bring about revival.

**anabolic** \an′əbäl′ik\ Denoting any substance that increases the rate of metabolism in a cell or organism.

**anabolism** \ənab′əlizm\ [Gk *anabol(ē)* a thing thrown upward, a carrying up and over + -ISM] The metabolic process in which simple substances are synthesized into more complex compounds. Compare CATABOLISM. Adj. anabolic.

**anacampsis** \an′əkamp′sis\ [Gk *anakampsis* a bending back, reflection] Reflection, especially of light or sound.

**anacamptometer** \an′əkamptäm′ətər\ An instrument for measuring reflexes.

**anacardic acid** $C_{22}H_{32}O_3$. A component of the seeds of *Anacardium occidentale* that has been used as an anthelmintic.

**anacidity** \an′əsid′itē\ [Gk *an-* priv. + ACIDITY] Lack of normal gastric acid secretion. **gastric a.** ACHLORHYDRIA.

**anaclasis** \ənak′ləsis\ [ANA- + -CLASIS] Rupture or ankylosis of a joint by force.

**anaclitic** \an′əklit′ik\ [Gk *anaklitik(os)* fitted for leaning upon] Dependent on another for gratification of bodily needs. See also ANACLITIC DEPRESSION.

**anacrotic** \an′əkrät′ik\ [Gk *anakrot(ein)* to lift up and strike together + -IC] **1** Relating to the upstroke of the arterial pulse. **2** ANADICROTIC.

**anacrotism** \ənak′rətizm\ The condition or characteristic of a pulse that is anacrotic (anadicrotic). Also *anadicrotism.*

**anacusis** \an′əkyoo′sis\ [Gk *an-* priv. + ACU-[2] + -SIS] Profound or total loss of hearing.

**anadenia** \an′ədē′nē·ə\ [Gk *an-* priv. + ADEN- + -IA] **1** A congenital absence of glands. **2** The lack of glandular function of a specified region or type. *Obs.*

**anadicrotic** \an′ədīkrät′ik\ [ANA- + Gk *dikrot(os)* double-beating + -IC] Describing a pulse with a double upstroke characterized by a prominent notch on the ascending limb of the pulse tracing. It is characteristic of aortic stenosis. Also *anacrotic.*

**anadicrotism** \an′ədik′rətizm\ ANACROTISM.

**anadipsia** \an′ədip′sē·ə\ [ANA- + -DIPSIA] Extreme thirst.

**anaemia** *Brit.* ANEMIA.

**anaerobe** \aner′ōb\ [Gk *an-* priv. + AERO- + Gk *bios* (way of) life] Any organism able to grow in the absence of air. Those of medical interest derive energy from fermentation. Others found in nature derive energy by anaerobic respiration (with nitrate or sulfate instead of oxygen as electron acceptor) or by photosynthesis. Compare AEROBE. Adj. anaerobic. **facultative a.** An organism able to grow either in the presence or absence of air. • Although this is the usual term for such strains, they can equally be considered facultative aerobes. **obligate a.** An organism able to grow only in the absence of air. Many species not only fail to grow but are rapidly killed in the presence of air because they lack superoxide dismutase.

**anaerobic** \an′erōb′ik\ **1** Able to live without oxygen. **2** Denoting an oxygen-free environment.

**anaerobiosis** \an′ərōbī·ō′sis\ [Gk *an-* priv. + AERO- + BIOSIS] Life processes taking place in the absence of molecular oxygen, particularly growth under anaerobic culture conditions. In deep cultures (e.g. commercial fermentations), competition between diffusion and utilization of oxygen provides for anaerobiosis in the depths. Solid media cultures in the laboratory are incubated in a container from which the oxygen has been removed.

**anaerogenic** \an′ərōjen′ik\ [Gk *an-* priv. + AERO- + -GENIC] Not producing gas as a product of metabolism, as certain bacteria.

**anaerosis** \an′erō′sis\ [Gk *an-* priv. + AEROSIS] A state of airlessness.

**anaesthesia** \an′esthē′zhə\ *Brit.* ANESTHESIA.

**anaesthetic** \an′esthet′ik\ *Brit.* ANESTHETIC.

**anaesthetist** *Brit.* ANESTHETIST.

**anagen** \an′əjən\ [Gk *anagen(nan)* (from *ana-* up, anew, RE- + *gennan* to beget, generate) to regenerate] The growth phase of the cycle of activity of the hair follicle. Compare CATAGEN, TELOGEN.

**anagenesis** \an′əjen′əsis\ [ANA- + GENESIS] The regeneration or repair of tissue or parts. *Obs.*

**anákhré** \an′akrā′\ [native West African, big nose] GOUNDOU.

**anal** \ā′nəl\ [*an(us)* + -AL] Pertaining to or located near the anus.

**analbuminemia** \an′albyoominē′mē·ə\ The absence of albumin from blood plasma or serum.

**analeptic** \anəlep′tik\ [Gk *analēptikos* (from *analambanein* to take up, retrieve, restore, from *ana* up + *lambanein* to take) restorative] **1** Stimulating the central nervous system, particularly with the property of improving the strength and vigor of cerebral activity. **2** An analeptic agent.

**analgecize** \anal′jəsīz\ To produce analgesia in by means of drugs or local anaesthetic agents. *Obs.*

**analgesia** \an′əljē′zē·ə\ [Gk *analgēsia* (from *an-* priv. + *algēsis* sense of pain) insensitivity] Loss of the sense of pain, as that produced by the injection of local anesthetic agents or by systemic drugs such as the opioids, or resulting from disease interrupting pain pathways in the central or peripheral nervous system. Also *alganesthesia.* **audio a.** AUDIOANALGESIA. **conduction a.** Loss of pain in certain regions of the body due to sensory denervation by pharmacologic agents. **congenital a.** A rare congenital nervous system defect, becoming apparent in early childhood as an inability to appreciate the pain of any injury, the most frequent being lesions of skin and mucous membrane. The tongue, lips, and fingers are bitten and chewed. The ordinary scrapes and bruises of childhood are much more severe and very often complicated by sepsis. Bone pain and abdominal pain are not felt, with serious consequences in the event of infection or fracture. Emotional disturbance may arise from this unnatural state. Avoidance of trauma is learned very gradually. The condition is probably inherited as an autosomal recessive trait. **continuous caudal a.** The continuous infusion of anesthetic solution via the caudal canal within the epidural space to relieve the pain of labor by blocking pain pathways of the lumbar and sacral nerve. **electrical a.** Transcutaneous or perineural stimulation produced by a low intensity, sine-wave current, used to relieve various pain syndromes. **hysterical a.** Loss of pain sensibility resulting from hysteria and not from organic disease. Examples include total hemianesthesia, or loss of pain sensation in a limb with an upper border or level corresponding to the position of a joint. **narcolocal a.** Lack of sensitivity to pain in a localized area or region following the administration of preanesthetic medication. **obstetrical a.** Relief of pain during labor. Techniques may include systemically given opioids, conduction analgesia, and psychologic approaches. **perineural a.** Analgesia produced by infiltration of local anesthetic solution around a nerve. Also *paraneural analgesia.* **relative a.** A form of incomplete general anesthesia in which consciousness remains while pain sensations are lost or reduced to an acceptable level. It is brought about by the inhalation of a mixture of nitrous oxide and oxygen or systemically given opioids. **serial caudal a.** Analgesia in the sacral area produced by serial injection of local anesthetic solution into the sacral epidural canal. **spinal a.** Analgesia below the level of the injection produced by the injection of local anesthetic agents or of other substances with more prolonged or even permanent effects, such as phenol or alcohol, into the spinal subarachnoid space.

**analgesic** \an′aljē′sik\ **1** Causing loss of sensitivity to pain without loss of consciousness. **2** An analgesic drug. For defs. 1 and 2 also *analgetic, antinociceptive.*

**analgetic** \an′aljet′ik\ ANALGESIC.

**analgia** \anal′jə\ [Gk *an-* priv. + -ALGIA] Absence of pain sensibility.

**analgic** \anal′jik\ Lacking sensitivity to pain.

**anality** \ānal′itē\ The anal elements of psychosexual development.

**analog** \an′əläg\ **1** Pertaining to data in the form of continuously variable physical quantities as contrasted to digital data in the form of discrete states. **2** Pertaining to representation of physical variables such as blood pressure by more convenient variables such as voltage. **3** ANALOGUE.

**analogous** \ənal′əgəs\ [Gk *analogos* proportionate, conformable, equivalent. See also ANALOGY.] With respect to parts and organs of different animals or plants, of like function but of unlike origin and development, e.g., the eyes of squids and vertebrates. Compare HOMOLOGOUS.

**analogue** \an′əläg\ [French (from Gk *analogia* proportion, analogy, from ANA- + Gk *logos* word, speech), analogous, similar] **1** A substance that is similar in molecular structure and chemical properties to another. Analogues of drugs or metabolites may have biologic action by binding to the enzymes and receptors that bind the natural compounds. **2** An organ or part of an animal or plant with like function but unlike structure and origin as that of another, such as the wing of a bird and the wing of a moth. Also *analog.* Compare HOMOLOGUE. **homologous a.** An organ or part that is similar in both structure and function to another. **metabolic a.** A chemical compound that has a structure similar to, but not identical with, that of a metabolite whose biologic function it can mimic or interfere with.

**analogy** \ənal′əjē\ [Gk *analogia* (from *ana-* thorough + *logos* reckoning, reason) correspondence, relation, proportion] Similarity in function between organs or parts of different animals and plants, whether or not the organs or parts compared are homologous. Compare HOMOLOGY.

**analphalipoproteinemia** \anal′fəlip′ōprōtēnē′mē·ə\ Congenital absence of serum $\alpha$-lipoprotein, resulting in deficiency of the high density lipoprotein fraction and accumulation of cholesteryl esters in tissues. The disease is inherited as an autosomal recessive, and the homozygote is characterized by enlargement of the tonsils, liver, and spleen; multiple orange or yellow spots or plaques of the pharyngeal and rectal mucosa; corneal opacity; and peripheral neuropathy. There is absence or near-absence of plasma $\alpha$-lipoproteins and also of pre-$\beta$-lipoproteins, and marked reduction in plasma concentrations of apolipoproteins A-I and A-II. Also *Tangier disease, hypoalphalipoproteinemia.*

**analysis** \ənal′isis\ [Gk (from *analyein* to unloose, undo, dissolve, resolve, from *ana-* up, through, thoroughly + *lyein* to loose, loosen; see also LYSIS) dissolution, solution, analysis] **1** Determination of the composition or the quantity or concentration of a material. **2** PSYCHOANALYSIS. **3** In electroencephalography, estimation or recording of the individual components of a complex waveform in terms of frequency and amplitude. **acoustic a. of speech** The process by which the complex sounds of speech are analyzed and categorized through the use of multiple acoustic filters with the results displayed graphically over time. **activation a.** Determination of the chemical elements present in a sample by irradiating it with neutrons and determining the characteristics of the induced radioactivity. **antigenic a.** Identification of the set of antigens used to classify types within a bacterial species. **bite a.** OCCLUSAL ANALYSIS. **blood gas a.** The measurement of oxygen and carbon dioxide levels in arterial or venous blood, usually expressed as partial pressure of the gases and often combined with a pH determination using the same sample. **child a.** Classical psychoanalysis in which the techniques have been modified so that they may be utilized in the therapy of children. Free association, dream interpretation, and transference neurosis must all be altered for use with children. Play therapy is a tactic employed by most child analysts in place of techniques normally used with adults. **cluster a.** In epidemiology, statistical methods for detecting significant nonrandom association of events in space and time, such as an unusual aggregation of cases of a rare disease in an area over a period. **decision a.** A problem-solving technique in which individual components contributing to a complex decision are defined and arranged in a sequence of decision points. Numerical values are assigned to the probability and to the consequences of each outcome. **direct a.** An unorthodox modification of psychoanalytic technique in which the therapist confronts the patient with immediate interpretations of the patient's behavior based on hunches about what that behavior might mean rather than on the free associations of the patient. **discriminant a.** A statistical technique which enables an individual observation to be assigned to one of two or more classes with a minimum probability of error. It makes use of a "discriminant function" derived in the first place from a large number of observations of individuals of known classification. **displacement a.** COMPETITIVE BINDING TECHNIQUE. **distributive a.** Treatment utilizing the therapist's interpretations which are distributed along the various lines indicated as being significant by the patient's symptoms, developmental history, personality traits, and current behavior. **ego a.** Psychoanalytic treatment based on a psychology of normal development rather than a psychology of conflict. Emphasis is placed on ego defenses, object relations, and internalization, and their contribution to structuralization of the personality. Also *structural analysis.* **end-group a.** Determination of the residue present at the end of a linear macromolecule, especially of a protein, a polynucleotide, or a polysaccharide. **factor a.** A statistical technique whereby a large number of variables in experimental or observational data are reduced to weights, or loadings, on a smaller number of hypothetical variables called factors, so as to account as fully as possible for the interrelationships found in the original data. **Feather a.** A method for determining the range in aluminum of beta particles emitted by a radionuclide of interest. It involves plotting the counting rate in a detector against sheet thickness in a series of aluminum absorbers, followed by comparing this curve with one similarly obtained with a standard emitter such as bismuth 210. **fluctuation a.** The demonstration, by the statistics of the frequency of mutants in parallel cultures, that phage or drugs only select, and do not direct, mutations. **Fourier a.** The process of analyzing a usually periodic temporal waveform by separating it into a series of harmonically related frequencies of known amplitude and phase. **gastric a.** HISTAMINE STIMULATION TEST. **isotope dilution a.** See under ISOTOPE DILUTION. **multivariate a.** In statistics, any method of data analysis capable of handling simultaneously a number of independent variables, such as blood pressure, serum cholesterol, smoking history, and body weight, in a group of persons being investigated for coronary artery disease. Examples of multivariate methods would be multiple regression techniques, multiple logistic functions, or factor analysis. **nearest neighbor a.** In the study of the sequence of any heteropolymer, any technique used in determining the frequency with which one specific monomeric unit occurs next to another specific one. Also *nearest neighbor sequence analysis.* **nearest neighbor base frequency a.** A nearest neighbor analysis of polynucleotides, such as DNA or RNA. **nearest neighbor sequence a.** NEAREST NEIGHBOR ANALYSIS. **occlusal a.** The study and evaluation of the occlusion of the teeth, particularly in cases of malocclusion. Study casts, anatomical articulators, and articulating paper may be used. Also *bite analysis.* **orthodox a.** CLASSIC PSYCHOANALYSIS. **path coefficient a.** In population genetics, an analytic method used in animal breeding, in the analysis of cause and effect in a system of correlated variables, and in theoretic population genetics whereby diagrammatic representations depict statistical relationships among related individuals. **probit a.** A statistical method of predicting survival that takes into account the graded severity of the injury and associated complicating problems. **ridit a.** A statistical technique for analyzing discrete data arranged in ordered categories. The only assumption made is that the categories represent intervals of some underlying continuous distribution, but its nature need not be specified. For example, patients suffering from a disease might be categorized as being mildly, moderately, severely, or very severely affected. The number in each category is transformed to a ridit which may then be compared with the distribution of ridits in a reference group. **saturation a.** COMPETITIVE BINDING TECHNIQUE. **sequential a.** A statistical technique based on sequential sampling. The units or groups of units that form the sample are drawn one at a time in sequence, and the cumulative result up to and including the last selection decides whether sampling is to continue or whether the hypothesis under test can be rejected. **stop-flow a.** A technique for evaluating the absorptive or secretory capability of cells lining a tubular or ductal system through which fluid normally flows. The flow of fluid is first halted by producing a block to outflow. Time is then allowed for equilibration between the luminal contents and the lining cells. Finally, interference to outflow is suddenly removed under circumstances which permit a rapid flow of fluid from the system, and small serial samples of the outflow are collected in rapid sequence. The nature and concentration of solutes in the samples is believed to be indicative of the differing absorptive and secretory characteristics of the lining cells that surrounded the fluid during the stand-still period. **structural a.** EGO ANALYSIS. **tetrad a.** An examination of the four products of meiosis of a single primary gametocyte, usually for analysis of crossing over. This is possible only in eukaryotes, such as yeast and fungi, in which the meiotic products remain together following division. **transactional a.** A form of psychotherapy that recognizes the importance of understanding the interplay between therapist and patient as a basic step in interpreting the interactions between the patient and others, that is, in apprehending external social reality. A recognition of the repetitive nature of maladaptive aspects of the patient's behavior and of emotional elements influencing their genesis leads to improved self-understanding and control of behavior. **tubeless gastric a.** DIAGNEX BLUE TEST. **a. of variance** A statistical technique for apportioning the total variance into components associated with various classifications or factors regarded as being sources of variation in the data. The subsequent analysis involves comparisons between these components. **vector a.** The analysis of entities characterized by direction in space as well as magnitude.

**analyst** \an′əlist\ A therapist who specializes in psychoanalysis; a psychoanalyst.

**analyte** \an′əlīt\ Any material or chemical substance subjected to analysis.

**analytic** \an′əlit′ik\ Psychoanalytic.

**analyzer** \an′əlī′zər\ In electroencephalography, an electronic instrument designed to break down, in a continuous or intermittent fashion, complex cerebral rhythms into their individual components, and to determine the amplitude and frequency of these components. Also *analyser* (British spelling). **amino acid a.** An apparatus for determining the amount of amino acids present in samples, usually hydrolysates of proteins. Most such devices separate the amino acids by chromatography on sulfonated polystyrene resins and then measure the colored product each produces after reaction with ninhydrin at a high temperature. **amino acid sequence a.** An instrument for determining the serial amino acid composition of a protein or peptide. **auditory a.** See under SENSORY ANALYZER. **blood gas a.** An instrument for determining the partial pressure of various gases dissolved in blood. **centrifugal fast a.** An analytic instrument composed of discrete reaction units radially arranged in a centrifuge head. Centrifugal force mixes the samples and reagents and propels them into a ring of cuvets, which passes through the light beam of a spectrophotometer that is capable of multiple rapid absorbance readings. **frequency a.** An instrument that separates a temporal waveform into its component frequencies and displays them as a function of time. **image a.** A device that registers and classifies, according to a predetermined program, the component aspects of photographic, microscopic, or projected images. **kinetic a.** An analytic instrument that measures the rate of change of absorbance of a reaction mixture over time, either continuously or at very frequent intervals. It is used especially for enzyme analyses. **oxygen gas a.** A device that measures the partial pressure or dissolved content of oxygen in a gaseous or liquid mixture. It is used especially to determine the oxygen partial pressure of blood or the oxygen saturation of blood hemoglobin. **pulse-height a.** An instrument designed to count gamma and other energies selectively, assuming that pulse heights are proportional to energies. An electronic window has adjustable sill and top, and only pulses with heights between the two are allowed to go through to the counter. Thus unwanted energies, often scatter counts, can be excluded. Also *pulse-height spectrometer.* **sensory a.** According to Pavlov and other experimental behaviorists, those regions in the nervous system capable of interpreting sensory signals from the environment that enter the brain through afferent pathways and of differentiating from this sensory information those signals that are of significance to the organism and of eliminating those that are not meaningful. Several types of sensory analyzers were said to exist in the nervous system, examples of which are the visual analyzer for the interpretation of visual stimuli and the auditory analyzer that functions to differentiate acoustic stimuli. **visual a.** See under SENSORY ANALYZER. **voice a.** An electronic instrument for displaying the frequency content of the voice as a function of time. It is used to diagnose speech disorders or to identify a particular speaker. **voice stress a.** A device permitting a graphic tracing to be made of certain speech sounds not detectable by the human ear. Normal voice tremor is suppressed by action of the autonomic nervous system when the speaker is under stress. **wave a.** An instrument that performs a Fourier analysis of a temporal waveform and displays the frequency content.

**anamnesis** \an'amnē'sis\ [Gk *anamnēsis* (from *ana-* up, back, RE- + *mnēsis* memory) a recalling to mind, reminiscence] The clinical history obtained from the patient; the patient's recollections of the events preceding his or her illness. **associative a.** A type of psychiatric history-taking or interviewing that attempts to make the patient aware of the relationship between his symptoms and his emotional life. Typically, the patient is encouraged to give more and more details about the interpersonal and intrapsychic events surrounding the appearance of symptoms.

**anamnestic** \an'amnes'tik\ [Gk *anamnēstikos* recalling the past] **1** Pertaining to anamnesis. **2** Of or relating to immunologic memory.

**anamorphosis** \an'əmôrfō'sis\ [Gk *anamorphōsis* a re-formation] **1** A progression in the evolution of a species. **2** An improvement in shape. **dioptric a.** The use of parallel prisms to change the shape of an image.

**ananabolic** \anan'əbäl'ik\ Unable to carry on anabolic metabolism.

**anancasm** \an'ankaz'm\ [Gk *anankasma* a forcing, compelling] A feeling or action that a subject feels to be forced upon him and which he feels incapable of controlling, such as is seen in obsession or compulsion.

**anangioplasia** \anan'jē·ōplā'zhə\ [Gk *an-* priv. + ANGIO- + -PLASIA] Congenitally small or absent blood vessels.

**anaphase** \an'əfāz\ The stage of mitosis or meiosis in which the chromosomes move from the equatorial plate toward the poles of the cell. Anaphase starts with division of the centromere. Because they are being pulled by a spindle fiber attached to their kinetocores, the chromosomes assume a V-shape. As the chromosomes move toward the poles, the poles move farther apart due to pushing of the spindle fibers which are not attached to chromosomes.

**anaphia** \anā'fē·ə\ [Gk *an-* priv. + *haph(ē)* sense of touch + -IA] Loss or reduction of the sense of touch. *Obs.* Also *anhaphia*. Adj. anaptic.

**anaphoresis** \an'əfôrē'sis\ *Obs.* ANHIDROSIS.

**anaphoretic** \an'əfôret'ik\ [Gk *an-* priv. + *(di)aphoretic*] ANTIPERSPIRANT.

**anaphrodisiac** \an'afrōdiz'ē·ak\ **1** Tending to reduce sexual desire. **2** An anaphrodisiac agent.

**anaphylactic** Of or relating to anaphylaxis.

**anaphylactogen** \an'əfīlak'təjən\ *Obs.* ALLERGEN.

**anaphylactoid** \an'əfīlak'toid\ Like anaphylaxis; having characteristics of anaphylaxis.

**anaphylactotoxin** \an'əfīlak'tōtäk'sin\ A product of complement activation capable of inducing anaphylaxis. Also *anaphylatoxin, anaphylotoxin*.

**anaphylaxis** \an'əfilak'sis\ [ANA- (upward, heightened, intensified) + Gk *phylaxis* guard, defense (from *phylax* a guard, sentinel, protector)] An acute or exaggerated allergic response in a sensitized host following injection of or exposure to a foreign protein or other substance. It may be induced experimentally in animals but also occurs in humans. The reaction is caused by release of histamine or other vasoreactive substances when antigen combines with antibody, predominantly IgE, on the surface of basophils or mast cells. Symptoms include edema, diarrhea, bleeding, vomiting, shock, bronchospasm, and respiratory distress. Also *anaphylactic reaction*. Adj. anaphylactic. **active a.** Any anaphylactic reaction that occurs in an individual with preformed antibodies to the inciting antigen. Compare PASSIVE ANAPHYLAXIS. **active cutaneous a.** A local reaction in skin, usually a wheal and flare reaction, occurring in response to antigen injected intradermally in an individual with skin-sensitizing antibodies specific for that antigen. It is often used to test for sensitivity to individual antigens. **generalized a.** SYSTEMIC ANAPHYLAXIS. **heterocytotropic a.** Passive anaphylaxis induced with heterocytotropic antibodies. Also *heterologous anaphylaxis*. **homocytotropic a.** Passive anaphylaxis induced with homocytotropic antibodies. Also *homologous anaphylaxis*. **inverse a.** **1** REVERSE PASSIVE ANAPHYLAXIS. **2** An inaccurate term for FORSMANN SHOCK. **local a.** Anaphylaxis in which the reaction is localized at the site where antigen is encountered. Examples include the site of injection in a skin test, as in passive cutaneous anaphylaxis; or the respiratory tract, as in the case of inhaled antigens. **passive a.** Anaphylaxis in which the sensitizing antibody (usually IgE) is injected into the subject either locally into the skin or systemically, and in which the anaphylactic reaction is then provoked by the administration of antigen. Compare ACTIVE ANAPHYLAXIS. **passive cutaneous a.** The transfer of skin-sensitizing antibodies, now identified as IgE, from one individual to another of the same species. Following intradermal injection of serum, antigen is injected intravenously and the site at which circulating antigen combines with cell-fixed antibody exhibits a wheal and flare reaction. Evans blue dye has been used in animals as an indicator for location and size of the reacting area. **reverse passive a.** An immunologically mediated reaction occurring when an animal is injected with antibodies to antigens occurring on its own tissues. The test example is the injection of anti-Forssman antibodies into guinea pigs, which causes severe endothelial damage. The antibodies responsible are not IgE and the reaction is not one of anaphylaxis. It is a cytotoxic reaction (type II of Coombs and Gell reactions). Also *inverse anaphylaxis, reverse anaphylaxis*. **systemic a.** Anaphylaxis in which the antigen is introduced into the circulation. The reaction involves many tissues although it may affect a particular organ or kind of tissue, depending upon the species, and may cause shock. Also *generalized anaphylaxis*.

**anaphylotoxin** \an'əfī'lətäk'sin\ ANAPHYLACTOTOXIN.

**anaplasia** \an'əplā'zhə\ [ANA- + -PLASIA] A process or state of a neoplasm characterized by the loss of normal cellular differentiation, tissue organization, and function. The degree of anaplasia, or deviation from the normal, has been used to grade tumors, such as bladder carcinomas. Also *dedifferentiation*.

**anaplastic** \an'əplas'tik\ Characterized by an extreme degree of anaplasia, as *anaplastic carcinoma of the thyroid*.

**anaplasty** \an'əplas'tē\ [ANA- + -PLASTY] Plastic or reconstructive surgery. *Outmoded.* Also *anaplastic surgery*.

**anaplerosis** \an'əplerō'sis\ [Gk *ana-* up + *plērōsis* a filling] Any plastic surgical procedure in which tissue is transplanted to fill in a defect and thus make the contour of the defective part more normal. *Outmoded.* Adj. anaplerotic.

**anaplerotic** \an'əplerät'ik\ Describing a reaction that effects the new formation of an intermediate of the tricarboxylic acid cycle, in order to maintain the intracellular concentration of it (or of another such intermediate) as those intermediates are utilized for biosynthesis.

**anapnea** \anap'nē·ə\ [Gk *anapnoia*, also *anapnoē* (from *anapnein* to breathe again) recovery of breath] The restoration of breathing. Adj. anapneic.

**anapnometer** \an′apnäm′ətər\ *Obs.* SPIROMETER.

**anarithmia** \an′ərith′mē·ə\ [Gk *an-* priv. + *arithm(os)* a number + -IA] Inability to count or to use numbers. *Obs.*

**anarthria** \anärth′rē·ə\ [New L, from Gk *an-* priv. + *arthr(oun)* (from *arthron* a joint) to articulate + -IA] Inability to speak, due not to any defect of the conceptualization of speech, but solely to loss of the ability to articulate. Phonation may be unaffected. The loss of articulation can be due to paralysis (upper or lower motor neuron), dystonia, or apraxia of the articulatory muscles. Dysarthria is a less severe disorder of articulation. **a. literalis** An inability to articulate letters.

**anasarca** \an′əsär′kə\ [Med L, from Gk *anasarka hydrōpa*, accus. of *anasarx hydrōps* (from *ana* throughout + *sarka*, accus. of *sarx* flesh + *hydrōps* dropsy) generalized dropsy] Severe edema involving the entire body and including marked swelling of subcutaneous tissues and the accumulation of fluid in serous cavities. Also *hyposarca*. Adj. anasarcous.

**anaschistic** \an′askis′tik\ [ANA- + Gk *schist(os)* (from *schizein* to split, cleave) divided, cloven + -IC] Splitting longitudinally: used especially of bivalent chromosomes during meiosis.

**anastigmatic** \an′astigmat′ik\ Free from astigmatism.

**anastole** \ənas′tōlē\ [Gk *anastolē* (from *anastellein* to go back, retire) a pulling back, withdrawal] A retraction of the edges of a wound.

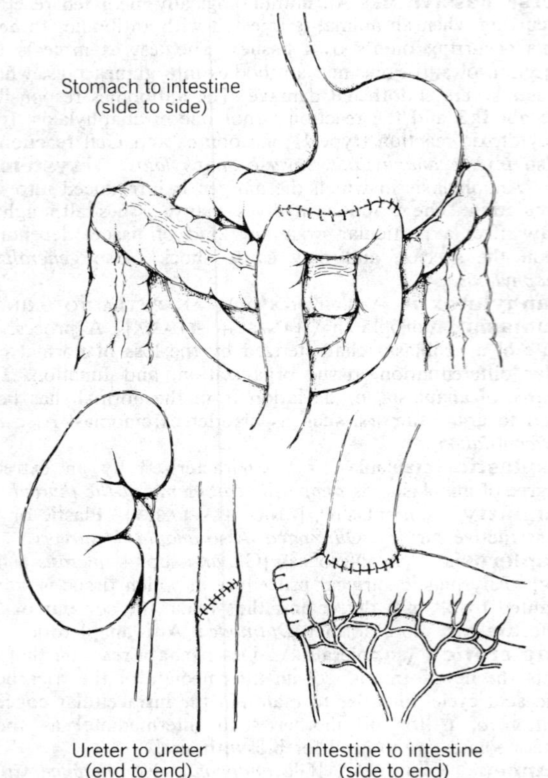


**Surgical anastomoses**

**anastomose** \ənas′tōmōs\ [back formation from ANASTOMOSIS] To create a communication between two separate structures.

**anastomosis** \ənas′təmō′sis\ [Gk *anastomōsis* (from *anastomoun* to open up, make patent, from *stoma* mouth) provision of an opening, inosculation, outlet] (*pl.* anastomoses.) **1** A natural juncture between similar structures, such as blood vessels or nerves. **2** A surgical joining of two, usually tubular, structures, such as two ends of a divided intestinal tract, blood vessels, or nerves. Also *inosculation*. Adj. anastomotic. **antiperistaltic a.** An anastomosis of two tubular structures to reestablish luminal continuity in such a way that the normal flow in one segment is contrary to that in the other. **aorticopulmonary a.** A communication between the aorta and pulmonary artery, either occurring naturally or resulting from a surgical or pharmacological intervention. It is used as a palliative treatment for complex cyanotic congenital heart disease. **a. around elbow joint** RETE ARTICULARE CUBITI. **a. around knee joint** **1** RETE ARTICULARE GENUS. **2** RETE PATELLARIS. **arterial a.** **1** The direct communication between two or more medium-sized arteries, such as in the circulus arteriosus cerebri, the anastomoses around various joints, and the anastomoses between branches of the intestinal arteries. **2** RETE ARTERIOSUM. **a. arteriolovenularis** [NA] A communication between a side branch of an arteriole and a venule, usually having a wide caliber, a muscular wall, and a precapillary sphincter by contraction of which the channel is closed and the blood is forced through an adjacent capillary system. When the short, shunting vessel is open, the blood short-circuits the capillary bed, thereby regulating capillary blood flow. In various parts of the body direct connections also exist between smaller arteries and corresponding veins, shunting blood in a similar fashion. Also *arteriolovenular anastomosis, anastomosis arteriovenosa, arteriovenous anastomosis.* **Billroth a.** BILLROTH'S OPERATION. **Clado's a.** The anastomosis between the appendicular and ovarian arteries in the infundibulopelvic ligament, or suspensory ligament of the ovary. **crucial a.** One of a series of anastomoses between the gluteal region and the knee joint, located at the back of the upper thigh in the region of the greater trochanter of femur and basically comprising four vessels in the rough form of a cross; the transverse branches of the medial and lateral circumflex femoral arteries that anastomose superiorly with the inferior gluteal artery and inferiorly with the first perforating branch of the profunda femoris artery. Also *cruciate anastomosis.* **direct transperitoneal ureterocolic a.** The surgical connection of a divided ureter to the colon through the posterior parietal peritoneum. **end-to-end a.** An anastomosis between the ends of two separate structures, as arteries or veins. **end-to-side a.** SIDE-TO-END ANASTOMOSIS. **esophagojejunal a.** The surgical reestablishment of luminal continuity, as by suturing, between the jejunum and the esophagus following a total gastrectomy. **faciohypoglossal a.** A surgical operation of joining the proximal end of the divided hypoglossal nerve in the neck to the distal end of the facial nerve, divided at its point of emergence from the stylomastoid foramen. The operation restores much of the muscular function of the face when performed within a year after damage to the intracranial portion of the facial nerve. Also *hypoglossal-facial-nerve anastomosis.* **Galen's a.** RAMUS COMMUNICANS NERVI LARYNGEI SUPERIORIS CUM NERVO LARYNGEO INFERIORI. **genicular a.** RETE ARTICULARE GENUS. **Haight a.** A double-layered anastomosis designed to prevent leakage from an esophageal anastomosis that has been performed in cases of esophageal atresia. **hypoglossal-facial-nerve a.** FACIOHYPOGLOSSAL ANASTOMOSIS. **Hyrtl's a.** HYRTL'S LOOP. **intermesenteric arterial a.** An occasional anastomosis between a large branch arising from the superior mesenteric artery or the middle colic artery at its root and the inferior mesenteric artery or its left colic branch. It is usually situated close to or within the paraduodenal fold, running parallel to the marginal artery of the colon. Also *Riolan's arc, intermesenteric arterial arch.* **intersubcardinal a.** One or more vessels in the embryo linking the subcardinal veins and lying ventral to the aorta. Eventually it becomes part of the left renal vein of the adult. Also *preaortic anastomosis.* **intestinal a.** The surgical establishment of a connection between two loops of intestine to provide luminal continuity. **isoperistaltic a.** An anastomosis of two tubular structures, usually intestine, so as to maintain luminal continuity in the natural direction of peristalsis for both segments. **lymphaticovenous a.** The surgical construction of a communication between the venous system and the lymphatic system. It is usually performed, using microsurgical techniques, in an extremity for the treatment of lymphedema. Also *lymphaticovenous shunt.* **meningeal arterial anastomoses** Junctions without intervening arterioles or capillaries between small cerebral cortical arteries lying deep to the pia mater. **nerve a.** The surgical operation of joining divided nerves to permit regeneration of nerve fibers. **portacaval a.** The surgical creation of a communication between the inferior vena cava and the portal vein or their tributaries with the purpose of relieving portal hypertension. Also *portosystemic anastomosis.* **postcostal a.** A longitudinal anastomosing vessel in the neck region of the embryo, one on each side, which links the upper seven intersegmental arteries and eventually becomes the vertebral artery. **post-transverse a.** Communication between the posterior branches of the dorsal segmental arteries of the embryo, behind the transverse processes of the vertebrae. The vertebral artery arises from a longitudinal anastomosis between the vertical branches of these segmental communications. **precapillary a.** An anastomosis between small arteries before they become capillaries. **precostal a.** A longitudinal anastomosis joining together certain embryonic intersegmental arteries and developing into the thyrocervical and costocervical trunks of the adult. **pyeloileocutaneous a.** A surgical connection of the renal pelvis to an isolated loop of ileum, from which a stoma is created for external drainage of urine. **rectosigmoid a.** The anastomosis between the various branches of the superior rectal artery that are given off prior to its termination into right and left branches. Branches of the anastomosis supply the region of the rectosigmoid junction and may also anastomose with the most distal sigmoid artery to form part of the marginal artery of the colon. Also *artery of Drummond, rectosigmoid artery.* **Roux-en-Y a.** Any Y-shaped anastomosis involving the small intestine. **Schmiedel's anastomoses** Anastomoses between the tributaries of the inferior vena cava and those of the portal system. **side-to-end a.** An anastomosis created between the end of one structure and the side of another. Also *end-to-side anastomosis.* **side-to-side a.** An anastomosis created between the sides of two structures being joined. **splenorenal a.** An anastomosis between the splenic and renal arteries or the splenic and renal veins. **Sucquet-Hoyer a.** SUCQUET-HOYER CANAL. **sutureless a.** Surgical anastomosis of nerves without the aid of sutures. The method usually employs plasma clot and a conduit to promote growth of nerve fibers between ends of nerves. **terminoterminal a.** END-TO-END ANASTOMOSIS. **transureteroureteral a.** The surgical anastomosis of the end of one ureter to the wall of the opposite ureter. **triple a.** **1** Any anastomosis, however created, that provides direct luminal continuity among three tubular structures. **2** The surgical reconstruction of luminal continuity following Whipple's operation. **ureteroileocutaneous a.** The anastomosis of the end of a ureter to an isolated loop of ileum that is linked to the outside of the body by a fistula, thus establishing external drainage. **ureterotubal a.** A surgical procedure in which a portion of fallopian tube is substituted for ureter. **ureteroureteral a.** An anastomosis that joins one part of a ureter with another part of the same ureter. **ventriculocisternal a.** TORKILDSEN SHUNT.

**anastral** \anas′trəl\ Without asters: used of achromatic figures.

**anatomical** \an′ətäm′əkəl\ [Gk *anatomik(os)* (from *anatomē* dissection; see ANATOMY) relating to or skilled in anatomy + -AL] **1** Pertaining to anatomy, or the structural organization of an organism. **2** Characterizing a purely structural or morphological feature of the body, without reference to clinical, surgical, or physiological considerations, as in *anatomical neck, anatomical dead space.* For defs. 1 and 2 also *anatomic.*

**anatomism** \ənat′əmizm\ [*anatom(y)* + -ISM] The theoretical concept that the phenomena of life in organized bodies are due to their structure.

**anatomist** \ənat′əmist\ [*anatom(y)* + -IST] One who is professionally involved in or a specialist in the science of anatomy.

**anatomopathology** \ənat′əmōpathäl′əjē\ The anatomic aspects of pathology.

**anatomy** \ənat′əmē\ [Late L *anatomia*, from Gk *anatomē* dissection, from *anatemnein* to dissect, cut up, from *ana-* up, thoroughly + *temnein* to cut] **1** The science of the structural organization of any organism, whether plant or animal. **2** The macroscopic structural organization of a part or body, usually determined by means of dissection. **3** Morphology; the study of the shape and underlying pattern of organisms. **applied a.** The practical application of anatomic knowledge to the diagnosis and treatment (including surgical techniques) of clinical conditions. **artificial a.** The study of structures and their relationships by means of models or other manufactured articles. **clastic a.** Artificial anatomy using models or drawings on superposed plastic sheets in removable layers depicting successively deeper structures. **comparative a.** The systematic comparison of bodily structures and their functions in all living organisms. **corrosion a.** The study of anatomy by means of special preparations wherein an organ or part is corroded by chemicals and removed after certain vessels, ducts, or parts are treated so as to withstand the corrosive action, preserving their form, e.g., corrosive removal of lung tissue to display the distribution of the bronchial tree and pulmonary vessels. **cross-sectional a.** The study of anatomy, especially the interrelation of regional structures, by the preparation of transverse, sagittal, or other sections of parts of the body. **descriptive a.** The description of the structure of tissues, organs, and parts as observed, either macroscopically or microscopically, without necessarily referring to their functions. The *Nomina Anatomica* has been formulated on this basis. Also *systematic anatomy.* **developmental a.** The branch of embryology concerned primarily with the development of structure, tissues, and organs, rather than with, for example, biochemical, genetic, or experimental aspects. **general a.** The combined gross and microscopic anatomy of the organs, tissues, and fluids of the body. **gross a.** The study of the structural organization of the different parts of an organism by means of dissection and with the unaided eye. Also *macroscopic anatomy.* **histologic a.** HISTOLOGY. **macroscopic a.** GROSS ANATOMY. **medical a.** The application of anatomic knowledge to the location, diagnosis, and treatment of medical disorders. **microscopic a.** HISTOLOGY. **minute a.** HISTOLOGY. **morbid a.** ANATOMIC PATHOLOGY. **pathological a.** ANATOMIC PATHOLOGY. **physiologic a.** The study of the structure of organs and tissues in relation to their normal functions. **practical a.** The study of anatomy by means of dissection and demonstration. **radiological a.** The study of normal bodily parts and their interrelations by using radiologic techniques. **regional a.** The study of structures in distinct regions of the body, isolated for descriptive convenience or on a functional basis, such as the head, the limbs, and the abdomen, or subdivisions of these such as the shoulder region, the brachial region, the gluteal region, etc. **surface a.** The study of the markings and bony points on the surface of the body, particularly in relation to underlying and deeper structures, e.g. the outline of the heart and location of its valves projected to the surface of the chest. **surgical a.** The study of the anatomy of a region of the body with particular emphasis on concepts important to the diagnosis and treatment of surgically correctable disease. **systematic a.** **1** The study of an organism's structures grouped into functional systems, such as respiratory, endocrine, digestive, nervous, circulatory, etc., without regard to specific regions. Also *systemic anatomy.* **2** DESCRIPTIVE ANATOMY. **topographic a.** The study of an organism's structures in relation to their neighboring structures as revealed by dissection, light and electron microscopy, or other techniques. For example, in gross anatomy, the relationships of nerves, blood vessels, and lymph nodes to a particular muscle, ligament, etc.

**anatoxin** \an′ətäk′sin\ TOXOID. **a.-Ramon** DIPHTHERIA TOXOID.

**anatoxireaction** \an′ətäksirē·ak′shən\ [ANA- + *toxi(coid)* + REACTION] MOLONEY TEST.

**anatricrotic** \an′ətrīkrät′ik\ Pertaining to a pulse wave with three identifiable notches on the upstroke.

**anatropia** \an′ətrō′pē·ə\ [ANA- + -TROPIA] Abnormal symmetrical binocular upturning of the eyes. Also *anotropia.* Adj. anatropic.

**anazolene sodium** $C_{26}H_{16}N_3Na_3O_{10}S_3$. 4′-Anilino-8-hydroxy-1,1′-azo-naphthalene-3,5′,6-trisulfonic acid trisodium salt, a dye that is used to evaluate cardiovascular function and measure plasma volume. Also *Coomassie blue.*

**AnCC** anodal closure contraction.

**-ance** \-əns\ [L *-antia* (from *-ans,* gen. *-antis,* pres. part. ending of verbs ending in *-are* + -IA) noun suffix denoting action, process, quality, state, or amount] A noun suffix denoting action, state, or condition.

**anchiroid** \ang′kəroid\ ANKYROID.

**anchorage** \ang′kərij\ The use of a tooth or other anatomical part as a base from which to push or pull other teeth. **cervical a.** A form of extraoral anchorage using the back of the neck as a base. Force is transmitted to the teeth by means of elastic and cords. **intermaxillary a.** The use of teeth in the opposite jaw as a base for anchorage. Also *maxillomandibular anchorage.* **intramaxillary a.** The use of teeth in the same jaw as a base for anchorage. Also *simple anchorage.* **maxillomandibular a.** INTERMAXILLARY ANCHORAGE. **occipital a.** The use of the cranium as anchorage by means of a headcap and elastic bands. **reciprocal a.** The use of two teeth or groups of teeth as bases for each other so that both move in the required, opposite directions. **simple a.** INTRAMAXILLARY ANCHORAGE.

**anchylo-** \ang′kilō-\ ANKYLO-.

**ancipital** \ansip′itəl\ Two-headed; two-edged.

**anciroid** \an′səroid\ ANKYROID.

***Ancistrodon*** \ansis′trədän\ *AGKISTRODON.*

**ancon** \ang′kän\ [Gk *ankōn* elbow] CUBITUS.

**anconad** \ang′kənad\ Toward the elbow.

**anconeus** \angkō′nē·əs\ [New L (from Gk *ankōn* elbow) pertaining to the elbow] See under MUSCULUS ANCONEUS.

**anconitis** \ang′kōnī′tis\ [Gk *ankōn* the bend or hollow of the arm, the elbow + -ITIS] An inflammation of the elbow joint.

**anconoid** \ang′kənoid\ Resembling an elbow.

**ancylo-** \an′silō-\ ANKYLO-.

***Ancylostoma*** \an′siläs′təmə\ [New L (from Gk *ankylo(s)* crooked, curved + *stoma* mouth)] A genus of bloodsucking intestinal nematodes (family Ancylostomatidae) commonly known as hookworms, of veterinary and medical importance as a cause of anemia. Adult parasites attach to the villi of the duodenum by paired sets of ventral teeth or cutting plates and suck blood. Eggs passed in feces develop in a few days into infective third-stage larvae in moist, sandy soil. Entry to the host is percutaneous, though infection by *A. duodenale,* the human Old World hookworm, may also be acquired orally. ***A. americanum*** *NECATOR AMERICANUS.* ***A. braziliense*** A species parasitic in the intestines of dogs and cats. In humans it may occur as cutaneous larva migrans (creeping eruption), caused by the wandering of larvae unable to complete their migration and development in the abnormal host. ***A. caninum*** The cosmopolitan hookworm of dogs. It is also capable of producing cutaneous larva migrans in humans. In pups or kittens, heavy infections with these worms may cause severe iron-deficiency anemia. ***A. duodenale*** The European or Old World hookworm, the common hookworm of humans in temperate areas of Europe and Asia, especially in the Mediterranean region. It is the principal cause of human ancylostomiasis. Also *Sclerostoma duodenale, Uncinaria duodenalis.*

**Ancylostomatidae** \an′silästō′mətədē′\ [ANCYLOSTOMA + *t* + -IDAE] The family of hookworm nematodes, including the important genera *Ancylostoma* and *Necator,* worldwide in distribution among many mammalian hosts, including humans. The worms are especially common in carnivores, where they typically attach to villi in the anterior small intestine, aided by cutting teeth or plates. They suck blood continuously, causing significant anemia in heavy infections, especially among young animals or humans. Also *Ancylostomidae.*

**ancylostome** \ansil′ästōm\ A member of the family Ancylostomatidae or of the genus *Ancylostoma.*.

**ancylostomiasis** \an′siləstōmī′əsis\ [*ancylostom(e)* + -IASIS] A disease caused by infection with nematodes (hookworms) of the genus *Ancylostoma* or *Necator.* The normal habitat in man is the small intestine, especially the jejunum. In humans, a moderate or heavy, chronic infection with *Ancylostoma duodenale* or *Necator americanus* is characterized by microcytic, hypochromic anemia, emaciation, hypoalbuminemia, and varying degrees of edema. Physical, mental, or sexual retardation may be present in chronically infected children. Mild infections may be asymptomatic. Also *ankylostomiasis.* **cutaneous a.** A localized erythema and dermatitis produced by ancylostome hookworm larvae as they penetrate the skin. Itching, often called ground itch or dew itch, can be severe, especially after sensitizing exposures. In man, the ankles, feet, and areas between the toes are commonly affected. Also *ancylostomiasis cutis, ancyclostome dermatitis.*

**Ancylostomidae** \an′silästäm′idē\ ANCYLOSTOMATIDAE

**Anders** [James Meschter *Anders,* U.S. physician, 1854–1936] Anders disease. See under ADIPOSIS TUBEROSA SIMPLEX.

**Andersch** [Carl Samuel *Andersch,* German anatomist, 1732–1777] **1** Andersch ganglion. See under GANGLION INFERIUS NERVI GLOSSOPHARYNGEI. **2** Andersch nerve. See under NERVUS TYMPANICUS.

**Andersen** [Dorothy Hansine *Andersen,* U.S. pediatrician, 1901–1963] Andersen's disease. See under GLYCOGEN STORAGE DISEASE IV.

**Anderson** [John F *Anderson,* U.S. physician, born 1873] Anderson and Goldberger test. See under TEST.

**Anderson** [Roger *Anderson,* U.S. orthopedic surgeon, 1891–1971] **1** Anderson's operation. See under ANDERSON'S AMPUTATION. **2** Roger-Anderson pin fixation appliance. See under ROGER-ANDERSON EXTRAORAL SPLINT.

**andr-** \andr-\ ANDRO-.

**Andrews** [George Clinton *Andrews,* U.S. dermatologist, born 1891] Andrews disease. See under PUSTULOSIS PALMARIS ET PLANTARIS.

**andriatrics** \an′drē·at′riks\ [ANDR- + -IATRICS] The branch of medicine dealing with diseases of men, such as those of the male genitalia. Also *andriatry.*

**andrin** \an′drin\ The androgens of the testis, as testosterone and $\Delta^4$-androstenedione. *Seldom used.*

**andro-** \an′drō-\ [Gk *anēr* (genitive *andros*) a man] A combining form meaning man, male. Also *andr-.*

**androblastoma** \-blastō′mə\ [ANDRO- + BLASTOMA] Any of a group of uncommon ovarian and testicular tumors containing Sertoli and Leydig cells of varying degrees of maturity. Indifferent gonadal cells of embryonal appearance are present in certain cases. Most are virilizing, but some are estrogenic or inactive. Subtypes of well-differentiated forms include tubular androblastoma, tubular androblastoma with lipid storage, Sertoli-Leydig cell tumor, and Leydig cell tumor. Tumors of intermediate and poor differentiation occur. They are more apt to be malignant. The well-differentiated forms are almost always benign. **tubular a.** A well-differentiated androblastoma composed of Sertoli cells forming well-defined tubules. Also *Sertoli cell tumor, tubular adenoma of Pick, testicular adenoma.*

**androcyte** \an′drəsīt\ [ANDRO- + -CYTE] SPERMATID.

**androgalactozemia** \-gəlak′təzē′mē·ə\ [ANDRO- + GALACTO- + Gk *zēmia* loss] Lactation from the male breast.

**androgen** \an′drəjən\ [ANDRO- + -GEN] Any hormone that induces masculinization in either sex, as some of the steroid hormones secreted by the testis (testosterone), the adrenal cortex (androst-4-ene-3,20-dione), or the ovary; $C_{19}$ steroid hormones. Also *androgenic hormone.* **adrenal a.** Any of the C-19 steroid hormones secreted by the normal adrenal in both sexes, as $\Delta^4$-androstenedione, dehydroepiandrosterone, or 11$\beta$-hydroxyandrostenedione. The chief precursors of urinary 17-ketosteroids, they are secreted in excess in the various forms of adrenal virilism.

**androgenesis** \-jen′əsis\ The development of a haploid organism containing only paternal chromosomes, occurring when the maternal nucleus disintegrates in the fertilized egg before fusion (syngamy) with the paternal nucleus. Also *patrogenesis.*

**androgenic** \-jen′ik\ [ANDRO- + -GENIC] Inducing masculinization or virilization in either sex.

**androgenicity** \-jənis′itē\ The quality of having a masculinizing or virilizing action, a property of androgenic hormones.

**androgenization** \andräj′ənīzā′shən\ Excessive androgen production in the female or the clinical state of virilization resulting from it or from the administration of androgen.

**androgenous** \andräj′ənəs\ **1** Referring to the birth of male offspring. **2** Pertaining to the preferential production of male offspring.

**androgone** \an′drəgōn\ [ANDRO- + Gk *gonē* seed] A spermatogenic cell.

**androgyne** \an′drəjīn\ [Gk *androgyn(os)* (from *anēr,* gen. *andros,* a man + *gynē* a woman) a hermaphrodite] FEMALE PSEUDOHERMAPHRODITE.

**androgynic** \-jin′ik\ Pertaining to androgyny; having both male and female characteristics.

**androgynous** \andräj′ənəs\ [Gk *androgynos* (from *anēr,* gen. *andros* a man, male + *gynē* a woman, female) a hermaphrodite] Having or exhibiting both male and female characteristics.

**androgynus** \andräj′ənəs\ [L, from Gk *androgynos.* See ANDROGYNOUS.] FEMALE PSEUDOHERMAPHRODITE.

**android** \an′droid\ [ANDR- + -OID] Like a male; manlike.

**andrology** \andräl′əjē\ [ANDRO- + -LOGY] The study of the male morphology and diseases of the male reproductive system.

**andromedotoxin** \andräm′ədōtäk′sin\ $C_{31}H_{50}O_{10}$. A toxic substance present in the leaves and bark of various species in the plant genera *Andromeda, Kalmia,* and *Rhododendron.* It stimulates the parasympathetic nervous system and causes labored respiration, hypotension, convulsions, and cardiac paralysis.

**andromerogone** \-mer′əgōn\ [ANDRO- + MERO-[1] + Gk *gonē* seed, offspring] An embryo that develops from the portion of an egg containing the male pronucleus. The embryo therefore only contains paternally derived chromosomes. Also *andromerogon, androgenone.*

**andromerogony** \-meräg′ənē\ [ANDRO- + MERO-[1] + -GONY] The development of an andromerogone.

**androphile** \an′drəfīl\ [ANDRO- + -PHILE] ANTHROPOPHILIC.

**androphilic** \-fil′ik\ [ANDRO- + -PHILIC] ANTHROPOPHILIC.

**androphilous** \andräf′iləs\ ANTHROPOPHILIC.

**androstane** The parent hydrocarbon of many androgenic $C_{19}$ steroids. It contains all the rings of cholesterol and the angular methyl carbons C-18 and C-19, but no side chain on C-17. Also *etiocholane* (obs.).

**androstanediol** Usually androstane-3,17-diol, a metabolite of certain androgens. Since natural steroids are derived from cholesterol, which has a 3-hydroxyl group, and removal of the side chain on C-17 leaves an oxygen in its place, the natural compound is 3,17. This compound could be formed by reduction of the main natural androgen, testosterone.

**androstanedione** One of the androgenic steroids, usually androstane-3,17-dione. This could be formed from testosterone by hydrogenating its 4(5) double bond and oxidizing the CHOH group at C-17 to CO′.

**androstenediol** Usually androst-4-ene-3,17-diol, which is a compound formed from testosterone by reduction of its 3-carbonyl group to —CHOH—.

**androstenedione** $C_{19}H_{26}O_2$. 4-Androstene-3,17-dione. A major component of the adrenal androgen and an ovarian secretory product. It is converted to estrone in the periphery and ultimately excreted in the urine as more polar 17-ketosteroids, chiefly androsterone and etiocholanolone. It is a metabolite of testerone formed by oxidation at C-17, and, like testerone, it is androgenic.

**androsterone** \andräs′tərōn\ $C_{19}H_{30}O_2$. 3α-Hydroxy-5α-androstan-17-one. A major metabolite of testosterone and androstenedione, found in the plasma and urine of men and women. Its biologic potency as an androgen is a fraction of that possessed by testosterone.

**AnDTe** anodal duration tetanus.

**-ane** [arbitrary alteration of -ENE, -INE, and -ONE] A suffix indicating a saturated hydrocarbon.

**anecdotal** \an′əkdō′təl\ Based on casual observation rather than systematic study or controlled scientific experimentation. ⟨"Only a dozen cases in the medical literature link liver toxicity to a combination of alcohol and acetaminophen. But anecdotal findings and speculation about interactions have fueled suspicion that a relation is often missed." —*Medical World News,* 8 Aug. 1980, 48.⟩

**anechoic** \an′ekō′ik\ [Gk *an-* priv. + *echoic*] Echo-free.

**anelectrotonus** \an′ilekträt′ənəs\ A state of reduced excitability in an excitable tissue due to hyperpolarization in the region of an anode during the passage of an electric current.

# anemia

**anemia** \ənē′mē·ə\ [New L *anaemia,* from Gk *anaimia* (from *an-* priv. + *(h)aim(a)* blood + -IA) blood deficiency] An abnormal decrease in the concentration of erythrocytes, concentration of hemoglobin, or hematocrit which may result from decreased production or increased loss or destruction of erythrocytes, often accompanied by characteristic signs and symptoms including pallor, asthenia, and dyspnea. Also *hypemia* (obs.), *hyphemia* (obs.), *oligocythemia* (obs.). **achlorhydric a.** ACHYLIC ANEMIA. **achrestic a.** Any progressive macrocytic anemia, resembling pernicious anemia but not responsive to vitamin $B_{12}$. In most instances it is a preleukemic syndrome. *Imprecise.* Also *Israels-Wilkinson anemia.* **achylic a.** Iron deficiency anemia in association with achlorhydria. *Obs.* Also *anemia achylica, achlorhydric anemia, Faber syndrome.* **acquired sideroachrestic a.** REFRACTORY SIDEROBLASTIC ANEMIA. **acquired sideroblastic a.** REFRACTORY SIDEROBLASTIC ANEMIA. **Addison's a.** PERNICIOUS ANEMIA. **Addison-Biermer a.** PERNICIOUS ANEMIA. **addisonian a.** PERNICIOUS ANEMIA. **ancylostome a.** A form of chronic microcytic hypochromic anemia resulting from hookworm disease. In humans it is caused by *Ancylostoma duodenale* or *Necator americanus.* It often accompanies malnutrition, especially in children. Also *Egyptian chlorosis, tropical chlorosis.* **aplastic a.** A serious and usually lethal blood disorder in which all cellular elements of blood and bone marrow are reduced in number due to failure of blood cell precursors to reproduce. Also *atrophic anemia, anhemopoietic anemia, aplastic myelosis.* **arctic a.** POLAR ANEMIA. **asiderotic a.** IRON DEFICIENCY ANEMIA. **atrophic a.** APLASTIC ANEMIA. **autoimmune hemolytic a.** Acquired hemolytic anemia in which the direct antiglobulin test is positive, thus demonstrating antibodies bound to the patient's erythrocytes. Also *autoimmune hemolytic disease.* **Baghdad spring a.** *Seldom used* FAVISM. **Banti's a.** Anemia accompanied by splenomegaly, leukopenia and often thrombocytopenia. It is part of the Banti syndrome. ***Bartonella* a.** A hemolytic anemia that accompanies the febrile stage (Oroya fever) of bartonellosis. **Biermer's a.** PERNICIOUS ANEMIA. **Biermer-Ehrlich a.** PERNICIOUS ANEMIA. Also *quintan fever, Meuse fever, shinbone fever, Volhynia fever, Wolhynia fever, His-Werner disease, Werner-his disease, quintana fever.* **chlorotic a.** CHLOROSIS. **a. of chronic disease** A mild-to-moderate anemia that is typically microcytic, or hypochromic and microcytic, and develops in association with malignancies or chronic inflammatory disorders such as rheumatoid arthritis. The disorder is caused by impairment in the recycling of iron from phagocytic digestion of hemoglobin to newly forming erythrocytic precursors. Also *simple chronic anemia.* **congenital aplastic a.** FANCONI'S ANEMIA. **congenital dyserythropoietic a.** A moderately severe life-long anemia with onset in infancy, due to abnormal formation and structure of erythrocyte precursors in bone marrow. Several types have been described, of which three are well recognized as congenital dyserythropoietic anemia types I, II, and III. Type I is inherited as an autosomal recessive disorder characterized by hemolytic anemia, macrocytosis, and erythrocyte fragmentation, and by bone marrow changes of megaloblastoid maturation of erythrocyte precursors, many of which are binucleate, and occasional pairs of normoblasts with internuclear chromatin bridges. Type II, the most common type, is inherited as an autosomal recessive disorder characterized by anemia, poikilocytosis, and bone marrow that displays many binucleate or multinucleate erythroid precursors. Erythrocytes exhibit high titers for i and I antigens, and the acid serum (Ham's) test is positive. Type II is also called HEMPAS (for hereditary erythroblastic multinuclearity with positive acid serum test). Type III is inherited as an autosomal dominant disorder characterized by anemia, macrocytosis, and marked multinuclearity of very large erythrocyte precursors in bone marrow. Erythrocytes exhibit high titers of i and I antigens. Type IV is a variant of type II, from which it differs in that the acid serum test is negative. Abbr. CDA **congenital Heinz-body a.** UNSTABLE HEMOGLOBIN HEMOLYTIC ANEMIA. **congenital hemolytic a.** HEREDITARY SPHEROCYTOSIS. **congenital hypoplastic a.** FANCONI'S ANEMIA. **congenital microcytic a.** THALASSEMIA. **congenital nonspherocytic hemolytic a.** Any of several hereditary hemolytic anemias which are not associated with spherocytosis. Included are hereditary hemolytic anemias due to deficiencies of erythrocyte enzymes or due to unstable hemoglobins. **congenital pernicious a.** A rare anemia of infancy due to lack of secretion of intrinsic factor by the stomach and the inability to absorb vitamin $B_{12}$ from dietary sources. In this disorder the anemia is macrocytic and megaloblastic, and has all the other features of pernicious anemia except that there is normal formation of hydrochloric acid in the stomach and there is no gastric atrophy. The disorder is inherited and is autosomal recessive. Only homozygotes are affected. **constitutional aplastic a.** FANCONI'S ANEMIA. **Cooley's a.** THALASSEMIA MAJOR. **Coombs-negative immune hemolytic a.** Hemolytic anemia associated with non-IgG immunoglobulin (such as complement or IgM) on the erythrocyte surface. **cow's milk a.** Iron deficiency anemia of infancy or early childhood due to prolonged use of bovine milk feeding without iron supplementation. In many cases there may be a sensitivity reaction of the intestine to nonheated whole cow's milk, with consequent malabsorption syndrome and intestinal bleeding. **crescent cell a.** SICKLE CELL ANEMIA. **cytogenic a.** PERNICIOUS ANEMIA. **Diamond-Blackfan a.** Congenital anemia due to failure of the bone marrow to produce red blood cells. Also *congenital pure red cell aplasia, Diamond-Blackfan syndrome.* **dilution a.** A reduction in hemoglobin concentration, erythrocyte count, or hematocrit of blood that is due to an increase in the volume of plasma in the circulating blood rather than to a reduction in the total number of erythrocytes or total hemoglobin content of the blood. It is a relative or spurious anemia. **dimorphic a.** An anemia characterized by the presence of two populations of erythrocytes, each presenting a different appearance in a stained blood film. **drepanocytic a.** SICKLE CELL ANEMIA. **Dresbach's a.** SICKLE CELL ANEMIA. **drug-induced hemolytic a.** Any hemolytic anemia that follows and is due to exposure to drugs such as penicillin, antimalarials, sulfones, sulfonamides, or $\alpha$-methyldopa. Some drug-induced hemolytic anemias, such as those due to penicillin or $\alpha$-methyldopa, have an immune basis. Some are due to the direct toxic effect of the drug, as with sulfones. Some drugs, such as antimalarials or sulfonamides, induce hemolysis in persons whose erythrocytes are deficient in glucose-6-phosphate dehydrogenase. **elliptocytic a.** HEREDITARY ELLIPTOCYTOSIS. **enzyme deficiency hemolytic a.** Any of several hereditary disorders in which there is accelerated destruction of erythrocytes in consequence of reduced activity of an enzyme of the erythrocyte. Most common of these disorders are glucose-6-phosphate dehydrogenase deficiency and pyruvate kinase deficiency. **erythroblastic a. of childhood** THALASSEMIA MAJOR. **Faber's a.** ACHYLIC ANEMIA. **familial erythroblastic a.** THALASSEMIA MAJOR. **familial microcytic a.** THALASSEMIA. **Fanconi's a.** A hereditary often fatal anemia that begins in infancy or early childhood and is accompanied by leukopenia, thrombocytopenia, skeletal anomalies and growth retardation. The bone marrow is hypocellular or aplastic. Inheritance is autosomal recessive. Also *congenital hypoplastic anemia, constitutional aplastic anemia, congenital aplastic anemia, constitutional infantile panmelopathy, congenital pancytopenia, Fanconi's pancytopenia, Fanconi syndrome, erythrogenesis imperfecta.* **febrile pleiochromic a.** THROMBOTIC THROMBOCYTOPENIC PURPURA. **fish tapeworm a.** A macrocytic and megaloblastic anemia caused by the fish tapeworm, *Diphyllobothrium latum,* and attributed to the high level of vitamin $B_{12}$ absorption by this parasite. The condition often occurs in Finland where *D. latum* infection is common, and is acquired by eating raw or partially cooked freshwater fish. **folic acid deficiency a.** Anemia that results from lack of folates. Also *Will's anemia.* **fragmentation hemolytic a.** Hemolytic anemia caused by excessive turbulence of erythrocyte flow which ruptures or fragments the cells, as in severe valvular heart disease or complicated cardiac valve replacement. **globe cell a.** SPHEROCYTIC ANEMIA. **goat's milk a.** Iron deficiency anemia occurring in infancy or early childhood as a result of prolonged feeding of goat's milk without iron supplementation. **ground itch a.** An anemia associated with high levels of hookworm infection and chronic hookworm disease. See also ANCYLOSTOMIASIS. **Heinz-body a.** 1 Any anemia in which Heinz bodies occur in a large proportion of erythrocytes. 2 UNSTABLE HEMOGLOBIN HEMOLYTIC ANEMIA. **hemolytic a.** Any anemia that is characterized by accelerated destruction of erythrocytes. Also *icterohemolytic anemia.* **hemolytic a. of pregnancy** A rare hemolytic anemia occurring during pregnancy. The disorder remits following delivery, but may relapse with subsequent pregnancies. In some cases the cause is autoimmunity. **hemorrhagic a.** Anemia that is due to blood loss. When blood loss is acute or recent, the erythrocytes are normocytic and normochromic. When blood loss is chronic, iron deficiency anemia results, and erythrocytes are often microcytic and hypochromic. **hereditary hypochromic a.** HEREDITARY SIDEROBLASTIC ANEMIA. **hereditary megaloblastic a.** Megaloblastic anemia that is due to any of several hereditary disorders, such as intestinal malabsorption of vitamin $B_{12}$ (the Imerslund syndrome), hereditary methylmalonic acidurias, the Lesch-Nyhan syndrome, hereditary orotic aciduria, and deficiency of enzymes of folate metabolism, among others. **hereditary nonspherocytic hemolytic a.** Any hereditary hemolytic disorder in which erythrocytes do not appear to be spherocytic in blood films. **hereditary sideroblastic a.** A rare hereditary anemia characterized by hypochromic, microcytic erythrocytes, often by elliptocytes and target cells in blood films and ringed sideroblasts in bone marrow films stained for iron by the Prussian blue method. The disorder occurs almost exclusively in males because it is X-chromosome-linked. Also *sex-linked hypochromic anemia of Rundles and Falls, hereditary hypochromic anemia, anemia hypochromica siderochestica hereditaria, Rundles-Falls syndrome.* **Herrick's a.** SICKLE CELL ANEMIA. **hookworm a.** Iron deficiency anemia due to gastrointestinal blood loss caused by hookworm infestation of the intestine. **hyperchromic a.** Anemia characterized by increased mean corpuscular hemoglobin concentration and seen only in hereditary spherocytosis. **a. hypochromica siderochestica hereditaria** HEREDITARY SIDEROBLASTIC ANEMIA. **hypochromic microcytic a.** Any anemia in which erythrocytes are smaller and paler than normal. Included are thalassemias, iron deficiency anemia, sideroblastic anemias, and the anemia of chronic disease. **hypoferric a.** IRON DEFICIENCY ANEMIA. **hypoplastic a.** Anemia due to reduction in the amount of hematopoietic tissue in the bone marrow; a mild form of aplastic anemia. **icterohemolytic a.** HEMOLYTIC ANEMIA. **idiopathic hypochromic a.** *Obs.* IRON DEFICIENCY ANEMIA. **idiopathic microcytic a.** *Obs.* IRON DEFICIENCY ANEMIA. **immunohemolytic a.** Any hemolytic anemia that is due to the presence in blood of an antibody. The antibody may react directly with components of the erythrocyte membrane, as in autoimmune hemolytic anemia; the antibody may react with an erythrocyte-hapten complex, as in penicillin-induced immunohemolytic anemia; or the erythrocyte may be lysed due to precipitation of antigen-antibody immune complexes on the erythrocyte membrane in an "innocent bystander" reaction. **iron deficiency a.** Anemia that results from decreased hemoglobin formation as a consequence of an insufficient amount of iron in the body. The anemia, when mild, usually has no characteristic morphologic features, but when the blood hemoglobin concentration declines to less than 10 g/dl, erythrocyte microcytosis (mean cell volume less than 80 femtoliters) is characteristic. Also *sideropenic anemia, hypoferric anemia, asiderotic anemia, chronic hypochromic anemia* (obs.), *idiopathic hypochromic anemia* (obs.), *idiopathic microcytic anemia* (obs.), *Witts anemia* (obs.). See also CHLOROSIS. **Israels-Wilkinson a.** ACHRESTIC ANEMIA. **juvenile pernicious a.** The very rare occurrence of pernicious anemia during the second decade of life. The few reported cases have had all the features of pernicious anemia that occurs in adults. The disorder is not known to be familial or hereditary. **lead a.** An anemia that is due to ingestion of lead. The erythrocytes in this condition may be hypochromic, and basophilic stippling of erythrocytes is usually pronounced. The anemia may be hemolytic because of inhibition of pyrimidine-5′-nucleotidase, or may have the features of a sideroblastic anemia because of inhibition of enzymes of heme synthesis. **Lederer's a.** An acute hemolytic anemia of unknown cause that remits spontaneously. Also *Lederer-Brill anemia, Lederer's disease.* **Leishman's a.** The anemia that accompanies kala-azar. **leukoerythroblastic a.** MYELOPHTHISIC ANEMIA. **lysolecithin hemolytic a.** Hemolytic anemia that follows envenomation with a toxin that converts lecithin to lysolecithin, as with some snake venoms. **macrocytic a.** Any anemia in which the average erythrocyte is larger than normal, i.e. the mean erythrocyte volume is 100 fl or greater. Also *megalocytic anemia.* **macrocytic achylic a.** PERNICIOUS ANEMIA. **malignant a.** PERNICIOUS ANEMIA. **Mediterranean a.** THALASSEMIA MAJOR. **megaloblastic a. due to anticonvulsant therapy** A macrocytic anemia with megaloblastic erythropoiesis observed in persons who are treated with drugs such as dilantin for the control of epilepsy. **megaloblastic a. of infancy** Any of several disorders that cause megaloblastic erythropoiesis and anemia during the first few years of life. The causes include dietary folate deficiency, intestinal malabsorption (as in sprue), congenital inability of the stomach to form intrinsic factor (congenital pernicious anemia), congenital cobalamin malabsorption (Imerslund syndrome), congenital deficiency of transcobalamin II, any of several methylmalonic acidurias, and other rare disorders. Many of these conditions are associated with severe neurologic disorders and some are accompanied by metabolic ketoacidosis. **megaloblastic a. of pregnancy** A macrocytic anemia occurring during the course of pregnancy due to deficiency of either dietary folic acid or of vitamin $B_{12}$. In western countries the former is the usual cause, and vitamin $B_{12}$ deficiency is rare. Among vegetarians, as in India, dietary vitamin $B_{12}$ deficiency is a common cause of this disorder. **megalocytic a.** MACROCYTIC ANEMIA. **meniscocytic a.** SICKLE CELL ANEMIA. **microangiopathic hemolytic a.** A hemolytic anemia caused by microvasculitis, especially as a result of deposition of fibrin within small blood vessels. **microcytic a.** Anemia characterized by abnormally small erythrocytes. **microdrepanocytic a.** SICKLE CELL ANEMIA. **microelliptopoikilocytic a. of Rietti, Greppi, and Micheli** THALASSEMIA MINOR. **miners' a.** An anemia resulting from ancylostomiasis and found among miners, first observed in central Europe. It is associated with fecally contaminated soil containing hookworm larvae in the mine shafts or other areas of continual soil contact. Also *tunnel anemia, tunnel disease.* **myelophthisic a.** An anemia that is accompanied by the presence of nucleated erythrocyte precursors and immature granulocytes in the peripheral blood. It is seen most often as a result of fibrosis of the bone marrow or invasion of the bone marrow by metastatic carcinoma. Also *leukoerythroblastic anemia, myelopathic anemia.* **myelosclerotic a.** The anemia of myelofibrosis or osteosclerosis. **nonspherocytic hemolytic a.** Any hemolytic anemia not characterized by spherocytes in the blood. **normochromic a.** Any anemia with normal mean corpuscular hemoglobin concentration. **normochromic normocytic a.** Any anemia in which erythrocytes have normal hemoglobin content and normal volume. **nutritional a.** Any anemia due to dietary inadequacy or intestinal malabsorption. Also *hematodystrophy.* **nutritional macrocytic a.** Any anemia characterized by abnormally large erythrocytes, due to dietary or malabsorptive deficiency of vitamin $B_{12}$ or folic acid. **nutritional megaloblastic a.** Anemia characterized by megaloblastic erythrocyte precursors, due to deficiency of vitamin $B_{12}$ or folate. **osteosclerotic a.** Anemia due to impairment of erythropoiesis by osteosclerosis. **ovalocytary a.** HEREDITARY ELLIPTOCYTOSIS. **pernicious a.** A megaloblastic anemia resulting from impaired intestinal absorption of vitamin $B_{12}$ due to insufficient availability of intrinsic factor. This anemia, found most commonly in older adults, is often accompanied by glossitis, gastric mucosal atrophy and achlorhydria, antibodies against gastric parietal cells or intrinsic factor, and neurologic signs. Also *Addison's anemia, Addison-Biermer anemia, addisonian anemia, Biermer's disease, Biermer's anemia, Biermer-Ehrlich anemia, cytogenic anemia, malignant anemia, Runeberg's anemia, Runeberg's disease, macrocytic achylic anemia, neuroanemia* (obs.). **phenylhydrazine a.** Anemia due to destruction of erythrocytes following ingestion of phenylhydrazine. It is caused by oxidation and denaturation of hemoglobin with production of Heinz bodies. Erythrocytes with hexose monophosphate pathway enzyme deficiencies are particularly susceptible. **physiologic a.** The normal fall in hemoglobin concentration observed in infants at about two months of age, reflecting the switch from fetal to adult hemoglobin and placental to pulmonary oxygenation. **polar a.** Anemia of unknown cause accompanying chronic exposure to cold. It is initially microcytic but later normocytic. Also *arctic anemia.* **posthemorrhagic a. of newborn** Anemia in newborn due to hemorrhage into the placenta during delivery. **primaquine-sensitive a.** Episodic hemolytic anemia following ingestion of primaquine or related antimalarial drugs, due to X-linked recessive inheritance of erythrocyte glucose-6-phosphate dehydrogenase deficiency. **pyridoxine-responsive a.** A rare variety of sideroblastic anemia that is ameliorated by pyridoxine. It is seen in males. **pyruvate-kinase deficiency a.** Hemolytic anemia due to deficiency of erythrocyte pyruvate kinase. **radiation a.** Aplastic or hypoplastic anemia which may occur after excessive exposure to ionizing radiation. Also *roentgen-ray anemia, x-ray anemia.* **a. refractoria sideroblastica** SIDEROBLASTIC ANEMIA. **refractory a.** Any anemia that is not ameliorated by hematinic supplementation. **refractory a. with excess blasts** A disorder characterized by anemia or pancytopenia, and by hypercellular bone marrow, with granulocytic hyperplasia and an increase in the proportion of myeloblasts and progranulocytes, but not in excess of 30% of bone-marrow cells. The disorder is usually fatal within one or two years, commonly following transition to acute nonlymphocytic leukemia. Also *refractory anemia with myeloblastosis.* Abbr. RAEB **refractory megaloblastic a.** Anemia characterized by megaloblastic erythrocyte precursors in the bone marrow and unresponsive to treatment with vitamin $B_{12}$ or folic acid. **refractory a. with myeloblastosis** REFRACTORY ANEMIA WITH EXCESS BLASTS. **refractory sideroblastic a.** A sideroblastic anemia that does not respond to treatment with large doses of pyridoxine, or to withdrawal of exposure to drugs or toxic substances. Also *anemia refractoria sideroblastica, acquired sideroblastic anemia, acquired sideroachrestic anemia.* **roentgen-ray a.** RADIATION ANEMIA. **Runeberg's a.** PERNICIOUS ANEMIA. **scorbutic a.** Anemia due to lack of vitamin C. **secondary sideroblastic a.** Any sideroblastic anemia that results from exposure of a person to drugs or toxic substances such as lead, isoniazid, cycloserine, or ethanol. **sex-linked hypochromatic a. of Rundles and Falls** HEREDITARY SIDEROBLASTIC ANEMIA. **sickle cell a.** **1** HOMOZYGOUS HEMOGLOBIN S DISEASE. **2** Any severe disorder due to formation of sickle cells, including homozygous hemoglobin S disease, hemoglobin S-C disease, hemoglobin S-D disease, hemoglobin S-O-Arab disease, and hemoglobin S-$\beta$-thalassemia. Also *Herrick's anemia, crescent cell anemia, drepanocytic anemia, Dresbach's anemia, meniscocytic anemia, meniscocytosis, sickle cell disease, sicklemia, microdrepanocytic anemia.* **sideremic a.** Any anemia associated with increased concentration of iron in serum, including sideroblastic anemia and thalassemia major. **sideroblastic a.** Any anemia that is associated with numerous ringed sideroblasts in the bone marrow. Also *sideroachrestic anemia.* **sideropenic a.** IRON DEFICIENCY ANEMIA. **simple chronic a.** ANEMIA OF CHRONIC DISEASE. **slaty a.** Anemia associated with cyanosis, usually the effect of a drug such as acetanilid or dapsone that may cause both hemolytic anemia and methemoglobinemia or sulfhemoglobinemia. The slate gray appearance of the face is due to the presence of methemoglobin of sulfhemoglobin in the blood. **spherocytic a.** Any anemia in which spherocytes are present in large numbers in the blood as determined by examination of a blood film. Spherocytes are characteristically found in the hemolytic anemias that result from extensive thermal burns, in autoimmune hemolytic disorders, and in hereditary spherocytosis. Also *globe cell anemia.* **splenic a.** Anemia, often associated with leukopenia and thrombocytopenia, in cases of congestive splenomegaly (the Banti syndrome) consequent to portal vein hypertension. Also *anemia splenetica.* **target cell a.** Any anemia in which target cells are numerous in the blood. Included are thalassemias, many hemoglobinopathies, and anemias associated with chronic liver disease. **thrombotic microangiopathic hemolytic a.** THROMBOTIC THROMBOCYTOPENIC PURPURA. **toxic a.** Any anemia due to destructive effects of chemicals, bacteria, biologic products, and other materials upon erythrocytes, or due to the effects of such substances upon production of erythrocytes by the bone marrow. **toxic hemolytic a.** Any hemolytic anemia that results from ingestion of drugs or chemicals that injure erythrocytes, from venoms of snakes or arthropods, or from hemolysins released by bacteria. **traumatic a.** Anemia that results from injury to soft tissues with extravasation of blood at the site of injury. In burns it begins on the fourth or fifth day as a consequence of heat damage to cell membranes and to a deficiency of serum and membrane lipid, which shortens the half-life. Burned cells transfused into normal patients regain a normal half-life. **triose-phosphate isomerase deficiency a.** A very rare hereditary hemolytic anemia due to deficiency of the enzyme triose-phosphate isomerase in the erythrocytes. The condition is of autosomal recessive inheritance and has been associated with mental retardation. **tropical a.** Any anemia that occurs in a person living in tropical areas. The most common causes are iron deficiency, as a consequence of blood loss from helminthiasis, and folate deficiency due to intestinal malabsorption (tropical macrocytic anemia). **tunnel a.** MINERS' ANEMIA. **unstable hemoglobin hemolytic a.** Any hemolytic anemia that is due to the presence of an unstable hemoglobin, such as hemoglobin Köln, hemoglobin Zürich, hemoglobin H, or others. Also *congenital Heinz body anemia, Heinz body anemia.* **Wills a.** FOLIC ACID DEFICIENCY ANEMIA. **Witts a.** *Obs.* IRON DEFICIENCY ANEMIA. **x-ray a.** RADIATION ANEMIA.

**anemic** \ənē′mik\ Lacking the normal quantity of erythrocytes or hemoglobin in the blood; having anemia.

**anemo-** \ənem′ō-, an′əmō-\ [Gk *anemos* wind] A combining form meaning wind.

**anemometer** \an′ēmäm′ətər\ [ANEMO- + -METER] An instrument for measuring the velocity of air flow.

**anemopathy** \an′ēmäp′əthē\ [ANEMO- + -PATHY] A disease associated with exposure to high winds.

**anencephalia** \an′ensefā′lyə\ ANENCEPHALY.

**anencephaly** \an′ensef′əlē\ [Gk *anenkephal(os)* (from *an-* priv. + *enkephalos* brain) brainless + -Y] The absence of a major portion of the cerebral and/or cerebellar hemispheres owing to erosion of the exposed brain tissue secondary to absence of the usual coverings that make up the cranial vault. The primary malformation is failure of closure of the cephalic part of the embryonic neural tube, which allows everted brain tissue to remain exposed on the surface of the head. Fetal movements within the confined space of the surrounding membranes and uterus wear away the friable tissues, leaving only tangled blood vessels covering the basal ganglia and brainstem. Also *anencephalia.*

**anenterous** \anen′tərəs\ [Gk *an-* priv. + ENTER- + -OUS] Lacking an alimentary canal, as in the cestodes.

**anephric** \anef′rik\ Lacking kidneys at birth, as in bilateral renal agenesis.

**anepiploic** \anep′iplō′ik\ Possessing no epiploon, or omentum.

**anergia** \anur′jə\ ANERGY.

**anergic** \anur′jik\ Of or characterized by anergy.

**anergy** \an′ərjē\ [Gk *anergia* (from *an-* priv. + *erg(on)* work + -IA) idleness] **1** Absent immunological reactivity (usually delayed hypersensitivity skin reactions) to an antigen to which the host has been exposed in a way that would raise positive reactions in a normal subject. Anergy can be found to PPD in subjects known to have encountered the tubercle bacillus, to ubiquitous antigens like *Candida,* or to skin painting with dichloronitrobenzene. Also *anergia.* **2** Lack of energy. **negative a.** Anergy to the products of an infectious organism which is accompanied by low clinical resistance to the organism. The anergy to PPD seen in miliary tuberculosis is regarded as an example of negative anergy. **positive a.** Anergy to the products of an infectious organism which is accompanied by high clinical resistance to the organism. The anergy to PPD found in sarcoidosis is regarded as an example of positive anergy. **specific a.** A loss of reactivity to a specific antigen while retaining normal reactivity to other antigens.

**aneroid** \an′eroid\ [French *anéroïde* (from Gk *a-* priv. + *nēr(os)* wet, damp + French *-oïde* -OID) concerning a barometer with an empty box] Containing no fluid: said of an instrument, as a type of sphygmomanometer, which operates without fluid.

**anerythropsia** \an′irithräp′sē·ə\ [Gk *an-* priv. + ERYTHR- + -OPSIA] PROTANOPIA.

**anesthekinesia** \anes′thēkīnē′zhə\ [Gk *an-* priv. + *aisthē(sis)* perception, sensation + *kinēs(is)* movement + -IA] **1** Motor paralysis accompanied by reduction or loss of sensibility. **2** Loss of the sensation of movement of a limb or organ. Seldom used in this sense. Also *anesthecinesia.*

# anesthesia

**anesthesia** \an′esthē′zhə\ [New L *anaesthesia,* from Gk *anaisthēsia* (from *an-* priv. + *aisthēsis* perception, sensation) insensibility] **1** Partial or complete loss of all forms of sensation such as cold, heat, pain, or touch, attributable to a lesion of the nervous system. Conventionally, the term *anesthesia* is more often used to identify loss of touch sensation, *analgesia* loss of pain sensibility. Also *atactilia.* **2** The use of inhalational or local agents to produce anesthesia. For defs. 1 and 2 also *anaesthesia* (British spelling). **ambulatory a.** Anesthesia used for minor operations, usually in low-risk patients who enter a facility for only one day. **basal a.** The injection of sedatives, opioids, or anesthetics, enterally or parenterally, to reduce consciousness short of general anesthesia. Also *basal narcosis.* **bulbar a.** Loss of cutaneous sensibility due to a brainstem lesion. **carbon dioxide absorption a.** CLOSED-CIRCUIT ANESTHESIA. **caudal a.** The injection of a local anesthetic through the sacrococcygeal ligament into the sacral and spinal epidural spaces. Also *caudal block, sacral block.* **closed-circuit a.** Inhalation anesthesia in which the anesthetic gas is continuously rebreathed while carbon dioxide exhaled by the patient is removed by an absorption apparatus. Also *carbon dioxide absorption anesthesia, closed-system anesthesia.* **compression a.** Anesthesia due to compression of a nerve. **conduction a.** Anesthesia in a local area by the injection of an anesthetic agent into the region of the nerve whose conductivity from the area is to be interrupted; nerve block. Also *nerve blocking anesthesia, nerve-trunk anesthesia.* **continuous caudal a.** The intermittent injection of a local anesthetic into the sacral canal via an indwelling catheter or needle. **continuous spinal a.** The intermittent injection of a local anesthetic into the subarachnoid space via an indwelling catheter or needle. **crossed a.** Loss of cutaneous sensation in a pattern seen in some brainstem lesions, in which there is anesthesia of the face on one side and of the trunk and limbs on the opposite side. **dissociated a.** Loss of the senses of temperature and pain, with preservation of the sense of touch. Also *dissociation symptom.* **electrical a.** An experimental method of producing narcosis by application of direct or alternating current via electrodes applied to the skull. Also *electroanesthesia.* **endobronchial a.** Anesthesia induced by the release of a gaseous mixture through a tube inserted into a bronchus. Also *one-lung anesthesia.* **endotracheal a.** Anesthesia induced by the release of a gaseous mixture into the lungs through a tube placed in the trachea. **epidural a.** The injection of a local anesthetic, via the back, into the spinal epidural space. It is used to anesthetize spinal nerves from the tenth thoracic through the fifth sacral nerve, depending on the technique utilized. Also *epidural block, peridural anesthesia.* **facial a.** Anesthesia of the skin of the face, usually attributable to a lesion of the trigeminal nerve or of one of its divisions or branches. **field block a.** Anesthesia produced in a local area by multiple injections of an anesthetic agent around the circumference of the area, thus creating a barrier against afferent sensation from the circumscribed area. Also *field block.* **gas-oxygen-ether a.** An anesthetic condition brought about by the inhalation of a mixture of nitrous oxide, oxygen, and diethyl ether vapor. **general a.** A narcosis produced with inhalation or intravenous agents, or both. Compare LOCAL ANESTHESIA. **girdle a.** Segmental anesthesia occurring in a ring or girdle around the trunk caused by a lesion of the posterior nerve roots, or intercostal nerves. **glove a.** Anesthesia of the hand, involving approximately the area which would be covered by a glove. The causes are similar to those of stocking anesthesia. **glove and stocking a.** Loss of touch sensation in the periphery of the limbs approximately corresponding to the areas covered by gloves and socks (or stockings), seen in many varieties of sensory or sensorimotor polyneuropathy. **gustatory a.** AGEUSIA. **hyperbaric spinal a.** Motor and sensory anesthesia below a specified level of the spine, produced by injecting into the spinal fluid an agent having a baricity greater than that of cerebrospinal fluid. The location of the heavy solution is controlled by tilting the patient's body or head up or to one side, thus bathing specific nerves to produce the desired effect. Also *hyperbaric anesthesia.* **hypobaric spinal a.** Motor and sensory anesthesia above a specified level of the spine, produced by injecting into the spinal fluid an agent having a baricity less than that of cerebrospinal fluid. The location of the light solution is controlled by allowing it to rise to a specific level to produce the desired effect. This is used in anesthetizing the uppermost parts of the body. **hypotensive a.** The deliberate lowering of blood pressure with intravenous drugs or general anesthetics in order to decrease blood loss during an operation. **hypothermic a.** Increasing degrees of narcosis induced as the body is deliberately cooled below 30°C. This is done to protect vital organs against ischemia. **infiltration a.** Local anesthesia produced by the injection of an anesthetic agent through the skin. The agent infiltrates the region and anesthetizes numerous peripheral nerve endings. **inhalation a.** Analgesia or narcosis resulting from inhalation of an anesthetic gas or vapor into the lungs. **insufflation a.** The delivery of anesthetic gases or vapors in oxygen via the nose, mouth, or trachea, in volumes sufficient to avoid rebreathing of the mixture and carbon dioxide accumulation. **intercostal a.** Anesthesia produced by the injection of an anesthetic agent about an intercostal nerve, thus causing a loss of dermatomal sensation distal to the point of injection. Also *intercostal block.* **intraosseous a.** Anesthesia of a tooth produced by drilling a narrow tunnel, about the width of a hypodermic needle, through the cortex of the alveolar bone, then injecting local anesthetic with a short needle through this tunnel into the cancellous bone. The drilling of the tunnel is rendered painless by infiltration anesthesia. **intravenous a.** A narcosis produced by an injection of general anesthetic solutions into a vein. **intravenous regional a.** The intravenous injection of a local anesthetic into an extremity that has been rendered bloodless by wrapping it with an Esmarch bandage and by applying a pneumatic tourniquet. **isobaric spinal a.** Anesthesia produced by the injection of an anesthetic solution with baricity equal to that of cerebrospinal fluid. Also *isobaric solution, normobaric solution.* **local a.** Anesthesia confined to one part of the body, such as the leg, arm, or cervical region. Also *regional anesthesia, regional block.* Compare GENERAL ANESTHESIA. **nasotracheal a.** A general anesthesia induced via a tracheal tube passed through the nose and pharynx. **nerve blocking a.** CONDUCTION ANESTHESIA. **nerve-trunk a.** CONDUCTION ANESTHESIA. **neurolept a.** General anesthesia induced with a combination of inhaled nitrous oxide and several intravenous agents, including analgesics, sedatives, and compounds used in dissociative anesthesia with or without a neuromuscular blocker. Such a state of anesthesia serves to minimize the stress of harmful reflexes and trauma. **olfactory a.** ANOSMIA. **one-lung a.** ENDOBRONCHIAL ANESTHESIA. **orotracheal a.** A general anesthesia induced via a tube passed through the mouth into the trachea. **paracervical block a.** Injection of a local anesthetic paracervically to block visceral afferent pain fibers of Frankenhäuser's ganglia. The technique is used to relieve the pain of uterine contractions during labor or to relieve pain associated with mechanical cervical dilatation or dilatation and curettage. **paravertebral block a.** The injection of a local anesthetic beside the spinal vertebral column in order to anesthetize emerging spinal or sympathetic nerves. Also *paravertebral block.* **peridural a.** EPIDURAL ANESTHESIA.

**pudendal block a.** The injection of an anesthetic into an area near the pudendal nerve in order to anesthetize the perineum. **rectal a.** The rectal instillation of anesthetic agents, in liquid or vapor form, in order to induce basal or general anesthesia. **regional a.** LOCAL ANESTHESIA. **saddle block a.** A subarachnoid or spinal anesthesia induced in the distribution of the second through the fifth sacral nerves. **segmental a.** Anesthesia occurring in the cervical, thoracic, lumbar, or sacral spinal segments. **semiclosed circuit a.** An anesthesia breathing system wherein most of the gas mixture is rebreathed and the remainder is vented into the atmosphere. **semiopen a.** A method of anesthesia whereby approximately half the amount of anesthetic exhaled is rebreathed while the remainder is released into the atmosphere. **sexual a.** FRIGIDITY. **spinal a.** The injection of a local anesthetic, via the back, into the lumbar subarachnoid space. Also *subarachnoid anesthesia.* **splanchnic a.** The interruption of nerve impulse conduction in the autonomic plexuses supplying the abdominal viscera. Also *splanchnic block.* **stocking a.** Anesthesia in the area covered by a stocking or sock. When occurring in a single limb with an abrupt transition between the areas of normal and impaired sensation, especially when the "level" corresponds to a joint, this may be a hyster ical phenomenon. When present in both lower limbs, with a gradual transition from impaired to normal areas of sensory perception, and especially when there are similar findings (glove anesthesia) in the upper limbs, it is usually indicative of polyneuropathy. **subarachnoid a.** SPINAL ANESTHESIA. **surgical a.** Local or general anesthesia induced for the performance of an operation. **tactile a.** Loss or reduction of the sense of touch. **thalamic hyperesthetic a.** Anesthesia of the limbs or trunk, usually unilateral and associated with hyperpathia in the anesthetic area, and resulting from a contralateral thalamic lesion. **thermal a.** Loss of temperature sensation. **topical a.** The application of a local anesthetic to the surface of any of the mucous membranes. **total a.** Anesthesia involving all sensory modalities. **total spinal a.** The inadvertent anesthetic block of all spinal segments with resulting respiratory paralysis. Also *total spinal block.* **twilight a.** Sleep produced with premedicants or basal anesthetics, formerly employed in obstetrics. *Outmoded.* **unilateral a.** Anesthesia restricted to one side of the body. **visceral a.** Loss of visceral sensation.

**anesthesiologist** \an′esthē′zē·äl′əjist\ A physician trained in the administration of anesthetics, treatment of pain, and use of life-support systems. • See note at ANESTHETIST.

**anesthesiology** \an′esthē′zē·äl′əjē\ [*anesthesi(a)* + *o* + -LOGY] The medical specialty concerned with anesthesia.

**anesthesognosia** \an′esthē′zägnō′zhə\ [*anesthes(ia)* + *o* + Gk *gnōs(is)* knowledge + -IA] *Seldom used* TACTILE AGNOSIA.

**anesthetic** \an′esthet′ik\ [Gk *anaisthētos* (from *an-* priv. + *aisthēsis* perception, sensation) insensible + -IC] **1** Relating to or characterized by a state of anesthesia; of or marked by loss of sensation. **2** Causing local or general anesthesia. **3** An anesthetic agent. **general a.** An anesthetic used to produce narcosis. It can be administered rectally or intravenously or it can be inhaled in a gas or vapor form. **local a.** An injectable or topical substance inducing anesthesia in the part of the body where it is applied by causing an interruption in nerve impulse conduction. **topical a.** Any anesthetic agent used for anesthetizing the surface of a mucous membrane. **volatile a.** An anesthetic in liquid form which evaporates to a vapor at an ambient temperature and pressure.

**anesthetist** \ənes′thətist\ An individual who administers an anesthetic. • In the United States, an anesthetist may be a nurse or technician rather than a physician specializing in anesthesiology (anesthesiologist). In Great Britain, South Africa, New Zealand, Japan, and India, only physicians provide anesthetics. In Japan and India, all anesthetists are specialists, hence are anesthesiologists. In New Zealand, anesthetics are provided either by an anesthesiologist or by a general practitioner (commonly called a *GP anesthetist*) who also functions as a part-time anesthetist.

**anesthetization** \ənes′thətīzā′shən\ [*anesthetiz(e)* + -ATION] The process leading to a state of local or general anesthesia.

**anesthetize** \ənes′thətīz\ [*anesthet(ic)* + -IZE] To induce local or general anesthesia in.

**anethopath** \anē′thəpath\ [Gk *an-* priv. + *etho(s)* manners, habit, custom + -PATH] PSYCHOPATH.

**aneugamy** \anyoo′gəmē\ The formation of an aneuploid zygote by union of gametes, either one or both of which failed to become haploid during meiosis.

**aneuploid** \an′yooploid\ [Gk *an-* priv. + EUPLOID] **1** Possessing a chromosome number other than an exact multiple of the haploid number. An aneuploid organism may be monosomic, with one less than the diploid number of chromosomes, or trisomic, with one more than the diploid number. **2** A cell or organism so characterized. Compare EUPLOID.

**aneuploidy** \an′yooploi′dē\ [Gk *an-* priv. + EUPLOIDY] The condition in which a somatic or gametic nucleus does not contain an exact multiple of a haploid set of chromosomes. Compare EUPLOIDY.

**aneurilemmic** \ənʸʊr′ilem′ik\ Lacking a neurilemmal sheath.

**aneurin** THIAMIN.

**Aneuroform** A fast-drying resinous material for encasing an intracranial aneurysm. A proprietary name.

**aneurogenic** \ənʸʊr′əjen′ik\ [Gk *a-* priv. + NEURO- + -GENIC] Lacking or failing to develop nerve fibers, as in a limb.

**aneurysm** \an′yʊrizm\ [Gk *aneurysma* (from ANA- + *eurys* wide) a dilatation] A saccular or fusiform outpouching of a layer or layers of an arterial wall, found usually in the elderly and thought to arise from a systemic collagen synthetic or structural defect. **abdominal a.** An aneurysm of the abdominal portion of the aorta, usually located below the renal arteries and almost always caused by atherosclerosis. **acute a.** An aneurysm which has developed abruptly. **ampullary a.** SACCULAR ANEURYSM. **aortic sinusal a.** An aneurysm of one of the aortic sinuses. It is usually congenital but may be the consequence of infection, as in syphilis or infective endocarditis. It tends to rupture into the chambers of the right side of the heart, resulting in a left-to-right shunt and a continuous murmur. Also *aneurysm of the sinus of Valsalva.* **arteriovenous a.** An aneurysmal connection between an artery and a vein. **arteriovenous pulmonary a.** An aneurysm arising from an arteriovenous fistula in the lung. **atherosclerotic a.** An aneurysm of an artery caused by advanced atherosclerosis. It often involves the abdominal portion of the aorta, though any atherosclerotic artery can be affected. **bacterial a.** MYCOTIC ANEURYSM. **berry a.** A small, saccular aneurysm arising at bifurcation points of cerebral arteries of the circle of Willis. It develops at gaps in the medial muscle, is connected to the artery by a narrow neck, and may rupture, causing subarachnoid hemmorhage. Also *brain aneurysm, cerebral aneurysm.* **cardiac a.**

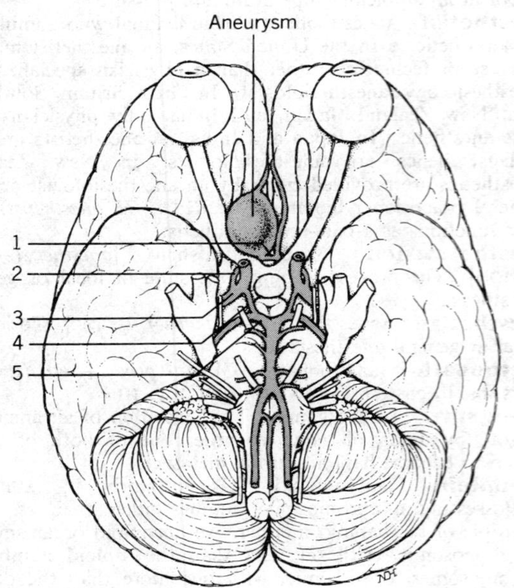


**Berry aneurysm** (showing arteries of circle of Willis: (1) anterior communicating; (2) anterior cerebral; (3) internal carotid; (4) posterior communicating; (5) basilar)

An aneurysm affecting the heart muscle, usually as a consequence of myocardial infarction but sometimes arising from other causes, such as trauma. **caroticocavernous a.** A fistulous communication between the internal carotid artery and the investing cavernous venous sinus. **cerebral a.** BERRY ANEURYSM. **Charcot-Bouchard a.** A minute, often multiple, saccular or fusiform aneurysm of arterioles and small arteries of the cerebral cortex and basal ganglia. Their rupture is believed to be the cause of massive cerebral hemorrhages in hypertensive individuals. Also *miliary aneurysm*. **cirsoid a.** A collection of tortuous, dilated, and interconnecting blood vessels. Also *racemose aneurysm, cirsoid varix, diffuse arterial ectasia*. **cylindroid a.** A fusiform aneurysm of approximately uniform diameter throughout its length. Also *tubular aneurysm*. **dissecting a.** *Incorrect* ARTERIAL DISSECTION. • Though widely used, *dissecting aneurysm* confuses two different pathological processes, aneurysm and dissection. **embolic a.** An aneurysm resulting from ischemic damage to the arterial wall caused by the lodging of an embolus. **false a.** An aneurysm, usually saccular, whose wall is formed by compressed perivascular soft tissue. It is usually caused by transmural rupture of the vessel wall as a result of trauma, or may follow an improperly sutured vascular incision. Also *aneurysmal hematoma*. **fusiform a.** An elongated aneurysm that gradually widens and then tapers to the diameter of the uninvolved vessel. **hernial a.** An aneurysm that results from damage to the outer coats of the vessel so that its wall is composed of the intima projecting through the interrupted outer media and adventitia. **infective a.** An aneurysm arising as a result of infection. **innominate a.** An aneurysm of the brachiocephalic trunk. **intracavernous a.** An aneurysm of the intracavernous segment of the internal carotid artery. Also *subclinoid aneurysm*. **intracranial a.** The dilatation or evagination of an intracranial blood vessel, usually an artery, the result of trauma or disease of the vessel wall. **intrathoracic a.** An aneurysm found within the thorax and usually arising from the aorta. Common causes include syphilis, atherosclerosis, and the Marfan syndrome. **lateral a.** An aneurysm that protrudes from one side of the vessel. **medical a.** An aneurysm which, due to its inaccessible location, is not amenable to surgical therapy. **miliary a.** CHARCOT-BOUCHARD ANEURYSM. **mycotic a.** An aneurysm caused by damage to the vessel wall by either bacteria or fungi. Most frequently it results from impaction of an infected embolus in the context of infective endocarditis. Occasionally, the infection may have spread from a nearby abscess. Also *bacterial aneurysm*. **Park's a.** An arteriovenous aneurysm connecting an artery with two veins. **peripheral a.** An aneurysm involving a small arterial branch. **phantom a.** A pulsating artery mistaken for an aneurysm on physical examination. **racemose a.** CIRSOID ANEURYSM. **saccular a.** An eccentric aneurysm affecting only a portion of the circumference of the vessel, connected to it by a relatively narrow neck and having a saclike shape. Most often these aneurysms result from trauma or syphilitic or mycotic involvement of the aorta or other large arteries. Also *ampullary aneurysm*. **silent a.** An aneurysm that has not caused any symptoms. **a. of the sinus of Valsalva** AORTIC SINUSAL ANEURYSM. **subclinoid a.** INTRACAVERNOUS ANEURYSM. **syphilitic a.** An aneurysm of the aortic arch, and less commonly the descending thoracic aorta, due to syphilitic aortitis. Such an aneurysm is large and often saccular, and may erode surrounding structures such as the spine, sternum, esophagus, and trachea. **thoracic a.** An aneurysm involving the ascending, arch, and descending thoracic portions of the aorta or less commonly, the pulmonary artery and its major branches. **thoracoabdominal aortic a.** Aneurysmal degeneration of both the descending thoracic and the suprarenal abdominal aortae. **traumatic a.** A false aneurysm due to blunt or penetrating injury. **true a.** An aneurysm whose wall is composed of stretched remnants of all the coats of the vessel wall. **tubular a.** CYLINDROID ANEURYSM. **venous a.** An aneurysm involving a vein. **ventricular a.** An aneurysm affecting either of the cardiac ventricles, most commonly the left, as a result of myocardial infarction.

**aneurysmal** \an′yʊriz′məl\ Resembling or pertaining to an aneurysm. Also *aneurysmatic*.

**aneurysmectomy** \an′yʊrizmek′təmē\ [ANEURYSM + -ECTOMY] The excision of an aneurysm.

**aneurysmography** \an′yʊrizmäg′rəfē\ [ANEURYSM + *o* + -GRAPHY] Radiography of an aneurysm after opacification.

**aneurysmoplasty** \an′yʊriz′məplas′tē\ [ANEURYSM + *o* + -PLASTY] A plastic surgical procedure on an aneurysm and the adjacent parts of an artery, with the intent to reduce or obliterate the aneurysm and restore more normal circulation through the artery.

**aneurysmorrhaphy** \an′yʊrizmôr′əfē\ [ANEURYSM + *o* + -RRHAPHY] **1** An intrasaccular aortic graft insertion to treat aneurysm. **2** An operative technique used to reduce or obliterate an aneurysmal sac by suturing. *Outmoded*.

**ANF** antinuclear factor (antinuclear antibody).

**angei-** \an′jē-\ ANGIO-.

**angeial** \anjē′əl\ [ANGEI- + -AL] VASCULAR.

**Anger** [Hal *Anger*, U.S. electrical engineer, born 1920] Anger camera. See under GAMMA CAMERA.

**angi-** \an′jē-\ ANGIO-.

**angiectasia** \an′jē·ektā′zhə\ [ANGI- + ECTASIA] An enlargement or lengthening of a blood vessel. Also *angiectasis, hemangiectasia.* **congenital dysplastic a.** KLIPPEL-TRENAUNAY-WEBER SYNDROME.

**angiectasis** \an′jē·ek′təsis\ [ANGI- + ECTASIS] ANGIECTASIA.

**angiectatic** \an′jē·ektat′ik\ Related to or effected by angiectasia. Also *angioectatic.*

**angiectomy** \an′jē·ek′təmē\ [ANGI- + -ECTOMY] The removal of all or part of a blood vessel.

**angiitis** \an′jē·ī′tis\ [ANGI- + -ITIS] Inflammation of a blood vessel. Also *angitis.* **granulomatous a.** A rare autoimmune disorder of small cerebral arteries, giving rise to symptoms and signs of focal cerebral dysfunction, epileptic seizures, and sometimes spinal cord involvement. **necrotizing a.** Inflammation of a blood vessel associated with fibrinoid necrosis, as in polyarteritis nodosa.

**angina** \anjī′nə\ [L (from *angere* to stifle, choke), the quinsy, a sore throat] **1** Severe sore throat with the implied quality of choking. • An old-fashioned term derived from the archaic word for quinsy and employed from early times for many distressing conditions of the throat and adjacent parts. It is encountered still in this sense in such terms as *Vincent's angina* and *Ludwig's angina.* **2** ANGINA PECTORIS. **3** Any of various diseases or conditions characterized by painful or cramping spasms. **abdominal a.** INTESTINAL ANGINA. **agranulocytic a.** Severe throat pain accompanied by mucosal ulceration in a patient with marked deficiency of neutrophils in the blood. Also *neutropenic angina.* **benign croupous a.** HERPANGINA. **Bretonneau's a.** PHARYNGEAL DIPHTHERIA. **a. capitis** HEADACHE. **cardiac a.** ANGINA PECTORIS. **a. cordis** ANGINA PECTORIS. **a. cruris** Intermittent claudication affecting the leg. *Outmoded.* **decubitus a.** Angina pectoris occurring in the recumbent position. Also *angina decubitus.* **a. diphtheritica** PHARYNGEAL DIPHTHERIA. **exertion a.** Angina pectoris precipitated by exercise or exertion. Also *angina of effort.* **fusospirochetal a.** VINCENT'S ANGINA. **hippocratic a.** *Outmoded* RETROPHARYNGEAL ABSCESS. **hypercyanotic a.** Angina pectoris occurring in patients with severe cyanotic heart disease. **intestinal a.** Abdominal pain caused by ischemia of mesenteric arterial flow, usually occurring after meals. Also *abdominal angina.* **a. inversa** PRINZMETAL'S ANGINA. **Ludwig's a.** A virulent infection of the cellular tissues surrounding the submandibular salivary glands, producing a brawny swelling beneath the chin and in the floor of the mouth. It may lead to respiratory obstruction due to subglottic edema. **necrotic a.** *Obs.* GANGRENOUS PHARYNGITIS. **neutropenic a.** AGRANULOCYTIC ANGINA. **a. parotidea** *Obs.* MUMPS. **a. pectoris** A strangling sensation or heavy chest discomfort, often radiating to the arms, especially the left, and usually precipitated by exertion. In current usage, the term implies a cardiac ischemic origin. Most commonly the consequence of coronary atherosclerosis, it may be due to a number of disorders, including coronary artery spasm and aortic stenosis. Also *angina cordis, cardiac angina, angina, Elsner's asthma, stenocardia, anginal syndrome.* **Plaut's a.** *Obs.* VINCENT'S ANGINA. **preinfarction a.** Angina pectoris which has preceded myocardial infarction. Also *acute coronary insufficiency, coronary intermediate syndrome, coronary failure syndrome, preinfarction syndrome* (outmoded). • The term is often inappropriately used for unstable angina, but it can only properly be applied retrospectively, when infarction has occurred. **Prinzmetal's a.** A variant of angina pectoris in which this symptom occurs at rest and is accompanied by elevation of the ST segments. It is now thought to be due to coronary arterial spasm, either in isolation or complicating coronary atherosclerosis. Also *angina inversa, variant angina pectoris.* **pseudomembranous a.** VINCENT'S ANGINA. **ulceromembranous a.** VINCENT'S ANGINA. **unstable a.** Angina pectoris that has recently become more severe or more frequent, being precipitated by less exertion or at rest. Also *acute coronary insufficiency, coronary intermediate syndrome, coronary failure syndrome, preinfarction syndrome* (outmoded). See also PREINFARCTION ANGINA. **variant a. pectoris** PRINZMETAL'S ANGINA. **Vincent's a.** An infection of the tonsil, associated with ulceration and membrane formation. The causative organisms include the bacillus *Fusobacterium fusiformis* and the spirochete *Borrelia vincenti,* which also affect the gums and mouth (necrotizing ulcerative gingivitis). Epidemics may occur, particularly in schools and camps. Also *fusospirochetal angina, pseudomembranous angina, ulceromembranous angina, trench throat, Vincent's disease, Plaut's angina* (obs.). See also NECROTIZING ULCERATIVE GINGIVOSTOMATITIS.

**anginal** \an′jinəl\ Pertaining to angina pectoris.

**anginoid** \an′jinoid\ Resembling angina pectoris; angina-like.

**angio-** \an′jē·ō-\ [Gk *angeion* vessel] A combining form denoting a vessel, especially a blood vessel. Also *angei-, angi-.*

**angioaccess** \an′jē·ō·ak′səs\ Any technique that provides chronic, readily available contact with the vascular system. It may be arterial or venous, or by means of an arteriovenous communication.

**angioarchitecture** \-är′kətek′chər\ VASCULATURE.

**angioblast** \an′jē·ōblast′\ [ANGIO- + BLAST] An embryonic cell type that gives rise to a blood vessel. Angioblasts appear early in human development, at the primitive streak stage, in the body stalk and wall of the yolk sac as blood islands. At first solid, these islands hollow out to form tubes of endothelium containing primitive blood cells. Also *vasoformative cell.* Adj. angioblastic.

**angioblastema** \-blastē′mə\ [ANGIO- + BLASTEMA] Aggregates of mesenchymal cells in the embryo that give rise to primitive blood vessels and the first blood cells.

**angioblastoma** \-blastō′mə\ [ANGIO- + BLASTOMA] HEMANGIOBLASTOMA. **retinal a.** A vascular malformation of the retina, seen in cerebroretinal angiomatosis (Lindau-von Hippel disease). It is visible with the ophthalmoscope.

**angiocardiograph** \-kär′dē·əgraf′\ A roentgenogram obtained during angiocardiography. Also *angiocardiogram.*

**angiocardiography** \-kär′dē·äg′rəfē\ [ANGIO- + CARDIOGRAPHY] Radiography of the heart and great vessels after injection of contrast medium into a vein, one of the cardiac chambers, or the aorta. Also *cardioangiography.* **gas a.** Angiocardiography with the use of a water-soluble gas, such as nitrous oxide or carbon dioxide, as the contrast medium. **rapid biplane a.** Angiocardiography done with special x-ray apparatus which permits the making of radiographs in two planes at right angles to each other, the radiographs for each plane being made in rapid succession either alternating with or simultaneous with those of the other plane. **retrograde a.** Radiographic examination of the heart after the injection of a radiopaque agent in the left ventricle through a catheter which has been placed in the aorta. This study permits the evaluation of left to right cardiac shunts, mitral regurgitation, and aortic stenosis or insufficiency. **right-sided a.** Sequential opacification of the superior vena cava, right atrium, right ventricle, pulmonary arteries, and pulmonary veins by means of an automatic film changer or motion-picture film after the injection of a bolus of contrast material, usually into a peripheral arm vein or into the superior vena cava by percutaneous catheter through an arm vein. Sometimes the inferior vena cava is catheterized via femoral vein approach, in which case contrast material enters the right atrium. **selective a.** Roentgenography of the heart and great vessels during the injection of contrast medium through a catheter, the tip of which has been placed in a specific great vessel or chamber of the heart.

**angiocinematography** \-sin′əmətäg′rəfē\ [ANGIO- + CINEMATOGRAPHY] Radiography of vessels or of the heart, with recording of the image on motion-picture film, thus permitting the study of motion. It is especially useful in the study of coronary arteries and the chambers of the heart.

**angioclast** \an′jē·ōklast′\ *Obs.* HEMOSTAT.

**angiocyst** \an′jē·ōsist′\ [ANGIO- + CYST] An island of mesenchymatous tissue in the embryo endowed with the ability to form blood cells. The best recognized are the islands of Wolff and Pander, situated in the outer mesenchymatous layer which surrounds the endoderm of the yolk sac. Also *angioblastic cyst.*

**angiodermatitis** \-dur′mətī′tis\ Dermatitis involving damage to the small blood vessels of the skin.

**angiodysplasia** \-displā′zhə\ Ectasia, dilatation, and tortuosity of capillaries and small veins within the mucosa and submucosa of the right colon, especially the cecum. The rupture of these vessels is a major cause of intestinal hemorrhage in elderly individuals.

**angiodystrophia** \-distrō′fē·ə\ ANGIODYSTROPHY. **a. ovarii** Angiodystrophy of the blood vessels of the ovary.

**angiodystrophy** \-dis′trəfē\ [ANGIO- + DYSTROPHY] A vascular disorder arising from nutritional deficiency. Also *angiodystrophia.*

**angioectatic** \-ektat′ik\ ANGIECTATIC.

**angioedema** \-ēdē′mə\ **1** ANGIONEUROTIC EDEMA. **2** GIANT URTICARIA. **hereditary a.** An autosomal dominant disorder characterized by episodic, usually self-limited attacks of peripheral edema, abdominal pain, and potentially fatal laryngeal edema. It is caused by a deficiency of complement $C_1$ esterase inhibitor. Treatment with androgen derivatives can prevent attacks in most cases. Also *$C_1$ esterase inhibitor deficiency, hereditary edema, hereditary angioneurotic edema* (outmoded).

**angioelephantiasis** \-el′əfantī′əsis\ [ANGIO- + ELEPHANTIASIS] Edema and hypertrophy associated with excessive angiomatosis.

**angioendothelioma** \-en′dəthē′lē·ō′mə\ [ANGIO- + ENDOTHELIOMA] A benign vascular tumor composed mainly of capillaries with prominent endothelial cells. It most commonly occurs in the head and neck area of children. Also *benign hemangioendothelioma.*

**angioendotheliomatosis** \-en′dəthē′lē·ō′mətō′sis\ The presence of malignant tumors of vascular origin occurring most frequently on the face and scalp of elderly men. **a. proliferans** A condition characterized by multiple benign lesions arising as a result of hyperplasia of the endothelial cells that line the blood vessels.

**angiofibroma** \-fībrō′mə\ [ANGIO- + FIBROMA] A benign tumor composed of vessels and fibrous tissue. Also *angiofibroblastoma* (outmoded), *hemangiofibroma.* **a. contagiosum tropicum** A skin disease, reported in Brazil, consisting of red papules that enlarge to form nodules. **intranasal a.** An angiofibroma presenting as an intranasal tumor. There are two well-recognized varieties: the juvenile angiofibroma and the bleeding polypus of the nasal septum. **juvenile a.** An uncommon tumor arising at the back of the nose adjacent to the sphenopalatine foramen and, although benign, liable to erode adjacent structures and spread along anatomical pathways, particularly into the nasopharynx. It occurs almost exclusively in young males and the necessary surgery is made difficult by the extreme vascularity of the lesion.

**angiogenesis** \-jen′əsis\ [ANGIO- + GENESIS] The development of blood vessels, either in the embryo or during repair, healing, and regeneration.

**angiogenic** \-jen′ik\ **1** Forming blood vessels during development. **2** Originating from vascular elements, as a neoplasm.

**angiograph** \an′jē·ōgraf′\ A radiograph obtained during angiography. Also *angiogram.*

**angiography** \an′jē·äg′rəfē\ [ANGIO- + -GRAPHY] Radiologic examination of vessels after the injection of a contrast agent. **aortic arch a.** Radiographic visualization of the aortic arch and its branches. It is usually achieved by the injection of contrast medium into the arch through a catheter inserted via a femoral artery. **carotid a.** Angiography of the common carotid artery and its branches. **cerebral a.** Radiologic examination of the arteries and veins of the brain after the injection of a radiopaque agent. Also *cerebral arteriography.* **coronary a.** The radiographic visualization of the coronary arteries, usually selectively, after injection of contrast medium through specially designed catheters. **digital subtraction a.** Angiography in which the x-ray images are digitized so that images taken before the introduction of a contrast agent can be computer subtracted from ones taken with a contrast agent, thus greatly enhancing the visibility of the contrast agent. **emission a.** RADIONUCLIDE ANGIOGRAPHY. **intravenous renal a.** Radiologic examination of the arteries of the kidney after the injection of a radiopaque agent into a vein. **orbital a.** Radiography of the vessels of the orbit which is obtained during carotid arteriography. In order to study the orbital veins it is necessary to inject the internal angular vein of the eye. **pulmonary a.** Radiographic visualization of the pulmonary vessels after the injection of a radiopaque agent, usually into the superior or inferior vena cava, right atrium, or pulmonary artery. **radionuclide a.** The visualization of blood vessels by injecting a source of gamma radiation into the bloodstream and observing the area of interest by scintigraphy. The method works well with cerebral vessels and also with thrombosed or varicose veins, portal veins, lymphatics, and others. Also *emission angiography.* **spinal cord a.** Angiographic demonstration of the blood vessels of the spinal cord. **vertebral a.** Angiographic demonstration of a vertebral artery, the basilar artery, and their branches, carried out by direct injection or catheterization of a vertebral artery.

**angiohemophilia** \-hē′məfil′yə\ An ill-defined tendency to bleed. Most cases originally so described were probably of von Willebrand's disease. *Obs.*

**angiohydrography** \-hidräg′rəfē\ HYDROANGIOGRAPHY.

**angioid** \an′jē·oid\ [ANGI- + -OID] Resembling a blood vessel; having the appearance of a blood vessel.

**angiokeratoma** \-ker′ətō′mə\ [ANGIO- + KERATOMA] A vascular malformation characterized by the combination of ectasia of superficial dermal vessels with some degree of hyperkeratosis, which results in a warty telangiectatic lesion. Also *angiokeratosis.* **a. corporis diffusum** An X-linked inborn error of glycosphingolipid metabolism due to deficiency of the enzyme α-galactosidase A. The catabolism of glycolipids is interrupted by the inability to cleave a terminal galactose residue, and neutral glycolipids accumulate in lysosomes, particularly in endothelial cells. Clinically, males develop acroparesthesia, hypohidrosis, episodic hyperpyrexia, angiokeratoma characterized by telangiectic lesions on the lower half of the body, a distinctive corneal dystrophy, cardiac hypertrophy, proteinuria, and progressive renal failure, with death in the third or fourth decade unless hemodialysis is begun. Female heterozygotes often have milder symptoms and signs and usually develop renal disease. Also *Fabry's disease, Fabry syndrome, Anderson-Fabry disease, α-galactosidase deficiency.* **a. of the scrotum** Small angiomatous papules of the scrotum. They first appear at adolescence and affect as much as 20 percent of the population in old age. The same condition can occur in the vulva, usually in old age.

**angiokeratosis** \-ker'ətō'sis\ ANGIOKERATOMA.

**angioleukitis** \-lookī'tis\ LYMPHANGITIS.

**angiolipoma** \-lipō'mə\ [ANGIO- + LIPOMA] A lipoma containing a prominent number of blood vessels. Also *nevoid lipoma, telangiectatic lipoma.*

**angiologia** \-lō'jə\ [ANGIO- + -LOGIA] [NA] The nomenclature of the constituent parts of the entire cardiovascular system.

**angiology** \an'jē·äl'əjē\ [ANGIO- + -LOGY] The branch of science concerned with blood vessels and lymph vessels.

**angiolymphangioma** \-limfan'jē·ō'mə\ [ANGIO- + LYMPHANGI- + -OMA] A benign tumor composed of blood vascular and lymphatic vascular components.

**angiolymphitis** \-limfī'tis\ LYMPHANGITIS.

**angiolysis** \an'jē·äl'isis\ [ANGIO- + LYSIS] Retrogression, obliteration, and disappearance of certain blood vessels during embryonic life. It is an important process in the rearrangement of blood vessels, leading eventually to the establishment of the definitive vascular pattern.

**angioma** \an'jē·ō'mə\ [ANGI- + -OMA] A benign vascular tumor composed of blood or lymphatic vessels. See also HEMANGIOMA, LYMPHANGIOMA. **arteriovenous a.** An agglomeration of tortuous and dilated blood vessels with multiple communications between arteries and veins. **arteriovenous a. of brain** An arteriovenous angioma within the cerebrum, the cerebellum, or the brainstem. **capillary a.** CAPILLARY HEMANGIOMA. **cavernous a.** CAVERNOUS HEMANGIOMA. **cerebral a.** An arteriovenous angioma of the cerebrum. **cherry a.** A bright red, small dome-shaped angioma. Although such angiomas appear in increasing frequency with advancing age, no significant systemic associations can be made. Also *De Morgan spot, Campbell de Morgan spot.* **a. cutis** An angioma of the skin. Also *hemangioma hypertrophicum cutis.* **fissured a.** GRANULOMA FISSURATUM. **hereditary hemorrhagic a.** Hereditary multiple angiomas or telangiectatic lesions associated with hemorrhages. **hypertrophic a.** An angioma with endothelial proliferation. **infectious a.** ANGIOMA SERPIGINOSUM. **a. pigmentosum atrophicum** *Obs.* XERODERMA PIGMENTOSUM. **plane a.** TELANGIECTATIC ANGIOMA. **sclerosing a.** *Incorrect* DERMATOFIBROMA. **senile a.** SIMPLE ANGIOMA. **a. serpiginosum** A rare nevoid malformation of the dermal blood vessels that usually appears in childhood as grouped red puncta on the limbs. Also *infectious angioma.* **simple a.** A common vascular malformation on the trunk in the middle-aged and elderly, characterized by domed, bright red papules. Also *senile angioma.* **spider a.** SPIDER TELANGIECTASIS. **spinal a.** An angioma within the spinal canal. Such angiomas may be within or outside the medulla. **stellate a.** SPIDER TELANGIECTASIS. **strawberry a.** STRAWBERRY NEVUS. **telangiectatic a.** A circumscribed nevoid malformation of the dermal capillaries that is not elevated above the normal surface of the skin. Also *plane angioma.* **tuberous a.** A subcutaneous cavernous hemangioma. **a. venosum racemosum** The swellings apparent in severe venous varicosity. *Obs.*

**angiomatoid** \an'jē·äm'ətoid\ [ANGIOMA + *t* + -OID] Resembling an angioma.

**angiomatosis** \-mətō'sis\ [ANGIOMA + *t* + OSIS] HEMANGIOMATOSIS. **cephalotrigeminal a.** STURGE-WEBER SYNDROME. **congenital dysplastic a.** A vascular tumor of developmental origin in which associated tissues are also found to be abnormal, as with overgrowth of bone seen in Klippel-Trenaunay syndrome or calcification of the cerebral cortex in Sturge-Weber syndrome. **diffuse corticomeningeal a.** VAN BOGAERT-DIVRY SYNDROME. **encephalofacial a.** STURGE-WEBER SYNDROME. **encephalotrigeminal a.** STURGE-WEBER SYNDROME. **hemorrhagic familial a.** HEREDITARY HEMORRHAGIC TELANGIECTASIA. **hepatic a.** PELIOSIS HEPATIS. **oculoencephalic a.** STURGE-WEBER SYNDROME. **a. retinae** Capillary neoplasms of the retina as occur in the von Hippel-Lindau syndrome. Also *hemangiomatosis retinae, hemangioblastoma retinae, hemangiogliomatosis retinae.* **Sturge-Weber encephalotrigeminal a.** STURGE-WEBER SYNDROME.

**angiomatous** \an'jē·äm'ətəs\ Pertaining to or resembling an angioma.

**angiomyolipoma** \-mī'ōlipō'mə\ [ANGIO- + MYO- + LIPOMA] A benign tumor of hamartomatous nature consisting of a mixture of adipose tissue, thick-walled vascular structures, and smooth-muscle elements. It is generally unencapsulated. The tumor arises in the renal cortex and is sometimes a feature of the tuberous sclerosis complex. Also *hemangiomyolipoma, lipomyohemangioma.* **renal a.** A benign tumor consisting of adipose tissue, smooth muscle, and blood vessels which may involve the kidneys. It may be asymptomatic or grow sufficiently large to cause displacement of the kidney and distortion of the calices. It may be associated with tuberous sclerosis. Also *renal hamartoma.*

**angiomyoma** \-mī·ō'mə\ [ANGIO- + MYOMA] A benign, well-circumscribed and frequently tender or painful tumor, consisting of convoluted thick-walled vessels associated with bundles of well-differentiated smooth muscle elements. The tumor occurs most commonly in the wrist and ankle region. Also *vascular leiomyoma.*

**angiomyoneuroma** \-mī'ōnʸʊrō'mə\ [ANGIO- + MYO- + NEUROMA] GLOMUS TUMOR.

**angiomyosarcoma** \-mī'ōsärkō'mə\ [ANGIO- + MYO- + SARCOMA] A sarcoma containing vascular and muscular components.

**angiomyxoma** \-miksō'mə\ [ANGIO- + MYXOMA] An angioma of the placenta which extends into the myxomatous tissue of the umbilical cord.

**angionecrosis** \-nekrō'sis\ Necrosis of blood vessel walls.

**angioneurectomy** \-nʸʊrek'təmē\ [ANGIO- + NEURECTOMY] The excision of blood vessels and nerves together, usually a conglomeration of blood vessels and nerves as in a glomus tumor.

**angioneuroedema** \-nʸʊr'ō·ēdē'mə \ ANGIONEUROTIC EDEMA.

**angioneuroma** \-nʸʊrō'mə\ [ANGIO- + NEUROMA] *Outmoded* GLOMUS TUMOR.

**angioneuromyoma** \-nʸʊr'ōmī·ō'mə \ [ANGIO- + NEURO- + MYOMA] *Outmoded* GLOMUS TUMOR.

**angioneuropathy** \-nʸʊräp'əthē\ Any form of neuropathy in which one or more nerves (cranial or peripheral) are damaged as a consequence of ischemia resulting from occlusive or inflammatory vascular disease.

**angioneurotic** \-nʸurät′ik\ Of or involving the blood or lymph vessels and the nerves. See under EDEMA.

**angio-osteohypertrophy** \-äs′tē·ōhīpur′trəfē\ KLIPPEL-TRENAUNAY-WEBER SYNDROME.

**angioparalysis** \-pəral′isis\ VASOMOTOR PARALYSIS.

**angioparesis** \-pərē′sis\ [ANGIO- + PARESIS] Diminished tone of the blood vessels.

**angiopathy** \an′jē·äp′əthē\ [ANGIO- + -PATHY] Any disorder of blood vessels.

**angioplasty** \an′jē·ōplas′tē\ [ANGIO- + -PLASTY] The reconstruction or restructuring of a blood vessel by operative means or by nonsurgical techniques such as balloon dilatation or laser. **balloon a.** A nonoperative technique to relieve vascular stenoses or occlusions, in which a double-lumen balloon-tipped catheter is inserted percutaneously into an artery or vein and advanced under x-ray control until the catheter tip has passed across the vessel occlusion or stenosis. At this point the balloon is inflated, forcing the vessel blockage open. The technique may be used for peripheral arteries, the coronary circulation, veins, and various vascular grafts. Also *balloon dilatation, percutaneous transluminal angioplasty.* **patch a.** An operative technique to relieve an arterial stenosis by performing a longitudinal arteriotomy through the site of the stenosis and then suturing into the resulting elliptical defect a patch of autogenous tissue or prosthetic material. **percutaneous transluminal a.** BALLOON ANGIOPLASTY. **percutaneous transluminal coronary a.** A technique used to compress atherosclerotic coronary stenoses in which an inflatable balloon-tipped catheter is passed into and across the lesion, thus increasing coronary artery blood flow.

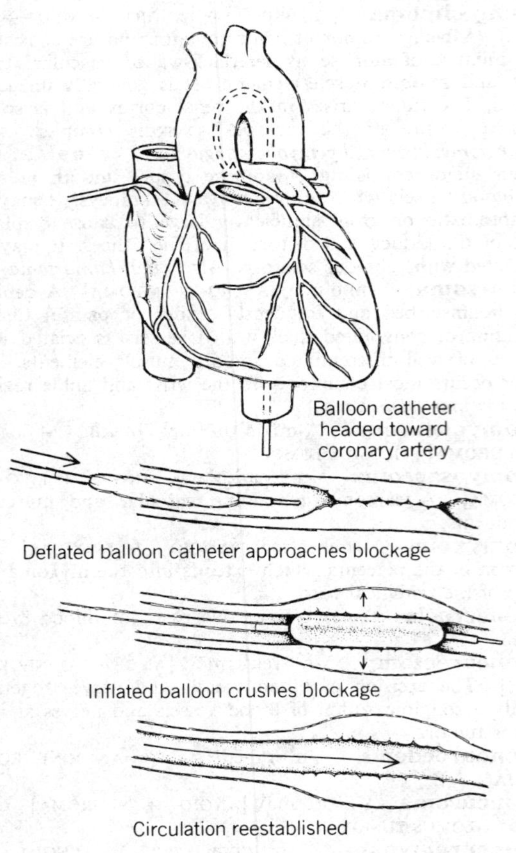


**Balloon angioplasty**

**angiopoiesis** \-poi·ē′sis\ [ANGIO- + -POIESIS] The process of blood vessel formation.

**angiopoietic** \-poi·et′ik\ Pertaining to angiopoiesis.

**angiopressure** \an′jē·ōpresh′ər\ Compression of a vessel to stop bleeding.

**angiorrhaphy** \an′jē·ôr′əfē\ [ANGIO- + -RRHAPHY] The repair of a blood vessel, usually by suture. **arteriovenous a.** The suturing of an artery and a vein to produce an arteriovenous fistula.

**angiosarcoma** \-särkō′mə\ [ANGIO- + SARCOMA] A highly malignant, vascular tumor which contains irregular anastomosing vascular channels lined by neoplastic, enlarged endothelial cells. It may occur in soft tissues or viscera, such as the liver. Also *malignant hemangioendothelioma, hemangiosarcoma.*

**angioscope** \an′jē·ōskōp′\ [ANGIO- + -SCOPE] A type of microscope used for observing capillary blood vessels.

**angioscopy** \an′jē·äs′kəpē\ [ANGIO- + -SCOPY] The visualization of small vessels by an angioscope.

**angioscotoma** \-skōtō′mə\ [ANGIO- + SCOTOMA] One of the very fine, linear field defects produced by the retinal blood vessels.

**angiospasm** \an′jē·ōspazm′\ VASOSPASM. **coronary a.** Spasm of the coronary arteries.

**angiostrongyliasis** \-strän′jəlī′əsis\ Infection with nematodes of the genus *Angiostrongylus.* Several species are recognized in rodents and other mammals. Light infections in man by the rodent lungworm, *A. cantonensis,* may be asymptomatic. In cases of overt disease, however, symptoms include meningoencephalitis and high eosinophilia of the cerebrospinal fluid and blood. See also EOSINOPHILIC MENINGITIS.

***Angiostrongylus*** \-strän′jiləs\ [New L, from ANGIO- + Gk *strongylos* round] A genus of metastrongyle lung nematodes that are parasitic in rats, dogs, and foxes. Accidental infection of humans with *A. cantonensis* or *A. malaysienensis* may result in eosinophilic meningoencephalitis. ***A. cantonensis*** A species of lungworm found in rats in the Pacific basin. It is acquired through ingestion of an intermediate host, land snails or slugs. Adults live in the rodent pulmonary arteries after an earlier period of development on the surface of the brain. Eggs hatch in the lung tissues and the larvae migrate to the mouth and are swallowed and passed in feces. Snails or slugs become infected through ingestion of feces of infected rats. Humans may become infected from ingestion of infected snails or slugs or from freshwater crustacea that have fed on infected mollusks, possibly including fish that serve as transport hosts. Raw vegetables fed on by infected snails or slugs may also contain larvae. The worms cannot complete their normal development in a human host but can cause angiostrongyliasis or eosinophilic meningoencephalitis. ***A. costaricensis*** *MORERASTRONGYLUS COSTARICENSIS.*

**angiostrophe** \an′jē·äs′trəfē\ [ANGIO- + Gk *strophē* a turning, twist] The twisting of the cut end of a vessel to stop hemorrhage. *Obs.* Also *angiostrophy* (obs.).

**angiotelectasis** \-telek′təsis\ [ANGIO- + TELE-[2] + Gk

*ektasis* a stretching out] Dilatation of arterioles, capillaries or venules.

**angiotensin** The octapeptide Asp-Arg-Val-Tyr-Ile-His-Pro-Phe. It is released from a plasma protein by proteinase action and is powerfully hypertensive, stimulating the smooth muscle of blood vessels. It also evokes aldosterone release from the adrenal cortex. It is sometimes designated angiotensin II to distinguish it from its precursor, angiotensin I, which possesses an extra two C-terminal residues. Also *angiotonin, adrenoglomerulotropin.* **a. I** The N-terminal decapeptide of angiotensinogen. It is released by the action of the enzyme renin. A further enzyme can act on it to release its C-terminal dipeptide and leave angiotensin II, the highly active pressor peptide. Also *proangiotensin.* **a. II** See under ANGIOTENSIN.

**angiotensinase** A proteolytic enzyme (EC 3.4.99.3) capable of splitting angiotensin (angiotensin II) at its Tyr-Ile bond to form two tetrapeptides and thereby inactivating it. Also *hypertensinase.*

**angiotensinogen** The plasma protein, an $\alpha_2$-globulin, from which angiotensin is released by proteolysis. Also *renin substrate, hypertensinogen.*

**angiotome** \an′jē·ōtōm′\ [ANGIO- + -TOME] A segment of an embryo or a block of embryonic tissue supplied by a blood vessel. Also *vascular segment.*

**angiotomography** \-təmäg′rəfē\ Radiologic examination which combines tomography and angiography.

**angiotomy** \an′jē·ät′əmē\ [ANGIO- + -TOMY] Incision of a blood vessel.

**angiotonic** \-tän′ik\ VASOTONIC.

**angiotonin** ANGIOTENSIN.

**angiotribe** \an′jē·ōtrīb′\ [ANGIO- + Gk *tribē* a rubbing, grinding away] A strong forceps equipped with a screw mechanism used to control hemorrhage from a blood vessel. *Obs.* Also *vasotribe.*

**angitis** \anjī′tis\ ANGIITIS.

**Angle** [Edward Hartley *Angle,* U.S. dentist, 1855–1930] **1** Angle's classification of malocclusion. See under CLASSIFICATION. **2** See under BAND, SPLINT.

# angle

**angle** The shape formed by the meeting of two lines or planes, or the space enclosed by them; angulus. **a. of aberration** The angle between the true and apparent positions of a celestial body as subtended at the eye of the observer. **acromial a.** ANGULUS ACROMIALIS. **acromial a. of scapula** ANGULUS LATERALIS SCAPULAE. **alpha a.** The angle between the visual axis and the optic axis. **Alsberg's a.** The angle at the apex of Alsberg's triangle. **alveolar a.** The angle at which a line passing through prosthion and subspinale meets the Frankfort plane. Some authorities use nasospinale instead of subspinale. **anomaly a.** The angle between the normal line of sight (visual axis) and the abnormal direction of alignment of an eye with macular suppression and selective use of a nonmacular portion of the retina for fixation. **anterior costal a.** A slight bend in the shaft of each of the second to tenth ribs that occurs a short distance from the anterior extremity. *Outmoded.* **anterior inferior a. of parietal bone** ANGULUS SPHENOIDALIS OSSIS PARIETALIS. **anterior a. of petrous portion of temporal bone** ANGULUS ANTERIOR PYRAMIDIS OSSIS TEMPORALIS. **anterior superior a. of parietal bone** ANGULUS FRONTALIS OSSIS PARIETALIS. **anterior vesicourethral a.** The angle formed by the anterior border, or junction of the inferolateral surfaces, of the urinary bladder and the urethra. **auriculo-occipital a.** The angle formed where lines from the auricular point to lambda and to the opisthion meet. **axial line a.** Any line angle parallel to the long axis of a tooth. **basal a.** The angle formed by a line drawn along the clivus with a line drawn along the planum sphenoidale on a lateral skull radiograph. The normal angle is about 130°. An angle of 150° or more is consistent with platybasia. **Bennett a.** The angle between the sagittal plane and the path of a point in the advancing condyle during lateral mandibular excursion. **biorbital a.** The angle formed by the meeting of lines extended posteriorly along the orbital axes. **Böhler's a.** An angle indicating the configuration of the calcaneus, measured from a roentgenogram of the lateral projection of the heel, with a normal value in the range of 28°–40° and being decreased with compression fractures of the bone. The angle is formed by the intersection of two lines, one line being drawn from the posterosuperior aspect of the talocalcaneal joint to the posterosuperior margin of the calcaneus, and the other line from the posterosuperior aspect of the talocalcaneal joint to the superior articular aspect of the calcaneocuboid joint. **Boogaard's a.** The angle formed by a line drawn along the clivus with a line drawn from the posterior margin of the foramen magnum to the clivus. This angle should normally measure 119°–136°. **Bull's a.** The angle, which may be measured on a lateral radiograph of the craniovertebral junction, between a line that is a direct posterior extension of the hard palate and one drawn horizontally through the body of the atlas vertebra. An angle of more than 10–15 degrees suggests a tilting of the body of the atlas with probable invagination into the base of the skull, or basilar impression. **cardiohepatic a.** The angle formed by the upper border of the liver and the right side of the heart. **cardiophrenic a.** The angle between the border of the heart and diaphragm, as demonstrated on posteroanterior radiographs of the chest. On a radiograph this is indistinguishable from the cardiohepatic angle. **carrying a.** The angle formed by the axis of the arm and the axis of the forearm in the extended, supinated position. It is easily measured on a radiograph. **cavosurface a.** A cavity angle formed by the junction of a wall of the cavity and the surface of the tooth. **cephalic a.** Any one of several angles formed by intersecting lines passing through selected craniometric points on the cranium and face. **cerebellopontine a.** A region of the brain situated in the posterior cranial fossa bounded laterally by the petrous part of the temporal bone, medially by the cerebellum and pons, above by the tentorium cerebelli, and below by the floor of the posterior fossa. It is the site of angle tumors and often of tremors of the eighth cranial nerve. **collodiaphyseal a.** The angle formed at the junction of the long axis of the shaft of the femur with that of the femoral neck. **condylar a.** The angle between the plane of the clivus and that of the foramen magnum. **a. of convergence** The angle between the visual axes of the two eyes. **coronary a.** ANGULUS FRONTALIS OSSIS PARIETALIS. **costal a.** ANGULUS COSTAE. **costophrenic a.** The angle formed at the junction of the pleura costalis and the pleura diaphragmatica. **costovertebral a.** The acute angle formed at the junction of the twelfth rib and the vertebral column on each side. **craniofacial a.** **1** The angle formed at the sphenoidale by the intersection of the nasion-sphenoidale and the basion-sphenoidale lines. **2** The angle formed at the midpoint of the sphenoethmoid suture between lines to that point from the subnasal point and the basion. **critical a.** The minimum angle of incidence at which a light ray incident on an interface between two media of different indexes of refraction, from the side with the higher index, is totally reflected with none of the light refracted into the other medium. **cusp a.** The angle made by the surface of a cusp of a tooth with a vertical line bisecting the cusp or with the plane perpendicular to this line at the tip. **Daubenton's a.** The angle at the opisthion between a line from the basion and a line from the nasion. **a. of deviation** The angle between an incident and refracted light ray. **duodenojejunal a.** FLEXURA DUODENOJEJUNALIS. **epigastric a.** The angle formed at the xiphisternal articulation between the body of the sternum and the xiphoid process. **ethmocranial a.** The angle at the junction of the basicranial axis and the extension of the plane of the cribiform plate of the ethmoid bone. Also *ethmoid angle.* **facial a.** The inferoposterior angle at the intersection of the Frankfort plane and the facial plane. **a. of femoral torsion** The angle formed between the transverse axis of the head of the femur and the transverse axis of the lower extremity of the femur. It is normally about 15° in adults and much larger in infancy. **filtration a.** ANGULUS IRIDOCORNEALIS. **Frankfort-mandibular plane a.** The angle between the Frankfort plane and the mandibular plane. **frontal a. of parietal bone** ANGULUS FRONTALIS OSSIS PARIETALIS. **gamma a.** The angle between the center of rotation of the eye and the center of the pupil, when projected to the fixation point. **gonial a.** The angle between a tangent to the lowe r border and a tangent to the posterior border of the mandible. **ileocolic a.** The wide angle between the terminal ileum and the ascending colon at the entrance of the ileum into the posteromedial aspect of the junction of the cecum and the ascending colon. **a. of incidence** The angle between the direction of propagation of a wave incident on an interface between two media and the normal to the interface at the point of incidence. **incisal guidance a.** The angle in the sagittal plane between a line drawn from the incisal edges of the maxillary and mandibular central incisors in centric occlusion and the occlusal plane. **incisal mandibular plane a.** The angle at which a line through the long axis of a lower central incisor tooth meets the mandibular plane, as measured on a lateral radiograph. **a. of inclination** 1 COLLODIAPHYSEAL ANGLE. 2 INCLINATIO PELVIS. **inferior a. of duodenum** FLEXURA DUODENI INFERIOR. **inferior a. of scapula** ANGULUS INFERIOR SCAPULAE. **infrasternal a. of thorax** ANGULUS INFRASTERNALIS THORACIS. **inner a. of eye** ANGULUS OCULI MEDIALIS. **iridial a.** ANGULUS IRIDOCORNEALIS. **iridocorneal a.** ANGULUS IRIDOCORNEALIS. **a. of iris** ANGULUS IRIDOCORNEALIS. **a. of jaw** ANGULUS MANDIBULAE. **kappa a.** The angle between the visual axis and the pupillary axis, measured where they intersect at the nodal point of the eye. **lambda a.** The angle between the visual axis and the pupillary axis, measured where they intersect at the pupil. **lateral a. of cerebellum** The rounded lateral border of the cerebellar hemisphere, marked by the horizontal fissure and forming the boundary between the superior and inferior cerebellar surfaces. **lateral a. of eye** ANGULUS OCULI LATERALIS. **lateral a. of scapula** ANGULUS LATERALIS SCAPULAE. **line a.** The angle at the meeting place of two planes. **a. of Louis** ANGULUS STERNI. **a. of Ludwig** ANGULUS STERNI. **a. of mandible** ANGULUS MANDIBULAE. **mandibular a.** ANGULUS MANDIBULAE. **manubriosternal a.** ANGULUS STERNI. **mastoid a. of parietal bone** ANGULUS MASTOIDEUS OSSIS PARIETALIS. **medial a. of eye** ANGULUS OCULI MEDIALIS. **medial a. of scapula** ANGULUS SUPERIOR SCAPULAE. **meter a.** A measure of the amount of convergence that is identical to the number of diopters of accommodation required for the stipulated distance. For example, at 25 cm, emmetropic eyes must accommodate 4 diopters and are said to have 4 meter angles of convergence. **a. of minimum deviation** The smallest amount by which a beam of monochromatic light is deflected on passing through a prism, as in a spectroscope. **a. of mouth** Either of the extremities of the oral fissure. **nasal a. of eye** ANGULUS OCULI MEDIALIS. **neck shaft a.** The angle at the junction of the neck of the femur and the shaft of the femur, used as an index to determine the degree of varus or valgus deformity at the hip. **occipital a.** ANGULUS OCCIPITALIS OSSIS PARIETALIS. **occipital a. of parietal bone** ANGULUS OCCIPITALIS OSSIS PARIETALIS. **olfactive a.** The angle between the plane of the cribriform plate of the ethmoid bone and the basicranial axis. Also *olfactory angle.* **optic a.** VISUAL ANGLE. **outer a. of eye** ANGULUS OCULI LATERALIS. **parietal a.** The angle formed at the junction of two lines, one on each side of the skull, drawn tangential to the ends of the transverse bizygomatic diameter and the maximum frontal diameter. The angle is zero when the lines are parallel, and negative if they diverge. **parietal a. of sphenoid bone** MARGO PARIETALIS ALAE MAJORIS. **a. of pelvis** INCLINATIO PELVIS. **pelvivertebral a.** 1 The angle formed between the plane of the superior pelvic aperture and the general line of the trunk. 2 INCLINATIO PELVIS. **phrenopericardial a.** CARDIOPHRENIC ANGLE. **a. of polarization** The angle between the plane of polarization of a light (or other transverse) wave and a specified reference plane. **posterior inferior a. of parietal bone** ANGULUS MASTOIDEUS OSSIS PARIETALIS. **posterior a. of petrous portion of temporal bone** MARGO POSTERIOR PARTIS PETROSAE OSSIS TEMPORALIS. **posterior superior a. of parietal bone** ANGULUS OCCIPITALIS OSSIS PARIETALIS. **prism a.** The angle formed at the apex of a prism. **a. of pubis** ANGULUS SUBPUBICUS. **QRS-T a.** The spatial angle in electrocardiography between the QRS area vector and the T area vector when the mean direction and magnitude of the areas are plotted for the frontal plane of the body. It is quite constant in normal hearts. **a. of reflection** The angle between the direction of propagation of a reflected wave and the normal to the reflecting surface at the point of reflection. **a. of refraction** The angle between the direction of propagation of a refracted wave and the normal to the refracting surface at the point of refraction. **a. of rib** ANGULUS COSTAE. **sacrovertebral a.** The prominent angle formed anteriorly at the articulation between the base of the sacrum and the fifth lumbar vertebra and rounded by the intervening disk, which is much thicker in front than behind. **scattering a.** The angle by which the direction of motion of a particle is changed in the process of collision with another particle. **sinodural a.** The angle of solid bone in the posterosuperior corner of the mastoid cavity between the plates of dense bone investing the lateral sinus posteriorly and part of the middle cranial fossa above. **solid a.** The solid bone in the angle formed by the three semicircular canals, as encountered, in the course of mastoid surgery, medial to the mastoid antrum. **sphenoid a.** ANGULUS SPHENOIDALIS OSSIS PARIETALIS. **sphenoidal a. of parietal bone** ANGULUS SPHENOIDALIS OSSIS PARIETALIS. **squint a.** The angle between the two optic axes of an individual with strabismus. **sternal a.** ANGULUS STERNI. **sternoclavicular a.** The angle formed by the junction of the manubrium sterni and the medial (sternal) end of the clavicle. **a. of sternum** ANGULUS STERNI. **subcostal a.** ANGULUS INFRASTERNALIS THORACIS. **subpubic a.** ANGULUS SUBPUBICUS. **substernal a.** ANGULUS INFRASTERNALIS THORACIS. **superior a. of duodenum** FLEXURA DUODENI SUPERIOR. **superior a. of petrous portion of temporal bone** MARGO SUPERIOR PARTIS PETROSAE OSSIS TEMPORALIS. **superior a. of scapula** ANGULUS SUPERIOR SCAPULAE. **a. of supination** The degree of rotation of the forearm from full pronation to full supination. **temporal a.** ANGULUS OCULI LATERALIS. **tentorial a.** The angle formed by the plane of the tentorium cerebelli meeting the basicranial axis. **a. of torsion** 1 The angle of rotation of the eye about the anteroposterior or sagittal axis, indicating the extent of the deviation of the primary vertical meridian of the eye when out of the primary position. Accordingly, rotation inward or outward, as the twelve o'clock position on the cornea moves nasally or temporally, is referred to as intorsion and extorsion, respectively. 2 The angle formed between the axes of any two different portions of a long bone. **uterine a.** The portion of the uterus where the fallopian tube enters the endometrial cavity. **venous a.** 1 The angle formed by the junction of the internal jugular and subclavian veins. Also *angulus venosus.* 2 In neuroradiology, the angle formed by the thalamostriate vein at its junction with the internal cerebral vein behind the anterior column of the fornix, usually marking the apex of the posterior superior limits of the interventricular foramen. It varies considerably with projection. **vesicourethral a.** Either the anterior or the posterior vesicourethral angle. **visual a.** The size of the angle produced at the eye by the two sides of an object under observation. Also *optic angle.* **Welcker's a.** ANGULUS SPHENOIDALIS OSSIS PARIETALIS. **xiphoid a.** The angle formed on either side of the xiphoid process at its junction with the seventh costal cartilage.

**angle-former** An instrument used to make bevels in cavity preparation.

**angor** \ang′gôr\ [L (from *angere* to stifle, choke), the quinsy, a sore throat, a strangling] Intense distress; angina. **a. animi** Fear of impending doom. **a. nocturnus** PAVOR NOCTURNUS.

**ångström** \ang′strəm, ông′-\ [after Anders Jonas *Ångström,* Swedish astronomer and physicist, 1814–1874] A unit of length equal to $10^{-10}$ meter, used especially to express the wavelengths of electromagnetic radiation. Originally the ångström was defined in terms of the red cadmium line, the line being given a wavelength of exactly 6438.4696 ångströms under specified conditions. Symbol: Å • This term is often spelled *angstrom.* **reciprocal å.** A unit of wave number of electromagnetic waves. Symbol: $Å^{-1}$

***Anguillula stercoralis*** \ang·gwil′yələ stur′kərā′lis\ *STRONGYLOIDES STERCORALIS.*

**angular** \ang′gyələr\ Pertaining to or shaped like an angle; bent at a point.

**angulation** \ang′gyəlā′shən\ [L *angulatus* (past part. of *angulare* to make a bend or angle) bent,angled + *-io* -ION] A deviation from a straight line. It may be seen in the malunion of a fracture or at a joint.

**anguli** \ang′gyəlī\ Plural of ANGULUS.

**angulus** \ang′gyələs\ [L (akin to Gk *ankylos* bent, crooked) a corner, angle] An angulation in or of a structure or part; angle. **a. acromialis** [NA] The prominent junction of the thick lateral border of the acromion with the inferior lip of the crest of the spine of the scapula, forming a subcutaneous bony landmark. Also *acromial angle.* **a. anterior pyramidis ossis temporalis** The anterior angle or border of the petrous part of the temporal bone, divided into two parts: a lateral, joined to the squama at the petrosquamous suture, and a medial, for articulation with the greater wing of the sphenoid bone. Also *anterior angle of petrous portion of temporal bone.* **a. costae** [NA] A sharp curve on the external surface of a rib, a short distance outwards from the tubercle where the shaft turns sharply outwards and forwards, while twisting on its long axis. A prominent linear marking here provides attachment for a tendon of the iliocostalis muscle. The distance between tubercle and angle is increasingly greater from the second to the tenth ribs. Also *angle of rib, costal angle.* **a. frontalis ossis parietalis** [NA] The anterior superior angle of the quadrangular parietal bone, corresponding to the junction of the sagittal and coronal sutures at bregma. Also *anterior superior angle of parietal bone, coronary angle, frontal angle of parietal bone.* **a. inferior scapulae** [NA] The thick, ridged angle formed by the meeting of the medial and lateral borders of the scapula. Attached to it posteriorly is the teres major muscle, while anteriorly is the lower mass of the serratus anterior muscle. Normally, the angle may be palpable subcutaneously, and usually it lies at the level of the seventh to eighth ribs posteriorly. Also *inferior angle of scapula.* **a. infrasternalis thoracis** [NA] The angle formed at the xiphisternal joint by the sloping, joined cartilages of the seventh to tenth ribs on each side of the anterior aspect of the outlet or inferior opening of the bony thorax. Also *subcostal angle, infrasternal angle of thorax, substernal angle.* **a. iridocornealis** [NA] The acute angle at the periphery of the anterior chamber of the eye, of which the inner, posterior side is formed by the anterior margin of the iris at its attachment to the ciliary body and the outer, anterior side by the trabecular meshwork at the sclerocorneal junction. Aqueous humor of the anterior chamber drains through this angle. Also *iridocorneal angle, angle of iris, iridial angle, filtration angle.* **a. lateralis scapulae** [NA] The angle at the junction of the lateral and superior borders of the scapula, constituting the head of the scapula and bearing the glenoid cavity on its free surface to form the shoulder joint with the head of the humerus. Also *lateral angle of scapula, condyle of scapula, acromial angle of scapula.* **a. ludovici** ANGULUS STERNI. **a. mandibulae** [NA] The angle formed at the junction of the inferior border and the posterior border of the ramus of the mandible. Posteriorly, the stylomandibular ligament attaches to it, while medially it is part of the attachment of the medial pterygoid muscle and laterally is part of the attachment of the masseter muscle. It is easily palpable under the skin. Also *angle of jaw, gonial angle, mandibular angle, angle of mandible.* **a. mastoideus ossis parietalis** [NA] The blunted posteroinferior angle of the parietal bone that articulates with the occipital bone and the mastoid portion of the temporal bone, the junction being called the asterion. Its inner surface is grooved by the end of the transverse sinus and the beginning of the sigmoid sinus. Also *posterior inferior angle of parietal bone, mastoid angle of parietal bone, mastoid margin of parietal bone.* **a. medialis scapulae** ANGULUS SUPERIOR SCAPULAE. **a. occipitalis ossis parietalis** [NA] The rounded posterosuperior angle of the quadrangular parietal bone, located at lambda, the meeting point of the lambdoid and sagittal sutures. Also *posterior superior angle of parietal bone, occipital angle of parietal bone, occipital angle.* **a. oculi lateralis** [NA] The acute angle at the lateral extremity of the palpebral fissure between the upper and lower eyelids. Also *lateral angle of eye, external canthus, lateral canthus, outer canthus, temporal angle, outer angle of eye.* **a. oculi medialis** [NA] The rounded angle at the medial extremity of the palpebral fissure between the upper and lower eyelids. Also *medial angle of eye, nasal angle of eye, medial canthus, inner canthus, internal canthus, inner angle of eye.* **a. oris** [NA] The lateral junction of the lips surrounding the orifice of the mouth; the angle of the mouth bounded by the labial commissure. Also *junction of the lips.* **a. sphenoidalis ossis parietalis** [NA] The acute anteroinferior angle of the parietal bone that fits the interval between the frontal bone and the greater wing of the sphenoid bone along the coronal and sphenoparietal sutures respectively. The internal surface is grooved, and sometimes canalized, by the anterior division of the middle meningeal vessels. Also *sphenoid angle, anterior inferior angle of parietal bone, Welcker's angle, sphenoidal angle of parietal bone, sphenoidal margin of parietal bone.* **a. sterni** [NA] The prominent anterior angulation produced at the articulation between the manubrium and gladiolus (body) of the sternum, and opposite the sternochondral junction of the second rib. It is an important surface landmark. Also *angulus ludovici, angle of Louis, angle of Ludwig, sternal angle, angle of sternum, manubriosternal angle.* **a. of stomach** INCISURA ANGULARIS GASTRICA. **a. subpubicus** [NA] The angle at the apex of the pubic arch that is formed by the converging ischiopubic rami meeting below the symphysis pubis. The angle is usually considerably larger in females than in males. Also *angle of pubis, subpubic angle, subpubic arch, arch of pelvis.* **a. superior pyramidis ossis temporalis** MARGO SUPERIOR PARTIS PETROSAE OSSIS TEMPORALIS. **a. superior scapulae** [NA] The angle formed at the junction of the superior and medial borders of the scapula, to which muscles are attached. Also *angulus medialis scapulae, medial angle of scapula, superior angle of scapula.* **a. venosus** VENOUS ANGLE.

**anhaphia** \anhā′fē·ə\ ANAPHIA.

**anhaptoglobinemia** \anhap′təglō′binē′mē·ə\ The absence of haptoglobin in blood or serum. It is commonly observed in persons who have had hemolysis. Congenital anhaptoglobinemia commonly occurs in some ethnic groups and is presumed to be a genetic trait.

**anhedonia** \an′hēdō′nē·ə\ [Gk *an-* priv. + *hēdon(ē)* enjoyment + -IA] Inability to derive pleasure from day-to-day activities that the normal person finds pleasurable. It may appear as one of the earliest complaints in schizophrenia.

**anhemopoiesis** \an′hemәpoi·ē′sis\ The lack of blood formation, as in aplastic anemia.

**anhidrosis** \an′hidro′sis\ [Gk *an-* priv. + HIDROSIS] A deficient production of sweat. Also *anaphoresis.* **postmiliarial a.** Anhidrosis following miliaria profunda. Also *heat anhidrosis, thermogenic anhidrosis.*

**anhidrotic** \an′hidrät′ik\ **1** Of or relating to anhidrosis. **2** An agent that causes anhidrosis. For defs. 1 and 2 also *anidrotic.*

**anhistic** \anhis′tik\ [Gk *an-* priv. + HIST- + -IC] Lacking organic tissue structure.

**anhydration** \an′hīdrā′shən\ DEHYDRATION.

**anhydremia** \an′hīdrē′mə\ [Gk *an-* priv. + HYDR- + -EMIA] The state of decreased water content of the blood.

**anhydride** [*anhydr(o)-* + -IDE] A chemical compound arising by reaction of two acid groups with loss of water. If the acids are carboxylic the compound has the formula R—CO—O—CO—R′.

**anhydro-** \an′hīdrō-, anhī′drō-\ [Gk *anydro(s)* (from *an-* priv. + (*hydōr* water) without water] A combining form signifying the removal of the elements of water from a compound. It is used particularly with the names of carbohydrates, since residues of such sugars (anhydro sugars) occur in living organisms.

**anhydrous** \anhī′drəs\ [Gk *an-* priv. + HYDR- + -OUS] Free of water: used especially of a salt that does not contain water of crystallization but can do so.

**Anichkov** [Nikolay Nikolaevich *Anichkov*, Russian pathologist, born 1885] Anichkov cell, Anichkov's myocyte. See under CARDIAC HISTIOCYTE.

**anideus** \ənid′ē·əs\ [New L, from Gk *aneideos* (from *an-* priv. + *eidos* form) formless] A fetus or a parasitic twin lacking all or most of the usual morphologic features.

**anidrotic** \an′idrät′ik\ ANHIDROTIC.

**anileridine** $C_{22}H_{28}N_2O_2$. 1-(*p*-Aminophenethyl)-4-phenylisonipecotic acid ethyl ester, a narcotic analgesic used for the relief of moderate-to-severe pain.

**aniline** Ph—$NH_2$. Phenylamine. It is prepared from benzene by nitration and subsequent reduction. It is a much weaker base than aliphatic amines (P*K* 4.6). It is used in organic synthesis and as an intermediate in dyestuff manufacture. **a. fuchsin** A solution of acid fuchsin in aniline water that is used to stain mitochondria.

**aniline gentian violet** Gentian violet dissolved in aniline water. It was originally employed as a biological stain, but its use has been superceded by that of crystal violet, one of its constituents.

**aniline red** BASIC FUCHSIN.

**anilism** \an′əlizm\ Acute poisoning by aniline, its homologues, or many of its derivatives. Its clinical manifestation is cyanosis in mucous membranes, conjunctivae, lips, ear lobes, and nail beds, caused by elevated levels of methemoglobin in the blood. Also *anilinism.*

**anima** \an′imə\ [L (akin to Gk *anemos* the wind) air, breath, spirit, vital principle] **1** In Jung's terminology, the soul or inward-directed part of the psyche. **2** The feminine soul of a man. **a. mundi** The theory that all of nature's phenomena are derived from an animistic, activating spirit.

**animal** [L (from *anim(a)* + *-al* neut. noun suffix; see ANIMA) a living creature, animal] Any organism of the animal kingdom (Animalia). Such organisms require oxygen and organic nutrients for existence and are usually capable of independent motion. Animals are distinguished from plants by the lack of chlorophyll and the presence of cell membranes rather than cell walls. **bulbopontine a.** DECEREBRATE ANIMAL. **control a.** An animal serving as a standard with which test animals subjected to an experimental procedure can be compared in order to permit a valid assessment of the effects of the procedure concerned. **decerebrate a.** An animal on which the brainstem has been transected between the inferior and superior colliculi, leaving the pons and medulla oblongata connected to the spinal cord. Also *bulbopontine animal.* **decorticate a.** An animal which has sustained removal of the cerebral cortex. **experimental a.** An animal subjected to scientific experiment, especially one manipulated or treated in a manner to be compared with a control animal that is left untreated. **Long-Lukens a.** An animal whose pancreas and adrenal glands have been removed. *Outmoded.* **spinal a.** Any animal whose spinal cord has been completely transected. The transection may occur at any level. **thalamic a.** An animal with its cerebrum transected immediately rostral to the thalamus.

**animalcule** \an′əmal′kyool\ [New L *animalcul(um)*, dim. of L *animal* animal] A protozoan or minute metazoan organism. *Older term.*

**animus** \an′əməs\ [L (akin to ANIMA) the mind, soul, consciousness, character] In Jung's terminology, the masculine soul of a woman.

**anion** \an′ī·ən\ [Gk *anion*, neut. sing. of *aniōn*, pres. part. of *anienai* to go up] An ion carrying one or more negative charges. Compare CATION.

**anionic** \an′ī·än′ik\ Denoting molecules or groups that possess a negative charge and are therefore attracted towards the anode on electrophoresis.

**aniridia** \an′īrid′ē·ə\ [Gk *an-* priv. + IRID- + -IA] The developmental absence of most of the iris. Its base is present upon the ciliary body and commonly compromises the aqueous outflow mechanism. Also *irideremia*.

**anis-** \an′is-, anīs-\ ANISO-.

**anisakiasis** \an′isəkī′əsis\ An infection of the lining of the stomach, less frequently the mucosa of the small intestine, and rarely, of other organs, by larvae of the family Anisakidae, ascaroid parasites of marine fish. In the case of an accidental human infection, it may cause ulcers and eosinphilic granulomas of the stomach and of the small intestine. It is often mistaken for carcinoma, ulcers, or an appendicitis. Infection occurs through ingestion of raw or undercooked marine fish. The normal final hosts for these larvae are marine fish-eating birds and mammals.

***Anisakis*** \an′isā′kis\ [ANIS- + Gk *akis* a point, barb, sting] A genus of parasitic nematodes, the larvae of which are found in marine fish. The adult worms are intestinal parasites of toothed whales, porpoises, and dolphins. Larvae, when ingested by humans in undercooked or raw fish, may cause anisakiasis.

**anischuria** \an′iskyoo′rē·ə\ [Gk *an-* priv. + *isch(ein)* to hold, restrain + -URIA] Inability to retain urine in the bladder.

**aniseikonia** \an′isīkō′nēə\ [ANIS- + Gk *eikōn* image + -IA] A size difference in the images seen by the two eyes. Also *anisoiconia*. Adj. aniseikonic.

**anisergy** \anis′ərjē\ [*anis-* + *erg(o)-* + -Y] Differences in blood pressure in different parts of the cardiovascular system. Also *anisopiesis*.

**anisic acid** $C_8H_8O_3$. 4-Methoxybenzoic acid. An acid from anethole, the phenolic ether in anise oil and fennel oil. It has been used as a carminative, antiseptic, and antipyretic agent.

**aniso-** \anī′sō-\ [Gk *anisos* (*an-* priv. + *isos* equal) unequal] A combining form meaning unequal, unlike. Also *anis-*.

**anisochromasia** \-krōmā′zhə\ ANISOCHROMIA.

**anisochromatic** \-krōmat′ik\ Exhibiting anisochromia.

**anisochromia** \-krō′mē·ə\ Variability in the intensity of color of erythrocytes in stained blood films. *Seldom used.* Also *anisochromasia*.

**anisocoria** \-kôr′ē·ə\ [ANISO- + *cor(e)-* + -IA] Unequal diameters of the pupils of the two eyes.

**anisocytosis** \-sītō′sis\ [ANISO- + *-cyt(e)* + -OSIS] Variability of size of cells, especially of erythrocytes. Compare ISOCYTOSIS.

**anisodactyly** \-dak′təlē\ A condition in which the corresponding digits on either side of the body are of unequal length.

**anisodiametric** \-dī·əmet′rik\ Having different diameters in different directions, as an egg.

**anisodont** \anī′sədänt\ [ANISO- + -DONT] Having teeth of more than one type.

**anisoiconia** \-īkō′nē·ə\ ANISEIKONIA.

**anisomastia** \-mas′tē·ə\ [ANISO- + MAST- + -IA] Inequality in the size of the breasts.

**anisomelia** \-mē′lyə\ [ANISO- + MEL-[1] + -IA] An inequality of limb length between corresponding pairs in the same individual.

**anisometropia** \-metrō′pē·ə\ [Gk *anisometr(os)* (from ANISO- + *metr(on)* measure) incommensurate + -OPIA] Unequal optical focus of the two eyes. Adj. anisometropic.

**anisomorphous** \-môr′fəs\ [ANISO- + MORPH- + -OUS] Varied or irregular in morphology; heteromorphous. Also *anisomorphic*.

**anisophoria** \-fôr′ē·ə\ [ANISO- + -PHORIA] An imbalance between the muscles of the two eyes such as to cause differing vertical alignments of the visual axes in the horizontal planes.

**anisopiesis** \-pī·ē′sis\ ANISERGY.

**anisopoikilocytosis** \-poi′kilōsītō′sis\ [ANISO- + POIKILO- + *-cyt(e)* + -OSIS] Greater than normal variability in size and shape of erythrocytes.

**anisorhythmia** \-riTH′mē·ə\ [ANISO- + RHYTHM + -IA ] An irregularity of the heart in which there is lack of coordination between atrial and ventricular activity.

**anisosmotic** \anī′säzmät′ik\ Differing in osmotic pressure or in the concentration of osmotically active particles.

**anisosthenic** \anī′səsthen′ik\ Differing in strength.

**anisotonic** \-tän′ik\ Varying in tension or tonicity.

**anisotropic** \-träp′ik\ [ANISO- + -TROPIC[1]] Having different physical properties when measured in different directions, such as the refractive index of a crystal or the electrical resistance of muscle. Also *anisotropal*.

**ankle** [Middle English *ankel*, from Old Norse (akin to Gk *ankylos* bent and L *angulus* corner)] **1** The region at the junction of the leg and the foot. **2** ARTICULATIO TALOCRURALIS. **tailors' a.** An adventitious bursa that forms at the lower end of the fibula as a result of the pressure exerted on the lateral malleolus when sitting on the floor in a cross-legged position.

**ankylo-** \ang′kilō-\ [Gk *ankylē* (akin to *ankylos* bent, crooked, and *ankōn* elbow) the bend or bending of a joint, a bent or stiffened joint, a noose, thong, frenum] A combining form meaning (1) stiff, fixed, ankylosed; (2) fused, tied, closed. Also *anchylo-, ancylo-*.

**ankyloblepharon** \-blef′ərän\ [Gk (from ANKYLO- + BLEPHARON) adhesion of the eyelids] A fusion of the margins of the eyelids, resulting in partial or complete closure of the interpalpebral opening.

**ankylocolpos** \-käl′pəs\ [ANKYLO- + Gk *kolpos* bosom, womb, fold] **1** The absence of the vagina as a result of fusion of the vaginal walls, hence secondary to surgery or injury. **2** Congenital agenesis of the vagina. This is not to be confused with imperforate vagina, which usually involves only the hymen.

**ankylodactyly** \-dak′təlē\ SYNDACTYLY.

**ankyloglossia** \-gläs′ē·ə\ [Gk *ankyloglōss(os)* (from ANKYLO- + *glōssa* tongue) tongue-tied + -IA] TONGUE-TIE.

**ankyloproctia** \-präk′tē·ə\ [ANKYLO- + PROCT- + -IA] Stenosis or atresia of the anus, usually of developmental origin.

**ankylosed** \ang′kilōzd\ Characterized by an ankylosis.

**ankyloses** \ang′kilō′sēz\ Plural of ANKYLOSIS.

**ankylosis** \ang′kilō′sis\ [Gk *ankylōsis* (from *ankylē* a bend, noose; see ANKYLO-) stiffening of a joint, a tie or adhesion of a part] A stiffness or immobilization of a joint as a result of injury, disease, or surgical intervention. **artificial a.** ARTHRODESIS. **bony a.** A rigid joint whose cavity is replaced by bone. Also *true ankylosis*. **capsular a.** Joint stiffness due to capsular shortening and thickening. **cricoarytenoid a.** Fibrous or bony ankylosis of the cricoarytenoid joint. It is usually the result of severe infection of the larynx, particularly tuberculosis or late syphilis when complicated by perichondritis, or of various kinds of trauma. It is now a rare disease. **dental a.** An abnormal condition in which the dentin is in contact with the bone, there being no periodontal ligament present in the area concerned. The condition is usually associated with root resorption following replantation or transplantation, or with retained and submerged deciduous teeth. **extra-articular a.** The ankylosis of a joint that is caused by a bony bar outside the joint capsule which adjoins adjacent bones. **extracapsular a.** A stiffness of a joint owing to the rigidity of structures lying outside the joint capsule. **fibrous a.** The reduced mobility of a joint due to intervening fibrous tissue. Also *pseudankylosis, spurious ankylosis, false ankylosis, ligamentous ankylosis, pseudoankylosis.* **intracapsular a.** A stiffness of a joint following disease or injury, or resulting from a complication of a surgical procedure. Also *intra-articular ankylosis.* **ligamentous a.** FIBROUS ANKYLOSIS. **operative a.** ARTHRODESIS. **partial a.** A bony bridge that crosses part of a joint. **spurious a.** FIBROUS ANKYLOSIS. **a. of the stapes** Ankylosis of the tympanostapedial syndesmosis, occurring frequently in cases of otosclerosis and tympanosclerosis. **true a.** BONY ANKYLOSIS. **unsound a.** A condition in which a joint that has been stiffened by disease is capable of slight movement.

**ankylostomiasis** \-stōmī′əsis\ ANCYLOSTOMIASIS.

**ankylotic** \ang′kilät′ik\ Of or relating to ankylosis.

**ankylotomy** \ang′kilät′əmē\ [ANKYLO- + -TOMY] The relief of ankyloglossia (tongue-tie) by division of the frenulum linguae.

**ankylurethria** \ang′kilʸūrē′thrē·ə\ [*ankyl(o)-* + URETHR- + -IA] Stenosis or atresia of the urethra, usually of developmental origin.

**ankyrism** \ang′kərizm\ An articulation formed by the hooking of one bone on another.

**ankyroid** \ang′kəroid\ In the shape of a hook. Also *anchiroid, anciroid.*

**anlage** \än′lägə\ [German (from *anlegen* to lay out, put on, install, apply, from *an-* on + *legen* to lay) a laying-out, installation, outline, plan] The first indication, usually as a group of cells starting to differentiate or becoming arranged in a definite pattern or outline, of a developing structure, organ, or part. Also *inceptus.* • Although *primordium* has a similar meaning in embryology, *anlage* is generally used for a theoretically earlier stage before even the recognizable or primordial features of an organ or part have appeared. **lateral thyroid a.** The primordium in the embryo of the lateral lobe of the thyroid gland. The ventral part of the fourth pharyngeal pouch was once thought to contribute to the lateral lobe, but this has been disputed, at least as regards contribution of glandular tissue. **vesicourethral a.** The precursor region of the bladder and urethra resulting from the division of the embryonic cloaca by the cloacal septum into a ventral vesicourethral portion and a dorsal rectal portion.

**ANLL** acute nonlymphocytic leukemia.

**Annandale** [Thomas *Annandale,* Scottish surgeon, 1838–1907] See under OPERATION.

**annectent** \ənek′tənt\ Joined to; connected with.

**annelid** \an′əlid\ A member of the phylum Annelida.

**Annelida** \ənel′idə\ A phylum of segmented worms including the earthworms and leeches.

**annexectomy** \an′eksek′təmē\ ADNEXECTOMY.

**annihilation** \ənī′əlā′shən\ The destruction of positive and negative subatomic particles of similar mass by direct combination, producing corresponding energy release. Positrons interact with ordinary electrons, and two annihilation photons of 0.511 MeV each are released.

**annular** \an′yələr\ Pertaining to, forming, or shaped like a ring.

**annulate** \an′yəlāt\ Characterized by, comprised of, or surrounded by rings or ringlike structures.

**annulet** \an′yəlit\ [irreg. from Middle French *annelet, anelet,* dim. of *anel* ring, from L *anel(lus),* dim. of *annulus, anulus* ring] **1** A small ring. **2** A thin, colored ring on the surface of or surrounding some organs.

**annuli** \an′yəlī\ Plural of ANNULUS.

**annuloplasty** \an′yəlōplas′tē\ [*annul(us)* + *o* + -PLASTY] Repair of an incompetent heart valve, usually the mitral valve.

**annulorrhaphy** \an′yəlôr′əfē\ [*annul(us)* + *o* + -RRHAPHY] The surgical suture of a ringlike defect, such as the surgical repair of the deep inguinal ring or external inguinal ring during a hernioplasty.

**annulospiral** \an′yəlōspī′rəl\ Describing an afferent nerve ending in which the sensory nerve fibers encircle intrafusal muscle fibers in the muscle spindle.

**annulotomy** \an′yəlät′əmē\ [*annul(us)* + *o* + -TOMY] An incision or division of an annulus: used especially of a cardiac valve annulus.

**annulus** \an′yələs\ [Med L spelling variant of *anulus,* dim. of *anus* ring. (The *nn* spelling has sometimes been rationalized on the false supposition that the word is derived from *annus* year, circuit.)] **1** A ring or ring-shaped structure. Also *anulus.* **2** The dense ring at the junction of the middle piece and the principal piece in advanced spermatids and many immature spermatozoa. Also *terminal ring, ring centriole.* **a. ciliaris** *Outmoded* ORBICULUS CILIARIS. **a. conjunctivae** [NA] A narrow region of epithelial thickening at the junction of the limbus corneae and the bulbar conjunctiva. Also *annulus of conjunctiva, conjunctival ring.* **a. femoralis** [NA] The oval abdominal opening or base of the conical femoral canal, its transverse diameter measuring about 1.25 cm, and normally closed by some condensed extraperitoneal fatty tissue, called the femoral septum, containing a lymph node and covered by parietal peritoneum. The ring is bounded in front by the inguinal ligament, behind by the fascia of the pectineus muscle, medially by the lacunar ligament, and laterally by the femoral vein. It is larger in females than in males. Also *femoral ring, crural ring* (outmoded). **a. fibrocartilagineus membranae tympani** [NA] The thickened margin at the periphery of the circular tympanic membrane, attached to the tympanic sulcus at the medial end of the osseus part of the external acoustic meatus. Also *fibrocartilaginous ring of tympanic membrane, Gerlach's annular tendon, annular ring of Gerlach.* **annuli fibrosi cordis** [NA] Dense fibrous rings that surround the atrioventricular, aortic, and pulmonary trunk orifices of the heart. Those surrounding the atrioventricular orifices provide attachment for the muscle fibers of the atria and ventricles and for the atrioventricular valves, while those surrounding the arterial orifices generally serve as a transition between the muscular cardiac walls on the one side and the fibrous tissue of the arterial walls on the other side. At the aortic orifice the fibrous ring forms three thickened notches at the lower end of the aortic sinuses. Also *fibrous rings of heart, Lower's rings.* **a. fibrosus disci intervertebralis** [NA] The laminated peripheral portion of each intervertebral disk, comprising a wider inner zone of fibrocartilage and a narrower outer zone of fibrous tissue, and surrounding the pulpy inner core of the disk. The laminae form incomplete rings overlapping each other, and are connected by strong fibrous cords in a complex fashion so as to strengthen the tissue and to permit rotatory compression. Also *annulus fibrosus fibrocartilaginis intervertebralis, fibrous ring of intervertebral disk.* **a. inguinalis profundus** [NA] The oval internal opening of the inguinal canal where the transversalis fascia is invaginated to permit the passage of the spermatic cord in the male or the round ligament of the uterus in the female. It is located at the midinguinal point about 1.25 cm above the inguinal ligament and is related medially to the inferior epigastric vessels, and to the interfoveolar ligament when present. Its long axis is vertical, varying in size but usually larger in males than in females. Also *deep inguinal ring, internal inguinal ring.* **a. inguinalis superficialis** [NA] The triangular hiatus in the aponeurosis of the external oblique muscle situated above and lateral to the crest of the pubis, through which passes the spermatic cord in the male or the round ligament of the uterus in the female and the ilioinguinal nerve in both sexes. Its narrow base is the pubic crest, while its sloping sides or margins are thickened by the lateral (inferior) crus and the medial(superior) crus. Also *superficial inguinal ring, external inguinal ring* (outmoded). **a. iridis major** [NA] A delicately striated broad concentric zone situated on the anterior surface of the iris and on the outer side of a concentric zigzag line about 1.5 mm from the pupillary margin of the iris. Also *greater ring of iris, greater circle of iris, ciliary ring of iris, ciliary zone* (outmoded). **a. iridis minor** [NA] A coarsely striated narrow concentric zone situated on the anterior surface of the iris, bordering the pupil and on the inner side of a concentric zigzag line about 1.5 mm from the pupillary margin of the iris. Also *lesser ring of iris, lesser circle of iris.* **a. ovalis** LIMBUS FOSSAE OVALIS. **a. sclerae** *Outmoded* SCHWALBE'S RING. **a. tendineus communis** [NA] A fibrous ring situated posteriorly within the orbit and attached to the superior, inferior, and medial margins of the optic canal, the medial part of the superior orbital fissure, and a tubercle on the edge of the greater wing of the sphenoid bone. It provides origin for the four rectus muscles of the eye, and through it pass the optic nerve, the ophthalmic artery, the two divisions of the oculomotor nerve, the nasociliary nerve, the abducent nerve and, occasionally, either one or both ophthalmic veins. Also *common tendinous ring, Zinn's ring, Zinn's ligament, aponeurosis of Zinn, zonular ligament, tendon of Zinn.* **a. tracheae** A ring of hyaline cartilage of the trachea. **a. tympanicus** [NA] An incomplete bony ring representing the tympanic part of the temporal bone that is partly fused with the squamous part at birth. It is deficient superiorly, and its medial concave aspect has a sulcus for the attachment of the peripheral margin of the tympanic membrane. After birth it grows laterally and posteriorly as a fibrocartilaginous plate to form the tympanic part of the bone. Also *tympanic annulus, tympanic ring, tympanic bone.* **a. umbilicalis** [NA] A variably shaped opening in the midline of the anterior abdominal wall that transmits the umbilical vessels, urachus, and, up to the third month of fetal life, the vitelline stalk. A few days after birth the opening closes, leaving a firm, skin-covered, fibrous ring or nodular scar in the linea alba, the umbilicus or navel, to the deep surface of which the obliterated vessels and urachus remain attached. Also *umbilical ring.* **Vieussens a.** **1** LIMBUS FOSSAE OVALIS. **2** ANSA SUBCLAVIA.

**ano-** \ā′nō-\ [L *anus* ring, anus] A combining form denoting the anus.

**AnOC** anodal opening contraction.

**anochromasia** \an′əkrōmā′zhə\ [New L, from L *an(us)* ring + *o* + *chroma(t)-* + -IA] An artifact in the appearance of erythrocytes on stained blood films, in which hemoglobin appears concentrated in a ring at the periphery, leaving a sharply demarcated, transparent central disk. Also *ring artifact, pessary ring artifact.*

**anociassociation** \ənō′sē·əsō′sē·ā′shən\ [Gk *a-* priv. + NOCI- + *association*] The practice of using an anesthetic agent to block noxious stimuli such as pain from reaching the brain of a patient during or after an operation in which general anesthesia is used, as a means of preventing circulatory shock.

**anococcygeal** \ā′nōkäksij′ē·əl\ Pertaining to the anus and the coccyx.

**anocutaneous** \-kyootā′nē·əs\ Pertaining to the anus and the skin.

**anodal** \anō′dəl\ Having to do with an anode.

**anode** \an′ōd\ [Gk *anodos* (from *an(a)* up + *(h)odos* a way) the way up, ascent] **1** In an x-ray tube, the metallic target, usually tungsten, on which the electron stream impinges. **2** A positive electrode. Also *positive pole.* **3** The collecting electrode of a photomultiplier tube. **4** The plate of a vacuum tube. Chiefly a British usage. **hooded a.** The anode of an x-ray tube in which the target is mounted at the bottom of a hollow metal tube to diminish secondary emission of x rays. **rotating a.** An x-ray tube target in the form of a disk which rotates at high speed during the exposure.

**anodontia** \an′ōdän′shə\ [Gk *anodont(os)* (from *an-* priv. + *odous*, gen. *odontos* tooth) toothless + -IA] Congenital absence of the teeth. It may be partial or total. Also *anodontism.* **a. vera** The congenital absence of all teeth. It is usually associated with an absence or deficiency of the epidermal glands.

**anodontism** ANODONTIA.

**anodyne** \an′ədīn\ [Gk *anōdyn(os)* (from *an-* priv. + *odyn(ē)* pain, distress) free from pain, allaying pain] A medication that relieves pain. The drug may be a narcotic analgesic or a non-narcotic agent such as aspirin. Also *acesodyne.*

**anogenital** \ā′nōjen′ətəl\ Pertaining to the anus and the genitalia.

**anomalad** \ənäm′əlad\ *Outmoded* SEQUENCE. **Robin a.** *Outmoded* ROBIN SEQUENCE.

**anomalo-** \ənäm′əlō-\ [Gk *anōmalos* (*an-* priv. + *homalos* even) irregular] A combining form meaning irregularity, anomaly.

**anomaloscope** \əmän′əlōskōp′\ [ANOMALO- + -SCOPE] A device that permits the subjective mixing of various proportions of red and green to match a standard yellow color, used to evaluate the variations of red-green color blindness.

**anomalous** \ənäm′ələs\ [Gk *anōmalos* (from *an-* priv. + *(h)omalos* even, regular) uneven, irregular] Outside the norm: used especially of specific defects.

**anomaly** \ənäm′əlē\ [Gk *anōmalia* (from *anōmalos* irregular) inconsistency, irregularity, abnormality] Any structure, function, or state outside the usual range of variation from the norm. **Alder-Reilly a.** An anomaly of leukocytes in which numerous, large, violet or red-violet granules (Alder-Reilly bodies) are in the cytoplasm, most commonly of neutrophils, but sometimes in monocytes or lymphocyte cytoplasm as well. The granules are about 0.1 μm in diameter, slightly larger than toxic granulations. The anomaly commonly accompanies mucopolysaccharidoses such as the Hurler syndrome, but may occur independently. Also *Alder's anomaly, Alder's constitutional granulation anomaly.* **Alius-Grignaschi a.** CONGENITAL MYELOPEROXIDASE DEFICIENCY. **Chédiak-Higashi a.** A fatal, hereditary, autosomal recessive disorder of lysosomes and melanosomes, characterized by the presence of giant lysosomal granules in all leukocytes, Döhle bodies in granulocytes, giant melanosomes in dermal epithelium, infiltration of tissues by histiocytes, albinism, neurologic disorders, lymphadenopathy, hepatomegaly, splenomegaly, anemia, leukopenia, thrombocytopenia, and radiographic signs of bone-marrow expansion. The disorder occurs in other mammalian species as well as in humans. Also *Chédiak-Steinbrinck-Higashi anomaly* (used especially in Europe), *Chédiak-Higashi syndrome, Chédiak-Itigashi disease, Béguez César disease, Steinbrinck's anomaly.* **Chiari a.** A congenital malformation of the hindbrain with excessive elongation of the cerebellar tonsils, which descend below the foramen magnum on either side of the medulla and upper spinal cord. Because of consequent interference with the circulation of the cerebrospinal fluid, hydrocephalus or syringomyelia or both may result. When there is an associated spina bifida in the lumbar region, this combination is called the Arnold-Chiari deformity. **chromosomal a.** CHROMOSOMAL ABERRATION. **congenital a.** An organ, region, or an individual that is anomalous from birth. • The term is usually applied to structural rather than functional abnormalities, although it may be applied in a generic sense to syndromes or associations of defects. **craniovertebral anomalies** A group of malformations or disorders of development of the brain or skull or both affecting the region of the craniovertebral junction. They include the Chiari anomaly, platybasia, and other anomalies in and around the foramen magnum. **developmental a.** An anomaly that arises at any time during the developmental span between conception and maturity at puberty or adulthood. • This term is preferred to *congenital anomaly* because it does not limit its scope to those anomalies evident at birth, and it is applied equally to functional as well as structural abnormality. **Ebstein's a.** A developmental defect of the heart in which the septal and mitral leaflets of the tricuspid valve are displaced downward into the right ventricle, dividing it into an "atrialized" part and an apical ventricular component which supports the pulmonary trunk. Also *Ebstein's malformation.* **fetal a.** **1** Any developmental anomaly seen in a fetus or newborn infant. **2** A developmental anomaly known to have originated during the fetal period of development, as distinct from the embryonic period. **Freund's a.** A narrowing of the upper thorax as a result of the shortening of the first rib and its cartilage. It was once considered a predisposition to tuberculosis because of the resulting defective expansion at the apex of the lung. **Hegglin's a.** MAY-HEGGLIN ANOMALY. **Jordan's a.** The presence of multiple lipid globules in the cytoplasm of most granulocytes and monocytes, appearing as vacuoles on blood films stained with the Wright stain. The condition is probably inherited in an autosomal recessive manner, and it appears to be harmless. **May-Hegglin a.** An autosomal dominant hereditary anomaly of leukocytes and platelets, characterized by large basophilic inclusions that resemble Döhle bodies in the cytoplasm of neutrophils, and by thrombocytopenia, giant or bizarrely shaped platelets, and unusually large platelet granules. Platelet function abnormalities may also be present, and affected persons may have a bleeding tendency. Also *Hegglin's anomaly.* **morning glory a.** The funnel-shaped crumpling of a retinal detachment associated with severe contraction of abnormal adherent vitreous structure. This is a characteristic feature of the very serious vitreoretinal problem, massive vitreous retraction. **Pelger-Huët a.** A hereditary anomaly of segmentation of nuclei of granulocytes, in which nearly all neutrophils are either band forms or bilobed in the configuration of pince-nez spectacles. In addition, nuclear chromatin is very condensed, resulting in numerous prominent clefts of unstained parachromatin. The anomaly is quite common, occurring in about one person in 3000. It has no adverse effect on health and does not impair neutrophil function. It is transmitted as an autosomal dominant trait. A few homozygotes have been recognized, whose neutrophils show no segmentation, i.e. all their neutrophils are myelocytes. Homozygous Pelger-Huët anomaly is also without adverse consequence or impaired function of neutrophils. In rabbits, Pelger-Huët anomaly of neutrophils is associated with severe skeletal abnormalities. Also *Pelger-Huët nuclear anomaly, Pelger's anomaly.* **Peters a.** ANTERIOR CHAMBER CLEAVAGE SYNDROME. **Pierre Robin a.** ROBIN SEQUENCE. **Poland's a.** A combination of unilateral defects in an upper quadrant of the body, most often involving syndactyly and the absence of the pectoralis minor and the sternal portion of the pectoralis major muscles. It occasionally includes the absence of the nipple and areola, rib defects, and hypoplasia of the hand or of the entire arm. Also *Poland syndrome.* **Rieger's a.** RIEGER SYNDROME **Shone's a.** The combination of parachute mitral valve with supravalvular ring of the left atrium, subaortic stenosis, and coarctation of the aorta. Also *Shone syndrome.* **Steinbrinck's a.** CHÉDIAK-HIGASHI ANOMALY. **Uhl's a.** A congenital anomaly characterized by the absence of the myocardium of the right ventricle, which is otherwise normal. Composed only of epicardium and endocardium, the wall of the ventricle is paper thin. **Undritz a.** An inherited condition in which 17 percent or more of mature neutrophiles have five or more nuclear lobes. It is an autosomal condition manifested in heterozygotes, without adverse clinical effect. Also *hereditary hypersegmentation of neutrophils.*

**anomer** \an′əmər\ The isomer of a sugar or glycoside that differs from the original in the configuration at the carbon atom that is potentially a carbonyl group. The anomers of a sugar interconvert via ring opening. Those of a glycoside cannot do so until the glycoside is hydrolyzed. Adj. anomeric.

**anomia** \ənō′mē·ə\ [Gk *a-* priv. + *(o)nom(a)* a name + -IA] A type of aphasia in which the patient can recognize objects, but is unable to name them or to relate a name to a specific object.

**anomie** \an′əmē\ [French (from Gk *anomia* lawlessness, from *a-* priv. + *nom(os)* law + *-ia* -IA), absence of law or organization] ALIENATION.

**anonychia** \an′ōnik′ē·ə\ [Gk *an-* priv. + ONYCH- + -IA] The congenital absence of one or more nails.

**anonyma** \ənän′əmə\ [Late L *anonyma* (fem. of *anonymus,* from Gk *anōnymos* unnamed, from *an-* priv. + *onyma,* also *onoma* name) innominate] Nameless; innominate. • Formerly applied to the innominate artery and vein, which are now called brachiocephalic trunk and vein respectively.

**anopelvic** \ā′nōpel′vik\ Pertaining to the anus and the pelvis.

***Anopheles*** \ənäf′əlēz\ [Gk *anōphelēs* (from *an-* priv. + *ōphelein* to help) useless, hurtful] A genus of mosquitoes (family Culicidae, subfamily Anophelinae) with palpi as long as the proboscis, and spotted wings. The eggs are laid singly, with characteristic floats. In most species, the female assumes an angled posture when biting. Many species are important as vectors of human and other mammalian malaria, filariasis, and some arboviral diseases. ***A. albimanus*** The primary vector of malarial agents in Panama. Its distribution includes Mexico, Ecuador, Colombia, Venezuela, and the West Indies. ***A. balabacensis*** *ANOPHELES DIRUS.* ***A. culicifacies*** An important vector of malaria-causing plasmodia throughout much of the Indo-Persian region, including Sri Lanka. ***A. darlingi*** An important vector of malarial agents in an area extending from Central America to Argentina. ***A. dirus*** An important vector of malarial agents in most of mainland southeast Asia north of 8° latitude. Also *Anopheles balabacensis, Cenopheles balabacensis.* ***A. freeborni*** A species widely distributed in the United States throughout the Rocky Mountains, New Mexico, and the Pacific Coast. It was a malarial vector in California during the gold rush. Endemic cases no longer occur but the possibility remains of re-establishing foci of infection derived from imported cases. ***A. funestus*** One of the more important vectors in tropical western Africa of plasmodia causing malaria in humans. ***A. gambiae*** A primary vector of plasmodia that cause human malaria in tropical Africa. It has also caused epidemic outbreaks when accidentally introduced, and subsequently eliminated, in Brazil near Natal and in upper Egypt. It is now considered a species complex consisting of six separate species: *A. melas,* a saltwater species in western Africa, *A. merus,* a saltwater island species in eastern Africa, the true *A. gambiae* (species A) in humid areas, *A. arabiensis* (species B) in more arid savannahs and steppes, and two relict species designated C and D. ***A. labranchiae*** An important vector in the Mediterranean region of human malarial agents. ***A. maculipennis*** A species that was formerly a major vector of malarial agents in Europe and southwest Asia. It originally included other mosquitoes that are now assigned to separate species making up the *A. maculipennis* complex, including *A. messeae* in the northern Palearctic region, *A. melanoon* (with its subspecies *A. melanoon subalpinus*) in southern Europe, the Caucasus, and Iran, *A. labranchiae* in Italy, Spain, and north Africa, *A. stroparvus* in more northerly Europe, and *A. sacharovi* in the Soviet Union, Italy, Austria, Syria, Jordan, and Israel. American species in the complex include *A. quadrimaculatus, A. earlei, A. freeborni, A. occidentalis,* and *A. aztecus.* The *A. maculipennis* complex was one of the first to be investigated and divided into species on the basis of minor differences in egg floats and bloodsucking habits such as degree of preference for human blood and of entry into houses. ***A. pseudopunctipennis*** A widely distributed species ranging from the southern United States to Argentina. It is an important vector of malaria in northern and western South America. ***A. quadrimaculatus*** A species, belonging to the *A. maculipennis* complex, which was the principal malarial vector in the southern, eastern, and central United States before about 1930 when malaria was eliminated as an endemic disease in this country. ***A. superpictus*** An important malaria vector in parts of the Indo-Persian region including Iraq, Oman, Iran, Afghanistan, Pakistan, India, and Sri Lanka.

**anophelicide** \ənäf′əlisīd′\ An agent lethal to anopheline mosquitoes.

**anophelifuge** \ənäf′əlifyooj′\ An agent that prevents the bite or acts as a repellent of mosquitoes of the genus *Anopheles.*

**Anophelinae** \ənäf′əlī′nē\ A subfamily of mosquitoes in the family Culicidae which contains a number of genera, including the type genus, *Anopheles,* some 90 species of which can serve as vectors of human malaria.

**anopheline** \ənäf′əlīn\ Of or belonging to the mosquito subfamily Anophelinae or the genus *Anopheles.*

**anophelism** \ənäf′əlizm\ The infestation or continued presence of anopheline mosquitoes in a given geographic area.

**anophthalmia** \an′äfthal′mē·ə\ [Gk *an-* priv. + *ophthalm(os)* eye + -IA] The complete failure of an eye to develop, except for tiny rudiments usually present on histopathologic examination. It may be caused by a lack of optic primordia or secondarily from degeneration of a poorly formed optic vesicle or cup.

**anopia** \anō′pē·ə\ [Gk *an-* priv. + -OPIA] Absence of one or both eyes or of vision.

**anoplasty** \ā′nōplas′tē\ A plastic surgical procedure on the anus, usually with the intent of restoring or improving fecal continence.

**Anoplura** \an′əploo′rə\ [Gk *anopl(os)* unarmed + *oura* tail] An insect order of some 490 species of sucking lice, which are mostly ectoparasites of mammals. Physical characteristics include absence of wings, a dorsoventrally flattened body, and legs adapted for clinging to hairs and feathers. Genera of medical importance are principally *Pediculus* and *Pthirus.*

**anopsia** \anäp′sē·ə\ [Gk *an-* priv. + -OPSIA] Loss of vision. • This term is usually used in combination, as in *hemianopsia.*

**anorchia** \anôr′kē·ə\ ANORCHISM.

**anorchid** \anôr′kid\ A genetic male without testes.

**anorchism** \anôr′kizm\ [Gk *anorch(os)* (from *an-* priv. + *orchis* testicle) lacking testicles + -ISM] The congenital absence of one or both testes in a genetic male. Also *anorchia, anorchidism.*

**anorectal** \ā′nōrek′təl\ Relating to the anus and rectum. Also *rectoanal.*

**anorectic** \an′ôrek′tik\ [Gk *anorekt(os)* without appetite + -IC. See ANOREXIA.] **1** Having no appetite; suffering from anorexia. **2** One who suffer from anorexia. **3** Pertaining to anorexia. **4** A substance that reduces the appetite. For defs. 1–4 also *anorexic, anoretic.*

**anorectocolonic** \ā′nōrek′tōkōlän′ik\ Pertaining to the anus, the rectum, and the colon.

**anorectoplasty** \-rek′tōplas′tē\ A plastic surgical operation on the anus and rectum.

**anorectum** \-rek′təm\ The anus and the rectum combined.

**anoretic** \an′ôret′ik\ ANORECTIC.

**anorexia** \an′ôrek′sē·ə\ [Gk (from *an-* priv. + *orex(is)* yearning, desiring + -IA), lack of appetite] A lack of appetite or desire for food. **hysterical a.** ANOREXIA NERVOSA. **a. nervosa** An eating disorder of unknown etiology characterized by fear of becoming obese, disturbed body image, inability to maintain body weight within the normal range (exemplified by significant weight loss), and, in females, amenorrhea. Over 90% of cases occur in females, with onset in adolescence. Death by starvation may occur in as many as 20% of cases. Also *hysterical anorexia, pseudoanorexia* (seldom used) .

**anorexiant** \an′ôrek′sē·ənt\ A substance that causes depression of appetite, such as a drug used to aid weight reduction; an anorectic drug.

**anorexic** \an′ôrek′sik\ ANORECTIC.

**anorexigenic** \an′ôrek′səjen′ik\ [*anorexi(a)* + -GENIC] Having the ability to depress the appetite and so facilitate weight reduction.

**anorgasmy** \an′ôrgaz′mē\ ORGASTIC IMPOTENCE.

**anorthopia** \an′ôrthō′pē·ə\ [Gk *an-* priv. + ORTH- + -OPIA] METAMORPHOPSIA.

**anoscope** \ā′nōskōp\ [ANO- + -SCOPE] PROCTOSCOPE.

**anosmia** \anäz′mē·ə\ [New L, from Gk *an-* priv. + *osmē* odor + -IA] Loss of the sense of smell, usually due either to disease of the olfactory mucosa with damage to olfactory end-organs, or to lesions of the olfactory nerve fibers and tracts. A common cause is head injury with division of olfactory nerve fibers as they traverse the cribriform plate of the ethmoid bone. Also *olfactory anesthesia*. Adj. anosmic. **a. gustatoria** Impairment of the sense of flavor (a combination of smell and taste) in a patient with anosmia.

**anosognosia** \anō′sägnō′sē·ə\ [Gk *a-* priv. + *noso(s)* disease + *-gnōs(is)* knowledge + -IA] A disorder of the body image marked by a denial of illness. It is usually due to a nondominant parietal lobe lesion. For example, the patient with a hemiplegia may deny that the paralyzed limbs belong to him and may even attempt to throw them out of bed. Adj. anosognosic.

**anospinal** \ā′nōspī′nəl\ Pertaining to the anus and the spinal cord.

**anosteoplasia** \ənäs′tē·ōplā′zhə\ [Gk *an-* priv. + OSTEO- + -PLASIA] Abnormal bone development.

**anostosis** \an′ästō′sis\ [Gk *an-* priv. + OSTOSIS] Defective or nonexistent bone development.

**anotropia** \an′ətrō′pē·ə\ [Gk *anō* up, upward + -TROPIA] ANATROPIA.

**anotus** \anō′təs\ [Gk *an-* priv. + OT- + L *-us*, masc. sing. noun suffix] An embryo, fetus, or postnatal individual without development of all or most of the usual auricular structures and frequently, to a greater or lesser extent, the components of the middle and inner ears. *Seldom used.*

**anovaginal** \ā′nōvaj′ənəl\ Pertaining to the anus and the vagina.

**anovaria** \an′ōver′ē·ə\ ANOVARISM.

**anovarism** \anō′verizm\ [Gk *an-* priv. + *ovar(io)-* + -ISM] Absence of ovaries. Also *anovaria*.

**anovular** \anäv′yələr\ [Gk *an-* priv. + OVULAR] Pertaining to the condition of anovulation. Also *anovulatory*.

**anovulation** \an′ävyəlā′shən\ [Gk *an-* priv. + OVULATION] Failure to release an ovum.

**anovulatory** \anäv′yələtôr′ē\ ANOVULAR.

**anoxaemia** *Brit.* ANOXEMIA.

**anoxemia** \an′äksē′mē·ə\ [Gk *an-* priv. + *ox(ygen)* + -EMIA] Lack of oxygen in the arterial blood. Adj. anoxemic.

**anoxia** \anäk′sē·ə\ [Gk *an-* priv. + *ox(ygen)* + -IA] Lack of oxygen in the circulating blood or in the tissues. Adj. anoxic. **altitude a.** ALTITUDE SICKNESS. **anoxic a.** Absence of oxygen supply to tissues due to absence of oxygen in the blood. The term is used interchangeably, but incorrectly, for hypoxic hypoxia. **cerebral a.** Loss or impairment of the oxygen supply to the brain, however caused. The pathologic changes so produced may be focal or generalized, depending upon the pathogenetic mechanism involved. **diffuse cerebral a.** Cerebral anoxia affecting the entire brain. **fetal a.** Reduction of oxygen levels in the fetus below the normal range. If uncorrected, this condition can lead to fetal distress during labor, damage to the central nervous system, even fetal death. **histotoxic a.** A condition in which a tissue is unable to utilize oxygen. It may result from such causes as narcotics ingestion or cyanide poisoning. **myocardial a.** Absence of oxygen supply to the myocardium. **stagnant a.** A deficiency in oxygen due to stagnation of blood flow rather than to deficiency of oxygen tension in the blood.

**anoxic** \anäk′sik\ Of or relating to anoxia.

**ansa** \an′sə\ [L, a handle, hook, loop] A structure shaped like a loop or an arch. Also *loop*. **a. of atlas** The loop formed by the ventral ramus of the first cervical spinal nerve as it joins the ascending branch of the second cervical nerve in front of the transverse process of the atlas and behind the internal jugular vein. It sends a branch to the hypoglossal nerve to form the radix superior of the ansa cervicalis. *Outmoded.* **a. of axis** The loop formed by the descending branch of the ventral ramus of the second cervical spinal nerve where it joins the ascending branch of the third cervical nerve, between the longus capitis and levator scapulae muscles. It gives off the radix inferior of the ansa cervicalis. . *Outmoded.* **a. cervicalis** [NA] A loop in the cervical plexus formed by a cranial ramus arising from the $C_1$ and $C_2$ spinal nerves and a caudal ramus from $C_2$ and $C_3$. The cranial ramus (radix superior ansae cervicalis) initially travels with the hypoglossal nerve. The ansa supplies strap muscles of the neck. Also *ansa hypoglossi, loop of hypoglossal nerve*. **a. of Drobnick** The fibers of the cervical sympathetic trunk that pass in front of and behind the inferior thyroid artery at the approximate level of the middle cervical ganglion, when it is present. *Outmoded.* **a. of Galen** RAMUS COMMUNICANS NERVI LARYNGEI SUPERIORIS CUM NERVO LARYNGEO INFERIORE. **gastric a.** The connection between the transverse colon and the greater curvature of the stomach by the greater omentum. *Outmoded.* **a. of Haller** RAMUS COMMUNICANS NERVI FACIALIS CUM NERVO GLOSSOPHARYNGEO. **Henle's a.** LOOP OF HENLE. **a. hypoglossi** ANSA CERVICALIS. **a. of Laignel-Lavastine** The celiac branch of the posterior vagal trunk that joins the medial edge of the left celiac ganglion, serving as an afferent to the celiac plexus. *Outmoded.* **a. lenticularis** An efferent axonal bundle emerging from the pallidal portion of the lenticular nucleus and extending through the medial internal capsule to join the fasciculus lenticularis entering the rostral portion of the thalamic ventral nuclear group. Also *lenticular loop*. **a. of Maubrac** The communication between the lateral series of deep branches of the cervical plexus and the accessory nerve in the substance of the sternocleidomastoid muscle. *Outmoded.* **a. nephroni** LOOP OF HENLE. **ansae nervorum spinalium** Looping communications between adjacent spinal nerves. Also *loops of spinal nerves*. **a. peduncularis** A myelinated axonal bundle extending from the thalamus through the inferior thalamic peduncle below the lenticular nucleus into the amygdaloid nuclei and contiguous zones of the temporal lobe and hypothalamus. Also *peduncular ansa of Gratiolet, Reil's ansa, peduncular loop*. **a. sacralis** The loop formed by the two sympathetic trunks as they meet at the ganglion impar anterior to the coccyx. *Seldom used.* **simple a.** An ansa that links antagonist muscles. *Outmoded.* **a. of the stapes** The horseshoe-shaped arch formed by the anterior and posterior crura of the stapes. *Outmoded.* **a. subclavia** [NA] A bundle of sympathetic fibers which, descending in front of and beneath the subclavian artery, connects the middle cervical ganglion with the inferior. It is collateral to the main sympathetic trunk that courses behind the artery to connect these ganglia, and has no special function or embryologic significance. Also *ansa of Vieussens, subclavian loop, loop of Vieussens, Vieussens annulus*. **a. vitellina** A looped venous sinus related to the yolk sac of the early human embryo and communicating with the umbilical veins. **a. of Wrisberg** RAMI CELIACI NERVI VAGI.

**ansae** \an′sē\ Plural of ANSA.

**ansamycin** [L *ansa* loop + -MYCIN] RIFAMYCIN.

**ansate** \an′sāt\ **1** Possessing a loop- or handlelike appendage. **2** In the shape of a loop. Also *ansiform*.

**anserine** $N^{\alpha}$-($\beta$-alanyl)-$N^{\pi}$-methylhistidine, a peptide found in muscle. Its function is unknown. It may act as a buffer.

**ansiform** \an′sifôrm\ ANSATE.

**ansotomy** \ansät′əmē\ [*ans(a)* + *o* + *-tomy*] The surgical division of an ansa.

**Anstie** [Francis Edmund *Anstie*, English physician, 1833–1874] Anstie's rule. See under ANSTIE'S LIMIT.

**ant-** \ant-\ ANTI-.

**Antabuse** A proprietary name for disulfiram.
**antacid** \antas′id\ [ANT- + ACID] Any of various medications taken orally to neutralize gastric acid and pepsin enzyme, providing a protective coating to the mucosa of the esophagus, stomach, and duodenum.
**antagglutinin** \ant′əgloo′tinin\ [ANT- + *agglutin(ation)* + -IN] A substance isolated from the seminal fluid of animals which has been shown to prevent the autoagglutination of washed spermatozoa.
**antagonism** \antag′ənizm\ A state of opposition or competition, especially a state in which a force or action and countervailing force or action tend to neutralize each other, as muscles, drugs, or disease processes. Also *counteraction.* **bacterial a.** The ability of certain bacterial species to inhibit the growth of others, through competition for food or release of toxic products. This interaction is especially important in the gastrointestinal tract, where suppression of major normal flora by antimicrobial agents allows overgrowth of normally minor components.
**antagonist** \antag′ənist\ [Gk *antagōnistēs* (from *antagōnizesthai* to struggle against, from ANT- + *agōn* contest) opponent] **1** An agent that opposes the action of another. **2** ANTAGONISTIC MUSCLE. **adrenergic a.'s** Substances that oppose or nullify the actions of sympathetic nerves or their transmitters. **alpha-adrenergic a.** ALPHA BLOCKER. **beta-adrenergic a.** BETA BLOCKER. **calcium a.** CALCIUM CHANNEL BLOCKER. • This term is not recommended. **insulin a.** Any of several substances that oppose the biologic actions of insulin, such as cortisol, growth hormone, and glucagon. Circulating materials neutralize the action of insulin directly by behaving as antibodies. **metabolic a.** ANTIMETABOLITE. **narcotic a.** A compound that binds to opiate receptors but produces little or no agonistic, morphinelike action.
**antanalgesia** Increased sensitivity to pain due to the property of certain drugs of lowering pain thresholds.
**antarthritic** \ant′ärthrit′ik\ ANTIARTHRITIC.
**antasthmatic** \ant′azmat′ik\ **1** Relieving or preventing asthma. **2** A remedy or preventative for asthma.
**antazoline** $C_{17}H_{19}N_3$. 4,5-Dihydro-*N*-phenyl-*N*-(phenylmethyl)-*1H*-imidazole-2-methanamine, an antihistaminic agent of relatively short duration in activity. It has weak local anesthetic and anticholinergic actions, as well. It is usually administered orally as the hydrochloride salt. The phosphate salt has been used in eye drops to treat ocular allergies. Also *imidamine.*
**ante-** \an′tē-, an′ti-\ [L *ante* before] A prefix meaning before, as in time, order, or position.
**antebrachial** \-brā′kē·əl\ Pertaining to the forearm or antebrachium. Also *antibrachial* (incorrect).
**antebrachium** \-brā′kē·əm\ [NA] The region of the upper limb between the elbow and wrist joints. Also *forearm.* Also *antibrachium* (incorrect).
**antecardium** \-kär′dē·əm\ PRECORDIUM.
**antecedent** \-sē′dənt\ **1** Preceding. **2** PRECURSOR. **plasma thromboplastin a.** FACTOR XI. Abbr. PTA
**ante cibum** [L *ante* before + *cibum,* accus. sing. of *cibus* food] Before food, i.e., before meals: used in prescription order writing to direct that the medicine be taken before regular meals.
**antecubital** \-kyoo′bitəl\ In front of the elbow region (cubitus).
**anteflexed** \an′tēflekst\ Bent forward; in a state of anteflexion.
**anteflexion** \-flek′shən\ A forward bend or curvature, as in part of an organ, e.g., a forward bending of the body of the uterus at its junction with the cervix.
**antegrade** \an′tēgrād\ ANTEROGRADE.
**antemetic** \ant′emet′ik\ ANTIEMETIC.
**ante mortem** \an′tē môr′təm\ [L *ante* before + *mortem,* accus. of *mors* death] Preceding death.
**antemortem** \-môr′təm\ [from the phrase ANTE MORTEM] Pertaining to or occurring in the period preceding death.
**antenatal** \-nā′təl\ [ANTE- + NATAL] Occurring before birth.
**antepartal** \-pär′təl\ ANTEPARTUM.
**antepartum** \-pär′təm\ [ANTE- + L *partum,* accus. of *partus* (from *partus,* past part. of *parere* to bring forth young) a birth, delivery] Occurring before the onset of labor. Also *antepartal.*
**anteposition** \-pəzish′ən\ Displacement of the uterus towards the symphysis pubis.
**ante prandium** [L *ante* before + *prandium* lunch] Before dinner: used in prescription writing.
**anteprostate** \-präs′tāt\ GLANDULA BULBOURETHRALIS.
**anteprostatic** \-prästat′ik\ In front of the prostate gland.
**antepulsion** \-pul′shən\ *Outmoded* ANTEROPULSION.
**antepyretic** Before the onset of fever.
**anterethic** **1** Reducing irritation; soothing: used of a medication. **2** An anterethic agent.
**anteriad** \antir′ē·əd\ Towards the front of the body; anteriorly.
**anterior** \antir′ē·ər\ [L, comparative of *ante* before] **1** Pertaining to the foreparts of a body or to the front surface of a body or part. **2** Situated in a forward position with respect to other comparable structures or parts. Also *anticus* (older term). • In human anatomy, *anterior* is used with reference to the "anatomical position" and corresponds roughly to *ventral.*
**antero-** \an′tərō-\ [New L, from L *anter(ior)*] A combining form meaning anterior or forward.
**anteroclusion** \-kloo′zhən\ [ANTERO- + *(oc)clusion*] MANDIBULAR PROGNATHISM.
**anterodorsal** \-dôr′səl\ In embryology, pertaining to the dorsal aspect of the head. *Outmoded.*
**anteroexternal** \-ikstur′nəl\ Located in or to the front and the outer side or the outer surface.
**anterograde** \an′tərōgrād′\ [ANTERO- + L *grad(i)* to step] **1** Proceeding forward or in the normal direction of flow or current. Also *antegrade.* **2** Pertaining to time subsequent to a given event, as *anterograde amnesia.* Compare RETROGRADE.
**anteroinferior** \-infir′ē·ər\ Located or passing in front and below.
**anterointerior** \-intir′ē·ər\ Located in front and internally.
**anterointernal** \-intur′nəl\ Located in front and to the inner aspect or medial side.
**anterolateral** \-lat′ərəl\ Located in front and to the side away from the midline of a body.
**anteromedial** \-mē′dē·əl\ Located in front and toward the inner side or the midline of a body.
**anteromedian** \-mē′dē·ən\ Located in front and in the midline or median plane.
**anteroparietal** \-pərī′ətəl\ Located forward in or on the wall of a cavity.
**anteroposterior** \-pästir′ē·ər\ Pertaining to both front and back, usually when referring to a direction or distance from front to back of the body or part. Also *ventroposterior.*
**anteropulsion** \-pul′shən\ [ANTERO- + PULSION] A motor defect in which walking tends to become progressively faster, a characteristic of Parkinson's disease. The patient's pace becomes so accelerated that he may lose his balance

and fall forward. Also *propulsion, antepulsion* (outmoded). Compare RETROPULSION.

**anteroseptal** \-sep′təl\ Located in front of a septum, specifically the atrioventricular septum of the heart.

**anterosuperior** \-səpir′ē·ər\ Located in front and above or cranially.

**anterotransverse** \-trans′vurs\ Pertaining to the front and transverse part of a structure.

**anteroventral** \-ven′trəl\ Located in front and towards the ventral surface.

**anteversion** \-vur′zhən\ The forward angulation or tilting of a structure.

**anthelix** \ant′hēliks\ [Gk *anthelix* (from ANT- + HELIX) the inner curvature of the ear] [NA] The narrow curved ridge of auricular cartilage of the external ear lying anterior and parallel to the posterior part of the helix and forming the posterior rim of the concha of the auricle. Superiorly it splits into two crura that are separated by the triangular fossa. Also *antihelix.*

**anthelminthic** \ant′helmin′thik\ ANTHELMINTIC.

**anthelmintic** \ant′helmin′tik\ [ANT- + Gk *helmins,* gen. *helminthos,* a worm + -IC] **1** Capable of killing or expelling helminths, especially intestinal parasitic worms. Also *anthelminthic, antihelmintic.* **2** An agent used to kill or expel helminths; a vermifuge. Also *helminthagogue.*

**anthelotic** **1** Effective against corns. **2** An athelotic agent.

**anthemorrhagic** \ant′hemôraj′ik\ ANTIHEMORRHAGIC.

**antherpetic** \ant′hərpet′ik\ **1** Acting to oppose or inhibit herpes. **2** An antherpetic agent.

**anthiolimine** $C_{12}H_9Li_6O_{12}S_3Sb$. 2,2′,2″ [Stibilidynetris-(thio)]trisbutanedioic acid hexalithium salt, a trivalent antimonial agent that has been used for the treatment of schistosomiasis. Also *antimony lithium thiomalate, lithium antimoniothiomalate.*

**anthracene** $C_{14}H_{10}$. The hydrocarbon formed by the fusion of three benzene rings in a line. It is found in coal tar.

**anthracic** \anthras′ik\ **1** Pertaining to anthrax. **2** Resembling anthrax; anthracoid.

**anthraco-** \an′thrəkō-\ [Gk *anthrax,* gen. *anthrakos* a coal. See ANTHRAX.] A combining form meaning (1) coal, carbon; (2) carbuncle, anthrax.

**anthracoid** \an′thrəkoid\ [*anthrac(o)-* + -OID] **1** Resembling anthrax. **2** Resembling a carbuncle.

**anthracoma** \an′thrəkō′mə\ [*anthrac(o)-* + -OMA] CARBUNCLE.

**anthraconecrosis** \-nekrō′sis\ The combination of carbon deposition and tissue necrosis, usually seen in the lungs. It may indicate tuberculosis complicating anthracosilicosis.

**anthracosilicosis** \-sil′ikō′sis\ Pneumoconiosis comprising both anthracosis and silicosis.

**anthracosis** \an′thrəkō′sis\ [*anthrac(o)-* + -OSIS] **1** A blackened condition of a tissue, especially that of the lung caused by accumulation of coal dust. **2** COAL WORKERS' PNEUMOCONIOSIS.

**anthracotic** \an′thrəkät′ik\ Relating to or affected by anthracosis.

**anthralin** 1,8,9-Anthratriol. An odorless, yellow crystalline powder used in topical medications in the treatment of psoriasis and other chronic dermatoses. Also *dithranol* (British usage).

**anthramycin** An anticarcinogenic substance produced by *Streptomyces refuineus.* Also *refuin.*

**anthranilic acid** *O*-Aminobenzoic acid. It is an intermediate in the biosynthesis of tryptophan.

**anthraquinone** A substance related to anthracene by oxidation of the central benzene ring to the *p*-quinone structure. It is an intermediate in the manufacture of dyestuffs and is related to natural dyes, such as alizarin.

**anthrax** \an′thraks\ [Gk, a coal, ember, carbuncle (red precious stone), malignant pustule] A usually fatal, acute infectious zoonosis which occurs in herbivorous animals, especially ruminants (cattle, sheep, goats), as a result of ingestion of spores of *Bacillus anthracis* from soil. The disease may be transmitted to man by direct inoculation with spores from infected animal hair, hide, bristles, or bone or from finished products (wool, brushes, bone meal) containing infected animal material or by inhalation of airborne spores. Cutaneous anthrax is the form most commonly seen in man, with a fatality rate of less than 5 percent with appropriate treatment. The case-fatality ratio without treatment is about 20 percent. Inhalation anthrax, intestinal anthrax, and cerebral anthrax in man are usually fatal, even when treated, with death precipitated by toxemia and shock. Also *milzbrand, carbuncular fever, splenic fever, splenic apoplexy, cacanthrax.* **cerebral a.** Anthrax marked by cerebral symptoms which result when bacilli invade the brain. This condition sometimes complicates inhalation or intestinal anthrax and is usually fatal, even when treated, with death precipitated by toxemia and shock. **cutaneous a.** A form of anthrax caused by introduction of the anthrax bacillus into minor skin abrasions or superficial wounds and characterized by an erythematous papular skin lesion (malignant pustule) that undergoes necrosis, resulting in the formation of a dark eschar surrounded by intense nonpitting edema. It is the form of anthrax most commonly seen in man, with a fatality rate of less than 5 percent with appropriate treatment. **inhalation a.** Anthrax of the respiratory tract resulting from inhalation of spores of the anthrax bacillus contaminating dust or animal hair. The illness occurs in two stages. Symptoms are initially nonspecific, resembling those of an upper respiratory tract infection, and seem to subside after a few days. The second stage of illness follows, with sudden development of severe respiratory distress, mediastinal node involvement, massive subcutaneous edema of the chest and neck, and shock. Death usually occurs within 24 hours of onset of the acute phase. **intestinal a.** A severe, usually fatal form of anthrax caused by the introduction of the anthrax bacillus into the intestinal tract, usually as a result of ingestion of contaminated raw or undercooked meat, and which may be characterized by fever, vomiting, abdominal pain, and bloody diarrhea. Death is precipitated by toxemia and shock. **pulmonary a.** INHALATION ANTHRAX.

**anthrone** 9,10-Dihydro-9-oxoanthracene. Its molecule consists of two benzene rings joined twice, once through a carbonyl, CO, group, and once more, *ortho* on each ring to the first join, by a methylene, $CH_2$, group. It is a tautomer of 9-hydroxyanathracene. It reacts with sugars (hexoses, aldopentoses, and derivatives) in sulfuric acid to give a blue-green color.

**anthropo-** \an′thrəpō-\ [Gk *anthrōpos* man, mankind] A combining form meaning man, human.

**anthropogenic** \-jen′ik\ Produced by or resulting from human activities. Also *anthropogenous.*

**anthropogenous** \an′thrəpäj′ənəs\ ANTHROPOGENIC.

**anthropoid** \an′thrəpoid\ [Gk *anthrōpoeidēs* (from *anthrōpo(s)* a human being + *-eidēs* -like, -OID) manlike, resembling humans] **1** Relating to or characteristic of the primate suborder Anthropoidea. **2** A member of the Anthropoidea. **3** Resembling human beings. **4** Apelike; characteristic of the anthropoid apes. *Popular.*

**Anthropoidea** \an′thrəpoi′dē·ə\ [New L, from ANTHROPOID] A suborder of the mammalian order Primates that comprises the families Cebidae (New World monkeys), Callithricidae (marmosets), Cercopithecidae (Old World monkeys), Pongidae (gibbons, gorillas, chimpanzees, and orangutans) and Hominidae (man). The Anthropoidea are distinguished from the Prosimii or lower primates, which include lemurs, lorises, and tarsiers.

**anthropologic** \-läj′ik\ Pertaining to anthropology.

**anthropology** \an′thrəpäl′əjē\ [ANTHROPO- + -LOGY] The scientific study of the human species and its near ancestors, with particular attention to the variability and development of human traits and ways of life in different populations and environments. **cultural a.** The anthropological study of human group attributes that are acquired and transmitted by learning, such as social organization, technologies, language, customs, traditions, religion, art, and the like. **forensic a.** The application of anthropological methods to medicolegal problems of individual identification. **hematological a.** The study of the constituents of the blood with reference to the differential distribution of blood groups, hemoglobin types, and other variables among human populations. **pathological a.** The study of disease in man from the viewpoint of its differential distribution among human groups. **physical a.** The study of the physical characteristics of human beings and their ancestors, and of the variability of these characteristics among and within identifiable groups. **social a.** The anthropological study of human societies, with particular reference to kinship systems, social roles, tribal organization, community structure, classes and castes, political, economic, and religious institutions, and the like. **zoological a.** Anthropology with particular reference to man's place in the animal kingdom, and with special emphasis on comparison with other primates.

**anthropometric** \-met′rik\ Pertaining to anthropometry.

**anthropometry** \an′thrəpäm′ətrē\ [ANTHROPO- + -METRY] **1** The measurement of the human body or its separate parts to determine the range and extent of the variability of its dimensions, such as height, limb lengths, skin fold thickness, and others. **2** The use of quantitative methods in any branch of anthropology. **forensic a.** The measurement of the human body from the viewpoint of helping to determine individual identity for medicolegal purposes. **nutritional a.** Measurement of the human body for the purpose of helping to determine nutritional status.

**anthropomorphic** \-môr′fik\ [ANTHROPO- + MORPH- + -IC] **1** Conceived or represented as having human characteristics. **2** Characterized by anthropomorphism.

**anthropomorphism** \-môr′fizm\ The attribution to animals or other nonhuman entities of the physical, mental, or emotional characteristics of human beings.

**anthroponosis** \-nō′sis\ [ANTHROPO- + *(zoo)nosis.* See ZOONOSIS.] A disease caused by an agent originally found in other vertebrates than man that has become adapted to man alone and is not found in other vertebrate hosts, though it may continue to have a life cycle involving invertebrate intermediate hosts. Urban cutaneous leishmaniasis caused by *Leishmania tropica tropica* is a possible example, though occasional infection in dogs has been reported. Adj. anthroponotic.

**anthropophilic** \-fil′ik\ [ANTHROPO- + -PHILIC] Thriving in a human environment or preferring humans as hosts: said of parasites that show specificity for humans as opposed to other species, or of any flora or fauna that benefits from human activities. Also *anthropophilous, androphilous, androphile, androphilic.* Compare ZOOPHILIC.

**anthropozoonosis** \-zō′ənō′sis\ [ANTHROPO- + ZOONOSIS] An infection acquired by humans that is maintained in nature by animals. Compare ZOOANTHROPONOSIS.

**anthropozoophilic** \-zō′əfil′ik\ Attracted more or less equally to humans and to some other kinds of animal host: said, for example, of certain kinds of mosquitoes.

**anti-** \an′tē-, an′tī-, an′ti-\ [Gk, opposite, against] A prefix meaning (1) opposing, counteracting, as in *antitoxin, anti-inflammatory*; (2) counteractive, defensive, as in *antidote, antibody*; (3) opposite or facing its counterpart, as in *antitragus*; (4) opposite or reversed with respect to some property of its counterpart, as in *antiparticle*; (5) complementary to, as in *anticodon.* Also *ant-.*

**antiabortifacient** \-abôr′təfā′shənt\ A substance that counteracts the action of an abortifacient.

**antiadrenergic** \-ad′renur′jik\ **1** Acting or tending to block sympathetic, or adrenergic, activity. **2** Any drug that counteracts the action of epinephrine or blocks conduction at adrenergic nerve terminals.

**antiamebic** \-əmē′bik\ **1** Having a destructive or suppressive effect on amebas. **2** An agent used to destroy or suppress parasitic amebas.

**antianemic** \-anē′mik\ **1** Preventing or correcting anemia. **2** Any antianemic substance, such as vitamin $B_{12}$.

**antianginal** \-an′jinəl\ **1** Alleviating angina pectoris. **2** A drug that alleviates angina pectoris.

**antianopheline** \-ənäf′əlīn\ Acting against or destructive to anopheline mosquitoes.

**antiantibody** \-an′tibäd′ē\ An antibody that reacts specifically with antibody when this is combined with antigen but that fails to react with the antibody alone or when it is aggregated by heat. Antiantibodies are rarely found in human serum. When they do occur, it is generally in the very old. Also *anti-immune body, anti-immune substance.*

**antiarachnolysin** \-ar′aknäl′əsin\ An antitoxin that counteracts arachnolysin, the hemolytic principle in spider venoms.

**antiarrhythmic** \-əriTH′mik\ **1** Capable of suppressing or preventing an arrhythmia. **2** An agent used to suppress or prevent an arrhythmia.

**antiarthritic** \-ärthrit′ik\ **1** Tending to counteract the effects of arthritis or provide relief from its symptoms. **2** An antiarthritic drug or treatment. Also *antarthritic.*

**antiatherogenic** \-ath′ərōjen′ik\ [ANTI- + ATHEROGENIC] Preventing or combating the development of atheromatous lesions.

**antibacterial** \-baktir′ē·əl\ Impairing the reproduction or survival of bacteria.

**antibechic** \-bek′ik\ [ANTI- + BECHIC] ANTITUSSIVE.

**antibiotic** \-bī·ät′ik\ [ANTI- + Gk *biōtik(os)* pertaining to life] Any of a number of substances, varying widely in structure and mode of action, produced by one microorganism and inhibitory or lethal to a second type of microorganism. Most antibiotics are produced by sporulating organisms late in their culture cycle. **broad-spectrum a.** An antibiotic active against a wide variety of genera of bacteria, usually including both Gram-negative and Gram-positive species. Such antibiotics include chloramphenicol, tetracycline, and some β-lactams. **β-lactam a.** A group of fungal products, including the penicillins and the cephalosporins, that contain a 4-membered β-lactam ring. These compounds cause lysis of growing bacteria by irreversibly inhibiting the enzymes that form cross-links between the peptide side-chains in the peptidoglycan. This reaction, and also the susceptibility of the antibiotics to inactivation by β-lactamases, depend on the high-energy C-N bond of the β-lactam ring. **macrolide a.** Any antibiotic whose molecule contains a large ring of atoms and is a lactone. The mold that makes such substances condenses together eight $C_3$-units derived from methylmalonyl-CoA. **polyene a.** Any antibiotic whose molecule contains many double bonds, usually as a stretch of conjugated double bonds in a large ring. Such antibiotics are used particularly against fungal infections, and they disrupt cell membranes.

**antiblennorrhagic** \-blen′ôraj′ik\ **1** Of or relating to the treatment of gonorrhea. **2** An agent that reduces the quantity of mucus secreted.

# antibody

**antibody** \an′tibäd′ē\ [transl. of German *Antikörper* (by ellipsis from *antitoxischer Körper* antitoxic "body" or substance) a counteractive substance] A protein molecule formed by the immune system which reacts specifically with the antigen that induced its synthesis. All antibodies are immunoglobulins. Also *immune body, preventive substance* (outmoded), *sensitizer, substance sensibilisatrice, sensitizing substance.* **agglutinating a.** An antibody that acts to aggregate particulate antigens; agglutinin. **albumin agglutinating a.** Agglutinin which has the property of inducing clumping of red blood cells when suspended in a medium containing albumin in a concentration of 22–30 g/dl. **anaphylactic a.** Any antibody capable of inducing an anaphylactic reaction. Usually an IgE antibody bound to surface receptors of tissue basophils causes the reaction, but there may also be IgE with the same specificity present and measurable in the circulation. **anti-A a.** Antibody that reacts with red cells carrying the A antigen, causing agglutination. Agglutinating anti-A antibodies are usually of the IgM class. Anti-A antibodies are found in the sera of subjects of blood groups O and B. Also *anti-A agglutinin.* **anti-B a.** Antibody that reacts with red cells carrying the B antigen, causing agglutination. Agglutinating anti-B antibodies are usually of the IgM class. Anti-B antibodies are found in the sera of subjects of blood groups O and A. Also *anti-B agglutinin.* **anti-D a.** Immune globulin capable of agglutinating or sensitizing red blood cells that bear the D antigen of the Rhesus blood group system. **anti-DNA a.** An antibody to either native (double-stranded) or denatured (single-stranded) DNA. The former is found in high quantity virtually only in patients with systemic lupus erythematosus. **anti-GBM a.** Antibody to the glomerular basement membrane, a complement-fixing autoantibody that is a common cause of glomerulonephritis and renal failure. It is also conspicuous in the Goodpasture syndrome. **anti-kidney antibodies** Antibodies formed against kidney cells or glomerular or tubule basement membranes. They are seen in certain abnormal conditions such as Goodpasture's disease or following renal transplantation. They may be raised in experimental animals. **anti-M a.** Antibody that reacts with red cells carrying the M antigen, causing agglutination. Also *anti-M agglutinin.* **anti mitochondrial a.** An autoantibody that is reactive with mitochondria originating from humans or many other species, its presence in serum being demonstrated by indirect immunofluorescence. High titers characteristically occur in biliary cirrhosis and may accompany other inflammatory or destructive diseases of the liver. **antinuclear a.** Any of several antibodies which interact with elements of cell nuclei. Antinuclear antibodies are found typically in the serum of patients with systemic lupus erythematosus and less frequently in other connective-tissue diseases. They are detected most usually by immunofluorescence or peroxidase techniques. Also *LE factor, LE cell factor, lupus erythematosus factor.* **anti-P a.** Antibody that reacts with red cells bearing the P blood group antigen, causing agglutination. Also *anti-P agglutinin.* **anti-Rh a.** Antibody to the Rh group of antigens found on human erythrocytes. Anti-Rh antibodies may be synthesized either by an Rh− mother with an Rh+ fetus or an Rh− patient who receives a transfusion of Rh+ blood. Agglutinating anti-Rh antibodies are of IgM class. IgG anti-Rh antibodies can cross the placenta and cause hemolytic disease of the newborn. Also *anti-Rh agglutinin.* **anti-S a.** Antibody that reacts with red cells bearing the S blood group antigen. Also *anti-S agglutinin.* **anti-smooth muscle a.** An autoantibody that is reactive with cytoplasmic constituents of smooth muscle from many species. It characteristically occurs in patients with chronic active hepatitis or, less often, in biliary cirrhosis, viral hepatitis, or infectious mononucleosis. Indirect immunofluorescence is used to demonstrate its presence in serum. **antithyroglobulin a.** One of the four autoantibodies often detected in certain thyroid diseases, primarily Hashimoto's thyroiditis but also in Graves disease and primary hypothyroidism. It is interpreted as evidence for an autoimmune pathogenesis in these disorders. Also *thyroglobulin antibody.* **autoimmune a.** *Older term* AUTOANTIBODY **basement membrane a.** An antibody which reacts specifically with antigens present in the basement membrane of tissues. Such antibodies are seen in certain forms of glomerulonephritis, such as Goodpasture's disease. **bivalent a.** An antibody with two antigen combining sites. **blocking a.** Antibody whose presence prevents or inhibits another form of immunologic reactivity. Anaphylactic reactions due to IgE antibody can be prevented by IgG blocking antibodies that compete for the antigen and prevent it from cross-linking cell-bound IgE. In tumor immunology, blocking antibodies have been described that prevent T cell-mediated lysis of tumor cells. Also *inhibiting antibody.* • In transplantation immunology, *blocking antibody* is used as a synonym for *enhancing antibody.* **cell-bound a.** An antibody which can react by its Fc region to Fc receptors on cells, and which can there bind antigen. The cross-linking by antigen of cell-bound antibody produces biologically important effects. **CF a.** COMPLEMENT-FIXING ANTIBODY. **cold a.** An antibody that binds antigen sufficiently strongly to produce an observable effect (usually agglutination or complement fixation) only at temperatures below 37°C. **cold-reacting a.** An antibody which optimally combines with antigen at temperatures below normal physiologic temperatures. **complement-fixing a.** An antibody, usually of the IgG or IgM type, which binds complement upon reacting with an antigen. Also *CF antibody.* **complete a.** An antibody which by virtue of its multivalence can directly agglutinate red blood cells or other particles. Compare INCOMPLETE ANTIBODY. **coprecipitating a.** An antibody that will not itself precipitate the antigen with which it reacts but which will be incorporated into a precipitate when the antigen is precipitated by other antibodies. Most monoclonal antibodies to monomeric antigens behave in this way. **cross-reacting a.** An antibody that reacts with antigenic determinants on molecules other than those used to raise the antibody. In most cases the cross-reaction is with chemically related groups on recognizably similar molecules. Thus antisera raised against a serum protein from one species will cross-react with the homologous protein from related species. Occasionally unexpected cross-reactions occur between apparently unrelated antigens. Unusually an antibody may react more strongly with an antigen other than that used to immunize it (heteroclytic reaction). **cytophilic a.** CYTOTROPIC ANTIBODY. **cytotoxic a.** An antibody which damages antigen-bearing cells, usually in the presence of complement. **cytotropic a.** An antibody, usually IgE, that binds to tissue cells that have surface receptors for the Fc fragment of the immunoglobulin. The bound antibody retains its capacity to combine with antigen and the occurrence of an antigen-antibody reaction stimulates the subjacent cell to release the contents of its granules or to engage in enhanced phagocytic activity. Also *cytophilic antibody, skin-sensitizing antibody.* **Donath-Landsteiner a.** An antibody which binds at low temperatures to the P blood group antigens on the patient's own red cells and causes hemolysis on warming. It is seen in patients with paroxysmal cold hemoglobulinuria. Also *Donath-Landsteiner cold autoantibody.* **enhancing a.** An antibody that can prevent rejection of an allogeneic graft. Enhancing antibodies are directed against the Ia (or D region) antigens of the major histocompatibility complex. These antigens are found on antigen-presenting cells in organ grafts and antibodies to them inhibit antigen presentation. **fluorescein-labeled a.** An antibody that has been covalently linked with fluorescein, usually in the form of isiothiocyanate. It is used extensively in immunofluorescence tests. Also *fluorescent antibody.* **Forssman a.** Antibody to the Forssman antigen. **H a.** 1 Antibody directed against the H antigens of bacterial flagella. 2 An antibody against H antigen (H substance), the precursor of blood groups A and B. Anti-H antibody is formed by subjects with the rare Bombay phenotype and reacts with all human erythrocytes (other than the Bombay type) but most strongly with those of blood group O. **heat-labile a.** An antibody that is denatured or made nonfunctional by heating at 56°C. **hepatitis B core a.** The antibody to the core antigen of hepatitis B virus. It usually develops during or shortly before the symptomatic disease occurs, and it persists throughout life. It is a useful marker for previous hepatitis B infection, because it does not develop after immunization with hepatitis B vaccine. **hepatitis B e a.** The antibody to the e antigen of hepatitis B virus. It normally develops during or after the convalescent phase of the disease and signals the elimination of e antigen from the circulation. It does not develop after immunization with hepatitis B vaccine. **hepatitis B surface a.** The antibody to the surface antigen of hepatitis B virus ($HB_sAg$). It develops well after convalescence from infection, lasts lifelong, and confers protection against subsequent infection. Hepatitis B vaccine is designed to elicit high titers of this antibody. **heterocytotropic a.** An antibody that binds by its Fc region to receptors on mast cells of species other than its own. Heterocytotropic antibodies are usually of IgG class and their binding to mast cells is stable for only a few hours. They are detected by the passive cutaneous anaphylaxis reaction. Also *xenocytophilic antibody.* Compare REAGINIC ANTIBODY. **heterogenetic a.** HETEROPHIL ANTIBODY. **heteroligating a.** HYBRID ANTIBODY. **heterophil a.** 1 Any antibody that reacts with heterophil antigens, especially with the Forssman antigen. Also *heterogenetic antibody.* 2 A human IgM antibody that agglutinates sheep red blood cells present in the serum during several immune-mediated diseases, including infectious mononucleosis. The heterophil antibody characteristic of infectious mononucleosis due to Epstein-Barr virus can be absorbed from serum by beef red cells but not by guinea pig kidney or other sources of the Forssman antigen. **homocytotropic a.** REAGINIC ANTIBODY. **humoral a.** Antibody found in the serum. **hybrid a.** A bivalent antibody in which the two antigen-binding sites are of different specificities. Thought not to occur in nature, such antibodies can be produced artificially from different immunoglobulin fragments or by cell-fusion techniques. Also *heteroligating antibody.* **immune a.** Antibody produced as a result of deliberate immunization with a variety of substances, including blood group antigens after transfusion, as opposed to natural antibodies. Compare NATURAL ANTIBODY. **immunosorbent a.** See under IMMUNOADSORPTION. **incomplete a.** An antibody that coats the surface of erythrocytes or bacteria but does not agglutinate them. Incomplete antibodies are usually of the IgG class. Their inability to agglutinate is not due to univalency. Cells treated with enzymes to remove sialic acid can often be agglutinated by incomplete antibodies. **inhibiting a.** BLOCKING ANTIBODY. **isoimmune a.** ALLOANTIBODY. **maternal antibodies** Antibodies, in the fetal blood (predominantly IgG) which have been produced by the mother and transmitted by the placenta. **monoclonal a.** An antibody secreted by a single clone of antibody-producing cells. Such antibodies have the same combining site, the same light chain, and the same immunoglobulin class, subclass, and allotype, and their production in tissue culture by the hybridoma technique has enormously expanded the availability of highly characterized and specific antibodies of far-reaching practical and experimental importance. Monoclonal antibodies are occasionally found in human disease, as in cold hemolytic antibody disease, or after immunization of experimental animals, as with bacterial polysaccharides, but most antibody formation *in vivo* is highly polyclonal. Monoclonal antibodies are also used widely for the isolation and purification of proteins, on a preparative and industrial scale. **natural a.** Antibody found in the serum of animals who have not been deliberately exposed to the antigen with which the antibody results. Since animals kept from birth in a rigorously antigen-free environment remain hypogammaglobulinemic, it can be assumed that natural antibodies arise from unintentional exposure to antigens. Compare IMMUNE ANTIBODY. **neutralizing a.** An antibody which decreases the infectious titer or detoxifies when complexed with the infectious agent or homologous toxin. **O a.** 1 An antibody directed against the somatic O antigen of Gram-negative bacteria. 2 An antibody directed against the O blood group. It may appear naturally following transfusions of incompatible blood. **opsonizing a.** An antibody whose activity is measured by its capacity to opsonize the particulate antigen with which it reacts. Opsonization may be produced by the antibody binding alone, usually IgG antibodies, or by complement fixation. Also *immune opsonin.* **precipitating a.** *Outmoded* PRECIPITIN. **protective a.** An antibody responsible for protective immunity to an infectious agent. **reaginic a.** Antibody responsible for acute anaphylactic reactions (type 1 hypersensitivity reaction). Reaginic antibody is usually of IgE class and its characteristic property is to bind to IgE Fc receptors on mast cells of their own species. The stability of its binding, lasting many days, allows it to be detected by the Prausnitz-Küstner reaction. When it is cross-linked on the mast cell surface by reaction with antigen, degranulation of the mast cell occurs with release of the mediators (histamine, leukotrienes, platelet activating factor, and eosinophil chemotactic factor) that produce anaphylaxis. IgE Fc receptors also occur on macrophages and the reaction of these with IgE antibodies to parasites bound on the parasite surface cause the parasite to be killed. Some IgG antibodies can also act as reaginic antibodies. Also *homocytotropic antibody, reagin, atopic reagin.* Compare HETEROCYTOTROPIC ANTIBODY. **Rh a.** Immunoglobulin capable of agglutinating or sensitizing red blood cells bearing antigens of the Rhesus blood group system. Also *Rh antiserum.* **saline agglutinating a.** An antibody that agglutinates red blood cells in the presence of physiological salt solutions alone: used especially in blood grouping serology. It is usually of IgM class. **skin-sensitizing a.** CYTOTROPIC ANTIBODY. **T a.** An antibody often present in normal human serum which reacts with the T antigen present on erythrocytes. The T antigen is only exposed after treatment of red cells with neuraminidase. Also *T agglutinin, Thomsen antibody, Thomsen-Friedenreich antibody.* **thyroglobulin a.** ANTITHYROGLOBULIN ANTIBODY. **thyroid microsomal antibodies** Autoantibodies against an antigen present in actively secreting thyroid epithelial cells, detectable by immunofluorescence testing or agglutination of particles coated with antigen. Thyroid microsomal antibodies are present in virtually all patients with Hashimoto's thyroiditis and in 85 percent of patients with Graves disease, regardless of the functional state of the thyroid. The antibodies are also found in 10 percent of healthy adults. **treponema-immobilizing a.** An antibody found in the serum of patients with syphilis (whether active or postinfectious) and active against the antigens of *Treponema pallidum.* In the presence of complement, the serum immobilizes a suspension of motile living *Treponema* organisms. It is highly specific for syphilis and does not give the false positive indications seen in the Wassermann reaction. **univalent a.** An antibody which has only one antigen binding site. Univalent antibodies probably do not occur *in vivo* but are frequently made by the hybridoma technique where the two Fab arms of the FgG molecule may have different light chains. They can also be produced from rabbit FgG by limited proteolyns (FabC fragments). • This term was formerly and erroneously used to describe antierythrocyte antibodies that failed to agglutinate erythrocytes. **Vi a.** An antibody directed against a surface antigen of strains of *Salmonella typhi,* believed to be associated with virulence (hence the abbreviation *Vi*). The antigen blocks access of agglutinating antibodies to the O antigen. **warm a.** An antibody, usually to erythrocytes, which binds antigen at 37°C and may lyse erythrocytes *in vivo* without a drop in body temperature. **Wassermann a.** An antibody present in the serum of most subjects with syphilis. It reacts with a cardiolipin, usually obtained from ox heart. The reaction is the basis of the Wassermann test for syphilis, which depends on the fixation of complement by the antibody in the presence of the lipid antigen. The antibody may give false positive reactions in other abnormal states. **xenocytophilic a.** HETEROCYTOTROPIC ANTIBODY.

**antibrachial** \-brā′kē·əl\ *Incorrect* ANTEBRACHIAL.

**antibrachium** \-brā′kē·əm\ *Incorrect* ANTEBRACHIUM.

**antibromic** **1** Deodorizing. **2** A deodorant or any deodorizing agent.

**antibubonic** \-bʸoobän′ik\ **1** Acting against bubonic plague. **2** An agent effective against bubonic plague.

**anticachectic** **1** Counteracting cachexia. **2** An agent that relieves or prevents cachexia.

**anticalculous** \-kal′kyələs\ Capable of preventing lithiasis or dissolving calculi already formed.

**anticarcinogen** \-kärsin′əjən\ A substance acting against a carcinogen or carcinogenic effect. Adj. anticarcinogenic.

**anticardium** \-kär′dē·əm\ PRECORDIUM.

**anticarious** \-kar′ē·əs\ Preventing or retarding the development of dental caries. Also *anticariogenic.*

**antichlorotic** \-klôrät′ik\ **1** Preventing or correcting chlorosis. **2** Any substance which prevents or corrects chlorosis.

**anticholinergic** \-kō′linur′jik\ Counteracting the action of acetylcholine: used especially of drugs which block conduction at cholinergic nerve endings. Also *cholinolytic.*

**anticipate** \antis′ipāt\ To occur earlier than expected according to the normal pattern, as a disease or symptom.

**anticipation** \antis′ipā′shən\ The appearance of a hereditary disease at a progressively earlier age in successive generations. This has been thought to occur in myotonic dystrophy, in certain types of hereditary tremor, in Huntington's disease, and in some forms of hereditary ataxia. However, the existence of this phenomenon has not been proved conclusively, and is assumed by some to be an artifact due in part to improved means of detection and increased awareness.

**anticlinal** \-klī′nəl\ [ANTI- + CLIN- + -AL] **1** Forming a ridge in which strata lean against each other, inclining in opposite directions. **2** Having an upright spine toward which spines on both sides incline.

**anticnemion** \an′tik·nē′mē·än\ SHIN.

**anticoagulant** \-kō·ag′yələnt\ **1** Interfering with or preventing normal blood clotting. Also *anticoagulative.* **2** A substance that prevents or retards coagulation, such as the drugs warfarin or heparin or an abnormal antibody. Also *decoagulant.* **circulating a.** A serum factor, probably an autoantibody, which interferes with normal blood clotting, sometimes found in patients with systemic lupus erythematosus, or myeloma, or in postpartum patients.

**anticoagulative** \-kō·ag′yəlā′tiv\ ANTICOAGULANT.

**anticodon** The sequence in a transfer RNA that pairs with a specific codon in messenger RNA on the ribosome.

**anticomplementary** \-käm′pləmen′terē\ Capable of inactivating or consuming complement on its own: said especially of serums being tested for antibody by complement fixation tests and which consume the added complement even in the absence of antigen. Anticomplementary activity can be due to the presence of immune complexes or of immunoglobulin aggregates; of antibodies reacting with components of the complement source; or of enzymes that destroy complement activity.

**anticonceptive** \-kənsep′tiv\ CONTRACEPTIVE.

**anticonvulsant** **1** Acting to prevent or control convulsions, as a drug. **2** An anticonvulsant agent. For defs. 1 and 2 also *anticonvulsive.*

**anticurare** An agent that prevents or reverses the effects of curare on skeletal muscle.

**anticus** \antī′kəs\ *Older term* ANTERIOR.

**antidepressant** \-dipres′ənt\ **1** Tending to counteract the effects of depression; alleviating or inhibiting depression. **2** An agent used to treat depression. For defs. 1 and 2 also *euphoriant.*

**antidiabetic** \-dī′əbet′ik\ **1** Counteracting or inhibiting the effects of diabetes mellitus. **2** An antidiabetic agent.

**antidiarrheal** \-dī′erē′əl\ **1** Counteracting diarrhea. **2** An agent used to treat diarrhea. For defs. 1 and 2 also *antidiarrheic.*

**antidiuresis** \-dī′yŏorē′sis\ [ANTI- + DIURESIS] Decreased urine excretion as a result of a number of causes, including dehydration, secretion or administration of antidiuretic hormone, acute renal failure, and any condition in which edema is forming.

**antidiuretic** \-dī′yŏoret′ik\ **1** Tending to decrease urinary volume. **2** An agent or mechanism that decreases urinary volume, as *antidiuretic hormone.*.

**antidotal** \-dō′tl\ [*antidot(e)* + -AL] Counteracting the

action of a poison. Also *antidotic.*
**antidote** \an′tidōt\ [Gk *antidotos* (from ANTI- + *didōnai* to give) given as a remedy, an antidote, remedy] Any means of neutralizing or counteracting the effects of a poison. **chemical a.** A chemical designed to react with a poison to form an innocuous compound or block the effect of the poison at the site of action. **mechanical a.** A mechanical procedure used to counteract the action of a poison. **physiologic a.** An agent which counteracts the action of a poison by inducing an opposite biological effect. **universal a.** An activated charcoal preparation that effectively adsorbs many chemicals, including drugs, in acute poisoning. It is usually administered in the form of a slurry or a mixture of charcoal, magnesium oxide, and tannic acid.
**antidotic** \-dät′ik\ ANTIDOTAL.
**antidromic** \-dräm′ik\ [Gk *antidrom(ein)* (from ANTI- + *dromos* course, race) to run in a contrary direction + -IC] Conducting in a direction opposite to that physiologically normal for an axon or nerve.
**antidysenteric** \-dis′ənter′ik\ **1** Acting against dysentery. **2** An agent effective against dysentery.
**antieczematic** \-ek′səmat′ik\ **1** ANTIECZEMATOUS. **2** A drug used to treat eczema.
**antieczematous** \-eksem′ətəs\ Tending to alleviate or inhibit eczema, as a drug. Also *antieczematic.*
**antiemetic** \-imet′ik\ [ANTI- + EMETIC] **1** Having the effect of suppressing vomiting. **2** An agent used to suppress vomiting. For defs. 1 and 2 also *antiemitic.*
**antienzyme** \-en′zīm\ An antibody which complexes specifically with an enzyme.
**antiepileptic** \-ep′ilep′tik\ **1** Acting to prevent or control epileptic seizures, as a drug or dietary measure. **2** An antiepileptic agent, especially a drug such as hydantoin.
**antierotica** Medications that reduce sexual desire.
**antierythrocyte** \-irith′rəsīt\ Any substance, such as an antibody, that reacts with erythrocytes or impairs their function or survival in circulation.
**antifebrile** ANTIPYRETIC.
**antifibrillatory** \-fībril′ətôr′ē\ **1** Having the capability of stopping or preventing fibrillation of the atria or ventricles. **2** An agent used to stop or prevent fibrillation.
**antifibrinolysin** \-fī′brinäl′isin\ An inhibitor of the fibrinolytic process.
**antifilarial** \-filer′ē·əl\ **1** Destructive to filariae. **2** An agent that destroys or is harmful to filariae.
**antiflatulent** \-flat′yələnt\ **1** Tending to decrease or prevent flatulence. **2** An antiflatulent agent.
**antifolate** Any drug that acts by interfering with the biosynthesis or metabolism of folic acid. Inhibitors of dihydrofolate reductase are particularly important examples, and are used in cancer chemotherapy.
**antifungal** \-fung′gəl\ **1** Killing or inhibiting the growth of fungi, as an antibiotic. **2** Any antifungal substance. For defs. 1 and 2 also *antimycotic.*
**antigalactic** \-gəlak′tik\ [ANTI- + GALACTIC] Reducing the secretion of milk by the breast.
**antigametocyte** \-gəmē′təsīt\ An agent or substance that is destructive to gametocytes of sporozoan parasites, such as malarial parasites.

# antigen

**antigen** \an′təjən\ [*anti(body)* + -GEN] Any substance which can elicit in a vertebrate host the formation of specific antibody or the generation of a specific population of lymphocytes reactive with that substance. Antigens may be protein or carbohydrate, lipid or nucleic acid, or contain elements of all or any of these as well as organic or inorganic chemical groups attached to protein or other macromolecule. Whether a material is an antigen in a particular host depends on whether the material is foreign to the host and also on the genetic makeup of the host, as well as on the dose and physical state of the antigen. Also *immunogen.* **A a.** $IV^2$-α-fucosyl-$IV^3$-α-N-acetylgalacosaminylneolactotetraosylceramide. A blood-group antigen whose presence determines the A blood type if the codominant allele at the ABO locus is A or H, and the AB blood type if the codominant allele is B. A antigens are components of the membranes of erythrocytes and other cells and are highly immunogenic. A antigens can be detected in saliva and other body fluids of secretors. They can also be extracted from tissue cells by ethanol. Also *A substance, blood group A glycolipid.* **accessible a.** Any of those antigens anatomically available *in vivo* for reaction with antibodies or with lymphocytes. These are antigens in the extracellular fluid or on the surfaces of cells or basement membranes which are in contact with the general extracellular fluid. **allergic a.** *Outmoded* ALLERGEN. **allogeneic a.** ALLOANTIGEN. **alpha a. of adenovirus** An antigen associated with the hexon structural protein of adenoviruses and which has group specificity and cross-reacts by the complement fixation test with the hexon of adenoviruses of most species of animals. **Au a.** HEPATITIS B SURFACE ANTIGEN. **Australia a.** HEPATITIS B SURFACE ANTIGEN. **autologous a.** An antigen that can give rise to an immune response in the individual from whom it comes. **B a.** $IV^2$-α-fucosyl-$IV^3$-α-galactosylneolactotetraosylceramide. A blood-group antigen whose presence determines the B blood type if the codominant allele at the ABO locus is B or H, and the AB blood type if the codominant allele is A. B antigens are components of the membranes of erythrocytes and other cells and are highly immunogenic. B antigens can be detected in saliva and other body fluids of secretors. They can also be extracted from tissue cells by ethanol. Also *B substance, blood group B glycolipid.* **beef heart a.** An antigen produced by extracting normal beef heart tissue with absolute alcohol, used in the Wassermann test. **beta a. of adenovirus** An antigen associated with the penton base structural protein of adenoviruses which has intra-subgroup as well as some weak group-reactive specificities. It exhibits a toxinlike activity which detaches infected cells from their glass or plastic substrate. **blood-group a.** A blood cell membrane component capable of inducing formation of an antibody. **C a.** A carbohydrate somatic antigen found in the cell walls of pneumococci and streptococci. Also *C substance.* **carbohydrate a.'s** Polysaccharides, from bacterial or other cells, that act as complete antigens or as haptens. **carcinoembryonic a.** An antigen found normally in the fetal gut, and as a glycoprotein derived from colon, lung and other endodermal adenocarcinomas. Its appearance in the serum of smokers and patients with inflammatory bowel disease makes it of limited diagnostic value. It can be detected in tissue sections of a number of adenocarcinomas. Abbr. CEA **chick embryo a.** YOLK SAC ANTIGEN. **common acute lymphocytic leukemia a.** An antigen present on the cell membrane of leukemic lymphoblasts in 70 percent of patients with acute lymphocytic leukemia and in a small proportion of patients with the acute "blast" phase of chronic granulocytic leukemia. **common enterobacterial a.** A deep-seated envelope antigen common to a wide variety of enteric bacteria, and possibly of significance in resistance to infection. Also *Kunin antigen.* Abbr. CEA **complement-fixing a.** An antigen that is detected by complement fixation. Viral complement-fixing antigens are usually internal and group- or family-specific rather than type- or strain-specific. **complete a.** An antigen capable of reacting with an antibody as well as inducing its formation, as distinguished from a hapten. **cross-reacting a.** An antigen that shares determinants with another antigen and hence reacts with antibody to the latter antigen. **D a.** The most commonly immunogenic antigen within the Rhesus blood group system. Individuals negative for this antigen are commonly referred to as being Rh-negative. **delta a. of adenovirus** An antigen of adenoviruses which is subgroup-specific and is located in the shaft, or rod, probably near the junction between the fiber and penton. **E a.** An antigen in the Rhesus blood group system. **e a.** See under HEPATITIS B E ANTIGEN. **epsilon a. of adenovirus** An antigen of adenoviruses which is type-specific and is part of the hexon. **F a.** FORSSMAN ANTIGEN. **fetal a.'s** Those antigens which are present during early fetal life and either are not present or are not recognized during adult life. These antigens may re-emerge to be recognized as foreign by the immune system during a disease process or may re-emerge on the surface of transformed cells. **flagellar a.** H ANTIGEN. **Forssman a.** A widely distributed heterophil antigen present on the tissues of many species and which, when injected, induces the formation of hemolysin for sheep erythrocytes. The antigenic determinant is believed to be a polysaccharide and was originally found in guinea pig kidneys. Also *F antigen, Forssman's lipoid.* **gamma a. of adenovirus** An antigen of adenoviruses which is located on the fiber and is type-specific. **group-specific a.** 1 An antigen shared by a group of related species, especially bacteria. Compare SPECIES-SPECIFIC ANTIGEN. 2 An antigenic determinant shared by a group of related compounds, such as the O antigens of various salmonella species. **H a.** 1 A blood-group antigen related to the ABO and Lewis blood groups. It is the precursor substance on which the products of the A and B blood-group genes act to produce the A and B antigens (or substances). H antigen is present on nearly all human erythrocytes and is found at highest concentration on those of blood group O. H antigen is an oligosaccharide, terminating in lactose, linked to proteins in erythrocyte and other cell membranes. A or B alleles at the ABO locus direct addition of *N*-acetylgalactosamine or galactose, respectively, to the H antigen. Presence of this antigen on erythrocytes depends on two loci. An H allele must be present at the Bombay locus to enable conversion of a precursor to the H antigen. (In the rare Bombay phenotype, H antigen is not formed and in consequence A and B antigens cannot be expressed. However, these subjects make anti-H antibodies.) An O allele (an amorph) must be present at the ABO locus to prevent further modification. Individuals who are homozygous or heterozygous for the Se allele at the secretor locus secrete H antigen in saliva. Also *H substance, released substance.* 2 Antigen of a bacterial flagellum. In enterobacteria the H antigen types, designated by small letters or by numbers, are used for classification. Also *flagellar antigen.* **H-2 a.** See under TRANSPLANTATION ANTIGEN. **hepatitis a.** HEPATITIS B SURFACE ANTIGEN. **hepatitis-associated a.** HEPATITIS B SURFACE ANTIGEN. **hepatitis B core a.** An antigen associated with the core of the hepatitis B virion. Free virus cores do not appear in serum but the core of the intact virion (Dane particle) can be rendered accessible to antibody by detergent. Antibody to the core antigen appears early in hepatitis B virus infection and persists at high titer while the infection lasts. Low levels are found for years afterward. Abbr. $HB_cAg$ **hepatitis B e a.** An antigen of hepatitis B virus whose presence in the serum has been associated with infectivity of serum and its ability to transmit hepatitis. Antibody to e antigen in the serum of hepatitis B virus carriers is associated with low infectivity of serum. Abbr. HBeAg **hepatitis B surface a.** A viral antigen found in the serum of patients with serum hepatitis due to hepatitis B virus infection, in a proportion of patients who have recovered from hepatitis B virus infection, and in a number of subjects who are carriers of the virus without obvious associated disease. Hepatitis B surface antigen represents surplus, noninfectious, virus coat material and is seen in the electron microscope as spherical particles of 22 nM diameter or tubules of 22 nM $\times$ 40–400 nM. Also *Australia antigen, hepatitis antigen, hepatitis-associated antigen, Au antigen, SH antigen, serum hepatitis antigen.* Abbr. HBsAg **heterophil a.** An antigen of essentially carbohydrate specificity that occurs on cell surfaces in many different species not necessarily taxonomically related. The Forssman antigen is a typical heterophil antigen. Also *heterogenetic antigen.* **Hikojima a.** One of three serotypes of *Vibrio cholerae,* the other serotypes being Inaba and Ogawa antigens. **histocompatibility a.** Any of the genetically determined antigens present on the cells of most tissues. In tissue allografting, absence of an immune response by a potential donor to the recipient's antigen demonstrates histocompatibility. **HLA a.** One of a group of inherited cell antigens that determine tissue compatibility in man; the human transplantation antigen. They comprise a highly polymorphic group of alleles controlled by a region of chromosome 6 and its four loci, and are expressed in nearly all nucleated cells. **homologous a.** ALLOANTIGEN. **H-Y a.** A minor histocompatibility antigen which is coded for on the Y chromosome and which allows female animals to reject grafts from syngeneic males. **I a.** A carbohydrate antigen present on the erythrocytes of the great majority of human adults, and also of rabbits. The antigen is not developed until after birth. Umbilical cord erythrocytes are negative for the I antigen and express instead an alternative specificity designated i. I antigens are the principal antigens against which cold agglutinins are directed. Also *I substance.* **Ia a.** A surface antigen of mouse cells, such as B lymphocytes and macrophages, that is determined by the IA gene of the major histocompatibility gene locus. Antibodies to the mouse Ia antigen cross-react with an antigen on human B lymphocytes which is, therefore, called "Ia-like antigen." The homologous antigenic specificity in humans is HLA-DR. **Inaba a.** One of three serotypes of *Vibrio cholerae,* the other serotypes being Hikojima and Ogawa antigens. **incomplete a.** HAPTEN. **isophile a.** *Outmoded* ALLOANTIGEN. **K a.'s** Blood cell membrane components capable of reacting specifically with anti-K antibodies. See also KELL BLOOD GROUP. **Kunin a.** COMMON ENTEROBACTERIAL ANTIGEN. **Kveim a.** See under KVEIM-SILTZBACH TEST. **lens a.'s** Proteins in the lens of the eye, of significance because they are inaccessible to the normal immune response. **Ly a.'s** Antigens present on the surface of T lymphocytes (designated Lyt) and B lymphocytes (designated Lyb) and that determine the functions of the cells. **M a.** 1 M PROTEIN. 2 The matrix protein antigen found in many enveloped viruses, which may serve to stabilize the lipid envelope. **major histocompatibility a.'s** See under MAJOR HISTOCOMPATIBILITY COMPLEX. **Mitsuda a.** LEPROMIN. **mumps skin test a.** A preparation of inactivated mumps virus that is injected intradermally as a skin test for prior immunizing exposure to mumps virus. The test has largely been replaced by those for serum antibodies. **NP a.** A nucleoprotein antigen found in viruses that have helical symmetry. **nuclear a.** Any antigen found in the cell nucleus: often used of such antigens to which autoantibodies are formed in systemic lupus erythematosus and related diseases. They include DNA nucleoprotein and its constituents, RNA nucleoproteins, and some nucleic acid free protein antigens. **O a.** The polysaccharide antigen of the lipopolysaccharide layer of Gram-negative bacterial cell walls. **Ogawa a.** One of three serotypes of *Vibrio cholerae,* the other serotypes being Hikojima and Inaba antigens. **organ-specific a.** An antigen present on a given tissue and which is specific for that organ. Organ-specific antigens may share antigenic determinants with the same tissues from other species but also contain antigens which are specific for that individual of the species. **P a.** A human blood group antigen having three variants: $P_1$, $P_2$, and $P^r$. **partial a.** HAPTEN. **pollen a.** The antigenic component of plant pollens concerned in the pathogenesis of hay fever. It is employed in tests for and hyposensitization of pollen allergies. **protective a.** The antigen involved in contributing towards the increased resistance of the host against an infecting organism. It thus stimulates the production of protective antibody responsible for immunity and is important in vaccination. **public a.'s** HIGH FREQUENCY BLOOD GROUP. **R a.** The somatic antigen of rough (R) variants of Gram-negative bacteria. **recall a.** An antigen eliciting a secondary immune response. **Rh a.** Any one of an allelic system of glycosphingolipids of the erythrocyte membrane that strongly stimulate antibody formation when introduced into the blood of persons lacking these substances. Formerly, antibody stimulation in this manner was the most common cause of hemolytic disease of the newborn. Several distinct Rh antigens are recognized. The erythrocytes of most people have one of the following antigens, designated by either of two nomenclature systems, as $Rh_0$ or CDe, $R_1$ or CDe, $R_2$ or cDE, $Rh_z$ or CDE. The blood of such people is said to be Rh positive. When these antigens are lacking, the blood is said to be Rh negative because the erythrocytes then have the rh or ce substance, which is usually not antigenic. Also *Rhesus antigen, Rhesus factor, Rh factor.* • *Rh* stands for *Rhesus,* since this system was first identified in rhesus monkeys. **S a.** One of numerous antigenetic determinants of the MNSs blood group. **self a.** AUTOANTIGEN. **serum hepatitis a.** HEPATITIS B SURFACE ANTIGEN. **SH a.** HEPATITIS B SURFACE ANTIGEN. **Sm a.** A nuclear antigen present in active chromatin, resistant to both DNAase and RNAase, to which antibodies are found in the serum of about 20 percent of patients with systemic lupus erythematosus. Antibody to Sm antigen is considered to be specific for the diagnosis of systemic lupus erythematosus. **somatic a.** Any antigen located within a bacterial cell, not in a capsule or in flagella. **species-specific a.** An antigen present in a species but not in closely related ones, used especially to classify bacteria. Compare GROUP-SPECIFIC ANTIGEN. **surface a.** Any of a large number of antigens that are on the surface of cells, such as the Ia antigen of lymphocytes or the AB, Kell, MNS, and other antigens of erythrocytes. **SV 40 T a.** A tumor antigen which is an early protein synthesized by simian virus 40 in transformed cells and in tumors induced by the virus. **T a.** **1** TUMOR ANTIGEN. **2** A minor antigen of the cell walls of streptococci. **3** TRANSPLANTATION ANTIGEN. **4** An autoantigen exposed on human erythrocytes following treatment with neuraminidase. Also *Thomas antigen.* **theta a.** An alloantigen on the surface of mouse T lymphocytes as well as on cells of the central nervous system. Its two allelic forms are designated Thy 1.1 and Thy 1.2. Also *thy 1 antigen.* **Thomas a.** T antigen. **thy 1 a.** THETA ANTIGEN. **thymus dependent a.** An antigen which requires an immune response from thymus-derived lymphocyte (T lymphocyte) in order to elicit an immune response in B lymphocytes which then mature into antibody-forming cells. **thymus independent a.** An antigen which does not require T lymphocyte participation to elicit an immune response in B lymphocytes. Animals lacking a thymus can respond to these antigens. Also *T independent antigen.* **T independent a.** THYMUS INDEPENDENT ANTIGEN. **tissue-specific a.** An antigen specific for a given tissue and not found in other tissues. Tissue-specific antigens have been described for most tissues, as in the colon, bladder, and various endocrine glands. In the central nervous system a series of tissue-specific antigens have been described which are specific for different cell types. Thus galactocerebroside is specific for oligodendrocytes and glial acidic fibrillary protein for astrocytes. **transplantation a.** Any of various molecules on cell surfaces that can give rise to the immunologically mediated rejection of the tissue bearing them when this is grafted into an allogeneic recipient. The most important transplantation antigens are those coded in the major histocompatibility complex (HLA in man and H-2 in mice) but there are a variety of others. **tumor a.** Any of various proteins that papovaviruses or oncogenic adenoviruses produce in cells but do not incorporate into the virions. Also *T antigen.* **tumor-specific a.** An antigen found in a tumor cell and absent in the corresponding normal tissue cells. Abbr. TSA **tumor-specific transplantation a.** Antigen present on a tumor cell surface that elicits an immune response, in a syngeneic animal or the tumor-bearing animal itself, which leads to the rejection of the tumor but has no effect on the normal cells from which the tumor arose. **VDRL a.** See under VDRL TEST. **Vi a.** A labile polysaccharide surface antigen forming a thin capsular layer in many salmonellae. The Vi antigen of *Salmonella typhi,* a homopolymer of *N*-acetyl galactosaminuronic acid, is important in virulence and is required for effectiveness in a vaccine. **viral capsid a.** An antigen which is part of the protein coat surrounding the nucleic acid of a virus. In enveloped viruses with helical symmetry, the capsid antigen is bound to nucleic acid, forming a nucleocapsid protein. In enveloped or naked viruses with icosahedral symmetry, the capsid is in the form of a protein coat surrounding the nucleic acid. There may be several capsid antigens of a virus. **yolk sac a.** An antigenic material prepared from chick embryos that are infected with *Chlamydia trachomatis.* It is used in tests for lymphogranuloma venereum. Also *chick embryo antigen.*

**antigenic** \-jen′ik\ Having the character or properties of an antigen; pertaining to antigens.

**antigenicity** \-jənis′itē\ IMMUNOGENICITY.

**antigerminal** \-jur′minəl\ Pertaining to that pole of an ovum opposite the germinal pole.

**antiglobulin** \-gläb′yəlin\ Antibody directed to immunoglobulins, usually those of a different species. Commonly used in antiglobulin testing (direct or indirect).

**antigoitrogenic** \-goi′trəjen′ik\ **1** Acting to stop or retard the development of goiter. **2** An antigoitrogenic agent.

**antigonadotropin** \-gän′ədōtrō′pin\ An agent that counteracts or inhibits the action of gonadotropic hormones. Also *antigonadotrophin.*

**anti HBc** Antibody to hepatitis B core antigen.

**anti HBs** Antibody to hepatitis B surface antigen.
**antihelix** \-hē′liks\ ANTHELIX.
**antihelmintic** \-helmin′tik\ ANTHELMINTIC.
**antihemorrhagic** \-hem′ôraj′ik\ **1** Tending to stop or prevent bleeding. **2** An agent that is used to stop or prevent bleeding. For defs. 1 and 2 also *anthemorrhagic.*
**antihidrotic** \-hīdrät′ik\ ANTIPERSPIRANT.
**antihistamine** Any agent that can prevent, reduce, or oppose the pharmacologic effects of histamine.
**antihistaminic** A therapeutic agent that blocks or impedes the effects of histamine by competing for the $H_1$ receptors related to allergies or the $H_2$ receptors involved in gastric acid secretion.
**antihydropic** Denoting a medication used to treat the accumulation of fluid in the tissues, i.e. dropsy, or edematous states.
**antihyperglycemic** **1** Reducing blood glucose levels from elevated values, as insulin does in the treatment of diabetes mellitus. **2** An antihyperglycemic medication.
**antihypertensive** \-hī′pərten′siv\ **1** Acting to lower high blood pressure. **2** An agent that lowers high blood pressure.
**antihypotensive** \-hī′pōten′siv\ **1** Counteracting hypotension. **2** An agent that counteracts hypotension.
**anti-infective** \-infek′tiv\ **1** Preventing or acting against infection. Also *anti-infectious.* **2** An agent that prevents or acts against infection.
**anti-inflammatory** **1** Suppressing or reducing inflammation. **2** An anti-inflammatory agent.
**anti-insulin** \-in′s$^y$əlin\ **1** Acting to counteract or inhibit the action of insulin. **2** An anti-insulin material.
**antileprotic** \-leprät′ik\ **1** Acting against leprosy. **2** An agent effective against leprosy.
**antileukemic** \-lookē′mik\ **1** Preventing leukemia or effective in its treatment. **2** Any antileukemic substance.
**antileukocytic** \-loo′kəsit′ik\ **1** Able to damage, impair the function of, or destroy leukocytes. **2** Any antileukocytic agent.
**antilewisite** DIMERCAPROL. **British a.** DIMERCAPROL. Abbr. BAL
**antilipemic** Denoting an agent that reduces elevated blood levels of lipids or lipoproteins.
**antilipotropic** \-lip′əträp′ik\ Opposing the formation of fat.
**antilithic** \-lith′ik\ **1** Preventing or slowing down the formation of calculi. **2** An agent that prevents or slows down the formation of calculi.
**antilobium** \-lō′bē·əm\ *Outmoded* TRAGUS.
**antiluetic** \-loo·et′ik\ ANTISYPHILITIC.
**antilymphocytic** \-lim′fəsit′ik\ **1** Able to damage, impair the function of, or destroy lymphocytes. **2** Any antilymphocytic agent.
**antimeningococcic** \-mening′gōkäk′sik\ **1** Acting against *Neisseria meningitidis..* **2** An agent effective against *Neisseria meningitidis..*
**antimenorrhagic** \-men′ôraj′ik\ [ANTI- + -MENORRHAGIC] Describing measures used to diminish menstrual flow.
**antimesenteric** \-mes′ənter′ik\ Denoting the side of the intestine which is opposite to the side with attachment to the mesentery.
**antimetabolite** A chemical that resembles a specific metabolite in structure and replaces or competes with the metabolite's role, and may thus modify or interfere with a metabolic pathway. Also *metabolic antagonist.*
**antimicrobial** \-mīkrō′bē·əl\ **1** Acting to kill or inhibit growth and multiplication of microbes. **2** An agent which kills or inhibits the growth and multiplication of microbes. For defs. 1 and 2 also *antimicrobic.*
**antimicrobic** \-mīkrō′bik\ ANTIMICROBIAL.
**antimitotic** \-mītät′ik\ **1** Interfering with or retarding the normal processes of mitosis. **2** A compound having such an effect and used to inhibit cell multiplication, as in chemotherapy for leukemia. Also *spindle poison.*
**antimongoloid** \-mäng′gəloid\ Marked by a downward slant of the outer aspect of the eyes, a feature of a number of syndromes. The condition occurs when the outer canthus of the palpebral fissure is lower than the inner, the opposite of a mongoloid appearance.
**antimony** Element number 51, having atomic weight 121.75. Antimony is a brittle, flaky metal, sometimes found native. Two stable isotopes occur in nature and numerous short-lived radioisotopes are known. Antimony is used chiefly as an alloying metal. Many of its compounds are toxic. Symbol: Sb
**antimony lithium thiomalate** ANTHIOLIMINE.
**antimony sodium tartrate** $Na(SbO)C_4H_4O_6 \cdot {}^1/_2 H_2O$. A crystalline salt of antimony used in treatment of trypanosomiasis and schistosomiasis and administered intravenously. It has the same schistosomicidal activity as the potassium salt and is claimed to be less toxic. Also *tartar emetic, sodium antimonyltartrate.*
**antimorph** \an′tēmôrf\ A mutant gene that tends to counteract the effect of its allele.
**antimorphic** \-môr′fik\ Tending to counteract the normal or wild-type genetic effect.
**antimuscarinic** **1** Having the ability to counteract the effects of muscarine and similar alkaloids, e.g., atropine. **2** An antimuscarinic agent.
**antimutagen** \-myoo′təjən\ Any factor that reduces the rate of spontaneous or induced mutation, either by rendering DNA less susceptible to alteration, interfering with the action of a mutagen, or promoting repair of DNA changes before they become fixed.
**antimycotic** \-mīkät′ik\ ANTIFUNGAL.
**antinarcotic** **1** Counteracting the effect of narcotics. **2** An antinarcotic agent.
**antinatriuresis** \-nā′trēyoorē′sis\ Decreased urinary excretion of sodium.
**antinauseant** \-nô′sē·ənt\ An agent that eliminates or relieves nausea.
**antineoplastic** \-nē′ōplas′tik\ [ANTI- + NEOPLASTIC] Acting against a neoplasm.
**antineuralgic** \-n$^y$Ural′jik\ [ANTI- + NEURALGIC] Relieving or preventing neuralgic pain: used especially of drugs or remedies.
**antineuritic** \-n$^y$Urit′ik\ [ANTI- + NEURITIC] Denoting a drug or remedy which prevents or relieves neuritis or neuropathy. Thus vitamin $B_1$ has been called the antineuritic vitamin since $B_1$ deficiency can cause polyneuropathy.
**antineurotoxin** \-n$^y$Ur′ətäk′sin\ [ANTI- + NEUROTOXIN] Any substance that delays, alleviates, or prevents the action of a neurotoxin.
**antinociceptive** \-nō′sisep′tiv\ **1** Tending to reduce the perception and behavioral effects of nociceptive stimuli. **2** ANALGESIC.
**antinuclear** \-n$^y$oo′klē·ər\ Forming a complex with or reacting with the nucleus of a cell.
**antioncotic** \-ängkät′ik\ [ANTI- + ONCOTIC] Acting against a tumor. *Obs.*
**antiovulatory** \-äv′yələtôr′ē\ [ANTI- + OVULATORY] Inhibiting the occurrence of ovulation.
**antiparallel** \-par′ələl\ Being parallel in position but opposite in direction, as two lines. The two strands of DNA

are so described, since the chains in the helix run in opposite directions.

**antiparalytic** \-par′əlit′ik\ Preventing, combating, or relieving paralysis: used especially of drugs, remedies, or therapeutic methods.

**antiparasympathomimetic** \-par′əsim′pəthōmimet′ik\ Denoting a drug, remedy, or method that counteracts or prevents the action of parasympathomimetic drugs.

**antipathogenic** \-path′əjen′ik\ **1** Acting against a pathogen. **2** An agent effective against a pathogen.

**antipedicular** \-pedik′yələr\ **1** Destructive of blood-sucking lice, especially those of the genus *Pediculus*.. **2** An agent that is destructive of blood-sucking lice; antipediculotic.

**antipediculotic** \-pedik′yəlät′ik\ **1** Effective against pediculosis; antipedicular. **2** An agent used in the treatment of pediculosis.

**antiperiodic** \-pir′ē·äd′ik\ **1** Acting against the periodic recurrence of symptoms or disease: used particularly with reference to recurrent fevers, as of malaria. **2** An agent used to prevent or alleviate the periodic recurrence of symptoms or disease.

**antiperistalsis** \-per′istal′sis\ RETROGRADE PERISTALSIS.

**antiperistaltic** \-per′istal′tik\ **1** Opposing or reducing peristaltic action. **2** An antiperistaltic agent. **3** Of or relating to antiperistalsis (retrograde peristalsis).

**antiperspirant** \-pur′spərənt\ An agent that has an inhibitory action on sweating. Also *antisudorific, anaphoretic, antihidrotic*.

**antiphagocytic** \-fag′əsit′ik\ Impeding the action of a phagocyte; preventing or slowing the rate of phagocytosis.

**antiphlogistic** Denoting a medication that prevents or corrects inflammation.

**antiphthiriac** \-thir′ē·ak\ **1** Destructive to blood-sucking lice; antipedicular. **2** An agent that is destructive to blood-sucking lice. See also ANTIPTHIRIAC.

**antiphthisic** \an′tifthiz′ik, an′tētiz′ik\ **1** Acting against tuberculosis, especially pulmonary tuberculosis. **2** An agent effective against tuberculosis, especially pulmonary tuberculosis.

**antiplasmin** \-plaz′min\ Any inhibitor of plasmin's fibrinolytic activity. The chief one is $\alpha_2$-antiplasmin.

**antiplasmodial** \-plazmō′dē·əl\ **1** Destructive or harmful to plasmodia. **2** An agent used to destroy plasmodia.

**antiplastic** \-plas′tik\ **1** Able to slow cellular division, especially that of the bone marrow. **2** Preventing or minimizing cicatrix formation. An obsolete usage. **3** Any antiplastic agent.

**antiplatelet** \-plāt′lət\ Designating a drug or antibody that reduces the number of platelets in the blood or diminishes their function.

**antipneumococcic** \-n$^y$oo′mōkäk′sik\ **1** Acting against *Streptococcus pneumoniae*.. **2** An agent effective against *Streptococcus pneumoniae*..

**antipodal** \antip′ədəl\ [*antipod(es)* + -AL] Situated on directly opposite sides of a cell or body.

**antipode** \an′tēpōd\ [back-formation from *antipodes*, from Gk *antipodes* (from *anti-* ANTI- + *podes*, pl. of *pous* foot) with feet opposite] An exact opposite.

**antiport** A transporter that exchanges one molecule or ion across a biologic membrane for another of the same or a different substance.

**antipraxia** A condition in which symptoms seem to be inconsistent or contradictory.

**antipraxy** The theory that the effect of a large dose of a drug should be completely opposite to that of a small dose of the same drug.

**antiprostate** \-präs′tāt\ GLANDULA BULBOURETHRALIS.

**antiprothrombin** \-prōthräm′bin\ Any anticoagulant which slows or prevents the conversion of prothrombin to thrombin.

**antipruritic** \-proorit′ik\ **1** Capable of relieving itching (pruritus). **2** A substance that relieves itching.

**antipsoriatic** \-sō′rē·at′ik\ **1** Acting against psoriasis. **2** An agent effective in treating psoriasis.

**antipsychotic** \-sīkät′ik\ NEUROLEPTIC.

**antipthiriac** \-thir′ē·ak\ **1** Destructive of lice of the genus *Pthirus*. **2** An agent effective against lice of the genus *Pthirus*. See also ANTIPHTHIRIAC.

**antipyogenic** \-pī′əjen′ik\ [ANTI- + PYOGENIC] **1** Acting against the production of pus. **2** An agent effective against the production of pus.

**antipyresis** The treatment of fever by the administration of drugs that lower body temperature.

**antipyretic** [ANTI- + PYRETIC] **1** Preventing or reducing fever. Also *antifebrile, febrifugal*. **2** An agent that prevents or reduces fever. Also *febrifuge, antithermic, febricide*.

**antirachitic** \-rəkit′ik\ **1** Preventing rickets. **2** Any substance having antirachitic characteristics. This includes any food that contains vitamin D, such as fish liver oil.

**antireticular** \-rətik′yələr\ Any substance or condition which inhibits the function of the reticuloendothelial system.

**antirheumatic** \-roomat′ik\ **1** Acting to counteract or palliate the effects of rheumatic disease. **2** An antirheumatic agent.

**antirickettsial** \-riket′sē·əl\ **1** Acting against rickettsiae. **2** An agent effective against rickettsiae.

**antisaluresis** \-sal′yoorē′sis\ Decreased urinary excretion of salts.

**antiscabietic** \-skā′bē·et′ik\ **1** Effective in the treatment of scabies. Also *antiscabious*. **2** An agent that is used against *Sarcoptes scabiei* in the treatment of scabies.

**antischistosomal** \-skis′təsō′məl\ **1** Destructive or harmful to schistosomes. **2** An agent capable of destroying or otherwise affecting the viability of schistosomes.

**antiscorbutic** \-skôrbyoo′tik\ **1** Preventing scurvy **2** Any substance having antiscorbutic characteristics. This includes any food that contains vitamin C, such as citrus fruit.

**antiseborrheic** \-seb′ôrē′ik\ **1** Tending to reduce the flow of sebum from the skin. **2** An agent used in the management of seborrheic dermatitis.

**antisecretory** \-sek′rətôr′ē\ Acting to stop or diminish secretion. Also *secretoinhibitory*.

**antiself** \an′tēself\ [ANTI- + *self*] In immunology, antibodies or lymphocytes reacting with the host's own antigens. ⟨"Perhaps these [multiple sclerosis] patients have an inborn error of immunologic perception, which permits the elaboration of antiself antibodies in the brain in response to the presence of an otherwise irrelevant virus" —Lewis Thomas, *The Youngest Science*, 1983, p. 73.⟩

**antisense** \an′tēsens\ Pertaining to the chain of the DNA double helix of a transcribed region of a chromosome that is *not* transcribed. The antisense DNA chain has the same nucleotide sequence (except for substitution of dTMP for UMP) as the mRNA.

**antisepsis** \-sep′sis\ The use of an antiseptic to reduce the number of viable bacteria on a surface.

**antiseptic** \-sep′tik\ [ANTI- + SEPTIC] **1** Pertaining to or capable of effecting antisepsis. **2** A substance capable of inhibiting or killing infectious agents, usually on a body surface. For defs. 1 and 2 also *colyseptic* (seldom used).

**antiserum** \an′tisir′əm\ A serum that contains antibodies, usually as a result of injection or transfusion of antigen or the result of infection or immunization. Also *immune serum.* **heterologous a.** An antibody directed against antigens found in another species. **homologous a.** An antibody directed against antigens found in the same species. **monospecific a.** A serum containing antibody reacting with only one antigen. **monovalent a.** A serum containing antibodies to one type of organism or only one antigen. Also *monovalent serum, monospecific serum.* **nerve growth factor a.** A substance consisting of antibodies to nerve growth factor and which when used either *in vivo* or *in vitro* negates the effects of nerve growth factor. **polyvalent a.** A serum containing antibodies directed against a number of different antigens. Also *polyvalent serum, multipartial serum.* **rabies a.** A preparation of native animal serum containing antibodies to the rabies virus. It is used, in conjunction with rabies vaccine, for the prevention of rabies in patients who have received bites in areas such as the head and neck from animals known or suspected of being rabid. **Rh a.** RH ANTIBODY. **therapeutic a.** A serum used in the treatment of a specific infection or disease.

**antisialagogue** \-sī·al′əgäg\ [ANTI- + SIALAGOGUE] An agent that suppresses the flow or the formation of saliva.

**antisialic** \-sī·al′ik\ Suppressing or decreasing the secretion of saliva.

**antisocial** \-sō′shəl\ [ANTI- + SOCIAL] **1** Characterized by avoidance of interpersonal relationships. **2** Manifesting behavior that violates the laws, rules, or moral or ethical code of one's culture indicating an antisocial and/or amoral personality.

**antispasmodic** \-spazmäd′ik\ [ANTI- + SPASMODIC] **1** Denoting a drug, remedy, or method that reduces activity in or relieves spasmodic contraction of unstriated muscle in the wall of the gastrointestinal tract or in blood vessels. **2** Any drug that reduces spasticity. An imprecise usage.

**antispastic** \-spas′tik\ Denoting a drug, remedy, or method that reduces or relieves spasticity.

**antispermotoxin** \-spur′mətäk′sin\ A substance that interferes with the action of a spermotoxin. Adj. antispermotoxic.

**antistaphylococcic** \-staf′əlōkäk′sik\ **1** Acting against staphylococci. **2** An agent effective against staphylococci.

**antisternum** \-stur′nəm\ A portion or area of the back opposite the sternum.

**antistreptococcic** \-strep′təkäk′sik\ **1** Acting against streptococci. **2** An agent effective against streptococci.

**antistreptolysin O** An antibody directed against the hemolysin, streptolysin O. Antistreptolysin O titers are raised in patients with rheumatic fever. Abbr. ASO

**antisudorific** \-soo′dôrif′ik\ ANTIPERSPIRANT.

**antisyphilitic** \-sif′ilit′ik\ **1** Of or relating to the treatment of syphilis. **2** A substance employed in the treatment of syphilis. For defs. 1 and 2 also *antiluetic.*

**antitetanolysin** \-tet′ənäl′isin\ An antibody that inhibits tetanolysin.

**antithenar** \antith′ənär\ **1** Located opposite the palm or the sole. **2** HYPOTHENAR.

**antithermic** ANTIPYRETIC.

**antithrombin** \-thräm′bin\ Any of several phenomena or plasma proteins that diminish the activity or concentration of thrombin during or following coagulation. The best characterized is antithrombin III, which is a single-chain normal plasma glycoprotein of 68 000 MW that combines with and neutralizes serum proteases, especially thrombin and factor Xa but also factors IXa, XIa, XIIa, and VII. Antithrombin I is the phenomenon of thrombin inhibition due to adsorption of thrombin by fibrin. Antithrombin II is a plasma protein that is a cofactor required for inhibition of thrombin by heparin. Antithrombin IV has properties like antithrombin III and is probably the same substance. Antithrombin V is the phenomenon of diminished thrombin activity in rheumatoid arthritis. Antithrombin VI is the phenomenon of thrombin inhibition by proteolytic "split products" of fibrinogen degradation.

**antithromboplastin** \-thräm′bəplas′tin\ An inhibitor of thromboplastin.

**antithrombotic** \-thrämbät′ik\ **1** Preventing the formation of thrombi. **2** An agent for dissolving thrombi.

**antithyroid** \-thī′roid\ [ANTI- + THYROID] Counteracting or inhibiting the function or hormonal secretion of the thyroid gland, or the effects of thyroid hormones. Also *antithyroidal.*

**antithyrotoxic** \-thī′rətäk′sik\ Counteracting the toxic effects of thyroid hormone, especially of excessive amounts of thyroid hormones, as in hyperthyroidism or hormonal overdose.

**antitonic** \-tän′ik\ **1** Reducing muscle tone. **2** Blocking or reducing the action of a drug or remedy used as a tonic.

**antitoxic** \-täk′sik\ [ANTI- + TOXIC] Counteracting the effect of a poison; relating to antitoxin.

**antitoxin** \-täk′sin\ [ANTI- + TOXIN] An antibody whose activity is measured by its ability to neutralize the toxic activity of the antigen to which it is raised. Antitoxins are commonly antibodies to bacterial toxins such as diphtheria or tetanus toxins. **botulism a.** A sterile, aqueous solution of the antibodies which neutralize toxin types A, B, and E of *Clostridium botulinum* and are used in the prevention and treatment of botulism. The trivalent antitoxin is of equine origin and is available in the United States only from the U.S. Centers for Disease Control. Subjects must be tested for sensitivity to horse serum before the antitoxin is given. The risk of hypersensitivity reactions is 9 percent, with anaphylaxis at 2 percent and serum sickness at 4 percent. Also *botulinum antitoxin, botulinus antitoxin, perfringens antitoxin, bivalent gas gangrene antitoxin, antibotulinus serum.* **bovine a.** Antitoxin prepared from cow serum instead of from horse serum, for use in subjects hypersensitive to horse serum. ***Crotalus* a.** A serum used in the treatment of poisoning by the venom of rattlesnakes of the genus *Crotalus.*. Also *anticrotalus serum.* **diphtheria a.** A sterile, aqueous solution of the antitoxic globulins isolated from the blood plasma or serum of a healthy horse immunized against the toxins of *Corynebacterium diphtheriae* and used in the prevention and treatment of diphtheria. Subjects must be tested for sensitivity to equine serum before the antitoxin is given. Also *antidiphtheria serum, Behring serum, Roux serum.* **gas gangrene a.** ANTI-GAS-GANGRENE SERUM. **perfringens a.** BOTULISM ANTITOXIN. **scarlet fever *Streptococcus* a.** A sterile prepration of immunoglobulins derived from the serum of healthy animals which have been immunized against the streptococci that cause scarlet fever. ***Staphylococcus* a.** A sterile preparation of immunoglobulins derived from the serum of healthy animals immunized against species of staphylococci. **tetanus a.** A sterile, aqueous solution of the antitoxic globulins isolated from the blood plasma or serum of a healthy human being, horse, or cow that has been immunized against the toxin of *Clostridium tetani.* It is used in the prevention and treatment of tetanus. Also *antitetanus serum.* **tetanus-perfringens a.** A serum prepared against the toxins of *Clostridium tetani* and *C. perfringens,* agents of tetanus and gas gangrene, respectively.

**antitragicus** \-traj′ikəs\ MUSCULUS ANTITRAGICUS.

**antitragus** \-trā′gəs\ [Gk *antitragos* (from *anti-* ANTI- + *tragos* he-goat, part of the ear) the part of the ear opposite the tragus. See TRAGUS.] [NA] A small tubercle projecting upward above the lobule of the auricle of the external ear and at the lower end of the anthelix. It lies opposite the anteriorly situated tragus and is separated from it by the intertragic incisure.

**antitreponemal** \-trep′ənē′məl\ **1** Destructive or harmful to *Treponema* organisms. **2** An agent capable of destroying *Treponema* organisms.

**antitrismus** \-triz′məs\ [ANTI- + TRISMUS] A disorder in which there is spasmodic or continuous contraction of the muscles which hold open the mouth and depress the lower jaw so that the mouth cannot be closed. Compare TRISMUS.

**antitrope** \an′tētrōp\ [ANTI- + -TROPE] One of a pair of bilaterally symmetrical organs or appendages of an organism, each being a mirror image of the other, e.g., the forelimbs or hindlimbs of a quadruped. Adj. antitropic.

**$\alpha_1$-antitrypsin** \-trip′sin\ Any of a group of glycoproteins migrating in the $\alpha_1$ region on serum protein electrophoresis and capable of inhibiting trypsin and such other proteolytic enzymes as elastase and collagenase. The levels rise nonspecifically in inflammation and with estrogen administration. Deficiency states, which are associated with development early in life of emphysema and/or cirrhosis, are determined by protease inhibitor (Pi) genes, of which M is the normal allele and Z and S are the most common abnormal forms.

**antituberculotic** \-tʸubur′kyəlät′ik\ An antituberculous agent.

**antituberculous** \-tʸubur′kyələs\ Acting against *Mycobacterium tuberculosis.*. Also *antituberculotic.*

**antitumor** \-tʸoo′mər\ [ANTI- + TUMOR] Describing activity against the growth, development, or spread of a tumor.

**antitumorigenic** \-tʸoomôr′ijen′ik\ [ANTI- + TUMORIGENIC] Acting against tumor development.

**antitussive** \-tus′iv\ [ANTI- + TUSSIVE] **1** Preventing or relieving coughing. **2** A remedy or medication that prevents or relieves coughing. For defs. 1 and 2 also *antibechic.*

**antivenene** \-ven′ēn\ ANTIVENIN.

**antivenereal** \-vənir′ē·əl\ **1** Opposing or counteracting venereal disease. **2** Any drug or treatment administered for the prophylaxis or cure of venereal disease. **3** Any drug or potion with anaphrodisiac properties.

**antivenin** \-ven′in\ [ANTI- + *ven(om)* + -IN] An antitoxin used to counteract animal venom, especially snake venom. Also *antivenom.* Also *antivenene.* **polyvalent crotaline a.** A sterile, lyophilized, polyvalent preparation of antivenom globulins from horse serum after immunization against four different pit viper species: *Crotalus atrox* (Western diamondback rattlesnake); *C. adamateus* (Eastern diamondback rattlesnake); *C. durissus terrificus* (South American rattlesnake); and *Bothrops atrox* (South American fer-de-lance).

**antivenom** \-ven′əm\ ANTIVENIN.

**antiviral** \-vī′rəl\ Destroying or counteracting viruses.

**antivirotic** \-vīrät′ik\ **1** Active against viruses or a virus; antiviral. **2** An antiviral agent.

**antivivisection** \-viv′isek′shən\ [ANTI- + VIVISECTION] Opposition to the use of living animals in biologic research.

**Anton** [Gabriel *Anton,* German neuropsychiatrist, 1858–1933] **1** Anton syndrome. See under SYMPTOM. **2** Anton-Babinski syndrome. See under SYNDROME.

**Antoni** [Nils Ragner Eugen *Antoni,* Danish neurologist, 1887–1968] See under NEURILEMMOMA.

**antral** \an′trəl\ Pertaining to an antrum.

**antrectomy** \antrek′təmē\ [*antr(um)* + -ECTOMY] An excision of an antrum, especially of the stomach.

**antritis** \antrī′tis\ [*antr(o)-* + -ITIS] **1** Inflammation of any antrum. **2** MAXILLARY SINUSITIS.

**antro-** \an′trō-\ [L *antrum* (from Gk *antron* cave) cave] A combining form denoting antrum.

**antroatticotomy** \-at′ikät′əmē\ ATTICOANTROTOMY.

**antrobuccal** \-buk′l\ Involving both the maxillary sinus and the cheek, or situated between them.

**antroduodenectomy** \-dʸoo′ōdenek′təmē\ Surgical resection of the pyloric antrum and the contiguous portion of the proximal duodenum.

**antromycosis** \-mīkō′sis\ [ANTRO- + MYCOSIS] Infection of the maxillary sinus with any species of fungus, particularly *Aspergillus* and *Candida.* Noninvasive and invasive varieties are recognized. The latter produces bone destruction and sometimes involvement of the orbit, and so needs to be differentiated from malignant disease.

**antronasal** \-nā′zəl\ Situated between or involving both the maxillary sinus and the interior of the nose.

**antroneurolysis** \-nʸuräl′isis\ Submucosal dissection to denervate the entire pyloric antrum.

**antrophore** [ANTRO- + -PHORE] A soluble, medicated bougie used in the treatment of disease in any cavity or canal, particularly the urethra.

**antrorse** \antrôrs′\ Turned forward and upward.

**antroscope** \an′trəskōp\ [ANTRO- + -SCOPE] A modified rigid fiberscope used for inspecting the interior of the maxillary sinus. It is passed through a broad straight cannula inserted into the maxillary sinus from beneath the inferior nasal concha.

**antrostome** \an′trəstōm\ [ANTRO- + Gk *stom(a)* mouth] A surgical opening, intended to persist, between the maxillary sinus and the inferior meatus of the nose. It is created to improve drainage in cases of chronic maxillary sinusitis.

**antrostomy** \anträs′təmē\ An operation creating an antrostome. **intranasal a.** Antrostomy in which the surgical approach is from within the nose. **radical maxillary a.** CALDWELL-LUC OPERATION.

**antrotomy** \anträt′əmē\ [ANTRO- + -TOMY] An operation to gain access to the interior of the maxillary sinus. **sublabial a.** An antrotomy in which the opening is created beneath the upper lip. It is performed as a means of exploring the antrum, of gaining access to structures beyond it, or as a step in more radical procedures.

**antrotympanic** \-timpan′ik\ Pertaining to the tympanic cavity and the mastoid antrum.

**antrotympanitis** Otitis media occurring most markedly in the tympanic and antral compartments of the middle ear. *Seldom used.*

**antrum** \an′trəm\ [L (from Gk *antron* cave, cavern), cave, cavern] (*pl.* antra) **1** A cavity or hollow within a bone. **2** A normal dilatation within certain hollow organs, such as the pyloric end of the stomach. **cardiac a.** PARS ABDOMINALIS ESOPHAGI. **duodenal a.** AMPULLA DUODENI. **ethmoid antra** *Outmoded* SINUS ETHMOIDALES. **a. folliculare** The cavity in a tertiary ovarian follicle that is filled with liquor follicularis and has a stratified epithelial lining of follicular cells thickened on one side by the cumulus oophorus. Also *follicular space.* **a. of Highmore** SINUS MAXILLARIS. **a. mastoideum** [NA] The large air sinus in the petrous part of the temporal bone communicating anteriorly by the aditus ad antrum with the epitympanic recess and posteriorly with some mastoid air cells that separate it from the sigmoid sinus. Its medial wall is related to the posterior semicircular canal, while the lateral wall is formed by the postmeatal process of the squamous part of the temporal bone. Its floor is perforated by foramina that communicate with mastoid air cells below, while the temporal lobe of the cerebrum rests on its roof. Also *mastoid antrum, mastoid cavity, Valsalva's antrum.* **maxillary a.** SINUS MAXILLARIS. **a. pyloricum** [NA] The dilated portion of the pyloric part of the stomach, situated between the angular incisure and the sulcus intermedius, which separate it from the body of the stomach and the pyloric canal respectively. Also *pyloric antrum, antrum of Willis, lesser cul-de-sac.* **tympanic a.** ANTRUM MASTOIDEUM. **Valsalva's a.** ANTRUM MASTOIDEUM. **a. of Willis** ANTRUM PYLORICUM.

**anuclear** \ān$^{y}$oo′klē·ər\ Without a cell nucleus, as an erythrocyte. Also *non-nucleated, anucleate.*

**anucleolar** \ā′n$^{y}$ooklē′ələr\ Lacking a nucleolus. Also *anucleolate.*

**ANUG** acute necrotizing ulcerative gingivitis.

**anulus** \an′yələs\ ANNULUS.

**anuresis** \an′yoorē′sis\ [Gk *an-* priv. + -URESIS] ANURIA.

**anuretic** \an′yooret′ik\ **1** Relating to or characterized by anuria. **2** Any agent or state that produces anuria.

**anuria** \ən$^{y}$oo′rē·ə\ [Gk *an-* priv. + -URIA] The absence of urine formation. It may result from urethral obstruction, bilateral cortical necrosis, or severe poststreptoccal acute glomerulonephritis. Oliguria of less than 200 ml per day is often erroneously referred to as anuria. Also *anuresis.* Adj. anuric, anuretic. **compression a.** The anuria of the crush syndrome. *Rare.* **obstructive a.** Cessation of urine flow usually caused by bilateral ureteral obstruction, or unilateral ureteral obstruction if only one kidney is functional. Bilateral renal arterial obstruction can also cause anuria. Also *postrenal anuria.* **prerenal a.** Cessation of urine flow secondary to decreased blood flow, either functional, as in shock or heart failure, or organic, as in renal artery occlusion. **renal a.** Cessation of urine flow caused by a disease of the kidney.

**anus** \ā′nəs\ [L, a ring, anus] The terminal orifice of the digestive tract, at the distal end of the anal canal and opening externally in the cleft between the buttocks. It is surrounded by wrinkled skin and is closed by sphincters. Also *archos* (outmoded). **artificial a.** A surgically created outlet of the intestinal stream other than the natural structure. Examples include any colostomy, ileostomy, or, more frequently, anal reconstruction necessitated by agenesis or incontinence. **imperforate a.** Absence of an external anal orifice on the perineum. It is usually secondary to failure of the embryonic proctodeal membrane to rupture, sometimes associated with anomalous partitioning of the embryonic cloaca, with the result that the anal canal or the rectum may be diverted to the urethra or vagina, or simply end blindly. Also *anal atresia, aproctia.* **a. vesicalis** A rectal opening into the urinary bladder. When of congenital origin, it is usually associated with an imperforate anus and is the result of incomplete development of the embryonic urorectal septum which normally partitions the cloaca into urogenital sinus and anorectal canal. **vulvovaginal a.** Anomalous location of the anus onto the vulva or vagina. When of congenital origin, it is usually associated with imperforate anus and is the result of incomplete development of the embryonic urorectal septum, which normally partitions the cloaca into urogenital sinus and anorectal canal. Also *anus vestibularis.*

**anvil** INCUS.

**anxiety** \angzī′itē\ [L *anxietas* (from *anxius* strained, stifled, from *anxus* past part. of *angere* to stifle, choke) anxiety] An unpleasant sensation consisting of a feeling of impending danger, apprehensive self-absorption, tense expectancy, a sense of uncertainty and powerlessness, and many physiologic manifestations of the body's readiness for emergency reactions, such as palpitations, sweating, and trembling. Unlike fear, anxiety is a response to an unreal, imagined, or unidentifiable danger. Also *neurotic anxiety.* **castration a.** Fear of genital loss or injury resulting in a castration complex. In psychoanalytic psychology, castration anxiety is considered to be one of the typical danger situations that occur in sequence in the developing child. It appears at 2½–3 years and persists to some degree throughout life, in the unconscious. For some psychoneurotic patients, it remains the major danger against which all their ego defenses are erected and around which their symptoms are developed. **existential a.** The malaise, fear, and dread experienced when one becomes aware of the prospect of nonbeing, nothingness, or death. The deep human concern with whether one can find a meaningful, satisfying, and fulfilling life is a necessary aspect of the dreadful encounter with nothingness, according to existentialist philosophy. **neurotic a.** ANXIETY. **separation a.** Anxiety provoked in a child by actual or threatened separation from the mother or mother-substitute. It is usually characterized by irritability, crying, and other signs of distress and protest. More often than not, it is a normal and expected reaction. **signal a.** In psychoanalytic psychology, the ego's defensive reaction to the threat that an id impulse will cross the repressive barrier and create a danger situation. The aroused anxiety signals the pleasure principle that danger is imminent, and the pleasure principle comes to the support of the ego in inhibiting or diverting the id impulse. The characteristic danger situations that provoke signal anxiety in the psychoneurotic subject are those that were passed through during early development: separation or loss of the love object during the first 1½ years of life, loss of love during the second year, castration or other body injury beginning at 2½–3 years, and the superego's punishment of guilt after the age of five or six.

**anxiolytic** \ang′zē·əlit′ik\ **1** Capable of preventing, reducing, or eliminating anxiety. **2** Any agent used in alleviating anxiety, such as benzodiazepine derivatives, antihistamine derivatives, and sedative drugs.

**AO** anodal opening.

**AOC** anodal opening contraction.

**AOCl** anodal opening clonus.

**aorta** \ā·ôr′tə\ [New L, from Gk *aortē* (akin to *aeirein* to raise, suspend) a great vessel, aorta, bronchus, knapsack; lit. something suspended or hanging, as the descending aorta seems to hang from the arch] [NA] The largest vessel of the systemic arterial system, from which the main arteries carrying oxygenated blood arise and subdivide into smaller and smaller vessels. Its orifice of origin is in the base of the left ventricle, from which it is separated by a valve, and it is divided for descriptive purposes into ascending aorta, arch of aorta, and descending aorta, the latter having thoracic and abdominal parts. It terminates in front of the fourth lumbar vertebra by bifurcating into the two common iliac arteries. Also *arteria aorta.* **abdominal a.** PARS ABDOMINALIS AORTAE. **a. abdominalis** PARS ABDOMINALIS AORTAE. **a. ascendens** PARS ASCENDENS AORTAE. **ascending a.** PARS ASCENDENS AORTAE. **bicuspal a.** A congenital anomaly in which the aortic orifice of the left ventricle possesses only two semilunar cusps, or valvules. **buckled a.** KINKED AORTA. **a. descendens** PARS DESCENDENS AORTAE. **descending a.** PARS DESCENDENS AORTAE. **descending thoracic a.** PARS THORACICA

AORTAE. **dextroposed a.** OVERRIDING AORTA. **dorsal a.** 1 The major artery of vertebrates that supplies arterial blood to the whole body except for the head and, in some species, the forelimbs. It originates from the systemic arch and runs caudad just ventral to the vertebral column to end as the caudal artery. In fishes, it arises from the arteries that drain the gills. 2 PARS DESCENDENS AORTAE. **dorsal embryonic a.** A large artery formed by fusion of the caudal portions of the paired primitive aortas of the embryo. It gives rise to the adult descending thoracic aorta, abdominal aorta, and median sacral artery. **double a.** A cardiovascular malformation in which both embryonic dorsal aortae persist as a vascular ring about the trachea and esophagus. Differential growth after birth may cause the ring to produce relative constriction of the trachea and esophagus, resulting in dysphagia and stridor. **dynamic a.** A markedly pulsating abdominal aorta, usually observed during radiological examination, as in fluoroscopic screening. **kinked a.** A distortion of the aortic arch at the isthmus just beyond the origin of the left subclavian artery that does not significantly obstruct the lumen and is usually recognized on radiological examination. Also *buckled aorta.* **left a.** The left dorsal aorta in the early embryo that fuses with the right one caudal to the developing heart to form a single channel that becomes the descending aorta of the adult. **overriding a.** A congenital anomaly, found with associated conditions in the tetralogy of Fallot, in which the aorta is so large in proportion to the narrowed pulmonary trunk that it pushes over to the right and arises astride the interventricular defect, receiving blood from both ventricles. Also *dextroposed aorta.* **palpable a.** An abdominal aorta that can be palpated easily through the anterior abdominal wall in a thin person. **pericardial a.** The portion of the ascending aorta invested, with the pulmonary trunk, by a tubular reflection of the serous pericardium, the posterior reflection forming the transverse sinus. *Outmoded.* **primitive a.** Either of a symmetrical pair of arteries formed during the third week in human embryos in mesoderm flanking the sides of the notochord and continued into the dorsolateral parts of the aortic arch arteries. The caudal portions soon fuse to form the dorsal aorta. The cranial portions do not fuse and in the head region become the internal carotid arteries which supply the brain. **a. sacrococcygea** *Outmoded* ARTERIA SACRALIS MEDIANA. **thoracic a.** PARS THORACICA AORTAE. **a. thoracica** PARS THORACICA AORTAE. **ventral a.** A vessel formed as a result of bifurcation of the cephalic end of the truncus arteriosus of the embryo. It supplies an arch artery to each of the branchial arches.

**aortae** \ā·ôr′tē\ Plural of AORTA.

**aortic** \ā·ôr′tik\ Of or pertaining to the aorta. Also *aortal.*

**aorticopulmonary** \ā·ôr′təkōpul′məner′ē\ Pertaining to the aorta and the pulmonary trunk or arteries. Also *aortopulmonary, aorticopulmonic.*

**aorticorenal** \ā·ôr′təkōrē′nəl\ Pertaining to the aorta and the kidney or kidneys.

**aortitis** \ā′ôrtī′tis\ [*aort(a)* + -ITIS] Inflammation of the aorta. In the past, it was most commonly due to syphilis, but this etiology has become rare in many countries. It may also occur due to giant cell arteritis, as part of Takayasu's disease, and in association with ankylosing spondylitis, and Reiter syndrome. **Döhle-Heller a.** SYPHILITIC AORTITIS. **rheumatic a.** Aortitis due to any of several rheumatic diseases, such as ankylosing spondylitis, Takayasu's arteritis, or rheumatic fever. **rheumatoid a.** Inflammation or nodule formation due to rheumatoid arthritis and affecting the aorta and/or the aortic valve. **syphilitic a.** Aortitis as a result of syphilis. Although aortic invasion starts early, its clinical presentation is a feature of tertiary syphilis. It is chiefly manifested by aortic regurgitation, stenosis of the coronary ostia, and aneurysm formation affecting the thoracic and especially the ascending aorta. Also *Döhle-Heller aortitis, Döhle disease, Heller-Döhle disease.* **ulcerous a.** An aortitis with ulceration.

**aortoarteritis** \ā·ôr′tō·är′terī′tis\ Arteritis of the aorta and the large arteries that is characterized by segmental stenoses and dilatations.

**aortocaval** \ā·ôr′tōkā′vəl\ Of or relating to processes that involve both the aorta and the vena cava, such as an aortocaval fistula.

**aortogram** \ā·ôr′təgram\ [*aort(a)* + *o* + -GRAM] A radiograph obtained during aortography.

**aortography** \ā′ôrtäg′rəfē\ [*aort(a)* + *o* + -GRAPHY] Radiographic examination of the aorta during and immediately after injection of a radiopaque agent into the aorta. **abdominal a.** Radiographic examination of the aorta, between the diaphragm and bifurcation, after the injection of a radiopaque agent. **intravenous a.** Radiographic examination of the aorta after its opacification by contrast medium injected into a peripheral vein. **retrograde a.** Radiographic study of the aorta after the intra-aortic injection of a contrast agent through a catheter which has been introduced into the aorta from a peripheral artery. **thoracic a.** Radiographic examination of the ascending aorta, aortic arch, and descending thoracic aorta after the injection of a radiopaque material. **translumbar a.** Radiologic examination of the abdominal aorta after the injection of a radiopaque agent through a catheter or needle which has been placed directly into the aorta percutaneously through the left flank.

**aortopathy** \ā′ôrtäp′əthē\ [*aort(a)* + *o* + -PATHY] Any disease affecting the aorta.

**aortoptosis** \ā′ôrtäptō′sis\ The downward displacement of the abdominal aorta, which can occur with visceroptosis.

**aortopulmonary** \ā·ôr′tōpul′məner′ē\ AORTICOPULMONARY.

**aortorrhaphy** \ā′ôrtôr′əfē\ [*aort(a)* + *o* + -RRHAPHY] Surgical repair of the aorta.

**aortosclerosis** \ā·ôr′tōsklerō′sis\ [*aort(a)* + *o* + SCLEROSIS] Arteriosclerosis affecting the aorta.

**aortotomy** \ā′ôrtät′əmē\ [*aort(a)* + *o* + -TOMY ] An aortic incision.

**AOS** anodal opening sound.

**AOTe** anodal opening tetanus.

**AP** 1 anterior pituitary. 2 angina pectoris. 3 arterial pressure. 4 anteroposterior.

**A-P** In radiology, the anteroposterior projection.

**ap-¹** \ap-\ APO-.

**ap-²** \ap-, əp-\ AD-.

**apallesthesia** \apal′esthē′zhə\ [A-¹ + PALLESTHESIA] PALLANESTHESIA.

**apancrea** \āpan′krē·ə\ [A-¹ + *pancre(as)* + *-(i)a*] An absence of the pancreas due to developmental failure. *Rare.*

**apancreatic** \āpan′krē·at′ik\ Characterized by the absence of the pancreas.

**aparalytic** \āpar′əlit′ik\ [Gk *a-* priv. + PARALYTIC] Without paralysis, or unaffected by paralysis.

**apathy** \ap′əthē\ [Gk *apatheia* insensibility to suffering, apathy] A pronounced indifference to one's surroundings and an absence of any evident feeling or emotion.

**apatite** A mineral containing the ions $Ca^{2+}$ and $PO_4^{3-}$ in the ratio 5:3, and also a univalent anion. That anion is often $OH^-$, in which case it is known as hydroxylapatite and occurs in bones and teeth. Replacement of $OH^-$ by $F^-$ strengthens it.

**apazone** $C_{16}H_{20}N_4O_2$. 5-(Dimethylamino)-9-methyl-2-propyl-1*H*-pyrazolo [1,2-a] [1,2,4] benzotriazine-1,3(2*H*)-dione, an anti-inflammatory analgesic drug whose properties resemble those of aspirin. It is used in the treatment of rheumatoid arthritis and osteoarthritis. Also *azapropazone*.

**APC** Acetylsalicylic acid, phenacetin, and caffeine, a combination of agents in many headache and cold tablets.

**APE** anterior pituitary extract.

**ape** Any of various large, tailless, nonhuman primates, especially one of the family Pongidae. **anthropoid a.** A primate of the family Pongidae; a chimpanzee, gorilla, orangutan, or gibbon. **great a.** An anthropoid ape of the subfamily Ponginae; a gorilla, orangutan, or chimpanzee.

**apellous** \āpel′əs\ [Gk *a-* priv. + L *pell(is)* the skin + -OUS] Circumcised; without a prepuce.

**apepsia** \āpep′sē·ə\ [Gk (from *a-* priv. + *peps(is)* cooking, digestion + -IA) indigestion] Absence of the digestive functions.

**apepsinia** \ā′pepsin′ē·ə\ Absence of secretion of pepsin by the stomach.

**aperient** \əpir′ē·ənt\ [L *aperiens*, gen. *aperientis*, pres. part. of *aperire* to open] A mild purgative or laxative. Also *aperitive*.

**aperiosteal** \āper′ē·äs′tē·əl\ Of or relating to a bone that is not enveloped in periosteum.

**aperitive** \əper′itiv\ [French *apéritif* (from L *aperire* to open) a stimulant to the appetite] **1** Having a stimulating effect on the appetite. **2** An appetite stimulant. **3** APERIENT.

**Apert** [Eugène *Apert*, French pediatrician, 1868–1940] **1** Apert syndrome, Apert's disease. See under ACROCEPHALOSYNDACTYLY. **2** See under SKULL. **3** Apert-Crouzon syndrome. See under ACROCEPHALOSYNDACTYLY TYPE II.

**apertura** \ap′ərt$^y$oo′rə\ [L (from *apertus*, past part. of *aperire* to open + *-ura* -URE), an opening] An opening or hole. Also *aperture*. **a. externa aqueductus vestibuli** [NA] A small slitlike orifice behind and lateral to the opening of the internal acoustic meatus near the center of the posterior surface of the petrous part of the temporal bone. The terminal part of the saccus endolymphaticus protrudes through the orifice into the posterior cranial fossa. Also *external aperture of aqueduct of vestibule, fissure of aqueduct of vestibule, external orifice of aqueduct of vestibule.* **a. externa canaliculi cochleae** [NA] A small foramen on the inferior surface of the petrous part of the temporal bone near the junction with the posterior surface and located below the internal acoustic meatus at the apex of a small triangular depression containing the inferior ganglion of the glossopharyngeal nerve in front of the medial portion of the jugular fossa. The foramen leads into the cochlear canaliculus and transmits the perilymphatic duct into a tubular prolongation of the dura mater that turns into the foramen so that a communication is established between the scala tympani and the subarachnoid space. Also *external aperture of canaliculus of cochlea, external opening of aqueduct of cochlea.* **a. lateralis ventriculi quarti** [NA] The opening on either side between the lateral recess of the fourth ventricle and the subarachnoid space. At its margins, the ependyma joins the pia mater. A tuft of the choroid plexus usually protrudes through it. Also *lateral aperture of fourth ventricle.* **a. mediana ventriculi quarti** [NA] A single midline opening in the roof of the fourth ventricle through which the ventricle communicates with the cerebellomedullary cistern. Also *median aperture of fourth ventricle, arachnoid foramen.* **a. pelvis inferior** [NA] The rhomboid lower opening of the true or lesser pelvis, bounded anteriorly by the ischiopubic rami, held together in the midline by the inferior pubic ligament, the posterior sides being the sacrotuberous ligaments, with the coccyx in the midline. Also *inferior aperture of minor pelvis, inferior pelvic strait, outlet of pelvis, pelvic outlet, inferior opening of pelvis.* **a. pelvis superior** [NA] The rounded or oval upper opening of the true, or lesser, pelvis, its boundaries forming the pelvic brim, comprising the terminal lines in front and at the sides and continuing through the sacral promontory posteriorly. Also *superior aperture of minor pelvis, pelvic plane of inlet, aditus pelvis* (outmoded), *first parallel pelvic plane, superior pelvic strait, pelvic inlet, pelvic brim, superior opening of pelvis, plane of inlet of pelvis.* **a. piriformis** [NA] The pear-shaped anterior bony aperture of the nasal cavities, wider below than above and bounded by the nasal bones and the maxillae. Also *bony anterior nasal aperture, piriform aperture, piriform opening, nasal opening of facial skeleton.* **a. sinus frontalis** [NA] The opening in the floor of the frontal sinus, lateral to the nasal spine and anterior to the ethmoidal notch and leading into the frontonasal canal, which ends in the anterior part of the middle meatus of the nasal cavity. Also *aperture of frontal sinus.* **a. sinus sphenoidalis** [NA] A rounded opening on each side of the sphenoidal crest in the upper part of the anterior wall of each sphenoidal sinus through which it communicates with the sphenoethmoidal recess of the nasal cavity. Also *aperture of sphenoid sinus, opening of sphenoidal sinus.* **a. thoracis inferior** [NA] The outlet of the skeleton of the thorax, wider in the transverse diameter than anteroposteriorly and closed by the diaphragm. It extends from the twelfth thoracic vertebra posteriorly along the costal arch to the infrasternal angle anteriorly, and the sides are formed by the twelfth and eleventh ribs. Also *inferior aperture of thorax, inferior thoracic aperture, thoracic outlet, lower thoracic opening, inferior thoracic opening.* **a. thoracis superior** [NA] The kidney-shaped inlet of the thoracic skeleton, its anteroposterior diameter being about one half the transverse diameter. It has a plane that inclines downwards and forwards from the first thoracic vertebra posteriorly to the top of the manubrium sterni anteriorly, the sides being formed by the first ribs. Also *superior aperture of thorax, superior thoracic aperture, thoracic inlet, superior thoracic opening, upper thoracic opening.* **a. tympanica canaliculi chordae tympani** [NA] A small orifice lateral to the pyramidal eminence in the posterior wall of the tympanic cavity through which the chorda tympani nerve emerges to pass forward across and behind the tympanic membrane from which it is separated by the handle of the malleus. The nerve is accompanied through the orifice by a branch of the stylomastoid artery. Also *tympanic aperture of canaliculus of chorda tympani.*

**aperturae** \ap′ərt$^y$oo′rē\ Plural of APERTURA.

**aperture** \ap′ərchər\ **1** APERTURA. **2** An opening or the diameter of such an opening, as in a lens to admit light. **angular a.** The angle formed by lines drawn from the focal point of a lens to diametrically opposed points on its periphery. Also *aperture of lens.* **bony anterior nasal a.** APERTURA PIRIFORMIS. **coded-image a.** A collimating device that provides a gamma camera with a series of overlapping pinhole images of a small organ such as the heart. The complete set is stored and decoded by computer to construct tomographic slices parallel to the camera's crystal. **external a. of aqueduct of vestibule** APERTURA EXTERNA AQUEDUCTUS VESTIBULI. **external a. of canaliculus of cochlea** APERTURA EXTERNA CANALICULI COCHLEAE. **a. of frontal sinus** APERTURA SINUS

FRONTALIS. **a. of glottis** RIMA GLOTTIDIS. **inferior a. of glottis** CAVITAS INFRAGLOTTICA. **inferior a. of minor pelvis** APERTURA PELVIS INFERIOR. **inferior thoracic a.** APERTURA THORACIS INFERIOR. **inferior a. of thorax** APERTURA THORACIS INFERIOR. **a. of larynx** ADITUS LARYNGIS. **lateral a. of fourth ventricle** APERTURA LATERALIS VENTRICULI QUARTI. **a. of lens** ANGULAR APERTURE. **median a. of fourth ventricle** APERTURA MEDIANA VENTRICULI QUARTI. **numerical a.** A calculation that describes the resolving power and light-gathering properties of a lens. It is the product of the refractive index of the medium through which the object is viewed times the sine of one half the angle of aperture of the lens. Abbr. NA **orbital a.** ADITUS ORBITAE. **piriform a.** APERTURA PIRIFORMIS. **posterior nasal a.** CHOANA. **a. of sphenoid sinus** APERTURA SINUS SPHENOIDALIS. **spinal a.** FORAMEN VERTEBRALE. **spurious a. of facial canal** *Outmoded* HIATUS CANALIS NERVI PETROSI MAJORIS. **superior a. of minor pelvis** APERTURA PELVIS SUPERIOR. **superior thoracic a.** APERTURA THORACIS SUPERIOR. **superior a. of thorax** APERTURA THORACIS SUPERIOR. **tympanic a. of canaliculus of chorda tympani** APERTURA TYMPANICA CANALICULI CHORDAE TYMPANI.

**apex** \ā′peks\ [L, a point, top, summit] (*pl.* apices) The pointed tip, extremity, or summit of a conical or triangular structure. **a. auriculae** [NA] A pointed projection on the outer or upper margin of the ear in lower mammals, corresponding to the tuberculum auriculae in humans. **a. of bladder** APEX VESICAE URINARIAE. **a. capitis fibulae** [NA] A rough eminence projecting upwards from the lateral side of the posterior surface of the head of the fibula on which the tendon of insertion of the biceps femoris muscle is split in two by the fibular collateral ligament. Also *styloid process of fibula.* **a. cartilaginis arytenoideae** [NA] The pointed superior process of the pyramid-shaped arytenoid cartilage that curves upwards, backwards, and medially to articulate with the corniculate cartilage in the free edge of the aryepiglottic fold that is attached to the apex. **a. cordis** [NA] The rounded apex of the cone-shaped left ventricle of the heart, located at the junction of the left and inferior borders of the heart and pointing to the left, anteriorly, and downwards. On the surface of the chest it is located clinically in the fifth left intercostal space just within the midclavicular line about 9 cm ($3^1/_2$ in) from the midline. Also *apex of heart.* **a. cornus posterioris medullae spinalis** [NA] On cross sections of the spinal cord, a crescentic or angular stratum of large neurons capping the substantia gelatinosa of the dorsal horn, sometimes including the substantia as well. Also *zona spongiosa.* **a. of heart** APEX CORDIS. **a. linguae** [NA] The pointed, rounded most anterior extremity of the tongue at the junction of the two free margins and usually resting against the incisor teeth. Also *apex of tongue, tip of tongue.* **a. of lung** APEX PULMONIS. **a. nasi** [NA] The most distal, angulate free extremity of the external nose. Also *tip of nose.* **a. ossis sacri** [NA] The blunted distal extremity of the sacrum that has an oval facet for articulation with the coccyx. Also *apex of sacrum, tip of sacral bone.* **a. partis petrosae ossis temporalis** [NA] The rough, irregular anteromedial end of the petrous part of the temporal bone that fits into the angular interval between the basilar part of the occipital bone and the posterior border of the greater wing of the sphenoid bone. It is characterized by the anterior opening of the carotid canal for the exit of the internal carotid artery, and it forms the posterolateral border of the foramen lacerum. Also *apex of petrous portion of temporal bone.* **a. patellae** [NA] The pointed inferior extremity of the triangular patella bone that provides the proximal attachment of the ligamentum patellae. Also *apex of patella.* **a. of petrous portion of temporal bone** APEX PARTIS PETROSAE OSSIS TEMPORALIS. **a. prostatae** [NA] The inferior, distal slightly narrowed portion of the conical chestnut-shaped prostate gland that rests upon the superior fascia of the urogenital diaphragm just above the sphincter urethrae. It contains the terminal part of the prostatic urethra. Also *apex of prostate gland.* **a. pulmonis** [NA] The conical, rounded upper extremity of each lung which lies in the plane of the thoracic inlet and extends up about one inch above the middle third of the clavicle. The cervical pleura covers it and lies between it and the suprapleural membrane. Also *apex of lung.* **a. radicis dentis** [NA] The tip of the root of a tooth most distal from the crown, perforated by one or more foramina for the entry of nerves and nutrient vessels into the pulp canal. Also *root apex, root tip.* **a. of sacrum** APEX OSSIS SACRI. **a. of tongue** APEX LINGUAE. **a. vesicae urinariae** [NA] The narrowed anterior part of the urinary bladder at the junction of its superior and inferolateral surfaces that extends towards the upper part of the symphysis pubis and has the median umbilical ligament, or remnant of the urachus, connecting it to the umbilicus behind the anterior abdominal wall. Also *apex of bladder.*

**apexcardiogram** \ā′pekskär′dē·ōgram′ \ **1** The graphic recording of cardiac movement in the region of the apex beat. **2** Any graphical recording of the movements of the heart against the chest wall.

**apexcardiography** \ā′pekskär′dē·äg′rəfē\ The technique of recording apexcardiograms.

**Apgar** [Virginia *Apgar,* U.S. anesthesiologist, 1909–1974] **1** Apgar scale. See under APGAR TEST. **2** See under SCORE.

**APH** anterior pituitary hormone (adenohypophysial hormone).

**aph-** \af-\ APO-.

**aphacia** \əfā′shə\ APHAKIA.

**aphacic** \əfā′sik\ APHAKIC.

**aphagia** \əfā′jə\ [Gk *a-* priv. + -PHAGIA] Unwillingness or inability to eat.

**aphagopraxia** \əfā′gōprak′sē·ə\ DYSPHAGIA.

**aphake** \af′āk\ An individual with aphakia: used in reference to persons who have had cataractous lenses removed.

**aphakia** \əfā′kē·ə\ [A-[1] + *phak(o)-* + -IA] Absence of the crystalline lens of the eye. Also *aphacia.* Adj. aphakic, aphakial.

**aphakic** \əfā′kik\ Pertaining to or characterized by aphakia; lacking a crystalline lens. Also *aphakial, aphacic.*

**aphalangia** \ā′fəlan′jē·ə\ [Gk *a-* priv. + *phalang(es)* + -IA] The absence of one or more phalanges in one or more fingers and toes.

**aphalgesia** \af′aljē′zē·ə\ HAPHALGESIA.

# aphasia

**aphasia** \əfā′zhə\ [Gk *aphasia* (from *a-* priv. + *phasis* speech, from *phanai* to speak + -IA) speechlessness] A change in, or loss of, the ability to use or understand spoken or written language, usually attributable to a cerebral lesion and occurring in the absence of any defect of phonation or articulation. Aphasia can be classified into two main forms, motor (expressive) aphasia and sensory (receptive) aphasia. **acoustic a.** WERNICKE'S APHASIA. **acoustic amnestic a.** NOMINAL APHASIA. **amnemonic a.** NOMINAL APHASIA. **amnesic a.** NOMINAL APHASIA. **amnestic a.** NOMINAL APHASIA. **anosmic a.** Inability to describe smell sensation in words. *Seldom used.* **apractic a.** BROCA'S APHASIA. **association a.** CONDUCTION APHASIA. **associative a.** CONDUCTION APHASIA. **auditory a.** WERNICKE'S APHASIA. **Broca's a.** Aphasia characterized by loss of the ability to express thoughts in words even though understanding of spoken and written language is intact. When the condition is complete the patient may be mute. Less severe forms are marked by hesitancy in spontaneous speech, poverty of words at the patient's command, and sometimes the repetition of isolated words or of expletives, and dysarthria is common. Usually there is associated agraphia. As the lesion responsible is in Broca's area, at the posterior end of the inferior frontal gyrus of the dominant hemisphere, there is often a contralateral hemiparesis, affecting predominantly the face and hand, due to involvement of the contiguous motor cortex. Also *expressive aphasia, motor aphasia, cortical motor aphasia, efferent motor aphasia, apractic aphasia, frontocortical aphasia, nonfluent aphasia, pure word dumbness, logaphasia, kinetic motor aphasia.* **central sensory a.** WERNICKE'S APHASIA. **color name a.** Aphasia manifested by inability to name colors. Also *amnesic color blindness.* **combined a.** Two or more types of aphasia occurring in the same patient. **commissural a.** CONDUCTION APHASIA. **complete a.** Total loss of the ability to express thoughts in language and to understand spoken and written language. **conduction a.** Aphasia characterized by fluency in spontaneous speech with paraphasia (use of incorrect words), and by normal or nearly normal comprehension of spoken language but markedly impaired repetition of words and phrases, usually with difficulty in naming people and objects. There may be associated apraxia of facial and limb movement. The condition is due to a lesion of the pathways joining Broca's and Wernicke's areas, usually in the suprasylvian or subsylvian regions. Also *association aphasia, associative aphasia, commissural aphasia, frontolenticular aphasia, lenticular aphasia, transcortical sensory aphasia, subcortical aphasia.* **cortical a.** Any form of aphasia due to a cortical lesion. *Outmoded.* **cortical motor a.** BROCA'S APHASIA. **cortical sensory a.** SENSORY APHASIA. **crossed a.** Aphasia occurring in a left-handed person due to a left hemisphere lesion or in a right-handed person due to one of the right hemisphere. **efferent motor a.** BROCA'S APHASIA. **expressive a.** BROCA'S APHASIA. **expressive-receptive a.** GLOBAL APHASIA. **finger a.** FINGER AGNOSIA. **fluent a.** Any sensory aphasia, such as jargon aphasia, in which there is a fluent but meaningless flow of words. **frontocortical a.** BROCA'S APHASIA. **frontolenticular a.** CONDUCTION APHASIA. **functional a.** Aphasia due to hysteria. Also *pseudoaphasia.* **gestural a.** AMIMIA. **gibberish a.** JARGON APHASIA. **global a.** Defects of all those processes, both expressive and receptive, which contribute to speech or to verbal communication. Also *total aphasia, expressive-receptive aphasia.* **graphic motor a.** AGRAPHIA. **graphomotor a.** AGRAPHIA. **impressive a.** SENSORY APHASIA. **jargon a.** A type of sensory or receptive aphasia characterized by deformation and transposition of syllables and words, or the use of correctly formed but inappropriate words, making speech unintelligible. Also *literal paraphasia, jargonorrhea, jargonaphasic logorrhea, gibberish aphasia, choreic paraphasia* (obs.), *jumbled speech.* Also *jargonaphasia.* **kinetic motor a.** BROCA'S APHASIA. **lenticular a.** CONDUCTION APHASIA. **a. lethica** NOMINAL APHASIA. **Lichtheim's a.** A variant of Broca's aphasia, with total loss of spontaneous speech, but retention of the ability to repeat words which the patient learns and/or of the ability to indicate with the fingers the number of syllables in the word of which he is thinking. *Seldom used.* **mixed a.** Any aphasia in which there is a combination of expressive (motor) and receptive (sensory) deficits. The most severe form is global aphasia. **monoglot asphasia** Loss by a polyglot patient of the ability to speak one language. **motor a.** BROCA'S APHASIA. **musical a.** AMUSIA. **nominal a.** A form of aphasia characterized by inability to recall words, especially the names of people or objects. Understanding of spoken and written language, writing from dictation, reading aloud, and repetition are unimpaired, and the word which is wanted may be uttered in spontaneous speech. The affected individual is able to recognize the object or person and may be able to demonstrate the use to which the object is put, even if he cannot name it. The causal lesion is usually in the dominant posterior temporal or parietal region. Also *amnesic aphasia, anomic aphasia, amnemonic aphasia, acoustic amnesic aphasia, aphasia lethica, amnestic aphasia, lethologica.* **nonfluent a.** BROCA'S APHASIA. **parieto-occipital a.** Alexia combined with apraxia. *Obs.* **paroxysmal a.** Any form of aphasia characterized by recurring and transient episodes, resulting either from jacksonian epilepsy due to cortical lesion, from recurrent cerebral ischemia, as in migraine or transient cerebral ischemic attacks, or from other recurring episodes of cerebral dysfunction. **posterior a.** Any sensory or receptive aphasia due to a lesion of the dominant temporoparietal cortex. Also *temporoparietal aphasia.* **puerperal a.** Aphasia developing during pregnancy, labor, or the puerperium. **pure motor a.** A restricted form of Broca's aphasia with severe impairment of the ability to express thoughts in words, in the absence of any defect of understanding of spoken or written language or of the ability to write. Often the patient has very few words at his command; these are produced hesitantly or repetitively and there is often severe agrammatism. Speech may be telegraphic (telegrammatism) or reduced to stereotypic utterances (stereotypy). Often there is severe associated dysarthria with contralateral facial weakness and hemiplegia. Also *subcortical motor aphasia, verbal aphasia* (outmoded). • In the past this name has often been given incorrectly to anarthria resulting from a cerebral lesion. **receptive a.** SENSORY APHASIA. **semantic a.** A form of aphasia marked by lack of recognition of the full significance of words and phrases. The patient often finds it difficult to understand the significance of a narrative or to draw logical conclusions from a particular sequence of thoughts and he may leave phrases unfinished. Often there is associated difficulty in interpreting maps and plans, with evidence of topographical agnosia. This is probably a complex disorder in which mild receptive aphasia is associated with other features of parietal lobe dysfunction. **sensory a.** Any of those forms of aphasia in which there is inability to understand spoken speech (word deafness), writing or printed words (word blindness) or gestures (receptive amimia), or to distinguish musical sounds (receptive amusia). Also *receptive aphasia, cortical sensory aphasia, impressive aphasia.* **subcortical a.** CONDUCTION APHASIA. **subcortical motor a.** PURE MOTOR APHASIA. **syntactical a.** Any form of aphasia in which syntax is impaired. Examples include loss of prepositions or other connecting words (agrammatism) or the use of words in an incorrect sequence. Also *agrammaphasia* (seldom used), *pseudoagrammatism*. **tactile a.** Nominal aphasia manifested by inability to name objects which are placed in the hand even though they are recognized by touch. **temporoparietal a.** POSTERIOR APHASIA. **total a.** GLOBAL APHASIA. **transcortical a.** Aphasia with retention of the ability to repeat words on dictation although spontaneous speech and understanding of words may both be impaired. It is a specific variety of conduction aphasia due to a lesion of the pathway joining Broca's and Wernicke's areas. **transcortical sensory a.** CONDUCTION APHASIA. **verbal a.** *Outmoded* PURE MOTOR APHASIA. **visual a.** ALEXIA. **Wernicke's a.** A common form of sensory or receptive aphasia due to a lesion in Wernicke's area of the dominant temporal lobe, usually in the posterior part of the first and second temporal gyri. There is severe inability to understand spoken words either individually or in phrases and sentences, with difficulty in repeating words on dictation. Spontaneous speech is, however, fluent but inappropriate in that the patient uses incorrect words (paraphasia) or else uses them in the wrong sequence, so that he speaks in jargon, but articulation is usually normal. Reading and writing are usually severely impaired. Because of the situation of the lesion a hemianopia or contralateral homonymous quadrantic field defect is often present. Also *acoustic aphasia, auditory aphasia, central sensory aphasia, logasthenia* (outmoded), *logokophosis* (outmoded).

**aphasiac** \əfā′zē·ak\ An aphasic individual.

**aphasic** \əfā′zik\ Relating to aphasia.

**aphasiologist** \əfā′zē·äl′əjist\ [*aphasiolog(y)* + -IST] One who studies disorders in speaking and writing language.

**aphasiology** \əfā′zē·äl′əjē\ [*aphasi(a)* + *o* + -LOGY] The study of disorders associated with speaking or writing language.

**aphasmid** \āfaz′mid\ [Gk *a-* priv. + PHASMID] A nematode lacking phasmids, the caudal sensory organs. The class formerly including these nematodes, Aphasmidia, is now given the name Adenophorea.

**apheresis** \əfer′əsis\ [Gk *aphairesis* (from *aphairein* to remove, withdraw, from *apo-* apart, off + *hairein* to take, seize) removal] HEMAPHERESIS. • This term, or the linguistically incorrect variant *pheresis*, is used in combination to indicate components being separated out, as *leukapheresis, plasmapheresis, plateletpheresis*.

**aphonia** \afō′nē·ə\ [Gk *aphōnia* (from *a-* priv. + *phōnē* sound of the voice) speechlessness] A variety of dysphonia in which the voice is completely lost or reduced to a whisper. Although organic disease, for example bilateral complete laryngeal paralysis, may produce it, the common cause is functional. **hysterical a.** Aphonia due to hysteria, with the result that the subject cannot speak, except in a whisper, but can cough, as in the case of the professional singer who loses his voice before an important engagement. Also *functional aphonia*. **a. paralytica** Aphonia due to bilateral complete laryngeal paralysis. *Outmoded.*

**aphonic** \afän′ik\ **1** A subject with aphonia. **2** Affected by aphonia.

**aphose** \afōz′\ [Gk *a-* priv. + *phōs* light, luminosity] SCOTOMA.

**aphosphorosis** \āfäs′fōrō′sis\ [A-[1] + *phosphor(us)* + -OSIS] A rare syndrome caused by a depletion of body phosphorus, as results from chronic and excessive use of insoluble antacids. It causes anorexia, malaise, weakness, skeletal pain, hemolytic anemia, granulocyte dysfunction, hypercalcemia, and production of renal calculi. It is easily cured by cessation of the medication causing the syndrome and a diet rich in phosphorus.

**aphrenia** \əfrē′nē·ə\ [Gk *a-* priv. + PHREN- + -IA] **1** *Obs.* MENTAL RETARDATION. **2** *Obs.* DEMENTIA.

**aphrodisiac** \af′rōdiz′ē·ak\ [Gk *aphrodisiak(os)* (from *aphrodisia*, neut. pl. of *aphrodisios* pertaining to love or venery, after *Aphroditē* goddess of love, L *Venus*) pertaining to sexual love] **1** Tending to stimulate sexual desire. **2** An aphrodisiac agent.

**aphtha** \af′thə\ Singular of APHTHAE.

**aphthae** \af′thē\ [Gk *aphthai* thrush] **1** Small, superficial, and often painful ulcers, especially of the mouth or pharynx, sometimes of the genitalia, characteristically multiple and often recurrent. Also *aphthous ulcers*. See also APHTHOUS STOMATITIS. **2** The lesions of thrush. *Older term.* **Bednar's a.** A pair of shallow ulcers about 1 cm in diameter, one on either side of the median raphe of the hard palate of infants. It is probably traumatic from friction of unsuitable teats or faulty feeding practice. It is a rare condition. **Behçet a.** BEHÇET SYNDROME. **cachectic a.** Ulcerative stomatitis in cachectic or debilitated patients, especially children, when attention to oral hygiene has been neglected. *Rare.* **contagious a.** FOOT-AND-MOUTH DISEASE. **epizootic a.** FOOT-AND-MOUTH DISEASE. **a. epizooticae** FOOT-AND-MOUTH DISEASE. **a. febriles** Aphthae occurring in conjunction with a fever. **malignant a.** FOOT-AND-MOUTH DISEASE. **Mikulicz a.** PERIADENITIS MUCOSA NECROTICA RECURRENS. **recurrent scarring a.** PERIADENITIS MUCOSA NECROTICA RECURRENS. **a. tropicae** Oral ulceration which produces whitish spots in the mouth and which may accompany tropical disorders, especially tropical sprue. Such disorders are usually associated with gross vitamin deficiencies of the B group. The administration of vitamin B supplements is combined with treatment of the underlying condition.

**aphthoid** \af′thoid\ APHTHOUS.

**aphthosa** \afthō′sə\ [New L, short for *febris aphthosa* aphthous fever] FOOT-AND-MOUTH DISEASE.

**aphthosis** \afthō′sis\ [*aphth(a)* + -OSIS] Any condition marked by the development of aphthae. **Touraine's a.** BEHÇET SYNDROME.

**aphthous** \af′thəs\ **1** Characterized by the occurrence or presence of aphthae. **2** Resembling aphthae. Also *aphthoid*.

**aphtovirus** \af′tōvī′rəs\ [*apht(hae)* + *o* + VIRUS ] A rhinovirus that causes foot-and-mouth disease (aphthous fever).

**apic-** \ā′pik-, ap′ik-, ā′pis-\ [L *apex*, gen. *apicis*, point, top, summit] A combining form meaning apex, apical. Also *apici-, apico-*.

**apical** \ap′ikəl\ Pertaining to or located at or near the apex of a structure.

**apicectomy** \ā′pisek′təmē\ APICOECTOMY.

**apices** \ap′isēz\ Plural of APEX.

**apici-** \ā′pisē-\ APIC-.

**apicilar** \āpis′ilər\ Attached to or located at the apex of a structure.

**apicitis** \ā′pisī′tis\ Inflammation of or involving an apex. **orbital a.** TOLOSA-HUNT SYNDROME.

**apico-** \ā′pikō-, ap′ikō-\ APIC-.

**apicoectomy** \ā′pikō·ek′təmē\ [APICO- + -ECTOMY] The surgical removal of the apex of a tooth root. It is carried out when conventional root canal treatment is impossible or unsuccessful. Also *apicectomy, apiectomy, root resection*.

**apicolysis** \ā′pikäl′isis\ [APICO- + LYSIS] A surgical procedure to collapse the apex of the lung, as formerly used in treatment of pulmonary tuberculosis.

**Apicomplexa** \ap′ikämplek′sə\ [New L, from *api(cal) complex*] A phylum of protozoa, all species of which are parasitic and are characterized by the so-called apical complex of organelles (polar rings, rhoptries, micronemes, conoid, and subpellicular microtubules) present at some stage of development. Cilia are absent and sexuality is by syngamy. It includes the class Sporozoea with the gregarines, coccidia (including the malarial parasites and related organisms), and the piroplasms. It was formerly considered a subphylum but was raised to phylum status in 1980.

**apicostomy** \ā′pikäs′təmē\ [APICO- + -STOMY] A form of surgical drainage in which the apex of a tooth root is exposed.

**apiectomy** \ā′pi·ek′təmē\ APICOECTOMY.

***Apiochaeta ferruginea*** \ā′pē·äkē′tə fer′oojin′ē·ə\ See under MEGASELIA.

**apiotherapy** \ā′pē·ōther′əpē\ [L *api(s)* bee + *o* + THERAPY] The therapeutic use of bee venom. In some parts of the world it is used to treat rheumatoid arthritis. Also *melissotherapy.*

**apisin** \ā′pisin\ BEE VENOM.

**A.P.L.** A preparation of urinary human chorionic gonadotropin. A proprietary name.

**aplacental** \ā′pləsen′təl\ **1** Lacking a placenta. **2** Any animal lacking a placenta.

**aplanatic** \ap′lənat′ik\ [Gk *a-* priv. + *planat(os)* (Doric variant of *planētos*) wandering, irregular, from *plan(asthai)* to wander, be irregular + -IC] Characterizing an optical system that is free of coma and spherical aberration.

**aplasia** \əplā′zhə\ [New L (from Gk *a-* priv. + *plas(is)* a forming, from *plassein* to form, + -IA), formlessness] The incomplete development of an organ or tissue. Rudimentary or primordial structures may be recognizable. Compare AGENESIS, DYSPLASIA, HYPOPLASIA. **a. axialis corticalis congenita** CEREBRAL DIFFUSE SCLEROSIS. **a. axialis extracorticalis congenita** PELIZAEUS-MERZBACHER DISEASE. **congenital pure red cell a.** DIAMOND-BLACKFAN ANEMIA. **a. cutis congenita** A developmental defect, sometimes of genetic origin, in which the skin is absent at birth, usually from sharply circumscribed areas of the vertex but occasionally from elsewhere on the scalp or on the limbs. The subcutis is often also missing. **germinal a.** GONADAL DYSGENESIS. **germinal cell a.** SERTOLI-CELL-ONLY SYNDROME. **lobular a.** A failure in development of the kidney characterized by a reduction of reniculi and calyces to five or less. Also *lobular hypoplasia.* **nuclear a.** Lack or impairment of development of one or more nuclei. **thymic a.** Congenital absence of the thymus, as seen in the DiGeorge syndrome. **thymic-parathyroid a.** DIGEORGE SYNDROME.

**aplastic** \āplas′tik\ [Gk *aplast(os)* (from *a-* priv. + *plassein* to form) unformed + -IC] **1** Characterized by failure of normal formation, development, or regeneration. **2** In embryology, denoting a cell or primordium not yet exhibiting signs of differentiation into more advanced cell or structure type.

**apleuria** \əplʊr′ē·ə\ [Gk *apleur(os)* without ribs + -IA] A developmental absence of one or more ribs, often associated with absence of the transverse process of the corresponding vertebra.

**apnea** \apnē′ə\ [Gk *apnoia* (from *a-* priv. + *pnoē* wind, breath) absence of breath] The absence or cessation of breathing. Adj. apneic. **chemoreceptor a.** Apnea caused by the administration of oxygen in the presence of central respiratory depression due to hypercarbia or opioids. When hypoxia causes peripheral chemoreceptors in the carotid body to maintain respiration reflexively, the administration of oxygen may remove the peripheral anoxic stimulus to breathing and thus produce apnea. **deglutition a.** The reflex inhibition of respiration, usually expiration, that takes place during swallowing. **hypersomnia sleep a.** OBSTRUCTIVE SLEEP APNEA. **induced a.** Apnea caused by the deliberate use of drugs acting on the central nervous system, as with opioids, or on the peripheral nervous sytem, as with neuromuscular blockers. **initial a.** Failure by a newborn infant to establish a sustained respiratory pattern within two minutes after birth. **a. in newborn** APNEA NEONATORUM. **late a.** Cessation of respiration for one minute or more by a newborn after sustained respiration has been established. **a. neonatorum** Failure of the initiation and maintenance of respiration in the newborn due to the effects of fetal anoxia on the nervous system. The initial failure (primary apnea) is succeeded by a phase of gasping. If recovery does not ensue, then, after a last spontaneous gasp, the infant enters a critical and potentially fatal stage (secondary or terminal apnea). Recovery is still possible by assisted respiration. Also *apnea in newborn.* **obstructive sleep a.** Episodes of apnea occurring during deep sleep due to inspiratory obstruction by the relaxed walls of the oropharynx. It is eventually relieved when increasingly strong inspiratory efforts succeed in drawing air past the obstruction to the accompaniment of a loud snore. **postanesthesia a.** PSEUDOCHOLINESTERASE DEFICIENCY. **primary a.** See under APNEA NEONATORUM. **secondary a.** See under APNEA NEONATORUM. **terminal a.** See under APNEA NEONATORUM. **traumatic a.** Absence of breathing following injury.

**apneumia** \apnʸoo′mē·ə\ [Gk *a-* priv. + PNEUM- + -IA] The developmental absence of one or both lungs.

**apneusis** \apnʸoo′sis\ [Gk *a-* priv. + PNEUSIS] Prolonged breath-holding at full inspiration. Adj. apneustic.

**apnoea** \apnē′ə\ *Brit.* APNEA.

**apo-** \ap′ō-\ [Gk *apo* (*aph-* as prefix before Gk aspirated vowel) away from, off, after] **1** A prefix meaning (1) separate; (2) derived or formed from. **2** In biochemistry, a prefix denoting an enzyme from which a cofactor, usually a tightly bound one, has been removed. The apo- enzyme is often catalytically inactive. Also *ap-*, *aph-*.

**apoatropine** $C_{17}H_{21}NO_2$. 1$\alpha$*H*,5$\alpha$*H*-tropan-3$\alpha$-ol atropate, the anhydride of atropine that is found with atropine in the belladonna root. It has limited use as an antispasmodic agent. Also *atropanine.*

**apochromat** \-krōmat′\ APOCHROMATIC OBJECTIVE.

**apochromatic** \-krōmat′ik\ Corrected for spherical and chromatic aberration: said of microscope objectives that are constructed of fluorite lenses combined to correct chromatic aberration for three colors and to compensate for spherical aberration when used with an appropriate ocular.

**apocope** \əpäk′əpē\ [Gk *apokopē* a cutting off] *Outmoded* AMPUTATION.

**apocoptic** \-käp′tik\ Resulting from an amputation.

**apocrine** \ap′əkrīn, ap′əkrin\ [Gk *apokrin(ein)* (from *apo-* apart, away + *krinein* to separate) to separate out, secrete] Of or relating to a gland which provides, or a secretion which contains, not only fluid but also cellular granules. Compare ECCRINE.

**apocrinitis** \-krinī′tis\ [*apocrin(e)* + -ITIS] Inflammation of an apocrine sweat gland. *Rare.*

**apocrustic** **1** Having astringent and repellent properties. **2** An apocrustic agent.

**apodia** \əpō′dē·ə\ [Gk *a-* priv. + POD- + -IA] The developmental absence of one or both feet. Also *apody, ectropody.*

**apoenzyme** The protein part of an enzyme, lacking any prosthetic group, coenzyme, or activating metal ion. Also *apoferment.*

**apoferritin** The protein part of ferritin, without the iron it can bind.

**apogee** \ap′əjē\ The highest point, such as that of a fever or the most severe stage in the progress of a disease; crisis.

**apolar** \āpō′lər\ Without poles, as a nerve cell without processes.

**apolipoprotein** \ap′ōlip′əprō′tēn\ The lipid-free, protein component of a lipoprotein. Apolipoproteins are important in the transport of lipids in plasma. Apolipoprotein A-I (Apo A-I) is a single amino acid chain of 28 300 MW and is the major protein moiety of high density lipoprotein (HDL) that also contains triglycerides and cholesterol. Apo A-I is an activator of lecithin:cholesterol acyl transferase (LCAT). Apolipoprotein A-II (Apo A-II) is a dimer of identical amino acid chains of 17 000 MW. It also binds both cholesterol and triglycerides and is a minor component of HDL. Apolipoprotein A-III (Apo A-III, also called Apo D) is a protein of 32 000 MW. It is a minor component of HDL. Apolipoprotein B (Apo B) is a protein of 240 000 or 335 000 MW. It is the major protein component of chylomicrons, intermediate density lipoproteins (IDL), very low density lipoproteins (VLDL) and low density lipoproteins (LDL). Apolipoprotein C-I (Apo C-I) is a protein of 6500 MW which is a minor component of VLDL and HDL and is also an activator of plasma LCAT. Apolipoprotein C-II (Apo C-II) is a single amino acid chain protein of 8800 MW that is a minor component of VLDL and certain HDL subfractions and is an activator of plasma lipoprotein lipase that hydrolyzes triglycerides of chylomicrons and VLDL to glycerol and free fatty acids. Apolipoprotein C-III (Apo C-III) is the major protein moiety of VLDL and is a minor component of HDL. It is a single amino acid chain protein of 8750 MW. Most ApoC-III is in the HDL fraction and about 25% is in the VLDL fraction. Apolipoprotein E (Apo E) is a single chain or dimer protein of about 37 000 MW. It forms part of all plasma lipoprotein classes but principally VLDL, and its plasma concentration is closely correlated with plasma triglyceride concentrations.

**apomixis** \-mik′sis\ [APO- + Gk *mixis* a mixing, intercourse] Asexual reproduction by the development of monoploid gametes in the absence of sexual reproductive processes. The equivalent form of reproduction in animals is parthenogenesis. Adj. apomyxic.

**apomorphine** \-môr′fin\ An alkaloid that is derived from morphine by removing a molecule of water.

**apomorphine hydrochloride** $C_{17}H_{18}ClNO_2$. A derivative of morphine, used as an expectorant, emetic, and hypnotic.

**aponeurectomy** \-nʸurek′təmē\ [*aponeur(osis)* + -ECTOMY] An excision of an aponeurosis.

**aponeurorrhaphy** \-nʸurôr′əfē\ [APO- + NEURO- + -RRHAPHY] FASCIORRHAPHY.

**aponeuroses** \-nʸurō′sēz\ Plural of APONEUROSIS.

**aponeurosis** \ap′ōnʸoorō′sis\ [Gk *aponeurōsis* (from APO- + Gk *neuron* a tendon) end of a muscle where it becomes a tendon] [NA] A broad tendinous sheet of dense connective tissue that is associated with the attachment of a muscle and is often thin and flat. It usually comprises several layers, the collagen fibers of each of which are parallel but in a different direction from those of adjacent layers. Also *aponeurotic membrane*. **abdominal a.** The conjoined aponeuroses of the oblique and transverse muscles of the anterior abdominal wall. **bicipital a.** APONEUROSIS MUSCULI BICIPITIS BRACHII. **clavicoracoaxillary a.** FASCIA CLAVIPECTORALIS. **crural a.** FASCIA CRURIS. **Denonvilliers a.** SEPTUM RECTOVESICALE. **epicranial a.** GALEA APONEUROTICA. **extensor a.** EXTENSOR EXPANSION. **a. of external oblique muscle of abdomen** The broad membranous sheet of strong fibrous tissue that is the continuation of the upper and middle fleshy muscle fibers of the external oblique muscle of the abdomen. It is found along a curved vertical line extending from the ninth costal cartilage to the anterior superior iliac spine. The fibers are directed downward and forward to end in the linea alba and to intermingle with the fibers of the opposite side as well as becoming attached to the upper margin of the pubic symphysis, the pubic crest, and pubic tubercle and the anterior superior iliac spine. Between the latter two bony points it forms the inguinal ligament. **femoral a.** FASCIA LATA FEMORIS. **a. of insertion** The flattened expansion serving as the tendon of insertion of a muscle. Also *fascia of insertion*. **a. of internal oblique muscle of abdomen** The strong membranous sheet of fibrous tissue that is the anterior continuation of the fleshy muscle fibers of the internal oblique muscle of the abdomen, except for the lowest fibers which form the conjoint tendon. The upper two thirds splits into two layers at the lateral margin of the rectus abdominis muscle to help form the rectus sheath and end at the medial margin in the linea alba. The lower one third does not split but passes with the aponeuroses of the external oblique and transversus abdominis muscles in front of the rectus abdominis. **a. of investment** The connective tissue fascia that encloses a muscle or group of muscles. When there is considerable movement between muscles, the fascia is composed of loose areolar tissue, possibly to facilitate movement. *Outmoded.* Also *investing fascia*. **a. linguae** [NA] The dense lamina propria of the mucous membrane of the dorsum of the tongue, fused with the interstitial connective tissue between the muscle bundles and providing attachment for the intrinsic muscles. It contains elastic fibers and the branches of many blood and lymphatic vessels and nerves, as well as glands. Also *lingual aponeurosis, lingual corium*. **lumbar a.** FASCIA THORACOLUMBALIS. **a. musculi bicipitis brachii** [NA] A broad fibrous sheet in the cubital fossa, given off the medial side of the tendon of biceps brachii muscle, which passes obliquely downwards and medially superficial to the brachial artery and deep to the median cubital vein to fuse with the deep fascia covering the origins of the forearm flexor muscles. Also *bicipital aponeurosis, bicipital fascia, lacertus fibrosus musculi bicipitis brachii, semilunar fascia*. **a. of occipitofrontal muscle** GALEA APONEUROTICA. **a. of origin** The flattened expansion serving as the tendon of origin of a muscle. **a. palatina** [NA] A thin fibrous sheet in the anterior two-thirds of the soft palate, formed by the flattened tendon of insertion of the tensor veli palatini muscle and attached to the posterior margin and adjacent inferior surface of the hard palate. In the midline it splits to enclose the musculus uvulae and it provides attachment for all the other muscles of the soft palate, which it supports. On its inferior surface are mucous glands. Also *palatine aponeurosis, palatopharyngeal aponeurosis* (outmoded). **a. palmaris** [NA] The thick triangular portion of deep fascia in the palm of the hand, the apex of which is continuous with the flexor retinaculum and also receives the tendon of the palmaris longus muscle superficially. Its base flares out into four slips, the superficial fibers of which reach the skin of the palm and fingers while the deeper fibers join the fibrous flexor sheaths. It is continuous medially and laterally with fascia over the hypothenar and thenar eminences, respectively, and from each border of the aponeurosis a septum passes dorsally to the first and fifth metacarpal bones dividing the contents of the palm into three compartments of clinical importance. It is firmly bound to the overlying skin, while deep to it are the flexor tendons of the fingers, blood vessels, and nerves. Also *palmar fascia, volar fascia, Dupuytren's fascia.* **perineal a.** MEMBRANA PERINEI. **pharyngeal a.** FASCIA PHARYNGOBASILARIS. **pharyngobasilar a.** FASCIA PHARYNGOBASILARIS. **a. plantaris** [NA] The deep fascia of the sole of the foot, divided into a thick central and thinner medial and lateral portions that are continuous with each other. The central portion is narrow posteriorly where it is attached to the calcaneal tuberosity, and wider distally where it divides into five processes, one to each toe. Similar to the aponeurosis palmaris, it sends septa from its sides deep into the sole to divide the muscles into three compartments. The medial and lateral portions cover subjacent muscles, for which they provide partial origin, and are continuous around the sides of the foot with the fascia of the dorsum of the foot. Also *plantar fascia, plantar aponeurosis.* **Sibson's a.** MEMBRANA SUPRAPLEURALIS. **subscapular a.** FASCIA SUBSCAPULARIS. **superficial perineal a.** FASCIA DIAPHRAGMATIS PELVIS INFERIOR. **superior perineal a.** FASCIA DIAPHRAGMATIS PELVIS SUPERIOR. **a. of superior surface of levator ani muscle** FASCIA DIAPHRAGMATIS PELVIS SUPERIOR. **temporal a.** FASCIA TEMPORALIS. **a. of vasti muscles** A fibrous expansion extending from an aponeurosis of insertion that is attached to the deep surface of the lower part of the vastus medialis and lateralis muscles. Each one blends with and reinforces the fibrous capsule of the knee on the corresponding side. That of the vastus lateralis also blends with the iliotibial tract and forms the retinaculum patellae laterale, while that of the vastus medialis forms the retinaculum patellae mediale. Some fibers of each expansion crisscross superficial to the patella, attaching to opposite sides of the upper end of the tibia. **a. of Zinn** ANNULUS TENDINEUS COMMUNIS.

**aponeurositis** \-nʸur'əsī'tis\ [*aponeuros(is)* + -ITIS] Inflammation of an aponeurosis as is seen in palmar or plantar fasciitis.

**aponeurotic** \-nʸurät'ik\ Pertaining to or resembling an aponeurosis.

**aponeurotome** \-nʸur'ətōm\ [*aponeuro(sis)* + -TOME] An instrument for cutting aponeuroses.

**aponeurotomy** \-nʸurät'əmē\ [*aponeuro(sis)* + -TOMY] The surgical incision of an aponeurosis.

**apophlegmatic** \-flegmat'ik\ EXPECTORANT.

**apophysary** \əpäf'əser'ē\ APOPHYSEAL.

**apophysate** \əpäf'əsāt\ Bearing an apophysis.

**apophyseal** \-fəzē'əl\ Relating to an apophysis. Also *apophysiary, apophysial, apophysary.*

**apophyseopathy** \-fiz'ē·äp'əthē\ Any disease or injury of an apophysis.

**apophyses** \əpäf'əsēz\ Plural of APOPHYSIS.

**apophysial** \-fiz'ē·əl\ APOPHYSEAL.

**apophysiary** \-fiz'yerē\ APOPHYSEAL.

**apophysis** \əpäf'isis\ [Gk (from *apophyein* to send out, produce, from *phyein* to grow) an outgrowth, process] Any outgrowth or bony protrusion, such as a tubercle or tuberosity, that is connected to and forms a part of a bone. It usually has muscle and tendon attached to it. **basilar a.** PARS BASILARIS OSSIS OCCIPITALIS. **calcaneal a.** The epiphysis of the posterior extremity of the calcaneus. **a. cerebri** CORPUS PINEALE. **a. helicis** SPINA HELICIS. **a. of Ingrassia** ALA MINOR OSSIS SPHENOIDALIS. **odontoid a.** DENS AXIS. **pterygoid a.** PROCESSUS PTERYGOIDEUS OSSIS SPHENOIDALIS. **a. of Rau** PROCESSUS ANTERIOR MALLEI.

**apophysitis** \əpäf'əsī'tis\ An inflammation or fragmentation of a bony apophysis. **a. tibialis adolescentium** OSGOOD-SCHLATTER DISEASE.

**apoplasmatic** \ap'ōplazmat'ik\ Describing a cellular product which forms a constituent part of the tissues of an organism, such as the matrix of bone and the fibers of connective tissue.

**apoplectic** \-plek'tik\ [Gk *apoplēktikos* of or disabled by apoplexy] Pertaining to apoplexy.

**apoplectiform** \-plek'tifôrm\ Resembling apoplexy. Also *apoplectoid.*

**apoplexy** \ap'əplek'sē\ [Gk *apoplēxia* (from *apoplēssein* to cripple by a stroke, from *apo-* apart, asunder + *plēssein* to strike, smite) apoplexy, paralysis] A sudden episode of impairment of cerebral function leading rapidly to coma, generally the result of a cerebrovascular accident. Intracerebral hemorrhage is the commonest cause, but occasionally massive cerebral infarction due to thrombosis or embolism may have the same effect. *Imprecise.* Also *cerebral stroke, apoplexia, apoplectic shock, apoplectic stroke.* Adj. apoplectic. **adrenal a.** Acute adrenocortical insufficiency owing to abrupt and massive hemorrhage into or infarction of the adrenal glands, as in the Waterhouse-Friderichsen syndrome. **bulbar a.** A cerebrovascular accident due to hemorrhage into or infarction of the brainstem. **capillary a.** Hemorrhage into the brain or into some other organ due to bleeding from capillaries. **cerebellar a.** A cerebrovascular accident due to hemorrhage into or infarction of a cerebellar hemisphere. **cerebral a.** A cerebrovascular accident due to intracerebral hemorrhage or massive infarction in one cerebral hemisphere. **delayed a.** A cerebrovascular accident following days or weeks after a head injury. Also *traumatic late apoplexy.* **embolic a.** A cerebrovascular accident resulting from embolic infarction of the brain. **fulminating a.** Apoplexy of explosive onset rapidly followed by coma and death. **heat a.** HEATSTROKE. **ingravescent a.** Apoplexy of gradual onset. **ovarian a.** Hemorrhage into the ovary. **pituitary a.** A syndrome of intense headache of sudden onset often followed by coma and subarachnoid hemorrhage and sometimes by unilateral blindness or a third nerve palsy due to massive infarction of or hemorrhage into the pituitary or a pituitary tumor. **placental a.** Sudden failure of placental function, usually due to premature separation of the placenta from the uterine wall, with hemorrhage and subsequent formation of a subplacental hematoma. **pontine a.** The syndrome resulting from hemorrhage into or infarction of the pons. Also *pontile apoplexy.* **spasmodic a.** A transient cerebral ischemic attack once thought to be due to spasm of a cerebral artery. *Obs.* **spinal a.** The clinical syndrome resulting from spontaneous hemorrhage into the spinal cord or from spinal subarachnoid hemorrhage. **splenic a.** ANTHRAX. **traumatic late a.** DELAYED APOPLEXY. **urethral a.** URETHRORRHAGIA. **uterine a.** ABRUPTIO PLACENTAE. **uteroplacental a.** COUVELAIRE UTERUS.

**apoprotein** A protein, which usually occurs with a nonprotein substance attached, from which this nonprotein part has been removed.

**aporepressor** \-ripres'ər\ A polypeptide, the product of a repressor gene, that must be activated, usually by combination with a small molecular weight corepressor, to enable binding to the operator locus and regulation of the activity of adjacent genes.

**apositia** \-sish'ē·ə\ [APO- + Gk *sit(os)* food + -IA] *Obs.* ANOREXIA.

**aposthia** \əpäs'thē·ə\ [Gk *a-* priv. + *posth(ē)* the foreskin + -IA] A developmental absence of the prepuce.

**apothanasia** \-thānā′zhə\ [APO- + Gk *thana(tos)* death + *s* + -IA] The lengthening or extension of life.

**apothecary** \əpäth′əker′ē\ [Late L *apothecarius* (from *apotheca*, from Gk *apothēkē* a store, repository, from *apotithenai* to lay away, store + L *-arius* dealer, keeper) a storekeeper] *Older term* PHARMACIST.

**apothem** \ap′əthem′\ [APO- + Gk *them(a)* (from *tithenai* to put, place) a deposit] A dark precipitate in vegetable infusions and decoctions, formed on exposure to air. Also *apotheme*.

**apozem** \ap′əzem′\ [Gk *apozema* (from *apozein* to boil off, throw off by fermenting) a decoction, potion] A medicated decoction. Also *apozema, apozeme*.

**apparatus** \ap′ərat′əs, ap′ərā′təs\ [L (from *apparare* to equip, outfit, from *ad-* to, for + *parare* to prepare, supply) preparation, equipment] A complex of structures such as tissues, organs, or parts, or occasionally specialized cells, that are associated by common functions and/or origins. **absorption a.** A device, used in measuring gases, that absorbs a gas or some constituent from a mixture and estimates the quantity either from properties of the absorbed material or from the reduced residual volume remaining after absorption. **acoustic a.** AUDITORY APPARATUS. **attachment a.** The supporting tissues of a tooth, taken as a whole. They include the gingiva, cementum, periodontal ligament, and alveolar bone. **auditory a.** The numerous organs and structures comprising the organ of hearing, essentially the various parts of the ear, including the labyrinthus cochlearis and perilympha within the labyrinthus osseus and the connections of the cochlear portion of the vestibulocochlear nerve. Also *acoustic apparatus*. **Barcroft's a.** WARBURG'S APPARATUS. **Benedict a.** BENEDICT-ROTH APPARATUS. **Benedict-Knipping a.** A recording spirometer used to study metabolic activity by measuring both oxygen consumption and carbon dioxide production. Oxygen consumption is determined by the descent of a spirometer bell. The generated carbon dioxide, which has been absorbed in an alkaline solution, is liberated by the addition of acid and measured by the ascent of the spirometer bell. Also *Knipping's apparatus*. **Benedict-Roth a.** A spirometer used for measuring oxygen consumption. The subject breathes in and out of a tank of oxygen through a tube containing soda lime, which removes the carbon dioxide in the expired air. Also *Benedict apparatus*. **biliary a.** BILIARY TRACT. **cerebellovestibular a.** The neural pathway by which the vestibular organs and their medullary nuclei act in coordination with the cerebellum to regulate balanced movement. **chromatic a.** The deeply staining masses of chromosomes associated with the spindle fibers during cell division. **ciliary a.** CORPUS CILIARE. **Desault's a.** DESAULT'S BANDAGE. **a. digestorius** [NA] The mouth, pharynx, and alimentary tract and their associated glands and organs, which are concerned with digestion, absorption, and excretion of food products. Also *digestive apparatus, systema digestorium, digestive organs, digestive system, alimentary system*. **genital a. of the female** The organa genitalia feminina externa and the organa genitalia feminina interna. **genitourinary a.** APPARATUS UROGENITALIS. **Golgi a.** A cytoplasmic organelle which is composed of a number of flattened sacs resembling smooth endoplasmic reticulum. The sacs are often cup-shaped and located near the nucleus, the open side of the cup generally facing toward the cell surface. The function of the Golgi apparatus is to accept vesicles from the endoplasmic reticulum, to modify the contents, and to distribute the products to other parts of the cell or to the cellular environment. Also *Golgi complex*. See also DICTYOSOME. **a. of Goormaghtigh** JUXTAGLOMERULAR APPARATUS. **Haldane a.** A chamber formerly used for studying the metabolic activity of small animals, especially the constituent gases of respiration. Also *Haldane's chamber*. **Hodgen's a.** HODGEN SPLINT. **Horsley-Clarke a.** STEREOTAXIC APPARATUS. **hyoid a.** In comparative anatomy, an articulated chain of bones or cartilages that extends from the base of the skull to the base of the tongue and usually develops from the hyoid visceral arch, from the ventral part of which the hyoid bone develops in humans. In humans, the term is loosely used to include the parts of the hyoid bone and its attachments to the base of the skull, namely, the stylohyoid ligament and styloid process. **inhalation anesthesia a.** Any device employed to induce general anesthesia, as an anesthesia machine, a full-face mask, a respiratory airway, an endotracheal tube, or a mechanical ventilator. **inhalation therapy a.** Any device utilized to improve pulmonary function, as a full-face mask, an endotracheal airway, a mechanical ventilator, or anything which supplies oxygen. **juxtaglomerular a.** A complex at the vascular pole of the renal glomerulus. The afferent arteriole, which contains juxtaglomerular cells, lies adjacent to a short section of distal tubule (the macula densa), in which the nuclei are larger and more closely packed than normal. In the angle between the arteriole and macula densa lie the lacis cells, which resemble the juxtaglomerular cells. They merge with the mesangium of the glomerular tuft. The whole complex is associated with renin production and may monitor glomerular blood flow according to the contents of the distal tubule. Also *periarterial pad* (obs.), *polar cushion of the glomerulus, juxtaglomerular body, apparatus of Goormaghtigh*. **Kirschner's a.** A device used to apply skeletal traction to a fractured limb. It consists of a wire (Kirschner wire), passed through the bone, to which traction is applied via a metal stirrup. **Knipping's a.** BENEDICT-KNIPPING APPARATUS. **Krogh's a.** **1** A microtonometer designed to measure gas tensions in blood. A small bubble of air is allowed to equilibrate in a stream of blood, after which it is transferred to a special capillary tube for gaseous analysis. **2** A simple recording spirometer in which the subject breathes in and out of a mouthpiece connected by valves to a recording tank spirometer that contains soda lime. **a. lacrimalis** [NA] The structures dealing with the secretion and transport of tears from the eyes to the nose, including the lacrimal glands, lacrimal ducts, lacrimal sac, and nasolacrimal duct. Also *lacrimal apparatus*. **lens a.** The lens of the eye, its capsule, and the zonula ciliaris. *Outmoded*. **locomotor a.** The structures that permit movement of the body and its parts, such as the skeleton, articulations, and muscles. **masticating a.** MASTICATORY APPARATUS. **masticatory a.** All of the structures involved in mastication, including the teeth, jaws, temporomandibular joint, muscles of mastication, tongue, and the associated nervous system. Also *masticating apparatus, stomatognathic system*. **mitotic a.** A nuclear structure, present only during cell division when it can be seen cytologically, that is composed of microtubules, RNA, and mucolipids. Together they constitute the asters, spindle, and matrix. Also *achromatic figure, mitotic figure*. **a. of Perroncito** PERRONCITO'S PHENOMENON. **pilosebaceous a.** A hair follicle and its sebaceous gland. **reproductive a.** The genital organs of the male and female. **a. respiratorius** [NA] An interconnected series of air passages, cavernous organs, and cells that permit the introduction of oxygen, the exchange of gases, and the removal of carbon dioxide from the body as well as, in humans, the production of speech. The anatomical components involved include the external nose and nasal cavity, the oral cavity and pharynx, paranasal sinuses, larynx, trachea, bronchi, lungs, and thoracic cavity, as well as the muscles related to their activities. Also *respiratory apparatus, systema respiratorium, respiratory system, respiratory tract.* **rocking a.** ROCKING BED. **Scholander a.** A modified Haldane gas analysis apparatus designed to measure the carbon dioxide and oxygen content in volumes of gas of one milliliter or less. It is often used in studies of gas exchange in small mammals and invertebrates. **sound-conducting a.** The various parts of the external and middle ear that collect and conduct sound waves to the inner ear, where they are converted to nerve impulses in the afferent fibers of the cochlear part of the vestibulocochlear nerve for transmission to the auditory pathways in the central nervous system. **spindle a.** A microtubular structure that extends from pole to pole during mitosis or meiosis. It appears to be organized by the centrioles, and functions in alignment and movement of chromosomes. **spine a.** A spikelike projection from the surface membrane of a neuronal dendritic process that contains parallel rows of endoplasmic reticulum and forms the postsynaptic portion of one variety of synaptinemal complex. **stereotaxic a.** An instrument used for precise placement of devices into the brain for purposes of recording, stimulation, injection, or destruction. Localization of any brain site is made by utilizing three coordinates: rostral-caudal, medial-lateral, and dorsal-ventral. Also *Horsley-Clarke apparatus, stereotaxic instrument.* **a. suspensorius lentis** *Outmoded* ZONULA CILIARIS. **suspensory a. of the pleura** Those muscle fibers and tendinous bundles that spread out from the scalenus anterior and medius muscles, as well as the scalenus minimus when present, and that attach on and strengthen the suprapleural membrane. *Outmoded.* Also *Sebileau suspensory ligaments.* **Taylor's a.** TAYLOR SPLINT. **Tiselius a.** A device for separating proteins or other charged molecules in a solution by electrophoresis wihout the use of solid support media. Migration of the charged molecules in an electric field is determined by measuring changes in refractive index of the solution. **a. urogenitalis** [NA] The customary combination of the organs concerned with the secretion and excretion of urine and those associated with reproduction in males and females. Also *urogenital apparatus, genitourinary apparatus, urogenital system, genitourinary system, systema urogenitale, genitourinary tract, urogenital tract.* **vestibular a.** The structures in the internal ear, namely, the utricle, sacculus, and ampullae of the semicircular ducts, that contain specialized sensory receptors perceiving and conveying information to the vestibular part of the vestibulocochlear nerve concerning the position of the head in space, either static or under linear or angular acceleration or deceleration. **vocal a.** In humans, the structures within the respiratory apparatus, particularly the components of the larynx, that are concerned specifically with phonation, or the production of speech. **Warburg's a.** A device used to measure oxygen consumption and carbon dioxide production of small portions of tissue under controlled temperature conditions. Also *Warburg vessel, Barcroft's apparatus.* **Zander a.** A system of levers and pulleys designed to provide manipulation and exercises for the trunk and limbs.

**append-** \əpend-\ [L *appendere* (from *ad-* to, onto + *pendere* to weigh) to suspend, hang] A combining form meaning appendage or appendix. Also *appendo-*.

**appendage** \əpen′dij\ [L *append(ix)* an addition + -AGE] **1** A structural protrusion. **2** A protruding body part such as a limb, mouth part, antenna, or tentacle. **atrial a.** AURICULA ATRIALIS. **auricular a.** **1** A small fleshy or cutaneous tab located anterior to the auricle of the ear. It may be associated with a branchial fistula, cyst, sinus, or other vestige of the first branchial groove of the early embryo. Also *preauricular appendage.* **2** AURICULA ATRIALIS. **caudal a.** A visible extension of the vertebral column beyond its usual termination in humans, forming a tail-like structure below the sacrum and above the anus. It probably represents supernumerary caudal somites or vertebral segments which fail to degenerate during fetal life. If not amputated at birth, it may attain a length of several centimeters. **cutaneous a.'s** Collectively, the pilosebaceous follicles and the sweat glands. **drumstick a.** A small (1.5 μm diameter) body containing sex chromatin extruded from the nucleus of human polymorphonuclear leukocytes in about 2% of females and 0.2% of males. With its attachment to the nucleus by a thin stalk, the body resembles a drumstick. Also *drumstick.* **a. of epididymis** APPENDIX OF THE EPIDIDYMIS. **epiploic a.'s** APPENDICES EPIPLOICAE. **a.'s of the eye** ORGANA OCULI ACCESSORIA. **a.'s of the fetus** FETAL ADNEXA. **fibrous a. of liver** APPENDIX FIBROSA HEPATIS. **left auricular a.** AURICULA SINISTRA. **ovarian a.** Either the epoöphoron or the paroöphoron, usually the former since the latter is rarely found in the adult. **preauricular a.** AURICULAR APPENDAGE. **right auricular a.** AURICULA DEXTRA. **testicular a.** APPENDIX TESTIS. **a. of the testis** APPENDIX TESTIS. **uterine a.'s** The ovaries, uterine tubes, and ligaments of the uterus. Also *adnexa uteri.* **a. of ventricle of larynx** SACCULUS LARYNGIS. **vermicular a.** APPENDIX VERMIFORMIS. **vesicular a.'s of epoöphoron of Morgagni** *Obs.* APPENDICES VESICULOSAE EPOÖPHORI.

**appendectomy** \ap′əndek′təmē\ [APPEND- + -ECTOMY] The surgical removal of the vermiform appendix. **auricular a.** The excision of the right or left atrial appendage of the heart.

**appendic-** \əpen′dik-, əpen′dis-\ APPENDICO-.

**appendiceal** \-isē′əl, -dish′əl\ Pertaining to an appendix. Also *appendical.*

**appendices** \əpen′disēz\ Plural of APPENDIX.

**appendicitis** \əpen′disī′tis\ [APPENDIC- + -ITIS] Inflammation of the vermiform appendix. It is of unknown etiology, but luminal obstruction by a variety of processes is present in approximately 70 percent of cases of acute appendicitis. The condition is typically marked by abdominal pain and often accompanied by nausea, vomiting, and fever. Localized abdominal tenderness is an essential finding. Treatment is almost invariably surgical. Complications may include peritonitis, abscess formation, and pylephlebitis. **actinomycotic a.** Appendicitis caused by *Actinomyces israelii.*. **acute obstructive a.** Appendicitis of acute onset with obstruction of the lumen of the appendix, usually by a fecalith. **amebic a.** Appendicitis caused by *Entamoeba histolytica,* with obstruction of the appendiceal lumen by the edematous bowel wall infested with the parasite. **gangrenous a.** Appendicitis complicated by gangrene, resulting from decreased blood supply. **helminthic a.** Appendicitis caused by helminths; verminous appendicitis. **lumbar a.** Appendicitis in an appendix that is posteriorly displaced, lying behind or below the cecum. **nonobstructive a.** Appendicitis without obstruction of the lumen. **obstructive a.** A clinical entity characterized by severe cramping abdominal pain which mimics the colic of small bowel obstruction but which is due to acute appendicitis without obstruction. **perforating a.** Appendicitis complicated by perforation of the appendix. **stercoral**

**a.** Appendicitis resulting from fecal concretion. **subperitoneal a.** Appendicitis in an appendix that is buried under the peritoneum. **verminous a.** Appendicitis caused by parasitic worms.

**appendico-** \əpen′dikō-\ [L *appendix*, gen. *appendicis* an appendage, attachment. See APPENDIX.] A combining form meaning appendix, especially the vermiform appendix. Also *appendic-*.

**appendicocecostomy** \-sēkäs′təmē\ [APPENDICO- + CECO- + -STOMY] The creation of a connection between the vermiform appendix and the cecum.

**appendicocele** \əpen′dəkōsēl′\ [APPENDICO- + -CELE[1]] A hernia containing the vermiform appendix.

**appendicoenterostomy** \-en′təräs′təmē\ [APPENDICO- + ENTERO- + -STOMY] The surgical establishment of a communication between the appendix and the small intestine.

**appendicolithiasis** \-lithī′əsis\ [APPENDICO- + LITHIASIS] A condition characterized by concretions in the vermiform appendix. Also *appendolithiasis.*

**appendicolysis** \əpen′dəkäl′isis\ [APPENDICO- + LYSIS] The surgical division of periappendicular adhesions.

**appendicostomy** \əpen′dəkäs′təmē\ [APPENDICO- + -STOMY] The creation of a stoma by securing the extremity of the vermiform appendix to the anterior abdominal wall. Also *Weir's operation.*

**appendicular** \ap′əndik′yələr\ **1** Of or relating to limbs or appendages. **2** Of or relating to an appendix; appendiceal.

**appendix** \əpen′diks\ [L (from *appendere* to suspend, hang, from *ad-* to, onto + *pendere* to weigh) an appendage, attachment, adjunct] (*pl.* appendices) **1** [NA] An accessory or dependent part attached to the main part of a structure. **2** APPENDIX VERMIFORMIS. **auricular a.** AURICULA ATRIALIS. **cecal a.** APPENDIX VERMIFORMIS. **ensiform a.** PROCESSUS XIPHOIDEUS. **a. of the epididymis** A mesonephric remnant that is occasionally present on the head of the epididymis. Also *appendage of epididymus, pedunculated hydatid, pedunculated hydatid of Morgagni.* **epiploic appendices** APPENDICES EPIPLOICAE. **appendices epiploicae** [NA] Small, peritoneum-covered projections of fat attached to the external free surface of the whole large intestine except the cecum, appendix vermiformis, and rectum. Also *epiploic appendices, epiploic appendages.* **a. fibrosa hepatis** [NA] An occasional fibrous band, situated in the left triangular ligament at the left extremity of the left lobe of the liver in the adult, that is the atrophied remnant of the larger left lobe in the child and may contain atrophied bile ducts. Also *fibrous appendix of liver, fibrous appendage of liver.* **a. morgagnii** **1** One of the appendices vesiculosae epoöphori. Also *hydatid of Morgagni.* **2** APPENDIX TESTIS. **pelvic a.** An appendix that has descended into the pelvis. When acutely inflamed in a woman, a pelvic appendix can simulate an ovarian abscess or cyst. **a. testis** [NA] A remnant of the upper end of the atrophied embryonic paramesonephric, or Müllerian, duct. It is represented as a tiny oval, sessile structure attached to the upper extremity of the testis just inferolateral to the head of the epididymis. Also *hydatid of Morgagni, sessile hydatid, testicular appendage, appendix morgagnii, nonpedunculated hydatid, appendage of the testis, sessile hydatid of Morgagni.* **a. of ventricle of larynx** SACCULUS LARYNGIS. **a. vermiformis** [NA] A narrow, worm-shaped tube which arises from the posteromedial wall of the cecum at a point where the three taeniae coli of the cecum and ascending colon converge and fuse with its longitudinal muscle fibers. Its direction and position vary considerably but it is commonly postcecal or retrocolic and it is usually connected by a short, falciform mesoappendix to the lower part of the mesentery of the ileum. It contains a considerable amount of lymphoid tissue in the submucosa. Also *vermiform appendix, vermicular appendage, vermiform process, cecal appendix, vermix, appendix.* **appendices vesiculosae epoöphori** [NA] A persistent group of tubules at the cranial end of the atrophied embryonic female mesonephros, represented by one or more small pedunculated vesicles or cysts connected to the fimbriae of a uterine tube or to an adjacent broad ligament. Also *vesicular appendages of epoöphoron of Morgagni, morgagnian cysts, vesicular appendices.*

**appendo-** \əpen′dō-\ APPEND-.

**appendolithiasis** \-lithī′əsis\ APPENDICOLITHIASIS.

**appetite** [L *appetitus* (from *appetitus*, past part. of *appetere* to desire from AP- + *petere* to seek) a longing] A desire to satisfy a need, especially a physiologic need as that for food. Also *orexia, orexis.* **perverted a.** PICA.

**appetitive** \ap′iti′tiv\ [Middle French *appetitif* (from L *appetit(us)* appetite + *-ivus* -IVE) pertaining to appetite] Of or relating to attraction; attractive. *Outmoded.*

**applanate** \ap′lənāt\ [Med L *applanat(us)*, past part. of *applanare* (from L *ap-* to + Late L *planare* to flatten, from L *planus* flat, level) to flatten] Horizontally flattened.

**applanation** \ap′lənā′shən\ [*applanat(e)* + -ION] The act of flattening or the condition of being flattened, as the cornea with an applanation tonometer.

**applanometer** \ap′lənäm′ətər\ [Med L *applan(are)* to flatten + *o* + -METER ] A device intended to measure the amount of flattening induced by pressure upon a spherical surface.

**apple** / **Adam's a.** *Popular* PROMINENTIA LARYNGEA. **devil's a.** STRAMONIUM. **Indian a.** MANDRAKE. **May a.** MANDRAKE. **a. of Peru** STRAMONIUM. **thorn a.** STRAMONIUM.

**appliance** \əplī′əns\ [English *apply* (from Middle English *applien*, from Old French *aplier* to apply, attach to, from L *applicare*, from *ap-* to + *plicare* to fold) + -ANCE] **1** A device performing a particular function, as to provide stability or support or to produce a structural change. **2** A device for moving, retaining, or splinting teeth. **Begg a.** LIGHT ROUND-WIRE APPLIANCE. **Bimler a.** An activator with a wire framework joined to acrylic wings and pads. **craniofacial a.** A device used to immobilize and/or reduce fractures of the facial bones. It may be external, utilizing headcaps or skeletal pins, or internal, using circumferential or suspension wiring. **crown of thorns a.** A device for the stabilization of complex facial bone fractures consisting of a metallic halo which is affixed to the skull by pointed set screws, and from which fixation rods, traction wires, and other devices can be supported. **Crozat a.** A removal orthodontic appliance made of wire. **edgewise a.** A fixed orthodontic appliance using arch wire of rectangular section instead of round. **fixed a.** An appliance, usually orthodontic, that is fixed to the teeth and is not removable by the patient. Also *permanent appliance.* **Frankel a.** An orthodontic appliance designed to relieve adverse pressures on soft tissues and direct the growth of the jaws. **functional a.** ACTIVATOR. **Hawley a.** A removable orthodontic retainer in which anterior teeth are held between a labial bow and the palatal base, extended on to the palatal surfaces of the teeth. Also *Hawley retainer.* **labiolingual a.** A fixed orthodontic appliance using stiff labial and lingual arch wires, fixed to the first molars, as the base for springs which are used to move other teeth. **light round-wire a.** A fixed orthodontic appliance using fine labial arch wires which are bent in between attachments to form springs and loops. Also *Begg appliance.* **monobloc a.** A removable orthodontic appliance in which the upper and lower bases are rigidly joined together. **multibanded a.** A fixed orthodontic appliance using bands on teeth other than first molars. Frequently all the teeth in an arch are banded. **occlusal overlay a.** BITE GUARD. **orthodontic a.** An appliance used to move teeth. It is used chiefly during the growth period but may also be used for adults. Also *regulating appliance.* **permanent a.** FIXED APPLIANCE. **pin and tube a.** A fixed orthodontic appliance using an arch wire with vertical ends that are fitted into tubes attached to bands on molar teeth. **regulating a.** ORTHODONTIC APPLIANCE. **retaining a.** RETAINER. **Roger-Anderson pin fixation a.** ROGER-ANDERSON EXTRAORAL SPLINT. **speech a.** A device to help speech where it is defective because of disease. Examples are obturators and electronic vibrators. **universal a.** A fixed orthodontic appliance using twin arch wires, one of which is round and the other flat.

**application / new drug a.** In the United States, an application to the FDA to permit more extensive evaluation of a drug in a wider range of patients. It follows the required pharmacological and toxicological tests in animals, and investigational clinical testing in selected patients. Abbr. NDA

**applicator** A device used to apply remedies to particular locations and parts of the patient. **beam-therapy a.** A cone or collimator attached to the exit port of a radiotherapy machine to define the size and shape of the radiation beam. **sandwich-mold a.** A device to deliver radiation therapy to the surface of a body part, usually to a tumor on the surface. It consists of two components, each containing radioactive material, placed on either side of the lesion being treated. **sonic a.** A transducer assembly designed for local therapeutic application of ultrasonic energy. **surface a.** An appliance, containing a source of radioactive material, which is applied to the surface of the body for a determined duration to provide radiation treatment.

**applied** Serving practical ends, as *applied science.*

**appliqué** \ap′likā′\ [French, past part. of *appliquer* to apply] ACCOLÉ FORM.

**appose** \apōz′\ [French *appose(r)* (from *ap-* AP-[2] + *poser* to place, put, from L *paus(a)* a pause, stop, stay) to apply, put on] To place or bring together or side by side, as the edges of a wound.

**appraisal** \əprā′zəl\ **health risk a.** An appraisal of whether an individual has a greater than average risk of illness or death compared with others the same age and sex, given what is known about the individual's physical and mental state, habits, and life style, with the object of advising the subject on ways to improve his or her prospects of life and health. Also *health hazard appraisal.* Abbr. HRA

**approach** A surgically created avenue of access to an organ or bodily part. **idiographic a.** The intensive study of a single case or individual instance. **nomothetic a.** The studying of general principles or laws of behavior, based on many observations made of many individuals. **transcranial a.** A frontal or temporal craniotomy in order to expose the brain, especially the hypophysis and the region about it. **transnasal a.** Exposure of the hypophysis through a nasal speculum, as in performing excision of the gland or a tumor. The sphenoid sinus is traversed and the floor of the sella turcica excised, usually with the aid of a surgical microscope and microsurgical instruments. The approach is also used for stereotaxic devices introduced into the sella turcica via the nares and guided by fluoroscopy. **transseptal a.** Transnasal exposure of the sella turcica. The retracting speculum is introduced through the space provided by reflection of the septal mucosa. Usually the initial incision is made beneath the upper lip. **transthoracic a.** Exposure through the thoracic cavity of vertebrae, intervertebral disks, intervertebral foramina, or the spinal canal.

**approximal** **1** Situated in the proximity of a structure or close together. **2** Facing an adjacent tooth: said of the surface of a tooth. For defs. 1 and 2 also *proximal, approximate.*

**approximate** \(1) əpräk′səmāt; (2) əpräk′səmit\ [Late L *approximat(us),* past part. of *approximare* to come near, from L *ap-* AP-[2] + *proximare* to come near to] **1** To bring into contiguity or apposition. **2** APPROXIMAL.

**approximator** \əpräk′səmā′tər\ An instrument employed to bring together anatomical structures. **rib a.** An instrument that brings together two ribs to permit surgical closure of the intercostal space. **skin-edge a.** An instrument that apposes the edges of a wound to permit surgical repair.

**APR** anterior pituitary reaction.

**apractic** \əprak′tik\ APRAXIC.

**apractognosia** \əprak′tägnō′zhə\ [Gk *aprakto(s)* effecting nothing, unmanageable + *gnōs(is)* knowledge + -IA] Inability to use objects because of lack of recognition of their nature and function. Also *apraxic agnosia.* **geometric a.** Loss of the ability to recognize and interpret geometric shapes due to a lesion of the parieto-occipital region of the dominant hemisphere, usually resulting in constructional apraxia, and often associated with agnosia for colors, alexia, and hemianopia.

**apraxia** \əprak′sē·ə\ [Gk *apraxia* (from *a-* priv. + *prassein,* also *prattein* to do, achieve + -IA) inaction] An inability to carry out skilled, purposive, and coordinated motor activity in the absence of paralysis of the part which would normally perform the movement required. The motor pathways involved in the movement concerned are intact and it is the conceptualization of the movement which is impaired. Adj. apraxic, apractic. • Although *apraxia* and *dyspraxia* are often used interchangeably, *apraxia* implies total loss rather than impairment of this particular skill. **agnosic a.** Apraxia due to agnosia. The inability to carry out the movement results from failure to recognize and interpret the sensory information upon which its performance depends. **akinetic a.** Apraxia, often limited to one limb or part of a limb, such as the hand, due to inability to interpret afferent kinesthetic information. **classic a.** KINETIC APRAXIA. **congenital a.** DEVELOPMENTAL APRAXIA. **constructional a.** A type of apraxia in which the patient is unable to draw from memory or from a model, or to construct simple or complex shapes with matchsticks or building blocks. In mildly afflicted patients, only the ability to draw in perspective may be lost. The capacity to make gestures and to recognize geometric symbols and objects is retained. This type of apraxia is one component of the Gerstmann syndrome. Also *geometric apraxia, optic apraxia, visual apraxia.* **cortical a.** KINETIC APRAXIA. **developmental a.** A syndrome in which there is delay in the development or acquisition of motor skills. It is one form of the clumsy child syndrome. Also *congenital apraxia.* **geometric a.** CONSTRUCTIONAL APRAXIA. **ideomotor a.** A type of apraxia involving derangement of simple actions carried out in order. These actions are modified, curtailed, or confused with other gestures, without any impairment of involuntary or reflex activity. This type of apraxia, which is due to an inability to express ideas by gesture, is closely related to amimia, and may manifest itself in one limb or other restricted part of the body such as the lips and tongue. Also *ideokinetic apraxia, transcortical apraxia.* **kinetic a.** Apraxia for skilled movements, usually of a limb or part of a limb such as the hand. Also *motor apraxia* (outmoded), *limb-kinetic apraxia, classic apraxia, cortical apraxia, innervation apraxia* (seldom used), *kinesthetic apraxia.* **oculomotor a.** Inability to move the eyes voluntarily in a given direction when reflex and random eye movements are intact. Also *ocular motor apraxia, Cogan syndrome.* **optic a.** CONSTRUCTIONAL APRAXIA. **sensory a.** Inability to perform a movement involving the use of a tool, instrument, or other object, because of inability to appreciate its size, shape, and purpose. **tongue a.** Inability to move or protrude the tongue voluntarily or on command in an individual who can involuntarily use the tongue, as in licking the lips. **transcortical a.** IDEOMOTOR APRAXIA. **trunk a.** Apraxia involving particularly movements which require the use of the muscles of the trunk. **visual a.** CONSTRUCTIONAL APRAXIA.

**apraxic** \əprak′sik\ Relating to apraxia. Also *apractic.*

**aprobarbital** $C_{10}H_{14}N_2O_3$. 5-(1-Methylethyl)-5-(2-propenyl)-2,4,6(1*H*,3*H*,5*H*)-pyrimidinetrione, an orally administered barbiturate with sedative and hypnotic properties. Its chronic use may lead to habituation or addiction.

**aproctia** \əpräk′shə\ [Gk *a-* priv. + PROCT- + -IA] IMPERFORATE ANUS.

**apron** [formerly, with article, *a napron*; from Old French *naperon*, dim. of *nape* cloth, from L *mappa* napkin] An article of protective clothing worn over one's clothes in the front of the body. **lead-rubber a.** An apron, made of a lead-impregnated rubber, worn as protection against scattered radiation by persons performing radiologic procedures.

**aprosexia** \ap′rəsek′sē·ə\ [Gk *aprosexia* (from *a-* priv. + *prosechein* to turn one's mind to) heedlessness] A condition characterized by a shortened attention span. **Guye's a.** Aprosexia combined with restlessness and irritability in children with nonsuppurative otitis media and nasal obstruction, usually considered due to adenoids.

**aprosody** \āpräs′ədē\ [Gk *a-* priv. + English *prosody*] Lack of fluctuation in the tempo and pitch of spoken words resulting in flat, monotonous speech.

**aprosopia** \ap′rəsō′pē·ə\ [Gk *aprosōp(os)* (from *a-* priv. + *prosōpon* face) faceless + -IA] The developmental absence of all or most characteristic facial features.

**aprotic** \aprō′tik\ [Gk *a-* priv. + *prot(on)* + -IC] Neither yielding nor combining with protons (with a given strength of base or acid): used of solvents, especially polar solvents, since the latter dissolve salts, and the anions of these salts are much more reactive as nucleophiles if the solvent is aprotic and so cannot form hydrogen bonds with them.

**APT** alum precipitated toxoid.

**aptitude** \ap′tət^y^ood\ [Med L *aptitudo* (from L *aptus* adapted, suitable) fitness] The constitutional substrate or inherent potential which allows an individual to acquire, after training, some general or particular kind of skill or knowledge, such as the producing of music.

**aptyalia** \ap′tī·ā′lyə\ [A- + PTYAL- + -IA] ASIALIA.

**aptyalism** \aptī′əlizm\ ASIALIA.

**APUD** [acronym for: (high) *a*(*mine* content) + (high) *p*(*recursor*) *u*(*ptake* from the ambient medium) + (presence of) *d*(*ecarboxylase*)] See under APUD CELLS.

**apudoma** \ap′ədō′mə\ [from *APUD (cells)* + -OMA] A tumor consisting of APUD cells located usually in the gut, less commonly in the pancreatic islets, adrenal medulla, pituitary and thyroid glands, and perhaps elsewhere. It often secretes one or more hormones or amines, as gastrin, calcitonin, and serotonin. It is implicated in the pathogenesis of multiple endocrine neoplasia Type I and Type II.

**apulmonism** \āpul′mənizm\ [Gk *a-* priv. + PULMON- + -ISM] A developmental absence of all or part of one or both lungs.

**apulosis** \ap′yoolō′sis\ [Gk *apoulōsis* (from *apouloun* to cicatrize, scar over, from *ap(o)-*, completive prefix, + *oulē* a scar) cicatrization] **1** CICATRIX. **2** CICATRIZATION.

**apulotic** \ap′yoolät′ik\ [Gk *apoulōtikos* causing to scar over. See APULOSIS.] CICATRIZANT.

**apurinic acid** DNA from which purines, but not pyrimidines, have been removed by mild acid hydrolysis.

**apus** \ā′pəs\ [New L (from Gk *apous* without foot or feet, from *a-* priv. + *pous* foot)] The developmental absence of one or both feet. It was once thought to be the result of intrauterine amputation associated with amniotic bands and adhesions.

**apyetous** \əpī′ətəs\ APYOGENOUS.

**apyknomorph** \əpik′nəmôrf′\ [Gk *apykno(s)* not dense or thick + *morph(ē)* form] A cell that has a loose, open chromatin pattern within the nucleus.

**apyogenous** \ā′pī·äj′ənəs\ [Gk *a-* priv. + PYO- + -GENOUS] Having no pus; not producing pus. Also *apyetous, apyous.*

**apyretic** \ā′pīret′ik\ [Gk *apyret(os)* (from *a-* priv. + *pyretos* fever) free from fever + -IC] AFEBRILE.

**apyrexia** \ā′pīrek′sē·ə\ [Gk (from *a-* priv. + *-pyrex-*, aorist stem of *pyressein* to have a fever + -IA) freedom from fever] The absence of a fever.

**apyrexial** \ā′pīrek′sē·əl\ AFEBRILE.

**apyrimidinic acid** A segment of deoxyribonucleic acid from which all of the pyrimidine bases have been chemically removed.

**aq.** *aqua* (L, water).

**aq. ad.** *aquam ad* (L, water to: used in directions for compounding prescriptions to indicate that water should be added to a specified volume).

**aq. dest.** *aqua destillata* (L, distilled water).

**aq. pur.** *aqua pura* (L, pure water).

**Â QRST** manifest mean QRST axis.

**aq. tep.** *aqua tepida* (L, tepid water).

**aqua** \ä′kwə\ [L, water] Water. **a. amnii** AMNIOTIC FLUID. **a. calcis** LIME WATER. **a. camphorae concentrata** CONCENTRATED CAMPHOR WATER. **a. cinnamomi** CINNAMON WATER. **a. fortis** NITRIC ACID. **a. labyrinthi** *Outmoded* PERILYMPHA. **a. menthae piperitae** PEPPERMINT WATER. **a. menthae viridis** SPEARMINT WATER. **a. oculi** HUMOR AQUOSUS. **a. pericardii** *Outmoded* PERICARDIAL FLUID. **a. rosae** ROSE WATER.

**aquae** \ā′kwē\ Plural of AQUA.

**aquaeductus** \ak′wəduk′təs\ AQUEDUCTUS.

**aqueduct** \ak′wədukt′\ [L *aquaeductus* (from *aquae*, gen. of *aqua* water + *ductus* a leading, from *ductus*, past part. of *ducere* to lead) aqueduct] AQUEDUCTUS. **cerebral a.** AQUEDUCTUS CEREBRI. **a. of cerebrum** AQUEDUCTUS CEREBRI. **a. of cochlea** AQUEDUCTUS COCHLEAE. **cochlear a.** AQUEDUCTUS COCHLEAE. **a. of Cotunnius** AQUEDUCTUS VESTIBULI. **fallopian a.** CANALIS FACIALIS. **a. of Fallopius** CANALIS FACIALIS. **a. of mesencephalon** AQUEDUCTUS CEREBRI. **a. of midbrain** AQUEDUCTUS CEREBRI. **a. of Sylvius** *Outmoded* AQUEDUCTUS CEREBRI. **ventricular a.** *Outmoded* AQUEDUCTUS CEREBRI. **a. of vestibule**

1 AQUEDUCTUS VESTIBULI. 2 DUCTUS ENDOLYMPHATICUS.

**aqueductus** \ak′wəduk′təs\ A tubular channel, canal, or conduit. Also *aqueduct, aquaeductus.* **a. cerebri** [NA] A narrow, ependyma-lined canal, 15 mm in length, connecting the third to the fourth ventricle. It is a midbrain structure, with the tectum mesencephali lying dorsal to the plane of the canal and the tegmentum ventral to it. In developmental and comparative anatomy it is known as the mesocele. Also *cerebral aqueduct, aqueduct of cerebrum, aqueduct of midbrain, ventricular aqueduct, canal of the midbrain, aqueduct of mesencephalon, aqueduct of Sylvius* (outmoded), *aqueductus Sylvii* (outmoded), *iter a tertio ad quartum ventriculum, iter of Sylvius, mesocoelia* (obs.), *sylviduct* (rare). **a. cochleae** [NA] A series of reticular perilymphatic cells with communicating intercellular clefts that lines the bony cochlear canaliculus, forming a communication between the perilymphatic space of the scala tympani and the subarachnoid space. Also *cochlear aqueduct, ductus perilymphaticus, perilymphatic duct, aqueduct of cochlea, periotic duct.* **a. Sylvii** *Outmoded* AQUEDUCTUS CEREBRI. **a. vestibuli** [NA] A bony canal extending from a large aperture in the medial wall of the vestibule of the internal ear to the posterior surface of the petrous part of the temporal bone and containing a prolongation of the membranous labyrinth, the ductus endolymphaticus, and its terminal closed saccus endolymphaticus, and small blood vessels. Also *aqueduct of vestibule, aqueduct of Cotunnius, canal of Cotunnius.*

**aqueous** \ā′kwē·əs\ 1 Containing, consisting of or resembling water: used especially of solutions, to indicate that the solvent is water. 2 HUMOR AQUOSUS.

**aquiparous** \akwip′ərəs\ [L *aqu(a)* water + *i* + *par(ere)* to bear young, beget, produce + -OUS] Producing a watery secretion. Also *aquiducous.*

**AR** 1 aortic regurgitation. 2 artificial respiration.

**Ar** Symbol for the element, argon.

**-ar** \-ər\ [L *-aris* (alternative of *-alis* after word ending in el sound)] A suffix meaning of or belonging to.

**ara-A** VIDARABINE.

**araban** ARABINAN.

**arabinan** A polysaccharide formed of arabinose residues and occurring in plants. Also *araban.*

**arabinose** An aldopentose sugar, the 2-epimer of ribose. L-Arabinose is a bacterial metabolite, and derivatives of both it and of D-arabinose occur widely in plants.

**2-araboketose** RIBULOSE.

**arachidonic acid** $CH_3$—$[CH_2]_4$—CH=CH—$CH_2$—CH=CH—$CH_2$—CH=CH—$CH_2$—CH=CH—$[CH_2]_3$—COOH. 5,8,11,14-Icosatetraenoic acid. An essential unsaturated fatty acid formed in animals from unsaturated-acids, such as linolenic acid, found in plants. Arachidonic acid is found only in animal fats, as in egg yolk and liver. It is a precursor of prostaglandins and thromboxanes.

**arachn-** \ərakn-\ ARACHNO-.

***Arachnia propionica*** \ərak′nē·ə präp′ē·än′əkə\ A species of actinomycete intermediate in properties between *Actinomyces* and *Propionibacterium* and able to cause typical actinomycotic lesions.

**arachnid** \ərak′nid\ [ARACHN- + -ID[1]] A member of the class Arachnida.

**Arachnida** \ərak′nidə\ [ARACHN- + New L *-ida,* plural in form from L *-ides,* patronymic suffix] A class of arthropods of the subphylum Chelicerata, which includes mites, ticks, spiders, scorpions, and related forms. Many of the most important parasites and vectors of human and animal pathogens are included in this large assemblage.

**arachnidism** \ərak′nidizm\ A morbid condition resulting from the bite of an arachnid, which may include ascending motor paralysis and destruction of peripheral nerve endings. Also *spider poisoning, arachnoidism, araneism.* See also LATRODECTISM, LOXOSCELISM.

**arachnitis** \ar′aknī′tis\ [ARACHN- + -ITIS] ARACHNOIDITIS.

**arachno-** \ərak′nō-\ [Gk *arachnē* spider's web or *arachnēs* spider] A combining form denoting (1) spider; (2) the arachnoidea. Also *arachn-.*

**arachnodactylia** \-daktil′yə\ ARACHNODACTYLY.

**arachnodactyly** \-dak′təlē\ The long thin fingers and toes seen in certain dysplasias such as the Marfan syndrome. Also *spider finger, dolichostenomelia, acromacria, arachnodactylia.* **congenital contractural a.** The autosomal dominant variation of the Marfan syndrome, characterized by limb contractures, arachnodactyly, and scoliosis.

**arachnogastria** \-gas′trē·ə\ SPIDER BELLY.

**arachnoid** \ərak′noid\ [Gk *arachnoeidēs* (from *arachnē* a spider, spider's web + *-eidēs* -like, -OID) cobweblike] 1 Having the appearance or texture of a spider's web. 2 Denoting the arachnoidea. Also *arachnoidal.* 3 ARACHNOIDEA.

**arachnoidea** \ar′aknoi′dē·ə\ [New L, short for *membrana arachnoidea* arachnoid membrane. See ARACHNOID.] [NA] The middle of the three layers of the meninges covering the brain and spinal cord. Its smooth external surface is closely applied to the dura mater, while the inner, roughened surface is separated from the pia mater by the subarachnoid space. In some locations the space is crossed by fine trabeculae. Also *arachnoid, arachnoid membrane, meningion* (obs.), *meningium* (obs.). Adj. arachnoid.

**arachnoideae** \ar′aknoi′di·ē\ Plural of ARACHNOIDEA.

**arachnoidism** \ərak′noidizm\ ARACHNIDISM.

**arachnoiditis** \ərak′noidī′tis\ [ARACHNOID + -ITIS] 1 Inflammation of the arachnoid membrane. Also *arachnitis.* 2 Any process of acute, subacute or chronic inflammation, scarring, proliferative or granulomatous process in the arachnoid membrane, whether primary or secondary, whether isolated or associated with damage to contiguous nervous tissues. Types of arachnoiditis, designated according to their situation, include optochiasmatic, basal, spinal, and many other forms. **adhesive a.** A chronic, sterile inflammatory fibrous reaction of the spinal cord membranes resulting in progressive obliteration of subarachnoid space, spinal fluid blockage, cord ischemia, and sensory and motor deficits. The condition may follow trauma, aseptic meningitis, or injection of foreign substances into the subarachnoid space. **basal a.** Arachnoiditis involving the arachnoid membranes around the base of the brain and basilar artery. Also *basilar arachnoiditis.* **a. of the cerebral hemispheres** Arachnoiditis involving particularly the arachnoid over the convexity of the cerebral hemispheres. **cisternal a.** Basal arachnoiditis involving particularly the basal subarachnoid cisterns. **opticochiasmatic a.** Arachnoiditis of the basal arachnoid, most severe around the optic nerves and chiasm. It gives rise to variable visual field defects, sometimes with unilateral or bilateral central scotomata, leading to optic atrophy. These clinical manifestations result either from compression of the optic nerves or chiasm or from ischemia due to scarring or proliferation of the arachnoid. Sometimes there is resultant arachnoid cyst formation, and the cyst, containing cerebrospinal fluid, may also cause compression. The condition may be due to syphilitic or other forms of granulomatous inflammatory change, such as sarcoidosis, or it may follow meningitis or subarachnoid hemorrhage, but many cases are unexplained. **a. of the posterior cerebral fossa** Arachnoiditis in the posterior fossa, which may cause intermittent or progressive communicating hydrocephalus, multiple cranial nerve palsies, or, if it develops in the outlet foramina of the fourth ventricle or cisterna magna, syringomyelia. **spinal a.** Arachnoiditis in the spinal canal giving rise to symptoms and signs of compression of the spinal cord and/or of spinal nerves and roots. A tuberculous form has been described, occurring especially in India, and in such cases the cerebrospinal fluid usually shows an excess of cells and protein, and tubercle bacilli may be isolated. In the idiopathic variety, the fluid is more often normal but its protein content may be raised and, if severe, a spinal block may occur, with a positive Queckenstedt's test and a marked rise in protein. Myelography usually shows a patchy hold-up of the contrast medium. Arachnoid cysts of developmental origin, filled with cerebrospinal fluid, may occur over the posterior aspect of the dorsal spinal cord, giving evidence of progressive cord compression. **spinal adhesive a.** Chronic adhesive arachnoiditis involving particularly the spinal arachnoid.

**arachnolysin** \ar′aknäl′isin\ [ARACHNO- + LYSIN] The active hemolytic component of spider venom.

**arachnopia** \ar′aknō′pē·ə\ *Obs.* LEPTOMENINGES.

**Aran** [François Amilcar *Aran*, French physician, 1817–1861] Aran-Duchenne amyotrophy, Aran-Duchenne muscular atrophy, Aran-Duchenne disease. See under PROGRESSIVE MUSCULAR ATROPHY.

**Araneida** \ar′ənē′idə\ [L *arane(us)* (from Gk *arachnēs* spider) a spider + *-ida*, suffix for taxonomic orders] An order of Arachnida which includes the spiders, many of which are of medical or veterinary importance. Also *Araneae.*

**araneism** \ərā′nē·izm\ ARACHNIDISM.

**araneous** \ərā′nē·əs\ [L *arane(us)* (from Gk *arachnaios* of spiders, like a spider's web) pertaining to spiders + -OUS] Cobweblike; arachnoid.

**Arantius** [*Arantius* (Giulio Caesar Aranzio), Italian anatomist and physician, 1530–1589] **1** Duct of Arantius, canal of Arantius. See under DUCTUS VENOSUS. **2** Nodules of Arantius. See under NODULI VALVULARUM SEMILUNARIUM VALVAE AORTAE. **3** Arantius ligament. See under LIGAMENTUM VENOSUM.

**araphia** \ərā′fē·ə\ [Gk *a-* priv. + *rhaph(ē)* a seam, suture + -IA] STATUS DYSRHAPHICUS.

**arb.** arbitrary.

**arbor** \är′bər\ [L, tree] A structure or part having branches like a tree. **a. bronchialis** [NA] The structural and functional unit formed by the bronchi and their branches or rami. Also *bronchial tree.* **a. vitae** A pattern of dendritic branching resembling the branching pattern of the evergreen tree of this name, e.g., cerebellar Purkinje cell dendrites.

**arbores** \ärbôr′ēz\ Plural of ARBOR.

**arborescent** \är′bôres′ənt\ Branching; treelike.

**arborization** \är′bôrīzā′shən\ [ARBOR + *-iz(e)* + -ATION] A branching pattern in the termination of a nerve fiber, as of an axon in a central tract, the axon of a free nerve ending in subcutaneous tissue, or a motoneuron in muscle. **cervical mucus a.** The occurrence of a fernlike pattern when uterine cervix mucus is allowed to dry for ten minutes on a glass slide and is then examined microscopically. It is indicative of the presence of estrogen, which alters the concentration of sodium chloride in the mucus. In humans, this pattern is seen in the proliferative phase of the menstrual cycle, between the seventh and 18th day, and in the presence of leaking amniotic fluid. Also *fern phenomenon, fern-leaf crystallization, ferning.*

**arborvirus** \är′bôrvī′rəs\ ARBOVIRUS.

**arbovirus** \är′bōvī′rəs\ [*ar(thropod)-bo(rne)* + VIRUS] Any of a heterogeneous group of RNA-containing viruses that are transmitted between humans, or between animals and humans, by arthropod vectors. No longer a useful category in the classification of viruses, the group includes members of the families Bunyaviridae, Togaviridae, Reoviridae, and Rhabdoviridae. Also *arborvirus, arbor virus.*

**ARC** **1** AIDS-related complex. See under ACQUIRED IMMUNE DEFICIENCY SYNDROME. **2** abnormal retinal correspondence.

**arc** \ärk\ [L *arcus* a bow] A segment of a curve, especially of a circumference. **autonomic reflex a.** An involuntary response of smooth or cardiac muscle or glands, in which the efferent part of the reflex arc is conveyed by sympathetic or parasympathetic nerves. **dorsal venous a.** Any of the following: (1) rete venosum dorsale manus; (2) rete venosum dorsale pedis; (3) arcus venosus dorsalis pedis. **epiploic a. of Haller and Barkow** The anastomosis between the omental branches of the right and left gastro-omental arteries, which lie between the layers of the greater omentum. The largest branch of each artery anastomoses near the margin of attachment of the greater omentum to the greater curvature of the stomach. **external marginal a. of Zuckerkandl** GYRUS SUBCALLOSUS. **mercury a.** An electric discharge that makes luminous a mercury vapor within a glass or quartz tube. It is a source of ultraviolet rays. **neural a.** A pathway consisting of two or more neurons, requiring an afferent and an efferent fiber. **nuclear a.** The concentric configuration

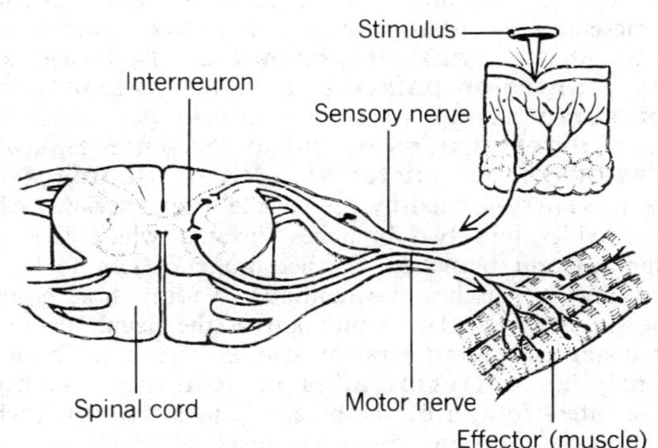


**Reflex arc**

of the fibrae lentis. *Outmoded.* **reflex a.** A neural arc of varying complexity underlying a relatively consistent autonomic or somatic motor response. Also *reflex circuit.* **retruded a. of closure** The path of closure with the condyles in their most posterior positions. **Riolan's a.** **1** INTERMESENTERIC ARTERIAL ANASTOMOSIS. **2** MARGINAL ARTERY OF COLON. **3** The series of arterial arches formed by anastomoses between adjacent branches of the jejunal and ileal arteries. **4** The part of the marginal artery of the colon that connects the middle with the left colic arteries within the transverse mesocolon. **5** The arch formed by the transverse mesocolon. Also *Riolan's arch, Riolan's arcade.* **sensorimotor a.** Any neural arc that includes an afferent side with input from a sense organ and an efferent side that activates striated muscle, including segmental reflexes and input-output circuits at suprasegmental levels.

**arcade** \ärkād′\ [French (from Provençal *arcada* an opening in form of an arch, from L *arcus* a bow), a wall opening whose upper part is an arch] An arched channel or passage; a series of arches. **anomalous mitral a.** A congenital anomaly in which the chordae tendineae from both papillary muscles are attached to the central portion of the anterior leaf of the mitral valve. It may result in mitral stenosis or regurgitation. **arterial a.'s** Anastomoses between side branches of adjacent arteries forming loops or arches, such as between the distal branches of the jejunal and ileal arteries in the mesentery, and the anterior and posterior arcades on the head of the pancreas. **Flint's a.** ARTERIAE ARCUATAE RENIS. **Riolan's a.** RIOLAN'S ARC.

**arcanum** A secret medication or nostrum.

**arcesis** [Gk *arkesis* (from *arkein* to ward off) help, service] A drug or dietary constituent that increases an individual's resistance to diseases.

# arch

**arch** \ärch\ [Old French *arche* (from L *arcus* a bow) an arch] **1** A wire or parallel wires made to conform to the dental arch. **2** In anatomy, any curved or bowlike structure; arcus. **abdominothoracic a.** ARCUS COSTALIS. **alveolar a. of mandible** ARCUS ALVEOLARIS MANDIBULAE. **alveolar a. of maxilla** ARCUS ALVEOLARIS MAXILLAE. **anastomotic a.** Arteries or veins joining end to end to form arches, as in the palm, sole of the foot, and mesentery. **anterior a. of atlas** ARCUS ANTERIOR ATLANTIS. **anterior carpal a.** PALMAR CARPAL ARCH. **anterior palatine a.** ARCUS PALATOGLOSSUS. **a. of aorta** ARCUS AORTAE. **aortic a.** ARCUS AORTICUS. **arterial a.'es of colon** See under MARGINAL ARTERY OF COLON. **arterial a.'es of ileum** Arches in the mesentery formed by the parallel ileal arteries, each of which divides into two branches distally, which then join similar adjacent branches. Further branches join to form a second series of arches and continue to form three or more further arches near the termination of the ileum. From the most distal arch, short straight arteries extend to the ileum to supply it. **arterial a.'es of jejunum** Arches in the mesentery formed by the parallel jejunal arteries, each of which divides into two branches distally, which then join similar adjacent branches. Further branches form a second series of arches, there being only one arch in the upper part of the mesentery. Short straight arteries pass to the jejunum from the arch nearest to the intestine. **arterial a.'es of kidney** ARTERIAE ARCUATAE RENIS. **axillary a.** PECTORODORSALIS MUSCLE. **a. of azygos vein** ARCUS VENAE AZYGOU. **basal a.** APICAL BASE. **branchial a.** Each of a series of bars of mesenchymal tissue arranged dorsoventrally between the pharynx and the cervical ectoderm of embryos and separated more or less completely by the branchial (pharyngeal) clefts and pouches. The arch arteries run through them and the cranial neural crest tissue penetrates them. In man the mesoderm of the branchial arches gives rise to the "visceral" skeleton and its striated muscle. Also *pharyngeal arch, postaural arch, postoral arch, cervical arch, visceral arch.* **cervical a.** BRANCHIAL ARCH. **a.'es of Corti** A series of epithelial arches formed by the convex heads of the obliquely sloping, long outer pillars or rods of Corti overlying and fitting into concavities on the heads of the converging, shorter inner pillar cells, forming the roof of the inner tunnel of Corti in the spiral organ. **cortical a.'es of the kidney** LOBULI CORTICALES RENIS. **costal a.** ARCUS COSTALIS. **a. of cricoid cartilage** ARCUS CARTILAGINIS CRICOIDEAE. **crural a.** LIGAMENTUM INGUINALE. **deep crural a.** The downward extension of the transversalis fascia from the region of the deep inguinal ring to strengthen the anterior part of the femoral sheath, from which transversely arched fibers splay out laterally towards the anterior superior iliac spine and medially behind the rectus abdominis muscle, while some descend behind the conjoint tendon to the pecten pubis. It may be absent, poorly defined, or a thickened band. Also *iliopubic tract, Thompson's ligament, tractus iliopubicus* (outmoded). **deep palmar a.** ARCUS PALMARIS PROFUNDUS. **deep palmar arterial a.** ARCUS PALMARIS PROFUNDUS. **deep palmar venous a.** ARCUS VENOSUS PALMARIS PROFUNDUS. **deep plantar a.** ARCUS PLANTARIS PROFUNDUS. **dental a.** The curved arrangement of the teeth in the maxilla or mandible. Also *arcus dentalis.* **dorsal carpal a.** RETE CARPALE DORSALE. **dorsal venous a. of foot** ARCUS VENOSUS DORSALIS PEDIS. **dorsal venous a. of the hand** RETE VENOSUM DORSALE MANUS. **dorsal a. of wrist** RETE CARPALE DORSALE. **double aortic a.** The persistence of both fourth embryonic aortic arches, which form a vascular ring encircling the trachea and esophagus. The arches may persist as arterial structures, or part of the circle may become atretic and be represented as a fibrous cord. See also PERSISTENT RIGHT AORTIC ARCH. **epiphyseal a.** The roof plate of the embryonic diencephalon from which the epiphysis or pineal body develops. **fallen a.'es** A flattening of the longitudinal and transverse arches of the foot. **fibrous a. of soleus muscle** ARCUS TENDINEUS MUSCULI SOLEI. **a.'es of the foot** The natural longitudinal and transverse concave arches produced by the plantar aspect of tarsal and metatarsal bones and their binding ligaments. The curved architectural design provides the mechanisms required for the special functions of the human foot in erect posture, namely, support of weight and locomotion. **gill a.** That structure in a vertebrate embryo which develops in the wall of the pharynx between successive gill clefts. **glossopalatine a.** ARCUS PALATOGLOSSUS. **Haller's a.'es** Ligamentum arcuatum laterale and ligamentum arcuatum mediale. **hyoid a.** The second branchial arch in embryos of which the mesenchyme gives rise to the stapes and the hyoid cartilaginous chain. The nerve of this arch is the seventh cranial (facial) nerve. Also *Reichert's arch, stylostapedian arch.* **hyothyroid a.** The third mesodermal pharyngeal arch which gives rise among other structures to the thyrohyal, precursor of the greater cornu of the hyoid bone. The nerve of this arch is the glossopharyngeal. Also *thyrohyoid arch.* **iliopectineal a.** ARCUS ILIOPECTINEUS. **inferior dental a.** ARCUS DENTALIS INFERIOR. **inferior palpebral a.** ARCUS PALPEBRALIS INFERIOR. **intermesenteric arterial a.** INTERMESENTERIC ARTERIAL ANASTOMOSIS. **ischiopubic a.** ARCUS PUBIS. **jugular venous a.** ARCUS VENOSUS JUGULARIS. **Langer's axillary a.** **lateral lumbocostal a.** LIGAMENTUM ARCUATUM LATERALE. **lateral lumbocostal a. of Haller** LIGAMENTUM ARCUATUM LATERALE. **longitudinal a. of foot** ARCUS PEDIS LONGITUDINALIS. **malar a.** ARCUS ZYGOMATICUS. **mandibular a.** The first visceral arch of the splanchnocranium, which forks into a more rostral maxillary process and a more caudal mandibular process, and develops into most of the lower part of the face as well as the zygomatic bones, the squamous part of the temporal bones, and the incus and malleus of the middle ear.

**marginal a. of lower eyelid** ARCUS PALPEBRALIS INFERIOR. **marginal a. of upper eyelid** ARCUS PALPEBRALIS SUPERIOR. **medial lumbocostal a.** LIGAMENTUM ARCUATUM MEDIALE. **medial lumbocostal a. of Haller** LIGAMENTUM ARCUATUM MEDIALE. **nasal a.** The angular arch formed by the nasal process of the maxilla on each side and the nasal bones between them. **neural a.** The arch formed in the primitive segmental sclerotome of an embryo which flanks the neural tube and eventually becomes the vertebral arch of an adult vertebra. **neural a. of vertebra** ARCUS VERTEBRAE. **orbital a. of frontal bone** **palatal a.** The concavity of the roof of the mouth formed by the maxillary and palatine bones. **palatine a.** The arch formed by the palatoglossus muscle on each side and the soft palate at the top. **palatoglossal a.** ARCUS PALATOGLOSSUS. **palatopharyngeal a.** ARCUS PALATOPHARYNGEUS. **palmar carpal a.** An anastomosis at the lower border of the pronator quadratus muscle between the transversely directed palmar carpal branches of the radial and ulnar arteries, joined by a branch from the anterior interosseous artery and recurrent branches from the deep palmar arch. It supplies the anterior aspects of the radiocarpal and carpal joints. Also *anterior carpal arch.* **paraphyseal a.** The arched part of the roof of the embryonic telencephalon from which the paraphysis arises. **parieto-occipital a.** ARCUS PARIETO-OCCIPITALIS. **a. of pelvis** 1 ANGULUS SUBPUBICUS. 2 ARCUS PUBIS. **persistent right aortic a.** The presence in a fetus or postnatal individual of the right fourth aortic arch of the embryo, instead of or in addition to the left fourth arch. If only the right arch persists, the aortic arch crosses the right rather than the left bronchus (right sided aortic arch); if both arches persist, double aortic arch is the result. The phenomenon is usually associated with other cardiovascular malformations but may be expected as a component of situs inversus. **pharyngeal a.** BRANCHIAL ARCH. **pharyngopalatine a.** ARCUS PALATOPHARYNGEUS. **plantar a.** ARCUS PLANTARIS PROFUNDUS. **plantar arterial a.** ARCUS PLANTARIS PROFUNDUS. **plantar venous a.** ARCUS VENOSUS PLANTARIS. **popliteal a.** LIGAMENTUM POPLITEUM ARCUATUM. **posterior a. of atlas** ARCUS POSTERIOR ATLANTIS. **posterior carpal a.** RETE CARPALE DORSALE. **posterior palatine a.** ARCUS PALATOPHARYNGEUS. **posterior a. of vertebra** ARCUS VERTEBRAE. **prepancreatic a.** A fairly constant anastomosis in front of the head of the pancreas between the right branch of the dorsal pancreatic artery and a small left branch of the anterior superior pancreaticoduodenal artery. **primitive costal a.'es** Curvatures formed by the developing ribs in an embryo. The costal processes of the primitive vertebral arches grow laterally in the embryonic thoracic region to form a series of primitive costal arches. **pubic a.** ARCUS PUBIS. **pulmonary a.** ARCUS AORTICUS. **Reichert's a.** HYOID ARCH. **rhinencephalic a.** GYRUS CINGULI. **right aortic a.** A congenital anomaly found in about 20% of cases of the tetralogy of Fallot in which the right aortic arch persists, resulting in a complete reversal of the aortic arch and its branches, and may or may not be accompanied by a situs inversus. In some cases of persistence of part of the right dorsal aorta, the aorta appears to divide near its origin and reunite so that the esophagus and trachea pass between the branches, a condition normal in reptiles. There are many other variations involving partial or complete persistence. **Riolan's a.** RIOLAN'S ARC. **saddle a.** A form of palatal arch in which the lateral sides appear to bulge downwards. This may occur with an excessively arched palate, found in some congenital anomalies involving the face. Also *saddle-shaped arch.* **Salus a.** The arch formed by a vein crossing a retinal artery, as observed in arteriosclerosis. **Shenton's a.** SHENTON'S LINE. **subpubic a.** 1 ARCUS PUBIS. 2 ANGULUS SUBPUBICUS. **superciliary a.** ARCUS SUPERCILIARIS. **superficial palmar a.** ARCUS PALMARIS SUPERFICIALIS. **superficial palmar arterial a.** ARCUS PALMARIS SUPERFICIALIS. **superficial palmar venous a.** ARCUS VENOSUS PALMARIS SUPERFICIALIS. **superficial plantar a.** ARCUS PLANTARIS SUPERFICIALIS. **superior dental a.** ARCUS DENTALIS SUPERIOR. **superior palpebral a.** ARCUS PALPEBRALIS SUPERIOR. **supraorbital a. of frontal bone** MARGO SUPRAORBITALIS OSSIS FRONTALIS. **systemic a.** The fourth aortic arch in vertebrates and vertebrate embryos. It allows blood to flow between the ventral and dorsal aortae, thus supplying the trunk and limbs with arterial blood. In adult amphibians and reptiles, both the right and left systemic arches persist, whereas adult birds retain only the right arch and adult mammals only the left arch. **tendinous a.** ARCUS TENDINEUS. **tendinous a. of levator ani muscle** ARCUS TENDINEUS MUSCULI LEVATORIS ANI. **tendinous a. of lumbodorsal fascia** LIGAMENTUM LUMBOCOSTALE. **tendinous a. of pelvic fascia** ARCUS TENDINEUS FASCIAE PELVIS. **tendinous a. of soleus muscle** ARCUS TENDINEUS MUSCULI SOLEI. **thyrohyoid a.** HYOTHYROID ARCH. **transverse a. of foot** ARCUS PEDIS TRANSVERSALIS. **trapezoidal a.** A mild form of tapering arch with straight buccal segments and a shallowly curved anterior segment. **Treitz a.** A vascular arch formed by the ascending branch of the left colic artery and the inferior mesenteric vein, which lies deep to a peritoneal fold, usually coinciding with the paraduodenal fold, located between the fourth, or ascending, part of the duodenum and the medial margin of the left kidney. Also *vascular arch of Treitz.* **U-shaped a.** A dental arch in which the buccal segments are parallel and the anterior segment is curved so that there is not a sudden change of direction at the canines. **venous a.'es of kidney** VENAE ARCUATAE RENIS. **a. of vertebra** ARCUS VERTEBRAE. **visceral a.** BRANCHIAL ARCH. **zygomatic a.** ARCUS ZYGOMATICUS.

**arch-** \ärk-\ ARCHI-.

**Archaebacteria** \är′kēbaktir′ē·ə\ [Gk *archai(os)* very ancient, primeval + BACTERIA] A group of bacteria, including methanogens and some halophiles, that appear to be relics of very primitive organisms. They lack muramic acid and glyceryl esters, their ribosomal RNA differs markedly in nucleotide sequence from that of eubacteria and has some homology to that of eukaryotes.

**archaic** \ärkā′ik\ [Gk *archaïk(os)* (from *archa(ios)* ancient + *-ikos* -IC; from *archē* a beginning) antiquated, old-fashioned] Ancestral or ancient: used of a structure or organ, or a part thereof, that has a considerable evolutionary age.

**arche-** \är′kē-\ ARCHI-.

**archencephalon** \är′kensef′əlän\ [ARCH- + ENCEPHALON] A portion of the embryonic neural tube which extends beyond the anterior extremity of the notochord and gives rise to the suprasegmental centers and to the rhinencephalon. It exhibits virtually no evidence of a metameric constitution. Also *primitive brain.*

**archenteron** \ärken′tərän\ [ARCH- + ENTERON] The primary embryonic cavity which in many forms appears at gastrulation by invagination of the vegetal cells to form a provisional stomach which communicates temporarily with the exterior by the blastopore. Also *gastrulation cavity, gastrocoele, primitive gut, primitive stomach.*

**archi-** \är′kē-\ [Gk *archē* a beginning] A combining form meaning primitive, original, first. Also *arch-, arche-*.

**archicerebellum** \är′kēserəbel′əm\ [ARCHI- + CEREBELLUM] FLOCCULONODULAR LOBE.

**archicortex** \är′kēkôr′teks\ [ARCHI- + CORTEX] [NA] The phylogenetically oldest part of thecerebral cortex and the earliest to differentiate in development. The hippocampus, dentate gyrus, and subiculum are generally accepted as the major constituents, but there is some basis for dispute. Also *archipallium*.

**archicyte** \är′kēsīt\ [ARCHI- + -CYTE] The zygote at the stage when its nucleus can first be observed and before cleavage has begun.

**archigastrula** \är′kēgas′trələ\ Theoretically, a gastrula in its most primitive (phylogenetic) form of development. It is exhibited more or less in cephalochordates and certain invertebrates.

**archigonocyte** \är′kēgän′əsīt′\ [ARCHI- + GONOCYTE] The first cell of a fertilized ovum which becomes a primordial germ cell, distinguished from a somatic cell by the persistence of its embryonic characteristics. Thus it is totipotent. Also *primordial germ cell, primordial gonocyte*.

**archil** CUDBEAR.

**archimorula** \är′kēmôr′yələ\ [ARCHI- + MORULA] A mass of cells, resembling a mulberry, resulting from division of the single-celled archicyte and forming before the appearance of the archigastrula.

**archinephron** \är′kēnef′rän\ [ARCHI- + NEPHRON] One of the individual units of the pronephros. Adj. archinephric.

**archipallium** \är′kēpal′ē·əm\ [ARCHI- + PALLIUM] ARCHICORTEX. Adj. archipallial.

**architectonics** \är′kitektän′iks\ The pattern of structural organization, or architectural arrangement, of a tissue, organ, or part.

**archo-** \är′kō-\ [Gk *archos* the anus or rectum] A combining form denoting the rectum.

**archos** \är′kəs\ *Outmoded* ANUS.

**arcual** \är′kyoo·əl\ Pertaining to an arch.

**arcualia** \är′kyoo·ā′lyə\ [L *arcu(s)* a bow + L *-alia*, neut. pl. of *-alis* -AL] Double pairs of cartilaginous nodules in the mesodermal sheath surrounding the vertebrate notochord. One pair develops dorsolaterally to become the neural arch, the other dorsoventrally to form the hemal arch.

**arcuate** \är′kyoo·āt\ [L *arcuat(us)*, past part. of *arcuare* (from *arcus* a bow, arch) to bend in the form of a bow] In the shape of a curved bow; arched.

**arcuation** \är′kyoo·ā′shən\ [L *arcuatio* (from *arcuatus*, past part. of *arcuare* to bend in the form of a bow) a structure consisting of arches, arcade] A bend or curvature that is usually abnormal.

**arcula** \är′kyələ\ *Outmoded* ORBITA.

**arcus** \är′kəs\ [L, a bow, arch] (*pl.* arcus) [NA] Any structure in the form of an arch or arc. **a. alveolaris mandibulae** [NA] The curved superior margin of the alveolar part of the body of the mandible, hollowed out by the sockets for the roots of the sixteen lower teeth around which the gingiva is attached. Also *alveolar arch of mandible, alveolar border of mandible, alveolar margin of mandible*. **a. alveolaris maxillae** [NA] The curved, thick inferior surface of the alveolar process of the maxilla, hollowed out by the sockets for the roots of the sixteen upper teeth around which the gingiva is attached. Also *alveolar arch of maxilla, alveolar border of maxilla, alveolar surface of maxilla, alveolar margin of maxilla*. **a. anterior atlantis** [NA] The slender arch of atlas that links its lateral masses anteriorly and that presents a median tubercle anteriorly for attachment of the anterior longitudinal ligament and a posterior facet for articulation with the dens of axis. Also *anterior arch of atlas*. **a. aortae** [NA] The continuation of the ascending aorta in the superior mediastinum, commencing behind the right sternal angle, where it ascends towards the left and posteriorly and then runs downwards on the left of the vertebral column to the fourth thoracic vertebra, where it ends by continuing as the descending aorta. It arches across the right pulmonary artery and the left bronchus, lying to the left of the trachea and esophagus. From its upper convexity arise the brachiocephalic, left common carotid, and left subclavian arteries. Also *arch of aorta*. **a. aorticus** Any of six arches in the embryo (designated I–VI) connecting the ventral and dorsal aortae on each side, the first passing through the mandibular arch and the succeeding arches developed in corresponding branchial arches. With the exception of the fifth arch, which hardly appears in humans, they develop craniocaudally, the earlier ones disappearing by the time the caudal ones are developed. The first disappears entirely; only the dorsal part of the second remains as the stem of the stapedial artery; the third forms the internal carotid and links up with the common carotid and external carotid arteries, which derive from the aortic sac; the fourth on the right side becomes the proximal part of the right subclavian artery, while on the left it forms the aortic arch between the left common carotid and left subclavian arteries; and the sixth takes part in the development of the pulmonary trunk and arteries and the ductus arteriosus. Also *aortic arch, pulmonary arch*. **a. cartilaginis cricoideae** [NA] The narrow anterior arch of the cricoid cartilage that has the cricothyroid muscle attached to its anterior and lateral surfaces on either side. At its junction with the lamina on each side is the articular facet for articulation with the inferior cornu of the thyroid cartilage. Also *arch of cricoid cartilage*. **corneal a.** ARCUS SENILIS. **a. costalis** [NA] The arch formed by the articulated costal cartilages of the seventh through tenth ribs forming the anterior sides of the inferior thoracic aperture leading up to the infrasternal angle. Also *costal arch, arcus costarum* (outmoded), *abdominothoracic arch*. **a. dentalis** DENTAL ARCH. **a. dentalis inferior** [NA] The parabolic curve formed by the teeth in the lower jaw, especially in the occlusal view. Also *inferior dental arch*. **a. dentalis superior** [NA] The elliptic curve formed by the teeth in the upper jaw, especially in the occlusal view. Also *superior dental arch*. **a. iliopectineus** [NA] A septum of fused iliac and psoas fasciae that stretches between the inguinal ligament and the hip bone, specifically its iliopectineal eminence dividing the space deep to the inguinal ligament into lacuna musculorum laterally and lacuna vasorum medially. Also *iliopectineal arch, iliopectineal ligament, ligamentum iliopectineale, iliopectineal fascia, iliac fascia, iliopectineal septum*. **a. inguinalis** LIGAMENTUM INGUINALE. **a. juvenilis** A corneal ring comparable in appearance to arcus senilis but occurring in younger people, often associated with lipoidal degenerations of the blood-vessel walls; a lipoidal infiltration of the peripheral corneal stroma, separated from the sclera by a zone of clear cornea. Also *arcus presenilis, anterior embryotoxon*. **a. lumbocostalis lateralis** LIGAMENTUM ARCUATUM LATERALE. **a. lumbocostalis medialis** LIGAMENTUM ARCUATUM MEDIALE. **a. palatoglossus** [NA] The anterior arch of the fauces, extending from the inferior surface of the soft palate to the side of the tongue on each side of the oropharyngeal isthmus and formed by the palatoglossus muscle covered by mucous membrane. Between it and the palatopharyngeal arch posteriorly is the tonsillar sinus containing the palatine tonsil. It is involved in the mechanism of deglutition. Also *palatoglossal arch, glossopalatine* *arch, anterior palatine arch, anterior pillar of fauces, anterior column of fauces.* **a. palatopharyngeus** [NA] The prominent posterior arch of the fauces, extending from the side of the uvula to the side of the pharynx on each side of the oropharyngeal isthmus and formed by the palatopharyngeus muscle covered by mucous membrane. Between it and the palatoglossal arch anteriorly is the tonsillar sinus containing the palatine tonsil. It is involved in the mechanism of deglutition. Also *palatopharyngeal arch, arcus pharyngopalatinus, pharyngopalatine arch, posterior palatine arch, posterior pillar of fauces, posterior column of fauces.* **a. palmaris profundus** [NA] An arterial arch formed by the terminal part of the radial artery anastomosing with the deep palmar branch of the ulnar artery deep to the adductor pollicis muscle and the digital flexor tendons and lumbrical muscles and superficial to the proximal ends of the metacarpal bones and interosseous muscles. It gives off three palmar metacarpal arteries, three perforating branches, and recurrent branches. Also *deep palmar arterial arch, deep palmar arch.* **a. palmaris superficialis** [NA] An arterial arch formed by the terminal part of the ulnar artery either alone or by anastomosing with either the superficial palmar branch of the radial artery or the arteria radialis indicis. It is covered by the palmar aponeurosis and the palmaris brevis muscle and lies on the flexor tendons of the fingers and the lumbrical muscles, the branches of the median nerve, and the flexor digiti minimi muscle. It gives off three common palmar digital arteries. Also *superficial palmar arterial arch, superficial palmar arch.* **a. palpebralis inferior** [NA] An arch formed along the margin of the tarsus in the lower eyelid by the inferior medial palpebral artery, a branch of the ophthalmic artery, which anastomoses at the lateral end of the eyelid with the lower of the two lateral palpebral branches of the lacrimal artery and with the transverse facial artery. Also *inferior palpebral arch, marginal arch of lower eyelid.* **a. palpebralis superior** [NA] An arch formed along the margin of the tarsus in the upper eyelid by the superior medial palpebral artery, a branch of the ophthalmic artery, which anastomoses with the supraorbital artery and, at the lateral end of the upper eyelid, with the upper of the two lateral palpebral branches of the lacrimal artery and with the zygomatico-orbital branch of the superficial temporal artery. Also *superior palpebral arch, marginal arch of upper eyelid.* **a. parieto-occipitalis** On those human brains in which the parieto-occipital sulcus extends onto the laterosuperior margin of the cerebral hemisphere, the curved gyrus around the end of the sulcus formed by continuation of the superior parietal lobule with occipital cortex. Also *parieto-occipital arch.* **a. pedis longitudinalis** The longitudinal curvature of the foot, formed by seven tarsal and five metatarsal bones and maintained normally by binding ligaments, supporting intrinsic muscles, and the tendons of extrinsic muscles of the foot. The posterior pillar of the arch is the calcaneal tuberosity; the summit is the weight-bearing talus bone, and the anterior pillar is formed by the heads of metatarsals. The arch is divided into a pars medialis and a pars lateralis. Also *longitudinal arch of foot.* **a. pedis transversalis** [NA] The transverse concavity under the foot that comprises a series of arches usually described as a single unit in the shape of a half-dome, the highest part being deep to the proximal part of the metatarsus and adjoining the distal tarsal bones, namely, the three cuneiform bones and the cuboid bone. Bound together by ligaments, the arch is supported by the intrinsic muscles and some extrinsic muscles of the foot, particularly the tendon of the peroneus longus muscle. Also *transverse arch of foot.* **a. pharyngopalatinus** ARCUS PALATOPHARYNGEUS. **a. plantaris profundus** [NA] The deep arch in the sole of the foot formed by the lateral plantar artery coursing from the base of the fifth metatarsal bone across the interosseous muscles to the first interosseous space, where it anastomoses with the deep plantar artery. Also *plantar arterial arch, deep plantar arch, plantar arch.* **a. plantaris superficialis** [NA] An occasional arterial arch that is formed by an enlarged superficial branch of the medial plantar artery joining the lateral plantar artery between the plantar aponeurosis and the flexor digitorum brevis muscle. Also *superficial plantar arch.* **a. posterior atlantis** [NA] The thick arch posterior to the vertebral foramen of the atlas that links the lateral masses, behind each of which it has a wide groove on its superior surface for the vertebral artery and first cervical nerve. Between them, the arch attaches the posterior atlanto-occipital membrane superiorly and the ligamenta flava inferiorly. At its apex is the small posterior tubercle for the attachment of the ligamentum nuchae. Also *posterior arch of atlas.* **a. presenilis** ARCUS JUVENILIS. **a. pubis** [NA] The arch below the bodies and symphysis of the pubis formed by the ischiopubic ramus on each side. It is equivalent to the sides of the angulus subpubicus. Also *arch of pubis, pubic arch, ischiopubic arch, arch of pelvis, subpubic arch.* **a. senilis** A ring-shaped degenerative lipoidal deposit in the peripheral corneal stroma, separated from the sclera by a narrow clear interval, occurring usually in middle age or later. It is of no systemic significance. Also *gerontoxon, corneal arcus, gerontotoxon.* **a. superciliaris** [NA] Either of two bilateral curved ridges of bone above and almost parallel to the supraorbital margin, meeting the other in a rhomboid elevation, the glabella, in the median line above the frontonasal suture. Above each arch is a shallow depression that separates it from the frontal tuberosity. The arches are usually more prominent in males. Also *superciliary arch, superciliary ridge, supraorbital ridge.* **a. tendineus** **1** [NA] A white fibrous arch attached to bone or to muscle and protecting vessels and nerves passing deep to it. **2** [NA] A thickened linear ridge of fascia over a muscle providing attachment for ligaments and muscle fibers. Also *tendinous arch.* **a. tendineus fasciae pelvis** [NA] A thickened white band in the superior fascia of the pelvic diaphragm along a line extending from the lower part of the pubic symphysis to the spine of the ischium, usually located about 2.5 cm below the arcus tendineus of the levator ani muscle. Anteriorly it blends with the tissue, or lateral ligament, supporting the urinary bladder, and posteriorly it is continuous with the uterosacral ligaments. Also *tendinous arch of pelvic fascia, white line of pelvic fascia.* **a. tendineus musculi levatoris ani** [NA] The thickened band of origin of the levator ani muscle from the obturator fascia, extending from a variable anterior attachment (usually either the obturator membrane or the body of pubis medial to it) to the spine of ischium posteriorly, where it corresponds to the attachment of the arcus tendineus fasciae pelvis. The arch of levator ani marks the junction between the intra- and extrapelvic portions of the obturator fascia. Also *tendinous arch of levator ani muscle.* **a. tendineus musculi solei** [NA] A fibrous arch between the tibial and fibular origins of the soleus muscle, from which some fibers of the muscle arise and deep to which the tibial nerve and popliteal vessels pass. Also *fibrous arch of soleus muscle, tendinous arch of soleus muscle.* **a. venae azygou** [NA] The convex arch formed by the azygos vein at the level of the fourth thoracic vertebra as it passes forward above the root of the right lung from the posterior mediastinum to the superior vena cava. The arch ends in the superior vena cava just before the latter passes through the pericardium. Its convexity faces upwards. Also *arch of azygos vein.* **a. venosus dorsalis pedis** [NA] A superficial venous arch across the dorsum of the foot near the bases of the metatarsal bones formed by the dorsal metacarpal veins, which receive the dorsal digital and the intercapitular veins. It communicates proximally with the dorsal venous rete and ends medially and laterally in the great and small saphenous veins respectively. Also *dorsal venous arch of foot.* **a. venosus jugularis** [NA] A large communicating vein in the suprasternal space between the right and left anterior jugular veins that receives tributaries from the inferior thyroid veins. Also *jugular venous arch.* **a. venosus palmaris profundus** [NA] The venae comitantes of the deep palmar arterial arch, lying on the proximal ends of the metacarpal bones and interossei deep to the flexor tendons of the fingers and receiving the palmar metacarpal veins corresponding to the arteries. Branches from the medial and lateral sides join similar branches from the superficial palmar venous arch to form the ulnar and radial veins respectively. Also *deep palmar venous arch, deep volar venous arch* (outmoded). **a. venosus palmaris superficialis** [NA] The venae comitantes of the superficial palmar arterial arch, lying deep to the palmar aponeurosis and receiving the common palmar digital veins. Branches from the medial and lateral sides join similar branches from the deep palmar venous arch to form the ulnar and radial veins respectively. Also *superficial palmar venous arch.* **a. venosus plantaris** [NA] The venae comitantes of the deep plantar arterial arch, lying on the interossei and deep to the flexor tendons of the toes and receiving the four plantar metatarsal veins. The arch drains along the lateral plantar artery, and the veins join the superficial venous rete to form the posterior tibial veins. Also *plantar venous arch.* **a. vertebrae** [NA] The posterior or dorsal arch of a typical vertebra, enclosing the vertebral foramen. It comprises a vertical narrow part, the pedicle, which extends back from the body of the vertebra on each side of the foramen, and behind this a broad, flat lamina that roofs over the foramen. The arch supports paired transverse and superior articular and inferior articular processes, and a single spinous process projecting backward. Also *arch of vertebra, neural arch of vertebra, posterior arch of vertebra.* **a. zygomaticus** [NA] The arch on the lateral side of the skull formed by the forward-projecting zygomatic process of the temporal bone meeting the temporal process of the zygomatic bone at an oblique suture. Deep to it passes the tendon of the temporalis muscle, the fascia of which is attached to its upper border, while the lower border gives origin to the masseter muscle. Also *malar arch, zygomatic arch, zygoma.*

**ardanesthesia** \är′danesthē′zhə\ *Seldom used* THERMOANESTHESIA.

# area

**area** [L a piece of ground, open space, area] (*pl.* areae, areas) **1** A particular part of a larger surface or of a region. **2** A circumscribed space. **3** A designated part of an organ having or related to a special function. **acoustic a.** AUDITORY AREA. **a. acustica** AREA VESTIBULARIS. **anterior hypothalamic a.** REGIO HYPOTHALAMICA ANTERIOR. **anterior intercondylar a. of tibia** AREA INTERCONDYLARIS ANTERIOR TIBIAE. **aortic a.** The area of the chest wall over the inner end of the right second costal cartilage where murmurs, especially systolic murmurs, deriving from the aortic valve are often well heard. **apical a.** **1** APICAL BASE. **2** An area of radiolucency adjacent to the apex of a tooth. **arterial baroreceptor a.** A region in the walls of the great arteries in the thorax that contains nerve endings sensitive to stretch induced by alterations in transmural intra-arterial blood pressure. It is important in the physiologic control of systemic blood pressure. **association a.'s** Those areas of cerebral cortex situated next to a primary projection area that mediate higher degrees of perception, interpretation, and related motor behavior. **associative a.** Any area of the central nervous system consisting of interneurons interposed between main afferent and efferent circuits. **asthmagenic a.** TRIGGER AREA OF NOSE. **auditory a.** Those regions of the cerebral cortex concerned with the reception and interpretation of sounds. In man, the area includes portions of the anterior transverse temporal gyrus, the superior temporal gyrus (including Heschl's gyrus), and adjacent postcentral gyrus (Brodmann's area 41). Also *acoustic area, auditory cortical area, auditory projection area.* **auditory association a.** The cortical association area for audition. Histologically it corresponds to Brodmann's area 42. **auditory cortical a.** AUDITORY AREA. **auditory projection a.** AUDITORY AREA. **auditory psychic a.** The primary auditory area of the cerebral cortex in the superior temporal convolution in the human brain and the contiguous auditory cortex of ill-defined limits. It includes Heschl's gyrus. **autonomic a.** Any region of the central nervous system, especially regions of the medulla and hypothalamus, principally concerned with autonomic regulation. **axial a.** An area on a limb in which there is a gap in the orderly numerical sequence of dermatomic areas. **Bamberger's a.** A region near the inferior angle of the left scapula where, upon percussion, pericardial effusion can be detected by cardiac dullness. **bare a. of liver** AREA NUDA HEPATIS. **beam a.** The cross-sectional area of a beam of sound, light, particles, etc. **Betz cell a.** The motor region of the cerebral cortex containing large, pyramidal neurons, found principally in the precentral gyrus of primates. **bleeding a. of nasal septum** KIESSELBACH'S AREA. **body surface a.** A measurement of the outer surface of the body derived from one of several formulas, such as the Du Bois formula or Meeh's formula. Body surface area is a key factor in calculating body heat loss. The surface area of an adult of 70 kg is equal to about 1.76 $m^2$. That of a newborn infant is equal to about 0.2 $m^2$. Also *total body surface.* **Broca's motor speech a.** The triangular and opercular portions of the inferior frontal gyrus of the cerebral cortex, corresponding to Brodmann's area 44 and involved in the motor control of verbal expression. Damage to the area on the left side in most individuals results in aphasia of spoken and written language. Also *motor speech area, first motor speech area, Broca center, Broca's convolution, cortical speech area, speech center, Broca's gyrus.* **Brodmann's a.'s** The individual sectors of a morphological parcellation of the various regions of the cerebral cortex based on cytoarchitecture. Based on anatomic criteria devised by the German anatomist K. Brodmann, this attempt at functional classification is currently the one most widely used. Also *Brodmann's cortical areas.* **buccopharyngeal a.** The region of the embryo which gives rise to the buccopharyngeal membrane. **cardiogenic a.** CARDIOGENIC PLATE. **a. centralis** A region at the optical center of the retina measuring 5–6 mm in diameter and containing the macula retinae. **central speech a.** WERNICKE CENTER. **a. choroidea**

The region in the embryonic third ventricle of the brain where the choroid plexus will develop. **cingulate a.** The area of the cerebral cortex overlying the cingulate gyrus and its isthmus. **a. cochleae** [NA] A rounded depressed area situated anteriorly below the transverse crest of the bony vertical plate separating the fundus of the internal acoustic meatus from the cochlea and vestibule of the internal ear. The area is pierced by the numerous openings of the tractus spiralis foraminosus through which the branches of the cochlear nerve pass. Also *cochlear area of internal acoustic meatus.* **Cohnheim's a.'s** An artifactitious grouping of myofibrils that is seen when older techniques of preparing transverse sections of skeletal muscle cells are used. **contact a.** The meeting place of two adjacent teeth or restorations. Also *contact point, point of proximal contact.* **cortical a.** Any functionally or architecturally distinctive zone of cerebral cortex. See illustration at CORTEX CEREBRI. **cortical gustatory a.** The area of cerebral cortex receiving input from the taste pathways. It is hidden within the lateral fissure in man. Also *gustatory area.* **cortical motor a.** The area of cerebral cortex controlling movement, principally the precentral and postcentral gyri in primates. Also *excitomotor area* (rare), *psychomotor area* (outmoded), *zona rolandica.* **cortical oculomotor a.** An area of cerebral cortex that can be excited to elicit eye movements, chiefly the frontal adversive field. Also *cortico-oculocephalogyric area.* **cortical olfactory a.** The areas of cerebral cortex involved in olfactory sensibility, consisting of the terminal zones of the olfactory tract and their secondary connections, including the olfactory tubercle and the prepiriform and periamygdaloid cortex. **cortical 4S a.** HINES STRIP AREA. **cortical sensory a.** 1 Any sector of cerebral cortex receiving a specific sensory input. 2 SOMATOSENSORY AREA. **cortical speech a.** BROCA'S MOTOR SPEECH AREA. **cortical tactile a.** Any of the several somatotopic representations of the tactile receptors within the cerebral cortex, mapped electrophysiologically. **cortical visual a.** 1 Any of the several retinotopic representations of the cerebral cortex determined electrophysiologically. 2 PRIMARY VISUAL AREA. **cortico-oculocephalogyric a.** CORTICAL OCULOMOTOR AREA. **cribriform a. of renal papilla** AREA CRIBROSA PAPILLAE RENALIS. **a. cribrosa papillae renalis** [NA] The apex of a renal papilla which is pierced by ten to forty openings of the terminal papillary ducts (of Bellini). Also *cribriform area of renal papilla.* **a. cribrosa superior** *Outmoded* AREA VESTIBULARIS SUPERIOR. **denture foundation a.** STRESS-BEARING AREA. **depressor a.** The area of the medullary vasomotor center which when stimulated lowers the heart rate and blood pressure. **dermatomic a.** DERMATOME. **donor a.** DONOR SITE. **effective reflecting a.** That area of a reflector of ultrasound from which an echo is received by the transducer. **embryonic a.** 1 The segmental portion of the egg in partial or incomplete cleavage, as in reptiles or birds, already formed of two layers and which gives rise to the embryo. It is surrounded at the periphery by the area vasculosa, a region where the blood vessels form. 2 A region of the blastocyst where the embryo will develop. Also *area germinativa.* **entorhinal a.** That part of the cortical area of the parahippocampal gyrus that is medial to the rhinal fissure. **excitable a.** Any cortical area that when artifically stimulated elicits a motor response. **excitomotor a.** *Rare* CORTICAL MOTOR AREA. **extrapyramidal motor a.** The electrically excitable zone of the frontal cerebral cortex from which movements can be elicited after interruption of the pyramidal tract. **eye a.** FRONTAL EYE FIELD. **a. of facial nerve** AREA NERVI FACIALIS. **first motor speech a.** BROCA'S MOTOR SPEECH AREA. **a. Foreli** H FIELDS OF FOREL. **frontal a.** The area of the cerebral cortex in front of the central sulcus, comprising that on the orbital and medial surfaces of the frontal lobe. **fronto-orbital a.** PREFRONTAL AREA. **fusion a.** PANUM'S AREA. **areae gastricae** [NA] Numerous small elevated areas, 1–6 mm in diameter, separated by furrows on the surface of the gastric mucous membrane and comprising many small gastric pits, or foveolae, between the plicae villosae. Several gastric glands open into each pit. **genital a.'s** Areas of the nasal mucosa that occasionally become engorged and even bleed during menstruation, probably due to the effects of estrogen. Also *genital spot.* **a. germinativa** EMBRYONIC AREA. **glove a.** The cutaneous surface of the hand and arm which would be covered by a glove and in which loss of sensation due to hysteria may be observed. **gustatory a.** CORTICAL GUSTATORY AREA. **Hines strip a.** A narrow zone of brain cortex lying between Brodmann's areas 4 and 6 which upon stimulation leads to reduced muscular tone and when ablated results in spasticity. Also *cortical 4S area.* **hinge a.** The part of an immunoglobulin molecule where the three arms of the immunoglobulin come together and which contains disulfide bonds between the heavy chains. **a. hypothalamica lateralis** [NA] The zone of fiber bundles and scattered neurons lying external to the more medial tier of discrete nuclei. Rostrally, it continues into the preoptic area. Also *lateral hypothalamic area.* **inferior vestibular a. of internal acoustic meatus** AREA VESTIBULARIS INFERIOR. **a. intercondylaris anterior tibiae** [NA] The wide, triangular nonarticular area on the proximal end of the tibia that lies between the superior articular surfaces of the condyles and anterior to the intercondylar eminence. The anterior horns of the menisci and the anterior cruciate ligament are attached here. Also *anterior intercondylar area of tibia, anterior intercondylar fossa of tibia.* **a. intercondylaris posterior tibiae** [NA] The narrow, grooved nonarticular surface on the proximal end of the tibia that lies between the superior articular surfaces of the condyles and posterior to the intercondylar eminence. The posterior horn of the medial meniscus and the posterior cruciate ligament are attached here. Also *posterior intercondylar area of tibia, posterior intercondylar fossa of tibia.* **intercondylar a.'s of tibia** The rough elongated areas between the superior articular facets on the proximal end of the tibia, divided into anterior and posterior areas by the intercondylar eminence, or spine of tibia. **interglobular a.'s** INTERGLOBULAR SPACES. **intermediate hypothalamic a.** REGIO HYPOTHALAMICA INTERMEDIA. **Kiesselbach's a.** The anterior part of the nasal septum where the mucous membrane contains a rich vascular network that is a common site for epistaxis and where varicosities may occur. Also *Little's area, bleeding area of nasal septum, Kiesselbach space.* **Laimer-Haeckerman a.** A potentially weak small triangular area on the posterior pharyngeal wall opposite a gap between the horizontal cricopharyngeus and the oblique thyropharyngeus fibers of the inferior constrictor muscle of the pharynx. During swallowing, the latter fibers are propulsive while the former have a sphincteric action so that failure of relaxation may lead to herniation of the pharyngeal mucosa posteriorly through the intermuscular gap. **language a.** Any cortical area involved in the understanding or execution of oral or written language. **lateral hypothalamic a.** AREA HYPOTHALAMICA LATERALIS. **Little's a.** KIESSELBACH'S AREA. **a. lunata** *Obs.* LOB-

ULUS SEMILUNARIS INFERIOR. **a. medullovasculosa** A tangled mass of residual blood vessels seen in rachischisis after the neural tissue which formerly surrounded them has been eroded away by intrauterine movement. **mirror a.** The illuminated portion of the surface of the cornea or crystalline lens as seen by the technique of specular reflection. **mitral a.** The area in the region of the apex beat where the sounds and murmurs deriving from the mitral valve are usually best heard. **mitral valve a.** The cross-sectional area of the orifice of the mitral valve when open. **motor a.** Any region of the central nervous system controlling movement, as the cortical motor area. **motor speech a.** BROCA'S MOTOR SPEECH AREA. **a. nervi facialis** [NA] A round area through which the facial nerve enters the facial canal above the transverse crest of the bony vertical plate at the lateral end, or fundus, of the internal acoustic meatus. Also *area of facial nerve, radial fossa.* **a. nuda hepatis** [NA] The triangular area on the right side of the posterior surface of the liver which is not covered by peritoneum and is bounded by the groove for the inferior vena cava on the left, the superior and inferior layers of the coronary ligament above and below respectively, and the right triangular ligament at its apex. It is attached to the diaphragm by areolar tissue, and is in direct contact with the right suprarenal gland. Also *bare area of liver.* **olfactory a.** RHINENCEPHALON. **optic a.** The site in the embryo which will give rise to the eye. **oval a. of Flechsig** FASCICULUS SEPTOMARGINALIS. **Panum's a.** The extent of the receptor field in a retina capable of contributing to binocular vision in cooperation with a corresponding point in the opposite retina. Also *fusion area.* **parastriate a.** The area of occipital cerebral cortex (Brodmann's areas 18 and 19) contiguous with the area striata, or primary visual area. Also *secondary visual cortex.* **a. paraterminalis** GYRUS SUBCALLOSUS. **parolfactory a. of Broca** AREA SUBCALLOSA. **Patrick's trigger a.'s** Any one of several areas on the skin of the face or the mucous membrane of the tongue and oral cavity in which a stimulus may provoke the painful spasms of idiopathic trigeminal neuralgia. **a. perforata** SUBSTANTIA PERFORATA. **pericruciate a.** The gyrus surrounding the cruciate sulcus in the cerebral cortex of carnivores, containing a large portion of the sensorimotor cortical area. **peristriate a.** The nonstriated cerebral cortex (Brodmann's area 19) that borders upon the parastriate cortex on medial and lateral surfaces of the occipital lobe. It is thought to be involved in voluntary ocular movements that accompany visual fixation. **piriform a.** PIRIFORM CORTEX. **portal a.** PORTAL CANAL. **postcentral a.** Sensory cortex (Brodmann's areas 3, 1, and 2) covering the postcentral gyrus, including surfaces of the gyrus facing the central and medial longitudinal fissures. Also *postrolandic area.* **post dam a.** POSTERIOR PALATAL SEAL AREA. **posterior hypothalamic a.** REGIO HYPOTHALAMICA POSTERIOR. **posterior intercondylar a. of tibia** AREA INTERCONDYLARIS POSTERIOR TIBIAE. **posterior palatal seal a.** The area, at the junction of the hard palate and soft palate, where a posterior palatal seal between an upper denture and the roof of the mouth is usually made. Also *post dam area.* **postrolandic a.** POSTCENTRAL AREA. **precentral motor a.** PRIMARY CORTICAL MOTOR AREA. **precommissural a.** AREA SUBCALLOSA. **prefrontal a.** The cortex of the frontal lobe lying anterior to the motor area on the lateral surface and extending onto the orbital surface. Well developed only in primates, this area is involved in higher intellectual and emotional functions. Also *fronto-orbital area.* **premotor a.** A strip of cerebral cortex (Brodmann's area 6) lying in front of the primary cortical (precentral) motor area and extending medially to the sulcus cinguli. Stimulation tends to elicit general movement patterns, in part mediated through projection to the precentral area. It has no Betz cells. Also *premotor cortex, prerolandic motor area.* **preoptic a.** The median region of the lamina terminalis between the optic chiasma above and the anterior commissure below. Its nuclei project to the hypothalamus and exhibit sexual dimorphism. **prepiriform a.** PREPIRIFORM CORTEX. **prerolandic motor a.** PREMOTOR AREA. **pressor a.** A portion of the brainstem vasomotor complex of nuclei that upon activation elicits increases in heart rate and blood pressure. **pressoreceptive a.'s** Regions in the medulla oblongata involved in reflex regulation of blood pressure. **pressure a.** 1 An area of skin, generally over bony prominences, that is subject to necrosis of the skin and underlying tissues due to patient immobilization. 2 PRESSURE POINT. **pretectal a.** The zone of tectal mesencephalon lying between the superior colliculi and the thalamus. It receives fibers from the optic tract, lateral geniculate body, and parietal cortex and projects to the tegmentum. It is associated with the visual pupillary and accommodative mechanisms. Also *pretectal region, pretectum.* **primary a.'s** Sensory projection areas of the cerebral cortex that receive a relatively direct input from some sensory tract. The pathway is usually interrupted only by a thalamic relay. **primary cortical motor a.** The precentral gyrus of the cerebral cortex (Brodmann's area 4), from which movements can be elicited with the weakest electrical stimuli. Also *precentral motor area, rolandic area.* **primary cortical receptor a.'s** The principal sectors of cerebral cortex representing each of the sensory systems. **primary motor a.** The precentral motor cortex rostral to the central sulcus, including Brodmann areas 4, 6, and 8. **primary receptive a.** Any area of cerebral cortex constituting the largest and earliest recognized representation of a given sense organ. **primary visual a.** That portion of the visual area of the occipital lobe cortex to which visual pathways project. It corresponds to the histologically defined area striata. Also *cortical visual area.* **projection a.'s** Areas of cerebral cortex that receive input from specific sensory systems. Primary and secondary areas are distinguished, the primary having the more direct connections. **psychomotor a.** *Outmoded* CORTICAL MOTOR AREA. **pulmonary a.** The part of the chest wall that overlies the lung. **pulmonary valve a.** 1 That precordial site, in the second intercostal space to the left of the sternum, where the pulmonary valve sound or murmur can best be heard. 2 The cross-sectional area of the pulmonary valve, as calculated from the cardiac output and the pressure gradient across the valve. **receptive a.** Any sector of cerebral cortex receiving an organized sensory pathway. **recipient a.** RECIPIENT SITE. **relief a.** That part of the stress-bearing area under a denture where the pressure is reduced because of relative hardness or increased sensitivity. **rolandic a.** PRIMARY CORTICAL MOTOR AREA. **rugae a.** The anterior portion of the palate where the mucosal surface has several transverse ridges on each side of the median raphe, producing a corrugated appearance. *Outmoded.* Also *rugae zone.* **saddle a.** The part of an edentulous ridge covered by a denture base (saddle). **segmental a.** DERMATOME. **self-cleansing a.** An area of a tooth where, because of the action of mastication, plaque is less likely to accumulate. **sensitive a.** The zone from which a neuron can be excited. Also *receptive field.* **sensorimotor a.** The precentral and postcentral areas of the primate cerebrum or, in lower animals, the equivalent primary sensory and motor cortical areas. **sensory a.** Any cerebral cortical area involved in sensory projection and perception of sensation, especially the postcentral gyrus. **septal a.** In subprimates, the thick medial wall of the cerebral hemisphere situated anterior and superior to the lamina terminalis and anterior commissure. In higher primates, it is represented by the septum pellucidum, area subcallosa and gyrus subcallosus (gyrus paraterminalis.). **silent a.** A region of cerebral cortex from which movements cannot be elicited by electrical stimulation. **somatosensory a.** A cortical zone (Brodmann's areas 3, 1, and 2) along the postcentral gyrus involved in the reception of cutaneous, proprioceptive, and visceral sensation. Also *somatic sensory area, somesthetic area, cortical sensory area.* **stress-bearing a.** The part of the residual alveolar ridge and palate used to support a full or partial denture. Also *denture-bearing area, stress-supporting area, denture foundation.* **a. striata** The area of cortex (Brodmann's area 17) bordering the calcarine fissure distinguished by the presence of the line of Gennari. It is the primary projection area for vision, and corresponds anatomically to the primary visual area. Also *striate cortex, calcarine cortex.* **strip a.** One of several narrow zones bordering certain cortical areas (Brodmann's areas 4, 8, 2, 19, and 24), the stimulation of which abolishes resistance to externally imposed movements or suppresses movements resulting from the stimulation of motor areas. • The term is often used specifically to designate cortex bordering Brodmann's area 4. **a. subcallosa** [NA] The part of the medial cerebral cortex located ventral to the corpus callosum and rostral to the anterior commissure. It is a portion of the more inclusive septal area. Also *precommissural area, parolfactory area of Broca.* **superior vestibular a. of internal acoustic meatus** AREA VESTIBULARIS SUPERIOR. **supplementary motor a.** Any cortical area, other than the primary motor area (Brodmann's area 4) and the primary frontal eye field, that upon stimulation elicits body or facial movements. **suppressor a.** Striplike sectors of cerebral cortex from which evoked movements can be suppressed by the local application of strychnine. These areas have been shown to be based mainly on artifactitious observations. **temporal a.** The area above the level of the zygomatic arch that extends forward to the eye. **thenar a.** 1 THENAR. 2 THENAR SPACE. **thymus-dependent a.** Those portions of the peripheral lymphoid organs which are characterized by a population of thymus-dependent lymphocytes (T lymphocytes), as the paracortical areas of lymph nodes, internodular zone of Peyer's patches, and the centers of the malpighian corpuscle of the spleen. Also *traffic area.* **thymus-independent a.** A zone within a peripheral lymphoid organ which is populated by lymphocytes derived from the bone marrow rather than those of thymic origin. **traffic a.** THYMUS-DEPENDENT AREA. **triangular a.** The forward continuation of the frontonasal process which elevates to form the bridge and apex of the nose. **tricuspid a.** The area of the fourth left intercostal space at the left sternal edge where the sounds and murmurs deriving from the tricuspid valve are often best heard. **tricuspid valve a.** The cross-sectional area of the orifice of the open tricuspid valve. **trigger a.** A surface area of the body the stimulation of which causes the onset of pain that is perceived in the region of stimulation, or elsewhere, as in referred pain. The cutaneous trigeminal zones are the trigger area, for example, from which an attack of trigeminal neuralgia can be produced by light contact. Also *trigger zone.* Compare TRIGGER POINT. **trigger a. of nose** A clinical reference to the posterior one third of the nasal septum. Also *asthmagenic area.* **vagus a.** TRIGONUM NERVI VAGI. **a. vasculosa** The plexuses of blood vessels in the wall of the yolk sac in humans. **ventral tegmental a. of Tsai** A diffuse zone of cells and fibers in rostral midbrain extending laterally from the interpeduncular fossa beneath the red nucleus and rostrally into caudal hypothalamus. Bilateral lesions produce catalepsy or narcolepsy while stimulation may produce respiratory changes. **a. vestibularis** [NA] A trapezoidal area extending laterally from the sulcus limitans on the floor of the fourth ventricle. It lies over the vestibular nuclei and is crossed by the striae medullares. Also *vestibular area, area acustica, ala alba medialis* (obs.), *auditory triangle, trigonum acustici, external white wing, acoustic tubercle* (outmoded), *tuberculum acusticum, amygdaloid tubercle of Schwalbe* (outmoded). **a. vestibularis inferior** [NA] A small central area, with a number of foramina for nerve twigs to the saccule, situated below the transverse crest on the bony vertical plate separating the fundus of the internal acoustic meatus from the internal ear. Also *inferior vestibular area of internal acoustic meatus, area cribrosa media.* **a. vestibularis superior** [NA] A small rounded depression with several foramina for nerve twigs to the utricle and the ampullae of the anterior and lateral semicircular ducts, situated behind the area nervi facialis above the transverse crest on the bony vertical plate separating the fundus of the internal acoustic meatus from the internal ear. Also *superior vestibular area of internal acoustic meatus, area cribrosa superior.* **visual a.** The cortical area over the lateral and medial surfaces of the occipital lobe that is functionally involved in vision. See also PRIMARY VISUAL AREA. **visuosensory a.** The portion of the visual cortical area concerned with the projection and perception of visual stimuli. **Wernicke's a.** WERNICKE CENTER.

**areflexia** \ā′riflek′sē·ə\ [Gk *a-* priv. + REFLEX + -IA] Absence of reflexes. Adj. areflexic. **isolated a.** Loss of deep tendon reflexes in the absence of any other evidence of neurological disease or dysfunction. This may be constitutional and unexplained, but more often it is an early manifestation of disease, such as tabes dorsalis or polyneuropathy, in which other signs have not yet appeared. It is commonly observed in association with the myotonic pupil (the Holmes-Adie syndrome).

**arenavirus** \ərē′nəvī′rəs\ [L *arena* sand + VIRUS, with reference to the dense granules likened to sand inside their virion] Any of the pleomorphic, enveloped viruses containing single-stranded RNA and belonging to the genus *Arenavirus,* family Arenaviridae. Included are lymphocytic choriomeningitis virus, Lassa virus, and the Tacaribe group (Tacaribe, Junín, Mapucho, and others).

**areola** \ərē′ōlə\ [L (dim. of *area* an open space), a small open space] (*pl.* areolae) 1 Any small interstice in a tissue. 2 The portion of the iris that borders the pupil of the eye. 3 AREOLA MAMMAE. **a. mammae** [NA] The pigmented ring around the nipple. Also *areola of nipple, areola of mammary gland, areola papillaris.* **primary a.** Any of the spaces formed by the degeneration of cartilage cells in cartilage undergoing ossification. **second a.** A ring which surrounds the areola mammae during pregnancy.

**areolae** \ərē′ōlē\ Plural of AREOLA.

**areolar** \ərē′ōlər\ 1 Resembling an areola. 2 Pertaining to an areola of any sort. 3 Descriptive of a tissue or other structure containing numerous interstices.

**areolate** \ərē′ōlāt\ Characterized by the presence of areolae.

**areolitis** \er′ē·ōlī′tis\ [*areol(a)* + -ITIS] An inflammation of the areola of the nipple.

**areometer** \er′ē·äm′ətər\ HYDROMETER.
**Arey** [Lesley Brainerd *Arey,* U.S. anatomist, born 1891] See under RULE.
**Arg** Symbol for arginine.
**arg** *argentum* (L, silver).
**argamblyopia** \är′gamblē·ō′pē·ə\ [Gk *arg(os)* idle + AMBLYOPIA] SUPPRESSION AMBLYOPIA.
***Argas*** \är′gəs\ A genus of soft ticks which are ectoparasitic on birds, bats, reptiles, and insectivores, and which sometimes attack humans. Some of these ticks are strongly flattened, with distinct margins and a leathery folded integument. They have characteristic minute "buttons," with a pit, and sensory hair.
**argasid** \ärgas′id\ **1** Of or belonging to the family Argasidae. **2** A tick of the family Argasidae; a soft tick.
**Argasidae** \ärgas′idē\ [*Argas* + -IDAE] A family of soft-bodied ticks of the superfamily Ixodoidea, characterized by a leathery, wrinkled, mamillated integument and differentiated from hard ticks by lack of a scutum. The family includes approximately 140 species and four genera: *Argas, Ornithodoros, Otobius* and *Antricola.* Several members are of medical or veterinary importance as vectors of relapsing fever in birds and mammals.
**argentaffin** \ärjen′təfin\ [L *argent(um)* silver + *affin(is)* akin or inclined to] Having the property of being stained by silver solutions without the addition of an external reducing agent. Also *argentophilic.*
**argentaffinoma** \ärjen′təfinō′mə\ [ARGENTAFFIN + -OMA] See under CARCINOID.
**argentation** \är′jəntā′shən\ [*argent(o)-* + -ATION] The use of an ammoniacal silver nitrate solution to stain specific structures within tissues.
**argento-** \ärjen′tō-\ [L *argentum* silver] A combining form denoting silver.
**argentophilic** \är′jəntōfil′ik\ ARGENTAFFIN.
**arginase** An enzyme (EC 3.5.3.1) that hydrolyzes arginine to urea and ornithine. It is the final step in the pathway of urea production in the liver. Also *canavanase* (obs.).
**arginine** $NH_2$—C(=NH)—NH—$[CH_2]_3$—CH($NH_2$)COOH. An amino acid that has a strongly basic side chain (p$K$ 12.5) so that it is positively charged in proteins. It is an essential in the diet for young mammals, because it and ornithine, with which it is rapidly interconvertible in urea synthesis, are not rapidly formed from other dietary sources. In bacteria and fungi it is made from glutamic acid.
**arginine glutamate** $C_{11}H_{23}N_5O_6$. L-Glutamic acid compound with L-arginine, an agent that is given intravenously in the treatment of ammonia intoxication that results from liver disease or liver failure.
**argininemia** \är′jəninē′mē·ə\ A disturbance of the urea cycle due to a deficiency of the enzyme arginase, which converts arginine to ornithine and urea. It results in hyperammonemia and increased urinary excretion of dibasic amino acids and cysteine. Patients may have spastic diplegia, seizures, and severe mental retardation.
**arginine oxytocin** An analogue of oxytocin with arginine at position 8, in place of leucine. It is chemically identical to arginine vasotocin.
**arginine vasopressin** The characteristic octapeptide form of vasopressin found in the supraopticoneurohypophysial unit of most mammals except for the pig family, which has lysine vasopressin. The peptide is arranged into a five-member S—S bonded ring with a three-member side chain in which arginine occupies the position next to the terminal glycinamide.
**arginine vasotocin** The supraopticoneurohypophysial peptide of nonmammalian vertebrates, present in all lower vertebrates studied. Its function may be chiefly as a vasopressor and in regulating the secretion of the adenohypophysis. The chemical structure is identical to that of arginine oxytocin, and also to that of arginine vasopressin except that isoleucine replaces phenylalanine in the five-member ring.
**argininosuccinate** $N^{\omega}$-(1,2-Dicarboxyethyl)-arginine. It is an intermediate in the synthesis of arginine from citrulline and aspartate in the process of urea synthesis in the liver.
**argininosuccinic acid** $N^{\omega}$- (1,2-Dicarboxyethyl) arginine, an intermediate in the urea cycle. It is formed by reaction between aspartate and citrulline with concomitant hydrolysis of ATP, and is transformed into arginine and fumarate. It can appear in the urine if argininosuccinate lyase is genetically defective.
**argininosuccinicaciduria** \är′jənin′əsuksin′ikas′idoo′rē·ə\ A genetic disease, transmitted as an autosomal recessive, due to a deficiency of arginosuccinase. It is characterized by mental retardation, ataxia, seizures, hepatic dysfunction, and friable hair. Argininosuccinate appears in the urine, while argininosuccinate, citrulline, and sometimes ammonia are increased in plasma and cerebrospinal fluid.
**argon** Element number 18, having atomic weight 39.948. It is a colorless, odorless, inert gas. It constitutes about 0.94% of the atmosphere. There are three naturally occurring, stable isotopes, argon 40 being predominant. Symbol: Ar
**Argonz** [J. *Argonz,* Argentinian physician, flourished 20th century] Argonz-del Castillo syndrome. See under SYNDROME.
**Argyll Robertson** [Douglas Moray Cooper Lamb *Argyll Robertson,* Scottish ophthalmologist, 1837–1909] **1** Pseudo-Argyll Robertson syndrome. See under ADIE SYNDROME. **2** Argyll Robertson pupil sign. See under ARGYLL ROBERTSON PUPIL. **3** See under SIGN.
**argyremia** \är′jərē′mē·ə\ [Gk *argyr(os)* silver + -EMIA] The presence of silver in the blood.
**argyria** \ärjir′ē·ə\ [Gk *argyr(os)* silver + -IA ] A deep, ash-gray discoloration of the skin and conjunctiva resulting from chronic exposure to silver or silver salts. Also *argyrism, silver poisoning.* **a. nasalis** Argyria of the nasal lining.
**argyrism** \är′jərizm\ ARGYRIA.
**Argyrol** A proprietary name for mild silver protein
**argyrophil** \arjī′rəfil\ [Gk *argyro(s)* silver + -PHIL] Having the property of being stained by silver solutions only in the presence of an external reducing agent.
**arhinencephaly** \ā′rīnənsef′əlē\ ARRHINENCEPHALY.
**-aria** \-er′ē·ə\ [New L (from L *-arius,* suffix forming nouns and adjectives)] A noun suffix forming generic and group names.
**Arias-Stella** [Javier *Arias-Stella,* Peruvian pathologist, flourished 20th century] Arias-Stella cells. See under CELL.
**ariboflavinosis** \ārī′bəflā′vinō′sis\ [Gk *a-* priv. + RIBOFLAVIN + -OSIS] The syndrome characteristic of riboflavin deficiency. The symptoms include angular cheilitis, cheilosis, seborrheic dermatitis, most marked in and around the nasolabial and nasobuccal folds, vascularization of the cornea, and glossitis (magenta tongue).
**-aric** [by analogy from *saccharic (acid)*] In chemistry, a suffix used with *acid* to replace *-ose* in the name of an aldose to form the name of the corresponding aldaric acid, such as glucaric acid.
**Arlt** [Carl Ferdinand Ritter von *Arlt,* Austrian ophthalmologist 1812–1887] **1** See under LINE, OPERATION. **2** Arlt sinus. See under RECESS.
**ARM** artificial rupture of the (fetal) membranes.

**arm** [Old English *earm* (akin to L *armus* arm and shoulder, forequarter of animal) the arm (including upper and forearm)] **1** The region of the upper limb between the shoulder and elbow; brachium. **2** The entire upper limb. A popular usage. **3** Any armlike piece or appendage. **4** In cytogenetics, either of the regions of a chromosome on either side of the centromere that extends to the telomere. It is designated short (*p*, for petite) or long (*q*), based on relative length. **5** A projection from or extension of the framework of a removable partial denture. **glass a.** A tendon injury to the biceps or supraspinatus muscle leading to a painful upper arm and sometimes resulting in subdeltoid bursitis. *Popular.* **Krukenberg's a.** A V-shaped stump, usually created following the amputation of the hand, in which the distal radius and ulna are separated and covered by skin to give a limited but mobile clawlike appendage. Also *Krukenberg's hand.* **prolapsed a.** A form of transverse lie of the fetus where the shoulder becomes impacted into the maternal pelvis and the fetal arm delivers through the uterine cervix. **reciprocal a.** An arm placed against a tooth to counter the force exerted by a clasp on the same tooth, in order to maintain the position of the tooth and so the efficiency of the clasp. **scanning a.** In an ultrasound imaging instrument, the device on which the transducer is mounted.

**armamentarium** \är′məmenter′ē·əm\ [L (from *armament(a)* implements, utensils + *-arium* -ARY), an arsenal, armory] The resources of the health practitioner, considered collectively, that can be brought to bear in the practice of medicine, including equipment and instrumentation, books, drugs, and diagnostic and therapeutic procedures.

**Armanni** [Luciano *Armanni,* Italian pathologist, 1839–1903] **1** Armanni-Ebstein cells. See under CELL. **2** Armanni-Ebstein change. See under CHANGE. **3** Armanni-Ebstein lesion. See under LESION.

**armpit** FOSSA AXILLARIS.

**Armstrong** [Charles *Armstrong,* U.S. surgeon, born 1886] Armstrong's disease. See under LYMPHOCYTIC CHORIOMENINGITIS.

**Arndt** [Rudolf Gottfried *Arndt,* German psychiatrist, 1835–1900] See under LAW.

**Arneth** [Joseph *Arneth,* German physician, 1873–1955] **1** See under CLASSIFICATION. **2** Arneth's count. See under FORMULA.

**Arnold** [Julius *Arnold,* German pathologist, 1835–1915] **1** Arnold-Chiari deformity. See under DEFORMITY. **2** Arnold's bodies. See under BODY.

**Arnold** [Philipp Friedrich *Arnold,* German anatomist, 1803–1890] **1** Arnold's bundle. See under TRACTUS FRONTOPONTINUS. **2** Arnold's ganglion, splanchnic ganglion of Arnold. See under GANGLION OTICUM. **3** Arnold's ganglion. See under GLOMUS CAROTICUM. **4** Arnold's innominate canal. See under CANALICULUS INNOMINATUS. **5** Arnold's canal, mastoid canaliculus of Arnold's nerve. See under CANALICULUS MASTOIDEUS. **6** Arnold's nerve. See under RAMUS AURICULARIS NERVI VAGI. **7** Bigeminate ligaments of Arnold. See under LIGAMENTA TARSOMETATARSALIA DORSALIA.

**aromatic** \ar′ōmat′ik\ **1** Having a pleasant odor; fragrant, as certain herbs and spices. **2** Possessing properties shown by benzene, such as having alternate double bonds (which are delocalized, so that several of the bonds are intermediate between double and single bonds), and showing greater stability than that calculated for localized double bonds.

**arrachement** \äräshmäN′\ [French (from L *eradicare* to uproot), a pulling up from the earth, removable by force, a tearing out] Removal of an opaque lens capsule.

**array** \ərā′\ An orderly arrangement or display of elements or components. **annular a.** An ultrasonic transducer array made up of ring-shaped elements arranged concentrically. **linear a.** An ultrasonic transducer array made up of rectangular elements in a line. **linear switched a.** A linear ultrasound transducer array operated by applying voltage pulses to groups of elements sequentially. Also *linear sequenced array.* **phase steered a.** A linear ultrasound transducer array operated by applying voltage pulses to all elements, but with small time differences or delays, providing a means of electronic sector scanning and focusing. **transducer a.** An ultrasonic transducer assembly containing more than one transducer element used for electronic scanning or focusing.

**arrector** \arek′tər\ [New L (from L *arrectus* erected, past part. of *arrigere* to erect, raise, from AD- + L *regere* to direct + *-or* -OR), that which raises] ERECTOR.

**arrectores** \ar′ektôr′ēz\ Plural of ARRECTOR.

**arrest** [French *arrêter* (from AD- + L *restare* to remain, resist) to stop or hold someone] **1** To stop; to slow down or hinder. **2** A cessation or interference. **cardiac a.** Complete loss of the mechanical function of the heart. It is most commonly due to ventricular fibrillation, though it can also result from asystole or cardiac rupture. It is often sudden but can occur gradually. **circulatory a.** Complete cessation of circulation of the blood, usually due to cardiac arrest, or obstruction to the circulation such as massive pulmonary embolism. **deep transverse a.** A condition during labor in which the fetal head presents with the sagittal suture in the transverse diameter of the maternal pelvis. This condition is associated with a prolonged second stage of labor and often with an android maternal pelvis. Also *transverse arrest.* **developmental a.** A pause, either permanent or temporary, in any developmental process. It can be part of the normal pattern of development, or may be brought about by extraneous factors, giving rise to abnormality. **epiphyseal a.** The bony fusion of the epiphysis with the metaphysis. It occurs at skeletal maturity or prematurely, owing to injury or disease of or surgery on the growth plate. **maturation a.** Failure of blood cells to develop beyond early stages of development, a characteristic of acute leukemias. **metaphase a.** Any stoppage of the cell cycle in metaphase. The technique is useful for synchronizing cell growth once the arresting agent, such as colchicine, is removed, or for preparing a cytologic study of nuclear chromosomes. **pelvic a.** Failure of the presenting part of the fetus to traverse the maternal pelvis during labor. **sinus a.** Cessation of activity of the sinuatrial node. It is usually transient. Ventricular activity may continue because of an atrioventricular nodal or ventricular pacemaker. Also *sinus standstill.* **transverse a.** DEEP TRANSVERSE ARREST.

**arrhaphia** \ərā′fē·ə\ [Gk *a-* priv. + *-rrhaph(y)* + -IA] STATUS DYSRHAPHICUS.

**Arrhenius** [Svante August *Arrhenius,* Swedish physicist and chemist, 1859–1927] See under EQUATION.

**arrheno-** \er′ənō-, ərē′nō-\ [Gk *arrhēn* male] A combining form meaning male.

**arrhenoblastoma** \-blastō′mə\ [ARRHENO- + BLASTOMA] Androblastoma, especially if ovarian and accompanied by masculinization. Also *arrhenoma, testiculoma ovarii, adenoma ovarii testiculare.*

**arrhinencephaly** \ā′rīnənsef′əlē\ [A-[1] + *rhinencephal(on)* + -Y] Absence of the rhinencephalon, a part of the midbrain anterior to the hypothalamus and concerned with smell and primitive feelings. Also *arhinencephaly.*

**arrhinia** \ərin′ē·ə\ [Gk *arhin* (from *a-* priv. + *rhis,* gen. *rhinos,* the nose) without a nose + -IA] Absence of the external nose.
**arrhythmia** \əriTH′mē·ə\ [Gk *arrhythm(os)* (from *a-* priv. + *rhythmos* rhythm) without rhythm + -IA] Any variation from normal, regular rhythm, especially cardiac rhythm. **nodal a.** An arrhythmia deriving from abnormalities of atrioventricular nodal function. **nonphasic sinus a.** Sinus arrhythmia in which there is no phasic variation in relation to respiration. **phasic a.** Respiratory arrhythmia. See under SINUS ARRHYTHMIA. **respiratory a.** See under SINUS ARRHYTHMIA. **sinus a.** A cyclical change in heart rate as a result of changes in discharge rate of the sinus node. It is usually a result of variations in vagal tone related to respiration, the heart rate increasing during inspiration and decreasing during expiration. It is found especially in children and young adults. Also *sinus dysrhythmia.* **vagal a.** A disturbance of rhythm as a result of vagal activity. See also SINUS ARRHYTHMIA.
**arrhythmic** \əriTH′mik\ Characterized by arrhythmia.
**Arroyo** [Carlos F. *Arroyo,* U.S. physician, 1892–1928] Arroyo sign. See under ASTHENOCORIA.
**arsenate** Any polyatomic anion with arsenic as the central atom, or any of its condensation products, or an ester of any of these forms: usually denoting $AsO_4^{3-}$ or its partially protonated forms. Used in biochemistry as an analogue of phosphate, its esters are readily formed and hydrolyzed. See also ARSENOLYSIS.
**arsenic** \är′sənik\ Element number 33, having atomic weight 74.92. Several allotropic forms exist, the most stable being a gray, very brittle, crystalline, semimetallic substance. Its compounds, which are very poisonous, are used in agricultural insecticides and poisons. Symbol: As **white a.** $As_4O_6$. Arsenic(III) oxide. *Outmoded.*
**arsenical** \ärsen′ikəl\ Any of several drugs containing arsenic, originally developed to combat infections by protozoa. The best known arsenical is arsphenamine, once used to treat syphilis.
**arsenicalism** \ärsen′ikəlizm\ A condition resulting from the accumulation of arsenic in the tissues due to chronic exposure to arsenicals. Signs and symptoms are malaise, fatigue, gastrointestinal disturbances, hyperpigmentation, altered hematopoiesis, and liver and kidney degeneration. See also ARSENIC POISONING.
**arsenite** Either of the ions $AsO_2^-$ or $AsO_3^{3-}$ or any of the highly toxic salts containing them. Because of the high affinity of the ion for dihydrolipoyl groups, these salts inhibit the biologic oxidation of 2-oxoacids.
**arsenization** Treatment with an arsenical medication.
**arsenobenzene** Any of several substances including arsphenamine and related arsenicals used in the treatment of syphilis and other spirochetal diseases.
**arsenoceptor** \ärsen′əsep′tər\ [*arsen(ic)* + *o* + *(re)ceptor*] A receptor site on a cell surface to which arsenic can attach, as in arsenical action against trypanosomes.
**arsenolysis** \är′sənäl′isis\ The process of breaking a bond by reaction with arsenate. It usually leads to hydrolysis, since esters of arsenic acid hydrolyze spontaneously. In studies of carbohydrate metabolism, this process is particularly applied to the acyl-enzyme of glyceraldehyde-3-phosphate dehydrogenase, which naturally reacts with phosphate to give acyl phosphate and free enzyme. Arsenate can replace phosphate, giving arsenolysis.
**arsenoresistant** \ärsen′ərizis′tənt\ Resistant to arsenicals, particularly arsphenamine used in the treatment of syphilis.
**arsenous hydride** ARSINE.
**arsenoxide** A compound containing the —As=O group. Such a compound is likely to be toxic because of its high affinity for dihydrolipoyl groups.
**arsine** $AsH_3$. A highly poisonous gas that may be formed when nascent hydrogen is produced in the presence of arsenic or arsenic-bearing substances. The boiling point is −55°C. It has a slight garlicky odor and produces hemolysis and renal failure. Also *hydrogen arsenide, arsenous hydride, arseniuretted hydrogen, hemolytic gas.*
**arsphenamine** $C_{12}H_{14}As_2Cl_2N_2O_2$. Arsenphenolamine hydrochloride. An organoarsenical compound formerly used for the treatment of syphilis. Also *Ehrlich 606, salvarsan.*
**artefact** \är′təfakt\ *Brit.* ARTIFACT.
**arterenol** NOREPINEPHRINE.
**arteri-** \ärtir′ē-\ ARTERIO-.

# arteria

**arteria** \ärtir′ē·ə\ [See ARTERY.] (*pl.* arteriae) A tubular vessel conducting blood away from the heart to the tissues that is usually relatively thick-walled, elastic, and muscular. Also *artery.* **arteriae alveolares superiores anteriores** [NA] Branches of the infraorbital artery from the third part of the maxillary artery that descend through the anterior alveolar canals to supply the upper canine and incisor teeth and the mucous membrane of the maxillary sinus. Also *anterior superior alveolar arteries, anterior dental arteries.* **a. alveolaris inferior** [NA] A branch of the first part of the maxillary artery that enters the mandibular foramen between the ramus of mandible and the sphenomandibular ligament to supply the lower teeth, chin (via the mental branch), and part of the mucous membrane of the mouth (via the lingual branch). Also *inferior alveolar artery, inferior dental artery, mandibular artery.* **a. alveolaris superior posterior** [NA] A branch from the third part of the maxillary artery in the pterygopalatine fossa that divides into branches, some of which enter the alveolar canals to supply the upper molar and premolar teeth and the mucous membrane of the maxillary sinus, while others continue on the alveolar process to supply the gums. Also *posterior superior alveolar artery, posterior dental artery.* **a. anastomotica** A connection between the orbital portion of the ophthalmic artery and the middle meningeal artery, i.e., between circulations of the internal and external carotid arteries. It passes between the orbit and the middle cranial fossa by way of the orbital fissure or through a separate foramen. When the ophthalmic branch from the internal carotid fails to develop, as happens normally in some animals and occasionally in humans, this anastomosis is the main pathway of blood to the retina. **a. angularis** [NA] The terminal part of the facial artery after the superior labial artery branches off. It ascends to the medial angle of the eye, supplies the ala of the nose, lacrimal sac, and orbicularis oculi muscle, and anastomoses with the infraorbital artery and the dorsal nasal branch of the ophthalmic artery. Also *angular artery.* **a. aorta** AORTA. **a. appendicularis** [NA] A branch of the inferior branch of the ileocolic artery that descends behind the termination of the ileum and runs in the mesoappendix, at first near and then in its free border, to supply the vermiform appendix. Also *appendicular artery, vermiform artery.* **arteriae arcuatae renis** Branches of the interlobar arteries of the kidney that diverge at the

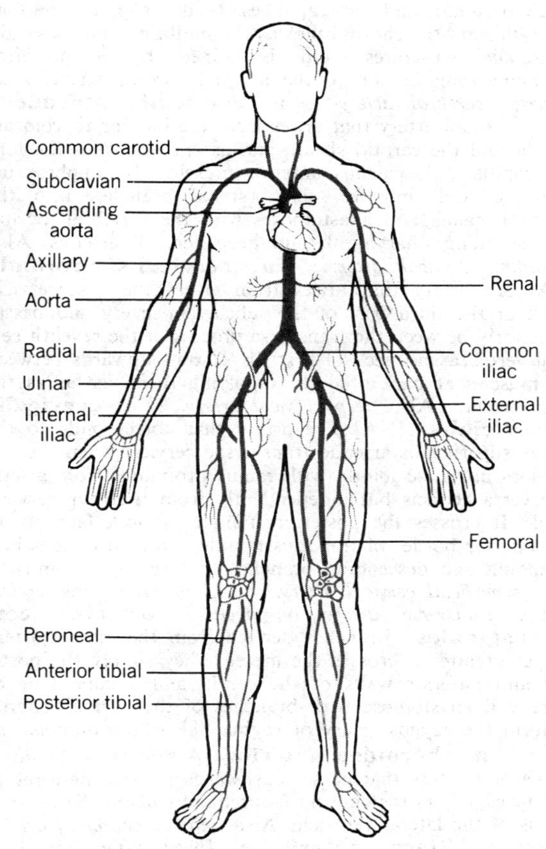


**Major arteries of the body**

corticomedullary junction at right angles to the direction of the interlobar arteries to form arches over the bases of the pyramids. They give off a radial series of interlobular arteries. Also *arteriae arciformes renis, arcuate arteries of kidney, Flint's arcade, arterial arches of kidney.* **a. arcuata pedis** [NA] An artery given off by the dorsalis pedis artery opposite the medial cuneiform, passing laterally over the bases of the metatarsal bones to anastomose with lateral tarsal and lateral plantar arteries. Its branches are the second, third, and fourth dorsal metatarsal arteries. Also *arcuate artery of foot, arcuate artery.* **a. auditiva interna** ARTERIA LABYRINTHI. **a. auricularis posterior** [NA] A small branch of the external carotid artery, arising opposite the tip of the styloid process to ascend on the process under cover of the parotid gland and end in the groove between the mastoid process and the cartilage of the auricle by dividing into auricular and occipital branches. Besides supplying the digastric, stylohyoid, and sternocleidomastoid muscles and the parotid gland, it gives rise to the stylomastoid artery. Also *posterior auricular artery.* **a. auricularis profunda** [NA] A small branch of the first part of the maxillary artery that ascends in the parotid gland behind the temporomandibular joint, which it supplies, and then pierces the wall of the external acoustic meatus to supply its inner lining and the outer aspect of the tympanic membrane. Also *deep auricular artery.* **a. axillaris** [NA] The continuation of the subclavian artery at the outer border of the first rib, extending through the axilla and along the medial side of the arm as far as the lower border of the teres major muscle, where it becomes the brachial artery. Its branches are the superior thoracic, thoracoacromial, lateral thoracic, subscapular, and the anterior and posterior circumflex humeral arteries. Also *axillary artery.* **a. basilaris** [NA] A single trunk formed at the base of the skull from the junction of the two vertebral arteries and extending from the lower to the upper border of the pons in its ventral groove. It terminates by dividing into two posterior cerebral arteries. Also *basilar artery, basilar trunk.* **a. brachialis** [NA] The continuation of the axillary artery at the lower border of the tendon of the teres major muscle coursing down the medial side of the arm to the front of the elbow joint midway between the humeral epicondyles, just distal to which it terminates by bifurcating into the radial and ulnar arteries. Also *brachial artery, humeral artery.* **a. brachialis superficialis** [NA] A fairly common variation that arises from either the axillary artery or the brachial artery just beyond its origin and remains superficial to the brachial muscles until it divides into the radial and ulnar arteries in the elbow region. Also *superficial brachial artery.* **a. buccalis** [NA] A small branch of the second part of the maxillary artery that runs forward with the buccal nerve between the medial pterygoid muscle and the tendon of insertion of the temporalis muscle on to the superficial aspect of the buccinator muscle, which it supplies, anastomosing with branches of the facial and infraorbital arteries. Also *buccal artery, buccinator artery.* **a. bulbi penis** [NA] A short, wide branch of the internal pudendal artery in the male that pierces the transversus perinei profundus muscle and the inferior fascia of the urogenital diaphragm and enters the bulb of the penis. A branch goes to the bulbourethral gland. Also *artery of bulb of penis, arteria bulbi urethrae, bulbourethral artery.* **a. bulbi vestibuli vaginae** [NA] A branch of the internal pudendal artery in the female that supplies the erectile tissue of the bulbus vestibuli and vagina. Also *artery of bulb of vestibule of vagina.* **a. canalis pterygoidei** [NA] An artery that usually branches off the third part of the maxillary artery in the pterygopalatine fossa but often arises from the greater palatine artery, and usually runs backward through the pterygoid canal for distribution to the mucous membrane of the upper part of the pharynx, auditory tube, tympanic cavity, and sphenoidal sinus. Also *artery of pterygoid canal, vidian artery.* **a. carotis communis** [NA] The major artery to the head and neck. On the left side it arises at an intrathoracic level from the aortic arch, and on the right by bifurcation of the brachiocephalic trunk behind the right sternoclavicular joint. Midway up the neck it terminates by branching into the external and internal carotid arteries. It usually has no other major branches. At its termination the vessel wall has a dilatation, the carotid sinus. Also *common carotid artery, carotid artery.* **a. carotis externa** [NA] The terminal branch of the common carotid artery that supplies the external structures of the head. It branches into the superior thyroid, ascending pharyngeal, lingual, facial, occipital, and posterior auricular branches and, terminally, the superficial temporal and maxillary arteries. These branches supply the face, skull and scalp, upper neck, pharynx, nose, and some deep areas of the ear. It also supplies the meninges of the anterior and middle cranial fossae. Also *external carotid artery.* **arteriae caroticotympanicae arteriae carotidis internae** [NA] Small branches given off by the internal carotid artery that pierce the wall of the carotid canal in the petrous part of the temporal bone to enter the tympanic cavity to anastomose with the anterior tympanic branch of the maxillary artery and the stylomastoid artery. Also *caroticotympanic arteries, rami caroticotympanici arteriae carotidis internae* (outmoded). **a. carotis interna** [NA] A terminal branch of the common carotid artery, arising at the level of the upper border of the thyroid cartilage. Through ophthalmic, posterior communicating, anterior and middle cerebral, tympanic, and minor branches it supplies the orbital contents, the forehead, internal and external surfaces of the nose, the pituitary gland, the trigeminal ganglion, and the tympanum in part, as well as the forebrain and portions of its choroid plexuses. Also *internal carotid artery.* **a. caudae pancreatis** [NA] One of the several pancreatic branches of the splenic artery, distributed to the tail of the pancreas. Also *caudal pancreatic artery.* **a. cecalis anterior** [NA] A branch of the inferior branch of ileocolic artery that supplies the anterior part of the cecum. Also *anterior cecal artery.* **a. cecalis posterior** [NA] A branch of the inferior branch of ileocolic artery that supplies the posterior part of the cecum. Also *posterior cecal artery.* **arteriae centrales anteromediales arteriae cerebri anterioris** A group of small branches from the anterior cerebral artery that penetrates the anterior perforated substance to supply the rostrum of the corpus callosum, the anterior part of the putamen and caudate nucleus, as well as the septum pellucidum. Also *arteriae thalamostriatae anteromediales arteriae cerebri anterioris* (outmoded). **a. centralis retinae** [NA] A branch of the ophthalmic artery which, after piercing the dural sheath about one centimeter behind the eyeball, runs in the center of the optic nerve to the optic papilla. There it bifurcates into superior and inferior, lateral and medial branches. These furnish essentially all the blood supply of the retina. Also *central retinal artery, artery of Zinn* (obs.). **a. cerebelli inferior anterior** [NA] A branch from the initial part of the basilar artery that supplies the anteroinferior surface of the cerebellum. Commonly, it forms a loop directed toward the internal auditory meatus, and gives rise to the labyrinthine artery. Also *anterior inferior cerebellar artery.* **a. cerebelli inferior posterior** [NA] A branch from the intracranial portion of the vertebral artery that passes around the medulla to reach the inferior surface of the cerebellum. It supplies these structures and the choroid plexus of the fourth ventricle. Also *posterior inferior cerebellar artery.* **a. cerebelli superior** A major branch of the basilar artery that supplies the superior surface of the cerebellum, the lamina quadrigemina, the pineal body, and the adjacent choroid plexus. In some animals it may arise from the posterior cerebral artery. Also *superior cerebellar artery.* **arteriae cerebri** [NA] The major blood vessels supplying the cerebral cortex; the anterior, middle, and posterior cerebral arteries. Also *cerebral arteries, arteries of cerebrum.* **a. cerebri anterior** [NA] A terminal branch of the internal carotid artery which, passing upward and backward around the rostrum and body of the corpus callosum, sends branches to the basal ganglia, the choroid plexus of the lateral ventricle, deep diencephalic structures, and the medial and, to a limited extent, lateral aspects of the frontal and parietal lobes. Also *anterior cerebral artery.* **a. cerebri media** [NA] A terminal branch of the carotid artery which, passing into the lateral fissure, ramifies over the insula and adjacent portions of the orbital frontal, parietal, and temporal cortices. Near its origin it sends central (striate) branches to the corpus striatum and internal capsule. Also *middle cerebral artery, sylvian artery.* **a. cerebri posterior** [NA] One of the branches formed by the midline bifurcation of the basilar artery. Passing around the cerebral peduncle, the artery reaches the tentorial surface of the cerebrum, where it sends branches to the temporal, occipital, and parietal lobes. It also supplies the corpus callosum, the choroid plexus, the midbrain, and basal diencephalic structures, and is joined by a posterior communicating branch to the internal carotid artery. Also *posterior cerebral artery.* **a. cervicalis ascendens** [NA] A small artery that arises from the inferior thyroid artery behind the carotid sheath and ascends between the longus capitis and scalenus anterior muscles. It supplies surrounding neck muscles, sends spinal branches into the vertebral canal, and anastomoses with the vertebral, occipital, ascending pharyngeal, and deep cervical arteries. Also *ascending cervical artery.* **a. cervicalis profunda** [NA] An artery that arises from either the costocervical trunk or the third part of the subclavian artery and passes posteriorly between the transverse process of the seventh cervical vertebra and neck of first rib. It runs upwards between the muscles at back of neck, supplying them, as far as the axis vertebra. Also *deep cervical artery.* **a. cervicalis superficialis** [NA] The artery that corresponds to the ramus superficialis arteriae transversae cervicis when the latter does not arise jointly with ramus profundus from arteria transversa cervicis but independently from the thyrocervical trunk. It crosses the posterior triangle of neck laterally to the anterior border of trapezius muscle, where it divides into ascending and descending branches that supply the muscle. Also *superficial cervical artery, superficial transverse cervical artery, transverse artery of neck.* **arteriae cervicovaginales** Branches derived from the uterine artery just at or after it crosses the ureter. They supply the posterior and anterior walls of the cervix and vagina. One or more will anastomose with branches of the vaginal arteries to form the azygos artery of vagina. Also *cervicovaginal arteries.* **a. choroidea anterior** A branch of the internal carotid artery that passes backwards toward the cerebral peduncles, enters the choroid fissure, and ends in the choroid plexus of the lateral ventricle. Also *anterior choroidal artery.* **arteriae ciliares anteriores** [NA] Arteries, derived from muscular branches of the ophthalmic artery, that course with tendons of the rectus muscles to the front of the eyeball, where they form a circumcorneal vascular zone deep to the conjunctiva, and then perforate the anterior part of the sclera to anastomose with long posterior ciliary arteries. Also *anterior ciliary arteries.* **arteriae ciliares posteriores breves** [NA] About eight arteries that arise from the ophthalmic artery or its branches and follow the optic nerve to the back of the eyeball, where they branch and pierce the sclera around the nerve and supply the choroid coat and ciliary processes. They anastomose with branches of the central artery and with long posterior and anterior ciliary arteries. Also *short ciliary arteries, short posterior ciliary arteries, branches of short posterior ciliary arteries.* **arteriae ciliares posteriores longae** [NA] Two branches of the ophthalmic artery that pierce the posterior part of the sclera and run between the sclera and choroid to the attached margin of the iris, where each divides into an upper and lower branch that anastomoses with a corresponding branch from the opposite side and with anterior ciliary arteries to form the circulus arteriosus iridis major. Also *long ciliary arteries, long posterior ciliary arteries.* **a. circumflexa anterior humeri** [NA] A small artery that may arise either in common with the posterior circumflex humeral artery or separately, from the third part of the axillary artery. It partly encircles the surgical neck of humerus deep to the coracobrachialis, biceps brachii, and deltoid muscles to end by anastomosing with the posterior circumflex humeral artery. It also sends a branch along the intertubercular sulcus to supply the shoulder joint and humeral head. Also *anterior circumflex humeral artery.* **a. circumflexa femoris lateralis** [NA] A large artery that usually arises from the lateral side of the profunda femoris artery and passes laterally on the iliopsoas and vastus intermedius muscles and deep to the sartorius and rectus femoris muscles, where it divides into ascending, transverse, and descending branches. Also *lateral circumflex femoral artery.* **a. circumflexa femoris medialis** [NA] An artery that arises either from the profunda femoris artery or femoral artery. It runs posteriorly through muscles, winding around the medial side of the proximal part of shaft of femur and giving off its ascending, transverse, and acetabular branches that supply the adductor and obturator externus muscles and hip joint. Also *medial circumflex femoral artery.* **a. circumflexa iliaca profunda** [NA] A branch of the external iliac artery that originates just above the inguinal ligament, behind which it ascends laterally to the anterior superior iliac spine. After piercing the transversalis fascia it runs along the inner lip of the iliac crest before it ascends between the transversus abdominis and internal oblique muscles to anastomose with the iliolumbar and superior gluteal arteries, as well as with the ascending branch of the lateral circumflex femoral, and lumbar and inferior epigastric arteries. Also *deep circumflex iliac artery.* **a. circumflexa iliaca superficialis** [NA] A small cutaneous branch of the femoral artery that pierces the fascia lata just below the inguinal ligament, along which it runs to the iliac crest. Its branches supply skin and superficial inguinal lymph nodes and anastomose with deep circumflex iliac, superior gluteal, and lateral circumflex femoral arteries. Also *superficial circumflex iliac artery.* **a. circumflexa posterior humeri** [NA] A large artery that arises from the third part of the axillary artery at the lower border of the subscapularis muscle and runs posteriorly with the axillary nerve through the quadrangular space and around the surgical neck of humerus to end deep to the deltoid muscle by supplying it, the shoulder joint and surrounding muscles, and anastomosing with the anterior circumflex humeral and profunda brachii arteries and small arteries on the acromion. Also *posterior circumflex humeral artery.* **a. circumflexa scapulae** [NA] A fairly large branch of the subscapular artery that hooks around the lateral border of scapula to enter the infraspinous fossa under cover of the teres minor muscle, where it gives off two branches: one, the infrascapular artery, runs in the subscapular fossa to supply the subscapularis muscle and anastomose with deep branch of transverse cervical and suprascapular arteries; the other branch continues down the lateral border to the inferior angle and anastomoses with deep branch of transverse cervical artery. Also *circumflex artery of scapula.* **a. colica dextra** [NA] A branch of the superior mesenteric artery that may occasionally arise by a common trunk with the ileocolic artery. It runs behind the peritoneum to the right, and near the ascending colon it divides into an ascending branch that anastomoses with the middle colic artery and a descending branch that anastomoses with the ileocolic artery. These anastomotic arches supply the upper two-thirds of the ascending colon and right colic flexure. Also *right colic artery, right superior colic artery* (outmoded). **a. colica media** [NA] A branch of the superior mesenteric artery that arises just below the pancreas, where it passes forward between layers of the transverse mesocolon, dividing into right and left branches that anastomose with the right and left colic arteries respectively to supply the transverse colon. Also *middle colic artery, accessory superior colic artery, transverse colic artery* (outmoded). **a. colica sinistra** [NA] The first branch of inferior mesenteric artery that runs behind the peritoneum and in front of the psoas major muscle to the left, where it divides into ascending and descending branches. These anastomose with middle colic and highest sigmoid arteries, respectively, to supply the left half of transverse colon and descending colon. Also *left colic artery, left superior colic artery.* **a. collateralis media** [NA] The larger of the two terminal branches of profunda brachii artery that runs downward behind the humerus through the triceps muscle to participate in the anastomosis around the elbow joint. Also *middle collateral artery.* **a. collateralis radialis** [NA] A terminal branch or continuation of the profunda brachii artery deep to the lateral head of triceps that runs with the radial nerve to pierce the lateral intermuscular septum and pass in front of the lateral epicondyle of humerus to anastomose with the radial recurrent artery. Also *radial collateral artery, collateral radial artery.* **a. collateralis ulnaris inferior** [NA] A branch of the brachial artery that arises in front of the brachialis muscle just above the medial epicondyle of humerus. Here it gives off branches that run down in front of the medial epicondyle to anastomose with the anterior ulnar recurrent, while it turns posteriorly behind the medial epicondyle, anastomosing with the middle collateral artery above the olecranon fossa and with the superior ulnar collateral and posterior ulnar recurrent arteries behind the epicondyle. Also *inferior ulnar collateral artery, anastomotica magna artery, supratrochlear artery.* **a. collateralis ulnaris superior** [NA] An artery that arises just below the midarm either from the brachial artery or the profunda brachii artery. It joins the ulnar nerve on the medial head of triceps muscle, accompanying it to the gap between medial epicondyle of humerus and olecranon and ending in the flexor carpi ulnaris muscle by anastomosing with posterior ulnar recurrent and inferior ulnar collateral arteries. Also *superior ulnar collateral artery, inferior profunda artery.* **a. comes nervi phrenici** ARTERIA PERICARDIACOPHRENICA. **a. comitans nervi ischiadici** [NA] A long, thin branch of the inferior gluteal artery that arises outside the pelvis and runs on the sciatic nerve, pierces it, and descends in it to the lower part of the thigh. Also *accompanying artery of ischiadic nerve, companion artery to sciatic nerve, sciatic artery.* **a. comitans nervi mediani** [NA] A long, thin branch of the anterior interosseous artery that arises proximally in the forearm and joins the median nerve, supplying it. It usually divides into an anterior terminal and a posterior terminal branch, the former passing deep to the pronator quadratus muscle and ending in the palmar carpal arch, while the latter pierces the interosseous membrane above the wrist and joins the dorsal carpal rete. Also *median artery, median artery of forearm.* **a. communicans anterior cerebri** [NA] A short, unpaired connection between the two anterior cerebral arteries near their origin. It completes the circle of Willis anteriorly. Also *anterior communicating artery of cerebrum.* **a. communicans posterior cerebri** [NA] A small artery connecting the internal carotid with the posterior cerebral artery. It contributes to the formation of the circle of Willis, and sends fine branches to the optic tract, crus cerebri, interpeduncular region, and hippocampal gyrus. Also *posterior communicating artery of cerebrum.* **arteriae conjunctivales anteriores** [NA] Branches of the anterior ciliary artery that run to the bulbar conjunctiva at the corneoscleral junction. Also *anterior conjunctival arteries.* **arteriae conjunctivales posteriores** [NA] Branches of the superior and inferior palpebral arches, formed by medial palpebral arteries between the orbicularis oculi muscle and the tarsal plate near the free margin of eyelid, that supply the conjunctival fornix and lacrimal caruncle. Also *posterior conjunctival arteries.* **a. coronaria dextra** [NA] An artery of the heart that arises from the right anterior aortic sinus of the ascending aorta and enters the right side of coronary sulcus, which it

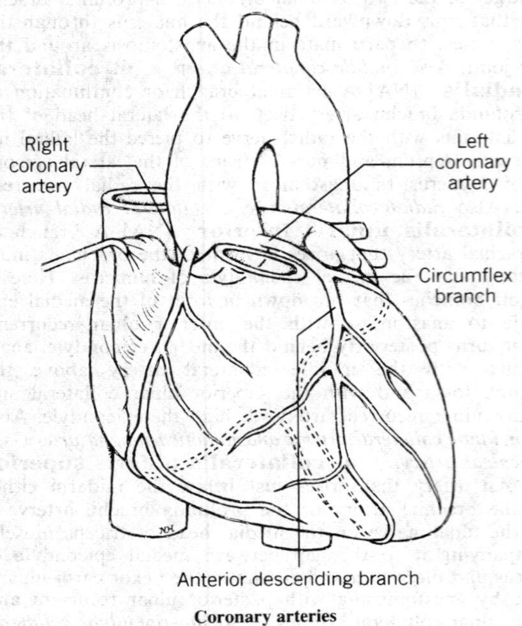


**Coronary arteries**

follows to the inferior surface. It turns left on the back of the heart to the posterior interventricular sulcus, where it anastomoses with the left coronary artery. Also *right coronary artery of heart.* **a. coronaria sinistra** [NA] An artery of the heart that arises from the left posterior aortic sinus of the ascending aorta and runs for a short distance between the left auricle and the pulmonary trunk, where it ends by dividing into two principal branches, the ramus circumflexus and ramus interventricularis anterior, which supply branches to both ventricles, the left atrium, the anterior two-thirds of the interventricular septum, and the sinuatrial node. Also *left coronary artery of heart, left auricular artery.* **a. cremasterica** [NA] A branch of the inferior epigastric artery that joins the ductus deferens and the genital branch of the genitofemoral nerve through the inguinal canal, supplying the cremaster muscle and coverings of the spermatic cord and anastomosing with the testicular artery. In the female, it is called the artery of round ligament of uterus. Also *cremasteric artery, arteria spermatica externa, external spermatic artery.* **a. cystica** [NA] The artery of the gallbladder that usually arises from the right branch of the hepatic artery in the cystic triangle, running downwards along the neck of the gallbladder to divide into superficial and deep branches, the former supplying the free surface and the latter the hepatic surface of gallbladder, as well as the adjacent liver. Branches also supply hepatic ducts and part of the common bile duct. Also *cystic artery.* **a. deferentialis** ARTERIA DUCTUS DEFERENTIS. **a. descendens genicularis** [NA] An artery that arises from the femoral artery just before it enters the opening in the adductor magnus. After giving off a saphenous branch, it descends to the medial side of the knee, where it anastomoses with the medial superior genicular artery. Also *arteria genus descendens, descending genicular artery, anastomotica magna artery.* **arteriae digitales dorsales manus** [NA] Collateral branches of dorsal metacarpal arteries of hand that run on and supply the adjacent dorsal sides of the index, middle, ring, and little fingers and anastomose with the deep palmar arch near their origins and with proper palmar digital branches of the superficial palmar arch. Also *dorsal digital arteries of hand, digital arteries of the finger.* **arteriae digitales dorsales pedis** [NA] Collateral branches of second, third, and fourth dorsal metatarsal arteries that arise at the clefts of the second, third, fourth, and fifth toes and course along their adjacent sides, supplying them. Also *dorsal digital arteries of foot, digital arteries of the toes.* **arteriae digitales palmares communes** [NA] Three arteries that arise from the convexity of the superficial palmar arch and run towards the webs of fingers on the second, third, and fourth lumbrical muscles, where each receives a corresponding palmar metacarpal artery before dividing into a pair of proper palmar digital arteries. Also *common palmar digital arteries, arteriae digitales volares communes, common volar digital arteries, ulnar metacarpal arteries.* **arteriae digitales palmares propriae** [NA] Collateral branches of the three common palmar digital arteries that run along and supply adjoining sides of index, middle, ring, and little fingers and end in a plexiform way beneath the pulp of the finger and around the matrix of the nail. Each has two dorsal branches to anastomose with dorsal digital arteries and supply the dorsum of the middle and distal phalanges. Also *proper palmar digital arteries, arteriae digitales volares propriae, collateral digital arteries, proper volar digital arteries, digital arteries of the fingers.* **arteriae digitales plantares communes** [NA] Arteries that arise from a superficial plantar arch when it is present, and extend to the toes to join plantar metatarsal arteries. In this variation, the common plantar digital arteries replace the more common small superficial digital branches of the medial plantar artery. Also *common plantar digital arteries.* **arteriae digitales plantares propriae** [NA] Collateral branches of plantar metatarsal arteries (usually four) that arise at the clefts of toes and supply their adjacent sides. The branch for the medial side of the first toe usually arises from the first plantar metatarsal artery, while that for the lateral side of the fifth toe is usually a separate branch from the lateral side of the plantar arch, but it may arise from the fourth plantar metatarsal artery. Also *proper plantar digital arteries, digital arteries of the toes.* **arteriae digitales volares communes** ARTERIAE DIGITALES PALMARES COMMUNES. **arteriae digitales volares propriae** ARTERIAE DIGITALES PALMARES PROPRIAE. **a. dorsalis clitoridis** [NA] One of the terminal branches of the internal pudendal artery in the female that pierces the inferior fascia of the urogenital diaphragm and runs forwards on the dorsum of the clitoris to terminate in its glans and prepuce. Also *dorsal artery of clitoris.* **a. dorsalis nasi** [NA] The lower of the terminal branches of the ophthalmic artery that pierces the orbital septum above the medial palpebral ligament and gives off a lacrimal branch to the sac before dividing into two branches that descend on the dorsum of nose, one anastomosing with the angular artery and the other with the lateral nasal branch of facial artery. Also *dorsal artery of nose, dorsal nasal artery.* **a. dorsalis pedis** [NA] The continuation of the anterior tibial artery extending from a point midway between the malleoli in front of the ankle joint to the proximal end of the first intermetatarsal space, where it terminates in two branches, the first dorsal metatarsal and deep plantar arteries. During its course it gives off lateral tarsal, medial tarsal, and arcuate arteries. Also *dorsal artery of foot, dorsalis pedis artery.* **a. dorsalis penis** [NA] One of the terminal branches of the internal pudendal artery in the male that pierces the inferior fascia of the urogenital diaphragm and ascends between crus penis and pubic symphysis to gain the dorsum of penis, along which it runs between dorsal nerve and deep dorsal vein to end in the glans and prepuce. It also supplies the skin of the penis. Also *dorsal artery of penis.* **a. dorsalis scapulae** [NA] A branch arising from the third part of the subclavian artery or, in about one third of cases, from the transverse cervical artery near the anterior margin of the trapezius muscle. It passes laterally either through or in front of brachial plexus, in front of the scalenus medius, and then deep to the levator scapulae and the rhomboideus muscles along the length of the vertebral border of the scapula. Also *dorsal scapular artery, deep branch of transverse cervical artery, transverse cervical artery, posterior scapular artery, arteria scapularis dorsalis, descending scapular artery.* **a. ductus deferentis** [NA] A small, thin artery that arises either from the anterior division of the internal iliac artery or the superior vesical artery and accompanies the ductus deferens to the testis, where it supplies the epididymis and anastomoses with the testicular artery. It also gives branches to the seminal vesicles and the ureter. It is homologous to the uterine artery of the female. Also *artery of ductus deferens, deferential artery, arteria deferentialis, deferent artery.* **a. epigastrica inferior** [NA] A branch of the external iliac artery that arises just above the inguinal ligament and ascends obliquely medial to the deep inguinal ring towards the rectus abdominis muscle. It pierces the transversalis fascia to pass in front of the arcuate line into the rectus sheath behind the muscle. It ends by anastomosing with the superior epigastric artery and lower posterior intercostal arteries. Also *inferior epigastric artery.* **a. epigastrica superficialis** [NA] A branch of the femoral artery that arises just below the inguinal ligament, pierces the fascia cribrosa and ascends superficial to the middle of the inguinal ligament to end near the umbilicus. It gives branches to superficial inguinal lymph nodes and subcutaneous fascia and skin, and anastomoses with branches of the inferior epigastric and superficial circumflex iliac arteries. Also *superficial epigastric artery.* **a. epigastrica superior** [NA] A terminal branch of the internal thoracic artery that arises at the level of the sixth intercostal space, descends between the sternal and costal origins of diaphragm to enter the rectus sheath, in which it anastomoses with inferior epigastric artery. It supplies the skin and muscles of the anterior abdominal wall and diaphragm, and anastomoses with the hepatic artery via the falciform ligament. Also *superior epigastric artery.* **arteriae episclerales** [NA] Branches of anterior ciliary arteries that supply the ocular bulb both anteriorly and posteriorly. Also *episcleral arteries.* **a. ethmoidalis anterior** [NA] A branch of the ophthalmic artery which, arising just distal to the optic canal, crosses through the cone of extraocular muscles, enters an ethmoid foramen, passes between the cribriform plate and the dura, enters the nasal roof, and finally appears beneath the skin on the bridge of the nose. Also *anterior ethmoidal artery.* **a. ethmoidalis posterior** [NA] A small, inconstant branch of the ophthalmic artery that leaves the orbit through the posterior ethmoidal foramen and sends branches to the posterior ethmoidal air sinuses before entering the cranial cavity, where it sends a meningeal branch to the dura mater, and nasal branches that pass through the cribriform plate to supply the upper part of the nasal cavity, the pharynx, and the sphenoidal sinus. Also *posterior ethmoidal artery.* **a. facialis** [NA] A tortuous artery that arises from the external carotid artery in the carotid triangle. At first medial to the ramus of the mandible, it becomes superficial as it hooks around the inferior border of the mandible anterior to the masseter muscle and moves behind the angle of the mouth to become the angular artery in the groove between nose and eye. Also *facial artery, arteria maxillaris externa, external maxillary artery.* **a. femoralis** [NA] The continuation of the external iliac artery that extends from the midinguinal point along the anteromedial side of the thigh to the junction of the middle and lower thirds of the thigh, where it passes through an opening in the adductor magnus muscle to become the popliteal artery. Also *femoral artery, crural artery.* **a. fibularis** [NA] A large branch of the posterior tibial artery, arising just below the lower border of the popliteus muscle, running along the medial border of the fibula deep to the flexor hallucis longus, and terminating as lateral calcaneal branches on the calcaneus. Just above the tibiofibular syndesmosis it gives off a perforating branch that pierces the interosseous membrane into the anterior compartment of the leg, where it joins in the lateral malleolar network but may replace the dorsalis pedis artery. Also *peroneal artery, fibular artery, arteria peronea.* **a. frontalis** ARTERIA SUPRATROCHLEARIS. **a. frontobasalis lateralis** [NA] A branch of the insular, or horizontal, part of the middle cerebral artery that ramifies over the lateral aspect of the inferior, or orbital, surface of the frontal lobe and supplies the inferior and lateral aspects of the frontal lobe. Also *ramus orbitofrontalis lateralis, rami orbitales arteriae cerebri mediae* (outmoded), *inferior lateral frontal branch of middle cerebral artery* (outmoded), *lateral frontobasal artery.* **a. frontobasalis medialis** [NA] A branch, usually the first, of the pars postcommunicalis of the anterior cerebral artery. It ramifies over the adjacent medial surface of the cerebral hemisphere and the medial aspect of the inferior surface of the frontal lobe and supplies the medial basal region of the frontal lobe, including the olfactory lobe, bulb, and tract; gyrus rectus, and internal orbital gyrus. Also *medial frontobasal artery, medial orbitofrontal artery, ramus orbitofrontalis medialis, rami orbitales arteriae cerebri anterioris* (outmoded), *inferior frontal artery.* **a. gastrica dextra** [NA] A branch of the common hepatic artery that intrudes between the two layers of lesser omentum in the pyloric region and runs to the left along the lesser curvature of stomach to anastomose with the left gastric artery. It supplies the pylorus and gives numerous anterior and posterior branches to the stomach. Occasionally it gives off a supraduodenal artery. Also *right gastric artery, right coronary artery of stomach, pyloric artery.* **arteriae gastricae breves** [NA] A series of small arteries given off either by the terminal part of the splenic artery or left gastro-omental artery that enter the gastrosplenic ligament and supply the greater curvature and fundus of stomach, anastomosing with left gastro-omental and left gastric arteries. Also *short gastric arteries, vasa brevia.* **a. gastrica sinistra** [NA] The smallest branch of the celiac trunk that runs cranially and to the left behind the omental bursa. At the cardiac end of stomach it gives off esophageal branches and passes downwards along the lesser curvature of stomach between the layers of lesser omentum. Also *left gastric artery, left coronary artery of stomach.* **a. gastroduodenalis** [NA] A short, sturdy branch of the common hepatic artery that descends with the common bile duct behind the first part of the duodenum, at the lower border of which it terminates in two branches, the right gastro-omental and superior pancreaticoduodenal arteries. In its course it gives off the retroduodenal artery and small branches to the pyloric part of the stomach and to the pancreas. Also *gastroduodenal artery.* **a. gastro-omentalis dextra** [NA] The larger of two terminal branches of the gastroduodenal artery that turns to the left along the greater curvature of stomach between layers of greater omentum, terminating by anastomosing with the left gastro-omental artery. It has a pyloric branch and many branches to the greater omentum and both surfaces of the stomach. Also *right gastroepiploic artery, right inferior gastric artery, right gastro-omental artery.* **a. gastro-omentalis sinistra** [NA] The largest branch of the splenic artery that arises near its termination and runs downward to the right through the gastrosplenic ligament to the greater curvature of stomach between the layers of greater omentum to anastomose with the right gastro-omental artery. It supplies a large branch to the greater omentum and branches to both surfaces of the stomach. Also *left gastroepiploic artery, left inferior gastric artery, left gastro-omental artery.* **a. genu inferior lateralis** ARTERIA INFERIOR LATERALIS GENUS. **a. genu inferior medialis** ARTERIA INFERIOR MEDIALIS GENUS. **a. genu media** ARTERIA MEDIA GENUS. **a. genus descendens** ARTERIA DESCENDENS GENICULARIS. **a. genu superior lateralis** ARTERIA SUPERIOR LATERALIS GENUS. **a. genu superior medialis** ARTERIA SUPERIOR MEDIALIS GENUS. **a. glutea inferior** [NA] The larger of the two terminal branches of the anterior division of the internal iliac artery. It leaves the pelvis posteriorly between the upper sacral nerves and below the piriformis muscle in the greater sciatic foramen. It runs with the sciatic nerve deep to the gluteus maximus and down the back of the thigh, supplying the skin and anastomosing with the first perforating, medial circumflex femoral, and lateral circumflex femoral arteries in the cruciate anastomosis. Also *inferior gluteal artery, sciatic artery.* **a. glutea superior** [NA] The largest branch of the posterior division of the internal iliac artery, that runs posteriorly between the lumbosacral trunk and the first sacral nerve, leaving the pelvis through the greater sciatic foramen above the piriformis muscle. Deep to the gluteus maximus it divides into a superficial and a deep branch. Inside the pelvis it supplies the piriformis and obturator externus muscles and the hipbone. Also *superior gluteal artery.* See also RAMUS SUPERFICIALIS ARTERIAE GLUTEAE SUPERIORIS, RAMUS PROFUNDUS ARTERIAE GLUTEAE SUPERIORIS. **arteriae helicinae penis** [NA] Those branches of the deep and dorsal arteries of penis that enter the cavernous spaces in a coiled, convoluted form. They are dilated and give off small capillaries to supply the trabecular structure of the erectile tissue. They have thick circular muscle and thickened longitudinal valvelike structures, which regulate the cavernous spaces during erection. At the end of erection these arteries contract and express the blood slowly into the venous plexus. Also *helicine arteries of penis, arteries of Mueller, helicine arteries.* **a. hemorrhoidalis inferior** ARTERIA RECTALIS INFERIOR. **a. hemorrhoidalis media** ARTERIA RECTALIS MEDIA. **a. hemorrhoidalis superior** ARTERIA RECTALIS SUPERIOR. **a. hepatica communis** [NA] A branch of the celiac trunk that runs to the right and forward behind the lesser sac and below its opening to reach the upper border of the first part of the duodenum. Here, after giving off the gastroduodenal artery, it becomes the proper hepatic artery, which enters the free border of the lesser omentum. Also *common hepatic artery, hepatic artery.* **a. hepatica propria** [NA] The continuation of the common hepatic artery after the gastroduodenal artery leaves it, when it enters the free edge of the lesser omentum to join the portal vein and common bile duct and ascends to the porta hepatis, where it terminates as the right and left hepatic arteries. It commonly gives off the right gastric artery at its origin. Also *proper hepatic artery, hepatic funiculus of Rauber, hepatic artery, middle hepatic artery* (outmoded and incorrect). **a. hyaloidea** [NA] HYALOID ARTERY. **a. hypogastrica** ARTERIA ILIACA INTERNA. **a. hypophysialis inferior** [NA] A branch of the cavernous part of the internal carotid artery that divides into medial and lateral branches. These branches anastomose with similar branches from the opposite side to form an arterial ring around the neural or posterior lobe of the hypophysis. The ring gives off central branches which form sinusoids within the substance of the lobe. Also *inferior hypophyseal artery.* **a. hypophysialis superior** [NA] A branch of the cerebral part of the internal carotid artery that runs below and behind the optic chiasma to the pituitary infundibulum and the median eminence of hypothalamus, forming a plexus with the opposite branch on their external surfaces. Most of its branches penetrate the glandular and nervous tissue to end in capillary tufts adjacent to bundles of nerve axons in the infundibulum. Some branches enter the upper surface of the anterior lobe and anastomose with the inferior hypophyseal arteries, supplying the anterior lobe. Also *superior hypophyseal artery.* **arteriae ileales** [NA] The lower branches of the left, convex side of the superior mesenteric artery that supply the ileum, except for its terminal part. Each vessel divides and subdivides, anastomosing with adjacent branches to form a series of arcades, the terminal one of which sends straight arteries to encircle the intestine. Also *ileal arteries, arteriae ileae.* **a. ileocolica** [NA] The large branch that arises distally from the right, concave side of the superior mesenteric artery and runs downward to divide into a superior and an inferior branch. The superior branch anastomoses with the right colic artery, while the inferior branch, or continuation of the artery, anastomoses with the termination of the superior mesenteric artery and gives off ascending, or colic, anterior and posterior cecal, appendicular, and ileal branches. Also *ileocolic artery, inferior right colic artery.* **a. iliaca communis** [NA] One of two terminal branches of the abdominal aorta that arises on the left of the fourth lumbar vertebra. Each artery diverges at an angle of about 65° from the other and descends to terminate opposite the lumbosacral junction by bifurcating into external and internal iliac arteries. The right branch is longer than the left and crosses the commencement of the inferior vena cava. It gives branches to the peritoneum, ureter, psoas major muscle, adjacent connective tissue, and lymph nodes. Also *common iliac artery.* **a. iliaca externa** [NA] The larger of the two terminal branches of the common iliac artery that runs along the superior aperture of the minor pelvis medial to the psoas major muscle until it reaches the midinguinal point, where it passes deep to the inguinal ligament as the femoral artery. It gives off deep circumflex iliac and inferior epigastric arteries, and branches to the psoas major muscle and lymph nodes. Also *external iliac artery, anterior iliac artery.* **a. iliaca interna** [NA] A terminal branch of the common iliac artery that arises in front of the sacroiliac joint and runs down into the minor pelvis to the superior border of the greater sciatic foramen, where it branches. It supplies the walls and viscera of the pelvis, the gluteal region, and perineum. Also *internal iliac artery, arteria hypogastrica, hypogastric artery, posterior pelvis artery.* **a. iliolumbalis** [NA] A branch of the posterior division of the internal iliac artery that ascends behind the common iliac artery to the medial border of the psoas major muscle and the superior aperture of the minor pelvis, where it divides into iliac and lumbar branches. Also *iliolumbar artery, small iliac artery.* See also RAMUS ILIACUS ARTERIAE ILIOLUMBALIS, RAMUS LUMBALIS ARTERIAE ILIOLUMBALIS. **a. inferior lateralis genus** [NA] A branch of the popliteal artery that runs laterally over the popliteus and deep to the gastrocnemius, fibular collateral ligament, and tendon of biceps femoris to the front of the knee, where its branches anastomose with the lateral superior genicular, medial inferior genicular, anterior tibial recurrent, posterior tibial recurrent, and circumflex fibular arteries. Also *lateral inferior genicular artery, arteria genu inferior lateralis, inferior lateral geniculate artery.* **a. inferior medialis genus** [NA] A branch of the popliteal artery that runs downward and medially over the popliteus muscle deep to the gastrocnemius muscle and tibial collateral ligament to the front of the knee, where it anastomoses with the medial superior genicular and lateral inferior genicular arteries, as well as with the saphenous branch of the descending genicular artery and the anterior tibial recurrent artery. It supplies the popliteus muscle, proximal end of tibia, and knee joint. Also *medial inferior genicular artery, arteria genu inferior medialis, inferior medial geniculate artery.* **a. infraorbitalis** [NA] A branch of the third part of the maxillary artery that arises in the pterygopalatine fossa and accompanies the infraorbital nerve through the infraorbital groove, canal, and foramen to emerge on the face, where it terminates as labial, nasal, and palpebral branches. It anastomoses with branches of the facial, ophthalmic, and transverse facial arteries, and during its course gives off orbital branches to muscles, and anterior alveolar branches. Also *infraorbital artery.* **arteriae intercostales posteriores I et II** [NA] Branches of the superior intercostal artery given off in the first and second intercostal spaces anterior to the neck of the adjacent rib. Their course is similar to that of the lower intercostal spaces. Each gives off a dorsal branch to muscles and a spinal branch into the vertebral canal. Also *posterior intercostal arteries I and II.* **arteriae intercostales posteriores III–XI** [NA] Usually nine pairs of arteries that arise from the dorsal aspect of the thoracic aorta and diverge to right and left over the bodies of vertebrae to reach the lower intercostal spaces. Each artery ascends between pleura and internal intercostal membrane to the costal groove at the angle of the corresponding rib, where it joins a vein and nerve to run anteriorly between the intercostalis intimus and internal intercostal muscles. Near the sternum it anastomoses with a branch of the internal thoracic or musculophrenic artery. The lowest two posterior intercostals proceed into the abdominal wall to anastomose with the subcostal, superior epigastric, and lumbar arteries. Also *posterior intercostal arteries III–XI, aortic intercostal arteries* (outmoded). **a. intercostalis suprema** [NA] A branch of the costocervical trunk that runs downward into the thorax anterior to neck of first rib and deep to the pleura. It gives off the first posterior intercostal artery and then may continue over neck of second rib as the second posterior intercostal artery to the second intercostal space. Also *highest intercostal artery, superior intercostal artery.* **arteriae interlobares renis** [NA] Secondary subdivisions of the primary anterior and posterior branches of the renal artery that penetrate the renal columns between the pyramids as far as the junction between cortex and medulla, where they divide dichotomously into arcuate arteries. Also *interlobar arteries of kidney.* **arteriae interlobulares hepatis** [NA] Branches of the terminal hepatic artery ramifying in the portal canals between the hepatic lobules and either entering the lobules to join the venous sinusoids or providing minute branches to supply the structures in the portal canals. Also *interlobular arteries of liver.* **arteriae interlobulares renis** [NA] Branches of arcuate arteries and the terminal ends of arcuate arteries that run vertically from the bases of renal pyramids to the surface of the cortex, where they may give off perforating arteries to anastomose with a plexus on the renal capsule. Most interlobular arteries give off afferent glomerular arteries in the cortex. Also *interlobular arteries of kidney, radiate arteries of kidney.* **a. interossea anterior** [NA] A terminal branch of the common interosseous artery that arises at the upper border of the interosseous membrane, anterior to which it proceeds deep to the flexor digitorum profundus and flexor pollicis longus muscles, which it supplies. It terminates at the upper border of the pronator quadratus as anterior terminal and posterior terminal branches. Its branches include the median artery and the nutrient artery to radius. Also *anterior interosseous artery, volar interosseous artery, palmar interosseous artery.* **a. interossea communis** [NA] A short, thick branch that arises from the ulnar artery just beyond its origin and runs down and posteriorly between the flexor digitorum profundus and the flexor pollicis longus until it reaches the proximal border of the interosseous membrane, where it terminates as anterior and posterior interosseous arteries. Also *common interosseous artery.* **a. interossea posterior** [NA] A terminal branch of the common interosseous artery that runs posteriorly between the proximal border of the interosseous membrane and the oblique ligament into the posterior compartment of the forearm. It proceeds between the deep and superficial layers of muscles, supplying them, down to the distal fifth, where it anastomoses with the posterior terminal branch of the anterior interosseous artery that pierces the interosseous membrane, and with the dorsal carpal arch. Proximally it gives off the interosseous recurrent artery, which ascends to join the rete articulare cubiti. Also *posterior interosseous artery, arteria interossea dorsalis, dorsal interosseous artery of forearm, posterior interosseous artery of forearm.* **a. interossea recurrens** [NA] A branch that arises from the posterior interosseous artery in the supinator muscle and ascends deep to the anconeus to the gap between the olecranon and lateral epicondyle of humerus, where it anastomoses with the middle collateral, inferior ulnar collateral, and posterior ulnar recurrent arteries. Also *interosseous recurrent artery, recurrent interosseus artery.* **arteriae intestinales** The approximately 15 arteries that arise from the left, convex side of the superior mesenteric artery and run in the mesentery to be distributed to the jejunum and most of the ileum. Each divides into two, and these unite with adjacent branches to form arcades that subdivide again and again until there are three or more arcades from which straight arteries proceed to supply the intestine. Proximally, in the jejunum, there is only one arcade, while distally, in the ileum, there are many complex arches with short, straight arteries. Also *intestinal arteries.* **arteriae jejunales** [NA] The proximal intestinal arteries that arise from the left side of the superior mesenteric artery. They run in parallel fashion in the mesentery, and each branches into two. These branches unite to form an arcade from which long, straight arteries proceed to the intestinal wall. More distally, the arcades subdivide to form two or more arcades from which shorter straight arteries proceed. They also supply lymph nodes and other tissues in the mesentery. Also *jejunal arteries.* **a. labialis inferior** [NA] A branch of the facial artery that arises at the angle of the mouth and runs tortuously in the orbicularis oris muscle of the lower lip to anastomose with the artery of the opposite side, and with the submental, sublabial, and mental arteries. It supplies the lower lip muscles, mucous membrane, and labial glands. Also *inferior labial artery.* **a. labialis superior** [NA] A branch that arises from the facial artery slightly higher than the inferior labial artery. After passing deep to the zygomaticus major muscle, it enters the upper lip and follows a course and distribution similar to that of inferior labial artery, but anastomoses only with its opposite counterpart. It gives off a branch to the nasal septum and to ala of nose. Also *superior labial artery.* **a. labyrinthi** [NA] A long, slender artery that arises from either the basilar artery or the anterior inferior cerebellar artery at the lower part of the pons. It joins the facial and vestibulocochlear nerves through the internal acoustic meatus to enter the internal ear, where it supplies the entire membranous labyrinth. Its branches are the vestibular, vestibulocochlear, and cochlear arteries. Also *labyrinthine artery, artery of labyrinth, internal auditory artery, arteria auditive interna.* **a. lacrimalis** [NA] A large branch that arises from the ophthalmic artery near the back of the orbit. It follows the lateral rectus muscle with the lacrimal nerve and supplies the lacrimal gland before it pierces the orbital septum above the lateral palpebral ligament, where it ends as the lateral palpebral arteries, which help to form the palpebral arches. It gives ciliary branches to the bulb, recurrent meningeal branches to anastomose with the middle meningeal artery, and zygomatic branches to the face and temporal fossa. Also *lacrimal artery.* **a. laryngea inferior** [NA] A branch of the inferior thyroid artery, usually of its ascending branch, that ascends in the tracheoesophageal groove with the recurrent laryngeal nerve and enters the larynx below the inferior pharyngeal constrictor muscle to supply the muscles and mucous membrane of the larynx. It anastomoses with its opposite fellow and with the superior laryngeal artery. Also *inferior laryngeal artery.* **a. laryngea superior** [NA] A branch of the superior thyroid artery that passes forward deep to the posterior margin of the thyrohyoid muscle and pierces the thyrohyoid membrane with the internal laryngeal nerve to supply the muscles and mucous membrane of the larynx and the inferior constrictor of pharynx. It anastomoses with its opposite fellow, and with the inferior laryngeal artery and cricothyroid branch of superior thyroid artery. Also *superior laryngeal artery.* **a. lienalis** ARTERIA SPLENICA. **a. ligamenti teretis uteri** [NA] A small branch of the inferior epigastric artery in females that corresponds to the cremasteric artery in males and accompanies and supplies the round ligament of the uterus through the inguinal canal to the labium majus. It anastomoses with branches of the external pudendal arteries. Also *artery of round ligament of uterus.* **a. lingualis** [NA] A branch of the external carotid artery that first lies superficial in the carotid triangle, runs upwards, and then loops forward on the middle pharyngeal constrictor muscle to gain the deep surface of the hyoglossus muscle. After running along the upper border of the hyoid bone, it turns sharply upward, giving off the sublingual artery and continuing as the deep lingual artery. It also has a suprahyoid branch and dorsal lingual branches. Also *lingual artery.* **a. lobi caudati** [NA] Either of two arteries, one arising from the left hepatic artery and one from the right hepatic artery, that supply the left and right parts, respectively, of the caudate lobe of the liver. Branches supply individual segments of the lobe. There may be a weak anastomosis between the right and left vessels. Also *artery of caudate lobe, spigelian artery.* **arteriae lumbales** [NA] Arteries, usually four on each side, that arise in series with posterior intercostal arteries from the posterior aspect of the abdominal aorta opposite the bodies of the first four lumbar vertebrae. The right lumbar arteries are longer than the left. They run posteriorly and laterally on the corresponding vertebral bodies and into muscles of the posterior abdominal wall, ramifying between the transversus abdominis and internal abdominal oblique muscles. They anastomose with the lower posterior intercostal, subcostal, iliolumbar, deep circumflex iliac, and inferior epigastric arteries. They supply the muscles of the abdominal wall, and each gives off vertebral branches to the vertebral bodies, a dorsal branch, and a spinal branch. Also *lumbar arteries.* **arteriae lumbales ima** [NA] A commonly present fifth pair of lumbar arteries that may arise from the median sacral artery or aorta or the common iliac arteries. It runs laterally deep to the latter vessels and may supply the psoas major and iliacus muscles and anastomose with the iliolumbar, deep circumflex iliac, and fourth lumbar arteries. It has dorsal and spinal branches. Also *lowest lumbar arteries, fifth lumbar arteries.* **a. lusoria** A developmental abnormality of the arch arteries resulting in a large vessel, usually the left subclavian artery, developing in a retroesophageal position and causing dysphagia by pressure on neighboring structures. **a. malleolaris anterior lateralis** [NA] A branch of either the anterior tibial artery or the dorsalis pedis artery that runs laterally deep to the extensor digitorum longus tendons to the lateral malleolus, where it anastomoses with the perforating peroneal artery and the lateral tarsal branch of the dorsalis pedis artery, as part of the lateral malleolar network. Also *anterior lateral malleolar artery, external malleolar artery, lateral anterior malleolar artery.* **a. malleolaris anterior medialis** [NA] A branch that arises proximal to the ankle joint from either the anterior tibial artery or the dorsalis pedis artery and runs deep to the tibialis anterior muscle to join the medial malleolar rete by anastomosing with branches of the posterior tibial artery. Also *anterior medial malleolar artery, internal malleolar artery, medial anterior malleolar artery.* **a. mammaria interna** ARTERIA THORACICA INTERNA. **a. masseterica** [NA] A small branch of the second part of the maxillary artery, arising medial to neck of mandible and passing through the mandibular notch, to end in the masseter muscle. It anastomoses with masseteric branches of the facial and transverse facial arteries. Also *masseteric artery.* **a. maxillaris** [NA] The larger of two terminal branches of the external carotid artery. Arising deep in the parotid gland opposite the neck of the mandible, its course is divided into three parts. The mandibular portion gives off the deep auricular, anterior tympanic, inferior alveolar, and middle meningeal arteries, and accessory meningeal branches. The pterygoid portion gives off the masseteric and buccal arteries, and deep temporal and pterygoid branches. The pterygopalatine portion gives off the posterior superior alveolar, infraorbital, greater palatine, and sphenopalatine arteries, the artery of the pterygoid canal, and pharyngeal branches. Also *maxillary artery, internal maxillary artery, deep facial artery.* **a. maxillaris externa** ARTERIA FACIALIS. **a. media genus** [NA] A small branch of popliteal artery that pierces the oblique popliteal ligament posteriorly to enter the knee joint and supply the synovial membrane and cruciate ligaments. Also *middle genicular artery, arteria genus media.* **a. meningea anterior** A small branch of the anterior ethmoidal artery that supplies the meninges of the anterior cranial fossa in the vicinity of the cribriform plate. Also *anterior meningeal artery.* **a. meningea media** [NA] A branch of the third part of the maxillary artery that ascends vertically deep to the medial pterygoid muscle to enter the middle cranial fossa through the foramen spinosum. It courses a groove of the greater wing of the sphenoid bone and terminates in the frontal (anterior) and parietal (posterior) branches, which spread between the dura mater and the internal cranial surface, supplying both and extending up to the vertex to anastomose with branches from the opposite side and with the anterior and posterior meningeal arteries. It also gives off ganglionic branches, a petrosal branch, the superior tympanic artery, and perforating or temporal branches that anastomose with deep temporal arteries. Also *middle meningeal artery.* **a. meningea posterior** [NA] A branch or continuation of the ascending pharyngeal artery that enters the posterior cranial fossa through the jugular foramen, supplying the dura mater and bone. Branches may also enter through the foramen lacerum and the hypoglossal canal. Also *posterior meningeal artery.* **a. mesenterica inferior** [NA] An unpaired branch of the abdominal aorta arising from its anterior surface at the level of the third lumbar vertebra. It runs to the left and downward, behind the peritoneum, crosses the left common iliac artery, and descends into the pelvis between layers of sigmoid mesocolon as the superior rectal artery. It supplies the large intestine from the left half of the transverse colon to the rectum. It gives off the left colic and sigmoid arteries. Also *inferior mesenteric artery.* **a. mesenterica superior** [NA] An unpaired branch of the abdominal aorta that arises from its front surface at the level of the first lumbar vertebra behind the head of the pancreas. It runs forward over the left renal vein, uncinate process of pancreas, and the third part of the duodenum to enter the root of the mesentery, which it follows in an arc, convexity to the left, to the terminal part of the ileum, where it anastomoses with ileal branches of the ileocolic artery and ileal arteries. It supplies all of the small intestine (except the upper half of the duodenum), cecum, ascendng colon, and the right half of the transverse colon. Its branches are the inferior pancreaticoduodenal, jejunal, ileal, middle colic, right colic, and ileocolic arteries. Also *superior mesenteric artery.* **arteriae metacarpales dorsales** [NA] Four arteries on the dorsum of the hand, three from the dorsal carpal arch, and one directly from the radial artery. The second, third, and fourth dorsal metacarpal arteries run on corresponding dorsal interosseous muscles to the webs of the fingers, where each ends in two dorsal digital branches. The first dorsal metacarpal artery arises from the radial artery on the first dorsal interosseous muscle, and divides into two branches for adjacent sides of the thumb and index finger. Also *dorsal metacarpal arteries.* **arteriae metacarpales palmares** [NA] Three or four branches of the deep palmar arch that run on the interosseous muscles to the webs of the fingers, where they terminate by joining the palmar common digital arteries. They supply interosseous muscles, bones, and the second to fourth lumbrical muscles. Also *palmar metacarpal arteries, palmar intermetacarpal arteries, volar metacarpal arteries, palmar interosseous arteries.* **arteriae metatarsales dorsales** [NA] Arteries on the dorsum of the foot, the first arising from the dorsalis pedis artery and the second, third, and fourth from the arcuate artery. They run over the dorsal interosseous muscles to the clefts of the toes, where each divides into two dorsal digital branches for adjoining toes. At the proximal end of the second, third, and fourth interosseous spaces, each receives a posterior perforating branch from the plantar arch, while distally each receives an anterior perforating branch from the plantar metatarsal arteries. Also *dorsal metatarsal arteries.* **arteriae metatarsales plantares** [NA] Usually four branches that arise from the plantar arch and run distally in four intermetatarsal spaces on corresponding interosseous muscles. When they reach the clefts of the toes, each divides into two proper plantar digital arteries and here each gives off an anterior perforating branch. Also *plantar metatarsal arteries, common digital arteries of foot.* **arteriae musculares arteriae ophthalmicae** [NA] A variable number of arteries that arise from either a common trunk of the the ophthalmic artery or the artery itself and accompany the branches of the oculomotor nerve in the orbital cavity to supply the muscles of the bulb. The inferior arteries give off most of the anterior ciliary arteries. Also *arteries to orbital muscles.* **a. musculophrenica** [NA] A terminal branch of the internal thoracic artery that runs laterally posterior to the costal cartilages of the false ribs to the ninth rib, where it lies between the transverse thoracic and the internal abdominal oblique muscles and anastomoses with the ninth to eleventh posterior intercostal arteries. It gives off anterior intercostal arteries to the seventh to ninth spaces, and branches to the pericardium, diaphragm, and abdominal wall muscles. Also *musculophrenic artery.* **arteriae nasales posteriores laterales** [NA] Branches given off by the sphenopalatine artery in the superior nasal meatus that ramify over the meatuses and conchae and anastomose with nasal branches of the greater palatine artery and with ethmoidal arteries and supply branches to the paranasal sinuses. Also *posterior lateral nasal arteries, branches of sphenopalatine artery to conchae and meatuses.* **arteriae nasales posteriores, laterales et septi** Arteriae nasales posteriores laterales and rami septales posteriores. *Outmoded.* Also *lateral and septal posterior nasal arteries, posterior septal arteries.* **a. nutricia** [NA] An artery of variable size that supplies a bone and its medullary cavity. It usually enters through a nutrient foramen. Also *nutrient artery, medullary artery, nutrient vessel.* **arteriae nutriciae humeri** [NA] Branches of the brachial and deep brachial arteries that enter the medullary cavity of the humerus. The former pierces the brachialis muscle to enter a foramen near the middle of the humerus, while the latter branch enters a foramen posterior to the deltoid tuberosity. Also *nutrient arteries of humerus.* **a. nutricia fibulae** [NA] A nutrient artery that arises from the upper third of the fibular artery and passes downward into the fibula. Also *nutrient artery of fibula.* **a. nutricia tibiae** [NA] A large artery that arises from the upper part of the posterior tibial artery and gives off some muscular branches to the tibialis posterior muscle before piercing it to enter the nutrient canal just below the soleal line of the tibia. Within the bone it divides into two branches, one coursing towards the upper extremity and the other to the distal end. Also *nutrient artery of tibia.* **a. obturatoria** [NA] Usually a branch of the anterior division of the internal iliac artery that runs anteriorly deep to the peritoneum to pass through the obturator canal above the superior part of the obturator membrane, and divides into terminal anterior and posterior branches. These are deep to the obturator externus muscle. Inside the pelvis it has iliac, or nutrient, vesical, and pubic branches. Also *obturator artery.* **a. obturatoria accessoria** [NA] An obturator artery that arises from either the inferior epigastric or the external iliac artery due to the enlargement of a small anastomosis that normally exists between the pubic branches of the inferior epigastric and the obturator artery. Its presence may be of consequence in a femoral hernia. Also *accessory obturator artery, abnormal obturator artery.* **a. occipitalis** [NA] A large branch of the external carotid artery, arising posteriorly where the hypoglossal nerve hooks around it. It runs upward to the gap between the mastoid process of the temporal bone and the transverse process of atlas, deep to the sternocleidomastoid muscle. It ramifies in the scalp in the parieto-occipital region. It has muscular branches to adjacent muscles, meningeal branches to the dura mater of the posterior cranial fossa, an auricular branch to the ear, a mastoid branch to the skull and dura mater, occipital branches to the scalp, and a descending branch that sets up a collateral circulation between the external carotid and subclavian arteries. Also *occipital artery.* **a. ophthalmica** [NA] A branch of the internal carotid artery that arises just anterior to the cavernous sinus and enters the orbital cavity through the optic canal along with the optic nerve. It crosses the nerve to the medial orbital wall, and terminates beneath the trochlea as supratrochlear and dorsal nasal arteries. Its other branches to the orbit and adjacent structures are the lacrimal, supraorbital, posterior ethmoidal, anterior ethmoidal, and medial palpebral arteries, while branches to the muscles and bulb of the eye are the central artery of retina, short posterior ciliary, long posterior ciliary, anterior ciliary, and muscular arteries. Also *ophthalmic artery.* **a. ovarica** [NA] One of a pair of slender branches from the front of the abdominal aorta that arise just below the renal arteries and run downward and laterally behind the peritoneum and anterior to the ureter and psoas major muscle. It descends into the pelvis medially across the common iliac artery into the suspensory ligament of the ovary and the broad ligament of the uterus. It terminates by entering the mesovarium and giving branches to the ovary, some of which anastomose with the uterine artery. Its other branches are the ureteral, infundibular, and tubal to the uterine tube, where it anastomoses with the uterine artery. Also *ovarian artery, tubo-ovarian artery, aortic uterine artery.* **a. palatina ascendens** [NA] The first branch of the facial artery, ascending on the lateral wall of the pharynx deep to the medial pterygoid muscle to the base of the skull, where it ends in two branches. The palatine branch loops over the upper border of the superior pharyngeal constrictor and descends to the soft palate, supplying it and the palatine glands and anastomosing with other palatine arteries. The other branch pierces the superior constrictor to supply the palatine tonsil and the auditory tube, anastomosing with the tonsillar and ascending pharyngeal arteries. Also *ascending palatine artery.* **a. palatina descendens** [NA] A branch of the third part of the maxillary artery that descends in the pterygopalatine fossa into the greater palatine canal along with the greater palatine nerve, where it gives off lesser palatine arteries. When it emerges from the greater palatine foramen, medial to the third molar, it becomes the greater palatine artery. Also *descending palatine artery.* **arteriae palatinae minores** [NA] Branches given off by the descending palatine artery in the greater palatine canal that descend through the lesser palatine foramina to supply the soft palate and palatine tonsil, where they anastomose with tonsillar branches of the facial, lingual, and ascending pharyngeal arteries. Branches given off in the canal also pierce and supply the lateral nasal wall. Also *lesser palatine arteries.* **a. palatina major** [NA] The continuation of the descending palatine artery after it emerges through the greater palatine foramen. It runs anteriorly along the alveolar process of the maxilla to the incisive canal, in which it anastomoses with the nasopalatine branch of the sphenopalatine artery. Branches supply the palatine glands, gingiva, and mucous membrane of palate. Also *greater palatine artery.* **arteriae palpebrales laterales** [NA] Two terminal branches of the lacrimal artery that run medially in the upper and lower eyelids, anastomosing with medial palpebral arteries to form the superior and inferior palpebral arches. Also *lateral palpebral arteries.* **arteriae palpebrales mediales** [NA] Two branches, superior and inferior, of the ophthalmic artery that arise at the trochlear of the superior oblique muscle. One runs above and one below the medial palpebral ligament to the free edge of each eyelid, where they anastomose with the lateral palpebral and other arteries to form the superior and inferior palpebral arches. The inferior branch also supplies the nasolacrimal duct. Also *medial palpebral arteries.* **a. pancreatica dorsalis** [NA] A branch of the splenic artery that occasionally arises from the celiac trunk or the superior mesenteric or common hepatic arteries. It supplies branches to the neck and body of the pancreas, and at the lower border of the pancreas it divides into left and right branches, the former being the inferior pancreatic artery. The right branch runs to the anterior surface of the neck, supplies the uncinate process, and runs across the head of the pancreas to form a prepancreatic arcade by anastomosing with the anterior superior pancreaticoduodenal artery. Also *dorsal pancreatic artery.* **a. pancreatica inferior** [NA] The left branch of the dorsal pancreatic artery that runs along the inferior border of the pancreas to its tail, where it often embeds itself and anastomoses with arteria caudae pancreatis and arteria pancreatica magna that supply the left side of the body and tail of the pancreas. Also *inferior pancreatic artery, transverse pancreatic artery.* **a. pancreatica magna** [NA] A branch of the splenic artery that penetrates the pancreas in its left half and sends branches to the left and right along the pancreatic duct. They anastomose with other branches to the pancreas, supplying mostly its tail. Also *great pancreatic artery.* **arteriae pancreaticoduodenales inferiores** [NA] Two branches, anterior and posterior, that usually arise from the superior mesenteric artery by a common stem at the upper border of the third part of the duodenum and supply the head of the pancreas. The anterior branch runs between the head of the pancreas and the duodenum anteriorly, while the posterior branch runs across the back of the pancreatic head toward the common bile duct. They anastomose with the anterior superior and posterior superior pancreaticoduodenal arteries respectively. The anterior branch also supplies the lower half of the duodenum. Also *inferior pancreaticoduodenal arteries, duodenal arteries.* **a. pancreaticoduodenalis superior anterior** [NA] A terminal branch of the gastroduodenal artery that arises at the lower border of the superior part of the duodenum and descends on the anterior surface of the groove between the head of the pancreas and the duodenum, supplying both. Inferiorly it anastomoses with the anterior branch of the inferior pancreaticoduodenal artery. Also *right inferior pancreaticoduodenal artery* (outmoded). **a. pancreaticoduodenalis superior posterior** [NA] A major branch of the gastroduodenal artery that usually arises at the upper border of the superior part of the duodenum and runs to the right and downwards on the back of the head of the pancreas, supplying it and the adjacent duodenum. Inferiorly it anastomoses with the posterior branch of the inferior pancreaticoduodenal artery. It also supplies the common bile duct as it crosses the duct. Also *right superior pancreaticoduodenal artery* (outmoded). **arteriae parietales anterior et posterior** [NA] Two cortical branches of the middle cerebral artery. The anterior parietal artery ascends from the lateral cerebral sulcus to the area of the intraparietal sulcus, and the posterior parietal artery extends posterosuperiorly from the sulcus. They are distributed to the postcentral gyrus, the lower part of the superior parietal lobule, and the whole of the inferior parietal lobule on the lateral surface of the cerebral hemisphere. Also *parietal branches of middle cerebral artery.* **a. parieto-occipitalis** [NA] The parieto-occipital branch of the middle cerebral artery. One of the terminal cortical branches of the middle cerebral artery that emerges over the posterior bank of the lateral sulcus onto the lateral surface of the cerebral cortex, courses posteriorly, and supplies the transitional region of cerebral cortex between the parietal and occipital lobes. **arteriae perforantes** [NA] Branches, usually four, of the deep femoral artery that perforate the adductor brevis and the adductor magnus close to the linea aspera of the femur so as to supply the posterior muscles of the thigh and the vastus lateralis muscle. They anastomose with each other in loops, and the first also joins the cruciate anastomosis. Also *perforating arteries, perforating branches of profunda femoris artery.* **a. pericardiacophrenica** [NA] A long, thin branch of the internal thoracic artery that arises at the first rib and descends with the phrenic nerve between pleura and pericardium to the diaphragm. Its branches supply the pericardium, pleura, diaphragm, and phrenic nerve, and it anastomoses with musculophrenic and inferior phrenic arteries. Also *pericardiacophrenic artery, arteria comes nervi phrenici, superior phrenic artery.* **a. perinealis** [NA] A branch of the internal pudendal artery that pierces the urogenital diaphragm to run in the superficial perineal space to the scrotum or labia majora, where it terminates in the posterior scrotal or labial branches. Also *perineal artery, arteria perinei, superficial perineal artery.* **a. peronea** ARTERIA FIBULARIS. **a. pharyngea ascendens** [NA] A long, variable branch of the external carotid artery that ascends vertically along the pharynx and deep to the internal carotid artery to the base of the skull. It gives off the inferior tympanic artery, posterior meningeal artery, pharyngeal branches to constrictor muscles, palatine branches to soft palate and tonsil, and prevertebral branches to deep structures. Also *ascending pharyngeal artery.* **a. phrenica inferior** [NA] Either of the first paired branches of the abdominal aorta arising opposite the first lumbar vertebra. They ascend and supply the diaphragm and suprarenal glands. Each has an anterior branch that anastomoses with the pericardiacophrenic artery, and a posterior branch that gives off superior suprarenal arteries and anastomoses with lower intercostal arteries. Also *inferior phrenic artery, great phrenic artery, diaphragmatic artery.* **arteriae phrenicae superiores** [NA] A small pair of arteries arising from the thoracic aorta just above the diaphragm, the upper surface of which they supply and where they anastomose with the pericardiacophrenic and musculophrenic arteries. Also *superior phrenic arteries, superior diaphragmatic arteries.* **a. plantaris lateralis** [NA] The larger of two terminal branches of the posterior tibial artery that runs from the medial process of the calcaneal tuberosity obliquely to the base of the fifth metatarsal bone, where it turns medially and deeply to the proximal part of the first interosseous space, where it anastomoses with the deep plantar branch of the dorsalis pedis artery, forming the plantar arch. Its branches are the plantar metatarsal and perforating arteries. Also *lateral plantar artery, external plantar artery.* **a. plantaris medialis** [NA] The smaller of two terminal branches of the posterior tibial artery that runs anteriorly along the medial side of the sole of the foot to the base of the first metatarsal bone, where it continues along the medial side of the big toe, anastomosing with the first plantar metatarsal artery. It gives off superficial digital branches that join the first, second, and third plantar metatarsal arteries, and it gives off deep branches to the muscles, joints, and skin on the medial side of the sole. Also *medial plantar artery, internal plantar artery.* **a. plantaris profunda arteriae dorsalis pedis** [NA] The terminal branch of the dorsalis pedis artery, which descends into the sole of the foot at the proximal end of the first interosseous space between the heads of the first dorsal interosseous muscle. It anastomoses with the lateral plantar artery to form the deep plantar arch. Also *deep plantar artery.* **a. poplitea** [NA] The continuation of the femoral artery, extending from the opening in the adductor magnus across the floor of the popliteal fossa to the lower border of the popliteus muscle, where it terminates as the anterior and posterior tibial arteries. Its branches are the sural arteries, superior muscular arteries to the hamstrings and adductor magnus, cutaneous branches to the skin on the back of the leg, and genicular arteries. Also *popliteal artery.* **a. princeps pollicis** [NA] A branch, given off by the radial artery as it turns medially across the palm, that runs along the first metacarpal bone deep to the flexor pollicis longus tendon to the base of the first proximal phalanx, where it terminates as two palmar digitals of the thumb. Also *principal artery of thumb, princeps pollicis artery.* **a. profunda brachii** [NA] The largest branch of the brachial artery that arises at the lower border of the teres major muscle and runs laterally behind the humerus in the spiral groove for radial nerve deep to the triceps muscle, where it terminates as the radial collateral and middle collateral arteries. Its other branches are the nutrient branch to the humerus and the deltoid branch to triceps and deltoid muscles, anastomosing with the posterior circumflex humeral artery. Also *deep brachial artery, superior profunda artery, profunda brachii artery.* **a. profunda clitoridis** [NA] A branch of the internal pudendal artery in females that pierces the inferior fascia of the urogenital diaphragm posteriorly and enters the crus of the clitoris to supply the corpus cavernosum. Also *deep artery of clitoris.* **a. profunda femoris** [NA] The largest branch of the femoral artery, which arises from its posterolateral aspect and descends posterior to the femoral artery and vein and adductor longus muscle to end by perforating the adductor magnus muscle as the fourth perforating artery in the hamstrings. Its branches are the medial femoral circumflex, lateral femoral circumflex, perforating arteries, and muscular branches to adductors and hamstrings. Also *deep femoral artery, profunda femoris artery.* **a. profunda linguae** [NA] The tortuous terminal portion, or continuation, of the lingual artery, extending from the anterior border of the hyoglossus muscle to the tip of the tongue. It runs along the genioglossus muscle under the mucous membrane, gives off vertical branches to dorsum of tongue, and anastomoses with its opposite artery both through the septum and at the tip of the tongue. Also *deep lingual artery, ranine artery.* **a. profunda penis** [NA] One of the terminal branches of the internal pudendal artery in males that pierces the inferior fascia of the urogenital diaphragm posteriorly, enters the crus penis, and runs centrally in the corpus cavernosum, supplying it. Also *deep artery of penis, artery to corpus cavernosum.* **arteriae pudendae externae** [NA] Branches of the femoral artery that arise just below the inguinal ligament and are usually described in two groups, superficial, and deep. The superficial branches pierce the cribriform fascia and ascend over the pubis to supply the skin over the lower abdomen. One branch passes on to the penis or clitoris, to anastomose at the prepuce with the dorsal artery. Also *external pudendal arteries.* **a. pudenda interna** [NA] The smaller of two terminal branches of the anterior division of the internal iliac artery that supplies the external genitalia. It leaves the pelvis below the piriformis muscle, entering the gluteal region, where it crosses the sacrospinous ligament and passes into the ischiorectal fossa. After its course in the pudendal canal, it goes through the superficial and deep perineal spaces, terminating as the deep artery of the penis or clitoris and the dorsal artery of the penis or clitoris. Also *internal pudendal artery, internal pudic artery.* **a. pulmonalis dextra** [NA] The right terminal branch of the pulmonary trunk that arises at about the level of the sternal angle and runs horizontally under the arch of the aorta and behind the ascending aorta and the superior vena cava to the hilus of the lung, where it divides into the anterior and interlobar trunks. The anterior trunk supplies the bronchopulmonary segments of the superior lobe of the lung while the interlobar trunk supplies those of the middle and inferior lobes. The anterior trunk gives off apical, anterior descending, posterior descending, and posterior ascending arteries. The middle lobe artery has medial and lateral segmental branches. The branches of the interlobar trunk to lower lobe segments are the superior (apical), subsuperior (subapical), medial basal (cardiac), anterior basal, lateral basal, and posterior basal. Also *right pulmonary artery.* **a. pulmonalis sinistra** [NA] The left terminal branch of the pulmonary trunk. It is shorter than the right branch, pierces the pericardium, is attached to the aortic arch by the ligamentum arteriosum, and runs horizontally anterior to the descending aorta and left bronchus. In the hilus of the lung it divides into two branches, one for each lobe of the lung. In general, the distribution of its branches is similar to that of the right. The branches to the superior lobe are apical, posterior, anterior descending, anterior ascending, and lingual. Those to the inferior lobe are the superior (apical), subsuperior (subapical), anterior basal, medial basal, posterior basal, and lateral basal. Also *left pulmonary artery.* **a. radialis** [NA] The smaller of two terminal branches of the brachial artery, which arises in the cubital fossa and runs downward, curving laterally, to the styloid process of the radius. Its branches may be grouped regionally: in the forearm are the radial recurrent, muscular, superficial palmar, and palmar carpal branches; at the wrist are the dorsal carpal and first dorsal metacarpal; and in the hand the princeps pollicis, radialis indicis, palmar metacarpal, recurrent, and proximal perforating branches. Also *radial artery.* **a. radialis indicis** [NA] A branch of the radial artery given off as the latter turns medially across the palm. It runs distally along the radial side of the index finger, at the tip of which it anastomoses with the proper digital artery. In the palm it anastomoses with the princeps pollicis artery. Also *radial artery of index finger, volar radial artery of index finger.* **a. radicularis magna** An especially large, anterior radicular branch of one of the lower thoracic or upper lumbar intersegmental arteries, usually on the left side. It may supply, in man, two-thirds of the blood supply to the spinal cord. Also *great ventral radicular artery, artery of Adamkiewicz.* **arteriae rectae spuriae** Branches of efferent arterioles of glomeruli located in the corticomedullary zone that pass downward to supply the collecting tubules and loops of Henle of the renal pyramids. **arteriae rectae verae** ARTERIOLAE RECTAE RENIS. **a. rectalis inferior** [NA] A branch of the internal pudendal artery that pierces the fascia of the pudendal canal and breaks up into branches that cross the ischiorectal fossa, supplying the skin, and the levator ani and external anal sphincter muscles. They anastomose with the middle and superior rectal arteries and the gluteal and perineal arteries. Also *inferior rectal artery, inferior hemorrhoidal artery, arteria hemorrhoidalis inferior.* **a. rectalis media** [NA] A branch of the anterior division of the internal iliac artery that runs across the pelvic floor to the middle part of the rectum to supply it and anastomose with the superior and inferior rectal arteries. It also gives branches to the vagina in the female, and to the seminal vesicles and ampulla of the ductus deferens in the male. Also *arteria hemorrhoidalis media, middle hemorrhoidal artery, middle rectal artery.* **a. rectalis superior** [NA] The continuation of the inferior mesenteric artery that descends into the pelvis between layers of sigmoid mesocolon. Opposite the third sacral vertebra it bifurcates, with a branch descending on either side of the rectum. Their branches pierce the wall and descend deep to the mucous membrane to the internal sphincter, where they anastomose with inferior and middle rectal arteries in a series of loops. Also *superior rectal artery, superior hemorrhoidal artery, arteria hemorrhoidalis superior, dorsal rectal artery* (outmoded). **a. recurrens radialis** [NA] A branch of the radial artery that arises just below the elbow joint and curves laterally across the supinator to divide into branches that supply adjacent muscles and the elbow joint and anastomose with the radial collateral branch of the deep brachial and interosseous recurrent arteries. Also *radial recurrent artery.* **a. recurrens tibialis anterior** [NA] A branch of the anterior tibial artery that ascends over the lower lateral side of the knee joint to anastomose with the inferior and the superior lateral genicular arteries. It supplies the tibialis anterior muscle and the knee joint. Also *anterior tibial recurrent artery.* **a. recurrens tibialis posterior** [NA] A branch that arises in the popliteal fossa, usually from the anterior tibial artery but sometimes from the posterior tibial artery. It ascends to the oblique popliteal ligament to supply it, the popliteus muscle, knee joint, and the superior tibiofibular joint. It anastomoses with the inferior medial genicular artery. Also *posterior tibial recurrent artery, posterior fibular recurrent artery* (outmoded). **a. recurrens ulnaris** [NA] Either of two branches, anterior and posterior, arising separately or from a common stem from the medial side of the ulnar artery, that supplies adjacent muscles, elbow joint, and ulnar nerve, and joins the rete articularis cubiti. Also *ulnar recurrent artery.* **a. renalis** [NA] Either of a pair of arteries that arises from the lateral aspect of the abdominal aorta at about the level of the second lumbar vertebra and runs laterally and horizontally anterior to crus of diaphragm and the psoas major muscle, and posterior to the renal vein. Near the hilum of the kidney, it divides either into anterior and posterior divisions (or trunks) or into four to five branches that penetrate the kidney in a segmental fashion. Other branches are the inferior suprarenal artery, the capsular, or perirenal, arteries, and a ureteral branch. Also *renal artery, emulgent artery.* **arteriae renis** [NA] The four or five segmental, or lobar, branches of the anterior and posterior divisions of the renal artery that divide within the kidney to provide interlobar arteries within the renal columns. These give off arcuate, interlobular, and perforating arteries in sequence. Also *renal arteries, arteries of kidney.* **arteriae retroduodenales** [NA] One or more branches of the gastroduodenal artery that arise and run posterior to the first part of the duodenum, supplying it, the common bile duct, and the adjacent head of the pancreas. Also *retroduodenal arteries.* **arteriae sacrales laterales** [NA] Two arteries, superior and inferior, that arise separately or occasionally from a single trunk from the posterior division of the internal iliac artery. The larger, superior branch enters the first anterior sacral foramen, gives off branches to the bone and the contents of the sacral canal, passes through the posterior sacral foramen to supply the skin and muscles over the sacrum, and anastomoses with the gluteal arteries. The inferior branch descends on the pelvic aspect of the sacrum to the coccyx to anastomose with the median sacral artery and branches from opposite side. The inferior branch gives off spinal branches through the second, third, and fourth anterior sacral foramina that anastomose with each other in the sacral canal and follow a course similar to that of the superior lateral sacral artery. Also *lateral sacral arteries.* **a.**

**sacralis mediana** [NA] A branch of the abdominal aorta that arises from its posterior aspect just above the bifurcation of the aorta and descends in the midline anterior to the lower lumbar vertebrae, sacrum, and coccyx. It may give off the lowest, or fifth, lumbar artery, and has lateral sacral branches that anastomose with lateral sacral arteries. It may have rectal branches that anastomose with rectal arteries. Also *median sacral artery, middle sacral artery, arteria sacralis media, aorta sacrococcygea* (outmoded), *caudal artery, coccygeal artery, sacrococcygeal artery.* **a. scapularis dorsalis** ARTERIA DORSALIS SCAPULAE. **a. segmenti anterioris** [NA] One of two main branches of the right hepatic artery that supplies the anterior segment of right internal lobe of liver and ends by dividing into branches to the superior and inferior hepatic areas. Also *anterior segmental artery, right ventral paramedian artery.* **a. segmenti anterioris inferioris** [NA] The branch of the lower branch of the anterior division of the renal artery that supplies the parenchyma of the anterior part of the lower segment of the kidney. Also *anterior inferior segmental artery.* **a. segmenti anterioris superioris** [NA] The branch of the anterior division of the renal artery that supplies the parenchyma of the anterior superior segment of the kidney. Also *anterior superior segmental artery.* **a. segmenti inferioris** [NA] The lower branch of the anterior division of the renal artery that supplies the lower segment of the kidney by an anterior and a posterior branch. Also *inferior segmental artery.* **a. segmenti lateralis** [NA] A branch of the left hepatic artery that divides into two branches, supplying the left dorsocranial and left ventrocaudal subsegments of the lateral segment of the left internal lobe of liver. Also *lateral segment artery.* **a. segmenti medialis** [NA] A branch of the left hepatic artery that divides intrahepatically into branches that supply the parenchyma of the quadrate lobe and the cranial portion of left paramedian subsegment of left internal lobe of liver. At its termination it gives off a branch to the ligamentum teres. Also *medial segmental artery, left ventral paramedian artery, middle hepatic artery, artery of segment IV of liver* (outmoded). **a. segmenti posterioris** 1 [NA] The posterior division of the renal artery, that enters the posterior aspect of the renal sinus, arches over the upper calix and then downward, giving off branches to the posterior segment, or the whole posterior aspect, of the kidney. 2 [NA] Either of two main branches of the right hepatic artery that supplies the posterior segment of right internal lobe of liver, and ends by dividing into cranial and caudal branches to the corresponding subsegments. Also *right dorsocaudal artery, right lateral hepatic artery* (outmoded) *For defs. 1 and 2* also *posterior segmental artery.* **a. segmenti superioris** [NA] The upper branch of the anterior division of the renal artery that divides into apical and lateral branches to supply the apical and upper (anterior) segments of the kidney. Also *superior segmental artery.* **arteriae sigmoideae** [NA] Branches from the lateral aspect of the inferior mesenteric artery that run downwards and to the left behind the peritoneum towards and supplying the sigmoid colon, where they branch and unite to form arcades that anastomose superiorly with the descending branch of the left colic artery and inferiorly with the superior rectal artery. Thus, a continuous marginal artery is formed along the border of the colon. Also *sigmoid arteries, inferior left colic arteries.* **a. spermatica externa** ARTERIA CREMASTERICA. **a. sphenopalatina** [NA] The terminal branch of the pterygopalatine portion of the maxillary artery that passes through the sphenopalatine foramen into the nasal cavity, where it divides into posterior lateral nasal branches and posterior septal branches. It anastomoses with the greater palatine and ethmoid arteries. Also *sphenopalatine artery, nasopalatine artery, posterior lateral nasal arteries, posterior septal arteries.* **a. spinalis anterior** An unpaired blood vessel lying along the ventral median fissure of the spinal cord. It originates superiorly (or rostrally) by a junction of branches from the two vertebral arteries, and at lower levels it receives several radicular branches from the vertebral, intercostal, and lumbar arteries. Also *anterior spinal artery.* **a. spinalis posterior** [NA] A branch of the vertebral artery which, arising within the vertebral canal, bifurcates to pass upward along the posterolateral sulcus of the lower medulla and downward to adjacent segments of the spinal cord. Superiorly, it joins and often arises from the posterior inferior cerebellar artery. Inferiorly, it is continuous with the dorsolateral spinal artery. Also *arteria spinalis dorsalis, posterior spinal artery.* **a. splenica** [NA] The largest branch of the celiac trunk that runs to the left along the posterosuperior border of the pancreas to the spleen. At first it is retroperitoneal, crossing the left crus of diaphragm, and then it becomes tortuous and grooves the superior border of the pancreas, gaining its ventral surface near its tail. Here it divides into superior and inferior terminal branches, which enter the splenorenal ligament and subdivide into splenic branches to the hilus and poles. There are many other branches, including the pancreatic, short gastric, and left gastro-omental arteries. The branches are involved in numerous anastomoses. Also *splenic artery, arteria lienalis.* **a. sternocleidomastoidea** RAMI STERNOCLEIDOMASTOIDEI ARTERIAE OCCIPITALIS. **a. stylomastoidea** [NA] A branch of the posterior auricular artery that penetrates the stylomastoid foramen where it joins the facial nerve. It gives off the posterior tympanic artery to the tympanic membrane, mastoid branches to mastoid air cells, and a stapedial branch to supply the stapedius, stapes, secondary tympanic membrane, and tympanic cavity. Also *stylomastoid artery.* **a. subclavia** [NA] The major artery to the upper extremity. Through its branches, it supplies also the shoulder (dorsal scapular and thyrocervical branches), portions of the thoracic wall (costocervical and internal thoracic branches), neck (thyrocervical branch), and brain structures within the posterior fossa (vertebral branch). On the right side it arises by bifurcation of the innominate artery and on the left it springs directly from the aortic arch. Also *subclavian artery.* **a. subcostalis** [NA] Either member of the lowest pair of parietal branches of the thoracic aorta, in series with the posterior intercostal arteries. Each runs anteriorly along the lower border of the twelfth rib, with the subcostal nerve, to enter the plane between the transverse abdominal and internal abdominal oblique muscles, where it anastomoses with superior epigastric, posterior intercostal, and lumbar arteries. Also *subcostal artery.* **a. sublingualis** [NA] Any of the terminal branches of the lingual artery that run on the genioglossus muscle and deep to the mylohyoid muscle to the sublingual gland, supplying these structures. It continues under the mucosa of the frenulum to anastomose with the artery of the opposite side and the submental artery. It also supplies the mucous membrane of the floor of the mouth and gingiva. Also *sublingual artery.* **a. submentalis** [NA] The largest of the cervical branches of the facial artery that arises anterior to the submandibular gland and runs on the mylohyoid muscle along the lower border of the mandible to the symphysis menti, where it ends in superficial and deep branches. The former branch anastomoses with the inferior labial artery, while the deep branch runs on bone and supplies the lower lip, anastomosing with the mental and inferior labial arteries. In its course it supplies the surrounding muscles and the submandibular lymph nodes, and anastomoses with sublingual and mylohyoid arteries. Also *submental artery.* **a. subscapularis** [NA] The largest branch of the axillary artery, that arises at and runs along the lower border of the subscapularis muscle, supplying muscles of the posterior wall of the axilla, lymph nodes, and the serratus anterior muscle. About three centimeters from its origin, it ends by dividing into the circumflex scapular and thoracodorsal arteries. Also *subscapular artery.* **a. sulci centralis** [NA] A cortical branch of the terminal part of the middle cerebral artery that arises in the lateral sulcus and ascends to ramify in the pia mater over the central sulcus. Its anterior branches supply the precentral gyrus whereas posterior branches supply the postcentral gyrus. Also *artery of central sulcus, rolandic artery* (outmoded), *artery of fissure of Rolando* (outmoded) . **a. sulci precentralis** [NA] A branch of the terminal part of the middle cerebral artery. It usually courses upward on the lateral surface of the cerebral cortex within the precentral sulcus, supplying the posterior portions of the superior, middle, and inferior frontal gyri anteriorly and the precentral gyrus posteriorly. Also *artery of precentral sulcus.* **a. superior lateralis genus** [NA] A branch of the popliteal artery that runs above the lateral condyle of femur and deep to the tendon of biceps femoris muscle, and divides into superficial and deep branches. The former supplies the vastus lateralis and anastomoses with the descending branch of the lateral circumflex femoral and lateral inferior genicular arteries, while the latter supplies the femur and knee joint and anastomoses with the medial inferior genicular and descending genicular arteries. Also *lateral superior genicular artery, arteria genu superior lateralis.* **a. superior medialis genus** [NA] A branch of the popliteal artery that runs medially over the medial condyle of femur deep to the hamstrings and tendon of adductor magnus. It divides into two branches, one supplying the vastus medialis muscle and anastomosing with the medial inferior genicular and descending genicular arteries. The other branch supplies the knee joint and patella and anastomoses with the lateral superior genicular artery. Also *medial superior genicular artery, arteria genu superior medialis.* **a. supraduodenalis** [NA] One or two inconstant branches that may arise from either the retroduodenal or the gastroduodenal artery or from branches of the hepatic artery. It supplies the first part of the duodenum and may anastomose with adjacent arteries. Also *supraduodenal artery.* **a. supraorbitalis** [NA] A branch of the ophthalmic artery that joins the supraorbital nerve and runs anteriorly between the periosteum and the levator palpebrae superioris muscle to the supraorbital foramen, through which it passes to end in superficial and deep branches. These supply the muscles, skin, and pericranium of the forehead and anastomose with branches of the superficial temporal, facial, lateral palpebral, and transverse facial arteries. Also *supraorbital artery.* **arteriae suprarenales superiores** [NA] Branches of the paired inferior phrenic arteries, or of their posterior branches, that supply the suprarenal gland on either side. Also *superior suprarenal arteries.* **a. suprarenalis inferior** [NA] Any of several small branches of the renal artery that enter and supply the posterior and inferior surfaces of the suprarenal gland. They may also arise from other neighboring vessels. Also *inferior suprarenal artery, inferior capsular artery.* **a. suprarenalis media** [NA] One or more branches arising from the abdominal aorta on each side near the origin of the renal artery. It usually runs obliquely upward across the crus of the diaphragm to the suprarenal gland, where it divides into several branches to supply the front and back surfaces of the gland. Also *middle suprarenal artery, middle capsular artery, aortic suprarenal artery.* **a. suprascapularis** [NA] An artery that arises from the thyrocervical trunk or in common with transverse cervical artery that runs laterally deep to and parallel to the clavicle to the base of the coracoid process, where it passes superficial to the transverse ligament of the scapula and deep to the supraspinatus muscle. It goes around the neck of the scapula and deep to the infraspinatus muscle, where it anastomoses with the circumflex scapular and descending scapular arteries. Also *suprascapular artery, arteria transversa scapulae, transverse scapular artery.* **a. supratrochlearis** [NA] A terminal branch of the ophthalmic artery that pierces the orbital septum at the medial angle of the orbit and ascends deep to the orbicularis oculi muscle, supplying it and anastomosing with the supraorbital artery and branches from the opposite side. It supplies the skin and periosteum. Also *supratrochlear artery, arteria frontalis, frontal artery, internal frontal artery.* **arteriae surales** [NA] Two large branches, medial and lateral, that arise from the popliteal artery behind the knee joint and supply the gastrocnemius, soleus, and plantaris muscles and give cutaneous branches to skin and fascia of the calf. Also *sural arteries.* **arteriae tarsales mediales** [NA] A few branches of the dorsalis pedis artery that join the medial malleolar network and supply the bones and joints on the medial side of the foot. Also *medial tarsal arteries, medial tarsal branches.* **a. tarsalis lateralis** [NA] A branch of the dorsalis pedis artery that arises opposite the talus bone and runs laterally deep to the extensor digitorum brevis, which it supplies. It anastomoses with the lateral malleolar, perforating peroneal, arcuate, and lateral plantar arteries and supplies bones and joints. Also *lateral tarsal artery.* **arteriae temporales profundae** Two branches, anterior and posterior, of the second part of the maxillary artery that ascend deep to the temporalis muscle, supplying it, the pericranium, and bone, and anastomose with the middle temporal and lacrimal arteries. Also *deep temporal arteries.* **a. temporalis anterior** [NA] A cortical branch of the middle cerebral artery that emerges from the lateral sulcus onto the lateral surface of the temporal lobe to be distributed to the anterior part of the superior and middle temporal gyri, including the temporal pole. It often anastomoses with the temporal branches of the posterior cerebral artery. Also *anterior temporal artery.* **a. temporalis media** [NA] A branch of the superficial temporal artery that arises opposite the zygoma and pierces the temporal fascia and muscle, supplying them and anastomosing on bone with the deep temporal arteries. Also *middle temporal artery.* **a. temporalis posterior** [NA] A cortical branch of the insular part of the middle cerebral artery that leaves the posterior part of the lateral sulcus by crossing the external aspect of the superior temporal gyrus and then the middle temporal gyrus to end opposite the preoccipital sulcus. It supplies the posterior parts of the superior, middle, and inferior temporal gyri. Also *posterior temporal artery.* **a. temporalis superficialis** [NA] The smaller of two terminal branches of the external carotid artery, arising in the parotid gland and ascending between the posterior zygomatic root and the external acoustic meatus (where it can be palpated to determine the pulse), above which it terminates in a frontal and a parietal branch. Also *superficial temporal artery.* **a. testicularis** [NA] One of a pair of branches of the abdominal aorta that descends over the psoas major muscle and behind the peritoneum to the deep inguinal ring, where it joins the ductus deferens in the spermatic cord through the inguinal canal to supply the testis. Also *testicular artery, funicular artery, internal spermatic artery.* **ar-**

**teriae thalamostriatae anteromediales arteriae cerebri anterioris** ARTERIAE CENTRALES ANTEROMEDIALES ARTERIAE CEREBRI ANTERIORIS. **a. thoracalis lateralis** ARTERIA THORACICA LATERALIS. **a. thoracalis suprema** ARTERIA THORACICA SUPERIOR. **a. thoracica interna** [NA] A branch of the first part of the subclavian artery. Its cervical portion runs forward and medially over the cupola of pleura behind the medial end of the clavicle to the cartilage of the first rib, where the thoracic portion starts. It runs down behind the costal cartilages just lateral to the sternum to the level of the sixth interspace, where it terminates as the superior epigastric and musculophrenic arteries. Its other branches are the pericardiacophrenic, mediastinal, sternal, thymic, pericardial, anterior intercostal, perforating, and lateral costal. Also *internal thoracic artery, arteria mammaria interna, internal mammary artery.* **a. thoracica lateralis** [NA] An artery that arises from either the axillary artery, subscapular artery, or thoracoacromial artery and descends along the lower border of the pectoralis minor muscle to the chest wall to supply the second to fifth intercostal spaces. It also supplies the axillary lymph nodes and adjacent muscles, and, in females, the mammary gland. Also *lateral thoracic artery, arteria thoracalis lateralis, lateral mammary artery, external mammary artery.* **a. thoracica superior** [NA] A small branch of either the first part of the axillary artery or the thoracoacromial artery that supplies the muscles of the first intercostal space, including the serratus anterior. Also *highest thoracic artery, arteria thoracalis suprema, superior thoracic artery, arteria thoracica suprema* (outmoded). **a. thoracoacromialis** [NA] A short branch of the second part of the axillary artery that perforates the clavipectoral fascia and divides into clavicular, pectoral, deltoid, and acromial branches. Also *thoracicoacromial artery.* **a. thoracodorsalis** [NA] A terminal branch and continuation of the subscapular artery that runs along the latissimus dorsi and subscapularis muscles, supplying both. It anastomoses with the circumflex scapular and descending scapular arteries, and sends branches to supply the thoracic wall on the medial side of the axilla. Also *thoracodorsal artery.* **a. thyroidea ima** [NA] An occasional artery that may arise either from the brachiocephalic trunk or arch of the aorta, or from adjacent vessels. It ascends anterior to the trachea to supply medial aspects of both lobes of the thyroid gland. Also *thyroidea ima artery, lowest thyroid artery, Neubauer's artery, middle thyroid artery, thyroidea ima.* **a. thyroidea inferior** [NA] The largest branch of the thyrocervical trunk which ascends between the carotid sheath and prevertebral fascia to the level of the cricoid cartilage, where it turns medially to enter the thyroid sheath just below its center. Its branches are the parathyroid branches; the inferior laryngeal artery; the pharyngeal, esophageal, tracheal, and muscular branches; and the tracheosoephageal artery. Also *inferior thyroid artery.* **a. thyroidea superior** [NA] A branch of the external carotid artery that arches downward deep to the infrahyoid muscles, supplying them, to the superior pole of the thyroid gland, where it ramifies and anastomoses with the inferior thyroid artery, forming an important collateral channel between the external carotid and subclavian arteries. Its branches include the infrahyoid branch, sternocleidomastoid artery, superior laryngeal artery, cricothyroid branch, and muscular branches. Also *superior thyroid artery.* **a. tibialis anterior** [NA] The smaller terminal division of the popliteal artery that passes between tibia and fibula over the interosseous membrane to the anterior compartment of the leg, in which it descends between muscles to the ankle joint where, midway between the malleoli, it becomes the dorsalis pedis artery. Its branches are the posterior tibial recurrent artery, anterior tibial recurrent artery, anterior medial malleolar artery, anterior lateral malleolar artery, muscular branches to the anterior compartment muscles, and an occasional fibular branch. Also *anterior tibial artery.* **a. tibialis posterior** [NA] The larger terminal division of the popliteal artery that runs obliquely down the back of the leg between superficial and deep muscles to the ankle joint where, deep to the flexor retinaculum and midway between the medial malleolus and the calcaneal tuberosity, it terminates as medial and lateral plantar arteries. Its branches are the peroneal artery, tibial nutrient artery, posterior medial malleolar artery, communicating branch, medial calcaneal branches, an occasional fibular branch, as well as branches to adjacent muscles and to the skin of the medial side of the leg. Also *posterior tibial artery.* **a. transversa cervicis** [NA] An artery that arises either from the thyrocervical trunk, from a common trunk with the suprascapular artery, or as a branch of the dorsal scapular artery. It runs laterally over the scalenus anterior muscle and obliquely across the posterior triangle of the neck at a higher level than the suprascapular artery to the trapezius muscle, where it ends in two branches, the ramus superficialis and ramus profundus. Also *transverse cervical artery, transverse artery of neck.* **a. transversa facialis** [NA] A branch of either the superficial temporal artery or the external carotid artery that arises in and supplies the parotid gland and runs transversely across the masseter muscle, supplying it and the parotid duct below, to end in the buccinator muscle. It anastomoses with the infraorbital, facial, and buccal arteries. Also *transverse facial artery, transverse artery of face.* **a. transversa scapulae** ARTERIA SUPRASCAPULARIS. **a. tympanica anterior** [NA] A branch that arises from the first part of the maxillary artery, either independently or in common with the deep auricular artery. It ascends through the petrotympanic fissure to join the chorda tympani nerve and supplies the mucosa of tympanum and tympanic membrane, around which it forms a vascular circle with the posterior tympanic artery. Also *anterior tympanic artery, glaserian artery.* **a. tympanica inferior** [NA] A small branch of the ascending pharyngeal artery that passes through a small canaliculus in the petrous portion of the temporal bone and into the tympanic cavity, where it anastomoses with other tympanic arteries. Also *inferior tympanic artery.* **a. tympanica posterior** [NA] A branch of the stylomastoid artery that arises in the facial canal and goes with the chorda tympani nerve to the posterior part of the tympanic membrane, to anastomose with the anterior tympanic artery and form a vascular circle around the membrane. Also *posterior tympanic artery.* **a. tympanica superior** [NA] A branch of the middle meningeal artery that passes into the canal for the tensor tympani muscle, supplying it and the mucosa of the canal. It may penetrate the tympanum through the petrosquamous suture and anastomose with other tympanic arteries. Also *superior tympanic artery.* **a. ulnaris** [NA] The larger of two terminal branches of the brachial artery that arises at the apex of the cubital fossa and runs downward and medially, at first deep to the flexor muscles but becoming comparatively superficial at the wrist, where it enters the palm superficial to the flexor retinaculum and lateral to the pisiform bone. It runs laterally deep to the palmar aponeurosis to form the superficial palmar arch by anastomosing with a branch from the radial artery. Its branches are the anterior and posterior ulnar recurrent, common interosseous, palmar carpal, dorsal carpal, deep palmar, and common palmar digital arteries, and muscular branches in the forearm. Also *ulnar artery.* **a. umbilicalis** [NA] UMBILICAL ARTERY. **a. urethralis** [NA] A small branch of the internal pudendal artery that pierces the inferior fascia of the urogenital diaphragm and enters the corpus cavernosum penis, in which it remains as far as glans penis. It supplies urethra and erectile tissue. Also *urethral artery.* **a. uterina** [NA] A branch of the anterior division of the internal iliac artery in females that runs downward and medially to the cervix uteri, where it ascends along the lateral wall of the uterus between layers of the broad ligament to the uterine tube. It turns laterally to the ovary, to end in an anastomosis with the ovarian artery. It gives branches to cervix, vagina (forming the azygos artery of vagina), the body and fundus of the uterus, the uterine tube, and round ligament of uterus. It is the homologue of the deferential artery in males. Also *uterine artery, fallopian artery.* **a. vaginalis** [NA] An artery in females that usually arises from the anterior division of the internal iliac artery but may be a branch of the uterine artery, and that corresponds to the inferior vesical artery in males. It sends branches to the fundus of urinary bladder, the vagina (to form azygos artery of vagina), and bulb of vestibule. Also *vaginal artery.* **a. vertebralis** [NA] The first and largest branch of the subclavian artery. It ascends through the transverse foramina of all cervical vertebrae except the seventh. On the posterior arch of the atlas, it pierces the posterior atlanto-occipital membrane and enters the foramen magnum to reach the posterior border of the pons, where it unites with the vertebral artery of the opposite side to form the basilar artery. It has spinal branches, and muscular branches that are deep to the cervical and suboccipital muscles. In the skull, it has posterior meningeal and bulbar branches, and it branches into the anterior spinal, posterior spinal, and posterior and inferior cerebellar arteries. Also *vertebral artery.* **arteriae vesicales superiores** [NA] Several branches of the nonobliterated umbilical artery that supply the superior portion of urinary bladder. They anastomose with branches of the opposite side and with the inferior vesical artery. They give branches to the urachus and its peritoneal fold and to the ureter. They may give off an artery to the ductus deferens. Also *superior vesical arteries.* **a. vesicalis inferior** [NA] An artery that may arise in common with the middle rectal artery or with other branches of the anterior division of the internal iliac artery, running to the junction of prostate and bladder and giving off branches to the bladder, prostate, seminal vesicles, and adjacent part of the ureter. Also *inferior vesical artery.* **a. zygomatico-orbitalis** [NA] A branch of the superficial temporal artery that may arise from the middle temporal artery and that runs along the upper border of the zygoma in the temporal fascia to supply the orbicularis oculi muscle and anastomose with the lacrimal and palpebral branches of the ophthalmic artery. Also *zygomatico-orbital artery.*

**arteriae** \ärtir′i·ē\ Plural of ARTERIA.

**arterial** \ärtir′ē·əl\ Of or relating to arteries. Also *arterious.*

**arterialization** \ärtir′ē·əlīzā′shən\ The conversion by oxygenation of venous blood to arterial blood. **a. of portal vein** A method that theoretically restores hepatic perfusion following an end-to-side portocaval shunt. An arterial graft is anastomosed to the distal (hepatic) portal vein or one of its branches.

**arteriarctia** \ärtir′rē·ärk′tē·ə \ [ARTERI- + L *arct(us)* strait, narrow + -IA] A narrowing of an artery. Also *arterioarctia.*

**arteriectopia** \ärtir′ē·ektō′pē·ə \ [ARTERI- + ECTOPIA] Development of an artery in an abnormal anatomic site, or persistence in such a site beyond the time of expected regression.

**arterio-** \ärtir′ē·ō-\ [Gk *artēria* artery, windpipe] A combining form denoting artery. Also *arteri-.*

**arterioarctia** \-ärk′tē·ə\ ARTERIARCTIA.

**arteriogenesis** \-jen′əsis\ [ARTERIO- + GENESIS] In embryology, the process of development and formation of the arteries and arterial pattern as exhibited in the adult.

**arteriograph** \ärtir′ē·əgraf′\ [ARTERIO- + -GRAPH] A radiograph obtained during arteriography. Also *arteriogram.*

**arteriography** \är′tirē·äg′rəfē\ [ARTERIO- + -GRAPHY] Radiographic examination of an artery or arteries after the injection of a radiopaque contrast agent. **axillary a.** Radiographic study of the arterial system of the upper extremity, especially the branches of the axillary artery, after the injection of a radiopaque contrast agent into the axillary artery. **carotid a.** Radiographic study of the carotid circulation after the injection of a radiopaque agent into the common, external, or internal carotid artery. **catheter a.** Roentgenography of vessels after their opacification by contrast medium introduced through a catheter inserted in an artery. **cerebral a.** CEREBRAL ANGIOGRAPHY. **cine coronary a.** Cineradiography of the coronary arteries during their opacification with contrast medium. **completion a.** OPERATIVE ARTERIOGRAPHY. **coronary a.** Radiologic study of the coronary arteries after the injection of a contrast agent into these vessels through a catheter introduced into the aorta. **femoral a.** Radiologic examination of the arterial system of the lower extremity after the injection of a radiopaque contrast agent into the femoral artery. **operative a.** An arteriography that is performed in the operating room following the completion of an arterial reconstructive procedure. It is intended to rule out the presence of technical defects. Also *completion arteriography.* **renal a.** Radiographic examination of the renal artery and its branches after the injection of a radiopaque contrast agent through a catheter placed selectively in the renal artery. **selective a.** Roentgenography of a specific artery and its branches after the injection of radiopaque contrast medium through a catheter, the tip of which is in that artery. **selective renal a.** Roentgenography of the renal artery and its branches after the injection of radiopaque contrast medium directly into the renal artery, usually via a catheter, the tip of which has been maneuvered into the lumen of the artery. **spinal a.** Roentgenography of vessels of the spinal cord after their opacification by contrast medium injected into a feeding artery. **vertebral a.** Radiographic study of the vertebral artery circulation after the injection of a radiopaque agent into the vertebral artery.

**arteriola** \ärtir′ē·ō′lə\ [New L, dim. of *arteria* artery] (*pl.* arteriolae) [NA] The smallest of the arteries, usually having a relatively thick, muscular wall. They are seldom visible macroscopically. Also *arteriole.* **arteriolae ellipsoideae** [NA] SHEATHED ARTERIES. **a. glomerularis afferens** [NA] An arteriole that usually arises from an interlobular artery, occasionally from an interlobar or an arcuate artery, and ends in a glomerulus in the renal cortex. Also *afferent glomerular arteriole, afferent arteriole, vas afferens arteriae interlobularis, vas afferens glomeruli, afferent vessel of glomerulus, afferent artery of glomerulus, artery of glomerulus, preglomerular arteriole.* **a. glomerularis efferens** [NA] An arteriole that arises from a renal glomerulus and then divides to form the peritubular capillary plexus around and between the proximal and distal convoluted tubules. Also *efferent glomerular arteriole, efferent arteriole, vas efferens arteriae interlobularis, vas efferens* *glomeruli, efferent vessel of glomerulus, efferent artery of glomerulus, revehent artery, postglomerular arteriole.* **a. macularis inferior** [NA] The lower branch of the central artery of retina that arises at the optic papilla and supplies the inferior portion of the macula retinae. It has nasal and temporal branches. Also *inferior macular arteriole, inferior macular artery.* **a. macularis superior** [NA] The upper branch of the central artery of the retina that arises at the optic papilla and supplies the superior portion of the macula retinae. It has nasal and temporal branches. Also *superior macular arteriole, superior macular artery.* **a. medialis retinae** [NA] A minute vessel supplying the medial portion of the retina between the superior and inferior nasal portions. Also *medial arteriole of retina.* **a. nasalis retinae inferior** [NA] The nasal branch of the inferior macular arteriole that supplies the lower medial portion of the retina. Also *inferior nasal arteriole of retina.* **a. nasalis retinae superior** [NA] The nasal branch of the superior macular arteriole that supplies the upper medial portion of the retina. Also *superior nasal arteriole of retina.* **a. precapillaris** METARTERIOLE. **arteriolae rectae renis** [NA] Branches of the arcuate arteries of the renal corticomedullary zone that pass down into the pyramids to supply their tubules. Occasionally they arise from interlobular arteries. Also *straight arteries of kidney, straight arterioles of kidney, arteriae rectae verae, straight medullary arteries, vasa recta.* **a. temporalis retinae inferior** [NA] The temporal branch of the inferior macular arteriole that supplies the lower lateral portion of the retina. Also *inferior temporal arteriole of retina.* **a. temporalis retinae superior** [NA] The temporal branch of the superior macular arteriole that supplies the upper lateral portion of the retina. Also *superior temporal arteriole of retina.* **arteriolae vaginatae** SHEATHED ARTERIES.

**arteriolae** \ärtir′ē·ō′lē\ Plural of ARTERIOLA.

**arteriolar** \ärtir′ē·ō′lər\ Resembling an arteriole or pertaining to an arteriole or arterioles.

**arteriole** \ärtir′ē·ōl\ [New L *arteriola.* See ARTERIOLA.] ARTERIOLA. **afferent a.** ARTERIOLA GLOMERULARIS AFFERENS. **afferent glomerular a.** ARTERIOLA GLOMERULARIS AFFERENS. **central a.** An arteriole which occupies the malpighian follicle of the spleen. **efferent a.** ARTERIOLA GLOMERULARIS EFFERENS. **efferent glomerular a.** ARTERIOLA GLOMERULARIS EFFERENS. **ellipsoid a.'s** SHEATHED ARTERIES. **inferior macular a.** ARTERIOLA MACULARIS INFERIOR. **inferior nasal a. of retina** ARTERIOLA NASALIS RETINAE INFERIOR. **inferior temporal a. of retina** ARTERIOLA TEMPORALIS RETINAE INFERIOR. **Isaacs-Ludwig a.** An occasional branch of the afferent glomerular arteriole that communicates directly with the peritubular capillary plexus. **medial a. of retina** ARTERIOLA MEDIALIS RETINAE. **postglomerular a.** ARTERIOLA GLOMERULARIS EFFERENS. **precapillary a.** METARTERIOLE. **preglomerular a.** ARTERIOLA GLOMERULARIS AFFERENS. **sheathed a.'s** SHEATHED ARTERIES. **straight a.'s of kidney** ARTERIOLAE RECTAE RENIS. **superior macular a.** ARTERIOLA MACULARIS SUPERIOR. **superior nasal a. of retina** ARTERIOLA NASALIS RETINAE SUPERIOR. **superior temporal a. of retina** ARTERIOLA TEMPORALIS RETINAE SUPERIOR.

**arteriolith** \ärtir′ē·əlith′\ [ARTERIO- + -LITH] A calcified structure in an artery or thrombus.

**arteriolitis** \ärtir′ē·əlī′tis\ [*arteriol(e)* + -ITIS] Inflammation of arterioles. Also *trichodarteriitis* (obs.).

**arteriology** \ärtir′rē·äl′əjē\ [ARTERIO- + -LOGY] The study of arteries and their diseases.

**arteriolonecrosis** \ärtir′ē·ō′lənekrō′sis\ Necrotic changes in arterioles.

**arteriolosclerosis** \ärtir′ē·ō′ləsklerō′sis\ Arteriosclerosis primarily involving the arterioles, with little lipid deposition but much luminal encroachment by intimal proliferation and vessel-wall fibrosis. Also *arteriolar sclerosis.*

**arteriolosclerotic** \ärtir′ē·ō′ləsklerät′ik\ Characterized by or relating to arteriolosclerosis.

**arteriolovenous** \ärtir′ē·ō′ləvē′nəs\ Relating to both arterioles and veins.

**arteriolovenular** \ärtir′ē·ō′ləven′yələr\ Relating to both arterioles and venules.

**arterionephrosclerosis** \-nef′rəsklerō′sis\ Arteriosclerosis of the renal artery branches, characterized by fibrosis, thickening and duplication of the elastic lamina, and intimal proliferation. If the lumen is sufficiently narrowed, ischemia of the involved segments of parenchyma will lead to atrophy and scarring of the kidney, with gradual loss of renal function. The condition is commonly seen in diabetes mellitus. Also *arteriosclerotic nephritis, arterial nephrosclerosis, benign nephrosclerosis.*

**arteriopathy** \är′tirē·äp′əthē\ [ARTERIO- + -PATHY] Any pathological state of the arteries. **hypertensive a.** Collectively, arterial lesions occurring in association with arterial hypertension. These include medial hypertrophy, duplication of the internal elastic lamina, intimal thickening, hyaline arteriosclerosis, and, in malignant hypertension, fibrinoid necrosis. **idiopathic medial a.** A nonarteriosclerotic occlusive arterial disease that is characterized by the degeneration of the arterial media and thought occasionally to result in aneurysm formation, as, for example, of the carotid artery. **Takayasu's a.** Nonarteriosclerotic arteritis that especially involves the brachiocephalic vessels and the aortic arch. It is characterized by signs of cerebral and upper extremity ischemia.

**arteriopressor** \-pres′ər\ [ARTERIO- + PRESSOR] Causing arterial constriction, with a resulting increase in blood pressure.

**arteriorenal** \-rē′nəl\ Pertaining to the arteries of the kidney.

**arteriorrhaphy** \ärtir′ē·ôr′əfē\ [ARTERIO- + -RRHAPHY] Incision of an artery, exposing its cavity.

**arteriorrhexis** \ärtir′ē·ôrek′sis\ [ARTERIO- + -RRHEXIS] Rupture of an artery.

**arteriosclerosis** \ärtir′ē·ōsklerō′sis\ [ARTERIO- + SCLEROSIS] Any of the various pathologic states associated with thickening and loss of elasticity in arterial walls. The most common of these is atherosclerosis, involving lipid deposition which is uncharacteristic of other forms of arteriosclerosis such as Mönckeberg sclerosis and arteriolosclerosis. Also *hardening of the arteries, arterial sclerosis, arteriocapillary sclerosis, vascular sclerosis.* **cerebral a.** Sclerosis of the cerebral arteries. In the larger intracranial arteries, the condition is usually due to atheroma which may lead to thrombosis and occlusion or embolism of arteries leading to cerebral infarction (stroke). Sclerosis of smaller vessels (arteriolosclerosis) is more often associated with or consequent upon arterial hypertension. Diffuse arteriosclerosis may lead to pseudobulbar palsy or arteriosclerotic "parkinsonism" or to multi-infarct (arteriosclerotic) dementia. **coronary a.** Thickening of the coronary arteries, usually atherosclerotic. **diffuse a.** Arteriosclerosis affecting both large and small vessels. **hyaline a.** Thickening of the wall of small arteries and arterioles, with varying degrees of luminal stenosis. It results from the deposition of an amorphous, eosinophilic substance probably derived from insudation of plasma proteins. It is seen in diabetes mellitus, hypertension, and in elderly individuals. **hypertensive a.** The arteriosclerosis which often complicates hypertensive disease. **infantile a.** INFANTILE ARTERITIS. **intimal a.** Thickening of the intima of arteries due to smooth-muscle-cell proliferation and fibrosis. It is characteristic of the aging process in arteries. **medial a.** MÖNCKEBERG SCLEROSIS. **Mönckeberg's a.** MÖNCKEBERG SCLEROSIS. **a. obliterans** Arteriosclerosis which results in obliteration of small arteries. Also *atherosclerosis obliterans.* **peripheral a.** Arteriosclerosis affecting blood vessels of the extremities. **presenile a.** Arteriosclerosis of unknown cause occurring at a relatively early age. **retinal a.** Arteriosclerosis of the retinal arteries, which can be observed with an ophthalmoscope.

**arteriosclerotic** \-sklerät′ik\ Relating to or affected by arteriosclerosis.

**arteriosity** \ärtir′ē·äs′itē\ The quality or state of being arterial, or the degree to which something is arterial, as the structure of blood vessels that is characteristic of arteries, or the relatively high oxygen saturation of blood that is characteristic of that in arteries.

**arteriospasm** \ärtir′ē·əspazm′\ Spasm affecting an artery; vasospasm of an artery.

**arteriospastic** \-spas′tik\ Relating to or affected by arteriospasm.

**arteriosympathectomy** \-sim′pəthek′təmē\ PERIARTERIAL SYMPATHECTOMY.

**arteriotomy** \ärtir′ē·ät′əmē\ [ARTERIO- + -TOMY] An opening into an artery.

**arteriotony** \ärtir′ē·ät′ənē\ [ARTERIO- + *ton(o)-* + -Y] ARTERIAL PRESSURE.

**arterious** \ärtir′ē·əs\ ARTERIAL.

**arteriovenous** \-vē′nəs\ Relating to or affecting both an artery and a vein. Abbr. AV, A-V

**arteritides** \är′tirit′idēz\ Plural of ARTERITIS.

**arteritis** \är′təri′tis\ [*arter(i)-* + -ITIS] An inflammatory disorder of an artery, frequently associated with systemic autoimmune conditions, allergic reactions, and toxic responses to chemicals. **coronary a.** An inflammatory disorder of a coronary artery, which may be due to a connective tissue disorder such as polyarteritis nodosa or giant cell arteritis. Also *coronaritis.* **cranial a.** Arteritis affecting one of the cranial blood vessels, especially temporal arteritis. **giant cell a.** Arteritis in which the arteries are affected by an inflammatory process characterized by multinucleate giant cells. It occurs in two main forms, temporal arteritis and Takayasu's arteritis. Also *granulomatous arteritis.* **Horton's a.** TEMPORAL ARTERITIS. **infantile a.** Diffuse arteritis and arteriosclerosis seen in infants and young children, usually resulting from congenital syphilis or chronic nephritis. Also *infantile arteriosclerosis.* **necrotizing a.** 1 POLYARTERITIS NODOSA. 2 Any arteritis involving necrosis. **a. nodosa** POLYARTERITIS NODOSA. **rheumatic a.** Arteritis associated with rheumatic fever. Although widely present during infection, it seldom leads to recognizable disorders. **rheumatoid a.** A form of necrotizing vasculitis sometimes seen in patients with rheumatoid arthritis. It involves small- to medium-sized blood vessels and may be indistinguishable from polyarteritis nodosa. **syphilitic a.** Arteritis in tertiary syphilis, mainly affecting the aorta. See also SYPHILITIC AORTITIS. **Takayasu's a.** An obliterative arteritis of unknown etiology, characterized by granulomatous lesions of medium-sized and large arteries, especially the aorta and other major arteries of the aortic arch and sometimes the pulmonary artery. Young women in Asia and Africa are most commonly affected. Cerebral symptoms and absent radial pulses result from involvement of the brachiocephalic trunk or its branches. Also *Takayasu's disease, Takayasu syndrome, Martorell syndrome, pulseless disease.* **temporal a.** A giant cell arteritis that particularly affects the elderly, especially women. It has a predilection for the temporal artery, but is often more widespread. Fever and a high erythrocyte sedimentation rate are usually present. There is considerable risk of blindness. It is strongly associated with polymyalgia rheumatica. Also *Horton's arteritis.* **a. umbilicalis** Septic inflammation of the umbilical artery in the neonate.

# artery

**artery** \är′tərē\ [L *arteria,* from Gk *artēria* (akin to *aortē* AORTA) a large artery or other tubular anatomic structure, esp. trachea or bronchus] ARTERIA. **abnormal obturator a.** ARTERIA OBTURATORIA ACCESSORIA. **accessory meningeal a.** A branch of the maxillary artery that, passing through the foramen ovale, supplies the dura and bone in the vicinity as well as the trigeminal ganglion. However, its main distribution is extracranial, to the pterygoid and tensor veli palatini muscles, the proximal part of the mandibular nerve, and the otic ganglion. **accessory obturator a.** ARTERIA OBTURATORIA ACCESSORIA. **accessory phrenic a.** An inconstant artery that arises from the abdominal aorta below the inferior phrenic arteries, or occasionally from the celiac artery, and is distributed to the fleshy part of the crura of the diaphragm. **accessory superior colic a.** ARTERIA COLICA MEDIA. **accompanying a. of ischiadic nerve** ARTERIA COMITANS NERVI ISCHIADICI. **accompanying a. of vein of Marshall** A small atrial branch of the circumflex branch of the left coronary artery of the heart that accompanies the oblique vein of the left atrium. **acetabular a.** 1 RAMUS ACETABULARIS ARTERIAE OBTURATORIAE. 2 RA-

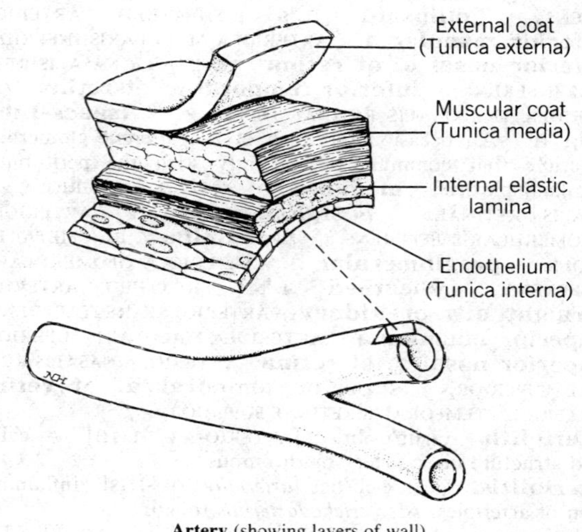


**Artery** (showing layers of wall)

MUS ACETABULARIS ARTERIAE CIRCUMFLEXAE FEMORIS MEDIALIS. **acromial a.** Any of three arteries: (1) ramus acromialis arteriae thoracoacromialis; (2) ramus acromialis arteriae suprascapularis; (3) ramus acromialis transversae scapulae. **a. of Adamkiewicz** ARTERIA RADICULARIS MAGNA. **adipose arteries of kidney** RAMI CAPSULARES ARTERIAE RENALIS. **afferent a. of glomerulus** ARTERIOLA GLOMERULARIS AFFERENS. **anastomotica magna a.** 1 ARTERIA COLLATERALIS ULNARIS INFERIOR. 2 ARTERIA DESCENDENS GENICULARIS. **angular a.** ARTERIA ANGULARIS. **a. of angular gyrus** A vessel, often the largest, that branches from the terminal (cortical) part of the middle cerebral artery and courses posteriorly to supply the supramarginal and angular gyri on the lateral surface of the parietal lobe of the cerebral cortex. **anonymous a.** TRUNCUS BRACHIOCEPHALICUS. **anterior auricular arteries** RAMI AURICULARES ANTERIORES ARTERIAE TEMPORALIS SUPERFICIALIS. **anterior bronchial arteries** RAMI BRONCHIALES ARTERIAE THORACICAE INTERNAE. **anterior cecal a.** ARTERIA CECALIS ANTERIOR. **anterior cerebral a.** ARTERIA CEREBRI ANTERIOR. **anterior choroidal a.** ARTERIA CHOROIDEA ANTERIOR. **anterior ciliary arteries** ARTERIAE CILIARES ANTERIORES. **anterior circumflex humeral a.** ARTERIA CIRCUMFLEXA ANTERIOR HUMERI. **anterior communicating a. of cerebrum** ARTERIA COMMUNICANS ANTERIOR CEREBRI. **anterior conjunctival arteries** ARTERIAE CONJUNCTIVALES ANTERIORES. **anterior dental arteries** ARTERIAE ALVEOLARES SUPERIORES ANTERIORES. **anterior ethmoidal a.** ARTERIA ETHMOIDALIS ANTERIOR. **anterior iliac a.** ARTERIA ILIACA EXTERNA. **anterior inferior cerebellar a.** ARTERIA CEREBELLI INFERIOR ANTERIOR. **anterior inferior segmental a.** ARTERIA SEGMENTI ANTERIORIS INFERIORIS. **anterior intercostal arteries** RAMI INTERCOSTALES ANTERIORES ARTERIAE THORACICAE INTERNAE. **anterior interosseous a.** ARTERIA INTEROSSEA ANTERIOR. **anterior interventricular a.** RAMUS INTERVENTRICULARIS ANTERIOR ARTERIAE CORONARIAE SINISTRAE. **anterior labial arteries** RAMI LABIALES ANTERIORES ARTERIAE PUDENDAE EXTERNAE. **anterior labial arteries of vulva** RAMI LABIALES ANTERIORES ARTERIAE PUDENDAE EXTERNAE. **anterior lateral malleolar a.** ARTERIA MALLEOLARIS ANTERIOR LATERALIS. **anterior medial malleolar a.** ARTERIA MALLEOLARIS ANTERIOR MEDIALIS. **anterior median arteries** A large number (250–300) of penetrating branches arising from the anterior spinal artery that enter the anterior median fissure of the spinal cord to supply the substance of the anterior and lateral horns, the central gray, and the base of the posterior horn of the spinal cord. Also *sulcal branches of anterior spinal artery.* **anterior mediastinal arteries** RAMI MEDIASTINALES ARTERIAE THORACICAE INTERNAE. **anterior meningeal a.** ARTERIA MENINGEA ANTERIOR. **anterior parietal a.** See under ARTERIAE PARIETALES ANTERIOR ET POSTERIOR. **anterior perforating arteries** RAMI PERFORANTES ARTERIAE THORACICAE INTERNAE. **anterior pericardiac arteries** Branches of the internal thoracic artery that arise at the level of the lower margin of the first rib and descend to the anterior surface of the pericardium, supplying it. They may be quite large, their size usually being inversely proportional to that of the pericardiacophrenic artery. **anterior scrotal arteries** RAMI SCROTALES ANTERIORES ARTERIAE PUDENDAE EXTERNAE. **anterior segmental a.** ARTERIA SEGMENTI ANTERIORIS. **anterior septal a.** 1 RAMUS SEPTI NASI ARTERIAE LABIALIS SUPERIORIS. 2 One of the rami interventriculares septales arteriae coronariae sinistrae. **anterior spinal a.** ARTERIA SPINALIS ANTERIOR. **anterior superior alveolar arteries** ARTERIAE ALVEOLARES SUPERIORES ANTERIORES. **anterior superior segmental a.** ARTERIA SEGMENTI ANTERIORIS SUPERIORIS. **anterior temporal a.** ARTERIA TEMPORALIS ANTERIOR. **anterior tibial a.** ARTERIA TIBIALIS ANTERIOR. **anterior tibial recurrent a.** ARTERIA RECURRENS TIBIALIS ANTERIOR. **anterior transverse a. of wrist** 1 The transverse anastomosis on the anterior surface of the carpus between the palmar carpal branches of the radial and ulnar arteries. 2 RAMUS CARPALIS PALMARIS ARTERIAE RADIALIS. 3 RAMUS CARPALIS PALMARIS ARTERIAE ULNARIS. **anterior tympanic a.** ARTERIA TYMPANICA ANTERIOR. **anterior ulnar recurrent a.** RAMUS ANTERIOR ARTERIAE RECURRENTIS ULNARIS. **anterolateral central arteries** Vessels branching from the sphenoidal part of the middle cerebral artery, comprising ten to fifteen delicate vessels and divided into medial and lateral striate branches. The vessels penetrate the anterior perforated substance and supply the globus pallidus, caudate nucleus, putamen, internal capsule, and a part of the lateral aspect of the thalamus. Also *anterolateral thalamostriate arteries.* **aortic intercostal arteries** *Outmoded* ARTERIAE INTERCOSTALES POSTERIORES (III–XI). **aortic suprarenal a.** ARTERIA SUPRARENALIS MEDIA. **aortic uterine a.** ARTERIA OVARICA. **appendicular a.** ARTERIA APPENDICULARIS. **arch a.** Anastomosis uniting the ventral aorta to one of the two primitive dorsal aortae. Between the third and sixth week of development in man six pairs of arterial arches appear successively, corresponding to each of the branchial arches visible on the lateral aspect of the cervicocephalic region. The two more cranial pairs (first and second) of arch arteries begin to dwindle by the time the third has been established. The fifth pair is difficult to identify and disappears. The third, fourth, and sixth eventually form the essential constituents of the great arteries of the systemic and pulmonary systems. The left sixth arch artery contributes anteriorly to form the left pulmonary artery and posteriorly to the ductus arteriosus which diverts the pulmonary circulation, functionally useless in the embryo, to the systemic circulation. This posterior portion retrogresses at birth when respiratory movements are established. Abnormally it may persist as patent ductus arteriosus. **arcuate a.** 1 ARTERIA ARCUATA PEDIS. 2 Any of the arcuatae arteriae renis. **arcuate a. of foot** ARTERIA ARCUATA PEDIS. **arcuate arteries of kidney** ARTERIAE ARCUATAE RENIS. **ascending cervical a.** ARTERIA CERVICALIS ASCENDENS. **ascending palatine a.** ARTERIA PALATINA ASCENDENS. **ascending pharyngeal a.** ARTERIA PHARYNGEA ASCENDENS. **axial a.** The primary arterial trunk of an embryonic limb. **axillary a.** ARTERIA AXILLARIS. **azygos arteries of vagina** Two median longitudinal arteries, one in front of and one behind the vagina, that are formed by branches of the uterine artery anastomosing with branches of the vaginal arteries from the internal iliac artery. **basilar a.** ARTERIA BASILARIS. **brachial a.** ARTERIA BRACHIALIS. **brachiocephalic a.** TRUNCUS BRACHIOCEPHALICUS. **bronchial arteries** RAMI BRONCHIALES AORTAE THORACICAE. **buccal a.** ARTERIA BUCCALIS. **buccinator a.** ARTERIA BUCCALIS. **bulbourethral a.** ARTERIA BULBI PENIS. **a. of bulb of penis** ARTERIA BULBI PENIS. **a. of bulb of vestibule of vagina** ARTERIA BULBI VESTIBULI VAGINAE. **calcarine a.** RAMUS CALCARINUS ARTERIAE OCCIPITALIS MEDIALIS. **callosomarginal a.** A vessel that arises from the anterior cerebral artery near the genu of the corpus callosum on the medial surface of the cerebral hemisphere. It gives off a number of branches that supply the cingulate gyrus and other gyri on the medial surface of the frontal and parietal lobes. **capsular arteries** RAMI CAPSULARES ARTERIAE RENALIS. **caroticotympanic arteries** ARTERIAE CAROTICOTYMPANICAE ARTERIAE CAROTIDIS INTERNAE. **carotid a.** ARTERIA CAROTIS COMMUNIS. **caudal a.** ARTERIA SACRALIS MEDIANA. **caudal pancreatic a.** ARTERIA CAUDAE PANCREATIS. **a. of caudate lobe** ARTERIA LOBI CAUDATI. **celiac a.** TRUNCUS COELIACUS. **central retinal a.** ARTERIA CENTRALIS RETINAE. **a. of central sulcus** ARTERIA SULCI CENTRALIS. **cerebral arteries** ARTERIAE CEREBRI. **a. of cerebral hemorrhage** LENTICULOSTRIATE ARTERY. **arteries of cerebrum** ARTERIAE CEREBRI. **cervicovaginal arteries** ARTERIAE CERVICOVAGINALES. **a. of Charcot** LENTICULOSTRIATE ARTERY. **a. of Charpy** The third perforating branch of the internal thoracic artery which supplies the medial part of the mammary gland. **circumflex fibular a.** RAMUS CIRCUMFLEXUS FIBULARIS ARTERIAE TIBIALIS POSTERIORIS. **circumflex a. of scapula** ARTERIA CIRCUMFLEXA SCAPULAE. **coccygeal a.** ARTERIA SACRALIS MEDIANA. **Cohnheim's a.** END ARTERY. **coiled arteries** RAMI HELICINI ARTERIAE UTERINAE. **collateral digital arteries** ARTERIAE DIGITALES PALMARES PROPRIAE. **collateral radial a.** ARTERIA COLLATERALIS RADIALIS. **a. to colliculi** A small circumferential branch of the posterior cerebral artery which supplies the superior and inferior colliculi. It arises from the posterior cerebral artery as the latter vessel encircles the brainstem. **common carotid a.** ARTERIA CAROTIS COMMUNIS. **common digital arteries of foot** ARTERIAE METATARSALES PLANTARES. **common femoral a.** The portion of the femoral artery proximal to the origin of the deep femoral artery. **common hepatic a.** ARTERIA HEPATICA COMMUNIS. **common iliac a.** ARTERIA ILIACA COMMUNIS. **common interosseous a.** ARTERIA INTEROSSEA COMMUNIS. **common palmar digital arteries** ARTERIAE DIGITALES PALMARES COMMUNES. **common plantar digital arteries** ARTERIAE DIGITALES PLANTARES COMMUNES. **common volar digital arteries** ARTERIAE DIGITALES PALMARES COMMUNES. **companion a. to sciatic nerve** ARTERIA COMITANS NERVI ISCHIADICI. **conal a.** Either the ramus coni arteriosi arteriae coronariae dextrae or the ramus coni arteriosi arteriae coronariae sinistrae. **conducting arteries** Large arteries that conduct blood from the heart to medium sized, or distributing, arteries. Their tunica media is very elastic and the wall is comparatively thin for the size of vessel. **copper-wire arteries** Exaggerated reflection from retinal arteries seen in arteriosclerosis. **corkscrew arteries** Tortuous arteries seen in the macular region of the ocular fundus. **cornual a.** One of the small arteries that, entering radially from surface vessels, supply the gray matter of the spinal cord. It is designated posterior, anterior, or lateral according to the cornu it enters. **a. to corpus cavernosum** ARTERIA PROFUNDA PENIS. **cortical arteries** The following vessels: (1) pars terminalis arteriae cerebri mediae; (2) pars postcommunicalis arteriae cerebri anterioris; (3) pars terminalis arteriae cerebri posterioris; and (4) arteriae interlobulares renis. **costocervical a.** TRUNCUS COSTOCERVICALIS. **cremasteric a.** ARTERIA CREMASTERICA. **cricothyroid a.** RAMUS CRICOTHYROIDEUS ARTERIAE THYROIDEAE SUPERIORIS. **crural a.** ARTERIA FEMORALIS. **cystic a.** ARTERIA CYSTICA. **deep auricular a.** ARTERIA AURICULARIS PROFUNDA. **deep brachial a.** ARTERIA PROFUNDA BRACHII. **deep cervical a.** ARTERIA CERVICALIS PROFUNDA. **deep circumflex iliac a.** ARTERIA CIRCUMFLEXA ILIACA PROFUNDA. **deep a. of clitoris** ARTERIA PROFUNDA CLITORIDIS. **deep descending cervical a.** The deep branch of descending branch of occipital artery that runs down the semispinalis capitis and cervicis muscles, anastomosing with the deep cervical branch of the costocervical trunk and with the vertebral artery. **deep external pudendal arteries** See under ARTERIAE PUDENDAE EXTERNAE. **deep facial a.** ARTERIA MAXILLARIS. **deep femoral a.** ARTERIA PROFUNDA FEMORIS. **deep lingual a.** ARTERIA PROFUNDA LINGUAE. **deep palmar a.** RAMUS PALMARIS PROFUNDUS ARTERIAE ULNARIS. **deep a. of penis** ARTERIA PROFUNDA PENIS. **deep plantar a.** ARTERIA PLANTARIS PROFUNDA ARTERIAE DORSALIS PEDIS. **deep temporal arteries** ARTERIAE TEMPORALES PROFUNDAE. **deep volar metacarpal a.** RAMUS PALMARIS PROFUNDUS ARTERIAE ULNARIS. **deferent a.** ARTERIA DUCTUS DEFERENTIS. **deferential a.** ARTERIA DUCTUS DEFERENTIS. **deltoid a.** 1 RAMUS DELTOIDEUS ARTERIAE THORACOACROMIALIS. 2 RAMUS DELTOIDEUS ARTERIAE PROFUNDAE BRACHII. **deltopectoral a.** *Outmoded* RAMUS DELTOIDEUS ARTERIAE THORACOACROMIALIS **a. of dentate nucleus** A terminal branch of the superior cerebellar artery that penetrates deep into the cerebellum, along the superior cerebellar peduncle, to the dentate nucleus, which it penetrates. **descending genicular a.** ARTERIA DESCENDENS GENICULARIS. **descending palatine a.** ARTERIA PALATINA DESCENDENS. **descending scapular a.** ARTERIA DORSALIS SCAPULAE. **diaphragmatic a.** ARTERIA PHRENICA INFERIOR. **digital arteries of the finger** 1 ARTERIAE DIGITALES DORSALES MANUS. 2 ARTERIAE DIGITALES PALMARES PROPRIAE. **digital arteries of the toes** 1 ARTERIAE DIGITALES DORSALES PEDIS. 2 ARTERIAE DIGITALES PLANTARES PROPRIAE. **distributing arteries** The most numerous class of arteries in the body, extending between conducting arteries and arterioles. They are of medium size, have a tunica media of the muscular type, and distribute blood to tissues and organs, regulating the volume of blood according to functional needs. Also *muscular arteries.* **dorsal carpal a.** Either ramus carpalis dorsalis arteriae radialis or ramus carpalis dorsalis arteriae ulnaris. **dorsal a. of clitoris** ARTERIA DORSALIS CLITORIDIS. **dorsal digital arteries** Either the arteriae digitales dorsales manus or the arteriae digitales dorsales pedis. **dorsal digital arteries of foot** ARTERIAE DIGITALES DORSALES PEDIS. **dorsal digital arteries of hand** ARTERIAE DIGITALES DORSALES MANUS. **dorsal a. of foot** ARTERIA DORSALIS PEDIS. **dorsal interosseous a. of forearm** ARTERIA INTEROSSEA POSTERIOR. **dorsalis pedis a.** ARTERIA DORSALIS PEDIS. **dorsal metacarpal arteries** ARTERIAE METACARPALES DORSALES. **dorsal metatarsal arteries** ARTERIAE METATARSALES DORSALES. **dorsal nasal a.** ARTERIA DORSALIS NASI. **dorsal a. of nose** ARTERIA DORSALIS NASI. **dorsal pancreatic a.** ARTERIA PANCREATICA DORSALIS. **dorsal a. of penis** ARTERIA DORSALIS PENIS. **dorsal rectal a.** *Outmoded* ARTERIA RECTALIS SUPERIOR. **dorsal scapular a.** ARTERIA DORSALIS SCAPULAE. **dorsal a. of tongue** RAMI DORSALES LINGUAE ARTERIAE LINGUALIS. **dorsomedian a. of spinal cord** One of a series of arteries that pass inward along the dorsal septum of the spinal cord. **a. of Drummond** 1 RECTOSIGMOID ANASTOMOSIS. 2 MAR-

GINAL ARTERY OF COLON. **a. of ductus deferens** ARTERIA DUCTUS DEFERENTIS. **duodenal arteries** ARTERIAE PANCREATICODUODENALES INFERIORES. **efferent a. of glomerulus** ARTERIOLA GLOMERULARIS EFFERENS. **emulgent a.** ARTERIA RENALIS. **end a.** An artery that does not anastomose with any other and conveys the only blood to an area, such as the central artery of retina. Also *terminal artery, Cohnheim's artery, telangion.* **a. of epididymis** A branch, or occasionally several branches, of the testicular artery that supplies the epididymis and anastomoses with the deferential artery at both the head and the tail of the epididymis as well as with the cremasteric artery. **episcleral arteries** ARTERIAE EPISCLERALES. **esophageal arteries** RAMI ESOPHAGEALES AORTAE THORACICAE. **external carotid a.** ARTERIA CAROTIS EXTERNA. **external iliac a.** ARTERIA ILIACA EXTERNA. **external malleolar a.** ARTERIA MALLEOLARIS ANTERIOR LATERALIS. **external mammary a.** 1 ARTERIA THORACICA LATERALIS. 2 RAMI MAMMARII LATERALES ARTERIAE THORACICAE LATERALIS. **external maxillary a.** ARTERIA FACIALIS. **external plantar a.** ARTERIA PLANTARIS LATERALIS. **external pudendal arteries** ARTERIAE PUDENDAE EXTERNAE. **external spermatic a.** ARTERIA CREMASTERICA. **facial a.** ARTERIA FACIALIS. **a. of the facial nerve** A small branch of the stylomastoid artery that accompanies the extracranial part of the facial nerve. **fallopian a.** ARTERIA UTERINA. **femoral a.** ARTERIA FEMORALIS. **fetal umbilical arteries** The vessels which carry deoxygenated blood from the fetus back to the placenta via the umbilical cord. Normally, there are two such vessels. **fibular a.** ARTERIA FIBULARIS. **fifth lumbar arteries** ARTERIAE LUMBALES IMA. **first palmar metacarpal a.** The occasional common trunk of origin of arteria princeps pollicis and arteria indicis radialis. Also *first palmar interosseous artery.* **a. of fissure of Rolando** *Outmoded* ARTERIA SULCI CENTRALIS. **frontal a.** ARTERIA SUPRATROCHLEARIS. **funicular a.** ARTERIA TESTICULARIS. **gastroduodenal a.** ARTERIA GASTRODUODENALIS. **glaserian a.** ARTERIA TYMPANICA ANTERIOR. **a. of glomerulus** ARTERIOLA GLOMERULARIS AFFERENS. **greater palatine a.** ARTERIA PALATINA MAJOR. **great pancreatic a.** ARTERIA PANCREATICA MAGNA. **great phrenic a.** ARTERIA PHRENICA INFERIOR. **great ventral radicular a.** ARTERIA RADICULARIS MAGNA. **helicine arteries** 1 ARTERIAE HELICINAE PENIS. 2 RAMI HELICINI ARTERIAE UTERINAE. **helicine arteries of penis** ARTERIAE HELICINAE PENIS. **hepatic a.** 1 ARTERIA HEPATICA COMMUNIS. 2 ARTERIA HEPATICA PROPRIA. **Heubner's a.** The recurrent branch of the anterior cerebral artery that supplies the anterior part of the caudate nucleus, the anterior one third of the putamen, and the inferior half of the anterior limb of the internal capsule. Thrombosis of this vessel causes paralysis of the contralateral face and upper limb. **highest intercostal a.** ARTERIA INTERCOSTALIS SUPREMA. **highest thoracic a.** ARTERIA THORACICA SUPERIOR. **humeral a.** ARTERIA BRACHIALIS. **hyaloid a.** The continuation of the central artery of the retina as a branch which in early embryos runs along the groove of the optic stalk, enters the back of the optic cup by the optic fissure, and extends to the back of the lens to supply its vascular tunic. This tunic degenerates before birth, and the hyaloid artery also disappears, but its course is marked by the persistence of the hyaloid canal. Also *arteria hyaloidea.* **hybrid arteries** Short transitional areas between large, elastic conducting arteries and medium-sized, muscular arteries of distribution. **hyoid a.** RAMUS SUPRAHYOIDEUS ARTERIAE LINGUALIS. **hypogastric a.** ARTERIA ILIACA INTERNA. **hypophyseal a.** Any of the four branches of the internal carotid artery that supply the hypophysis cerebri, including the superior and inferior hypophyseal arteries. **ileal arteries** 1 ARTERIAE ILEALES. 2 ARTERIAE INTESTINALES. **ileocolic a.** ARTERIA ILEOCOLICA. **iliolumbar a.** ARTERIA ILIOLUMBALIS. **incisor a.** A terminal branch of the inferior alveolar artery that runs in the mandibular canal from the level of the first premolar tooth anteriorly below the incisor teeth to the midline, where it anastomoses with the artery of the opposite side. It supplies the mandible and root sockets and sends branches into the pulp canals of the teeth along its course. **inferior alveolar a.** ARTERIA ALVEOLARIS INFERIOR. **inferior capsular a.** ARTERIA SUPRARENALIS INFERIOR. **inferior dental a.** ARTERIA ALVEOLARIS INFERIOR. **inferior epigastric a.** ARTERIA EPIGASTRICA INFERIOR. **inferior esophageal arteries** RAMI ESOPHAGEALES ARTERIAE GASTRICAE SINISTRAE. **inferior frontal a.** ARTERIA FRONTOBASALIS MEDIALIS. **inferior gluteal a.** ARTERIA GLUTEA INFERIOR. **inferior hemorrhoidal a.** ARTERIA RECTALIS INFERIOR. **inferior hypophyseal a.** ARTERIA HYPOPHYSIALIS INFERIOR. **inferior labial a.** ARTERIA LABIALIS INFERIOR. **inferior laryngeal a.** ARTERIA LARYNGEA INFERIOR. **inferior lateral geniculate a.** ARTERIA INFERIOR LATERALIS GENUS. **inferior lateral sacral a.** See under ARTERIAE SACRALES LATERALES. **inferior left colic arteries** ARTERIAE SIGMOIDEAE. **inferior macular a.** ARTERIOLA MACULARIS INFERIOR. **inferior medial geniculate a.** ARTERIA INFERIOR MEDIALIS GENUS. **inferior mesenteric a.** ARTERIA MESENTERICA INFERIOR. **inferior pancreatic a.** ARTERIA PANCREATICA INFERIOR. **inferior pancreaticoduodenal arteries** ARTERIAE PANCREATICODUODENALES INFERIORES. **inferior phrenic a.** ARTERIA PHRENICA INFERIOR. **inferior profunda a.** ARTERIA COLLATERALIS ULNARIS SUPERIOR. **inferior rectal a.** ARTERIA RECTALIS INFERIOR. **inferior right colic a.** ARTERIA ILEOCOLICA. **inferior segmental a.** ARTERIA SEGMENTI INFERIORIS. **inferior suprarenal a.** ARTERIA SUPRARENALIS INFERIOR. **inferior thyroid a.** ARTERIA THYROIDEA INFERIOR. **inferior thyroid a. of Cruveilhier** RAMUS CRICOTHYROIDEUS ARTERIAE THYROIDEAE SUPERIORIS. **inferior tympanic a.** ARTERIA TYMPANICA INFERIOR. **inferior ulnar collateral a.** ARTERIA COLLATERALIS ULNARIS INFERIOR. **inferior vesical a.** ARTERIA VESICALIS INFERIOR. **infracostal a.** RAMUS COSTALIS LATERALIS ARTERIAE THORACICAE INTERNAE. **infraorbital a.** ARTERIA INFRAORBITALIS. **infrascapular a.** See under ARTERIA CIRCUMFLEXA SCAPULAE. **inguinal arteries** RAMI INGUINALES ARTERIAE FEMORALIS. **innominate a.** TRUNCUS BRACHIOCEPHALICUS. **interlobar arteries of kidney** ARTERIAE INTERLOBARES RENIS. **interlobular arteries of kidney** ARTERIAE INTERLOBULARES RENIS. **interlobular arteries of liver** ARTERIAE INTERLOBULARES HEPATIS. **internal auditory a.** ARTERIA LABYRINTHI. **internal carotid a.** ARTERIA CAROTIS INTERNA. **internal deep circumflex a.** RAMUS PROFUNDUS ARTERIAE CIRCUMFLEXAE FEMORIS MEDIALIS. **internal frontal a.** ARTERIA SUPRATROCHLEARIS. **internal iliac a.** ARTERIA ILIACA INTERNA. **internal malleolar a.** ARTERIA MALLEOLARIS ANTERIOR MEDIALIS. **internal mammary a.** ARTERIA THORACICA INTERNA. **internal maxillary a.** ARTERIA MAXILLARIS. **internal**

**plantar a.** ARTERIA PLANTARIS MEDIALIS. **internal pudendal a.** ARTERIA PUDENDA INTERNA. **internal pudic a.** ARTERIA PUDENDA INTERNA. **internal spermatic a.** ARTERIA TESTICULARIS. **internal thoracic a.** ARTERIA THORACICA INTERNA. **interosseous recurrent a.** ARTERIA INTEROSSEA RECURRENS. **interpapillary a. of kidney** *Outmoded* SEGMENTAL ARTERY OF KIDNEY. **interventricular septal arteries** Rami interventriculares septales arteriae coronariae dextrae and rami interventriculares septales arteriae coronariae sinistrae. **intestinal arteries** ARTERIAE INTESTINALES. **jejunal arteries** ARTERIAE JEJUNALES. **arteries of kidney** ARTERIAE RENIS. **Kugel's a.** A branch of the right coronary artery supplying the atrioventricular node. **labial a.** Either arteria labialis inferior, arteria labialis superior, or one of either rami labiales anteriores or rami labiales posteriores. **a. of labyrinth** ARTERIA LABYRINTHI. **labyrinthine a.** ARTERIA LABYRINTHI. **lacrimal a.** ARTERIA LACRIMALIS. **lateral anterior malleolar a.** ARTERIA MALLEOLARIS ANTERIOR LATERALIS. **lateral circumflex femoral a.** ARTERIA CIRCUMFLEXA FEMORIS LATERALIS. **lateral frontobasal a.** ARTERIA FRONTOBASALIS LATERALIS. **lateral inferior genicular a.** ARTERIA INFERIOR LATERALIS GENUS. **lateral mammary a.** 1 ARTERIA THORACICA LATERALIS. 2 RAMI MAMMARII LATERALES ARTERIAE THORACICAE LATERALIS. **lateral palpebral arteries** ARTERIAE PALPEBRALES LATERALES. **lateral plantar a.** ARTERIA PLANTARIS LATERALIS. **lateral posterior malleolar arteries** RAMI MALLEOLARES LATERALES ARTERIAE FIBULARIS. **lateral sacral arteries** ARTERIAE SACRALES LATERALES. **lateral segmental a.** ARTERIA SEGMENTI LATERALIS. **lateral and septal posterior nasal arteries** ARTERIAE NASALES POSTERIORES, LATERALES ET SEPTI. **lateral spinal a.** A longitudinally directed artery lying in the base of the denticulate ligament. **lateral striate arteries** Central branches of the middle cerebral artery that ascend in the external capsule along the lateral aspect of the lentiform nucleus, and then bend medially to traverse the internal capsule and supply the caudate nucleus. **lateral superior genicular a.** ARTERIA SUPERIOR LATERALIS GENUS. **lateral tarsal a.** ARTERIA TARSALIS LATERALIS. **lateral thoracic a.** ARTERIA THORACICA LATERALIS. **lateral thymic arteries** RAMI THYMICI ARTERIAE THORACICAE INTERNAE. **left auricular a.** *Outmoded* ARTERIA CORONARIA SINISTRA. **left colic a.** ARTERIA COLICA SINISTRA. **left coronary a. of heart** ARTERIA CORONARIA SINISTRA. **left coronary a. of stomach** ARTERIA GASTRICA SINISTRA. **left gastric a.** ARTERIA GASTRICA SINISTRA. **left gastroepiploic a.** ARTERIA GASTRO-OMENTALIS SINISTRA. **left gastro-omental a.** ARTERIA GASTRO-OMENTALIS SINISTRA. **left inferior gastric a.** ARTERIA GASTRO-OMENTALIS SINISTRA. **left inferior pancreaticoduodenal a.** *Outmoded* RAMUS ANTERIOR ARTERIAE PANCREATICODUODENALIS INFERIORIS. **left lateral hepatic a.** See under ARTERIA SEGMENTI LATERALIS. **left marginal a. of heart** RAMUS MARGINALIS SINISTER CORDIS. **left pulmonary a.** ARTERIA PULMONALIS SINISTRA. **left superior colic a.** ARTERIA COLICA SINISTRA. **left superior pancreaticoduodenal a.** *Outmoded* RAMUS POSTERIOR ARTERIAE PANCREATICODUODENALIS INFERIORIS. **left ventral paramedian a.** ARTERIA SEGMENTI MEDIALIS. **lenticulostriate a.** A particularly large member of the anterolateral group of striate arteries arising from the middle cerebral artery. It is the artery of the brain most susceptible to rupture. Also *artery of cerebral hemorrhage, artery of Charcot.* **lesser palatine arteries** ARTERIAE PALATINAE MINORES. **lingual a.** ARTERIA LINGUALIS. **long ciliary arteries** ARTERIAE CILIARES POSTERIORES LONGAE. **long posterior ciliary arteries** ARTERIAE CILIARES POSTERIORES LONGAE. **lowest lumbar arteries** ARTERIAE LUMBALES IMA. **lowest thyroid a.** ARTERIA THYROIDEA IMA. **lumbar arteries** ARTERIAE LUMBALES. **mandibular a.** ARTERIA ALVEOLARIS INFERIOR. **marginal a. of colon** A fairly constant artery linking a series of connecting arcades produced by anastomoses of branches of the major vessels supplying the large intestine. Typically it commences with the colic branch of the ileocolic artery and ends at the sigmoid arteries. Occasionally, secondary arcades intervene between it and the colon. It gives off straight arteries to supply the colon. Also *Riolan's arc, artery of Drummond.* **masseteric a.** ARTERIA MASSETERICA. **mastoid a.** 1 Any of the rami mastoidei arteriae auricularis posterioris. 2 RAMUS MASTOIDEUS ARTERIAE OCCIPITALIS. **maxillary a.** ARTERIA MAXILLARIS. **medial anterior malleolar a.** ARTERIA MALLEOLARIS ANTERIOR MEDIALIS. **medial calcaneal arteries** RAMI CALCANEI ARTERIAE TIBIALIS POSTERIORIS. **medial circumflex femoral a.** ARTERIA CIRCUMFLEXA FEMORIS MEDIALIS. **medial frontobasal a.** ARTERIA FRONTOBASALIS MEDIALIS. **medial inferior genicular a.** ARTERIA INFERIOR MEDIALIS GENUS. **medial orbitofrontal a.** ARTERIA FRONTOBASALIS MEDIALIS. **medial palpebral arteries** ARTERIAE PALPEBRALES MEDIALES. **medial plantar a.** ARTERIA PLANTARIS MEDIALIS. **medial posterior malleolar arteries** RAMI MALLEOLARES MEDIALES ARTERIAE TIBIALIS POSTERIORIS. **medial segmental a.** ARTERIA SEGMENTI MEDIALIS. **medial superior genicular a.** ARTERIA SUPERIOR MEDIALIS GENUS. **medial tarsal arteries** ARTERIAE TARSALES MEDIALES. **median a.** ARTERIA COMITANS NERVI MEDIANI. **median a. of forearm** ARTERIA COMITANS NERVI MEDIANI. **median sacral a.** ARTERIA SACRALIS MEDIANA. **mediastinal arteries** RAMI MEDIASTINALES PARTIS THORACICAE AORTAE. **medullary a.** ARTERIA NUTRICIA. **medullary arteries of brain** 1 Sprigs of the vertebral and posterior inferior cerebellar arteries that penetrate radially into the substance of the medulla. 2 Branches of cortical arteries that supply the white matter of the cerebral hemispheres. **medullary spinal a.** A branch of a segmental spinal artery which travels over a spinal root to terminate in the vasa corona of the cord. It does not normally send direct branches to the root. Only a few unpaired medullary spinal arteries are found along the length of spinal cord, one being the arteria radicularis magna. Compare RADICULAR ARTERY. **mental a.** RAMUS MENTALIS. **middle capsular a.** ARTERIA SUPRARENALIS MEDIA. **middle cerebral a.** ARTERIA CEREBRI MEDIA. **middle colic a.** ARTERIA COLICA MEDIA. **middle collateral a.** ARTERIA COLLATERALIS MEDIA. **middle genicular a.** ARTERIA MEDIA GENUS. **middle hemorrhoidal a.** ARTERIA RECTALIS MEDIA. **middle hepatic a.** 1 An inconstant branch of the proper hepatic artery that supplies the quadrate lobe. It may replace the branch to this area normally arising from the arteria segmenti medialis. 2 An outmoded and incorrect term for ARTERIA HEPATICA PROPRIA. 3 ARTERIA SEGMENTI MEDIALIS. **middle meningeal a.** ARTERIA MENINGEA MEDIA. **middle rectal a.** ARTERIA RECTALIS MEDIA. **middle sacral a.** ARTERIA SACRALIS MEDIANA. **middle suprarenal a.**

ARTERIA SUPRARENALIS MEDIA. **middle temporal a.** ARTERIA TEMPORALIS MEDIA. **middle thyroid a.** ARTERIA THYROIDEA IMA. **arteries of Mueller** ARTERIAE HELICINAE PENIS. **muscular arteries** DISTRIBUTING ARTERIES. **musculophrenic a.** ARTERIA MUSCULOPHRENICA. **mylohyoid a.** RAMUS MYLOHYOIDEUS ARTERIAE ALVEOLARIS INFERIORIS. **nasopalatine a.** ARTERIA SPHENOPALATINA. **Neubauer's a.** ARTERIA THYROIDEA IMA. **nutrient a.** ARTERIA NUTRICIA. **nutrient a. of fibula** ARTERIA NUTRICIA FIBULAE. **nutrient arteries of humerus** ARTERIAE NUTRICIAE HUMERI. **nutrient a. of tibia** ARTERIA NUTRICIA TIBIAE. **obliterated hypogastric a.** LIGAMENTUM UMBILICALE MEDIALE. **obturator a.** ARTERIA OBTURATORIA. **occipital a.** ARTERIA OCCIPITALIS. **omphalomesenteric a.** A large arterial trunk that is present in embryos to supply the alimentary tract. The trunk is formed by fusion of several ventral branches from the dorsal aorta and at first is distributed to the midgut and yolk sac. Later it becomes the artery of the yolk sac stalk, and persists after birth as the superior mesenteric artery. **ophthalmic a.** ARTERIA OPHTHALMICA. **a. of the optic chiasma** A branch, often divided into two, of the anterior cerebral artery that supplies part of the optic chiasma. The median zone receives branches from the internal carotid arteries via the stalk of the hypophysis cerebri. **arteries to orbital muscles** ARTERIAE MUSCULARES ARTERIAE OPHTHALMICAE. **ovarian a.** ARTERIA OVARICA. **palatine a.** Any of four arteries: (1) arteria palatina ascendens; (2) arteria palatina descendens; (3) arteria palatina major; (4) arteria palatina minor. **palmar carpal a.** Either ramus carpalis palmaris arteriae radialis or ramus carpalis palmaris arteriae ulnaris. **palmar intermetacarpal arteries** ARTERIAE METACARPALES PALMARES. **palmar interosseous a.** ARTERIA INTEROSSEA ANTERIOR. **palmar interosseous arteries** ARTERIAE METACARPALES PALMARES. **palmar metacarpal arteries** ARTERIAE METACARPALES PALMARES. **paramedian arteries** The short central branches of the anterior spinal arteries of the vertebral artery, the pontine branches of the basilar artery, and branches of the posterior communicating artery that penetrate the brainstem, the pons, or mesencephalon adjacent to or in the midline. **parotid a.** 1 RAMUS PAROTIDEUS ARTERIAE AURICULARIS POSTERIORIS. 2 RAMUS PAROTIDEUS ARTERIAE TEMPORALIS SUPERFICIALIS. **penicilli arteries** PENICILLI SPLENIS. **perforating arteries** ARTERIAE PERFORANTES. **perforating arteries of foot** RAMI PERFORANTES ARTERIARUM METATARSALIUM PLANTARIUM. **perforating arteries of hand** RAMI PERFORANTES ARTERIARUM METACARPALIUM PALMARIUM. **perforating arteries of internal mammary a.** RAMI PERFORANTES ARTERIAE THORACICAE INTERNAE. **perforating peroneal a.** RAMUS PERFORANS ARTERIAE FIBULARIS. **pericallosal a.** The portion of the anterior cerebral artery that continues posteriorly along the sulcus of the corpus callosum on the medial surface of the cerebral cortex beyond the point where the callosomarginal artery branches from the main trunk. • It is sometimes simply referred to as the continuation of the anterior cerebral artery. **pericardiacophrenic a.** ARTERIA PERICARDIACOPHRENICA. **perineal a.** ARTERIA PERINEALIS. **peroneal a.** ARTERIA FIBULARIS. **phrenicopericardial a.** A branch of the lateral branch of the inferior phrenic artery that traverses the diaphragm through the point of penetration of the phrenic nerve and supplies the diaphragmatic aspect of the fibrous pericardium and the connective tissue binding it to the diaphragm. **plantar metatarsal arteries** ARTERIAE METATARSALES PLANTARES. **popliteal a.** ARTERIA POPLITEA. **postcentral a. of optic nerve** A collateral branch of the central artery of the retina that accompanies the central artery to the point where the latter bends forwards at the center of the optic nerve. The collateral branch then passes backwards towards the optic foramen. It supplies the macular fibers in this portion of its course. **posterior auricular a.** ARTERIA AURICULARIS POSTERIOR. **posterior cecal a.** ARTERIA CECALIS POSTERIOR. **posterior cerebral a.** ARTERIA CEREBRI POSTERIOR. **posterior cervical a.** RAMUS DESCENDENS ARTERIAE OCCIPITALIS. **posterior circumflex humeral a.** ARTERIA CIRCUMFLEXA POSTERIOR HUMERI. **posterior communicating a. of cerebrum** ARTERIA COMMUNICANS POSTERIOR CEREBRI. **posterior conjunctival arteries** ARTERIAE CONJUNCTIVALES POSTERIORES. **posterior dental a.** ARTERIA ALVEOLARIS SUPERIOR POSTERIOR. **posterior descending coronary a.** RAMUS INTERVENTRICULARIS POSTERIOR ARTERIAE CORONARIAE DEXTRAE. **posterior ethmoidal a.** ARTERIA ETHMOIDALIS POSTERIOR. **posterior fibular recurrent a.** *Outmoded* ARTERIA RECURRENS TIBIALIS POSTERIOR. **posterior inferior cerebellar a.** ARTERIA CEREBELLI INFERIOR POSTERIOR. **posterior intercostal arteries I and II** ARTERIAE INTERCOSTALES POSTERIORES I ET II. **posterior intercostal arteries III-XI** ARTERIAE INTERCOSTALES POSTERIORES III–XI. **posterior interosseous a.** ARTERIA INTEROSSEA POSTERIOR. **posterior interosseous a. of forearm** ARTERIA INTEROSSEA POSTERIOR. **posterior interventricular a.** RAMUS INTERVENTRICULARIS POSTERIOR ARTERIAE CORONARIAE DEXTRAE. **posterior labial arteries of vulva** RAMI LABIALES POSTERIORES ARTERIAE PUDENDAE INTERNAE. **posterior lateral nasal arteries** 1 ARTERIAE NASALES POSTERIORES LATERALES. 2 ARTERIA SPHENOPALATINA. **posterior medial malleolar arteries** RAMI MALLEOLARES MEDIALES ARTERIAE TIBIALIS POSTERIORIS. **posterior median arteries** Certain penetrating branches derived from the plexus of arteries on the dorsal surface of the spinal cord which enter the posterior median sulcus to supply the medial parts of the dorsal column. **posterior mediastinal arteries** RAMI MEDIASTINALES PARTIS THORACICAE AORTAE. **posterior meningeal a.** ARTERIA MENINGEA POSTERIOR. **posterior parietal a.** See under ARTERIAE PARIETALES ANTERIOR ET POSTERIOR. **posterior pelvic a.** ARTERIA ILIACA INTERNA. **posterior pericardiac arteries** RAMI PERICARDIACI AORTAE THORACICAE. **posterior scapular a.** ARTERIA DORSALIS SCAPULAE. **posterior scrotal arteries** RAMI SCROTALES POSTERIORES ARTERIAE PUDENDAE INTERNAE. **posterior segmental a.** ARTERIA SEGMENTI POSTERIORIS. **posterior septal arteries** 1 RAMI SEPTALES POSTERIORES. 2 ARTERIAE NASALES POSTERIORES, LATERALES ET SEPTI. **posterior spinal a.** ARTERIA SPINALIS POSTERIOR. **posterior sternal arteries** RAMI STERNALES ARTERIAE THORACICAE INTERNAE. **posterior superior alveolar a.** ARTERIA ALVEOLARIS SUPERIOR POSTERIOR. **posterior temporal a.** ARTERIA TEMPORALIS POSTERIOR. **posterior tibial a.** ARTERIA TIBIALIS POSTERIOR. **posterior tibial recurrent a.** ARTERIA RECURRENS TIBIALIS POSTERIOR. **posterior tympanic a.** ARTERIA TYMPANICA POSTERIOR. **posterior ulnar recurrent a.** RAMUS POSTERIOR ARTERIAE RECURRENTIS ULNARIS. **a. of precentral sulcus** ARTERIA SULCI PRECENTRALIS. **princeps pollicis a.** ARTERIA PRINCEPS POLLICIS. **principal a. of thumb** ARTERIA

PRINCEPS POLLICIS. **profunda brachii a.** ARTERIA PROFUNDA BRACHII. **profunda femoris a.** ARTERIA PROFUNDA FEMORIS. **proper hepatic a.** ARTERIA HEPATICA PROPRIA. **proper palmar digital arteries** ARTERIAE DIGITALES PALMARES PROPRIAE. **proper plantar digital arteries** ARTERIAE DIGITALES PLANTARES PROPRIAE. **proper volar digital arteries** ARTERIAE DIGITALES PALMARES PROPRIAE. **pterygoid arteries** RAMI PTERYGOIDEI ARTERIAE MAXILLARIS. **a. of pterygoid canal** ARTERIA CANALIS PTERYGOIDEI. **pubic a.** 1 RAMUS PUBICUS ARTERIAE EPIGASTRICAE INFERIORIS. 2 RAMUS PUBICUS ARTERIAE OBTURATORIAE. **pulmonary a.** TRUNCUS PULMONALIS. **a. of the pulp** The first and longest portion of the penicilli splenis in the red pulp of the spleen. **pyloric a.** ARTERIA GASTRICA DEXTRA. **radial a.** ARTERIA RADIALIS. **radial collateral a.** ARTERIA COLLATERALIS RADIALIS. **radial a. of index finger** ARTERIA RADIALIS INDICIS. **radial recurrent a.** ARTERIA RECURRENS RADIALIS. **radiate arteries of kidney** ARTERIAE INTERLOBULARES RENIS. **radicular a.** A small branch of a spinal artery that supplies a spinal root and accompanies it into the spinal canal. It may arise distally, or centrally from the vasa corona of the cord. **ranine a.** ARTERIA PROFUNDA LINGUAE. **rectosigmoid a.** RECTOSIGMOID ANASTOMOSIS. **recurrent interosseous a.** ARTERIA INTEROSSEA RECURRENS. **renal a.** ARTERIA RENALIS. **renal arteries** ARTERIAE RENIS. **retrocostal a.** RAMUS COSTALIS LATERALIS ARTERIAE THORACICAE INTERNAE. **retroduodenal arteries** ARTERIAE RETRODUODENALES. **revehent a.** ARTERIOLA GLOMERULARIS EFFERENS. **right colic a.** ARTERIA COLICA DEXTRA. **right coronary a. of heart** ARTERIA CORONARIA DEXTRA. **right coronary a. of stomach** ARTERIA GASTRICA DEXTRA. **right dorsocaudal a.** ARTERIA SEGMENTI POSTERIORIS. **right gastric a.** ARTERIA GASTRICA DEXTRA. **right gastroepiploic a.** ARTERIA GASTRO-OMENTALIS DEXTRA. **right gastro-omental a.** ARTERIA GASTRO-OMENTALIS DEXTRA. **right inferior gastric a.** ARTERIA GASTRO-OMENTALIS DEXTRA. **right inferior pancreaticoduodenal a.** 1 *Outmoded* ARTERIA PANCREATICODUODENALIS SUPERIOR ANTERIOR. 2 See under ARTERIAE RETRODUODENALES. **right lateral hepatic a.** *Outmoded* ARTERIA SEGMENTI POSTERIORIS. **right marginal a. of heart** RAMUS MARGINALIS DEXTER CORDIS. **right pulmonary a.** ARTERIA PULMONALIS DEXTRA. **right superior colic a.** *Outmoded* ARTERIA COLICA DEXTRA. **right superior pancreaticoduodenal a.** *Outmoded* ARTERIA PANCREATICODUODENALIS SUPERIOR POSTERIOR. **right ventral paramedian a.** ARTERIA SEGMENTI ANTERIORIS. **Riolan's a.** A variant of the middle colic artery, the origin of which may be from either the celiac artery, the superior mesenteric artery, or the dorsal pancreatic artery. It takes part in the marginal artery of the colon. **rolandic a.** *Outmoded* ARTERIA SULCI CENTRALIS. **a. of round ligament of hip joint** RAMUS ACETABULARIS ARTERIAE CIRCUMFLEXAE FEMORIS MEDIALIS. **a. of round ligament of uterus** ARTERIA LIGAMENTI TERETIS UTERI. **sacrococcygeal a.** ARTERIA SACRALIS MEDIANA. **sciatic a.** 1 ARTERIA COMITANS NERVI ISCHIADICI. 2 ARTERIA GLUTEA INFERIOR. **screw arteries** RAMI HELICINI ARTERIAE UTERINAE. **a. of the scrotal septum** One of the terminal posterior scrotal branches of the perineal artery. It supplies the median septum scroti. **segmental a. of kidney** One of the primary terminal branches of the anterior and posterior rami of the renal artery that supply the vascular segments of the kidney. Arteria segmenti superioris, arteria segmenti anterioris superioris, arteria segmenti anterioris inferioris, and arteria segmenti inferioris are supplied by the ramus anterior, and arteria segmenti posterioris by the ramus posterior. Also *interpapillary artery of kidney* (outmoded). **a. of segment IV of liver** *Outmoded* ARTERIA SEGMENTI MEDIALIS. **septal a.** A branch of the superior labial artery that supplies the nasal septum and anastomoses with septal branch of the sphenopalatine artery. **septal arteries of heart** Branches from the right coronary and left coronary arteries to the interatrial and interventricular septa of the heart; namely, rami atriales and rami interventriculares septales, respectively. **sheathed arteries** The second portion of the penicilli arteriae lienalis in the red pulp of the spleen that has a characteristic spindle-shaped thickening (Schweigger-Seidel sheath) of its wall, formed by a condensation of reticular cells and macrophages. Also *ellipsoid arterioles, sheathed arterioles, arteriolae ellipsoideae, arteriolae vaginatae.* **short ciliary arteries** ARTERIAE CILIARES POSTERIORES BREVES. **short gastric arteries** ARTERIAE GASTRICAE BREVES. **short posterior ciliary arteries** ARTERIAE CILIARES POSTERIORES BREVES. **sigmoid arteries** ARTERIAE SIGMOIDEAE. **silver-wire arteries** Arteries that when seen with an opthalmoscope resemble light reflected from a silver wire. They are associated with hypertension. **small iliac a.** ARTERIA ILIOLUMBALIS. **somatic arteries** Intersegmental branches of the embryonic dorsal aorta which supply the body wall. **sphenopalatine a.** ARTERIA SPHENOPALATINA. **spigelian a.** ARTERIA LOBI CAUDATI. **spinal arteries** A set of arteries comprising: (1) rami spinales arteriae vertebralis; (2) rami spinales arteriae cervicalis ascendentis; (3) rami spinales arteriae intercostalis suprema; (4) ramus spinalis arteriarum lumbalium; (5) rami spinales arteriarum sacralium lateralium; (6) ramus spinalis arteriae subcostalis; (7) ramus spinalis rami dorsalis arteriarum intercostalium posteriorum III-XI; (8) ramus spinalis rami lumbalis arteriae iliolumbalis. **spiral arteries** RAMI HELICINI ARTERIAE UTERINAE. **splenic a.** ARTERIA SPLENICA. **sternal arteries** RAMI STERNALES ARTERIAE THORACICAE INTERNAE. **sternocleidomastoid a.** 1 RAMI STERNOCLEIDOMASTOIDEI ARTERIAE OCCIPITALIS. 2 RAMUS STERNOCLEIDOMASTOIDEUS ARTERIAE THYROIDEAE SUPERIORIS. **straight arteries of kidney** ARTERIOLAE RECTAE RENIS. **straight medullary arteries** ARTERIOLAE RECTAE RENIS. **striate arteries** Central branches of the middle cerebral artery and to a small extent the anterior cerebral artery which pierce the anterior perforated substance to supply the corpus striatum and internal capsule. Also *rami striati arteriae cerebri mediae.* **stylomastoid a.** ARTERIA STYLOMASTOIDEA. **subclavian a.** ARTERIA SUBCLAVIA. **subcostal a.** ARTERIA SUBCOSTALIS. **sublingual a.** ARTERIA SUBLINGUALIS. **submental a.** ARTERIA SUBMENTALIS. **subscapular a.** ARTERIA SUBSCAPULARIS. **sulcal arteries** VENTROMEDIAN ARTERIES. **superficial antebrachial a.** See under ARTERIA BRACHIALIS SUPERFICIALIS. **superficial brachial a.** ARTERIA BRACHIALIS SUPERFICIALIS. **superficial cervical a.** ARTERIA CERVICALIS SUPERFICIALIS. **superficial circumflex iliac a.** ARTERIA CIRCUMFLEXA ILIACA SUPERFICIALIS. **superficial epigastric a.** ARTERIA EPIGASTRICA SUPERFICIALIS. **superficial external pudendal arteries** See under ARTERIAE PUDENDAE EXTERNAE. **superficial femoral a.** The portion of the femoral artery distal to the origin of the deep femoral artery. **superficial medial a. of foot** RAMUS SUPERFICIALIS

ARTERIAE PLANTARIS MEDIALIS. **superficial palmar a.** RAMUS PALMARIS SUPERFICIALIS ARTERIAE RADIALIS. **superficial perineal a.** ARTERIA PERINEALIS. **superficial temporal a.** ARTERIA TEMPORALIS SUPERFICIALIS. **superficial transverse cervical a.** 1 RAMUS SUPERFICIALIS ARTERIAE TRANSVERSAE CERVICIS. 2 ARTERIA CERVICALIS SUPERFICIALIS. **superficial transverse perineal a.** An artery that arises from the perineal artery, near the base of the urogenital diaphragm, and runs medially on the inferior surface of the superficial transverse perineal muscle to anastomose with its fellow from the opposite side, the posterior scrotal artery and the inferior rectal arteries. It supplies the area between the anus and the end of the membranous urethra, including the bulbospongiosus and the external anal sphincter muscles. **superficial volar a.** RAMUS PALMARIS SUPERFICIALIS ARTERIAE RADIALIS. **superior cerebellar a.** ARTERIA CEREBELLI SUPERIOR. **superior diaphragmatic arteries** ARTERIAE PHRENICAE SUPERIORES. **superior epigastric a.** ARTERIA EPIGASTRICA SUPERIOR. **superior gluteal a.** ARTERIA GLUTEA SUPERIOR. **superior hemorrhoidal a.** ARTERIA RECTALIS SUPERIOR. **superior hypophyseal a.** ARTERIA HYPOPHYSIALIS SUPERIOR. **superior intercostal a.** ARTERIA INTERCOSTALIS SUPREMA. **superior labial a.** ARTERIA LABIALIS SUPERIOR. **superior laryngeal a.** ARTERIA LARYNGEA SUPERIOR. **superior lateral sacral a.** See under ARTERIAE SACRALES LATERALES. **superior macular a.** ARTERIOLA MACULARIS SUPERIOR. **superior mesenteric a.** ARTERIA MESENTERICA SUPERIOR. **superior phrenic a.** 1 ARTERIA PERICARDIACOPHRENICA. 2 ARTERIAE PHRENICAE SUPERIORES. **superior profunda a.** ARTERIA PROFUNDA BRACHII. **superior rectal a.** ARTERIA RECTALIS SUPERIOR. **superior segmental a.** ARTERIA SEGMENTI SUPERIORIS. **superior sternocleidomastoid a.** RAMUS STERNOCLEIDOMASTOIDEUS ARTERIAE THYROIDEAE SUPERIORIS. **superior suprarenal arteries** ARTERIAE SUPRARENALES SUPERIORES. **superior thoracic a.** ARTERIA THORACICA SUPERIOR. **superior thyroid a.** ARTERIA THYROIDEA SUPERIOR. **superior tympanic a.** ARTERIA TYMPANICA SUPERIOR. **superior ulnar collateral a.** ARTERIA COLLATERALIS ULNARIS SUPERIOR. **superior vesical arteries** ARTERIAE VESICALES SUPERIORES. **supraduodenal a.** ARTERIA SUPRADUODENALIS. **supraorbital a.** ARTERIA SUPRAORBITALIS. **suprarenal arteries** The arteriae suprarenales superiores, arteria suprarenalis media, and arteria suprarenalis inferior. **suprascapular a.** ARTERIA SUPRASCAPULARIS. **supratrochlear a.** 1 ARTERIA SUPRATROCHLEARIS. 2 ARTERIA COLLATERALIS ULNARIS INFERIOR. **sural arteries** ARTERIAE SURALES. **sylvian a.** ARTERIA CEREBRI MEDIA. **terminal a.** 1 The caudal portion of the anterior spinal artery running along the filum terminale. 2 END ARTERY. **testicular a.** ARTERIA TESTICULARIS. **thalamogeniculate arteries** Four to six central branches of the posterior cerebral artery supplying the posterolateral and posterosuperior parts of the thalamus and the lateral geniculate nucleus. Also *rami thalamici arteriae cerebri posterioris.* **thalamoperforate arteries** Thalamic branches, included among the posterolateral central branches of the posterior cerebral artery, that perforate the thalamus to supply its lateral and posterior parts. **thoracicoacromial a.** ARTERIA THORACOACROMIALIS. **thoracodorsal a.** ARTERIA THORACODORSALIS. **thymic arteries** RAMI THYMICI ARTERIAE THORACICAE INTERNAE. **thyroidea ima a.** ARTERIA THYROIDEA IMA. **tonsillar a.** RAMUS TONSILLARIS ARTERIAE FACIALIS. **transverse cervical a.** 1 ARTERIA TRANSVERSA CERVICIS. 2 ARTERIA DORSALIS SCAPULAE. **transverse colic a.** *Outmoded* ARTERIA COLICA MEDIA. **transverse a. of face** ARTERIA TRANSVERSA FACIALIS. **transverse facial a.** ARTERIA TRANSVERSA FACIALIS. **transverse a. of neck** 1 ARTERIA TRANSVERSA CERVICIS. 2 RAMUS SUPERFICIALIS ARTERIAE TRANSVERSAE CERVICIS. 3 ARTERIA CERVICALIS SUPERFICIALIS. **transverse pancreatic a.** ARTERIA PANCREATICA INFERIOR. **transverse scapular a.** ARTERIA SUPRASCAPULARIS. **tubo-ovarian a.** ARTERIA OVARICA. **ulnar a.** ARTERIA ULNARIS. **ulnar metacarpal arteries** ARTERIAE DIGITALES PALMARES COMMUNES. **ulnar recurrent a.** ARTERIA RECURRENS ULNARIS. **umbilical a.** One of the two arteries contained within the umbilical cord which convey blood from the fetus to the allantochorionic placenta. In the early stage, they are direct continuations of the primitive dorsal aorta, but later in fetal life they come to arise from the internal iliac artery. Also *arteria umbilicalis.* **urethral a.** ARTERIA URETHRALIS. **uterine a.** ARTERIA UTERINA. **vaginal a.** ARTERIA VAGINALIS. **venous arteries** VENAE PULMONALES. **ventral splanchnic arteries** The segmental branches given off from the embryonic dorsal aorta which supply the digestive tube. **ventromedian arteries** Branches of the anterior spinal artery that enter the anterior medial fissure and pass alternately to left and right portions of the central gray. Also *sulcal arteries.* **vermiform a.** ARTERIA APPENDICULARIS. **vertebral a.** ARTERIA VERTEBRALIS. **vidian a.** ARTERIA CANALIS PTERYGOIDEI. **vitelline a.** An embryonic artery that supplies the yolk sac. At first there are two. They fuse to give rise eventually to the superior mesenteric artery of the adult. **volar interosseous a.** ARTERIA INTEROSSEA ANTERIOR. **volar metacarpal arteries** ARTERIAE METACARPALES PALMARES. **volar radial a. of index finger** ARTERIA RADIALIS INDICIS. **a. of Zinn** ARTERIA CENTRALIS RETINAE. **zygomatico-orbital a.** ARTERIA ZYGOMATICO-ORBITALIS.

**arthr-** \ärthr-\ ARTHRO-.

**arthralgia** \ärthral′jə\ [ARTHR- + -ALGIA] Joint pain with objective findings of heat, redness, tenderness to touch, loss of motion, or swelling. Compare ARTHRITIS. **acromegalic a.** Arthralgia caused by the joint abnormalities of acromegaly. **nonspecific a.** SYPHILITIC ARTHRITIS. **periodic a.** Intermittent arthralgia that recurs at predictable time intervals. **a. saturnina** Severe pain in joints due to gout caused by chronic lead poisoning.

**arthralgic** \ärthral′jik\ Pertaining to or having arthralgia.

**arthrectomy** \ärthrek′təmē\ [ARTHR- + -ECTOMY] The surgical removal of a joint.

**arthrempyesis** \är′thrempī·ē′sis\ [ARTHR- + Gk *empyēsis* suppuration] *Obs.* PYARTHROSIS.

**arthresthesia** \är′thresthē′zhə\ [ARTHR- + -ESTHESIA] Position and joint sensibility; the ability to perceive movement at a joint.

**arthrifuge** A drug or any other treatment for the relief of gout.

**arthritic** \ärthrit′ik\ Pertaining to or having arthritis.

**arthritides** \ärthrit′idēz\ Plural of ARTHRITIS.

**arthritis** \ärthrī′tis\ [Gk (from *arthron* a joint) of the joints, as in *arthritis nosos* joint disease] Any abnormality of a joint in which objective findings of heat, redness, swelling, tenderness, loss of motion, or deformity are present. The term is usually qualified by an adjective describing the cause, such as rheumatoid, gouty, infectious, or post-traumatic. Compare ARTHRALGIA. Adj. arthritic. **acromegalic a.** Osteoarthritis associated with acromegaly, due mainly to cartilaginous overgrowth. **acute rheumatic a.** Arthritis occurring in patients with acute rheumatic fever. **atrophic a.** OSTEOARTHRITIS. **bacterial a.** Infectious arthritis due to infection with a bacterium, as opposed to a virus, mycobacterium, or fungus. **Bekhterev's a.** ANKYLOSING SPONDYLITIS. **blennorrhagic a.** GONOCOCCAL ARTHRITIS. **chronic inflammatory a.** Inflammatory arthritis of prolonged duration, either infectious or noninfectious. In the latter case, rheumatoid arthritis is often implied. **chronic villous a.** A form of chronic inflammatory arthritis in which the synovium is markedly hypertrophied, forming villi on pathologic examination, as in rheumatoid arthritis. **chylous a.** Arthritis in which synovial fluid appears milky and contains chylomicra. It is usually attributed to obstruction of draining lymphatic vessels, and may involve lymph obstruction by filarial worms. **colitic a.** Any of several forms of inflammatory arthritis of the colon occurring in association with ulcerative colitis or Crohn's disease. The two major forms are an axial arthritis characterized by sacroileitis and ankylosing spondylitis and a peripheral arthritis principally involving large joints. **cricoarytenoid a.** Arthritis of the cricoarytenoid joint occurring rarely as a complication of a variety of acute and chronic infections of the larynx but particularly in rheumatoid disease where an incidence as high as 30 percent has been reported. The symptoms include local pain, hoarseness and, in advanced cases, dyspnea and stridor. **crystal a.** Any of those forms of arthritis characterized by the presence of crystals within leukocytes found in synovial fluid during an attack. Three spontaneous forms occur in man: gout (monosodium urate crystal), pseudogout (calcium pyrophosphate dihydrate crystal), and hydroxyapatite disease (hydroxyapatite crystal). Crystalline antibiotics or corticosteroids injected into joints can also cause a transient crystal arthritis. **degenerative a.** OSTEOARTHRITIS. **dysenteric a.** ENTEROPATHIC REACTIVE ARTHRITIS. **enteropathic reactive a.** Arthritis presumed to be precipitated by immunologic mechanisms in response to infection by enteric pathogens such as *Shigella flexneri, Salmonella* spp., *Yersinia enterocolitica*, or *Campylobacter fetus*. It may be acute or chronic, aseptic or septic, migratory or nonmigratory, monoarticular or polyarticular, and may involve any joint but most often affects knees and ankles. Most patients who develop arthritis following *Shigella, Salmonella, Yersinia*, or *Campylobacter* gastroenteritis have the specific histocompatibility antigen HLA B27. Some patients may manifest other symptoms permitting definite diagnosis of the Reiter syndrome. Also *dysenteric arthritis, postinfectious arthritis.* **exudative a.** Inflammatory arthritis from any cause. **fungal a.** Infectious arthritis caused by a fungus. In the United States the most common causative infections are histoplasmosis and coccidioidomycosis. Also *arthritis fungosa, mycotic arthritis.* **gonococcal a.** Arthritis resulting from disseminated infection with *Neisseria gonorrhoeae* and classically characterized by acute onset of migratory polyarthritis which subsequently localizes in one or more joints, tenosynovitis, and vesicopustular skin lesions. Also *blennorrhagic arthritis, urethral arthritis, gonorrheal arthritis, gonorrheal rheumatism.* **gouty a.** GOUT. **hemophilic a.** Arthritis, especially of large joints, that occurs in the course of hemophilia after hemorrhage into joints. **hemorrhagic a.** Arthritis in which hemorrhage is demonstrated within the joint fluid. It most commonly occurs in hemophiliac, traumatized, or anticoagulated patients. **hypertrophic a.** Arthritis associated with new bone growth such as the osteophytes of osteoarthritis. **infectious a.** Arthritis due to an identifiable microbiologic agent. Also *infectional arthritis.* **juvenile rheumatoid a.** A form of arthritis, distinct from the adult type of rheumatoid arthritis, usually occurring in children and often, but not always, characterized by high fever and rash as in Still's disease. Juvenile rheumatoid arthritis generally does not give positive tests for rheumatoid factor or rheumatoid nodules. **Lyme a.** LYME DISEASE. **Marie-Strümpell a.** ANKYLOSING SPONDYLITIS. **menopausal a.** Arthritis occurring at about the time of the female menopause. No specific menopausal arthritis is recognized, but rather other forms of arthritis, such as degenerative or rheumatoid, may occur in this age group. **mixed a.** Simultaneous osteoarthritis and rheumatoid arthritis. **a. mutilans** Extremely destructive arthritis, often characterized by conspicuous osteolysis, occurring characteristically in psoriatic arthritis and sometimes in rheumatoid arthritis. **mycotic a.** FUNGAL ARTHRITIS. **neurogenic a.** NEUROGENIC ARTHROPATHY. **a. nodosa** Osteoarthritis with Heberden's nodes. **nondeforming a.** Inflammatory arthritis that subsides without causing permanent change, such as is seen in rheumatic fever and lupus erythematosus. **noninflammatory a.** Arthritis in which the physical findings of inflammation are absent and the joint fluid, when examined, shows a low leukocyte count, good viscosity, and good mucin clot test. Usually osteoarthritis or traumatic arthritis is implied, as distinguished from inflammatory forms such as rheumatoid, infectious, or crystal arthritis. Also *arthrosis.* **ochronotic a.** A degenerative, progressive arthritis, occurring in alkaptonuria, that is characterized by the deposition of black pigment, polymers of homogentisic acid, in articular cartilage. The spine is usually affected first, followed by the knees and hips. Also *ochronotic arthropathy.* **palindromic a.** Episodic severe inflammatory arthritis occurring with prolonged intervals of no abnormality. Many authorities believe that palindromic arthritis is one of the ways in which rheumatoid arthritis is first manifest. **patellar-femoral a.** A form of arthritis, generally traumatic or degenerative osteoarthritis, that involves the joint interface between the posterior surface of the patella and the intercondylar aspect of the femur. **periosteal a.** Joint degeneration that is accompanied by a periosteal reaction, as seen in the small bones of the foot in Martin's disease. **postinfectious a.** ENTEROPATHIC REACTIVE ARTHRITIS. **proliferative a.** Inflammatory arthritis with synovial proliferation. **psoriatic a.** Any of several forms of arthritis, often involving the distal interphalangeal joints or the spine, occurring in persons with psoriasis. Also *arthropathia psoriatica, psoriatic arthropathy.* **purulent a.** PURULENT SYNOVITIS. **pyogenic a.** Arthritis due to infection by a pyogenic bacterium, characterized by high counts of white blood cells in the synovial fluid. **rheumatoid a.** A common form of chronic inflammatory arthritis of unknown cause, not associated with a known infection. It is a multisystem disease with protean manifestations and is characterized most often by sustained inflammation of multiple joints. The histology of the inflamed joints is characterized by the formation of pannus. The disease is associated with the presence of autoantibodies to IgG (the rheumatoid factors). **rheumatoid a. of spine** *Outmoded* ANKYLOSING SPONDYLITIS. **senescent a.** OSTEOARTHRITIS. **a. sicca** Inflammatory arthritis without much exudation. **suppurative a.** Inflammatory arthritis with marked exudation of inflammatory cells into the joint fluid. Infection is usually assumed to be present. **syphilitic a.** 1 Arthritis due to primary infection of the joint by *Treponema pallidum*. 2 Neuropathic arthritis due to tabes dorsalis. For defs. 1 and 2 also *syphilitic arthropathy, nonspecific arthralgia.* **tuberculous a.** Arthritis occurring as a result of tuberculous infection of a joint, and marked by chronic inflammation, effusion, and, later, ankylosis. Also *arthrocace, white tumor.* **uratic a.** GOUT. **urethral a.** GONOCOCCAL ARTHRITIS. **a. urethritica** The arthritis of the Reiter syndrome. **venereal a.** The arthritis of the Reiter syndrome. **villous a.** PIGMENTED VILLONODULAR SYNOVITIS. **viral a.** Arthritis due to infection by a virus, such as hepatitis virus B or that of rubella.

**arthro-** \är′thrō-\ [Gk *arthron* joint] A combining form meaning (1) joint; (2) articulation in speech. Also *arthr-*.

**arthrocace** \ärthräk′əsē\ [ARTHRO- + Gk *kakē* badness] TUBERCULOUS ARTHRITIS.

**arthrocentesis** \-sentē′sis\ [ARTHRO- + -CENTESIS] The puncture of a joint with a needle for the purpose of removing joint fluid.

**arthroclasia** \-klā′zhə\ [ARTHRO- + -CLASIA] The surgical disruption of an ankylosis to permit joint motion.

**arthroclisis** \-klī′sis\ [ARTHRO- + -CLISIS] The presence or the production of ankylosis of a joint. Also *arthrokleisis.*

***Arthroderma*** \-dur′mə\ [ARTHRO- + Gk *derma* skin] A genus of the family Gymnoascaceae, class Ascomycetes, which is the perfect (sexual) stage of the form-genus *Trichophyton.* This genus constitutes a medically important group of dermatophytes.

**arthrodesia** \-dē′zhə\ ARTHRODESIS.

**arthrodesis** \ärthräd′əsis\ [ARTHRO- + -DESIS] A surgical procedure consisting of the obliteration of a joint space with creation of a bony fusion so that no movement can occur at the joint. Also *operative ankylosis, artificial ankylosis, syndesis, arthrodesia.* **extra-articular a.** The fusion of a joint by insertion of a bone graft extracapsularly across the bones that make up the joint.

**arthrodia** \ärthrō′dē·ə\ [Gk *arthrōdia* (from *arthrōdēs* articulated, well-knit, from *arthron* a joint) a gliding or arthrodial joint] ARTICULATIO PLANA.

**arthrodial** \ärthrō′dē·əl\ Resembling or pertaining to an arthrodia (articulatio plana).

**arthrodysplasia** \-displā′zhə\ [ARTHRO- + DYSPLASIA] The abnormal development of one or more skeletal joints. **hereditary a.** NAIL-PATELLA SYNDROME.

**arthroempyesis** \-empī·ē′sis\ [ARTHRO- + Gk *empyēsis* suppuration] PYARTHROSIS.

**arthroereisis** \-ərī′sis\ [ARTHRO- + Gk *ereisis* (from *ereidein* to press a thing against, prop, fix firmly) a pressing or pushing a thing against] 1 A surgical procedure that limits the amount of motion possible in a joint which has become excessively mobile as a result of paralysis. 2 Restoration of stability to a flail joint. For defs. 1 and 2 also *arthrorisis.*

**arthrogram** \är′thrəgram\ [ARTHRO- + -GRAM] A radiograph obtained during arthrography. Also *arthrograph.*

**arthrography** \ärthräg′rəfē\ [ARTHRO- + -GRAPHY] Radiologic examination of a joint after the injection of a radiopaque agent and/or gas into the joint. Also *hydropneumogony* (obs.). **air a.** ARTHROPNEUMOROENTGENOGRAPHY.

**arthrogryposis** \-gripō′sis\ [ARTHRO- + GRYPOSIS] A congenital malformation in which the limb joints are fixed in contracture, usually in extension. The condition is observable at birth or in the neonatal period. **congenital multiple a.** A congenital rigidity or relative immobility of the joints, particularly of the limbs, with atrophy of the associated muscles, fibrosis of the joint capsules, and often the absence of those motor neurons in the spinal cord that normally innervate the affected muscles. Talipes and scoliosis are common symptoms. The etiology is controversial, but recent evidence suggests destruction of motor neurons to the affected limbs during the second or third trimester. Also *arthrogryposis syndrome, amyoplasia congenita, myodystrophia fetalis, arthrogryposis multiplex, arthrogryposis multiplex congenita.*

**arthrohyal** \-hī′əl\ [ARTHRO- + HYAL] A cartilaginous element in the hyoid chain of the embryo, derived from the posterior region of Reichert's cartilage (second branchial arch), and placed between the tympanohyal and the stylohyal with which it unites. In man it is incorporated in the styloid process of the temporal bone.

**arthrokatadysis** \-kətad′isis\ PROTRUSIO ACETABULI.

**arthrokleisis** \-klī′sis\ ARTHROCLISIS.

**arthrolith** \är′thrəlith\ [ARTHRO- + -LITH] A stone, as of urate or calcium, occurring in a joint.

**arthrologia** \-lō′jə\ [ARTHRO- + -LOGIA] 1 [NA] The nomenclature dealing with joints and ligaments. 2 ARTHROLOGY.

**arthrologic** \-läj′ik\ Pertaining to arthrology.

**arthrology** \ärthräl′əjē\ [ARTHRO- + -LOGY] The branch of science dealing with the joints and ligaments of the body. Also *syndesmology, syndesmologia* (outmoded), *arthrologia, synosteology.*

**arthrolysis** \ärthräl′isis\ [ARTHRO- + LYSIS] The surgical freeing of adhesions within a joint.

**arthromeningitis** \-men′injī′tis\ SYNOVITIS.

**arthrometer** \ärthräm′ətər\ [ARTHRO- + -METER] An instrument for measuring the extent of joint movement.

**arthrometry** \ärthräm′ətrē\ [ARTHRO- + -METRY] The theory and practice of measuring the range of motion of joints.

**arthro-ophthalmopathy** \-äf′thalmäp′əthē\ [ARTHRO- + OPHTHALMOPATHY] STICKLER SYNDROME.

**arthro-osteo-onychodysplasia** NAIL-PATELLA SYNDROME.

**arthropathia** \-path′ē·ə\ [ARTHRO- + -PATHIA] ARTHROPATHY. **a. psoriatica** PSORIATIC ARTHRITIS.

**arthropathology** \-pathäl′əjē\ The study of the anatomic pathology of joints.

**arthropathy** \ärthräp′əthē\ [ARTHRO- + -PATHY] Any joint disease. Also *arthropathia.* **Charcot's a.** NEUROGENIC ARTHROPATHY. **degenerative vertebral a.** DEGENERATIVE SPONDYLOSIS. **diabetic a.** Neuropathic arthropathy due to diabetic neuropathy. **dislocating a.** Degenerative arthrosis of a joint following repeated dislocations. **disuse a.** Joint stiffness and premature degeneration owing to prolonged disuse or immobilization. **gonococcal a.** Arthropathy that usually affects a large joint, such as the knee, and caused by a gonococcal infection. **Heberden's a.** See under HEBERDEN'S NODES. **hemophilic a.** The abnormalities seen in joints of hemophiliacs after repeated episodes of spontaneous bleeding. Initially they consist of siderotic synovitis, and in later stages, secondary gross degeneration of the articular cartilage and bone. **neurogenic a.** Degenerative or destructive arthropathy involving one or several joints, resulting from repeated unnoticed trauma occurring when there is loss of the appreciation of pain sensation. It is seen particularly in syringomyelia, when the shoulder and/or elbow are most often involved, in tabes dorsalis, when the spinal column, hip, knee, ankle, or foot are affected, or in severe sensory neuropathy when the changes are most evident in the joints of the fingers, hands, toes, and feet. The affected joints are swollen and show an abnormal range of movement. Radiographs show progressive destruction of joint surfaces, and even of the ends of long bones. Also *neurogenic arthritis, Charcot's joint, Charcot's arthropathy, neurarthropathy, neuroarthropathy.* **ochronotic a.** OCHRONOTIC ARTHRITIS. **osteopulmonary a.** HYPERTROPHIC PULMONARY OSTEOARTHROPATHY. **palindromic a.** A recurrent pain and swelling in joints that is of unknown etiology. **psoriatic a.** PSORIATIC ARTHRITIS. **pyrophosphate a.** An articular disease of unknown etiology characterized by the deposition of calcium pyrophosphate dihydrate crystals in articular cartilage and synovium. The affected joints develop an acute synovitis which, after repeated episodes, evolves into an osteoarthritis. **stationary a.** NEUROGENIC ARTHROPATHY. **syphilitic a.** SYPHILITIC ARTHRITIS. **tabetic a.** Neurogenic arthropathy in tabes dorsalis. Also *tabetic osteoarthropathy.*

**arthrophyte** \är′thrəfīt\ [ARTHRO- + Gk *phyt(on)* a plant, tree] An abnormal substance such as cartilage or a bone fragment or calculus present within a joint.

**arthroplasty** \är′thrōplas′tē\ [ARTHRO- + -PLASTY] **1** The surgical creation of a new or artificial joint where an ankylosis exists. **2** A plastic surgical operation to change the contours or mechanics of a joint, with the intent of improving function. Adj. arthroplastic. **allograft a.** A plastic operation performed on any joint, utilizing alloplastic materials. Also *alloarthroplasty.*

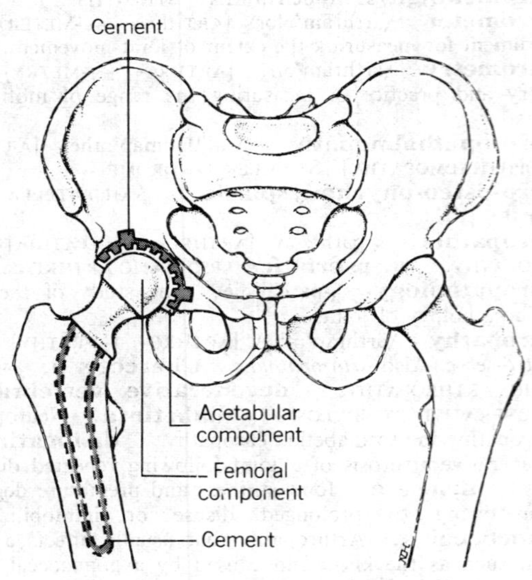


**Arthroplasty** (total hip joint replacement)

**arthropneumoroentgenography** \-nʸoo′mōrent′genäg′rəfē\ [ARTHRO- + PNEUMO- + ROENTGENOGRAPHY] Roentgenography of a joint following the injection of a gas into it, such as air or carbon dioxide. Also *air arthrography, arthropneumography.*

**arthropod** \är′thrəpäd\ [ARTHRO- + -POD] Any member of the phylum Arthropoda.

**Arthropoda** \ärthräp′ədə\ [New L (from ARTHRO- + -POD) joint-legged animals] An enormous phylum of invertebrates characterized by a chitinous exoskeleton, a segmented body, paired segmented legs, an open circulatory system, complex musculature, and a complete digestive tract. It is the largest phylum of the kingdom Animalia and contains eight classes, the most ubiquitous being Arachnida, Crustacea, and, the largest of all animal classes, the Insecta.

**arthropyosis** \-pī-ō′sis\ PYARTHROSIS.

**arthrorisis** \-rī′sis\ ARTHROEREISIS.

**arthrosclerosis** \-sklerō′sis\ Sclerosis of a joint.

**arthroscope** \är′thrəskōp\ [ARTHRO- + -SCOPE] An instrument utilizing fiberoptics and permitting visualization of the inside of a joint by joint puncture through a small incision.

**arthroscopy** \ärthräs′kəpē\ [ARTHRO- + -SCOPY] The visualization of the insides of joints with the aid of an arthroscope.

**arthrosis** \ärthrō′sis\ [ARTHR- + -OSIS] NONINFLAMMATORY ARTHRITIS. **a. deformans** OSTEOARTHRITIS. **temporomandibular a.** Osteoarthritis of the temporomandibular joint.

**arthrosteitis** \är′thrästē·ī′tis\ [ARTHR- + OSTEITIS] An inflammation of the bony components of a joint.

**arthrostomy** \ärthräs′təmē\ ARTHROTOMY.

**arthrotome** \är′thrətōm\ [ARTHRO- + -TOME] A surgical instrument for incising a joint.

**arthrotomy** \ärthrät′əmē\ [ARTHRO- + -TOMY] The surgical incision of a joint. Also *arthrostomy, synosteotomy.*

**arthrotropia** \-trō′pē·ə\ [ARTHRO- + Gk *trop(ē)* a turn, change + -IA] A twisted or turned state of a limb.

**arthrotropic** \-träp′ik\ [ARTHRO- + -TROPIC[1]] Having a propensity to affect joints, as certain viral infections; joint-seeking.

**arthroxesis** \ärthräk′səsis\ [ARTHRO- + Gk *xesis* a scraping] The scraping of an articular cartilage.

**Arthus** [Nicolas Maurice *Arthus,* French bacteriologist, 1862–1945] **1** Arthus phenomenon. See under REACTION. **2** Passive Arthus reaction. See under REACTION. **3** Reverse passive Arthus reaction. See under REACTION.

**articular** \ärtik′yələr\ [L *articularis* (from *articulus* a joint) pertaining to joints] Pertaining to a joint or affecting the joints.

**articularis cubiti** \ärtik′yəler′is koo′bitī\ SUBANCONEUS.

**articulate** \ärtik′yəlāt\ **1** Having joints; jointed. **2** To bring together or join so as to form a joint, allowing movement between the parts. **3** To produce (intelligible sounds) with the organs of speech. **4** Capable of producing the sounds of speech. **5** Able to speak easily or clearly; fluent in speech.

**articulated** \ärtik′yəlāt′id\ Connected by one or more joints; jointed.

# articulatio

**articulatio** \ärtik′yəlā′shō\ [L (from *articulus* a joint, small joint, dim. of *artus,* pl., joints, limbs, parts, akin to Gk *arthron* a joint) a jointed structure] (*pl.* articulationes) [NA] The junction of two or more bones or segments to form more or less movable parts. Also *joint, junctura ossium, osseous junction, articulus, junctura* (outmoded). **a. acromioclavicularis** [NA] A plane joint between the medial margin of the acromion of scapula and the lateral end of the clavicle. Also *acromioclavicular joint, acromioclavicular articulation.* **a. atlantoaxialis lateralis** One of a pair of plane joints between the inferior facet of the lateral mass of the atlas and the superior facet of the axis on each side. Also *lateral atlantoaxial articulation.* **a. atlantoaxialis mediana** [NA] A pivot joint between the dens axis and a ring formed by the anterior arch of atlas anteriorly and the transverse ligament of atlas posteriorly. Also *median atlantoaxial articulation, Cruveilhier's joint.* **a. atlanto-occipitalis** [NA] Either of a pair of ellipsoid joints formed by a condyle of the occipital bone and a superior articular facet of the lateral mass of the atlas on each side. Also *atlanto-occipital articulation, craniovertebral articulation, occipital articulation, occipitoatlantal articulation, Cruveilhier's joint, atlanto-occipital joint.* **a. bicondylaris** [NA] A synovial joint in which two distinct, rounded condyles articulate with two opposing concave surfaces (as in the knee joints) in such manner that most of the movement is in one plane, and rotation is rather limited. Also *condylar articulation, condylar joint, condyloid joint* (imprecise), *condylarthrosis.* **a. calcaneocuboidea** [NA] A saddle-shaped joint between the anterior surface of the calcaneus bone and the proximal surface of the cuboid bone. Also *calcaneocuboid articulation, calcaneocuboid joint.* **a. capitis costae** [NA] Any of several usually plane, or gliding, joints between the heads of the typical ribs and articular facets on the contiguous margins of bodies of adjacent thoracic vertebrae and the intervertebral disks between them. Also *articulation of head of rib, capitular articulation, costocentral articulation, capitular joint.* **articulationes carpi** [NA] The articulationes intercarpales and articulatio radiocarpalis. Also *carpal articulations.* **articulationes carpometacarpales** [NA] The plane joints between the distal carpal bones and the bases of the second, third, fourth, and fifth metacarpal bones. Also *carpometacarpal articulations, metacarpocarpal articulations, carpometacarpal joints.* **a. carpometacarpalis pollicis** [NA] The saddle-shaped, separate articulation between the trapezium bone and the base of the first metacarpal bone. Also *carpometacarpal articulation of thumb, first carpometacarpal articulation.* **a. cartilaginea** A type of joint in which the adjacent bony surfaces or margins are united by intervening cartilage, either hyaline or fibrocartilage. Movement is very slight. There are two varieties, namely, synchondrosis and symphysis. Also *junctura cartilaginea, amphiarthrosis* (outmoded), *slightly movable articulation, slightly movable joint, cartilaginous joint.* **articulationes cinguli membri inferioris** The joints of the lower limb, or pelvic, girdle comprising the sacroiliac articulations and the symphysis pubis. Also *articulations of girdle of inferior member, juncturae cinguli membri inferioris.* **articulationes cinguli membri superioris** The joints of the upper limb, or pectoral, girdle comprising the acromioclavicular and sternoclavicular articulations. Also *articulations of girdle of superior member, juncturae cinguli membri superioris.* **a. composita** [NA] A synovial joint in which more than two skeletal elements are involved. Also *composite articulation, composite joint, compound articulation, compound joint.* **a. condylaris** ARTICULATIO ELLIPSOIDEA. **articulationes costochondrales** [NA] The cartilaginous joints between the lateral ends of costal cartilages and the anterior end of their corresponding ribs. Also *costochondral articulations, costochondral joints.* **a. costotransversaria** [NA] A gliding joint between the articular facet on the tubercle of a rib and the articular facet on the corresponding transverse process of a vertebra. This is absent on the eleventh and twelfth ribs. Also *costotransverse articulation, articulation of tubercle of rib, costotransverse joint.* **articulationes costovertebrales** [NA] The joints of the ribs with the vertebral column, comprising articulatio capitis costae and articulatio costotransversaria. Also *costovertebral articulations, costovertebral joints.* **a. coxae** [NA] The ball-and-socket joint between the rounded head of the femur and the cup-shaped acetabulum of the hipbone. Also *articulation of hip, coxal articulation, femoral articulation, hip joint, hip.* **a. cricoarytenoidea** [NA] The synovial joint between the oval articular surface on the base of the arytenoid cartilage and the superior margin of the lamina of the cricoid cartilage, held together by a loose fibrous capsule strengthened by the posterior cricoarytenoid ligament and permitting gliding and rotational movements that produce alterations in the position and tension of the vocal cords. Also *cricoarytenoid articulation, cricoarytenoid joint.* **a. cricothyroidea** [NA] The synovial joint between each inferior cornu of the thyroid cartilage and each side of the cricoid cartilage, each joint having a fibrous capsule and strengthening accessory ligaments. Gliding and rotational movements are permitted, producing changes in position and tension of the vocal cords. Also *cricothyroid articulation, cricothyroid joint.* **a. cubiti** [NA] The compound joint between the distal end of the humerus and the proximal ends of the radius and ulna, comprising the articulatio humeroradialis and the articulatio humeroulnaris. It is continuous with the articulatio radioulnaris proximalis. Also *cubital articulation, cubital joint, articulation of elbow, elbow joint.* **a. cuneocuboidea** [NA] A plane synovial joint that is situated between the relatively flat adjacent cartilage-covered surfaces of the lateral cuneiform and cuboid bones. The articular capsule and synovial cavity are continuous with those of the cuneonavicular joint. The bones are connected by plantar, dorsal, and interosseous ligaments. This joint, as well as the articulations between the cuneiform bones, may be considered part of the cuneonavicular articulation, as one articular capsule and cavity is common to all. Movement is limited to a small amount of gliding and rotation during inversion and eversion of the foot. Also *cuneocuboid joint.* **a. cuneonavicularis** [NA] The compound plane joint between the distal surface of the navicular bone and the proximal surfaces of the three cuneiform bones. Also *cuneonavicular articulation, cuneonavicular joint.* **a. ellipsoidea** [NA] A biaxial joint that has an oval convex surface articulating with an oval concavity, as in the radiocarpal joint. Also *ellipsoidal articulation, ellipsoidal joint, articulatio condylaris.* **a. fibrosa** A joint in which the opposing bony surfaces or margins are very close together, being united by intervening fibrous tissue or ligament, and in which no appreciable movement is permitted. There are three varieties, namely, syndesmosis, sutura, and gomphosis. Also *junctura fibrosa, synarthrosis, immovable joint, immovable articulation.* **a. genus** [NA] A compound condylar joint comprising two condyloid joints between the two femoral condyles and the superior articular surfaces of the tibia with the intervening menisci, as well as the articulation between the patella and the patellar surface of the femur. Also *articulation of knee, knee joint.* **a. humeri** [NA] The simple spheroid joint between the hemispherical head of the humerus and the shallow, concave glenoid cavity of the scapula. Also *articulation of shoulder, articulation of humerus, shoulder joint.* **a. humeroradialis** [NA] The simple, spheroid portion of the cubital articulation that involves the capitulum of humerus articulating with the depression on the head of radius. Also *humeroradial articulation, humeroradial joint.* **a. humeroulnaris** [NA] The simple, hinge portion of the cubital articulation that involves the trochlea of humerus articulating with the trochlear notch of ulna. Also *humeroulnar articulation, humeroulnar joint.* **a. incudomallearis** [NA] The saddle-shaped joint between the elliptical facet on the head of the malleus and the body of the incus, situated in the epitympanic recess. Also *incudomalleolar articulation, incudomalleolar joint.* **a. incudostapedia** [NA] A ball-and-socket joint between the rounded lentiform process of the long process of the incus and the hollowed head of the stapes, enclosed by a fibroelastic capsule lined by synovial membrane. Also *incudostapedial articulation, incudostapedial joint.* **articulationes intercarpales** [NA] The joints between and within the proximal and distal rows of carpal bones. Also *intercarpal articulations, intercarpal joints.* **articulationes interchondrales** [NA] The simple plane joints between the fifth through tenth costal cartilages, in series at their contiguous surfaces where they bend upward toward the sternum. Also *interchondral articulations of ribs, intercostal articulations, interchondral joints.* **articulationes intercuneiformes** [NA] The plane synovial joints between the relatively flat, apposed articular surfaces of the three cuneiform bones of the foot. Their articular capsules and synovial cavities are continuous with the cuneocuboid and cuneonavicular joints. The bones are held together by plantar, dorsal, and interosseous ligaments. Movements are limited to some gliding and rotation on each other during inversion and eversion of the foot. Also *intercuneiform joints.* **articulationes intermetacarpales** [NA] The simple plane joints between the adjacent sides of the bases of the second through fifth metacarpal bones. Also *intermetacarpal articulations, articulations of metacarpal bones, intermetacarpal joints.* **articulationes intermetatarsales** [NA] The simple plane joints between the adjacent sides of the bases of the five metatarsal bones. Also *intermetatarsal articulations, articulations of metatarsal bones.* **articulationes interphalangeales manus** [NA] The simple hinge joints between the phalanges of each finger. Also *interphalangeal articulations of hand, interphalangeal articulations of fingers, articulations of digits of hand, articulations of fingers.* **articulationes interphalangeales pedis** [NA] The simple hinge joints between the phalanges of each toe. Also *interphalangeal articulations of foot, interphalangeal articulations of toes, articulations of digits of foot, articulations of toes.* **articulationes intertarseae** The joints that unite the tarsal bones, comprising the subtalar articulation, talocalcaneonavicular articulation, calcaneocuboid articulation, and cuneonavicular articulation. Also *intertarsal articulations, tarsal joints.* **a. lumbosacralis** [NA] The joint between the bodies of the fifth lumbar vertebra and the first sacral vertebra, united by a thick, wedge-shaped intervertebral disk to which the anterior and posterior longitudinal ligaments are fused. The joint is strengthened by the ligamenta flava and the supraspinous and interspinous ligaments, which are also associated with the right and left zygapophysial joints between the two bones. Also *junctura lumbosacralis, lumbosacral joint.* **articulationes manus** The various joints between and within the wrist, carpus, metacarpus, and fingers. Also *articulations of hand.* **a. mediocarpalis** [NA] The compound irregular joint between the distal articular surfaces of the bones of the proximal row of carpal bones and the proximal articular surfaces of the bones of the distal row. Also *mediocarpal articulation, mediocarpal joint, midcarpal joint.* **articulationes membri inferioris liberi** The joints of the bones of the lower limb, comprising the hip, knee, tibiofibular, ankle, and foot joints. Also *articulations of free inferior limb, articulations of free inferior member.* **articulationes membri superioris liberi** The articulations of the bones of the upper limb, comprising the shoulder, elbow, radioulnar, wrist, and hand joints. Also *articulations of free superior member, articulations of free superior limb.* **articulationes metacarpophalangeales** [NA] The simple ellipsoid joints between the oval, concave bases of the proximal phalanges and the rounded heads of the five metacarpal bones. Also *metacarpophalangeal articulations, metacarpophalangeal joints.* **articulationes metatarsophalangeales** [NA] The simple ellipsoid joints between the oval, concave bases of the proximal phalanges and the rounded heads of the five metatarsal bones. Also *metatarsophalangeal articulations, metatarsophalangeal joints.* **articulationes ossiculorum auditus** [NA] Articulatio incudomallearis, articulatio incudostapedia, and syndesmosis tympanostapedia. Also *articulations of auditory ossicles.* **a. ossis pisiformis** [NA] The simple, plane synovial joint between the pisiform bone and the underlying triquetral bone. Also *articulation of pisiform bone, pisocuneiform articulation, pisotriquetral joint.* **articulationes pedis** [NA] The various joints between and within the ankle, tarsus, metatarsus, and toes. Also *articulations of foot.* **a. plana** [NA] A synovial joint that involves opposing articular surfaces that are flat or slightly curved, and that permits mainly gliding movements, such as the intermetatarsal joints. Also *plane articulation, arthrodia, gliding articulation, plane joint, gliding joint, arthrodial joint, adarticulation, planiform diarthrosis.* **a. radiocarpalis** [NA] The biaxial ellipsoid joint between the distal end of the radius and the inferior surface of the articular disk proximally, and the scaphoid, lunate, and triquetral bones distally. Also *radiocarpal articulation, wrist joint, radiocarpal joint.* **a. radioulnaris distalis** [NA] The simple trochoid joint in which the rounded head of the ulna articulates with the ulnar notch of the radius and the head of the ulna abuts distally on an articular disk. Also *distal radioulnar articulation, inferior radioulnar articulation, inferior cubitoradial articulation, inferior radioulnar joint.* **a. radioulnaris proximalis** [NA] The simple trochoid joint in which the circumferential articular surface of the head of the radius articulates with the radial notch of the ulna within the annular ligament of radius. Also *proximal radioulnar articulation, superior radioulnar articulation, superior radioulnar joint.* **a. sacrococcygea** [NA] A symphysis between the lowest piece of the sacrum and the base of the coccyx, with a thin disk of fibrocartilage interposed between them and resembling any other intervertebral joint. Occasionally the disk is replaced by a synovial joint and the coccyx becomes freely movable. The joint is surrounded by ventral, superficial dorsal, deep dorsal, and lateral sacrococcygeal ligaments. Also *sacrococcygeal joint, sacrococcygeal articulation, junctura sacrococcygea, coccygeal joint, sacroccygeal symphysis* (outmoded), *sacrococcygeal synchondrosis* (outmoded). **a. sacroiliaca** [NA] The simple, irregular synchondrosis on each side that binds the lower limb girdle to the axial skeleton at the auricular surfaces of the sacrum and the ilium. Also *sacroiliac articulation, sacroiliac symphysis* (outmoded), *iliosacral articulation, sacroiliac joint.* **a. sellaris** [NA] A synovial joint in which the opposing surfaces are reciprocally concavoconvex, as in the carpometacarpal articulation of the thumb. It is a biaxial joint. Also *sellar articulation, sellar joint, saddle joint, reciprocal articulation, saddle articulation, saddle-shaped joint.* **a. simplex** [NA] A synovial joint in which only two bones participate. Also *simple articulation, simple joint.* **a. spheroidea** [NA] A synovial joint in which a somewhat spherical head of a bone fits into a cup-shaped cavity, permitting multiaxial movement. Examples are the hip and shoulder joints. Also *spheroidal articulation, spheroidal joint, ball-and-socket articulation, ball-and-socket joint, multiaxial joint, polyaxial joints, enarthrodial joint, enarthrosis.* **a.**

**sternoclavicularis** [NA] The somewhat saddle-shaped gliding joint formed by the medial end of the clavicle, the superolateral clavicular notch of the manubrium sterni, and the cartilage of the first rib. The joint is completely divided by an articular disk. Also *sternoclavicular articulation, sternoclavicular joint.* **articulationes sternocostales** [NA] The joints between the medial ends of the costal cartilages of the true, or first seven, ribs and the concavities on the lateral margins of the sternum. The first cartilage is joined by a synchondrosis, but the remainder are joined by synovial joints, the cavities of which are often absent especially in the lower joints. The articular surfaces are covered by fibrocartilage and are held together by fibrous capsules fused to the radiate sternocostal ligaments as well as by intra-articular ligaments. The seventh costal cartilage also has anterior and posterior costoxiphoid ligaments. Gliding movements provide considerable mobility during respiration. Also *sternocostal articulations, costosternal articulations, sternochondral articulations, chondrosternal articulations, sternocostal joints.* **a. subtalaris** [NA] A simple ellipsoid and gliding joint between the concave posterior calcaneal facet on the inferior surface of the talus and the convex posterior facet on the upper surface of the calcaneus. Also *subtalar articulation, articulatio talocalcanea, calcaneoastragaloid articulation, posterior talocalcanean joint, subtalar joint.* **a. synovialis** A joint that is usually freely mobile and has the contiguous bony surfaces covered by hyaline cartilage, and occasionally fibrocartilage, held together by a fibrous capsule lined inside by a synovial membrane and strengthened outside by ligaments. In some locations the joint is completely or partially divided by a synovium-lined articular disk, or meniscus. Occasionally a bony surface within the capsule is deepened by a rim of fibrocartilage, or labrum. The bony surfaces are characterized by a low coefficient of friction, their movements being facilitated by a nutrient lubricant, or synovial fluid. This type of joint includes most of the joints of the body and is divided into several varieties, both simple and complex, according to the shapes of the articular surfaces and the kind of movements permitted. Also *synovial joint, synovial articulation, junctura synovialis, diarthrosis, freely movable joint, freely movable articulation, abarthrosis, diarthrodial joint, perarticulation.* **a. talocalcanea** ARTICULATIO SUBTALARIS. **a. talocalcaneonavicularis** [NA] A compound, multiaxial joint in which the rounded head of the talus articulates with the posterior concave surface of the navicular bone, while the anterior and middle calcaneal facets on the inferior surface of neck and head of talus fit on corresponding articular facets on the upper surface of the calcaneus and on the upper surface of the plantar calcaneonavicular ligament. Also *talocalcaneonavicular articulation, talocalcaneonavicular joint, anterior talocalcanean joint.* **a. talocruralis** [NA] A compound hinge joint in which the malleolar articular surface of the fibula, the inferior and malleolar articular surfaces of the tibia, and the inferior transverse tibiofibular ligament form a deep socket that receives the body of the talus. Also *talocrural joint, talocrural articulation, talotibiofibular joint, ankle joint, mortise joint, ankle.* **a. talonavicularis** The ellipsoid joint between the talus bone and the navicular bone, a portion of the transverse tarsal joint. Also *talonavicular articulation.* **a. tarsi transversa** [NA] A compound, irregular joint formed by the talonavicular portion of the talocalcaneonavicular articulation and the calcaneocuboid joint. The two joints are usually separated but the distal bones move as a unit on the proximal ones. Also *transverse tarsal articulation, transverse tarsal joint, Chopart's articulation, Chopart's joint, midtarsal joint.* **articulationes tarsometatarsales** [NA] Three plane joints between the bones of the tarsus and the metatarsus, comprising a medial joint between the medial cuneiform and first metatarsal bones; an intermediate joint between the intermediate and lateral cuneiform bones proximally and the second and third metatarsal bones distally; and a lateral joint between the cuboid bone proximally and the fourth and fifth metatarsal bones distally. Also *tarsometatarsal articulations, Lisfranc's joints, cuneometatarsal joints, tarsometatarsal joints.* **a. temporomandibularis** [NA] A compound condylar joint formed by the articular tubercle and anterior portion of the mandibular fossa of the temporal bone superiorly and the condyle of the mandible inferiorly. An articular disk divides the joint into separate upper and lower parts. The movements of this articulation are combinations of hinge and sliding motion. Rotational movements involve the joints of both sides acting synchronously. Together they act as a bicondylar joint. Also *temporomandibular articulation, temporomandibular joint, mandibular articulation, jaw joint, mandibular joint.* **articulationes thoracis** [NA] Numerous joints situated between the ribs and the vertebral column and the sternum as well as between some of the ribs themselves and between the manubrium, body, and xiphoid process of the sternum. They include articulationes costovertebrales, articulatio capitis costae, articulatio costotransversaria, articulationes sternocostales, articulationes costochondrales, articulationes interchondrales, and synchondroses sternales. Also *joints of thorax.* **a. tibiofibularis** **1** [NA] A simple plane joint between the articular surface of the head of the fibula and the fibular facet on the lateral condyle of the tibia. Also *superior tibiofibular joint.* **2** A syndesmosis tibiofibularis that receives an occasional upward extension of the articular cavity of the talocrural articulation. For defs. 1 and 2 also *tibiofibular articulation, tibiofibular joint.* **a. trochoidea** [NA] A uniaxial joint in which either a central bony cylinder rotates within a surrounding osteoligamentous ring, as in the proximal radioulnar joint, or the ring rotates around the cylinder, as in the median atlantoaxial joint. Also *trochoid articulation, trochoid joint, pivot articulation, pivot joint, rotary joint, helicoid ginglymus, lateral ginglymus, diarthrosis rotatoria, trochoides.* **articulationes vertebrales** [NA] The numerous joints situated between the various components of the vertebral column, namely, articulationes zygapophysiales, articulatio lumbosacralis, articulatio sacrococcygea, and symphysis intervertebralis. Also *joints of the vertebral column.* **articulationes zygapophysiales** [NA] Synovial joints of the plane variety between the articular processes of adjoining vertebrae, held together by fibrous capsules. The accessory ligaments include ligamenta flava, interspinous, supraspinous, and intertransverse ligaments between the laminae, spines, and transverse processes of the vertebrae. Also *juncturae zygapophyseales, zygapophysial joints, interarticular joints.*

# articulation

**articulation** \ärtik′yəlā′shən\ [L *articulatio.* See ARTICULATIO.] **1** A movable or fixed joint between bones. Also *syntaxis.* **2** See under DENTAL ARTICULATION. **3** The movements of oral and pharyngeal speech apparatus in the production of speech sounds. Compare PHONATION. **acromioclavicular a.** ARTICULATIO ACROMIOCLAVICULA-

RIS. **atlanto-occipital a.** ARTICULATIO ATLANTO-OCCIPITALIS. **atloid a.** The attachment of the base of the skull to the spinal column. **a.'s of auditory ossicles** ARTICULATIONES OSSICULORUM AUDITUS. **balanced a.** BALANCED OCCLUSION. **ball-and-socket a.** ARTICULATIO SPHEROIDEA. **calcaneoastragaloid a.** ARTICULATIO SUBTALARIS. **calcaneocuboid a.** ARTICULATIO CALCANEOCUBOIDEA. **capitular a.** ARTICULATIO CAPITIS COSTAE. **carpal a.'s** ARTICULATIONES CARPI. **carpometacarpal a.'s** ARTICULATIONES CARPOMETACARPALES. **carpometacarpal a. of thumb** ARTICULATIO CARPOMETACARPALIS POLLICIS. **chondrosternal a.'s** ARTICULATIONES STERNOCOSTALES. **Chopart's a.** ARTICULATIO TARSI TRANSVERSA. **cochlear a.** COCHLEAR JOINT. **composite a.** ARTICULATIO COMPOSITA. **compound a.** ARTICULATIO COMPOSITA. **condylar a.** ARTICULATIO BICONDYLARIS. **congruent a.** A joint in which the opposing surfaces correspond in curvature and form. **costocentral a.** ARTICULATIO CAPITIS COSTAE. **costochondral a.'s** ARTICULATIONES COSTOCHONDRALES. **costosternal a.'s** ARTICULATIONES STERNOCOSTALES. **costotransverse a.** ARTICULATIO COSTOTRANSVERSARIA. **costovertebral a.'s** ARTICULATIONES COSTOVERTEBRALES. **coxal a.** ARTICULATIO COXAE. **craniovertebral a.** ARTICULATIO ATLANTO-OCCIPITALIS. **cricoarytenoid a.** ARTICULATIO CRICOARYTENOIDEA. **cricothyroid a.** ARTICULATIO CRICOTHYROIDEA. **cubital a.** ARTICULATIO CUBITI. **cuneonavicular a.** ARTICULATIO CUNEONAVICULARIS. **dental a.** The relationship of occluding surfaces of the mandibular teeth, whether natural or artificial, with those of the maxillary teeth during jaw movement. Also *dynamic occlusion, gliding occlusion*. **a.'s of digits of foot** ARTICULATIONES INTERPHALANGEALES PEDIS. **a.'s of digits of hand** ARTICULATIONES INTERPHALANGEALES MANUS. **distal radioulnar a.** ARTICULATIO RADIOULNARIS DISTALIS. **a. of elbow** ARTICULATIO CUBITI. **ellipsoidal a.** ARTICULATIO ELLIPSOIDEA. **false a.** PSEUDARTHROSIS. **femoral a.** ARTICULATIO COXAE. **a.'s of fingers** ARTICULATIONES INTERPHALANGEALES MANUS. **first carpometacarpal a.** ARTICULATIO CARPOMETACARPALIS POLLICIS. **a.'s of foot** ARTICULATIONES PEDIS. **a.'s of free inferior limb** ARTICULATIONES MEMBRI INFERIORIS LIBERI. **a.'s of free inferior member** ARTICULATIONES MEMBRI INFERIORIS LIBERI. **freely movable a.** ARTICULATIO SYNOVIALIS. **a.'s of free superior limb** ARTICULATIONES MEMBRI SUPERIORIS LIBERI. **a.'s of free superior member** ARTICULATIONES MEMBRI SUPERIORIS LIBERI. **a.'s of girdle of inferior member** ARTICULATIONES CINGULI MEMBRI INFERIORIS. **a.'s of girdle of superior member** ARTICULATIONES CINGULI MEMBRI SUPERIORIS. **gliding a.** ARTICULATIO PLANA. **a.'s of hand** ARTICULATIONES MANUS. **a. of head of rib** ARTICULATIO CAPITIS COSTAE. **hinge a.** GINGLYMUS. **a. of hip** ARTICULATIO COXAE. **humeroradial a.** ARTICULATIO HUMERORADIALIS. **humeroulnar a.** ARTICULATIO HUMEROULNARIS. **a. of humerus** ARTICULATIO HUMERI. **iliosacral a.** ARTICULATIO SACROILIACA. **immovable a.** ARTICULATIO FIBROSA. **incongruent a.** A joint articulation that has irregular surfaces. **incudomalleolar a.** ARTICULATIO INCUDOMALLEARIS. **incudostapedial a.** ARTICULATIO INCUDOSTAPEDIA. **inferior cubitoradial a.** ARTICULATIO RADIOULNARIS DISTALIS. **inferior radioulnar a.** ARTICULATIO RADIOULNARIS DISTALIS. **intercarpal a.'s** ARTICULATIONES INTERCARPALES. **interchondral a.'s of ribs** ARTICULATIONES INTERCHONDRALES. **intercostal a.'s** ARTICULATIONES INTERCHONDRALES. **intermetacarpal a.'s** ARTICULATIONES INTERMETACARPALES. **intermetatarsal a.'s** ARTICULATIONES INTERMETATARSALES. **interphalangeal a.'s of fingers** ARTICULATIONES INTERPHALANGEALES MANUS. **interphalangeal a.'s of foot** ARTICULATIONES INTERPHALANGEALES PEDIS. **interphalangeal a.'s of hand** ARTICULATIONES INTERPHALANGEALES MANUS. **interphalangeal a.'s of toes** ARTICULATIONES INTERPHALANGEALES PEDIS. **intertarsal a.'s** ARTICULATIONES INTERTARSEAE. **a. of knee** ARTICULATIO GENUS. **lateral atlantoaxial a.** ARTICULATIO ATLANTOAXIALIS LATERALIS. **mandibular a.** ARTICULATIO TEMPOROMANDIBULARIS. **median atlantoaxial a.** ARTICULATIO ATLANTOAXIALIS MEDIANA. **mediocarpal a.** ARTICULATIO MEDIOCARPALIS. **a.'s of metacarpal bones** ARTICULATIONES INTERMETACARPALES. **metacarpocarpal a.'s** ARTICULATIONES CARPOMETACARPALES. **metacarpophalangeal a.'s** ARTICULATIONES METACARPOPHALANGEALES. **a.'s of metatarsal bones** ARTICULATIONES INTERMETATARSALES. **metatarsophalangeal a.'s** ARTICULATIONES METATARSOPHALANGEALES. **occipital a.** ARTICULATIO ATLANTO-OCCIPITALIS. **occipitoatlantal a.** ARTICULATIO ATLANTO-OCCIPITALIS. **patellofemoral a.** FEMOROPATELLAR JOINT. **petro-occipital a.** SYNCHONDROSIS PETRO-OCCIPITALIS. **phalangeal a.'s** Either articulationes interphalangeales manus or articulationes interphalangeales pedis. **a. of pisiform bone** ARTICULATIO OSSIS PISIFORMIS. **pisocuneiform a.** ARTICULATIO OSSIS PISIFORMIS. **pivot a.** ARTICULATIO TROCHOIDEA. **plane a.** ARTICULATIO PLANA. **proximal radioulnar a.** ARTICULATIO RADIOULNARIS PROXIMALIS. **a. of pubis** SYMPHYSIS PUBICA. **radiocarpal a.** ARTICULATIO RADIOCARPALIS. **radioulnar a.** Either articulatio radioulnaris proximalis or articulatio radioulnaris distalis. **reciprocal a.** ARTICULATIO SELLARIS. **sacrococcygeal a.** ARTICULATIO SACROCOCCYGEA. **sacroiliac a.** ARTICULATIO SACROILIACA. **saddle a.** ARTICULATIO SELLARIS. **sellar a.** ARTICULATIO SELLARIS. **a. of shoulder** ARTICULATIO HUMERI. **simple a.** ARTICULATIO SIMPLEX. **slightly movable a.** ARTICULATIO CARTILAGINEA. **spheroidal a.** ARTICULATIO SPHEROIDEA. **sternochondral a.'s** ARTICULATIONES STERNOCOSTALES. **sternoclavicular a.** ARTICULATIO STERNOCLAVICULARIS. **sternocostal a.'s** ARTICULATIONES STERNOCOSTALES. **subtalar a.** ARTICULATIO SUBTALARIS. **superior radioulnar a.** ARTICULATIO RADIOULNARIS PROXIMALIS. **synovial a.** ARTICULATIO SYNOVIALIS. **talocalcaneonavicular a.** ARTICULATIO TALOCALCANEONAVICULARIS. **talocrural a.** ARTICULATIO TALOCRURALIS. **talonavicular a.** ARTICULATIO TALONAVICULARIS. **tarsometatarsal a.'s** ARTICULATIONES TARSOMETATARSALES. **temporomandibular a.** ARTICULATIO TEMPOROMANDIBULARIS. **tibiofibular a.** 1 ARTICULATIO TIBIOFIBULARIS. 2 SYNDESMOSIS TIBIOFIBULARIS. **a.'s of toes** ARTICULATIONES INTERPHALANGEALES PEDIS. **transverse tarsal a.** ARTICULATIO TARSI TRANSVERSA. **trochoid a.** ARTICULATIO TROCHOIDEA. **a. of tubercle of rib** ARTICULATIO COSTOTRANSVERSARIA.

**articulationes** \ärtik′yəlā′shē·ō′nēz\ Plural of ARTICULATIO.

**articulator** \ärtik′yəlā′tər\ A device with a hinge or hinges to simulate the opening and closing of the mouth. Casts of the upper and lower dental arches are attached to the arms of the articulator. Also *dental articulator, occluder.*

**adjustable a.** An anatomic articulator in which all the inclines of the simulated temporomandibular articulation and incisal guide can be altered. **anatomic a.** An articulator that simulates the sliding movements of the temporomandibular articulation as well as the hinge movements. **dental a.** ARTICULATOR. **plain-line a.** An articulator that simulates only the hinge movement of the temporomandibular articulation. Also *hinge articulator.*

**articulatory** \ärtik′yələtôr′ē\ **1** Having to do with the joints or articulations. **2** Pertaining to the enunciation of speech.

**articulo** \ärtik′yəlō\ [L *(in) articulo* at the moment of crisis. *In articulo mortis* means on the brink of death.] A crisis; a turning point. **a. mortis** See under IN ARTICULO MORTIS.

**articulus** \ärtik′yələs\ ARTICULATIO.

**artifact** \är′tifakt\ [a variant of *artefact,* from L *arte* by skill or art, ablative of *ars* art + *factum* a thing made, from neut. sing. of *factus,* past part. of *facere* to make] Any record or image obtained in the course of applying a medical diagnostic technique which is not representative of the structures under study but is adventitious. Adj. artifactual. **mosaic a.** A hexagonally patterned artifact of intercellular material often seen in microscopic examinations of skin scrapings that have been cleaned with potassium hydroxide solution. **pessary ring a.** ANOCHROMASIA. **ring a.** ANOCHROMASIA.

**aryepiglottic** \ar′ē·ep′iglät′ik\ Pertaining to both the arytenoid cartilage and the epiglottis. Also *arytenoepiglottic* (seldom used), *aryepiglottidean.*

**aryepiglottidean** \ar′ē·ep′iglätid′ē·ən\ ARYEPIGLOTTIC.

**-ary** \-erē\ [L*-aria* (fem.), *-arium* (neut.), from *-arius* (masc.), adjectival suffix forming noun suffix] A noun suffix denoting a person or thing connected or associated with.

**aryl** \ar′il\ [*ar(omatic)* + -YL] A group derived from an aromatic hydrocarbon by removal of a hydrogen atom, e.g. phenyl. Thus aniline, Ph—$NH_2$, is an example of an arylamine.

**arylesterase** The enzyme (EC 3.1.1.2) that catalyzes the hydrolysis of acylated phenols. It is found in mammalian tissues.

**arylsulfatase** Any enzyme that catalyzes the hydrolysis of a phenyl sulfate to a phenol and sulfate. They are classified as EC 3.1.6.1, although groups with different specificities exist. Among their substrates are estrogen sulfates, and they occur in mammalian tissues as well as in microorganisms.

**arytena** \ar′itē′nə\ [Gk *arytaina* ladle, vessel used as a liquid measure] A structure shaped like a ladle or pitcher.

**arytenoepiglottic** \arit′ēnō·ep′iglät′ik\ *Seldom used* ARYEPIGLOTTIC.

**arytenoid** \ar′itē′noid\ [Gk *arytainoeidēs* (from *arytain(a)* a ladle + *-eidēs* -like, -OID shaped like or suggestive of ladle] **1** Shaped like a ladle or pitcher. **2** Pertaining to specific cartilages and muscles of the larynx.

**arytenoidectomy** \ar′itēnoidek′təmē\ [ARYTENOID + -ECTOMY] Excision of the arytenoid cartilage, as performed for the relief of bilateral abductor paralysis of the larynx.

**arytenoideus** \ar′itēnoi′dē·əs\ Musculus arytenoideus obliquus and musculus arytenoideus transversus considered together.

**arytenoidopexy** \ar′itənoi′dōpek′sē\ [ARYTENOID + *o* + -PEXY ] An operation for fixing the arytenoid cartilage so as to abduct the vocal cord in cases of bilateral abductor paralysis of the larynx.

**aryvocalis** \ar′ēvōkā′lis\ [*ary(tenoid)* + L *vocalis* vocal] Some deep fibers of the musculus vocalis that are inserted into the vocal ligament. Also *aryvocalis muscle of Ludwig, Ludwig's muscle.*

**AS** **1** aortic stenosis. **2** arteriosclerosis.

**As** astigmatism.

**as** *auris sinistra* (L, left ear).

**as-** \as-, əs-\ AD-.

**asacria** \əsā′krē·ə\ [Gk *a-* priv. + *sacr(um)* + -IA] The developmental absence of the sacrum.

**asafetida** An oleogum resin obtained from the rhizome and roots of *Ferula asafetida* and related members of the family Umbelliferae. The disagreeable odor has been the basis for its use as an animal repellent, but it is also used as a condiment and food flavoring agent, as well as an expectorant in the treatment of bronchitis.

**asbestiform** \asbes′tifôrm\ Characterized by an asbestoslike fibrous structure.

**asbestos** \asbes′təs\ [L (from Gk, not quenched, unquenchable, from *a-* priv. + *sbestos* quenched) an unquenchable mineral, apparently confused with Gk *amiantos lithos* an incombustible mineral, asbestos] A fibrous silicate which occurs naturally in two forms, as amphiboles (such as crocidolite asbestos) and as serpentines (such as chrysotile), which are widely used in making tiles, roofing, gutters, etc., and for insulation and fireproofing. Exposure to asbestos dust can cause asbestosis and lung cancer. The amphiboles are the main cause of mesothelial tumors of the pleura and peritoneum, which are highly malignant and invariably fatal. **blue a.** CROCIDOLITE ASBESTOS. **chrysotile a.** CHRYSOTILE. See under ASBESTOS. Also *white asbestos.* **crocidolite a.** A form of asbestos having a lavender blue color and fibers that can be spun. It is regarded as the main cause of mesothelial tumors, which are invariably fatal. Its use in industry has been severely restricted because of its carcinogenicity. Also *blue asbestos.* **white a.** CHRYSOTILE.

**asbestosis** \as′bestō′sis\ Bilateral, diffuse, interstitial fibrosis of the lungs resulting from inhalation of asbestos fibers. It has a delayed onset after years of exposure and is characterized by dyspnea, finger clubbing, and bilateral crepitations heard at the lung bases. Also *amianthosis, asbestos pneumoconiosis.*

**ascariasis** \as′kərī′əsis\ [*Ascar(is)* + -IASIS] Disease resulting from infection with ascarid worms, especially members of the species *Ascaris lumbricoides.* Infestation of the gastrointestinal tract may produce nonspecific symptoms, especially diarrhea and anorexia. As part of the life cycle of the worm involves passage through the lung, a pneumonia with eosinophilia may occur. Treatment with pyrantel pamoate or mebendazole is generally successful. Also *ascariosis.*

**ascaricide** A drug or agent destructive of intestinal roundworms of the genus *Ascaris.* Also *lumbricide* (obs.).

**ascarid** \as′kərid\ [Gk *askar(is)* intestinal worm + -ID[1]] **1** Of or belonging to the family Ascarididae. **2** A nematode of the family Ascarididae.

**Ascaridae** \asker′idē\ ASCARIDIDAE.

**Ascarididae** \as′kerid′idē\ [ASCARID + -IDAE] An important family of large nematodes parasitizing the small intestines of man and other mammals and of birds. Genera of medical or veterinary interest include *Ascaris, Toxocara, Parascaris, Lagochilascaris,* and *Toxascaris.*. Also *Ascaridae.*

**ascariosis** \as′kerē·ō′sis\ ASCARIASIS.

***Ascaris*** \as′kəris\ [Gk *askaris* intestinal worm] A genus of large, heavy-bodied nematodes parasitic in the small intestine of man and other vertebrates. The life cycle is direct via infectious eggs with no intermediate host being required. About 15 species have been described from mammals. ***A. lumbricoides*** The giant intestinal roundworm of man, one of the most widely prevalent of human helminths, occurring in tropical as well as many temperate regions of the world. Light infection is usually asymptomatic, but moderate to severe burdens may cause loss of appetite, as well as colic and nervous symptoms. The abdomen protrudes in heavy infections, particularly in children. Adult worms may be stimulated to migrate up the esophagus, into orifices such as the ampulla of Vater, or through an eroded portion of the gut wall. ***A. vermicularis*** *Older term* ENTEROBIUS VERMICULARIS.

**ascendens** \asen′dəns\ [L, pres. part. of *ascendere* to ascend] Moving upward; ascending.

**ascensus** \asen′səs\ [L, a going up, place for ascending] An ascent; an abnormally high position. **a. uteri** An abnormally high position of the uterus.

**ascertainment** \as′ərtān′mənt\ The method of locating or selecting individuals (probands) or families having a particular heritable trait. **complete a.** Any method of ascertainment that identifies all individuals or families having a particular genetic trait in a population. Also *complete selection.* **incomplete a.** Any method of ascertainment that identifies some but not all individuals having a particular genetic trait in a given population. Incompleteness may be: an integral feature of a study due to large population size, in which case random sampling techniques are used; a consequence of insensitivity of detection methods or noncooperation of individuals at risk; or a result of inadequate study design. Examples are truncate ascertainment, single ascertainment, and multiple ascertainment. Also *incomplete selection.* **multiple a.** Any selection process in which more than one affected sib may be detected, but not all affected individuals are probands. It is a situation intermediate to truncate and single ascertainment. Also *multiple selection.* **single a.** Any method of identifying families affected by a rare (usually recessive) heritable condition in which the probability of detecting the family is proportionate to the number of affected individuals in the sibship. Also *single selection.* **truncate a.** A method of ascertainment that identifies only families having at least one person having a particular genetic trait. The probability of a family being detected is independent of its size and of the number of affected sibs. Also *truncate selection.*

**Asch** [Morris Joseph *Asch*, U.S. laryngologist, 1833–1902] See under FORCEPS, SPLINT.

**Ascher** [Karl Wolfgang *Ascher*, Czech-born U.S. ophthalmologist, 1887–1971] See under SYNDROME.

**Aschheim** [Selmar *Aschheim*, German obstetrician and gynecologist, 1878–1965] Aschheim-Zondek hormone. See under LUTEINIZING HORMONE.

**Aschner** [Bernhardt *Aschner*, Austrian physician, 1883–1960] Aschner's reflex, Aschner's phenomenon. See under OCULOCARDIAC REFLEX.

**Aschoff** [Ludwig *Aschoff*, German pathologist, 1866–1942] **1** Rokitansky-Aschoff sinuses of the gallbladder. See under SINUS. **2** Aschoff cell. See under CELL. **3** Aschoff's node, node of Aschoff and Tawara. See under NODUS ATRIOVENTRICULARIS. **4** Aschoff's nodules. See under ASCHOFF BODIES.

**ascia** \as′ē·ə\ [L, an axe (the bandage so called from the shape of the folds)] A reversed spiral bandage.

**ASCII** [*A(merican) S(tandard) C(ode for) I(nformation) I(nterchange)*] A 7-bit computer code for transmitting a set of 128 characters including upper- and lowercase letters, numerals, special symbols, and control codes.

**ascites** \əsī′tēz\ [Late L, from Gk *askitēs* dropsy, ascites, from *askos* a leather bag, wineskin, paunch] The intraperitoneal accumulation of watery fluid in the nature of a transudate, with a specific gravity of approximately 1.010 and a protein content of less than 3 percent. It is most commonly a complication of cirrhosis of the liver, and has a complex pathogenesis that includes portal hypertension, hypoalbuminemia, and retention of sodium and water. The abdomen may be greatly distended by the accumulation of many liters of fluid and the patient will have breathing difficulty. Also *abdominal dropsy, peritoneal dropsy, hydroperitoneum, seroperitoneum.* **bile a.** CHOLEPERITONEUM. **bloody a.** HEMORRHAGIC ASCITES. **chyliform a.** CHYLOPERITONEUM. **chylous a.** CHYLOPERITONEUM. **dialysis a.** A persistent ascites of unknown etiology that occurs during the course of chronic hemodialysis. Ascites also may occur during chronic peritoneal dialysis, usually subsiding weeks to months after the patient is switched to hemodialysis. **exudative a.** Ascites in which the fluid is not a transudate but an exudate. **fatty a.** CHYLOPERITONEUM. **gelatinous a.** Ascites associated with mucinous tumors of the ovary. **hemorrhagic a.** Ascites in which the fluid is grossly bloody. This is seen when the patient suffers from a bleeding diathesis or has a metastatic cancer invading the peritoneal cavity. Also *bloody ascites.* **hydremic a.** Ascites in which the fluid is unusually watery. It may occur in cases of malnutrition with severe hypoproteinemia. **milky a.** CHYLOPERITONEUM. **nephrogenic a.** Ascites caused by a renal disorder, as in the nephrotic syndrome. **a. praecox** Ascites which appears earlier than peripheral edema in constrictive pericarditis. **pseudochylous a.** Ascites characterized by cloudy or milky fluid resembling chyle but containing no lipids. **transudative a.** The typical form of ascites, in which the fluid is a transudate, i.e., has a specific gravity of approximately 1.010.

**ascitic** \əsit′ik\ Pertaining to ascites.

**ascitogenous** \as′ētäj′ənəs\ Causing ascites.

**Ascoli** [Alberto *Ascoli*, Italian serologist, 1877–1957] See under TREATMENT.

**Ascoli** [Maurizio *Ascoli*, Italian pathologist, 1876–1958] **1** Ascoli's reaction. See under TEST. **2** Ascoli's test. See under MIOSTAGMIN REACTION.

**ascorbate** \as′kôrbāt, askôr′bāt\ A substance derived from ascorbic acid.

**ascorbate oxidase** A copper-containing enzyme (EC 1.10.3.3), found in plants, that catalyzes the reaction in which one oxygen molecule oxidizes two molecules of ascorbic acid to dehydroascorbic acid. Also *ascorbic acid oxidase.*

**ascorbic acid** L-*threo*-2,3-Dehydrohexono-1,4-lactone. Its lack in primates and guinea pigs causes the deficiency disease scurvy (hence the name *ascorbic*), but it can be synthesized by most other mammals. It is easily destroyed by oxidation. Biologically it acts as a coreductant in several oxidations that use molecular oxygen. One of these is involved in forming the cross-links of collagen, and this is deficient in scurvy. It occurs in high concentrations in citrus fruits. In the animal body its concentration is high in the adrenal cortex, and it is discharged into the blood when steroid hormones are secreted under the influence of adrenocorticotropin. See also VITAMIN C.

**ascorbic acid oxidase** ASCORBATE OXIDASE.

**ascorbyl palmitate** L-Ascorbic acid-6-palmitate. An ester derivative of ascorbic acid that is more lipid-soluble than ascorbic acid but has the same reductive properties as the vitamin. These physical properties of the ester extend the range of applications of ascorbic acid as a preservative and antioxidant.

**ascosin** An antibiotic produced by *Streptomyces canescens*, with activity against yeasts and some filamentous fungi but none against bacteria.

**ASD** atrial septal defect.

**-ase** [by analogy from *diastase*, the prototype of enzymes. See DIASTASE.] A suffix indicating an enzyme. Added to the name of a substance it usually indicates an enzyme that hydrolyzes that substance. Thus proteinases hydrolyze proteins and asparaginase hydrolyzes asparagine.

**asecretory** \asē′krətôr′ē\ Not secreting.

**asemia** \āsē′mē·ə\ [Gk *a-* priv. + *sēm(a)* sign + -IA] Inability to use or to understand signs, gestures, or written or printed language. This disorder may be due to a lesion of the cerebral cortex or psychogenic in origin. It is a combination of amimia and alexia. *Outmoded.*

**asemognosia** \ā′semägnō′zhə\ [Gk *a-* priv. + *sēm(a)* sign + *gnōs(is)* knowledge + -IA] LOGAGNOSIA.

**asepsis** \əsep′sis\ [Gk *a-* priv. + SEPSIS] **1** The absence of microorganisms from a given environment. **2** The use of measures aimed at avoiding the contamination of previously disinfected objects, substances, persons, and places, such as operating theaters.

**aseptate** \āsep′tāt\ [Gk *a-* priv. + SEPTATE] Lacking septa, or dividing walls, as in fungal hyphae.

**aseptic** \əsep′tik\ [Gk *a-* priv. + SEPTIC] Characterized by asepsis; free of infective agents.

**aseptic acid** A mixture of boric acid, hydrogen peroxide, and salicylic acid in water, formerly used as an antiseptic solution.

**asexual** \āsek′shoo·əl\ [Gk *a-* priv. + SEXUAL] Having a sexless form of reproduction; without sex.

**AsH** Symbol for hyperopic astigmatism.

**ash** [Old English *asce*, akin to L *arere* to be dry, become dry] The residue of minerals and their oxides that remains after the combustion of biologic or other materials.

**ASHD** arteriosclerotic heart disease.

**Asherman** [Joseph G. *Asherman*, Czech gynecologist, born 1889] See under SYNDROME.

**ashing** \ash′ing\ The process of converting an organic substance into inorganic materials as a prelude to analyzing its content of certain elements. It is often done "wet," or in solution, as by treating with sulfuric acid and oxidizing agents.

**asialia** \ā′sī·ā′lyə\ [Gk *a-* priv. + SIAL- + -IA] Absence of saliva. Also *aptyalia, aptyalism.*

**asiderosis** \ā′sidərō′sis\ [Gk *a-* priv. + *sider(o)-* + -OSIS] A marked, abnormal decrease of iron deposits in the body.

**as-if** See under AS-IF PERSONALITY.

**asjike** \äsjī′kē\ BERIBERI.

**Askanazy** [Max *Askanazy*, German pathologist, 1865–1940] Askanazy cell. See under HÜRTHLE CELL.

**ASL** antistreptolysin.

**AsM** Symbol for myopic astigmatism.

**Asn** Symbol for asparagine.

**ASO** **1** arteriosclerosis obliterans. **2** antistreptolysin O.

**asoma** \āsō′mə\ [Gk *a-* priv. + SOMA] (*pl.* asomata) A fetus or embryo with a rudimentary or formless body attached to a recognizable but often abnormal head. Also *asomus.*

**asomata** \āsō′mətə\ Plural of ASOMA.

**asomatognosia** \āsō′mətägnō′zhə\ [Gk *a-* priv. + SOMATO- + Gk *gnōs(is)* knowledge + -IA] Inability of a patient to recognize a part of his body, such as a paralyzed limb, as belonging to him. Compare DYSSOMATOGNOSIA.

**asomus** \āsō′məs\ (*pl.* asomata) ASOMA.

**asonia** \āsō′nē·ə\ [Gk *a-* priv. + L *son(us)* a sound, note + -IA] AMUSIA.

**Asp** Symbol for aspartic acid.

**asp** [L and Gk *asp(is)* asp] Any of several small, venomous Old World snakes in the family Viperidae, including the Egyptian asp (*Cerastes vipera*) and the European asp (*Vipera aspis*).

**aspalasoma** \as′paləsō′mə\ [Gk *aspala(x)* mole rat + SOMA] A fetus or embryo with eventration of the lower abdomen combined with a condition resembling exstrophy of the bladder in which the digestive, urinary, and sexual organs open separately.

**asparaginase** An enzyme (EC 3.5.1.1) that hydrolyzes asparagine to aspartic acid and ammonia. It is used in the treatment of leukemia, because it destroys asparagine, which is required by mammalian cells, especially when they are growing rapidly.

**asparagine** $NH_2$—CO—$CH_2$—CH($NH_2$)COOH. One of the 20 amino acids incorporated into proteins. It occurs in high concentration as free amino acid in many plants. It is not essential in the diet, as it is easily made from oxaloacetate.

**aspartame** \aspär′tām, as′pərtām\ The dipeptide ester Asp-Phe-OMe. It has a much sweeter taste than sucrose and is used as an artificial sweetener. When heated it develops a sour taste and so cannot be used for cooking or baking but is ideally suited for warm or cold foods and beverages.

**aspartate** Any of the salts, ions, or esters of aspartic acid, especially the ion predominating in neutral solution, $^-$OOC—$CH_2$—CH(—$NH_3^+$)—$COO^-$. The aspartate residue is the deprotonated form of the aspartic residue, and is —NH—CH(—$CH_2$—$COO^-$)—CO—. **a. family** The amino acids that derive all or part of their carbon from aspartate. They include methionine, homoserine, threonine, diaminopimelate, and (in bacteria) lysine.

**aspartate aminotransferase** The enzyme (EC 2.6.1.1) that catalyzes the reaction of aspartate with 2-oxoglutarate to give glutamate and oxaloacetate. It contains pyridoxal phosphate. Its concentration in blood may be raised in liver and heart diseases that are associated with damage to those tissues. Also *glutamate oxaloacetate transaminase* (previous name).

**aspartate carbamoyltransferase** The enzyme (EC 2.1.3.2) that catalyzes transfer of a carbamoyl group from carbamoyl phosphate onto the amino group of aspartate. The reaction is a step in pyrimidine synthesis and is inhibited by CTP. Also *aspartate transcarbamylase.*

**aspartate kinase** The enzyme (EC 2.7.2.4) that catalyzes transfer of a phospho group from ATP to aspartate, forming 4-phosphoaspartate. This reaction makes possible the subsequent reduction of the acyl group to form phosphate and aspartate semialdehyde, a precursor in the biosynthesis of threonine, lysine, methionine and isoleucine in bacteria. Also *aspartokinase.*

**aspartate transcarbamylase** ASPARTATE CARBAMOYLTRANSFERASE.

**aspartic acid** HOOC—$CH_2$—CH(—$NH_2$)—COOH. One of the twenty amino acids incorporated in proteins. It is central to amino acid metabolism, being the source of one of the nitrogen atoms in the biosynthesis of urea. It is readily synthesized in the body and is therefore not essential in the diet.

**aspartocin** An antibacterial substance produced by *Streptomyces griseus* that is active against Gram-positive bacteria.

**aspartokinase** ASPARTATE KINASE.

**aspartylglycosaminuria** \aspär′təlglī′kōsam′inoo′rē·ə\ An autosomal recessive defect of glycoprotein catabolism resulting in urinary excretion of 2-acetamido-1-($\beta$′-1-aspartamido)-1,2-dideoxyglucose. The phenotype of homozygotes includes severe mental retardation, coarse facies, cranial asymmetry, scoliosis, periodic hyperactivity, impaired motor function, and vacuolated lymphocytes. The specific enzymopathy is unclear.

**aspect** 1 The surface or part that faces in a specified direction. 2 A particular appearance or look. **dorsal a.** The surface of a structure or of the body that faces towards the dorsum, or back. **ventral a.** The surface of a structure or of the body facing towards the ventral, or front, side of the body.

**asper** \as′pər\ [L, rough, rugged] Rough.

**aspergilli** \as′pərjil′ī\ Plural of ASPERGILLUS.

**aspergillic acid** $C_{12}H_{20}N_2O_2$. 6-Sec-butyl-1-hydroxy-3-isobutyl-2(1*H*)pyrazinone. An antibiotic produced by *Aspergillus flavus* that inhibits the growth of the tubercle bacillus.

**aspergillin** 1 An allomelanin produced by mature spores of *Aspergillus niger.* 2 Any of a number of antibiotic substances isolated from *Aspergillus.* An imprecise and ambiguous term.

**aspergilloma** \as′pərjilō′mə\ A lesion of pulmonary aspergillosis, in which *Aspergillus fumigatus* or *A. niger* grow into a mycelial ball-like mass within a lung cavity, ectatic bronchus, or, less commonly, within the pleural space. Also *fungus ball.*

**aspergillomycosis** \as′pərjil′ōmīkō′sis\ ASPERGILLOSIS.

**aspergillosis** \as′purjilō′sis\ [*Aspergill(us)* + -OSIS] A condition caused by hypersensitivity to or invasive infection with *Aspergillus* species, notably *A. fumigatus* and *A. niger.* Infection may be chronic and granulomatous, or acute and associated with severe necrotizing inflammation. Local hypersensitivity reactions occur especially in the lungs. Also *aspergillomycosis.* **aural a.** Aspergillosis of the ear with one of a number of fungi of the genus *Aspergillus,* especially *A. niger.* The external ear is the site of the disease in the majority of cases. See also OTOMYCOSIS. **pulmonary a.** Infection of the lung with *Aspergillus* fungi. See also ASPERGILLOMA.

**aspergillotoxicosis** \as′pərjil′ōtäk′sikō′sis\ ASPERGILLUS TOXICOSIS.

***Aspergillus*** \as′purjil′əs\ [Med L (from L *aspergere* to sprinkle, scatter), a sprinkler] A form-genus of imperfect fungi (Deuteromycetes) some species of which are known to cause infections in humans and animals. It includes many mold species, some with black spores, as the pathogenic *A. niger,* found in the external auditory meatus; a blue mold in *A. glaucus* on fruit; and yellowish spores by the pathogenic *A. flavescens.* Antibiotics are produced by several species including *A. clavatus* (clavacin), *A. flavus* (aspergillic acid), *A. fumigatus* (fumigacin, fumigatin), *A. parasiticus* (penicillin II), *A. terreus* (citrinin). Several others are pathogenic, but the majority of *Aspergillus* species are harmless molds and contaminants. ***A. flavus*** A species which produces flavotoxins when grown on cereal grains. It has also been implicated as a causal agent of varying kinds of aspergillosis, for example, of the external ear. ***A. fumigatus*** A thermotolerant fungus that is a primary agent of pulmonary aspergillosis. It grows well on compost and cereal grains, creating a hazard for humans, birds, and animals when the spores are inhaled. ***A. parasiticus*** A worldwide species of fungus which often infests peanuts, soybeans, and other cereal grains either when growing or stored as seeds or prepared animal feed. Some strains produce aflatoxins which cause aflatoxicosis in many animal species. The aflatoxins are also considered to be potent causes of liver cancer.

**aspergillus** \as′pərjil′əs\ (*pl.* aspergilli) Any fungus which belongs to the form-genus *Aspergillus.*

**aspermatism** \āspur′mətizm\ [Gk *a-* priv. + SPERMAT- + -ISM] Inability to secrete or inability to ejaculate semen. Also *aspermia.*

**aspermatogenesis** \āspur′mətōjen′əsis\ [Gk *a-* priv. + SPERMATOGENESIS] Failure to produce spermatozoa.

**aspermia** \āspur′mē·ə\ ASPERMATISM.

**asphalgesia** [Gk *asph(e)* them + ALGESIA ] A burning sensation experienced on touching objects while in a hypnotic state.

**asphyctic** \asfik′tik\ Relating to or in a state of asphyxia.

**asphyxia** \asfik′sē·ə\ [Gk (from *a-* priv. + *sphyx(is)* pulse, from *sphyzein* to throb, beat) stoppage of the pulse (which was also its original meaning in English)] Failure or prevention of the respiratory process due either to obstruction of air flow to the lungs or to lack of oxygen in the inspired air. **autoerotic a.** SEXUAL ASPHYXIA. **blue a. in the newborn** The state of an infant who does not breathe spontaneously at birth and is oxygen depleted but sufficiently reactive to respond to stimulation or breathe spontaneously after a variable delay. Also *asphyxia livida.* Compare WHITE ASPHYXIA IN THE NEWBORN. **fetal a.** A condition in which the fetus has an inadequate oxygen supply due to such circumstances as umbilical cord prolapse with compression, placental separation, or the use of certain drugs during labor. Also *intrauterine asphyxia.* **intrauterine a.** FETAL ASPHYXIA. **a. livida** BLUE ASPHYXIA IN THE NEWBORN. **a. neonatorum** The state of an infant who does not breathe spontaneously at birth. *Imprecise.* **a. pallida** WHITE ASPHYXIA IN THE NEWBORN. **sexual a.** Accidental ligature strangulation occurring during autoerotic sexual acts, typically by young males who attempt to induce mild cerebral hypoxia during masturbation by binding their lower extremities, external genitalia, and neck. The cerebral hypoxia is thought to enhance the satisfaction of masturbation. Death occurs when the victim loses consciousness before he can release the ligatures. The weight of the body continues to tighten them, producing asphyxial death by strangulation. Also *autoerotic asphyxia.* **symmetric a.** RAYNAUD'S PHENOMENON. **traumatic a.** Asphyxia resulting from injury, especially that which causes upper airway obstruction or inhalation of blood, vomit, or other material. **white a. in the newborn** The state of an infant who does not breathe spontaneously at birth and is nonreactive, limp, and pallid from vasoconstriction of the skin. Also *asphyxia pallida.* Compare BLUE ASPHYXIA IN THE NEWBORN.

**asphyxiant** \asfik′sē·ənt\ 1 Asphyxiating; asphyxia-producing. 2 An agent capable of causing asphyxia. **chemical a.** Any gas which does not exclude oxygen from the lungs but exerts a chemical action either on the blood, preventing oxygen transportation, or on the tissues, preventing them from using oxygen. Included in this category are carbon monoxide, which acts on the blood, cyanides, which act on the tissues, and hydrogen sulfide, which paralyzes the respiratory center. Chemicals which produce methemoglobinemia and prevent release of oxygen from blood are also considered chemical asphyxiants. **simple a.** Any gas which does not act as a poison but causes asphyxiation by displacing oxygen in the atmosphere. Common simple asphyxiants are nitrogen, methane, helium, and carbon dioxide. They are hazardous only in high concentrations in confined spaces. Some, such as carbon dioxide, have other systemic effects.

**asphyxiate** \asfik′sē·āt\ 1 To bring about asphyxia in. 2 To undergo asphyxia.

**asphyxiation** \asfik′sē·ā′shən\ The process of bringing about or undergoing asphyxia.

**aspidospermine** $C_{22}H_{30}N_2O_2$. 1-Acetyl-17-methoxyaspido-spermidine. A basic compound from the bark of *Aspidosperma quebrachoblanco.* It is used as a respiratory stimulant.

**aspirate** \as′pirāt\ [See ASPIRATION.] **1** To remove by suction. **2** Material obtained by a process of suction.

**aspiration** \as′pirā′shən\ [L *aspiratio* (from *aspiratus,* past part. of *aspirare* to breathe upon) a blowing, respiration] **1** Withdrawal from an enclosed space by the application of a partial vacuum. **2** The act of drawing into the lungs. **endometrial a.** Removal of the endometrial lining of the uterus with a cannula and a device to apply suction. **meconium a.** Aspiration of meconium into the lungs at birth. **vacuum a.** Removal of the uterine contents and the uterine lining with a cannula and a device to apply suction.

**aspirator** \as′pirā′tər\ [*aspirat(e)* + -OR] Any apparatus used to create suction to withdraw material from the body. **Dieulafoy's a.** A syringe fitted with a two-way tap so that fluid may be drawn into the syringe through one channel and expelled through the other.

**aspirin** [German, from *A(zetyl)* acetyl + *Spir(säure)* salicylic acid + -IN] $C_9H_8O_4$. A white crystalline powder commonly used as an analgesic and antipyretic agent. Also *acetylsalicylic acid, acetosal, sulfacetic acid.* **aluminum a.** An aluminum salt containing about 80% aspirin. It is a chewable, more palatable form of aspirin.

**asplenia** [Gk *asplēn(os)* (from *a-* priv. + *splēn* spleen) without spleen + -IA] An absence of the spleen. **functional a.** Loss of splenic function with intact spleen.

**asplenic** \āsplen′ik\ Referring to or characterized by absence of the spleen or of splenic function.

**asporogenic** \as′pôrōjen′ik\ [Gk *a-* priv. + SPORO- + -GENIC] Neither originating from nor forming spores. Also *asporogenous.*

**asporogenous** \as′pôräj′ənəs\ ASPOROGENIC.

**assault** [French *assaut* (from AS- + L *saltus,* past part. of *salire* to leap) action of assailing] **1** A threat or intentional attempt to inflict bodily injury on another. • Technically, the application of force to the body of another with production of injury is *battery.* **2** In medical jurisprudence, any procedure, treatment, or operation performed on a patient without obtaining appropriate informed consent. **criminal a.** An unlawful attempt to inflict bodily injury on another or a threat to inflict bodily injury on another under such circumstances where there is demonstrated ability to execute the threat and the threat produces realistic fear of immediate peril. **felonious a.** An assault of sufficient magnitude and extremity that, if the attempt at or threat of bodily injury were executed, the perpetrator would be subject to the punishment of a felony. **indecent a.** An assault upon a member of the opposite sex in which indecent liberties are taken without the consent of and against the will of the injured party, but without an intent to commit rape.

**assay** [French *essayer* (from L *exagium* a weighing) to make a try at, assay, test] The measurement of the concentration of a substance, especially by specific chemical, enzymatic, or immunologic reaction, or by biologic effect on an organism. **biological a.** BIOASSAY. **competitive protein binding a.** An assay method based on the limited number of binding sites on a carrier substance, and the fact that labeled and unlabeled ligands are equally bound. When the unknown hormone or other substance occupies some of the binding sites, the number of free sites is then often determined, with the help of a radioactive tracer. The difference between the total number of sites and those left free indicates the amount of the unknown substance. **complement binding a.** Any technique in which the concentration of an analyte is determined through its effect on an immunologic reaction whose end point is the initiation of the complement sequence. **enzyme-linked immunosorbent a.** A quantitative technique in which either the antigen or antibody can be measured by using an indicator antibody with an enzyme that has accurately quantifiable activity. The enzyme-tagged indicator antibody can be either an antiglobulin reagent, which attaches to the antibody, or an antibody that is specific for the antigenic material under study. Either the antigen or antibody is fixed to a solid phase immunosorbent, and then allowed to interact with the complementary material. Abbr. ELISA **immune a.** IMMUNOASSAY. **immunoradiometric a.** RADIOIMMUNOASSAY. **Limulus a.** An assay for endotoxin that is based on coagulation of the blood of the horseshoe crab *Limulus polyphemus.* **microbiologic a.** A technique for quantifying metabolically active materials, such as folic acid and vitamins, by measuring their effect on the growth of standardized preparations of microorganisms. **radiometric a.** The quantitative determination of one or more components of a substance by means of a radiolabeled substance introduced into the system. **radioreceptor a.** An *in vitro* test for the presence of receptors on a cell surface, performed by radiolabeling an aliquot of the ligand for which the receptor is specific and measuring the amount of radioactivity that the cell can bind. It is used especially to study actions of hormones or drugs on target cells.

**assembly** / **cell a.** An hypothesized functional organization of neurons serving as a temporary and self-maintained complex circuit, set in motion by repeated experience or practice, and constituting the basic unit of perception or thought. Stimulation of any part of the assembly, whether directly by sensory excitement or indirectly by an associative connection with another such unit, is held to re-establish activity in the whole. **transducer a.** An ultrasonic transducer element and damping and matching materials assembled in a case.

**assessment** / **psychological a.** An evaluation of the level of overall psychological functioning characteristic of an individual through use of psychological tests, observations, inventories, and interviews. The principal components that contribute to overall functioning, such as cognition, motivation, interests, special talents, or limitations, are appraised separately. However, an equal emphasis must be given to their particular configuration or unique synthesis, since behavior as a whole is necessarily cumulative and integrated within a total system.

**assident** \as′idənt\ [L *assidens,* gen. *assidentis,* pres. part. of *assidere* (from *as-* AS- + *sedere* to sit) to sit nearby, be near at hand] Present in most but not all cases of a disease: said of a symptom.

**assimilation** \əsim′əlā′shən\ [L *assimilatio* (from *assimilatus,* past part. of *assimilare* to make like, from AS- + *similis* like) a making alike] **1** The incorporation of substances into tissue following digestion. **2** The learning process whereby newly acquired information about objects, persons, or events is interpreted and understood within the framework of existing knowledge, called schema. **genetic a.** The selection, resulting in genetic fixation, of a phenotype that originally seemed advantageous only in a limited environment.

**assistant** / **dental a.** A person who assists a dentist in the practice of dentistry, performing a variety of functions including clinical, clerical, reception, laboratory, and, usually, radiographic work. Also *dental auxiliary, dental extender* (used only in the United States), *dental surgery assistant* (British usage). • In New Zealand, dental assistants are not permitted to do radiographic work. **dental surgery a.** The British term for DENTAL ASSISTANT. **physician a.** A person specially trained to perform medical tasks, under a physician's supervision, that might otherwise be performed by the physician. Also *physician extender.* Abbr. PA

**Assmann** [Herbert *Assmann,* German internist, 1882–1950] Assmann's tuberculous infiltrate. See under FOCUS.

**association** [Med L *associatio* (from L *associare* to join, from AS- + L *socius* a companion) association] **1** A connection established between two psychological phenomena, such as ideas or feelings, as the result of experience or learning. **2** In statistics, a condition in which two attributes, or values of two variables, occur together either more frequently (positive association) or less frequently (negative association) than would be expected by chance. **3** A group of individuals or collective entities collaborating for a common purpose. **clang a.** A shift in the content of thought based upon the sound of a word rather than its meaning, for example, skipping suddenly from talking about religious preoccupations to talking about experiences in the theater because of the similarity of the sounds "pray" and "play." Also *klang association.* **controlled a.** See under CONTROLLED ASSOCIATION TEST. **free a. 1** The reporting of everything and anything that goes through the mind by a psychoanalytic patient. Dreams, mistakes of everyday life, and apparently nonsensical or irrelevant thoughts provide a rich source of stimuli for associations, which are used by the analyst in making interpretations to the patient. **2** See under FREE ASSOCIATION TEST. **individual practice a.** An arrangement, sometimes a form of health maintenance organization, under which community practitioners participate in a prepaid health care plan and agree to provide services to the plan's enrollees in return for a defined, usually fee-for-service, payment. **klang a.** CLANG ASSOCIATION.

**associus** \əsō′sē·əs\ [L *as-* AS- + *socius* associated] Associated; joined with.

**assortment** [French *assortiment* (from AS- + L *sors,* gen. *sortis,* a part, share) a sorting] During meiosis, the distribution, usually random, to gametes of one chromosome of each pair (in anaphase of the first meiotic division) and one chromatid of each bivalent (in anaphase of the second meiotic division). **independent a.** As described by Mendel's second law, the random distribution of chromosomes, in anaphase of the first meiotic division, or of chromatids, in anaphase of the second meiotic division, relative to the products of meiosis. It brings about the random distribution of nonalleles, but linkage creates a less than completely independent assortment of nonalleles. **random a.** The random segregation at meiotic anaphase of homologues.

**assumption of risk** See under RISK.

**astasia** \astā′zhə\ [Gk *a-* priv. + *stas(is)* + -IA] Inability to stand upright, because of motor incoordination, in the absence of paralysis. This condition is almost always accompanied by abasia. Adj. astatic.

**astasia-abasia** \astā′zhə-abā′zhə\ Astasia accompanied by abasia. Also *abasia-astasia.*

**astatic** \astat′ik\ Relating to astasia.

**astatine** Element number 85, a halogen which was represented by a gap below iodine in the periodic table until it was synthesized in 1940 by bombarding bismuth with alpha particles. Twenty isotopes have been identified, all of them alpha particle emitters, the most stable being astatine 210. The isotopes of mass numbers 215, 217, 218, and 219 exist in nature as products of radioactivity in equilibrium with their parent isotopes of uranium and thorium. It is estimated that less than an ounce is present in the lithosphere at any one time. Chemically, astatine is believed to be very similar to iodine. The reported mass numbers of the isotopes range from 200 to 219, and the half-lives from about .0003 seconds to 8.3 hours. Symbol: At

**asteatosis** \as′tē·ətō′sis\ OLIGOSTEATOSIS.

**aster** [Gk *astēr* a star] **1** A microscopic radiate or star-like formation. **2** The structure with radiating filaments that surrounds the centrosome or centriole of a cell during mitosis or meiosis. Also *kinosphere.* Adj. astral. **sperm a.** Cytoplasm briefly assuming an astral form before retraction in contact with the male pronucleus after fertilization of an ovum. The phenomenon is less apparent in mammals than in other animals.

**astereocognosy** \əstir′ē·əkäg′nəsē\ [Gk *a-* priv. + *stereo(s)* solid, stiff + L *cognos(cere)* to learn, know + -Y] TACTILE AGNOSIA.

**astereognosis** \əstir′ē·ägnō′sis\ [Gk *a-* priv. + STEREO- + Gk *gnōsis* knowledge] TACTILE AGNOSIA.

**asterion** \astir′ē·än\ [Gk *asterion,* neut. of *asterios* (from *astēr* a star) like a star, starry] [NA] The point of meeting of the lambdoid, parietomastoid, and occipitomastoid sutures.

**asterixis** \as′tərik′sis\ [Gk *a-* priv. + *stērixis* (from *stērizein* to be firmly fixed) a fixed position] A form of recurrent tremor of the upper limbs, seen best with the arms held outstretched, and reminiscent of a bird flapping its wings. This is seen particularly in hepatic encephalopathy. Also *flapping tremor, flap.*

**asternal** \āstur′nəl\ **1** Without a sternum. **2** Not related or joined to the sternum.

**asteroid** \as′təroid\ Star-shaped.

**asthenia** \asthē′nē·ə\ [Gk *astheneia* (from *a-* priv. + *sthen(os)* strength + -IA) weakness] A nonspecific symptom characterized by loss of energy and strength and a feeling of weakness. It usually accompanies chronic debilitating conditions such as infectious diseases and cancer. Adj. asthenic. **bulbospinal a.** *Incorrect* MYASTHENIA GRAVIS. **muscle a.** MYASTHENIA. **myalgic a.** BENIGN MYALGIC ENCEPHALOMYELITIS. **neurocirculatory a.** A functional disturbance of the circulatory system, a component of an anxiety state. Features include fatigue, submammary pain, and tachycardia. An imprecise and old fashioned term. Also *effort syndrome, Da Costa syndrome, irritable heart, soldier's heart.* **neurotic a.** NEURASTHENIA.

**asthenic** \asthen′ik\ Characterized by asthenia.

**asthenocoria** \asthē′nəkôr′ē·ə\ [Gk *a-* priv. + STHENO- + *cor(e)-* + -IA] The condition in which the pupillary reflexes are reduced in amplitude or speed; weak contraction of the pupil in response to reflexes such as is seen in adrenal insufficiency. Also *Arroyo sign.*

**asthenopia** \as′thənō′pē·ə\ [Gk *asthen(ēs)* weak + -OPIA] A poorly defined subjective condition in which fatigue or discomfort is attributed to some fault of the eyes, in the absence of obvious organic cause of the symptoms; undue fatigue of apparently healthy eyes. Also *visus debilitas.* Adj. asthenopic.

**asthenospermia** \as′thənōspur′mē·ə\ [Gk *astheno(s)* without strength + SPERM + -IA] Lack of normal motility and vitality of spermatozoa.

**asthma** \az′mə\ [Gk (irreg. from *azein* to pant, breathe hard; akin to *aēnai* to blow) panting, asthma] A usually chronic condition characterized by dyspneic episodes, especially such a condition caused by airway constriction, as bronchial asthma. **allergic a.** Asthma resulting from an allergic reaction to an inhaled substance. **atopic a.** Asthma occurring in an individual who is constitutionally predisposed to develop allergic responses to common environmental substances. **bronchial a.** Asthma resulting from variable narrowing of bronchi and bronchioles due to smooth muscle spasm, inflammation or edema of the bronchial mucous membranes, and overproduction of mucus. Also *spasmodic asthma* (outmoded). **carders' a.** BYSSINOSIS. **cardiac a.** A condition characterized by acute attacks of dyspnea with wheezing, resembling bronchial asthma but resulting from a left-sided cardiac disorder associated with a rise in left atrial and pulmonary venous and capillary pressure. Also *cardiasthma, cardioasthma, Rostan's asthma.* **cotton-dust a.** BYSSINOSIS. **diisocyanate a.** Asthma resulting from inhalation of diisocyanate chemicals. **dust a.** Asthma provoked by inhalation of dust. **Elsner's a.** ANGINA PECTORIS. **essential a.** INTRINSIC ASTHMA. **extrinsic a.** Asthma caused by external or environmental factors. **food a.** Asthma resulting from adverse reactions to foods. **infective a.** Asthma associated with infection. **intrinsic a.** Asthma for which no extrinsic cause can be found. Also *essential asthma.* **isocyanate a.** Asthma resulting from inhalation of isocyanate fumes. **millers' a.** A lung condition caused by exposure to allergens in grain or flour. One recognized cause is the grain weevil, *Sitophilus granarius.*. **miners' a.** An obsolete and incorrect term for COAL WORKERS' PNEUMOCONIOSIS. • The condition was called asthma because sufferers were short of breath **nervous a.** Asthma attributed to emotional causes. **platinum a.** Asthma occurring among workers exposed to the complex salts of platinum during their manufacture or in photographic processing, metal refining, or electroplating. It is an allergic condition associated with rhinitis and urticaria. **pollen a.** Asthma due to inhaled pollens and therefore seasonal. **printers' a.** A condition caused by exposure to gum acacia and other gums sprayed in isopropyl-alcohol solution onto sheets to prevent colors from contaminating the next sheet. The gum is a potent allergen and has caused asthma in as many of 50% of workers exposed. **reflex a.** Asthma caused by a reflex response to a stimulus. **Rostan's a.** CARDIAC ASTHMA. **silo workers' a.** SILO-FILLERS' DISEASE. **spasmodic a.** *Outmoded* BRONCHIAL ASTHMA. **strippers' a.** BYSSINOSIS. **true a.** A dyspneic condition caused by spasmodic airway narrowing (specifically, bronchial asthma) as distinguished from other conditions with which this has sometimes been confused such as emphysema or pneumoconiosis.

**asthmatic** \azmat′ik\ [Gk *asthmatikos* panting, suffering from asthma] Having or relating to asthma.

**asthmatoid** \az′mətoid\ Having characteristics resembling those of asthma.

**astigmatic** \as′tigmat′ik\ Pertaining to or affected by astigmatism.

**astigmatism** \əstig′mətizm\ [Gk *a-* priv. + *stigma*, gen. *stigmat(os)* a mark, spot + -ISM] An optical condition in which the lens system is unable to focus light rays to a point, but rather produces two linear foci at right angles to each other. This is due to unequal spherical strength in different meridians of the lens. Adj. astigmatic. **a. against the rule** Astigmatism in which the section of least curvature is within 30° of vertical. Also *inverse astigmatism.* **compound a.** Astigmatism in which the astigmatic meridians are either both myopic or both hyperopic. **corneal a.** Astigmatism in which astigmatic error is attributable to faults in the cornea. **direct a.** ASTIGMATISM WITH THE RULE. **hyperopic a.** Astigmatism in which one astigmatic meridian is hyperopic and the other is emmetropic or hyperopic. Also *hypermetropic astigmatism.* **inverse a.** ASTIGMATISM AGAINST THE RULE. **irregular a.** The uneven optical distortion resulting when optical surfaces are not uniform spherocylinders. The astigmatic meridians may not be at right angles to each other or one meridian may vary in dioptric strength. **lenticular a.** Astigmatism in which astigmatic error is due to optical faults in the lens of the eye. **mixed a.** Astigmatism in which one astigmatic meridian is myopic and the other is hyperopic. **myopic a.** Astigmatism in which one astigmatic meridian is myopic and the other is emmetropic or myopic. **oblique a.** Astigmatism in which the astigmatic axes lie midway between vertical and horizontal. **regular a.** Astigmatism in which the two astigmatic meridians are at right angles to each other. **retinal a.** A subjective response in which the various visual meridians are of differing clarity, despite full correction of optical astigmatism. This is explained by the hypothesis that photoreceptors are not uniformly distributed. **a. with the rule** Astigmatism in which the section of least curvature is within 30° of horizontal. Also *direct astigmatism.*

**astigmatometer** \as′tigmətäm′ətər\ ASTIGMOSCOPE.

**astigmatometry** \as′tigmətäm′ətrē\ ASTIGMOMETRY.

**astigmatoscope** \as′tigmat′əskōp\ ASTIGMOSCOPE.

**astigmometer** \as′tigmäm′ətər\ ASTIGMOSCOPE.

**astigmometry** \as′tigmäm′ətrē\ [*astigm(atism)* + *o* + -METRY] The measurement of astigmatism by means of an astigmoscope. Also *astigmatometry.*

**astigmoscope** \astig′məskōp\ A device capable of detecting and measuring astigmatism. Also *astigmometer, astigmatometer, astigmatoscope.*

**astomia** \əstō′mē·ə\ [Gk *a-* priv. + STOM- + -IA] The developmental absence of the mouth.

**Aston** [Francis William *Aston*, English physicist and chemist, 1877–1945] See under RULE.

**astr-** \astr-\ ASTRO-.

**astragalar** \astrag′ələr\ [*astragal(us)* + -AR] *Outmoded* TALAR.

**astragalectomy** \as′tragəlek′təmē\ TALECTOMY.

**astragalus** \astrag′ələs\ [Gk *astragalos* any of various bones, esp. the ankle bone] TALUS.

**astringe** [L *astringe(re)* (from *a(d)-*, as intensifying prefix, + *stringere* to draw tight) to bind close, tighten] To display astringent properties and prevent the discharge of a secretion after topical application.

**astringent** [See ASTRINGE.] **1** Having styptic properties, or the ability to stop secretions or bleeding from the skin or tissues. Also *constringent.* **2** An astringent agent.

**astro-** \as′trə-\ [Gk *astron* star] A combining form meaning star, star-shaped.

**astroblast** \as′trəblast\ [ASTRO- + -BLAST] A precursor cell that gives rise to an astrocyte. Also *astrocytoblast.*

**astroblastoma** \-blastō′mə\ [ASTROBLAST + -OMA] A very rare brain tumor composed of cells with the morphology of astroblasts. Astroblastic cells may be seen in astrocytomas and in glioblastomas. The diagnosis of astroblastoma should be restricted to pure growths of this type. There is controversy over this as a clinicomorphologic entity.

**astrocyte** \as′trōsīt′\ [ASTRO- + -CYTE] A cell comprising one of the major categories of neuroglia, characterized by relatively large size, ample cytoplasm, microfilaments, and extensive radiating processes. Astrocytes are found in both the gray and white matter of the central nervous system. Also *Cajal cell, phalangeal cell of Deiters, Deiters cell* (outmoded), *spider cell* (outmoded). Adj. astrocytic. **atypical a.** A modified astrocytic glial cell that is usually

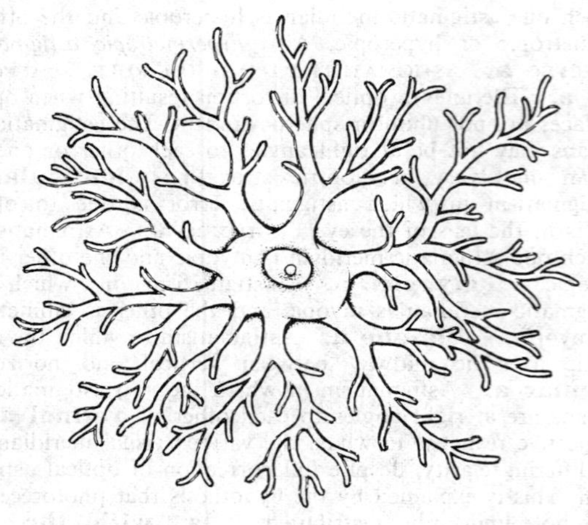
Astrocyte

found in specialized sites such as the cerebellar cortex, the retina, and the posterior lobe of the pituitary. **fibrous a.** Any of the stellate glial cells whose cell bodies and fibrous, filament-possessing processes are found in the white matter of the brain and spinal cord. **protoplasmic a.** 1 An astrocytic glial cell present within the gray matter and possessing numerous cytoplasmic processes ramifying between the neurons, axons, and blood vessels. Also *protoplasmic neuroglia.* 2 A glial cell with swollen, acidophilic cytoplasm and an eccentric nucleus. Such cells are characteristic of injured nervous tissue and certain tumors. Also *gemistocyte, gemistocytic cell.*

**astrocytoblast** \-sī′təblast\ ASTROBLAST.

**astrocytoma** \as′trōsītō′mə\ [*astrocyt(e)* + -OMA] A central nervous system tumor composed predominantly of astrocytes. A number of subtypes have been described, including fibrillary astrocytoma, protoplasmic astrocytoma, and gemistocytic astrocytoma. These astrocytomas are usually slow growing but may evolve into anaplastic forms. Also *astroglioma, astroma, astrocytic glioma.* **anaplastic a.** An astrocytoma of one of the recognized subtypes with areas of anaplasia. It may focally resemble a glioblastoma. **a. diffusum** A widely infiltrating astrocytoma within the brain or spinal cord. **a. fibrillare** FIBRILLARY ASTROCYTOMA. **fibrillary a.** An astrocytoma with many intracytoplasmic fibrils. Also *astrocytoma fibrillare.* **gemistocytic a.** An astrocytoma composed mainly of large, plump cells with abundant eosinophilic cytoplasm. Also *gemistocytoma.* **pilocytic a.** An astrocytoma composed predominantly of fusiform cells with long, wavy fibrillary processes. Most of these occur in children and young adults and are slow growing with little tendency to anaplasia. Cystic forms occur particularly in the cerebellum. Pilocytic astrocytoma of juvenile type and optic nerve glioma are forms of pilocytic astrocytoma. **a. protoplasmaticum** PROTOPLASMIC ASTROCYTOMA. **protoplasmic a.** An astrocytoma with few or no cytoplasmic fibrils. The cells are often large, with abundant cytoplasm. Also *astrocytoma protoplasmaticum.*

**astrocytomatosis cerebri** \-sī′təmətō′sis ser′əbrī\ GLIOMATOSIS CEREBRI.

**astrocytosis** \-sītō′sis\ A focal increase in the number of astrocytes, usually as a result of injury to the central nervous system.

**astroglia** \asträg′lē·ə\ Neuroglia of the astrocytic type; a tissue of astrocytes.

**astroglioma** \as′träglē·ō′mə\ ASTROCYTOMA.

**astrogliosis** \as′träglī·ō′sis\ GLIOSIS.

**astroma** \astrō′mə\ ASTROCYTOMA.

**astrophobia** \-fō′bē·ə\ [ASTRO- + -PHOBIA] Fear of the stars or heavens.

**astrosphere** \as′trəsfēr\ [ASTRO- + SPHERE] The set of radiating cytoplasmic fibrils which extend from the centrosphere during mitosis or meiosis. The astrosphere may or may not contain a centriole.

**Astrup** [Poul *Astrup,* Danish chemist, born 1915] Micro-Astrup method. See under METHOD.

**Asx** A symbol for an amino acid that gives aspartic acid after hydrolysis. Hence it may be either aspartic acid or asparagine beforehand. It is used especially in peptide sequences.

**asyllabia** \ā′silā′bē·ə\ [Gk *a-* priv. + *syllab(le)* + -IA] A restricted form of aphasia or alexia in which the patient is able to recognize individual letters, but is unable to form or to decipher syllables.

**asylum** [L, from Gk *asylon* (from *a-* priv. + *sylē* right of seizure) a refuge, sanctuary] An institution for the shelter and care of those unable to care for themselves. *Older term.*

**asymbolia** \asimbō′lē·ə\ [A-[1] + *symbol* + -IA] Inability to understand and interpret symbols such as words, numbers, gestures, signs, diagrams, or musical notes, or even occasionally other sensory information. A somewhat imprecise collective term, embracing features of alexia, amimia, amusia, and visual agnosia. Also *asymboly.* **a. for pain** A rare form of agnosia for pain sensation, usually of constitutional origin. The peripheral and central pathways concerned with the recording and conduction of pain sensation are intact, as is the perception of other forms of sensation. The patient fails to appreciate the painful character of a sensation which is normally painful and reacts inadequately or not at all. **tactile a.** TACTILE AGNOSIA.

**asymboly** \asim′bəlē\ ASYMBOLIA.

**asymmetrical** \ā′simet′rikəl\ 1 Displaying asymmetry. 2 Denoting molecules lacking such elements of symmetry as would render them achiral.

**asymmetry** \āsim′ətrē\ [Gk *asymmetria* (from *a-* priv. + *symmetria* SYMMETRY) disproportion] 1 Lack of symmetry. 2 Disproportion or absence of correspondence between like organs or parts on the left and right sides of an organism. **encephalic a.** A discrepancy in the size or configuration of the cerebrum or lateral ventricles of the two sides. It is usually a birth defect, but may result from a neoplasm or hydrocephalus.

**asymphytous** \əsim′fətəs\ Not fused; separate.

**asymptomatic** \ā′simptəmat′ik\ Being without symptoms; symptom-free.

**asynapsis** \āsinap′sis\ DESYNAPSIS.

**asynchronism** \āsin′krōnizm\ A state of asynchrony as in incoordination of movement.

**asynchronous** \āsin′krōnəs\ Pertaining to or characterized by asynchrony.

**asynchrony** \āsin′krōnē\ [Gk *a-* priv. + SYNCHRONY] Absence of synchrony, especially in movement. Adj. asynchronous.

**asynclitism** \əsin′klitizm\ [Gk *a-* priv. + SYNCLITISM] A form of transverse position of the presenting fetal vertex during labor where the sagittal suture is tilted anteriorly or posteriorly rather than being midway between the symphysis and the sacral promontory. Also *biparietal obliquity.* **anterior a.** A form of asynclitism where the sagittal suture of the presenting fetal vertex is tilted towards the sacral promontory. The anterior parietal bone is palpated vaginally. Also *Nägele's obliquity.* **posterior a.** A form of asynclitism where the sagittal suture of the presenting fetal vertex is tilted towards the symphysis. The posterior parietal bone is palpated vaginally. Also *Litzmann's obliquity.*

**asynechia** \ā'sinē'kē·ə\ Lack of continuity of structure in an organ.

**asynergia** \ā'sinur'jə\ ASYNERGY. **a. major** Severe incoordination producing a markedly ataxic gait.

**asynergic** \ā'sinur'jik\ Describing or pertaining to asynergy.

**asynergy** \āsin'urjē\ [Gk *a-* priv. + SYNERGY] Sequential and jerky performance of the various movements which make up an action, a feature of cerebellar incoordination, as distinguished from a smoothly synchronous and coordinated manner of performance. Also *decomposition of movements, asynergia.* **axial a.** Asynergy affecting the muscles of the head and trunk. **axioappendicular a.** Asynergy affecting the head, trunk, and limbs. **progressive cerebellar a.** DYSSYNERGIA CEREBELLARIS MYOCLONICA. **progressive locomotor a.** TABES DORSALIS. **truncal a.** CENTRAL ATAXIA. **verbal a.** An abnormal manner of speaking which results from uncoordinated neuromotor activity of the vocal tract or speech apparatus in chorea.

**asynovia** \ā'sinō'vē·ə\ Deficient production of synovial fluid by the synovial membrane.

**asyntaxia** \ā'sintak'sē·ə\ [Gk, (from *a-* priv. + *syntaxis* order, arrangement) disorder, disarray] The failure of embryonic development to proceed in the normal sequence or to completion. **a. dorsalis** A type of abnormal development in which failure of coordination of embryologic processes results in failure of closure of the neural groove.

**asystemic** \ā'sistem'ik\ Not systemic.

**asystole** \āsis'təlē\ [Gk *a-* priv. + SYSTOLE] Absence of systolic activity in the heart; cardiac standstill. Also *Beau syndrome.*

**asystolic** \ā'sistäl'ik\ Pertaining to or characterized by asystole.

**At** Symbol for the element, astatine.

**at-** \at-, ət-\ AD-.

**ATA** alimentary atoxic aleukia.

**-ata** [New L (from L *-ata*, neut. pl. of *-atus* -ATE)] A combining form meaning those having such a property or properties: used in zoologic taxa.

**Atabrine** A proprietary name for quinacrine hydrochloride.

**atactic** \ətak'tik\ ATAXIC.

**atactiform** \ətak'tifôrm\ Resembling ataxia.

**atactilia** \ā'taktil'yə\ ANESTHESIA.

**ataractic** [Gk *a-* priv. + *taraktikos* disturbing, from *tarassein* to disturb] **1** Producing peace or tranquility of mind. **2** An ataractic agent; a tranquilizer. For defs. 1 and 2 also *ataraxic.*

**ataralgesia** \at'eraljē'sēə\ NEUROLEPTANALGESIA.

**ataraxic** ATARACTIC.

**atavism** \at'əvizm\ [L *atav(us)* (from *at(ta)* father or grandfather + *avus* grandfather) a great-great-great-grandfather, remote ancestor, forefather + -ISM] The appearance of a heritable character present in remote ancestors but presumed lost because of its absence in more recent direct ancestors. It may be caused by recombination, homozygosity of recessive genes, effects of modifying genes, or environmental factors. The descendant showing the characteristic is sometimes called a throw-back. Also *reversion.*

**atavistic** \at'əvis'tik\ Characterized by a reversion to a phenotype not present for several preceding generations.

**ataxia** \ətak'sē·ə\ [Gk (from *a-* priv. + *taxis* order, arrangement, from *tassein* to draw up, arrange) disorder, irregularity] Unsteadiness, incoordination or disorganization of movements in the absence of paralysis. In sensory ataxia, the disorder is secondary to impairment of position and joint sense in the affected part, in cerebellar ataxia to loss of the normal cerebellar influence upon motor activity. Also *amyotaxia, dyssynergia, dyssynergy, ataxy.* Adj. ataxic. **acute cerebellar a.** Ataxia developing acutely due to a cerebellar lesion, often of inflammatory or demyelinating type. **acute cerebellar a. of infancy** Severe cerebellar ataxia of acute onset in infancy, often with fever. The affected infant is severely ataxic, often with total inability to walk or even to sit unsupported, and the eyes may show opsoclonus or severe nystagmus. The cerebrospinal fluid may be normal or may show a slight pleocytosis. The condition usually resolves spontaneously within a few weeks and is believed to be a form of acute postinfective encephalomyelitis predominantly involving the cerebellum. **acute tabetic a.** Sensory ataxia developing acutely in tabes dorsalis. **alcoholic a.** Ataxia occurring in chronic alcoholism. This may be sensory, due to alcoholic polyneuropathy, or of the central or truncal type, due to alcoholic cerebellar degeneration. **Briquet's a.** Hysterical unsteadiness of gait, often accompanied by hysterical sensory loss in the lower limbs. **Bruns frontal a.** Unsteadiness in walking, resembling central cerebellar ataxia, with a tendency to stagger from side to side, sometimes with astasia-abasia. The condition occurs as a consequence of extensive lesions, often bilateral, of the frontal lobes. Some authorities believe that this syndrome is due to an apraxia of gait. Also *frontal ataxia, frontal lobe ataxia.* **bulbar a.** Ataxia due to a lesion of central cerebellar connections in the pons or medulla oblongata. **central a.** Ataxia of gait occurring in lesions of central cerebellar structures (the vermis and roof nuclei or paleocerebellum). The affected patients stagger from side to side, walk on a wide base, and have difficulty in stopping and in turning, but so-called classical cerebellar signs such as dysmetria and past-pointing may not be present in the limbs. Also *truncal ataxia, truncal asynergy, equilibratory ataxia.* **cerebellar a.** Ataxia caused by malformation or damage to the cerebellum and/or the cerebellar tracts and connections. When midline cerebellar structures, such as the vermis, are involved, this gives rise to central ataxia. Involvement of one cerebellar hemisphere (the neocerebellum) or of its connections results in a tendency to deviate to the affected side on walking, with incoordination, dysmetria, adiadochokinesia, past-pointing, and sometimes intention tremor in the limbs on the side of the lesion, and nystagmus on looking to the affected side. Bilateral or severe unilateral lesions cause a typical cerebellar dysarthria. **cerebellofugal degeneration a.** DYSSYNERGIA CEREBELLARIS MYOCLONICA. **cerebral a.** Ataxia due to cerebral, as distinct from cerebellar, lesions. **cervical a.** Ataxia of sensory type resulting from a lesion of the cervical portion of the spinal cord. **a. cordis** *Obs.* ATRIAL FIBRILLATION. **dentate cerebellar a.** DYSSYNERGIA CEREBELLARIS MYOCLONICA. **diphtheritic a.** Sensory ataxia in diphtheritic polyneuropathy. **dynamic a.** KINETIC ATAXIA. **equilibratory a.** CENTRAL ATAXIA. **familial a.** HEREDITARY ATAXIA. **family a.** HEREDITARY ATAXIA. **Ferguson-Critchley type of a.** A rare form of hereditary ataxia, usually beginning between the ages of 30 and 45 years, in which the affected individuals manifest clinical features such as optic atrophy, nystagmus, cerebellar ataxia, and corticospinal tract signs resembling those of multiple sclerosis. **Friedreich's a.** FRIEDREICH'S DISEASE. **frontal a.** BRUNS FRONTAL ATAXIA. **frontal lobe a.** BRUNS FRONTAL ATAXIA. **hereditary a.** A group of progressive inherited disorders of the nervous system of unknown etiology of which cerebellar ataxia and degeneration is generally one clinical and pathological feature. However, other genetically-determined diseases of the nervous system, such as hereditary spastic paraplegia, in which there is no cerebellar involvement, are often classified for convenience in this group. Also *familial ataxia, family ataxia.* **hereditary cerebellar a.** MARIE'S HEREDITARY CEREBELLAR ATAXIA. **Holmes a.** PRIMARY PROGRESSIVE CEREBELLAR DEGENERATION. **Holmes type cerebellar a.** PRIMARY PROGRESSIVE CEREBELLAR DEGENERATION. **hysteric a.** Ataxia of gait, or any other movement, due to hysteria and not to organic disease. **kinetic a.** Ataxia which becomes increasingly evident during voluntary movement, especially of the limbs. Also *dynamic ataxia, limb-kinetic ataxia.* **labyrinthic a.** VESTIBULAR ATAXIA. **labyrinthine a.** VESTIBULAR ATAXIA. **Leyden's a.** DIABETIC PSEUDOTABES. **limb a.** Ataxia involving the limbs more severely than the trunk. Also *nonequilibratory ataxia.* **limb-kinetic a.** KINETIC ATAXIA. **locomotor a.** TABES DORSALIS. **Marie's hereditary cerebellar a.** Any of the forms of hereditary ataxia of late onset and comparatively slow progression, marked by progressive cerebellar ataxia of the trunk and limbs, usually with no evidence of involvement of other motor or sensory pathways, but in rare cases characterized by associated features of corticospinal tract involvement, or by optic atrophy and retinitis pigmentosa. Also *Nonne-Marie syndrome, Marie sclerosis, hereditary cerebellar ataxia.* **motor a.** Ataxia which only becomes evident during purposive movement. **nonequilibratory a.** LIMB ATAXIA. **nutritional spinal a.** TROPICAL ATAXIC NEUROPATHY. **ocular a.** NYSTAGMUS. **polyneuritic spinocerebellar a.** Any form of spinocerebellar ataxia associated with polyneuropathy, as in Refsum's disease. **postural a.** STATIC ATAXIA. **professional a.** OCCUPATIONAL CRAMP. **pseudotabetic a.** Sensory ataxia, as seen in severe cases of polyneuritis, such as diabetic pseudotabes. **psychomotor a.** GENERAL PARESIS. **Sanger Brown a.** A variety of hereditary ataxia, one of the spinocerebellar degenerations. The affected patients usually show evidence of progressive cerebellar ataxia, optic atrophy, and signs of bilateral corticospinal tract degeneration. **sensory a.** Ataxia of one or more limbs or of gait resulting not from cerebellar disease or dysfunction but from loss of proprioceptive sensation in the extremities, with consequential severe impairment of motor control. **spinal a.** Ataxia caused by lesions of the spinal cord, involving either the posterior columns (sensory ataxia) or the spinocerebellar tracts (cerebellar ataxia). **spinocerebellar a.** 1 Any of those forms of hereditary ataxia in which cerebellar dysfunction gives rise to clinical manifestations. 2 Any of the acquired forms of cerebellar degeneration including those which may complicate remote carcinoma. **static a.** Swaying or unsteadiness, evident when the patient stands upright. Also *postural ataxia.* **truncal a.** CENTRAL ATAXIA. **vestibular a.** Ataxia caused by damage to the labyrinths or their central vestibular connections. Also *labyrinthine ataxia, labyrinthic ataxia.*

**ataxiagram** \ətak′sē·əgram′\ [ATAXIA + -GRAM] A line drawn by a subject with ataxia in the writing hand, demonstrating deviation from the intended direction.

**ataxia-telangiectasia** \ətak′sē·ə-telan′jē·ektā′zhə\ An autosomal recessive disorder characterized by progressive cerebellar ataxia beginning in childhood, oculocutaneous telangiectases, oculomotor apraxia, an immunologic defect accounting for recurrent sinopulmonary infection, hypoplasia of the thymus, and a susceptibility to lymphatic malignancy. The basic biochemical defect is unknown, but cultured cells from patients are prone to radiation-induced chromosome breaks and rearrangements because of a defect in DNA repair. Also *Louis-Bar syndrome, Louis-Bar disease, ataxia-telangiectasia syndrome.*

**ataxic** \ətak′sik\ Describing or pertaining to ataxia. Also *atactic.*

**ataxiophemia** \ətak′sē·əfē′mē·ə\ *Outmoded* CEREBELLAR DYSARTHRIA.

**ataxophemia** \ətak′səfē′mē·ə\ *Outmoded* CEREBELLAR DYSARTHRIA.

**ataxospastic** \ətak′səspas′tik\ [*atax(ia)* + *o* + SPASTIC] Describing a combination of spasticity and ataxia. *Obs.*

**ataxy** \ətak′sē\ ATAXIA.

**-ate** \-āt, -it, -ət\ [L *-atus,* past part. ending of verbs of first conjugation, denoting acted upon, acting, office or function] A suffix meaning (1) having a (specified) feature, as *flagellate* (having flagella); (2) a result or product of a (specified) process, as *hemolysate, filtrate*; (3) an anion or ester derived from a (specified) acid, as *ascorbate*; (4) to become, cause to become, produce, or bring about, as *pupate, pronate, salivate, asphyxiate*; (5) to treat or process with, as *fluoridate, oxygenate.*

**atelectasis** \at′əlek′təsis\ [New L, from *atel(o)-* + ECTASIS] A state of airlessness, and hence reduced volume, especially of the lung. **absorption a.** SECONDARY ATELECTASIS. **compression a.** Atelectasis due to compression, usually from a tumor or from fluid or air in the pleural space. **congestive a.** ADULT RESPIRATORY DISTRESS SYNDROME. **discoid a.** FLEISCHNER LINE. **a. in the newborn** 1 See under PRIMARY ATELECTASIS. 2 See under SECONDARY ATELECTASIS. **lobar a.** Atelectasis involving one lobe of the lung. **a. of the middle ear** Collapse of the tympanic membrane as the result of persisting negative pressure in the middle ear, usually as a consequence of eustachian tube malfunction. In advanced cases the membrane becomes atrophic and closely applied to the medial wall of the tympanic cavity, including the long process of the incus and the stapes, so that the tympanic cavity ceases to be air-containing. There is usually a previous history of secretory otitis media. **obstructive a.** Atelectasis resulting from blockage of a bronchus or of bronchioles leading to the affected part of the lung. **platelike a.** FLEISCHNER LINE. **postnatal asphyxia a.** RESPIRATORY DISTRESS SYNDROME OF NEWBORN. **primary a.** A state of complete airlessness of the alveoli of the lung at birth, resulting from inadequate inspiratory effort, failure of assisted ventilation, or bronchial obstruction. **resorption a.** SECONDARY ATELECTASIS. **secondary a.** Atelectasis that occurs after initial lung expansion: usually applied to the neonatal period. It may be due to weakness of inspiratory effort, lack of surfactant, or bronchial or bronchiolar obstruction from inhaled meconium, blood, or mucus. When air is absorbed and not replenished the alveolus collapses. This tends to be a patchy condition throughout the lung. Also *absorption atelectasis, resorption atelectasis.* **segmental a.** Atelectasis affecting a given segment or segments of the lung.

**atelectatic** \at′əlektat′ik\ Relating to or in a state of atelectasis.

**ateleiosis** \ətē′lē·ō′sis\ [Gk *atelei(a)* (from *a-* priv. + *tel-*

*(os)* an end + *-eia* -IA) incompleteness + -OSIS] Dwarfism resulting from anterior pituitary insufficiency in childhood, associated with normal gonadal maturation, normal development of secondary sexual characteristics, and normal thyroidal and adrenocortical function. Reproductive ability is often unimpaired. Also *ateleiotic dwarfism, sexual ateleiotic dwarfism, ateliosis.*

**ateleiotic** \ətē′lē·ät′ik\ **1** Characterized by or pertaining to ateleiosis. **2** Imperfectly developed; incomplete. Also *atelic, ateliotic.*

**atelic** \ətē′lik\ ATELEIOTIC.

**ateliosis** \ətē′lē·ō′sis\ ATELEIOSIS.

**ateliotic** \ətē′lē·ät′ik\ ATELEIOTIC.

**atelo-** \at′əlō-\ [Gk *atelēs* (*a-* priv. + *telos* end) incomplete, without end] A combining form meaning incomplete, imperfect.

**atelocardia** \-kär′dē·ə\ [ATELO- + CARDIA] Incomplete cardiac development.

**atelocephalus** \-sef′ələs\ [ATELO- + -CEPHALUS] An embryo, fetus, or newborn infant with atelocephalia, that is, with an incomplete head.

**atelocheilia** \-kī′lyə\ [ATELO- + *cheil-* + -IA ] A faulty development of the lips.

**atelocheiria** \-kī′rē·ə\ [ATELO- + *cheir-* + -IA ] A faulty development of the hand.

**ateloencephaly** \-ensef′əlē\ [ATELO- + ENCEPHAL- + -Y] The incomplete or faulty embryonic development of the brain.

**ateloglossia** \-gläs′ē·ə\ [ATELO- + Gk *glōssa* tongue + -IA] An incomplete development of the tongue.

**atelognathia** \at′əlägnā′thē·ə\ [ATELO- + GNATH- + -IA ] The incomplete development of the jaw.

**atelokinesia** \-kīnē′zhə\ *Seldom used* TREMOR.

**atelomyelia** \-mī·ē′lyə\ [ATELO- + MYEL- + -IA] The incomplete or deficient development of the spinal cord.

**atelopodia** \-pō′dē·ə\ [ATELO- + -POD + -IA] The incomplete or imperfect development of the feet.

**ateloprosopia** \-prōsō′pē·ə\ [ATELO- + PROSOP- + -IA] An incomplete or imperfect development of the face that is usually of prenatal onset.

**atelorachidia** \at′əlôrakid′ē·ə\ [New L, from ATELO- + Gk *rhachis* the back, spine + -IA] The incomplete development of the vertebral column.

**athelia** \əthē′lyə\ [Gk *a-* priv. + THEL- + -IA] The developmental absence of one or both nipples.

**athermanous** \əthur′mənəs\ [French *athermane* (from Gk *a-* priv. + *thermē*) absorbing calorific radiations + -OUS] Not permeable to radiant heat.

**athermic** \əthur′mik\ AFEBRILE.

**athero-** \ath′ərō-\ [See ATHEROMA.] A combining form meaning atheroma.

**atheroembolism** \-em′bōlizm\ Embolism of the contents of an atheromatous plaque.

**atherogenesis** \-jen′əsis\ [ATHERO- + GENESIS] Formation of atheromatous material in arteries.

**atherogenic** \-jen′ik\ [ATHERO- + -GENIC] Giving rise to atheromas; causing or tending to cause atherogenesis.

**atheroma** \ath′ərō′mə\ [Gk *athērōma* (from *athērē* gruel, porridge) a tumor containing porridgelike matter] A disorder of arterial walls characterized by degenerative changes, deposition of lipid, proliferation of smooth muscle cells, and fibrosis. **cerebral a.** Atheroma of the arteries supplying blood to the brain.

**atheromatosis** \-mətō′sis\ [ATHEROMA + *t* + -OSIS] Widespread atheromatous arterial disease.

**atheromatous** \ath′ərō′mətəs\ Pertaining to or affected by atheroma.

**atherosclerosis** \-sklerō′sis\ [ATHERO- + SCLEROSIS] Atheromatous disease in which the atheromatous plaque is complicated by fibrosis and calcification. Also *arterial lipoidosis, nodular sclerosis.* **coronary a.** Atherosclerosis of the coronary arteries. **a. obliterans** ARTERIOSCLEROSIS OBLITERANS.

**atherosclerotic** \-sklerät′ik\ Pertaining to or associated with atherosclerosis.

**athetoid** \ath′ətoid\ Relating to athetosis, as *athetoid movements* or *athetoid cerebral palsy.*

**athetosis** \ath′ətō′sis\ [New L (from Gk *athetos* without fixed position, from *a-* priv. + *tithenai* to place + -OSIS)] A form of involuntary movement which is repetitive, slow, and writhing, or undulating in character. Such movements are predominantly seen in the hands and feet, but proximal limb muscles are also involved. They may be associated with decreased tone in antagonistic muscles during movement. Stimulation and emotion bring about an increase in athetotic movements, whereas they may be reduced by rest and cease during sleep. Athetosis is most often seen in cases of cerebral palsy, and it results from lesions in the corpus striatum. Similar movements may, however, occur in hepatolenticular degeneration and in various forms of leukodystrophy and may represent a side-effect of treatment with levodopa in cases of parkinsonism. Also *athetoid spasm.* Adj. athetotic, athetosic. **bilateral a.** DOUBLE ATHETOSIS. **double a.** Athetosis involving all four limbs, usually seen in cases of cerebral palsy and associated with prenatal or perinatal damage to the corpus striatum. Sometimes similar manifestations occur in inherited metabolic disorders of the nervous system, such as lipidosis or leukodystrophy. Also *Hammond syndrome* (seldom used), *Hammond's disease, bilateral athetosis, Vogt's disease.* **posthemiplegic a.** Athetosis developing in the weak or paralyzed limbs following hemiplegia, usually due to a cerebrovascular accident. **pupillary a.** HIPPUS. **unilateral a.** Athetosis affecting only one side of the body.

**athrepsia** \əthrep′sē·ə\ [Gk *a-* priv. + *threps(is)* (from *trephein* to feed, nourish) a feeding, nourishing + -IA] MARASMUS.

**athrocytosis** \ath′rōsītō′sis\ [Gk *athro(os)* assembled, collected + *-cyt(e)* + -OSIS] The process of absorption of macromolecules into renal tubular cells from the tubular lumen.

**athrophagocytosis** \ath′rōfag′əsītō′sis\ Phagocytosis of nonnutrient material.

**athymia** \əthim′ē·ə\ [Gk *a-* priv. + *thym(us)* + -IA] **1** Absence of the thymus. Also *athymism, athymismus.* **2** *Obs.* MELANCHOLIA. **3** *Obs.* DEMENTIA.

**athyreosis** \əthī′rē·ō′sis\ [Gk *a-* priv. + *thyre(o)-* + -OSIS] *Seldom used* HYPOTHYROIDISM. • The term is a misnomer, since it means literally a total absence of thyroid function

**athyreotic** \əthī′rē·ät′ik\ *Seldom used* HYPOTHYROID. • See note at *athyreosis.*

**athyroidism** \əthī′roidizm\ [Gk *a-* priv. + THYROID + -ISM] *Seldom used* HYPOTHYROIDISM. • See note at *athyreosis.*

**-ation** \-ā′shən\ [L verb-stem ending *-a-* + noun-forming suffix *-tio*, gen. *-tionis*] A noun suffix denoting an action, process, or result.

**atlantal** \ətlan′təl\ Pertaining to the atlas.

**atlanto-** \ətlan′tō-\ [Gk *atlas*, gen. *atlantos* the atlas] A combining form denoting the atlas.

**atlantoaxial** \-ak′sē·əl\ Pertaining to the atlas and the axis. Also *atloaxial, atloaxoid, atlantoepistrophic, odontoatlantal.*

**atlantobasilaris internus** A variant of the longus capitis muscle, occurring in about five percent of cases, in which the muscle extends from the anterior tubercle of the atlas to the base of the skull.

**atlantodidymus** \-did′iməs\ [ATLANTO- + -DIDYMUS] Conjoined twins consisting of one body and one neck with two heads, or substantial parts thereof. Also *atlodidymus.*

**atlantoepistrophic** \-ep′isträf′ik\ *Outmoded* ATLANTOAXIAL.

**atlantoid** \ətlan′toid\ Of or pertaining to the atlas bone.

**atlantomastoid** \-mas′toid\ Pertaining to the atlas and the mastoid process of the temporal bone.

**atlanto-occipital** \-äksip′itəl\ Pertaining to the atlas and the occipital bone. Also *atloido-occipital.*

**atlanto-odontoid** \-ōdän′toid\ Pertaining to the atlas bone and the odontoid process of axis.

**atlas** [Med L, from Gk, after *Atlas,* the Titan of Greek mythology who supported the heavens on his shoulders (as the first vertebra supports the skull)] **1** The first vertebra in amniote vertebrates, located next to the skull. As part of the atlas-axis complex, it affords the head of higher vertebrates greater freedom of movement. **2** [NA] In humans, a unique vertebra that lacks a body and spinous process. It comprises two solid lateral masses joined in front by a short anterior arch and behind by a longer posterior arch. The superior articular facets articulate with the condyles of the skull, whereas the inferior facets articulate with the axis. The dens axis fits between the lateral masses, permitting rotational movements of the head.

**atloaxial** \at′lō·ak′sē·əl\ ATLANTOAXIAL.

**atloaxoid** \at′lō·ak′soid\ ATLANTOAXIAL.

**atlodidymus** \at′lōdid′iməs\ ATLANTODIDYMUS.

**atloido-occipital** \atloi′dō·äksip′itəl\ ATLANTO-OCCIPITAL.

**atm** Symbol for standard atmosphere.

**atmo-** \at′mə-\ [Gk *atmos* steam, vapor] A combining form denoting vapor or gas.

**atmolysis** \atmäl′isis\ [ATMO- + LYSIS] **1** The separation of gases by exploitation of their differing diffusibilities. **2** The disintegration of organic tissue by contact with the fumes of volatile fluids.

**atmos** atmosphere *Popular.*

**atmosphere** \at′məsfir\ **standard a.** An international reference pressure defined as 101 325 pascals exactly. It was originally defined as 760 millimeters of mercury; the difference is within 1 part in $10^7$. It is no longer used as a unit of pressure. Also *normal atmosphere* (outmoded), *standard pressure.* Symbol: atm

**atmospherization** \atmäs′ferīzā′shən\ The oxygenation of venous blood.

**at no** atomic number.

**atom** \at′əm\ [Gk *atomos* (from *a-* priv. + *tom-,* noun and adj. stem of *temnein* to cut, divide) individual, indivisible] The smallest particle of an element that can exist. It consists of a positively charged nucleus and the electrons around it. **asymmetric carbon a.** A carbon atom carrying four different groups. It has no plane of symmetry and therefore makes chiral a molecule that contains it, unless it is accompanied by a compensating atom of the opposite chirality. **Bohr a.** A conception of the atom in which the neutrons and protons are located in a tiny central nucleus, with a diameter one ten thousandth of the atom. Electrons are held within the atom but outside of the nucleus, confined to orbital locations around the nucleus analogous to planetary orbits around the sun. **excited a.** A neutral atom that is temporarily unstable because one or more of its electrons occupy orbits too far from the nucleus for normal stability. They settle down into place, emitting their excess energy as x rays, fluorescence, or phosphorescence. **g a.** GRAM-ATOM. **radiating a.** An atom that discharges excess energy, either by a nuclear change, effecting a more stable proton-neutron configuration, or by shifting its electrons into lower-energy orbits. **recoil a.** An atom that is recoiling from a collision with an energetic particle or photon, for example after a photoelectric interaction. Often the recoil is negligible, but must be nonzero in order to conserve momentum.

**atomic** \ətäm′ik\ Of or relating to an atom.

**atomizer** \at′əmī′zər\ A device used to create a jet of spray.

**atonia** \ətō′nē·ə\ [Gk (from *atonos* slack, from *a-* priv. + *tonos* tension) slackness, debility] **1** Lack of tone; weakness or reduction in the normal tone of a tissue or an organ. Also *atonicity, atony.* **2** Loss of energy or force. Adj. atonic.

**atonia-astasia** \ətō′nē·ə·astā′zhə\ FÖRSTER'S DIPLEGIA.

**atonic** \ətän′ik\ Lacking muscle tone, as a relaxed muscle.

**atonicity** \at′ōnis′itē\ ATONIA.

**atony** \at′ənē\ ATONIA. **chronic intestinal a.** IDIOPATHIC INTESTINAL PSEUDO-OBSTRUCTION. **muscle a.** MYATONIA. **a. of the uterus** Failure of the uterus to contract maximally after delivery of the baby and placenta. This results in heavy uterine bleeding. Also *metratonia.*

**atopic** \ətäp′ik\ [Gk *atop(os)* (from *a-* priv. + *topos* place) out of place, unwonted + -IC] Predisposing to the development of diseases associated with excessive IgE antibody formation.

**atopognosia** \ətäp′ägnō′zhə\ [Gk *a-* priv. + TOPO- + Gk *gnōs(is)* knowledge + -IA] Inability to localize a sensory stimulus correctly in extrapersonal space. Also *atopognosis.*

**atopy** \at′əpē\ [Gk *atopia* (from *atopos;* see ATOPIC) a being out of place, oddness] An abnormal, immediate hypersensitivity to certain common allergens, such as house dusts, animal dander, and pollen, that is related to the production of the IgE antibody, reagin. The predisposition for hypersensitivity involving the production of reagin is believed to be inherited. Also *atopic allergy, intrinsic allergy, atopic hypersensitivity.*

**-ator** \-ātər\ [L *-atus* past-part. termination of first-conjugation verbs + *-or,* a suffix denoting an agent, doer, performer] A combining form meaning one who performs an act, agent.

**atoxic** \ətäk′sik\ [Gk *a-* priv. + TOXIC] **1** Not toxic. **2** Not caused by or associated with a toxin.

**atoxigenic** \ətäk′səjen′ik\ Not producing toxins.

**ATP** adenosine triphosphate.

**ATPase** Adenosine triphosphatase, an enzyme that hydrolyzes ATP to ADP and phosphate. For many such enzymes the natural process is accompanied by some other process, such as the relative movement of myosin and actin rods responsible from muscular contraction or the pumping of ions across membranes. Such ion pumps include one for pumping sodium out of cells and potassium in, one for pumping calcium into sarcoplasmic reticulum to terminate muscular contraction, and one capable of pumping hydrogen ions. This last process, when driven backwards in mitochondria and bacteria, allows electrochemical gradients of hydrogen ions to be used for ATP synthesis.

**atractoid** \ətrak′toid\ Spindle-shaped.

**atractylic acid** A poisonous glycoside from *Atractylis gummifera* L. It produces convulsions and interferes with nerve conduction and the citric acid cycle. Also *atractyloside, atractyligenin.*

**atractyligenin** \atrak′təlijen′in\ ATRACTYLIC ACID.
**atractyloside** \at′rəktil′ōsīd\ ATRACTYLIC ACID.
**atransferrinemia** \ātrans′ferinē′mē·ə\ The absence or severe deficiency of transferrin, inherited as an autosomal recessive trait and resulting in severe iron deficiency anemia and hemosiderosis. Also *transferrin deficiency.*
**atraumatic** \ā′trômat′ik\ [Gk *a-* priv. + TRAUMATIC] Causing or likely to cause little or no physical or psychological injury. For example, a spinal tap is said to be atraumatic if it does not introduce red blood cells into the fluid.
***Atrax*** \ā′traks\ A genus of venomous, funnel-web mygalomorph spiders (family Dipluridae) of Australia. Important species include *A. formidabilis,* the tree funnel-web spider, and *A. robustus.* A number of fatalities have been attributed to the bite of the male of the latter species, which is particularly aggressive.
**atresia** \ətrē′zhə\ [Gk *a-* priv. + *trēs(is)* perforation (from *tetranein* to perforate) + -IA] The developmental failure to form a lumen or orifice such as a hollow or tubular viscus or sphincters and external openings of such viscera, or the acquired, usually cicatricial, closure of such lumina or openings. **anal a.** IMPERFORATE ANUS. **a. of the aorta** Absence of any patent communication between the ascending aorta, usually grossly hypoplastic, and the ventricular mass. In rare cases, a segment of the aortic arch is represented by a fibrous chord. **aortic valve a.** The presence of an imperforate valve membrane blocking the communication between the ventricular mass and the ascending aorta. **acquired a. of the external auditory meatus** Meatal atresia resulting from injury to or disease of the external ear. The injury may be accidental, such as results from burns, or surgical, as in mastoidectomy. The disease, usually inflammatory, includes chronic external otitis. **biliary a.** The developmental occlusion of any of the major biliary ducts. **choanal a.** Occlusion of one or both choanae, whether congenital or acquired. Both are rare, the latter more so than the former. The bilateral congenital condition gives rise to serious difficulty with respiration and feeding from the moment of birth. The acquired condition may complicate severe trauma, particularly war wounds, late syphilis, tuberculosis, or diphtheria. **congenital a. of the external auditory canal** Congenital absence of the external auditory canal or canals, usually associated with deformity or absence of the external ear, often with middle-ear abnormalities and rarely with cochlear aplasia. It may be one feature of a congenital syndrome, as in the Treacher-Collins syndrome. **a. of the external auditory canal** Failure of the external auditory canal to form (congenital atresia) or, later, closure of the canal due to disease or injury (acquired atresia). Also *meatal atresia.* **follicular a.** The failure of a graafian follicle to mature. Also *atresia folliculi.* **a. folliculi** FOLLICULAR ATRESIA. **a. iridis** ATRETOPSIA. **meatal a.** ATRESIA OF THE EXTERNAL AUDITORY CANAL. **mitral a.** A lesion of the mitral valve such that it prevents communication between an atrium and the underlying ventricular mass. It may be produced either by an imperforate valve membrane or by complete absence of the atrioventricular connection. It usually affects the morphologically left atrium. **pulmonary a.** The developmental failure of an opening or passage to form in the pulmonary artery, usually at the level of the pulmonary valve. **pulmonary valve a.** The presence of an imperforate pulmonary valve membrane blocking the entry to the pulmonary trunk. **tricuspid a.** A lesion of the morphologically tricuspid valve which prevents communication between an atrium and the ventricular mass. It may be produced either by an imperforate valve membrane or by complete absence of the atrioventricular connection. **tricuspid valve a.** The presence of an imperforate valve membrane blocking the communication between an atrium and the ventricular mass. It usually affects the morphologically right atrium. **vaginal a.** Incomplete development of the vagina, which can manifest itself as a narrowing or shortening, or by presence of transverse septae.
**atret-** \ətrēt-\ ATRETO-.
**atretic** \ətret′ik\ [ATRET- + -IC] Having an occluded lumen, orifice, or valve of developmental origin.
**atreto-** \ətrē′tō-\ [Gk *atrētos* (*a-* priv. + *trētos* pierced through) not perforated] A combining form meaning lacking an opening, usually of development causation; imperforate. Also *atret-.*
**atretoblepharia** \-blefer′ē·ə\ [ATRETO- + BLEPHAR- + -IA] Incomplete separation of the margins of the upper and lower eyelids, which are originally fused in the embryo and normally separate during embryonic development.
**atretocephalia** \-sefā′lyə\ [ATRETO- + CEPHAL- + -IA] The absence of the usual orifices of the head.
**atretocormia** \-kôr′mē·ə\ [ATRETO- + Gk *korm(os)* the trunk of a tree + -IA] The absence of one or more of the usual orifices of the body.
**atretocystia** \-sis′tē·ə\ [ATRETO- + CYST- + -IA ] The absence of one or more of the openings into and from the bladder.
**atretogastria** \-gas′trē·ə\ [ATRETO- + GASTR- + -IA] A lack of the usual openings into and from the stomach.
**atretometria** \-mē′trē·ə\ [ATRETO- + METR- + -IA ] An absence of the usual openings into or from the uterus.
**atretopsia** \ā′trētäp′sē·ə\ [ATRET- + -OPSIA] The absence of the pupillary opening. Also *atresia iridis.*
**atreturethria** \ətrē′t$^y$Urē′thrē·ə\ The absence of the usual opening of the urethra. Compare HYPOSPADIAS.
**atria** \ā′trē·ə\ Plural of ATRIUM.
**atrial** \ā′trē·əl\ Pertaining to an atrium. Also *auricularis.*
**atrialized** \ā′trē·əlīzd′\ Incorporated into a cardiac atrium, for example as part of the right ventricle in Ebstein's anomaly or as the venae cavae in normal embryogenesis.
**atrichia** \ətrik′ē·ə\ [Gk *atrich(os)* hairless + -IA. See ATRICHOUS.] The absence of hair, especially the congenital lack of hair.
**atrichous** \ətrik′əs\ [Gk *atrichos* (from Gk *a-* priv. + *thrix,* gen. *trichos,* the hair) without hair] **1** In bacteria, lacking flagella. **2** Being without hair.
**atrio-** \ā′trē·ō-\ [L *atrium* entrance hall or chamber] A combining form denoting atrium.
**atriomegaly** \-meg′əlē\ [ATRIO- + -MEGALY] Enlargement of one or both atria of the heart.
**atrionector** \-nek′tər\ NODUS SINUATRIALIS.
**atrioseptoplasty** \-sep′təplas′tē\ The reconstruction or realignment of the interatrial septum.
**atriotomy** \ā′trē·ät′əmē\ [ATRIO- + -TOMY] An incision of the right or left atrium of the heart.
**atrioventricular** \-ventrik′yələr\ Pertaining both to atrial and to ventricular chambers of the heart, usually implying progression from the atria to the ventricles. Also *auriculoventricular.* Abbr. AV, A-V
**atrioventricularis communis** COMMON ATRIOVENTRICULAR CANAL.
**atriplicism** \ətrip′lisizm\ [L *atriplex,* gen. *atriplicis* (adaptation of Gk *atraphaxus* orach, *Atriplex rosea*), a kitchen herb, orach + -ISM] A morbid condition, usually of the fingers, characterized by painful swelling and sometimes gangrene, resulting from eating the spinachlike greens of *Atriplex littoralis.*.
**atrium** \ā′trē·əm\ [L, entrance hall, chamber] (*pl.* atria)

1 A chamber or vestibule connected to or providing access to another chamber, space, or vessel. 2 An atrium of the heart. **a. alveolare** [NA] One of the spaces between the termination of the alveolar ducts and the alveolar sacs in the lung. Some authorities consider it to be merely a terminal expansion of an alveolar duct. **common a.** A developmental defect of the interatrial septum in which two atria remain as a single chamber that receives blood from both the systemic and the pulmonary veins. Also *single atrium.* **a. cordis** [NA] One of the two thin-walled muscular chambers of the heart that lie above, behind, and slightly to the right of the thicker-walled ventricles. They are separated from each other internally by the interatrial septum, and each is continuous with its ventricle through an atrioventricular orifice protected by a valve. Each possesses an auricular appendage. Also *atrium of heart, auricle, auricula* (outmoded). **a. dextrum** [NA] The atrium of the heart that lies to the right and in front of the left atrium, receiving blood from the superior and inferior venae cavae and the coronary sinus and transmitting it to the right ventricle through the right atrioventricular orifice guarded by the tricuspid valve. Cephalad to the orifice and projecting to the left from the anterosuperior surface is the right auricle. Also *right atrium.* **a. of heart** ATRIUM CORDIS. **a. of infection** The point of entry of infecting organisms. **a. meatus medii** [NA] A shallow depression in the lateral wall of the nasal cavity continuous with the anterior portion of the middle meatus and located above the vestibule and below the agger nasi. Also *atrium of middle meatus of nose.* **primitive a.** A portion of the cardiac tube in embryos represented by a single cavity situated behind the bulboventricular region. At its ventral extremity it communicates with the ventricle by the atrioventricular canal. **right a.** ATRIUM DEXTRUM. **single a.** COMMON ATRIUM. **a. sinistrum** [NA] The atrium of the heart lying to the left of and partly posterior to the right atrium and receiving on its right and left sides the openings of the right and left upper and lower pulmonary veins respectively. The blood entering it is pumped into the left ventricle through the left atrioventricular orifice guarded by the mitral valve. Projecting anteriorly from its upper left part is the left auricle.

**atropanine** APOATROPINE.

**atrophia** \ətrō′fē·ə\ [New L, from Gk (from *atrophein* to waste away from lack of nourishment, from *a-* priv. + *trephein* to support, nourish) lack of nourishment, wasting away] ATROPHY. **a. mesenterica** TABES MESENTERICA. **a. musculorum lipomatosa** PSEUDOHYPERTROPHIC MUSCULAR DYSTROPHY. **a. senilis** SENILE ATROPHY. **a. striata et maculosa** Linear and macular atrophy of sun-damaged skin. Also *atrophoderma striatum et maculatum.* **a. testiculi** TESTICULAR ATROPHY. **a. unguium** A reduction in the size and a thinning of the nail plate which may lead to complete loss of the nail and replacement with scar tissue. It may be congenital or acquired, as can be seen in a lichen planus infection. *Rare.*

**atrophic** \əträf′ik\ Indicating atrophy.

**atrophie** \ätrōfē′, at′rəfē\ ATROPHY. **a. blanche** A clinical syndrome caused predominantly by hypostatic congestion and characterized by white atrophic macules, telangiectases, and small painful ulcers, most frequently seen on the skin of the lower extremities of middle-aged and older women. Also *white atrophy.*

**atrophoderma** \at′rōfədur′mə\ [Gk *atropho(s)* atrophying + -DERMA] CUTANEOUS ATROPHY. **follicular a.** Atrophy confined to the perifollicular dermis. It gives rise to dimplelike follicular depressions. **idiopathic a. of Pasini and Pierini** A superficial form of morphea, characterized by the development of plaques, mainly on the trunk. Also *Pasini-Pierini syndrome.* **macular a.** MACULAR ATROPHY. **neuritic a.** The smooth, glazed state of denervated skin. **a. striatum et maculatum** ATROPHIA STRIATA ET MACULOSA. **vermiculate a. of the cheeks** A form of keratosis pilaris atrophicans in which follicular plugs on the cheeks are followed by reticulate atrophy when these are shed. Also *folliculitis ulerythematosa reticulata.*

# atrophy

**atrophy** \at′rəfē\ [New L *atrophia.* See ATROPHIA.] 1 A wasting or shrinking of a cell, tissue, organ, or part of an organism after it has developed completely and achieved its full size. It may result from a decreased workload, ischemia, disuse, or lack of endocrine stimulation. Also *atrophia, atrophie.* 2 To cause or undergo atrophy; waste away. **acute infantile spinal muscular a.** WERDNIG-HOFFMANN DISEASE. **acute yellow a. of the liver** The pathologic findings in the liver following fulminant hepatitis: a small liver of soft consistency with red-brown discoloration from bile staining. Microscopically there is extensive degeneration of liver cells leaving a residual framework of collapsed reticulin with some sparing of parenchymal cells in the periportal facies. Also *hepatodystrophy, Rokitansky's disease.* **alveolar a.** A gradual diminution of the size of the alveolar bone after the extraction of the teeth. **Aran-Duchenne muscular a.** PROGRESSIVE MUSCULAR ATROPHY. **arthritic a.** A wasting of the muscles associated with a joint damaged by an arthritic process. **blue a.** Atrophy marked by bluish pigmentation that follows the self-administration of drugs by injection. **bone a.** OSTEOPOROSIS. **brown a.** The brownish pigmentation of certain organs due to the intracellular accumulation of lipofuscin, seen in association with atrophy. This condition is characteristically seen in old people, in severe starvation, and in wasting diseases. The organs principally involved are the heart, liver, and spleen. **cardiac a.** Atrophy of the myocardium, usually associated with cachexia or senility. Also *acardiotrophia* (obs.), *atrophic heart.* **cerebellar a. of late onset and cortical type** Atrophy of the cerebellar cortex, usually affecting particularly the vermis. Onset may be after the age of 70 years, and the condition is characterized by central ataxia with dysarthria and shaky writing. In some cases there is also progressive spasticity due to degeneration of the corticospinal tracts. The condition is now classified as one of the hereditary ataxias and is closely related to primary progressive cerebellar degeneration. Also *lamellär cerebellar atrophy.* **cerebral a.** Any condition resulting in atrophy of the cerebral hemispheres. Also *phrenatrophia* (outmoded). **Charcot-Marie a.** CHARCOT-MARIE-TOOTH DISEASE. **Charcot-Marie-Tooth a.** CHARCOT-MARIE-TOOTH DISEASE. **circumpapillary chorioretinal a.** A ring of visible sclera surrounding the optic disk due to the atrophy of aging. Also *peripapillary senile halo, senile halo.* **circumscribed a. of the brain** 1 Any condition in which there is atrophy of one area of the brain without involvement of other areas. 2 PICK'S DISEASE. **compensatory a.** Regression of one of a pair or all but one of a group of endocrine organs when the other gland secretes an excessive amount of their common hormone, as contralateral atrophy of the adrenal cortex in the presence of a functioning adrenocortical adenoma, or regression of the three remaining parathyroid glands in the face of a secretory adenoma of the fourth gland. **compression a.** PRESSURE ATROPHY. **correlated a.** Atrophy of a part of the body as a consequence of the excision or destruction of a functionally related structure. **corticostriatospinal a.** CORTICOSTRIATOSPINAL DEGENERATION. **Cruveilhier's a.** PROGRESSIVE MUSCULAR ATROPHY. **cutaneous a.** Atrophy of the skin. Also *atrophoderma.* **cyanotic a. of the liver** Liver atrophy resulting from ischemic hepatitis. **degenerative a.** Atrophy of a tissue or organ due to degeneration of its component cells. **Dejerine-Thomas a.** OLIVOPONTOCEREBELLAR DEGENERATION. **denervated muscle a.** NEUROGENIC ATROPHY. **disuse a.** A wasting of soft tissues, along with osteoporosis, that is secondary to disuse. Also *inactivity atrophy.* **Eichhorst's a.** A progressive form of muscular dystrophy affecting mainly the muscles of the lower limb and giving rise to clawing of the toes. **endometrial a.** Menopausal endometrium in which there is a significant diminution in glands and stroma, with occasional cystic glandular formation. **essential a. of iris** A rare, progressive wasting of the iris characterized by thinning and perforation in multiple locations, displacement of the pupil, and damage to the trabecular meshwork with resultant glaucoma. **facial a.** PROGRESSIVE UNILATERAL FACIAL ATROPHY. **facioscapulohumeral a.** FACIOSCAPULOHUMERAL MUSCULAR DYSTROPHY. **familial spinal muscular a.** Any of the forms of spinal muscular atrophy that occur in infancy, childhood, and adult life and which are genetically determined. **fat replacement a.** Atrophy of subcutaneous fat, its replacement by inflammatory cells, and its subsequent replacement by scar tissue. **fatty a.** The replacement of atrophic tissue by fat, such as the fatty infiltration of muscle in certain forms of muscular dystrophy. Also *adipositas ex vacuo.* **Fazio-Londe a.** An inherited form of neuropathic muscular atrophy occurring in infancy or early childhood and affecting predominantly the cranial nerves. The condition may be related to Werdnig-Hoffmann disease. **gastric a.** A type of atrophy characteristic of atrophic gastritis in which there is complete loss of the normal gastric glands with thinning of the mucosa. There may be variable amounts of infiltration by lymphocytes, plasma cells, and occasional eosinophils. **gauntlet a.** Atrophy of the distal muscles of the forearm and hand, as seen in cases of Charcot-Marie-Tooth disease. **general a.** Wasting away of the tissues of the body as occurs in starvation. **gingival a.** A gradual diminution in height of the gingiva not associated with inflammation or trauma. Its occurrence is in dispute. **gray a.** SECONDARY OPTIC ATROPHY. **hemifacial a.** PROGRESSIVE UNILATERAL FACIAL ATROPHY. **hemilingual a.** HYPOGLOSSAL ATROPHY. **hereditary optic a.** LEBER'S OPTIC ATROPHY. **Hoffmann's a.** WERDNIG-HOFFMANN DISEASE. **hypoglossal a.** Wasting of one half of the tongue due to a lesion of the hypoglossal nerve of the corresponding side. Also *hemilingual atrophy.* **inactivity a.** DISUSE ATROPHY. **inanition a.** Prolonged nutrient loss due to diarrhea, as might be caused by abuse of laxatives. **infantile a.** MARASMUS. **inflammatory a.** Atrophy of portion of an organ as a result of pressure exerted by an inflammatory exudate or by granulation tissue. **interstitial a.** The loss of bone mineral without the loss of the collagenous fibrous architecture of bone. **ischemic muscular a.** VOLKMANN'S ISCHEMIC CONTRACTURE. **Jadassohn's macular a.** Macular atrophy following macular erythema of the trunk, upper arms, and thighs. **juvenile familial muscular a.** A progressive form of spinal muscular atrophy, of autosomal recessive inheritance, usually beginning in childhood, adolescence, or early adult life, and as a rule first involving proximal muscles in the upper and lower limbs. Hypertrophy of the calves is common. Progression is usually gradual. Evidence of corticospinal tract involvement is generally absent, and clinically the condition may closely resemble that of muscular dystrophy of the Duchenne or limb-girdle type, less often of the facioscapulohumeral type. Also *pseudomyopathic spinal muscular atrophy, Kugelberg-Welander disease, juvenile spinal muscular atrophy, juvenile muscular atrophy, Kugelberg-Welander syndrome.* **lactation a.** Hyperinvolution of the uterus associated with breast feeding. **lamellar cerebellar a.** CEREBELLAR ATROPHY OF LATE ONSET AND CORTICAL TYPE. **Landouzy-Dejerine a.** FACIOSCAPULOHUMERAL MUSCULAR DYSTROPHY. **Leber's optic a.** An ocular disorder characterized by progressive loss of central vision resulting from degeneration of the optic nerve and papillomacular bundle. Males are almost exclusively affected. Onset of central vision loss is variable but usually occurs in the early third decade. The mode of inheritance is unlear. Women transmit the trait while men usually do not. The disorder is likely heterogeneous. Also *hereditary optic atrophy, von Leber's atrophy.* **lobar a.** PICK'S DISEASE. **macular a.** Cutaneous atrophy confined to small circumscribed patches. Also *macular atrophoderma.* **muscular a.** Atrophy of skeletal muscle due to any cause. The commonest causes are disuse, denervation, or primary disease of muscle (myopathy). Also *myophagism, myophagia.* **myelopathic a.** PROGRESSIVE MUSCULAR ATROPHY. **myelopathic muscular a.** Atrophy of muscles secondary to disease of the spinal cord. **myopathic a.** Wasting of muscles due to primary disease or dysfunction of skeletal muscle, not consequent upon any lesion of the central or peripheral nervous system; myopathy. **myotonic a.** DYSTROPHIA MYOTONICA. **neurogenic a.** Atrophy of skeletal muscle resulting from any lesion or disease of the lower motor neurons. Also *denervated muscle atrophy, neural atrophy.* **neurotrophic a.** Any muscular atrophy due to disease or dysfunction of motor nerves. **numeric a.** Atrophy caused by decrease in the number of elements in a tissue or organ. **olivopontocerebellar a.** One of the group of hereditary ataxias, usually of dominant inheritance, due to combined degeneration of the cerebellum, olivary nuclei, and pontine tracts and nuclei. The onset of the condition is usually in middle life, with progressive dysarthria, cerebellar ataxia, static tremor of the limbs resembling that of parkinsonism, and signs of corticospinal tract degeneration. Dementia is not uncommon in affected individuals. Five main types are known, but some subjects, especially sporadic cases, defy classification. **olivorubrocerebellar a.** A form of hereditary ataxia resembling olivopontocerebellar atrophy clinically but in which, pathologically, degeneration is found also to involve the central cerebellar and red nuclei. **optic a.** Death of all or part of the optic nerve fibers, recognizable by ophthalmoscopic identification of typical pallor of the optic disk and usually by peripheral constriction of the visual field, confirmed by perimetry. **pallidal a.** JUVENILE PARALYSIS AGITANS. **paraneoplastic cerebellar a.** Atrophy and degeneration of the cerebellar cortex, particularly involving the Purkinje cells, and of spinocerebellar tracts leading to a subacute cerebellar syndrome, associated with the presence of extracranial malignant disease. The pathogenesis of the condition has not been elucidated. Also *paraneoplastic subacute cerebellar degeneration, spinocerebellar degeneration compli-*

*cating carcinoma.* **Parrot's a. of the newborn** MARASMUS. **pathologic a.** Extreme atrophy of an organ or part, making it no longer viable. **periodontal a.** A gradual change in the supporting structures of the teeth following the extraction of an opposing tooth or disuse. The changes include osteoporosis, narrowing of the periodontal ligament space, and change in direction of the collagen fibers of the ligament. **peroneal a.** CHARCOT-MARIE-TOOTH DISEASE. **peroneal muscular a.** CHARCOT-MARIE-TOOTH DISEASE. **physiologic a.** SENILE ATROPHY. **Pick's convolutional a.** PICK'S DISEASE. **Pick's gyral a.** PICK'S DISEASE. **pigmentary a.** Atrophy of an organ or part associated with accumulation of a pigment in its cells. For example, lipofuscin deposition in cardiac myocytes imparts a brownish color to the myocardium of old people. **postmenopausal a.** The shrinking of the uterus in the postmenopausal period. **post-traumatic a. of bone** POST-TRAUMATIC OSTEOPOROSIS. **pressure a.** Atrophy of an organ or part caused by mechanical compression of a tumor, hematoma, or other expanding mass. Also *compression atrophy.* **primary optic a.** A type of optic atrophy in which ophthalmoscopically visible gliotic or pigmentary changes are absent. This results from damage to the deeper portions of the axons of the optic nerve, which may be affected anywhere between the exit of the retinal vessels from the optic nerve (about one centimeter behind the eye) and the lateral geniculate body (the end of this axon). **progressive diffuse cerebrocortical a.** ALPERS SYNDROME. **progressive facial a.** ROMBERG'S PROGRESSIVE FACIAL HEMIATROPHY. **progressive muscular a.** A form of motor neuron disease presenting as progressive muscular atrophy due to degeneration of anterior horn cells in the spinal cord. The condition commonly begins with wasting, weakness, and fasciculation of the small muscles of the hand, less often in the feet and legs, but may begin in any muscle or muscle group. Also *Aran-Duchenne amyotrophy, Cruveilhier's atrophy, myelopathic atrophy, Aran-Duchenne disease, Aran-Duchenne muscular atrophy, creeping palsy, atrophic muscular paralysis, creeping paralysis, Cruveilhier's paralysis, wasting paralysis, Duchenne syndrome.* **progressive neural a.** Atrophy of muscles due to disease of motor nerves. **progressive neural muscular a.** Any of a group of inherited neuropathies in which there is progressive muscular wasting and weakness and in which the primary pathological change is one of peripheral nerves rather than anterior horn cells in the spinal cord. The neuropathic varieties of peroneal muscular atrophy are examples. Also *progressive neuromuscular atrophy, progressive neuropathic muscular atrophy.* **progressive nuclear muscular a.** Any form of progressive muscular atrophy resulting from degeneration of the motor nuclei of the brainstem or of the anterior horns of the spinal cord, including the inherited forms of spinal muscular atrophy, as well as the muscular wasting which occurs in adult motor neuron disease. *Imprecise.* Also *progressive nuclear amyotrophy.* **progressive a. of the skin** Cutaneous atrophy that accompanies old age. Also *senile cutaneous atrophy.* **progressive spinal muscular a. of infancy** WERDNIG-HOFFMANN DISEASE. **progressive unilateral facial a.** An inherited condition characterized by progressive atrophy of the soft tissues of half of the face. It is accompanied by controlateral sensory jacksonian epilepsy, trigeminal neuralgia, and changes in the eyes and hair. In approximately 5 percent of cases there is also atrophy of half of the body. Also *hemifacial atrophy, unilateral facial atrophy, facial atrophy.* **pseudohypertrophic muscular a.** DUCHENNE TYPE MUSCULAR DYSTROPHY. **pseudomyopathic spinal muscular a.** JUVENILE FAMILIAL MUSCULAR ATROPHY. **pulp a.** A gradual diminution, associated with advancing age, in the number of cells of the dental pulp. **red a.** Atrophic changes secondary to congestion. **renal a.** A decrease in kidney substance involving the size and weight of all its elements. Also *atrophic kidney.* **rheumatic a.** Muscular or osseous atrophy due to rheumatic disease. **scapuloperoneal muscular a.** A form of progressive spinal muscular atrophy in which the muscular weakness and wasting begins in and often remains restricted to the periscapular and to the peroneal and anterior tibial groups of muscles. **Schweninger-Buzzi macular a.** Macular atrophy in which the protruding atrophic lesions, as large as 2 cm in diameter, can be readily indented with the fingers. No clinically evident inflammatory changes precede its onset. **secondary optic a.** A type of optic atrophy in which the changes caused by previous damage to the optic disk itself are visible. These changes include gliotic proliferation upon the disk and disruption of surrounding pigment. Also *gray atrophy.* **senile a.** Atrophy associated with normal aging. Also *physiologic atrophy, atrophia senilis.* **senile cutaneous a.** PROGRESSIVE ATROPHY OF THE SKIN. **serous a.** Atrophy of adipose tissue and its replacement by serous fluid. Often seen in cases of extreme malnutrition associated with rapid weight loss. **simple a.** Decrease in size of an organ or tissue not associated with any other changes. **spinopontine a.** A rare variety of hereditary ataxia of autosomal dominant inheritance giving progressive ataxia, nystagmus, dysarthria, hyperreflexia, and extensor plantar responses and in which there is degeneration of the nuclei of the basis pontis, cerebellar peduncles, and long tracts in the spinal cord. **striate a. of the skin** STRIAE ATROPHICAE. **subacute yellow a.** A form of liver atrophy similar to acute yellow atrophy but in which there is somewhat less cellular collapse and loss of hepatic architecture. **Sudeck's a.** POST-TRAUMATIC OSTEOPOROSIS. **syphilitic spinal muscular a.** A rare condition in which syphilitic meningomyelitis gives a clinical picture superficially similar to that of spinal muscular atrophy. Also *syphilitic progressive spinal muscular atrophy.* **testicular a.** Shrinking of a testis, due to any of various physiologic or pathologic causes. Also *atrophia testiculi, orchiatrophy, orchidatrophia, orchidatrophy.* **Tooth's a.** CHARCOT-MARIE-TOOTH DISEASE. **toxic a.** Tissue or organ atrophy associated with infectious diseases and presumed to result from the deleterious effects of toxins released by microbes. **traction a.** STRIAE ATROPHICAE. **traumatic a.** Decreased mass of a whole or part of a patient resulting from injury. Severe catabolism and malnutrition may decrease the whole body muscle mass by 30 percent prior to death. **tubular a.** A shrinkage or loss of renal tubule cells secondary to ischemia, tubule obstruction, or direct toxic injury. The tubules may be collapsed, dilated, or even normal in size, with cuboidal or flattened epithelial cells characterized by pale, vacuolated cytoplasm, decreased organelles, and sparse shortened microvilli in proximal tubules. The basement membranes of chronic atrophied tubules often are thickened. In advanced atrophy tubule cells may disappear. **unilateral facial a.** PROGRESSIVE UNILATERAL FACIAL ATROPHY. **vascular a.** Atrophy resulting from inadequate blood supply. **von Leber's a.** LEBER'S OPTIC ATROPHY. **Werdnig-Hoffmann a.** WERDNIG-HOFFMANN DISEASE. **white a.** ATROPHIE BLANCHE. **yellow a.** 1 See under ACUTE YELLOW ATROPHY OF THE LIVER. 2 See under SUBACUTE YELLOW ATROPHY.

**atropine** $C_{17}H_{23}NO_3$. An alkaloid obtained from *Atropa belladonna* with anticholinergic activity. It is used systemically to produce relaxation of smooth muscles in various organs, and is given locally in the eye to dilate the pupil and paralyze the ciliary muscle for accommodation. **fungal a.** A toxin similar to muscarine. It is found in *Amanita muscaria* and can cause death in man and animals if ingested in large quantities. Atropine is antidotal.

**atropine methylbromide** METHYLATROPINE HYDROBROMIDE.

**atropine methyl nitrate** $C_{18}H_{26}N_2O_6$. The methonitrate salt of atropine. It is a quaternary ammonium salt with properties like those of atropine, but is highly ionized in the body fluids and less effective on the central nervous system. It is used primarily to treat congenital pyloric stenosis and pylorospasm in infants. Also *methylatropine nitrate.*

**atropine oxide hydrochloride** $C_{17}H_{23}NO_4 \cdot HCl$. A preparation of atropine used to treat gastric ulcers and spasm of the gastrointestinal tract.

**atropine salicylate** A salt form of atropine that is soluble in water and in alcohol. It has the same uses as atropine sulfate.

**atropine sulfate** The sulfate salt of atropine, which has appreciable solubility in water. It is the most commonly used form of atropine for eye ointments, eye drops, injectable preparations, and tablets.

**atropinism** \at′rəpīnizm\ [*atropin(e)* + -ISM] Poisoning due to atropine. Also *atropism.*

**atropinization** The effects resulting from treatment with atropine, or the administration of atropine to achieve those effects.

**atropism** \at′rōpizm\ ATROPINISM.

**ATS** antitetanus serum (tetanus antitoxin).

**attachment** [French *attachement* (from Old French *estache* a post, akin to Old English *staca* a stake, + *-ment* -MENT) attachment] A fastening or connection of one part to another, as a tendon or ligament to bone. **bar a.** A fixed bar between two or more teeth or roots for supporting and retaining a removable denture. **epithelial a.** The biologic mechanism uniting epithelial cells of the junctional epithelium to the tooth surface. The morphologically recognizable components are hemidesmosomes and the internal basement lamina. **frictional a.** PRECISION ATTACHMENT. **intracoronal a.** A precision attachment in which the female portion lies entirely within the contour of the abutment tooth. Also *internal attachment, intracoronal retainer.* **key-and-keyway a.** *Outmoded* PRECISION ATTACHMENT. **muscle-tendon a.** The junction between the ends of muscle fibers and the tendinous processes where the sarcolemma covering the cone-shaped ends of the muscle fibers fuses with the ends of the collagenous bundles of the perimysium that are continuous with those of the tendon. Also *myotendinal junction.* **precision a.** A frictional fastener for a fixed or removable partial denture or bridge. It usually consists of male and female portions which fit together, the female being in the natural tooth and the male in the prothesis. Also *frictional attachment, key and keyway attachment* (outmoded).

**attack** An acute episode of disease or disordered function, such as a seizure, faint, or stroke. **adversive a.** An attack of focal epilepsy in which there is involuntary turning of the head and eyes to the opposite side. It is due to a unilateral frontal-lobe lesion. Also *Vulpian's conjugate deviation.* **anxiety a.** A sudden onset of anxiety that often mounts to panic proportions. **apnea a.'s** Prolonged pauses occurring in expiration in some newborn infants, particularly if premature. Such periods may last 20 seconds or longer before breathing begins again, either spontaneously or after gentle stimulation. When there is a risk of dangerous anoxia, an apneic monitor should be considered. Prolonged or frequent apneic attacks call for intervention. **apoplectiform a.** A stroke or cerebral vascular accident; an attack of apoplexy. • In the past this term has also been used to identify other acute disorders of cerebral function resembling a stroke, such as a congestive attack of general paresis. **cataplectic a.** CATAPLECTIC CRISIS. **centrencephalic a.** An epileptic attack which begins with loss of consciousness and in which the abnormal discharge starts in the upper brainstem. **cerebellar a.** TONIC CEREBELLAR ATTACK. **cyclical epileptic a.'s** Epileptic attacks arising spontaneously at more or less regular and foreseeable intervals. In most cases, cyclical seizures do not seem to be associated with any obvious predisposing factor, and their periodicity, which is governed by unknown biological mechanisms, seems to be significant only when analyzed statistically. More rarely, there is an obvious factor in connection with their periodicity, either diurnal rhythms, as in sleep epilepsy, or the menstrual cycle (catamenial epilepsy). **decerebrate a.** TONIC CEREBELLAR ATTACK. **drop a.** An episode of sudden falling, due to "giving way of the knees," without any alteration of consciousness, occurring most often in the middle-aged and elderly. The attacks have been attributed to brainstem ischemia due to vertebrobasilar insufficiency, but this has been disputed. They may be very frequent and troublesome, and rarely respond to any form of treatment. They are not epileptic. Also *drop seizure.* **epileptic a.** An episode of cerebral dysfunction resulting from a hypersynchronous, self-maintained neuronal discharge, which may involve both hemispheres (generalized epilepsy), one cerebral hemisphere (unilateral epilepsy) or part of a hemisphere (partial epilepsy). **epileptiform a.** An attack resembling epilepsy but different in etiology and character, such as a transient cerebral ischemic attack. **focal a.** An epileptic attack arising in a specific area of the brain, usually due to a focal organic lesion. **heart a.** A sudden cardiac disorder, especially an episode of myocardial infarction. **major epileptic a.** An attack of epilepsy with loss of consciousness and a tonic-clonic (convulsive) phase. **myoclonic a.** MYOCLONUS. **nonepileptic vagal a.** WHITE BREATH-HOLDING. **posterior a.** TONIC CEREBELLAR ATTACK. **subclinical epileptic a.** SUBCLINICAL EPILEPSY. **tonic a.** TONIC CONVULSION. **tonic cerebellar a.** A type of attack marked by sudden hyperextension of the body in opisthotonus, with the eyeballs rolled upwards, and generally occurring without loss of consciousness. The attack may last for several minutes. This condition is usually observed in patients with tumors in the posterior cerebral fossa, and is usually accompanied by increased intracranial pressure. Also *posterior crisis, posterior attack, cerebellar attack, decerebrate crisis, decerebrate attack.* **transient carotid ischemic a.** An episode of transient cerebral ischemia involving that part of the brain supplied by the internal carotid artery. **transient ischemic a.** An episode of transient ischemia of the brain or brainstem producing symptoms of neurologic dysfunction which may last for minutes or hours, and then subsides completely but shows a tendency to recur. Most are due to recurrent microembolism, some to hemodynamic causes. Abbr. TIA Also *transient cerebral ischemia.* **uncinate a.** An attack of focal epilepsy due to an abnormal discharge, and usually a focal lesion, arising in the uncinate gyrus of the temporal lobe. Typically the attack begins with an olfactory or gustatory aura which may be succeeded by other manifestations of temporal lobe epilepsy, including fear, anxiety, déjà vu, and/or jamais vu. **unilateral epileptiform a.** Transient motor or sensory manifestations confined to one half of the body and due to a contralateral cerebral lesion. Most such episodes should be classified as attacks of focal or jacksonian epilepsy, while those which resemble but are different etiologically from epilepsy, such as transient cerebral ischemia, should be identified according to their causation. **vasovagal a.** An unusual form of attack, characterized by gastric, respiratory, and cardiac discomfort with slowing of the pulse, pallor, and sometimes with impaired consciousness. Some are probably syncopal, some emotional, and some epileptic. *Outmoded.* Also *Gowers disease, Gowers syndrome.*

**attention** An adjustment made by the sense organs, central nervous system, and the body's postural mechanisms to maximize the clearness of a particular stimulus or situation. This focusing lends vividness to selected aspects of mental experience, while inhibiting the action of others, to produce a state of optimal responsiveness in behavior.

**attenuant** An agent that dilutes or weakens the virulence of a pathogenic organism or the effects of a drug.

**attenuated** \əten′yoo·ā′tid\ Having decreased virulence: used especially of live virus vaccines. Attenuation is achieved either through selection of less virulent mutants or through physiologic alteration by exposure to unfavorable conditions.

**attenuation** \əten′yoo·ā′shən\ A reduction in power, intensity, activity, or virulence, as of a wave as it passes through a medium, of an electric quantity as it passes through an attenuator, or of a live virus vaccine by selection of less virulent mutants or by exposure to unfavorable conditions.

**attenuator** \əten′yoo·ā′tər\ An electrical device that reduces the amplitude of a voltage or current, with essentially no distortion of the waveform.

**attic** [French *attique* (from L *atticus* of Attica) a top storey, upper compartment] RECESSUS EPITYMPANICUS. **tympanic a.** RECESSUS EPITYMPANICUS.

**atticoantral** \at′ikō·an′trəl\ Of or relating to the recessus epitympanicus and the antrum mastoideum of the middle ear.

**atticoantrotomy** \at′ikō·anträt′əmē\ The surgical exposure of the atticoantral region of the middle ear, by way of the external auditory meatus. The operation entails removing the outer epitympanic wall and the posterosuperior wall of the deep part of the meatus so as to expose the epitympanic and antral contents with a view to eradicating disease. Also *antroatticotomy.*

**atticotomy** \at′ikät′əmē\ [ATTIC + *o* + -TOMY] The surgical exposure of the epitympanum of the middle ear, performed in order to explore the epitympanum and, if possible, eradicate disease. **transmeatal a.** An atticotomy performed through the intact external auditory meatus.

**attitude** [French (from Italian *attitudine* posture, disposition, from L *aptitudo* fitness) posture, attitude] **1** Position of the body; posture. **2** The relative position of the fetus *in utero.* **3** A relatively stable set of dispositions for the individual to respond in characteristic ways to stimuli; a mental set. Attitudes are determined both by culture and from individual experience. **abstract a.** The ability to conceptualize and to think symbolically. It involves voluntarily assuming a mental set, shifting voluntarily from one aspect of a situation to another, extracting a general rule from a series of discrete events, organizing and planning ahead in time, and assuming an attitude to the merely possible. Abstraction ability and the ability to shift back and forth as needed between the abstract attitude and the concrete attitude are indicators of cerebral integrity that are likely to be impaired early on in the course of any brain disorder. Also *categorical attitude.* **a. of combat** PUGILISTIC ATTITUDE. **deflexion a.** A form of cephalic presentation of the fetal head where, due to deflexion of the head, either a brow or face presentation occurs. **Devergie's a.** A posture in death marked by flexed elbows and knees, extended ankles, and closed fingers. **discobolus a.** The attitude assumed by an individual standing with his arms extended sideways, when a cold caloric stimulus is applied to one ear. Reflex action causes the arm on the stimulated side to fall while the other arm rises. **fetal a.** The relationship of the various parts of the body of a fetus to each other. Normally, the fetal attitude is characterized by moderate flexion of all the joints, with the head flexed upon the abdomen and chest. **forced a.** An unusual or abnormal position of an extremity or part of the body resulting from a neurological or musculoskeletal condition. **pugilistic a.** Postmortem flexion of the elbows, knees, hips, and neck, mimicking the defensive posture of a boxer, with fists clenched. It is seen in burned, usually charred, bodies and is caused by the stiffening and shortening of muscle fibers by heat. Also *attitude of combat.*

**atto-** \at′ō-\ [Danish *atten* eighteen] A prefix denoting $10^{-18}$: used with SI units. Symbol: a

**attractant** \ətrak′tənt\ Any agent that stimulates the approach of some type of organism, such as pheromones or other baits that attract insects or other pests to poisons or traps.

**attraction** The power or process by which bodies are drawn together. **capillary a.** CAPILLARITY. **electric a.** A force of attraction resulting from the property of being electrically charged.

**attribute** \at′rəbyoot\ A qualitative characteristic of an individual or group, such as sex or blood group, as opposed to a quantitative value, such as body weight or blood pressure level.

**attrition** \ətrish′ən\ **1** The action or process of rubbing or wearing away. **2** The mechanical wearing down of biting surfaces of the teeth from mastication, characterized by differential wear of dentin and enamel.

**at vol** atomic volume.

**Atwater** [Wilbur Olin *Atwater,* U.S. scientist, 1844–1907] Atwater's chamber, Atwater-Benedict chamber, Atwater-Benedict calorimeter. See under ATWATER'S CALORIMETER.

**at wt** atomic weight.

**AU** **1** antitoxin unit. **2** *aures unitas* (L, both ears together). **3** *aures uterque* (L, each ear).

**Au** Symbol for the element, gold.

**Au-antigenemia** \an′təjənē′mē·ə\ The presence of hepatitis B virus surface antigen (formerly called Australia antigen) in the blood.

**Aub** [Joseph Charles *Aub,* U.S. physician, 1890–1973] Aub-Dubois standards. See under DUBOIS STANDARD.

**Aubert** [Hermann *Aubert,* German physiologist and psychologist, 1826–1892] See under PHENOMENON.

***Auchmeromyia luteola*** \ôkmer′ōmī′yə loo′tē·ō′lə\ A fly common in Africa south of the Sahara desert. The larva, known as the Congo floor maggot, sucks the blood of persons sleeping on the floor or on low beds. It can cause considerable discomfort, but is not involved in the transmission of any known disease agent.

**audio-** \ô′dē·ō-\ [L *audire* to hear] A combining form meaning hearing.

**audioanalgesia** \-an′aljē′zē·ə\ The delivery of certain sound waves or music via earphones to reduce the sensation of pain during dental or surgical procedures. Also *audio analgesia.*

**audiogenic** \-jen′ik\ [AUDIO- + -GENIC] Occurring as a result of exposure to sound.

**audiogram** \ô′dē·əgram′\ [AUDIO- + -GRAM] A chart, produced by an audiometer, recording the auditory threshold of the individual being tested. The chart can be produced manually or by a printer. **Bekesy a.** The audiogram obtained using the Bekesy audiometer. It is characterized by a continuous zigzag line plotting the auditory threshold from low to high frequency. Also *self-recording audiogram*. **cortical a.** The audiogram resulting from cortical-evoked response audiometry. **pure tone a.** An audiogram in which the threshold for pure tone stimuli is charted in decibels of hearing level down the vertical axis, the horizontal axis being the frequency which is usually measured in octave steps from 125 Hz to 8 kHz. **self-recording a.** **1** An audiogram that results from a semiautomatic pure tone audiometer. It is used for hearing screening in industry. **2** BEKESY AUDIOGRAM. **serial a.** One of a sequence of audiograms charting variation of auditory threshold in an individual over a period of time. **speech a.** The graphic display of an individual's ability to perceive the words or sentences of standardized, recorded speech material. It is usually charted by percentage accuracy against intensity.

**audiologist** \ô′dē·äl′əjist\ [*audiolog(y)* + -IST] An individual involved in the diagnosis, assessment, management, education, or rehabilitation of the hearing-impaired. • This is an imprecise term as it is applied variously to a physician specializing in audiologic medicine, an audiologic scientist or technician, an educational audiologist, or a trained retailer of hearing aids.

**audiology** \ô′dē·äl′əjē\ [AUDIO- + -LOGY] The scientific study of hearing in man and other animals, including the effects of deranged function, and frequently also including aspects of the education and rehabilitation of the hearing-impaired. Compare ACOUSTICS.

**audiometer** \ô′dē·äm′ətər\ [AUDIO- + -METER] The instrumentation used to measure auditory acuity and to establish the hearing threshold for pure tones, modulated tones, or other stimuli, or speech material. **Bekesy a.** A pure tone audiometer in which the tone is progressively changed across the usual frequency range, the intensity being continuously controlled by the subject so that it remains just audible. **evoked response a.** Electrophysiologic instrumentation required for the administration of trains of auditory stimuli, and the amplifying and computer facilities required for the subsequent signal processing, as a means of determining auditory response. **Langenbeck's noise a.** An audiometer used to determine aspects of suprathreshold hearing function. A noise of predetermined intensity is presented and the intensity at which pure tones are just heard produces the supraliminal noise audiometric curve. **pure tone a.** An instrument used universally in the measurement of hearing, generating pure tones of specified frequencies and intensities, usually at octave or half-octave intervals and in 5 dB increments, calibrated according to international standards. **semiautomatic pure tone a.** A pure tone audiometer in which tone of the stimulus is changed automatically after a short period of time to one an octave higher. The intensity varies continuously, either increasing or decreasing, and is controlled by the subject in an effort to maintain the loudness at a just perceptible level.

**audiometric** \-met′rik\ Having to do with the measurement of auditory acuity.

**audiometrician** \-mətrish′ən\ A person trained to measure auditory threshold, and, usually, to carry out a wide variety of other audiologic investigations. Also *audiologic technician, physiological measurement technician in audiology* (British usage).

**audiometry** \ô′dē·äm′ətrē\ [AUDIO- + -METRY] The measurement of auditory acuity in order to determine the hearing threshold. **air-conduction a.** Audiometry involving the determination of pure-tone auditory threshold for air-borne sounds and usually involving the use of earphones. **Bekesy a.** Audiometry using the Bekesy audiometer. **bone-conduction a.** Audiometry for determining pure tone auditory threshold, using a bone conduction transducer. **brainstem-evoked response a.** Audiometry involving the detection and measurement of changes in electric potential arising from the auditory stimulation of the cochlea and its neural connections to the midbrain. Also *brainstem-evoked audiometry* (incorrect). **clinical a.** Audiometry involving the clinical use of a tuning fork, voice, and pure tone audiometry as appropriate. **cortical-evoked response a.** Audiometry involving the detection of time-related changes of electrical potential emanating from the cortex in response to a train of auditory, usually tonal, stimuli of appropriate intensity. Also *cortical audiometry*. Abbr. CERA **electric response a.** Audiometry involving the detection of changes of electric potential in the neural structures subserving audition induced by audible sound stimuli. Also *evoked response audiometry*. Abbr. ERA **electrodermal a.** PSYCHOGALVANIC SKIN RESPONSE AUDIOMETRY. **evoked response a.** ELECTRIC RESPONSE AUDIOMETRY. **impedance a.** The measurement of middle-ear function using the impedance bridge. • This is an incorrect term since it is not necessarily an auditory threshold which is measured. **industrial a.** The routine measurement of hearing threshold of workers in heavy industry and other employment where there are high ambient noise levels. **localization a.** Audiometry involving the use of the localization response in the infant and younger child as an indicator that a free-field sound stimulus of known intensity has been heard. **psychogalvanic skin response a.** A technique, now little used, for measuring hearing by gauging alteration in the electric resistance of the subject's skin consequent upon a mild electric shock administered with the auditory stimulus. Also *electrodermal audiometry, PGSR audiometry, psychogalvanic audiometry*. **pure tone a.** The technique by which the pure tone audiogram is obtained. **self-recording a.** The use of a semiautomatic pure tone audiometer, usually for screening in industry. Also *self-screening audiometry*.

**audiovisual** \-vizh′oo·əl\ Making use of both hearing and sight.

**audit** \ô′dit\ **medical a.** Detailed retrospective review and evaluation of medical records by a skilled staff to assess the care that was provided.

**audition** [L *auditio* (from *auditus*, past part. of *audire* to hear) the sense or sensation of hearing] The process, use, or sense of hearing. **thought a.** A hallucination that one's own thoughts are being spoken or broadcast by another. Also *thought echoing*.

**auditorius** \ô′ditôr′ē·əs\ NERVUS VESTIBULOCOCHLEARIS.

**auditory** \ô′ditôr′ē\ Pertaining to audition.

**auditosensory** \ô′ditōsen′sərē\ Describing or pertaining to the auditory receptive area of the temporal cortex.

**Auerbach** [Leopold *Auerbach*, German anatomist, 1828–1897] **1** Auerbach's node. See under GANGLION. **2** Auerbach's plexus. See under PLEXUS MYENTERICUS.

**Aufricht** [Gustave *Aufricht*, U.S. surgeon, 1894–1972] See under SPECULUM.

**AUG** acute ulcerative gingivitis.

**Auger** [Pierre Victor *Auger*, French physicist, born 1899]

See under EFFECT, ELECTRON.

**augmentor** \ôgmen′tər\ Serving to increase the force and excursion of heart muscle contractions, as nerve cells or their axons.

**augnathus** \ôgnā′thəs\ [Gk *au* again + *gnathos* jaw, esp. lower jaw] An embryo, fetus, or infant with a doubled mandibular arch or lower jaw.

**aula** \ô′lə\ [L, forecourt of a Greek house, inner court] The most anterior or rostral portion of the third ventricle. *Seldom used.*

**auliplexus** \ô′liplek′səs\ The part of the choroid plexus extending into the aula. *Obs.*

**aura** \ôr′ə\ [Gk, breeze, breath, gasp, aura] **1** Any sensation or feeling which precedes an attack of epilepsy whether the latter is focal or generalized in character. These warning sensations in fact constitute a part of the attack. Thus affective (fear, anxiety), sensory (visual, auditory, gustatory, olfactory, or somatic), epigastric, and many other types of aura have been described and their character may be helpful in identifying the site of origin of the epileptic discharge, which may then remain localized to give a focal seizure or may spread more widely and produce a major attack. **2** Any of the prodromal or warning symptoms of an attack of migraine which may include a variety of visual, sensory and, less often, motor symptoms due to ischemia of the retina, cerebral cortex, or brainstem which result from the initial phase of arterial constriction occurring in this condition. Adj. aural. **auditory a.** An aura in which the subject hears sounds, either complex and formed, such as bells, music, etc., or crude and unorganized. **autonomic a.** AUTONOMIC EPILEPSY. **dysmnesic a.** DYSMNESIC EPILEPSY. **epileptic a.** Any aura occurring in an attack of epilepsy. Also *abortive epilepsy.* **generalized somatic a.** GENERALIZED EPILEPTIC SOMATIC SENSATION. **gustatory a.** *Incorrect* PRIMARY GUSTATORY EPILEPSY. **hallucinatory a.** *Incorrect* EPILEPTIC HALLUCINATION. **illusional a.** EPILEPTIC ILLUSION. **intellectual a.** The transient state of dreaminess, detachment, or depersonalization which may constitute the aura of an attack of temporal lobe epilepsy. **kinesthetic a.** Any sensation of movement of a part or of the whole of the body occurring at the onset of an epileptic attack before consciousness is lost. Also *motor aura.* **myoclonic a.** Myoclonic jerking preceding a major epileptic seizure. **neuralgic a.** Any painful sensation occurring as a part of the aura or primary manifestations of an attack of focal somatosensory epilepsy. Also *neuralgiform aura.* **paramnesic a.** DYSMNESIC EPILEPSY. **primary auditory a.** PRIMARY AUDITORY EPILEPSY. **psychic a.** *Incorrect* PSYCHIC EPILEPSY. **reminiscent a.** An intellectual aura in which there is also a sensation of déjà vu. **sensory a.** PRIMARY SOMATOSENSORY EPILEPSY. **somatosensory a.** PRIMARY SOMATOSENSORY EPILEPSY. **a. vertiginosa** VERTIGINOUS EPILEPSY. **vertiginous a.** VERTIGINOUS EPILEPSY. **visceral a.** AUTONOMIC EPILEPSY. **visual a.** Any aura in which the subject experiences visual hallucinations, whether formed and complex or unformed and crude. See also PRIMARY VISUAL EPILEPSY.

**aural**[1] \ôr′əl\ [L *aur(is)* ear + -AL] Of, relating to, or received by the ear.

**aural**[2] \ôr′əl\ [*aur(a)* + -AL] Relating to or characteristic of an aura.

**auramine O** \ôr′əmin\ A yellow dye that fluoresces under appropriate excitation. Because it penetrates the cell wall of acid-fast organisms, it is used with rhodamine B to stain fixed preparations of tubercle bacilli. It is also used as a stain of DNA and as a skin antiseptic. Also *canary yellow.*

**aurantiasis** \ôr′əntī′əsis\ [New L *aurant(ius)* orange-colored + -IASIS] HYPERCAROTENEMIA.

**aurantiogliocladin** $C_{10}H_{12}O_4$. 2,3-Dimethoxy-5,6-dimethyl-*p*-benzoquinone. An antibiotic substance found in *Gliocladium* species.

**Aureomycin** A proprietary name for chlortetracycline hydrochloride.

**aures** \ôr′ēz\ Plural of AURIS.

**auri-**[1] \ôr′ē-, ôri-\ [L *auris* ear] A combining form denoting the ear.

**auri-**[2] [L *aurum* gold] A combining form denoting gold, especially gold(III).

**auriasis** \ôrī′əsis\ CHRYSIASIS.

**auric** \ôr′ik\ [L *aur(um)* gold + -IC] Related to gold. • This term was previously used exclusively for the Au(III) state.

**auricle** \ôr′ikl\ [L *auricula.* See AURICULA.] **1** AURICULA. **2** ATRIUM CORDIS. **accessory a.** A cervical auricle, or a poorly formed external ear on the neck, usually over the sternomastoid muscle and probably related to the groove of one of the ectodermal clefts. Cartilage is sometimes present but the "ear" is seldom more than an annoying cutaneous projection. Also *cervical auricle.* **left a. of heart** AURICULA SINISTRA. **right a. of heart** AURICULA DEXTRA.

**auricula** \ôrik′yələ\ [L (dim. of *auris* the ear), lobe of the ear] **1** [NA] The irregularly shaped fibrocartilaginous plate that is covered with skin and projects from each side of the head, having a concave lateral surface of eminences and depressions and serving as part of the external ear to collect and channel the vibrations of sound waves to the tympanic membrane. Also *auricle, pinna, ala auris.* **2** AURICULA ATRIALIS. **3** *Outmoded* ATRIUM CORDIS. **a. atrialis** [NA] A small pouchlike muscular appendage projecting from the anterosuperior surface of each atrium of the heart, the right one being conical and the left one more elongated, more curved, and narrower than the right. Also *atrial appendage, auricular appendage, auricula, auricular appendix.* **a. dextra** [NA] The small pouchlike muscular projection from the anterosuperior part of the right atrium of the heart, extending to the left to cover the base of the ascending aorta medially. Its interior is ridged by a lacework of pectinate muscles continuous with those on part of the atrium. Also *right auricle of heart, right auricular appendage.* **a. sinistra** [NA] The long, narrow, and curved muscular projection from the anterosuperior part of the left atrium of the heart, extending over the left side of the origin of the pulmonary trunk. Its inner surface has a meshwork of pectinate muscles, and it is separated from the atrium by a slight constriction. Also *left auricle of heart, left auricular appendage.*

**auriculae** \ôrik′yəlē\ Plural of AURICULA.

**auricular** \ôrik′yələr\ **1** Of or relating to the auricle or the ear in general. Also *pinnal, auricularis.* **2** *Outmoded* ATRIAL. **3** Pertaining to an auricula atrii.

**auricularis** \ôr′ikyəler′is\ **1** AURICULAR. **2** ATRIAL.

**auriculectomy** \ôrik′yəlek′təmē\ Excision of the auricle.

**auriculotemporal** \ôrik′yəlōtem′pərəl\ Having to do with the auricle of the external ear as well as with the adjacent temporal region. Also *temporoauricular.*

**auriculoventricular** \ôrik′yəlōventrik′yələr\ ATRIOVENTRICULAR.

**auriform** \ôr′ifôrm\ [AURI-[1] + -FORM] Shaped like an ear.

**aurin** \ôr′in\ **1** A colored compound, derived from triphenylmethane, that is used as a pH indicator and as stain for tubercle bacilli. Dark red with greenish metallic luster in its crystalline state, it changes from yellow to purplish red at a pH 6.8 to 8.2. Also *corallin.* **2** ROSOLIC ACID.

**aurinarium** A suppository or bougie for the outer ear, usually having a cocoa-butter base.

**aurintricarboxylic acid** A chelating agent with high affinity for beryllium, which has been used to treat beryllium poisoning. The ammonium salt is used to measure aluminum.

**auris** \ôr′is\ [L, the ear] The organ of hearing or vestibulocochlear organ, comprising auris externa, auris media, and auris interna; the ear. **a. externa** [NA] The outer portion of the vestibulocochlear organ, comprising the auricle, or pinna, and the external acoustic meatus and conducting sound waves to the tympanic membrane, which separates it from the middle ear. Also *external ear, outer ear* (seldom used). **a. interna** [NA] The innermost portion of the vestibulocochlear organ that comprises two parts, namely, the bony labyrinth within the petrous part of the temporal bone consisting of the vestibule, cochlea, and three semicircular canals, within which is the second part, the membranous labyrinth consisting of the saccule and utricle in the vestibule, the duct of the cochlea, and the three semicircular ducts. The branches of the vestibulocochlear nerve ramify in the walls of the membranous labyrinth, within which is endolymph and surrounding which is the perilymph. Also *internal ear, inner ear.* **a. media** [NA] The irregular cavity lined by mucoperiosteum, filled with air, and extending medially from the tympanic membrane to the lateral wall of the internal ear in the petrous part of the temporal bone. It may be divided into cavitas tympanica, adnexa mastoidea, and tuba auditiva. The latter connects it anteriorly to the nasopharynx, while it communicates posteriorly with the mastoid antrum through the aditus ad antrum. Also *middle ear.* • Formerly it was regarded synonymous with cavitas tympanica (or cavum tympani), but this is now considered to be only part of the middle ear.

**auriscope** \ôr′iskōp\ [AURI-[1] + -SCOPE] OTOSCOPE.

**aurist** \ôr′ist\ *Older term* OTOLOGIST.

**auro-** [L *aurum* gold] A combining form denoting gold, especially gold(I).

**aurochromoderma** \ôr′ōkrō′mədur′mə\ CHRYSIASIS.

**aurotherapy** \ôr′ōther′əpē\ CHRYSOTHERAPY.

**aurothioglucose** A water-soluble compound of gold containing about 50% gold. It has been used in the treatment of rheumatoid arthritis and some related diseases such as nondisseminated lupus erythematosus.

**aurothioglycanide** $\alpha$-Auromercaptoacetanilid. An organic form of gold that is practically insoluble in water, ether, and chloroform. It is equivalent to sodium aurothiomalate in effectiveness and toxicity. Also *aurothioglycolanilide.*

**aurothiomalate disodium** $C_4H_3AuNa_2O_4S.H_2O$. A water-soluble gold salt used in the treatment of rheumatoid arthritis. Also *gold sodium thiomalate, sodium aurothiosuccinate.*

**aurothiosulfate** $Na_3Au(S_2O_3)_2$. A water-soluble gold salt that has been used for the treatment of rheumatoid arthritis.

**auscultate** \ôs′kultāt\ To examine (a patient) by auscultation; to subject to auscultation. Also *auscult.*

**auscultation** \ôs′kultā′shən\ [L *auscultatio* (from *auscultare* to listen, from *aus-*, variant of *aur(is)* ear, + *-c(u)l-*, variant of *-cli-* as in *(in)cli(nare)* to incline, bend down) attentive listening, lit., bending an ear] A physical examination by listening, with or without a stethoscope, usually to the lungs, heart, abdomen, or peripheral vessels. **direct a.** Auscultation without a stethoscope. Also *immediate auscultation.* **obstetric a.** Auscultation of the fetal heart during pregnancy or labor.

**auscultatory** \ôskul′tətôr′ē\ Of or relating to auscultation; perceived by auscultation.

**Austin Flint** [*Austin Flint,* U.S. physician, 1812–1866] Austin Flint phenomenon. See under MURMUR.

**Australoid** \ôs′trəloid\ **1** Characterized by or similiar to the physical features of the aboriginal peoples of Australia, or of Australasia (Australia, New Guinea, and Melanesia). **2** An individual having such physical features.

**Australopithecinae** \ôstrā′lōpith′əsī′nē\ [*Australopithec(us),* a genus, + *-inae,* a suffix used for zoological subfamilies] The zoological subfamily that contains the fossil "apemen," "man-apes," and "near-men" from the Plio-Pleistocene, first discovered in 1924 at Taung in the Republic of South Africa. Their known range has been extended by subsequent finds to east Africa, including such sites as Olduvai Gorge in Tanzania, Koobi Fora in Kenya, and Hadar in Ethiopia.

**australopithecine** \ôstrā′lōpith′əsin\ **1** Belonging or pertaining to the Australopithecinae. **2** A member of the Australopithecinae.

***Australopithecus*** \ôstrā′lōpith′əkəs\ [New L, from L *austral(is)* southern + Gk *pithēkos* ape, monkey] A genus of the Australopithecinae that includes groups of south and east African fossil hominids.

***Austrobilharzia*** \ôs′trōbilhär′zē·ə\ [New L (from L *auster* the south + *BILHARZIA*] A genus of blood flukes in the family Schistosomatidae. They are parasitic in aquatic birds and are used experimentally to infect other birds. Several species are implicated in human cercarial dermatitis (swimmer's itch).

**aut-** \ôt-\ AUTO-.

**autarcesis** \ôtär′səsis\ [Gk *autarkē(s)* (from *aut(os)* self + *arkein* to ward off) strong enough, independent + -SIS] NATURAL IMMUNITY.

**autecious** \ôtē′shəs\ [AUT- + Gk *oiki(a)* a dwelling + -OUS] Requiring only one host to complete the life cycle: a characteristic of many parasites. Also *autoecious, autecic, autoecic, homecious, homoecious.* Compare HETERECIOUS.

**autism** \ô′tizm\ [AUT- + -ISM] Thinking and behavior which shows a preoccupation with the self to the relative exclusion of the outside world, which may in time seem unreal to the subject. Also *autosynnoia.* **akinetic a.** *Obs.* CATATONIC STUPOR. **early infantile a.** A pervasive developmental disorder with onset before 30 months of age, consisting of self-absorption, inability to relate to others, auditory avoidance simulating deafness and avoidance of eye contact, many language disturbances such as echolalia and metaphoric language, an anxious and obsessive desire to maintain the status quo, highly repetitive play, predilection for rhythmic movements such as rocking and whirling, a peculiar attachment to isolated objects, and a sensual preoccupation with surfaces. Motor development and skills are hardly impaired. When intelligence is innately high a very gradual improvement to near normal can be expected. Also *childhood autism, infantile autism, Kanner syndrome, childhood schizophrenia.* Adj. autistic.

**autistic** \ôtis′tik\ Characterized by autism.

**auto-** \ô′tō-\ [Gk *autos* self] A prefix meaning self, arising from within rather than from without. Also *aut-.*

**autoagglutination** \-əgloo′tənā′shən\ The agglutination of particles such as erythrocytes or platelets when suspended in one's own plasma or serum without addition of antiserum or other substances.

**autoagglutinin** \-əgloo′tinin\ An autoantibody giving rise to agglutination, usually of erythrocytes.

**autoallergic** \-əlur′jik\ AUTOIMMUNE.

**autoallergization** \-əlur′jīzā′shən\ The act or process by which autoallergy is produced.
**autoallergy** \-al′ərjē\ AUTOIMMUNITY.
**autoanalyzer** \-an′əlīzər\ An instrument that uses continuous-flow technology to perform automated chemical testing. Specimens are aspirated into tubing and kept separate by a bolus of air or inert solution. Sample fractions and reagents, separated by air bubbles, flow continuously through appropriate equipment for the establishment of reactions and photometric determination of end points.
**autoantibody** \-an′tibäd′ē\ [AUTO- + ANTIBODY] An antibody that reacts with a component of the tissues of the animal making the antibody. Also *autoimmune antibody* (older term). **cold a.** An autoantibody that is active only at temperatures below 37°C. **Donath-Landsteiner cold a.** DONATH-LANDSTEINER ANTIBODY. **incomplete a.** An autoantibody to erythrocytes found at low titer in normal subjects that can be detected even at reduced temperatures only by its ability to initiate complement activation and that cannot by itself agglutinate erythrocytes. **warm a.** An autoantibody that binds to cells such as erythrocytes at 37°C.
**autoanticomplement** \-an′tēkäm′pləment\ IMMUNOCONGLUTININ.
**autoantigen** \-an′təjən\ [AUTO- + ANTIGEN] A tissue component of a subject that produces an immune response (autoantibodies) within the subject. Also *self antigen*. Adj. autoantigenic.
**autoaudible** \-ô′dibl\ Audible to oneself: used especially of sounds arising within the components of the middle or inner ear or vascular and other sounds arising more distantly in the body.
**autobacteriophage** \-baktir′ē·əfāj′\ An autogenous bacteriophage; a phage obtained from the patient under treatment.
**autobiotic** \-bī·ät′ik\ [AUTO- + BIOTIC] Describing any substance produced by a cell which influences the activities of that cell.
**autocatalytic** Denoting a process whose product is a catalyst for the process, so that once initiated the process rapidly accelerates.
**autocholecystectomy** \-kō′lēsistek′təmē\ [AUTO- + CHOLECYSTECTOMY] Spontaneous infolding of the gallbladder into the intestine followed by separation from its attachments and passage of the organ out through the intestinal tract.
**autochthonous** \ôtäk′thənəs\ [Gk *autochthōn* (from *auto-* self + *chthōn* land, earth) indigenous, native + -OUS] **1** Native to a particular habitat; aboriginal. **2** Describing a tissue graft transplanted to a new site on the same individual. *Seldom used.*
**autocinesis** \-sīnē′sis\ AUTOKINESIS.
**autoclave** \ô′tōklāv\ [French (from *auto-* AUTO- + L *clav(is)* a key) orig., a pressure lock] An automatically regulated apparatus for the sterilization of objects by steam under pressure.
**Autoclip** A surgical clip applied with an automatic staple. It is usually employed for wound closure in place of a suture. A proprietary name.
**autocytolysis** \-sītäl′isis\ AUTOLYSIS.
**autocytolytic** \-sī′təlit′ik\ AUTOLYTIC.
**autodepilation** \-dep′ilā′shən\ AUTOEPILATION.
**autodigestion** \-dijes′chən\ AUTOLYSIS.
**autodiploid** \-dip′loid\ Having two chromosomes or sets of chromosomes that arose from reduplication of a haploid chromosome or set. Examples of autodiploid bodies are ovarian teratomas and intrauterine moles.
**autoechopraxia** \-ek′ōprak′sē·ə\ [AUTO- + ECHOPRAXIA] Purposeless repetition of a stereotyped movement.
**autoecic** \ôtē′sik\ AUTECIOUS.
**autoecious** \ôtē′shəs\ AUTECIOUS.
**autoeczematization** \-ekzem′ətīzā′shən\ SECONDARY SPREAD.
**autoepilation** \-ep′ilā′shən\ A spontaneous loss of hair. Also *autodepilation.*
**autoeroticism** \-irät′isizm\ [AUTO- + EROTICISM] **1** In psychoanalytic psychology, the earliest stage in the development of object relationships where the self is the only object recognized and the infant does not differentiate between self and nonself. **2** Self-stimulation, especially masturbation. For defs. 1 and 2 also *autoerotism, autosexualism.*
**autoerythrophagocytosis** \-irith′rəfag′əsītō′sis\ The ingestion of autologous erythrocytes by macrophages.
**autofluorescence** \-floo′əres′əns\ Fluorescence brought on by substances naturally present in a tissue. Also *natural fluorescence.*
**autofundoscope** \-fun′dəskōp\ AUTO-OPHTHALMOSCOPE.
**autogamous** \ôtäg′əməs\ Pertaining to or characterized by autogamy.
**autogamy** \ôtäg′əmē\ [AUTO- + Gk *gam(os)* marriage + -Y] A form of self-fertilization. In one type of autogamy, nuclear division occurs without cytokinesis, the two resulting nuclei reuniting to form a synkaryon. In other cases, closely related cells conjugate. In some species of Protozoa the unicellular organism divides into two daughter gametes which undergo a period of nuclear maturation before they fuse. Also *automixis.*
**autogeneic** \-jənē′ik\ AUTOGENOUS.
**autogenesis** \-jen′əsis\ SPONTANEOUS GENERATION. Adj. autogenetic, autogenic.
**autogenous** \ôtäj′ənəs\ [Gk *autogen(ēs)* sprung from the same stock + -OUS] **1** Originating within an individual, as a bacterial vaccine derived from a patient's own bacterial flora or tissue transferred from one site to another within the same subject. Also *autogeneic.* **2** Capable of autogeny, as certain kinds of mosquito.
**autogeny** \ôtäj′ənē\ [AUTO- + -GEN + -Y] The maturation of eggs in a female insect without benefit of any special type of feeding to supply particular nutrients, as in certain mosquitos which can reproduce successfully without the female's blood meal that is required in most species.
**autograft** \ô′təgraft\ [AUTO- + GRAFT] Tissue or an organ transplanted from one site to another within or on the same individual. Also *autotransplant, autologous graft* (older term).
**autografting** \ô′təgrafting\ The transplantation of an autograft. Also *autotransplantation, autoplasty.*
**autohemagglutination** \-hem′əgloo′tinā′shən\ Clumping of the red cells of an individual in whose serum the agglutinin is found.
**autohemagglutinin** \-hem′əgloo′tinin\ Antibody capable of clumping red blood cells of an individual in whose serum it is found.
**autohemic** \-hē′mik\ Dependent upon the presence of autologous blood.
**autohemolysin** \-hēmäl′isin\ Antibody capable of destroying red blood cells of an individual in whose serum it is found. Also *autohemopsonin* (obs.).
**autohemolysis** \-hēmäl′isis\ Accelerated destruction of a person's own red blood cells. Adj. autohemolytic.
**autohemopsonin** \-hem′äpsō′nin\ *Obs.* AUTOHEMOLYSIN.
**autohemotherapy** \-hē′məther′əpē\ Treatment of disease by means of autotransfusion.

**autohistoradiograph** \-his′tərā′dē·əgraf′\ AUTORADIOGRAPH.
**autoimmune** \-imyoon′\ Marked by the state of autoimmunity; having the property of responding immunologically to tissues of one's own body. Also *autoallergic.*
**autoimmunity** \-imyoo′nitē\ [AUTO- + IMMUNITY] A condition characterized by cell-mediated or humoral immunologic response to antigens of one's own body. This occasional departure from the usual recognition of self and nonself by the immune system contributes to a variety of diseases. Also *autoallergy.*
**autoimmunization** \-im′yənīzā′shən\ Any act or process by which autoimmunity is produced.
**autoinfection** \-infek′shən\ [AUTO- + INFECTION] Infection by an organism already located in or on the body or transferred from one area of the body to another.
**autoinflation** \-inflā′shən\ VALSALVA MANEUVER.
**autoinfusion** \-infyoo′zhən\ The use of bandages or other pressure devices applied to the extremities to force venous blood toward the heart in patients with blood loss.
**autoinoculation** \-inäk′yəlā′shən\ [AUTO- + INOCULATION] Inoculation with organisms already present in or on the body; self-inoculation.
**autointoxication** \-intäk′sikā′shən\ [AUTO- + INTOXICATION] **1** INTESTINAL INTOXICATION. **2** AUTOTOXICOSIS. **intestinal a.** INTESTINAL INTOXICATION.
**autokinesis** \-kīnē′sis\ [AUTO- + KINESIS] Voluntary activity or movement. Also *autokinesia.* Also *autocinesis.*
**autoleukoagglutinin** \-loo′kō·əgloo′tinin\ Antibody capable of clumping white blood cells of an individual in whose serum it is found.
**autologous** \ôtäl′əgəs\ [AUTO- + *-logous* as in *homologous*] **1** Deriving from the same individual. Also *autochthonous.* **2** Obtained from the same individual as that providing the other constituents of the experiment or study: said especially of serum, tissue, cells, etc., under immunologic study. Compare HOMOLOGOUS.
**autology** \ôtäl′əjē\ [AUTO- + -LOGY] The science of understanding oneself; self-analysis. *Seldom used.*
**autolysate** \ôtäl′isāt\ The substances produced in the process of tissue autolysis.
**autolysis** \ôtäl′isis\ [AUTO- + LYSIS] The disintegration of cells and tissues by the degradative action of lysosome-derived hydrolytic enzymes of dead cells. The process begins within minutes of death as these enzymes are activated by the acidosis caused by decreased oxidative metabolism. Autolysis, a postmortem phenomenon, may be distinguished from necrosis, which it resembles, by the absence of inflammatory response. Also *autocytolysis, autodigestion.*
**autolysosome** \-lī′səsōm\ [AUTO- + LYSOSOME] A membrane-bound cytoplasmic organelle which results from the fusion of a lysosome and an autophagosome.
**autolytic** \-lit′ik\ Capable of or indicating autolysis. Also *autocytolytic.*
**autolyze** \ô′təlīz\ To induce or to undergo autolysis.
**Automatic Clinical Analyzer** An automated anaylzer that performschemical analyses by means of prepackaged pouches of reagents dispensed for single tests on individual serum specimens. A proprietary name. Abbr. ACA
**automatism** \ôtäm′ətizm\ [Gk *automatismos* (from *automatos* acting freely or spontaneously, from AUTO- + *-matos,* akin to L *mens,* gen. *mentis* mind, will) a spontaneous or accidental occurrence] **1** Behavior that is not under the control of the will, as a reflexive response. **2** Apparently goal-directed activity that is not, in fact, under the conscious, voluntary control of the subject. It occurs in epilepsy, catatonia, and fugue states. For defs. 1 and 2 also *automatic action, automatic behavior.* **ambulatory alcoholic a.** BLACKOUT. **command a.** Obedience to an order without any critical judgment. It may occur in hypnosis and in catatonic schizophrenia. **epileptic a.** Any form of automatism occurring either as the sole manifestation or as one part of an attack of epilepsy. Though apparently conscious the patient is unaware of the actions involved and has no recollection of them subsequently. Depending upon the site of origin of the epileptic discharge, such automatic activities include chewing and swallowing movements, changes in facial expression, mimicry and gestures, verbalization (words, phrases, sentences, or repetitive utterances) and even complex organized movements, such as undressing, walking, and, in rare instances, violent behavior. Such automatism is common in temporal lobe epilepsy and may occur at the onset of the attack or in postictal confusional states (postepileptic automatism). **postepileptic a.** Automatism following an attack of epilepsy. Also *postictal automatism.* **vigil ambulatory a.** VIGILAMBULISM.
**automaton** \ôtäm′ətän\ [L (from Gk, neut. of *automatos* spontaneous; see AUTOMATISM) an automatic contrivance] (*pl.* automata) A machine, such as a robot, that exhibits living qualities such as observation, effort, and decision, or that follows preset instructions.
***Automeris io*** \ôtäm′ərisī′ō\ The Io moth. The larva, which is a spiny green caterpillar with a red lateral stripe, can cause a stinging (urticating) dermatitis if handled.
**automixis** \-mik′sis\ [AUTO- + Gk *mixis* a mixing, intercourse] AUTOGAMY.
**autonomic** \-näm′ik\ [Gk *autonom(os)* independent + -IC. See AUTONOMOUS.] Functioning independently of the will; not under voluntary control: said of that part of the nervous system which regulates the activities of blood vessels, secretory glands, and viscera. It comprises parasympathetic and sympathetic components.
**autonomotropic** \-näm′əträp′ik\ Relating to or important in the control of the autonomic nervous system.
**autonomous** \ôtän′əməs\ [Gk *autonom(os)* (from AUTO- + *nomos* law) independent + -OUS] Independent and self-governing to the extent that the organism is able to act on the basis of endogenous forces and not only in response to external influences.
**auto-ophthalmoscope** \-äfthal′məskōp\ An ophthalmoscope with which an examiner may view his own eye. Also *autophthalmoscope, autofundoscope.*
**auto-oxidation** Oxidation spontaneously occurring in the presence of air and not requiring catalysts. Also *autoxidation.*
**autopathic** \-path′ik\ *Seldom used* IDIOPATHIC.
**autopathy** \ôtäp′əthē\ IDIOPATHY.
**autophagia** \-fā′jə\ [Gk *autophag(os)* (from *auto-* self + *phagein* to eat) self-devouring + -IA] **1** The biting or eating of one's own flesh. **2** The intracellular digestion of endogenous material of the cell within a lysosome. Also *autophagy.* **3** The recycling of the body of its own tissue during starvation.
**autophagosome** \-fag′əsōm\ [Gk *autophago(s)* self-devouring + English *-some* as in *lysosome*] A membrane-limited cytoplasmic body from which autolysis develops. It is a lysosome containing degenerating cellular organelles. Also *cytolysosome.*
**autophagy** \ôtäf′əjē\ AUTOPHAGIA.
**autopharmacology** The regulation of body functions by the activity of natural, endogenous chemical constituents of the tissues.
**autophene** \ô′təfēn\ A character that is produced by the

genes of the cell, tissue, or organism expressing the phenotype. Such characters behave autonomously on transfer or transplantation to a different genetic milieu. Compare ALLOPHENE.

**autophilia** \-fil′yə\ [AUTO- + -PHILIA] **1** EGOMANIA. **2** NARCISSISM.

**autophony** \ôtäf′ənē\ [AUTO- + PHON- + -Y] A condition in which the patient is aware of the sound of his voice or of his pulse amplified, as it seems, within his head. This is usually associated with certain disorders of the middle and external ear. Adj. autophonous.

**autophotograph** \-fō′təgraf\ AUTORADIOGRAPH.

**autophthalmoscope** \ô′täfthal′məskōp\ AUTO-OPHTHALMOSCOPE.

**autoplasty** \ô′təplas′tē\ AUTOGRAFTING. **peritoneal a.** Peritonization using tissue from the peritoneum of the same patient.

**autoploid** \ô′təploid\ [AUTO- + -PLOID] Having two or more chromosomes or sets of chromosomes that arose from reduplication of a haploid chromosome or set. Also *autopolyploid*.

**autopodium** \-pō′dē·əm\ [New L, from AUTO- + Gk *podion* small foot] The most distal part of a developing limb. It comprises the rudiments of the carpal and tarsal bones, metacarpals and metatarsals, and the phalanges, and will eventually become the hand or the foot.

**autopolyploid** \-päl′əploid\ AUTOPLOID.

**autoprothrombin** \-prōthräm′bin\ [AUTO- + PROTHROMBIN] Any of several of the prothrombin-related clotting factors. **a. I** FACTOR X. **a. II** FACTOR IX. **a. IIa** PROTEIN C. **a. C** THROMBOKINASE.

**autopsy** \ô′täpsē\ [Gk *autopsia* (from *autopt(ein)* to see for oneself, witness, from *aut(o)-* self + *opt-*, *ops-* sight, seeing) ascertainment by inspection] The examination, after death, of an animal body, usually human, with the intent of determining the cause of death, the extent of a disease or injuries, the effect of therapy, and the existence of any previously unrecognized antemortem pathologic conditions. Also *necropsy, sectio cadaveris, thanatopsy, postmortem*. **forensic a.** MEDICOLEGAL AUTOPSY. **medicolegal a.** An autopsy performed with the objective of reconstructing events and circumstances which preceded death and which involved the deceased. The important concerns of a medicolegal autopsy include determination of the cause of death, absolute identification of the deceased, establishment of the time of death, collection and preservation of evidence, discovery of preexisting pathologic conditions, and establishing the manner of death. Also *forensic autopsy*. **psychological a.** The gathering of information concerning the lifestyle, habits, personality traits, character, and frame of mind of an individual who has died violently, particularly by suicide. The information is used to determine the motive for and/or the manner and circumstances of death.

**autoradiograph** \-rā′dē·əgraf′\ A radiograph obtained from exposure of photographic film or plate to tissue, cells, or other objects containing radionuclides. Also *autohistoradiograph, autophotograph, autoradiogram*.

**autoradiography** \-rā′dē·äg′rəfē\ [AUTO- + RADIOGRAPHY] The technique of recording on a photographic emulsion the radiations emitted by radioactive material in the object being studied.

**autoregulation** \-reg′yəlā′shən\ [AUTO- + REGULATION] An intrinsic mechanism for self-adjustment, as for example that which leads to the maintenance of a constant blood flow to a tissue despite wide variation in perfusion pressure. **heterometric a.** Regulation by mechanisms controlling ventricular contractility which depend on the length of the myocardial fibers at the end of diastole. **homeometric a.** Regulation by mechanisms controlling ventricular contractility which are independent of the length of the myocardial fibers at the end of diastole.

**autoreinfection** \-rē′infek′shən\ Self-reinfection; autoinfection.

**autoreinfusion** \-rē′infyoo′zhən\ AUTOTRANSFUSION.

**autoreproduction** \-rē′prəduk′shən\ The process by which a prokaryotic organism, a eukaryotic cell, a virus, a chromosome, or a DNA molecule replicates itself by utilizing precursors found within the cell.

**autoscopy** \ôtäs′kəpē\ [AUTO- + -SCOPY] The phenomenon of seeing one's double, usually in the form of a hazy face and upper torso that mimic one's own gestures and expressions. It may be a symptom of temporoparietal pathology. Also *autoscopic hallucination*.

**autosensitization** \-sen′sətīzā′shən\ Sensitization of the body's own tissues, often through priming with autoantigens. **erythrocyte a.** See under AUTOERYTHROCYTE SENSITIZATION SYNDROME.

**autosensitize** \-sen′sətīz\ To make sensitive to the body's own tissues; subject to autosensitization. Also *isosensitize*.

**autosexing** \ô′tōsek′sing\ A technique, used in experimental and agricultural genetics, in which alleles of genes which are located on a sex chromosome and which have phenotypic effects that appear early in life are introduced so that males and females can be distinguished at an earlier stage than possible in wild populations.

**autosexualism** \-sek′shoo·əlizm\ [AUTO- + SEXUAL + -ISM ] AUTOEROTICISM.

**autosite** \ô′təsīt\ [AUTO- + *(para)site*] The more nearly normal of unequal conjoined twins, to which the parasite is attached. Also *host*.

**autosomal** \-sō′məl\ Pertaining to an autosome; not associated with a sex chromosome.

**autosomatognosis** \-sō′mətägnō′sis\ [AUTO- + SOMATO- + Gk *gnōsis* knowledge] A patient's lack of awareness of a bodily defect, as in the phantom limb of the amputee.

**autosome** \ô′təsōm\ [AUTO- + *(chromo)some*] Any chromosome that occurs in the nucleus except for the sex chromosomes or accessory chromosomes. Human somatic cells ordinarily have 22 pairs of autosomes. Also *euchromosome* (obs.).

**autosplenectomy** \-splenek′təmē\ [AUTO- + SPLENECTOMY] Marked atrophy of the spleen as a result of repeated infarcts with almost complete disappearance of the splenic pulp and replacement by fibrous tissue containing iron and calcium deposits. It is typically seen in sickle cell anemia.

**autostimulation** \-stim′yəlā′shən\ Immunization of an animal with autoantigenic material.

**autosuggestion** \-sugjes′chən\ A mental set adopted without critical awareness and originating within the mind of the individual himself rather than with another. Also *self-suggestion*.

**autosympathectomy** \-sim′pəthek′təmē\ [AUTO- + SYMPATHECTOMY] A permanent peripheral arterial dilatation resulting from destruction of sympathetic nerve function by an endogenous process, such as the neuropathy that accompanies diabetes mellitus.

**autosynapsis** \-sinap′sis\ [AUTO- + SYNAPSIS] The pairing at meiosis of chromosomes derived from the same parent. It occurs only in polyploid or aneuploid organisms. Also *autosyndesis*.

**autosynnoia** \-sinoi′ə\ [AUTO- + Gk *synnoia* (from *synnoein* to think deeply upon) deep thought, meditation] **1** Self-preoccupation to such a degree that no attention is paid to the outside world. 2 AUTISM.

**autotechnicon** \-tek′nikän\ An automated device that is used to transfer tissue blocks through dehydrating and clearing agents prior to embedding in paraffin wax.

**autotherapy** \-ther′əpē\ Treatment of oneself.

**autotomography** \-təmäg′rəfē\ [AUTO- + TOMOGRAPHY] A technique of body section roentgenography in which the part being radiographed is rotated instead of the usual technique of moving the x-ray tube and the x-ray film. The plane demonstrated is that of the axis of rotation. Adj. autotomographic.

**autotomy** \ôtät′əmē\ [AUTO- + -TOMY] Fission, as of a cell.

**autotopagnosia** \-täp′agnō′zhə\ [AUTO- + TOPAGNOSIA] A disorder of the body image, due to a lesion of the parietal cortex in the nondominant hemisphere, characterized by inability to relate the parts of one's own body to extrapersonal space, often with consequent loss of topographical orientation. Sometimes the affected individual is also unable to identify and interrelate the parts of the body in another individual or in a model. Also *body-image agnosia, Pick syndrome.*

**autotoxicosis** \-täk′sikō′sis\ Poisoning by harmful substances generated within the body itself. *Seldom used.* Also *autointoxication.*

**autotoxin** \-täk′sin\ Any harmful substance generated within the body. *Rare.*

**autotransformer** \-transfôr′mər\ A stepup or stepdown voltage transformer in which the primary and secondary coils have some of their windings in common.

**autotransfusion** \-transfyoo′zhən\ The transfusion of blood into the subject from whom it was obtained or from whom it has escaped, as from bleeding. Also *autoreinfusion.*

**autotransplant** \-trans′plant\ AUTOGRAFT.

**autotransplantation** \-trans′plantā′shən\ AUTOGRAFTING.

**autotroph** \ô′tətrōf\ [Gk *autotrophos* (from *auto-* self + *trophos* feeding, nourishing) self-nourishing] An organism that can use carbon dioxide as a general source of carbon and hence can grow without organic compounds. Some (i.e. chemotrophs) derive the required energy by chemosynthesis, such as the oxidation of hydrogen of hydrogen sulfide, and others by photosynthesis. Compare HETEROTROPH.

**autotrophic** \-träf′ik\ 1 Of or relating to an autotroph. 2 Denoting the mode of nutrition characterizing autotrophs.

**autotuberculin** \-t$^y$ubur′kyəlin\ 1 Tuberculin prepared from cultures of a patient's own sputum. 2 Tuberculin derived from a patient's tuberculous lesion and absorbed by that patient's body. Also *autogenous tuberculin.*

**autotuberculinization** \-t$^y$ubur′kyəlinīzā′shən\ Absorption by the patient's body of products of metabolized *Mycobacterium tuberculosis* from the patient's own tuberculous lesions.

**autovaccination** \-vak′sinā′shən\ Injection of an autovaccine into the body.

**autovaccine** \-vaksēn′\ A bacterial vaccine derived from cultures obtained from the patient's own tissues or secretions.

**autoxidation** AUTO-OXIDATION.

**autozygous** \-zī′gəs\ [AUTO- + ZYG- + -OUS] Homozygous at a given genetic locus because of inbreeding, a consequence of having both alleles descended from one allele at that locus in an ancestor. The characteristic can be present in a single individual or multiple individuals who share a common ancestor.

**aux-** \ôks-\ AUXO-.

**auxano-** \ôk′sənō-\ [Gk *auxanein* to augment, increase, make grow] AUXO-.

**auxanodifferentiation** \ôk′sənōdif′ərен′shē·ā′shən\ [AUXANO- + DIFFERENTIATION] The appearance of specific function in a developing organ.

**auxanography** \ôks′anäg′rəfē\ [AUXANO- + -GRAPHY] The study of variations in chemical or environmental conditions that affect the growth rate of bacteria. A culture plate is examined to determine the effects of the substituents on growth of an organism. The procedure can be used to characterize either the substitutent elements or the organism.

**auxesis** \ôksē′sis\ [Gk *auxēsis* growth, increase] 1 Normal growth. 2 Growth caused by an increase in cell size without an increase in cell numbers. For defs. 1 and 2 also *auxetic growth.*

**auxetic** \ôkset′ik\ Of the nature of auxesis.

**auxiliary** \ôksil′yərē\ [L *auxiliaris* (from *auxilium* help, assistance, support, from *augere* to amplify, reinforce) helpful, reinforcing] 1 Capable of functioning as a substitute; supporting. 2 Subordinate or supplementary. 3 ADMINICULUM. **dental a.** DENTAL ASSISTANT. **torquing a.** In an orthodontic appliance, a spring designed to cause rotation of a tooth.

**auxiliomotor** \ôksil′ē·əmō′tər\ Aiding or helping to initiate movement or motion.

**auxin** [AUX- + -IN] A substance that induces plant cell growth. It is now known to be indole-3-acetic acid, although other substances, called auxins a and b, were once thought to be responsible for the growth-promoting effect.

**auxiometer** \ôk′sē·äm′ətər\ AUXOMETER.

**auxo-** \ôk′sō-\ [Gk *auxein* to increase] A combining form meaning growth, increase. Also *aux-, auxano-.*

**auxocardia** \-kär′dē·ə\ CARDIOMEGALY.

**auxocyte** \ôk′sōsīt\ [AUXO- + -CYTE] A cell concerned in growth or reproduction, as an oocyte, spermatocyte, or sporocyte in the early stages of development.

**auxodrome** \ôk′sōdrōm\ [AUXO- + Gk *drom(os),* a course, a running] The course of a child's growth plotted on a grid.

**auxometer** \ôksäm′ətər\ [AUXO- + -METER] A device to measure the magnification produced by a lens. Also *auxiometer.*

**auxotonic** \-tän′ik\ [AUXO- + TONIC] Contracting against strengthening resistance, as a muscle that is working against a weight of increasing heaviness.

**auxotroph** \ôk′sōtrōf\ [AUXO- + Gk *trophos* feeder, nourishing] A microbial strain with a special growth requirement due to a block in a biosynthetic pathway. The auxotroph may be a mutant but similar growth requirements also occur in organisms found in nature. If the block is incomplete the auxotroph is termed "leaky." See also AUXOTROPHIC MUTANT.

**auxotrophic** \-träf′ik\ [AUXO- + -TROPHIC] Requiring one or more specific growth factors in addition to general sources of material and energy.

**AV** 1 atrioventricular. 2 arteriovenous. 3 aortic valve.

**A-V** 1 atrioventricular. 2 arteriovenous.

**av** 1 average. 2 avoirdupois.

**availability** / **physiologic a.** The extent to which the pharmaceutic or nutritive ingredient of a drug or food substance can actually be assimilated and made available to the body in a biologically active state, in contrast to the quantity of those ingredients present in the substance administered. Also *biologic availability.*

**avalanche** AVALANCHE IONIZATION. **Townsend a.** AVALANCHE IONIZATION.

**avalvular** \āval′vyələr\ Lacking valves.
**avascular** \āvas′kyələr\ [Gk *a-* priv. + VASCULAR] Not supplied with vessels or not possessing a vascular system.
**avascularization** \āvas′kyəler′īzā′shən\ [AVASCULAR + *-iz(e)* + -ATION] The interruption of the vascular supply to organs or tissue.
**avdp** avoirdupois.
**Avellis** [Georg *Avellis,* German laryngologist, 1864–1916] Avellis hemiplegia, Avellis syndrome, Avellis-Longhi syndrome. See under AVELLIS PARALYSIS.
**average** ARITHMETIC MEAN. **moving a.** Any of a set of values which are substituted for the successive terms of an ordered series with the object of eliminating random fluctuations. The moving average of a given term is the arithmetical mean of a stated number, usually odd, of terms on either side of the given term. **spatial a. temporal a.** See under SPATIAL AVERAGE TEMPORAL AVERAGE INTENSITY. Abbr. SATA **spatial peak temporal a.** See under SPATIAL PEAK TEMPORAL AVERAGE INTENSITY. Abbr. SPTA **time weighted a.** The average obtained by adding the values recorded at measured time intervals, multiplying the total by that time interval, and dividing the product by the total time over which observations are taken.
**averaging / spike-triggered a.** A technique in which the advent of a propagated potential from a single muscle unit or nerve cell can trigger the sweep of an electronic averaging device. It makes possible the extraction of faint signals from a background of random noise. **time a.** Electronic manipulation of a signal to present an average display over a preselected time.
**avermectin** \ā′vurmek′tin\ One of a group of potent antiparasitic drugs active against many nematodes and arthropods. Considered an experimental anthelmintic for human parasites, it blocks synaptic transmission from interneurons to motor neurons. The avermectins have been proposed for use in treatment and prophylaxis against onchocerciasis.
**aversive** \əvur′siv\ [L *avers(us)* turned away, averse + -IVE] Causing to avoid, dislike, or turn away from.
**aviadenovirus** \ā′vē·ad′ənōvī′rəs\ [L *avi(s)* bird + ADENOVIRUS] Any of the adenoviruses of the genus *Aviadenovirus* that are isolated from birds. Ten distinct serotypes have been identified. All members of the genus share a common cross-reacting antigen absent in the mastadenoviruses. The virions are naked, ether-resistant, icosahedral particles, 70–80 nm in diameter, and contain a linear, double-stranded DNA genome with a mass of 20–25 million daltons.
**avidin** A protein in egg white. It can bind a biotin molecule tightly (dissociation constant $10^{-15}$ M) to each of its four subunits. Since it also binds biotin groups in enzymes, its ability to inhibit carboxylases and transcarboxylases is used to detect their dependence on biotin.
**avidity** \əvid′itē\ [L *aviditas* (from *avid(us)* greedy, from *avere* to long for, + *-itas* -ITY) greediness] The overall tendency of the antibodies in a particular antiserum to combine with a complex antigen. It depends on the number and variety of determinants on the antigen and on the intrinsic affinity of each for various antibodies in the serum. Symbol: $K_a$
**avirulent** \āvir′yələnt\ Lacking virulence: used especially of mutant strains of an ordinarily pathogenic organism. The loss of virulence may be only partial.
**avitaminosis** \āvī′təminō′sis\ [Gk *a-* priv. + VITAMIN + -OSIS] *Imprecise* HYPOVITAMINOSIS. **conditioned a.** Vitamin deficiency due to impaired absorption of the vitamin in question. Something in the diet or physiology of the subject may impair absorption. For example, alcohol impairs folate absorption, and vitamin $B_{12}$ absorption is impaired by achlorhydria. **a. D** 1 RICKETS. 2 OSTEOMALACIA.
**avitaminotic** \āvī′təminät′ik\ Causing a vitamin deficiency. For example, alcohol is avitaminotic in that it impairs folate absorption.
**avivement** \avēvmäN′\ [French *avive(r)* (from L *viv(us)* living, fresh) to make fresher or more alive + French *-ment* -MENT] The débridement of nonviable or contaminated tissue from the edges of a wound prior to surgical closure.
**Avogadro** [Amadeo *Avogadro,* Italian chemist, 1776–1856] See under LAW, CONSTANT, NUMBER.
**avoidance** 1 DENIAL. 2 Avoidance conditioning. See under CONDITIONING. **phobic a.** Keeping away from a feared object or situation, as seen in a person with a phobic disorder.
**avoirdupois** \av′ərdəpoiz′\ See under AVOIRDUPOIS WEIGHT.
**avulsion** \əvul′shən\ [L *avulsio* (from *avulsus,* past part. of *avellere* to pull off, tear away) a pulling off, tearing away] 1 A forceful disruption or separation, as of a nerve, tissue, or body part. Also *exoresis.* 2 The displacement of a tooth from its socket to the extent that the periodontal ligament fiber bundles are severed. **complete scalp a.** See under SCALP AVULSION. **incomplete scalp a.** See under SCALP AVULSION. **nerve a.** The separation or disruption of a nerve by traction. Also *neurexeresis.* **scalp a.** The forceful circumferential separation of the skin of the head from the skull. It may be either a complete avulsion or a partial one. In a complete avulsion, the portion of the skull from the hairline to the neck is involved, whereas in a partial avulsion less than the entire scalp is disrupted. Such trauma is frequently caused by entrapment of long hair in machinery or by a tangential blow to the scalp. **tooth a.** Traumatic removal of a tooth, its root, and, sometimes, part of its bony attachment.
**awakening / delayed a.** SLEEP PARALYSIS.
**awu** atomic weight unit (atomic mass unit).
**ax** 1 axis. 2 axillary.
**Axenfeld** [Karl Theodor Paul Polykarpus *Axenfeld,* German ophthalmologist, 1867–1930] 1 Morax-Axenfeld bacillus. See under BACILLUS. 2 See under SYNDROME, LOOP. 3 Morax-Axenfeld conjunctivitis. See under ANGULAR CONJUNCTIVITIS. 4 Axenfeld-Krukenberg spindle. See under KRUKENBERG SPINDLE.
**axenic** \āzen′ik\ [Gk *a-* priv. + *xen(o)-* + -IC] Lacking bacterial flora: used especially of small laboratory animals that have been delivered by cesarean section and raised in sterile chambers. Also *germ-free.*
**axes** \ak′sēz\ Plural of AXIS.
**axial** \ak′sē·əl\ Situated in or pertaining to the axis of an organism, an organ, or a part.
**axiation** \ak′sē·ā′shən\ [*axi(s)* + -ATION] The development of an axis in an embryo or structure. This is one of the fundamental patterns of organization in biological structures.
**axifugal** \aksif′yəgəl\ Directed away from an axis or axon towards the periphery. Also *axofugal.*
**axil** \ak′sil\ *Outmoded* FOSSA AXILLARIS.
**axilemma** \ak′silem′ə\ AXOLEMMA.
**axilla** \aksil′ə\ [L, dim. of prehistoric L *axla* (later *ala*) a wing, shoulder joint, armpit; akin to Old English *eaxl* shoulder] (*pl.* axillae) FOSSA AXILLARIS.
**axillae** \aksil′ē\ Plural of AXILLA.
**axillary** \ak′siler′ē\ 1 Pertaining to or situated near the axilla. 2 Referring to the angle between an organ or structure and its axis, as in *axillary shoot.*
**axio-** \ak′sē·ə-\ [*axi(s)* + *o*] A combining form denoting an axis, especially, in dentistry, the long axis of the tooth: often used in combination with terms such as buccal, labial, and gingival, to describe the angles used in cavity preparation.

**axion** \ak′sē·än\ [prob. irreg. for Gk *axōn* axis] The brain and spinal cord. *Obs.*

**axiopodium** \ak′sē·əpō′dē·əm\ AXOPODIUM.

**axipetal** \aksip′ətəl\ Directed toward an axis or axon. Also *axopetal.*

**axis** [L (akin to Gk *axōn* an axle, axis) an axle, axis, pivot] **1** The straight line passing through a body or structure, on which it rotates. **2** In anatomy, a line through the body or an organ or a structure around which the parts are more or less symmetrically arranged. It may also be applied to the short stem of an artery, such as the celiac artery, before it divides into its branches, and to the vertebral column. **3** [NA] The second cervical vertebra, distinguished by the dens projecting vertically from its body. It articulates superiorly with the atlas, which rotates on it. Also *epistropheus.* **anteroposterior a.** **1** A sagittal or vertical axis of movement of the eyeball through the axis opticus. **2** In electrocardiography, the axis perpendicular to the frontal plane. **basifacial a.** A line joining the subnasal point and the midpoint of the sphenoethmoidal suture. Also *facial axis.* **brain a.** *Seldom used* BRAINSTEM. **a. bulbi externus** [NA] An imaginary line extending from the anterior pole at the center of the anterior curvature of the cornea to the posterior pole at the central point on the posterior curvature of the sclera. **a. bulbi internus** [NA] An imaginary line on the optic axis of the eye extending from the midpoint on the posterior surface of the cornea to the anterior surface of the retina just anterior to the posterior pole. Also *internal axis of eye, axis oculi interna.* **celiac a.** TRUNCUS COELIACUS. **cell a.** An imaginary line running through the poles of a cell. **cephalocaudal a.** LONG AXIS OF BODY. **cerebrospinal a.** The central nervous system; the brain and spinal cord. Also *neural axis, encephalospinal axis.* **condylar a.** A line joining the two condyles of the mandible and around which the mandible rotates during part of the act of opening the jaws. Also *condyle chord, condyle cord.* **condyle a.** The line around or along which a condyle of a bone rotates within a joint. **conjugate a.** *Outmoded* CONJUGATE DIAMETER. **costocervical arterial a.** TRUNCUS COSTOCERVICALIS. **craniocaudal a.** EMBRYONIC AXIS. **craniofacial a.** BASAL PLATE. **dorsoventral a.** Any anteroposterior line in the median plane at right angles to the long axis of the body. **embryonic a.** An imaginary longitudinal line extending from the cephalic tip to the caudal end of an embryo seen from above. It establishes the left and right sides of embryos and indicates their essential bilateral symmetry. It is only at gastrulation that the embryonic axis can be discerned from the establishment of the prochordal plate and the primitive streak. Also *craniocaudal axis.* **encephalospinal a.** CEREBROSPINAL AXIS. **facial a.** BASIFACIAL AXIS. **frontal a.** An imaginary transverse line passing through the center of the eyeball. **hinge a.** An imaginary line joining the condyles of the mandible and about which rotation occurs during the very earliest part of the opening movement. Also *mandibular axis.* **horizontal a.** A transverse axis through the geometric center of the eyeball in relation to which the center of the cornea moves upwards and downwards. **a. lentis** [NA] A line connecting the anterior and posterior poles, or central points, of the crystalline lens surfaces in the eye. **long a.** An imaginary line passing through or parallel to the greatest length of an object. Also *longitudinal axis.* **long a. of body** The line passing from head to tail of the body around which its weights are most symmetrically distributed. Also *cephalocaudal axis.* **longitudinal a.** LONG AXIS. **mandibular a.** HINGE AXIS. **neural a.** CEREBROSPINAL AXIS. **normal a.** The electrical axis of the heart within normal limits, usually between −30° and +110° in adults. **opening a.** An imaginary line about which the mandible rotates when opening wide, when the sliding movement of the temporomandibular articulations allows the condyles to move forward at the same time as further hinge movement is taking place. The position of the opening axis is approximately at a line joining the lingulae. **optic a.** An imaginary line passing through the centers of the cornea and of the lens of an eye. **optical a.** The continuous line passing through the centers of curvature of the two surfaces of a lens. Also *principal axis.* **a. opticus** [NA] A line joining the anterior pole, or center of anterior curvature, of the eyeball to the posterior pole, or center of posterior curvature. This line usually differs slightly from the visual axis. **a. pelvis** [NA] An imaginary curved line originating from the midpoint of the superior pelvic aperture, passing at right angles to its plane, through the midpoint of the minor pelvis, to the midpoint of the inferior pelvic aperture, at right angles to its plane. The line tends to follow the anterior profile of the sacrum and coccyx, viewed laterally. Also *pelvic axis.* **pituitary-adrenocortical a.** The interrelation between anterior pituitary and adrenocortical function, including the negative feedback inhibition system that regulates the secretion of pituitary adrenocorticotropin. Rising concentrations of circulating glucocorticoids selectively inhibit pituitary release of adrenocorticotropin, whereas subnormal circulating titers of adrenocorticosteroids allow augmented adrenocorticotropic hormone (ACTH) production, which in turn stimulates the adrenal cortex to increased secretion of all adrenocortical steroids. Negative feedback inhibition by plasma cortisol concentration is distinct from and partly independent of the neuroendocrine regulation of ACTH secretion by hypothalamic corticotropin-releasing factor. **pituitary-gonadal a.** The interrelation between pituitary and gonadal function, the negative feedback inhibition system that regulates the secretion of pituitary follicle-stimulating hormone (FSH) and luteinizing hormone (LH) and of estrogens and progesterone in the female and testosterone in the male. Rising concentrations of circulating gonadal steroids selectively inhibit pituitary release of gonadotropins, whereas subnormal circulating titers of the gonadal steroids allow augmented gonadotropin production, which in turn stimulates the gonads to increased secretion of sex hormones. It is distinct from and partly independent of the neuroendocrine regulation of gonadotropin secretion by hypothalamic gonadotropin-releasing hormone. **pituitary-thyroid a.** The interrelation between anterior pituitary and thyroid function, the negative feedback inhibition system that regulates the secretion of pituitary thyrotropin (TSH) and thyroid hormone. Rising concentrations of circulating thyroxine ($T_4$) or triiodothyronine ($T_3$) selectively inhibit pituitary release of thyrotropin, whereas subnormal circulating titers of the thyroid hormones allow augmented thyrotropin production, which in turn stimulates the thyroid to increased secretion of $T_4$ and $T_3$. It is distinct from and partly independent of the neuroendocrine regulation of TSH secretion by hypothalamic thyrotropin-releasing hormone. **principal a.** OPTICAL AXIS. **pupillary a.** A line perpendicular to the iris plane and originating from the center of the pupil. **right a.** The electrical axis of the heart directed more to the right than normally, that is, greater than +110° in adults. **sagittal a.** The anteroposterior axis around which the working condyle is considered to rotate during lateral mandibular movements. **T a.** The electrical axis of the T wave of the electrocardiogram. **a. of uterus** An imaginary line passing through the longest longitudinal diameter of the uterus. **vertical a.** 1 The axis of the mean cardiac vector when it is directed vertically. 2 The line around which the working condyle rotates in a horizontal plane during lateral excursions of the lower jaw. **vertical a. of eye** A cephalad-caudad oriented line through the center of rotation of an eye, serving as the axis of rotation for adduction and abduction of the eye. **visual a.** An imaginary line that passes, through the center of the pupil, from the object observed to the macula lutea of the retina. Also *visual line, linea visus.*

**axo-** \ak′sō-\ [Gk *axōn* an axis] A combining form meaning (1) axon, axonal; (2) axis, axial. Also *axono-*.

**axo-axonic** \ak′sō·aksän′ik\ Designating the synaptic or other type of contact of one axon with another.

**axodendrite** \-den′drīt\ [AXO- + DENDRITE] A dendrite, usually unmyelinated, arising as a side branch from a neuron's axon.

**axofugal** \aksäf′yəgəl\ AXIFUGAL.

**axoid** \ak′soid\ Resembling or pertaining to the axis, or second cervical vertebra. Also *axoidean.*

**axolemma** \-lem′ə\ [AXO- + Gk *lemma* a husk, skin] The delicate plasma membrane lying between the axon and the myelin sheath in peripheral nerves. It is considered part of the neuron plasma membrane. Also *axilemma, Mauthner sheath, Mauthner's membrane.*

**axolysis** \aksäl′isis\ [AXO- + LYSIS] Disappearance of axons as a result of direct local injury or death of the parent neurons.

**axometer** \aksäm′ətər\ [AXO- + -METER] A device for locating the optical center of an optical lens.

**axon** \ak′sän\ [Gk *axōn* (akin to L *axis* axle, axis) an axle, axis] 1 A neuronal process that conducts impulses away from the cell body. It is usually the major process of the cell. 2 Any of the fibers in a nerve, spinal root, or central tract. Some of these fibers conduct impulses toward the cell body (e.g., the axon of a dorsal root ganglion cell). For defs. 1 and 2 also *neuraxon, axis cylinder, axone, Deiter's process, neuraxis, nerve fiber, neuron* (obs.). 3 COLUMNA VERTEBRALIS. Adj. axonal. **giant a.** An especially large axon found coursing longitudinally along the central nervous system in various worms, arthropods, and cephalopods. Some are huge for an axon (to 1000 μm in diameter), but in other species they are large only in relation to the other neurons. They make possible rapid, nearly simultaneous excitation of a series of body segments. Giant axons and the neurons possessing such axons in cephalopods have been used extensively in studies of axonal conduction and membrane properties. Also *giant fiber.* **group Ia a.** PRIMARY AFFERENT. **naked a.** An unmyelinated axon. **unmyelinated a.'s** UNMYELINATED FIBERS.

**axonapraxis** \-əprak′sis\ NEURAPRAXIA.

**axone** \ak′sōn\ AXON.

**axoneme** \ak′sōnēm\ [AXO- + Gk *nēm(a)* thread, yarn] 1 The axial core of a chromosome. 2 The central core or shaft of a flagellum or cilium, which is composed of nine peripheral fibers and two central fibers. It arises from a basal granule, the point of origin of the flagellum or cilium. In a spermatazoon, it traverses the neck, body, and tail and is probably responsible for motility. Also *axial filament, protofilament.*

**axono-** AXO-.

**axonometer** \ak′sänäm′ətər\ [AXONO- + -METER] A device for determining the axis of a cylindrical lens.

**axonotmesis** \ak′sänätmē′sis\ [AXONO- + Gk *tmēsis* a cutting, parting] A traumatic lesion of a peripheral nerve producing dissolution of continuity of axons without loss of continuity of the nerve sheath, so that spontaneous regeneration may ultimately take place.

**axonotomy** \ak′sänät′əmē\ [AXONO- + -TOMY] The experimental procedure of cutting the axon of a nerve cell.

**axopetal** \aksäp′ətəl\ AXIPETAL.

**axoplasm** \ak′sōplazm\ [AXO- + -PLASM] The semifluid substance or neuroplasm of an axon. Adj. axoplasmic.

**axopodium** \-pō′dē·əm\ [New L, from AXO- + Gk *podion* small foot] (*pl.* axopodia) A long, needlelike, usually fixed pseudopodium containing a stiff axial filament consisting of a bundle of fibrils originating near the center of the body. It is typically found in free-living aquatic amebas of the class Heliazoa. Also *axiopodium.*

**axostyle** \ak′sōstīl\ [AXO- + Gk *styl(os)* pillar] A long supporting rod extending the length of the body of some flagellate protozoans and often protruding from the posterior end. There may be one or several and they may be rigid or filamentous, depending on the species. They serve as an endoskeleton and perhaps also for locomotion.

**Ayala** [A. G. *Ayala,* Italian neurologist, 1878–1943] Ayala's equation, Ayala's index. See under AYALA'S QUOTIENT.

**Ayer** [James Bourne *Ayer,* U.S. neurologist, born 1882] Ayer-Tobey test. See under TOBEY-AYER TEST.

**Ayerza** [Abel *Ayerza,* Argentinian physician, 1861–1918] Ayerza syndrome. See under DISEASE.

**Ayre** [James Ernest *Ayre,* U.S. gynecologist, born 1910] See under BRUSH.

**Ayre** [Philip *Ayre,* English anesthetist, flourished 20th century] See under TUBE.

**az-** AZO-.

**azacosterol hydrochloride** $C_{25}H_{44}N_2O \cdot 2HCl$. A hypocholesterolemic steroidal agent which also has been used as an antifertility chemical to control nuisance birds, such as pigeons.

**azacyclonol** $C_{18}H_{21}NO$. α,α-Diphenyl-4-piperidinemethanol. A tranquilizer formerly used in the treatment of schizophrenia. Also *γ-pipradol.*

**8-azaguanine** Guanine in which C-8 and H-8 are replaced by a nitrogen atom. If administered to organisms it can be incorporated into nucleic acids and then interferes with protein synthesis.

**azaguanine** $C_4H_4N_6O$. 8-Azaguanine. A purine antimetabolite resembling guanine that retards the growth of some tumors in mice. Also *guanazolo, triazologuanine.*

**azamethonium** \az′əmethō′nē·əm\ PENTAMETHAZENE.

**azamethonium bromide** A ganglionic blocking agent similar in its action to hexamethonium bromide. It has been used as an antihypertensive drug and to lower the blood pressure to reduce bleeding during surgical operations.

**azaperone** $C_{19}H_{22}FN_3O$. A tranquilizer used in veterinary medicine as a sedative and hypnotic.

**azapetine phosphate** $C_{17}H_{20}NO_4P$. An α-adrenergic blocking agent similar to tolazoline. It has been used to treat hypertension and peripheral vascular disease.

**azapropazone** APAZONE.

**azaribine** 2-β-D-Ribofuranosyl-as-triazine-3,5(2*H*,4*H*)-dione-2′,3′,5′-triacetate. It has been used in the treatment of psoriasis, mycosis fungoides, and polycythemia vera. It is hydrolyzed to azauridine in the body by deacetylation.

**azaserine** $C_5H_7N_3O_4$. L-Serine diazoacetate (ester). An antibiotic, derived from a *Streptomyces* species, that inhibits purine synthesis.

**azathioprine** $C_9H_7N_7O_2S$. 6[(1-Methyl-4-nitroimidazol-5-yl)thio] purine. A derivative of 6-mercaptopurine, which is used as an immunosuppressive drug. It is being evaluated in the treatment of systemic lupus erythematosis, leukemia, rheumatoid arthritis, and several other conditions.

**6-azauridine** $C_8H_{11}N_3O_6$. 2-β-D-Ribofuranosyl-1,2,4-triazine-3,5(2H,4H)-dione. A pyrimidine antimetabolite effective against psoriasis, mycosis fungoides, and polycythemia vera.

**azepinamide** $C_{13}H_{18}ClN_3O_3S$. An orally effective hypoglycemic agent of the sulfonylurea class.

**azetepa** $C_8H_{14}N_5OPS$. *PP*-Di(aziridin-l-yl)-*N*-ethyl-*N*-1,3,4-thiadiazol-2-ylphosphinamide. An antimetabolite with antineoplastic properties.

**azethreonam** AZTREONAM.

**azide** The ion $N_3^-$, one of its salts, or an organic molecule containing the $—N_3$ group. Many of the salts are explosive. Because of its high affinity for iron(III), $N_3^-$ inhibits electron transport, and sodium azide is thus used to prevent bacterial growth in solutions for biochemical work.

**azidothymidine** ZIDOVUDINE. Abbr. AZT

**azo** [from the combining form AZO-] Designating any compound of the type R—N=N—R. Thus Ph—N=N—Ph is called azobenzene. If the R groups differ, the compound can be named by designating R—N=N— as a group. For example, Ph—N=N— is phenylazo. Aliphatic azo compounds of the type R—N=N—H are generally highly unstable and readily decompose to R—H and gaseous nitrogen. Aromatic azo compounds are often synthesized from diazonium coupling reactions. They are of commercial importance as dyes and coloring materials.

**azo-** [French *azote* (from Gk *a-* priv. + *zōē* life) nitrogen] A combining form indicating substitution of nitrogen for carbon in a compound. For a more detailed explanation of usage see AZO. Also *az-*.

**azobilirubin** \ā'zōbil'iroo'bin\ The pinkish purple compound that is produced by the reaction of conjugated bilirubin with diazotized sulfanilic acid in van den Bergh's test.

**azocarmine** \ā'zōkär'min\ Any of several red or bluish red acid dyes that are used in compound stains, especially for microscopic examination of connective tissue.

**azoic** \āzō'ik\ [Gk *azō(os)* (from *a-* priv. + *zōē* life) lifeless + -IC] Devoid of organic life.

**azole** \az'ōl\ Any heterocyclic compound containing an aromatic five-membered ring with at least one nitrogen atom. The simplest azole is pyrrole. Azoles that contain more than one nitrogen atom are diazoles, such as imidazole (1,3-diazole), triazoles, and tetrazole.

**azomethine** IMINE.

**azomycin** $C_3H_3N_3O_2$. 2-Nitro-1*H*-imidazole. An antibiotic compound produced by an unidentified *Streptomyces* species. It is active *in vitro* against *Bacillus subtilis, Escherichia coli, Shigella dysenteriae,* and a variety of other organisms.

**azoospermia** \āzō'əspur'mē·ə\ [Gk *a-* priv. + ZOO- + SPERM + -IA] Absence of spermatozoa in the semen. Also *azoospermatism*.

**azotemia** \az'ōtē'mē·ə\ [French *azot(e)* nitrogen + -EMIA] An abnormal increase in concentration of urea or other nitrogenous substances in the blood plasma. Also *hyperazotemia, nitremia*. See also UREMIA. **prerenal a.** Azotemia in presence of normal renal function. Also *extrarenal azotemia, nonrenal azotemia.*

**AZT** **1** azidothymidine (zidovudine). **2** Ascheim-Zondek test.

**aztreonam** $C_{13}H_{17}N_5O_8S_2$. 2-[[[1-(2-Amino-4-thiazolyl)-2-[(2-methyl-4-oxo-1-sulfo-3-azetidinyl)amino]-2-oxoethylidene]amino]oxy]-2-methylpropanoic acid. A synthetic antibiotic with a monocyclic beta-lactam nucleus. It is active against Gram-negative bacteria, including *Pseudomonas aeruginosa.* Cross-reactivity of allergic reactions with penicillins and cephalosporins may occur with only a low frequency, as these are structurally different from aztreonam. It is administered either intravenously or intramuscularly. Also *azethreonam.*

**azul** \az'ool\ [Spanish, blue] PINTA.

**azure** \azh'ər\ [Old French *azur,* from Med L *azzurum,* from Arabic *al-lazward,* from Persian *lājward* lapis lazuli or its color] Any of the violet-blue basic dyes of the thiazin series that are used as stains for microscopic examination of cells and tissues. **a. II** A mixture of azure dyes and methylene blue that is used in Giemsa stains and in stains to demonstrate intracellular organisms. **a. B** $C_{15}H_{16}N_3SCl$. A violet-blue basic dye sometimes used in compound stains, especially in Giemsa stains and stains for Negri bodies. It is useful in distinguishing RNA from DNA.

**azuresin** \azh'oorez'in\ See under DIAGNEX BLUE TEST.

**azurin** A mixture of theobromine acetate and sodium salicylate that has been used as a diuretic medication.

**azurophil** \azhoo'rəfil\ Any cell, particle, or granule which stains preferentially with blue aniline dyes. Also *azurophile.*

**azurophilia** \azh'oorəfil'yə\ An affinity for blue dyes.

**azurophilic** \azh'oorəfil'ik\ Capable of staining or combining with blue aniline dyes: used especially of cytoplasmic granules in peripheral blood leukocytes.

**azyges** \əzī'jēz\ OS SPHENOIDALE.

**azygogram** \az'igəgram\ A roentgenogram obtained during azygography.

**azygography** \az'igäg'rəfē\ [*azygo(s)* + -GRAPHY] Radiographic examination of the azygos vein after the injection of a contrast medium. This can be done in a retrograde fashion, by means of a catheter introduced into the azygos vein where it enters the superior vena cava, or in an anterograde fashion, by the intraosseous injection of the contrast medium into the marrow space of the left eighth or ninth ribs.

**azygos** \az'igəs\ [Gk (from *a-* priv. + *zyg(on)* yoke, crossbar) unwed, unpaired] AZYGOUS.

**azygous** \āzī'gəs, az'igəs\ [Gk *azyg(os)* unpaired + -OUS. See AZYGOS.] Single; unpaired, as of a structure or part. Also *azygos.*

**azymic** \azim'ik, azī'mik\ Not containing an enzyme.

# B

**B** 1 Symbol for the unit, bel. 2 Symbol for the element, boron. 3 Symbol for the quantity, magnetic induction, expressed in teslas. 4 Symbol for asparagine or aspartic acid without specifying which. 5 bacillus.

***β*** 1 The second letter of the Greek alphabet, beta. 2 A symbol designating the second atom from a reference center in the structural model of a molecule. Thus the *β*-carbon of a carboxylic acid is C-3, the carboxyl group being C-1.

**Ba** Symbol for the element, barium.

**Baastrup** [Christian Ingerslev *Baastrup*, Danish radiologist, 1885–1950] Baastrup's disease, Baastrup syndrome. See under KISSING SPINES.

**Babbitt** [Isaac *Babbitt*, U.S. inventor, 1799–1862] See under METAL.

**Babcock** [Harriett *Babcock*, U.S. psychologist, flourished 20th century] See under SENTENCE.

**Babcock** [William Wayne *Babcock*, U.S. surgeon, 1872–1963] Jackson-Babcock operation. See under BABCOCK'S OPERATION.

**Babès** [Victor *Babès*, Rumanian bacteriologist, 1854–1926] 1 Babès-Ernst corpuscles, Babès-Ernst granules. See under BABÈS-ERNST BODIES. 2 Babès nodes, Babès nodules. See under BABÈS TUBERCLES.

***Babesia*** \babē′zhə\ [after Victor *Babès*, Rumanian bacteriologist, 1854–1926 + -IA] A genus of sporozoan intracellular parasites of the family Babesiidae, order Piroplasmida, that inhabit red blood cells of many mammals including cattle and humans. They are transmitted by ixodid or argasid ticks. Many species are agents of babesiosis (piroplasmosis), an economically important disease of domestic animals in many parts of the world. Also *Piroplasma, Babesiella, Nuttallia, Pyroplasma, Pyrosoma.* ***B. bigemina*** An etiologic agent of bovine babesiosis, an important disease in much of the world, transmitted principally be the tick *Boophilus annulatus.* The disease has not existed in the United States since 1939. • *B. bigemina* was the first pathogen of vertebrates discovered to be arthropod-borne. This was established in 1893 when Smith and Kilbourne demonstrated that Texas fever (bovine babesiosis) was transmitted by ticks. ***B. microti*** A species found in voles (genus *Microtus*) and other wild rodents, widespread in North America and transmitted by the northern deer tick, *Ixodes dammini,* which feeds on rodents, white-tailed deer, and occasionally on humans. It is responsible for outbreaks of human babesiosis on Martha's Vineyard, Nantucket, and nearby coastal areas of New England.

***Babesiella*** \babē′sē·el′ə\ *BABESIA.*

**babesiosis** \babē′sē·ō′sis\ [*Babesi(a)* + -OSIS] A disease of various domestic and wild mammals and sometimes humans, caused by any one of numerous species of *Babesia.* The organism inhabits red cells and is transmitted by ticks. Human infection is sometimes asymptomatic but may cause malaise, fever, chills, and myalgia, with mild hepatosplenomegaly and mild to severe hemolytic anemia. In splenectomized patients, the disease may progress to renal failure and death. Also *piroplasmosis* (obs.).

**Babinski** [Joseph François Felix *Babinski*, French neurologist, 1857–1932] 1 Pseudo-Babinski sign. See under SIGN. 2 Anton-Babinski syndrome. See under SYNDROME. 3 Babinski-Fröhlich syndrome. See under FRÖHLICH SYNDROME. 4 Babinski-Vaquez syndrome. See under BABINSKI SYNDROME. 5 See under LAW, PSEUDOSIGN. 6 Babinski's test. See under SIGN. 7 Babinski-Nageotte syndrome. See under SYNDROME. 8 Babinski's phenomenon, Babinski reflex, Babinski's toe sign. See under EXTENSOR PLANTAR RESPONSE.

**baby** [prob. akin to *babble*] A child between birth and the age of achievement of walking, about 14 months; an infant. **blue b.** An infant or child cyanotic since birth because of developmental defects of the heart or lungs that result in incomplete oxygenation of the blood. The condition is most commonly due to transposition of the great arteries or the tetralogy of Fallot. **collodion b.** A newborn infant whose skin is shiny, translucent, and appears tightly drawn over the face and other parts of the body. This collodionlike appearance is due to persistence of the epitrichial layer of epidermis beyond its normal disappearance in the sixth month of gestation. After birth the abnormal layer cracks and begins desquamation, often resulting in ichthyosis lamellaris. Complete recovery may follow. **test-tube b.** The product of an *in vitro* fertilization with subsequent intrauterine implantation. A popular term.

**Bachman** [George William *Bachman*, U.S. pathologist, born 1890] Bachman reaction. See under TEST.

**Bacillaceae** \bas′əlā′si·ē\ [*Bacill(us)* + -ACEAE] A family of Gram-positive sporulating bacilli, including particularly the aerobic or facultative genus *Bacillus* and the anaerobic *Clostridium.*

**bacillaemia** *Brit.* BACILLEMIA.

**bacillary** \bas′əler′ē\ 1 Of, pertaining to, or caused by bacilli: used especially to distinguish bacterial from amebic dysentery. 2 Rod-shaped; bacilliform.

**bacillemia** \bas′əlē′mē·ə\ The presence of bacilli in the blood.

**bacilli** \bəsil′ī\ Plural of BACILLUS.

**bacilliform** \bəsil′ifôrm\ Having the shape of a bacillus; rod-shaped.

**bacillin** An antibiotic substance isolated from *Bacillus subtilis,* which is active against both Gram-positive and Gram-negative bacteria.

**bacillosis** \bas′əlō′sis\ [*bacill(us)* + -OSIS] An infection caused by bacilli.

**bacilluria** \bas′əloo′rē·ə\ [*bacill(us)* + -URIA] 1 A condition in which bacilli are present in the urine. 2 The presence of any bacteria in the urine.

***Bacillus*** \bəsil′əs\ A genus of large, Gram-positive, aerobic, spore-forming, rod-shaped bacteria. ***B. abortus*** *Obs. BRUCELLA ABORTUS.* ***B. anthracis*** A large, aerobic, Gram-positive, nonmotile, sporulating bacillus, the cause of anthrax in domestic animals and occasionally in man. Seen in the blood of dying sheep in 1850, it was the first bacterium shown to cause disease. ***B. botulinus*** *Obs. CLOSTRIDIUM BOTULINUM.* ***B. dysenteriae*** *Obs. SHIGELLA DYSENTERIAE.* ***B. enteritidis*** *Obs. SALMONELLA ENTERITIDIS.* ***B. fusiformis*** *Obs. FUSOBACTERIUM FUSIFORMIS.* ***B. licheniformis*** A species similar to *B. subtilis* but also denitrifying and fermentative, forming butanediol and glycerol. It forms irregular, lumpy colonies. ***B. mallei*** *Outmoded PSEUDOMONAS MALLEI.* ***B. megaterium*** A rather large bacillus (diameter, 1.5–3 μm) that forms poly-*β*-hydroxybutyrate. ***B. melitensis***

*Obs.* BRUCELLA MELITENSIS. ***B. oedematiens*** *Obs.* CLOSTRIDIUM NOVYI. ***B. pyocyaneus*** *Obs.* PSEUDOMONAS AERUGINOSA. ***B. subtilis*** An aerobic, nonfermentative, slender, spore-forming, Gram-positive bacillus. It forms butanediol but no poly-$\beta$-hydroxybutyrate. It is of historical importance as the hay bacillus at the center of the controversy over spontaneous generation and in the resulting discovery of bacterial spores. ***B. tetani*** *Obs.* CLOSTRIDIUM TETANI. ***B. typhosus*** *Obs.* SALMONELLA TYPHI.

**bacillus** \bəsil′əs\ [Late L, variant of L *bacillum* (dim. of *baculum* a rod, staff, akin to Gk *baktron* a stick, cudgel; see BACTERIUM) a small stick, rod] (*pl.* bacilli) **1** Any rod-shaped bacterium. **2** Any organism of the genus *Bacillus*, as well as numerous organisms that have been reclassified under other genus names. **Bang's b.** *BRUCELLA ABORTUS.* **Battey b.** *MYCOBACTERIUM INTRACELLULARE* • The bacillus is named after *Battey*, a tuberculosis hospital in Rome, Georgia. **Bordet-Gengou b.** *BORDETELLA PERTUSSIS.* **butter b.** SMEGMA BACILLUS. **Calmette-Guérin b.** An avirulent strain of *Mycobacterium bovis*, cultured many years to diminish its pathogenicity. Abbr. BCG **colon b.** An organism of the species *Escherichia coli.* **diphtheria b.** *CORYNEBACTERIUM DIPHTHERIAE.* **Döderlein's b.** Any of various lactobacilli that have been isolated from the human vagina. **Ducrey's b.** *HAEMOPHILUS DUCREYI.* **dysentery b.** SHIGELLA. **enteric bacilli** Gram-negative rods cultured aerobically from the intestinal contents or stool. The bacteroides, which are obligate anaerobes, are excluded. *Ambiguous.* **Friedländer's b.** *Older term KLEBSIELLA PNEUMONIAE.* **fusiform b.** Any Gram-negative, slender, anaerobic, rod-shaped bacterium with tapered ends, such as a member of the genus *Fusobacterium.* **gas b.** A bacillus, *Clostridium perfringens*, that forms copious gas in gangrenous tissue. **Hansen's b.** *Older term* LEPROSY BACILLUS. **hay b.** See under *BACILLUS SUBTILIS.* **Hofmann's b.** *CORYNEBACTERIUM PSEUDODIPHTHERITICUM.* **influenza b.** Any bacillus of the species *Haemophilus influenzae.* **Johne's b.** *MYCOBACTERIUM PARATUBERCULOSIS.* **Klebs-Löffler b.** *CORYNEBACTERIUM DIPHTHERIAE.* **Koch-Weeks b.** *HAEMOPHILUS AEGYPTIUS.* **leprosy b.** An organism of the species *Mycobacterium leprae*, the cause of human leprosy. Also *Hansen's bacillus* (older term). **Morax-Axenfeld b.** An organism of the species *Moraxella lacunata. Outmoded.* **paracolon bacilli** A group of nonpathogenic enterobacteria closely related to *Escherichia coli. Obs.* **Pfeiffer's b.** *HAEMOPHILUS INFLUENZAE.* **plague b.** See under *YERSINIA PESTIS.* **smegma b.** An organism of the species *Mycobacterium smegmatis.* Also *butter bacillus.* **tetanus b.** *CLOSTRIDIUM TETANI.* **timothy hay b.** A microorganism of the species *Mycobacterium phlei.* **tubercle b.** An organism of the species *Mycobacterium tuberculosis.* **typhoid b.** An organism of the species *Salmonella typhi.* **Vincent's b.** *FUSOBACTERIUM FUSIFORMIS.* **vole b.** An organism of the species *Mycobacterium microti.* **Welch's b.** *Obs. CLOSTRIDIUM PERFRINGENS.*

**bacitracin** An antibiotic obtained from Tracy-I strain of *Bacillus subtilis* and used only topically. It inhibits cell wall synthesis and is effective against a variety of Gram-positive cocci and bacilli, including *Neisseria, Haemophilus influenzae*, and *Treponema pallidum.* At higher concentrations it inhibits the growth of *Actinomyces* and *Fusobacterium.*

**back** The posterior surface of the trunk of the body; dorsum. **flat b.** A loss of normal thoracic kyphosis. Also *hollow back.* **functional b.** A backache for which no obvious pathologic cause may be discerned. **hollow b.** FLAT BACK. **hump b.** A deformity of the back due to scoliosis or kyphosis. Also *hunch back.* **old man's b.** Degenerative spondylitis affecting the lumbar region. **poker b.** POKER SPINE. **saddle b.** LORDOSIS. **static b.** A backache, usually of the lower back, arising from postural strain. **sway b.** LORDOSIS.

**backbleeding** The amount of retrograde bleeding noted within a vessel when it is proximally occluded. It is used clinically as a general index of distal vessel patency and collateral blood flow.

**backbone** COLUMNA VERTEBRALIS.

**backcross** In experimental genetics, the mating of an offspring that is heterozygous at a locus or loci with an individual, often a parent, that is homozygous at the locus or loci at issue. Also *backcross mating.*

**backflow** A flowing in a direction opposite that of normal or expected. **pyelolymphatic b.** The drainage of the contrast medium during retrograde pyelography or intravenous urography medially through lymphatic vessels to the periaortic lymph nodes, appearing as opacified small vessels extending toward the renal hilus and probably representing the lymphatic drainage of pyelosinus backflow. Also *pyelolymphatic reflux.* **pyelorenal b.** Reflux of a contrast medium during retrograde pyelography or intravenous urography from the ureter into lymphatics draining into the renal parenchyma, specifically into the periaortic lymph nodes (pyelolymphatic backflow), the renal sinus (pyelosinus backflow), the tubules (pyelotubular backflow), or veins (pyelovenous backflow). Also *pyelorenal reflux.* **pyelosinus b.** The extension of the contrast medium during retrograde pyelography or an intravenous urography from the pelvicaliceal system into the surrounding fat of the renal sinus, apparently through microruptures of caliceal fornices due to increased intracaliceal pressure as occurs with acute ureteral obstruction. Also *pyelosinus reflux, pyelosinus extravasation.* **pyelotubular b.** The extension of the contrast medium during retrograde pyelography in a retrograde fashion into the collecting ducts, as evidenced by fine lines from a calix into its papilla. Also *pyelotubular reflux.* **pyelovenous b.** The entry of the contrast medium during retrograde pyelography or intravenous urography into the renal venous system, visualized most commonly in arcuate veins. It is usually the result of rupture of a caliceal fornix into the sinus or into lymphatic channels. Also *pyelovenous reflux.*

**backing** A flat metal plate used to attach a facing to a denture or bridge.

**backlighting** [*back* + *lighting*] RETROILLUMINATION.

**backscatter** Any radiation, as of photons, ultrasound waves, etc., that is scattered back in the general direction of the source. Also *backscattered radiation.*

**backward** **1** Toward the back; posteriorly. **2** Directed or moving in a reverse direction, as a flow of fluid.

**bacteraemia** *Brit.* BACTEREMIA.

**bacteremia** \bak′tərē′mē·ə\ [*bacter(ia)* + -EMIA] The presence of bacteria in the blood. Also *bacteriemia.* **puerperal b.** The presence of bacteria in the bloodstream of the mother following delivery of an infant.

**bacteremic** \bak′tərē′mik\ Pertaining to or caused by bacteremia.

**bacteri-** \baktir′ē-\ BACTERIO-.

**bacteria** \baktir′ē·ə\ Plural of BACTERIUM.

**bacterial** \baktir′ē·əl\ Pertaining to, belonging to, or resulting from bacteria.

**bactericidal** \bak′tərisī′dl\ Capable of causing a rapid decrease in viability of bacteria through physical or chemical action. Also *cidal.* Compare BACTERIOSTATIC.

**bactericide** \baktir′əsīd\ Any agent that rapidly decreases the viability of bacteria. **specific b.** BACTERIOLYSIN.

**bactericidin** \bak′tərisī′din\ Any substance lethal to bacteria. Also *bacteriocidin.*

**bacterid** \bak′tərid\ A widespread eruption attributed to hematogenic dissemination from an infective focus of bacterial antigens in a sensitized subject. Also *bacteride.*

**bacteriemia** \bak′təri·ē′mē·ə\ BACTEREMIA.

**bacterio-** \baktir′ē·ō-\ [New L *bacterium.* See BACTERIUM.] A combining form denoting bacteria. Also *bacteri-.*

**bacteriocidin** \-sī′din\ BACTERICIDIN.

**bacteriocin** \bak′tərē·ō′sin\ A protein substance that is produced by a specific strain of bacteria and exerts a lethal effect on closely related strains. Colicins and pyocins are bacteriocins produced by *Escherichia coli* and *Pseudomonas aeruginosa* respectively.

**bacteriocinogen** \-sin′əjən\ A plasmid that codes for the production of a bacteriocin.

**bacteriologist** \baktir′ē·äl′əjist\ A scientist who specializes in bacteriology.

**bacteriology** \baktir′ē·äl′əjē\ [BACTERIO- + -LOGY] The branch of science concerned with bacteria. It is a branch of the broader field of microbiology, and it can be divided into many subspecialties, such as agricultural, medical, industrial, systematic, diagnostic, soil, or marine. Adj. bacteriologic. **medical b.** The branch of bacteriology concerned with the microorganisms found in humans in states of health and disease. **systematic b.** The branch of bacteriology concerned with the classification of bacteria. It has the twofold objective of establishing a determinative key and determining taxonomic (evolutionary) relationships.

**bacteriolysin** \baktir′ē·äl′isin\ An antibody that causes bacteriolysis. Also *specific bactericide.*

**bacteriolysis** \baktir′ē·äl′isis\ [BACTERIO- + LYSIS] A process that damages the bacterial cell envelope and allows the leakage of the intracellular constituents. It is often used to refer to the action of antibody plus complement on Gram-negative bacteria. **immune b.** Lysis of Gram-negative bacteria by the action of antibody and complement.

**bacteriolytic** \-lit′ik\ Capable of causing lysis of bacteria.

**bacteriophage** \baktir′ē·ōfāj′\ [BACTERIO- + -PHAGE] Any virus that infects bacteria. Also *phage.* **mature b.** A bacteriophage in the form of a complete, infectious virion resulting from assemblage of the various components. **temperate b.** A bacteriophage capable of stable multiplication in a bacterium without killing it, usually through lysogenation. **vegetative b.** A bacteriophage in the stage of intracellular multiplication. With temperate phages, this multiplication leads to indefinite persistence of phage DNA in host cells. With virulent phages, it leads to the death of host cells at the end of the vegetative cycle. **virulent b.** A bacteriophage that is unable to become a prophage, but multiplies vegetatively and kills the host cell at the end of the growth cycle.

**bacteriophagology** \-fagäl′əjē\ The study of bacteriophages. Also *phagology* (seldom used).

**bacteriophytoma** \-fītō′mə\ [BACTERIO- + PHYT- + -OMA] A mass or tumor caused by a bacterium.

**bacteriosis** \baktir′ē·ō′sis\ [*bacteri(a)* + -OSIS] An infection or disease caused by bacteria.

**bacteriostasis** \baktir′ē·äs′təsis\ [BACTERIO- + -STASIS] The state of bacterial cells that are no longer growing, either because they have reached the stationary phase or because a bacteriostatic agent has been added.

**bacteriostat** \baktir′ē·əstat′\ A chemical agent that causes bacteriostasis.

**bacteriostatic** \-stat′ik\ [BACTERIO- + -STATIC] **1** Capable of inhibiting bacterial growth without rapid loss of viability. Compare BACTERICIDAL. **2** Pertaining to or exhibiting bacteriostasis.

**bacteriotropin** \-trō′pin\ An immunoglobulin that binds to bacteria, rendering them susceptible to phagocytosis; an opsonin specific to bacteria.

***Bacterium*** \baktir′ē·əm\ A formerly broad genus, most of whose members are now distributed among many other genera, including *Escherichia, Salmonella,* and *Shigella.* ***B. actinomycetemcomitans*** A small, Gram-negative, anaerobic coccobacillus of doubtful pathogenicity, found in the frequently mixed infections in actinomycotic lesions. ***B. typhosum*** *Obs.* *SALMONELLA TYPHI.*

**bacterium** \baktir′ē·əm\ [New L, from Gk *baktērion* (akin to L *bacillum* a small stick, rod), dim. of *baktron* a stick, cudgel] (*pl.* bacteria) Any member of the class of prokaryotic organisms. They divide by binary fission and have a single chromosome, no nuclear envelope, and usually a characteristic rigid peptidoglycan cell wall. Bacteria are the smallest organisms, having an average diameter of 1 μm. Most are free-living, some live in or on animals or plants, and a few are obligatory intracellular parasites. Also *schizomycete* (obs.), *fission fungus* (obs.). Adj. bacterial. **blue-green bacteria** CYANOBACTERIA. **Dar es Salaam b.** A serotype of *Salmonella.* **lactic acid bacteria** Bacteria that ferment sugars primarily to lactic acid, or to lactic and acetic acids and carbon dioxide. They include the genera *Lactobacillus, Leuconostoc,* and *Streptococcus.* They are responsible for the souring of milk and other foods. Because of their stable, complex growth requirements lactic acid bacteria have been useful in bioassays and in the discovery of vitamins. They are commercially important in cheese

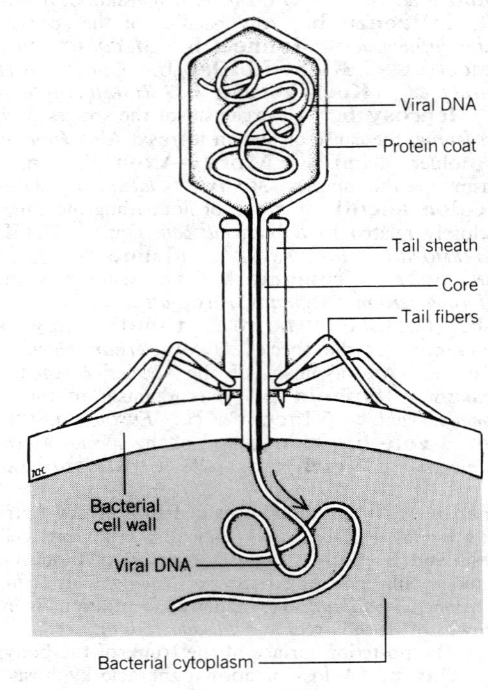


**Bacteriophage**

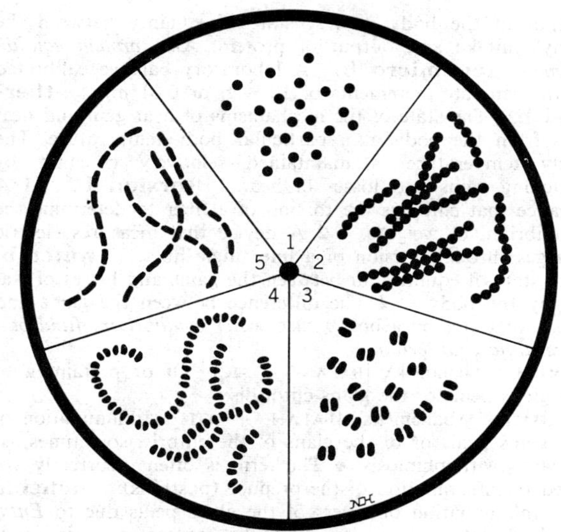


Bacteria (1) Cocci; (2) staphylococci; (3) diplococci; (4) streptococci; (5) bacilli.

production and in the fermentation of plant material, such as ensilage or sauerkraut. **propionic acid bacteria** A group of bacteria that ferment lactic acid to propionic acid. This group includes *Propionibacterium acnes*, found on skin, and organisms responsible for the holes in Swiss cheese. **resistant bacteria** 1 Bacteria that are not susceptible to commonly used antibiotics. 2 Bacteria that are not sensitive to a specific antibiotic against which they are tested. **sulfur b.** Any bacterium that can oxidize inorganic sulfur compounds.

**bacteriuria** \baktir′ēyoo′rē·ə\ [*bacteri(a)* + -URIA] The presence of bacteria in the urine. More than $10^5$ organisms per ml of recently excreted urine are indicative of a urinary tract infection. Also *bacteruria*.

**bacteroid** \bak′təroid\ Any member of the genera *Bacteroides* or *Fusobacterium*. Also *bacteroides*.

**Bacteroidaceae** \bak′təroidā′si·ē\ [*bacter(i)-* + -OID + -ACEAE] A family of bacteria that includes the genera *Bacteroides* and *Fusobacterium*. These bacteria often develop atypical shapes.

***Bacteroides*** \bak′təroi′dēz\ A genus of strictly anaerobic, mostly nonmotile, Gram-negative rod-shaped bacteria which are the preponderant flora of the vertebrate gut but are not detected in the usual aerobic plate culture. The butyric fermentation is not as prominent as in the clostridia. Bacteroides are important causes of sepsis in patients with weakened defenses or damaged tissues. Species designations are in a state of flux. ***B. corrodens*** A species often isolated from the oral cavity. Colonies produce a typical pitting of the agar culture medium. ***B. fragilis*** The species most prevalent in human infections but not in the normal flora. ***B. fusiformis*** *Older term* FUSOBACTERIUM FUSIFORMIS. ***B. melaninogenicus*** A species frequently encountered in mixed infections in abscesses and Vincent's angina. It forms a dark pigment that fluoresces in ultraviolet light of relatively long wavelength, and can be seen in purulent discharges as well as in colonies.

**bacteroides** \bak′təroi′dēz\ BACTEROID.

**bacteroidosis** \bak′təroidō′sis\ [*Bacteroid(es)* + -OSIS] Infection by bacteria of the genus *Bacteroides*..

**bacteruria** \bak′təryoo′rē·ə\ BACTERIURIA.

**bactoprenol** \bak′təpren′əl\ Undecaprenol pyrophosphate, a $C_{55}$ polyisoprene derivative in bacterial membranes that transfers precursor units to the peptidoglycan and the O chain of the lipopolysaccharide.

**badge** / **film b.** A small package of metal or plastic, worn by personnel and containing a film sensitive to particulate or electromagnetic radiation. It can be used to evaluate the total amount of ionizing radiation to which an individual has been exposed over a known time. Also *film dosimeter, thermoluminescent dosimetry badge*.

**Baer** [Karl Ernst von *Baer*, Estonian naturalist and embryologist, 1792–1876] **1** See under PLANE. **2** Baer's law, law of von Baer. See under LAW. **3** Baer's vesicle. See under VESICULAR OVARIAN FOLLICLE. **4** Theca of follicle of von Baer. See under THECA EXTERNA.

**Bäfverstedt** [Bo Erik *Bäfverstedt*, Swedish physician, born 1905] Bäfverstedt syndrome. See under BENIGN LYMPHOCYTOMA CUTIS.

**bag** / **bolus b.'s** Bags containing tissue-equivalent material, used in radiotherapy for dose build-up or attenuation. **colostomy b.** A plastic or rubber appliance that is sealed to the skin to cover a colostomy stoma. It provides a reservoir for feces and protection for the stoma. **Douglas b.** A distensible gas-tight bag used to collect expired air. **ileostomy b.** A rubber or plastic appliance fitted over an ileostomy and secured to the skin with a removable adhesive. It is used for collection of stoma drainage, whether fecal material or urine, from an ileal conduit. **micturition b.** A device for collecting urine of patients with urinary incontinence. **nuclear b.** The nuclei aggregated in the central portion of intrafusal muscle fibers of a muscle spindle. See also NUCLEAR BAG FIBER. **Perry b.** An ileostomy bag with a small latex cuff reinforced with a stiff plastic ring. It is usually secured with a belt. **Petersen's b.** An inflatable rubber bag that is introduced into the rectum to elevate the bladder anteriorly during suprapubic bladder surgery. **Politzer's b.** A strong piriform rubber bag used to inflate the middle ear in politzerization and eustachian catheterization. **reservoir b.** A device in an anesthesia breathing circuit which serves to collect expired gas that is not vented into the atmosphere. Such a reservoir has a fixed rate of gas inflow and is capable of compensating for variations in respiratory demand. **testicular b.** SCROTUM. **Tucker dilatable b.** A balloonlike structure mounted at the end of a long metal tube and inflatable from a syringe filled with water, used for dilating esophageal strictures, particularly in the cricopharyngeal and esophagogastric regions. **Voorhees b.** A rubber bag that can be inflated with water, used for dilating the pregnant cervix. **b. of waters** The amniotic fluid and fetal membranes. *Popular*. **Whitmore b.** An ileostomy bag used for drainage of urine from an ileal conduit. The end of the bag contains a valve or stopcock to permit emptying of urine without removing the bag from the stoma.

**Baillarger** [Jules Gabriel François *Baillarger*, French neurologist, 1809–1890] **1** See under LAYER. **2** Baillarger syndrome, Frey-Baillarger syndrome. See under AURICULOTEMPORAL SYNDROME. **3** Baillarger's band, Baillarger stripes, Baillarger striations, striae of Baillarger. See under BAILLARGER'S LINES.

**Bainbridge** [Francis Arthur *Bainbridge*, English physiologist, 1874–1921] Bainbridge reflex. See under EFFECT.

**Baker** [James Porter *Baker*, U.S. physician, born 1902] Charcot-Weiss-Baker syndrome. See under CAROTID SINUS SYNDROME.

**Baker** [William Morrant *Baker*, English surgeon, 1839–1896] Baker cyst. See under POPLITEAL BURSITIS.

**BAL** British antilewisite.

**balan-** \bal′ən-\ BALANO-.

**balance** **1** A device to determine weight by achieving spatial equilibrium between a weight of known mass and the unknown quantity. Determination may employ pans suspended at each end of a beam, or it may be based on elastic deformation of a spring. **2** A state of equilibrium or functionally appropriate proportion among constituents. **3** The measured relationship between input and output of a substance. **acid-base b.** The state of acid and base gains and losses by the body at a particular hydrogen ion concentration. The body pH is maintained relatively constant by matching gains and losses of acid and base. Also *acid-base equilibrium*. **analytical b.** A laboratory balance calibrated for accurate discrimination of small increments of weight. The beam and the weight pans are supported on knife edges. **calcium b.** **1** The difference between the calcium intake and the calcium output of a subject. **2** A state of equilibrium in the intake and output of calcium. Up until about 30 years of age, the body is said to be in positive calcium balance with more calcium being deposited in the skeleton than is being liberated. After that time, the body goes into slight negative balance. Extreme negative calcium balance occurs in certain conditions such as osteoporosis. **carbon b.** **1** A quantitative description of the comparative state of the carbon intake and output of the body. **2** A state of equality between the body's intake and output of carbon. Also *carbon equilibrium*. **electrolyte b.** **1** A state of equilibrium in the intake and output of electrolytes by the body. **2** The difference between the intake and the output of electrolytes by a body. **energy b.** A condition in which caloric intake equals energy output, as in the normal adult, thus maintaining a stable body weight. Also *body equilibrium, calorie equilibrium*. **fluid b.** WATER BALANCE. **glomerulotubular b.** **1** The adjustment of the rate of renal tubular solute reabsorption by the majority of nephrons functioning at or below their maximum reabsorptive capacity so that reabsorption equals the rate of the filtration of the solute by the glomerulus of the same nephron. **2** The reabsorption in the proximal tubules of the kidney of a constant proportion of the sodium and water filtered by the glomeruli despite wide variations in glomerular filtration rate. **heat b.** **1** The difference between the heat produced and the heat lost by a system, such as the human body. **2** A state of equilibrium between the production of heat and the loss of heat. **metabolic b.** **1** A state of equilibrium between the overall anabolic and catabolic processes of the body. **2** The difference between the overall anabolic and catabolic processes in a subject. Also *metabolic equilibrium*. **microchemical b.** A laboratory balance calibrated to discriminate microgram increments such as $10^{-6}$ g or 0.001 mg. **mineral b.** **1** A state of equilibrium between the intake and output of minerals by the body. **2** The difference between the mineral intake and the mineral output of a body. **nitrogen b.** **1** A state of equilibrium between the intake and output of nitrogen by the body. **2** The difference between the nitrogen intake and the nitrogen output of a subject. Also *nitrogen equilibrium*. **protein b.** **1** A quantitative description of the comparative state of the protein intake and output of the body. **2** A state of equality between the body's intake and output of protein. Also *protein equilibrium*. **semimicro b.** A laboratory balance calibrated to discriminate increments of $10^{-5}$ g, or 0.01 mg. **thermal b.** The state of the mechanisms of heat gain and heat loss from the body at a particular body temperature. The body temperature is maintained relatively constant by matching gains and losses of heat. **torsion b.** **1** A balance that employs the torsion of a fiber to determine the equilibrium of weights. **2** A device that measures electric charges through torsion of a fine single fiber. **water b.** **1** A state of equilibrium between the gains and losses of water by the body. **2** The difference between the gains and losses of water by a body. Also *water equilibrium, fluid balance, fluid equilibrium*.

**balanic** \bəlan′ik\ [BALAN- + -IC] Of or pertaining to the glans penis or the glans clitoridis.

**balanitis** \bal′ənī′tis\ [BALAN- + -ITIS] Inflammation of the glans penis or of the glans of the clitoris, sometimes associated with phimosis. • The term is often incorrectly applied to inflammation of the prepuce (posthitis). **amebic b.** Inflammation or ulcers of the glans penis due to *Entamoeba histolytica* and thought to be contracted during anal intercourse with someone with amebic dysentery. **b. circinata** A usually painless form of balanitis associated with the Reiter syndrome. Also *circinate balanitis*. **erosive b.** An acute inflammation of the glans penis and prepuce with ulceration and the discharge of copious purulent material, occurring in persons with some degree of phimosis. It is usually caused by Vincent's bacillus or by nonspecific treponemata. **gangrenous b.** Balanitis due to combinations of anaerobic bacteria and characterized by progressive ulcerative lesions and a foul discharge. It causes rapid destruction of the glans penis and possibly the rest of the external genitalia. Also *phagedenic balanitis, balanoposthomycosis, Corbus disease*. **plasma cell b.** A nonmalignant chronic inflammatory disorder of the glans penis characterized clinically by a velvety red lesion and histologically by a gross infiltrate of plasma cells; a form of Zoon's erythroplasia. **b. xerotica obliterans** A late stage of lichen sclerosus et atrophicus of the penis. Also *Stühmer's disease, kraurosis penis*.

**balano-** \bal′ənō-\ [Gk *balanos* acorn] A combining form denoting the glans penis or glans clitoridis. Also *balan-*.

**balanoblennorrhea** \-blen′ôrē′ə\ [BALANO- + BLENNORRHEA] An inflammation of the external surface of the glans penis. Also *balanorrhea*.

**balanocele** \bal′ənōsēl′\ [BALANO- + -CELE[1]] Protrusion of the glans penis through a disrupted prepuce.

**balanoplasty** \bal′ənōplas′tē\ [BALANO- + -PLASTY] A restorative or reconstructive operation on the glans penis.

**balanoposthitis** \-pästhī′tis\ [BALANO- + Gk *posth(ē)* prepuce + -ITIS] Inflammation of the mucous membrane of the glans penis and prepuce.

**balanoposthomycosis** \-päs′thōmīkō′sis\ [BALANO- + Gk *posth(ē)* prepuce + *o* + MYCOSIS] GANGRENOUS BALANITIS.

**balanorrhagia** \bal′ənôrā′jə\ [BALANO- + -RRHAGIA] Balanitis in which there is a discharge of pus.

**balanorrhea** \bal′ənôrē′ə\ BALANOBLENNORRHEA.

**balantidial** \bal′əntid′ē·əl\ Of or pertaining to the parasitic ciliate *Balantidium*..

**balantidiasis** \bal′əntidī′əsis\ An intestinal infection due to *Balantidium coli*. Also *balantidiosis, balantidosis*.

***Balantidium*** \bal′əntid′ē·əm\ [New L (from Gk *balantidion*, dim. of *balantion* a bag, pouch)] A genus of ciliate protozoans consisting primarily of free-living forms but with a few species which are parasitic in animals, including humans.

**balantidosis** \bal′əntidō′sis\ BALANTIDIASIS.

**Balbiani** [Edouard-Gerard *Balbiani,* French biologist, 1823–1899] See under RING.

***Balbiania*** \bal′bē·ā′nē·ə\ *SARCOCYSTIS.*

**balbuties** \balboo′shi·ēz\ [New L, irreg. from L *balbutire* to stammer] *Obs.* STUTTERING.

**baldness** Partial or total absence of hair on the scalp, as in calvities or alopecia. **common male b.** CALVITIES.

**Balint** [Rezsoe *Balint,* Hungarian physician, 1874–1929] See under SYNDROME.

**Ball** [Sir Charles Bent *Ball,* Irish surgeon, 1851–1916] Ball's valves. See under VALVULAE ANALES.

**ball** / **chondrin b.** An encapsulated, ball-like mass of cells found in hyaline cartilage. **fatty b. of Bichat** CORPUS ADIPOSUM BUCCAE. **food b.** A bezoar usually found in the stomach and composed of partially digested or undigested food material such as pits, seeds, or citrus pith. **b. of the foot** The plantar aspect of the foot opposite the heads of the metatarsals, where they are padded by a thick mass of fibrofatty tissue. It is especially important in locomotion, as it supports the weight of the body when the heel is raised. **fungus b.** ASPERGILLOMA. **hair b.** TRICHOBEZOAR. **b. of thumb** THENAR.

**Ballance** [Charles Alfred *Ballance,* English surgeon, 1857–1936] See under SIGN.

**Ballantyne** [John William *Ballantyne,* Scottish pathologist, 1861–1923] See under SYNDROME.

**Ballet** [Gilbert *Ballet,* French neurologist, 1853–1916] See under SIGN.

**balling** The aggregation of erythroblast nuclei into dense, concentrated masses, characteristic of erythropoietic maturation.

**Ballingall** [George *Ballingall,* English surgeon, 1780–1855] Ballingall's disease. See under MYCETOMA.

**ballism** \bal′izm\ [Gk *ballismos* (from *ballizein* to dance, jump, from *ballein* to throw, tumble) a jumping about] Choreiform or other crude, disorganized movements of one or more limbs. Also *ballismus.*

**ballistic** \bəlis′tik\ **1** Pertaining to ballistics. **2** Characterizing movements intitiated by propulsion and further modified only by external factors such as friction, impact, and gravity; not guided or controlled.

**ballistics** \bəlis′tiks\ [L *ballist(a)* (from Gk *ballein* to hurl) engine for throwing stones or darts + -ICS] The science concerned with the propulsion, flight, and effects of projectiles, especially their impact on living or inanimate objects. **drug b.** The measurement of the physical size, shape, and weight, and the categorization of the texture and color of tablets, capsules, ampules, and other vehicles and containers known or suspected to contain drugs and chemicals manufactured illicitly. **forensic b.** That field within ballistics primarily concerned with the recovery and positive identification of fired bullets and expended cartridge cases. Positive identification requires the determination that the bullets in question were fired through a unique weapon, to the exclusion of all other weapons. Also *firearms identification.* **wound b.** The field within ballistics concerned with the type and magnitude of injury or deformity produced by the impact of a projectile on a target and its subsequent course through the target until it comes to rest. Important considerations include the size and shape of the entrance wound, production of secondary projectiles such as bone fragments, depth of penetration, and severity of the wound. For experimental work, the targets are usually animals or gelatin blocks.

**ballistocardiogram** \bəlis′təkär′dē·əgram′\ The recording made by a ballistocardiograph.

**ballistocardiograph** \bəlis′təkär′dē·əgraf′\ An instrument which provides graphic representation of the movements of the body imparted by the ballistic forces associated with cardiac contraction and ejection of blood and with the deceleration of blood flow through the large blood vessels. It was formerly used for estimating cardiac output and other aspects of cardiac function.

**balloon** An inflatable device that can be inserted in a body cavity to provide support or to enclose a tube or catheter. **Hunter b.** A device that is used for occlusion of the inferior vena cava to prevent the formation of a pulmonary embolism. It uses a percutaneously-inserted balloon-tipped catheter, the balloon of which can be inflated and detached when at the proper site. **pilot b.** A small balloon connected to the inflating line of a cuff on the endotracheal tube during anesthesia or respiratory assistance. When the cuff is inflated, the pilot balloon serves to indicate the air pressure of the cuff.

**ballooning** The marked swelling of epidermal cells, with loss of intercellular bridges, that is characteristic of some viral infections of the skin.

**ballottement** \bəlät′mənt, balôtmäN′\ [French (from *ballott(er)* to roll around, toss about, shake, from Old French *ballotte* a little ball, + *-ment* -MENT) a rolling around, tossing about, shaking] A maneuver in physical examination in which an organ or mass deep to the surface is pushed so as to rebound palpably against the wall of the containing space, especially a fluid-filled space, as in ascites. In obstetrics, the maneuver is utilized to palpate a fetus in the amniotic cavity. Also *repercussion.* **abdominal b.** Ballottement in which an intra-abdominal viscus or mass is displaced by one examining hand into the direction of the other hand in order to assess size and texture. Also *indirect ballottement.* **external b.** Ballottement elicited by palpation of the fetus on abdominal examination. This finding is most evident when the fetus presents as a breech. **indirect b.** ABDOMINAL BALLOTTEMENT. **internal b.** Ballottement elicited by vaginal examination of a pregnant woman. This finding is evident from the second trimester through the early third trimester of pregnancy. **kidney b.** A method of bimanual palpation of a kidney, consisting of the placing of one hand in the lumbar region to support the kidney while pressing rapidly inward with the other hand, which is placed on the lateral hypochondrium, opposite the supporting hand. Also *renal ballottement.*

**balneotherapy** \bal′nē·əther′əpē\ [*balne(um)* + *o* + THERAPY] The use of baths for the treatment of injuries and diseases.

**balneum** \bal′nē·əm\ [L (from Gk *balaneion* bathing room), a bath, bathing room; pl. *balnea,* public baths] A bath or a place for bathing.

**Baló** [Jozsef Matthias *Baló,* Hungarian neurologist, born 1896] Baló's concentric encephalitis, Baló syndrome, Baló's concentric sclerosis. See under BALÓ'S DISEASE.

**balsam** \bôl′səm\ [L *balsamum,* from Gk *balsamon* balsam, prob. from Semitic (akin to Assyrian *bašāmu* balsam and Hebrew *bōsem* spice, perfume)] A fragrant, resinous, or oleoresinous exudate from any of various plants. Balsams contain a high proportion of benzoic and/or cinnamic acids or their esters. **Canada b.** A microscopial mounting medium made from an oleoresin obtained from *Abies balsamea.* The oleoresin is known to cause contact dermatitis in some cases. **friars' b.** COMPOUND BENZOIN TINCTURE. **Holland b.** JUNIPER TAR. **Peruvian b.** A mixture of volatile oil and resin that is obtained from the trunks of the trees *Myroxylon pereirae* and *M. balsamum* of the family Leguminosae. The balsam, which contains cinnamein, is used externally as a stimulant and antiseptic and internally as an expectorant. Also *Indian balsam.* **silver b.** JUNIPER TAR. **Turlington's b.** COMPOUND BENZOIN TINCTURE. **Wade's b.** COMPOUND BENZOIN TINCTURE.

**balsamic** 1 Pertaining to or resembling balsam. 2 Soothing: said of medicines.

**Bamberger** [Eugen *Bamberger,* Austrian physician, 1858–1921] Marie-Bamberger syndrome, Marie-Bamberger disease, Bamberger-Marie disease. See under HYPERTROPHIC PULMONARY OSTEOARTHROPATHY.

**Bamberger** [Heinrich von *Bamberger,* Austrian physician, 1822–1888] 1 See under AREA. 2 Bamberger sign. See under ALLOESTHESIA. 3 Bamberger's disease. See under INFANTILE MASSIVE SPASM.

**Bancroft** [Joseph *Bancroft,* English physician, 1836–1894] 1 See under FILARIA. 2 Bancroftian filariasis. See under BANCROFT'S FILARIASIS.

**bancroftiasis** \ban′kräfti′əsis\ BANCROFT'S FILARIASIS.

**band** / **A b.** One of the broad dark bands that traverse skeletal and cardiac muscle fibers and correspond to highly ordered, longitudinal arrangements of myosin filaments. These bands stain darkly with hematoxylin and anisotropically with polarized light. Also *A disk, Q disk, transverse disk, anisotropic disk, anisotropous disk, anisotropic band.* **amniotic b.'s** Bands of tissue formed during intrauterine life between amnion and fetus or across the amniotic cavity. They have been considered a cause of fetal deformity, but are more likely a result of degenerative processes. **angiomesenteric b.** An occasional bandlike constriction produced by tight stretching of the superior mesenteric artery as it crosses the transverse part of the duodenum. **Angle b.** A clamp band used in orthodontics, with the clamp on the lingual side. **anisotropic b.** A BAND. **anogenital b.** A median ridge which develops in the cloacal region of the embryo, marking the formation of the primitive perineum. **anterior b. of colon** TAENIA LIBERA. **atrioventricular b.** FASCICULUS ATRIOVENTRICULARIS. **Baillarger's b.'s** BAILLARGER'S LINES. **Bekhterev's b.** BEKHTEREV'S LAYER. **b. of Broca** The part of the embryonic rhinencephalon which eventually becomes a fiber tract crossing the area parolfactoria. The tract used to be known as Broca's diagonal band. **Büngner's b.'s** Encircling bands formed around regenerating nerve fibers by the Schwann cells. Also *ledbänder.* **cholecystoduodenal b.** CYSTICODUODENAL LIGAMENT. **Clado's b.** LIGAMENTUM SUSPENSORIUM OVARII. **confidence b.** CONFIDENCE INTERVAL. **contoured b.** Any noncylindrical band, particularly one made bulbous in order to fit a tooth closely. **dentate b.** GYRUS DENTATUS. **diagonal b.** A fiber strip rostral to the optic tract at the posterior boundary of the olfactory tubercle, containing the large nucleus of the band of Broca. Also *bandaletta diagonalis of Broca, olfactory station of Broca, diagonal band of Broca.* **episternal b.** The transverse band of tissue lying cranial to the developing sternum and from which the interclavicular ligament is derived. **Essick cell b.** CORPUS PONTOBULBARE. **forbidden b.** In a solid, a range of energies from which electrons are exluded. **free b. of colon** TAENIA LIBERA. **G b.'s** The darkly stained regions seen in chromosomes that have been treated in cytologic preparations with Giemsa stain at an alkaline pH. **genitomesenteric b.** An occasional peritoneal fold extending from the antimesenteric border of the terminal ileum across the cecum either to the right iliac fossa or to the inguinal ring. It may produce downward kinking of the terminal ileum. Also *Lane's band.* **Gennari's b.** A conspicuous horizontal (tangential) band or stripe of myelinated intracortical fibers visible in the cerebral convolutions forming the walls of the calcarine fissure and coursing parallel to the surface of the visual cortex, corresponding to the outer line of Baillarger. Also *line of Gennari, stripe of Gennari, Gennari's layer, stria of Gennari.* **Giacomini's b.** The rostral tip of the dentate gyrus of the hippocampus extending over the uncus. Also *frenulum of Giacomini.* **H b.** A band that transversely bisects the A band of skeletal muscles. It appears pale upon staining and disappears during contraction. **Henle's b.** Fibers of the transversus abdominis aponeurosis that occasionally pass behind the rectus abdominis below the arcuate line of the rectus sheath. **His b.** FASCICULUS ATRIOVENTRICULARIS. **horny b.** BAND OF TARINUS. **b.'s of Hunter-Schreger** SCHREGER'S LINES. **I b.** One of the lightly staining bands that traverses skeletal and cardiac muscle fibers and corresponds to the actin filament zone. The I band narrows during muscle contraction and, in contrast to the A band, rotates polarized light only to a minor degree. Also *isotropic fiber, I disk, isotropic disk, J disk.* **iliotibial b.** TRACTUS ILIOTIBIALIS. **b. of Kaes-Bekhterev** *Outmoded* BEKHTEREV'S LAYER. **Ladd's b.'s** Bands or cords of connective tissue that reach from the right upper quadrant to the right colon. When congenital colonic malrotation has occurred, these bands span the upper abdomen transversely and have been implicated in duodenal obstruction. **Lane's b.** GENITOMESENTERIC BAND. **Leonardo's b.** TRABECULA SEPTOMARGINALIS. **limbic b.'s** Two muscular bands, a superior and an inferior, which develop in the wall of the right atrium of the embryonic heart. They become involved in the formation of the tuberculum intervenosum and the sinus septum. **lip furrow b.** LABIAL LAMINA. **M b.** A line that lies across the center of the H band of skeletal muscles and corresponds to the zone where fine strands interconnect with adjacent myosin filaments. Also *M disk.* **Maissiat's b.** TRACTUS ILIOTIBIALIS. **matrix b.** A band used to contain and mold a plastic dental restoration during its placement and setting, and subsequently removed. **Meckel's b.** That part of the anterior ligament of the malleus that extends from the anterior process and neck of the malleus through the petrotympanic fissure to the spine of the sphenoid bone. Also *Meckel's ligament.* **mesocolic b.** TAENIA MESOCOLICA. **moderator b.** TRABECULA SEPTOMARGINALIS. **omental b.** TAENIA OMENTALIS. **omphalomesenteric b.** A dense band or cord of connective tissue bridging the umbilicus and distal ileum. It it an abnormal remnant of the omphalomesenteric duct. **orthodontic b.** An open-ended metal cylinder cemented around the crown of a tooth as an anchorage for an orthodontic appliance. **Parham b.** A metal band used to internally fix long bone fractures. The band is placed at the fracture site to hold the fragments in apposition. **b. of Reil** 1 TRABECULA SEPTOMARGINALIS. 2 RIBBON OF REIL. **retention b.** MUSCULUS SUSPENSORIUS DUODENI. **b.'s of Schreger** SCHREGER'S LINES. **Sebileau's b.'s** Occasional fibromuscular fasciculi extending from the neck of the first rib and the anterior tubercle of the seventh cervical vertebra and attached to the suprapleural membrane. **Soret b.** An absorption band at about 400 nm, characteristic of porphyrins. **sternal b.** STERNAL BARS. **b. of Tarinus** The rostral portion of the stria terminalis extending to the septal region. Also *horny band.* **valence b.** In a solid, a range of energies that valence electrons may occupy. **Vicq d'Azyr's b.** The horizontal band of thin, myelinated fibers in the outer granular layer of the area striata of human cerebral cortex. **Z b.** A thin, darkly staining band that bisects the I bands of skeletal muscles. It appears to represent an anchor point for the actin filaments. Also *Z line, Krause line, thin disk, Z disk, intermediate disk.* **zonular b.** ZONA ORBICULARIS ARTICULATIONIS COXAE.

**bandage** [French (from *bande* a band, ribbon; from Germanic, akin to English *bind,* + -AGE) binding, bandage] **1** Any artificial covering for a wound; a dressing. **2** Any wrap or strapping, usually of gauze, used to protect, cover, or immobilize an injured or diseased part. See also entries under DRESSING and GAUZE. **3** To cover with gauze or other material. **adhesive b.** ADHESIVE ABSORBENT DRESSING. **barrel b.** A roller or folded triangular bandage for the support of a fractured jaw. **compression b.** A dressing that applies pressure to the covered area. It is used to prevent edema, stop bleeding, or hold a skin graft firmly in place. **demigauntlet b.** A bandage applied over the hand without coverage of the fingers. Also *demigauntlet.* **Desault's b.** A bandage that binds the elbow to the side of the body, with a pad placed in the axilla. Also *Desault's apparatus.* **figure-of-8 b.** A bandage in which the turns cross each other in a configuration resembling the figure 8. **Fricke's b.** A wrapping for the scrotum used in the treatment of epididymitis and orchitis. **gauntlet b.** A glovelike bandage covering the hand and all fingers. Also *gauntlet.* **reversed b.** A bandage in which the roller is inverted or half-twisted at each turn, creating a smooth fit to the limb. **roller b.** ROLLER. **Sayre's b.** An adhesive plaster bandage utilized to support and immobilize a fractured clavicle. **Scultetus b.** A rectangular bandage with the edges cut into numerous tails that may be wrapped around the injured part and fixed individually with safety pins or by other means. Also *scultetus.* **spica b.** A figure-of-eight bandage usually applied to joint areas such as the shoulder and thorax, thigh and pelvis, or thumb and hand. Also *spica.* **Velpeau's b.** A bandage used to support the arm in fractures of the clavicle.

**bandaletta** \ban′dəlet′ə\ **b. diagonalis of Broca** DIAGONAL BAND.

**banding** / **chromosome b.** In producing a karyotype, the process of using any of a variety of enzymes, stains, and chemical manipulations to produce differentially stained or fluorescent regions, which are oriented perpendicularly to the long axis of each chromosome. The regions are consistent for all like chromosomes of an organism, and they can be used to specifically identify each chromosome. **G b.** In cytogenetics, the preparation of a karyotype by treatment with Giemsa stain. **pulmonary artery b.** In the operative management of congenital heart disease, restriction of the lumen of the pulmonary artery over a short segment of its length by binding it with inelastic material, thereby raising the blood pressure in the right ventricle and diminishing left-to-right shunting through a coexisting ventricular defect. Banding will also have the effect of diminishing pulmonary blood flow and reducing the likelihood that pulmonary hypertension will develop.

**Bandl** [Ludwig *Bandl,* German obstetrician, 1842–1892] Bandl's ring. See under PATHOLOGIC RETRACTION RING.

**bandwidth** **1** The range of frequencies or wavelengths over which a device is intended to operate. **2** For amplifiers, the difference between the upper and lower frequency at which the response is 0.707 of the midband response.

**Bang** [Bernard Laurits Frederik *Bang,* Danish veterinarian, 1848–1932] Bang's bacillus. See under *BRUCELLA ABORTUS.*

**Bangerter** [Alfred P. D. *Bangerter,* Swiss ophthalmologist, born 1909] Bangerter's method. See under PLEOPTICS.

**bank** A facility for storing and maintaining in a viable state certain kinds of tissues, organs, or other biologic materials for tranfusions, transplantations, inseminations, or other uses. **blood b.** A repository for blood collected from donors, to be used at a later time by recipients. Blood banks are maintained by individual hospitals or, in many cases, by whole communities for use in several hospitals. **eye b.** A system of obtaining and distributing available donor corneas to the surgeons performing corneal transplantation. **skin b.** A repository for the preparation, preservation, and storage of donor skin. **sperm b.** A facility where sperm is stored in a frozen state for use in artificial insemination.

**Banti** [Guido *Banti,* Italian pathologist, 1852–1925] See under DISEASE, SYNDROME, ANEMIA.

**BAO** basal acid output.

**baptisin** A glycoside obtained from the dried root of *Baptisia tinctoria* (wild indigo), an herbaceous plant native to North America that has been used to treat fevers and has purgative properties.

**bar[1]** [Old French *barre* bar, from Med L *barra* bar, barrier] **1** Any oblong part that bridges a gap between structures or obstructs a passage. **2** A rigid metal wire or casting connecting two or more parts of a partial denture. **arch b.** A thick wire, bent to fit the buccal or lingual surface of the dental arch and serving as the basis for a splint or orthodontic appliance. **b. of bladder** PLICA INTERURETERICA. **House b.** The vertical bony partition between area nervi facialis and area vestibularis superior in the fundus of the internal acoustic meatus. It is a critical landmark for identifying the facial nerve in the translabyrinthine surgical approach to the internal acoustic meatus. **hyoid b.'s** The two cartilaginous bars of the second branchial arch which become part of the hyoid bone. **interureteric b.** PLICA INTERURETERICA. **Kennedy b.** CONTINUOUS BAR RETAINER. **labial b.** A metal bar, part of a partial denture running labially to the teeth, at the level of the gingiva, and connecting the parts of the denture which carry replacement teeth. **lumbrical b.** A component of a hand orthosis used to prevent extension of the second to fifth proximal phalanges. **median b.** A fibrotic fold of abnormal connective tissue, stretched across the trigone of the bladder at its neck, that may produce fibrous contracture and obstruction of the urethral orifice. Also *Mercier's barrier, valvula prostatica.* **Mercier's b.** PLICA INTERURETERICA. **metatarsal b.'s** Shoe inserts at the level of the metatarsals, used to maintain the position of the foot and prevent contractures of the toes following injury or burns of the foot. **palatal b.** A metal bar used in a partial upper denture formed to fit the palate, connecting the parts of the denture which carry replacement teeth. **Passavant's b.** A rounded horizontal ridge on the posterior pharyngeal wall produced by the palatopharyngeal sphincter, especially well observed when the soft palate is elevated during swallowing. Also *Passavant's cushion, Passavant's pad, Passavant's ridge, pharyngeal ridge.* **sternal b.'s** The paired anterior cartilages in the region of the embryonic thorax which unite to form the sternum. Also *sternal band.* **sublingual b.** A major connector joining two bases of a partial denture. It is placed on the floor of the mouth. **terminal b.** A line, stainable with iron hematoxylin, that is situated apparently between adjacent epithelial cells near their luminal borders. It is now known to correspond to the junctional complex seen by electron microscopy, which consists of a tight junction followed by an intermediate junction and then one or more desmosomes. **thyroid b.** One of the cartilaginous masses which in the embryo gives rise to half of the thyroid cartilage.

**bar[2]** [Gk *bar(os)* (akin to *barys* heavy) weight, pressure] A unit of pressure equal to $10^5$ pascals, 100 kilopascals; a popular, noncoherent unit used in conjunction with SI. Symbol: bar

**bar-** \bar-\ BARO-.

**baragnosia** \bar′agnō′zhə\ [BAR- + Gk *agnōsia* a not knowing] Inability to assess the weight of objects. Also *abarognosia, baragnosis, baroagnosis.*

**baralyme** \bar′əlīm\ A combination of barium hydroxide and sodium hydroxide used as a carbon dioxide absorber when gases are rebreathed in an anesthesia breathing circuit.

**baranesthesia** \bar′anesthē′zhə\ [BAR- + ANESTHESIA] Loss of deep pressure sensation.

**Bárány** [Robert *Bárány,* Austrian physician, 1876–1936] See under DRUM, TEST, BOX.

**barba** \bär′bə\ [L] [NA] BEARD.

**barbeiro** \bärbā′roo\ [Portuguese, barber] A cone-nose bug of the species *Panstrongylus megistus.*

**barbital** 5,5-Diethylbarbituric acid. A barbiturate. Also *barbitone, malonal.*

**barbitalism** \bär′bətälizm\ BARBITURISM.

**barbitone** BARBITAL.

**barbituism** \bär′bichoo·izm\ BARBITURISM.

**barbiturate** \bärbich′ərāt\ Any of the substituted derivatives of barbituric acid, whose molecule is a six-membered ring containing two —NH— groups, derived from the condensation of urea with malonic acid or its esters. Barbiturates are anesthetics and depressants of the central nervous system. Biochemically, they inhibit electron transport in the respiratory chain between NADH and cytochromes.

**barbituric acid** $C_4H_4N_2O_3$. A crystalline substance, melting at 248°C with decomposition. It is a tautomer of 2,4,6-trihydroxypyrimidine, soluble in hot water and in dilute acids and alkalies. Its numerous derivatives substituted in the 5-position (barbiturates) have hypnotic (sedative) properties. Also *malonylurea.*

**barbiturism** \bär′bichərizm\ A clinical condition caused by the chronic use of barbital or its derivatives and characterized by irritability and impairment of intellectual, sensory, and motor functions. Also *barbitalism, barbituism, barbital poisoning, barbiturate poisoning.*

**barbula** \bär′byələ\ [L, dim. of *barba* beard] HAIR TUFT.

**Barclay** [Alfred Ernest *Barclay,* English radiologist, 1876–1949] See under NICHE.

**Barcroft** [Sir Joseph F *Barcroft,* English physiologist, 1872–1947] Barcroft's apparatus. See under WARBURG'S APPARATUS.

**Bard** [Louis *Bard,* French physician, 1857–1930] Bard-Pic syndrome. See under SYNDROME.

**Bard** [Philip *Bard,* U.S. psychologist, 1898–1945] Cannon-Bard theory of emotions. See under THEORY.

**Bardet** [Georges *Bardet,* French physician, born 1885] Bardet-Biedl syndrome. See under SYNDROME.

**bare** Without medical malpractice insurance. A term used only in the U.S. ⟨"Dr. Rogers, who practices bare and is still representing himself in two other malpractice suits." —*Medical World News,* 18 Aug. 1980, 31.⟩

**baresthesia** \bar′esthē′zhə\ [BAR- + ESTHESIA] PRESSURE SENSE.

**baresthesiometer** \bar′esthē′zē·äm′ətər\ [BAR- + ESTHESIO- + -METER] An instrument used for measuring cutaneous pressure perception. *Seldom used.*

**barhypesthesia** \bar′hīpesthē′zhə\ [BAR- + HYP- + -ESTHESIA] Impairment of deep pressure sensation.

**bariatrics** \bar′ē·at′riks\ [*bar(o)-* + -IATRICS] The study of obesity and its treatment.

**baric** \bar′ik\ **1** Of or relating to barium. **2** Pertaining to atmospheric weight or pressure.

**baricity** \baris′itē\ The weight or density of a substance in comparison to a different substance at similar conditions of temperature and atmospheric pressure.

**baritosis** \bar′itō′sis\ [*bari(um)* + *t* + -OSIS] The presence of small, radiographically dense nodules in the lungs due to inhalation of barium-containing dust, usually from barium ores. These nodules produce no harmful effects. Also *barytosis.*

**barium** \bar′ē·əm\ Element number 56, having atomic weight 137.33. Barium is a soft alkaline earth metal resembling calcium chemically. Seven stable isotopes occur in nature, and numerous short-lived radioisotopes are known. The valence is 2. Barium salts are electron-dense and are thus useful in radiology. All of the water-soluble and acid-soluble compounds of barium are poisonous. The carbonate has been used as a rat poison. Symbol: Ba

**barium sulfate** A salt of low solubility. It is used in radiology as a contrast agent for examination of the gastrointestinal tract.

**barium titanate** $BaTiO_3$. A ceramic piezoelectric material used in ultrasonic transducers.

**bark** The outer covering of the woody parts of a plant, tree, or shrub, including all tissues outside the cambium. **bearberry b.** CASCARA SAGRADA. **chittam b.** CASCARA SAGRADA. **chittem b.** CASCARA SAGRADA. **chittim b.** CASCARA SAGRADA. **cinchona b.** CINCHONA. **druggists' b.** The dried bark of *Cinchona calisaya* and other *Cinchona* species that contain up to 14 percent quinine. It is usually prescribed in the form of an extract. **eleuthera b.** An aromatic bitter obtained from the bark of *Croton eluteria.* **grape b.** An alcoholic extract of the dried bark of *Guarea rusbyi.* It is used as an expectorant or, in larger doses, as an emetic. **Jesuits' b.** CINCHONA. **Persian b.** CASCARA SAGRADA. **Peruvian b.** CINCHONA. **purshiana b.** CASCARA SAGRADA. **quillaia b.** PANAMA WOOD. **sacred b.** CASCARA SAGRADA. **soap b.** PANAMA WOOD.

**Barkan** [Otto *Barkan,* U.S. ophthalmologist, 1887–1958] Barkan's operation. See under GONIOTOMY.

**Barker** [Arthur Edward James *Barker,* English surgeon, 1850–1916] See under POINT.

**Barkman** [Ake *Barkman,* Swedish internist, flourished 20th century] See under REFLEX.

**Barkow** [Hans Karl Leopold *Barkow,* German anatomist, 1798–1873] See under LIGAMENT.

**Barlow** [John B. *Barlow,* South African cardiologist, flourished 20th century] See under SYNDROME.

**Barlow** [Thomas *Barlow,* English physician, 1845–1945] Barlow's disease. See under INFANTILE SCURVY.

**Barnes** [Robert *Barnes,* English obstetrician, 1817–1907] See under ZONE, CURVE.

**baro-** \bar′ō-\ [Gk *baros* weight] A combining form meaning (1) weight; (2) atmospheric pressure. Also *bar-.*

**baroagnosis** \-agnō′sis\ BARAGNOSIA.

**baroceptor** \-sep′tər\ BARORECEPTOR.

**barodontalgia** \-däntal′jə\ [BAR- + ODONTALGIA] AERODONTALGIA.

**barometer** \bəräm′ətər\ [BARO- + -METER] An instrument that measures atmospheric pressure.

**baropacer** \bar′ōpā′sər\ A device for the continuous or repetitive stimulation of baroreceptors.

**baroreceptor** \-risep′tər\ A sense organ responsive to the stretch of large vessel walls signaling blood pressure.

These pressure receptors are found in the aortic arch, carotid sinus, vena cava, and cardiac auricle, and serve to regulate reflex control of blood pressure and heart rate. Also *baroceptor, pressoreceptor.*

**barosensitive** \-sen′sətiv\ Pressure sensitive.

**barosinusitis** \-sī′nəsī′tis\ SINUS BAROTRAUMA.

**barostat** \bar′ōstat\ [BARO- + -STAT] A structure which, because of its ability to sense pressure, is involved in the feedback mechanisms ensuring stability of pressure, as in the baroreceptors of the carotid sinus.

**barotalgia** \bar′ōtal′jə\ [BAR- + OTALGIA] Pain in the middle ear due to a difference in pressure between that in the middle ear and that in the surrounding atmospheric pressure.

**barotitis** \-tī′tis\ [BAR- + OTITIS] OTITIC BAROTRAUMA. **b. media** BAROTRAUMATIC OTITIS MEDIA.

**barotrauma** \bar′ōtrô′mə\ [BARO- + TRAUMA] Noninfective inflammatory changes produced in the ear or in one or more of the paranasal sinuses by uncorrected barometric pressure difference between the environmental atmosphere and the gases, normally air, within the cavity concerned. Usually the internal pressure is lower than that of the atmosphere outside. The condition is liable to occur during flight, particularly descent, deep sea diving, subaqua swimming and in patients undergoing radiotherapy in hyperbaric oxygen, especially when concurrent rhinitis causes congestion of the sinus ostia or of the eustachian tube. **b. of the ear** OTITIC BAROTRAUMA. **odontalgia b.** AERODONTALGIA. **otitic b.** The effect of barotrauma on the ear. The middle ear is usually involved (barotraumatic otitis media), the involvement of the inner ear (barotraumatic otitis interna) occurring only rarely. Also *barotrauma of the ear, barotraumatic otitis, barotitis.* **sinus b.** Barotrauma of one or more of the paranasal sinuses. In contrast with other kinds of sinusitis, the frontal sinus may be involved in the absence of involvement of the maxillary sinus. Facial pain is the leading symptom, sometimes accompanied by blood-stained nasal discharge. Also *barosinusitis, barotraumatic sinusitis.*

**Barr** [Murray Llewellyn *Barr,* Canadian histologist, born 1908] See under BODY.

**Barr** [Yvonne M. *Barr,* English virologist, flourished 20th century] Epstein-Barr virus. See under VIRUS.

**Barraquer** [Ignacio *Barraquer,* Spanish ophthalmologist, 1884–1965] See under OPERATION.

**Barraquer** [José Antonio *Barraquer,* Spanish physician, born 1852] Barraquer-Simons syndrome. See under PROGRESSIVE LIPODYSTROPHY.

**Barré** [Jean Alexandre *Barré,* French neurologist, born 1880] **1** Barré's pyramidal sign. See under SIGN. **2** Barré-Guillain syndrome, Guillain-Barré polyneuritis, Guillian-Barré-Strohl syndrome, Landry-Guillain-Barré syndrome. See under GUILLAIN-BARRÉ SYNDROME. **3** Guillain-Barré reflex. See under SOLE-TAP REFLEX.

**Barrett** [Norman Rupert *Barrett,* English surgeon, born 1903] See under ESOPHAGUS, ULCER.

**barrier** **1** An obstacle to the free movement of materials, as from one organ or system to another, as in the blood-brain barrier. **2** Difficulty or inability to relate to others, such as the schizophrenic subject's difficulties in forming interpersonal relationships. **3** In projective methods, designating a response emphasizing the periphery or delimitation of a percept. **architectural b.** Any feature of a building or other structure that makes it inaccessible to disabled persons, as, for example, the lack of ramps or elevators as a barrier to persons in wheelchairs. **blood-aqueous b.** A little-understood anatomical-physiological system whereby the ciliary epithelium in the orbit regulates the functions of the ciliary body by serving as a lipid membrane in permitting selective filtration, secretion, and diffusion of substances, and by providing passage of fluids in both directions between the aqueous chamber and the bloodstream. Also *blood-ocular fluid barrier.* **blood-brain b.** The normal state of limited exchange between the lumen of the brain capillaries on the one hand and the cerebrospinal fluid and extracellular fluid of the brain on the other. It is thought to be maintained by a continuous band of tight junctions between endothelial cells of the capillaries. Also *blood-cerebrospinal fluid barrier, blood-cerebral barrier, blood-cortical barrier, blood-spinal fluid barrier, Held's limiting membrane.* **blood-ocular fluid b.** BLOOD-AQUEOUS BARRIER. **blood-spinal fluid b.** BLOOD-BRAIN BARRIER. **blood-thymus b.** The state of limited exchange between the lumen of the thymic capillaries and the thymic tissue. It is thought to be maintained by the interposition of a sheet of epithelial cells between the capillaries and the thymic lobules. **energy b.** In a reaction that does not occur spontaneously because the energy level of the reactants is not adequate to allow the reaction to start, the difference between the energy content of the reactants and the energy level needed to allow the reaction to start. Energy supplied to effect the reaction is called the activation energy. Enzymes are capable of reducing the energy barrier. **gastric mucosal b.** The state of resistance of the gastric mucosa to digestion by the acid and pepsin in the gastric chyme. It is thought to be due at least in part to the properties of the gastric mucous layer and its contained bicarbonate secretion. **Mercier's b.** **1** PLICA INTERURETERICA. **2** MEDIAN BAR. **placental b.** The cellular and connective tissue membrane that normally everywhere intervenes between the maternal and fetal circulations in the placenta. It is composed of both maternal and fetal elements arranged in layers, the number of layers varying in different animal groups. Where all layers are present the barrier is said to be epitheliochorial. Endotheliochorial and hemochorial barriers have reduced numbers of layers. The placental barrier prevents mixing of maternal and fetal blood cells and is also important in that it allows passage of gases and certain ions but limits transfer of substances with high molecular weight. **primary protective b.** A wall or other barrier which is exposed to a direct beam of radiation and is sufficiently thick to reduce the exposure to a permissible level. **secondary protective b.** A barrier which receives mainly scattered radiation and reduces it to a permissible exposure level.

**Barsony** [Theodor *Barsony,* German physician, 1887–1942] Barsony-Teschendof syndrome. See under DIFFUSE ESOPHAGEAL SPASM.

**Bartholin** [Caspar *Bartholin,* II, Danish anatomist, 1655–1738] **1** Bartholinian abscess. See under ABSCESS. **2** Bartholin's gland. See under GLANDULA VESTIBULARIS MAJOR. **3** Bartholin's duct. See under DUCTUS SUBLINGUALIS MAJOR.

**bartholinitis** \bär′tōlinī′tis\ [*Bartholin('s ducts)* + -ITIS] Inflammation of the greater vestibular glands.

**Bartholomew** [Rudolph A. *Bartholomew,* U.S. obstetrician, 1886–1969] See under RULE.

**Barton** [Alberto L. *Barton,* Peruvian physician, 1871–1950] Bartonia bodies. See under BODY.

**Barton** [John Rhea *Barton,* U.S. surgeon, 1794–1871] See under FORCEPS, OPERATION, FRACTURE.

***Bartonella*** \bär′tənel′ə\ [after Alberto L. *Barton,* Peruvian physician, 1871–1950] A genus of small, Gram-negative, rod-shaped bacteria that parasitize red blood cells. The principal human pathogen is *B. bacilliformis.* ***B. bacilliformis*** A minute, rickettsialike, Gram-negative, Giemsa-staining organism with an unusual tropism for erythrocytes. It grows slowly in semisolid agar containing hemoglobin. It produces a commonly fatal disease (bartonellosis) along the Pacific slope of the Andes, and is transmitted by sandflies.

**bartonellemia** \bär′tənelē′mē·ə\ Septicemia caused by *Bartonella bacilliformis.*

**bartonelliasis** \bär′tənelī′əsis\ BARTONELLOSIS.

**bartonellosis** \bär′tənelō′sis\ [*Bartonell(a)* + -OSIS] An infectious disease of man caused by *Bartonella bacilliformis* and transmitted by the sandfly. It is seen in Andean mountain valleys of Peru, Columbia, and Ecuador. Manifestations are an acute, febrile illness with hemolytic anemia (Oroyo fever) followed by granulomatous skin lesions known as verruga peruana. The incubation period is about three weeks. Bone pain and hepatosplenomegaly are other clinical features. If untreated, there is a 10–40 percent mortality rate. Also *bartonelliasis, Carrión's disease.*

**Bartter** [Frederic Crosby *Bartter,* U.S. physiologist, born 1914] **1** Bartter-Schwartz syndrome. See under SCHWARTZ-BARTTER SYNDROME. **2** See under SYNDROME.

**Barwell** [Richard *Barwell,* English surgeon, 1826–1916] See under OPERATION.

**bary-** \bar′i-\ [Gk *barys* heavy, difficult] A combining form meaning heavy, difficult, dull.

**baryesthesia** \-esthē′zhə\ [BARY- + ESTHESIA] PRESSURE SENSE.

**baryglossia** \-gläs′ē·ə\ [Gk *baryglōss(os)* (from *barys* heavy + *glōssa* the tongue) chattering wearily + -IA] Indistinct speech due to a disorder of the tongue itself or of the nerves supplying it.

**barylalia** \-lā′lyə\ [BARY- + Gk *lalia* a talking, babbling] Indistinct, slow speech from any cause. The most frequent cause is a lesion in the central nervous system, as in general paresis and senile dementia.

**barymazia** \-mā′zhə\ [BARY- + *maz(o)-* + -IA] MAMMARY HYPERTROPHY.

**baryta** Barium oxide. It is obtained by heating barium carbonate.

**barytosis** \-tō′sis\ BARITOSIS.

**barytron** \bar′iträn\ *Outmoded* MESON.

**basad** \bā′sad\ [*bas(e)* + -AD] Toward the base of a structure.

**basal** \bā′səl\ Pertaining to or situated adjacent to a base of a structure or organ.

**basaloid** \bā′səloid\ Having a superficial resemblance to the cells comprising the basal layer of the epidermis.

**basaloma** \bā′səlō′mə\ BASAL CELL CARCINOMA.

**base** [French (from L *basis*; see BASIS) a pedestal, foundation, base, main ingredient, mordant for a dye, alkali] **1** The lowest, most dependent, or supporting part; foundation; basis. **2** A substance that can combine with protons. The protonated form is the conjugate acid of the base. ● If the term is unqualified, this meaning is usually intended, and it may be specified as a Brønsted base. **3** A substance that combines with another by donating electrons to form the bond between them. This form of base, where the other substance is not a proton, is termed a Lewis base. **4** The purines adenine and guanine and the pyrimidines uracil, cytosine, and thymine, or their derivatives, as they occur bound to sugars in nucleic acids. **apical b.** That portion of the jawbones supporting the apical regions of the roots of the teeth. After extraction of the teeth the alveolar process tends to be resorbed but the apical base persists. Also *basal arch, apical area.* **b. of bladder** FUNDUS VESICAE URINARIAE. **b. of brain** FACIES INFERIOR CEREBRI. **Brønsted b.** A substance that can combine with the ion $H^+$, as distinguished from a Lewis base. **buffer b.** A proton acceptor that minimizes changes in the pH of a solution when acid is added. **cement b.** A layer of dental cement under the principal restorative material in a restoration, used for heat insulation, to reduce the amount of expensive precious metal used, or to fill in undercuts. **b. of cerebrum** FACIES INFERIOR HEMISPHERII CEREBRI. **conjugate b.** The base derived from a particular acid by dissociation of a proton. **cranial b.** Either basis cranii externa (norma basilaris) or basis cranii interna. **data b.** DATABASE. **denture b.** The part of a denture which rests on the oral mucosa and to which artificial teeth are attached. Also *saddle.* **extension b.** A base, constituting part of a partial denture, which is not supported by a tooth at one end. Also *free-end base, free-end saddle.* **b. of finger** The junction of the finger with the palm at the level of the metacarpophalangeal joint and approximately at that of the webs of the fingers. **free-end b.** EXTENSION BASE. **b. of heart** BASIS CORDIS. **b. of iris** MARGO CILIARIS IRIDIS. **Lewis b.** A substance that can combine with other substances (Lewis acids) by donating the electrons that form the bond between them. Unlike a Brønsted base, the substances bound are not restricted to the ion $H^+$. **b. of lung** BASIS PULMONIS. **b. of metatarsal** BASIS METATARSALIS. **b. of nail** RADIX UNGUIS. **ointment b.** A semisolid material used to hold medications in suspension or solution for external application. **b. pair** Bases in the two complementary strands of the molecules of DNA or RNA which are paired by hydrogen bonding between them across the axis of the helix. Because of their spatial configuration, adenine always pairs with thymine (in DNA) or uracil (in RNA) and cytosine always pairs with guanine. **b. of phalanx of finger** BASIS PHALANGIS DIGITORUM MANUS. **b. of phalanx of toe** BASIS PHALANGIS DIGITORUM PEDIS. **b. of prostate** BASIS PROSTATAE. **rare b.'s** Nucleoside phosphates, other than adenosine, cytidine, guanosine or uridine, incorporated into tRNA molecules. Rare bases include ribosylthymine, 5,6-dihydrouridine, 5-ribosyluracil, inosine, and 1-methylguanosine. These bases are important in establishing the unique spatial organization of the tRNA molecule. **record b.** BASEPLATE. **b. of renal pyramid** BASIS PYRAMIDIS RENALIS. **b. of sacrum** BASIS OSSIS SACRI. **Schiff b.** IMINE. **b. of skull** BASIS CRANII. **b. of stapes** BASIS STAPEDIS. **temporary b.** BASEPLATE. **time b.** The time coordinate on a display. **trial b.** BASEPLATE. **whole blood buffer b.** The sum of all buffer anions in the blood capable of binding protons within the tolerable limits of body pH, normally equal to 45–50 $mEq\,l^{-1}$. It is used as an index of nonrespiratory alteration in acid-base balance. **whole body buffer b.** The sum of all buffer anions in the body capable of binding protons within the tolerable limits of body pH. **wobble b.** The base of the third residue in a codon, often replaceable by another base without change of the tRNA bound by the mRNA containing it, and hence without change of the amino acid incorporated under its direction.

**Basedow** [Karl Adolph von *Basedow,* German physician, 1799–1854] See under GOITER.

**baseline** The horizontal line traced when no difference of potential is being recorded. Also *isoelectric line, isoelectric level.* **Reid's b.** BASE LINE.

**baseosis** \bā′sē·ō′sis\ [BASE + -OSIS] ALKALOSIS.

**baseplate** **1** A temporary form representing the base of a denture and used for making recordings of jaw relations, for arranging artificial teeth, or for trial placement in the mouth. It is usually made of shellac, wax, or acrylic resin. Also *record base, temporary base, trial base*. Also *base plate*. **2** That portion of the bladder surrounding the opening into the urethra, acting as a floor during filling and becoming a cone-shaped funnel during voiding.

**bases** \bā′sēz\ Plural of BASIS.

**bas-fond** \bäfôN′\ [French (from *bas* low, from Late L *bassus* low + *fond* bottom, lowest part, from L *fundus* bottom), low, sunken land, level of the sea bottom] Fundus, particularly that of the urinary bladder.

**basi-** \bā′sē-, bā′si-\ [Gk *basis* a stepping, walk, place whereon one steps, pedestal] A combining form denoting (1) base; (2) step, gait. Also *basio-, baso-*.

**basial** \bā′sē·əl\ **1** Pertaining to the basion. **2** Relating to a base.

**basialveolar** \bā′sē·alvē′ələr\ Of or pertaining to both the basion and the alveolar point, particularly the distance measured between them. Also *basioalveolar*.

**basibranchial** \-brang′kē·əl\ Arising from the ventral ends or sides of the branchial arch skeleton, usually giving rise to an unpaired skeletal structure, such as the body of the hyoid bone.

**basicity** \bāsis′itē\ A measure of basic property, usually p*K*.

**basicranial** \-krā′nē·əl\ Pertaining to the base of the skull.

**basidio-** \bəsid′ē·ō-\ [New L *basidium* (from Gk *bas(is)* a base + New L *-idium*, diminishing suffix)] A combining form denoting a basidium.

***Basidiobolus*** \bəsid′ē·äb′ələs\ [New L *basidium*, dim. of Gk *basis* a base + L *bolus* (from Gk *bōlos* clod, lump) morsel, piece] A genus of fungi that are primarily saprobic, but which includes at least one species known to be a human pathogen. ***B. ranarum*** A species of fungus which causes subcutaneous phycomycosis. It is present as a saprophyte in the intestinal tract of beetles, frogs, toads, and lizards. It has been described in east and west Africa and in Indonesia.

**basidiospore** \bəsid′ē·əspôr\ [BASIDIO- + SPORE] A fungal spore borne on the outside of a basidium, following karyogamy and meiosis.

**basidium** \bəsid′ē·əm\ [New L, dim. of Gk *basis* a base] (*pl.* basidia) A fungal structure bearing on its distal clublike surface a definite number of basidiospores, typically four, that are usually formed following karyogamy and meiosis.

**basifacial** \bā′sifā′shəl\ Of or pertaining to the lower portion of the face.

**basihyal** \-hī′əl\ [BASI- + HYAL] The body of the hyoid bone. Also *basihyoid*.

**basilad** \bas′ilad\ In the direction of the base or basal part of a structure or organ.

**basilar** \bas′ilər\ Near or pertaining to the base or basal part of a structure or organ.

**basilaris cranii** \bas′iler′is krā′nē·ī\ The bones of the base of the skull that support the brain and form the cranial fossae.

**basilateral** \bā′silat′ərəl\ Pertaining to the base and side or sides of a structure or part. Also *basolateral*.

**basilemma** \-lem′ə\ [BASI- + LEMMA] BASEMENT MEMBRANE.

**basilic** \bəsil′ik\ [Arabic *bāsilīq*, perh. from a pseudo-Greek variant (confused with Gk *basilikos* royal) of Med L *basilaris* basilar, basal: the basilic vein was associated, for bloodletting purposes, with parts of the body below the head, as opposed to the cephalic vein, which was supposed to connect with the head] Pertaining to or designating the vena basilica.

**basiloma** \bas′ilō′mə\ BASAL CELL CARCINOMA.

**basilomental** \bas′ilōmen′təl\ Pertaining to the basilar part of the occipital bone and the chin region.

**basilopharyngeal** \bas′ilōfərin′jē·əl\ Relating to the basilar part of the occipital bone and the pharynx.

**basin / kidney b.** A kidney-shaped basin used for the collection of sputum and other body fluids.

**basio-** \bā′sē·ō-\ BASI-.

**basioalveolar** \bā′sē·ō·alvē′ələr\ BASIALVEOLAR.

**basioccipital** \bā′sē·äksip′ətəl\ Of or pertaining to the basilar process of the occipital bone.

**basioglossus** \bā′sē·ōgläs′əs\ The fibers of the hyoglossus muscle of the tongue that arise from the body of the hyoid bone.

**basion** \bā′sē·än\ [New L, irreg. from Gk *basis* base] A craniometric point situated at the center of the anterior edge of the foramen magnum.

**basiotic** \bā′sē·ō′tik\ [BASI- + OTIC] **1** Pertaining to the basal plate, basiotic bone, and the otic capsule in the developing skull. **2** Relating to the basion.

**basiotribe** \bā′sē·ōtrīb′\ [BASIO- + Gk *tribē* a rubbing, grinding away] BASILYST.

**basipharyngeal** \-fərin′jē·əl\ Pertaining to the lower surface of the postsphenoid bone and the pharynx below.

**basipresphenoid** \-prēsfē′noid\ Of or pertaining to the basisphenoid and presphenoid bones and their centers of ossification.

**basirhinal** \-rī′nəl\ Of or relating to the base of the brain and the nose.

**basis** [L and Gk, a base, pedestal] The lower, fundamental, and often the broadest part of an organ or structure, usually opposite its apex; base. **b. capituli** See under CAPITULUM. **b. cartilaginis arytenoideae** [NA] The concave base of the pyramidal arytenoid cartilage of the larynx, having a smooth facet that rests upon and articulates with the upper border of the lamina of cricoid cartilage. **b. cerebri** **1** The inferior aspect of the forebrain exclusive of midbrain and hindbrain. **2** FACIES INFERIOR CEREBRI. **b. cochleae** [NA] The base of the conical bony cochlea of the internal ear that lies upon the internal acoustic meatus. **b. cordis** [NA] The ill-defined base of the cone-shaped heart that is formed by the two atria, the left to a larger extent than the right, lying between the proximal parts of the great vessels. The base faces backward and to the right, where it is separated from the fifth to ninth vertebrae (the precise number depending on whether posture is recumbent or erect) by the pericardium, esophagus, aorta, and right pulmonary veins. Also *base of heart*. **b. cranii** The sloping floor or base of the skull. It comprises the basis cranii externa and the basis cranii interna. Also *base of skull*. **b. cranii externa** **1** [NA] The outer, or inferior, surface of the base of the skull, having an irregular oval outline. It comprises portions of the maxilla and the palatine, temporal, zygomatic, vomer, sphenoid, and occipital bones. It is perforated by vessels and nerves (including the spinal cord) leading to and from the brain, and gives attachment to muscles, tendons, and ligaments. Anteriorly it is joined to the bones of the face, and the condyles of the mandible articulate with it. **2** *Imprecise* NORMA BASILARIS. **b. cranii interna** [NA] The inner, or superior, surface of the base of the skull, forming the floor of the cranial cavity on which the brain and its vessels and membranes rest. The surface slopes downward and backward in humans and is divided into the fossa cranii anterior, fossa cranii media, and fossa cranii posterior. The bones involved include parts of the frontal, ethmoid, sphenoid, temporal, and occipital bones. The base is perforated by vessels and nerves (including the spinal cord) leading to and from the brain. **b. encephali** FACIES INFERIOR CEREBRI. **b. glandulae suprarenalis** FACIES RENALIS GLANDULAE SUPRARENALIS. **b. mandibulae** [NA] The lower border, or base, of the body of the mandible that extends posteriorly and laterally from the symphysis menti to the ramus, meeting the latter at the level of the third molar tooth. Also *inferior border of mandible.* **b. metacarpalis** [NA] The expanded end, or base, of each metacarpal bone that articulates with one or more bones of the distal carpal row as well as with the bases of adjacent metacarpal bones. The exception is the base of the isolated first metacarpal (thumb), which does not articulate with the second metacarpal base. **b. metatarsalis** [NA] The irregularly expanded end, or base, of each metatarsal bone that articulates with one or more bones of the distal row of the tarsus as well as with the bases of adjacent metatarsal bones. Also *base of metatarsal.* **b. modioli** [NA] The broad base of the modiolus, or conical central axis of the bony cochlea, that appears at the lateral end of the internal acoustic meatus. It corresponds to the cochlear area and is perforated by fibers of the cochlear nerve. **b. ossis sacri** [NA] The complex structure composed centrally of the superior, or cranial, surface of the first sacral vertebra and the alae on each side of it, and posteriorly the upper triangular opening of the sacral canal, with a large superior articular process laterally for articulation with the inferior articular processes of the fifth lumbar vertebra. Through the wedge-shaped intervertebral disk, the sacral body articulates with the body of the fifth lumbar vertebra, forming the sacrovertebral angle. The anterior projecting edge of the sacral body forms the promontory. Also *base of sacrum.* **b. patellae** [NA] The thick superior border, or base, of the triangular patella, to which is attached the part of the quadriceps femoris muscle derived from the rectus femoris and vastus intermedius muscles. Also *superior border of patella.* **b. pedunculi cerebri** CRUS CEREBRI. **b. phalangis digitorum manus** [NA] The slightly expanded proximal end, or base, of each phalanx of the fingers. The proximal phalanx has a single concavity for articulation with the rounded head of a corresponding metacarpal, while the bases of the middle and distal phalanges have double facets. They provide attachment for muscles, tendons, and ligaments. Also *proximal extremity of phalanx of finger, base of phalanx of finger.* **b. phalangis digitorum pedis** [NA] The slightly expanded proximal end, or base, of each phalanx of the toes. The proximal phalanx has a single concavity for articulation with the corresponding head of the metatarsal, while the bases of the middle and distal phalanges have double facets. The bases provide attachment for muscles, tendons, and ligaments. Also *proximal extremity of phalanx of toe, base of phalanx of toe.* **b. prostatae** [NA] The vesical aspect, or base, of the prostate gland that faces cranially and lies against the neck of the urinary bladder. The urethra enters the base near its anterior border, and the ejaculatory duct pierces it posteriorly. Also *base of prostate.* **b. pulmonis** [NA] The semilunar, concave base of the lung, related through the pleura to the convex superior surface of the diaphragm, which separates the left lung from the left lobe of the liver, the gastric fundus, and the spleen, and the right lung from the right lobe of the liver. Also *base of lung.* **b. pyramidis renalis** [NA] The base of the conical renal pyramid of the medulla of the kidney that faces the outer surface, or cortex. Also *base of renal pyramid.* **b. stapedis** [NA] The flattened, oval base, or footplate, of the stapes that is fixed to the rim of the fenestra vestibuli of the tympanic cavity by the annular ligament. Also *base of stapes, foot plate, footplate.*

**basisphenoid** \-sfē′noid\ [BASI- + SPHENOID] An important component of the cartilaginous base of the embryonic skull. It gives rise to the posterior part of the body of the adult sphenoid bone. Also *basisphenoid bone.*

**basitemporal** \-tem′pərəl\ Of or pertaining to the lower aspect of the temporal bone.

**basivertebral** \-vur′təbrəl\ Pertaining to or located within the body of a vertebra.

**basket / fiber b.'s** The supportive meshworks of fibers (extensions of Müller's fibers) that support the bases of rods and cones in the retina. Collectively, they form the membrana limitans externa.

**baso-** \bā′sō-\ BASI-.

**basocyte** \bā′sōsīt\ [BASO- + -CYTE] BASOPHIL.

**basocytopenia** \-sī′təpē′nē·ə\ An abnormal decrease in circulating basophilic leukocytes.

**basocytosis** \-sītō′sis\ BASOPHILIC LEUKOCYTOSIS.

**basograph** \bā′sōgraf\ [BASO- + -GRAPH] An instrument that graphically records abnormalities of gait.

**basolateral** \-lat′ərəl\ **1** Denoting the amygdaloid nuclei, one of the two major subdivisions of the corpus amygdaloideum. **2** BASILATERAL.

**basophil** \bā′sōfil\ [BASO- + -PHIL] **1** Any cell with cytoplasm that stains with basic dyes. Also *basophilic cell, basocyte.* **2** A polymorphonuclear leukocyte that has a small number (for example, 10–30) of prominent purple or black cytoplasmic granules when stained by Romanowsky dyes. The granules contain histamine and chondroitin sulfate. An increase in the number of basophils in blood is characteristic of chronic granulocytic leukemia, but may also be observed following infections such as pertussis, measles, tuberculosis, and hepatitis. For defs. 1 and 2 also *basophile.* **3** BASOPHILIC.

**basophilia** \bā′sōfil′yə\ [BASO- + -PHILIA] **1** An affinity for basic dyes, such as that exhibited by the cell nucleus for hematoxylin. **2** An elevated count of basophilic leukocytes in the peripheral blood. It is seen in allergies and in myxedema, and particularly in chronic granulocytic leukemia. **3** The persistence of blue cytoplasmic staining of peripheral blood erythrocytes, as seen in cases of severe anemia with increased erythropoietic activity. For defs. 2 and 3 also *basophilism.* **pituitary b.** BASOPHIL ADENOMA. **punctate b.** BASOPHILIC STIPPLING OF ERYTHROCYTES.

**basophilic** \bā′sōfil′ik\ **1** Exhibiting a blue color when stained by Romanowsky-type stains such as the Wright stain. Also *basophil.* **2** Having a large number of basophil granulocytes. For defs. 1 and 2 also *basophilous.*

**basophilism** \bāsäf′ilizm\ BASOPHILIA. **Cushing's b.** CUSHING'S DISEASE. **pituitary b.** BASOPHIL ADENOMA.

**basophilous** \bāsäf′iləs\ BASOPHILIC.

**basoplasm** \bā′sōplazm\ Basophilic cytoplasm.

**basosquamous** \-skwā′məs\ Exhibiting differentiation toward both squamous and basal cells.

**Bass** [Charles Cassedy *Bass,* U.S. physician, born 1875] Bass-Watkins test. See under TEST.

**Bassen** [Frank Albert *Bassen,* U.S. physician, born 1903] Bassen-Kornzweig disease, Bassen-Kornzweig syndrome. See under ABETALIPOPROTEINEMIA.

**Bassini** [Edoardo *Bassini,* Italian surgeon, 1846–1924] See under OPERATION.

**bassorin** A polysaccharide constituent of tragacanth and certain other plant gums that swells in water to yield a mucilagenous gel. It has found limited use as an ingredient of selected dermatologic preparations.

**Bastedo** [Walter Arthur *Bastedo,* U.S. physician, 1873–1952] See under RULE.

**Bastian** [Henry Charlton *Bastian*, English neurologist, 1837–1915] See under SYNDROME.

**Bateman** [Thomas *Bateman*, English physician, 1778–1821] Bateman's disease. See under MOLLUSCUM CONTAGIOSUM.

**bath / alternant-contrast b.** CONTRAST BATH. **cabinet b.** A hot air bath in which the patient is placed in a cabinet. **contrast b.** Alternating immersion of a limb in hot and cold water. Also *alternant-contrast bath.* **infrared b.** A form of radiant heat therapy in which a cradle containing an infrared-generating apparatus is placed over the part to be treated. **kinetotherapeutic b.** A bath within a unit that allows underwater exercises. **needle b.** A bath in which a shower of very fine jets of water is sprayed onto the body part being treated. **oxygen b.** A bath in which oxygen is dissolved in the bath water. **paraffin b.** Immersion of a body part in warm liquid paraffin to provide even distribution of superficial heat. It is primarily used in the treatment of arthritis of the hands or feet, and was formerly used in the treatment of burns. **sauna b.** A Finnish style hot air bath, usually taken in a specially constructed room built of wood and equipped with a device capable of raising air temperature to levels adequate to induce profuse sweating. In the classic sauna bath the skin is mildly beaten with branches from birch or cedar trees, and the bather is immediately exposed to cold after emerging from the sauna. **sitz b.** A bath in which the patient sits in a tub, immersing only the hips and buttocks. **transcutan b.** A bath containing dissolved therapeutic agents that are absorbed through the skin, the heated water enhancing absorption. **water b.** A container of water that is held at a constant temperature. It is used to provide a temperature-controlled environment for immersing vessels of fluid or other objects.

**bathesthesia** \bath′esthē′zhə\ BATHYESTHESIA.

**bathmotropic** \bath′mōträp′ik\ [Gk *bathmo(s)* a step, stair + -TROPIC] Influencing the excitability of muscle or nervous tissue. Increased responsiveness is considered positively bathmotropic and decreased responsiveness negative.

**batho-** \bath′o-\ [Gk *bathos* depth, height] A combining form meaning depth.

**bathochromic** Denoting a shift to longer wavelength, usually of an absorption band in a spectrum. This reflects a smaller difference in energy between the excited and ground states.

**bathy-** \bath′i-\ [Gk *bathys* deep, high] A combining form meaning deep.

**bathyaesthesia** *Brit.* BATHYESTHESIA.

**bathyanesthesia** \-an′esthē′zhə\ [BATHY- + ANESTHESIA] Loss of sensibility in the deeper structures of the body. *Outmoded.*

**bathyesthesia** \-esthē′zhə\ [BATHY- + ESTHESIA] Deep or pressure sensibility. Also *bathesthesia.*

**Batson** [Oscar Vivian *Batson*, U.S. otolaryngologist, born 1894] System of Batson, Batson's plexus. See under VERTEBRAL-VENOUS SYSTEM.

**battarism** \bat′ərizm\ [See BATTARISMUS.] *Seldom used* STUTTERING.

**battarismus** \bat′ərizməs\ [New L, from Gk *battarismos* a stuttering] *Seldom used* STUTTERING.

**Batten** [Frederic Eustace *Batten*, English opththalmologist, 1865–1918] Batten's disease. See under JUVENILE CEROID-LIPOFUSCINOSIS.

**battering / baby b.** A British usage for CHILD ABUSE. **child b.** CHILD ABUSE.

**battery** **1** A device that converts chemical energy to electric current. **2** Two or more cells electrically connected to produce electric current. **3** A series of procedures, such as tests given for diagnosis of disease or psychological tests. **4** Repeated severe beatings or recurrent infliction of other injuries. **test b.** A series of psychological tests administered at the same time, usually of a related and overlapping kind, that are intended to measure a particular trait, ability, or special form of defect, such as, organic brain damage. In some batteries, the levels of performance achieved on individual tests are combined into a single composite score.

**Battle** [William Henry *Battle*, English surgeon, 1855–1936] **1** See under SIGN. **2** Battle-Jalaguier-Kammerer incision. See under BATTLE'S INCISION.

**baud** \bôd\ [after Jean M. *Émile Baud(ot)*, French engineer, 1845–1903] In digital data transmission, the number of signal elements per second. When each element carries one bit, the baud rate is numerically equal to bits per second.

**Baudelocque** [Jean Louis *Baudelocque*, French surgeon and obstetrician, 1746–1810] Baudelocque's diameter, Baudelocque's line. See under EXTERNAL CONJUGATE.

**Bauhin** [Gaspard *Bauhin*, Swiss botanist and anatomist, 1560–1624] **1** Bauhin's glands. See under GLANDULA LINGUALIS ANTERIOR. **2** Bauhin's valve. See under VALVA ILEOCECALIS.

**Baumès** [Pierre Prosper François *Baumès*, French physician, 1791–1871] Baumès law, Colles-Baumès law. See under COLLES LAW.

**Baumgarten** [Paul Clemens von *Baumgarten*, German pathologist, 1848–1928] **1** Cruveilhier-Baumgarten murmur. See under MURMUR. **2** Baumgarten's glands. See under GLAND. **3** Baumgarten syndrome. See under CRUVEILHIER-BAUMGARTEN SYNDROME.

**bay** An anatomic depression, recess, or inlet containing liquid. **lacrimal b.** The slightly concave contour of the eyelids medial to the punctae.

**Bayle** [Antoine Laurent Jesse *Bayle*, French physician, 1799–1858] Bayle's disease. See under GENERAL PARESIS.

**Bazett** [Henry Cuthbert *Bazett*, English physician and physiologist, 1885–1950] See under FORMULA.

**Bazin** [Antoine Pierre Ernest *Bazin*, French dermatologist, 1807–1877] **1** Bazin's disease. See under ERYTHEMA INDURATUM. **2** See under ULCER.

**BBA** born before arrival (of a doctor, midwife, etc.).

**BBB** bundle branch block.

**BBT** basal body temperature.

**BC** **1** bone conduction (used in hearing tests). **2** birth control.

**BCAF** basophil chemotaxis augmentation factor.

**BCF** basophil chemotactic factor.

**BCG** bacille Calmette-Guérin (Calmette-Guérin bacillus).

**b.d.** *bis die* (L, twice a day).

**BE** **1** barium enema. **2** base excess. **3** bacterial endocarditis.

**Be** Symbol for the element, beryllium.

**bead / rachitic b.'s** RACHITIC ROSARY.

**beading / b. of the ribs** RACHITIC ROSARY.

**beak** The straight or curved, hard, horny, anterior continuation of the mouth of birds. **parrot's b.** The radiographic appearance of a syndesmophyte adjacent to a degenerative intervertebral disk. **b. of sphenoid bone** ROSTRUM SPHENOIDALE.

**beaker** A cylindrical glass container with a pouring lip that is used in laboratories for storing, mixing, or heating liquids.

**Beale** [Lionel Smith *Beale*, English physician, 1828–1906] Beale's ganglion cells. See under CELL.

**beam** A stream of photons or particles that are moving in the same direction. **broad b.** In radiology and radiation protection, a beam of radiation whose cross section is large enough so that photons which are scattered by a barrier or other material in the beam contribute to the measured intensity of the beam. Compare NARROW BEAM. **electron b.** A bundle of high-speed electrons. **narrow b.** In radiology and radiation protection, a beam whose cross section is small enough so that any photons which are scattered by a barrier or other material in the beam will be scattered out of the beam. Compare BROAD BEAM. **neutron b.** A flow of neutrons, generally of fast neutrons. **useful b.** In radiology, that part of the primary radiation beam which emerges from the source after collimation.

**bearberry** UVA URSI.

**Beard** [George Miller *Beard*, U.S. physician, 1839–1883] Beard's disease. See under NEURASTHENIA.

**beard** The growth of terminal hair on the chin and cheeks that is induced by androgenic stimulation. Also *barba.*

**bearwood** CASCARA SAGRADA.

**beat** 1 To pulsate; throb. 2 A pulsation or throb; stroke. **apex b.** The pulsation which is visible or palpable on the chest wall, resulting from the impact of the apex of the left ventricle as it rotates forward during systole. As a physical sign it is sometimes defined as the point of maximum thrust but also as the lowest and leftmost point at which a definite thrust can be felt. It is usually located in the fifth left intercostal space within the midclavicular line, but may be displaced by chest deformity or heart or lung disease. Also *apex impulse, apical impulse.* **atrial b.** The impulse arising from the atrium. See also A WAVE. **automatic b.** Ectopic beat arising as a consequence of automatic activity and not conducted from elsewhere in the heart. **capture b.** An atrial beat conducted to the ventricles, or a ventricular beat conducted to the atria; a phase of atrioventricular dissociation. Also *interference beat.* **ciliary b.** The rhythmic, coordinated movement of cilia on the surface of a cell. The basal body, or centriole, serves to regulate the processes involved. **combination b.** FUSION BEAT. **coupled b.'s** Cardiac beats occurring in pairs, usually a sinus beat followed by a ventricular premature beat. **dependent b.** FORCED BEAT. **dropped b.** The absence of a single beat. See also MOBITZ BLOCK. **echo b.** See under RECIPROCAL RHYTHM. **ectopic b.** A beat which arises from outside the sinuatrial node. **escape b.** An ectopic beat which arises after the next anticipated beat of sinus origin, indicating the escape of an ectopic pacemaker from sinuatrial node control. **forced b.** An ectopic beat which arises as a result of an impulse from another source, such as by artificial stimulation. Also *dependent beat.* **fusion b.** A superimposition of an ectopic beat on an impulse originating in the sinuatrial node. Also *combination beat, mixed beat, summation beat.* **heart b.** See under HEARTBEAT. **idioventricular b.** An ectopic beat arising in the venticle without an impulse from higher up in the conducting system. **interference b.** CAPTURE BEAT. **mixed b.** FUSION BEAT. **paired b.'s** Beats occurring in pairs, either as in coupled beats, or as pairs of ectopic beats. **premature b.** A beat occurring earlier than the next anticipated beat of sinuatrial origin. **reciprocal b.** See under RECIPROCAL RHYTHM. **retrograde b.** A beat which causes atrial contraction as a result of conduction of an impulse retrogradely by the atrioventricular node. **summation b.** FUSION BEAT. **ventricular fusion b.** A superimposition of a ventricular ectopic beat on a ventricular impulse of sinuatrial origin. **ventricular premature b.** A ventricular ectopic beat which occurs prior to the next anticipated beat of sinuatrial origin.

**Beau** [Joseph Honoré Simon *Beau*, French physician, 1806–1865] 1 Beau syndrome. See under ASYSTOLE. 2 Beau's lines. See under LINE.

**becanthone hydrochloride** $C_{22}H_{29}ClN_2O_2S$. 1-[[2[Ethyl(2-hydroxy-2-methylpropyl)amino]ethyl]-amino]-4-methylthioxanthen-9-one hydrochloride. An antischistosomal agent.

**Beccaria** [Augusto *Beccaria*, Italian physician, flourished in the 20th century] See under SIGN.

**bechic** \bek′ik\ [Gk *bēx*, gen. *bēchos*, a cough + -IC] 1 Of or relating to coughing. 2 An agent that induces or promotes coughing.

**Beck** [Carl *Beck*, German-born U.S. surgeon, 1856–1911] Beck's method. See under GASTROSTOMY.

**Beck** [Claude Schaeffer *Beck*, U.S. surgeon, 1894–1971] Beck I operation, Beck II operation. See under OPERATION.

**Becker** [Samuel William *Becker*, U.S. physician, 1894–1964] See under NEVUS.

**Beckmann** [Ernst Otto *Beckmann*, German chemist, 1853–1923] See under THERMOMETER.

**Béclard** [Pierre Augustin *Béclard*, French anatomist and surgeon, 1785–1825] 1 Point of Béclard. See under POINT. 2 See under SIGN, TRIANGLE.

**beclomethasone dipropionate** $C_{28}H_{37}ClO_7$. 9-Chloro-11β,17,21-trihydroxy-16β-methylpregna-1,4-diene-3,20-dione dipropionate, a synthetic glucocorticoid agent used to treat chronic bronchial asthma by aerosol inhalation and topically for some allergic skin diseases.

**becquerel** \bekrel′, bek′ərel′\ [after Antoine Henri *Becquerel*, French physicist, 1852–1908] The special name for the SI derived unit of activity (of a radionuclide) equal to one per second, $1s^{-1}$. In terms of the former unit, curie, it equals approximately $2.70 \times 10^{-11}$ curies. Symbol: Bq

**bed** 1 A piece of furniture for sleeping or lying on; a measure of capacity or utilization in hospitals and other inpatient facilities, one bed corresponding to one patient. 2 In anatomy, a supporting layer, base, or matrix. **air b.** A bed provided with an inflatable mattress. **air fluidized b.** A bed in which a large volume of air passes through millions of tiny silicone beads. It thereby equalizes pressure on all parts of the body and helps to prevent pressure sores. **capillary b.** The total mass of capillaries in a part or the whole of the body or the volume of blood contained within them. **circle b.** A bed whose frame is so designed that a patient can be intermittently turned from front to back. With this device the patient is turned head over feet rather than from side to side. **collateral vascular b.** The mass of vessels involved in the provision of collateral circulation. **Gatch b.** A bed that is articulated between the hips and knees and with a foot board so that patients can be cared for in the semisitting position. **metabolic b.** A bed designed to facilitate the collection of feces and urine for evaluation and quantification in metabolic balance studies. **mud b.** A bed with a mattress of very fine silicates, designed to distribute pressure evenly over all body parts and thereby prevent pressure sores. **nail b.** MATRIX UNGUIS. **placental b.** BASAL PLATE OF WINCKLER **plaster b.** A plaster of Paris mold that supports the trunk and lower limbs and is used in diseases and injuries of the spine. **rocking b.** A mechanically operated bed for the treatment of pulmonary insufficiency. Alternating head-up and head-down positions cause the diaphragm to rise and fall with the movement of the abdominal contents, thereby improving alveolar ventilation. Also *rocking apparatus.* **Sanders b.** A rocking bed used to im-

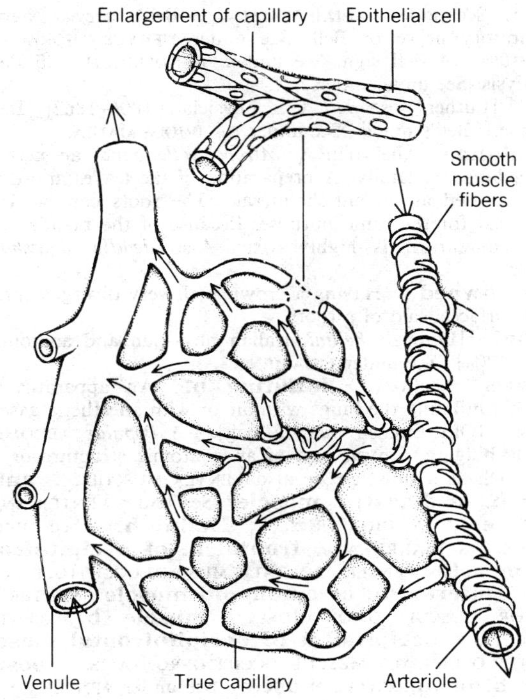


**Capillary bed**

prove circulation in chronic occlusive arterial disease. **stomach b.** The organs and structures forming the posterior relations of the stomach through the omental bursa, namely, the diaphragm, left suprarenal gland and front of upper pole of the kidney, splenic artery, anterior surface of pancreas, left colic flexure, transverse mesocolon, and transverse colon. In addition, the spleen is related through the greater sac. **vascular b.** The total mass of the vessels, arterial, capillary, and venous, supplying an organ or the whole body.

**bedbug** Any of various hemipterous insects that infest human habitations and feed on human blood, especially those of the family Cimicidae. The common bedbug of temperate regions is *Cimex lectularius.* Also *chinch.* Also *bed bug.* **Mexican b.** An assassin bug of the species *Triatoma sanguisuga.* Also *flying bedbug, Texas bedbug.* **oriental b.** A bedbug of the species *Cimex hemipterus.* **Texas b.** MEXICAN BEDBUG.

**bedewing** \bidʸoo′ing\ [Middle English *bedewen,* from *be-,* prefix denoting on, around, over + *dew,* from Old English *dēaw* dew] Corneal epithelial edema resulting from corneal decompensation, as from endothelial dystrophy or acute glaucoma.

**bedfast** BEDRIDDEN.

**bedpan** A vessel used for urination and defecation of a person confined to bed.

**bedridden** Confined to bed by one's condition. Also *bedfast.*

***Bedsonia*** \bedsō′nē·ə\ *Obs.* *CHLAMYDIA.*

**bedsore** An ulceration usually occurring over prominent body surfaces, such as vertebral spines, heels, knees, or sacrum, produced by prolonged pressure on the part as sometimes occurs with bedridden patients. Also *decubitus ulcer, decubital ulcer, pressure sore, chronic decubitus, decubitus chronicus, decubital gangrene, pressure gangrene, hospital gangrene.*

**bedwetting** Nocturnal urinary incontinence in children. See under ENURESIS.

**Beer** [August *Beer,* German physicist, 1825–1863] Beer-Lambert law. See under BEER'S LAW.

**beeswax** YELLOW WAX. **bleached b.** WHITE WAX. **unbleached b.** YELLOW WAX.

**beetle** An insect of the order Coleoptera. **blister b.** A beetle of the family Meloidae. Beetles of this family contain a vesicant substance, cantharidin, which can blister the skin. See also CANTHARIDES. Also *blister bug.*

**Beevor** [Charles Edward *Beevor,* English neurologist, 1854–1908] See under SIGN.

**Begbie** [James *Begbie,* Scottish physician, 1798–1869] Begbie's disease. See under GRAVES DISEASE.

**Begg** [P. Raymond *Begg,* Australian orthodontist, born 1898] Begg appliance. See under LIGHT ROUND-WIRE APPLIANCE.

**Béguez César** [Antonio *Béguez César,* Cuban physician, flourished 20th century] Béguez César disease. See under CHÉDIAK-HIGASHI ANOMALY.

**behaving** Descriptive of an animal free to act spontaneously or in response to environmental stimuli, usually with the connotation that parameters of behavior or nervous activity are being monitored.

**behavior** [formerly *behavour,* from Middle English *behav(en)* (from *be-,* intensive prefix + *have*) to behave + *-our,* suffix denoting activity] Any of the activities of a human or animal that can be observed directly by others, or which can be made systematically observable by the use of special transducers or procedural strategies. **adaptive b.** **1** A behavioral response that enhances survival. **2** A behavioral adjustment that helps an individual interact more efficiently with environmental stimuli. **attachment b.** Behavior resulting from actual or threatened severance of bonds between child and parent. It is manifested by stranger anxiety at the age of six to eight months, and above this age by distressful crying, anxiety, anger, searching for and demanding the return of the lost parent, as seen most patently in the small child abruptly separated from the mother. Older children may express some of these feelings verbally or in their behavior at the loss of or separation from a parent for whatever reason. **automatic b.** AUTOMATISM. **collective b.** That behavior which people collectively exhibit in a group but which they would not exhibit individually. **displacement b.** Behavior of a substitute kind evoked where the appropriate consummatory response to a situation is blocked or prevented, particularly if two fixed action patterns of response are simultaneously aroused that are in conflict. **impulsive b.** Any behavior that is classified as a disorder of impulse control, such as pathologic gambling, kleptomania, and explosive disorders. In some classificatory systems, drug and alcohol abuse and the paraphilias are also included as impulse disorders. General characteristics of such disorders are an ego-syntonic impulse which has an element of irresistibility, a feeling of increasing tension preceding the act, which is then followed by pleasure or relief, and a minimal distortion of the original impulse. **instinctive b.** Those unlearned, complex, and organized patterns of behavior that are goal-directed and biologically adaptive for a given species, and which have been determined primarily by genetic factors, for example, the nest building behavior of birds. **respondent b.** Behavior that is primarily controlled by the nature of the specific stimulus that elicits it, rather than by any effect that it might have on the environment. It is this form of behavioral response, similar to that governed by reflex action, that serves as the basis for establishing the classical (Pavlovian) conditioned response. **species-specific b.** Those patterns of behavior that are characteristic of most members of the same species when faced with similar circumstances. These often complex and stereotyped behaviors appear to be universal, invariant, and unlearned, thus contributing, along with anatomical structures and other shared attributes, to the definition of a particular species.

**behaviorism** \bihāv′yərizm\ [BEHAVIOR + -ISM] The school of psychology which holds that only overt behavior, i.e. that observable by another person, can serve as the subject matter for psychology. Behavior can be studied and understood without any reference to conscious experience or use of mentalistic constructs. Also *behavioristic psychology.*

**behaviour** *Brit.* BEHAVIOR.

**behaviourism** *Brit.* BEHAVIORISM.

**Behçet** [Halushi Behçet, Turkish dermatologist, 1889–1948] Behçet triple symptom complex, Adamantiades-Behçet syndrome. See under BEHÇET SYNDROME.

**Behr** [Carl *Behr,* German ophthalmologist, 1876–1943] See under DISEASE.

**Behring** [Emil Adolf von *Behring,* German bacteriologist, 1854–1917] **1** Behring serum. See under DIPHTHERIA ANTITOXIN. **2** See under LAW.

**BEI** butanol-extractable iodine.

**Beigel** [Hermann *Beigel,* German physician, 1830–1879] Beigel's disease. See under WHITE PIEDRA.

**bejel** \bej′el\ [Arabic] Endemic, nonvenereal syphilis caused by *Treponema pallidum* and occurring in childhood. The disease is rapidly vanishing, but foci remain in the eastern Mediterranean, southern Africa, southeastern Asia, and the western Pacific. Also *nonvenereal syphilis.*

**Bekesy** [Georg von *Bekesy,* Hungarian-born U.S. biophysicist, 1899–1972] **1** See under AUDIOMETRY, AUDIOGRAM, AUDIOMETER. **2** Bekesy calibration. See under PURE TONE CALIBRATION.

**Bekhterev** [Vladimir Mikhailovich *Bekhterev,* Russian neurologist, 1857–1927] **1** See under REACTION, SYMPTOM, REFLEX. **2** Bekhterev's reflex. See under NASAL REFLEX. **3** Bekhterev's arthritis, Bekhterev spondylitis, Bekhterev syndrome. See under ANKYLOSING SPONDYLITIS. **4** Bekhterev's band, band of Kaes-Bekhterev, layer of Kaes-Bekhterev, stria kaesbekhterevi, stripe of Kaes-Bekhterev. See under BEKHTEREV'S LAYER. **5** Bekhterev's nucleus. See under NUCLEUS VESTIBULARIS SUPERIOR. **6** Bekhterev's tract. See under TRACTUS TEGMENTALIS CENTRALIS. **7** Mendel-Bekhterev sign. See under SIGN. **8** Bekhterev-Mendel reflex, Bekhterev's reflex. See under MENDEL-BEKHTEREV REFLEX.

**bel** \bel\ [after Alexander Graham *Bell,* Scottish-born U.S. physicist, 1847–1922] A unit expressing the ratio between powers $P_1$ and $P_2$, used especially in communication and acoustic sciences, equal to $\log_{10}P_1/P_2$. Symbol: bel • In general, only the unit *decibel* is used.

***Belascaris*** \bəlas′kəris\ *TOXOCARA.*

**belch** [Middle English *belchen,* from Old English *bealcian* to splutter forth] See under ERUCTATION.

**belemnoid** \belem′noid\ [Gk *belemn(on)* dart + -OID ] **1** Shaped like a dart. **2** A styloid process.

**Belfield** [William Thomas *Belfield,* U.S. surgeon, 1856–1929] Belfield's operation. See under VASOTOMY.

**Bell** [Charles *Bell,* Scottish anatomist, 1774–1842] **1** Bell's law. See under BELL-MAGENDIE LAW. **2** Bell spasm. See under FACIAL SPASM. **3** Bell's nerve, external respiratory nerve of Bell. See under NERVUS THORACICUS LONGUS. **4** Bell sign. See under PHENOMENON. **5** Bell's paralysis. See under PALSY.

**Bell** [Luther Vose *Bell,* U.S. physician, 1806–1862] Bell's delirium, Bell's mania. See under DELIRIOUS MANIA.

**belladonna** \bel′ədän′ə\ *Atropa belladonna,* an herb of the Solanaceae family. A preparation of the leaves and dried tops is used as an anticholinergic. The roots can be dried and used for the same purpose. Because of the plant's atropine content, it is highly toxic. Also *deadly nightshade, dwale.*

**bell-crowned** Having a crown with very divergent proximal surfaces: said of a tooth.

**Bellini** [Lorenzo *Bellini,* Italian physician and anatomist, 1643–1704] See under LIGAMENT.

**bellows** \bel′ōz\ **inflating b.** An apparatus for forcibly inflating the lungs with air or with anesthetic gases.

**belly** [Old English *bælg* a bag] **1** *Popular* ABDOMEN. **2** The bulging, central part of an anatomic structure or organ such as a muscle. See also VENTER MUSCULI. **anterior b. of digastric muscle** See under VENTER ANTERIOR MUSCULI DIGASTRICI. **Delhi b.** See under TRAVELERS' DIARRHEA. **frontal b. of occipitofrontal muscle** VENTER FRONTALIS MUSCULI OCCIPITOFRONTALIS. **inferior b. of omohyoid muscle** VENTER INFERIOR MUSCULI OMOHYOIDEI. **muscle b.** VENTER MUSCULI. **occipital b. of occipitofrontal muscle** VENTER OCCIPITALIS MUSCULI OCCIPITOFRONTALIS. **posterior b. of digastric muscle** See under VENTER POSTERIOR MUSCULI DIGASTRICI. **spider b.** An abdomen with very prominent superficial venous pattern, as may be seen in portal hypertension or inferior vena cava obstruction. Also *arachnogastria.* **superior b. of omohyoid muscle** VENTER SUPERIOR MUSCULI OMOHYOIDEI.

**bellybutton** UMBILICUS.

**belonoid** \bel′ənoid\ [Gk *belon(ē)* needle + -OID] Shaped like a needle.

**belonoskiascopy** \bel′ənōskī·as′kəpē\ [Gk *belon(ē)* a needle + *o* + SKIA- + -SCOPY] A subjective method of refraction consisting of observation of the movement of a narrow bar across the pupil.

**bemegride** $C_8H_{13}NO_2$. 4-Ethyl-4-methyl-2,6-piperidinedione. An analeptic drug which has been used as an antagonist in the treatment of barbiturate poisoning.

**benactyzine** $C_{20}H_{25}NO_3$. α-Hydroxy-α-phenylbenzeneacetic acid 2-(diethylamino)ethyl ester, an orally administered compound with anticholinergic activity that acts as a tranquilizer. Usually the hydrochloride of the compound is used.

**Benadryl** A proprietary name for diphenhydramine hydrochloride.

**benanserin hydrochloride** $C_{19}H_{23}ClN_2O$. 1-Benzyl-2-methyl-5-methoxytryptamine hydrochloride, a synthetic structural analogue of serotonin with strong antagonistic properties. It is of historic interest in connection with the early stages of research that established the functional importance of serotonin in the central nervous system.

**benapryzine hydrochloride** $C_{21}H_{27}NO_3{\cdot}HCl$. 2-(Ethylpropylamine)ethyl benzilate hydrochloride.An anticholinergic drug with limited usefulness in the treatment of parkinsonism. It is usually given together with levodopa and amantadine for this purpose.

**Bence Jones** [Henry *Bence Jones,* English physician, 1814–1873] **1** Bence Jones cylinders. See under CYLINDER. **2** See under PROTEINURIA. **3** Bence Jones body, Bence Jones globulin, Bence-Jones monoclonal immunoglobulin. See under BENCE JONES PROTEIN.

**bend** A flexure or curve that appears during the early development of an embryo. **head b.** CEPHALIC FLEXURE. **iliac b. of ureter** The angulation in the ureter at the point where it crosses the iliac vessels and descends into the true pelvis. **neck b.** CERVICAL FLEXURE.

**bendazac** $C_{16}H_{14}N_2O_3$. [(1-benzyl-1*H*-indazol-3-yl-)oxy]acetic acid. An anti-inflammatory compound used topically for the treatment of dermatitis, eczema, and other skin disorders.

**Bender** [Lauretta *Bender*, U.S. psychiatrist, born 1897] See under TEST.

**bendrofluazide** BENDROFLUMETHIAZIDE.

**bendroflumethiazide** $C_{15}H_{14}F_3N_3O_4S_2$. 3-Dihydro-3-(phenylmethyl)-6-(trifluoromethyl)-2*H*-1,2,4-benzo-thiadiazine-7-sulfonamide 1,1-dioxide. An antihypertensive and diuretic agent of the thiazide class that is used for the treatment of hypertension. Also *bendrofluazide, benzydroflumethiazide.*

**bends** One of the early manifestations of decompression sickness. It is characterized by limb and joint pains. **labyrinthine b.** Sudden deafness, vertigo, and tinnitus following too rapid decompression, occurring in decompression sickness.

**Benedek** [Ladislaus *Benedek*, Austrian neurologist, 1887–1945] See under REFLEX.

**Benedict** [Francis Gano *Benedict*, U.S. chemist and physiologist, 1870–1957] **1** Atwater-Benedict calorimeter, Atwater-Benedict chamber. See under ATWATER'S CALORIMETER. **2** Harris and Benedict standard. See under STANDARD.

**Benedict** [Stanley Rossiter *Benedict*, U.S. chemist, 1884–1936] See under METHOD.

**Benedikt** [Moritz *Benedikt*, Austrian physician, 1835–1920] See under SYNDROME.

**beneficiary** \benʹəfishʹərē\ A person who receives insurance benefits or who is covered by a health care prepaid plan.

**benefit** **1** A sum of money payable to an insurance policyholder, or to a provider of services to the policyholder, for expenses or costs resulting from a loss covered by the policy. **2** The services provided under the terms of a service type insurance policy. **indemnity b.'s** Health insurance policy benefits that pay cash rather than provide health care services for losses such as illness and injury. Benefits are usually paid to the enrollee although they may be assigned to the provider. **service b.'s** Health insurance benefits which provide services rather than cash benefits to the beneficiary and under which payment is made directly to the provider of service for covered services to an eligible enrollee. There may still be coinsurance, deductible, and other provisions which require the patient to pay a portion of the charges directly.

**Benemid** A proprietary name for probenecid.

**benethamine penicillin G** The *N*-benzyl-2-phenylethylamine salt of penicillin G. It has low solubility in water and is used for intramuscular injection to provide prolonged effective concentrations of the antibiotic in the blood and tissues. Also *benzethamine penicillin.*

**benign** \binīn\ [L *benignus* (from *bene* well (adverb) + root of *gignere* to beget, generate) kind, generous] **1** Relatively mild; likely to have a favorable outcome: said of an illness. **2** Not malignant; not having the potential for metastasis: said of a neoplasm. For defs. 1 and 2 also *benignant.*

**benjamin** \benʹjəmən\ BENZOIN.

**Bennett** [Edward Hallaran *Bennett*, Irish surgeon, 1837–1907] See under DISLOCATION, FRACTURE.

**Bennett** [John Hughes *Bennett*, English physician, 1812–1876] Bennett's disease. See under LEUKEMIA.

**Bennett** [Norman Godfrey *Bennett*, English dental surgeon, 1870–1947] See under ANGLE, MOVEMENT.

**benorterone** $C_{19}H_{28}O_2$. 17-$\beta$-Hydroxy-17-methyl-B-norandrost-4-en-3-one. An antiandrogenic steroid that has been used in the treatment of acne and idiopathic hirsutism.

**benoxinate hydrochloride** $C_{17}H_{28}N_2O_2 \cdot HCl$. A local anesthetic used in ophthalmology to obtain surface anesthesia by installation in the conjunctiva.

**benperidol** $C_{22}H_{24}FN_3O_2$. A tranquilizer with actions like those of haloperidol.

**Bensley** [Robert Russell *Bensley*, Canadian-born U.S. anatomist, 1867–1956] Bensley specific granules. See under GRANULE.

**Benson** [Arthur H. *Benson*, English ophthalmologist, 1860–1912] Benson's disease. See under ASTEROID HYALOSIS.

**bentonite** An aluminosilicate clay. It is used as a suspending agent for medicaments and as an inhibitor of nucleases.

**bentonite magma** 5% colloidal hydrated aluminum silicate. It is used in pharmaceutical preparations in this concentration (w/w) in water as a suspending agent, and has also been used in the past as a bulk laxative.

**benzaldehyde** $C_6H_5CHO$. A colorless liquid with a characteristic odor like that of bitter almonds. It is used as a flavoring agent in oral medications. Also *artificial essential oil of almond.*

**benzalkonium chloride** A mixture of alkylbenzyldimethylammonium chlorides of the general composition $[C_6H_5CH_2N(CH_3)_2 \cdot R]Cl$, with R representing alkyl groups from $C_8H_{17}$ to $C_{18}H_{37}$. The mixed quaternary ammonium compounds are used as a disinfectant on skin surfaces and mucous membranes against many types of bacteria, viruses, fungi, yeasts, and protozoa. It is also used as a preservative in eye drops and ophthalmologic medicine containers.

**benzamine hydrochloride** $\beta$-EUCAINE.

**benzathine penicillin G** A salt form of a combination of penicillin G and *N,N*-dibenzylethylenediamine in the ratio of 2:1. It is a white, crystalline complex of penicillin with a sustained action time. The preparation is employed for both oral and parenteral administration of penicillin as an antibiotic. Also *N,N'-dibenzylethylenediamine penicillin.*

**benzazoline hydrochloride** TOLAZOLINE HYDROCHLORIDE.

**benzcurine iodide** GALLAMINE TRIETHIODIDE.

**benzene** \benʹzēn\ $C_6H_6$. A hydrocarbon found in coal tar. Its molecule is a regular hexagon of CH groups. It is the simplest aromatic compound. **b. ring** In organic chemistry, a ring composed of six carbon atoms linked by alternate single and double bonds or, more exactly by two electrons in $\sigma$ orbitals and one in a $\pi$ orbital. Also *benzene nucleus.*

**benzene hexachloride** HEXACHLOROCYCLOHEXANE. **gamma b.** LINDANE.

**benzestrofol** ESTRADIOL BENZOATE.

**benzethamine penicillin** BENETHAMINE PENICILLIN G.

**benzethonium chloride** $C_{27}H_{42}ClNO_2$. *N,N*-Dimethyl-*N*-[2-[2-[4-(1,1,3,3-tetramethylbutyl)phenoxy]ethoxy]ethyl]-benzene-methanaminium chloride, a synthetic quaternary ammonium compound used as a topical anti-infective agent and as a preservative in some medicinal preparations.

**benzhexol hydrochloride** TRIHEXYPHENIDYL HYDROCHLORIDE.

**benzhydramine hydrochloride** DIPHENHYDRAMINE HYDROCHLORIDE.

**benzidine** The substance formed from biphenyl, Ph—Ph, by substituting an amino group on each ring *para* to the junction. It has been shown to be carcinogenic, but was formerly used extensively in testing for blood, which catalyzes its oxidation to form blue compounds. It also gives its name to the benzidine rearrangement, in which it is formed from *N,N'*-diphenylhydrazine, Ph—NH—NH—Ph.

**benzimidazole** A substance whose molecule contains benzene and imidazole rings with two common atoms. It is a purine analogue and is part of the coenzyme $B_{12}$ molecule.

**benzocaine** $C_9H_{11}NO_2$. Ethyl aminobenzoate. A white, crystalline powder, slightly soluble in water. It is applied topically as a local anesthetic to the skin and mucous membranes.

**benzoctamine** $C_{18}H_{19}N$. 9-(Methylaminomethyl)-9,10-dihydro-9,10-ethanoanthracene. It is used as a sedative and muscle relaxant, generally in the form of the hydrochloride.

**benzodepa** $C_{12}H_{163}O_3P$. [Bis(1-aziridinyl)-phosphenyl]carbamic acid phenylmethyl ester. It is used as an antineoplastic agent.

**benzodiazepine** Any of the active, central nervous system depressants that have a common structure of a seven-member, heterocyclic diazo ring fused with a benzene ring. They all have a 5-aryl or 5-cyclohexenyl substitution. Representative drugs include chlordiazepoxide, diazepam, and lorazepam, which are used as sedatives and antianxiety drugs.

**benzodioxan** Any of a class of α-adrenergic blocking agents of which piperoxan is the most important member.

**benzogynestryl** ESTRADIOL BENZOATE.

**benzoic acid** Ph—COOH. The simplest aromatic acid. It is derived from coal tar by oxidation of toluene.

**benzoin** Ph—CO—CHOH—Ph. A resin obtained from the cut stem of species of Styracaceae, especially *Styrax benzoin, S. parallelonerus,* and *S. tonkinensis.* The resin has antiseptic properties and is used in the treatment of certain skin disorders. It is also used as an expectorant. Also *gum benjamin, gum benzoin, benjamin.*

**benzolism** \ben′zōlizm\ BENZENE POISONING.

**benzonatate** $C_{30}H_{53}NO_{11}$. 4-(Butylamino)benzoic acid 3,6,9,12,15,18,21,24,27-nonaoxaoctacos-1-yl ester. A pale, viscous liquid that has been administered orally as an antitussive medication. Also *benzononatine.*

**benzopurpurine** Any of a group of azo dyes that are used as the red, acid stain in polychrome mixtures and as pH indicators, turning from purple in highly acid conditions to red at a pH range of 1.2 to 4.0. Also *ozamin.*

**benzopyrene** Either of two substances, benzo[a]pyrene and benzo[e]pyrene, according to how the extra benzene ring is fused to the 4-ring structure of pyrene. Benzo[a]pyrene occurs in coal tar and is carcinogenic. Also *benzpyrene.*

**benzoquinone** A substance whose molecule is a six-membered ring of two CO groups, in positions 1,2 (*ortho*) or 1,4 (*para*) and two —CH═CH— groups. It can be reduced to a phenol containing two hydroxyl groups.

**benzoquinonium chloride** $C_{34}H_{50}Cl_2N_4O_2$. 2,5-Bis(3-diethylaminopropylamino)-benzoquinone bis(benzylchloride). It is a synthetic neuromuscular blocking agent which has been used as a skeletal muscle relaxant drug.

**benzothiadiazides** THIAZIDES.

**benzoyl** The group Ph—CO—, derived from benzoic acid. Symbol: Bz

**benzoyl ecgonine** $C_6H_5COC_9H_{14}O_3N$. An ester of ecgonine that is found in Peruvian coca leaves or is prepared from cocaine. It is a central nervous system stimulant with actions like those of caffeine.

**benzoylmethylecgonine** COCAINE.

**benzphetamine hydrochloride** $C_{17}H_{21}N{\cdot}HCl$. *N*,α-Dimethyl-*N*-(phenylmethyl)benzeneethenamine hydrochloride. A sympathomimetic amine resembling amphetamine in its actions. It is used in the treatment and control of obesity as an anorexiant. It is given orally.

**benzpyrene** BENZOPYRENE.

**benzpyrinium bromide** $C_{15}H_{17}BrN_2O_2$. 3-[[(Dimethylamino)-carbonyl]oxy]-1-(phenylmethyl)pyridinium bromide. An anticholinesterase drug with cholinergic effects much like those of neostigmine.

**benzthiazide** $C_{15}H_{14}ClN_3O_4S_3$. 6-Chloro-3-[[(phenylmethyl)thio]methyl]2*H*-1,2,4-benzothiadiazine-7-sulfonamide 1,1-dioxide. A compound with diuretic and antihypertensive properties. It is given orally.

**benztropine mesylate** $C_{21}H_{25}NO{\cdot}C_4O_3S$. *endo*-3-(Diphenylmethoxy)-8-azabicyclo[3.2.1]octane methanesulfonate. A compound with anticholinergic activity. It is also an antihistaminic and it has local anesthetic properties. It has been used in the treatment of parkinsonism. It may be given orally, intramuscularly or intravenously.

**benzydamine hydrochloride** $C_{19}H_{24}ClN_3O$. 1-Benzyl-3-(3-dimethylaminopropoxy)indazole. It is used as an analgesic, antipyretic and an anti-inflammatory drug.

**benzydroflumethiazide** BENDROFLUMETHIAZIDE.

**benzyl** The group Ph—$CH_2$—. Symbol: Bzl

**benzyl benzoate** $C_{14}H_{12}O_2$. A compound occurring naturally as a volatile oil in several balsams. It has been used in topical medications to control scabies and as a pharmaceutical aid in the preparation of dimercaprol for injection.

**benzyloxycarbonyl** The group Ph—$CH_2$—O—CO—. This was the first group to be widely used in peptide synthesis to protect the amino group of one amino acid when coupling it to the amino group of another. Because of the stability of the benzyl carbocation, anhydrous acid will remove it, and it can also be removed by reduction. It acylates the amino group and so removes its nucleophilic nature, but is not so electron-withdrawing as to lead to racemizing reactions. Also *carbobenzoxy.* Abbr. Cbz, Z

**benzylpenicillin** PENICILLIN G.

**benzylpenicillin potassium** PENICILLIN G POTASSIUM.

**benzylpenicillin procaine** PROCAINE PENICILLIN G.

**benzylpenicillin sodium** PENICILLIN G SODIUM.

**benzyl succinate** $(C_6H_5—CH_2—O—CO—CH_2)_2$. The dibenzyl ester of succinic acid, used as an antispasmodic agent for smooth muscle.

**bepascum** CALCIUM BENZAMIDOSALICYLATE.

**bephenium** *N,N*-Dimethyl-*N*-(phenoxyethyl)benzenemethanaminium pamoate. A compound used as an anthelmintic agent in veterinary medicine. It is given as the pamoate or hydroxynaphthoate salt forms.

**Béraneck** [Edmond *Béraneck,* Swiss bacteriologist, 1859–1920] See under TUBERCULIN.

**Berardinelli** [Waldemar *Berardinelli,* Argentinian physician, 1903–1956] Berardinelli syndrome. See under SEIP SYNDROME.

**Béraud** [Brune Jean Jacques *Béraud,* French surgeon, 1823–1865] **1** Valvule of Béraud. See under VALVE. **2** See under LIGAMENT.

**berberine** An alkaloid derived from *Hydrastis canadensis* that is used as an antimalarial, carminative, and febrifuge. It is also used in dressings for the treatment of external ulcers. Also *umbellatine.*

**berberine bisulfate** $C_{20}H_{18}NO_4{\cdot}HSO_4$. An acid salt of berberine, a 2% solution of which has been used to promote healing in cases of cutaneous leishmaniasis.

**Berger** [Hans *Berger,* German neurologist, 1873–1941] Berger's rhythm. See under ALPHA RHYTHM.

**Berger** [Jean *Berger*, French nephrologist, flourished 20th century] Berger's disease. See under MESANGIAL IGA/IGG GLOMERULONEPHRITIS.

**Berger** [Paul *Berger*, French surgeon, 1845–1908] Berger's amputation. See under OPERATION.

**Bergmann** [Ernst von *Bergmann*, German surgeon, 1836–1907] Bergmann cells. See under CELL.

**Bergmann** [Gottlieb Heinrich *Bergmann*, German neurologist and anatomist, 1781–1860] Bergmann's fibers. See under FIBER.

**Bergmeister** [Otto *Bergmeister*, Austrian physician, 1845–1918] See under PAPILLA.

**Bergonié** [Jean-Alban *Bergonié*, French physician, 1857–1925] Bergonié-Tribondeau law. See under LAW.

**beriberi** \ber′ēber′ē\ [Singhalese (from *beri* weakness) extreme weakness] A nutritional deficiency disease caused by a prolonged deficiency in the intake of the water-soluble vitamin, thiamin (vitamin $B_1$). Deficiency of other members of the vitamin B complex is often coexistent. Beriberi is a major public health problem when highly polished rice is a common nutrient. It occurs sporadically in alcoholics and in chronic malabsorption. Major clinical types are atrophic beriberi, wet beriberi, and infantile beriberi. The disease is preventable with adequate intake of thiamin. Treatment consists of thiamin supplements together with other B-complex vitamins. Also *perneiras* (Brazilian), *Ceylon sickness, endemic polyneuritis, polyneuritis endemica, panneuritis endemica, rice disease, hinchazón* (Cuban), *inchação* (Brazilian), *loempe, neuritis multiplex endemica, asjike.* **atrophic b.** Beriberi in which muscular weakness, atrophy and sensory loss due to polyneuropathy dominate the clinical picture. Neurologic features include numbness and burning sensations in the feet, followed by limb weakness. Also *dry beriberi, paralytic beriberi.* **infantile b.** Manifestations of thiamine deficiency in infants breast-fed by women with thiamine deficiency. The women themselves may not have symptoms when their breast-fed babies develop typical signs. The peripheral neuropathy has a predilection in infants for the optic nerve, causing loss of vision; for the third nerve, causing ptosis; and for the recurrent laryngeal nerve, causing hoarseness. Encephalopathy may give rise to convulsions, coma, and death. Also *taon* (Philippine term). **paralytic b.** ATROPHIC BERIBERI. **wet b.** A form of beriberi characterized chiefly by cardiovascular manifestations with a dilated heart and with edema resulting from congestive heart failure. Also *wet dropsy.*

**berkelium** \burk′lē·əm\ A very rare, unstable element of the actinide series, having atomic number 97 and atomic weight 247. The first berkelium identified was produced in a cyclotron by bombarding americium 241 with helium ions. Eight isotopes have been described. Berkelium resembles other actinide elements in having a tendency to accumulate in bone. Half-lives range from 4 hours to 1400 years. Symbol: Bk

**Berkow** [Samuel Gordon *Berkow*, U.S. surgeon, born 1899] See under SCALE.

**Berkson** [Joseph *Berkson*, U.S. biometrician, born 1899] See under BIAS.

**Berlin** [Rudolf *Berlin*, German oculist, 1833–1897] See under DISEASE.

**Bernard** [Claude *Bernard*, French physiologist, 1813–1878] **1** Claude Bernard-Horner syndrome, Bernard-Horner syndrome, Bernard syndrome, Horner-Bernard syndrome. See under HORNER SYNDROME. **2** See under PUNCTURE. **3** Bernard's duct. See under DUCTUS PANCREATICUS ACCESSORIUS.

**Bernard** [Jean *Bernard*, French hematologist, born 1907] Bernard-Soulier syndrome. See under SYNDROME.

**Bernhardt** [Martin *Bernhardt*, German neurologist, 1844–1915] Bernhardt's disease, Bernhardt-Roth syndrome, Bernhardt's paresthesiae. See under MERALGIA PARESTHETICA.

**Bernheim** [Hippolyte-Marie *Bernheim*, French psychologist, 1840–1919] **1** See under SYNDROME. **2** Bernheim therapy. See under HYPNOTHERAPY.

**Berry** [Sir James *Berry*, Canadian surgeon, 1860–1946] Berry's ligament. See under LIGAMENTUM THYROHYOIDEUM LATERALE.

**Bertin** [Exupère Joseph *Bertin*, French anatomist, 1712–1781] **1** Bertin's bones, Bertin's ossicles. See under CONCHA SPHENOIDALIS. **2** Renal columns of Bertin. See under COLUMNAE RENALES. **3** Bertin's ligament. See under LIGAMENTUM ILIOFEMORALE.

**Bertolotti** [Mario *Bertolotti*, Italian physician, born 1876] See under SYNDROME.

**Bertrand** [Ivan Georges *Bertrand*, French neurologist, 1863–1965] **1** Van Bogaert-Bertrand disease. See under CANAVAN'S DISEASE. **2** Canavan-van Bogaert-Bertrand disease. See under VAN BOGAERT'S FAMILIAL AXONAL SPONGY DEGENERATION.

**berylliosis** \bəril′ē·ō′sis\ [*bervlli(um)* + -OSIS] A disease resulting from the inhalation or accidental implantation of beryllium. Exposure to beryllium dust or vapors from beryllium salts is a modern industrial hazard that can manifest itself either as an acute disorder that is generally self-limited when exposure is discontinued, or as a chronic illness characterized by granulomatous fibrosis of the lungs, and less frequently involvement of the skin, subcutaneous tissue, lymph nodes, liver, and other structures. The chronic illness carries with it a high morbidity, due primarily to pulmonary fibrosis. The characteristic granulomas are of the hard, or noncaseating, variety, resembling those seen in sarcoidosis. Also *beryllium poisoning.*

**beryllium** \beril′ē·əm\ Element number 4, having atomic weight 9.0122. One of the lightest metals, beryllium has specific gravity 1.848. The only natural isotope is beryllium 9. It is transparent to x rays and has a low neutron capture cross-section. It has several technologic applications, notably in nuclear reactors. Beryllium and its salts are highly toxic. Symbol: Be

**berythromycin** $C_{37}H_{67}NO_{12}$. 12-Deoxyerythromycin. An antibacterial and antiamebic agent. Also *erythromycin B.*

**Besnier** [Ernest *Besnier*, French dermatologist, 1831–1909] **1** Besnier's prurigo. See under FLEXURAL PRURIGO. **2** Besnier-Boeck disease. See under SARCOIDOSIS.

**Best** [Franz *Best*, German pathologist, 1878–1920] **1** Best's carmine stain. See under STAIN. **2** Best's macular degeneration, vitelliform degeneration of Best, Best disease. See under VITELLIFORM MACULAR DEGENERATION.

**bestiality** \bes′chē·al′itē\ A type of paraphilia characterized by the use of animals as the preferred or only way by which to achieve sexual excitement. Also *zoophilia.*

**beta** \bā′tə, bē′tə\ The name of the second letter of the Greek alphabet. Symbol: $\beta$

**betacism** \bā′təsizm\ [Gk *bēta* second letter of the alphabet + *c* + -ISM] A disorder of speech in which the consonant *b* receives excessive emphasis and other consonants may be pronounced as *b.*

**betahistine hydrochloride** $C_8H_{12}N_2 \cdot 2HCl$. *N*-Methyl-2-pyridineethanamine dihydrochloride. A drug with histaminelike actions. It is administered orally as a vasodilator to control the frequency of episodes of vertigo in patients with Menière's disease.

**betaine** $Me_3N^+—CH_2—COO^-$. Trimethylammonioacetate. The product of methylation of glycine. The name is used for substitution products and so for the whole class of zwitterionic substances containing quaternary nitrogen. It is an intermediate in the catabolism of choline, which can be oxidized to form it.

**betaine hydrochloride** $C_5H_{12}ClNO_2$. 1-Carboxy-*N,N,N*-trimethyl-methanaminium hydrochloride, the oxidation product of choline in which the alcohol is oxidized to a carboxylic acid. It has been used as a lipotropic factor to supply a source of methyl groups.

**betamethasone** $C_{22}H_{29}FO_5$. 9α-Fluoro-16β-methylprednisolone. A very potent, anti-inflammatory glucocorticoid. It is used topically and orally as a long-acting steroidal agent.

**betamethasone acetate** The 21-acetate ester derivative of betamethazone, which has the same properties and uses as the parent drug. It is used in combination with the sodium phosphate ester to give both rapid action and sustained release intramuscularly or intra-articularly.

**betamethasone benzoate** The 17-benzoate ester of betamethasone. It has the same properties and uses as the parent drug, and it is applied topically in creams, gels, and lotions.

**betamethasone dipropionate** The 17,21-dipropionate ester of betamethasone. It has the same properties and uses as the parent drug. It is used topically in creams, ointments, and lotions, and as a 0.1% solution in aerosol form.

**betamethasone sodium phosphate** The disodium salt of the 21-phosphate ester of betamethasone. It has the same actions and properties as the parent drug. It is used as an injectable suspension, usually in combination with the acetate ester, for sustained release of the steroid.

**betamethasone valerate** The 17-valerate ester of betamethasone. It has the same properties and uses as the parent drug. It is applied topically in the form of creams, ointments, lotions, and an aerosol.

**betazole hydrochloride** $C_5H_9N_3{\cdot}2HCl$. 1*H*-Pyrazole-3-ethanamine dihydrochloride. A histamine analogue which stimulates the stomach to secrete hydrochloric acid. It is used in diagnostic tests of gastric secretion and given intramuscularly or subcutaneously. Also *gastramine.*

**bethanechol chloride** $C_7H_{17}ClN_2O_2$. 2-[(Aminocarbonyl)oxy]-*N,N,N*-trimethyl-1-propanaminium chloride. It is a cholinergic drug used to treat gastric retention following postoperative urinary retention, postoperative abdominal distention and vagotomy. It is given subcutaneously or orally.

**bethanidine sulfate** $C_{10}H_{15}N_3{\cdot}\frac{1}{2}H_2SO_4$. *N,N*-Dimethyl-*N*-(phenylmethyl)guanidine sulfate 2:1. It is an adrenergic blocking agent used in the treatment of malignant essential hypertension.

**between-brain** *Obs.* DIENCEPHALON.

**Betz** [Vladimir Aleksandrovich *Betz,* Russian anatomist, 1834–1894] **1** See under AREA. **2** Betz cells. See under CELL.

**Bevan** [Arthur Dean *Bevan,* U.S. surgeon, 1861–1943] See under OPERATION.

**Bevan Lewis** [William *Bevan Lewis,* English physiologist, 1847–1929] Bevan Lewis cells. See under BETZ CELLS.

**bevel** \bev′əl\ [possibly Middle French, from Old French *baïf* with open mouth] The angled margin of a cavity in a tooth prepared for a gold filling.

**bex** \beks\ [Gk *bēx* (gen. *bēchos*) a cough] COUGH. **b. convulsiva** PERTUSSIS.

**bexia** \beshē′ə\ [alteration of Portuguese *bexiga* (from L *vesica* bladder) bladder, vesicle, pock, pox, smallpox] ALASTRIM.

**beziehungswahn** \betsē′ungs·vän′\ [German *Beziehung* reference + *Wahn* erroneous opinion, presumption] A paranoid state characterized by a preponderance of ideas of reference. **sensitiver b.** A paranoid state with hypersensitivity and ideas of reference, often an outgrowth of the subject's feeling that he has done something contrary to his own moral or ethical standards.

**bezoar** \bē′zôr\ [Arabic *bāzahr* bezoar, from Persian *bādzahr, pādzahr* bezoar, from *pād* protecting against + *zahr* poison] An agglomeration of food or foreign material in the intestinal tract of animals, including man. It may be classified according to primary constituent, as trichobezoar (hair) or phytobezoar (plant material), but may fall into a miscellaneous category of intragastric bodies, including fungal agglomerations, food boli, chemical concretions, and foreign bodies.

**Bezold** [Albert von *Bezold,* German physiologist, 1838–1868] **1** See under GANGLION. **2** Bezold-Jarisch reflex, Bezold-Jarisch effect. See under BEZOLD REFLEX.

**Bezold** [Friedrich *Bezold,* German otologist, 1842–1908] **1** See under MASTOIDITIS. **2** See under ABSCESS.

**BFP** biologic false positive.

**Bi** Symbol for the element, bismuth.

**bi-**[1] \bī-\ [L prefix *bi-* (related to *bis, bis-; bis-* before s, c, or vowel) two, doubly] A prefix meaning two or twice, doubly. Also *bis-, bin-*.

**bi-**[2] \bī-\ BIO-.

**Bial** [Manfred *Bial,* German physician, 1870–1908] See under TEST, REAGENT.

**bialamicol hydrochloride** $C_{28}H_{40}N_2O_2{\cdot}2HCl$. 3,3′-bis[(diethylamino)methyl]-5,5′-di-(2-propenyl)[1,1′-biphenyl]-4,4′-diol dihydrochloride. An antiamebic drug, formerly administered orally for the treatment of acute or chronic amebiasis. Also *biallylamicol* (obs.).

**Bianchi** [Giovanni Battista *Bianchi,* Italian anatomist, 1681–1761] Bianchi's nodules. See under NODULI VALVULARUM SEMILUNARIUM VALVAE AORTAE.

**biarticular** \bī′ärtik′yələr\ Involving two joints; diarthric.

**biarticulate** \bī′ärtik′yəlāt\ Comprising two joints or having a double joint.

**bias** \bī′əs\ [French and Middle French *biais* (from Gk *epikarsios* crosswise, at an angle) oblique] In statistics, any of those influences that distort the representative quality of results. A systematic error on the part of the observer is often the cause of bias. **Berkson's b.** A systematic bias in the distribution of disease among hospital patients which may invalidate the findings of case-control studies in which the controls are drawn from a population of hospitalized patients. **Neyman's b.** A form of bias which arises in epidemiologic investigations of diseases having a long natural history and which is due to the elimination of the possibility of inclusion, as cases in case-control studies of patients who had died of the disease under study.

**Biasotti** [Alfredo *Biasotti,* Argentinian physician, born 1903] Houssay-Biasotti syndrome. See under HOUSSAY SYNDROME.

**biauricular** \bī′ôrik′yələr\ **1** Pertaining to the two auricles of the ears. **2** Referring to a diameter measured in cephalometry. Also *binauricular.*

**biaxial** \bī·ak′sē·əl\ Possessing two axes around which completely independent movements can take place, as in an ellipsoidal joint.

**bib.** *bibe* (L, drink).

**biballism** \bībal′izm\ [BI- + BALLISM] A very rare syndrome marked by violent, disorganized, involuntary movements of the whole body, corresponding to bilateral hemiballismus or unusually violent senile chorea.

**Biber** [Hugo *Biber,* Swiss physician, 1864–1918] Biber-Haab-Dimmer dystrophy. See under LATTICE DYSTROPHY OF THE CORNEA.

**biblio-** \bib′lē·ō-\ [Gk *biblion* book] A combining form meaning book.

**bibulous** \bib′yələs\ Absorbent.

**bicameral** \bīkam′ərəl\ Having two compartments or divisions.

**bicapsular** \bīkap′sʸələr\ Possessing two capsules, as a joint.

**bicarbonate** [BI-[1] + CARBONATE] The ion $HCO_3^-$ and its salts. It is the main form of carbon dioxide in solution at neutral pH. **plasma b.** The bicarbonate ion concentration of plasma, normally about 28 mEq/l. Also *blood bicarbonate, alkali reserve, alkaline reserve.* **standard b.** The portion of plasma bicarbonate that is derived from nonrespiratory sources. It reflects the sum of metabolic reactions that affect bicarbonate level, measured as the bicarbonate concentration after blood has been equilibrated at 37°C to $PCO_2$ of 40 mm of mercury. Normal values are 21 to 25 mEq/l. When $PCO_2$ is normal, the actual and standard bicarbonate values are equal. Deviations from the normal limits signify a metabolic acid-base disturbance.

**bicarbonatemia** \bīkär′bōnātē′mē·ə\ HYPERBICARBONATEMIA.

**bicardiogram** \bīkär′dē·əgram′\ The electrocardiographic complex formed by the combined activity of the right and left atria. *Obs.*

**bicellular** \bīsel′yələr\ **1** Made up of two cells. **2** Having two compartments.

**bicephalus** \bīsef′ələs\ DICEPHALUS.

**biceps** \bī′seps\ [L (from *bi-* two + *-ceps,* combining form from *caput* head), two-headed] A muscle possessing two heads. **b. brachii** MUSCULUS BICEPS BRACHII. **b. femoris** MUSCULUS BICEPS FEMORIS.

**Bichat** [Marie François Xavier *Bichat,* French anatomist, physician, and biologist, 1771–1802] **1** Bichat's foramen. See under CISTERNA VENAE MAGNAE CEREBRI. **2** Cerebral fissure of Bichat, fissure of Bichat. See under FISSURA TRANSVERSA CEREBRI. **3** Bichat's fatty body of cheek, Bichat's fat pad, fatty ball of Bichat, Bichat's protuberance. See under CORPUS ADIPOSUM BUCCAE. **4** Bichat's membrane. See under HENLE'S FENESTRATED MEMBRANE. **5** Bichat's tunic. See under TUNICA INTERNA VASORUM.

**bicipital** \bīsip′ətəl\ Having two heads, or origins, or denoting a two-headed (biceps) muscle.

**Bickel** [Gustav *Bickel,* German physician, flourished late 19th century] Bickel's ring. See under TONSILLAR RING.

**biconcave** \bīkän′kāv\ [BI- + CONCAVE] Referring to an optical lens that is concave on both sides.

**biconvex** \bīkän′veks\ [BI- + CONVEX] Referring to an optical lens that is convex on both sides.

**bicornis** \bīkôr′nis\ Having two points, horns, or hornlike projections. Also *bicornuate, bicornate, bicornous, bicornute.*

**bicoudate** \bī′koodāt\ Having two angles or bends.

**bicuspid** \bīkus′pid\ [New L *bicuspis,* gen. *bicuspidis,* two-pointed, a two-pointed tooth, from L *bi-* two + *cuspis* a point] **1** Having two cusps or points. **2** A tooth having two cusps. In man the eight bicuspids, two in each segment, are immediately in front of the molar teeth and behind the cuspids (canine teeth). Also *premolar, bicuspid tooth, premolar tooth.*

**bicuspidization** \bīkus′pidīzā′shən\ An operative procedure in which the normally tricuspid aortic valve is converted into a valve with two cusps.

**b.i.d.** *bis in die* (L, twice a day).

**bidactyly** \bīdak′təlē\ [BI- + DACTYL + -Y] A developmental absence of the three medial digits with only the first and fifth represented. It is an extreme degree of the lobster-claw deformity.

**Bidder** [Friedrich H. *Bidder,* German anatomist, 1810–1894] Bidder's ganglia. See under VENTRICULAR GANGLIA.

**bidentate** \bīden′tāt\ Having two teeth: used especially of chelation in which two atoms of a chelating agent bind to a single metal ion.

**biduotertian** \bid′yoo·ōtur′shē·ən\ [L *bidu(us)* (from *bi-* two + *dies* day) of two days + *o* + TERTIAN] Characterizing a quotidian fever cycle in vivax malaria in which two broods are present and a tertian cycle has not yet been established.

**biduous** \bid′yoo·əs\ Continuing for two days.

**Bielschowsky** [Max *Bielschowsky,* German neurologist, 1869–1940] **1** Bielschowsky-Jansky syndrome, Bielschowsky's disease, Bielschowsky-Jansky disease, Bielschowsky-Dollinger syndrome, Jansky-Bielschowsky type ceroid-lipofuscinosis. See under LATE INFANTILE CEROID-LIPOFUSCINOSIS. **2** Bielschowsky's method. See under STAIN. **3** Scholz-Bielschowsky-Henneberg diffuse cerebral sclerosis. See under METACHROMATIC LEUKODYSTROPHY.

**Biemond** [A. *Biemond,* French neurologist, flourished 20th century] **1** Biemond syndrome type I. See under BIEMOND SYNDROME. **2** Biemond syndrome type II. See under BIEMOND SYNDROME.

**Bier** [August Karl Gustav *Bier,* German physician, 1861–1949] **1** Bier's passive hyperemia. See under TREATMENT. **2** See under BLOCK.

**Biermer** [Anton *Biermer,* German physician, 1827–1892] Biermer's anemia, Biermer's disease, Addison-Biermer anemia. See under PERNICIOUS ANEMIA.

**Biett** [Laurent Théodore *Biett,* Swiss dermatologist, 1781–1840] Collarette of Biett. See under BIETT'S COLLAR.

**bifascicular** \bī′fasik′yələr\ Involving two fascicles, in particular, two of the three fascicles deriving from the atrioventricular trunk, or bundle of His: the right bundle and the anterior and posterior branches of the left bundle. In a bifascicular block, for example, conduction is blocked in two of the three fascicles.

**bifid** \bī′fid\ [L *bifid(us)* (from *bi(s)* twice + *fid-,* stem of *findere* to split) split or divided into two parts] Split or divided into two, usually equal parts by a median cleft.

***Bifidobacterium*** \bif′idōbaktir′ē·əm\ A genus of Gram-positive, anaerobic, heterofermentative rods, classified in the family Actinomycetaceae. The cells are pleomorphic and they form short branches under some conditions. They are prominent, along with lactobacilli, in the feces of milk-fed infants. Also *Lactobacillus bifidus* (obs.).

**bifixate** \bīfik′sāt\ [BI- + FIXATE] To fixate binocularly; perceive in focus with both eyes.

**bifocal** \bīfō′kl\ [BI- + FOCAL] A spectacle lens with two focal distances utilized for the correction of presbyopia. The inferior portion of the lens is usually focused for near work, while the upper portion serves distance vision.

**bifocals** BIFOCAL GLASSES.

**biforate** \bīfôr′āt\ Possessing two openings, foramina, or perforations.

**bifurcate** \bīfur′kāt\ Forked; having two prongs or branches.

**bifurcatio** \bī′fərkā′shō\ [Med L, bifurcation. See BIFURCATION.] A division or branching of one structure into two. Also *bifurcation.* **b. tracheae** [NA] The site of division of the trachea into the two principal bronchi, one for each lung, usually seen just to the right of the midline opposite the fifth thoracic vertebra. Also *bifurcation of trachea.*

**bifurcation** \bī′fərkā′shən\ [L *bifurc(us)* two-pronged + -ATION] **1** BIFURCATIO. **2** The place at which the roots of a two-rooted tooth separate. **b. of bundle of His** The point of division of the atrioventricular bundle into the right and left crura, at the upper border of the muscular part of the interventricular septum of the heart. **b. of trachea** BIFURCATIO TRACHEAE.

**Bigelow** [Henry Jacob *Bigelow,* U.S. surgeon, 1818–1890] **1** Bigelow's ligament. See under LIGAMENTUM ILIOFEMORALE. **2** Bigelow septum. See under CALCAR FEMORALE.

**bigemina** \bījem′ənə\ BIGEMINY.

**bigeminal** \bījem′ənəl\ [Late L *begemin(us)* doubled + -AL. See BIGEMINY.] Double or twin, as pulse occurring in pairs.

**bigeminum** \bījem′ənəm\ [Late L, neut. sing. of *bigeminus* doubled, from BI- + L *geminus* double, twin] Either the superior or the inferior colliculiof the corpora quadrigemina of a fetus.

**bigeminy** \bījem′inē\ [Late L *bigemin(us)* double, duplicated (from BI- + *geminus* twin) + -Y] The occurrence of phenomena in pairs, particularly, pairs of cardiac beats in which the first is of sinuatrial origin and the second of ectopic origin, usually ventricular. It may result in a coupled pulse, but the second beat may be so weak that it is impalpable, giving the impression of bradycardia. Also *bigemina.* **atrial b.** Bigeminy in which an atrial ectopic beat follows a beat of sinuatrial origin. **atrioventricular nodal b.** Bigeminy in which an ectopic beat of atrioventricular nodal origin follows each sinus beat. Also *nodal bigeminy.* **escape-capture b.** Bigeminy in which the first of two beats in an escape beat and the second is a conducted sinus beat. **nodal b.** ATRIOVENTRICULAR NODAL BIGEMINY. **reciprocal b.** Bigeminy in which an atrioventricular nodal beat is followed by a reciprocal beat. **ventricular b.** Bigeminy in which the first beat is of sinuatrial origin and the second ventricular.

**bigerminal** \bījur′minəl\ [BI- + GERMINAL] Pertaining to two germs or two ova.

**Bignami** [Amico *Bignami,* Italian physician, 1862–1929] Marchiafava-Bignami disease. See under MARCHIAFAVA-BIGNAMI SYNDROME.

**bi-ischial** \bī·is′kē·əl\ Pertaining to both ischial tuberosities. Also *bituberal.*

**bilateral** \bīlat′ərəl\ Having, affecting, or pertaining to the two sides, especially the two symmetrical or opposite sides of an organ or the body.

**bilateralism** \bīlat′ərəlizm\ BILATERAL SYMMETRY.

**bilayer** \bī′lā·ər\ A double layer. **lipid b.** The structure found in most biologic membranes, in which two layers of lipid molecules are so arranged that their hydrophobic parts interpenetrate, whereas their hydrophilic parts form the two surfaces of the bilayer.

**bile** \bīl\ [L *bilis* bile] A fluid secreted by the liver and discharged into the duodenum where it is integral in the digestion and absorption of fats. Normal bile output by the liver is 800–1000 ml per day. Bile salts solubilize triglyceride fats to allow their absorption, and the absorption of some vitamins, into the intestine. Bile is the main route of excretion for bilirubin, cholesterol, some hormonal products, and some drugs and poisons. The alkalinity of bile is in part responsible for neutralization of the duodenal contents. Control of bile secretion is complex. Secretin produces an increase in bile flow. The reabsorption of bile salts from the intestine stimulates the liver to produce more bile. Also *gall, fel.* See also HEPATIC BILE. **cystic b.** Bile contained within the gallbladder. It is more concentrated than hepatic bile because of the reabsorbtion of electrolytes and water by the gallbladder wall. Unlike hepatic bile, cystic bile may be yellow, green, or brown in color. Also *gallbladder bile.* **hepatic b.** The straw-colored, viscid fluid secreted by the liver cells into the bile ducts. It is an alkaline isotonic mixture composed of mucin, bile acids, lecithin, cholesterol, bilirubin, protein, and several electrolytes. The fraction of hepatic bile that is stored in the gallbladder is converted into cystic bile, which is more concentrated. **milk of calcium b.** A thick puttylike bile containing a high concentration of calcium. Its presence may cause the gallbladder to appear completely opaque on plain x-ray films of the abdomen. The calcium usually exists as the carbonate, but may be associated with phosphate or bilirubin. Also *limy bile.* **ox b.** See under OX BILE EXTRACT. **white b.** Pigment-free gallbladder fluid that occurs when the cystic duct is obstructed.

***Bilharzia*** \bilhär′zē·ə\ [after Theodor Maximilian *Bilharz,* German helminthologist and physician, 1825–1862 + -IA] A former name for *SCHISTOSOMA.*

**bilharzial** \bilhär′zē·əl\ [*Bilharzi(a)* + -AL] SCHISTOSOMAL.

**bilharziasis** \bil′härzī′əsis\ [after Theodor *Bilharz,* German helminthologist and physician, 1825–1862 + -IASIS] SCHISTOSOMIASIS.

**bilharzioma** \bilhär′zē·ō′mə\ [*Bilharzi(a)* + -OMA] A tumor of the urinary bladder, caused by or containing schistosomes, or associated with schistosomiasis of the bladder.

**bilharziosis** \bilhär′zē·ō′sis\ [See BILHARZIASIS.] SCHISTOSOMIASIS.

**bili-** \bil′i-\ [L *bilis* bile] A combining form denoting bile.

**biliary** [BILI- + -ARY] Relating to bile or to the structures in which the bile is contained or transported.

**bilidigestive** \-dijes′tiv\ [BILI- + DIGESTIVE] Referring to the biliary and intestinal tracts, or to the part of the digestive system in which bile is involved.

**bilifaction** \-fak′shən\ CHOLEPOIESIS.

**biligenesis** \-jen′əsis\ CHOLEPOIESIS.

**biligenic** \-jen′ik\ [BILI- + -GENIC] Bile-producing; cholepoietic.

**biligulate** \bilig′yəlāt\ Having two tonguelike structures or processes.

**Bili-Labstix** A strip impregnated with reagents for performing chemical tests on urine. A proprietary name.

**bilin** \bil′in\ The parent compound of linear tetrapyrroles. It contains four pyrrole rings joined by three —CH= groups. Natural bilins, such as biliverdin, are formed in the breakdown of heme, and they are colored.

**bilious** \bil′yəs\ **1** Relating to or associated with bile. **2** Characterized by or affected with biliousness.

**biliousness** \bil′yəsnəs\ **1** An excess of bile. **2** A symptom complex of nausea, vomiting, abdominal pain, headaches, and constipation, attributed to liver dysfunction.

**bilirachia** \-rā′kē·ə\ The presence of bilirubin in the cerebrospinal fluid giving it a xanthochromic appearance. It may result from increased plasma levels of direct bilirubin with a normal blood-brain barrier or from increased plasma levels of indirect bilirubin associated with increased permeability of the blood-brain barrier.

**bilirubin** \-roo′bin\ [BILI- + L *rub(er)* red + -IN] A red reduction product of the green compound biliverdin. Formed in heme catabolism, it is transported to the liver where it is glycosylated and secreted into the bile.

**bilirubinaemia** *Brit.* BILIRUBINEMIA.

**bilirubinemia** \-roo′binē′mē·ə\ [BILIRUBIN + -EMIA] The presence of bilirubin in the blood, a normal condition. *Seldom used.*

**bilirubinuria** \-roo′binoo′rē·ə\ [BILIRUBIN + -URIA] The excretion of bilirubin in the urine, which causes the urine to be dark brown in color. In high concentration, bilirubin may stain casts.

**biliuria** \-yoo′rē·ə\ [BILI- + -URIA] The presence of bile or bile salts in the urine.

**biliverdin** The first linear tetrapyrrole formed in heme catabolism, a 1,19,21,24-tetrahydro-1,19-dioxobilin. It has CO groups at the ends of the molecule where the fourth bridge carbon of heme has been removed. It is converted by reduction into bilirubin.

**billion** \bil′yən\ **1** In the United States, one thousand million; $10^9$. **2** In Great Britain, one million million; $10^{12}$. • Since the 1970s, especially in financial contexts, *billion* has been used increasingly in Britain with the meaning one thousand million, or $10^9$. The traditional British term for $10^9$ is *milliard.* In Australia and, since the 1970s, in New Zealand, a *billion* refers to $10^9$. In Japan the official translation of *billion* is $10^9$.

**Billroth** [Christian Albert Theodor *Billroth,* German surgeon, 1829–1894] **1** Billroth hypertrophy. See under ADULT HYPERTROPHY OF THE PYLORUS. **2** Billroth's disease. See under TRAUMATIC MENINGOCELE. **3** Billroth anastomosis. See under OPERATION. **4** Billroth's cords. See under SPLENIC CORDS. **5** Billroth strand. See under TRABECULA OF SPLEEN.

**bilobate** \bīlō′bāt\ Divided into or having two lobes. Also *bilobed.*

**bilobular** \bīläb′yələr\ Divided into or having two lobules. Also *bilobulate.*

**bilocular** \bīläk′yələr\ [BI-[1] + *locul(us)* + -AR] Divided into or having two compartments, cavities, or cells. Also *biloculate.*

**biloculation** \bīläk′yəlā′shən\ [*bilocul(ar)* + -ATION] The condition of having or being divided into two compartments or cavities.

**bimalar** \bīmā′lər\ Pertaining to the two malar, or zygomatic, bones, or the distance between them.

**bimalleolar** \bī′malē′ələr\ Involving or pertaining to the medial and lateral malleoli.

**bimanual** \bīman′yoo·əl\ [BI- + MANUAL] Involving the use of both hands.

**bimastoid** \bīmas′toid\ Of or pertaining to the two mastoid processes of the temporal bones.

**bimaxillary** \bīmak′siler′ē\ Of, pertaining to, affecting, or extending between the maxilla and the mandible.

**bin-** [L *bini* two each, double] BI-[1].

**binangle** \bin′angl\ [BIN- + *angle*] Of an instrument, having a shank with two angles in it.

**binary** \bī′nərē\ **1** Of or consisting of two. **2** Having two possibilities, such as on or off, 1 or 0.

**binasal** \bīnā′zəl\ [BI-[1] + NASAL] Pertaining to the nasal visual field of both eyes.

**binaural** \bīnôr′əl\ [BIN- + AURAL] **1** Pertaining to both ears. Also *binotic.* **2** Having two ears.

**binauricular** \bī′nôrik′yələr\ BIAURICULAR.

**bind** **1** To wrap, as with bandages. **2** In chemistry, to effect or enter into combination; to combine with (another substance) or to cause to enter into a combination, usually reversibly. **bipolar double b.** A double bind characteristic of family interaction in which two conflicting messages emanate from two people, usually the mother and father, thus serving to confuse the child or children. **double b.** A dilemma in which the subject is presented with mutually contradictory messages or injunctions by another person. No matter which alternative is chosen, the subject errs or offends by not having chosen the other one. The double bind is often a characteristic of the relationship between schizophrenic individuals and others in the patient's family and has been proposed as a causative factor of schizophrenia. **unipolar double b.** A double bind in which one parent gives the child or children contradictory messages.

**binder** A bandage or girdle utilized to support relaxed abdominal musculature following childbirth. Also *abdominal binder, obstetric binder.*

**Binet** [Alfred *Binet,* French psychologist, 1857–1911] **1** Binet's test. See under BINET-SIMON TEST. **2** Stanford-Binet test. See under STANFORD-BINET INTELLIGENCE SCALE.

**Bing** [Albert *Bing,* German otologist, 1844–1922] See under SIGN, TEST.

**Bing** [Jens *Bing,* Danish physician, born 1916] Bing-Neel syndrome. See under SYNDROME.

**Bing** [Paul Robert *Bing,* German neurologist, 1878–1956] See under REFLEX.

**binging** \bin′jing\ Binge eating. See under BULIMIA.

**binocular** \bənäk′yələr, bī-\ [BIN- + OCULAR] Pertaining to the use of both eyes together to achieve a cerebral synthesis of the visual stimuli.

**binotic** \binō′tik\ [BIN- + OTIC] BINAURAL.

**binovular** \bināv′yələr\ [BIN- + OVULAR] Derived from two separate ova or eggs, as *binovular twins.* Also *biovular.*

**Binswanger** [Otto *Binswanger,* German psychiatrist, 1852–1929] Binswanger's encephalitis. See under DISEASE.

**binuclear** \bīnʸoo′klē·ər\ [BI- + NUCLEAR] Having two nuclei: used especially of a cell. Also *binucleate.*

**binucleolate** \bī′nʸooklē′əlāt\ Having two nucleoli.

**bio-** \bī′ō-\ [Gk *bios* life] A combining form denoting life. Also *bi-*[2].

**bioaccumulation** \-əkyoo′myəlā′shən\ The accumulation of chemicals by organisms present in the environment, most often expressed as the ratio of the concentration of a chemical in the organism to that in the medium, usually water. A high partition coefficient and resistance to degradation are the principal factors responsible for high bioaccumulation ratio values. Also *biomagnification, biconcentration, biologic magnification.*

**bioacoustics** \-əkoo′stiks\ The study of the production and characteristics of sound in relation to living organisms.

**bioactive** \-ak′tiv\ Having an effect on living tissue; characterized by bioactivity.

**bioactivity** \-aktiv′itē\ The process by which some organism or chemical, such as an enzyme, has an effect on or creates a response in living tissue.

**bioassay** [BIO- + ASSAY] The quantitative estimation of the amount or potency of a substance such as a drug, antibiotic, hormone, vitamin, etc. based upon its production of a specific type of biological activity or response, either *in vivo* or *in vitro,* compared with that induced by a standard substance or preparation. The method can also be used to identify or measure the toxicity of a pollutant or other substance in an environment, through the controlled observation of its effects on selected animals. Also *biological assay, biological monitoring.*

**bioavailability** \-əvā′ləbil′itē\ The extent to which an agent can be utilized by a biologic target tissue.

**bioblast** \bī′ōblast\ [BIO- + -BLAST] A hypothetical unit of living matter capable of dividing, growing, and stimulating cell function.

**biochemistry** \-kem′istrē\ [BIO- + CHEMISTRY] The study of the chemical components of living matter, the reactions they undergo, and the energetic changes that accompany such reactions. Hence it represents the study of life at the molecular level.

**biocompatibility** \-kəmpat′əbil′itē\ The capability of a prosthesis implanted in the body to exist in harmony with tissue without causing deleterious changes such as fibrous capsule formation, wear, and infection.

**bioconcentration** \-kän′səntrā′shən\ BIOACCUMULATION.

**biocycle** \bī′ōsīkl\ [BIO- + CYCLE] BIORHYTHM.

**biocytin** The amide formed between the carboxyl group of biotin and the ϵ-amino group of lysine. A residue of biocytin is the form in which biotin occurs in enzymes that contain it. Biocytin occurs naturally in yeast.

**biocytinase** \-sī′tənās\ The enzyme that cleaves biocytin to biotin and lysine.

**biodialysis** \-dī·al′isis\ [BIO- + DIALYSIS] The process of separating crystalloid from colloid substances by passage through biologic tissue that functions as a semipermeable membrane.

**biodynamics** \-dīnam′iks\ [BIO- + DYNAMICS] The study of the force and motion of living matter. Also *vitodynamics.*

**bioelectric** \-ilek′trik\ Pertaining to electrical phenomena occurring in living tissues or organs. Also *electrobiologic.*

**bioelectricity** The electric phenomena inherent in living cells or tissues, consisting of the electric potentials observed in nerve and muscle tissues.

**bioelectronics** The application of electronic techniques to the problems of biology and medicine.

**bioenergetics** \-en′ərjet′iks\ The study of energy changes in living organisms.

**bioengineering** \-en′jənir′ing\ BIOMEDICAL ENGINEERING.

**bioethics** \-eth′iks\ The study of the ethical implications in modern medical and surgical practice and in biomedical research. Adj. bioethical.

**biofeedback** \-fēd′bak\ [BIO- + FEEDBACK] A technique permitting an individual to gain control over internal physiologic processes, such as heart rate or blood-pressure level, of which he is ordinarily unaware, by arranging for these to produce easily perceived stimuli which can be monitored, for example, by audible tones.

**bioflavonoid** \-flā′vənoid\ Any of a group of compounds found widely in plants that have an effect on the fragility and permeability of small blood vessels, increasing the resistance of capillaries to rupture. Most are derivatives of 2-phenyl benzopyrone. Also *vitamin P, permeability vitamin.*

**biogenesis** \-jen′əsis\ [BIO- + GENESIS] The view that organisms develop only from pre-existent living material, and are not spontaneously generated from nonliving material. Adj. biogenetic.

**biogeography** \-jē·äg′rəfē\ The effects of geographical features on animal and plant life. Also *chorology.*

**bioglass** \bī′ōglas\ A ceramic-glass material used as a bone prosthesis. Living bone fuses with it because chemically it resembles hydroxyapatite.

**biohazard** \bī′ōhaz′ərd\ [BIO- + HAZARD] The likelihood that, under the conditions being experienced, a microbiological organism, disease vector, or physical or chemical agent will produce adverse health effects in human beings or some other target species as a result of ingestion, inhalation, transcutaneous absorption, or other form of exposure, association, or contact between the pathogenic or toxic agent and its target.

**biohydraulic** \-hīdrô′lik\ Pertaining to the movement of aqueous fluids through living tissue.

**biokinetics** \-kīnet′iks\ The branch of science that pertains to the study of activity in living organisms.

**biologicals** Therapeutic preparations derived or obtained from living organisms, such as sera, vaccines, and antitoxins. **lyophilized b.** Biologicals preserved or stored by freeze-drying *in vacuo* to obtain a dry, powder form.

**Biological Stain Commission** A nonprofit corporation that provides standardized specifications for stains and certifies the performance of marketed stains.

**biology** \bī·äl′əjē\ [BIO- + -LOGY] The science concerned with the study of life and living organisms. **cell b.** CYTOLOGY. **descriptive b.** BIOPHYSIOGRAPHY. **mathematical b.** BIOMETRY. **molecular b.** A branch of biology concerned with the properties of specific molecules and the interactions between molecules in the living organisms in which they occur. **population b.** A branch of biologic science that incorporates elements of genetics, ecology, ethology, and taxonomy in the study of how organisms interact.

**biolysis** \bī·äl′isis\ [BIO- + LYSIS] The decomposition of organic matter by the action of living organisms.

**biomagnification** \-mag′nəfəkā′shən\ BIOACCUMULATION.

**biomechanics** \-məkan′iks\ The application of mechanics to the structures of living animals, especially to the forces on the skeleton caused by the muscles and gravity and resulting movements of the locomotor system. Also *animal mechanics.*

**biomedical** \-med′əkl\ **1** Biologic and medical, as *biomedical sciences.* **2** Of or having to do with medicine considered in the context of the biological sciences, with emphasis on its relationship to the basic sciences underlying clinical practice. **3** Of or relating to biomedicine.

**biomedicine** \-med′əsin\ The application of the principles of the biologic sciences to the study and practice of medicine.

**biometry** \bī·äm′ətrē\ [BIO- + -METRY] The application of statistical methods to biologic phenomena; mathematical analysis of biologic data. Also *mathematical biology.*

**biomicroscope** \-mī′krəskōp\ [BIO- + MICROSCOPE] A microscope equipped with sharply focused slit illumination, allowing detailed inspection of living transparent structures, as found in the eye. Also *keratoiridoscope.* **slit-lamp b.** A biomicroscope for the clinical examination of eyes under magnification, illuminated by a narrow collimated light.

**biomicroscopy** \-mīkräs′kəpē\ The examination of living transparent tissue, as of the eye, by means of a biomicroscope.

***Biomphalaria*** \bī′ämfəler′ē·ə\ [*bi(o)-* + *omphal(o)-* + -ARIA] A medically important genus of freshwater pulmonate snails that includes the major intermediate hosts of human schistosomiasis mansoni. Several species occur in Africa, South America, the Caribbean, Saudi Arabia, and Yemen. This genus includes the former genera *Planorbina, Taphius, Armigerus, Australorbis* and *Tropicorbis,* the diagnostic features of which were not sufficient to separate them, in accordance with a ruling by the International Commission on Zoological Nomenclature in 1965. ***B. alexandrina*** The principal snail intermediate host of *Schistosoma mansoni* in Egypt, Saudi Arabia, and Yemen. Also *Planorbis boissyii* (former name). ***B. glabrata*** An important species occurring in South America and some Caribbean islands, where it is the chief intermediate host of *Schistosoma mansoni.* It is also widely used in laboratory research on this and other species of trematodes.

**bionecrosis** \-nəkrō′sis\ NECROBIOSIS.

**bionics** \bī·än′iks\ [*bi-* (as in *biologic*) + *-onics* (as in *electronics*)] The study of the characteristics and functions of living systems in order to develop mathematical, computer, or physical models which simulate parallel phenomena. These models might suggest new techniques and devices in engineering.

**bionomics** \-näm′iks\ [BIO- + NOM- + -ICS] ECOLOGY.

**bionomy** \bī·än′əmē\ [BIO- + *nom(o)-* + -Y ] The body of scientific laws governing vital processes and functions.

**-biont** \-bē·änt, -bī′änt\ [alteration of Gk *biount(os),* gen. of *biōn,* pres. part. of *biōnai* or *bioun* to live] A combining form designating an organism that lives in a (specified) way or environment.

**biophage** \bī′ōfāj\ [BIO- + -PHAGE] An organism that subsists on living matter.

**biophagous** \bī·äf′əgəs\ Characterized by feeding on living matter.

**biopharmaceutics** The science of pharmaceutical agents, their dosage, and the relationship of dosage to the onset, amplitude, and duration of the resulting drug action.

**biophotometer** \-fōtäm′ətər\ A device for measurement of dark adaptation of the eye.

**biophylaxis** \-fəlak′sis\ The nonspecific defense mechanisms of the body, such as phagocytosis and vascular reactions of the inflammatory process.

**biophysics** \-fiz′iks\ [BIO- + PHYSICS] The application of the principles and methods of physics and physical chemistry to the study of biologic phenomena.

**biophysiography** \-fiz′ē·äg′rəfē\ That branch of biology that deals with the description of organs and structures. Also *descriptive biology.*

**bioplasia** \-plā′zhə\ [BIO- + -PLASIA] The formation of tissue through the conversion of food energy.

**bioplasm** \bī′ōplazm\ PROTOPLASM.

**biopolymer** Any polymeric substance, such as a protein, a polysaccharide, or a nucleic acid, that is produced by a living organism.

**biopotential** \-pəten′shəl\ BIOELECTRIC POTENTIAL.

**biopsy** \bī′äpsē\ [BI-[2] + *-opsy* as in *autopsy*] **1** The removal from the living body of a small portion of tissue for diagnosis by microscopic examination. **2** The tissue removed for this purpose. **aspiration b.** The removal of cells or tissue fragments by needle and syringe, usually for the preparation of a smear rather than of histologic sections. **biochemical b.** Diagnostic chemical analysis of small samples of tissue done in conjunction with histopathologic evaluation. Chemical analysis of tissues may be performed to confirm diagnoses made morphologically. For example, the presence of specific hormones or metabolites can be characteristic of certain neoplasms and therefore aid in their detection. **chorionic villus b.** An experimental biopsy of placental tissue during the first trimester of pregnancy as a means of detecting genetic abnormality in the fetus. **cytological b.** A procedure in which a sample of individual cells is obtained from solid tissue by scraping, irrigation, or suction aspiration. **endoscopic b.** The removal of a sample of tissue through any of various types of endoscope. **excisional b.** The surgical removal of an unidentified lesion, including all of the abnormal tissue and a margin of surrounding normal tissue. Also *total biopsy.* **incisional b.** The excision of part of a lesion without disturbing the surrounding normal tissue. **needle b.** A biopsy obtained by needle puncture. **nerve b.** The surgical removal of a portion of a peripheral nerve trunk to establish a diagnosis of leprosy. The procedure is rarely required except in suspected cases of pure neural leprosy. **open b.** A biopsy done during surgery. **punch b.** A diagnostic surgical procedure in which a small core of representative tissue is removed for analysis. Also *trephine biopsy.* **ring b.** A surgical procedure in which a cylindrical section of a representative tissue is removed for diagnostic purposes. **scalene lymph node b.** Biopsy of a lymph node from the scalene region at the root of the neck. These nodes may be involved without palpable enlargement, especially in cases of sarcoidosis or lung cancer. **sponge b.** A cytological biopsy in which a small piece of sponge is used to pick up a sample of individual cells from an epithelial surface. **sternal b.** A biopsy of the sternum to study the bone marrow. **total b.** EXCISIONAL BIOPSY. **trephine b.** PUNCH BIOPSY. **wound b.** A biopsy of the surface of a wound, generally performed to check the state of the granulation tissue or to assess the degree of infection or inflammation.

**biopterin** A stereoisomer of 2-amino-6-(1,2-dihydroxypropyl)-4-hydroxypteridine. Its reduced forms act as coenzymes of hydroxylation by molecular oxygen, as in the conversion of phenylalanine into tyrosine, in which a tetrahydrobiopterin is concomitantly converted into the dihydro compound. Other pterins can replace it in this reaction.

**bioptic** \bī·äp′tik\ Pertaining to biopsy.

**biorbital** \bī·ôr′bitəl\ Pertaining to both orbits or the distance between them.

**Biörck** [Gunnar Carl Wilhelm *Biörck,* Swedish physician, born 1916] Biörck-Thorson syndrome, Biörck syndrome. See under CARCINOID SYNDROME.

**biorheology** \-rē·äl′əjē\ [BIO- + RHEOLOGY] The study of the movement and deformation of the matter constituting living organisms.

**biorhythm** \bī′ōriTHm\ [BIO- + RHYTHM] A cycle of change that occurs in a biologic organism. Also *biocycle, biologic rhythm.*

**bioscience** \bī′ōsī′əns\ The branch of natural science that deals with organisms and living matter; biology considered in the context of the natural sciences. Adj. bioscientific.

**bioscopy** \bī·äs′kəpē\ [BIO- + -SCOPY] The examination of vital functions such as respiration, heart beat, and pulse to determine whether or not an individual is alive. *Seldom used.*

**biosis** \bī·ō′sis\ [Gk *biōsis* way of life] Life; vitality.

**biostatics** \-stat′iks\ The scientific study of the relationship of function to structure in organisms.

**biostatistics** \-statis′tiks\ [BIO- + *statistics*] **1** The application of statistical methods to the description of vital phenomena and the analysis of biological data. **2** *Outmoded* VITAL STATISTICS.

**biosynthesis** \-sin′thəsis\ The process of synthesis, in living organisms, of compounds from simpler precursors.

**Biot** [Camille *Biot,* French physician, born 1878] Biot sign, Biot's breathing. See under RESPIRATION.

**biotaxis** \-tak′sis\ [BIO- + Gk *taxis* arrangement, order] The influence or attraction between one cell or organism and another, which contributes to the organization of living cells. Also *biotaxy.*

**biotechnology** \-teknäl′əjē\ The application of the biological sciences, especially genetics, to technologic or industrial uses. ⟨"DNA research and other new strategies in biotechnology are developing so rapidly that no one can forecast their future." —*New York Times,* 27 Jan. 1980, 1.⟩

**biotelemetry** \-telem′ətrē\ Detection of function, activity, or location of a human or animal and transmission, usually by radio, to a remote location where data are recorded.

**biotic** \bī·ät′ik\ Pertaining to living matter.

**biotin** A substance whose molecules consist of two 5-membered rings, one a thiolane ring, the other formed by fusion of the side opposite the sulfur of this ring to an —NH—CO—NH— group. The thiolane ring carries a pentanoic acid side chain, and in several proteins this is linked by an amide bond to the ϵ-amino group of lysine to form biocytin, which participates in many biologic carboxylations. It reacts with ATP and carbon dioxide to convert one of its —NH— groups into —N(—$COO^-$)—, and the carbon dioxide thus "fixed" is subsequently transferred to an appropriate recipient. It is a vitamin for many animals, including man. Humans require a few micrograms daily, and it is readily formed in the large intestine by the endogenous flora. For this reason it is difficult to produce biotin deficiency in humans by withholding it from the diet, but deficiency can result from excessive consumption of raw egg white, which contains avidin. Symptoms of biotin avitaminosis are dry skin, anemia, and hypercholesterolemia. Also *anti-egg-white factor, factor H, factor S, skin factor, factor W, coenzyme R* (outmoded), *vitamin H*.

**biotinyl** The acyl group that is derived from biotin by removing —OH from its carboxyl group. This is the form in which biotin is found in some proteins (e.g. some carboxylating enzymes), such a group being a substituent on lysine. **b. enzyme** An enzyme containing the biotinyl group, as a result of acylation by biotin of a lysine residue. Biotin is normally in this form as the prosthetic group in enzymes that have used it, and it reacts with carbon dioxide in carboxylation reactions. The reactive part of the biotin can move between the active center responsible for carboxylating it and the one where it donates carbon dioxide because of the length of the arm made up of biotin and the side chain of the lysine residue.

**biotomy** \bī·ät′əmē\ [BIO- + -TOMY] *Older term* VIVISECTION.

**biotoxicology** \-täk′səkäl′əjē\ The study of poisonous substances produced or derived from living plant or animal organisms.

**biotoxin** \-täk′sin\ [BIO- + TOXIN] Any poison produced in the cells, tissues, or fluids of a living plant or animal organism.

**biovular** \bī·äv′yələr\ BINOVULAR.

**bipalatinoid** A two-compartment medicinal capsule that dissolves in the stomach and releases the two components, which then interact and produce their therapeutic effects.

**biparasitic** \bī′parəsit′ik\ HYPERPARASITIC.

**biparasitism** \bīpar′əsitizm\ HYPERPARASITISM.

**biparental** \bī′pəren′təl\ Derived from separate parents of opposite sex; of diecious origin. Also *duoparental*.

**biparietal** \bī′pərī′ətəl\ Pertaining to the two parietal bones of the skull.

**bipartite** \bīpär′tīt\ Comprising or divided into two parts or subdivisions.

**bipennate** \bīpen′āt\ [BI- + PENNATE] Resembling a feather that is bilaterally symmetrical along a central line, as a muscle with fibers converging on each side of a central tendon. Also *bipenniform*. Compare UNIPENNATE.

**biperforate** \bīpur′fôrāt\ Having two perforations or foramina.

**biperiden** $C_{21}H_{29}NO$. α-5-Norbornen-2-yl-α-phenyl-1-piperidinepropanol. An anticholinergic drug used in the treatment of parkinsonism and in the control of extrapyramidal disorders due to such drugs as the phenothiazines.

**biperiden hydrochloride** The hydrochloride form of biperiden, used orally for the same indications as biperiden.

**biperiden lactate** The lactate form of biperiden, suitable for parenteral administration for the same indications as biperiden.

**biphasic** \bīfā′zik\ Having two phases.

**biphenamine** $C_{19}H_{23}NO_3$. β-Diethylaminoethyl-2-hydroxy-3-phenylbenzoate. An agent used, as the hydrochloride, as an antiseborrheic medication, a topical anesthetic, and an antibacterial and antifungal agent.

**biphetamine** A combination in equal proportions of dextroamphetamine and amphetamine in capsules. It has limited value in the treatment of obesity. Tolerance develops to the anorectic effect, and drug dependency is a potential hazard.

**BIPM** Bureau International des Poids et Mesures (International Bureau of Weights and Measures).

**bipolar** \bīpō′lər\ **1** Having two poles or opposite extremities, as some bacterial and other cells. **2** Denoting neurons having a major dendrite entering at one pole and an axon leaving the cell directly opposite. **3** Denoting the common form of stimulating electrode having two active contact surfaces or poles, or therapeutic techniques or devices delivering stimuli through bipolar contacts. Also *dipolar*.

**bipolarity** \bī′pōlar′itē\ AMBIVALENCE.

**bipotentiality** \bī′pəten′shē·al′itē\ [BI- + POTENTIAL + -ITY] The capacity in embryology of cells or organs to pursue one or the other of two possible lines of development: used especially in the context of sexual differentiation. Adj. bipotential. **b. of the gonad** The ability of the embryonic gonad to become either a testis or an ovary depending on circumstances or stimuli. The indifferent stage of the embryonic gonad has the cell types to provide the supporting elements of either sex. The essential effect on the differentiating gonad is due to the genetic constitution of the germ cells as well as to hormonal and other influences.

**biramous** \bīrā′məs\ Having or comprising two branches.

**Bird** [Golding *Bird*, English physician, 1814–1854] See under TREATMENT.

**birefringence** \bī′rəfrin′jəns\ [BI-[1] + *refring(ent)* + -ENCE. See REFRINGENT.] **1** The property of certain crystalline materials of exhibiting different indexes of refraction for light waves polarized in mutually perpendicular planes. **2** The splitting of a light wave into two waves having mutually perpendicular polarizations and traveling at different speeds, as a result of the difference in indexes of refraction. Also *double refraction*. **crystalline b.** Birefringence due to the regular asymmetrical arrangement of bonds between ions or molecules. Also *intrinsic birefringence*. **flow b.** Birefringence resulting from the orientation of anisotropic molecules, or of certain kinds of suspended particles, as a result of internal stress in a flowing liquid. Also *streaming birefringence*. **form b.** Birefringence produced by the orientation of asymmetrical submicroscopic particles in a regular pattern, in a surrounding medium that has a different refractive index. **intrinsic b.** CRYSTALLINE BIREFRINGENCE. **strain b.** The birefringence observed in isotropic structures of tissues exerting tension, or subjected to pressure, as embryonic tissue, or muscle tissue. **streaming b.** FLOW BIREFRINGENCE.

**birhinia** \bīrin′ē·ə\ [BI- + RHIN- + -IA] The apparent division of the external nose into two parts by a cleft or depression in the sagittal plane, giving the appearance that the nostrils are separated laterally, as is sometimes seen in ocular hypertelorism. True duplication of the nose is not known to occur in the absence of some degree of cephalopagus.

**Birkett** [John *Birkett*, English surgeon, 1815–1904] See under HERNIA.

**Birnberg** [Charles H. *Birnberg*, U.S. obstetrician and gynecologist, born 1900] See under BOW.

**birth** [Middle English *birthe, burde*, from Old Norse *byrth* birth, akin to Old English *byrde, gebyrde* birth and German *Geburt* birth] The process of being born; the separation of a fetus from its internal existence in a mother. Adj. natal. **breech b.** The vaginal birth of a fetus with the buttocks or feet as the presenting part. **complete b.** The total birth of a fetus, followed by severing of the umbilical cord between the mother and the fetus. **cross b.** TRANSVERSE LIE. **dead b.** STILLBIRTH. **head b.** CEPHALIC PRESENTATION. **immature b.** Birth of an infant weighing over 500 grams but less than 1000 grams and having a reduced chance of survival. *Seldom used.* **live b.** The complete expulsion or extraction from its mother of a product of conception irrespective of the duration of pregnancy, which after such separation, breathes or shows any other evidence of life, such as beating of the heart, pulsation of the umbilical cord, or definite movement of voluntary muscles, whether or not the umbilical cord has been cut or the placenta is attached. Each such product of conception is considered live-born. • This definition was adopted by the World Health Assembly in 1950 and is valid internationally. However, in general usage, the term applies primarily to fetuses beyond 20 weeks' duration of gestation from the first day of the last menstrual period. **multiple b.'s** Deliveries yielding more than one offspring in species ordinarily producing one. **partial b.** Delivery of part but not all of the fetus. **post-term b.** Delivery of a fetus after a gestation period of more than 42 weeks. **premature b.** Delivery of a fetus after a gestation period of between 20 and 38 weeks. Infants born during this interval usually weigh between 500 g and 2499 g. **spontaneous breech b.** Delivery of a fetus in the breech presentation without the use of traction or oxytocic drugs. **total b.'s** The sum of the number of live births and stillbirths occurring in a given population during a given period. It is the denominator for calculating the stillbirth rate and the perinatal mortality rate.

**birthing** Delivery or parturition. An informal term. **alternative b.** Any of several methods in which childbirth is carried out in a homelike setting usually without the use of medication or most obstetric instruments.

**birthmark** A nevus of congenital origin. It may be vascular in nature or result from excessive pigmentation. **strawberry b.** STRAWBERRY NEVUS.

**birthweight** The body weight at birth, used as an indicator of developmental maturity and viability. Birthweights above 2.5 kg are considered to be normal. Any values below this for whatever reason are associated with an increased death rate. Over 50 percent of babies born weighing less than 1.5 kg do not survive one week. Babies above 2 kg have a good chance of survival.

**bis-** \bis-\ BI-[1].

**bisacodyl** 4,4′-(2-Pyridylmethylene)diphenol diacetate. A relatively gentle laxative, commonly used by oral or rectal routes of administration for constipation. **b. tannex** A combination of bisacodyl and tannin. It is used as a colonic evacuant and as an effective ingredient of cleansing enemas.

**bisacromial** \bis′əkrō′mē·əl\ Of or pertaining to both acromial processes of the scapula.

**bisalbuminemia** \bisal′byoonē′mē·ə\ A condition in which two electrophoretically distinct albumins exist simultaneously in the serum of an affected individual. It is known to have a genetic basis. Also *para-albuminemia.*

**bisaxillary** \bisak′səler′ē\ Of or pertaining to both axillae.

**bischloromethyl ether** A highly carcinogenic compound, more potent than its analogue, chloromethyl ether. It is found as a contaminant in the production of resins. Its carcinogenic activity has been confirmed by animal experimentation and an increased risk of lung cancer in exposed workers.

**Bischof** [W. *Bischof,* German neurosurgeon, flourished in the 20th century] Bischof's myelotomy. See under COMMISSURAL MYELOTOMY.

**Bischoff** [Theodor Ludwig Wilhelm *Bischoff,* German anatomist and physiologist, 1807–1882] Bischoff's crown. See under CORONA RADIATA.

**biscuit** [French (from BIS- + French *cuit,* past part. of *cuire* to cook, fire, from L *coquere* to cook), biscuit] In dentistry, fired porcelain before it is glazed.

**biseptate** \bīsep′tāt\ Possessing two partitions.

**bisexual** \bīsek′shoo·əl\ [BI-[1] + SEXUAL] Having anatomic or behavioral characteristics of both sexes. Also *ambisexual.* Compare HERMAPHRODITIC.

**bisexuality** \bī′sekshoo·al′itē\ The quality of having elements of both sexes. It can have physical or psychological manifestations. Also *ambisexuality.*

**bisiliac** \bīsil′ē·ak\ Of or pertaining to both iliac bones or corresponding parts of them.

**Bismarck** [Prince Otto Edward Leopold von *Bismarck-Schoenhausen,* German statesman, 1815–1898] See under BROWN.

**bismuth** \biz′məth\ A metallic element of atomic number 83, atomic weight 208.98. It has various industrial uses. Some compounds are used in cosmetics and medicine. Symbol: Bi **b. magma** MILK OF BISMUTH. **milk of b.** Bismuth hydroxide and bismuth subcarbonate combined in water to contain between 5.2 and 5.8 percent bismuth trioxide. It is used orally as an antacid and topically for the treatment of skin irritations. Also *bismuth magma.* **precipitated b.** A finely divided, purified preparation of metallic bismuth, used in several medicinal forms of bismuth, including preparations suitable for intramuscular injection. It has been essentially replaced by penicillin in the treatment of syphilis.

**bismuth aluminate** $Al_6Bi_2O_{12}\cdot 10H_2O$. A compound whose decahydrate salt is a light powder which is nearly insoluble in water. It has been used as an antacid.

**bismuth and ammonium citrate** A solution containing the equivalent of 5–6% of $Bi_2O_3$, prepared by dissolving bismuth citrate in dilute ammonia solution. It has been used as an antacid.

**bismuth crystal violet** Bismuth crystal violet solution (gentian violet) in which the crystal violet is maintained at an 0.5% concentration in glycerin and water and serves as a bacteriostatic solution. It is used as a topical medication.

**bismuth iodide** $BiI_3$. A compound of bismuth that has been used in combination with emetine in the treatment of intestinal amebiasis.

**bismuth oxychloride** BiOCl. An odorless, tasteless, white powder insoluble in water. It was formerly used intramuscularly in the treatment of syphilis and yaws, and has been given by mouth as an antacid.

**bismuth oxysalicylate** BISMUTH SALICYLATE.

**bismuth salicylate** $C_6H_4OH.CO(BiO)$. A white, basic salt containing approximately 58% bismuth. It is insoluble in water, alcohol, and ether, and it has been given intramuscularly as a suspension in oil in the treatment of syphilis and yaws, and orally in the treatment of intestinal disorders. Also *bismuth subsalicylate, bismuth oxysalicylate.*

**bismuth sodium tartrate** A neutral, white powder containing 35–42% bismuth. It has been used in the treatment of syphilis, yaws, and several other diseases.

**bismuth sodium triglycollamate** $C_{24}H_{28}BiN_4Na_7O_{25}$. A double salt combination of sodium bismuthyl triglycollamate and disodium triglycollamate. It is used in the treatment of lupus erythematosus.

**bismuth subcarbonate** A white, odorless, tasteless powder containing 80–82.5% bismuth in the form of the carbonate salt. It was used orally as an antacid, and has been also used externally in the treatment of mild skin irritations.

**bismuth subgallate** An insoluble, yellow, odorless, tasteless powder containing 46–52% bismuth. It has been used topically as a dusting powder and was formerly used orally in the treatment of gastrointestinal diseases.

**bismuth subsalicylate** BISMUTH SALICYLATE.

**bismuth violet** An antiseptic solution for external use, containing dilute bismuth crystal violet.

**bisobrin lactate** $C_{32}H_{48}N_2O_{20}$. *meso*-1,1′-Tetramethylene bis[1,2,3,4-tetrahydro-6,7-dimethoxyisoquinoline] di-lactate. A fibrinolytic agent.

**bisoxatin acetate** 2,2-Bis(*p*-hydroxyphenyl)-2*H*-1,4-benzoxazin-3(4*H*)-one diacetate. An agent used as a laxative.

**2,3-bisphosphoglyceric acid** *P*—O—$CH_2$—CH(—O—*P*)—COOH. A cofactor in the enzymatic interconversion of 2- and 3-phosphoglyceric acids. This reaction occurs in the breakdown of sugars and in gluconeogenesis via the Embden-Meyerhof pathway. The substance also binds to hemoglobin, stabilizing its deoxygenated form. An increase in its concentration in erythrocytes occurs as part of the mechanism of human adaptation to high altitudes.

**bistable** \bī′stābl\ Having two stable states, as certain electronic circuits.

**bistephanic** \bī′stefan′ik\ Pertaining to both stephanions or, usually, to the shortest distance measured between them. This diameter often corresponds to the maximum breadth of the frontal bone.

**bistratal** \bīstrā′tl\ Having two layers or strata.

**bisulfate** *Obs.* ACID SULFATE.

**bit** [*b(inary) (dig)it*] A unit of computer information representing one binary digit. **check b.** A redundant bit appended to a group of bits to make the sum of the bits always odd or always even to enable error detection.

**bite** 1 A record in modeling material of the relationship of the upper and lower dental arches in occlusion. 2 The pressure developed in closing the jaws. **balanced b.** BALANCED OCCLUSION. **close b.** 1 An abnormally large overbite. 2 A small distance between the maxillary and mandibular arches. Also *deep bite.* **closed b.** 1 OVERCLOSURE. 2 An abnormally large overbite. **convenience b.** ACQUIRED ECCENTRIC OCCLUSION. **cross b.** CROSSBITE. **deep b.** CLOSE BITE. **edge-to-edge b.** EDGE-TO-EDGE OCCLUSION. **locked b.** LOCKED OCCLUSION. **normal b.** NORMAL OCCLUSION. **open b.** Occlusion in which a number of opposing teeth cannot be brought into contact in any position of the mandible. **raised b.** An increased vertical relation brought about accidentally or deliberately by a dental prosthesis or other restoration. It is occasionally caused by overeruption of posterior teeth in chronic periodontitis. **rest b.** A record of the jaws in the rest relation. **stork b.** Any of the marks found on the forehead and nape of the neck of some newborn infants, due to fine capillary angiomas. They fade in a few months. Also *capillary flame, erythema nuchae.* **underhung b.** MANDIBULAR PROGNATHISM. **wax b.** A maxillomandibular record made by interposing wax between the upper and lower teeth. **X-b.** CROSSBITE.

**bite-block** OCCLUSION RIM.

**bitegauge** BITE GAUGE.

**bitemporal** \bītem′pərəl\ Of or pertaining to both temporal bones or both temples or, in anthropometry, to the diameter measured between the posterior ends of the two zygomatic processes, approximating the biauricular diameter.

**biteplane** A sloping biteplate, arranged to move the opposing teeth in a horizontal direction as well as vertically. Also *bite plane.*

**biteplate** An orthodontic appliance having a flat surface arranged to come into contact with opposing teeth in advance of the general closure, in order to depress these teeth relative to the others. Also *bite plate.*

**bite-wing** An intraoral x-ray film with a flat horizontal paper projection which is held between upper and lower cheek teeth during exposure. It is used chiefly for diagnosing proximal caries. • This term was formerly a trade name.

**bithionol** $C_{12}H_6Cl_4O_2S$. 2,2′-Thiobis(4,6-dichlorophenol). An anti-infective agent active against bacteria, molds, and yeast.

**bithionolate sodium** $C_{12}H_4Cl_4Na_2O_2S$. The sodium salt of bithionol. It is used for the same purposes as bithionol.

**bithionol sulfoxide** The sulfoxide derivative of bithionol. It is used as an anti-infective agent.

***Bithynia*** \bithin′ē·ə\ [ancient country of Asia Minor] BULIMUS ***B. fuchsiana*** *BULIMUS FUCHSIANUS*

***Bitis*** \bī′tis\ [New L] A genus of venomous snakes in the family Viperidae. Found in Africa, they are characterized by sluggish movement, a short thick body, and a heart-shaped head.

**Bitot** [Pierre A. *Bitot*, French physician, 1822–1888] Bitot spots, Bitot's patches. See under SPOT.

**bitrochanteric** \bī′trōkənter′ik\ Pertaining to the greater trochanters of the femurs or the greater and lesser trochanters of a single femur.

**bitropic** \bīträp′ik\ [BI-[1] + -TROPIC[1]] Attracted to, or having an affinity for, two different tissues or organs: said especially of certain parasites.

**bitters** A tonic or infusion of bitter-tasting substances prepared from any of a wide variety of plants and acting as an appetite or digestive stimulant by exciting the taste buds and stimulating the excretion of saliva and gastric juices. Those plants that have been used for bitters include *Acorus calamus,* sweet flag; *Aristolochia serpentaria* and *A. reticulata,* snakeroot; *Cinchona*; various *Gentiana* species, such as gentian; *Humulus lupulus,* hops; *Panax quinquefolium,* American gingeng; *Quassia amara,* Suriname quassia; and *Sabatia angularis,* American centaury. Also *amara.* **aromatic b.** Bitters that are effective as a flavoring substance because of their content of volatile oils.

**Bittner** [John Joseph *Bittner*, U.S. biologist, 1904–1961] Bittner milk factor. See under MOUSE MAMMARY TUMOR VIRUS.

**bituberal** \bītʸoo′bərəl\ BI-ISCHIAL.

**bitumen** \bitʸoo′mən\ [L (prob. from Gaulish) tar, asphalt, bitumen] A black, resinous residue produced in the distillation and purification of petroleum and coal. It has been used as a component of dermatological preparations for chronic skin diseases. **sulfonated b.** Bitumen that has been sulfonated and neutralized by adding ammonium sulfate. It has the same uses as bitumen.

**bituminosis** \bitʸoo′minō′sis\ [*bitumin(ous coal)* + -OSIS] COAL WORKERS' PNEUMOCONIOSIS.

**biuret** [BI-[1] + *ure(a)* (assimilated to the obsolescent suffix *-uret,* from New L *-uretum* compound of, -IDE[1])] $NH_2$—CO—NH—CO—$NH_2$. A compound formed by heating urea. See also BIURET TEST.

**bivalent** \bī′vālənt, bīvā′lənt\ 1 Having two valences: used of chemical groups. 2 Having two charges: used of ions. For defs. 1 and 2 also *divalent.* 3 In cytogenetics, characterizing the state of two chromosomes held in apposition by chiasmata during prophase of the first meiotic division. Normally the two chromosomes are a pair of homologues (homomorphic bivalent). Alternatively, the two chromosomes may be partly nonhomologous (heteromorphic bivalent). **4** Having two combining sites for antigen: said of antibodies.

**biventer** \bī′ventər\ [BI- + VENTER] **1** DIGASTRIC. **2** A digastric anatomic structure, usually a muscle. **b. cervicis** MUSCULUS SPINALIS CAPITIS.

**biventral** \bīven′trəl\ DIGASTRIC.

**biventricular** \bī′ventrik′yələr\ Pertaining to or affecting both ventricles of the heart.

**bivitelline** \bī′vītel′in\ [BI- + VITELLINE] Possessing two yolks.

**bixin** $C_{25}H_{30}O_4$. 6,6′Diapo-ψ,ψ-carotenedioic acid monomethyl ester. A carotenoid carboxylic acid isolated from the seeds of *Bixa orellana*, a tropical American and West Indian evergreen. It has been used as a yellow coloring material in foods, such as vegetable oils, and in pharmaceutical preparations.

**bizygomatic** \bī′zīgōmat′ik\ Pertaining to the most lateral or prominent point on each zygomatic arch or, in anthropometry, to the measured distance (bizygomatic breadth) between these two points.

**Bizzozero** [Guilio Cesar *Bizzozero*, Italian physician, 1846–1901] Bizzozero's corpuscle, Bizzozero cell. See under PLATELET.

**Bjerrum** [Jannik Peterson *Bjerrum*, Danish ophthalmologist, 1827–1892] See under SCOTOMETER, SCREEN.

**Bjerrum** [Jannik Petersen *Bjerrum*, Danish ophthalmologist, 1851–1920] Bjerrum sign. See under SCOTOMA.

**Björnstad** [R. *Björnstad*, Danish physician, flourished 20th century] See under SYNDROME.

**Bk** Symbol for the element, berkelium.

**Black** [Greene V. *Black*, U.S. dentist, 1836–1915] See under CLASSIFICATION.

**black** **1** Reflecting very little or no light; denoting the darkest color. **2** Such a color; the color of coal. **animal b.** ANIMAL CHARCOAL. **bone b.** ANIMAL CHARCOAL. **ivory b.** ANIMAL CHARCOAL. **Paris b.** ANIMAL CHARCOAL. **Sudan b. B** A fat stain that is used for demonstrating simple fats and myelin. It has also been used for staining leukocyte granules and the Golgi apparatus.

**blackbody** An ideal thermal radiator that completely absorbs all radiation falling on it and for a given temperature emits the maximum possible thermal radiation.

**Blackfan** [Kenneth D. *Blackfan*, U.S. physician, 1883–1941] Diamond-Blackfan syndrome. See under DIAMOND-BLACKFAN ANEMIA.

**blackfly** A fly of the family Simuliidae. Also *buffalo gnat*. Also *black fly*.

**blackhead** COMEDO.

**blackout** **1** A loss of vision before loss of consciousness caused by inadequate cerebral perfusion, as due to postural hypotension or positive gravitational forces encountered in aerial maneuvers. **2** Amnesia for one's behavior during a drinking episode, characteristic of moderately advanced alcoholics. Also *ambulatory alcoholic automatism*.

**bladder** [Old English *blædre*] **1** A hollow distensible sac; especially, an organ that serves as a receptacle for a liquid or gas; vesica. **2** Specifically, the urinary bladder. See under VESICA URINARIA. **chyle b.** CISTERNA CHYLI. **encysted b.** A condition of the bladder in which a communicating cyst of the urachus forms a vesical diverticulum. **fasciculated b.** A thick-walled bladder having ridges on the inner wall formed by hypertrophied muscle bundles, often associated with the presence of cellulae or diverticula. This condition develops in the presence of chronic urinary outflow obstruction (usually prostate hypertrophy) or neurogenic bladder dysfunction. Also *trabeculated bladder*. **gall b.** See under VESICA BILIARIS. **hypertonic b.** A bladder characterized by an exaggeration of its muscle tonicity caused by a local irritation or inflammation or a spinal cord lesion. **irritable b.** Bladder dysfunction manifested by urge to urinate, frequent urination, and nocturia. The condition may be secondary to an irritative focus within the bladder such as a bladder stone, a bladder tumor, interstitial cystitis, or urinary infection. **nervous b.** An irritable bladder, characterized by urinary frequency and urgency to void, in the absence of documented underlying pathology. *Popular*. **sacculated b.** A bladder having cellulae or diverticula, congenital or acquired, protruding through the muscle fibers of the bladder wall. It is most often seen in conjunction with the bladder wall thickening or trabeculation (fasciculated bladder) associated with urinary outflow obstruction or neurogenic bladder dysfunction. **spinal shock b.** A reaction of the bladder to injury of the spinal cord, characterized by the absence of reflex activity below the level of the lesion. During this period, which may last several weeks, often referred to as the phase of spinal shock, the bladder is areflexic, frequently developing urinary retention and requiring continual or intermittent catheterization for purposes of urinary drainage. After the phase of spinal shock has passed, the bladder may become hyperreflexic. **trabeculated b.** FASCICULATED BLADDER. **urinary b.** VESICA URINARIA.

**bladderworm** CYSTICERCUS.

**blade** A wide, expanded, relatively flat portion, as of a bone. **Foregger b.** A straight laryngoscope blade attached to a light source, for tracheal intubation. **Macintosh b.** The special tongue blade of the Macintosh laryngoscope. **shoulder b.** SCAPULA.

**bladevent** \blād′vent\ In dentistry, a type of blade endosteal implant with perforated blades so that new bone can form in the spaces and so provide positive retention.

**Blainville** [Henri Marie Ducrotay *Blainville*, French zoologist and anthropologist, 1778–1850] Blainville ears. See under EAR.

**Blair** [Vilray Papin *Blair*, U.S. surgeon, 1871–1955] **1** See under KNIFE. **2** Blair-Brown graft. See under SPLIT-SKIN GRAFT.

**Blakemore** [Arthur Hendley *Blakemore*, U.S. surgeon, 1879–1970] Sengstaken-Blakemore tube. See under TUBE.

**Blalock** [Alfred *Blalock*, U.S. surgeon, 1899–1965] **1** Blalock-Taussig operation. See under BLALOCK'S OPERATION. **2** Blalock-Hanlon operation. See under OPERATION.

**Blandin** [Philippe Frédéric *Blandin*, French surgeon, 1798–1849] **1** Blandin's ganglion. See under GANGLION SUBMANDIBULARE. **2** Sublingual ganglion of Blandin. See under GANGLION SUBLINGUALE. **3** Blandin's gland, Blandin and Nuhn gland, anterior lingual gland of Blandin and Nuhn. See under GLANDULA LINGUALIS ANTERIOR.

**blank** In laboratory analysis, an aliquot of inactive material or reagents that is used to provide a baseline against which the analytical end point of the active components can be compared.

**blanket** A covering or coating layer. **hypothermic b.** A blanket, usually of rubber, that contains cold water flowing through tubing for carrying away body heat and inducing hypothermia. **mucus b.** The layer of mucus covering mucous membranes, particularly ciliated mucous membrane, in which the layer is moved continuously in the direction of the beat of the cilia.

**blast**[1] [Gk *blastos* a bud] BLAST CELL.

**blast**[2] [Old English *blaest* (akin to *blāwan* to blow) from common Germanic] An explosion with its associated shock wave. **bechic b.** The rush of air through the bronchi, trachea, and larynx caused by coughing.

**blast-** \blast-\ BLASTO-.

**-blast** \-blast\ [Gk *blastos* bud, germ] A combining form meaning (1) a structure or tissue involved in early embryonic development; (2) a formative, undifferentiated, or precursor cell.

**blastema** \blastē′mə\ [Gk *blastēma* (from *blastanein* to sprout, grow; akin to *blastos* bud, germ) a shoot, offshoot] A tissue or group of cells which, as a result of the complex process of embryonic induction, and following cellular migration and differentiation, give rise either to a complete organ or part of an organ. **metanephric b.** One of the two elements, the other being the ureteric bud, from which the metanephros develops. It forms in the caudal part of the nephrogenic cord and gives origin to the nephros or excretory part of the metanephros. In rare cases a part of the metanephric blastema may undergo malignant transformation to form a nephroblastoma (Wilms tumor). Also *metanephrogenic blastema.*

**blastin** \blas′tin\ A substance which nourishes cells or stimulates their growth.

**blasto-** \blas′tō-\ [Gk *blastos* bud, germ] A combining form meaning bud, germ, relating to early growth or development. Also *blast-.*

**blastocele** \blas′təsēl\ BLASTOCOELE.

**blastocoele** \blas′təsēl\ [BLASTO- + -COELE] The cavity of a blastula. Also *segmentation cavity, cleavage cavity.* Also *blastocele.*

**blastocyst** \blas′təsist\ [BLASTO- + CYST] The modified blastula of mammals. It consists of a hollow sphere of cells which results from the process of cleavage, and is formed at the late morula stage when fluid passes into the intercellular spaces between the inner and outer layers of cells. The blastocyst is divided into two parts, an outer layer of small slightly flattened cells, the trophoblast (trophoblastic ectoderm), and an inner cell mass consisting of a small group of larger polyhedral cells contained within the trophoblastic vesicle. The cavity of the blastocyst (blastocoele) separates the trophoblast from the inner cell mass except for the small area where they are in contact. Also *embryonic sac, blastodermic vesicle.*

**blastoderm** \blas′tōdurm′\ [BLASTO- + -DERM] In mammals, the outer layer of cells of the blastula surrounding a cavity, the blastocoele. The blastoderm lines the zona pellucida, and its cells, the blastomeres, are formed as the result of cleavage of the fertilized ovum. Also *membrana germinativa.* **embryonic b.** The part of the blastoderm giving rise to the embryo proper. **extraembryonic b.** The part of the blastoderm which gives rise to the membranes rather than the embryo proper. **trilaminar b.** The stage of development in which the embryo is represented by the three primary layers: the ectoderm, the mesoderm, and the entoderm. This results from the process of gastrulation which takes place during the first hours of incubation, such as in birds. The primitive streak appears within about 10 hours, and Hensen's node within about 15 hours. The three germ layers are established by about 20 hours. The process of gastrulation is completed when the three layers are established.

**blastodisk** \blas′tədisk\ [BLASTO- + DISK] A flattened convex plate of embryonic blastodermal cells (blastomeres) present on the surface of the yolk in ova with a large amount of that substance and which undergo incomplete cleavage, as in the avian egg. **bilaminar b.** A developmental stage of the blastodisk when only ectoderm and endoderm can be identified.

**blastogenesis** \-jen′əsis\ [BLASTO- + GENESIS] **1** Reproduction by budding; asexual reproduction. **2** The transmission of inherited characters by the germ plasm. **3** The early stage of development of an embryo with the formation of the blastoderm. Adj. blastogenetic, blastogenic.

**blastoma** \blastō′mə\ [BLAST- + -OMA] **1** A tumor of embryonic type, as a retinoblastoma, nephroblastoma, hepatoblastoma, or neuroblastoma. **2** *Obs.* NEOPLASM. **pulmonary b.** A lung tumor composed of immature pulmonary epithelial and stromal elements. The degree of malignancy is variable. It occurs in adults as well as children. Also *pneumoblastoma.*

**blastomere** \blas′təmir\ [BLASTO- + -MERE] One of the cells into which the egg divides following the first or subsequent cleavage mitoses, and before obvious cell differentiation begins. Also *cleavage cell, segmentation cell.* **formative b.** One of the blastomeres destined to give rise to the embryo rather than to the trophoblast.

**blastomerotomy** \-mirät′əmē\ [*blastomer(e)* + *o* + -TOMY] Destruction of a blastomere or blastomeres. Also *blastotomy.*

***Blastomyces*** \blas′tōmī′sēz\ [BLASTO- + Gk *mykēs* mushroom, fungus] An obsolete genus of yeastlike, monilial fungi that included *Paracoccidioides* and the imperfect stage of *Ajellomyces (B. dermatitidis).* ***B. dermatitidis*** The form-species of the fungus which is the etiologic agent of (North American) blastomycosis. It is actually the imperfect stage of *Ajellomyces dermatitidis.*

**blastomycete** \-mīsēt′\ [BLASTO- + *-mycete(s)*] Any fungus of the genera *Paracoccidioides* or *Blastomyces.*

**blastomycin** \-mī′sin\ A sterile filtrate from a broth culture of *Blastomyces dermatitidis.* It is used in intradermal tests.

**blastomycosis** \-mīkō′sis\ [*Blastomyc(es)* + -OSIS] **1** A granulomatous, suppurative, slowly progressing infectious disease caused by the fungus *Blastomyces dermatitidis.* There are two main clinical presentations, systemic blastomycosis and cutaneous blastomycosis. The disease usually begins as a respiratory infection with cough, pleural chest pain, fever, chills, malaise, anorexia, and weight loss. The infection may subsequently disseminate to the skin, bones, and internal genitalia. It is found in North America, several African countries, and in Latin America. Also *Gilchrist's disease, North American blastomycosis, Gilchrist's mycosis.* **2** See under SOUTH AMERICAN BLASTOMYCOSIS **Brazilian b.** SOUTH AMERICAN BLASTOMYCOSIS. **cutaneous b.** A mycotic infection of the skin caused by *Blastomyces dermatitidis* (North American blastomycosis) or *Paracoccidioides brasiliensis* (South American blastomycosis). The portal of entry is usually the lung, spores being inhaled from contaminated soil, or mouth. The South American variety has a predilection for mucocutaneous junctions. The lesions are crusted in character. Also *dermatitis blastomycotica.* **European b.** CRYPTOCOCCOSIS. **North American b.** BLASTOMYCOSIS. **South American b.** A chronic infectious disease caused by the fungus *Paracoccidioides brasiliensis* and found in most South American countries and as far north as Mexico. The disease is characterized by ulcerated, granulomatous lesions of the oral and nasal mucosa, pharynx, larynx, vocal cords, and skin; by lymphadenopathy; by nodular visceral lesions, especially in the lungs; and by respiratory symptoms, including dyspnea, cough, and purulent or bloody sputum. Also *paracoccidioidomycosis, Brazilian blastomycosis, Lutz-Splendore-Almeida disease, Almeida's disease,* *paracoccidioidal granuloma.* **systemic b.** Blastomycosis of either the North American or South American variety that may involve most organs in the body through dissemination of the infection. The causative organisms are identical to those producing cutaneous blastomycosis. The infecting organisms enter the body through the mouth or through the lungs by inhalation.

**blastomycotic** \-mīkät′ik\ Pertaining to blastomycosis.

**blastoneuropore** \-n^yŭr′əpôr\ A transient aperture formed by the fusion of the blastopore and the neuropore in certain embryos.

**blastopore** \blas′təpôr\ [BLASTO- + PORE] In mammalian embryos, an opening or pit resulting from the inward migration of the embryonic ectodermal cells situated at the cephalic extremity of the primitive streak (Hensen's node or the primitive knot). A cord of cells known as the notochordal or head process migrates from Hensen's node between the ectoderm and endoderm. The invagination of the blastopore then extends into the notochordal process to form the notochordal or archenteric (later neurenteric) canal. During gastrulation in nonmammalian miolecithal eggs the blastopore is the circular opening where the outer layer of cells or ectoderm is continuous with the invaginated endoderm.

**blastotomy** \blastät′əmē\ [BLASTO- + -TOMY] BLASTOMEROTOMY.

**blastula** \blas′tyələ\ [New L, dim. of Gk *blastos* a bud, shoot, sucker] The usually spherical structure produced by cleavage of a fertilized egg. It follows the morula stage and consists of a single layer of cells (blastoderm) surrounding a fluid-filled cavity (blastocoele).

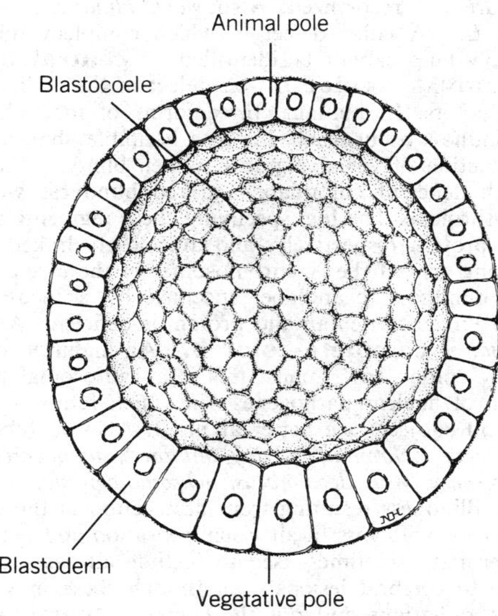


**Blastula** (hemisected)

**blastulae** \blas′tyəlē\ Plural of BLASTULA.

**blastulation** \blas′tyəlā′shən\ The conversion of a morula to a blastula by the development of a more or less regular central cavity (blastocoele). In the human species this occurs on about the fourth day of development, shortly after the ovum passes from the oviduct into the uterine cavity. In man as in other mammals the blastula is somewhat modified into a blastocyst, and shortly after its formation the zona pellucida is lost at the start of implantation.

**Blatin** [Marc *Blatin*, French physician, born 1878] Blatin sign. See under HYDATID THRILL.

***Blatta*** \blat′ə\ The type genus of the cockroach family Blattidae, the most widespread and economically important species being the oriental cockroach, *Blatta orientalis.*

***Blattella germanica*** \blatel′ə jərman′ikə\ The so-called German cockroach, probably the most widely distributed and universally common cockroach.

**Blattidae** \blat′idē\ [L *blatt(a)* a cockroach + -IDAE] A family of cockroaches that includes some important domiciliated pests of humans such as *Blatta orientalis,* the oriental cockroach, and *Periplaneta americana,* the American cockroach. The genus *Supella* includes other important pest insects in this family.

**bleaching** The removal of discoloration, as from a tooth with oxygenating agent and sometimes heat. It may be carried out internally in the case of nonvital teeth or externally for vital teeth.

**bleb** \bleb\ [onomatopoeic, from making a bubble with the lips] **1** A fluid filled space that is either within or beneath the epidermis and is usually greater than 1 cm in diameter. Compare BULLA, VESICLE. **2** An evagination of an intracellular membrane. **nuclear b.** A fingerlike extension of the outer nuclear membrane which may pinch off to form a vesicle. The sites of the nuclear bleb may represent sites of new membrane formation, with the vesicles coalescing to form endoplasmic reticulum or Golgi membranes.

**bleed** / **nose b.** EPISTAXIS.

**bleeder** **1** Any person or animal with a tendency to bleed. **2** A blood vessel from which blood escapes in a surgical field.

**bleeding** **1** The extravasation of blood from transected or partially transected vessels. **2** Purposeful removal of blood from the circulation; phlebotomy. **dysfunctional uterine b.** Abnormal painless bleeding which occurs in the absence of obvious pathology, usually caused by anovulation. **functional b.** Bleeding associated with normal menses. **implantation b.** Bleeding during early pregnancy from eroded uterine blood vessels at the site of implantaton of the fertilized ovum. Also *placentation bleeding.* **midcyclical b.** Uterine bleeding which occurs around the time of ovulation. **occult b.** Bleeding, especially from the gastrointestinal tract, in amounts too small for its evidence to be detected with the naked eye. **placentation b.** IMPLANTATION BLEEDING. **postmenopausal b.** Bleeding from the genital tract which occurs at least six months after a menopause. **punctate b.** **1** Capillary bleeding. **2** Brisk bleeding from the dermal vascular plexus used as an end point to ensure bed viability during the tangential excision and grafting of a burn wound.

**blenno-** \blen′ō-\ [Gk *blennos* mucus] A combining form denoting mucus. Also *blenn-.*

**blennogenic** \blen′əjen′ik\ MUCIGENOUS.

**blennogenous** \blenäj′ənəs\ MUCIGENOUS.

**blennorrhagia** \blen′ôrā′jə\ [BLENNO- + -RRHAGIA] **1** GONORRHEA. **2** BLENNORRHEA.

**blennorrhea** \blen′ôrē′ə\ [BLENNO- + -RRHEA] A conjunctival inflammation resulting in mucoid discharge. Adj. blennorrheal. **b. neonatorum** Any form of conjunctivitis in the newborn, but especially gonococcal ophthalmia.

**blennorrhoea** *Brit.* BLENNORRHEA.

**bleomycin** A group of glycopeptide antibiotics isolated from *Streptomyces verticillus* and having antineoplastic activity. They are divided into bleomycins A and B, depending upon differences in their terminal amines.

**bleomycin sulfate** The sulfates of a mixture of related glycopeptide antibiotics from *Streptomyces verticillus* or by synthesis. These include bleomycins $A_2$ and $B_2$ and related components that copurify with them. The agent is given parenterally and is used as an antineoplastic drug against squamous cell carcinoma, Hodgkin's disease, other lymphomas, and malignant neoplasms of the testis.

**blephar-** \blef′ər-\ BLEPHARO-.

**blepharadenitis** \blef′ərad′ənī′tis\ [BLEPHAR- + ADENITIS] Inflammation of eyelid glands, such as the meibomian glands, the Zeis glands, or the Moll glands.

**blepharal** \blef′ərəl\ [BLEPHAR- + -AL] Pertaining to the eyelid.

**blepharectomy** \blef′ərek′təmē\ [BLEPHAR- + -ECTOMY] Surgical removal of part or all of an eyelid.

**blepharism** \blef′ərizm\ [BLEPHAR- + -ISM] BLEPHAROSPASM.

**blepharitis** \blef′ərī′tis\ [BLEPHAR- + -ITIS] Inflammation of the eyelid. Also *lippa, lippitude*. Adj. blepharitic. **b. angularis** Inflammation of the lateral canthi. **marginal b.** Inflammation of the apposing edges of the eyelids. Also *blepharitis marginalis, echinophthalmia, tylosis ciliaris, granular lid, blepharitis ciliaris.* **seborrheic b.** The presence of scaly and greasy flakes deposited along the eyelid margins. Also *blepharitis squamosa, squamous seborrheic blepharitis.* **b. ulcerosa** Inflammation of the eyelids of sufficient severity to cause local areas of tissue necrosis. Also *ulcerative blepharitis, psorophthalmia.*

**blepharo-** \blef′ərō-\ [Gk *blepharon* eyelid] A combining form denoting (1) the eyelid; (2) cilia. Also *blephar-*.

**blepharoadenoma** \-ad′ənō′mə\ [BLEPHARO- + ADENOMA] An epithelial tumor of the eyelids.

**blepharochalasis** \-kal′əsis\ [BLEPHARO- + Gk *chalasis* a slackening, loosening] A redundancy and drooping of the skin folds of the upper eyelids. Also *blepharodermachalasis.*

**blepharoclonus** \blef′əräk′lōnəs\ [BLEPHARO- + CLONUS] Clonic intermittent opening and closing of the eyelids.

**blepharocoloboma** \-käl′əbō′mə\ [BLEPHARO- + COLOBOMA] A notch or fissure of the eyelid. It may be of developmental origin, in which case it is likely to be associated with an oblique facial cleft, or it may be of pathologic or traumatic origin.

**blepharoconjunctivitis** \-känjungk′tivī′tis\ Associated inflammation of both the eyelid margins and the conjunctiva.

**blepharodermachalasis** \-dur′məkal′əsis\ BLEPHAROCHALASIS.

**blepharodiastasis** \-dī·as′təsis\ [BLEPHARO- + DIASTASIS] An inability to close the eyelids or to close them completely.

**blepharon** \blef′ərän\ [Gk, eyelid] PALPEBRA.

**blepharopachynsis** \-pakin′sis\ The thickening of an eyelid as a result of a pathologic condition.

**blepharophimosis** \-fimō′sis\ [BLEPHARO- + PHIMOSIS] The inability to open the eyelids to the usual degree.

**blepharoplast** \blef′ərōplast′\ [BLEPHARO- + -PLAST] BASAL BODY.

**blepharoplasty** \blef′ərōplas′tē\ [BLEPHARO- + -PLASTY] Surgical correction of an eyelid deformity. Also *tarsoplasty, tarsoplasia.*

**blepharoptosis** \-tō′sis\ [BLEPHARO- + PTOSIS] Downward displacement of an upper eyelid.

**blepharorrhaphy** \blef′ərôr′əfē\ [BLEPHARO- + -RRHAPHY] **1** Surgical repair of an eyelid wound. **2** TARSORRHAPHY.

**blepharospasm** \blef′ərōspazm′\ [BLEPHARO- + SPASM] Involuntary contraction of the orbicularis oculi, resulting in firm closure of both eyes. Also *nictitating spasm, winking spasm, spasmus nictitans.* **essential b.** Blepharospasm occurring in the absence of disease of the eye or the sensory afferent fibers from the eye and cornea. **symptomatic b.** Blepharospasm due to an organic nervous disorder such as postencephalitic parkinsonism.

**blepharosphincterectomy** \-sfingk′tərek′təmē\ [BLEPHARO- + SPHINCTER + -ECTOMY] Excision of a portion of the orbicularis oculi muscle, performed for the relief of severe blepharospasm.

**blepharostat** \blef′ərōstat′\ [BLEPHARO- + -STAT] A surgical instrument for holding an eyelid.

**blepharotomy** \blef′ərät′əmē\ [BLEPHARO- + -TOMY] The surgical cutting of an eyelid, as to drain an abscess. Also *tarsotomy.*

**Blessig** [Robert *Blessig*, German physician, 1830–1878] **1** See under GROOVE. **2** Blessig cyst, Blessig's lacunae. See under CYST.

**blind** [Old English, from common Germanic] **1** Unable to see; without the power of sight. **2** Closed at one end; having no separate outlet, as *a blind gut* (the cecum), *a blind fistula.*. **color b.** Affected by color blindness; unable to distinguish certain hues.

**blindgut** CAECUM.

**blindism** \blīn′dizm\ Any stereotyped hand or body movement, such as rubbing the eyes or flapping the hands, that occurs in a child with impaired vision when the child is anxious or feels under pressure to perform.

**blindness** [Old English *blind* + -NESS] The inability to see; lack of the power of sight. See also AMAUROSIS, LEGAL BLINDNESS. **amnesic color b.** COLOR NAME APHASIA. **apperceptive b.** VISUAL AGNOSIA. **blue b.** A color defect in which spectral colors corresponding to short wavelengths are not recognized. Also *violet blindness.* **blue-yellow b.** A color defect in which complementary blue and yellow hues cannot be identified. **central b.** CENTRAL SCOTOMA. **color b.** A defect in the ability to distinguish colors. In humans, three forms of monochromatic color blindness occur, each due to a heritable abnormality in the production of visual pigment. Green blindness is associated with deficient chloralabe and red blindness with deficient erythrolabe. The loci specifying these pigments are deutan and protan, respectively, and are closely linked distally on the long arm of the X chromosome. In the rare condition of blue blindness, cyanolabe, specified by a locus that is probably linked to deutan and protan, is deficient. Also *color amblyopia.* **complete color b.** An inability to distinguish any colors. In humans, this is an autosomal recessive condition of unclear pathogenesis in which retinal cones are absent and subjects see better at night. Also *achromatopsia, achromatopia, achromatism, day blindness, monochromatism, monochromasy, visus decoloratus, achromatognosia.* **cortical b.** Blindness resulting from destruction of the occipital visual cortex, with loss of all visual sensation and perception. • The term is sometimes used to include all cases of blindness due to cerebral lesions even though these may involve the optic radiations and not the cortex. **cortical psychic b.** VISUAL AGNOSIA. **day b.** **1** HEMERALOPIA. **2** COMPLETE COLOR BLINDNESS. **flash b.** Temporary inability to see after exposure to an intensely bright light due to inactivation of the photopigments. **flight b.** A blindness that occurs without loss of consciousness in pilots of aircraft during sudden turns at high speed, when the eyes or brain are temporarily deprived of blood. **hysterical b.** Blindness resulting from hysteria in the absence of any physical abnormality of the eye or visual pathways. Also *mind blindness, psychanopsia.* **legal b.** A legally defined degree of loss of vision that qualifies the individual for certain social benefits. A common stipulation in the United States is 20/200 or less corrected distant acuity or 20 degrees or less of visual field. In the United Kingdom the legal definition is "so blind as to be unable to perform work for which eyesight is essential." (National Insurance Act, 1948). • Although definitions of *legal blindness* vary in different jurisdictions, definitions comparable to that of the United States obtain in Canada, Australia, India, and Japan (although in Japan the definition stipulates 10 degrees or less of visual field). In South Africa, the definition is similar to that used in the United Kingdom. **letter b.** A specific form of word blindness in which the patient is unable to recognize printed or written letters. **mind b.** 1 HYSTERICAL BLINDNESS. 2 *Obs.* VISUAL AGNOSIA. **musical b.** A form of alexia marked by the inability to recognize and interpret musical notations. Also *musical alexia, receptive amusia, note blindness.* **night b.** NYCTALOPIA. **note b.** MUSICAL BLINDNESS. **object b.** Visual agnosia for objects. **psychic b.** VISUAL AGNOSIA. **pure word b.** Alexia affecting the ability to read words. "Interior language" is retained, reading being the only language modality to be lost. The patient can write spontaneously and to dictation but cannot read what he has written. He may also have difficulty in identifying shapes, or orienting lines, and cannot understand the structure and form of letters. Copying is carried out with great difficulty and is always incomplete, with mistakes with regard to letters and to lines, whereas spontaneous writing is unimpaired. Also *geometric alexia, isolated alexia, occipital alexia, optic alexia, pure alexia, alexia without aphasia, sensory alexia, symbolic alexia, verbal alexia, Wernicke subcortical opticoagnosia.* **red b.** A form of faulty color vision in which spectral colors corresponding to long wavelengths are not recognized. **red-green b.** Defective color vision affecting red and green recognition. This may include protanopia, deuteranopia, protanomaly, and deuteranomaly. **river b.** Blindness resulting from onchocerciasis. See also OCULAR ONCHOCERCIASIS. **sign b.** Visual agnosia for signs or gestures. It is a form of visual asymbolia. **snow b.** Temporary visual loss due to corneal epithelial damage by ultraviolet light reflected from the surface of snow. Also *niphablepsia, ophthalmia nivialis.* **solar b.** Visual loss from corneal damage by ultraviolet or retinal damage by infrared or visible rays of sunlight. Also *sun blindness.* **sun b.** SOLAR BLINDNESS. **text b.** ALEXIA. **twilight b.** The inability of the eyes to function normally in the mesopic range of adaptation. **word b.** 1 A type of alexia or restricted form of receptive aphasia marked by the inability to recognize and interpret written words or signs, although the individual letters are recognized. Also *typholexia.* 2 ALEXIA.

**blink** [Middle English *blenken* to flinch; of obscure origin] A reflex closure of the eyelids in response to sudden movement within the visual field close to the face or on sudden exposure to bright light.

**blister** [Middle English; akin to Old English *blæst* blast] 1 A fluid-filled space either within or beneath the epidermis. 2 To form a blister. **burn b.** A blister formed following a partial thickness burn. **fever b.** COLD SORE. **Marochetti's b.'s** Small blisters which occur on the underside of the tongue in rabies. **water b.** A blister that is filled with a clear fluid. *Popular.*

**bloater / blue b.** A patient with cyanosis and congestive heart failure resulting from chronic obstructive pulmonary disease. An informal term. Compare PINK PUFFER.

**Bloch** [Bruno *Bloch,* Swiss dermatologist, 1878–1933] 1 Bloch's method for dopa oxidase. See under METHOD. 2 Bloch-Sulzberger syndrome. See under INCONTINENTIA PIGMENTI.

# block

**block** 1 An obstruction or hindrance to passage. 2 Inhibition of normal flow, action, or conduction. 3 An interruption in nerve impulses or electrical signals. See also BLOCKING. **affect b.** An inability to express emotions adequately and appropriately. It stems from inhibition and is seen especially in obsessive-compulsive neurotics and schizophrenics. **alveolar-capillary b.** Impairment of the passage of oxygen or similar gases across the alveolocapillary membrane. It may be the result of various conditions including, for example, diffuse interstitial pulmonary fibrosis. **anesthetic b.** The interruption of nerve impulses by injection of an anesthetic agent around a nerve to produce temporary or long-lasting sensory loss. **anode b.** The electrical stimulation block of nerve or muscle impulse conduction at the anode due to a reduced depolarization, hyperpolarization of the cell membrane. Also *anodal block, anodic block, hyperpolarization block.* **anterograde b.** A block in the conduction of the electrical impulse on its route from the sinuatrial node to the ventricles. **arborization b.** Block of the conduction impulse within the cardiac ventricles, possibly due to block in the ramifications of Purkinje fibers. **articular b.** A condition whereby a joint cannot achieve its full range of movement owing to an intra-articular obstruction. **atrioventricular b.** Block of conduction between the cardiac atria and ventricles. **Bier b.** A technique of regional anesthetic administration in which the veins of an extremity distal to a suprasystolic tourniquet are filled with a local anesthetic solution. **brachial b.** A regional block in which an upper extremity is anesthetized by infiltrating its three major nerves with a local anesthetic agent at the axilla. **bundle branch b.** Heart block affecting one of the two branches of the atrioventricular bundle. Also *interventricular block.* **caudal b.** CAUDAL ANESTHESIA. **cerebrospinal-fluid b.** Obstruction of the subarachnoid space, preventing the normal circulation of cerebrospinal fluid. **complete heart b.** Complete cessation of conduction from the atria to the ventricles. Also *complete atrioventricular dissociation.* **cryogenic b.** The reduction of tissue activity by means of local cooling. **entrance b.** A heart block which prevents depolarization or inactivation of an ectopic pacemaker. Thus, provided there is no exit block, the ectopic pacemaker can continue to initiate the effective impulses while being protected because of a unidirectional blockade. It is a feature of parasystole. Also *protective block.* **epidural b.** EPIDURAL ANESTHESIA. **exit b.** The blocking of transmission from a cardiac pacemaker to surrounding tissue. An exit block may occur with any of the potential pacemaking tissues of the heart and also with artificial pacemakers. **field b.** FIELD BLOCK ANESTHESIA. **first-degree atrioventricular b.** A form of block in which all impulses are transmitted abnormally slowly between the atria and ventricles, associated with prolongation of the P-R interval. **ganglionic b.** Interruption of synaptic transmission in ganglia that may be caused by local anesthesia or by drugs which block the action of neurotransmitters. While this term can refer to such a mechanism involving any ganglion it most often refers to the sympathetic ganglia in the autonomic nervous system. **heart b.** Slowing or obstruction to conduction of impulses through the normal conducting tissues of the heart, applied particularly to atrioventricular conduction, through the atrioventricular node and bundle. **high degree atrioventricular b.** A second- or third-degree atrioventricular block. **hyperpolarization b.** ANODE BLOCK. **incomplete heart b.** Heart block which is less than complete. **incomplete left bundle branch b.** Loss of conduction in part of the left bundle branch. **incomplete right bundle branch b.** A condition in which conduction is partially but not completely blocked in the right bundle branch, often characterized by a QRS complex showing an rSr pattern less than 0.12 seconds in duration. It may be due to delay in conduction within the ventricle rather than within the bundle branch itself. **intercostal b.** INTERCOSTAL ANESTHESIA. **interventricular b.** BUNDLE BRANCH BLOCK. **intra-atrial b.** Impaired conduction through the atria, often associated with broadening and bifid appearance of P waves. **intraspinal b.** The obstruction of the subarachnoid space by any compressive lesion in the spinal canal. **intraventricular b.** Impaired conduction through the ventricles either because of bundle branch block or block within the ventricular tissue. **left bundle branch b.** Heart block affecting the left bundle branch, associated with broadening of the QRS complex to 0.12 seconds or more. **manometric b.** Absence of increase in distal cerebrospinal fluid pressure, as measured by a spinal manometer, when intracranial pressure is temporarily increased by compression of the jugular veins. Obstruction of the spinal subarachnoid space is implied. **meningeal b.** Interruption of the free flow of cerebrospinal fluid in the subarachnoid space due either to compression or meningeal adhesions. **Mobitz b.** Either of two types of second-degree atrioventricular block involving dropped beats. Type 1, usually resulting from a block in the atrioventricular nodal tissues, is a Wenckebach block, with progressive prolongation of the P-R interval until a ventricular beat is dropped, the cycle then repeating itself. Type 2, usually due to a block in both bundle branches, is marked by intermittent dropped beats without progressive prolongation of the P-R interval. Also *Mobitz-type atrioventricular dissociation.* **nerve b.** An interruption of a nerve's impulses, usually by injection of an anesthetic agent about a nerve. **neuromuscular b.** A spontaneous or therapeutic interruption in the transmission of nerve impulses to muscle, as may be caused by local anesthesia or disease. **paravertebral b.** PARAVERTEBRAL BLOCK ANESTHESIA. **partial b.** A disorder of cardiac conduction in which some beats are conducted and others are not. **partial atrioventricular b.** Partial block affecting atrioventricular conduction. **peri-infarction b.** An intraventricular conduction defect associated with a myocardial infarct. **portal b.** Obstruction of the portal vein. **protective b.** ENTRANCE BLOCK. **regional b.** LOCAL ANESTHESIA. **retrograde b.** Impairment of conduction in a retrograde direction, that is, from ventricle or junctional tissues to the atria. **right bundle branch b.** Defective conduction through the right branch of the atrioventricular bundle. **sacral b.** CAUDAL ANESTHESIA. **second-degree atrioventricular b.** Atrioventricular block in which some impulses are conducted to the ventricles while others are not; partial atrioventricular block. Also *second-degree heart block.* **segmental b.** A spinal, epidural, or peripheral nerve block confined to a specific or limited number of dermatomes. **sinuatrial b.** A conduction defect in which there is partial or complete blockade of impulses leaving the sinuatrial node of the heart. Also *sinoauricular block.* **sphenopalatine ganglion b.** Application of a topical anesthetic to the sphenopalatine ganglia (ganglia pterygopalatina). See also SYMPATHICOTHERAPY. **spinal subarachnoid b.** **1** An obstruction in the spinal canal causing closure of the spinal subarachnoid space. **2** Spinal anesthesia produced with an anesthetic agent injected into the subarachnoid space. For defs. 1 and 2 also *spinal block.* **splanchnic b.** SPLANCHNIC ANESTHESIA. **stellate b.** An interruption of the efferent and afferent impulses traversing the ganglion cervicothoracicum (stellate ganglion) to and from the head, neck, hands, and heart, produced by an injection of an anesthetic agent. **subarachnoid b.** An obstruction of the subarachnoid space about the brain or spinal cord, usually caused by a tumor, inflammation, or hematoma. **sympathetic b.** An interruption in the conduction of nerve impulses in any part of the thoracolumbar division of the autonomic nervous system, produced by administering a local anesthetic. **third-degree heart b.** Complete heart block, there being no conduction of impulses from the atria to the ventricles. **total spinal b.** TOTAL SPINAL ANESTHESIA. **unidirectional b.** A block in which impulses are blocked from traveling in one direction along a conduction pathway but not in the opposite direction. It is a characteristic component of reentry. **ventricular b.** Obstruction of any part of the ventricular system of the brain, preventing normal circulation of ventricular fluid. It is usually caused by a tumor in the third or fourth ventricle, or by neoplastic or atretic occlusion of the iter, the foramen of Luschka, or the foramen of Magendie. Such obstruction, if unrelieved, results in hydrocephalic dilatation of all lumina anterior to the block. **vertebral b.** The inability of one vertebra to move in relation to its neighbor because of articular pathology or muscle spasm. **Wenckebach b.** A form of partial heart block in which there is a progressive prolongation of conduction from one site to another, until one beat is not conducted, following which conduction restarts with a further episode of progressive prolongation, and the cycle is repeated. It usually occurs as a Mobitz block, type 1, a second-degree atrioventricular block in which there is progressive prolongation of the P-R interval over a number of beats until one ventricular beat is dropped. Also *Wenckebach's phenomenon.* **Wilson b.** Right bundle branch block associated with a tall R wave in lead I and a broad, low-voltage S wave.

**blockade** \bläkād′\ Transient interruption of the activity of a functional system, usually by a chemical substance. **adrenergic b.** Chemical inhibition of sympathetic effector responses and related catecholamine release. **cholinergic b.** Chemical inhibition of cholinergic synapses, including those in autonomic ganglia, parasympathetic postganglionic effectors, and myoneural junctions. **lymphatic b.** Obstruction of the vessels that normally permit lymph to flow from peripheral regions to the thoracic duct and right lymphatic duct and from there into the venous circulation. Such obstruction may be due to tumors, microfilariae, surgery, or other causes, and commonly results in persistent swelling of the extremity that is distal to the site of obstruction. **neuromuscular b.** Failure of excitation of muscle contraction by an impulse descending its motor axon due to failure to invade the motor endplates, failure to transmit effectively across the neuromuscular synapse, or insensitivity of receptor sites on the muscle-fiber membrane. **reticuloendothelial b.** The state of the cells of the reticuloendothelial system following parenteral administration of quantities of inert particles, as of carbon or iron. The mononuclear phagocytic cells of the reticuloendothelial system engulf these particles and thus phagocytosis is temporarily suspended. **sympathetic b.** Chemical inhibition of synaptic activity in sympathetic ganglia whereby postganglionic neurons are not excited.

**blockage** \bläk′ij\ A blocked condition or place. **renal b.** 1 Obstruction of the renal pelvis or ureter, interfering with passage of urine. 2 *Obs.* ACUTE RENAL FAILURE.

**blocker** A pharmacologic agent whose mechanism of action depends upon prevention of a normal or usual action of a pathway or receptor. **alpha b.** 1 Any of a class of drugs that block the alpha-adrenergic receptor. These are further classified by their relative selectivity in blocking $\alpha_1$ and $\alpha_2$ receptors. Drugs in this class are used in the treatment of pheochromocytoma and to acutely lower blood pressure. 2 Any agent capable of blocking the binding and effect of agonists at alpha-adrenergic receptors. For defs. 1 and 2 also *alpha-adrenergic antagonist.* **beta b.** 1 Any of a class of drugs that block the beta-adrenergic receptor. These are further classified by their relative selectivity in blocking $\beta_1$ or $\beta_2$ receptors. Depending on their pharmacologic action, drugs in this class are used for the treatment of angina, hypertension, cardiac arrhythmias, glaucoma, and hyperthyroidism. 2 Any agent capable of blocking the binding and effect of agonists at alpha-adrenergic receptors. For defs. 1 and 2 also *beta-adrenergic antagonist.* **bronchial b.** A balloon used for the occlusion of a bronchus during endobronchial anesthesia. The anesthetic is administered through only one lung in order to allow the other lung to collapse for surgery or to prevent spillage of secretions from an infected lung. **calcium channel b.** 1 Any agent that tends to block the movement of calcium ions through a pore in the membrane known as the calcium channel. 2 Any of a class of drugs that block the movement of calcium ions through the calcium channel. Blockage of this channel alters the polarization of the membrane as well as the intracellular levels of calcium. Calcium channel blockers are used in the treatment of angina, cardiac arrhythmias, hypertension, and cerebral vasospasm. For defs. 1 and 2 also *calcium antagonist* (not recommended). **neuromuscular b.** Any drug given for muscle paralysis during general anesthesia. It acts at the neuromuscular junction either by competition with acetylcholine, as tubocurarine, or by extended depolarization, as succinylcholine. **starch b.** An agent that is supposed to inhibit the natural breakdown of starch in the gut into smaller absorbable molecules. As a result the starch, as well as the calories it contains, is excreted in the stool in an unutilized form. To date, starch blockers have been shown to be limited value in weight reduction and may have undesired side-effects if used on a long-term basis.

**blocking** 1 Capable of interrupting or inhibiting. 2 Interruption; inhibition; blockage. 3 In clinical encephalography, the temporary interruption of a cerebral rhythm, brought about by a sudden stimulus. The most frequent example is temporary blockage of the alpha rhythm by sensory excitation (usually visual), as when the subject opens his eyes. **alpha b.** 1 The inhibition of transmission at alpha-adrenergic nerve endings, as by means of drugs. 2 The inhibition of the alpha (9–11/sec) rhythm of a cortical electroencephalogram and its replacement by another type of rhythm, usually a faster, low-voltage rhythm. **b. of thought** A sudden stoppage in the train of thought, often a manifestation of schizophrenia. Also *thought deprivation, thought withdrawal, sejunction.*

**blood** [Old English *blōd,* akin to German *Blut* blood, prob. to Old English *blōwan* to bloom] The red fluid that circulates in arteries, capillaries, and veins. It consists of plasma and several sorts of cells, especially erythrocytes, leukocytes, and platelets. **arterial b.** Blood that is within arteries or has been obtained from an artery, as by arterial puncture. **banked b.** Blood which has been obtained from a donor, treated with anticoagulants and preservatives, and stored until needed for transfusion. **cord b.** Blood contained within the umbilical cord. **defibrinated b.** Blood from which the fibrin has been removed during coagulation. **laky b.** Blood which has undergone partial or complete hemolysis. **occult b.** Blood present in amounts too small to be detected with the naked eye. **oxalated b.** Blood anticoagulated by the addition of oxalate. **peripheral b.** The blood in systemic circulation that is remote from the heart. **sludged b.** Red cell clumping and sedimentation *in vivo* with resultant obstruction of smaller vessels. Shock is often causative. **splanchnic b.** The blood in that part of the visceral circulation innervated by the splanchnic nerves, such as the vascular beds of the liver, spleen, and gut. **strawberry-cream b.** Blood with sufficient hyperlipidemia to cause lightening of its normal color. **venous b.** Blood flowing in veins. It has lost oxygen and gained carbon dioxide by passing through metabolically active tissue. **whole b.** Blood that has not been separated into its components such as leukocytes, red blood cells, plasma, or platelets.

**Bloodgood** [Joseph Colt *Bloodgood,* U.S. surgeon, 1866–1935] Bloodgood's disease. See under CYSTIC MASTOPATHY.

**blood group** A phenotype defined by any one of the many erythrocyte antigenic structures that are identifiable by agglutination with specific antisera or plant lectins, or by lysis when exposed to specific antisera. All blood groups are genetically determined. Many are highly polymorphic and organized in series of allotypes, with most series specified by alleles at one or more closely linked genetic loci. The relative importance of blood groups in blood transfusion incompatibilities, maternal-fetal incompatibilities, and organ transplantation is largely determined by their immunogenicity. The ABO and Rh series of blood groups are highly immunogenic and, in humans, are the blood groups specified in the common blood type of the individual. Blood groups are useful medicolegally, as in excluding paternity, and in genetic and anthropologic investigations. **A b.** That blood group within the ABO blood group system which confers A antigen on the cytoplasmic membrane of erythrocytes and most other cells. The A gene codes for an enzyme *N*-acetyl-D-galactosaminyltransferase. Persons of this blood group develop, during infancy, the antibody to the antithetical antigen B. **AB b.** The blood group within the ABO blood group system which confers both A and B antigens on the cytoplasmic membrane of erythrocytes and most other cells. Persons of this blood group do not develop antibodies to A or B antigen. **ABO b.** See under ABO BLOOD GROUP SYSTEM. **Auberger b.** An antigen which is inherited in an autosomal dominant fashion with a frequency in French and English populations of 82% and which appears to be independent of ABO, MNSs, P, Rh, Duffy, Kidd, Lewis, and Lutheran blood group systems. **B b.** That blood group within the ABO blood group system which confers B antigen on the cytoplasmic membrane of erythrocytes and most other cells. The B gene codes for an enzyme D-galactosyltransferase. Persons of this blood group develop, during infancy, the antibody to the antithetical antigen-A. **Bombay b.** See under BOMBAY PHENOTYPE. **Cartwright's b.** Red blood cell antigen ($Yt^a$ and $Yt^b$) defined by their reactivity with anti-$Yt^a$ and anti-$Yt^b$ sera. **CDE b.** An Rh erythrocyte antigen alternatively called

$Rh_z$. See under RH ANTIGEN. **Diego b.** Red blood cell antigens ($Di^a$ and $Di^b$) defined by their reactivity with anti-$Di^a$ and anti-$Di^b$ sera. $Di^a$ is found in most Mongoloid people, and especially in American Indians. $Di^b$ is common in all ethnic groups. **Dombrock b.** Red blood cell antigens ($Do^a$ and $Do^b$) defined by their reactivity with anti-$Do^a$ and anti-$Do^b$ sera. **Duffy b.** Red blood cell antigens, mainly $Fy^a$ and $Fy^b$, defined by their reactivity with anti-$Fy^a$ andanti-$Fy^b$ sera and characteristically inactivated by enzymes such as papain or ficin. **high frequency b.** Blood cell membrane components found in 95% or more of individuals tested. Also *public antigens.* **I b.** Red blood cell antigens (I antigens and i antigens) characteristically defined by their reactivity at 4°C with anti-I and anti-i sera. They are found in adult red cells (I antigens) and fetal red cells (i antigens) in more than 99% of those subjects tested. **Kell b.** A human blood group consisting of a series of codominant antigens that are determined by alleles at a locus probably on the short arm of chromosome 2. Its expression is partially determined by the Kell blood group precursor locus (symbolized Xk), which is linked to chronic granulomatous disease on the distal short arm of the X chromosome. It was first detected through antiserum produced by a woman named Kell, and the Cellano and Sutter blood groups were shown to be related antigenically and determined by the same locus. The most common allotypes are KK, Kk, kk and $K^-k^-$, the latter's apparent absence of a Kell antigen being determined by a silent allele. Because of the immunogenicity of the Kell antigens, this blood group is second only to ABO and Rh in clinical importance. **Kidd b.** A human blood group, consisting of two codominant antigens (Jk(a) and Jk(b)), that is determined by alleles at a single locus (symbolized Jk) which is mapped to the proximal short arm of chromosome 2. A rare, silent allele occurs most often in Asians. The antigens are moderately immunogenic and occasionally are associated with delayed hemolytic transfusion reactions or hemolytic disease of the newborn. It is named for the patient discovered producing the antiserum. **Lewis b.** A system of soluble antigens ($Le^a$ and $Le^b$) present in plasma and body fluids which are adsorbed to the erythrocyte membrane. The Lewis genes interact with the secretor genes responsible for the secretion of A, B, and H antigens. **low frequency b.** Blood cell membrane components which occur in the general population with a frequency of less than 1%. **Lutheran b.** A human blood group, consisting of two codominant antigens (Lu(a) and Lu(b)), that is determined by alleles at the Lutheran locus (symbolized LU), which is linked to the secretor locus on chromosome 19. Rare alleles, including an amorph, exist. Of low immunogenicity, this group rarely causes transfusion reactions. It is named for a multiply transfused patient first discovered with the antiserum. **MNSs b.** A human blood group, consisting of four codominant antigens (M, N, S, and s), that is determined by alleles at two closely linked loci (symbolized MN and Ss) which are mapped to the long arm of chromosome 4. Rare alleles, including amorphs, exist. Of low immunogenicity, this group rarely causes transfusion reactions. **O b.** That blood group within the ABO blood group system which is characterized by the absence of A or B antigen on the cytoplasmic membrane of erythrocytes and other cells. Persons of this blood group develop, during infancy, antibodies to A and B antigens. **P b.** A system of human erythrocyte antigens which are related chemically and/or which crossreact to anti-P antibodies. Two series of antigens exist and are determined by separate genetic loci: the $P_1$ series (originally P+) are paraglobosides; the $P_2$ series includes $P_2$ ($T_{j2a3}$) and p ($T_{j2a53}$), both globosides, and $p^k$, a trihexosylceramide. **Rh b.** A complex series of primate erythrocyte antigens that is determined by an unknown number of tightly linked genes which map as a single locus (symbolized Rh) to the distal short arm of human chromosome 1. The series was originally determined by immunizing rabbits to erythrocytes from rhesus monkeys. At least one antigen, denoted Rh2 or Rho(D), is highly immunogenic and is responsible for most cases of severe hemolytic disease in newborns, a disorder preventable by prior passive immunization of Rh-negative women. Also *rhesus blood group.* See also HEMOLYTIC DISEASE OF THE NEWBORN, ERYTHROBLASTOSIS FETALIS. **Sutter b.** An erythrocyte antigen defined by a reaction to an antibody designated $Is^a$. It is inherited as a dominant trait. It occurs in about 20 percent of American blacks and is rare in other groups. **Xg b.** Erythrocyte antigen controlled by an X-linked locus. $Xg^a$ antigen is present in 66% of northern European males and 85% of the females of the same ethnic group.

**bloodletting** The drawing of blood for a therapeutic purpose. *Older term.*

**bloodstream** The circulating blood within the vascular system. Also *blood stream.*

**blood type** The phenotype of erythrocyte antigens in a given individual, determined by the pattern of erythrocyte reaction with antisera specific for various antigens. In humans, it usually refers to the phenotype of the ABO and Rh series of blood group antigens. See also BLOOD GROUP.

**Bloom** [David *Bloom,* U.S. dermatologist, born 1892] See under SYNDROME.

**Blount** [Walter Putnam *Blount,* U.S. orthopedist, born 1900] Blount's disease. See under OSTEOCHONDROSIS DEFORMANS TIBIAE.

**blowfly** Any of various flies in the family Calliphoridae, such as bluebottle and greenbottle flies, whose larvae develop in rotting meat or sometimes in sores or necrotic tissues of living animals. Also *blow fly.*

**BLS** basic life support.

**blue** [Middle English and French *bleu,* Old French *blou* (of Germanic origin) blue, German *blau* blue] **1** A color of the visible spectrum falling between green and purple. **2** A substance, usually a stain or dye, that is blue in appearance, or that produces a cytochemical reaction resulting in blue staining. For chemical names including *blue,* see under the chemical name. **C. brilliant b.** BRILLIANT CRESYL BLUE. **Coomassie b.** ANAZOLENE SODIUM. **Evans b.** $C_{34}H_{24}N_6Na_4O_{14}S_4$. A brown, green, or bluish green odorless powder used to measure blood volume by intravenous injection. **indigo b.** INDIGO. **Nile b.** A stain that is used to differentiate phospholipids from neutral fat in tissue. **Prussian b.** $Fe_4[Fe(CN)_6]_3$. Iron(III) hexacyanoferrate(II), (previously known as ferric ferrocyanide). It is formed as a blue precipitate when iron(III) salts are mixed with hexacyanoferrate(II), and also when iron(II) salts are mixed with hexacyanoferrate(III). Its formation has been used as a test for iron (the Perls test). **Victoria b.** Any of several basic dyes of the diphenylnaphthylmethane series that are used in staining microorganisms and in stains for elastic tissue.

**Blumberg** [Jacob Moritz *Blumberg,* German gynecologist and surgeon, 1873–1955] See under SIGN.

**Blumenbach** [Johann Friedrich *Blumenbach,* German zoologist and anthropologist, 1752–1840] Blumenbach's clivus, clivus blumenbachii. See under CLIVUS.

**Blumenthal** [Ferdinand *Blumenthal,* German physician, born 1870] Blumenthal's disease. See under ERYTHROLEUKEMIA.

**Blumer** [George *Blumer,* U.S. physician, 1858–1940] See under SHELF.
**blush** [Old English *blyscan* to redden, prob. akin to *blȳsa* a torch] An involuntary vasodilatation most apparent in the face and neck. It is evidenced by a redness of the skin and often occurs as a response to embarrassment. **angiographic b.** A localized zone of relative radiodensity appearing during the venous phase of an angiography, such as may be seen in a meningioma during cerebral angiography or in a renal carcinoma during renal angiography.
**BM** bowel movement.
**BMA** British Medical Association.
**BMG** benign monoclonal gammopathy (monoclonal gammopathy of undetermined significance).
**BMR** basal metabolic rate.
**BNA** Basle Nomina Anatomica.
**board** **1** A flat piece of wood or other resistant material having proportionately greater length than width. **2** A body of officials, as that establishing standards for a discipline or specialty. **alphabet b.** A board on which the letters of the alphabet are displayed, to be used by a patient with inability to speak but who can construct words and sentences by pointing to the board. Also *communication board.* **back b.** SPINE BOARD. **communication b.** ALPHABET BOARD. **exercise b.** A board with a smooth surface to permit gliding-type exercises by a weakened limb. Talcum powder is often applied to the board to further reduce friction. Also *powder board.* **powder b.** EXERCISE BOARD. **specialty b.** An organization that certifies physicians or other health care professionals as specialists or subspecialists in a particular field of practice. **spine b.** An inflexible board placed on a stretcher under the back of a patient with a suspected spine injury. Also *back board.* **transfer b.** A wooden board used in transferring a patient to and from a wheelchair to a bed, car, or another chair.
**board certified** Certified as having passed an examination given by a specialty board after attaining board eligible status: said of a physician or other health care professional.
**board eligible** Eligible for specialty board examination, having met certain specified criteria such as prior training requirements: said of a physician or other health care professional.
**Boari** [Achille *Boari,* Italian surgeon, flourished late 19th century–early 20th century] See under OPERATION.
**Boas** [Ismar Isidor *Boas,* German physician, 1858–1938] See under ALGESIMETER, POINT, SIGN.
**Bochdalek** [Vincenz Alexander *Bochdalek,* Czech anatomist, 1801–1883] **1** Canal of Bochdalek. See under THYROGLOSSAL DUCT. **2** See under GANGLION, CANAL. **3** Bochdalek's pseudoganglion. See under PLEXUS DENTALIS SUPERIOR. **4** Bochdalek's gap. See under PLEUROPERICARDIAL HIATUS. **5** Valvule of Bochdalek. See under BOCHDALEK'S VALVE.
**Bock** [August Carl *Bock,* German anatomist, 1782–1833] **1** Bock's nerve. See under RAMUS PHARYNGEUS GANGLII PTERYGOPALATINI. **2** Bock's ganglion. See under INFERIOR CAROTID GANGLION.
**Bockhart** [Max *Bockhart,* German dermatologist, 1883–1921] See under IMPETIGO.
**Bodechtel** [Gustav *Bodechtel,* German physician, born 1899] Bodechtel-Guttmann disease. See under SUBACUTE SCLEROSING PANENCEPHALITIS.
**bodenplatte** \bō′dənplät′ə\ [German *Boden* floor + *Platte* plate] FLOOR PLATE.
**Bodian** [David *Bodian,* U.S. anatomist, born 1910] See under METHOD.
***Bodo*** \bō′dō\ The type genus of the family Bodonidae, order Kinetoplastida. Its members are found in stagnant water, feces, and urine. These small flagellates have two anterior flagella, one directed forward, and one trailing. Also *Prowazekia.* ***B. caudatus*** A coprozoic species associated with human feces and stagnant water. ***B. saltans*** A species of flagellate protozoans known as springing monads. They have been found in skin lesions and ulcers. ***B. urinarius*** A species occurring in human urine.

# body

**body** [Old English *bodig*] **1** The entire animal frame with head, organs, and extremities. **2** The principal or central part of an organism, organ, or structure. **3** A small organ; an organelle. **4** Any small discrete mass of material. **accessory b.** An argentophil body, probably analogous to the lamellar bodies seen with the electron microscope, in the area of the neck of the developing spermatozoon. Such structures have been considered to arise as the result of nuclear shrinkage during spermiogenesis. **acetone b.** KETONE BODY. **adipose b. of cheek** CORPUS ADIPOSUM BUCCAE. **adipose b. of ischiorectal fossa** CORPUS ADIPOSUM FOSSAE ISCHIOANALIS. **adipose b. of orbit** CORPUS ADIPOSUM ORBITAE. **adrenal b.** GLANDULA SUPRARENALIS. **Alder bodies** Alder-Reilly bodies. See under ALDER-REILLY ANOMALY. **Alder-Reilly bodies** See under ALDER-REILLY ANOMALY. **Amato bodies** DÖHLE BODIES. **amygdaloid b.** CORPUS AMYGDALOIDEUM. **amyloid bodies** CORPORA AMYLACEA. **anti-immune b.** ANTIANTIBODY. **aortic bodies** CORPORA PARA-AORTICA. **apical b.** ACROSOME. **Arnold's bodies** Erythrocyte fragments, especially large pieces of membrane, in the peripheral blood. **asbestos bodies** Asbestos fibers coated with iron, glycosaminoglycans, and sometimes calcium. They are seen in the sputum and lesions of interstitial pulmonary fibrosis caused by asbestos inhalation. Also *ferruginous bodies.* **Aschoff bodies** Submiliary granulomatous lesions which, when found in the myocardium, are characteristic of acute rheumatic carditis and pathognomonic of rheumatic fever. They occur in the proximity of blood vessels, and consist of an eosinophilic central area surrounded by various cellular elements. Also *Aschoff's nodules.* See also ASCHOFF CELL. **asteroid b.** Star-shaped eosinophilic intracytoplasmic inclusions found within vacuoles of multinucleated giant cells. These bodies are most commonly seen in sarcoid granulomas but may be observed in other granulomatous conditions, especially berylliosis. **Auer bodies** Rod-shaped structures approximately 5$\mu$ long by 0.5$\mu$ wide, in the cytoplasm of leukemic myeloblasts, formed by coalescence of lysosomal granules. Auer bodies are acidophilic and thus appear red with Romanowsky-type stains. When present, they indicate an acute granulocytic leukemia. Auer bodies also are positive by peroxidase stain. Also *Auer rods.* **Babès-Ernst bodies** Polymetaphosphate granules, which stain metachromatically with methylene blue. They are found in various bacteria, yeasts, and protozoa, and are useful in the recognition of *Corynebacterium diphtheriae.* Also *Babès-Ernst corpuscles, Babès-Ernst granules.* **bacillary bodies** Iron-containing cytoplasmic inclusions seen in various stages of erythrocyte development, indicative of hemoglobin synthesis and related to punctate basophilia. These granular, Feulgen-negative inclusions, seen most commonly in erythrocytic precursors in the bone marrow, are usually related to hemolytic anemia and may be seen following splenectomy. **Barr b.** In mammalian somatic cells in interphase, a condensed clump of chromatin located subjacent to the nuclear membrane in the homogametic sex. In humans, it corresponds to the inactive X chromosome found in normal XX females and in males who have two or more X chromosomes in addition to the Y chromosome. The number of Barr bodies per cell equals one less than the number of X chromosomes. Also *sex chromatin, X chromatin, X chromatin body.* **Bartonia bodies** Organisms of the species *Bartonella bacilliformis.* **basal b.** A minute, elongated or thickened organelle, as in protozoa, from which the axoneme of each flagellum or cilium emerges. It is structurally identical to the centriole and is thought to be derived from its replication products. Also *basal granule, basal corpuscle, blepharoplast, kinetosome.* **Bence Jones b.** BENCE JONES PROTEIN. **Bichat's fatty b. of cheek** CORPUS ADIPOSUM BUCCAE. **Cabot's ring bodies** CABOT'S RINGS. **Call-Exner b.** A small area of cystic liquefaction between ovarian follicular cells that often contains some eosinophilic material and represents a characteristic feature of a granulosa cell tumor. **carotid b.** GLOMUS CAROTICUM. **cavernous b. of clitoris** CORPUS CAVERNOSUM CLITORIDIS. **cavernous b. of penis** CORPUS CAVERNOSUM PENIS. **cell b.** The cytoplasm which surrounds the nucleus of a cell. **central b.** CENTRIOLE. **chromaffin b.** PARAGANGLION. **ciliary b.** CORPUS CILIARE. **Civatte bodies** Colloid bodies occurring in the epidermis, usually in lichen planus. **b. of clitoris** CORPUS CLITORIDIS. **colloid bodies** Hyaline bodies representing degenerated cells seen in the epidermis in lichen planus and lupus erythematosus and in the fundus of the eye in senile retinal degeneration. These bodies are not specific of any particular disease. **compressible cavernous bodies** Portosystemic anastomoses in the wall of the lower end of the esophagus and of the anal canal that are susceptible to varicosities that may project into and decrease the size of the lumen of the organs at these sites. **Councilman bodies** Round to oval, homogeneous, eosinophilic bodies found in the liver in acute toxic or viral hepatitis. They represent necrotic hepatocytes which have shrunken and condensed, and are often found within Kupffer cells that have phagocytized them, or in the space of Disse, or within sinusoids. Their presence is useful in the diagnosis of acute hepatitis. Also *Councilman lesion.* **Cowdry's type A inclusion bodies** Rounded, acidophilic masses of amorphous material which displace the chromatin of the cell nucleus to the periphery of the nucleus. The presence of these bodies is suggestive of infection with cytomegalovirus, herpes simplex, adenovirus, or subacute sclerosing panencephalitis virus (measles virus). **Cowdry's type B inclusion bodies** Small, indistinct, particulate, round, or oval bodies found in the cell nucleus or cytoplasm. They are less reliable than Cowdry's type A inclusion bodies as indicators of antecedent viral infections. *Seldom used.* **cytoid bodies** Globular structures resembling cell nuclei seen in retinal nerve fibers damaged by ischemia. They represent swollen axons with degenerated cytoplasmic organelles and are the histologic counterpart of the cotton-wool spots of the retina. **Deetjen's b.** PLATELET. **demilune b.** A crescentic figure containing hemoglobin, seen in blood films of persons with malaria, and believed to be a portion of a partially lysed erythrocyte. See also GLASS BODY. **Döhle bodies** Cytoplasmic particles that are approximately 1.0 $\mu$m in diameter, are pale blue by Romanowsky stain, and are found in neutrophils, especially in persons with infections or other toxic states. Döhle bodies are commonly accompanied by toxic granulation of neutrophils. They are composed of aggregates of endoplasmic reticulum. Also *Döhle inclusion bodies, Amato bodies, trypochetes.* **Donné's bodies** COLOSTRUM CORPUSCLES. **Donovan bodies** Large mononuclear cells containing *Calymmatobacterium granulomatis (Donovania granulomatis),* found in lesions of granuloma inguinale. Upon staining with the Wright stain, the bacilli are blue with pink capsules. **Dutcher b.** A clear vacuolelike inclusion in the nucleus of a plasma cell. Dutcher bodies are composed of immunoglobulins. They may be seen in plasma cells of bone marrow in both benign and malignant conditions. **Ehrlich's hemoglobinemic bodies** HEINZ BODIES. **elementary b.** A virus particle, especially as viewed by electron microscopy. **Elschnig bodies** Translucent globules upon the lens capsule following extracapsular cataract extraction. These represent aberrant development of new lens fibers. Also *Elschnig's pearls.* **Elzholz bodies** Myelinlike bodies seen at the polar end of Schwann cell nuclei in degenerating and regenerating myelinated nerves. **embryoid b.** A structure resembling an embryo. It is seen in germ cell tumors, such as embryonal carcinoma, teratoma, and polyembryoma. **b. of epididymis** CORPUS EPIDIDYMIDIS. **epithelial bodies** *Obs.* PARATHYROID GLANDS. **falciform b.** The elongate infective sporozoite of malaria concentrated in the infected mosquito's salivary glands prior to injection into a host. *Older term.* **fatty b. of acetabular fossa** A mass of fatty tissue which is covered by synovial membrane and that is lodged in the acetabular fossa of the hip joint. **fatty b. of orbit** CORPUS ADIPOSUM ORBITAE. **ferruginous bodies** ASBESTOS BODIES. **b. of fornix** CORPUS FORNICIS. **fuchsin bodies** RUSSELL BODIES. **b. of gallbladder** CORPUS VESICAE BILIARIS. **Gamna-Favre bodies** MIYAGAWA BODIES. **Gamna-Gandy bodies** Small foci of fibrosis admixed with iron and calcium salts resulting from the organization of previous perivascular hemorrhages. Their color can range from a yellowish brown to a rust texture. These bodies occur primarily in the spleen in association with congestive splenomegaly, sickle cell disease, and hemochromatosis. Also *Gamna nodules, Gandy-Gamna nodules, siderotic nodules.* **geniculate b.** Either of the protuberances of the caudal thalamus, the corpus geniculatum laterale or the corpus geniculatum mediale. **Giannuzzi's b.** DEMILUNE OF GIANNUZZI. **glass b.** The pale, transparent, hemoglobin-free portion of a partially lysed erythrocyte seen in blood films of persons with malaria. On one margin of a glass body is a crescentic demilune body that contains the remaining hemoglobin. **glomus bodies** GLOMIFORM GLANDS. **Golgi b.** DICTYOSOME. **Guarnieri bodies** Intracytoplasmic inclusions seen predominantly in epithelial cells of tissues infected by vaccinia virus or smallpox virus. These inclusions are generally acidophilic, are best visualized in Giemsa stain, and are composed of large ovoid virions. Also *Guarnieri's corpuscles, Paschen's corpuscles, Paschen's granules, Guarnieri's inclusions.* **habenular b.** HABENULA. **Hassall's b.** HASSALL'S CORPUSCLE. **Hassall-Henle bodies** Hyaline deposits observed on the posterior surface of Descemet's membrane at the corneal margins, associated with senescence. Also *Hassall-Henle warts, guttae opthalmicae, cornea guttata.* **Heinz bodies** Cytoplasmic inclusions seen in erythrocytes of patients with abnormal hemoglobin and certain enzyme deficiencies such as glucose-6-phosphate dehydrogenase deficiency. These bodies are composed of oxidized, precipitated, and degraded hemoglobin and their presence favors erythrophagocytosis in splenic sinuses. Also *Heinz granules, Ehrlich's hemoglobinemic bodies.* **hematoxylin bodies** Small, poorly defined bodies that readily take up hematoxylin stain, seen occasionally in fixed tissues of patients with systemic lupus erythematosus. These basophilic masses are presumed to be the remains of whole nuclei that have been exposed to anti-nuclear antibodies. These nuclei swell, lose their chromatin pattern, and are extruded. When seen in histologic section, the bodies are pathognomonic of systemic lupus erythematosus. **b. of Highmore** MEDIASTINUM TESTIS. **Hollenhorst bodies** HOLLENHORST PLAQUE. **Howell-Jolly bodies** Small, usually spherical, basophilic bodies no larger than one micron, occasionally found within circulating erythrocytes in a variety of pathologic conditions. They have the appearance of pyknotic nuclei on Wright-stained peripheral blood smears, are Feulgen positive, and are thought to represent degraded nuclear material resulting from abnormal mitosis. They are characteristically seen following splenectomy or in association with hemolytic anemias, hyposplenism, and megaloblastic anemias. Also *Howell's bodies, Jolly's bodies, nuclear particles, chromatin particles.* **hyaline bodies** Intracytoplasmic deposits of homogeneous eosinophilic material associated with a variety of pathologic as well as physiologic conditions. When observed in renal tubular epithelium, these inclusions represent proteinaceous material that has been resorbed from the tubular lumen. This material generally represents the accumulation of excessive amounts of protein that cannot be metabolized or transported from the cells. **hyaline bodies of the pituitary** Globules of neurosecretory material that are located within the posterior lobe of the pituitary gland. **hyaloid b.** CORPUS VITREUM. **b. of hyoid bone** CORPUS OSSIS HYOIDEI. **b. of ilium** CORPUS OSSIS ILII. **immune b.** ANTIBODY. **inclusion bodies** Intranuclear or intracytoplasmic accumulation of viral particles seen with the light microscope in cells infected with herpes, smallpox, rabies, and other diseases. **infrapatellar fatty b.** CORPUS ADIPOSUM INFRAPATELLARE. **infundibular b.** NEUROHYPOPHYSIS. **intravertebral b.** CORPUS VERTEBRAE. **b. of ischium** CORPUS OSSIS ISCHII. **Jolly's bodies** HOWELL-JOLLY BODIES. **juxtaglomerular b.** JUXTAGLOMERULAR APPARATUS. **juxtarestiform b.** A myelinated axon bundle in the medial portions of the inferior cerebellar peduncle primarily containing connections between cerebellum and vestibular nuclei. **ketone b.** Any of the substances: acetone, 3-hydroxybutyric acid, and 3-oxobutyric acid (acetoacetic acid). These accumulate in the blood when acetyl-CoA is produced in the liver more rapidly than it can be oxidized, as in diabetes and starvation. Also *acetone body.* **Lafora's bodies** The characteristic histopathologic change of familial myoclonic epilepsy, consisting of intracytoplasmic structures measuring 1-20 $\mu$M found in neurons of the basal ganglia, dentate nucleus, and other areas of the central nervous system. These bodies are round, concentric masses with dense irregular cores and a fibrillary appearance under the electron microscope. **Lallemand-Trousseau bodies** BENCE JONES CYLINDERS. **lateral geniculate b.** CORPUS GENICULATUM LATERALE. **Laveran bodies** Malarial parasites as they appear in their blood-infecting stages. *Older term.* Also *Laveran's corpuscles.* **Leishman-Donovan b.** *Older term* AMASTIGOTE. **lenticular b.** *Obs.* NUCLEUS LENTIFORMIS. **Lewy bodies** Eosinophilic inclusions in the cytoplasm of pigmented neurons, primarily in the substantia nigra and locus ceruleus, seen in Parkinson's disease. **Lieutaud's b.** TRIGONUM VESICAE. **Lindner's initial bodies** MIYAGAWA BODIES. **Luschka's b.** GLOMUS COCCYGEUM. **Luse bodies** Irregular transversely banded structures that can be seen by electron microscopy between the constituent cells of neurolemmas. They are thought to be composed of fibrous, long spaced collagen. **b. of Luys** *Outmoded* NUCLEUS SUBTHALAMICUS. **Mallory's bodies** Large, homogeneous, eosinophilic, irregular eccentric masses found in the cytoplasm of hepatocytes. These bodies are characteristic but not pathognomonic of alcoholic liver disease. Ultrastructurally, they are composed of actin-like filaments associated with rough endoplasmic reticulum. **malpighian b. of kidney** CORPUSCULUM RENALE. **malpighian bodies of spleen** FOLLICULI LYMPHATICI SPLENICI. **mamillary b.** CORPUS MAMILLARE. **b. of mandible** CORPUS MANDIBULAE. **b. of maxilla** CORPUS MAXILLAE. **medial geniculate b.** CORPUS GENICULATUM MEDIALE. **medullary b. of cerebellum** CORPUS MEDULLARE CEREBELLI. **medullary b. of vermis** CORPUS MEDULLARE CEREBELLI. **Michaelis-Gutmann bodies** Laminated microspherules containing calcium and iron, seen in malakoplakia. **Miyagawa bodies** Intracytoplasmic inclusions of variable size seen within macrophages and other cells infected with *Chlamydia trachomatis* in conditions such as lymphogranuloma venereum and trachoma. These bodies represent developmental stages of the microorganism. Also *Gamna-Favre bodies, Lindner's initial bodies.* **molluscum bodies** The intracytoplasmic inclusion bodies characteristic of molluscum contagiosum. Also *molluscous corpuscles.* **Mott bodies** Translucent, globular, eosinophilic, intracytoplasmic bodies seen within plasma cells in multiple myeloma. They represent retained immunoglobulin secreted by the tumor cells. **multivesicular b.** A cytoplasmic structure that appears as a vacuole containing numerous tiny vesicles. It forms from a lysosome by an inward budding of the limiting membrane of the lysosome. **b. of nail** CORPUS UNGUIS. **Negri bodies** Intracytoplasmic, eosinophilic inclusion bodies seen in neurons infected with the rabies virus. These inclusions are found in all neurons but most frequently in those of Ammon's horn of the hippocampus and are the most characteristic histologic feature of rabies. **Nissl bodies** NISSL SUBSTANCE. **no-threshold bodies** NO-THRESHOLD SUBSTANCES. **olivary b.** OLIVA. **pacchionian bodies** GRANULATIONES ARACHNOIDEALES. • The term especially denotes the large ones found in older individuals. **pampiniform b.** EPOÖPHORON. **b. of pancreas** CORPUS PANCREATIS. **para-aortic bodies** CORPORA PARA-AORTICA. **parabasal b.** An organelle found in flagellate protozoans. Its morphology varies greatly among the genera, though it is part of the kinetic complex and associated with flagellar movement. It is closely associated with the nucleus and is connected by a fine filament to the basal granule, which lies at the origin of the flagellum. **parabigeminal b.** A region located ventrolateral to the inferior colliculus, composed of transversely or obliquely coursing fibers among which are scattered groups of nerve cells collectively known as the parabigeminal nucleus. Some of the fibers in the parabigeminal body are corticopontine fibers from the cerbral cortex, while certain of the neurons forming the parabigeminal nucleus course to lateral nuclei in the pons. **paraphyseal b.** PARAPHYSIS. **parolivary bodies** Nuclei olivaris accessorius medialis and dorsalis. See under NUCLEUS OLIVARIS ACCESSORIUS MEDIALIS, NUCLEUS OLIVARIS ACCESSORIUS DORSALIS. **pearly bodies** EPITHELIAL PEARLS. **penile b.** CORPUS PENIS. **b. of penis** CORPUS PENIS. **perineal b.** CENTRUM

TENDINEUM PERINEI. **pheochrome bodies** CORPORA PARA-AORTICA. **phi bodies** Peroxidase-positive rod-shaped or spindle-form cytoplasmic structures found in leukemic myeloblasts when stained for peroxidase. Phi bodies are not visualized on Wright or other Romanowsky stain. They have the same significance as Auer bodies. **Pick bodies** Cytoplasmic argentophilic bodies found in neurons of the frontal cortex of the brain in cases of Pick's disease. **pineal b.** CORPUS PINEALE. **pituitary b.** PITUITARY GLAND. **polar b.** One of the small rudimentary cells formed during the specialized nuclear divisions that result in the maturation of a mammalian ovum. Each contains half the number of chromosomes characteristic for the species and very scanty cytoplasm. It derives the name polar because the body is pinched off at the animal pole of the maturing ovum. The first polar body is formed when the primary oocyte divides at the first maturation division, a reductional division, to give rise to a haploid secondary oocyte. This event occurs in the ovarian follicle and the polar body is extruded from the ovum but retained within the zona pellucida. The second polar body is formed at the second maturation, or equational, division usually just before or at the time of fertilization. The first polar body may itself divide mitotically to give a total of three polar bodies. They all eventually degenerate but in rare cases may be fertilized before doing so. **postbranchial b.** ULTIMOBRANCHIAL BODY. **presegmenting b.** PRESEGMENTER. **primitive perineal b.** The lower end of the wedgelike cloacal septum where it meets the cloacal membrane and forms a distinct ridge across the future perineal region of the embryo. **psammoma bodies** Spherical, laminated deposits of calcified material generally seen in both benign and malignant epithelial neoplasms, such as papillary carcinoma of thyroid and certain serous papillary tumors of ovary. They measure 50–200 $\mu$ in diameter. Similarly mineralized deposits are also seen in the meninges associated with meningiomas, and occasionally within the choroid plexus. Also *sand bodies.* **pseudolutein b.** CORPUS ATRETICUM. **psittacosis inclusion bodies** Intracellular colonies of *Chlamydia psittaci* found in infected cells during the course of psittacosis. **b. of pubis** CORPUS OSSIS PUBIS. **pyknotic bodies** Shrunken hyperchromatic fragments of nuclear material from polymorphonuclear neutrophils. They are found in cells degenerating from senescence or in severe infections, and may be seen in feces of individuals with colonic microabscesses. **quadrigeminal bodies** CORPORA QUADRIGEMINA. **b. of radius** CORPUS RADII. **Reilly bodies** Alder-Reilly bodies. See under ALDER-REILLY ANOMALY. **Renaut's bodies** Poorly staining granular deposits seen in degenerating nerve fibers in association with muscular dystrophy. **residual b.** A whorl of myelin figures in the cytoplasm, thought to represent the final stage in the process of lysosome degradation. **residual b. of Regnaud** A mass of degenerating cell material and lipid left over after differentiation of the sperm tail during spermiogenesis. **restiform b.** PEDUNCULUS CEREBELLARIS INFERIOR. **reticulate b.** The intracellular stage in the life cycle of chlamydiae. **b. of rib** CORPUS COSTAE. **rice bodies** Small, hard bodies predominantly found within joints and probably representing organized fragments of torn cartilage or cartilagenous metaplasia of synovial tissue. These structures are occasionally found in tendon sheaths and bursae. **Rosenmüller's b.** EPOÖPHORON. **Russell bodies** Globular intracytoplasmic deposits of acidophilic material within plasma cells. These hyaline inclusions stain deeply with fuchsin dye and are frequently observed in neoplastic plasma cells as well as plasma cells involved in chronic inflammatory reactions. The material in these cells is inspissated immunoglobulin. Also *fuchsin bodies, Russell corpuscles.* **sand bodies** PSAMMOMA BODIES. **Sandström's bodies** PARATHYROID GLANDS. **Savage's perineal b.** CENTRUM TENDINEUM PERINEI. **Schaumann bodies** Nodular lesions within a sarcoid granuloma, thought to be diagnostic of sarcoidosis. **Schmorl b.** SCHMORL'S NODULE. **semilunar b.** DEMILUNE OF GIANNUZZI. **b. of sphenoid** CORPUS OSSIS SPHENOIDALIS. **spongy b. of male urethra** CORPUS SPONGIOSUM PENIS. **spongy b. of penis** CORPUS SPONGIOSUM PENIS. **b. of sternum** CORPUS STERNI. **b. of stomach** CORPUS GASTRICUM. **striate b.** CORPUS STRIATUM. **supracardial bodies** CORPORA PARA-AORTICA. **suprapericardial b.** ULTIMOBRANCHIAL BODY. **suprarenal b.** GLANDULA SUPRARENALIS. **b. of sweat gland** CORPUS GLANDULAE SUDORIFERAE. **Symington's b.** LIGAMENTUM ANOCOCCYGEUM. **b. of talus** CORPUS TALI. **threshold bodies** THRESHOLD SUBSTANCES. **thyroid b.** *Outmoded* THYROID GLAND. **b. of tibia** CORPUS TIBIAE. **tingible b.** A densely basophilic mass that represents residual nuclear material from rapidly dividing immature cells of the germinal center of lymph nodes. These are engulfed by macrophages, where they appear as multiple cytoplasmic inclusions of varying size and shape. **b. of tongue** CORPUS LINGUAE. **touch bodies** CORPUSCULA TACTUS. **trachoma bodies** Intracytoplasmic inclusions found within conjunctival epithelium in acute trachomatous infection. They are composed of the infective agent, *Chlamydia trachomatis,* in various stages of development. **trapezoid b.** CORPUS TRAPEZOIDEUM. **Trousseau-Lallemand bodies** BENCE JONES CYLINDERS. **turbinated b.** A turbinate bone, or concha, and its neighboring tissues, especially the concha nasalis. **b. of ulna** CORPUS ULNAE. **ultimobranchial b.** A structure derived from the fifth pharyngeal (branchial) pouch and which in early embryonic life is situated just above the pericardium. Normally it disappears but it may persist as an anomaly. Also *suprapericardial body, postbranchial body.* **b. of uterus** CORPUS UTERI. **Verocay bodies** Foci of cells in a neurilemmoma with nuclei in palisades at each end of a fiber bundle. **b. of vertebra** CORPUS VERTEBRAE. **vertebral b.** CORPUS VERTEBRAE. **b. of Vicq d'Azyr** SUBSTANTIA NIGRA. **Virchow-Hassall b.** HASSALL'S CORPUSCLE. **vitreous b.** CORPUS VITREUM. **wolffian b.** MESONEPHROS. **X chromatin b.** BARR BODY. **yellow b. of ovary** CORPUS LUTEUM. **zebra bodies** Cytoplasmic inclusions which have a striped zebralike appearance under the electron microscope and are typically found in certain cortical neurons in patients with cœroid-lipofuscinosis. **Zuckerkandl's b.** PARAGANGLION.

**body-rocking** Monotonous rhythmic movements seen in infants, children, and mentally subnormal or disturbed adults, performed in a variety of postures, from recumbency to standing. They appear to be a way of relieving tension and anxiety or of shutting off all impressions from the outer world by maintaining a kind of pleasurable self-stimulation. Blind children are prone to rock, lacking the distraction and interest of the visual world, and institutionalized children rock from boredom, emptiness, and loneliness. Rocking is often a form of generalized hyperactivity in organic brain dysfunction at any age.

**Boeck** [Caesar Peter Moeller *Boeck*, Norwegian dermatologist, 1845–1917] Boeck sarcoid, Boeck's disease, Besnier-Boeck disease, Hutchinson-Boeck syndrome, Hutchinson-

Boeck disease, Besnier-Boeck-Schaumann disease. See under SARCOIDOSIS.

**Boeck** [Karl Wilhelm *Boeck*, Norwegian dermatologist, 1808–1875] Danielssen-Boeck disease. See under SARCOIDOSIS.

**Boerhaave** [Hermann *Boerhaave*, Dutch physician, 1668–1738] **1** See under SYNDROME. **2** Boerhaave's glands. See under SWEAT GLANDS.

**Bogomolets** [Aleksandr Alexsandrovich *Bogomolets*, Russian endocrinologist and physiologist, 1881–1946] Bogomolets serum. See under ANTIRETICULAR CYTOTOXIC SERUM.

**Bogros** [Annet Jean *Bogros*, French anatomist, 1786–1823] See under SPACE.

**Bogrov** [Sergei Livovich *Bogrov*, Russian anatomist, born 1878] Fibers of Bogrov. See under FIBER.

**Bohr** [Christian *Bohr*, Danish physiologist, 1855–1911] See under EFFECT, EQUATION.

**Bohr** [Niels H. D. *Bohr*, Danish physicist, 1885–1962] See under ATOM, THEORY.

**boil** [earlier *bile*, from Old English *bȳl, bȳle*] *Popular* FURUNCLE. **Aleppo b.** CUTANEOUS LEISHMANIASIS. **Baghdad b.** CUTANEOUS LEISHMANIASIS. **blind b.** A furuncle that does not suppurate. **Delhi b.** CUTANEOUS LEISHMANIASIS. **Madura b.** MYCETOMA. **saltwater b.** An ulcer occurring on the hands and forearms of fishermen, usually caused by the continuous exposure of an abrasion to seawater. Also *seawater boil.* **shoe b.** OLECRANON BURSITIS.

**bol.** *bolus* (L, a pill), used in prescription writing.

**bolenol** $C_{20}H_{32}O$. 19-Nor-17$\alpha$-pregn-5-en-17-ol. An anabolic steroid.

**Bollinger** [Otto von *Bollinger*, German pathologist, 1843–1909] Bollinger's granules. See under GRANULE.

**Bollman** [Jesse Louis *Bollman*, U.S. physiologist, born 1896] Mann-Bollman fistula. See under FISTULA.

**bolometer** \bōläm′ətər\ [Gk *bol(ē)* (from *ballein* to throw) a throw, stroke + *o* + -METER] **1** An instrument for measuring the force of cardiac contractions. **2** An extremely sensitive instrument for measuring radiant heat.

**Bolton** [Joseph Shaw *Bolton*, English neurologist, 1867–1946] **1** Bolton point. See under POINT. **2** Bolton plane, Broadbent-Bolton plane. See under NASION-POSTCONDYLARE PLANE. **3** See under TRIANGLE.

**bolus** \bō′ləs\ [L (from Gk *bōlos* clod, lump), morsel, piece] **1** A pharmaceutical preparation in the form of a spherical mass to be swallowed. **2** A chewed, rounded mass of food ready to be swallowed. **b. alba** KAOLIN.

**bombard** To expose to a beam of charged particles or other ionizing radiation.

**bombesin** \bämbē′sin\ A gastrointestinal polypeptide comprising 14 amino acids which causes antral gastrin release and stimulation of gastric acid secretion, and also acts upon the vasculature, gallbladder, pancreas, lung, and urinary tract.

**bond** [Middle English *bond, band* (from Old Norse, akin to Old English *bend* fetter) binding force] The mode of combination of atoms within a molecule. Chemical reactions depend largely on the breaking and formation of bonds. **conjugated double b.'s** Pi bonds whose pi orbitals overlap. They are usually alternate double bonds. This allows transmission of electronic effects affecting reactivity through the molecule. **disulfide b.** A covalent bond formed between two sulfur atoms. The resulting structure is found particularly in extracellular proteins, joining half-cystine residues formed by the oxidation of cysteine. It endows protein molecules with some rigidity and is particularly abundant in the proteins of hair. A disulfide is easily reduced to two thiol groups. Lipoic acid is an example of biologically important disulfide. Also *disulfide bridge.* **glycosidic b.'s** The bond formed between a sugar and alcohol (often another sugar) in a glycoside, the bond from C to O-R in —O—C(—O—R)(—R′)—. It is much less stable than a normal ether bond, and can be broken by acids and enzymes, thanks to the presence of the other oxygen atom in the grouping. **hydrogen b.** A bond formed between one atom, usually nitrogen, oxygen, or fluorine, and the hydrogen atom bonded to another such electronegative atom. It is largely electrostatic in origin, depending on the charge distribution of the bonding structures. It is important in the structure of water, proteins, and nucleic acids, and accounts for the high boiling point of water ($H_2O$) in comparison, for example, with the gas $H_2S$. **hydrophobic b.** The tendency of nonpolar groups to aggregate, as if by mutual attraction, when placed in water. No actual bond exists, but the groups have affinity for each other, rather than for water. **ionic b.** The attraction between ions of opposite charge. **isopeptide b.** A covalent amide bond between amino-acid residues in peptides and proteins other than between C-1 of one residue and N-2 of another. The commonest is between the side chains of lysine and glutamic acid. Isopeptide bonds are important in structural proteins such as keratin and fibrin. **pi b.** A bond between two atoms in which the electron pair has two regions of electron density on opposite sides of the line between the atoms. The C═O group, for example, contains two bonds between carbon and oxygen, one of which is a pi bond. Like other pi bonds it is easily polarized, as when a nucleophile approaches the carbon atom at the start of an addition reaction. **sigma b.** A bond between two atoms in which the electron pair is distributed about the line between the two atoms in a radially symmetrical manner, with maximal electron density on the line. Single bonds are normally sigma bonds, and one bond of a double or triple bond is also.

**bonding** The process by which mother and newborn infant develop a strong mutual attachment through repeated contact involving the senses of sight, hearing, touch, and smell. ⟨"Bonding and breast-feeding are inextricably related." —*Medical World News*, 5 Feb. 1979, 77⟩ **direct b.** The fixation of an orthodontic attachment directly to the surface of a tooth without the use of a band. Special techniques, such as the acid etch, are employed.

**Bondy** [Gustav *Bondy*, Austrian otologist, flourished 20th century] Bondy mastoidectomy, Bondy operation. See under MODIFIED RADICAL MASTOIDECTOMY.

# bone

**bone** [Old English *bān*, from common Germanic (akin to German *Bein* leg) a bone] **1** A specialized connective tissue in which lamellae of helically arranged collagen fibers are held together by a ground substance impregnated with inorganic salts to provide hardness and rigidity to the tissue which remains plastic; bony tissue. **2** Any of the component units of the skeleton, composed of this tissue; os. **accessory b.** A supernumerary nodule of bone, or ossicle, occasionally observed in radiograms, usually of the wrist and foot bones. **accessory cuboid b.** A supernumerary ossicle that extends posterolaterally from the cuboid bone, forming a tubercle. **accessory multangular b.**

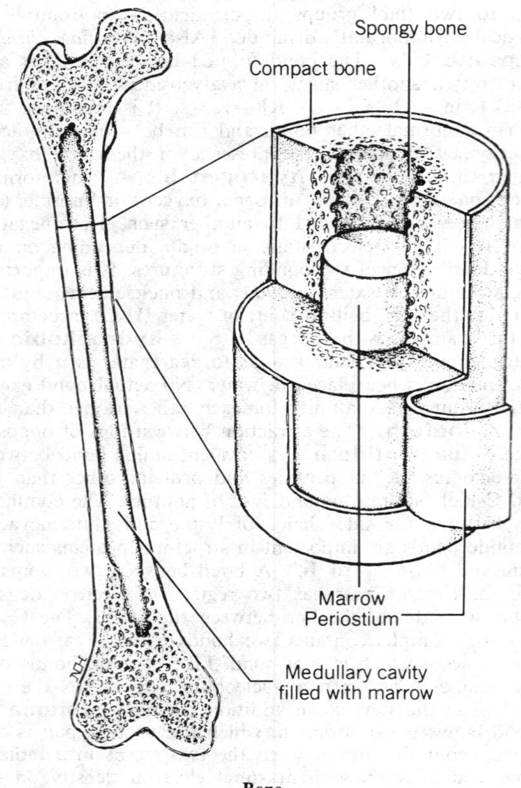


**Bone**

OS CENTRALE. **acetabular b.** OS ACETABULI. **acromial b.** ACROMION. **alar b.** OS SPHENOIDALE. **alisphenoid b.** ALA MAJOR OSSIS SPHENOIDALIS. **alveolar b.** The bone surrounding the roots of the teeth. **alveolar b. proper** The bony wall of the alveolus, comprising a relatively thin perforated plate adjacent to the root. It consists of cancellous bone (with the incorporation of Sharpey's fibers forming bundle bone) except where the socket involves part of the cortical plate. **ankle b.** TALUS. **astragaloid b.** TALUS. **back b.** COLUMNA VERTEBRALIS. **basal b.** That part of the mandible or maxilla that supports the alveolar bone. **basihyal b.** 1 The body of the hyoid bone. 2 The basal, or median, ventral plate of the hyoid arch. **basilar b.** PARS BASILARIS OSSIS OCCIPITALIS. **basioccipital b.** PARS BASILARIS OSSIS OCCIPITALIS. **basiotic b.** A small supernumerary piece of bone representing in the fetus the anterior part of the basilar apophysis of the occipital bone which is developed from an additional center of ossification (basiotic center) distinct from the basioccipital center. It is only rarely present. **basipresphenoid b.** The ossification centers giving rise to the presphenoid portion of the sphenoid bone. **basisphenoid b.** BASISPHENOID. **Bertin's b.'s** CONCHA SPHENOIDALIS. **blade b.** SCAPULA. **breast b.** STERNUM. **bregmatic b.** OS PARIETALE. **Breschet's b.'s** OSSA SUPRASTERNALIA. **bundle b.** 1 The portion of alveolar bone that receives the perforating collagen fibers of Sharpey that cross the periodontal ligament. 2 The compact bone containing bundles of Sharpey's fibers passing from the periosteum in the region of tendinous or ligamentous attachments. See also LAMELLAR BONE. **cancellous b.** SUBSTANTIA SPONGIOSA OSSIUM. **capitate b.** OS CAPITATUM. **carpal b.'s** OSSA CARPI. **cartilage b.** ENDOCHONDRAL BONE. **cavalry b.** RIDERS' BONE. **central carpal b.** OS CENTRALE. **b.'s of cerebral cranium** OSSA CRANII. **cheek b.** OS ZYGOMATICUM. **coccygeal b.** OS COCCYGIS. **collar b.** CLAVICULA. **compact b.** SUBSTANTIA COMPACTA OSSIUM. **cortical b.** SUBSTANTIA CORTICALIS OSSIUM. **costal b.** OS COSTALE. **cotyloid b.** OS ACETABULI. **cranial b.'s** OSSA CRANII. **b.'s of cranium** OSSA CRANII. **cribriform b.** OS ETHMOIDALE. **cubital b.** OS TRIQUETRUM. **cuboid b.** OS CUBOIDEUM. **cuckoo b.** OS COCCYGIS. **cuneiform b. of carpus** OS TRIQUETRUM. **ear b.'s** OSSICULA AUDITUS. **ectethmoid b.'s** The labyrinths or lateral masses of the ethmoid bone that contain the sinuses. **endochondral b.** Bone formed by endochondral ossification, from primary centers of ossification appearing at specific times during development within the shaft of a preformed cartilaginous model. Secondary centers appear at the ends of long bones, again mainly at specific times after birth, and fuse with the bone developed from the primary center. Also *cartilage bone.* **epactal b.'s** OSSA SUTURALIA. **epihyal b.** An ossified ligament of the styloid or mastoid processes of the temporal bone. **epipteric b.** A sutural bone that develops in the region of the pterion. Also *Flower's bone, pterion ossicle.* **episternal b.'s** OSSA SUPRASTERNALIA. **ethmoid b.** OS ETHMOIDALE. **exercise b.** Bone that has arisen in a muscle or a tendon as a result of excessive exercise. **exoccipital b.** PARS LATERALIS OSSIS OCCIPITALIS. **exocranial wormian b.** A sutural bone that involves only the outer table of the skull. **external cuneiform b.** OS CUNEIFORME LATERALE. **b.'s of face** OSSA FACIEI. **facial b.'s** OSSA FACIEI. **fetal b.** PRIMARY BONE. **femoral b.** FEMUR. **fibular b.** FIBULA. **b.'s of fingers** OSSA DIGITORUM MANUS. **first cuneiform b.** OS CUNEIFORME MEDIALE. **flank b.** OS ILII. **flat b.** OS PLANUM. **Flower's b.** EPIPTERIC BONE. **fourth turbinate b.** CONCHA NASALIS SUPREMA. **frontal b.** OS FRONTALE. **funny b.** The sulcus between the medial epicondyle of the humerus and the olecranon process of the ulna where the ulnar nerve is accessible to external pressure and if rolled, compressed or jarred, produces a peculiar sensation. **Goethe's b.** 1 A large sutural bone at the junction of the sagittal and lambdoid sutures. 2 OS INCISIVUM. **greater multangular b.** OS TRAPEZIUM. **hamate b.** OS HAMATUM. **heel b.** CALCANEUS. **heterotopic b.** 1 Any bone that is not a part of the axial or appendicular skeleton, such as the os penis and os cordis. 2 Bone formation or calcification occurring in an abnormal location, most commonly seen in muscle (myositis ossificans) or tendon following severe trauma or burns. **highest turbinate b.** CONCHA NASALIS SUPREMA. **hip b.** OS COXAE. **hyoid b.** OS HYOIDEUM. **iliac b.** OS ILII. **inca b.** OS INTERPARIETALE. **incarial b.** OS INTERPARIETALE. **incisive b.** OS INCISIVUM. **inferior spongy b.** *Outmoded* CONCHA NASALIS INFERIOR. **inferior turbinate b.** CONCHA NASALIS INFERIOR. **innominate b.** *Outmoded* OS COXAE. **intermaxillary b.** OS INCISIVUM. **intermediate cuneiform b.** OS CUNEIFORME INTERMEDIUM. **internal cuneiform b.** OS CUNEIFORME MEDIALE. **interparietal b.** OS INTERPARIETALE. **intrachondrial b.**

Bone tissue that arises within cartilage which has undergone calcification, as is seen in the otic capsule. **ischial b.** OS ISCHII. **jaw b.** JAWBONE. **jugal b.** OS ZYGOMATICUM. **Krause b.** OS ACETABULI. **lacrimal b.** OS LACRIMALE. **lamellar b.** Mature cortical bone in which the collagen fibers are arranged in parallel rows around osteons. Also *lamellated bone.* **lateral cuneiform b.** OS CUNEIFORME LATERALE. **lesser multangular b.** *Outmoded* OS TRAPEZOIDEUM. **lesser trapezium b.** OS TRAPEZOIDEUM. **lingual b.** OS HYOIDEUM. **long b.** OS LONGUM. **lower jaw b.** MANDIBULA. **b.'s of lower limb** OSSA MEMBRI INFERIORIS. **lunate b.** OS LUNATUM. **malar b.** OS ZYGOMATICUM. **mastoid b.** PROCESSUS MASTOIDEUS OSSIS TEMPORALIS. **maxillary b.** MAXILLA. **maxilloturbinal b.** CONCHA NASALIS INFERIOR. **medial cuneiform b.** OS CUNEIFORME MEDIALE. **membrane b.** Bone developed by intramembranous ossification, from centers of ossification appearing directly in embryonic connective tissue without any development within a cartilaginous model. This type of ossification occurs in the cranial vault and in the facial bones. **mesethmoid b.** The most anterior bone of the braincase of primates, rodents, and carnivores, anterior to the presphenoid bone. **mesocuneiform b.** OS CUNEIFORME INTERMEDIUM. **metacarpal b.'s** OSSA METACARPI I–V. **metatarsal b.'s** OSSA METATARSI I–V. **middle cuneiform b.** OS CUNEIFORME INTERMEDIUM. **middle turbinate b.** CONCHA NASALIS MEDIA. **mosaic b.** The characteristic histologic appearance of bone that is affected by Paget's disease. It often reflects increased bone turnover and irregular ossification. **nasal b.** OS NASALE. **navicular b.** OS NAVICULARE. **navicular b. of foot** OS NAVICULARE. **navicular b. of hand** OS SCAPHOIDEUM. **nonlamellated b.** WOVEN BONE. **occipital b.** OS OCCIPITALE. **odontoid b.** DENS AXIS. **orbitosphenoidal b.** ALA MINOR OSSIS SPHENOIDALIS. **palate b.** OS PALATINUM. **palatine b.** OS PALATINUM. **parietal b.** OS PARIETALE. **pelvic b.** OS COXAE. **perichondral b.** Bone formed by ossification in a membranous perichondrium and laid down on the surface of cartilage, especially in long bones. **periosteal b.** The lamina of cartilage cells and osteoblasts on the surface of developing long bones that becomes separated from the subjacent cartilage or bone to form the periosteum or perichondrium, the deeper layer of which remains potentially osteogenic. **petrosal b.** PARS PETROSA OSSIS TEMPORALIS. **petrous b.** PARS PETROSA OSSIS TEMPORALIS. **phalangeal b.'s of foot** OSSA DIGITORUM PEDIS. **phalangeal b.'s of hand** OSSA DIGITORUM MANUS. **Pirie's b.** An accessory tarsal bone occasionally seen near the head of the talus. **pisiform b.** OS PISIFORME. **pneumatic b.** OS PNEUMATICUM. **postsphenoidal b.** The posterior part of the sphenoid bone prior to the eighth month of fetal life. It includes two centers of ossification for the body of the sphenoid behind the tuberculum sellae and two for the alisphenoid, or medial part of each greater wing. The postsphenoid usually unites with the presphenoid before birth. **prefrontal b.** PARS NASALIS OSSIS FRONTALIS. **prefrontal b. of von Bardeleben** PROCESSUS FRONTALIS MAXILLAE. **preinterparietal b.** Fused additional centers of ossification that may occur in front of the interparietal part of the occipital bone and fuse with it. The centers of ossification may fuse and remain separate from the interparietal bone, thereby forming a sutural bone. **premaxillary b.** OS INCISIVUM. **presphenoidal b.** The anterior part of the sphenoid bone prior to the eighth month of fetal life. It is developed from two cartilaginous centers in front of the tuberculum sellae and from two centers for the orbitosphenoids, or lesser wings of the sphenoid. They unite at about the fourth month and fuse with each other across the midline at about the time the presphenoid fuses with the postsphenoid. **primary b.** A type of bone which first appears when bone is being formed in the fetus of mammals, in new bone formation at fractures, and in some bony growths. It is similar to bone in some adult lower vertebrates and also to that in some bones of marine mammals. Primary bone has an indistinct trabecular structure, more or less closely knit, and devoid of obvious lamellae but with a coarse-fibered matrix. Also *fetal bone.* **primitive b.** WOVEN BONE. **pterygoid b.** PROCESSUS PTERYGOIDEUS OSSIS SPHENOIDALIS. **pubic b.** OS PUBIS. **pyramidal b.** OS TRIQUETRUM. **radial b.** RADIUS. **radial carpal b.** OS SCAPHOIDEUM. **resurrection b.** OS SACRUM. **reticulated b.** WOVEN BONE. **riders' b.** A localized ossification of the distal end of the adductor magnus muscle at the insertion into the adductor tubercle of the femur. It is sometimes seen in horseback riders. Also *cavalry bone.* **Riolan's b.'s** RIOLAN'S OSSICLES. **rudimentary b.** A bone which does not fully develop into adult life either because it is vestigial in an evolutionary sense or because of interference with its growth. **sacral b.** OS SACRUM. **scaphoid b.** OS SCAPHOIDEUM. **scaphoid b. of hand** OS SCAPHOIDEUM. **scapular b.** SCAPULA. **scroll b.'s** The conchae nasalis inferior, media, superior, and suprema. **secondary b.** Parallel or concentric lamellae, with the fibers arranged longitudinally and circumferentially, that constitute typical osteons and replace woven-fibered bone. **secondary cuboid b.** The lateral portion of the navicular bone, which is quite separated from the rest of the bone and is sometimes fused to the cuboid bone. It is rarely independent in the human foot. **second cuneiform b.** OS CUNEIFORME INTERMEDIUM. **semilunar b.** OS LUNATUM. **septal b.** Either septa interalveolaria or septa interradicularia. **sesamoid b.'s** OSSA SESAMOIDEA. **sesamoid b.'s of foot** OSSA SESAMOIDEA PEDIS. **sesamoid b.'s of hand** OSSA SESAMOIDEA MANUS. **sesamoid b. of lateral head of gastrocnemius muscle** A sesamoid bone occasionally located in the origin of the lateral head of the gastrocnemius muscle behind the lateral femoral condyle. **shank b.** **1** TIBIA. **2** In quadrupeds, the medial supporting bone between the knee joint and ankle joint. **shin b.** TIBIA. **short b.** OS BREVE. **sieve b.** LAMINA CRIBROSA OSSIS ETHMOIDALIS. **b.'s of skull** OSSA CRANII. **solid b.** SUBSTANTIA COMPACTA OSSIUM. **sphenoid b.** OS SPHENOIDALE. **sphenoidal turbinate b.** CONCHA SPHENOIDALIS. **sphenoturbinal b.** CONCHA SPHENOIDALIS. **spoke b.** RADIUS. **spongy b.** SUBSTANTIA SPONGIOSA OSSIUM. **squamo-occipital b.** The squamous part of the fetal occipital bone comprising a membranous upper, or interparietal, portion and a cartilaginous lower, or supraoccipital, portion. **squamosal b.** **1** PARS SQUAMOSA OSSIS TEMPORALIS. **2** A membrane bone of the vertebrate skull, varying in shape and size in different species and forming part of the posterior side wall of the cranium. In zoology, it is usually referred to simply as "the squamosal." **squamous b.** PARS SQUAMOSA OSSIS TEMPORALIS. **stirrup b.** STAPES. **subperiosteal b.** Bone laid down by osteoblasts of the deeper osteogenetic layer of the periosteum during the growth of bone. **superior turbinate b.** CONCHA NASALIS SUPERIOR. **supernumerary b.** A bone in excess of the usual number of its kind, particularly in segmentally arranged bones such as ribs and vertebrae. **suprainterparietal b.** A sutural bone occurring occasionally in the posterior part of the sagittal suture. **supraoccipital b.** The lower portion of the squamous part of the occipital bone that extends between the supreme nuchal line and the foramen magnum and abuts laterally on the petromastoid. This area ossifies in cartilage, and its external surface provides attachment for nuchal muscles and ligaments. **suprasternal b.'s** OSSA SUPRASTERNALIA. **supreme ethmoid b.** CONCHA NASALIS SUPREMA. **supreme nasal b.** CONCHA NASALIS SUPREMA. **supreme turbinate b.** CONCHA NASALIS SUPREMA. **sutural b.'s** OSSA SUTURALIA. **tabular b.** OS PLANUM. **tarsal b.'s** OSSA TARSI. **temporal b.** OS TEMPORALE. **thigh b.** FEMUR. **third cuneiform b.** OS CUNEIFORME LATERALE. **b.'s of toes** OSSA DIGITORUM PEDIS. **trabecular b.** SUBSTANTIA SPONGIOSA OSSIUM. **trapezium b. of Lyser** OS TRAPEZOIDEUM. **trapezoid b. of Lyser** OS TRAPEZIUM. **triangular b.** OS TRIQUETRUM. **triangular b. of tarsus** OS TRIGONUM. **triquetral b.** OS TRIQUETRUM. **turbinate b.** Any of four bones: (1) concha nasalis inferior; (2) concha nasalis media; (3) concha nasalis superior; (4) concha nasalis suprema. **tympanic b.** 1 ANNULUS TYMPANICUS. 2 PARS TYMPANICA OSSIS TEMPORALIS. **ulnar carpal b.** OS TRIQUETRUM. **unciform b.** OS HAMATUM. **uncinate b.** OS HAMATUM. **upper jaw b.** MAXILLA. **b.'s of upper limb** OSSA MEMBRI SUPERIORIS. **vomer b.** See under VOMER. **whirl b.** PATELLA. **wormian b.'s** OSSA SUTURALIA. **wormian b. of the fontanels** A sutural bone which develops at the site of a fontanel. *Outmoded.* **wormian b.'s of the sutures** OSSA SUTURALIA. **woven b.** Immature, prenatal, spongy bone containing interconnected vascular spaces around which the bundles of osteocollagenous fibers form an irregular nonlamellated network with scattered lacunae. This type of bone is rapidly replaced by mature bone but some persists in adults in the lining of tooth sockets, the osseous labyrinth, and near cranial sutures. It is also found in normal repair of bone and in rapidly growing bone tumors. Also *nonlamellated bone, primitive bone, reticulated bone.* **xiphoid b.** 1 PROCESSUS XIPHOIDEUS. 2 *Outmoded* STERNUM. **zygomatic b.** OS ZYGOMATICUM.

**bonelet** \bōn′lət\ A tiny bone, or ossicle.

**bone-salt** HYDROXYAPATITE.

**Bonnet** [Amedée *Bonnet,* French surgeon, 1802–1858] See under CAPSULE.

**Bonnot** [Edmond *Bonnot,* U.S. anatomist, flourished late 19th–early 20th century] Bonnot's gland. See under INTERSCAPULAR GLAND.

**boomslang** \bōm′släng\ [Afrikaans (from *boom* tree + *slang* snake) a tree snake] A venomous, arboreal snake of the species *Dispholidus typus,* found in southern Africa.

**booster** BOOSTER DOSE.

**boot** / **air b.** An air splint used as a temporary orthosis, usually for a lower limb. **pneumatic b.** A device to effect extrinsic limb compression by an inclusive pneumatic system, sudden deflation of which is accompanied by reactive hyperemia in the limb. Abnormalities of this response may be demonstrated by Doppler pressures or radionuclide scanning. **Unna's paste b.** A paste of gelatin, glycerin, and zinc oxide applied to the leg, which is then covered with a spiral bandage. Paste is added to the bandage and then more bandaging and paste until rigidity is achieved. It is used in the treatment of stasis ulcers, stasis eczema, and varicose veins. Also *Unna's boot.*

**Boothby** [Walter Meredith *Boothby,* U.S. medical researcher, 1880–1953] See under BLB MASK.

**borborygmus** \bôr′bərig′məs\ [Gk *borborygmos* a rumbling, from *borborizein* to rumble] (*pl.* borborygmi) Abdominal rumbling; sounds which occur due to the passage of gas through the intestines.

**bordeaux B** \bôrdō′\ CERASINE.

**border** The edge, margin, or delimitation of a surface, structure, or tissue; margo. **b. of acetabulum** LABRUM ACETABULARE. **alveolar b. of mandible** ARCUS ALVEOLARIS MANDIBULAE. **alveolar b. of maxilla** ARCUS ALVEOLARIS MAXILLAE. **anterior b. of liver** MARGO INFERIOR HEPATIS. **anterior b. of pancreas** MARGO ANTERIOR PANCREATIS. **anterior b. of radius** MARGO ANTERIOR RADII. **anterior b. of tibia** MARGO ANTERIOR TIBIAE. **brush b.** The closely packed microvilli which line the luminal surface of the proximal convoluted tubules and which facilitate absorption. Also *striated border, border fibrils.* **external b. of tibia** FACIES LATERALIS TIBIAE. **inferior b. of liver** MARGO INFERIOR HEPATIS. **inferior b. of mandible** BASIS MANDIBULAE. **inferior b. of pancreas** MARGO INFERIOR PANCREATIS. **inferior b. of spleen** MARGO INFERIOR SPLENIS. **interosseous b. of fibula** MARGO INTEROSSEUS FIBULAE. **interosseous b. of radius** MARGO INTEROSSEUS RADII. **interosseous b. of tibia** MARGO INTEROSSEUS TIBIAE. **interosseous b. of ulna** MARGO INTEROSSEUS ULNAE. **lacrimal b. of maxilla** MARGO LACRIMALIS MAXILLAE. **lambdoid b. of occipital bone** MARGO LAMBDOIDEUS SQUAMAE OCCIPITALIS. **lateral b. of humerus** MARGO LATERALIS HUMERI. **lateral b. of scapula** MARGO LATERALIS SCAPULAE. **left b. of heart** *Outmoded* FACIES PULMONALIS CORDIS. **medial b. of foot** MARGO MEDIALIS PEDIS. **medial b. of forearm** MARGO MEDIALIS ANTEBRACHII. **medial b. of humerus** MARGO MEDIALIS HUMERI. **medial b. of tibia** MARGO MEDIALIS TIBIAE. **orbital b. of sphenoid bone** FACIES ORBITALIS ALAE MAJORIS. **b. of oval fossa** LIMBUS FOSSAE OVALIS. **peripheral b. of iris** MARGO CILIARIS IRIDIS. **posterior b. of fibula** MARGO POSTERIOR FIBULAE. **posterior b. of petrous portion of temporal bone** MARGO POSTERIOR PARTIS PETROSAE OSSIS TEMPORALIS. **posterior b. of radius** MARGO POSTERIOR RADII. **posterointernal b. of fibula** CRISTA MEDIALIS FIBULAE. **right b. of heart** MARGO DEXTER CORDIS. **striated b.** BRUSH BORDER. **superior b. of patella** BASIS PATELLAE. **superior b. of petrous portion of temporal bone** MARGO SUPERIOR PARTIS PETROSAE OSSIS TEMPORALIS. **superior b. of scapula** MARGO SUPERIOR SCAPULAE. **superior b. of spleen** MARGO SUPERIOR SPLENIS. **vermilion b.** The external, reddish mucosal portion of the lips that is continuous with the intraoral mucosa of the vestibule and ends anteriorly at the junction with the skin of the lips. The upper and lower borders surround the oral fissure, meeting at the corners, or commissures, of the mouth. The reddish color is imparted by the underlying capillaries. Also *vermilion zone, vermilion transitional zone, red margin.*

**borderline** Having some but not all of the properties that would justify such a classification, as *borderline hypertension, a borderline schizophrenic.* • The word often conveys the sense of progression toward the condition cited, which is apt to occur unless corrective action is taken.

**Bordet** [Jules Jean Baptiste Vincent *Bordet,* Belgian bacteriologist, 1870–1961] 1 Bordet-Gengou agar. See under AGAR. 2 Bordet-Gengou bacillus. See under *BORDETELLA PERTUSSIS.* 3 Bordet and Gengou reaction. See under COMPLEMENT FIXATION.

***Bordetella*** \bôr′dətel′ə\ [after J. J. B. V. *Bordet,* Belgian bacteriologist, 1870–1961] A genus of small, nonmotile, Gram-negative bacilli whose principal species is *B. pertussis. B parapertussis* and *B. bronchiseptica* also can cause disease in man. ***B. parapertussis*** An occasional cause of whooping cough. It is differentiated from *Bordetella pertussis* by its cultural and serologic reactions. ***B. pertussis*** A small, nonmotile, Gram-negative, aerobic bacillus which causes whooping cough. It attaches specifically to ciliated bronchial epithelium, producing a dermonecrotic exotoxin that is also a lymphocytosis-promoting factor. The toxin activates adenylate cyclase, but with a different specificity from cholera and other enterotoxins. Growth requirements are simple but the organism is delicate, and growth is promoted by agents that bind fatty acids. It is usually cultured on Bordet-Gengou agar, which contains fresh sheep blood. Also *Bordet-Gengou bacillus.*

**Bordier** [Leonard Henri *Bordier,* French physician, born 1863] Bordier-Fränkel sign. See under SIGN.

**boric acid** $H_3BO_3$. A white crystalline powder, or white crystals slightly greasy to the touch, odorless, melting at 185°C with decomposition. It is soluble in water, ethanol, and glycerol, slightly soluble in acetone. A weak acid (p*K* 9.2), in alkali it adds OH— to form $B^-(OH)_4$ rather than loses a proton. On heating to 100°C it loses a molecule of water to form metaboric acid. It is a weak, nonirritant antiseptic, but is not bacteriocidal. It is not harmless, and its application to wounds and sores can lead to damage. Its medicinal preparations are (3%) boric acid solution and 10% boric acid in petroleum jelly.

**Born** [Gustav Jacob *Born,* German anatomist, 1851–1900] Born method of wax plate reconstruction. See under METHOD.

**bornyl salicylate** SALIT.

**borocaine** PROCAINE BORATE.

**boron** Element number 5, having atomic weight 10.81. Boron is a nonmetal existing either as a hard, lustrous, crystalline solid or as an amorphous brownish black powder. The two naturally occurring isotopes have mass numbers 10 and 11. Boron is never found free but in numerous compounds. The valence is 3. Some boron compounds act as cumulative poisons. Symbol: B

**borosalicylic acid** A mixture of one part boric acid and two parts salicylic acid. It has been used as an antiseptic ingredient in washes and ointments.

***Borrelia*** \bôrel′yə\ [after Amédée *Borrel,* French bacteriologist, 1867–1936] A genus of spirochetes many species of which cause relapsing fever. They are larger and more loosely coiled than *Treponema* and are easily seen when stained with aniline dyes. Some strains grow, very slowly, in complex media under anaerobic conditions. In addition to *B. recurrentis,* many species may be transmitted to man from lower animals by ticks of the genus *Ornithodoros,* causing endemic relapsing fever. In relapsing fever, circulating antibody agglutinates the organisms and prevents further multiplication. Each succeeding wave of relapse is due to the emergence of an antigenic variant. Also *Entomospira.* ***B. burgdorferi*** The spirochete that causes Lyme disease. It is transmitted to humans by the tick *Ixodes dammini.* ***B. duttoni*** A species of *Borrelia* that has been a frequent cause of endemic relapsing fever in Africa. ***B. recurrentis*** The spirochete that causes epidemic relapsing fever. It is spread among humans by the body louse *Pediculus humanus.*

**Borsieri** [Giovanni Battista *Borsieri* de Kanifeld, Italian physician 1725–1785] Borsieri sign. See under LINE.

**boss** [Old French *boce* hump, swelling] A rounded protuberance or projection from a surface. **frontal b.** TUBER FRONTALE. **parietal b.** The prominent portion of the lateral aspect of the parietal bone. **sanguineous b.** CAPUT SUCCEDANEUM.

**bosselated** \bäs′əlātid\ Bearing many bosses; covered with bosses; knobby.

**bosselation** \bäs′əlā′shən\ **1** A boss or knobby eminence. **2** The condition of having many bosses or of becoming covered with bosses.

**bossing** The formation or presence of bosses; bosselation. **b. of the cranium** Prominences on the central portion, or dome, of the frontal and parietal bones in infancy. It is sometimes due to rickets, which causes thickening of the outer table of the bones. It may also result from chronic severe anemias of infancy, in which overactive and hypertrophied hemopoietic tissue expands the marrow cavity and causes new bone to be laid down as a reactive process. The malformed cranium is sometimes known as a hot cross bun skull. Also *frontal bossing.*

**Bostock** [John *Bostock,* English physician, 1773–1846] Bostock's catarrh. See under HAY FEVER.

**Boston** [Leonard Napoleon *Boston,* U.S. physician, 1871–1931] Boston sign. See under EYELID LAG.

**bot** \bät\ [prob. from Low German; akin to Dutch *bot*] A botfly larva.

**Botallo** [Leonardo *Botallo,* Italian physician, 1530–1600] **1** Ligament of Botallo. See under LIGAMENTUM ARTERIOSUM. **2** Ganglion of duct of Botallo. See under NODUS LIGAMENTIS ARTERIOSI.

**botfly** \bät′flī\ Any myiasis-producing fly whose larvae are called bots, especially one of the genus *Gasterophilus* which produces enteric myiasis in horses. Also *bot fly.* **human b.** A fly of the species *Dermatobia hominis.*

**bothria** \bäth′rē·ə\ Plural of BOTHRIUM.

***Bothriocephalus*** \bäth′rē·ōsef′ələs\ [*bothri(um)* + -CEPHALUS] A genus in the cestode family Bothriocephalidae, order Pseudophyllidea, frequently found infecting freshwater fish in North America. ***B. mansoni*** *SPIROMETRA MANSONI* ***B. mansonoides*** *SPIROMETRA MANSONOIDES*

**bothrium** \bäth′rē·əm\ [New L (from Gk *bothrion* a small pit, hole)] (*pl.* bothria) One of a pair of sucking grooves located on the dorsal and ventral surfaces of the scolex of most members of the cestode order Pseudophyllidea.

***Bothrops*** \bäth′räps\ [Gk *bothr(os)* a pit, trench + *ōps* face, eye] A genus of venomous snakes of the family Viperidae, subfamily Crotalinae, found in South America and on islands in the Caribbean Sea. ***B. atrox*** A pit viper of South and Central America known as the fer-de-lance. It is a major cause of snakebite in South America. An adult produces about 80–200 mg of venom, while a lethal dose for humans is estimated at 50 mg. An antivenin is generally available.

**botogenin** A precursor used in the synthesis of pharmacologically active steroids. It is isolated from a tuber, *Dioscorea mexicana,* the Mexican yam. Also *gentrogenin.*

**botryoid** \bät′rē·oid\ [Gk *botry(s)* a bunch of grapes + -OID] Having a grapelike appearance, as in sarcoma botryoides.

***Botryomyces*** \bät′rē·əmī′sēz\ [Gk *botry(s)* a bunch of grapes + *o* + -MYCES] The organism once believed to cause botryomycosis.

**botryomycoma** \bät′rē·əmīkō′mə\ [*Botryomyc(es)* + -OMA] A chronic granulomatous response to bacterial infection, characterized by a cutaneous or subcutaneous swelling. The bacteria involved are usually staphylococci or species of *Pseudomonas.*

**botryomycosis** \bät′rē·əmīkō′sis\ [*Botryomyc(es)* + -OSIS] An infection caused by staphylococci (or, rarely, Gram-negative rods) and characterized by cutaneous (or, rarely, visceral) granulomatous lesions with suppurative foci containing granules. The infection occurs in horses, cattle, camels, and man. Adj. botryomycotic.

**Böttcher** [Arthur *Böttcher*, German anatomist, 1831–1889] **1** Charcot-Böttcher crystalloids. See under CRYSTALLOID. **2** Böttcher's ganglion. See under GANGLION SPIRALE COCHLEAE. **3** Böttcher space. See under SACCUS ENDOLYMPHATICUS.

**bottle** / **wash b.** **1** A bottle used to direct delivery of a stream of liquid. It is constructed either with two tubes in the cap, such that blowing into one causes emission from the other, or with flexible sides such that squeezing the container produces flow. **2** A bottle containing liquid through which gas is passed for purification.

**bottom** / **weavers' b.** Chronic ischial bursitis caused by constant pressure on the bone by sitting on a hard surface.

**bottromycin** \bät′rəmī′sin\ An antibiotic with a substituted tetrapeptide ring. It inhibits protein synthesis.

**botuliform** \bätyoo′lifôrm\ Shaped like a sausage.

**botulin** \bät′yəlin\ *Seldom used* BOTULINUM TOXIN.

**botulism** \bät′yəlizm\ [L *botul(us)* a sausage + -ISM] A paralytic, often fatal illness caused by *Clostridium botulinum*, different strains of which produce several immunologically distinct botulinum toxins. Types A, B, and E account for most human botulism, while types C and D are associated with botulism in animals, especially cattle, ducks, and chickens. Most human cases result from ingestion of food contaminated with the preformed toxin. See also BOTULISM FOOD POISONING. **food-borne b.** BOTULISM FOOD POISONING. **infant b.** *Clostridium botulinum* infection in otherwise healthy infants, usually 3–20 weeks of age, producing the floppy infant syndrome. First reported in 1976, the disease is not well understood. Most features of its pathogenesis and the mechanisms of recovery are unknown. The clinical syndrome is thought to result from production *in vivo* of botulinum toxin. The *C. botulinum* organism and the toxin (type A or B) are both demonstrable in the stool and may persist in the gut for weeks after the infant recovers. Affected infants are afebrile and, after a brief prodromal period of constipation, develop depression of the sucking and gag reflexes, an altered cry, cranial nerve deficits, generalized muscle weakness, hypotonia, and areflexia. Nearly 50 percent suffer respiratory arrest. Most infants recover completely with only intensive supportive care. Because many patients are already recovering when the diagnosis is made, antitoxin is only rarely used and its role in treatment is unclear. Respiratory arrest due to infant botulism is thought to account for some cases of sudden infant death syndrome. **wound b.** A rare form of botulism resulting from toxin production by *Clostridium botulinum* (type A or B) infecting a traumatic wound. The clinical syndrome that develops 7–14 days after the injury is virtually identical to that seen in botulism food poisoning, although the wound infection may produce fever. Treatment is the same as for botulism food poisoning.

**bouba** \bō′bə\ **1** A Portuguese term for MUCOCUTANEOUS LEISHMANIASIS. **2** A Portuguese term for YAWS.

**Bouchard** [Charles Jacques *Bouchard*, French physician, 1837–1915] **1** Bouchard's nodules. See under BOUCHARD'S NODES. **2** Charcot-Bouchard aneurysm. See under ANEURYSM.

**bouffée** \bUfā′\ A transient attack or episode. **b. délirante** An acute psychotic episode or series of episodes, often schizophrenic, in reaction to a severely disturbing experience or situation. The prognosis of such a disorder is favorable.

**bougie** \boozhē′\ [French (from *Bougie* or *Bugia*, Algeria, source of candle wax), candle] A flexible, slender, cylindrical instrument for insertion into tubular body canals, used for such purposes as exploration, dilatation, calibration, application of medication, and guidance for the passage of other instruments. **b. à boule** A bougie with a bulbous tip, used especially for calibration of the urethra. Also *bulbous bougie*. **Hurst's b.'s** A series of mercury-weighted, blunt-tipped bougies with graded diameters used for dilation of esophageal strictures. **Maloney b.'s** A series of mercury-weighted, tapered-tipped bougies with graded diameters used for dilation of esophageal strictures. **wax-tipped b.** A bougie with a wax tip, used to establish the presence of a urethral or ureteral stone.

**bougienage** \boojēnäzh′\ [BOUGIE + *n* + -AGE] Treatment of a narrowed or constricted segment of a tubular organ by introduction of a bougie, as in dilatation of a urethral or esophageal stricture. Also *bouginage*.

**Bouillaud** [Jean Baptiste *Bouillaud*, French physician, 1796–1881] **1** See under SIGN. **2** Bouillaud's disease. See under RHEUMATIC HEART DISEASE.

**Bouin** [Pol Andre *Bouin*, French histologist, 1870–1962] Bouin's fixative, Bouin solution. See under FLUID.

**boulimia** \boolim′ē·ə\ BULIMIA.

**boundary** Anything serving as a limit. **ego b.** The hypothesized delimitation between the ego and nonego. The inner ego boundary is the line between the ego and the unconscious. The external ego boundary is the line between the ego and the outer world and determines the degree to which objects are perceived as real or familiar.

**bouquet** \bookā′\ [French, from older *bosquet* thicket, from Old French *boschet*, dim. of *bosc, bois* forest] A structure or part suggesting the shape of a bunch or bouquet of flowers. **b. of Riolan** RIOLAN'S NOSEGAY.

**Bourgery** [Marc-Jean *Bourgery*, French anatomist and surgeon, 1797–1849] Bourgery's ligament. See under LIGAMENTUM POPLITEUM OBLIQUUM.

**Bourneville** [Désiré-Magloire *Bourneville*, French neurologist, 1840–1909] Bourneville's phakomatosis, Bourneville syndrome, Bourneville-Pringle syndrome, Bourneville's disease, Bourneville-Brissaud disease. See under TUBEROUS SCLEROSIS.

**bout** / **periodic drinking b.'s** A type of alcoholism manifested in recurrent paroxysmal episodes of alcohol overindulgence during which the alcoholic drinks for days or weeks. Following recovery from one such episode, the alcoholic may remain abstinent for weeks or months before the next episode. Also *binge drinking, dipsomania, epsilon alcoholism, paroxysmal alcoholism, periodic drinking*.

**bouton** \bootôN′\ [French (from *bouter* to push, sprout) a bud, sprout, button, pimple] **1** A small knoblike structure; especially, an end foot of an axon. **2** A papule, pimple, or boil. **b. en passage** A bouton located along the course of the axon, as distinguished from one at the axon's terminal. **b. terminal** END FOOT.

**boutonneuse** \bootônœz′\ [French (from *bouton* button, pimple, papule + *-euse*, fem. of *-eux* adjectival suffix) pimply, papular] BOUTONNEUSE FEVER.

**boutonnière** \bootônyer′\ [French (from *bouton* a button) a buttonhole] An incision into a membrane, resembling a buttonhole.

**Bouveret** [Leon *Bouveret*, French physician, 1850–1929] **1** Bouveret's disease, Bouveret syndrome. See under PAROXYSMAL TACHYCARDIA. **2** See under SYNDROME, SIGN, UL-

CER. **3** Bouveret-Duguet ulcer. See under ULCER.

**bow** [Middle English *bowe,* from Old English *boga*] An instrument or device shaped like a bow. **Birnberg b.** A polyethylene intrauterine contraceptive device shaped like a figure eight. **cupid's b.** The line formed by the junction of the skin and the vermilion border at the center of the upper lip. **hypochordal b.** The structure at the blastemal stage that connects the vertebral ends of two costal processes of the upper three or four developing cervical vertebrae to each other anteriorly. It persists only in the atlas where it chondrifies, becomes ossified during the first postnatal year, and forms the anterior arch of the atlas and also the anterior tips of its lateral masses. **labial b.** A bow-shaped wire on the anterior portion of an orthodontic appliance. It may contact the labial surfaces of the anterior teeth or occasionally, in the upper jaw, be high in the labial sulcus and carry fine-wire springs. **Logan b.** A steel U-shaped bow, fastened with adhesive tape to both cheeks of an infant during the postoperative period of a cleft lip repair, used to prevent tension on the suture line during facial movements.

**Bowditch** [Henry Pickering *Bowditch,* U.S. physiologist, 1840–1911] **1** Bowditch phenomenon. See under STAIRCASE PHENOMENON. **2** Bowditch's law. See under ALL-OR-NONE LAW.

**bowel** [Middle English *bouel,* from Old French *buele* intestine, from Med L *botellum* intestine, from L *botellus,* dim. of *botulus* sausage] INTESTINE.

**Bowen** [John Templeton *Bowen,* U.S. dermatologist, 1857–1941] **1** Bowen's disease of the penis. See under DISEASE. **2** Bowen's precancerous dermatosis. See under BOWEN'S DISEASE.

**bowenoid** \bō′wənoid\ [after John Templeton *Bowen,* American dermatologist, 1857–1941 + -OID] Resembling Bowen's disease.

**bowl / mastoid b.** The bowl-shaped excavation in the mastoid process, created at mastoidectomy, particularly when the excavation communicates with the external auditory meatus as in radical or modified radical mastoidectomy.

**bowleg** GENU VARUM. **nonrachitic b.** OSTEOCHONDROSIS DEFORMANS TIBIAE.

**Bowman** [Sir William *Bowman,* English ophthalmologist, anatomist, and physiologist, 1816–1892] **1** See under MEMBRANE, SPACE. **2** Bowman's disk. See under DISK OF STRIATED MUSCLE FIBERS. **3** Bowman's capsule. See under CAPSULA GLOMERULI. **4** Bowman's gland. See under GLANDULA OLFACTORIA. **5** Bowman's tubes. See under CORNEAL TUBES. **6** Bowman's lamina, Bowman's layer, lamina elastica anterior bowmani. See under LAMINA LIMITANS ANTERIOR CORNEAE. **7** Bowman's muscle. See under MUSCULUS CILIARIS.

**box / Barany's b.** A small metal box containing a machine producing high intensity noise that masks all other sounds when placed against the ear. It is used in certain hearing tests. **black b.** A usually complicated electronic device of hidden or unspecified design which does however perform a known function or have a fixed input-output relationship. **Blair suction b.** A hand-held instrument consisting of an oblong metal box having a slit-like aperture on one surface and a nipple for attaching a vacuum hose on another. It is used for lifting, stretching, and stabilizing the skin while harvesting split-thickness grafts freehand. *Obs.* **glove b.** An enclosed space used to manipulate objects or materials that should be isolated from the general laboratory environment. The operator places his or her hands in gloves that are sealed into openings in the glass protective partition to prevent contact between the operator and the material but permit manipulation through the flexible gloves. **Hogness b.** A region along the eukaryotic DNA molecule which serves as the site of recognition and attachment of RNA polymerase, located about 25 base pairs upstream from the point of the start of transcription. **homeo b.** A short (several hundred nucleotides or less), highly conserved nucleotide sequence common to multiple homoeotic genes. **hot air b.** HOT-BOX. **obstruction b.** A device used for estimating the strength of various drives in experimental animals by indicating how much of a specified noxious stimulation will be endured to reach a goal; for example, by counting the number of crossings made of an electrically charged grid in a given time period in order to reach food or a female in estrus, or to retrieve pups. **Pribnow b.** A region along the prokaryotic DNA molecule which serves as a recognition site and point of attachment for RNA polymerase, located about 10 base pairs upstream from the point of the beginning of transcription. Also *TATA box.* **Skinner b.** An enclosure in which an animal, as a pigeon, is placed in order to perform some instrumental act, such as pressing a bar or pecking at a spot. The behavior must be learned for the animal to obtain a reward, typically a food pellet. Control of extraneous environmental influences is made possible, and the acquisition of the instrumental response can be related to the schedule of reinforcement in effect. **TATA b.** PRIBNOW BOX. **voice b.** LARYNX.

**boxidine** $C_{19}H_{20}F_3NO$. 1-[2-[[4′-(trifluoromethyl)-4-biphenyl]oxy]ethyl]pyrrolidine. An agent with anticholesterolemic activity. It also blocks the synthesis of adrenal steroids.

**boxing** The attachment of a vertical wall to the margin of a dental impression in order to contain the liquid plaster when casting.

**Boyden** [Edward Allen *Boyden,* U.S. anatomist, 1886–1977] **1** See under TEST. **2** Sphincter of Boyden. See under MUSCULUS SPHINCTER DUCTUS CHOLEDOCHI.

**Boyle** [Robert *Boyle,* Irish-born British physicist and chemist, 1627–1691] See under LAW.

**Bozeman** [Nathan *Bozeman,* U.S. surgeon, 1825–1905] **1** Bozeman's operation. See under HYSTEROCYSTOCLEISIS. **2** See under POSITION.

**BP** **1** blood pressure. **2** British Pharmacopoeia.

**bp** boiling point.

**BPL** $\beta$-propiolactone

**Bq** Symbol for the unit, becquerel.

**Br** Symbol for the element, bromine.

**Braasch** [William F. *Braasch,* U.S. urologist, 1878–1975] See under CATHETER.

**brace** [Old French (from L *brachia,* pl. of *brachium* the arm, from Gk *brachiōn* the arm), the two arms, a measure of five feet, a grasp] An external orthosis used to influence the growth of underlying musculoskeletal structures or to hold a deformity in the corrected position but allowing movement of the joints and, in the lower extremity, weight bearing. **Boston b.** A modular polypropylene body jacket that is used in the conservative treatment of scoliosis. **dropfoot b.** A brace that prevents plantar flexion of a foot with weakened dorsiflexors. **Klenzak b.** A double-bar foot-ankle brace used to prevent footdrop. A spring-assisted ankle joint produces ankle dorsiflexion. **Knight b.** A brace used to support the trunk and consisting of lateral and posterior rigid or semirigid uprights and a wide abdominal component. **Knight-Taylor b.** A back brace that adds shoulder straps to a Knight brace, more adequately to prevent motion of the thoracolumbar spine. **Lenox Hill b.** A hinged brace that supports the knee when it has been rendered unstable by ligamentous injuries. **Milwaukee b.** MOE BRACE. **Moe b.** A body brace extending into the cervical region. It is used in the conservative treatment of scoliosis. Also *Milwaukee brace.* **Taylor b.** A trunk brace with rigid uprights, shoulder straps, abdominal support, and a pelvic band, used to prevent flexion of the thoracolumbar spine.

**bracelet** Any of the transverse creases in the skin on the front of the wrist. **Nageotte's b.'s** Paranodal transverse bands on the surface of myelinated axons of peripheral nerves. Also *spiny bracelets.*

**Brachet** [Jean Louis *Brachet,* French physician, born 1789] Brachet mesolateral fold. See under MESOLATERAL FOLD.

**brachi-** \brā′kē-, brā′ki-\ BRACHIO-.

**brachia** \brā′kē·ə\ Plural of BRACHIUM.

**brachial** \brā′kē·əl\ Of or relating to the arm, or brachium.

**brachialgia** \brā′kē·al′jə\ [BRACHI- + -ALGIA] Pain in the arm.

**brachiform** \brā′kifôrm\ Shaped or bent like an arm.

**brachio-** \brā′kē·ō-\ [L *brachium* or *bracchium* (from Gk *brachiōn* arm) arm] A combining form denoting arm. Also *brachi-.*

**brachiocephalic** Pertaining to or involving the arm and the head.

**brachiocubital** \-kyoo′bitəl\ Pertaining to or involving the arm and the elbow or forearm.

**brachiocyrtosis** \-sirtō′sis\ A deformity of the arm. Also *brachiocyllosis.*

**brachium** \brāk′ē·əm\ [L (from Gk *brachiōn* the arm), the arm] (*pl.* brachia) **1** [NA] The region between shoulder and elbow. **2** A structure or formation resembling an arm. **anterior conjunctival b.** BRACHIUM COLLICULI SUPERIORIS. **b. colliculi caudalis** BRACHIUM COLLICULI INFERIORIS. **b. colliculi inferioris** [NA] The myelinated axon bundle extending from beneath the inferior colliculus to the thalamic medial geniculate body. Also *brachium of inferior colliculus, brachium quadrigeminum inferius, brachium colliculi caudalis.* **b. colliculi rostralis** BRACHIUM COLLICULI SUPERIORIS. **b. colliculi superioris** [NA] The large myelinated extension of the optic tract caudal to the thalamus ending in the superior colliculus. Also *anterior conjunctival brachium, brachium of superior colliculus, brachium quadrigeminum superius, brachium colliculi rostralis, prebrachium.* **b. conjunctivum cerebelli** PEDUNCULUS CEREBELLARIS SUPERIOR. **b. of inferior colliculus** BRACHIUM COLLICULI INFERIORIS. **b. opticum** The surface markings made by bundles of fibers passing from the corpora quadrigemina to the optic thalamus. **b. pontis** PEDUNCULUS CEREBELLARIS MEDIUS. **b. quadrigeminum inferius** BRACHIUM COLLICULI INFERIORIS. **b. quadrigeminum superius** BRACHIUM COLLICULI SUPERIORIS. **b. of superior colliculus** BRACHIUM COLLICULI SUPERIORIS.

**Bracht** [Erich Franz *Bracht,* German obstetrician, born 1882] See under MANEUVER.

**brachy-** \brak′ē-\ [Gk *brachys* short] A combining form meaning short.

**brachybasia** \-bā′zhə\ [BRACHY- + *bas(i)-* + -IA] A slow shuffling gait with short steps (march à petits pas) seen in Parkinson's disease and also in arteriosclerotic "parkinsonism," and due to diffuse cerebral softening resulting usually from widespread arteriosclerosis in hypertensive subjects.

**brachycephalic** \-səfal′ik\ Having a short, broad head, with a cephalic index greater than 80; characterized by brachycephaly.

**brachycephaly** \-sef′əlē\ [BRACHY- + CEPHAL- + -Y] Shortness and broadness of the head, with a cephalic index greater than 80. These proportions are common in certain populations, and may also occur as a developmental abnormality in inherently dolichocephalic or mesocephalic individuals, as from premature closure of the coronal suture.

**brachychilia** \-kī′lē·ə\ [BRACHY- + CHIL- + -IA] A condition in which the lips are too short to permit comfortable closure of the mouth. Also *brachycheilia.*

**brachycnemia** \brak′ēk·nē′mē·ə\ [BRACHY- + Gk *knēm(ē)* the leg + -IA] An abnormal shortness of the legs, of either developmental or traumatic origin.

**brachydontia** \-dän′shə\ [BRACHY- + *-(o)dontia*] The abnormal shortness of one or more teeth.

**brachyesophagus** \-esäf′əgəs\ [BRACHY- + ESOPHAGUS] Abnormal shortness of the esophagus. It is often seen with diaphragmatic hernia in which the stomach is displaced into the thorax.

**brachyglossal** \-gläs′əl\ [BRACHY- + GLOSSAL] Characterized by an abnormally short tongue.

**brachygnathia** \-nā′thē·ə\ [BRACHY- + GNATH- + -IA] MICROMANDIBLE.

**brachymetacarpia** \-met′əkär′pē·ə\ [BRACHY- + *metacarp(al)* + -IA] An abnormal shortness of one or more metacarpals. It usually affects the fourth and fifth metacarpals.

**brachymetapody** \-mətap′ədē\ [BRACHY- + META- + -POD + -Y] A shortness of metacarpals and/or metatarsals, with a resulting apparent shortness of associated digits.

**brachymetatarsia** \-met′ətär′sē·ə\ [BRACHY- + *metatars(al)* + -IA] The abnormal shortness of one or more metatarsals.

**brachymetropia** \-metrō′pē·ə\ [BRACHY- + Gk *metr(on)* a measure + -OPIA] MYOPIA.

**brachymetropic** \-mətrō′pik\ MYOPIC.

**brachymorphic** \-môr′fik\ [BRACHY- + MORPH- + -IC] Relatively short and broad in body build.

**brachyphalangia** \-fəlan′jə\ [BRACHY- + *phalang(es)* + -IA] An abnormal shortness of one or more phalanges.

**brachypodous** \brəkip′ədəs\ [BRACHY- + -POD + -OUS] Marked by abnormally short feet.

**brachyradiotherapy** \-rā′dē·əther′əpē\ BRACHYTHERAPY.

**brachyrhinia** \-rin′ē·ə\ [BRACHY- + RHIN- + -IA] An unusual degree of shortness of the nose.

**brachyrhyncus** \-ring′kəs\ [BRACHY- + Gk *rhynchos* snout, bill, beak] An abnormal flatness or recession of the central portion of the face as is seen in cyclopia or certain facial clefts.

**brachyskelic** \-skel′ik\ Having abnormal shortness of one or more legs. Also *brachyskelous.*

**brachytherapy** \-ther′əpē\ [BRACHY- + THERAPY] Treatment by radiation from a sealed source that is implanted or attached to the surface of the body. Also *brachyradiotherapy.* **interstitial b.** Brachytherapy involving insertion of a sealed source into or near a tumor or other lesion to be irradiated. Needles or seeds may be used, containing radium, radon, cobalt 60, or other radioactive substances. **intracavitary application b.** INTRACAVITARY RADIOTHERAPY.

**bracket** An orthodontic attachment to a tooth by means of a band or adhesive cement for connection to an orthodontic appliance.

**brady-** \brad′ē-\ [Gk *bradys* slow] A combining form meaning slow.

**bradyarrhythmia** \-əriTH′mē·ə\ An arrhythmia in which the ventricular rate is abnormally slow, usually less than 60 beats per minute.

**bradyarthria** \-är′thrē·ə\ [BRADY- + ARTHR- + -IA] Abnormally slow speech due to disease or dysfunction of the nervous system. Also *bradylalia, bradyglossia.*

**bradyauxesis** \-ôksē′sis\ [BRADY- + AUXESIS] The slower growth of one part of a structure or organism compared with that of the whole structure or whole organism; a form of heterauxesis.

**bradycardia** \-kär′dē·ə\ [BRADY- + -CARDIA] A slow heart rate, usually defined as less than 60 beats per minute in adults. **fetal b.** A drop in the baseline fetal heart rate to a level below 120 beats per minute. To be classified as bradycardia, the drop must be sustained for ten minutes or longer. **nodal b.** Bradycardia in which the pacemaker of the heart is situated in the atrioventricular nodal region rather than in the sinuatrial node. **physiologic b.** Bradycardia occurring in the absence of cardiac disease. Also *true bradycardia.* **sinus b.** Bradycardia resulting from an abnormally slow discharge from the sinuatrial node. **true b.** PHYSIOLOGIC BRADYCARDIA. **vagal b.** A slow heart rate as a consequence of vagal overactivity. **ventricular b.** Slow ventricular rate, usually associated with advanced atrioventricular block.

**bradycardic** \-kär′dik\ Characterized by or relating to bradycardia.

**bradycinesia** \-sīnē′zhə\ BRADYKINESIA.

**bradygenesis** \-jen′əsis\ [BRADY- + GENESIS] The lengthening of certain stages in embryonic development. Compare TACHYGENESIS.

**bradyglossia** \-gläs′ē·ə\ [BRADY- + GLOSS- + -IA ] BRADYARTHRIA.

**bradykinesia** \-kīnē′zhə\ [BRADY- + KINESIA] Abnormal slowness of voluntary movement, often associated with a diminution of the range of movement, typically seen in parkinsonism. Also *bradykinesis, bradypragia* (seldom used), *bradycinesia.*

**bradykinetic** \-kinet′ik\ Pertaining to or exhibiting bradykinesia.

**bradykinin** \-kī′nin\ The 9-residue peptide Arg-Pro-Pro-Gly-Phe-Ser-Pro-Phe-Arg, which is released by proteinases from a plasma globulin. It acts as a vasodilator and relaxant of smooth muscle.

**bradylalia** \-lā′lyə\ [BRADY- + -LALIA] BRADYARTHRIA.

**bradypnea** \brad′ip·nē′ə, brad′ēnē′ə\ [BRADY- + -PNEA] Abnormally slow breathing.

**bradypragia** \-prā′jə\ [BRADY- + Gk stem *prag-*, from *prassein* to do, practice + -IA] *Seldom used* BRADYKINESIA.

**bradyrhythmia** \-riTH′mē·ə\ [BRADY- + RHYTHM + -IA ] **1** BRADYCARDIA. **2** In electroencephalography, slowing down of the frequency of the dominant electrical activity of the brain to less than that of the alpha rhythm, that is, to less than 8 Hz.

**bradytachycardia** \-tak′ikär′dē·ə\ A disorder of heart rhythm and conduction in which the patient experiences episodes of bradycardia (usually sinus in origin) and tachycardia (frequently due to atrial tachycardia, flutter, or fibrillation). See also BRADYCARDIA-TACHYCARDIA SYNDROME.

**bradytrophic** \-träf′ik\ Causing decreased activity in living organisms.

**bradyzoite** \-zō′īt\ [BRADY- + *zo(o)-* + -ITE] An asexual stage, in which tissue cysts are formed, in the development of certain coccidian parasites.

**Bragg** [Sir William Henry *Bragg*, English physician, 1862–1942] **1** Bragg-Gray principle. See under PRINCIPLE. **2** See under PEAK.

**braille** \brāl\ [after Louis *Braille*, French educator, 1809–1852] A system of printing or writing for the blind by which configurations of raised dots represent letters and can be read by feeling with the fingers.

**Brain** [Walter Russell *Brain*, English physician, 1895–1966] See under REFLEX.

**brain** [Old English *brægen*] **1** In chordates, the enlarged rostral portion of the neuraxis serving functions of special sense reception, autonomic and somatic motor control, sensory perception, and other higher mental processes. Developmentally it consists of the rhombencephalon, mesencephalon, and prosencephalon, all of which are enclosed within the cranium. Also *encephalon.* **2** In invertebrates, the enlarged and specialized rostralmost ganglion of the central nervous system. **cyclopean b.** CYCLENCEPHALY. **isolated b.** ENCÉPHALE ISOLÉ. **olfactory b.** RHINENCEPHALON. **primitive b.** ARCHENCEPHALON. **respirator b.** The brain of a patient after brain death when respiration and cardiac function are being artificially maintained. **thalamic b.** *Obs.* DIENCEPHALON. **visceral b.** *Outmoded* LIMBIC SYSTEM. **wet b.** CEREBRAL EDEMA.

**braincase** The cranial part of the skull containing the brain; neurocranium.

**brain-damaged** See under BRAIN-DAMAGED CHILD.

**brain dead** Marked by or designating the termination of brain function, as evidenced by the loss of all reflexes and electrical activity of the brain. See also BRAIN DEATH.

**brainstem** The central core of the brain, including in sequence the medulla oblongata, pons, and midbrain. The diencephalon is sometimes included. Also *brain axis.*

**branch** [Old French *branche* (from Late L *branca* a claw, paw, perhaps from Celtic) a branch, limb] RAMUS. **bundle b.** One of the branches of the bundle of His; crus dextrum fasciculi atrioventricularis or crus sinistrum fasciculi atrioventricularis. **b.'es of the bundle of His** The crus dextrum fasciculi atrioventricularis and crus sinistrum fasciculi atrioventricularis. **gluteal b. of MacAlister** The first muscular branch of the internal pudendal artery. It arises just as it enters the ischioanal fossa, where the branch pierces the sacrotuberous ligament and supplies the gluteus maximus muscle. **b.'es of suprascapular artery to supraspinatus muscle** Branches of the suprascapular artery that arise after it crosses the superior transverse ligament and enters the supraspinous fossa. There they supply the supraspinatus muscle. **sural communicating b.** A branch of the lateral cutaneous nerve of the calf that crosses the lateral head of the gastrocnemius to join the sural nerve. It may descend to the heel as a separate branch. **thenar b. of median nerve** The short nerve that arises either from the lateral side of the median nerve or in common with the palmar digital nerves just distal to the flexor retinaculum, where it divides into the muscular branches to the thenar muscles. **b.'es of vertebral artery** See under ARTERIA VERTEBRALIS.

**branchial** \brang′kē·əl\ [L *branchi(ae)* gills + -AL] Pertaining to or resembling gills, as in *branchial cleft.*

**branching** Formation of an offshoot, division, or ramus from a parent structure such as a vessel or nerve. When division is equal, the type of branching is called a bifurcation.

**branchiogenic** \brang′kē·ōjen′ik\ [L *branchi(ae)* gills + *o* + -GENIC] **1** Gill-forming; forming a branchial arch or a branchial cleft. **2** Originating from a branchial arch or a branchial cleft. Also *branchiogenous.*

**branchiomere** \brang′kyōmir′\ A segment of the splanchnic mesoderm from which the branchial arches are developed, situated between two branchial clefts. Each branchiomere is covered on its outer surface with ectoderm and on its inner surface with endoderm.

**Brandt** [Thure *Brandt*, Swedish physician, 1819–1895] See under TREATMENT.

**Bras** [Gerrit *Bras*, Indonesian pathologist, flourished 20th century] Stuart-Bras syndrome. See under SYNDROME.

**brash** \brash\ [Scottish dialect] HEARTBURN. **water b.** A sour taste occurring at the back of the mouth due to accumulation of a salty fluid, often occurring in association with heartburn.

**Braune** [Christian Wilhelm *Braune*, German anatomist, 1831–1892] **1** Braune's ring. See under PATHOLOGIC RETRACTION RING. **2** Braune's canal. See under PARTURIENT CANAL. **3** Braune's muscle. See under MUSCULUS PUBORECTALIS. **4** Superior intercostal vein of Braune. See under VEIN.

**Braun von Ferwald** [Richard *Braun von Fernwald*, Austrian obstetrician, born 1866] See under SIGN.

**Bravais** [Louis *Bravais*, French physician, flourished 19th century] Bravais-jacksonian epilepsy. See under JACKSONIAN EPILEPSY.

**Braxton Hicks** [John *Braxton Hicks*, English gynecologist, 1823–1897] **1** Hicks version. See under BRAXTON HICKS VERSION. **2** Hicks contractions. See under BRAXTON HICKS CONTRACTIONS. **3** Hicks sign. See under BRAXTON HICKS SIGN.

**Bray** [Charles William *Bray*, U.S. otologist, born 1904] **1** Wever-Bray effect. See under COCHLEAR MICROPHONIC POTENTIAL. **2** Wever-Bray phenomenon. See under COCHLEAR MICROPHONICS.

**breadth** \bredth\ **b. of accommodation** RANGE OF ACCOMMODATION. **bizygomatic b.** The measured distance between the most prominent, lateral points on the zygomatic arches, used mainly in anthropometry.

**break** / **chromatid b.** Any discontinuity in a chromatid, usually defined cytologically. It is generally recognized in metaphase cells in which one of the two chromatids of the chromosome is interrupted. **isochromatid b.** Any discontinuity at the same locus in both sister chromatids of a chromosome, usually defined cytologically. It is generally described in metaphase cells. The result is often fusion to form one dicentric and one acentric chromosome. **single chain b.** NICK. **single strand b.** NICK.

**breakage and reunion** The process by which crossing over occurs, in which chromatids of homologous chromosomes break and fuse end-to-end with their homologue during meiosis.

**breakoff** A type of depersonalization reported by aviators flying alone at high altitudes, consisting of an uncomfortable feeling of being detached from the earth. This feeling is sometimes elaborated into a generalized fear of flying.

**breast** [Old English *brēost* breast] **1** The front of the chest or thorax. **2** MAMMA. **broken b.** MAMMARY ABSCESS. **caked b.** A lactating breast in which the milk duct is temporarily blocked, causing hardness in that area of the breast. **chicken b.** PECTUS CARINATUM. **cystic b.** CYSTIC MASTOPATHY. **gathered b.** MAMMARY ABSCESS. **keeled b.** PECTUS CARINATUM. **male b.** MAMMA MASCULINA. **pigeon b.** PECTUS CARINATUM. **shotty b.** CYSTIC MASTOPATHY. **supernumerary b.'s** POLYMASTIA.

**breath** [Old English *bræth* odor, breath] **1** The air which enters and leaves the lungs during respiration. **2** A single cycle of inhalation and exhalation. **lead b.** A metallic odor of the breath from lead poisoning. Also *saturnine breath, halitus saturninus.* **liver b.** FETOR HEPATICUS. **saturnine b.** LEAD BREATH.

**Breathalyzer** A breath analyzer used to detect the presence of alcohol in the body. A proprietary name.

**breath-holding** Any of various forms of syncope common in children aged one to four years, precipitated by a sudden hurt or shock felt as an insult. • *Breath-holding* usually refers to the phenomenon described under *blue breath-holding,* but many syncopal attacks of childhood do not fit exactly the symptoms of either *blue breath-holding* or *white breath-holding.* The term *breath-holding* is in fact a misnomer for cessation of breathing in expiration. Also *reflex hypoxic crisis.* **blue b.** The commonest form of syncope in children aged one to four years, precipitated by any sudden shock, hurt, surprise, or disappointment, felt as an insult and with a strong element of self-pity. After spending his breath on one long cry, the child goes into a period of apnea, in expiration, lasting 10 to 20 seconds, becomes cyanosed and may lose consciousness, probably as a result of diminished venous return to the heart. Some stiffening or twitching may then be seen. The color and consciousness return in about half a minute. The attacks are not epileptic and recovery is invariable. Also *reflex anoxic crisis.* **white b.** A form of syncope in children precipitated by any sudden hurt or shock felt as an insult. Such children suffer a vagus-mediated cardiac arrest, which may last from 2 to 20 seconds or even longer, causing cerebral anoxia from which a brief tonic to clonic seizure may ensue. The attacks are not epileptic and recovery is invariable. Also *reflex anoxic seizure, nonepileptic vagal attack.*

**breathing** The inhalation and exhalation (of air or other gas) in the process of respiration. **apneustic b.** Breathing characterized by long periods of breath-holding at full inspiration. **ataxic b.** Irregular breathing with random deep and shallow breaths. It is a rare manifestation of lesions of the medulla oblongata. **autonomous b.** A rare syndrome due to lesions of the cervicomedullary junction in which there is paralysis of the chest and limbs with retention of spontaneous breathing but without the ability to take a breath or stop breathing voluntarily. **Biot's b.** See under BIOT'S RESPIRATION. **bronchial b.** Abnormally harsh and clear breath sounds heard on auscultation over a consolidated lung. **Cheyne-Stokes b.** See under CHEYNE-STOKES RESPIRATION. **continuous positive pressure b.** A technique of artificial assisted ventilation in which the airway pressure is greater than atmospheric pressure throughout the respiratory cycle. **diaphragmatic b.** A type of breathing in which the diaphragm contributes predominantly to respiratory movement. **glossopharyngeal b.** A type of breathing adopted by some people with severe weakness of the respiratory muscles, in which air is gulped or "swallowed" into the lungs, using the muscles of the pharynx. Also *frog breathing.* **intermittent positive pressure b.** A technique of artificial assisted ventilation in which air is forced into the lungs by the intermittent raising of its pressure above atmospheric pressure. **Kussmaul b.** KUSSMAUL RESPIRATION. **mouth-to-mouth b.** MOUTH-TO-MOUTH RESUSCITATION. **periodic b.** Breathing characterized by periods of shallow respiration or apnea interspersed with periods of hyperpnea. **shallow b.** Breathing in which there are abnormally small respiratory excursions and hence low tidal volume. **suppressed b.** Breathing of an abnormally slow, shallow, or halting pattern, usually adopted to avoid or reduce pain caused by breathing. **vesicular b.** Breathing characterized by the auscultatory sounds of healthy lungs.

**Breda** [Achille *Breda*, Italian dermatologist, 1850–1933] **1** Breda's disease. See under MUCOCUTANEOUS LEISHMANIASIS. **2** Breda's disease. See under YAWS.

**breech** [Old English *brec* breeches, pl. of *broc,* which also means breeches] The nates, or buttocks. **frank b.** See under FRANK BREECH PRESENTATION.

**breeding** / **selective b.** ARTIFICIAL SELECTION. **b. true** A state in which the appearance in offspring of a phenotype is apparently unaltered from that present in the parents.

**bregma** \breg′mə\ [Gk *bregma* upper part of the head] A craniometric point situated at the junction of the frontal bone and the two parietal bones. Also *sinciput.* Adj. bregmatic.

**bregmatodymia** \breg′mətōdim′ē·ə\ [Gk *bregma,* gen. *bregmatos,* top of the head + *(di)dym(os)* double, a twin + -IA] A condition in which equal conjoined twins are fused at the bregma, where the sagittal and coronal sutures of the respective skulls meet.

**bremsstrahlung** \bremz′shträ′lʊng\ [German *Brems(e)* a brake, braking, drag + *Strahlung* radiation] Electromagnetic radiation generated when an electron is decelerated, losing energy that reappears in the form of photons. One form of x rays originates in this process, being given off when high-speed electrons strike the target in an x-ray tube. Also *braking radiation.*

**Brennemann** [Joseph *Brennemann,* U.S. pediatrician, 1872–1944] See under SYNDROME.

**Brenner** [Fritz *Brenner,* German pathologist, born 1877] See under TUMOR.

**brepho-** \bref′ō-\ [Gk *brephos* embryo] A combining form meaning embryo, newborn.

**brephoplasty** \bref′ōplas′tē\ [BREPHO- + -PLASTY] Transplantation to an animal of tissue originating from an embryo or from a newborn of the same species. Also *brephoplastic graft.*

**Breschet** [Gilbert *Breschet,* French anatomist, 1784–1845] **1** Breschet's bones. See under OSSA SUPRASTERNALIA. **2** Breschet's canals. See under CANALES DIPLOICI. **3** Breschet's veins. See under VENAE DIPLOICAE. **4** Breschet's hiatus. See under HELICOTREMA.

**Brescia** [Michael J. *Brescia,* U.S. nephrologist, born 1933] Brescia-Cimino fistula. See under RADIOCEPHALIC FISTULA.

**Bretonneau** [Pierre Fidele *Bretonneau,* French physician, 1778–1862] Brettoneau's angina, Brettoneau's disease. See under PHARYNGEAL DIPHTHERIA.

**bretylium tosylate** $C_{18}H_{24}BrNO_3S$. 2-Bromo-*N*-ethyl-*N,N*-dimethyl-benzenemethanaminium 4-methylbenzene sulfonate. An adrenergic blocking agent used in the treatment of hypertension and as an antiarrhythmic drug in certain types of ventricular tachycardia.

**Breuer** [Josef *Breuer,* Austrian physician, 1842–1925] Hering-Breuer reflex. See under REFLEX.

**brevi-** \brev′i-\ [L *brevis* short] A combining form meaning short.

**brevicollis** \-käl′is\ [New L, from L *brevi(s)* short + *collum* neck] An abnormal shortness of the neck.

**breviflexor** \-flek′sər\ Any short flexor muscle.

**brevium** \brē′vē·əm\ URANIUM $X_2$.

**Bricker** [Eugene M. *Bricker,* U.S. urologist, born 1908] See under OPERATION.

**bridge** [Old English *bricg* a bridge] **1** Any tissue or process joining two parts of an organ or linking a space; pons. **2** The upper, bony part of the nose. **3** A dental prosthesis attached to one or more abutment teeth and which cannot be readily removed by the wearer. Also *fixed partial denture, bridgework* (popular). **4** A protoplasmic strand linking two cells. **anaphase b.** The stretching of a dicentric chromosome between the two poles of the spindle, during anaphase of mitosis or meiosis. Injuries to chromosomes, which may be caused by radiation, allow fusion of broken chromosomes fragments, occasionally yielding dicentric chromosomes. **arteriolovenular b.** An arterial capillary connecting an arteriole to a venule. **Bellevue b.** A scrotal support consisting of tape placed across the anterior upper thighs, used in treating epididymitis. **cantilever b.** A dental bridge which has a pontic unsupportedat one end. Also *extension bridge.* **cell b.'s** CROSS-BRIDGES. **chromatid b.** A structure formed during anaphase of mitosis or meiosis when only one of the daughter strands of a dicentric chromosome has its centromeres pulled to opposite poles. **chromosome b.** A structure formed during anaphase of mitosis or meiosis when a dicentric chromosome spans the gap between the separating cell poles because its centromeres are being pulled to opposite poles. **cytoplasmic b.** A temporary cytoplasmic connection joining one blastomere with another. There is also a tendency for some dividing type B spermatogonia and spermatocytes to keep contact through a narrow cytoplasmic bridge which may contribute to the formation of abnormal spermatozoa with two heads or two tails. **dentin b.** A layer of calcified material, more or less resembling dentin, which may be formed as a seal at the surface of the pulp after pulpotomy or pulp exposure. **disulfide b.** DISULFIDE BOND. **extension b.** CANTILEVER BRIDGE. **fixed b.** A bridge with at least one attachment cemented to an abutment tooth. Also *stationary bridge.* **Gaskell's b.** *Outmoded* FASCICULUS ATRIOVENTRICULARIS. **impedance b.** A four-arm electric circuit that converts impedance changes in one of the arms to voltage changes at the output. It is used for detecting breathing-caused impedance changes in the lung. **intercellular b.'s** CROSS-BRIDGES. **malleus-footplate b.** In tympanoplasty, a graft or prosthesis fashioned to bridge the gap between the malleus and the stapes footplate. It is implanted when the stapes superstructure and the incus have been destroyed or their remnants removed. **malleus-stapes b.** In tympanoplasty, a graft or prosthesis fashioned to bridge the gap between the malleus and the intact stapes. It is implanted after the removal or destruction of the incus. **b. of the nose** The interorbital or upper part of the dorsum of the nose, formed by the nasal bones. Also *ponticulus nasi* (outmoded). **stationary b.** FIXED BRIDGE. **Wheatstone b.** A diamond-shaped electric circuit in which each of the four arms is a resistor. Voltage is applied top to bottom. When the output voltage measured side to side is zero, the bridge is balanced, which permits calculation of an unknown resistor from knowledge of the other three. This circuit is also used in transducers in which changes in resistance generate proportional changes in the output voltage.

**bridgework** *Popular* BRIDGE.

**bridle** \brī′dl\ FRENUM.

**Briggs** [Lloyd Vernon *Briggs,* U.S. psychiatrist, 1863–1941] See under LAW.

**Bright** [Richard *Bright,* English physician, 1789–1858] See under DISEASE.

**Brill** [Nathan Edwin *Brill,* U.S. physician, 1860–1925] **1** Brill-Symmers disease. See under NODULAR LYMPHOSARCOMA. **2** Brill-Zinsser disease. See under BRILL'S DISEASE.

**brim** / **pelvic b.** APERTURA PELVIS SUPERIOR.

**Brinkerhoff** [William Carey *Brinkerhoff,* U.S. physician, 1861–1974] See under SPECULUM.

**Briquet** [Pierre *Briquet,* French physician, 1796–1881] See under ATAXIA, SYNDROME.

**brisement** \brēzmäN′\ [French (from *briser* to break, from Gaulish) a breaking] The breaking or tearing of a structure. **b. forcé** The forcible breaking of a bony ankylosis.

**Brissaud** [Edouard *Brissaud,* French neurologist,

1852–1909] Bourneville-Brissaud disease. See under TUBEROUS SCLEROSIS.

**British Pharmaceutical Codex** A publication of the Pharmaceutical Society of Great Britain that supplements the British Pharmacopoeia with additional information on official drugs, other medicinal substances, and prescription mixtures.

**British Pharmacopoeia** A pharmacopeia published periodically under the direction of the General Medical Council. All the drugs included are considered to be "official" agents. Abbr. BP

**brittle** [Middle English *britel*, akin to Old English *breotan* to break to pieces] Difficult to control: said of diabetes mellitus; marked by abrupt swings between ketoacidosis and hypoglycemia.

**broach** \brōch\ A fine, tapering wire used in root-canal treatment. **barbed b.** A broach with many fine barbs, used for removing tooth pulp.

**Broadbent** [Sir William Henry *Broadbent*, English physician, 1835–1907] **1** See under SIGN, LAW. **2** Broadbent-Bolton plane. See under NASION-POSTCONDYLARE PLANE.

**broad-spectrum** Possessing antibiotic activity against a wide variety of Gram-positive and Gram-negative bacteria.

**Broca** [Pierre Paul *Broca*, French surgeon and neurologist, 1824–1880] **1** See under AMNESIA, FISSURE, APHASIA, POUCH. **2** Broca's plane. See under VISUAL PLANE. **3** Parolfactory area of Broca. See under AREA SUBCALLOSA. **4** Broca's convolution, Broca's region. See under GYRUS FRONTALIS INFERIOR. **5** Broca's convolution. See under BROCA'S MOTOR SPEECH AREA. **6** Bandaletta diagonalis of Broca, olfactory station of Broca. See under DIAGONAL BAND. **7** Grand lobe limbique of Broca. See under LIMBIC LOBE.

**Brock** [Sir Russell Claude *Brock*, English surgeon, born 1903] **1** Brock's operation, Brock's procedure, Brock technique, Brock's infundibulectomy. See under TRANSVENTRICULAR CLOSED VALVOTOMY. **2** Brock syndrome. See under MIDDLE LOBE SYNDROME.

**Brockenbrough** [E. C. *Brockenbrough*, U.S. surgeon, born 1930] See under SIGN.

**Brocq** [Louis Anne Jean *Brocq*, French dermatologist, 1856–1928] **1** See under PSEUDOPELADE. **2** Lupoid sycosis of Brocq. See under SYCOSIS.

**brocresine** (Aminooxy)-6-bromo-*m*-cresol. A histamine decarboxylase inhibitor. It has been used to treat pruritis and chronic urticaria.

**Brödel** [Max *Brödel*, German-born U.S. medical artist, 1870–1941] **1** See under LINE. **2** Brödel's white line. See under LINE.

**Broders** [Albert Compton *Broders*, U.S. pathologist, 1885–1964] Broders index. See under CLASSIFICATION.

**Brodie** [Sir Benjamin Collins *Brodie*, English surgeon, 1783–1862] **1** See under ABSCESS. **2** Brodie's tumor. See under CYSTOSARCOMA PHYLLODES. **3** Brodie's knee. See under DISEASE.

**Brodie** [Charles Gordon *Brodie*, Scottish anatomist, 1786–1818] Brodie's ligament. See under TRANSVERSE HUMERAL LIGAMENT.

**Brodmann** [Korbinian *Brodmann*, German neurologist, 1868–1918] Brodmann's cortical areas. See under BRODMANN'S AREAS.

**brom-** \brōm-\ [Gk *brōmos* stench] **1** A combining form indicating the presence of bromine as a principal element of a chemical compound. **2** A combining form meaning stench, foul smell. Also *bromo-*.

**broma-** \brō′mə-\ [Gk *brōma*, gen. *brōmatos* food] A combining form meaning food. Also *bromato-*.

**bromatherapy** \brō′məther′əpē\ [BROMA- + THERAPY] DIET THERAPY.

**bromato-** [Gk *brōma*, gen. *brōmatos* food] BROMA-.

**bromatotherapy** \brō′mətōther′əpē\ DIET THERAPY.

**bromatotoxin** A toxin that forms in spoiled food from the activity of fermentative bacteria.

**bromazepam** $C_{14}H_{10}BrN_3O$. 7-Bromo-1,3-dihydro-5-(2-pyridyl)-2H-1,4-benzodiazepin-2-one. It is a minor tranquilizer.

**bromchlorenone** 6-Bromo-5-chloro-2-benzoxazotinone. A fungicidal agent that is used topically.

**bromelain** \brō′məlān\ A trypsinlike proteolytic enzyme concentrate produced from the juice of *Ananas comosus*, pineapple. It is used medically to reduce inflammation and edema, and to facilitate tissue repair. Also *plant protease concentrate, bromelin.*

**bromethol** TRIBROMOETHANOL SOLUTION.

**bromhexine hydrochloride** $C_{14}H_{20}Br_2N_2{\cdot}HCl$. 2-Amino-3,5-dibromo-*N*-cyclohexyl-*N*-methylbenzenemethanamine monohydrochloride. A compound which has the ability to decrease the viscocity of sputum. It is used as an expectorant and an agent to lower the mucus content of respiratory secretions.

**bromhidrosis** \brōm′hidrō′sis\ [BROM- + HIDR- + -OSIS] Foul-smelling sweat which usually originates in the axillary apocrine sweat glands. Also *bromidrosis, kakidrosis, osmidrosis, fetid sweat.*

**bromide** Any compound of bromine, especially with one other element, including salts and hence also the ion formed by adding an electron to a bromine atom.

**bromidism** \brō′midizm\ BROMIDE POISONING.

**bromidrosis** \brō′midrō′sis\ BROMHIDROSIS.

**bromindione** 2-(4-Bromophenyl)indone-1,3-dione. A compound with anticoagulant properties. It has actions much like those of phenylindanedione.

**bromine** \brō′mēn\ [French *brom(e)* (from Gk *brōmos* stench) + -INE] Element number 35, having atomic weight 79.909. The two naturally occurring, stable isotopes have mass numbers 79 and 81. Numerous short-lived unstable isotopes have been identified. A member of the halogen group of elements, bromine is a heavy, reddish brown liquid that vaporizes at room temperature and boils at 58.78°C. Both liquid and vapor are toxic and destructive of tissue. Valences are 1, 3, 5, and 7. It is rarely found in biologic compounds, though a brominated tyrosine is found in sponges. Symbol: Br

**bromine 82** A radioisotope of bromine, emitting beta and gamma radiation. It is used in the study of electrolytic exchange and extracellular body water measurements. Physical half-life is 36 hours. Symbol: $^{82}Br$

**brominism** \brō′minizm\ A condition resulting from excessive exposure to bromine or its compounds. The signs and symptoms are acne, headache, fetid breath, and drowsiness. Also *bromism.*

**bromization** **1** The addition or introduction of bromine or bromides. **2** The administration of very large doses of bromides.

**bromized** Treated with bromides or bromine-containing medications.

**bromo-** \brō′mə-\ BROM-.

**bromocriptine** \-krip′tīn\ 2-Bromo-α-ergocryptine, an ergot derivative which is a dopamine receptor agonist. It is used in the treatment of acromegaly, nonpuerperal galactorrhea, and in some cases of pituitary-dependent Cushing syndrome.

**5-bromodeoxyuridine** The analogue of thymidine in which the methyl group is replaced by a bromine atom. It has antiviral action, especially against herpesviruses. Abbr. BUDR

**bromodiphenhydramine hydrochloride** $C_{17}H_{20}BrNO \cdot HCl$. *β*-(*p*-Bromobenzhydryloxy)ethyldimethylamine hydrochloride. It is used as an antihistaminic medication.

**bromoiodism** \-ī′ōdizm\ [*brom(ine)* + *o* + *iod(o)-* + -ISM] Poisoning by bromine and iodine or their compounds.

**bromomania** \-mā′nē·ə\ [*brom(ide)* + *o* + -MANIA] The symptoms of chronic intoxication with bromide compounds, including central nervous system depression, delirium, hallucinations, ataxia, incoordination, blurred vision, and disturbances of color perception. Also *bromide psychosis.*

**bromomenorrhea** \-men′ôrē′ə\ [BROMO- + MENORRHEA] Menstruation characterized by an offensive odor.

**bromomethane** \-meth′ān\ METHYL BROMIDE.

**bromophenol blue** \-fē′nôl\ A dye and indicator of the sulfonphthalein group, with four bromide substituents. It changes from yellow to blue over the pH range 3.0 to 4.6. As an acid dye it can be used to demonstrate protein amino groups. Also *bromphenol blue, tetrabromophenol blue.*

**bromothymol blue** A dye and indicator of the sulfonphthalein group. It changes from yellow, through green at neutrality, to blue in alkaline solutions over the pH range 6.0 to 7.6. It can be used as a vital dye and as a stain for fungus infection of plants. Also *bromthymol blue, dibromothymolsulfonphthalein.*

**5-bromouracil** \-yoo′rəsil\ An analogue of thymine in which the methyl group is replaced by an atom of bromine. This molecule can replace thymine in deoxyribonucleic acid, where it is mutogenic. It can be used as a density marker for newly synthesized DNA chains.

**brompheniramine maleate** $C_{16}H_{19}BrN_2 \cdot C_4H_4O_4$. The maleate salt of brompheniramine. It is used as an antihistaminic agent.

**bromphenol blue** BROMOPHENOL BLUE.

**Bromsulphalein** A proprietary name for sulfobromophthalein sodium. Abbr. BSP

**bromthymol blue** BROMOTHYMOL BLUE.

**bronch-** \brängk-\ BRONCHO-.

**bronchi** \bräng′kī\ Plural of BRONCHUS.

**bronchi-** \bräng′kē-\ BRONCHO-.

**bronchia** \bräng′kē·ə\ Plural of BRONCHIUM.

**bronchial** \bräng′kē·əl\ Of or pertaining to the bronchi and/or their branches.

**bronchiectasia** \-ektā′zhə\ BRONCHIECTASIS.

**bronchiectasic** \-ektā′zik\ BRONCHIECTATIC.

**bronchiectasis** \-ek′təsis\ [BRONCHI- + ECTASIS] Abnormal dilatation of bronchi. Also *bronchiectasia.* **capillary b.** Bronchiectasis involving the smaller, peripheral portions of the bronchial tree. **cylindrical b.** A form of bronchiectasis in which the dilated bronchi retain parallel walls. **cystic b.** A form of bronchiectasis in which bronchi are irregularly dilated, resulting in cystlike dilatations. **dry b.** Bronchiectasis without production of sputum. **fusiform b.** A pattern of bronchiectasis in which the ends of bronchi are dilated. **saccular b.** A pattern of bronchiectasis in which localized dilatations of bronchi form irregular saclike cavities. Also *varicose bronchiectasis.*

**bronchiectatic** \-ektat′ik\ Relating to or characterized by bronchiectasis. Also *bronchiectasic.*

**bronchiloquy** \brängkil′əkwē\ [BRONCHI- + L *loqu(i)* to speak + -Y] Abnormal conduction of the sound of the voice on auscultation over consolidated lung tissue.

**bronchiocele** \bräng′kē·əsēl′\ BRONCHOCELE.

**bronchiogenic** \bräng′kē·əjen′ik\ BRONCHOGENIC.

**bronchiole** \bräng′kē·ōl\ BRONCHIOLUS. **alveolar b.'s** BRONCHIOLI RESPIRATORII. **lobular b.** TERMINAL BRONCHIOLE. **respiratory b.'s** BRONCHIOLI RESPIRATORII. **terminal b.** One of about six subdivisions, or branchings, of a small bronchiole that enters a single lung lobule and that has a complete circular muscle coat that controls the air passage. Each one branches into respiratory bronchioles. Also *lobular bronchiole.*

**bronchioli** \brängkī′əlī\ Plural of BRONCHIOLUS.

**bronchiolitis** \-ōlī′tis\ [*bronchiol(o)-* + -ITIS] Inflammation of the bronchioles. **acute b.** Bronchiolitis from an acute infection, usually by respiratory syncytial virus, principally affecting infants and causing severe breathlessness and wheezing. **acute obliterating b.** Acute bronchiolitis causing obstruction and obliteration of bronchioles. **b. fibrosa obliterans** A process of fibrotic scarring and hence obstruction of bronchioles of the lung. It may follow severe pneumonia but in many cases the cause is unknown.

**bronchiolo-** \brängkī′əlō-, bräng′kē·əlō-\ [New L *bronchiolus,* dim. of BRONCHUS] A combining form denoting bronchiole.

**bronchiolus** \brängkī′ələs\ [New L, dim. of BRONCHUS] One of the numerous subdivisions of the intrapulmonary secondary bronchi in which the diameter diminishes to 1 mm or less, cartilage is absent, epithelial cells are cuboidal, and smooth muscle and elastic fibers course in the walls of collagenous connective tissue. Also *bronchiole.* **bronchioli respiratorii** [NA] Subdivisions of terminal bronchioles, short tubes with a diameter of 0.5 mm or less, with a few alveoli budding from thin walls, each communicating with two or more alveolar ducts that end in alveoli and alveolar sacs. Also *respiratory bronchioles, alveolar bronchioles.*

**bronchiostenosis** \bräng′kē·əstenō′sis\ BRONCHOSTENOSIS.

**bronchitic** \brängkit′ik\ Relating to or characterized by bronchitis.

**bronchitis** \brängkī′tis\ [BRONCH- + -ITIS] Inflammation of the bronchi. **acute b.** Acute, usually infective, inflammation of bronchi causing cough and sputum production. **acute laryngotracheal b.** An acute, usually infective, inflammatory condition involving bronchi, larynx, and trachea, with severe breathlessness and wheezing. **acute suppurative b.** Acute inflammation of the bronchi with formation of pus. **Castellani's b.** BRONCHOSPIROCHETOSIS. **chronic b.** Chronic inflammation of bronchi resulting in cough, sputum production, and often progressive breathlessness. It is generally caused by cigarette smoking. **dry b.** Bronchitis without production of sputum. **fibrinous b.** Bronchitis with fibrinous exudate in bronchi which may form a cast of portions of the bronchial tree. Also *membranous bronchitis, plastic bronchitis, pseudomembranous bronchitis.* **hemorrhagic b.** BRONCHOSPIROCHETOSIS. **membranous b.** FIBRINOUS BRONCHITIS. **b. obliterans** Bronchitis resulting in obliteration of smaller branches of the bronchial tree. **plastic b.** FIBRINOUS BRONCHITIS. **pseudomembranous b.** FIBRINOUS BRONCHITIS. **suffocative b.** Bronchitis causing severe obstruction to air flow in the lungs. **summer b.** Bronchitis occurring primarily in summer; probably allergic asthma.

**bronchium** \bräng′kē·əm\ [New L, from Gk *bronchion* a bronchus, dim. of *bronchos* windpipe] (*pl.* bronchia) One of the subdivisions of a bronchus, but larger than a bronchiole.

**broncho-** \bräng′kō-\ [Gk *bronchos* windpipe] A combining form denoting bronchus. Also *bronch-, bronchi-.*

**bronchoalveolar** \-alvē′ələr\ BRONCHOVESICULAR.

**bronchoaspergillosis** \-as′pərjilō′sis\ Involvement of the bronchi by an *Aspergillus* fungal infection, producing either an allergic or nonallergic inflammatory bronchitis.

**bronchocele** \bräng′kōsēl\ [BRONCHO- + -CELE[2]] A localized dilatation in a bronchus. Also *bronchiocele.*

**bronchoconstriction** \-kənstrik′shən\ Narrowing of a bronchus caused by contraction of bronchial smooth muscle.

**bronchoconstrictor** \-kənstrik′tər\ 1 Causing bronchoconstriction. 2 An agent that causes bronchoconstriction.

**bronchodilatation** \-dil′ətā′shən\ 1 Dilatation of a bronchus; the relaxation of a bronchoconstriction. Also *bronchodilation.* 2 A dilatation in a bronchus.

**bronchodilator** \-dīlā′tər\ 1 Causing dilatation of bronchi. 2 An agent that causes dilatation of bronchi.

**bronchoegophony** \-ēgäf′ənē\ EGOPHONY.

**bronchoesophageal** \-esäf′əjē′əl\ Pertaining to both bronchi and the esophagus, as in the case of a fistula between these structures.

**bronchoesophagoscopy** \-esäf′əgäs′kəpē\ Endoscopic examination of the tracheobronchial tree and the esophagus.

**bronchofiberscope** \-fī′bərskōp\ FIBEROPTIC BRONCHOSCOPE.

**bronchogenic** \-jen′ik\ [BRONCHO- + -GENIC] Arising in, or spreading from, a bronchus. Also *bronchiogenic, bronchogenous.*

**bronchogram** \bräng′kəgram\ A roentgenogram obtained during bronchography.

**bronchography** \brängkäg′rəfē\ Radiography of the bronchial tree after opacification by the instillation of a suitable contrast material into the trachea or into a bronchus.

**broncholith** \bräng′kəlith\ [BRONCHO- + -LITH] A calculus within a bronchus. It is usually a residue of previous tuberculosis. Also *bronchial calculus.*

**broncholithiasis** \-lithī′əsis\ A condition characterized by multiple broncholiths in the lungs.

**bronchomalacia** \-malā′shə\ A condition of unknown cause in which the walls of bronchi are abnormally soft.

**bronchomotor** \-mō′tər\ Capable of modifying the state of contraction of a bronchial muscle.

**bronchomycosis** \-mīkō′sis\ A fungal infection of the bronchi.

**bronchophony** \brängkäf′ənē\ [BRONCHO- + Gk *phōn(ē)* sound, voice + -Y] The auscultatory sound of the voice characteristically heard over an area of consolidation in the lung. Also *bronchial voice.* **pectoriloquous b.** An abnormally clear voice sound heard on auscultation of the lungs when the patient whispers, usually over solid or cavitated lung. Also *whispered bronchophony.*

**bronchoplasty** \bräng′kəplas′tē\ Any plastic operation on a bronchus.

**bronchopleural** \-plur′əl\ Pertaining to or involving a bronchus and the pleura or pleural cavity.

**bronchopneumonia** \-n$^{y}$oomō′nē·ə\ Inflammation of the lung producing patchy and often widespread consolidation. It is most frequently of infectious etiology, and is the most common x-ray manifestation of bacterial pneumonia. Also *bronchial pneumonia, lobular pneumonia, catarrhal pneumonia.* **influenzal b.** Bronchopneumonia occurring during or soon after an influenza infection. Rarely caused by the influenza virus, it usually results from a secondary bacterial infection. **inhalation b.** Bronchopneumonia resulting from inhalation of substances harmful to the lungs.

**bronchopneumonic** \-n$^{y}$oomän′ik\ Relating to bronchopneumonia.

**bronchopulmonary** \-pul′mōner′ē\ Relating to the bronchi and lungs.

**bronchorrhea** \bräng′kôrē′ə\ [BRONCHO- + -RRHEA] Abnormally profuse watery secretion from the bronchi.

**bronchoscope** \bräng′kəskōp\ [BRONCHO- + -SCOPE] An instrument for examining the interior of the tracheobronchial tree for diagnostic and therapeutic purposes including the aspiration of secretions and the removal of foreign bodies and biopsy specimens. A flexible fiberoptic bronchoscope is in widespread use in addition to the traditional rigid instrument. **fiberoptic b.** A flexible bronchoscope making use of fiberoptics to transmit light and images. The controllable tip facilitates examination of the remote parts of the bronchial tree. Also *bronchofiberscope.*

**bronchoscopy** \brängkäs′kəpē\ [BRONCHO- + -SCOPY] The examination of the interior of the tracheobronchial tree through a bronchoscope.

**bronchospasm** \bräng′kəspazm\ [BRONCHO- + SPASM] Bronchoconstriction of a spasmodic nature. Also *bronchial spasm.*

**bronchospirochetosis** \-spī′rōkētō′sis\ Infectious hemorrhagic bronchitis associated with spirochetal infection. Also *Castellani's bronchitis, Castellani's disease, hemorrhagic bronchitis, bronchopulmonary spirochetosis.*

**bronchospirometer** \-spīräm′ətər\ A type of spirometer used in bronchospirometry.

**bronchospirometry** \-spīräm′ətrē\ A technique for obtaining spirometric measurements from one lung or one lobe of a lung, by passing a cuffed tube into a bronchus. Also *bronchoscopic spirometry.* **differential b.** A technique of obtaining spirometric measurements from two parts of the lung for comparison between them.

**bronchostenosis** \-stenō′sis\ A local narrowing of a bronchus. Also *bronchial stenosis, bronchiostenosis.*

**bronchostomy** \brängkäs′təmē\ [BRONCHO- + -STOMY] An opening in a bronchus that communicates with the skin through the chest wall.

**bronchotomy** \brängkät′əmē\ [BRONCHO- + -TOMY] Incision of a bronchus.

**bronchotracheal** \-trā′kē·əl\ Of or pertaining to the bronchi and the trachea. Also *tracheobronchial.*

**bronchovesicular** \-vesik′yələr\ Pertaining to the bronchi and the pulmonary alveoli. Also *vesiculobronchial, bronchoalveolar.*

**bronchus** \bräng′kəs\ [New L (from Gk *bronchos* windpipe)] (*pl.* bronchi) [NA] One of the large conducting air passages of the lungs, commencing at the bifurcation of the trachea and terminating in the bronchioles. The extrapulmonary bronchus has a structure similar to that of the trachea, with incomplete rings of fibrocartilage united by connective tissue and smooth muscle. The wall of an intrapulmonary bronchus is completely surrounded by cartilage plates that become more irregular with subsequent subdivisions of each bronchus until they disappear when the bronchioles commence. The outermost layer of the bronchial wall has dense connective tissue containing many elastic fibers. The muscle layer comprises interlacing bundles. The mucosa is similar to that of the trachea. With repeated subdivisions, the bronchial walls become thinner. The primary bronchi divide into secondary, or lobar, bronchi, which in turn divide into tertiary, or segmental, bronchi and subsegmental bronchi to the bronchopulmonary segments. **apical b.** 1 *Imprecise* BRONCHUS SEGMENTALIS APICALIS [SUPERIOR] (B VI). 2 BRONCHUS SEGMENTALIS APICALIS (B I). **extrapulmonary b.** BRONCHUS PRINCIPALIS [DEXTER ET SINISTER]. **intermediate b.** That portion of the right principal bronchus that is situated immediately distal to the inferior border of the superior lobar bronchus and proximal to the superior border of the middle lobar bronchus. **intrapulmonary b.** Any of the bronchi located between the termination of the primary bronchi and the commencement of the bronchioles, comprising the secondary and segmental bronchi. **left apical b.** 1 The apical bronchus of the bronchus segmentalis apicoposterior (B I + II) of the superior lobe of the left lung. 2 The bronchus segmentalis apicalis (B VI) of the left inferior lobe. **left dorsal b.** The posterior bronchus of the bronchus segmentalis apicoposterior (B I + B II) of the superior lobe of the left lung. **left superior ventral b.** The left bronchus segmentalis anterior (B III). **lingular b.** The caudal division of the left superior lobe bronchus. It descends into the lingula and divides into the bronchus lingularis superior (B IV) and bronchus lingularis inferior (B V). **b. lingularis inferior (B V)** [NA] The branch of the lingular bronchus, or caudal division, of the left superior lobe bronchus that supplies the inferior lingular bronchopulmonary segment (S V). Also *inferior lingular bronchus.* **b. lingularis superior (B IV)** [NA] The branch of the lingular bronchus, or caudal division, of the left superior lobe bronchus that supplies the superior lingular bronchopulmonary segment (S IV). Also *superior lingular bronchus.* **bronchi lobares** [NA] The terminal divisions of the primary right and left bronchi that supply the lobes of the lungs. There are three on the right (bronchus lobaris superior dexter, bronchus lobaris medius dexter, bronchus lobaris inferior dexter) and two on the left (bronchus lobaris superior sinister, bronchus lobaris inferior sinister), each of which in turn divides into segmental bronchi. Also *lobar bronchi, secondary bronchi.* **main b.** BRONCHUS PRINCIPALIS [DEXTER ET SINISTER]. **principal b.** BRONCHUS PRINCIPALIS [DEXTER ET SINISTER]. **b. principalis [dexter et sinister]** [NA] One of the two terminal divisions of the trachea, each (right and left) passing to the hilum of the corresponding lung, where each divides into intrapulmonary, or lobar, bronchi. The structure of the extrapulmonary bronchi is almost the same as that of the trachea but changes when they enter the lungs. Also *primary bronchus, principal bronchus, main bronchus, extrapulmonary bronchus.* **right apical b.** The bronchus segmentalis apicalis [superior] (B VI) of the right lung. **right ventral b.** The right bronchus segmentalis anterior (B III). **secondary bronchi** BRONCHI LOBARES. **segmental bronchi** BRONCHI SEGMENTALES. **bronchi segmentales** [NA] The primary branches of the lobar bronchi that are distributed to the functionally independent units of lung tissue, the bronchopulmonary segments, where they subdivide repeatedly until they become the narrow, fine bronchioles. Also *segmental bronchi.* **b. segmentalis anterior (B III)** [NA] The branch of the superior lobe bronchus of each lung that runs anteroinferiorly to supply the anterior bronchopulmonary segment (S III). It gives off a lateral and an anterior branch. In the left lung, where the superior lobe bronchus has only two branches, compared to three in the right lung, the cranial branch gives off the anterior segmental bronchus (B III) before continuing as the apicoposterior segmental bronchus (B I + II). In the right lung, the anterior segmental bronchus derives directly from the superior lobe bronchus. Also *anterior bronchus.* **b. segmentalis apicalis (B I)** [NA] A branch of the superior lobe bronchus that runs superolaterally toward the apex of the lung to supply the apical bronchopulmonary segment (S I). It has an apical and an anterior branch. Also *apical bronchus.* **b. segmentalis apicalis [superior] (B VI)** [NA] A branch from the posterior aspect of the inferior lobe bronchus of each lung that passes posteriorly to supply the superior bronchopulmonary segment (S VI) of the inferior lobe of the lung. Also *superior segmental bronchus, apical bronchus* (imprecise), *bronchus of Nelson.* • The term *bronchus segmentalis apicalis* has become firmly established in the vocabulary of thoracic surgeons, and their decision has been to retain an "apical bronchus" for both the apex of the lung (*bronchus segmentalis apicalis*) and for the "apex" of the inferior lobe of the lung. However, the *Nomina Anatomica* refers to the latter as *bronchus segmentalis apicalis [superior] (B VI)* in the hope that the alternative term *superior* will in time replace *apicalis* in reference to the lower lobe of both lungs. **b. segmentalis apicoposterior (B I + B II)** [NA] The continuation of the cranial division of the left superior lobe bronchus that supplies the apicoposterior bronchopulmonary segment (S I + S II). It ends in apical and posterior branches. Also *apicoposterior bronchus.* **b. segmentalis basalis anterior (B VIII)** [NA] The branch of the anteromedial stem of the inferior lobe bronchus of each lung that passes to the anterior basal bronchopulmonary segment (S VIII). In the left lung it usually arises in common with the medial basal segmental bronchus (B VII), but it may arise independently from the left inferior lobe bronchus. Also *anterior basal bronchus.* **b. segmentalis basalis lateralis (B IX)** [NA] The branch of the posterolateral stem of the inferior lobe bronchus of each lung that descends laterally to supply the lateral basal bronchopulmonary segment (S IX). It arises in common with the posterior basal segmental bronchus (B

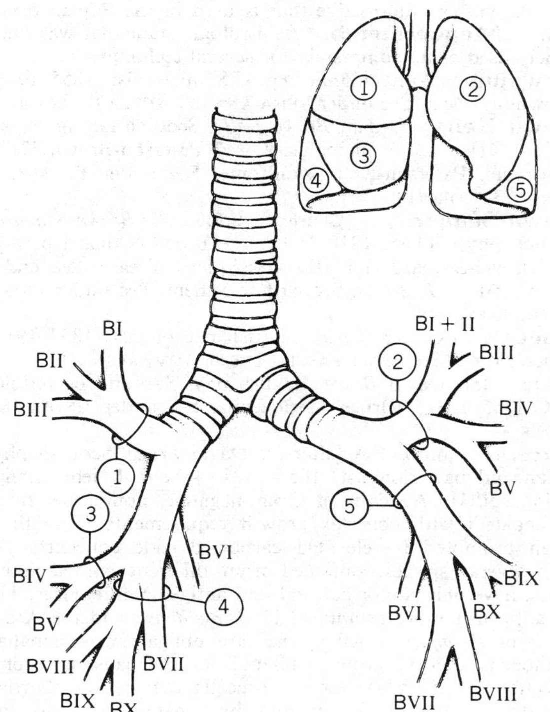


**Segmental bronchi** Right lung: (BI) apical, (BII) posterior, (BIV) lateral, (BV) medial. Left lung: (BI + II) apicoposterior, (BIV) superior lingular, (BV) inferior lingular. Both lungs: (BIII) anterior, (BVI) superior, (BVII) medial basal, (BVIII) anterior basal, (BIX) lateral basal, (BX) posterior basal. Lobes of lung supplied: (1) right superior, (2) left superior, (3) right middle, (4) right inferior, (5) left inferior.

X). Also *lateral basal bronchus.* **b. segmentalis basalis medialis [cardiacus] (B VII)** [NA] The branch of the inferior lobe bronchus that descends inferomedially to supply the medial basal bronchopulmonary segment (S VII), a small area below the hilum of the lung. In the left lung, B VII arises in common with the anterior basal segmental bronchus (B VIII) from the anteromedial stem, or division, of the left inferior lobe bronchus. In a small number of cases it arises independently from the left inferior lobe bronchus. Also *medial basal bronchus.* **b. segmentalis basalis posterior (B X)** [NA] The branch of the posterolateral stem of the inferior lobe bronchus of each lung that descends posteriorly to supply the posterior basal bronchopulmonary segment (S X). It arises in common with the lateral basal segmental bronchus (B IX). Also *posterior basal bronchus.* **b. segmentalis lateralis (B IV)** [NA] The division of the middle lobe bronchus that supplies the lateral segment (S IV) of the middle lobe of the right lung. Also *lateral bronchus.* **b. segmentalis medialis (B V)** [NA] The division of the middle lobe bronchus that supplies the medial segment (S V) of the middle lobe of the right lung. Also *medial bronchus.* **b. segmentalis posterior (B II)** [NA] The branch of the right superior lobe bronchus that runs posterolaterally to supply the posterior bronchopulmonary segment (S II), which is the posteroinferior portion of the right superior lobe. Also *posterior bronchus.* **stem b.** The continuation of the left and right primary bronchi of the primitive lungs, following the formation of two lateral bronchi on the right side and one on the left. It forms the lower lobes of the lungs. **subapical b.** A small supplementary bronchus that arises from the posterior surface of the inferior lobe bronchus. It may be included in the posterior part of the apical bronchus of the inferior lobe of either lung. It is present in about one third of left lungs.

**Brønsted** [Johannes N. *Brønsted,* Danish chemist, 1879–1947] See under ACID, BASE.

**Brooke** [Henry Ambrose Grundy *Brooke,* English dermatologist, 1854–1919] Brooke's tumor. See under TRICHOEPITHELIOMA.

**broth** [Middle and Old English] A rich liquid culture medium for bacteria. See also AGAR, CULTURE MEDIUM, MEDIUM, CULTURE. **carbohydrate b.** A liquid culture medium consisting of peptone and beef extract, with a single sugar and a pH indicator that demonstrates acid production if the sugar is fermented. A series of broths with different sugars is used to establish the fermentative properties of bacteria. **dextrose b.** A liquid enrichment medium composed of a beef extract and tryptone base with added dextrose that is used for cultivating microorganisms, especially streptococci and meningococci. Also *sugar broth.* **heart infusion b.** A tryptone and beef heart broth used as a general purpose medium for cultivating microorganisms and as a basal medium to which carbohydrates or red blood cells can be added. Also *heart infusion agar.* **infusion b.** A bacteriologic culture medium, used especially for fastidious pathogens, that is enriched with the constituents extracted from meat by hot water. **lauryl sulfate b.** A selective culture medium of tryptone and lactose that is used to detect coliform organisms in water, foods, and dairy products. Sodium lauryl sulfate inhibits the growth of organisms other than coliforms. **nitrate b.** A liquid culture medium containing beef extract, peptone, and potassium nitrate, used in classifying microorganisms according to their capacity to reduce nitrate to nitrite. **nutrient b.** A general-purpose agar or broth medium that contains beef extract, peptones, and sodium chloride. Because it does not contain additives such as blood or serum it will support growth only of nonfastidious organisms. Also *nutrient culture medium.* **selenite b.** An enrichment liquid medium of tryptone, lactose, and sodium selenite that permits the growth of enteric pathogens, especially species of *Salmonella,* and inhibits growth of nonpathogenic coliform bacilli. After incubation, samples are streaked on diagnostic solid media. **Stuart b.** STUART TRANSPORT MEDIUM. **sugar b.** DEXTROSE BROTH.

**brow** [Old English *brū,* akin to Gk *ophrys* brow] **1** FRONS. **2** The superciliary arch; the eyebrow region. **olympic b.** The protruding forehead seen in congenital syphilis.

**Brown** [Charles Leonard *Brown,* U.S. physician, born 1899] Brown-Symmers disease. See under ACUTE INFANTILE ENCEPHALOPATHY.

**Brown** See under DENIS BROWN.

**Brown** [H. W. *Brown,* U.S. ophthalmologist, born 1898] Brown sheath syndrome. See under SUPERIOR OBLIQUE TENDON SHEATH SYNDROME.

**Brown** [James Barrett *Brown,* U.S. plastic surgeon, 1899–1971] **1** See under DERMATOME. **2** Blair-Brown graft. See under SPLIT-SKIN GRAFT.

**Brown** [Robert *Brown,* English botanist, 1773–1858] Brownian-Zsigmondy movement. See under BROWNIAN MOVEMENT.

**brown** **1** A color combining red, yellow, and black; the color of chocolate. **2** A substance, usually a stain or dye, that is brown in appearance, or that produces a cytochemical reaction resulting in brown staining. For chemical names including *brown,* see under the chemical name. **Bismarck b.** A synthetic diazo dye that is used in the Papanicolaou test. **Manchester b.** A histologic stain that was once widely used as a counterstain for several techniques.

**Browning** [William *Browning,* U.S. anatomist, 1855–1941] Browning's vein. See under VENA ANASTOMOTICA INFERIOR.

**Brown Kelly** [Adam *Brown Kelly,* Scottish laryngologist, 1865–1941] **1** See under SIGN. **2** Paterson-Brown Kelly syndrome, Paterson-Kelly syndrome. See under PLUMMER-VINSON SYNDROME.

**Brown-Séquard** [Charles Edouard *Brown-Séquard,* French physiologist, 1818–1894] **1** Brown-Séquard paralysis, Brown-Séquard sign, Brown-Séquard disease. See under SYNDROME. **2** Brown-Séquard treatment. See under ORGANOTHERAPY.

**Bruce** [Alexander *Bruce,* Scottish neurologist, 1854–1911] Bruce's tract. See under FASCICULUS SEPTOMARGINALIS.

**Bruce** [Sir David *Bruce,* English physician and bacteriologist, 1855–1931] Bruce's septicemia. See under UNDULANT FEVER.

***Brucella*** \broosel'ə\ [after Sir David *Bruce,* Scottish physician and bacteriologist, 1855–1931 + *-ella* L fem. diminishing suffix] A genus of Gram-negative, nonmotile, small coccobacilli with complex growth requirements. Growth is often promoted by elevated carbon dioxide concentration. The several species, obtained from different animal reservoirs, have only minor cultural and antigenic differences. The M antigen is more prominent in *B. melitensis* and the A antigen in *B. abortus.* All species are obligatory mammalian pathogens, able to grow in phagocytes and causing chronic infection. ***B. abortus*** A brucella that causes abortion in cattle. It may be shed in milk by apparently healthy animals and is thereby transmitted to man, in whom it causes an infection that may be acute, relapsing, chronic, or subclinical. Also *Bang's bacillus, Bacillus abortus.* ***B. melitensis*** A brucella obtained from the milk and urine of apparently healthy goats. It was the first brucella to be identified as the cause of human infection. It causes Malta fever. Also *Bacillus melitensis* (obs.). ***B. neotomae*** A brucella obtained from the desert wood rat. ***B. ovis*** A brucella obtained from sheep. ***B. suis*** A brucella obtained from swine. It occasionally infects humans.

**brucella** \broosel′ə\ Any organism of the genus *Brucella.*

**Brucellergen** A nucleoprotein of brucella, used in a skin test for delayed hypersensitivity to the organism. A trade name.

**brucellin** \broosel′in\ A combined preparation from the three species of *Brucella,* used in skin testing for brucellosis.

**brucellosis** \broo′səlō′sis\ [*Brucell(a)* + -OSIS] A generalized infectious disease caused by bacteria of the genus *Brucella* and transmitted from cattle, goats, swine, and other domestic mammals to man by contact or by ingestion of milk from an infected animal. The human disease, also known as undulant fever, is characterized by fever, headache, and malaise. The most common forms of human brucellosis are Malta fever, caused by *B. melitensis,* primarily a pathogen of goats, and abortus fever, caused by *B. abortus,* which is primarily responsible for contagious abortion in cattle.

**Bruch** [Karl Wilhelm Ludwig *Bruch,* German anatomist, 1819–1884] **1** Bruch's membrane, Bruch's layer. See under COMPLEXUS BASALIS CHOROIDEAE. **2** Bruch's glands. See under GLAND.

**brucine** $C_{23}H_{26}N_2O_4$. A toxic polycyclic alkaloid. Since it is a chiral base, crystallization of brucine salts has been used to separate enantiomeric acids.

**Brücke** [Ernst Wilhelm von *Brücke,* German physiologist, 1819–1892] **1** Brücke's fibers, fibrae meridionales brückei. See under FIBRAE MERIDIONALES MUSCULI CILIARIS. **2** See under MUSCLE.

**Brudzinski** [Josef von *Brudzinski,* Polish physician, 1874–1917] **1** Brudzinski sign. See under NUCHAL SIGN. **2** Brudzinski's reflex. See under SIGN.

**Brug** [S. L. *Brug,* Dutch parasitologist, born 1879] See under FILARIA.

***Brugia*** \broo′jə\ [after S. L. *Brug,* Dutch parasitologist, born 1879] A genus of filaria chiefly from southeast Asia, formerly included in the genus *Wuchereria.* Species include *B. malayi, B. pahangi, B. patei, B. guyanensis,* and *B. beaveri.* The latter two were the first described from the New World. Human infections are reported from several species, though only *B. malayi* is of medical importance. ***B. malayi*** A species of mosquito-transmitted filarial worms found in southeast Asia, eastern India, and Sri Lanka. Chronic infection may lead to elephantiasis of the extremities. Also *Wuchereria malayi, Filaria malaya* .

**bruise** [Middle English *bruis(en)* (influenced by Old French *bruisier*) to bruise, from Old English *brȳsan* to crush, pound] CONTUSION.

**bruit** \brʏ·ē′, broo′ē\ [French, a sound, noise] An auscultatory sound or murmur, especially one arising from the heart or vessels. • The term is now used primarily to describe murmurs over peripheral vessels. **aneurysmal b.** A murmur heard over an aneurysm. **carotid b.** A murmur heard over the carotid artery. **cranial b.** A bruit which can be heard at any point over the cranium. **b. de canon** An abnormally loud first heart sound heard intermittently in complete atrioventricular block when atrial contraction immediately precedes ventricular contraction. At other times in this condition the first heart sound may be abnormally soft. **b. de choc** An abrupt and loud second heart sound. *Obs.* **b. de craquement** A cracking sound associated with pericardial or pleural disease. **b. de cuir neuf** A creaking sound, as of new leather, due to pericardial or pleural friction. **b. de galop** GALLOP RHYTHM. **b. de moulin** MILL WHEEL MURMUR. **b. de pot fêlé** CRACKED-POT SOUND. **b. de rappel** A double sound resembling two beats on a drum, due to splitting of the second sound or to a second sound followed by an opening snap. **b. de Roger** A loud holosystolic murmur at the left sternal edge due to a small ventricular septal defect (maladie de Roger). Also *Roger's bruit.* **b. de tambour** The noise suggestive of a bass drum of the aortic second sound in syphilitic aortitis. Also *bruit de tabourka, timbre métallique.* **false b.** The artifactual production of a bruit by the stethoscope or in the ear of the auscultator. **Roger's b.** BRUIT DE ROGER. **spinal b.** A bruit which can be heard over the spinal column. **systolic b.** SYSTOLIC MURMUR.

**Brunn** [Albert von *Brunn,* German anatomist, 1849–1895] **1** Brunn's epithelial nests. See under NEST. **2** See under MEMBRANE.

**Brunner** [Johann Conrad von *Brunner,* Swiss anatomist, 1653–1727] Brunner's glands. See under GLANDULAE DUODENALES.

**Bruns** [Ludwig *Bruns,* German neurologist, 1858–1916] See under ATAXIA, SIGN, SYNDROME.

**Brunschwig** [Alexander *Brunschwig,* U.S. surgeon, 1901–1969] Brunschwig's operation. See under PELVIC EXENTERATION, BRUNSCHWIG'S OPERATION.

**brush** **1** An instrument consisting of bristles or other flexible wirelike material set in a backing or handle and used especially for cleaning or the application of a substance. **2** Any structure or part likened to a brush, as it consists of a dense cluster of hairs or hairlike projections. **Ayre b.** A surgical instrument made of flexible bristles attached to a flexible handle, used to collect a sample of gastric mucus for diagnostic cytologic analysis. **electrical b.** A usually compact carbon block that contacts the rotating commutator on the armature of an electric motor or generator for conducting current to or from it. **Haidinger's b.'es** Radiating entoptic lines extending to either side of fixation, induced by viewing polarized light. Rotation of the plane of polarization causes a corresponding rotation of the brushes. **b.'es of Ruffini** A sensory ending appearing as a skein of branches within a cutaneous papilla. Also *organ of Ruffini, terminal cylinders.* **stomach b.** A surgical instrument with bristles and a long flexible handle used to sample superficial gastric mucosal cells for cytologic diagnostic purposes.

**Brushfield** [Thomas *Brushfield,* English physician, 1858–1937] **1** Brushfield spots. See under SPOT. **2** Brushfield-Wyatt syndrome, Brushfield-Wyatt disease. See under STURGE-WEBER SYNDROME.

**brushing** / **bronchial b.** A technique of collecting material abraded from the surface of a bronchus or bronchial lesion by passing a fine brush through a bronchoscope.

**brushite** The mineral $CaHPO_4{\cdot}2H_2O$, which may be prepared as a precipitate on mixing $CaCl_2$ and $Na_2HPO_4$ solutions under controlled conditions. It may be converted into hydroxylapatite for protein adsorption by heating with alkali.

**Bruton** [Ogden Carr *Bruton,* U.S. pediatrician, born 1908] Bruton type agammaglobulinemia, Bruton's disease. See under INFANTILE SEX-LINKED HYPOGAMMAGLOBULINEMIA.

**bruxism** \bruk′sizm\ [irreg. from Gk *brych(ein)* to bite, grind or gnash the teeth + -ISM] A grinding or gnashing of the teeth in sleep. It produces distinctive polished wear facets on opposing teeth and may aggravate periodontal disease. Also *night grinding.*

**bruxomania** [*brux(ism)* + *o* + MANIA ] A nervous disorder characterized by grinding of the teeth. Also *brychomania.*

**bry-** \brī-\ BRYO-.
**Bryant** [Sir Thomas *Bryant*, English surgeon, 1828–1914] See under TRACTION, LINE.
**bryo-** \brī'ə-\ [Gk *bryon* moss] A combining form denoting moss. Also *bry-*.
**BS** 1 breath sound(s). 2 blood sugar. 3 bowel sound.
**BSER** brainstem-evoked response audiometry.
**B.Th.U.** British thermal unit (the traditional British abbreviation).
**BTU** British thermal unit (used in the U.S., Canada, South Africa, and Japan).
**Btu** British thermal unit (the preferred U.S. abbreviation; not used in Canada).
**buba** \b^y oo'bə\ [American Spanish, pustule, small tumor] 1 A South American Spanish term for MUCOCUTANEOUS LEISHMANIASIS. 2 A South American Spanish term for YAWS. **b. madre** MOTHER YAW.
**bubas braziliana** \b^y oo'bəs braz'ilyan'ə\ MUCOCUTANEOUS LEISHMANIASIS.
**bubble** 1 A spheroidal envelope of liquid enclosing gas. 2 A gas-filled space within a liquid. 3 An auscultatory sound produced by or suggestive of bubbles. 4 A plastic, tentlike enclosure in which a patient who is particularly susceptible to infection can be maintained in a germ-free environment. *Popular*.
**bubo** \b^y oo'bō\ [Med L, from Gk *boubōn* the groin, a swelling in the groin] A swollen, inflamed lymph node, particularly in the neck, axilla, or groin. Adj. bubonic. **bullet b.** The hard bubo of primary syphilis. **chancroidal b.** Inguinal adenitis associated with chancroid. Also *virulent bubo*. **climatic b.** LYMPHOGRANULOMA VENEREUM. **indolent b.** A chronic bubo showing no tendency to suppurate. **malignant b.** A bubo associated with bubonic plague. Also *pestilential bubo*. **nonvenereal b.** The adenitis of lymphogranuloma venereum that arises from a source other than syphilis. **pestilential b.** MALIGNANT BUBO. **primary b.** Syphilitic inguinal adenitis that is not preceded by a visible primary genital lesion. **strumous b.** LYMPHOGRANULOMA VENEREUM. **syphilitic b.** A bubo symptomatic of inguinal adenitis associated with primary syphilis. **tropical b.** LYMPHOGRANULOMA VENEREUM. **virulent b.** CHANCROIDAL BUBO.
**bubonadenitis** \b^y oo'bänad'ənī'tis\ Acute, painful inflammation of inguinal or axillary lymph nodes seen in association with syphilis, chancroid, and lymphogranuloma venereum.
**bubonic** \b^y oobän'ik\ Characterized by buboes.
**bubonocele** \b^y oobän'ōsēl\ [Gk *boubōnokēlē* (from *boubōn* the groin + *kēlē* a hernia) an inguinal hernia] A swelling in the groin due to an inguinal or femoral hernia.
**bucca** \buk'ə\ [L, the mouth, a cheek] (*pl.* buccae) [NA] The side of the face forming the lateral wall of the oral vestibule. It is composed of the buccinator muscle covered by fascia, a thick pad of fat, and molar glands, the whole lined internally with mucous membrane; the cheek. Also *mala, gena*.
**buccal** \buk'l\ [L *bucc(a)* cheek + -AL] Relating to or in the direction of the cheek: in dentistry, said especially of the surface of a tooth facing the cheek or lips. Also *genal*.
**bucco-** \buk'ō-, buk'ə-\ [L *bucca* cheek] A combining form denoting cheek.
**buccocclusion** \buk'əkloo'zhən\ [*bucc(o)-* + OCCLUSION] Buccoversion of a group of teeth.
**buccocervical** \-sur'vikəl\ 1 Of or relating to the cheek and the neck. 2 Pertaining to the buccal surface of the neck of a molar or premolar tooth. For defs. 1 and 2 also *cervicobuccal*.
**buccofacial** \-fā'shəl\ Pertaining to the outer aspect of the cheek.
**buccolabial** \-lā'bē·əl\ Pertaining to the buccal cavity and the lips.
**buccolingual** \-ling'gwəl\ Referring to the buccal and the lingual aspects of the alveolus or of a tooth.
**buccoversion** \-vur'zhən\ [BUCCO- + VERSION] Deviation of a tooth from the normal arch toward the cheek.
**Buchner** [Hans Ernst Angass *Buchner*, German bacteriologist, 1850–1902] See under TUBERCULIN, EXTRACT.
**Buck** [Gurdon *Buck*, U.S. surgeon, 1807–1877] 1 Buck's fascia. See under FASCIA PENIS PROFUNDA. 2 See under OPERATION. 3 Buck's traction. See under EXTENSION.
**buckling** Overcrowding of the anterior teeth. **scleral b.** An operation for retinal detachment which infolds a ridge of sclera to enhance apposition between retina and choroid.
**Bucky** [Gustav P. Bucky, German-born U.S. roentgenologist, 1880–1963] 1 Bucky's rays. See under RAY. 2 Potter-Bucky grid, Bucky grid, Potter-Bucky diaphragm, Bucky-Potter diaphragm. See under BUCKY DIAPHRAGM.
**buclizine hydrochloride** $C_{28}H_{33}ClN_2 \cdot 2HCl$. 1-[(4-Chlorophenyl)phenylmethyl]-4-[[4-(1,1-dimethylethyl phenyl]-methyl]piperazine dihydrochloride. An antihistaminic agent used to relieve nausea from motion sickness.
**Bucy** [Paul Clancy *Bucy*, U.S. neurologist, born 1904] Klüver-Bucy syndrome. See under SYNDROME.
**bud** [of uncertain origin] In embryology, an outgrowth having the appearance of a small rounded mass which has the potential for growth and differentiation. **appendage b.** LIMB BUD. **appendicular b.** In human embryos of about 12 mm crown-rump length (39 days), a small conical projection that develops on the caudal limb of the umbilical loop of the midgut near its apex. The basal part of the conical projection gives rise to the cecum and the apical part to the appendix. The appendix appears as a bud (appendicular) at the apex of the conical projection, but there is no clear boundary line between the cecum and appendix. **bronchial b.** One of the numerous outgrowths from the lateral and stem bronchi in the embryonic lungs. Bronchial buds become the air passages of the respective lobes of the lungs. **dorsal pancreatic b.** An embryonic outgrowth which appears on the dorsal wall of the duodenum, in somite embryos, opposite but slightly cranial to the hepatic diverticulum. It grows rapidly and extends dorsocranially into the mesoduodenum to the left of the vitelline veins. Following rotation of the duodenum the dorsal pancreas extends into the dorsal mesogastrium. In human embryos of about 12 mm crown-rump length, the dorsal and ventral pancreatic primordia fuse to form a single organ, the dorsal pancreas giving origin to the body, the upper part of the head, and the tail. The duct of the dorsal pancreas forms the distal part of the main pancreatic duct (duct of Wirsung), while the duct of the ventral pancreas forms the proximal part. The connection between the dorsal pancreatic duct and the duodenum usually retrogresses, but may persist as an accessory duct (duct of Santorini). **end b.** The compact mass of cells at the caudal end of an early embryo formed from the primitive knot and the shortened primitive streak. It eventually gives rise to the lower part of the trunk and to the tail if one is to be formed. Also *tail bud*. **epidermal b.** Any of the ectodermal structures derived from the epithelium of the skin (epidermis) which gives rise to hair, nails, and the epithelial cells of the sweat and sebaceous glands and of the mammary glands. **epithelial b.** The ring of

epithelial outgrowth surrounding a skin appendage during the healing of a deep dermal burn. Coalescence of these rings restores epithelial cover over the burned surface. Also *skin bud, skin island.* **gustatory b.** CALICULUS GUSTATORIUS. **hepatic b.** A diverticulum from the foregut that gives rise to the liver and its ducts. The secretory cells of the liver and associated glands are derived from embryonic endoderm while the muscular and connective tissue elements are derived from visceral mesoderm and from the mesoderm of the septum transversum. Also *hepatic diverticulum.* **left pancreatic b.** An embryonic endodermal outgrowth analogous to the ventral or right pancreatic bud. Its existence has been questioned by some embryologists. When anomalous remnants persist, it may give rise to an accessory pancreas connected to the duodenum by an accessory duct, or to the anatomical anomaly in which the pancreas completely surrounds the duodenum (annular pancreas). **limb b.** A protrusion on the body wall of an embryo. It is caused by a dense mass of mesenchyme covered by epithelium and marks the site of the formation of one of the forelimbs or hindlimbs. Also *appendage bud.* **liver b.** An endodermal diverticulum which grows out from the embryonic foregut. It gives rise to the parenchyma of the liver, the ducts of the liver, the bile duct, the cystic duct, and the gallbladder. **lung b.** An outgrowth of endoderm from the floor of the embryonic foregut just caudal to the pharyngeal pouches. It gives rise eventually to the trachea and the bronchial tree. Soon after its appearance, the lung bud bifurcates into two primary bronchi. **mammary b.** Any of the small epithelial projections developing from the mammary line which are the precursors of the mammary glands. **placental syncytial b.'s** SYNCYTIAL SPROUTS. **right pancreatic b.** VENTRAL PANCREATIC BUD. **skin b.** EPITHELIAL BUD. **tail b.** END BUD. **taste b.** CALICULUS GUSTATORIUS. **tooth b.** The early, knoblike stage of a tooth germ. **ureteric b.** An outgrowth from the caudal part of the mesonephric duct (wolffian duct) near its junction with the cloaca, and from which develops the collecting tubules, the calyces, the pelvis, and ureter. It is one of the two elements which gives rise to the metanephros, the other being the metanephric blastema. Also *ureteric diverticulum.* **b. of urethra** *Outmoded* BULBUS PENIS. **vascular b.** The protrusion which marks the earliest stage of formation of a new blood vessel from one already in existence. **ventral pancreatic b.** An embryonic outgrowth which arises, slightly later than the dorsal pancreatic bud, in the angle below the hepatic rudiment. Its cavity usually communicates with that of the hepatic diverticulum, but it may open separately into the duodenum. With rotation of the duodenum its original ventral surface is now directed to the right, so that the ventral pancreas now extends into the mesoduodenum, being separated from the dorsal pancreas by a part of the left vitelline vein which becomes the portal vein. The ventral pancreas is represented by the lower part of the head of the pancreas following fusion of the two primordia. The duct of the ventral pancreas forms the proximal part of the main pancreatic duct (duct of Wirsung). Also *right pancreatic bud.*

**Budd** [George *Budd,* English physician, 1808–1882] Budd-Chiari disease, Budd's disease. See under BUDD-CHIARI SYNDROME.

**budding** **1** A form of unequal asexual division in which a segment, branch, or bud is formed and subsequently forms a copy of the parent, either as a part of a colony or linear chain or as a separate individual organism. See also SEGMENTATION, STROBILATION, GEMMATION. **2** In embryology, the appearance of a small excrescence or protuberance, such as a limb bud, or vascular bud, which has the potential for differentiation and growth into a more complex structure, such as a limb or a new blood vessel.

**Budge** [Julius Ludwig *Budge,* German physiologist, 1811–1888] Budge center. See under ERECTION CENTER.

**Budin** [Pierre Constant *Budin,* French gynecologist, 1846–1907] **1** See under PELVIMETER. **2** Budin's joint. See under SYNCHONDROSIS INTRAOCCIPITALIS POSTERIOR.

**BUDR** 5-bromodeoxyuridine.

**Buerger** [Leo *Buerger,* U.S. physician, 1879–1943] Buerger's disease. See under THROMBOANGIITIS OBLITERANS.

**Buergi** [Emil *Buergi,* Swiss pharmacologist, born 1872] Buergi's theory. See under HYPOTHESIS.

**bufa-** \bʸoo′fə-\ BUFO-.

**bufadienolide** [from L *bufo* toad] A $C_{24}$ steroid whose side chain on position 17 consists of a six-membered, doubly unsaturated lactone. Various bufadienolides, hydroxylated on C-3 and sometimes on C-5 and C-14, are found in toad poisons and in plants and have action on the heart.

**bufagin** $C_{24}H_{32}O_5$. A toxic steroid with cardiostimulatory properties that is found in the dermal secretions of toads such as *Bufo agua.* Also *bufagenin.*

**bufanolide** The parent compound of bufadienolide, consisting of androstane with a six-membered lactone ring on C-17, formed from a 1-(hydroxymethyl)-3-carboxypropyl group.

**buffer** [*buff* (to strike) + -ER] A system that keeps relatively constant the concentration of some constituent, such as hydrogen ions. It consists of some substance (A) capable of binding the constituent to be kept constant (L), part of it bound (AL) and part free (A). If the concentrations of AL and A both greatly exceed that of L, the concentration of free L will change relatively little when L is added to or removed from the solution. Unqualified the word usually means a hydrogen-ion buffer, a mixture of an acid and its conjugate base. Metal buffers are also widely used. See also entries under chemical names. **bicarbonate b.** A solution of a weak acid, carbonic acid, and its salt, bicarbonate, capable of limiting changes in hydrogen ion concentration following the addition of acid or base. It is a quantitatively important component of the body's buffer systems uniquely linked to the respiratory system which controls the acid element of the buffer through its effect on $PCO_2$. **veronal acetate b.** A buffer solution that contains sodium barbitone and sodium acetate and that is used in Palade's fixative. Also *veronal buffer.*

**buffering** The resisting of a change in acidity or basicity in a solution when an acid or alkali is added.

**bufo-** \bʸoo′fō-\ [L *bufo* toad] A combining form denoting toad. Also *bufa-.*

**buformin** $C_6H_{15}N_5$. *N*-Butylimidocarbonimidic diamide. A biguanidine oral hypoglycemic agent.

**bufotoxin** \bʸoo′fōtäk′sin\ $C_{40}H_{60}N_4O_{10}$. The principle toxin of the venom of the common European toad, *Bufo vulgaris.* Also *vulgarobufotoxin.*

**bufylline** AMBUPHYLLINE.

**bug** **1** Any insect of the order Hemiptera. **2** Popularly, any of various insects or other small arthropods. **assassin b.** Any of various bugs of the hemipteran family Reduviidae, named for their insect predatory activities. Some occasionally bite humans with a painful but not highly toxic effect. Some species of the subfamily Triatominae, however, are vectors of *Trypanosoma cruzi.* **bed b.** BEDBUG. **blister b.** BLISTER BEETLE. **cocaine b.** Formication occurring in cocaine users. **cone-nose b.** Any of various bloodsucking bugs of the subfamily Triatominae of the family Reduviidae. Several species are medically important as vectors of Chagas disease. **harvest b.** HARVEST MITE. **kissing b.** Any of various bloodsucking bugs of the family Reduviidae, so called from their habit of biting on the face, especially about the mouth. **red b.** RED MITE.

**Buhl** [Ludwig von *Buhl,* German pathologist, 1816–1880] Buhl-Dittrich law. See under LAW.

**bulb** [L *bulbus.* See BULBUS.] BULBUS. **aortic b.** BULBUS AORTAE. **b. of corpus cavernosum** BULBUS PENIS. **b. of corpus spongiosum** BULBUS PENIS. **dental b.** DENTAL PAPILLA. **duodenal b.** 1 PARS SUPERIOR DUODENI. 2 AMPULLA DUODENI. **b. of eye** BULBUS OCULI. **gustatory b.** *Outmoded* CALICULUS GUSTATORIUS. **b. of hair** BULBUS PILI. **b. of the heart** BULBUS CORDIS. **inferior b. of internal jugular vein** BULBUS INFERIOR VENAE JUGULARIS. **inferior b. of jugular vein** BULBUS INFERIOR VENAE JUGULARIS. **jugular b.** 1 BULBUS INFERIOR VENAE JUGULARIS. 2 BULBUS SUPERIOR VENAE JUGULARIS. **b.'s of Krause** CORPUSCULA BULBOIDEA. **b. of lateral ventricle** BULBUS CORNUS POSTERIORIS. **olfactory b.** BULBUS OLFACTORIUS. **onion b.** A globular structure found around myelinated axons and composed of proliferated Schwann cells and collagen fibers. It represents a nonspecific tissue reaction following myelin and axonal degeneration, as seen in many peripheral neuropathies including hereditary motor and sensory neuropathy, leprosy, and Refsum's disease. **b. of ovary** The mass of interwoven veins and smooth muscle fibers in the mesovarium. Also *Rouget's bulb.* **b. of penis** BULBUS PENIS. **b. of posterior horn** BULBUS CORNUS POSTERIORIS. **Rouget's b.** BULB OF OVARY. **sinovaginal b.** Any of the bilateral posterior endodermal evaginations of epithelial cells from the urogenital sinus close to the attachment of the mesonephric ducts. At full development, the bulb fuses with the caudal end of the vaginal cord to form the vaginal plate. The site of origin of the evagination is the location of the future hymeneal orifice. **spinal b.** MEDULLA OBLONGATA. **superior b. of jugular vein** BULBUS SUPERIOR VENAE JUGULARIS. **taste b.** *Outmoded* CALICULUS GUSTATORIUS. **b. of urethra** BULBUS PENIS. **vaginal b.** 1 The solid epithelial plate that forms the lower vaginal wall and arises from either the fused paramesonephric ducts or the urogenital sinus. 2 BULBUS VESTIBULI VAGINAE. **b. of vestibule** BULBUS VESTIBULI VAGINAE. **b. of vestibule of vagina** BULBUS VESTIBULI VAGINAE. **b. of vestibule of vulva** Two elongated masses of erectile tissue located on either side of the vaginal orifice and joined in front by a narrow band. Embryologically, they correspond to the corpora spongiosa of the male. **vestibulovaginal b.** BULBUS VESTIBULI VAGINAE.

**bulb-** \bulb-\ [L *bulbus* (from Gk *bolbos* a bulb, bulbous root) a bulb, bulbous root] A combining form meaning bulb, bulbar. Also *bulbo-.*

**bulbar** \bul′bər\ 1 Pertaining to a bulb. 2 Denoting the medulla oblongata.

**bulbi** \bul′bī\ Plural of BULBUS.

**bulbiform** \bul′bifôrm\ In the shape of a bulb. Also *bulboid.*

**bulbitis** \bulbī′tis\ [BULB- + -ITIS] Inflammation of the male urethra at the point where it is surrounded by the bulbus penis.

**bulbo-** \bul′bō-\ BULB-.

**bulbocapnine** $C_{19}H_{19}NO_4$. 10-Methoxy 1,2-(methylenedioxy)-6a$\alpha$-aporphin-11-ol, an alkaloid obtained from the roots of *Corydalis cava.* It serves to inhibit reflex and motor activity of striated muscle, and it is used therapeutically in the treatment of tremors and of Menière's disease.

**bulbocavernosus** \-kav′ərnō′səs\ MUSCULUS BULBOSPONGIOSUS.

**bulbogastrone** \-gas′trōn\ A material of unknown chemical structure extractable from duodenal mucosa, which can inhibit gastrin-mediated gastric acid secretion but fails to stimulate secretion by the pancreas.

**bulboid** \bul′boid\ BULBIFORM.

**bulbomembranous** \-mem′brənəs\ Pertaining to the membranous portion of the urethra and the spongy portion of the bulbus penis.

**bulbonuclear** \-n^y^oo′klē·ər\ Pertaining to the gray nuclei of the brainstem.

**bulbopontine** \-pän′tīn\ [BULBO- + PONTINE] 1 Pertaining to both the pons and the medulla oblongata. 2 Denoting projections from the medulla oblongata to the pons.

**bulbospinal** \-spī′nəl\ [BULBO- + *spinal (cord)*] Denoting fibers descending from the medulla oblongata to the spinal cord.

**bulbospongiosus** \-spän′jē·ō′səs\ MUSCULUS BULBOSPONGIOSUS.

**bulbourethral** \-yoorē′thrəl\ Pertaining to the bulbous part of the male urethra, situated between the anterior penile (or pendulous) part and the posterior prostatic and membranous parts.

**bulbous** \bul′bəs\ 1 Having the appearance and characteristics of a bulb. 2 Developing from or bearing a bulb.

**Bulbulian** [Arthur H. *Bulbulian,* Turkish-born U.S. medical researcher, born 1900] BLB MASK. See under MASK.

**bulbus** \bul′bəs\ [L (from Gk *bolbos* bulb, bulbous root), bulb, bulbous root] A spheroidal, or enlarged, part of an organ or structure. Also *bulb.* **b. aortae** [NA] An oval dilatation of the ascending aorta as it leaves the heart where the aortic sinuses, localized internal bulgings, are situated. Also *aortic bulb.* **b. caroticus** SINUS CAROTICUS. **b. cordis** The most cranial part of the primitive heart of the embryo, a dilated region of the embryonic cardiac tube between the ventricle and the truncus arteriosus. The bulbus cordis is divided by a spiral aorticopulmonary septum formed by the growth and fusion of the bulbar ridges. In the human embryo, fusion occurs in the eighth week of development and the septum divides the bulbus cordis into the aorta, which later communicates with the left ventricle, and the pulmonary artery, which communicates with the right ventricle. Also *bulb of the heart, Loetwig's ganglion.* **b. cornus posterioris** [NA] A prominence on the medial wall of the posterior horn of the lateral ventricle marking the position of the forceps major of the corpus callosum. Also *bulb of lateral ventricle, bulb of posterior horn.* **b. inferior venae jugularis** [NA] A dilatation of the internal jugular vein just above its termination where it joins the subclavian vein to form the brachiocephalic vein. Just above the bulb the internal jugular vein possesses a pair of valves. Also *inferior bulb of jugular vein, jugular bulb, inferior bulb of internal jugular vein, sinus of jugular vein.* **b. oculi** [NA] The spherical ball that forms the peripheral organ of sight and is situated in the orbital cavity, where it is separated from the fatty body by its fascial sheath. It extends between the anterior and the posterior poles and comprises three tunics and their contents, namely, the fibrous tunic consisting of the sclera and cornea, the vascular tunic consisting of the choroid, ciliary body, and iris, and the nervous tunic forming the retina. Its anterior segment houses the anterior and posterior chambers, while the posterior segment contains the vitreous chamber. Its movements are produced by the extraocular muscles. Also *bulb of eye, eyeball, orb* (seldom used). **b. olfactorius** [NA] A flattened, oval neural appendage of the cerebral hemisphere, representing a diverticulum of the primitive rhinencephalon and mediating olfaction. Lying largely above the medial margin of the orbital plate of the frontal bone, and below the gyri recti and frontalis, it receives olfactory bundles passing through the ethmoid cribiform plate. After the signals they carry are processed through several strata of neurons, the output is relayed to the olfactory tract. The bulb and the tract constitute the first cranial nerve. Also *olfactory bulb, olfactory tubercle, Morgagni's tubercle, ofactory ganglion.* **b. penis** [NA] The oval enlargement of the corpus spongiosum at the radix of the penis where it abuts against the inferior aspect of the inferior fascia of the urogenital diaphragm, being pierced here by the urethra, and where it lies in the groove between the crura of the penis. Anteriorly it tapers to become continuous with the corpus spongiosum. Also *bulb of corpus spongiosum, bulb of penis, bulb of corpus cavernosum, bulbus urethrae, bulb of urethra, bud of urethra* (outmoded). **b. pili** [NA] The expanded tip of the root of a hair that is embedded in the follicle and has its base invaginated by the vascular papilla. It is composed of polyhedral cells. Also *bulb of hair.* **b. superior venae jugularis** [NA] A dilatation of the internal jugular vein at its origin from the sigmoid sinus at the base of the skull. It is located in the posterior part of the jugular foramen and just below the floor of the tympanic cavity. Also *superior bulb of jugular vein, Heister's diverticulum, jugular bulb.* **b. urethrae** BULBUS PENIS. **b. vestibuli vaginae** [NA] A mass of erectile tissue on each side of the vaginal orifice situated on the inferior fascia of the urogenital diaphragm and covered by the bulbospongiosus. Each is connected to the other anteriorly by the narrow pars intermedia bulborum, and to the glans clitoridis. The bulbs are the homologue of the bulbus penis and corpus spongiosum of the male. Also *bulb of vestibule of vagina, vestibulovaginal bulb, vaginal bulb, bulb of vestibule, bulbus vestibuli.*

**bulimia** \b$^y$oolim′ē·ə\ [Gk *boulimia* (from *bou(s)* ox, cow + *lim(os)* hunger) ravenous hunger] **1** A ravenous or insatiable appetite for food. Also *hyperphagia, adephagia* (obs.), *cynorexia* (seldom used), *lycorexia, hyperorexia, bulimorexia, phagomania, polyorexia, polyphagia, sitomania* (outmoded), *sitiomania* (obs.). **2** An eating disorder marked by rapid consumption of large amounts of food, often of minimal nutritional value, in a short period of time. Such eating (binge eating) is typically episodic and recurrent, accompanied by awareness that the overeating is abnormal, by fear that eating cannot be stopped voluntarily, and by depressed mood and self-deprecating thoughts after each binge. Each binge is usually terminated by abdominal pain, induced vomiting, or social interruption of the secret eating pattern. For defs. 1 and 2 also *boulimia*. Adj. bulimic.

**bulimorexia** \b$^y$oolim′ôrek′sē·ə\ BULIMIA.

***Bulimus*** \b$^y$oolī′məs\ [New L, prob. from Gk *boulimos* great hunger, from *bous* a cow, ox + *limos* hunger, famine] A genus of freshwater snails in the subfamily Buliminae with an ovate, 10-mm shell, thickened peristome, and a thick calcareous concentric operculum. Also *Bithynia..* ***B. fuchsianus*** An oriental snail species, medically important as an intermediate host for the Chinese liver fluke, *Clonorchis sinensis..* Also *Bithynia fuchsiana..* ***B. leachii*** A medically important species widely distributed in central and eastern Europe and Siberia. It is the first intermediate host of the liver fluke *Opisthorchis felineus,* a fish-borne parasite infecting dogs, cats, and humans.

***Bulinus*** \b$^y$oolī′nəs\ A genus of freshwater snails of the family Planorbidae found in Africa, southern Europe, and the Middle East. They are intermediate hosts of important human and animal trematodes, including several *Schistosoma* species. ***B. africanus*** A widespread species (subgenus *Physopsis*), of African planorbid snails. In Zimbabwe, Mozambique, and South Africa it serves as the intermediate host of *Schistosoma haematobium* and *S. rodhaini.* In Zaire it is the intermediate host of *S. intercalatum* of humans. In South Africa, Transvaal, and Zimbabwe it is the host of *S. matthei* of cattle, sheep, and goats. In Zambia it carries *S. leiperi,* which infects various ungulates. Also *Physopsis africana.* ***B. truncatus*** A north and east African freshwater snail, certain strains of which are of great medical importance as the chief intermediate hosts of human schistosomiasis haematobia.

**Bull** [James William Douglas *Bull,* English neuroradiologist, born 1911] See under ANGLE.

**bull.** *bulliat* (L, let it boil).

**bulla** \bʊl′ə\ [L, a bubble or any bubblelike protuberance] (*pl.* bullae) **1** A fluid-filled space that is either within or beneath the epidermis and is usually greater than 2 cm in diameter. Compare BLEB, VESICLE. **2** Any pathologic bubble-like space within a tissue. **3** A bulging or bulbous anatomic structure. **emphysematous b.** A thin-walled air-containing space within the lung resulting from emphysema. **b. ethmoidalis** [NA] A bulging of the middle ethmoidal air cells, or sinuses, producing a rounded projection of the medial wall of the ethmoidal labyrinth into the lateral wall of the middle meatus of the nasal cavity under cover of the middle nasal concha. Anteroinferior to it is the long, narrow hiatus semilunaris. The sinuses open on or above the bulla into the nasal cavity. Also *ethmoid bulla, ethmoidal bulla of nasal cavity, ethmoidal bulla of ethmoidal bone.*

**bullae** \bʊl′ē\ Plural of BULLA.

**bullectomy** \bʊlek′təmē\ [*bull(a)* + -ECTOMY] Surgical removal of a bulla, especially of an emphysematous bulla of the lung.

**bullosis** \bʊlō′sis\ [*bull(a)* + -OSIS] A condition characterized by the presence of bullae. *Rare.* **b. diabeticorum** A disorder of the skin in uncontrolled diabetes mellitus in which bullae appear, usually on the feet and ankles.

**bullous** \bʊl′əs\ Marked by the presence of bullae.

**bumps** / **goose b.** GOOSE FLESH. **pump b.** Bony exostoses of the upper, outer border of the os calcis. The condition may be associated with bursitis, inflammation, and callosity, and it is believed to be caused by continuous attrition from ill-fitting shoes. *Popular.*

**BUN** blood urea nitrogen.

**bunamidine hydrochloride** $C_{25}H_{38}N_2O{\cdot}HCl$. *N,N*-Dibutyl-4-(hexyloxy)-1-naphthalenecarboximidamide hydrochloride. It is used as an anthelmintic agent.

**bundle** [Middle English *bundel,* from Middle Dutch *bondel,* dim. of *bond* a group, from *binden* to bind] A more or less distinct group of fibers, either nervous or muscular; fasciculus. **aberrant b.'s** Fascicles that leave the pyramidal tract in its course along the pons and medulla to project to motor nuclei of the cranial nerves. **Arnold's b.** TRACTUS FRONTOPONTINUS. **atrioventricular b.** FASCICULUS ATRIOVENTRICULARIS. **A-V b.** FASCICULUS ATRIOVENTRICULARIS. **axial b. of muscle spindle** The central fascicle of intrafusal fibers coursing through the encapsulated portion of a muscle spindle, usually to protrude beyond the poles of the capsule. In different animal species and muscles it may contain from one to twelve intrafusal fibers, and in certain pathological conditions dozens of fibers. **basis b.'s** *Outmoded* FASCICULI PROPRII. **central tegmental b.** TRACTUS TEGMENTALIS CENTRALIS. **cir-**

**cumolivary b. of the pyramid** A fasciculus of fibers which leaves the cerebral pyramid to pass inferiorly and then upward around the caudal pole of the inferior olive to synapse on cells in a nucleus (nucleus of the circumolivary bundle) formed during development by migration of cells from the rhombic lip of the fourth ventricle, as do the cells of the pontine nuclei. The circumolivary bundle and its nucleus therefore belong to the corticopontine projection system. **cleidoepitrochlear b. of deltoid muscle** A very inconstant supernumerary bundle of the deltoid muscle that arises from the clavicle, courses on outside of the cephalic vein, and terminates as a slim tendon on the medial epicondyle of the humerus. **comb b.** A tract extending forward from the substantia nigra to the globus pallidus and putamen. Interdigitation with fibers of the internal capsule give it a comblike appearance. Also *nigrostriatal tract.* **crossed olivocochlear b.** OLIVOCOCHLEAR BUNDLE OF RASMUSSEN. **fundamental b.'s** *Obs.* FASCICULI PROPRII. **ground b.'s of Flechsig** FASCICULI PROPRII. **b. of Helweg** *Seldom used* TRACTUS OLIVOSPINALIS. **b. of His** FASCICULUS ATRIOVENTRICULARIS. **inferior longitudinal b.** FASCICULUS LONGITUDINALIS INFERIOR CEREBRI. **inferior occipitofrontal b.** FASCICULUS OCCIPITOFRONTALIS INFERIOR. **Keith's b.** NODUS SINUATRIALIS. **Kent's b.** FASCICULUS ATRIOVENTRICULARIS. **Kent-His b.** FASCICULUS ATRIOVENTRICULARIS. **Killian's b.** PARS CRICOPHARYNGEA MUSCULI CONSTRICTORIS PHARYNGIS INFERIORIS. **lateral pontine b.** A composite fasciculus of descending fibers that leaves the cerebral peduncle to terminate in the pontine gray matter. **main b.** The proximal portion, or truncus, of the fasciculus atrioventricularis, extending from its origin to its division into crura. *Outmoded.* **mamillotegmental b.** The tract containing axons from the mamillary bodies that terminate in the dorsal and ventral tegmental nuclei (of Gudden). **marginal b.** TRACTUS DORSOLATERALIS. **medial forebrain b.** A myelinated axon bundle prominent in most vertebrates that arises from basal septal and olfactory regions and projects to the hypothalamus, the midbrain tegmentum, and brainstem autonomic nuclei. **medial longitudinal b.** FASCICULUS LONGITUDINALIS MEDIALIS. **Meynert's b.** FASCICULUS RETROFLEXUS. **Monakow's b.** TRACTUS RUBROSPINALIS. **muscle b.** A group, or fasciculus, of muscle fibers surrounded by perimysium. **olfactory b.** TRACTUS OLFACTORIUS. **olivocochlear b. of Rasmussen** Efferent fibers that originate in or caudal to the superior olivary nucleus, emerging with the contralateral vestibular nerve and crossing to the cochlear nerve to terminate on hair cells of the organ of Corti and possibly the vestibular organ. They modify the threshold of sensory responses. Also *bundle of Rasmussen, Rasmussen's nerve fibers, bundle of Oort, crossed olivocochlear bundle.* **oval b.** A nerve tract in the embryonic posterior funiculus of the spinal cord, situated in the peripheral part of the alar lamina between the posterior horn and the posterointermediate septum, which is the rudiment of the fasciculus cuneatus (column of Burdach). **oval b. of Flechsig** FASCICULUS SEPTOMARGINALIS. **papillomacular b.** The ganglion cell axons extending from the macula to the optic disk. **Pick's b.** Aberrant fibers of the pyramidal tract that pass through the medulla oblongata on a plane above the pyramids. **posterior accessory b. of posterior cruciate ligament** An occasional variant of the posterior meniscofemoral ligament in which a portion splits off and ascends either in front of or behind the posterior cruciate ligament. **posterior longitudinal b.** FASCICULUS LONGITUDINALIS MEDIALIS. **precommissural b.** TRACTUS OLFACTORIUS. **predorsal b.** *Obs.* TRACTUS TECTOSPINALIS. **b. of Probst** In a human brain in which the corpus callosum has failed to develop, a longitudial bundle of fibers coursing along the medial wall of the hemisphere. It contains fascicles leaving the fornix and parietofrontal association fibers. **proprius b.'s of spinal cord** FASCICULI PROPRII. **b. of Rasmussen** OLIVOCOCHLEAR BUNDLE OF RASMUSSEN. **respiratory b.** *Obs.* TRACTUS SOLITARIUS. **b. of Schultze** *Obs.* FASCICULUS INTERFASCICULARIS. **Schütz b.** *Obs.* FASCICULUS LONGITUDINALIS DORSALIS. **solitary b.** TRACTUS SOLITARIUS. **b. of Stanley Kent** FASCICULUS ATRIOVENTRICULARIS. **subcallosal b.** FASCICULUS SUBCALLOSUS. **superior longitudinal b.** FASCICULUS LONGITUDINALIS SUPERIOR CEREBRI. **tendon b.** A group, or fascicle, of parallel collagenous fibers held together by connective tissue and continuous with the endomysium and perimysium of muscle. **thalamomamillary b.** FASCICULUS MAMILLOTHALAMICUS. **Thorel's b.** A number of myocardial fibers of the right atrium extending from the sinuatrial node around the medial side of the orifice of the inferior vena cava to the atrioventricular node. They do not constitute a specialized pathway connecting the two nodes, as was formerly believed. **transverse b.'s of palmar aponeurosis** FASCICULI TRANSVERSI APONEUROSIS PALMARIS. **Türck's b.** 1 TRACTUS TEMPOROPONTINUS. 2 TRACTUS CORTICOSPINALIS VENTRALIS. **uncinate b.** FASCICULUS UNCINATUS. **b. of Vicq d'Azyr** *Outmoded* FASCICULUS MAMILLOTHALAMICUS.

**bungarotoxin** \bung′gərōtäk′sin\ A neurotoxic substance isolated from the venom of the elapid snake *Bungarus multicinctus,* the banded krait of Taiwan. It produces neuromuscular block by binding with acetylcholine receptors.

***Bungarus*** \bung′gərəs\ A genus of venomous snakes of the family Elapidae; the kraits.

**Bunge** [Gustav von *Bunge,* German physiologist, 1844–1920] See under LAW.

**Bunge** [Richard *Bunge,* German surgeon, born 1870] Bunge's amputation. See under APERIOSTEAL AMPUTATION.

**Büngner** [Otto van *Büngner,* German neurologist, 1858–1905] Büngner's bands. See under BAND.

**buniodyl** $C_{15}H_{15}I_3NNaO_3$. 2-[[2,4,6-Triiodo-3-[(1-oxobutyl)amino]phenyl]methylene]butanoic acid monosodium salt, an iodine-containing radiopaque contrast medium used to visualize the gallbladder and the biliary tract.

**bunion** [prob. from Middle English *boni, bony* a swelling, from Middle French *bugne* a bump, swelling] An abnormal prominence of the medial side of the first metatarsal head, with exostosis formation, adventitious bursa, and callosity formation in association with valgus displacement of the great toe. **tailors' b.** BUNIONETTE.

**bunionectomy** \bun′yənek′təmē\ The excision of a bunion.

**bunionette** \bun′yənet′\ A localized swelling at the lateral or dorsal aspect of the fifth metatarsophalangeal joint, caused by an inflammatory bursa overlying prominent bony points. Also *tailors' bunion.*

**Bunnell** [Walls Willard *Bunnell,* U.S. physician, born 1902] 1 Paul-Bunnell reaction. See under PAUL-BUNNELL TEST. 2 Paul-Bunnell-Davidsohn test. See under TEST.

**bunodont** \byoo′nōdänt\ [Gk *boun(os)* hill, mound + -ODONT] Having rounded cusps: said of teeth.

**bunolol hydrochloride** $C_{17}H_{25}NO_3{\cdot}HCl$. 5-[3-[(1,1-Dimethylethyl)amino]-2-hydroxy-propoxy]-3,4-dihydro-1(2*H*)-naphthalenone hydrochloride. It is used as a $\beta$-adrenergic blocking agent. It has pharmacologic effects similar to those of propranolol.

**Bunsen** [Robert Wilhelm Eberhard *Bunsen,* German chemist, 1811–1899] See under BURNER.

***Bunyaother*** \bun′yə·uTH′ər\ A pseudogenus to which viruses in the Bunyaviridae family are provisionally assigned when they have not been classified in a recognized genus.

**Bunyaviridae** \bun′yəvī′ridē\ A family of arthropod-borne RNA viruses. The virions are 90–100 nm in diameter and enveloped. The family includes one established genus, *Bunyavirus,* and a number of viruses of uncertain classification.

**bunyavirus** \bun′yəvī′rəs\ [from *Bunya(mwera) virus*] Any of a large group of RNA viruses belonging to the *Bunyavirus* genus of the family Bunyaviridae. Transmitted person-to-person by arthropod vectors (mosquitoes, sandflies, and ticks), many of them produce febrile systemic disease or meningoencephalitis in humans. Bunyaviruses of medical importance include those of the California encephalitis group, major causes of mosquito-borne encephalitis in the United States; Oropouche virus, causing mosquito-borne febrile illness in Amazonian Brazil; group C bunyaviruses and the sandfly fever group, agents of acute febrile illnesses in Central and South America; Rift Valley fever virus, causing disease in man and sheep in south and east Africa; and Crimean hemorrhagic fever virus of the Congo-Crimean hemorrhagic fever group, agent of tick-borne Crimean hemorrhagic fever in humans.

**buphthalmos** \b[y]oofthal′məs\ [Gk *bou(s)* bullock, cow, ox + *(o)phthalmos* eye] Enlargement of the eye due to increased intraocular fluid pressure during infancy or gestation. Also *buphthalmia, buphthalmus, congenital glaucoma, hydrophthalmos, hydrophthalmus, hydrophthalmia, infantile glaucoma.*

**bupivacaine hydrochloride** $C_{18}H_{28}N_2O \cdot HCl$. dl-1-Butyl-2′,6′-pipecoloxylidine hydrochloride, a local anesthetic with an amide linkage and a long duration of action. It is used primarily as a regional nerve block and epidural block by injection.

**buquinolate** $C_{20}H_{27}NO_5$. 4-Hydroxy-6,7-bis-(2-methylpropoxy)-3-quinolinecarboxylic acid, ethyl ester. It is used as an antibacterial (coccidiostat) for poultry.

**bur** [Middle English *burre,* akin to Old English *byrst* a bristle] Any of various small drills used in dentistry. Also *burr.* **diamond b.** A bur with a spherical head coated with diamond paste, designed for fitting handpieces driven by electric or pneumatic motors. It is used in various kinds of ear surgery, particularly in microsurgery.

**buramate** $C_{10}H_{13}NO_3$. 2-Hydroxyethyl benzylcarbamate. It is used as a tranquilizer and as an anticonvulsant drug.

**Burchard** [H. *Burchard,* German chemist, flourished 19th century] Burchard-Liebermann test, Liebermann-Burchard reaction, Burchard-Liebermann reaction. See under LIEBERMANN-BURCHARD TEST.

**Burdach** [Karl Friedrich *Burdach,* German physiologist and anatomist, 1776–1847] **1** Burdach's fibers. See under FIBER. **2** See under FISSURE. **3** Burdach's tract, column of Burdach, cuneate fasciculus of Burdach, fasciculus of Burdach. See under FASCICULUS CUNEATUS BURDACHI. **4** Funiculus cuneatus Burdachi. See under FASCICULUS CUNEATUS MEDULLAE OBLONGATAE. **5** Nucleus of Burdach's column. See under NUCLEUS CUNEATUS.

**Bureau International des Poids et Mesures** \bYrō′ eNternasyônal′ dā pwä ā məzYr′\ The international laboratory of weights and measures at Sèvres, France, under the authority of the Conférence Géneral des Poids et Mesures and supervised by the Comité International des Poids et Mesures. Abbr. BIPM

**Buren** [William Holme van *Buren,* U.S. surgeon, 1819–1883] Van Buren's disease. See under PEYRONIE'S DISEASE.

**buret** \byUret′\ [French *burette* (dim. of Old French *buire, buie* a pitcher, from Frankish) a cruet, buret] A graduated container, usually of glass, with a stopcock or other device that allows delivery of a measured quantity of liquid. Also *burette.*

**Bürger** [Max *Bürger,* German physician, born 1885] Bürger-Grütz syndrome. See under FAMILIAL HYPERLIPOPROTEINEMIA TYPE I.

**Burk** [Dean *Burk,* U.S. biochemist, born 1904] Lineweaver-Burk equation. See under LINEWEAVER-BURK PLOT.

**Burkitt** [Denis Parsons *Burkitt,* English physician active in Uganda, born 1911] Burkitt's tumor. See under LYMPHOMA.

**burn** [Old English *byrnan* to be on fire, combined with *bærnan* to set afire] A lesion caused by contact with a hot substance, flame, explosion, harsh chemical, or electricity. The depth of the injury is proportional to the heat of the agent and the duration of exposure. A first degree burn causes erythema and may cause epithelial sloughing in five to seven days. A partial thickness burn usually blisters and will heal spontaneously in one to seven weeks. A full thickness burn destroys all regenerative elements and must be skin grafted or heal by cicatrix. Many chemicals, usually acids or bases, can cause lesions of similar depth. Electricity, as current meets resistance in the skin, develops high temperatures and creates areas of tissue necrosis that are usually full thickness and may involve deeper tissues. **arc b.** An electrical burn caused by the passage of electricity jump-

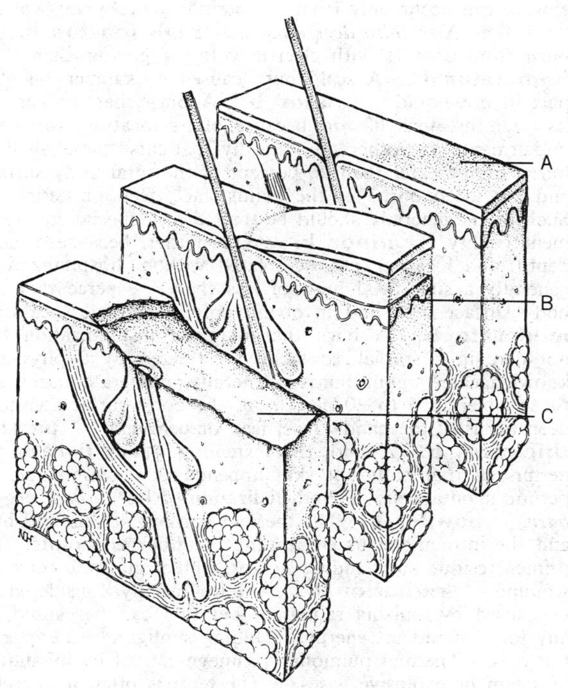


**Burns** (A) First degree; (B) partial thickness; (C) full thickness.

ing from the source to the conductor through the air. **brush b.** A lesion resembling a burn caused by violent friction which abrades the skin to a variable depth proportional to the severity of the friction. Also *abrasion, friction burn.* **circumferential b.** A burn encompassing the entire circumference of a part. Such burns are particularly treacherous if they occur as full thickness burns because loss of skin elasticity may compromise distal circulation as edema formation continues. **closed space b.** A flame burn occurring in a confined space, where smoke does not readily escape into the outdoors. Smoke inhalation frequently complicates such burns. **coagulation b.** A full thickness burn that denatures all the dermal protein. **corneal b.** Thermal damage to the cornea, usually found with flash or explosive burns or in patients who are unconscious and cannot protect the corneas by closing their eyes. **deep dermal b.** A burn with a depth that extends to the deep layer of the dermis. Such burns will heal spontaneously if infection is prevented, but take longer than three weeks to do so and usually produce noticeable scarring. **dermal b.** Any burn whose depth extends into, but not through, the dermis. **electrical b.** A burn caused by the passage of electricity from a source through the victim to a ground. Current limited to 220 volts usually burns only the skin, but high voltage creates severe underlying damage to any tissue in its path. It usually causes an entrance and an exit wound. **first degree b.** A superficial burn, involving the epidermis only. Such burns provoke erythema but never blisters, are quite painful, and heal without scarring in three to five days. **flash b.** A burn of short duration and high intensity caused by the explosion of gases or vapors, or from an electrical discharge. **fourth degree b.** A burn extending in depth to subcutaneous or deeper tissues. **friction b.** BRUSH BURN. **full thickness b.** A burn encompassing the full thickness of the dermis, so that wound closure can occur only from the periphery or by surgical intervention. Also *third degree burn.* **high tension b.** A burn from contact with electric voltages greater than 220. **immersion b.** A scald burn caused by submersion of a part in hot liquid. **major b.** A burn that, because of its size, threatens life or, because of its location, threatens impairment. In otherwise healthy patients these include burns over greater than 20 percent of the total body surface and any deep burns of the hands, face, feet, or perineum. Such burns generally should be treated in a specialized treatment facility. **minor b.** A burn that, because of size, depth, and location, can be treated without hospitalization, generally a superficial burn of less than five percent of the body surface area and involving only nonkinetic locations. **moderate b.** A burn that requires hospitalization but not care in a specialized facility if treated by a physician knowledgeable about burns. Generally, moderate burns are those covering 5 to 20 percent of the body surface without deep burns of the hands, face, feet, or perineum. **partial thickness b.** A burn that extends partially through the dermis so that sufficient skin appendages remain viable to permit spontaneous re-epithelialization. Also *second degree burn.* **powder b.** The thermal burning of skin and hair and the intracutaneous embedding of unburned powder and primer residue surrounding a close-range, gunshot entrance wouund. **radiation b.** A burn usually considered to be caused by ionizing radiation, but that can be caused by any form of radiant energy, including sunlight. **respiratory b.** Thermal pulmonary damage caused by inhalation of steam or explosive gases. • The term is often incorrectly used to describe pulmonary complications resulting from smoke inhalation. **second degree b.** PARTIAL THICKNESS BURN. **superficial b.** A partial thickness burn whose depth will permit spontaneous epithelialization in less than three weeks. Such burns generally heal without excessive scarring or impairment of function. Also *superficial dermal burn.* **thermal b.** Any burn resulting from heat in contrast to chemicals or radiation. **third degree b.** FULL THICKNESS BURN.

**burner** The source of flame in a lamp or heating apparatus. **Bunsen b.** A standard gas burner for laboratory use in which air mixes with the gas stream through lateral openings in the column prior to the point of ignition, creating a hot, nearly smokeless flame.

**Burnett** [Charles Hoyt *Burnett,* U.S. physician, born 1913] Burnett syndrome. See under MILK-ALKALI SYNDROME.

**Burnett** [Sir William *Burnett,* Scottish physician, 1779–1861] See under SOLUTION.

**burn-in** 1 The operation of a device prior to its normal use to stabilize its characteristics and identify early failures. 2 To apply extra exposure to portions of a photograph to increase its density.

**burnisher** \bur′nishər\ An instrument with rounded working surfaces used in dentistry to polish metal surfaces, to stretch margins of cast restorations, or to contour matrices.

**Burns** [Allan *Burns,* Scottish anatomist, 1781–1813] Burns ligament. See under MARGO FALCIFORMIS HIATUS SAPHENUS.

**Burow** [Karl August *Burow,* German surgeon, 1809–1874] 1 Burow's triangles. See under TRIANGLE. 2 Burow solution. See under ALUMINUM ACETATE SOLUTION. 3 See under VEIN.

**burr** BUR.

# bursa

**bursa** \bur′sə\ [Late L (from Gk *byrsa* hide, leather, wineskin) a bag, purse] (*pl.* bursae) 1 A sac or pouchlike anatomic structure. 2 [NA] BURSA SYNOVIALIS. **adventitious b.** A bursa which forms in response to pressure or friction over a bony point. Also *adventitial bursa.* **b. anserina** [NA] The bursa between the tibial collateral ligament of knee joint and the tendons of the sartorius, gracilis, and semitendinosus muscles near their insertions. Also *anserine bursa.* **b. of biceps brachii muscle** 1 VAGINA TENDINIS INTERTUBERCULARIS. 2 BURSA CUBITALIS INTEROSSEA. **b. bicipitoradialis** [NA] A bursa between the tendon of insertion of the biceps brachii muscle and the smooth anterior surface of the radial tuberosity. Also *bicipitoradial bursa.* **b. of calcaneal tendon** BURSA TENDINIS CALCANEI. **Calori's b.** An inconstant bursa located between the arch of the aorta and the trachea. **common peroneal b.** VAGINA MUSCULORUM PERONEORUM COMMUNIS. **copulatory b.** A male sexual appendage at the posterior end of certain nematodes, used for attachment to the female during copulation. It is characteristic of hookworms and other strongyloid nematodes. Also *bursa copulatrix.* **b. cubitalis interossea** [NA] A bursa frequently found between the tendon of the biceps brachii muscle and the ulna and neighboring muscles. Also *interosseous cubital bursa.* **deep infrapatellar b.** BURSA INFRAPATELLARIS PROFUNDA. **epiploic b.** RECESSUS INFERIOR OMENTALIS. **b. of Fabricius** A sac or pocket formed by the posterodorsal wall of the cloaca of chickens. It forms the primary lymphoid organ for the development of B lymphocytes and in this way is analagous to the thymus, which is the primary organ for T lymphocytes. In mammals the fetal liver has the functions performed by the bursa of Fabricius in birds. **Fleischmann's b.** BURSA SUBLINGUALIS. **b. of flexor carpi radialis muscle** VAGINA SYNOVIALIS TENDINIS MUSCULI FLEXORIS CARPI RADIALIS. **gluteal intermuscular bursae** BURSAE INTERMUSCULARES MUSCULORUM GLUTEORUM. **b. of great toe** A bursa, located between the indistinct facets on the bases of the first and second metatarsal bones, that replaces the weak interosseous fibers usually connecting the two bases. The bursa is occasionally replaced by a true intermetatarsal joint. **b. iliopectinea** [NA] A large bursa between the iliopsoas tendon anteriorly and the iliopubic eminence and the capsule of the hip joint posteriorly. It may communicate with the cavity of the hip joint. Also *iliopectineal bursa.* **inferior subtendinous b. of biceps femoris muscle** BURSA SUBTENDINEA MUSCULI BICIPITIS FEMORIS INFERIOR. **infracardiac b.** A small, closed, supradiaphragmatic, mesothelial cavity in the embryo lying between the esophagus and the right lung bud. It is a cranial extension of the right pneumatoenteric recess which will become the primitive lesser sac of the peritoneal cavity. The extension can become closed off and persist in the adult. **b. infrahyoidea** [NA] A bursa occasionally present below the body of the hyoid bone between the sternohyoid muscles anteriorly and the thyrohyoid membrane posteriorly. It may be present on either side of the median line or fused in the midline. Also *infrahyoid bursa.* **b. infrapatellaris profunda** [NA] A bursa between the ligamentum patellae and the upper part of the front of the tibia. Also *deep infrapatellar bursa.* **bursae intermusculares musculorum gluteorum** [NA] The intermuscular gluteal bursae, including those between the tendon of insertion of the gluteus maximus muscle and the origin of the vastus lateralis muscle. Also *gluteal intermuscular bursae.* **intertubercular b.** VAGINA TENDINIS INTERTUBERCULARIS. **b. intratendinea olecrani** [NA] A bursa occasionally found within the tendon of the triceps brachii near its insertion. Also *intratendinous bursa of olecranon.* **b. ischiadica musculi glutei maximi** [NA] A small bursa, often absent, located between the ischial tuberosity and the gluteus maximus muscle. Also *ischial bursa of gluteus maximus muscle.* **b. ischiadica musculi obturatoris interni** [NA] A large bursa between the tendon of the obturator internus muscle and the cartilage-lined lesser sciatic notch where the tendon makes a right-angle bend. Also *ischial bursa of internal obturator muscle.* **ischial b. of gluteus maximus muscle** BURSA ISCHIADICA MUSCULI GLUTEI MAXIMI. **ischial b. of internal obturator muscle** BURSA ISCHIADICA MUSCULI OBTURATORIS INTERNI. **b. of latissimus dorsi muscle** BURSA SUBTENDINEA MUSCULI LATISSIMI DORSI. **multilocular b.** A bursa containing many compartments, or loculi. **b. musculi bicipitis femoris superior** [NA] A bursa located between the common tendon of origin of the long head of the biceps femoris and semitendinosus muscles and the origin of the semimembranosus muscle and the ischial tuberosity. Also *superior bursa of biceps femoris muscle.* **b. musculi coracobrachialis** [NA] A bursa frequently found between the tendon of the coracobrachialis muscle, the subscapularis muscle, and the coracoid process. Also *coracobrachial bursa, subcoracoid bursa.* **b. musculi extensoris carpi radialis brevis** [NA] A small bursa between the tendon of insertion of the extensor carpi radialis brevis muscle and the back of the base of the third metacarpal. **b. musculi obturatoris interni** Either bursa ischiadica musculi obturatoris interni or bursa subtendinea musculi obturatoris interni. **b. musculi piriformis** [NA] A small bursa often present between the tendons of the piriformis and superior gemellus muscles and the femur. Also *bursa of piriform muscle.* **b. musculi semimembranosi** [NA] A large bilocular bursa with one sac extending between the semimembranosus muscle, the medial head of the gastrocnemius muscle, and the knee joint, while the other sac lies between the tendon of insertion of the semimembranosus muscle and the medial condyle of tibia. The bursa may communicate with the cavity of the knee joint. Also *bursa of semimembranosus muscle.* **b. musculi tensoris veli palatini** [NA] A bursa interposed between the tendon of the tensor veli palatini muscle and the pterygoid hamulus, around which the tendon hooks at right angles. Also *bursa of tensor veli palatini muscle.* **b. musculi thyrohyoidei** A bursa often present between the thyrohyoid muscle, the greater cornu of hyoid bone, and the underlying thyrohyoid membrane. **b. omentalis** [NA] A large, irregularly shaped potential recess of the serous peritoneal cavity situated posterior to the stomach and lesser omentum and extending superiorly to the liver and diaphragm and inferiorly into the greater omentum. Also *omental bursa, lesser peritoneal cavity, lesser sac of peritoneal cavity, omental sac, epiploic cavity, epiploic sac.* **b. ovarica** A peritoneal recess situated between the ovary and the mesosalpinx. **b. of pectoralis major muscle** A bursa frequently located between the tendon of insertion of the pectoralis major muscle and the tendon of the long head of the biceps brachii muscle. **b. pharyngealis** [NA] A small, median, inconstant blind sac in the base of the pharyngeal tonsil, surrounded on each side by prominent folds of diffuse lymphoid tissue that spread laterally and forwards from it. It is the remnant of the pouch of Luschka in the embryo. Also *pharyngeal bursa, Thornwaldt's cyst, middle pharyngeal recess.* **b. of piriform muscle** BURSA MUSCULI PIRIFORMIS. **bursae prepatellares** The bursae in front of the patella, comprising the bursa subcutanea prepatellaris, bursa subfascialis prepatellaris, and bursa subtendinea prepatellaris. Only the first of these is constant. Usually only one exists, but when more than one occurs they usually communicate freely. Also *prepatellar bursae.* **radial b.** VAGINA TENDINIS MUSCULI FLEXORIS POLLICIS LONGI. **b. retrohyoidea** [NA] A bursa interposed between the anterior surface of the thyrohyoid membrane and the concave posterior surface of the body of the hyoid bone. Also *retrohyoid bursa.* **retromammary b.** Any of several expanded loose connective tissue spaces between the fascia on the posterior surface of the mammary gland and the underlying pectoral fascia, giving the appearance of a serous sinus. **rider's b.** An adventitious bursa that forms on the inner side of the knee in horseback riders. **sacral b.** BURSA SUBCUTANEA SACRALIS. **b. of semimembranosus muscle** BURSA MUSCULI SEMIMEMBRANOSI. **b. subacromialis** [NA] A large bursa between the acromion and coracoacromial ligament superiorly and the tendon of insertion of the supraspinatus muscle on the greater tubercle of the humerus inferiorly. It may extend distally to join the subdeltoid bursa deep to the deltoid muscle, and it may communicate with the shoulder joint cavity. Also *subacromial bursa.* **subacromiodeltoid b.** A large bursa that results from the confluence of the subdeltoid and subacromial bursae. **b. subcoracoidea** An occasional bursa that becomes isolated from the subtendinous bursa of the subscapularis muscle, close to the base of coracoid process of scapula. Also *subcoracoid bursa.* **b. subcutanea** A synovial sac located deep to the skin, usually over bone. Also *subcutaneous synovial bursa.* **b. subcutanea acromialis** [NA] A flat bursa superficial to the acromion of scapula and deep to the skin. Also *subcutaneous acromial bursa.* **b. subcutanea calcanea** [NA] A bursa between the inferior surface of the calcaneus and the skin of the plantar aspect of the foot. Also *subcutaneous calcaneal bursa.* **b. subcutanea infrapatellaris** [NA] A bursa between the skin and the distal part of the ligamentum patellae and the adjacent tuberosity of tibia. Also *subcutaneous infrapatellar bursa.* **b. subcutanea malleoli lateralis** [NA] A bursa between the skin and the distal part of the lateral malleolus of fibula. Also *subcutaneous bursa of lateral malleolus.* **b. subcutanea malleoli medialis** [NA] A bursa between the skin and the underlying medial malleolus of tibia. Also *subcutaneous bursa of medial malleolus.* **b. subcutanea olecrani** [NA] A bursa between the skin and the posterior surface of the olecranon process of the ulna. Also *subcutaneous bursa of olecranon.* **b. subcutanea prepatellaris** [NA] A bursa between the skin and the lower half of the patella and the proximal half of ligamentum patellae. It is associated with the condition known as housemaid's knee. Also *subcutaneous patellar bursa.* **b. subcutanea prominentiae laryngealis** [NA] A bursa, usually found in males, between the skin and the anterior prominence of the thyroid cartilage of the larynx. Also *subcutaneous bursa of prominence of larynx.* **b. subcutanea sacralis** A subcutaneous bursa resulting from pressure, usually found in the elderly, posterior to the sacrococcygeal articulation or to the spines of the lower sacral vertebrae. Also *sacral bursa.* **b. subcutanea trochanterica** [NA] A subcutaneous bursa overlying the greater trochanter of the femur. Also *subcutaneous trochanteric bursa.* **b. subcutanea tuberositatis tibiae** [NA] A bursa anterior to the tibial tuberosity, covered by skin only or by skin and crural fascia. Also *subcutaneous bursa of tuberosity of tibia.* **subcutaneous acromial b.** BURSA SUBCUTANEA ACROMIALIS. **subcutaneous calcaneal b.** BURSA SUBCUTANEA CALCANEA. **subcutaneous infrapatellar b.** BURSA SUBCUTANEA INFRAPATELLARIS. **subcutaneous b. of lateral malleolus** BURSA SUBCUTANEA MALLEOLI LATERALIS. **subcutaneous b. of medial malleolus** BURSA SUBCUTANEA MALLEOLI MEDIALIS. **subcutaneous b. of olecranon** BURSA SUBCUTANEA OLECRANI. **subcutaneous patellar b.** BURSA SUBCUTANEA PREPATELLARIS. **subcutaneous b. of prominence of larynx** BURSA SUBCUTANEA PROMINENTIAE LARYNGEALIS. **subcutaneous synovial b.** BURSA SUBCUTANEA. **subcutaneous trochanteric b.** BURSA SUBCUTANEA TROCHANTERICA. **subcutaneous b. of tuberosity of tibia** BURSA SUBCUTANEA TUBEROSITATIS TIBIAE. **b. subdeltoidea** [NA] A bursa between the deltoid muscle and the capsule of the shoulder joint, fused with the tendons of the supraspinatus, infraspinatus, and teres minor muscles (the rotator cuff). It is usually continuous with the subacromial bursa. Also *subdeltoid bursa.* **b. subfascialis prepatellaris** [NA] An inconstant bursa located between the fascia lata and the underlying patella and partly covered by fibers of the quadriceps femoris tendon. Also *subfascial prepatellar bursa.* **b. sublingualis** An occasional serous bursa located deep to the floor of the mouth between the mucosa and the genioglossus muscle near the median line. Also *Fleischmann's bursa.* **b. submuscularis** A synovial sac located deep to a muscle, usually overlying a bone, tendon, or ligament. Also *submuscular synovial bursa.* **b. subtendinea** A synovial sac separating a tendon from another structure. **bursae subtendineae musculi sartorii** [NA] Bursae located between the tendons of sartorius, gracilis, and semitendinosus muscles. Occasionally one or more may be in communication with the bursa anserina. Also *subtendinous bursae of sartorius muscle.* **b. subtendinea iliaca** [NA] A bursa between the tendon of insertion of the iliopsoas muscle and the lesser trochanter of femur. Also *subtendinous iliac bursa.* **b. subtendinea musculi bicipitis femoris inferior** [NA] A bursa between the tendon of the biceps femoris muscle and the underlying fibular collateral ligament of the knee joint. Also *inferior subtendinous bursa of biceps femoris muscle.* **b. subtendinea musculi gastrocnemii lateralis** [NA] A bursa frequently present between the tendon of origin of the lateral head of the gastrocnemius muscle and the posterior aspect of the capsule of knee joint. It may communicate with the joint cavity. Also *subtendinous bursa of lateral head of gastrocnemius muscle.* **b. subtendinea musculi gastrocnemii medialis** [NA] A bursa present between the tendon of origin of the medial head of the gastrocnemius muscle, the underlying medial condyle of femur, and the capsule of the knee joint. It often communicates with the bursa of the semimembranosus muscle and the cavity of the knee joint. Also *subtendinous bursa of medial head of gastrocnemius muscle.* **b. subtendinea musculi infraspinati** [NA] A bursa between the tendon of the infraspinatus muscle and the capsule of the shoulder joint or, in some instances, the greater tubercle of humerus. Also *subtendinous bursa of infraspinatus muscle.* **b. subtendinea musculi latissimi dorsi** [NA] A bursa located in the axilla between the tendons of the latissimus dorsi and teres major muscles where they cross each other. Also *bursa of latissimus dorsi muscle.* **b. subtendinea musculi obturatoris interni** [NA] A bursa between the tendon of insertion of the obturator internus muscle and the posterior aspect of the capsule of the hip joint. Also *subtendinous bursa of internal obturator muscle.* **b. subtendinea musculi subscapularis** [NA] A bursa deep to the tendon of the subscapularis muscle at the glenoid border and the adjacent neck of scapula. It communicates with the cavity of the shoulder joint. Also *subtendinous bursa of subscapularis muscle.* **b. subtendinea musculi teretis majoris** [NA] A bursa posterior to the tendon of insertion of the teres major muscle at the medial lip of the intertubercular groove of humerus. Also *subtendinous bursa of teres major muscle.* **b. subtendinea musculi tibialis anterioris** [NA] A bursa between the tendon of the tibialis anterior muscle and the medial surface of the medial cuneiform bone of tarsus. Also *subtendinous bursa of anterior tibial muscle.* **b. subtendinea musculi trapezii** [NA] A bursa between the tendon of insertion of the trapezius muscle and the medial end of the spine of scapula. Also *bursa of trapezius muscle.* **b. subtendinea musculi tricipitis brachii** [NA] An inconstant bursa between the tendon of insertion of the triceps muscle and the middle facet of the posterior surface of the olecranon process of ulna, above which the posterior capsular ligament is attached. **b. subtendinea prepatellaris** [NA] An inconstant bursa between the flattened tendon of the quadriceps femoris muscle and the front of the patella. Also *subtendinous prepatellar bursa.* **subtendinous b. of anterior tibial muscle** BURSA SUBTENDINEA MUSCULI TIBIALIS ANTERIORIS. **subtendinous iliac b.** BURSA SUBTENDINEA ILIACA. **subtendinous b. of infraspinatus muscle** BURSA SUBTENDINEA MUSCULI INFRASPINATI. **subtendinous b. of internal obturator**

**muscle** BURSA SUBTENDINEA MUSCULI OBTURATORIS INTERNI. **subtendinous b. of lateral head of gastrocnemius muscle** BURSA SUBTENDINEA MUSCULI GASTROCNEMII LATERALIS. **subtendinous b. of medial head of gastrocnemius muscle** BURSA SUBTENDINEA MUSCULI GASTROCNEMII MEDIALIS. **subtendinous prepatellar b.** BURSA SUBTENDINEA PREPATELLARIS. **subtendinous bursae of sartorius muscle** BURSAE SUBTENDINEAE MUSCULI SARTORII. **subtendinous b. of subscapularis muscle** BURSA SUBTENDINEA MUSCULI SUBSCAPULARIS. **subtendinous b. of teres major muscle** BURSA SUBTENDINEA MUSCULI TERETIS MAJORIS. **superior b. of biceps femoris muscle** BURSA MUSCULI BICIPITIS FEMORIS SUPERIOR. **supernumerary b.** A bursa that does not occur over a recognized anatomical structure. **b. suprapatellaris** [NA] A large bursa between the posterior surface of the quadriceps femoris muscle and the anterior surface of the lower end of the femur. It usually communicates with the knee joint and occasionally with the subtendinous bursa of the medial head of the gastrocnemius muscle and the semimembranosus bursa. Also *suprapatellar bursa.* **b. synovialis** [NA] A sac of synovial membrane supported by dense irregular connective tissue and containing a film of synovial fluid, found interposed between two structures and permitting them to move freely over each other without friction. It may be simple or multilocular, and may be subcutaneous, subfascial, submuscular, or subtendinous. Also *synovial bursa.* **synovial trochlear b.** VAGINA SYNOVIALIS MUSCULI OBLIQUI SUPERIORIS. **b. tendinis calcanei** [NA] A bursa between the calcanean tendon (Achilles tendon) and the upper part of the posterior surface of the calcaneus. Also *bursa of calcaneal tendon.* **b. of tensor veli palatini muscle** BURSA MUSCULI TENSORIS VELI PALATINI. **b. of testes** SCROTUM. **b. of trapezius muscle** BURSA SUBTENDINEA MUSCULI TRAPEZII. **bursae trochantericae musculi glutei medii** [NA] Two bursae deep to the gluteus medius muscle, including a small, constant bursa overlying the anterolateral surface of the greater trochanter of femur and, posteriorly, a small bursa between the gluteus medius and piriformis muscles. Also *trochanteric bursae of gluteus medius muscle.* **b. trochanterica musculi glutei maximi** [NA] A large, multilocular bursa between the fascial tendon of the gluteus maximus muscle and the posterior part of the lateral surface of the greater trochanter of the femur and the proximal part of the origin of the vastus lateralis muscle. Also *trochanteric bursa of gluteus maximus muscle.* **b. trochanterica musculi glutei minimi** [NA] A large bursa between the tendon of insertion of the gluteus minimus muscle and the anterior surface of the greater trochanter of femur. Also *trochanteric bursa of gluteus minimus muscle.* **trochanteric b. of gluteus maximus muscle** BURSA TROCHANTERICA MUSCULI GLUTEI MAXIMI. **trochanteric bursae of gluteus medius muscle** BURSAE TROCHANTERICAE MUSCULI GLUTEI MEDII. **trochanteric b. of gluteus minimus muscle** BURSA TROCHANTERICA MUSCULI GLUTEI MINIMI. **ulnar b.** VAGINA SYNOVIALIS COMMUNIS MUSCULORUM FLEXORUM.

**bursae** \bur′sē\ Plural of BURSA.

**bursate** \bur′sāt\ Characterized by a copulator bursa: applied primarily to strongyle nematodes.

**bursectomy** \bərsek′təmē\ [*burs(a)* + -ECTOMY] The surgical excision of a bursa.

**bursitis** \bursī′tis\ [*burs(a)* + -ITIS] A swelling and inflammation of a bursal sac. Also *bursal synovitis.* **Achilles b.** An inflammatory swelling of the bursa about the distal end of the Achilles tendon. Also *achillobursitis, calcaneal bursitis, retrocalcaneobursitis, retrocalcaneal bursitis, calcaneal osteochondritis, Haglund's deformity, Haglund's disease, Swediaur's disease, Albert's disease.* **adhesive b.** ADHESIVE CAPSULITIS. **calcaneal b.** ACHILLES BURSITIS. **calcific b.** Bursitis accompanied by the deposition of hydroxyapatite within the bursa. **ischial b.** Inflammation and swelling over the bursa of the ischial tuberosity characterized by severe pain over the center of the buttock, often radiating down the back of the leg. The pain worsens when the subject is seated. **olecranon b.** Inflammation and swelling of the bursa over the olecranon process. The condition is found in horses as well as humans. Also *shoe boil, capped elbow, miners' elbow, student's elbow.* **omental b.** Inflammation of the peritoneal surface of the omental bursa. **pharyngeal b.** TORNWALDT'S BURSITIS. **popliteal b.** A swelling behind the knee that is caused by synovial fluid escaping posteriorly from the capsule to form a synovial lined sac. Also *Baker cyst.* **prepatellar b.** Inflammation of the bursa in front of the patella with fluid accumulation within it. **retrocalcaneal b.** ACHILLES BURSITIS. **scapulohumeral b.** CALCIFIC TENDINITIS. **subacromial b.** CALCIFIC TENDINITIS. **subdeltoid b.** CALCIFIC TENDINITIS. **Tornwaldt's b.** Chronic postnasal pharyngitis consequent on infection of the pharyngeal bursa. Pus in the bursa may become encysted leading to eventual scar formation and nasopharyngeal stenosis. Also *pharyngeal bursitis, Tornwaldt's disease.*

**bursolith** \bur′səlith\ [*burs(a)* + *o* + -LITH ] A calculus or any loose body within a bursa.

**burst** In the electroencephalogram, a wave form of short duration which stands out from the background activity. **bilaterally synchronous b.** A relatively short burst of generalized, sometimes recurring, high-voltage potentials in the electroencephalogram, such as the spike-wave complex, which are seen particularly in patients with epilepsy.

**Burton** [Henry *Burton*, English physician, 1799–1849] **1** Burton's line. See under LEAD LINE. **2** See under SIGN.

**Buschke** [Abraham *Buschke*, Polish-born German dermatologist, 1868–1943] **1** Buschke scleredema. See under SCLEREDEMA. **2** Tumor of Buschke-Loewenstein. See under TUMOR. **3** Busse-Buschke disease, Buschke's disease. See under CRYPTOCOCCOSIS. **4** Buschke-Ollendorff syndrome. See under DISSEMINATED LENTICULAR DERMATOFIBROSIS.

**bushmaster** [*bush* + *master*] A large, venomous snake, *Lachesis mutus,* found in South America.

**Busquet** [Paul *Busquet*, French physician, 1866–1930] See under DISEASE.

**Busse** [Otto Emil Franz Ulrich *Busse*, German pathologist, 1867–1922] Busse-Buschke disease. See under CRYPTOCOCCOSIS.

**busulfan** $C_6H_{14}O_6S_2$. Tetramethylene di(methanesulfonate). An antineoplastic, alkylating drug used primarily in the treatment of granulocytic leukemia.

**butabarbital** 5-*sec*-Butyl-5-ethylbarbituric acid. A sedative and hypnotic. Its duration of action is intermediate. Also *butabarbitone, butobarbitone.*

**butabarbital sodium** $C_{10}H_{15}N_2NaO_3$. 5-Ethyl-5-(1-methylpropyl)-2,4,6(1*H*,3*H*,5*H*)-pyrimidinetrione sodium salt, a barbiturate with sedative and hypnotic properties. It is administered orally.

**butabarbitone** BUTABARBITAL.

**butacaine sulfate** 3-(Dibutylamino)-propanol-4-aminobenzoate sulfate. A local anesthetic often used in the eye.

**butacetin** $C_{12}H_{17}NO_2$. 4′-*tert*-Butoxyacetanilide. It is used as an antidepressant agent and an analgesic drug.

**butadiazamide** $C_{12}H_{14}ClN_3O_2S_2$. *N*-(5-Butyl- 1,3,4-thiadiazol-2-yl)-*p*-chlorobenzenesulfonamide. A hypoglycemic agent given orally.

**butalbital** $C_{11}H_{16}N_2O_3$. 5-(2-Methylpropyl)-5-(2-propenyl)-2,4,6 (1*H*,3*H*,5*H*)-pyrimidinetrione. An intermediate-acting barbiturate given orally as a sedative. Also *isobutylallylbarbituric acid.*

**butallylonal** $C_{11}H_{15}BrN_2O_3$. 5-(2-Bromo-2-propenyl)-5-(1-methylpropyl)2,4,6(1*H*,3*H*,5*H*)-pyrimidinetrione. A hypnotic agent with actions of an intermediate-acting barbiturate. It was once widely used.

**butamben** $C_{11}H_{15}NO_2$. *N*-Butyl-*p*-aminobenzoate, an ester with local anesthetic activity. It is used topically in ointments or dusting powders by direct application to skin lesions, such as burns. Also *butyl aminobenzoate.*

**butane** $CH_3—CH_2—CH_2—CH_3$. The saturated hydrocarbon with a chain of four carbon atoms in its molecule. The term is sometimes extended to include 2-methylpropane. • In systematic nomenclature, the linear hydrocarbon, of which 2-methylpropane is an isomer, is meant.

**butaperazine** 2-Butyryl-10-[3-(4-methyl-1-piperazinyl)-propyl]phenothiazine. An antipsychotic agent effective in the treatment of psychiatric disorders. It is used in schizophrenia and given orally.

**butaperazine maleate** The maleate ester derivative of butaperazine. It is used for the same indications as butaperazine.

**butaprobenz** $(C_{18}H_{30}N_2O_2)_2 \cdot H_2SO_4$. *p*-Aminobenzoyldibutylaminopropanol sulfate. A local anesthetic with properties like those of cocaine. It is given subcutaneously in conjunction with adrenalin to produce a limited vasoconstrictor response and localize the region of anesthesia.

**butethal** $C_{10}H_{16}N_2O_3$. 5-Butyl-5-ethyl-2,4,6(1*H*,3*H*,5*H*)-pyrimidine trione. A barbiturate which acts by way of a metabolic intermediate. It is administered orally as a sedative.

**butethamine hydrochloride** $C_{13}H_{20}N_2O_2 \cdot HCl$. 2-[(2-Methylpropyl)amino]ethanol-4-aminobenzoate (ester)hydrochloride. An anesthetic agent used to produce nerve block in dentistry.

**buthiazide** $C_{11}H_{16}ClN_3O_4S_2$. 6-Chloro-3,4-dihydro-3-isobutyl-2*H*-1,2,4-benzothiadiazine-7-sulfonamide 1,1-dioxide. A thiazide drug used as an antihypertensive and diuretic agent.

***Buthus*** \byoo′thəs\ A genus of highly venomous scorpions found in North Africa, Egypt, Ethiopia, Somalia, and parts of Spain and France.

**butobarbitone** BUTABARBITAL.

**butoxamine hydrochloride** $C_{15}H_{25}NO_3 \cdot HCl$. α-[1-[(1,1-Dimethylethyl)amino]-2,5-dimethoxybenzenemethanol hydrochloride. A drug with antilipemic activity that inhibits the mobilization of fatty acids.

**butriptyline hydrochloride** $C_{21}H_{27}N \cdot HCl$. ±-10,11-Dihydro-*N*,*N*,*β*-trimethyl-5*H*-dibenzo[*a*,*d*]cycloheptene-5-propylamine hydrochloride. A tricyclic antidepressant drug.

**butt** [Middle English *butt(en)* to drive, thrust, from Old French *buter* to thrust, from Germanic *botan* to thrust] To place side by side so as to meet.

**butterfly** 1 An insect of the order Lepidoptera, distinguished from moths by possession of simple club-shaped antennae. The form of a butterfly with outstretched wings gives rise to the names of various objects suggestive of this form. 2 A piece of wing-shaped tape used to approximate surgically or traumatically incised skin. 3 A large wad of wing-shaped absorbent material used in gynecological surgery. 4 A skin flap used to obtain coverage of a defect by advancement of the flaps. 5 BUTTERFLY ERUPTION.

**buttock** [Old English *buttuc* end, akin to English *butt*] See under NATES.

**button** A round, protuberant form, such as a lesion, anatomic structure, or surgical device. **Aleppo b.** CUTANEOUS LEISHMANIASIS. **belly b.** *Popular* UMBILICUS. **Biskra b.** CUTANEOUS LEISHMANIASIS. **bone b.** A circular fragment of bone removed with a trephine. **oriental b.** CUTANEOUS LEISHMANIASIS. **Panje voice b.** TRACHEOESOPHAGEAL FISTULA VOICE BUTTON PROSTHESIS. **peritoneal b.** A short, collared tube connecting the peritoneal cavity and the skin. It is inserted to drain peritoneal fluid. **synaptic b.** END FOOT. **terminal b.** END FOOT.

**buttonhole** A short incision into an organ or tissue. It may be created inadvertently during dissection of a nearby structure as, for example, a buttonhole in the skin during subcutaneous dissection.

**butyl** \byoo′til\ 1 In systematic nomenclature, the group $CH_3—CH_2—CH_2—CH_2—$. 2 Any of the isomers of this group. Particularly important among these is the tertiary butyl group $Me_3C$. The stability of its carbocation and steric hindrance to displacement of the attached group give it properties different from those of most alkyl groups.

**butyl aminobenzoate** BUTAMBEN.

**butylparaben** $C_{11}H_{14}O_3$. 4-Hydroxybenzoic acid butyl ester. It is used as an antifungal medication, and added to a variety of drug preparations as a pharmaceutic preservative.

**butyr-** \byoo′tər-\ [L *butyrum* (from Gk *boutyron* butter) butter] A combining form denoting butter. Also *butyro-*.

**butyraceous** 1 Buttery in texture. 2 Containing a substance of the consistency of butter.

**butyric acid** $CH_3—CH_2—CH_2—COOH$. Butanoic acid. It occurs with other lower fatty acids in the milk of some mammals, esterified with glycerol, and is a characteristic component of butter.

**butyro-** \byoo′tərō-\ BUTYR-.

**butyroid** \byoo′təroid\ [BUTYR- + -OID] Resembling butter, especially in consistency.

**butyryl-CoA dehydrogenase** One of the enzymes (EC 1.3.99.2) responsible for fatty acid oxidation. It acts on the acyl-CoA molecules of shorter length to transfer hydrogen to an acceptor and thus leave the substrate with a 2,3 double bond. It is a flavoprotein.

**Bychowski** [Zygmunt *Bychowski*, Polish physician, died 1935] Grasset-Bychowski sign. See under GRASSET'S PHENOMENON.

**bypass** \bi′pas′\ 1 To pass blood or other fluid via an autologous or prosthetic conduit around an area of obstruction. 2 Any conduit that is capable of creating such a passage around an obstruction. **aortocoronary b.** CORONARY BYPASS. **aortoiliac b.** A technique of revascularization of the lower extremities wherein a prosthetic graft circumvents atherosclerotic stenoses or occlusions in the distal aorta or iliac arteries, linking the aorta and the common or external iliac arteries. **axillo-axillary b.** An operative technique used to connect the left and right axillary arteries by using a subcutaneous prosthetic graft. It is usually performed to relieve arm ischemia due to innominate or subclavian artery stenosis or occlusion. **axillofemoral b.** An extra-anatomic bypass in which a long graft from the axillary artery is used to revascularize one or both lower extremities. **cardiopulmonary b.** The support of the circulation by a heart-lung machine, as used in open-heart surgery. **carotid-subclavian b.** An operative

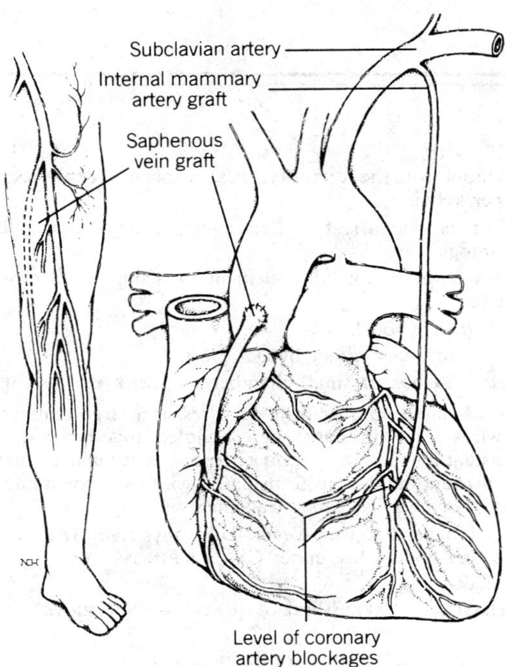


**Completed double coronary bypass**

technique to connect the common carotid and subclavian arteries, either by direct anastomosis or by autogenous or prosthetic graft material. It is used to relieve arm ischemia due to innominate or proximal subclavian artery stenosis or occlusion. **coronary b.** A technique of revascularization of the ischemic heart wherein coronary artery stenoses or occlusions are bypassed by segments of vein, artery, or prosthetic graft from the proximal aorta. Also *aortocoronary bypass.* **extra-anatomic b.** The revascularization of an ischemic organ or limb by means of a bypass graft that is constructed through routes not followed by the anatomic paths of large axial arteries. For example, an ischemic leg can be revascularized by a graft tunneled subcutaneously from the opposite femoral artery or the ipsilateral axillary artery. **femoropopliteal b.** The anastomosis of a vascular graft to the femoral and popliteal arteries in order to bypass occlusive disease in the superficial femoral artery. **ileojejunal b.** An operation for treatment of morbid obesity in which the proximal jejunum is anastomosed to the distal ileum or colon, thereby excluding the greater portion of the small intestine in the digestive process. **infrapopliteal b.** The revascularization of a lower extremity by means of a vein or prosthetic graft carried to the tibial or pedal vessels. ***in situ* b.** A technique of arterial revascularization that uses a nearby vein. The vein is left in its anatomic position and its valves rendered incompetent to permit passage of arterial blood flow. ***in situ* saphenous vein b.** An *in situ* bypass that uses the saphenous vein for femoral-popliteal or femoral-tibial reconstruction to provide revascularization of the lower extremity. **left heart b.** Diversion of the flow of blood from the pulmonary veins or left atrium directly to the aorta using a pump or extracorporeal system. **obturator b.** A graft of autogenous or prosthetic material passed from the common, external, or internal iliac artery through the obturator foramen and the posterior thigh to the mid- or distal superficial femoral artery. It is usually performed in order to bypass arterial infection in the ipsilateral groin. **partial b.** The diversion of a portion of the blood flowing through an organ or vessel. **percutaneous biliary b.** The drainage of bile from the liver by means of a plastic tube or catheter inserted percutaneously into the liver. It is performed in cases of obstructive jaundice, usually due to unresectable cancer. **right heart b.** The diversion of the flow of blood from the venae cavae into the pulmonary artery. **subclavian-subclavian b.** An operative technique used to connect the right and left subclavian arteries in which an autogenous or prosthetic graft is tunneled through the anterior neck. It is usually performed to relieve arm ischemia due to innominate or proximal subclavian artery stenosis or occlusion.

**byssaceous** \bisā′shəs\ Made up of fine threads or filaments, like flax.

**byssinosis** \bis′inō′sis\ [Gk *byssin(os)* made of *byssos* a fine yellow flax, the linen made from it, akin to Hebrew *bûtz*; + -OSIS] An occupational respiratory disease of cotton, flax, soft-hemp, and sisal workers, characterized by symptoms of chest tightness at the beginning of the work week. It is caused by exposure to dust emitted in preparatory processes. Byssinosis may eventually lead to chronic obstructive pulmonary disease and severe disability. Also *carders' asthma, cotton-dust asthma, strippers' asthma, flax-dressers' disease, hemp-workers' disease.*

**byte** \bīt\ A group of binary digits usually of eight bits, operated on as a group.

**Bywaters** [Eric George Lapthorne *Bywaters*, English physician, born 1910] Bywaters syndrome. See under ACUTE TUBULAR NECROSIS.

# C

**C.** 1 Calorie. 2 closure. 3 contraction.
**°C** 1 Symbol for the unit, degree Celsius. 2 Symbol for the unit, degree centigrade.
**$C_{CR}$** creatinine clearance.
**$C_{IN}$** inulin clearance.
**C1** The first component of complement. It is made up of three components (C1q, C1r, and C1s) which combine as macromolecular complex *in vivo* in the presence of calcium ions. C1 is activated by reaction with antigen-antibody complexes to form $\overline{C1}$, a protease which cleaves C2 and C4. (The bar over a component denotes enzymatic activity).
**C2** The second component of complement, although it reacts third in the classical complement pathway sequence. It is heat labile at 56°C and is the zymogen of serine protease. C2 binds to C4b (both in solution and cell-bound) in the presence of magnesium ions and is then split by $\overline{C1}$ to give C4b,2b, the C3 converting enzyme of the classical pathway and C2a. Deficiencies of C2 are known to occur in Caucasians and are linked to the MHC locus.
**C3** The third component of complement. C3 is the major complement component in quantity and is central to the complement pathways. It belongs to the family of proteins (C4,C3,C5 and α2 macroglobulin) that are inactivated by nitrogen nucleophiles. It is cleaved by the C3-converting enzymes into two fragments: C3a, which is an anaphylactotoxin; and C3b, which can bind covalently to acceptor molecules by an ester or amide bond. Fixed C3b reacts with receptors on phagocytic cells and is an important opsonin. Also *beta-1C globulin* (obs.).
**C4** The fourth component of complement. It is a member of the protein family (C4,C3,C5 and α2 macroglobulin) that is inactivated by nitrogen nucleophiles. It is cleaved by $\overline{C1}$ into C4a, a weakly anaphylactotoxic fragment; and C4b, which can bind to acceptor molecules by ester or amide bonds. Also *beta-1E globulin* (obs.).
**C5** The fifth component of complement. It belongs to the same protein family as C3 and C4 but has lost the capacity to form covalent bonds with acceptor molecules. It is cleaved by the C3-converting enzymes (but only when the C5 is bound to C3b) to give C5a, a powerful anaphylactotoxin; and C5b, the fragment which initiates the membrane attack pathway. Also *beta-1F globulin* (obs.).
**C6** The sixth component of complement. C6 combines stoichiometrically with C5b to give C5b,6 a stable complex which can react with C7 to produce C5,6,7, which has a short-lived membrane binding site and can thereby bind to cells.
**C7** The seventh component of complement. C7 combines with C5b,6 to give C5b,6,7, a complex with a short-lived membrane binding site, which can bind to cells and there fixes the site of the complement lesion.
**C8** The eighth component of complement. It is made up of two distinct subcomponents: the C8β chain and the C8α-γ chain, which combine noncovalently. C8 combines with C5,6,7, the C8β reacting before C8α-γ.
**C9** The ninth component of complement. C9 combines with C5b,6,7,8 and is polymerized by this complex to form, most usually, a circular torus which gives the complement lesion its characteristic morphology.
**c** Symbol for centi-: used with SI units.
**c.** 1 calorie. 2 centum (L, one hundred). 3 *cum* (L, with).
**c̄** *cum* (L, with).
*C* Symbol for the quantity, heat capacity, expressed in joules per kelvin.
**CA** 1 cardiac arrest. 2 coronary artery. 3 cancer. 4 chronologic age.
**Ca** 1 Symbol for the element, calcium. 2 cancer. 3 cathode.
**ca.** *circa* (L, about).
**CABG** coronary artery bypass graft.
**cabinet** A box or small chamber. **heat c.** HOT-BOX.
**cable** A small number of large wires or a large number of small wires, each insulated and bundled together with an outer insulating sheath. **coaxial c.** A tubular insulated shield surrounding a central insulated wire used for minimizing losses for high-frequency transmission.
**Cabot** [Richard Clarke *Cabot*, U.S. physician, 1868–1939] Cabot's ring bodies. See under CABOT'S RINGS.
**cac-** \kak-\ CACO-.
**cacanthrax** \kakan′thraks\ [CAC- + ANTHRAX] ANTHRAX.
**CaCC** cathodal closure contraction.
**Cacchione** [Aldo *Cacchione*, Italian physician, flourished 20th century] De Sanctis-Cacchione syndrome. See under SYNDROME.
**cacesthesia** \kak′esthē′zhə\ [CAC- + ESTHESIA] Any form of disordered or abnormal sensation. *Outmoded.* Also *kakesthesia.*
**cachectic** \kəkek′tik\ Pertaining to or suffering from cachexia.
**cachet** \ka′shā′\ [French (from *cacher* to hide, press, from L *coactare* to constrain), a small engraved seal, mark, imprint] A disk-shaped capsule for enclosing a powder dose of medicine that has an unpleasant taste.
**cachexia** \kəkek′sē·ə\ [Gk *kachexia* (from *kak(os)* bad + *hex(is)* bodily state, habit + -IA) poor condition, a poor state of health] General wasting, feebleness, inanition, and emaciation, usually associated with severe chronic disease or malnutrition. Also *cachexy.* **addisonian c.** Weight loss and generalized wasting due to primary adrenocortical insufficiency (Addison's disease). Also *adrenal cachexia.* **amyotrophic c.** An appearance resembling that of cachexia and resulting from severe muscular atrophy, as in motor neuron disease. **c. aphthosa** *Outmoded* TROPICAL SPRUE. **cardiac c.** Cachexia as a consequence of heart disease. **exophthalmic c.** GRAVES DISEASE. **Grawitz c.** A poorly defined, relentlessly progressive, fatal wasting disorder of the elderly which resembles pernicious anemia but lacks the characteristic hematologic abnormalities. **c. hypophysiopriva** The general wasting of advanced, severe, and untreated panhypopituitarism, now rarely seen. It is characterized by weight loss, emaciation, the signs and symptoms of secondary gonadal, thyroidal, and adrenocortical failure, and results in death. Also *hypophysial cachexia, pituitary cachexia.* **hypothalamic pituitary c.** A syndrome clinically similar to cachexia hypophysiopriva but resulting from a primary lesion in the hypothalamus with secondary failure of the anterior pituitary and tertiary deficiency of the gonads, thyroid, and adrenal cortex. **neurogenic c.** Cachexia complicating a

chronic nervous or mental condition. Also *psychogenic cachexia, nervous cachexia* (obs.). **pituitary c.** CACHEXIA HYPOPHYSIOPRIVA. **psychogenic c.** NEUROGENIC CACHEXIA. **saturnine c.** A state of malnutrition with loss of weight from excessive exposure to lead or its compounds. **thyrotoxic c.** *Obs.* GRAVES DISEASE. **tropical c.** A general state of marked ill health resulting from exposure to tropical conditions, usually over a very long period. There may be malnutrition accompanied by anemia, wasting, and possibly chronic liver disease. Intestinal parasites, tropical malabsorption, malaria, or other chronic infections may be responsible for the condition, but it is usually caused by a combination of several factors. *Outmoded.*

**cachexy** \kəkek′sē\ CACHEXIA.

**caco-** \kak′ə-\ [Gk *kakos* bad] A combining form meaning bad. Also *cac-, kako-, kak-.*

**cacogenic** \-jen′ik\ Leading to or pertaining to genetic deterioration through bad sexual selection.

**cacogeusia** \-joo′sē·ə, -gyoo′zhə\ [CACO- + Gk *geus(is)* a tasting, sense of taste + -IA] A variety of dysgeusia in which an unpleasant taste is noticed in the absence of the corresponding stimulus. Among the causes are psychological disturbances and temporal lobe epilepsy in which gustatory aura of this kind may occur.

**cacolalia** \-lā′lyə\ [CACO- + -LALIA] COPROLALIA.

**cacorhythmic** \-riTH′mik\ Characterized by irregular rhythm.

**cacosmia** \kakäz′mē·ə\ [CACO- + *osm(o)-*[2] + -IA] A perversion of the sense of smell in which unpleasant odors are perceived in the absence of the corresponding stimulus. Also *kakosmia.*

**cacothenic** \-then′ik\ Pertaining to genetic deterioration attributable to environmental factors.

**cacuminal** \kakyoo′minəl\ Uppermost; highest; most superior.

**CAD** coronary artery disease.

**cadaver** \kədav′ər\ [L (from *cadere* to fall, die in battle), a corpse] A dead animal or, more especially, human body. • In common medical use, *cadaver* refers to human bodies prepared by embalming technique for medical studies.

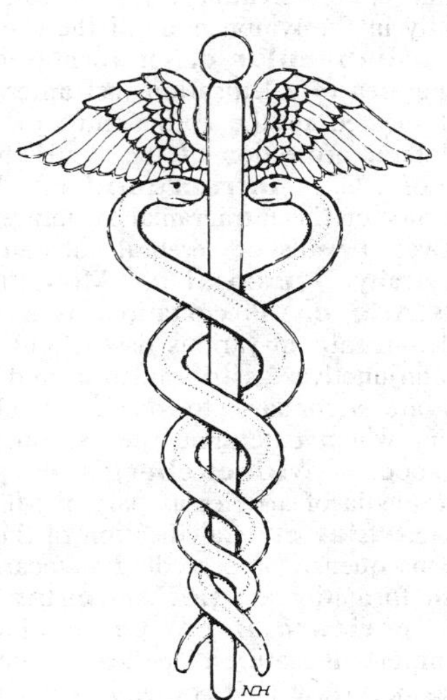

Caduceus

**cadaverine** $H_2N—[CH_2]_5—NH_2$. Pentamethylenediamine. A poisonous, syrupy, foul-smelling substance arising by decarboxylation of lysine in bacteria and in decomposing flesh. It is a skin irritant and possible sensitizing agent.

**cadaverous** \kədav′ərəs\ Resembling or characteristic of a cadaver.

**cadmium** \kad′mē·əm\ Element number 48, having atomic weight 112.41. Cadmium is a soft, bluish white metal that occurs combined in zinc and other ores. There are eight natural stable isotopes, the most abundant having mass numbers 112 and 114. Numerous radioactive isotopes are known. Cadmium has numerous technologic applications. Since cadmium and its compounds are toxic, long-term exposure of workers represents a serious industrial hazard if adequate safeguards are not adopted. Symbol: Cd

**CaDTe** cathodal duration tetanus.

**caduca** \kədoo′kə\ [L, fem. of *caducus* falling, ready to fall] DECIDUA.

**caduceus** \kədoo′sē·əs\ [L, also *caduceum,* alteration of Doric Gk *karykeion,* Attic Gk *kērykeion,* Ionic Gk *kērykēïon* a herald's wand, usu. with two serpents wound around it] The winged staff of the god Hermes, oppositely entwined by a pair of snakes, the symbol of a herald. It used as an emblem of medicine by many organizations. Compare STAFF OF AESCULAPIUS.

**cae-** \sē-, se-\ For words beginning *cae-*, see also under CE-.

**caecostomy** *Brit.* CECOSTOMY.

**caecum** \sē′kəm\ [L *(intestinum) caecum* blind intestine, from *caecus* blind] **1** [NA] The large, blind sac that forms the commencement of the large intestine below the entrance of the terminal ileum, above which it is continuous with the ascending colon. The vermiform appendix projects from its posteromedial wall. It is situated in the right iliac fossa at a level above the lateral half of the inguinal ligament. Also *blind gut, blindgut, caput coli, blind intestine, typhlon* (obs.). **2** Any blind pouch or tube that ends in a cul-de-sac. For defs 1 and 2 also *cecum.* **c. cupulare ductus cochlearis** [NA] The terminal blind sac at the apical turn of the cochlear duct just beyond the hamulus of the spiral lamina where it is attached to the cupula cochleae and forms part of the boundary of the helicotrema. Also *cupular cecum of cochlear duct, lagena.* **c. vestibulare ductus cochlearis** [NA] The small, blind sac forming the commencement of the cochlear duct adjacent to the orifice of the ductus reuniens and occupying the cochlear recess of the vestibule. Also *vestibular cecum of cochlear duct.*

**caecus** \sē′kəs\ [L, blind] A blind pouch.

**caeno-** \sē′nō-, sē′nə-\ CENO-[3].

**caeruloplasmin** *Brit.* CERULOPLASMIN.

**caesarean** \sizer′ē·ən\ See under CESAREAN SECTION.

**cafard** \käfär′\ [French, cockroach; *avoir le cafard* to feel low] MELANCHOLIA.

**caffeine** \kafēn′, kaf′ē·in\ [French *caféine,* from *café* coffee + -INE] $C_8H_{10}N_4O_2$. A bitter white crystalline xanthine that is soluble in water. It is a central nervous system stimulant that is slightly diuretic and a mild vasodilator. It may be used as an antidote to hypnotic drugs. It is found in various plant products: chocolate (*Theobroma cacao*), coffee (*Coffea arabica*), guarana (*Paullinia* sp.), kola (*Cola nitida*), maté (*Ilex paraguayensis*), and tea (*Thea sinensis*).

**caffeinism** \kafē′nizm\ [CAFFEIN + -ISM] A condition resulting from the ingestion of excessive amounts of caffeine. The symptoms are tachycardia, dyspepsia, irritability, and insomnia.

**Caffey** [John *Caffey,* U.S. pediatrician, 1895–1966] Caffey's disease, Caffey syndrome, Caffey-Silverman syndrome. See under INFANTILE HYPEROSTOSIS.

**cage** Any structure serving to enclose or confine, especially one with walls of mesh or struts. **Faraday c.** An enclosure, usually of wire, intended to exclude electromagnetic interference when recording electrical activity from a biological preparation. **rib c.** *Popular* COMPAGES THORACIS.

**cahincic acid** $C_{40}H_{64}O_{18}$. A glycoside from the cahinca root, *Chiococca racemosa*. It is used as a cathartic and as a diuretic medication. Also *cahinic acid, caincic acid.*

**caino-** \kī'nə-\ CENO-[1].

**Cairns** [Sir Hugh William Bell *Cairns*, English surgeon, born 1896] See under SYNDROME.

**Cajal** [Santiago Ramón y *Cajal*, Spanish histologist, 1852–1934] **1** See under METHOD, CELL. **2** Cajal cell. See under ASTROCYTE.

**cajeputol** EUCALYPTOL.

**cajuputene** $C_{10}H_{16}$. The characteristic ingredient of cajuput oil. The aromatic liquid is used as an anthelmintic agent and as an ingredient in some ointments and liniments.

**Cal** **1** Symbol for the unit, Calorie. **2** Symbol for the unit, calorie. An incorrect symbol in this sense.

**calabashcurarine** An alkaloid with properties like those of tubocurarine but differing somewhat in pharmacologic properties.

**calamine** A pink powder composed of zinc oxide or basic zinc carbonate and a small amount of ferric oxide. It is used as a topical protectant or astringent in the form of a powder, lotion, cream, or ointment. Also *lapis calaminaris.*

**calamus scriptorius** The tapering inferior extremity of the fourth ventricle, bordered on its sides by the two clavae and bridged caudally by the obex. The entrance of the central canal is at the tip of the calamus. • The name derives from the fancied resemblance of the structure to the tip of a reed pen (Latin, "writing pen").

**calc-** \kalk-, kals-\ [L *calx,* gen. *calcis,* lime, stone, limestone] A combining form meaning calcium or lime. Also *calci-, calco-.*

**calcaneal** \kalkā'nē·əl\ Pertaining or belonging to the calcaneus. Also *calcanean.*

**calcaneoapophysitis** \kalkā'nē·ō·əpäf'əzī'tis\ Inflammation of the soft parts of the heel at the point of insertion of the Achilles tendon.

**calcaneodynia** \kalkā'nē·ōdin'ē·ə \ Pain in the heel or calcaneus. Also *calcanodynia.*

**calcaneus** \kalkā'nē·əs\ [Late L, alteration of L *calcaneum* (from *calx,* gen. *calcis,* heel, foot) heel, hinder part of the foot] [NA] The largest bone of the tarsus. Its long axis is directed anteriorly, superiorly, and laterally, and it articulates with the talus, which rests on it, and with the cuboid bone anteriorly. Its posterior projection forms the heel, which serves as a lever for the action of the calf muscles attached to it, and it forms the posterior pillar of the medial longitudinal arch. Also *calcaneum, heel bone, os calcis.*

**calcanodynia** \kal'kənōdin'ē·ə\ CALCANEODYNIA.

**calcar** \kal'kär\ [L (from *calx,* gen. *calcis,* heel), a spur, cock's spur] A spur or spurlike process; a sharp projection from a structure. **c. avis** A linear protuberance marking the position of the calcarine fissure along the medial wall of the posterior horn of the lateral ventricle. Also *pes hippocampi minor, unguis avis, unguis ventriculi lateralis cerebri.* **c. femorale** A strengthening slim vertical plate of bone within the femur that extends from the inner compact bone at the upper end of linea aspera into the spongy bone of the neck, fusing with its posterior wall and the adjacent spongy bone of the greater trochanter and strengthening this region. Also *Bigelow septum.* **c. pedis** CALX.

**calcarine** \kal'kerin\ **1** Pertaining to a calcar, especially the calcar avis. **2** Spur-shaped.

**calcariuria** \kalkar'ēyoo'rē·ə\ [L *calcari(us)* pertaining to lime + -URIA] The urinary excretion of lime salts. *Seldom used.*

**calcaroid** \kal'karoid\ **1** Describing a localized deposit found in the brain substance in various degenerative disorders. It resembles an area of calcification but contains no calcium. **2** A calcaroid deposit.

**calci-** \kal'sē-\ CALC-.

**calcicosis** \kal'sēkō'sis\ [CALCI- + *-cosis,* by analogy with *(sili)cosis*] Pneumoconiosis or any lung condition resulting from inhalation of marble or chalk dust, occurring among workers in the mining, quarrying, and shaping of stone or other products. Pure calcium carbonate does not cause pneumoconiosis, but impurities in the stone, such as quartz, can do so.

**calciferol** Any of various compounds that have vitamin D activity, such as cholecalciferol or ergocalciferol, and that are derived from sterols by breaking ring B at the 9-10 bond. They possess a 5,7,10(19) conjugated system of double bonds.

**calcification** \kal'sifikā'shən\ [L *calx,* gen. *calcis,* lime, stone, limestone + -FICATION] The deposition of calcium salts within organic tissue. Also *calcium infiltration, calcareous infiltration.* **aortic c.** Deposition of calcium in the wall of the aorta, a characteristic feature of arteriosclerosis. **conjunctival metastatic c.** The deposition of calcium phosphate microcrystals in the superficial conjunctival layers of the eye. This condition may occur in patients with advanced renal failure who have increased serum inorganic phosphate but whose serum calcium may be normal or even decreased. While the deposits usually are asymptomatic, they may cause the irritation called "the red eyes of renal failure." **coronary c.** Calcification in the walls of the coronary arteries. **dystrophic c.** A focal form of calcification characterized by deposition of hydroxyapatite crystals in previously damaged tissues such as heart valves, scars, old foci of tuberculosis, and atheromatous plaques. The pathogenesis is unclear, but unrelated to disturbances of calcium metabolism. The serum calcium is normal. **eggshell c.** In radiology, a thin circumferential layer of calcification, seen characteristically in the lymph node of the chest in a patient with silicosis. **habenular c.** In roentgenography of the head, a midline area of calcification just anterior to the pineal body and located in the epithalamus of the brain. As seen on the lateral projection of the skull, the calcification has the shape of a C. **intracranial c.** The deposition of calcium in any of the intracranial structures, as the dura mater, blood vessel walls or cerebral substance. It may be visible radiologically. **medial c.** MÖNCKEBERG SCLEROSIS. **metastatic c.** Precipitation, as a result of renal disease, of calcium salts in various tissues and organs including tendons, conjunctiva, gastric mucosa, and arterial walls. Precipitations are secondary to decreased blood pH and serum albumin, which determine the saturation of calcium salts in the blood. **Mönckeberg's c.** Deposition of calcium in the media of arteries as part of Mönckeberg sclerosis. **myocardial c.** Calcification of the myocardium, usually the consequence of preceding myocardial infarction with aneurysm formation. **periarticular c.** CALCIFIC TENDINITIS. **pericardial c.** Calcification of the pericardium, an important feature of pericardial constriction and also sometimes occurring as a consequence of rheumatic pericarditis without producing constriction. **pulmonary c.** The presence or accumulation of calcium salts in lung tissues. **valvular c.** Calcification of the apparatus of a cardiac valve.

**calcified** \kal′səfīd\ Containing deposits of calcium salts.

**calcination** \kal′sənā′shən\ [Middle French (from *calcin(er)* to change a substance into lime by fire, from L *calx*, gen. *calcis*, lime, + Old French *-ation* -ATION), a changing into lime by fire] The application of heat to remove all traces of water and other volatiles so as to produce a dry powder.

**calcinosis** \kal′sinō′sis\ [L *calcin(are)* (from *calx*, gen. *calcis*, lime) to make lime + -OSIS] Any of various pathologic conditions characterized by the deposition of calcium salts in tissues. Also *calcium thesaurismosis*. **c. circumscripta** A condition marked by localized areas of calcinosis cutis. **intervertebral c.** Calcium deposits in the intervertebral disks. Also *Verse disease, chondritis intervertebralis calcarea*. **tumoral c.** A tumorlike lesion containing calcium and proteinaceous material. **c. universalis** Dystrophic calcification of the skin and subcutaneous tissues seen most commonly in patients with dermatomyositis and rarely in those with scleroderma. It is characterized by numerous large deposits of calcium which may also involve muscles and tendons.

**calcio-** \kal′sē·ō-\ [New L *calcium*, from L *calx*, gen. *calcis*, lime, stone, limestone] A combining form denoting calcium.

**calciokinesis** \kal′sē·ōkīnē′sis\ The mobilization of stored calcium.

**calciorrhachia** \kal′sē·ôrā′kē·ə\ [CALCIO- + Gk *rhach(is)* the back, backbone + -IA] The presence of calcium in the cerebrospinal fluid.

**calcipenia** \kal′səpē′nē·ə\ An absence or insufficiency of calcium in the diet.

**calcipexis** CALCIPEXY.

**calcipexy** \kal′səpek′sē\ [CALCI- + -PEXY] The fixation of calcium in tissues. Also *calcipexis*.

**calciphile** \kal′səfīl\ [CALCI- + -PHILE] Having an affinity for calcium salts.

**calciphylaxis** \kal′səfīlak′sis\ [CALCI- + Gk *phylaxis* guarding, protection] The experimentally induced formation of ectopic calcified tissue consequent to a challenging agent administered to a prepared host in which a hypersensitive state has been induced. Adj. calciphylactic. **systemic c.** The generalized deposition of calcium salts in tissues following the intravenous or intraperitoneal administration of an antigen in a sensitive individual. **topical c.** A localized deposition of calcium following the subcutaneous administration of an antigen in a sensitized individual.

**calcite** A crystalline form of calcium carbonate. It occurs in many rocks, and has the optical property of double refraction. Two slabs bonded together form a Nicol prism.

**calcitonin** \kal′sətō′nin\ A 32-amino-acid polypeptide which functions as a hypocalcemic hormone in mammals. It is synthesized in and secreted by the parafollicular cells (C cells) of the thyroid in man and by the ultimobranchial body in species such as teleosts and amphibians. Its importance in regulating human serum calcium concentration is not firmly established. It may have an important influence on phosphate metabolism and calcium absorption and distribution. It is secreted in excess by the thyroid gland if affected by certain medullary carcinomas, as in multiple endocrine neoplasia Type II. Also *thyrocalcitonin*. **synthetic c.** A completely synthesized form of salmon calcitonin that has the same amino acid composition and sequence as that isolated from the natural source. It is given by intramuscular or subcutaneous injection for idiopathic hypercalcemia and osteitis deformans. Also *salcatonin*.

**calcitriol** \kal′sətrī′ôl\ 1,25-DIHYDROXYCHOLECALCIFEROL.

**calcium** \kal′sē·əm\ [L *calx*, gen. *calcis*, lime, stone, limestone + *-ium*, New L suffix] Element number 20, having atomic weight 40.08. An abundant alkaline earth metal, it forms over three percent of the earth's crust, always in combined form. Six stable isotopes occur in nature. The valence is 2. The calcium ion is one of the principal cations regulating biologic processes. Calcium is a component of bones, teeth, shells, and leaves. It is required in several enzymes, such as the lipases. Symbol: Ca

**calcium 45** A radioisotope of calcium emitting purely beta radiation. It has been employed in mineral metabolism research. Its soft beta radiation makes it suitable for autoradiography but does not permit scintigraphy *in vivo*. Physical half-life is 165 days. Symbol: $^{45}Ca$

**calcium acetylsalicylate carbamide** CALCIUM CARBASPIRIN.

**calcium alginate** The calcium salt of alginic acid, a polyuronic acid composed of D-mannuronic acid and L-guluronic acid. It is used as an absorbable hemostatic agent, in dressings to pack bleeding wounds, and in treatment of epistasis.

**calcium aminosalicylate** The calcium salt of *p*-aminosalicyclic acid, used in the treatment of tuberculosis, usually in combination with streptomycin.

**calcium benzamidosalicylate** $(C_{14}H_{10}NO_4)_2Ca\cdot5H_2O$. Calcium 4-benzamido-2-hydroxybenzoate pentahydrate. A cream-colored, odorless, almost tasteless powder. It is slowly hydrolyzed in the body to yield prolonged levels of aminosalicylate, and is used in the treatment of tuberculosis. Also *calcium benzoylpas, bepascum*.

**calcium benzoate** The calcium salt of benzoic acid. It is used as a preservative in foods.

**calcium benzoylpas** CALCIUM BENZAMIDOSALICYLATE.

**calcium carbaspirin** $C_{19}H_{18}CaN_2O_9$. A white, amorphous powder that has analgesic and antipyretic properties like aspirin. Also *calcium acetylsalicylate carbamide, carbasalate calcium*.

**calcium carbimide** $CCaN_2$. A powder or crystalline solid that is nearly insoluble in water but hydrolyzes to calcium hydrogen cyanamide. The cyanamide ions inhibit enzymes that metabolize acetaldehyde. Also *calcium cyanamide*. **citrated c.** A mixture of one part of highly purified calcium carbimide (calcium cyanamide) with two parts by weight of citric acid. It inhibits the metabolism of acetaldehyde formed from ethanol and causes unpleasant symptoms if alcoholics consume any quantity of alcohol. It is similar in this respect to disulfiram.

**calcium cyanamide** CALCIUM CARBIMIDE.

**calcium cyclamate** The calcium salt of cyclamic acid. It, and the sodium salt, have been used as non-nutritive sweeteners in foods. Although still permitted in some countries, cyclamates have been banned in the United States by the Food and Drug Administration since 1969.

**calcium disodium edetate** EDETATE CALCIUM DISODIUM.

**calcium disodium ethylenediaminetetraacetate** EDETATE CALCIUM DISODIUM.

**calcium disodium versenate** EDETATE CALCIUM DISODIUM.

**calcium gluceptate** $C_{14}H_{26}CaO_{16}$. A formulation of calcium that is suitable for intramuscular or intravenous administration as a treatment for hypocalcemic tetany. Also *calcium hexahydroxyheptonate*.

**calcium hydroxide** $Ca(OH)_2$. A white powder with a slightly bitter, alkaline taste. It is used in the form of a solution. Also *slaked lime*.

**calcium lactate** $C_6H_{10}CaO_6 \cdot 5H_2O$. The calcium salt of lactic acid, used as a calcium supplement.

**calcium novobiocin** The calcium salt of novobiocin. It has the actions and uses of novobiocin and is suitable for administration of novobiocin as a liquid suspension.

**calcium pantothenate** The calcium salt of pantothenic acid, often used in vitamin supplements.

**calcium phosphate** A compound containing calcium and the phosphate radical, $PO_4$. Calcium phosphate, which is utilized in a monobasic, dibasic, and tribasic form, is used both as an antacid and a calcium supplement.

**calcium sodium lactate** A combination of calcium and sodium lactates containing 7.5–8.5% calcium and 8.5–10% sodium. It is used for the same indications as calcium lactate, and the presence of sodium lactate is said to increase its solubility.

**calciuria** \kal'sēyoo'rē·ə\ [CALCI- + -URIA] The renal excretion of calcium. **induced c.** Urinary calcium excretion as modified by a standard calcium load, a maneuver used in the differential diagnosis of absorptive hypercalciuria vs. normocalcemic hyperparathyroidism. In the former, urinary calcium concentrations are normal but increase at a rapid rate after calcium load. In the latter, concentrations are raised and increase somewhat after the load. There are also differences in urinary cyclic AMP response in the two conditions.

**calco-** \kal'kə-\ CALC-.

**calcodynia** \kal'kədin'ē·ə\ PAINFUL HEEL.

**calcospherite** \kal'kəsfir'īt\ One of the small, globular, basophilic bodies seen in tissues affected by calcification, usually of the dystrophic type.

**calculi** \kal'kyəlī\ Plural of CALCULUS.

**calculifragous** \kal'kyəlif'rəjəs\ [L *calculi*, pl. of *calculus* (dim. of CALX) a pebble, + *frag(osus)* full of broken stones, fragile + -OUS] Pertaining to the breaking up of a bladder stone.

**calculogenesis** \kal'kyəlōjen'əsis\ The formation of calculi.

**calculosis** \kal'kyəlō'sis\ LITHIASIS.

**calculous** \kal'kyələs\ Affected by or pertaining to calculus.

**calculus** \kal'kyələs\ [L (dim. of *calx*, gen. *calcis*, limestone, a stone), a pebble, small stone] (*pl.* calculi) A solid structure or concretion formed in a pre-existing body cavity such as the gallbladder or the renal pelvis and often composed of organic and inorganic salts. Calculi are usually multiple, spherical, and pebblelike, although they may acquire the shape of the cavity in which they developed. **alternating c.** A calculus which on cross-section is characterized by successive layers of different materials. Also *combination calculus.* **articular c.** A calculus within a joint. Also *joint calculus.* **biliary c.** GALLSTONE. **blood c.** Calcification in an old blood clot. Also *hemic calculus.* **branched c.** STAGHORN CALCULUS. **bronchial c.** BRONCHOLITH. **calcareous renal c.** A renal calculus composed of calcium salts which probably developed by nucleation of a nidus from supersaturated urine. The nidus enlarges by crystal and epitaxial growth, and by crystal aggregation. Calculus formation is enhanced by hypercalciuria and hyperoxaluria. However, in a few instances calcareous renal calculi are formed in the presence of normocalciuria. Also *calcareous kidney stone.* **cardiac c.** A calcified mass of necrotic tissue or blood clot in a wall or valve of the heart. Also *cardiolith.* **cholesterol c.** A large, usually single gallstone that is composed primarily of pure cholesterol. It is pale yellow, usually radiolucent, and has a radiating crystalline and glistening appearance on cross section. Also *metabolic stone.* **combination c.** ALTERNATING CALCULUS. **cystic c.** A calculus in the urinary bladder or the gallbladder. **cystine c.** A renal calculus formed by the concretion of cystine crystals. This is the only feature of cystinuria that leads to clinical manifestations of urinary tract obstruction, or of infection. **decubitus c.** A urinary tract calculus resulting from the hypercalciuria of prolonged bed rest. **dental c.** Mineralized microbial plaque attached to and covering the enamel and/or root surfaces of the teeth. Two types may be differentiated according to position during formation in relation to the gingival margin, supragingival and subgingival dental calculus. Subgingival calculus is darker in color owing to the incorporation of blood pigments. The inorganic components of dental calculus include calcium phosphate, calcium carbonate, and magnesium phosphate in a mucopolysaccharide matrix. Of mainly apatite structure, dental calculus incorporates desquamated cells, remnants of leukocytes, and food debris in addition to the filamentous organisms of plaque. Also *tartar.* **fusible c.** A calculus composed of a mixture of triple and calcium phosphates. **gonecystic c.** SPERMATIC CALCULUS. **hemic c.** BLOOD CALCULUS. **joint c.** ARTICULAR CALCULUS. **lacrimal c.** DACRYOLITH. **lacteal c.** A calculus in a breast ductule. **mammary c.** Calcification within the breast. **matrix c.** A white or yellow urinary calculus consisting of a matrix of mucoprotein and sulfated mucopolysaccharide, and including also calcium salts. **nasal c.** RHINOLITH. **noncalcareous renal c.** A renal calculus composed of cystine, uric acid, or struvite. Also *noncalcareous renal stone.* **oxalate c.** A calculus in the urinary tract formed from calcium oxalate. Such formations may occur independently of hyperoxaluria. **pancreatic c.** A concretion within the duct of the pancreas. Also *pancreatolith, pancreolith.* **phosphate c.** A calculus in the urinary tract, composed of calcium phosphate and often including urates, which may be hard or friable. **preputial c.** PREPUTIAL CONCRETION. **primary renal c.** A calculus associated with an apparently normal urinary tract and usually composed of calcium oxalate or

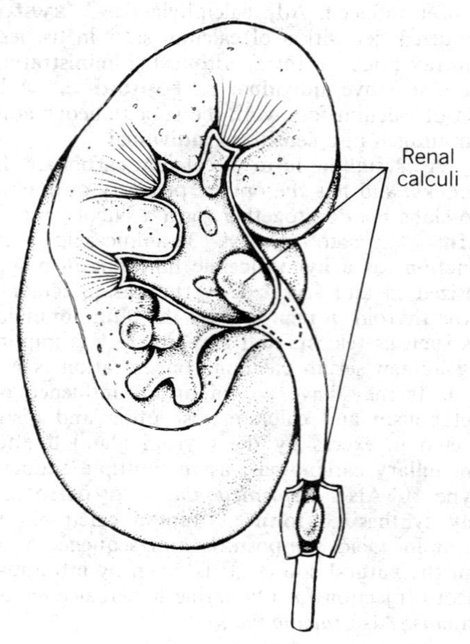

urates. **c. of the prostate** A small calculus in a prostatic duct, consisting mainly of calcium carbonate and calcium phosphate and formed by the deposition of calcareous material in the corpora amylacea. Also *prostatolith, prostatic calculus.* **renal c.** Any of the hard concretions varying in size from a tiny particle to staghorn calculi which may fill the renal pelvis. Ninety percent are calcium, the remainder being composed mainly of cystine, uric acid, or struvite. Small calculi may be passed for years without symptoms, while larger ones may cause renal colic, hematuria, or ureteral or pelvic obstruction leading to hydronephrosis or infection. Also *kidney stone, nephrolith.* **secondary renal c.** A calculus formed secondary to obstruction and infection and usually composed of ammonium magnesium phosphates. **serumal c.** SUBGINGIVAL CALCULUS. **spermatic c.** A calculus formed in a seminal vesicle. Also *gonecystic calculus.* **staghorn c.** A large renal calculus that fills a calix or the pelvis and calices, thus having the appearance of a staghorn. Also *branched calculus.* **struvite c.** A renal calculus composed of struvite, usually associated with urinary tract infections due to urea-splitting bacteria such as some strains of *Proteus, Pseudomonas, Klebsiella, E. coli,* and *Staphylococcus.* Urease produced by these bacteria catalyzes the hydrolysis of urea to ammonium and hydroxyl ions. Thus, the urine is alkaline and has a high ammonium content. Trivalent phosphate ion also is increased due to greater dissociation of phosphate at a high pH. These factors favor a supersaturated state of the infected urine with respect to struvite. Therapy is directed toward the infection, which unfortunately may be difficult to eradicate. Also *struvite stone.* **subgingival c.** Calculus in a gingival sulcus or periodontal pocket. It is usually harder and darker than supragingival calculus. Also *serumal calculus, serumal tartar.* **supragingival c.** Calculus on the visible surface of a tooth. It is usually softer and lighter in color than subgingival calculus. **tonsillar c.** TONSILLOLITH. **urate c.** URIC ACID CALCULUS. **ureteral c.** A calculus in the ureter, usually having been formed in the kidney but only rarely in situ. It usually produces colic. Also *ureteric calculus, ureteral stone.* **uric acid c.** A renal calculus composed of uric acid. Uric acid calculi are radiolucent. They form in acid urine, and may be prevented by maintaining the urine pH alkaline. They frequently complicate conditions characterized by hyperuricemia and hyperuricosuria, such as gout, or several hematologic disorders including polycythemia. However, more than half the instances of uric acid calculi occur in the absence of hyperuricemia or hyperuricosuria. Also *urate calculus, urate stone.* **urinary c.** A calculus anywhere in the urinary tract. Also *urolith.* **uterine c.** A calcified structure within the uterus. Also *uterolith.* **vesical c.** A calculus in the urinary bladder. Calculi developing there as a result of urinary stasis, infection (e.g., bacteria or schistosomiasis), or the presence of a foreign body are termed primary vesical calculi. Those having reached the bladder from the ureter or kidney are termed secondary vesical calculi. Also *cystolith, bladder stone.* **vesicoprostatic c.** A calculus of the prostate that continues into the bladder. **xanthine c.** A renal calculus formed of xanthine, occurring in children with the rare disorder, xanthinuria. The calculus is radiolucent. Also *xanthic calculus.*

**Caldani** [Leopoldo Marcantonio *Caldani,* Italian anatomist, 1725–1813] See under LIGAMENT.

**Caldwell** [E. W. *Caldwell,* U.S. radiologist, 1870–1918] See under PROJECTION.

**Caldwell** [George W. *Caldwell,* U.S. physician, 1834–1918] Caldwell-Luc operation. See under OPERATION.

**Caldwell** [William Edgar *Caldwell,* U.S. obstetrician, 1880–1943] Caldwell-Moloy classification. See under CLASSIFICATION.

**calef.** **1** *calefactus* (L, warmed). **2** *calefac* (L, make warm).

**calefacient** An agent that brings a sense of warmth to the area it medicates.

**calf** [Old Norse *kālfi* the calf] The bulging fleshy region at the back of the leg below the knee; sura.

**caliber** \kal′ibər\ [French *calibre* (from Arabic *qālib* a mold, form, last) bore diameter] The internal diameter of a tube.

**calibrate** \kal′ibrāt\ [*calib(e)r* + -ATE] **1** To graduate or adjust (a measuring instrument) by comparison to a known standard. **2** To ascertain the internal diameter of by using a calibrator.

**calibration** \kal′ibrā′shen\ [*calib(e)r* + -ATION] The measurement of amplitude and duration in standard units in electroencephalography and clinical neurophysiology. Electroencephalographic recordings include calibration marks that indicate the specific voltage of a particular vertical amplitude of the wave form and the corresponding unit of time equivalent to the duration of the wave in a horizontal direction. **pure tone c.** Calibration of a pure tone audiometer by adjusting frequency and intensity outputs.

**calibrator** \kal′ibrātər\ [*calib(e)r* + -ATOR] An instrument used to determine the internal diameter of a tubular structure. **dose c.** A low-sensitivity ionization chamber constructed with a well suitable for checking the intense gamma emissions involved in shipments of some radioactive materials, eluates from laboratory generators of radioactive materials, therapeutic doses, and so on, all too energetic for typical counting equipment.

**caliceal** \kal′isē′əl\ Pertaining to a calix or calices. Also *calyceal.*

**calicectasis** \kā′lisek′təsis\ PYELOCALIECTASIS.

**calicectomy** \kal′isek′təmē\ [CALIX (pl., *calices*) + -ECTOMY] The surgical removal of a renal calix. Also *caliectomy.* Also *calycectomy.*

**calices** \kal′isēz\ Plural of CALIX.

**calicine** \kal′isin\ Similar to or related to a calix. Also *calycine.*

**caliculi** \kəlik′yəlī\ Plural of CALICULUS.

**caliculus** \kəlik′yələs\ [L (dim. of *calix* cup) a small cup] (*pl.* caliculi) A small, cup-shaped, bulbous structure resembling the closed calyx of a flower. Also *calycle.* Also *calyculus.* **c. gustatorius** [NA] One of the numerous ovoid or conical aggregations or buds of specialized oral stratified epithelial cells serving as the peripheral gustatory organ. The cells are either receptor gustatory or supporting cells having synapselike contacts with the terminal gustatory fibers of the chorda tympani, glossopharyngeal, and vagus nerves. The buds are located mostly on the surface of the tongue, especially on the walls of the vallate and foliate papillae but also on the fungiform papillae, soft palate, palatoglossal arches, epiglottis, and posterior wall of the oropharynx. They are most numerous in newborn infants, whereafter many atrophy, especially on the back of the tongue and the epiglottis. Also *taste bud, taste bulb* (outmoded), *gustatory bud, gustatory bulb* (outmoded), *Schwalbe's corpuscle, taste corpuscle.*

**caliectasis** \kal′i·ek′təsis\ [*cali(x)* + ECTASIS] PYELOCALIECTASIS.

**caliectomy** \kal′i·ek′təmē\ CALICECTOMY.

**californium** A transuranic element of atomic number

98. The 12 known isotopes have mass numbers from 242 to 253. All are emitters of alpha particles, with half-lives ranging from 3.7 minutes to approximately 800 years. It was first produced in 1949 as californium 244 (half-life approximately 19 minutes), by alpha bombardment of curium 242 at the University of California. Californium 252, with a half-life of 2.65 years, undergoes spontaneous fission and is a very strong neutron emitter. This isotope in trace amounts has some industrial uses. Symbol: Cf

**caliper** \kal′ipər\ [alteration of *caliber.* See CALIBER.] **1** A rigid orthosis that gives external support to weakened or deformed limbs. Also *caliper splint.* **2** Any of various instruments having a pair of adjustable, curved legs that can be set against opposing surfaces or at two specific points on a surface for the precise measurement of the distance between them, often used to measure an inside or outside diameter: usually used in the plural. **skinfold c.'s** An instrument used to measure skinfold thickness at various sites on the body as a means of assessing total body fat and nutritional status of a person. Measurements are made at four sites: triceps of the arm, subscapular, biceps of the arm, and iliac crest. Using the total value from these sites, body fat content may be ascertained from standard tables. **ultrasonic c.'s** Markers on the display of an ultrasound imaging instrument which are used for measuring size of or distance between objects. **walking c.** A lower limb orthosis, usually constructed of leather with metal struts, that is used to facilitate walking.

**calix** \kā′liks\ [L, a cup, vessel] (*pl.* calices, calyces) A cup-shaped organ or cavity. Also *calyx.* **major renal calices** CALICES RENALES MAJORES. **minor renal calices** CALICES RENALES MINORES. **calices renales** The subdivisions of the renal pelvis, which usually divides into two major calices, each of which in turn divides into several cup-shaped minor calices that terminate in relation to one or more conical renal papillae through which the urine enters the renal pelvis. Also *renal calices.* **calices renales majores** [NA] The two or three principal branches of the renal pelvis within the renal sinus, each of which in turn divides into several minor calices. Also *major renal calices.* **calices renales minores** [NA] The several branches of each of the major calices of the renal pelvis, each of which has an indented and expanded cuplike end that fits tightly around one to three renal papillae, the apices of which are pierced by the openings of the collecting tubules. Also *minor renal calices.*

**Calkins** [Leroy Adelbert *Calkins,* U.S. obstetrician, 1894–1960] See under SIGN.

**Call** [Friedrich von *Call,* Austrian physician, 1844–1917] Call-Exner body. See under BODY.

**CALLA** common acute lymphocytic leukemia antigen.

**Callahan** [John R. *Callahan,* U.S. endodontist, 1853–1918] Callahan's method. See under CHLOROPERCHA METHOD.

**Calleja** [Camilo *Calleja,* Spanish anatomist, died 1913] Islands of Calleja, Calleja's islets. See under ISLAND.

**callicrein** KALLIKREIN.

***Calliphora*** \kalif′ərə\ [New L, from Gk *kalli-* beauty + *-phor(os)* -bearing] A genus of blowflies, many of which (bluebottles) are of a metallic blue color and have larvae that feed on decaying organic material, including dead animals and meat scraps. Some species are obligatory or facultative parasites, depositing their eggs in wounds or body openings. ***C. vomitoria*** The common bluebottle fly, which deposits its eggs in decaying debris, in superficial wounds or in and around body orifices. The larvae produce myiasis in domestic animals of the affected part. Also *Musca vomitoria.*

**Calliphoridae** \kal′ifôr′idē\ [*Calliphor(a)* + -IDAE] A large family of muscoid flies. Most species are saprophytic, larvating in animal carcasses, but some are primary flesh invaders or secondary invaders of sores, causing myiasis. Some species also transmit microorganisms on the hair of their legs. Genera include *Auchmeromyia, Calliphora, Chrysomyia, Cordylobia, Cochliomyia, Lucilia, Phaenicia, Phormia,* and others.

***Callitroga*** \kal′itrō′gə\ COCHLIOMYIA. ***C. hominivorax*** *COCHLIOMYIA HOMINIVORAX.*

**callosal** \kəlō′səl\ Of or denoting the corpus callosum.

**callosity** \kəläs′itē\ [L *callositas* (from *callos(us)* full of calluses + *-itas* -ITY) callousness, hardening of the skin] A circumscribed thickening of the skin, particularly the horny layer, in response to repeated pressure or friction. Also *callus.*

**callosomarginal** \kəlō′sōmär′jənəl\ Pertaining to corpus callosum and medial frontal gyri.

**callosum** \kəlō′səm\ [L *callosum,* neut. of *callosus* hard, tough] CORPUS CALLOSUM.

**callous** \kal′əs\ **1** Having the properties of a callosity. **2** Marked by calluses.

**callus** \kal′əs\ [L, hard skin, callus] **1** The hard new tissue that collects around the ends of fractured bones in the healing process and eventually becomes bone in forming a new union. **2** CALLOSITY. **central c.** A callus seen between the medullary cavities of a broken bone. Also *internal callus, myelogenous callus.* **definitive c.** A callus that has become ossified into mature bone. Also *intermediate callus, permanent callus.* **ensheathing c.** A callus that surrounds a fracture and is laid down by the periosteum. Also *external callus.* **intermediate c.** DEFINITIVE CALLUS. **internal c.** CENTRAL CALLUS. **myelogenous c.** CENTRAL CALLUS. **permanent c.** DEFINITIVE CALLUS. **provisional c.** A callus that is formed in the medullary cavities of broken bones and is later resorbed when definitive callus is established.

**calmative** **1** Sedative or calming; reducing excitement. **2** A calmative agent.

**Calmette** [Léon Charles Albert *Calmette,* French bacteriologist, 1863–1933] **1** Calmette's test. See under REACTION. **2** See under SERUM, TUBERCULIN. **3** Calmette-Guérin bacillus. **4** See under BACILLUS. **5** Calmette's vaccine. See under BCG VACCINE.

**calmodulin** A protein of 148 residues, found in most animal cells, with four binding sites for $Ca^{2+}$ions. These sites bind the calcium by carboxylate groups of aspartate residues, and have dissociation constants of .06–1 μM. Its change of conformation when the calcium is bound affects the activity of many enzymes, allowing it to respond to changes in $[Ca^{2+}]$. Important among these are phosphodiestereases that hydrolyze nucleoside 3′,5′-cyclic phosphates. It is a constituent of phosphorylase kinase, in which its binding of calcium activates the enzyme during muscular contraction.

**calomel** $Hg_2Cl_2$. Dimercury(2+) chloride. It has very low solubility in water. A suspension of it in contact with metallic mercury gives an electrode with a fixed potential, often used as a reference electrode. Much less toxic than mercury(II) compounds, it was once used medicinally. Also *mercurous chloride, hydrargyri subchloridum.*

***Calomys*** \kal′ōmis\ A genus of South American field mice, some of which are reservoir hosts of arenaviruses such as Junín virus (found in *C. laucha, C. musculinus*) and Machupo virus (in *C. callosus*).

**calor** \kā′lôr, kal′ər\ [L, heat] Heat, as a natural element of the body. **c. febrilis** The hot sensation experienced by febrile patients. **c. innatus** The natural heat of the

body. **c. internus** The internal heat or warmth of the body.
**Calori** [Luigi *Calori,* Italian anatomist, 1807–1896] See under BURSA.
**calori-** \kal′əri-, kəlôr′i-\ [L *calor* heat] A combining form meaning heat.
**caloric** \kəlôr′ik\ [CALOR + -IC] **1** Of or relating to heat. **2** Pertaining to a calorie.
**caloricity** \kal′ôris′itē\ [CALORIC + -ITY] The capacity of an animal to generate heat.
**Calorie** \kal′ôrē\ [See CALORIE.] A unit of quantity of heat, used to express the energy value of food, equal to 1000 $cal_{15}$; 4.1855 kilojoules, approximately. Also *kilogram-calorie, large calorie, food calorie.* Symbol: Cal
**calorie** \kal′ôrē\ [French, from L *calor* heat] A unit of quantity of heat, the quantity of heat required to raise the temperature of 1 gram of water by 1°C under specified conditions. One calorie equals 4.2 joules, approximately. Also *standard calorie, small calorie* (obs.). Also *calory.* Symbol: cal **15°C c.** The unit of heat equal to the heat required to raise the temperature of one gram of water from 14.5°C to 15.5°C at one atmosphere pressure; 4.1855 joules, approximately. Also *gram-calorie, microcalorie* (outmoded). Symbol: $cal_{15}$ **food c.** CALORIE **International Table c.** A unit of quantity of heat defined as 4.1868 joules exactly. Also *I. T. calorie.* Symbol: $cal_{IT}$ **large c.** CALORIE. **small c.** *Obs.* CALORIE. **standard c.** CALORIE. **thermochemical c.** A unit of quantity of heat defined as 4.184 joules exactly. Symbol: $cal_{th}$
**calorifacient** \kəlôr′ifā′shənt\ Producing heat; calorific: used especially of foods.
**calorific** \kal′ôrif′ik\ [L *calorificus* (from *calori-* heat- + *-ficus* -making] Producing or capable of producing heat.
**calorigenic** \kəlôr′ijen′ik\ [CALORI- + -GENIC] Producing heat. Also *calorigenetic.*
**calorimeter** \kal′ôrim′ətər\ [CALORI- + -METER] An instrument that measures the heat liberated by a process such as combustion or metabolism. **Atwater's c.** A chamber used to measure the heat produced by human subjects. It has insulated walls internally lined with water-filled pipes. The current of water is arranged to maintain a constant temperature of the inner wall. With a knowledge of water flow and the temperature of the water entering and leaving the chamber, it is possible to measure the heat production of a subject within the chamber. The chamber is ventilated by a current of air. The expired air is conducted out of the chamber and its water and carbon dioxide content measured. Also *Atwater-Benedict calorimeter, Atwater chamber, Atwater-Benedict chamber.* **bomb c.** An apparatus used to measure the oxidizable energy present in a food. A sample is burned in an oxygen-filled container and the heat evolved is determined by measuring the increase in temperature of a known quantity of water in which the container is immersed. It represents the total energy content of a food, even though not all this energy is available to the body. **compensating c.** A two-chamber system used to measure the heat production of animals. The conduction and radiation heat loss from the animal's chamber is calculated by comparison with heat loss from an identical chamber in which hydrogen is burned at a suitable rate. **respiration c.** An apparatus for measuring the gaseous exchange and heat production of a living organism.
**calorimetry** \kal′ôrim′ətrē\ [CALORI- + -METRY] The measurement of heat absorption or heat production. **direct c.** The measurement of heat production by monitoring temperature changes. **indirect c.** The determination of heat production by observing the quantity of oxygen consumed and calculating its heat equivalent. The energy equivalent of oxygen may be assumed to be 20 kilojoules per liter, or it may be calculated on the basis of the nutrients consumed or of the respiratory quotient. **partitional c.** A determination of the allocation of heat loss from the body by source, such as conduction, convection, radiation, and evaporation.
**caloripuncture** \kal′ôripungk′chər\ A puncture achieved by the application of heat.
**caloritropic** \kəlôr′iträp′ik\ [CALORI- + -TROPIC[1]] THERMOTROPIC.
**calory** \kal′ôrē\ CALORIE.
**Calot** [Jean-François *Calot,* French surgeon, 1861–1944] See under OPERATION, TREATMENT, TRIANGLE.
**calpain** A calcium-activated, intracellular proteinase. Its proteolytic action activates some cellular enzymes, such as certain protein kinases.
**calpastatin** A protein of molecular mass about 70 kDa that binds and inhibits calpain.
**cal·s$^{-1}$** Symbol for the unit, calorie per second.
**calvaria** \kalver′ē·ə\ [L (from *calv(a)* skull, scalp, from *calvus* bald) skull, cranium] The upper, domelike part of the cranium that encloses and protects the brain, comprising the upper parts of the frontal, parietal, and occipital bones. Also *calvarium* (incorrect), *cranium cerebrale, skullcap, skull cap, roof of skull.* Compare CRANIUM.
**calvarial** \kalver′ē·əl\ Pertaining to the calvaria.
**calvarium** \kalver′ē·əm\ *Incorrect* CALVARIA.
**Calvé** [Jacques *Calvé,* French surgeon, 1875–1954] **1** Calvé's disease. See under VERTEBRA PLANA. **2** Calvé-Perthes disease, Legg-Calvé-Perthes disease. See under PERTHES DISEASE.
**calvities** \kalvish′i·ēz\ [L, (from *calvus* bald) baldness] The bitemporal and frontovertical loss of hair characteristic of ordinary baldness in males and abnormal androgenetic baldness in females. Also *androgenetic alopecia, common male baldness, male pattern alopecia.*
**calx** \kalks\ [L (gen. *calcis*), heel] (*pl.* calces) [NA] The rounded protuberance forming the posterior end of the foot; the heel. Also *calcar pedis.*
**calyceal** \kal′isē′əl\ CALICEAL.
**calycectasis** \kal′isek′təsis\ PYELOCALIECTASIS.
**calycectomy** \kal′isek′təmē\ CALICECTOMY.
**calyces** \kal′isēz\ Plural of CALYX.
**calycine** \kal′isin\ CALICINE.
**calycle** \kal′ikl\ CALICULUS.
**calyculus** \kəlik′yələs\ CALICULUS.
***Calymmatobacterium granulomatis*** \kəlim′ətōbaktir′ē·əm gran′yəlō′mətis\ A short, Gram-negative, nonmotile, facultative, encapsulated, nutritionally exacting bacillus. It causes granuloma inguinale. In the lesions, Donovan bodies are pathognomonic. Also *Donovania granulomatis.*
**calyx** \kā′liks\ [L, from Gk *kalyx* a shell, husk, pod of fruit, calyx of flower; in L often confused with *calix* cup] CALIX.
**cambendazole** $C_{14}H_{14}N_4O_2S$. An odorless, white crystalline solid, practically insoluble in water. It is used in veterinary medicine as an anthelmintic agent.
**cambium** \kam′bē·əm\ [New L (from Med L, a supposed alimentary humor, from Late L, exchange) the growth layer in the stems and roots of vascular plants] In anatomy, the deep layer of the periosteum that lies adjacent to the bone in adults.
**camera** [L (from Gk *kamara* anything with vaulted or arched cover), a vault, arched ceiling or roof, chamber] **1** Any device that records still or moving images on a photographic film or plate. **2** Any of several electronic scan-

ning and imaging devices, such as a gamma camera, that enable radiation patterns to be visualized on a cathode-ray tube, computer printout, photographic film, etc. **3** Any enclosed space, cavity, or chamber. **Anger c.** GAMMA CAMERA. **c. anterior bulbi** [NA] The anterior portion of the anterior segment of the eyeball, situated between the cornea anteriorly and the lens and iris posteriorly. It contains aqueous humor that drains through the iridocorneal angle at its periphery. It communicates with the posterior chamber through the pupil. Also *anterior chamber of eye, camera oculi anterior* (outmoded), *camera oculi major.* **electron diffraction c.** A camera that is capable of receiving the focused image of an electron diffraction pattern. **gamma c.** A device used to visualize the distribution of a gamma-emitting radionuclide in the body of a patient or in some other opaque body. A large-diameter (25 cm) sodium iodide scintillation crystal views the patient through a parallel-hole or pinhole collimator. An array of photomultipliers behind the crystal monitors the scintillations and, through electronic circuitry, informs a cathode-ray output tube as to where each scintillation occurs. The cathode ray then twinkles at the indicated location. A photographic time exposure of the cathode-ray face therefore produces an image of the distribution of the radionuclide. These devices and their more recent derivatives have proven invaluable in the application of radioactivity to medicine. Also *Anger camera, radionuclide camera, scintillation camera, static imaging device.* **c. lucida** An optical device that uses prisms, mirrors, and sometimes a microscope to project a virtual image on a plane so it can be traced. **c. obscura** A dark box containing a lens and screen used for viewing, tracing, or making photographs of external objects. **c. oculi** Either camera anterior bulbi or camera posterior bulbi. **c. oculi anterior** *Outmoded* CAMERA ANTERIOR BULBI. **c. oculi major** CAMERA ANTERIOR BULBI. **c. oculi minor** CAMERA POSTERIOR BULBI. **c. oculi posterior** *Outmoded* CAMERA POSTERIOR BULBI. **positron c.** An imaging device designed for use with positron emitters because their annihilation radiation offers some advantages. **c. posterior bulbi** [NA] The triangular posterior portion of the anterior segment of the eyeball, situated between the iris anteriorly, the lens and vitreous body posteriorly, and the ciliary body laterally. Peripherally the ciliary processes projecting between the zonular fibers produce most of the aqueous humor filling it. It communicates with the anterior chamber through the pupil. Also *posterior chamber of eye, camera oculi posterior* (outmoded), *camera oculi minor.* **powder c.** An x-ray diffraction camera for the analysis of a powdered specimen. **c. pulpi** PULP CHAMBER. **radionuclide c.** GAMMA CAMERA. **scintillation c.** GAMMA CAMERA. **c. vitrea bulbi** [NA] The large space occupying the posterior four-fifths of the eyeball and extending between the lens anteriorly and the concavity of the retina posteriorly. It is filled with the vitreous body. Also *vitreous chamber.* **x-ray c.** An apparatus in which a beam of x rays is used to analyze the structure of a crystal by recording the pattern of diffracted x rays on a film.

**camerae** \kam′ərē\ Plural of CAMERA.

**Cammann** [George Philip *Cammann,* U.S. physician, 1804–1863] Cammann stethoscope. See under BINAURAL STETHOSCOPE.

**cAMP** cyclic adenosine monophosphate (adenosine 3′,5′-cyclic phosphate).

**Campbell** [William Francis *Campbell,* U.S. physician, 1867–1926] Campbell's ligament. See under SUSPENSORY LIGAMENT OF AXILLA.

**Camper** [Peter *Camper,* Dutch physician and anatomist, 1722–1789] **1** Camper's plane. See under LINE. **2** Camper's chiasm, chiasma tendinosum camperi. See under CHIASMA TENDINUM DIGITORUM MANUS. **3** Camper's ligament. See under DIAPHRAGMA UROGENITALE. **4** See under FASCIA, LINE.

**camphor** \kam′fər\ [Med L *camphora* (from Arabic *kāfūr* camphor) camphor] $C_{10}H_{16}O$. Any of a group of alcoholic or ketonic, bicyclic terpenes obtained primarily from the evergreen tree *Cinnamomum camphora.* It is a colorless or white substance with a distinctive odor and pungent, aromatic taste. It occurs as crystals, granules, or masses, and is used topically as a rubefacient. It has antiseptic, carminative, mildly irritating, and stimulating properties. Also *gum camphor, camphora.* **carbolated c.** A mixture of 1.5 parts camphor, one part phenol, and one part alcohol. It has been used an an antiseptic dressing for wounds. **carbolic c.** A mixture containing three parts camphor and one part phenol. It has been used to treat toothaches and athlete's foot, but must not be applied to extensive areas or to the face. Also *phenol camphor.* **gum c.** CAMPHOR. **mentholated c.** A mixture of equal parts camphor and menthol, used as a local counterirritant and in inhalers or in water for inhalation for acute bronchitis. Also *peppermint camphor.* **phenol c.** CARBOLIC CAMPHOR. **salol c.** An oily preparation containing two parts camphor and three parts salol (phenyl salicylate). It has been used as a local antiseptic medication. **thyme c.** THYMOL. **turpentine c.** TERPIN.

**camphora** \kamfôr′ə\ CAMPHOR.

**camphoraceous** Containing or resembling camphor.

**camphorism** \kam′fôrizm\ Poisoning from ingestion or injection of camphor. The symptoms are vomiting, clonic convulsions, delirium, respiratory failure, coma, and death.

**camphor salicylate** A solid mixture of 84 parts camphor and 65 parts salicylic acid. It is used externally as an ingredient of ointments for various skin diseases.

**campimeter** \kampim′ətər\ [L *camp(us)* a flat plain, open field + *i* + -METER] An examining surface used for measurement of the visual field.

**campimetry** \kampim′ətrē\ [L *camp(us)* a level surface, open field + *i* + -METRY] The measurement of the field of vision.

**campospasm** \kam′pōspazm\ CAMPTOCORMIA.

**campto-** \kamp′tō-\ [Gk *kamptos* bent] A combining form meaning bent.

**camptocormia** \-kôr′mē·ə\ [CAMPTO- + Gk *korm(os)* trunk of a tree, log + -IA] A syndrome, consisting of anterior bending of the trunk that produces an apelike posture, persistent lumbar pain, and sexual impotence. Often there is a history of trauma or hysteria. Also *camptospasm, campospasm.*

**camptodactylia** \-daktil′yə\ CAMPTODACTYLY.

**camptodactylism** \-dak′təlizm\ CAMPTODACTYLY.

**camptodactyly** \-dak′təlē\ [CAMPTO- + DACTYL- + -Y] A fixed flexion deformity of one or more fingers. Also *camptodactylia, camptodactylism.*

**camptospasm** \kamp′tōspazm\ CAMPTOCORMIA.

**camptothecin** $C_{20}H_{16}N_2O_4$. 4-Ethyl-4-hydroxy-1*H*-pyrano-[3′,4′:6,7]indolizino[1,2-b]quinoline-3,14(4H,12*H*)-dione. A compound having antileukemic and anticancer properties, found in the shrub *Camptotheca acuminata* of the family Nyssaceae.

**campus** [L, field, plain] **c. of Wernicke** WERNICKE'S TRIANGLE.

***Campylobacter fetus*** \kam′pəlōbak′tər fē′toos\ A spirally curved Gram-negative rod, with polar flagellum, that can utilize amino acids but not carbohydrates. It causes abortions in cattle and serious infections in debilitated humans. Also *Vibrio fetus* (obs.).

**campylobacteriosis** \kam′pəlōbak′tərē·ō′sis\ Infection with *Campylobacter fetus*..

**campylognathia** \kam′pəlōnā′thē·ə\ [Gk *kampylo(s)* bent, curved + GNATH- + -IA] A curved deformity of the jaw associated with a cleft of the lip.

**Camurati** [Mario *Camurati*, Italian physician, 1896–1948] Camurati-Engelmann disease. See under PROGRESSIVE DIAPHYSEAL DYSPLASIA.

# canal

**canal** [French, from L *canalis* (irreg. from *canna* a reed, pipe; see CANNULA) a channel, conduit, trough] A tubular space, channel, or structure; canalis. **abdominal c.** CANALIS INGUINALIS. **accessory palatine c.'s** CANALES PALATINI MINORES. **accessory root c.** A fine canal running from the main root canal to the periodontal ligament. It is found near the apex and, in multi-rooted teeth, at the furcations. Also *branching canal, collateral pulp canal, lateral canal.* **adductor c.** CANALIS ADDUCTORIUS. **Alcock's c.** CANALIS PUDENDALIS. **alimentary c.** CANALIS ALIMENTARIUS. **alveolar c.'s of maxilla** CANALES ALVEOLARES MAXILLAE. **alveolodental c.'s** CANALES ALVEOLARES MAXILLAE. **anal c.** CANALIS ANALIS. **anterior alveolar c.'s** CANALES ALVEOLARES MAXILLAE. **anterior c. of chorda tympani** The small bony canal that lies at the medial end of the petrotympanic fissure and conducts the chorda tympani out of the tympanic cavity anterior to the handle of the malleus. **anterior condylar c.** CANALIS HYPOGLOSSI. **anterior condyloid c.** CANALIS HYPOGLOSSI. **anterior ethmoidal c.** One of two grooves in the superior surface of the ethmoidal labyrinth that are converted into anterior and posterior canals by the frontal bone articulation. The anterior canal opens on the inner wall of the orbit at the foramen ethmoidale anterius, and transmits the anterior ethmoidal vessels and nerve. **anterior palatine c.** 1 CANALIS INCISIVUS. 2 FORAMEN INCISIVUM. **anterior semicircular c.** CANALIS SEMICIRCULARIS ANTERIOR. **c. of Arantius** DUCTUS VENOSUS. **Arnold's c.** CANALICULUS MASTOIDEUS. **Arnold's innominate c.** CANALICULUS INNOMINATUS. **atrioventricular c.** A narrow portion of the embryonic primitive cardiac tube through which the primitive or common atrium communicates with the primitive ventricle during the second to fourth weeks of intrauterine life. After development of the ventral and dorsal endocardial cushions, the canal becomes first a common atrioventricular opening. After fusion of the cushions to form the septum intermedium, this opening becomes divided into a left biscupid or mitral orifice and a right tricuspid orifice, each with their valves. Failure of development at one of these stages gives rise to cardiac anomalies described as persistence of the atrioventricular or atrial canal, and persistence of the common atrioventricular canal or ostium commune. These malformations are frequently accompanied by anomalies of development of the interatrial and intraventricular septa and of the mitral and triscupid valves. **auricular c.** 1 MEATUS ACUSTICUS EXTERNUS. 2 The atrioventricular canal in the embryonic heart. **basipharyngeal c.** CANALIS VOMEROVAGINALIS. **biliary c.** DUCTULUS BILIFER. **birth c.** PARTURIENT CANAL. **c. of Bochdalek** 1 A small canal that extends obliquely through the tympanic membrane and opens on its outer surface. 2 THYROGLOSSAL DUCT. **bony c.'s of ear** LABYRINTHUS OSSEUS. **bony semicircular c.'s** CANALES SEMICIRCULARES OSSEI. **branching c.** ACCESSORY ROOT CANAL. **Braune's c.** PARTURIENT CANAL. **Breschet's c.'s** CANALES DIPLOICI. **calciferous c.'s** Canals of lime salts found in cartilage undergoing calcification. **caroticotympanic c.'s** CANALICULI CAROTICOTYMPANICI. **carotid c.** CANALIS CAROTICUS. **carpal c.** CANALIS CARPI. **c.'s of cartilage** Vascular canals found in cartilage undergoing ossification. **caudal c.** CANALIS SACRALIS. **central c. of modiolus** CANALES LONGITUDINALES MODIOLI. **central c. of spinal cord** CANALIS CENTRALIS MEDULLAE SPINALIS. **central c. of Stilling** CANALIS HYALOIDEUS. **central c. of vitreous** CANALIS HYALOIDEUS. **cerebrospinal c.** The cavity in the embryo within the developing brain and spinal cord. **cervical c.** CANALIS CERVICIS UTERI. **cervicoaxillary c.** The tubelike fascial investment of the axillary vessels and trunks of the brachial plexus passing from the supraclavicular fossa into the apex of the axilla. The canal is bounded anteriorly by the middle third of the clavicle, posteriorly by the superior border of the scapula, and medially by the first rib. **cervicouterine c.** CANALIS CERVICIS UTERI. **c. of the cervix** CANALIS CERVICIS UTERI. **chordal c.** NOTOCHORDAL CANAL. **c. of chorda tympani** CANALICULUS CHORDAE TYMPANI. **ciliary c.'s** SPATIA ANGULI IRIDOCORNEALIS. **Civinini's c.** ITER CHORDAE ANTERIUS. **Cloquet's c.** CANALIS HYALOIDEUS. **cochlear c.** CANALIS SPIRALIS COCHLEAE. **collateral pulp c.** ACCESSORY ROOT CANAL. **common atriopventricular c.** A single or common canal between the atrial and ventricular chambers of the heart, seen normally in the early stages of cardiac embryology but sometimes persisting to give rise to cardiac anomalies. Also *atrioventricularis communis, canalis communis.* See also ATRIOVENTRICULAR CANAL. **condylar c.** CANALIS CONDYLARIS. **condyloid c.** CANALIS CONDYLARIS. **connecting c.** The arched connecting tubule between a distal convolution of a renal tubule and a collecting tubule. **corneal c.** One of the spaces that lies between the trabeculae at the margin of the posterior limiting membrane of the cornea. Aqueous humor drains through these canals on its way back to the venous system. **c. of Corti** CUNICULUS INTERNUS. **c. of Cotunnius** 1 AQUEDUCTUS VESTIBULI. 2 Aqueductus vestibuli and canaliculus cochleae as a continuous channel. **craniopharyngeal c.** A canal in the developing cartilaginous sphenoid that contains the hypophysial diverticulum. Although it is usually obliterated by the third month of intrauterine life, it may persist as a canal between the anterior part of the hypophysial fossa of the sphenoid bone and the exterior, possibly at the junction of the palate and nasal septum. Some authorities believe that the canal is unrelated to the development of the anterior lobe of the pituitary, and that it is caused by the development of blood vessels. **craniovertebral c.** The continuous cavity within the cranium and the vertebral column that contains the brain, the spinal cord, and the meninges and related structures. **crural c.** CANALIS FEMORALIS. **crural c. of Henle** CANALIS ADDUCTORIUS. **dentinal c.'s** DENTINAL TUBULES. **digestive c.** CANALIS ALIMENTARIUS. **diploic c.'s** CANALES DIPLOICI. **Dorello's c.** An occasional osseofibrous canal or foramen, formed partly by the petrosphenoidal ligament, located at the apex of the petrous part of the temporal bone and the side of the dorsum sellae, and transmitting the abducent nerve as it enters the cavernous sinus. It may also transmit the inferior petrosal sinus. **c. of epididymis** DUCTUS EPIDIDYMIDIS. **ethmoidal c.'s** FORAMINA ETHMOIDALIA. **eustachian c.** TUBA AUDITIVA. **external acoustic c.** MEATUS ACUSTICUS EXTERNUS. **external auditory c.** MEATUS ACUSTICUS EXTERNUS. **external semicircular c.** CANALIS SEMICIRCULARIS LATERALIS. **facial c.** CANALIS FACIALIS. **fallopian c.** CANALIS FACIALIS. **femoral c.** CANALIS FEMORALIS. **Ferrein's c.** RIVUS LACRIMALIS. **flexor c.** CANALIS CARPI. **ganglionic c.** CANALIS SPIRALIS MODIOLI. **gastric c.** CANALIS GASTRICUS. **genital c.** The genital passages of the female urogenital apparatus. Also *genital duct.* **greater palatine c.** CANALIS PALATINUS MAJOR. **gubernacular c.** 1 One of a pair of embryonic structures consisting of a fold of peritoneum, later to become the inguinal canal, and containing the gubernaculum testis. 2 A channel passing from the crypt of an unerupted successional tooth toward the surface of the alveolar bone. It opens on the lingual aspect of a deciduous incisor or a canine but usually within the socket of a deciduous molar. **c. of Guidi** CANALIS PTERYGOIDEUS. **gynecophoric c.** A lengthwise ventral groove in a male schistosome worm in which the female is clasped in a copulatory embrace. **hair c.** The tubular epidermic channel in the hair follicle that contains the root of the hair. **Hannover's c.** SPATIUM ZONULARE. **haversian c.** The central canal of an osteon, the cylindrical unit of structure of compact bone. It contains a neurovascular bundle, the vessels of which are usually capillaries and postcapillary venules that are closely associated with the loose connective tissue that fills the canal. The nerve fibers are usually nonmyelinated. The canal is surrounded by concentrically arranged lamellae of bone which vary in number and thickness. Also *canalis centralis osteoni, haversian space, Leeuwenhoek's canal.* **Henle's c.** LOOP OF HENLE. **Hensen's c.** DUCTUS REUNIENS. **c. of Hering** CHOLANGIOLE. **hernial c.** The passageway through which a hernia passes. **Hirschfeld's c.'s** INTERDENTAL CANALS. **Holmgren-Golgi c.'s** ENDOPLASMIC RETICULUM. **Huguier's c.** ITER CHORDAE ANTERIUS. **Hunter's c.** CANALIS ADDUCTORIUS. **Huschke's c.** A canal or foramen present in the floor of the bony part of the external auditory meatus, near the tympanic ring, during the first five years of childhood, but which may persist through life. **hyaloid c.** CANALIS HYALOIDEUS. **hypoglossal c.** CANALIS HYPOGLOSSI. **hypophyseal c.** MEDIAN CRANIOPHARYNGEAL CANAL. **iliac c.** LACUNA MUSCULORUM. **incisive c.** CANALIS INCISIVUS. **inferior dental c.** CANALIS MANDIBULAE. **infraorbital c.** CANALIS INFRAORBITALIS. **inguinal c.** CANALIS INGUINALIS. **interdental c.'s** Nutrient canals passing vertically between anterior teeth and visible in radiographs. Also *Hirschfeld's canals.* **interlobular biliary c.** One of the ducts that carries bile through the portal tract system to the main hepatic ducts. **internal acoustic c.** MEATUS ACUSTICUS INTERNUS. **internal auditory c.** MEATUS ACUSTICUS INTERNUS. **intersacral c.'s** FORAMINA INTERVERTEBRALIA OSSIS SACRI. **intestinal c.** The part of the alimentary canal located between the pyloric end of the stomach and the anus; intestinum. Also *intestinal tract.* **intracytoplasmic c.** One of the deep invaginations of the surface membrane of a cell. These canals are lined by numerous microvilli and are seen particularly in the parietal cells of the gastric mucosa. Also *plasmatic canal.* **intralobular biliary c.** DUCTUS INTERLOBULARIS BILIFER. **Jacobson's c.** CANALICULUS TYMPANICUS. **c. for Jacobson's nerve** CANALICULUS TYMPANICUS. **lacrimal c.** CANALIS NASOLACRIMALIS. **lateral c.** ACCESSORY ROOT CANAL. **lateral inferior vomerobasilar c.** CANALIS PALATOVAGINALIS. **lateral semicircular c.** CANALIS SEMICIRCULARIS LATERALIS. **lateral superior vomerobasilar c.** CANALIS VOMEROVAGINALIS. **Lauth's c.** SINUS VENOSUS SCLERAE. **Leeuwenhoek's c.** HAVERSIAN CANAL. **lesser palatine c.'s** CANALES PALATINI MINORES. **longitudinal c.'s of modiolus** CANALES LONGITUDINALES MODIOLI. **Löwenberg's c.** DUCTUS COCHLEARIS. **lumbrical c.'s of Kanavel** Tubular extensions of the lumbrical fascial sheaths that form distal diverticula of the midpalmar and thenar spaces of the palm of the hand. **mandibular c.** CANALIS MANDIBULAE. **median craniopharyngeal c.** A canal situated, in the fetus, in the center of the sphenoidal cartilage at the base of the chondrocranium, developing at about the 14 mm stage in man. This canal, through which passes the pharyngeal stalk of the hypophysis, is obliterated by ingrowth of the surrounding cartilage. Rarely (in about 10%) it persists into the newborn period, and very exceptionally (0.29% of cases) into adult life, when either a small collection of veins or the pharyngeal stalk of the hypophysis may pass through it. Occasionally only one of these orifices may persist: either the superior, at the center of the pituitary fossa, or the inferior, situated 2 or 3 mm behind the posterior part of the vomer and above the spheno-occipital suture, on the inferior aspect of the body of the sphenoid. Also *hypophyseal canal.* **medullary c.** NEURAL CANAL. **membranous semicircular c.'s** DUCTUS SEMICIRCULARES. **mental c.** One of the two terminal branches of the mandibular canal that commence below the root of the second lower premolar tooth and turn upwards and laterally to end at the mental foramen. **c. of the midbrain** AQUEDUCTUS CEREBRI. **c.'s of modiolus** 1 CANALES LONGITUDINALES MODIOLI. 2 CANALIS SPIRALIS MODIOLI. **musculotubal c.** CANALIS MUSCULOTUBARIUS. **nasal c.** CANALIS NASOLACRIMALIS. **nasolacrimal c.** CANALIS NASOLACRIMALIS. **nasopalatine c.** CANALIS INCISIVUS. **neural c.** 1 The central cavity of the neural tube of the embryo. Also *medullary canal.* 2 CANALIS VERTEBRALIS. **neurenteric c.** A canal which appears shortly after gastrulation and communicates between the caudal extremity of the neural tube and the hindgut (archenteron) of the embryo. The canal represents the blastopore and the notochordal canal. It is encountered in some vertebrate species but missing in others. **notochordal c.** A temporary canal that develops during mammalian gastrulation in the anterior extremity of the primitive streak. This invagination of the blastopore extends into the notochordal process to form the notochordal canal. This canal is continuous with the amniotic cavity which is itself temporarily in communication with the yolk sac cavity. Also *chordal canal.* **c. of Nuck** See under PERITONEOVAGINAL CANAL. **nutrient c. of bone** An oblique channel that passes through the cortex of a bone to reach the medullary cavity. It normally carries a nutrient artery and vein that supply the bony tissue and bone marrow. Also *canalis nutricius ossis.* **obstetric c.** PARTURIENT CANAL. **obturator c.** CANALIS OBTURATORIUS. **obturator c. of pubic bone** SULCUS OBTURATORIUS OSSIS PUBIS. **olfactory c.** A primitive nasal cavity in an embryo once the nasal pit has deepened and come to communicate with the mouth cavity through the primitive posterior naris to form a canal. **omphalomesenteric c.** The endoblastic tube connecting the midgut of the embryo with the umbilical vesicle (yolk sac). A free communication persists with the yolk sac until the late somite stage. Eventually it is represented only by a narrow vitellointestinal duct. This duct is normally obliterated and loses its connection with the apex of the original midgut loop before this returns to the abdominal cavity. Occasionally part or all of it may persist. In the commonest anomaly of this type the proximal part of the duct persists to form Meckel's diverticulum. It is present in about 2 percent of the population and is attached to the ileum about 2 feet from the ileocecal junction. Ectopic gastric mucosa or pancreatic tissue may be found in its wall. Also *vitelline duct, yolk stalk (used chiefly in the U.S.).* **optic c.** CANALIS OPTICUS. **orbital c.'s** FORAMINA ETHMOIDALIA. **osseous cochlear c.** The bony canal containing the duct of the cochlea. **osseous eustachian c.** CANALIS MUSCULOTUBARIUS. **palatomaxillary c.** CANALIS PALATINUS MAJOR. **palatovaginal c.** CANALIS PALATOVAGINALIS. **parturient c.** The passage through which the fetus passes at birth, comprising the uterus, the vagina, and the vulva. Also *birth canal, obstetric canal, Braune's canal.* **pelvic c.** The space between the superior strait and the inferior strait of pelvis, bounded by the hip bones on the sides and the sacrum posteriorly. **peritoneovaginal c.** A diverticulum of the peritoneal membrane which extends into the inguinal canal. It accompanies the round ligament of the uterus (ligamentum teres uteri) in the female (where it is also called *canal of Nuck*), and is usually completely obliterated by the fourth month of intrauterine life. In the male, where it is also called *processus vaginalis testis,* it accompanies the testis (and gubernaculum testis) in its descent into the scrotum. In the adult, the region which partially surrounds the testis is termed the tunica vaginalis testis. If the processus remains patent in the male it may provide a channel for a "congenital" type of indirect or oblique form of inguinal hernia. Also *vaginoperitoneal canal, vaginal process, processus vaginalis peritonei, saccus vaginalis, vaginal sac.* **perivascular c.** A lymphatic channel that accompanies a blood vessel. **persistent common atrioventricular c.** A persistent single or common canal between the atrial and ventricular chambers of the heart as seen normally in early stages of cardiac embryology. The proximate cause is thought to be failure of the atrioventricular endocardial cushions to appear or to fuse in the sagittal plane of the embryonic atrioventricular canal. **Petit's c.** SPATIUM ZONULARE. **pharyngeal c.** CANALIS PALATOVAGINALIS. **pharyngotracheal c.** The upper end of the tracheobronchial or laryngotracheal groove in the floor of the embryonic pharynx after the groove has developed into a tube. It becomes a canal which communicates with the developing pharynx and becomes partially surrounded by cartilages to give rise to the definitive larynx with an opening into the pharynx called the glottis. **plasmatic c.** INTRACYTOPLASMIC CANAL. **pleural c.'s** Parts of the embryonic coelomic cavity which extend from the pericardial cavity, on each side of the developing pharynx, to join the peritoneal cavity. Each canal becomes invaginated by the ipsilateral lung bud and contributes to the definitive pleural cavity. Each becomes separated from the pericardial and peritoneal cavities by the formation of the pleuropericardial and pleuroperitoneal membranes respectively. Also *pericardioperitoneal canals.* **pleuropericardial c.** A canal or duct linking each pleural canal with the developing pericardial cavity. it becomes closed off by growth of the pleuropericardial fold. **pleuroperitoneal c.** Each of a pair of passages in the embryo connecting the primitive pleural and peritoneal cavities. These communications are eventually closed by the pleuroperitoneal membranes (the pillars of Uskow) which form the paired dorsal portions of the diaphragm. The anterior margins of the latter are continuous with the posterolateral edge of the central tendinous portion. Occasionally these communications may persist and are the likely origin of certain types of congenital diaphragmatic hernias, as of the pleuropericardial hiatus. **portal c.** One of many channels at the periphery of the lobules of the liver containing fine branches of the portal vein, the hepatic artery, and the bile duct, accompanied by a network of lymphatics. Also *portal area, canalis portalis, Kiernan spaces.* **posterior alveolar c.** One of the canales alveolares maxillae. **posterior c. of chorda tympani** CANALICULUS CHORDAE TYMPANI. **posterior condylar c.** CANALIS CONDYLARIS. **posterior dental c.'s** CANALES ALVEOLARES MAXILLAE. **posterior ethmoidal c.** One of two grooves in the superior surface of the ethmoidal labyrinth that are converted into anterior and posterior canals by the frontal bone articulation. The posterior canal opens on the inner wall of the orbit at the foramen ethmoidale posterius, and transmits the posterior ethmoidal vessels and nerve. **posterior palatine c.'s** CANALES PALATINI MINORES. **posterior semicircular c.** CANALIS SEMICIRCULARIS POSTERIOR. **pterygoid c.** CANALIS PTERYGOIDEUS. **pterygopalatine c.** 1 CANALIS PALATINUS MAJOR. 2 CANALIS PALATOVAGINALIS. **pudendal c.** CANALIS PUDENDALIS. **pulp c.** ROOT CANAL. **pyloric c.** CANALIS PYLORICUS. **recurrent c.** CANALIS PTERYGOIDEUS. **c.'s of Rivinus** DUCTUS SUBLINGUALES MINORES. **root c.** A tapering extension of the pulp chamber into the root of a tooth. It contains pulp tissue and the vessels and nerves that supply the main body of the pulp in the pulp chamber. Also *pulp canal, canalis radicis dentis.* **Rosenthal's c.** CANALIS SPIRALIS COCHLEAE. **sacculoutricular c.** DUCTUS UTRICULOSACCULARIS. **sacral c.** CANALIS SACRALIS. **Scarpa's c.'s** CANALIS INCISIVUS. • The term denotes specifically the median canals. **Schlemm's c.** SINUS VENOSUS SCLERAE. **semicircular c.'s** CANALES SEMICIRCULARES OSSEI. **serous c.** LYMPHATIC CAPILLARY. **sheathing c.** The channel for the processus vaginalis peritonei. **Sondermann's c.'s** Occasional conical projections of the endothelium of the inner wall of the sinus venosus sclerae. **sphenopalatine c.** 1 CANALIS PALATOVAGINALIS. 2 CANALIS PALATINUS MAJOR. **sphenopharyngeal c.** CANALIS PALATOVAGINALIS. **spinal c.** CANALIS VERTEBRALIS. **spiral c. of cochlea** CANALIS SPIRALIS COCHLEAE. **spiral c. of modiolus** CANALIS SPIRALIS MODIOLI. **spiral c. of Rosenthal** CANALIS SPIRALIS COCHLEAE. **spiroid c.** CANALIS FACIALIS. **Stensen's c.** DUCTUS PAROTIDEUS. **c. of Stilling** CANALIS HYALOIDEUS. **subsartorial c.** CANALIS ADDUCTORIUS. **Sucquet-Hoyer c.** Cutaneous arteriolovenular anastomoses found in the digits. Also *Sucquet-Hoyer anastomosis.* **superior maxillary c.** FORAMEN ROTUNDUM OSSIS SPHENOIDALIS. **superior semicircular c.** CANALIS SEMICIRCULARIS ANTERIOR. **supraorbital c.** The incisura and foramen supraorbitalis. **tarsal c.** SINUS TARSI. **c. for tensor tympani muscle** SEMICANALIS MUSCULI TENSORIS TYMPANI. **Theile's c.** SINUS TRANSVERSUS PERICARDII. **thymopharyngeal c.** An epithelial canal present in the embryo, formed by the migration of thymic precursors originating in the third and fourth branchial pouches. Abnormally it may persist, and may be the site of aberrant lobules of thymic tissue in the neck or upper mediastinum. **Tourtual's c.** CANALIS PALATINUS MAJOR. **tubal c.** SEMICA-

NALIS TUBAE AUDITIVAE. **tubotympanal c.** The dorsal portion or wing of the first pharyngeal pouch, which also probably incorporates part of the dorsal wing of the second pouch. It differentiates to form the auditory, or eustachian, tube and its lateral end forms the middle ear, or tympanum. Also *tubotympanic canal, tubotympanic recess.* **tympanic c.** CANALICULUS TYMPANICUS. **tympanic c. of cochlea** SCALA TYMPANI. **umbilical c.** The communication between the intraembryonic coelom and extraembryonic coelom, which persists for some time in the umbilical cord. It lodges the vitellointestinal duct and accommodates the midgut loop when it protrudes into the cord between the sixth and the tenth week of gestation. **uterocervical c.** CANALIS CERVICIS UTERI. **uterovaginal c.** A midline channel which develops in the urogenital septum in embryos of about 23 mm crown-rump length. This septum is formed by the fusion of the two paramesonephric (müllerian) ducts. It eventually differentiates to form the uterus and the vagina. **utriculosaccular c.** DUCTUS UTRICULOSACCULARIS. **vaginal c.** The cavity of the vagina. Also *vulvouterine canal.* **vaginoperitoneal c.** PERITONEOVAGINAL CANAL. **Van Hoorne's c.** DUCTUS THORACICUS. **Velpeau's c.** CANALIS INGUINALIS. **ventricular c.** CANALIS GASTRICUS. **vertebral c.** CANALIS VERTEBRALIS. **vesicourethral c.** That part of the urogenital sinus above the openings of the mesonephric ducts which gives rise to the bladder and part of the urethra. **vestibular c.** In the female embryo, the part of the urogenital sinus which gives rise to the vestibule. **vestibular c. of cochlea** SCALA VESTIBULI. **vidian c.** CANALIS PTERYGOIDEUS. **Volkmann's c.'s** The bony canals that connect adjacent haversian canals with each other and with the bone surface. A neurovascular bundle is normally present within these canals. **vomerine c.** CANALIS VOMEROVAGINALIS. **vomerovaginal c.** CANALIS VOMEROVAGINALIS. **vulvar c.** VESTIBULUM VAGINAE. **vulvouterine c.** VAGINAL CANAL. **c.'s of Walther** DUCTUS SUBLINGUALES MINORES. **c.'s of Wearn** Capillary beds of the sinusoidal variety located in the muscular wall of the heart. **c. of Wirsung** DUCTUS PANCREATICUS. **zygomaticofacial c.** FORAMEN ZYGOMATICOFACIALE. **zygomatico-orbital c.** See under FORAMEN ZYGOMATICO-ORBITALE. **zygomaticotemporal c.** FORAMEN ZYGOMATICOTEMPORALE.

**canales** \kənā′lēz\ Plural of CANALIS.

**canalicular** \kan′əlik′yələr\ Pertaining to or resembling a canaliculus.

**canaliculi** \kan′əlik′yəlī\ Plural of CANALICULUS.

**canaliculitis** \kan′əlik′yəlī′tis\ [*canalicul(us)* + -ITIS] Inflammation of the lacrimal canaliculus.

**canaliculization** \kan′əlik′yəlīzā′shən\ [*canalicul(i)* + *-iz(e)* + -ATION] The formation of small channels (canaliculi).

**canaliculorhinostomy** \kan′əlik′yəlôrīnäs′təmē\ *Outmoded* DACRYOCYSTORHINOSTOMY.

**canaliculus** \kan′əlik′yələs\ [L (dim. of *canalis* a groove, channel), a small groove or channel] (*pl.* canaliculi) A very narrow, fine canal or channel. In bone, canaliculi form a network in the hard interstitial substance, linking all the lacunae into a system of cavities. **auricular c.** CANALICULUS MASTOIDEUS. **bile c.** CANALICULUS BILIFER. **c. bilifer** [NA] One of the very fine bile ducts that form a network between the liver cells from which microvilli protrude into the lumen of the ducts throughout the parenchyma. At the periphery of the hepatic lobules they join to form the ductuli biliferi or the intralobular bile ductules, which enter the interlobular bile ducts in the portal canals. Also *bile canaliculus, bile capillary.* **canaliculi caroticotympanici** [NA] Passages in the wall of the carotid canal near the apex of the petrous part of the temporal bone that transmit communicating twigs from the carotid plexus to the tympanic plexus. Also *caroticotympanic canals, caroticotympanic foramina, caroticotympanic tubules.* **c. chordae tympani** [NA] A minute canal in the posterior wall of the tympanic cavity that extends from the facial canal, near its termination, to the tympanic cavity, which it penetrates close to the posterior border of the tympanic membrane. The canaliculus conveys the chorda tympani branch of the facial nerve to the medial surface of the tympanic membrane. Also *canal of chorda tympani, canalis chordae tympani, iter chordae posterius, posterior canal of chorda tympani.* **c. cochleae** [NA] One of the three openings in the bony canal of the cochlea that extends to the upper border of the jugular foramen on the inferior surface of the petrous part of the temporal bone. The minute canal is occupied by the perilymphatic duct and a sleevelike prolongation of the dura mater, establishing a communication between the scala tympani and the subarachnoid space. It also transmits a small vein to join the inferior petrosal sinus. Also *canaliculus of cochlea.* **canaliculi dentales** DENTINAL TUBULES. **haversian canaliculi** CANALICULI OF OSTEOCYTES. **incisor c.** INCISIVE DUCT. **c. innominatus** An occasional canal that opens on the medial side of the foramen spinosum of the sphenoid bone and transmits the lesser petrosal nerve from the tympanic plexus to the otic ganglion. Also *innominate canaliculus, Arnold's innominate canal.* **intercellular canaliculi** The tiny canals that are lined by small microvilli and are situated between adjacent secretory cells such as the serous salivary gland cells. **c. lacrimalis** [NA] A fine, angulated canal in each eyelid that commences at the punctum on the edge of the eyelid and runs medially to end in the lacrimal sac at the upper end of the nasolacrimal duct; the lacrimal duct. **c. mastoideus** [NA] A minute canal that commences on the lateral wall of the jugular fossa, passes laterally through the temporal bone, and terminates by opening in the tympanomastoid fissure. It transmits the auricular branch of the vagus nerve to the front of the mastoid process, where it divides into two branches. Also *auricular canaliculus, mastoid canaliculus, Arnold's canal.* **canaliculi of osteocytes** The fine channels that interconnect the osseous lacunae with each other and with the vascular supply, thereby providing nutrition to the osteocytes. Also *haversian canaliculi.* **Thiersch c.** Any of the small channels found in reparative tissue that transport nutrients. They are the precursors of vascular tissue. **c. tympanicus** [NA] The minute canal that transmits the tympanic branch of the glossopharyngeal nerve from its inferior ganglion up to the tympanic cavity, where it divides to form the tympanic plexus on the surface of the promontory. The entrance to the canaliculus is on the bony ridge dividing the opening of the carotid canal from the jugular fossa on the inferior surface of the petrous part of the temporal bone. Also *tympanic canaliculus, canal for Jacobson's nerve, Jacobson's canal, tympanic canal.*

**canalis** \kənā′lis\ [L, a channel, conduit. See CANAL.] (*pl.* canales) A canal or narrow tubular channel. **c. adductorius** [NA] A triangular aponeurotic tunnel in the middle third of the anteromedial aspect of the thigh extending from the apex of the femoral triangle to the opening in the adductor magnus muscle. The canal transmits the femoral vessels, deep lymphatics, and the saphenous nerve. Also *adductor canal, crural canal of Henle, Hunter's canal, subsartor-*

*ial canal, canalis subsartorialis.* **c. alimentarius** That part of the digestive apparatus that includes the tubular passage of the esophagus, the stomach, the small intestine, and the large intestine. Also *alimentary canal, alimentary tract, digestive canal, digestive tract, enteron.* **canales alveolares maxillae** [NA] Fine canals piercing the posterior wall of the maxillary sinus and appearing as ridges on its walls for the transmission of nerves and vessels, which may be divided into anterior and posterior, to the molar and premolar teeth. Also *alveolar canals of maxilla, posterior dental canals, alveolodental canals, anterior alveolar canals, posterior alveolar canals, canales alveolares.* **c. analis** [NA] The terminal segment of the alimentary canal, commencing at the level of the urogenital diaphragm as a continuation of the rectum after passing through the pelvic diaphragm and ending at the anus. Also *anal canal.* **c. basipharyngeus** CANALIS VOMEROVAGINALIS. **c. caroticus** [NA] A channel through the petrous part of the temporal bone that transmits the internal carotid artery and its plexus of sympathetic nerves and veins from the base of the skull to its interior. The external opening is on the inferior aspect of the posterolateral part of the bone, from which the canal passes upward and forward, and then upward within the bone, exiting at the apex of the petrous part of the temporal bone over the foramen lacerum, where the artery enters the middle cranial fossa. Also *carotid canal.* **c. carpi** [NA] An osseofibrous tunnel between the flexor retinaculum anteriorly and the concave arch that is formed by the carpal bones and ligaments posteriorly, through which the flexor tendons and the median nerve pass from the forearm to the palm and digits. It is a common site of compression of the median nerve, producing palsy referred to as the carpal tunnel syndrome. Also *carpal canal, carpal tunnel, flexor canal, flexor tunnel.* **c. centralis medullae spinalis** [NA] A tenuous canal extending throughout the length of the spinal cord and continuing above into the medulla oblongata, where it enlarges to merge with the fourth ventricle. It is located centrally within the gray matter, is lined by ependyma, and contains a minute amount of cerebrospinal fluid. Developmentally, it represents the lumen of the neural tube. Also *central canal of spinal cord, syringocoele, ventricle of cord.* **c. centralis osteoni** HAVERSIAN CANAL. **c. cervicis uteri** [NA] A channel, about 2.5 cms in length, connecting the cavity of the body of the uterus at the internal os to the vaginal cavity at the external os. The canal is broader at its center than at its ends, and its anterior and posterior walls have a longitudinal mucosal ridge from which palmate folds ascend laterally (plicae palmatae). Also *canal of the cervix, cervical canal, cervicouterine canal, uterocervical canal.* **c. chordae tympani** CANALICULUS CHORDAE TYMPANI. **c. communis** COMMON ATRIOVENTRICULAR CANAL. **c. condylaris** [NA] An occasional canal leading from the condylar fossa posterior to the jugular process and the occipital condyle to the groove of the sigmoid sinus on the interior of the skull. It transmits the condylar emissary vein from the sinus to the veins in the suboccipital triangle. Also *condylar canal, condyloid canal, posterior condyloid foramen, posterior condylar canal.* **canales diploici** [NA] Channels in the diploë of the cranial bones providing passage for the large diploic veins, the walls of which are thin and without valves. Also *Breschet's canals, diploic canals.* **c. facialis** [NA] A bony channel traversing the temporal bone from the internal acoustic meatus to the stylomastoid foramen on the inferior surface. It conducts the facial nerve. Early in its course the canal is related to the vestibular portion of the inner ear, and then makes a sharp bend posteriorly (the geniculum canalis facialis), after which it runs on the wall of the tympanic cavity. Also *facial canal, fallopian aqueduct, fallopian canal, aqueduct of Fallopius, spiroid canal.* **c. femoralis** [NA] The medial compartment of the funnel-shaped femoral sheath that has the base of the lacunar ligament medially, the femoral vein laterally, the inguinal ligament anteriorly, and the pectineus muscle and fascia posteriorly. Also *femoral canal, crural canal.* **c. gastricus** [NA] The longitudinal gastric mucosal folds (plicae gastricae) that form a regular, grooved channel along the lesser curvature of the stomach. When the stomach is distended, these ridges tend to flatten or disappear. Also *ventricular canal, gastric canal, magenstrasse, canalis ventriculi.* **c. hyaloideus** [NA] A fine channel extending through the vitreous body of the vitreous chamber of the eye from the optic disk to the center of the posterior surface of the lens. In embryonic life, it runs horizontally and straight, transmitting the hyaloid artery. In the adult, it follows a wavy, curved course. Also *hyaloid canal, central canal of Stilling, central canal of vitreous, Cloquet's canal, canal of Stilling.* **c. hypoglossi** [NA] A short canal that commences in the posterior cranial fossa at a foramen above the anterior part of the occipital condyle and terminates externally, anterolateral to the condyle. It transmits the hypoglossal nerve, a meningeal branch of the ascending pharyngeal artery, and a small emissary vein or a venous plexus that connects the sigmoid sinus to the internal jugular vein. Also *hypoglossal canal, anterior condyloid canal, anterior condyloid foramen, anterior condylar canal.* **c. incisivus** [NA] One of a number of canals that lead from foramina in the median incisive fossa, located anteriorly in the bony palate and posterior to the incisor teeth, to the floor of the nasal cavity. The lateral canals transmit the terminations of the sphenopalatine artery which anastomose with branches of the greater palatine artery to the nose. Also *incisive canal, anterior palatine canal, nasopalatine canal, Scarpa's canals.* **c. infraorbitalis** [NA] A canal deep to the orbital surface of the maxilla in the floor of the orbit, commencing as a groove, or sulcus, at the posterior border and terminating at the infraorbital foramen on the anterior surface of the body of the maxilla just below the lower margin of the orbit and superior to the canine fossa. The canal transmits the infraorbital nerve and vessels. Also *infraorbital canal.* **c. inguinalis** [NA] In the adult, an oblique tunnel in the lower anterior abdominal wall, commencing internally at the deep inguinal ring situated just above the middle of the inguinal ligament and terminating externally at the superficial inguinal ring situated just above and lateral to the pubic crest. The canal transmits the spermatic cord in the male, the round ligament of uterus in the female, and the ilioinguinal nerve in both sexes. Also *inguinal canal, abdominal canal, Velpeau's canal.* **canales longitudinales modioli** [NA] Canals that tunnel the modiolus and conduct cochlear nerves and vessels to the middle and apical turns of the cochlea. Also *longitudinal canals of modiolus, canals of modiolus, central canal of modiolus.* **c. mandibulae** [NA] A channel traversing the ramus and body of the mandible, commencing at the mandibular foramen situated near the middle of the medial surface of the ramus and terminating at the mental foramen on the external surface of the body opposite the second premolar tooth. The canal transmits the inferior alveolar vessels and nerves. Also *mandibular canal, inferior dental canal.* **c. musculotubarius** [NA] The combination of two parallel grooves, one above the other, separated by a thin curved plate of bone, the septum canalis musculotubarii, located at the anterior part of the angle of junction of the petrous and the squamous parts of the temporal bone, and converted into canals by the overlying tympanic plate. The upper canal, semicanalis musculus tensoris tympani, transmits the tensor tympani muscle to the tympanic cavity, while the lower, semicanalis tubae auditivae, is the bony part of the auditory tube permitting air communication between the tympanic cavity and the pharynx. Also *musculotubal canal, osseous eustachian canal.* **c. nasolacrimalis** [NA] A groove in the nasal surface of the maxilla, directed downward, posteriorly, and laterally into the inferior meatus of the nose, and converted into a canal by the lacrimal bone and inferior nasal concha. The canal runs just medial to the maxillary sinus, and contains the nasolacrimal duct. Also *nasolacrimal canal, nasal canal, lacrimal canal.* **c. nutricius ossis** NUTRIENT CANAL OF BONE. **c. obturatorius** [NA] A canal bounded below by the ligamentous superior border of the obturator membrane and above by the medially directed obturator groove at the superior end of the lateral border of the pubic bone. It is traversed by the obturator vessels and nerve coursing between the pelvis and thigh. Also *obturator canal.* **c. opticus** [NA] A short, circular passage at the posteromedial apex of the pyramidal orbit, located between the roots of the lesser wing of the sphenoid bone, and transmitting the optic nerve and the ophthalmic artery to the orbit. Also *optic canal, foramen opticum ossis sphenoidalis* (outmoded), *optic foramen of sphenoid bone.* **canales palatini minores** [NA] Canals that branch from the greater palatine canal close to the junction between the lamina of the pterygoid process and the horizontal plate of the palatine bone. They transmit the lesser (posterior and middle) palatine nerves and arteries to supply the uvula, tonsil, and soft palate. Also *lesser palatine canals, canales palatini, accessory palatine canals, posterior palatine canals.* **c. palatinus major** [NA] A communicating passage between the lower end of the pterygopalatine fossa and the roof of the mouth, located at the junction of the posterior surface of the maxilla with the perpendicular plate of the palatine bone. The canal transmits the anterior palatine nerve and the descending palatine artery. Also *greater palatine canal, canalis pterygopalatinus, pterygopalatine canal, palatomaxillary canal, sphenopalatine canal, Tourtual's canal.* **c. palatovaginalis** [NA] A passage formed between the vaginal process of the medial pterygoid plate and the sphenoidal process of the palatine bone and the body of the sphenoid bone. It transmits pharyngeal branches of the sphenopalatine artery and of the sphenopalatine ganglion to the roof of the nasopharynx. Also *palatovaginal canal, canalis pharyngeus, pharyngeal canal, lateral inferior vomerobasilar canal, pterygopalatine canal, sphenopalatine canal, sphenopharyngeal canal.* **c. portalis** PORTAL CANAL. **c. pterygoideus** [NA] A canal running in an anteroposterior direction at the junction of the medial pterygoid plate with the body of the sphenoid. It conducts the nerve of the pterygoid canal to the sphenopalatine ganglion and a branch of the pterygopalatine division of the maxillary artery. Also *pterygoid canal, vidian canal, canal of Guidi, recurrent canal.* **c. pterygopalatinus** CANALIS PALATINUS MAJOR. **c. pudendalis** [NA] A fibrous tunnel usually formed by a splitting of the obturator fascia and extending in the lateral wall of the ischiorectal fossa from the lesser sciatic foramen to the posterior margin of the urogenital diaphragm. The canal transmits the internal pudendal vessels and nerves and some of their branches. Also *pudendal canal, Alcock's canal.* **c. pyloricus** [NA] A subdivision of the pyloric portion of the stomach, the proximal part being the antrum, a dilatation just distal to the body of the stomach and the angular notch, and the distal part being the short constricted pyloric canal which ends at, but does not include, the sphincter of the pylorus. Frequently the antrum cannot be distinguished from the canal. Also *pyloric canal.* **c. radicis dentis** ROOT CANAL. **c. reuniens** DUCTUS REUNIENS. **c. sacralis** [NA] That portion of the vertebral canal that extends from the first sacral vertebra to the hiatus sacralis, where the laminae of the fourth and fifth sacral vertebrae are incomplete. Also *sacral canal, caudal canal.* **canales semicirculares ossei** [NA] Three semicircular canals located postero-

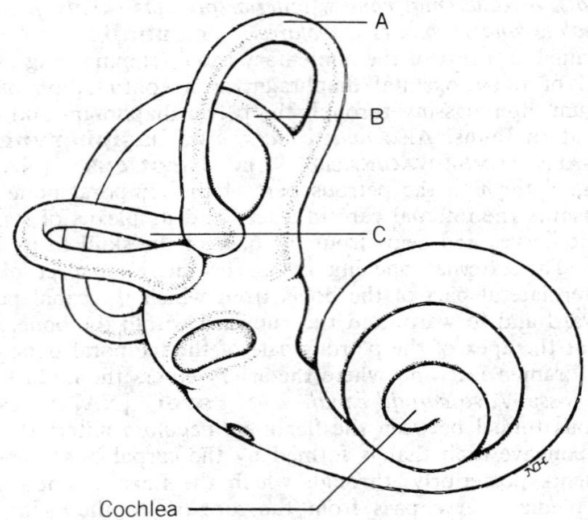


**Semicircular canals** (A) Superior; (B) posterior; (C) lateral.

superior to and opening into the vestibule of the internal ear, each being two-thirds of a circle and lying at right angles to the other two. These bony canals, measuring about 1 mm in diameter, contain membranous ducts, and each one has one end dilated as an ampulla. They are designated anterior, lateral, and posterior. Also *semicircular canals, bony semicircular canals.* **c. semicircularis anterior** [NA] A bony canal in the petrous part of the temporal bone, lying in the vertical plane at right angles to the long axis of that bone and above the vestibule. Its anterolateral end is ampullated and its other end joins the end of the posterior semicircular canal to form the common limb, or crus commune, which opens into the vestibule. Also *anterior semicircular canal, superior semicircular canal.* **c. semicircularis lateralis** [NA] The shortest of the three canals in the petrous part ofthe temporal bone, lying in the horizontal plane at right angles to the other two canals, with its ampulla opening in the vestibule close to that of the anterior canal. Also *lateral semicircular canal, external semicircular canal.* **c. semicircularis posterior** [NA] The longest of the three semicircular canals, lying in the vertical plane, arched posteriorly almost parallel to the posterior surface of the petrous part of the temporal bone. Its inferior, ampullated end opens into the vestibule, while its superior extremity opens into the crus commune. Also *posterior semicircular canal.* **c. spinalis** CANALIS VERTEBRALIS. **c. spiralis cochleae** [NA] A canal about 30 mm long that makes two and one-half turns around the conical central bony axis, or modiolus, of the cochlea. By means of a thin plate, the osseous spiral lamina, which projects out from the modiolus like the thread of a screw, the canal is partly subdivided into an upper passage, the scala vestibuli, and a lower passage, the scala tympani. Also *spiral canal of cochlea, cochlear ca-*

*nal, Rosenthal's canal, spiral canal of Rosenthal.* **c. spiralis modioli** [NA] The spiral passage in the attached margin of the osseous spiral lamina of the modiolus, containing the sensory spiral ganglion of the cochlea. The minute canals of the tractus spiralis foraminosus bend outwards, enlarge, and fuse with the spiral canal. Also *spiral canal of modiolus, canals of modiolus, ganglionic canal.* **c. subsartorialis** CANALIS ADDUCTORIUS. **c. ventriculi** CANALIS GASTRICUS. **c. vertebralis** [NA] The continuous canal formed by the total series of vertebral foramina of the articulated vertebral column in which is found the spinal cord and its membranes, the spinal nerve roots, blood vessels, and the posterior longitudinal ligament. Also *vertebral canal, spinal canal, tubus vertebralis, neural canal, canalis spinalis.* **c. vomerovaginalis** [NA] The sagittally oriented canal between the superior surface of the vaginal process of the medial pterygoid plate and the ala of the vomer on either side that transmits branches of the sphenopalatine vessels and the pterygopalatine ganglion toward the incisive foramen and nasal septum. Also *vomerovaginal canal, canalis basipharyngeus, basipharyngeal canal, vomerine canal, lateral superior vomerobasilar canal.*

**canalization** \kan′əlīzā′shən\ **1** The formation of channels. **2** A form of developmental homeostasis that buffers the developmental processes of an organism against environmental or genetic perturbations, thus creating little variation in phenotype.

**Canavan** [Myrtelle May *Canavan*, U.S. neuropathologist, 1879–1953] **1** Canavan's diffuse sclerosis, Canavan spongy degeneration, Canavan-van Bogaert-Bertrand disease. See under VAN BOGAERT'S FAMILIAL AXONAL SPONGY DEGENERATION. **2** See under DISEASE.

**canavanase** *Obs.* ARGINASE.

**cancellated** \kan′səlātid\ CANCELLOUS.

**cancellous** \kan′sələs\ [L *cancell(i)* (dim. of earlier *cancri* grillwork, barrier, pl. of *cancer*, prob. variant of *carcer* prison) latticework, grating + -OUS] Referring to a honeycomblike, spongy, or reticular structure, particularly of bony tissue. Also *cancellated.*

**cancer** [L (akin to Gk *karkinos* a crab, cancer) a crab, an eating ulcer, cancer] An uncontrolled proliferation of cells which usually destroys and invades adjacent tissues, metastasizes, and follows a fatal course if untreated. Cancer cells typically have structural abnormalities of size, shape, staining qualities, and number of chromosomes. Cancerous tissue often resembles recognizable tissues, such as glands or epidermis, but is usually abnormally organized, showing evidence of insufficient differentiation and haphazard growth. Cancer cells function abnormally in qualitative and quantitative ways. They may produce mucus but retain it, they may produce fetal antigens, and they may secrete normal or inappropriate hormones. Carcinomas and sarcomas are more specific forms of cancer. Cancer also includes diffuse nontumor-forming neoplastic processes such as leukemias. Also *malignant tumor.* • *Cancer* is often imprecisely used synonymously with *carcinoma,* as *cancer in situ.* **arsenic c.** A cancer which occurs as an occupational risk in workers exposed to arsenic compounds in the manufacture of arsenical sheep dips, in mining, and in the smelting of metal ores that contain arsenic compounds, or by exposure to a contaminated water supply. The lungs and skin are the most commonly affected sites. Arsenic cancer of the skin also occurs in patients treated with arsenical mixtures for psoriasis and other skin conditions. **asbestos c.** A cancer caused by exposure to asbestos. It is usually a mesothelioma of the pleura or a carcinoma of the lung. It is not asbestosis. **3,4-benzpyrene c.** Cancer caused by exposure to 3,4-benzpyrene which is a constituent of coal-tar derivatives and shale oil. It occurs or has occurred among chimney sweeps (chimney sweeps' cancer) and those who handle tar and pitch. Its characteristic sites of occurrence are the skin of the eyelids, ears, face, and scrotum. Also *pitch cancer, pitch-workers' cancer.* **betel c.** A squamous cell carcinoma of the buccal mucosa, found in persons who chew a mixture of betel nut and tobacco. Also *buyo cheek cancer.* **buyo cheek c.** BETEL CANCER. • *Buyo* is a local name for betel in the Philippine Islands. **chimney sweeps' c.** A squamous cell carcinoma of the skin of the scrotum of chimney sweeps, due to the deposition of carcinogens at this site. This is one of the oldest recognized forms of occupational cancer. Also *soot cancer, carcinoma asbolicum.* **chromate c.** Cancer of the lungs which occurs among workers making chromates from chrome ore. It may also occur in the chrome-color industry. The risk is considered highest in persons handling monochromates. **chutta c.** A cancer of the palate developing as a result of smoking an Indian cigar (called a chutta) with the lighted end inside the mouth. **claypipe c.** A carcinoma of the lip associated with smoking clay pipes. **colloid c.** MUCINOUS CARCINOMA. **contact c.** A cancer developing after contact with another cancer. **corset c.** CANCER EN CUIRASSE. **dermoid c.** *Obs.* SQUAMOUS CELL CARCINOMA. **c. à deux** Cancers occurring at about the same time in two people who live together. **encephaloid c.** A cancer with a soft consistency like that of brain, due to high cellular content with a paucity of stroma. Said of some breast carcinomas. **c. en cuirasse** A scirrhous breast carcinoma which causes the skin of the thorax to be rigid and fixed to underlying structures. Also *corset cancer, carcinoma en cuirasse.* **glandular c.** ADENOCARCINOMA. **green c.** *Obs.* CHLOROMA. **c. in situ** CARCINOMA IN SITU. **kangri c.** A localized squamous cell cancer of the skin, occurring on the abdomen or thighs in Kashmir and Tibet, where people carry baskets of hot coals (kangri stoves) under their clothes to keep warm. **latent c.** **1** A cancer which has not caused symptoms. **2** A cancer found unexpectedly at autopsy. Also *incidental cancer, subclinical cancer.* **metastatic c.** METASTASIS. **mineral oil c.** A skin cancer which arises from prolonged and continuous contact with mineral oils. It has had a high incidence among mule-spinners in the cotton industry who come in contact with shale oil used in oiling the spindles. The common site of occurrence is the scrotum. It also occurs among workers exposed to mineral oil in engineering, as well as among gunsmiths. Also *paraffin cancer, shale oil cancer, mule-spinners' cancer, shale-workers' cancer, mule-spinners' disease.* **mule-spinners' c.** MINERAL OIL CANCER. **multicentric c.** A cancer presumed to have multiple sites of origin. **nickel c.** A cancer of the lungs and ethmoid bone, found in workers refining nickel from ores containing metallic arsenides. Arsenic is suspected as the cause, but nickel in the form of nickel carbonyl is also suspect. **occult c.** A cancer which has not caused symptoms at its primary site but manifests itself in metastases or in secondary phenomena, such as migratory thrombophlebitis. **osteoblastic c.** A primary or secondary cancer in bone which is associated with abnormal ossification. Metastatic prostate carcinoma is the most typical form. **osteolytic c.** A cancer producing bone destruction. **paraffin c.** MINERAL OIL CANCER. **pitch c.** 3,4-BENZPYRENE CANCER. **pitch-workers' c.** 3,4-BENZPYRENE CANCER. **primary c.** A cancer at its site of origin, as opposed to a metastatic or secondary cancer. **radiologists' c.** A squamous cell carcinoma of the skin, often multicentric, developing in professional persons repeatedly exposed to x rays. Also *x-ray cancer.* **radium c.** A cancer that occurs in persons exposed to radium and its compounds in the production of radioactive substances and in therapeutic radium laboratories. In the past it was found among workers painting luminous dials. It may occur as cancer of the lung and sarcoma of bone. **rodent c.** BASAL CELL CARCINOMA. **Schneeberg c.** A type of lung carcinoma related to inhalation of dust rich in radioactive uranium, first observed among the workers in the Schneeberg mines of Saxony. **scirrhous c.** SCIRRHOUS CARCINOMA. **shale oil c.** MINERAL OIL CANCER. **shale-workers' c.** MINERAL OIL CANCER. **smokers' c.** A carcinoma of the bronchus due to tobacco smoking, particularly cigarettes. Other cancers associated with smoking are of the larynx, lip, mouth, esophagus, and pharynx. Those of the lip and mouth may be associated with pipe smoking. **soot c.** CHIMNEY SWEEPS' CANCER. **tar c.** A squamous cell carcinoma of the skin caused by continued exposure to tar and tar products. **ulcer c.** A carcinoma developing in a preexisting chronic ulcer such as one found in the stomach or skin. **ulcerated c.** A malignant tumor, usually a carcinoma, whose surface is necrotic, often with a centrally depressed crater. The skin and alimentary tract are common sites for this lesion. **vinyl chloride c.** An angiosarcoma of the liver occurring among workers who have had heavy exposures to vinyl-chloride monomer in the production of polyvinyl chloride. **x-ray c.** RADIOLOGISTS' CANCER.

**canceremia** \kan′sərē′mē·ə\ The presence of cancer cells in the blood. Also *carcinemia.*

**cancericidal** \kan′sərisī′dl\ Causing destruction of cancer cells. Also *cancerocidal.*

**cancerigenic** \kan′sərijen′ik\ CARCINOGENIC.

**cancerization** \kan′sərīzā′shən\ Development of cancer.

**cancerocidal** \kan′sərōsī′dl\ CANCERICIDAL.

**cancerogenic** \kan′sərōjen′ik\ CARCINOGENIC.

**cancerologist** \kan′səräl′əjist\ A specialist in cancerology; an oncologist.

**cancerology** \kan′səräl′əjē\ The study of cancer. Also *cancrology.* • This term is less commonly used than *oncology,* the study of tumors.

**cancerosis** \kan′sərō′sis\ [CANCER + -OSIS] A cancer that is widely disseminated throughout the body. • The terms *carcinomatosis* and *sarcomatosis* are more often used.

**cancerostatic** \kan′sərōstat′ik\ [CANCER + *o* + -STATIC] Capable of halting the growth of a cancer.

**cancerous** \kan′sərəs\ Of or relating to cancer.

**cancer-ulcer** \kan′sər-ul′sər\ 1 An ulcerated cancer. 2 A cancer developing in an ulcer.

**cancriform** \kang′krifôrm\ [L *cancri,* gen. of *cancer* cancer + -FORM] Resembling a cancer in appearance.

**cancroid** \kang′kroid\ [L *cancer,* gen. *cancri,* + -OID] 1 Resembling a cancer. 2 A squamous cell carcinoma of the skin.

**cancrology** \kangkräl′əjē\ CANCEROLOGY.

**cancrum** \kang′krəm\ [New L, prob. from English CANKER] Canker. **c. nasi** Gangrenous infection spreading from the nasal mucous membrane to the tissues around the nose, most commonly seen in undernourished children after a debilitating illness, such as measles. Also *gangrenous rhinitis.* **c. oris** Gangrenous ulceration of the soft tissues in and around the mouth, and capable of spreading to involve the full thickness of the lips and cheeks. It develops from necrotizing ulcerative gingivitis in children 2–6 years of age who are malnourished or recovering from infectious diseases. An infarct presents on the surface of the face when the spreading destruction from within the mouth arrests the blood supply to the area. Response to antibiotic therapy is good but scar contraction and trismus are complications of healing. Also *oral gangrene, acute necrotizing stomatitis, gangrenous stomatitis, necrotizing ulcerative stomatitis, stomatonecrosis, stomatonoma (seldom used).* See also NECROTIZING ULCERATIVE GINGIVOSTOMATITIS.

**candela** \kan′dələ\ [L, a light, candle] The SI base unit of luminous intensity. It is the luminous intensity, in a given direction, of a source emitting a monochromatic radiation of a frequency of $540 \times 10^{12}$ hertz, of which the energy in that direction is 1/683 watt per steradian. Also *new candle* (obs.). Symbol: cd **c. steradian** LUMEN.

**candicidin** A mixture of polyene antibiotic substances obtained from *Streptomyces* species and having fungistatic and fungicidal activity against *Candida.* It is used to treat vaginal candidiasis.

***Candida*** \kan′didə\ [L, fem. of *candidus* glowing, of a shining white, clear] A form-genus of fungi in the family Cryptococcaceae, order Moniliales. They are considered yeastlike, but no sexual reproductive mechanisms are known, thereby causing this genus to be retained in the form-class Deuteromycetes. Some species are known to be human

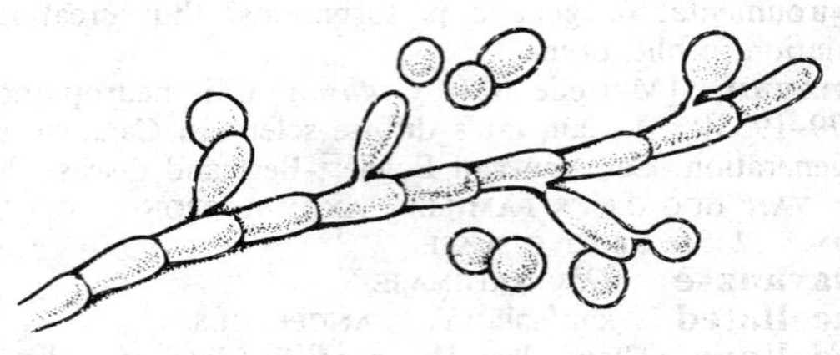

Candida

pathogens. Also *Monilia* (older term). ***C. albicans*** A common species of imperfect fungi normally found in the skin and alimentary flora. It can cause serious disease, including various forms of candidiasis, when the microbial flora is deranged by antibiotics or other conditions. Also *thrush fungus.* ***C. tropicalis*** A form-species of fungus implicated with both endocarditis and septicemia.

**candidal** \kan′didəl\ Pertaining or belonging to a member of the form-genus *Candida..* Also *monilial* (incorrect).

**candidemia** \kan′didē′mē·ə\ Septicemia caused by *Candida.*

**candidiasis** \kan′didī′əsis\ [*Candid(a)* + -IASIS] An infection of any part of the body with a yeast of the genus *Candida,* usually *Candida albicans.* Also *candidosis, moniliasis* (older term). **cutaneous c.** An infection of the skin, especially moist sites, with a yeast of the genus *Candida,* usually *Candida albicans.* It is characterized by minute white subcorneal pustules, erythema, and peeling as well as the appearance of satellite lesions. **endocardial c.** Endocarditis caused by infection with a fungus of the genus *Candida.* **oral c.** THRUSH.

**candidid** \kan′didid\ CANDIDIDE.

**candidide** \kan′didīd\ An allergic reaction, usually of the skin, to a *Candida* infection in another part of the body. Candidides have often been diagnosed on scanty evidence and are not as well-defined as dermatophytides. Also *candidid.*

**candidosis** \kan′didō′sis\ CANDIDIASIS.

**candidulin** \kandid′yəlin\ A crystalline antibacterial

agent derived from a member of mycobacteria (not including *Mycobacterium tuberculosis*) as well as from other bacteria.

**candiru** \kandiroo′\ [Portuguese *candiru* (from Tupi)] Small urophilous catfish found in the Amazon River that are feared by swimmers for their possible entry into the vagina of females or urethra of males, invading the urethra and bladder. Cystitis and urethritis are said to result from irritation caused by dead fish.

**candle** [L *candela* (from *candere* to glow, shine) candle] **1** A cylinder of wax or tallow, often tapered, enclosing a wick that when ignited provides light. **2** A cylindrical filter of unglazed porcelain or diatomaceous earth, formerly used for filtering out bacteria. An obsolete usage. **Chamberland c.** A filter of unglazed porcelain, formerly used for preparing bacteria-free filtrates. **new c.** *Obs.* CANDELA.

**candle-guttering** \-gut′əring\ The pneumoencephalographic appearance of irregular protrusions into the cerebral ventricles in patients with tuberous sclerosis. • The protrusions suggest blobs of wax on a burning candle.

**cane** / **broad-based c.** A cane with three or four points to provide a wide base of support. **glider c.** A cane with wheels on the inner legs permitting gliding of the cane on the floor.

**canescent** \kānes′ənt\ [L *canescens*, gen. *canescentis*, pres. part. of *canescere* (from *canere* to be white, from *canus* gray like ashes, white, hoary) to become white or gray] Becoming gray.

**canine** \kā′nīn\ [L *caninus* (from *canis* dog) pertaining to dogs] **1** The third tooth in each quadrant starting from the midline. It has the longest root of all the teeth and a conical crown terminating in a point which is gradually worn down by physiologic attrition. Also *canine tooth, cuspid.* **2** Relating to dogs and allied animals of the genus *Canis.*

**caniniform** \kānīn′ifôrm\ Shaped like a canine tooth.

**caninus** \kānī′nəs\ MUSCULUS LEVATOR ANGULI ORIS.

**canities** \kānish′i·ēz\ [L (from *canus* grayish, hoary), whiteness, grayness of hair] A graying or whitening of the hair.

**canker** \kang′kər\ [Middle English *canker, cancre,* from Norman French *cancre,* from L *cancer* crab, cancer, ulcer] A spreading ulceration, particularly of the mouth.

**canna** \kan′ə\ [L, from Gk *kanna* a reed. See CANNULA.] A reed or stick, as in *canna major, canna minor.* **c. major** *Outmoded* TIBIA. **c. minor** *Outmoded* FIBULA.

**cannabinol** A compound containing two benzene rings fused to a six-membered ring containing oxygen. It is a component of cannabis. It is less active pharmacologically than its tetrahydro derivative, from which it is formed by dehydrogenation to produce one of the benzene rings.

**cannabis** \kan′əbis\ [L, from Gk *kannabis* (akin to prehistoric Germanic *hanipiz,* whence Old English *haenep,* English *hemp*) hemp] A plant of the species *Cannabis sativa.* Its leaves and pistillate flowering tops are variously prepared as marihuana, hashish, and hashish oil, which are hallucinogenic and intoxicating because of their tetrahydrocannabinol content. Also *Indian hemp, American hemp, hemp.*

**cannibalism** \kan′əbəlizm\ **1** The act or practice of eating members of one's own species. Its causes and functions are not always well understood, but in some species it occurs as a population control mechanism when density is high. **2** Phagocytosis of one cancer cell by another, usually seen in highly malignant and anaplastic tumors.

**Cannon** [Walter Bradford *Cannon,* U.S. physiologist, 1871–1945] **1** See under POINT, RING, THEORY. **2** Cannon's law of denervation. See under LAW. **3** Cannon-Bard theory of emotions. See under THEORY.

**cannula** \kan′yələ\ [L, dim. of *canna,* a reed, pipe, from Gk *kanna* a reed, prob. from Semitic; akin to Hebrew *qāneh,* a reed, stalk] A semirigid or rigid plastic or metal tube inserted into the lumen of a vessel, duct, or cavity. Also *canula.* **infusion c.** A cannula used for the instillation of fluid into a cavity, duct, or a blood vessel. **irrigation c.** A cannula used to introduce and often also withdraw an irrigating solution called a jet wash. Such a cannula is used for endometrial cytology. **Karman c.** A plastic tube with a flexible tip used to perform a suction abortion. Also *Karman catheter.* **perfusion c.** A cannula containing channels that provide continuous flow into and out of a cavity, vessel, or duct. **ventricular c.** A specially devised needle or tube with a stylet, used for removal of ventricular fluid and for injections into the ventricles. **washout c.** A tube or catheter that is inserted into a blood vessel and can be irrigated without removal from the vessel.

**cannulate** To introduce a cannula into.

**cannulation** \kan′yəlā′shən\ The introduction of a cannula.

**canth-** \kanth-\ CANTHO-.

**canthal** \kan′thəl\ Pertaining to a canthus, the lateral or medial angle between the upper and lower eyelids.

**cantharic acid** $C_{10}H_{12}O_4$. A crystalline acid obtained from cantharidin by heating with hydriodic acid.

**cantharidal** Containing or pertaining to cantharides. Also *cantharidial.*

**cantharides** A preparation of dried blister beetles, *Cantharis (Lytta) vesicatoria.* The active substance, cantharidin, is a potent vesicant and the agent has limited application externally as an irritant and blistering medication. Historically, it has been claimed to be an aphrodisiac because of its irritating effects on the genitourinary tract if taken orally. Also *Spanish fly* (popular), *muscae hispanicae.*

**cantharidial** CANTHARIDAL.

**cantharidism** \kanther′idizm\ A morbid condition caused by absorption or ingestion of cantharides. Symptoms are blistering of the skin, severe gastroenteritis, nephritis, and possibly death.

***Cantharis vesicatoria*** \kan′tharis ves′ikətôr′ē·ə\ A species of blister beetle found in Spain and southern France during early summer; the so-called Spanish fly. The vesicant preparation cantharides, also known as Spanish fly, is made from the dried beetles. Also *Lytta vesicatoria.*

**canthectomy** \kanthek′təmē\ [CANTH- + -ECTOMY] Surgical excision of tissue located at the junction of the eyelids.

**canthi** \kan′thī\ Plural of CANTHUS.

**canthitis** \kanthī′tis\ [CANTH- + -ITIS] Inflammation of a canthus.

**cantho-** \kan′thō-\ [Gk *kanthos* corner of the eye] A combining form denoting the canthus. Also *canth-.*

**cantholysis** \kanthäl′isis\ [CANTHO- + LYSIS] The horizontal splitting of the lateral canthus or the severance of the lateral palpebral ligament.

**canthoplasty** \kan′thəplas′tē\ [CANTHO- + -PLASTY] A plastic surgical operation on the medial or lateral canthus of the eye to change its shape or position or to reconstruct it.

**canthorrhaphy** \kanthôr′əfē\ [CANTHO- + -RRHAPHY] Partial closure, by suturing, of the internal or external canthus of the eye. The usual purpose is to shorten the palpebral fissure.

**canthotomy** \kanthät′əmē\ [CANTHO- + -TOMY] A horizontal cut extending the palpebral aperture, often used to aid the exposure of the eye during cataract surgery.

**canthus** \kan′thəs\ [New L, from Gk *kanthos* outer rim

of a wheel, corner of the eye] (*pl.* canthi) The lateral or medial angle of the palpebral aperture. Adj. canthal. **external c.** ANGULUS OCULI LATERALIS. **internal c.** ANGULUS OCULI MEDIALIS. **inner c.** 1 ANGULUS OCULI MEDIALIS. 2 COMMISSURA PALPEBRARUM MEDIALIS. **c. inversus** Caudal displacement of the medial canthus of the eye. **lateral c.** 1 ANGULUS OCULI LATERALIS. 2 COMMISSURA PALPEBRARUM LATERALIS. **medial c.** 1 ANGULUS OCULI MEDIALIS. 2 COMMISSURA PALPEBRARUM MEDIALIS. **outer c.** 1 ANGULUS OCULI LATERALIS. 2 COMMISSURA PALPEBRARUM LATERALIS.

**Cantor** [Meyer O. *Cantor,* U.S. surgeon, born 1907] See under TUBE.

**canula** \kan′yələ\ CANNULA.

**cap** An artificial dental crown. *Popular.* **abduction c.** A device of leather or canvas to support the arm in abduction. **acrosomal c.** ACROSOME. **anterior head c.** A covering of the anterior portion of the head of a spermatozoon. **bishop's c.** AMPULLA DUODENI. **chin c.** CHIN CUP. **cradle c.** A greasy crust frequently present on an infant's scalp; seborrhea of the scalp in infants. *Popular.* Also *milk crust, milk scall.* **Dumas c.** An occlusive cervical cap used for contraception. **duodenal c.** AMPULLA DUODENI. **dutch c.** A contraceptive cervical diaphragm. **enamel c.** The first formed enamel at the tip of a growing cusp. **fibrin c.** HYALINE LESION. **fibrinoid c.** HYALINE LESION. **knee c.** PATELLA. **metanephrogenic c.** A part of the metanephric blastema which comes into relation with each ampulla of the branching collecting system derived from the ureteric bud. Each cap subsequently divides into two small spheres of cells, and others form the blastemal cap for successive subdivisions of the ampulla. Each cap forms a vesicle which develops into the proximal and distal convoluted tubules, the glomerulus, and the loop of Henle of a single nephron. The first vesicles appear at the end of the seventh week. The renal vesicles may fail to join the collecting tubules, and, if widespread, this condition may give rise to congenital polycystic kidneys. Also *metanephric cap.* **phrygian c.** The characteristic radiologic appearance of a congenital deformity of the gallbladder in which a folding of the mucosa or of the entire gallbladder wall, extends partially across the lumen. **polar c.** A specialized region of the cytoplasm seen near the centrosome of a dividing cell in higher plants. The polar cap is believed to be the site of spindle formation. **postnuclear c.** A covering of the posterior portion of the head of a spermatozoon. Also *posterior head cap.* **pulp c.** A small concavoconvex disk placed over a pulp exposure to hold therapeutic agents in place and to protect the exposure from pressure. **skull c.** CALVARIA.

**CAP** catabolite activator protein.

**cap.** 1 *capsula* (L, capsule). 2 *capiat* (L, let him take).

**capacitance** \kəpas′itəns\ [*capacit(y)* + -ANCE] 1 The property of an isolated conductor, or of an arrangement of conductors, of permitting the storage of electrical charge by the establishment of appropriate potentials or potential differences. 2 The measure of that property, given by the ratio of the magnitude of the stored charge to the magnitude of the potential (difference). **membrane c.** The storage of a static electric charge in a membrane constituting the principal component of membrane reactance opposing the flow of current and thus a determinant of the time constant; its measurement is important for estimating ion conductances.

**capacitation** \kəpas′itā′shən\ A change which takes place in the mature spermatozoon whereby it acquires the ability to fertilize an ovum. This process usually occurs within the female genital tract, though it may also be induced experimentally *in vitro* in suitable tissue culture medium, and is characterized by the loss of the acrosome cap and an increase in respiratory metabolism.

**capacitor** \kəpas′itər\ A device for storing electricity, usually made of parallel conductors separated by air, plastic, ceramic, or mica. Also *condenser* (outmoded).

**capacity** [French *capacité* (from L *capacitas* capacity, from *capax* able to hold) power to contain] 1 The ability to hold, receive, or retain. 2 A measure of such ability, as an amount or volume of a substance that a structure can hold or retain. **antigen binding c.** The quantitative aspects of the reaction of an antibody with its antigen, reflecting the specificity of antigen and antibody and the molecular forces that hold antigen and antibody together. **carbon monoxide diffusing c.** The diffusing capacity of carbon monoxide across the alveolocapillary membrane. This is a useful test of the gas exchange function of the lung. It is expressed by the following ratio:

$$\frac{\text{Volume of CO absorbed per minute}}{\text{Alveolar CO tension — mean pulmonary capillary CO tension}}$$

Abbr. DCO **diffusing c.** A measure of the ability of a substance to traverse from alveolar air to pulmonary capillary blood or vice versa. Also *diffusion capacity.* See also CARBON MONOXIDE DIFFUSING CAPACITY, OXYGEN DIFFUSING CAPACITY. **forced vital c.** The volume of air that is expired from full inspiration using maximal effort and speed. In some patients with obstructive pulmonary disease, excessive positive expiratory pressure may lead to air trapping so that the forced vital capacity is less than the vital capacity obtained by slow expiration. Abbr. FVC Also *forced expired volume.* **functional residual c.** The volume of air remaining in the lungs at the end of a quiet expiration. It comprises the expiratory reserve volume together with the residual volume. Also *stationary air* (obs.), *functional residual air* (obs.). **heat c.** THERMAL CAPACITY. **inspiratory c.** The maximum volume that can be inspired into the lungs after a normal expiration. It encompasses the tidal volume and the inspiratory reserve volume. **iron binding c.** The maximum ability of serum proteins to bind iron, expressed as μg/dl or mmol/l of iron that is protein-bound following addition of Fe(III) to a serum specimen. Normal values are approximately 250 μg/dl to 450μg/dl. Total iron binding capacity (TIBC) reflects transferrin content of serum. It is often increased in iron deficiency states and in pregnancy. It is decreased when there is infection, malignancy, inflammatory disease, hepatic cirrhosis, nephrotic syndrome, and in the very rare hereditary condition atransferrinemia. **maximal breathing c.** MAXIMUM BREATHING CAPACITY. **maximal respiratory c.** MAXIMUM BREATHING CAPACITY. **maximal tubular excretory c.** The maximum rate at which the tubule cells can actively transfer a substance from the peritubular fluid into the tubular lumen. Also *maximal tubular secretory capacity.* **maximal tubular reabsorptive c.** The maximum rate at which the tubule cells can actively transfer a substance from the tubular lumen to the peritubular fluid. **maximal tubular secretory c.** MAXIMAL TUBULAR EXCRETORY CAPACITY. **maximum breathing c.** The maximum volume of air that can be voluntarily ventilated in one minute. Also *maximal breathing capacity, maximal respiratory capacity, respiratory capacity, maximum voluntary ventilation.* Abbr. MBC. **maximum lung c.** TOTAL LUNG CAPACITY. **mental c.** The potential for the development of any mental ability or mental function as determined by native, or constitutional, factors. **oxygen c.** The maximum volume of oxygen that can be taken up by a tissue in the presence of excess oxygen. **oxygen diffusing c.** The diffusing capacity of oxygen across the alveolocapillary membrane. It is expressed by the following ratio:

$$\frac{\text{Volume of oxygen absorbed per minute}}{\text{Alveolar oxygen tension — mean pulmonary capillary } O_2 \text{ tension}}$$

Abbr. $DO_2$ **respiratory c.** MAXIMUM BREATHING CAPACITY. **testamentary c.** The state of mental competence legally necessary for the making of a will. **thermal c.** 1 The amount of heat required to raise the temperature of a body 1°C. 2 The product of mass and specific heat, expressed in joules or calories. For defs. 1 and 2 also *heat capacity.* **timed vital c.** The volume of air expired in a stated time interval, divided by the total expired volume. The most frequently used time interval is one second. This ratio is expressed as $FEV_1/FVC$. Vital capacity may be normal but timed vital capacity abnormal in diseases associated with increased airway resistance. A one-second-time timed vital capacity of less than 75 percent indicates airway obstruction. **total lung c.** The volume of air in the lung at full inflation. Also *maximum lung capacity.* Abbr. TLC **vital c.** The maximum volume of air that can be expired from the lungs after a full inspiration, usually measured by spirometry. Abbr. VC

**Capgras** [Jean Marie Joseph *Capgras,* French psychiatrist, 1873–1950] Capgras symptom. See under SYNDROME.

***Capillaria*** \kap′iler′ē·ə\ [New L, from L *capillus* a hair, filament] The type genus of the aphasmid nematode subfamily Capillariinae, family Trichuridae (or Capillariidae). There are some 37 species parasitic in fish, 13 in amphibia, 13 in reptiles, 104 in birds, and 84 in mammals. The species *C. philippinensis* is a significant agent of disease in humans. Also *Hepaticola, Trichosoma.* ***C. philippinensis*** The causative agent of human intestinal capillariasis (Philippine capillariasis). Although clearly not well adapted to the human host, this nematode is able to reproduce within the intestinal mucosa.

**capillariasis** \kap′ilərī′əsis\ [*Capillar(ia)* + -IASIS] Any infection by nematodes of the genus *Capillaria.* Also *hepaticoliasis.* **intestinal c.** 1 Any intestinal infection by nematodes of the genus *Capillaria.* 2 A disease of humans apparently limited to central Luzon in the Philippines and Thailand, caused by *C. philippinensis.* It may occur in epidemics. It is thought to result from infected, raw, freshwater fish bearing the larval nematodes. Small rodents may be alternative hosts. The adult worms produce a severe inflammatory reaction in the small intestine. The worms appear to reproduce in the intestinal mucosa, a condition that can result in a massive, protein-wasting, malabsorptive enteropathy, leading to death in some cases. Thiabendazole and mebendazole are of value in treatment. Also *Philippine capillariasis.*

**capillarioscopy** \kap′iler′ē·äs′kəpē\ A method of examining the structure of a capillary network of a tissue *in vivo* by using a microscope. Also *microangioscopy.*

**capillaritis** \kap′ilerī′tis\ [*capillar(y)* + -ITIS] Inflammation of capillaries.

**capillarity** \kap′iler′itē\ The surface forces that cause fluids to move along capillary tubing. Also *capillary attraction.*

**capillary** \kap′iler′ē\ [L *capill(us)* a hair, the hair of the head, the filaments of plants + -ARY] 1 Hairlike or pertaining to a hair. 2 Having a lumen of very small size: said of vessels and tubes. 3 Pertaining to the dynamics of liquids in very small vessels or tubes, as *capillary attraction.* 4 A vessel, especially a blood or lymph vessel, of the smallest size. 5 VAS CAPILLARE. **arterial c.** METARTERIOLE. **arteriolar c.** METARTERIOLE. **bile c.** CANALICULUS BILIFER. **glomerular c.** One of the blood capillaries contained within the renal glomerulus. **junctional c.** METARTERIOLE. **lymphatic c.** One of the numerous hairlike vessels in most tissues, the wall of which consists of a single layer of endothelial cells, that form a network draining the lymph and join each other to form larger vessels by adding connective tissue coats to the endothelium. It resembles a blood capillary but the basement membrane is often absent. In different tissues its structure and the size of its lumen may vary. Also *lymph capillary, serous canal.* **Meigs capillaries** Capillaries situated in the myocardium. **peritubular c.** One of the capillary blood vessels connecting the descending and ascending vasa recti of the renal medulla. These capillaries lie between and around the loops of Henle and collecting ducts, and they are lined by a fenestrated endothelium. **secretory capillaries** A narrow channel between two adjacent secretory cells that carries the secretion to the main ductular system. **sinusoidal capillaries** Large capillaries, usually more than 10 $\mu$m wide, that anastomose irregularly with each other and have thin walls without adventitia. They are normally found in many organs, including liver, adrenal and spleen. **venous c.** A minute vessel that drains a capillary network and joins other venous capillaries to form venules. Also *postcapillary, venula postcapillaris.*

**capilli** \kapil′ī\ [See CAPILLUS.] (*sing.* capillus) [NA] The hair of the scalp.

**capillovenous** \kap′ilōvē′nəs\ Involving or connecting capillaries and veins.

**capillus** \kapil′əs\ [L (possibly irreg. from *cap(itis)* of the head + *pilus* a hair) a hair, filament, hair of the head] Singular of CAPILLI.

**capistration** \kap′istrā′shən\ [L *capistratus,* past part. of *capistrare* to muzzle] PHIMOSIS.

**capita** \kap′itə\ Plural of CAPUT.

**capital** [L *capital(is)* (from *caput,* gen. *capitis,* the head + *-alis* -AL) pertaining to the head] 1 Of or relating to the head. 2 Pertaining to the head of the femur.

**capitate** \kap′itāt\ 1 Head-shaped; possessing a rounded end. 2 OS CAPITATUM.

**capitatum** \kap′itā′təm\ OS CAPITATUM.

**capitellum** \kap′itel′əm\ [Late L, a little head, dim. of L *caput* the head] CAPITULUM HUMERI.

**capitula** \kapit′yələ\ Plural of CAPITULUM.

**capitular** \kapit′yələr\ Of or pertaining to a capitulum.

**capitulum** \kəpit′yələm\ [L (dim. of *caput* head), a little head] 1 A small head or small rounded eminence on a bone for articulation with another bone. 2 CAPITULUM HUMERI. **c. costae** CAPUT COSTAE. **c. fibulae** CAPUT FIBULAE. **c. humeri** [NA] The globular portion of the humeral condyle, located on the anterior and inferior aspects of the distal extremity of the humerus, lateral to the trochlea and medial to the lateral epicondyle. It articulates with the concavity on the proximal aspect of the head of the radius to form the humeroradial joint. Also *capitulum of humerus, capitellum, capitulum, little head of humerus, eminence of humerus.* **c. mallei** CAPUT MALLEI. **c. processus condyloidei mandibulae** CAPUT MANDIBULAE. **c. ulnae** CAPUT ULNAE.

**Caplan** [Anthony *Caplan,* British physician, 1907–1976] Caplan's nodules. See under CAPLAN SYNDROME.

**capno-** \kap′nō-\ [Gk *kapnos* smoke] A combining form

meaning (1) smoke; (2) carbon dioxide. Also *capn-*.
**capnohepatography** \kap′nōhep′ətäg′rəfē\ [CAPNO- + HEPATOGRAPHY] Radiography of the liver containing gas in its vascular tributaries after the intravenous administration of carbon dioxide. This procedure is seldom used.
**capnophilic** \-fil′ik\ [CAPNO- + -PHILIC] Growing best with added carbon dioxide; said of bacteria.
**capobenate sodium** The sodium salt of capobenic acid. It has antiarrhythmic properties.
**capobenic acid** $C_{16}H_{23}NO_6$. 6-[(3,4,5-Trimethoxybenzoyl)amino]hexanoic acid. A white, odorless powder, practically insoluble in water. The pharmacologic properties of its sodium salt have been studied, and in this form it has antiarrhythmic properties.
**capping** Localization to the polar areas of a cell surface of membrane determinants that had been evenly distributed on the cell surface before interaction with specific antigen. This step follows patching and usually precedes internalization of the surface components. **pulp c.** The covering of an exposed pulp with inert or therapeutic material to maintain its vitality.
**Capps** [Joseph Almarin *Capps*, U.S. physician, 1872–1964] Capps sign. See under REFLEX.
**capreomycin** An antibiotic isolated from certain strains of *Streptomyces capreolus.* It has antitubercular properties with bacteriostatic and bacteriocidal activity.
**capreomycin sulfate** The sulfate salt of the antibiotic capreomycin.
**capric acid** $CH_3—[CH_2]_8—COOH$. Decanoic acid. It is one of the natural fatty acids, but of slightly shorter chain length than those predominating in most natural lipids.
**capriloquism** \kapril′əkwizm\ [L *capr(a)* she-goat + *i* + *loqu(i)* to speak + -ISM] EGOPHONY.
**caproic acid** *Outmoded* HEXANOIC ACID. • This name has been abandoned because of its similarity with the names *capric* and *caprylic acids.*
**caprylic acid** *Outmoded* OCTANOIC ACID.
**caps-** \kaps-\ [L *capsa* chest, box] A combining form meaning box, boxlike. Also *kaps-*.
**capsaicin** $C_{18}H_{27}O_3N$. A crystalline substance, the pungent principle of the oleoresin found in capsicum. It may cause contact dermatitis.
**capsicin** An oleoresin obtained from capsicums. It is used as the active ingredient in external counterirritants, and in dilute forms internally as a carminative agent.
**capsicism** The habitual use of capsicum.
**capsicum** \kap′sikəm\ The dried fruit of various species of *Capsicum* of the Solanaceae family. Varieties of *C. annuum* include Bombay and Natal capsicums, Louisiana sport pepper, paprika, and tabasco pepper. *C. frutescens* yields African chillies and Cayenne pepper. A tincture of the fruit is used as a carminative. The irritant value of the dried fruits originates with their pungent phenolic constituent capsaisin. Capsicum is used externally as an ointment, plaster, or medicated wool in which it serves as a counterirritant, and in poultices to relieve toothache.
**capsid** The protein coat of a virion, composed of large multimeric proteins, which closely surrounds the nucleic acid. The capsid is constructed by assembling its component capsomeres according to a rigorous geometric pattern. The number of capsomeres in any one capsid depends on the shape of that capsid and is dictated by the laws of crystallography. Thus, icosahedral capsids may contain 12, 32, 42, 79, 92 . . ., but no intermediate numbers of capsomeres.
**capsomere** An oligomeric protein subunit of a viral capsid, comprising five or six monomers in pentagonal and hexagonal capsomeres, respectively. In either type, the monomers form polygonal rings with central holes of diameter as large as about 40 Å.
**capsotomy** \kapsät′əmē\ CAPSULOTOMY.
**capsul-** \kap′s^yəl-\ [L *capsula* (dim. of *capsa* a chest, box) a little chest or box] A combining form meaning a capsule. Also *capsuli-, capsulo-*.
**capsula** \kap′s^yələ\ [L (dim. of *capsa* a chest, box), a little chest or box] (*pl.* capsulae) **1** A fatty, fibrous, cartilaginous or membranous tissue that covers, connects, or envelops a structure, organ, or part. Also *capsule.* **2** TUNICA ADVENTITIA. **c. adiposa** A capsule or sheath composed mostly of fat. **c. adiposa renis** [NA] A layer of fatty tissue completely surrounding the fibrous capsule of the kidney and continuing into the renal sinus through the hilum. Also *adipose capsule of kidney, adipose capsule, fatty capsule of kidney.* **c. articularis** [NA] A sleevelike sac attached to the circumference of the articular margins of the component bones of a synovial joint, enclosing, usually completely, the joint cavity. It may be loose or tight, permitting free movement, and is strengthened by surrounding ligaments or accessory bands. The wall of the capsule comprises two layers, an outer fibrous membrane (membrana fibrosa) and an inner synovial membrane (membrana synovialis). Also *articular capsule, joint capsule, synovial capsule.* **c. articularis coxae** The strong but loose ligamentous sac that is firmly attached some distance from the acetabulum and its lip, except anteriorly at the outer margin of the labrum, while inferiorly it is joined to the transverse ligament and adjacent bone as far as the obturator membrane. Also *capsule of hip joint, capsular ligament of hip joint.* **c. articularis cricoarytenoidea** [NA] The loose synovium lined sac attached to the margins of the articular surfaces between the cricoid cartilage and the arytenoid cartilage. Also *cricoarytenoid articular capsule.* **c. articularis cricothyroidea** [NA] The synovium lined sac attached to the margins of the thyroid articular surface on the lateral aspect of the cricoid cartilage and the articular surface on the inferior cornu of the thyroid cartilage. Accessory bands strengthen the capsule. Also *cricothyroid articular capsule.* **c. articularis genus** A thin, loose, but strong sac enclosing the cavity of the knee joint and strengthened by strong bands fused with it. Also *capsule of knee joint.* **c. articularis humeri** A loose sac attached to the complete circumference of the glenoid cavity of the scapula beyond the glenoid labrum and to the anatomic neck of the humerus. Also *articular capsule of humerus, articular capsule of shoulder joint.* **c. cordis** PERICARDIUM. **c. externa** [NA] The thin, slightly curved layer of white matter lying between the lateral aspect of the lentiform nucleus and the claustrum. It contains fibers descending from the frontoparietal operculum of theinsula en route to subthalamic areas, and also fibers from the anterior commissure. Also *capsula externa nuclei lentiformis, external capsule.* **c. extrema** [NA] The thin layer of white matter between, and coterminous with, the claustrum and the cortex of the insula. Also *extreme capsule.* **c. fibrosa** A fibrous sheath or capsule surrounding an organ or structure. **c. fibrosa glandulae thyroideae** [NA] A fibrous capsule that encloses the thyroid gland and sends fibers into its substance. It is attached by a loose areolar layer to the visceral fascia. Also *fibrous capsule of thyroid gland, capsula glandulae thyreoideae.* **c. fibrosa perivascularis** [NA] A fibrous sheath surrounding the hepatic triad of the bile duct, the portal vein, and the hepatic artery from the porta hepatis throughout their branchings in the liver. Also *perivascular fibrous capsule, fibrous capsule of liver, Glisson's capsule.* **c. fibrosa renis** [NA] A strong but thin fi-

brous membrane enveloping the surface of the kidney, dividing at the hilum into two layers, one penetrating the hilum to line the walls of the renal sinus, and the other ensheathing the vessels and nerves before they enter the hilum. The fibrous capsule is surrounded by the adipose capsule. Also *fibrous capsule of kidney, tunica fibrosa renis* (outmoded), *perinephric capsule.* **c. glandulae thyreoideae** CAPSULA FIBROSA GLANDULAE THYROIDEAE. **c. glomeruli** The spherical, expanded commencement of a renal tubule, the wall of which is invaginated by a small glomerulus of convoluted capillary blood vessels. Between the glomerulus (adherent to the inner layer) and the outer layer of the capsule is the urinary space continuous with the lumen of the proximal convoluted tubule. Also *capsule of glomerulus, Bowman's capsule, glomerular capsule.* **c. interna** [NA] A massive, fan-shaped, and laterally concave tract formed by afferent and efferent fibers converging from widespread areas of the cerebral cortex to form the cerebral peduncle. The lentiform nucleus fills the hollow, being separated by the anterior limb of the capsule from the head of the caudate nucleus, and by its posteroinferior parts from the thalamus. Also *internal capsule.* **c. lentis** [NA] LENS CAPSULE.

**capsulae** \kap′sʸəlē\ Plural of CAPSULA.

**capsular** \kap′sʸələr\ Pertaining to, resembling, or belonging to a capsule.

**capsulation** The packaging of a medication in a capsule of gelatin or some other soluble material.

# capsule

**capsule** \kap′sʸəl\ [L *capsula.* See CAPSULA.] **1** A gelatinous sheath containing a dose of a drug. **2** CAPSULA. **3** In radiotherapy, a small metallic tube, 1–2 cm in length, in which is sealed a radioactive substance such as radium or cesium 137. It is applied to the body surface or within body cavities. **4** A loose, gelatinous layer surrounding certain bacteria, having a sharply defined or a diffuse boundary. Most bacterial capsules are made of polysaccharides with short repeating units, but some are polypeptides. In many pathogens the capsules antagonize phagocytosis and are essential for virulence. **accessory adrenal c.'s** GLANDULAE SUPRARENALES ACCESSORIAE. **acoustic c.** OTIC CAPSULE. **adherent c.** A sac surrounding and inseparable from the surface of an organ or part. **adipose c. 1** An enveloping sac composed mostly of fatty tissue. **2** CAPSULA ADIPOSA RENIS. **adipose c. of kidney** CAPSULA ADIPOSA RENIS. **adrenal c.** GLANDULA SUPRARENALIS. **anthrax c.** A polypeptide of D-glutamic acid, formed by *Bacillus anthracis* under elevated $CO_2$ concentration. **articular c.** CAPSULA ARTICULARIS. **articular c. of humerus** CAPSULA ARTICULARIS HUMERI. **articular c. of shoulder joint** CAPSULA ARTICULARIS HUMERI. **atrabiliary c.** GLANDULA SUPRARENALIS. **auditory c.** OTIC CAPSULE. **biopsy c.** A capsule or tabletlike device that is ingested and, when passing through the small intestine, excises and retains a small amount of jejunal mucosa for analysis after the device has passed through the fecal stream. This remains an experimental technique. **Bonnet's c.** The anterior portion of vagina bulbi. **Bowman's c.** CAPSULA GLOMERULI. **brood c.** One of the daughter colonies floating in hydatid fluid within the primary hydatid cyst. **cartilage c.** A condensation of cartilaginous matrix around a lacuna. **cartilaginous ear c.** CAPSULE OF THE LABYRINTH. **cricoarytenoid articular c.** CAPSULA ARTICULARIS CRICOARYTENOIDEA. **cricothyroid articular c.** CAPSULA ARTICULARIS CRICOTHYROIDEA. **Crosby c.** A peroral instrument for intestinal mucosa biopsy. It consists of a cylindrical capsule that holds by suction a portion of mucosa, which is cut off by a spring-activated knife. **crystalline c.** *Outmoded* LENS CAPSULE. **decavitamin c.** A capsule that contains at least 1.2 mg of vitamin A, 10 μg of vitamin D, 70 mg of ascorbic acid, 10 mg of calcium pantothenate, 1 μg of cyanocobalamin, 50 μg of folic acid, 20 mg of niacinamide, 2 mg of pyridoxine hydrochloride, 2 mg of riboflavin, 2 mg of thiamine hydrochloride or equivalent thiamine mononitrate, and an appropriate form of α-tocopherol. It is used as a multivitamin dietary supplement. **dental c.** PERIODONTIUM. **enteric c.** A capsule resistant to digestion under the acidic conditions of the stomach and intended to be digested in the intestine. **external c.** CAPSULA EXTERNA. **extreme c.** CAPSULA EXTREMA. **fatty c. of kidney** CAPSULA ADIPOSA RENIS. **fibrous articular c.** MEMBRANA FIBROSA CAPSULAE ARTICULARIS. **fibrous c. of corpora cavernosa of penis** TUNICA ALBUGINEA CORPORUM CAVERNOSORUM. **fibrous c. of graafian follicle** THECA EXTERNA. **fibrous c. of kidney** CAPSULA FIBROSA RENIS. **fibrous c. of liver 1** CAPSULA FIBROSA PERIVASCULARIS. **2** TUNICA FIBROSA HEPATIS. **fibrous c. of spleen** TUNICA FIBROSA SPLENIS. **fibrous c. of testis** TUNICA ALBUGINEA TESTIS. **fibrous c. of thyroid gland** CAPSULA FIBROSA GLANDULAE THYROIDEAE. **formalized c.** An enteric capsule prepared by dipping in formaldehyde solution and then drying. Also *glutoid capsule.* **Glisson's c. 1** CAPSULA FIBROSA PERIVASCULARIS. **2** TUNICA FIBROSA HEPATIS. **glomerular c.** CAPSULA GLOMERULI. **c. of glomerulus** CAPSULA GLOMERULI. **glutoid c.** FORMALIZED CAPSULE. **c. of heart** PERICARDIUM. **hepatobiliary c.** CAPSULA FIBROSA PERIVASCULARIS. **hexavitamin c.** A multivitamin capsule containing not less than 1.5 mg of vitamin A, 10 μg of vitamin D, 75 mg of ascorbic acid, 2 mg of thiamine hydrochloride or the equivalent thiamine mononitrate, 3 mg of riboflavin, and 20 mg of niacinamide. It is used as a dietary supplement. **c. of hip joint** CAPSULA ARTICULARIS COXAE. **internal c.** CAPSULA INTERNA. **joint c.** CAPSULA ARTICULARIS. **c. of knee joint** CAPSULA ARTICULARIS GENUS. **c. of the labyrinth** The cartilaginous shell which, in the embryo, differentiates in the mesenchyme which surrounds the epithelial labyrinth. It develops into the bony labyrinth of the adult. Also *cartilaginous ear capsule.* **lens c.** The transparent, elastic membrane closely surrounding the lens, thicker in front than behind. The fibers of the ciliary zonule are attached to it, in front and behind the equator of the lens. In the embryo, it is the mesoderm immediately adjacent to the developing lens. By the second month of human development it becomes vascularized and is called the vascular capsule of the lens, the anterior portion being termed the pupillary membrane. The posterior part is supplied by the hyaloid artery and the anterior part by the anterior ciliary artery. The vessels of the lens capsule normally atrophy before birth but vascularization may persist in certain forms of congenital cataract. Also *capsula lentis, phacocyst, periphacus, periphakus.* **nasal c.** The cartilages that surround the embryonic nasal region and that develop into the bones and cartilages of the nose. Also *olfactory capsule.* **olfactory c.** NASAL CAPSULE. **optic c.** The embryonic precursor of the sclera of the eye. **otic c.** A mesodermal condensation which surrounds the otocyst, or membranous labyrinth, of the internal ear. It chondrifies and finally ossifies to contribute to the petrous temporal bone. Also *acoustic capsule, auditory capsule.* **perinephric c.** CAPSULA FIBROSA RENIS. **periotic c.** The mesenchyme surrounding the embryonic otocyst. At first it is relatively dense and becomes chondrified. With increase in size of the membranous labyrinth, the adjacent part of the cartilage becomes dedifferentiated to form loose, periotic bone. Eventually periotic, or perilymphatic, spaces appear in this tissue and come to surround the membranous labyrinth. **perivascular fibrous c.** CAPSULA FIBROSA PERIVASCULARIS. **radiotelemetry c.** ENDORADIOSONDE. **serous c. of spleen** TUNICA SEROSA SPLENIS. **sympathoblastic c.** A grouping of sympathoblasts (sympathicoblasts) which are sited at the periphery of a central acidophilic zone formed by their intertwined fibrillar processes. This type of histologic appearance is often seen in the sympathetic nervous system of the embryo, and in sympathoblastomas. According to some authors, sympathoblastic capsules can also be encountered in nephroblastomas. **synovial c.** **1** CAPSULA ARTICULARIS. **2** MEMBRANA SYNOVIALIS CAPSULAE ARTICULARIS. **telemetry c.** ENDORADIOSONDE. **Tenon's c.** VAGINA BULBI. **c. of thymus** A delicate layer of fibrous tissue that surrounds each lobe of the thymus and sends septa inwards to incompletely divide the lobe into irregular lobules.

**capsulectomy** \kap′sʸəlek′təmē\ [*capsul(e)* + -ECTOMY] The surgical excision of a capsule. **renal c.** Excision of a renal capsule.

**capsuli-** \kap′sʸəli-\ CAPSUL-.

**capsulitis** \kap′sʸəlī′tis\ [*capsul(a)* + -ITIS] Inflammation of a capsule, as the capsule of a joint or a lens. **adhesive c.** Marked restriction of joint motion due to fibrosis in an area of prior capsulitis, most commonly seen in the shoulder. Also *adhesive bursitis.* **hepatic c.** PERIHEPATITIS.

**capsulo-** \kap′sʸələ-\ CAPSUL-.

**capsuloplasty** \kap′sʸələplas′tē\ [CAPSULO- + -PLASTY] An operation to repair, reduce, or change the shape of a joint capsule, or to replace a missing part or all of a joint capsule.

**capsulorrhaphy** \kap′sʸəlôr′əfē\ [CAPSULO- + -RRHAPHY] The repair of a torn joint capsule by suturing, especially to prevent recurring dislocations.

**capsulotome** \kap′sʸələtōm′\ [CAPSULO- + -TOME] A surgical instrument for cutting the capsule of the crystalline lens.

**capsulotomy** \kap′sʸəlät′əmē\ [CAPSULO- + -TOMY] The incision of the capsule of a structure, as of a joint to gain access to the joint or to relieve contracture or, of the lens as part of a cataract operation. Also *capsotomy.* **renal c.** Incision of a renal capsule.

**captodiamine hydrochloride** A sedative and muscle relaxant agent used in the treatment of anxiety and tension. Also *captodiame hydrochloride.*

**captopril** $C_9H_{15}NO_3S$. 1-(3-Mercapto-2-methyl-1-oxopropyl)-L-proline. The first orally active angiotensin converting enzyme inhibitor developed. It is used in the treatment of hypertension and congestive heart failure. Side effects include bone marrow suppression, rash, and fever.

**capture** **1** The trapping and retention by an atomic nucleus of an additional particle, such as an orbital electron in one form of isobaric decay or a neutron in a reactor. Capture often causes instability, with consequent decay, fission, or gamma radiation. **2** The trapping and retention by an atom or ion of an additional electron, either from a free condition or from another atom or ion. **ventricular c.** The normally conducted heart beat which ends a period of atrioventricular dissociation.

**caput** \kap′ət\ [L (akin to prehistoric Germanic *haubud-*; Old English *hēafod*) head] **1** The upper extremity of the human body, consisting of cranium and face, and containing the brain, and the organs of vision, smell, taste and hearing; the head. **2** The proximal, anterior, or superior extremity, usually expanded or globular, of any body, organ, part, or structure. **3** CAPUT MUSCULI. **c. breve musculi bicipitis brachii** [NA] The short head of the biceps brachii muscle that arises by a flat tendon from the tip of the coracoid process of scapula, together with the coracobrachialis muscle. Also *short head of biceps brachii muscle, medial head of biceps brachii muscle, coracoradialis.* **c. breve musculi bicipitis femoris** [NA] The short head of the biceps femoris muscle that arises by tendinous fibers from the lateral lip of the linea aspera of femur, the proximal two-thirds of the lateral supracondylar ridge, and the lateral intermuscular septum. It joins the long head in a common tendon of insertion. Also *short head of biceps femoris muscle.* **c. coli** CAECUM. **c. costae** [NA] The expanded vertebral, or posterior, extremity of a rib, usually having two convex articular facets separated by a crest. The first, tenth, eleventh, and twelfth ribs usually have only a single facet that articulates with a single vertebra. Also *head of rib, capitulum costae.* **c. deformatum** COXA PLANA. **c. distortum** TORTICOLLIS. **c. epididymidis** [NA] The expanded upper extremity of the epididymis that rests upon the superior pole of the testis, with which it is directly connected by the efferent ductules of the testis. Also *head of epididymis.* **c. fibulae** [NA] The expanded, rounded proximal extremity of the fibula, having a medial circular surface that articulates with the lateral condyle of the tibia and a pointed apex posteriorly for the attachment of the arcuate popliteal ligament and part of the tendon of the biceps femoris muscle. Also *head of fibula, capitulum fibulae.* **c. galeatum** A fetal head that is covered with a caul at the time of birth. **c. humerale musculi flexoris carpi ulnaris** [NA] The humeral head of the flexor carpi ulnaris muscle, arising from the common flexor tendon on the lower anterior surface of the medial epicondyle of the humerus. Also *humeral head of flexor carpi ulnaris muscle.* **c. humerale musculi flexoris digitorum sublimis** CAPUT HUMEROULNARE MUSCULI FLEXORIS DIGITORUM SUPERFICIALIS. **c. humerale musculi pronatoris teretis** [NA] The humeral head of the pronator teres muscle, arising from the upper half of the anterior surface of the medial epicondyle of the humerus, the medial intermuscular septum, and the overlying deep fascia. Also *humeral head of pronator teres muscle.* **c. humeri** [NA] The nearly hemispherical proximal extremity of the humerus, directed medially, posteriorly, and superiorly to articulate with the glenoid cavity of the scapula. Also *head of humerus.* **c. humeroulnare musculi flexoris digitorum superficialis** [NA] The humeroulnar head of the flexor digitorum superficialis muscle that arises from the common tendon on the medial epicondyle of the humerus, the medial border of the coronoid process of ulna, and the ulnar collateral ligament, and from the intermuscular septum between it and overlying muscles. It is continuous with and fused to the fleshy radial head, forming a common belly. Also *caput humerale musculi flexoris digitorum sublimis, humeral head of flexor digitorum sublimis muscle, humeroulnar head of flexor digitorum superficialis.* **c. laterale musculi gastrocnemii** [NA] The lateral head of the gastrocnemius muscle, arising from the lateral surface of the lateral condyle of the femur and a portion of the adjacent lateral supracondylar line, as well as from the capsule of the knee joint. An aponeurosis develops on its posterior surface, and it remains separate from the medial head until they join the soleus muscle to form the tendo calcaneus. Occasionally the lateral head may be absent. Also *lateral head of gastrocnemius muscle.* **c. laterale musculi tricipitis brachii** [NA] The lateral head of the triceps brachii muscle, arising by a flattened tendon from the upper lateral portion of the posterior surface of the humerus, from the point of insertion of the teres minor muscle down to the radial groove at the lateral border of the humerus, the fibers converging toward the common tendon of insertion. Also *lateral head of triceps brachii muscle, lateral head of triceps muscle.* **c. longum musculi bicipitis brachii** [NA] The long head of the biceps brachii muscle, arising by a bifurcated tendon from the supraglenoid tuberosity and the posterior part of the glenoid labrum of the scapula, passing across the front of the head of the humerus within the capsule of the shoulder joint, and then down the intertubercular groove under the transverse humeral ligament, up to which point the tendon is surrounded by a sheath of synovial membrane. Also *long head of biceps brachii muscle.* **c. longum musculi bicipitis femoris** [NA] The long head of the biceps femoris muscle, arising by a tendon common to it and the semitendinosus muscle from the inferomedial facet on the upper area of the ischial tuberosity, and from the sacrotuberous ligament. Also *long head of biceps femoris muscle.* **c. longum musculi tricipitis brachii** [NA] The long head of the triceps brachii, arising by a flat tendon from the infraglenoid tuberosity of the scapula and partly attached to the capsule of the shoulder joint. The muscle fibers descend superficial to the medial head and medial to the lateral head to fuse with them in a common tendon of insertion. Also *long head of triceps brachii muscle, long head of triceps muscle, medial head of triceps muscle.* **c. mallei** [NA] The rounded upper extremity of the malleus, located in the epitympanic recess and articulating posteriorly with the incus. Also *head of malleus, capitulum mallei.* **c. mandibulae** [NA] The oval proximal expansion of the condylar process of the mandible, having its long axis transverse to the ramus and covered by fibrocartilage for articulation with the mandibular fossa and the intervening fibrous articular disk. Also *head of mandible, capitulum processus condyloidei mandibulae, head of condyloid process of mandible.* **c. mediale musculi gastrocnemii** [NA] The medial head of the gastrocnemius muscle, arising above and posterior to the medial condyle of femur, from an area on the popliteal surface of the femur just above and from the capsule of the knee joint. Also *medial head of gastrocnemius muscle.* **c. mediale musculi tricipitis brachii** [NA] The medial head of the triceps brachii muscle that arises from the triangular area on the posterior surface of the humerus below the radial groove and from the medial and lateral intermuscular septa. Also *medial head of triceps brachii muscle.* **c. metacarpalis** [NA] The rounded, distal extremity of a metacarpal bone that is covered with cartilage for articulation with the base of the proximal phalanx. A prominent tubercle and fossa are located on each side of the head for the attachment of a collateral ligament of the metacarpophalangeal joint. The prominence of the knuckles is produced by the metacarpal heads. Also *head of metacarpal bone.* **c. metatarsale** [NA] The expanded convex distal extremity of a metatarsal bone, the articular surface of which extends further on the plantar than on the dorsal surface. The sides of the head are flattened, but have a tubercle and depression for the attachment of a collateral ligament of the metatarsophalangeal joint. Also *head of metatarsal bone.* **c. musculi** [NA] The tendinous or fleshy attachment of origin of a muscle, usually to the least movable bone in a particular movement, especially where there is more than one site of origin producing more than one such tendinous or fleshy portion of that muscle. Also *head of muscle, caput.* **c. obliquum musculi adductoris hallucis** [NA] The oblique head of the adductor hallucis muscle that arises from the bases of the second, third, and fourth metatarsal bones and from the sheath of the peroneus longus muscle. Its medial part blends with the flexor hallucis brevis and is attached to the lateral sesamoid of the big toe, while the lateral part joins the transverse head for attachment to the lateral sesamoid and the base of the first phalanx of the big toe. Also *oblique head of adductor hallucis muscle.* **c. obliquum musculi adductoris pollicis** [NA] The oblique head of the adductor pollicis muscle that arises from the flexor retinaculum, the capitate bone, and the bases of the second and third metacarpals. It converges on the transverse head to form a tendon that is inserted into the ulnar side of the base of the proximal phalanx of the thumb. Also *oblique head of adductor pollicis muscle.* **c. ossis femoris** [NA] The smooth, globular hemisphere at the proximal extremity of the femur that articulates with the acetabulum. It is covered with articular cartilage except at the fovea capitis femoris, where the ligament of the head of femur is attached. Also *head of femur, head of thigh bone.* **c. pancreatis** [NA] The expanded right extremity of the pancreas, which is flattened anteroposteriorly and situated within the concavity of the duodenum. The inferior and left part is curved posterior to the superior mesenteric vessels to form the uncinate process. Posteriorly the head is demarcated on the left by the formation of the portal vein, by the superior mesenteric and splenic veins. This surface is also grooved by the bile duct and related mainly to the inferior vena cava behind it. Also *head of pancreas.* **c. phalangis digitorum manus** [NA] Any of the slightly expanded distal articular extremities of the proximal and middle phalanges of the medial four fingers and the proximal phalanx of the thumb. They resemble pulleys, grooved in the center and elevated at each side, and articulate with the base of the more distal phalanx. Also *head of phalanx of fingers.* **c. phalangis digitorum pedis** [NA] Any of the slightly expanded, pulley-shaped distal extremities of the proximal and middle phalanges of the lateral four toes and the proximal phalanx of the hallux. Each articulates with the base of the adjoining, more distal phalanx. Also *head of phalanx of toes.* **c. planum** COXA PLANA. **c. quadratum** An abnormally shaped, angular head owing to frontal and parietal skull bosses. It is sometimes seen in rickets. **c. radiale musculi flexoris digitorum superficialis** [NA] The radial head of the flexor digitorum superficialis muscle that arises from the anterior oblique line and lower part of the anterior border of the radius. Also *radial head of flexor digitorum superficialis muscle.* **c. radii** [NA] The expanded, disklike proximal extremity of the radius, having a depression superiorly for articulation with the capitulum of the humerus, and an articular circumference that is wider medially, for articulation with the radial notch of the ulna, while the rest is surrounded by the proximal part of the annular ligament. Also *head of radius.* **c. stapedis** [NA] The laterally-directed, rounded projection of the stapes, connected by its neck to the two crura and having a cartilage-covered depression for articulation with the lentiform process of the incus. Also *head of stapes.* **c. succedaneum** A caplike projection on the fetal scalp due to edema secondary to pressure during labor. Also *sang-*

*uineous boss.* **c. tali** [NA] The large, rounded anterior end of the talus. Also *head of talus, head of astragalus.* **c. transversum musculi adductoris hallucis** [NA] The transverse head of the adductor hallucis muscle that arises from the capsules of the third, fourth, and fifth metatarsophalangeal joints and joins the tendon of insertion of the oblique head into the base of the proximal phalanx of the big toe. Also *transverse head of adductor hallucis muscle.* **c. transversum musculi adductoris pollicis** [NA] The transverse head of the adductor pollicis muscle that arises from the palmar ridge of the third metacarpal bone and from the deep palmar fascia. It is inserted with the oblique head by a tendon into the ulnar side of the base of the proximal phalanx of the thumb. Also *transverse head of adductor pollicis muscle.* **c. ulnae** [NA] The small, rounded articular process at the distal end of the ulna that lies adjacent to its styloid process, the articular disk being attached between the two, thereby excluding the inferior flat surface of the head from the radiocarpal joint. The articular circumference of the head fits into the ulnar notch of the radius to form the distal radioulnar joint. Also *head of ulna, capitulum ulnae.* **c. ulnare musculi flexoris carpi ulnaris** [NA] The ulnar head of the flexor carpi ulnaris muscle that arises from the medial side of the olecranon, the upper two-thirds of the posterior border of the ulna, and the intermuscular septum between it and flexor digitorum superficialis. Also *ulnar head of flexor carpi ulnaris muscle.* **c. ulnare musculi pronatoris teretis** [NA] The ulnar head of the pronator teres muscle that arises from the medial side of the coronoid process of the ulna and joins the humeral head at an acute angle. Also *ulnar head of pronator teres muscle, coronoid head of pronator teres muscle.*

**Carabelli** [Georg C. *Carabelli*, Austrian dentist, 1787–1842] Carabelli tubercle. See under CUSP.

**caramiphen edisylate** $C_{38}H_{60}N_2O_{10}S_2$. 1-Phenylcyclobentanecarboxylic acid 2-(diethylamino)ethyl ester 1,2-ethanedisulfonate (2:1), a weak anticholinergic drug used as an antitussive agent. It is given orally.

**caramiphen hydrochloride** $C_{18}H_{27}NO_2 \cdot HCl$. 2-Diethylaminoethyl-1-phenyl-cyclopentane-1-carboxylate hydrochloride. A white, crystalline powder with a slight odor and a bitter taste. It is a weak anticholinergic agent, and is used as a spasmolytic drug for diseases of the basal ganglia, such as parkinsonism.

**carat** [Arabic *qīrāt* (from Gk *keration* fruit of the locust tree, carob) a bean, weight of four grains] *Popular* METRIC CARAT. **metric c.** A unit of mass or weight equal to $2 \times 10^{-4}$ kilogram, or 200 milligrams: used especially for commercial dealings in precious stones, diamonds, and pearls. Also *carat* (popular). Symbol: MC (British usage)

**carate** \keräʹtē\ PINTA.

**carbachol** $C_6H_{15}ClN_2O_2$. 2-[(aminocarbonyl)oxy]-*N,N,N*-trimethylethanaminium chloride. A hygroscopic, crystalline powder with cholinergic properties. It has been applied topically to the conjunctiva for the treatment of glaucoma. Also *choline chloride carbamate, carbamylcholine, carbocholine.*

**carbamate** A salt or ester of carbamic acid containing the $NH_2COO$ group. The esters are urethanes and are hypnotics.

**carbamazepine** $C_{15}H_{12}N_2O$. 5-Carbamoyl-5*H*-dibenz[*b,f*]azepine. An effective anticonvulsant drug for the treatment of generalized tonic-clonic seizures and for partial seizures with complex symtomatology. It resembles phenytoin in its anticonvulsant spectrum of activity.

**carbamide** *Obs.* UREA.

**carbamino** An unstable complex of carbon dioxide with an amine R—$NH_2$ to form R—NH—COOH.

**carbaminohemoglobin** The normal complex of hemoglobin with carbon dioxide that transports carbon dioxide in the blood by the reversible formation of —NH—$CO_2^-$ at the terminal amino groups of hemoglobin.

**carbamoyl** The group $NH_2$—CO—. Also *carbamyl.*

**carbamoylaspartic acid** $NH_2$—CO—NH—CH(COOH)—$CH_2$—COOH. A compound formed by the reaction between aspartate and carbamoyl phosphate in the pathway of pyrimidine biosynthesis. The enzyme responsible, aspartate carbamoyltransferase, is inhibited allosterically by CTP and is therefore active only when pyrimidines are needed by the organism.

**carbamoylation** \kärbamʹō·ilāʹshən\ The reaction of the N-terminal valine of hemoglobin with cyanate, resulting in attachment of the carbamoyl group to the amino group of valine. Carbamoylation of hemoglobin S prevents it from sickling when deoxygenated.

**carbamoyl phosphate** $NH_2$—CO—O—$PO_3H_2$. The donor of carbamoyl groups in the formation of citrulline during urea biosynthesis and in the formation of *N*-carbamoyl aspartate during pyrimidine biosynthesis.

**carbamoyl-phosphate synthetase** Any enzyme that forms carbamoyl phosphate with the concomitant hydrolysis of ATP. Two such enzymes are known: one (EC 6.3.4.16) uses ammonia and carbon dioxide as substrates and is responsible for the synthesis in mammalian liver mitochondria which leads to urea formation; the other (EC 6.3.5.5) uses glutamine and carbon dioxide, and is involved in the synthesis of carbamoyl phosphate that occurs in bacteria as a step in pyrimidine biosynthesis.

**carbamoyltransferase** Any enzyme that transfers the carbamoyl group —CO—$NH_2$. One such enzyme, ornithine carbamoyltransferase, is important in the biosynthesis of citrulline from ornithine in the formation of urea. Another, aspartate carbamoyltransferase, is important in the formation of *N*-carbamoylaspartate in the biosynthesis of pyrimidines. Also *transcarbamoylase.*

**carbamyl** CARBAMOYL.

**carbamylcholine** CARBACHOL.

**carbasalate calcium** CALCIUM CARBASPIRIN.

**carbasus** \kärʹbəsəs\ [L, from Gk *karpasos* flax, linen, cotton] Cotton or gauze. *Obs.*

**carbenicillin** $C_{17}H_{18}N_2O_6S$. 6[(Carboxyphenylacetyl)-amino]-3,3-dimethyl-7-oxo-4-thia-1-azabicyclo[3.2.0]heptane-2-carboxylic acid. A broad spectrum, semisynthetic penicillin that is acid-labile and must be given parenterally.

**carbetapentane citrate** $C_{26}H_{39}NO_{10}$. 1-Phenylcyclopentanecarboxylic acid 2-(2-diethylaminoethoxy)ethyl ester citrate salt, an antitussive agent used to treat coughs due to infections of the upper respiratory tract. It is given orally.

**carbidopa** $C_{10}H_{14}N_2O_4 \cdot H_2O$. S-α-Hydrazino-3,4-dihydroxy-α-methylbenzenepropanoic acid monohydrate. A peripheral decarboxylase inhibitor which is given with levodopa to permit more of the latter to cross the blood-brain barrier and to be decarboxylated to dopamine in the brain. It also reduces the degree of peripheral decarboxylation of dopa and the resulting effects of dopamine released there. It is given orally.

**carbimazole** $C_7H_{10}N_2O_2S$. An antithyroid drug consisting of a carbethoxy derivative of methimazole, to which it is metabolized in man.

**carbinol** *Obs.* METHANOL. • This name was used mainly for substituted derivatives.

**carbinoxamine maleate** $C_{20}H_{23}ClN_2O_5$. 2-[(4-Chlorophenyl)-2-pyridinylmethoxy]-*N,N*-dimethylethanamine maleate, an antihistaminic drug that is used to treat allergic conditions. It is given orally.

**carbobenzoxy** BENZYLOXYCARBONYL.

**carbocation** \kär′bəkat′ī′ən\ A cation whose positive charge is located to a significant degree on one or more carbon atoms. Such cations are normally unstable and exist only as reaction intermediates.

**carbochloral** CARBOCLORAL.

**carbocholine** CARBACHOL.

**carbocloral** $C_5H_8Cl_3NO_3$. Ethyl(2,2,2-trichloro-1-hydroxyethyl)carbamate. A hypnotic prepared from chloral and urethane. Also *carbochloral.*

**carbocromen** CHROMONAR HYDROCHLORIDE.

**carbodiimide** HN═C═NH. A substance of which the parent compound is unknown, probably because it tautomerizes to $H_2N$═CN. The substituted carbodiimides R—N═C═N—R are of great importance as coupling agents in synthesizing peptides and phosphate esters. Thus, a carboxylic acid R′—COOH reacts with R—N═C═N—R to form R—N═C(—NH—R)—O—CO—R′ in which the acyl group is reactive and which will react with an amine R″—$NH_2$ to form R′—CO—NH—R″ and a substituted urea R—NH—CO—NH—R.

**carbohydrate** \kär′bəhī′drāt\ Any of the sugars and their condensation products, the oligosaccharides and polysaccharides. They are hydrolyzed by acid to sugars, and have the general formula $C_x(H_2O)_y$. Related compounds may also be classed as carbohydrates. **C c.** An antigen that is extracted from the cell walls of streptococci by hot acid or formamide or enzymatically and is detected in a precipitin reaction. This antigen forms the basis for the Lancefield classification.

**carbolfuchsin** \kär′bəlfook′sin\ A solution of phenol (carbolic acid) and basic fuchsin that is used to stain acid-fast microorganisms. See also ZIEHL-NEELSEN STAIN. **Ziehl-Neelsen c.** ZIEHL-NEELSEN STAIN.

**carbolic acid** *Outmoded* PHENOL.

**carbolism** \kär′bōlizm\ Poisoning from the ingestion of phenol. The average fatal dose is 15 grams but as little as 1.0 gram may cause nausea, vomiting, circulatory collapse, tachypnea, convulsions, and death.

**carbomycin** $C_{42}H_{67}NO_{16}$. An antibiotic chemical derived from the growth media of *Streptomyces halstedii.* It is effective against most Gram-positive bacteria.

**carbon** \kär′bən\ [L *carbo,* gen. *carbonis* (prob. akin to *cremare* to burn, cremate) charcoal] A nonmetallic element having atomic number 6 and atomic weight 12.011. Carbon is widely dispersed in the universe, both native and in compounds. Three allotropes (graphite, diamond, and an amorphous form) exist, and a fourth (so-called white carbon) has been reported. There are seven known isotopes, ranging in mass number from 10 to 16. The most abundant is carbon 12, a stable isotope that forms 98.89% of naturally occurring carbon. The other stable isotope, carbon 13, has a natural abundance of 1.11%. Traces of radioactive carbon 14 occur in the atmosphere as a result of the transmutation of nitrogen by solar radiation. Chemically, carbon has to a unique degree the ability to form long chains and stable rings, giving rise to millions of organic compounds of which living organisms are composed. Valences are 2, 3, and 4. Symbol: C **radioactive c.** Any radioactive isotope of carbon, the most common being carbon 14, with a half-life of 5730 years. Also *radiocarbon.*

**carbon 12** A stable isotope of carbon, comprising 98.89% of naturally occurring carbon. It is used as a standard in certain definitions, as of the mole and the dalton. Symbol: $^{12}C$

**carbon 14** A radioactive isotope of carbon, emitting only beta radiation. The presence of carbon 14 as a component of natural carbon permits the determination of the age of organic fossil matter. It is also used medically in hormone radioassays and to label fats for absorption studies. Physical half-life is 5730 years. Symbol: $^{14}C$

**carbonate** \kär′bənāt\ **1** The ion $CO_3^-$ and salts that contain it. **2** Any anion of which carbon is the central atom. **3** Any ester of carbonic acid.

**carbonate dehydratase** The enzyme (EC 4.2.1.1) that catalyzes the hydration of carbon dioxide to form carbonic acid as well as the reverse reaction. It is a zinc-containing enzyme particularly abundant in blood and in gastric mucosa. Dehydration of carbonic acid is catalyzed in the proximal but not the distal tubules of the kidney. Carbonate dehydratase in the proximal tubule cell brush borders reduces the gradient against which protons are secreted, and thus is important in the reabsorption of bicarbonate. Carbonate dehydratase is inhibited by acetazolamide. It has very great catalytic efficiency, catalyzing the reaction at almost the diffusion-controlled rate limit. Also *carbonic anhydrase.*

**carbon dioxide** O═C═O. The end product of catabolism of most of the carbon ingested by animals. It is used as chief nutrient by green plants in photosynthesis and by photosynthetic and autotrophic bacteria. Relatively small amounts can be used for certain important reactions in animals, many of which are catalyzed by biotin-containing enzymes (as in the carboxylation of acetyl-coenzyme A, methylmalonyl-coenzyme A, and pyruvate) and all of which involve nucleophilic attack on the carbon atom. **solid c.** Carbon dioxide in solid, crystalline form. It does not melt but sublimes at atmospheric pressure at −78.5°, and is used as a coolant. It is also used to treat some types of skin disorders. Also *dry ice.*

**carbonic anhydrase** CARBONATE DEHYDRATASE.

**carbon monoxide** CO. A highly poisonous, odorless, tasteless gas, formed when carbon-containing material burns with restricted access of oxygen. It forms an explosive mixture with air. It is formed biologically from the formyl group of formyltetrahydrofolate in the gas gland of the marine organism the Portuguese man-of-war, and also by some bacteria. It has a high affinity for metal atoms and ions. It is toxic by inhalation since it competes with oxygen in binding with hemoglobin and certain respiratory enzymes, thereby resulting in diminished availability of oxygen in tissues. Also *sweet gas.*

**carbon tetrachloride** $CCl_4$. Tetrachloromethane. It is used as a refrigerant, in fire extinguishers, as a grain fumigant, and in dry cleaning. It is toxic because it damages cell membranes. Its ingestion by humans often results in liver damage. See also CARBON TETRACHLORIDE POISONING.

**carbonyl** The group CO, either when bivalent in an organic compound or occurring (as carbon monoxide) as a ligand to a metal atom.

**carboxybiotin** The form of biotin in many carboxylases after it has reacted with carbon dioxide and ATP with carboxylation of the biotin and hydrolysis of the ATP. The carboxylate group replaces hydrogen on one of the nitrogen atoms of the biotin to form a labile compound which can transfer this group to acceptors.

**carboxydismutase** The original name for RIBULOSE-BISPHOSPHATE CARBOXYLASE.

**γ-carboxyglutamic acid** A tricarboxylic amino acid that is characteristic of the N-terminal region of vitamin K-dependent coagulation factors such as prothrombin, factor VII, factor X, and proteins C, S, and Z. The terminal γ-carboxyglutamic acid is formed by carboxylation of glutamic acid, as a post-translational event, in the presence of vitamin

K. This modification enables these proteins to bind calcium ions. Symbol: Gla

**carboxyhemoglobin** Hemoglobin with carbon monoxide bound to its iron(II) atom. Because the binding is so tight, it is easily formed from hemoglobin at low concentrations of carbon monoxide, so that blood loses its power of carrying oxygen, but it slowly dissociates when carbon monoxide is removed. It has a characteristic cherry-red color.

**carboxyhemoglobinemia** \kärbäk′sēhem′əglō′bin-ē′mē·ə\ An abnormal increase in the amount of carboxyhemoglobin in the blood. *Imprecise.*

**carboxyl** —C(=O)—OH. A group which arises when primary alcohols or aldehydes are oxidized. It occurs in weak acids, of p*K* typically about 5, and is very stable.

**carboxylase** Any enzyme that catalyzes the reaction X—H + $CO_2$ ⇌ X—COOH. Carboxylases may catalyze the reaction directly (as does the phosphoenolpyruvate carboxylase of plants and bacteria, which yields oxaloacetate and inorganic phosphate), or involve *N*-carboxybiotin as intermediate (in which case they concomitantly convert ATP into ADP and orthophosphate).

**carboxylation** The replacement of a hydrogen atom by a carboxyl group. **reductive c.** The process of fixing carbon dioxide by incorporating it in a carboxyl group that is then reduced. In photosynthesis and chemosynthesis, ribulose diphosphate is thus converted to phosphoglyceric acid, and some anaerobic bacteria can convert acetate to pyruvate.

**carboxylesterase** An enzyme that catalyzes the hydrolysis of esters of carboxylic acids (as distinct from esters of other acids, such as phosphoric). Also *aliesterase.*

**carboxylic acid** Any substance that is an acid by virtue of containing a carboxyl group.

**carboxyl-terminal** C-TERMINAL.

**carboxyltransferase** Any enzyme that catalyzes the reaction R—H + R′—COOH → R—COOH + R′—H. The one characterized is methylmalonyl-CoA carboxyltransferase, which contains a biotinyl group to transfer the carbon dioxide and is important in the metabolism of fatty acids with an odd number of carbon atoms.

**carboxy-lyase** Any enzyme catalyzing a reaction of the type R—COOH ⇌ R—H + $CO_2$. Such enzymes include pyruvate decarboxylase (found in plants and microorganisms, which produces acetaldehyde, the precursor of ethanol) and histidine decarboxylase (responsible for histamine formation in higher animals).

**carboxymethyl** The group HOOC—$CH_2$—. It may be introduced into proteins using iodoacetate, when cysteine residues become residues of *S*-carboxymethylcysteine.

**carboxypeptidase** Any enzyme that hydrolyzes the final peptide bond of a peptide or protein and thus releases the amino acid represented in the substrate by a residue with a free carboxyl group. Carboxypeptidases occur among digestive enzymes. They are useful in determining peptide sequences. Carboxypeptidase A is a zinc protein and removes most neutral C-terminal residues, but not proline. Carboxypeptidase B removes C-terminal lysine or arginine.

**carbromal** $C_7H_{13}BrN_2O_2$. *N*-(Aminocarbonyl)-2-bromo-2-ethylbutanamide, a white crystalline powder with sedative properties. It is given orally.

**carbuncle** \kär′bungkl\ [L *carbunculus* (dim. of *carbo* coal, charcoal) a small coal, carbuncle] **1** A deep infection of a group of contiguous hair follicles with *Staphylococcus aureus,* accompanied by intense inflammatory changes in the surrounding and underlying tissues, and resulting in the formation of an abscess. **2** A large pustule or abscess from any of various causes, especially cutaneous anthrax. For defs. 1 and 2 also *anthracoma, carbunculus.* **malignant c.** Malignant pustule. See under CUTANEOUS ANTHRAX. **renal c.** RENAL ABSCESS.

**carbunculus** \kärbungk′yələs\ CARBUNCLE.

**carbutamide** 4-Amino-*N*-[(butylamino)-carbonyl]-benzenesulfonamide. It is both a sulfonamide and a urea. It has hypoglycemic action.

**Carcassone** [Bernard Gauderic *Carassone,* French surgeon, flourished 18th century] Carcassone's ligament, perineal ligament of Carcassone. See under MEMBRANA PERINEI.

**carcin-** \kär′sən-\ CARCINO-.

**carcinectomy** \kär′sənek′təmē\ [CARCIN- + -ECTOMY] A surgical procedure in which all or part of an epithelial malignant tumor, or carcinoma, is removed. Also *carcinomectomy, carcinosectomy.*

**carcinemia** \kär′sənē′mē·ə\ CANCEREMIA.

**carcino-** \kär′sənō-\ [Gk *karkinos* crab, cancer] A combining form denoting cancer. Also *carcin-.*

**carcinoembryonic** \-em′brē·än′ik\ [CARCINO- + EMBRYONIC] Relating to features present in both carcinomatous and embryonic tissues, as *carcinoembryonic antigen..*

**carcinogen** \kär′sinōjən\ [CARCINO- + -GEN] A cancer-causing substance or action. **direct-reacting c.** A substance that does not require metabolic activation to be carcinogenic. Direct-reacting carcinogens can be formed in the host from procarcinogens such as nitrosamine. Also *primary carcinogen.*

**carcinogenesis** \-jen′əsis\ [CARCINO- + GENESIS] The causation of cancer.

**carcinogenic** \-jen′ik\ [CARCINO- + -GENIC] Capable of causing cancer. Also *cancerigenic, cancerogenic.*

**carcinogenicity** \-jənis′itē\ [CARCINO- + -GENIC + -ITY] The ability to cause cancer.

**carcinoid** \kär′sinoid\ [CARCIN- + -OID] A tumor of the diffuse endocrine system, derived from Kulchitsky-type cells. The typical or classical carcinoid is also known as the enterochromaffin carcinoid or argentaffinoma because of the strong affinity of the tumor cells for silver, using argentaffin and argyrophil staining techniques. The most frequent site for these tumors is the appendix and, less often, the small intestine and cecum. All carcinoids are considered to be malignant on pathologic grounds, but the malignancies are usually of low grade, particularly in those of the appendix, which may be benign clinically. Carcinoids may produce 5-hydroxytryptamine (serotonin), kallikrein, somatostatin, glucagon, gastrin, etc. Large tumors may be associated with the carcinoid syndrome, (diarrhea, vasomotor changes, and fibrosis of the endocardium). Carcinoids less commonly arise in the bronchus, thymus, stomach, pancreas, and urogenital tract. Also *Kulchitsky cell carcinoma.* **bronchial c.** A carcinoid arising in the wall of a bronchus. • The term *bronchial adenoma* has been used as a synonym but should be discouraged because this tumor is not benign, though it may show a low degree of malignancy. **enterochromaffin c.** The classical carcinoid as found in the appendix and other midgut sites, strongly positive with argentaffin techniques. **G-cell c.** GASTRINOMA.

**carcinology** \kär′sənäl′əjē\ [CARCINO- + -LOGY] *Seldom used* ONCOLOGY.

**carcinolysin** Any chemical or agent that has the capability of destroying cancer cells.

**carcinolysis** \kär′sənäl′isis\ [CARCINO- + LYSIS] Destruction of cancer cells.

**carcinolytic** \-lit′ik\ Capable of destroying cancer cells.

# carcinoma

**carcinoma** \kär′sinō′mə\ [New L, from Gk *karkinōma* a spreading sore, ulcer, cancer, from *karkinos* a crab] (*pl.* carcinomas, carcinomata) A malignant epithelial tumor. This is the most frequent form of cancer. Also *epithelioma.* Adj. carcinomatous. **acinar c.** ACINAR ADENOCARCINOMA. **acinar cell c.** ACINAR ADENOCARCINOMA. **acinous c.** ACINAR ADENOCARCINOMA. **adenoid cystic c.** A malignant tumor having a characteristic cribriform appearance with duct cells and myoepithelial cells arranged around small cystic spaces. It occurs mainly in the salivary glands, including the minor salivary glands of the mouth and upper respiratory tract. The tendency to spread along perivascular and perineural planes makes surgical eradication difficult. Also *adenocystic carcinoma, carcinoma adenoides cysticum, cribriform carcinoma, cylindroma* (outmoded). **adenoid squamous cell c.** A squamous cell carcinoma with glandlike structures. **c. adenomatosum** ADENOCARCINOMA. **adenosquamous c.** A tumor in which adenocarcinomatous and squamous carcinomatous components are both present. Also *adenoepithelioma.* **alveolar cell c.** BRONCHIOLOALVEOLAR CARCINOMA. **c. of the ampulla of Vater** An adenocarcinoma of the mucosa of the ampulla of Vater. It is typically papillary and causes obstruction to bile outflow. **anaplastic c.** 1 A carcinoma with tumor cells showing considerable pleomorphism, hyperbasophilia of nuclei, and numerous, often abnormal, mitoses. • In this sense, the term *anaplastic* can be applied to a differentiated carcinoma, such as an anaplastic squamous cell carcinoma. 2 UNDIFFERENTIATED CARCINOMA. • In this sense it is better to use *undifferentiated* than *anaplastic* owing to confusion with sense 1. **anaplastic thyroid c.** A highly malignant, poorly differentiated neoplasm of the thyroid typically occurring after age 50. It metastasizes early and widely, fails to take up iodine, is stony hard in consistency, and characteristically leads to death within a few months after diagnosis. **apocrine c.** A carcinoma of apocrine glands or apocrine epithelium. **argentaffin c.** The typical form of carcinoid. **c. asbolicum** CHIMNEY SWEEPS' CANCER. **c. of the auricle** Carcinoma arising on or involving the pinna. Two types occur: squamous cell carcinoma and basal cell carcinoma. Except in advanced cases, the treatment is surgical excision. **basal cell c.** A locally invasive, slowly spreading tumor, which rarely metastasizes, arising in the epidermis or hair follicles, and in which, in particular, the peripheral cells usually simulate the basal cells of the epidermis. These tumors are specially common on the faces of elderly persons. A variety of histologic patterns occurs, such as solid, cystic, or adenoid. Keratin and melanin may be present. Subtypes which have been described include the superficial multicentric type, with multiple foci of tumor; morphea type, with small strands embedded in desmoplastic stroma, which may be more aggressive than the other types; and fibroepithelial type, with branching cords of tumor cells surrounding stroma. Also *rodent ulcer, basiloma, basaloma, carcinoma basocellulare, rodent cancer, hair-matrix carcinoma, Krompecher's carcinoma, basal cell epithelioma, Krompecher's tumor.* **basaloid c.** A squamous cell carcinoma with histologic features resembling basal cell carcinoma. It typically occurs at the cloacogenic zone of the anal canal. **c. basocellulare** BASAL CELL CARCINOMA. **basosquamous c.** A carcinoma having histologic features of both basal cell carcinoma and squamous cell carcinoma. Also *basosquamous cell carcinoma, intermediary carcinoma, intermediate-cell carcinoma, metatypical carcinoma, basisquamous epithelioma.* **betel-nut c.** A squamous cell carcinoma of the oral mucosa due to chewing betel nut or a mixture in which betel nut is a component. It is common in parts of Southeast Asia. **branchiogenic c.** Any carcinoma arising from remnants of branchial epithelium, usually squamous cell carcinoma. **bronchioloalveolar c.** An uncommon form of adenocarcinoma of the lung with tall tumor cells lining the alveolar septa usually resulting in a minimum of destruction of parenchyma despite extensive spread of tumor along air spaces. Mucus production by the tumor cells may be considerable. Metastases beyond the lung are usually late in developing. Also *alveolar cell carcinoma, bronchiolar carcinoma, carcinomatoides alveogenica multicentrica.* **burn scar c.** A squamous cell carcinoma developing in a neglected or chronically irritated burn scar. Also *Marjolin's ulcer, warty ulcer.* **cerebriform c.** MEDULLARY CARCINOMA. **chorionic c.** CHORIOCARCINOMA. **clear cell c.** RENAL CELL CARCINOMA. **cloacogenic c.** 1 A carcinoma of cloacal origin. 2 A carcinoma arising in the cloacogenic zone of the anal canal. It may have a variety of growth patterns and cell forms, including basaloid, transitional, and squamous. **colloid c.** MUCINOUS CARCINOMA. **corpus c.** Carcinoma of the body of the uterus. **cribriform c.** 1 ADENOID CYSTIC CARCINOMA. 2 The cribriform pattern of intraductal carcinoma of the breast. • Because of the double usage this term is not recommended. **c. cuniculatum** A well-differentiated, verrucous, hyperkeratotic carcinoma of the skin, typically arising on the sole of the foot in males. Local recurrence is common and can be very extensive. Also *epithelioma cuniculatum.* **cylindric cell c.** An adenocarcinoma whose cells are tall and cylindrical. Also *cylindrical carcinoma.* **desmoplastic c.** SCIRRHOUS CARCINOMA. **duct c.** A carcinoma arising in a duct, as of the breast. **ductal papillary c.** A duct carcinoma with a papillary growth pattern. **c. durum** SCIRRHOUS CARCINOMA. **embryonal c.** A malignant germ cell tumor of the testis and less commonly of the ovary, composed of tumor cells of primitive epithelial appearance. Growth patterns may be acinar, tubular, papillary, or solid. Also *undifferentiated malignant teratoma, anaplastic malignant teratoma.* **embryonal c. of the testis** A highly malignant germ cell tumor of the testis of primitive epithelial appearance. **c. en cuirasse** CANCER EN CUIRASSE. **endometrioid c.** A nonuterine carcinoma having the histologic appearance of a carcinoma of the endometrium. It is typically found in the ovary. **epibulbar c.** A carcinoma of the bulbar conjunctiva, typically starting at the limbus. **epidermoid c.** SQUAMOUS CELL CARCINOMA. **erysipeloid c.** A metastatic carcinoma of the skin that resembles the cutaneous infection of erysipelas. It is most often seen in association with primary breast cancer. **exophytic c.** A carcinoma growing into the space above its originating surface in a papillary manner. **c. ex ulcere** A carcinoma arising in an ulcer, as of the stomach or skin. **fibrosing basal cell c.** MORPHEA TYPE BASAL CELL CARCINOMA. **follicular c.** A thyroid carcinoma with growth patterns and cells resembling those seen in mature or developing thyroid glands. No papillary structures should be present. Follicular carcinoma is usually more malignant than the papillary type. **fungating c.** A carcinoma whose gross growth pattern resembles a fungus as it projects from the surface, as of the colon or the stomach. **gelatiniform c.** MUCINOUS CARCINOMA. **gelatinous c.** MUCINOUS CARCINOMA. **giant cell c.** A carcinoma containing numerous large, multinucleated, pleomorphic, and bizarre tumor giant cells. The most frequent sites are the thyroid and lung. It is highly malignant. Also *carcinoma gigantocellulare.* **glandular c.** ADENOCARCINOMA. **glottic c.** Carcinoma of the larynx located on the vocal fold or folds and accounting for well over 50% of such cases. The outlook at this site is much better than with carcinoma elsewhere in the larynx, with some 80% of early stage cases remaining free of disease five years after treatment. **granular cell c.** A carcinoma with cells containing prominent cytoplasmic granules. **granulosa cell c.** GRANULOSA CELL TUMOR. **hair-matrix c.** BASAL CELL CARCINOMA. **hepatocellular c.** A malignant tumor of the liver composed of cells resembling hepatocytes. The tumor cells are typically arranged as trabeculae, but acinar and scirrhous patterns may also occur. Bile production is specific for this tumor but is not a constant feature. Growth along blood vessels is characteristic. In adults, hepatocellular carcinoma is frequently associated with cirrhosis. In children, cirrhosis is usually absent. Also *liver cell carcinoma, hepatocarcinoma, hepatoma, malignant hepatoma.* **Hürthle cell c.** A follicular type of thyroid carcinoma with large oxyphilic cells having abundant eosinophilic cytoplasm similar to that found in oncocytes. Also *oncocytic carcinoma, oxyphilic carcinoma.* **hyaline c.** *Obs.* MUCINOUS CARCINOMA. **hypernephroid c.** RENAL CELL CARCINOMA. **inflammatory c.** A carcinoma of the breast with edema, hyperemia, tenderness, and rapid enlargement, usually associated with extensive invasion of dermal lymphatics by tumor. Also *carcinoma mastitoides.* **c. in situ** A lesion of epithelial tissue with the cellular and architectural features of cancer but without evidence of invasion into supporting stroma. It is most commonly encountered in the uterine cervix and skin, but is also seen in bronchial epithelium, esophagus, and vagina. It may occur in glandular epithelium like that of the endometrium, stomach, and colon. Also *intraepithelial carcinoma, intraepidermal carcinoma, intraepidermal epithelioma, cancer in situ, preinvasive carcinoma.* **intermediary c.** BASOSQUAMOUS CARCINOMA. **intermediate-cell c.** BASOSQUAMOUS CARCINOMA. **intraepidermal c.** CARCINOMA IN SITU. **intraepithelial c.** CARCINOMA IN SITU. **intrahepatic bile duct c.** CHOLANGIOCARCINOMA. **islet cell c.** A rare tumor of the islets of Langerhans which can produce insulin (insulinoma) or glucagon (glucagonoma). The degree of malignancy is usually low. Benign forms, islet cell adenomas, are more frequent. Also *malignant nesidioblastoma.* **Krompecher's c.** BASAL CELL CARCINOMA. **Kulchitsky cell c.** CARCINOID. **c. of the larynx** Carcinoma occurring in the glottic, subglottic, and supraglottic regions of the larynx as well as in the marginal zone between the larynx and laryngopharynx, that is, on the suprahyoid portion of the epiglottis and the aryepiglottic folds. Between 96 and 98 percent are squamous cell carcinomas and most are well-differentiated. **liver cell c.** HEPATOCELLULAR CARCINOMA. **lobular c.** An invasive carcinoma of the breast originating in the intralobular ductules. **lobular c. in situ** A lobular carcinoma of the breast without stromal invasion. The intralobular ductules are filled and distended by tumor cells. **lymphoepithelial c.** LYMPHOEPITHELIOMA. **c. mastitoides** INFLAMMATORY CARCINOMA. **medullary c.** **1** A carcinoma with little stroma, composed of tumor cells showing no specific organization. **2** A carcinoma which grossly is bulky and soft with the consistency of marrow or brain. Also *cerebriform carcinoma, encephaloma.* **3** A carcinoma of the thyroid with functional and structural characteristics of parafollicular cells (C cells). This type of tumor may have amyloid in its stroma and may produce calcitonin. Also *carcinoma medullare, carcinoma molle, medullary thyroid carcinoma, parafollicular thyroid carcinoma.* **medullary breast c.** A carcinoma of the breast with large cells showing no structural organization, little fibrous stroma, good demarcation, and often lymphoid infiltration. The prognosis appears to be better than for the usual duct carcinoma of the breast. **medullary thyroid c.** MEDULLARY CARCINOMA. **Merkel cell c.** A malignant tumor of the skin thought to arise from neuroreceptor (Merkel) cells. It is composed of small cells with little cytoplasm, growing as sheets or trabeculae. Mitotic activity is high. Electron microscopy shows the cells to contain dense-core (neurosecretory) granules. Also *Merkel cell tumor, trabecular carcinoma of the skin.* **metatypical c.** BASOSQUAMOUS CARCINOMA. **c. molle** MEDULLARY CARCINOMA. **morphea type basal cell c.** A basal cell carcinoma with nests and strands of tumor cells embedded in a heavily fibrosed stroma. Also *fibrosing basal cell carcinoma, morpheic epithelioma.* **mucinous c.** An adenocarcinoma which produces and retains massive amounts of mucus which is usually visible to the naked eye. The mucus accumulates extracellularly in glandular and cystic spaces and may be extravasated into the stroma. It is most often seen in tumors of the colon and ovary. Mucinous carcinoma should not be confused with mucus-secreting carcinoma. The former indicates massive secretion. Many adenocarcinomas secrete smaller amounts of mucus. Also *mucinous adenocarcinoma, mucoid adenocarcinoma, colloid carcinoma, colloid cancer, gelatiniform carcinoma, gelatinous carcinoma, hyaline carcinoma* (obs.), *mucoid carcinoma, carcinoma muciparum, carcinoma mucocellulare, mucous carcinoma, carcinoma mucosum, carcinoma myxomatodes, pseudomucinous carcinoma of the ovary, colloma* (obs.), *colloid tumor.* **mucocellular c.** SIGNET RING CELL CARCINOMA. **c. mucocellulare** MUCINOUS CARCINOMA. **mucoepidermoid c.** A malignant tumor containing squamous cells, mucus-type glandular cells, and cells of intermediate type. These may be separated or intimately juxtaposed. The degree of malignancy varies from low to high. It is most often seen in the salivary glands but occurs at other sites, such as the lung. **mucoid c.** MUCINOUS CARCINOMA. **c. mucosum** MUCINOUS CARCINOMA. **mucous c.** MUCINOUS CARCINOMA. **c. myxomatodes** MUCINOUS CARCINOMA. **nasopharyngeal c.** Carcinoma arising in the mucous membrane of the nasopharynx. It is usually undifferentiated and may have a prominent lymphoid cell infiltrate among the tumor cells, in which case the term *lymphoepithelial carcinoma* is appropriate. It is particularly common among those of southern Chinese origin. Abbr. NPC **nonencapsulated sclerosing c.** SCLEROSING CARCINOMA OF THE THYROID. **oat cell c.** **1** SMALL CELL CARCINOMA. **2** A subtype of small cell carcinoma composed of uniform cells slightly larger than lymphocytes with sparse cytoplasm and dense nuclei. It typically occurs in the lung. **occult c.** A carcinoma whose primary site is unknown or symptomless but which manifests itself from its secondary deposits or secondary phenomena. Also *carcinoma occulta.* **oncocytic c.** HÜRTHLE CELL CARCINOMA. **oxyphilic c.** HÜRTHLE CELL CARCINOMA. **c. of the pancreas** A malignant neoplasm of exocrine pancreatic epithelium. It may be solid or cystic, ductal or acinar, glandular, mucinous, adenosquamous, squamous, or undifferentiated. **papillary c.** A carcinoma with tumor cells growing on stromal stalks. It is most commonly seen in transitional cell carcinomas of the bladder and as a special form of thyroid cancer. Also *papillocarcinoma.* **papillary c. of the ovary** A common form of ovarian cancer with tumor cells arranged in a papillary manner in cystic structures or on the surface. It is more frequent in the serous type than in the mucinous form of ovarian carcinoma. Also *serous papillary cystadenocarcinoma.* **papillary serous c.** A papillary carcinoma of the ovary with serous-type cells. **papillary thyroid c.** A malignant neoplasm of the thyroid which has a papillary growth pattern. It comprises about half of all thyroid carcinomas. It is commoner in females, and may occur at any age but is often seen in children and young adults, sometimes associated with a history of cervical radiotherapy in childhood. It does not take up iodine. It can become more malignant with advancing age, spreading locally, and metastasizing relatively late. Treatment with thyroid hormone retards tumor growth in some cases. It is considered to be less malignant than follicular thyroid carcinoma. **parafollicular thyroid c.** MEDULLARY CARCINOMA. **polypoid c.** A carcinoma with a growth pattern of one or more fingerlike projections extending upward from its origin. **postcricoid c.** Carcinoma, almost always squamous cell carcinoma, arising in the laryngopharynx at its junction with the esophagus, that is, posterior to the cricoid cartilage. There is a statistically significant association with the Plummer-Vinson syndrome. In contrast with other varieties of carcinoma of the laryngopharynx, the incidence is higher in women than in men. **preinvasive c.** CARCINOMA IN SITU. **prickle cell c.** SQUAMOUS CELL CARCINOMA. **c. with productive fibrosis** SCIRRHOUS CARCINOMA. **pseudomucinous c. of the ovary** MUCINOUS CARCINOMA. **pyriform fossa c.** The most common variety of carcinoma to arise in the laryngopharynx, usually in the groove between the medial and lateral walls of the pyriform fossa. The great majority, almost always squamous cell carcinomas, occur in men. **renal cell c.** A carcinoma with cells resembling those of renal cortex. The tumor cells are of renal tubular origin and have clear cytoplasm due to abundant glycogen. Their cell membranes are often clearly defined. Cells with granular cytoplasm may also occur in renal cell carcinomas. Also *clear cell carcinoma, adenocarcinoma of kidney, renal adenocarcinoma, Grawitz tumor, hypernephroma, hypernephroid carcinoma, epinephroma, clear cell tumor.* **scirrhous c.** An adenocarcinoma, which has a small number of tumor cells in relation to an abundant amount of dense collagenous stroma. The tumor cells are isolated and dispersed throughout the fibrous component, and the tumor is consequently firm. The breast is the most frequent site for this tumor. Also *carcinoma with productive fibrosis, scirrhoma, scirrhus, desmoplastic carcinoma, carcinoma durum, scirrhous adenocarcinoma, scirrhous cancer.* **sclerosing c. of the thyroid** A variety of papillary carcinoma of the thyroid characterized by abundant scar tissue, small size, and relatively favorable prognosis. Also *nonencapsulated sclerosing carcinoma.* **c. of the scrotum** A malignant tumor of the skin of the scrotum, typically of squamous cell type. It is one of the oldest recognized forms of occupational cancer, namely, chimney sweeps' cancer. Also *carcinoma scroti.* **sebaceous c.** A carcinoma of the sebaceous glands. The tumor cells secrete lipid. **seminal c.** SEMINOMA. **signet ring cell c.** An adenocarcinoma characterized by a prominent component of isolated cells distended with mucus. The nucleus is typically pushed to one side to give the signet ring effect. This tumor is most frequently seen in the stomach and is highly malignant. Also *mucocellular carcinoma.* **c. simplex** An undifferentiated carcinoma without a distinctive microscopic pattern. **small cell c.** A highly malignant tumor of the lung, composed of small, darkly staining cells with scant cytoplasm. The cells may be round, ovoid, or fusiform. It is more common in cigarette smokers than in others. Though radiosensitive, it is difficult to cure because of early metastatic spread. The tumor is associated with ectopic hormone production, especially of ACTH. Also *oat cell carcinoma.* **spindle cell c.** A carcinoma, usually of squamous cell type, which contains a prominent component of undifferentiated spindle-shaped cells. This results in a sarcomalike appearance. This tumor is seen mostly in the esophagus and hypopharynx. **spinous cell c.** SQUAMOUS CELL CARCINOMA. **squamous cell c.** A carcinoma composed of stratified squamous epithelium. Keratin may be present and intercellular bridges can often be found. This tumor type is the most frequent form of carcinoma in the skin, oral mucosa, esophagus, larynx, bronchus, uterine cervix, and vagina. Also *epidermoid carcinoma, prickle cell carcinoma, spinous cell carcinoma, squamous carcinoma, squamous cell epithelioma, dermoid cancer* (obs.). **sweat gland c.** A malignant tumor of sweat glands. This type of tumor appears less frequently than the sweat gland adenomas, and can resemble various portions of the sweat gland apparatus. **teratoid c.** TERATOCARCINOMA. **trabecular c.** A carcinoma with cells arranged in elongated, often anastomosing, groups. This growth pattern is seen most often in hepatocellular carcinoma and some follicular carcinomas of the thyroid. **trabecular c. of the skin** MERKEL CELL CARCINOMA. **transitional cell c.** A carcinoma with cells resembling transitional epithelium of the urinary tract. **undifferentiated c.** A malignant epithelial tumor which does not show evidence of specific tissue differentiation, such as squamous or glandular features. Also *anaplastic carcinoma.* **c. of the urinary bladder** A malignant neoplasm of the bladder mucosa usually of transitional cell type, less commonly squamous or glandular, frequently displaying a papillary growth pattern. The squamous cell type is associated with schistosomiasis of the bladder and is common in Egypt and Iraq. **V2 c.** A transplantable carcinoma of rabbits originating from the malignant transformation of a Shope papilloma. Also *VX2 carcinoma.* **verrucous c.** A well-differentiated, slow-growing, squamous cell carcinoma with a pronounced overgrowth of warty vertical folds. It shows minimal cell atypia and has a pushing rather than an invasive border. It usually grows in the oral cavity or upper respiratory tract. **VX2 c.** V2 CARCINOMA.

**carcinomata** \kär′sənō′mətə\ Plural of CARCINOMA.

**carcinomatoides alveogenica multicentrica** \-mətoi′dēz alvē′əjen′ikə mul′tisen′trikə\ BRONCHIOLOALVEOLAR CARCINOMA.

**carcinomatosis** \-mətō′sis\ [CARCINOMA + *t* + -OSIS ] A carcinoma that is widely disseminated throughout the body. Also *carcinosis, epitheliomatosis.* **c. of the meninges** Diffuse dissemination of metastatic carcinoma throughout the cerebrospinal subarachnoid space. **c. pleurae** Diffuse secondary (metastatic) growth of carcinoma on the pleural surfaces.

**carcinomatous** \kär′sənäm′ətəs\ Of or relating to carcinoma.

**carcinomectomy** \-mek′təmē\ CARCINECTOMY.

**carcinosarcoma** \-särkō′mə\ A rare, single tumor containing carcinomatous and sarcomatous components. Spindle cell transformation and stromal metaplasia in a carcinoma may mimic a carcinosarcoma. It occurs in a variety of organs. **embryonal c.** 1 A carcinosarcoma composed of embryonal-type tissues. 2 *Obs.* NEPHROBLASTOMA. **Flexner-Jobling c.** A transplantable carcinosarcoma of rats. **Walker c. 256** WALKER SARCOMA.

**carcinosectomy** \-sek′təmē\ CARCINECTOMY.

**carcinosis** \kär′sənō′sis\ CARCINOMATOSIS.

**carcinostatic** \-stat′ik\ [CARCINO- + -STATIC] Capable of arresting the growth of a carcinoma.

**card-** \kärd-\ CARDIO-.

**cardelmycin** NOVOBIOCIN.

**Carden** [Henry Douglas *Carden*, English surgeon, died 1872] See under AMPUTATION.

**cardenolide** Any of the $C_{23}$ steroids whose side chain on C-17 consists of the lactone of 4-hydroxybut-2-enoic acid joined by its C-3. They have a *cis* junction of rings C and D, and hydroxyl groups at C-3 and C-14, and they may have other hydroxyl groups. Their glycosides, including digoxin, occur in plants and are used as arrow poisons and therapeutically for their action on the heart.

**cardi-** \kär′dē-\ CARDIO-.

**cardia** \kär′dē·ə\ [Gk *kardia* heart] 1 PARS CARDIACA GASTRIS. 2 OSTIUM CARDIACUM. 3 *Outmoded* COR. 4 The region of the heart. An outmoded usage. **c. of stomach** PARS CARDIACA GASTRIS.

**cardia-** \kär′dē·ə-\ CARDIO-.

**-cardia** \-kär′dē·ə\ [CARD- + -IA] A combining form denoting a condition of the heart.

**cardiac** \kär′dē·ak\ [Gk *kardiak(os)* pertaining to the heart] 1 Pertaining to the heart. 2 Pertaining to the esophageal end, or opening, of the stomach. Also *cardiacus.*

**cardial** \kär′dē·əl\ Of or relating to the cardia of the stomach.

**cardialgia** \kär′dē·al′jə\ [GK *kardialgia* (from *kardi(a)* ostium cardiacum + *alg(os)* pain + -IA) heartburn] 1 HEARTBURN. 2 Pain in the heart or in the area of the heart.

**cardiant** An agent that stimulates the heart.

**cardiasthma** \kär′dē·az′mə\ CARDIAC ASTHMA.

**cardiectasis** \kär′dē·ek′təsis\ [CARDI- + ECTASIS] DILATATION OF THE HEART.

**cardiectomy** \kär′dē·ek′təmē\ [CARDI- + -ECTOMY] A surgical procedure in which the gastric cardia, that part of the stomach surrounding the esophagus, is removed.

**cardio-** \kär′dē·ō-\ [Gk *kardia* heart] A combining form denoting (1) the heart; (2) the ostium cardiacum. Also *card-, cardi-, cardia-.*

**cardioactive** \-ak′tiv\ Having an effect upon the heart: said especially of drugs.

**cardioangiography** \-an′jē·äg′rəfē\ ANGIOCARDIOGRAPHY.

**cardioangiology** \-an′jē·äl′əjē\ [CARDIO + ANGIO- + -LOGY] Study of the heart and blood vessels.

**cardioaortic** \-ā·ôr′tik\ Pertaining to the heart and aorta.

**cardioarterial** \-ärtir′ē·əl\ Pertaining to the heart and arteries.

**cardioasthma** \-az′mə\ CARDIAC ASTHMA.

**cardiocentesis** \-sentē′sis\ PARACENTESIS CORDIS.

**cardiochalasia** \-kalā′zhə\ [CARDIO- + CHALASIA] Relaxation of the cardiac, or lower esophageal, sphincter, often responsible for gastresophageal reflux or unexplained vomiting, especially in children.

**cardiocirrhosis** \-sirō′sis\ Cirrhosis of the liver resulting from longstanding right-sided heart failure.

**cardiodynamic** \-dīnam′ik\ Pertaining to the kinetic aspects of heart function. Also *cardiokinetic.*

**cardioesophageal** \-ēsäf′əjē′əl\ Pertaining to the junction of the esophagus and stomach, or to the esophagus and the cardia of the stomach.

**cardiogenesis** \-jen′əsis\ [CARDIO- + GENESIS] Formation and development of the heart in the embryo.

**cardiogenic** \-jen′ik\ [CARDIO- + -GENIC] 1 Originating in the heart; resulting from cardiac function or malfunction. 2 Relating to cardiogenesis; giving rise to the embryonic heart.

**cardiogram** \kär′dē·ōgram′\ [CARDIO- + -GRAM] Any type of graphic record of heart action or sounds, especially an electrocardiogram. See also APEXCARDIOGRAM, ECHOCARDIOGRAM, PHONOCARDIOGRAM, VECTORCARDIOGRAM. **esophageal c.** A record of the contraction of the left atrium made by a sensing device behind it in the esophagus. **precordial c.** KINETOCARDIOGRAM. **vector c.** VECTORCARDIOGRAM.

**cardiograph** \kär′dē·ōgraf′\ [CARDIO- + -GRAPH] An instrument for recording cardiograms.

**cardiography** \kär′dē·äg′rəfē\ [CARDIO- + -GRAPHY] Any technique of graphically recording heart action or sounds; the production of cardiograms. **apex c.** See under APEXCARDIOGRAPHY. **radionuclide c.** A scintigraphic procedure used for evaluation of cardiac function, determined by studying the movements of radioactive blood, containing labeled albumin or red cells in the cardiac chambers. Data are recorded with a gamma camera over the precordium. Also *gamma cardiography, radiocardiography, emission cardiography.* **ultrasonic c.** ECHOCARDIOGRAPHY. **vector c.** VECTORCARDIOGRAPHY.

**cardiohepatic** \-həpat′ik\ Pertaining to the heart and liver.

**cardioid** \kär′dē·oid\ Resembling a heart.

**cardioinhibitor** An agent that inhibits the activity of the heart.

**cardiokinetic** \-kinet′ik\ CARDIODYNAMIC.

**cardiokymography** \-kīmäg′rəfē\ The technique of recording on x-ray film changes in the outline of the beating heart.

**cardiolipin** Diphosphatidylglycerol. The molecule contains three glycerol residues, linked end to end through phosphaste groups, and four fatty acyl groups. It is present in mitochondrial and bacterial membranes.

**cardiolith** \kär′dē·ōlith′\ [CARDIO- + -LITH] CARDIAC CALCULUS.

**cardiologist** \kär′dē·äl′əjist\ A physician who specializes in the diagnosis and treatment of heart disease.

**cardiology** \kär′dē·äl′əjē\ [CARDIO- + -LOGY] The study of the heart and its diseases.

**cardiolysis** \kär′dē·äl′isis\ The division of adhesions between the heart and surrounding structures, usually the pericardium.

**cardiomalacia** \-məlā′shə\ A softening of heart muscle, usually due to extensive necrosis. Also *softening of the heart.*

**cardiomegalia** \-məgā′lyə\ CARDIOMEGALY.

**cardiomegaly** \-meg′əlē\ [CARDIO- + -MEGALY] Enlargement of the heart, due either to myocardial hypertrophy, chamber dilatation, or both. Also *cardiomegalia, macrocardia, megacardia, megalocardia, auxocardia.* **idiopathic c.** Cardiac enlargement whose cause is unknown.

**cardiomelanosis** \-mel′ənō′sis\ A condition in which deposits of melanin are found in the muscle fibers of the heart.

**cardiometer** \kär′dē·äm′ətər\ [CARDIO- + -METER] An instrument for measuring the size of the heart, or the force of its contractions.

**cardiometry** \kär′dē·äm′ətrē\ [CARDIO- + -METRY] The measurement of the size of the heart or its force of contraction.

**cardiomyoliposis** \-mī′ōlipō′sis\ Deposits of fat in heart muscle fibers, seen in certain conditions such as anemia, chronic alcoholism, and phosphorus poisoning. Also *fatty cardiomyopathy* (imprecise).

**cardiomyopathy** \-mī·äp′əthē\ [CARDIO- + MYOPATHY] Heart muscle disease, especially primary or idiopathic disease of the myocardium, as distinguished from diseases secondary to the common disease processes of atherosclerosis, hypertension, valvular heart disease, or pulmonary heart disease. Also *myocardiopathy, myopathia cordis, myocardosis, myocardiosis.* **alcoholic c.** Cardiomyopathy resulting from chronic alcoholism. It usually leads to heart failure with low cardiac output. Some cases, with thiamin deficiency, are characterized initially by a high cardiac output. Also *alcoholic myocardiopathy.* **Becker's c.** The myocardial component of the Becker (late-onset) type of X-linked muscular dystrophy. **beer-drinker's c.** A form of congestive heart failure resulting from the consumption of large quantities of beer to which cobalt had been added for the purpose of enhancing its foaming quality. Also *beer heart.* **familial c.** Cardiomyopathy occurring in families and usually inherited as a mendelian dominant, and characterized by muscular hypertrophy with fibrosis, cardiac arrhythmias, and premature death. **fatty c.** 1 Fatty infiltration and encasement of the heart in the very obese. 2 *Imprecise* CARDIOMYOLIPOSIS. **hypertrophic c.** A cardiomyopathy of unknown etiology characterized by extreme hypertrophy of the ventricular walls and especially the septum. It may cause obstruction of the outflow of the left ventricle and, occasionally, the right. Also *Corvisart's disease.* **nephropathic c.** Cardiomyopathy resulting from kidney disease. **nonobstructive hypertrophic c.** A disease characterized by hypertrophy, and later fibrosis, of heart muscle, especially that of the left ventricle, without known cause. There is no obstruction to ejection of blood. **obstructive hypertrophic c.** A disease characterized by hypertrophy, and later fibrosis, of heart muscle, especially the interventricular septum. Unlike the nonobstructive form, hypertrophy of the muscle of the outflow tract obstructs ejection of blood from the ventricle. Also *obstructive cardiomyopathy.* See also IDIOPATHIC HYPERTROPHIC SUBAORTIC STENOSIS. **thyrotoxic c.** The abnormal state of the heart muscle in some cases of hyperthyroidism, leading to disturbances of rhythm and heart failure. **toxic c.** The pathologic effects on heart muscle of poisons or toxins of any kind.

**cardiomyotomy** \-mī·ät′əmē\ An operation for the relief of achalasia of the cardia when more conservative treatment has failed. A long incision is made through the muscular wall down to, but not through, the mucous membrane at the cardioesophageal junction. Also *Heller's operation, esophagocardiomyotomy, esophagomyotomy, Heller esophagomyotomy.*

**cardionector** \-nek′tər\ CONDUCTION SYSTEM OF THE HEART.

**cardionephric** \-nef′rik\ CARDIORENAL.

**cardiopaludism** \-pal′yədizm\ A form of falciparum malaria causing myocardial ischemia due to capillary emboli from malaria-infected red cells.

**cardiopathic** \-path′ik\ [CARDIO- + -PATH + -IC ] Pertaining to or characterized by disease of the heart.

**cardiopathy** \kär′dē·äp′əthē\ [CARDIO- + -PATHY] Disease of the heart.

**cardiopericardiopexy** \-per′ikär′dē·ōpek′sē\ The promotion of adhesions between the heart and the pericardium in order to increase collateral blood flow to an ischemic myocardium.

**cardiopericarditis** \-per′ikärdi′tis\ MYOPERICARDITIS.

**cardioplasty** \kär′dē·ōplas′tē\ ESOPHAGOGASTROPLASTY.

**cardioplegia** \-plē′jə\ [CARDIO- + -PLEGIA] Iatrogenic arrest of the heart by the use of cold or chemical substances to protect the myocardium during ischemia, a technique employed in cardiopulmonary bypass surgery.

**cardioplegic** \-plē′jik\ Having the effect of suspending or suppressing the heart's contractions: said of methods or substances such as hypothermia, electric shock, or drugs, used for immobilizing the heart to facilitate surgical treatment.

**cardiopneumatic** \-n$^y$oomat′ik\ Pertaining to heart and respiration.

**cardiopneumograph** \-n$^y$oo′məgraf\ An instrument that graphically records cardiopneumatic movements.

**cardiopneumonopexy** \-n$^y$oomän′ōpek′sē\ [CARDIO- + PNEUMONO- + -PEXY] An operative procedure to provide collateral blood supply to heart muscle by forming vascular adhesions between the left lung and the myocardium.

**cardioptosia** \kär′dē·ōtō′zhə\ [CARDIO- + *-ptos(is)* + -IA] DROP HEART.

**cardioptosis** \kär′dē·ōtō′sis\ [CARDIO- + -PTOSIS] DROP HEART.

**cardiopulmonary** \-pul′məner′ē\ Pertaining to or involving both heart and lungs. Also *cardiopulmonic, pneumocardial.*

**cardiopuncture** \-pungk′chər\ PARACENTESIS CORDIS.

**cardiorenal** \-rē′nəl\ Pertaining to or involving both heart and kidneys. Also *cardionephric.*

**cardiorrhaphy** \kär′dē·ôr′əfē\ [CARDIO- + -RRHAPHY] A suture of cardiac defects.

**cardiospasm** \kär′dē·ōspazm′\ ACHALASIA OF THE CARDIA. **tropical c.** A sequela of Chagas disease seen chiefly in southern South America, characterized by megaesophagus with dysphagia. It is caused either by direct action of the parasite *Trypanosoma cruzi* on the parasympathetic ganglia or by toxic substances it produces. The colon, duodenum, or other tubular organs may also be affected. Also *entalação, tropical dysphagia, Chagas disease of the esophagus.*

**cardiotachometer** \-təkäm′ətər\ An instrument used for cardiotachometry.

**cardiotachometry** \-təkäm′ətrē\ Continuous and usually prolonged recording of the speed of the heart beat.

**cardiotomy** \kär′dē·ät′əmē\ [CARDIO- + -TOMY] 1 Surgical incision of the heart. 2 Incision into the proximal or cardiac end of the stomach.

**cardiotonic** 1 Having a tonic or stimulatory effect on the heart. 2 A cardiotonic agent.

**cardiotopography** \-tōpäg′rəfē\ The descriptive anatomy of the heart and surrounding region.

**cardiotoxic** \-täk′sik\ Having a deleterious or poisonous effect upon the function of the heart through damage to its muscle or conduction system.

**cardiovalvulotome** \-val′vyələtōm′\ VALVULOTOME.

**cardiovalvulotomy** \-val′vyəlät′əmē\ VALVOTOMY.

**cardiovascular** \-vas′kyələr\ Pertaining to or comprising the heart and blood vessels.

**cardiovectography** \-vektäg′rəfē\ VECTORCARDIOGRAPHY.

**cardioversion** \-vur′zhən\ [CARDIO- + VERSION] The restoration of sinus rhythm by electric shock using a defibrillating instrument.

**cardiovert** \kär′dē·ōvurt′\ To subject (the heart rhythm or the patient) to cardioversion.

**cardioverter** \-vur′tər\ [CARDIO- + *(re)verter*] A defibrillator that produces a discharge synchronized to the R wave of the electrocardiogram for terminating atrial arrhythmias.

**cardiovirus** \-vī′rəs\ A member of the *Cardiovirus* genus in the Picornaviridae family. The genus comprises two groups, the encephalomyocarditis (EMC) viruses and the encephalomyelitis viruses. Mice are the most common natural hosts but some cardioviruses have been isolated from a wide variety of mammals, including humans. The virions are naked, ether-resistant particles with icosahedral symmetry, 20–30 nm in diameter. They contain a single segment of single-stranded linear RNA which acts as a message.

**carditis** \kärdī′tis\ [CARD- + -ITIS] Inflammation of the heart. **acute rheumatic c.** Inflammation of endocardium, myocardium, or pericardium as part of the systemic inflammatory process of rheumatic fever and representing an immune response to streptococcal infection. Weakening the heart's action at the time, its healing often causes chronic disease of the valves later. **streptococcal c.** Acute inflammation of the heart, especially the myocardium, directly due to the damaging effect of toxins derived from streptococcal bacteria in the throat or elsewhere. **verrucous c.** VERRUCOUS ENDOCARDITIS.

**care** / **acute c.** Health care for one episode of illness or injury. Compare LONG-TERM CARE. ● In the United Kingdom, *acute care* generally refers to short-term care for the acutely ill. In India, it refers to immediate care, not the whole episode. **ambulatory c.** Health services by a hospital or other health facility to patients who are not confined to the facility and who return to their homes after treatment; outpatient care. **continuity of c.** The extent to which a patient's health care is obtained from the same source of services over a period of time or for a specific episode of illness. **custodial c.** Board, room, and other personal assistance services, generally provided on a long-term basis. Such care is usually provided in boarding homes. In psychiatry, custodial care involves protection and monitoring of the patient or protection of others from the patient's destructive potential as a major component. It may include active medical intervention, but most often it is needed for chronically ill patients whose level of function is unlikely to change appreciably for the better, even though they may require continuing drug treatment and milieu therapy in order to prevent or retard further deterioration. **extended c.** LONG-TERM CARE. **family c.** The placement of a chronically mentally ill patient in a family setting, usually with unrelated guardians, as part of the rehabilitation phase of treatment. The Gheel colony in Antwerp, Belgium, is a well-known organized system of family care. **foster c.** The nurture of an infant or child by a person or persons other than the natural parents. If undertaken for payment, legislation in most countries demands certain standards of living and of competence of the fosterer. Foster parents have no legal parental rights over the child. Fostering is usually on a short-term basis, i.e., weeks or months, to answer a family crisis. Long-term fostering is also practiced, i.e., up to adolescence or adulthood and sometimes with a view to eventual adoption. Groups of children may be fostered in homes for that purpose. ● In India and South Africa, foster care is not subject to legislative control and is arranged privately. **home health c.** Health services rendered in the patient's usual place of residence, often provided to aged, disabled, or sick individuals who do not need institutional care. Services may be specialized or general primary care and may be offered by a variety of providers, including visiting nurses and representatives of home health agencies. **intensive c.** Hospital care for the most seriously ill utilizing advanced technology and specially trained personnel. **long-term c.** Health services provided on a long-term basis, required by persons who are chronically ill, aged, disabled, or retarded, in an institution or at home. Long-term care is commonly provided in nursing homes and mental hospitals. In psychiatry, long-term care is designed to maintain the patient at the highest level of functioning possible within the limitations imposed by chronic mental illness. Such services may include custodial care within a mental hospital, partial hospitalization, outpatient care, or a spectrum of domiciliary settings ranging from highly structured skilled nursing homes through halfway houses to satellite housing with minimal supervision. Also *extended care, long-stay care*. Compare ACUTE CARE. **nursing c.** Health care intended to assist an individual who is sick or well in the performance of those activities contributing to health that the individual would perform unaided if he or she had the necessary strength, will, or knowledge. Nursing care may also be provided to contribute to the comfort and serenity of a patient who is dying, and is commonly provided to assist other health professionals, as physicians. **primary c.** Basic health services for day-to-day care of the patient provided by physicians and other providers and requiring the lowest level of technology and special expertise by comparison with secondary and tertiary care. **progressive patient c.** A system of organizing patient care in which patients are grouped together in units depending on their need for care as determined by their degree of illness rather than by traditional factors such as medical or surgical specialty. The three usual levels of care are intensive, intermediate, and minimal or self care. **secondary c.** The intermediate level of care provided by specialists such as internists and general surgeons, usually on referral by primary care providers. At this level the technology is not as sophisticated or the skills as specialized as in tertiary care. **skilled nursing c.** Nursing care which, as defined in legislation in the United States under entitlement programs, generally requires a higher level of training than that of a nurse's aide. **tertiary c.** The most highly specialized level of health care services, characterized by highly trained specialists and frequently by highly sophisticated technologies.

**Carey Coombs** [*Carey* Franklin *Coombs*, English physician, 1879–1932] See under MURMUR.

**caries** \kar′ēz, kar′i·ēz\ [L, rot, decay] **1** Focal resorption or destruction of the calcified structure of a bone, resulting in softening and formation of a cavity. **2** See under DENTAL CARIES. **arrested c.** Dental caries of which the progress has been stopped either spontaneously or because of intervention. In enamel a brown discoloration is seen, the area of decalcification having been recalcified by salts from the saliva. Arrested caries may occur in dentin if the overlying enamel is lost. Dentin which had been softened by caries becomes hard and appears brown. **central c.** The existence of chronic abscess cavities within bone, as seen in osteomyelitis. **dental c.** Localized and progressive destruction of teeth by bacterial action. Microorganisms in dental plaque change sugars into acids which demineralize the subsurface of enamel immediately below the plaque. Proteolytic bacteria follow and attack the organic matrix of the enamel, and later the dentin, where the carious process proceeds more rapidly. Ultimately the pulp is reached and pulpitis, then necrosis, follow. The frequency of sugar consumption seems to be more important in the causation of dental caries than the total amount. It is principally a disease of childhood and adolescence. In old age dental caries commences in the cementum of the roots of teeth which have been exposed by gingival recession. It does not occur in periodontal pockets. Also *dental decay.* **dry c.** Caries of joints and the ends of bones caused by tuberculosis and characterized by a lack of suppuration. Also *caries sicca.* **rampant c.** Rapidly advancing and widespread dental caries, particularly at the cervical parts of the teeth. It may be due to frequent sugar consumption or to diminution in salivary flow following radiotherapy of the head and neck. **recurrent dental c.** Caries in previously sound enamel at the margin of a restoration. **secondary c.** 1 Dental decay attacking the inner surface of enamel from the rapidly spreading caries in the underlying dentin. 2 Dental decay occurring at the margin of a restoration. **senile dental c.** Caries on the roots of the teeth exposed by gingival recession in old age. **c. sicca** DRY CARIES. **spinal c.** TUBERCULOSIS OF SPINE. **c. tuberculosa** Caries of bone caused by tuberculosis.

**carina** \kərē′nə\ [L, keel or bottom of a ship] 1 A ridge or keel-shaped structure or projection. 2 The region of the sternum to which the pectoral muscles are attached, as found in bats, moles, and all except flightless birds. **c. tracheae** [NA] The ridge between the proximal ends of the two principal bronchi, formed by a triangular downward projection from the middle of the inferior border of the lowest tracheal cartilage. It is semilunar in an anteroposterior direction and may be supplemented or replaced by fibrous tissue. Also *carina of trachea.* **c. urethralis vaginae** [NA] The crestlike projection produced by columna rugarum anterior vaginae in the distal part of the anterior wall of the vagina where it lies immediately posterior to the urethra. Also *urethral carina of vagina, vaginal carina, Luschka's tubercle, urethral ridge.*

**carinae** \kərī′nē\ Plural of CARINA.

**carinate** \kar′ənāt\ Pertaining to or resembling a carina.

**carination** \kar′ənā′shən\ [*carin(a)* + -ATION] A ridged or keel-shaped part.

**cario-** \kar′e·ō-\ [L *caries* decay] A combining form denoting caries.

**cariogenesis** \-jen′əsis\ The process of caries formation.

**cariogenic** \-jen′ik\ [CARIO- + -GENIC] Producing or tending to produce caries.

**cariogenicity** \-jənis′itē\ The state of being cariogenic; the production of or tendency to produce caries.

**cariosity** \kar′ē·äs′itē\ The condition of being carious.

**cariostatic** \-stat′ik\ [CARIO- + -STAT + -IC] Tending to slow down or arrest the caries process.

**carious** \kar′ē·əs\ Characterized by caries.

**carisoprodol** A skeletal muscle relaxant drug, closely related chemically to meprobamate. Also *isopropyl meprobamate.*

**Carlens** [Eric *Carlens,* Swedish physician, born 1908] See under TUBE.

**carmalum** \kärmal′əm\ A histologic stain containing carmine or carminic acid and alum. It is used especially to stain nuclei.

**Carman** [Russell Daniel *Carman,* U.S. physician, 1875–1926] Carman meniscus sign. See under MENISCUS SIGN.

**carminative** \kärmin′ətiv\ [Med L *carminativum* (from *carminare* to clean out, orig., to card wool, from L *carmen* a wool card) a medicine for "diluting and relaxing the gross humors"] 1 Tending to prevent the formation or cause the expulsion of gas in the alimentary tract. 2 A carminative agent; an agent used to relieve flatulence.

**carmine** \kär′min\ A natural dye extracted from the cochineal insect *Coccus cacti* using aluminum hydroxide. It is used for staining in bulk, particularly for embryologic specimens. Its staining properties may be enhanced by the addition of mordants, and its solubility increases in acidic and alkaline solutions. Synthetic formulations of the dye have also been prepared. Also *carmine red, carminum.*

**carneous** \kär′nē·əs\ Fleshy.

**carnitine** $Me_3N^+—CH_2—CHOH—CH_2—COO^-$. 3-Hydroxy-4-trimethylammoniobutyrate. Carnitine crosses the inner mitochondrial membrane by a transport system which also accepts its $O^3$-acyl derivatives. Fatty acids enter mitochondria for oxidation in this form, after transfer to the hydroxyl group of carnitine from the thiol group of coenzyme A. Also *vitamin* $B_T$.

**carnivore** \kär′nivôr\ [L *carnivorus* (from *caro,* gen. *carnis,* flesh + *vorare* to eat) meat-eating] 1 Any member of the mammalian order Carnivora, which includes dogs, cats, bears, badgers, racoons, civets, and hyenas. 2 Any meat-eating animal. Adj. carnivorous.

**carnivorous** \kärniv′ərəs\ [*carnivor(e)* + -OUS] Pertaining to a diet of flesh; meat-eating. Also *zoophagic, zoophagous.*

**Carnochan** [John Murray *Carnochan,* U.S. surgeon, 1817–1887] See under OPERATION.

**carnosine** $N^\alpha$-$\beta$-Alanylhistidine. A dipeptide found in muscle. Its function is not known, though it may act as a buffer. It occurs with anserine, its derivative by methylation on the imidazole ring.

**carnosinemia** \kär′nōsinē′mē·ə\ A congenital abnormality of amino acid metabolism resulting in abnormally increased concentrations of carnosine in the blood, mental retardation, and seizures.

**Carnot** [Nicolas Leonard Sadi *Carnot,* French physicist, 1796–1832] Carnot's function. See under CARNOTIC FUNCTION.

**carotene** Any of several $C_{40}$ hydrocarbons whose molecules are composed of eight isoprene units joined in such a manner that the orientation of these units is reversed in the center of the molecule. $\beta$-Carotene has one particular symmetrical structure and possesses vitamin A activity. Asymmetrical carotenes having one end of their molecule like $\beta$-carotene also have vitamin A activity. Because of the conjugated polyene structure, carotenes are brightly colored (usually orange-red) plant pigments. Also *previtamin H.*

**$\beta$-carotene** $\beta,\beta$-Carotene. A yellow-solid, practically insoluble in water, used as a yellow coloring in foods and a precursor of vitamin A. An increase in intake of $\beta$-carotene causes a yellow skin pigmentation which decreases photosensitivity in patients with erythropoietic protoporphyria.

**carotenemia** \kar′ōtənē′mē·ə\ *Imprecise* HYPERCAROTENEMIA.

**carotenoid** A carotene or any of its oxygenated derivatives.

**carotenosis** \kar′ōtenō′sis\ HYPERCAROTENEMIA.

**caroticoclinoid** \kərät′ikōklī′noid\ Pertaining to the internal carotid artery and a clinoid process of the sphenoid bone.

**caroticotympanic** \kərät′ikōtimpan′ik\ Pertaining to the carotid canal and the tympanum, especially in reference to vessels and canaliculi.

**carotid** \kərät′id\ [Gk (pl.) *karōtides* (akin to *karōtikos* stupefying, soporific, from *karoun* to stun, stupefy) the carotid arteries; so called (according to Galen) because pressure applied over them can cause loss of consciousness] Pertaining to the common carotid artery or, less commonly, to the internal carotid or external carotid artery.

**carotinemia** \kar′ōtinē′mē·ə\ *Imprecise* HYPERCAROTENEMIA.

**carotinoderma** \kərät′inōdur′mə\ The yellow pigmentation of the skin that can accompany carotinemia.

**carotinosis** \kar′ōtinō′sis\ HYPERCAROTENEMIA.
**carp-**[1] \kärp-\ CARPO-[1].
**carp-**[2] \kärp-\ CARPO-[2].
**carpal** \kär′pl\ Of or pertaining to the carpus, or wrist. Also *carpale.*
**carpectomy** \kärpek′təmē\ [CARP-[1] + -ECTOMY] A surgical procedure in which all or part of one or more wrist bones is removed.
**Carpenter** [George Alfred *Carpenter,* English physician, 1859–1910] Carpenter syndrome. See under ACROCEPHALOPOLYSYNDACTYLY.
**carphology** \kärfäl′əjē\ [Gk *karpho(s)* bits of wool + -LOGY] Aimless plucking at the clothes or bedcoverings as seen in delirious states and the degenerative dementias. Also *carphologia, floccillation.*
**carpo-**[1] \kär′pō-\ [Gk *karpos* wrist] A combining form denoting the carpus. Also *carp-*[1].
**carpo-**[2] \kär′pō-\ [Gk *karpos* fruit] A combining form denoting fruit. Also *carp-*[2].
**carpocarpal** \kär′pōkär′pl\ **1** Pertaining or relating to two parts of the carpus. **2** Denoting the joint between the proximal and the distal carpal rows.
**carpometacarpal** \kär′pōmet′əkär′pl\ Pertaining to both the carpus and the metacarpus.
**carpopedal** \kär′pōped′əl\ Pertaining to or affecting the carpus and the foot, or the wrists and the feet.
**carpophalangeal** \kär′pōfā′lan′jē·əl\ Pertaining to both the carpus and the phalanges.
**carpoptosis** \kär′päptō′sis\ [CARPO- + PTOSIS] WRIST-DROP.
**Carpue** [Joseph Constantine *Carpue,* English surgeon, 1764–1846] Carpue's operation, Carpue's rhinoplasty. See under INDIAN RHINOPLASTY.
**Carpule** A rubber-stoppered glass vial which fits into a metal injector and is used to administer a unit dosage of local anesthetic. A proprietary name.
**carpus** \kär′pəs\ [L (from Gk *karpos* wrist), the wrist] [NA] The region between the distal ends of the forearm bones and the proximal border of the hand, approximately the bases of the metacarpals. The region includes the eight carpal bones (ossa carpi) and their binding ligaments, capsules, blood vessels, nerves, and attachments. Also *wrist.* **c. curvus** MADELUNG'S DEFORMITY.
**Carr** [Francis Howard *Carr,* English chemist, born 1874] Carr-Price test. See under TEST.
**Carrel** [Alexis *Carrel,* French surgeon and biologist active in the United States, 1873–1944] **1** See under PATCH, FLASK. **2** Carrel-Lindbergh pump. See under PUMP.
**carrier** **1** A person who harbors and releases pathogenic organisms without manifesting symptoms of the disease associated with the pathogen. A carrier may thus infect others without exhibiting any signs of the disease transmitted. **2** VECTOR. **3** An individual who may transmit a given trait genetically without expressing it phenotypically; commonly, an individual who is heterozygous for a recessive gene which in the homozygous state produces abnormality or disease. **4** A substance that receives a chemical group in one reaction and passes it on in another reaction. $NAD^+$, for example, can act as a hydrogen carrier and hemoglobin as an oxygen carrier. **5** A compound used in conjunction with another substance, such as a drug, to facilitate transmission of the latter. **6** A macromolecule that binds with a hapten, thus producing an immune response. Also *schlepper.* **7** An insurer or underwriter. **active c.** A carrier excreting a specific organism during a time of observation. **amalgam c.** A device for conveying to a tooth cavity small quantities of freshly prepared amalgam, which is plastic and nonadhesive and therefore not easily picked up. **chronic c.** A carrier who harbors a specific organism over a long period of time. A chronic typhoid carrier, for example, is defined as a person known to harbor *Salmonella typhi* for one year or more. **closed c.** A carrier who is noninfectious. **contact c.** A carrier subsequent to identifiable contact with a known case. **convalescent c.** A carrier who continues to excrete a specific organism after the disease has ceased to be clinically apparent. **electron c.** An intermediate in a cellular metabolic pathway that reversibly gains or loses an electron or electrons, as a flavoprotein or cytochrome. **enteric c.** A carrier in whom a specific organism persists in the intestinal tract. Also *intestinal carrier.* **gallbladder c.** A carrier in whom a specific organism persists in the gallbladder. **gametocyte c.** An individual whose red blood cells contain malarial gametocytes and who can therefore infect feeding *Anopheles* vectors. **healthy c.** A carrier without past or present clinical manifestations of a disease. **hemophilia c.** A female who has an allele determining either hemophilia A or hemophilia B on an X chromosome. **incubation c.** A carrier who excretes a specific organism during the incubation period of a disease. **intermittent c.** A carrier who excretes a specific organism at intervals but is shown to be free of the organism at other times. **intestinal c.** ENTERIC CARRIER. **isotopic c.** A carrier incorporating a stable isotope of a radiotracer. It is often used when the desired amount of the tracer is too minute for practical chemical handling. Thus the radiotracer signals the progress of the stable isotope through a series of chemical or metabolic reactions. **ligature c.** A surgical instrument designed to facilitate the placement of surgical sutures prior to tying. **temporary c.** A carrier who excretes a specific organism for a brief period of time, as after recovery from a disease. **urinary c.** A carrier in whom a specific organism persists in the urinary tract and is excreted in the urine.
**Carrión** [Daniel A. *Carrión,* Peruvian medical student, 1850–1886] Carrión's disease. See under BARTONELLOSIS.
**Carteaud** [Alexandre *Carteaud,* French physician, born 1897] Gougerot-Carteaud syndrome. See under CONFLUENT AND RETICULATE PAPILLOMATOSIS.
**Carter** [Henry Vandyke *Carter,* English physician, 1831–1907] See under MYCETOMA.

# cartilage

**cartilage** \kär′tilij\ [L *cartilago* cartilage, gristle] A relatively nonvascular, specialized connective tissue comprising cartilage cells, young chondroblasts, and mature chondrocytes, occupying lacunae in a matrix of amorphous ground substance surrounding a network of collagen fibers. Cartilage is divided, according to the nature of the contained fibers of the matrix, into hyaline cartilage, white fibrocartilage, and yellow or elastic fibrocartilage. During early fetal life, the major part of the skeleton is cartilaginous, but most of it is slowly replaced by bone. In the adult, cartilage is found primarily in joints, the walls of the thorax, and in tubular structures such as the larynx, trachea, bronchi, nose, and ears. Cartilage receives its nutrition by diffusion from nearby capillary networks found outside the investing perichondrium. It is both resilient and elastic, and able to resist compressive and shearing forces and undergo continued growth. Also *cartilago, gristle.* **accessory nasal c.'s** CARTILAGINES NASALES ACCESSORIAE. **c. of acoustic meatus** CARTILAGO MEATUS ACUSTICI. **annular c.** *Outmoded* CARTILAGO CRICOIDEA. **aortic c.** The second costal cartilage on the right side. **arthrodial c.** CARTILAGO ARTICULARIS. **articular c.** CARTILAGO ARTICULARIS. **arytenoid c.** CARTILAGO ARYTENOIDEA. **c. of auditory tube** CARTILAGO TUBAE AUDITIVAE. **auricular c.** CARTILAGO AURICULAE. **basal c.** BASAL PLATE. **basilar c.** The cartilage that fills the foramen lacerum at the apex of the petrous part of the temporal bone. Also *fibrocartilago basalis, basal fibrocartilage.* **branchial c.** The cartilaginous rod present in each branchial arch. The rods develop into or contribute to important bony structures such as the mandible and hyoid bone, or they persist in cartilaginous form as the thyroid cartilage. **calcified c.** A step in the process of endochondral ossification occurring just prior to bone formation. **cellular c.** A primitive or early stage in developing cartilage during which there is a high ratio of cells to matrix. Also *parenchymatous cartilage.* **central c.** *Outmoded* NUCLEUS LENTIS. **circumferential c.** **1** LABRUM GLENOIDALE. **2** LABRUM ACETABULARE. **conchal c.** CARTILAGO AURICULAE. **condylar c.** A secondary cartilage, appearing about the twelfth week of intrauterine life and extending from the head of the mandible downwards and anteriorly into the ramus. It is the main center of mandibular ramus growth, the upper end beneath the fibrous articular surface persisting until about the twenty-fifth year of life. **connecting c.** The cartilage in a cartilaginous joint in which there is restricted movement. Also *interosseous cartilage, uniting cartilage.* **corniculate c.** CARTILAGO CORNICULATA. **costal c.** CARTILAGO COSTALIS. **cricoid c.** CARTILAGO CRICOIDEA. **cuneiform c.** CARTILAGO CUNEIFORMIS. **diarthrodial c.** CARTILAGO ARTICULARIS. **ectethmoid c.** One of the paired lateral parts of the cartilaginous ethmoid in the fetal nasal capsule, in which ossification commences in the fourth month of intrauterine life and gives rise to the labyrinth of the ethmoid bone. **elastic c.** ELASTIC FIBROCARTILAGE. **embryonic c.** Cartilaginous tissue, with an epithelioid appearance, characterized by the presence of small chondroblasts which are loaded with glycogen and very closely packed together. The thin matrix of basic material which separates them comprises only precollagenous and collagenous fibrils covered in a little chondromucoid. Originally derived from mesenchyme, this tissue subsequently develops into fetal cartilage, then adult cartilage, or forms the cartilage model for bone formation. **ensiform c.** PROCESSUS XIPHOIDEUS. **epactal c.'s** *Outmoded* CARTILAGINES NASALES ACCESSORIAE. **epiglottic c.** CARTILAGO EPIGLOTTICA. **epiphyseal c.** The new cartilage produced by the epiphysis on the distal side of the zone of growth cartilage in long bones. **episternal c.** A small cartilage on each side of the ventral aspect of the embryonic thorax which contributes to the lateral portion of the developing manubrium sterni. **eustachian c.** CARTILAGO TUBAE AUDITIVAE. **c. of external acoustic meatus** CARTILAGO MEATUS ACUSTICI. **external semilunar c. of knee joint** MENISCUS LATERALIS ARTICULATIONIS GENUS. **fetal c.** A specialized type of fibrous connective tissue which forms most of the temporary skeleton of the embryo. It provides a model in which most of the bones develop and constitutes an important part of the growth mechanism of the organism. **floating c.** A piece of articular cartilage that has become detached, after trauma, from the femoral condyles or the undersurface of the patella. **greater alar c.** CARTILAGO ALARIS MAJOR. **growth c.** A zone of cartilage between the epiphysis and metaphysis, or shaft, of all bones other than skull bones and clavicles. Growth of the skeleton is brought about by the formation of new cartilage matrix and cells by the epiphysis, thus adding continually to the thickness of the zone from the distal side, while on the proximal side the conversion of cartilage into bone takes place by ossification processes in the shaft. When the growth cartilage is entirely converted to bone at the end of puberty, growth ceases. **hyaline c.** A form of cartilaginous tissue in which the matrix is composed almost entirely of mucopolysaccharide with minimal connective tissue fiber content. It appears semitranslucent or glassy and has a low coefficient of friction, making it suitable for articular surfaces. **inferior c. of nose** CARTILAGO ALARIS MAJOR. **interarticular c.** DISCUS ARTICULARIS. **interarytenoid c.** CARTILAGO SESAMOIDEA. **intermediary c.** OSSIFYING CARTILAGE. **internal semilunar c. of knee joint** MENISCUS MEDIALIS ARTICULATIONIS GENUS. **interosseous c.** CONNECTING CARTILAGE. **intervertebral c.'s** DISCI INTERVERTEBRALES. **investing c.** CARTILAGO ARTICULARIS. **Jacobson's c.** CARTILAGO VOMERONASALIS. **laryngeal c.'s** CARTILAGINES LARYNGIS. **laryngeal c. of Luschka** CARTILAGO SESAMOIDEA. **lateral nasal c.** CARTILAGO NASI LATERALIS. **lesser alar c.'s** CARTILAGINES ALARES MINORES. **lower lateral c.** CARTILAGO ALARIS MAJOR. **Luschka's c.** CARTILAGO SESAMOIDEA. **mandibular c.** MECKEL'S CARTILAGE. **meatal c.** CARTILAGO MEATUS ACUSTICI. **Meckel's c.** The cartilaginous rod that develops in the first branchial arch. It subsequently becomes interrupted and contributes to part of the mandible as well as the malleus, and probably the incus, among the auditory ossicles. The line of continuity between mandible and malleus is represented by the sphenomandibular and anterior malleolar ligaments. Also *mandibular cartilage.* **mesethmoid c.** The medial portion of the cartilaginous ethmoid in the fetal nasal capsule, in which ossification occurs in the first year after birth to form the perpendicular plate and crista galli. **minor c.'s** *Outmoded* CARTILAGINES NASALES ACCESSORIAE. **minor alar c.'s** CARTILAGINES ALARES MINORES. **c. of Morgagni** CARTILAGO CUNEIFORMIS. **mucronate c.** *Outmoded* PROCESSUS XIPHOIDEUS. **nasal c.'s** CARTILAGINES NASI. **c. of nasal septum** CARTILAGO SEPTI NASI. **ossifying c.** The cartilage formed in the embryo which is converted in the course of development to bone and becomes a part of the skeleton, as opposed to other types of cartilage which do not become ossified. Also *temporary cartilage, precursory cartilage, intermediate cartilage.* **palpebral c.'s** TARSAL PLATES. **parachordal c.'s** A pair of cartilages (right and left) which develop by chondrification of the condensed ectomeninx immediately caudal to the hypophysis in the region of the lost cranial portion of the notochord. These cartilaginous centers appear during the second month of intrauterine life, and it is in this region that the bony hypoglossal canals develop. **paranasal c.** Cartilage developing around the nasal region of the fetus, giving rise to the inferior nasal concha and most of the ethmoid. **paraseptal c.** CARTILAGO VOMERONASALIS. **parenchymatous c.** CELLULAR CARTILAGE. **periotic c.** Cartilage surrounding the developing otocyst or otic vesicle. As the otocyst forms, it becomes surrounded by mesoderm of otic capsule which chondrifies. Subsequently the cartilage ossifies to contribute to the petrous part of the temporal bone. **permanent c.** Cartilage that persists and does not ossify. **precricoid c.** CARTILAGO SESAMOIDEA. **precursory c.**

OSSIFYING CARTILAGE. **Reichert's c.** The cartilage which appears in the mesenchymatous condensation of the second (hyoid) arch. This gives rise to the stapes, the styloid process, the stylohyoid ligament, and the lesser cornu and upper part of the body of the hyoid bone on each side. **reticular c.** ELASTIC FIBROCARTILAGE. **Santorini's c.** CARTILAGO CORNICULATA. **semilunar c.'s of knee** SIGMOID CARTILAGES. **septal c. of nose** CARTILAGO SEPTI NASI. **sesamoid c. of larynx** CARTILAGO SESAMOIDEA. **sesamoid c.'s of nose** 1 CARTILAGINES NASALES ACCESSORIAE. 2 CARTILAGINES ALARES MINORES. **sesamoid c. of vocal ligament** CARTILAGO SESAMOIDEA. **sigmoid c.'s** The meniscus lateralis articulationis genus, together with the meniscus medialis articulationis genus. **slipping rib c.** A costal cartilage that rubs against another, thus causing pain. **spheno-basilar c.** A cartilaginous junction between the sphenoid and the basilar part of the occipital bone. It does not ossify until age 18 to 25 years, which may still allow a small degree of growth of the base of the skull in early adult life. **spheno-occipital c.** The cartilage of the spheno-occipital synchondrosis which usually ossifies at about 20 years of age. **sternal c.** CARTILAGO COSTALIS. **supra-arytenoid c.** *Outmoded* CARTILAGO CORNICULATA. **supra-scapular c.** SUPRASCAPULA. **synarthrodial c.** The cartilage in any fibrous or cartilaginous joint. **tarsal c.'s** TARSAL PLATES. **temporary c.** OSSIFYING CARTILAGE. **tendon c.** Cartilage which differentiates where a tendon is inserted into a bone, or in a tendon where it crosses a bone. In the latter case, the cartilage is usually temporary and ossifies at a later stage to form a sesamoid bone, such as the pisiform bone in the tendon of the flexor carpi ulnaris. **thyroid c.** CARTILAGO THYROIDEA. **tracheal c.'s** CARTILAGINES TRACHEALES. **triquetral c.** 1 CARTILAGO ARYTENOIDEA. 2 DISCUS ARTICULARIS ARTICULATIONIS RADIOULNARIS DISTALIS. **triquetrous c.** 1 CARTILAGO ARYTENOIDEA. 2 DISCUS ARTICULARIS ARTICULATINIS RADIOULNARIS DISTALIS. **triradiate c.** A star-shaped cartilage formed by the union of the three plates placed between the centers of ossification in the hip bone. **triticeal c.** CARTILAGO TRITICEA. **tubal c.** CARTILAGO TUBAE AUDITIVAE. **uniting c.** CONNECTING CARTILAGE. **upper nasal c.** CARTILAGO NASI LATERALIS. **vomerian c. of Hirschfeld** CARTILAGO VOMERONASALIS. **vomerian c. of Huschke** CARTILAGO VOMERONASALIS. **vomerine c.** CARTILAGO VOMERONASALIS. **vomeronasal c.** CARTILAGO VOMERONASALIS. **Weitbrecht's c.** DISCUS ARTICULARIS ARTICULATIONIS ACROMIOCLAVICULARIS. **Wrisberg's c.** CARTILAGO CUNEIFORMIS. **xiphoid c.** PROCESSUS XIPHOIDEUS. **Y c.** The triradiate, Y-shaped, epiphyseal cartilage that separates the ilium, ischium, and pubis in the acetabulum. Ossification in it commences around puberty and is completed between 20 and 25 years of age. **yellow c.** ELASTIC FIBROCARTILAGE.

**cartilagines** \kär′tilaj′inēz\ Plural of CARTILAGO.

**cartilaginification** \kär′tiləjin′ifikā′shən\ CHONDRIFICATION.

**cartilaginiform** \kär′tiləjin′ifôrm\ CARTILAGINOID.

**cartilaginoid** \kär′tilaj′inoid\ Resembling cartilage. Also *cartilaginiform*.

**cartilaginous** \kär′tilaj′inəs\ Pertaining to or composed of cartilage.

**cartilago** \kär′tilā′gō\ [L, gen. *cartilaginis*, cartilage, gristle] CARTILAGE. **cartilagines alares minores** [NA] A variable number of small platelike cartilages situated in the fibrous membrane attaching the posterior margin of the greater alar cartilage to the frontal process of the maxilla. Also *lesser alar cartilages, minor alar cartilages, sesamoid cartilages of nose.* **c. alaris major** [NA] A thin, flexible plate of cartilage situated bilaterally at and forming the tip of the nose. It is acutely bent to form a medial crus, or septal process, that takes part in the septum mobile nasi, and a lateral crus that occupies the anterior and superior portion of the ala. Also *greater alar cartilage, inferior cartilage of nose, lower lateral cartilage.* **c. articularis** [NA] Hyaline cartilage that usually covers and adheres to the articular surface of a bone in a synovial joint. It is smooth, flexible, elastic, and variable in thickness in different joints and within a joint. Also *articular cartilage, investing cartilage, arthrodial cartilage, diarthrodial cartilage.* **c. arytenoidea** [NA] One of a pair of pyramid-shaped cartilages articulated by their bases to the superior border of the lamina of the cricoid cartilage on which they rest. The upward projecting apex of each articulates with the corniculate cartilage in the aryepiglottic fold, while the anteriorly projecting vocal process gives attachment to the vocal ligament and the laterally projecting muscular process has two intrinsic laryngeal muscles attached to it. Also *arytenoid cartilage, triquetral cartilage, triquetrous cartilage.* **c. auriculae** [NA] A plate of fibrocartilage with depressions and eminences that produce the characteristic appearance and shape of the auricle of the external ear. It is absent on the lobule, deficient between the crus helicis and the tragus, and has two fissures. Also *auricular cartilage, conchal cartilage, fibrocartilage of the auricle.* **c. corniculata** [NA] One of a pair of conical nodules of elastic fibrocartilage that articulates with the apex of an arytenoid cartilage, to which it is sometimes fused in the aryepiglottic fold of mucous membrane. Also *corniculate cartilage, Santorini's cartilage, supra-arytenoid cartilage* (outmoded), *corniculum, corniculum laryngis, corpora santoriana.* **c. costalis** [NA] A flattened bar of hyaline cartilage extending anteriorly from the sternal end of each rib. Also *costal cartilage, sternal cartilage, costicartilage, cartilaginous extremity of rib.* **c. cricoidea** [NA] An unpaired cartilage shaped like a signet ring at the lower end of the larynx, comprising a quadrangular lamina posteriorly, on which rest the arytenoid cartilages, and a narrow arch anteriorly. On each side is an articular facet for the inferior cornu of the thyroid cartilage that lies above it. Its lower margin is connected to the first tracheal ring by the cricotracheal ligament. Its inner surface is lined by mucous membrane. Also *cricoid cartilage, annular cartilage.* **c. cuneiformis** [NA] One of a pair of rodlike nodules of elastic fibrocartilage, each lying anterior to the corniculate cartilage in the aryepiglottic fold and producing an elevation on the surface of the mucous membrane. Also *cuneiform cartilage, Morgagni's tubercle, Wrisberg's cartilage, cartilage of Morgagni.* **c. epiglottica** [NA] An unpaired leaf-shaped plate of fibrocartilage that is partly covered by mucous membrane anteriorly, connecting it to the base of the tongue, while from its lateral margins the mucosa continues as the aryepiglottic folds forming the aditus laryngis. Also *epiglottic cartilage.* **c. epiphysialis** [NA] A layer or plate of specialized hyaline cartilage located in a growing bone between the shaft, or diaphysis, and the extremity, or epiphysis. It permits growth in length of the bone until it has reached its characteristic size, when the cartilage ossifies and the bone is said to have reached maturity. Also *epiphysial cartilage, epiphysial plate, growth plate, epiphyseal disk.* **cartilagines laryngis** [NA] The cartilages providing the framework of the larynx, comprising the unpaired thyroid, cricoid, and epiglottic cartilages and the paired arytenoid, corniculate, and cuneiform cartilages, as well as some inconstant sesamoid cartilages. Also *laryngeal cartilages.* **c. meatus acustici** [NA] The trough-shaped tube of fibrocartilage, incomplete posterosuperiorly, that forms the lateral portion of the external acoustic meatus. Laterally it is continuous with the cartilage of the auricle, while medially it is firmly connected by fibrous tissue to the lateral lip of the osseous portion. Also *cartilage of acoustic meatus, cartilage of external acoustic meatus, meatal cartilage.* **cartilagines nasales accessoriae** [NA] An inconstant number of small cartilaginous plates situated in the angular interval between each greater alar and lateral nasal cartilage and above the lesser alar cartilages. Also *accessory nasal cartilages, epactal cartilages, minor cartilages* (outmoded), *sesamoid cartilages of nose.* **cartilagines nasi** [NA] The cartilages situated about the piriform-shaped nostrils and constituting part of the framework of the external nose, comprising the paired lateral nasal and greater alar cartilages; the variable lesser alar, accessory nasal, and vomeronasal cartilages; and the unpaired median cartilage of the nasal septum. Also *nasal cartilages.* **c. nasi lateralis** [NA] A triangular cartilage situated on either side of and partly fused anteriorly to the cartilage of the nasal septum. Also *lateral nasal cartilage, upper nasal cartilage.* **c. septi nasi** [NA] A thin quadrilateral plate of cartilage forming the anterior part of the nasal septum, wedged posteriorly between the anterior margins of the perpendicular plate of the ethmoid bone and the vomer. Also *cartilage of nasal septum, septal cartilage of nose.* **c. sesamoidea** 1 [NA] One of a pair of supernumerary cartilaginous nodules constantly present in some mammals but only occasionally found in humans at the lateral side of the arytenoid cartilages. Each is connected to the arytenoid and corniculate cartilages by small elastic ligaments. 2 [NA] Minute unpaired nodules of cartilage deep to the pharyngeal submucosa over the cricopharyngeal ligament. Also *interarytenoid cartilage, precricoid cartilage.* 3 An inconstant cartilaginous nodule in the anterior part of the vocal ligament. Also *laryngeal cartilage of Luschka, Luschka's cartilage, sesamoid cartilage of vocal ligament.* • The variant *sesamoid cartilage of larynx* applies to all three senses above. 4 CARTILAGO TRITICEA. **c. thyroidea** [NA] The largest cartilage of the larynx, composed of two quadrangular plates or laminae that fuse anteriorly at and below the angulated laryngeal prominence or Adam's apple, above which the plates are separated by the superior thyroid notch. The external surface provides attachment for muscles while the internal surface is lined by mucous membrane and is related to the vocal apparatus. Also *thyroid cartilage.* **cartilagines tracheales** [NA] Sixteen to twenty narrow incomplete rings of hyaline cartilage occupying about two-thirds of a circle with their free posterior ends linked together by elastic and smooth muscle fibers, forming the flexible framework of the trachea. They are set horizontally one above the other and separated by narrow gaps filled by elastic fibrous membranes, or annular ligaments, continuous with the perichondrium of each cartilage. They are lined internally by mucous membrane. Also *tracheal cartilages, tracheal rings.* **c. triticea** [NA] A small nodule of cartilage occasionally present in the lateral thyrohyoid ligament of the larynx. It may become calcified. Also *triticeal cartilage, corpus triticeum, corpusculum triticeum, cartilago sesamoidea, triticeous nodule, triticeum, triticeous node.* **c. tubae auditivae** [NA] A troughlike plate of cartilage bent into medial and lateral laminae closed laterally and inferiorly by a membranous lamina to form the framework of the cartilaginous portion of the auditory tube and located in a groove between the greater wing of the sphenoid bone and the petrous part of the temporal bone. Posteriorly it is firmly attached to the osseous portion while anteriorly it opens into the lateral wall of the pharynx just behind the inferior nasal concha. Also *cartilage of auditory tube, tubal cartilage, eustachian cartilage.* **c. vomeronasalis** [NA] A strip of cartilage on each side of the anterior end of the inferior margin of the cartilage of the nasal septum, attached to it and to the maxilla anteriorly and to the vomer posteriorly. Also *vomeronasal cartilage, Jacobson's cartilage, vomerine cartilage, paraseptal cartilage, vomerian cartilage of Hirschfeld, vomerian cartilage of Huschke.*

**cartilagotropic** \kär′tilā′gəträp′ik\ Tending to turn into cartilage.

**caruncle** \kär′ungkl\ [L *caruncula.* See CARUNCULA.] CARUNCULA. **hymenal c.'s** CARUNCULAE MYRTIFORMES. **lacrimal c.** CARUNCULA LACRIMALIS. **Morgagni's c.** LOBUS MEDIUS PROSTATAE. **morgagnian c.** LOBUS MEDIUS PROSTATAE. **myrtiform c.'s** CARUNCULAE MYRTIFORMES. **salivary c.** CARUNCULA SUBLINGUALIS. **sublingual c.** CARUNCULA SUBLINGUALIS. **urethral c.** A small red eminence on the mucous membrane of the urinary meatus in women.

**caruncula** \kərung′kyələ\ [L (dim. of *caro* flesh), a little piece of flesh, small protuberance of flesh] (*pl.* carunculae) A small fleshy nodule or eminence. Also *caruncle.* **carunculae myrtiformes** The numerous mucous membrane projections of the hymen that surround the vaginal orifice after its rupture. Also *hymenal caruncles, myrtiform caruncles, carunculae hymenales.* **c. lacrimalis** [NA] A small, rounded fleshy body that occupies the lacus lacrimalis in the medial angle of the eye. Also *lacrimal caruncle.* **c. mammillaris** *Outmoded* TRIGONUM OLFACTORIUM. **c. sublingualis** [NA] A small rounded elevation, at the apex of which is the orifice of the submandibular duct and sometimes also the orifice of the major sublingual duct, on each side of the frenulum linguae in the floor of the mouth. Also *sublingual caruncle, caruncula salivaris* (outmoded), *sublingual papilla, salivary caruncle.*

**carunculae** \kərung′kyəlē\ Plural of CARUNCULA.

**caruncular** \kərung′kyələr\ Pertaining to or resembling a caruncle.

**Carus** [Carl Gustav *Carus,* German physiologist, 1789–1869] Circle of Carus. See under CURVE.

**carver** An instrument with a sharp blade used for carving the wax patterns of a cast restoration or amalgam while in a plastic state.

**caryo-** \kar′ē•ō-, kar′yə-\ KARYO-.

**Casal** [Gaspar *Casal,* Spanish physician, 1691–1759] Casal's collar. See under NECKLACE.

**Casamino acids** The amino acids constituting casein, obtained by enzymatic hydrolysis. A complete set of the amino acids is obtained partly in the form of short peptides, including those that are destroyed in acid hydrolysis, such as glutamine and tryptophan. A proprietary name.

**cascade** \kaskād′\ [French, from Italian *cascata* a cascade, from *cascare* to fall, from assumed Vulgar L *casicare* to fall, from L *casus,* past part. of *cadere* to fall] A series of events in which an initial stage triggers a second that then triggers a third, and so on, in sequence, until some final state is reached. **extrinsic coagulation c.** See under CASCADE HYPOTHESIS OF COAGULATION. **intrinsic coagulation c.** See under CASCADE HYPOTHESIS OF COAGULATION.

**cascading** \kaskā′ding\ A technique such as an electronic counter or amplifier that utilizes several stages combined in series to obtain an effect, separation, or signal gain greater than that possible with a single stage.

**cascara** \kaskar′ə\ [Spanish *cáscara* rind, husk, bark] CASCARA SAGRADA. **c. sagrada** The dried bark of *Rhamnus purshiana*, extracts of which are used as purgatives. Also *bearberry bark, chittam bark, chittem bark, chittim bark, sacred bark, cascara, purshiana bark, Persian bark, bearwood.*

**case** 1 An instance of disease, injury, or other abnormal condition. 2 A subject cited as having a disease, injury, or other abnormal condition; patient. • This usage is regarded by some as objectionable, though it is common. **coroner's c.** An unexplained death legally requiring investigation to determine the cause and the manner of death. • The exact criteria defining such cases vary among different jurisdictions but generally include any sudden, unexpected, suspicious, or violent death, or death unattended by a physician. **index c.** In epidemiology, the first case of a given disease in a population or group to come to notice even though it may not have been the first case to have occurred in that population or group, such as the first known case of tuberculosis in a family. The first patient studied is called the proband. **primary c.** In epidemiology, the first case of an infectious disease to occur in a population or group, such as the first case of measles in a school. **secondary c.** In epidemiology, a case of infectious disease occurring in a person exposed to infection from a primary case.

**caseation** \kā′sē·ā′shən\ 1 Precipitation of casein or accumulation of a cheeselike material. 2 CASEOUS NECROSIS.

**case-control** Employing an epidemiologic technique based on a study of cases in which the disease to be studied already exists, used especially when randomized studies cannot be performed.

**casein** [L *case(us)* cheese + -IN] One of several milk proteins, of molecular mass 20–30 kDa. $\alpha$-Casein, $\beta$-casein, $\gamma$-casein, and $\kappa$-casein have been distinguished, and some of these show genetic variation. They are rich in phosphoserine residues.

**casein hydrolysate** \kā′sē·in hīdräl′isāt, kā′sēn\ Casein that is produced by enzymatic or acidic hydrolysis of a protein into its constituent amino acids. The hydrolysis is not complete when enzymatic degradation is used and some peptides remain. As a result, however, the product is more palatable. It contains only L-amino acids, and while some loss of all amino acids occurs during hydrolysis, tryptophan losses are most significant. Casein hydrolysate is added to various foods to enrich them with protein and it is often used as a base for liquid protein preparations.

**case-mix** CASE MIX. See under MIX.

**caseous** \kā′sē·əs\ [L *caseus* cheese] 1 Cheesy; curdlike. 2 Relating to or resulting from caseation.

**caseum** \kā′sē·əm\ [L (also *caseus*), cheese] A material that resembles cottage cheese in consistency and that forms as a result of tuberculous necrosis of tissue.

**caseworm** \kās′wurm\ 1 CADDIS WORM. 2 CASE WORM.

**Casoni** [Tomaso *Casoni,* Italian physician, 1880–1933] Casoni skin test. See under REACTION.

**Casselberry** [William Evans *Casselberry,* U.S. laryngologist, 1858–1916] See under POSITION.

**Casser** [Giulio *Casser* (Casseri), Italian anatomist, 1556–1616] 1 Casser's ligament, casserian ligament. See under LIGAMENTUM MALLEI LATERALE. 2 Casser's muscle. See under LIGAMENTUM MALLEI ANTERIUS. 3 Casser's perforated muscle. See under MUSCULUS CORACOBRACHIALIS.

**cassette** 1 A small cartridge containing magnetic tape for use in any of various electronic devices. 2 In radiology, an aluminum or plastic frame in which an unexposed x-ray film is sandwiched between two fluorescent intensifying screens.

**Cassidy** [Maurice Alan *Cassidy,* English physician, flourished early 20th century] Cassidy syndrome, Cassidy-Scholte syndrome. See under CARCINOID SYNDROME.

**cast** [Middle English (from *casten* to throw, from Old Norse *kasta* to throw) a throw, something thrown or cast off, or the form in which it is cast off] 1 A rigid dressing used to immobilize the trunk or limbs in instances of fractures, dislocations, and other injuries. It is usually made with a bandage impregnated with plaster of Paris. 2 The mold of a segment of a tubular structure such as a bronchiole or a renal tubule, formed from hardened material clogging the lumen and which may be expelled, as in sputum or urine; especially, a urinary cast. 3 *Popular* STRABISMUS. **bacterial c.** A urinary cast from a pyelonephritic kidney and which contains bacteria. **blood c.** RED BLOOD CELL CAST. **broad c.** A cast approximately four times as broad as the usual cast, formed in a collecting tubule. The presence in urine of large numbers reflects end-stage renal disease. **broad epithelial cell c.** A broad cast into which epithelial cells have been incorporated, reflecting advanced renal parenchymal disease. **coma c.** A urinary cast with highly refractile granules. Coma casts were formerly considered a sign of impending coma of diabetes. **decidual c.** An accumulation of degenerating decidua passed from the uterus of a patient with an ectopic pregnancy. Also *endometritis tuberosa papulosa.* **dental c.** A replica of dental and oral structures made by pouring liquid plaster into an impression of them, allowing the plaster to set, and removing the impression. Also *dental model.* **epithelial cell c.** A cast in which epithelial cells have been incorporated, reflecting renal parenchymal disease. **false c.** A formed element in the urinary sediment that looks like a cast, but is not. It is often composed of mucus fibers or aggregations of crystals. Also *pseudocast.* **fatty c.** A cast that contains fatty material, indicating tubular fatty change, and common in the urine of patients with the nephrotic syndrome of any cause. **fibrinous c.'s** Casts containing fibrin. These are readily demonstrable by immunofluorescent techniques in renal tubules, and reflect glomerular damage. Fibrinous casts in the urine are refractile and dark yellow. **granular c.** A cast characterized by the presence of fine or coarse granules, representing degeneration of cells, usually tubular, previously incorporated into the cast. Granular casts reflect parenchymal renal disease. **hair c.** TRICHOBEZOAR. **hyaline c.** A clear, slightly refractile cylinder best seen in the urinary sediment upon microscopic examination under low lighting. Hyaline casts are composed mainly of Tamm-Horsfall protein, a mucoprotein of tubular origin, but also may contain other serum proteins. Their rate of formation depends on the degree of proteinuria, and the urine flow rate and pH. They dissolve rapidly at alkaline pH. Although usually associated with renal parenchymal disease, occasionally a few or even a moderate number of hyaline casts appear in normal urine. **leukocyte c.** A cast which incorporates leukocytes from the kidney, and which indicates the presence of an infectious or inflammatory disease of the kidney. As the cast passes through an inflamed lower urinary tract additional leukocytes may adhere to it. Also *pus cast.* **pigmented c.'s** Casts which are brown when associated with hemoglobinuria, and gray-yellow when associated with jaundice, reflecting renal parenchymal disease in either case. **plaster of Paris c.** An external splint made of plaster of Paris used to support underlying tissues during the healing process. **pus c.** LEUKOCYTE CAST. **red blood cell c.** A cast that incorporates one or more red blood cells which originated from glomerular damage or, rarely, from peritubular hemorrhage. The red cells in the cast may be individually distinct, or a homogeneous orange-red color. Red cell casts always reflect glomerular disease. Also *blood cast.* **refractory c.** A cast fabricated with materials that resist high temperatures without disintegrating. **renal c.** URINARY CAST. **tube c.** *Obs.* URINARY CAST. **urate c.** An aggregation of urates that is shaped like a urinary cast. **urinary c.** A cylindrical proteinaceous mold of renal tubules, often incorporating elements of intact or degenerating cells. Formation depends in part on pH and protein content of urine

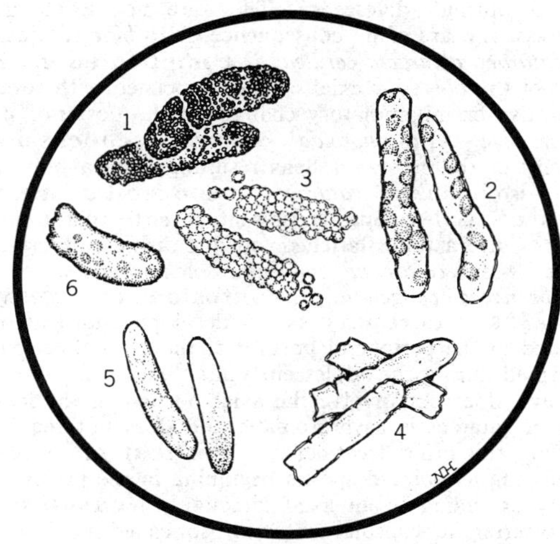


**Urinary casts** (1) Coarse granular casts; (2) epithelial cell casts; (3) red blood cell casts; (4) waxy casts; (5) hyaline casts; (6) casts with pyocytes.

and rate of urine flow, and in part on presence of glomerular, interstitial, or tubular lesions in the kidneys. Major types are hyaline, which consist largely of Tamm-Horsfall mucoprotein; coarsely or finely granular; red cell; white cell; and broad or waxy. Occasional hyaline casts are seen in normal urine. After strenuous exercise, normal persons may excrete small numbers of all the above types of cast except broad or waxy, which are indicative of advanced renal disease. Also *renal cast, tube cast* (obs.). **waxy c.** A cast in which cellular elements have degenerated into waxy-appearing material, reflecting advanced renal parenchymal disease.

**Castellani** [Sir Aldo *Castellani,* Italian physician, 1879–1971] **1** See under TREATMENT. **2** Castellani-Low symptom. See under SYMPTOM. **3** Castellani's bronchitis, Castellani disease. See under BRONCHOSPIROCHETOSIS. **4** Castellani's vaccine. See under TYPHOID AND PARATYPHOID VACCINE.

**casting** The process by which a substance is cast in a mold or the object so shaped and solidified. **vacuum c.** The formation of an object by pouring plastic material into a mold and creating a vacuum behind it so the plastic is pulled against the walls of the mold.

**Castle** [William Bosworth *Castle,* U.S. physician, born 1897] Castle's factor. See under INTRINSIC FACTOR.

**castrate** \kas′trāt\ [L *castrat(us),* past part. of *castrare* to cut, geld, castrate] To deprive of gonadal function by surgical or, rarely, chemical means.

**castration** \kastrā′shən\ [L *castratio* (from *castratus,* past part. of *castrare* to cut, geld, castrate) castration] Surgical excision of the testicles or ovaries. In males, this operation results in the loss of ability to produce sperm. In females, the operation eliminates the production of ova and the occurrence of estrus. Castration has been used to control certain neoplasms, primarily prostatic adenocarcinoma, and carcinoma of the breast. Compare ANORCHISM, CRYPTORCHIDISM. **female c.** A surgical procedure in which a bilateral oophorectomy is performed, resulting in sterility. **radiologic c.** Destruction of the hormonal functions of the gonads by the use of ionizing radiation. Gametogenesis is more sensitive to gamma rays than is hormone secretion.

**castroid** \kas′troid\ An individual having the characteristics of one who has been castrated; eunuchoid.

**casualty** \kazh′oo·əltē\ Incapacitation or loss of useful service of an individual by death, injury, illness, or other cause: used especially, often in the plural, of military combatants killed, wounded, or missing, or of a civilian population suffering a natural disaster.

**CAT** computerized axial tomography.

**cat-** \kat-\ CATA-.

**cata-** \kat′ə-\ [Gk *kata* (*kath-* as prefix before aspirated Gk words or elements) down] A prefix meaning down, against. Also *kata-, cat-, kat-, cath-, kath-.*

**catabasis** \kətab′əsis\ [Gk *katabasis* (from *katabainein* to go down) a going down] The period of abatement of a disease. Adj. catabatic.

**catabiosis** \-bī·ō′sis\ [CATA- + BIOSIS] **1** Any activity in a living tissue that influences physically related tissue. **2** Normal cellular senescence.

**catabolin** \kətab′əlin\ Mediator produced by mononuclear blood cells in immune reaction that causes the breakdown of connective tissue matrix. It is believed to be identical to interleukin-1.

**catabolism** \kətab′əlizm\ [Gk *katabol(ē)* a throwing down + -ISM] The metabolic process in which complex compounds are broken down into simpler substances. Also *regression, devolution* (seldom used), *involution.* Also *katabolism.* Compare ANABOLISM.

**catacrotic** \-krät′ik\ [CATA- + Gk *krot(os)* a beat + -IC] Characterized by having one or more notches, or small upward waves, on the descending limb: said of a pulse or pulse wave.

**catadicrotic** \-dīkrät′ik\ [CATA- + DICROTIC] Characterized by having two notches, or small upward waves, on the descending limb: said of a pulse or pulse wave.

**catadidymus** \-did′iməs\ [CATA- + -DIDYMUS] Twin embryos, fetuses, or newborn infants united at the head and/or the thorax but doubled in the inferior regions.

**catagen** \kat′əjən\ [CATA- + *-gen* as in *anagen*] The involutionary phase of the cycle of activity of the hair follicle. Compare ANAGEN, TELOGEN.

**catagenesis** \-jen′əsis\ [CATA- + GENESIS] Biologic regression.

**catagmatic** \kat′agmat′ik\ Capable of healing a broken bone.

**catalase** \kat′əlās\ A heme-containing enzyme (EC 1.11.1.6) that is found in the microbodies (peroxisomes) of animal cells and that catalyzes the reaction $2H_2O_2 \rightleftharpoons 2H_2O + O_2$. Its iron is normally in the III state.

**catalepsy** \kat′əlep′sē\ [Gk *katalēpsis* (from *katalambanein* to seize, hold down, repress, stop, from *lambanein* to grasp) seizure, holding, stoppage, catalepsy] A condition marked by posturing or prolonged maintenance of physical attitudes, as in the waxy flexibility of some catatonic schizophrenics who often appear to be in a trancelike state or the rigid posturing of some patients with frontocerebellar lesions. Also *stupor vigilans.* Adj. cataleptic.

**catalogia** \-lō′jə\ [CATA- + -LOGIA] VERBIGERATION.

**catalysis** \kətal′isis\ [Gk *katalysis* (from *katalyein* to dissolve, resolve, settle, make peace, from *lyein* to loose, dissolve) resolution, settlement (as by arbitration)] The phenomenon of acceleration of a reaction by a substance that is not destroyed in the reaction. Since simultaneous destruction of the catalyst may occur, catalysis may often be inferred if several molecules of reactant are transformed at an accelerated rate for each molecule of the catalyst added. **superacid c.** Catalysis by a metal ion of charge greater than unity. It is more effective than catalysis by $H^+$ because of the greater electron attraction of the greater charge on the ion.

**catalyst** \kat′əlist\ [Gk *kataly(tēr)* an arbitrator + English *-(i)st.* See also CATALYSIS.] A substance that participates in a reaction and thereby increases its rate without being destroyed or incorporated into the products. Catalysts may be inorganic, as is platinum in hydrogenations, or organic, as are certain proteins (enzymes) in biologic systems.

**catalyze** \kat′əlīz\ To act as a catalyst of (a chemical reaction).

**catamenia** \-mē′nē·ə\ [Gk *katamēnia* (neut. pl. of *katamēnios* monthly, from *kata-,* intensive prefix + *mēn* month) monthlies] MENSES.

**catamenial** \-mē′nē·əl\ Pertaining to the catamenia; menstrual.

**catamenogenic** \-men′ōjen′ik\ Resulting in menstruation.

**cataphoresis** \-fôrē′sis\ ELECTROPHORESIS.

**cataphrenia** \-frē′nē·ə\ [CATA- + PHREN- + -IA] PSEUDODEMENTIA.

**cataphylaxis** \-fīlak′sis\ [CATA- + Gk *phylaxis* guarding, protection] **1** The concentrated movement of leukocytes and antibodies to the site of an infection. **2** The collapse of the body's natural resistance to infection. For defs. 1 and 2 also *kataphylaxis.*

**cataplectic** \-plek′tik\ Relating to or characteristic of cataplexy.

**cataplexie du réveil** \kätäpleksē′ dʏ rāvā′ē\ SLEEP PARALYSIS.

**cataplexy** \kat′əpleksē\ [Gk *kataplēx(is)* (from *kataplēssein* to strike down, from *kata* down + *plēssein* to strike) amazement, consternation + -Y] A paroxysmal disorder of postural tone in which in response to an emotional stimulus, such as pleasure, laughter, anger, or excitement, there is sudden loss of function of some or all of the voluntary muscles. Consciousness and awareness are preserved throughout the attack. The condition usually occurs in association with narcolepsy, and is believed to be due to hypersensitivity of one part of the reticular inhibitory system. It bears no relationship to epilepsy. Adj. cataplectic.

**catapophysis** [CAT- + APOPHYSIS] A process of bone or of brain tissue. *Outmoded.*

# cataract

**cataract** \kat′ərakt\ [L *cataracta,* earlier *catarractes,* from Gk *katarrhaktēs* (from *katarrhēgnynai* to burst forth, rush down) waterfall, water gate, portcullis; in Med L also window grating, applied in fig. sense to the eye condition] Any opacity of the crystalline lens, regardless of whether it affects visual acuity or has any clinical significance. Also *cataracta.* Adj. cataractous. **arborescent c.** A cataract having a branching shape. **atopic c.** A cataract associated with severe chronic atopic dermatitis. **axial c.** A cataract located on the line of sight. **axiliary c.** An elongated lens opacity oriented anteroposteriorly in the center of the lens. **blue c.** CERULEAN CATARACT. **blue dot c.** CERULEAN CATARACT. **bottlemakers' c.** HEAT-RAY CATARACT. **brunescent c.** An advanced nuclear cataract of a reddish brown color. Also *cataracta brunescens.* **capsular c.** An opacity of the capsule of the crystalline lens. **capsulolenticular c.** An opacity of both capsule and crystalline lens. **cerulean c.** Small blue punctate lens opacities located in the deep cortex in the lamellae formed during adolescence. They are not axial, do not progress, and are of no consequence. Also *blue cataract, blue dot cataract, cataracta cerulea.* **complicated c.** A cataract of the posterior axial cortex, associated with severe degenerative or inflammatory changes of the posterior portion of the eye. Also *choroidal cataract.* **concussion c.** Opacity of the crystalline lens resulting from a blow to the eye. Also *contusion cataract.* **congenital membranous c.** A lens opacity present at birth that transforms the lens into a thin, flattened, opaque disk of abnormal lens tissue. Also *cataracta congenita membranacea, cataracta membranacea congenita.* **contusion c.** CONCUSSION CATARACT. **coronary c.** A developmental lens opacity situated in the peripheral portion of the crystalline lens that is formed during the adolescent years. Since it is nonprogressive and does not involve the axial portion of the lens, this type of cataract is asymptomatic and does not require surgery or any other treatment. **cortical c.** A cataract developing as pointed spokes beginning in the periphery and slowly extending in an axial direction. **cupuliform c.** A posterior subcapsular cataract, so called because of its concave shape. **cystic c.** FLUID CATARACT. **diabetic c.** A cataract occurring as a complication of diabetes mellitus. **dry-shelled c.** HYPERMATURE CATARACT. **electrical c.** A premature cataract developing months or a few years after a high voltage electrical burn of the body. If the electrical burn involves the head, the incidence may be as high as 30 percent. **embryonal nuclear c.** A congenital cataract in which opacity occurs only in the embryonal nucleus of the lens. **fibroid c.** PSEUDOPHAKIA FIBROSA. **floriform c.** A radiating axial congenital cataract with a fanciful resemblance to flower petals. **fluid c.** A lens opacity in which the cortex has liquefied. Also *cystic cataract.* **fusiform c.** A central cataract oriented in an axial direction. Also *spindle cataract.* **glassblowers' c.** HEAT-RAY CATARACT. **glaucomatous c.** Punctate cortical opacities due to nutritional damage sustained at the time of an attack of angle closure glaucoma. **gray c.** An opacity occupying the entire crystalline lens or at least its anterior portion so that the pupil appears grossly gray in color. **green c.** *Obs.* GLAUCOMA. **hard c.** A cataract with an extremely dense nucleus. **heat-ray c.** A condition occurring in persons exposed through their work to infra-red rays. It is characterized in its early stages by changes in the posterior pole of the lens. Changes later spread to the rest of the lens cortex. Also *bottlemakers' cataract, glassblowers' cataract, puddlers' cataract, glassblowers' disease.* **heterochromic c.** A cataract associated with heterochromic cyclitis. **hypermature c.** A far advanced cataract in which shrinkage of the lens occurs. Also *cataracta aridosiliquata, overripe cataract, dry-shelled cataract.* **immature c.** An early stage of cataract in which there is a slight increase of fluid within the cortical fibers. **infantile c.** Opacity in one or both lenses occurring in infancy. Some cataracts may begin and progress after birth, others may be congenital, as because of rubella, or due to an embryopathy. Many congenital forms are inherited as an autosomal dominant trait. Cataracts are associated with a large number of diseases or syndromes which may be grouped under intraocular infection or disease; inborn errors of metabolism; trauma; drugs, including oxygen in prematurity; and radiation and chromosomal aberration. **intumescent c.** A markedly swollen, opaque lens. **irradiation c.** Opacity of the crystalline lens resulting from epithelial damage by radiation, as by x ray, ultrasonic waves, ultraviolet, or infrared. **juvenile c.** A lens opacity developing in middle or late childhood, sometimes progressing from an infantile cataract, sometimes arising *de novo.* **lamellar c.** A developmental cataract in which the opacity is limited to a layer of developing lens fibers corresponding to a particular period of growth. Portions of the lens formed at an earlier or later time may be entirely clear. Also *zonular cataract.* **lenticular c.** An opacity of the lens that does not affect its capsule. **mature c.** An advanced cataract in which the cortex has become opaque and soft. **membranous c.** An atrophic cataract that has a very thin anteroposterior diameter. **milky c.** A cataract in which the cortex has liquefied. **morgagnian c.** A cataract in which a dense nuclear remnant has gravitated to the bottom of milky fluid representing the completely liquefied cortex. **nuclear c.** An opacity of the central portion of the crystalline lens. Also *nuclear sclerosis.* **occupational c.** Any cataract of which one's occupation places one at risk. This can occur as a result of trauma, electric shock, exposure to infra-red heat or ionizing radiation, and possibly from handling dinitrophinol and dinitro-orthocresol. **overripe c.** HYPERMATURE CATARACT. **perinuclear c.** A cataract of the deep cortical lens fibers, surrounding the lens nucleus. **peripheral c.** A cataract of the equatorial periphery of the lens, leaving the axis clear. **polar c.** A cataract that develops in an area around the anterior or posterior pole of the lens. **puddlers' c.** HEAT-RAY CATARACT. **punctate c.** Lens opacities consisting of multiple small faults distributed throughout the lens cortex. **pyramidal c.** A polar cataract in which the opacity has a conical shape. **radiation c.** A cataract resulting from exposure to ionizing radiation. **reduplication c.** A collar-button shape of axial cataract, the two portions being located subcapsularly and in the deeper cortex. **ripe c.** A lens opacity with enough cortical liquefaction to permit easy extracapsular extraction. **secondary c.** A recurrent cataract following incomplete surgical removal or extensive lens injury. **sedimentary c.** A partially liquefied cataract with gravitational displacement of its contents. **senile c.** A lens opacity occurring spontaneously in an older person. **siliculose c.** A shrunken and calcified lens opacity. Also *siliquose cataract.* **Soemmering's ring c.** A secondary growth of lens opacity after incomplete cataract extraction. Lens material re-forms from the equatorial epithelium, resulting in a ring-shaped opacity. Also *Soemmering's ring.* **soft c.** A cataract with a nucleus that can easily be fragmented during surgical removal. **spindle c.** FUSIFORM CATARACT. **stationary c.** A cataract that does not increase in extent or density. **stellate c.** A cataract of radiating shape because it conforms to the pattern of lens fiber distribution. **subcapsular c.** An opacity located directly internal to the lens capsule. **sunflower c.** A cataract associated with copper poisoning, located anteriorly and shaped like a disk (corresponding to the pupil) surrounded by a large ovoid pattern resembling petals. **sutural c.** A congenital cataract with opacities distributed along the sites of the embryonic sutures of the lens. **zonular c.** LAMELLAR CATARACT.

**cataracta** \kat′ərak′tə\ CATARACT. **c. aridosiliquata** HYPERMATURE CATARACT. **c. brunescens** BRUNESCENT CATARACT. **c. cerulea** CERULEAN CATARACT. **c. congenita membranacea** CONGENITAL MEMBRANOUS CATARACT. **c. membranacea congenita** CONGENITAL MEMBRANOUS CATARACT.

**cataractogenic** \kat′ərak′təjen′ik\ [CATARACT + *o* + -GENIC] Capable of inducing opacification of the crystalline lens.

**cataractous** \kat′ərak′təs\ Associated with or of the nature of cataracts.

**catarrh** \kətär′\ [Gk *katarrhoos* (from *katarrheein* to drip, flow down, from *kata* down + *rhein* to flow) flowing down, a downflow, catarrh] A condition of the mucous membranes, particularly those of the upper respiratory tract, characterized by inflammation and conspicuous, mainly mucinous discharge. *Popular.* Also *rheuma* (obs.). **autumnal c.** HAY FEVER. **Bostock's c.** *Obs.* HAY FEVER. **epidemic c.** Upper-respiratory-tract infection in the course of such epidemic illnesses as influenza. *Older term.* **postnasal c.** The accumulation of secretions in the nasopharynx. It is a symptom common to a number of upper respiratory inflammatory diseases. *Imprecise.* **spring c.** VERNAL CONJUNCTIVITIS. **summer c.** *Seldom used* HAY FEVER. **vernal c.** Hay fever occurring in the spring due to the pollens of the early flowering trees and plants. *Rare.*

**catarrhal** \kətär′əl\ Liable to cause or characterized by catarrh.

**Catarrhina** \-rī′nə\ [Gk *katarrhina,* neut. pl. of *katarrhin* (from *kata* down + *rhis,* gen. *rhinos,* nose, in pl. *rhines* nostrils) long-nosed, hooknosed] CERCOPITHECOIDEA.

**catarrhine** \kat′ərīn\ Of or relating to the primate family Cercopithecoidia (Catarrhina).

**catastrophe** \kətas′trəfē\ **error c.** An accumulation of faulty or error proteins within a cell, causing failure of the cell's specific function and thought to be due to template failure, possibly associated with cellular aging. Also *Orgel phenomenon, Orgel's hypothesis.*

**catatasis** \kətat′əsis\ [Gk *katatasis* (from *kateinein* to stretch) a stretching, esp. for setting broken or dislocated bones] The longitudinal traction of a limb or structure to reduce a fracture or dislocation.

**catatonia** \kat′ətō′nē·ə\ [CATA- + *ton(o)-* + -IA] **1** A subtype of schizophrenia characterized by prominent alterations in muscle tone or motor reactivity such as stupor, negativism, posturing, rigidity, or agitation. **2** The abnormality of muscle tone seen in catalepsy. For defs. 1 and 2 also *catatony* (obs.).

**catatonic** \-tän′ik\ Characterized by or manifesting elements of catatonia.

**catatonoid** \kətat′ənoid\ Resembling or mimicking catatonia.

**catatony** \kətat′ənē\ *Obs.* CATATONIA.

**catatropia** \-trō′pē·ə\ [CATA- + -TROPIA] Downward deviation of one eye.

**catechol** \kat′əkôl\ *O*-Dihydroxybenzene. It is easily oxidized to form a quinone. Many catechols, such as dopa, are biologically important.

**catecholamine** A compound containing an *o*-catechol nucleus and an amine group on a chain of two carbon atoms *m* and *p* to the phenolic hydroxyl groups. It is thus related to epinephrine. Several are sympathomimetic; several are precursors or metabolites of epinephrine. Also *adrenergic amine.*

**catechol methyl ether** GUAIACOL.

**catechol *O*-methyltransferase** The enzyme (EC 2.1.1.6) that catalyzes methylation of catechols on a phenolic oxygen by transfer of a methyl group from *S*-adenosylmethionine. It is found in plasma, the liver, and the kidneys, and probably catalyzes the initial step in physiological inactivation of the circulating catecholamines, epinephrine and norepinephrine. Abbr. COMT

**catechu** A dried, aqueous extract of the leaves and young shoots of *Uncaria gambier (Rubiaceae),* a climbing shrub cultivated in the East Indies. It is an astringent, and is used in the treatment of diarrhea. Also *gambir, pale catechu.* **pale c.** CATECHU.

**catelectrotonus** \kat′ilekträt′ənəs\ [CAT- + ELECTRO- + TONUS] A state of reduced threshold in excitable tissue in the vicinity of a cathodal electrode.

**catenated** \kat′ənā′tid\ [L *catenat(us),* past part. of *catenare* to chain, join by a chain + English *-ed,* suffix denoting past part.] Joined like the links in a chain by being in the form of closed rings with one passing through another.

**catenulate** \kəten′yəlāt\ [Late L *catenul(a),* dim. of L *catena* a chain + -ATE] Chainlike; composed of individual units joined in a linear arrangement: characteristic of certain protozoan colonies and fungal spore groupings. Also *catenoid.*

**catgut** An absorbable surgical suture material obtained from the treated and preserved connective tissues of animals. Also *catgut suture, surgical gut.* **carbolized c.** Catgut derived from the connective tissues of animals and treated with phenol, now obsolete. **chromic c.** Catgut that has been heated with chromium trioxide to increase its strength and durability. Also *chromicized catgut.*

**cath-** \kath-\ CATA-.

**cath** **1** cathartic. **2** catheter.

**catha** \kath′ə\ The freshly dried leaves of *Catha edulus,* an evergreen shrub native to northeastern Africa and Arabia. It is chewed and ingested for an effect of euphoria and general excitement. Tea prepared from the leaves, and the oil expressed from the seeds, are also stimulating. This plant is a source of the alkaloid cathine (norpseudoephedrine). Also *khat.*

**cathaeresis** CATHERESIS.

**catharometer** \kath′əräm′ətər\ [Gk *katharo(s)* clean, pure, true + -METER] An instrument that measures and records the thermal conductivity of air.

**catharsis** \kəthär′sis\ [Gk *katharsis* (from *kathairein* to cleanse, from *katharos* clean) a cleansing, purge] **1** The expulsion of feces aided by an osmotic, irritant or stimulant agent taken orally or by enema; purgation. **2** The reexperiencing of repressed memories with their associated emotions so that they no longer need be released in disguised form as symptoms; the therapeutic discharge of repressed material and its associated affect. Also *psychocatharsis* (outmoded).

**cathartic** \kəthär′tik\ **1** Causing or promoting catharsis. **2** An agent which causes or promotes movement of the bowels. **bulk c.** A cathartic derived from natural or semisynthetic polysaccharides or cellulose derivatives which acts by adding bulk to and hydrating the feces. **lubricant c.** A cathartic which acts by hydrating and thereby lubricating the feces. **saline c.** A cathartic consisting of magnesium salts, sulfates, phosphates, or tartrates which acts by retaining water in the intestinal lumen by osmotic forces. Also *saline purgative.* **stimulant c.** A cathartic which acts by stimulating bowel motility and secretion of fluid and electrolytes from the colonic mucosa.

**cathartic acid** An active ingredient in senna that has laxative properties. Also *cathartinic acid.*

**cathepsin** An intracellular proteinase, usually situated in lysosomes. Originally, only enzymes with an acid pH optimum were designated cathepsins, but now various other enzymes are included.

**catheresis** [Gk *kathairesis* (from *kathairein* to take down) a putting down, reducing] Weakness or prostration caused by a medication. Also *cathaeresis.*

**catheretic** **1** Mildly caustic. **2** Causing weakness or prostration: used of medicines.

**catheter** \kath′ətər\ [Gk *katheter̄* (from *kathie(nai)* to send down, reach by sounding, from *kat(a)* down + *hienai* to send + *-tēr,* agentive suffix) something inserted, a catheter] A long, thin, hollow surgical instrument, usually flexible and with one or more lumina, that is inserted into a body cavity, such as the bladder, for the purpose of drainage or for the administration of diagnostic or therapeutic agents. **balloon c.** A catheter with two lumens, the tip of which is equipped with a collapsible balloon. The balloon is inflated after insertion into a vessel in order to extract a thrombus or embolus, or, occasionally, to occlude blood flow. **Braasch bulb c.** A surgical catheter with a spherical tip and a long firm base. It serves the dual purpose of dilatation and calibration. **cardiac c.** A long, fine, flexible tube, usually radiopaque, designed for insertion into a peripheral blood vessel through which it can then be manipulated under x-ray control into the heart. There it is used for registration of pressures, sampling of blood, or rapid injection of radiopaque substances which will outline the

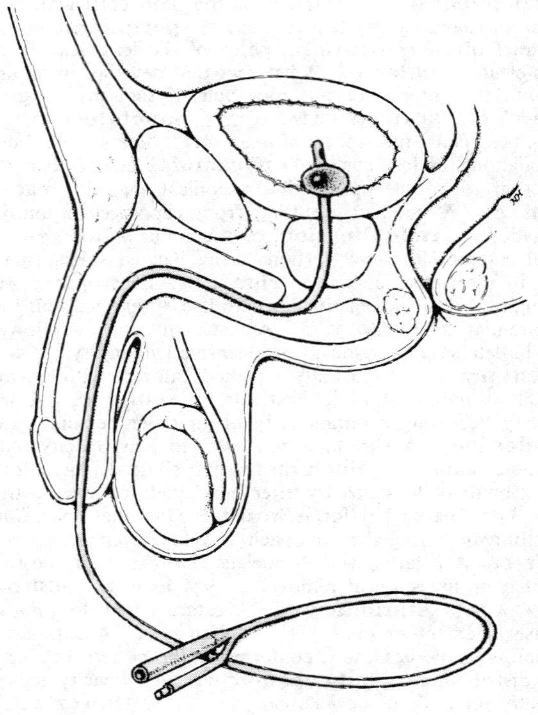

Foley catheter

chambers and blood vessels of the heart. Also *intracardiac catheter.* **coaxial counterflow single needle blood access c.** A catheter with two lumens for use in single-needle hemodialysis. One of the lumens is used to withdraw blood from the subject, the other to return blood from the dialyzer. **de Pezzer c.** A self-retaining catheter with a bulbous tip. **double-current c.** A surgical catheter with two lumina, one for injection and one for drainage of the irrigating solution. Also *two-way catheter.* **eustachian c.** A catheter having a slightly curved beak and a length of approximately 15 cm. It is available in several sizes. It is used in performing eustachian catheterization. **filiform-tipped c.** A catheter whose leading end is initially very slender and flexible so as to facilitate passage through a constricted, angulated, or obstructed tubular structure. Also *whip catheter.* **flexible c.** A catheter of soft rubber. Also *Nélaton's catheter, soft catheter.* **Fogarty c.** One of a variety of catheters that are tipped with inflatable balloons of varying diameters and that are widely used to remove thrombi or emboli from blood vessels. The deflated balloon is passed beyond the obstructing material, inflated, and then withdrawn along with its entrapped thrombus or embolus. **Foley c.** A self-retaining catheter held in place in the urinary bladder with an inflated balloon. **indwelling c.** A catheter held in place within the bladder. **intracardiac c.** CARDIAC CATHETER. **Karman c.** KARMAN CANNULA. **Nélaton's c.** FLEXIBLE CATHETER. **opaque c.** A catheter made of material that is opaque to x rays. **oropharyngeal c.** A catheter inserted through the nose into the oropharynx, usually for delivery of oxygen. **Robinson c.** A straight catheter with several openings, used to drain the urinary bladder. **self-retaining c.** A catheter, such as a Foley catheter, which is so constructed that it will remain in place. **soft c.** FLEXIBLE CATHETER. **spiral-tip c.** A catheter with a slightly eccentric filiform tip. **Swan-Ganz c.** A multilumen, flow-directed, flexible catheter floated into the pulmonary artery using an inflatable balloon at the tip. By thermodilution techniques, repetitive measurements of cardiac output can be performed. The device can also be used to measure pulmonary capillary wedge pressure and to sample mixed venous blood. **Tenckhoff peritoneal c.** A permanently implanted catheter designed for long-term peritoneal dialysis, either periodic or chronic ambulatory. The catheter is inserted into the peritoneal cavity after passing through a subcutaneous tunnel in the anterior abdominal wall. The portion of the catheter remaining within the tunnel contains one or two cuffs of woven or felt Dacron material from which fibroblastic ingrowth anchors the catheter and forms a barrier to bacteria. **Texas c.** CONDOM URINAL. **tracheal c.** A plastic catheter for aspirating secretions from the lower airways after anesthesia and in the tracheostomized patient. **two-way c.** DOUBLE-CURRENT CATHETER. **ventricular c.** A small-caliber, rubber or plastic tube used for temporary or more prolonged removal of ventricular fluid or for injections into the ventricles. **whip c.** FILIFORM-TIPPED CATHETER. **whistle-tip c.** A catheter with a terminal opening and a subterminal side opening. **winged c.** A self-retaining catheter that is held in place by two projections at its end.

**catheterization** \kath′ətərīzā′shən\ [CATHETER + *-iz(e)* + -ATION] The insertion of a catheter. Also *catheterism.* **cardiac c.** The procedure of inserting a cardiac catheter through a peripheral blood vessel into the heart, most often for diagnostic, less often for therapeutic, purposes. **eustachian c.** The introduction of an eustachian catheter into the pharyngeal opening of the eustachian tube through the nose or, rarely, through the mouth. It is performed as a means of examining or treating a diseased middle-ear cleft. Using Politzer's bag and the auscultation tube, deductions may be made relating to tubotympanic health or disease. Moreover, with the addition of these two instruments, the technique may be used to inflate the middle ear or to pass medicated vapors or fluids into it. The use of this technique has declined in recent years. **hepatic vein c.** The procedure of passing a catheter through a peripheral vein into the inferior vena cava and thence a variable distance into a hepatic vein. Pressures may then be recorded, blood samples collected and, more rarely, radiopaque fluids injected to visualize the anatomy of the liver. **laryngeal c.** The passage of a catheter through the rima glottidis with the object of either aspirating secretions from the tracheobronchial airway or administering anesthetics. **retrourethral c.** Insertion of a catheter into the urethra through an incision of the bladder. **suprapubic c.** Passage of a catheter above the pubic arch directly into the bladder. **transseptal c.** A method of catheterization of the left side of the heart. A cardiac catheter is passed through a femoral vein into the right atrium. A long needle, curved at the end, is passed through the catheter to lodge in the foramen ovale which it then pierces. The catheter is then passed over the needle into the left atrium and the needle is withdrawn.

**catheterize** \kath′ətərīz\ To insert a catheter into.

**catheterostat** \kath′ətərōstat′\ [CATHETER + *o* + -STAT] A long, thin apparatus used for storing, cleaning, and sterilizing catheters.

**cathetometer** \kath′ətäm′ətər\ An instrument which aids in the reading of graduated instruments such as burets and thermometers.

**cathexis** \kəthek′sis\ [Gk *kathexis* (from *katechein* to hold, keep back) a holding, keeping hold of] The concentration of psychic energy upon a particular object. Also *emotional investment.*

**cathine** NORPSEUDOEPHEDRINE.

**cathisophobia** \kath′isōfō′bē·ə\ [Gk *kathis(is)* a sitting down + *o* + -PHOBIA] AKATHISIA.

**cathodal** \kath′ōdəl\ Pertaining to the cathode.

**cathode** \kath′ōd\ [Gk *kathodos* (from *kata* down + *hodos* path, way) a going down] **1** In a vacuum tube such as an x-ray tube, the heated electrode from which electrons are ejected. **2** A negative electrode. Also *negative pole.* **photo c.** A structure inside a photocell, photomultiplier tube, or image amplifier tube, which emits electrons when struck by light photons.

**catholicon** [Gk *katholikon*, neut. sing. of *katholikos* general, universal] A panacea; a remedy for all diseases.

**cation** \kat′ī·ən\ [Ionic Gk *kation*, neut. sing. of *katiōn*, pres. part. of *katienai* to go down] An ion carrying a positive charge, thus moving toward the cathode in electrophoresis. Also *kation.* Compare ANION.

**cationic** \kat′ī·än′ik\ Of or relating to a cation; possessing positive charge.

**catoptrics** \kətäp′triks\ [Gk *katoptr(on)* a mirror + -IC + *s*] The study of the physics of light reflection.

**catoptroscope** \kətäp′trəskōp\ [Gk *katoptro(n)* a mirror + -SCOPE] An instrument used to examine objects by means of reflected light.

**Caucasoid** \kô′kəsoid\ **1** Characterized by or similar to the physical features of the "Caucasian" or "white" peoples of Europe and Asia. **2** An individual having such physical features. • The term *Caucasian* was adopted as a name for the race because Blumenbach used a woman from the Caucasus as his example of the type in 1795.

**cauda** \kô′də\ [L, the tail of an animal] [NA] In human anatomy, any tapering tail-like structure. Also *tail.* **c. epididymidis** [NA] The narrow, pointed inferior extremity of the epididymis, continuous with the body above and attached anteriorly to the lower pole of the testis by loose connective tissue and a reflection of the tunica vaginalis. It contains the tightly coiled ductus epididymidis, which increases in thickness here and becomes continuous with the ductus deferens. Also *tail of epididymis.* **c. equina** [NA] The bundle of spinal roots and filum terminale descending from the lumbosacral enlargement of the cord, through the subarachnoid space, to successive dural exits of the spinal nerves. The configuration results from differential growth of the spinal cord and the vertebral canal. **c. helicis** [NA] A pointed, tail-like process at the posteroinferior extremity of the cartilage of the helix of the ear that is separated below from the antitragus by the deep antitragohelicine fissure. Also *tail of helix.* **c. pancreatis** [NA] The narrow, triangular left extremity of the pancreas which is situated between the two layers of the splenorenal ligament with the splenic vessels. It usually is in contact with the gastric surface of the spleen. Also *tail of pancreas.*

**caudad** \kô′dad\ [L *caud(a)* the tail + -AD] Toward the tail or caudal end of the body. Also *caudalward.* Compare CEPHALAD, CRANIAD.

**caudae** \kô′dē\ Plural of CAUDA.

**caudal** \kô′dəl\ **1** Pertaining to a cauda or tail. **2** At or toward the tail end of the body. **3** Relatively near the tail end as compared with other structures of the same kind nearer the head; in human anatomy, commonly equivalent to *inferior.* Compare CRANIAL.

**caudalis** \kôdā′lis\ [New L (from L *caud(a)* tail + *-alis* -AL) pertaining to a tail] Caudal.

**caudalward** \kô′dəlwərd\ CAUDAD.

***Caudamoeba sinensis*** \kô′dəmē′bə sinen′sis\ ENTAMOEBA HISTOLYTICA.

**caudate** \kô′dāt\ [Med L *caudat(us)* (from L *caud(a)* tail) tailed] **1** Possessing or shaped like a tail. **2** Pertaining to the nucleus caudatus. **3** NUCLEUS CAUDATUS.

**caudatum** \kôdā′təm\ *Seldom used* NUCLEUS CAUDATUS.

**caudex** \kô′deks\ [L (also *codex*), the stem or trunk of a tree] A stemlike or stalklike structure. **c. cerebri** *Obs.* PEDUNCULUS CEREBRI.

**caudocephalad** \kô′dōsef′əlad\ In a direction from the tail toward the head.

**caul** \kôl\ [Middle French *cale* (from Frankish *skala* shell) a bonnet, hairnet, net] Amniotic membranes sometimes covering the fetal head at birth. Also *cowl, pileus, veil.*

**caumesthesia** \kô′mesthē′zhə\ [Gk *kaum(a)* burning heat + -ESTHESIA] A condition in which the patient feels a sense of burning heat although neither his own temperature nor the ambient temperature are particularly high. *Seldom used.*

**causalgia** \kôzal′jə\ [Gk *kaus(is)* heat, burning + -ALGIA] A specific syndrome of severe and peculiarly unpleasant, burning pain, often associated with smooth, shiny skin and profuse sweating in the affected part and with hypersensitivity to touch and temperature which follows an incomplete lesion of a peripheral nerve, usually the median or ulnar. The exact pathogenesis of the condition is unknown, but it is frequently improved by sympathectomy. Also *thermalgia.*

**causation** \kôzā′shən\ An act or agency by which a result is produced. **legal c.** A legal doctrine requiring the establishment of the fact that an effect, result, or condition was caused by a specific, identifiable action or acts. In tort law (including cases of medical malpractice), it must be proved that the event or series of events causing injury to the plaintiff would not have occurred, if not for some action of the defendant. Establishing proof of causation does not in itself constitute proof of liability, since breach of duty must also be proved before a defendant can be held liable.

**cause** [L *causa* cause] Something that brings about a change; that which produces an effect. **constitutional c.** Any inherent feature of bodily makeup that is responsible for producing some effect. **contributory c. of death** Any significant condition, disease, injury, or morbid state, contributing to the death of a person but not related to the causal sequence specified by the underlying cause of death. • *Contributory cause of death,* like *underlying cause of death,* is an internationally recognized term. **exciting c.** Any act, event, or other factor that can be shown to be causally related to the production of a particular result or condition. **external c.** In medical statistics, any of those causes of death which are classified in the International Classification of Diseases as accidents, poisonings, or violence. **immediate c.** In a succession of causes leading to a result or effect, the final cause which, in and of itself and without additional intervening causes, directly produces the given result, as in death due to peritonitis arising as a complication of a gunshot wound to the abdomen. Peritonitis is the immediate cause of death, and the gunshot wound is the proximate cause. **local c.** A cause which is restricted to the anatomic site or area where its effect is produced. **precipitating c.** A cause that initiates a series of events leading to an effect but which does not, in and of itself, produce the effect. Also *ultimate cause.* **predisposing c.** An antecedent condition or factor which makes an individual more susceptible to a particular effect. **proximate c.** **1** That cause which, in the absence of any other efficient intervening cause, is directly responsible for producing an effect and without which the effect would not have occurred. • *Proximate cause of death* is equivalent to *underlying cause of death,* the preferred term in international usage. **2** In medical malpractice, the negligent act or conduct that initiates a series of events leading to the production of an injury even when some other agent produces the injury, or that negligent act or conduct which immediately precedes and directly produces the injury. For defs. 1 and 2 also *primary cause.* **remote c.** A secondary, predisposing, or precipitating cause, i.e., one that contributes to but is not directly or immediately responsible for the final effect. **secondary c.** A nonessential cause that adds to or enhances the effect of a primary or proximate cause. **specific c.** A cause which produces a specific effect and which is the only cause capable of producing that effect. **ultimate c.** PRECIPITATING CAUSE. **underlying c. of death** A disease or injury which initiated the train of morbid events leading directly to death, or the circumstances of the accident or violence which produced the fatal injury. The underlying cause is to be distinguished from the immediate cause, for example hypostatic pneumonia developing in a patient with a fractured femur, and from the contibutory causes of death which may be recorded on the death certificate. See also PROXIMATE CAUSE, IMMEDIATE CAUSE. • *Underlying cause of death* is an internationally recognized term equivalent to *proximate cause of death.*

**caustic** \kôs′tik\ [Gk *kaustikos* (from *kaiein* to burn) causing burning, corrosive, inflammatory] **1** Capable of eating away tissue; destructive by a corrosive or burning effect: used especially of alkalies which, being largely dissociated in water, produce a high concentration of $OH^-$ ions. **2** A caustic agent or substance. **3** The surface constituted by all the foci of a reflecting or refracting surface. For a rotationally symmetric surface, it is the envelope of the exit rays of an entrance beam parallel to the axis of symmetry. Also *focal surface.* **lunar c.** TOUGHENED SILVER NITRATE.

**cauter** \kô′tər\ CAUTERY.

**cauterant** \kô′tərənt\ Any material that is caustic or destructive of viable tissue.

**cauterization** \kô′tərīzā′shən\ [*cauter(y)* + -IZE + -ATION] The use of a cautery or caustic agent to medically or surgically treat a lesion or to stop bleeding. **c. by points** A surgical technique in which a fine probe bearing a cauterizing agent is used to heat deep, small areas. Also *punctuate cauterization.* **cold c.** The use of carbon dioxide snow for cauterization. **punctuate c.** CAUTERIZATION BY POINTS.

**cautery** \kô′tərē\ [L *cauteri(um)* (from Gk *kautērion* branding iron, from *kaiein* to burn) branding iron] **1** The destruction or searing of viable tissue by an agent such as heat, electricity, or caustic chemical. **2** An agent that effects cautery. Also *cauter.* **button c.** A process in which a disk-shaped iron is used as a cauterizing agent. Also *Corrigan's cautery.* **chemical c.** CHEMOCAUTERY. **cold c.** CRYOCAUTERY. **Corrigan's c.** BUTTON CAUTERY. **electric c.** A machine equipped with a wire tip through which a high-voltage electric current is passed to destroy or cut tissue or to coagulate the ends of bleeding vessels and thus obtain hemostasis. Also *galvanic cautery, galvanocautery.* **gas c.** A surgical device that uses a fine jet of burning gas to destroy tissue. **potential c.** Cauterization by means of an escharotic agent without the application of heat or electricity. Also *virtual cautery.* **Ziegler c.** A cautery method used in the treatment of mild degrees of ectropion often associated with old age.

**cava** \kā′və\ **1** Plural of CAVUM. **2** Fem. of L *cavus* hollow.

**caval** \kā′vəl\ Pertaining to a vena cava.

**cavascope** \kav′əskōp\ [L *cava* a cavity + -SCOPE] An illuminating instrument used for viewing a body cavity.

**cave** CAVUM.

**caveola** \kav′ē·ō′lə\ [New L, dim. of L *cavea* an enclosure] MICROPINOCYTOTIC VESICLE.

**cavern** [L *caverna.* See CAVERNA.] **1** An abnormal cavity, usually of the lung and resulting from caseous necrosis due to tuberculosis. **2** CAVERNA. **c.'s of corpora cavernosa of penis** CAVERNAE CORPORUM CAVERNOSORUM PENIS. **c.'s of corpus spongiosum** CAVERNAE CORPORIS SPONGIOSI. **Schnabel's c.'s** Spaces between the nerve fibers in an optic nerve atrophic because of nutritional changes.

**caverna** \kavur′nə\ [L (from *cavus* hollow), cave, cavern] (*pl.* cavernae) A small enclosed space or cavity. Also *cavern.* **cavernae corporis spongiosi** [NA] The dilatable intercommunicating vascular spaces separated from each other by fine trabeculae and lined by endothelium that is continuous with that of the veins draining this network in the corpus spongiosum penis. They comprise its erectile tissue, which surrounds the urethra traversing it. Also *caverns of corpus spongiosum.* **cavernae corporum cavernosorum penis** [NA] The dilatable intercommunicating vascular spaces separated from each other by trabeculae, forming a network in the corpora cavernosa penis and comprising their erectile tissue. They are lined by non-fenestrated endothelium continuous with that of the veins draining the network. Also *caverns of corpora cavernosa of penis.*

**cavernitis** \kavərnī′tis\ [*(corpus) cavern(osum)* + -ITIS] Inflammation of the corpus cavernosum of the penis. **fibrous c.** PEYRONIE'S DISEASE.

**cavernoma** \kav′ərnō′mə\ CAVERNOUS HEMANGIOMA. **c. lymphaticum** CAVERNOUS LYMPHANGIOMA.

**cavernositis** \kav′ərnōsī′tis\ CAVERNITIS.

**cavernostomy** \kav′ərnäs′təmē\ [CAVERN + *o* + -STOMY] A surgical procedure in which a body cavity is opened, usually to provide drainage, as in the case of a lung abscess.

**cavernous** \kav′ərnəs\ **1** Characterized by or containing cavities. **2** Resulting from the presence of cavities; characteristic of cavitation, as *cavernous voice sounds.*

**cavitary** \kav′iter′ē\ Pertaining to or possessing a cavity or cavities.

**cavitas** \kav′itəs\ [L (from *cavus* hollow), a state of hollowness] [NA] A hollow space or concavity in an organ, part, or structure, often designating only a potential space; cavity. **c. abdominalis** The large, continuous space in the trunk below the thoracic cavity, usually divided anatomically into the abdominal cavity proper and the pelvic cavity, or true pelvis. The superior boundary is the respiratory diaphragm, and inferiorly the abdominal cavity ends at the superior aperture of the true pelvis. Anteriorly and laterally are the muscular and fascial abdominal walls, while posteriorly are the lumbar vertebrae and their muscles, ligaments, and fasciae. The cavity is lined by a serous membrane, the parietal peritoneum, and contains the organs of the digestive system, the kidneys and suprarenal glands, the spleen, and their related structures, as well as the abdominal aorta, inferior vena cava, and their branches and tributaries. Also *abdominal cavity, cavum abdominis.* **c. articularis** [NA] The space filled with fluid enclosed within the synovial membrane lining the fibrous capsule and between the contiguous articular surfaces of a synovial joint. Also *articular cavity, cavum articulare* (outmoded), *joint cavity.* **c. conchae** [NA] The deep, hollowed portion of the concha of the auricle below the crus helicis. The space leads into the external acoustic meatus. Also *cavity of concha, cavum conchae.* **c. dentis** PULP CHAMBER. **c. epiduralis** [NA] The space between the dural sac that encloses the spinal cord and roots and the wall of the vertebral canal. It contains the epidural fat, arteriolar tissue, and a plexus of veins. Also *cavum epidurale* (outmoded), *epidural cavity, epidural space, extradural space.* **c. glenoidalis** [NA] The concave, piriform depression in the head, or lateral angle, of the scapula, covered with articular cartilage and deepened by the labrum glenoidale to receive the head of the humerus in the shoulder joint. Also *glenoid cavity, glenoid fossa.* **c. infraglottica** [NA] The cone-shaped lower part of the laryngeal cavity, extending from the rima glottidis to the lower border of the cricoid cartilage where it becomes continuous with the trachea. It is narrow above and wide below. Also *infraglottic cavity, cavum infraglotticum, subglottis* (outmoded), *inferior aperture of glottis.* **c. laryngis** [NA] The space within the tubular air passage in front of the pharynx and extending from the aditus laryngis at the root of the tongue to the trachea opposite the lower border of the cricoid cartilage. Also *laryngeal cavity, cavum laryngis.* **c. medullaris ossium** [NA] A large, spongelike space enclosed within the compact bone of the shaft, or diaphysis, of a long bone that communicates with the intertrabecular spaces at the ends of the bone. The cavity is lined by a vascularized, condensed areolar tissue, the endosteum, and contains the bone marrow. Also *medullary cavity of bones, marrow cavity, cavum medullare ossium, medullary cavity, medullary space, marrow space.* **c. nasi** [NA] The cavity of the peripheral olfactory organ and respiratory passage that extends from the nostrils of the external nose to the choanae communicating posteriorly with the nasal part of the pharynx. It is divided into right and left halves by the nasal septum, each side being bounded by a roof, floor, and medial and lateral walls, and divided into vestibular, olfactory, and respiratory regions. The lateral wall is characterized by four projecting conchae, lateral to and below each of which is a space, or meatus. The roof is partly formed by the cribriform plate of the ethmoid bone, while the floor is the upper surface of the hard palate. The mucous membrane lining the cavity is continuous with that of the paranasal sinuses that open into it. Also *nasal cavity, cavum nasi.* **c. nasi ossea** [NA] The bony skeleton of the nasal cavity, the roof of which comprises the nasal and frontal bones, the cribriform plate of the ethmoid, and the body of the sphenoid bone, while the floor is formed by the superior surface of the bony palate. Also *bony cavity of nose, cavum nasi osseum.* **c. oris** [NA] The space bounded by the lips anteriorly, the cheeks laterally, the hard and soft palates superiorly, and a mucosa-lined muscular floor occupied by the tongue. Posteriorly it is continuous with the oropharynx, through the isthmus faucium. It is divided into an outer part, vestibulum oris, and a larger, inner part, cavitas oris propria, which are lined by mucous membrane. Also *oral cavity, cavum oris, mouth cavity.* **c. oris propria** [NA] The part of the mouth bounded externally by the teeth, gums and alveolar arches and leading back to the isthmus of the fauces. The floor is formed by the tongue and sublingual mucosa while the roof consists of the hard and soft palate. Also *oral cavity proper, cavum oris proprium.* **c. pelvis** [NA] The space enclosed by the pelvic bones and lying between the superior aperture of the pelvis, or inlet, above and the pelvic diaphragm, or outlet, below. It is lined by parietal peritoneum, and contains the pelvic viscera. Also *pelvic cavity, cavum pelvis.* **c. pericardialis** [NA] The potential space between the opposed visceral and parietal layers of the closed serous pericardium of the heart, containing a film of fluid permitting free movement of the heart within the pericardial sac. Also *pericardial cavity, cavum pericardii.* **c. peritonealis** [NA] The potential space between the parietal and visceral layers of peritoneum. Also *peritoneal cavity, cavum peritonaei, cavum peritonei, greater peritoneal cavity, greater sac of peritoneum.* **c. pharyngis** [NA] The space in the upper part of the digestive tube, situated behind the nasal cavity, the mouth, and the larynx, with each of which it is continuous, and extending from the base of the skull to the level of the lower border of the cricoid cartilage opposite the sixth cervical vertebra, where it becomes continuous with the space within the esophagus. Also *cavity of pharynx, cavum pharyngis, pharyngeal cavity.* **c. pleuralis** [NA] The potential serous space between the visceral and the parietal pleura of each lung. Normally the two layers of pleura are in contact with each other. Also *pleural cavity, cavum pleurae* (outmoded)*, pleural sac, pleural space.* **c. subarachnoidea** [NA] The space between the subarachnoid membrane, which is closely applied to the dura mater, and the pia mater, which closely follows the contours of the brain. Over the cerebral convolutions the space is a mere slit, while over gross irregularities of the brain and beyond the end of the spinal cord it is enlarged to form cisterns. The space is filled with cerebrospinal fluid. Also *subarachnoid cavity, Magendie space, meningeal space, pia-arachnoid space, subarachnoid space, cavum subarachnoidale.* **c. thoracis** [NA] The upper part of the body cavity, surrounded by the thoracic walls and bounded above by the neck at the supraclavicular plane and below by the respiratory diaphragm separating it from the abdominal cavity. It is divided into the right and left pleural cavities, with the mediastinum between them. Also *cavum thoracis, cavum pectoris, thoracic cavity.* **c. tympanica** [NA] The space in the middle ear, lined by mucous membrane, that is continuous with that of the auditory tube anteriorly and the mastoid antrum posteriorly. Crossing the space are the articulated auditory ossicles extending from the tympanic membrane laterally to the fenestra vestibuli medially. Also *tympanic cavity, cavity of middle ear, cavum tympani.* • The term was formerly synonymous with auris media, but now considered to be only part of it. **c. uteri** [NA] The space between the anterior and posterior walls of the uterus. It is small and slitlike in the normal, nonpregnant female, in whom the walls are in close apposition. Its broad base is in the fundus between the internal openings of the uterine tubes, while its apex is at the internal os of the uterus, through which it is continuous with the canal of the cervix. Also *uterine cavity, cavum uteri.*

**cavitates** \kav′itā′tēz\ Plural of CAVITAS.

**cavitation** \kav′itā′shən\ **1** The formation of a cavity or cavities. **2** The production and dynamics of bubbles in a sound field. **c. of the septum pellucidum** The formation of a cyst in the septum pellucidum. This is often associated with the punch-drunk syndrome.

# cavity

**cavity** [L *cavitas.* See CAVITAS.] A hollow space or concavity in an organ, part, or structure, often designating only a potential space; cavitas. **abdominal c.** CAVITAS ABDOMINALIS. **allantoic c.** The cavity of the allantois, filled with allantoic fluid. The allantois varies in size in different animal types. **amniotic c.** The closed sac between the embryo and the amnion containing the amniotic fluid. In man the cavity arises in the early postimplantation period (by day $7^1/_2$) by cavitation within the inner cell mass, and separates the embryonic ectoderm from the overlying trophoblast tissue. The amnion develops from cells of the embryonic ectoderm and adjacent cytotrophoblast to form a domelike layer of flat epithelium overlying the embryonic disk and continuous on all sides with its margin. The amniotic cavity is a closed one except for a short time when it communicates with the secondary yolk sac and, later, with the hindgut, through the notochordal canal. At term the amniotic cavity contains about 0.5 liters of amniotic fluid. **anterior mediastinal c.** MEDIASTINUM ANTERIUS. **articular c.** CAVITAS ARTICULARIS. **bony c. of nose** CAVITAS NASI OSSEA. **buccal c.** **1** VESTIBULUM ORIS. **2** A cavity on the buccal surface of a tooth. **cleavage c.** BLASTOCOELE. **coelomic c.** COELOM. **complex c.** A cavity involving more than one surface of a tooth. It may be either a carious cavity or, more often, a prepared cavity. Also *compound cavity.* **c. of concha** CAVITAS CONCHAE. **cotyloid c.** ACETABULUM. **cranial c.** The space enclosed by the cranial bones and containing the brain, its membranes, and related structures. **dental c.** A carious lesion or hole in a tooth. **ectoplacental c.** FALSE AMNION. **epidural c.** CAVITAS EPIDURALIS. **epiploic c.** BURSA OMENTALIS. **external oral c.** VESTIBULUM ORIS. **false amniotic c.** FALSE AMNION. **gastrulation c.** ARCHENTERON. **glandular c.** The central lumen of an exocrine gland into which its secretion is discharged. **glenoid c.** CAVITAS GLENOIDALIS. **glenoid c. of scapula** CAVITAS GLENOIDALIS. **greater peritoneal c.** CAVITAS PERITONEALIS. **greater sigmoid c. of ulna** INCI-

SURA TROCHLEARIS ULNAE. **infraglottic c.** CAVITAS INFRAGLOTTICA. **ischiorectal c.** FOSSA ISCHIOANALIS. **joint c.** CAVITAS ARTICULARIS. **laryngeal c.** CAVITAS LARYNGIS. **laryngopharyngeal c.** PARS LARYNGEA PHARYNGIS. **lesser peritoneal c.** BURSA OMENTALIS. **lesser sigmoid c. of ulna** INCISURA RADIALIS ULNAE. **marrow c.** CAVITAS MEDULLARIS OSSIUM. **mastoid c.** ANTRUM MASTOIDEUM. **Meckel's c.** CAVUM TRIGEMINALE. **medullary c.** CAVITAS MEDULLARIS OSSIUM. **medullary c. of bones** CAVITAS MEDULLARIS OSSIUM. **c. of middle ear** CAVITAS TYMPANICA. **mouth c.** CAVITAS ORIS. **nasal c.** CAVITAS NASI. **nerve c.** *Popular* PULP CHAMBER. **oral c.** CAVITAS ORIS. **oral c. proper** CAVITAS ORIS PROPRIA. **orbital c.** ORBITA. **pelvic c.** CAVITAS PELVIS. **pericardial c.** CAVITAS PERICARDIALIS. **pericardiopleuroperitoneal c.** The communication present at a very early stage of embryonic development when the pericardial cavity (within the septum transversum) has not yet been isolated from the pleuroperitoneal cavity. The separation of the pleural from the pericardial cavity occurs somewhat later with closure of the pleuroperitoneal canals by the pleuroperitoneal membranes (the pillars of Uskow). **peritoneal c.** CAVITAS PERITONEALIS. **pharyngeal c.** CAVITAS PHARYNGIS. **pharyngolaryngeal c.** PARS LARYNGEA PHARYNGIS. **pharyngonasal c.** PARS NASALIS PHARYNGIS. **pharyngo-oral c.** PARS ORALIS PHARYNGIS. **c. of pharynx** CAVITAS PHARYNGIS. **pleural c.** CAVITAS PLEURALIS. **popliteal c.** FOSSA POPLITEA. **posterior mediastinal c.** MEDIASTINUM POSTERIUS. **prepared c.** A dental cavity which has been prepared for the placement of a restoration by the removal of caries and other procedures intended to enhance the retention and prolong the life of the restoration. **primary amniotic c.** A cavity resulting from the separation of the trophoblast from the inner cell mass. On its trophoblastic side, this cavity is lined by flattened cells, the amnioblasts, possibly derived from the trophoblast. The floor of the cavity is formed by the ectodermal layer of the embryonic disk. **primary nasal c.** A blind sac in the embryo resulting from invagination of the nasal pits and the surrounding ectoderm. The nasal pits are the result of invagination of the paired olfactory, or nasal, placodes on the ectoderm of the face. The paired primary nasal cavities are separated by the midline nasal septum, which grows backwards to fuse with the palate. **primary oral c.** The primitive buccal or mouth cavity in the embryo before the nasal cavity has developed and after the rupture of the buccopharyngeal membrane. **pulp c.** PULP CHAMBER. **c. of Retzius** SPATIUM RETROPUBICUM. **Rosenmüller's c.** RECESSUS PHARYNGEUS. **secondary nasal c.** The embryonic nasal cavity after the palate has developed. **secondary oral c.** The oral cavity after the development of the palate in the embryo. **segmentation c.** BLASTOCOELE. **c. of septum pellucidum** CAVUM SEPTI PELLUCIDI. **serous c.** Any closed cavity in the body that is lined by a serum-secreting cellular membrane. Examples include the pericardial cavity and the peritoneal cavity. **sigmoid c. of radius** INCISURA ULNARIS RADII. **smooth surface c.** A cavity that does not arise from a pit or fissure, including proximal cavities and labial or lingual cavities that do not arise from the labial or lingual pits. Occlusal cavities are excluded because they always arise from pits or fissures. **somite c.** MYOCOELE. **splanchnic c.** VISCERAL CAVITY. **Stafne's c.** A developmental invagination of the mandible containing submandibular salivary gland tissue. Radiologically it resembles a cyst cavity. **subarachnoid c.** CAVITAS SUBARACHNOIDEA. **subdural c.** SPATIUM SUBDURALE. **thoracic c.** CAVITAS THORACIS. **trigeminal c.** CAVUM TRIGEMINALE. **tympanic c.** CAVITAS TYMPANICA. **uterine c.** CAVITAS UTERI. **visceral c.** 1 A body cavity containing viscera and related structures, such as the abdominal cavity and the pelvic cavity. 2 The coelomic cavity or one of its derivative cavities, such as the pleural cavity and the peritoneal cavity. Also *splanchnic cavity.*

**cavography** \kavägʹrəfē\ [*(vena) cav(a)* + *o* + -GRAPHY] Roentgenography of the inferior or superior vena cava during opacification by contrast medium.

**cavosurface** \kavʹōsurʹfəs\ Relating to the surface of the tooth and the internal surface of the cavity: used particularly to describe the line angle where the two surfaces meet.

**cavovalgus** \kavʹōvalʹgəs\ TALIPES CAVOVALGUS.

**cavum** \kāʹvəm\ [L (from *cavus* hollow), a hollow, cavity] An enclosed space or cavity in an organ or a part of the body. Also *cave.* **c. abdominis** CAVITAS ABDOMINALIS. **c. articulare** *Outmoded* CAVITAS ARTICULARIS. **c. conchae** CAVITAS CONCHAE. **c. dentis** PULP CHAMBER. **c. epidurale** CAVITAS EPIDURALIS. **c. infraglotticum** CAVITAS INFRAGLOTTICA. **c. laryngis** CAVITAS LARYNGIS. **c. mediastinale anterius** MEDIASTINUM ANTERIUS. **c. mediastinale posterius** MEDIASTINUM POSTERIUS. **c. medullare ossium** CAVITAS MEDULLARIS OSSIUM. **c. nasi** CAVITAS NASI. **c. nasi osseum** CAVITAS NASI OSSEA. **c. oris** CAVITAS ORIS. **c. oris proprium** CAVITAS ORIS PROPRIA. **c. pectoris** CAVITAS THORACIS. **c. pelvis** CAVITAS PELVIS. **c. pericardii** CAVITAS PERICARDIALIS. **c. peritonaei** CAVITAS PERITONEALIS. **c. peritonei** CAVITAS PERITONEALIS. **c. pharyngis** CAVITAS PHARYNGIS. **c. pleurae** *Outmoded* CAVITAS PLEURALIS. **c. pleuropericardiale** The combined pleural and pericardial components of the coelom. **c. psalterii** A recess of the cavum septi pellucidi extending between the inferior surface of the corpus callosum and the arch of the fornix, sometimes as far as the splenium. It does not communicate with the ventricular system. Also *Verga space, Verga's ventricle, sixth ventricle.* **c. pulpae** PULP CHAMBER. **c. septi pellucidi** [NA] A slitlike space between the two laminae of the septum pellucidum. It is not homologous with the ventricles, and does not communicate with them. Also *cavity of septum pellucidum, pseudocele, pseudoventricle, rhomboid sinus, ventriculus quintus, fifth ventricle.* **c. subarachnoideale** CAVITAS SUBARACHNOIDEA. **c. subdurale** SPATIUM SUBDURALE. **c. thoracis** CAVITAS THORACIS. **c. trigeminale** [NA] An evagination of the subarachnoid cavity of the posterior fossa along the fifth nerve and nearer portions of the trigeminal ganglion. Thus, it passes over the crest of the petrous pyramid, and lies deep to the dura lining the anterior fossa. Also *trigeminal cavity, Meckel's cavity, Meckel's space.* **c. tympani** CAVITAS TYMPANICA. **c. uteri** CAVITAS UTERI. **c. veli interpositi** An extension of the subarachnoid cistern sometimes found extending into the tela choroidea ventriculi quarti. **c. vesicouterinum** EXCAVATIO VESICOUTERINA.

**Cazenave** [Pierre-Louis-Alphee *Cazenave,* French dermatologist, 1802–1877] 1 Cazenave's disease. See under LUPUS ERYTHEMATOSUS. 2 Cazenave's disease. See under PEMPHIGUS FOLIACEUS. 3 Cazenave's vitiligo. See under ALOPECIA AREATA.

**Cb** Symbol for the element, colobium, now called niobium.

**CBC** complete blood count.

**CBF** cerebral blood flow.
**CBG** corticosteroid-binding globulin.
**cc** Symbol for the unit, cubic centimeter.
**CCC** cathodal closure contraction.
**CCK** cholecystokinin.
**CCU** coronary care unit. ⟨"By 1967, the nation could boast more than 300 CCUs; by 1976 there were 6,500." —*Medical World News,* 2 Oct. 1978, 50⟩
**CD** conjugata diagonalis (diagonal conjugate).
**$CD_{50}$** mean curative dose.
**Cd** Symbol for the element, cadmium.
**cd** Symbol for the unit, candela.
**CDC** Centers for Disease Control.
**cDNA** DNA synthesized by RNA-directed DNA polymerase as a copy of RNA, usually isolated mRNA. It therefore differs in sequence from eukaryotic chromosomal DNA by the absence of introns. It may be used as a probe for the presence of the gene coding for a particular protein by testing for its hybridization with chromosomal DNA.
**CDP** Symbol for cytidine diphosphate.
**CDPcholine** CYTIDINE DIPHOSPHATE CHOLINE.
**Ce** Symbol for the element, cerium.
**CEA** carcinoembryonic antigen.
**ceasmic** \sē·az′mik\ [Gk *keasm(a)* a chip + -IC] Having or appearing to have embryonic fissures persisting into postnatal life.
**cecal** \sē′kəl\ **1** Of or pertaining to the cecum. **2** Ending in a blind sac.
**cecectomy** \sēsek′təmē\ [*cec(um)* + -ECTOMY] The surgical removal of the cecum. Also *typhlectomy.*
**Cecil** [Arthur Bond *Cecil,* U.S. surgeon, born 1885] **1** See under OPERATION. **2** Cecil-Culp repair of hypospadias. See under REPAIR.
**cecitis** \sēsī′tis\ [*cec(um)* + -ITIS] Inflammation of the cecum.
**ceco-** \sē′kō-\ [L *caecus* blind; *caecum* blind gut] A combining form meaning (1) cecum, caecum; (2) blind.
**cecocele** \sē′kōsēl\ A sliding hernia in which the wall of the cecum forms part of the hernia sac.
**cecocentral** \-sen′trəl\ [CECO- + *central*] Pertaining to the area between the blind spot and the fixation point. Also *centrocecal.*
**cecocolon** \-kō′lən\ The cecum and the colon considered as a single functional unit.
**cecocolopexy** \-kō′ləpek′sē\ [CECO- + COLO- + -PEXY ] A surgical procedure in which the cecum and the colon are suspended to prevent ptosis or volvulus.
**cecocolostomy** \-kōläs′təmē\ COLOCECOSTOMY.
**cecocystoplasty** \-sis′təplas′tē\ [CECO- + CYSTO- + -PLASTY] Augmentation of bladder capacity by sewing in a patch of cecum.
**cecofixation** \-fiksā′shən\ CECOPEXY.
**cecoileostomy** \-il′ē·äs′təmē\ [CECO- + ILEO- + -STOMY] A surgical procedure creating an opening between the cecum and the ileum following a resection or bypass procedure. It may rarely occur spontaneously from trauma, inflammation, or a neoplasm.
**cecopexy** \sē′kōpek′sē\ [CECO- + -PEXY] A surgical procedure in which the cecum is suspended to prevent ptosis or torsion. Also *cecofixation.*
**cecoplication** \-plīkā′shən\ [CECO- + PLICATION] A surgical procedure in which the cecal wall is fixed in place to prevent volvulus in a redundant colon.
**cecosigmoidostomy** \-sig′moidäs′təmē\ [CECO- + SIGMOID + *o* + -STOMY] A surgical procedure creating an opening between the cecum and the sigmoid colon following a resection or bypass procedure. Rarely, it may result from trauma, inflammation, or a neoplasm.
**cecostomy** \sēkäs′təmē\ [CECO- + -STOMY] A surgical procedure creating an opening between the cecum and the skin, thus diverting the fecal stream. It may rarely result spontaneously from trauma, inflammation, or a neoplasm.
**cecotomy** \sēkät′əmē\ [CECO- + -TOMY] An incision into the cecum. It is usually produced surgically, but it may result from trauma.
**cecum** \sē′kəm\ CAECUM. **cupular c. of cochlear duct** CAECUM CUPULARE DUCTUS COCHLEARIS. **vestibular c. of cochlear duct** CAECUM VESTIBULARE DUCTUS COCHLEARIS.
**cefaclor** $C_{15}H_{14}ClN_3O_4S{\cdot}H_2O$. 7-(D-2-amino- 2-phenylacetamido)-3-chloro-3-cephem-4-carboxylic acid monohydrate, a semisynthetic antibacterial agent of the second generation cephalosporin family. It is employed therapeutically in the treatment of infections by *Haemophilus influenzae* as well as some Gram-negative bacilli, and it may also be used for some types of otitis media. It is administered orally.
**cefadroxil** $C_{16}H_{17}N_3O_5S{\cdot}H_2O$. 7-[D-(-)-α-Amino-α-(4-hydroxyphenyl)-acetamido]-3-methyl-3-cephem-4-carboxylic acid monohydrate, a synthetic antibacterial agent of the first generation cephalosporin family of drugs. It is effective against many Gram-positive bacterial species as well as *Escherichia coli, Klebsiella pneumoniae,* and *Proteus* strains. It is given orally.
**cefamandole** $C_{18}H_{18}N_6O_5S_2$. A cephalosporin antibiotic claimed to be highly effective against *Enterobacter* species and *Haemophilus influenzae.* It is used for the treatment of Gram-negative microorganisms that are resistant to other cephalosporins.
**cefatrizine** $C_{18}H_{18}N_6O_5S_2$. 7-[D-α-Amino-α-(4-hydroxyphenyl)acetamido]-3-(1,2,3-triazol-4(5)-ylthiomethyl)-3-cephem-4-carboxylic acid, an orally effective semisynthetic antibiotic of the cephalosporin family.
**cefazolin sodium** $C_{14}H_{13}N_8NaO_4S_3$. 7-(1-(1*H*)-tetrazolylacetamido)-3-[2-(5-methyl-1,3,4-thiadiazolyl)thiomethyl]$\Delta^3$-cephem-4-carboxylic acid sodium salt. A semisynthetic antibiotic that is derived from 7-aminocephalosporanic acid. It has the same actions and uses as cephaloridine, and it is given parenterally.
**cefmetazole** $C_{15}H_{17}N_7O_5S_3$. 7-[[[(Cyanomethyl)thio] acetyl]amino]-7-methoxy-3-[[(1-methyl-1*H*-tetrazol-5-yl)thio] methyl]-8-oxo-5 thia-1-azabicyclo[4.2.0]oct-2-ene-2-carboxylic acid, a semisynthetic antibacterial agent derived from cephamycin C.
**cefonicid** $C_{18}H_{18}N_6O_8S_3$. 7-[(Hydroxyphenylacetyl)amino]-8-oxo-3-[[[1-(sulfomethyl)-1*H*-tetrazol-5-yl]thio]methyl]-5-thio-1-azabicyclo[4.2.0]oct-2-ene-2-carboxylic acid. A semisynthetic antibacterial agent of the cephalosporin family. It is long lasting and effective against a wide variety of bacterial species. Structurally similar to cefamandole, it is given intramuscularly and intravenously.
**cefoperazone** $C_{25}H_{27}N_9O$. 7-[D-(-)-α-(4-Ethyl-2,3-dioxo-1-piperazinecarboxamido)-α-(4-hydroxyphenyl)acetamido]-3-[[(1-methyl-1-1*H*-tetrazol-5-yl)- thio]methyl]-3-cepham 4-carboxylic acid, a semisynthetic antibacterial agent of the piperazine-cephalosporin type (third generation). It is effective against *Pseudomonas* and a number of Gram-negative bacilli. It is administered intramuscularly or intravenously.
**ceforanide** $C_{20}H_{21}N_7O_6S_2$. 7-[[[2-(Aminomethyl)phenyl]-acetyl]-amino]- 3-[[[1-(carboxymethyl)- 1*H*- tetrazol- 5-yl]thio]-methyl]-8-oxo-5-thia-1-azabicyclo[4.2.0]oct-2-ene- 2-carboxylic acid. A semisynthetic broad spectrum antibiotic of the cephalosporin family. It is relatively long-acting and it

is administered intramuscularly or intravenously.

**cefotaxime** $C_{16}H_{17}N_5O_7S_2$. 7-[2-(2-Amino-4-thiazolyl)-2-methoxyiminoacetamido]cephalosporanic acid, a semisynthetic antibacterial agent of the cephalosporin family. It has high activity against many Gram-negative bacilli. The sodium salt form has good penetration of the blood-brain barrier to the cerebrospinal fluid. It is given by intramuscular or intravenous injection.

**cefotiam** $C_{18}H_{23}N_9O_4S_3$. 7-β-[2-(Aminothiazol-4-yl)acetamido]-3-[[[1-(2-dimethylaminoethyl)-1*H*-tetrazol-5-yl]thio]methyl]-ceph-3-em-4-carboxylic acid, a broad spectrum semisynthetic antibacterial agent of the cephalosporin group. It is similar to cephmandole in activity, and it is highly effective against *Staphylococcus aureus, S. pneumoniae,* and *S. pyrogenes.* It has a short half-life.

**cefoxitin** $C_{16}H_{17}N_3O_7S_2$. A cephalosporin antibiotic with greater activity than cephalothin against Gram-negative organisms. It is also more resistant against the β-lactamases of Gram-negative organisms, and particularly effective against *Bacteroides fragilis.*

**cefsulodin** $C_{22}H_{20}N_4O_8S_2$. 7-(α-Sulfophenylacetamido)-3-(4′-carbamoylpyridinium)methyl-3-cephen-4-carboxylate, a semisynthetic antibacterial agent of the cephalosporin class of drugs. It is effective against *Pseudomonas.*

**ceftizoxime** $C_{13}H_{13}N_5O_5S_2$. (6R,7R)-7-[2-2-Amino-4-thiazolyl)-glyoxylamido]-8-oxo-5-thia-1-azabicyclo[4.2.0]oct-2-ene-2-carboxylic acid $7^2$-(*Z*)-(O-methyloxime), a semisynthetic antibacterial agent of the cephalosporin family. It has a wide spectrum of activity and is given intramuscularly or intravenously.

**ceftriaxone** $C_{18}H_{18}N_8O_7S_3$. 7-[[(2-Amino-4-thiazolyl)(methoxyimino)acetyl]amino]-8-oxo-3-[[(1,2,5,6-tetrahydro-2-methyl-5,6-dioxo-1,2,4-triazin-3-yl)thio]methyl]-5-thia-1-azabicyclo[4.2.0]oct-2-ene-2-carboxylic acid. A semisynthetic third-generation cephalosporin antibiotic. It has a broad spectrum of activity against both Gram-positive and Gram-negative bacteria. Because of its relatively long half-life of approximately eight hours, the dosing interval of 12 or 24 hours is less frequent than for many cephalosporins. It is administered either intravenously or intramuscularly.

**cefuroxime** $C_{16}H_{16}N_4O_8S$. 3-[[(Aminocarbonyl)oxy]methyl]-7-[[2-furanyl(methoxyimino)acetyl]amino]-8-oxo-5-thia-1-azabicyclo[4.2.0]oct-2-ene-2-carboxylic acid, a semisynthetic antibacterial agent of the cephalosporin family.

**Cel.** Celsius.

**cel** Celsius. An obsolete abbreviation.

**cel-**[1] \sēl-\ CELO-[1].

**cel-**[2] \sēl-\ COELO-.

**-cele**[1] \-sēl\ [Gk *kēlē* hernia, swelling.] A combining form meaning (1) hernia; (2) swelling, tumor.

**-cele**[2] \-sēl\ -COELE.

**Celestin** [Felix *Celestin,* French physician, born 1900] See under TUBE.

**celiac** \sē′lē·ak\ [L *coeliacus,* from Gk *koiliakos* (from *koilia* abdominal cavity) of or pertaining to the bowels] Pertaining to the abdominal cavity or abdominal viscera. Also *coeliac.*

**celiectomy** \sē′lē·ek′təmē\ [*celi(o)-* + -ECTOMY] A surgical incision into the abdominal cavity.

**celio-** \sē′lyō-\ [Gk *koilia* the hollow of the belly, cavity] A combining form denoting the abdomen. See also COELO-.

**celiocentesis** \-sentē′sis\ ABDOMINOCENTESIS.

**celiocolpotomy** \-kälpät′əmē\ [CELIO- + COLPO- + -TOMY] A surgical incision into the abdominal cavity through the vagina. Also *celioelytrotomy, vaginal celiotomy.*

**celioelytrotomy** \-el′ēträt′əmē\ [CELIO- + ELYTRO- + -TOMY] CELIOCOLPOTOMY.

**celioenterotomy** \-en′terät′əmē\ LAPAROENTEROTOMY.

**celiogastrotomy** \-gasträt′əmē\ LAPAROGASTROTOMY.

**celiohysterectomy** \-his′tərek′təmē\ [CELIO- + HYSTERECTOMY] ABDOMINAL HYSTERECTOMY.

**celiomyomectomy** \-mī′əmek′təmē\ [CELIO- + MYOMECTOMY] ABDOMINAL MYOMECTOMY.

**celiomyomotomy** \-mī′əmät′əmē\ [CELIO- + MYOMOTOMY] A surgical incision into a muscular tumor approached through the abdominal wall. Also *laparomyomotomy.*

**celioparacentesis** \-par′əsentē′sis\ ABDOMINOCENTESIS.

**celiopyosis** \-pī·ō′sis\ [CELIO- + PY- + -OSIS] Pus in the abdominal cavity, as in purulent peritonitis.

**celiorrhaphy** \sē′lē·ôr′əfē\ [CELIO- + -RRHAPHY] LAPARORRHAPHY.

**celiotomy** \sē′lē·ät′əmē\ [CELIO- + -TOMY] An incision into the abdominal cavity. Usually produced surgically, it may also, but rarely, result from penetrating trauma. Also *abdominal section, laparotomy* (imprecise). **vaginal c.** CELIOCOLPOTOMY. **ventral c.** An incision through the anterior abdominal wall. It is usually produced surgically but it can result from penetrating trauma as well. Also *ventrotomy.*

# cell

**cell** [L *cella.* See CELLA.] **1** The fundamental unit of which all organisms are composed, consisting of a mass of protoplasm contained within a plasma membrane. The protoplasm, in a eukaryotic cell, is divided into a nucleus and cytoplasm. The cytoplasm contains a variety of organelles including mitochondria, ribosomes, lysosomes, plastids, granules, lipid vacuoles, etc. Cells are varied in size, shape, and degree of differentiation. **2** A small closed, or nearly closed, compartment. For defs. 1 and 2 also *cellula, cellule.* **A c.** ALPHA CELL. **Abbe-Zeiss counting c.** THOMA-ZEISS COUNTING CHAMBER. **absorption c.** A clear glass cylinder used to hold a solution for determination of its absorption spectrum. **absorptive c. of intestine** One of the columnar cells that covers the surface of intestinal villi. Such cells are specialized for absorption, having a brush border composed of microvilli on the free surface. **acid c.** OXYNTIC CELL. **acidophilic c.** EOSINOPHIL. **acoustic hair c.'s** AUDITORY CELLS. **activated reticular c.** A cell that was once believed to be an antigen-stimulated histiocyte but which is in fact a reactive lymphocyte, or immunoblast. **adipose c.** FAT CELL. **adventitial c.** PERICYTE. **agranular c.** A cell that has no cytoplasmic granules. **air c.** **1** One of the air-filled cavities found within the ethmoid bone and the mastoid process. **2** ALVEOLUS. **air c.'s of auditory tube** CELLULAE PNEUMATICAE TUBAE AUDITIVAE. **air c.'s of Mosher** Ethmoidal air cells that are occasionally present beneath the ethmoidal bulla and open into the middle ethmoidal cells. **albuminous c.** SEROUS CELL. **alpha c.** **1** Any of the cells scattered throughout the islets of Langerhans which synthesize, store, and secrete glucagon. The secretory granules are stainable with eosin and azocarmine and as seen by electron microscopy appear round with a closely applied membranous sac and an electron-dense center. **2** An eosinophil of the anterior pituitary.

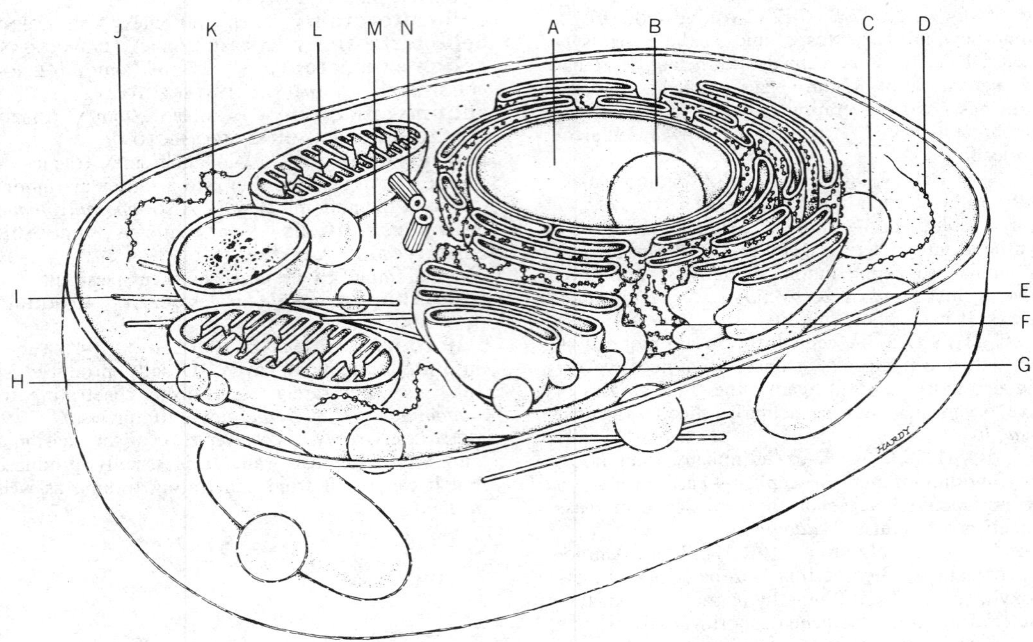


**Eukaryotic cell** (A) Nucleus; (B) nucleolus; (C) secretory vacuole; (D) polysome; (E) smooth endoplasmic reticulum; (F) rough endoplasmic reticulum; (G) Golgi apparatus; (H) peroxisome; (I) cytoskeleton; (J) cell membrane; (K) lysosome; (L) mitochondrion; (M) cytoplasm; (N) centriole.

For defs. 1 and 2 also *A cell.* **alveolar c.** PNEUMOCYTE. **Alzheimer c.'s** Abnormal astrocytes that develop in response to various forms of brain injury. There are two types: type I cells are usually seen around infarcts and have dark nuclei and well defined cytoplasms, and type II cells are usually associated with systemic conditions that result in high blood ammonia levels, such as cirrhosis of the liver. They are characterized by large pale nuclei with thick and irregular nuclear membranes. Their cytoplasm is not apparent on routine stains. **amacrine c.** **1** A neuron that lacks a main process or axon, having dendrites only. Such cells are found in the inner nuclear lamina of the retina. Also *amacrine.* **2** SPONGIOBLAST. **ameboid c.** A cell that moves by projecting and retracting pseudopodia. Amebas move in this way, as do leukocytes. Also *locomotive cell.* **amphophilic c.** A cell containing cytoplasm that stains readily with either acid or basic dyes. **anaplastic c.** An undifferentiated cell, i.e., one lacking the morphologic and functional characteristics permitting its recognition, characteristic of malignant neoplasms. **Anichkov c.** CARDIAC HISTIOCYTE. **anterior ethmoidal air c.'s** CELLULAE ANTERIORES ETHMOIDALES. **anterior horn c.** A motoneuron, either skeletomotor or fusimotor in type, located in the anterior horn of the spinal cord. **apocrine c.** A secretory cell in which a portion of the cytoplasm is lost and becomes a part of the secretion, as a cell in the mammary and sebaceous glands. **apolar c.** A type of neuron found in the embryo which characteristically has neither processes nor poles. **APUD c.'s** A group of diversified cells apparently specialized for the synthesis and release of polypeptides and amines. They are located throughout the alimentary tract including the pancreas, the central nervous system (hypothalamus, neurohypophysis, pineal), thyroid (C cells), adrenal medulla, carotid body, lungs, urinary tract and skin. They are implicated in the secretion of gastrin, somatostatin, secretin, enteroglucagon, other gastrointestinal hormones, and perhaps the pancreatic islet cell hormones. **argentaffin c.** A cell that can be stained by silver solutions without the addition of an external reducing agent. Such cells form a part of the diffuse endocrine system. Also *Kulchitsky cell.* **argyrophilic c.** A cell that can be stained by silver solutions only in the presence of an external reducing agent. **Arias-Stella c.'s** A typical glandular proliferation of the endometrium associated with ectopic pregnancy. **Armanni-Ebstein c.'s** Cells with marked cytoplasmic vacuolization due to an excess of glycogen. This reversible lesion does not affect function and is characteristic of diabetes mellitus. Cells most commonly affected include those of the proximal convoluted tubules of the kidney, hepatocytes, and beta cells of the islets of Langerhans. **Aschoff c.** The typical cell found in Aschoff bodies in rheumatic fever. It is a large, elongated cell with one or more vesicular nuclei. The chromatin has a characteristic pattern, with a central rod from which thin fibrils radiate towards the nuclear membrane. **Askanazy c.** HÜRTHLE CELL. **auditory c.'s** The epitheliocytus sensorius pilosus internus and epitheliocytus sensorius pilosus externus. Also *acoustic hair cells.* **autologous lymphokine activated killer c.'s** Lymphocytes taken from a subject and cultured *in vitro* in high concentrations of interleukin-2. Such cells acquire the characteristics of natural killer cells and show preferential cytotoxicity against certain malignant cells. They have been reinfused into the host subject as a form of nonspecific immunotherapy against cancer. **B c.** **1** B LYMPHOCYTE. **2** BETA CELL. **balloon c.'s** Enlarged, swollen, and degenerated cells with greatly increased cytoplasmic mass, a change commonly seen in hepatocytes in acute viral hepatitis. **band c.** BAND NEUTROPHIL. **basal c.** A cell of the lower layer of the epidermis. Also *basilar cell.* **basal c. of taste bud** EPITHELIOCYTUS BASALIS GUSTATORIUS. **basilar c.** BASAL CELL. **basket c.** 1 A cell of the molecular layer of the cerebellar cortex. It has a horizontal axon that, passing across the long axis of the folium, sends out branches, each of which breaks up into a mesh of fibrils or basket surrounding the body of a Purkinje cell. 2 SMUDGE CELL. 3 MYOEPITHELIAL CELL. **basophilic c.** BASOPHIL. **basophilic c. of anterior lobe of the hypophysis** A cell that stains strongly with basic dyes and may represent either a thyrotropic or a gonadotropic cell. Some also include corticotrophic cells in this category. **battery c.** A single compartment of a galvanic battery, which contains electrolyte and two electrodes. Also *electrochemical cell.* **beaker c.** GOBLET CELL. **Beale's ganglion c.'s** The bipolar cells of the cardiac parasympathetic ganglia. One process is straight and the other convoluted. **Bergmann c.'s** Specialized astrocytic glial cells of the cerebellum. Their cell bodies are lined up in a row some distance beneath the surface, and have apical processes that pass vertically outward and then ramify beneath the pia. **berry c.** MORULA CELL. **beta c.** The insulin-secreting cell of the pancreatic islets of Langerhans, comprising as much as 80 percent of the islet cells in the normal adult human being. It can be stained specifically with aldehyde fuchsin for light microscopy. Also *B cell.* **Betz c.'s** Giant pyramidal cells in Brodmann's area 4, especially the hindlimb area on the medial aspect of the precentral gyrus. Their axons pass through the medullary pyramids. Also *giant pyramidal cells, Bevan Lewis cells* (obs.). **biochemical fuel c.** A battery cell that uses biologic compounds as fuel and usually oxygen as the oxidizer. For example it might use bodily energy sources to power a pacemaker. **bipolar c.** A neuron having two processes that leave the cell body at opposite poles. They occur, for example, in the retina, and in the vestibular and cochlear ganglia. **bipolar retinal c.** Any of the retinal nerve cells located between the ganglion cells and the rods and cones. **bite c.** KERATOCYTE. **Bizzozero c.** PLATELET. **bladder c.'s** Distended epithelial cells present in embryonic digits of the limbs. Also *Zander cells.* **blast c.** The earliest recognizable precursor of the major blood cell types. Blast cells are usually larger than differentiated cells, 15–20 microns in diameter, and lack cytoplasmic granules. Their nuclear chromatin is fine or unclumped and nucleoli are usually prominent. Also *blast.* See also MYELOBLAST, LYMPHOBLAST. **bloated c.** GITTER CELL. **blood c.'s** Any formed elements normally found in circulating blood, including erythrocytes, leukocytes, and platelets. **body c.** SOMATIC CELL. **bone c.** OSTEOCYTE. **bony ethmoidal c.** An air cell of the ethmoid bone. **border c.** OXYNTIC CELL. **bristle c.'s** The epitheliocytus sensorius pilosus internus and epitheliocytus sensorius pilosus externus of the spiral organ and cellula sensoria pilosa of the vestibular labyrinth of the internal ear. Also *hair cells.* **bronchic c.'s** ALVEOLI PULMONIS. **brood c.** A mother cell which gives rise to a cluster of daughter cells. **brush bipolar c.** FLAT BIPOLAR CELL. **bulliform c.** Thin-walled cells located in the plant epidermis which cause rolling, folding, or opening of leaves in response to changes in turgor pressure. **burr c.** ECHINOCYTE. **C c.** Any of the cells which secrete calcitonin and are situated in the tissues between the thyroid follicles in the thryoid gland. Also *parafollicular cell, interfollicular cell, clear cell, light cell of thyroid.* **Cajal c.** 1 One of the astrocytes arranged horizontally in the cerebral cortex. 2 ASTROCYTE. **cameloid c.** ELLIPTOCYTE. **cardiac failure c.'s** Hemosiderin-laden macrophages found in the lungs of patients with long-standing left-sided heart failure. Their presence indicates prior episodes of pulmonary edema associated with extravasation of red blood cells. **cartilage c.** CHONDROCYTE. **castration c.'s** Vacuolated basophilic cells in the anterior pituitary after gonadectomy and in gonadal deficiency. As in the postmenopausal state, the gonadotropin-secreting cells are those affected. **caudate c.'s** Glial cells having tail-like extensions whose appearance has been compared to that of a comet. They occur in gray matter. **central c.** PEPTIC CELL. **central sensory c.** A neuron within the central nervous system that carries impulses originating in a sensory organ. **centrifugal bipolar c.** A cell form in the inner nuclear layer of the retina believed to be a developmental stage of an amacrine cell. Also *Polyak's i-type cell.* **chief c.** 1 In the parathyroid glands, the cell that is responsible for the synthesis and secretion of a parathyroid hormone. Also *principal cell.* 2 A zymogenic cell of the gastric mucosa. **chromaffin c.** A cell that secretes and stores catecholamines and gives off a yellow-brown color after exposure to an aqueous solution of a chromium salt. Such cells are innervated by preganglionic sympathetic nerve fibers. Also *pheochrome cell.* **chromophobe c.** One of the cell types in the adenohypophysis whose cytoplasm has a weak affinity for both acidic and basic dyes. **ciliated c.** A cell with one or more cilia protruding from its surface. **Clara c.'s** Cells present in bronchi and bronchioles which may be concerned with secretion of pulmonary surfactant. **clear c.** 1 CLEAR CELL OF THE PARATHYROID GLAND. 2 C CELL. **clear c. of the parathyroid gland** A chief cell of the parathyroid gland that has an excess of clear cytoplasm. It is seen in hyperplasia and adenoma formation. Also *water-clear cell, clear cell.* **cleavage c.** BLASTOMERE. **clump c.** A melanin-containing neuroectodermal cell of the iris. **cochlear c.'s** The specialized sensory cells of the spiral organ, including the auditory cells connected to the cochlear division of the vestibulocochlear nerve. *Outmoded.* **columnar c.** An epithelial cell that is taller than its width as seen in histologic sections. **commissural c.** Any of the cells in the gray matter of the spinal cord whose axons travel in commissures to the contralateral side. **committed c.** A lymphocyte, after exposure to antigen, that is delegated to differentiate to either immunologic memory cells or to cells producing antibody. **companion c.** A long, spindle-shaped, nucleated parenchymal cell associated with a sieve-tube cell in the phloem of an angiosperm, arising from unequal division of a mother cell. The large sieve-tube cell loses most of its protoplasm and is maintained by secretions from the small companion cell. **compound granule c.** GITTER CELL. **cone c.** RETINAL CONE. **cone bipolar c.** A vertically oriented nerve cell of the internal nuclear lamina with a dendrite contacting the base of a cone and an axon that synapses on one or more ganglion cells. **conjunctival c.** A modified stratified squamous cell that forms part of the conjunctival epithelium. **connective tissue c.'s** Those cells that produce the intercellular matrix or ground substance and fibers of connective tissue. **c.'s of Corti** The various neurosensory or acoustic hair cells of the spiral organ in the internal ear, including the epitheliocytus sensorius pilosus internus and epitheliocytus sensorius pilosus externus. **corticotropic c.** One of the cells of the anterior lobe of the hypophysis that secretes adrenocorticotropic hormone. They are small cells, with sparse secretory granules, and have been variably classified in acidophilic, basophilic, and chromophobe categories because of their poor staining properties. Also *corticotroph*. **crescent c.** DEMILUNE CELL. **cribrate c.** A cell with an attenuated sheet of cytoplasm that is perforated by numerous sievelike pores to permit the rapid transport of large volumes of fluid. **cuboidal c.** An epithelial cell that is approximately square when examined in histologic sections. **cytomegalic c.'s** The characteristic cells of cytomegalic inclusion disease. They are large (25–40 μm in diameter), contain prominent nuclei, and have intranuclear and intracytoplasmic inclusion bodies. **cytotoxic c.** *Imprecise* NATURAL KILLER CELL. **D c.** DELTA CELL. **daughter c.** One of the cells resulting from the division of a mother cell. **decidual c.'s** Endometrial stromal cells enlarged into round or polygonal shapes due to pregnancy. The nucleus is vesicular, while the cytoplasm is a pale, basophilic shade. **deep c.** MESANGIAL CELL. **Deiters c.** 1 *Outmoded* ASTROCYTE. 2 EPITHELIOCYTUS PHALANGEUS EXTERNUS. **delta c.** One of the endocrine cells of the islets of Langerhans. They have been shown to contain both gastrin and somatostatin. Also *D cell*. **demilune c.** A serous cell that is located at the periphery of a mucous acinus in the submandibular salivary gland. It secretes via a fine channel into the central lumen of the acinus. Also *cell of Giannuzzi, crescent cell*. **dendritic c.** A cell with numerous ramifying cytoplasmic processes that is situated within lymphoid tissue and between adjacent lymphoid cells. The dendritic cell is concerned with the presentation of antigenic stimuli to the lymphoid system. **diffuse ganglion c.** A retinal ganglion cell having a single thick dendrite that branches at several levels of the inner plexiform layer and forms contacts with bipolar cells. **diploid c.** See under DIPLOID. **displaced ganglion c.** A retinal cell having the appearance of a ganglion cell but located in the internal nuclear layer. **dome c.'s** EPITRICHIUM. **Dorothy Reed c.'s** STERNBERG-REED CELLS. **Downey c.** ATYPICAL LYMPHOCYTE. **dust c.** ALVEOLAR MACROPHAGE. **EAC rosette forming c.** A cell that forms a rosette configuration with adherent erythrocytes when the cell is incubated with erythrocytes coated with IgM antibody and complement. This phenomenon demonstrates the presence of receptors for complement on the cell surface, a characteristic of B-lymphocytes. **ectoblastic c.** An undifferentiated embryonic cell destined to become a definitive ectodermal cell, recognized by its position in an early embryo and by its cytochemical and cytoplasmic characteristics. **ectodermal c.** One of the cells composing the outermost of the three primary germ layers, ectoderm, mesoderm, endoderm, that appear superimposed one above another at an early stage in development of an embryo. Definitive ectodermal cells are present at completion of gastrulation and eventually give rise to the epidermis of the skin and its derivatives, and also contribute to the development of teeth, the hypophysis, the anal canal and probably to certain other structures. **electrochemical c.** BATTERY CELL. **electromotive force c.** A battery cell that contains an anode, a cathode, and an electrolyte and produces an electromotive force between the electrodes. **embryonal c.'s** 1 Early embryonic cells which have not yet started to differentiate. 2 Cells formed as a result of cleavage of the fertilized ovum. **embryonic c.** 1 Any cell, usually undifferentiated, from an early embryo or found in a similar state elsewhere. 2 A cell resulting from cleavage of a fertilized ovum which as yet shows no obvious indication of its fate other than its participation in the formation of a part of an embryo. **emigrated c.** A leukocyte which has passed through the capillary wall into the extravascular fluid. **enamel c.** AMELOBLAST. **end c.** A cell that has lost the capacity for cell division and has become fully differentiated. Neurons and skeletal muscle cells are regarded as end cells. **endothelial c.** One of the flattened cells that line vascular channels of various sizes. The cytoplasm is normally permeable in capillaries and is fenestrated in the renal glomerulus, intestinal villi, endocrine glands, and the pancreas. **enterochromaffin c.'s** One of the scattered, and usually solitary, hormone-secreting cells of the stomach, pancreas, and intestine that contain gastrin, 5-hydroxytryptamine, and other vasoactive peptides. **ependymal c.'s** Glial cells, pyramidal or cuboidal in shape, which line the central canal of the spinal cord and the ventricles and choroid plexuses of the brain. **epiblastic c.** Any of the cells formed after subdivision of the embryonic ectoderm (ectoblast) into neuroblast and epiblast, which give rise to the epidermis and its derivatives, the skin and its associated glands. *Outmoded*. **epithelial c.** A cell that forms part of a covering or lining of a body surface. **epithelioid c.** The principal cell of granulomas. It is characterized by abundant pale pink cytoplasm, hence the resemblance to epithelial cells that gives it its name. Epithelioid cells are modified macrophages and are typically seen in such granulomatous inflammations as tuberculosis, schistosomiasis, and sarcoidosis. **E-rosette forming c.** A cell to which several sheep erythrocytes adhere, when the cell is incubated with the erythrocytes, resulting in a rosette configuration. The phenomenon is characteristic of T-lymphocytes. **erythroid c.** Any erythrocyte or erythrocyte precursor. **eta c.** A cell found in the lining of hepatic sinusoids that is thought to be related to the development of hepatic fibrosis in disease states. **ethmoidal c.'s** CELLULAE ETHMOIDALES. **faggot c.** A myeloblast that contains in its cytoplasm a large number of Auer rods, e.g. 5–20, arranged in bundles. Faggot cells are characteristic of acute progranulocytic leukemia. **c.'s of Fañanás** Protoplasmic astrocytes of distinctive form found in the deeper portion of the molecular layer of the cerebellar cortex. Their short, feathery branches are directed toward the surface. Also *gliocytus radiatus, glia of Fañanás*. **fat c.** A connective tissue cell with the capacity to make and store neutral fat within a cytoplasmic vacuole. When depleted of fat, the cell may be difficult to differentiate from a fibroblast. Also *lipocyte, adipose cell, adipocyte*. **fatty granule c.** A microglial cell that contains lipid vacuoles. **Ferrata c.** HEMOHISTIOBLAST. **fiber c.** 1 Any cell with attenuated and elongated cytoplasm. *Ambiguous*. 2 A large, elongated cell that is found in cervical smear preparations and is suggestive of the presence of invasive carcinoma of the cervix. **fixed c.** A macrophage of connective tissue which is attached to the fibers of the reticulum, usually a highly specialized cell. **flagellate c.** A motile cell having a flagellum or flagella. **flat bipolar c.** A cell in the retinal internal nuclear layer that connects cones with all types of ganglion cells. Also *brush bipolar cell*. **foam c.** A histiocyte filled with lipid droplets which give it a foamy appearance. It is the characteristic cell of a xanthoma. Also *xanthoma cell*. **follicle c.'s** 1 Flattened or low, cuboidal, epithelial cells surrounding the ovum in a primary follicle. With growth of the follicle, they become the granulosa cells in the membrana granulosa. Also *follicular cells*. 2 In lymphoid tissue, cells which form the primary and secondary follicles. **follicular center c.** Any of a series of B lymphocytes normally present in the germinal center of lymph nodes. Also *germinal center cell.* See under LARGE CLEAVED FOLLICULAR CENTER CELL, LARGE UNCLEAVED FOLLICULAR CENTER CELL, SMALL CLEAVED FOLLICULAR CENTER CELL, SMALL NONCLEAVED FOLLICULAR CENTER CELL. **foot c.** GLOMERULAR EPITHELIAL CELL. **foreign-body giant c.** A multinucleated giant cell formed by coalescence and fusion of macrophages in response to a foreign body which it phagocytoses and attempts to destroy. **free c.** A macrophage that originated from a primitive reticular cell, usually having a spindle or a flattened shape and located in loose connective tissue. However it can become a rounded motile cell and travel in the circulatory system to other connective-tissue areas. **fuchsinophil c.** A cell that stains selectively with either acid or basic fuchsin. **fusiform c.** SPINDLE CELL. **G c.** One of the individually distributed cells in the pyloric and upper small intestinal glands that secretes gastrin. These cells form part of the diffuse endocrine, or APUD, system. **ganglion c.** A neuron, or cell body of a neuron, located in an autonomic or sensory ganglion. Also *gangliocyte.* **ganglion c. of retina** The cell body of the axon of the optic nerve, located on the vitreal side of the retina. **Gaucher c.** An enlarged histiocyte filled with glucocerebroside. It is the characteristic cell of Gaucher's disease and is found throughout the reticuloendothelial system, especially in the bone marrow, spleen, liver, and lymph nodes. The cytoplasm is textured, having the appearance of crumpled tissue paper, and stains with PAS. **gemistocytic c.** PROTOPLASMIC ASTROCYTE. **generative c.** One of the two cells of a pollen grain, the one which divides to produce the microgametophyte, the other being the tube cell. **germ c.** Any cell of an organism whose function is reproduction, in contrast to the vegetative cells that are primarily concerned with growth and nutrition. They exist in two forms, gametes (ova and spermatozoa) and spores. Also *reproductive cell, germinal cell.* **germinal center c.** FOLLICULAR CENTER CELL. **ghost c.** ERYTHROCYTE GHOST. **c. of Giannuzzi** DEMILUNE CELL. **giant c.** **1** A large, multinucleate cell. **2** A fused mass of macrophages as is seen in foreign-body reactions and tuberculoid granulomas. **3** A neoplastic cell in which nuclear division occurred but was not followed by cytoplasmic division. **giant bipolar c.** A large bipolar cell of the retina having dendrites that synapse with several cones and rods. **giant ganglion c.** A particularly large and diffuse ganglion cell found in areas surrounding the central portion of the retina. **giant pyramidal c.'s** BETZ CELLS. **Gierke c.'s** The small, darkly-staining, Golgi type II neurons of the substantia gelatinosa of the spinal cord. **gitter c.** A lipid-laden microglial phagocyte commonly seen at the edge of healing brain infarcts. These cells phagocytize lipid previously contained by necrotic or degenerating brain cells. Also *compound granule cell, bloated cell.* See also MICROGLIA. **glandular c.** An epithelial cell that is specialized for secretion and is usually arranged with others in a secretory unit or gland. **glial c.'s** NEUROGLIAL CELLS. **glitter c.'s** Polymorphonuclear leukocytes whose cytoplasmic granules exhibit brownian movement on microscopic examination of urine sediment, a characteristic of pyelonephritis. **glomerular capsular c.** A cell that lines the inner aspect of the glomerular capsule (Bowman's capsule). **glomerular epithelial c.** Any of the epithelial cells of the visceral wall of the renal glomerulus having footlike processes (pedicels) by which they are attached to the glomerular basement membrane. Also *podocyte, foot cell.* **glomus c.** A modified smooth muscle cell that forms part of the contractile mechanism of a glomus arteriovenous anastomosis. **goblet c.** A mucous cell that has a large cytoplasmic vacuole such that its overall shape resembles a flask or goblet. Also *beaker cell.* **Golgi c.'s** Either Golgi type I neurons or Golgi type II neurons. See under NEURON. **gonadotropic c.** A type of basophilic cell in the anterior pituitary that secretes gonadotropic hormone and undergoes characteristic changes after gonadectomy or in gonadal deficiency states. It is not certain whether this cell is of one type, secreting FSH and LH, or of two types, with one secreting FSH and the other LH. **Goormaghtigh c.'s** JUXTAGLOMERULAR CELLS. **granular c.** A cell of the granular layer of the epidermis. **granule c.'s** The minute neurons found in immense numbers in the granular layer of the cerebellar cortex. Their axons ascend to the molecular layer, where they bifurcate to form the parallel fibers. The clawlike dendritic terminals receive input from mossy fibers. **granulosa c.** Any of the cells surrounding the female germ cell within developing ovarian follicles. **granulosa-lutein c.'s** LUTEIN CELLS. **grape c.** MORULA CELL. **great alveolar c.** TYPE II PNEUMOCYTE. **guard c.** One of two crescent-shaped chlorophyll-containing cells bordering a pore in the epidermis of plants. Changes in turgor of the pair of cells regulate the opening or closing of the pore. The two guard cells plus the opening make up the stoma. **gustatory c.'s** The several cell types that comprise a taste bud, including epitheliocytus sensorius gustatorius, epitheliocytus sustentans, and epitheliocytus basalis. They are stimulated by substances in solution that enter the porus gustatorius and reach the sensory surface. **gyrochrome c.** A neuron having its chromophil substance arranged in rings. *Seldom used.* **hair c.'s** BRISTLE CELLS. **hairy c.** See under LEUKEMIC RETICULOENDOTHELIOSIS. **haploid c.** See under HAPLOID. **heart-failure c.'s** Iron-containing alveolar macrophages in the lung of patients with heart failure. Also *heart-disease cells, heart-lesion cells.* **heckle c.** PRICKLE CELL. **HEK c.'s** Human embryo kidney cells, used in tissue culture. **HEL c.'s** Human embryo lung cells, used in tissue culture. **HeLa c.'s** A line of tissue culture cells derived from a squamous cell carcinoma of the uterine cervix. • *HeLa* is an acronym based on the donor's name. **helmet c.** A schizocyte in the shape of a helmet. **helper c.** Any of a subclass of T lymphocytes that facilitate immune responses such as conversion of B lymphocytes to plasma cells. In normal blood approximately two-thirds of T lymphocytes are helper cells. They are identified by surface antigen specificities $OKT_4$ and Leu-3a in addition to the general T lymphocyte surface antigens. Also *inducer cell, helper T lymphocyte.* Compare SUPPRESSOR CELL. **hemopoietic c.** A cell of blood or bone marrow or other blood-forming tissue that is capable of dividing to form additional blood or bone-marrow cells. **Hensen c.'s** Five or six rows of columnar cells on the outer side of Deiters cells, or epitheliocytus phalangeus externus, which comprise some of the supporting cells at th e lateral end of the spiral organ. Microvilli are present on their free surfaces, and near the cecum cupulare they contain fat globules. **hepatic c.** LIVER CELL. **hilus c.** A modified ovarian stromal cell that is normally found in the region of the hilus of the ovary. It corresponds in form and function to the Leydig cell of the testis. Also *sympathicotrophic cell, sympathotropic cell.* **Hodgkin c.'s** STERNBERG-REED CELLS. **Hofbauer c.'s** Circular or ellipsoid cells present in the chorionic villi of human placentae. They are fetal in origin and possibly function as motile histiocytes, may play some role in fetal nutrition, possess vacuoles, and may also have a secretory activity. **horizontal c.'s** The multipolar neurons in the third (Polyak) layer of the retina. They have a long process that makes synaptic contacts with both the spherules of rods and the pedicles of cones, and several short processes having junctions either on cone pedicles (cone horizontal cells) or on rod spherules (rod horizontal cells). Also *horizontal neurons.* **horn c.** 1 A ganglion cell from the anterior or posterior horn of the spinal cord. 2 An epithelial cell which has lost its nucleus, the ultimate product of the process of keratinization in the epidermis. Horn cells are eventually shed as invisible particles. **Hortega c.'s** MICROGLIA. **hot c.** A heavily shielded area in which highly radioactive materials are manipulated by remote control, the operator watching what he is doing through a thick window. The arrangement minimizes the operator's exposure to radiation. **Hürthle c.** A large cell sometimes found in the thyroid gland, having eosinophilic, granular cytoplasm. Also *oxyphil cell, Askanazy cell.* **hyperchromatic c.** A cell that has an increased affinity for stains compared with normal cells of the same type: usually used in reference to the increased staining ability of the nucleus in the presence of DNA. **I c.** 1 IMMUNOCYTE. 2 A fibroblastic cell containing cytoplasmic inclusions characteristic of mucolipidosis II. **immunocompetent c.** IMMUNOCYTE. **immunologically competent c.** IMMUNOCYTE. **incasing c.** *Outmoded* EPITHELIOCYTUS SUSTENTANS GUSTATORIUS. **indifferent c.** UNDIFFERENTIATED CELL. **individual bipolar c.** MONOSYNAPTIC BIPOLAR CELL. **inducer c.** HELPER CELL. **inflammatory c.** Any cell which is active in the inflammatory response to a foreign particle, such as a neutrophil. **inner hair c.** EPITHELIOCYTUS SENSORIUS PILOSUS INTERNUS. **inner phalangeal c.** EPITHELIOCYTUS PHALANGEUS INTERNUS. **intercalary c.** A small cell type located between the main columnar cells of the fallopian tube epithelium. It may represent a precursor of the columnar cells. Also *peg cell, intercalated cell.* **intercapillary c.** MESANGIAL CELL. **interfollicular c.** C CELL. **internuncial c.** INTERNEURON. **interstitial c.'s of Leydig** LEYDIG CELLS. **interstitial c.'s of the testis** LEYDIG CELLS. **islet c.'s** Any of the several types of cells comprising the islets of Langerhans of the pancreas. **juvenile c.** METAMYELOCYTE. **juxtaglomerular c.'s** Modified smooth muscle cells which are found in the media of the afferent arteriole as it enters the renal glomerulus. These cells contain secretory granules of renin and form part of the juxtaglomerular apparatus. Also *Goormaghtigh cells, juxtaglomerular epitheliod cells* (seldom used). **K c.** NATURAL KILLER CELL. **killer c.** NATURAL KILLER CELL. **Kulchitsky c.** ARGENTAFFIN CELL. **Kupffer c.** One of the phagocytic cells that contributes toward the formation of an endothelial lining of the liver sinusoids. Also *von Kupffer cell, stellate cell of liver.* **Kurloff c.** A cell found in the peripheral blood and lymphoid system of guinea pigs that are pregnant or treated with estrogen. It contains a large body which is PAS positive and is postulated to be a modified lymphocyte of unknown function. **L c.'s** A strain of mouse cells maintained in cell cultures. They are useful for growing a number of viruses. **lacis c.** A modified smooth muscle cell found in the juxtaglomerular apparatus of the kidney. **lacrimoethmoid c.'s** Some anterior ethmoidal air cells lying deep to the lacrimal bone where the posterosuperior part of its nasal surface articulates with the ethmoid bone. **Langerhans c.** A dendritic cell of the epidermis that is seen in hematoxylin and eosin sections as a high level clear cell. Although it was once thought to be related to the melanocytes of the basal layer, this theory has been rejected.

**Langhans c.** 1 One of the cells of the cytotrophoblast (Langhans layer) of the placental chorionic villi. 2 See under LANGHANS GIANT CELL. **Langhans giant c.** A multinucleated giant cell formed by the coalescence of epithelioid macrophages and measuring up to 50 $\mu$m in diameter. These cells, which contain several dozen nuclei arranged in a characteristic horseshoe pattern, are a feature of certain forms of chronic granulomatous inflammation such as that of tuberculosis, schistosomiasis, and leprosy. **large cleaved follicular center c.** A type of B lymphocyte that is normally present in the germinal center of lymph nodes and is regarded as an intermediate stage between small cleaved and small noncleaved follicular center cells, in the transformation of a lymphocyte to immunoblast and plasma cell. It is approximately 12 micrometers in diameter, its nucleus has deep foldings or clefts, chromatin is clumped, and cytoplasm may have immunoglobulin inclusions. The cytoplasm is not pyroninophilic. Also *centrocyte, germinocyte.* **large noncleaved follicular center c.** A type of B lymphocyte that is normally present in the germinal center of lymph nodes and is regarded as the immediate precursor of the B immunoblast. It is approximately 15–20 microns in diameter, its nucleus lacks folding or clefts, chromatin is finely dispersed, and 1–3 prominent nucleoli are present, usually close to the margin of the nucleus. The cytoplasm is pyroninophilic and more abundant than in other follicular center cells. Following this stage of activation, the follicular center cell becomes an immunoblast and migrates out from the lymph node follicle. Also *centroblast, germinoblast.* **LE c.** A neutrophil or macrophage that has phagocytized the damaged nucleus of another cell, seen in peripheral blood smears of patients with systemic lupus erythematosus who have circulating antinuclear antibodies. Also *lupus erythematosus cell.* **Leclanché c.** The common flashlight battery, which has a carbon anode and zinc cathode. **Leishman's chrome c.'s** Blood leukocytes containing phagocytosed malaria pigment. *Obs.* **lepra c.'s** Lipid-laden macrophages seen in the tissues of patients suffering from lepromatous leprosy. Their cytoplasm is foamy, and is filled with round masses of acid-fast bacilli. Also *Virchow cells.* **Leydig c.'s** Testosterone-secreting cells of the testicular connective tissues that contain rod-shaped crystalloids with rounded or pointed ends, abundant agranular endoplasmic reticulum, phospholipids, cholesterol, and vacuoles containing fat. The number of cells varies with age and disease. Also *interstitial cells of the testis, interstitial cells of Leydig.* **light c. of thyroid** C CELL. **littoral c.** The flattened mesothelial cell which forms the lining of sinuses in lymph nodes and bone marrow. Also *lining cell.* **liver c.** One of the parenchymal cells of the liver, which are arranged in a series of laminae to form the liver lobules. Also *hepatic cell, hepatocyte.* **locomotive c.** AMEBOID CELL. **lupus erythematosus c.** LE CELL. **luteal c.** A constituent cell of a corpus luteum, containing a yellow pigment, lutein, and capable of secreting the hormone progesterone. These cells are derived from the granular layer of the ovarian follicle. **lutein c.'s** Granular lipid-containing cells of the ovarian follicles that produce the corpus luteum of the ovary. Also *granulosa-lutein cells.* **lymph c.** LYMPHOCYTE. **lymphoblastic plasma c.** PLASMABLAST. **lymphoid c.** LYMPHOCYTE. **macroglial c.'s** MACROGLIA. **malpighian c.** PRICKLE CELL. **Martinotti's c.** A fusiform cell found in various layers of the cerebral cortex. **mast c.** A connective tissue cell commonly found adjacent to blood vessels and in the lymphatic system, skin, lung, and other tissues. Mast cells are approximately 20 microns in diameter and have cytoplasm filled by numerous (30–100) prominent metachromatic granules that stain black or purplish black with Romanowsky dyes. The granules contain heparin and histamine, and are involved in urticarial reactions. Mast cells are markedly increased in urticaria pigmentosa. Also *labrocyte, mastocyte.* • Mast cells (German *Mastzellen*) are so called because their cytoplasmic granules, originally thought to contain stored nutrients, were likened to mast, that is, acorns, nuts, etc. used to fatten livestock. **mastoid c.'s** CELLULAE MASTOIDEAE. **matrix c.'s** 1 The basal cells of the lobules of sebaceous glands. 2 The cells of the hair matrix. **medullary interstitial c.** A cell in the connective tissue of the renal medulla that contains secretory granules of prostaglandin. **medulloepithelial c.** A neuroepithelial cell found in the primitive neural tube. In contact with the internal limiting membrane and having no relation with the external limiting membrane these cells divide rapidly by mitosis and assume a rounded appearance. It is likely that these cells represent the stem cells which will give rise to neuroblast tissue. Alternatively, they may remain undifferentiated within the neuroglial or neuronal tissue. **melanotropic c.** One of the cells in the pars intermedia region of the anterior lobe of the pituitary that secrete melanocyte-stimulating hormone. **memory c.** Any of a subclass of lymphocytes which, long after the original immune response, retain the ability to proliferate and differentiate when antigen is encountered again. See also IMMUNOLOGIC MEMORY. **Merkel c.** MENISCUS TACTUS. **Merkel-Ranvier c.** MELANOCYTE. **mesangial c.** Any of the modified smooth muscle cells that form the central branching structure of the renal glomerular tuft. The mesangial cells produce and are surrounded by a matrix of basement-membranelike material. Also *intercapillary cell, deep cell.* **mesenchymal c.'s** Cells comprising the packing tissue between the other germ layers in an embryo. They are nonepithelial cells with amoeboid characteristics which come to lie between the epithelial cells and the coelomic cavity lining. They are predominantly of mesodermal origin but ectoderm can give rise to them either directly or by way of the neural crest, and it is also possible that to a more limited extent endoderm does so also. A collection of mesenchymal cells is referred to as mesenchyme. **mesothelial c.'s** Cells of mesodermal origin that form the lining epithelium of the pleural pericardial and peritoneal cavities. **Mexican hat c.** TARGET ERYTHROCYTE. **Meynert c.'s** Pyramidal neurons of that part of the cerebral cortex related to the calcarine fissure. **microglial c.'s** MICROGLIA. **middle ethmoidal air c.'s** CELLULAE MEDII ETHMOIDALES. **midget bipolar c.** Any of the monosynaptic, bipolar retinal nerve cells located between the foveal cones and the ganglion cells. Each of these synapses on a single midget ganglion cell. **migratory c.** WANDERING CELL. **Mikulicz c.** A foamy histiocyte found in the chronic granulomatous lesions of the nose and nasopharynx of patients with rhinoscleroma. It contains numerous Gram-negative bacilli of the species *Klebsiella rhinoscleromatis.* **mitral c.** A second-order neuron of the olfactory pathway. Located in the fourth layer of the olfactory bulb, it has superficially directed apical dendrites that contact incoming olfactory nerve fibers, and at its other pole an axon that passes into the olfactory tract. • The term derives from the fancied resemblance of the soma to a bishop's mitre. **monocytoid c.** A cell that resembles a monocyte. **monosynaptic bipolar c.** A cone bipolar cell that synapses on a single ganglion cell. Also *individual bipolar cell.* **monosynaptic ganglion c.** A retinal ganglion cell found adjacent to the fovea. Its single dendrite usually embraces the terminals of a single midget bipolar cell, thereby mediating transmission from a single cone. **mop bipolar c.** ROD BIPOLAR CELL. **morula c.** A plasma cell that contains numerous cytoplasmic globules, thus resembling a cluster of grapes. The globules are composed of immunoglobulins. Morula cells are seen commonly in bone marrow of multiple myeloma, but they also occur in benign conditions. Also *berry cell, grape cell, mulberry cell.* **mossy c.** A protoplasmic astrocyte having a large cell body and numerous branching processes. **mother c.** A cell which undergoes division, giving rise to two or more cells (daughter cells). Also *parent cell.* **motile c.** A cell that is capable of movement. **motor c.** MOTONEURON. **Mott c.** A type of Russell body seen in the inflammatory infiltrate of rhinoscleroma. **mouth c.'s** Detached squamous epithelial cells recovered in the sputum. **mucous c.** An epithelial cell that synthesizes and secretes mucin. **mucous neck c.** A mucus-secreting cell that is situated particularly in the region of the necks of gastric glands. **mulberry c.** MORULA CELL. **Müller c.'s** See under SUSTENTACULAR TISSUE. **multipolar c.** A neuron with multiple processes that extend out from the cell body. Such cells are seen most often in the central nervous system. **mural c.** A nucleated cell lining the walls of the retinal capillaries. **muscle c.** A mesenchymal cell that is highly specialized for contraction. Also *myocyte.* **myeloid c.** Any leukocyte of the granulocytic series. **myeloma c.** A neoplastic plasma cell that proliferates and replaces the bone marrow of patients with multiple myeloma. **myoepithelial c.** A contractile cell of epithelial origin found at the periphery of a secretory acinus or duct. Also *basket cell.* **myogenic c.** MYOBLAST. **myoid c.** Any cell that resembles a skeletal muscle cell and thus may be contractile or contain contractile proteins. **natural killer c.** A large lymphocyte with azurophilic cytoplasmic granules. Natural killer cells comprise a minor fraction of the lymphocytes of normal blood. They are directly cytotoxic to other cells. Some schemes represent them as being a separate class of lymphocytes rather than being T lymphocytes. They are identified by surface antigen specificity Leu-7. Also *killer cell, killer lymphocyte, cytotoxic cell* (imprecise), *K cell, NK cell.* **nerve c.** 1 NEURON. 2 The cell body of a neuron, particularly as seen in a histologic section. **neuroepithelial c.'s** Epithelioid cells adapted in various ways for the reception of specific sensory stimuli, such as olfactory cells, taste cells, and hair cells of the ear. **neuroepithelial taste c.** EPITHELIOCYTUS SENSORIUS GUSTATORIUS. **neuroglial c.'s** The supportive cells of the central nervous system, including the ependyma, astrocytes, and oligodendroglia of ectodermal origin, and the microglia of mesodermal origin. Also *glial cells.* **neurosecretory c.** A cell derived from neuroectoderm and capable of secreting one or more of a variety of biologically active amines that may exert their effects either locally or at a distant site. **neurosensory c.** The most primitive type of neuron to form in an early embryo. **neutrophilic c.** NEUTROPHIL. **nevus c.** The principal cell component of nevi, found in the epidermis, the dermis, or both. It is similar to a melanocyte, but lacks dendritic projections. **niche c.** TYPE II PNEUMOCYTE. **Niemann-Pick c.** An enlarged histiocyte filled with sphingomyelin. It is the characteristic cell of Niemann-Pick disease and is found throughout the reticuloendothelial system as well as in the gastrointestinal tract and lungs. The cytoplasm of these cells is finely vacuolated or foamy, and stains positively with fat stains. Also *Pick's cell.* **NK c.** NATURAL KILLER CELL. **normal c.** Any cell that occurs naturally in an organ or tissue without distortion caused by disease. **nucleated c.** Any cell that contains a nucleus. **nucleated red blood c.** Any nucleated erythrocyte precursor. **null c.** NUL LYMPHOCYTE. **nurse c.'s** SERTOLI CELLS. **oat c.'s** Small, round or oval cells with little or no visible cytoplasm that constitute the main component of oat cell carcinoma of the lung. This cell is believed to be derived from the argentaffin, or Kulchitsky, cell of the bronchial mucosa. **olfactory c.'s** Spindle-shaped, modified bipolar nerve cells evenly distributed between the supporting cells of the olfactory epithelium in the roof of the nasal cavity. Each cell body has a dendritic process reaching the surface where it swells to form an olfactory vesicle which has clusters of long cilia. The unmyelinated axon of each cell extends into the lamina propria where the axons form bundles or fila olfactoria which pierce the cribriform plate of the ethmoid bone to enter the olfactory bulb of the brain. **oligodendroglial c.** One of the glial cells of the central nervous system responsible for the formation of myelin sheaths around axons. It has few cytoplasmic processes. **Opalski c.** A large rounded cell with a large nucleus and finely granular or foaming cytoplasm which stains a light rose color with Nissl stains. The cell is found in various parts of the basal ganglia in patients with Wilson's disease and is thought by some to be specific for this condition. **osseous c.** OSTEOCYTE. **osteochondrogenic c.** A cell that is capable of differentiating toward either an osteoblast or a chondroblast. **osteogenic c.** OSTEOBLAST. **outer hair c.** EPITHELIOCYTUS SENSORIUS PILOSUS EXTERNUS. **outer phalangeal c.** EPITHELIOCYTUS PHALANGEUS EXTERNUS. **owl's eye c.'s** Cells that are infected by a cytomegalovirus: used especially in reference to desquamated renal tubular epithelium. **oxyntic c.** A large, rounded cell with eosinophilic cytoplasm, found at intervals along the body of a gastric gland. These cells secrete acid into the lumen of the gastric glands. Also *parietal cell, border cell, acid cell.* **oxyphil c.** **1** HÜRTHLE CELL. **2** In the parathyroid glands, a cell type distinct from the chief cell, appearing in man around puberty and having a small pyknotic nucleus and intensely eosinophilic granular cytoplasm. **packed red blood c.'s (human)** The sedimented erythrocytes of human blood, free of plasma. The concentrated preparation of cells is used in transfusions to replace the loss of these cellular elements. **Paget c.'s** Large, pale-staining cells, often with mucin-filled vacuoles, occurring in the epidermis in mammary and extramammary Paget's disease. **palatine air c.** An air sinus enclosed in the orbital process of the palatine bone. **Paneth c.** A zymogenic cell with eosinophilic cytoplasmic granules that is found at the bottom of the glandulae intestinales. **parafollicular c.** C CELL. **paraluteal c.** THECAL CELL. **paralutein c.** THECAL CELL. **parent c.** MOTHER CELL. **parietal c.** OXYNTIC CELL. **pathologic c.** Any abnormal cell that appears in the course of a disease or pathologic process. **pavement c.** A flattened epithelial or squamous cell. **peg c.** INTERCALARY CELL. **peptic c.** A zymogenic cell in a gastric gland. Also *central cell.* **pericapillary c.** PERICYTE. **perineurial c.** A cell of the perineurium that forms a delicate membrane that ensheathes bundles of individual nerve fibers. **peripheral sensory c.** A neuron within the peripheral nervous system that carries the impulses that originated in a sensory receptor. **peritoneal exudate c.** Any cell present in a peritoneal exudate following various infections, often elicited for experimental purposes by the injection of irritant substances such as paraffin or peptone broth. The early states of the exudate contain mostly neutrophils and, later, macrophages and lymphocytes. The lavaged cells from the peritoneum are then used in immunologic experiments. **perivascular c.** PERICYTE. **perivascular glial c.'s** MICROGLIA. **pessary c.** A strikingly hypochromic erythrocyte, in which stainable cytoplasm is concentrated in a thin peripheral rim, usually a technical artifact. **petrosal c.'s** Air cells extending inwards into the petrous part of the temporal bone often as far as the petrosal apex. **phalangeal c.** Either epitheliocytus phalangeus externus or epitheliocytus phalangeus internus. **phalangeal c. of Deiters** **1** EPITHELIOCYTUS PHALANGEUS EXTERNUS. **2** ASTROCYTE. **phantom c.** ERYTHROCYTE GHOST. **pheochrome c.** CHROMAFFIN CELL. **physaliferous c.'s** The characteristic cell of chordomas. It is composed of abundant greatly vacuolated cytoplasm and vesicular nucleus and is probably derived from notochordal rests. **Pick's c.** NIEMANN-PICK CELL. **pigment c.** A cell that bears pigment granules in the cytoplasm. Also *chromatocyte.* **pigment c. of iris** Any of the cells comprising the melanin-bearing neural ectoderm on the posterior surface of the iris. **pigment c. of skin** MELANOCYTE. **pineal c.** PINEALOCYTE. **plaque-forming c.'s** Antibody-forming cells detected by the production of small zones (or plaques) of hemolysis in the hemolytic plaque test. **plasma c.** The cell which synthesizes, stores, and secretes immunoglobulin. The plasma cell is usually ovoid, with an eccentric nucleus. The chromatin is arranged like the spokes of a wheel. The cytoplasm is strongly basophilic due to an abundance of RNA and of endoplasmic reticulum. Plasma cells arise from the terminal differentiation of B lymphocytes. Also *plasmacyte, plasmocyte.* **pluripotent c.** A cell that retains the ability to differentiate in more than one direction. **PNH c.'s** Red cells characteristically found in patients with paroxysmal nocturnal hemoglobinuria. PNH cells typically lyse in acidified serum, or in the presence of thrombin or sucrose in water solution. **Polyak's i-type c.** CENTRIFUGAL BIPOLAR CELL. **polychromatic c.** An erythrocyte precursor with mixed acidophilic and basophilic cytoplasmic staining. Also *polychromatophil cell, polychromatophil, polychromophil, polychromatocyte.* **polyhedral c.** A cell that bears a polyhedral shape as a result of being closely packed with similar cells. **polysynaptic ganglion c.** A ganglion cell whose dendrites spread widely to contact from several to hundreds of bipolar cells. Unistratified, diffuse, and displaced subtypes are recognized. **posterior ethmoidal air c.'s** CELLULAE POSTERIORES ETHMOIDALES. **postmitotic c.** A cell type that can no longer divide by mitosis, and cannot be replaced from a stem cell population. Aging in multicellular organisms is attributed to changes in these cells, sometimes specifically to those molecules in postmitotic cells that do not turn over, such as nuclear deoxyribonucleic acid. **pregnancy c.** Any of the chromophobe cells of the pituitary observed in pregnant women. **pregranulosa c.'s** Precursors of the membrana granulosa cells found in the ovarian cortical region before they have become arranged as an envelope surrounding an oocyte and are then called primitive granulosa cells. Some authorities consider pregranulosa cells to be derived from the covering epithelium of the ovary. **prickle c.** A cell of the malpighian layer of the epidermis. Also *heckle cell, malpighian cell.* **primary embryonic c.** An undifferentiated cell from a very young embryo, capable of developing into a definitive cell type. **primitive reticular c.** A cell type which forms a network by its processes, making contacts with those of other cells of its kind. This cellular network also includes reticular fibers. It is found as a stroma in bone marrow and in lymphatic tissue. **primordial germ c.** ARCHIGONOCYTE. **principal c.** CHIEF CELL. **pulmonary epithelial c.** PNEUMOCYTE. **Purkinje c.'s** Very large and characteristic neurons of the middle layer of the cerebellar cortex. They have a drop-shaped body topped by a dense trellislike ramification of dendrites extending through the molecular layer in a direction transverse to the long axis of the folium. Synaptic connections, each of distinctive form, are made by parallel fibers, climbing fibers, and basket cells. The single axon ends in a central cerebellar nucleus where its effect is inhibitory. Also *Purkinje's corpuscles* (obs.). **pyknotic c.** A dying cell that contains a contracted, dense, and often distorted nucleus. **pyramidal c.** Any neuron whose cell body has a pyramidal or conical shape. The best known and most numerous examples are the pyramidal cells of the neocortex and hippocampus. Pyramidal cells are characterized by small lateral dendrites and a basal dendrite directed toward the cortical surface, and a large apical axon that may remain within cortical layers or enter the medullary substance. Also *pyramidal neuron.* See also STELLATE CELLS. **pyroninophilic blast c.** IMMUNOBLAST. **red c.** ERYTHROCYTE. **red blood c.** ERYTHROCYTE. **c. of the red nucleus** A constituent cell of the red nucleus in the midbrain. These cells give rise to the rubrospinal tract. **Reed-Sternberg c.'s** STERNBERG-REED CELLS. **regeneration c.** A cell with morphological features that indicate rapid growth following tissue damage. The cytoplasm is likely to be basophilic due to a high RNA content and the nucleus enlarged with a prominent nucleolus. **renal tubular c.** A cell that lines the tubular part of a nephron. **Renshaw c.'s** Interneurons in the ventromedial portion of the spinal cord believed to have an exclusively inhibitory effect on spinal motor neurons. These cells were originally thought to be short-axoned neurons and representative inhibitory cells throughout the central nervous system, a conception which has not stood the test of time. **reproductive c.** GERM CELL. **responder c.** See under ONE-WAY MIXED LYMPHOCYTE CULTURE. **resting c.** A cell which is not undergoing mitosis or meiosis. Often much synthetic activity is occurring in such a cell. *Outmoded.* Also *vegetative cell.* See also INTERPHASE. **resting wandering c.** FIXED MACROPHAGE. **reticular c.** HISTIOCYTE. **reticuloendothelial c.** HISTIOCYTE. **reticulum c.** HISTIOCYTE. **rhagiocrine c.** MACROPHAGE. **rod c.** Any of the retinal visual cells serving scotopic vision. **rod bipolar c.** A retinal bipolar cell whose profusely branching dendrite contacts several rod spherules while its unbranched axon synapses on one to four ganglion cells. Also *mop bipolar cell.* **Rouget c.** PERICYTE. **S c.'s** Mucoid cells in the anterior lobe of the pituitary gland which contain a protein rich in sulfurs and cysteine. **Sala c.'s** Star-shaped connective tissue cells related to sensory nerve endings in the pericardium. **satellite c.** 1 Any of the reactive neuroglial cells surrounding a damaged sensory ganglion cell. 2 A small, unspecialized cell intimately applied to the surface of extra- and intrafusal fibers of skeletal muscle. Such cells have the potential to form new fibers in regenerating muscle and possibly in muscle hypertrophy. **satellite c.'s of skeletal muscle** Small cells derived from myoblasts that are present at the periphery of skeletal muscle cells and persist into adult life. They may contribute to the limited regeneration of which skeletal muscle is capable. Also *sarcoplasts.* **scavenger c.** PHAGOCYTE. **Schwann c.** 1 A cell that produces the myelin sheath over one internode of a myelinated axon, or that in unmyelinated fibers envelops the bundle of naked axons. Also *nerve corpuscle* (older term). 2 The nucleus and perinuclear cytoplasm of such a cell. **secondary c.** A battery cell that can either supply electric energy or be recharged: a storage battery. **segmentation c.** BLASTOMERE. **segmented c.** SEGMENTED NEUTROPHIL. **seminal c.** Any of the cells that line a seminal tubule, including both Sertoli cells and the cells involved in spermatogenesis. **sensitized c.** 1 A cell which has been exposed to a specific antigen and is capable of showing an immune response if and when that antigen is reintroduced. 2 A cell which has been coated with antibody. **sensory c.** Any neuron whose axon, or more exactly dendrite, innervates a sensory receptor. The cell body may be in a dorsal root ganglion, peripherally located ganglion of a cranial nerve, or the mesencephalic ganglion of the trigeminal nerve. **septal c.** TYPE II PNEUMOCYTE. **serous c.** An exocrine cell whose function is to elaborate a watery, protein-rich fluid usually containing an enzyme. Also *albuminous cell, serozymogenic cell.* **Sertoli c.'s** Tall columnar cells in the seminiferous tubules of the testis, attached proximally to the basement membrane and reaching distally toward the lumen of the tubule. The Sertoli cells have large pale nuclei with conspicuous nucleoli. They anchor, protect, and possibly nourish the developing spermatids. Also *nurse cells, columns of Sertoli.* **sexual c.'s** Immature germ cells of either the testis or ovary that are the anlage of the mature spermatozoa or ova. **Sézary c.** The characteristic cell of the Sézary syndrome. This neoplastic T lymphocyte is primarily found in the skin lesions and peripheral blood and has a deeply indented, cerebriform nucleus and scanty cytoplasm. **shadow c.** ERYTHROCYTE GHOST. **sickle c.** An erythrocyte deformed into a crescent shape by tactoids formed by polymerization of hemoglobin S. Also *meniscocyte, drepanocyte.* See also SICKLE CELL ANEMIA. **signet-ring c.** A cell with a large, single cytoplasmic vacuole that displaces the nucleus to one side. This cell is seen in certain mucin-producing adenocarcinomas, most commonly those of the stomach. **skein c.** RETICULOCYTE. **small cleaved follicular center c.** A type of B lymphocyte that is normally present in the germinal center of lymph nodes and is regarded as the precursor of other types of follicular center cells. It is a small lymphocyte, approximately eight micrometers in diameter, and its nucleus has clumped chromatin and an indentation or cleft. The cytoplasm is not pyroninophilic. Also *centrocyte, germinocyte.* **small noncleaved follicular center c.** A type of B lymphocyte that is normally present in the germinal center of lymph nodes and is regarded as an intermediate stage between large cleaved and large noncleaved follicular center cells. It is approximately 12 micrometers in diameter, its nucleus lacks foldings or clefts, chromatin is finely dispersed, and 1–3 prominent nucleoli are present. The cytoplasm is basophilic and pyroninophilic. Also *centroblast, germinoblast.* **smooth muscle c.** A muscle cell in which the actin and myosin filaments are relatively unstructured so that cross-striations are not produced. These cells are associated with visceral structures and can be stimulated via the autonomic nervous system. **smudge c.** Any of the remnants of disrupted cells that appear as purple smudges in Romanowsky-stained blood films, especially in chronic lymphocytic leukemia. Also *basket cell.* **somatic c.** An uncommitted cell of the body wall of an embryo. Also *body cell.* **somatotropic c.** One of the cells of the anterior lobe of the hypophysis that secretes growth hormone. They are large cells and they stain specifically with Orange G. They are included in the acidophilic category of cells. Also *somatotropin producing cell.* **sperm c.** SPER-

MATOZOON. **spermatogenic c.'s** Cells that are the anlage of sperm. **spermatogonial c.** An undifferentiated germ cell near the wall of the seminiferous tubule. Through repeated mitotic divisions a population of primary spermatocytes is produced. **spider c.** **1** *Outmoded* ASTROCYTE. **2** PERICYTE. **spindle c.** A cell with the shape of a spindle: usually descriptive of relatively undifferentiated connective tissue cells. Also *fusiform cell.* **splenic c.** Any of the constituent cells of the spleen. **spur c.** ACANTHOCYTE. **squamous c.** A flattened epithelial cell that is usually arranged in layers to form a protective stratified squamous epithelium. Also *bridge corpuscle.* **squamous alveolar c.** TYPE I PNEUMOCYTE. **stab c.** BAND NEUTROPHIL. **staff c.** BAND NEUTROPHIL. **standard c.** A precision battery cell used in a potentiometer to make accurate voltage measurements. **static balance receptor c.** A sensory hair cell in the macula of the utricle that forms part of the membranous labyrinth of the inner ear. **stellate c.'s** **1** Any star-shaped cells. Also *sternzellen.* **2** Cells of the molecular layer of the cerebellum having unmyelinated, horizontally oriented axons. Those adjacent to the Purkinje cell layer are larger and are usually called basket cells. **3** Cells of the cerebral cortex, particularly layer IV, having a polygonal shape, multiple radiating dendrites, and an axon that may be short and ramify near the cell body or longer and enter the medullary substance. The latter are called stellate pyramidal cells or star pyramids, so called from their resemblance to pyramidal cells. Giant stellate cells are found along the calcarine fissure. **stellate c. of liver** KUPFFER CELL. **stellate pyramidal c.'s** See under STELLATE CELLS. **stem c.** A primitive cell which divides to produce a line of differentiated cells, as a primitive blood cell which precedes the blast stage, or a spermatogonial cell. **Sternberg-Reed c.'s** Giant cells with abundant cytoplasm and multilobular or multiple nuclei. Bilobed nuclei may assume a mirror-image form. Nucleoli are large, round, and acidophilic, usually one per nuclear segment. The identification of these cells is considered necessary for a diagnosis of Hodgkin's disease. Also *Hodgkin cells, Dorothy Reed cells, Reed-Sternberg cells.* **stimulator c.** See under ONE-WAY MIXED LYMPHOCYTE CULTURE. **stippled c.** An erythrocyte that exhibits basophilic stippling when stained with the Wright stain or with some other Romanowsky-type stain. **strap c.** One of the characteristic shapes taken by cells of rhabdomyosarcomas. This cell is elongated, has an abundant eosinophilic cytoplasm that may show cross striations, and is generally of uniform width. **stroma c.** A connective tissue cell that forms the skeletal framework of an organ. **supporting c.'s** Various cells that usually form a solid but flexible protective framework for adjacent specialized cells in organs such as the maculae, the spiral organ of the internal ear, the olfactory organ in the nasal cavity, and the gustatory organ in the mouth and pharynx. In the internal ear they are basically slender, columnar cells with a round nucleus at the lower end, and they contain bundles of tonofibrils. In the spiral organ they include the inner and outer pillar cells, the inner and outer phalangeal or hair cells, border cells, and the cells of Hensen and Claudius. Also *sustentacular cells.* **supporting c. of taste bud** EPITHELIOCYTUS SUSTENTANS GUSTATORIUS. **suppressor c.** Any of a subclass of T lymphocytes that inhibit immune responses such as conversion of B lymphocytes to plasma cells. In normal blood approximately one-third of T lymphocytes are suppressor cells. They are identified by surface antigen specificities $OKT_8$ and Leu-3a in addition to the general T lymphocyte surface antigens. Also *suppressor T lymphocyte.* Compare HELPER CELL. **sustentacular c.'s** SUPPORTING CELLS. **sustentacular c. of taste bud** EPITHELIOCYTUS SUSTENTANS GUSTATORIUS. **sympathetic c.** A cell that forms part of the sympathetic outflow of the autonomic nervous system. The sympathetic postganglionic nerve fibers normally secrete epinephrine and norepinephrine. **sympathetic formative c.** SYMPATHOBLAST. **sympathicotrophic c.** HILUS CELL. **sympathochromaffin c.'s** A syncytium of cells in the embryo which develops into either small cells (sympathoblasts), which become transformed into sympathetic nerve cells, or large chromaffin cells, which separate from the others and aggregate to form chromaffin organs such as para-aortic bodies (paraganglia) and the medulla of the suprarenal. Also *sympathogonia.* **sympathotropic c.** HILUS CELL. **syncytial c.** A multinucleate cell that is formed by mitosis without subsequent cytoplasmic division. **synovial c.** A specialized connective tissue cell that lines a synovial or joint cavity and contributes to the synovial fluid. **T c.** T LYMPHOCYTE. **tadpole c.'s** Large cells that resemble the shape of a tadpole, with hyperchromatic large nuclei: used especially in cytology to describe smears that are seen in malignancies. **tailed red c.** DACRYOCYTE. **tanned red c.'s** Red blood cells, usually from nonhuman mammals, that are treated with tannic acid so that their surface will adsorb soluble antigens or antibodies. They are used to produce agglutination as the end point of a reaction between a soluble antigen and a soluble antibody. **tapetal c.** A cell in the tapetal layer of the choroid in the eye of carnivores. **target c.** **1** TARGET ERYTHROCYTE. **2** Any cell that is affected by a substance such as a hormone or drug directed at that cell. **tart c.** A macrophage that contains a second nucleus, representing an ingested cell that has yet to undergo significant change in its nuclear structure. **taste c.'s** Epithelioid cells grouped in the center of a taste bud that are sensitive to chemical stimuli associated with taste. These cells, of which there are two morphologic types, synapse with afferent axons. They bear a few microvilli, but the so-called gustatory hairs seen in light microscopy are mainly found on supporting cells surrounding the taste cells. **taste receptor c.** EPITHELIOCYTUS SENSORIUS GUSTATORIUS. **teardrop c.** DACRYOCYTE. **tendon c.'s** Fibroblasts that secrete the collagenous fibers of tendinous tissue and remain embedded within the structure of the resultant tendon. Also *tendon corpuscles.* **theca interna c.** A modified ovarian stromal cell situated in the inner layer of the fibrocellular sheath around a developing ovarian follicle. **thecal c.** A modified ovarian stromal cell forming part of the fibrocellular sheath around a developing ovarian follicle. It contributes to the formation of the corpus luteum and is derived from a theca interna cell. Also *theca-lutein cell, paraluteal cell, paralutein cell.* **Thoma-Zeiss counting c.** THOMA-ZEISS COUNTING CHAMBER. **thymus-dependent c.** T LYMPHOCYTE. **thymus-derived c.** T LYMPHOCYTE. **thyrotropic c.** One of the cells of the anterior lobe of the hypophysis which secretes thyroid stimulating hormone. The secretory granules are basophilic and stain selectively with aldehyde fuchsin. Also *thyrotroph.* **Tiselius electrophoresis c.** A component of the optical system employed in moving boundary electrophoresis. It is used to contain and isolate the separable components. **totipotential c.** An undifferentiated cell capable of developing into any kind of cell. The fertilized egg is totipotential. **Touton giant c.** A multinucleated giant cell whose many nuclei are centrally placed and surrounded by a pale, lipid-rich rim of cytoplasm, characteristically found in histiocytomas and xanthomas. **transitional c.** 1 A cell that forms part of a transitional epithelium, especially the urinary epithelium. 2 A cell of the transitional zones in the anal canal, esophagogastric junction, and nasopharynx, where squamous epithelium changes to columnar epithelium. **tubal air c.'s** CELLULAE PNEUMATICAE TUBAE AUDITIVAE. **tube c.** A spermatogonium which is in contact with the inside of a seminiferous tubule of the testis. **tubular c.** An epithelial cell that lines a tubule, as the proximal and distal tubules of the kidney. **Türk c.** An atypical circulating form of plasma cell seen in patients with various disorders, most commonly lymphocytosis, chronic infections, and leukemoid reactions. These cells have characteristics of both plasma cells and lymphocytes, yet retain similarities to blast cells. Also *Türk's irritation leukocyte.* **tympanic c.'s** CELLULAE TYMPANICAE. **type I c.** TYPE I PNEUMOCYTE. **type II c.** TYPE II PNEUMOCYTE. **Tzanck c.** A degenerated keratinocyte, round or globoid in shape, that has lost its connections with neighboring cells in the epidermis. It is characteristic of pemphigus. **undifferentiated c.** A cell which has an embryonic appearance and which exhibits no evidence of differentiation. Also *indifferent cell.* **unipolar c.** UNIPOLAR NEURON. **unit c.** The smallest portion of a crystal that, by repetition, gives the whole structure of the crystal. **vacuolated c.** A cell that contains small spaces or cavities within its cytoplasm. **c.'s of van Gehuchten** *Obs.* GOLGI TYPE II NEURONS. **van Hansemann c.'s** Large, occasionally multinucleated histiocytes with granular cytoplasm and commonly containing Michaelis-Guttmann bodies found in the lamina propria of the urinary bladder and other tissues affected by malakoplakia. **vasoformative c.** ANGIOBLAST. **vegetative c.** RESTING CELL. **Vero c.'s** A serially propagated heteroploid cell line derived from African green monkey kidney cells used widely for virus isolation. **vestibular hair c.'s** Numerous sensory hair cells located in the macula sacculi, macula utriculi, and crista ampullaris of the vestibular labyrinth of the internal ear. They are of two types: the epitheliocytus piriformis is piriform-shaped with a rounded base containing a nucleus and a short neck, and the epitheliocytus columnaris is cylindrical with a central nucleus and a prominent Golgi apparatus. On their free surfaces are numerous stereocilia or "hairs" and a single kinocilium, all of which are embedded in either the membrana statoconiorum of the maculae or the cupula gelatinosa of the ampullary crest, in which changes of pressure or tension due to movements of the head will stimulate the hair cells. Also *cellula sensoria pilosa.* **Virchow c.'s** 1 LEPRA CELLS. 2 CORNEAL CORPUSCLES. **visual c.'s** The rods and cones of the retina. **von Kupffer c.** KUPFFER CELL. **wandering c.** A cell that is capable of moving about in tissues, as a free macrophage, lymphocyte, or plasmacyte. Also *migratory cell.* **Warthin-Finkeldey c.** A multinucleated giant cell found in the tissues of patients with measles during the prodromal and early stages of the disease. The nuclei are closely packed and may number several dozen. The tissues affected include lymph nodes, nasopharyngeal lymphoid tissue, lung, and vermiform appendix. **water-clear c.** CLEAR CELL OF THE PARATHYROID GLAND. **white c.** LEUKOCYTE. **white blood c.** LEUKOCYTE. **wing c.'s** Broad, flat cells at an intermediate depth in the corneal epithelium. **xanthoma c.** FOAM CELL. **Zander c.'s** BLADDER CELLS. **zymogenic c.** A cell that contains secretory granules filled with digestive enzymes.

**cella** \sel′ə\ [L (akin to *celare* to hide, conceal) a cell, compartment, cubicle] An enclosed space, compartment, or cell.

**cellae** \sel′ē\ Plural of CELLA.

**cell-free** Describing material derived from living organisms when it contains no complete cells, all cells having been broken in extracting the material from them.

**celliferous** \selif′ərəs\ Productive of cells.

**celloidin** \seloi′din\ An alcohol and ether solution of cellulose nitrate or cellulose acetate used in embedding tissue for microscopic sections. Also *photoxylin.*

**cellu-** \sel′yə-\ CELLULO-.

**cellul-** \sel′yəl-\ CELLULO-.

**cellula** \sel′yələ\ [L (dim. of *cella* a cell, compartment, cubicle) a little cell] (*pl.* cellulae) CELL. **cellulae anteriores ethmoidales** The anterior group of air cells in the ethmoidal labyrinth that communicate with the ethmoidal infundibulum, curving forward and upward from the middle nasal meatus. Occasionally the infundibulum ends blindly in front by forming some anterior air cells. Also *anterior ethmoidal air cells.* **cellulae ethmoidales** [NA] The small, honeycomblike air spaces in the labyrinth of the ethmoid bone, divided into anterior, middle, and posterior groups of cells and lined by a mucous membrane continuous with that of the nasal cavity. They comprise the sinus ethmoidalis. Also *ethmoidal cells.* **cellulae mastoideae** [NA] The honeycomblike air spaces in the mastoid process of the petrous part of the temporal bone that are usually divided into three groups, two of which contain air and communicate with the middle ear through the aditus ad antrum. The third, located at the apex of the mastoid process, contains marrow. Also *mastoid cells.* **cellulae medii ethmoidales** The middle group of air cells in the ethmoidal labyrinth that are covered laterally by the orbital place of the labyrinth. Medially they produce the bulging bulla ethmoidalis, projecting into the lateral wall of the middle nasal meatus. The cells open into the meatus on the surface of or just above the bulla. Also *middle ethmoidal air cells.* **cellulae pneumaticae tubae auditivae** [NA] Air spaces, or cells, that occasionally extend either from the floor of the tympanic cavity or medially from the mastoid process into the petrous part of the temporal bone below the auditory tube in relation to the carotid canal. Also *air cells of auditory tube, cellulae pneumaticae tubariae* (outmoded), *tubal air cells.* **cellulae posteriores ethmoidales** The posterior group of air cells in the ethmoidal labyrinth that opens into the superior nasal meatus. Also *posterior ethmoidal air cells.* **c. sensoria pilosa** VESTIBULAR HAIR CELLS. **cellulae tympanicae** [NA] Air cells in the thin lower part of the anterior wall of the tympanic cavity that separates the latter from the carotid canal. They may extend into the floor of the cavity, closely related to the superior jugular bulb. Also *tympanic cells.*

**cellulae** \sel′yəlē\ Plural of CELLULA.

**cellular** \sel′yələr\ 1 Pertaining to, derived from, or composed of cells. 2 Containing numerous compartments or chambers.

**cellularity** \sel′yəler′itē\ The proportion of a tissue or mass that consists of cells, as opposed to fibers and ground substance.

**cellulase** An enzyme that catalyzes the hydrolysis of $\beta$1,4-linked glucose units in cellulose and related polysaccharides. It is not present in higher animals but is present in plants, some bacteria, and invertebrates such as protozoa and snails. Colonization of the gut by such organisms is therefore of vital importance to the nutrition of ruminant animals.

**cellule** \sel′yool\ [French, from L *cellula.* See CELLULA.] CELL.

**celluli-** CELLULO-.
**celluliferous** \sel′yəlif′ərəs\ [CELLULI- + -FEROUS] Carrying or producing small cells.
**cellulitis** \sel′yəlī′tis\ [CELLUL- + -ITIS] A diffuse form of acute inflammation that characteristically involves loose connective tissue of subcutaneous regions. **anaerobic c.** Inflammation of cellular tissue, usually subcutaneous tissue, caused by anaerobic bacteria. Gas is frequently produced in the tissue by the infecting organism. **dissecting c.** Cellulitis spreading between layers of infected tissues. **gangrenous c.** Cellulitis culminating in the death of tissue. **gaseous c.** Cellulitis associated with gas formation in tissues and often caused by anaerobic bacteria. This type of cellulitis is also seen in diabetics infected with aerobic enteric bacilli. **indurated c.** Inflammation of connective tissue, in which with passage of time increased collagen has formed, leading to hardness. **orbital c.** Infection of the tissues contained within the bony orbit, exclusive of the eye. **pelvic c.** *Rare* PARAMETRITIS. **periurethral c.** Inflammation of the loose subcutaneous and cellular tissue surrounding the urethra. **streptococcus c.** Cellulitis caused by streptococci. It usually involves the skin and often presents as erysipelas.
**cellulo-** \sel′yəlō-\ [L *cellula* a small cell, compartment] A combining form meaning (1) cell, cellular; (2) loose connective tissue. Also *cellu-, cellul-, celluli-*.
**celluloneuritis** \-n$^y$ŏorī′tis\ [CELLULO- + NEURITIS] Inflammation of peripheral nerves, due to spread of inflammation from surrounding soft tissue. *Seldom used.* Also *neuronitis, celluloradiculoneuritis.* **acute anterior c.** *Obs.* GUILLAIN-BARRÉ SYNDROME.
**celluloradiculoneuritis** \-radik′yəlōn$^y$ŏorī′tis\ [CELLULO- + RADICULO- + NEURITIS] CELLULONEURITIS.
**cellulosa** \sel′yəlō′sə\ [New L, short for *tunica cellulosa* cellular tunic] An investing layer of cells.
**cellulose** \sel′əlōs\ [CELLUL- + -OSE[2]] The main structural polysaccharide of the cell walls of plants and hence the major constituent of wood and cotton. Its molecules consist of long chains of $\beta$1,4-linked D-glucopyranoside units. **microcrystalline c.** A partially depolymerized form of cellulose prepared from purified wood cellulose by acid hydrolysis. It is used as a filler in tablets and in the preparation of other formulations of pharmaceutical agents. **oxidized c.** An absorbable form of cellulose prepared by oxidizing cellulose with nitrogen dioxide, used as a local hemostatic packing. It is gradually and completely absorbed.
**cellulose acetate** A cellulose resin that is partially esterified by treatment with acetic acid and can be processed into transparent, translucent, or opaque films. It is used especially as a support medium in electrophoretic procedures.
**cellulose acetate phthalate** A free-flowing white powder prepared by combining a reduction product of phthalic anhydride and a partial acetate ester form of cellulose. The product is used as a tablet-coating agent.
**cellulotoxic** \-täk′sik\ [CELLULO- + TOXIC] Toxic to cells.
**celo-[1]** \sē′lō-\ [Gk *kēlē* hernia] A combining form meaning tumor or hernia. Also *cel-*.
**celo-[2]** \sē′lō-\ COELO-.
**celom** \sē′ləm\ COELOM.
**celomic** \sēläm′ik\ COELOMIC.
**celoscope** \sē′lōskōp\ [CELO-[2] + -SCOPE] An instrument used to examine the abdominal cavity. Also *coeloscope.*
**celosomia** \sē′lōsō′mē·ə\ [CELO-[1] + Gk *sōm(a)* body + -IA] A developmental defect characterized by incomplete closure of the anterior body wall, resulting in herniation, to variable degrees, of thoracic and abdominal viscera. The sternum, sternal ends of ribs, and muscular body wall are usually defective or poorly developed.
**celothel** \sē′lōthel′\ MESOTHELIUM.
**celothelium** \sē′lōthē′lē·əm\ MESOTHELIUM.
**celotomy** \sēlät′əmē\ [CELO-[1] + -TOMY] HERNIOTOMY.
**celovirus** \sē′lōvī′rəs\ [from *c(hicken) e(mbryo) l(ethal) o(rphan)* + VIRUS] An aviadenovirus that is lethal for chicken embryos. Also *CELO virus.*
**celozoic** \sē′lōzō′ik\ COELOZOIC.
**Celsius** \sel′sē·əs\ [after Anders *Celsius,* Swedish astronomer, 1701–1744] See under DEGREE, SCALE, THERMOMETER.
**cement** \siment′\ [L *caementum.* See CEMENTUM.] **1** A substance forming a bond between two surfaces. **2** CEMENTUM. **black copper c.** A zinc phosphate cement containing cupric oxide. It is used mainly in splint fixation and the cementation of orthodontic bands. **calcium hydroxide c.** A lining material for deep cavities in teeth. One formula contains calcium hydroxide powder in a methyl cellulose base. **glass-ionomer c.** A dental cement formed when aluminum ions from an acid-leachable glass cross link with a poly (alkenyl acid) in aqueous solution. The aluminum cations form ionic bonds with the negatively charged hydroxyapatite of enamel and the collagen of dentin. The cement can be used as material for filling erosion cavities with minimal tooth preparation, and as a luting medium for gold and porcelain restorations. **intercellular c.** A thin layer of material that helps to bind together adjacent cells. Also *cementin.* **muscle c.** A connective tissue matrix that lies between adjacent smooth muscle cells. **oxyphosphate c.** A dental cement used for luting or as a base. The powder is mainly zinc oxide and the liquid is mainly a solution of phosphoric acid. **polycarboxylate c.** A dental cement containing zinc oxide and polycarboxylic acid. **silicate c.** A cement used for the restoration of anterior teeth. The powder is chiefly acid-soluble glass and the liquid is chiefly a solution of phosphoric acid. Also *synthetic porcelain.* **silicophosphate c.** A cement used for restorations and luting, consisting of a mixture of silicate and oxyphosphate cements. **zinc oxide and eugenol c.** A dental cement used chiefly as a temporary filling. The powder is zinc oxide and the liquid is eugenol (oil of cloves). It sets slowly unless an accelerator is added. Also *zinc-eugenol cement.*
**cementicle** \simen′tikl\ [*cement(um)* + English suffix *-icle*] A small mineralized body occasionally found in the periodontal ligament, sometimes attached to the cementum.
**cementin** \simen′tin\ [CEMENT + -IN] INTERCELLULAR CEMENT.
**cemento-** \simen′tə-\ [L *caementum* (for *caedimentum;* from *caedere* to cut) mortar, rough unhewn stones, rubble] A combining form denoting cementum.
**cementoblast** \simen′təblast\ [CEMENTO- + -BLAST] A differentiated type of mesoderm cell which is found in the immediate vicinity of the cementum and plays an active part in its formation. During cementogenesis some of these cells may be completely surrounded by the cementum, and are then referred to as cementocytes. They are large cuboidal cells with a spheroid or ovoid nucleus.
**cementoblastoma** \-blastō′mə\ CEMENTOMA.
**cementocyte** \simen′təsīt\ One of the cells similar to osteocytes lying within lamellae of cementum around a tooth root. Also *cement corpuscle.*

**cementogenesis** \-jen′əsis\ The process of the formation of the dental cementum, analagous to osteogenesis. It occurs by apposition, often rhythmically, of thin successive layers of cementum. During its formation the cementum is bordered by a layer of cells (cementoblasts). A fine layer of nonmineralized cementum (cementoid) can sometimes be discerned on the surface. During cementogenesis, some cementoblasts can be included in the cementum (chiefly in the apical third of the root) to become cementocytes.

**cementoid** \simen′toid\ [CEMENT + -OID] The uncalcified, most recently formed layer of cementum.

**cementoma** \sim′əntō′mə\ [*cement(o)-* + -OMA] A dysplastic or neoplastic lesion in which the bone around the apices of vital teeth is replaced first by a fibrous type of connective tissue and then by an osteocementoid tissue (periapical osteofibrosis or periapical osteofibroma). The cementoma appears as an irregular radiopaque area in the bone, surrounding the apices of the roots of teeth. During its early stages of development this anomaly appears radiolucent, although pulpal testing will elicit a positive response. This aberration is classified as an odontogenic tumor. Also *cementoblastoma.*

**cementopathia** \-path′ē·ə\ A theory that a pathologic condition of the cementum causes chronic periodontal disease.

**cementosis** \sim′əntō′sis\ [*cement(o)-* + -OSIS] A localized, abnormal deposition of cementum. Also *hypercementosis.*

**cementum** \simen′təm\ [L *caementum* (from *cae(dere)* to strike, break, smash + *-mentum,* noun-forming suffix) broken stones or rubble used in making concrete or mortar] A thin layer of calcified tissue covering and firmly attached to the dentin of the tooth root. It may be thicker at the apex of the tooth, particularly in later life. There are two main types, cellular and acellular. In some animals, cementum also forms an external layer on the crown. Also *crusta petrosa dentis, crusta radicis, bony substance of tooth, substantia ossea dentis, cement.* **acellular c.** The cementum covering approximately the coronal two thirds of a root. No cementocytes are present. **cellular c.** The cementum covering approximately the apical third of a root or repaired resorption areas, and containing cementocytes. Also *osteocementum.* **primary c.** The cementum present on a tooth root on eruption. Layers of secondary cementum may subsequently be added physiologically or pathologically. **secondary c.** Cementum laid down after the primary layer, which is present at eruption.

**ceno-**[1] \sē′nō-\ [Gk *kainos* new, fresh] A combining form meaning new, recent. Also *caino-, kaino-.*

**ceno-**[2] \sē′nō-\ [Gk *koinos* shared in common] A combining form meaning common, shared. Also *coeno-, kaino-, coino-, koino-.*

**ceno-**[3] \sē′nō-\ [Gk *kenos* empty] A combining form meaning empty, emptiness. Also *caeno-, keno-.*

**cenobium** \sēnō′bē·əm\ COENOBIUM.

**cenogenesis** \sē′nōjen′əsis\ [CENO-[1] + GENESIS] Embryonic development in which the appearance of new features occurs as an adaptive response to environmental conditions.

***Cenopheles balabacensis*** \sēnäf′əlēz bal′əbəsen′sis\ *ANOPHELES DIRUS.*

**cenosite** \sē′nōsīt\ [CENO-[2] + Gk *sitos* food] A commensal organism that can live apart from its host. Also *coinosite.*

# center

**center** [Med French *centre,* from L *centrum* center, the fixed point of a pair of compasses, from Gk *kentron* fixed point of compasses, sharp point, sting, goad, akin to *kentein* to sting, stab, goad] **1** The middle part of a body, part, or organ. **2** A point at or around which something becomes organized, as in *center of ossification.* **3** A collection of nerve cells associated with a particular function. **4** A facility serving a community or a particular group or specializing in a particular service, as in *day center.* **acoustic c.** AUDITORY CENTER. **active c.** ACTIVE SITE. **anospinal c.** Those segments of the sacral spinal cord ($S_2$–$S_5$) mediating the contraction and relaxation of the levator ani and external anal sphincter muscles that are used during defecation. **apneustic c.** An area in the lateral pontine tegmentum that through medullary centers under its control mediates the Hering-Breuer reflex and is capable of inhibiting the expiration phase of respiration. **appetite c.** FEEDING CENTER. **association c.** **1** The regions of cerebral cortex intercalated between the sensory and motor areas, and believed to mediate complex integrative functions. **2** Any aggregate of interneurons. **auditopsychic c.** The region of the cerebral cortex (part of Brodmann's area 22) involved in the interpretation of words, sounds, and music. **auditory c.** Areas of the superior temporal gyrus essential for recognition of words (Brodmann's area 42) and musical recall (areas 22 and 38). Also *acoustic center.* **auditory word c.** WERNICKE CENTER. **basioccipital c.** One of the centers of ossification (in cartilage) of the occipital which gives rise to the basilar portion of that bone. In man it appears about the sixth week of intrauterine life. Also *basilar center.* **basiotic c.** A supernumerary center of ossification of the occipital situated in front of the basioccipital center and giving rise to the basiotic bone of the fetus. **basisphenoid c.** The two pairs of ossification centers for the body of the sphenoid bone. They appear in cartilage, an anterior or presphenoid pair appearing about the ninth week of gestation and a posterior or postsphenoid pair appearing about the fourth month. Each pair consolidates into a single center and the presphenoid and postsphenoid centers fuse about the eighth month of gestation. **Béclard's ossification c.** A secondary ossification center in the epiphysial cartilage at the lower end of the femur which appears during the ninth month of intraembryonic life in man. **birthing c.** A facility other than a hospital for the delivery of babies. Birthing centers are usually intended to provide a more homelike environment than most hospital obstetric suites. **brain c.** **1** Any cortical area that serves in the integration and coordination of a specific function. **2** Any deep-lying group of neurons and neuropil performing a specific function. **Broca c.** BROCA'S MOTOR SPEECH AREA. **Budge c.** ERECTION CENTER. **bulbar respiratory c.** Cell groups in the medulla oblongata involved in respiratory reflexes, including those in the region of nucleus and tractus solitarus and surrounding cells of the reticular formation (dorsal medullary respiratory center), and the nucleus ambiguus and surrounding reticular formation (ventral medullary respiratory center). **burn c.** A multidisciplinary facility dedicated to the care of burn victims. • In some contexts a burn center is distinguished from a burn unit by implying responsibility for education and research about burns in addition to its clinical purpose. However, in common usage the two terms are often regarded as synonymous. **cardiac c.** Any of various regions of the medulla and hypothalamus where stimulation causes acceleration (cardioaccelerating center) or slowing (cardioinhibitory center) of the heart. **cardioaccelerating c.** A region in the reticular formation of the medulla (part of the cardiac center) where central influences tending to increase the heart rate are integrated. **cardioinhibitory c.** Any area of the brain stem mediating the slowing of the heart rate through increase in tonic vagal outflow and/or decrease in sympathetic outflow, especially the vagal dorsal motor nucleus in the medulla (part of the cardiac center). **cardiovascular c.** Any of various regions of the medulla and hypothalamus governing the nervous control and tonus of the vascular system, including heart rate, blood pressure, and peripheral blood flow. Also *vascular center, vasomotor center, vasotonic center.* **chondrification c.** A site where cartilage is first laid down, especially in the embryo and fetus. **ciliospinal c.** The pupillodilator center in the lower cervical and first or second thoracic segments of the spinal cord. **convergence c.** Any area in the brain capable of coordinating convergence of the eyes in those animals in which this is possible, e.g., in primates a cortical area bordering the rostral limit of the frontal eye field. The nucleus of Perlia adjacent to the oculomotor nucleus has been proposed as the site of this function in man and in other species where it is found, but this is unproven. **coordination c.** Any more or less circumscribed region in the central nervous system where elements of a complex activity, primarily motor or autonomic, are correlated to yield a purposeful behavioral response. **costal c.** Each of two anterolateral centers of ossification of a vertebra. They correspond to the pleural arch and become a rib in the thoracic region, the anterior part of the transverse process of a cervical vertebra, the costal process (incorporated into the transverse process) of a lumbar vertebra, and the anterior portion of the lateral part of the sacrum. **coughing c.** The region of the medulla containing the vagal motor nuclei from which coughing can be elicited by electrical stimulation. **defecation c.** A center at sacral levels of the spinal cord concerned with coordination of the components of defecation, including contraction of the sigmoid colon, rectum, and abdominal muscles, and relaxation of the anal sphincters. **deglutition c.** An area in the medulla including cells of the motor nuclei of the fifth, ninth, tenth, and twelfth cranial nerves controlling the sequentially programed movements of the tongue, soft palate, pharynx, and upper esophagus involved in swallowing. **dentary c.** A center of ossification, comparable to that giving rise to the dentary in reptiles, appearing about the seventh week of human intrauterine life lateral to Meckel's cartilage and developing into a bony plate. From it a shelf grows upwards to support the tooth germs, and posteriorly an ascending process arises. **ejaculation c.** A region at lumbosacral levels of the spinal cord concerned with coordination of the sympathetic and parasympathetic activity involved in ejaculation and other genital reflexes. Also *spinogenital center.* **erection c.** A bilaterally located center at the $S_{2-4}$ level of the spinal cord, which mediates erection of the penis or clitoris. Also *genital center, genitospinal center, Budge center.* **eupraxic c.** Any brain center concerned with the coordinated performance of willed, purposeful movement. **exoccipital c.** Each of the two symmetric centers of ossification of the occipital which give rise to the lateral parts (or masses) of that bone. **facial c.** The portion of the primary sensorimotor cortical area, located far laterally along the precentral gyrus, that governs facial movements. **feeding c.** A heterogenous cluster of cells in the lateral hypothalamus that serve to trigger the sensation of hunger and feeding behavior when stimulated by low blood glucose or certain endocrine secretions or when excited by electrical stimulation. Also *hunger center, appetite center.* **Flemming c.** GERMINAL CENTER. **foot clonus c.** The locus at spinal cord $L_5$–$S_2$ levels mediating the ankle jerk and clonus on one side. *Seldom used.* **genital c.** ERECTION CENTER. **genitospinal c.** ERECTION CENTER. **germinal c.** A lymphoid follicle that has been stimulated by one or more antigens and contains a pale central zone where proliferation of lymphocytes and macrophages containing nuclear debris can be identified. Also *germinal follicle, Flemming center, reaction center.* **glossokinesthetic c.** The cortical area on the posterior extent of the frontal gyrus that controls tongue movements and the articulation of sounds. **glycogenic c.** A region in the floor of the lower part of the fourth ventricle, injury to which results in glycosuria. **gustatory c.** Any of several brain structures thought to mediate the sensation of taste, including the gustatory nucleus in the medulla, the nucleus ventralis posteromedialis of the thalamus, portions of the hypothalamus, and antero-inferior portions of the sensorimotor cortex and limen insulae (Brodmann's area 53). **hunger c.** FEEDING CENTER. **hypothalamic c.'s** The nuclei of the hypothalamus, which are mainly concerned with the regulation of autonomic activity. The anterior and middle nuclei are chiefly involved in the control of the parasympathetic system, and the posterior nuclei are involved in the control of the sympathetic system. **ideomotor c.** Any center in the cerebral cortex involved in the coordination of ideomotor activities such as speech, especially Broca's motor speech area. **inactivation c.** A hypothetical region of a mammalian X chromosome that functions to inactivate the entire chromosome, both during random X inactivation and when autosomal loci are translocated to the X. **inhibitory c.** Neuronal regions the stimulation of which causes the cessation or inhibition of activity. They may be defined either according to position, as cerebral, cerebellar, spinal, or according to their particular function, as cardioinhibitory. **interim accommodation c.** HALFWAY HOUSE. **interparietal c.** Each of two symmetrical centers of ossification of the occipital which, after rapid fusion, give rise to the superior portion of the squamous part of that bone. This part may remain separate throughout life as the interparietal bone. **c. of Kerckring** A supernumerary center of ossification, situated between the suboccipital center and the foramen magnum, and giving rise to the ossicle of Kerckring, or opisthionic element. **kinesthetic c.** Regions involved in the perception of movement or position of parts of the body, lying in the cortex surrounding the central fissure in man, principally the postcentral gyrus. **kinetic c.** CENTROSOME. **Kronecker c.** CARDIOINHIBITORY CENTER. **Lumsden c.** PNEUMOTAXIC CENTER. **mastication c.** **1** The part of the motor area in the precentral gyrus involved in coordinating movements of the jaws. **2** The motor nucleus of the trigeminal nerve. **medical c.** A large health care facility which usually includes a hospital and provides more complex care and a wider range of services than a traditional community hospital. It is also characterized by specialized services provided on a referral basis. **medullary c.** See under CENTRUM SEMIOVALE. **medullary c. of cerebellum** CORPUS MEDULLARE CEREBELLI. **micturition c.** The bilateral center in the sacral spinal cord coordinating micturition, including the contraction of the bladder's detrusor muscle and relaxation of its smooth and striated sphincters. Activity in sympathetic, parasympathetic, and somatic motor outflows is involved. Also *vesical center, vesicospinal center.* **motor c.** Any part of the central nervous system from which electric stimulation can elicit skeletal muscle contraction, principally the precentrl gyrus motor cortex and the motor neurons of the brain stem and spinal cord. **negative reward c.** PUNISHMENT CENTER. **olfactory c.** Any area in the brain contributing to the organization of the sense of smell, as the area subcallosa, tuberculum olfactorum, and nucleus of the diagonal band. **optical c.** The point in a lens or system of lenses such that a ray of light passing through it is unchanged in direction. **orbitosphenoid c.** The center of ossification for the lesser wing of the sphenoid bone. One center appears on each side of the developing skull lateral to the optic foramen about the ninth week of fetal life. **c. of ossification** A point where ossification starts in any bone. Those in the shaft or body, the primary centers, appear mostly before birth and go on growing until full adult size is reached at physical maturity. Secondary ossification centers are formed in the epiphyses, mostly from birth onwards, to form the bony features at the upper and lower ends of long bones. The centers appear at particular ages and show sex and other differences. Primary and secondary centers fuse when growth ceases. Hormones and other factors control the activity of the centers. **pacemaker c.** **1** The cardiovascular center of the medulla. **2** An aggregate of neurons displaying inherent rhythmicity. **panting c.** A region in the hypothalamus the stimulation of which induces panting. It occupies the lateral hypothalamic area from the rostral pole of the ventromedial nucleus caudally into the midbrain tegmentum. Also *polypneic center.* **parturition c.** An area in the lumbosacral spinal cord serving to initiate and coordinate the autonomic and somatic efferent discharge and resultant muscular activity of the uterus in labor and associated contractions of abdominal muscles. **phrenic c.** CENTRUM TENDINEUM. **plantar reflex c.** The connections at the $S_{1-2}$ level of the spinal cord that mediate the plantar reflex. **pneumotaxic c.** A group of cells in the rostral pons that inhibit rhythmic inspiration independently of the vagus nerves when the expiratory center of the medulla is excited. Also *Lumsden center.* **poison control c.** An organized facility that provides information about poisons, emergency treatments, and poison control. **polypneic c.** PANTING CENTER. **pontine c. for lateral gaze** PARABDUCENT NUCLEUS. **punishment c.** Any area in the brain whose stimulation characteristically produces discomfort and pain in animal or man. Such sites include the gray matter surrounding the aqueduct of Sylvius and the periventricular structures of thalamus and hypothalamus. Also *negative reward center.* **reaction c.** GERMINAL CENTER. **rectovesical c.** An area in the gray matter of the sacral spinal cord comprising the micturition center and the defecation center. **respiratory c.** Any of several interrelated centers in the pons and medulla that regulate respiration, including the pneumotaxic, apneustic, and medullary respiratory centers. **reward c.** Any of several areas in the septum, ventromedial hypothalamic nuclei and medial forebrain bundle of the brain which, on being stimulated, give a sensation of pleasure. **rotation c.** The axis about which a body segment rotates. **salivary c.** A region of the medulla from which salivation can be elicited by electrical stimulation, comprising the region of the solitary nuclei in the floor of the fourth ventricle and the motor neurons of the seventh and ninth cranial nerves forming the superior and inferior salivatory nuclei respectively. Also *salivation center.* **satiety c.** A group of cells in the ventromedian hypothalamus governing the sensation of satiety and intake of food. Its stimulation suppresses eating, while a lesion there leads to hyperphagia. **semioval c.** See under CENTRUM SEMIOVALE. **sensory c.** Any cortical region or nucleus at higher levels of the brain serving the reception, integration, and perception of sensory stimuli. **sex-behavior c.** The nucleus ventromedialis hypothalami, especially with reference to its supposed role in controlling sexual behavior. **somatosensory c.'s** Those regions of the central nervous system involved in somatic sensation, largely determined by electrophysiologic mapping of tactile evoked activity and including principally the dorsal column nuclei of the medulla, the nuclei of the ventral thalamic group, and the postcentral gyrus of the cerebral cortex. **speech c.** BROCA'S MOTOR SPEECH AREA. **spinal cardioaccelerator c.** A center at thoracic levels ($T_{1-4}$) of the spinal cord, where sympathetic outflow producing acceleration of the heart is organized. **spinogenital c.** EJACULATION CENTER. **splenial c.** An ossification center which takes part in the formation of the inner plate of the mandible. **spoken-word c.** WERNICKE CENTER. **suboccipital c.** One of the centers of ossification of the occipital which give rise to the inferior part of the squamous portion of that bone. **sudorific c.** **1** The center in the anterior hypothalamus controlling sweating. **2** Any center in the medulla oblongata or spinal cord involved in autonomic nervous control over sweating. For defs. 1 and 2 also *sweat center.* **swallowing c.** The center in the medulla oblongata, near or including the nucleus ambiguus and the vagal nuclei, that coordinates the act of swallowing. **sweat c.** SUDORIFIC CENTER. **taste c.** GUSTATORY CENTER. **tendinous c.** CENTRUM TENDINEUM. **thermoregulatory c.** Any of those regions of the hypothalamus controlling heat conservation and heat loss. **thirst c.** A group of cells anterior to the hunger center in the lateral hypothalamus that control sensations of thirst. **trophic c.** Any neuronal aggregate whose activity is essential for the maintenance of a peripheral structure or part of the body. **vascular c.** CARDIOVASCULAR CENTER. **vasomotor c.** CARDIOVASCULAR CENTER. **vasotonic c.** CARDIOVASCULAR CENTER. **vesical c.** MICTURITION CENTER. **vesicospinal c.** MICTURITION CENTER. **visual c.** Any region of the central nervous system receiving direct or indirect projection from the retina, including the lateral geniculate body, the superior colliculus, and especially the area striata of the visual cerebral cortex. **visuopsychic c.** The area of cerebral cortex (Brodmann area 18) bordering the visual cortex and serving the integration and interpretation of visual stimuli. **vital c.'s** Those areas or functions of the lower brain stem essential for respiration, circulation, and therefore maintenance of life. **vomiting c.** A region in the medulla where electric or pharmacologic stimulation induces vomiting, considered to be the center for the coordination of vomiting reflexes. **Wernicke c.** The cortical area involved in the recognition of spoken words and calls. It covers portions of the supramarginal, angular, superior, and middle temporal gyri, and inlcudes Brodmann's areas 39 and 40. Also *Wernicke's area, Wernicke zone, auditory word center, spoken-word center, central speech area.* **winking c.** A pontine area coordinating the winking reflex. It is located near to, and includes in part, the nucleus nervi facialis.

**Centers for Disease Control** A United States government agency charged with the prevention and control of disease. Before 1973, the agency was known as the Communicable Disease Center and was concerned with the prevention and control of communicable and vector-borne diseases. Abbr. CDC

**centesis** \sentē′sis\ [Gk *kentēsis* (from *kentein* to prick, pierce) a puncturing] Any procedure in which a needle is introduced into a body cavity to aspirate fluid or gas for diagnostic or therapeutic purposes; paracentesis.

**-centesis** \-sentē′sis\ [Gk *kentēsis.* See CENTESIS.] A combining form meaning a puncturing or piercing.
**centi-** \sen′tə-\ [L *centum* one hundred] A combining form denoting (1) $10^{-2}$, one hundredth: used with SI units; (2) one hundred. Symbol: c
**centigrade** \sen′təgrād\ [CENTI- + GRADE] **1** A unit of plane angular measure equal to 0.01 grade, $10^{-4}$ right angle, or $10^{-4} \times \pi/2$ radian. **2** See under CENTIGRADE SCALE.
**centiliter** \sen′təlē′tər\ [CENTI- + LITER] A unit of volume or capacity equal to 0.01 liter, $10^{-5}$ cubic meter, or 10 cubic centimeters; 0.338 (US) fluid ounce. Symbol: cl
**centimeter** \sen′timē′tər\ [CENTI- + METER] A unit of length equal to 0.01 meter; 10 millimeters; 0.3937 inch. Symbol: cm **conventional c. of mercury** A unit of pressure equal to 10 conventional millimeters of mercury; $1.333\ 22 \times 10^3$ pascals; 1.333 22 kilopascal. Symbol: cmHg **conventional c. of water** A unit of pressure equal to 10 conventional millimeters of water; 98.0665 pascals. Symbol: $cmH_2O$ **conventional c. of water-second per liter** A unit of resistance to flow, especially of airways, equal to $9.806\ 65 \times 10^4$ pascals second per meter cubed, or $9.806\ 65 \times 10^{-2}$ kilopascals second per liter. Symbol: $cmH_2O \cdot s/l$, $cmH_2O \cdot s \cdot l^{-1}$ **cubic c.** A unit of volume equal to $10^{-6}$ cubic meter, or 1 milliliter; 0.061 cubic inch. Symbol: $cm^3$ **c. of mercury** See under CONVENTIONAL CENTIMETER OF MERCURY. **c. of water** See under CONVENTIONAL CENTIMETER OF WATER.
**centimorgan** \sen′təmôr′gən\ One one-hundredth of a morgan. It has a corrected crossover frequency of one percent. Also *map unit, crossover unit.*
**centinem** \sen′tənem′\ A unit of nutrition equal to 0.01 nem.
**centr-** \sentr-\ CENTRO-.
**centra** \sen′trə\ Plural of CENTRUM.
**centrad** \sen′trad\ [CENTR- + -AD] In the direction of the center or a center, particularly the center of the body.
**centrage** \sen′trij\ [CENTR- + -AGE] Perfect optical alignment of an optical system.
**central** **1** Being or relating to a center. **2** Chief; dominant; controlling.
**centralis** \sentrā′lis\ [L (from *centr(um)* center + *-alis* -AL), central] In the middle or at the center; central.
**centraxonial** \sen′traksō′nē·əl\ Having the axis in the median plane.
**centre** \sen′tər\ *Brit.* CENTER.
**centrencephalic** \sen′trensəfal′ik\ Relating to the center of the encephalon, especially the brainstem and its bilateral, integrative functions.
**centri-** \sen′tri-\ CENTRO-.
**centric** \sen′trik\ [CENTR- + -IC] Designating any position of the mandible where the condyles are in a bilaterally balanced position.
**centriciput** \sentris′iput\ The central region of the head or scalp, midway between the occiput and sinciput. Also *midhead.*
**centrifugal** \sentrif′ʸəgl\ [CENTRI- + L *fug(a)* a fleeing, flight + -AL] **1** Tending to move away from the center, especially in a circular path directed radially outward. **2** Conducting or directed away from the central nervous system; efferent.
**centrifugation** \sentrif′yəgā′shən\ The use of a centrifuge to separate materials of differing densities. **cesium chloride gradient c.** Analytical ultracentrifugation in which the materials to be separated are placed in a tube containing a cesium chloride solution that is highly concentrated at the bottom and progressively less concentrated near the top. During centrifugation the constituents sink through the cesium chloride until they reach the level at which their density matches that of the cesium chloride solution. **density gradient c.** Ultracentrifugation in which a solution that is used as a suspending medium manifests a density gradient in the direction of centrifugal force, thus enhancing the separation of materials that remain at a solute concentration level equal to their own density. **differential c.** A method of centrifugation in which cellular organelles are separated on the basis of sedimentation velocity. When the homogenate is first centrifuged, the fastest sedimenting organelles form a pellet in the bottom of the tube. If the supernatant fluid is removed, the pellet can be resuspended and repelleted to purify the preparation. The initial supernatant fluid is then centrifuged at a higher speed, thus pelleting a group of organelles which sediment less rapidly. **zonal c.** Centrifugation in which different substances form different zones, which may be separately removed from the centrifuge tube. Usually the separation is based on different sedimentation velocities, so that the different materials have moved different distances into a density gradient when the centrifuge is stopped.
**centrifuge** \sen′trifyooj′\ [CENTRI- + L *fugere* to flee] **1** A device for rapid rotation of an object around a central axis, subjecting the contents to centrifugal force and enhancing the separation of suspended particles or mingled fluids according to their relative densities. **2** To subject to centrifugation. **human c.** A device that suspends human or animal subjects at the end of a long, motor-driven arm, permitting controlled rotation and application of acceleration and deceleration forces.
**centrilobular** \sen′triläb′yələr\ Of or relating to the central part of a lobule of an organ, such as the liver. Also *centrolobular.*
**centriole** \sen′trē·ōl\ [CENTRI- + -OLE] A hollow cylindrical body found in the cytoplasm of the cell, about 0.4 μm long and 0.15 μm in diameter. Frequently centrioles occur in pairs at right angles to one another near the nuclear envelope. The wall of the centriole is composed of nine sets of microtubules. Generally each set is a triplet with the three tubules lying in the same plane and embedded in a dense granular matrix. Centrioles are responsible for organizing the spindle apparatus. Centrioles are found in animal cells and lower plant cells but they have not been observed in higher plant cells. The basal body of a cilium or flagellum has a structure identical with that of a centriole. Also *central body.* **anterior c.** PROXIMAL CENTRIOLE. **distal c.** The centriole located farther from the nucleus in a spermatozoon, the other being the proximal centriole. **proximal c.** The centriole located near the nucleus in the midpiece of a spermatozoon, the other being the distal centriole. Also *anterior centriole.* **ring c.** ANNULUS.
**centripetal** \sentrip′ətəl\ [CENTRI- + L *pet(ere)* to seek + -AL] **1** Tending to move toward the center, especially in a circular path directed radially inward. **2** Conducting or directed toward the central nervous system; afferent.
**centro-** \sen′trə-\ [Gk *kentron* the stationary point of a pair of compasses. See also CENTER.] A combining form meaning center, central. Also *centr-.*
**centroacinar** \-as′inər\ Pertaining to that portion of a gland closest to the centrally located duct.
**centroblast** \sen′trəblast\ **1** SMALL NONCLEAVED FOLLICULAR CENTER CELL. **2** LARGE NONCLEAVED FOLLICULAR CENTER CELL.
**centrocecal** \-sē′kəl\ CECOCENTRAL.
***Centrocestus*** \-ses′təs\ A genus of minute flukes in the family Heterophyidae, found in fishes, cats, dogs, and hu-

mans. The metacercariae are found in fishes and pass to the final host when the transport hosts is ingested.

**centrocyte** \sen′trəsīt\ [CENTRO- + -CYTE] 1 LARGE CLEAVED FOLLICULAR CENTER CELL. 2 SMALL CLEAVED FOLLICULAR CENTER CELL.

**centrodesmus** \-des′məs\ [CENTRO- + Gk *desmos* band, bond] The band of achromatic fibrils which connects the two centrosomes in the early stages of meiosis or mitosis. Also *centrodesmose.*

**centrolecithal** \-les′ithəl\ [CENTRO- + LECITH- + -AL] Describing an egg in which the yolk is centrally located and surrounded by a peripheral layer of protoplasm, such as is found in the arthropods. Segmentation of such eggs is superficial.

**centrolobular** \-läb′yələr\ CENTRILOBULAR.

**centromere** \sen′trəmir\ [CENTRO- + -MERE] The usually single region of a chromosome with which spindle fibers associate during mitosis or meiosis. In metaphase chromosomes, the centromere is constricted and its location determines a standard classification scheme of the karyotype (acrocentric, metacentric, etc.). The centromere is largely constitutive heterochromatin which stains darkly with Giemsa (G- and C-banding) and relatively poorly by reverse techniques (R-banding). Lack of a centromere leads to random distribution to daughter cells, and usually to loss of the chromosome. Presence of two centromeres (dicentric chromosome) can lead to anaphase bridges or to chromosome breakage. Also *kinetochore, kinomere.* Symbol: cen

**centromeric** \-mer′ik\ Pertaining to the centromere.

**centronucleus** \-n$^y$oo′klē·əs\ AMPHINUCLEUS.

**centro-osteosclerosis** \-äs′tē·əsklerō′sis\ OSTEOSCLEROSIS MYELOFIBROSIS.

**centrosclerosis** \-sklerō′sis\ OSTEOSCLEROSIS MYELOFIBROSIS.

**centrosome** \sen′trəsōm\ [CENTRO- + *som(a)*] A specialized area of cytoplasm, usually close to the nucleus of a cell, within the fertilized ovum that plays an important part in mitosis. It appears as a clear zone with the centrioles located near its center. Also *cytocentrum, centrosphere, kinetic center.*

**centrum** \sen′trəm\ [L, center. See CENTER] 1 A center. 2 CORPUS VERTEBRAE. **c. medianum of Luys** NUCLEUS MEDIALIS CENTRALIS THALAMI. **c. medullare** See under CENTRUM SEMIOVALE. **c. semiovale** 1 The expanse of white matter seen in a horizontal section through a cerebral hemisphere at a level above the corpus callosum. Also *centrum ovale minor.* 2 The expanse of white matter in a horizontal section through the corpus callosum, comprising the centrum semiovale of each hemisphere together with the corpus callosum. Also *centrum ovale majus, centrum ovale.* For defs. 1 and 2 also *medullary center, centrum medullare, semioval center.* **c. tendineum** [NA] The trefoil-shaped, aponeurotic tendon of insertion of the respiratory diaphragm, situated at the center of the dome-shaped muscle just below the pericardium to which it is partly fused. The inferior vena cava passes through it to the right atrium. Also *central tendon of diaphragm, centrum tendineum diaphragmatis, tendinous center, phrenic center, trefoil tendon, tendo cordiformis* (outmoded), *van Helmont's mirror* (outmoded), *speculum helmontii* (outmoded), *intermediate tendon* (outmoded) . **c. tendineum diaphragmatis** CENTRUM TENDINEUM. **c. tendineum perinei** [NA] A fibromuscular mass, or body, situated in the median plane separating the anal canal from the membranous part of the urethra and the bulb of the penis in the male, and from the lower end of the vagina in the female. Extensions of all the muscles of the region decussate through it and many are attached there. Also *central tendon of perineum, perineal body, Savage's perineal body.* **c. vertebrae** 1 CORPUS VERTEBRAE. 2 The primary ossification center that appears dorsal to the notochord for the development of the major part, or centrum, of the body of a vertebra, except for the dorsolateral portions, which are extensions from the vertebral arch centers.

***Centruroides*** \sen′trooroi′dēz\ A genus of scorpions found in tropical and subtropical areas of the western hemisphere. Some species are venomous. Among the better known members of the genus are *C. suffusus,* the Durango scorpion, and *C. sculpturatus,* a dangerous species found in Arizona.

***Cenurus*** \senyoo′rəs\ *COENURUS.*

**cenurus** \senyoo′rəs\ COENURUS.

**cephacetrile** A cephalosporin antibiotic used parenterally and having an antibiotic spectrum similar to that of cephalothin.

**cephal-** \sef′əl-\ CEPHALO-.

**cephalad** \sef′əlad\ [CEPHAL- + -AD] Toward the head or cephalic end of the body. Compare CAUDAD.

**cephalalgia** \sef′əlal′jə\ [Gk *kephalgia* (from *kephal(ē)* head + *alg(os)* pain + -IA) a headache] Headache; pain in the head. Also *cephalgia, cephalodynia.* Adj. cephalalgic. **histamine c.** MIGRAINOUS NEURALGIA. • This was once thought to be due to the release of histamine with consequential effects upon the extracranial arteries. **pharyngotympanic c.** GLOSSOPHARYNGEAL NEURALGIA.

**cephalematocele** \sef′əlēmat′ōsēl\ CEPHALOHEMATOCELE.

**cephalematoma** \sef′əlem′ətō′mə\ CEPHALOHEMATOMA.

**cephalexin** $C_{16}H_{17}N_3O_4S{\cdot}H_2O$. D-7-(2-Amino-2-phenylacetamido)-3-methyl-8-oxo-5-thia-1-azabicyclo[4.2.0]oct-2-ene-2-carboxylic acid. A semisynthetic antibiotic derived from cephalosporin C. Cephalexin is effective against many types of Gram-positive and Gram-negative bacteria. It is given orally to treat many kinds of infections in the organs and tissues.

**cephalgia** \sefal′jə\ CEPHALALGIA.

**cephalhematocele** \sef′əlhēmat′ōsēl\ CEPHALOHEMATOCELE.

**cephalhematoma** \sef′əlhē′mətō′mə\ CEPHALOHEMATOMA.

**cephalhydrocele** \sef′əlhī′drəsēl\ [CEPHAL- + HYDROCELE] Accumulation of serous fluid, usually cerebrospinal fluid, between the scalp and the cranium. **traumatic c.** Accumulation of cerebrospinal fluid beneath the scalp as a result of fracture of the skull.

**cephalic** \sefal′ik\ [Gk *kephalikos* (from *kephal(ē)* head) of or for the head] 1 Relating to the head. 2 Pertaining to the superior or cranial portion of any anatomical structure.

**cephalin** Any of the phosphatidylethanolamines and phosphatidylserines found especially in the tissues of the central nervous system. They contain a primary amino group, in distinction from phosphatidylcholines, which do not. *Outmoded.*

**cephalization** \sef′əlīzā′shən\ [CEPHAL- + *-iz(e)* + -ATION] Progressive development of the structures and functions of the head, as of the embryo.

**cephalo-** \sef′əlō-\ [Gk *kephalē* head] A combining form denoting the head. Also *cephal-.*

**cephalocathartic** 1 Clearing the head by causing the discharge of mucus from the nasal passages. 2 An agent that clears the head or treats disorders of the head.

**cephalocaudad** \-kô′dad\ From the cephalic to the caudal end; from head to tail.

**cephalocaudal** \-kô′dəl\ Pertaining to or directed toward both the head and the tail, usually used in reference to the long axis of the body.

**cephalocele** \sefal′ōsēl\ ENCEPHALOCELE.

**cephalocyst** \sef′əlōsist′\ [CEPHALO- + CYST] The larval cyst of a taenioid tapeworm, especially the hydatid cyst of *Echinococcus granulosus.*.

**cephalodidymus** \-did′iməs\ [CEPHALO- + Gk *didymos* double, a twin] **1** DICEPHALUS. **2** An individual exhibiting any of several varieties of duplicitas anterior.

**cephalodymus** \sef′əläd′iməs\ [CEPHALO- + Gk *(di)-dymos* double, a twin] CEPHALOPAGUS.

**cephalodynia** \-din′ē·ə\ [CEPHAL- + -ODYNIA] CEPHALALGIA.

**cephalogenetic** \-jənet′ik\ [CEPHALO- + GENETIC] Describing the region of the fertilized embryo which gives rise to the head.

**cephaloglycin** $C_{18}H_{19}N_3O_6S$. 7-(D-α-Aminophenylacetamido)cephalosporanic acid. One of the cephalosporin antibiotics, with antibacterial activity similar to that of the broad-spectrum penicillins. It is given orally.

**cephalogram** \sef′əlōgram′\ A roentgenogram of the head, obtained for measurement of its dimensions.

**cephalogyric** \-jī′rik\ [CEPHALO- + GYR- + -IC] Pertaining to movements in which the head turns involuntarily.

**cephalohematocele** \-hēmat′ōsēl\ [CEPHALO- + HEMATOCELE] A swelling caused by the extension of blood from an intracranial source through a congenital or traumatically caused opening in the skull. Also *cephalematocele, cephalhematocele.*

**cephalohematoma** \-hē′mətō′mə\ [CEPHALO- + HEMATOMA] A tumor or swelling caused by a collection of extravasated blood beneath the pericranium. It usually results from trauma and often indicates an underlying skull fracture. Also *cephalematoma, cephalhematoma.* **c. deformans** A prominence of the skull resulting from calcification at the site of a subpericranial hemorrhage. **c. in newborn** The collection of sanguineous fluid over one or both parietal bones and occasionally over the occipital bone, due to subperiostial hemorrhage occurring under the stresses of the passage of the head through the birth canal.

**cephalomegaly** \-meg′əlē\ An increase in the size of the head; macrocephaly.

**cephalomelus** \sef′əläm′ələs\ [CEPHALO- + Gk *melos* limb] A malformed embryo, fetus, or newborn infant with an appendage resembling an arm or leg growing from the head.

**cephalomenia** \-mē′nē·ə\ [CEPHALO- + Gk *mēn* a month + -IA] Vicarious menstruation from the head, usually due to endometriosis.

**cephalomeningitis** \-men′injī′tis\ *Seldom used* MENINGOENCEPHALITIS.

**cephalometric** \-met′rik\ Pertaining to cephalometry.

**cephalometry** \sef′əläm′ətrē\ [CEPHALO- + -METRY] The measurement of the dimensions of the head in living individuals. **fetal c.** Measurement of the fetal skull. **radiographic c.** The measurement of the dimensions of the head by radiographic methods. **ultrasonic c.** The use of ultrasonography to measure biparietal diameters or other fetal measurements. The technique is used to detect certain fetal abnormalities or fetal age.

**cephalomotor** \-mō′tər\ Pertaining to or producing movements of the head.

**cephalonia** \sef′əlō′nē·ə\ Macrocephaly with brain hypertrophy.

**cephalopagus** \sef′əläp′əgəs\ [CEPHALO- + -PAGUS] Equal conjoined twins joined at the head. Also *cephalodymus, symphocephalus, sycephalus, monocranius, monocephalus, syncephalus.* **c. occipitalis** Equal conjoined twins joined at the occipital region of the head. **c. parasiticus** Unequal conjoined twins in which the parasitic member consists largely of a reduced head attached to the cranial region of the host. **c. parietalis** Equal conjoined twins joined at the parietal region of the head.

**cephalopathia splanchnocystica** \-path′ē·ə splangk′nəsis′tikə\ A familial condition involving bilateral renal cysts and central nervous system malformations. Also *Michel syndrome.*

**cephalopelvic** \-pel′vik\ Pertaining to the relationship between measurements of the fetal skull and measurements of the maternal pelvis.

**cephalopelvimetry** \-pelvim′ətrē\ [CEPHALO- + PELVIMETRY] Clinical, sonographic, or radiologic measurements of the fetal skull and maternal pelvis.

**cephaloplegia** \-plē′jə\ [CEPHALO- + -PLEGIA] **1** Paralysis of the head muscles. **2** Paralysis of the neck muscles, leading to inability to hold up the head.

**cephalorachidian** \-rākid′ē·ən\ [CEPHALO- + RACHIDIAN] Pertaining to the skull and vertebral column. Also *cephalorhachidian.*

**cephaloridine** $C_{19}H_{17}N_3O_4S_2$. (6*R-trans*)-1-[[2-Carboxy-8-oxo-7-[(2-thienylacetyl)amino]-5-thia-1-azabicyclo[4.2.0]oct-2-en-3-yl]methyl]pyridinium hydroxide inner salt. A semisynthetic antibiotic from cephalosporin C. It is effective against many Gram-negative and Gram-positive bacteria. It is given intramuscularly or intravenously.

**cephalosporin** Any of several penicillinase-resistant antibiotics isolated from the fungus *Cephalosporium* and related structurally to the penicillins. Like the penicillins they are derived from an acyl-Cys-Val peptide, and are cyclized to form the strongly acylating β-lactam ring. They differ, however, in that the thiol group of the cysteine residue has reacted with C-4 rather than C-3 of the valine, so that the β-lactam ring is fused to a six-membered tetrahydrothiazine ring, instead of to a five-membered thiaxolidine ring as in the penicillins. They act by inhibiting the peptide cross-linking of bacterial cell-wall formation. Most of the cephalosporins used therapeutically are semisynthetic derivatives of cephalosporin C. **c. C** $C_{16}H_{21}N_3O_8S$. 7-(D-5-Amino-5-carboxyvaleramido)-3-(hydroxymethyl)-8-oxo-5-thia-1-azabicyclo[4.2.0]-oct-2-ene-2-carboxylic acid acetate. An antibacterial steroid derived from *Cephalosporium acremonium.* The drug serves as a precursor for many semisynthetic antibiotics, such as cephalothin, cephalexine, and cephaloridine. These are effective against many Gram-positive and Gram-negative bacterial infections. **c. N** D-(4-Amino-4-carboxybutyl)penicillin. An antibiotic produced by *Cephalosporium salmosynnematum.* It is effective against most Gram-negative species of bacteria and was formerly used for the treatment of typhoid fever and gonorrhea. Also *penicillin N, adicillin, synnematin.* **c. P** $C_{33}H_{50}O_8$. A steroidal antibacterial agent that contains as many as five components ($P_1$, $P_2$, $P_3$, $P_4$, and $P_5$). $P_1$, 6α,16β-Bis(acetyloxy)-3α,7β-dihydroxy-29-nordammara-17(20),24-dien-21-oic acid, is considered to be the most active of the five components.

**cephalosporinase** \-spôr′inās\ A β-lactamase that hydrolyzes cephalosporins.

***Cephalosporium*** \-spôr′ē·əm\ [CEPHALO- + -SPORIUM] A form-genus of imperfect fungi considered to be causal agents of mycetoma.

**cephalostat** \sef′əlōstat′\ [CEPHALO- + -STAT] An apparatus for holding the head in a standard position during radiography, used chiefly in dental radiology.

**cephalotetanus** \-tet′ənəs\ CEPHALIC TETANUS.

**cephalothin** $C_{16}H_{16}N_2O_6S_2$. 6*R-trans*-3-[(Acetyloxy) methyl] -8-oxo-7- [(2-thienylacetyl)amino] -5-thia- 1-azabicyclo [4.2.0]-oct-2-ene-2-carboxylic acid. A synthetic analogue of cephalosporin C which is effective against many types of Gram-positive and Gram-negative bacteria.

**cephalothin sodium** $C_{16}H_{15}N_2NaO_6S_2$. 7-(2-Thienylacetamido)cephalosporanic acid, a bactericidal agent with the same spectrum of activity as cephaloridine. It is not well-absorbed from the gastrointestinal tract and is given intramuscularly or by intravenous injection.

**cephalothoracoiliopagus** \-thō′rəkō·il′ē·äp′əgəs\ Equal conjoined twins with union in the cephalic, thoracic, and iliac regions.

**cephalothoracopagus** \-thō′rəkäp′əgəs\ [CEPHALO- + THORACO- + -PAGUS] SYNADELPHUS. **c. dibrachius** A cephalothoracopagus in which only two upper extremities are evident, in contrast with a cephalothoracopagus having four fully or partially developed upper-limb structures. **c. disymmetros** A cephalothoracopagus in which there are two equally developed faces. They are usually directed laterally, although there may be a degree of fusion between the right side of one and the left side of the other. **c. monosymmetros** A cephalothoracopagus in which one face is well developed. Rudiments of a second face may be present on the opposite side of the fused head.

**cephalothorax** \-thō′raks\ That part of the body of an arachnid or higher crustacean which consists of the union or fusion of the head with one or more thoracic segments.

**cephalotropic** \-träp′ik\ [CEPHALO- + -TROPIC[1]] Showing an affinity for brain tissue, such as a centrally active drug.

**cephaloxia** \sef′əläk′sē·ə\ [*cepha(lo)*- + Gk *lox(os)* slanting + -IA] TORTICOLLIS.

**-cephalus** \-sef′ələs\ [New L, from Gk *kephalē* head] A combining form denoting a (specified) type or condition of the head, especially a developmental abnormality of the head.

**cephamycin** \sef′əmī′sin\ Any of a group of antibiotics closely related to the cephalosporins but produced by streptomycetes rather than by fungi.

**cephapirin sodium** $C_{17}H_{16}N_3NaO_6S_2$. 3-[(Acetyloxy)methyl]-8-oxo-7-[[(4-pyridinylthio)-acetylamino]-5-thia-1-azabicyclo-[4.2.0]oct-2-ene-2-carboxylic acid monosodium salt. A semisynthetic antibiotic from cephalosporin-C that is used for the treatment of infections of the respiratory tract and the genitourinary system, and for infections of the tissues and blood. It is administered intramuscularly and intravenously. It is effective against a variety of Gram-negative and Gram-positive bacteria.

**cephradine** A cephalosporin used both orally and parenterally. Its antimicrobial action is similar to that of cephalexin.

**ceptor** \sep′tər\ *Outmoded* RECEPTOR. **chemical c.** CHEMORECEPTOR. **contact c.** MECHANORECEPTOR. **distance c.** DISTANCE RECEPTOR. **nerve c.** Any receptor that transmits information toward the neuronal cell body or toward the central nervous system.

**CERA** cortical-evoked response audiometry.

**ceramics** \siram′iks\ **dental c.** The art and science of making dental restorations or parts thereof in porcelain.

**ceramide** An N-acylated sphingoid, usually sphingosine. The acyl group is usually derived from a fatty acid of 18 to 26 carbon atoms. It occurs in combination with phosphocholine in sphingomyelin, which is present in cell membranes.

**ceramide trihexoside** The sphingolipid that accumulates in keratoma corporis diffusum (Fabry's disease) as result of deficiency of the enzyme $\alpha$-galactosidase.

**cerasine** \ser′əsin\ **1** $C_{10}H_7{\cdot}N{=}N{\cdot}C_{10}H_4(SO_2ONa)_2OH$. A red azo dye that is used as a cytoplasmic stain and as a coloring agent for pharmaceutic preparations. Also *bordeaux red, fast red B, bordeaux B.* **2** A cerebroside from brain tissue that is composed of galactose, sphingosine, and lignoceric acid.

***Cerastes*** \səras′tēz\ A small genus of venomous snakes of the family Viperidae, order Squamata, found in desert regions of northern Africa. It includes the common sand viper (*C. vipera*) and the horned viper, or asp (*C. cerastes*). The venom of these snakes has a strong hemolytic effect.

**cerat-** \ser′ət-\ KERATO-.

**cerate** \sir′āt\ [L *ceratum* (from *cera* wax) wax salve] A medical preparation for external application, containing wax to make it flexible but less likely to melt like an ointment when spread. Also *ceratum.* **blistering c.** A plaster containing cantharides to produce blisters on the skin. Also *cantharides cerate.* **lead subacetate c.** A cerate composed of lead subacetate, camphor, lanolin, and paraffin. **simple c.** A cerate composed of benzoinated lard and white wax. **Turner c.** CALAMINE OINTMENT.

**ceratectomy** \ser′ətek′təmē\ KERATECTOMY.

**ceratin** \ser′ətin\ KERATIN.

**ceratitis** \ser′ətī′tis\ KERATITIS.

**cerato-** \ser′ətō-\ KERATO-.

**ceratocricoid** \-krī′koid\ Pertaining to the inferior horn of the thyroid cartilage and the cricoid cartilage, or to the cricothyroid articulation. Also *keratocricoid.*

**ceratocricoideus** MUSCULUS CERATOCRICOIDEUS.

**ceratoglossus** \-gläs′əs\ [CERATO- + *(hyo)glossus*] The larger, posterior part of the hyoglossus muscle that is attached to the greater cornu of the hyoid bone. *Outmoded.*

**ceratohyal** \-hī′əl\ The part of the hyoid bone which develops from the middle of the second branchial arch cartilage (the stylohyoid ligament) attached above to the tip of the styloid process of the temporal bone and below to the lesser horn of the hyoid bone. Rarely it may become ossified. Also *keratohyal.*

**ceratopharyngeus** \-ferin′jē·əs\ PARS CERATOPHARYNGEA MUSCULI CONSTRICTORIS PHARYNGIS MEDII.

***Ceratophyllus*** \ser′ətäf′ələs\ A genus of fleas found on fowl, rodents, dogs, cats, and humans. The genus includes the western chicken flea, *C. niger.* ***C. fasciatus*** *NOSOPSYLLUS FASCIATUS.*

**Ceratopogonidae** \-pōgän′idē\ [CERATO- + Gk *pōgōn* a beard + -IDAE] A dipteran family of small gnats or biting midges. Three genera members of which attack warm-blooded animals, including humans, are *Culicoides, Lasiohelea,* and *Leptoconops.*

**ceratum** CERATE.

**cercaria** \sərkar′ē·ə\ [Gk *kerk(os)* the tail of an animal + -ARIA] (*pl.* cercariae) The swimming larval form of digenetic trematodes. They leave the first intermediate host, usually a snail, and encyst in or on a transport or second intermediate host, or penetrate directly through the skin of the final host, as in schistosomes. The anterior portion, or body, of the cercaria has suckers, a mouth, an alimentary system and other systems, and genital primordia. To it is attached the lashing propulsive organ, or tail, which varies widely in form in different species.

**cercaricidal** Having a destructive effect on cercaria, the free-swimming larval forms of trematodes.

**cerci** \sur′sī\ Plural of CERCUS.

**cerclage** \serkläzh′\ [French (from *cercl(e)* circle, from L *circus* circle + *-age* -AGE), act of circling] A technique for correction of retinal detachment in which an equatorial encirclement compresses the outer coats of the eye inward to approximate the retina.

**cercocyst** \surʹkəsist\ [Gk *kerko(s)* tail + *kyst(is)* sac, bladder] The tailed cysticercoid of certain cyclophyllidean cestodes such as *Hymenolepis nana*, that develops within the villus of the vertebrate host. Also *cercocystis*.

**cercoid** \surʹkoid\ CYSTICERCOID.

**cercomer** \surʹkəmər\ [Gk *kerko(s)* tail + *mer(os)* part] A tail-like appendage of certain larval stages of tapeworms, often containing the six hooklets used by the hexacanth to claw into the intermediate host in which the next larval stage develops. Examples are the procercoid of the order Pseudophyllidea and the cysticercoid larvae of taenioid cestodes such as *Hymenolepis.*.

***Cercomonas hominis*** PENTATRICHOMONAS HOMINIS.

**Cercopithecoidea** \surʹkōpithʹēkoiʹdē·ə \ [New L, from *Cercopithec(us)*, a genus of African monkeys, + *-oidea*, a suffix used for zoological superfamilies] The superfamily of primates that contains Old World monkeys, the great apes, and humans. In these primates the nostrils open downward and the tail, when present, is not prehensile. Also *Catarrhina*. Adj. cercopithecoid, catarrhine.

**cercosporamycosis** \sərkäsʹpərəmīkōʹsis\ [New L, from *Cercospora*, a genus, + MYCOSIS] A rare, mycotic disease found in Indonesia, and caused by the fungus *Cercospora apii*, a plant pathogen, later reidentified as *Mycocentrospora acerina*. Verrucose nodules with confluent patches on the face, extension to the nasal cavities, and destruction of the turbinates and nasal septum have been described. There may be dissemination of the disease to other areas.

**cercus** \surʹkəs\ [Gk *kerkos* a tail] (*pl.* cerci) A hairlike or bristlelike sensory appendage, usually one of a bilateral pair, at the posterior end of insects such as cockroaches and of certain other arthropods.

**cerebellar** \serʹəbelʹər\ Of or relating to the cerebellum.

**cerebelli-** \serʹəbeli-\ CEREBELLO-.

**cerebellitis** \serʹəbelīʹtis\ [*cerebell(um)* + -ITIS] Inflammation of the cerebellum, of any cause, giving rise to a cerebellar syndrome, such as acute cerebellar ataxia of infancy. **acute c.** CEREBELLAR ENCEPHALITIS.

**cerebello-** \serʹəbelʹō-\ [L *cerebellum* (dim. of *cerebrum* brain)] A combining form denoting the cerebellum. Also *cerebelli-*.

**cerebelloretinal** \-retʹənəl\ Pertaining to the cerebellum and retina.

**cerebellorubrospinal** \-rooʹbrəspīʹnəl\ Denoting a major pathway of influence from the cerebellum comprised of outflow from central cerebellar nuclei on one side, passing over the superior cerebellar peduncle to the red nucleus on the other side, and after relay there, descending the rubrospinal tract.

**cerebellospinal** \-spīʹnəl\ Pertaining to the cerebellum and spinal cord.

**cerebellothalamic** \-thalamʹik\ Pertaining to the cerebellum and thalamus.

**cerebellovestibular** \-vestibʹyələr\ Pertaining to the cerebellum and vestibular apparatus and their central connections.

**cerebellum** \serʹəbelʹəm\ [L (dim. of *cerebrum* the brain) a small brain] [NA] The larger portion of the hindbrain. It takes the form of two fissured and foliated hemispheres interconnected by a vermis. The latter anteroventrally forms the roof of the fourth ventricle, while laterally three pairs of robust brachia connect afferent and efferent tracts to the brainstem. It also receives input from the viscera and special senses and contributes to motor coordination generally. Also *micrencephalon* (obs.), *opisthencephalon* (rare), *parencephalon* (seldom used).

**cerebr-** \serʹəbr-, sərēʹbr-\ CEREBRO-.

**cerebral** \serʹəbrəl, sərēʹbrəl\ Of or relating to the cerebrum.

**cerebri-** \sərēʹbri-, serʹəbri-\ CEREBRO-.

**cerebriform** \sərebʹrifôrm\ Resembling the appearance of the brain or brain tissue.

**cerebro-** \serʹəbrə-, sərēʹbrə-\ [L *cerebrum* brain] A combining form denoting the brain or cerebrum. Also *cerebr-*, *cerebri-*.

**cerebrocardiac** \-kärʹdē·ak\ Pertaining to the cerebrum and the heart.

**cerebrocerebellar** \-serʹəbelʹər\ Pertaining to the cerebrum and cerebellum.

**cerebrocuprein** SUPEROXIDE DISMUTASE.

**cerebrohyphoid** \-hīʹfoid\ Resembling brain tissue.

**cerebromacular** \-makʹyələr\ MACULOCEREBRAL.

**cerebromalacia** \-məlāʹshə\ ENCEPHALOMALACIA.

**cerebromedullary** \-medʹyələrʹē\ CEREBROSPINAL.

**cerebromeningeal** \-meninʹjē·əl\ Affecting or pertaining to the brain and its meninges.

**cerebromeningitis** \-menʹinjīʹtis\ [CEREBRO- + MENINGITIS] MENINGOENCEPHALITIS.

**cerebro-ocular** \-äkʹyələr\ Affecting or pertaining to the brain and the eye.

**cerebropathy** \serʹəbräpʹəthē\ [CEREBRO- + -PATHY] Any disease or dysfunction of the brain. Also *cerebropathia*, *cerebrosis* (outmoded).

**cerebropontine** \-pänʹtīn\ Affecting or pertaining to the cerebrum and pons. Also *cerebropontile*.

**cerebropsychosis** \-sīkōʹsis\ [CEREBRO- + PSYCHOSIS] Mental illness due to organic disease of the brain.

**cerebrorachidian** \-rākidʹē·ən\ CEREBROSPINAL.

**cerebroretinal** \-retʹənəl\ Affecting or pertaining to the brain and retina.

**cerebroside** \serʹəbrəsīdʹ\ [CEREBRO- + *(galacto)side*] A hexose derivative of a ceramide, formed from it by transfer of the hexosyl group to the primary alcohol group from UDP-glucose or UDP-galactose as donor. Galactose is the main sugar residue in the cerebrosides of brain and myelin. Cerebrosides containing glucose are abundant in the cell membranes of spleen and liver. They accumulate in Gaucher's disease. Also *Gaucher lipid*.

**cerebrosidosis** \-sīdōʹsis\ Any disease characterized by a defect in lipid metabolism that causes an abnormal accumulation of cerebroside. The best-known disorder of this category is Gaucher's disease, and another is Krabbe's disease.

**cerebrosis** \serʹəbrōʹsis\ [CEREBR- + -OSIS] *Outmoded* CEREBROPATHY.

**cerebrospinal** \-spīʹnəl\ Affecting or pertaining to the brain and spinal cord. Also *cerebrorachidian*, *encephalospinal*, *encephalorachidian*, *cerebromedullary*.

**cerebrospinant** 1 Acting upon the brain and spinal cord. 2 A cerebrospinant agent.

**cerebrostomy** \serʹəbräsʹtəmē\ [CEREBRO- + -STOMY] The creation of an opening between the cerebral ventricles and the subarachnoid space or of an external opening from the ventricles.

**cerebrotomy** \serʹəbrätʹəmē\ [CEREBRO- + -TOMY] The dissection of the brain substance.

**cerebrotyphus** \-tīʹfəs\ [CEREBRO- + TYPHUS] *Incorrect* TYPHOID ENCEPHALITIS. • This term is hallowed by use, but incorrect, as the word *typhus* should be used to designate a specific rickettsial infection which may also produce cerebral complications.

**cerebrovascular** \-vasʹkyələr\ Pertaining to the blood vessels or circulation of the brain.

**cerebrum** \serʹəbrəm, sərēʹbrəm\ [L (akin to Gk *kara*

head and *kranion* skull) the brain] **1** [NA] In the adult, those brain components derived from the embryonic telencephalon, including the cerebral hemispheres, rhinencephalon, and basal ganglia. **2** All parts of the brain above the tentorium, or the entire brain. An outmoded usage.

**cerecloth** \sir′klăth\ [L *cer(a)* wax + English *cloth*] An antiseptic cloth impregnated with wax.

**cereolus** [L, a small taper, dim. of *cereus* a wax taper] A medicated bougie for installation into the urethra.

**cerevisia** \ser′əviz′ē·ə\ [L (from Gaulish) ale, beer] Any brewed malt liquor, such as beer or ale.

**cerevisiae** \ser′əviz′i·ē\ Genitive of CEREVISIA. **c. fermentum siccatum** DRIED YEAST.

**cerium** \sir′ē·əm\ Element number 58, having atomic weight 140.12. It is the most abundant of the lanthanide series of elements and the second most reactive, after europium. Cerium(IV) compounds are used as oxidizing agents, as in the decarboxylation of 2-oxoacids. Symbol: Ce

**cero-** \sir′ō-\ [L *cera* (akin to Gk *kēros*) wax] A combining form denoting wax.

**ceroid lipofuscin** A chemically heterogeneous, variably pigmented, autofluorescent lipid deposit in neuronal and visceral cells. Accumulation occurs in vacuoles formed by fusion of lysosomes with endocytic vesicles. To a mild degree a histologic concomitant of aging, excessive accumulation due to inborn errors of metabolism occurs in the group of disorders called ceroid lipofuscinoses.

**ceroid-lipofuscinosis** \sē′roid-lip′ōfusinō′sis\ **1** The accumulation of excessive amounts of ceroid lipofuscin in cells, primarily of the central nervous system (neuronal ceroid-lipofuscinosis) and certain cells of the viscera, usually due to an inborn error of metabolism. **2** A group of rare hereditary disorders, differentiated by age of onset and characterized by progressive ataxia, intellectual deterioration, seizures, autosomal recessive inheritance, and abnormal accumulation of ceroid lipofuscin in the central nervous system. **adult c.** A type of ceroid-lipofuscinosis in which cerebellar ataxia or extrapyramidal signs begin in adulthood, intellectual deterioration is mild and protracted, and visual loss does not occur. The fundamental defect is unclear. In most cases inheritance is autosomal recessive, but some dominant pedigrees have been noted. Also *Kufs type ceroid-lipofuscinosis, Kufs disease, late juvenile cerebromacular degeneration, late onset cerebral sphingolipidosis.* **Finnish type c.** INFANTILE CEROID-LIPOFUSCINOSIS. **Hagberg-Santavuori variant of c.** INFANTILE CEROID-LIPOFUSCINOSIS. **infantile c.** A type of ceroid-lipofuscinosis in which onset of psychomotor deterioration, hypotonia, myoclonus, and visual deterioration due to optic atrophy occurs in the first 18 months of life, and death soon follows. The cause is unclear, and the disease is more common in Finland than elsewhere. Also *Santavuori type ceroid-lipofuscinosis, Finnish type ceroid-lipofuscinosis, Hagberg-Santavuori variant of ceroid-lipofuscinosis.* **Jansky-Bielschowsky type c.** LATE INFANTILE CEROID-LIPOFUSCINOSIS. **juvenile c.** A type of ceroid-lipofuscinosis in which progressive visual and intellectual deterioration, spasticity, and ataxia begin between the ages of five and ten years, and survival may extend to late adolescence. The diagnosis is often suggested by the ophthalmologist on the basis of retinal pigmentary degeneration. Also *Batten's disease, Spielmeyer-Vogt disease, Vogt-Spielmeyer disease.* **Kufs type c.** ADULT CEROID-LIPOFUSCINOSIS. **late infantile c.** A type of ceroid-lipofuscinosis in which the same signs as in the infantile form are first noted between one and four years of age and death occurs within 2–6 years of onset. Also *Jansky-Bielschowsky type ceroid-lipofuscinosis, Bielschowsky's disease, Bielschowsky-Dollinger syndrome, Bielschowsky-Jansky syndrome, Bielschowsky-Jansky disease, Jansky-Bielschowsky disease.* **Santavuori type c.** INFANTILE CEROID-LIPOFUSCINOSIS.

**ceroplasty** \sir′ōplas′tē\ [CERO- + -PLASTY] The manufacture of anatomic wax models.

**certifiable** \sur′təfī′əbəl\ Capable of being certified, as a case of infectious disease that is required to be reported or a case of mental disorder sufficiently extreme to warrant confinement.

**certificate** A legal document affirming that something is true or valid. **birth c.** The registration document used for officially recording a birth. **death c.** A reporting form used for the legally required notification of appropriate governmental authorities of an individual's death, the time and date it occurred, and its cause. An internationally agreed form of medical certificate of cause of death is published in the *International Classification of Diseases* (WHO).

**certification** **1** The act or process of certifying; specifically, the act or process by which a governmental or nongovernmental agency or organization evaluates and recognizes an individual, institution, or educational program as meeting certain predetermined standards. **2** The formal written declaration of a fact, such as the registration of a birth or the specification of the cause of death on a death certificate. **3** The process of completing the necessary legal documents for commitment of a patient to a mental hospital. Laws differ by jurisdiction regarding authorization for involuntary hospitalization. **preadmission c.** Review of the need for proposed inpatient health care services prior to the time of admission to the institution, required by some insurers as a condition of coverage of the admission.

**certify** **1** To issue a determination that an individual, program, or institution has met certain specified criteria and standards. **2** To document the need for involuntary hospitalization or commitment to a specified treatment program or institution.

**ceruloplasmin** \seroo′ləplaz′min\ A plasma glycoprotein $\alpha$-globulin of approximate molecular weight 132 000, containing six copper atoms per molecule and serving as an electron acceptor in the oxidation of plasma iron from Fe(II) to Fe(III) and possibly in other reactions. A low plasma concentration of ceruloplasmin is characteristic of Wilson's disease, but its role in this disorder is uncertain.

**cerumen** \seroo′mən\ [New L, from Gk *kēroumenos* (from *kēros* beeswax, wax) formed of wax] The brownish, waxy secretion of the tubular ceruminous glands, modified sweat glands situated mostly in the cartilaginous portion of the external acoustic meatus. Also *earwax, sordes aurium* (obs.). **impacted c.** An accumulated mass of earwax, firmly lodged in the external auditory meatus and resisting removal. It is likely to produce a degree of hearing impairment. Also *ceruminal impaction.*

**ceruminal** \seroo′mənəl\ CERUMINOUS.

**ceruminolysis** \seroo′minäl′isis\ Dissolution of earwax in the external acoustic meatus.

**ceruminolytic** \seroo′minōlit′ik\ Pertaining to or producing ceruminolysis.

**ceruminoma** \seroo′minō′mə\ A tumor, usually slow growing, involving the ceruminous glands of the external acoustic meatus.

**ceruminosis** \seroo′minō′sis\ Abnormal or excessive secretion of earwax.

**ceruminous** \seroo′minəs\ Of or pertaining to cerumen. Also *ceruminal.*

**cervic-** \sur′vik-, sur′vis-\ CERVICO-.

**cervical** \sur′vikəl\ [CERVIC- + -AL] Pertaining to the

neck, or the neck of any organ or structure.

**cervicalgia** \sur′vikal′jə\ [CERVIC- + -ALGIA] Pain in the neck. Also *trachelodynia, cervicodynia.*

**cervicalis** \sur′vikā′lis\ Cervical.

**cervicectomy** \sur′visek′təmē\ [CERVIC- + -ECTOMY] TRACHELECTOMY.

**cervicispinal** \sur′visispī′nəl\ Affecting or pertaining to the neck and spinal cord.

**cervicitis** \sur′visī′tis\ [CERVIC- + -ITIS] Inflammation of the uterine cervix. Also *trachelitis.* **granulomatous c.** Granulomatous inflammation of the cervix, usually caused by tuberculosis, syphilis, or lymphogranuloma venereum.

**cervico-** \sur′vikō-\ [L *cervix* (genitive *cervicis*) neck] A combining from meaning neck or cervix. Also *cervic-.*

**cervicoauricular** \-ôrik′yələr\ Pertaining to the neck and the ear or the auricle of the ear.

**cervicobrachial** Pertaining to the neck and the arm.

**cervicobrachialgia** \-brā′kē·al′jə\ [CERVICO- + BRACHIALGIA] Pain in the neck and arm.

**cervicobuccal** \-buk′əl\ BUCCOCERVICAL.

**cervicocolpitis** \-kälpī′tis\ [CERVICO- + COLPITIS] Inflammation of the cervix and vagina. **c. emphysematosa** An acute inflammation of the cervix and vagina caused by gas-forming bacteria and characterized by the presence of submucosal gas-filled spaces.

**cervicodorsal** Pertaining to the neck and the back.

**cervicodynia** \-din′ē·ə\ [CERVIC- + -ODYNIA] CERVICALGIA.

**cervicohumeral** \-hyoo′mərəl\ Pertaining to or involving the neck and the arm.

**cervicolingual** \-ling′gwəl\ LINGUOCERVICAL.

**cervicomuscular** \-mus′kyələr\ Pertaining to or affecting the muscles of the neck.

**cervicoplasty** \sur′vikōplas′tē\ [CERVICO- + -PLASTY] Plastic surgery on the cervix of the uterus or on the neck.

**cervicovaginitis** \-vaj′inī′tis\ [CERVICO- + VAGINITIS] Inflammation of the cervix and vagina.

**cervicovesical** \-ves′ikəl\ Pertaining to the uterine cervix and bladder.

**cervix** \sur′viks\ [L (akin to *cerebrum* brain) the nape, neck] (*pl.* cervices) **1** The region of the body between the head and the trunk; collum. **2** A narrowed part of an organ or structure; especially, one adjoining a part called the corpus (body) or the caput (head). For defs. 1 and 2 also *neck.* **3** CERVIX UTERI. **c. of axon** The point of constriction of a myelinated axon where its myelin sheath begins. **c. columnae posterioris** A part of the posterior columns of the spinal cord just posterior to the central gray commissure where the fiber tracts seem in transverse section to be slightly constricted. **c. cornu** The neck or origin of the posterior horn of spinal cord gray matter. **c. dentis** NECK OF TOOTH. **double c.** A congenital malformation in which there are two uterine cervices, probably most often associated with some degree of failed union of the two paramesonephric ducts of the embryo. **incompetent c.** A condition characterized by painless dilatation of the uterine cervix during the second trimester of pregnancy. If not treated successfully, the condition leads to rupture of the fetal membranes followed by delivery of an immature fetus. **c. uteri** [NA] The narrow, cylindrical lower portion of the uterus, demarcated from the body on the surface by the isthmus, which is opposite the internal os of the uterus. It projects into the anterior wall of the proximal end of the vagina, forming the fornices. The supravaginal portion is separated from the bladder anteriorly by fibrous connective tissue, or parametrium, and from the rectum posteriorly by the rectouterine pouch. It contains a spindle-shaped passage, canalis cervicis uteri, extending from the internal os of the uterus to the external os in the vagina. Also *neck of uterus, cervix, uterine neck.* **c. vesicae** [NA] That portion of the urinary bladder surrounding the internal urethral meatus by which the bladder communicates with the urethra. It is located in the angle formed by the fundus and the inferolateral surface of the bladder. It is the lowest and most fixed part of the bladder, and lies a little behind the lower part of the symphysis pubis. Also *neck of urinary bladder.*

**CES** central excitatory state.

**cesarean** \sizer′ē·ən\ [after Gaius Julius *Caesar,* Roman general and statesman, 100–44 B.C., who is thought to have been born in this manner] CESAREAN SECTION.

**cesium** \sē′zē·əm\ Element number 55, having atomic weight 132.9. The element is a liquid at room temperature (melting point, 28.4°C). It is the most electropositive of the alkali metals. Valence is 1. It reacts violently with cold water, the hydroxide being the strongest base known. Cesium is used to catalyze the hydrogenation of certain organic compounds and it has a few other specialized applications. Symbol: Cs

**cesium 137** A radioactive element emitting beta radiation. Because its ever-present daughter, barium 137m, emits a valuable 662-KeV gamma photon, cesium 137 is used as a performance standard to calibrate scintillation counters and scanners. It is also used in intracavitary radiotherapy and implants. Physical half-life is 30 years. Symbol: $^{137}Cs$

**Cestan** [Raymond *Cestan,* French physician, 1872–1934] **1** Cestan syndrome. See under CESTAN-CHENAIS SYNDROME. **2** Dutemps-Cestan sign, Dupuy-Dutemps and Cestan sign. See under CESTAN SIGN. **3** Cestan-Raymond syndrome, Raymond-Cestan syndrome. See under SUPERIOR PONTINE SYNDROME.

**cesticidal** Effective against flatworms (cestodes).

**Cestoda** \sestō′də\ [New L, alter. of *Cestoidea*] A subclass of Cestoidea comprising the true tapeworms, which typically have a segmented or strobilate body and attach themselves to their host by means of a scolex. Adult forms are intestinal parasites of vertebrates. Recent classifications divide the subclass into ten orders, of which Cyclophyllidea and Pseudophyllidea are of particular medical interest. Also *Eucestoda.*

**cestode** \ses′tōd\ **1** A member of the subclass Cestoda; a segmented tapeworm. **2** Any member of the class Cestoidea; a cestoid.

**cestodiasis** \ses′tōdī′əsis\ Any infection or disease due to a cestode.

**cestodology** \ses′tōdäl′əjē\ [*cestod(e)* + *o* + -LOGY] The scientific study of tapeworms.

**cestoid** \ses′toid\ [L *cest(us)* a belt, girdle (from Gk *kestos* embroidered, the embroidered girdle of Aphrodite) + -OID] **1** Any member of the class Cestoidea, including but not confined to the true tapeworms in the subclass Cestoda. **2** Tapewormlike; cestodelike.

**Cestoidea** \sestoi′dē·ə\ [CESTOID + New L *-ea,* class suffix] A class of Platyhelminthes that includes the subclasses Cestoda (true or segmented tapeworms) and Cestodaria (unsegmented tapeworms). All are characterized by absence of a digestive tract or mouth throughout their life cycle.

**cetrimide** Any quaternary ammonium bromide, principally hexadecyltrimethylammonium bromide, $CH_3$—$[CH_2]_{15}$—$N^+(CH_3)_3Br^-$.

**cetylpyridinium chloride** $C_{21}H_{38}ClN$. 1-Hexadecylpyridinium chloride, a white powder used as a topical disinfectant and a preservative in certain pharmaceuticals.

**CF** 1 calibration factor. 2 cardiac failure. 3 cystic fibrosis. 4 Christmas factor (factor IX). 5 carbolfuchsin. 6 citrovorum factor (folinic acid). 7 complement fixation.

**Cf** Symbol for the element, californium.

**CFA** 1 complete Freund's adjuvant (Freund's complete adjuvant). 2 complement-fixation antibody.

**cff** critical fusion frequency (critical flicker fusion frequency).

**CFT** complement fixation test.

**CGL** chronic granulocytic leukemia.

**cGMP** cyclic guanosine monophosphate.

**CGS** centimeter-gram-second system.

**CH** crown-heel.

**CHAD** cold hemolytic antibody disease.

**Chaddock** [Charles Gilbert *Chaddock*, U.S. neurologist, 1861–1936] Chaddock's reflex. See under SIGN.

**Chadwick** [James Read *Chadwick*, U.S. gynecologist, 1844–1905] See under SIGN.

**Chagas** [Carlos Ribeiro Justiniano *Chagas*, Brazilian physician, 1879–1934] **1** See under MYOCARDITIS. **2** Chagas disease of the esophagus. See under TROPICAL CARDIOSPASM. **3** Chagas-Cruz disease. See under CHAGAS DISEASE.

**chagoma** \shəgō′mə\ [*Chag(as disease)* + -OMA] The skin lesion occurring in Chagas disease, following the bite of the vector reduviid bug.

**chain** [Old French *chaiene* (from L *catena* chain) a chain] **1** A covalently linked linear sequence of atoms, usually carbon, or of larger residues such as nucleotides. **2** A linear series of cells held together by incomplete fission. It is formed normally by streptococci and by some other organisms when wall synthesis is impaired. **A c.** A particular chain of a protein molecule. For example, the A chain of insulin is the 21-residue chain containing four half-cystine residues (originally so called because oxidation of these residues to cysteic acid left it the more acidic of the two chains). **alpha (α) c.** One of the two polypeptide chains present in nearly all human hemoglobins. It is combined with ε chains in hemoglobin Gower 2 (embryonic), with two γ chains in hemoglobin F, and with two β chains or two δ chains in adult hemoglobin A or $A_2$, respectively. The α chain contains 141 amino acids encoded by the α globin gene loci that are on the short arm of human chromosome 16. Mutations at the α loci give rise to hemoglobin variants or α-thalassemias. **amino-acid side c.** The part of an amino-acid molecule designated R in the formula $NH_3^+$—CHR—$COO^-$. It is so called because it is not in the main chain of atoms in a polypeptide. Polypeptides differ in the order of side chains of their constituent amino-acid residues. **beta (β) c.** One of the two polypeptide chains present in hemoglobin in two copies each. It contains 146 amino acids and is encoded by the β gene in a complex of globin loci (non-alpha globin cluster) on the short arm of human chromosome 11. Mutations at the β locus give rise to many variant hemoglobins, including hemoglobins S and C. **delta (δ) c.** The heavy chain portion of the IgD immunoglobulin. *Older term.* **electron transport c.** The series of electron carriers, contained in a mitochondrial or other membrane, by which reducing equivalents are passed from a reductant such as NADH to an oxidant such as dioxygen, or the reactions by which this process occurs. This electron passage is normally accompanied by pumping of hydrogen ions through the membrane, which may lead to ATP formation. **epsilon (ε) c.** The heavy chain portion of the IgE immunoglobulin. *Older term.* **food c.** The path followed by nutrients, including trace elments, and sometimes accompanied by toxicants, in moving from one organism to another or one species of organism to another. **gamma (γ) c.** The heavy chain portion of the IgG immunoglobulin. *Older term.* **H c.** HEAVY CHAIN. **heavy c.** The heavier of the two pairs of polypeptide chains that constitute the immunoglobulin molecule, having a molecular mass of 50 000–70 000 daltons and comprising approximately 440–560 amino acid residues. Five classes of heavy chains exist, designated alpha (α), delta (δ), epsilon (ε), gamma (γ), and mu (μ), distinguished by amino acid sequences in the 75–80% of the chain not involved in antibody specificity. These sequences determine the biologic and serologic characteristics of the immunoglobulin molecules. Immunoglobulin molecules are classified by the specific pair of heavy chains they possess, with the letters A, D, E, G, and M representing those molecules containing α, δ, ε, γ, and μ chains, respectively. Also *H chain.* **hemolytic c.** The complex of erythrocyte, antierythrocyte antibody, and complement that leads to hemolysis in cold antibody autoimmune hemolytic disorders. **immunoglobulin c.** Any of the polypeptide chains which comprise an immunoglobulin molecule. **J c.** A polypeptide chain which enables the formation of polymers in IgM and certain IgA molecules. **kappa (κ) c.** One of the two types of light polypeptide chains (22 000 daltons) which make up part of an immunoglobulin molecule, the other being the lambda chain. Human kappa chains bear the Inv allotype marker. **L c.** LIGHT CHAIN. **lambda (λ) c.** One of the two types of light polypeptide chains (22 000 daltons) which make up part of an immunoglobulin molecule, the other being the kappa chain. **light c.** The lighter of the two pairs of polypeptide chains that constitute the immunoglobulin molecule, having a molecular mass of approximately 23 000 daltons and comprising approximately 220 amino acid residues. In an immunoglobulin molecule, each light chain is attached by disulfide bonds to one heavy chain, just above the hinge region at which the two heavy chains are linked. Two types of light chains exist, kappa (κ) and lambda (λ), characterized by different amino acid sequences in that portion of the chain not involved in antibody specificity. In man, approximately two thirds of immunoglobulin molecules have two κ chains and one third have two λ chains. Also *L chain.* **mu (μ) c.** The heavy chain component of the immunoglobulin IgM. **nascent polypeptide c.** A polypeptide in the process of translation, which is still attached at its C-terminal end to a ribosome by means of a tRNA molecule. **ossicular c.** OSSICULA AUDITUS. **respiratory c.** The electron transport chain involved in respiration. **side c.** Part of the molecule not on the main chain of atoms. As applied to an amino acid R—CH($NH_2$)COOH it means R, since this is the portion not forming part of the peptide backbone in a residue —NH—CHR—CO—. **sympathetic c.** TRUNCUS SYMPATHICUS. **T c.** SECRETORY PIECE. **transport polypeptide c.** SECRETORY PIECE.

**chair** / **birthing c.** A special chair in which a woman in labor sits in order to utilize the forces of gravity to assist progress in labor and facilitate vaginal delivery. ⟨"A new reclining chair has replaced the old obstetrical table at Memorial Hospital here. . . . The birthing chair, as it's called" —*Medical World News*, 5 Mar. 1979, 30⟩ **growing c.** A chair with changeable or modifiable construction for a growing child. **pendular c.** A chair which rotates around a vertical axis, alternating between a clockwise and anticlockwise direction at precisely controlled rates. It is used in the analysis and diagnosis of vestibular disorders.

**chalasia** \kəlā′zhə\ [Gk *chalas(is)* (from *chalan* to make loose or slack) a letting loose, relaxing + -IA] Relaxation of a muscle or muscle group previously in a state of contraction, especially at the cardioesophageal sphincter or in voluntary muscles which have contracted synergistically.

**chalastodermia** [Late Gk *chalasto(s)* (from Gk *chalan* to loosen, slacken) loose + -DERMIA] CUTIS LAXA.

**chalazia** \kəlā′zē·ə\ Plural of CHALAZION.

**chalazion** \kəlā′zē·än\ [Gk (dim. of *chalaza* a clump, knot) a small lump or cyst] A chronic granulomatous cyst of a meibomian gland of the eyelid. Situated within the tarsal plate, this lesion is visible on the conjunctival surface of the eyelid, which distinguishes a chalazion from a superficial mass of the eyelid.

**chalcitis** \kalsī′tis\ [Gk *chalk(os)* copper + -ITIS] Deposits of copper within the tissues. Also *chalkitis.*

**chalcomycin** One of the macrolide antibiotics, capable of inhibiting protein synthesis.

**chalcosis** \kalkō′sis\ [Gk *chalk(os)* copper + -OSIS] A deposit of particles of copper in the lungs, a finding of no clinical significance. **c. oculi** Copper deposits within the eye, usually due to a retained intraocular copper foreign body. An almost pathognomonic feature is the sunflower cataract, a central disk of opacity of the anterior lens capsule corresponding to the pupil area, with surrounding petal-like opacities extending into the peripheral capsule. Also *chalcosis lentis, ocular chalcosis.*

**chalkitis** \kalkī′tis\ CHALCITIS.

**challenge** 1 The administration of antigen/allergen to a previously sensitized individual in order to induce an immune response. 2 To test (immunity) by such a challenge or subject to a challenge.

**chalone** \kal′ōn\ Any of a group of polypeptides or glycoproteins that inhibit mitosis in the tissues in which they are formed. They are tissue-specific, but are very similar from one species to another. Mitotic supression by chalones is reversible without apparent harm to the cells. Adj. chalonic.

**chaluni** \chaloo′nē\ PITTED KERATOLYSIS.

**chamber** An enclosed space; a compartment; an atrium. **Abbe-Zeiss counting c.** THOMA-ZEISS COUNTING CHAMBER. **acoustic c.** A room or specially designed enclosure in which a very high level of sound attenuation is achieved and in which sound reflection and reverberation are minimal. It may be used for the measurement of hearing or for the measurement of the performance of acousticophysical instrumentation. **air-equivalent ionization c.** An ionization chamber having walls made of a material, often a plastic, having atoms whose average proton number is close to the average for air. Over the energy range for which it is designed, the chamber then behaves much as a standard air chamber would, and for convenience the former can be made much smaller. **altitude c.** A chamber in which reduced barometric pressures can be artificially produced. It is used to simulate the effects of high altitude. **anterior c. of eye** CAMERA ANTERIOR BULBI. **aqueous c.** The camera anterior bulbi and camera posterior bulbi considered together. **Atwater c.** ATWATER'S CALORIMETER. **Atwater-Benedict c.** ATWATER'S CALORIMETER. **Boyden c.** A device for observing and quantifying chemotaxis, consisting of two chambers separated by a micropore filter. Chemotactic material is placed in one chamber and cells in the other. The rate of migration of cells into the filter membrane indicates the intensity of chemotactic response. **cardiac c.'s** CHAMBERS OF THE HEART. **counting c.** HEMOCYTOMETER. **decompression c.** A chamber in which raised barometric pressures can be produced and gradually reduced. It is used in the prevention and treatment of decompression sickness. **c.'s of eye** The camera anterior bulbi, camera posterior bulbi, and camera vitrea bulbi. **free-air ionization c.** An air-wall ionization chamber designed for standardizing x-ray beams. The beam is collimated to prevent it from striking the walls, and the electrode configuration is such that the volume from which ions are collected is predictable. The ion current is then related to x-ray intensity. **Haldane's c.** HALDANE APPARATUS. **c.'s of the heart** The right and left atria and the right and left ventricles of the heart. Also *cardiac chambers.* **hyperbaric c.** A closed, airtight space in which air pressure may be raised above normal atmospheric pressure, used in the treatment of decompression sickness (caisson disease) and, with the administration of oxygen at hyperbaric pressures, in the treatment of carbon monoxide poisoning and of gas gangrene. **ionization c.** A gas-filled chamber containing a charged electrode that will attract ions generated in the gas by entering radiation. The rate of discharge can then measure the intensity of the radiation, or the amount of discharge can measure the quantity. **multiwire proportional c.** A radiation detector filled with xenon at pressures ranging from one to ten atmospheres. It is an excellent detector for spatial resolution of gamma ray distributions for photon energies between 25 and 140 keV. **Petroff-Hauser counting c.** A device permitting the enumeration of the bacterial cells in a fixed volume under the microscope. **pocket c.** A cigar-sized ionization chamber that can be worn on the person. It operates on the condenser-discharge principle, being given an initial charge and then clipped into a pocket for a known time. The amount of discharge measures the person's radiation exposure. Also *pocket dosimeter.* **posterior c. of eye** CAMERA POSTERIOR BULBI. **pronephrotic c.** The central cavity of the rudimentary nephrotomes of the pronephros. The primordium of the pronephros can be identified in the 8-somite human embryo (22nd day) but it completely regresses by the beginning of the fifth week. The human pronephros possesses no glomeruli and is probably functionless. **pulp c.** The central space in the crown of a tooth that accommodates the main part of the pulp. It is continuous with the root canals but apart from this it is a totally enclosed space. Also *camera pulpi, cavitas dentis, nerve cavity* (popular), *cavum coronale, cavum dentis, cavum pulpae, pulp cavity.* **rabbit-ear c.** A system of transparent plates that are placed over a hole punched in a rabbit's ear to observe the cells or tissue growing into the space between the plates. Also *Sandison-Clark chamber.* **relief c.** A space made between part of the fitting surface of a denture and the underlying tissue for the purpose of relieving pressure on that part of the underlying tissue, which is called the relief area. **Sandison-Clark c.** RABBIT-EAR CHAMBER. **thimble ionization c.** A small ionization chamber containing a central pin as one electrode and thimble-shaped cap whose inner surface forms the other electrode. **Thoma-Zeiss counting c.** An apparatus consisting of a chamber 0.1 mm in depth, with a counting surface that is divided into 0.05 mm squares. It is used to count blood cells. Also *Abbe-Zeiss counting chamber, Thoma-Zeiss counting cell, Abbe-Zeiss counting cell.* **vitreous c.** CAMERA VITREA BULBI. **Zappert's c.** HEMOCYTOMETER.

**Chamberlain** [W. Edward *Chamberlain,* U.S. radiologist, 1891–1947] See under LINE.

**Chamberland** [Charles Edouard *Chamberland,* French bacteriologist, 1851–1908] See under CHAMBERLAND CANDLE.

**Chamberlen** [Peter *Chamberlen,* English obstetrician, 1560–1631] See under FORCEPS.

**chancebone** \chans′bōn\ OS ISCHII.

**chancre** \shang′kər\ [French (from L *cancer* crab, cancer) ulcer] **1** A syphilitic ulcer developing at the site of invasion of *Treponema pallidum.* **2** A cutaneous ulcer of certain other diseases, such as chancroid, tularemia, or sporotrichosis. **erosive c.** A primary lesion of syphilis marked by superficial ulceration only. **fungating c.** A lesion in which fungal hypha cells are intermingled with host cells. **hard c.** A primary sore of syphilis. Also *initial syphilitic lesion, syphilitic ulcer.* **hunterian c.** A primary sore of syphilis that is characterized by marked induration, with oozing of serum or crusting. **mixed c.** A lesion due to syphilis and a coexistent venereal infection, usually chancroid. **c. redux** A recurrence of ulceration at site of a primary syphilitic chancre. Also *recurrent chancre.* **soft c.** CHANCROID. **sporotrichotic c.** An inflammed skin lesion at an inoculation site in the subcutaneous mycosis sporotrichosis. **sulcus c.** An ulcerous form of pseudochancre in the coronal sulcus of the penis. Such ulcers are always indurated, whether due to syphilis or other disease. **true c.** The primary lesion of syphilis. Also *primary sore.* **tularemic c.** The primary lesion of tularemia of man, usually seen on the fingers or hands. The lesion begins as a papule that becomes a pustule which ruptures to form an ulcer up to 2 cm in diameter, after which the regional lymph nodes become swollen, inflamed, and painful. The uncomplicated illness in untreated patients runs its course in two weeks to several months. Therapy with streptomycin is promptly effective.

**chancroid** \shang′kroid\ [*chancr(e)* + -OID] An acute, localized, sexually transmitted disease caused by the Gram-negative bacillus *Haemophilus ducreyi,* clinically characterized by tender, usually painful ulcers in the genital region which may heal spontaneously or erode deeply into tissues. About half of the affected patients develop inguinal lymphadenitis. Also *soft sore, venereal ulcer, ulcus venereum, soft chancre.*

**chancrous** \shang′krəs\ **1** Imitating chancre. **2** Characterized by the presence of chancre.

**Chandler** [Fremont Augustus *Chandler,* U.S. orthopedic surgeon, 1893–1954] See under DISEASE.

**change / Alzheimer's neurofibrillary c.** A proliferation of neurofibrillary tangles with a neuronal perikaryon, seen as a characteristic histologic feature in cerebral neurons in Alzheimer's disease but also observed in apparently normal individuals in late life. **Armanni-Ebstein c.** Excessive intracellular deposits of glycogen, as seen in patients with diabetes mellitus. **fatty c.** An abnormal accumulation of neutral fat within parenchymatous cells, occurring mostly in the liver but also in the kidney and heart. By itself a reversible lesion, fatty change occurs in response to many types of cell injury. The prototype is the greatly enlarged liver caused by excessive alcoholic intake. Such livers may double their weight, are grossly yellow and greasy, and microscopically the hepatocytes are overloaded with cytoplasmic lipid droplets that displace the nucleus. Remarkably, abstention results in reversal of the change, whereas continued alcohol consumption may lead to cirrhosis of the liver. Also *fatty metamorphosis.* **free energy c.** The change in free energy in a reaction. In biology this is usually the change in Gibbs energy in the reaction. The fall in Gibbs energy is the maximum useful work the reaction can do under conditions of constant temperature and pressure. Symbol: $\Delta G$ **harlequin color c.** A transitory vasomotor disturbance in the newborn in which there is flushing of the skin of one entire side of the body and blanching of the other, with a sharp demarcation down the midline of the face and trunk. It lasts for a few minutes or hours and has no pathologic significance. The pattern can be reversed by turning the baby over, when the pink underside becomes the blanched upper side. Also *harlequin sign, harlequin flush.* **hydropic c.** An advanced form of cloudy swelling in which the excess water accumulated in the cell cytoplasm appears as visible vacuoles. It is seen in the cells of the proximal convoluted tubules of the kidney, in hepatocytes, and in myocardial cells in certain infections; in carbon tetrachloride poisoning; and in hypokalemia. **tubular hydropic c.** TUBULAR EDEMA.

**channel** [Old French *chanel, canel,* from L *canalis* groove, trough, trench] **1** A groove or passageway, as for the transmission of impulses or fluid. **2** A small opening or pore in an excitable membrane through which ions can move, such as a calcium channel. **3** In electroencephalography, the electrical activity of the brain as recorded between a pair of electrodes applied to the scalp by means of a pen on moving paper. Machines in common use have from 8 to 20 channels which can record simultaneously the electrical activity from many parts of the brain. **blood c.'s** Passages without an endothelial lining permitting blood circulation, usually found in granulation tissue. **central c.** *Outmoded* METARTERIOLE. **collector c.'s** The communicating vessels joining the canal of Schlemm to the intrascleral veins, functioning to permit escape of aqueous humor from the eye into the bloodstream. **c. of Haller** A narrowing of the cardiac tube in an embryo at the point where the bulbus cordis becomes separated from the primitive ventricle, marked externally by the bulboventricular sulcus and internally by the bulboventricular ridge. Also *primary interventricular foramen.* **lymph c.'s** LYMPHATIC SINUSES. **perineural c.** PERIVASCULAR SPACE. **perivascular c.** PERIVASCULAR SPACE. **thoroughfare c.** The distal end of a metarteriole traversing the capillary bed to end directly in a venule. This serves as a low-resistance channel for increasing the blood flow, and is found in such sites as the skin, ear, and mesenteries. Also *preferential channel.*

**chaotropic** \kā′ōträp′ik\ [Gk *chao(s)* unformed mass + -TROPIC[1]] Denoting a substance that destroys the order of water when dissolved in it and thereby raises the solubility of hydrophobic substances in the solution. Chaotropic agents are often large anions, such as thiocyanate and perchlorate. A chaotropic series is a listing of substances in the order of their chaotropic power.

**Chaoul** [Henri *Chaoul,* German radiologist, 1888–1964] See under THERAPY, TUBE.

**character** [L (from Gk *charaktēr,* impress or stamp on a person or thing, likeness), a mark set upon any thing, a style of writing or speaking] **1** A distinctive feature, trait, or property; attribute, as *secondary sex characters.* Also *characteristic.* **2** The distinctive attributes of a person, including innate endowment and constitutional factors as well as the habitual attitudes and traits that have developed as a result of experience or training, the totality of a person's relationship to his environment and his ego-syntonic style of relating to others, and the constellation of defense mechanisms that a person automatically and customarily employs to maintain psychosocial stability. Also *personality, personality type.* • Historically, *character* implied an emphasis on the nature of the subject, while *personality* emphasized experiential, interpersonal factors. **acquired c.** A phenotype produced by environmental influences. **anal c.** COMPULSIVE PERSONALITY. **compound c.** A phenotype produced by two or more genes. **dominant c.** DOMINANT TRAIT. **epileptic c.** A group of behavioral and personality characteristics once believed to be identifiable in epileptic subjects. Patients with psychosis, and with affective and personality disorders, may suffer from epilepsy, which can also be a manifestation of organic brain disease which may in turn cause behavioral changes. Patients with severe and frequent attacks of epilepsy may also suffer brain damage as a direct consequence of the attacks. Also *epileptic temperament, epileptoid personality, explosive personality.* ● Even though most authorities agree that no specifically epileptic character can be identified, the term continues to be used and implies one or more of the following features: rigidity, egocentricity, religiosity, and explosive outbursts of emotion. **mendelian c.** A phenotype that is determined solely or predominantly by a gene or genes at a specific locus on the chromosome. In humans, such characters may be autosomal dominant, autosomal recessive, or X-linked. Also *unit character.* **monogenic c.** Any phenotypic feature determined by a single gene locus, the inheritance of such characters being in accord with mendelian laws. Also *single gene trait.* **polygenic c.** Any phenotypic feature determined by many genes. Such characters are often quantitatively variable and their inheritance does not follow mendelian laws. **primary sex c.'s** The distinctive gonadal or genital characters of each sex, as the testis in the male and the ovary in the female. They are the gametogenic and hormone-secreting organs of the male or female sex which are responsible for the development of secondary sex characters. **psychotic c.** A character which typifies an individual with residual or latent symptoms of schizophrenia but with no gross break with reality. *Imprecise.* **quantitative c.** A polygenic character whose variability can be specified metrically. It is inherited in a multifactorial mode, with the genetic component determined by many genes. **recessive c.** RECESSIVE TRAIT. **secondary sex c.'s** The extragonadal characters specific for maleness or femaleness, such as phallic growth and breast development; the features other than those involving gametogenesis and secretion of the sex hormones. **sex-influenced c.** A phenotype determined primarily by an autosomal locus but whose manifestations differ between sexes. Also *sex-conditioned character.* **sex-limited c.** A character that is expressed in only one sex. The gene determining the character may be on either an autosome or a sex chromosome. **sex-linked c.** A phenotype determined by a gene located on a sex chromosome. **unit c.** MENDELIAN CHARACTER.

**characteristic** CHARACTER. **film c.'s** Properties of a film, such as contrast and speed, which are often shown as a plot of the film density versus the logarithm of the exposure. **receiver operating c.'s** The characteristics of a curve (ROC curve) that depicts how the number of false-positive and true-positive results on a test changes as the threshold criteria change. Measures of performance, such as sensitivity and specificity, can give misleading results when diagnostic tests are compared unless there is a means to take into account variability of the criterion level used. Abbr. ROC

**charbon** \shärbôN'\ [French (from L *carbo* a coal, charcoal), coal] ANTHRAX.

**charcoal** Carbon obtained from organic matter by drawing off volatile compounds, as by charring wood in an airless environment. **animal c.** Charcoal produced by the destructive distillation of bones and other animal tissues. Also *bone black, animal black, ivory black, Paris black.* **dextran coated c.** An adsorbent material commonly used in radioimmunoassays to remove free antigen from a reaction mixture that contains both free and bound antigen. **purified animal c.** A purified form of animal charcoal, produced by the incomplete combustion of animal bone and other animal tissues.

**Charcot** [Jean-Martin *Charcot,* French neurologist, 1825–1893] **1** See under SIGN, TRIAD, FOOT, SYNDROME. **2** Charcot's joint, Charcot's arthropathy. See under NEUROGENIC ARTHROPATHY. **3** Charcot's hand. See under PREACHER'S HAND. **4** Charcot-Böttcher crystalloids. See under CRYSTALLOID. **5** Charcot's fever, Charcot's intermittent fever. See under INTERMITTENT HEPATIC FEVER. **6** Erb-Charcot disease. See under SYPHILITIC SPASTIC PARAPLEGIA. **7** Charcot-Weiss-Baker syndrome. See under CAROTID SINUS SYNDROME. **8** Charcot's disease. See under OPHTHALMOPLEGIC MIGRAINE. **9** Charcot's disease. See under TABETIC ARTHROPATHY. **10** Charcot's disease, Charcot-Marie atrophy, Charcot-Marie-Tooth atrophy, Charcot-Marie-Tooth-Hoffmann syndrome. See under CHARCOT-MARIE-TOOTH DISEASE. See under CHARCOT-LEYDEN CRYSTALS. **11** Charcot syndrome. See under INTERMITTENT CLAUDICATION. **12** Charcot syndrome. See under AMYOTROPHIC LATERAL SCLEROSIS.

**charge** **1** A quantity of electricity. **2** A cost or expense. **electron c.** The quantity of elemental negative electricity of the electron, equal to $1.6 \times 10^{-19}$ coulomb or $4.8 \times 10^{-10}$ esu. **ionic c.** The product of the electron charge and the valence of the ion under consideration. It is the total charge caused by gain or loss of electrons by the neutral atom. **specific electron c.** A charge of the electron divided by its mass.

**Charles** [Jacques-Alexandre-Cesar *Charles,* French physicist, 1746–1823] See under LAW.

**Charles** [Sir R. Haverlock *Charles,* English surgeon, flourished 20th century] See under OPERATION.

**charleyhorse** [prob. from the name of a lame horse] Pain or spasm in a muscle following a contusion. *Popular.*

**Charlin** [C. Carlos *Charlin,* Chilean physician, 1886–1945] See under SYNDROME.

**charpie** \shär'pē\ LINT.

**charring** \chär'ing\ A surgical procedure in which damaged or abnormal tissue is converted to carbon residue.

**chart** [L *charta.* See CHARTA.] A diagrammatic, graphic, or tabular presentation of data. **Amsler's c.'s** A grid of white lines upon a black background, used to detect metamorphopsia (visual distortion). **E-type c.** SNELLEN CHART. **exposure c.** In radiology, a set of x-ray factors and exposure times for radiography of different parts or thicknesses of the patient. **flow c.** A diagram utilizing symbols such as rectangles, diamonds, and circles, with lines connecting them, to represent a step-by-step sequence through a procedure or computer program. **Landolt ring c.** A visual acuity chart for illiterate individuals, consisting of broken rings resembling the letter C with the break oriented in different directions. **Snellen c.** The commonly used distant visual acuity chart comprising letters of various sizes. The individual being examined is tested on his perception of letters of smaller and smaller size to determine the level of visual acuity. Also *E-type chart.*

**charta** [L (from Gk *chartēs* a leaf of paper made from separate papyrus layers), papyrus] A piece of paper coated or saturated with an active agent or compound. In some instances the paper is burned and the medicated smoke inhaled as a means of treatment.

**chartreusin** $C_{32}H_{32}O_{14}$. An antibiotic from *Streptomyces chartreusis,* with tuberculostatic activity.

**chartula** A small piece of paper suitable for wrapping a dose of a medicinal powder or drug.

**chasma** \kaz'mə\ [Gk (from *chainein* to yawn) a gulf, chasm] A large opening; a cleft or chasmlike orifice. Also *chasmus.*

**Chassaignac** [Pierre Marie Edouard *Chassaignac*, French surgeon 1804–1879] Chassaignac's tubercle. See under TUBERCULUM ANTERIUS VERTEBRAE CERVICALIS VI.
**Chauffard** [Anatole Marie Emile *Chauffard*, French physician, 1855–1932] **1** Chauffard-Still syndrome, Still-Chauffard syndrome. See under CHAUFFARD SYNDROME. **2** Minkowski-Chauffard syndrome. See under HEREDITARY SPHEROCYTOSIS.
**chaulmoogric acid** 13-(Cyclopent-2-enyl)-tridecanoic acid. A $C_{18}$ fatty acid which occurs in chaulmoogra oil (hydnocarpus oil) and has been used in treating leprosy.
**Chaussier** [François *Chaussier*, French physician, 1746–1828] See under SIGN.
**CHD** **1** congenital heart disease. **2** coronary heart disease.
**ChE** cholinesterase.
**check** / **delta c.** A quality control procedure that scrutinizes the differences in measured values of the same analyte between one analysis and the next.
**checkerboard** PUNNETT SQUARE.
**Chédiak** [Moises *Chédiak*, French physician, flourished mid-20th century] Chédiak-Higashi disease, Chédiak-Steinbrinck-Higashi anomaly. See under CHÉDIAK-HIGASHI ANOMALY.
**cheek** [Middle English *cheke* jawbone, cheek, from Old English *cece,ceace, ceoke* jawbone, akin to Dutch *kaak* jaw, cheek] The fleshy part of the face forming the lateral wall of the oral cavity; bucca. Adj. buccal. **cleft c.** Any of several varieties of facial cleft in which the cheek or lateral face bears an embryonic fissure from the failure of facial processes to fuse properly, as in genal cleft.
**cheekbone** OS ZYGOMATICUM.
**cheek-tooth** A molar or premolar.
**cheil-** \kīl-\ CHEILO-.
**cheilectomy** \kīlek′təmē\ [CHEIL- + -ECTOMY] The excision of a lip or edge of tissue. It is usually the result of surgery but it may result from penetrating trauma as well.
**cheilectropion** \kī′lektrō′pē·än\ Eversion of the lip, usually as the result of the contraction of cutaneous scar tissue.
**cheilitis** \kīlī′tis\ [CHEIL- + -ITIS] An inflammation of the lips. Also *cheilosis.* Also *chilitis.* **actinic c.** SOLAR CHEILITIS. **allergic c.** Inflammation and swelling of the lips resulting from a delayed hypersensitivity to a specific antigen such as a perfume in lipstick. **angular c.** Inflammation of the lips leading to chronic fissures at the commissures of the lips. It is a feature of a variety of general and local disorders including certain deficiency diseases, infections, and problems which result in salivary spillage at the corners of the mouth. Also *angular stomatitis, perlèche, commissural cheilitis.* **apostematous c.** CHEILITIS GLANDULARIS. **commissural c.** ANGULAR CHEILITIS. **exfoliative c.** A chronic, superficial, inflammatory disorder of the lips characterized by repeated exfoliation. **c. glandularis** A chronic cheilitis resulting from enlargement and secondary infection of heterotopic salivary glands in the lips. Also *myxadenitis labialis, apostematous cheilitis.* **granulomatous c.** Intermittent edema of the upper or lower lip, becoming persistent and chronic. Focal granulomata are present. **impetiginous c.** Impetigo of the lips, usually seen in children. **mycotic c.** A chronic fungal infection of the lips. The commonest form is an infection of the angles of the mouth with *Candida albicans.* **solar c.** Acute inflammatory changes or chronic degenerative changes of the lips induced by exposure to sunlight. Also *actinic cheilitis.*
**cheilo-** \kī′lō-\ [Gk *cheilos* lip, edge, rim] A combining form denoting the lip. Also *cheil-, chil-, chilo-.*
**cheiloalveoloschisis** \-al′vē·əläs′kisis\ [CHEILO- + ALVEOLO- + -SCHISIS] A cleft lip with a defective maxilla so that the premaxilla tends to be separated from the remainder of the maxilla and the palate. It may be unilateral or bilateral, partial or complete.
**cheilognathoglossoschisis** \-nath′əgläsäs′kisis\ [CHEILO- + GNATHO- + GLOSSO- + -SCHISIS] A midline cleft of the lower jaw in which the lower lip, the mandible, and the tongue may be cleft or hypoplastic to varying degrees. This does not represent persistence of an embryonic facial fissure but probably is the result of incomplete anastomoses of vascular supplies from the two sides of the face.
**cheilognathopalatoschisis** \-nath′əpal′ətäs′kisis\ CHEILOGNATHOURANOSCHISIS.
**cheilognathoprosoposchisis** \-nath′əpräs′ōpäs′kisis\ [CHEILO- + GNATHO- + PROSOPO- + -SCHISIS] An oblique facial cleft combined with a cleft of the lip and jaw.
**cheilognathoschisis** \-nathäs′kisis\ [CHEILO- + GNATHO- + -SCHISIS] A condition characterized by a cleft lip and jaw.
**cheilognathouranoschisis** \-nath′əyoo′rənäs′kisis\ [CHEILO- + GNATHO- + URANO- + -SCHISIS] A condition characterized by a cleft lip, jaw, and palate.
**cheiloplasty** \kī′lōplas′tē\ [CHEILO- + -PLASTY] An operation to change the shape or contour of one or both lips or to repair a defect in the lips. Also *labioplasty.*
**cheilorrhaphy** \kīlôr′əfē\ [CHEILO- + -RRHAPHY] An operation involving suturing of a lip, especially the repair of a congenitally cleft lip.
**cheiloschisis** \kīläs′kisis\ [CHEILO- + -SCHISIS] CLEFT LIP.
**cheilosis** \kīlō′sis\ CHEILITIS. **angular c.** Inflammation of the corner of the mouth. It is commonly caused by bacterial or fungal infection.
**cheilostomatoplasty** \-stōmat′ōplas′tē\ Surgical repair of a defect of the lips and mouth, especially a defect resulting from injury or the removal of a neoplasm.
**cheilotomy** \kīlät′əmē\ [CHEILO- + -TOMY] An incision usually into the lip, or, rarely, into an edge or ridge of tissue.
**cheir-** \kīr-\ CHEIRO-.
***Cheiracanthium*** \kī′rəkan′thē·əm\ *CHIRACANTHIUM.*
**cheiralgia** \kīral′jə\ [CHEIR- + -ALGIA] Pain and paresthesiae in the hand. **c. paresthetica**
**cheiro-** \kī′rō-\ [Gk *cheir* hand, hand and arm] A combining form denoting the hand. Also *cheir-, chir-, chiro-.*
**cheirobrachialgia** \-brā′kē·al′jə\ [CHEIRO- + BRACHIALGIA] Pain in the hand and arm. *Obs.* Also *chirobrachialgia.*
**cheirocinesthesia** \-sin′esthē′zhə\ CHEIROKINESTHESIA.
**cheirognostic** \kī′rägnäs′tik\ [CHEIRO- + Gk *gnōstik(os)* (from *gnōstos* known, from *gignōskein* to perceive, learn) relating to knowledge] **1** Able to distinguish or recognize one's own or another's hand or parts of the hand. **2** Able to distinguish between right and left. *Obs.* Also *chirognostic.*
**cheirokinesthesia** \-kin′esthē′zhə\ [CHEIRO- + KINESTHESIA] The sense of awareness of movements of the hand, as in writing. Also *cheirocinesthesia.* Adj. cheirokinesthetic.
**cheiromegaly** \-meg′əlē\ [CHEIRO- + -MEGALY] Enlargement of one or both hands, such as may be seen in syringomyelia. Also *megalocheiria, pseudoacromegaly* (seldom used). Also *chiromegaly.*
**cheiropodalgia** \-pōdal′jə\ [CHEIRO- + PODALGIA] Pain in the extremities. *Obs.* Also *chiropodalgia.*
**cheirospasm** \kī′rōspazm\ [CHEIRO- + SPASM] A spasm of the muscles of the hand. Also *chirospasm.*
**chelate** \kē′lāt\ [Gk *chēl(ē)* claw, pincer + -ATE] A

complex formed between a metal ion and a chelating agent. Such complexes are highly stable and often met in analysis.

**chelation** \kēlā′shən\ [*chelat(e)* + -ION] The binding of a metal ion by more than one group. See also CHELATING AGENT.

**chelicera** \kelis′ərə\ [New L, from Gk *chēl(ē)* claw, talon + *i* + *ker(as)* horn] (*pl.* chelicerae) One of the paired anterior appendages characteristic of arachnids. Together with the pedipalpi (and the hypostome in ticks and some mites) they constitute the mouth parts. In spiders they bear fangs with venom ducts, and in ticks and parasitic mites they are adapted for cutting and piercing.

**chelidon** \kel′idän\ [Gk *chelidōn* the swallow (from the resemblance of the shape of the tail), the hollow above the bend of the elbow] FOSSA CUBITALIS.

**cheloid** \kē′loid\ [Gk *chēlē* a hoof, talon, claw + -OID] KELOID.

**cheloidosis** \kē′loidō′sis\ **1** The hereditary tendency to form keloids. **2** The presence of keloids.

**chemasthenia** \kem′asthē′nē·ə\ Any debilitating condition involving the chemical processes of the body.

**chemiatry** \kemī′ətrē\ IATROCHEMISTRY.

**chemical** **1** Denoting the properties dealt with in the science of chemistry. **2** Concerning chemistry. **3** Any substance of specified atomic or molecular composition; especially, such a substance when used in laboratory and industrial processes. **radiomimetic c.** A substance with effects on living organisms like those of ionizing radiation, such as mutagenic effects.

**chemico-** \kem′əkō-\ CHEMO-.

**chemicocautery** \-kô′terē\ CHEMOCAUTERY.

**chemio-** \kem′ē·ō-\ CHEMO-.

**chemiotaxis** \-tak′sis\ CHEMOTAXIS.

**chemiotherapy** CHEMOTHERAPY.

**chemist** **1** A specialist or expert in chemistry. **2** The British term for PHARMACIST.

**chemistry** [Gk *chēmeia* (prob. from root of *chymenos,* Epic aorist part. of *cheein* to pour) alchemy, chemistry] **1** The science that deals with the structure of matter in terms of molecules, atoms and particles, and of the reactions that occur between elements or molecules, whether spontaneously or under the effects of physical agents. **2** The collection of chemical properties of an element or of organic or mineral compounds, as *blood chemistry.* **analytical c.** The chemical determination of the nature and composition of elements in mixtures or compounds. **clinical c.** **1** Chemical analysis of substances important in human health and disease. **2** The branch of laboratory medicine that uses chemical analysis for diagnostic tests. **forensic c.** The specialized application of the theories and practices of chemistry to the solution of legal problems, particularly criminal problems. The especially prominent disciplines of chemistry include qualitative and quantitative analysis, organic chemistry, and physical chemistry. **histologic c.** HISTOCHEMISTRY. **organic c.** The chemistry of carbon compounds, particularly those that contain hydrogen and carbon-carbon bonds. **pharmaceutical c.** The branch of organic chemistry that is concerned with the synthesis and preparation of compounds that have beneficial pharmacologic effects on disease, or that have diagnostic value. Also *pharmacochemistry.* **physical c.** The branch of chemistry that deals with the physics of chemical changes. **radiation c.** The branch of chemistry that deals with the chemical effects produced by high levels of ionizing radiation. Corrosion, aging, decomposition, etc., are subjects of interest.

**chemo-** \kē′mō-, kem′ō-\ [Gk *chēmeia* alchemy, chemistry] A combining form meaning chemistry, chemical. Also *chemico-, chemio-.*

**chemoautotroph** \-ô′təträf\ CHEMOLITHOTROPH.

**chemoautotrophic** \-ô′təträf′ik\ CHEMOLITHOTROPHIC.

**chemobiotic** Having a combination of therapeutic properties for chemotherapeutic and antibiotic objectives.

**chemocautery** \-kô′terē\ [CHEMO- + CAUTERY] The destruction of tissue by the application of a chemical such as phenol. Also *chemical cautery, chemicautery.*

**chemoceptor** \kem′ōsep′tər\ CHEMORECEPTOR.

**chemocoagulation** \-kō·ag′yəlā′shən\ The use of chemicals to coagulate, i.e., destroy, tissue.

**chemodectoma** \-dektō′mə\ [CHEMO- + Gk *dekt(ēs)* (from *dechesthai* to accept, receive) receiver, receptor + -OMA] PARAGANGLIOMA.

**chemodifferentiation** \-dif′ərenshē·ā′shən\ The chemical changes which precede any obvious cellular changes associated with cytodifferentiation during early embryonic development. These chemical changes are sometimes recognizable histochemically.

**chemoimmunology** \-im′yənäl′əjē\ IMMUNOCHEMISTRY.

**chemokinesis** \-kīnē′sis\ The stimulation of activity in living organisms by chemical means. Adj. chemokinetic.

**chemolithotroph** \-lith′əträf\ A bacterium that can grow by $CO_2$ fixation at the expense of purely inorganic reactions, such as the oxidation of $H_2$ or $H_2S$ by $O_2$ or $Fe^{3+}$. Also *chemoautotroph.*

**chemolithotrophic** \-lith′əträf′ik\ Relating to a chemolithotroph. Also *chemoautotrophic.*

**chemomorphosis** \-môrfō′sis\ [CHEMO- + MORPHO- + -SIS] Chemically induced change in form or developmental stage.

**chemonucleolysis** \-nʸoo′klē·äl′isis, -nʸoo′klē·ōlī′sis\ Injection of a sclerosing fluid into a spinal intervertebral disk as a method of treating prolapse of the disk.

**chemoorganotroph** \-ôr′gənōträf′\ An organism that utilizes organic compounds as the source of its material and energy; heterotroph.

**chemopallidectomy** \-pal′idek′təmē\ [CHEMO- + PALLIDECTOMY] Destruction of the globus pallidus by injecting a chemical.

**chemopallidothalamectomy** \-pal′idōthal′amek′təmē\ [CHEMO- + PALLIDO- + THALAMECTOMY] Destruction of the globus pallidus and the thalamus by injecting a chemical.

**chemopallidotomy** \-pal′idät′əmē\ [CHEMO- + PALLIDOTOMY] Partial destruction of the globus pallidus by injecting a chemical.

**chemoprophylaxis** \-prō′filak′sis\ [CHEMO- + PROPHYLAXIS] The prevention of development, activation, or spread of a specific disease by administration of a chemical agent. Also *chemoprevention.* **local c.** Application of an antimicrobial agent directly to a wound or mucosal surface in order to prevent microbial colonization and subsequent infection.

**chemoreceptor** \-risep′tər\ [CHEMO- + RECEPTOR] A sense organ excited by specific chemical substances and changes in their concentration, e.g., gustatory, olfactory, and carotid body receptors. Also *chemoceptor, chemical ceptor.*

**chemoresistant** \-rezis′tənt\ Descriptive of a tumor or tissue that is relatively resistant to damage by a chemotherapeutic drug or regime.

**chemosensitive** \-sen′sitiv\ Responsive to a chemical change in the environment. Also *chemosensory.*

**chemoserotherapy** Treatment combining drug therapy with serum.

**chemosis** \kēmō′sis\ [Gk *chēmōsis* (from *chēmē* a clam or cockle) a swelling of the conjunctiva around the cornea] A marked inflammation or swelling of the bulbar conjunctiva, which may be so severe as to protrude from the eyelids; edema and redness of the conjunctiva. Adj. chemotic.

**chemostat** \kem′ōstat\ [CHEMO- + -STAT] A device that permits cultivation of microbes under constant conditions by providing inflow of medium and outflow of culture at the same rate, the density of the growth being set by some limiting nutrient.

**chemosterilant** \-ster′ilənt\ A chemical used to control pests, especially insects, by causing reproductive sterility in their population. Several aziridinyl compounds, tepa, metepa, and apholate, have been studied as insect chemosterilants.

**chemosterilization** \-ster′ilīzā′shən\ Reproductive sterilization of noxious pests, especially insects, by chemical means. See also CHEMOSTERILANT, STERILANT.

**chemosuppression** \-supresh′ən\ The use of a drug to suppress an infection below the clinical level.

**chemosurgery** \-sur′jərē\ The destruction of abnormal tissues with chemical agents, used especially for tissues that are neoplastic, inflammatory, or necrotic. **Mohs c.** A method of treating skin cancers wherein the tumor is fixed before excision with zinc chloride paste. After the tumor is excised, it is examined microscopically, and with the aid of a previously drawn diagram of the excised portion of the tumor, the location of any remaining tumor is easily identified and subsequently removed in the same fashion. Also *Mohs surgery.*

**chemotactic** \-tak′tik\ Of or characterized by chemotaxis. Also *chemotropic.*

**chemotaxis** \-tak′sis\ [CHEMO- + TAXIS] A directional migration of a living organism due to a chemical stimulus. Also *chemiotaxis, chemotropism.* **leukocyte c.** The unidirectional migration of leukocytes towards a chemical attraction generated within an inflammatory focus. Neutrophils migrate within 90 minutes, and macrophages do so more slowly. The principal chemical attractants are bacterial products and components of the complement system, particularly C3 and C5 fragments.

**chemothalamectomy** \-thal′əmek′təmē\ [CHEMO- + THALAMECTOMY] Destruction of the thalamus by injecting a chemical.

**chemothalamotomy** \-thal′əmät′əmē\ [CHEMO- + THALAMOTOMY] Partial destruction of the thalamus by injecting a chemical.

**chemotherapeutic** Related to chemotherapy.

**chemotherapy** [CHEMO- + THERAPY] The treatment of disease with chemical compounds or drugs. Also *chemiotherapy, chemotherapeutics, histochemotherapy.* **topical c.** Local application of a chemically active agent, such as an antimicrobial drug, to prevent or treat infection in wounds, or an antitumor drug, used in some skin cancers.

**chemotic** \kēmät′ik\ Pertaining to or affected by chemosis.

**chemotransmitter** \-transmit′ər\ **1** A chemical substance, released at the presynaptic nerve terminal when a nerve impulse arrives, which produces a response in an effector cell, often by combining with a specific receptor upon the postsynaptic cell surface. **2** Any chemical substance which conveys a message from one part of the body to another.

**chemotropic** \-träp′ik\ CHEMOTACTIC.

**chemotropism** \kēmät′rōpizm\ CHEMOTAXIS.

**Chenais** [Louis J. *Chenais,* French physician, 1872–1950] Cestan-Chenais syndrome. See under SYNDROME.

**chenodeoxycholic acid** 3$\alpha$,7$\alpha$-dihydroxy-5$\beta$-cholanic acid. A mammalian bile acid found largely conjugated with taurine and glycine.

**cherubism** \cher′oobizm\ [*cherub* + -ISM] An uncommon hereditary disease of the jaws, probably of autosomal dominant inheritance. It becomes manifest in early childhood as progressive, painless, symmetrical swelling of the jaws though usually only of the mandible. The child's face assumes a cherubic appearance. Once believed to be a type of fibrous dysplasia, it is now considered a separate entity. Also *familial fibrous dysplasia of the jaws, disseminated juvenile fibrous dysplasia of the jaws, familial fibrous swelling of the jaws.*

**Chervin** [Claudius *Chervin,* French educator, 1824–1896] Chervin's method. See under TREATMENT.

**chest** [Old English *cist,* from common Germanic, from L *cista* a box, chest, from Gk *kistē* a box, chest] The upper part of the trunk between the neck and the abdomen; thorax. **alar c.** FLAT CHEST. **barrel c.** A cylindrical chest with a marked increase of the anteroposterior diameter that changes little during respiration. It is characteristic of emphysema. Also *emphysematous chest, barrel-shaped thorax.* **blast c.** A syndrome of pulmonary contusion resulting from the sudden increase in ambient pressure during an explosion, as in an air-blast injury. **emphysematous c.** BARREL CHEST. **fissured c.** The failed closure of the thoracic wall in the sternal region. It is usually associated with ectopia cordis. **flail c.** A condition in which part of the chest wall moves independently of the rest of the chest, usually as a result of trauma. Also *pendelluft chest, stove-in chest.* **flat c.** An abnormality in which the thorax is flattened from front to back. Also *alar chest.* **funnel c.** PECTUS EXCAVATUM. **hourglass c.** A thorax exhibiting narrowing of the central region, such as may be seen in rickets. **keeled c.** PECTUS CARINATUM. **paralytic c.** A long narrow chest with marked prominence of the ribs owing to atrophy of adjacent muscles. **pendelluft c.** FLAIL CHEST. **phthinoid c.** PTERYGOID CHEST. **pigeon c.** PECTUS CARINATUM. **pterygoid c.** A long and narrow chest characterized by obliquity of the lower ribs, which may reach the iliac crest, backward projecting scapulae, and a tendency to pectus excavatum. Also *phthinoid chest.* **rachitic c.** The shape of the chest seen in rickets, characterized by protuberant sternum, incurving of the lower ribs, and beading of the ribs at the costochondral junctions. **stove-in c.** FLAIL CHEST.

***Cheyletiella parasitivorax*** \kī′letyel′ə par′əsī′tēvôr′aks\ An ectoparasitic mange mite of cats, dogs, rabbits, and humans. The mange of dogs that has been attributed to this species, however, is now thought to be caused by *C. yasguri,* that of cats by *C. blakei,* both species causing a scurfy, pruriginous dermatitis and an itching dermatitis in humans who handle infected pets. The true *C. parasitivorax* is associated with infestation of rabbits.

**Cheyne** [John *Cheyne,* Scottish physician active in Ireland, 1777–1836] Cheyne-Stokes breathing. See under CHEYNE-STOKES RESPIRATION.

**CHF** congestive heart failure.

**Chiari** [Hans *Chiari,* Czech physician, 1851–1916] **1** See under NET, ANOMALY. **2** Budd-Chiari disease, Chiari's disease, Chiari syndrome. See under BUDD-CHIARI SYNDROME.

**Chiari** [Johann Baptist *Chiari,* Austrian physician, 1817–1854] Chiari-Frommel disease, Frommel-Chiari syndrome. See under CHIARI-FROMMEL SYNDROME.

**chiasm** \kī′azm\ [Gk *chiasma.* See CHIASMA.] CHIASMA. **Camper's c.** CHIASMA TENDINUM DIGITORUM MANUS. **c. of digits of hand** CHIASMA TENDINUM DIGITORUM MANUS. **optic c.** CHIASMA OPTICUM. **tendinous c. of flexor digitorum sublimis muscle** CHIASMA TENDINUM DIGITORUM MANUS.

**chiasma** \kī·az′mə\ [Gk, a crossed pair of lines as in the Gk letter chi (X)] (*pl.* chiasmata) **1** In anatomy, a decussation of two structures, such as nerves or tendons. Also *chiasm.* **2** In cytogenetics, the region of contact between homologous chromosomes during meiosis. **3** Any intersection or crossing of two lines. **c. opticum** [NA] A flattened, X-shaped body visible anterior to the tuber cinereum. It consists of converging optic nerves anteriorly, the diverging optic tracts passing backward, and a crossing of some fibers from one side to the other. The proportion of optic nerve fibers that cross differs among animals. In man, fibers from the nasal half of each retina cross. Also *optic chiasma, optic commissure, commissura optica, optic decussation.* **c. tendinum digitorum manus** [NA] The passage of a tendon of the flexor digitorum profundus muscle through an oval gap produced by the splitting, rejoining, and decussation of the flattened tendon of the corresponding flexor digitorum superficialis muscle tendon opposite the proximal phalanx. Also *chiasm of digits of hand, tendinous chiasm of flexor digitorum sublimis muscle, Camper's chiasm, chiasma tendinosum camperi* (outmoded).

**chiasmal** \kī·az′məl\ CHIASMIC.

**chiasmata** \kī·az′mətə\ Plural of CHIASMA.

**chiasmic** \kī·az′mik\ Pertaining to or resembling a chiasma. Also *chiasmatic, chiasmal.*

**chiasmometer** \kī′azmäm′ətər\ [*chiasm(a)* + *o* + -METER] A device to measure the distance between the centers of rotation of the two eyes. Also *chiastometer.*

**chickenpox** VARICELLA.

**chief of service** The person, often a physician, in charge of a specific type of service in a health care facility. A term used chiefly in the U.S., Canada, and South Africa. • It is understood in the United Kingdom but rarely used. It is not used in Australia, New Zealand, India, or Japan. In New Zealand, *head of department* is the preferred usage for this sense.

**chief of staff** The person in charge of all health care professionals in a provider organization, such as the physician in charge of the medical staff in a hospital. A term used chiefly in the U.S. and Japan. • The term is not used in the United Kingdom, Australia, New Zealand, or India. In South Africa, *medical superintendent* is preferred, and in New Zealand *chairman of staff* is used in this sense.

**Chievitz** [Johan Henrik *Chievitz,* Danish anatomist, 1850–1901] See under ORGAN.

**chigger** \chig′ər\ [African, akin to Wolof *chiga*] The six-legged larva of a trombiculid mite. This is the skin-inhabiting, parasitic stage of the mite, which is generally minute and red in color, and feeds on serous elements of the host's tissue. The species that attack humans usually produce a wheal, which is followed by intense itching and commonly by a secondary dermatitis. Some species, such as *Leptotrombidium akamushi,* are vectors of scrub typhus. Also *harvest mite (British), red bug, kedani (Japanese).*

**chignon** \shēnyôN′\ [French (alteration of Middle French *chaignon* a chain, the nape of the neck, from L *catena* a chain), an arrangement of hair at the back of the neck] WHITE PIEDRA.

**chigoe** \chig′ō\ [Spanish *chigo* (of Carib origin) a sand flea] A flea of the species *Tunga penetrans.* Also *sand flea, chigoe flea, chigger flea, jigger flea, jigger, chigo.*

**chikungunya** \chik′ʊng·gʊn′yə\ [Makonde (language of southeastern Tanzania) (from *kungunya(la)* to curl or fold up) something that causes one to double up with pain] An illness resembling dengue caused by an alphavirus (chikungunya virus) and spread by mosquitoes, usually *Aedes* species. It is characterized by sudden onset of fever, chills, severe incapacitating joint pain and, usually, a maculopapular rash. Epidemics have occurred in Africa, India, and Southeast Asia. In Thailand a variant of the disease with hemorrhagic manifestations has been described. Also *chikungunya fever.*

**chil-** \kīl-\ CHEILO-.

**Chilaiditi** [Demetrios *Chilaiditi,* Austrian physician, born 1883] See under SYNDROME.

**chilblain** \chil′blān\ [*chil(l)* + *blain,* from Old English *blegen* inflammatory sore, blister] A lesion resulting from a vascular response to a combination of low temperatures and humidity. Chilblains are characterized by dull erythema, itching, pain, and swelling and occur mainly on the fingers, toes, and ears. Also *perniosis.*

**child** [Old English *cild*] **1** In pediatrics, a person between the age of infancy and puberty, that is, between about one and 14 years of age. **2** In demography, a person who has not yet reached the age of puberty. **atypical c.** A child with a pervasive developmental disorder consisting of defective ego development, withdrawal, and many autistic traits. Unlike other autistic children the atypical child usually possesses above average motor ability, grace and agility, and talent in some capacity which is exploited. The talent may be in musical appreciation or performance, acrobatic skill, constructing ability, or even a bizarre verbal ability, such that the atypical child makes better use of the environment than is possible for other autistic children. **autistic c.** See under EARLY INFANTILE AUTISM. **battered c.** A child who has been physically or sexually abused, or both, by a parent or caretaker. Injuries may be secondary to intentional acts of omission or failure to provide, or to repeated and excessive beatings. See also BATTERED CHILD SYNDROME. **brain-damaged c.** A child exhibiting any of various symptoms indicative of injury to brain tissue. Symptoms include impairment of perception, comprehension, learning capacity, abstract reasoning, and judgment; lack of perseverance; distractability; emotional impulsiveness and overreaction with loss of control when suddenly disappointed or surprised; poor tolerance of frustration; visual, auditory, or kinesthetic impairment; motor disabilities that range from clumsiness to moderate or severe palsy; and proneness to seizures. **ego deviant c.** A child with a pervasive developmental disorder such as early infantile autism. **newborn c.** See under NEONATE.

**childbirth** The process of giving birth to a child.

**childhood** The time of an individual's life from birth to the beginning of adolescence.

**childproof** Designed with the safety of children in mind, as a medication container that cannot be easily opened by a child.

**children-ever-born** The number of children born as of a given date by a woman aged 15 years or over. This information is often collected at the time of a census. The number per 1000 women aged 50 years and over is equal to the completed family size.

**chilitis** CHEILITIS.

**chill** [Old English *cele,* akin to *ceald* cold] **1** A sense of coldness. It may be associated with compulsive shivering, teeth chattering, gooseflesh, and skin pallor that result from exposure to moisture or cold, or from an imminent feverish illness. **2** A mild, nonspecific, feverish illness. **brass c.** METAL-FUME FEVER. **braziers' c.** METAL-FUME FEVER. **spelters' c.** METAL-FUME FEVER. **urethral c.** A chill or cold sensation resulting from the introduction of a catheter. This may be the result of bacteremia caused by the catheterization. **zinc c.** METAL-FUME FEVER.

**chilo-** \kī′lō-\ CHEILO-.

**chilomastigiasis** \-mas′tijī′əsis\ Infection by protozoans of the genus *Chilomastix,* which are found in man and swine but are nonpathogenic. Also *chilomastixiasis, chilomastosis, tetramitiasis.*

***Chilomastix*** \-mas′tiks\ [CHILO- + Gk *mastix* a whip] A genus of flagellate protozoans (order Retortamonadida, class Zoomastigophorea) parasitic in the intestine of vertebrates. ***C. mesnili*** A species found in the human colon and cecum. A common commensal, it causes no significant harm to the human host. It is suspected of being an occasional cause of diarrhea in children, but this has not been established. Also *Tetramitus mesnili.*

**chilomastixiasis** \-mas′tiksī′əsis\ CHILOMASTIGIASIS.

**chilomastosis** \-mastō′sis\ CHILOMASTIGIASIS.

**chilopa** \kīlō′pə\ ONYALAI.

**chimera** \kīmir′ə, kimir′ə\ [L *chimaera,* from Gk *chimaira* a monster in Gk myth represented as a composite of goat, lion, and serpent] An organism composed of two or more genetically distinct cell types. Chimeras can arise through a variety of spontaneous and experimental processes including mutation, mixing of blood cell precursors during dizygous twin pregnancy, mixing of dispersed cells of the early embryo, or grafting tissue from one organism to a zygote of different genotype. **heterologous c.** In experimental genetics, a chimera formed by cells or tissues from two different species. **homologous c.** A chimera formed by cells or tissues from organisms of the same species but different genotype. It occurs in humans most commonly when the blood of dizygous twins mixes *in utero.* **irradiation c.** RADIATION CHIMERA. **isologous c.** A chimera formed by cells or tissues from two different organisms that have the same genotype. Such a case is difficult to recognize in humans, but it might occur when the blood of monozygous twins mixes *in utero.* **radiation c.** An organism displaying immunologic characteristics of both host and donor following whole-body irradiation to neutralize an immune response to the donor's cells, as in a bone marrow graft. Also *irradiation chimera.* **tetraparental c.** An animal derived from four parents. This is achieved by fusing two allogeneic early blastocysts and reimplanting the fusion product in the uterus. Tetraparental chimeras allow the relative effects of genetic constitution and early environment of the development of immunologic tolerance and reactivity to be studied.

**chimerism** \kīmer′izm\ [*chimer(a)* + -ISM] The existence in an individual organism of more than one genetically distinct stable cell line of the same species. In humans, spontaneous chimerism occurs most often when blood cells from one dizygous twin mix with the co-twin *in utero.* Chimerism also results from any organ transplantation other than one between identical twins. **blood group c.** Having two stable, genetically distinct lines of blood cells, which can often be distinguished based on differences in blood group antigens. In humans, this most often arises when blood cells from one dizygous twin mix with the co-twin *in utero.*

**chin** [Old English *cinn,* akin to L *gena* jaw, cheek] The eminence below the mouth produced by the arched anterior part of the body of the mandible projecting beyond the alveolar process; mentum. **double c.** A prominent fatty or fleshy fold under the chin.

**chincap** CHIN CUP.

**chinch** \chinch\ [Spanish *chinche* (from L *cimex,* gen. *cimicis,* bug, bedbug) bedbug] BEDBUG.

**chiniofon** The sodium salt of 7-iodo-8-oxyquinoline-5-sulfonic acid, given with sodium bicarbonate. It is used to kill amebas in the intestinal tract.

**chir-** \kīr-\ CHEIRO-.

***Chiracanthium*** \kī′rəkan′thē·əm\ A cosmopolitan genus of small spiders with whitish abdomens, some species of which are poisonous. The bite can cause local tissue destruction and a slight fever. Also *Cheiracanthium.*

**chiral** \kī′rəl\ [CHIR- + -AL] Not superposable with its mirror image. To be chiral a structure must lack both a plane of symmetry and a center of symmetry. A carbon atom attached to four different groups forms a chiral center.

**chirality** \kīral′itē\ [CHIRAL + -ITY] The property possessed by an object, e.g. a molecule, if it differs from its mirror image.

**chirismus** \kīriz′məs\ [New L (from Gk *cheir* the hand + *-ismos* -ISM)] Spasm involving the hand. *Obs.*

**chiro-** \kī′rō-\ CHEIRO-.

**chirobrachialgia** \-brā′kē·al′jə\ CHEIROBRACHIALGIA.

**chirognostic** \kī′rägnäs′tik\ CHEIROGNOSTIC.

**chiromegaly** \-meg′əlē\ CHEIROMEGALY.

**chiropodalgia** \-pōdal′jə\ CHEIROPODALGIA.

**chiropodical** \-pō′dikəl\ Of or relating to chiropody (podiatry).

**chiropodist** \kīräp′ōdist\ [CHIRO- + -POD + -IST] PODIATRIST.

**chiropody** \kīräp′ōdē\ [CHIRO- + -POD + -Y] PODIATRY.

**chiropractic** \-prak′tik\ [CHIRO- + Gk *praktik(os)* fit for doing, able] A therapeutic system based on the doctrine that the nervous system largely determines the state of health and which utilizes manipulation, particularly of the spinal column.

**chiropractor** \-prak′tər\ A practitioner of chiropractic.

**chirospasm** \kī′rōspazm\ CHEIROSPASM.

**chirurgeon** \kīrur′jən\ [See SURGEON.] *Obs.* SURGEON.

**chirurgery** \kīrur′jərē\ [See SURGERY.] *Obs.* SURGERY.

**chisel** In dentistry, a hand instrument for cleaving enamel. **binangled c.** A chisel with two angles in its shank, for use in hard-to-reach places. **periodontal c.** A chisel scaler used with a pushing action.

**chi-square** \kī′-skwer′\ In statistics, a random variable derived from observations made on a random sample and having a known probability function. It is widely used to test for differences between two independently derived proportions, for homogeneity within a set of proportions, and for the goodness of fit between observations and their predicted or expected values. Symbol: $\chi^2$

**chitin** \kī′tin\ $C_{30}H_{50}O_{19}N_4$. A tough, insoluble polysaccharide that is the main constituent of the arthropod exoskeleton. It is also found in certain fungi.

**chitinase** An enzyme that hydrolyzes the glycosidic bonds in chitin, attacking them randomly.

**chitinous** \kī′tinəs\ Pertaining to or composed of chitin.

**chitoneure** \kī′tōnyʊr′\ [Gk *chitōn* shirt, tunic + *neur(on)*] The sheathing of axons in a nerve, formed collectively by the perineurium, endoneurium, and axonal neurilemmas. *Outmoded.*

**chlamydemia** \klam′idē′mē·ə\ The presence in the blood of chlamydial organisms.

***Chlamydia*** \klamid′ē·ə\ [New L, from Gk *chlamydion,* dim. of *chlamys,* gen. *chlamydos* a cloak, mantle] The sole genus of the family Chlamydiaceae, consisting of tiny, prokaryotic, obligately intracellular parasites, classified as a special type of bacterium. In their unique developmental cycle, multiplication occurs in a noninfectious, fragile, reticulate body, up to 1000 nm in diameter, which releases infectious elementary bodies. These are Gram-negative spheres of 300 nm diameter, specialized for survival outside the host cell. *Chlamydia* have a smaller genome than most bacteria. They depend on the host cell for ATP and many biosynthetic products, and they can be grown *in vivo* or in tissue culture. They are causative agents of the psittacosis-lymphogranuloma-trachoma disease group. Also *Bedsonia* (obs.), *Miyagawanella* (obs.). ***C. psittaci*** An infectious agent in a wide variety of birds. The infection is often latent but may give rise to active disease under stress. Organisms are shed in feces and discharges and remain infective in dust. In man the infection (ornithosis) also varies widely in severity. There is a marked immunologic cross-reactivity with *C. trachomatis.* • The specific name derives from the initial belief that the organism was restricted to psittacine birds (parrots). ***C. trachomatis*** A species restricted to humans. It is the cause of trachoma and, in developed countries, the much milder inclusion conjunctivitis, often transmitted from asymptomatic infection of the genital tract. It is a major cause of nongonococcal urethritis and of more serious infections of various parts of the genital tract, and is the cause of lymphogranuloma venereum. The relation of strain differences to this wide range of pathogenesis is not well established. The species is differentiated from *C. psittaci* by its susceptibility to sulfadiazine and by its producing glycogen in sufficient quantity to be detected by iodine stain.

**chlamydia** \klamid′ē·ə\ (*pl.* chlamydiae) Any member of the genus *Chlamydia.*

**chlamydiae** \klamid′i·ē\ Plural of CHLAMYDIA.

**chlamydial** \klamid′ē·əl\ Pertaining to or characteristic of members of the genus *Chlamydia.*

**chlamydiosis** \klamid′ē·ō′sis\ Any chlamydial infection.

**chlamydospore** \klam′idōspôr′\ [Gk *chlamys,* gen. *chlamydos,* a horseman's short cloak or mantle + SPORE] A thick-walled, intercalary, and terminal fungal hyphal cell that generally functions as a resting spore. Fungi that produce chlamydospores are often implicated in dermatophytosis.

**chloasma** \klō·az′mə\ [Gk, variant of *chlōrasma* (from *chlōros* green) greenness] MELASMA. **c. gravidarum** MELASMA GRAVIDARUM.

**chlor-** \klôr-\ CHLORO-.

**chloracetic acid** Any of the derivatives of acetic acid in which the hydrogens are replaced with one (mono-), two (di-), or three (tri-) chlorine atoms. Monochloroacetic acid, for example, is a keratolytic agent that is used to remove warts and corns.

**chloral** $Cl_3C—CHO$. 2,2,2-Trichloroacetaldehyde. It is a highly reactive aldehyde and remains hydrated (chloral hydrate) as $Cl_3C—CH(OH)_2$ on crystallization. It is hypnotic.

**chloral hydrate** $CCl_3—CH(OH)_2$. Since chloral is an extremely reactive aldehyde, it has a high affinity for all nucleophiles, including water. Hence the hydrate is a stable compound, and although it is interconvertible with the free aldehyde in aqueous solution, equilibrium greatly favors the hydrate, which is the only form easily isolable as a crystalline compound. It was formerly used medicinally as a soporific.

**chloralism** \klôr′əlizm\ A condition resulting from the excessive use of chloral, which may lead to confusion, incoordination, ataxia, respiratory distress, and coma. See also CHLORAL HYDRATE POISONING.

**chloralize** To treat with chloral hydrate.

**chlorambucil** $C_{14}H_{19}Cl_2NO_2$. 4-[Bis(2-chloroethyl-amino]benzenebutanoic acid, an antineoplastic, alkylating agent that is used in the treatment of chronic lymphocytic leukemia, malignant lymphomas, and Hodgkin's disease.

**chloramine-T** The sodium salt of *N*-chloro-*p*-toluenesulfonamide. It is remarkable in that the ammonia molecule becomes an acid strong enough to form a stable sodium salt when substituted by both chloro and tosyl groups. The substance is a mild chlorinating and oxidizing agent, used for disinfection.

**chloramphenicol** \-amfen′ikôl\ $C_{11}H_{12}C1_2N_2O_5$. An antibiotic produced synthetically and from cultures of *Streptomyces venezuelae.* It is used as an antibacterial agent, especially against salmonellae, and as an antirickettsial agent.

**chloramphenicol palmitate** The palmitate ester of chloramphenicol. It is used to avoid the bitter taste of chlorpromazine, and is hydrolyzed into the biologically active antibiotic by intestinal and tissue lipases.

**chlorate** A salt of chloric acid.

**chlorbutol** $CCl_3—CMe_2—OH$. A compound smelling of camphor, used as a mild antiseptic.

**chlorcyclizine hydrochloride** $C_{18}H_{22}Cl_2N_2$. 1-[(4-Chlorophenyl)phenylmethyl]-4-methylpiperazine hydrochloride, an antihistaminic drug that is given orally.

**chlordecone** \klôr′dēkōn\ $C_{10}C_{10}O$. A nondegradable polychlorinated ketone formerly used as an insecticide under the proprietary name Kepone, and having toxic effects on humans and marine life. Neurologic symptoms and sterility were among the effects noted in a poisoning episode in Virginia in 1974–1975.

**chlordiazepoxide hydrochloride** $C_{16}H_{15}Cl_2N_3O$. 7-Chloro-*N*-methyl-5-phenyl-3*H*-1,4-benzodiazepin-2-amine 4-oxide hydrochloride. A benzodiazepine tranquilizer that is used in the treatment of tension and anxiety states. It is given orally, intravenously, or intramuscularly.

**chlorhexidine gluconate** $C_{22}H_{30}Cl_2N_{10}·2C_6H_{12}O_7$. 1,1′-Hexamethylenebis[5-(4-chlorophenyl)biguanide]digluconate, a 20% aqueous solution which is used, after dilution, as a disinfectant in solutions, creams, and gels.

**chlorhydria** \-hī′drē·ə\ [CHLOR- + HYDR- + -IA] The presence of gastric acid secretion.

**chloride** **1** The ion $Cl^-$ or a salt that contains it. Although the chloride ion has a very low affinity for $H^+$, so that HCl is a strong acid, it is fairly nucleophilic in reactions at saturated carbon. **2** A chloro compound in organic chemistry, such as an acid chloride. **3** Chlorine in combination with a more electropositive element, as iodine chloride.

**chloridemia** \-idē′mē·ə\ HYPERCHLOREMIA.

**chlorinated** \klôr′inā′tid\ **1** Having hydrogen replaced by chlorine: used especially of a chemical compound. **2** Having chlorine in solution: used especially of water with chlorine added as a disinfectant.

**chlorine** \klôr′ēn\ Element number 17, having atomic weight 35.453. At ordinary temperatures, elemental chlorine is a greenish yellow poisonous gas with a penetrating odor. Liquid chlorine boils at −34.6°C. It is soluble in water and is used throughout the world to produce safe drinking water. Chemically a very active member of the halogen group of elements, chlorine is never found free in nature. Valences are 1, 3, 5, and 7. Chlorine ions are the principal cellular and extracellular anions in living organisms. Many compounds of chlorine, especially synthetic organic compounds, are highly toxic or carcinogenic or both, and have become very troublesome environmental pollutants. Symbol: Cl

**chlorisondamine chloride** $C_{14}H_{20}Cl_6N_2$. 4,5,6,7-Tetrachloro-1,3-dihydro-2-methyl-2-[2-(trimethylammonio)ethyl]-2*H*-isoindolium dichloride, a bis-quaternary ammonium derivative with ganglionic blocking properties. It is used therapeutically as an antihypertensive drug.

**chlormezanone** $C_{11}H_{12}ClNO_3S$. 2-(4-Chlorophenyl)tetrahydro-3-methyl-4*H*-1,3-thiazin-4-one 1,1 dioxide, a white, crystalline powder with tranquilizing and muscle relaxant properties. It is given orally.

**chloro-** \klôr′ō-, klôr′ə-\ [Gk *chlōros* light green] **1** A combining form designating the replacement of hydrogen by chlorine. **2** A combining form meaning green, especially pale green. Also *chlor-*.

**chlorobutanol** $C_4H_7Cl_3O$. 1,1,1-Trichloro-2-methyl-2-propanol, a colorless or white crystalline solid that has an odor resembling camphor. It has been used as an antimicrobial agent in pharmaceutical solutions and as a sedative in veterinary medicine.

**chlorodinitrobenzene** \-dīnī′trōben′zēn\ DICHLORONITROBENZENE.

**chloroform** \klôr′əfôrm\ $CHCl_3$. Trichloromethane. A volatile liquid used as a solvent and once used as an anesthetic. It is toxic to inhale, causing liver damage. It is also used as a reagent in organic synthesis. **liniment of c.** A mixture of chloroform and camphor liniment in equal amounts. It has been used externally as a rubefacient.

**chlorogenic acid** $C_{16}H_{18}O_9$. One of the components of the widely distributed caffetannins from coffee, maté, tobacco, cinchona, and nux vomica. Chemically it is the depside formed by acylation of quinic acid on O-3 with caffeic acid.

**chloroguanide hydrochloride** PROGUANIL HYDROCHLORIDE.

**chloroleukemia** \-lookē′mē·ə\ CHLOROMA.

**chloroma** \klôrō′mə\ [CHLOR- + -OMA] A variant of acute granulocytic leukemia, or occasionally of chronic granulocytic leukemia, in which green circumscribed tumors composed of leukemic cells occur; a form of granulocytic sarcoma. Also *chloroleukemia, green cancer* (obs.).

***P*-chloromercuribenzoate** $Cl—Hg—C_6H_4—COO^-$. A compound used in protein chemistry as a reagent for thiols. In solution, the chloride can leave the mercury atom and be replaced by hydroxide or, with great affinity, thiolate. Since the whole molecule is somewhat hydrophobic, it often reacts with thiol groups in proteins that are not accessible to most charged, or polar, reagents.

**chloromethane** $CH_3Cl$. A gas at ordinary temperature, but easily liquefied under pressure. It is an anesthetic, but is not usable because of its high toxicity. It is used in the chemical industry as a methylating agent. Chronic occupational exposure may produce a staggering gait, difficulty in speech, nausea, dizziness, and blurred vision. Acute exposure has similar effects with a shorter latency period. Coma and convulsions may also occur. Also *methyl chloride*.

**chloropenia** \-pē′nē·ə\ HYPOCHLOREMIA.

***p*-chlorophenol** PARACHLOROPHENOL.

**chlorophyll** \klôr′əfil\ [CHLORO- + Gk *phyllon* a leaf] The green plant and algal pigment that exists in five different forms of a porphyrin nucleus chelated with magnesium. It is an electron donor in photosynthesis. It has limited use as a deodorant. Also *chlorophyl* (outmoded spelling). **c. a** $C_{55}H_{72}O_5N_4Mg$. A blue-green chlorophyll that is universal in both higher plants and algae. It is a cyclic, tetrapyrrolic molecule containing a magnesium atom. It has absorption peaks in organic solvents at wavelengths of 420 and 660 nm. **c. b** $C_{55}H_{70}O_6N_4Mg$. A yellowish green chlorophyll found in plants and the algal divisions Chlorophycophyta and Euglenophycophyta. In contrast with chlorophyll a, it has a —CHO group on the third carbon instead of $—CH_3$. It has absorption peaks in organic solvents at wavelengths of 453 and 642 nm. **c. c** A chlorophyll found in algae of the divisions Bacillariophycophyta, Chrysophycophyta, Cryptophycophyta, Phaeophycophyta, and Pyrrophycophyta. It has absorption peaks in organic solvents at wavelengths of 425 to 625 nm. It consists of two closely related compounds. **c. d** $C_{54}H_{70}MgN_4O_6$. A chlorophyll found in algae of the division Rhodophycophyta. In organic solvents it has absorption peaks at wavelengths of 450 and 690 nm. Also *2-desvinyl-2-formyl chlorophyll a*.

**chloropia** \klôrō′pē·ə\ CHLOROPSIA.

**chloroplast** \klôr′ōplast\ [CHLORO- + -PLAST] A photosynthetic organelle found in eukaryotic cells. Also *chloroplastid*.

**chloroprocaine hydrochloride** $C_{13}H_{20}Cl_2N_2O_2$. 4-Amino-2-chlorobenzoic acid 2-diethylaminoethyl ester hydrochloride, a local anesthetic with properties like those of procaine.

**chloropsia** \klôräp′sē·ə\ [*chlor(o)-* + -OPSIA] Green vision, as may occur in digitalis poisoning. Also *chloropia*.

**chloropyrilene citrate** CHLOROTHEN CITRATE.

**chloroquine** $C_{18}H_{26}ClN_3$. $N^4$-(7-Chloro-4-quinolinyl)-$N',N'$-diethyl-1,4-pentanediamine. An aminoquinoline derivative with antimalarial activity. It is particularly effective against intraerythrocytic forms of the malarial parasite.

**chloroquine hydrochloride** The hydrochloride salt of chloroquine that is available for parenteral administration to patients unable to tolerate oral therapy. It is used to treat extraintestinal amebiasis.

**chlorosis** \klôrō′sis\ [CHLOR- + -OSIS] Iron deficiency anemia supposedly characterized by a greenish yellow pallor, especially in young women. Also *chlorotic anemia, green sickness*. **Egyptian c.** ANCYLOSTOME ANEMIA. **tropical c.** ANCYLOSTOME ANEMIA.

**chlorosulfonic acid** $Cl—SO_2—OH$. A yellow liquid that reacts violently with water, fuming in air; $d_4^{20} = 1.753$. The freezing point is −80°C, and the boiling point, 152°C. It is used as a condensing agent and to make sulfate esters, sulfones and saccharin.

**chlorothen citrate** $C_{14}H_{18}ClN_3S$, $C_6H_8O_7$. *N*-(5-Chlorothen-2-yl)-$N',N'$-dimethyl-*N*-pyrid-2-ylethylenediamine dihydrogen citrate. A white, crystalline powder, soluble in water and alcohol, practically insoluble in chloroform and ether. It is an oral antihistaminic agent. Also *chloropyrilene citrate*.

**chlorothiazide** $C_7H_6ClN_3O_4S_2$. 6-Chloro-2*H*-1,2,4-benzothiadiazine-7-sulfonamide 1,1-dioxide, a white crystalline powder with diuretic properties. Administered orally, it is used to treat various conditions that can lead to edema. edema.

**chloroxine** $C_9H_5Cl_2NO$. 5,7-Dichloro-8-quinolinol, a synthetic anti-infective agent that is structurally related to many other substituted 8-hydroxyquinoline compounds. It is used to treat dandruff and seborrheic dermatitis of the scalp by external application only.

**chlorpheniramine** $C_{16}H_{19}ClN_2$. γ-(4-Chlorophenyl)-*N,N*-dimethyl-2-pyridinepropanamine, a potent antihistaminic agent with a relatively short duration of three to six hours. It is generally given orally as the maleate.

**chlorphenoxamine hydrochloride** $C_{18}H_{23}Cl_2NO$. 2-[1-(4-Chlorophenyl)-1-phenylethoxy]-*N,N*-dimethylethanamine hydrochloride. It is an anticholinergic agent used in the treatment of Parkinson's disease, and it is given orally.

**chlorpromazine** $C_{17}H_{19}ClN_2S$. 2-Chloro-10-(3-dimethylaminopropyl)phenothiazine. The prototype phenothiazine antipsychotic drug. It has tranquilizing properties, reduces spontaneous motor activity, has antiemetic activity, and alters the body temperature control mechanisms.

**chlorpropamide** $C_{10}H_{13}ClN_2O_3S$. 4-Chloro-*N*-[(propylamino)carbonyl]benzenesulfonamide, an oral hypoglycemic agent of the sulfonurea class. It is given orally in the treatment of diabetes.

**chlorprothixene** $C_{18}H_{18}ClNS$. 3-(2-Chloro-9*H*-thioxanthen-9-ylidene)-*N,N*-dimethyl-1-propanamine, a psychotropic drug of the thioxanthene class. It is used as a tranquilizer and to control symptoms in psychotic patients and is given orally or by intramuscular injection.

**chlorquinaldol** $C_{10}H_7Cl_2NO$. 5,7-Dichloro-2-methyl-8-quinolinol. An oxyquinoline derivative with antibacterial and antifungal properties. It is used topically, usually in an ointment or cream form, to treat minor skin infections.

**chlortetracycline** \klôr′tetrəsī′klēn\ $C_{22}H_{23}ClN_2O_8$. A broad-spectrum antibiotic biosynthesized by *Streptomyces aureofaciens.*

**chlorthalidone** $C_{14}H_{11}ClN_2O_4S$. 2-Chloro-5-(1-hydroxy-3-oxo-1-isoindolinyl)benzenesulfonamide. A variant form of the benzothiadiazine diuretics with the same type of action on the kidney. It is used as a diuretic and antihypertensive medication.

**chloruresis** \klôr′yoorē′sis\ [*chlor(ide)* + -URESIS] The excretion of greater than normal amounts of chloride in the urine.

**chloruretic** \klôr′yooret′ik\ **1** Any condition or drug that increases urinary chloride excretion. **2** Pertaining to chloruresis.

**chloruria** \klôryoo′rē·ə\ [*chlor(ide)* + -URIA] The excretion of chloride in the urine.

**chlorzoxazone** $C_7H_4ClNO_2$. 5-Chloro-2(3*H*)-benzoxazololone, a muscle relaxant drug chemically unrelated to mephenesin but similar in its pharmacological properties. It is given orally.

**choana** \kō′ənə\ [Gk *choanē*, a funnel, a funnel-shaped hollow] (*pl.* choanae) [NA] An oval aperture on each side of the posterior border of the nasal septum, communicating each nasal fossa with the nasal pharynx. The bony constituents of these openings are the choanae osseae, comprising on each side the horizontal plate of the palatine bone below, the base of the skull above, and laterally the medial pterygoid plate. They are separated from each other by the posterior border of the vomer in the median plane. Also *posterior naris, postnaris, posterior nasal aperture, internal naris* (outmoded). **choanae osseae** The bones forming the framework of each choana. Also *bony choanae.* **primitive c.** One of two internal nasal orifices in the embryo. The nasal cavities, which initially are blind sacs, overlie the roof of the front part of the primitive mouth and are separated from it only by membranes. The membranes thin and rupture during the seventh week of human gestation to create the primitive choanae. The openings are closed subsequently by formation of the palate and are supplanted by the secondary, or definitive, choanae, which open into the pharynx. Also *primary choana.* **secondary c.** The definitive choana in the embryo established by the extension posteriorly of the original nasal cavities due to the formation of the definitive palate by the fusion of the palatal shelves. Growth of the nasal septum and fusion with the cephalic surface of the hard palate establishes the two separate choanae, continuous with the pharynx posteriorly.

**choanae** \kō′ānē\ Plural of CHOANA.

**choanate** \kō′ənāt\ Possessing a funnel-like opening, or infundibulum.

**choice / germinal c.** The selection of germ cells from individuals with specific characteristics to be used in selective breeding, either immediately or in the future. It is a method advocated by some for positive eugenics in humans. **object c.** The choice of one person or object which is elevated to the status of most significant other for the subject at any particular time. The apparent choice may be largely forced on the subject by reason of immaturity and physical dependence, but at other times the subject may consciously select an object, based on determining or predisposing factors, in order to gain gratification.

**choke** [Old English *acēocian* to strangle] **1** To obstruct breathing by occluding the respiratory airways at a site between the mouth and the tracheal bifurcation. **2** To obstruct air or fluid flow. **ophthalmovascular c.** PAPILLEDEMA.

**choking** Sudden inability to breathe due to acute obstruction of the pharynx, larynx, or trachea.

**chol-** \kōl-, käl-, kəl-\ CHOLE-.

**cholagogic** Having the action of a cholagogue.

**cholagogue** [CHOL- + -AGOGUE] A compound that stimulates the flow of bile, particularly by contraction of the gallbladder.

**cholane** 17-(1-Methylbutyl)-androstane. The parent hydrocarbon of the bile acids.

**cholangeitis** \kō′lanjē·ī′tis\ CHOLANGITIS.

**cholangiectasis** \kōlan′jē·ek′təsis\ [*cholangi(o)-* + ECTASIS] Dilatation of the bile ducts, usually as a result of obstruction. Also *cholangiectasia.*

**cholangio-** \kəlan′jē·ō-, kōlan′jē·ō-\ [CHOL- + ANGIO-] A combining form meaning bile duct.

**cholangioadenoma** \-ad′ənō′mə\ INTRAHEPATIC BILE DUCT ADENOMA.

**cholangiocarcinoma** \-kär′sənō′mə\ [CHOLANGIO- + CARCINOMA] An intrahepatic malignant tumor composed of cells resembling those of biliary epithelium. Unlike hepatocellular carcinoma, cholangiocarcinoma is infrequently associated with cirrhosis. Also *intrahepatic bile duct carcinoma, malignant cholangioma.*

**cholangioenterostomy** \-en′təräs′təmē\ [CHOLANGIO- + ENTERO- + -STOMY] A surgical procedure creating a connection between a bile duct and the small intestine, usually performed for relief of an absolute or relative obstruction of the distal bile duct. The connection is only rarely the result of inflammatory or neoplastic disease, or trauma.

**cholangiogastrostomy** \-gasträs′təmē\ [CHOLANGIO- + GASTRO- + -STOMY] A surgical procedure that creates a connection between a bile duct and the stomach. This may also result from neoplastic, inflammatory, or traumatic disease, occurring spontaneously, but this is rare.

**cholangiography** \kōlan′jē·äg′rəfē\ [CHOLANGIO- + -GRAPHY] Radiographic examination of the biliary ducts after their opacification by a suitable contrast medium administered intravenously, injected directly through the liver percutaneously or at the time of surgery, or after endoscopic cannulation of the ampulla of Vater. **cystic duct c.** Roentgenographic study of the biliary system after instillation of contrast medium into the cystic duct during biliary surgery. **intravenous c.** Radiographic examination of the common bile duct and gallbladder after the intravenous administration of a radiopaque agent which is selectively taken up by the liver and excreted into the biliary system. **operative c.** Cholangiography done at the time of surgical exposure of the gallbladder or biliary ducts. **percutaneous transhepatic c.** Roentgenography of the biliary ducts after their opacification by a water-soluble positive contrast medium injected through a thin needle, the tip of which has been placed in a bile duct after percutaneous puncture of the liver. Also *percutaneous cholangiography, transhepatic cholangiography.* **T-tube c.** Cholangiography by the instillation of contrast medium into the stem of a T-tube whose arms are in the common bile duct.

**cholangiohepatitis** \-hep′ətī′tis\ [CHOLANGIO- + HEPATITIS] Pyogenic inflammation, often caused by obstruction, involving the extrahepatic bile ducts and ascending into the intrahepatic biliary system and liver parenchyma. It may be caused by liver flukes, such as *Fasciola hepatica, F. gigantica,* or *Clonorchis sinensis.*

**cholangiohepatoma** \-hep′ətō′mə\ A combined hepatocellular carcinoma and cholangiocarcinoma.

**cholangiojejunostomy** \-jəjoonäs′təmē\ [CHOLANGIO- + JEJUNO- + -STOMY] A surgical procedure that creates a connection between a bile duct and the proximal part of the small intestine, usually performed to relieve a relative or absolute bile duct obstruction. This connection rarely results from neoplastic, traumatic, or inflammatory disease, occurring spontaneously. **intrahepatic c.** A surgical procedure creating an opening between a bile duct within the substance of the liver and the proximal part of the small intestine. It is most often done to relieve a partial or complete distal bile duct obstruction that is of benign or malignant etiology.

**cholangiole** \kōlan′jē·ōl\ [*cholangi(o)-* + -OLE] One of the small, thin-walled ductules that connect the bile canaliculi to the interlobular bile ducts. It is now considered part of the ductuli biliferi. Also *canal of Hering.*

**cholangiolitis** \kōlan′jē·ōlī′tis\ [*cholangiol(e)* + -ITIS] Inflammation of the small intrahepatic biliary radicles. Adj. cholangiolitic.

**cholangioma** \kōlan′jē·ō′mə\ [*cholangi(o)-* + -OMA] INTRAHEPATIC BILE DUCT ADENOMA. • Usage without the adjective *benign* should be discouraged, as it may be misused for a malignant tumor (cholangiocarcinoma). **benign c.** INTRAHEPATIC BILE DUCT ADENOMA. **malignant c.** CHOLANGIOCARCINOMA.

**cholangioscopy** \kōlan′jē·äs′kəpē\ CHOLEDOCHOSCOPY.

**cholangiostomy** \kōlan′jē·äs′təmē\ [CHOLANGIO- + -STOMY] A surgical procedure that creates an opening in the bile duct, for purposes of internal drainage. It usually involves insertion of a T tube if the drainage is to be external, as in the case of a common duct exploration.

**cholangiotomy** \kōlan′jē·ät′əmē\ [CHOLANGIO- + -TOMY] A surgical incision into a bile duct, usually for the purpose of exploration and/or drainage of the biliary tree.

**cholangitis** \kō′lanjī′tis\ [*cholang(io)-* + -ITIS] Inflammation of the intrahepatic or extrahepatic biliary ducts, most commonly associated with choledocholithiasis. Also *cholangeitis.* **acute suppurative c.** Acute pyogenic inflammation of the bile ducts, often seen in conjunction with distal obstruction by a common bile duct stone. **nonsuppurative c.** Inflammatory destruction of the interlobular and septal bile ducts, as occurs in primary biliary cirrhosis. **primary sclerosing c.** A fibrosing inflammation of unknown origin involving segments of the extrahepatic bile ducts with or without involvement of the intrahepatic ducts, which results in progressive narrowing and obliteration of the bile duct lumens. **secondary sclerosing c.** A fibrosing inflammation of the bile ducts caused by obstruction at a site distal to the inflammation.

**cholanic acid** The parent structure from which bile acids may be named. It may be considered to be derived from cholesterol by removal of the 3-hydroxyl group, saturation of the double bond, and removal of the end of the side chain leaving C-24 as a carboxyl group. Two structures are thus derived, according to the stereochemistry with which the 5,6 double bond is saturated. Of these, 5$\beta$-cholanic acid, with the 5-H in the $\beta$-position, i.e. toward the viewer in the conventional way of drawing steroid formulas, and with an angle between the planes of rings A and B, is the one from which most bile acids are derived.

**cholanopoiesis** \kō′lənōpoi·ē′sis\ [*cholan(ic)* + *o* + -POIESIS] The formation of bile acids, their conjugates, and salts by the liver.

**chole-** \kō′lə-\ [Gk *cholē* gall, bile] A combining form denoting bile. Also *chol-, cholo-.*

**cholecalciferol** The form of vitamin D obtained by irradiating 7-dehydrocholesterol. It may be formed by the action of light on the skin, which explains the beneficial effect of sunlight in the prevention of rickets. It contains ring B of cholesterol broken and a conjugated 5,7,10(19)-triene system. Also *vitamin* $D_3$.

**cholecyst-** CHOLECYSTO-.

**cholecystagogue** \-sis′təgäg\ [CHOLECYST- + -AGOGUE] An agent that stimulates contraction of the gallbladder.

**cholecystectasia** \-sis′tektā′zhə\ [CHOLECYST- + ECTASIA] Dilatation of the gallbladder.

**cholecystectomy** \-sistek′təmē\ [CHOLECYST- + -ECTOMY] The surgical removal of the gallbladder and its contents. It may be done because of inflammatory disease, stone disease, or, rarely, for neoplastic processes. It may be combined with a common bile duct exploration.

**cholecystenteric** \-sis′tenter′ik\ [CHOLECYST- + ENTERIC] Pertaining to a communication or relation between the gallbladder and the luminal gastrointestinal tract.

**cholecystenteroanastomosis** \-sisten′tərō·ənas′təmō′sis\ [CHOLECYST- + ENTERO- + ANASTOMOSIS] A surgical connection between the gallbladder and the small intestine, usually the proximal jejunum. This is frequently done to bypass an obstructed biliary tree, if the cystic duct is patent and the obstruction is distal. It may result from inflammatory or neoplastic diseases or occur spontaneously, but this is rare. Also *cholecystoenteroanastomosis, enterocholecystostomy.*

**cholecystenterostomy** \-sisten′təräs′təmē\ [CHOLECYST- + ENTERO- + -STOMY] A surgical anastomosis of the gallbladder to the small intestine. Also *cholecystoenterostomy, cholecystenterorrhaphy.*

**cholecystgastrostomy** \-sist′gasträs′təmē\ [CHOLECYST- + GASTRO- + -STOMY] A surgical procedure that creates a connection between the gallbladder and the stomach. It may result spontaneously, though rarely, from inflammatory, neoplastic, or traumatic processes as well. Also *cholecystogastrostomy.*

**cholecystic** \-sis′tik\ [CHOLECYST- + -IC] Of or relating to the gallbladder.

**cholecystis** \-sis′tis\ [New L, from CHOLE- + CYSTIS ] VESICA BILIARIS.

**cholecystitis** \kō′lēsistī′tis\ [CHOLECYST- + -ITIS] Inflammation of the gallbladder. It may be acute or chronic, is most commonly associated with cholelithiasis, and causes pain in the right upper quadrant of the abdomen. **c. cystica** ADENOMYOMATOSIS OF THE GALLBLADDER. **emphysematous c.** A form of cholecystitis in which the gallbladder wall contains gas as a manifestation of infection by gas-producing bacteria. Also *cholecystitis emphysematosa, pneumocholecystitis, gaseous cholecystitis, gaseous pericholecystitis.* **c. glandularis proliferans** ADENOMYOMATOSIS OF THE GALLBLADDER.

**cholecystnephrostomy** \-sist′nəfräs′təmē\ [CHOLECYST- + NEPHRO- + -STOMY] A surgical procedure that creates a connection between the gallbladder and a kidney, usually the renal pelvic kidney. It may result, though rarely, from inflammatory, neoplastic, or traumatic causes as well. Also *cholecystonephrostomy.*

**cholecysto-** [CHOLE- + CYSTO-] A combining form meaning gallbladder. Also *cholecyst-.*

**cholecystocele** \-sis′təsēl\ [CHOLECYSTO- + -CELE] A cystic dilatation of the gallbladder which may be congenital or result from inflammation.

**cholecystocholangiogram** \-sis′təkōlan′jē·ōgram′\ A roentgenogram of the gallbladder and bile ducts after their opacification by a contrast medium, administered either orally or intravenously or by direct injection at the time of surgery.

**cholecystocolostomy** \-sis′təkōläs′təmē\ [CHOLECYSTO- + COLO- + -STOMY] A surgical procedure creating an opening between the gallbladder and the large intestine, usually the hepatic flexure or right transverse colon. It may result, though rarely, from inflammatory, neoplastic, or traumatic causes occurring spontaneously. Also *colocholecystostomy, cholecystocolotomy.*

**cholecystoduodenostomy** \-sis′təd$^y$oo′ōdēnäs′təmē\ [CHOLECYSTO- + DUODENO- + -STOMY] A surgical procedure that creates an opening between the gallbladder and the duodenum. It is usually done for relief of a distal biliary obstruction but it can result from trauma. Also *duodenocholecystostomy, duodenocystostomy.*

**cholecysto-endysis** \-sis′tō·en′disis\ [CHOLECYSTO- + Gk *endysis* a putting on, entering] CHOLECYSTOTOMY.

**cholecystoenteroanastomosis** \-sis′tō·en′tərō·ənas′təmō′sis\ CHOLECYSTENTEROANASTOMOSIS.

**cholecystoenterostomy** \-sis′tō·en′təräs′təmē\ CHOLECYSTENTEROSTOMY.

**cholecystoenterotomy** \-sis′tō·en′tərät′əmē\ [CHOLECYSTO- + ENTEROTOMY] A surgical incision into the intestine and the gallbladder. Also *enterocholecystotomy.*

**cholecystogastrostomy** \-sis′təgasträs′təmē\ CHOLECYSTGASTROSTOMY.

**cholecystography** \-sistäg′rəfē\ Radiographic visualization of the gallbladder after the oral administration of tetraiodophenothalein compounds. Also *Graham's test, gallbladder function test.* **post fatty meal c.** BOYDEN'S TEST.

**cholecystoileostomy** \-sis′tō·il′ē·äs′təmē\ [CHOLECYSTO- + ILEO- + -STOMY] A surgical procedure creating an opening between the gallbladder and the distal small intestine. Although it is usually created surgically, it may result from traumatic, neoplastic, or inflammatory causes as well.

**cholecystojejunostomy** \-sis′təjējoonäs′təmē\ [CHOLECYSTO- + JEJUNO- + -STOMY] A surgical anastomosis of the gallbladder to the jejunum.

**cholecystokinin** \-sis′təkī′nin\ A 33-residue peptide hormone secreted by the duodenal and upper jejunal mucosa. It stimulates the gallbladder to contract and release pancreatic enzymes and bile. It is found also in cells of the hypothalamus and may participate in the regulation of appetite. Deranged metabolism of the hormone occurs in Zollinger-Ellison syndrome, exocrine pancreatic insufficiency, celiac disease, and perhaps in some cases of irritable bowel syndrome. Also *pancreozymin.* Abbr. CCK

**cholecystolithotomy** \-sis′təlithät′əmē\ [CHOLECYSTO- + LITHOTOMY] The surgical removal of the stones from within the cavity of the gallbladder. It is usually associated with a cholecystectomy or cholecystostomy. Also *cholelithotomy.*

**cholecystolithotripsy** \-sis′təlith′ətrip′sē\ [CHOLECYSTO- + LITHOTRIPSY] A surgical procedure in which the stones within the gallbladder are crushed. It is usually associated with a cholecystectomy or cholecystostomy. Also *cholelithotripsy.*

**cholecystonephrostomy** \-sis′tənəfräs′təmē\ CHOLECYSTNEPHROSTOMY.

**cholecystopathy** \-sistäp′əthē\ [CHOLECYSTO- + -PATHY] Any disorder of the gallbladder.

**cholecystopyelostomy** \-sis′təpī′əläs′təmē\ [CHOLECYSTO- + PYELO- + -STOMY] A surgical procedure creating an opening between the gallbladder and the renal pelvis. The opening may occur spontaneously from inflammatory, neoplastic, or traumatic etiologies, but this is rare.

**cholecystorrhaphy** \-sistôr′əfē\ [CHOLECYSTO- + -RRHAPHY] The suturing of an opening in the gallbladder, usually an opening resulting from an incision or rupture.

**cholecystostomy** \-sistäs′təmē\ [CHOLECYST- + -OSTOMY] A surgical procedure creating an opening between the gallbladder and the skin. It is usually accomplished by placing a tube in the gallbladder. The procedure is most often performed if an inflammatory biliary tract disease is present and a cholecystectomy is unsafe.

**cholecystotomy** \-sistät′əmē\ [CHOLECYSTO- + -TOMY] An opening into the gallbladder that is usually surgically created. It may, however, result from inflammatory, neoplastic, or traumatic etiologies. Also *cholecysto-endysis, cystifellotomy, laparocholecystotomy.*

**choledoch-** \kōled′ək-\ CHOLEDOCHO-.

**choledochal** Pertaining to the ductus choledochus, or common bile duct.

**choledochectomy** \kō′lədäkek′təmē\ [CHOLEDOCH- + -ECTOMY] A surgical procedure in which all or part of the common bile duct is excised. It may be performed for neoplastic, traumatic or inflammatory disease, and it is associated in most cases with a choledochoenterostomy.

**choledochendysis** \kō′lədäken′disis\ [CHOLEDOCH- + Gk *endysis* an entering] CHOLEDOCHOTOMY.

**choledochitis** \kō′lədäkī′tis\ [CHOLEDOCH- + -ITIS] Inflammation of the common bile duct.

**choledocho-** \kōled′əkō-\ [Gk *cholēdochos* (from *cholē* bile + *dechesthai* to accept, receive) containing bile] A combining form denoting the common bile duct.

**choledochocholedochostomy** \-kōled′əkäs′təmē\ [CHOLEDOCHO- + CHOLEDOCHO- + -STOMY] A surgical procedure that creates an opening between two segments of the common bile duct, usually after resection of a small segment of bile duct for stricture, neoplasm, or trauma. Also *choledochodochorrhaphy.*

**choledochocystostomy** \-sistäs′təmē\ [CHOLEDOCHO- + CYSTO- + -STOMY] A surgical procedure creating an opening between the gallbladder and the common bile duct. Rarely, such an opening may result spontaneously from trauma, inflammation, or a neoplastic disease process.

**choledochodochorrhaphy** \-däkôr′əfē\ CHOLEDOCHOCHOLEDOCHOSTOMY.

**choledochoduodenostomy** \-d$^y$oo′ōdēnäs′təmē\ [CHOLEDOCHO- + DUODENO- + -STOMY] A surgical procedure that creates an opening between the common bile duct and the duodenum. It is usually created for distal bile duct obstruction. Rarely, it may result spontaneously from a neoplastic, inflammatory, or traumatic disease process.

**choledochoenterostomy** \-en′teräs′təmē\ [CHOLEDOCHO- + ENTERO- + -STOMY] A surgical procedure that creates an opening between the common bile duct and the small intestine. It is usually performed to relieve relative or absolute stricture of the distal bile duct, but it may result spontaneously from trauma, inflammatory disease, or neoplasm.

**choledochogastrostomy** \-gasträs′təmē\ [CHOLEDOCHO- + GASTRO- + -STOMY] A surgical procedure to create an opening between the common bile duct and the stomach. It may result spontaneously from trauma, neoplasm, or inflammatory disease, but such occurrences are rare.

**choledochography** \kōled′əkäg′rəfē\ [CHOLEDOCHO- + -GRAPHY] Radiography of the common bile duct which has been opacified by an appropriate contrast medium.

**choledochohepatostomy** \-hep′ətäs′təmē\ [CHOLEDOCHO- + HEPATO- + -STOMY] The surgical procedure that creates an opening between the common bile duct and some part of the intrahepatic biliary tree.

**choledochoileostomy** \-il′ē·äs′təmē\ [CHOLEDOCHO- + ILEO- + -STOMY] A surgical procedure to create an opening between the common bile duct and the distal portion of the small bowel. Rarely, such an opening may occur spontaneously as a result of trauma or neoplastic or inflammatory disease.

**choledochojejunostomy** \-jējoonäs′təmē\ The surgical opening of communication between the common bile duct and the proximal portion of the small bowel. It is usually created to bypass relative or absolute obstruction of the distal bile duct, which can be of inflammatory, traumatic, or neoplastic origin.

**choledocholith** \kōled′əkōlith′\ [CHOLEDOCHO- + -LITH] A common bile duct calculus.

**choledocholithiasis** \-lithī′əsis\ [CHOLEDOCHO- + LITHIASIS] A condition in which calculi are present in the bile ducts.

**choledocholithotomy** \-lithät′əmē\ [CHOLEDOCHO- + LITHOTOMY] A surgical procedure in which the common bile duct is explored and stones are removed.

**choledocholithotripsy** \-lith′ətrip′sē\ [CHOLEDOCHO- + LITHOTRIPSY] A surgical procedure in which the common bile duct is explored and stones within the duct are crushed to permit their passage through the ampulla.

**choledochonephroscope** \-nef′rōskōp\ An endoscopic instrument that is used to visualize the interior of the kidney collecting system or the common bile duct. The instrument can also be used for stone manipulation.

**choledochoplasty** \kōled′əkōplas′tē\ [CHOLEDOCHO- + -PLASTY] An operation on the common bile duct, especially one to restore a lumen of adequate size in an area of stricture.

**choledochorrhaphy** \kōled′əkôr′əfē\ [CHOLEDOCHO- + -RRHAPHY] Suture repair of an incised, torn, or divided common bile duct.

**choledochoscope** \kōled′əkōskōp′\ A flexible fiberoptic instrument which allows intraoperative visualization of the biliary tract lumen. It is used primarily to detect bile duct stones or tumors.

**choledochoscopy** \kōled′əkäs′kəpē\ Visualization of the lumen of the extrahepatic bile ducts during surgery by use of a choledochoscope. Also *cholangioscopy*.

**choledochostomy** \kōled′əkäs′təmē\ [CHOLEDOCHO- + -STOMY] A surgical procedure creating an opening into the common bile duct in order to facilitate drainage and/or exploration of the duct.

**choledochotomy** \kōled′əkät′əmē\ [CHOLEDOCHO- + -TOMY] An incision into the common bile duct, created either surgically or as a result of trauma. Also *choledochendysis*.

**choledochus** \kōled′əkəs\ [Gk *cholēdochos* containing bile] DUCTUS CHOLEDOCHUS.

**cholehemothorax** \-hē′məthôr′aks\ CHOLOHEMOTHORAX.

**cholelith** \kō′ləlith\ [CHOLE- + -LITH] GALLSTONE.

**cholelithiasis** \-lithī′əsis\ A condition marked by the presence of stones in the gallbladder. Also *chololithiasis*.

**cholelithic** \-lith′ik\ [CHOLE- + LITH- + -IC] Of or relating to gallstones. Also *chololithic*.

**cholelithotomy** \-lithät′əmē\ CHOLECYSTOLITHOTOMY.

**cholelithotripsy** \-lith′ətrip′sē\ CHOLECYSTOLITHOTRIPSY.

**cholemia** \kōlē′mē·ə\ [CHOL- + -EMIA] The presence of bile salts and pigments in the systemic circulation. *Seldom used.* **familial c.** GILBERT SYNDROME.

**cholemic** \kōlē′mik\ Describing the appearance imparted to serum by the presence of excess bile pigments.

**choleperitoneum** \-per′itōnē′əm\ [CHOLE- + PERITONEUM] The presence of bile in the peritoneal cavity. Also *bile ascites*.

**choleperitonitis** \-per′itōnī′tis\ [CHOLE- + PERITONITIS] BILE PERITONITIS.

**cholepoiesis** \-poi·ē′sis\ [CHOLE- + -POIESIS] The process by which the liver synthesizes and secretes bile salts or other substances which comprise the bile. Also *bilifaction, biligenesis, cholopoiesis*.

**cholepoietic** \-poi·et′ik\ Referring to the formation of bile. Also *biligenetic, chologenetic*.

**cholera** \käl′ərə\ [Gk (of uncertain origin; perhaps akin to *cholē* bile or to *cholades* intestines) an intestinal disorder usually causing diarrhea] **1** A contagious disease caused by *Vibrio cholerae*, which produces a toxin that alters the water and electrolyte fluxes toward secretion in the upper intestinal tract, thereby causing a profuse, watery diarrhea resulting in severe dehydration and electrolyte imbalance. The disease is endemic in southeast Asia and India and epidemic globally. It is commonly transmitted in contaminated drinking water. Also *Asiatic cholera, indoloemia*. **2** See under EUROPEAN CHOLERA. **Asiatic c.** CHOLERA. **bilious c.** EUROPEAN CHOLERA. **dry c.** CHOLERA SICCA. **European c.** An acute gastroenteritis of uncertain etiology, usually characterized by bilious diarrhea and prevalent in southern Europe especially in the summer and early autumn. *Obs.* Also *bilious cholera*. • This dubious disease entity, originally known simply as *cholera*, lent its name to "Asiatic" cholera, a specific and much more severe disease, when the latter was epidemic in Europe at various times in the 19th century. Now only the "Asiatic" disease is normally referred to as *cholera*. **c. fulminans** CHOLERA SICCA. **c. infantum** INFANTILE GASTROENTERITIS. **pancreatic c.** VERNER-MORRISON SYNDROME. **c. sicca** Fatal cholera in which death is not preceded by vomiting and diarrhea. Also *dry cholera, cholera fulminans, cholera siderans*.

**choleragen** \käl′ərəjən\ CHOLERA TOXIN.

**choleraic** \käl′ərā′ik\ Pertaining to cholera.

**choleresis** \käl′ərē′sis\ [CHOLE- + *r* + -ESIS] Bile secretion by the liver.

**choleretic** \käl′əret′ik\ **1** Concerning bile secretion (choleresis). **2** An agent that promotes bile secretion by the liver.

**choleriform** \käl′erifôrm′\ Resembling cholera; cholera-like.

**cholerrhagia** \käl′ərā′jə\ [CHOLE- + -RRHAGIA] Excessive biliary flow.

**cholerrhagic** \käl′əraj′ik\ [CHOLE- + *-rrhag(ia)* + -IC] Pertaining to biliary flow.

**cholestane** $C_{27}H_{46}$. The parent hydrocarbon of the sterols. Its molecule consists of four fused rings, three being cyclohexane rings and one a cyclopentane ring, bearing two methyl groups at ring junctions, and bearing a 1-methylheptyl group on the five-membered ring. The name once designated 5$\alpha$-cholestane (with the name *coprostane* reserved for 5$\beta$-cholestane) but it is no longer restricted to one configuration at C-5.

**cholestasis** \-stā′sis\ [CHOLE- + -STASIS] Impairment of bile flow at any level from the canaliculus to the duodenum. The clinical condition resulting therefrom, characterized by icterus and pruritus, is due to the accumulation in blood and tissues of substances normally secreted in bile, particularly bilirubin, bile salts, and cholesterol. Also *cholestasia* (seldom used). **familial intrahepatic c.** BYLER'S DISEASE.

**cholesteatoma** \kō′ləstē·ətō′mə\ [irreg. from *choleste(rol)* (orig. regarded as the characteristic substance contained in the lesion) + -OMA, and assimilated in form to *steatoma*] **1** A variety of chronic otitis media, of which the principal feature is the occurrence, in the epitympanic or antral region of the middle ear, of a cystlike lesion lined with keratinizing stratified squamous epithelium and packed with keratin arranged in concentric sheets. From this focus, the disease may spread widely through the temporal bone, damaging the sound-conducting mechanism and leading sometimes to one or more intracranial complications, often of a serious nature. Cholesteatoma has been subdivided into primary and secondary varieties. The only treatment for cholesteatoma is surgery. • This particular condition is designated as acquired cholesteatoma to differentiate it from rare congenital cholesteatoma. **2** The cystlike lesion packed with keratin, occurring in cases of cholesteatoma. For defs. 1 and 2 also *cholesteatoma auris.* **3** A cystlike tumor containing keratin. Also *pearl tumor.* Adj. cholesteatomatous. **intracranial c.** A benign congenital tumor of ectodermal origin, arising usually from the skull or its diploë and compressing adjacent structures of the brain. The manifestations of such tumors depend upon their location. **paranasal sinus c.** **1** CHRONIC CASEOUS SINUSITIS. **2** A rare variety of sinusitis in which squamous metaplasia of the sinus lining is followed by the accumulation within the sinus of the products of desquamation. • This usage is misleading as this is not a true cholesteatoma **primary acquired c.** The variety of cholesteatoma that arises in the attic or posterosuperior quadrant of the tympanum with nothing to suggest predisposing middle-ear suppuration. Also *primary cholesteatoma.* **secondary acquired c.** The variety of cholesteatoma in which there is evidence of preceding chronic otitis media, usually in the form of a perforation. It is often a large perforation of the pars tensa membranae tympani. Also *secondary cholesteatoma.*

**cholesteatosis** \-stē′ətō′sis\ CHOLESTEATOMA.

**cholesteremia** \kōles′tərē′mē·ə\ HYPERCHOLESTEROLEMIA.

**cholesterinemia** \kōles′tərinē′mē·ə\ HYPERCHOLESTEROLEMIA.

**cholesterinosis** \kōles′tərinō′sis\ CHOLESTEROSIS.

**cholesterinuria** \kōles′tərinoo′rē·ə\ CHOLESTEROLURIA.

**cholesterohistechia** \kōles′tərōhistek′ē·ə \ *Obs.* CHOLESTEROSIS.

**cholesterol** \kōles′tərôl\ [earlier *cholesterin,* from French *cholestérine* (from Gk *cholē* bile + Gk *ster(eos)* solid + French *-ine* -IN) lit., solidified bile substance, as in gallstones; with -IN replaced by -OL to show the hydroxyl group] Cholest-5-en-3$\beta$-ol. The $\beta$ in the name signifies that the hydroxyl group is towards the viewer when the steroid skeleton is drawn in the conventional way. The atom O-3 is introduced during the cyclization step in biosynthesis when lanosterol is formed, to be converted subsequently into cholesterol. Cholesterol and its esters are important in giving rigidity to animal cell membranes, and it also serves as a precursor for bile acids and steroid hormones. **radioiodinated c.** Cholesterol that has been labeled with radioactive iodine, e.g. iodocholesterol I 125. It is used in metabolic studies.

**cholesterol acyltransferase** The enzyme (EC 2.3.1.26) responsible for forming esters of cholesterol by transferring an acyl group, which normally contains a *cis* double bond, from coenzyme A.

**cholesterolemia** \kōles′tərälē′mē·ə \ [CHOLESTEROL + -EMIA] The presence of cholesterol in the blood, a normal condition.

**cholesterol esterase** The enzyme (EC 3.1.1.13) responsible for hydrolyzing esters of cholesterol and some other sterols to liberate the sterol and fatty acid.

**cholesterolestersturz** \kōles′təräles′tərstʊrts′\ [German *Cholesterol* cholesterol + *Ester* ester + *Sturz* a fall, tumble] A reduction in the proportion of cholesterol esters to cholesterol in blood.

**cholesterolosis** \kōles′tərälō′sis\ CHOLESTEROSIS. **c. of the gallbladder** A condition seen in the gallbladder of multiparous women, characterized by yellow flecks of lipid that decorate the mucosa. Microscopically, cholesterol-filled histiocytes accumulate beneath a normal epithelium. There is usually minimal to moderate evidence of inflammation, and cholesterol is found in high concentration in the bile.

**cholesteroluria** \kōles′tərälooʹrē·ə\ [CHOLESTEROL + -URIA] The excretion of increased amounts of cholesterol in the urine, characteristic of patients with nephrotic syndrome, in whose urine cholesterol esters are present in oval fat bodies. Also *cholesterinuria.*

**cholesterosis** \kōles′tərō′sis\ [*cholester(ol)* + -OSIS] Excessive or abnormal deposition of cholesterol in tissues, such as the cutaneous xanthomas of familial hypercholesterolemia. *Rare.* Also *cholesterolosis, cholesterinosis, cholesterohistechia* (obs.). **c. cutis** *Seldom used* XANTHOMA.

**cholestyramine resin** A copolymer of styryl-divinylbenzene containing strongly basic quaternary ammonium groups, used to chelate bile acids in the intestinal tract and prevent reabsorption of excessive bile acids.

**cholic** \kō′lik\ [CHOL- + -IC] Pertaining to bile.

**cholic acid** 3$\alpha$,7$\alpha$,12$\alpha$-Trihydroxy-5$\beta$-cholanic acid. One of the principal acids in mammalian bile, it is found in conjugation with taurine and glycine.

**choline** \kō′lēn\ $Me_3N^+—CH_2—CH_2—OH$. 2-Hydroxyethyltrimethylammonium. It is important as a constituent of phosphatidylcholine in membranes and of the neurotransmitter acetylcholine. It is formed by methylation of glycinol (ethanolamine, 2-aminoethanol) by *S*-adenosylmethionine. Also *transmethylation factor.*

**choline acetyltransferase** An enzyme (EC 2.3.1.6) that catalyzes the reaction acetyl-CoA + choline ⇌ CoA + *o*-acetylcholine. It effects the biosynthesis of the neurotransmitter acetylcholine. Also *choline acetylase* (outmoded).

**choline chloride carbamate** CARBACHOL.

**choline kinase** An enzyme (EC 2.7.1.32) that catalyzes the reaction: ATP + choline ⇌ ADP + *O*-phosphocholine, and thus phosphorylates choline. This is a preliminary to its reaction with CTP to expel pyrophosphate and form CDPcholine, which can react with diacylglycerol to form the phosphatidylcholine of phospholipids.

**cholinephosphotransferase** An enzyme (EC 2.7.8.2) that catalyzes the reaction: CDPcholine + 1,2-diacylglycerol ⇌ CMP + phosphatidylcholine. It is responsible for the incorporation of choline into phospholipids.

**cholinergic** \kō′linur′jik\ [*cholin(e)* + *erg(o)-* + -IC] Denoting a synapse, nerve terminal, or aggregate of neurons for which the principal neurotransmitter is acetylcholine. Also *cholinogenic, cholinoreactive.*

**choline salicylate** $C_{12}H_{19}NO_4$. 2-Hydroxy-*N,N,N*-trimethylethanaminium salt with 2-hydroxybenzoic acid (1:1), the choline salt of salicylic acid. It has the analgesic, antipyretic properties of salicylic acid and is given orally.

**cholinesterase** Any enzyme that catalyzes the hydrolysis of esters of choline. There are two main types. The first (acetylcholinesterase) is relatively specific for esters of acetic acid. The second type, which is sometimes called pseudocholinesterase, hydrolyzes butyrylcholine faster than acetylcholine and is found in plasma. **true c.** ACETYLCHOLINESTERASE.

**cholinoceptive** \kō′linōsep′tiv\ Reactive to acetylcholine: used especially of receptor sites, usually on the surface of effector cells, with which acetylcholine unites to produce an effect, or to which inhibitors of acetylcholine can bind to block the cell's responses.

**cholinogenic** \kō'linōjen′ik\ CHOLINERGIC.

**cholinolytic** \kō'linōlit′ik\ ANTICHOLINERGIC.

**cholinomimetic** \kō'linōmimet′ik\ Having actions resembling those of acetylcholine, but not actually mediated by that substance.

**cholinoreactive** \kō'linôrē·ak′tiv\ CHOLINERGIC.

**cholinoreceptors** \kō'linôrisep′tərs\ Receptor sites, located on cells of effectors innervated by cholinergic nerve fibers, that respond to acetylcholine released from these parasympathetic fibers. Compare CHOLINERGIC RECEPTOR.

**cholo-** \kō'lə-\ CHOLE-.

**chologenetic** \-jənet′ik\ CHOLEPOIETIC.

**cholohemothorax** \-hē'məthôr′aks\ Cholothorax with added blood. Also *cholehemothorax*.

**chololithiasis** \-lithī′əsis\ CHOLELITHIASIS.

**chololithic** \-lith′ik\ CHOLELITHIC.

**cholopoiesis** \-poi·ē′sis\ CHOLEPOIESIS.

**cholothorax** \-thôr′aks\ The presence of bile in the pleural cavity. It may result from a fistula across the diaphragm connecting an inflamed, distended gallbladder or bile ducts with the right pleural cavity.

**choluria** \kōloo′rē·ə\ [CHOL- + -URIA] The excretion of bile or bile pigments in the urine. Bile itself does not circulate or enter the urine. The dark color of urine, the yellow foam upon shaking, and the chemical reactions result from the presence of conjugated bilirubin.

**chondr-** \kändr-\ CHONDRO-.

**chondral** \kän′drəl\ Pertaining to or consisting of cartilage; cartilaginous.

**chondralloplasia** \kän'dralōplā′zhə\ CHONDRODYSTROPHY.

**chondrectomy** \kändrek′təmē\ [CHONDR- + -ECTOMY] The removal of cartilage, either by surgery or as a result of trauma.

**chondri-** \kän'drē-\ CHONDRIO-.

**chondric** \kän′drik\ Pertaining to cartilage.

**chondrification** \kän'drifikā′shən\ [CHONDRI- + -FICATION] The process of turning into cartilage. Also *cartilaginification*.

**chondrio-** \kän'drē·ō-\ [Gk *chondrios* (dim. of *chondros,* a grain) a small grain] A combining form meaning grain, granular. Also *chondri-*.

**chondritis** \kändrī′tis\ [CHONDR- + -ITIS] Any inflammatory disorder of cartilage. **costal c.** COSTOCHONDRITIS. **ear c.** Inflammation of the cartilage of the external ear. It is most often seen as a form of pressure necrosis after burns to the ear. It can generally be prevented by avoidance of pressure on the ear. **c. intervertebralis calcarea** INTERVERTEBRAL CALCINOSIS.

**chondro-** \kän'drō-\ [Gk *chondros* a grain, granule; cartilage] A combining form denoting cartilage. Also *chondr-*.

**chondroblast** \kän′drōblast\ CHONDROPLAST.

**chondroblastoma** \-blastō′mə\ [CHONDROBLAST- + -OMA] A relatively rare, benign tumor, characterized by highly cellular and relatively undifferentiated tissue with chondroblastlike cells together with giant cells of osteoclast type. Only small amounts of intercellular matrix are usually present. This is a lesion of the epiphyses of long bones adjacent to the cartilage plate. The tumor usually occurs in patients under 20 years of age. Also *Codman's tumor, epiphyseal chondroblastoma, calcifying giant cell tumor, epiphyseal chondromatous giant cell tumor.*

**chondrocalcinosis** \-kal'sinō′sis\ The presence within a joint cartilage of radiologically or crystographically demonstrable calcium, usually as calcium pyrophosphate dihydrate. Also *pseudogout* (incorrect). **articular c.** Inflammation of a joint resulting from the deposition of calcium pyrophosphate crystals in the articular cartilage and synovial fluid. It affects the knee and other large joints and occurs typically in association with metabolic diseases such has hemochromatosis, diabetes mellitus, and Wilson's disease.

**chondroclasis** \-klā′sis\ [CHONDRO- + -CLASIS] The resorption of cartilage, such as occurs during endochondral ossification.

**chondroclast** \kän′drōklast\ [CHONDRO- + -CLAST] A multinucleate giant cell that is considered to be responsible in part for resorption of cartilaginous tissue.

**chondrocranium** \-krā′nē·əm\ That part of the skull where ossification is preceded by chondrification. It is confined chiefly to the base of the skull, whereas the sides and vault of the skull are ossified directly in connective tissue by membranous ossification.

**chondrocyte** \kän′drōsīt\ [CHONDRO- + -CYTE] The formative cell of cartilaginous tissue. The cells lay down the cartilaginous matrix around them, thereby creating a series of spaces, or lacunae, in which the chondrocytes persist. Also *cartilage corpuscle, cartilage cell.*

**chondrodermatitis** \-dur'mətī′tis\ [CHONDRO- + DERMATITIS] **1** An inflammation of skin and cartilage. **2** CHRONIC NODULAR CHONDRODERMATITIS OF THE HELIX. **chronic nodular c. of the helix** A tender chronic inflammatory nodule of the margin of the helix that involves the dermis and the underlying perichondrial connective tissue. Also *chondrodermatitis nodularis chronica helicis, chondrodermatitis, Winkler's disease.*

**chondrodysplasia** \-displā′zhə\ [CHONDRO- + DYSPLASIA] CHONDRODYSTROPHY. **genotypic c.** ENCHONDROMATOSIS. **hyperplastic c.** HYPERPLASTIC CHONDRODYSTROPHY. **metaphyseal c., McKusick type** An autosomal recessive syndrome, most commonly found in Old Order Amish populations, characterized by short-limbed dwarfism; fine, sparse hair; and an immune deficiency that increases susceptibility to chicken pox and malignancy. Also *cartilage-hair hypoplasia, cartilage-hair hypoplasia syndrome.* **c. punctata** Either of two congenital skeletal dysplasias that share punctate calcifications in the epiphyses of the long bones and vertebral processes. An autosomal dominant form, known as the Conradi syndrome, Conradi's disease, Conradi-Hünermann syndrome, or Hünermann's disease, is associated with asymmetric limb shortening, depressed nasal bridge, and scoliosis. In a minority of cases cataracts, contractures, and ichthyosiform skin lesions are present. The autosomal recessive form, called the rhizomelic type, is characterized by severe rhizomelic dwarfism, coronal clefts in the vertebrae, a high frequency of cataracts and skin changes, and death in infancy. Dominant and X-linked recessive forms probably exist as well, the former being lethal in hemizygous males. Also *chondrodystrophia fetalis calcificans, stippled epiphyses syndrome.* **rhizomelic type c. punctata** See under CHONDRODYSPLASIA PUNCTATA. **unilateral c.** A disorder of cartilage growth in which portions of the epiphyseal plate of tubular bones become incorporated in mature bone. These enchondromas later resume growth, causing expansion of the bone with a liability to spontaneous fracture and crippling deformities. The condition is usually unilateral and may be associated with cataracts. Chondrosarcoma develops in ten percent of affected subjects. Also *Ollier's disease, multiple congenital enchondromas, Ollier's osteochondromatosis.*

**chondrodystrophia** \-distrō′fē·ə\ CHONDRODYSTROPHY. **c. fetalis** *Outmoded* ACHONDROPLASIA. **c. fetalis calcificans** CHONDRODYSPLASIA PUNCTATA.

**chondrodystrophy** \-dis′trəfē\ [CHONDRO- + DYSTROPHY] A condition characterized by abnormal development of cartilage, particularly of the limb epiphyses, resulting in stunted growth of the limbs and short stature (chondrodystrophic dwarfism), but with normally developed skull and spine. Also *Conradi-Raap syndrome, chondrodystrophia, chondrodysplasia, chondralloplasia.* **hyperplastic c.** Chondrodystrophy characterized by overgrowth of the epiphyses. Also *hyperplastic chondrodysplasia.* **hypoplastic c.** Chondrodystrophy characterized by vacuolated bone and irregular development of the epiphyses. **hypoplastic fetal c.** An inexact and outmoded term for ACHONDROPLASIA. **c. malacia** The abnormal development of cartilage accompanied by a softening of the growth plate.

**chondroepiphyseal** \-ep′ifizē′əl\ Pertaining to the epiphyseal cartilage or cartilages.

**chondroepiphysitis** \-ep′ifizī′tis\ An inflammation of the epiphyseal growth plates.

**chondrogenesis** \-jen′əsis\ The formation of cartilaginous tissue. Also *chondrosis.*

**chondrogenic** \-jen′ik\ [CHONDRO- + -GENIC] Of or related to cartilage formation. Also *chondrogenetic.*

**chondroglossus** \-gläs′əs\ MUSCULUS CHONDROGLOSSUS.

**chondrohypoplasia** \-hī′pōplā′zhə\ *Obs.* HYPOCHONDROPLASIA.

**chondroitin** A polysaccharide composed of alternate residues of *N*-acetylgalactosamine and glucuronic acid, linked as —GlcA($\beta$1-3)GalNAC($\beta$1-4)—. It occurs in the cornea.

**chondroitin sulfate** A glycosaminoglycan composed of alternate residues of $\beta$-D-glucuronic acid, glycosylated on O-4, and $\beta$-D-*N*-acetylgalactosamine 4- or 6-sulfate, glycosylated on O-3. Both chondroitin 4-sulfate and chondroitin 6-sulfate occur, and are a major constituent of cartilage.

**chondroitin sulfate B** DERMATAN SULFATE.

**chondrolipoma** \-lipō′mə\ A benign tumor of the mesenchyme that contains both cartilaginous and lipomatous tissue.

**chondrology** \kändräl′əjē\ [CHONDRO- + -LOGY] The scientific study of cartilage.

**chondrolysis** \kändräl′isis\ [CHONDRO- + LYSIS] The degeneration of cartilage cells which are then replaced by bone during intracartilaginous ossification or necrosis of articular cartilage, particularly of the hip.

**chondroma** \kändrō′mə\ [CHONDR- + -OMA] (*pl.* chondromas, chondromata) A relatively common, benign tumor characterized by the formation of mature cartilage, often involving the short tubular bones of the hands and feet. It is usually situated centrally (enchondroma) but may be periosteal or juxtacortical in location. **c. of lung** A relatively common tumorlike lesion with nodules of cartilage admixed with fibrous and adipose tissues, often intermingled with bronchial epithelium. It is considered to be a hamartoma rather than a true neoplasm. It rarely produces symptoms but because of its density appears on radiographs. Also *chondromatous hamartoma.* **medullary c.** ENCHONDROMA. **true c.** ENCHONDROMA.

**chondromalacia** \-məlā′shə\ [CHONDRO- + MALACIA] A softening of the articular cartilage. **c. fetalis** A condition in which the fetus is born dead with characteristically soft and pliable limbs due to softening of the epiphyseal cartilage. Also *fetal chondromalacia.* **c. of the larynx** LARYNGOMALACIA. **c. patellae** Chondromalacia that is limited to the posterior aspect of the patella and associated with patellofemoral pain. The condition occurs mainly in adolescents and young adults. Also *patellar chondromalacia.*

**chondromatosis** \-mətō′sis\ [CHONDROMA + *t* + -OSIS] The formation of multiple small chondromas. **synovial c.** A condition in which cartilaginous loose bodies are formed by cartilage metaplasia of the synovial lining of joints and tendon sheaths. Also *synovial osteochondromatosis.*

**chondromatous** \kändräm′ətəs\ Pertaining to or having the characteristics of cartilage.

**chondromere** \känd′rōmir\ [CHONDRO- + -MERE] One of the segmentally arranged cartilaginous precursors of the vertebrae in the developing vertebral column.

**chondrometaplasia** \-met′əplā′zhə\ A pathological condition in which metaplastic change occurs in the chondroblasts.

**chondromyoma** \-mī·ō′mə\ [CHONDRO- + MYOMA] A benign tumor of mesenchyme that contains both cartilage and muscle elements.

**chondromyxofibroma** \-mik′səfībrō′mə\ CHONDROMYXOID FIBROMA.

**chondromyxoma** \-miksō′mə\ CHONDROMYXOID FIBROMA.

**chondro-osteodystrophy** \-äs′tē·ōdis′trəfē\ OSTEOCHONDRODYSPLASIA.

**chondropathy** \kändräp′əthē\ [CHONDRO- + -PATHY] Any disease or injury of cartilage.

**chondrophyte** \kän′drōfīt\ A cartilaginous outgrowth that occurs at a joint.

**chondroplast** \kän′drōplast\ A cell which produces cartilage. Also *chondroblast.*

**chondroplasty** \kän′drōplas′tē\ [CHONDRO- + -PLASTY] An operation to change the size or shape of one or more cartilages, or to repair a torn or displaced cartilage.

**chondroporosis** \-pôrō′sis\ [CHONDRO- + POROSIS] The formation of sinuses with cartilage. It is a process that can occur during normal ossification.

**chondrosarcoma** \-särkō′mə\ [CHONDRO- + SARCOMA] A relatively common, malignant tumor found chiefly in adults and characterized by the formation of cartilage, but not of bone, by the tumor cells. The pelvis, ribs, shoulder, femur, and humerus are common sites, and central location in bones is typical. Calcification and endochondral ossification frequently occur in chondrosarcomas, but bone formation by the tumor cells is seen only in osteosarcoma. Adj. chondrosarcomatous. **juxtacortical c.** A chondrosarcoma arising from the external surface. This type appears to have a better prognosis than the usual central form. **mesenchymal c.** A rare, malignant tumor containing more or less differentiated cartilage together with highly vascular spindle-cells or round-celled "mesenchymal" tissue. Also *chondrosarcoma myxomatodes.*

**chondroseptum** \-sep′təm\ The cartilage of the nasal septum.

**chondrosis** \kändrō′sis\ [CHONDR- + -OSIS] CHONDROGENESIS.

**chondroskeleton** \-skel′ətən\ **1** A cartilaginous skeleton, as in the embryo and in certain fishes. **2** The portion of the adult skeleton composed of cartilage.

**chondrosternal** \-stur′nəl\ **1** Pertaining to costal cartilage and the sternum. **2** Pertaining to sternal cartilage.

**chondrosternoplasty** \-stur′nōplas′tē\ [CHONDRO- + STERNO- + -PLASTY] The conversion of a funnel chest or pigeon chest to a more normal contour by operating on the costal cartilages adjacent to the sternum and then transposing the sternum in the desired direction. Also *costosternoplasty.*

**chondrotomy** \kändrät′əmē\ [CHONDRO- + -TOMY] An incision into cartilage.

**chondrotrophic** \-träf′ik\ Relating to the growth of cartilage.

**chondroxiphoid** \-zī′foid\ Pertaining to the xiphoid process.

**CHOP** A chemotherapy regimen that includes cyclophosphamide, hydroxyurea, vincristine (Oncovin), and prednisone.

**Chopart** [François *Chopart,* French surgeon, 1743–1795] **1** Chopart's articulation, Chopart's joint. See under ARTICULATIO TARSI TRANSVERSA. **2** Chopart's operation. See under CHOPART'S AMPUTATION. **3** Chopart's operation. See under MEDIOTARSAL AMPUTATION. **4** Ligament of Chopart. See under LIGAMENTUM BIFURCATUM.

**Chopra** [Sir Ram Nath *Chopra,* Indian physician and pharmacologist, born 1882] Chopra's antimony test. See under CHOPRA ANTIMONY REACTION.

**chorangioma** \kôran′jē·ō′mə\ CHORIOANGIOMA.

**chord / condyle c.** CONDYLAR AXIS.

**chord-** \kôrd-\ CHORDO-.

**chorda** \kôr′də\ [L (from Gk *chordē* a cord, string of gut), a gut, intestine] (*pl.* chordae) Any cord or tendinous structure. **c. dorsalis** NOTOCHORD. **c. gubernaculum** A cord of dense mesenchyme stretching between the transverse bend in the embryonic genital ridge and the inguinal crest on the adjoining abdominal wall that later forms the lower part of the gubernaculum testis or of the round ligament of the uterus. **c. obliqua** [NA] A strong, narrow band that runs obliquely superior to the interosseous membrane of the forearm, extending from the lateral margin of the tuberosity of the ulna to the tuberosity of the radius and the line below it as far as the interosseous margin. The posterior interosseous vessels run posteriorly between it and the interosseous membrane. It is occasionally absent. Also *oblique cord, oblique ligament, Weitbrecht's cord, Weitbrecht's ligament, Cooper's ligament, oblique ligament of elbow joint, round ligament of elbow joint, oblique ligament of forearm, oblique ligament of Cooper, oblique ligament of superior radioulnar joint, oblique cord of elbow joint.* **c. spermatica** *Outmoded* FUNICULUS SPERMATICUS. **c. spinalis** *Older term* MEDULLA SPINALIS. **chordae tendineae cordis** [NA] Fibrous cords that attach each cusp of the two atrioventricular valves to papillary muscles of the corresponding ventricle of the heart. The cords vary in thickness and are usually branched. Also *tendinous cords.* **c. tympani** [NA] A derivative of the nervus intermedius which leaves the main nerve in the facial canal to enter the middle ear cavity, crosses the handle of the malleus, exits the skull through the petrotympanic fissure, and joins the lingual branch of the mandibular nerve. Its parasympathetic fibers synapse in submandibular and sublingual ganglia, while other fibers mediate taste over the anterior two-thirds of the tongue. Also *tympanichord.* Adj. tympanichordal. **c. umbilicalis** UMBILICAL CORD. **c. vertebralis** The notochord; the primitive backbone. • The term is sometimes incorrectly used for the spinal cord.

**chordae** \kôr′dē\ Plural of CHORDA.

**chordamesoderm** \kôr′dəmez′ədurm\ [CHORDA + MESODERM] In embryos possessing three germ layers, a layer that develops between the ectoblast and the endoblast, originating from cells of the germinal disk which invaginate along the primitive streak to Hensen's node (at its cephalic extremity). It comprises two groups of cells: an axial component which forms the notochord (which ultimately regresses in all but the most primitive vertebrates, such as *Amphioxus* and cyclostomes); and two lateral components which constitute the mesoblast.

**Chordata** \kôrdā′tə\ [CHORD- + -ATA] The phylum of animals characterized by the presence, at some stage of development, of a dorsal hollow nerve cord, a notochord, and gill slits or gill pouches. Chordata is usually considered to include the subphyla Urochordata, Cephalochordata, and Vertebrata. The Hemichordata are also included by some taxonomists.

**chordate** \kôr′dāt\ [CHORD- + -ATE] **1** Any member of the phylum Chordata. **2** Possessing a notochord.

**chordee** \kôrdē′\ [French *cordée,* fem. of *cordé* (from Gk *chordē* a string of gut, cord, a sausage) corded] An abnormal downward curvature of the penis, most apparent on erection, due to hypospadias or to infection of the urethra, as in gonorrhea. Also *chordeic penis, chordurethritis, gryposis penis.*

**chorditis** \kôrdī′tis\ [CHORD- + -ITIS] **1** CHORDITIS VOCALIS. **2** Inflammation of the spermatic cord. **c. nodosa** VOCAL NODULES. **c. vocalis** Any inflammatory condition of the vocal cord or cords. Also *chorditis.*

**chordo-** \kôr′dō-\ [Gk *chordē* cord, string of gut] A combining form meaning cord, as the spinal cord or notochord. Also *chord-.*

**chordoma** \kôrdō′mə\ [CHORD- + -OMA] A tumor characterized by a lobular arrangement of tissue, made up of highly vacuolated cells (physaliphorous cells) and mucoid intercellular material. Chordomas are restricted to the axial skeleton, especially at the sacral and spheno-occipital regions. They are believed to arise from notochordal tissue. Chordomas are slow growing but infiltrate adjacent structures and are often fatal. Metastases are uncommon. Adults are usually affected. Also *chordoblastoma, chordoepithelioma, chordosarcoma, notochordoma.*

**chordopexy** \kôr′dōpek′sē\ CORDOPEXY.

**chordosarcoma** \-särkō′mə\ [CHORDO- + SARCOMA] CHORDOMA.

**chordoskeleton** \-skel′ətən\ [CHORDO- + SKELETON] The skeletal elements formed about the notochord.

**chordotomy** \kôrdät′əmē\ [CHORDO- + -TOMY] An incision into the spinal cord to interrupt a fasciculus, usually in the spinothalamic tract in the quadrant anterior to the attachment of the dentate ligament, for the relief of pain distally. Also *cordotomy.*

**chordurethritis** \kôrd′yoorəthrī′tis\ [*chord(o)-* + URETHRITIS] CHORDEE.

**chorea** \kôrē′ə\ [Gk *choreia* a dancing, choral dance] A form of involuntary movement marked by fine, disorganized, and random movements of the extremities, usually the hands and feet, and involving the proximal limb and trunk muscles to a lesser extent. There is often associated facial grimacing with movements of the tongue. The muscles are hypotonic, the knee jerks often pendular, and there is a typical exaggeration of associated movements during volitional activity. Chorea may be rheumatic (Sydenham's chorea) or inherited, as in Huntington's disease. In both forms the principal pathologic changes are in the caudate nuclei. Choreiform movements may also occur in many other diseases or as an effect of various neuroleptic drugs. Also *St. Modestus disease, periodic jactitation, morbus saltatorius, paralysis vacillans, St. Anthony's disease.* **acute c.** SYDENHAM'S CHOREA. **atonic c.** PARALYTIC CHOREA. **chronic c.** HUNTINGTON'S DISEASE. **chronic progressive hereditary c.** HUNTINGTON'S DISEASE. **c. cordis** Involvement of the heart in rheumatic chorea. **c. cruciata** Chorea involving in an irregular or asymmetrical way the two halves of the body, for example, the right foot and left hand. *Seldom used.* **dancing c.** CHOREOMANIA. **degenerative c.** HUNTINGTON'S DISEASE. **diaphragmatic c.** DIAPHRAGMATIC TIC. **c. dimidiata** HEMICHOREA. **epidemic c.** CHOREOMANIA. **c. festinans** *Obs.* PARALYSIS AGITANS. **c. gravidarum**

Chorea occurring in a pregnant woman. **c. gravis** Severe chorea giving rise to dysphagia, impaired nutrition, and sometimes exhaustion. **habit c.** TIC. **hemilateral c.** HEMICHOREA. **hemiplegic c.** HEMICHOREA. **hereditary c.** HUNTINGTON'S DISEASE. **Huntington's c.** HUNTINGTON'S DISEASE. **hysterical c.** Choreiform movements occurring as a result of hysteria rather than as symptoms of true chorea. The movements sometimes resemble gestures or actions associated with the patient's occupation. **infective c.** SYDENHAM'S CHOREA. **jumping c.** CHOREOMANIA. **juvenile c.** SYDENHAM'S CHOREA. **limp c.** Severe chorea attended by weakness, immobility, and hypotonia of the limbs. **c. minor** SYDENHAM'S CHOREA. **c. mollis** A mild form of Sydenham's chorea. **c. nocturna** Chorea in which the movements continue during sleep. **c. nutans** Chorea in the limbs, associated with jerky head movements or rhythmic nodding of the head. **one-sided c.** HEMICHOREA. **paralytic c.** Chorea which is so severe that the affected limb or limbs appear to be paralyzed. Thus severe hemichorea may simulate hemiplegia. Also *atonic chorea.* **polymorphous c.** GILLES DE LA TOURETTE SYNDROME. **posthemiplegic c.** Choreic movements developing in the paretic limbs following hemiplegia or hemiparesis. Also *postparalytic chorea.* **prehemiplegic c.** Hemichorea occurring as an antecedent of hemiplegia or hemiparesis. **rheumatic c.** SYDENHAM'S CHOREA. **saltatory c.** INFANTILE MASSIVE SPASM. **senile c.** Choreiform movements, usually of the limbs, developing suddenly or insidiously in patients over the age of 60 years having no family history of Huntington's disease. When unilateral, the condition may represent a mild form of hemiballismus. The condition is usually associated with cerebral softening, often a lacunar state due to arteriosclerosis, in the region of the subthalamic nuclei. **Sydenham's c.** Chorea which appears to be due to a rheumatic affliction of the brain, often following streptococcal infection. Pathological evidence is scanty, as death from the disease is exceptionally rare, but usually the changes are minimal with scattered inflammatory cell infiltration and cell loss in the corpus striatum. The condition is commonest in children, adolescents, and young adults who show not only choreic movements of the face, tongue, and extremities but also emotional lability and typical exaggeration of associated movements during voluntary activity. Sometimes the condition affects predominantly one arm and leg (hemichorea) and it may appear for the first time in pregnancy (chorea gravidarum) and may then recur in subsequent pregnancies. The patient usually recovers in one to four months, but emotional lability may persist much longer and relapses may follow upper respiratory tract infection. Rheumatic heart disease is an occasional sequel. Also *simple chorea, infective chorea, rheumatic chorea, chorea minor, St. Vitus dance, St. Guy's chorea, Breutsch's disease, rheumatic encephalopathy, acute chorea, juvenile chorea, infectious myoclonia.* **tetanoid c.** Choreic movements accompanying progressive lenticular degeneration. **unilateral c.** HEMICHOREA.

**choreic** \kôrē′ik\ Pertaining to or suffering from chorea. Also *choreal, choreatic.*

**choreiform** \kôrē′ifôrm\ [Gk *chore(a)* + *i* + -FORM] Resembling the movements of chorea. Also *choreoid.*

**choreoathetosis** \kôr′ē·ō·ath′ətō′sis\ Involuntary movements showing features of both chorea and athetosis. Adj. choreathetotic. **paroxysmal familial c.** MOUNT SYNDROME. **paroxysmal kinesogenic c.** Recurring choreoathetosis of unknown etiology in which the involuntary movements are generally precipitated by voluntary movement. The condition may respond to anticonvulsant drugs. Also *periodic dystonia.*

**choreoid** \kôr′ē·oid\ CHOREIFORM.

**choreomania** \kôr′ē·ōmā′nē·ə\ [*chore(a)* + *o* + -MANIA] A disorder prevalent in the Middle Ages, often affecting large numbers of individuals in relatively closed communities, in which bizarre patterns of involuntary movement (hysterical chorea) superficially resembling chorea occurred. Also *dancing chorea, epidemic chorea, jumping chorea, jumping disease, dancing mania, choromania* (obs.), *tarantism, tarentism, jumping sickness* (outmoded).

**chorio-** \kôr′ē·ō-\ A combining form meaning (1) chorion; (2) choroid.

**chorioadenoma destruens** \-ad′ənō′mə des′troo·əns\ A lesion in which a hydatidiform mole invades the wall of the uterus and may produce secondary deposits in other sites. Avascular chorionic villi must be identified for this diagnosis. Infiltration of the myometrium can lead to necrosis, hemorrhage and inflammation. Invasion of vessels may give rise to metastases, usually in the lungs and vagina. Also *chorioadenoma, invasive hydatidiform mole, invasive mole, malignant mole, malignant hydatidiform mole, metastisizing mole.*

**chorioallantois** \-əlan′tō·is\ [CHORIO- + ALLANTOIS] An extraembryonic structure derived from the union of the chorion and the allantois which, especially in reptiles and birds, plays an important role in gas exchange. In these vertebrates it is a membrane apposed to the eggshell. In many mammals it gives rise to the placenta. Also *chorioallantoic membrane.*

**chorioamnionic** \-am′nē·än′ik\ [CHORIO- + AMNIONIC] AMNIOCHORIONIC.

**chorioamnionitis** \-am′nē·ənī′tis\ [CHORIO- + AMNION + -ITIS] Inflammation of the fetal membranes as a result of infection, usually bacterial infection.

**chorioangiofibroma** \-an′jē·ōfībrō′mə\ [CHORIO- + ANGIOFIBROMA] An angiofibroma of the placenta.

**chorioangioma** \-an′jē·ō′mə\ [CHORIO- + ANGIOMA] A hemangioma of the placenta. Also *chorangioma.*

**chorioangiopagus parasiticus** \-an′jē·äp′əgəs par′əsit′ikəs\ OMPHALOSITE.

**chorioblastoma** \-blastō′mə\ [CHORIO- + BLASTOMA] CHORIOCARCINOMA.

**choriocapillaris** \-kap′iler′is\ LAMINA CHOROIDOCAPILLARIS.

**choriocarcinoma** \-kär′sənō′mə\ [CHORIO- + CARCINOMA] A malignant neoplasm consisting of proliferating trophoblast invading, destroying, and multiplying in the maternal tissues. It typically occurs in the uterus but may in rare cases arise in the ovary or fallopian tube. It may follow any form of pregnancy, normal, ectopic, or abortion, but most often is preceded by hydatidiform mole. Necrosis and hemorrhage are characteristic. Microscopically, cytotrophoblast and syncytiotrophoblast are present. No chorionic villi are seen. Chorionic gonadotrophin is elevated in blood and urine. Frequently lutein cysts are in the ovaries. It is highly malignant if untreated. Also *chorioepithelioma, chorioblastoma, chorionic carcinoma, chorioma, chorionic epithelioma, deciduocellular sarcoma, chorionepithelioma, deciduoma malignum, deciduosarcoma, tropoblastic malignant teratoma, syncytioma malignum, trophoblastoma.* **c. of the testis** The most malignant but least frequent germ cell testicular tumor, composed of syncytiotrophoblastic and cytotrophoblastic cells. Chorionic gonadotrophin is elevated in serum and urine. It may occur in a pure form or mixed with other germ cell elements.

**chorioepithelioma** \-ep′ithē′lē·ō′mə\ [CHORIO- + EPITHELIOMA] CHORIOCARCINOMA.

**choriogenesis** \-jen′əsis\ The formation and development of the chorion.

**chorioid** \kôr′ē·oid\ CHOROIDEA.

**chorioidea** \kôr′ē·oi′dē·ə\ CHOROIDEA.

**chorioiditis** \kôr′ē·oidī′tis\ CHOROIDITIS.

**chorioma** \kôr′ē·ō′mə\ CHORIOCARCINOMA.

**choriomeningitis** \-men′injī′tis\ [CHORIO- + MENINGITIS] **1** Inflammation of the meninges and of the chor .d plexus. **2** See under LYMPHOCYTIC CHORIOMENINGITIS. **lymphocytic c.** An acute infection due to the lymphocytic choriomeningitis virus, an arenavirus. It presents after a 5–10 day incubation period with fever and influenzalike symptoms. A brief period of improvement is followed by onset of headache and recurrence of fever, and some patients develop meningitis in this second phase of illness. The illness, including the meningitis, usually resolves spontaneously but does on rare occasions progress to encephalomyelitis, which can be fatal. Cerebrospinal fluid shows a marked lymphocytic pleocytosis but only a slight rise, if any, in protein content. The disease is usually spread by house mice, which serve as a reservoir of infection and contaminate food or other household objects with urine and droppings, but some cases have resulted from contact with hamsters or guinea pigs. Person-to-person spread has not been demonstrated. Also *Armstrong's disease, Wallgren's aseptic meningitis, epidemic serous meningitis, acute benign lymphocytic meningitis, curable serous meningitis, acute curable juvenile subarachnoiditis* (seldom used). Abbr. LCM

**chorion** \kôr′ē·än\ [Gk, afterbirth] The outermost of the fetal membranes of mammals, formed from extraembryonic somatopleuric mesoderm and the overlying trophoblast. The trophoblast divides into an outer syncytiotrophoblast and an inner cytotrophoblast. The chorion varies greatly in its size and characteristics but is essential in that it develops villi, engaged in fetal-maternal exchange, which become incorporated into a placenta. It is sometimes called the serosa in reptiles and birds. Also *chorionic vesicle, chorionic sac.* Adj. chorial, chorionic. **c. avillosum** CHORION LAEVE. **c. frondosum** The villus-bearing part of the chorion, which eventually becomes the fetal part of the placenta. During early stages the whole chorion is more or less covered with villi but later the chorion laeve appears, lacking villi. Also *shaggy chorion, chorion villosum.* **c. laeve** The part of the chorion that becomes devoid of villi. It forms on the side of the chorionic sac opposite to where the placenta forms. Also *chorion avillosum.* **primitive c.** The chorion after mesoderm has been added to the trophoblast and before development of the primary chorionic villi. **shaggy c.** CHORION FRONDOSUM. **c. villosum** CHORION FRONDOSUM.

**chorionepithelioma** \kôr′ē·änep′ithē′lē·ō′mə\ [CHORION + EPITHELIOMA] CHORIOCARCINOMA.

**chorionic** \kôr′rē·än′ik\ Relating to or derived from the chorion, as *chorionic gonadotropin.*

**chorionitis** \kôr′ē·änī′tis\ *Obs.* SCLERODERMA.

**chorioplaque** \kôr′ē·ōplak′\ A multinuclear giant cell that is present in certain cellular infiltrations in the skin.

**chorioretinal** \-ret′inəl\ Pertaining to the choroid and the retina.

**chorioretinitis** \-ret′inī′tis\ [CHORIO- + RETINITIS] Inflammation involving both the choroid and the retina. Because of their thinness and proximity, any inflammation is apt to involve both layers. However, the primary site may be in one or the other tissue. For example, *Toxoplasma* organisms are found exclusively within the retina, whereas *Histoplasma* affect the choroid. Inflammation may result from infection with, among other agents, cytomegalovirus, herpesvirus, *Treponema pallidum, Mycobacterium tuberculosis, Toxoplasma gondii,* or *Histoplasma capsulatum.* Also *choroidoretinitis.*

**chorioretinopathy** \-ret′inäp′əthē\ [CHORIO- + RETINOPATHY] A disorder of both the choroid and the retina.

**chorismate** The anion of chorismic acid. In plants, fungi, and bacteria, it is an intermediate in the biosynthesis of the aromatic amino acids phenylalanine, tyrosine, and tryptophan. It thus stands at a branch point of biosynthesis. Its molecule consists of 1,2,5,6-tetradehydro-3,4-dihydroxycyclohexanecarboxylic acid, substituted on O-3 with a 1-carboxyethenyl group.

**chorismic acid** 3-(1-Carboxyvinyloxy)-4-hydroxycyclohexa-1,5-diene-1-carboxylic acid. It is a precursor of prephenic acid in the pathway of biosynthesis of tryptophan, phenylalanine, and tyrosine in plants and bacteria.

**chorista** \kôris′tə\ [Gk *chōrista*, neut. pl. of *chōristos* separable] A small aggregate of tissue which is histologically normal within itself but is in an abnormal location, as ectopic bits of adrenal imbedded within a kidney.

**choristoma** \kôr′istō′mə\ [Gk *chōrist(os)* separable + -OMA] A collection of heterotopic tissues which grow as a tumor or tumorlike lesion. For example, a choristoma of the intestine may be simply a mass of ectopic pancreatic tissue. A choristoma of the conjunctiva may contain lacrimal gland, cartilage, smooth muscle, and skin appendages. Also *choristoblastoma, aberrant rest.* Compare HAMARTOMA, TERATOMA.

**choroid** \kôr′oid\ [Gk *choroeidēs*, alter. of *chorioeidēs* (from *chorio(n)* afterbirth, fetal membrane + *-eidēs* -like, -OID) chorionlike] **1** Resembling the chorion or other vascular or villous membrane, as in *choroid plexus.* **2** CHOROIDEA. **c. proper** SUBSTANTIA PROPRIA CHOROIDEAE.

**choroid-** \kôr′oid-\ CHOROIDO-.

**choroidea** \kôroi′dē·ə\ [New L, short for *tunica* (or *membrana*) *choroidea*, transl. of Gk *chorioeides chitōn* choroid tunic or membrane. See also CHOROID.] [NA] The thin vascular membrane that lies between the inner surface of the sclera and the pigmented layer of the retina over the posterior five sixths of the eyeball. Posteriorly it is pierced by the optic nerve, where it is fused to the sclera, and anteriorly it extends to the ora serrata retinae. It is the posterior portion of the uveal tract, the anterior portion being composed of the ciliary body and the iris. It consists of an outer vascular lamina, an intermediate choroidocapillary lamina, and an inner basal complex or layer. Also *choroid, chorioid, chorioidea.* Adj. choroidal.

**choroidectomy** \kôr′oidek′təmē\ [*choroid (plexus)* + -ECTOMY] Excision of the choroid plexus. This procedure is sometimes used for the treatment of hydrocephalus.

**choroideremia** \kôr′oiderē′mē·ə\ [CHOROID- + Gk *erēmia* absence] A sex-linked, recessive, degenerative condition in which the choroidal structure becomes severely atrophic, exposing the underlying sclera to ophthalmoscopic view. Carrier females can be recognized by the presence of punctuate scattering of pigment within the peripheral fundus. Also *tapetochoroidal dystrophy, progressive tapetochoroidal dystrophy.*

**choroiditis** \kôr′oidī′tis\ [CHOROID- + -ITIS] Inflammation of the choroid. Also *chorioiditis, posterior uveitis.* ● Older usage of *choroiditis* included a variety of degenerative changes more properly referred to as *choroidopathy.* **anterior c.** Inflammation of the periphery of the choroid. **areolar c.** An inflammation or degeneration of the choroid in which multiple depigmented areas develop, beginning at the posterior pole. **areolar central c.** An inflammatory or degenerative depigmentation of the posterior ocular fundus. Also *Förster's choroiditis, Förster's disease.* **central c.** Inflammation of the posterior pole of the fundus. **Doyne's familial honeycombed c.** DOYNE HONEYCOMB DEGENERATION OF RETINA. **exudative c.** An inflammatory or degenerative disease of the choroid, characterized by an outpouring of proteinaceous debris. **Förster's c.** AREOLAR CENTRAL CHOROIDITIS. **c. guttata senilis** DOYNE HONEYCOMB DEGENERATION OF RETINA. **Jensen's c.** A severe, juxtapapillary chorioretinitis resulting in damage to optic nerve fibers and a consequential visual-field defect. **metastatic c.** Hematogenous spread of infection to the choroid, as in syphilis, tuberculosis, or pyemia. **senile macular exudative c.** SENILE DISCIFORM DEGENERATION. **c. serosa** GLAUCOMA. **Tay's c.** DOYNE HONEYCOMB DEGENERATION OF RETINA.

**choroido-** \kəroi′dō-\ [See CHOROID.] A combining form meaning choroid. Also *choroid-*.

**choroidocyclitis** \-sīklī′tis\ [CHOROIDO- + CYCL- + -ITIS] UVEITIS.

**choroidoiritis** \-īrī′tis\ [CHOROIDO- + *ir(is)* + -ITIS] UVEITIS.

**choroidopathy** \kôr′oidäp′əthē\ [CHOROIDO- + -PATHY] Degenerative or traumatic changes of the choroid, as distinguished from choroidal inflammation. At times this clinical distinction may be difficult to make. **areolar c.** A degenerative change of the choroid characterized by the development of large atrophic areas in the posterior fundus. Also *central areolar choroidal sclerosis.* **central serous c.** A slight accumulation of fluid in the macular region of the eye, lying between the retinal pigment epithelium and the outer segments. It is due to a leakage through the pigment epithelium of unknown etiology. A relative central scotoma results, but usually resolves spontaneously within a few months. Also *central angiospastic retinitis, retinitis centralis serosa, central serous retinopathy, central angiospastic retinopathy.* **guttate c.** DOYNE HONEYCOMB DEGENERATION OF RETINA.

**choroidoretinitis** \-ret′inī′tis\ CHORIORETINITIS.

**chorology** \kôräl′əjē\ BIOGEOGRAPHY.

**choromania** \kôr′ōmā′nē-ə\ *Obs.* CHOREOMANIA.

**Chotzen** [F. *Chotzen,* German physician, flourished 20th century] Chotzen syndrome. See under ACROCEPHALOSYNDACTYLY TYPE III.

**Christ** [J. *Christ,* German physician, flourished early 20th century] Christ-Siemens syndrome. See under ANHIDROTIC ECTODERMAL DYSPLASIA.

**Christensen** [Erna *Christensen,* Danish neurologist, 1906–1967] Christensen-Krabbe disease, Christensen-Krabbe progressive infantile cerebral poliodystrophy. See under KRABBE'S DISEASE.

**Christian** [Henry Asbury *Christian,* U.S. internist, 1876–1951] **1** Christian-Weber disease, Weber-Christian disease, Weber-Christian syndrome, Christian's disease. See under RELAPSING FEBRILE NONSUPPURATIVE PANNICULITIS. **2** Christian's disease, Schüller-Christian disease, Christian syndrome, Hand-Schüller-Christian syndrome, Schüller-Christian syndrome. See under HAND-SCHÜLLER-CHRISTIAN DISEASE.

**Christmas** [Stephen *Christmas,* English hospital patient of 20th century] Christmas disease. See under HEMOPHILIA B.

**Chrobak** [Rudolf *Chrobak,* Austrian gynecologist, 1843–1910] See under TEST.

**chrom-** \krōm-\ CHROMO-.

**chromaffin** \krō′məfin, krōmaf′in\ [*chrom(ium)* + L *affin(is)* akin or inclined to] Having an affinity with chromium salts, especially dichromates, such as to stain brown or yellowish brown by forming a precipitate containing chromium oxide; pheochrome. Substances which react in this way include epinephrine, particularly in adrenal medullary cells, and 5-hydroxytryptoamine, or serotonin, particularly in interochromaffin cells and in certain brainstem neurons. Catecholamines such as norepinephrine and dopamine, though related to epinephrine, do not yield a strong chromaffin reaction.

**chromaffinity** \krō′mafin′itē\ An affinity with chromium salts that characterizes certain cells and causes them to stain brown or yellowish brown.

**chromaffinoma** \krō′mafinō′mə\ [CHROMAFFIN + -OMA] **1** A tumor of cells giving the chromaffin reaction. Also *chromaffinoblastoma.* **2** PHEOCHROMOCYTOMA. **medullary c.** A pheochromocytoma of the adrenal medulla.

**chromaffinopathy** \krō′mafinäp′əthē\ Any pathologic condition of chromaffin tissue, as of the adrenal medulla or glomus jugulare.

**chroman** The substance whose molecule consists of a benzene ring substituted at adjacent atoms with an $—O—[CH_2]_3—$ group, forming a second six-membered ring. It is part of the flavonoid structure, common in plant products, including flower pigments, built up from cinnamic acid.

**chromaphil** \krō′məfil\ CHROMOPHIL.

**chromargentaffin** \krōm′ärjen′təfin\ Staining with chromium salts and also taking up silver: used especially of cells of the mucous coat of the alimentary canal.

**chromat-** \krō′mət-\ CHROMO-.

**chromate** Any anion containing chromium as a central atom, e.g., tetrafluorooxochromate(V) for $CrF_4O^-$. Unqualified it usually means the ion $CrO_4^{2-}$, which is converted into dichromate, $Cr_2O_7^{2-}$, in acid solution. It is an oxidizing agent.

**chromatic** \krōmat′ik\ [Gk *chrōmatikos* (from *chrōma* color) pertaining to color] Of or relating to color, the possession of color, or the ability to produce color.

**chromatid** \krō′mətid\ [CHROMAT- + -ID$^2$] One of the two longitudinal subunits into which chromosomes divide during mitosis or meiosis. The two chromatids are held together by the centromere.

**chromatin** \krō′mətin\ [CHROMAT- + -IN] A molecule composed of DNA, RNA, and protein, located in the cell, and having an affinity for basic stains. Chromatin also exhibits a positive Feulgen reaction. The chromatin may be dispersed or gathered into discrete packets (chromosomes). The chromatin makes up the genetic material of the cell. Also *chromoplasm.* See also HETEROCHROMATIN, EUCHROMATIN. Adj. chromatinic. **sex c.** BARR BODY. **X c.** BARR BODY.

**chromatin-negative** \krō′mətin-neg′ətiv\ Not containing sex chromatin (Barr bodies), as the nuclei of most male mammalian cells.

**chromatinolysis** \krō′mətinäl′əisis\ CHROMATOLYSIS.

**chromatin-positive** \krō′mətin-päs′ətiv\ Containing sex chromatin (Barr bodies), as the nuclei of most autosomal female mammalian cells.

**chromatism** \krō′mətizm\ [CHROMAT- + -ISM] Chromatic aberration of an optical lens.

**chromato-** \krō′mətō-\ CHROMO-.

**chromatoblast** \krōmat′əblast\ [CHROMATO- + -BLAST] A cell that can differentiate into a chromatophore.

**chromatocinesis** \-sīnē′sis\ CHROMATOKINESIS.

**chromatocyte** \krōmat′əsīt\ [CHROMATO- + -CYTE] PIGMENT CELL.

**chromatogenous** \krō′mətäj′ənəs\ Producing pigmentation or color.

**chromatogram** \krōmat′əgram\ [CHROMATO- + -GRAM] **1** The support, usually paper, on which substances have been separated by chromatography and made visible including, if necessary, by staining. **2** A diagram of a chromatographic separation, such as a graph of a concentration against the volume of an effluent from a column.

**chromatograph** \krōmat′əgraf\ [CHROMATO- + -GRAPH] **1** To submit to chromatography. **2** An instrument used in chromatographic analysis.

**chromatography** \krō′mətäg′rəfē\ [CHROMATO- + -GRAPHY] The process of separating substances according to the differences in their partition coefficients between two phases (solid-liquid, liquid-liquid, or liquid-gas), in which one phase moves relative to the other, and each substance in the sample moves with it at a fraction of its speed of movement equal to the fraction of time that the molecules spend in that phase. • The term derives from the fact that colored substances were originally separated as colored bands that moved at different speeds down a column. **affinity c.** Chromatography of proteins on an adsorbent designed to contain groups that bind particular proteins because they resemble ligands for which the proteins have natural affinity. **antibody affinity c.** The separation of different antigens in a solution by the use of various antibodies on immunoabsorbent columns. The converse process is also used, and immobilized antigens on a column may be employed to separate mixtures of antibodies. Also *analytical immunofiltration.* **electric c.** ELECTROPHORESIS. **filter paper c.** PAPER CHROMATOGRAPHY. **gas c.** Chromatography that uses an inert gas as the moving phase. **gas-liquid c.** Chromatography in a column with a gas as the moving phase and a liquid, usually held on a solid support, as the stationary phase. The partition between phases thus depends on the volatility of the substances being separated. It is particularly useful for hydrocarbons and lipid derivatives. Abbr. GLC **gel filtration c.** Chromatography in which substances separate according to their molecular size. The stationary phase consists of gel particles, and the substances being separated can, as their molecular size decreases over a certain range, penetrate an increasing fraction of the gel water. Hence they partition increasingly in favor of the stationary gel water as opposed to the moving interstitial water, and so move along the column at decreasing velocities. Also *gel permeation chromatography, molecular-sieve chromatography.* **high-pressure liquid c.** Chromatography with a liquid mobile phase in which the stationary phase is very finely divided and a high pressure is used to achieve rapid separations with good resolution. Also *high-performance liquid chromatography.* **ion-exchange c.** Chromatography on an ion exchanger, such as an ion-exchange resin or a substituted cellulose derivative. It is particularly useful for charged substances, such as amino acids on a sulfonated polystyrene resin, where the substances may separate by reason of the partition differences determined by nonionic forces, such as the retardation of valine relative to glycine by hydrophobic forces. **molecular-sieve c.** GEL FILTRATION CHROMATOGRAPHY. **paper c.** Chromatography on a sheet of paper. The paper acts as a support for a stationary liquid phase as well as allowing a mobile liquid phase to pass through it by capillarity. Also *filter paper chromatography.* **partition c.** Chromatography in which the stationary phase and the moving phase are immiscible fluids. The substances being separated partition differently between them, and move at different rates because they spend different fractions of the time in the moving phase. **thin-layer c.** Chromatography on a thin layer of solid phase, or on a solid support for a liquid phase. This form of chromatography has the advantage of usually being rapid, although only small amounts of material can be handled. Abbr. TLC **two-dimensional c.** Chromatography in one direction along a sheet of support, often paper, and then in a second direction at right angles to the first. Often, by using a different pair of phases in the second dimension, separations can be achieved with two systems that could not be achieved by either alone. Alternatively, the same system can be used in both dimensions, but some of the substances have undergone a specific modification between the two separations.

**chromatokinesis** \-kīnē′sis\ [CHROMATO- + KINESIS] Movement of chromatin to produce a variety of forms. Also *chromatocinesis.*

**chromatology** \krō′mətäl′əjē\ [CHROMATO- + -LOGY] The scientific study of color.

**chromatolysis** \krō′mətäl′isis\ [CHROMATO- + LYSIS] The change that occurs in the Nissl substance of a neuron when its axon is cut or damaged. It is characterized by dispersion of Nissl substance and displacement of the nucleus with accompanying swelling of the cell body. Also *chromatinolysis, tigrolysis, chromolysis.* **central c.** The disappearance of chromatin or its displacement peripherally in the cytoplasm of neuronal cell bodies (perikarya) in the central nervous system secondary to lesions of their axons.

**chromatometer** [CHROMATO- + -METER] COLORIMETER.

**chromatophil** \krō′mətōfil′\ CHROMOPHIL.

**chromatophile** \krō′mətōfīl′\ CHROMOPHIL.

**chromatophilia** \-fil′yə\ [CHROMATO- + -PHILIA] The characteristic of combining readily with cytoplasmic stains.

**chromatophore** \krō′mətōfôr′\ One of two types of pigment-containing cells: the melanophores, which contain melanin pigment and are usually responsible for the color of the dermis or epidermis of animals, and the iridiophores, which contain iridescent reflecting pigments associated with the dermis of poikilotherms and the irises of birds. Also *chromatoplast, pigmentophore.*

**chromatophorotropic** \-fôr′əträp′ik\ Influencing the migration of pigment cells, or the pigment within cells, toward a specific tissue layer.

**chromatoplasm** \krō′mətōplazm′\ The colored or pigmented material of the protoplasm of a pigmented cell.

**chromatoplast** \krō′mətōplast′\ CHROMATOPHORE.

**chromatopsia** \krō′mətäp′sē·ə\ [CHROMAT- + -OPSIA] An abnormal subjective perception of color, as may occur following cataract extraction or in digitalis poisoning. Also *chromopsia, chrotopsia.*

**chromatoptometry** \krō′mətäptäm′ətrē\ The evaluation of color vision.

**chromatosis** \krō′mətō′sis\ [CHROMAT- + -OSIS] PIGMENTATION.

**chromatotaxis** \-tak′sis\ [CHROMATO- + TAXIS] The attraction and destruction of chromatin by substances in the cell nucleus, while the cell body remains intact.

**chromatotropism** \krō′mətät′rəpizm\ CHROMOTROPISM.

**chromaturia** \krō′mətoo′rē·ə\ [CHROMAT- + -URIA] Excretion of abnormally colored urine. *Seldom used.*

**chrome** [Gk *chrōm(a)* color] *Obs.* CHROMIUM. • This term is still used in specific contexts, often to denote a substance containing chromium or in the names of certain pigments.

**chrome hematoxylin** A hematoxylin solution, which includes a chromium salt as a mordant. It is used in the Weigert-Pal technique for staining myelin.

**chromhidrosis** \krōm′hidrō′sis\ [CHROM- + HIDR- + -OSIS] The production of colored sweat. Also *chromidrosis.*

**chromidium** \krōmid′ē·əm\ (*pl.* chromidia) A pigment granule or fibril in the cytoplasm of the cell. Adj. chromidial.

**chromidrosis** \krō′midrō′sis\ CHROMHIDROSIS.

**chromium** \krō′mē·əm\ Element number 24, having atomic weight 51.996. It is a gray, lustrous, corrosion-resistant metal. Valences are 2, 3, and 6. All chromium compounds are colored and all are toxic. Traces of chromium are essential to higher animals, and rats raised in a chromium-free environment show abnormalities related to insulin utilizatin. Also *chrome* (obs.). Symbol: Cr

**chromium 51** A radioactive isotope of chromium, emitting gamma rays, most commonly used to label red blood cells for red cell survival determination or to label damaged red blood cells for spleen imaging. Its half-life is 27.8 days. Symbol: $^{51}$Cr

**chromo-** \krō′mō-\ [Gk *chrōma* (genitive *chrōmatos*) color] A combining form meaning color, stain, or pigment. Also *chrom-, chromato-.*

***Chromobacterium*** \-baktir′ē·əm\ A Gram-negative, aerobic or facultative, rod-shaped bacterium that produces a violet pigment. It is frequently present in soil and water and is occasionally pathogenic.

**chromoblast** \krō′mōblast\ [CHROMO- + -BLAST] The precursor of a pigment cell.

**chromocenter** \krō′mōsen′tər\ [CHROMO- + CENTER] KARYOSOME.

**chromocyte** \krō′mōsīt\ [CHROMO- + -CYTE] A pigmented or colored cell.

**chromogen** \krō′mōjən\ [CHROMO- + -GEN] **1** Any compound that can yield a colored derivative, usually in an enzymatic reaction. **2** A species, especially of *Mycobacterium,* that forms colored (yellow to orange) colonies. **Porter-Silber c.'s** Substances that give a yellow color with phenylhydrazine in sulfuric acid. They are steroids containing the 17,21-dihydroxy-20-oxo- grouping, and include cortisol, the hormone predominating in human adrenocortical secretion.

**chromogenic** \-jen′ik\ [CHROMO- + -GENIC] Capable of forming a colored substance under specified conditions, as in a chemical assay.

**chromogranin** An acidic protein of molecular mass 77 kDa, found in chromaffin granules.

**chromolysis** \krōmäl′isis\ CHROMATOLYSIS.

**chromoma** \krōmō′mə\ [CHROM- + -OMA] *Obs.* MALIGNANT MELANOMA.

**chromomere** \krō′mōmir\ [CHROMO- + -MERE] A region of a chromosome distinguished cytogenetically by a difference in diameter, condensation, or staining properties. It is most readily viewed in prophase of mitosis or meiosis or in polytene chromosomes. The functional significance of chromomeres is unclear.

**chromometer** \krōmäm′ətər\ COLORIMETER.

**chromomycosis** \-mīkō′sis\ A chronic disease of the skin and subcutaneous tissues caused by a variety of different dematiaceous fungi that gain entrance into puncture and trauma sites and result in warty outgrowths and ulcers of the exposed sites. Also *verrucose dermatitis, verrucous eczema.*

**chromonar hydrochloride** $C_{20}H_{28}ClNO_5$. A coumarin derivative with coronary vasodilator properties. It has been used to prevent attacks of angina pectoris. Also *carbocromen.*

**chromonucleic acid** DEOXYRIBONUCLEIC ACID.

**chromophil** \krō′mōfil\ [CHROMO- + -PHIL] A cell or cytoplasmic structure that readily combines with cytoplasmic stains. Also *chromaphil, chromatophil, chromatophile, chromophile.*

**chromophobe** \krō′mōfōb\ [CHROMO- + Gk *phob(os)* fear] A cell that does not take a stain or that stains only very weakly; especially, a cell of the anterior pituitary gland, which stains weakly due to sparse cytoplasmic granules.

**chromophobia** \-fō′bē·ə\ [CHROMO- + -PHOBIA] Inability or limited ability of a cell, organelle, or tissue to stain.

**chromophore** \krō′məfôr\ [CHROMO- + -PHORE] The group or groups in a molecule which absorb visible or ultraviolet radiation. They are usually unsaturated groups such as —CH═CH—, —N═N—, or —C(═O)—, and are particularly likely to give color when conjugated.

**chromophose** \krō′mōfōs\ [CHROMO- + PHOSE] A sensation of a colored spot in or in front of the eye.

**chromoplasm** \krō′mōplazm\ CHROMATIN.

**chromoplast** \krō′mōplast\ [CHROMO- + -PLAST] A pigmented plastid, such as a chloroplast, found in the cytoplasm of plant cells and certain protozoa, usually distinguished from the chlorophyll-containing chloroplastid. Also *chromoplastid.*

**chromoprotein** A colored protein, such as hemoglobin.

**chromopsia** \krōmäp′sē·ə\ CHROMATOPSIA.

**chromoretinography** \-ret′inäg′rəfē\ Photography of the ocular fundus in color.

**chromoscopy** \krōmäs′kəpē\ [CHROMO- + -SCOPY] The measurement of color vision.

**chromosome** \krō′məsōm\ [German *Chromosom* (from CHROMO- + *-som* -SOME) lit., a readily staining body] In any cell, a structure that contains DNA encoding genetic information inherited from the parents. Prokaryotes, mitochondria, and chloroplasts have a single, circular chromosome. Eukaryotic cells have a characteristic number of chromo-

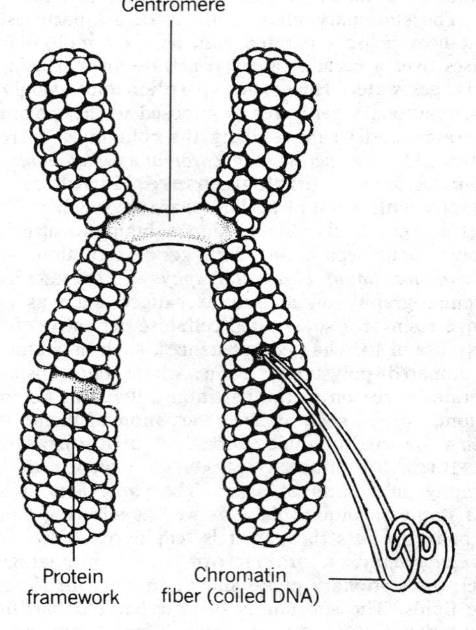


**Chromosome**

somes, with a complex organization including histones and nonhistone proteins as well as DNA. Eukaryotic chromosomes are enclosed in the cell nucleus, and their structure goes through a cycle of major changes during mitosis or meiosis. Adj. chromosomal. **accessory c.'s** Any of the structures in the nucleus of the cell in plants or animals that are cytologically definable as chromosomes but are not part of the usual complement of autosomal and sex chromosomes of the organism. They rarely contain genetic information of importance to the organism, and they are usually relatively small and heterochromatic. They do not form chiasmata with the autosomes or the sex chromosomes and are often eliminated or undergo nondisjunction at meiosis or mitosis. They may be rare or present in nearly all members of a population of a species. Different individuals may possess as many as 30 or more per cell. Also *supernumerary chromosomes, odd chromosomes* (outmoded), *B chromosomes.* **acentric c.** A chromosome lacking a centromere. **acrocentric c.** A chromosome in which the centromere is close to one end such that one arm is much longer than the other. The short arm of human acrocentric chromosomes (Group D, encompassing chromosomes 13, 14, and 15; and Group G, encompassing chromosomes 21 and 22) may have satellites associated. Also *subtelocentric chromosome.* **B c.'s** ACCESSORY CHROMOSOMES. **bivalent c.** See under BIVALENT. **daughter c.** Either of the two chromatids that moves to the opposite pole of the spindle and segregates to daughter cells or gametes. **dicentric c.** A chromosome with two centromeres. **fragile X c.** One portion of a long arm of an X chromosome which, on culture in a folate-deficient medium, is recognizable as fragile. Its presence in a male leads to X-linked mental deficiency. **giant c.** 1 See under POLYTENE CHROMOSOME. 2 See under LAMPBRUSH CHROMOSOMES. **heteromorphic c.** ALLOSOME. **heterotypical c.** ALLOSOME. **homologous c.** One of a pair of chromosomes that has the same linear sequence of genetic loci, possesses similar cytologic structure, and pairs during meiosis. Also *homologue.* **lampbrush c.'s** A large chromosome found in the diplotene stage of the primary oocyte of certain vertebrates and in spermatocytes of *Drosophila.* These chromosomes have a central axis from which numerous pairs of loops project, giving the appearance of a lampbrush or test-tube brush. These chromosomes may be larger than the polytene chromosomes of Diptera. **late replicating X-c.** A mammalian X-chromosome that replicates later in the period of DNA synthesis in the interphase cycle than do the autosomes and the X-chromosome that is active in transcription. It constitutes the Barr body in interphase nuclei. **m-c.** MITOCHONDRIAL CHROMOSOME. **metacentric c.** A chromosome having the centromere near the middle, resulting in nearly equal lengths of the arms. In humans, this includes chromosomes of groups A and F. Also *mediocentric chromosome.* **mitochondrial c.** A circular DNA molecule within a mitochondrion that encodes polypeptides, rRNA, and tRNA that function predominantly in the organelle. It is the basis for maternal inheritance. In mammals, the double-helical molecule encodes 37 structural genes and is not bound by histones. Its nucleotide sequence is completely determined and its genetic code differs slightly from that of the nuclear chromosomes. Also *m-chromosome.* **mitotic c.** Any nuclear chromosome of a cell in mitosis, as opposed to interphase. Chromosomes in some phases of mitosis, such as metaphase or prophase, are examined in cytogenetics and are used to construct karyotypes. **monocentric c.** A chromosome that has one centromere, which is the normal state of human chromosomes. **nonhomologous c.'s** Chromosomes that contain different linear sequences of genetic loci, are morphologically dissimilar, and do not predictably pair at meiosis. Also *nonhomologues.* **nucleolar c.'s** Any chromosome cytologically associated with a nucleolus. Such chromosomes contain a nucleolar organizer region and ribosomal RNA genes. **odd c.'s** *Outmoded* ACCESSORY CHROMOSOMES. **Philadelphia c.** A small, acrocentric human chromosome that lacks parts of its long arm and that is found in the clone of cells apparently causing chronic granulocytic leukemia. The deleted chromosome has been shown to be 22, with the missing portion translocated usually to chromosome 9. Symbol: $Ph^1$ **polytene c.** One of the specialized chromosomes of the salivary glands of certain insects, such as members of the fruit fly genus *Drosophila.* The chromosomes divide repeatedly to produce the so-called giant salivary chromosomes, of great value in genetic mapping studies. **ring c.** 1 Any chromosome that morphologically appears as a ring, without discernible telomeres. These may be aberrant and meiotically unstable, as they are in humans, or they may occur normally from two terminal chiasmata during diakinesis. 2 The circular DNA molecule of many bacteria and viruses. **sex c.** A chromosome that has a major sex-determining role. In animals one sex, the homogametic sex, has a homologous pair of sex chromosomes. The other sex, the heterogametic sex, has one of these homologues and a morphologically and genetically distinct second sex chromosome. In humans, the female has two X chromosomes and the male one X and one Y chromosome. Also *idiochromosome, heterosome (rarely used).* **somatic c.** Any chromosome present in or isolated from somatic cells. **submetacentric c.** A chromosome having the centromere between the midpoint and one of the ends such that the centromeric index is between 25 and 45. In humans this includes chromosomes of groups B, C, and E. **subtelocentric c.** ACROCENTRIC CHROMOSOME. **supernumerary c.'s** ACCESSORY CHROMOSOMES. **telocentric c.** A chromosome with its centromere at the morphologic end. **W c.** In species in which the female is heterogametic, the chromosome that is limited to the female. **X c.** One of the sex chromosomes found in many species. In humans, it is relatively large, metacentric, and a member of the C group. **Y c.** One of the sex chromosomes found in some species. In humans it is small, acrocentric, and a member of the G group. Its long arm usually fluoresces after cytologic staining with quinacrine. **Z c.** In species in which the female is heterogametic, the chromosome present in both sexes.

**chromospermism** \-spur′mizm\ [CHROMO- + SPERM + -ISM] A condition of coloration of the sperm.

**chromotropic** \-träp′ik\ Being drawn toward or attracted by a pigment.

**chromotropism** \krōmät′rəpizm\ [CHROMO- + TROPISM] The movement or orientation of motile organisms toward, or in response to, a specific color or pigment. Also *chromatotropism.*

**chron-** \krän-\ CHRONO-.

**chronaxy** \krō′naksē\ [CHRON- + Gk *axi(a)* worth, value] The minimum duration of electric current required to induce muscular contraction at a voltage of two times the rheobase (i.e. threshold voltage). Also *chronaxia, chronaxie.*

**chronic** \krän′ik\ [Gk *chronikos* (from *chron(os)* time + *-ikos* -IC) pertaining to time] Of or characterized by extended duration and typically by slow development or a pattern of recurrence: said especially of a disease. Compare ACUTE.

**chronicity** \krōnis′itē\ The condition of being chronic.

**chrono-** \krän′ō-, krän′ə-, krō′nō-\ [Gk *chronos* time] A combining form denoting time. Also *chron-*.

**chronobiology** \-bī·äl′əjē\ The study of the effect of time passage on living systems.

**chronograph** \krän′əgraf\ [CHRONO- + -GRAPH] A device that records the passage of time through prespecified intervals.

**chronometry** \krōnäm′ətrē\ [CHRONO- + -METRY] The measurement of time.

**chronomyometer** \-mī·äm′ətər\ An instrument for measuring the chronaxy of muscle.

**chronophobia** \-fō′bē·ə\ [CHRONO- + -PHOBIA] Pathologic fear of the passing of time or of its immensity. This is a common type of stress reaction observed in prison inmates serving long sentences.

**chronoscope** \krän′əskōp\ [CHRONO- + -SCOPE] A device that measures and records extremely short intervals of elapsed time, as, for example, the time of transmission of an electrical impulse.

**chronotropism** \krōnät′rəpizm\ [CHRONO- + TROPISM] **1** An alteration in the rate of a recurring phenomenon. **2** An alteration in heart rate. Adj. chronotropic.

**chrotopsia** \krōtäp′sē·ə\ CHROMATOPSIA.

**chrys-** \kris-\ CHRYSO-.

**chrysalis** \kris′əlis\ (*pl.* chrysalides, chrysalises) A pupa, of a butterfly or other insect, with a relatively rigid integument and without a cocoon. Also *chrysalid*.

**chrysarobin** Purified Goa powder, which is used in ointments to treat skin disorders such as psoriasis. The major active ingredient is chrysophenolanthanol.

**chrysiasis** \krisī′əsis\ [*chrys(o)-* + -IASIS] Deposition of gold within tissues, in light-exposed areas of skin and sclera. It may visibly occur in the cornea and conjunctiva, as following gold therapy for arthritis. Also *chrysosis, auriasis, aurochromoderma, chrysoderma*.

**chryso-** \kris′ō-\ [Gk *chrysos* gold] A combining form denoting gold. Also *chrys-*.

**chrysoderma** \-dur′mə\ CHRYSIASIS.

***Chrysomyia*** \-mī′yə\ [CHRYSO- + Gk *myia* a fly] A genus of flies of the family Calliphoridae, causing myiasis in animals and man, and found in Africa, parts of Asia, Australia, and New Guinea. ***C. bezziana*** A species of calliphorid flies widespread in Africa, Asia, and islands of the Indian and Pacific oceans. The larvae are often found in wounds of man and other animals, causing severe myiasis. Cattle are particularly often affected, many fatally. Also *Cochliomyia bezziana*. ***C. macellaria*** *COCHLIOMYIA MACELLARIA*.

**chrysophanic acid** $C_{15}H_{10}O_4$. 1,8-Dihydroxy-3-methylanthraquinone. A golden yellow powder, insoluble in water, but soluble in alkalies. It is used in dermatology in the treatment of psoriasis and eczema. It occurs free and also combined in cascara, senna, and rhubarb. Also *rhubarb yellow, lapathin*.

***Chrysops*** \kris′äps\ [Gk *chrysōps* (from *chrys(os)* gold + *ōps* eye) gold-colored] A genus of *Musca*-sized tabanid biting flies including the deer flies and mangrove (or mango) flies. ***C. dimidiata*** A species that is an intermediate host of *Loa loa* in southwestern Africa; the mangrove (or mango) fly. ***C. discalis*** A deer fly that is a vector of tularemia in the western United States. ***C. silacea*** An important vector of *Loa loa* in tropical Africa.

**chrysosis** \krisō′sis\ CHRYSIASIS.

**chrysotherapy** \-ther′əpē\ [CHRYSO- + THERAPY] The use of gold salts for therapy. Also *aurotherapy*.

**chrysotile** \kris′ōtīl\ $Mg_3(Si_2O_5)(OH_4)$. Hydrated magnesium silicate, a form of asbestos occurring in serpentine rock. It is widely distributed in many countries and represents more than 90% of the world's asbestos production. It can be distinguished from other varieties of asbestos by its color, which ranges from white to grey-green. If inhaled as dust it can cause asbestosis and carcinoma of the lung. Also *chrysotile asbestos, white asbestos*.

**chunk** A unit of material carried momentarily in short-term memory. Owing to a limited capacity, only a relatively few items can be held, and these only briefly. Organizing the material into meaningful chunks, such as words or already familiar number sequences, much increases the ability to process information. The digit series 14921066 broken into chunks of 1492 and 1066 reduces substantially the number of items to be carried in the short-term memory phase.

**churganja** \chərgän′jə\ MARIHUANA.

**Chvostek** [Franz *Chvostek*, Austrian surgeon, 1835–1884] Chvostek symptom, Chvostek-Weiss sign, Schultze-Chvostek sign. See under CHVOSTEK SIGN.

**chyl-** \kīl-\ CHYLO-.

**chyle** \kīl\ [Gk *chylos* juice, chyle] The fluid in the intestinal lymph vessels involved in absorption from the lumen of the gut.

**chylemia** \kīlē′mē·ə\ The presence of chyle in blood.

**chyli-** \kī′lē-\ CHYLO-.

**chylifacient** \-fā′shənt\ **1** An agent promoting the formation of chyle. **2** Capable of promoting the formation of chyle. Also *chylifactive, chylificatory*.

**chyliferous** \kīlif′ərəs\ Containing or conveying chyle.

**chylificatory** \kīlif′ikətôr′ē\ CHYLIFACIENT.

**chyliform** \kī′lifôrm\ Resembling chyle; chylelike.

**chylo-** \kī′lō-, kī′lə-\ [Gk *chylos* juice, chyle] A combining form denoting chyle. Also *chyl-, chyli-*.

**chylocele** \kī′ləsēl\ [CHYLO- + -CELE[1]] The excess flow of chyle into the tunica vaginalis area of the testis, commonly seen in testicular filariasis.

**chylocyst** \kī′ləsist\ CISTERNA CHYLI.

**chyloderma** \-dur′mə\ [CHYLO- + Gk *derma* skin] FILARIAL ELEPHANTIASIS.

**chylomediastinum** \-mē′dē·astī′nəm\ The presence of chyle in the mediastinum, usually caused by malignant or traumatic disruption of lymphatics.

**chylomicron** \-mī′krän\ [CHYLO- + Gk *mikron*, neut. of *mikros* small] A lipoprotein particle that is less dense than water and with a diameter of 75–600 nm. It consists principally of triacylglycerol, but it also contains small amounts of cholesterol, phospholipids, and apoproteins. Formed in the epithelial cells of the small intestine, chylomicrons are the means whereby dietary fat is absorbed. They first enter the lymph fluid and are emptied into blood via the thoracic duct. The triacylglycerol is released from the chylomicrons by the enzyme lipoprotein lipase, found largely in liver and adipose tissue. Also *lipomicron*.

**chylomicronemia** \-mī′krānē′mē·ə\ The presence of excessive numbers of chylomicrons in the blood, which give a turbid appearance to plasma at body temperature. Also *hyperchylomicronemia*.

**chylopericarditis** \-per′ikärdī′tis\ [CHYLO- + PERICARDITIS] Inflammation of the pericardium resulting from the presence of chyle in it. See also CHYLOPERICARDIUM.

**chylopericardium** \-per′ikär′dē·əm\ The presence of chyle in the pericardium, usually due to obstruction or trauma to the thoracic duct.

**chyloperitoneum** \-per′itōnē′əm\ The presence of chyle in the peritoneal cavity, resulting from anomalies, injuries, or obstruction of the thoracic duct. Also *chylous ascites, chyliform ascites, fatty ascites, milky ascites*.

**chylopleura** \-plUr′ə\ CHYLOTHORAX.

**chylorrhea** \kī′lôrē′ə\ [CHYLO- + -RRHEA] **1** Discharge of chyle into the bowel lumen, often seen in intestinal lymphangiectasia. **2** Discharge of chyle to an external surface, as after transection of the thoracic duct in the neck.

**chylosis** \kīlō′sis\ [CHYL- + -OSIS] The production and metabolism of chyle.

**chylothorax** \-thôr′aks\ Accumulation of chyle in the pleural space. It usually occurs when the thoracic duct is interrupted by trauma or obstructed by tumor. Compare CHYLOPLEURA, CHYLOUS HYDROTHORAX.

**chylous** \kī′ləs\ Relating to or containing chyle.

**chyluria** \kīloo′rē·ə\ [CHYL- + -URIA] The presence of chyle in the urine. Chyluria results from rupture of lymphatics into the renal pelvis in the presence of obstruction of the upper abdominal or thoracic lymph flow due to any cause. The presence of chyle causes the urine to appear milky. Also *lymphuria, chylous urine, galacturia* (obs.). **c. tropica** The presence of chyle in the urine resulting from lymphatic obstruction around the urinary system and caused by infection with the filarial nematodes *Wuchereria bancrofti* and *Brugia malayi.*

**chymase** *Obs.* CHYMOSIN.

**chyme** \kīm\ [Gk *chym(a)* (from *chein* to pour) a liquid] The semifluid contents in the lumen of the upper gastrointestinal tract that is formed from ingested food.

**chymopapain** Any of a few related cysteine proteinases (EC 3.4.22.6) found in papaya latex but different from papain.

**chymosin** An acid proteinase (EC 3.4.23.4), similar to pepsin, found in the stomach of young animals. Also *rennin* (obs.), *chymase* (obs.), *pexin.*

**chymotrypsin** A proteinase (EC 3.4.21.1) formed in the intestine from the enzymatically inactive precursor chymotrypsinogen by proteolysis. It reacts with peptides, most rapidly if a hydrophobic residue contributes the CO group of the —CO—NH— bond being split, to release amine and become acylated on one of its serine residues (chymotrypsin is therefore classed as a serine proteinase). Nearby histidine and aspartate residues assist nucleophilic attack by this serine by removing a hydrogen ion from it. The acyl enzyme is then hydrolyzed. Chymotrypsin contains disulfide bonds. Several forms exist according to the number of peptide bonds in it that have been split in addition to the one whose splitting is necessary for the activation of chymotrypsinogen. Much of its sequence is the same as those of other serine proteinases, both digestive, such as trypsin, and not, such as thrombin. **c. alpha** A proteolytic enzyme isolated as chymotrypsinogen from bovine pancreas and activated to chymotrypsin. It is used in ophthalmology to dissect the zonule of the lens in intracapsular cataract extraction, and externally for enzymatic débridement of exudates around burns and ulcerated tissue. **sterile c.** A sterile solution of chymotrypsin that has been used in cataract operations to loosen the lens by dissolving the zonular fibers.

**chymotrypsinogen** The enzymatically almost inactive precursor of chymotrypsin secreted by the pancreas. Cleavage by trypsin of the Arg-Ile bond between residues 15 and 16 converts it into chymotrypsin.

**chymotryptic** Concerning chymotrypsin: used especially of reactions catalyzed by it, as in *chymotryptic splitting,* or the products of such reactions, such as the peptides produced on treatment of a protein with the enzyme.

**CI** **1** color index. **2** *Colour Index.* **3** coronary insufficiency.

**Ci** curie.

**Ciaccio** [Gino Giuseppi Vincenzo *Ciaccio,* Italian anatomist, 1824–1901] Ciaccio's glands. See under GLANDULAE LACRIMALES ACCESSORIAE.

**cib.** *cibus* (L, food).

**cibisotome** \sibis′ōtōm\ CYSTITOME.

**cicatrices** \sik′ətrī′sēz\ Plural of CICATRIX.

**cicatricial** \sik′ətrish′l\ Pertaining to a scar. Also *uletic* (obs.).

**cicatrix** \sik′ətriks, sikā′triks\ [L, a scar] (*pl.* cicatrices) A scar; fibrous material composed of collagen and ground substance, produced in the healing of a wound. Also *apulosis.* **brain c.** A scar in the brain. **filtering c.** The surface scar on an eye that has had glaucoma surgery to permit aqueous humor to escape to a subconjunctival location. **hypertrophic c.** A scar with an overgrowth of fibrous tissue. **manometric c.** A healed perforation of the pars tensa membranae tympani, which, because of the absence of the supporting fibrous layer, moves in or out with variations of intratympanic air pressure. **meningocerebral c.** An area of scarring involving both the meninges and brain substance. It is often a result of a penetrating wound which causes the meninges to adhere to the brain surface.

**cicatrizant** \sikat′rizənt\ [Med L *cicatrizans,* gen. *cicatrizantis,* pres. part. of *cicatrizare* to scar, from L *cicatrix* scar] An agent capable of causing scar formation. Also *apulotic, synulotic.*

**cicatrization** \sik′ətrizā′shən\ [*cicatr(ix)* + *-iz(e)* + -ATION] The process of scar evolution associated with wound contraction. Also *epulosis* (seldom used), *apulosis, ulosis.*

**cicatrize** \sik′ətrīz\ To heal in a way that results in the formation of a scar.

**cicutism** \sik′yətizm\ [*Cicut(a)* + -ISM] Poisoning from water hemlock (*Cicuta* sp.). The symptoms are convulsions, dilated pupils, cyanosis, and coma.

**CID** cytomegalic inclusion disease.

**cidal** \sī′dl\ BACTERICIDAL.

**-cide** \-sīd\ [L *-cida* -killer and *-cidium* the killing of, from *caedere* to cut down, kill] A combining form meaning (1) something that kills or destroys (a specified kind of organism), as in *insecticide;* (2) the killing or destruction of (something specified), as in *homicide.*

**CIE** counterimmunoelectrophoresis.

**ciguatera** \sē′gwəter′ə\ [Spanish, from Taino, prob. from *cigu(a)* a sea snail + Spanish *-era,* fem. noun suffix] A form of poisoning due to the ingestion of certain marine tropical fish. Symptoms may include gastrointestinal disturbances, muscular weakness, and disturbances in the central nervous system. Also *siguatera.*

**cilia** \sil′ē·ə\ Plural of CILIUM.

**ciliaris** \sil′ē·er′is\ MUSCULUS CILIARIS.

**ciliariscope** \sil′ē·er′iskōp\ [*ciliar(y body)* + *i* + -SCOPE] A device to examine the ciliary body by means of a corneal contact lens.

**ciliarotomy** \sil′ē·erät′əmē\ [*ciliar(y body)* + *o* + -TOMY] Surgical incision of the ciliary body.

**ciliary** \sil′ē·er′ē\ Pertaining to or resembling the eyelashes or any cilia or hairlike processes: usually used in reference to structures in the orbit, as *ciliary ganglion* and *ciliary process.*

**ciliastatic** \sil′ē·əstat′ik\ [CILIA + -STAT + -IC] Serving to impair or arrest the motility of cilia, especially the cilia of the respiratory mucosa. Certain drugs and drying of the mucosa can have a ciliastatic effect.

**Ciliata** \sil′ē·ā′tə\ [L *cili(um)* eyelash, eyelid + -ATA] A former class of protozoa of the subphylum (now phylum) Ciliophora, which bear cilia or structures related to cilia, such as cirri or membranelles, throughout the life cycle. These protozoans typically contain two nuclei, a vegetative macronucleus and a genetic micronucleus. *Paramecium* and *Balantidium* are examples. Also *Infusoria* (outmoded).

**ciliate** \sil′ē·āt\ **1** CILIATED. **2** An organism which possesses cilia.

**ciliated** \sil′ē·ā′tid\ Having cilia.

**ciliation** \sil′ē·ā′shən\ **1** The development of eyelashes. **2** The formation or development of cilia. **3** A state characterized by the possession of cilia.

**ciliocytophoria** \sil′ē·ōsī′təfôr′ē·ə\ Widespread destruction of the ciliated epithelium of the bronchi in association with an infection such as viral pneumonia.

**Ciliophora** \sil′ē·äf′ərə\ [*cili(um)* + *o* + New L *-phora*, neut. pl. of Gk *-phoros*, suffix denoting bearing, carrying] A phylum of protozoa, consisting mostly of free-living species, which possess cilia or compound ciliary organelles during some stage of their development. A few species, such as *Balantidium coli*, are parasitic. The group was formerly considered a subphylum of the phylum Protozoa, but recently was elevated to phyletic rank, with three classes, Kinetofragminophorea (including *Balantidium*), Oligohymenophorea (*Tetrahymena, Paramecium*), and Polymenophorea (*Stentor, Euplotes*).

**cilioscleral** \sil′ē·ōsklir′əl\ Pertaining to the ciliary body and the overlying sclera.

**ciliospinal** \sil′ē·ōspī′nəl\ [*cili(ary)* + *o* + *spinal*] Pertaining to the center located at the lower cervical and upper first or second thoracic segments where sympathetic control over pupillary dilatation originates. • As neither the ciliary body nor the ciliary ganglion is involved in this action, the term is a misnomer.

**ciliotomy** \sil′ē·ät′əmē\ [*cili(ary)* + *o* + -TOMY] A cutting of the ciliary body or ciliary nerve.

**ciliotoxicity** The property of a drug or other agent of impeding the ciliary motility of cells, such as those lining the respiratory tract.

**cilium** \sil′ē·əm\ [L, eyelash, eyelid] (*pl.* cilia) **1** An eyelash; one of the short, thick hairs attached in two or three rows along the free edge of the eyelids, the upper hairs curving upward and the lower hairs downward. They grow to a fixed length, live for about three months, and are then replaced. **2** The free edge of the eyelid. An outmoded usage. **3** A long slender microscopic process extending from a cell surface and capable of rhythmic motion. It extends from a centriole just inside the plasma membrane and is composed of nine doublets of microtubules around the periphery with two single central microtubules. **olfactory c.** One of the cilial processes projecting from the free border of a receptor cell in the olfactory epithelium.

**cillosis** \silō′sis\ [New L, from *cill-* as in *(os)cill(ation)* + -OSIS] Trembling of an eyelid, especially spasmodic movement of the upper lid but also the much more common benign myokymia of the lower eyelid. *Seldom used.* Also *cillo.* Adj. cillotic.

**cimetidine** $C_{10}H_{16}N_6S$. *N*-Cyano-*N′*-methyl-*N″*-[2-[[(5-methyl-1*H*-imidazol-4-yl)methyl]thio]ethyl]guanidine, an effective antagonist of histamine $H_2$-receptors. It inhibits gastric secretion of hydrochloric acid by all stimuli and is a frequently used medication for the treatment of peptic ulcers. It is usually given orally but can be administered intravenously.

***Cimex*** \sī′meks\ [L, a bug, bedbug] A genus of bedbugs of the family Cimicidae, in the order Hemiptera. These bloodsucking bugs, with a characteristic disagreeable pungent odor, are notorious associates of humans, frequenting mattresses and crevices near sleeping quarters, and biting at night. The two best known human associates are *C. lectularius*, the common bedbug, which is cosmopolitan in distribution, and *C. hemipterus*, which is more frequently found in the tropics. ***C. hemipterus*** A species widespread in both hemispheres but especially prevalent in the tropics, where it is a serious parasite of humans in their dwellings. It also feeds on the blood of domestic fowl and certain bats. It is morphologically and biologically similar to *C. lectularius*. ***C. lectularius*** The common bedbug of temperate climates. Though associated with humans over the centuries, it appears not to have become a vector of any pathogen.

**Cimicidae** \simis′idē\ [L *cimex*, gen. *cimicis*, a bug, bedbug + -IDAE] A family of wingless, bloodsucking insects in the suborder Heteroptera, order Hemiptera, which are commonly known as bedbugs. Medically important genera include *Cimex, Haematosiphon, Leptocimex*, and *Oeciacus*.

**Cimino** [James E. *Cimino*, U.S. nephrologist, born 1928] Brescia-Cimino fistula. See under RADIOCEPHALIC FISTULA.

**cin-** \sin-\ KINE-.

**cinanesthesia** \sin′anesthē′zhə\ KINANESTHESIA.

**cinching** \sin′ching\ [Spanish *cincha* (from L *cingulum* a girdle, belt, from *cingere* to gird) a girth, cinch + -ING] The surgical shortening of a muscle, especially an extraocular muscle, by plication.

**cinchona** \sinkō′nə\ The root and stem bark of several species of *Cinchona* and their hybrids, rich sources of the quinoline alkaloids quinine, quinidine, cinchonine, and cinchonidine. *C. calisaya* yields calisaya, yellowbark, or calisaya bark; *C. pelletierana* produces cusco bark, and *C. lancifolia* yields Cartagena bark. Also *cinchona bark, Peruvian bark, Jesuits' bark, quinaquina* (older term), *quinquina*.

**cinchonic** Pertaining to or derived from cinchona.

**cinchonic acid hydrochloride** CINCHONINE DIHYDROCHLORIDE.

**cinchonidine hydrochloride** $C_{19}H_{22}N_2O$. A drug with antimalarial properties. It also has effects on the heart similar to those of quinidine, but to a lesser degree.

**cinchonine** $C_{19}H_{22}N_2O$. A white, crystalline alkaloid with a bitter taste, obtained from cinchona bark. It is used as an antimalarial agent, like quinine.

**cinchonine dihydrochloride** $C_{19}H_{22}ON_2{\cdot}2HCl$. A white, crystalline salt that is soluble in water. Also *cinchonic acid hydrochloride*.

**cinchonism** An illness produced by excessive or prolonged treatment with cinchona or cinchona bark alkaloids, such as quinine. The toxic symptoms include tinnitus, rash, nausea, mental and cardiac disturbances, and failure of the circulatory or respiratory systems. Also *quininism*.

**cinchopen** $C_{16}H_{11}NO_2$. 2-Phenyl-4-quinoline carboxylic acid. An agent with analgesic and antipyretic properties like aspirin. The incidence of serious hepatotoxicity with this drug has practically eliminated its use.

**cinclisis** \sin′klisis\ Rapid repetitive movement of a part of the body.

**cine-** \sin′ə-, sin′ē-\ KINE-.

**cineangiocardiography** \-an′jē·ōkär′dē·äg′rəfē\ Motion picture recording of angiocardiography, usually by recording successive fluoroscopic images.

**cineangiogram** \-an′jē·ōgram′\ The filmed record taken during cineangiography.

**cineangiograph** \-an′jē·ōgraf′\ The camera used for cineangiography.

**cineangiography** \-an′jē·äg′rəfē\ Motion picture recording of angiography, usually by recording successive fluoroscopic images.

**cinedensigraphy** \-densig′rəfē\ [CINE- + L *dens(us)* dense + *i* + -GRAPHY] The recording of the movements of body structures by using x rays and radiation detectors.

**cine-esophagogram** \-esäf′əgōgram\ A motion picture record of the esophagus while the patient is swallowing a

contrast agent, usually barium.
**cinefluorography** \-floo′əräg′rəfē\ [CINE- + FLUOROGRAPHY] CINERADIOGRAPHY.
**cinefluoroscopy** \-floo′əräs′kəpē\ A motion picture recording of fluoroscopy. *Seldom used.*
**cinematics** \-mat′iks\ KINEMATICS.
**cinematography** \-mətäg′rəfē\ [*cinemat(ic)* + *o* + -GRAPHY] CINERADIOGRAPHY.
**cinematoradiography** \-mat′ôrā′dē·äg′rəfē\ CINERADIOGRAPHY.
**cineole** EUCALYPTOL.
**cinephlebography** \-flebäg′rəfē\ [CINE- + PHLEBO- + -GRAPHY] The motion picture recording of successive fluoroscopic images of a vein or veins after the injection of contrast medium.
**cineradiography** \-rā′dē·äg′rəfē\ [CINE- + RADIOGRAPHY] The recording with motion pictures of successive fluoroscopic images. Also *cinefluorography, cinematography, cinematoradiography, roentgenocinematography.*
**cinerea** \sinir′ē·ə\ [L, fem. of *cinereus* ashy] SUBSTANTIA GRISEA.
**cinesalgia** \sin′esal′jə\ KINESALGIA.
**cinesi-** \sin′əsē-, sīnē′sē-\ KINESIO-.
**cinesio-** \sīnē′sē·ō-\ KINESIO-.
**cineso-** \sīnē′sō-\ KINESIO-.
**cineto-** \sinet′ō-, sīnē′tō-\ KINETO-.
**cingula** \sin′gyələ\ Plural of CINGULUM.
**cingulate** \sin′gyəlāt\ Pertaining to or resembling a cingulum.
**cingule** \sin′gyool\ CINGULUM.
**cingulotomy** \sin′gyəlät′əmē\ [*cingul(ate gyrus)* + *o* + -TOMY] An undercutting of the gray matter of the cingulate gyrus to disconnect it from the cortex. This procedure is a form of psychosurgery for the treatment of psychosis.
**cingulum** \sin′gyələm\ [L, a girdle, cincture] (*pl.* cingula) **1** A girdlelike or beltlike structure, usually partially or totally encircling another structure. Also *girdle.* **2** [NA] A bundle of fibers in the white matter of the gyrus cinguli which follows the curve of the corpus callosum from the anterior perforated substance to the hippocampal gyrus. For defs 1 and 2 also *cingule.* **3** CINGULUM DENTIS. **c. athleticum** A band of telangiectatic venules encircling the chest in a pattern that is related to the insertions of the diaphragm. It is supposedly a consequence of severe physical strain. **c. dentis** [NA] An inverted V-shaped, horizontal ridge near the base, neck, or gum margin of the lingual surface of the crowns of the upper incisor teeth. It is rarely visible on the lower incisors. Also *basal ridge, cingulum.* **c. extremitatis inferioris** CINGULUM MEMBRI INFERIORIS. **c. extremitatis superioris** CINGULUM MEMBRI SUPERIORIS. **c. hemispherii** *Outmoded* GYRUS CINGULI. **c. membri inferioris** [NA] The irregular bony ring at the lower end of the trunk, formed by the two innominate bones, joined at the symphysis pubis anteriorly and articulated with the sacrum posteriorly, serving to conduct stresses from the axial skeleton to the lower limbs, to protect the pelvic viscera, and to act as a birth canal in mammals. Also *cingulum extremitatis inferioris, pelvic girdle, hip girdle, girdle of inferior extremity.* **c. membri superioris** [NA] The incomplete bony ring formed by the clavicle and the scapula articulating with each other at the acromioclavicular joint and with the trunk at the sternoclavicular joint. It attaches and supports the upper limb at the shoulder joint. Also *cingulum extremitatis superior, shoulder girdle, pectoral girdle, thoracic girdle, girdle of superior extremity, upper limb girdle.*
**cinnabar** MERCURIC SULFIDE.
**cino-** \sin′ō-, sī′nō-\ KINO-.
**cinology** \sinäl′əjē\ KINESIOLOGY.
**cinometer** \sinäm′ətər\ KINESIMETER.
**cion** \sī′än\ [Gk *kiōn* uvula] *Outmoded* UVULA.
**cionectomy** [*cion(o)-* + -ECTOMY] UVULOTOMY.
**ciono-** \sī′ōnō-\ [Gk *kiōn* column, uvula] A combining form denoting the uvula. Also *kiono-.*
**circadian** \sur′kədē′ən, surkā′dē·ən\ [L *circa* about, around + *di(em)*, accus. sing. of *dies* day + English *-an*, suffix denoting of or pertaining to] Characterized by or describing a rhythm or recurring period of biological activity of roughly 24 hours. Although theoretically linked to the day-night cycle, it has been shown to persist even when day-night clues are removed.
**circellus** \sərsel′əs\ [L, dim. of *circes* a circle or ring] A small circle or ring.
**circinate** \sur′sināt\ [L *circinatus* (from *circinus* a curved line) made circular, rounded] Having an annular, coiled, or circular configuration.
**circle** [L *circulus.* See CIRCULUS.] **1** A geometric figure in the form of a continuous curved line everywhere equidistant from the center. **2** CIRCULUS. **arterial c. of cerebrum** CIRCULUS ARTERIOSUS CEREBRI. **arterial c. of optic nerve** CIRCULUS VASCULOSUS NERVI OPTICI. **arterial c. of Willis** CIRCULUS ARTERIOSUS CEREBRI. **c. of Carus** CURVE OF CARUS. **defensive c.** A state of reciprocal inhibition or antagonism between two pathologic conditions in the same subject, so that each tends to limit the development of the other. **greater arterial c. of iris** CIRCULUS ARTERIOSUS IRIDIS MAJOR. **greater c. of iris** ANNULUS IRIDIS MAJOR. **c. of Hovius** A circular anastomosis of the ciliary veins in the sclera at the sclerocorneal junction. Also *circulus venosus hovii* (outmoded). **Huguier c.** An arterial anastomosis between the right and left uterine arteries occasionally present around the isthmus of the uterus. **lesser arterial c. of iris** CIRCULUS ARTERIOSUS IRIDIS MINOR. **lesser c. of iris** ANNULUS IRIDIS MINOR. **Robinson's c.** A vascular circle in the abdomen, formed by anastomosis of the aorta and the common iliac, hypogastric, ovarian, and uterine arteries. **vascular c. of optic nerve** CIRCULUS VASCULOSUS NERVI OPTICI. **venous c. of mammary gland** PLEXUS VENOSUS AREOLARIS. **c. of Willis** CIRCULUS ARTERIOSUS CEREBRI. **c. of Zinn** CIRCULUS VASCULOSUS NERVI OPTICI.
**circuit** \sur′kit\ [L *circuitus* (from *circuire* to go around, from *circu(m)* around + *ire* to go) a going round, a circuit] **1** A network of electronic components providing a path of electric current or magnetic flux. **2** Any closed path or course, often circular. **active c.** An electric circuit whose output depends on the control of power from a source. Amplifiers, oscillators, and logic circuits are active. Resistors, transformers, and diodes are passive. **analog c.** An electronic circuit in which voltages vary continuously, as differentiated from a digital circuit in which voltages exist only at discrete levels. **Bain c.** A breathing circuit for general anesthesia. There is a high gas flow and an expiratory valve to prevent carbon dioxide rebreathing. **breathing c.** The route followed by inhaled and exhaled anesthetic gases in an anesthesia breathing system. **coincidence c.** A pulse-handling circuit with two inputs, so designed that it produces an output pulse only if two input pulses arrive at the same time. Such circuits are particularly useful in the detection and imaging of the annihilation radiation that always accompanies positron emission. **constant potential c.** An electronic circuit used to maintain a voltage at a constant value. **full-wave c.**

An electronic circuit which inverts half of each cycle of an alternating electrical current, resulting in two pulses per cycle, each having the same polarity. **integrated c.** An electronic circuit contained in a tiny chip of silicon. Such circuits are capable of great complexity and high reliability. **logic c.** A two-state electronic circuit that performs the symbolic logic functions such as AND, NOT, OR, NAND, and NOR. Input and output states (levels) are logical 1 (high) usually at +5 V, or logical 0 (low) usually at 0 V. See also LOGIC. **Magill-Mapleson c.** A breathing circuit for general anesthesia. There is a high gas flow and an expiratory valve to prevent carbon dioxide rebreathing. **open c.** An electric circuit that has a break in the conductor so that current cannot pass. **Papez c.** The neuronal circuit constituting the limbic brain which involves the hippocampus, fornix, mammillary body and anterior thalamic nuclei. **quenching c.** An inhibiting circuit that prepares a Geiger-Müller tube for repeated ionizing events. It prevents prolongation of avalanche ionization, or a spontaneous repetitive discharge, by promptly though briefly lowering the anode voltage as soon as a genuine pulse has been passed on to the scaler. **reflex c.** REFLEX ARC. **reverberating c.** A type of neuronal pathway possessing feedback loops, usually described to exist in the brain, that allow the perpetuation of neuronal activity. Certain thalamocortical pathways have been described as reverberating circuits. **scaling c.** A circuit that produces an output pulse for a preselected number of input pulses. In a flip-flop, or binary scaler, the ratio is 1:2. In a decade scaler it is 1:10, and so on.

**circulation** [Med L *circulatio* (from *circulari* to move in a circle, from L *circulare* to make circular) movement in a circle, the making of a circuit] **1** Movement in a circle or circuit, that is, back to the starting point, especially movement of blood through veins, heart, arteries and capillaries. **2** Movement of body fluid, as blood in the vascular system, lymph in the lymphatic system, or interstitial fluid in the interstitial spaces. **allantoic c.** FETAL CIRCULATION. **assisted c.** Circulation augmented by mechanical means, such as electromechanical pumps, in treatment of circulatory insufficiency of the limbs. **chorionic c.** PRIMARY EMBRYONIC CIRCULATION. **collateral c.** An alternative set of blood vessels through which blood may be diverted when an obstruction occurs in the normal blood supply. **compensatory c.** Any alternative pathway by which blood circulation can be maintained when an obstruction occurs, as by collateral vessels. **coronary c.** The blood flow through the blood vessels of the heart. **cross c.** Perfusion of blood from one animal to another through a connection between the two vascular systems. **embryonic c.** PRIMARY EMBRYONIC CIRCULATION. **enterohepatic c.** A recurring cycle in which a substance that is absorbed from the lumen of the gut passes to the liver as an element of the blood and is then re-excreted into the gut as an element of the bile. **extracorporeal c.** Circulation of blood outside the body through a heart-lung machine for oxygen-carbon dioxide exchange or through an artificial kidney for dialysis of compounds normally excreted by the kidney. **fetal c.** Circulation of the blood within the vascular system of the fetus. The deoxygenated blood from the fetus passes to the placenta through the umbilical arteries, and the oxygenated blood is returned to the fetus via the umbilical vein. Also *umbilical circulation, allantoic circulation.* **greater c.** SYSTEMIC CIRCULATION. **hypophyseoportal c.** The portal system of veins which surrounds the stalk of the pituitary gland and carries hormones

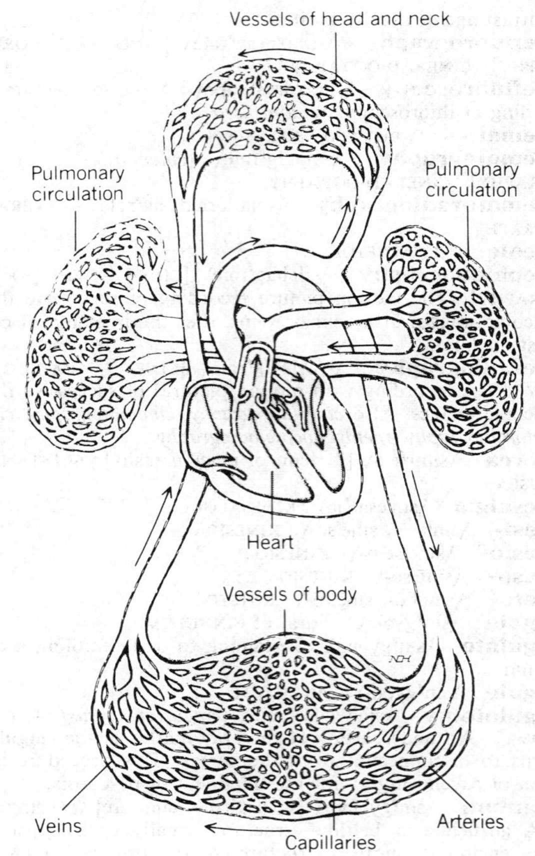


**Circulation of blood**

between the hypothalamus and the posterior lobe of the pituitary. **intervillous c.** The circulation of maternal blood through the intervillous spaces of the human placenta. **lesser c.** PULMONARY CIRCULATION. **omphalomesenteric c.** VITELLINE CIRCULATION. **plasmatic c.** In grafting, the diffusion of plasma through the blood vessels of the graft before they have established continuity with the blood vessels of the recipient site. This is a process that usually lasts around 48 hours, and on which the graft depends for its survival. **portal c.** **1** Any blood vascular system that intervenes between the capillary networks of two organs before the blood returns to the heart. **2** The circulation of blood from the gastrointestinal tract and spleen to the liver, through the portal vein. **primary embryonic c.** The first circulation by which the earliest nutriment and oxygen is conveyed to the embryo. It is almost entirely extraembryonic, within the yolk sac, connecting stalk and chorion. The precocious development of the embryonic heart and blood vessels is correlated with the rapid enlargement of the chorionic sac at this time. Also *chorionic circulation, embryonic circulation.* **pulmonary c.** The blood vascular system between the right ventricle and the left atrium, which includes the pulmonary arteries, capillaries, and veins. Its major function is to allow oxygen uptake and carbon dioxide excretion. Also *lesser circulation.* **systemic c.** The blood vascular system between the left ventricle and the right atrium. Also *greater circulation.* **thebesian c.** The circulation provided by the venae cardiacae minimae (thebesian veins). **umbilical c.** FETAL CIRCULATION. **vertebral-basilar c.** That part of the cerebral circulation that consists of the vertebral and basilar arteries and their branches. **vitelline c.** The circulatory system of the fetus which develops in the blood vessels of the wall of the yolk sac. Also *omphalomesenteric circulation.*

**circulus** \sur′kyələs\ [L (dim. of *circus* a thing of circular form), a circle] A ringlike structure, usually used in reference to the arrangement of arteries and veins. Also *circle.* **c. arteriosus cerebri** [NA] A channel of anastomosed vessels encircling the chiasmatic and hypophysial regions at the base of the brain, and made up of the internal carotid and anterior, middle, and posterior cerebral arteries of both sides and the anterior and posterior communicating arteries. Also *arterial circle of cerebrum, circle of Willis, arterial circle of Willis, circulus arteriosus willisi, circulus willisii.* **c. arteriosus iridis major** [NA] A circular anastomosis between the anterior and the long and short posterior ciliary arteries in the ciliary body along the attached margin of the iris. Also *greater arterial circle of iris.* **c. arteriosus iridis minor** [NA] An incomplete vascular circle near the free margin of the iris, formed by branches of the greater arterial circle of the iris. Some scholars consider these vessels to be venous. Also *lesser arterial circle of iris.* **c. arteriosus willisi** CIRCULUS ARTERIOSUS CEREBRI. **c. articularis vasculosus** CIRCULUS VASCULOSUS. **c. umbilicalis** An anastomosis in the extraperitoneal tissue around the umbilicus between small branches of the superior and inferior epigastric arteries and the urachal branches of the superior vesical arteries. *Outmoded.* **c. vasculosus** [NA] A looped anastomosis of blood vessels located at the articular margins of the bones in a joint, representing the terminations of the vessels of the synovial membrane. Also *circulus articularis vasculosus.* **c. vasculosus nervi optici** [NA] An arterial circle formed by an anastomosis of branches of the short posterior ciliary arteries in the sclera around the entrance of the optic nerve. The anastomosis communicates with pial arteries supplying the nerve and with twigs of the central artery of the retina. Also *vascular circle of optic nerve, arterial circle of optic nerve.* **c. venosus** PLEXUS VENOSUS AREOLARIS. **c. venosus hovii** *Outmoded* CIRCLE OF HOVIUS. **c. venosus ridleyi** *Outmoded* SINUS CIRCULARIS. **c. willisii** CIRCULUS ARTERIOSUS CEREBRI.

**circum-** \sur′kəm-\ [L *circum* around] A prefix meaning around, about, surrounding.

**circumanal** \-ā′nəl\ [CIRCUM- + ANAL] Situated or occurring around the anus. Also *perianal.*

**circumarticular** \-ärtik′yələr\ Encircling a joint; periarticular; periarthric.

**circumaxillary** \-ak′siler′ē\ Around the axilla; periaxillary.

**circumbuccal** \-buk′l\ Around or encircling the mouth.

**circumbulbar** \-bul′bər\ [CIRCUM- + BULBAR] Pertaining to the area surrounding the eyeball.

**circumcallosal** \-kəlō′səl\ Arching over the corpus callosum.

**circumcision** \-sizh′ən\ [Late L *circumcisio* (from L *circumcidere* to cut around, circumcize, from *circum* around + *caedere* to cut) circumcision] **1** The operation of cutting off the end of the foreskin of the penis. This has been performed by many peoples of the world from time immemorial, as a sacrificial rite among Jews and Moslems, or as a mark of initiation into manhood. It is also widely practiced in some countries or communities for reasons merely of hygiene, most of which are dubious. **2** The excision of parts of the external genitalia of female children in some cultures. There is no medical indication for circumcision in females. **female c.** Surgical incision into the prepuce of the clitoris. **pharaonic c.** The practice of suturing or clasping the prepuce or labia majora of women to prevent sexual intercourse. Although associated with significant health hazards, this form of female circumcision is practiced in many regions of Africa.

**circumclusion** \-kloo′zhən\ [CIRCUM- + *(oc)clusion*] The surgical occlusion of an artery by means of a circumferential wire and a short pin.

**circumcorneal** \-kôr′nē·əl\ [CIRCUM- + CORNEAL] Surrounding the cornea.

**circumcrescent** \-kres′ənt\ [CIRCUM- + CRESCENT] Growing over and around an object.

**circumference** \surkum′fərəns\ [L *circumferentia.* See CIRCUMFERENTIA.] CIRCUMFERENTIA. **arm c.** A measure used in pediatrics to assess nutritional status, reflecting both caloric adequacy and muscle mass. The circumference of the upper midarm is measured with a soft tape measure. The midarm muscle circumference can then be calculated by subtracting the product of 3.14 and the skinfold (in cm) to account for arm fat. The result is plotted on a reference graph. Patients with values below normal are likely to be severely malnourished. The measure has been widely used to diagnose protein-calorie malnutrition. **articular c. of head of radius** CIRCUMFERENTIA ARTICULARIS RADII. **articular c. of head of ulna** CIRCUMFERENTIA ARTICULARIS CAPITIS ULNAE.

**circumferentia** \surkum′fəren′shə\ [L (from CIRCUM + *ferens,* gen. *ferentis,* pres. part. of *ferre* to bear), a bearing around, circumference] The outer limit or periphery of a rounded structure or body. Also *circumference.* **c. articularis capitis ulnae** [NA] The convex articular surface on the lateral side of the head of the ulna that articulates with the ulnar notch of the radius. Also *articular circumference of head of ulna, circumferentia articularis capituli ulnae.* **c. articularis radii** [NA] The portion of the disk-shaped head of the radius, wider on the medial aspect, that articulates with the radial notch of the ulna and is encircled by the annular ligament. Also *articular circumference of head of radius.*

**circumflex** \sur′kəmfleks\ [L *circumflex(us),* past part. of *circumflectere* (from *circum-* around + *flectere* to bend, bow, turn) to bend or wind about] In the form of an arc of a circle; bow-shaped, especially with reference to the passage, arrangement, or formation of certain structures, such as blood vessels and nerves. Also *circumflexus.*

**circuminsular** \-in′syələr\ Encircling or situated at the periphery of the cerebral insula.

**circumlental** \-len′təl\ [CIRCUM- + L *lens* (gen. *lentis*) lentil + -AL] Surrounding the crystalline lens.

**circumnuclear** \-n$^y$oo′klē·ər\ PERINUCLEAR.

**circumolivary** \-äl′iver′ē\ Located around the periphery of the nucleus olivaris.

**circumpennate** \-pen′āt\ CIRCUMPENNATE MUSCLE.

**circumstantiality** \-stan′shē·al′itē\ [L *circumstanti(a)* (from *circumstans, circumstantis,* pres. part. of *circumstare* to stand round, surround) a standing round, circumstance + -AL + -ITY] Speech or thinking characterized by unnecessary overdetailing that impedes rather than promotes communication. It has been reported in schizophrenia and also in epileptic dementia and obsessional disorders.

**circumvallate** \-val′āt\ [L *circumvallat(us),* past part. of *circumvallare* (from *circum-* around + *vallare* to fortify) to surround with a rampart, fortify] Surrounded by a trench or fossa or by a ridge as, for example, the circumvallate papillae on the tongue.

**circumvascular** \-vas′kyələr\ PERIVASCULAR.

**circumvolute** \-väl′yoot\ [L *circumvolut(us),* past part. of *circumvolvere* (from *circum-* around + *volvere* to wind or turn around, roll along, revolve) to roll around] Twisted or folded around.

**circumvolutio** \-vōloo′sho\ [Med L, from L *circumvolutus.* See CIRCUMVOLUTE.] A structure or tissue twisted or folded into a tortuous shape; a convolution, or gyrus. **c. cristata** LIMBIC LOBE.

**cirrhogenous** \siräj′ənəs\ Inducing or resulting in cirrhosis.

**cirrhosis** \sirō′sis\ [Gk *kirrh(os)* tawny + -OSIS] A chronic disease of the liver characterized by nodular regeneration of hepatocytes and diffuse fibrosis. It is caused by parenchymal necrosis followed by nodular proliferation of the surviving hepatocytes. The regenerating nodules and accompanying fibrosis interfere with blood flow through the liver and result in portal hypertension, hepatic insufficiency, jaundice, and ascites. Also *fibroid induration, granular induration.* **acholangic biliary c.** Cirrhosis of the liver associated with complete failure of development of the biliary tree. **alcoholic c.** LAENNEC CIRRHOSIS. **biliary c.** Cirrhosis of the liver resulting from biliary tract obstruction, either intrahepatic or extrahepatic. Also *obstructive cirrhosis.* See also PRIMARY BILIARY CIRRHOSIS, SECONDARY BILIARY CIRRHOSIS. **biliary c. of children** A cirrhosis of the liver which follows prolonged obstruction of the bile duct system and is due to partial or complete atresias, congenital malformation of the bile duct, cysts, inspissated bile, or chronic cholangitis. Histologically, small bile duct proliferation, enlargement and medial hypertrophy of the hepatic arteries, and diffuse fibrosis are found in the biliary fasciculi. Later there is loss of liver parenchyma and fibrosis spreads to the whole organ. Terminal liver failure ensues often by the age of six months. Surgical exploration of the biliary system occasionally reveals an obstruction that can be relieved. **cardiac c.** A chronic, fibrotic condition of the liver resulting from long-standing chronic, passive congestion and right-sided heart failure. It is characterized by delicate fibrosis of the central veins, extending into the surrounding sinusoids. Hepatocellular regeneration and nodular transformation rarely occur, and thus this condition is usually not a true cirrhosis. **congenital hepatic c.** CONGENITAL HEPATIC FIBROSIS. **cryptogenic c.** Cirrhosis of unknown etiology. This category accounts for approximately 25 percent of all cases of cirrhosis seen today. **Glisson's c.** A fibrous thickening of the liver capsule caused by old peritonitis or longstanding ascites. It is not actually a cirrhosis. **Hanot c.** PRIMARY BILIARY CIRRHOSIS. **hepatic c.** CIRRHOSIS OF THE LIVER. **Indian childhood c.** A form of liver cirrhosis that occurs in children in India, now thought to be caused by ingestion of copper derived from milk stored in copper or brass vessels. It is frequently fatal. **Laennec c.** Cirrhosis precipitated by alcohol abuse and characterized histologically as a fibrotic process extending between portal tracts and enclosing single lobules which may be replaced by regeneration nodules. Also *portal cirrhosis, Laennec's disease, alcoholic cirrhosis.* **c. of the liver** A chronic diffuse end-stage hepatic disease state with multiple etiologies, characterized histologically by evidence of present or past hepatic cell necrosis, diffuse fibrosis, and regenerating nodules. Sequelae include failure of parenchymal cell function and interference with normal hepatic blood flow. Clinical features include ascites and varices as a consequence of portal hypertension, jaundice, coagulopathy, and encephalopathy. Also *chronic interstitial hepatitis, hepatic cirrhosis, hepatocirrhosis.* **c. of the lung** *Obs.* DIFFUSE INTERSTITIAL PULMONARY FIBROSIS. **macronodular c.** A form of cirrhosis characterized by large, regenerating nodules usually measuring one centimeter in diameter separated by irregular, broad bands of fibrous tissue. This morphologic type of cirrhosis is characteristic of viral cirrhosis and the cirrhosis of Wilson's disease, but may also be seen in the advanced stages of most other forms of cirrhosis. **metabolic c.** Cirrhosis associated with a systemic metabolic disorder, such as Wilson's disease or hemochromatosis. **micronodular c.** Cirrhosis characterized by small, regenerating nodules measuring less than one centimeter and usually 2-4 mm in diameter. The nodules are separated by thin, delicate fibrous bands. The prototype micronodular cirrhosis is that seen in association with excessive alcoholic intake. **monolobular c.** *Seldom used* PRIMARY BILIARY CIRRHOSIS. **multilobular c.** *Seldom used* POSTNECROTIC CIRRHOSIS. **obstructive c.** BILIARY CIRRHOSIS. **pericholangiolitic c.** PRIMARY BILIARY CIRRHOSIS. **periportal c.** POSTNECROTIC CIRRHOSIS. **pigment c.** Cirrhosis associated with hemochromatosis. The liver is fibrotic and has a chocolate brown color due to the heavy deposition of hemosiderin within hepatocytes, Kupfer cells, and scar tissue. Hepatocellular carcinoma complicates pigment cirrhosis in 10 to 20 percent of patients. Also *pigmentary cirrhosis.* **portal c.** LAENNEC CIRRHOSIS. **posthepatitic c.** Cirrhosis which results from antecedent acute or chronic active hepatitis. **postnecrotic c.** Cirrhosis which develops as a consequence of viral or toxic hepatitis and is characterized pathologically as lobular necrosis with collapse of the reticular framework and the development of fibrous bands which demarcate large regenerating nodules. Also *multilobular cirrhosis* (seldom used), *periportal cirrhosis.* **primary biliary c.** A biliary cirrhosis of unknown etiology that chiefly affects middle-aged women. It is characterized pathologically by a spectrum of features including inflammatory destruction of intrahepatic bile ducts, granulomas, bile duct proliferation, cholestasis, portal fibrosis, and cirrhosis. Clinically it may be asymptomatic or present with pruritus, jaundice, hypercholesterolemia, or xanthoma, and progress to the usual sequelae of cirrhosis. Also *Hanot cirrhosis, Hanot syndrome, Hanot's disease, monolobular cirrhosis* (seldom used). **pulmonary c.** DIFFUSE INTERSTITIAL PULMONARY FIBROSIS. **secondary biliary c.** Cirrhosis of the liver caused by prolonged partial or total biliary obstruction. Recognized causes include congenital biliary atresia, obstruction from gallstones, or malignant obstruction. **stasis c.** Cirrhosis resulting from intrahepatic vascular congestion, as in cardiac cirrhosis and the Budd-Chiari syndrome. **syphilitic c.** Cirrhosis associated with congenital or tertiary syphilis. Rarely seen today, it results from perisinusoidal fibrosis and confluence of gummas. Spirochetes are usually demonstrable. Healing of the gummas results in their replacement by deep scars that divide the organ into parenchymal masses of irregular size and shape. This appearance is known as hepar lobatum. **vascular c.** Cirrhosis resulting from obstruction, usually thrombotic, of the hepatic and, less commonly, the portal veins.

**cirrhotic** \sirät′ik\ Pertaining to or affected by cirrhosis.

**cirri** \sir′ī\ Plural of CIRRUS.

**cirrus** \sir′əs\ [L, a lock or tuft of hair] (*pl.* cirri) The sensory or locomotor organ formed from a tuft of fused cilia found in some ciliate protozoa.

**cirs-** \surs-\ CIRSO-.
**cirso-** \sur′sō-\ [Gk *kirsos* dilated vein, varix] A combining form meaning varix. Also *cirs-*.
**cirsocele** \sur′sōsēl\ VARICOCELE.
**cirsoid** \sur′soid\ [CIRS- + -OID] Resembling a varix; varicoid.
**cirsophthalmia** \sur′säfthal′mē·ə\ [CIRS- + OPHTHALMIA] Varicosity of the conjunctival blood vessels.
**cis** \sis\ [L *cis* on this side of (as to place or time)] **1** Having the configuration of being on the same side, in chemistry usually referring to two groups on the same side of a double bond or of a ring. **2** In genetics, having both wild-type alleles of two linked, heterozygous loci on the same chromosome. See also COUPLING. Compare TRANS.
***cis-*** [L *cis* on this side of (as to place or time)] A stereochemical prefix indicating that two groups of a molecule are in the cis configuration.
**cistern** \sis′tərn\ [L *cisterna*. See CISTERNA.] CISTERNA. **anterolateral cerebellar c.** The subarachnoid space at the site of the cerebellopontine angle. Within it are found the trigeminal, facial, vestibulocochlear, glossopharyngeal, and vagus nerves. **basal c.** CISTERNA INTERPEDUNCULARIS. **cerebellomedullary c.** CISTERNA CEREBELLOMEDULLARIS. **c. of the chiasma** CISTERNA CHIASMATIS. **chiasmatic c.** CISTERNA CHIASMATIS. **chyle c.** CISTERNA CHYLI. **c. of the corpus callosum** CISTERNA CORPORIS CALLOSI. **c. of fossa of Sylvius** CISTERNA FOSSAE LATERALIS CEREBRI. **great c.** CISTERNA CEREBELLOMEDULLARIS. **c. of the great cerebral vein** CISTERNA VENAE MAGNAE CEREBRI. **interpeduncular c.** CISTERNA INTERPEDUNCULARIS. **c. of the lateral fossa** CISTERNA FOSSAE LATERALIS CEREBRI. **lumbar c.** The enlargement of the subarachnoid space extending from the end of the spinal cord (in man, at the second lumbar vertebra) to the caudal termination of the arachnoid-dural sac (at level $S_2$). It contains the cauda equina, and is the objective in a lumbosacral spinal tap. Also *cisterna lumbalis.* **c. of Pecquet** CISTERNA CHYLI. **pontine c.** The shallow expanse of subarachnoid space bounded by the pons and medulla behind and the bony clivus in front. It communicates superiorly with the interpeduncular cistern, inferiorly with the spinal subarachnoid space, and inferolaterally with the cisterna cerebellomedullaris. It is traversed by the basilar artery. Also *cisterna pontis.* **posterior c.** CISTERNA CEREBELLOMEDULLARIS. **subarachnoidal c.'s** CISTERNAE SUBARACHNOIDEALES. **superior c.** CISTERNA VENAE MAGNAE CEREBRI. **supracallosal c.** CISTERNA CORPORIS CALLOSI.
**cisterna** \sistur′nə\ [L (from *cista* a box), a hollow place underground for holding water, cistern] (*pl.* cisternae) **1** [NA] An enclosed space, usually a dilatation in a drainage pattern, that serves as a reservoir for body fluids, such as lymph and cerebrospinal fluid. Also *cistern.* **2** One of a group of membrane-enclosed sacs in the cell cytoplasm, often flattened and arranged in a stack (e.g., Golgi cisternae). **c. ambiens** CISTERNA VENAE MAGNAE CEREBRI. **c. basalis** CISTERNA INTERPEDUNCULARIS. **c. caryothecae** PERINUCLEAR SPACE. **c. cerebellomedullaris** [NA] An expansion of the subarachnoid space lying between the inferior surface of the cerebellum, the dorsal surface of the medulla and, posteroinferiorly, the arachnoid sheet bridging these. Inferiorly, it is continuous with the spinal subarachnoid space. In the surgical procedure of a suboccipital cisternal tap it is approached with a cannula through the posterior atlanto-occipital membrane. Also *cerebellomedullary cistern, posterior cistern, cisterna magna, great cistern, postcisterna.* **c. chiasmatis** [NA] The enlargement of the subarachnoid space centered on the optic chiasma and extending upward to the rostrum of the corpus callosum. Prechiasmatic and postchiasmatic portions are sometimes distinguished. Also *cistern of the chiasma, chiasmatic cistern.* **c. chyli** [NA] A saccular dilatation at the commencement of the thoracic duct that is joined by the right and left lumbar and the intestinal lymphatic trunks. It is usually on the right side of the abdominal aorta and in front of the bodies of the first and second lumbar vertebrae. Also *ampulla chyli, chyle cistern, chylocyst, cistern of Pecquet, receptaculum chyli* (outmoded), *receptaculum pecqueti* (outmoded), *chyle bladder.* **c. corporis callosi** A long, curved cistern above the superior surface of the corpus callosum and beneath the lower margin of the falx cerebri. The anterior cerebral arteries pass along it. Also *supracallosal cistern, cistern of the corpus callosum.* **c. fossae lateralis cerebri** [NA] The enlargement of the subarachnoid space formed where the arachnoid crosses the lateral cerebral fissure. It contains the middle cerebral artery. Also *cistern of the lateral fossa, cistern of fossa of Sylvius, cisterna sulci lateralis, cisterna valleculae lateralis cerebri.* **Golgi cisternae** The flattened platelike sacules that form into stacks to make the Golgi apparatus. The peripheral regions of the cisternae are often expanded and may contain pores or fenestrations. **c. interpeduncularis** [NA] The dilatation of the subarachnoid space occupying the fossa between the cerebral peduncles and uncal gyri of the temporal lobe. The mammillary bodies protrude from its roof and portions of the circle of Willis lie in the floor. Also *interpeduncular cistern, cisterna intercruralis profunda, basal cistern, cisterna basalis.* **c. laminae terminalis** The extension of the cistern of the optic chiasm lying rostral to the lamina terminalis. **c. lateralis pontis** That portion of the pontine cistern extending dorsolaterally into the cerebellopontine angle. **c. lumbalis** LUMBAR CISTERN. **c. magna** CISTERNA CEREBELLOMEDULLARIS. **c. perilymphatica** The perilymphatic space in the vestibule of the internal ear adjacent to the inner orifice of the cochlear canaliculus through which the scala tympani communicates with the subarachnoid space. *Outmoded.* **c. pontis** PONTINE CISTERN. **cisternae subarachnoideales** [NA] Enlargements of the subarachnoid space formed where the arachnoid, crossing between prominences of the brain, diverges from the pia mater, which follows the brain contours. In the lumbar region, a cistern is formed where the spinal cord ends short of the arachnoid-dural sac. Also *subarachnoidal cisterns, subarachnoidal sinuses.* **c. sulci lateralis** CISTERNA FOSSAE LATERALIS CEREBRI. **c. valleculae lateralis cerebri** CISTERNA FOSSAE LATERALIS CEREBRI. **c. venae magnae cerebri** The subarachnoid space bounded by the splenium of the corpus callosum, the lamina quadrigemina, and the superior surface of the cerebellum. It is a landmark for locating the great cerebral vein and the pineal body. Also *cistern of the great cerebral vein, cisterna ambiens, superior cistern, Bichat's foramen.*
**cisternae** \sistur′nē\ Plural of CISTERNA.
**cisternography** \sis′tərnäg′rəfē\ [*cistern(a)* + *o* + -GRAPHY] The demonstration of the anatomical spaces occupied by the cerebrospinal fluid and of the circulation kinetics of cerebrospinal fluid by means of intrathecally administered radioactive tracers or contrast agents.
**cistron** \sis′trän\ [CIS + *tr(ans)* + -ON] A segment of a chromosome that encodes a single product, either a polypeptide chain or an RNA molecule. This is a rigorous functional definition of a gene, introduced in microbiology and based on the ability of mutations in different genes to complement each other in trans (i.e. on different copies of a chromosome

in the same cell) but not in cis.

**Citelli** [Salvatore *Citelli*, Italian laryngologist, 1875–1947] See under SYNDROME.

**citrase** *Obs.* CITRATE LYASE.

**citratase** *Obs.* CITRATE LYASE.

**citrate** \sit′rāt, sī′trāt\ Any salt of citric acid. It is produced as a by-product of carbohydrate metabolism and is readily broken down by the body to produce energy.

**citrate lyase** A bacterial enzyme (EC 4.1.3.6) that catalyzes the reaction: citrate ⇌ acetate + oxaloacetate. The equilibrium of this reaction favors breakdown of citrate. Also *citrase* (obs.), *citrate aldolase* (obs.), *citratase* (obs.).

**citrate synthase** The enzyme (EC 4.1.3.7) that catalyzes the reaction: oxaloacetate + acetyl-CoA + $H_2O$ ⇌ citrate + CoA. Its equilibrium greatly favors citrate synthesis, as the hydrolysis of the enzyme-bound intermediate citryl-CoA is difficult to reverse under physiologic conditions. The enzyme is responsible for the entry of 2C-units into the citric acid cycle. Also *citrogenase* (obs.), *condensing enzyme* (outmoded).

**citric acid** HOOC—$CH_2$—C(OH)(COOH)—$CH_2$—COOH. A tricarboxylic acid which is soluble in water and forms colorless crystals. It is particularly abundant in citrus fruits, but is also present as an intermediate of aerobic metabolism in most tissues. It occupies a key position in the breakdown of fats and carbohydrates, since both these pathways yield the acetyl groups of acetyl-CoA, which are incorporated into citrate via citrate synthase before being oxidized. It is used as a diuretic, an anticoagulant, and as a preventive of scurvy. It is also used as a flavoring agent in confectionery, beverages, and other food products.

***Citrobacter*** \sit′rōbak′tər\ An enterobacterium closely related to *Escherichia coli* but able to use citrate as sole carbon source. It comprises the former *Escherichia freundii* and the Bethesda-Ballerup group of paracolon organisms. It is primarily free-living, but is occasionally found in the normal enteric bacteria and in infections.

**citrogenase** *Obs.* CITRATE SYNTHASE.

**citrulline** $H_2N$—CO—NH—$[CH_2]_3$—CH($NH_2$)COOH. An intermediate in the synthesis of urea in the liver. It is formed by transfer of a carbamoyl group from carbamoyl phosphate onto ornithine.

**citrullinemia** \sit′rulinē′mē·ə\ A metabolic disorder involving the urea cycle, in which a block in the formation of arginosuccinic acid from citrulline results from deficiency of the enzyme arginosuccinic acid synthetase. Citrulline and ammonia accumulate in the blood, the degree of ammonemia determining the severity of clinical symptoms. An acute neonatal form with very high ammonia levels results in coma and death in a few days. A chronic form with postprandial ammonemia is marked by episodic severe vomiting, coma, and seizures, with microcephaly and severe mental retardation. There is also a much milder form with no hyperammonemia.

**citrullinuria** \sit′rulinoo′rē·ə\ The increased urinary excretion of citrulline in citrullinemia, a condition characterized by mental retardation, vomiting, hypotonia and intermittent hyperammonemia. It is due to a deficiency of arginosuccinic acid synthetase, its transmission probably an autosomal recessive.

**citruria** \sitroo′rē·ə\ [*citr(ate)* + -URIA] The presence of citrate in urine. Renal citrate metabolism is related to pH regulation by the kidney. Its oxidation may provide energy for sodium reabsorption. Citrate excretion decreases during acidosis and increases during alkalosis.

**Civatte** [Achille *Civatte*, French dermatologist, 1877–1956] Civatte bodies. See under BODY.

**Civiale** [Jean *Civiale*, French surgeon, 1792–1867] Civiale's operation. See under LITHOLAPAXY.

**Civinini** [Filippo *Civinini*, Italian anatomist, 1805–1844] **1** Civinini's canal. See under ITER CHORDAE ANTERIUS. **2** Ligament of Civinini. See under LIGAMENTUM PTERYGOSPINALE. **3** Civinini spine, Civinini's process. See under PROCESSUS PTERYGOSPINOSUS.

**Cl** Symbol for the element, chlorine.

**cladiosis** \klad′ē·ō′sis\ CLADOSPORIOSIS.

**Clado** [Spiro *Clado*, Turkish-born French gynecologist, 1862–1920] See under ANASTOMOSIS.

**cladosporiosis** \klad′ōspôr′ē·ō′sis\ [*Cladospori(um)* + -OSIS] Infection by any organism of the genus *Cladosporium*.. Also *cladiosis.*

***Cladosporium*** \klad′ōspôr′ē·əm\ A form-genus of pigmented fungi, some of which are known agents of chromomycosis.

**clairvoyance** [French *clair* (from L *clarus* clear, from *calare* to call) clear + French *voyance* (from *voir* to see, from L *videre* to see) a preternatural gift of seeing past, future, and absent or invisible objects] The hypothetical ability to see or to perceive mentally, without use of the eyes as organs of sense, objective events or persons distant in place or time.

**clamoxyquin dihydrochloride** $C_{17}H_{26}ClN_3O$. 5-Chloro-7-[[[(3-diethylamino) propyl]amino]methyl]-8-quinolinoldihydrochloride, a quinoline derivative that has been used as an antiamebic drug.

**clamp** [Middle English, from Middle Dutch *klampe* clamp] An instrument for compressing tissue. **anastomosis c.** A surgical instrument designed to provide simultaneous noncrushing occlusion and apposition of two vessels while anastomosis is performed. **bone c.** A surgical instrument designed to support, retract, or stabilize

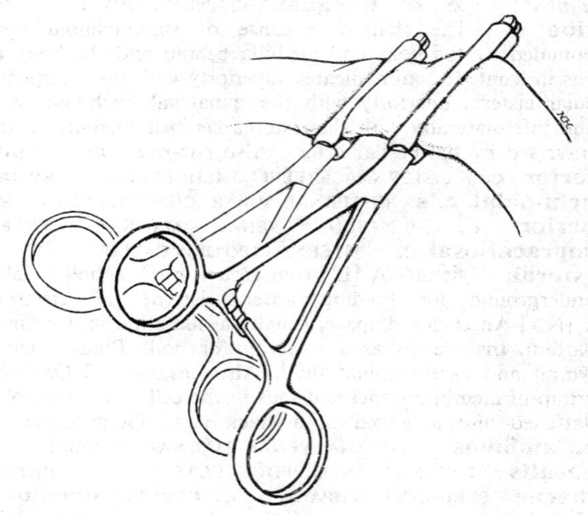

Anastomosis clamps

bone during an orthopedic procedure. Also *bone-holding clamp.* **cervical punch biopsy c.** A surgical instrument designed to obtain small samples of tissue from the uterine cervix for the purpose of histologic and cytologic analysis. **Crile's c.** A surgical instrument with rubber-coated jaws that provide gentle, noncrushing compression of vascular structures during an anastomosis; a heavy hemostat. **crushing c.** Any of various surgical instruments designed to provide firm compression of tissues grasped without regard to the ultimate survival of the tissue between the jaws. **Crutchfield c.** A screw clamp used for gradual occlusion of the carotid artery in the neck. The stem of the clamp, which extends through the neck wound, is detached when occlusion of the artery is completed. **Doyen's c.** A surgical instrument with two flexible jaws designed to provide noncrushing compression. It is usually used to establish hemostasis during gastrointestinal surgery. **fenestrated c.** A surgical clamp with multiple small holes or a single large hole in each jaw. It is designed to provide compression of the tissues grasped. **gingival c.** A rubber dam clamp that retracts the gingiva. **hemostatic c.** A surgical device designed to occlude or compress tissues or vessels in order to control their bleeding. **lever-compression c.** A surgical instrument with relatively long handles and short jaws that is designed to provide extremely firm compression of tissues. **Martel's c.** A clamp frequently used in bowel surgery to provide crushing compression of the distal segment of bowel. **microvascular c.** A noncrushing clamp, usually with pressure-calibrated jaws, that is used to occlude tiny blood vessels while they are being anastomosed under the operating microscope. **occlusion c.** A surgical instrument designed to compress a hollow structure, such as a blood vessel, duct, or section of the gastrointestinal tract, without damaging the tissue grasped. **Payr c.** A double-handled instrument that occludes a segment of the gastrointestinal tract, such as the pylorus, during surgery. **pedicle c.** A scissorlike instrument with curved blades and a long handle that is designed to compress a pedicle during surgery. **Potts c.'s** A curved clamp designed to apply gentle, noncrushing compression to vascular structures. **rubber dam c.** A spring clip placed on a tooth to hold a rubber dam in place. **Selverstone c.** A clamp similar to the Crutchfield clamp. **towel c.** TOWEL CLIP. **vascular c.** Any of a variety of noncrushing clamps that are used to occlude blood vessels without causing gross tissue damage. **voltage c.** A technique in which the potential across a biological membrane can be instantaneously changed and maintained at some predetermined value. This allows membrane ionic conductance to be measured as a function of time at different fixed potentials. **Willett's c.** WILLETT FORCEPS.

**clap** [Middle English *clap(er)* a brothel, earlier a rabbits' burrow, from Old French *clapier* (from Old Provençal *clapier* a rabbits' burrow, from *clap* a heap of stones) a hole hollowed out by rabbits] *Popular* GONORRHEA.

**clapotement** \kläpôtmäɴ′\ [French (onomatopoeic), a lapping of water] SUCCUSSION SOUNDS.

**clapping** A form of percussive massage using flat or slightly curved hands. It is a technique sometimes used in physical therapy to encourage expectoration.

**Clara** [Max *Clara*, Austrian anatomist, born 1899] Clara cells. See under CELL.

**Clark** [Alfred Joseph *Clark*, U.S. pharmacologist, 1885–1941] Clark's body area rule. See under RULE.

**Clark** [Alonzo *Clark*, U.S. physician, 1807–1887] See under SIGN.

**Clark** [Cecil Henry Douglas *Clark*, English chemist, flourished 20th century] See under RULE.

**Clark** [Earl Perry *Clark*, U.S. biochemist, born 1892] Clark-Collip method. See under METHOD.

**Clark** [Eliot *Clark*, U.S. anatomist, 1881–1963] Sandison-Clark chamber. See under RABBIT-EAR CHAMBER.

**Clark** [Guy Wendell *Clark*, U.S. biochemist, born 1887] See under TEST.

**Clark** [Leland C. *Clark*, Jr., U.S. biochemist, born 1918] See under ELECTRODE.

**Clarke** [Cecil *Clarke*, English physician, flourished 20th century] Hadfield-Clarke syndrome. See under CLARKE-HADFIELD SYNDROME.

**Clarke** [Jacob Augustus Lockhart *Clarke*, English anatomist, physician and neurologist 1817–1880] **1** Dorsal nucleus of Clarke, Clarke's column of spinal cord. See under NUCLEUS DORSALIS CLARKII. **2** Nucleus of Clarke's column, Clarke's nucleus, posterovesicular column of Clarke. See under NUCLEUS THORACICUS. **3** Clarke's collateral bundle. See under BUNDLE. **4** Clarke-Monakow nucleus. See under NUCLEUS CUNEATUS ACCESSORIUS.

**-clasia** \-klā′zhə\ [Gk *klasis* (from *klan* to break, break into pieces) fracture, breakage + *-ia*, L and Gk abstract noun suffix] A combining form meaning the act or condition of breaking up, disintegration.

**-clasis** \-kləsis\ -CLASIA.

**clasmatocyte** \klazmat′əsīt\ *Older term* MACROPHAGE.

**clasmatosis** \klaz′mətō′sis\ [Gk *klasma*, gen. *klasmatos*, a fragment, piece broken off + -OSIS] The fragmentation or breaking off of parts of a cell.

**clasmocytoma** \klaz′məsītō′mə\ *Obs.* HISTIOCYTIC LYMPHOMA.

**clasp** [Middle English *claspe, clapse*, prob. akin to Old English *clyppan* to clasp, embrace] An elongated metal projection from the base, used to attach a dental appliance to a natural tooth by embracing it or by impinging on an undercut. **Adam's c.** A wire clasp incorporating two arrowheads, used for orthodontic appliances. **circumferential c.** A clasp encircling more than half of the circumference of a tooth. **continuous c.** CONTINUOUS BAR RETAINER. **wrought c.** A clasp made of wire that has been drawn, making it stronger.

**class** [L *class(is)* a class, division] **1** A group whose members share a common characteristic not possessed by other entities. **2** A taxonomic group ranking between phylum (or division) and order. **form-c.** See under FORM.

**classification** [French (from *class(e)* a class, from L *class(is)* a division, order + *i* + French *-fication* -FICATION), a classifying, being classified] A system used to organize various conditions, structures, or processes into categories based on certain shared characteristics. **Angle's c. of malocclusion** A classification of the various types of malocclusion, based largely on the mesiodistal relations in occlusion of the first molars: (class 1) arches in normal anteroposterior relation with the first molars in normal occlusion; (class 2) lower arch in posterior relation to the upper arch, (division 1) labioversion of upper anterior teeth, (subdivision) unilateral protrusion of upper anterior teeth, (division 2) labioversion of upper lateral incisor teeth, with linguoversion of upper central incisors, (subdivision) unilateral condition; (class 3) anterior relationship of lower arch to upper arch, (subdivision) unilateral condition. This classification is now considered to be too crude, and many other classifications based on it, but with additional divisions and subdivisions, have been used. But it is still, in its original form, a basic worldwide means of communication in orthodontics. ⟨Angle, Edward Hartley, *Malocclusion of the Teeth*, Philadelphia, 1907.⟩ **Arneth c.** A classification of neutrophils according to the number of lobes of their nuclei. The percentages of neutrophils with 1, 2, 3, 4, 5, etc. nuclear lobes are tabulated. In normal blood, neutrophils with 3 to 4 lobes predominate. Neutrophils with 6 or more lobes are said to be hypersegmented. If a greater than normal percent of neutrophils have 1 or 2 nuclear lobes, a young population of neutrophils is present, and neutrophils are said to be "left-shifted." Neutrophils having 5 or more lobes are older; a blood film containing many neutrophils with 5 or more lobes is said to be "right-shifted." Left-shifted neutrophils are characteristic of acute bacterial infections; right-shifted neutrophils are characteristic of pernicious anemia or folate deficiency. See also COOKE'S CRITERION. **bacterial c.** A system of bacterial nomenclature that serves primarily as a determinative key. It is also arranged on classical taxonomic lines (with orders, families, genera, and species), intended to reflect phylogenetic relationships. However, the criteria are not as sharp as for higher organisms, because species are not defined in terms of interfertility boundaries, and various criteria of closeness, such as morphology, physiology, and DNA composition and sequence, are not always consistent. **Berman c. of pelves** A functional classification of the maternal pelvis based on pelvic size and shape and predictive of the course of labor. **Black's c.** A system of classifying cavities based on the type of cavity preparation required, originally consisting of five classes, to which a sixth has been added. Class 1 comprises cavities beginning in structural defects of the teeth, as in pits and fissures. Class 2 comprises cavities in proximal surfaces of bicuspids and molars. Class 3 comprises cavities in proximal surfaces of cuspids and incisors that do not involve removal and restoration of the incisal angle. Class 4 comprises cavities in proximal surfaces of cuspids and incisors that require removal and restoration of the incisal angle. Class 5 comprises cavities in the gingival third (not pit cavities) of the labial, buccal, or lingual surfaces of the teeth. Class 6, an addition to Black's original classification, comprises cavities on incisal edges and cusp tips of the teeth. **Broders c.** The grouping of histologic specimens of cancer by the degree of differentiation shown by the cells as a guide to the malignancy of the tumor: (Grade I) one-fourth of the cells are undifferentiated (three-fourths being differentiated), (Grade II) one half of the cells are undifferentiated, (Grade III) three-fourths of the cells are undifferentiated, and (Grade IV) all cells are undifferentiated. Also *Broders index*. **Caldwell-Moloy c.** A method of classifying the female pelvis based on anterior-posterior and tranverse measurements of the inlet of the pelvis. The pelvic types include: android, anthropoid, gynecoid, and platypelloid. **Child c.** A clinical and biochemical grading system for hepatic cirrhosis. It was originally used as a means for prognostication in patients undergoing emergency portocaval shunting for bleeding varices. It is based on determinations of serum albumin and bilirubin levels and the presence of ascites, encephalopathy, and signs of malnutrition. **Dukes c.** The grouping of cases of colorectal carcinoma by the extent of spread in resected specimens, used as a guide to prognosis: (1) tumors not spread beyond muscle layers, called Class A; (2) tumors spread to pericolic or perirectal tissues but without lymph node involvement, called Class B; (3) cases with metastases in lymph nodes, called Class C. **French-American-British c.** A classification of acute leukemia into three subtypes for acute lymphocytic leukemia and six subtypes for acute nonlymphocytic leukemia, on the basis of morphology as determined on a Wright stain of a blood film. Using L to indicate lymphocytic forms and M to indicate the nonlymphocytic forms, the classification is as follows: L1 is acute lymphocytic leukemia in which small lymphoblasts with regular nuclei, scanty cytoplasm, and inconspicuous nucleoli predominate; L2 is acute lymphocytic leukemia in which lymphoblasts with abundant cytoplasm, prominent nucleoli, and cleaved or indented nuclei predominate; and L3 is acute lymphocytic leukemia in which lymphoblasts are large, have abundant deeply basophilic cytoplasm with prominent vacuolation, and nucleoli are prominent. The L3 lymphoblast has features of lymphoblasts in Burkitt's lymphoma. M1 is acute granulocytic leukemia in which myeloblasts show no differentiation and no cytoplasmic granules; M2 is acute granulocytic leukemia with early progranulocytes present as well as myeloblasts; M3 is acute progranulocytic leukemia, in which the predominant cells contain primary granules and many cells contain bundles or "faggots" of Auer rods; M4 is acute myelomonocytic leukemia in which most of the myeloblasts have cytoplasmic features like those of monocytes; M5 is acute ("Schilling type") monocytic leukemia in which the abnormal cells are large, with little or no cytoplasmic granularity, nuclei are elongated and folded, and nucleoli are prominent; M6 is erythroleukemia (DiGuglielmo's disease), in which myeloblasts are increased in bone marrow and erythroid precursors are markedly increased, megaloblastoid, and bizarre. Also *FAB classification*. **Goldstein's c.** A classification system for the different types of aphasia, based upon anatomical, psychological, or clinical criteria. The classification discriminates between expressive speech defects, such as anarthria, peripheral motor aphasia or cortical motor aphasia; receptive speech defects, such as peripheral sensory aphasia or central sensory aphasia; central aphasia, such as conduction aphasia; amnesic aphasia, transcortical aphasia, and speech defects attributable to damage to nonverbal mental processes. **Griffith's c.** The classification of group A streptococci based on their ability to agglutinate in the presence of specific antiserum, in distinction to the Lancefield classification in which precipitin reactions are the end point. **Head's c.** Classification of aphasia into four clinical types: verbal aphasia, syntactical aphasia, nominal aphasia, and semantic aphasia. **Kauffmann-White c.** A classification of salmonellas based on their O (lipopolysaccharide) and H (flagellar) antigens. **Keith-Wagener-Barker c.** A classification of hypertensive retinopathy employing four grades of severity. Grade I is ophthalmoscopically unrecognizable; Grade II shows minimal vascular changes; Grade III manifests definite arteriolar constriction; Grade IV manifests optic disk edema. **Kennedy c.** A classification of partial edentulousness related to denture design: (class 1) bilateral extension base, (class 2) unilateral extension base, (class 3) bounded saddle or saddles, and (class 4) anterior saddle crossing the midline. Each class has modifications numbered according to additional tooth loss. **Kiel c.** A classification of malignant non-Hodgkin's lymphomas according to cell type into the following groups: lymphoblastic, Burkitt's type; lymphoblastic, convoluted cell and unclassified types; centrocytic; centroblastic/centrocytic; centroblastic; immunoblastic; predominantly small cleaved cell; lymphocytic, B- and T- types, and lymphoplasmacytic. In this classification, centrocytes correspond to well-differentiated follicular center lymphocytes and centroblasts to histiocytes or undifferentiated, large, noncleaved, follicular center cells. **Kleist's c.** Classification of the different types of aphasia, based upon an analysis of the receptive and expressive components of speech. The classification comprises, from the motor point of view, mutism with regard to spoken sounds (anarthric speech), and mutism for words, sounds, and phrases. From the sensory point of view, it comprises deafness to verbal sounds (classical verbal deafness), verbal deafness (Wernicke's cortical aphasia), deafness for names, and deafness for phrases (paragrammatism). **Kraepelin's c.** The subdivision of functional psychoses on the basis of their natural history into manic-depressive psychoses, which do not show deterioration, and dementia praecox, where progression to a profound dementia is characteristic. At the time of the classification's inception (1896), involutional melancholia was in a separate category, but it was later placed alongside manic-depressive psychoses as a type of affect psychosis. **Lancefield c.** An immunologic classification of streptococci into groups A to O, based on the C carbohydrate of the cell wall. This antigen is detected by a precipitin reaction as the end point. Group A streptococci are the most important human pathogens. **Landsteiner c.** A classification of blood types, according to the presence of antigens of the ABO system on erythrocyte membranes, as blood group A, B, AB, or O. **Lukes-Butler c.** A classification of Hodgkin's disease according to histologic features, as (1) lymphocytic and histiocytic, nodular or diffuse; (2) nodular sclerosis; (3) mixed; (4) diffuse fibrosis; and (5) reticular. The classification has been simplified by classifying according to (1) lymphocyte predominance; (2) nodular sclerosis; (3) mixed cellularity; and (4) lymphocytic depletion. This simplified four-group classification (the Rye classification) has been widely adopted. **Lukes-Collins c. of lymphoma** A classification of malignant lymphomas according to (a) whether the principal cell is a B lymphocyte or T lymphocyte, and (b) the morphology of the cell. The B-cell lymphomas are subclassified as small lymphocytic; plasmacytoid lymphocytic; follicular center cell, small cleaved, large cleaved, small noncleaved, or large noncleaved; and B-cell immunoblastic sarcoma. The T-cell lymphomas are subclassified as convoluted lymphocytic, T-cell immunoblastic sarcoma, and histiocytic. **Luria's c.** Classification of the forms of aphasia into aphasia caused by phonetic disintegration, aphasia resulting in disturbance in communication and understanding, aphasia caused by successive loss of synthesis of components in a regular sequence, and frontal aphasia caused by loss of the ability to regulate speech. **New York Heart Association c.** **1** A graded classification of disability due to heart disease. Class I: Heart disease present but no symptoms with ordinary physical activity. Class II: No symptoms at rest or with mild exertion. Class III: Comfortable at rest but symptoms develop with even mild exertion. Class IV: Incapable of any exertion without symptoms, which may also be present at rest. **2** A graded classification of therapeutic regimes appropriate to heart disease of differing severity. Class A: Physical activity need not be restricted. Class B: Severe or competitive exertion is inadvisable. Class C: Some restrictions on ordinary physical activity are advised. Class D: Ordinary physical activity should be markedly restricted. Class E: Complete rest in bed or chair is needed. **Papanicolaou c.** The grouping of cytological specimens according to degrees of cellular abnormalities for the detection of malignancy: (class I) absence of atypical or abnormal cells (negative for malignancy); (class II) atypical cells but no evidence of malignancy (negative); (class III) cells suggestive but not conclusive of malignancy (suspicious); (class IV) cells strongly suggestive of malignancy (positive); and (class V) cells conclusive of malignancy (positive). **Rappaport c.** A classification of malignant non-Hodgkin's lymphomas according to cell type (lymphocyte or histiocyte) and histologic pattern (nodular or diffuse). Four principal categories are defined: diffuse lymphocytic, diffuse histiocytic, nodular lymphocytic, and nodular histiocytic. The classification is expanded by defining degree of differentiation (maturation) of lymphocytes into the subtypes nodular poorly-differentiated lymphocytic, nodular mixed, nodular histiocytic, diffuse well-differentiated lymphocytic, diffuse poorly-differentiated lymphocytic, diffuse mixed, and diffuse histiocytic. **Rye c. of Hodgkin's disease** See under LUKES-BUTLER CLASSIFICATION. **Schilling c.** A classification of neutrophils according to whether their nuclei are segmented into lobes connected by a filament of chromatin. Those with non-segmented nuclei are designated "bands" or "stabs," and all those with segmented nuclei are tabulated together. An increase in the number of bands is characteristic of acute bacterial infections. See also COOKE'S CRITERION. **TNM c.** A classification of malignant tumors by extent of disease, expressed in respect to the primary tumor (T), the presence of regional lymph node metastasis (N), and distant metastasis (M). **c.'s of tumors** Any of several systems for categorizing tumors. The classification may be by site and behavior, as the WHO International Classification of Diseases (ICD); by histology, as the WHO International Histological Classification of Tumours; by extent of disease, (clinical stage), as the UICC's TNM classification (T = tumor, N = lymph nodes, M = metastases); or by differentiation of tumor cells, as the classification of Broders. The WHO coding system, ICD-O, provides rubrics for site, behavior, histology and differentiation compatible with the classifications listed above. **White's c.** A method of classifying diabetes mellitus during pregnancy in order to predict the obstetric and fetal outcome of the pregnancy. The classification takes into account the age at onset of the disease and its duration, severity, and complications. The scale goes from class A, or gestational diabetes, through class F, which represents patients who have diabetes complicated by a serious form of nephropathy, to classes G, H, R, and T, representing many other clinical conditions that are inimical to normal gestation in diabetes. **Wullstein c.** A classification of the modes of sound transmission across the middle ear after surgical reconstruction or after spontaneous healing following otitis media. It is used as a guide in planning tympanoplasty.

**class-interval** \-in'tərvəl\ The range of values determining a group in a classification of statistical data. For example, if the number of deaths in a series were classified by the age groups 0–4, 5–9, and 10–14 years, the class-interval would be five years.

**-clast** \-klast\ [Gk *-klastēs* (from *klan* to break, break into pieces), suffix denoting one who or that which breaks] A combining form denoting something, as a surgical implement, used to break or crush (something specified).

**clastic** \klas'tik\ [Gk *klast(os)* (verbal of *klan* to break, break into pieces) broken into pieces + -IC] Separable into parts, as an anatomic model.

**clastogenic** \klas'təjen'ik\ Capable of or predisposing to the breakage of chromosomes.

**clathrate** \klath'rāt\ [L *clathrat(us),* past part. of *clathrare* to furnish with a lattice, from *clathri* lattices] A complex in which an atom or molecule of one substance is surrounded by a crystal lattice of another.

**Claude** [Henri *Claude,* French psychiatrist, 1869–1945] **1** See under SIGN. **2** Claude and Lhermitte syndrome. See under HYPOTHALAMIC SYNDROME. **3** Claude's red nucleus syndrome, Claude syndrome. See under INFERIOR RED NUCLEUS SYNDROME.

**claudication** \klô'dikā'shən\ [L *claudicatio,* from *claudicare* to limp, be lame, from *claudus* lame] Lameness or limping, often associated with pain. **intermittent c.** Cramplike pain and weakness in muscles, most often those of the calf with consequent lameness. Symptoms develop progressively with walking and disappear with rest. It is due usually to atherosclerotic narrowing of the arteries of supply. Also *Charcot syndrome, angiosclerotic paroxysmal myasthenia.* **intermittent c. of the cauda equina** Pain and paresthesia, often succeeded by sensory loss, motor weakness, and loss of reflexes, arising in the motor and sensory distribution of lumbar or sacral roots after the patient has walked some distance. These symptoms disappear after a few minutes' rest. The neurologic signs, which are sometimes minimal but are accentuated by walking, are those of a cauda equina syndrome. The condition is caused by ischemia of the cauda equina due to intervertebral disk prolapse or lumbar canal stenosis, and the symptoms are usually relieved by surgical decompression. Also *pseudoclaudication syndrome, Verbiest syndrome.* **intermittent spinal c.** Intermittent symptoms of spinal cord dysfunction, such as weakness, paresthesiae, and sphincter disturbance, brought on by exertion. When symptoms are present, signs such as hyperreflexia, an extensor plantar response, or sensory loss may be present but disappear after rest. The condition is precipitated by ischemia of the spinal cord caused by arterial disease, usually atheroma, and may presage subsequent spinal cord infarction due to occlusion of the anterior or posterior spinal arteries. **venous c.** Intermittent claudication due to obstruction in veins.

**claudicatory** \klô′dikətôr′ē\ Of or relating to claudication.

**claustra** \klôs′trə\ Plural of CLAUSTRUM.

**claustrophobia** \klôs′trəfō′bē·ə\ [L *claustr(um)* a bolt, bar, place shut up + -PHOBIA] Pathologic fear of being confined in a small place such as an elevator or automobile.

**claustrum** \klôs′trəm\ [L (akin to *clausus,* past. part. of *claudere* to close) a bolt, bar, barrier] (*pl.* claustra) [NA] A thin sheet of gray matter coextensive with the insula on one side and the putamen on the other, though separated from the latter by the external capsule. It has zones associated primarily with the insular cortex (insular claustrum) and with the prepiriform and adjacent cortex (prepiriform or temporal claustrum). Also *claustral layer.* **c. gutturis** *Outmoded* PALATUM MOLLE. **c. oris** *Outmoded* PALATUM MOLLE.

**clausura** \klôsoo′rə\ [L, a closure, lock, bolt] The congenital failure to form an opening or passageway.

**clava** \klā′və\ [L, a club] **1** An anatomical structure resembling the end of a club. **2** TUBERCULUM NUCLEI GRACILIS.

**clavate** \klā′vāt\ [New L *clavat(us)* (from L *clav(a)* a club + *-atus* -ATE) club-shaped] Club-shaped; gradually thickening at one end.

**clavation** \klavā′shən\ [L *clav(a)* a club + -ATION ] GOMPHOSIS.

**clavicle** \klav′ikl\ CLAVICULA.

**clavicotomy** \klav′ikät′əmē\ [*clavic(le)* + *o* + -TOMY] A surgical procedure in which the clavicle is either cut or divided, usually in order to gain exposure of deeper structures.

**clavicula** \klavik′yələ\ [L (dim. of *clavis* key, akin to *claudere* to close) a bolt, fastener, key; anatomic use originated in New L by assimilation in meaning to the related Gk word *kleis* (gen. *kleidos*) a key, fastener, bolt, bar, collarbone] [NA] An elongated, S-shaped subcutaneous long bone stretching horizontally above the first rib from the manubrium sterni and first costal cartilage, with which it forms the sternoclavicular joint, to the acromion of the scapula, where it forms the acromioclavicular joint. Its medial two-thirds is triangular in shape and convex anteriorly, while the lateral one-third is flat above and below and concave anteriorly. As part of the shoulder girdle, it serves as a prop to the shoulder, enabling the upper limb to move freely away from the trunk. Also *clavicle, collar-bone, collar bone.* Adj. clavicular.

**claviculectomy** \klavik′yəlek′təmē\ [New L *clavicul(a)* clavicle + -ECTOMY] A surgical procedure in which part or all of the clavicle is resected.

**clavipectoral** \klav′ikōpek′tôrəl\ Pertaining to the clavicle and the chest or pectoral region.

**clavus** \klā′vəs\ [L (akin to *claudere* to shut), a nail, wart, callous excrescence] CORN.

**claw / griffin c.** CLAW HAND.

**clawhand** CLAW HAND.

**clay** A material that is a common component of soils. It has a latticed molecular structure, is usually aluminosilicate, and often is able to exchange ions. Clays suspended in water can be vehicles for medicaments.

**clearance** A calculated figure representing the volume of plasma which, on one circulatory passage through the kidneys, could be completely cleared of its load of a solute. Expressed as ml/min, it reflects the glomerular filtration rate, and is calculated from the formula:

$$C = \frac{[U] \cdot V}{[P]},$$

where $C$ is clearance rate, $[U]$ is the concentration of the solute in urine, $[P]$ is the concentration of solute in plasma, and $V$ is the rate of urine flow in ml/min. Correction factors for body surface area and for rates of solute production and tubular absorption or secretion may be applied. **blood-urea c.** UREA CLEARANCE. **creatinine c.** A measurement of the rate at which the kidneys remove creatinine from the blood. It is a fairly reliable indicator of the glomerular filtration rate, except if severe renal disease exists or if there is an exogenous source of creatinine. **endogenous creatinine c.** A clinically useful approximation of the glomerular filtration rate. Creatinine production is roughly proportional to muscle mass. Creatinine in man is secreted by the tubules which makes its clearance higher than the actual glomerular filtration rate, but noncreatinine chromogen is included in the usual methods of measurement of creatinine in blood, which makes the clearance lower than the actual filtration rate. The two errors tend to make the endogenous creatinine clearance close to the glomerular filtration rate, but the relationship is variable, especially in the diseased kidney. **fractional c. of dextran** The fraction of dextran filtered at the glomerulus that appears in the urine, calculated by dividing the dextran excretory rate by the glomerular filtration rate. The fractional clearance of dextrans is a function of the effective dextran molecular radius. The fractional clearances of dextrans with different effective radii are used to estimate the preselectivity of the glomerular capillaries. **fractional free water c.** The fraction of the volume of glomerular filtrate represented by the free water clearance. It is related to the fractional urine flow. **free water c.** The amount of water excreted in the urine in excess of the amount necessary to make the urine isosmotic with the plasma. Free water clearance in ml per minute is the difference between the urine flow and the osmolal clearance. When the osmolal clearance exceeds the urine flow, the free water clearance has a negative value. **immune c.** IMMUNE ELIMINATION. **interocclusal c.** INTEROCCLUSAL DISTANCE. **inulin c.** The calculated minimum volume of plasma that contains the quantity of inulin (a polymer of fructose of molecular weight 5000) excreted in the urine in one minute when the concentration of plasma inulin is maintained at a steady value. Inulin is freely filtered at the renal glomerulus and is neither reabsorbed nor excreted by the renal tubules so that its clearance value is a measure of glomerular filtration rate. **osmolar c.** The virtual volume of plasma cleared of osmotically active substances in milliosmoles per minute. **plasma c.** The virtual amount of plasma from which could be cleared the amount of a substance that appears in the urine per minute, calculated from the formula for clearance. **plasma iron c.** The time required for the disappearance from the plasma of 50% of an injected dose of radioactive iron, normally about 60–90 minutes. **sodium *p*-aminohippuric acid c.** The clearance of *p*-aminohippurate (PAH), as calculated from the clearance formula. At low plasma concentrations, PAH clearance gives an excellent approximation of renal plasma flow. At high concentrations, PAH clearance can be used to calculate maximal rate of proximal tubular transport. See also EFFECTIVE RENAL PLASMA FLOW. **urea c.** The clearance of urea, an endogenous solute, from renal blood flow, as calculated from the clearance formula. At urine flow rates about 2 ml/min, it gives a reasonably good indication of the glomerular filtration rate, but it is now largely supplanted by creatinine clearance, which is more reliable and simpler to apply. Also *blood-urea clearance.* **whole body c.** The sum of the individual clearances of a substance by the various organs and tissues of the body. For example, in the case of a substance that is eliminated by renal excretion and hepatic biotransformation, the whole body clearance is the sum of renal and hepatic clearance.

**clearer** CLEARING AGENT.

**cleavage** \klē′vij\ [Middle English *cleve(n)*, from Old English *clēofan* + -AGE ] The progressive segmentation (cytokinesis) of the fertilized ovum following sequential mitotic divisions. The overall volume of the cytoplasm remains unchanged during successive divisions, but the cleavage products (blastomeres) become smaller and smaller. This stage of early development precedes the blastula stage. **accessory c.** A type of peripheral cleavage resulting from polyspermy and occurring in telolecithal eggs. The yolk is concentrated towards the vegetal pole of the ovum. **adequal c.** Cleavage resulting in blastomeres of almost equal size. **bilateral c.** EQUAL CLEAVAGE. **complete c.** HOLOBLASTIC CLEAVAGE. **discoidal c.** MEROBLASTIC CLEAVAGE. **equal c.** Cleavage that results in the formation of blastomeres equal in size, as exhibited in cephalochordates, marsupials, and placental mammals. Also *regular segmentation, bilateral cleavage.* **holoblastic c.** Cleavage characterized by complete division of the mass of the fertilized egg to form the blastomeres. Also *complete segmentation, complete cleavage.* **incomplete c.** MEROBLASTIC CLEAVAGE. **indeterminate c.** Cleavage in which individual blastomeres do not have a predetermined fate as to the development of a specific tissue or organ. **meroblastic c.** Cleavage of the ovum in which only the nuclei and the nucleated cytoplasm divide, while the cellular cytoplasm (vitellus) undergoes little or no division. It is found in fish, reptiles, and birds. Also *partial segmentation, incomplete cleavage.* **unequal c.** Cleavage in which the blastomeres are unequal in size, those of the vegetal pole remaining larger than those of the animal pole, as exhibited in protostomes, lower fishes and amphibians. Also *unequal segmentation.*

**cleft** [Middle English *clift*, from Old English *clyft*, past part. of *cleofan* to cleave, split] A fissure or interval, which may be normal or abnormal. In the latter it is often of developmental origin, representing failed or incomplete union of primordia from different sources or locations, as with facial clefts. **anal c.** CRENA ANI. **branchial c.'s** Clefts situated between the branchial arches which result in communication between the cavity of the pharynx and the exterior. They result from the disappearance of the closing membranes made by the union of the bottom of the ectobranchial pouches with the endobranchial pouches. They remain open in lower vertebrates and gills develop on their borders. In higher vertebrates and in man, they are more or less imperfectly open and then only during embryonic stages. In rare instances they can persist and give rise to fistulas, cysts, and sinus tracts in adult forms. Also *branchial fissures, visceral clefts.* **cholesterol c.** An elongated defect in a tissue section that represents the site of a cholesterol crystal that has been dissolved during the preparative procedures. **coelomic c.** The split in the lateral mesoderm resulting in the formation of the coelom and the somatopleure and splanchnopleure. **corneal c.** CORNEAL FISSURE. **facial c.** Any of several grooves, fissures, or scars on the face due to incomplete closure of the normal fissures that separated various facial processes during the embryonic period. **fetal c.** A cleft in the developing optic cup. Also *choroidal cleft.* **first visceral c.** The hyomandibular or first branchial cleft of the embryo formed by the breakdown of the membrane between the first ectodermal groove and the first endodermal pouch. In aquatic vertebrates internal gills develop on the walls of the cleft. In man the first cleft becomes obliterated in its ventral portion but its dorsal portion forms the lining of the external auditory meatus. **genal c.** A transverse or lateral facial cleft or scar due to the incomplete union of the maxillary process with the mandibular arch of the embryo. It is usually associated with macrostomia. Also *lateral facial cleft.* **genital c.** A midline ectodermal invagination derived from original proctodeum between the labioscrotal swellings. Initially it is separated from the urogenital sinus by the urogenital membrane, but the latter breaks down and continuity is established. The cleft remains in the female to form the vestibule of the vagina but in the male it is obliterated by fusion of the scrotal swellings. **gill c.** An ectodermal invagination or groove separating adjacent branchial arches and corresponding to each pharyngeal pouch from which, in mammals, it is separated by a membrane. In fishes and in tadpole stages of amphibia the membrane breaks down between the gills. Also *pharyngeal cleft, pharyngeal slit, gill slit.* **gingival c.** A localized absence of gingiva, exposing part of the root surface. Also *cleft gingiva.* **gluteal c.** CRENA ANI. **hyobranchial c.** A groove situated immediately caudal to the second, or hyoid, arch in the embryonic pharyngeal region. Also *hyoid cleft, posthyoidean cleft, second branchial groove* (used especially in the U.S.). **hyomandibular c.** The groove between the first, or mandibular, and second, or hyoid, pharyngeal arches. In mammals, the cleft becomes the external auditory meatus. **intergluteal c.** CRENA ANI. **intratonsillar c.** *Outmoded* FOSSA SUPRATONSILLARIS. **Lanterman's c.'s** SCHMIDT-LANTERMAN INCISURES. **Larrey's c.** MORGAGNI'S FORAMEN. **lateral facial c.** GENAL CLEFT. **c. of the mandible** A midline fissure or lesser defect in the mandibular region, variously involving the mandible, chin, and lower lip. It is thought to result from incomplete union at the midline of the embryonic first branchial arches. **Maurer's c.'s** MAURER'S DOTS. **median facial c.** A midline cleft of the face due to failed or incomplete development of both medial nasal processes and a consequent failure to unite with the tips of the respective maxillary processes. As a result the prolabium of the upper lip is incomplete or absent. Also *median cleft of the maxilla.* **middle-ear c.** The narrow, air-containing cleft within the head, some 6.5 cm long in the adult, comprising, in sequence, the eustachian tube, the tympanic cavity, the mastoid antrum, and the mastoid air cells. Also *tubotympanic cleft.* **natal c.** CRENA ANI. **oblique facial c.** A facial cleft, groove, or scar that crosses the upper lip to the nostril then continues to the lower lid of the same side. It results from incomplete closure of the oronasal and the naso-optic grooves of the embryo. The underlying cause is probably the improper union of the maxillary process with both medial and lateral nasal processes of the same side. Also *facial coloboma*. **orbitonasal c.** A deep cleft in the embryonic face separating the lateral (external) nasal process and the maxillary process. Its abnormal persistence gives rise to the oblique facial cleft. Also *naso-optic groove*. **pharyngeal c.** GILL CLEFT. **posthyoidean c.** HYOBRANCHIAL CLEFT. **primary synaptic c.** SYNAPTIC TROUGH. **pudendal c.** RIMA PUDENDI. **Santorini's c.'s** INCISURAE CARTILAGINIS MEATUS ACUSTICI. **Schmidt-Lanterman c.'s** SCHMIDT-LANTERMAN INCISURES. **Stillman's c.** A very narrow gingival cleft at one time thought, mistakenly, to be caused by occlusal trauma to the adjacent tooth. **submucous c.** A palatal cleft concealed by intact mucoperiosteum. **synaptic c.** The narrow cleft or gap between a terminal bouton and the postsynaptic dendritic process. Neurotransmitter substances are released into it. **tubotympanic c.** MIDDLE-EAR CLEFT. **visceral c.'s** BRANCHIAL CLEFTS. **vulval c.** RIMA PUDENDI.

**cleido-** \klī′dō-\ [Gk *kleis*, gen. *kleidos* a bolt, bar, key, collarbone. See also CLAVICULA.] A combining form denoting the clavicle. Also *cleid-, clid-, clido-*.

**cleidocostal** \-käs′təl\ Pertaining to the clavicle and a rib or the ribs.

**cleidocranial** \-krā′nē·əl\ Pertaining to the clavicle or clavicles and the cranium.

**cleidohumeral** \-hyoo′mərəl\ Pertaining to the clavicle and the humerus.

**cleidohyoid** \-hī′oid\ Pertaining to the clavicle and the hyoid bone.

**cleidomastoid** \-mas′toid\ Pertaining to the clavicle and the mastoid process.

**cleido-occipital** \-äksip′ətəl\ Pertaining to the clavicle and the occiput.

**cleidorrhexis** \-rek′sis\ [CLEIDO- + -RRHEXIS] CLEIDOTOMY.

**cleidoscapular** \-skap′yələr\ Pertaining to or involving the clavicleand the scapula.

**cleidosternal** \-stur′nəl\ STERNOCLAVICULAR.

**cleidotomy** \klīdät′əmē\ [CLEIDO- + -TOMY] The intentional division of the fetal clavicle in order to allow delivery of the shoulders. Also *cleirorrhexis*.

**-cleisis** \-klī′sis\ [Gk *klēisis* (from *kleiein* to close) a shutting up, closing] A combining form meaning a closure or welding. Also *-clisis, -kleisis*.

**clemastine** $C_{21}H_{26}ClNO$. 2-[2-[1-(4-Chlorophenyl)-1-phenylethoxy]ethyl]-1-methylpyrrolidine, a compound used as an antihistaminic in the form of its hydrogen fumarate salt. It is used to treat allergic skin disorders and allergic rhinitis.

**clemizole** $C_{19}H_{20}ClN_3{\cdot}HCl$. 1-(*p*-Chlorobenzyl)-2-(1-pyrrolidinyl-methyl)benzimidazole. An antihistaminic drug with little anticholinergic activity but having moderate sedative effects. It is also used to form a repository form of penicillin G, as a salt of benzylpenicillinic acid.

**clemizole penicillin** The clemizole salt of penicillin G, which is a long-acting form of penicillin. Clemizole has antihistaminic properties, so these effects are also exerted along with the slow release of the drugs.

**cleptomania** \klep′təmā′nē·ə\ KLEPTOMANIA.

**Clérambault** [Gaetan-Henri-Alfred-Edouard-Leon-Marie Gatian de *Clérambault*, French psychiatrist, 1872–1934] Clérambault-Kandinsky syndrome. See under CLÉRAMBAULT-KANDINSKY COMPLEX.

**Cléret** [M. *Cléret*, French physician, flourished early 20th century] Launois-Cléret syndrome. See under FRÖHLICH SYNDROME.

**Clevenger** [Shobal Vail *Clevenger*, U.S. neurologist, 1843–1920] Clevenger's fissure. See under SULCUS TEMPORALIS INFERIOR.

**click** An abrupt, sharp, nonresonant sound, as that heard on auscultation. **ejection c.** A brief high-pitched sound heard at the onset of ejection of blood through the aortic or pulmonary valve, that is, very soon after the first heart sound. It occurs in patients in whom the valve is stenosed but mobile, or bicuspid, or when the vessel beyond is dilated. Also *ejection sound*. **mitral c.** OPENING SNAP. **systolic c.** Any of various sharp sounds, including ejection clicks, occurring during cardiac systole and due to a variety of causes, such as mitral valve prolapse and regurgitation, often trivial, or to causes outside the heart.

**clid-** \klīd-\ CLEIDO-.

**clido-** \klī′dō-\ CLEIDO-.

**cliff / visual c.** An apparatus for testing unlearned depth perception in young human or animal subjects. Two patterned surfaces are visible just below a sheet of heavy glass, one just below the glass and the other several feet below it. When placed on an opaque board at the line between those surfaces, the young subject will readily cross the "shallow" side but refuses to approach the "deep" side.

**climacteric** \klī′makter′ik, klīmak′tərik\ [L *climacter* (from Gk *klimaktēr* a step of a staircase, round of a ladder) a year of one's life at the close of which some great change is to befall the body] **1** The somatic and psychological signs and symptoms marking the cessation of reproductive life in women at menopause, associated with changes in the endocrine system. Menopausal symptoms include sudden sensation of heat and flushing of the face and torso, and vaginal dryness. Also *climacterium*. **2** A critical life period in men corresponding to that in which the climacteric occurs in women, but less well defined. It is often marked by nocturia, fatigue, indecisiveness, diminished sexual desire, and various degrees of erective or ejaculatory impotence. Also *male climacteric, male menopause*.

**climacterium** \klī′makter′ē·əm\ CLIMACTERIC. **c. praecox** PREMATURE MENOPAUSE.

**climactic** \klīmak′tik\ Of or relating to a climax.

**climax** \klī′maks\ [Gk *klimax* (from *klinein* to make a slope or slant) a staircase or ladder] **1** The moment of greatest severity in the course of a disease. **2** The acme of excitement in the sexual act; orgasm.

**clin-** \klin-\ CLINO-.

**clindamycin** \klin′damī′sin\ $C_{18}H_{33}ClN_2O_5S$. 7 (S)-Chloro-7-deoxylincomycin, a semisynthetic antibiotic derived from lincomycin and used to treat bacterial infections, especially those caused by anaerobes.

**clinic** [early modern French *clinique* clinical medicine (later, a place where this was taught or practiced), from L *clinice*, from Gk *klinikē (technē)* lit. bedside (technique), from *klinikos* pertaining to beds. See also CLINICAL.] **1** An outpatient or ambulatory care facility. **2** An outpatient facility associated with a hospital. **3** An outpatient facility that provides care for a specified group such as a pregnant women, well infants, or the indigent. **4** A period of medical instruction conducted at the bedside, or the place where such a session occurs. **ambulant c.** OUTPATIENT CLINIC. **outpatient c.** An ambulatory care clinic, usually associated with or located in a hospital or other inpatient facility. Also *ambulant clinic*. **screening c.** An ambulatory care provider organization which is designed to test or examine large numbers of patients for a specific disease or group of diseases, especially to find cases that were previously undiagnosed.

**clinical** \klin′ikəl\ [early modern English *clinic* (adj. and noun), from L *clinicus,* from Gk *klinikos* clinical, bedside, pertaining to beds (from *klinē* a bed, couch, from *klinein* to lean, recline) + -AL] **1** Based on or involving direct examination and care of patients, as at bedside. **2** Of or relating to a clinic.

**clinician** \klinish′ən\ [CLINIC + *-ian,* suffix denoting practitioner] A health care professional practitioner who is directly involved in the examination, treatment, or care of patients.

**clinico-** \klin′ikō-\ [Gk *klinikos* (from *klinē* a bed) pertaining to beds] A combining form meaning clinical.

**clinicogenetic** \-jənet′ik\ Pertaining to heritable or chromosomal disorders that have medical relevance.

**clinicopathologic** \-path′əläj′ik\ Pertaining to correlations between clinical signs and symptoms, and pathologic findings, as in *clinicopathologic conference.*

**clinicopathology** \-pathäl′əjē\ CLINICAL PATHOLOGY.

**Clinitest** A tablet that uses copper sulfate reduction to demonstrate the presence of reducing sugars in body fluids. A proprietary name.

**clino-** \klī′nō-, kli′nə-\ [Gk *klinein* (akin to *klinē* bed) to incline, bend, recline] A combining form meaning (1) bed; (2) reclining; (3) slant, slope, deflection. Also *clin-.*

**clinocephaly** \-sef′əlē\ [CLINO- + CEPHAL- + -Y] The abnormal contour of the skull in which the superior curvature is saddle-shaped instead of domed in lateral view.

**clinodactyly** \-dak′təlē\ [CLINO- + DACTYL- + -Y ] A congenital deflection of one or more digits from the central axis of the hand or foot. Also *clinodactylism.*

**clinoid** \klī′noid\ In the shape of or resembling a bed.

**clinometer** \klīnäm′ətər\ [CLINO- + -METER] A device to measure cyclotorsion.

**clinoscope** \klī′nəskōp\ [CLINO- + -SCOPE] A device to measure latent cyclotorsion.

**clinostatic** \-stat′ik\ [CLINO- + STAT-[1] + -IC] Occurring in the recumbent position.

**clioquinol** IODOCHLORHYDROXYQUIN.

**clip** A surgical device used primarily to approximate skin edges or to provide permanent occlusion of blood vessels during a surgical procedure. Usually made of metal, it is inserted with a special mechanical tool. **catheter c.** A clip used with a bladder catheter to prevent escape of urine. **dura c.** A malleable V-shaped or U-shaped wire that can be closed with a specially designed clamp to occlude a blood vessel. It is nonreactive in tissues and can be left in place permanently. **skin c.** A metal wire or ribbon used to approximate the edges of a wound in the skin. Also *Michel's clip.* **towel c.** An instrument used to attach surgical drapes to each other or to the patient in order to maintain a sterile field at the time of operation. Also *towel clamp, towel forceps.*

**cliseometer** \klis′ē·äm′ətər\ An instrument used for measuring the angle of inclination of the axis of the pelvis to the vertebral column. Also *kliseometer.*

**-clisis** \-klī′sis, -kləsis\ -CLEISIS.

**clition** \klit′ē·än\ In craniometry, the midpoint of the anterior border of the clivus.

**clitoralgia** \klit′əral′jə\ [*clitor(is)*+-ALGIA] Pain in the clitoris.

**clitoridectomy** \klit′əridek′təmē\ [New L *clitoris,* gen. *clitorid(is)* + -ECTOMY] A surgical resection of the clitoris.

**clitoriditis** \klit′əridī′tis\ CLITORITIS.

**clitorimegaly** \klit′ərimeg′əlē\ [*clitori(s)* + -MEGALY] MACROCLITORIS.

**clitoris** \klit′əris, klī′təris\ [New L, from Gk *kleitoris* clitoris (orig. lit. meaning prob. hillock, small eminence, akin to Gk *kleitys* hillside and *klinein* to incline)] [NA] In females, an erectile organ, homologous with the penis, situated behind the anterior commissure of the labia majora, where it is partially surrounded by folds of the labia minora, an anterior fold forming the prepuce over the glans and a posterior fold forming the frenulum. It arises from the ischiopubic rami by two crura that ascend towards the symphysis pubis, below which they are separated by a septum and bound together by dense fibrous tissue to form the corpora cavernosa of the corpus clitoridis, which is held to the symphysis by a suspensory ligament. The corpus turns downwards to end as the glans clitoridis. Also *coles femininus* (outmoded), *penis femineus* (outmoded), *penis muliebris* (outmoded). Adj. clitoral, clitoridean.

**clitoritis** \klit′ərī′tis\ [*clitor(is)* + -ITIS] Inflammation of the clitoris. Also *clitoriditis.*

**clitoromegaly** \klit′ərōmeg′əlē\ [*clitor(is)* + -MEGALY] Enlargement of the clitoris.

**clitorrhagia** \klit′ərā′jə\ [*clito(ris)* + -RRHAGIA] Bleeding from the clitoris.

**clival** \klī′vəl\ Pertaining to the clivus.

**clivus** \klī′vəs\ [L, a hill, slope] [NA] A sloping bony surface forming the anterior wall of the posterior cranial fossa and formed by the basilar part of the occipital bone and the posterior part of the body of the sphenoid bone, thereby extending from the foramen magnum between the jugular tubercles to the dorsum sellae. Resting on it are the medulla oblongata, the lower part of the pons, and the plexus of basilar sinuses. Also *clivus blumenbachii, Blumenbach's clivus.* **basilar c.** CLIVUS OSSIS OCCIPITALIS. **c. basilaris** CLIVUS OSSIS OCCIPITALIS. **Blumenbach's c.** CLIVUS. **c. blumenbachii** CLIVUS. **c. monticuli** DECLIVE. **c. ossis occipitalis** The lower, or posterior, part of the clivus, formed by the pars basilaris of the occipital bone. Also *basilar clivus, clivus basilaris.* **c. ossis sphenoidalis** The upper, or anterior, part of the clivus, formed by the posterior part of the body of the sphenoid bone, or dorsum sellae.

**CLL** chronic lymphocytic leukemia.

**cloaca** \klō·ā′kə\ [L, a sluice, sewer, drain] **1** The posteroventral pocket, found in most vertebrates, including monotremes but excluding all other mammals, which communicates with the exterior and into which the orifices of the digestive, urinary, and genital systems open. **2** A similar structure in mammalian embryos. **3** The respiratory, excretory, or reproductive duct at the end of the digestive tract in certain invertebrates. Adj. cloacal. **persistent c.** The continuation beyond normal fetal duration of a common vestibular chamber into which the urinary, genital, and digestive tracts empty. **ventral c.** The ventral part of the cloaca in an embryo as it becomes divided by the cloacal septum. The primitive bladder and the primitive urogenital sinus thus become demarcated.

**cloacogenic** \klō·ā′kəjen′ik\ [L *cloac(a)* sluice, floodgate, drain + *o* + -GENIC] Arising from the cloaca.

**clock** / **aging c.** The concept that genetic material is programed to stop the duplication of diploid cells after a set number of doublings or, in the case of postmitotic fixed cells, to impair cell functions so that the useful life of the cell comes to an end. **biological c.** A control system thought to be responsible for the various biorhythms. The popular notion of such a system is an oversimplification of a complex set of endogenous and exogenous factors that influence diverse biologic activities.

**clofazimine** $C_{27}H_{22}Cl_2N_4$. *N*,10-Bis(4-chlorophenyl)-2,10-dihydro-2-[(1-methylethyl)imino]-3-phenazinamine. An antibacterial drug used in the treatment of dapsone-resistant leprosy and tuberculosis. A reddish pigmentation of the skin is a major adverse reaction to this drug, limiting its use.
**clofibrate** $C_{12}H_{15}ClO_3$. 2-(4-Chlorophenoxy)-2-methylpropanoic acid ethyl ester. An anticholesterolemic agent used to reduce serum lipids.
**clomiphene citrate** A nonsteroid compound with weak estrogenic activity. It induces the release of a hypothalamic releasing hormone that in turn stimulates the release by the anterior pituitary of follicle stimulating hormone (FSH) and luteinizing hormone (LH). It is used to treat infertility in anovulatory women and any of the forms of hypogonadotropic hypogonadism in men.
**clon** \klän, klōn\ CLONE.
**clonal** \klō′nəl\ Of or pertaining to a clone.
**clonazepam** $C_{15}H_{10}ClN_3O_3$. 5-(2-Chlorophenyl)-1,3-dihydro-7-nitro-2*H*-1,4-benzodiazepin-2-one, a benzodiazepine antiepileptic drug that is useful in the treatment of myoclonic seizures in children. It is given orally.
**clone** \klōn\ [Gk *klōn* a young shoot, twig, sprout] A population of cells or organisms derived from a single cell or organism by asexual or vegetative propagation. All members of the clone have the same genetic information and are thus nearly identical with the parent cell or organism. Also *clon.* Adj. clonal. **forbidden c.** A clone of immunocompetent cells reactive to self antigens which, according to the clonal selection theory of immunity, should be eliminated in fetal life. It was suggested that autoimmune disease is caused by such forbidden clones arising by somatic mutation in adult life.
**clonic** \klän′ik\ **1** Of or describing clonus. **2** Describing the phase of an epileptic convulsion or the type of movement occurring in this phase, usually in the form of brief muscular contractions repeated at short, regular intervals.
**clonicotonic** \klän′ikōtän′ik\ Demonstrating or pertaining to alternating clonic and tonic contractions.
**clonidine** 2-(2,6-Dichloroanilino)-2-imidazoline. A drug used to treat hypertension. It acts centrally as an $\alpha$-adrenergic agonist.
**clonidine hydrochloride** $C_9H_{10}Cl_3N_3$. 2-(2,6-Dichloroanilino)-2-imidazoline hydrochloride, an antihypertensive medication that is given orally. It first stimulates $\alpha$-adrenergic receptors and then produces a blockade of $\alpha$-adrenergic peripheral receptors.
**clonism** \klän′izm\ [*clon(us)* + -ISM] A state of successive clonic contractions. Also *clonismus, clonospasm.*
**clonogenic** \klän′ōjen′ik\ [*clon(e)* + *o* + -GENIC] Derived from or consisting of a clone.
**clonograph** \klän′əgraf\ [*clon(us)* + *o* + -GRAPH] An instrument used for recording clonus.
**clonorchiasis** \klō′nôrkī′əsis\ [*Clonorch(is)* + -IASIS] An infection caused by the trematode parasite *Clonorchis sinensis* (Chinese or oriental liver fluke) in which the adult flukes infect the bile ducts. The disease occurs principally in China, Hong Kong, Korea, and Vietnam. Autochthonous cases have been reported from Hawaii and California. Treatment was previously unsatisfactory, but praziquantel gives satisfactory results. Also *clonorchiosis.*
***Clonorchis sinensis*** \klōnôr′kis sinen′sis\ The Chinese or Oriental liver fluke, a trematode of the family Opisthorchiidae which is common in the Far East. It is parasitic in the bile ducts of man and other fish-eating animals, such as cats and dogs. Infection results from eating raw, smoked, or undercooked freshwater fish in which the infective metacercariae are found. Cyprinoid fish serve as the principal second intermediate host. Several operculate snails are the first intermediate hosts in which the cercariae develop, which encyst in the fish host, forming infective metacercariae.
**clonospasm** \klän′ōspazm\ [Gk *klono(s)* violent motion, tumult + SPASM] CLONISM.
**clonus** \klō′nəs\ [New L (from Gk *klonos* violent motion as in battle, tumult)] **1** A repetitive, rhythmical contraction and relaxation such as that which may occur in one phase (clonic phase) of a convulsion, or the similar phenomenon which may be induced at a joint by stretching a muscle in a spastic limb or one showing hyperreflexia. **2** A sudden, transient muscular contraction involving movement of one or more parts of the body. **ankle c.** Clonus induced by the abrupt dorsiflexion of the foot, followed by continued stretching of the Achilles tendon. Also *foot clonus.* **toe c.** Clonus involving the great toe induced by sudden passive dorsiflexion. **wrist c.** Clonus in the forearm muscles induced by sudden passive flexion or extension of the wrist.
**clopamide** $C_{14}H_{20}ClN_3O_3S$. 3-(Aminosulfonyl)-4-chloro-*N*-(2,6-dimethyl-1-piperidinyl)benzamide. A diuretic agent with actions and uses like chlorothiazide. It is given orally.
**Cloquet** [Hippolyte *Cloquet,* French anatomist, 1787–1840] See under GANGLION.
**Cloquet** [Jules Germain *Cloquet,* French anatomist, 1790–1883] **1** Cloquet's hernia. See under PECTINEAL HERNIA. **2** See under PSEUDOGANGLION. **3** Cloquet's canal. See under CANALIS HYALOIDEUS. **4** Cloquet's gland. See under CLOQUET'S NODE. **5** Cloquet's ligament. See under RUDIMENT OF VAGINAL PROCESS.
**clorazepate dipotassium** $C_{16}H_{11}ClK_2N_2O_4$. 7-Chloro-2,3-dihydro-2,2-dihydroxy-5-phenyl-1*H*-1,4-benzodiazepine-3-carboxylic acid dipotassium salt, a compound used for the symptomatic relief of anxiety and for neuroses associated with anxiety symptoms as prominent components of the conditions. It is also used to alleviate symptoms of acute alcohol withdrawal. It is given orally.
**clorazepic acid** $C_{16}H_{13}ClN_2O$. An acid, usually administered as the dipotassium salt, with antianxiety properties much like diazepam. It is classed as a minor tranquilizer.
**clorophene** $C_{13}H_{11}ClO$. 4-Chloro-2-(phenylmethyl)-phenol, a clorinated disinfectant that is effective against a variety of bacteria and fungi.
**clortermine hydrochloride** $C_{10}H_{14}ClN{\cdot}HCl$. 2-Chloro-$\alpha$,$\alpha$-dimethyl-phenethylamine hydrochloride, an analogue of amphetamine with similar properties. It has been used in the treatment of obesity as an anorexic agent. It is given orally.
**Closs** [Karl *Closs,* Swedish physician, flourished 20th century] Danbolt-Closs syndrome. See under ACRODERMATITIS ENTEROPATHICA.
**clostridia** \klästrid′ē·ə\ Plural of CLOSTRIDIUM.
***Clostridium*** \klästrid′ē·əm\ [New L (from Gk *klōstēr* a thread, line, yarn, spindle + -IDIUM)] A genus of large, Gram-positive, anaerobic or aerotolerant, spore-forming bacilli commonly found in soil, mud, and the mammalian gastrointestinal tract. Various species are primarily proteolytic, saccharolytic, or both, and they accumulate various products of butyric fermentation and sometimes of propionic fermentation. Among the many species, a few cause disease under special conditions. ***C. botulinum*** A strictly anaerobic clostridium that causes botulism through formation of a powerful toxin of several types. There is also evidence of occasional colonization of the gastrointestinal tract of infants. The organism is widely distributed in soil and lake bottoms and on vegetation. The spores may survive and germinate in home-canned low-acid vegetables without detectable spoilage.

The toxin is destroyed by boiling the food before ingestion. Also *Bacillus botulinus* (obs.). See also BOTULINUM TOXIN. ***C. difficile*** A clostridium often present in the intestine. Its excessive growth, with its production of enterotoxin, is often responsible for the pseudomembranous colitis induced by antibiotics, especially clindamycin. ***C. histolyticum*** An aerotolerant clostridium found in wounds. It hydrolyzes collagen by secreting collagenase, and grows well on meat digest without sugar. ***C. novyi*** A clostridium found in wounds and feces. It grows poorly without carbohydrate. Several of the toxins involved have been identified. Also *Clostridium oedematiens* (obs.), *Bacillus oedematiens* (obs.). ***C. perfringens*** The major cause of gas gangrene, the bacteriology of which is often mixed. *C. perfringens* is nonmotile, rarely forms spores, and causes stormy fermentation of milk. Some clostridial wound infections spread rapidly in muscle resulting in gas gangrene. The organism produces many exotoxins, some of which are enzymes that hydrolyze tissue macromolecules. The $\alpha$-toxin is a lecithinase (phospholipase), whose attack on cell membranes has necrotizing and lethal effects. Strains that form an enterotoxin are also a frequent cause of food poisoning. Also *Clostridium welchii* (obs.), *Welch's bacillus* (obs.). ***C. septicum*** A histotoxic clostridium found in wound infections and in septicemia. ***C. sordellii*** A clostridium found in wounds. ***C. sporogenes*** A clostridium found in wounds that grows well on meat digest without carbohydrates. ***C. tertium*** An aerotolerant clostridium found in wounds and feces that ferments both protein and carbohydrate. ***C. tetani*** A highly motile (swarming), strictly anaerobic bacterium, widely distributed in soil and feces. It causes tetanus by contamination of wounds containing necrotic tissue. It often forms a spherical terminal spore that gives the cell a "drumstick" appearance. Not histotoxic, it ferments meat digest but not protein or sugars. It releases a powerful neurotoxin (tetanospasmin) during growth. Positive identification of the isolated organism requires demonstration of toxin formation. Also *Bacillus tetani* (obs.), *tetanus bacillus*. ***C. welchii*** *Obs.* *CLOSTRIDIUM PERFRINGENS.*

**clostridium** \klästrid′ē·əm\ (*pl.* clostridia) A bacillus of the genus *Clostridium*.

**closure** \klō′zhər\ [L *clausura* (from *clausus*, past part. of *claudere* to close + *-ura* -URE) a closing] A procedure, such as the repair of a surgical wound following surgery, in which two or more parts, at least one of which is movable, are brought together. **delayed primary c.** DELAYED PRIMARY SUTURE. **flask c.** In denture making, the pressing together of the two halves of a flask in order to force plastic material into the mold. **primary c.** A suture place at the time of the initial surgical procedure. Also *primary suture*. **velopharyngeal c.** Closing of the pharyngeal isthmus by elevation of the soft palate and contraction of the palatopharyngeal sphincter during the act of swallowing. **wound c.** The provision of an epithelial cover over a wound. It can be accomplished by approximating the wound edges, performing a skin graft, or allowing spontaneous healing from the edges.

**clot** 1 A solid or semisolid mass formed in or from a fluid medium; a coagulum or thrombus. 2 To form such a mass; coagulate. **agonal c.** A blood clot formed in the heart during the moments of dying. Also *agony clot*. **antemortem c.** A blood clot found in the heart or vascular tree at postmortem but which had formed there before death. **blood c.** THROMBUS. **chicken-fat c.** A postmortem clot in which the erythrocytes settled out before the clot formed. Such clots are brilliant yellow. **currant jelly c.** A postmortem clot that forms before the erythrocytes have sedimented. **laminated c.** A thrombus characterized by layering of fibrin, platelets, and erythrocytes. Thrombi developing antemortem tend to exhibit such layering, particularly when they form in aneurysms. **marantic c.** A blood clot which has formed in a severely malnourished individual with sluggish circulation. **plasma c.** Coagulated blood plasma used to effect union and healing of sectioned peripheral nerves not under tension. Also *plasma glue*. **postmortem c.** A blood clot that has formed after death in the heart or in a blood vessel. **Schede's c.** A collection of congealed blood and blood products that is allowed to form in an osseous cavity after resection of necrotic bone and surrounding tissue. **spiderweb c.** A delicate, weblike structure that forms in cerebrospinal fluid obtained from patients with tuberculous meningitis after the fluid has been in a test tube for a few hours at room temperature or at 37°C. **stratified c.** A thrombus made up of different colored layers. **white c.** WHITE THROMBUS.

**clotrimazole** $C_{22}H_{17}ClN_2$. 1-[(2-Chlorophenyl)diphenylmethyl]-1*H*-imidazole, a broad spectrum antifungal agent used topically.

**clouding of consciousness** Impaired orientation, perception, and awareness, suggestive of some organic disturbance of brain function. Also *mental fog*.

**cloxacillin** \kläk′səsil′in\ $C_{19}H_{18}ClN_3O_5S$. 5-Methyl-3-*o*-chlorophenyl-y-isoxazolylpenicillin. A semisynthetic, penicillinase-resistant penicillin which is used primarily to treat infections caused by penicillinase-producing staphylococci.

**clubbing** A proliferation of soft tissue about the terminal phalanges of the fingers or toes. The nails develop lateral and longitudinal curvatures. **c. of the calix** The absence of the normal caliceal cup on intravenous urography or retrograde pyelography, indicating increased back pressure, loss of the papilla, or scarring of the kidney due to chronic pyelonephritis. **c. of the fingers** The enlargement and expansion of the extremities of the fingers or toes. The nails develop lateral and longitudinal curvatures. It may occur congenitally or as part of a disease process such as chronic liver disease, chronic suppuration, bacterial endocarditis, and cyanotic heart disease.

**clubfoot** TALIPES.

**clubhand** TALIPOMANUS.

**clumping** The process of forming a cluster or mass composed of individual entities, as bacteria or cells; specifically, agglutination.

**cluneal** \kloo′nē·əl\ Pertaining to the clunis or clunes.

**clunes** \kloo′nēz\ (*sing.* clunis) NATES.

**clunis** \kloo′nis\ [L, a buttock] Singular of CLUNES.

**Clutton** [Henry H. *Clutton*, English surgeon, 1850–1909] See under JOINT.

**clysis** \klī′sis\ [Gk *klysis* (from *klyzein* to drench, wash out) a drenching, enema] The introduction of a solution into the body by some means other than through the mouth. **subeschar c.** The instillation of antibiotics directly into and under a cutaneous burn. Systemically administered antibiotics cannot be delivered to avascular tissue, but high levels can be achieved by this direct administration.

**clyster** [Gk *klystēr* (from *klyzein* to drench, wash out) an enema or enema syringe] *Older term* ENEMA.

**Cm** Symbol for the element, curium.

**cm** Symbol for the unit, centimeter.

**CM-cellulose sodium** Carboxymethylcellulose sodium, a bulk-forming laxative.

**CMF** The anticancer chemotherapeutic combination of cyclophosphamide, methotrexate, and fluorouracil.

**CMHC** community mental health center.

**CMI** cell-mediated immunity.
**CML** chronic myelogenous leukemia (chronic granulocytic leukemia).
**CMP** Symbol for cytidine monophosphate.
**c.m.s.** *cras mane sumendus* (L, to be taken tomorrow morning).
**c.n.** *cras nocte* (L, tomorrow night).
**cnemial** \nē′mē·əl\ [Gk *knēm(ē)* the leg between knee and ankle + English *-ial,* from L *i* + *-alis* -AL] Pertaining to the leg, especially the shin.
**cnemis** \nē′mis\ [Gk *knēmis* a greave, legging] The anterior part of the leg; the shin.
**Cnidaria** \nīder′ē·ə\ [Gk *knidē* a nettle, stinging mollusk + -ARIA] A subphylum of nematocyst-containing coelenterates.
**CNS** central nervous system.
**c.n.s.** *cras nocte sumendus* (L, to be taken tomorrow night).
**Co** Symbol for the element, cobalt.
**co-** \kō-, kə-\ [L prefix *co-*, variant of L prefix *com-* (from *cum* with). See COM-.] A prefix meaning together, with, jointly.
**CoA** coenzyme A.
**coacervate** A phase that separates from aqueous solution rich in a hydrated polymer.
**coadaptation** \kō′adaptā′shən\ Correlated adaptative changes occurring in two mutually dependent biological systems.
**coadunation** The combining of different substances into a uniform mixture. Also *coadunition.*
**coagglutination** \kō′əgloo′tinā′shən\ **1** The aggregation by a single antiserum of two distinct particulate antigens, only one being the sensitizing antigen. **2** The aggregation of guinea-pig erythrocytes by immune complexes between C4 of any species (other than guinea pig) and the appropriate anti-C4 antibodies.
**coagula** \kō·ag′yələ\ Plural of COAGULUM.
**coagulability** \kō·ag′yələbil′itē\ The potential of blood or plasma to clot.
**coagulant** \kō·ag′yələnt\ **1** Inducing clotting. **2** A substance that induces clotting, such as thrombin.
**coagulase** \kō·ag′yəlās\ An enzyme, excreted by *Staphylococcus aureus,* that converts prothrombin to thrombin and hence causes clotting of plasma. It may contribute to the formation of localized lesions by *S. aureus* and may be a factor in the greater virulence of *S. aureus* compared with coagulase-negative bacteria such as *S. epidermidis.* Also *staphylocoagulase.*
**coagulate** \kō·ag′yəlāt\ To undergo or cause to undergo coagulation.
**coagulation** \kō·ag′yəlā′shən\ [L *coagulatio* (from *coagulare* to curdle, congeal, from *coactus,* past part. of *cogere* to bring together) a curdling] The precipitation of fibrin from blood or plasma; clotting. The process depends upon the presence of calcium, phospholipid, and a cascade of plasma proteins acting sequentially. **disseminated intravascular c.** An acquired bleeding disorder that is the result of activation of the clotting mechanism within circulating blood. The condition may be caused by metastatic carcinomas, especially of the prostate, by abruptio placentae, by infections such as bacillary septicemia or meningococcemia, progranulocytic leukemias, and many other causes. The condition is characterized by thrombocytopenia, hypofibrinogenemia, and prolonged prothrombin time, prolonged partial thromboplastin time, and reduced activity of coagulation factors V, VII, VIII, IX, X, XI, and prothrombin. Also *defibrination syndrome, consumptive coagulopathy, consumptive thrombohemorrhagic disorder.* Abbr. DIC **electric c.** ELECTROCOAGULATION. **infrared c.** The destruction of tissue by infrared radiation, as for example a hemorrhoid. **intravascular c.** A pathologic process resulting in formation of blood clots in the circulating blood. It may be of a macroscopic form (thromboembolic disease) or it may be microscopic (disseminated intravascular coagulation).
**coagulative** \kō·ag′yəlā′tiv\ Capable of coagulating or causing coagulation; coagulable.
**coagulator** \kō·ag′yəlā′tər\ A surgical device designed to establish hemostasis by imparting either electric or light energy to the tissue.
**coagulogram** \kō·ag′yələgram′\ A recording, usually photoelectric, of the precipitation of fibrin from plasma during clotting.
**coagulopathy** \kō·ag′yəläp′əthē\ A disorder of the blood-clotting mechanism. **consumptive c.** DISSEMINATED INTRAVASCULAR COAGULATION.
**coaguloviscosimeter** \kō·ag′yəlōvis′kōsim′ətər\ A device that measures the changes in viscosity of blood or plasma during clotting.
**coagulum** \kō·ag′yələm\ A clot arising from blood or plasma as the result of coagulation or of heating. **closing c.** The fibrinous and cellular plug that seals off the initial entry point in the endometrium after the blastocyst has become completely embedded during interstitial implantation.
**coapt** \kō′apt\ [Late L *coapt(are)* (from L *co-* with + *apt(are)* to adapt to) to adjust or adapt to] To approximate two surfaces without tension.
**coaptation** \kō′aptā′shən\ [COAPT + -ATION] The approximation of two surfaces, as the edges of a wound.
**coarctate** \kō·ärk′tāt\ [See COARCTATION.] **1** To compress or press very close together, as in a surgical procedure in which two structures are mutually strengthened. **2** Compressed; pressed together.
**coarctation** \kō′ärktā′shən\ [L *coar(c)tatio* (from *coar(c)tare* to constrict, from *co-* together + *ar(c)tare* to tighten, from *artus* tight) tightening, constriction] Constriction or narrowing, especially of the aorta. **adult type c. of the aorta** Congenital localized constriction of the aorta, distal to the left subclavian artery, at or just distal to the point of insertion of the ductus arteriosus, the latter having closed normally. **c. of the aorta** The congenital partial or complete obliteration of the aorta above, opposite to, or just beyond the site of entry of the ductus arteriosus. In the preductal type there is considerable variation in its extent and in the involvement of other vessels. The postductal type is probably related to extension into the aortic wall of tissue derived from that surrounding the ductus arteriosus. This tissue contracts after birth to bring about stenosis of the ductus and, if present, of the aorta also. In severe coarctation, the blood pressure becomes high proximally and low distally. **infantile type c. of the aorta** A congenital narrowing of the aorta between the origin of the left subclavian artery and the entry of the ductus arteriosus. **reversed c.** A complication of the aortic arch syndrome in which, because the arteries to the arms become narrowed, the blood pressure is lower in them than in the legs.
**CoASH** A symbol for coenzyme A suitable for use in equations in which the SH group becomes acylated.
**coat** **1** A fibrous or other tissue forming the outer covering or sheath of an organ or structure. **2** One of the layers forming the lining or wall of a tubular or hollow structure or organ. See also TUNICA. **adventitial c.** TUNICA AD-

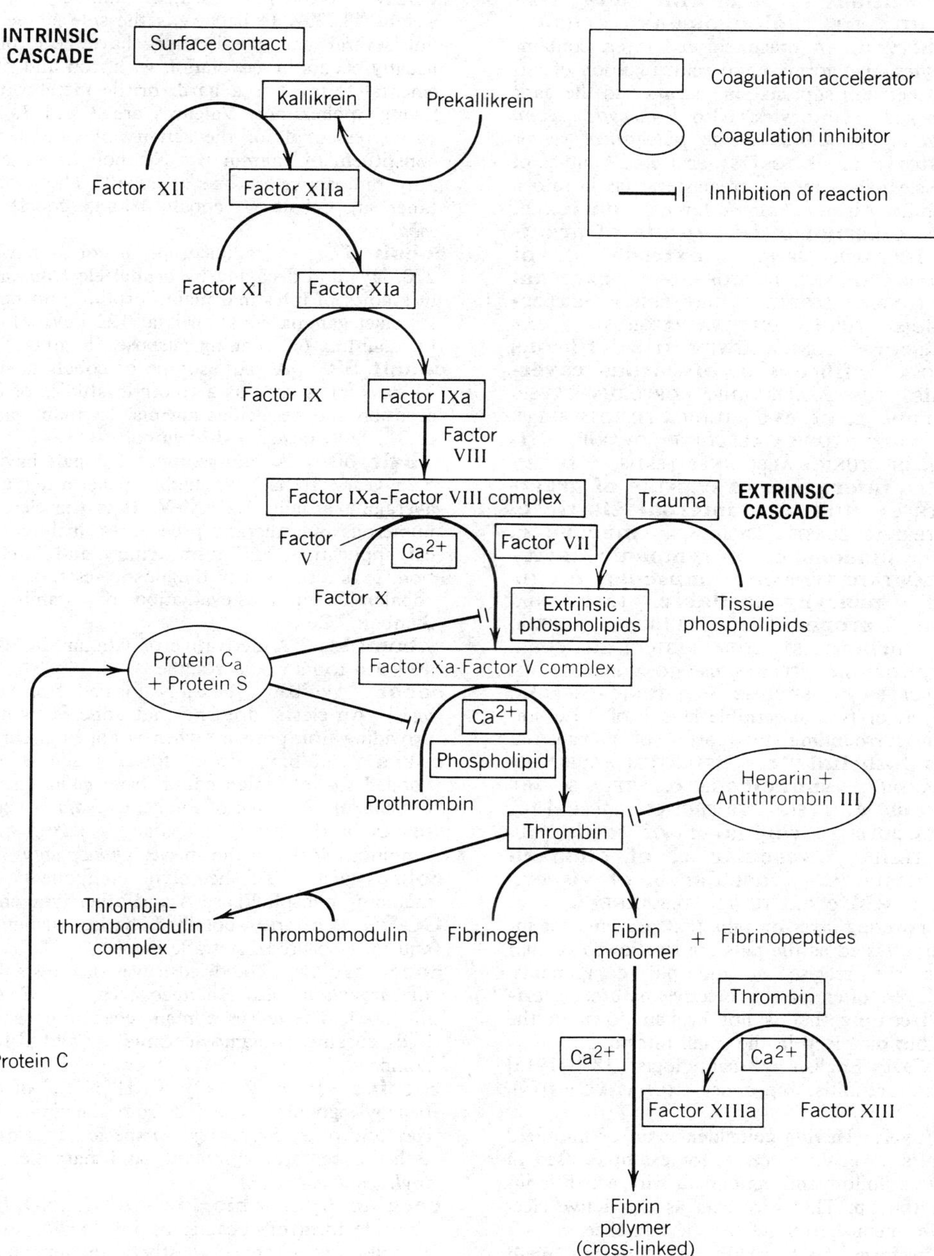


**The coagulation cascade**

VENTITIA. **adventitious c. of uterine tube** TELA SUBSEROSA TUBAE UTERINAE. **albugineous c.** TUNICA ALBUGINEA. **buffy c.** A cream-colored layer, containing mostly leukocytes, that forms upon centrifugation of anticoagulated blood between supernatant plasma and the dark red column of packed erythrocytes. Also *leukocytic cream, buffy crust, crusta inflammatoria, crusta phlogistica, yellow layer.* **cremasteric c. of testis** Scattered bundles of the cremaster muscle joined by the cremasteric fascia into a continuous membrane. Also *cremasteric layer.* **dartos c.** TUNICA DARTOS. **external c. of capsule of graafian follicle** THECA EXTERNA. **external c. of esophagus** TUNICA ADVENTITIA ESOPHAGI. **external c. of ureter** TUNICA ADVENTITIA URETERIS. **external c. of vessels** TUNICA EXTERNA VASORUM. **external c. of viscera** TUNICA ADVENTITIA. **fibrous c.** TUNICA FIBROSA. **fibrous c. of corpus cavernosum of penis** TUNICA ALBUGINEA CORPORUM CAVERNOSORUM. **fibrous c. of eye** TUNICA FIBROSA BULBI. **fibrous c. of ovary** TUNICA ALBUGINEA OVARII. **fibrous c. of testis** TUNICA ALBUGINEA TESTIS. **fuzzy c.** GLYCOCALYX. **internal c. of capsule of graafian follicle** THECA INTERNA. **internal elastic c. of artery** INTERNAL ELASTIC LAMINA. **mucous c.** TUNICA MUCOSA. **mucous c. of tympanic cavity** TUNICA MUCOSA CAVITATIS TYMPANI. **muscular c.** TUNICA MUSCULARIS. **pharyngobasilar c.** FASCIA PHARYNGOBASILARIS. **proper c.** TUNICA PROPRIA. **proper c. of corium** STRATUM RETICULARE CORII. **proper c. of pharynx** TELA SUBMUCOSA PHARYNGIS. **sclerotic c.** SCLERA. **serous c.** TUNICA SEROSA. **spore c.** A layer, or two discernible layers, of water-impermeable protein surrounding the cortex of a bacterial spore. **subendothelial c.** STRATUM SUBENDOTHELIALE ENDOCARDII. **submucous c.** TELA SUBMUCOSA. **subserous c.** TELA SUBSEROSA. **uveal c.** TUNICA VASCULOSA BULBI. **vaginal c. of testis** TUNICA VAGINALIS TESTIS. **vascular c. of stomach** TELA SUBMUCOSA GASTRICA. **vascular c. of viscera** TELA SUBMUCOSA. **white c.** TUNICA ALBUGINEA.

**coating** 1 A covering layer on pills that prevents the ingredients from being tasted as the pills are swallowed or that selectively delays the release of the pill components. 2 Any covering layer, often of a protective nature. **enteric c.** A pill coating that is not broken down in the stomach by acid, but dissolved in the small intestine.

**Coats** [George *Coats*, English ophthalmologist, 1876–1915] Coats disease, Coats retinitis. See under EXUDATIVE RETINITIS.

**coaxial** \kō·ak′sē·əl\ Having coincident axes or mounted on concentric shafts. A coaxial needle, for example, used in electromyography, is hollow and contains a wire which is insulated except at the tip. This wire acts as the active electrode and the outer metal barrel acts as the reference.

**cobalamin** The form of vitamin $B_{12}$ in which the cobalt atom in the center of the corrin ring has as fifth ligand, a nitrogen atom of the 5,6-dimethylbenzimidazole ribonucleotide that is joined to the ring through a side chain, but lacks a sixth ligand, R. Such a ligand is normally present. In vitamin $B_{12}$ R = CN, and in coenzyme $B_{12}$ R = 5-deoxyadenosyl. Methylcobalamin and hydroxocobalamin are other natural forms. **c. concentrate** The dry, partially purified material obtained from selected *Streptomyces* cultures, containing not less than 500 μg of cobalamin per gram. It is a relatively inexpensive, concentrated form of vitamin $B_{12}$, suitable for use in oral preparations of the vitamin.

**cobalt** \kō′bôlt\ Element number 27, having atomic weight 58.9332. Cobalt 59 is the sole stable natural isotope, but several unstable isotopes have been produced. Cobalt usually occurs in association with iron and nickel ores. In elemental form, it is a hard, brittle metal with important alloying applications. Valences are 2 and 3. Biologically, cobalt is essential for the activity of several enzymes. It is a constituent of vitamin $B_{12}$. Symbol: Co **radioactive c.** Any radioactive isotope of cobalt. Those of clinical importance are cobalt 57, cobalt 58, and cobalt 60. Also *radiocobalt.*

**cobalt 57** A radioisotope of cobalt having a half-life of 270 days and decaying by orbital electron capture. It is used in studies of intestinal malabsorption and pernicious anemia. Its chief gamma emission is at 122 keV, which is convenient for counting or scanning purposes. Symbol: $^{57}$Co

**cobalt 58** A radioisotope of cobalt having a half-life of 71 days. It is used as a tracer in studies of intestinal malabsorption and pernicious anemia. Its main gamma emission is at 811 keV, rather high. Symbol: $^{58}$Co

**cobalt 60** A radioisotope of cobalt having a half-life of 5.25 years. It has two highly penetrating gamma emissions averaging around 1.25 MeV. It is the element of choice in numerous radiotherapy procedures, including teletherapy, local application, and intracavitary and interstitial implantation. It is also used in diagnostic tests, as a label for cyanocobalamin for the evaluation of vitamin $B_{12}$ absorption. Symbol: $^{60}$Co

**cobamide** A derivative of vitamin $B_{12}$ that lacks a base attached to its ribose residue.

**coban** \kō′ban\ [Possibly formed from *co(hesive) ban(dage)*] An elastic dressing that adheres tightly to itself, thus providing firm pressure when wrapped circumferentially.

**cobra** \kō′brə\ [short for Portuguese *cobra de capelo* hooded snake, Indian cobra, from *cobra* snake, from L *colubra* snake] A snake of the genus *Naja,* a genus of venomous snakes in the family Elapidae. **king c.** A very large venomous snake of the species *Ophiophagus hannah.*

**cobralysin** The hemolytic components of cobra venom, including phospholipase A and other lytic enzymes.

**COBS** cesarean-obtained, barrier-sustained (used of rats and mice so bred). A trade name.

**coca** \kō′kə\ The dried leaves of the small trees or shrubs *Erythroxylum coca,* Huanuco coca, and *E. truxillense,* Truxillo coca. The leaves contain cocatannic acid and the alkaloids cocaine, cinnamoylcocaine, α- and β-truxilline, and ecgonine.

**cocaine** [*coca* + -INE] $C_{17}H_{21}NO_4$. An alkaloid, methylbenzoylecgonine, extracted from the leaves of *Erythroxylum coca* and other *Erythroxylum* species. It is used as a local anesthetic, cerebral stimulant, and narcotic. Also *benzoylmethylecgonine.*

**cocaine hydrochloride** $C_{17}H_{21}NO_4{\cdot}HCl$. The hydrochloride form of cocaine, having local anesthetic properties. It is used as a topical anesthetic for mucous membranes and other surfaces of the ear, nose, and throat, and in bronchoscopy. As with cocaine, its abuse leads to addiction.

**cocainism** \kōkā′nizm\ [*cocain(e)* + -ISM] Cocaine dependency with such evidence of cocaine intoxication as agitation, loquaciousness, overestimation of physical and mental capacities, tachycardia, sweating, and elevated blood pressure.

**cocainization** \kō′kānīzā′shən\ The use of cocaine in topical anesthesia.

**cocarboxylase** *Outmoded* THIAMIN PYROPHOSPHATE.

**cocarcinogen** \kōkär′sənəjən\ [CO- + CARCINOGEN] A substance or agent which has little or no carcinogenicity but can potentiate the effect of a carcinogen.

**cocarcinogenesis** \kōkär′sənōjen′əsis\ [CO- + CARCINOGENESIS] The reinforcement of carcinogenesis.

**cocci** \käk′sī\ Plural of COCCUS.

**Coccidia** \käksid′ē·ə\ A subclass of the protozoan class Sporozoea, phylum Apicomplexa, in which sporogony usually occurs in the same host, most commonly in the gut epithelial cells or associated gland cells of invertebrates and vertebrates.

**coccidia** \käksid′ē·ə\ [See COCCIDIUM.] Plural of COCCIDIUM.

**coccidial** \käksid′ē·əl\ Of or pertaining to coccidia. Also *coccidian.*

**coccidian** \käksid′ē·ən\ **1** A member of the order Eucoccidiida, subclass Coccidia, usually with reference to the genus *Eimeria.* **2** COCCIDIAL.

***Coccidioides immitis*** \käksid′ē·oi′dēz imī′tis\ The species of fungus that is the etiologic agent of coccidioidomycosis.

**coccidioidin** \käksid′ē·oi′din\ Antigen prepared from *Coccidioides immitis* and used for intradermal testing in the diagnosis of coccidioidomycosis.

**coccidioidoma** \käksid′ē·oidō′mə\ A tuberclelike lesion caused by the fungus *Coccidioides immitis* and found usually in the lungs. With time, the lesion undergoes fibrosis and calcification. Also *coccidioidal granuloma.*

**coccidioidomeningitis** \käksid′ē·oi′dōmen′injī′tis\ Meningitis resulting from infection by *Coccidioides immitis..*

**coccidioidomycosis** \käksid′ē·oi′dōmīkō′sis\ [*Coccidioid(es)* + *o* + MYCOSIS] A disease usually acquired by inhalation of the spores of *Coccidioides immitis* and often manifested by respiratory symptoms, pneumonia, or erythema nodosum. In most cases, the infection is benign and limited to the lungs. Also *coccidiomycosis, Posada-Wernicke disease, San Joaquin disease, San Joaquin fever, valley fever.* **disseminated c.** A severe, metastasizing infection caused by the hematogenous spread of *Coccidioides immitis* and involving the lungs, skin, viscera, bones, central nervous system, and other organs. **latent c.** Coccidioidomycosis in an individual whose previous medical history has no record of the disease, but for whom hypersensitivity tests result in a positive reaction. **primary extrapulmonary c.** Coccidioidomycosis which results from cutaneous inoculation with *Coccidioides immitis* and in which secondary lymphadenopathy is usual. Also *chancriform syndrome.*

**coccidiomycosis** \käksid′ē·ōmīkō′sis\ COCCIDIOIDOMYCOSIS.

**coccidiosis** \käk′sidē·ō′sis\ [*coccidi(a)* + -OSIS] A parasitic intestinal infection in animals, including poultry, and occasionally in man. It is caused by coccidia, usually *Isospora* or *Eimeria* species. It is characterized by severe enteritis with diarrhea or dysentery and tenesmus. In man, copious, watery, mucoid stools, anorexia, and nausea are symptomatic.

**coccidiostat** \käksid′ē·ōstat′\ Any of various chemical substances used to inhibit the development of coccidia infections in animals. A coccidiostat is often added to animal feed or drinking water.

***Coccidium*** \käksid′ē·əm\ [dim. of L *coccum* or *coccus* the scarlet berry, kermes berry, a scarlet cloth, from Gk *kokkos* a berry, kernel] A former genus of Coccidia which included organisms now classified as *Eimeria, Isospora,* and *Sarcocystis.* ***C. hominis*** *SARCOCYSTIS HOMINIS.*

**coccidium** \käksid′ē·əm\ [See *COCCIDIUM.*] (*pl.* coccidia) A protozoan organism of the subclass Coccidia.

**coccobacillus** \käk′ōbəsil′əs\ [*cocc(us)* + *o* + BACILLUS] A bacterium having the shape of a very short rod and often, under some conditions, a sphere. The rods are often linked as diplobacilli.

**cocculin** \käk′yəlin\ PICROTOXIN.

***Coccus*** \käk′əs\ A genus of scale insects in the family Coccidae, superfamily Coccoidea, order Hemiptera. Useful as the source of cochineal, kermes, and lac, these insects are on the other hand injurious to many economically important plants.

**coccus** \käk′əs\ [New L, from Gk *kokkos* a berry, kernel] (*pl.* cocci) A spherical or nearly spherical bacterium, grouped in some genera in pairs (diplococci), chains (streptococci), tetrads (sarcinae), or three-dimensional clusters (staphylococci). **pyogenic cocci** A group of predominantly invasive pathogens that tend to produce purulent lesions. They are rapidly destroyed when they are phagocytosed. They include streptococci, staphylococci, and neisseriae.

**coccyalgia** \käk′sē·al′jə\ COCCYDYNIA.

**coccydynia** \käk′sidin′ē·ə\ [*coccy(x)* + *-(o)dynia*] Persistent pain in the coccyx, whether spontaneous or following a fall on the buttocks. Also *coccyalgia, coccygalgia, coccygodynia, coccyodynia.*

**coccygeal** \käksij′ē·əl\ Relating to the os coccygis.

**coccygectomy** \käk′sijek′təmē\ [Gk *kokkyx,* gen. *kokkyg(os)* coccyx + -ECTOMY] Resection of the coccyx.

**coccygodynia** \käk′sigōdin′ē·ə\ COCCYDYNIA.

**coccygotomy** \käk′sigät′əmē\ [Gk *kokkyx,* gen. *kokkygo(s)* coccyx + *o* + -TOMY] An incision into the coccyx.

**coccyodynia** \käk′sē·ōdin′ē·ə\ COCCYDYNIA.

**coccyx** \käk′siks\ [L (from Gk *kokkyx* a cuckoo), a cuckoo, from the resemblance of the *os coccygis* to a cuckoo's beak] OS COCCYGIS.

**cochineal** \kät′chinēl\ [Old Spanish *cochinilla* cochineal, wood louse] A biological carmine dye and coloring agent made from dried, small scale insects, *Coccus cacti.*

**cochl.** *cochleare* (L, spoonful).

**cochl. amp.** *cochleare amplum* (L, heaping spoonful).

**cochlea** \käk′lē·ə\ [L (from Gk *kochlias* a snail with a spiral shell), a snail, periwinkle, snail shell] [NA] The anterior part of the bony labyrinth of the internal ear, lying anterior to the vestibule in the petrous part of the temporal bone and resembling a snail shell, comprising a base lying upon the internal acoustic meatus, and a cone-shaped central axis, or modiolus, around which a canal winds for two-and-a-half turns to the apex, or cupula, which is directed laterally. The bony canal contains a membranous tube, the cochlear duct, enclosing the spiral organ, in which the fibers of the cochlear nerve terminate and in which the sense of hearing is located. Also *acoustic labyrinth, bony cochlea.* **membranous c.** DUCTUS COCHLEARIS.

**cochlear** \käk′lē·ər\ Pertaining to the cochlea.

**cochleare** [L (from *cochlea* a snail), spoonful, spoon] A spoon: used in prescription writing. **c. amplum** A heaping spoonful: used in prescription writing. **c. magnum** A big spoon, i.e., a tablespoon: used in prescription writing. **c. medium** A medium-sized spoon, i.e., a dessertspoon: used in prescription writing. **c. minimum** The smallest spoon, i.e., a teaspoon: used in prescription writing. **c. modicum** A moderate spoon, i.e., a dessertspoon: used in prescription writing. **c. parvum** A small spoon, i.e., a teaspoon: used in prescription writing. **c. plenum** A full spoon, i.e., a tablespoon: used in prescription writing.

**cochleariform** \käk′lē·er′ifôrm\ In the shape of a spoon.

**cochleography** \käk′lē·äg′rəfē\ The study of events

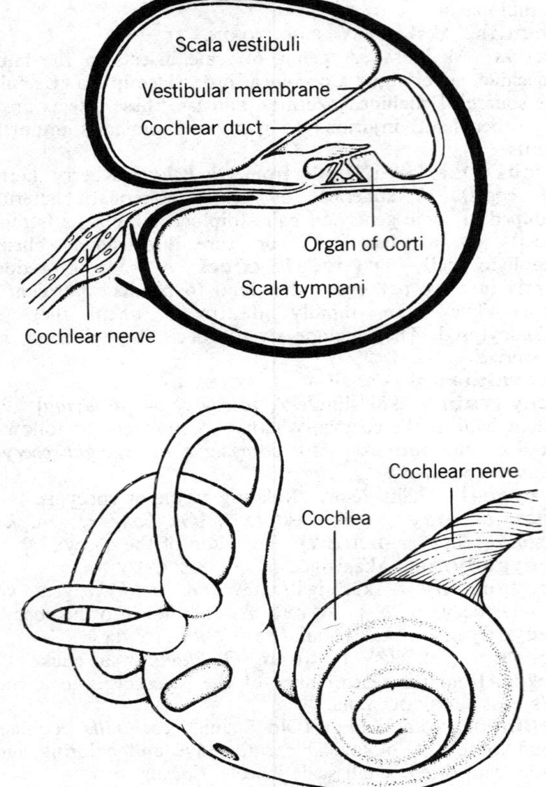


**Cochlea** (with cross-section)

arising in the cochlea and manifest as changes in electrical potential (electrocochleography) or as accoustic events emanating from the cochlea (acoustic cochleography). These intracochlear phenomena result from auditory stimulation and are used in the study of normal and disordered cochlear function. **acoustic c.** The investigation of the biomechanical status of the cochlea through the measurement and analysis of stimulated acoustic emissions. It is clinically useful in the detection of cochlear hearing disorders.

**cochleostomy** \käk′lē·äs′təmē\ [*cochle(a)* + *o* + -STOMY] Labyrinthectomy performed via the round window by opening the cochlear duct and puncturing the lamina spiralis ossea.

***Cochliomyia*** \käk′lē·ōmī′yə\ [Gk *kochli(as)* a snail, screw + *myia* a fly] The genus of myiasis-producing flesh flies in the family Calliphoridae; screwworm flies. Also *Callitroga*. ***C. americana*** *COCHLIOMYIA HOMINIVORAX*. ***C. bezziana*** *CHRYSOMYIA BEZZIANA*. ***C. hominivorax*** The primary screwworm fly, an obligate myiasis-producing parasite of considerable economic importance in animals. It is also a cause of epidemics of human myiasis in some areas in South America and Central America. The gravid females are strongly attracted to wounds and sores of animals during the warmest part of the day and lay their eggs in or near such sores. The screwworm larvae hatch quickly, burrow into the wound, and feed on the tissue. The fly is also a cause of nasopharyngeal myiasis in man. Control of this insect has been greatly aided by use of broad-scale distribution of irradiated male flies. Also *Callitroga hominivorax*. ***C. macellaria*** The secondary screwworm fly, usually a saprozoic scavenger. Its larvae may produce a secondary myiasis by developing in necrotic tissues, sores, and wounds. Also *Compsomyia macellaria, Chrysomyia macellaria*.

**cochl. mag.** *cochleare magnum* (L, tablespoonful).

**cochl. med.** *cochleare medium* (L, dessertspoonful).

**cochl. parv.** *cochleare parvum* (L, teaspoonful).

**Cock** [Edward *Cock*, English surgeon, 1805–1892] See under TUMOR.

**cockade** \käkād′\ [irreg. from *cocarde* (from Old French *coquarde* a vain person, from *coq* a cock, of onomatopoeic origin, from the similarity of the cockade to the cock's comb) an insigne worn on the head] A lesion with concentric zones of different colors, as in erythema multiforme.

**Cockayne** [Edward Alfred *Cockayne*, English physician, 1880–1956] **1** See under SYNDROME. **2** Weber-Cockayne epidermolysis bullosa. See under EPIDERMOLYSIS BULLOSA SIMPLEX OF HANDS AND FEET.

**cockroach** [Spanish *cucaracha*, irreg. from *cuca* a caterpillar] An insect belonging to one of the families Blattidae, Blattellidae, or Blaberidae of the order Dictyoptera (included in Orthoptera in some systems). The species *Blattella germanica* (the German cockroach), *Blatta orientalis* (the oriental cockroach), and *Periplaneta americana* (the so-called American cockroach) are all abundant in many or most parts of the world. Though they are notorious household pests and can spread bacteria and other agents by direct mechanical means, they appear not to be involved in the biologic transmission of any human disease. Also *roach*.

**cocktail** A drink containing several ingredients or drugs. **Rivers c.** A mixture of dextrose, thiamin chloride, and insulin dissolved in an isotonic saline solution. It has been used as a treatment for alcohol detoxication, and is given intravenously. Also *Philadelphia cocktail*.

**coconscious** \kōkän′shəs\ *Obs.* PRECONSCIOUS.

**coconsciousness** \kōkän′shəsnis\ **1** The mental processes of the dissociated personality that exist side by side with the primary personality. Also *double consciousness*. **2** The edge or fringe of consciousness.

**coct.** *coctio* (L, boiling).

**coction** \käk′shən\ [L *coctio* (from *coctus*, past part. of *coquere* to cook) a cooking] The act of cooking, boiling, or altering a substance by applying of heat.

**COD** cause of death.

**code** [L *codex* (for *caudex*) the trunk of a tree, a wooden tablet covered with wax for writing, book, writing] **1** Any system of symbols, characters, and rules devised to transmit information, such as that used to write a program for a digital computer. **2** A system or set of rules establishing a standard, as for professional conduct. **degenerate c.** A code in which each bit of information is potentially encoded by any one of two or more different symbols. The genetic code is degenerate because most amino acids are specified by more than one codon. **genetic c.** The system that defines the correspondence between nucleotide sequences in DNA and amino acid sequences in proteins. Each three successive nucleotides constitute a codon, or triplet, which is the fundamental unit of the code. Of the $4^3$ (or 64) codons, 61 specify an amino acid and three specify termination of the polypeptide chain. Also *genetic code dictionary, genetic information, genetic alphabet*.

**codehydrogenase** Either NAD or NADP, which act as the immediate electron acceptors for many enzymes that catalyze the removal of hydrogen from substrates. *Obs.*

**codeine** [French *codéine,* from Gk *kōde(ia)* bulb, head, capsule (of poppy) + -INE] $C_{18}H_{21}NO_3 \cdot H_2O$. 7,8-Didehydro-4,5-epoxy-3-methoxy-17-methylmorphinan-6-ol. A narcotic analgesic present in opium and made by methylation of morphine. It is a white, crystallined powder, used in oral medications as an antitussive agent and analgesic. Also *monomethylmorphine.*

**codeine phosphate** $C_{18}H_{21}O_3NH_3PO_4 \cdot H_2O$. The phosphate salt of codeine. It is a commonly used form of codeine, and is used for the same purposes.

**codeine sulfate** $C_{18}H_{21}O_3N)_2H_2SO_4 \cdot 5H_2O$. The sulfate salt of codeine. It is a commonly used form of codeine in medicinal preparations because of its greater water solubility.

**codeine valerianate** $C_{18}H_{21}O_3NC_4H_9COOH$. A valeric acid salt of codeine. It is used as an antispasmodic and hypnotic medication.

**codex** [L, a book, account book, ledger] (*pl.* codices) An authorized formulary or pharmacopeia containing information about officially recognized and other medical substances.

**Codivilla** [Alessandro *Codivilla,* Italian surgeon, 1861–1912] See under OPERATION.

**Codman** [Ernest Amory *Codman,* U.S. surgeon, 1869–1940] **1** Codman's tumor. See under CHONDROBLASTOMA. **2** See under SIGN, TRIANGLE.

**codominant** \kōdäm′inənt\ Pertaining to a pair of dissimilar alleles that are both expressed when present together at a particular locus, the individual being a compound heterozygote at that locus. In humans, the alleles at the ABO blood group locus are codominant; an individual heterozygous for the A and B alleles expresses both and the blood group is AB.

**codon** \kō′dän\ [*cod(e)* + -ON] The smallest unit of genetic material that can specify an amino acid residue in the synthesis of a polypeptide chain. The codon consists of three adjacent nucleotides. **amber c.** The codon UAG, which normally signifies polypeptide chain termination. Organisms with mutations producing this codon in place of one coding for an amino acid are known as amber mutants. The mutations can be suppressed by the presence of a tRNA that binds to this codon and inserts an amino acid, usually serine, glutamine, or tyrosine. • The student who first noticed this mutation was named Bernstein, which is the German word for amber. **initiator c.** A codon that directs the initiation of translation of messenger ribonucleic acid at the ribosome. AUG, GUG, and GUA are the initiator codons. The initiator establishes the proper "frame" for reading the entire message. Also *initiation codon.* **nonsense c.** A codon that does not code for any amino acid, usually one produced by mutation and causing polypeptide chain termination. **ochre c.** The codon UAA, which normally signifies polypeptide chain termination. Organisms with mutations producing this codon in place of one coding for an amino acid are known as ochre mutants. The mutations can be suppressed by the presence of a tRNA that binds to this codon and inserts an amino acid. **stop c.** TERMINATION SEQUENCE. **termination c.** TERMINATION SEQUENCE. **umber c.** The codon UGA, which normally signifies polypeptide chain termination. Organisms with mutations producing this codon in place of one coding for an amino acid are known as umber mutants. The mutations can be suppressed by the presence of a tRNA that binds to this codon and inserts an amino acid.

**coe-** \sē-\ For words beginning *coe-,* see also under CE-.

**coefficient** \kō′efish′ənt\ [CO- + L *efficiens* (gen. *efficientis,* pres. part. of *efficere* to bring to pass, effect) effecting] A numerical quantity which multiplies a function or an algebraic expression. **activity c.** The factor by which the concentration of a substance in solution must be multiplied to obtain its activity, or its partial molar Gibbs energy. The activity coefficient of a solute in dilute solution approaches unity. **atomic attenuation c.** The linear attenuation coefficient divided by the number of atoms per unit volume, expressed by the unit $cm^2/atom$. Also *total atomic attenuation cross-section.* **attenuation c.** The fraction of a beam of radiation (or sound) which is removed from the beam as it passes through an absorber, per unit absorber thickness (unit, $cm^{-1}$) or per unit area density (unit, $cm^2/g$). **biologic c.** The energy used by a body at rest. It is expressed as a proportion of the normal value for energy consumption at rest. **c. of consanguinity** COEFFICIENT OF INBREEDING. **diffusion c.** A proportionality constant which expresses the rate of diffusion of a substance. It represents the rate of transfer of the substance per unit concentration gradient. The value of the coefficient depends on molecular weight and chemical structure of the diffusing molecule, as well as the chemical composition and temperature of the solvent. Also *diffusion constant.* **distribution c.** PARTITION COEFFICIENT. **c. of friction** The ratio between the force required to move two surfaces across one another and the normal force holding the two surfaces in contact with each other. **Hill c.** A parameter in the Hill equation. It is the slope of the curve of log $(y/[1-y])$ against log $s$, where $y$ is the fractional saturation of a substance, such as an enzyme, with a ligand, and $s$ is the concentration of free ligand. It is a measure of the cooperativity of the binding, being unity for independent binding sites. It cannot exceed the number of ligand molecules bound by one molecule of binding agent. Symbol: $n_H$ **homogeneity c.** In radiology, the ratio of the first half-value layer to the second half-value layer of a radiation beam. **c. of inbreeding** **1** The probability, usually denoted by $F$, that an individual will be homozygous at a given genetic locus because a single allele was passed through both parents from a common ancestor. For the offspring of a consanguineous mating, $F$ is equal to one half the coefficient of relationship, $r$, of the parents. **2** The probability in a population that any individual will be homozygous at a given genetic locus because the parents share a common ancestor. For defs. 1 and 2 also *coefficient of consanguinity.* **intensity transmission c.** The ratio of transmitted intensity to incident intensity for a beam of particles or a wave that has passed through a boundary or set of boundaries between different media. **isometric c. of lactic acid** The ratio of the isometric tension produced by a muscle before it fatigues to the milligrams of lactic acid produced. **isotonic c.** The smallest concentration of a salt solution in which red cell hemolysis does not occur. **c. of kinship** COEFFICIENT OF RELATIONSHIP. **linear absorption c.** The fraction of the energy in a collimated beam of radiation that is deposited in an absorber, per unit absorber thickness. It is not identical with the linear attenuation coefficient if radiation is scattered outside the absorber. **linear attenuation c.** The fraction of photons removed from a collimated beam of radiation, per centimeter of thickness of the absorber on which the beam impinges. **mass absorption c.** The linear absorption coefficient divided by the density of the absorber, expressed as $cm^2/g$. **mass attenuation c.** The linear attenuation coefficient divided by the density of the absorber, expressed by the unit $cm^2/g$. Symbol: $\mu/P$ **Ostwald solubility c.** The number of milliliters of gas dissolved in a milliliter of liquid under conditions of one atmosphere partial pressure of the gas at the ambient temperature of the experiment. **partition c.** The ratio between concentrations of a substance in two phases at equilibrium. Also *distribution coefficient.* **phenol c.** The ratio of the disinfecting power of other phenolic compounds to that of phenol, under standard conditions. It is not readily applicable to other classes of disinfectants, whose action varies with a different power of the concentration. **reflection c.** The ratio of reflected amplitude or intensity to incident amplitude or intensity of a wave or beam of particles affected by a boundary between two media. **c. of relationship** 1 The probability, *r,* that two persons have in common a gene descended from the same ancestor. For the offspring of a consanguineous mating, the coefficient of inbreeding *F,* is one half the coefficient of relationship of the parents. 2 In two related persons, the proportion of all genes that are identical by descent. For defs. 1 and 2 also *coefficient of kinship.* **sedimentation c.** The velocity at which a particle, e.g. a protein molecule, sediments per unit acceleration of the centrifugal field to which it is subjected. It is often expressed in Svedberg units. Also *Svedberg coefficient, sedimentation constant.* Symbol: *s* **selection c.** A quantitative expression of the reproductive fitness of one genotype relative to another. In a stable population, the coefficient expresses the selective disadvantage of a mutant phenotype relative to the optimum individuals. The values of the coefficient range from one, for a genetic lethal, to zero, for a fitness equivalent to the optimal (usually the wild-type) phenotype. **Svedberg c.** SEDIMENTATION COEFFICIENT. **temperature c.** The factor by which the rate of a chemical reaction increases when the temperature rises by 10°C. It is, for reactions of conveniently measurable rates, typically about 2. High values are typical of protein denaturation reactions. **c. of utilization of oxygen** That portion of blood that gives up its oxygen as it passes through a tissue. **c. of variation** In statistics, the ratio of the standard deviation to the mean. It is an index of relative variation, and as such it allows comparisons between the degrees of dispersion of two or more series.

**coel-** \sēl-\ COELO-. • For words beginning *coel-,* see also under CEL-.

**coelarium** \sēler′ē·əm\ MESOTHELIUM.

**-coele** \-sēl\ [Gk *koilon* a hollow, cavity] A combining form meaning a hollow space, cavity. Also *-cele, -coel.*

**Coelenterata** \sēlen′terā′tə\ A phylum of invertebrates built around a body cavity, and including the hydras, corals, and jellyfish.

**coelenterate** \sēlen′terāt\ 1 Pertaining to the phylum Coelenterata. 2 A member of the phylum Coelenterata.

**coeliac** \sē′lē·ak\ CELIAC.

**coelio-** \sē′lyō-\ CELIO-.

**coeliocyesis** \-sī·ē′sis\ [COELIO- + Gk *kyēsis* pregnancy] ABDOMINAL PREGNANCY.

**coeliotomy** \sē′lē·ät′əmē\ *Brit.* CELIOTOMY.

**coelo-** \sē′lō-\ [Gk *koilos* hollow, *koilon* a body cavity] A combining form meaning hollow or cavity. Also *coel-, cel-, celo-.*

**coelom** \sē′ləm\ [Gk *koilōma* (from *koilos* hollow) a cavity] The cavity that develops in the embryo between the split layers of the lateral mesoderm. At first it is both extraembryonic and intraembryonic. The principal body cavities (pericardial, pleural, and peritoneal) develop from the intraembryonic portion, and are separated in higher vertebrates by the secondary development of the diaphragm. Also *coelomic cavity, celom.* **abdominal c.** The inferior part of the coelom in the embryo which gives rise to the peritoneal cavity. It is situated between the mesodermal somatopleure (lining the deep face of the abdominal wall) and the splanchnopleure (covering the viscera). These two plates are linked by a layer of coelomic epithelium, the future peritoneum. The abdominal coelom initially extends into the umbilical cord (as an umbilical hernia), but this regresses by about the tenth week when the midgut loop, having completed its rotation, returns to the abdominal cavity. **extraembryonic c.** The part of the coelom hollowed out in the mesoderm situated outside the embryo. The coelom extends into both the intraembryonic mesoderm, and the extraembryonic mesoderm, and the two parts are in continuity for a while. The extraembryonic coelom, at an earlier stage well-developed, shrinks slowly, proportional to the growth of the amnion. Also *exocoelom.*

**coelomic** \sēläm′ik\ Of or relating to the coelom. Also *celomic.*

**coeloscope** \sē′lōskōp\ CELOSCOPE.

**coelothel** \sē′lōthel\ MESOTHELIUM.

**coelothelium** \-thē′lē·əm\ MESOTHELIUM.

**coelozoic** \-zō′ik\ [COELO- + *zo(o)-* + -IC] Inhabiting body cavities: said especially of certain extracellular protozoan parasites. Also *celozoic.*

**coeno-** \sē′nō-\ CENO-.[2]

**coenobium** \sēnō′bē·əm\ [Late L, from Late Gk *koinobion,* noun from neut. sing. of Gk *koinobios* (from *koino(s)* shared in common + *bios* life, way of life) living in community] (*pl.* coenobia) A colony of independent organisms, cells, or units combined within a common membrane or enveloping structure. Also *cenobium.*

**coenurosis** \sēnyoorō′sis\ [*Coenur(us)* + -OSIS] A disease mainly of sheep and cattle and sometimes other herbivores, rarely, of man, caused by the larval encysted tapeworms (coenuri) of *Multiceps multiceps* and *M. serialis,* small taenioid tapeworms. The adult tapeworms live in large numbers, generally without pathology, in the small intestine of dogs and other canids. Also *coenuriasis, cenuriasis, cenurosis.*

***Coenurus*** \sēnyoo′rəs\ [*coen(o)-* + New L *-urus,* combining form from Gk *oura* tail] A former genus that included what are now recognized as the larval forms of tapeworms of the genus *Multiceps.* Also *Cenurus.*

**coenurus** \sēnyoo′rəs\ (*pl.* coenuri) The larval form of some taeniid tapeworms in the genus *Multiceps* in which a bladder containing several developing invaginated scoleces is formed. There are no free-floating daughter cyst colonies within the bladder as in hydatid cysts, and there are fewer scoleces. Also *cenurus.*

**coenzyme** \kō·en′zīm\ An organic substance of relatively low molecular mass (usually less than 1 kDa) required for an enzymatic reaction. It often proves to be a substrate for one enzyme which converts it into a form that is reconverted to the first by a second enzyme. It thus links two reactions, usually by transferring a group from one substance to another. **c. I** *Obs.* NICOTINAMIDE ADENINE DINUCLEOTIDE. **c. II** *Obs.* NICOTINAMIDE ADENINE DINUCLEOTIDE PHOSPHATE. **c. A** The coenzyme of acetylation, allowing sulfonamides to be acetylated by carrying acetyl and many other acyl groups as thioesters on its —SH group. Its molecule consists of adenosine 3′,5′-bisphosphate, with the 5′-phosphate joined in diphosphate linkage with that of pantetheine 4′-phosphate. Abbr. CoA **nucleotide c.** A coenzyme that is, in its chemical nature, a nucleotide. NAD and NADP are important nucleotide coenzymes. **c. Q** UBIQUINONE. **c. R** *Outmoded* BIOTIN.

**coeur** \kœr\ [French, heart] **c. en sabot** The appearance of the heart in the posteroanterior radiologic view in some cases of the tetralogy of Fallot, in which the apex is blunted and uplifted suggesting the toe of a wooden shoe (sabot). Also *sabot heart, wooden shoe heart.*

**coexcitation** \kō′eksitā′shən\ Excitation of more than one site at the same time; stimulation of more than one type of sensory receptor simultaneously.

**cofactor** \kō′fak′tər\ [CO- + FACTOR] A heat-stable, nonprotein substance necessary for optimal activity of some enzymes. It may be an inorganic ion or a more complex organic material. **c. V** FACTOR V. **platelet c. I** FACTOR VIII. **platelet c. II** FACTOR IX. **ristocetin c.** FACTOR VIIIR:AG.

**Coffey** [Robert Calvin *Coffey*, U.S. surgeon, 1869–1933] See under SUSPENSION, TECHNIQUE.

**Cogan** [David Glendenning *Cogan*, U.S. physician, born 1908] Cogan's disease. See under SYNDROME.

**cognition** \kägnish′ən\ [L *cognitio* (from *cognitus*, past part. of *cognoscere* to look at, learn, know) an examining, knowledge of a thing] The intellectual functions or ways of knowing and thinking, including the processes of perceiving, imagining, remembering, reasoning, and judging. Adj. cognitive.

**cognitive** \käg′nitiv\ Of or characteristic of cognition.

**cohesion** \kōhē′zhən\ [French *cohésion* (from L *cohaesus*, past part. of *cohaerere* to stick, hold fast together) cohesion] The sticking together of like objects to form a whole either by mutual attraction, as of molecules in a liquid, or by collision of growing tissues, as in the union of similar parts or organs in a plant.

**cohesive** \kōhē′siv\ **1** Marked by cohesion; sticking together. **2** In dentistry, tending to adhere and form a solid mass: said of pure gold used as a restorative material.

**Cohn** [Ferdinand Julius *Cohn*, German bacteriologist, 1828–1898] See under SOLUTION.

**Cohnheim** [Julius Friedrich *Cohnheim*, German pathologist, 1839–1884] **1** Cohnheim's areas. See under AREA. **2** Cohnheim's artery. See under END ARTERY. **3** Cohnheim's fields. See under FIELD.

**cohort** \kō′hôrt\ [L *cohors*, gen. *cohortis*, a troop, throng] In demography and epidemiology, a group of persons having experienced an event in common during the same time period. The concept is applied particularly in long-term studies.

**coil** A structure consisting of a series of loops or spirals. **choke c.** A number of turns of wire formed into a coil for providing electrical inductance. It passes direct current but limits or chokes off high-frequency alternating current. **chromosome c.** The spiral or helical coil formed by two or more chromonemata during mitosis or meiosis. The coiling transforms the functional form of the chromosome into the transport form. **induction c.** A spiral of insulated wire wound about an iron core. Sending a pulsating current through the coil induces a pulsating high voltage in a second coil wound around the first. Also *spark coil.* **paranemic c.** A chromosome coil in which the chromonemata are freely separable subunits. **plectonemic c.** A chromosome coil in which the chromosomal threads are intertwined and are inseparable. **random c.** The conformation of a polymeric molecule in which those angles of rotation between subunits that are not rigid are randomly distributed. Proteins approach such a conformation in solutions of those denaturing agents that solubilize them, such as urea. **relational c.** An arrangement of strands (chromatids or chromosomes) in which one is twisted about another, as in a rope. The strands are interlocked so that they can only be separated by uncoiling. Relational coiling is characteristic of sister chromatids during mitosis and paired homologous chromosomes during prophase of meiosis. **resistance c.** A coil of standardized electrical resistance (a resistor) used in electrical measuring circuits. **spark c.** INDUCTION COIL. **standard c.** A helical chromatin structure found in mitotic chromosomes, that appears similar to the coil of the meiotic chromosomes.

**coin-counting** PILL-ROLLING TREMOR.

**coindication** \kō′indikā′shən\ A second indication for therapeutic intervention along with the primary indication.

**coinfection** \kō′infek′shən\ An infection occurring simultaneously or jointly with another infection in the same host.

**coino-** \koi′nō-, sē′nō-\ CENO-[2].

**coinosite** \koi′nōsīt\ CENOSITE.

**coisogenic** \kō′īsōjen′ik\ Of or relating to congenic strains whose difference is limited to one locus. See also CONGENIC.

**Coiter** [Volcher *Coiter*, Dutch anatomist active in Italy, 1534–1600] See under MUSCLE.

**coition** \kō·ish′ən\ COITUS.

**coitus** \kō′itəs\ [L (past part. of *coire* to come together), coitus] Sexual union between male and female by insertion of the penis into the vagina. Also *sexual intercourse, pareunia, congressus, copulation, coition, sexual congress* (older term). Adj. coital. **c. interruptus** Withdrawal of the penis from the vagina before ejaculation as a method of contraception. Also *onanism.* **c. reservatus** Sexual intercourse in which the male delays orgasm until the female reaches climax, or indefinitely as a form of coitus interruptus.

**col** \kôl, käl\ [French (from L *collum* the neck, throat) a collar, depressed portion of a mountain ridge] The margin of interdental gingiva that fills the space below and partly around the contact area between the two spheroidal surfaces of adjacent teeth. Consequently there are lingual and buccal peaks of gingiva connected by the col, which resembles the sagging ridge of a ridge tent.

**col-** \käl-, kōl-, kəl-\ COM-.

**colat.** *colatus* (L, strained)

**colcemide** \kōl′səmīd\ A derivative of colchicine that inhibits formation of the mitotic spindle by reducing the size of the tubulin pool available for assembly.

**colchicine** \käl′chisin\ $C_{22}H_{25}NO_6$. A polycyclic alkaloid that blocks mitosis in metaphase by binding to spindle proteins and preventing separation of centromeres. It prevents the polymerization of tubulin, thus interfering with the formation of microtubules in the cytoplasm of a cell. It is used to treat gout and Hodgkin's disease, familial Mediterranean fever, and amyloidosis, and in cytogenetics to prepare metaphase karyotypes, in experimental genetics to synchronize cell cycles, and in horticulture to induce polyploidy. It is extremely poisonous.

**cold** / **common c.** A syndrome due to any one of a number of viruses, such as rhinoviruses, coronaviruses, parainfluenza viruses, or respiratory syncytial viruses. It is characterized by an acute, contagious upper respiratory tract infection, with rhinitis, pharyngitis, cough, and general indisposition. Also *acute catarrhal rhinitis, acute rhinitis.*

**cold-blooded** POIKILOTHERMIC.

**coldsore** COLD SORE.

**Cole** [Harold Newton *Cole*, U.S. dermatologist, 1884–1966] Zinser-Cole-Engman syndrome. See under DYSKERATOSIS CONGENITA.

**Cole** [Lewis Gregory *Cole*, U.S. radiologist, 1874–1954] See under SIGN.

**cole-** \käl′ə-\ COLEO-.

**colectomy** \kälek′təmē\ [*col(on)* + -ECTOMY] A resection of all or part of the large intestine. Also *laparocolectomy.*

**coleo-** \käl′ē·ō-\ [Gk *koleos* or *koleon* sheath] A combining form meaning sheath or vagina. Also *cole-*.

**coleocystitis** \-sistī′tis\ [COLEO- + CYSTITIS] An inflammatory condition of the vagina and the urinary bladder.

**Coleoptera** \käl′ē·äp′tərə\ [New L, neut. pl. of Gk *koleopteros* sheath-winged, from *koleo(s)*, also *koleo(n)* a sheath + *ptera* wings] The beetles, the largest order of insects, consisting of over 300 000 species. The order is characterized by horny elytra or wing covers, enclosing and protecting delicate folded membranous wings beneath them. This vast assemblage includes insects of a great range of habits and adaptations. Included are highly beneficial insects such as the ladybug beetles, and the destructive weevil beetles. Though some are mechanical transmitters of pathogens, few are biological vectors of direct medical importance. See also SCARABIASIS.

**colestipol hydrochloride** A basic anion-exchange resin composed of copolymers of diethylenetriamine and 1-chloro-2,3-epoxypropane hydrochloride. The product is essentially insoluble and given orally in the treatment of hypercholesterolemia. Its actions are like those of cholestyramine.

**colet.** *coletur* (L, let it be strained).

**colibacillosis** \kō′lēbas′ilō′sis\ Infection with *Escherichia coli*.

**colic** \(1) kō′lik; (2) käl′ik\ [Med L *colica (passio)* (from *colicus*, from Gk *kōlikos*, properly *kolikos*, pertaining to or affected with colic; see COLON) the colic "passion"] **1** Relating to or associated with the colon: used primarily in anatomic terms. **2** Any of various conditions characterized by abdominal pain, especially paroxysmal pain occurring in a crescendo-decrescendo pattern dependent upon visceral smooth-muscle peristalsis. Also *colica*. **appendicular c.** Colic which originates in the vermiform appendix and is precipitated by occlusion of the appendiceal lumen and consequent inflammation. Also *appendiceal colic, vermicular colic*. **biliary c.** Paroxysms of pain in the right hypochondrium which may radiate to the back and right shoulder, associated with nausea and sometimes vomiting, due to the passage of gallstones or other objects along the biliary tract. Also *hepatic colic, gallstone colic*. **bilious c.** Abdominal pain with a prominent component of emesis. **cystic c.** Acute abdominal pain originating in the bladder. **endemic c.** Severe abdominal pain, accompanied by diarrhea which occurs especially frequently in some parts of the tropics. Multiple pathogens are involved with marked geographic variations. **flatulent c.** Abdominal pain due to distention of the stomach or intestines with gas or air. **gallstone c.** BILIARY COLIC. **hepatic c.** BILIARY COLIC. **kidney c.** RENAL COLIC. **lead c.** Acute abdominal pain due to lead poisoning. This condition, seen among cider drinkers in Devonshire, England and wine drinkers in Poitou, France in the seventeenth century, was due to the consumption of the beverages prepared in vats or vessels contaminated with lead. **menstrual c.** DYSMENORRHEA. **milk c.** The colic occurring in lactose intolerance. **ovarian c.** Pain in the ovary, as in ovulation. **painters' c.** Lead colic from exposure to lead in paint. **pancreatic c.** Abdominal pain due to obstruction of the pancreatic ductal system. **renal c.** Paroxysmal pain caused by acute obstruction of the renal pelvis or ureter, usually induced by migration of a renal calculus or blood clot and usually lasting one hour or more. The pain may be localized in the lumbar region or radiate along the course of the ureter through the flank, hypogastrium, iliac fossa, and groin, and sometimes along the internal border of the thigh. It may be accompanied by bladder tenesmus and various reflex phenomena, such as nausea, vomiting, and even intestinal obstruction. Certain diseases, such as renal tumor, hydronephrosis, or acute pyelonephritis may cause pains that are similar to those of renal colic. Also *kidney colic*. **salivary c.** Colicky pain in the parotid or submandibular region, usually signaling the presence of a calculus obstructing a salivary duct. **stercoral c.** Abdominal pain due to an excessive accumulation of feces in the intestine. **tubal c.** Cramplike pain in an oviduct. **ureteral c.** Abdominal pain due to blockage of the ureter. **uterine c.** Cramplike pain in the uterus. **vermicular c.** APPENDICULAR COLIC. **verminous c.** Colic caused by intestinal worms. Also *worm colic*.

**colica** \käl′ikə\ [L, colic] *Seldom used* COLIC. **c. scortorum** DYSMENORRHEA.

**colicin** \käl′isin\ A protein released by some strains of *Escherichia coli* that is lethal to certain other strains. Various colicins, designated by capital letters, such as A, E3, or K, act as nucleases, membrane-damaging agents, etc. Colicins and colicinogens were the first recognized members of the broader class of bacteriocins and bacteriocinogens.

**colicinogen** \käl′isin′əjən\ A plasmid that codes for production of a colicin.

**colicinogenic** \käl′isin′əjen′ik\ Carrying a colicinogen: said of bacteria.

**colicky** \käl′ikē\ **1** Characteristic of or like colic. **2** Afflicted with colic.

**colicoplegia** \käl′ikōplē′jə\ [COLIC + *o* + -PLEGIA ] Colic and paralysis from lead poisoning.

**colicystitis** \käl′isistī′tis\ Cystitis caused by *Escherichia coli*.

**coliform** \käl′ifôrm\ [*(Escherichia) coli* + -FORM] **1** Designating Gram-negative, lactose-fermenting enteric bacilli. **2** In water bacteriology, designating organisms that are oxidase-negative and able to form acid and gas on a bile-salts medium.

**colinearity** \kōlin′ē·ar′itē\ The concept that the amino acid sequence of a peptide corresponds exactly to the sequence of the codons of the appropriate coding sequence (exon or cistron) of the gene specifying the peptide.

**coliphage** \käl′ifāj\ A bacteriophage whose host is *Escherichia coli*.

**coliplication** \kō′liplikā′shən\ COLOPLICATION.

**colipuncture** \kō′lipungk′chər\ [*col(on)* + *i* + PUNCTURE] COLOCENTESIS.

**colisepsis** \kō′lisep′sis\ [*(Escherichia) coli* + SEPSIS] An infection with *Escherichia coli* which is often severe and associated with bloodstream invasion.

**colistin** A cyclopolypeptide antibiotic produced by the soil bacterium *Bacillus (Aerobacillus) colistinus*. It is a broad-spectrum antibiotic, particularly effective against Gram-negative bacteria.

**colistin sulfomethate sodium** A form of colistin suitable for parenteral administration. It can be used topically, given in an aerosol for respiratory infections, or used for eye infections by subconjunctival injection. Also *sodium colistimethate*.

**colitides** \kōlit′idēz\ Plural of COLITIS.

**colitis** \kōlī′tis\ [*col(on)* + -ITIS] Inflammation of the colon. **amebic c.** Colonic inflammation caused by amebic infection; amebic dysentery. **balantidial c.** Inflammation of the colon caused by infection with *Balantidium coli*. **c. cystica profunda** A polypoid or intramural mass of the colon or rectum, composed of benign mucous cysts and associated with chronic proctitis. This is a non-neoplastic condition resulting from the continued secretion of mucous glands trapped in the submucosa and rarely deeper in the wall. Normal mucus-secreting cells find their way into the bowel wall along healing ulcerations and fissures. This benign condition must not be mistaken for an invasive mucin-producing adenocarcinoma. **c. cystica superficialis** Cystic transformation of the colonic mucosa seen occasionally in children dying from leukemia, tropical sprue and, especially, pellagra. **granulomatous c.** Granulomatous inflammation of the colon, as may be seen in Crohn's disease. **ischemic c.** Inflammation of the colon due to inadequacy of its blood supply, usually seen in the elderly in the absence of a demonstrable arterial occlusion. It is characterized clinically by abdominal pain and rectal bleeding, and may result in stricture. **mucous c.** *Outmoded* IRRITABLE BOWEL SYNDROME. **pseudomembranous c.** A form of pseudomembranous inflammation of the colon seen following antibiotic therapy, usually in postoperative patients. Although controversy remains regarding its etiology and pathogenesis, it is possible that broad-spectrum antibiotics allow the growth of clostridial organisms, which in turn release a toxin that causes the colonic lesion. This is characterized by patchy, superficial ulceration of the mucosa and a covering green yellow exudate composed of fibrin, neutrophils, and mucus. The antibiotics most commonly implicated are clindamycin and lincomycin, although it has been observed with many others. Also *membranous diarrhea, pseudomembranous enteritis, pseudomembranous enterocolitis.* **regional c.** Crohn's disease affecting the colon. Also *segmental colitis.* **spastic c.** *Outmoded* IRRITABLE BOWEL SYNDROME. **transmural c.** Colitis affecting all layers of the intestinal wall, as in Crohn's disease of the colon. **ulcerative c.** A chronic inflammatory disease of the colon, or of the colon and rectum, characterized clinically by diarrhea often with blood and mucus and crampy abdominal pain. Onset is often in the second or third decade but may be at any age, with a chronic relapsing and remitting course, or rarely a fulminant course resulting in toxic megacolon. Also *colitis ulcerativa* (seldom used). **uremic c.** Colitis seen in renal failure, often manifest clinically as colonic bleeding. Increased ammonia within the colon is the postulated cause.

**colitose** \käl′itōs\ 3,6-Dideoxy-L-galactose. A component of O antigen 35 in group O salmonellae. It was first isolated from *Escherichia coli.*

**colitoxemia** \kō′lētäksē′mē·ə\ [*(Escherichia) coli* + TOXEMIA] A toxic condition produced by the presence in the blood of *Escherichia coli* or its by-products.

**colla** \käl′ə\ Plural of COLLUM.

**collagen** \käl′əjən\ [Gk *kolla* glue + -GEN] An abundant protein of connective tissue that forms fibrils of great tensile strength. It has a peculiar helical structure, determined by its often repeated -Gly-Pro-Xaa- tripeptide sequence. Three polypeptide chains, each of 1000 residues, are twined to form a rod-shaped molecule, which packs regularly in a staggered fashion. Covalent cross-linking can strengthen the structure. It is secreted from the cell as a procollagen, after which extracellular enzymes cleave a piece from both the amino and carboxyl ends of the molecule to form collagen.

**collagenase** Any proteinase that catalyzes the hydrolysis of collagen. Some collagenases, such as *Clostridium histolyticum* collagenase (EC 3.4.24.3), are metalloproteinases and some, such as *Hypoderma* collegenase (EC 3.4.21.49) are serine proteinases.

**collagenation** \käl′əjenā′shən\ The formation of collagen within growing or healing tissue.

**collagenic** \käl′əjen′ik\ COLLAGENOUS.

**collagenoblast** \kälaj′ənōblast′\ A maturing fibroblast capable of producing collagen.

**collagenocyte** \kälaj′ənōsīt′\ A mature cell capable of producing collagen.

**collagenogenic** \kälaj′ənōjen′ik\ COLLAGENOUS.

**collagenolysis** \kälaj′ənäl′isis\ The degradation of collagen.

**collagenolytic** \kälaj′ənōlit′ik\ Capable of undergoing or producing collagenolysis.

**collagenoma** \kälaj′ənō′mə\ A tumorlike collection of mature collagen in the skin, generally arranged in bundles. It can occur in patients with tuberous sclerosis and is considered to be hamartomatous in nature. **familial cutaneous c.** DISSEMINATED LENTICULAR DERMATOFIBROSIS.

**collagenosis** \kälaj′ənō′sis\ COLLAGEN DISEASE. **reactive perforating c.** The formation of a papule with a central plug consisting of necrobiotic collagen. The papule appears as a response of the skin to significant trauma and is believed to be genetically induced.

**collagenous** \kälaj′ənəs\ Pertaining to or characterized by the production of collagen. Also *collagenogenic, collagenic.*

**collapse** [L *collaps(us),* past part. of *collabi* to fall together, fall in or down] **1** A state of prostration from physical or psychological cause, often characterized by cardiovascular collapse or shock. **2** A falling in of the walls of a structure or organ. **alveolar c.** The absence of air in the alveolar space, as in atelectasis caused by bronchial obstruction, or by compression as in pneumothorax. **cardiovascular c.** Failure of blood circulation due either to failure of the heart to pump effectively or of the arterioles to maintain tone, or to loss of blood volume, or a combination. Also *circulatory collapse.* **heat c.** Circulatory failure caused by overexposure to heat. See also HEAT EXHAUSTION. **c. of the lung** Loss of volume of the lung due to a reduced amount of air in the alveoli of one or more lobes or segments. **massive c.** Collapse of a whole lung or a large part of a lung.

**collar** [French *collier* (from L *collum,* also *collus* neck, throat) necklace] A band surrounding a neck. **abrasion c.** The abrasion which partially or completely surrounds the skin margin of a gunshot entrance wound. It is produced by the projectile or bullet as it stretches the skin surface when it perforates the skin. In appearance, it resembles reddish brown parchment and is concentric or eccentric depending upon the angle at which the projectile strikes the skin. Also *marginal abrasion, rim of abrasion.* **Biett's c.** The ring of scales developing around the papular lesion of secondary syphilis. Also *collarette of Biett.* **Casal's c.** CASAL'S NECKLACE **four-poster c.** A cervical brace with four adjustable uprights, used to reduce motion of the head and neck. **c. of pearls** VENEREAL COLLAR. **perichondral bony c.** The periosteal bony envelope which in the young embryo develops about the cartilaginous shaft of long bones. **periosteal bone c.** Thick periosteum that envelops immature long bones. **renal c.** In an embryo, a venous ring around the aorta below the origin of the superior mesenteric artery, formed by anastomotic channels between the subcardinals, supracardinals, azygous venous lines, and the subcentral veins. **venereal c.** Syphilitic leukoderma of the neck and shoulders. It is virtually pathognomonic of late syphilis. Also *collar of pearls, leukoderma colli,.*

**collar-bone** CLAVICULA.

**collarette** \käl′eret′\ [French *collerette* ruff] **1** A small circular or crescentic structure suggestive of a collar or ruff. **2** IRIS COLLARETTE. **c. of Biett** BIETT'S COLLAR. **iris c.** The zigzag line 1.5 mm from the pupillary margin on the anterior surface of the iris that separates the annulus iridis major from the annulus iridis minor. It marks the line of attachment of the pupillary membrane in the fetus. Also *iris frill, collarette.*

**collastin** \kōlas′tin\ Degenerate collagenous tissue.

**collateral** \kōlat′ərəl\ [Med L *collateral(is)* (from L *col-* with + *latus,* gen. *lateris,* the side + *-alis* -AL) parallel, side by side] **1** Being or situated to the side. **2** Subordinate; secondary. **3** Related or originating by divergence from a common source. **4** A parallel or anastomosing branch, as of a vessel; an alternate channel of circulation or communication. **5** In neuroanatomy, a side branch of an axon.

**Colles** [Abraham *Colles,* Irish surgeon, 1773–1843] **1** See under MOTHER, FRACTURE, LAW. **2** Colles fascia. See under MEMBRANOUS LAYER OF THE PERINEUM. **3** Reverse Colles fracture. See under FRACTURE. **4** Triangular ligament of Colles. See under MEMBRANA PERINEI. **5** Colles ligament. See under LIGAMENTUM REFLEXUM. **6** Colles space. See under SPATIUM PERINEI SUPERFICIALE.

**Collet** [Frederic Justin *Collet,* French laryngologist, born 1870] Collet syndrome. See under COLLET-SICARD SYNDROME.

**colliculectomy** \kōlik′yəlek′təmē\ [*collicul(us) (seminalis)* + -ECTOMY] Surgical removal of the colliculus seminalis.

**colliculi** \kōlik′yəli\ Plural of COLLICULUS.

**colliculitis** \kōlik′yəlī′tis\ [*collicul(us) (seminalis)* + -ITIS] Inflammation involving the colliculus seminalis.

**colliculus** \kōlik′yələs\ [L (dim. of *collis* a hill), a mound] A small conical mound or elevation. **c. abducentis** COLLICULUS FACIALIS. **c. of arytenoid cartilage** COLLICULUS CARTILAGINIS ARYTENOIDEAE. **c. cartilaginis arytenoideae** [NA] A small pointed eminence on the anterior margin and anterolateral surface overhanging the triangular pit of the arytenoid cartilage. Also *colliculus of arytenoid cartilage.* **c. facialis** [NA] A rounded swelling located on the medial eminence of the fourth ventricle at the midpontine level. It corresponds to the nucleus of the abducens nerve, and the internal genu of the facial nerve looping around the nucleus. Also *facial colliculus, facial hillock, facial eminence, eminentia facialis, eminentia abducentis, colliculus abducentis.* **c. inferior** [NA] The caudal elevation of the mesencephalic roof, containing a large auditory nucleus and its connections. Also *inferior colliculus.* **c. seminalis** [NA] An oval elevation on the urethral crest, about two-thirds down the prostatic urethra. The slitlike opening of the prostatic utricle is located on it in the median line. Also *seminal colliculus, verumontanum, seminal crest, seminal hillock, caput gallinaginis* (outmoded), *colliculus urethralis* (outmoded). **c. superior laminae quadrigeminae** [NA] Either of a pair of spherical elevations on the cranial part of the midbrain tectum. It receives fibers from the optic tract by way of the brachium colliculi superioris, and serves as a center for visual reflexes. Also *superior colliculus.* **c. urethralis** *Outmoded* COLLICULUS SEMINALIS.

**Collier** [James Stansfield *Collier,* English neurologist, 1870–1935] See under TRACT.

**colligative** \käl′igā′tiv\ Denoting any property of a solution that depends on the total molar concentration of solute particles, irrespective of their nature. Examples are the depression of freezing point and the osmotic pressure.

**collimation** \käl′imā′shən\ In radiology, the process of restricting the size of the radiation beam by means of lead or other radiation-absorbing diaphragms.

**collimator** \käl′imā′tər\ [New L *collimat(us),* past part. of *collimare,* variant of L *colineare* to aim or level something at + New L *-or* -OR] An apparatus fastened to an x-ray tube to limit the size of the x-ray beam to the field of interest. It may be a fixed cone or variable lead shutters, usually including a light beam to define the field. Also *localizer.*

**collinear** \kōlin′ē·ər\ [COL- + LINEAR] Centered along the same line: used of light or radiation beams.

**Collins** See under TREACHER COLLINS.

**colliotomy** \käl′ē·ät′əmē\ [Gk *koll(a)* glue + *i* + *o* + -TOMY] ADHESIOTOMY.

**Collip** [James Bertram *Collip,* Canadian biochemist, 1892–1965] Clark-Collip method. See under METHOD.

**collision** [L *collisio* (from *collisus,* past part. of *collidere* to strike one thing against another, from COL- + L *laedere* to strike against) a striking together] **1** Intrauterine contact between twins such that engagement of either one is prevented. *Older term.* **2** The interaction between two molecules (including atoms) or atomic or subatomic particles, as a photon and electron, as if the two were actually coming into contact. **elastic c.** A collision in which there is no transformation between kinetic energy and internal (excitation) energy of one or both of the colliding systems. **scattering c.** A collision in which an incident photon or other particle is deflected from its original path. Such a collision may be either inelastic or elastic. Also *scattering event.*

**collodion** \kəlō′dē·än\ [Gk *kollōdēs* gluelike] A preparation of nitrocellulose from which membranes for dialysis can be made. **hemostatic c.** STYPTIC COLLODION. **salicylic acid c.** A solution of 10 g of salicylic acid per 100 ml of flexible collodion. It is used to remove warts and corns. **simple c.** Nitrocellulose dissolved in a solution of alcohol and ether. **styptic c.** Collodion containing sufficient tannic acid to confer styptic properties to the preparation. Also *hemostatic collodion.*

**colloid** \käl′oid\ [Gk *koll(a)* glue + -OID] A substance that is in a state between that of a solution and an emulsion, where particles are suspended in a fluid medium. The suspended particles are larger than the crystalloid molecules that form solutions, but are not large enough to settle out under the influence of gravity. The colloidal particles have a diameter between 1 and 100 nm and are suspended in a dispersion medium. The particles are referred to as the disperse, internal, or discontinuous phase while the medium is the dispersion medium or the external or continuous phase. Protein solutions have many of the properties of colloids. **amyl c.** A preparation consisting of amyl hydride, ethanol, veratrine, aconitine and collodion. It is used as a coating to relieve pain. Also *anodyne colloid.* **thyroid c.** The colloid occurring within the thyroid follicles, consisting mainly of thyroglobulin.

**colloidal-S** A preparation of iron oxide formerly used parenterally in the treatment of infections.

**colloidopexy** \käloi′dōpek′sē\ The process of cellular inclusion of foreign colloidal material. Also *colloidopexia.*

**colloma** \kälō′mə\ [Gk *koll(a)* glue + -OMA] *Obs.* MUCINOUS CARCINOMA.

**collum** \käl′əm\ [L, the neck, throat] **1** The region of the body joining the head to the trunk; the neck or cervix. **2** Any necklike part of a structure or organ. Also *neck, trachelos.* **c. anatomicum humeri** [NA] A slight constriction or groove just distal to the margin of the head of the humerus and most obvious superiorly where it separates the articular surface from the tubercles. Its circumference provides attachment for the capsule of the shoulder joint. Also *anatomical neck of humerus, true neck of humerus, neck of humerus.* **c. chirurgicum humeri** [NA] The tapered junction of the proximal extremity and the shaft of the humerus, just distal to the tubercles, where fractures commonly occur and may involve the closely related axillary nerve and posterior circumflex humeral artery. Also *surgical* *neck of humerus.* **c. costae** [NA] The portion at the posterior end of a rib between its head and the tubercle located at the junction with the shaft. It is flattened dorsoventrally, and lies in front of the transverse process of the corresponding vertebra. Also *neck of rib.* **c. distortum** TORTICOLLIS. **c. femoris** COLLUM OSSIS FEMORIS. **c. folliculi pili** NECK OF HAIR FOLLICLE. **c. glandis penis** [NA] A curved, grooved constriction proximal to the corona glandis at the base of the glans penis. Also *neck of glans penis, neck of penis.* **c. humeri** The neck of the humerus, either collum anatomicum humeri or collum chirurgicum humeri. **c. mallei** [NA] The constriction between the rounded head of the malleus and the enlarged area where the manubrium and the processes are attached. The anterior ligament of the malleus is attached to it. Also *neck of malleus.* **c. mandibulae** [NA] The anteroposteriorly flattened upper end of the condylar process of the mandible just below its expanded ovoid head. Anteriorly it has a depression for the insertion of the lateral pterygoid muscle, while medially it is related to the auriculotemporal nerve and the maxillary artery. Also *neck of condylar process of mandible, neck of mandible, collum processus condyloidei mandibulae.* **c. ossis femoris** [NA] A stout, constricted column of bone connecting the head of the femur to the shaft, directed anteriorly, medially, and superiorly at an angle of 125° to the shaft in the adult. It is flat anteriorly, totally encapsulated, and joined to the shaft at the intertrochanteric line. The posterior surface, only the medial two-thirds of which is encapsulated, is concave, and sharply demarcated from the shaft by the raised intertrochanteric crest. The neck is perforated by large vascular foramina. Also *neck of femur, collum femoris.* **c. processus condyloidei mandibulae** COLLUM MANDIBULAE. **c. radii** [NA] The constricted part of the proximal extremity of the radius that joins the rounded head to the shaft just above the radial tuberosity. Its upper part is surrounded by the annular ligament. Also *neck of radius.* **c. scapulae** [NA] The inconspicuous narrowing between the lateral angle, or glenoid cavity, and the platelike body of the scapula that provides attachment to the capsule of the shoulder joint. Also *neck of scapula.* **c. tali** [NA] The constricted portion of the talus, anterior to its body and posterior to its rounded articular head. It is perforated superiorly by vascular foramina, while inferiorly it is grooved by the sulcus tali. Also *neck of talus, neck of ankle bone.* **c. valgum** TORTICOLLIS. **c. vesicae biliaris** [NA] The narrow, sinuous connection between the body of the gallbladder and the cystic duct. It is connected by areolar tissue to the liver at the right end of the porta hepatis, and its mucous membrane is thrown into oblique folds. It is constricted at its junction with the cystic duct. Also *neck of gallbladder, collum vesicae felleae.*

**collut.** *collutorium* (L, mouthwash).

**collutoria** \käl′ootôr′ē·ə\ Plural of COLLUTORIUM.

**collutorium** [L *collutus,* past part. of *colluere* to wash, rinse + *-orium* -ORY] COLLUTORY.

**collutory** A medicinal preparation used as a mouthwash or gargle. Also *collutorium.*

**collyria** \kälir′ē·ə\ Plural of COLLYRIUM.

**collyrium** \kälir′ē·əm\ [L (from Gk *kollyrion* eye salve), medicine for the eyes, eye salve] A liquid medication for instillation on the eye.

**colo-** \kō′lō-\ COLON-.

**coloboma** \käl′ōbō′mə\ [Gk *kolobōma* (from *kolobos* maimed, mutilated) a part cut off or missing] **1** Any defective or cleft part. **2** Any developmental defect of the eye and its parts. **atypical c.** A developmental notch in the ocular structures that is located elsewhere than at the six o'clock meridian of the embryonic choroid fissure. **c. auriculae** A cleft or notch on the earlobe. It may be either congenital or acquired. **bridge c.** A typical coloboma in which the midportion of the fetal fissure closes. **c. of the choroid** A defect in the choroid layer and, usually, of the retina at the approximate position of the fetal choroidal fissure in the embryonic optic cup. The retinal scotoma and the choroidal defect allow visualization of the sclera as a white patch or streak. **c. of the ciliary body** A congenital cleft or scar on the ciliary body at the approximate position of the embryonic optic fissure (choroidal fissure of eye). **facial c.** OBLIQUE FACIAL CLEFT. **Fuchs c.** A small crescentic defect in the choroid at the inferior edge of the optic disk. Also *congenital crescent of the choroid.* **c. iridis** A congenital notch or cleft on the inferior aspect of the iris. It may be associated with clefts or scars on the choroid and ciliary body. Also *coloboma of the iris.* **c. lentis** A peripheral indentation or irregular curvature on the lens, not directly associated with incomplete closure of the embryonic optic fissure (choroidal fissure of eye). **c. of the optic disk** A congenital cleft, furrow, or craterlike defect on the optic disk signifying incomplete formation of the optic nerve at the optic fissure (choroidal fissure of eye). Also *coloboma of the optic nerve, coloboma of the optic nerve entry.* **c. palpebrale** A notch on the lower lid marking incomplete closure of the embryonic naso-optic groove. **c. retinae** A congenital defect in the inferior part of the retina, representing incomplete closure of the embryonic optic fissure (choroidal fissure of eye). **c. of the vitreous** A congenital notch or groove in the inferior part of the vitreous body, which may become filled with mesoderm.

**colocecostomy** \-sēkäs′təmē\ [COLO- + CECO- + -STOMY] A surgical procedure creating an opening between the large intestine and the cecum, usually after a section of colon has been bypassed or resected. Such an opening may rarely result spontaneously from trauma or from inflammatory or neoplastic disease. Also *cecocolostomy.*

**colocentesis** \-sentē′sis\ [COLO- + -CENTESIS] A surgical procedure in which a small opening is made in the large intestine in order to withdraw fluid or gas. This is usually done to decompress a massively dilated large bowel. Also *colipuncture.*

**colocholecystostomy** \-kō′ləsistäs′təmē\ [COLO- + CHOLECYSTO- + -STOMY] CHOLECYSTOCOLOSTOMY.

**coloclysis** \kōläk′lisis\ Colonic irrigation.

**colocolic** \-käl′ik\ Relating or connecting different parts of the colon, as an anastomosis or fistulous tract.

**colocolostomy** \-kōläs′təmē\ [COLO- + COLOSTOMY] A surgical opening between two sections of the large intestine, usually following resection or bypass of a colonic segment. Such an opening may also result, though rarely, from a neoplasm, inflammation, or trauma.

**colocynth** \kō′lōsinth\ The dried pulp of the fully developed but unripe fruit of *Citrullus colocynthis.* It is used as a powerful cathartic. Also *colocynthis.*

**colocynthidism** \-sin′thidizm\ [Gk *kolokynthis,* gen. *kolokynthidos,* round gourd, cucurbita + -ISM] Poisoning from the use of colocynth, which may cause severe inflammation of the gastrointestinal tract, vomiting, watery and bloody stools, severe muscular pain, and collapse.

**colocynthis** COLOCYNTH.

**coloenteritis** \-en′terī′tis\ [COLO- + ENTERITIS] ENTEROCOLITIS.

**colofixation** \-fiksā′shən\ [COLO- + FIXATION] A surgical procedure in which a markedly redundant large intestine is suspended from the abdominal wall to prevent ptosis. Also *colopexy*.

**colohepatopexy** \-hep′ətōpek′sē\ [COLO- + HEPATO- + -PEXY] A surgical procedure in which the large intestine is fixed to the liver in order to prevent the formation of gastrohepatic adhesions.

**coloileal** \-il′ē·əl\ ILEOCOLIC.

**colitis** \kōläl′isis\ [COLO- + LYSIS] A surgical procedure in which all of the adhesions fixing the colon to the abdominal wall and other intra-abdominal viscera are lysed, or divided.

**colon** \kō′lən\ [L, from Gk *kolon* (sometimes confused with *kōlon* limb, member, as if meaning a "member" of the intestines) the colon] [NA] That portion of the large intestine extending from the cecum at the ileocolic junction to the rectum and comprising ascending, transverse, descending, and sigmoid portions. It is distinguished by haustra coli, taeniae coli, appendices epiploicae, and the absence of villi on its mucous membrane, which is raised into numerous crescentic folds corresponding to the intervals between the haustrations. **c. ascendens** [NA] The continuation of the cecum above the ileocecal valve, ascending along the right side of the abdominal cavity through the right lumbar and hypochondriac regions to the inferior surface of the liver, where it terminates in the right colic flexure. It is usually surrounded by peritoneum except for its posterior surface, which is in contact with the posterior abdominal wall. **c. descendens** [NA] The portion of the colon that extends downwards from the left colic flexure, through the left hypochondriac and lumbar regions, lateral to the left lateral plane, to the left iliac fossa, where it terminates as the sigmoid colon at the inlet of the true pelvis. It is covered by peritoneum in front and at the sides. Occasionally its posterior surface is attached to the posterior abdominal wall by a mesocolon. **giant c.** *Seldom used* MEGACOLON. **irritable c.** IRRITABLE BOWEL SYNDROME. **lead-pipe c.** A rigid, contracted, and nondistensible colon as evidenced on contrast studies. The appearance most often results from scarring in chronic ulcerative colitis. **redundant c.** A sigmoid colon of excessive length that results in hooking or coiling. It is usually of developmental origin. **c. sigmoideum** [NA] The portion of the colon that commences at the inlet of the true pelvis as the continuation of the descending colon and terminates as the rectum in the median plane in front of the third sacral vertebra. It is surrounded by peritoneum, its mesocolon being attached to the posterior pelvic wall. During its course it forms several bends resembling either an inverted V or an S. Its position and shape vary considerably. Also *sigmoid colon, sigmoid flexure of colon* (outmoded). **spastic c.** IRRITABLE BOWEL SYNDROME. **c. transversum** [NA] The portion of the colon that arches from the right colic flexure below the liver in the right lumbar region to the left colic flexure below the spleen in the left hypochondriac region. Its convexity faces inferiorly and its position and extent vary considerably. Most of it is surrounded by peritoneum, its mesocolon being attached to the anterior margin of the body of the pancreas. Also *transverse colon*.

**colon-** \kō′lən-\ [Gk *kolon* colon] A combining form denoting the colon. Also *colo-*.

**colonic** \kōlän′ik\ **1** Of or pertaining to the colon. **2** A colonic irrigation or enema.

**colonization** \käl′ənīzā′shən\ Implantation of a microbe at a site, such as multiplication of staphylococci in the anterior nares.

**Colonna** [Paul C. *Colonna*, U.S. orthopedic surgeon, 1892–1966] See under OPERATION.

**colonopathy** \kō′lōnäp′əthē\ [COLON- + *o* + -PATHY] Any colonic disease or disorder. Also *colopathy*.

**colonoscopy** \kō′lōnäs′kəpē\ [COLON- + *o* + -SCOPY] A procedure in which a long, flexible, fiberoptic instrument is used for the visualization and, if necessary, biopsy of the entire length of the large intestine. **fiberoptic c.** An endoscopy of the colon by means of a flexible fiberoptic device that is inserted transanally.

**colony** [L *colonia* (from *colonus* a farmer, settler, from *colere* to cultivate) a colony, farm] A compact mass of bacteria, usually derived by vegetative multiplication of a single cell, on the surface of a streaked or spread plate or in the depth of a pour plate of solid medium. **fried-egg c.** A colony characteristic of mycoplasmas on solid media, very thin at the periphery, and thicker and extending into the agar at the center. **G c.** GONIDIAL COLONY. **Gheel c.** A home-boarding system for mentally ill patients in existence since the 13th century in Gheel, Belgium. **glossy c.** A colony with a moist and shiny surface, associated with abundant capsule production. **gonidial c.** A drug-resistant dwarf colony of staphylococci that are selected by various antimicrobial agents. Their walls are probably defective, as in L-forms. Also *G colony*. **M c.** MUCOID COLONY. **matt c.** A flat colony, produced by partial drying or capsular hydrolysis of a glossy or mucoid colony. **mother c.** A colony at whose edge secondary colonies have arisen. **mucoid c.** A colony even moister than a glossy colony. Also *M colony*. **R c.** ROUGH COLONY. **rough c.** A colony with a dry, rough surface usually due to the absence of capsules on the bacteria. Also *R colony*. **S c.** SMOOTH COLONY. **satellite c.** A colony of an auxotroph fed by a neighboring colony of another strain, best observed with a heavy seeding of the former and well-isolated colonies of the latter. **secondary c.** A colony of distinct morphology appearing at the edge of an older colony, usually on prolonged incubation. It reflects a mutation to improved growth on the medium that is being depleted. **smooth c.** A colony with a smooth surface. With most bacteria it reflects the presence of a capsule, but with mycobacteria, smooth and rough colonies reflect differences in the waxy coat. Also *S colony*.

**colopathy** \kōläp′əthē\ COLONOPATHY.

**colopexostomy** \-peksäs′təmē\ [COLO- + *-pex(y)* + *o* + -STOMY] A surgical procedure in which the colon or large intestine is fixed to the anterior abdominal wall, and a colostomy created within the suspended segment of bowel.

**colopexotomy** \-peksät′əmē\ [COLO- + *-pex(y)* + *o* + -TOMY] A surgical procedure in which the large intestine is incised and then suspended from the abdominal wall to prevent ptosis.

**colopexy** \kō′lōpek′sē\ [COLO- + -PEXY] COLOFIXATION.

**colophony** \kōläf′ənē\ ROSIN.

**coloplication** \-plikā′shən\ [COLO- + PLICATION] An operation in which tucks are taken in the wall of a dilated colon to shorten it or to decrease the size of the lumen. Also *coliplication*.

**coloproctectomy** \-präktek′təmē\ [COLO- + PROCTECTOMY] The surgical removal of part or all of the large bowel and rectum. This procedure may be combined with an enterostomy or an anastomosis.

**coloproctitis** \-praktī′tis\ [COLO- + PROCTITIS] Proctocolitis; an inflammatory process involving both the colon and rectum. Also *colorectitis*.

**coloproctostomy** \-präktäs′təmē\ [COLO- + PROCTO- + -STOMY] A surgical opening created between the large bowel and the rectum, usually following rectosigmoid resection or bypass. Such an opening may occur spontaneously, but rarely, as a result of inflammation, trauma, or neoplastic disease. Also *colorectostomy.*

**coloptosis** \kō'läptō'sis\ [COLO- + -PTOSIS] Downward displacement or a lower than usual position of the colon, especially of the transverse portion.

**color** [L, color] A visually perceived quality of bodies or substances depending upon their emission or reflection of specific wavelengths of visible light. The longer visible wavelengths give the sensation of seeing a red color, whereas the shorter visible wavelengths make the body appear blue. **metameric c.'s** Seemingly identical colors that result from different combinations of chromatic stimuli. **pseudoisochromatic c.'s** Different colors that appear identical to a colorblind individual.

**color.** *coloretur* (L, let it be colored).

**colorblind** See under COLOR BLIND.

**colorblindness** See under COLOR BLINDNESS.

**colorectal** \-rek'təl\ Of or relating to both the colon and the rectum.

**colorectitis** \-rektī'tis\ [COLO- + RECT- + -ITIS ] COLOPROCTITIS.

**colorectostomy** \-rektäs'təmē\ [COLO- + RECTO- + -STOMY] COLOPROCTOSTOMY.

**colorimeter** \kul'ərim'ətər\ [COLOR + *i* + -METER] An instrument for determining the shade or intensity of color. Also *chromatometer, chromometer.* **photoelectric c.** A device that measures the intensity of color of a transparent solution by determining the amount of light incident on a photocell after passage through a calibrated filter. Also *electrophotometer.*

**colorimetry** \kul'ərim'ətrē\ [COLOR + *i* + -METRY] An analytic technique based on color as the measured end point. The measurement may be visual, photoelectric, or spectrophotometric. Adj. colorimetric.

**colorrhaphy** \kōlôr'əfē\ [COLO- + -RRHAPHY] The surgical repair of the colon by suturing in order to form a line of union.

**colorrhea** \kō'lôrē'ə\ [COLO- + -RRHEA] A mucous diarrhea originating predominantly from the colon. Also *colonorrhea.*

**colosigmoidostomy** \-sig'moidäs'təmē\ [COLO- + SIGMOID + -STOMY] A communication between the right, transverse, or left colon and the sigmoid colon. It is usually surgically created following a colonic resection or bypass, but it may result from an inflammatory or neoplastic fistular tract.

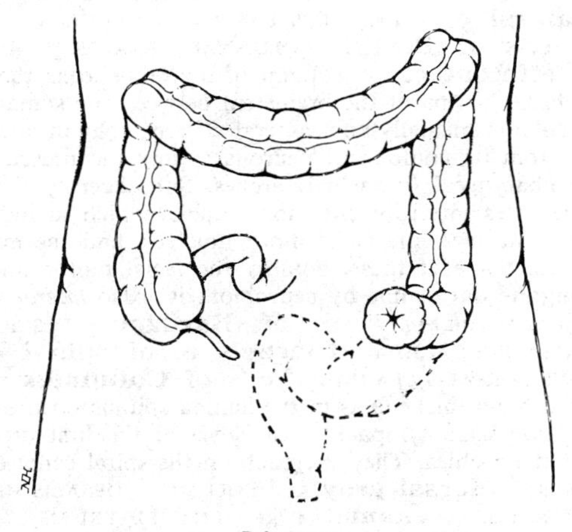
Colostomy

**colostomy** \kōläs'təmē\ [COLO- + -STOMY] The establishment of an opening between the colon and the skin. It is usually surgically created to divert the fecal stream, but it may be the result of an inflammatory or neoplastic fistular tract. **dry c.** A surgical procedure resulting in a communication between the large bowel and the skin that is not productive of feces and is therefore not diverting the colonic contents. A dry colostomy may occur, though rarely, as a result of a neoplasm, inflammation, or trauma. Also *mucus fistula.* **end c.** A colostomy in which the proximal end of the divided colon is exteriorized to form an artificial anus. **ileotransverse c.** A communication between the colon and the ileum. It is usually created surgically following right colon resection or bypass, but it may result from a neoplastic or inflammatory fistular tract. Also *ileotransversostomy.* **wet c.** A surgical procedure resulting in an opening between the large bowel and the skin that is productive of feces and is therefore diverting the colonic contents, as least in part. A wet colostomy may result, though rarely, from a neoplasm, inflammation, or trauma.

**colostrorrhea** \kōläs'trôrē'ə\ [*colostr(um)* + *o* + -RRHEA] The discharge or secretion of colostrum.

**colostrum** \kōlas'trəm\ [L, the first breast milk given after a birth] A yellow fluid produced by the mammary gland at the beginning of lactation. It is high in protein and immune substances and also has a growth factor that causes the newborn infant's intestines to grow in size so as to be ready to receive the mother's milk. Also *foremilk, neogala.* **c. gravidarum** The colostrum secreted during the several days just prior to delivery or immediately after delivery.

**colotomy** \kōlät'əmē\ [COLO- + -TOMY] An opening into the colon, usually surgically created for the purpose of inspection, polyp removal, or anastomosis. It may also result from neoplastic or inflammatory disease. Also *laparocolotomy.*

**colovaginal** \-vaj'ənəl\ Relating or connecting the colon with the vagina, as a fistula.

**colp-** \kälp-\ COLPO-.

**colpalgia** \kälpal'jə\ [COLP- + -ALGIA] COLPODYNIA.

**colpectasia** \käl'pektā'zhə\ [COLP- + Gk *ektas(is)* a stretching, distending + -IA] Distension of the vagina. Also *colpectasis.*

**colpectomy** \kälpek'təmē\ [COLP- + -ECTOMY] Partial or complete surgical excision of the vagina. Also *vaginectomy.*

**colpedema** \käl'pidē'mə\ [COLP- + EDEMA] Swelling of the vaginal wall.

**colpeurynter** \käl'pyoorin'tər\ [COLP- + Gk *euryn(ein)* to widen, dilate (from *eurys* wide) + *-tēr*, agentive suffix] METREURYNTER.

**colpeurysis** \käl'pyUr'isis\ [COLP- + Gk *eury(nein)* to widen, dilate (from *eurys* wide) + *-sis*, derivative noun suffix] Dilatation of the vagina by surgery.

**colpismus** \kälpis'məs\ VAGINISMUS.

**colpitis** \kälpī'tis\ [COLP- + -ITIS] Inflammation of the vagina. Adj. colpitic. **emphysematous c.** EMPHYSEMATOUS VAGINITIS. **c. granulosa** GRANULAR VAGINITIS. **c. mycotica** Fungal infection of the vagina, usually caused by *Candida albicans.*.

**colpo-** \käl'pō-\ [Gk *kolpos* bosom, womb, vagina] A combining form denoting the vagina. Also *kolpo-, colp-, kolp-*.

**colpocele** \käl′pōsēl\ [COLPO- + -CELE[1]] A hernia protruding into the vagina. Also *vaginocele.*

**colpoceliocentesis** \-sē′lē·ōsentē′sis\ CULDOCENTESIS.

**colpoceliotomy** \-sēlē·ät′əmē\ CULDOCENTESIS. **anterolateral c.** Surgical entry into the peritoneal cavity through an incision into the vagina and anterior cul-de-sac.

**colpocleisis** \-klī′sis\ [COLPO- + -CLEISIS] Surgical closure of the vagina, used in the treatment of uterine and vaginal prolapse.

**colpocystitis** \-sistī′tis\ [COLPO- + CYSTITIS] Inflammation of the vagina and urinary bladder.

**colpocystocele** \-sis′təsēl\ [COLPO- + CYSTOCELE] A weakening of the anterior vaginal wall and levator ani sling, which allows the bladder to protrude into the vagina.

**colpocystoplasty** \-sis′təplas′tē\ [COLPO- + CYSTOPLASTY] Surgical repair of a stretched or herniated vesicovaginal wall, or of a defect in the wall.

**colpocystotomy** \-sistät′əmē\ [COLPO- + CYSTOTOMY] An incision into the bladder through the wall of the vagina.

**colpocytogram** \-sī′təgram\ In vaginal cytology, an analysis of the cell types present. The information can be used to study the hormonal status of the patient.

**colpodynia** \-din′ē·ə\ [COLP- + -ODYNIA] Pain in the vagina. Also *colpalgia, vaginodynia.*

**colpoepisiorrhaphy** \-ipiz′ē·ôr′əfē\ Repair of an episiotomy.

**colpohyperplasia** \-hī′pərplā′zhə\ [COLPO- + HYPERPLASIA] The excessive growth of mucous membrane or formation of rugae in the vagina.

**colpohysterectomy** \-his′tərek′təmē\ VAGINAL HYSTERECTOMY.

**colpohysterotomy** \-his′tərät′əmē\ [COLPO- + HYSTEROTOMY ] A hysterotomy performed through a vaginal incision.

**colpomyomectomy** \-mī′əmek′təmē\ VAGINAL MYOMECTOMY.

**colpomyomotomy** \-mī′əmät′əmē\ [COLPO- + MYOMOTOMY] VAGINAL MYOMECTOMY.

**colpoparovariocystectomy** \-par′ōver′ē·ōsistek′təmē\ [COLPO- + *par(a)-* + OVARIO- + CYSTECTOMY] Surgical removal of an ovarian cyst through a vaginal incision.

**colpoperineorrhaphy** \-per′inē·ôr′əfē\ [COLPO- + PERINEORRHAPHY] Perineorrhaphy done through the vagina. Also *colpoperineoplasty, vaginoperineorrhaphy.*

**colpopexy** \käl′pōpek′sē\ [COLPO- + -PEXY] Surgical fixation in an elevated position of a descended vagina. The current approach is to produce a posterior fixation to the sacrospinous ligaments or sacrum. Also *vaginapexy, vaginopexy, vaginofixation.*

**colpoplasty** \käl′pōplas′tē\ [COLPO- + -PLASTY] Plastic surgical repair of the vagina, usually done to return the urethra, bladder, and rectum to their normal positions. Also *vaginoplasty, colporrhaphy, vaginofixation, elytroplasty.*

**colpopoiesis** \-poi·ē′sis\ [COLPO- + -POIESIS] The creation of a vagina, where none existed, by dissection and insertion of a split-skin graft.

**colpopolypus** \-päl′əpəs\ [COLPO- + L *polypus* polyp] (*pl.* colpopolypi) A polyp in the vagina. Also *elytropolypus.*

**colpoptosis** \käl′pōtō′sis\ Prolapse of the vagina.

**colporectopexy** \-rek′təpek′sē\ [COLPO- + RECTO- + -PEXY] Fixation of a prolapsed rectum in the normal position by suturing it to the vaginal wall.

**colporrhagia** \käl′pôrā′jə\ [COLPO- + -RRHAGIA] Vaginal bleeding.

**colporrhaphy** \kälpôr′əfē\ [COLPO- + -RRHAPHY] **1** Repair of a torn vagina. **2** COLPOPLASTY.

**colposcope** \käl′pōskōp\ [COLPO- + -SCOPE] An instrument inserted into the vagina for examination of the vagina and cervix by means of a magnifying lens. It is used primarily to identify abnormal vascular and epithelial patterns associated with early neoplasia.

**colpospasm** \käl′pōspazm\ VAGINISMUS.

**colpostat** \käl′postat\ [COLPO- + -STAT] A device for holding an instrument, such as a radium applicator, in place in the vagina.

**colpostenosis** \-stenō′sis\ [COLPO- + STENOSIS] Narrowing of the vagina.

**colpostenotomy** \-stenät′əmē\ [COLPO- + STENO- + -TOMY] A surgical incision into the vagina to relieve a stricture or narrowing produced by trauma, infection, or radiation, or occurring congenitally.

**colpotherm** \käl′pōthurm\ [COLPO- + Gk *therm(ē)* heat] A device for measuring the temperature of the vagina, proported to be useful for detecting ovulation.

**colpotomy** \kälpät′əmē\ [COLPO- + -TOMY] An incision into the vagina. Also *vaginotomy, culdotomy.* **posterior c.** A surgical incision in the posterior vagina to enter the cul-de-sac. It may be used for surgical sterilization, diagnosis, or treatment of ovarian or tubal disease.

**colpoureterocystotomy** \-yoorē′tərōsistät′əmē\ [COLPO- + URETERO- + CYSTOTOMY] A surgical incision for ureteral or urinary bladder disease made through the vagina.

**colpoureterotomy** \-yoorē′tərät′əmē\ [COLPO- + URETERO- + -TOMY] A surgical incision made through the vagina to correct a ureteral disorder such as stenosis or a calculus.

**colpoxerosis** \-zērō′sis\ [COLPO- + XEROSIS] Dryness of the vagina and vulva.

**Colubridae** \käloo′bridē\ [L *coluber,* gen. *colubris,* a snake, adder + -IDAE] A cosmopolitan family of mostly nonpoisonous or mildly poisonous snakes and some highly poisonous species. Venomous species have small, grooved fangs at the rear of the mouth. There are approximately 1000 species. Adj. colubrid.

**columbium** A term used mostly in commerce and technology for NIOBIUM. Symbol: Cb

**columella** \käl′yəmel′ə\ [L (dim. of *columna* column), a small column] A small anatomical columna. **c. fornicis** *Obs.* COLUMNA FORNICIS.

**columellae** \käl′yəmel′ē\ Plural of COLUMELLA.

**column** [L *columna.* See COLUMNA.] COLUMNA. **anal c.'s** COLUMNAE ANALES. **anterior c. of fauces** ARCUS PALATOGLOSSUS. **anterior gray c.** COLUMNA VENTRALIS MEDULLAE SPINALIS. **anterior rugal c. of vagina** COLUMNA RUGARUM ANTERIOR VAGINAE. **anterolateral c.** FUNICULUS LATERALIS MEDULLAE SPINALIS. **c.'s of Bertin** COLUMNAE RENALES. **branchial efferent c.** A column of motor neurons that lies in the basal lamina of the brainstem between the somatic efferent column medially and visceral efferent column laterally. Axons from its component neurons supply the musculature of the pharyngeal (branchial) arches. Subsequently the column becomes interrupted to form nuclei which include the gustatory nucleus, the facial motor nucleus, and the nucleus ambiguus. Some of these, notably the facial motor nucleus, may migrate out of line by neurobiotaxis. Also *lateral somatic efferent column.* **c. of Burdach** FASCICULUS CUNEATUS BURDACHI. **Clarke's c. of spinal cord** NUCLEUS DORSALIS CLARKII. **c.'s of Cotunnius** Longitudinal bony thickenings in the lamina spiralis on the inner wall of the scala tympani at the level of the first or basal turn of the cochlea. They encroach on the spiral canal of the modiolus. **dorsal gray c.** COLUMNA DORSALIS MEDULLAE SPINALIS. **enamel c.'s** ENAMEL PRISMS. **fat c.'s** Columns of fatty tissue that extend from the cutaneous connective tissue to the skin appendages. Also *columnae adiposae.* **c. of fornix** COLUMNA FORNICIS. **general somatic afferent c.** A column of neurons, in the alar lamina of the developing neural tube, where axons of primary sensory neurons relay general somatic sensations such as pain, touch, and thermal sense. Derivatives of the column include the dorsal gray horn of the spinal cord, the nuclei gracilis and cuneatus, and the sensory nuclei of the trigeminal nerve. **general somatic efferent c.** The column of neurons situated most medially in the basal lamina of the developing neural tube. The axons of these neurons supply musculature derived from somites. Derivatives of the column include ventral horn motor neurons of the spinal cord, oculomotor nuclei of the third, fourth, and sixth cranial nerves and the hypoglossal nucleus. **general visceral efferent c.** A column of neurons in the lateral part of the basal lamina of the developing neural tube. Its neurons constitute preganglionic elements of the parasympathetic and sympathetic nervous systems. Derivatives of the column in the brainstem include the Edinger-Westphal nucleus of the third cranial nerve, the salivatory nuclei of the seventh and ninth cranial nerves, and the dorsal motor nucleus of the vagus. In the spinal cord its derivatives lie in the intermediolateral column of the thoracolumbar and sacral regions. **c. of Goll** FASCICULUS GRACILIS MEDULLAE SPINALIS. **c. of Gowers** TRACTUS SPINOCEREBELLARIS VENTRALIS. **gray c.'s of spinal cord** COLUMNAE GRISEAE. **intermediolateral cell c.** COLUMNA INTERMEDIOLATERALIS. **ion exchange c.** A column of an ion exchanger, usually for use in chromatography. **lateral gray c.** COLUMNA LATERALIS MEDULLAE SPINALIS. **lateral somatic efferent c.** BRANCHIAL EFFERENT COLUMN. **lateral c. of spinal cord** COLUMNA LATERALIS MEDULLAE SPINALIS. **c.'s of Morgagni** COLUMNAE ANALES. **positive c.** The glowing ionized gas seen near the positive electrode of a partially evacuated tube when a high voltage is placed on the tube. *Seldom used.* **posterior c. of fauces** ARCUS PALATOPHARYNGEUS. **posterior gray c.** COLUMNA DORSALIS MEDULLAE SPINALIS. **posterior rugal c. of vagina** COLUMNA RUGARUM POSTERIOR VAGINAE. **posteromedian c.** COLUMNA POSTEROMEDIANA. **posterovesicular c. of Clarke** NUCLEUS THORACICUS. **rectal c.'s** COLUMNAE ANALES. **renal c.'s** COLUMNAE RENALES. **renal c.'s of Bertin** COLUMNAE RENALES. **c. of Rolando** EMINENTIA TRIGEMINA. **c.'s of rugae of vagina** COLUMNAE RUGARUM VAGINAE. **c.'s of Sertoli** SERTOLI CELLS. **somatic motor c.** The column or longitudinal alignment along the brain stem and spinal cord formed by motor nuclei of skeletal muscles, exclusive of the branchial musculature. **somatic sensory c.** Those portions of gray matter in the brainstem and spinal cord that are intimately related to sensory input from the body. **special somatic afferent c.** A column of neurons in the brainstem where primary sensory neurons of certain special senses relay. For the most part, this column comprises the cochlear and vestibular nuclei of the eighth cranial nerve. **spinal c.** COLUMNA VERTEBRALIS. **Stilling's c.** A group of small neurons extending beyond the rostral and caudal limits of the definitive nucleus dorsalis of Clarke. The term is sometimes restricted to the cervical group. **Türck's c.** TRACTUS CORTICOSPINALIS VENTRALIS. **c.'s of vagina** COLUMNAE RUGARUM VAGINAE. **ventral c. of spinal cord** COLUMNA VENTRALIS MEDULLAE SPINALIS. **vertebral c.** COLUMNA VERTEBRALIS. **visceral motor c.** The discontinuous column or alignment along the neuraxis of the central nuclei for autonomic outflow. At cord levels it is represented by the intermediolateral cell column, which is situated between columns relating to visceral sensory inflow and outflow to branchial arch derivatives where these are represented. In the brainstem, it includes the nucleus of Edinger-Westphal and the salivatory nuclei. Thus, the visceral motor column includes sympathetic and parasympathetic primary motoneurons to somatic structures as well as viscera. Also *visceral efferent column.* **visceral sensory c.** The longitudinal zone along the neuraxis, particularly in the developing nervous system, involved in the reception of sensory inflow from the viscera. In the cord it occupies the lateral, basal part of the dorsal horn, dorsal to the visceral motor column.

**columna** \kōlum′nə\ [L (akin to *columen, culmen* summit, top, zenith) a column or pillar] (*pl.* columnae) A pillar-like or cylindrical, often vertical or longitudinal, structure or formation. Also *column.* **columnae adiposae** FAT COLUMNS. **columnae anales** [NA] The five to ten vertical folds of mucous membrane that are unevenly spaced in the upper half of the anal canal and each of which contains a branch of the superior rectal artery and vein. They are more obvious in children than in adults. Enlargement of the veins may lead to primary internal hemorrhoids. Also *anal columns, rectal columns, columns of Morgagni, mucous folds of rectum.* **c. anterior medullae spinalis** COLUMNA VENTRALIS MEDULLAE SPINALIS. **c. dorsalis medullae spinalis** 1 [NA] The dorsal (posterior) sensory neuropil derived from the embryonic alar plate of the spinal cord, including the marginal layer, substantia gelatinosa, and nucleus proprius, or Rexed's layers 1 through 5. Also *dorsal gray column, posterior gray column, columna posterior medullae spinalis.* 2 FUNICULUS POSTERIOR MEDULLAE SPINALIS. **c. fornicis** [NA] That portion of the fornix which, continuing downward and forward from the body of the fornix, passes anterior to the foramen of Monro and enters the floor of the diencephalon. The columns on the two sides are at the posterior margin of the two laminae of the septum pellucidum. Also *column of fornix, pars libera columnae fornicis, anterior pillar of fornix.* **columnae griseae** [NA] Longitudinal ridges protruding from the central core of gray matter in the spinal cord, including a posterior (dorsal) column directed dorsolaterally, and an anterior (ventral) column. A less prominent lateral column is also present at thoracic and upper lumbar levels. Seen in cross-section, these columns are called horns, or cornua. Also *gray columns of spinal cord.* **c. intermediolateralis** [NA] A column of spindle-shaped or ovoid cells occupying the apical region of the lateral horn in the thoracic and upper lumbar segments of the spinal cord. These small motor neurons give rise to preganglionic sympathetic fibers which exit via the ventral roots and reach the various sympathetic ganglia as the rami communicantes albi. Also *nucleus intermediolateralis, lateral sympathetic nucleus, nucleus sympathicus lateralis, intermediolateral cell column, intermediolateral tract.* **c. lateralis medullae spinalis** 1 [NA] A lateral protrusion of the spinal gray matter. It is small relative to the dorsal and ventral columns and is restricted to the thoracic and upper lumbar segments. Also *lateral column of spinal cord, lateral gray column.* 2 FUNICULUS LATERALIS MEDULLAE SPINALIS. **c. posterior medullae spinalis** COLUMNA DORSALIS MEDULLAE SPINALIS. **c. posterolateralis** Fasciculus cuneatus medullae spinalis, along with its rostral continuation, the fasciculus cuneatus medullae oblongatae. **c. posteromediana** The fasciculus gracilis medullae spinalis, along with its rostral continuation, the fasciculus gracilis medullae oblongatae. Also *posteromedian column.* **co-**

**lumnae renales** [NA] The parts of the renal cortex that extend between adjacent pyramids towards the renal sinus. Also *renal columns, columns of Bertin, interpyramidal cortex, renal columns of Bertin.* **c. rugarum anterior vaginae** [NA] The median longitudinal ridge of mucous membrane on the anterior wall of the vagina from which several smaller ridges, or rugae, extend laterally and craniad on each side. Also *anterior rugal column of vagina.* **c. rugarum posterior vaginae** [NA] The median longitudinal ridge of mucous membrane on the posterior wall of the vagina from which several smaller ridges, or rugae, extend laterally and craniad on each side. Also *posterior rugal column of vagina.* **columnae rugarum vaginae** Columna rugarum anterior vaginae and columna rugarum posterior vaginae. Also *columns of rugae of vagina, columns of vagina.* **c. ventralis medullae spinalis** 1 [NA] The anterior column of spinal cord gray matter, consisting primarily of motonuclei of the skeletal musculature. Also *ventral column of spinal cord, anterior gray column, columna anterior medullae spinalis.* 2 FUNICULUS ANTERIOR MEDULLAE SPINALIS. **c. vertebralis** [NA] The axis of the skeleton situated dorsally in the median plane and supporting the skull superiorly in humans, while inferiorly it ends in the coccyx and is joined to the hip bones at the sacroiliac joints through which the weight of the body is transmitted to the lower limbs. It comprises a series of bony segments, or vertebrae, joined to each other by intervertebral disks, joints, and ligaments which permit a small amount of movement between two adjacent vertebrae but provide the column as a whole with considerable flexibility. It is divided regionally into cervical, thoracic, lumbar, sacral, and coccygeal portions, in the latter two of which the vertebrae are fused to form single bones, the sacrum and the coccyx, respectively. The column supports the trunk, provides attachment for muscles, and protects the spinal cord and nerve roots. Also *vertebral column, spinal column, backbone, back bone, spine, axon, vertebrarium, rachis.*

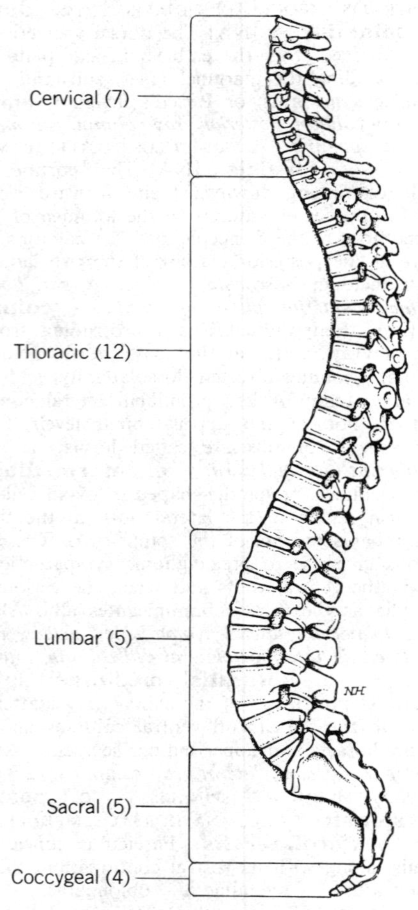


**Vertebral column**

**columnae** \kōlum′nē\ Plural of COLUMNA.

**colyseptic** \kō′lēsep′tik\ *Seldom used* ANTISEPTIC.

**com-** \käm-, kōm-, kəm-\ [L prefix *com-* (from *cum* with; *com-* is so used before *b, m, p,* and sometimes *f* but becomes *co-* before a vowel and before *th, w,* and sometimes other consonants; in L words *com-* became *co-* before a vowel, *h,* and *gn*; *com-* assimilates to *l* as *col-,* to *r* as *cor-,* and becomes *con-* before all other consonants) with, together, jointly] A prefix meaning together, with, jointly. Also *col-, con-, cor-.*

**coma**[1] \kō′mə\ [Gk *kōma* a deep sleep, lethargy] A loss of consciousness from which the patient cannot be roused. **agrypnodal c.** VIGIL COMA. **alcoholic c.** Coma induced by acute alcohol intoxication, usually over 400 mg/100 ml alcohol in the blood, and marked by rapid, light respiration, usually with tachycardia and hypotension. **apoplectic c.** Coma induced by cerebral, cerebellar, or brainstem hemorrhage, by embolism, or by cerebral thrombosis (apoplexy, or stroke). Loss of consciousness may be accompanied by signs indicating the site of the lesion, such as conjugate deviation of the head and eyes, tonal asymmetry, or unilateral extensor plantar response. **deanimate c.** Deep coma with loss of all somatic and autonomic reflex activity. The maintenance of life in such cases depends wholly upon supportive measures such as assisted respiration, and cardiac arrest will quickly follow if the respirator is stopped. This may be a transient state or it may be irreversible. In the latter case the electroencephalogram is usually isoelectric (completely flat). **deep c.** A profound state of coma, with abolition of all reflex responses and, frequently, severe respiratory and circulatory disturbance. **diabetic c.** The coma of severe diabetic ketoacidosis. **epileptic c.** Coma persisting after the tonic-clonic phase of a major epileptic convulsion. **hepatic c.** HEPATIC ENCEPHALOPATHY. **hyperosmolal c.** Coma resulting from any metabolic disorder associated with hyperosmolality of the blood. **hyperosmolar nonketotic c.** Coma in any disorder associated with hyperosmolality, with the exception of diabetic coma, in which there is also ketosis. **hypoglycemic c.** Coma resulting from hypoglycemia due either to insulin overdosage or to panhypopituitarism. **hypopituitary c.** Coma occurring in advanced, severe panhypopituitarism. It is generally associated with hypoglycemia owing to absence of growth hormone, thyroid hormone, and cortisol. **hypothermic c.** Coma due to hypothermia. **irreversible c.** Coma due to a condition of the brain from which no recovery is possible or in which there is no prospect of recovery of consciousness. **metabolic c.** Coma occurring in any metabolic disorder and in the absence of any demonstrable macroscopic physical abnormality of the brain. **myxedema c.** The coma of very severe hypothyroidism in the elderly. It is reversible in many cases, although formerly was always fatal. **postepileptic c.** Loss of consciousness persisting after an attack of epilepsy. **thyrotoxic c.** A coma marking the end stage of a thyrotoxic crisis. **uremic c.** Coma associated with the uremic state, possibly related to the accumulation of dialyzable toxic derivatives of aromatic amino acids. Dehydration and a brain pH less than 7.3 related to renal failure may also play important roles, as may cerebrovascular accidents. **vigil c.** A state of stupor in which the patient is mute and shows no purposive verbal or motor responses to stimuli although the eyes are open and give a false impression of alertness. Also *agrypnodal coma.*

**coma**[2] \kō′mə\ [L *coma* (from Gk *komē* hair of the head, foliage, tail of a comet) hair, foliage] An aberration of a lens arising from inequality of the magnification for different zones of the lens.

**comatose** \kō′mətōs\ [Gk *kōma,* gen. *kōmat(os)* coma + -OSE] Describing or pertaining to an individual in coma.

**comb** [Middle English, from Old English *camb*] A template which forms sample wells when pouring an electrophoretic gel.

**Comby** [Jules *Comby,* French pediatrician, 1853–1947] See under SIGN.

**comedo** \käm′idō, kəmē′dō\ [New L (from L, a glutton, from *comedere* to eat up, consume) a maggot or something suggestive of a maggot] (*pl.* comedones) A greasy plug in a sebaceous follicle composed of a mixture of keratin, sebum, and bacteria and capped by layer of melanin, which gives it a black appearance. Also *blackhead* (popular). **closed c.** MILIUM. **open c.** A mature comedo in which the orifice of the follicle is dilated by a mass of keratin. The impacted keratinous plug is capped by a layer of melanin that is usually visible to the naked eye. **polyporous comedones** Comedones that appear to be multiple but are in fact interconnected, sharing common openings. They occur mainly on the back, especially in cases of acne conglobata or in elderly males. **solar comedones** Comedones caused by prolonged exposure to sunlight. They occur mainly around the eyes and on the cheeks of elderly men, often in association with elastotic degeneration of the dermal collagen. Also *senile comedones.*

**comedocarcinoma** \käm′idōkär′sənō′mə\ [COMEDO + CARCINOMA] A carcinoma of the breast in which the ducts are occluded with tumor having a characteristic necrotic core. It has the appearance of paste in a tube.

**comedomastitis** \käm′idōmastī′tis\ [COMEDO + MASTITIS] A breast inflammation primarily involving the ducts.

**comedones** \käm′idō′nēz\ Plural of COMEDO.

**comes** \kō′mēz\ [L, companion, follower] (*pl.* comites) A blood vessel accompanying an artery, vein, or nerve.

**comitance** \käm′itəns\ [L *comit(ari)* (from *comes,* gen. *comitis* companion) to accompany, follow + -ANCE] A characteristic of strabismus in which the angle of deviation between the two eyes remains constant regardless of the direction of gaze. This indicates a supranuclear etiology of the strabismus, rather than an infranuclear or nuclear muscle paresis. Adj. comitant.

**comites** \käm′itēz\ Plural of COMES.

**comitial** \kəmish′əl\ [L *comitial(is morbus)* (from *comiti(a),* pl. of *comitium* a place of assembly, usu. in Rome, + *-alis* -AL + *morbus* disease, sickness) epilepsy, the falling sickness; hence *comitialis* relating to the *comitia*; as substantive, epilepsy, so called because its occurrence ended the *comitia*] EPILEPTIC.

**commensal** \kəmen′səl\ [Med L *commensal(is)* (from L *com-* with + *mens(a)* table + *-alis* -AL) pertaining to those who eat together] **1** Living on or within another organism without conferring benefit or harm. **2** An organism that lives on or within another organism without conferring benefit or harm. Also *commensal parasite.*

**commensalism** \kəmen′səlizm\ [COMMENSAL + -ISM] A symbiotic relationship in which the members of one species benefit from the association whereas those of the other species remain unaffected. **epizoic c.** PHORESIS.

**comminuted** \käm′inyoo′tid\ [L *comminut(us),* past part. of *comminuere* to lessen, break into small pieces + English *-ed*] Broken into fragments: used especially of multiple fractures of a bone.

**comminution** \käm′inyoo′shən\ [L *comminutus,* past part. of *comminuere* to lessen, break into small pieces] **1** The condition of being comminuted; broken into fragments. **2** The act of breaking into fragments or pulverizing.

**commissura** \käm′ishoo′rə\ [L (from *commissus,* past part. of *committere* to bring together), a jointure, a joining together] (*pl.* commissurae) **1** A juncture between corresponding anatomical parts, from each side, in or across the midplane of a body or part, such as the eyelids, cusps of a heart valve, and genital labia. **2** A midline crossing of a bundle of nerve fibers connecting similar structures on the two sides of the brain or spinal cord. **3** In the spinal cord, one of the bridges of gray matter that cross above and below the central canal. For defs. 1, 2, and 3 also *commissure.* Adj. commissural. See also DECUSSATION. **c. alba medullae spinalis** [NA] A zone of white fibers in the spinal cord passing from one side to the other ventral to the central canal. The gray commissure borders it dorsally and the median fissure ventrally. Also *anterior white commissure, ventral white commissure, commissure of white matter of cord.* **c. anterior cerebri** [NA] The anterior commissure of the telencephalon containing myelinated axons connecting the paired olfactory bulbs and connecting symmetrical zones of the frontal and temporal cortex. Also *anterior commissure, anterior commissure of cerebrum.* **c. anterior grisea medullae spinalis** The thin layer of gray matter situated ventral to the central canal of the spinal cord. **c. colliculorum anteriorum** The commissural fibers connecting homotopic regions of the paired superior colliculi. **c. colliculorum inferiorum** The midline axonal bundle connecting homotopic regions of the paired inferior colliculi. **c. fornicis** [NA] A bundle of fibers arising from the hippocampal fimbria and the posterior column of the fornix to cross to the opposite column and hippocampus. Its position marks the beginning of the body of the fornix, though less concentrated commissural fibers are found as far anterior as the septum pellucidum. Also *commissura hippocampi, hippocampal commissure, commissure of fornix, delta fornicis,.* **c. grisea medullae spinalis** **1** Any of the zones of neurons and nonmyelinated fibers bordering the ependyma immediately dorsal or ventral to the central canal. **2** The total of such connecting gray matter dorsal and ventral to the canal. **c. habenularum** [NA] A looping bundle of fibers connecting the two habenular nuclei and associated striae. It lies at the base of the dorsal lamina leading to the pineal body, hence above the posterior commissure. Also *commissure of habenulae.* **c. hippocampi** COMMISSURA FORNICIS. **c. inferior guddeni** GUDDEN'S COMMISSURE. **c. labiorum anterior** [NA] The junction of the labia majora anteriorly above the clitoris. Also *anterior commissure of labia.* **c. labiorum oris** [NA] The junction of the upper and lower lips, lateral to the corner of the mouth on each side of the oral fissure. Also *commissure of lips of mouth, junction of the lips.*

**c. labiorum posterior** [NA] The posterior boundary of the pudendal cleft where the posterior ends of the labia majora flatten and are joined to each other by skin of the perineum. Also *posterior commissure of labia.* **c. magna cerebri** CORPUS CALLOSUM. **c. optica** CHIASMA OPTICUM. **c. palpebrarum lateralis** [NA] The union of the upper and lower eyelids at the lateral angle of the eye. Also *lateral palpebral commissure, lateral commissure of eyelids, lateral canthus, outer canthus.* **c. palpebrarum medialis** [NA] The union of the upper and lower eyelids at the medial angle of the eye. The junction is more rounded and extended than the lateral angle so that it is not in contact with the eyeball, forming the lacus lacrimalis. Also *medial palpebral commissure, medial commissure of eyelids, medial canthus, inner canthus.* **c. posterior cerebri** [NA] A large bundle of fibers dorsal to the third ventricle entrance to the aqueduct, i.e., at the base of the inferior wall of the pineal recess. It is composed of crossing fibers from the posterior commissural nucleus of Darkschewitsch, the interstitial nucleus, the medial longitudinal fasciculus, and the habenular and other nearby nuclei. Also *posterior commissure.* **c. posterior medullae spinalis** The stratum of gray matter dorsal to the central canal connecting the central gray masses on the two sides of the cord. **c. superior meynerti** VENTRAL SUPRAOPTIC COMMISSURE. **c. supraoptica dorsalis** DORSAL SUPRAOPTIC COMMISSURE. **commissurae supraopticae** In the human brain, those fiber tracts crossing in the lamina terminalis dorsal to the optic tract and below the anterior commissure. They include the commissures of Ganser, Gudden, and Meynert, which for the most part designate decussations. Also *supraoptic commissures.*

**commissurae** \käm′isyoo′rē\ Plural of COMMISSURA.

**commissural** \kəmis′yərəl, käm′isyoo′rəl\ Pertaining to or having the appearance of a commissure.

**commissure** \käm′ishoor\ [French, from L *commissure.* See COMMISSURA.] COMMISSURA. **anterior c.** COMMISSURA ANTERIOR CEREBRI. **anterior c. of cerebrum** COMMISSURA ANTERIOR CEREBRI. **anterior hypothalamic c.** DORSAL SUPRAOPTIC COMMISSURE. **anterior c. of labia** COMMISSURA LABIORUM ANTERIOR. **anterior white c.** COMMISSURA ALBA MEDULLAE SPINALIS. **c. of the bulb** PARS INTERMEDIA BULBORUM. **chiasmatic posterior c.** VENTRAL SUPRAOPTIC COMMISSURE. **dorsal c. of the cerebellum** In an embryo, fibers crossing the roof of the fourth ventricle around which the corpus cerebelli will develop. *Seldom used.* **dorsal supraoptic c.** The more dorsal and anterior of the supraoptic commissures. Its fibers arise at hypothalamic and even midbrain loci, and after crossing pass to pallidum and subthalamus regions. Also *commissura supraoptica dorsalis, superior hypothalamic decussation, anterior hypothalamic decussation, anterior hypothalamic commissure, commissure of Ganser, superior supraoptic decussation, decussatio supraoptica dorsalis, superior commissure.* **Forel's c.** SUPRAMAMILLARY DECUSSATION. • It is distinct from Forel's decussation (ventral tegmental decussation). **c. of fornix** COMMISSURA FORNICIS. **c. of Ganser** DORSAL SUPRAOPTIC COMMISSURE. **great c.** CORPUS CALLOSUM. **Gudden's c.** Fibers of the ventral supraoptic commissure that course within the optic chiasma at one point in their pathway between the medial geniculate bodies on either side. Also *commissura inferior guddeni, intrachiasmatic commissure.* **c. of habenulae** COMMISSURA HABENULARUM. **hippocampal c.** COMMISSURA FORNICIS. **inferior c.** Fascicles of the two tractus solitarii that cross beneath the gracile fasciculi and above the central canal at the lower end of the medulla. **interthalamic c.** ADHESIO INTERTHALAMICA. **intrachiasmatic c.** GUDDEN'S COMMISSURE. **lateral c. of the cerebellum** In an embryo, fibers in the roof of the fourth ventricle which pass between the vestibular nuclei on the two sides. The flocculonodular lobe develops around it. **lateral c. of eyelids** COMMISSURA PALPEBRARUM LATERALIS. **lateral palpebral c.** COMMISSURA PALPEBRARUM LATERALIS. **c. of lips of mouth** COMMISSURA LABIORUM ORIS. **medial c. of eyelids** COMMISSURA PALPEBRARUM MEDIALIS. **medial palpebral c.** COMMISSURA PALPEBRARUM MEDIALIS. **Meynert's c.** VENTRAL SUPRAOPTIC COMMISSURE. **middle c. of cerebrum** *Obs.* ADHESIO INTERTHALAMICA. **optic c.** CHIASMA OPTICUM. **posterior c.** COMMISSURA POSTERIOR CEREBRI. **posterior c. of labia** COMMISSURA LABIORUM POSTERIOR. **superior c.** DORSAL SUPRAOPTIC COMMISSURE. **supraoptic c.'s** COMMISSURAE SUPRAOPTICAE. **ventral supraoptic c.** Fibers decussating immediately dorsal to the optic commissure and to some extent coursing within it. A variety of origins and destinations have been described for the fibers, including the lower brainstem, the midbrain tegmentum, and particularly the medial geniculate body. In submammals, some fibers connect the superior and inferior colliculi, and others are decussating tectothalamic, tectosubthalamic, and tectohypothalamic fascicles. Also *decussatio supraoptica ventralis, Meynert's commissure, commissura superior meynerti, suprachiasmatic decussation, inferior hypothalamic decussation, chiasmatic posterior commissure, ventral supraoptic decussation.* **ventral white c.** COMMISSURA ALBA MEDULLAE SPINALIS. **c. of the vestibule** PARS INTERMEDIA BULBORUM. **c.'s of vulva** The commissura labiorum anterior and the commissura labiorum posterior considered together. **c. of white matter of cord** COMMISSURA ALBA MEDULLAE SPINALIS.

**commissurorrhaphy** \käm′isyərôr′əfē\ [*commissur(e)* + *o* + -RRHAPHY] Suture closure of a commissure to decrease the size of the adjacent orifice.

**commissurotomy** \käm′isyərät′əmē\ [*commisur(e)* + *o* + -TOMY] **1** The division by surgical means of any commissure. **2** COMMISSURAL MYELOTOMY. **mitral c.** An incision or fracture of fused mitral valve commissures. It is usually performed to relieve mitral stenosis. Also *mitral valvotomy.*

**commitment** \kəmit′mənt\ [L *commit(tere)* (from *com-* together + *mittere* to send) to commit, consign + -MENT] The act of placing a patient into a hospital, especially a mental hospital, or under some other kind of protective custody, usually by way of certifying that the individual is unable to meet the demands of daily living or is a source of danger to himself or others. Compare VOLUNTARY ADMISSION.

**committee / tissue c.** A committee in a hospital which reviews and evaluates all surgery that is performed primarily using criteria related to pathological diagnosis and preoperative indications.

**commotio** \kämō′shō\ [L, a moving, commotion] Concussion or shock wave. *Seldom used.* **c. cerebri** CONCUSSION OF THE BRAIN. **c. retinae** Edema of the retina, usually affecting the macula, following ocular contusion. Also *concussion of the retina.* **c. spinalis** CONCUSSION OF THE SPINAL CORD.

**communicable** \kəmyoo′nəkəbəl\ Capable of being transmitted from one organism to another.

**Communicable Disease Center** The former name of the Centers for Disease Control.

**communication** **1** Information or ideas exchanged or transmitted from one party to another. **2** Access between two structures. 3 In anatomy, the linking or extension of a structure or part to another part or region. **arteriovenous c.** 1 An abnormal connection between artery and vein, without interposition of capillaries. 2 ARTERIOVENOUS SHUNT. **confidential c.** Personal and private information concerning an individual that is volunteered or discovered during a professional, confidential relationship and that the recipient is legally and ethically forbidden to divulge without the consent of the confiding individual, except under circumstances defined by law. In some jurisdictions, knowledge that an individual is a danger to society is a circumstance allowing a breach of confidentiality. **nonverbal c.** Those aspects of the communication of information between individuals that do not explicitly employ language, such as facial expression, gesture, body posture, proximity, and touching. Many of these signals serve to communicate the affective or attitudinal state of the individual and may be relatively unconscious and involuntary. **privileged c.** Confidential information received in the course of a confidential relationship that the recipient cannot be forced to divulge, as in a judicial proceeding, without the consent of the informant, except as defined by the applicable laws of the state or jurisdiction.

**communis** \kəmyoo′nis\ [L, common, general, ordinary] Common; possessed by several.

**community / therapeutic c.** 1 A psychiatric hospital or unit whose social organization is used as a primary tool in treatment, management, resocialization, and rehabilitation of its patients. 2 A drug-free residential program for rehabilitating drug addicts.

**comp.** *compositus* (L, a compound: used in pharmacy).

**compact** \kämpakt′\ Solid, compressed, and lacking spaces within, such as compact bone.

**compacta** \kämpak′tə\ STRATUM COMPACTUM ENDOMETRII.

**compaction** \kämpak′shən\ [L *compactio* (from *compingere* to fasten or join together) a putting or joining together] INTERLOCKING.

**compages thoracis** \kämpā′jēz thôrā′sis\ [L *compages* framework (from *compingere* to enclose, hold together) + *thoracis* of the thorax] [NA] The bony skeleton enclosing the thoracic cavity, comprising the thoracic vertebrae, ribs, costal cartilages, and sternum and having a superior aperture continuous with the neck and an inferior aperture closed by the diaphragm. It protects and supports the thoracic viscera, and functions during respiration. Also *rib cage* (popular).

**compartment** One of the areas partitioned off within a larger enclosed space; a separate section or chamber. **extracellular c.** A space within the body or within a tissue that is external to the cells. **intracellular c.** The space within the body or within a tissue which is occupied by the cells. **muscular c.** LACUNA MUSCULORUM.

**compartmentalization** \käm′pärtmen′təlīzā′shən\ 1 The partitioning of the protoplasm of a cell into compartments, each enclosed by a selectively permeable membrane. Cytoplasmic organelles, such as mitochondria, Golgi vesicles, and lysosomes, are examples of cellular compartments. Also *compartmentation.* 2 The unconscious defense mechanism of keeping separate different parts of the mental apparatus or character that ordinarily would be kept together.

**compatibility** 1 The capacity of two or more drugs when given together to act without producing adverse chemical interactions and without antagonizing the actions of any of the component agents. 2 The state of being compatible; the capacity to exist together without harmful consequences.

**compatible** [Med L *compatibilis* (from *com-* with + *pati* to tolerate) mutually tolerant, simultaneously tenable] 1 Exhibiting compatibility, as two drugs. 2 Capable of existing together without harmful consequences.

**compendium** (*pl.* compendiums, compendia) A comprehensive collection of important information in summary form on a large number of related items or topics. **drug c.** A comprehensive collection of essential, summary information on a large number of drugs, like a pharmacopoeia.

**compensation** \käm′pənsā′shən\ [L *compensatio* (from *com-* COM- + *pensatus,* past part. of *pensare* to weigh ) a balancing together] 1 The tendency of an organism to respond to impaired function or defect by a change in its activity that counterbalances the impairment or defect. 2 In neurophysiology, the more or less complete return of a behavioral, motor, or sensory function following a deficit caused by damage or dysfunction of a nervous structure normally instrumental to that function, e.g., the return of normal posture following labyrinthectomy. **attenuation c.** SWEPT GAIN. **Bekhterev c.** BEKHTEREV DECOMPENSATION. **dosage c.** The regulation of genes on sex chromosomes that results in the phenotype determined by the homogametic sex being similar to that of the heterogametic sex. In humans, inactivation of most of one of the X chromosomes in the female is the predominant mechanism. **electronic distance c.** SWEPT GAIN. **time gain c.** SWEPT GAIN. Abbr. TGC

**compensator** \käm′pənsā′tər\ In radiation therapy, a filter placed in the radiation beam to modify the dose distribution in the irradiated body.

**compensatory** \kämpen′sətôr′ē\ 1 Correcting or making up for an inferiority or loss, as through hypertrophy of tissue or increased functioning of the organ or system in question; having a counterbalancing effect. 2 Being a substitute for something that is unacceptable or unattainable.

**competence** \käm′pətəns\ [L *competentia* (from *competere* to fit, suit, from COM- + *petere* to seek) correspondence, suitability] 1 The ability to function normally. 2 In embryology, the attribute or ability to differentiate in response to inductors. The competence for neural induction is, for example, restricted to ectoderm and is present during a short period only. 3 In bacteriology, the ability to take up transforming DNA. 4 In forensic medicine, competency. **embryonic c.** The ability of a group of embryonic cells to respond normally to the influence of an inductor. **immunologic c.** IMMUNOCOMPETENCE.

**competency** \käm′pitənsē\ [*competenc(e)* + -Y. See COMPETENCE.] Sufficient mental ability of an individual to allow his participation in a judicial proceeding. A determination of competency is usually ordered by a court in preparation for an individual's acting as a witness or a defendant. **c. to stand trial** The ability of a defendant to understand the nature of the charges against him, to distinguish between pleas of guilty and not guilty, and to prepare a defense, instruct counsel, and challenge a juror. A term used chiefly in the U.S., Canada, New Zealand, and Japan.

**competition** The process by which one rather than the other of two possible reactions takes place. Thus, a binding site may be able to bind two different substances, but not simultaneously. Since only one of them may produce some effect, competition by the other for the site may have inhibitory consequences. Substances that bind at different sites may also show competition if binding at one site prevents binding at the other. Similar competition may occur between enzymes or receptors. **antigenic c.** In immunization, a response to one antigen in a mixture that is less than the response to the same antigen given alone.

**compimeter** \kämpim′ətər\ [L *compi(tum)* a place where two or more ways meet, a crossroad + -METER] TANGENT SCREEN.

**complaint** A disease or symptom, especially as reported by the patient on seeking medical treatment.

**complement** [L *complementum* (from COM- + root *ple* of L *complere* to fill up) what is added to complete a thing] The heat-labile constituent of normal (nonimmune) serum that is required in addition to specific antibody to bring about the immune lysis of erythrocytes or of certain bacteria. Complement is made up of about twenty distinct proteins which form in part two triggered enzyme cascades (the classical and alternative pathways) culminating in the activation of C3, and proceed to the formation of a self-associating, multimolecular complex (membrane attack complex or membrane attack complement pathway) which can insert into membranes and cause them to leak. In addition to its membrane-damaging properties, complement is an important inflammatory mediator system. Also *alexin* (obs.). See also COMPONENT OF COMPLEMENT under COMPONENT. **chromosome c.** The total set of nuclear chromosomes of an organism. In humans, the normal chromosome complement comprises 22 pairs of autosomes and 2 sex chromosomes. **component of c.** See under COMPONENT.

**complementarity** \käm′pləməntar′itē\ In families and other groups, the degree of balance that has been reached between the emotional needs of the individual members. **dominant c.** Complementation by two loci when each is heterozygous with the phenotype determined by the action and interaction of one allele at each locus. Compare RECESSIVE COMPLEMENTARITY. **recessive c.** Complementation by two loci when each is homozygous for alleles that separately determine recessive traits. The presence of heterozygosity for an allele at either locus that specifies a dominant trait suppresses the complementary phenotype. Compare DOMINANT COMPLEMENTARITY.

**complementary** \käm′pləmen′tərē\ **1** Serving to complete or to partially correct a deficiency. **2** Mutually supplying each other's lack, as the relationship that obtains between a dominant and submissive partner. **3** Describing a color which when mixed with another results in white. **4** Describing a color which is specific as an afterimage or contrast with another color.

**complementation** \käm′pləmentā′shən\ The restoration of a wild-type phenotype or function through interaction of two cells, chromosomes, or viruses, each of which is a genetic mutant at a different locus. In general, complementation occurs only between different genes (cistrons). **allelic c.** INTERGENIC COMPLEMENTATION. **interallelic c.** INTERGENIC COMPLEMENTATION. **intercistronic c.** Intergenic complementation in which the two mutant genes are not part of the same cistron. **intergenic c.** Complementation resulting from mutations occurring in two different genetic loci in diploid organisms. The process was first described in bacteria rendered partially diploid for at least the two loci at issue and in bacteriophage in which two strains, each carrying one of the mutations, separately infected a single bacterium. Also *allelic complementation, interallelic complementation.* **intracistronic c.** Intergenic complementation in which the two mutant genes are part of the same cistron. **intragenic c.** Complementation in diploid organisms resulting from the presence of different mutations at the same genetic locus. The two mutant alleles in some manner cancel their usual expression or lack thereof, resulting in at least partial restoration of the wild phenotype. ***in vitro* c.** **1** Complementation that occurs as a result of processes or manipulations outside the organism, as the production of a recombinant DNA molecule with a functional sequence from two mutant clones of DNA. **2** The metabolic reconstitution that takes place when two cell lines with similar or identical mutant phenotypes are fused.

**complex** \käm′pleks\ [L *complexus* (past part. of *complecti* to contain, surround, compass, from COM- + L *plectere* to twist, plait, bend) a compassing, encircling] **1** In electroencephalography, a group of recurring brain waves varying in amplitude and duration, but bearing a constant relation to one another, and having a constant shape and form. **2** In electrocardiography, a deflection composed of two or more components, as *QRS complex.* **3** An entity formed by combination of two or more molecules, often combining reversibly or noncovalently. **4** To form a complex with. **5** The aggregation of ideas or emotions of particular significance to the subject with associated ideas and affects. The resulting aggregate is typically repressed, in whole or in part, and exerts a determining or modifying influence on the subject's thoughts, feelings, actions, and personality. Also *constellation.* **6** See under IMMUNE COMPLEX. **abortive c.** A complex formed between an enzyme and one or more substrate molecules when this complex cannot proceed to form products. Examples include an enzyme that has bound a substrate incorrectly, and one that has bound two molecules of donor or acceptor in a transferase reaction instead of one of each. Compare PRODUCTIVE COMPLEX. **AIDS-related c.** See under ACQUIRED IMMUNE DEFICIENCY SYNDROME. **antigen-antibody c.** IMMUNE COMPLEX. **apical c.** A system of organelles, characteristic of sporozoan protozoa of the phylum Apicomplexa. Components of the system include polar ring or rings, conoid, micronemes, rhoptries, and subpellicular tubules present at some stage. **atrial c.** The portion of the electrocardiogram that represents electrical activation of the atria; the P wave. **basal lamina c. of choroid** COMPLEXUS BASALIS CHOROIDEAE. **Behçet triple symptom c.** BEHÇET SYNDROME. **castration c.** A complex distinguished by the fear of loss of or injury to the penis, typically associated with the phallic and oedipal phases of psychosexual development. See also CASTRATION ANXIETY. **Clérambault-Kandinsky c.** A delusional syndrome in which the central feature is a feeling that one's mind is controlled by some outside agency. Also *Clérambault-Kandinsky syndrome.* **diphasic c.** An electrocardiographic complex with both positive and negative deflections. **EAHF c.** The combination of eczema, asthma, and hay fever. **Eisenmenger's c.** A congenital malformation characterized by a combination of a ventricular septal defect together with overriding of the aortic valve. It should not be confused with the Eisenmenger syndrome, which is pulmonary vascular disease because of a left-to-right shunt. Also *Eisenmenger's tetralogy.* **Electra c.** The female form of the Oedipus complex. *Older term.* Also *father complex.* **equiphasic c.** An electrocardiographic complex in which positive and negative deflections are equal. **father c.** ELECTRA COMPLEX. **female Oedipus c.** See under OEDIPUS COMPLEX. **flocculonodular c.** FLOCCULONODULAR LOBE. **Friedmann's c.** BOXERS' ENCEPHALOPATHY. **Ghon c.** PRIMARY COMPLEX. **Golgi c.** GOLGI APPARATUS. **hapten-carrier c.** The whole antigenic structure resulting from the coupling of a hapten and a carrier. **hemoglobin-haptoglobin c.** The binding of a hemoglobin and haptoglobin molecule. Due to the high affinity between the two, plasma hemoglobin is not found in a free state until all free haptoglobin has been consumed, a situation caused by severe intravascular hemolysis. **immune c.** A macromolecular complex of antigen and antibody molecules bound together in a lattice. Soluble complexes found particularly in excess of antigen are small aggregates while large complexes are found at equivalence and are insoluble. Also *antigen-antibody complex.* **inferior olivary c.** The convoluted nucleus in the basal medulla overlying the corticospinal tract and lateral to the medial lemniscus. The complex consists of three nuclei: 1) a principal inferior, 2) a dorsal accessory, and 3) a medial accessory olivary nucleus. The axons of this nucleus project upon the cerebellum via the inferior cerebellar peduncle. **iron-dextran c.** IRON-DEXTRAN INJECTION. **jumped process c.** A dislocation of one or both zygapophysial joints between the articular processes of vertebrae. **junctional c.** See under TERMINAL BAR. **K c.** In electroencephalography, a slow-wave complex of high amplitude evoked by a sensory stimulus while the subject is asleep. **Lutembacher's c.** LUTEMBACHER SYNDROME. **major histocompatibility c.** A small region of the genome which is highly conserved in vertebrate evolution and codes for three classes of highly polymorphic molecules of immunologic interest. Class 1 products are the transplantation antigens having $\beta2$ microglobulin as their light chain. Only the heavy chain is coded in the major histocompatibility complex (MHC). Class 2 products are the transplantation antigens without $\beta2$ microglobulin. Both their $\alpha$ chains and $\beta$ chains are coded in the MHC. Class 3 products are complement components. In man, the MHC is on chromosome 6 and is called HLA (human lymphocyte antigens). Class 1 molecules are contained in HLA-A, HLA-B, HLA-C; Class 2 molecules in HLA-DR, HLA-DC (renamed DQ), and HLA-SB (renamed DP); Class 3 and HLA-DZ molecules are C2, factor B, and a duplicated locus for C4 (C4A and C4B). T lymphocytes recognize antigens only in the context of MHC (Class 1 or Class 2) molecules. There are many diseases susceptibility to which is associated with particular HLA antigens. Also *MHC complex.* Abbr. MHC **membrane attack c.** See under COMPLEMENT. **Meyenburg's c.'es** Microhamartomas of the biliary tract system composed of cystically dilated bile ducts lying in a fibrous tissue stroma, seen in polycystic disease of the liver in adults. **MHC c.** MAJOR HISTOCOMPATIBILITY COMPLEX. **oculomotor nuclear c.** The nuclear complex consisting of motor neurons innervating eye muscles supplied by the nervus oculomotorius (third cranial nerve). Also *oculomotor complex.* **Oedipus c.** That stage of infantile psychosexual development when the child's love of the opposite-sex parent and rivalry with the same-sex parent is at its height, typically at about five years of age. In psychoanalytic theory, the Oedipus complex is the nuclear concept of the neuroses and significantly influences adult sexuality. • The term alludes to the Oedipus of Greek mythology, who unwittingly killed his father and married his mother. *Oedipus complex* may be used to refer to a child of either sex. However, in contexts where a distinction is necessary, *female Oedipus complex* is sometimes used to avoid confusion with the term's original reference to male children exclusively. **Parkinson-dementia c.** A progressive degenerative disease of the central nervous system giving rise to features of both parkinsonism and dementia and sometimes associated with evidence of amyotrophic lateral sclerosis. It is endemic among the Chamorro people on the island of Guam and in some other areas of the Pacific. **primary c.** The combination of a circumscribed, tuberculous pulmonary lesion and extension of disease to regional lymph nodes. It is seen as an initial manifestation of tuberculosis, usually in children. Also *Ghon complex.* **productive c.** A complex between an enzyme and substrate(s) that can proceed to form products. Compare ABORTIVE COMPLEX. **QRS c.** The deflections of the electrocardiogram caused by depolarization of the ventricles, consisting of an upward, or positive, deflection (R) preceded and followed by negative deflections (Q and S). One or two of the three components may be absent. Also *ventricular depolarization complex.* See also Q WAVE, R WAVE, S WAVE. **QRST c.** The deflections of the electrocardiogram caused by depolarization and repolarization of the muscles of the ventricles during the course of ventricular systole. **ribosome-lamella c.** GRANULAR ENDOPLASMIC RETICULUM. **Schilder-Addison c.** ADRENOLEUKODYSTROPHY. **soluble c.** An antigen-antibody complex which does not go on to precipitate. Soluble complexes may be formed in either antigen or antibody excess rather than at equivalence. Complexes formed in the presence of complement are much more soluble than those formed in its absence. **spike-wave c.** In electroencephalography, a recurring wave form consisting of a single slow wave with an associated spike. Usually the slow wave and the spike are of consistent amplitude and bear a constant temporal relationship to each other. When these discharges occur at a frequency of 3 Hz, they are virtually diagnostic of epilepsy and are usually but not invariably associated with petit mal. Slower variants are less specific, as are irregular wave and spike discharges. **Steidele's c.** An absence of the aortic arch from birth. **symptom c.** A constellation of symptoms constituting a clinical syndrome. **synaptonemal c.** **1** The structure found between two homologous chromosomes that can be defined by electron microscopy at the region of a meiotic synapsis. It consists of two lateral elements that flank a central element. The lateral elements are interconnected with the central element by transverse filaments. The complex is 0.2 μm thick and runs the entire length of the chromosome. The coaxial complex is associated with the nuclear membrane. **2** The region of contact between one neuron and the next in a pathway. It includes the terminal bouton of the afferent fiber, the synaptic cleft, and the specialized area or postsynaptic membrane of the efferent fiber. **ternary c.** A complex of three components, especially that of an enzyme with both its substrates bound. **ureterotrigonal c.** URETEROVESICAL JUNCTION. **ventricular c.** The deflections of the electrocardiogram associated with ventricular systole; the QRST complex. **ventricular depolarization c.** QRS COMPLEX. **Wilks symptom c.** MYASTHENIA GRAVIS.

**complexion** [Old French *complexion* a mixing of humors, temperament, from L *complexio* a combination, from *complexus,* past part. of *complecti* to compass, encircle] The color and texture of the skin of the face.

**complexus** \kämplek′səs\ [L, a compassing, encircling] **1** An anatomical structure consisting of several parts. **2** MUSCULUS SEMISPINALIS CAPITIS. **c. basalis choroideae** [NA] The thin, innermost layer of the choroid proper, which was considered to be a homogeneous, glassy membrane prior to electron microscopy, but now has been shown to consist of two layers, namely, an external stratum elasticum comprising a dense network of elastic fibers continuous with the basement membrane of lamina choroidocapillaris and in contact with the neuroglia of the optic nerve fibers posteriorly, and a stratum fibrosum internally which is continuous with the basement membrane of the pigment cells of the retina and ends posteriorly at the optic disk. Both layers extend anteriorly into the ciliary body. Also *lamina basalis choroideae, Bruch's layer, Bruch's membrane, glassy membrane, Henle's membrane, Hovius membrane, basal lamina of choroid, posterior border lamella of Fuchs* (outmoded), *vitreous membrane, vitreous lamella, basal layer, basal lamina complex of choroid, entochoroidea.*

**compliance** \kəmplī′əns\ 1 Flexibility, as in an ability to yield to pressure. 2 The volume change resulting from the application of a unit change in pressure between the inside and outside of a hollow viscus. Compare ELASTANCE. 3 Disposition to follow a prescribed regimen or specific instructions, as those of a physician to a patient, as in *patient compliance.* **dynamic c.** Pulmonary compliance calculated during normal breathing without cessation of respiration. Compare STATIC COMPLIANCE. **motor c.** A state of oversubmissiveness or oversuggestibility of behavior, as in schizophrenic children who go limp in the lap of the examiner or move their entire body in response to a single touch on the palm. **pulmonary c.** Lung distensibility, measured as pressure required per unit increase of lung volume. **somatic c.** The degree to which a person's motor or organ functioning can express the energy of unconscious impulses, which can thus be converted into the physical symptoms of conversion hysteria or the somatoform disorders. **static c.** Pulmonary compliance calculated by measuring lung volumes and corresponding distending pressures at intervals during which breathing is interrupted transiently. Compare DYNAMIC COMPLIANCE.

**complicated** Characterized by complications, as a disease.

**complication** [Late L *complicatio* (from L *complicatus,* past part. of *complicare* to fold together, from *com-* with + *plicare* to fold) a folding together] A disease or other disorder that arises in a subject from a preexisting disorder, or which arises from an unrelated cause but aggrevates the preexisting disorder.

**component** \kəmpō′nənt\ A constituent part, especially, an integral or essential part. **c. of complement** The individual proteins that make up the complement system. Those components that are needed for the lysis of antibody-coated sheep erythrocytes by human or guinea-pig serum are denoted as C1–C9, although the reactive sequence is C1, C4, C2, C3, C5 . . . C9. (C denotes complement). This sequence comprises the components peculiar to the classical pathway: C1, C4, and C2; C3, which is common to all pathways; and the components of the membrane attack pathway C5–C9. The components peculiar to the alternative pathway are denoted as FB, FD, and properdin. (F denotes factor.) The control proteins are C1-inhibitor, FI, FH, C4-binding protein, and S-protein. Decay accelerating factor and the complement receptor CR1 are further control proteins that occur on cell membranes but not in plasma. **G c.** G FACTOR OF SPEARMAN. **plasma thromboplastin c.** FACTOR IX. Abbr. PTC **thromboplastic plasma c.** FACTOR VIII. **Woodbridge's c.'s of anesthesia** The four components which are considered essential in the general anesthetic state: sensory depression, motor blockade, unconsciousness, and suppression of reflex actions.

**composition** The proportion of substances in a mixture or of elements in a compound. **modeling c.** MODELING COMPOUND.

**compos mentis** \käm′pōs men′tis\ [L *compos* (from *com-* with + *potis* able, possible) able, master of + *mentis,* gen. of *mens* mind, reason] Sound of mind; denoting a state of health in which there is full control and use of one's mental faculties. Compare NON COMPOS MENTIS.

**compound** 1 A substance composed of different elements. 2 A combination of two or more ingredients, as in a pharmaceutical preparation. **APC c.** A preparation containing acetylsalicylic acid, phenacetin, and caffeine. **c. G-11** HEXACHLOROPHENE. **genetic c.** 1 A diploid genotype that is characterized by heterozygosity for two different mutant alleles. 2 A cell or organism that is heterozygous for two different alleles. The resulting phenotype is often intermediate to those of the mutant alleles when homozygous. Also *compound heterozygote, allozygote.* **Hurler-Scheie c.** MUCOPOLYSACCHARIDOSIS IH/S. **impression c.** MODELING COMPOUND. **isopropyl alcohol rubbing c.** A 70% solution of isopropyl alcohol in water which is used on the skin as a rubefacient. **methonium c.'s** A family of compounds, such as hexamethonium, which impede ganglionic neural impulses. Such agents are employed in the management of hypertension. **modeling c.** A thermoplastic material used for impressions and occlusal rims. Also *modeling composition, impression compound, modeling plastic.* **Reichstein's c. Q** *Older term* 11-DEOXYCORTICOSTERONE. **sulfonylurea c.'s** Isopropylthiodiazylsulfonilamide compounds that are closely related to the sulfonamide drugs, which lower the blood sugar levels and have been useful in the treatment of diabetes. Among them are acetohexamide, thiohexamide, tolbutamide, and chlorpropamide.

**compounding** The art of mixing drugs and drug ingredients to obtain a formula suitable as a medication for the purpose intended.

**compress** \(1) käm′pres; (2) kəmpres′\ [L *compressus* (from *compressus,* past part. of *comprimere* to press or squeeze together) a pressing together] 1 A pad of usually folded material applied to develop pressure on a body part. 2 To cause to undergo compression. **cribriform c.** A compress that is finely perforated to allow the escape of wound fluids. **fenestrated c.** A compress in which there are holes for escape of wound fluids and for visual inspection of the wound.

**compression** The application of pressure on a body, part of a body, a volume of gas, etc., resulting in increased compactness or density. **c. of the brain** CEREBRAL COMPRESSION. **cardiac c.** 1 Constant pressure upon the heart, as by fluid, exudate, or tumors in the pericardium, such that its proper relaxation is impeded. 2 CARDIAC MASSAGE. **c. of the cauda equina** Pressure on the cauda equina due to any process such as primary or secondary neoplasia, inflammation, or hemorrhage. **cerebral c.** The effect upon the cerebrum of any focal lesion, such as a tumor, abscess, or hemorrhage, which compresses the brain. Also *compression of the brain.* • The term is sometimes applied to intracranial hypertension, thus embracing various other processes such as cerebral edema, which increase the intracranial pressure. **digital c.** Pressure by fingers or thumb upon a wound that compresses a blood vessel to prevent bleeding. **jugular c.** The application of pressure by means of a digit or instrument to the internal jugular vein with consequent back pressure in the cerebral venous sinuses and an increase in the intracranial pressure which may be demonstrable by cerebrospinal fluid manometry. **c. of nerve roots** Injury to segmental spinal roots, and often also of spinal nerves, as they enter, traverse, or leave the neural foramina and the spinal cord, usually resulting from a herniated disk or an osteophyte. **renal artery c.** Compression of a main renal artery by a tumor or fibrous band. Depending on the degree of compression, hypertension, renal scarring, and renal functional impairment may result. **spinal c.** Pressure applied to the spinal cord by any process, such as primary or secondary neoplasia, inflammation or hemorrhage, and affecting its function. **sponge stick c.** The use of a sponge stick pressed vigorously upon a vessel to control hemorrhage. It is useful in the control and repair of an aortocaval fistula.

**compressor** An instrument, machine, or muscle which compresses. **aortic c.** A T-shaped device that is used to compress the abdominal aorta, thereby controlling or diminishing hemorrhage following trauma or aneurysm rupture. **c. naris** PARS TRANSVERSA MUSCULI NASALIS. **c. radicis penis** Fibers, usually anterior, of the bulbospongiosus muscle that spread over the root of the penis. *Outmoded.* **c. urethrae** See under MUSCULUS COMPRESSOR URETHRAE. **urethral c.** 1 Elastic metal forceps, covered with rubber, into which the penis is introduced to close the urethra in urinary incontinence or to retain a soluble drug or anesthetic in the urethra. 2 See under MUSCULUS COMPRESSOR URETHRAE. **c. vaginae** The musculus bulbospongiosus in the female. Also *constrictor vaginae* (outmoded). **c. venae dorsalis** 1 Occasional fasciculi of the ischiocavernosus muscle that pass anteriorly to the dorsal surface of the penis or clitoris. With reference to the penis it is also known as Houston's muscle. *Outmoded.* Also *pubocavernosus.* 2 Fibers of the bulbospongiosus muscle that usually insert into the fascia on the dorsum of the penis or clitoris superficial to the dorsal veins. *Outmoded.*

***Compsomyia macellaria*** \kämp'sōmī'yə mas'əler'ē·ə\ *COCHLIOMYIA MACELLARIA.*

**Compton** [Arthur Holly *Compton,* U.S. physicist, 1892–1962] See under ELECTRON, EFFECT, SCATTERING.

**compulsion** \kəmpul'shən\ [L *compulsus* (past part. of *compellere* to impel, move) impelled] An ego-alien impulse to perform an action, typically repetitively and ritualistically, even though the action is not pleasurable in itself and has no purpose other than to gain temporary relief of tension. Compulsions are obsessions in action and are a major feature of obsessive-compulsive neurosis. Also *compulsive act, compulsive action, forced act, imperious act.* **checking c.** FOLIE DU DOUTE. **repetition c.** A compulsion to repeat earlier actions even though they are painful. According to Freud, the death or destructive or aggressive instincts are under the control of the repetition-compulsion principle, whose major purpose is to restore the organism to an earlier condition.

**computer** [L *computare* to count, calculate] A machine that accepts data, processes it, and supplies the results. **analog c.** A computer that solves problems by setting up electric circuits that are analogous to the mathematical or physical problem. **digital c.** A stored-program computer that performs sequences of instructions on digital data.

**con-** \kän-, kōn-, kən-\ COM-.

**con A** CONCANAVALIN A.

**conalbumin** A protein of egg white. It binds iron(III) and has been identified with transferrin. The carbohydrate content differs between the egg and the serum forms. Also *ovotransferrin.*

**conarium** \kōner'ē·əm\ [New L, from Gk *kōnarion* (dim. of *kōnos* cone) the pineal gland] CORPUS PINEALE.

**conation** \kōnā'shən\ [L *conatio* (from *conari* to strive, undertake) an attempting, striving] The active part of the personality, which includes all striving, acting, and willing; those aspects of mind or behavior that are governed by impulses, wishes, drives, motives, appetites, or aversions. Adj. conative.

**concameration** \känkam'ərā'shən\ [L *concameratio* (from *concameratus,* past part. of *concamerare* to arch over, from *con-* with + *camera* an arched vault, ceiling, or roof) a vaulting, arched place] An arrangement of interconnecting cavities.

**concanavalin A** \kän'kanav'əlin\ A lectin produced in the jack bean, *Canavalin ensiformis.* It binds to all membrane glycoproteins containing α-glucoside or α-mannoside groups and can form clusters. It can also act as a mitogen, chiefly for T lymphocytes, and agglutinates many cell types. Also *con A.*

**concatemer** \känkat'əmir\ [Late L *concate(nare)* (from L *con-* with + *catena* a chain) to link together + Gk *mer(os)* a part] A structure consisting of a number of subunits connected end-to-end as in a chain or row, as a number of genes connected in a row.

**concatenate** \känkat'ənāt\ [Late L *concatenare* (from L *con-* with + *catena* a chain) to link or chain together] 1 To link together in a chain. 2 Having a linked structure, like a chain.

**Concato** [Luigi Maria *Concato,* Italian physician, 1825–1882] See under DISEASE.

**concave** \kän'kāv, känkāv'\ [L *concav(us)* hollow, concave] 1 Rounded and hollow, like part of the interior surface of a sphere. 2 In ophthalmology, pertaining to a negative lens or surface.

**concavity** \känkav'itē\ A hollowed-out, incurved area or depression on the surface of an organ or a structure.

**concavoconcave** \känkā'vōkän'kāv\ Concave on both sides, as an optical lens with negative power on both surfaces.

**concavoconvex** \känkā'vōkän'veks\ Concave on one side and convex on the other, as an optical lens with negative power on one side and positive power on the other.

**concentrate** [French *concentrer* (from CON- + L *centrum* center) to concentrate] 1 A drug preparation that has been increased in strength by evaporation or other means to remove a portion of the inactive liquid or components. 2 A preparation of a drug which is unusually rich in an active material, such as a vitamin. **liver c.** A concentrated preparation of dried mammalian liver which has been used in the past as replacement therapy in certain deficiency diseases, e.g., as a source of iron to stimulate hematopoiesis. **plant protease c.** BROMELAIN.

**concentrated** 1 Designating a substance in solution from which part of the solvent has been removed. 2 Describing a preparation containing a high proportion of the active compound.

**concentration** / **amount of substance c.** See under AMOUNT. **bicarbonate ion c.** The concentration in a fluid containing all bicarbonate compounds. It can be approximated directly, or it can be derived by subtracting from the total carbon dioxide concentration the product of the carbon dioxide partial pressure multiplied by a temperature-related coefficient, which relates carbon dioxide and carbonic acid content to the partial pressure of carbon dioxide. Direct measurement is used for extracellular fluids. For intracellular fluids the derived figure, which includes carbamino compounds and carbonate, may be more appropriate. **maximum allowable c.** The highest concentration of a harmful substance to which daily exposure for eight hours throughout one's working life will not cause any disease or other deviation from a normal state of health. This concept is used in the USSR to determine permissible levels of exposure for workplaces. Abbr. MAC **maximum urinary c.** The maximum concentration of solutes that can be achieved in the urine after 18 to 24 hours of fluid restriction. **mean corpuscular hemoglobin c.** The average hemoglobin concentration expressed in grams per deciliter of packed erythrocytes. It is calculated by dividing hemoglobin concentration (in grams per deciliter) by hematocrit. **minimum alveolar c.** The anesthetic concentration which at one atmosphere produces immobility in 50 percent of the subjects exposed to the noxious stimulus. It is used as a measure of general anesthetic potency. Abbr.

MAC **minimum inhibitory c.** The lowest concentration of an antibiotic agent which, when present in a nutrient culture medium, will prevent growth of a specific bacterial strain. Abbr. MIC **molar c.** A measure of concentration in an amount of substance (moles) per unit volume (liters). In SI units this is expressed as $mol \cdot l^{-1}$. Symbol: M **selective c.** The concentration of an isotope in an organ or tissue compared with that in other tissues or in the whole organism. **substance c.** AMOUNT OF SUBSTANCE CONCENTRATION. See under AMOUNT.

**concentric** \känsen′trik\ Having a common center.

**concept** \kän′sept\ [Med L *conceptus* (from L *concipere* to conceive, from CON- + *capere* to hold, seize) an idea, concept] A mental category, such as "animal," "home," or "gravity," obtained by recognizing, isolating, and then naming a property held in common by several elements originating from different sources. Although in a strict interpretation a concept is an idea of any entity, whether abstract or concrete, it is more often restricted to any broad organizing or explanatory principle or belief. Also *conception.* **no-threshold c.** The concept that no critical threshold dose exists which is completely free of effects, despite difficulties in measuring such effects. In radiology, diminishingly small doses of ionizing radiation have mutational, cell lethal, or DNA damaging effects of progressively less importance.

**conception** \känsep′shən\ [L *conceptio* (from *concipere* to catch, catch on, conceive, from CON- + *capere* to take, take hold) conception, inception of pregnancy, a concept] 1 The act or condition of becoming pregnant; the initiation of pregnancy. 2 The process of forming a concept. 3 CONCEPT.

**conceptive** \känsep′tiv\ 1 Capable of conceiving. 2 Pertaining to conception.

**conceptus** \kənsep′təs\ [L (from *concipere* to conceive) conception, the result of conception] The total products of conception, not just the embryo or fetus but everything derived from the fertilized egg, including the entire chorionic sac in early stages of pregnancy and the placenta with fetal membranes in later stages. Also *gestation sac.*

**concerted** \kənsur′tid\ Describing two steps in a chemical reaction if the energy barrier to their occurring together is less than that for either alone. Thus, for example, in the transfer of a methyl group from *S*-adenosylmethionine to ethanolamine in choline formation, bond formation between the N and C atoms is concerted with bond breakage between C and S atoms, since the former alone would make a 5-coordinate carbon atom, and the latter alone would make a 3-coordinate carbon atom, both highly unstable.

**concha** \käng′kə\ [L (from Gk *konchē* a mussel, mussel shell, any shell-like object) a shellfish, seashell] (*pl.* conchae) [NA] Any structure resembling the form of a shell, as the conchae of the auricle of the external ear and of the nasal cavity. **c. of auricle** CONCHA AURICULAE. **c. auriculae** [NA] A deep hollow on the lateral surface of the auricle of the external ear, partly surrounded posteriorly by the anthelix and having the tragus and the antitragus overlapping it anteriorly and inferiorly respectively. The cavity is partly divided by the crus helicis into the cymba conchae above it and the cavitas conchae below. Also *concha of auricle.* **c. lacrimalis** A thin, bony lamella, recurved anteriorly and inward, that forms the posterior margin of the lacrimal sulcus on the nasal surface of the maxilla. There it also elevates the anterior margin of the orifice of the maxillary sinus. It articulates with the lacrimal bone and helps to form the nasolacrimal canal. *Outmoded.* **c. nasalis** One of the horizontal bony projections of the lateral wall of the nasal cavity which is covered by mucous membrane and separates one nasal meatus from another above and/or below. Three are usually present, namely the concha nasalis superior, concha nasalis media, and concha nasalis inferior. A fourth, the concha nasalis suprema, is occasionally present. Also *nasal turbinate, turbinate.* **c. nasalis inferior** [NA] A thin, curved bony plate articulating with the nasal surface of the maxilla and the perpendicular plate of the palatine bone and overhanging the inferior nasal meatus of the lateral wall of the nasal cavity. Its lacrimal process helps to form the canal for the nasolacrimal duct, which opens under cover of its anterior portion. It lies horizontally and is covered by thick mucous membrane. Also *inferior spongy bone* (outmoded), *inferior turbinate bone, maxilloturbinal bone, infraturbinal, inferior turbinate.* **c. nasalis media** [NA] A large bony projection from the entire length of the medial surface of the ethmoidal labyrinth, extending posteriorly to articulate with the perpendicular plate of the palatine bone and having its concave lateral surface overhanging the middle meatus of the nasal cavity. It is covered by thick mucous membrane. Also *middle turbinate bone, middle nasal turbinate, mesoturbinal, mesoturbinate.* **c. nasalis superior** [NA] A bony plate projecting from the medial surface of the ethmoidal labyrinth, smaller than and lying above and behind the middle nasal concha, and overhanging the small, shallow superior nasal meatus. Posteriorly the superior concha is separated by the sphenoethmoidal recess from the anterior aspect of the body of the sphenoid bone. The mucous membrane covering it forms part of the specialized olfactory epithelium. Also *superior turbinate bone, superior nasal turbinate, supraturbinal.* **c. nasalis suprema** [NA] The smallest of the bony projections from the medial surface of the ethmoidal labyrinth, projecting from the posterosuperior part of the lateral nasal wall in the sphenoethmoidal recess and overlying the small, short supreme nasal meatus. The mucous membrane covering it forms part of the specialized olfactory epithelium. Also *supreme nasal concha, highest turbinate bone, supreme nasal bone, supreme ethmoid bone, fourth turbinate bone, Santorini's concha, supreme turbinate bone, turbinate of Santorini.* **nasoturbinal c.** AGGER NASI. **Santorini's c.** CONCHA NASALIS SUPREMA. **c. sphenoidalis** [NA] A paired, thin, cone-shaped, curved bony plate, the superior surface of which usually fuses with the anteroinferior surface of the body of the sphenoid bone before puberty. The inferior surface helps to form the posterior part of the roof of the nasal cavity and the upper boundary of the sphenopalatine foramen. The anterior vertical margin joins that of the opposite side at the sphenoidal crest in the midline. The base is in contact with the ethmoid bone, and may be fused to it to complete the posterior ethmoidal sinuses. The anterior wall is pierced by the opening of the sphenoidal sinus. Also *sphenoidal concha, sphenoturbinal bone, sphenoturbinal ossicles, sphenoidal turbinate bone, Bertin's bones, Bertin's ossicles, sphenoidal turbinals, sphenoid turbinate, Wistar's pyramids* (outmoded). **supreme nasal c.** CONCHA NASALIS SUPREMA.

**conchae** \käng′kē\ Plural of CONCHA.

**conchotome** \käng′kōtōm\ [*conch(a)* + *o* + -TOME] Any one of a variety of punch forceps designed for removing portions of the nasal conchae. Also *turbinotome.*

**conchotomy** \kängkät′əmē\ [*conch(a)* + *o* + -TOMY] TURBINOTOMY.

**concis.** *concisus* (L, cut).

**conclination** \kän′klinā′shən\ INTORSION.

**concoction** [L *concoctio* (from *concoctus,* past part. of *concoquere* to cook together, digest) a cooking together, digesting] A medicinal formulation of several ingredients, the combination of which is used to achieve some therapeutic objective.

**concomitant** \känkäm′itənt\ Occurring together; attending.

**concordance** \känkôr′dəns\ **1** The occurrence of a given phenotypic trait in both twins of a pair. **2** The occurrence of a given phenotype in both individuals or groups of individuals being examined. **3** Appropriate or normal connection between segments of the heart.

**concordant** \känkôr′dənt\ Of or relating to a concordance.

**concrescence** \känkres′əns\ [CON- + L *crescens,* pres. part. of *crescere* to grow] The joining together of two teeth by cementosis.

**concretio** \känkrē′shō\ [L (from CON- + L *cretus,* past part. of *crescere* to grow), a growing together] CONCRETION. **c. cordis** A condition in which the visceral and parietal layers of the pericardium are completely or nearly completely stuck together by fibrous and sometimes calcified adhesions. Also *concretio pericardii.* **c. pericardii** CONCRETIO CORDIS.

**concretion** \känkrē′shən\ [L *concretio.* See CONCRETIO.] Any mass of inorganic material formed in a hollow viscus or dilated gland or duct; a calculus. Also *concretio.* **preputial c.** A concretion formed by the accumulation of smegma and concentrated urinary salts under a tight prepuce. Also *acrobystiolith, preputial calculus, postholith.* **prostatic c.'s** Small masses that may form in the alveolus of the prostate. **tophic c.** TOPHUS.

**concretism** \känkrē′tizm\ [*concret(e)* + -ISM] CONCRETE THINKING.

**concretization** \känkrē′tīzā′shən\ [*concret(e)* + *-iz(e)* + -ATION] CONCRETE THINKING.

**concussion** \känkush′ən\ [L *concussio* (from *concussus,* past part. of *concutere* to shake, move violently) a shaking, concussion] A sudden and violent jarring or shaking resulting in injury to soft tissue, as to the brain. **acceleration c.** A concussion injury produced when a moving head forceably impacts a stationary object (as in a fall) or when a resting but freely movable head is forceably impacted (as by a blow). In either situation, the mobility of the head allows the impact to produce a rotary acceleration of intracranial contents, causing the brain to shift within its dural covering, thus producing the injury. Compare COMPRESSION CONCUSSION. **air c.** **1** A high pressure wave resulting from an explosion in air and of a degree sufficient to cause concussion of the brain. **2** The clinical syndrome resulting from an explosion in air. **c. of the brain** The sudden displacement of intracranial contents resulting from a blow on the head, characterized by temporary impairment of function of the brain and usually by momentary or brief loss of consciousness. Also *commotio cerebri.* **compression c.** A concussion injury produced when a moving force is applied to a resting head which is relatively immobile due to external support or fixation. The lack of mobility prevents rotary acceleration of the brain and injury is produced by local distortion and deformation of the skull as it resumes its original shape. A compression concussion requires much greater force than an acceleration concussion to produce an injury of the same magnitude. Compare ACCELERATION CONCUSSION. **c. of the labyrinth** Acoustic trauma involving impairment of hearing and tinnitus, resulting from a sudden extreme pressure change on the ears, for instance from a blow on the ear or exposure to a bomb blast. **c. of the retina** COMMOTIO RETINAE. **c. of the spinal cord** A transient disturbance in spinal cord function resulting from a transmitted impact as distinct from a direct physical injury. Also *commotio spinalis.*

**condensation** \kän′densā′shən\ **1** The transition from a gaseous to a liquid phase, or from a gas or liquid to a solid phase. **2** The process of rendering a material, such as dental amalgam, more compact by applying pressure. **3** The confluence of several elements into a single element that comes to represent all of its component parts. A single person in a dream, for instance, may represent the dreamer's father and, at the same time, the dreamer's employer, a hated rival, and an idealized hero.

**condenser** \kənden′sər\ **1** The system of lenses used to focus light upon an object subjected to microscopic examination. It may be part of the microscope itself or a separate apparatus associated with the light source. **2** Equipment used to lower the temperature of a material, as to convert a gas into the liquid phase or a liquid into a solid. **3** An instrument for compacting filling material into a prepared tooth cavity. Also *plugger.* **4** *Outmoded* CAPACITOR. **amalgam c.** A device used for condensing dental amalgam. **darkfield c.** A condenser with a central obstruction to a substage light source that produces a cone of light whose apex is focused upon the object to be examined. Only rays diffracted from the specimen will enter the objective lens, so the object appears brilliantly light against a dark background. **foil c.** A device used for condensing gold foil in a tooth filling. Also *gold plugger.*

**condition** [L *conditio* (variant of more correct *condicio,* from *condicere* to make an agreement with, from CON- + L *dicere* to say) a contract, agreement] **1** State or mode of being, especially state of health. **2** To train to respond in a particular way to a specified stimulus. **preexisting c.** An injury, disease, or other condition which existed in a health insurance policyholder prior to issuance of the policy and which is generally grounds for an exclusion from coverage of costs resulting from that condition. **standard c.'s** STANDARD TEMPERATURE AND PRESSURE.

**conditioner** / **tissue c.** A gel applied to the fitting surface of a denture as treatment of chronically inflamed and hyperplastic mucosa.

**conditioning** That form of simple learning in which a specified stimulus comes to elicit a particular behavioral response. Also *conditioning learning.* **avoidance c.** Operant conditioning in which the subject learns to make a response that serves to abort or avoid an aversive stimulus. Such responses come to be made at a signal indicating the threat of punishment, and are held to be maintained by the reduction of anxiety when the potentially painful situation is successfully avoided. **classical c.** A method of establishing conditioned responses achieved by pairing an indifferent or neutral stimulus with another stimulus that has a biologically based capability for arousing a response without a need for learning or prior experience. As the result of many pairings of the two stimuli, in a rigidly controlled experimental sequence, the once neutral stimulus will come to evoke the same, or a very similar, behavioral response as was initially evoked by the original biologically active stimulus. Also *Pavlovian conditioning, type S conditioning, respondent conditioning.* **higher-order c.** An extended variant of the classical conditioning procedure. The conditioned stimulus of one training series, such as the tone sounded with every presentation of food to a hungry dog, is then itself employed as if it was an unconditioned stimulus in a later training series. **instrumental c.** OPERANT CONDITIONING. **operant c.** Conditioning identified by instrumental acts, or responses made, that affect the environment in such a way as to bring about a reward or reinforcement for the experimental subject. The strengthening of a learned connection of this type is completely contingent on evoking a particular response. Unless that response is initiated, no reward is forthcoming. Also *instrumental conditioning, type R conditioning, reinforcement conditioning.* **Pavlovian c.** CLASSICAL CONDITIONING. **reinforcement c.** OPERANT CONDITIONING. **respondent c.** CLASSICAL CONDITIONING. **type R c.** OPERANT CONDITIONING. **type S c.** CLASSICAL CONDITIONING.

**condom** \kän′dəm\ [Origin unknown; the theory of an eponymous inventor named *Condom* or *Condon* has been shown to be apocryphal] A penile sheath of rubber or similar material worn during intercourse to prevent conception or infection.

**Condorelli** [Luigi *Condorelli,* Italian pathologist, born 1899] Condorelli syndrome. See under CONDORELLI'S ENCEPHALITIS.

**conduct** [L *conductus,* past part. of *conducere* to bring or lead together, conduct, from *con-* with + *ducere* to lead] To pass (a nerve impulse) along a nerve fiber or to propagate (an impulse) along an excitable membrane.

**conductance** \kənduk′təns\ The reciprocal of resistance in a DC circuit, expressed in siemens. Symbol: *G* **airway c.** Air flow rate in the respiratory tract divided by the pressure producing flow. It may be calculated during inspiration or expiration, or as the mean of the two. **input c.** The transmembrane conductance presented by a cell to an intracellularly delivered electrical impulse.

**conduction** \kənduk′shən\ The transmission or transfer of electricity, heat, sound, or nervous impulse through material or tissues. **aberrant c.** Abnormal pathway of travel of the excitatory impulse of the heart, especially through ventricular muscle. **accelerated c.** Abnormally rapid rate of travel of the excitatory impulse of the heart from atrium to ventricle, usually through an abnormal pathway as in the Wolff-Parkinson-White and short PR syndromes. **air c.** Transmission through the air as in the case of sound waves. This is the normal manner in which sound waves reach the tympanic membrane in the process of hearing. **anomalous c.** Abnormal, especially accelerated, conduction of the excitatory impulse of the heart. **anterograde c.** Conduction of the excitatory impulse of the heart in the normal forward direction from the atria to the ventricles. Also *forward conduction.* **antidromic c.** Electrically evoked nerve impulse conduction in the opposite direction from that elicited under physiologic circumstances. **atrial c.** INTRA-ATRIAL CONDUCTION. **atrioventricular c.** Passage of the excitatory impulse of the heart from the atria through specialized muscle fibers to the ventricles. It is represented by the P-R interval of the electrocardiogram. **avalanche c.** Activation of a large number of neurons by an impulse originally arising in a few or in a single neuron. **bone c.** The transmission of vibrations in the audiofrequency range through the bones of the skull to the cochlea, as, for instance, when a vibrating tuning fork is firmly applied to the mastoid process. Also *cranial conduction, osteotympanic conduction.* **cardiac c.** The conduction of the electrical impulse through the heart. See also CONDUCTION SYSTEM OF THE HEART. **concealed c.** Passage of an excitatory impulse of the heart through only part of the conducting tissue. It fails to excite ventricular activation, but may influence the timing and character of the next impulse. **cranial c.** BONE CONDUCTION. **decremental c.** Delayed or obstructed conduction of the activating impulse of the heart through a normal atrioventricular node due to progressive decline in the amplitude and in the rate of rise of the action potential of the fibers. It is seen when atrial rates are very high and sometimes with atrial premature beats. **delayed c.** Prolongation of the time taken by the activating impulse of the heart to travel from the atria to the ventricles, that is, more than 0.2 second for a normal heart rate; first-degree atrioventricular block. **ephaptic c.** Conduction of a nervous impulse from one nerve fiber or neuron to another through direct physical contact without an intervening synapse. **forward c.** ANTEROGRADE CONDUCTION. **intra-atrial c.** Conduction of the activating impulse of the heart along the walls of the atria, normally from sinoatrial to atrioventricular node, represented by the P wave of the electrocardiogram. Also *atrial conduction.* **intraventricular c.** Conduction of the activating impulse of the heart along the walls of the ventricles, represented by the QRS complex of the electrocardiogram. It normally spreads from the distal end of the main atrioventricular bundles (of His) along its two branches in the interventricular septum to end in the Purkinje network of subendocardial fibers at the base of the ventricles. Also *ventricular conduction.* **nerve c.** The passage of a nerve impulse along a process of a neuron. Also *nervous conduction.* **osteotympanic c.** BONE CONDUCTION. **retrograde c.** Conduction of the activating impulse of the heart in the opposite direction to normal, that is, from ventricles to atria, or from the atrioventricular node through the atria. Also *retroconduction.* **saltatory c.** Impulse conduction in myelinated axons believed to be discontinuous, "jumping" between successive nodes of Ranvier. **sound c.** The conveying of acoustic energy through air, fluid, biological tissues such as bone, or manufactured materials. **synaptic c.** Nerve impulse transmission across any type of synapse. **ventricular c.** INTRAVENTRICULAR CONDUCTION. **ventriculoatrial c.** Conduction from ventricles to atria; retrograde conduction.

**conductivity** \kän′duktiv′itē\ The ability of nerve and muscle to transmit a wave of excitation.

**conductor** **1** A material that transmits electricity, heat, or sound by direct molecular transfer. **2** A grooved director for guiding a surgical knife when slitting open a sinus or fistula.

**conduit** \kän′dʸoo·it\ A channel or passage. **ileal c.** A section of distal small bowel that is separated surgically with its blood supply intact to serve as a communication between the skin and the ureter following a cystectomy.

**conduplicate** \kändʸoo′plikit\ Folded lengthwise on itself, as a structure or posture, as that of a fetus with the knees drawn up against the head.

**conduplicato** \kändʸoo′plikā′tō\ Bent double, as the fetus *in utero.* **c. corporis** A form of transverse lie or shoulder presentation of a fetus. The fetus assumes a flexed position in which the knees are closely approximated to the thorax.

**condylar** \kän′dilər\ Pertaining to a condyle. Also *condylicus.*

**condylarthrosis** \kän′dilärthrō′sis\ ARTICULATIO BICONDYLARIS.

**condyle** \kän′dīl\ [French (from L *condylus* knuckle, from Gk *kondylos* knuckle), prominence of a joint] CONDYLUS. **extensor c. of humerus** EPICONDYLUS LATERALIS HUMERI. **external c. of femur** CONDYLUS LATERALIS FEMORIS. **external c. of humerus** EPICONDYLUS LATERALIS HUMERI. **external c. of tibia** CONDYLUS LATERALIS TIBIAE. **flexor c. of humerus** EPICONDYLUS MEDIALIS HUMERI. **c. of humerus** CONDYLUS HUMERI. **internal c. of femur** CONDYLUS MEDIALIS FEMORIS. **internal c. of humerus** EPICONDYLUS MEDIALIS HUMERI. **internal c. of tibia** CONDYLUS MEDIALIS TIBIAE. **lateral c. of femur** CONDYLUS LATERALIS FEMORIS. **lateral c. of humerus** EPICONDYLUS

LATERALIS HUMERI. **lateral c. of tibia** CONDYLUS LATERALIS TIBIAE. **c. of mandible** PROCESSUS CONDYLARIS MANDIBULAE. **mandibular c.** PROCESSUS CONDYLARIS MANDIBULAE. **medial c. of femur** CONDYLUS MEDIALIS FEMORIS. **medial c. of humerus** EPICONDYLUS MEDIALIS HUMERI. **medial c. of tibia** CONDYLUS MEDIALIS TIBIAE. **occipital c.** CONDYLUS OCCIPITALIS. **radial c. of humerus** EPICONDYLUS LATERALIS HUMERI. **c. of scapula** ANGULUS LATERALIS SCAPULAE. **third occipital c.** An inconstant precondylar tubercle, either single or bilateral, that is located just anterior to the anterior margin of the foramen magnum on the inferior surface of the basilar part of the occipital bone. It represents a manifestation of an occipital vertebra and it may either articulate with the anterior arch of the atlas or be fused to it. **ulnar c. of humerus** EPICONDYLUS MEDIALIS HUMERI.

**condylectomy** \kän′dilek′təmē\ [*condyl(e)* + -ECTOMY] The surgical removal of a condyle.

**condyli** \kän′dilī\ Plural of CONDYLUS.

**condylicus** \kändil′ikəs\ CONDYLAR.

**condyloid** \kän′diloid\ Resembling or pertaining to a condyle.

**condyloma** \kän′dilō′mə\ [Gk *kondylōma* (from *kondylos* a knuckle) a callosity, knob] (*pl.* condylomata) A wartlike tumor or growth which is the result of hypertrophy of the prickle-cell layer of the epidermis. Also *verruca mollusciformis.* **c. acuminatum** A sexually transmitted squamous cell papilloma of the anogenital region caused by one of several distinct strains of papovaviruses. It frequently occurs in grapelike clusters. Also *pointed condyloma, papilloma venereum, acuminate wart, verruca acuminata, genital wart.* **flat c.** A hypertrophic flattened papular lesion that occurs on the anogenital skin in the secondary stage of syphilis. Also *condyloma latum, mucous papule.* **pointed c.** CONDYLOMA ACUMINATUM. **c. subcutaneum** MOLLUSCUM CONTAGIOSUM.

**condylomata** \kän′dilō′mətə\ Plural of CONDYLOMA.

**condylomatosis** \kän′dilō′mətō′sis\ [CONDYLOMA + *t* + -OSIS ] A condition characterized by the presence of condylomata. Also *condylosis.*

**condylosis** \kän′dilō′sis\ CONDYLOMATOSIS.

**condylotomy** \kän′dilät′əmē\ A surgical incision or division of a condyle.

**condylus** \kän′diləs\ [L (from Gk *kondylos* a knuckle), a knuckle] A rounded articular process at an extremity of a bone. Also *condyle.* **c. humeri** [NA] That portion of the distal extremity of the humerus lying between the epicondyles and comprising the trochlea, capitulum, and related fossae, namely, the radial, coronoid, and olecranon. Also *condyle of humerus.* **c. lateralis femoris** [NA] One of the two expanded, rounded masses at the distal extremity of the femur, partly covered by articular cartilage for articulation with the patella and the lateral condyle of the tibia. Anteriorly it is united with the medial condyle by the patellar surface, while posteriorly they are separated by the deep, intercondylar fossa. Also *lateral condyle of femur, external condyle of femur.* **c. lateralis humeri** EPICONDYLUS LATERALIS HUMERI. **c. lateralis tibiae** [NA] One of two prominent masses forming the proximal extremity of the tibia that has an almost circular superior articular surface for the lateral condyle of the femur. Its medial border has the projecting lateral intercondylar tubercle centrally placed. It is subcutaneous anteriorly, and projects over the shaft posteriorly where, inferolaterally, it has a rounded articular facet for the head of the fibula. Also *lateral condyle of tibia, external condyle of tibia.* **c. medialis femoris** [NA] One of the two expanded, rounded masses at the distal extremity of the femur, partly covered by articular cartilage for articulation with the patella and the medial condyle of the tibia. Anteriorly it is united with the lateral condyle by the patellar surface, while posteriorly they are separated by the deep intercondylar fossa. Anteroposteriorly it is more curved than the lateral condyle, and its convex medial surface is easily palpated and bears the adductor tubercle for the insertion of the adductor magnus muscle. Also *medial condyle of femur, internal condyle of femur.* **c. medialis humeri** EPICONDYLUS MEDIALIS HUMERI. **c. medialis tibiae** [NA] One of two prominent masses forming the proximal extremity of the tibia that has an oval, concave superior articular surface for the medial condyle of the femur. At the center of its lateral border is the medial intercondylar tubercle. Also *medial condyle of tibia, internal condyle of tibia.* **c. occipitalis** [NA] One of two convex, kidney-shaped processes on the inferior surfaces of the lateral, or condylar, parts of the occipital bone on either side of the foramen magnum for articulation with the superior facets of the atlas. Also *occipital condyle.*

**cone** [L *conus.* See CONUS.] **1** A solid that tapers from a circular base to a point, or any object resembling such a solid in shape. **2** See under RETINAL CONE. **3** A cylindrical device attached to an x-ray tube to restrict the size of the radiation beam. **acrosomal c.** A body situated between the acrosomal granule and the nucleus of a developing spermatid. **adjusting c.'s** A system of measuring the distance between the visual axes of the two eyes by aligning two cones, open at their bases and tips, in front of the eyes. Since each visual axis must pass through the apex of the corresponding cone, the desired distance is easily ascertained by measuring the distance between the apices. **antipodal c.** The set of astral rays extending from the centriole, directed away from the equatorial plate, in a dividing cell. **arterial c.** CONUS ARTERIOSUS. **attraction c.** FERTILIZATION CONE. **cerebellar pressure c.** The result of compression of the cerebellar tonsils and vermis into a cone shape due to herniation of the brain into the foramen magnum. It results usually from increased intracranial pressure or from enlargement of the cerebellum, as from a tumor. **ectoplacental c.** ECTOPLACENTA. **elastic c. of larynx** CONUS ELASTICUS LARYNGIS. **ether c.** A device fitted over the face for administration of ether, utilizing the open-drop technique of inducing anesthesia. **fertilization c.** A small protruberance which develops on the surface of the ovum at the site of contact with the fertilizing spermatozoon. This region gradually engulfs the spermatozoon and then retracts, carrying the spermatozoon inwards. Also *attraction cone.* **graduated c.** A device used primarily in postmortem studies to measure the diameters of blood vessels and valve orifices. **growth c.** A slight bulbous expansion at the tip of a growing or regenerating axon. **gutta-percha c.** A long, narrow cone of gutta-percha used in endodontics for filling root canals. Cones are made in various standard widths and lengths. Also *gutta-percha point.* **Haller's c.'s** LOBULI EPIDIDYMIDIS. **c. of light** LIGHT REFLEX. **long c.** A cylindrical collimator attached to an x-ray tube to provide an anode-skin distance of 12 to 20 inches (30.5–50.8 cm). It is often used in roentgenography of parts of the skull, as in dental radiology. **medullary c.** CONUS MEDULLARIS. **ocular c.** The cone formed by rays of light entering through the pupil, the base being the cornea and the apex being on the retina. Also *visual cone.* **pilar c.** An invagination into the depth of the hair bud forming a cavity which rapidly fills with mesoblast cells which subsequently form the framework of the developing hair. The hair root is located deep in this flasklike depression in the corium and subcutaneous tissue, and its base, which rests upon and encloses the hair papilla, is expanded into the hair bulb. Growth of the hair results from continued multiplication of the epidermal cells around the papilla. **pulmonary c.** CONUS ARTERIOSUS. **retinal c.** One of the two types of specialized retinal photoreceptor processes. It is flask shaped and protrudes outward through the external limiting membrane at its junction with its cell body. The cones are most numerous in or near the macula retinae and absent over the optic disk. Also *cone cell, visual cone.* **short c.** A cylindrical collimator attached to an x-ray tube to provide an anode-skin distance of less than 12 inches (30.5 cm), usually about 8 inches (20.3 cm). It is used especially in dental radiology. **tentorial pressure c.** The distortion of the brain resulting from herniation of the medial portions of the temporal lobes into the tentorial opening, and due to increased supratentorial pressure. **terminal c. of spinal cord** CONUS MEDULLARIS. **treatment c.** In radiation therapy, an open-ended metallic cylinder attached to the exit port of the housing of the radiation source to limit the size of the radiation beam. It is used to diminish scatter of radiation as well as to define the source-to-skin distance. **twin c.'s** Binucleated retinal cones that result from the fusion of two adjacent cones. **vascular c.'s** LOBULI EPIDIDYMIDIS. **visual c.** **1** OCULAR CONE. **2** RETINAL CONE.

**cone-monochromat** \\-män′ōkrō′mat\\ An individual completely lacking in color discrimination ability because of an anomaly of function of the retinal cones.

**conexus** \\kənek′səs\\ [L (from *conectere* to fasten, join), a connection, union] CONNEXUS. **c. interthalamicus** ADHESIO INTERTHALAMICA.

**confabulation** \\kənfab′yəlā′shən\\ [Late L *confabulatio* (from L *confabulatus,* past part. of *confabulari* to talk together) a talking together] The act of filling memory gaps which have resulted from organically induced amnesia, with false stories that are believed by the subject and often maintained despite contradictory evidence. It is a characteristic symptom of Wernicke-Korsakoff psychosis and alcohol amnestic disorder. Also *fabrication.*

**confectio** CONFECTION.

**confection** [L *confectio* (from *conficere* to make or bring together, prepare) preparation, composition] A medicinal preparation that has been made sweet by the addition of sugar, honey, or syrup. Also *confectio.*

**conference** / **clinical-pathological c.** A teaching method, used in medical training, in which the instructing clinician is presented with the facts of an unfamiliar case in order to demonstrate to students the process of differential diagnosis. A pathologist then presents a diagnosis based on examination of tissue sections removed surgically or at autopsy. This diagnosis usually disproves or confirms the clinical one. Discussion of the case, its diagnosis, and its management follows. Abbr. CPC

**confertus** \\känfur′təs\\ [L, past part. of *confercire* to cram together] Close together; confluent; coalescing.

**confidentiality** \\kän′fiden′shē·al′itē\\ The right of a subject to control the disposition of information disclosed during the course of a professional relationship and the reciprocal obligation of the professional to ensure that no harm will befall the subject as a result of disclosures of such information. The conditions under which the obligation may or must be breached are usually determined by laws, which vary from one jurisdiction to another.

**configuration** \\känfig′yərā′shən\\ The form and arrangement of parts or groups that form a whole structure, as the spatial arrangement of atoms in a molecule. **cis c.** See under CIS. **trans c.** See under TRANS.

**conflict** [L *conflictus* (past part. of *confligere* to strike one thing against another) a striking together] A struggle between incompatible or contradictory forces, drives, impulses, or affects occurring within the subject, between the subject and others, or between internal and external demands. **intrapsychic c.** A struggle or opposition of interests between different parts of one person, as between the ego and superego.

**confluence** \\kän′floo·əns\\ CONFLUENS. **c. of sinuses** CONFLUENS SINUUM.

**confluens** \\kän′floo·enz\\ [L, pres. part. of *confluere* to flow together] The meeting place or junction of two or more flowing streams. Also *confluence.* **c. sinuum** [NA] The junction of the superior sagittal, straight, and occipital sinuses that bring venous blood from the brain with the two lateral sinuses that drain it away. The confluens is located over the internal occipital protuberance, where the sagittally oriented cerebellar and cerebral falces intersect the transversely directed tentorium cerebelli. Also *confluence of sinuses, torcular herophili.*

**confluent** \\kän′floo·ənt\\ Flowing together; merging.

**confocal** \\känfō′kl\\ PARFOCAL.

**conformation** \\kän′fôrmā′shən\\ [L *conformatio* (from *conformatus,* past part. of *conformare* to form, fashion) a forming or fashioning properly] The arrangement the atoms of a molecule assume in space. Different conformations interconvert without bond breakage.

**conformer** \\kənfôr′mər\\ **1** An oval device used to shape the contours of the eye socket after enucleation of an eye. **2** A particular molecule in one of the possible conformations that it can adopt. **neck c.** A splint made of synthetic and usually somewhat flexible material used to apply even pressure to a burn scar of the neck to prevent hypertrophic scarring and to maintain the submandibular angle, thus preventing the chin from being drawn toward the chest as the scar contracts.

**confrontation** \\kän′fräntā′shən\\ **1** The presentation of facts, observations, etc. by one individual, and insistence that another individual, the subject, give attention to the material presented. It is a typical technique of encounter group therapy but is used in other types of group and individual psychotherapy as well. **2** Any method of visual field examination in which the patient and examiner face one another and observe test objects (e.g., the examiner's finger) at various points in the area equidistant between them. The patient's responses are compared with the examiner's presumably normal vision to detect gross field defects.

**confusion** [L *confusio* (from *confusus,* past part. of *confundere* to mingle, mix, disturb, confuse) a mingling, confusion] Disorientation resulting from memory impairment, hallucinations, mistaken interpretation of events, and/or uncertainty about one's role or identity. **epileptic c.** A state of mental confusion occurring either during an attack of epilepsy, as in petit mal status or temporal lobe epilepsy, or after the attack has apparently ended (postepileptic confusion). **postepileptic c.** Confusion persisting after an attack of epilepsy.

**cong.** *congius* (L, gallon).

**congelation** \\kän′jəlā′shən\\ [L *congelatio,* from *congelatus,* past part. of *congelare* to freeze, congeal] FROSTBITE.

**congener** [L (from *con-* with + *gener* son-in-law), belonging to the same family] **1** Any member of a family of substances related in molecular or atomic structure. **2** Members of the same genus, as two species. Adj. congeneric.

**congenerous** \känjen′ərəs\ Having a common origin, cause, function, or action.

**congenic** \känjen′ik\ Of or relating to a strain that differs from the parental inbred strain at one restricted region of the genome. Congenic strains are developed in experimental genetics by selective breeding of highly inbred individuals. If the difference is limited to one locus, the strains are coisogenic.

**congenital** \känjen′ətəl\ [L *congenit(us)* born together with, from *con-* with + *genitus*, past part. of *gignere* to beget, bring forth + -AL] Being present at or from birth, with developmental origin implied. Also *congenitus, geneogenous, inborn.* • In current usage *developmental* is often preferred to *congenital* because the former refers to the total span of development, whether embryonic, fetal, or postnatal. *Congenital* implies that the condition originated prenatally and was manifest at birth, whereas a *developmental* condition, though originating before birth, need not be manifest at birth, but may appear at any time until the onset of adolescence.

**congestin** \kənjes′tin\ A highly poisonous material derived from the tentacles of sea anemones. It produces extensive dilatation of the splanchnic vessels and hemorrhage when injected into laboratory animals. Also *actinocongestin.*

**congestion** \kənjes′chən\ [L *congestio* (from *congerere* to accumulate, from CON- + *gerere* to carry, have) an accumulation] The accumulation of an excessive volume of fluid, especially blood, in an organ or part, as may occur in heart failure resulting from impaired venous drainage. **cerebral c.** CEREBRAL EDEMA. **circulatory c. in renal failure** A syndrome that occurs in either acute or chronic advanced renal failure, characterized by severe dyspnea, pulmonary edema, cardiomegaly, venous distension and gallop rhythm. In contrast to circulatory overload in cardiac failure, the cardiac output is normal or increased and the circulation time normal or decreased. Also *circulatory overload in renal failure.* **hypostatic c.** Accumulation of fluid in the lowest part of an organ due to the combined effect of gravity and impeded return of blood by the veins. **passive c.** VENOUS CONGESTION. **pulmonary c.** An excessive quantity of blood in the lungs, as in certain forms of heart failure. **rebound c.** Congestion in mucous membranes following vasoconstriction from locally applied epinephrine and certain other topical vasoconstrictors. It is probably related to altered vascular activity resulting from tissue hypoxia. Also *epinephrine reversal.* **renal c.** Increased amount of blood in renal veins and capillaries, usually due to congestive heart failure or renal vein obstruction. **venous c.** Congestion due to impeded return of blood by the veins, which may occur secondary to heart failure. Also *passive congestion.*

**congestive** \kənjes′tiv\ Characterized by or pertaining to congestion.

**conglobate** \kän′glōbāt\ [L *conglobat(us)*, past part. of *conglobare* to gather into a rounded form or ball] Clumped together into a rounded mass: said of some glands.

**conglobation** \kän′glōbā′shən\ **1** A clumping or forming together into a rounded mass. **2** A rounded mass or formation.

**conglomerate** \kən·gläm′ərāt\ **1** Massed together; forming a cluster of separate elements. **2** A heterogenous mass.

**conglutination** \kän·gloo′tinā′shən\ **1** The powerful agglutination of cells carrying iC3b on their surfaces by conglutinin. **2** The adhesion of tissues to each other. **c. of cervix** A condition in which, despite adequate uterine contractions during labor, the cervix fails to dilate.

**conglutinin** \kän·gloo′tinin\ A plasma protein found only in Bovidae and which acts as a specific ligand for cell-bound iC3b and therefore agglutinates complement-coated cells. Conglutinin is a polymeric, collagen-containing protein and binds to the carbohydrate moiety of iC3b only in the presence of calcium ions.

**conglutinogen** \kän·gloo′tinəjən\ The determinant exposed in cell-bound iC3b which reacts with bovine conglutinin. The determinant is carbohydrate and is similar or identical to a carbohydrate determinant found in yeast cell walls.

**congress** / **sexual c.** *Older term* COITUS.

**congressus** \kän·gres′əs\ [L (from *congressus*, past part. of *congredi* to come or go with, come together), a coming together, intercourse] COITUS.

**coni** \kō′nī\ Plural of CONUS.

**conic** \kän′ik\ Shaped like a cone. Also *conical.*

**coniism** \kō′nē·izm\ [*coni(um)* + -ISM] Poisoning from the consumption of conium, or poison hemlock. Symptoms are paralysis of the limbs, then the respiratory system, leading to unconsciousness and death.

**coning** \kō′ning\ **c. of the cervix** CONIZATION.

**coniocortex** \kō′nē·ōkôr′teks\ KONIOCORTEX.

**conium** \kō′nē·əm\ The dried, unripe fruit of the poison hemlock, *Conium maculatum*, in the family Umbelliferae (Apiaceae). Along with all other parts of its biennial plant, it is highly poisonous. Coniine, *N*-methyloconiine, conhydrine, coniic acid, ethylpiperidine, and pseudoconhydrine are among the constituents of the fruit. It has been used as a sedative, an antispasmodic, and an anodyne, and in the treatment of hemorrhoids.

**conization** \kän′īzā′shən\ A surgical removal of a cone-shaped piece of tissue from the cervix. A circular incision is made around the cervical os and then carried obliquely into the cervical canal. The purpose is to remove the cervical transformation zone, the site of cervical neoplasia. Also *coning of the cervix.*

**conjoined** [CON- + *joined*] United or fused peripherally so as to maintain some separate identity: said of monovular twins that represent incomplete separation into two during cleavage or early stages of embryogenesis.

**conjugant** \kän′jəgənt\ A member of a pair of organisms undergoing conjugation.

**conjugata** \kän′jəgā′tə\ [L (fem. of *conjugatus*, past part. of *conjugare* to yoke or join together), yoked or joined together] DIAMETER CONJUGATA. **c. diagonalis** DIAGONAL CONJUGATE. **c. vera** DIAMETER CONJUGATA. **c. vera obstetrica** OBSTETRIC CONJUGATE.

**conjugate** \kän′jəgət\ **1** Joined in pairs; coupled. **2** DIAMETER CONJUGATA. **anatomic c.** DIAMETER CONJUGATA. **available c.** OBSTETRIC CONJUGATE. **diagonal c.** The anteroposterior diameter of the inlet, or superior aperture, of the pelvis measured per vaginam between the midpoint of the sacral promontory and the lower border of the symphysis pubis. Also *conjugata diagonalis, false conjugate, diagonal conjugate diameter, conjugata diagonalis.* **effective c.** The anatomic conjugate in cases of spondylolisthesis, when it is measured from the symphysis pubis to the nearest lumbar vertebra. Also *false conjugate.* **external c.** The diameter measured between the depression under the spinous process of the fifth lumbar vertebra and the upper border of the symphysis pubis. Also *external conjugate diameter, Baudelocque's diameter, Baudelocque's line.* **false c.** **1** DIAGONAL CONJUGATE. **2** EFFECTIVE CONJUGATE. **c. of the inlet** DIAMETER CONJUGATA. **internal c.** DIAMETER CONJUGATA. **obstetric c.** The least anteroposterior diameter to be encountered during the passage of the fetal head through the inlet, or superior aperture, of the pelvis, measured by radiography between the sacral promontory and a point just below the upper margin of the symphysis pubis on its inner aspect. Also *obstetric conjugate diameter, available conjugate, conjugata vera obstetrica.* **obstetric c. of the outlet** The measurement of the conjugate of the outlet increased by the distance that the coccyx can be displaced posteriorly. **c. of the outlet** The anteroposterior diameter of the outlet, or inferior aperture, of the pelvis measured from the apex of the coccyx to the lower margin of the symphysis pubis. The lowest point of the sacrum is sometimes used instead of the coccyx. **true c.** DIAMETER CONJUGATA.

**conjugated** \kän′jəgā′tid\ In chemistry, describing double bonds (pi bonds) whose pi orbitals overlap. They are usually alternate double bonds. This allows transmission of electronic effects affecting reactivity through the molecule.

**conjugation** \kän′jəgā′shən\ [L *conjugatio* (from *conjugatus,* past part. of *conjugare* to join together ) a yoking or fastening together] **1** In biochemistry, a combination of different metabolites with certain molecules which favors their excretion. These molecules are mainly glucuronic acid and sulfuric acid, and occasionally amino acids. **2** The union and nuclear exchange between paired acellular organisms, as seen in protozoan ciliates or the passage of some or all DNA, as a replicated set, from a donor to a bacterial recipient.

**conjunctiva** \kän′jungktī′və\ [New L, short for *tunica* (or *membrana) conjunctiva* (from L *conjunctivus* conjunctive, connective, from *conjungere* to connect, unite, from *con-* together + *jungere* to yoke) a connective coat or membrane; so called because it is continuous over the inside of the eyelid and the outside of the eyeball] (*pl.* conjunctivae) TUNICA CONJUNCTIVA. Adj. conjunctival. **bulbar c.** TUNICA CONJUNCTIVA BULBI. **corneal c.** The part of the bulbar conjunctiva covering the cornea where it is reduced to only its epithelium. **ocular c.** TUNICA CONJUNCTIVA BULBI. **palpebral c.** TUNICA CONJUNCTIVA PALPEBRARUM. **scleral c.** The part of the bulbar conjunctiva that covers the sclera to which it is loosely connected and from which it is separated by loose areolar tissue and the anterior part of the bulbar sheath.

**conjunctivitis** \känjungk′tivī′tis\ [*conjunctiv(a)* + -ITIS] Inflammation of the conjunctiva. **actinic c.** Conjunctivitis caused by exposure to ultraviolet radiation, as from therapeutic lamps, klieg lights, and welding torches (welders' conjunctivitis). Also *ultraviolet ray ophthalmia, actinic ray ophthalmia, electric ophthalmia, klieg conjunctivitis.* **acute contagious c.** An epidemic form of conjunctival inflammation caused by *Haemophilus aegyptius* (Koch-Weeks bacillus) and characterized by a mucopurulent discharge. Also *pink eye, pinkeye, epidemic conjunctivitis, Koch-Weeks conjunctivitis.* **acute follicular c.** Infection of the conjunctiva characterized by follicle formation. It may be caused by an adenovirus, molluscum contagiosum virus, or other virus associated with conjunctivitis. **acute hemorrhagic c.** Acute inflammation of the conjunctiva with marked hemorrhage, due to infection with an enterovirus or a coxsackievirus. **angular c.** Conjunctivitis characterized by reddening of the canthi. Also *Morax-Axenfeld conjunctivitis.* **atopic c.** Inflammation of the conjunctiva associated with airborne allergens characteristic of atopy. **calcareous c.** Deposition of calcific nodules within conjunctival cysts. **caterpillar c.** Conjunctivitis nodosa caused by caterpillar hairs. Also *caterpillar ophthalmia.* **croupous c.** Conjunctival inflammation associated with pseudomembrane formation. **diphtheritic c.** Conjunctival infection with *Corynebacterium diphtheriae,* often with formation of a pseudomembrane. **diplobacillary c.** Conjunctival infection with the Morax-Axenfeld diplobacillus, *Moraxella lacunata.* **eczematous c.** PHLYCTENULAR CONJUNCTIVITIS. **Egyptian c.** TRACHOMA. **epidemic c.** ACUTE CONTAGIOUS CONJUNCTIVITIS. **follicular c.** Conjunctival inflammation associated with the presence of lymphoid follicles. **glare c.** Conjunctivitis from glare due to sunshine or to light reflection from snow. Also *solar ophthalmia.* **gonococcal c.** Conjunctivitis caused by *Neisseria gonorrhoeae.* Also *gonorrheal conjunctivitis, gonorrheal ophthalmia.* See also GONOCOCCAL OPHTHALMIA OF NEWBORN. **gonorrheal c.** GONOCOCCAL CONJUNCTIVITIS. **granular c.** TRACHOMA. **hypertrophic c.** A proliferative conjunctivitis in which large papillary excrescences form on the palpebral conjunctiva, especially on the upper lid. The usual cause is the allergic irritation of vernal conjunctivitis. **inclusion c.** An acute, purulent conjunctivitis caused by *Chlamydia trachomatis* and infecting newborn infants from passage through the mother's birth canal. Infection is also thought to be spread to older children and adults by infected swimming pool water. Also *paratrachoma.* **infantile purulent c.** Acute infection of the conjunctival sac giving rise to visible pus, due to a great variety of organisms or viruses. It is highly contagious and occurs from time to time in epidemic form in neonatal nurseries. Also *ophthalmia neonatorum.* See also GONOCOCCAL OPHTHALMIA OF NEWBORN. **infectious c.** Any conjunctivitis caused by microorganisms, regardless of whether or not it is contagious. **klieg c.** ACTINIC CONJUNCTIVITIS. **Koch-Weeks c.** ACUTE CONTAGIOUS CONJUNCTIVITIS. **larval c.** Conjunctivitis caused by fly larvae embedded in the eye. It is a form of myiasis. **c. medicamentosa** Allergic or toxic conjunctivitis caused by topical application of drugs. **membranous c.** A very severe conjunctivitis in which newly formed plaques of inflammatory debris are so firmly adherent to the conjunctiva that they leave a bleeding surface when removed. **meningococcus c.** Conjunctivitis caused by *Neisseria meningitidis..* **molluscum c.** Conjunctivitis that develops along with molluscum contagiosum of the margin of the eyelid. **Morax-Axenfeld c.** ANGULAR CONJUNCTIVITIS. **c. necroticans infectiosa** Infectious conjunctivitis accompanied by unilateral enlargement of parotid and submaxillary salivary glands. Also *Pascheff's conjunctivitis.* **c. nodosa** A focal inflammatory conjunctival reaction to imbedded caterpillar hairs or filaments of vegetation. Also *nodular conjunctivitis, ophthalmia nodosa.* **nodular c.** CONJUNCTIVITIS NODOSA. **Parinaud's c.** A syndrome of conjunctivitis, usually unilateral and follicular, accompanied by preauricular lymphadenopathy. The condition is seen in conjunction with tularemia, lymphogranuloma venereum, and cat-scratch fever. One of the pathogens, a filamentous bacterium, was formerly identified as a leptothrix but does not meet the present taxonomic requirements for *Leptotrichia..* Also *Parinaud syndrome, oculoglandular syndrome.* **Pascheff's c.** CONJUNCTIVITIS NECROTICANS INFECTIOSA. **phlyctenular c.** Inflammation characterized by a localized elevation of the conjunctiva, often also involving the cornea. The etiology may be tuberculosis or chronic bacterial allergy. Also *eczematous conjunctivitis, scrofular conjunctivitis.* **pseudomembranous c.** Severe conjunctivitis associated with an overlying, loosely adherent layer of inflammatory debris. **scrofular c.** *Obs.* PHLYCTENULAR CONJUNCTIVITIS. **shipyard c.** EPIDEMIC KERATOCONJUNCTIVITIS. **spring c.** VERNAL CONJUNCTIVITIS. **squirrel plague c.** TULAREMIC CONJUNCTIVITIS. **swimming pool c.** Acute conjunctivitis apparently acquired as a result of swimming. It is usually caused by an adenovirus (type 3). **trachomatous c.** TRACHOMA. **tularemic c.** Painful, purulent, usually unilateral conjunctivitis caused by *Francisella tularensis.* It is the principal manifestation of oculoglandular tularemia and may be accompanied by preauricular or cervical lymphadenopathy. Also *conjunctivitis tularensis, squirrel plague conjunctivitis.* **uratic c.** A chronic form of conjunctivitis complicating gout and resulting from the deposition of urate crystals. **vernal c.** An allergic conjunctivitis attributed to sensitivity to pollens from spring-blooming vegetation. Also *spring conjunctivitis, spring catarrh.* **Widmark's c.** A severe conjunctivitis localized in the inferior cul-de-sac.

**conjunctivodacryocystostomy** \kän′jungktī′vōdak′rē·ōsistäs′təmē\ A surgical opening between the inner canthus and the lacrimal sac, as required to bypass lacrimal canicular obstruction.

**conjunctivorhinostomy** \kän′jungktī′vōrīnäs′təmē\ A surgical opening between the inner canthus and the nasal cavity, as required to bypass lacrimal canicular and sac destruction.

**Conn** [Jerome W. *Conn,* U.S. physician, born 1907] Conn syndrome. See under PRIMARY ALDOSTERONISM.

**connatal** \kän′ātəl\ [CON- + NATAL[1]] Originating or acquired at birth.

**connection** / **intertendinous c.'s** CONNEXUS INTERTENDINEUS. **thalamostriate c.'s** THALAMOSTRIATE RADIATION.

**connector** 1 ADAPTER. 2 Something that connects; a link between separate parts or units. 3 A bar connecting components of a removable or fixed partial denture, or an implant.

**Connell** [Frank Gregory *Connell,* U.S. surgeon, 1875–1968] See under SUTURE.

**connexus** \känek′səs\ [L, *conexus.* See CONEXUS.] A connecting structure. Also *conexus.* **c. intertendineus** [NA] Three fibrous bands which are directed transversely or obliquely downwards and laterally and bind together the adjacent diverging tendons of the extensor digitorum muscle on the back of the hand. Also *intertendinous connections, juncturae tendinum, tendinous junctions.*

**conoid** \kō′noid\ 1 Cone-shaped or resembling a cone. 2 An organelle, part of the apical complex, that is found in developmental stages of protozoa of the phylum Apicomplexa. It is thought to be involved in penetration of the host cell by these sporozoan obligatory parasites. **Sturm's c.** The pathway of light between the two linear foci of a cylindrical lens.

**conquinine** QUINIDINE.

**Conradi** [Andreas Christian *Conradi,* Norwegian physician, 1809–1869] See under LINE.

**Conradi** [Erich *Conradi,* German physician, born 1882] Conradi's disease, Conradi syndrome, Conradi-Hünermann syndrome. See under CHONDRODYSPLASIA PUNCTATA.

**cons.** *conserva* (L, keep).

**consanguineous** \kän′sang·gwin′ē·əs\ Pertaining to or characterized by consanguinity.

**consanguinity** \kän′sang·gwin′itē\ [L *consanguinitas* (from *con-* with + *sanguis,* gen. *sanguin(is)* blood + *-itas* -ITY) blood relationship, kinship] The genetic, social, and legal relationship between individuals that is attributable to descent from a recent common ancestor; blood relationship. • *Consanguinity* is often used loosely to mean consanguineous marriage, consanguineous mating, or inbreeding. This usage is not recommended.

**consciousness** [L *conscius* (from *conscire* to be conscious) conscious, privy to, witness of + -NESS] A state of awareness; the ability to appreciate sensory stimuli and to conduct and control the processes of thought. Consciousness also embraces that form of mental experience which relates to knowledge, awareness, and appreciation of the self and surroundings. **double c.** COCONSCIOUSNESS.

**consensual** \känsen′shoo·əl\ [CON- + SENSUAL] Pertaining to a reflex response of one effector organ to the sensory stimulation of another organ, usually the contralateral one of a pair.

**consent** 1 In forensic medicine, to take part in illegal sexual intercourse without objection or resistance. 2 Competent, knowing, and voluntary agreement to a therapeutic or experimental procedure. **informed c.** A patient's or a legal guardian's consent to medical treatment, which is based on his or her genuine understanding of the nature of the illness, the purpose and potential success of treatment, the alternatives to treatment, the consequences of no treatment, and the inherent risks and potential hazards of treatment. A physician is legally obligated to fully disclose to his patient all information necessary to enable the patient to choose intelligently whether or not to accept treatment. • The term may also be used in connection with a subject's agreement to participate in a clinical experiment. *Informed consent* is recognized legally in the U.S., United Kingdom, Canada, Australia, New Zealand, and India.

**conservation** The protection, care, and supervision of the use of a resource, including a natural resource such as water. A term used in the U.S., Canada, and New Zealand. **c. of energy** See under CONSERVATION OF ENERGY PRINCIPLE. **hearing c.** The preservation of normal hearing and the prevention of hearing loss. Hearing conservation may apply to the individual who has middle-ear disease or is threatened by sensorineural hearing loss, as from ototoxic drugs, but it has been applied most widely to noise control, which is regulated through the individual wearing of sound-attenuation devices, through improved engineering and architectural design of rooms and buildings, and by appropriate legislative procedures.

**conservative** Designed to restore relatively satisfactory health or function while avoiding radical therapeutic or surgical measures; based on commonly accepted practice; not innovative or experimental. Compare RADICAL.

**conserve** A medicinal confection.

**consistency** \kənsis′tənsē\ [Med L *consistentia* (from L *consistens,* gen. *consistentis,* pres. part. of *consistere* to take a stand, agree + *-ia* -Y) consistency] In epidemiology, a criterion for judging postulated causal relationships, namely that the association is observed under differing circumstances and by different methods of study.

**consolidant** \kənsäl′idənt\ 1 An agent that causes healing or union. 2 Of or relating to healing or union.

**consolidation** \kənsäl′idā′shən\ 1 The replacement of air in a lung by material, usually inflammatory, so as to render this portion of the lung airless. It is a characteristic effect of pneumonia. 2 The theoretical process by which memory traces are converted into a form permitting long-term storage for prolonged or indefinite recall. The nature of the process is not understood, but such conditions as retroactive inhibition and retrograde amnesia warrant the conclusion that such a process exists.

**conspecific** \kän′spesif′ik\ [CON- + SPECIFIC] Belonging to the same species.

**conspergent** A dusting powder, such as starch, used to prevent pills or suppositories from sticking to each other.

**conspersus** [L, past part. of *conspergere* to sprinkle, from CON- + L *spargere* to scatter] A mixture of two or more finely divided substances, used externally as a dusting powder on the skin.

**constancy** \kän′stənsē\ [L *constantia* (from *constans,* gen. *constantis,* pres. part. of *constare* to stand, stand fast) steadiness + *-ia* -Y] Stability in personality, established in childhood and subsequently expressed as being characteristic of the individual's life-style. **object c.** The tendency for objects to be perceived in the same way despite wide variations in the physical stimuli received from them. For example, visual characteristics of objects will be perceived as constant under markedly altered conditions of illumination, distance, or position.

**constant** [L *constans,* gen. *constantis,* pres. part. of *constare* to stand, stand fast] A quantity whose value does not change during a particular process, but which may change for different initial and/or boundary conditions. **affinity c.** The equilibrium constant for the combination of two substances. It is the reciprocal of the dissociation constant for the reverse reaction. It has the dimensions of the reciprocal of concentration. **association c.** A measure of the degree to which two molecular species will reversibly associate at equilibrium. It is expressed as the concentration of the complex divided by the product of the concentrations of the two unbound species. Also *binding constant.* **Avogadro's c.** The value of the number of elementary particles per unit amount of substance. It is about $6.023 \times 10^{23}$ $mol^{-1}$. Symbol: $N_A$ **binding c.** ASSOCIATION CONSTANT. **catalytic c.** The rate constant for the transformation of an enzyme-substrate complex into products. It is the limiting velocity of an enzyme-catalyzed reaction divided by the concentration of enzyme. Symbol: $k_o$, $k_{cat}$ **decay c.** The probability of radioactive disintegration per unit time and per atom, a characteristic of each radionuclide. It is defined by the equation $dN/dt = -N\lambda$, where dN/dt represents the disintegration rate in a sample containing N atoms, and λ is the decay constant. The value of this constant is equal to 0.693 divided by the physical half-life. Also *disintegration constant, radioactive constant.* Symbol: λ **diffusion c.** DIFFUSION COEFFICIENT. **disintegration c.** DECAY CONSTANT. **dissociation c.** The ratio [A][B]/[AB], denoting the concentration of dissociated and undissociated forms of a molecule at equilibrium in a solution. The higher the value, the greater the tendency of that molecule to dissociate. It is used especially to describe the tendency of weak acids to yield hydrogen ion and the conjugate base. **dissociation c. of water** The ratio $[H^+][OH^-]/[H_2O]$. However, since $[H_2O]$ remains virtually constant at 55 M when water is the solvent, the constant is usually expressed as $[H^+][OH^-]$. Its value varies with temperature and is about $10^{-14}$ $M^2$. **equilibrium c.** The product of the concentration of the products of a reaction divided by the product of the concentrations of the reactants when the reaction is at equilibrium. Activities, i.e. idealized concentrations, may need to be substituted for concentrations in order that the quantity should prove to be constant. The equilibrium constant will be dimensionless if the reaction has the same number of product molecules as of reactant molecules, otherwise it will have dimensions of concentration raised to a positive or negative integral power. Symbol: Keq **equilibrium dose c.** The energy that would be absorbed by material surrounding a radionuclide if absorption were complete, per unit of accumulated activity. If $\Delta_i$ stands for emitted radiation of type *i*, then $\Delta_i = 2.13 N_i E_i$ in gram-rads per microcurie-hour, where $E_i$ is the average energy, measured in MeV, for *i*-type radiation emitted per disintegration, and $N_i$ is the fractional frequency of that radiation. For the total absorbed energy, $\Delta_i$ must be calculated for each type of emitted radiation, gamma rays, electrons, x rays, beta particles, and so on, and the results summed. **Faraday's c.** A value which represents the charge of one mole of singly-charged ions: $F = N_a e = 96\,489 \pm 2$ coulombs/mole, where $N_A$ = Avogadro's constant and $e$ = the electrical charge of the ion. **flotation c.** The solute density to which a lipoprotein localizes in density gradient ultracentrifugation. **gas c.** The constant *R* in the equation $PV + RT$, where *P* is the pressure exerted by unit amount of substance of an ideal gas, *V* is its volume, and *T* is its absolute temperature. The value of *R* is 8.3144 J $K^{-1}$ $mol^{-1}$, or 1.987 cal $K^{-1}$ $mol^{-1}$. **gravitational c.** The constant of proportionality in Newton's law of gravitation, equal to the gravitational force between any two particles of matter times the square of the distance between them, divided by the product of their masses; a universal constant equal to $6.672 \times 10^{-11}$ newton meter squared per kilogram squared. Also *newtonian constant.* Symbol: G **growth rate c.** The rate of increase in the number of cells in a culture divided by that number. This quotient is a constant for cell growth during the exponential phase. **Michaelis c.** An empirical constant that characterizes the way in which the velocity of an enzyme-catalyzed reaction depends on substrate concentration when this dependence follows Michaelis kinetics. It has the dimensions of a concentration, and is equal to the substrate concentration at which the velocity is half its limiting value. Symbol: $K_m$ See also MICHAELIS-MENTEN EQUATION. **newtonian c.** GRAVITATIONAL CONSTANT. **Planck's c.** $6.63 \times 10^{-27}$ erg-sec, a natural constant occurring in many physical formulas. For one, it is the constant of proportionality, *h*, relating the frequency, *ν*, of a photon, assuming that it is wavelike, to its contained energy: $E = h\nu$. **radioactive c.** DECAY CONSTANT. **rate c.** The constant *k* in the reaction: $v \rightleftharpoons k[A]_\alpha[B]_\beta...$, where *v* is the rate of reaction and [A], [B], etc., are the concentrations of reactants. Also *velocity constant.* **sedimentation c.** SEDIMENTATION COEFFICIENT. **specific gamma-ray c.** The exposure rate, in roentgens per hour, per millicurie at 1 cm from a very small gamma-emitting source, assuming that there is no scattering or attenuation. **specificity c.** The catalytic constant of an enzyme-catalyzed reaction divided by the Michaelis constant. The name derives from the fact that the rates of reaction of two different substrates competing for the same enzyme will be proportional to the products of substrate concentration and specificity constant for the two substrates. The specificity constant is also the apparent second-order constant for the reaction between enzyme and substrate at low substrate concentrations, i.e. when saturation of enzyme with substrate is negligible. **time c.** For the output of a first-order system (i.e., one that contains a single energy-storage element) forced by a step or an impulse, the time required to complete 63.2% (1 − 1/e) of the total rise (to a step increase) or decay (to a step decrease). The time constant is ~44% longer ($1/\log_e 2$) than the half-life. **velocity c.** RATE CONSTANT.

**constellation** \kän′stelā′shən\ [Late L *constellatio* (from *constellatus* starred, from L *con-* with + *stellatus,* past part. of *stellare* to be starry, from *stella* a star, planet) a constellation] COMPLEX.

**constipated** \kän′stipā′tid\ Affected by constipation. Also *costive.*

**constipation** \kän′stipā′shən\ [L *constipatio* (from *constipare* to crowd together, from *con-* together + *stipare* to pack, fill, crowd; akin to English *stiff*) crowding, congestion] The condition in which bowel movements are delayed or inadequate; undue retention of feces in the large intestine. Also *costiveness.*

**constituent** \kənstich′oo·ənt\ 1 Each of the different elements present in a compound. 2 A substance present in the composition of a mixture.

**constitution** [L *constitutio* (from *constituere* to establish, arrange, from CON- + *statuere* to erect, set up, from *stare* to stand) arrangement, disposition, organization] 1 The individual, physical makeup of a human being or other organism, determined by hereditary factors the specific effects of which are shaped by environmental influences. Constitution is often used to describe the quality of the body's essential strength or inner resources in the face of stress, disease, or the aging process. 2 The composition of a chemical compound. **lymphatic c.** Lymphoid hyperplasia. **XXX sex chromosome c.** TRIPLE-X CHROMOSOMAL ABERRATION. **XYY chromosome c.** A state of aneuploidy in which some or all of the cells of a human male have an extra Y chromosome. The phenotypic consequences are variable, from undetectable to tall stature, acne vulgaris, and learning disability. It occurs in one per 800 men and was once incorrectly associated with violent or aggressive behavior. Also *XYY syndrome* (incorrect).

**constitutional** [CONSTITUTION + -AL] 1 Biologically predetermined, or so fixed as to be relatively immutable and unvarying. 2 Involving the total organism; systemic.

**constrict** \kənstrikt′\ [See CONSTRICTION.] 1 To narrow or make smaller (an opening or lumen); reduce the capacity of (a space). 2 To squeeze or compress; force into a smaller space.

**constriction** \kənstrik′shən\ [L *constrictio* (from *constrictus*, past part. of *constringere* to bind together, tie up) a contraction, tying up] 1 The process of constricting or the condition of being constricted. 2 A constricted part or structure, as a blood vessel. 3 A sensation of tightness or compression. **congenital ring c.'s** A circumferential indentation of the distal part of the extremities of uniform depth in any given instance, but varying from one constriction to the next. It has been attributed to a mesodermal deficiency during intrauterine development but in fact the cause is unknown. In its most severe form it may result in autoamputation distal to the constriction. **duodenopyloric c.** PYLORIC CONSTRICTION. **primary c.** In cytogenetics, a constricted or condensed region of a chromosome associated with, and in part defining, the centromere. **pyloric c.** A circular groove on the outer surface of the stomach marking the position of the orifice of the pyloric sphincter and often containing the prepyloric vein (of Mayo). Also *duodenopyloric constriction, duodenopyloric groove.* **secondary c.** A constricted or condensed region of a chromosome not associated with the centromere. Most acrocentric chromosomes have secondary constrictions at the end of their short arms by which satellites are attached.

**constrictor** \kənstrik′tər\ That which constricts or squeezes a part, especially a muscle that contracts to narrow or squeeze a tubular organ or structure. **c. naris** PARS TRANSVERSA MUSCULI NASALIS. **c. radicis penis** The middle fibers of the bulbospongiosus muscle that encircle the bulb of the penis. *Outmoded.* **c. vaginae** *Outmoded* COMPRESSOR VAGINAE.

**constringent** ASTRINGENT.

**consult** 1 To confer with; seek advice from. 2 To act as a consultant.

**consultant** 1 An expert in a medical or surgical specialty who is called upon to give advice regarding the diagnosis or treatment of a patient, often by the patient's primary-care physician. 2 In Great Britain, a medical or surgical practitioner formally recognized as expert in a specialty and having an appointment in a hospital. ● In the U.S. and Canada, *consultant* is used only with the sense of def. 1. Usage in South Africa, Australia, New Zealand, and India accords with that of Britain.

**consultation** A meeting of physicians or medical specialists to determine a diagnosis or therapy or to evaluate the management of a patient, often with the end of recommending a particular course of action. **therapeutic c.** 1 A patient-oriented consultation in which a consultant, on the basis of direct examination of the patient or information from the primary therapist, or both, advises the therapist on the diagnosis, treatment, rehabilitation, or other management problems involving the patient. 2 A single session with a consultant which is considered to have benefited the patient.

**consumption** \kənsump′shən\ [L *consumptio* (from *consumere* to use up, exhaust, from *con-*, intensive or completive prefix, + *sumere* to take, take on) a wearing away, wasting away, consumption] 1 The process by which a quantity is used up. 2 A wasting disease of the body; specifically, pulmonary tuberculosis. An obsolete usage.

**consumptive** \kənsump′tiv\ [*consumpt(ion)* + -IVE] 1 Pertaining to pulmonary tuberculosis. 2 A person suffering from pulmonary tuberculosis. An obsolete usage.

**cont.** 1 content. 2 containing. 3 continue(d). 4 contra. 5 *contusus* (L, bruised).

**contact** [L *contactus* (from *contactus*, past part. of *contingere* to touch, from CON- + L *tangere* to touch, happen) a touching, contact] 1 A coming together or touching of two bodies or surfaces. 2 An exposure to a source of infection. 3 A person who has been exposed to a source of infection. **balancing c.** Contact between upper and lower dentures, or natural teeth on the side away from which the lower jaw has deviated. **centric c.** CENTRIC OCCLUSION. **deflective occlusal c.** A premature occlusal contact which causes an eccentric closure. Also *interceptive occlusal contact.* **occlusal c.** Contact of upper and lower teeth in habitual occlusion. **premature occlusal c.** A contact in premature interference. Also *prematurity.* **proximal c.** The contact between adjacent teeth or restorations in adjacent teeth. **working c.** Contact of dentures or natural teeth on the side to which the lower jaw has deviated.

**contactant** \käntak′tənt\ A substance capable of inducing a delayed hypersensitivity reaction on contact with the skin.

**contagion** \käntā′jən\ [L *contagio* (from *contingere* to contact, attain, stain, pollute, infect, from CON- + *tangere* to touch; influenced by *tingere* to stain) communication, contact, contagion] The transmission of an infectious disease from one person to another either by direct contact or indirectly by means of fomites.

**contagious** \kəntā′jəs\ [Late L *contagiosus.* See CONTAGION.] 1 Capable of being transmitted by direct or indirect contact from one person to another, as a disease. 2 Capable of transmitting an infectious disease to others.

**contagium** \käntā′jē·əm\ [L, contagion. See CONTAGION.] (*pl.* contagia) The causative agent of a contagious disease.

**contaminant** \kəntam′inənt\ 1 Anything that contaminates, as *food contaminant.* 2 An additional microorganism that is present in a culture incorrectly presumed to be pure. It may arise from inadequate initial purification or from inadequate aseptic technique in subsequent manipulations. Contaminants have been responsible for many misleading results in biochemical studies on microorganisms. **food c.** Any substance which is consumed but is not a food substance, a natural constituent of food, or a food additive, and trace amounts of which remain in the finished food after the processes of production, refinement, preparation, packaging, preservation, transport, and storage.

**contamination** \kəntam′inā′shən\ [L *contaminatio* (from *contaminare* to pollute, debase, prob. from CON- + root of *tangere* to touch) defilement, pollution] **1** The presence of any undesirable, unwanted, or defiling solid, liquid, or gaseous material in a substance or environment. **2** The presence of infectious matter or of undesirable, unwanted, or alien microorganisms in a microbiological culture, sterile preparation, wound, or in any other substance or environment. **3** The presence of unwanted radioactive material in a substance or environment in which it is alien or not naturally present. ● Some definitions of physical contamination may include qualifications as to the allowable quantities or to injurious effects, or may have a special connotation for quality control purposes, as in food hygiene. *Contamination* and *pollution* are often regarded as synonymous, but *contamination* is used more frequently with reference to specific situations, samples, or substances (including foods), whereas *pollution* is often used with a broader ecological connotation, such as in air, water, or soil pollution.

**content** [L *contentus* (from *contentus,* past part. of *continere* to contain, hold, from CON- + L *tenere* to hold) that which is kept or contained] Material contained or encompassed. **carbon dioxide c.** The concentration, in a fluid such as blood, of carbon dioxide plus concentrations of carbonic acid and bicarbonate that readily convert to carbon dioxide upon acidification of the fluid. The measurement is made by determining the volume of $CO_2$ gas generated per unit volume of fluid following addition of a strong acid. Normal values for human blood are 19 to 25 mmol/l for arterial blood and 23 to 30 mmol/l for venous blood. **catalytic c.** The catalytic amount of a component of a system divided by the mass of the system, expressed in katals per kilogram or moles per kilogram second. Symbol: $Z_c/m_s$ **effective radium c.** An amount of radium producing the same effects as a given quantity of radium in a container with a standard amount of wall filtration (usually 0.5 mm platinum). **equivalent radium c.** The quantity of an encapsulated radioactive material which gives the same gamma-ray exposure rate as a stated amount of radium. **polymorphism information c.** With respect to polymorphic genetic markers, a measure of the usefulness of a given marker in performing linkage analysis, measured on a scale of 0 (uninformative) to 1. It is an approximation of the frequency of heterozygotes for the marker in the population under study. Abbr. PIC

**contiguity** \kän′tigyoo′itē\ Close contact between adjacent cells, parts, or structures without being continuous or connected.

**contiguous** \käntig′yoo·əs\ Touching at the borders or edges; adjacent.

**contin.** *continuetur* (L, let it be continued).

**continence** \kän′tinəns\ [L *continentia* (from *continens,* gen. *continentis,* pres. part. of *continere* to contain, hold, from CON- + L *tenere* to hold) repression, restraint] Self-control, usually with respect to sexual indulgence, defecation, or urination.

**continuity** \kän′tin$^y$oo′itē\ The state of being uninterrupted or connected without a break.

**contortion** \kəntôr′shən\ [L *contortio* (from *contortus,* past part. of *contorquere* to twist violently around, to turn about) a turning or whirling about] **1** Writhing movements. **2** A distorted position of the trunk or limbs or of the features of the face.

**contour** \kän′toor\ [French (from CON- + L *tornare* to round with a lathe, from Gk *torneuein* to work with lathe and chisel), outline, circuit] A two-dimensional curve that represents the outline or shape of the body or a part. **equal loudness c.** The contour represented by a line joining together the differing intensity levels of those pure tone frequencies that are judged by the subject, being tested for auditory activity, to be all of the same loudness.

**contouring** \kän′tʊring\ The purposeful changing in shape of a structure. In plastic surgery, body contouring may involve a thigh lift, an abdominoplasty, reduction or augmentation mammoplasty, etc. **body c.** The performance of a cosmetic operation, or a series of such operations, on various parts of the torso and extremities to improve the contours of these areas. **occlusal c.** OCCLUSAL ADJUSTMENT.

**contra-** \kän′trə-\ [L *contra* opposite to, against] A prefix meaning against, opposite, contrary.

**contra-angle** [CONTRA- + ANGLE] Of instruments, having the working tip at or near the continuation of the axis of the handle, thus reducing the rotational force present when the tip is some distance away from that line.

**contra-aperture** \-ap′ərchər\ COUNTERINCISION.

**contraception** \-sep′shən\ [CONTRA- + *(con)ception*] The prevention of conception. **intrauterine c.** Contraception achieved by placing a device within the uterus. **rhythm c.** RHYTHM METHOD.

**contraceptive** \kän′trəsep′tiv\ [CONTRA- + *(con)ceptive*] **1** Designed to prevent conception, as a device, drug, or method. Also *anticonceptive.* **2** A device, drug, or method used to prevent conception. **barrier c.** Any form of contraception in which ascent of sperm into the uterine cervix is blocked by a barrier, such as a condom, diaphragm, or cervical cap. **combination oral c.** An oral contraceptive that combines an estrogen and progestogen in each tablet. Also *combined oral contraceptive pill.* **intrauterine c.** A device placed within the uterus to prevent pregnancy. **oral c.** A hormonal preparation taken orally to prevent conception, especially one taken by women to block ovulation and thus prevent pregnancy. Also *birth control pill.* **sequential oral c.** An oral contraceptive preparation in which the tablets for use during the first two weeks of a menstrual cycle contain only an estrogen while those for the last week of a cycle contain both an estrogen and a progestogen. Also *sequential oral pill.*

**contract** \kəntrakt′\ [L *contract(us),* past part. of *contrahere* to draw together] **1** To compress, shorten, or reduce in size, as muscle. **2** To develop or acquire, as a disease.

**contractile** \kəntrak′tīl\ [CONTRACT + -ILE] Capable of contraction, or contributing to the intracellular mechanism that produces a contraction.

**contractility** \kän′traktil′itē\ The ability of a tissue or cell organelle to shorten or develop tension when subjected to an appropriate stimulus. **galvanic c.** The ability of a muscle to contract in response to a direct current, often implying a lower threshold to direct than to alternating current stimuli, as seen in denervated muscle. **neuromuscular c.** Contractile capability of a muscle activated through its motor innervation, either by indirect stimulation via the muscle nerve or by direct contact with the muscle with resulting excitation of intramuscular nerve branches.

**contraction** [L *contractio* (from CON- + L *tractus,* past part. of *trahere* to draw, pull) a contracting, drawing together] **1** A reduction in size or bulk. **2** A reversible shortening of an excitable tissue, as muscle; specifically, a heartbeat. **3** A simultaneous shortening by agonist and antagonist muscles to hold a limb straight. **aerobic c.** Muscle contraction in which the immediate source of energy is the oxidation of fat and carbohydrates. It characterizes red muscles and the slow-oxidative type of muscle fiber. **anaerobic c.** Muscular contraction dependent for energy primarily on glycogenolysis. It is characteristic of pale muscles and the fast-glycolytic type of muscle fiber. **anisometric c.** ISOTONIC CONTRACTION. **anodal closure c.** In direct stimulation of muscle, a contraction in the vicinity of the anode when a DC current is applied. Also *anodal closing contraction.* **anodal opening c.** Contraction at the anode when a stimulus current is interrupted. **atrial c.** The normal coordinated shortening of the muscle fibers of the atrial chambers of the heart, whereby they expel blood into the ventricles. **automatic ventricular c.** A contraction caused by an activating impulse which has arisen spontaneously in the ventricle; a ventricular escape beat. It usually occurs when the sinuatrial impulse is abnormally slow. **bladder-neck c.** A congenital or acquired narrowing of the vesical outlet. It usually causes urinary obstruction, but may be asymptomatic. **blocked atrial c.** An atrial contraction which fails to stimulate a ventricular one owing to obstruction to passage of the activating impulse in or through the atrioventricular node to the ventricle. **Braxton Hicks c.'s** Uterine contractions during the latter half of pregnancy which do not occur in association with labor. In contrast to the contractions of labor, these contractions are usually painless and occur at irregular intervals. Also *false uterine contractions, Hicks contractions, Braxton-Hicks sign, Hicks sign.* **cardiac c.** The pumping action of the heart produced by shortening of the muscle fibers of its chambers. **carpopedal c.** CARPOPEDAL SPASM. **cathodal closure c.** Contraction at the cathode when a DC stimulus commences. Also *cathodal closing contraction.* **cathodal opening c.** Excitation of a muscle at the cathode when a DC stimulus current is interrupted. **cicatricial c.** The natural tendency of a maturing scar to become smaller. As it contracts, it pulls normal tissue with it until tension overcomes the force of contraction. **concentric c.** SHORTENING CONTRACTION. **false uterine c.'s** BRAXTON HICKS CONTRACTIONS. **faradic c.** Contraction in response to an alternating, repetitive, or transitory electrical stimulus applied directly to the muscle. **fibrillary c.** FIBRILLATION. **galvanic c.** Contraction of muscle induced by a directly applied constant-current stimulus. **Hicks c.'s** BRAXTON HICKS CONTRACTIONS. **hourglass c.** Contraction of the uterus in its midportion. **hunger c.'s** Powerful contractions of the stomach that occur two to three hours after the stomach has emptied and which last for about one half hour. They are repeated at intervals of two to three hours if food is not eaten. **isokinetic c.** Contraction in which a constant amount of force is produced throughout the range of the muscle's action or an affected joint's movement. Certain exercise machines are designed to require such contraction. **isometric c.** Contraction in a muscle that is prevented from changing its length, i.e., the distance from origin to insertion. Slight shortening of fibers within the muscle may still occur due to in-series elasticity or reorientation of fascicles. **isotonic c.** Muscular contraction in which force at the tendon remains constant. The muscle length may change. Also *amisometric contraction.* **isovolumetric c.** Contraction without reduction of volume, as in the beginning of contraction of a ventricle of the heart before the opening of the semilunar valve. **lengthening c.** Activation of a muscle while it progressively lengthens as a result of some external force. **myoclonic c.** MYOCLONUS. **myotatic c.** Contraction of a muscle produced by a sharp blow to its surface or tendon with a reflex hammer or other appropriate instrument. **palmar c.** DUPUYTREN'S CONTRACTURE. **paradoxical c.** A clinical sign in which electrical (faradic) stimulation over a muscle produces a contraction opposite to that expected. Thus, stimulation over a flexor muscle produces extension and vice versa. This phenomenon occurs because of partial or complete paralysis of the muscle being tested, due, as a rule, to a lesion of the lower motor neuron. The stimulus, applied with sufficient intensity, spreads to and stimulates normally innervated antagonistic muscles. **premature c.** Contraction of a chamber of the heart occurring before it is due, usually from an abnormal site of impulse formation; an extrasystole. **secondary c.** Contraction of a muscle in one limb of a frog produced when its nerve, placed across a muscle in the opposite limb, is excited by activation of that muscle. *Outmoded.* **segmentation c.** Irregular or rhythmic circular contractions of the small intestine that divide the intestine into a number of regular sections. **shortening c.** Muscle activation that occurs while the muscle is undergoing reduction in length. The shortening may be due to the contraction or be externally imposed in addition. Also *concentric contraction.* **tetanic c.** **1** TETANUS. **2** Contraction of muscle, motor unit, or muscle fiber with production of essentially unwavering force as induced by synchronous electrical stimulation at rates above the fusion frequency. Rest periods with stimulation are generally allowed before and after the period of stimulation, which therefore is limited. **tonic c.** Sustained force production by a muscle in response to repetitive stimuli or spontaneous nerve impulses. In vertebrate muscle, tonic contraction depends upon a continuing contraction by some or all of the motor units in response to asynchronous impulses in their axons. In some muscles of invertebrates, a catch mechanism in the myofibrillar apparatus may prolong the contraction state after initial nervous excitation. **tumultuous c.'s** Uterine contractions during labor which are of increased frequency and intensity as compared to the usual contractions of labor. **twitch c.** The momentary contraction of a skeletal muscle induced by a single stimulus applied to its motor nerve. **uterine c.** A contraction of the uterine musculature usually associated with pregnancy.

**contracture** \käntrak′chər\ [L *contractura* (from *contrahere* to draw together, unite, from CON- + *trahere* to draw, pull) a narrowing, tapering] **1** Permanent shortening of a skeletal muscle, due either to weakness or paralysis of the muscle at a time when its antagonists are strong, to progressive weakness and postural changes, as in muscular dystrophy or spinal muscular atrophy, or to disease processes giving rise to progressive fibrosis within the muscle or its tendon. **2** A wholly recoverable state of prolonged contraction of a skeletal muscle, either produced by repetitive electrical stimulation or occurring spontaneously, due to abnormal biochemical processes, usually after exertion, as in McArdle's disease. **3** Hysterical contraction of skeletal muscle in which the affected limb is held in an abnormal posture such as marked flexion of the fingers, with any attempt to extend the fingers evoking intense contraction of the flexors. **burn scar c.** The loss of joint mobility as a result of shortening of a burn scar over the joint. **Dupuytren's c.** A fibrous thickening of the palmar fascia that leads to progressive flexion deformities of the fingers, with the medial fingers more severely affected. Etiological factors include epilepsy and alcoholism. It can be associated with knuckle pads, contracture of the plantar fascia, and Peyronie's disease. Also *palmar contraction.* **extrapyramidal c.** Contracture or shortening of skeletal muscle occurring as a consequence of long-lasting extrapyramidal hypertonia (plastic or "cogwheel" rigidity) as seen in parkin-

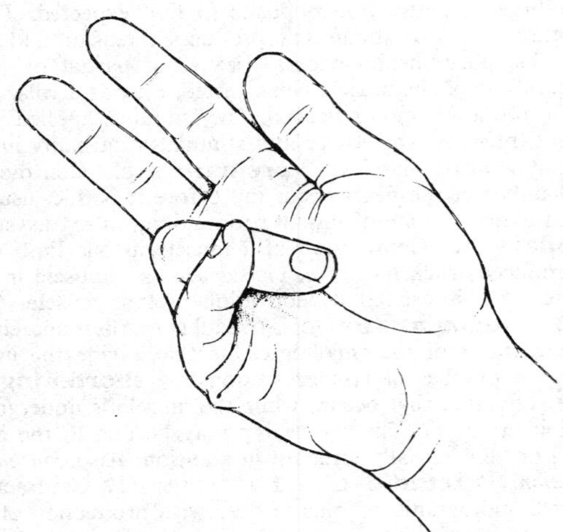

Dupuytren's contracture

sonism, especially the postencephalitic variety. • Sometimes this term is used, incorrectly, to identify extrapyramidal rigidity or hypertonia itself. **flexion c.** The loss of a joint's ability to extend fully. **functional c.** HYSTERICAL CONTRACTURE. **hypertonic c.** An irreversible shortening of muscles and tendons as a result of long-standing spasticity. **hysterical c.** Apparent contracture (such as gross flexion of the fingers which dig into the palm) with intense resistance when any attempt is made passively to overcome it (as by attempting to straighten the fingers), resulting not from organic disease but from hysteria. These contractures most often affect the hand or foot and often follow minor injury, especially where financial compensation is involved. Electromyography demonstrates continuous activity in the agonist muscles, and electrical stimulation of the antagonists may temporarily abolish the contracture. Also *functional contracture.* **ischemic c.** Permanent shortening of a muscle due to necrosis and replacement fibrosis following prolonged interference with the blood supply, as by injury, tourniquet, pressure of overtight bandage, or cold. **ischemic c. of the left ventricle** Irreversible contracture and necrosis of the left ventricle as a complication of cardiopulmonary bypass. Also *stony heart.* **muscle c.** A fibrosis and shortening of a muscle. It usually results in a limb deformity. **permanent c.** An irreversible shortening, as in the case of a joint that has lost range of motion due secondarily to soft tissue shortening. **veratrin c.** A prolonged contraction of skeletal muscle brought about by the intramuscular administration of veratrin. **Volkmann's ischemic c.** A syndrome of infarction and subsequent fibrous contracture of forearm flexor muscles usually resulting from damage to the brachial artery as a consequence of supracondylar fracture of the humerus. The contracture gives rise to flexion deformities in the hand and fingers. Also *Volkmann's paralysis, Volkmann's ischemic paralysis, Volkmann's contracture, ischemic muscular atrophy, Volkmann syndrome.*

**contraextension** \-iksten′shən\ COUNTEREXTENSION.

**contrafissure** \-fish′ər\ A fracture in a bone located opposite the site of impact. Also *counterfissure, contrafissura.*

**contraincision** \-insizh′ən\ COUNTERINCISION.

**contraindicant** \-in′dikənt\ **1** Being a contraindication; indicating that a particular course of treatment is inadvisable. **2** CONTRAINDICATION.

**contraindicate** \-in′dikāt\ To make inadvisable. ⟨"We support as much breast-feeding as possible . . . But we're also concerned about toxins that would contraindicate it." —*Medical World News,* 30 Mar. 1981, 7.⟩

**contraindication** \-in′dikā′shən\ Any fact or circumstance that renders a particular course of treatment inadvisable or undesirable. Also *contraindicant.*

**contralateral** \-lat′ərəl\ Pertaining to or located on the opposite side of a body or part. Also *heterolateral.*

**contrast** [French *contraste* (from CONTRA- + L *stare* to stand) opposition of feelings or effects] **1** A dissimilarity between two things made evident by comparing them. **2** In medical imaging, the differences in brightness in the images of the structures under study. **high c.** SHORT-SCALE CONTRAST. **long-scale c.** That degree of contrast in which the range of image densities is wide and great in number, and each density exhibits only a relatively small tonal difference from its neighbor. Also *low contrast.* **object c.** In nuclear medicine, the ratio of activity in a lesion to the activity surrounding a lesion, described mathematically as $(B-T)/B$, where $C$ is the object contrast, $B$ is the surrounding activity, and $T$ is the lesion activity. **radiographic c.** The difference in film density between different structures seen on a roentgenogram. **short-scale c.** That degree of radiographic contrast in which the range of image densities is small in number, and each density exhibits a large tonal difference from its neighbor. Also *high contrast.*

**contrastimulant** SEDATIVE.

**contrastimulism** The practice of employing contrastimulants as a therapeutic regimen.

**contrastimulus** \-stim′yələs\ Anything having a sedative effect.

**cont. rem.** *continuetur remedium* (L, let the remedy, i.e., the medication, continue).

**control** [French *contrôle* (from CONTRA- + L *rotula* a little wheel) a double register for verification] **1** A group or subject in an experiment or study serving as a standard from which another or other groups or subjects differ significantly in being exposed to the variable under study. The control functions as a means of isolating the variable under study by matching other factors with the experimental group in order to minimize the likelihood that such factors might have accounted for the results noted. For example, a group of persons known or considered likely to be free of a given disease may serve as a control for comparison with a group of patients (matched by age, sex, and other factors) known to have the disease, in order to explore an epidemiologic hypothesis. A control may also consist of a group suffering from a given disease and from whom a specific treatment has been withheld, to be compared with another group suffering from the same disease to whom the treatment is given, as a means of measuring the effectiveness of the treatment. A group of laboratory animals may constitute a control when compared with another group of like animals which have been subjected to an experimental treatment or used for standardizing a biological measurement. **2** To verify by employing a control: said especially of an experiment. **astigmatism c.** A control which adjusts the uniformity of focus over a display screen. **automatic gain c.** An electronic circuit that continuously readjusts the amplitude of an incoming signal so that it lies within prescribed limits. It is used in hearing aids, tape recorders, and radios.

Abbr. AGC **biologic c.** The restriction of populations of parasites, weeds, or other pests through the use of viruses, bacteria, insects, or other organisms. **birth c.** Any of various methods designed to enable people to avoid having children except when they intend to do so. Artificial contraceptive devices and sterilization are commonly used methods of birth control. Also *fertility regulation.* **chin c.** A system whereby the chin can be used to activate various self-help devices, as by quadriplegic patients. **Diack c.** A chemical indicator in tablet form hermetically sealed in a glass tube. When placed inside a steam sterilizer, it signals conditions adequate for sterilization by a change in appearance. **feedback c.** A self-regulatory system in which a change or event in a process affects the course of the process. For example, in numerous biological systems a cell product, upon reaching a particular threshold, will switch off its own synthesis. As the concentration of the cell product falls, the synthetic mechanism is restarted. **fine c.** The regulation of enzyme activity by feedback inhibition: used to emphasize the distinction from "coarse control," which is the regulation of the same process by varying the rate of enzyme synthesis. **multivalent c.** Control of formation of the enzymes of a branched biosynthetic pathway, requiring a mixture of the end products because all enter the leader peptide in the mechanism of regulation by attenuation. **noise c.** The various approaches adopted in engineering and architectural design which prevent or reduce the emission of high intensity noise. Noise control has application to specific industrial environments or to road traffic, aircraft, or other noise, as it applies to the general population. There is an increasing tendency to enforce such measures by legislation at the national level. **relaxed c.** A mutation in bacteria that prevents the repression of ribosomal RNA synthesis in response to deprival of a required amino acid. See also STRINGENT CONTROL. **Schick c.** A preparation of heat-inactivated toxin derived from *Corynebacterium diphtheriae* and used, in doses of 0.2 ml, as the control for the active unheated toxin injected in the Schick test. **stringent c.** The mechanism that coordinates ribosomal RNA synthesis with protein synthesis in bacteria. When translating ribosomes are deprived of a required amino acid they form quanosine 3′-diphosphate-5′-diphosphate which represses ribosomal RNA synthesis. In mutants resulting from relaxed control the ribosomes lack a protein required for synthesis of 3′-diphosphtate-5′-diphosphate. **synergic c.** The coordinating and integrating influence of the cerebellum upon voluntary movement. *Outmoded.* **tonic c.** Maintained nerve impulse or muscle activity. **vestibuloequilibratory c.** The contribution made by the vestibular apparatus to the maintenance of the body's equilibrium. **voluntary c.** Muscular action influenced by the will. Also *volitional control.*

**contuse** \käntooz′\ [L *contus(us),* past part. of *contundere* to bruise, crush, break] To bruise or cause a contusion.

**contusion** \käntoo′zhən\ [L *contusio* (from *contusus,* past part. of *contundere* to bruise, crush) a bruising, shattering] An injury in which the skin is not broken but underlying blood vessels are disrupted, causing a hematoma under the skin. At first it presents itself as a swelling, then becomes bluish black, then greenish, then yellowish, and then resolves. Also *bruise.* **brain c.** Disruption of small blood vessels and brain cells within the brain, following trauma. It may or may not be associated with skull fracture. **cerebral c.** Bruising of the brain as a result of closed head injury. The effects are more serious than in the case of concussion in that there is evidence of areas of hemorrhage into the brain substance. **contrecoup c.** CONTRECOUP INJURY. **c. of spinal cord** Bruising of the spinal cord due to physical injury.

**contusive** \käntoo′siv\ Producing a bruise or contusion.

**conular** \kän′yələr\ Conical.

***Conus*** \kō′nəs\ [L (from Gk *kōnos* a pine cone, cone), a cone] A genus of stinging or venomous mollusks (poison cone shells) in the family Conidae. The animal possesses a long proboscis armed with a harpoonlike, coiled tip of modified radular teeth and venom from a special gland and venom duct. The poison apparatus found in tropical waters of the Pacific are used to paralyze prey, usually other shellfish. The most dangerous of these brilliantly-colored, slow-moving, Indo-Pacific cone shells are *Conus geographus, C. tulipa, C. textile,* and *C. marmoreus. C. geographus* is generally considered the most venomous.

**conus** \kō′nəs\ [L (from Gk *kōnos* a pine cone, cone), a cone] (*pl.* coni) **1** A crescent-shaped area of exposed sclera adjacent to the optic disk. The exposure of the sclera is due to incomplete formation or degeneration of the overlying choroid and retinal pigment layer, hence, the appearance implies a developmental or degenerative condition. **2** In anatomy, a cone-shaped structure. **c. arteriosus** [NA] The smooth area above the supraventricular crest of the right ventricle related to the outflow of blood upwards to the pulmonary orifice. It represents a persistent part of the bulbus cordis of the embryo. Also *arterial cone, conus cordis* (outmoded), *infundibulum of heart, pulmonary cone, cardiac infundibulum, infundibulum.* **c. elasticus laryngis** [NA] A yellow elastic membrane attached inferiorly to the superior margin of the cricoid cartilage. It is thickened and subcutaneous anteriorly to form the median cricothyroid ligament, attached above to the inferior border of the thyroid cartilage in the midline. The superior margins of the paired lateral portions of the membrane are free, parallel, and thickened to form the vocal ligaments stretching horizontally between the thyroid angle and the vocal processes of the arytenoid cartilages. Also *membrana cricovocalis, cricovocal membrane, conus elasticus of larynx, elastic cone of larynx, cricothyroarytenoid ligament* (outmoded), *cricothyroid membrane, lateral part of cricothyroid ligament.* **coni epididymidis** LOBULI EPIDIDYMIDIS. **c. medullaris** [NA] The tapering caudal extremity of the spinal cord proper. Also *medullary cone, terminal cone of spinal cord, conus terminalis.* • The term is properly applied to acaudate species, like man.

**convalesce** \kän′vəles′\ To recover one's health following illness, injury, or surgery; be a convalescent.

**convalescence** \kän′vəles′əns\ [Late L *convalescentia,* from *convalescens.* See CONVALESCENT.] The recovery of health following illness, injury, or surgery.

**convalescent** \kän′vəles′ənt\ [L *convalescens,* gen. *convalescentis,* pres. part. of *convalescere* (from *con-*, intensive or completive prefix, + *valescere* to become strong or well, from *valere* to be strong or well) to recover strength or health] **1** Recovering one's health following illness, injury, or surgery. **2** A person who is convalescent.

**convection** \kənvek′shən\ [Late L *convectio* (from *convectus,* past part. of *convehere* to carry or bring together, convey) a carrying together, conveying] The transport of heat in liquids or gases by a circulatory movement related to the rising of heated, less dense particles and the sinking of cooled, more dense particles.

**convergence** \känvur′jəns\ [See CONVERGENT.] **1** The act or condition of coming together toward a point. **2** The simultaneous rotation of both eyes toward the midline, as occurs in the act of near gaze. **accommodative c.** Nasalward deviation of the eyes associated with focusing upon a near fixation point. **conjugate c.** TONIC CONVERGENCE. **far point of c.** The point of intersection of the visual axes when convergence is completely relaxed. **fusional c.** Convergence initiated by cerebral synthesis of the two ocular images. **near point of c.** The point of intersection of the visual axes when maximal convergence is exerted. **negative c.** DIVERGENCE. **positive c.** An increase in the amount of nasalward positioning of the eyes. **tonic c.** Convergence due to the normal state of partial contraction of the extraocular muscles. Also *conjugate convergence.*

**convergent** \kənvur′jənt\ [Late L *convergens,* gen. *convergentis,* pres. part. of *convergere* (from *con-* together + *vergere* to incline, slope) to approach a junction] **1** Tending to come together toward a point; characterized by convergence. **2** Denoting the condition in which both eyes are rotated toward each other.

**conversion** \kənvur′shən\ [L *conversio* (from *convertere* to turn upside down or around, from *con-,* intensive or completive prefix, + *vertere* to cause to turn) a rotation, revolution, transformation] **1** An unconscious mental mechanism by which emotional conflict is transformed into motor, visceral, or sensory physical manifestations, as in some forms of hysteria. Also *somatic conversion, somatization.* **2** TRANSMUTATION. **gene c.** The apparent conversion of one allele to another during meiosis. It is detected in situations in which the genotype of all gametes can be analyzed. For example, an individual heterozygous at locus *A* (*A*/*a*) would be expected to produce gametes that have *A* and *a* in equal frequencies. Gene conversion, due perhaps to unequal crossing over, would result in a 1:3 ratio of *A* to *a* gametes, or vice versa. **internal c.** The discharge of energy from an excited nucleus by ejection of an orbital electron from the atom, rather than by emitting a gamma photon. **lysogenic c.** The ability of a lysogenic phage genome to interact with a bacterial genome to alter the production of a given bacterial product or toxin. The best example is the lysogenic conversion to toxin production by diphtheria organisms following infection with lysogenic diphtherial bacteriophages. **Mantoux c.** The transition from a tuberculin-negative state to a tuberculin-positive state. The diagnosis is made on the basis of an intracutaneous injection of a tuberculin solution. The change indicates recent exposure to an infection with tubercle bacilli. Compare MANTOUX REVERSION. **phage c.** The ability of bacterial virus (phage) genome to interact with the bacterial genome so that a particular bacterial synthesis or product is under the genetic control of the phage genome. **somatic c.** **1** CONVERSION. **2** CONVERSION HYSTERIA. **wound c.** The process whereby a partial thickness cutaneous burn results in full thickness necrosis due to infection or local ischemia.

**convertase** \kənvur′tās\ Designating those proteinases of complement that convert one component into another. Thus complement component C3 convertase splits a peptide bond in component C3 to activate it.

**converter** \kənvur′tər\ A device that can transform signals from one mode to another, as from analog to digital, serial to parallel, or low frequency to high frequency. **analog-to-digital c.** An electronic circuit that converts an analog voltage or physical motion to a proportional digital number suitable for entry into a digital computer. **data c.** A machine that converts data in one form such as punch cards, magnetic tape, or paper tape to another form. **digital-to-analog c.** An electronic circuit that converts binary digital numbers into a proportional analog voltage. **scan c.** A device that stores a gray-scale image and allows it to be displayed on a television monitor. An analog scan converter stores image information as an electric charge distribution on a silicon target. A digital scan converter stores ultrasound echo amplitudes as a matrix of numbers.

**convertin** \kənvur′tin\ The activated form of factor VII, designated factor VIIa.

**convex** \kän′veks, känveks′\ [L *convexus* (akin to *convehere* to carry or bring together, convey) elevated, vaulted, convex] **1** Curving outward like part of the exterior surface of a sphere. **2** In ophthalmology, pertaining to a plus lens or surface. **low c.** Pertaining to a weak plus lens or surface.

**convexity** \känvek′sitē\ **1** The state of being convex. **2** An appearance of the surface of a cell, part, or organ that is evenly rounded or curved outwards. Compare CONCAVITY.

**convexobasia** \känvek′sōbā′zhə\ A deformity in which the occipital bone is inclined forward by the cervical spine. Such an abnormality may be seen in osteitis deformans.

**convexoconcave** \känvek′sōkänkāv′\ Convex on one side and concave on the other; pertaining to a lens having plus power on one surface, negative power on the other surface.

**convexoconvex** \känvek′sōkänveks′\ Convex on both sides; pertaining to a lens having plus power on both surfaces.

**convoluted** \kän′vōloo′tid\ Rolled together, one part on another; coiled; folded inward. Also *convolute.*

**convolution** \kän′vōloo′shən\ [L *convolutio* (from *convolutus,* past part. of *convolvere* to roll together, roll around, wind around) convolution] One of the tortuous elevations bordered by sulci, or fissures, that are characteristic of the cerebrum of higher and larger vertebrates. Such a convolution, or gyrus, consists of cortical gray matter overlying a medullary core of white matter. Also *convolutio.* Adj. convolutional. **Broca's c.** **1** GYRUS FRONTALIS INFERIOR. **2** BROCA'S MOTOR SPEECH AREA. **callosal c.** GYRUS CINGULI. **first temporal c.** GYRUS TEMPORALIS SUPERIOR. **Heschl's c.'s** HESCHL'S GYRI. **occipitotemporal c.** GYRUS OCCIPITOTEMPORALIS LATERALIS. **second temporal c.** GYRUS TEMPORALIS MEDIUS. **transitional c.'s** GYRI ANNECTENTES. **Zuckerkandl's c.** GYRUS SUBCALLOSUS.

**convolutional** \kän′vōloo′shənəl\ Denoting or having the characteristics of a convolution, or gyrus.

**convulsant** \kənvul′sənt\ Any drug, substance, or physical disturbance which can induce convulsions.

**convulsion** \känvul′shən\ [L *convulsio* (from *convulsus,* past part. of *convellere* to rend, shake loose, tear away, from CON- + L *vellere* to pluck, pull out) a rending, shaking, convulsion] Any involuntary contraction of skeletal muscle, especially the successive phases, occurring in a major epileptic seizure, of generalized tonic contraction of muscles and generalized clonic jerking following an initial loss of consciousness. Transient generalized clonic movements which occasionally occur in prolonged syncope or which may result from drugs are epileptiform and can also be characterized as convulsions, as can the attacks associated with fever and infection in infancy (febrile convulsions). Minor and focal attacks of epilepsy and myoclonus are not usually regarded as convulsions. **audiogenic c.** A convulsion precipitated by an auditory stimulus. **central c.** A convulsion resulting from a neuronal discharge arising in centrally situated structures in the brain. Also *essential convulsion.* **choreic c.** A myoclonic jerk superficially resembling a choreiform movement. **clonic c.** Any convulsion in which clonic muscular contractions occur. *Imprecise.* **essential c.** CENTRAL CONVULSION. **febrile c.'s** Convulsions precipitated by fever. Some infants show a tendency to convulse whenever they are febrile for any reason. While some of these continue to suffer spontaneous attacks of epilepsy as they grow older, many lose this tendency after the age of three and no longer require anticonvulsant drug therapy. Nevertheless, some such children show a slightly increased tendency to develop epilepsy in adult life. Major attacks of epilepsy in constitutionally predisposed individuals of any age may sometimes be precipitated by infective illness associated with pyrexia. Also *hyperthermic convulsions, hyperpyrexic convulsions.* **hypoglycemic c. in newborn** Generalized convulsions in infants, especially in males if their birth weight is low relative to the length of gestation, and if preeclamptic toxemia has complicated the pregnancy. It is characterized by twitchings, apnea attacks, cyanosis or pallor, reluctance to feed, limpness, and very low blood sugar. It can be fatal and carries high risks of severe brain damage unless the blood sugar level can be restored immediately. **hysterical c.'s** Convulsions resulting from hysteria and not from epilepsy or organic brain disease. These attacks are usually florid, bizarre and generally occur, as if for maximum effect, in front of an audience. Tongue-biting and incontinence do not occur initially but may ultimately accompany the attacks if the patient has been asked about these features repeatedly. **immediate post-traumatic c.** A seizure immediately following trauma to the brain, caused by direct brain injury or by cerebral hypoxia. **infantile c.** Any major epileptic attack occurring in infancy. • This term is used to embrace many types of attack occurring in infancy, including infantile massive spasm, febrile convulsions, and even nonepileptic phenomena such as syncope with transient convulsive jerking, and breath-holding attacks which differ greatly in prognosis and management. Though imprecise, this term is still widely used. **jackknife c.** INFANTILE MASSIVE SPASM. **lightning major c.** A relatively uncommon type of epileptic seizure in childhood characterized by a very sudden single clonic contraction of the muscles of the limbs, trunk, neck, and face. The child may be thrown forwards or backwards and may acquire a chronic contusion or ulcer on the occiput or forehead from many exact repetitions of the fall. Postictal unconsciousness is brief. The electroencephalogram shows a single massive spike in all leads at the moment of the attack. **local c.** An attack of focal or jacksonian epilepsy. **mimetic c.** TIC. **mimic c.** TIC. **puerperal c.** Seizures in women following labor, usually caused by eclampsia in the early puerperium, and by cerebral vein thrombosis in the second week of the puerperium. **salaam c.** INFANTILE MASSIVE SPASM. **simple febrile c.'s** Isolated attacks of major epilepsy occurring during a febrile illness without subsequent recurrence. *Seldom used.* **static c.'s** INFANTILE MASSIVE SPASM. **tetanic c.** 1 A tonic convulsion without loss of consciousness. 2 A generalized muscle spasm occurring in tetanus. **tonic c.** A convulsion giving rise to a state of continuous tonic contraction, without clonic jerking, sometimes being generalized, sometimes focal and then involving a single limb. A brainstem origin for these attacks is postulated. Also *tonic attack, tonic spasm, tetanic spasm* (seldom used). **toxic c.** A convulsion due to the effect of an endogenous or exogenous toxin on the nervous system. Also *toxic spasm.* **traumatic c.** TRAUMATIC SEIZURE. **uremic c.** A convulsion or seizure associated with uremia, either acute or chronic, usually of the generalized major motor type, although focal motor seizures, even without loss of consciousness, do occur. The reason for the lowered seizure threshold in uremia is not known. Convulsions due to hypertensive encephalopathy can be distinguished from those of uremia by the presence of papilledema and hypertensive retinopathy in the former but not the latter. Convulsions may also occur during hemodialysis as part of the dysequilibrium syndrome, and following very large doses of penicillin in the presence of decreased renal function.

**convulsive** \kənvul′siv\ Denoting, affecting, causing or pertaining to a convulsion. Also *convulsionary, convulsivant.*

**Cooke** [William Edmond *Cooke,* English physician, 1881–1939] See under CRITERION.

**Coolidge** [William David *Coolidge,* U.S. physicist, 1873–1974] Coolidge tube, Coolidge x-ray tube. See under TUBE.

**cooling / peritoneal c.** The experimental technique of reducing body temperature by perfusing the peritoneal cavity with a cool fluid. **pleural c.** The experimental technique of reducing body temperature by perfusing the pleural cavity with a cool fluid.

**Coombs** [Robin Royston Amos *Coombs,* English physician and pathologist, born 1921] 1 Direct Coombs test. See under DIRECT ANTIGLOBULIN TEST. 2 Coombs test. See under ANTIGLOBULIN TEST. 3 Indirect Coombs test. See under INDIRECT ANTIGLOBULIN TEST. 4 Coombs serum. See under ANTIGLOBULIN SERUM.

**Coons** [A. J. *Coons,* U.S. immunologist, born 1912] Coons fluorescent antibody method. See under METHOD.

**Cooper** [Sir Astley Paston *Cooper,* English anatomist and surgeon, 1768–1841] 1 Cooper's hernia. See under RETROPERITONEAL HERNIA. 2 Oblique ligament of Cooper, Cooper's ligament. See under CHORDA OBLIQUA. 3 Cooper suspensory ligaments. See under LIGAMENTA SUSPENSORIA MAMMARIA. 4 Cooper's ligament, inguinal ligament of Cooper, pectineal ligament of Cooper. See under LIGAMENTUM PECTINEALE. 5 Cooper's ligament hernioplasty. See under MCVAY'S OPERATION.

**cooperation** Coordinated action serving a common purpose. **T lymphocyte-B lymphocyte c.** The interaction of T lymphocytes with B lymphocytes in order to produce normal levels of antibody to thymus dependent antigens. This interaction may occur directly or through participation of macrophages. Also *T-B cell cooperation.* **T lymphocyte-T lymphocyte c.** An interaction between different subsets of T lymphocytes to control the immune responses. For example, the use of monoclonal T cell subset markers indicates that there are specific suppressor or helper functions in the T cell subsets.

**cooperative** \kō·äp′ərətiv\ Exhibiting cooperativity.

**cooperativity** \kō·äp′ərətiv′itē\ The effect in which one molecule assists the action of another. This is seen, for example, in cooperative binding, in which a second molecule of ligand binds more easily than the first. This situation can give rise to a sigmoid curve of saturation against concentration of free ligand. **negative c.** The phenomenon in which one molecule makes the action of another more difficult. It often applies to ligand binding by a protein, where binding at one site lowers the affinity of another site in the protein. **positive c.** The facilitation by one molecule of the effect of another, as in binding by a protein, where binding of one ligand molecule facilitates the binding of another. Such an effect may give a sigmoid curve of saturation against the concentration of free ligand, as shown for oxygen binding by hemoglobin.

**COP** A chemotherapy regimen that includes cyclophosphamide, vincristine (Oncovin), and prednisone.

**COPA** A chemotherapy regimen that includes cyclophosphamide, vincristine (Oncovin), prednisone, and doxorubicin (Adriamycin).

**coparaffinate** An anti-infective dermal medication prepared by mixing neutralized isoparaffinic acid with iso-octyl hydroxybenzyldialkyl amines.

**COPD** chronic obstructive pulmonary disease.

**Cope** [Sir Vincent Zachary *Cope*, English surgeon, born 1881] See under SIGN.

**copepod** \kō′pepäd\ [Gk *kōpē* oar + -POD] A member of the crustacean subclass Copepoda. Copepods are among the most abundant of aquatic invertebrates. Also *water flea* (popular).

**Copepoda** \kōpep′ədə\ [Gk *kōpē* a handle, oar + New L *-poda*, neut. pl. combining form from Gk *pous*, gen. *podos*, foot] A subclass of Crustacea included among the forms commonly called microcrustacea and constituting an essential link in the aquatic food chain from plants to animals. Some copepods are intermediate hosts of parasites, especially tapeworms, of fish and mammals, including the human parasites *Diphyllobothrium latum* and *Dracunculus medinensis.*

**coping** \kō′ping\ A simple cap, not tooth-shaped, but made to fit on a prepared tooth to accommodate an artificial crown or a bridge abutment. Also *thimble.*

**Coplin** [W. M. L. *Coplin*, U.S. physician, 1864–1928] See under JAR.

**copper** Element number 29, having atomic weight 63.546. It is a reddish, lustrous metal and a very good conductor of heat and electricity. Valences are 1 and 2. Copper compounds are toxic and are used in many agricultural poisons. Trace amounts of the element are essential in many enzyme systems in plants and animals. Copper is a key constituent in the oxygen transport systems of invertebrates. Symbol: Cu Adj. cupric.

**copperas** FERROUS SULFATE.

**copperhead** **1** A venomous snake of the New World, belonging to the genus *Agkistrodon.* **2** A venomous snake of Australia, *Denisonia superba.*

**copr-** \käpr-\ COPRO-.

**copremesis** \käp′rəmē′sis\ [COPR- + EMESIS] FECAL VOMITING.

**copro-** \käp′rə-\ [Gk *kopros* dung] A combining form meaning (1) feces; (2) filth. Also *copr-, kopro-, kopr-.*

**coproantibody** \-an′tēbäd′ē\ An antibody found in the intestinal tract and hence in the feces. It is mainly of the IgA type.

**coprolagnia** \-lag′nē·ə\ COPROPHILIA.

**coprolalia** \-lā′lyə\ [COPRO- + -LALIA] The use of obscene words or speech, sometimes appearing as a paraphilia or as an involuntary utterance as in the Gilles de la Tourette syndrome. Also *coprolalomania, coprophrasia, cacolalia, compulsive swearing, coprophilia, eschrolalia* (seldom used), *lalochezia* (seldom used), *scatologia.*

**coprolith** \käp′rəlith\ FECALITH.

**coprology** \käpräl′əjē\ [COPRO- + -LOGY] The scientific study and analysis of feces, usually for diagnostic purposes. Also *scatology, skatology.* Adj. coprologic.

**coproma** \käprō′mə\ [COPR- + -OMA] STERCOROMA.

***Copromastix prowazeki*** \-mas′tiks prō′wazek′ē\ *TETRAMITUS ROSTRATUS.*

***Copromonas*** \käpräm′ənas\ [COPRO- + Gk *monas* single, a unit] A genus of uniflagellate, elongate coprozoic protozoa (class Phytomastigophorea) found in the feces of toads, frogs, and humans. They feed on bacteria and encyst after pair fusion.

**coprophil** \käp′rəfil\ [COPRO- + -PHIL] Any microorganism, such as a bacterium, found living in excrement. Also *coprophile.*

**coprophile** \käp′rəfīl\ [COPRO- + -PHILE] COPROPHIL.

**coprophilia** \-fil′yə\ [COPRO- + -PHILIA] **1** Pathologic interest in feces or dirt. **2** A paraphilia in which excrement or dirt is a necessity for sexual gratification. Also *coprolagnia, scatophilia.* Adj. coprophilic, coprophilous. **3** COPROLALIA.

**coprophrasia** \-frā′zhə\ COPROLALIA.

**coproporphyria** \-pôrfir′ē·ə\ An autosomal dominant, hepatic form of porphyria that clinically resembles the acute intermittent form but has the distinct biochemical basis of a deficiency of the mitochondrial enzyme coproporphrinogen oxidase. Many heterozygotes for this deficiency are asymptomatic or have only psychiatric involvement, while others have severe, relapsing colic or constipation. A marked elevation only of coproporphrinogen in the feces is diagnostic.

**coproporphyrin** A porphyrin whose substituents are four methyl groups and four 2-carboxyethyl groups. It is an intermediate in heme biosynthesis and may be present in normal urine. Like other porphyrins, it can be excreted in increased amounts in congenital porphyrias.

**coprostasis** \käpräs′təsis\ [COPRO- + -STASIS] Fecal impaction in the intestine.

**coprozoa** \-zō′ə\ [COPRO- + Gk *zōa*, pl. of *zōon* living being, animal] (*sing.* coprozoon) Protozoa that live in excrement but not in the intestine of the organism that discharges it.

**copula** \käp′yələ\ [L, bond, band, bond of union] (*pl.* copulae, copulas) In anatomy, a narrow connecting part or structure. In embryology, a connecting structure or bond that forms in the midline, as the *lingual copula.* **lingual c.** A midline union in the floor of the embryonic pharynx of the ventral portions of the second visceral arches. Initially it lies in front of the hypobranchial eminence, but is soon overgrown from behind by third arch tissue and becomes buried. For this reason the lingual copula and the hypobranchial eminence are sometimes regarded as variant terms for the same entity. Also *copula linguae.*

**copulation** \käp′yəlā′shən\ [L *copulatio* (from *copulatus*, past part. of *copulare* to join together, couple) a union, coupling] COITUS.

**coq.** *coque* (L, boil).

**coq. in s. a.** *coque in sufficiente aqua* (L, boil in sufficient water).

**coq. s. a.** *coque secundum artem* (L, boil properly).

**coquille** \kôkē′ē, kôkēl′\ [French (from L *conchylium* a mussel, shellfish, from Gk *konchylion* a mussel or cockle), the calcareous shell of a mollusk] An inexpensive molded optical lens.

**cor** \kôr\ [L (gen. *cordis*, akin to Gk *kardia* and English *heart*) the heart] [NA] The hollow, chambered organ that serves as the muscular pump for the circulation of the blood; heart. Also *cardia* (outmoded). **acute c. pulmonale** Rapidly increasing distension and failure of the right ventricle resulting from acute pulmonary embolism. **c. adiposum** FATTY HEART. **c. biloculare** HEMICARDIA. **c. bovinum** Gross enlargement of the heart, especially of the left ventricle, in cases of aortic valve incompetence. Also *bovine heart, ox heart.* **c. dextrum** RIGHT HEART. **c. pseudotriloculare biatriatum** A malformed heart in which tricuspid atresia or double-inlet left ventricle during intrauterine life resulted in a rudimentary right ventricle and a dominant left ventricle. Consequently the heart functions as a three-chambered organ, the right ventricle being simply an outflow chamber. *Outmoded.* **c. pulmonale** Enlargement of the right side of the heart secondary to disease of the lungs or pulmonary circulation, including such causes as pulmonary vascular disease, emphysema, and disorders of the thoracic cage. It may be acute or chronic. **c. sinistrum** LEFT HEART. **c. triatrium** A congenital malformation in which an abnormal partition divides either the right or left atrium into two compartments. Most often it is the left atrium that is divided, usually with a proximal pulmonary venous compartment and a distal compartment communicating with the mitral valve and, typically, the right atrium through the foramen ovale. A divided right atrium is much rarer and is due to persistence of the embryonic valves of the sinus venosus. Also *cor triatriatum, cor triauriculare, triatrial heart.* **c. triloculare** A malformed heart in which either the interatrial or the interventricular septal structures have failed to develop, or else have developed minimally, leaving the atrial or ventricular segments essentially as a single chamber and the heart as a three-chambered organ. *Outmoded.* Also *three-chambered heart, trilocular heart.* **c. venosum** *Outmoded* RIGHT HEART.

**cor-** \kôr-\ COM-.

**coracidia** \kôr′əsid′ē·ə\ Plural of CORACIDIUM.

**coracidium** \kôr′əsid′ē·əm\ [Gk *korax*, gen. *korakos*, a crow, raven, thing hooked like a raven's bill + -IDIUM] (*pl.* coracidia) The first-stage swimming embryo of pseudophyllid and other cestodes with aquatic life cycles. It consists of a six-hooked oncosphere larva within a ciliated embryophore. When ingested by an appropriate kind of copepod as first intermediate host, the larva develops into a proceroid, the next larval stage in the tape worm's life cycle.

**coracoacromial** \kôr′əkō·əkrō′mē·əl\ Pertaining to the coracoid and acromial processes of the scapula. Also *acromiocoracoid.*

**coracobrachialis** \kôr′əkōbrā′kē·ā′lis\ MUSCULUS CORACOBRACHIALIS.

**coracoclavicular** \kôr′əkōklavik′yələr\ Pertaining to the coracoid process of the scapula and the clavicle.

**coracohumeral** \kôr′əkōyoo′mərəl\ Pertaining to the coracoid process of the scapula and the humerus.

**coracoid** \kôr′əkoid\ [Gk *korakoeidēs* (from *korax*, gen. *korako(s)* a raven + *-eidēs* -like, -OID) like a raven's beak] **1** CORONOID. **2** The coracoid process of the scapula.

**coracoiditis** \kôr′əkoidī′tis\ A painful condition that may follow an injury about the coracoid process and scapula. It is often associated with deltoid wasting.

**coracoradialis** \kôr′əkōrā′dē·ā′lis\ CAPUT BREVE MUSCULI BICIPITIS BRACHII.

**corallin** \kôr′əlin\ AURIN.

**Corbus** [Budd Clarke *Corbus*, U.S. urologist, 1876–1954] Corbus disease. See under GANGRENOUS BALANITIS.

**cord** [L *chorda* (from Gk *chordē* a string of gut, string of a lyre, sausage) an intestine, gut, string of a musical instrument] In anatomy, any long, rounded, stringlike structure; chorda. **Billroth's c.'s** SPLENIC CORDS. **condyle c.** CONDYLAR AXIS. **dental c.** The precursor of the enamel organ. **enamel c.** A chain of epithelial cells connecting the enamel organ to the dental lamina. Also *enamel septum.* **false vocal c.** PLICA VESTIBULARIS. **Ferrein's c.** PLICA VOCALIS. **ganglionated c.** *Seldom used* TRUNCUS SYMPATHICUS. **genital c.** Fused mesodermal folds formed in the embryo below the caudal edge of the mesonephric ridge and near the urogenital sinus giving rise to a transverse partition across the cavity of the pelvis. It contains the caudal portions of the mesonephric (wolffian) and paramesonephric (müllerian) ducts. Also *urogenital cord.* **germinal c.'s** Cords of cells in the embryonic gonads, providing the covering for oogonia in the ovary and giving rise to primitive seminiferous tubules in the testis. **gubernacular c.** A cord, which later becomes a fibromuscular bundle, lying within the peritoneal inguinal fold and extending from the lower pole of the testis to a site on the lower ventral abdominal wall that eventually becomes the scrotum. It traverses the region that will form the future inguinal canal when the abdominal muscles differentiate. This cord, which becomes the gubernaculum of the testis, plays some part in the descent of the testis. Also *chorda gubernaculum.* **hepatic c.'s** In histologic sections, the lines of hepatic parenchymal cells that radiate out from a central vein. This, in fact, represents a transected plate of liver cells. **c. of Hippocrates** TENDO CALCANEUS. **lateral c. of brachial plexus** FASCICULUS LATERALIS PLEXUS BRACHIALIS. **lumbosacral c.** TRUNCUS LUMBOSACRALIS. **medial c. of brachial plexus** FASCICULUS MEDIALIS PLEXUS BRACHIALIS. **medullary c.'s** Thin irregular strands of epithelial tissue within the medulla of the adult ovary. With the rete ovarii and the epoöphoron these constitute a group of rudimentary, nonfunctional homologues of the tubule and duct systems of the testis. The medullary cords, the rete ovarii, and the epoöphoron, respectively, are the homologues of the seminiferous and straight tubules, the rete testis, and the testicular ends of the efferent ductules. Also *primary sex cords.* **mesonephrogenic c.'s** In the embryo, the middle region of the nephrogenic cord, which is formed by the fusion of the nephrotome plates, giving rise to the mesonephros. **metanephrogenic c.'s** The caudal part of the nephrogenic cord which gives rise to the metanephros. The arrangement of these cords is much less clear than in the adjacent more cranial regions in which the pronephros and mesonephros developed. The metanephros gradually takes over the functions of the mesonephros as that organ becomes nonfunctional at the end of the fourth month. **nasolacrimal c.** In the embryo, a cord of epithelial tissue situated between the ciliary margin at the angle of the developing eye region and the mouth. It is related medially to the median nasal process and laterally to the maxillary process. The upper part of the cord gives rise to the nasolacrimal duct which grows actively and eventually terminates in the lateral wall of the nasal cavity below the inferior concha. **nephrogenic c.** A mass of tissue which develops by longitudinal fusion of the segmental junctional region, the intermediate mesoderm, which is situated between and connects the medial (paraxial) mesoderm and the lateral plate mesoderm in the early embryo and extends along most of its length. From this structure most of the excretory system develops. The most cranial segments collectively constitute the pronephros, the intermediate segments constitute the mesonephros, and the most caudal segments constitute the metanephros or definitive kidney. **nerve c.** A nerve bundle or trunk. *Seldom used.* **oblique c. of elbow joint** CHORDA OBLIQUA. **Pflüger's c.'s** A group of cells with connections to the covering ovarian epithelium that form the anlage of the ovarian follicular epithelium. The cords, also described as columns or tubules, are secondary features of female gonadal development. Also *ovarian tubes.* **posterior c. of brachial plexus** FASCICULUS POSTERIOR PLEXUS BRACHIALIS. **primary sex c.'s** MEDULLARY CORDS. **pronephrogenic c.** In the embryo, the cranial part of the nephrogenic cord that gives rise to the pronephros. **psalterial c.** STRIA VASCULARIS DUCTUS COCHLEARIS. **red pulp c.'s** SPLENIC CORDS. **rete c.'s** Mesenchymal cells of the embryonic gonadal medulla that ultimately develop into the rete testis or the rete ovarii. **spermatic c.** FUNICULUS SPERMATICUS. **spinal c.** MEDULLA SPINALIS. **splenic c.'s** Reticular strands around the venous sinuses, or red pulp, in the spleen. Also *Billroth's cords, red pulp cords.* **tendinous c.'s** CHORDAE TENDINEAE CORDIS. **testicular c.** FUNICULUS SPERMATICUS. **testis c.'s** Cords of cells that become recognizable in the primordium of the male gonad during the sixth week of gestation, when the primordium can be recognized as a testis. At first, these cords are attached to the covering coelomic epithelium but later they are cut off by the tunica albuginea. The cells of the testis cords probably differentiate into sustentacular cells of Sertoli. The primordial germ cells migrate into the cords and become intercalated among the sustentacular cells. **true vocal c.** PLICA VOCALIS. **umbilical c.** A flexible mucovascular structure which connects the umbilicus with the placenta and usually contains two umbilical arteries and a single vein. In the newborn it normally measures about 54 cm in length, but it can vary from 18 cm to 122 cm and about 1 cm to 1.5 cm in diameter. It is first formed during the fifth week of embryonic life and initially contains the yolk sac and body stalk with the enclosed allantois. The soft homogeneous intercellular substance of the cord is called Wharton's jelly. Also *chorda umbilicalis.* **urogenital c.** GENITAL CORD. **vocal c.** PLICA VOCALIS. **Weitbrecht's c.** CHORDA OBLIQUA. **c.'s of Willis** Fibrous bands that stretch transversely across the inferior angle of the superior sagittal sinus and partly cover the internal openings of the superior cerebral veins.

**cord-** \kôrd-\ For words beginning *cord-*, see also under CHORD-

**cordal** \kôr′dəl\ Pertaining to a cord, especially the true vocal cord.

**cordate** \kôr′dāt\ CORDIFORM.

**cordectomy** \kôrdek′təmē\ [CORD + -ECTOMY] **1** Excision of any cordlike structure, particularly a vocal cord. **2** Excision or resection of the spinal cord, as might be performed in an experimental animal or, rarely, in man to abolish a tumor or to interrupt reflexes.

**cordiform** \kôr′difôrm\ Heart-shaped. Also *cordate.*

**cordite** \kôr′dīt\ An explosive substance containing nitroglycerine. Workers making this substance may suffer from headaches, nausea, and vomiting. They develop a tolerance, which may be lost over the weekend. Such workers have a higher than expected mortality from acute myocardial infarction.

**corditis** \kôrdī′tis\ [CORD + -ITIS] FUNICULITIS.

**cordomesoblast** \kôr′dōmez′əblast\ CHORDAMESODERM.

**cordopexy** \kôr′dōpek′sē\ [CORD + *o* + -PEXY] An operation to improve the laryngeal airway, in cases of bilateral abductor paralysis of the larynx, by fixing one vocal cord in the abducted position. Also *chordopexy.*

**cordotomy** \kôrdät′əmē\ CHORDOTOMY.

**core** [Middle English] **1** The central or innermost part of an entity, as of an atom or protein molecule. **2** The central mass of necrotic tissue in a furuncle or other destructive inflammatory lesion. **3** In fingerprint patterns, the central ridge line forming the pattern. **spore c.** The protoplast of the bacterial spore. The resistance of its proteins to denaturation appears to be due to dehydration and to the presence of a high concentration of calcium dipicolinate.

**core-** \kôr′ə-\ [Gk *korē* pupil of the eye] A combining form denoting the pupil. Also *coro-.*

**coreclisis** \-klī′sis\ [CORE- + -CLISIS] Obliteration of the iris aperture. Also *coroclisis.*

**corectome** \kôrek′tōm\ [*cor(e)-* + EC- + -TOME ] A surgical instrument designed for cutting the iris.

**corectomedialysis** \kôrek′təmē′dē·al′isis\ [CORECTOME + DIALYSIS] An operation intended to center the pupil in the eye.

**corectopia** \kôr′ektō′pē·ə\ [Gk *kor(ē)* the pupil of the eye + *ektop(os)* out of the way + -IA] Displacement of the pupil from its usual central position, usually a developmental condition rather than the result of injury or inflammation.

**coredialysis** \-dī·al′isis\ [CORE- + DIALYSIS] Avulsion of the base of the iris.

**corediastasis** \-dī·as′təsis\ [CORE- + DIASTASIS] Dilatation of the pupil. Also *corodiastasis.*

**corelysis** \kôrel′isis\ [CORE- + LYSIS] Separation of anterior or posterior synechiae.

**coremorphosis** \-môrfō′sis\ [CORE- + Gk *morphōsis* a shaping] Surgical shaping of a pupillary opening in the iris.

**corenclisis** \kôr′enklī′sis\ [*cor(e)-* + EN- + -CLISIS] A filtering operation for glaucoma that maintains the patency of a limbal incision by including a fold of iris between the cut corneoscleral edges.

**coreoplasty** \kôr′ē·əplas′tē\ [CORE- + *o* + -PLASTY ] Surgical modification of the pupil. Also *coroplasty, corotomy.*

**corepexy** \kôr′əpek′sē\ [CORE- + -PEXY] The surgical repositioning of a pupil into its normal position.

**corepressor** \-pres′ər\ A metabolite that combines with a repressor protein and blocks the transcription of messenger ribonucleic acid. Neither the repressor protein nor the metabolite corepressor alone can prevent transcription.

**coretomedialysis** \kôr′ətōmē′dē·al′isis\ [CORE- + -TOME + DIALYSIS] PERIPHERAL IRIDECTOMY.

**coretomy** \kôret′əmē\ [CORE- + -TOMY] IRIDOTOMY.

**Corey** [Robert Brainard *Corey,* U.S. chemist, 1897–1971] Pauling-Corey helix. See under ALPHA HELIX.

**Cori** [Carl Ferdinand *Cori,* Czech-born U.S. biochemist, 1896–1984] Cori ester. See under GLUCOSE 1-PHOSPHATE.

**Cori** [Gerty Theresa Radnitz *Cori,* U.S. biochemist, 1896–1957] **1** Cori ester. See under GLUCOSE 1-PHOSPHATE. **2** Cori's disease. See under GLYCOGEN STORAGE DISEASE.

**corium** \kôr′ē·əm\ [L, the hide or skin of an animal, leather, bark of a tree, rind of a fruit, crust] DERMIS. **lingual c.** APONEUROSIS LINGUAE.

**corn** [Middle English and Old French *corne* horn, from L *cornu* the horn of a beast] **1** A localized callosity of the feet or fingers that occurs as a result of friction and pressure. **2** A condition of the equine foot, characterized by a focal area of swelling and discoloration of the sole in the angle between the wall and the bar. It results from a bruise which may become infected and causes pain and lameness. Also *clavus, hard corn, heloma.* **hard c.** CORN. **seed c.** A viral wart, especially a plantar wart. *Popular.* **soft c.** A localized soft thickening of the epidermis that occurs between the toes, usually between the fourth and fifth toes. It is often macerated and painful.

**cornea** \kôr′nē·ə\ [short for New L *cornea tunica* (from L *corneus* horny, made of horn) a horny coat or integument] [NA] The anterior, convex transparent part of the fibrous tunic of the eyeball, which provides structural strength, refractive power, and optical transmission. The anterior layer, the corneal epithelium, is continuous with that of the conjunctiva, whereas its deepest layer is the endothelium of the anterior chamber of the eye. Between these layers are the anterior limiting layer, the substantia propria, and the posterior limiting layer. The cornea is nonvascular. Adj. corneal, keratitic. **conical c.** KERATOCONUS. **c. farinata** The presence of small irregular opacities within the stroma of an older cornea as a benign condition. **flat c.** CORNEA PLANA. **c. globata** MEGALOCORNEA. **c. guttata** HASSALL-HENLE BODIES. **c. plana** A congenital reduced curvature of the cornea. Also *flat cornea.* **sugarloaf c.** KERATOCONUS. **c. verticillata** A benign corneal dystrophy in which vortices of curved lines are visible by biomicroscopy.

**corneal** \kôr′nē·əl\ Relating to or characteristic of the cornea.

**corneoblepharon** \kôr′nē·ōblef′ərən\ [*corne(a)* + *o* +

BLEPHARON] Adhesion between the cornea and the eyelids.
**corneoiritis** \kôr′nē·ō·īrī′tis\ [L *corne(a)* + *o* + IRITIS] Inflammation of both iris and cornea.
**corneosclera** \kôr′nē·ōsklir′ə\ TUNICA FIBROSA BULBI.
**corneoscleral** \kôr′nē·ōsklir′əl\ Pertaining to the cornea and the sclera.
**corneous** \kôr′nē·əs\ HORNY.
**Corner** [Edred Moss *Corner,* English surgeon, 1873–1950] Corner's tampon. See under PLUG.
**Corner** [George Washington *Corner,* U.S. anatomist, born 1889] Corner-Allen test. See under TEST.
**cornet** [Middle French *cornette,* dim. of *corne* horn, from L *cornu* horn of an animal] A bony layer.
**corneum** \kôr′nē·əm\ Either stratum corneum epidermidis or stratum corneum unguis.
**corniculate** \kôrnik′yəlāt\ **1** In the shape of a small horn. **2** Having horns or hornlike processes.
**corniculum** \kôrnik′yələm\ [L, a little horn, dim. of *cornu* horn of an animal] **1** A small cornu. **2** CARTILAGO CORNICULATA.
**cornification** \kôr′nifikā′shən\ KERATINIZATION.
**cornoid** \kôr′noid\ Resembling keratin.
**cornu** \kôr′n$^y$oo\ [L, horn of an animal] (*pl.* cornua) A structure in the shape of a horn; hornlike projection. Also *horn.* **c. Ammonis** HIPPOCAMPUS. • The term is named after Ammon, the ram-headed deity of ancient Egypt. **c. anterius medullae spinalis** [NA] The large, bulbous protrusion formed by the anterior column of central gray matter as seen in a cross-section of the cord. Also *anterior cornu, anterior horn of spinal cord, motor horn, ventral horn of spinal cord, cornu ventrale, ventricornu.* **c. anterius ventriculi lateralis** [NA] A recess of the lateral ventricle extending forward and laterally into the frontal lobe. Posterior to the interventricular foramen, it is continuous with the central part of the lateral ventricle. Also *anterior horn of lateral ventricle, frontal horn of lateral ventricle, precommissure, precornu.* **c. coccygeum** [NA] One of two upward projections from the posterior surface of the body of the first piece of the coccyx that articulate with the sacral cornua to enclose the last intervertebral foramen for the passage of the fifth sacral nerve. The cornu coccygeum is the homologue of the pedicle and superior articular process of a vertebra. Also *coccygeal horn.* **c. cutaneum** CUTANEOUS HORN. **c. descendens** CORNU INFERIUS VENTRICULI LATERALIS. **c. dorsale medullae spinalis** [NA] The posteriorly directed column of gray matter of the spinal cord as it appears in cross-section. Also *cornu posterius medullae spinalis, dorsal horn of spinal cord, posterior horn of spinal cord.* **c. inferius cartilaginis thyroideae** [NA] The caudal prolongation of the thick posterior margin of each lamina of the thyroid cartilage, curving medially to articulate by a rounded facet on its medial aspect with the articular surface of the cricoid cartilage to form the cricothyroid joint. Also *inferior horn of thyroid cartilage.* **c. inferius marginis falciformis** [NA] The sharp lower border of the falciform margin, or lateral border, of the hiatus saphenus, an oval opening in the fascia lata of the thigh situated just below the medial end of the inguinal ligament. The great saphenous vein hooks over the lower border to empty into the underlying femoral vein. Also *inferior horn of saphenous opening, inferior horn of falciform margin.* **c. inferius ventriculi lateralis** [NA] A large extension of the lateral ventricle that curves around the posterior end of the thalamus, and extends almost to the pole of the temporal lobe. Also *inferior horn of cerebrum, inferior horn of lateral ventricle, temporal horn of lateral ventricle, cornu temporale ventriculi lateralis, cornu descendens, underhorn.* **c. laterale medullae spinalis** [NA] A laterally directed protrusion of the spinal gray matter. It is small relative to the anterior and posterior cornua, and is restricted to the thoracic and upper lumbar segments. Also *lateral horn of spinal cord, lateral gray horn of spinal cord.* **c. majus ossis hyoidei** [NA] The larger of the two processes that project posterosuperiorly on each side of the body of the U-shaped hyoid bone, serving as an attachment for the thyrohyoid, hyoglossus, and digastric muscles, the middle constrictor of pharynx, and the thyrohyoid membrane, and ending posteriorly in a rounded tubercle to which the lateral thyrohyoid ligament is attached. Also *greater horn of hyoid bone.* **c. minus ossis hyoidei** [NA] The smaller of the two processes on each side of the body of the U-shaped hyoid bone that projects posterosuperiorly from the junction of the body and the greater horn. It is sometimes completely cartilaginous and connected to the greater horn by a synovial joint and to the body by fibrous tissue, giving attachment to the chondroglossus and middle constrictor muscle of the pharynx, while the stylohyoid ligament is attached to its apex. Also *lesser horn of hyoid bone, superior horn of hyoid bone* (outmoded). **c. posterius medullae spinalis** CORNU DORSALE MEDULLAE SPINALIS. **c. posterius ventriculi lateralis** [NA] A large recess of the lateral ventricle extending backward and medially into the occipital lobe. It is found only in anthropoids. Also *posterior horn of lateral ventricle, postcornu.* **c. sacrale** [NA] One of the two tubercles representing the inferior articular processes of the fifth sacral vertebra, located posteriorly and projecting caudally at the sides of the sacral hiatus to articulate with the coccygeal cornua, to which they are connected by ligaments. Also *sacral horn, coccygeal eminence.* **c. superius cartilaginis thyroideae** [NA] The long, upward prolongation of the thick posterior margin of each lamina of the thyroid cartilage, curving slightly inwards to its conical tip, to which is attached the lateral thyrohyoid ligament from the greater horn of the hyoid bone. Also *superior horn of thyroid cartilage.* **c. superius marginis falciformis** [NA] The well-defined upper extension of the falciform margin, or lateral border, of the hiatus saphenus, an oval opening in the fascia lata of the thigh situated just below the medial end of the inguinal ligament, that anchors to the pubic tubercle. Also *superior horn of saphenous opening, superior horn of falciform margin, ligament of Scarpa.* **c. temporale ventriculi lateralis** CORNU INFERIUS VENTRICULI LATERALIS. **c. uteri (dextrum/sinistrum)** [NA] The junction of the fundus and the upper end of the right and left lateral borders of the body of the uterus where the wall is pierced by the uterine tube. Also *lateral horn of uterus, uterine horn.* **c. ventrale** **1** CORNU ANTERIUS MEDULLAE SPINALIS. **2** CORNU ANTERIUS VENTRICULI LATERALIS.
**cornua** \kôr′n$^y$oo·ə\ Plural of CORNU.
**cornual** \kôr′n$^y$oo·əl\ Pertaining to a cornu. Also *cornuate.*
**coro-** \kôr′ō-\ CORE-.
**coroclisis** \kôr′ōklī′sis\ CORECLISIS.
**corodiastasis** \kôr′ōdī·as′təsis\ [CORO- + DIASTASIS] COREDIASTASIS.
**corometer** \kôräm′ətər\ [CORO- + -METER] PUPILLOMETER.
**corona** \kôrō′nə\ [L (from Gk *korōnē* a crow, raven, anything hooked like a crow's bill), a garland, wreath, crown] **1** Any crownlike or garlandlike projection or arrangement; a partially or completely encircling structure. **2** The highest part of an organ, structure, or part, such as the top of the head or the upper part of a tooth. Also *crown.* **c. capi-**

**tis** The crown, or topmost part, of the head. Also *crown of the head.* **c. ciliaris** [NA] An annular, crested region on the inner aspect of the ciliary body, surrounding the base of the iris and situated anterior to the annulus ciliaris. It is ridged by about eighty ciliary processes, between which are the smaller ciliary plicae and the hollows for the attachment of the zonular fibers. Also *ciliary crown.* **c. clinica** [NA] The part of the crown and root of a tooth visible outside the gingiva. Also *clinical crown, physiologic crown.* **c. dentis** [NA] The part of a tooth that is covered with enamel, separated from the root by the slightly constricted neck. Also *anatomic crown, crown of tooth.* **c. glandis penis** [NA] The projecting, rounded posterior margin of the glans penis, located anterior to the obliquely narrowed neck of the glans. **c. of glans penis** CORONA GLANDIS PENIS. **c. radiata** **1** [NA] The prominent crown of radiating fascicles passing from the internal capsule to widespread areas of the cerebral cortex. **2** A layer of columnar cells derived from the membrana granulosa of the ovarian follicle which lie radially arranged on the outside of the zona pellucida of the maturing oocyte. Their basal processes penetrate the zona, and probably supply nutriment to the oocyte. The corona cells are present after ovulation, but are dispersed after fertilization. Also *radiating crown.* **c. seborrheica** A red band along the upper border of the forehead and temples due to seborrheic dermatitis. *Seldom used.* **Zinn's c.** CIRCULUS VASCULOSUS NERVI OPTICI.

**coronad** \kôr′ōnad\ Toward any corona.

**coronae** \kôrō′nē\ Plural of CORONA.

**coronal** \kôr′ənəl, kərō′nəl\ **1** Pertaining to the crown of the head or any corona. **2** Directed or located in the side-to-side plane of the coronal suture or in a vertical plane parallel to it. Also *coronalis.*

**coronalis** \kôr′ənā′lis\ [NA] CORONAL.

**coronaritis** \kôr′ənərī′tis\ [*coronar(y + arter)itis*] CORONARY ARTERITIS.

**coronary** \kôr′əner′ē\ [L *coronari(us)* (from *coron(a)* a wreath, garland, ring, circle + *-arius* -ARY) pertaining to a wreath or circular shape] **1** Encircling; crownlike: said chiefly of certain anatomic structures. **2** Of or relating to the coronary blood vessels of the heart. **3** A heart attack resulting from coronary thrombosis. *Popular.* **café c.** An attack resembling coronary thrombosis, caused by sudden obstruction of the laryngotracheal tree by aspirated food.

**coronavirus** \kərō′nəvī′rəs\ [CORONA + VIRUS] Any member of the *Coronavirus* genus and Coronaviridae family, a group of enveloped RNA viruses that infect humans, chickens, turkeys, pigs, cattle, mice, rats, and cats. In humans they are an important cause of the common cold, particularly in the winter.

**coroner** \kôr′ənər\ [Middle English, a crown officer, from Anglo-French *coroune,* also *corone* crown, from L *corona* crown; + Anglo-French *-er* -ER] An elected, or occasionally, appointed official empowered to investigate sudden, unexpected, suspicious, and violent deaths occurring within his jurisdiction. In the United States, coroners are county officials. Qualifications for the position vary. Most jurisdictions, however, require a Doctor of Medicine degree. See also MEDICAL EXAMINER. • The term is also used in this sense in Australia, New Zealand, and South Africa. In Canada and India, coroners are always appointed, as in England and Wales, where coroners may be either medically or legally qualified. In Scotland the office is called *procurator fiscal.* In South Africa the corresponding office is held by *magistrates,* legal officials who do not have the degree of doctor of medicine.

**coronoid** \kôr′ənoid\ [Gk *korōn(ē)* a crow, something curved like a crow's bill + -OID ] **1** In the shape of a crow's beak, applied to certain bony processes and projections. Also *coracoid.* **2** Crown-shaped.

**coroparelcysis** \kôr′ōperel′sisis\ [CORO- + Gk *parelkysis* (from *par(a)-* aside, along + *(h)elkein* to draw, pull) protraction] Optical iridectomy, in which a new pupil is created adjacent to a central corneal scar.

**coroplasty** \kôr′ōplas′tē\ COREOPLASTY.

**corotomy** \kôrät′əmē\ [CORO- + -TOMY] COREOPLASTY.

**corpora** \kôr′pôrə\ Plural of CORPUS.

**corporal** \kôr′pərəl\ [L *corpor(alis)* (from *corpus,* gen. *corporis,* body + *-alis* -AL) pertaining to the body] Pertaining to or affecting the body.

**corporation** / **professional c.** A corporation formed by one or more practitioners for the purpose of rendering professional services that require legal authorization, such as a license. Professional corporations are common in medicine, law, accounting, architecture, and other fields, and, in the United States, may be organized under the law of most states. Practice as or in a professional corporation may entail tax benefits and other advantages, but typically does not affect professional responsibility, privilege, or malpractice liability. Abbr. PC

**corporeal** \kôrpôr′ē·əl\ Pertaining to or involving the body.

**corporic** \kôrpôr′ik\ Affecting the body as a whole or the body of an organ.

**corps** \kôr\ [French (from L *corpus* the body), the body] (*pl.* corps) A corpus; body. **c. ronds** The distinctive cells that are seen in the upper malpighian layer of the epidermis in keratosis follicularis. Their cytoplasm contains a large round dyskeratotic mass surrounded by a clear halo.

**corpse** \kôrps\ [variant of *corps,* from Middle English and Middle French *corps* body, from L *corpus* body] A dead body, especially a human body. • In common medical and medicolegal use, *corpse* refers to a body encountered or examined early in the postmortem interval, in contrast to *cadaver.*

# corpus

**corpus** \kôr′pəs\ [L (gen. *corporis*), the body, the flesh] (*pl.* corpora) **1** The entire body of a human or animal; the main body or mass of anything. **2** The main portion of a structure, part, or organ. **c. adiposum buccae** [NA] A pad of fat of varying thickness that provides the roundness of the cheeks of the face and is located deep to the muscles of expression and superficial to the buccinator muscle and its fascia. Also *adipose body of cheek, sucking pad, sucking cushion, suctorial pad, Bichat's fat pad, Bichat's protuberance, fatty ball of Bichat, buccal fat pad, Bichat's fatty body of cheek.* **c. adiposum fossae ischioanalis** [NA] Adipose connective tissue that fills the ischiorectal fossa. Also *adipose body of ischiorectal fossa.* **c. adiposum infrapatellare** [NA] A mass of fat in the knee joint, located at the base of the infrapatellar fold distal to the patella and separating the synovial membrane from the ligamentum patellae. Also *infrapatellar fatty body, infrapatellar fat pad, retropatellar fat pad.* **c. adiposum orbitae** [NA] The mass of fat situated behind the eyeball from which it is separated by the vagina bulbi. The fat lies around and between the extraocular muscles, nerves, and vessels. Also *adipose body of orbit, fatty body of orbit.* **c. albicans** An advanced retrogressive phase of the corpus luteum occurring weeks after ovulation, in which an amorphous convoluted hyalinized center is surrounded by cicatricial tissue. Also *corpus fibrosum, white scar of ovary, Willis gland.* **c. amygdaloideum** [NA] An almond-shaped gray mass located in the dorsomedial portion of the temporal lobe, in front of and above the tip of the inferior horn of the lateral ventricle. It is covered by the periamygdaloid cortex, and is continuous caudally with the uncus of the parahippocampal gyrus. It is usually divided into corticomedial and basolateral cell groups, which may in turn be further subdivided. Major sources of afferent fibers are the olfactory system, the diencephalon, and the neocortex of the inferior temporal gyrus. Efferent fibers project to the preoptic area, the ventral hypothalamus, the septal region, and the dorsomedial thalamus. Also *amygdaloid body, nucleus amygdalae, amygdaloid nucleus, amygdala.* **corpora amylacea** Round, eosinophilic masses found principally in dilated prostatic glands. They are composed of desquamated cells forming concentric lamellae around inspissated secretions composed of glycoprotein and mucoprotein. Also *amyloid bodies.* **c. atreticum** An ovarian follicle that has failed to mature. Also *atretic follicle, atretic ovarian follicle, anovular ovarian follicle, pseudolutein body.* **c. calcanei** The body of the calcaneus, no longer demarcated within the whole bone. **c. callosum** [NA] The great longitudinally arched commissure which connects the cortices of the cerebral hemispheres. It lies at the bottom of the longitudinal fissure at a distance beneath the cerebral falx, and is bordered by the gyrus cinguli. Farther laterally, it merges with the corona radiata and incidentally roofs the lateral ventricles. The posterior and anterior limits are thickened as the splenium and genu respectively, while the truncus corporis callosi fills in the interval. Extending inferiorly from the ventral recurved portion of the genu as far as the anterior commissure is the thin rostrum. Development is proportional to the relative volume of the neocortex, and is maximal in man. Also *great commissure, commissura magna cerebri, callosum.* **c. cavernosum clitoridis** [NA] One of two contiguous rods of erectile tissue surrounded by dense fibrous tissue and separated from each other by an incomplete fibrous septum where they form the body of the clitoris anteriorly, while posteriorly they diverge and each becomes connected to the ischiopubic ramus by a crus. Also *cavernous body of clitoris.* **c. cavernosum penis** [NA] One of two elongated masses of erectile tissue situated on each side and on the dorsum of the body of the penis and extending from the crus penis on each side to its cone-shaped distal end within the hollow inner aspect of the glans penis. Throughout most of their length both are surrounded by the tunica albuginea and separated by a median fibrous septum. They are grooved on their urethral surface by the corpus spongiosum penis, and on their dorsal surface by the deep dorsal vein of penis. Also *cavernous body of penis.* **c. cerebelli** [NA] The paleocerebellum and neocerebellum, that is, all portions of the cerebellum anterior to the posterolateral fissure, excluding the archicerebellum or flocculonodular lobe. **c. ciliare** [NA] A thickened part of the tunica vasculosa bulbi that is situated in front of the ora serrata retinae and joins the choroid to the iris. It forms the medial boundary of the iridocorneal angle of the anterior chamber. It consists of the corona ciliaris, processus ciliares, orbiculus ciliaris, and musculus ciliaris, and its main functions are to suspend the lens, act in accommodation of the eye, and take part in the production of aqueous humor. Its inner surface is lined by the two epithelial layers of the pars ciliaris retinae, the outer one of which is heavily pigmented. Also *ciliary body, ciliary apparatus.* **c. clitoridis** [NA] The body of the clitoris, located at the anterior end of the rima pudendi posterior to the symphysis pubis and partly covered by the anterior folds of the labia minora. It consists of two corpora cavernosa, and is held to the inferior border of the pubic arch by the suspensory ligament. Its anterior extremity is a fused, free, rounded tubercle forming the glans and composed of spongy erectile tissue. The clitoris is homologous with the penis but differs in that it is completely separate from the urethra. Also *body of clitoris.* **c. coccygeum** GLOMUS COCCYGEUM. **c. costae** [NA] The flattened, thin, curved and twisted shaft of a rib, extending from the tubercle to the anterior or sternal extremity. The external surface is convex, presents a marked angle posteriorly, and provides attachment for muscles, while the internal surface is concave and has the deep costal groove on its inferior border. Also *body of rib, shaft of rib.* **c. delicti** 1 The proven fact that a crime has been committed, as in a murder case, the established fact that the victim is dead and that he was murdered. 2 The physical entity upon which a crime has been committed, such as property that has been vandalized or the remains of a murder victim. **c. dentatum cerebelli** *Obs.* NUCLEUS DENTATUS CEREBELLI. **c. dentatum olivae** *Obs.* NUCLEUS OLIVARIS. **c. epididymidis** [NA] The portion of the C-shaped epididymis that lies along the posterior border of the testis, extending from the head, or caput, to the tail, or cauda, of the epididymis and containing the convolutions of the ductus epididymidis. It is separated from the lateral surface of the testis by the sinus of epididymis. Also *body of epididymis.* **c. femoris** CORPUS OSSIS FEMORIS. **c. fibrosum** CORPUS ALBICANS. **c. fibulae** [NA] The long shaft of the fibula, extending from the head to the lateral malleolus, or lower end. It is quadrangular in its upper three-fourths and triangular below. Its three borders and three surfaces are related to different groups of muscles, and one of the former has the interosseous membrane binding it to the tibia. Also *shaft of fibula.* **c. fimbriatum hippocampi** FIMBRIA HIPPOCAMPI. **c. fornicis** [NA] That portion of the fornix cerebri extending from the caudal level where the two fornices first communicate across the midline, rostrally to the interventricular foramen. At these levels it is continuous with the posterior and anterior pillars of the fornix respectively. Also *body of fornix.* **c. gastricum** [NA] The ill-defined major portion of the stomach, which extends from a horizontal plane through the cardiac orifice to an oblique plane through the angular notch. It connects the fundus of the stomach to the pyloric antrum. Also *body of stomach.* **c. geniculatum laterale** [NA] A nucleus or swelling of the metathalamus located lateral to the medial geniculate body. It receives impulses from the optic tract, and projects via the geniculocalcarine tract to the visual cortex. Also *lateral geniculate body.* **c. geniculatum mediale** [NA] A metathalamic eminence located lateral to the superior colliculus. It is formed by the medial geniculate nucleus, where activity arriving in the lateral lemniscus is relayed to the auditory radiation and cortex. Also *medial geniculate body.* **c. glandulae bulbourethralis** The body of the bulbourethral gland, no longer demarcated from the whole gland. **c. glandulae sudoriferae** The coiled secretory portion of a sweat, or sudoriferous, gland, located in the tela subcutanea or deep in the corium and opening by a duct either on the surface of the skin or into a hair follicle. Also *body of sweat gland.* **c. glandulare prostatae** PARENCHYMA PROSTATAE. **c. hemorrhagicum** A blood clot formed in the cavity left by rupture of a graafian follicle. **c.**

**highmori** MEDIASTINUM TESTIS. **c. humeri** [NA] The shaft of the humerus, situated between the surgical neck proximally and the condyle and epicondyles distally. It is almost cylindrical proximally and triangular distally, and presents three margins and three surfaces. Also *shaft of humerus.* **c. incudis** [NA] The main, somewhat cuboidal, part of the incus that has a concavoconvex surface anteriorly for articulation with the head of the malleus, and two projections, the short and the long crus, on the opposite aspect. **c. linguae** [NA] The major, oral part of the tongue anterior to the V-shaped groove, or terminal sulcus, located on the posterosuperior surface that separates it from the root posteriorly. The margins of the tongue meet anteriorly at the tip. The dorsum has a rough appearance produced by many small projections, the lingual papillae. Also *body of tongue.* **c. luteum** The yellow progesterone-secreting body formed in the ovary at the site of a ruptured ovarian follicle. Also *yellow body of ovary.* **c. luysii** NUCLEUS SUBTHALAMICUS. **c. mamillare** [NA] Either of two protuberances on the baseof the brain on each side of the interpeduncular recess, containing the mamillary nuclei of the posterior hypothalamus. Also *mamillary body, mamillary eminence, pars mamillaris hypothalami, mamillary tubercle of hypothalamus.* **c. mammae** [NA] The main mass of the breast excluding the skin, subcutaneous fat, and connective tissue and its deep attachments, and comprising the parenchyma or glandular tissue and ducts, and the stroma or connective tissue and fat that lie between and around the parenchyma, as well as blood and lymphatic vessels and nerves. The mass is conical or discoid in shape, being thickest opposite the nipple, and with a concave base resting on the deep fascia. A process, or axillary tail, extends into the axilla from the upper outer quadrant of the mass. **c. mandibulae** [NA] The horizontal, curved, horseshoe-shaped anterior part of the lower jaw bone that supports the lower teeth. The two halves, originally separate, are fused in the midline at the lower end of which is the mental protuberance, or chin, while the body ends posteriorly where it meets each ramus almost at a right angle. Also *body of mandible.* **c. maxillae** [NA] The pyramidal mass of each maxilla, hollowed by a large cavity, or sinus, and supporting the upper teeth. It has four surfaces (anterior, orbital, nasal, and infratemporal) as well as four processes (the frontal and zygomatic, extending from the superior part of the body, and the palatine and alveolar processes from the inferior part) whereby it takes part in the formation of the orbit, hard palate, and nasal cavity. Together, the maxillae occupy the central part of the face above the mandible. Also *body of maxilla.* **c. medullare cerebelli** [NA] The central, white matter of the cerebellum. In sagittal section, it appears as the arbor vitae. Also *medullary body of cerebellum, medullary body of vermis, medullary center of cerebellum, nucleus medullaris cerebelli.* **c. metacarpalis** [NA] The prismatic shaft of a metacarpal bone, curved longitudinally so the concave aspect is palmward and having three surfaces, a medial and a lateral for the origins of the interossei, separated by a median ridge, as well as a flat posterior surface, most of which is covered by the flat tendons of the extensor muscles. Also *shaft of metacarpal bone.* **c. metatarsalis** [NA] The longitudinally curved and tapering shaft of a metatarsal bone, concave plantarward and flattened from side to side to form three borders and three surfaces. Also *shaft of metatarsal bone.* **c. nuclei caudati** [NA] That portion of the caudate nucleus lying in the floor of the central part of the third ventricle. Rostrally and caudally it merges with the head and tail of the nucleus, respectively. **c. ossis femoris** [NA] The almost cylindrical shaft of the femur that commences distal to the tuberosities and ends at the condyles. Its longitudinal plane has a convexity anteriorly, while posteriorly it is strengthened by a projecting ridge, or linea aspera, that terminates in the distal third by dividing into the medial and lateral supracondylar ridges enclosing the triangular popliteal surface. Also *shaft of femur, corpus femoris.* **c. ossis hyoidei** [NA] The horizontal, central part of the U-shaped hyoid bone that lies just below the mandible and ends posteriorly in the greater and lesser horns on each side. It is shaped like an irregular quadrilateral, and flattened anteroposteriorly. Its anterior surface is convex forward for the attachment of several muscles, while the smooth concave posterior surface is separated from the epiglottis by the thyrohyoid membrane and a bursa. Also *body of hyoid bone.* **c. ossis ilii** [NA] The lower portion of the ilium lying below the broad wing, or ala, and forming the upper two-fifths of the acetabulum. Its internal surface forms part of the side wall of the pelvis minor and gives attachment to part of the obturator internus muscle. Also *body of ilium.* **c. ossis ischii** [NA] The major part of the ischium, exclusive of the ramus. Superiorly it forms two-fifths of the acetabulum and most of the acetabular fossa externally, while its smooth internal surface forms part of the wall of the pelvis minor and gives attachment to some of the obturator internus muscle. Posteriorly it has the spine of ischium for the attachment of the levator ani and coccygeus muscles, and the rough tuberosity for the origins of the hamstring muscles. Also *body of ischium.* **c. ossis pubis** [NA] The anteroposteriorly flattened anterior portion of the pubis that with its opposite fellow forms the symphysis pubis in the midline, while its lateral side forms part of the obturator foramen and has the superior ramus extending upwards and backwards to the acetabulum, and the inferior ramus running downwards and laterally to meet the ischial ramus. Its rough anterior surface provides attachment for muscles of the thigh; the posterior surface is related to the urinary bladder in the lesser pelvis; and the superior border forms the pubic crest for the attachment of abdominal wall muscles. Also *body of pubis.* **c. ossis sphenoidalis** [NA] The cubical, central mass of the sphenoid bone that contains two air sinuses separated by a septum and has the greater and lesser wings and the pterygoid processes attached to it. Its superior, or cerebral, surface has the hollow sella turcica to lodge the hypophysis cerebri, bounded posteriorly by a square plate of bone, the dorsum sellae, behind which the clivus slopes downward. The anterior surface has the sphenoidal crest forming part of the septum of the nose, while the inferior surface has a prominent ridge, the sphenoidal rostrum. Also *body of sphenoid.* **c. pampiniforme** EPOÖPHORON. **c. pancreatis** [NA] The central, triangular portion of the pancreas, extending transversely and slightly upwards from right to left on the posterior abdominal wall from the constricted neck, grooved posteriorly by the portal and superior mesenteric veins, to the tapering tail, where it comes in contact with the gastric surface of the spleen. It lies in the epigastric and left hypochondriac regions at the level of the first lumbar vertebra, and has anterior, posterior, and inferior surfaces separated by superior, anterior, and inferior margins. Also *body of pancreas.*

**corpora para-aortica** [NA] Aggregates of chromaffin cells embedded in a capillary plexus forming two elongated masses along each side of the abdominal aorta near the inferior mesenteric artery. Chemoreceptor endings monitoring blood gases are distributed in these bodies, and the chromaffin cells secrete noradrenalin. Also *organs of Zuckerkandl, para-aortic bodies, pheochrome bodies, aortic bodies, glomera aortica, aortic paraganglia, aortic glands, supracardial bodies.*

**c. paraterminalis** GYRUS SUBCALLOSUS. **c. penis** [NA] The cylindrical free portion of the penis, extending from the radix, or root, in the perineum to the tip of the glans and composed of the two corpora cavernosa and the single corpus spongiosum containing the urethra. It is completely surrounded by thin skin that is loosely connected by areolar tissue to the underlying fascial sheath and folded beyond the neck of the glans to form the prepuce. It is pendulous when flaccid but becomes erect when engorged with blood. Also *shaft of penis, body of penis, penile body.* **c. phalangis digitorum manus** [NA] The somewhat anteroposteriorly flattened oval shaft of each phalanx of the fingers, extending from the base to the head of each. Also *shaft of phalanx of fingers.* **c. phalangis digitorum pedis** [NA] The oval shaft of each phalanx of the toes, somewhat flattened anteroposteriorly and compressed from side to side at the center, extending from the base to the head of each. Also *shaft of phalanx of toes.* **c. pineale** [NA] A small, conical body attached by a stalk to the epithalamus and lying in the groove between the superior colliculi. It is reddish gray in color and weighs 100–180 mg in the adult human. It is composed of parenchymal and neuroglial cells, and is innervated by postganglionic nerve fibers arising in the cervical sympathetic ganglia. At least six neurotransmitters, including serotonin and norepinephrine, and four or more hormonal peptides, including somatostatin and oxytocin, are found in the pineal body, but only melatonin, which undergoes a nychthemeral cycle apparently in response to light-dark alternation, is secreted into the blood like a hormone. The precise hormonal functions of the corpus pineale in man are not known, but a role in light-dark response, salt and water metabolism, and regulation of the time of onset of puberty is postulated. The corpus pineale becomes important clinically when it impinges on adjacent structures, as in the Parinaud syndrome, or is associated with macrogenitosomia praecox, as in the Pellizzi syndrome. Also *pineal body, apophysis cerebri, epiphysis cerebri, pineal organ, pineal gland, conarium, pinus.* **c. pontobulbare** A ridge obliquely crossing the restiform body just caudal to the cochlear nuclei, containing neurons that receive input from the cerebral cortex and project to the cerebellum. It is a component of the pontocerebellar projection, which is well developed only in man. Also *Essick cell band.* **corpora quadrigemina** The four small swellings, called the two superior and two inferior colliculi, on the roof of the midbrain, behind the third ventricle and pineal body. They are involved with auditory and visual reflexes in mammals. Also *quadrigeminal bodies, quadrigemina.* **c. radii** [NA] The triangular shaft of the radius, extending from the tuberosity to the lower end with a gentle convexity directed laterally and presenting a sharp interosseous, or medial, margin and rounded anterior and posterior margins with three surfaces between them. It increases in thickness, becoming quadrilateral distally. Also *body of radius, shaft of radius.* **c. restiforme** PEDUNCULUS CEREBELLARIS INFERIOR. **corpora santoriana** CARTILAGO CORNICULATA. **c. spongiosum penis** [NA] An elongated cylindical mass of erectile tissue situated in the median groove on the undersurface of the tunica albuginea surrounding the corpora cavernosa penis. Proximally it forms the bulbus penis attached to the perineal membrane, and distally it expands to form the glans penis. It is surrounded by a fibrous sheath and is traversed by the spongy urethra. Also *spongy body of penis, spongy body of male urethra.* **c. spongiosum urethrae muliebris** A thin layer of spongy erectile tissue deep to the mucosa of the female urethra, consisting of a plexus of veins between an outer circular and an inner longitudinal layer of smooth muscle, as well as connective tissue with a predominance of elastin fibers. **c. sterni** [NA] The long, narrow, bladelike central portion of the sternum, extending from the manubrium above to the xiphoid process below, with costal notches along each lateral border for articulation with the costal cartilages of the second to seventh ribs. The rough anterior and the smooth posterior surfaces provide attachment for muscles. Also *body of sternum, midsternum, gladiolus.* **c. striatum** [NA] The principal subcortical mass of gray matter, constituting the largest portion of the basal ganglia. It consists of the caudate and lentiform nuclei. Also *striate body.* • It is called a striate body because of the interdigitation of myelinated fiber bundles piercing the nuclear masses. **c. subthalamicum** NUCLEUS SUBTHALAMICUS. **c. tali** [NA] The cuboidal part of the talus behind its neck, with a superior, or trochlear, surface for articulation with the tibia in the ankle joint, a lateral articular surface for the lateral malleolus, a medial articular surface for the medial malleolus, and an inferior articular surface resting on the calcaneus. Also *body of talus.* **c. tibiae** [NA] The sturdy triangular shaft of the tibia, extending from the tuberosity proximally to the lower end, tapering between the middle and distal thirds and then expanding again. It has anterior, medial, and interosseous margins with three surfaces in between, providing attachment for the leg muscles and their intermuscular septa. The anterior margin and the medial surface are subcutaneous. Also *body of tibia, shaft of tibia.* **c. trapezoideum** [NA] A large field of transversely oriented fascicles and interspersed nuclei located in the ventral tegmentum of the cranial medulla and adjacent pons. The fibers arise in the cochlear and trapezoid nuclei, cross, and then ascend into the lateral lemniscus. Also *trapezoid body, trapezoid.* **c. triticeum** CARTILAGO TRITICEA. **c. ulnae** [NA] The tapering shaft of the ulna, extending from the radial notch at the proximal extremity to the head distally, being triangular in its proximal three-fourths and cylindrical distally. It has interosseous, posterior, and anterior margins and three surfaces in between. Also *body of ulna, shaft of ulna.* **c. unguis** [NA] The main, exposed part of the nail, distal to the root and covered by the nail wall proximally along its sides, with its deep surface lying on the nail bed. It ends distally at the free border. Also *body of nail.* **c. uteri** [NA] The proximal two-thirds of the adult nongravid uterus, above and proximal to the narrow isthmus located at the level of the internal os of the uterus. The part above the plane of entrance of the uterine tubes is the fundus. The anterior, or vesical, surface is separated by the peritoneum from the urinary bladder, while the posterior, or intestinal, surface is related to the sigmoid colon. The cavity of the body is triangular in shape. Also *body of uterus.* **c. vertebrae** [NA] The mass of a vertebra anterior, or ventral, to the vertebral foramen and arch. It is generally cylindrical, but varies greatly in size and shape in different parts of the vertebral column. The rough superior and inferior surfaces are attached to intervertebral disks, and their margins are lipped. The sides have numerous vascular foramina, and in the thoracic region bear articular facets for ribs. Also *centrum, centrum vertebrae, body of vertebra, vertebral body, intravertebral body.* **c. vesicae biliaris** [NA] The part of the gallbladder between the rounded broad end, or fundus, and the bent, narrow neck situated near the right end of the porta hepatis. The upper surface is in contact with the liver, while the undersurface is related to the transverse colon's right side. Also *body of gallbladder.* **c. vesicae urinariae** [NA] The part of the urinary bladder situated between the base, or fundus, on the posterior surface and the apex, to which the median umbilical ligament is attached. **c. vitreum** [NA] The body of colorless, transparent gel that occupies the vitreous chamber in the posterior four-fifths of the eyeball. Anteriorly it is indented by the hyaloid fossa, against which the lens fits and from the center of which the hyaloid canal extends to the optic disk. It is about 99% water with some mucoprotein, hyaluronic acid, and salts, and it contains a meshwork of collagenous fibrils. Also *vitreous body, hyaloid body, vitreous, vitreum.* See also HUMOR VITREUS.

**corpuscallostomy** \kôr′pəskaläs′təmē\ The surgical procedure of craniocaudal section of the corpus callosum.

# corpuscle

**corpuscle** \kôr′pusl\ [L *corpusculum.* See CORPUSCULUM.] Any discrete, small structure, usually microscopic in size. Also *corpusculum.* **articular c.** CORPUSCULA ARTICULARIA. **axis c.** A pile of epithelioid cells and intermeshed axon terminals found at the center of a tactile corpuscle. **Babès-Ernst c.'s** BABÈS-ERNST BODIES. **basal c.** BASAL BODY. **Bizzozero's c.** PLATELET. **blood c.** Any blood cell. **bone c.** OSTEOCYTE. **bridge c.** SQUAMOUS CELL. **bulboid c.'s** CORPUSCULA BULBOIDEA. **cartilage c.** CHONDROCYTE. **cement c.** CEMENTOCYTE. **chyle c.** A lymphocyte present in chyle. **colostrum c.'s** Histiocytic cells present within colostrum that contain cytoplasmic fat globules. **concentrated human red blood c.** A human whole blood preparation that represents a concentrated suspension of red blood cells. The cells are obtained from donors within 14 days of use and have previously been cross-matched with the recipient. **concentric c.** HASSALL'S CORPUSCLE. **corneal c.'s** Stellate fibroblastic cells that lie between layers of dense fibrous tissue in the cornea. Also *Virchow cells, Virchow's corpuscles* (older term), *Toynbee's corpuscles* (older term). **Dogiel's c.'s** Encapsulated mechanoreceptor endings principally found in genital skin. **dust c.** PLATELET. **genital c.'s** CORPUSCULA GENITALIA. **ghost c.** ERYTHROCYTE GHOST. **Golgi c.** TENDON ORGAN. **Golgi-Mazzoni c.'s** GOLGI-MAZZONI ENDINGS. **Guarnieri's c.'s** GUARNIERI BODIES. **Hassall's c.** A small nest of concentrically arranged hyalinized epithelial cells in the medulla of the thymus. Also *thymus corpuscle, thymic corpuscle, Leber's corpuscle, concentric corpuscle, Virchow-Hassall body, Hassall's body.* **Hayem's elementary c.** PLATELET. **Krause's c.'s** CORPUSCULA BULBOIDEA. **lamellar c.'s** CORPUSCULA LAMELLOSA. **lamellated c.'s** CORPUSCULA LAMELLOSA. **Laveran's c.'s** LAVERAN BODIES. **Leber's c.** HASSALL'S CORPUSCLE. **lymphoid c.** LYMPHOCYTE. **malpighian c. of kidney** CORPUSCULUM RENALE. **malpighian c.'s of spleen** FOLLICULI LYMPHATICI SPLENICI. **Mazzoni's c.** A spherical sensory organ similar in structure to an end-bulb of Krause, but smaller and with a less profusely coiled axon terminal. **meconium c.'s** Enterocytes of the terminal ileum of a fetus that have become stained by meconium. **Meissner's c.'s** CORPUSCULA TACTUS. **Merkel's c.'s** Tactile end-organs found broadly distributed in the basal epidermis, in the form of disks of Merkel cells specialized to serve as slowly-adapting mechanoreceptors. **molluscous c.'s** MOLLUSCUM BODIES. **nerve c.** *Older term* SCHWANN CELL. **oval c.'s** CORPUSCULA TACTUS. **pacinian c.'s** A large, globular form of lamellar corpuscle found in the vicinity of joints, in tendon sheaths and interosseous membranes, in some subcutaneous locations, at the base of abdominal mesenteries, and near arteriovenous anastomoses. They are sensors for accelerating or velocity but in some sites possibly have other functions. Also *Vater's corpuscles, Vater-Pacini corpuscles, Pacini's corpuscles.* See also CORPUSCULA LAMELLOSA. **Paschen's c.'s** GUARNIERI BODIES. **phantom c.** ERYTHROCYTE GHOST. **Purkinje's c.'s** *Obs.* PURKINJE CELLS. **pus c.** PYOCYTE. **red c.** ERYTHROCYTE. **red blood c.** ERYTHROCYTE. **renal c.** CORPUSCULUM RENALE. **reticulated c.** RETICULOCYTE. **Ruffini's c.'s** Small, globular to cylindrical sensory organs that respond to pressure and warmth. They consist of a tangle of branches of a group II axon embedded in a granular matrix and surrounded by a thin capsule. They tend to be associated in clusters supplied by the single axon. They are found in finger pads, fascial planes, joint capsules, tendons, and tendon sheaths. Also *Ruffini's endings, spray endings, ball-of-thread endings.* **Russell c.'s** RUSSELL BODIES. **Schwalbe's c.** CALICULUS GUSTATORIUS. **shadow c.** ERYTHROCYTE GHOST. **splenic c.'s** FOLLICULI LYMPHATICI SPLENICI. **tactile c.'s** 1 CORPUSCULA TACTUS. 2 Receptors mediating the sense of touch. **taste c.** CALICULUS GUSTATORIUS. **tendon c.'s** TENDON CELLS. **terminal nerve c.'s** CORPUSCULA NERVOSA TERMINALIA. **thymic c.** HASSALL'S CORPUSCLE. **thymus c.** HASSALL'S CORPUSCLE. **touch c.'s** CORPUSCULA TACTUS. **Toynbee's c.'s** *Older term* CORNEAL CORPUSCLES. **Traube's c.** ERYTHROCYTE GHOST. **Valentin's c.'s** Minute amyloid inclusions occasionally seen in nervous tissue. **Vater's c.'s** PACINIAN CORPUSCLES. **Vater-Pacini c.'s** PACINIAN CORPUSCLES. **Virchow's c.'s** *Older term* CORNEAL CORPUSCLES. **white c.** LEUKOCYTE. **white blood c.** LEUKOCYTE.

**corpuscula** \kôrpus′kyələ\ Plural of CORPUSCULUM.

**corpuscular** \kôrpus′kyələr\ Of, pertaining to, or resembling corpuscles.

**corpusculum** \kôrpus′kyələm\ [L (dim. of *corpus* the body, the flesh), a little body, corpuscle] (*pl.* corpuscula) 1 CORPUSCLE. 2 A small aggregation of specialized cells, often of nervous tissue. **corpuscula articularia** Any of several types of encapsulated sensory receptors found in the fibrous capsule of a joint. Also *articular corpuscle.* **corpuscula bulboidea** [NA] Thinly lamellated, globular receptors consisting of a mass of epithelioid cells containing an intricate skein of branches from a single myelinated axon. They are found in skin and mucosal surfaces and are sensors of cold. Also *end-bulbs of Krause, bulbs of Krause, Krause's corpuscles, corpuscula bulbiformia, bulboid corpuscles.* **corpuscula genitalia** Encapsulated tactile or pressure receptors located beneath mucosal and modified skin areas of the genitalia, sometimes including receptors of the nipple and areola. Also *genital corpuscles, genital receptors.* **corpuscula lamellosa** Sensory receptors consisting of a distinctive multilaminated sheath surrounding a central core harboring the variously branched or unbranched naked terminal of a sensory axon. Recognized subtypes are pacinian, paciniform, and Herbst corpuscles. They are extremely sensitive to phasic changes in surrounding pressure. Also *lamellated corpuscles, lamellar corpuscles.* **corpuscula nervosa terminalia** The specialized terminal portions of somatic sensory axons, found principally in the cutaneous and dermal layers and surrounded by a corpuscular structure probably derived from Schwann cells. The specialized encapsulated structures are probably not involved in impulse transduction. Various types are included, such as pacinian, Herbst, Merkel's, and Meissner's corpuscles, Golgi tendon organs, and muscle spindles, each of which is believed to subserve a specific sensory submodality. Also *corpuscula nervorum terminalia, corpuscula nervosa incapsulata, terminal nerve corpuscles, encapsulated nerve endings*. Compare CORPUSCULUM NERVOSUM ACAPSULATUM. **c. nervosum acapsulatum** [NA] Any of an extensive array of unmyelinated axon terminals broadly distributed in the dermis, cornea, muscles, and viscera. The terminals rarely display bare or "free" zones of membrane, but are surrounded by only a thin Schwann cell process and appear to be exposed when examined by light microscopy. A role in pain perception has often been suggested for these fine axon terminals, but evidence indicates that this is not an exclusive function. The majority of these endings are believed to be polymodal nociceptors, but many are sensitive mechanoreceptors, possibly subserving tickle and itch sensations. Also *nonencapsulated ending, unencapsulated ending, free nerve ending* (imprecise). Compare CORPUSCULA NERVOSA TERMINALIA. **c. renale** [NA] The composite of the glomerulus and the capsula glomeruli, the latter being the most proximal part of the nephronum. It is one of more than a million small round masses situated in the renal cortex and columns. Also *renal corpuscle, malpighian body of kidney, malpighian corpuscle of kidney, corpusculum renis, acinus renis malpighii* (outmoded), *acinus renalis malpighii* (outmoded). **corpuscula tactus** **c. triticeum** CARTILAGO TRITICEA.

**correction** The act of changing conditions to remove error or reduce the effect of a fault, as of a defect of vision. **Yates c.** An adjustment required in the calculation of chi-square in a fourfold table to allow for the fact that the entries being integers are discontinuous whereas the underlying distribution on which the chi-square test is based is continuous.

**corrective** 1 Promoting a favorable change in the course of a disease or other abnormal condition. 2 An agent which when added to a drug strengthens its effectiveness.

**correlation** \kôr′əlā′shən\ [New L *correlatio* (from COR- + L *relatio* a carrying back, a telling, from *relatus*, past part. of *referre* to carry back)] In statistics, interdependence between two or more variables. When a change in one variable is accompanied by a change in the second variable in the same direction, the correlation is positive. If the second variable changes, but in a direction opposite to that of the first variable, the correlation is negative. **zero c.** The total absence of interrelationship between two variables.

**correspondence** \kôr′əspän′dəns\ [French *correspondance* (from *correspondre* to be in communication, from COR- + L *respondere* to promise in return, answer) correspondence] RETINAL CORRESPONDENCE. **anomalous retinal c.** A faulty binocular directional orientation, in which a parafoveal area in one eye assumes a straight-ahead value under conditions of binocular function. **harmonious retinal c.** An anomalous retinal correspondence in which the angular distance of the nonmacular fixing area from the fovea is the same as the angle of strabismus. **retinal c.** The relationship of paired receptors in the two retinas that have the same directional orientation. Also *correspondence*.

**Corrigan** [Sir Dominic John *Corrigan*, Irish physician, 1802–1880] 1 Corrigan's cautery. See under BUTTON CAUTERY. 2 Corrigan's disease. See under AORTIC REGURGITATION. 3 Corrigan's pulse. See under COLLAPSING PULSE.

**corrigent** [L *corrigens*, gen. *corrigentis*, pres. part. of *corrigere* to set right, moderate] 1 A drug or other agent that is added to a formula to correct another drug's action or side effect, or to decrease its strength, harshness, poor taste, or other undesired property. 2 Rendering milder.

**corrin** $C_{19}H_{22}N_4$. The substance representing the core of vitamin $B_{12}$, consisting of three dihydropyrroles and one tetrahydropyrrole joined in a ring, two directly and the others through —CH= bridges.

**corrinoid** Any substance related in structure to vitamin $B_{12}$. The molecules of such compounds contain four reduced pyrrole rings united into a macrocycle by links between the carbon atoms adjacent to their nitrogen atoms. Three such links are through =CH— bridges, which may in turn be methylated, whereas one is a direct chemical bond.

**corrugation** \kôr′əgā′shən\ [Med L *corrugatio* (from L *corrugatus*, past part. of *corrugare* to wrinkle) a corrugation, wrinkling] A folding of the scalp, as in cutis verticis gyrata.

**corrugator** \kôr′əgā′tər\ A muscle that puckers or wrinkles the skin.

**corset** A firm circumferential support around the chest or abdomen. It is commonly used in disorders of the spine. **Milwaukee c.** A trunk orthosis extending from the chin and occiput to the pelvic area, used to correct scoliotic curves of the spine.

**cort.** 1 cortex. 2 cortical.

**cortex** \kôr′teks\ [L (akin to *corium* hide, leather)] A distinctive external or investing layer of the substance of an organ or structure. Also *cortical layer*. Adj. cortical. **aberrant suprarenal c.** Glandulae suprarenales accessoriae that are composed of cortical tissue. **adrenal c.** CORTEX GLANDULAE SUPRARENALIS. **agranular c.** A cerebral cortical arrangement of cells and fibers in which the granular layers II and IV are relatively small, as seen in the precentral gyrus. **auditory c.** The zone of the superior temporal gyrus in man (Brodmann's areas 41 and 42), recipient of a cochlear projection via the thalamic medial geniculate body. Also *transverse gyri of Heschl*. **calcarine c.** AREA STRIATA. **c. cerebelli** [NA] The layer of gray

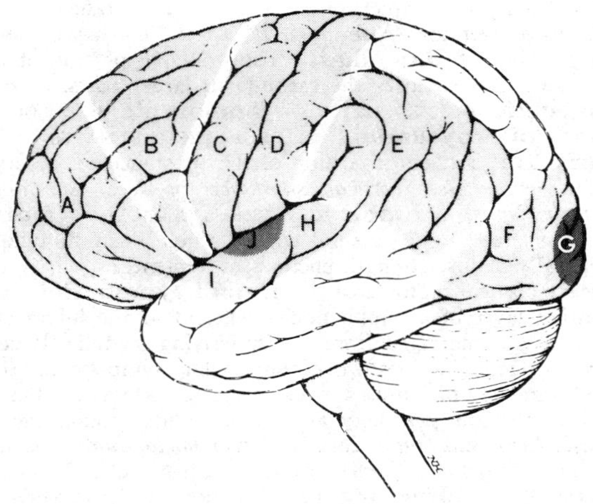


**Cerebral cortex** Major functional areas: (A) biological intelligence; (B) premotor; (C) somatomotor; (D) somatosensory; (E) bodily awareness; (F) visual psychic; (G) visual sensory; (H) speech understanding; (I) auditory psychic; (J) auditory sensory.

matter covering the folia of the cerebellum. It has a nearly uniform structure, consisting of an outermost stratum moleculare and an underlying stratum granulosum that includes the stratum gangliosum in which lie the Purkinje cells. Also *cerebellar cortex, substantia corticalis cerebelli.* **cerebral c.** CORTEX CEREBRI. **c. cerebri** [NA] The gray matter forming the outer layer of the cerebral hemispheres, extensively folded into fissures in most large mammals. Its superficial layer consists of axons, dendrites, and glia overlying two or more cellular layers bounded below by white matter. There are various schemes for classifying functional zones on the basis of cellular and fibrous architectural criteria. Also *pallium, cerebral cortex, brain mantle, substantia corticalis cerebri, mantle* (popular). Adj. pallial. **cingulate c.** GYRUS CINGULI. **driftwood c.** DYSTOPIC CORTICAL MYELINOGENESIS. **entorhinal c.** The large cortical field, corresponding to area 28 of Brodmann, interposed between the hippocampal formation and the neocortex, principally caudally contiguous with the area striata. It is a principal source of fibers to the hippocampus via the alvear and perforant paths. **eulaminate c.** *Older term* ISOCORTEX. **fetal c.** A deep layer of the fetal adrenal cortex, composed of large acidophil cells irregularly arranged in a network. Well developed during all of fetal life, it separates the medulla from the definitive cortex, which is itself not very thick. It disappears a few months after birth. Its shrinkage is related to the progressive maturation of the definitive cortex, which is completed about the second postnatal year in man. The fetal cortex seems to produce hormones which are metabolized to form estrogen by the placenta. Their production becomes dependent on the hypophysis from the fifth month of fetal life, as is shown by observations on some anencephalics. It is thought to participate in androgenic secretion and when overactive may cause masculinization of the genital ducts of a female fetus, or the precocious virilization of a male fetus. Also *X-zone, X zone, androgenic zone, fetal zone.* **frontal premotor c.** The rostral portion of the motor cortex (Brodmann's area 6), the principal site of proximal muscle representation. **c. glandulae suprarenalis** [NA] The extensive peripheral part of the suprarenal gland, yellowish in color and rich in lipids, with no chromaffin tissue. It comprises three zones of cells and produces more than three steroids. Also *adrenal cortex, interrenal system* (obs.). **c. of hair shaft** The principal portion of the hair shaft that encloses the medulla in larger hairs. **homogenetic c.** ISOCORTEX. **homotypic c.** ISOCORTEX. **interpyramidal c.** COLUMNAE RENALES. **c. lentis** The soft outer portion of the substance of the crystalline lens. Also *cortical substance of lens, substantia corticalis lentis.* **limbic c.** GYRUS CINGULI. **motor c.** Any area of the cerebral cortex which when stimulated electrically at low strength elicits a movement, especially the primary cortical motor area. **c. nodi lymphatici** The investing layer of a lymph node, deficient at the hilum and not clearly demarcated from the underlying medulla. It consists of a reticular meshwork surrounding lymphocytes that also forms lymph sinuses when arranged loosely. Afferent vessels enter the periphery at various points around the sinuses. Also *substantia corticalis lymphoglandulae, cortical substance of lymph nodes.* **nonolfactory c.** *Outmoded* ISOCORTEX. **olfactory c.** The area of basal cerebral cortex where the olfactory tract terminates, including the tuberculum olfactorium and the prepyriform and periamygdaloid cortices. **c. of ovary** A thick, dense, fibrous outer layer of the ovary that contains the ovarian follicles and corpora lutea and that surrounds the more vascular medulla. **periamygdaloid c.** The laminar, superficial portion of the amygdala and part of the termination cortex of the lateral olfactory tract. It is sometimes included in the pyriform cortex. Also *cortical nucleus of amygdala.* **piriform c.** **1** The cerebral cortex of the piriform gyrus of the temporal lobe. Also *piriform area.* **2** PREPIRIFORM CORTEX. **precentral motor c.** The electrically excitable cortex, rostral to the central sulcus, from which movements can be elicited. It corresponds to areas 4, 6, and 8 of Brodmann. **premotor c.** PREMOTOR AREA. **prepiriform c.** The three-layered sector of olfactory cerebral cortex at the junctional zone between the basal frontal and temporal lobes, delimited by cytoarchitectonic criteria. Also *prepiriform area, piriform cortex.* **c. renalis** [NA] The portion of the kidney which lies just deep to the fibrous capsule and comprises the pars radiata, pars convoluta and columnae renales. Also *renal cortex, cortex renis, cortical substance of kidney* (outmoded). **retrosplenial c.** The caudal continuation of the cingulate gyrus surrounding the splenium of the corpus callosum. It is part of the posterior limbic cortex, corresponding to area 29 of Brodmann. **secondary visual c.** PARASTRIATE AREA. **sensorimotor c.** The paracentral (rolandic) cortex of primates and pericruciate cortex of carnivores constituting the primary motor and somatosensory fields, considered as a unified entity because of their consistent contiguity and functional interaction. **somatosensory c.** Any area of the cerebral cortex related to the projection and initial stages in integration of somatic sensory stimuli; in man, the postcentral areas of the parietal lobe. **spore c.** A thick layer in the bacterial spore surrounding the core and containing a loosely crosslinked peptidoglycan. **striate c.** AREA STRIATA. **supplementary motor c.** See under GYRUS PARACENTRALIS. **thymic c.** The outer zones of the thymic lobules, which are composed of small lymphocytes that lie in a framework of branching reticular cells and fibers.

**Corti** [Alfonso Giacomo Gaspare *Corti,* Italian anatomist, 1822–1876] **1** Corti's ganglion. See under GANGLION SPIRALE COCHLEAE. **2** Arches of Corti. See under ARCH. **3** Canal of Corti, tunnel of Corti, inner tunnel of Corti. See under CUNICULUS INTERNUS. **4** Corti's auditory teeth, Corti's teeth. See under DENTES ACUSTICI. **5** Corti's membrane. See under MEMBRANA TECTORIA DUCTUS COCHLEARIS. **6** Cells of Corti. See under CELL.

**cortiadrenal** \kôr′tē·adrē′nəl\ CORTICOADRENAL.

**cortical** \kôr′təkəl\ Pertaining to or having the characteristics of a cortex.

**corticalization** \kôr′təkal′izā′shən\ The phylogenetic process tending to localize subcortical functions in the cortex. It includes the processes of encephalization and telencephalization.

**corticate** \kôr′tikāt\ Possessing a cortex.

**corticectomy** \kôr′tisek′təmē\ [*cortic(es),* pl. of CORTEX + -ECTOMY] TOPECTOMY.

**cortices** \kôr′tisēz\ Plural of CORTEX.

**corticifugal** \kôr′tisif′yəgəl\ Denoting or pertaining to neuronal pathways along which impulses travel from the cerebral cortex to other parts of the nervous system. Also *corticofugal.*

**corticipetal** \kôr′tisip′ətəl\ CORTICOAFFERENT.

**cortico-** \kôr′təkō-\ [L *cortex,* gen. *corticis,* bark, rind, shell] A combining form meaning cortex, cortical.

**corticoadrenal** \-adrē′nəl\ Pertaining to or arising from the cortex of the suprarenal gland; adrenocortical. Also *cortiadrenal.*

**corticoafferent** \-af′ərənt\ Denoting projections, either of sensory origin or from central nuclei, to the cerebral cortex. Also *corticipetal, corticopetal.*

**corticoautonomic** \-ō'tənäm'ik\ Describing or pertaining to those neuronal pathways from the cerebral cortex which influence the autonomic nervous system.

**corticobulbar** \-bul'bər\ Pertaining to projections from the cerebral cortex to the medulla oblongata.

**corticoefferent** \-ef'ərənt\ Describing or pertaining to corticofugal or effector neurons from the cerebral cortex.

**corticofugal** \kôr'tikäf'yəgəl\ CORTICIFUGAL.

**corticogram** \kôr'təkōgram'\ ELECTROCORTICOGRAM.

**corticoliberin** \-lib'ərin\ CORTICOTROPIN RELEASING HORMONE.

**corticomedullary** \-med'yəler'ē\ **1** Involving both the cortex and the medulla of an organ. **2** Proceeding from the cortex to the medulla.

**corticopetal** \kôr'təkäp'ətəl\ CORTICOAFFERENT.

**corticopontine** \-pän'tīn\ Pertaining to the cerebral cortex and pons, particularly the projection of cortical axons onto the ipsilateral pontine nuclei.

**corticopontocerebellar** \-pän'təser'əbel'ər\ Pertaining to a major projection from motor and other cortical areas to the opposite cerebellar cortex via a relay and crossing located in the pons.

**corticorubral** \-roo'brəl\ Pertaining to interrelations and projections between areas of the cerebral cortex and the red nucleus.

**corticospinal** \-spī'nəl\ Pertaining to the cerebral cortex and spinal cord, especially the functional projection or anatomic tract between them.

**corticosteroid** \-ster'oid\ **1** A steroid from the adrenal cortex. Its typical features are a $C_2$ side-chain (C-20 and C-21) on C-17, 11$\beta$ and 21-hydroxyl groups, a 20-oxo group and a conjugated 4-en-3-one system. This arrangement is found in corticosterone. • *Corticosteroid* is used especially of the $C_{21}$ steroid hormones that are clinically useful in treating allergic, inflammatory, and other diseases. **2** Any synthetic analogue of cortisol. For defs. 1 and 2 also *adrenocorticosteroid.*

**corticosterone** \kôr'təkäs'tərōn\ $C_{21}H_{30}O_4$. 11$\beta$,21-Dihydroxypregn-4-ene-3,20-dione, a steroid hormone found in the adrenal cortex of mammals. It is the main corticosteroid of the rat, and is present in human adrenocortical secretion, which contains cortisol, its 17-hydroxy derivative. Most mammals secrete a mixture of the two. It possesses life-maintaining properties in animals lacking a functional adrenal cortex but is less potent in inducing sodium retention than deoxycorticosterone.

**corticostriate** \-strī'āt\ Pertaining to interrelations between the cerebral cortex and the corpus striatum.

**corticotroph** \kôr'təkōträf'\ CORTICOTROPIC CELL.

**corticotrophic** \-träf'ik\ ADRENOCORTICOTROPIC.

**corticotrophin** \-träf'in\ ADRENOCORTICOTROPIC HORMONE.

**corticotropic** \-träp'ik\ ADRENOCORTICOTROPIC.

**corticotropin** \-träp'in\ ADRENOCORTICOTROPIC HORMONE.

**$\beta$-corticotropin** \-träp'in\ The 39-amino acid adrenocorticotropic hormone found in the anterior pituitary of man, pigs, sheep, and cattle. Its biologic activity resides in the amino acid sequence 1-24 at the *N*-terminal of the molecule. This sequence is the same for all these species, and only the sequence 25–33 is species-specific.

**cortisol** \kôr'təsôl\ $C_{21}O_5$. 11$\beta$,17$\alpha$,21-Trihydroxyprregn-4-ene-3,20-dione, a steroid hormone of the adrenal cortex of man and many other species. It is the principal corticosteroid in the human circulation. It increases output of glucose by the liver and glucose formantion from amino acids. It regulates the microcirculation, acts to maintain blood pressure, and exhibits anti-inflammatory action. It is used to treat allergic, inflammatory, and neoplastic diseases. Also *hydroxycortisone, 17-hydroxycorticosterone.*

**cortisone** \kôr'təsōn\ $C_{21}H_{28}O_5$. 17$\alpha$21-Dihydroxy-4-pregnene-3,11,20-trione, a steroid hormone with effects similar to those of cortisol. It is the product of oxidation of cortisol at C-11 from —CHOH— to —CO—. It is less active than cortisol for topical application, but can be converted into cortisol in the body.

**cortisone acetate** The acetate ester form of the glucocorticoid cortisone. It is a white, crystalline powder that is employed as an anti-inflammatory agent in the treatment of allergies and certain collagen diseases. It is used to correct certain adrenal cortical deficiencies. It can be given intramuscularly, orally, or topically.

**coruscation** \kôr'əskā'shən\ [Late L *coruscatio* (from L *coruscatus,* past part. of *coruscare* to glitter, flash) a flashing] A subjective sensation of flashing lights or glittering in front of the eyes.

**Corvisart** [Jean-Nicolas *Corvisart,* French physician, 1755–1821] **1** Corvisart's disease. See under HYPERTROPHIC CARDIOMYOPATHY. **2** See under DISEASE.

**corybantism** \kôr'iban'tizm\ [after Gk *Korybas,* gen. *Korybantis,* a priest who attended the nature goddess Cybele in dance and music, + -ISM] Wild and even maniacal delirium with severe hallucinations, sleeplessness, and generalized muscular twitching. Also *corybantiasm.*

**corynebacteriophage** \kôr'inēbaktir'ē·əfāj'\ A bacteriophage of *Corynebacterium* species.

***Corynebacterium*** \kôr'inēbaktir'ē·əm\ [Gk *korynē* a mace, club + BACTERIUM] A group of Gram-positive, mostly aerobic, nonsporulating rods that are often club-shaped and stain irregularly. They include a few human pathogens, many plant pathogens, and soil and water bacteria. They are not all closely related taxonomically, since G + C content ranges from 48% to 70%. The human parasites appear to be related taxonomically to *Mycobacterium* and *Nocardia,* since their cell walls are related chemically and serologically. ***C. acnes*** *Obs.* *PROPIONOBACTERIUM ACNES.* ***C. diphtheriae*** An aerobic, nonmotile, nonencapsulated corynebacterium that causes diphtheria. The cells in stained smears often form sharp angles with each other, and they contain polymetaphosphate granules (Babès-Ernst bodies) that stain metachromatically with methylene blue. In tellurite media the colonies are black. Mitis, gravis, and intermedius strains are differentiated by colonial morphology. Virulent strains form diphtheria toxin, coded for by a temperate phage ($\beta$-phage). Toxin formation is repressed by $Fe^{2+}$, interacting with a host repressor protein. Also *diphtheria bacillus, Klebs-Löffler bacillus.* ***C. hofmanni*** *CORYNEBACTERIUM PSEUDODIPHTHERITICUM.* ***C. minutissimum*** An organism isolated from lesions of erythrasma. ***C. ovis*** *CORYNEBACTERIUM PSEUDOTUBERCULOSIS.* ***C. pseudodiphtheriticum*** A nontoxigenic inhabitant of the human throat. It can be differentiated from *C. diphtheriae* by fermentation reactions. Also *Corynebacterium hofmanni, Hofmann's bacillus.* ***C. pseudotuberculosis*** A bacterium, very similar to *C. diphtheriae* morphologically, that forms a hemolytic and lethal toxin and causes caseous lymphadenitis of sheep and goats and ulcerative lymphangitis of horses. Also *Corynebacterium ovis.* ***C. pyogenes*** A species which is the common cause of numerous suppurative infections in cattle, sheep, goats, and swine. ***C. xerosis*** An inhabitant of the human conjunctival sac and skin. It can be differentiated from *C. diphtheriae* by fermentation reactions and lack of toxin formation.

**corynebacterium** \kôr′inēbaktir′ē·əm\ (*pl.* corynebacteria) Any microorganism of the genus *Corynebacterium.*

**coryneform** \kôrin′ifôrm, kôrī′nifôrm\ [Gk *korynē* a club, shepherd's staff + -FORM] Designating a group of Gram-positive, nonsporulating bacteria that form irregular, often curved rods, including principally the aerobic corynebacteria and the anaerobic propionibacters.

**coryza** \kôrī′zə\ [Gk *koryza* (from *korys* helmet, head + *zeein* to boil, seethe) a cold in the head, catarrh] ACUTE RHINITIS.

**cosmopolitan** \käs′məpäl′itən\ [Gk *kosmo(s)* order, world, universe + *polit(ēs)* citizen of a city or state + English *-an,* from L *-anus* adjectival suffix] Universally distributed; found in all major regions.

**costa** \käs′tə\ [L, rib, side] (*pl.* costae) **1** OS COSTALE. **2** BASAL ROD. **costae fluitantes** [NA] The eleventh and twelfth ribs, whose ventral tips are free and not attached to the costal cartilages above them. Also *floating ribs, vertebral ribs.* **costae spuriae** [NA] The lower five pairs of ribs, whose costal cartilages do not articulate directly with the sternum. Also *false ribs, vertebrochondral ribs, vertebral ribs, spurious ribs, abdominal ribs* (outmoded), *asternal ribs* (outmoded). **costae verae** [NA] The upper seven pairs of ribs that are connected by their costal cartilages directly to the sides of the sternum. Also *true ribs, vertebrosternal ribs, sternal ribs.* **c. fluctuans** One of the costae fluitantes. **c. fluctuans decima** A floating tenth rib.

**costae** \käs′tē\ Plural of COSTA.

**costal** \käs′təl\ [Med L *costal(is)* (from L *cost(a)* rib, side + *-alis* -AL) pertaining to a rib or side] Pertaining to a rib or ribs.

**costalgia** \kästal′jə\ [*cost(o)-* + -ALGIA] A pain originating in a rib.

**costalis** \kästā′lis\ [NA] Costal.

**costate** \käs′tāt\ [L *costat(us)* (from *cost(a)* rib, side + *-atus* -ATE) ribbed] **1** Possessing ribs; ribbed. **2** Having connecting structures.

**costectomy** \kästek′təmē\ [*cost(o)-* + -ECTOMY] Excision or resection of a rib.

**Costen** [James Bray *Costen,* U.S. otolaryngologist, 1895–1962] Costen syndrome. See under TEMPOROMANDIBULAR JOINT SYNDROME.

**costi-** \käs′tē-\ COSTO-.

**costicartilage** \käs′tēkär′təlij\ CARTILAGO COSTALIS.

**costicervical** \käs′tēsur′vikl\ Pertaining to the ribs and the neck.

**costiferous** \kästif′ərəs\ Rib-bearing, as of thoracic vertebrae.

**costive** \käs′tiv\ [Old French *costeve,* past part. of *costever* to crowd together, from L *constipare* (from *con-* together + *stipare* to press, crowd) to press or crowd together] **1** CONSTIPATED. **2** Tending to cause constipation. **3** An agent that causes constipation.

**costiveness** \käs′tivnis\ [COSTIVE + -NESS] **1** CONSTIPATION. **2** The tendency or capacity to cause constipation.

**costo-** \käs′tō-\ [L *costa* rib] A combining form denoting the ribs. Also *costi-.*

**costoabdominal** \-abdäm′ənəl\ Pertaining to the ribs and the abdomen.

**costocentral** \-sen′trəl\ COSTOVERTEBRAL.

**costocervicalis** \-sur′vikā′lis\ MUSCULUS ILIOCOSTALIS CERVICIS.

**costochondral** \-kän′drəl\ Pertaining to a rib and its costal cartilage or to ribs and costal cartilages.

**costochondritis** \-kändrī′tis\ Inflammation of the cartilages attached to the ribs, which results in pain and local tenderness over the anterior chest wall. Also *Tietze's disease, Tietze syndrome, costal chondritis, costochondral syndrome.*

**costocoracoid** \-kôr′əkoid\ Pertaining to the ribs and the coracoid process of the scapula.

**costodiaphragmatic** \-dī′əfragmat′ik\ COSTOPHRENIC.

**costogenic** \-jen′ik\ Emanating from a rib.

**costoinferior** \-infir′ē·ər\ Pertaining to the lower ribs.

**costolumbar** \-lum′bər\ LUMBOCOSTAL.

**costophrenic** \-fren′ik\ Pertaining to the ribs and the respiratory diaphragm. Also *phrenocostal, phrenicocostal, costodiaphragmatic.*

**costoplasty** \käs′tōplas′tē\ [COSTO- + -PLASTY] The surgical reduction of the rib hump seen in structural scoliosis.

**costopneumopexy** \-n^y^oo′mōpek′sē\ [COSTO- + PNEUMO- + -PEXY] The surgical procedure of anchoring the lung to a rib.

**costosternoplasty** \-stur′nōplas′tē\ [COSTO- + STERNO- + -PLASTY] CHONDROSTERNOPLASTY.

**costosuperior** \-səpir′ē·ər\ Pertaining to the upper ribs.

**costotome** \käs′tətōm\ [COSTO- + -TOME] A knife or shears designed for cutting through the ribs or costal cartilage.

**costotomy** \kästät′əmē\ [COSTO- + -TOMY] Resection or division of a rib or costal cartilage.

**costotransverse** \-transvurs′\ Pertaining to or between the ribs and the transverse processes of the vertebrae with which they articulate. Also *transversocostal.*

**costotransversectomy** \-trans′vərsek′təmē\ Excision of a proximal portion of a rib together with a transverse process of a vertebra.

**costovertebral** \-vur′təbrəl\ Pertaining to the ribs and the bodies of the vertebrae with which they articulate.

**costoxiphoid** \-zī′foid\ Pertaining to or connecting the ribs and the xiphoid process of the sternum.

**cosyntropin** \kō′sinträp′in\ A synthetic preparation of adrenocorticotropic hormone, comprising the N-terminal, 24-amino acid sequence which possesses nearly the same steroidogenic potency as the native 39-amino acid molecule ($ACTH^{1-39}$). Given intravenously or subcutaneously (250 $\mu$g), it probably causes fewer untoward effects than $ACTH^{1-39}$ when used to test adrenocortical responsivity or reserve.

**cot** The concentration of nucleic acid in moles per liter at time zero (0), multiplied by the length of time in seconds that reassociation has proceded.

**COTe** cathodal opening tetanus.

**cothromboplastin** \kōthräm′bəplas′tin\ FACTOR VII.

**cotransduction** \kō′transduk′shən\ The transfer of two or more closely linked genes, by means of bacteriophage, from a donor to a recipient bacterium.

**Cotte** [Gaston *Cotte,* French surgeon, 1879–1951] See under OPERATION.

**Cotting** [Benjamin Eddy *Cotting,* U.S. surgeon, 1812–1898] See under OPERATION.

**Cotton** [Aimé Auguste *Cotton,* French physicist, 1869–1951] See under EFFECT.

**cotton** The fibers of the capsules, or bolls, of one or more of the cultivated varieties of *Gossypium* species. The seeds of the plant yield cottonseed oil, which is composed of olein, palmitin, and stearin. The oil is used in liniments and in pharmaceuticals as a solvent. **absorbent c.** A naturally occurring fiber frequently used as a material for sterile dressings and surgical sponges. Also *cotton wool.* **capsicum c.** Absorbent cotton impregnated with methyl salicylate and capsicum.

**cottonmouth** WATER MOCCASIN.

**Cotugno** [Domenico Felice Antonio *Cotugno* (*Cotunnius*), Italian anatomist, 1736–1822] **1** Columns of Cotunnius. See under COLUMN. **2** Canal of Cotunnius. See under AQ-

DUCTUS VESTIBULI. **3** See under CANAL, SPACE. **4** Cotugno's disease. See under SCIATICA. **5** Nerve of Cotunnius. See under NERVUS NASOPALATINUS.

**co-twin** A member of a twin pair, regardless of zygosity.

**cotyle** \kät′ilē\ ACETABULUM.

**cotyledon** \kät′ilē′dän\ [Gk *kotylēdōn* a cup-shaped hollow or cavity] See under PLACENTAL COTYLEDON. **placental c.** One of the subdivisions or lobes of the human placenta seen on its maternal or uterine surface after expulsion of the organ at birth. There are 15 to 20 such cotyledons in a normal human placenta. When attached *in situ* to the uterine wall, the cotyledons or lobules are separated by maternal connective tissue that is partially shed on separation of the placenta after birth. Also *lobe of the placenta.*

***Cotylogonimus*** \kät′ilōgän′əməs\ [Gk *kotyl(ē)* a small cup + *o* + *gonimos* fruitful] *HETEROPHYES.*

**cotyloid** \kät′iloid\ **1** Cup-shaped. **2** Pertaining to the acetabulum; acetabular.

**cotylopubic** \kät′ilōpyoo′bik\ Pertaining to the acetabulum and the pubis.

**cotylosacral** \kät′ilōsā′krəl\ Pertaining to the acetabulum and the sacrum.

**cough** **1** To expel air suddenly and explosively from the lungs. **2** A sudden explosive expulsion of air from the lungs. It may be reflex or voluntary. **3** A persistent or transient condition characterized by coughing. For defs. 2 and 3 also *bex, tussis.* **barking c.** A staccato, barklike cough, characteristic of measles or tracheitis in children. **bovine c.** The low-pitched, hollow, blowing cough produced when one or both vocal cords are paralyzed in the cadaveric (paramedian) position. **brassy c.** A cough producing a high-pitched metallic sound, resulting from pressure on the trachea. **ear c.** A reflex cough caused by stimulation of the auricular branch of the vagus nerve. Characteristically it is caused by the use of instruments in cleaning the external ear. **extrapulmonary c.** Any cough not attributable to causes within the lungs. **hacking c.** A short, dry, frequently repeated cough. **paroxysmal c.** A cough that occurs in intermittent episodes or attacks. **productive c.** A cough that yields sputum. **reflex c.** A cough produced by stimulation of or dysfunction of nerve afferents apart from those of the respiratory tract, as of the external auditory meatus. **stomach c.** A reflex cough induced by disease or dysfunction of the stomach. Also *tussis stomachalis.* **trigeminal c.** A reflex cough attributed to irritation of the sensory branches of the maxillary divison of the trigeminal nerve in the nose, palate, or pharynx. **weavers' c.** Outbreaks of coughing or of asthma occurring among cotton-weavers as a result of exposure to molds in the size applied to the warp. In addition to mold allergens, vegetable allergens, such as tamarind seed, used for size have caused severe respiratory symptoms. **whooping c.** PERTUSSIS.

**coulomb** \koolām′, koo′lōm\ [after Charles Augustin de *Coulomb*, French physicist, 1736–1806] The special name for the SI derived unit of the quantity of electricity transported in one second by a current of one ampere, a measure of quantity of electricity, electric charge, and electric flux. Also *ampere-second.* Symbol: C **c. per kilogram** A unit of ionization exposure. For x-radiation or gamma radiation, the total electric charge of the ions of one sign produced when all the electrons liberated by photons in an elementary quantity of air are stopped in air, divided by the mass of the elementary quantity of air. Symbol: C/kg, $C{\cdot}kg^{-1}$ **c. per kilogram second** A unit of ionization exposure rate, equal to the ionization exposure in a given interval of time divided by that time. Symbol: C/(kg·s) or $C{\cdot}kg^{-1}{\cdot}s^{-1}$ • The alternative SI derived unit, ampere per kilogram, is identical with coulomb per kilogram second.

**coumermycin** \koo′mərmī′sin\ An antibiotic that inhibits DNA gyrase.

**coumestrol** $C_{15}H_8O_5$. 3,9-Dihydroxy-6*H*-benzofuro [3,2-*c*]-[1]benzopyran-6-one. An estrogenic compound that occurs naturally in certain species of plants such as *Trifolium repens*, strawberry clover.

**Councilman** [William Thomas *Councilman*, U.S. pathologist, 1854–1933] Councilman lesion. See under COUNCILMAN BODIES.

**counseling** A type of supportive or re-educative psychotherapy, including guidance in psychosocial situations that are not attributable to specific mental disorders. It consists of sympathetic listening and understanding which leads to self-help in dealing with social or occupational problems, such as personal relationships. **genetic c.** A clinical genetics service in which data about the medical and family history of the subject (the consultand) are combined with knowledge of human genetics to provide the consultand and his or her family with information about whether a hereditary condition is present, the potential for recurrence risks, the possible burden of the condition and its prognosis, and the options that are available for treatment and prevention of the condition. The service is best performed by a professional (the genetic counselor) who is specifically trained and certified, and who is sensitive to the psychosocial, cultural, religious, as well as genetic and medical aspects of the condition. **nondirective c.** Psychotherapeutic procedures centered on the client, in which the therapist provides only the most minimal direction, serving instead as one who listens with empathy and expresses a caring attitude and nonjudgmental understanding of the client's feelings and behavior. Also *client-centered therapy, nondirective therapy.*

**count** [French *compte* (from Late L *computus*, from L *computare* to count, compute, from COM- + L *putare* to think, count) calculation, number] The quantity of items in a sample, as of red blood cells or pollutant particles. **Addis c.** A quantification of the formed elements, such as red cells, white cells, protein, and casts, that are present in a 12-hour collection of urine. Serial counts indicate the temporal progression of renal disease. **Arneth's c.** ARNETH'S FORMULA. **bleeding point c.** An index of the severity of gingivitis and early chronic periodontitis. **blood c.** The determination of the number of erythrocytes, leukocytes, and platelets per volume unit of blood, utilizing a counting chamber of known size and accurate dilutions of whole blood. **complete blood c.** A combination of laboratory tests including hemoglobin, hematocrit, erythrocyte count, leukocyte count, and differential count. Also *hemogram, blood profile.* Abbr. CBC **differential c.** The relative number of various types of leukocytes, expressed as a percentage of the total leukocyte count. **dust c.** Any measure of the concentration of dust particles per unit volume of air, as of concentrations of fibrous material like asbestos in fibers per milliliter or of the concentration of dust particles roughly estimated from samples counted with a konimeter or optical dust indicator. The most commonly used unit for measuring dust concentrations is mass concentration, measured in milligrams per cubic meter, which has largely replaced particle counting but not fiber counting. **filament-nonfilament c.** The proportion of segmented to nonsegmented neutrophils in a blood sample. **leukocyte c.** The number of leukocytes of all types in a given volume of whole blood or other body fluid. Also *total white count.* **pollen c.** An estimate of the number of pollen particles in a standard volume of ambient air that is made to indicate the possible prevalence of hay fever or other allergic symptoms in susceptible people. **red cell c.** The number of erythrocytes in a given volume of whole blood. **reticulocyte c.** The percentage of erythrocytes which display basophilic reticulum after supravital staining. **ridge c.** In fingerprint patterns, the number of ridges crossed by a line drawn from the core of the pattern to the triradius. **Schilling blood c.** A differential neutrophil count which assigns neutrophil leukocytes to only four categories: segmented, staff (band), juvenile (metamyelocyte), and myelocyte. Also *staff count.* **staff c.** SCHILLING BLOOD COUNT. **total white c.** LEUKOCYTE COUNT.

**counter** An instrument that changes from one state to the next of a sequence of different states for each pulse of an input signal. **automated differential leukocyte c.** Any of several automated or semiautomated instruments that identify circulating blood leukocytes according to morphologic and/or biochemical characteristics and report them in accepted diagnostic categories as percentages of the total leukocytes present. **colony c.** A device to facilitate counting bacterial colonies, often by using a needle that activates a recording instrument at each contact. **Coulter c.** An electronic particle counter that estimates the size and number of particles in fluids. It is used especially for counting cells and platelets in blood and cells in other body fluids. A proprietary name. **crystal c.** A pulse counter that uses a scintillation crystal for the detector. **electronic cell c.** A device that determines the number of cells in liquid specimens by counting the voltage pulses generated by the decrease in resistance produced as cells pass through a calibrated aperture. **end-window c.** A Geiger-Müller counter having a thin window on the end of the counter tube, allowing beta particles to enter the tube and be counted. **gamma scintillation c.** An instrumentation system for detecting and counting photons from a radioactive source, usually composed of a sodium iodide crystal activated with thallium, a photomultiplier tube, and electronic devices for signal amplification, pulse-height analysis, and counting of signals. **gamma well c.** An instrumentation system for detecting and counting photons from a radioactive source, designed to achieve higher counting efficiency. A hole in the center of the thallium-activated sodium iodide crystal creates a well that collects a very high percentage of the gamma rays. **gas-flow c.** A modified Geiger-Müller tube with side tubes so that gas can be passed through the sensitive chamber. Such a tube can monitor, for example, $^{14}CO_2$ produced by the metabolism of an organism. **Geiger c.** GEIGER-MÜLLER COUNTER. **Geiger-Müller c.** An apparatus for the detection and measurement of radioactivity. It is composed of a gas-filled tube with two co-axial electrodes maintained with very high electrical fields, so that any gas ionization results in electrical discharge. Also *Geiger counter.* **immersion c.** A radiation detector designed to be immersed into a radioactive liquid. **liquid-flow c.** A radiation counter that contains a tube through the detector chamber for the measurement of the radioactivity in a liquid as it flows through the tube. **proportional c.** A counter using a gas-filled detector, usually of the Geiger-Müller type, operated with an applied voltage less than that required for ordinary Geiger-Müller operation but high enough so that substantial avalanche amplification can occur. In such a case the avalanche ionization remains localized in the general region of the original ion burst without spreading up and down the central wire, and the size of the output pulse is proportional to the number of ion pairs initially created. Since this number indicates the energy of the ionizing particle, pulse-height analysis can provide a spectrum of the entering energies. **scintillation c.** A device for the detection of alpha, beta, gamma, or x rays by use of fluorescent materials and photomultiplier tubes. The detector system consists of a crystal or liquid, a photomultiplier tube, and a preamplifier. These may be assembled as probes or well counters. For detection of alpha radiation, a zinc sulfide screen is used. For beta radiation, a scintillant liquid is used. For detection of x rays or gamma photons, a sodium iodide crystal activated with thallium is used. **whole-body c.** A gamma-ray counter whose detector with its shield is so designed that the radiation from the entire body of a patient or from any large source can be measured.

**counter-** \koun′tər-\ [French *contre* (from L *contra* against) against] A combining form meaning (1) opposed to or against; (2) corresponding or complementary.

**counteraction** \-ak′shən\ ANTAGONISM.

**counterbalance** \-bal′əns\ A force or condition offsetting another. **renal c.** The compensatory hypertrophy of a kidney or part of a kidney in response to the partial or total loss or removal of the other kidney. The hypertrophy occurs readily in infants and children, more slowly in adults, and may not be detectable in the elderly. Along with organic hypertrophy, renal function of the remaining kidney increases rapidly, so that several weeks to months after a nephrectomy renal function approaches normal.

**counterconditioning** \-kəndish′əning\ In behavior therapy, the formation by means of conditioning techniques, of an alternative response that is incompatible with or antagonistic to a maladaptive response in the subject's behavior.

**countercurrent** \-kur′ənt\ Flowing in an opposite direction to permit the exchange of chemicals or heat.

**counterdepressant** A drug or agent that reverses or antagonizes the depressant effects of another drug.

**counterextension** \-iksten′shən\ Application of a force on a limb in a proximal direction while another force is applied in the opposite direction. Also *contraextension.*

**counterfissure** \-fish′ər\ CONTRAFISSURE.

**counterimmunoelectrophoresis** \-im′yənō·ilek′trōfôrē′sis\ A technique for the rapid achievement of a precipitin line between an antigen and an antibody in a gel medium. The antigen and antibody must have different electrophoretic mobilities so that, when placed in suitably positioned wells, they move toward each other when electrical current is applied. The procedure is highly sensitive to small quantities of antigen or antibody because directed mobility achieves a greater concentration of reactants than unmodified diffusion. Also *immuno-osmophoresis, immunosmoelectrophoresis, counter electrophoresis, countercurrent electrophoresis, counter migration electrophoresis.* Also *counter immunoelectrophoresis.* Abbr. CIE

**counterincision** \-insizh′ən\ A second surgical incision, usually smaller than the first, made for purposes of better visualization, drainage, or manipulation of tissues during a surgical procedure. It is also used as a relaxing incision during hernia repair. Also *counteropening, counterpuncture, contraincision, contra-aperture.*

**counterirritant** \-ir′itənt\ **1** A substance that produces a superficial irritation to alleviate pain arising from deeper organs. **2** Producing or relating to counterirritation.

**counterirritation** \-ir′itā′shən\ A technique whereby pain or irritation in one part of the body is relieved by the application of a mildly painful or irritant stimulus elsewhere, usually on the skin.

**counteropening** \-ō′pəning\ COUNTERINCISION.
**counterphobia** \-fō′bē·ə\ The phobic person's seeking of the very situation that is feared.
**counterpoison** \-poi′zən\ Any substance used to counteract a poison.
**counterpulsation** \-pulsā′shən\ A method of augmenting an impaired circulation by means of a pump which is synchronized with the heart beat. See also INTRA-AORTIC BALLOON PUMP.
**counterpuncture** \-pungk′chər\ COUNTERINCISION.
**counter-rolling** \-rōl′ing\ See under OCULAR COUNTER-ROLLING REFLEX.
**countershock** \-shäk′\ A direct-current electric shock applied to the heart in order to terminate an abnormal rhythm, especially fibrillation.
**counterstain** \-stān′\ An additional stain that is used in microscopy to contrast with the primary or selective stain. Also *contrast stain, afterstain*.
**counterstroke** \-strōk′\ [*counter-* + *stroke*] CONTRECOUP INJURY.
**countertraction** \-trak′shən\ Traction applied in a direction opposite to another traction.
**countertransference** \-transfur′əns\ [COUNTER- + TRANSFERENCE] The effects of the therapist's unconscious needs and conflicts on his ability to understand and deal with the patient appropriately.
**counting** / **coincidence c.** The counting of pulses generated by ionizing events in more than one detector, but only if two or more arrive simultaneously at the input end of the system. This arrangement is useful in counting positron emitters in the presence of a troublesome background. The two annihilation photons are shot off simultaneously, and the coincidence circuit recognizes them as "good" counts. Background events arrive singly and are suppressed.
**coup** \koo\ [French (from L *colaphus* a blow or buffet with the fist, slap, from Gk *kolaphos* a box on the ear, a cuff), a blow, stroke] A blow, thrust, or impact. **c. de fouet** A sudden sharp pain in the calf associated with rupture of the plantaris muscle. **c. de sang** An imprecise and outmoded term for CEREBRAL EDEMA. **c. de soleil** SUNSTROKE.
**coupler** / **acoustic c.** An instrument approximating the human external ear canal in terms of volume and compliance. The output of an electromagnetic sound source, such as an earphone, is coupled to a microphone for calibration purposes. Also *artificial ear*.
**coupling** **1** In genetics, with reference to two linked, doubly heterozygous loci, the occurrence of both mutant alleles on one chromosome and the two wild-type alleles on the homologue. If A and B designate the wild-type alleles and a and b the mutants at two loci, then the genes are "in coupling" if A and B are on the same chromosome (AB/ab), that is, are in cis configuration. Also *coupling phase*. Compare REPULSION. **2** Alternating sinus and premature ectopic cardiac beats resulting usually in a regular succession of paired beats. **3** ADDITION. **contact c.** Acoustic coupling between a transducer and the skin through any of various media, such as water, oil, or gel. **electrochemical c.** The coupling of a chemical concentration gradient across a membrane with an opposing electrical potential or electrical charge. **excitation-contraction c.** The sequence of events from the electrical excitation of the cell membrane of a muscle fiber to the development of tension by the myofibrillar filaments. It includes the spread of excitation over the transverse tubules, release of $Ca^{++}$ions from the longitudinal tubules, and catalysis of the reactions that promote the sliding of actin and myosin filaments with respect to one another, and the resulting shortening of the sarcomere. **immersion c.** The coupling of an ultrasonic transducer to an object by immersing both in a bath of the coupling medium. **liquid c.** A coupling between a transducer and the skin through a liquid medium, either by immersion or through liquid-filled bags.
**Courtois** [Adolphe *Courtois*, French neurologist, born 1903] See under SIGN.
**Courvoisier** [Ludwig Georg *Courvoisier*, Swiss surgeon, 1843–1918] **1** See under LAW, SIGN. **2** Courvoisier-Terrier syndrome. See under SYNDROME.
**cousin** Any person related to another by descent through the brother or sister of a parent, grandparent, or of any ancestor. First cousins are the offspring of siblings, and second cousins are the offspring of first cousins.
**Coutard** [Henri *Coutard*, French roentgenologist, 1876–1950] See under METHOD.
**Couvelaire** [Alexandre *Couvelaire*, French obstetrician, 1873–1948] See under UTERUS.
**covalent** \kōvā′lənt\ [CO- + *valent*, back-formation from VALENCE] Formed by the sharing of at least one and usually a pair of electrons: used especially of chemical bonds between atoms.
**covariance** \kōver′ē·əns\ An index of the concomitant variation of two variables. Thus, if the height ($x$) and weight ($y$) of each of $N$ individuals are measured, the covariance of $x$ and $y$ is given by:

$$\text{cov}\,(x;y) = \frac{\Sigma\,(x - \bar{x})\,(y - \bar{y})}{N},$$

where $\bar{x}$ and $\bar{y}$ are the respective means and $\Sigma$ indicates summation.
**covariate** \kōver′ē·āt\ A variable known to be or suspected of being correlated with the dependent variable under study. For example, in an epidemiologic study of the relationship between cervical cancer and social class, age at first marriage might be a covariate.
**coverglass** COVER GLASS. See under GLASS.
**coverslip** COVER GLASS.
**Cowdry** [Edmund Vincent *Cowdry*, U.S. pathologist, 1888–1975] **1** Cowdry's type A inclusion bodies. See under BODY. **2** Cowdry's type B inclusion bodies. See under BODY.
**cowl** \kôl\ CAUL.
**Cowper** [William *Cowper*, English anatomist, 1666–1709] **1** See under CYST. **2** Cowper's gland. See under GLANDULA BULBOURETHRALIS. **3** Cowper's ligament. See under FASCIA PECTINEA.
**cowperitis** \kou′pərī′tis, koo′-\ [*(glands of) Cowper* + -ITIS] Inflammation of the bulbourethral glands of Cowper (Cowper's glands).
**cowpox** \kou′päks\ A mild eruptive skin disease of cattle caused by a poxvirus and affecting the teats and udders. The infecting virus can be transmitted to humans by skin contact with infected animals. See also VACCINIA.
**Cox** [Herald Rea *Cox*, U.S. virologist, born 1907] Cox vaccine. See under TYPHUS VACCINE.
**Cox** [Willelm Hendrik *Cox*, Dutch physician, 1861–1933] Cox modification of Golgi's corrosive sublimate method. See under METHOD.
**coxa** \käk′sə\ [L, hip, haunch] The hip or hip joint. **c. adducta** COXA VARA. **c. flexa** COXA VARA. **c. magna** A hip joint with an abnormally large femoral head. **c. plana** A hip joint with an abnormally flattened femoral head, commonly seen in Perthes disease. Also *caput planum, caput deformatum*. **c. valga** A defor-

mity of the upper end of the femur characterized by an increased angle between the femoral neck and shaft. **c. vara** A deformity of the upper end of the femur that is marked by a decreased angle between the femoral neck and shaft. Also *coxa flexa, coxa adducta.* **c. vara luxans** Coxa vara in combination with a dislocation of the femoral head.

**coxalgia** \käksal′jə\ [*cox(a)* + -ALGIA] Pain in the hip. **Mediterranean c.** Hip pain that is sometimes seen in cases of brucellosis.

**coxankylometer** \käksang′kiläm′ətər\ An instrument that measures the degree of deformity in a diseased hip joint.

**coxarthria** \käks′är′thrē·ə\ COXITIS.

**coxarthritis** \käks′ärthrī′tis\ COXITIS.

**coxarthropathy** \käks′ärthräp′əthē\ Any disease affecting the hip joint.

**coxarthrosis** \käks′ärthrō′sis\ Degenerative osteoarthrosis of the hip joint.

**coxcomb** \käks′kōm\ See under DES SYNDROME.

***Coxiella burnetii*** \käksyel′ə bərnet′ē·ī \ A rickettsial agent, the cause of Q fever. It differs from species of *Rickettsia* in that it is unusually stable outside host cells, it is acquired by humans by inhalation of material from infected animals rather than via a bite of an arthropod, and it shows no immunologic cross reaction. Also *Rickettsia burnetii* (obs.), *Rickettsia diaporica* (obs.).

**coxitis** \käksī′tis\ [*cox(a)* + -ITIS] Inflammation of the hip joint. Also *coxarthritis, coxarthria.* **c. fugax** Transient synovitis of the hip. Also *transient coxitis.* **senile c.** Osteoarthritis of the hip. **transient c.** COXITIS FUGAX.

**coxofemoral** \käk′sōfem′ərəl\ Pertaining to the hip or hip bone and the femur.

**coxotuberculosis** \käk′sōt^y^ubur′kyəlō′sis\ [*cox(a)* + *o* + TUBERCULOSIS] Tuberculosis of the hip joint.

**coxsackievirus** \käksak′ēvī′rəs\ [after *Coxsackie,* New York, home of patients from whom the virus was first recovered and identified.] Any of a group of RNA viruses belonging to the Picornaviridae family and the *Enterovirus* genus. Coxsackieviruses are divided into types A and B based on differing pathogenicity for newborn mice. There are six type B viruses and 23 type A viruses. They are major causes of viral meningitis, myopericarditis, exanthems, and other febrile syndromes in man. Also *Coxsackie virus.*

**cozymase** *Obs.* NICOTINAMIDE ADENINE DINUCLEOTIDE.

**CP** Chemically pure, generally accepted to mean that there are no chemicals present other than those stated which would affect its properties and reaction as a reagent or drug.

**CPAP** continuous positive airway pressure. **nasal C.** NASAL CONTINUOUS POSITIVE AIRWAY PRESSURE.

**CPC** clinicopathological conference.

**CPK** creatine kinase (once called creatine phosphokinase).

**cpm** counts per minute.

**CPR** cardiopulmonary resuscitation.

**CR** 1 complement receptor. 2 conditioned reflex.

**CR1** See under COMPLEMENT RECEPTOR.

**CR2** See under COMPLEMENT RECEPTOR.

**CR3** See under COMPLEMENT RECEPTOR.

**Cr** Symbol for the element, chromium.

**crab** 1 Any of a diverse group of crustaceans of the order Decapoda most typically characterized by a broad, flat cephalothorax and carapace. 2 *Popular* PUBIC LOUSE.

**Crabtree** [Herbert G. *Crabtree,* English physician and biochemist, flourished 20th century] See under EFFECT.

**cradle** A frame placed over an injured limb to keep bedding away from its surface or on which heating or cooling appliances may be mounted. **electric c.** A cradle with electric light bulbs or infrared emitters to warm the body part. Also *heat cradle.* **heat c.** ELECTRIC CRADLE.

**Crafts** [Leo Melville *Crafts,* U.S. neurologist, 1863–1938] See under TEST.

**Cramer** [Friedrich *Cramer,* German surgeon, 1847–1903] See under SPLINT.

**cramp** [Middle English *crampe,* from Old French *crampe* twisted, from the Germanic] 1 An involuntary, spasmodic, painful, muscular contraction. 2 Any spasmodic type of pain, such as intestinal cramp or colic. **accessory c.** *Outmoded* SPASMODIC TORTICOLLIS. • This was once thought erroneously to be due to a lesion of the spinal accessory nerve. **heat c.** A condition occurring in workers doing heavy physical work in hot climates or work environments and characterized by cramps in the calves spreading to the abdomen and upper limbs. It is caused by excessive loss of sodium chloride in sweat together with reduced sodium chloride levels following the drinking of water. It can be prevented by drinking fluids containing sodium chloride. **menstrual c.'s** DYSMENORRHEA. **muscle c.** A sudden, involuntary contraction of a group of muscle fibers, accompanied by severe local pain, with subsequent slow relaxation and cessation of pain. Cramp may be associated with fatigue, salt deficiency, or ischemia of muscle, but may also be troublesome nocturnally, especially in older subjects, without apparent cause. **nocturnal c.'s** Muscular cramps occurring in bed at night, often but not always during sleep. Also *recumbency cramps.* **occupational c.** Any of various disorders in which painful spasm develops in the muscles associated with the movements and activities required by a particular occupation, rendering the movements increasingly difficult to perform. The disorders are psychosomatic in origin and include writer's cramp, violin player's cramp, and many more. Also *occupational neurosis, professional cramp, professional neurosis, craft palsy, functional spasm, occupation spasm, craft neurosis.* **professional c.** OCCUPATIONAL CRAMP. **recumbency c.'s** NOCTURNAL CRAMPS. **seamstresses' c.** Occupational cramp in seamstresses, making it difficult to sew. Also *sewing spasm.* **stokers' c.'s** Heat cramps suffered by stokers, as those formerly tending steam boilers in ships, who must work in hot confined places. Also *miners' cramps.* **tailors' c.** Occupational cramp in tailors. Also *tailors' spasm.* **watchmakers' c.** Occupational cramp in watchmakers causing difficulty in repairing watches. **writers' c.** Painful cramp in the writing hand occurring during the course of writing. The condition, which is psychosomatic in origin, causes increasing spasm of the digits which hold the pen as the individual attempts to write, and the pen may be driven through the paper. No other movements or activities are affected. Also *graphospasm, scriveners' palsy, paralysis notariorum, writers' paralysis, lock spasm, writers' spasm.*

**Crampton** [Philip *Crampton,* Irish surgeon, 1777–1858] 1 See under LINE. 2 Crampton's muscle. See under BRÜCKE'S MUSCLE.

**crani-** \krā′nē-\ CRANIO-.

**craniad** \krā′nē·ad\ [CRANI- + -AD] 1 Toward the head or cephalic end of the body; cephalad. Compare CAUDAD. 2 Toward the cranium.

**cranial** \krā′nē·əl\ 1 Pertaining to the cranium. 2 In or toward the cranium or head. 3 Relatively near the head as compared with other structures of the same kind nearer the tail end; in human anatomy, commonly equivalent to *superior.* Compare CAUDAL.

**cranialis** \krā′nē·ā′lis\ Cranial.

**craniectomy** \krā′nē·ek′təmē\ [CRANI- + -ECTOMY] Excision of a part of the cranium. **linear c.** The excision of a strip of the cranium, as in the correction of a misshapen skull resulting from premature closure of cranial sutures.

**cranio-** \krā′nē·ō-\ [L *cranium* skull] A combining form denoting the cranium. Also *crani-*.

**craniocaudal** \-kô′dəl\ [CRANIO- + CAUDAL] Reaching from head to tail: used especially of a measurement of the length of an embryo or an animal.

**craniocele** \krā′nē·ōsēl′\ ENCEPHALOCELE.

**craniocerebral** \-ser′əbrəl\ Relating to the cranium and the cerebrum.

**craniocervical** \-sur′vikl\ Relating to the cranium and the neck.

**craniodidymus** \-did′iməs\ [CRANIO- + DI-[2] + -DYMUS] Conjoined twins having two heads but united throughout the trunk.

**craniofacial** \-fā′shəl\ Relating to the cranium and the face.

**craniofenestria** \-fənes′trē·ə\ [CRANIO- + L *fenestr(a)* a window + -IA] The incomplete ossification of the bones of the cranial vault such that the calvarium of a newborn infant or young child appears fenestrated. Areas of deficient ossification are within the confines of the usual bones, therefore they are distinct from the normal fontanelles and sutures. Also *craniolacunia, lacuna skull, lückenschädel.*

**craniolacunia** \-ləkoo′nē·ə\ [CRANIO- + L *lacun(a)* cavity + -IA] CRANIOFENESTRIA.

**craniomandibular** \-mandib′yələr\ Pertaining to the cranium and the mandible.

**craniomeningocele** \-mening′gōsēl\ [CRANIO- + MENINGOCELE] A protrusion through a defect in the scalp and skull of the cranial meninges.

**craniometric** \-met′rik\ Pertaining to craniometry.

**craniometry** \krā′nē·äm′ətrē\ [CRANIO- + -METRY] The study of the shape and dimensions of the skull, primarily the human skull, for anatomic or anthropological purposes. Measurements are taken between craniometric points, a set of standard defined points in terms of which all significant dimensions are thought to be derivable.

**craniopagus** \krā′nē·äp′əgəs\ [CRANIO- + -PAGUS] Conjoined twins united at the head. **c. frontalis** Conjoined twins united at the forehead. **c. occipitalis** Conjoined twins united at the occiput. Also *iniopagus, iniodymus, craniopagus posterior.* **c. parasiticus** Unequal, conjoined twins in which the smaller or incomplete twin is attached as a parasite to the occipital region of the more nearly normal twin. Also *epicomus, miodidymus.* **c. parietalis** A craniopagus in which conjoined twins are united at the parietal regions of their crania, one on its right side and the other on its left.

**craniopathy** \krā′nē·äp′əthē\ [CRANIO- + -PATHY] Any diffuse abnormality of the skull, especially one related to metabolic disease. *Seldom used.* **metabolic c.** METABOLIC ENCEPHALOPATHY.

**craniopharyngeal** \-fərin′jē·əl\ Pertaining to the cranium and the pharynx.

**craniopharyngioma** \-fərin′jē·ō′mə\ [CRANIO- + PHARYNGI- + -OMA] A tumor which appears to arise from vestigeal remnants of the craniopharyngeal pouch (Rathke's pouch). Among the histologic features are squamous epithelium lining cysts, ameloblastomatous tissue, and calcification. It typically occurs in the suprasellar or intrasellar regions, and projects into the third ventricle. It is locally destructive but does not metastasize. Children and young adults are primarily affected, but the tumor does present in older individuals. Also *Rathke's pouch tumor, Rathke's tumor, pituitary adamantinoma, pituitary ameloblastoma, craniopharyngeal duct tumor.*

**cranioplasty** \krā′nē·ōplas′tē\ [CRANIO- + -PLASTY] Repair of a congenital or acquired defect or deformity of the cranium.

**craniorachischisis** \-rəkis′kisis\ [CRANIO- + -RACHI + -SCHISIS] The failure of the neural tube to close in regions of both the brain and spinal cord. The condition is associated with secondary defects in the cranium and spinal column. **c. totalis** The failure of the neural tube to close throughout its length, occurring with associated defects in the usual overlying tissues. As a result the central nervous tissue is exposed throughout much or all of its length.

**craniosacral** \-sā′krəl\ **1** Pertaining to the cranium and the sacrum. **2** Pertaining to the parasympathetic autonomic system.

**cranioschisis** \krā′nē·äs′kisis\ [CRANIO- + -SCHISIS] The failure of the neural tube to close in the region of the brain. It is associated with secondary defects in the usual overlying skull and scalp so that varying degrees of the abnormal brain are exposed.

**craniospinal** \-spī′nəl\ Pertaining to the cranium and the spinal, or vertebral, column. Also *craniovertebral.*

**craniostenosis** \-stenō′sis\ The premature closure of the cranial sutures and fontanelles, resulting in a small, maldeveloped skull. Also *craniostosis.*

**craniosynostosis** \-sin′ästō′sis\ [CRANIO- + SYNOSTOSIS] Premature fusion of the cranial sutures, usually occurring before birth, and resulting in deformity of the skull. The fusion prevents the normal shape given to the cranium by the growth of the brain. Thus, fusion of the sagittal suture, the commonest form, prevents lateral growth and allows compensatory expansion forward and backward, giving a long, narrow shape of the head, sometimes with a ridge at the metopic suture line (scaphocephaly). Other forms seen are dolichocephaly, brachycephaly, acrocephaly, and oxycephaly. Asymmetrical forms also occur.

**craniotabes** \-tā′bēz\ A thinning or weakening of the skull bones of an infant of sufficient degree to allow indentation on pressure with the fingers or thumbs. It occurs in association with rickets, cleidocranial dysostosis, and prematurity.

**craniotome** \krā′nē·ōtōm′\ [CRANIO- + -TOME] An instrument for making an opening or a cut in the cranium.

**craniotomy** \krā′nē·ätəmē\ [CRANIO- + -TOMY] **1** An operation producing an opening in the cranium. **2** A puncturing of the fetal skull to allow drainage of its contents so that vaginal delivery can be accomplished.

**craniotopography** \-tōpäg′rəfē\ The study of the relations between the external landmarks of the skull and the meninges, brain structures, and vessels within.

**craniotympanic** \-timpan′ik\ Pertaining to the skull and the middle ear.

**craniovertebral** \-vur′təbrəl\ CRANIOSPINAL.

**cranium** \krā′nē·əm\ [Med L (from Gk *kranion* the upper part of the head, a helmet; akin to *kara* the head and to *korys* a helmet, the head), the skull] **1** [NA] The skull, excluding the mandible, comprising several bones immovably fixed at the sutures, serving as a protection for the brain and cerebral circulation as well as for special sense organs, and providing attachment for facial muscles of expression, masticatory muscles, and postural muscles, as of the neck and pharynx. Some anatomists equate the cranium with the whole skull, including the mandible, and divide it into cranium cerebrale and cranium viscerale, or facial bones. Also *skull.* **2** CRANIUM CEREBRALE. Compare CALVARIA. **c. bifidum** ENCEPHALOCELE. **c. bifidum occultum** A congenital defect in the cranium with no defect in the overlying scalp. It is said to occur independently of abnormality in the brain. **c. cerebrale** 1 That part of the skull that encloses the brain and is directly supported by the vertebral column. It is formed by the occipital, two parietal, two temporal, sphenoid, and ethmoid bones. Also *cranium, cerebral cranium.* 2 CALVARIA. See also OSSA CRANII. **c. viscerale** The facial skeleton that encloses the mouth and nose and helps to form, with the cerebral cranium, the orbit that encloses the eye. It includes the movable mandible and the hyoid bone that supports the tongue and is suspended from the base of the skull. Also *visceral cranium.* See also OSSA FACIEI.

**crast.** *crastinus* (L, for tomorrow).

**crater** [L, from Gk *kratēr* a mixing vessel, bowl, any hollow, crater] A localized, rimmed depression in the surface of a tissue.

**crateriform** Hollowed; shaped like a bowl.

**craterization** Saucerization of an osteomyelitic abscess within bone.

**craunology** CRENOLOGY.

**cravat** A triangular bandage folded from apex to base.

**Crawford** [Brian Hewson *Crawford,* English physiologist, flourished 20th century] Stiles-Crawford effect. See under EFFECT.

**crawling** FORMICATION.

**CRD** chronic respiratory disease.

**cream** 1 A substance, such as a pharmaceutical preparation, having the appearance and consistency of dairy cream, as *cream of magnesia.* 2 A thick, ointmentlike emulsion, usually applied to the skin for cosmetic, protective, or medicinal purposes. **aluminum hydroxide c.** An aqueous suspension containing colloidal aluminum hydroxide. It is used in the treatment of peptic ulcer. **antibiotic c.** Any one of various agents that are applied directly to a wound or burn to prevent bacterial infection. The agents, which are suspended in an ointment or cream base, include true antibiotics, chemicals, and metals. **barrier c.** Any of various preparations applied before work to exposed skin to prevent dermatitis and to facilitate skin cleansing after dirty work. These creams give only limited protection from substances which are harmful to the skin. **cold c.** A cream prepared, according to the USP formula, so that approximately 1000 g consists of spermaceti 125 g, white wax 120 g, mineral oil 560 g, sodium borate 5 g, and purified water 190 ml. It is applied topically as an emollient, and can be used alone or as a vehicle for medications. **leukocytic c.** BUFFY COAT. **c. of magnesia** A compound in which sufficient hydrated magnesium oxide is suspended in an aqueous solution to yield the equivalent of 7.9% magnesium hydroxide. Also *magnesium hydroxide mixture.* **c. of tartar** $C_4H_5KO_6$. A colorless or white, crystalline powder used most commonly as a cathartic. It also has diuretic properties, and was formerly used as a dusting powder in surgical gloves. Also *potassium bitartrate, potassium acid tartrate, cremor tartari.*

**crease** [earlier *creaste,* from Middle English *creste* crest, ridge of a roof] 1 In anatomy, a depressed line, or linear furrow, produced by a fold. 2 TANGENTIAL WOUND. **flexion c.** FLEXURE LINE. **gluteofemoral c.** SULCUS GLUTEALIS. **palmar c.** One of the flexure lines in the palm of the hand. **simian c.** SIMIAN LINE. **Sydney c.** SYDNEY LINE.

**creatine** \krē′ətin\ $H_2N—C(=NH)—NMe—CH_2—COOH$. *N*-Amidino-*N*-methylglycine. A compound present in vertebrate muscle. It is largely phosphorylated, the phosphocreatine providing the means of rephosphorylating ADP to form ATP. It is made by transfer of an amidino group from arginine to glycine, followed by methylation by *S*-adenosylmethionine.

**creatine kinase** The enzyme (EC 2.7.3.2) that catalyzes the reaction: ADP + phosphocreatine ⇌ ATP + creatine. By this reaction phosphocreatine acts as a reserve of high-energy phosphate and maintains the supply of ATP. Also *Lohmann's enzyme.*

**creatinemia** The presence of creatine in blood, plasma, or serum.

**creatine phosphate** *Incorrect* PHOSPHOCREATINE. • This substance is a phosphoramidate, not a phosphate.

**creatinine** The product of cyclization of creatine by lactam formation. Creatinine output is proportional to muscle amount and very constant. Urinary creatinine is measured to check completeness of urine collection, and its clearance to measure glomerular filtration rate.

**creatoxin** KREOTOXIN.

**Credé** [Karl Siegmund Franz *Credé,* German gynecologist and obstetrician, 1819–1892] 1 Credé's method. See under CREDÉ'S MANEUVER. 2 Credé method of expressing placenta. See under METHOD.

**creep** Further, slow lengthening of a muscle following the initial major lengthening in response to an imposed load.

**cremaster** [Gk *kremastēr* (from *kremannynai* to hang) a suspender, the muscle by which the testicles are suspended] MUSCULUS CREMASTER. Adj. cremasteric.

**cremor** [L, a decoction, gruel] Cream. **c. tartari** CREAM OF TARTAR.

**crena** \krē′nə\ [L, a cleft, notch] A cleft or notch. **c. ani** The cleft between the buttocks or nates, at the base of which the anus opens externally. Also *anal cleft, clunial cleft, gluteal cleft, natal cleft, crena clunium, intergluteal cleft, gluteal furrow.* **c. cordis** Both sulcus interventricularis anterior and sulcus interventricularis posterior.

**crenae** \krē′nē\ Plural of CRENA.

**crenate** \krē′nāt\ To form numerous tiny conical projections on the surface of (an erythrocyte), usually an effect of osmotic imbalance between the interior and exterior of the cell, as in a hypertonic solution.

**crenation** \krēnā′shən\ [L *crena* a cleft, notch + -ATION] Any of the tiny conical projections on the surface of a crenated erythrocyte. Also *crenulation.*

**crenocyte** \krē′nōsīt\ ECHINOCYTE.

**crenology** [Gk *krēn(ē)* a spring, well + *o* + -LOGY] The science of mineral waters and springs used for therapeutic purposes. Also *craunology.*

**crenulation** \kren′yəlā′shən\ CRENATION.

**creolin** A skin disinfectant solution containing a two percent solution of cresol or similar phenolic compound.

**creotoxin** \krē′ōtäk′sin\ KREOTOXIN.

**crepitant** \krep′itənt\ Producing an audible or palpable crackling.

**crepitation** \krep′itā′shən\ [Late L *crepitatio* (from L *crepitatus,* past part. of *crepitare* to crackle, rustle, rattle) a crackling, rattling] The grating or crackling noise which may be elicited by moving fractured bone ends or arthritic joints, or palpating soft tissues containing air. **articular c.** ARTICULAR CREPITUS.

**crepitus** \krep′itəs\ [L, a rattling, clashing, tinkling, rustling] 1 A crackling or grating sound produced in the body; crepitation. 2 The sound of flatus discharged from the intestine. **articular c.** The grating or grinding sound elicited when irregular joint surfaces move over each other. Also *articular crepitation, joint crepitus.* **bony c.** The gritty sound or sensation made by rubbing the ends of a fractured bone together. **joint c.** ARTICULAR CREPITUS. **c. uteri** The presence of gas within the substance of the uterus, usually secondary to infection caused by a gas-forming organism such as *Clostridium perfringens.*

**crescent** \kres′ənt\ [L *crescens,* gen. *crescentis,* pres. part. of *crescere* to grow, increase] **1** Resembling the shape of the visible part of the moon in its first quarter. **2** A form or structure having a crescent shape. **articular c.** MENISCUS ARTICULARIS. **blastoporal c.** A part of the dorsal lip of the embryo which invaginates during gastrulation, giving this region a crescentlike appearance. **cellular c.** A crescentic mass made up entirely of cells, as seen in the early stages of crescentic glomerulonephritis. **congenital c. of the choroid** FUCHS COLOBOMA. **epithelial c.** The proliferation and accumulation of cells in the inside of Bowman's capsule. They tend to displace the glomerular tuft, and thus acquire a semilunar shape. The presence of crescents within glomeruli is characteristic of crescentic glomerulonephritis, and indicates a severe form of glomerular damage. Although they are an important component of crescents, the epithelial cells of Bowman's capsule are not the only cells present. Recent evidence indicates a role for circulating mononuclear phagocytes in the origin and composition of the crescent. **fibrous c.** A crescent, composed almost entirely of connective tissue, indicating a late stage of crescentic glomerulonephritis. Fibrous crescents predominate when the patient's life has been prolonged by renal dyalysis. Also *fibrocellular crescent.* **c. of Giannuzzi** DEMILUNE OF GIANNUZZI. **malarial c.** The gametocyte stage of *Plasmodium falciparum.* Males or microgametocytes are round-ended, light-staining, with diffuse nuclear material. Females or macrogametocytes are sharp-ended and darker-staining, with a compact nucleus. Also *demilune.* **myopic c.** An area of exposed sclera adjacent to the optic disk in a nearsighted eye. **sublingual c.** The floor of the mouth below the tip of the tongue. The lingual frenum rises from the crescent at the midpoint.

**cresol** Any of the three isomeric hydroxytoluenes, i.e., *C*-methyl phenols. All are obtained from coal tar and are similar to phenol in properties.

**cresorcinol** $C_7H_8O_2$. 2,4-Dihydroxytoluene. A derivative of cresol with germicidal and antiseptic properties. It is used in aqueous solution to sterilize surgical equipment.

**cresoxydiol** MEPHENESIN.

**cresoxypropanediol** MEPHENESIN.

# crest

**crest** [L *crista.* See CRISTA.] **1** A linear prominence or ridge, usually hard or bony. **2** CRISTA. **3** A tuft or comb on the head of a bird or other animal. **acoustic c.** CRISTA AMPULLARIS. **acousticofacial c.** Part of the neural crest tissue associated with the seventh and eighth cranial nerves in the embryo. Initially it comprises a single mass on each side but it divides to form the geniculate ganglion of the seventh cranial nerve and the spiral and vestibular ganglia of the eighth cranial nerve. **alveolar c.** The margin of alveolar bone surrounding a tooth. **ampullar c.** CRISTA AMPULLARIS. **ampullary c.** CRISTA AMPULLARIS. **anterior c. of fibula** MARGO ANTERIOR FIBULAE. **anterior intertrochanteric c.** LINEA INTERTROCHANTERICA. **anterior lacrimal c.** CRISTA LACRIMALIS ANTERIOR. **anterior obturator c.** CRISTA OBTURATORIA. **anterior sphenoidal c.** CRISTA SPHENOIDALIS. **anterior c. of tibia** MARGO ANTERIOR TIBIAE. **arcuate c. of arytenoid cartilage** CRISTA ARCUATA CARTILAGINIS ARYTENOIDEAE. **articular sacral c.** CRISTA SACRALIS INTERMEDIA. **basal c.** CRISTA BASILARIS DUCTUS COCHLEARIS. **basilar c.** CRISTA BASILARIS DUCTUS COCHLEARIS. **basilar c. of occipital bone** TUBERCULUM PHARYNGEUM. **buccinator c.** CRISTA BUCCINATORIA. **cerebral c.'s of cranial bones** JUGA CEREBRALIA OSSIUM CRANII. **cervical c. of female urethra of Barkow** CRISTA URETHRALIS FEMININA. **c. of cochlear window** CRISTA FENESTRAE COCHLEAE. **conchal c. of maxilla** CRISTA CONCHALIS MAXILLAE. **conchal c. of palatine bone** CRISTA CONCHALIS OSSIS PALATINI. **deltoid c.** TUBEROSITAS DELTOIDEA HUMERI. **dental c.** In the embryo, a crest formed by the dental follicles within the substance of the jaw which encloses the developing teeth. **dermal c.'s** CRISTAE CUTIS. **ethmoidal c. of maxilla** CRISTA ETHMOIDALIS MAXILLAE. **ethmoidal c. of palatine bone** CRISTA ETHMOIDALIS OSSIS PALATINI. **external frontal c.** LINEA TEMPORALIS OSSIS FRONTALIS. **external occipital c.** CRISTA OCCIPITALIS EXTERNA. **external sacral c.** CRISTA SACRALIS LATERALIS. **falciform c.** CRISTA TRANSVERSA. **female urethral c.** CRISTA URETHRALIS FEMININA. **femoral c.** LINEA ASPERA FEMORIS. **fimbriated c.** PLICA FIMBRIATA. **frontal c.** CRISTA FRONTALIS. **ganglionic c.** A cellular band formed by a mass of specialized ectodermal cells and situated dorsolaterally to the neural tube. It develops in the lateral margin of the neural plate and, to a minor extent in the head region, from the placodes. It separates from the neural plate and comes to lie under it just before the neural tube closes. It gives rise to the ganglia associated with the cranial and spinal nerves and also to mesectoderm. Also *ganglion ridge.* **gingival c.** The extreme edge of the gingiva where the epithelium of the gingival sulcus meets the oral epithelium. **gluteal c.** TUBEROSITAS GLUTEA OSSIS FEMORIS. **c. of greater tubercle of humerus** CRISTA TUBERCULI MAJORIS. **c. of head of rib** CRISTA CAPITIS COSTAE. **iliac c.** CRISTA ILIACA. **iliopectineal c. of iliac bone** LINEA ARCUATA OSSIS ILII. **iliopectineal c. of pelvis** LINEA TERMINALIS PELVIS. **iliopectineal c. of pubis** EMINENTIA ILIOPUBICA. **c. of ilium** CRISTA ILIACA. **infratemporal c.** CRISTA INFRATEMPORALIS. **infundibuloventricular c.** CRISTA SUPRAVENTRICULARIS. **inguinal c.** The point on the ventral embryonic abdominal wall where the inguinal fold containing the gubernaculum testis passes through. Later the passage becomes elongated and oblique to form the inguinal canal. **c. of insertion** A rough linear ridge on the surface of a bone for the tendinous or aponeurotic insertion of a muscle. **intermediate sacral c.** CRISTA SACRALIS INTERMEDIA. **internal frontal c.** CRISTA FRONTALIS. **internal occipital c.** CRISTA OCCIPITALIS INTERNA. **intertrochanteric c.** CRISTA INTERTROCHANTERICA. **interureteric c.** PLICA INTERURETERICA. **c. of larger tubercle** CRISTA TUBERCULI MAJORIS. **lateral sacral c.** CRISTA SACRALIS LATERALIS. **c. of lesser tubercle** CRISTA TUBERCULI MINORIS. **malar c. of great wing of sphenoid bone** MARGO ZYGOMATICUS ALAE MAJORIS. **male urethral c.** CRISTA URETHRALIS MASCULINA. **marginal c.** CRISTA MARGINALIS. **c.'s of matrix of nail** CRISTAE MATRICIS UNGUIS. **medial c. of fibula** CRISTA MEDIALIS FIBULAE. **medial sacral c.** CRISTA SACRALIS MEDIANA. **mitochondrial c.'s** CRISTAE OF MITOCHONDRIA. **c.'s of nail bed** CRISTAE MATRICIS UNGUIS. **nasal c. of maxilla**

CRISTA NASALIS MAXILLAE. **nasal c. of palatine bone** CRISTA NASALIS OSSIS PALATINI. **nasopalatine c.** CRISTA PALATINA. **c. of neck of rib** CRISTA COLLI COSTAE. **neural c.** Each of two cellular longitudinal ectodermal bands (sometimes called lophoneuroepithelium) which become detached from the dorsolateral borders of the neural tube just prior to its closure (neurulation) and separation from the ectodermal roof. The bands are at first continuous but become segmented, paralleling the somitic metameres, and give rise to ganglion cells and fibers of the peripheral nervous system, and most of the peripheral cells of the autonomic nervous system. It probably also gives rise to the chromaffin cells, to part of the leptomeninges and connective tissue pigment cells (melanoblasts). Mesenchymal cells of the head and branchial arch cartilage cells are also probably derived from neural crest cells. **oblique c. of thyroid cartilage** LINEA OBLIQUA CARTILAGINIS THYROIDEAE. **obturator c.** CRISTA OBTURATORIA. **papillary c.'s** CRISTAE CUTIS. **pectineal c. of femur** LINEA PECTINEA FEMORIS. **pharyngeal c. of occipital bone** TUBERCULUM PHARYNGEUM. **posterior lacrimal c.** CRISTA LACRIMALIS POSTERIOR. **pubic c.** CRISTA PUBICA. **c. of pubis** CRISTA PUBICA. **c. of ridge** The highest linear elevation of a ridge. **sacral c.** CRISTA SACRALIS MEDIANA. **c. of scapular spine** The prominent posterior, subcutaneous border of the spine of the scapula to which muscles are attached and that is continuous laterally with the acromion, while medially it expands into a smooth triangular area at the medial margin of the scapula. **seminal c.** COLLICULUS SEMINALIS. **c. of smaller tubercle** CRISTA TUBERCULI MINORIS. **sphenoidal c.** CRISTA SPHENOIDALIS. **c. of spinous processes of sacrum** CRISTA SACRALIS MEDIANA. **spiral c.** LABIUM LIMBI VESTIBULARE LAMINAE SPIRALIS. **supinator c.** CRISTA MUSCULI SUPINATORIS. **c. of supinator muscle** CRISTA MUSCULI SUPINATORIS. **supramastoid c.** A thick ridge extending posteriorly from the root of the zygomatic process of the temporal bone, continuous with the temporal line above the external acoustic meatus, forming part of the posterior border of the temporal fossa, and providing attachment for the thick temporal fascia over the temporalis muscle. Also *crista supramastoidea.* **supraventricular c.** CRISTA SUPRAVENTRICULARIS. **temporal c. of frontal bone** LINEA TEMPORALIS OSSIS FRONTALIS. **terminal c. of right atrium** CRISTA TERMINALIS ATRII DEXTRI. **tibial c.** MARGO ANTERIOR TIBIAE. **transverse c.** 1 CRISTA TRANSVERSALIS. 2 CRISTA TRANSVERSA. **transverse c. of internal auditory meatus** CRISTA TRANSVERSA. **triangular c.** CRISTA TRIANGULARIS. **trigeminal c.** The part of the neural crest associated with the trigeminal nerve. It principally differentiates into the trigeminal or semilunar ganglion, though it has been suggested that the cranial part of the crest is incorporated into the midbrain to form the mesencephalic nucleus of the trigeminal. **c. of vestibule** CRISTA VESTIBULI. **zygomatic c. of great wing of sphenoid bone** MARGO ZYGOMATICUS ALAE MAJORIS.

**cresta** \kres′tə\ An organelle observed as a small, membranous, independently moving structure near the pelta of some trichomonads.

**crestomycin** PAROMOMYCIN.

**cresyl blue / brilliant c.** A basic dye of the oxazine group that is used to demonstrate the presence of reticulocytes in blood smears. It is also used as an indicator of oxidation-reduction status. Also *B. B. S. cresyl blue, 2 R. N. cresyl blue, C. brilliant blue.*

**cresyl violet** \kres′il\ A metachromatic synthetic dye that stains nuclei a violet color, plasma blue, and amyloid mucin and mast cell granules red.

**creta** \krē′tə\ [L, clay or chalk] Chalk. **c. praeparata** A ground and refined preparation of natural calcium carbonate. It has been used as an antacid and to treat diarrhea.

**cretinism** \krē′tinizm\ [French *crétinisme,* from Swiss French dialect *crétin* ("poor thing," lit., Christian) a cretin + *-isme* -ISM] Arrested physical and mental development resulting from failure of the fetal thyroid to secrete hormone *in utero;* congenital hypothyroidism. Many of the stigmata persist through infancy and childhood and into adult life unless thyroid hormone replacement therapy is immediately started. Patients exhibit dementia, stunted growth, typical lesions of the skull, bones, and soft tissues, sluggishness, and anemia. Laboratory indices reveal virtually total thyroid deficiency. Also *infantile hypothyroidism, myxedematous infantilism* (older term), *thyroid infantilism* (seldom used), *congenital myxedema.* **athyreotic c.** Cretinism owing to aplasia or dysplasia of the fetal thyroid. Also *sporadic nongoitrous cretinism, spontaneous cretinism, sporadic cretinism.* **endemic c.** Cretinism occurring with comparatively high frequency in a population or region, usually owing to defective diet (one lacking iodine or containing goitrogens). **nonendemic goitrous c.** Cretinism associated with goiter owing to any one of several inborn errors of thyroid hormone biosynthesis. The metabolic block prevents $T_4$ and $T_3$ synthesis. Pituitary hypersecretion of thyrotropin follows and the gland becomes hyperplastic (goitrous), but the block impedes elaboration of normal hormone with ensuing hypothyroidism. In the absence of inbreeding, transmission of the defect to offspring is unlikely. Also *sporadic goitrous cretinism.* **spontaneous c.** ATHYREOTIC CRETINISM. **sporadic c.** ATHYREOTIC CRETINISM. **sporadic goitrous c.** NONENDEMIC GOITROUS CRETINISM. **sporadic nongoitrous c.** ATHYREOTIC CRETINISM.

**Creutzfeldt** [Hans Gerhard *Creutzfeldt,* German psychiatrist, 1885–1964] Jakob-Creutzfeldt disease, Creutzfeldt-Jakob presenile encephalopathy, Creutzfeldt-Jakob syndrome. See under CREUTZFELDT-JAKOB DISEASE.

**crevice** \krev′is\ A small fissure; a crack in a surface. **gingival c.** GINGIVAL SULCUS.

**crevicular** \krevik′yələr\ Relating to a crevice, especially the gingival crevice (or sulcus).

**CRH** corticotropin-releasing hormone.

**crib** [Old English *cribb* a stall for oxen, akin to German *Krippe* crib, manger] 1 A removable orthodontic appliance. 2 A wire clasp used in removable appliances. **tongue c.** An appliance to discourage tongue thrust during swallowing.

**cribra** \krib′rə\ Plural of CRIBRUM.

**cribral** \krib′rəl\ 1 Pertaining to the cribrum. 2 Pertaining to any sievelike structure.

**cribrate** \krib′rāt\ CRIBRIFORM.

**cribriform** \krib′rifôrm\ Resembling a sieve; perforated by many small openings. Also *cribrate, cribrose.*

**cribrum** \krib′rəm\ [L (akin to *cernere* to sift) a sieve] (*pl.* cribra) LAMINA CRIBROSA OSSIS ETHMOIDALIS.

**Crick** [Francis Harry Compton *Crick,* English biochemist, born 1916] 1 Watson-Crick model. See under MODEL. 2 Watson-Crick helix. See under DOUBLE HELIX.

**cricoid** \krī′koid\ [Gk *krikoeidēs* (from *kriko(s)* a ring + *-eidēs* -OID) ring-shaped] 1 Resembling or shaped like a ring. 2 Denoting the cricoid cartilage.

**cricoidectomy** \krī′koidek′təmē\ Excision of the cricoid cartilage. Excision of the whole cartilage alone is never indicated but excision of the anterior arch may be required in operations for subglottic laryngeal stenosis.

**cricopharyngeus** \krī′kōfərin′jē·əs\ PARS CRICOPHARYNGEA MUSCULI CONSTRICTORIS PHARYNGIS INFERIORIS.

**cricothyroid** \krī′kōthī′roid\ Pertaining to the cricoid and thyroid cartilages.

**cricothyrotomy** \krī′kōthīrät′əmē\ [*cricothyro(id)* + -TOMY] An emergency operation for the relief of upper airway obstruction by way of a midline incision in the neck. The cricothyroid membrane is incised and the opening maintained with an oval-section laryngotomy tube. Modern practice is to regard it as a temporary expedient only pending the establishment of an elective tracheostomy. Also *laryngotomy, inferior laryngotomy, cricothyroidotomy* (seldom used), *intercricothyrotomy, thyrocricotomy.*

**cricotomy** \krīkät′əmē\ [*crico(id)* + -TOMY] Incision of the cricoid cartilage as a means of gaining access to the trachea for the emergency relief of upper airway obstruction. It has been abandoned as an intentional procedure as it results in severe subglottic stenosis.

**cricotracheotomy** \krī′kōtrā′kē·ät′əmē\ An outmoded procedure with the indications and objects of tracheotomy but in which the incision was carried upward through the cricoid cartilage as well as through the upper tracheal rings. It was found to carry the serious risk of subglottic stenosis and is therefore avoided as an intentional procedure. Also *laryngotracheotomy, tracheolaryngotomy.*

**Crigler** [John Fielding *Crigler*, Jr., U.S. physician, born 1919] Crigler-Najjar disease. See under SYNDROME.

**Crile** [George Washington *Crile*, U.S. surgeon, 1864–1943] See under CLAMP.

**criminalistics** \krim′inəlis′tiks\ FORENSIC SCIENCE.

**criminology** \krim′inäl′əjē\ The scientific study of criminal behavior, including its antecedents, determinants, modifiers, effects, responses to intervention, etc.

**crisis** \krī′sis\ [Gk *krisis* (from *krinein* to separate, judge, pronounce) a separating, deciding, crisis of a disease] **1** A point in the course of a disease marked by a sudden, sharp change, for better or worse; especially, such a turning point leading to a marked improvement and to a more favorable prognosis. **2** An abrupt intensification of a symptom, as a paroxysm. **addisonian c.** The syndrome that accompanies acute onset or aggravation of Addison's disease or other forms of adrenal insufficiency, resulting in lethargy, fever, vascular collapse, and often death. Also *acute adrenocortical insufficiency, adrenocortical crisis, adrenal crisis.* **adolescent c.** The physiologic and emotional changes that occur during adolescence and constitute a sudden demand on the ego for novel adaptational responses. **adrenal c.** ADDISONIAN CRISIS. **adrenocortical c.** ADDISONIAN CRISIS. **brainstem c.** A transient episode of brainstem dysfunction, as in vertebrobasilar insufficiency. **cataplectic c.** Abrupt, transient loss of postural tone of all or part of the musculature, usually arising in patients who also suffer from narcolepsy. Consciousness is not lost. Also *cataplectic attack.* **catathymic c.** A disorder of impulse control consisting of an isolated, sudden act of violence erupting from a background of intolerable tension. Also *isolated explosive disorder.* **celiac c.** A sudden worsening of the clinical state of an infant or child with celiac disease (gluten enteropathy) due to ingestion of wheat germ-containing food, even in minute amounts, in those in the process of recovery on a gluten-free diet. It is due to a further injury of the ileal mucosa by gluten and characterized by intestinal atony, gaseous distension, outpouring of fluid into the small bowel, dehydration, and collapse sometimes to the point of shock. X rays show distended loops of small intestine and fluid levels resembling paralytic ileus or intestinal obstruction. However, a laparotomy is contraindicated. **cholinergic c.** Increasing muscular weakness due to cholinergic paralysis of skeletal muscles. It usually is a result of overdosage with cholinergic drugs in myasthenia gravis. **decerebrate c.** TONIC CEREBELLAR ATTACK. **developmental c.** A sudden disturbance in psychosocial homeostasis related to demands for novel adaptational responses by the ego as a result of the physiologic and emotional changes of continuing development and maturation. One form of developmental crisis is adolescent crisis. **Dietl's c.** Sudden coliclike flank or abdominal pain associated with nausea and vomiting due to twisting or obstruction of a renal pedicle. **false c.** PSEUDOCRISIS. **febrile c.** The stage in a febrile disease when there is a sudden drop in temperature. **genital c. of newborn** The temporary presence of mammary hypertrophy, estrinization of the vaginal mucosa, and even scant menstrual discharge in a newborn female due to the transplacental acquisition of estrogen from the mother. **glaucomatocyclitic c.** An acute attack of moderately severe glaucoma in an eye suffering from uveitis so mild as to be almost inapparent. **hemolytic c.** A profound anemia resulting from sudden, massive erythrocyte destruction with inadequate erythropoietic response. It is an occasional occurrence in inherited abnormalities of the erythrocyte membrane, metabolism, or hemoglobin structure. **hypertensive c.** A sudden increase of blood pressure to a very high level associated with vomiting, severe headache, transient blindness, and rapid deterioration of renal function. Prompt hospitalization and control of hypertension are essential. **identity c.** A severe form of alienation characterized by loss of a sense of historical continuity and inability to accept the role the subject believes is expected of him or her. One type of identity crisis is reactive confusion. **laryngeal c.** An attack of laryngeal spasm in a case of tabes dorsalis. It is usually preceded by paraesthesia and cough and sometimes terminates in loss of consciousness. **myasthenic c.** Severe muscular weakness, often with respiratory paralysis, occurring as a result of myasthenia gravis. **nitritoid c.** A fainting episode following the intravenous injection of arsphenamine, with flushing of the face, difficult breathing, cough, and pain over the precordial region. The pulse is rapid and weak. The condition resembles that produced by poisoning with amyl nitrite. Also *nitritoid syndrome.* **oculogyric c.** An attack of involuntary upward conjugate deviation of the eyes, sometimes with retrocollis, lasting for minutes or, rarely, for hours, occurring in postencephalitic parkinsonism. Also *parkinsonian crisis.* **physiologic c.** Any sudden change that arises endogenously in the course of apparently normal development. It is observed frequently in childhood schizophrenia as a manifestation of embryonic neuronal plasticity and maturational lag. **posterior c.** TONIC CEREBELLAR ATTACK. **reflex anoxic c.** BLUE BREATH-HOLDING. **reflex hypoxic c.** BREATH-HOLDING. **salt-losing c.** A syndrome resembling those features of addisonian crisis that are due to mineralocorticoid (aldosterone) deficiency, a condition occurring in the course of the sodium-losing (salt-losing) form of congenital adrenocortical hyperplasia. Also *salt-depletion crisis.* **situational c.** A situation in which novel adaptational responses are occasioned by exposure to unfamiliar or unexpected conditions. Normal development and maturation are characterized by successful coping with potentially traumatic situations, such as separation, loss of love, physical punishment, or even annihilation. When such situations cannot be handled adequately they may serve as precipitants for the development of abnormal behavior patterns or other psychopathology. **tabetic c.** Any paroxysmal episode of pain, often associated with other evidence of dysfunction of the organ in which the pain appears to arise, occurring in a patient with tabes dorsalis. **thyrotoxic c.** A sudden and life-threatening exacerbation of the symptoms and signs of hyperthyroidism, particularly those associated with Graves' disease. It is usually marked by extraordinarily high fever, prostration, and coma. It is often precipitated by streptococcal pharyngitis or thyroid surgery. Also *thyroid crisis, thyroid storm, thyrotoxic storm.* **utricular crises** Drop attacks considered due to utricular otoliths.

**crispatura** \kris′pət^yoo′rə\ [L (from *crispare* to curl, pucker) a curling, puckering, wrinkling] Puckering or wrinkling, as of the skin.

**crista** \kris′tə\ [L (akin to *crinis* the hair of the head, a curl) a tuft or comb on the head of a bird, crest or plume on a helmet] (*pl.* cristae) An elevation, a ridge, or other linear structure projecting from a surface; a prominent border to a structure, more commonly with reference to a bone. Also *crest, ridge.* **c. ampullaris** [NA] The most prominent edge, or apex, of a triangular thickening of the membranous wall of each ampulla of the semicircular ducts of the internal ear, projecting into the lumen and containing the nerve endings of the ampullary branch of the vestibular division of the acoustic nerve. The epithelium comprises hair cells and supporting cells. Also *ampullary crest, acoustic crest, transverse septum of ampulla, ampullar crest, raphe of the ampulla.* **c. arcuata cartilaginis arytenoideae** [NA] A horizontal ridge on the anterolateral surface of the arytenoid cartilage, located between the triangular pit above, containing some mucous glands and the attachment of the vestibular ligament, and the oblong pit below for the vocalis muscle. Also *arcuate crest of arytenoid cartilage.* **c. basilaris ductus cochlearis** [NA] The inwardly projecting apex of the spiral ligament of the cochlea to which the outer edge of the basilar membrane is attached. Also *basal crest, basilar crest.* **c. buccinatoria** A faint linear ridge, extending from the base of the anterior border of the coronoid process of the mandible to the first molar tooth along the lateral aspect of the alveolar part, to which the buccinator muscle is attached. Also *buccinator crest.* **c. capitis costae** [NA] A transverse ridge that divides the articular surface of the head of a rib into two facets for articulation with the bodies of the two adjacent vertebrae, the ridge being attached to the intervening intervertebral disk. Also *crest of head of rib, interarticular ridge of head of rib.*

**cristae** \kris′tē\ Plural of CRISTA.

**cristal** \kris′təl\ Pertaining to a crest or ridge.

**cristate** \kris′tāt\ Ridged, with reference to bone or bony structures; having a crest or a crestlike structure, as on the head of some birds.

**cristobalite** \kristō′bəlīt\ [after Cerro San *Cristóbal,* Pachuca, Mexico + -ITE. Pachuca is extremely rich in mineral ores, esp. silver, mined since Aztec times] A form of silica used in refractory dental investments to increase thermal expansion.

**criterion** \krītir′ē·än\ [Gk *kritērion* (from *kritēs* a judge, arbiter, from *krinein* to separate, decide) a means for judging or trying, a standard, test] (*pl.* criteria) A standard against which different values can be compared. **Cooke's c.** The principle generally adopted for determining the number of nuclear lobes in a segmented neutrophil: each lobe must be separated from the rest of the nucleus by a fine strand of chromatin; otherwise it is not counted as a separate lobe. A nucleus is not considered segmented unless lobes are separated by one or more fine chromatin strands. **Jones criteria** A list of major and minor findings compiled for the purpose of diagnosing acute rheumatic fever. **Spiegelberg's criteria for ovarian pregnancy** Criteria for differentiating an ovarian pregnancy from other ectopic pregnancies. The criteria include the following: that the fallopian tube on the affected side be intact; that the fetal sac occupy the position of the ovary; that the ovary be connected to the uterus by the ovarian ligament; and that definite ovarian tissue be found in the wall of the pregnancy.

**crithidia** \krithid′ē·ə\ [New L, from Gk *krithidion,* dim. of *krithē* barley, barleycorn] *Outmoded* EPIMASTIGOTE.

**critical** [Gk *kritikos* (from *kritēs* a decider, judge) examining, judging + -AL ] **1** Of the nature of a crisis; of decisive importance in the course of a disease. **2** Being at a point or stage in a process indicating the imminence of a decisive change in condition.

**criticality** \krit′ikal′itē\ In a system containing fissionable material, the condition when the number of neutrons produced by fission is just equal to those lost by leakage or capture, and thus the system is capable of sustaining a chain reaction.

**CRM** cross-reacting material.

**Crohn** [Burrill Bernard *Crohn,* U.S. physician, born 1884] See under DISEASE.

**Cro-Magnon** \krō′-mag′nən\ Pertaining to a population of upper Pleistocene *Homo sapiens* typified by a specimen recovered in 1868 from Cro-Magnon near Les Eyzies, Dordogne, France.

**cromolyn sodium** $C_{23}H_{14}Na_2O_{11}$. 5,5′-[2-Hydroxy-1,3-propanediyl)bis(oxy)]bis-[4-oxo-4H-1-benzopyran-2-carboxylic acid] disodium salt. It is used in the treatment of allergic rhinitis and asthma, and is believed to act by interfering with the release of histamine.

**Crookes** [William *Crookes,* English chemist and physicist, 1832–1919] See under TUBE.

**CROS** contralateral routing of signals.

**Crosby** [William Holmes *Crosby,* Jr., U.S. physician, born 1914] See under CAPSULE.

**cross** **1** To mate two members of a breeding population, usually with the intent of producing offspring with particular genetic traits found in one or both of the parents. **2** The product of a mating between two organisms, most often a union arranged for specific genetic purposes. **3** Any object or structure characterized by the intersection of two oblong parts. **occipital c.** EMINENTIA CRUCIFORMIS.

**cross-absorption** \-absôrp′shən\ Addition of a strain of bacteria to antiserum in order to remove antibodies shared with another organism, leaving antibodies specific for the latter.

**crossbite** A tooth or group of teeth in abnormal lateral relation with the antagonistic teeth, while other adjacent teeth are in normal relation. Also *cross bite, X-bite.*

**crossbreed** **1** HYBRID. **2** To mate two individuals of different strains or species; hybridize.

**crossbreeding** HYBRIDIZATION.

**cross-bridges** In light microscopy, the appearance of zones of firm attachment between adjacent epidermal cells. It is due primarily to artifactual shrinkage. The attachments correspond to the desmosomes that are seen by electron microscopy. Also *intercellular bridges, cell bridges, prickles.*

**cross-dressing** TRANSVESTISM.

**cross-eye** ESOTROPIA.

**cross-feeding** Stimulation of the growth of one microorganism by a product excreted by another growing in the same medium. This phenomenon is often observed between parallel streaks of mutants blocked in different steps of the same pathway. Also *syntrophism.*

**cross-fire** A technique of radiotherapy in which multiple external radiation beams are aimed at the tumor or volume of tissue being treated, resulting in the highest concentration of radiation dose to the desired volume, with smaller doses of radiation given to multiple, other areas of the body. Also *cross-fire treatment.*

**crossfoot** TALIPES VARUS.

**crossing over** The process by which homologous chromosomes pair at homologous loci during meiosis or mitosis and interchange segments of DNA. The result in functional terms is the exchange of genetic information between chromosomes and the mixing of alleles derived from the two parents. It usually occurs reciprocally and during meiosis through the formation of chiasmata. Also *recombination, cross-over.* **unequal c.** The exchange of segments between homologous chromsomes at nonreciprocal locations due to improper pairing. It results in duplication of a portion of chromosome in one homologue and deletion of the same portion from the other homologue.

**cross-linking** The joining of chains of a polymer. Cross-linking often renders polymers insoluble. Thus ion-exchange resins based on sulfonated polystyrene usually contain units of divinylbenzene as cross-linking agents, since each such unit will be a member of two different chains. Likewise fibrin clots are stabilized by the enzymatic reaction of lysine residues in some chains with glutamine residues in others, with release of ammonia to introduce amide links between the chains.

**cross-matching** Testing for serologic compatibility between donor blood and blood of the prospective transfusion recipient. The major cross-match tests the recipient's serum against the donor's cells. The minor cross-match tests the donor's serum against the recipient's cells. Positive tests, which indicate incompatibility, are indicated by erythrocyte agglutination that is observed macroscopically or microscopically.

**cross-over** **1** CROSSING OVER. **2** A recombinant homologue. **3** Describing an experiment or study in which each of two matched groups alternately serves as control and experimental group. For example, one group may at first be subjected to a particular treatment that is withheld from the second group. Later, the treatment is withheld from the first group but given to the second. The cross-over study design may be regarded as a form of matching in which each subject serves as his or her own control.

**cross-reaction** **1** The interaction of an antigen with an antibody formed against a different antigen with which the first antigen shares closely related or common antigenic determinants. **2** An adverse reaction to a drug or chemical by a person previously sensitized to another related substance. Adj. cross-reactive.

**cross-section** **1** A two-dimensional representation of an anatomic or other structure, the plane usually being perpendicular to the long axis. **2** A representative sampling, as of a population. Symbol: $\sigma$ **capture c.** A measure of the probability that a particle striking an atomic nucleus will be captured. **nuclear c.** A measure of the probability that some nuclear reaction of interest will occur if the nucleus is struck by a particle or a photon. **total atomic attenuation c.** ATOMIC ATTENUATION COEFFICIENT.

**cross-sensitivity** \-sen′sitiv′itē\ Immunologic cross-reactivity detected in assays of hypersensitivity.

**cross-striations** \-strī·ā′shəns\ **1** Transverse lines or bands seen in striated muscle fibers. **2** Transverse lines in enamel prisms, visible in light microscopy, which may mark daily increments of growth.

**crosstalk** Signals coupling from one nerve to another such that impulses of one nerve fiber are conducted across the membranes of one nerve fiber to another as the result of ephaptic conduction.

**Crosti** [Agostino *Crosti,* Italian dermatologist, born 1896] Gianotti-Crosti syndrome. See under INFANTILE PAPULAR ACRODERMATITIS.

**crotalin** A protein occurring in rattlesnake venom. It was formerly used therapeutically in the treatment of certain forms of epilepsy.

**Crotalinae** \krō′talī′nē\ [New L, from the genus name *Crotalus.* See *CROTALUS.*] A subfamily of New World venomous snakes of the family Viperidae; the pit vipers. They are characterized by anterior fangs and special heat receptors bilaterally situated between the eye and the nostril. These receptors enable them to locate warm-blooded prey. Adj. crotaline.

**crotalotoxin** \krō′talətäk′sin\ A poisonous substance occurring in rattlesnake venom.

***Crotalus*** \krät′ələs\ [New L, from Gk *krotalon* a rattle, castanet] A New World genus of venomous snakes of the family Viperiadae, subfamily Crotalinae; the rattlesnakes. They are characterized by rattles formed from modified scales that adhere to the end of the tail. They are found in temperate to tropical regions.

**crotamiton** $C_{13}H_{17}NO$. *N*-ethyl-*N*-(2-methylphenyl)-2-butenamide. It is used chiefly as a scabicide and applied topically to the skin.

**crotch** \kräch\ [Middle English *croche, crucche* a crutch, from Old English *crycce* a staff] The angle or fork formed where the medial sides of the thighs join the trunk. *Popular.*

**crotonic acid** $CH_3—CH═CH—COOH$. (*E*)-But-2-enoic acid. Its thioesters are intermediates in the degradation and biosynthesis of fatty acids.

**crotonism** \krō′tōnizm\ Poisoning from ingestion of croton oil. Symptoms are severe gastrointestinal irritation, diarrhea, epigastric pain, prostration and collapse. Death has been reported from ingestion of as little as 20 drops.

**croton oil** A semidrying poisonous oil expressed from the seed of the small tree *Croton tiglium.* It was formerly used as a purgative, and is a powerful local irritant.

**croup** \kroop\ [Scots (prob. from Old English *krōpan* to cry aloud), to cry, speak, or cough hoarsely] A symptom complex occurring in children with various respiratory illnesses, having larynigitis in common, and comprising a characteristic brassy cough together with one or more of the following: inspiratory stridor, hoarseness, and signs of laryngeal respiratory obstruction. • Until the middle of the nineteenth century the term was used to signify a clinical entity, later recognized as consisting chiefly of cases of laryngeal diphtheria. **diphtheritic c.** LARYNGEAL DIPHTHERIA. **false c.** **1** LARYNGISMUS STRIDULUS. **2** LARYNGITIS STRIDULOSA. **pseudomembranous c.** *Obs.* LARYNGEAL DIPHTHERIA. **spasmodic c.** LARYNGITIS STRIDULOSA.

**croupous** \kroo′pəs\ Characterized by or relating to croup (in its older sense, now identified mainly as laryngeal diphtheria). *Obs.*

**croupy** \kroo′pē\ Resembling croup, usually referring to the cough characteristic of croup.

**Crouzon** [Octave *Crouzon,* French neurologist, 1874–1938] **1** Crouzon's disease, Crouzon syndrome. See under CRANIOFACIAL DYSOSTOSIS. **2** Apert-Crouzon syndrome. See under ACROCEPHALOSYNDACTYLY TYPE II.

**crown** [French *couronne* (from L *corona* a garland, wreath, crown) garland of flowers or leaves placed upon the head, mark of royalty or nobility] CORONA. **anatomic c.**

CORONA DENTIS. **artificial c.** A restoration involving the whole or a major part of the natural crown of a tooth. **Bischoff's c.** CORONA RADIATA. **cap c.** SHELL CROWN. **ciliary c.** CORONA CILIARIS. **clinical c.** CORONA CLINICA. **dowel c.** A complete crown replacing the whole of the natural crown and supported by a dowel fitted into the root canal of a nonvital tooth. Also *post crown.* **faced c.** VENEERED METAL CROWN. **c. of the head** CORONA CAPITIS. **physiologic c.** CORONA CLINICA. **post c.** DOWEL CROWN. **radiating c.** CORONA RADIATA. **shell c.** A complete crown of metal which does not fit the prepared tooth except at the neck. The intervening space is filled with cement when the crown is cemented in place. Also *cap crown.* **steel c.** A ready-made stainless steel crown used to restore deciduous molars or fractured permanent incisors in children. **c. of tooth** CORONA DENTIS. **veneered metal c.** A metal crown having all or part of its surface covered with porcelain or acrylic resin. Also *veneered crown, faced crown.*

**crown-heel** Relating to or describing a measurement of the height of an embryo or fetus taken from the vertex of the skull to its heel. At term, a human fetus attains an average crown-heel measurement of 47 cm or about 18.5 inches. Due to variations in length of fetal legs, this measurement is more variable and less accurate as an estimate of fetal age than the crown-rump measurement. Abbr. C.H.

**crowning** 1 The phase just prior to termination of the second stage of labor when the fetal scalp is fully visible in association with marked distension of the maternal perineum. 2 The fitting of an artificial crown on a tooth.

**CRP** C-reactive protein.

**CRT** cathode ray tube.

**cruces** \kroo′sēz\ Plural of CRUX.

**crucial** \kroo′shəl\ [L *crux* (gen. *crucis*) cross + -AL] Crossed; cross-shaped, as an incision.

**cruciate** \kroo′shē·āt\ [L *cruciat(us)*, past part. of *cruciare* (from *crux*, gen. *crucis*, a cross) to torture] Shaped like or resembling a cross.

**crucible** [Med L *crucibulum* (prob. from L *crux*, gen. *crucis*, a cross, from having four wicks in the form of a cross, + *-bulum* as in *turibulum* a censer) a crucible, small lamp, vessel for melting metals] A special vessel composed of heat-resistant material, used to hold a metal or other material that requires intense heat to be melted.

**cruciform** \kroo′sifôrm\ Shaped like a cross; cruciate.

**crude** Being in a raw, unpurified form; unrefined: used of drugs or chemicals.

**crufomate** $C_{12}H_{19}ClNO_3P$. Methylphosphoramidic acid 2-chloro-4-(1,1,-dimethylethyl)-phenyl methyl ester. It is employed in veterinary medicine as an antihelmintic agent.

**crunch** / **mediastinal c.** A grating or crunching sound heard on auscultation of the chest denoting the presence of air in the mediastinum. **xiphisternal c.** A grating or crunching sound that is audible or can be auscultated over the junction between the xiphoid process and the sternum.

**cruor** \kroo′ôr\ [L, coagulated blood] Clotted blood.

**crura** \kroo′rə\ Plural of CRUS.

**crural** \kroo′rəl\ Pertaining or belonging to the leg or to any crus.

**crureus** \kroorē′əs\ MUSCULUS VASTUS INTERMEDIUS.

**cruritis** \kroorī′tis\ [CRUS + -ITIS] PHLEGMASIA ALBA DOLENS.

**crurogenital** \kroo′rōjen′ətəl\ Pertaining to the thighs and the external genital organs.

**cruroscrotal** \kroo′rōskrō′təl\ Pertaining to the thighs and the scrotum.

**crurotomy** \krooråt′əmē\ [L *crus*, gen. *cruris*, the leg from knee to ankle + *o* + -TOMY] In otology, the surgical division of the crura of the stapes, as in stapedectomy. Also *crusotomy.*

**crus** \krus, kroos\ [L (gen. *cruris*) the leg from the knee to the ankle] (*pl.* crura) 1 [NA] The leg; specifically, the region between the knee and the ankle joints; the shank. 2 [NA] Any leglike part or organ. **c. I** LOBULUS SEMILUNARIS SUPERIOR. **c. II** LOBULUS SEMILUNARIS INFERIOR. **anterior c. of internal capsule** CRUS ANTERIUS CAPSULAE INTERNAE. **c. anterius capsulae internae** [NA] That portion of the internal capsule lying anterior to its genu. Nerve fascicles there, passing downward and backward, separate the head of the nucleus caudatus from the lentiform nucleus. Also *anterior limb of internal capsule, anterior crus of internal capsule, pars frontalis capsulae internae.* **c. anterius stapedis** [NA] The shorter and less curved of the two limbs that diverge from the neck of the stapes and are then connected distally by a flattened oval plate, or base, which is held to the margin of the fenestra vestibuli by the annular ligament. The limbs and plate thus constitute a "stirrup," or stapes. Also *anterior limb of stapes.* **crura anthelicis** [NA] The two ridged subdivisions of the anthelix that surround the fossa triangularis in the upper part of the auricle of the external ear. Also *limbs of anthelix.* **c. breve incudis** [NA] The short, peg-shaped process of the incus that projects posteriorly, to be attached by the posterior incudal ligament to the fossa incudis in the epitympanic recess. Also *short limb of incus.* **c. cerebelli ad pontem** *Obs.* PEDUNCULUS CEREBELLARIS MEDIUS. **c. cerebri** 1 [NA] A large bundle of fibers at the midbrain level passing caudally from cerebral cortical areas to destinations in the brainstem tegmentum, the basilar pons, and gray areas of the spinal cord (i.e., the corticotegmental, corticopontine, corticomedullary, and corticospinal tracts). The crus ends as these longitudinal tracts enter the basis pontis. Also *basis pedunculi cerebri.* 2 The pedunculus cerebri, including the fiber bundle, the tegmentum, and the substantia nigra separating them. Also *pes cerebri.* **c. clitoridis** [NA] The posterior extension of each corpus cavernosum clitoridis for attachment to the pubic and ischial rami on each side of the pubic arch. Also *crus of clitoris, root of clitoris.* **c. dextrum diaphragmatis** [NA] A broad, musculotendinous origin of the respiratory diaphragm, arising from the right anterolateral surfaces of the bodies and intervertebral disks of the upper three lumbar vertebrae and extending upwards so that its medial margin joins that of the left crus to form the median arcuate ligament, while the remaining fibers split around the esophageal opening and end in the central tendon of the diaphragm. See also CRURA DIAPHRAGMATIS, DIAPHRAGMA. **c. dextrum fasciculi atrioventricularis** [NA] The rounded right limb of the atrioventricular bundle which arises from its trunk at the upper border of the muscular part of the interventricular septum. It runs superficially in the right side of the septum, initially in the muscle and then subendocardially, towards the apex of the heart, where it enters the septomarginal trabecula. Then it passes into the anterior papillary muscle where it divides into a network of Purkinje fibers that ramify deep to the endocardium to all parts of the right ventricle. **crura of diaphragm** CRURA DIAPHRAGMATIS. **crura diaphragmatis** Crus dextrum diaphragmatis, crus sinistrum diaphragmatis and pars lumbalis diaphragmatis. **c. fasciculi atrioventricularis dextrum et sinistrum** The right and left limbs of the atrioventricular bundle that pass down superficially in the ventricular septum, one on each side. The right limb passes through the septomarginal trabecula to the anterior papillary muscle, where it breaks into a plexus of Purkinje fibers, while the left limb terminates similarly after dividing into two or more strands near the ventricular apex, where they subdivide and enter the papillary muscles. **c. fornicis** [NA] A band of white fibers that, leaving the body of the fornix, passes backward behind the posterior thalamus, curves forward to the hippocampus, and then spreads out to form the alveus and terminate as the fimbria. Also *crus of fornix, pars tecta columnae fornicis, posterior pillar of fornix.* **c. helicis** [NA] The anterior continuation of the helix that forms a prominent oblique ridge, dividing the deepest concavity, or concha, of the auricle of the external ear into an upper hollow, the cymba conchae, and a lower larger area, the cavum conchae. Also *crista helicis.* **c. laterale annuli inguinalis superficialis** [NA] The lateral, or inferior, margin of the superficial inguinal ring, stronger than the medial and composed of fibers of the inguinal ligament attached to the pubic tubercle. In the male, the fibers become grooved by the spermatic cord resting on it. **c. laterale cartilaginis alaris majoris** [NA] The oval outer limb of the greater alar cartilage that curves dorsally in the anterior part of the nasal ala on each side, articulating with the lateral nasal cartilage superiorly and connected to the nasal margin of the maxilla by dense fibrous and fatty tissue, maintaining the contour of each ala. It joins the medial crus at the tip of the nose at an angle of 30°. **c. longum incudis** [NA] The slender long process of the incus extending vertically downward, behind, and parallel to the handle of the malleus to end in a bent, rounded projection, the lentiform process, that articulates with the head of the stapes. Also *long limb of incus.* **c. mediale annuli inguinalis superficialis** [NA] A narrow band of the aponeurosis of the obliquus abdominis externus that forms the medial, or superior, margin of the superficial inguinal ring and is attached to the pubic crest and the front of the symphysis pubis, interweaving with the opposite crus. **c. mediale cartilaginis alaris majoris** [NA] The narrow medial plate of the greater alar cartilage that is acutely bent backwards on the lateral crus at the tip of the nose, where it is loosely attached by fibrous tissue to the medial crus of the opposite side and to the lower part of the septal cartilage, thereby aiding in the formation of the septum mobile nasi. **crura membranacea** [NA] Collectively, the ends, or limbs, of each semicircular duct that attach each duct to the utricle. Also *membranous crura.* **crura membranacea ampullaria ductus semicircularis** [NA] Localized spherical dilatations of one end of each of the three semicircular ducts, each lying within the ampulla of each corresponding bony canal. In each duct, the ampullary wall is thickened locally, projecting into the cavity as the crista ampullaris. **c. membranaceum commune ductus semicircularis** [NA] The common stem of the junction of the medial end of the superior semicircular duct and the upper end of the posterior duct opening into the utricle of the internal ear. **c. membranaceum simplex ductus semicircularis** [NA] The nonampullary end of the lateral semicircular duct entering the utricle. **membranous crura** CRURA MEMBRANACEA. **crura ossea** [NA] Collectively, the parts of the three bony semicircular canals of the internal ear that lodge correspondingly named ends of the membranous semicircular ducts, namely, crura ossea ampullaria, crus osseum commune, and crus osseum simplex. **crura ossea ampullaria** [NA] The dilated ends of the bony semicircular canals containing the crura membranacea ampullaria ductus semicircularis. **c. osseum commune** [NA] The part of the bony semicircular canals adjacent to the vestibule and containing the crus membranaceum commune ductus semicircularis. **c. osseum simplex** [NA] The extremity of the bony lateral semicircular canal containing the crus membranaceum simplex ductus semicircularis. **c. penis** [NA] The elongated posterior extension of each corpus cavernosum penis attached on each side to the pubic arch anterior to the ischial tuberosity, where it is covered by the ischiocavernosus muscle. **posterior c. of internal capsule** CRUS POSTERIUS CAPSULAE INTERNAE. **c. posterius capsulae internae** [NA] That portion of the internal capsule, posterior to the genu, that fans out and separates the thalamus medially from successively superior, posterior, and inferior aspects of the lentiform nucleus laterally. The crus connects cortical areas posterior to the central fissure to lower levels of the brain. Also *posterior crus of internal capsule, pars occipitalis capsulae internae.* **c. posterius stapedis** [NA] The posterior, longer, and more curved of the two limbs that diverge from the neck of the stapes and are connected distally by a flattened oval plate, or base, which is held to the fenestra vestibuli by ligaments. Also *posterior limb of stapes.* **c. sinistrum diaphragmatis** [NA] A musculotendinous origin of the respiratory diaphragm arising from the left anterolateral surfaces of the bodies and intervertebral disk of the upper two lumbar vertebrae and extending upwards so that its medial margin joins that of the right crus to form the median arcuate ligament, while the remaining fibers ascend to the central tendon of the diaphragm. See also CRURA DIAPHRAGMATIS, DIAPHRAGMA. **c. sinistrum fasciculi atrioventricularis** [NA] The flattened left limb of the atrioventricular bundle which arises from its trunk at the upper border of the muscular part of the interventricular septum. It runs superficially beneath the endocardium on the left side of the septum where it divides into two or more branches. These continue towards the apex of the heart where they subdivide further and enter the trabeculae carneae to reach the papillary muscles. In the papillary muscles they form networks of Purkinje fibers that ramify deep to the endocardium to all parts of the left ventricle. **stapedial crura** Crus anterius stapedis and crus posterius stapedis. **superior c. of cerebellum** PEDUNCULUS CEREBELLARIS SUPERIOR.

**crush** [Middle English *crushen,* from Old French *croissir* to break, gnash, from Germanic *krostjan* to gnash] To press between two opposing objects with sufficient force to cause injury. See also CRUSH INJURY.

**crusotomy** \kroosät′əmē\ CRUROTOMY.

**crust** [L *crusta.* See CRUSTA.] **1** A hard outer covering or coating. **2** Hardened, dried exudate or secretions. Also *crusta, incrustation.* **buffy c.** BUFFY COAT. **milk c.** CRADLE CAP.

**crusta** \krus′tə\ [L (akin to Gk *krystallos* clear ice, and *kryos* an icy cold), crust, rind, scab, shell] CRUST. **c. inflammatoria** BUFFY COAT. **c. petrosa dentis** CEMENTUM. **c. phlogistica** BUFFY COAT. **c. radicis** CEMENTUM.

**Crustacea** \krustā′shē·ə\ [New L, neut. pl. of *crustaceus* (from L *crusta* crust, rind, scab, shell + *-aceus* -ACEOUS) having a shell or crust] A class of the phylum Arthropoda characterized by two pairs of antennae, a body usually with two divisions (cephalothorax and abdomen), and biramous appendages. Most are aquatic and gill-breathing, including shrimps, lobsters, crabs, and a large assemblage of related forms.

**crustacean** \krustā′shē·ən\ **1** Pertaining to the class Crustacea. **2** A member of the class Crustacea, as a crab or lobster.

**crustae** \krus′tē\ Plural of CRUSTA.

**crutch** [Middle English *crucche,* from Old English *crycce* a staff] A walking aid, commonly but not necessarily used in a pair, whereby the weight of the body is borne primarily or entirely by the arms and shoulder girdle. It generally consists of a long upright, or a pair of uprights that converge at the distal end, with a crosspiece or cuff at the proximal end to fit the axilla or the arm, and a hand grip. **axillary c.** A crutch with a padded concave crosspiece at the proximal end which fits into the axilla; the most common type of crutch. **Canadian c.** A crutch which has at its proximal end a cuff to fit the arm at midlevel rather than a crosspiece to fit in the axilla. **perineal c.** A support on an operating table that is used to position the patient during a surgical procedure.

**Crutchfield** [William Gayle *Crutchfield,* U.S. surgeon, born 1900] See under TONGS.

**Cruveilhier** [Jean *Cruveilhier,* French anatomist, 1791–1874] **1** Cruveilhier-Baumgarten murmur. See under MURMUR. **2** Cruveilhier's atrophy, Cruveilhier's paralysis. See under PROGRESSIVE MUSCULAR ATROPHY. **3** Cruveilhier's fossa. See under FOSSA SCAPHOIDEA OSSIS SPHENOIDALIS. **4** See under SIGN. **5** Cruveilhier's joint. See under ARTICULATIO ATLANTOAXIALIS MEDIANA. **6** Cruveilhier's joint. See under ARTICULATIO ATLANTO-OCCIPITALIS. **7** Cruveilhier-Baumgarten syndrome. See under SYNDROME. **8** Cruveilhier's ulcer. See under GASTRIC ULCER. **9** Cruveilhier's fascia. See under FASCIA PERINEI SUPERFICIALIS. **10** Cruveilhier's plexus. See under POSTERIOR CERVICAL PLEXUS. **11** Cruveilhier's ligaments, glenoid ligaments of Cruveilhier. See under LIGAMENTA PLANTARIA ARTICULATIONUM METATARSOPHALANGEALIUM.

**crux** \kruks\ [L, a cross] A structure in the shape of a cross. **c. of heart** The site of intersection of the walls of the four chambers of the heart, corresponding externally to the junction of the atrioventricular and interventricular grooves.

**Cruz** [Oswaldo *Cruz,* Brazilian physician, 1871–1917] Chagas-Cruz disease, Cruz trypanosomiasis, trypanosomiasis cruzi. See under CHAGAS DISEASE.

**cry-** \krī-\ CRYO-.

**cryaesthesia** *Brit.* CRYESTHESIA.

**cryalgesia** \krī′aljē′sē·ə\ Pain induced by the application of cold.

**cryanesthesia** \krī′anesthē′zhə\ [CRY- + ANESTHESIA] Loss of perception of cold, as during hypothermia or from the application of freezing compounds.

**cryesthesia** \krī′esthē′zhə\ [CRY- + -ESTHESIA] Undue sensitivity to cold.

**crymo-** \krī′mō-\ [Gk *krymos* frost, icy chill] A combining form meaning cold.

**crymotherapy** \krī′mōther′əpē\ CRYOTHERAPY.

**cryo-** \krī′ō-\ [Gk *kryos* (adjective) icy cold, chill] A combining form meaning cold. Also *cry-.*

**cryoanesthesia** \-an′esthē′zhə\ The freezing of skin with ice, carbon dioxide snow, or the evaporation of ethyl chloride. It is used in preparing the skin for the surgical excision of superficial tumors, incisions, and drainage.

**cryobiology** \-bī·äl′əjē\ [CRYO- + BIOLOGY] The study of the low-temperature effects on living systems.

**cryocardioplegia** \-kär′dē·ōplē′jə\ The preservation of heart viability during cardiac operations by the external application of cold.

**cryocautery** \-kô′tərē\ [CRYO- + CAUTERY] Cautery by the application of extreme cold. Also *cold cautery.*

**cryocrit** \krī′ōkrit\ The proportion of a column of blood that is precipitated cryoprotein when blood from a person with a cryoprotein is centrifuged in a hematocrit tube at 25°C or less.

**cryode** \krī′ōd\ [Gk *kryos* icy cold, chill] CRYOPHAKE.

**cryoextraction** \-ikstrak′shən\ [CRYO- + EXTRACTION] Removal of a cataract by means of the attachment of a freezing probe to the moist lens surface.

**cryoextractor** \-ikstrak′tər\ [CRYO- + EXTRACTOR] CRYOPHAKE.

**cryofibrinogen** \-fībrin′əjən\ Altered plasma fibrinogen that precipitates from chilled plasma.

**cryofibrinogenemia** \-fībrin′ōjənē′mē·ə\ The presence of cryofibrinogen in the plasma.

**cryogen** \krī′ōjən\ [CRYO- + -GEN] An agent used to produce low temperatures.

**cryoglobulin** A globulin that precipitates on cooling.

**cryoglobulinemia** \-gläb′yəlinē′mē·ə\ **1** The occurrence of cryoglobulin in the blood plasma. **2** The clinical syndrome resulting from cold-induced reversible precipitation of cryoglobulin in susceptible blood vessels. For defs. 1 and 2 also *macrocryoglobulinemia.* **mixed c.** The presence of multiple cryoglobulins, often resulting from hepatic, renal, autoimmune, infections, or lymphoproliferative disease.

**cryohypophysectomy** \-hīpäf′isek′təmē\ [CRYO- + HYPOPHYSECTOMY] Ablation of the pituitary by freezing the gland *in situ.* It is accomplished by the introduction of a specially designed probe cooled by liquid nitrogen.

**cryometer** \krī·äm′ətər\ [CRYO- + -METER] A temperature measuring device adapted for use at very low temperatures.

**cryopallidectomy** \-pal′idek′təmē\ [CRYO- + PALLIDECTOMY] Destruction of the globus pallidus by cold, applied by means of a stereotaxic device. It is performed for the control of hypertonic disorders and adventitious movements of the body, as in parkinsonism.

**cryopexy** \krī′ōpek′sē\ [CRYO- + -PEXY] Reattachment of a detached retina by means of adhesions stimulated by the irritation of freezing.

**cryophake** \krī′ōfāk\ [CRYO- + *-phake* lens, from Gk *phak(os)* a lentil, lentil-shaped object + *e*] A surgical device having a small refrigerated tip that will freeze to the surface of a cataract, forming a bond that will permit intracapsular extraction. Also *cryoextractor, cryostylet, cryode.*

**cryoprecipitate** **1** Any precipitate that forms on cooling. **2** A plasma fraction that is obtained by freezing and then thawing normal human plasma. When frozen plasma is thawed slowly, the last proteins to dissolve include fibrinogen and factor VIII, and these make up the cryoprecipitate. After centrifugal concentration, it can be used in saline solution as an effective therapeutic agent for patients with classic hemophilia (factor VIII deficiency).

**cryoprecipitation** \-prisip′itā′shən\ The precipitation of material from solution by exposure to temperatures low enough to affect its solubility but not so low as to freeze the solvent. It is used especially to concentrate factor VIII from donor plasma for use as a transfusion product.

**cryopreservation** \-prez′ərvā′shən\ The preservation of viability of donor tissue by means of freezing techniques.

**cryoprobe** \krī′ōprōb\ [CRYO- + PROBE] A surgical instrument maintained at an extremely cold temperature that is used for freezing tissues, as in neurosurgical or ophthalmologic procedures.

**cryoprotein** \-prō′tēn\ Any plasma protein that results in gelling or solidification of plasma or serum upon cooling to less than 37°C.

**cryoscope** \krī′ōskōp\ [CRYO- + -SCOPE] An instrument used to determine a freezing point. It is used especially to measure the osmolality of solutions.

**cryospasm** \krī′ōspazm\ Muscular contraction induced by cold.

**cryostat** \krī′ōstat\ [CRYO- + -STAT] A refrigerated machine which contains a microtome. It is used to cut thin sections from quick frozen tissues and is used extensively in immunofluorescent studies.

**cryostylet** \krī′ōstī′lət\ [CRYO- + STYLET] CRYOPHAKE.

**cryosurgery** \-sur′jərē\ [CRYO- + SURGERY] Destruction of tissue by local freezing, used especially in neurosurgery, usually in the basal ganglia for relief of tremor or pain. It is performed by introducing liquid nitrogen through a needle directed by stereotaxy.

**cryothalamectomy** \-thal′amek′təmē\ [CRYO- + THALAMECTOMY] Destruction of the thalamus by freezing. The procedure is comparable to that employed in cryopallidectomy and is performed particularly in the caudal ventral lateral nucleus for relief of pain.

**cryotherapy** \-ther′əpē\ [CRYO- + THERAPY] The therapeutic use of cold. Also *crymotherapy, frigotherapy.*

**cryotome** \krī′ōtōm\ [CRYO- + -TOME] FREEZING MICROTOME.

**cryoultramicrotomy** \-ul′trəmīkrät′əmē\ [CRYO- + ULTRA- + MICRO- + -TOMY] The process of cutting ultrathin sections in a cryostat for use in electron microscopy.

**crypt** \kript\ [L *crypta.* See CRYPTA.] CRYPTA. **anal c.'s** SINUS ANALES. **dental c.** The space in the bone accommodating a developing tooth. **enamel c.** The primitive socket for a developing tooth germ within the fetal jaw, surrounded by the alveolar walls, filled with mesenchyme, and containing the enamel organ. **c.'s of Fuchs** CRYPTS OF IRIS. **Haller's c.'s** GLANDULAE PREPUTIALES. **c.'s of iris** Tiny holes in the surface and loose stroma of the annulus iridis minor through which vessels may be visible in the stroma. Also *crypts of Fuchs.* **c.'s of Lieberkühn** GLANDULAE INTESTINALES. **lingual c.'s** Deep tubular invaginations of surface epithelium into each follicle of the lingual tonsil, the lining of stratified squamous epithelium being surrounded by lymphatic tissue. Also *crypts of tongue.* **Littre's c.'s** 1 GLANDULAE PREPUTIALES. 2 GLANDULAE URETHRALES URETHRAE MASCULINAE. **Luschka's c.'s** 1 Aberrant bile ducts in the connective tissue layer of the wall of the gallbladder. Some may join bile ducts, but they do not open into the lumen of the gallbladder. Also *Luschka's ducts, Theile's glands.* 2 *Incorrect* ROKITANSKY-ASCHOFF SINUSES OF THE GALLBLADDER. **c. of Morgagni** 1 One of the sinus anales. 2 FOSSA NAVICULARIS URETHRAE. **mucous c.'s of duodenum** GLANDULAE DUODENALES. **multilocular c.** 1 A simple branched acinar gland. 2 The lobule of a compound acinar or tubuloacinar gland. **c.'s of palatine tonsil** FOSSULAE TONSILLARES TONSILLAE PALATINAE. **c.'s of pharyngeal tonsil** FOSSULAE TONSILLARES TONSILLAE PHARYNGEALIS. **synovial c.** An extension of synovial membrane beyond the fibrous membrane of the capsule, in the form of a pouch into which the articular cavity is expanded. **c.'s of tongue** LINGUAL CRYPTS. **tonsillar c.'s of palatine tonsil** CRYPTAE TONSILLARES TONSILLAE PALATINAE. **tonsillar c.'s of pharyngeal tonsil** CRYPTAE TONSILLARES TONSILLAE PHARYNGEALIS. **c.'s of Tyson** GLANDULAE PREPUTIALES.

**crypt-** \kript-\ CRYPTO-.

**crypta** \krip′tə\ [L (from Gk *kryptē* a vault, crypt, from *kryptein* to hide, cover), a grotto, cavern, vault] (*pl.* cryptae) A minute, tubular pit or recess on a free surface; a simple glandular tube. Also *crypt.* **cryptae mucosae** (*sing.* crypta mucosa.) GLANDULA MUCOSA. **cryptae mucosae duodeni** GLANDULAE DUODENALES. **cryptae tonsillares tonsillae palatinae** [NA] Ten to fifteen deep, narrow, or tubular recesses extending from openings, or fossulae, on the medial surface of the palatine tonsils. They penetrate most of the depth of the tonsils and are branched, ending blindly. Also *tonsillar crypts of palatine tonsil.* **cryptae tonsillares tonsillae pharyngealis** [NA] Expanded ducts that open either on the surface or into cleftlike invaginations of the pharyngeal tonsil. Although considered cryptlike, these ducts are not homologous to the tonsillar crypts of the palatine tonsil. Also *tonsillar crypts of pharyngeal tonsil, sulci of pharyngeal tonsil.* **cryptae urethrae muliebris** GLANDULAE URETHRALES URETHRAE FEMININAE.

**cryptae** \krip′tē\ Plural of CRYPTA.

**cryptectomy** \kriptek′təmē\ The surgical excision of a crypt or pitlike depression or recess, as seen in a tonsillectomy.

**cryptenamine** An antihypertensive agent derived from a nonaqueous extract of *Veratrum viride.* It is composed of several ester alkaloids, notably protoveratrines A and B, neogermetrine, and germerine.

**cryptenamine acetate** The acetate salt of cryptenamine. It is used in the treatment of hypertensive encephalopathy and eclampsia. It is given intravenously or intramuscularly.

**cryptenamine tannate** The tannate salt of cryptenamine, used therapeutically in the management of moderate to severe hypertension. It is given orally.

**cryptic** \krip′tik\ 1 Masked or occult; larvate: said of diseases or conditions with unnoticed or atypical manifestations. 2 Concealed or camouflaged: said of the larval or the adult stages in the life cycle of certain organisms. 3 Phenotypically very similar or indistinguishable: said of species or strains that cannot be identified morphologically.

**crypticity** \kriptis′itē\ [CRYPTIC + -ITY] The property of being hidden, usually applied to an enzyme present in a cell that does not manifest its presence because permeability barriers, or the absence of a transport protein, impede access to it by one of its substrates.

**cryptitis** \kriptī′tis\ Inflammation of a glandular crypt, especially in the rectum or anus.

**crypto-** \krip′tə-\ [Gk *kryptos* hidden] A combining form meaning (1) crypt; (2) hidden, secret, disguised. Also *crypt-, krypto-.*

**cryptocephalus** \-sef′ələs\ [CRYPTO- + -CEPHALUS] A fetus or newborn infant with an extremely small or poorly developed head.

**Cryptococcaceae** \-käkā′si·ē\ [*Cryptococc(us)* + -ACEAE] A form-family of asporogenous yeasts included in form-class Deuteromycetes. Many fungi of this group are human pathogens.

**cryptococcal** \-käk′əl\ Of or relating to cryptococcosis.

**cryptococcoma** \-käkō′mə\ [*Cryptococc(us)* + -OMA] A localized granuloma due to *Cryptococcus neoformans.* It heals by encapsulation and leaves no residual scar. Also *toruloma* (obs.).

**cryptococcosis** \-käkō′sis\ [*Cryptococc(us)* + -OSIS] A disease caused by the yeastlike fungus *Cryptococcus neoformans* which is frequently found in pigeon droppings in many parts of the world. Following the entry of spores via the respiratory tract, it produces in man an acute, subacute, or chronic disease involving the brain, meninges, lungs, skin, and other organs. The main focus of the infection is the central nervous system where it produces a severe and often fatal meningitis. The organism is best demonstrated in India ink preparations of cerebrospinal fluid. Amphotericin B is the usual agent used in treatment. Also *Buschke's disease, Busse-Buschke disease, torulosis, European blastomycosis.*

***Cryptococcus*** \-käk′əs\ [CRYPTO- + COCCUS] A form-genus of fungi that reproduce by budding and produce copious amounts of a slimelike polysaccharide encapsulation. *Cryptococcus neoformans* is pathogenic for man and other animals. ***C. neoformans*** A form-species of fungus which is the etiologic agent of cryptococcosis.

**cryptodeterminant** \-ditur′minənt\ INACCESSIBLE DETERMINANT.

**cryptodidymus** \-did′iməs\ [CRYPTO- + -DIDYMUS] Unequal, conjoined twins in which the smaller or parasitic one is concealed, to some degree, within the more nearly normal twin. Also *impacted twins.*

**cryptogenic** \-jen′ik\ Of unknown origin or etiology, as a disease. Also *cryptogenetic.* Compare PHANEROGENIC.

**cryptoleukemia** \-lookē′mē·ə\ ALEUKEMIC LEUKEMIA.

**cryptomenorrhea** \-men′ôrē′ə\ [CRYPTO- + MENORRHEA] Concealed menstruation, such as that seen with imperforate hymen or cervical obstruction.

**cryptophthalmia** \krip′täfthal′mē·ə\ A congenital absence of the palpebral fissure and the typical structure of eyelids, with the skin passing uninterruptedly over a microphthalmic or rudimentary eye. Also *ankyloblepharon totale.*

**cryptoplasmic** \-plaz′mik\ Having a concealed or inapparent causative agent: said of infections in which the infective organisms cannot be located.

**cryptoporous** \-pôr′əs\ Having imperceptible or obscure pores.

**cryptopyic** \-pī′ik\ [CRYPTO- + PY- + -IC ] Pertaining to or characterized by concealed suppuration.

**cryptorchid** \kriptôr′kid\ Of or having the characteristics of cryptorchidism.

**cryptorchidectomy** \krip′tôrkidek′təmē\ The surgical excision of one or both cryptorchid or undescended testes.

**cryptorchidism** \kriptôr′kidizm\ [CRYPT- + *orchid(o)-* + -ISM] A condition in which one or both testes have never descended into the scrotum. It is most often related to a developmental defect in the testis or its ligamentous attachments to the body wall, and it is associated in adult life with impaired fertility or sterility. Also *cryptorchism, retained testicle, undescended testicle, retained testis, undescended testis.* Compare ANORCHISM, CASTRATION.

**cryptorchidopexy** \kriptôr′kidōpek′sē\ ORCHIOPEXY.

**cryptorchism** \kriptôr′kizm\ CRYPTORCHIDISM.

**cryptosporidiosis** \-spôr′idē·ō′sis\ Infection with the protozoan parasite *Cryptosporidium.* It causes sporadic, self-limited diarrheal illness associated with mild systemic symptoms in normal children and adults but produces severe, intractable infection in immunocompromised patients, most notably those with acquired immune deficiency syndrome (AIDS) or hypergammaglobulinemia.

***Cryptosporidium*** \-sporid′ē·əm\ [New L (from CRYPTO- + New L *spor(a)* seed, spore + -IDIUM)] A genus of protozoan organisms that infect the gastrointestinal tract of various animal species and humans. It is now recognized as one of the pathogens observed in acquired immune deficiency syndrome. See also CRYPTOSPORIDIOSIS.

***Cryptostroma*** \-strō′mə\ A form-genus of imperfect fungi which, although relatively rare, causes cryptostromosis or maple-bark disease.

**cryptostromosis** \-strōmō′sis\ [*Cryptostrom(a)* + -OSIS] A form of allergic alveolitis resulting from a hypersensitivity reaction to spores of *Cryptostroma corticale.* See also MAPLE BARK DISEASE.

**cryptotia** \kriptō′shə\ [CRYPT + OT- + -IA] A congenital anomaly wherein the cartilage of the upper portion of the external ear remains buried beneath the scalp.

**cryptotoxic** Having toxic or harmful properties that are not readily apparent: most often used of solutions that may change from a nontoxic to a toxic state upon disruption of the colloidal balance or upon some other change of the physical properties of the solution.

**cryptozoite** \-zō′īt\ [CRYPTO- + Gk *zō(on)* a living being, animal + -ITE] The stage of the development of the malarial parasite, *Plasmodium,* that occurs in the hepatocyte (liver cell) from the sporozoite, which is inoculated by an infected mosquito. It is the first stage of liver schizogony in the exoerythrocytic cycle. The second generation of progeny are called metacryptozoites. This phase accounts for the incubation period of malaria and the relapses in that disease.

**crystal** [L *crystallum* (from Gk *krystallos* crystal, clear ice, from *kryos* an icy cold) crystal] A solid of regular shape which reflects the regular arrangement of its molecules or ions. **asthma c.'s** CHARCOT-LEYDEN CRYSTALS. **blood c.'s** Precipitated bile pigment found in tissue after hemorrhage and in plasma after hemolysis. **Charcot-Leyden c.'s** Colorless diamond-shaped or pointed proteinaceous crystals that are seen microscopically in body fluids with a high concentration of degenerating eosinophilic granulocytes, especially in the sputum of patients with allergic asthma and in the feces of patients with protozoal infections. Also *Charcot-Neumann crystals, asthma crystals.* **ear c.'s** STATOCONIA. **liquid c.** A liquid containing long molecules that change orientation with changes in temperature or electric field and modify the scattering or absorption of light. **rock c.** QUARTZ. **scintillation c.** Any crystal that has the photoelectric characteristics of absorbing photon energies and emitting light.

**crystallitis** \kris′təlī′tis\ [*crystall(ine lens)* + -ITIS] PHAKITIS.

**crystallization** \kris′təlīzā′shən\ The formation of crystals, a process often used to purify a substance. **fern-leaf c.** CERVICAL MUCUS ARBORIZATION.

**crystallography** \kris′təläg′rəfē\ [L *crystall(um)* crystal + *o* + -GRAPHY] The study of crystals. **x-ray c.** X-RAY DIFFRACTION.

**crystalloid** \kris′təloid\ A substance whose molecules are small, as opposed to a colloid. **Charcot-Böttcher c.'s** Slender crystals 10–25 $\mu$ long, usually found in Sertoli cells of the human testis, but not in other species.

**crystalluria** \kris′taloo′rē·ə\ The presence of crystals in the urine, as seen on microscopic examination of the urinary sediment. Alkaline urine may contain crystals of ammonium magnesium phosphates, ammonium urate, calcium carbonate, or calcium phosphate. Acid urine may contain crystals of calcium oxalate or uric acid. These are of little clinical significance, especially if urine has been standing or refrigerated. However, characteristic cystine crystals appear in the cystinurias, while leucine and tyrosine crystals may appear during aminoacidurias. Characteristic crystals also may be found in the urine of patients on sulfonamide drugs.

**Cs** Symbol for the element, cesium.

**CSF** 1 cerebrospinal fluid. 2 colony stimulating factor.

**CSM** cerebrospinal meningitis.

**CT** computerized tomography; computed tomography.

**ctenoids** \tē′noidz\ [Gk *ktenoeidēs* (from *kteis,* gen. *kteno(s)* a comb + *-eidēs* -OID) comblike] In the electroencephalogram, positive spikes with frequencies of the 6 Hz and 14 Hz.

***Ctenopsyllus segnis*** \tē′nōsil′əs seg′nis\ *LEPTOPSYLLA SEGNIS*

***Ctenus*** \tē′nəs\ See under *PHONEUTRIA*.

**C-terminal** Designating the end of a peptide chain where the residue —NH—CHR—COOH has a free carboxyl group. Also *carboxyl-terminal*.

**CTP** Symbol for cytidine triphosphate.

**Cu** Symbol for the element, copper.

**cu** cubic.

**cubeb** The dried, unripe fruits of *Piper cubeba*, containing an oil formerly used as a urinary tract antiseptic agent. It has also been used as a carminative, expectorant, and flavoring agent. Also *tailed pepper*.

**cubebism** A toxicity associated with the ingestion of cubeb, the dried, unripe fruit of *Piper cubeba*. The acute symptomology includes severe gastroenteritis.

**cubital** \kyoo′bitəl\ [L *cubitalis* (from *cubitus* the elbow or the forearm) of the elbow or forearm] Pertaining to the elbow, the ulna, or the forearm. Also *cubitalis*.

**cubitocarpal** \kyoo′bitōkär′pəl\ RADIOCARPAL.

**cubitoradial** \kyoo′bitōrā′dē·əl\ **1** Pertaining to the radius and the ulna. **2** Denoting the musculus pronator quadratus. *Outmoded*.

**cubitus** \kyoo′bitəs\ [L, the elbow, arm below the elbow] **1** [NA] The elbow or the part of the elbow anterior to the joint. Also *ancon*. **2** The elbow, forearm, and hand. Also *elbow region*. **3** ULNA. **c. valgus** A deformity of the elbow in which the forearm is inclined away from the midline when the upper limb is held in the anatomical position. **c. varus** A deformity of the elbow in which the forearm is inclined towards the midline with the palm facing forwards in the anatomical position. Also *gun stock deformity*.

**cuboid** \kyoo′boid\ **1** Shaped like a cube. Also *cuboidal*. **2** OS CUBOIDEUM.

**cuboidal** \kyooboi′dəl\ **1** CUBOID. **2** Consisting of cuboid elements. **3** Pertaining to the cuboid bone.

**cuboideonavicular** \kyooboi′dē·ōnavik′yələr\ Pertaining to the cuboid and navicular bones. Also *cubonavicular, naviculocuboid*.

**cuboides** \kyooboi′dēz\ OS CUBOIDEUM.

**cubonavicular** \kyoo′bōnavik′yələr\ CUBOIDEONAVICULAR.

**cucurbocitrin** A glucoside principle from the seeds of the common watermelon, *Cucurbita citrullus*. It is employed in the treatment of hypertension and is claimed to lower blood pressure by capillary dilatation.

**cudbear** A powdered preparation of lichens such as *Lecanora tartarea* or *Rocella tinctoria* used as a red coloring material for pharmaceutical preparations. It is lightened by the addition of acid and turns purplish with the addition of alkali, and is therefore sometimes used in pharmacy as a test for alkalies and acids. *R. tinctoria* and other species of lichen are the source of litmus. Also *orchil, archil, persio*.

**cue** [possibly from the *q* or *qu* of L *quando* when] **1** An aspect of the perceptual field which permits the recognition or discrimination of a particular stimulus. **2** Some signal received by the organism from the environment, not usually in the full center of attention, which guides or controls serial responses previously learned to reach some goal. **distance c.'s** Those aspects of sensory stimulation of the eye or ear which permit a perception of the relative distance of the stimulus source, usually beginning at twenty or more feet (13 m) away. For sound, these cues consist of relative intensity or the time difference of sound waves reaching the ears. For vision, distance cues include such aspects as object superposition, perspective, light, and shade.

**cuff** [Middle English *cuffe, coffe* glove, possibly an alteration of Middle French *coif, coiffe* woman's headdress] A wide encircling band containing a balloon which can be inflated to control the flow of a fluid passing through it by constricting or sealing the conveying vessel. Cuffs are used in sphygmomanometry, in the administration of anesthesia, and in providing respiratory assistance. **epithelial c.** The totality of the junctional epithelium surrounding a tooth. It was once thought that the cells were in close contact with the tooth but not actually attached. **rotator c.** The musculotendinous reinforcement of the fibrous capsule of the shoulder joint produced by the inserting fibers of the subscapularis muscle anteriorly, the supraspinatus muscle superiorly, and the infraspinatus and teres minor muscles posteriorly. Also *musculotendinous cuff*.

**cuffing** The perivascular inflammatory reaction, consisting of an accumulation of various leukocytes, seen in infectious, inflammatory, or autoimmune disease.

**cuirass** \kwiras′\ [French *cuirass(e)* (from L *coriacea* leathern, from *corium* hide, skin, bark) iron armor covering back and breast] A shell-like casing which is closely fitted around the thorax in treatment of weakness of the respiratory muscles, so that evacuation of air from within the cuirass causes expansion of the thorax and hence inhalation.

**cuj.** *cujus* (L, of which).

**cul-de-sac** \kul′dəsak′, kYdəsäk′ \ [French *cul* (from L *cul(us)* the fundament) the buttocks + French *de* of + *sac* (from L *sac(cus)* a bag) a bag] A pouchlike cavity or a tube closed at one end. **Douglas c.** EXCAVATIO RECTOUTERINA. **Gruber's c.** A lateral extension of the suprasternal space between the sternal part of the sternocleidomastoid muscle anteriorly and the middle layer of the deep cervical fascia posteriorly. It contains the termination of the anterior jugular vein, lymph nodes, and fat. Also *Gruber's fossa, sac of Gruber*. **inferior c.** The space between the lower bulbar conjunctiva and the palpebral conjunctiva of the lower lid. **lesser c.** ANTRUM PYLORICUM.

**culdocentesis** \kul′dōsentē′sis\ [*cul(-de-sac of) Do(uglas)*, + -CENTESIS] Placement of the needle of a fine catheter into the pouch of Douglas through the vaginal wall in order to aspirate fluid for diagnostic purposes. Also *colpoceliocentesis, colpoceliotomy, elytroceliotomy*.

**culdoplasty** \kul′dōplas′tē\ [*cul-(de-sac of) Do(uglas)* + -PLASTY] An operation to repair relaxation of the posterior fornix of the vagina.

**culdoscope** \kul′dōskōp\ An endoscope used in performing a culdoscopy.

**culdoscopy** \kuldäs′kəpē\ Visual examination of the uterus, oviducts, and ovaries using an instrument inserted through the cul-de-sac of Douglas and into the peritoneal cavity.

**culdotomy** \kuldät′əmē\ COLPOTOMY.

***Culex*** \kyoo′leks\ [L, a gnat, mosquito] A genus of mosquitoes found worldwide but more frequently in tropical areas. It includes over 2,000 species, many of which serve as vectors for a wide variety of diseases of humans, animals, and birds, including many arbovirus diseases and forms of avian malaria. ***C. nigripalpus*** A mosquito vector of eastern equine virus, St. Louis encephalitis virus, and others. ***C. pipiens*** A polytypic species of mosquito that includes the northern house mosquito or rainbarrel mosquito *C. pipiens pipiens*, and the southern house mosquito *C. pipiens quinquefasciatus*, both of which are worldwide in distribution. Many forms are capable of autogeny. Mosquitoes of this species invade houses freely and breed in nearby small bodies of water, especially in those with high organic pollution. They are vectors of the human filarial worm *Wuchereria bancrofti*, the dog heartworm *Dirofilaria immitis*, avian pox virus, avian malarial parasites, and probably also of St.

Louis and western encephalitis viruses. ***C. quinquefasciatus*** A mosquito vector of a number of Togaviridae and Bunyaviridae viruses, including St. Louis encephalitis virus, as well as avipoxvirus (avian poxvirus), the filarial parasite *Wuchereria bancrofti,* avian malaria, and the dog heartworm *Dirofilaria immitis.* This common pest mosquito breeds in sewage drains and pit latrines in Asia and Africa, especially in poor urban areas, where it is thought to be increasing in numbers and range. Also *Culex pipiens quinquefaciatus.* ***C. tarsalis*** An abundant species throughout the southern United States, reaching elevations up to 2700 meters (9000 feet). It is especially common in semiarid regions. It feeds chiefly on the blood of domestic and wild birds, but also on that of horses, cattle, and humans. It is one of the principal vectors of St. Louis and western equine encephalitis viruses. ***C. tritaeniorhynchus*** A widely distributed mosquito that is the most important vector in the Far East of Japanese encephalitis virus. It is also found in the Near East and in parts of Africa.

**Culicidae** \kyoolis′idē\ [L *culex,* gen. *culicis,* gnat + -IDAE] A family of the order Diptera, suborder Nematocera, which comprises the mosquitoes. It is divided into the subfamilies Culicinae, Anophelinae, and Toxorhynchitinae.

**culicidal** \kyoo′lisī′dəl\ Lethal to mosquitoes, especially culicine mosquitoes.

**culicide** \kyoo′lisīd\ [L *culex,* gen. *culi(cis)* a gnat, mosquito + -CIDE] An agent that kills mosquitoes, especially culicine mosquitoes.

**culicifuge** \kyoolis′ifyooj\ [L *culex,* gen. *culicis,* gnat + -FUGE] A repellent of mosquitoes and gnats.

**Culicinae** \kyoo′lisī′nē\ A subfamily of the mosquito family Culicidae. It includes medically important genera such as *Culex* and *Aedes.*

**culicine** \kyoo′lisīn\ Of or belonging to the mosquito subfamily Culicinae.

***Culicoides*** \kyoo′likoi′dēz\ [New L, from L *culex,* gen. *culicis* gnat + New L *-oides* -OID] A genus of tiny (0.6 to 5 mm long), fiercely biting gnats or midges of the family Ceratopogonidae. Some species are vectors of the nonpathogenic human filariae *Dipetalonema perstans* and *Mansonella ozzardi,* of *Onchocerca* of horses and cattle, and various viruses of domestic sheep and of fowl.

**culicosis** \kyoo′likō′sis\ [L *culex,* gen. *culic(is)* a gnat, mosquito + -OSIS] A dermatitis caused by the bites of *Culex* mosquitoes. The dermatitis is not transmitted by a bite but is a direct consequence of the inflammatory changes induced by many bites.

***Culiseta*** \kyoo′lisē′tə\ A genus of culicine mosquitoes. Nine species of the genus are found in North America. These mosquitoes are often domiciliated and are pests of cattle and horses. Also *Theobaldia* (former name). ***C. melanura*** A species of the eastern and central United States that transmits the viral agents of eastern and western equine encephalitis and probably serves as a maintenance host of eastern equine encephalitis.

**Cullen** [Thomas Stephen *Cullen,* U.S. gynecologist, 1868–1953] See under SIGN.

**culling** The identification and removal of specific objects, most often the removal of defective erythrocytes from the circulating blood by the spleen.

**culmen** \kul′mən\ [L (also *columen*; akin to *collis* hill), the highest point, summit, top] (*pl.* culmina) [NA] The superiorly bulging portion of the cerebellum between the primary fissure and the lobulus centralis, especially that part along the vermis. It includes lobules three to five of the vermis in Larsell's classification. Also *culmen monticuli, lobulus culminis.*

**culmina** \kul′minə\ Plural of CULMEN.

**Culp** [Ormond Skinner *Culp,* U.S. surgeon, 1910–1977] **1** See under URETEROPELVIOPLASTY. **2** Cecil-Culp repair of hypospadias. See under REPAIR.

**cultivation** \kul′tivā′shən\ The culture of cells, generally *in vitro,* by providing a nutrient medium and an environment which will permit growth and reproduction.

**culturable** \kul′chərəbl\ Able to grow and reproduce *in vitro.*

**culture** [L *cultura* (from *cultus,* past part. of *colere* to till, cultivate) culture, cultivation] **1** The product of the growth of an inoculum of microbial or other cells incubated in a suitable medium. See also CULTURE MEDIUM, MEDIUM, BROTH, AGAR. **2** To grow a microorganism under controlled conditions. **blood c.** **1** A liquid bacterial culture medium, for identification of specific pathogens causing bacteremia, containing brain suspension, dextrose, citrate, and peptones in meat infusion broth, buffered to pH 7.4 with phosphate. **2** Any attempted culture of microorganisms from blood. **cell c.** A population of disaggregated tissue cells maintained or propagated *in vitro.* Three basic types exist: primary cultures, diploid cell strains, and continuous cell lines. Animal cell cultures require a complex medium, serum factors, and elevated carbon dioxide. **chorioallantoic c.** The use of the chorioallantois of the developing chick embryo as a culture medium for the cultivation of microorganisms, cells, or tissues. **continuous c.** A microbial culture in an apparatus, such as a chemostat, in which fresh medium enters at a growth-limiting rate, displacing an equal volume of culture. The medium surrounding the growing cells, and the production of metabolites, are thus kept constant. **direct c.** The primary culture of microorganisms from a clinical specimen, as contrasted with subsequent subcultures of pure strains. **embryo c.** Any *in vitro* method for stimulating and supporting growth and development of an embryo. The embryo may originate from extracorporeal fertilization or from excision or collection from the reproductive tract of the biologic mother. **enrichment c.** A growth medium that contains nutrients that will be used by a desired microorganism better than by others that are not wanted. It thus increases (enriches) the proportion, in samples of soil, water, or other natural materials, of particular microorganisms. **histologic c. of wound sections** A method of burn wound culture whereby thin vertical sections of the burn are plated on culture medium and examined at 18 hours. The technique allows not only bacterial identification, but detects the level of invasion within the burn. **mixed lymphocyte c.** A technique to demonstrate the differences in surface antigenic composition between lymphocytes from two different individuals. Reactive T lymphocytes undergo immunoblastogenesis and multiplication when cultured in the presence of antigenically foreign cells. The level of blastogenesis is measured by the degree to which the cultured cells incorporate $^{14}$C- or $^{3}$H-labeled thymidine. HLA-D antigens are the predominant stimulus to reactivity. The culture is used to determine histocompatibility between donor and recipient in tissue transplantation and to type for HLA-D antigens. Abbr. MLC **one-way mixed lymphocyte c.** A modification of the mixed lymphocyte culture in which cells from one individual are treated with mitomycin or x-ray radiation to prevent blastogenesis. The treated cells serve only as an antigenic stimulus to the untreated cells. Treated cells are called stimulator cells, and untreated cells are called responder cells. **organ c.** Any *in vitro* method for, at a minimum, maintaining the viability of an organ or complex tissue that has been excised from a plant or animal. In some instances, the goal is to stimulate growth or differentiation in order to preserve function. **primary c.** Any *in vitro* method or system for maintaining viability or stimulating growth of cells or organs that have just been removed from the organism. **pure c.** A culture containing only one kind of microorganism, usually derived by subculture from a single colony on a plate. With an organism that might be a minor component of the original population, two successive single-colony isolations are necessary to eliminate contaminants. **quantitative c.** A culture method whereby a wound biopsy is taken, minced, weighed, and cultured in serial dilutions such that results can be reported as the number of organisms per gram of tissue. A culture containing $10^5$ or more implies significant infection of the tissue. **roller tube c.** A tissue culture placed in a roller tube and rotated and incubated on a roller drum, usually at 12 revolutions per hour. This system of incubation provides optimal conditions for growth of certain viruses, such as rhinoviruses. **shake c.** A liquid culture that is aerated by constant agitation during incubation. **slant c.** A culture in a tube of solid medium that is allowed to harden at an angle in order to provide a larger surface for inoculation. Also *slope culture* (British usage). **stab c.** A culture that has been inoculated with a needle in the depth of a tube of solid medium. Such cultures remain viable much longer than surface cultures, and they allow comparison of response to aerobic and to anaerobic conditions. **stock c.** Any culture preserved in a laboratory as a source of subcultures. **streak c.** A culture on the surface of a solid medium, streaked in such a way that diminishing population density will provide isolated colonies on some part of the plate. **surface c.** A superficial culture of a wound or burn obtained by direct application of a culture plate, or by rubbing a moistened swab over the wound. Such cultures provide qualitative but not quantitative information about the bacterial ecology. **synchronous c.** A culture in which all the cells are at approximately the same stage in the cycle of growth and division. In bacteria synchronization is conveniently achieved by using an inoculum of cells isolated from the usual heterogeneous population on the basis of uniform size. **tissue c.** A preparation of living cells that are growing *in vitro* and are supported by nutrient fluids. Also *cellular explant.* **type c.** A culture preserved in a culture collection in order to provide different investigators with the same strain.

**culture medium** A broth, agar, or tissue preparation that is used to detect the presence and enhance the growth of microorganisms. Also *medium.* See also AGAR, BROTH, MEDIUM, CULTURE. **agar c.** AGAR. **chocolate c.** Any microbiologic culture medium that contains blood heated so that it turns chocolate brown in color. **defined c.** A culture medium composed entirely of pure, defined chemicals, in contrast to the extracts of plant or animal material often used in diagnostic or large-scale cultivation. It is used especially for research, or to prepare vaccines free of adventitious antigens. **differential c.** A medium that contains dyestuffs or chemical constituents that cause colonies of different organisms to have different and distinctive appearances upon culturing. **enriched c.** A liquid or agar medium to which nutrients such as blood, serum, or peptones are added to enhance the growth of fastidious microorganisms such as *Neisseria* and *Haemophilus.* **eosin-methylthionine chloride c.** EOSIN-METHYLENE BLUE AGAR. **indicator c.** A culture medium containing an acid-base indicator, used to delineate growth and metabolic patterns of individual organisms. **litmus-milk c.** A culture medium that is prepared from skim milk and that contains litmus as a pH indicator. It is used to demonstrate many biochemical properties of growing bacteria. The fermentation of glucose and lactose produces an acid pH change, the proteolytic enzymes cause an alkaline pH change and a clearing of the opaque medium, coagulating enzymes produce solid casein curds, and the accompanying evolution of gas, results in "stormy clotting." Also *milk culture medium.* **Löffler's blood c.** A culture medium used to isolate diphtheria bacilli. It consists of infusion broth, beef serum, and whole egg. Also *Löffler serum agar, Löffler medium, Löffler serum.* **milk c.** LITMUS-MILK CULTURE MEDIUM. **N.N.N. c.** NOVY, MCNEAL AND NICOLLE MEDIUM. **nutrient c.** NUTRIENT BROTH. **peptone water c.** Peptone water used as an enrichment medium for the isolation of *Vibrio cholerae.* **selective c.** A culture medium containing substances that inhibit the growth of certain organisms while permitting or encouraging the growth of pathogens of diagnostic interest. **semisolid c.** MOTILITY TEST MEDIUM. **thioglycollate c.** A broth medium containing peptone, sodium chloride, thioglycollate, and cystine that is used for cultivating aerobic or anaerobic organisms. The thioglycollate and cystine maintain a low Eh, which permits the growth of strict anaerobic organisms. **Wilson-Blair c.** BISMUTH SULFITE AGAR.

**cumulative** Denoting the additive, combined effects of a number of ineffective doses of a drug that, in the aggregate, result in a pronounced effective response.

**cumuli** \kyoom′yəlī\ Plural of CUMULUS.

**cumulus** \kyoom′yələs\ [L, a heap, pile] [NA] A heap, or collection, of cells. **c. oophorus** A peninsulalike accumulation of granulosa cells surrounding the ovum of an ovarian follicle. Also *cumulus ovaricus, ovarian cumulus, discus oophorus.*

**cuneate** \kyoo′nē·āt\ [L *cuneatus,* past part. of *cuneare* to form into the shape of a wedge, from *cuneus* a wedge] Wedge-shaped. Also *cuneiform.*

**cunei** \kyoo′nē·ī\ Plural of CUNEUS.

**cuneiform** \kyoonē′ifôrm\ **1** CUNEATE. **2** Any of the cuneiform bones, such as os cuneiforme intermedium and the os cuneiforme laterale.

**cuneus** \kyoo′nē·əs\ [L, a wedge] [NA] A wedge-shaped lobule of cerebral cortex located on the medial surface of the occipital lobe and bounded by the parieto-occipital and calcarine sulci. Also *gyrus cunei, cuneate lobe.*

**cunicular** \kyoonik′yələr\ Pertaining to or characteristic of cuniculi.

**cuniculus** \kyoonik′yələs\ [L, a rabbit, mine, subterranean passage or hole] (*pl.* cuniculi) One of the serpiginous burrows made by pregnant *Sarcoptes scabiei* mites in the skin of a host. **c. internus** [NA] A triangular space in the spiral organ of Corti, the base of which is the zona arcuata of the basilar membrane. The sides are formed by the rows of the inner and outer rods, or pillar cells, which come into contact at the apex. Also *tunnel of Corti, canal of Corti.*

**cunnus** \kun′əs\ [L, the vulva] PUDENDUM FEMININUM.

**cup** In anatomy, a deep hollow space with rounded sides and edges. **chin c.** A device for forcing the chin in an upward and backward direction, consisting of elastic bands attached to a headcap. Also *chincap, chin cap.* **eye c.** EYECUP. **favus c.** SCUTULUM. **glaucomatous c.** An abnormal extent of excavation of the optic disk, caused by nerve fiber loss due to increased intraocular pressure. **Montgomery's c.'s** Large endometrial glands in the upper two thirds of the cervix uteri. **optic c.** **1** An indentation of the distal wall of the optic vesicle, brought about by rapid marginal growth, and producing a double-layered cup attached to the diencephalon by a tubular stalk (future optic nerve). This structure is first seen in the embryo during the third month. Of the two layers formed, the outer acquires pigment and develops into the pigmented layer of the retina. The inner layer then divides into a thicker posterior portion (pars optica retinae), which develops into the visual receptive portion of the adult retina, and a thinner anterior portion (pars caeca retinae). The inferior aspect of the optic stalk near its attachment to the optic cup develops a slight groove which becomes continuous distally with the fetal fissure. This subsequently closes and surrounds the blood vessels that pass to the optic cup. Non- or partial fusion of this tissue results in the condition known as coloboma. Also *ophthalmic cup, ocular cup.* 2 EXCAVATIO DISCI. **perilimbal suction c.** A device that exerts pressure upon the anterior sclera, just behind the cornea, used in order to block the escape of aqueous humor from the anterior chamber, thereby permitting study of the dynamics of aqueous outflow. **physiologic c.** EXCAVATIO DISCI.

**cupola** \kyoo′pōlə\ [Italian (from L *cupula* a cup-shaped object) cupola] CUPULA.

**cupping** 1 The application of a cupping glass to skin to draw the blood to the surface, formerly used after scarifying in bloodletting. 2 The process or fact of assuming a cup-like or concave shape. **c. of the calix** The concavity of the normal calix of the kidney as seen radiologically after opacification of the caliceal system, the concavity representing the impression by the renal pyramid. **pathologic c.** An excessively deepened optic disk, significant in that its cause is the loss of nerve fibers.

**cupric** \k$^y$oo′prik\ [Late L *cupr(um)* copper + -IC] Relating to copper(II).

**cupro-** [Late L *cupr(um)* (from L *aes cyprium* copper of Cyprus) copper] A combining form used to designate copper, especially at the center of a complex, and especially of copper(I). Also *cupr-.*

**cuproproteins** \k$^y$oo′prōprō′tēns\ A group of compounds, including hemocuprein, hepatocuprein, erythrocuprein, and cerebrocuprein, containing copper and zinc and having superoxide dismutase activity. Other cuproproteins include the soluble amine oxidases which are benzylamineoxidase (from pig plasma), spermine oxidase (from bovine plasma), diamine oxidase (from pig kidney), and a connective tissue amine oxidase (from bovine aorta).

**cuprous** \k$^y$oo′prəs\ [Late L *cupr(um)* + -OUS] Relating to copper(I).

**cupula** \kyoo′pyələ\ [L (dim. of *cupa* a large cask) a cup-shaped object, a little tub] An inverted cup-shaped or dome-shaped structure, usually at the apex of an organ or part. Also *cupola.* **c. of ampullary crest** CUPULA CRISTAE AMPULLARIS. **c. cochleae** [NA] The conical apex of the bony cochlea that points laterally toward the anterosuperior part of the medial wall of the tympanic cavity. Also *cupula of cochlea.* **c. cristae ampullaris** [NA] A thick, cylindrical, noncellular gelatinous mass into the base of which project the microvilli, stereocilia, and kinocilia of the hair cells and supporting cells of the ampullary crest of each semicircular duct. Its free apical border does not reach the opposite wall of the ampulla, and is displaced to one or other side by movement of the endolymph. It is similar to the membrana statoconiorum, but lacks statoconia. Also *cupula of ampullary crest.* **c. pleurae** [NA] The dome-shaped upward continuation of the costal pleura over the apex of the lung, extending from the medial border of the first rib into the root of the neck as high as the neck of the first rib. It is supported by the suprapleural membrane. Also *cupula of pleura, cervical pleura, pleural dome.*

**cupulae** \kyoo′pyəlē\ Plural of CUPULA.

**cupular** \kyoo′pyələr\ Cup-shaped; dome-shaped. Also *cupulate.*

**curage** \kyooräzh′\ CURETTAGE.

**curare** \k$^y$oorä′rē\ [mainland Carib *kurari*] A mixture of alkaloids, primarily curarine and related compounds, from the root-bark of several poisonous plants, the most important of these being *Strychnos toxifera* and *Chondodendron tomentosum.* The poison is used by South American hunters to paralyze game with arrow tips dipped in curare. The active principle, *d*-tubocurarine, is a nondepolarizing neuromuscular blocking agent used to obtain muscular relaxation during anesthesia. Also *curari.*

**curaremimetic** Having properties similar to those of curare.

**curari** CURARE.

**curariform** Having a pharmacologic action resembling that of curare.

**cure** [L *cura* care, attention] 1 Any prescribed course of treatment designed to restore health. 2 Treatment leading to a restoration of health. 3 Recovery from illness or injury. 4 To restore the health of; be the agent of recovery from illness or injury. **mind c.** *Popular* PSYCHOTHERAPY. **radical c.** 1 An operation that removes all traces of diseased tissue. 2 An operation that prevents recurrence of a condition.

**curet** \kyooret′\ CURETTE.

**curettage** \kyooretäzh′, kyUret′ij\ [French *curetage* cleaning with a curette] A surgical procedure, either diagnostic or therapeutic, in which a body cavity or tissue is scraped with a sharp curved instrument or aspirated with a cannula, as in *uterine curettage.* Also *curage, curettement.* **medical c.** Uterine bleeding induced by the sequential administration and withdrawal of hormones. **root c.** ROOT PLANING. **suction c.** A method of evacuating the contents of the uterus by aspiration with hollow cannulae of differing diameters following dilatation of the uterine cervix. It is most frequently used for management of first-trimester elective abortions or incomplete abortions.

**curette** \kyooret′\ [French (from *curer* to clean out) a scraper, spatula, curette] A surgical instrument with a curved spoonlike tip and long handle, designed for scraping a body cavity or tissue for diagnostic or therapeutic reasons. Also *curet.* **adenoid c.** One of a variety of instruments for removing the adenoids. It is introduced behind the soft palate into the nasopharynx where it is used to plane or scrape away the lymphoid tissue. **Beckmann's c.** An adenoid curette similar to Gottstein's curette but differing in that the triangular opening is replaced by a quadrilateral fenestra better suited to embrace the adenoid mass. **Delstanche's c.** A Gottstein curette modified by the addition of a hinged, toothed cage that serves to trap the removed tissue. **Gottstein's c.** The original ring-shaped adenoid curette. **Hartmann's c.** A modification of Gottstein's curette. The half-inch cutting blade forms the distal edge of a triangular fenestra set at right angles to the handle. **St. Clair Thomson's c.** A widely-used adenoid curette which combines the advantages of the quadrilateral fenestra of Beckmann's curette with the hinged cage of Delstanche's curette.

**curettement** \kyooret′mənt\ CURETTAGE.

**curie** \kyoo′rē\ [after Marie *Curie* (born Marja Sklodowska), Polish-French chemist and physicist, 1867–1934] A unit of radioactivity, the rate of nuclear transformations or transitions of a radionuclide or a radioactive source, defined since 1950 as equal to $3.7 \times 10^{10}$ per second exactly; $3.7 \times 10^{10}$ becquerels exactly. Before 1950 the curie was the disintegration rate of one gram of radium. Symbol: Ci

**curie-hour** \kyoo′rē-\ A unit of total number of nuclear

transformations or transitions occurring in one hour when a radionuclide or radioactive source has an activity of one curie; 1.332 × $10^{14}$ transformations. Symbol: Ci·h

**curium** \kyoo′rē·əm\ An artificially created element of the actinide series, having atomic number 96 and atomic weight 247. Thirteen isotopes are known. Curium 247 is the most stable, having a half-life of 16 million years. It is a chemically reactive, gray metal and is intensely radioactive. Readily absorbed into the body, it accumulates in the bones and destroys the erythrocyte-forming mechanism. Symbol: Cm

**Curling** [Thomas Blizard *Curling,* English surgeon, 1811–1888] See under ULCER.

**current** [L *currens* (gen. *currentis*), pres. part. of *currere* to run] **1** The flow of electricity through a circuit, as the flow of electrons in a metal or ions in an electrolyte. **2** A stream or flow of gas or liquid, as occurs in breathing or blood flow. **action c.** ACTION POTENTIAL. **after c. 1** AFTERCURRENT. **2** The positive current across a nerve membrane following the conducted action current. **alternating c.** A current that reverses periodically and has an average value of zero. **anelectrotonic c.** The extrinsic, passive electric current applied to cells or tissue at the anodal (positive) pole of a pair of stimulating electrodes, reducing excitability. Also *anodal current.* **anionic c.** The negative current across nerve and muscle membranes conveyed by an anion, principally chloride. **anodal c.** ANELECTROTONIC CURRENT. **ascending c.** CENTRIPETAL CURRENT. **axial c.** The central core of flowing blood. **blaze c.** The flow of electricity in tissues that results from mechanical stimulation. **catelectrotonic c.** Current emanating from an electrode of negative polarity. It reduces the threshold of excitable tissue. **centrifugal c.** An electric current with the positive pole near the center of the body and the negative source in the periphery. In nerve it refers to current flow between the cathode placed peripheral to the anode. Also *descending current.* **centripetal c.** An electric current passing through the body with a positive peripheral pole and a negative peripheral potential difference. In nerve it refers to the direction of current flow when the anode is peripheral to the cathode. Also *ascending current.* **combined c.** The summed current at the point in a circuit where branch circuits converge. **damped c.** A current whose magnitude gradually decreases as a result of dissipation of energy. **demarcation c.** INJURY CURRENT. • The term has the particular connotation of delineating the border between intact and injured tissue. **depolarization c.** An electrical current that tends to depolarize a charged, excitable membrane. **descending c.** CENTRIFUGAL CURRENT. **diphasic action c.** The current in a peripheral nerve accompanying the conducted diphasic action potential recorded from a single extra-axonal site. **direct c.** An electrical current which flows in one direction only. At high voltages it is used primarily in industries where electrolytic activity is desired and in powering electric trains. The human organism is about six times less sensitive to direct current than to alternating current. Injuries caused by direct current are much less common, but can be very severe. **electric c.** The motion of electric charge in a circuit or part of a circuit. **electrotonic c.** An extrinsic decremental current imposed upon a portion of a cell membrane or tissue, resulting in only passive change in the resting potential. **ephaptic c.** INTERAXONAL CURRENT. **fault c.** A current that flows from one conductor to ground or another conductor due to an abnormal connection such as a short circuit. **fulguration c.** A high frequency current producing a spark that is used for superficial desiccation and destruction of skin. **galvanic c.** A steady, nonpulsating direct current. It may be supplied from an electrostatic machine or a battery, or it may be produced as the rectified and filtered current from an alternator. **high-frequency c.** An alternating sinusoidal or pulsating current of relatively high frequency. The lower limit is variously taken as the maximum frequency encountered in physiological firing of nervous elements (200Hz), the frequency at which muscle no longer responds with a contraction (ca. 1000Hz), or the rate at which tissues are optimally heated (several kHz) therapeutically. **induced c.** A current caused by a change in the magnetic flux through the circuit resulting from a changing current in another circuit. Also *induction current.* **injury c.** A steady current flowing between a chemically or physically injured region on the surface membrane of muscle or nervous tissue and nearby normally polarized areas. Also *demarcation current.* **interaxonal c.** A passive electrotonic current derived from the extracellular potential field induced by an axonal action potential extending to adjacent axons. Also *ephaptic current.* **inverse c.** The current resulting from a voltage applied to a rectifier in the direction opposite to the normal flow. **ionization c.** The current flowing through a gas that has been ionized, such as by radiation. **monophasic action c.** The conducted nerve impulse recorded with one electrode placed at the crushed or cut end of a nerve and one along the nerve bundle. **nerve action c.** The current generated in the axon membrane by the conducted action potential. **oscillating c.** Electric current whose direction of flow reverses in a periodic or quasiperiodic fashion. **Oudin c.** An electric current used in diathermy that is of high frequency and higher voltage than that used for regular short wave diathermy treatment. **resting c.** The electrical current resulting from the potential difference measured between intracellular and extracellular electrodes. **rising c.** The active phase of cell membrane depolarization. **saturation c.** The current produced by an ionization chamber when the voltage across the chamber is high enough to collect all the ions without recombination. **sine-wave c.** An alternating current the wave shape of which is described by a sinusoidal function of time. **sinusoidal c.** An oscillating electrical current of sinusoidal waveform, usually with the implication that the current swings to either side of a net zero current baseline. Physiological stimulators often deliver this form of current. **static c.** The flow of charged particles from one physical body to another. Also *spark-gap current, static induced current.* **static-wave c.** The current occurring in a body that is suddenly discharged after the current has been raised to a high potential by an electrostatic machine. **undamped c.** A current of constant amplitude.

**Curschmann** [Heinrich *Curschmann,* German physician, 1846–1910] See under SPIRAL.

**Curtis** [Arthur Hale *Curtis,* U.S. gynecologist, 1881–1955] Curtis and Fitz-Hugh syndrome. See under FITZ-HUGH AND CURTIS SYNDROME.

**curvatura** \kur′vətyoo′rə\ [L (from *curvare* to bow, bend, curve) a bowing, bending] A gentle bend, or flexure, of a line or a linear surface of a structure. Also *curvature.* **c. gastrica major** [NA] The long, convexly curved left border of the stomach, directed anteroinferiorly and extending from the cardiac notch to the pylorus. It gives attachment to the gastrosplenic ligament and the two layers of the greater omentum containing the gastro-omental vessels. Also *greater curvature of stomach.* **c. gastrica minor** [NA] The short, concavely arched right border of the stomach, directed posterosuperiorly, extending from the cardiac orifice to the pylorus, and providing attachment to the two layers of the lesser omentum between which the left and right gastric vessels run. Also *lesser curvature of stomach.*

**curvature** \kur′vəchər\ [L *curvatura.* See CURVATURA.] CURVATURA. **anterior c.** KYPHOSIS. **backward c.** LORDOSIS. **compensatory c.** A flexible, nonstructural curvature of the spine, adjacent to a region of structural spinal deformity, that provides for the maintenance of trunk balance. **c. of field** A curved distortion of an image caused by an aberration of an optical system, as of a microscope. **greater c. of stomach** CURVATURA GASTRICA MAJOR. **hyperopia of c.** CURVATURE HYPEROPIA. See under HYPEROPIA. **lateral c.** SCOLIOSIS. **lesser c. of stomach** CURVATURA GASTRICA MINOR. **occlusal c.** CURVE OF OCCLUSION. **Petzval c.** The sum, over all the optical surfaces in an optical system, of the quantity $R(1/n'-1/n)$ for each surface, where $R$ is the radius of curvature of the surface and $n$ and $n'$ are the indices of refraction before and after the surface, respectively. **Pott's c.** An angular deformity of the spine due to tuberculous spondylitis. **c. of the spine** A normal or abnormal deviation from straight of the entire vertebral column. The normal curvature of the spine consists of lordosis of the cervical and lumbar areas and kyphosis at the thoracic area. Pathologic curvature of the spine consists of abnormal kyphosis and/or scoliosis.

**curve** [L *(linea) curva* (from *curvus* curved, not straight, akin to Gk *kyrtos* humped, convex) a curved line] **1** A line which deviates from a straight course in a continuous manner. **2** A surface which is not plane. **3** The graphic representation of a continuous mathematical function. **alignment c.** The curve of a line passing through the center of the occlusal surfaces of the upper or lower teeth, paralleling the dental arch. *Outmoded.* **audiometric c.** The line on an audiogram intersecting the frequencies at the threshold level of hearing. Also *audibility curve.* **Barnes c.** The anterior segment of a circle the center of which is the promontory of the sacrum. It generally corresponds to the pelvic outlet. **bell-shaped c.** NORMAL CURVE. **biphasic c.** DIPHASIC CURVE. **buccal c.** The curve of occlusion from the mesial surface of the first premolar to the distal surface of the third molar. **camel c.** A temperature or other curve showing two elevations separated by a depressed or normal phase. It is usually used to describe a double daily spike in temperature which is said to be common in gonococcal endocarditis and kala-azar. Also *saddleback temperature curve, dromedary curve* (incorrect). **c. of Carus** The curved line followed through the true pelvis by the presenting part of the fetus at birth and obtained by joining the axes of a number of pelvic planes. Also *circle of Carus.* **compensating c.** A curve of occlusion of dentures such that contact is maintained between the cusps of upper and lower posterior teeth in forward positions of the mandible. It is a concave curve when viewed from above. **cystometric c.** CYSTOMETROGRAM. **decay c.** A plot of the relative amount of specified radionuclide in a sample, as a function of time. Typically it is a straight line when plotted on a semilog grid. **dental c.** CURVE OF OCCLUSION. **diabetic glucose tolerance c.** The definitive diagnostic test for diabetes mellitus, the curve described by sequentially measured plasma glucose concentrations over time after the oral or intravenous administration of a standard quantity of glucose (50–100 grams). In diabetic subjects, most or all values for plasma glucose are higher than in normal subjects. **diphasic c.** A graphic representation on a single basis of two quantities having basically similar sinusoidal forms but differing in phase, such as the voltages in a two-phase electrical circuit. Also *biphasic curve.* **dose-response c.** A graphic correlation of the influence of a series of dose levels of an agent, such as ionizing radiation or a chemical, on a parameter which is influenced by it, such as cell viability, mutational frequency, or DNA damage. Also *dose-effect curve.* **dromedary c.** *Incorrect* CAMEL CURVE. • A misnomer based on confusion of the dromedary, which has one hump, with the two-humped Bactrian camel. **dye-dilution c.** A graph of the concentrations of a dye such as indocyanine green, measured over a period of time at a fixed point in the circulation after a known quantity of the dye has been very rapidly injected into the bloodstream. It is used in calculations of cardiac output, of arterial shunts in congenital heart disease, and of valvular regurgitation. **Frank-Starling c.** STARLING'S CURVE. **Friedman c.** A plot representing the extent of cervical dilatation or descent of the fetal head during labor and the elapsed time, represented in cm/hr, in order to determine whether or not labor is progressing satisfactorily. **gaussian c.** NORMAL CURVE. **Gompertz c.** See under GROWTH CURVE. **growth c.** A mathematical expression for the change in size, either increase or decrease, of a population with the passage of time. Three such curves are:

$$\text{Gompertz} \quad y = ka^{b^t};$$

$$\text{logistic} \quad y = \frac{k}{1 + e^{at}}; \text{ and}$$

$$\text{modified exponential} \quad y = k + ab^t;$$

where in each case $y$ is the size of the population at time $t$ and $a$, $b$, and $k$, are parameters. **indicator-dilution c.** A graph of the concentrations of a dye or other indicator such as cold water or a radioactive substance, measured over a period of time at a fixed point in the circulation after a known quantity of the indicator has been injected very rapidly into the bloodstream. See also DYE-DILUTION CURVE. **intracardiac pressure c.** A graphic record of the changes of pressure inside one of the chambers of the beating heart. **inverted-U c. of arousal** A graphic description of the influence of emotional arousal on performance. Mild arousal increases alertness, attention, and interest in carrying out the task at hand, thereby enhancing the quality of performance. Very strong emotional arousal, however, is intrusive and will likely produce some decrements in the quality of performance. The inverted U describes the fact that performance is optimal where moderate levels of emotional arousal obtain. **isoresponse c.** A line showing the locations from which a small radioactive source produces the same count rate in a collimated detector. **isovolume pressure-flow c.** A graph of instantaneous expiratory flows generated by varied expiratory pressures at fixed lung volume. **labial c.** The curve of occlusion between the distal surfaces of the canine teeth. **learning c.** A graphic representation of progress made in the ability to carry out a specified task as the result of practice. The number of trials is usually measured on the horizontal axis, and performance, in terms of the amount of material learned, errors made, etc., is represented on the vertical axis. **logistic c.** See under GROWTH CURVE. **luetic c.** The results seen in the colloidal gold test of cerebrospinal fluid from a subject with meningovascular syphilis. The color change is greatest in the last four or five of the ten tubes. **Monson c.** **1** A curve, concave upward and parallel to the coronal plane, which passes through the tips of the cusps of the molar teeth in the human dentition. 2 In prosthetic dentistry, a curve of occlusion where each cusp and incisal edge conform to a segment of the surface of a sphere 8 inches in diameter, with its center in the region of the glabella. **modified exponential c.** See under GROWTH CURVE. **normal c.** The frequency curve of a normal distribution. Also *gaussian curve, normal curve of distribution, normal probability curve, bell-shaped curve.* **c. of occlusion** An imaginary spheroidal surface against which the tips of the cusps of the teeth are in contact. Also *occlusal curvature, dental curve.* **oxyhemoglobin dissociation c.** A graph which displays the relationship between oxygen in combination with hemoglobin of blood and tension of oxygen to which that blood is exposed. Also *oxygen dissociation curve, oxygen-hemoglobin dissociation curve.* **paretic c.** The results seen in the colloidal gold test of cerebrospinal fluid from a subject with general paresis. The color change is greatest in the first four or five of the ten tubes. **photopic sensitivity c.** A graphic representation of relative luminous efficiency of high-intensity lights of different wavelength. The peak of luminous efficiency is obtained with yellow-green light of wavelength 560 nm. Also *photopic dominator curve.* **Price-Jones c.** A chart of the erythrocyte diameters obtained from a specimen of blood. By convention, diameter is plotted on the abcissa and percentage of the sample on the ordinate. **pulse c.** A graphic record of the pressure and volume changes in a pulse, especially arterial; a sphygmogram. **ROC c.** See under RECEIVER OPERATING CHARACTERISTICS. **saddleback temperature c.** CAMEL CURVE. **c. of Spee** The curve of occlusion of natural teeth extended posteriorly, where it coincides with the articular eminences. **Starling's c.** A graphic record of the response of cardiac stroke output to rises in atrial pressure, determined chiefly by return of blood in the veins. They rise together up to a certain point, after which the heart becomes overloaded, and as atrial pressure rises, cardiac output falls. Also *Frank-Starling curve.* **stress-strain c.** A curve plotting force versus deformation when stretching or compressing a body. **tension c.'s** The curvilinear arrangement of bony trabeculae that is believed to result from a direction of applied stresses. **titration c.** The curve plotting some measured characteristic of a solution, often its pH, against the amount of titrant added. **Wunderlich's c.** Irregular oscillations of temperature for several days before defervescence occurs in a patient with typhoid fever.

**cusec** cubic foot per second. *Popular.*

**Cushing** [Harvey Williams *Cushing,* U.S. neurosurgeon, 1869–1939] 1 See under MYOPATHY, SYNDROME, PHENOMENON. 2 Cushing's basophilism. See under DISEASE. 3 Cushing's operation. See under SUBTEMPORAL DECOMPRESSION. 4 Cushing syndrome medicamentosus. See under IATROGENIC CUSHING SYNDROME. 5 Cushing syndrome. See under PONTOCEREBELLAR ANGLE SYNDROME. 6 Ectopic Cushing syndrome. See under SYNDROME. 7 Rokitansky-Cushing ulcer, Cushing-Rokitansky ulcer. See under CUSHING'S ULCER. 8 Alcoholic pseudo-Cushing syndrome. See under SYNDROME. 9 Cushingoid face, cushingoid facies. See under MOON FACE.

**Cushing** [Hayward Warren *Cushing,* U.S. surgeon, 1854–1934] See under SUTURE.

**cushingoid** \kŭsh′ingoid\ [after Harvey Williams *Cushing,* U.S. neurosurgeon, 1869–1939 + -OID] Like the signs and symptoms of Cushing's disease or the Cushing syndrome.

**cushion** In anatomy, any soft or fleshy structure resembling a pad. **atrioventricular canal c.'s** ENDOCARDIAL CUSHIONS. **endocardial c.'s** Swellings in the dorsal and ventral walls of the atrioventricular canal of the embryonic heart. They eventually fuse to form the septum intermedium separating the right and left atrioventricular openings. Also *atrioventricular canal cushions.* **c. of epiglottis** TUBERCULUM EPIGLOTTICUM. **levator c.** TORUS LEVATORIUS. **Passavant's c.** PASSAVANT'S BAR. **polar c. of the glomerulus** JUXTAGLOMERULAR APPARATUS. **sucking c.** CORPUS ADIPOSUM BUCCAE.

**cusp** \kusp\ [L *cuspis.* See CUSPIS.] CUSPIS. **anterior c. of mitral valve** CUSPIS ANTERIOR VALVAE ATRIOVENTRICULARIS SINISTRAE. **anterior c. of tricuspid valve** CUSPIS ANTERIOR VALVAE ATRIOVENTRICULARIS DEXTRAE. **aortic c.** CUSPIS ANTERIOR VALVAE ATRIOVENTRICULARIS SINISTRAE. **Carabelli c.** An additional cusp sometimes occurring on the lingual surface of maxillary molars. Also *Carabelli tubercle.* **dorsal c. of mitral valve** CUSPIS POSTERIOR VALVAE ATRIOVENTRICULARIS SINISTRAE. **dorsal c. of tricuspid valve** CUSPIS POSTERIOR VALVAE ATRIOVENTRICULARIS DEXTRAE. **infundibular c. of tricuspid valve** CUSPIS ANTERIOR VALVAE ATRIOVENTRICULARIS DEXTRAE. **marginal c. of tricuspid valve** CUSPIS POSTERIOR VALVAE ATRIOVENTRICULARIS DEXTRAE. **medial c. of tricuspid valve** CUSPIS SEPTALIS VALVAE ATRIOVENTRICULARIS DEXTRAE. **plunger c.** A cusp which tends to force food particles past the contact area between two teeth in the opposite jaw. **posterior c. of mitral valve** CUSPIS POSTERIOR VALVAE ATRIOVENTRICULARIS SINISTRAE. **posterior c. of tricuspid valve** CUSPIS POSTERIOR VALVAE ATRIOVENTRICULARIS DEXTRAE. **right c. of mitral valve** CUSPIS ANTERIOR VALVAE ATRIOVENTRICULARIS SINISTRAE. **semilunar c.** VALVULA SEMILUNARIS. **septal c. of tricuspid valve** CUSPIS SEPTALIS VALVAE ATRIOVENTRICULARIS DEXTRAE. **shearing c.** One of the cusps of the teeth used for shearing food. These are the buccal cusps of maxillary cheek teeth, the lingual cusps of mandibular cheek teeth, and the tips of maxillary incisors and canines. **stamp c.** A cusp of a tooth which occludes with a fossa in the opposing dental arch. Generally, maxillary lingual cusps and mandibular buccal cusps are stamp cusps. **ventral c. of mitral valve** CUSPIS ANTERIOR VALVAE ATRIOVENTRICULARIS SINISTRAE. **ventral c. of tricuspid valve** CUSPIS ANTERIOR VALVAE ATRIOVENTRICULARIS DEXTRAE.

**cuspid** \kus′pid\ [L *cuspis,* gen. *cuspid(is)* a point, cusp] CANINE. • The term refers to the single-cusped (unicuspid) structure of the canine teeth in the human dentition, as distinguished from bicuspids and tricuspids.

**cuspis** \kus′pis\ [L, a point] (*pl.* cuspides) 1 A triangular leaflet of an atrioventricular valve, attached at its base to the annulus fibrosus, where it receives some atrial muscle fibers and capillaries. The remainder comprises dense connective tissue covered on each surface by endocardium. It differs from a valvula in that it has chordae tendineae attached to its apex, margins, and ventricular surface. 2 A conical projection on the occlusal surface of a tooth. For defs. 1 and 2 also *cusp.* **c. anterior valvae atrioventricularis dextrae** [NA] The anterior and largest of the three triangular cusps of the tricuspid valve, situated between the infundibulum and the atrioventricular orifice. Also *cuspis anterior valvulae tricuspidalis* (outmoded), *ventral cusp of tricuspid valve, infundibular cusp of tricuspid valve, anterior cusp of tricuspid valve.* **c. anterior valvae atrioventricularis sinistrae** [NA] The anterior and larger of the two triangular cusps of the mitral valve, situated anteriorly and to the right between the aortic and the atrioventricular orifices. The chordae tendineae are attached near its free margin. Also *aortic cusp, cuspis anterior valvulae bicuspidalis* (outmoded), *right cusp of mitral valve, ventral cusp of mitral valve, anterior cusp of mitral valve.* **c. anterior valvulae bicuspidalis** *Outmoded* CUSPIS ANTERIOR VALVAE ATRIOVENTRICULARIS SINISTRAE. **c. anterior valvulae tricuspidalis** *Outmoded* CUSPIS ANTERIOR VALVAE ATRIOVENTRICULARIS DEXTRAE. **c. dentis** The cusp of a tooth. **c. medialis valvulae tricuspidalis** *Outmoded* CUSPIS SEPTALIS VALVAE ATRIOVENTRICULARIS DEXTRAE. **c. posterior valvae atrioventricularis dextrae** [NA] The posterior cusp of the tricuspid valve, with chordae tendineae from the anterior and posterior papillary muscles attached to its apex, margins, and ventricular surface. Also *cuspis posterior valvulae tricuspidalis, dorsal cusp of tricuspid valve, marginal cusp of tricuspid valve, posterior cusp of tricuspid valve.* **c. posterior valvae atrioventricularis sinistrae** [NA] The posterior and smaller of the two cusps of the mitral valve, situated posteriorly in and to the left of the left atrioventricular orifice. Also *cuspis posterior valvulae bicuspidalis, dorsal cusp of mitral valve, posterior cusp of mitral valve.* **c. posterior valvulae bicuspidalis** *Outmoded* CUSPIS POSTERIOR VALVAE ATRIOVENTRICULARIS SINISTRAE. **c. posterior valvulae tricuspidalis** CUSPIS POSTERIOR VALVAE ATRIOVENTRICULARIS DEXTRAE. **c. septalis valvae atrioventricularis dextrae** [NA] The cusp of the tricuspid valve that is adjacent to the membranous part of the interventricular septum. Chordae tendineae from the posterior and septal papillary muscles are attached to it. Also *cuspis medialis valvulae tricuspidalis* (outmoded), *medial cusp of tricuspid valve, septal cusp of tricuspid valve.*

**cusums** \kyooʹsums\ [*cu(mulated) + sums*] Cumulated sums, employed in a powerful but simple technique for detecting changes in the trend of a sequence of values observed at regular intervals. Successive differences of the observations from some predetermined level are accumulated to give the series of cumulated sums (cusums) which, when plotted on an appropriate scale, give an early indication of any change in the average level of the variable under study. First developed in connection with quality control in industry, the method has applications in clinical medicine in monitoring, for example, the effect of therapy on blood pressure, respiratory function, and other such variables.

**cut** 1 To incise or divide (tissues or other materials) with a sharp instrument. 2 To diminish the concentration of by dilution. 3 In forensic medicine, an incised wound whose surface length is greater than its depth of penetration. Compare STAB WOUND.

**cutaneous** \kyootāʹnē·əs\ [Med L *cutaneus* (from L *cutis* skin) of the skin] Of or pertaining to the skin.

**cutdown** A small skin incision, usually over a vein or artery, that is made for rapid and direct establishment of vascular access.

**cuticle** \kyooʹtikl\ [L *cuticula,* dim. of *cutis* skin] 1 A fold of epidermis which overlaps the base of the nail; eponychium. Also *nail skin.* 2 The layer of overlapping cells that cover the hair. 3 The layer of cells lining the internal root sheath of the hair follicle. For defs. 1, 2, and 3 also *cuticula.* **dental c.** 1 Any of the cuticles or follicles found on teeth. *Imprecise.* 2 An organic nonmineralized layer of irregular width and distribution, frequently found between the internal basement lamina of the junctional epithelium and the tooth surface. Also *cuticula dentis.* **enamel c.** NASMYTH'S MEMBRANE. **Gottlieb's c.** PRIMARY CUTICLE. **keratose c.** The anterior lamella of the lamina vitrea, deposited by the retinal pigment cells. **primary c.** A thin homogeneous layer on the surface of enamel prior to eruption of the tooth, and after eruption seen histologically in the region of the gingival sulcus; the inner layer of Nasmyth's membrane. Also *Gottlieb's cuticle.* **prism c.** PRISM SHEATH. **c. of root sheath** The innermost cell layer of the internal root sheath. **secondary c.** The remains of oral epithelial cells which cover the primary cuticle as the tooth erupts. It is the only cuticle on exposed cementum.

**cuticula** \kyootikʹyələ\ (*pl.* cuticulae) CUTICLE. **c. dentis** DENTAL CUTICLE.

**cuticular** \kyootikʹyələr\ Pertaining to or consisting of cuticle.

**cutification** \kyooʹtifikāʹshən\ [L *cuti(s)* skin + -FICATION] 1 EPITHELIALIZATION. 2 The process of forming skin.

**cutireaction** \kyooʹtērē·akʹshən\ CUTANEOUS REACTION. **von Pirquet's c.** PIRQUET'S REACTION.

**cutis** \kyooʹtis\ [L (akin to Gk *kytos* container and Old English *hȳd* skin, hide) the skin] 1 [NA] The visible surface of the skin, which is a part of the integumentum commune. 2 The skin as a whole. **c. anserina** GOOSE FLESH. **c. hyperelastica** EHLERS-DANLOS SYNDROME. **c. laxa** A congenital laxness or overgrowth of skin which may appear to hang in folds. Also *dermachalasis, loose skin.* **c. vera** DERMIS.

**cutter / section c.** MICROTOME.

**cuvette** \kyoovetʹ\ [French (dim. of *cuve* tank, from L *cupa* a large cask, vat) bowl, basin] A small vessel, especially one with optical surfaces suitable for measurements of absorption of radiation in the visible or ultraviolet range.

**CV** 1 cardiovascular. 2 conjugate vera (conjugata). 3 coefficient of variation.

**CVA** 1 costovertebral angle 2 cerebrovascular accident

**CVD** color vision deviant (color deviant).

**CVO** conjugata vera obstetrica (obstetric conjugate).

**CVP** 1 central venous pressure. 2 A chemotherapy that includes cyclophosphamide, vinblastine, and prednisone.

**CVS** cardiovascular system.

**CW** continuous wave.

**Cx** 1 convex. 2 cervix.

**Cy** Symbol for cyanogen.

**cyan-** \sīʹən-\ CYANO-.

**cyanate** The ion $CNO^-$, or a salt containing it, or an ester of HO—CN. Cyanate ion reacts with $H^+$ and amine $R—NH_2$ to form $R—NH—CO—NH_2$. This reaction is slowly reversible, so that aqueous urea solutions contain ammonium cyanate after standing or heating, and hence can carbamoylate proteins.

**cyanhemoglobin** \sīʹənhēʹməglōʹbin\ The reaction product of hydrogen cyanide and hemoglobin, characterized by a brilliant red color.

**cyanide** \sīʹənīd\ 1 The ion $CN^-$, or a salt that contains it. The ion $CN^-$ has a high affinity for many metal ions, including the iron of cytochrome oxidase, and this accounts for its toxicity. 2 An organic compound containing the CN group; a nitrile.

**cyanmethemoglobin** \-met·hēʹməglōʹbin\ A relatively nontoxic compound formed by the binding of cyanide with methemoglobin. Also *cyanide methemoglobin.*

**cyano-** \sīʹənō-\ [Gk *kyanos* dark blue substance] A combining form meaning blue, bluish. Also *kyano-, cyan-, kyan-.*

**cyanobacteria** \-baktirʹē·ə\ [CYANO- + BACTERIA] (*sing.* cyanobacterium) A group of photosynthetic bacteria formerly known as cyanophytes or blue-green algae because their form of photosynthesis, unlike that of other photosynthetic bacteria, releases $O_2$ from $H_2O$. They have been reclassified because of their prokaryotic organization. Also *blue-green bacteria.*

**cyanocobalamin** Cobalamin with cyanide as a ligand to cobalt(III); vitamin $B_{12}$.

**cyanogen bromide** Br—CN. A powerful electrophile, used in protein chemistry in acid solution to break peptide chains on the C-terminal side of methionine residues, giving $Br^-$, Me—CH, and a C-terminal homoserine lactone.

**cyanolabe** \sī′ənōlāb′\ A visual pigment that absorbs blue light. Deficient synthesis, which is rare and an autosomal recessive trait in humans, results in blue color blindness.

**cyanophose** \sī′ənōfōs′\ A perception of blue color.

**cyanophytes** \sī′ənōfīts′\ See under CYANOBACTERIA.

**cyanopsia** \sī′ənäp′sē·ə\ [CYAN- + -OPSIA] A condition in which bluish vision is perceived. Also *cyanopia.*

**cyanopsin** \sī′ənäp′sin\ A photopigment characteristic of retinal cones.

**cyanosed** \sī′ənōzd, -nōst\ Manifesting cyanosis.

**cyanosis** \sī′ənō′sis\ [Gk *kyanōsis* (from *kyanos* dark blue) dark blue coloration] A bluish discoloration, particularly of the skin or mucous membranes, due to an excessive proportion of reduced hemoglobin in the blood, to stagnation of blood in capillaries of the skin or mucous membranes, or to the presence of methemoglobin, sulfhemoglobin, or other abnormal pigments. Adj. cyanotic. **c. bulbi** A dusky, bluish color of the white of the eye due to the presence of hemoglobin deficient in oxygen. **central c.** Cyanosis resulting from arterial desaturation, characteristic of right-to-left shunts within the heart or between the great arteries, or as a consequence of inadequate oxygenation of the blood in the lungs. **compression c.** A bluish discoloration of a region of the body due to venous obstruction, as from a mass compressing the superior vena cava, causing cyanosis of face, neck, and arms. **enterogenous c.** A bluish discoloration of the skin that is due to methemoglobinemia or sulfhemoglobinemia and is thought to be caused by absorption of nitrites or sulfides from the intestine. *Rare.* **false c.** A cyanosislike greyish discoloration of skin and mucous membranes that is not due to alteration of hemoglobin or low oxygen saturation of hemoglobin, but is due to the presence of pigments in the skin, such as the silver occurring in argyria or the iron and melanin in hemochromatosis. **peripheral c.** Cyanosis due to an excessive proportion of reduced hemoglobin in the capillaries and venules as a result of extreme oxygen extraction at the capillary level. It is usually associated with a low skin blood flow and vasoconstriction. **pulmonary c.** Cyanosis due to arterial oxygen desaturation caused by pulmonary disease. **c. retinae** A dusky, bluish color of the retina due to the presence of hemoglobin deficient in oxygen. **shunt c.** Cyanosis as a result of an intracardiac shunt or a shunt between the great arteries. **toxic c.** Cyanosis secondary to the formation of methemoglobin, resulting from the action of particular drugs and chemical agents, such as nitrites.

**cyanotic** \sī′ənät′ik\ Characterized by cyanosis.

**cyath.** *cyathus* (L, a glassful).

**cybernetics** \sī′bərnet′iks\ [Gk *kybernēt(ēs)* a steersman, governor + -ICS] The comparative study of communication and control systems in animal and machine, for example study of the digital computer as a possible model of brain function.

**cycl-** \sikl-, sīkl-\ CYCLO-.

**cyclamate** Any of the salts of cyclamic acid. These compounds are intensely sweet, but non-nutritive, and their use in foods has been attended by doubts about their safety. They are no longer permitted in foods in the United States.

**cyclamic acid** $C_6H_{11}$—NH—$SO_3H$. Cyclohexylsulfamidic acid.

**cyclandelate** $C_{17}H_{24}O_3$. α-Hydroxybenzeneacetic acid 3,3,5-trimethylcyclohexyl ester. A general smooth muscle relaxant drug with very weak antimuscarinic activity. Its pharmacological activity is much like that of papaverine, and it is used for its antispasmodic activity.

**cyclarthrodial** Related to or assocated with a cyclarthrosis.

**cyclarthrosis** \sik′lärthrō′sis\ A joint which allows rotation.

**cyclase** Any enzyme that catalyzes a cyclization.

**cycle** [Gk *kyklos* a ring, round, circle] **1** A recurrent sequence of phenomena, as in a physiological process, or the period of elapsed time in one such sequence. **2** In organic chemistry, a molecule or group of atoms in a closed chain (ring). If the chain is composed entirely of carbon atoms, it is a carbocycle. If composed of other atoms, especially oxygen, nitrogen, and sulfur, it is a heterocycle. **3** In biochemistry, a series of transformations undergone by a system such that the starting compound is re-formed and the balance corresponds to a simple reaction. **anovulatory c.** ANOVULATORY MENSTRUATION. **breakage-fusion-bridge c.** The abnormal cytogenetic process by which a dicentric chromosome is broken when its two centromeres are pulled to opposite poles during anaphase of mitosis or meiosis. After duplication, the fusion of the broken ends of sister chromatids results in another dicentric chromosome capable of repeating the cycle, with rearrangements, duplications, and deletions of genetic loci occurring as a result. Also *bridge-breakage-fusion-bridge cycle.* **carbon c.** The processes by which carbon circulates naturally, in which it is converted by photosynthesis from carbon dioxide into organic matter, and in which it is reconverted into carbon dioxide by the fermentative and oxidative actions of living organisms. **cardiac c.** The course of events in the heart between the onset of one heartbeat and the next, including atrial systole and diastole and ventricular systole and diastole. **cell c.** The sequence of events in dividing cells, generally divided into the following phases or periods: $G_1$, following mitosis and prior to DNA synthesis; S, the period of DNA synthesis; $G_2$, following DNA synthesis, M or D, the period during which division occurs. **chewing c.** MASTICATING CYCLE. **citric acid c.** TRICARBOXYLIC ACID CYCLE. **Cori c.** The sequence of reactions that links the production of lactic acid from glucose in skeletal muscles and its carriage via the blood to the liver, with its utilization to form glucose in that organ (gluconeogenesis). Also *glucose-lactate cycle.* **cytoplasmic c.** The stage in the life cycle of some parasites during which they live in the cytoplasm of host cells. **Embden-Meyerhof c.** EMBDEN-MEYERHOF PATHWAY. **endogenous c.** The period in the life cycle of a parasite which is passed within the body of the host. **endometrial c.** The succession of changes which the endometrium undergoes during each menstrual cycle. **estrous c.** The recurring episodes of sexual heat and reproductive receptivity in the adult female of most mammalian species other than humans. Occurring at more or less regular intervals, it is characterized by a pattern of rising and falling rates of secretion of estrogen and progesterone, with accompanying morphologic and functional changes in the secondary sex organs. The cycle is subdivided into proestrus, diestrus, estrus, and metestrus. **exogenous c.** The period in the life cycle of a parasite which is passed outside the final or definitive host. **fatty acid oxidation c.** The sequence of reactions involved in the β-oxidation of fatty acids to yield only acetylcoenzyme A if the starting material contains an even number of carbon atoms, or acetylcoenzyme A and one mol. of propionylcoenzyme A if it contains an odd number of carbon atoms. **futile c.** A cycle of reactions whose net effect is the hydrolysis of ATP or of a similar substance. An example is the conversion of fructose 6-phosphate into fructose 1,6-bisphosphate at the expense of ATP, and the subsequent hydrolysis of the bisphosphate to fructose 6-phosphate and inorganic phosphate. The two reactions that make up such a cycle are usually under controls such that conditions that activate one of them deactivate the other. Nevertheless, the futile cycle here described, which generates heat, can be important for this property, as in the flight of bumblebees. **glucose-lactate c.** CORI CYCLE. **glycine succinate c.** The reactions by which glycine and succinate react initially to form δ-aminolevulinic acid. Succinate is first converted into succinyl-CoA, which then reacts with glycine. These reactions were designated a cycle when it was thought that a major pathway of glycine breakdown went through them, and that the δ-aminolevulinic acid was degraded to succinate, in addition to its known role as a precursor of porphyrins. **glyoxylate c.** A pathway by which plants and microbes convert fatty acids into carbohydrate. The net reaction is the oxidation of two molecules of acetyl-CoA to form succinate and coenzyme A. It takes place by the action of isocitrate lyase to effect the aldol cleavage of isocitrate to glyoxylate and succinate. The glyoxylate then reacts with acetyl-CoA and water, under the influence of malate synthase, to yield malate and coenzyme A. The other reactions of the pathway are those of the citric acid cycle. The glyoxylate cycle plays a necessary role in the growth of microorganisms on $C_2$-compounds such as acetate and ethanol, in the microbial utilization of fatty acids, and in the conversion of fats into carbohydrates by fatty seeds (such as those of castor beans) during germination. The enzymes of the glyoxylate cycle in such seeds are contained in discrete intracellular bodies (glyoxysomes). The cycle does not occur in mammals. Also *glyoxylate pathway.* **hair c.** The regular sequence of anagen, catagen, and telogen (growth, involution, and rest) of the hair follicle. **Hodgkin c.** The sequence of events occurring in the regenerative linkage between membrane potential and membrane sodium permeability in excitable cells. Membrane depolarization increases membrane sodium permeability, which results in entry of sodium into the cell and further depolarization of the membrane. **Krebs c.** TRICARBOXYLIC ACID CYCLE. **Krebs-Henseleit c.** UREA CYCLE. **lactation c.** A sequence of stages during lactation which includes the filling of the breast with milk, the process of nursing and the consequent emptying of the breast, and a refractory period which follows nursing. **life c.** The cycle of reproductive and developmental stages through which individual organisms pass. **mammary c.** The rhythmic changes in breast tissue which correspond to variations in hormonal levels occurring during a menstrual cycle. **masticating c.** The cycle of movements of the mandible during mastication, consisting of opening, movement to the working side, cusp-to-cusp closure through the bolus, and completion of closure to centric occlusion along cusp paths. Also *chewing cycle.* **menstrual c.** A sequence of physiologic changes in the uterine endometrium of certain primates, including humans. It corresponds to variations in estrogen and progesterone secretion in relationship to the growth of an ovarian follicle, ovulation, and the brief persistence followed by regression of a corpus luteum. Unless pregnancy occurs, each cycle is terminated by menstruation. • In general usage, the term *menstrual cycle* covers all the bodily changes that accompany the ovarian and uterine cycles. **mitotic c.** MITOSIS. **mosquito c.** The developmental phase of the malarial parasite that takes place in the mosquito host. Also *Ross cycle.* **nasal c.** The normal variations in the degree of engorgement and secretory activity of the nasal lining occurring at intervals through the day in response to such factors as circadian hormonal activity, changes in temperature, humidity, posture, and emotional influences. **nitrogen c.** The circulation of nitrogen in nature, in which atmospheric

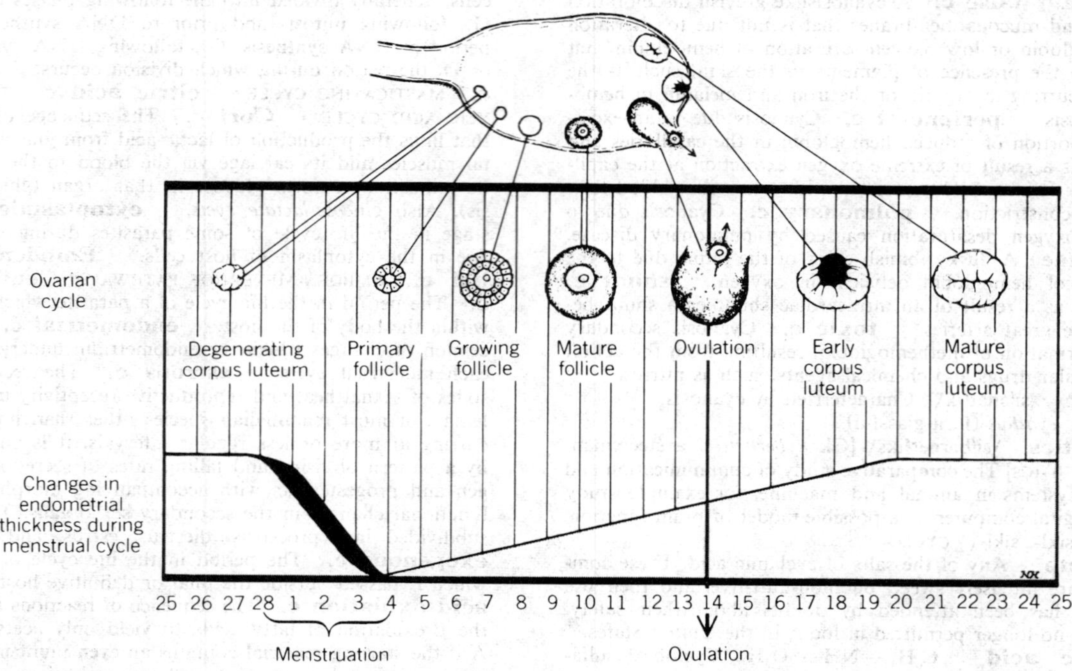


**The menstrual cycle**

dinitrogen is made available to plants by conversion into nitrates and nitrites in lightning flashes and by bacterial reduction to ammonia, and is regenerated by bacterial action on decaying organic matter. **oogenetic c.** OVARIAN CYCLE. **ornithine c.** *Outmoded* UREA CYCLE. **ovarian c.** A sequence of changes in the ovary starting with follicle development followed by ovulation, with subsequent development and regression of a corpus luteum if pregnancy does not ensue. Also *oogenetic cycle.* **pentose phosphate c.** A cyclic sequence of reactions in which carbons 1, 2, and 3 of glucose are oxidized to $CO_2$, with concomitant reduction of NADP. By a series of $C_2$- and $C_3$-transfer reactions, catalyzed by transketolase and transaldolase, two molecules of glucose 6-phosphate are regenerated for every three molecules that enter the sequence. Three molecules of $CO_2$ and one of glyceraldehyde 3-phosphate are also formed. As indicated by the name of the cycle, pentose phosphates are the immediate oxidation products that are formed from glucose 6-phosphate after loss of $CO_2$. These reactions of the cycle are responsible for the supply of pentose phosphates for nucleotide biosynthesis. A variant of this cycle (the Calvin cycle), which in effect operates in reverse, brings about the autotrophic fixation of $CO_2$. **c. per second** The SI derived unit of frequency, the frequency of a periodic phenomenon having a periodic time of one second. Symbol: c/s • It is now generally called *hertz.* **reproductive c.** The physiologic changes occurring in the female reproductive tract from the time of fertilization until delivery of the fetus. **Ross c.** MOSQUITO CYCLE. **sex c.** The set of physiologic changes that occur cyclically in the female reproductive tract of man and animals during the nonpregnant state. Also *sexual cycle.* **tricarboxylic acid c.** A sequence of ten enzymatic reactions by which, in effect, one molecule of acetate as acetyl-CoA is totally oxidized to two molecules of $CO_2$ and water. When coupled to the phosphorylation of ADP via the electron transport chain (oxidative phosphorylation), each turn of the cycle can be accompanied by the formation of 12 molecules of ATP from 12 molecules of ADP and 12 molecules of inorganic phosphate. The cycle is initiated by the condensation of acetyl-CoA with the $C_4$-dicarboxylic acid, oxaloacetate, to yield citrate. In the course of the subsequent reactions the oxaloacetate is regenerated. The cycle occurs in all organisms able to oxidize their food materials totally to $CO_2$ and water. The component enzymes are associated with cell membranes, and in eukaryotes they are usually compartmented in mitochondria. Component steps of the cycle are also important in making the carbon skeletons of many cell components, such as the glutamate and aspartate "families" of amino acids, pyrimidines, and pyrroles. These reactions occur also in anaerobes. This dual role of the cycle may pose problems to microorganisms living on single carbon sources. Also *Krebs cycle, citric acid cycle.* See also ANAPLEROTIC REACTION. **urea c.** A sequence of reactions, occurring in the liver of ureotelic animals, leading to the formation of urea, $CO(NH_2)_2$, which is excreted. The cycle is initiated by the reaction of carbamoyl phosphate with ornithine to form citrulline. This product reacts with aspartate to yield argininosuccinate (with concomitant cleavage of ATP to AMP and pyrophosphate) which, by elimination of fumarate, gives rise to arginine. The enzyme arginase hydrolyzes this amino acid to form urea and re-form the starting material, ornithine. All these reactions except the first occur in the cytoplasm of the liver cell. Also *Krebs-Henseleit cycle, ornithine cycle* (outmoded). **visual c.** The series of photopigments and degradation products that occur in the rods and cones following spectral stimulation.

**cyclectomy** \sīklek′təmē\ [CYCL- + -ECTOMY] Surgical removal of a portion of the ciliary body.

**cyclencephaly** \sī′klensef′əlē\ [CYCL- + Gk *enkephal(os)* the brain + -Y] The developmental fusion of the cerebral hemispheres with varying degrees of obliteration of the sagittal fissure. It is regularly present in cyclopia. Also *cyclopean brain.*

**cyclic** \sik′lik, sī′klik\ [Gk *kyklikos* (from *kyklos* circle, ring) circular] **1** Describing a chemical compound whose molecule contains at least one closed chain (ring) of atoms such as that of benzene. **2** Occurring in regular cycles, as a sequence of symptoms.

**cyclic adenosine monophosphate** ADENOSINE 3′,5′-CYCLIC PHOSPHATE. Abbr. cAMP

**cyclic AMP** ADENOSINE 3′,5′-CYCLIC PHOSPHATE.

**3′,5′-cyclic AMP synthetase** ADENYLATE CYCLASE.

**cyclic nucleotide** An enzymatically derived phosphate ester of a nucleoside in which the phosphate is bound cyclically to the 3′ and 5′ positions on the nucleoside pentose. There are two known physiologically important forms, cyclic AMP and cyclic GMP.

**cyclicotomy** \sī′klikät′əmē\ CYCLOTOMY.

**cyclic phosphate** The compound formed by esterification of two hydroxyl groups in a single molecule with the same residue of phosphoric acid.

**cyclitis** \siklī′tis\ [CYCL- + -ITIS] Inflammation of the ciliary body. **heterochromic c.** A mild inflammation of the anterior uveal tract associated with a relative sympathetic denervation and melanin pigment deficiency, usually affecting only one eye. Also *Fuchs syndrome.* **plastic c.** A severe inflammation of the anterior uveal tract that results in an outpouring of fibrinous debris into the aqueous humor. **serous c.** Inflammation of the anterior uveal tract that permits a fine suspension of plasma proteins to enter the aqueous humor.

**cyclization** \sī′klīzā′shən, sik′-\ [*cycl(e)* + *-iz(e)* + -ATION] A reaction in which two parts of a molecule combine so that a ring of atoms is formed within the molecule, sometimes with addition of another molecule to complete the ring.

**cyclizine** $C_{18}H_{22}N_2$. 1-Diphenylmethyl-4-methylpiperazine. An antihistaminic agent used as an antiemetic and to prevent motion sickness. It is usually given as the hydrochloride or lactate salt.

**cyclo-** \sī′klə-\ [Gk *kyklos* a ring, circle, circular motion] **1** A combining form meaning (1) circular or cyclical; (2) the ciliary body; (3) rotation, torsion. **2** A combining form indicating that a molecule, often of a hydrocarbon, contains a ring. Also *cycl-.*

**cycloartenol** A $C_{30}$ sterol, with a methylene group joined to C-9 and C-10 to form a cyclopropane ring. It is the first steroid made in the pathway by which squalene is converted into sterols in plants. (Lanosterol plays a similar role in animals.) It is made by isomerization of squalene 2,3-epoxide, which is also the precursor of animal sterols.

**cyclobarbital** $C_{12}H_{16}N_2O_3$. 5-(1-Cyclohexen-1-yl)-5-ethyl-2,4,6(1*H*,3*H*,5*H*)-pyrimidinetrione. A barbiturate which is short to intermediate-acting, with sedative and hypnotic activities. It is given orally.

**cyclobutanol** $CH_2—CH_2—CH_2—CH—OH$ (ring: first $CH_2$ bonded to CH). A secondary cyclic alcohol, having a boiling point of 123°C.

**cyclochoroiditis** \-kôr′oidī′tis\ [CYCLO- + CHOROID- + -ITIS] Inflammation of the entire uveal tract.

**cyclocryotherapy** \-krī′əther′əpē\ [CYCLO- + CRYOTHERAPY] Freezing of the ciliary body, performed to reduce

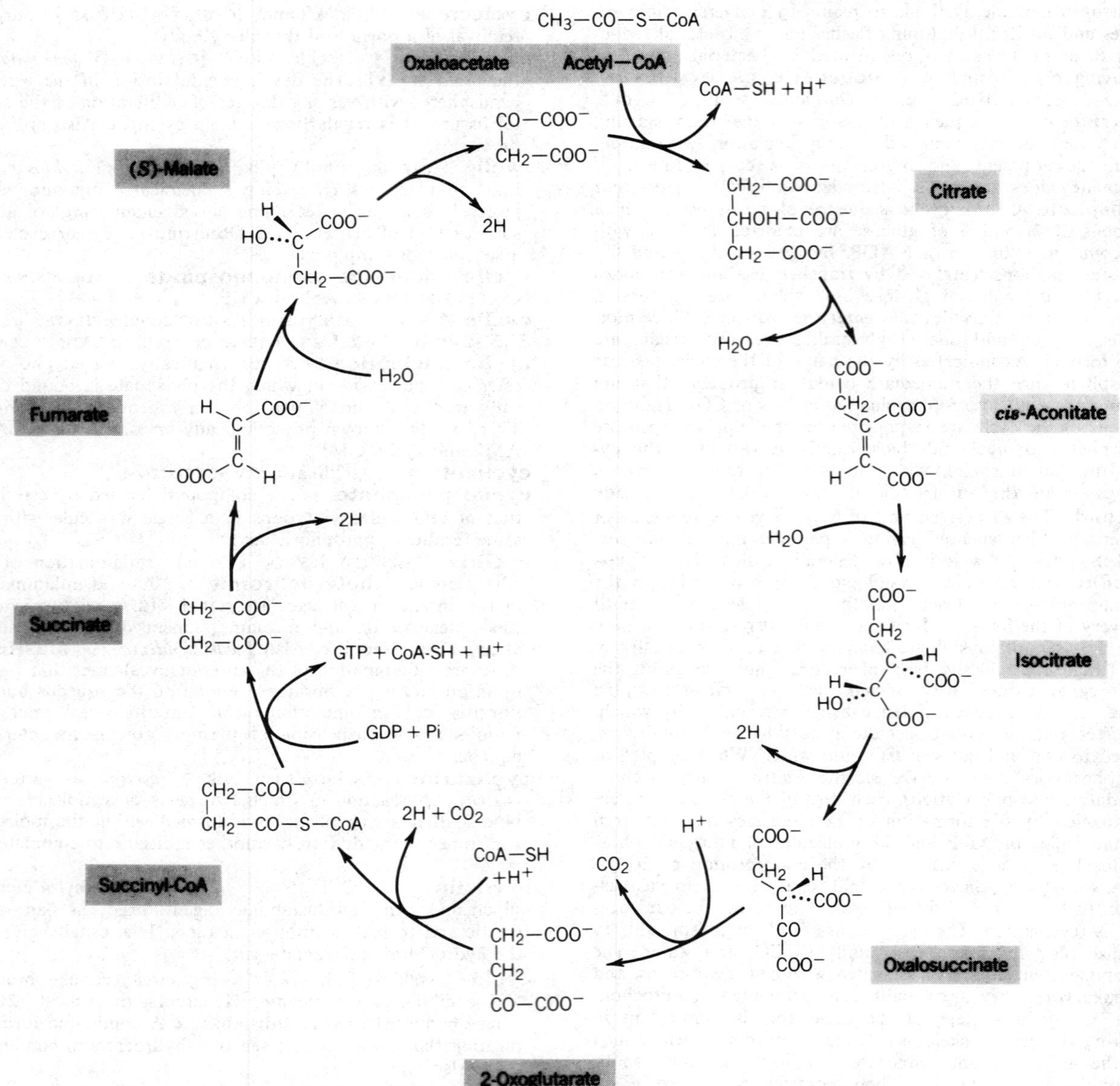


**The tricarboxylic acid cycle** The oxalosuccinate and aconitate remain largely enzyme-bound.

the secretion of aqueous humor in glaucoma.

**cyclodeviation** \-dē′vē·ā′shən\ [CYCLO- + DEVIATION] A torsional fault of eye position, due to rotation upon the anteroposterior axis.

**cyclodialysis** \-dī·al′isis\ [CYCLO- + DIALYSIS] The surgical separation of the ciliary body from the sclera, usually performed in treating glaucoma.

**cyclodiathermy** \-dī′əthur′mē\ Electrical destruction of the ciliary body, performed to reduce the secretion of aqueous humor in glaucoma.

**cycloduction** \-duk′shən\ The rotation of the eye around an anteroposterior axis.

**cycloelectrolysis** \-il′ekträl′isis\ [CYCLO- + ELECTROLYSIS] A glaucoma operation in which the rate of formation of aqueous humor is reduced by damaging the ciliary body with an electrical current.

**cycloheximide** \-hek′simīd\ An antibiotic obtained from certain strains of *Streptomyces griseus* that inhibits the peptidyl transfer reaction of protein synthesis in eukaryotic cells but not in prokaryotes or mitochondria.

**cycloid** \sī′kloid\ [CYCL- + -OID] Recurrent or periodic: used of both the acute, recurring, self-limited mood swings of manic-depressive or bipolar disorders and the less extreme alternations between self-satisfaction and general disaffection that are characteristic of cyclothymic personality.

**cycloisomerase** Any enzyme that catalyzes the addition to a double bond of another part of the substrate molecule, thus forming a ring. Such enzymes are classified as EC 5.5. An example is the enzyme that interconverts glucose 6-phosphate and inositol phosphate.

**cyclokeratitis** \-ker′ətī′tis\ [CYCLO- + KERAT- + -ITIS] Inflammation of both the ciliary body and the cornea. Also *Dalrymple's disease.*

**cyclomethycaine** $C_{22}H_{33}NO_3$. 4-(Cyclohexyloxy)benzoic acid 3-(2-methyl-1-piperidinyl)propyl ester. A local anesthetic usually employed as the hydrochloride or the sulfate. It acts on the skin and mucosa of the rectum and genitourinary tract, but is less effective on the mucous membranes of the mouth, nose, and eye. It is formulated in an aerosol, cream, ointment, jelly, and suppository.

**cyclo-oxygenase** An enzyme present in most cells that catalyzes the formation of the vasoactive prostaglandins thromboxane and prostaglandin $I_2$. The acetylation of cyclo-oxygenase by aspirin is the basis for aspirin's antiplatelet-aggregating role. Also *prostaglandin synthetase.*

**cyclopean** \-pē′ən\ [Gk *Kyklōpei(os)* pertaining to the Cyclopes + English *-an,* adjectival suffix] Pertaining to or marked by the anomaly of having a single midline eye: said of an embryo or fetus.

**cyclopentamine** $C_9H_{19}N$. *N,* α-Dimethylcyclopentaneethanamine, a sympathomimetic drug that produces relatively little central excitation and useful systemic pressor activity. It is used primarily for local application as a vasoconstrictor to the nasal mucous membranes or to the eye. It is usually used as the hydrochloride.

**cyclopentolate hydrochloride** $C_{17}H_{25}NO_3{\cdot}HCl$. α-(1-Hydroxycyclopentyl)benzene-acetic acid 2-(diethylamino)-ethyl ester hydrochloride, a synthetic, antimuscarinic agent with pharmacologic properties much like those of atropine. It is used only in the eye as a mydriatic and cycloplegic medication. It may be used in combination with a sympathomimetic agent.

**cyclophoria** \sī′klōfôr′ē·ə\ [CYCLO- + -PHORIA] A latent torsional deviation of the eyes. **negative c.** Cyclophoria with a tendency to torsion nasalward of the twelve o'clock positions of the eyes. Also *minus cyclophoria.* **positive c.** Cyclophoria with a tendency to torsion temporally of the twelve o'clock positions of the eyes. Also *plus cyclophoria.*

**cyclophosphamide** $C_7H_{15}Cl_2N_2O_2P$. *N,N*-Bis(2-chloroethyl)tetrahydro-2*H*-1,3,2-oxazaphosphorin-2-amine 2-oxide, an antineoplastic agent of the alkylating group, related to the nitrogen mustard mechlorethamine hydrochloride. It is used for treatment of leukemias, lymphomas, and other tumors responsive to nitrogen mustard therapy. It is given orally, but there is also a preparation suitable for injection.

**cyclophrenia** \-frē′nē·ə\ [CYCLO- + -PHRENIA] *Obs.* MANIC-DEPRESSIVE PSYCHOSIS.

**Cyclophyllidea** \-filid′ē·ə\ [CYCLO- + Gk *phyll(on)* a leaf + *-idea,* suffix used for higher taxonomic names] An order of tapeworms (subclass Cestoda) that includes most of the normal and accidental or incidental cestode parasites of humans and domestic animals. They are characterized by a scolex with four rounded suckers and frequently an apical rostellum, marginal genital pores, and compact follicular postovarian vitellaria. There is no uterine pore. The life cycle is complex, involving one or moreintermediate hosts. In a vertebrate first intermediate host, the larvae may be of the cysticercus, coenurus, hydatid, or strobilocercus type. In the invertebrate intermediate host a cysticercoid is found, and in the vertebrate second intermediate host the larva is usually of the plerocercoid type.

**cyclopia** \sīklō′pē·ə\ [*cyclop(s)* + -IA] A developmental defect in which the eyes and the optic tracts show varying degrees of fusion at the midsagittal plane. Secondary malformations affect the orbits, which are also united, and the nose, which usually has the form of a proboscis protruding from the forehead above the fused eye. It is usually associated with cyclencephaly. Also *cyclopean eye, synophthalmia.*

**cycloplegia** \-plē′jə\ [CYCLO- + -PLEGIA] Paralysis of accommodation, as might result from atropinization of the ciliary muscle. Adj. cycloplegic.

**cycloplegic** \-plē′jik\ **1** A parasympatholytic drug that blocks the innervation of the ciliary body. **2** Pertaining to cycloplegia.

**cyclopropane** \-prō′pān\ $C_3H_6$. A flammable gas with a garlic odor, which, when inhaled as a general anesthetic, produces all stages of surgical anesthesia. Its molecule consists of a ring of three —$CH_2$— groups. Also *trimethylene.*

**cyclops** \sī′kläps\ [L, from Gk *kyklōps* (from *kykl(os)* a circle + *ōps* an eye, face) one of the Cyclopes, a mythical race of one-eyed giants] An abnormal fetus or newborn infant with cyclopia. Also *monoculus, synophthalmus.*

**cycloserine** $C_3H_6N_2O_2$. D-4-Amino-3-isoxazolidinone. It is a naturally occurring antibiotic produced by *Streptomyces orchidaceus.* This agent is effective against a wide range of both Gram-positive and Gram-negative bacteria. It is used to treat tuberculosis and is given orally.

**cyclospasm** \sī′kləspazm\ [CYCLO- + SPASM] Continuing contraction of the musculature of the ciliary body. This causes discomfort with use of the eyes and may blur distant vision.

**cyclosporine** $C_{62}H_{111}N_{11}O_{18}$. An orally administered immunosuppressive agent obtained from the fungus *Tolypocladium inflatum.* Commonly used in organ transplantation, as it lacks significant myelotoxicity, it has made cardiac transplantation feasible. It appears to inhibit T cell formation and interleukin-2 production. Also *cyclosporin A.*

**cyclothiazide** $C_{14}H_{16}ClN_3O_4S_2$. A diuretic medication similar in its actions and uses to chlorothiazide.

**cyclothymia** \-thim′ē·ə\ [CYCLO- + -THYMIA] **1** *Imprecise* MANIC-DEPRESSIVE PSYCHOSIS. **2** A state characterized by the traits of the cyclothymic personality.

**cyclotia** \sīklō′shə\ SYNOTIA.

**cyclotome** \sī′klətōm\ [CYCLO- + -TOME] A surgical knife designed for incision of the ciliary body.

**cyclotomy** \sīklät′əmē\ [CYCLO- + -TOMY] A surgical incision of the ciliary body. Also *cyclicotomy.*

**cyclotorsion** \-tôr′shən\ [CYCLO- + TORSION] A rotary movement of the eye in a direction parallel to its equator. Also *wheel rotation.*

**cyclotron** \sī′kləträn\ A device to accelerate charged particles, such as protons or deuterons, to high energies. The particles follow a spiral path inside a vacuum chamber placed between the poles of a large magnet.

**cyclotropia** \sī′klōtrō′pē·ə\ [CYCLO- + -TROPIA] A form of strabismus in which the deviation consists of rotation around an anteroposterior axis. **negative c.** An ocular deviation in which extorsion is present in both eyes. Also *minus cyclotropia.* **positive c.** An ocular deviation in which intorsion occurs in both eyes. Also *plus cyclotropia.*

**cyclozoonosis** \-zō′ənō′sis\ A zoonosis caused by an organism which requires more than one vertebrate host for completion of its life cycle. For example, tapeworms of the genus *Taenia,* such as *T. saginata,* develop as larvae in cattle and other ruminants but live as adults in the human intestine.

**cycrimine hydrochloride** $C_{19}H_{30}ClNO$. α-Cyclopentyl-α-phenyl-1-piperidinepropanol hydrochloride, a drug with central anticholinergic effects similar to those of trihexyphenidyl. It is used to treat parkinsonism.
**Cyd** Symbol for cytidine.
**cyl.** 1 cylinder. 2 cylindrical lens.
**cylinder** [Gk *kylindros* a rolling, cylinder] 1 A solid object circular at top and bottom and having depth, as a disk or column. 2 CYLINDRICAL LENS. **axis c.** AXON. **Bence Jones c.'s** Gelatinous cylindrical masses seen in the seminal channels in the testis. Also *Lallemand-Trousseau bodies, Trousseau-Lallemand bodies.* **crossed c.'s** A device used in refraction and consisting of optical cylinders of equal but opposite strengths positioned with axes oriented at right angles to each other. **Ruffini c.'s** Corpuscular somatosensory terminals in the deep dermal layer and also found associated with hairs and joint capsules. Although once believed to be thermoreceptors, they are probably slowly-adapted sensitive mechanoreceptors. **terminal c.'s** BRUSHES OF RUFFINI.
**cylindroid** \silin′droid\ 1 Appearing or shaped like a cylinder. 2 A cast in the urine of various origins, similar to urinary casts in refractility and shape, except that one end tapers off into a thin tail. Cylindroids may appear in association with urinary casts or in otherwise normal urine from persons without kidney disease.
**cylindroma** \sil′indrō′mə\ 1 A tumor which appears to have cylinders of stroma surrounded by epithelial cells. The stroma typically has a myxoid appearance due to a high content of connective tissue mucins. Also *myxocylindroma.* 2 *Outmoded* ADENOID CYSTIC CARCINOMA. 3 *Outmoded* ECCRINE DERMAL CYLINDROMA. • The term has been rendered outmoded by its more specific designations. It is further not recommended since adenoid cystic carcinoma, a form of cylindroma, is malignant and eccrine dermal cylindroma is benign. **eccrine dermal c.** A benign lobulated sweat gland tumor with epithelial cell groups surrounded by a hyaline membrane. It occurs mainly on the scalp. Also *turban tumor, nevus epitheliomatocylindromatosus, cylindroma* (outmoded).
***Cylindrothorax melanocephala*** \sil′indrōthôr′aks mel′ənōsef′ələ\ An African blister beetle that secretes cantharidin, which can cause severe dermatitis on contact.
**cylindruria** \sil′indroo′rē·ə\ [Gk *kylindr(os)* a rolling, cylinder + -URIA] The excretion of urinary casts.
**cymba** \sim′bə\ [L (from Gk *kymbē* bottom of a drinking vessel), a small boat] A boat-shaped structure. **c. conchae auriculae** [NA] The hollow portion of the concha, above the crus of helix of the auricle of the external ear.
**cymbiform** \sim′bifôrm\ In anatomy, boat-shaped; scaphoid.
**cymbo-** \sim′bō-\ [L *cymba* (from Gk *kymbē* hollow vessel, boat) small boat] A combining form meaning boat-shaped.
**cymbocephaly** \sim′bōsef′əlē\ [CYMBO- + CEPHAL- + -Y ] A developmental deformity of the cranium in which there is concavity of the upper surface or curvature. It may appear prenatally or postnatally.
**cymograph** \sī′mōgraf\ KYMOGRAPH.
**cyn-** \sin-, sīn-\ CYNO-.
**cynanche** \sinan′kē\ [Gk *kynanchē* (from *kyōn*, gen. *kynos*, dog + *anchein* to press tight, esp. the throat, to strangle) a bad kind of sore throat, a dog collar] Severe sore throat often with incipient or existing respiratory obstruction. *Obs.* Also *synanche.*
**cyno-** \sī′nə-\ [Gk *kyōn* (genitive *kynos*) dog] A combining form meaning dog. Also *cyn-.*
**cynocephaly** \-sef′əlē\ [CYNO- + CEPHAL- + -Y] A developmental deformity of the head in which the cranium slopes backwards from the face in such manner as to suggest the head of a dog.
**cynodontism** \sī′nədäntizm\ The property of having a tooth form in which the pulp cavity is narrow. Compare TAURODONTISM.
**cynomolgus** \-mäl′gəs\ [New L, alteration of L *cynamolgus* a member of a Lybian tribe (from Gk *kynamolgos* a dog milker, from *kyōn* dog + *amolg(ē)* milking] A popular name for the monkey *Macaca fascicularis* (previously *M. irus*), frequently used in laboratory research. It is easier to handle than the rhesus, *M. mulatta.*. Also *crab-eating macaque.*
***Cynomyia*** \-mī′yə\ A genus of bluebottle flesh flies that deposit ova in decaying meat and open wounds, which can result in secondary myiasis.
**Cyon** [Elie de *Cyon*, Russian physiologist, 1843–1912] Cyon's nerve. See under AORTIC NERVE.
**cyproheptadine hydrochloride** $C_{21}H_{22}ClN$. 4-(5-*H*-Dibenzo[*a,d*]cyclohepten-5-ylidene)-1-methylpiperidine hydrochloride, a tricyclic antihistaminic agent that is useful in a variety of allergic conditions. It is used to treat pruritic dermatoses, and it is employed as an antihistaminic medication. It is given orally.
**cyrtoid** \sur′toid\ Having the curvature or shape of a hump.
**cyrtosis** \sərtō′sis\ [Gk *kyrtōsis* (from *kyrtos* convex, humped) a hump, convexity] 1 KYPHOSIS. 2 A bony deformity.
**Cys** Symbol for cysteine.

# cyst

**cyst** \sist\ [Gk *kystis* (from *kyein* to contain, be pregnant) the bladder, a bag, pouch] 1 Any closed cavity or sac lined by a definable epithelium or abnormal tissue and usually containing a fluid or other material. 2 A bladder. For defs. 1 and 2 also *cystis* (obs.). 3 A capsule or membranous protective sheath or covering of parasitic origin and enclosing a larval, resting, reproductive, or transmission stage of a parasite. Examples among helminths include hydatid cyst, among protozoa infective stages of *Entamoeba* and *Giardia* or tissue cysts enclosing progeny of such sporozoan parasites as *Toxoplasma* and *Sarcocystis.* **allantoic c.** A cystic swelling of the urachus. The latter, derived from the allantoic duct, usually retrogresses, but localized remnants of the endodermal lining may remain and become cystic. Also *urachal cyst.* **alveolar hydatid c.** A hydatid cyst formed by larvae of the tapeworm *Echinoccus multilocularis,* which grows by exogenous budding unconfined by an outer laminated membrane. The presence of this multilocular cyst, most common in the liver, is usually fatal in humans and animals. Microtine rodents (voles, lemmings, and the like) usually serve as the intermediate host bearing the cyst, and foxes as the normal final host. Also *multilocular hydatid cyst, Virchow's hydatid.* **amnionic c.** A cyst formed by the fusion of amniotic folds with accumulation of fluid. **aneurysmal bone c.** A tumorlike osteolytic lesion composed of blood-filled spaces separated by bony or fibrous trabeculae with osteoclasts. The lesion can develop rapidly and reach a large size. Also *aneurysmal giant cell tumor.* **angioblastic c.** ANGIOCYST. **antral c.** A mucous

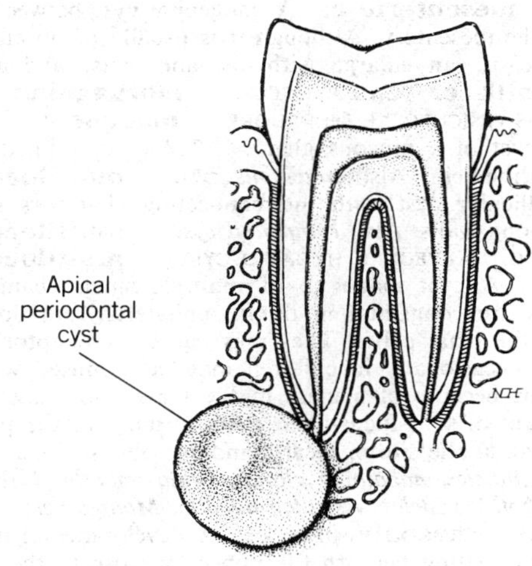


or retention cyst arising in the lining membrane of the maxillary sinus and sometimes expanding to fill the cavity of the sinus. **apical periodontal c.** A periodontal cyst arising at the apex of a tooth. Also *dental cyst, periapical cyst, apical cyst, root-end cyst.* **apoplectic c.** A cystic cavity formed by the organization of extravasated blood, especially in association with brain hemorrhage. **arachnoid c.** A sac of intracranial or spinal arachnoid membrane usually containing cerebrospinal fluid and often exerting pressure on the brain or spinal cord. It may be congenital or acquired. **Baker c.** POPLITEAL BURSITIS. **Blessig c.'s** A benign, microscopic cystic degeneration of the peripheral retina, almost universally present, even in children. Also *Iwanoff cysts, Blessig's lacunae.* **bone c.** **1** Any fluid-filled cyst within bone. Also *osteocystoma.* **2** TRAUMATIC BONE CYST. **branchial c.** A branchiogenous cyst, the least uncommon variety of which arises from the second branchial cleft and is present in the neck as a symptomless, smooth, rounded, usually fluctuant swelling below and behind the angle of the jaw. Also *branchial cleft cyst, cervical hydrocele.* **bronchial c.** BRONCHOGENIC CYST. **bronchogenic c.** A cyst of developmental origin derived from the bronchial tree. Also *bronchial cyst, bronchopulmonary cyst.* **bursal c.** A cyst occurring within a bursa. **cervical c.** Any one of a variety of cysts occurring in the neck of which the most prevalent are branchial and thyroglossal cysts. **chocolate c.** A cyst containing old, organized blood and clots. It is typically seen in the ovary where it results from cyclic bleeding from endometriosis. **choledochal c.** A congenital cystic dilatation of the common bile duct. Also *choledochus cyst.* **chyle c.** A focal dilatation of a lymphatic vessel filled with inspissated lymph, occasionally found in the mesentery. **colloid c.** A cyst lined with columnar and mucous epithelium and filled with a jellylike substance. Within the brain, it is invariably found in the anterior aspect of the third ventricle, where it may cause hydrocephalus and headaches. The lesion grows slowly and is amenable to surgical excision. **colloid c. of third ventricle** A congenital cyst believed to arise from the anlage of the paraphysis. It contains a gelatinous material and produces symptoms by intermittent blockade of one or more foramina of Monro, resulting in dilatation of the lateral ventricles. **compound c.** MULTILOCULAR CYST. **congenital c.'s of the kidney** A rare congenital anomaly manifested by the formation of single or multiple unilocular cysts in the renal parenchyma. The cysts do not communicate with the renal pelvis. They may be confused with parenchymal tumors. **congenital preauricular c.** A subcutaneous cyst developing in front of the ear from epithelial remnants of the first ectodermal branchial cleft. **congenital c. of the prostate** An unusual congenital cystic formation in the prostate due to a failure of communication between the mesonephric ducts and vesicourethral anlage. **congenital c. of the seminal vesicles** A rare, congenital, anomalous cystic lesion of the seminal vesicles which may produce bladder neck obstruction. **congenital c. of the urethra** A rare, congenital, cystic lesion of the urethra occurring at any point from the external meatus to the bladder outlet. It may cause urethral obstruction. **corpus luteum c.** An ovarian cyst formed by an accumulation of serous fluid within a persistent corpus luteum. **Cowper's c.** A cyst of one of the bulbourethral glands. **craniobuccal c.** RATHKE CYST. **craniopharyngeal duct c.** RATHKE CYST. **cutaneous c.** EPIDERMAL CYST. **cuticular c.** EPIDERMAL CYST. **daughter c.** A cyst present within the lumen of a larger cystic structure. It is exemplified by the brood capsules in the hydatid cyst of the tapeworm *Echinococcus granulosus.* Also *secondary cyst.* **dental c.** APICAL PERIODONTAL CYST. **dentigerous c.** A follicular cyst surrounding the crown of an unerupted tooth or, more rarely, surrounding an odontome. **dermoid c.** A cyst whose wall contains elements of skin, including a squamous epithelial lining, hair follicles, and sebaceous glands. Neuroectodermal, endodermal, and mesodermal components may also be present. It is considered to be a form of mature teratoma and may be found in a variety of organs but is especially common in the ovary, occurring much less frequently in the testis. In the skin, dermoid cysts are most common on the face in the region of the facial clefts. Also *dermoid, inclusion dermoid.* **dermoid c. with malignant transformation** TERATOMA WITH MALIGNANT TRANSFORMATION. **dilatation c.** A cyst formed by expansion of a pre-existing cavity. **distention c.** RETENTION CYST. **duplication c.** A localized duplication of the alimentary canal, attached to or originating from any part of the canal from the oral cavity to the anus. It may be spherical, with no lumenal continuity with the alimentary canal, or it may be tubular and have fistulalike continuity with the lumen of the adjacent gut. **echinococcus c.** HYDATID CYST. **endometrial implantation c.** A site of endometriosis, usually on the peritoneal surface, that has undergone cystic transformation due to local accumulation of secretions. **enteric c.** A congenital cyst lined by intestinal mucosa and sometimes the whole intestinal wall. These cysts may occur in two locations, the abdomen and the mediastinum. In the former they develop in close apposition to the alimentary canal and usually do not communicate with the lumen of the gut. They are more common in the posterior mediastinum, where they are usually attached to the esophagus and are often associated with vertebral malformations. **enterogenous mediastinal c.** PARAESOPHAGEAL CYST. **ependymal c.** A cyst arising from the ependymal lining of the ventricles of the brain or of the central canal of the spinal cord. **epidermal c.** A cyst lined with keratinizing stratified squamous epithelium. It is found most frequently in the skin. Also *cutaneous cyst, cuticular cyst, epidermal inclusion cyst, wen, Keratin cyst.* **epidermoid c.** A cyst lined with squamous stratified epithelium, but without associated cutaneous glands and hair, and containing keratin, often in concentric layers. It is commonly a cyst of the skin, as a sebaceous cyst, but also occurs at the base of the brain and in the middle-ear cleft (cholesteatoma). **c. of the epididymis** A benign cystic growth on the epididymis appearing either as a retention cyst containing spermatozoa or a simple, unilocular serous cyst. **epithelial c.** A cystic space lined by epithelium. **epoophoral c.** PAROVARIAN CYST. **eruption c.** A dentigerous cyst associated with an erupting tooth. **extra-axial leptomeningeal c.'s** Arachnoid cysts of developmental origin occurring in the posterior fossa of the skull in cases of the Dandy-Walker syndrome. **extravasation c.** A cyst resulting from hemorrhage into the tissues. **exudation c.** A cystic structure produced by the accumulation of excessive amounts of exudates or secretory fluids in a closed cavity. **false c.** PSEUDOCYST. **fissural c.** Any cyst formed by the proliferation of epithelium included within connective tissue present at union lines of bones, particularly in the oral region. **follicular c.** 1 A cyst resulting from the occlusion of a follicle, especially a graafian follicle that fails to rupture and is distended by serous fluid. 2 A cyst formed by a dental follicle. See under DENTIGEROUS CYST. **ganglion c.** SYNOVIAL GANGLION. **Gartner c.** A cystic enlargement of a remnant or small segment of Gartner's duct. Also *gartnerian cyst.* **gas c.** A cyst with gaseous contents, generally the result of bacterial gas production within a closed space. **germinal inclusion c.** An ovarian cyst formed by the invagination and isolation of small segments of the germinal epithelium from the ovarian surface. **globulomaxillary c.** A fissural cyst arising at the junction of the globular and maxillary processes. **glomerular c.** A renal cyst that contains a glomerulus in its cavity, occasionally present in polycystic renal disease. **hemorrhagic c.** A cystic structure formed by the organization of a hematoma, or the result of bleeding into a preexisting cyst. **hydatid c.** A cyst formed by the larval stage of tapeworms of the genus *Echinococcus.* Also *echinococcus cyst, proliferation cyst, hydatid.* See also UNILOCULAR HYDATID CYST, ALVEOLAR HYDATID CYST, ECHINOCOCCOSIS. **implantation c.** A cyst lined with stratified squamous epithelium that develops as a result of the displacement of epithelial tissue into neighboring structures. **inclusion c.** A cystic lesion found in connective tissue and epithelial tissue. **intracranial parasitic c.** Any cyst of parasitic origin, such as a hydatid cyst, occurring within the cranial cavity. **intrapituitary c.** A cyst developing within the pituitary gland. **Iwanoff c.'s** BLESSIG CYSTS. **keratin c.** EPIDERMAL CYST. **lacteal c.** GALACTOCELE. **laryngeal c.** Any cyst arising from any part of the larynx. Most are mucous or retention cysts arising occasionally from the mucosa of the epiglottis or the laryngeal ventricle or elsewhere. Rarely congenital laryngeal cysts may present at birth giving rise to life-threatening laryngeal obstruction. **lateral c.** PERIODONTAL CYST. **lutein c.** A cyst of the ovary formed from the corpus luteum. **median anterior maxillary c.** The commonest inclusion cyst of the maxilla, located near the incisive canal. It is lined by squamous epithelium or columnar ciliated epithelium, and probably originates from remnants of the nasopalatine duct. Also *median maxillary cyst, nasopalatine duct cyst, nasopalatine cyst.* **median palatal c.** A cyst arising in the midline of the hard palate from epithelium included along the line of fusion of the palatal processes of the maxillae. **meibomian c.** An enlargement of a meibomian gland within the tarsal plate of the eyelid. Also *tarsal cyst.* **mesenteric c.** A congenital cyst between the leaves of the mesentery. Although it is usually of no clinical significance, it can enlarge with age and cause abdominal pain. **milk c.** GALACTOCELE. **morgagnian c.'s** APPENDICES VESICULOSAE EPOÖPHORI. **mucous c.** 1 A retention cyst of a mucous gland. 2 Any cyst filled primarily with mucin. Also *mucinous cyst.* **multilocular c.** A follicular cyst with interconnecting chambers separated by bony walls. Also *compound cyst.* **multilocular hydatid c.** ALVEOLAR HYDATID CYST. **multilocular renal c.** A cyst made up of multiple small chambers. Such cysts are congenital in origin, unilateral, and do not open into the renal pelvis. They may cause no symptoms or harm, but occasionally in children may be confused with a renal tumor because of a mass in the flank and hematuria. **nabothian c.'s** Mucus-filled cysts formed on the portio of the cervix at the site of local glandular obstructions. Also *nabothian follicles, nabothian glands, ovula nabothi, Naboth's ovules, Naboth's vesicles, vesiculae nabothi, Montgomery's cups* (outmoded). **nasoalveolar c.** A developmental inclusion cyst presenting beneath the upper lip close to the midline in the alveolabial sulcus, or else adjacent to this locality in the floor of the nasal vestibule. Also *nasolabial cyst.* **nasolabial c.** NASOALVEOLAR CYST. **nasopalatine c.** MEDIAN ANTERIOR MAXILLARY CYST. **nasopalatine duct c.** MEDIAN ANTERIOR MAXILLARY CYST. **neural c.** Any developmental cyst arising in or in relation to the primitive neural canal. **neurenteric c.** A developmental teratomatous cyst arising in the posterior mediastinum or from the posterior abdominal wall in the midline and containing both neural and visceral elements. There is often an attachment to the spinal dura mater. **odontogenic c.** A cyst arising from odontogenic tissues, such as the dental lamina or the enamel organ. **oil c.** A cyst filled with oily material. It may result from degeneration of its lining cells or from alteration of its original contents such as sebum or lymph. **omental c.** A thin-walled cyst between the leaves of the omentum. It may be congenital, or acquired as a result of infection or trauma. **ovarian c.** A cyst of the ovary, usually implying a benign one. **paradental c.** PERIODONTAL CYST. **paraesophageal c.** A mediastinal reduplication cyst or inclusion cyst, originating from the dorsal foregut. It is attached to the wall of the esophagus or occasionally embedded within its wall. Also *enterogenous mediastinal cyst.* **c. of the paramesonephric duct** A congenital cystic dilatation of a remnant of the paramesonephric duct located in the perineal midline. **paranephric c.** A cyst located in the perirenal fat. **parapyelitic c.'s** Clusters of cysts, probably congenital, located near the upper ureters, which may cause deformity and compression of the renal pelvis, pain, obstruction, and infection. **paratracheal c.** A mediastinal bronchogenic cyst originating from the ventral foregut. It is located close to the trachea or main-stem bronchi. **paratubal c.** A cyst lying in the broad ligament adjacent to the uterine tube. It represents a remnant of the mesonephric duct or tubules. **parovarian c.** A cyst of the epoöphoron. Also *epoophoral cyst, paroophoritic cyst.* **pearl c.** A mass of epithelial cells growing within the anterior chamber or iris as a result of traumatic implantation of surface cells inside the eye. **periapical c.** APICAL PERIODONTAL CYST. **pericardial c.** A cyst arising from the pericardium, usually benign and containing clear fluid. Also *springwater cyst.* **periodontal c.** A cyst arising in the periodontal ligament from the epithelial rests. Also *lateral cyst, paradental cyst, radicular cyst, radiculodental cyst, root cyst.* **perirenal c.** A retroperitoneal cyst, occurring singly or multiply, possibly derived from the mesonephric ducts, usually on the left side and often associated with polycythemia. Perirenal cysts may attain a large size and are often felt as large masses which displace abdominal organs and cause pressure symptoms. **perisalpingian c.** The cystic dilatation of any of the remnants of the embryonic mesonephric ducts in the mesosalpinx between the ovary and the uterus. **phaeomycotic c.** A deeply pigmented (brown) subcutaneous granuloma caused by fungi of the form-genus *Phoma.*. **pilar c.** SEBACEOUS CYST. **piliferous c.** A dermoid cyst, especially one of the sacrococcygeal area. **pilonidal c.** PILONIDAL SINUS. **placental c.** A cystlike formation in the chorionic plate of the placenta, secondary to degeneration and liquefaction in the placental septa or at sites of intervillous fibrin. **porencephalic c.** A cyst within the cerebral substance communicating with the lateral ventricle. Some such cysts are congenital but most are a late sequel of head injury or infarction with resorption of the damaged cerebral substance. **post-traumatic leptomeningeal c.** A localized collection of cerebrospinal fluid surrounded by leptomeningeal adhesions and resulting from injury. **preauricular c.** A rarely occurring branchiogenous cyst located in front of the crus of helix of the external ear and usually associated with a preauricular sinus. **primordial c.** An odontogenic cyst arising from the enamel organ and replacing the tooth which would have been formed. **proliferation c.** HYDATID CYST. **pyelogenic renal c.** CALICEAL DIVERTICULUM. **radicular c.** PERIODONTAL CYST. **radiculodental c.** PERIODONTAL CYST. **Rathke c.** An epithelium-lined cyst in the sella turcica or between the sella and the nasopharynx. It is thought to represent a cystic dilatation of a remnant of the embryonic Rathke's pouch. Also *Rathke's cleft cyst, pituitary diverticulum cyst, Rathke's pouch cyst.* **renal c.** Any saclike structure containing fluid in a kidney. It may be single or multiple, simple or multilocular, of various origins, and may be innocuous or characteristic of medullary cystic or polycystic diseases. **residual c.** A cyst remaining after the extraction of a tooth or growing from cells left behind after the removal of a cyst. **retention c.** A cyst that results from obstruction to the normal outflow of a glandular secretion. Also *secretory cyst, distention cyst.* **retroperitoneal c.** Any cyst lying between the parietal peritoneum and the body wall, variously containing urine, lymph, blood, glandular secretions, or seromucinous material. Some may reach large size, as for example mesonephric and paramesonephric remnants. **root c.** PERIODONTAL CYST. **root-end c.** APICAL PERIODONTAL CYST. **sacral c.** A congenital cyst containing cerebrospinal fluid and developing within the sacral canal. Such cysts may extend into and erode the sacral bone and may also cause compression of sacral nerve roots. Also *Tarlov cyst, sacral perineurial cyst.* **Sampson c.** ENDOMETRIOMA. **sarcosporidian c.** SARCOCYST. **sebaceous c.** A common cyst containing keratin and formed by the obstruction of the duct of a sebaceous gland, as on the scalp. It is lined by squamouslike cells which swell as they approach the cavity and lose distinct cell borders. Also *pilar cyst, trichilemmal cyst, wen.* **secondary c.** DAUGHTER CYST. **secretory c.** RETENTION CYST. **seminal c.** A cyst containing semen, usually found in the testicle. **septal c.** CAVUM SEPTI PELLUCIDI. **sequestration c.** 1 A cyst originating in epithelial cells that have been driven or displaced into or beneath the dermis. 2 Any cyst arising from extraneous tissue sequestered anywhere in the body, or from ectopic embryonic cells that have been incorporated in the wrong site. **serous c.** A cyst filled with clear, serous fluid. **single c.** SOLITARY RENAL CYST. **soap c.** A cystic collection of yellow fatty matter in the breast. **solitary bone c.** A bone space of doubtful origin in the metaphyses of long bones of children. It may be empty or filled with fluid and have a thin connective-tissue lining. **solitary renal c.** A solitary cyst of the renal cortex, varying in size and containing fluid which resembles plasma transudate. A solitary renal cyst may be confused with a renal tumor. Also *single cyst.* **c. of the spermatic cord** A benign cyst of the funiculus spermaticus resulting from failure of obliteration of the processus vaginalis. **springwater c.** PERICARDIAL CYST. **steatoid c.** A small, cutaneous cyst formed by the accumulation of sebaceous material. **sublingual c.** *Seldom used* RANULA. **subsynovial c.** A local accumulation of synovial fluid adjacent to and arising from a joint. **synovial c.** SYNOVIAL GANGLION. **Tarlov c.** SACRAL CYST. **tarsal c.** MEIBOMIAN CYST. **thecal c.** A fluid distension of a tendon sheath. **theca-lutein c.** A follicular cyst of the ovary associated with hydatidiform mole, choriocarcinoma, and some pregnancies. The cyst is generally multiple and bilateral. It is produced by chorionic gonadotropin secreted by the trophoblastic tissue. Grossly, it is bluish and multilocular. Microscopically, the cyst shows marked luteinization of the theca interna zone. **thymic c.'s** Cystic structures within or along the route of embryonic descent of the thymus. They are sometimes lined by low, ciliated, columnar epithelia. **thyroglossal c.** The cystic dilatation of a remnant of the embryonic thyroglossal duct, located between the site of original thyroid invagination near the base of the tongue and the definitive location of the thyroid gland. Found usually in the young, it may be congenital or develop at any age, and grow slowly without symptoms. Rupture may result in a thyroglosssal fistula to mucous membrane or skin. **Tornwaldt c.** BURSA PHARYNGEALIS. **traumatic bone c.** An air space in a bone, usually the mandible. It is thought to be the result of injury causing extravasation of blood, followed by its resorption but without new bone replacement. Also *unicameral bone cyst, bone cyst.* **trichilemmal c.** SEBACEOUS CYST. **true c.** A cyst lined by epithelium and not resulting from dilatation of a previously existing cavity or duct. **tubo-ovarian c.** A cyst involving the fallopian tube and ovary. **tubular c.** The cylindrical dilatation of an occluded duct or tube. Also *tubulocyst.* **umbilical c.** VITELLOINTESTINAL CYST. **unicameral c.** UNILOCULAR CYST. **unicameral bone c.** 1 TRAUMATIC BONE CYST. 2 A solitary benign fluid-filled cyst that arises at the end of an immature long bone. **unilocular c.** A cystic structure having a single cavity. Also *unicameral cyst.* **unilocular hydatid c.** A cyst formed by *Echinococcus granulosus* containing a single fluid-filled cavity or loculus lined with a germinative interior layer and externally enclosed in a laminated protective membrane or sheath. The cyst is filled with hydatid fluid and the infective scoleces of immature worms (hydatid sand). **urachal c.** ALLANTOIC CYST. **urinary c.** A cyst that contains urine. **vitellointestinal c.** A cyst resulting from persistence of a segment of the vitelline duct. It is usually seen in infants and most commonly appears as a mass in the umbilicus. Also *umbilical cyst, vitelline cyst, enterocystoma.* **wolffian c.** Distention of any of the wolffian vestiges by a clear, serous fluid. The most common of these are the parovarian cysts that are remnants of the wolffian ducts, lined by a cuboidal or columnar epithelium.

**cyst-** \sist-\ CYSTO-.

**cystadenocarcinoma** \sistad′ənōkär′sinō′mə\ An adenocarcinoma containing grossly visible cystic cavities lined by tumor. Papillary neoplastic structures may project into the cysts (papillary cystadenocarcinoma). It is most frequently found in the ovary as a serous or mucinous tumor. Also *cystocarcinoma* (outmoded). **mucinous c.** A cystadenocarcinoma with mucin-producing epithelium. It is typically found in the ovary. Also *pseudomucinous cystadenocarcinoma, pseudomucinous cystocarcinoma.* **papillary c.** An adenocarcinoma with a papillary growth pattern and a prominent cystic nature. It typically occurs in the ovary. **pseudomucinous c.** MUCINOUS CYSTADENOCARCINOMA. **serous papillary c.** PAPILLARY CARCINOMA OF THE OVARY.

**cystadenofibroma** \sistad′ənōfībrō′mə\ An adenofibroma with a prominent cystic component.

**cystadenoma** \sis′tadənō′mə\ [CYST- + ADENOMA] An adenoma containing grossly visible epithelial lined cysts. It is typically found in the ovary, pancreas, and salivary glands. Also *adenocystoma, adenocele, cystoadenoma.* **c. cylindrocellulare celloides ovarii** MUCINOUS CYSTADENOMA OF THE OVARY. **mucinous c.** A cystadenoma with mucin-producing epithelium, typically found in the ovary. Also *pseudomucinous cystadenoma.* **mucinous c. of the ovary** An ovarian neoplasm occurring principally in middle life characterized by the formation of large, generally multiloculated cystic masses. This tumor is composed of nonciliated, tall, columnar mucous-secreting epithelium producing a gelatinous material rich in glycoproteins and mucin. Microscopically, the tumor cells have basal nuclei and mucous-filled cytoplasms. Also *cystadenoma cylindrocellulare celloides ovarii, colloid ovarian cystoma, colloid ovarian tumor.* **papillary c.** An adenoma with both papillary and cystic characteristics, especially an ovarian tumor. **papillary c. lymphomatosum** ADENOLYMPHOMA. **papillary serous c.** A serous cystadenoma with epithelium arranged as papillae. **c. phyllodes** CYSTOSARCOMA PHYLLODES. **pseudomucinous c.** MUCINOUS CYSTADENOMA. **serous c.** A cystadenoma of the ovary with serous epithelium.

**cystadenosarcoma** \sistad′ənōsärkō′mə\ *Obs.* CYSTOSARCOMA PHYLLODES.

**cystalgia** \sistal′jə\ [CYST- + -ALGIA] Pain in the urinary bladder. Also *cystodynia.*

**cystathionase** *Outmoded* CYSTATHIONINE γ-LYASE.

**cystathionine** HOOC—CH($NH_2$)—$CH_2$—S—$CH_2$—$CH_2$—CH($NH_2$)—COOH. A sulfur compound formed from serine and homocysteine. Cystathionine γ-lyase catalyzes its cleavage to cysteine, ammonia, and 2-oxobutyrate. These reactions lie on the pathway of the catabolism of methionine to succinyl-CoA.

**cystathionine γ-lyase** An enzyme (EC 4.4.1.1) that catalyzes the hydrolysis of cystathionine to form cysteine, ammonia, and 2-oxobutyrate. This enzyme is of widespread occurrence. Its action in mammals ensures that cysteine is not needed if the diet contains adequate methionine. It contains pyridoxal phosphate. Also *cystathionase* (outmoded).

**cystathionine β-synthetase** An enzyme (EC 4.2.1.22) that catalyzes the formation of cystathionine from serine and homocysteine. This step precedes the action of cystathionine γ-lyase in the mammalian pathway by which cysteine is synthesized.

**cystathioninuria** \sis′təthī′ōninoo′rē·ə\ **1** The abnormal urinary excretion of the amino acid cystathionine. **2** An autosomal recessive disorder in the metabolism of sulfur-containing amino acids caused by deficient activity of γ-cystathionase. The clinical effects in homozygotes are uncertain, and most such individuals are normal except for the urinary excretion of cystathionine.

**cystauchenotomy** \sis′tôkənät′əmē\ [CYST- + Gk *auchēn,* gen. *aucheno(s),* neck, throat + -TOMY] Incision of the bladder neck.

**cysteamine** MERCAPTOETHYLAMINE.

**cystectomy** \sistek′təmē\ [CYST- + -ECTOMY] **1** Partial or total removal of the urinary bladder or gallbladder. **2** Surgical removal of a cyst. **radical c.** Complete excision of the bladder and surrounding tissues, including the prostate, as in the treatment of cancer of the bladder. **simple c.** Surgical excision of the bladder.

**cysteic acid** $HO_3S$—$CH_2$—CH($NH_2$)—COOH. An acid formed by the oxidation of cysteine or cystine to the corresponding sulfonic acid. This oxidation may be performed on these residues in proteins before analysis to determine sequence or composition.

**cysteine** HS—$CH_2$—CH($NH_2$)COOH. One of the 20 amino acids that can be incorporated into proteins. Its side chain is slightly deprotonated at neutral pH (p$K$ about 9) to form one of the most nucleophilic groups in proteins. The thiol group of cysteine participates in the reaction of glyceraldehyde-3-phosphate dehydrogenase and of papain. In extracellular proteins, the cysteine residues are usually oxidized to cystine and so provide cross-linking between chains. Peptides containing cysteine are unstable to air, but cysteine residues in proteins are often in the interior of the molecules and this can make the proteins that contain them stable to air.

**cystencephalus** \sis′tensef′ələs\ A fetus or newborn infant with an extreme degree of internal hydrocephalus, such that the cerebral hemispheres are little more than a fluid-filled sac. The more extreme cases probably represent hydranencephaly instead of hydrocephalus.

**cysti-** \sis′tē-\ CYSTO-.

**cystic** \sis′tik\ **1** Relating to or characterized by cysts. **2** Relating to a bladder (urinary bladder or gallbladder).

**cysticerci** \sis′tisur′sī\ Plural of CYSTICERCUS.

**cysticercoid** \sis′tisur′koid\ [*cysticerc(us)* + -OID] The larval form of certain cyclophyllidean tapeworms found in its arthropod intermediate host, usually an insect. It differs from the cysticercus by the lack of a fluid-filled bladder and the presence of a cercomer, although as with other final-stage cestode larvae, it contains the scolex of the future mature tapeworm. Also *cercoid.*

**cysticercosis** \sis′tisərkō′sis\ [*cysticerc(us)* + -OSIS] A disease caused by cysticerci of the pork tapeworm (*Taenia solium*) in muscle, the central nervous system, the eye, heart, or subcutaneous tissues. An incidental form of parasitic infection in man, it is caused by the hatching of eggs in the intestine either directly from a concurrent infection or through ingestion of eggs in human feces. Brain involvement can result in jacksonian epilepsy and severe central nervous system damage from blockage of ventricular fluid or displacement of brain tissue. Praziquantel and corticosteroids have given promising therapeutic results. Also *cysticercus disease.* **c. with muscle hypertrophy** Multiple cysticerci in the voluntary muscles giving rise to myopathy and diffuse muscle hypertrophy. **racemose form c.** Multiple cysticerci clustered like a bunch of grapes. This form is sometimes found in the fourth cerebral ventricle where it gives rise to recurrent lymphocytic meningitis and hydrocephalus. **spinal c.** Cysticerci in the spinal canal or spinal cord.

***Cysticercus*** \sis′tisur′kəs\ [CYSTI- + Gk *kerkos* tail] A former taenioid genus including the bladderworms, which are now known to be the larval stage of cestodes of the genus *Taenia* and related forms. ● This generic name and the several specific names that it enters into are still sometimes used when it is convenient to do so. Sometimes they are printed in roman rather than italic type in recognition of their unofficial status, for example, Cysticercus bovis. ***C. bovis*** The larval form of *Taenia saginata,* a tapeworm of man, found as cysticerci in the muscles of cattle. ***C. cellulosae*** The larval form of *Taenia solium,* a tapeworm of man, found mainly in the muscles of pigs but also of dogs and man.

**cysticercus** \sis'tisur'kəs\ [See CYSTICERCUS.] (*pl.* cysticerci) The larval form of certain taenioid tapeworms, which consists of a scolex invaginated in a bladderlike, fluid-filled, pea-sized membranous sheath, encysted in various tissues of the mammalian intermediate host. Also *bladderworm, measle.*

**cysticolithectomy** \sis'tikō'lithek'təmē\ [CYSTIC + *o* + LITH- + -ECTOMY] Surgical removal of a gallstone by means of an incision in the cystic duct.

**cysticolithotripsy** \sis'tikōlith'ōtrip'sē\ [CYSTIC + *o* + LITHO- + -TRIPSY] The crushing of a stone in the cystic duct.

**cysticorrhaphy** \sis'tikôr'əfē\ [CYSTIC + *o* + -RRHAPHY ] A suturing of the cystic duct.

**cysticotomy** \sis'tikät'əmē\ [CYSTIC + *o* + -TOMY] Incision of the cystic duct.

**cystides** \sis'tidēz\ Plural of CYSTIS.

**cystido-** \sis'tədō-\ CYSTO-.

**cystidotrachelotomy** \-trā'kelät'əmē\ [CYSTIDO- + TRACHELO- + -TOMY] Incision of the bladder neck.

**cystifellotomy** \sis'tifelät'əmē\ [CYSTI- + L *fel,* gen. *fellis* gall, gall bladder, bile + *o* + -TOMY] CHOLECYSTOTOMY.

**cystiferous** \sistif'ərəs\ Denoting the presence of cysts.

**cystiform** \sis'tifôrm\ CYSTOID.

**cystine** HOOC—CH($NH_2$)—$CH_2$—S—S—$CH_2$—CH($NH_2$)—COOH. The disulfide formed by removal of hydrogen from the —SH groups of two molecules of cysteine. Its residues provide cross-links in proteins between polypeptide chains, and these contribute to the mechanical properties of many proteins, such as hair.

**cystinosis** \sis'tinō'sis\ A disease characterized by lysosomal accumulation of free cystine and its crystallization in reticuloendothelial cells in many tissues, including bone marrow, liver, spleen, lymph node, kidneys, retina, uvea, and conjunctiva. The disease probably is transmitted as an autosomal recessive. It is often associated with the Fanconi syndrome. Three clinical forms with different prognoses have been recognized: benign, intermediate, and nephrogenic. Also *cystine storage disease, Lignac's disease, Lignac-Fanconi syndrome.* **benign c.** A condition characterized by symptomless deposition of cystine in bone marrow, cornea, and leukocytes. The kidneys are spared and lifespan is normal. The diagnosis is usually made by eye examination. **intermediate c.** A slowly developing form of cystinosis with survival into the second and third decades. Serious disturbance of renal tubular function is a late development. **nephrogenic c.** A severe form of cystinosis characterized by renal tubule dysfunction, the Fanconi syndrome, and progressive renal failure leading to uremia before puberty. Polyuria and polydipsia may develop as early as six months, to be followed within a year by growth retardation, renal rickets, acidosis, and other manifestations of the Fanconi syndrome. A characteristic pigmentation of the peripheral retina becomes apparent within the first few weeks of life.

**cystinuria** \sis'tinoo'rē·ə\ **1** An abnormal urinary excretion of cystine. **2** Any of several autosomal recessive and probably allelic disorders in which transport defects of dibasic amino acids predispose to urolithiasis. They are designated cystinuria I, II, and III, and, with an overall prevalence of about 1 in 7000, they are one of the more common inborn errors of metabolism. Also *familial cystinuria.* **c. I** Cystinuria in which homozygotes excrete excessive cystine, lysine, arginine, and ornithine in the urine while heterozygotes excrete normal amounts. Intestinal transport of these dibasic amino acids is absent in homozygotes. **c. II** Cystinuria that, for homozygotes, is similar to cystinuria I, but for heterozygotes is characterized by a mildly elevated urinary excretion of cystine and lysine and some susceptibility to urolithiasis. **c. III** Cystinuria in which homozygotes have normal or mildly reduced intestinal transport of cystine and lysine and abnormal urinary excretion. Heterozygotes have a less marked reduction in urinary excretion and normal intestinal transport. **familial c.** CYSTINURIA.

**cystirrhagia** \sis'tirā'jə\ CYSTORRHAGIA.

**cystis** \sis'tis\ [Gk *kystis* (from *kyein* to contain, be pregnant) the bladder, a bag, pouch] *Obs.* CYST.

**cystitis** \sistī'tis\ [CYST- + -ITIS] Acute or chronic inflammation of the urinary bladder. **acute c.** A common acute inflammatory process of the mucosa and submucosa of the bladder, which may occur in association with infections of the urinary tract, such as those caused by *Escherichia coli.* **allergic c.** An acute or subacute irritation of the bladder mucosa due in some cases to angioedema of the bladder and urethra. **chronic interstitial c.** A pronounced intramural inflammatory process of the bladder, frequently associated with calculi or chronic supravesical disease. Also *interstitial cystitis, panmural cystitis, panmural fibrosis of the bladder.* **croupous c.** DIPHTHERITIC CYSTITIS. **c. cystica** Chronic cystitis characterized by the presence of small translucent cysts in the vesical mucosa, especially in the trigone. **diphtheritic c.** Cystitis resulting as a complication of infection from *Corynebacterium diphtheriae* and typically involving formation of a false membrane. Also *croupous cystitis.* **emphysematous c.** Cystitis characterized by gas-filled cysts in the bladder wall. Also *cystitis emphysematosa.* **eosinophilic c.** Inflammation of the urinary bladder accompanied by the presence of eosinophils in the urine. **exfoliative c.** Inflammation of the bladder with associated sloughing of the bladder wall. **c. follicularis** A chronic inflammation of the urinary bladder in which nodules containing masses of lymphocytes are present on the mucosal surface. **gangrenous c.** A progressive, particularly virulent infection of the bladder, producing edema, ischemia, and necrosis of the bladder mucosa. **c. glandularis** Chronic inflammation of the vesical mucosa with hyperplasia and formation of crypts resembling mucous glands. Also *glandular cystitis.* **incrusted c.** Chronic cystitis characterized by deposition of phosphatic and other inorganic salts on the inflamed bladder mucosa. **interstitial c.** CHRONIC INTERSTITIAL CYSTITIS. **mechanical c.** Inflammation of the bladder that is caused by irritation, as by a calculus. **panmural c.** CHRONIC INTERSTITIAL CYSTITIS. **c. papillomatosa** Cystitis in which papillomatous outgrowths occur on the bladder mucosa. **postpartum c.** Infection or inflammation of the urinary bladder of a mother following delivery of an infant. **ulcerative c.** A progressive infection of the bladder giving rise to sloughing and ulceration of large areas of the mucosa.

**cystitome** \sis'titōm\ [CYSTI- + -TOME] A surgical knife designed for incision into a cavity, especially one designed to open the capsule of the crystalline lens in cataract surgery. Also *cibisotome.*

**cysto-** \sis'tə-\ [Gk *kystis* sac, bladder] A combining form meaning cyst, sac, or bladder, especially the urinary bladder or the gallbladder. Also *cyst-, cysti-, cystido-.*

**cystoadenoma** \-ad′ənō′mə\ CYSTADENOMA.

**cystocarcinoma** \-kär′sənō′mə\ [CYSTO- + CARCINOMA] *Outmoded* CYSTADENOCARCINOMA. **pseudomucinous c.** MUCINOUS CYSTADENOCARCINOMA.

**cystocele** \sis′təsēl\ [CYSTO- + -CELE[1]] A defect of the pelvic supporting structures causing a prolapse of the bladder into the vagina, clinically manifested by varying degrees of frequency, urgency, incontinence, dysuria, and mechanical discomfort.

**cystocolostomy** \-kōläs′təmē\ [CYSTO- + COLO- + -STOMY] An operation creating a passage between the urinary bladder and the colon, causing urine to pass into the rectum.

**cystodynia** \-din′ē·ə\ [CYST + -ODYNIA] CYSTALGIA.

**cystoenterocele** \-en′tərōsēl′\ [CYSTO- + ENTEROCELE] Herniation of a part of the bladder and the intestine.

**cystoepiplocele** \-ēpip′lōsēl\ [CYSTO- + EPIPLOCELE] Herniation of a part of the bladder and the omentum.

**cystofibroma** \-fībrō′mə\ A fibroma with cysts. *Outmoded.* **c. papillare** CYSTOSARCOMA PHYLLODES.

**cystogastrostomy** \-gasträs′təmē\ [CYSTO- + GASTRO- + -STOMY] A surgical procedure in which a thick-walled, mature, pancreatic pseudocyst is anastomosed to the posterior wall of the stomach for purposes of drainage of the cyst.

**cystogenesis** \-jen′əsis\ The process and mechanism by which a cyst is formed. Also *cystogenia.*

**cystogram** \sis′təgram\ [CYSTO- + -GRAM] A radiograph of the urinary bladder after opacification by contrast medium, usually instilled into the bladder via a urethral catheter.

**cystography** \sistäg′rəfē\ [CYSTO- + -GRAPHY] **1** Radiography of the urinary bladder after opacification of its lumen by contrast medium instilled usually via a urethral catheter. **2** Radiography of a cyst after opacification of its lumen by contrast medium instilled usually via a needle. **voiding c.** Radiography of the region of the lower ureters, urinary bladder, and urethra while the patient is voiding, the urine having been opacified by intravenous urography or cystography.

**cystoid** \sis′toid\ [CYST + -OID] Having the shape and appearance of a cyst but lacking a true wall or capsule. Also *cystiform.*

**cystojejunostomy** \-jəjoonäs′təmē\ [CYSTO- + JEJUNOSTOMY] A surgical procedure in which a thick-walled, mature, pancreatic pseudocyst is anastomosed to a loop of jejunum for purposes of drainage of the cyst.

**cystolith** \sis′təlith\ [CYSTO- + -LITH] VESICAL CALCULUS.

**cystolithectomy** \-lithek′təmē\ [CYSTO- + LITHECTOMY] Removal of a calculus by means of a surgically created opening in the urinary bladder. Also *cystolithotomy.*

**cystolithiasis** \-lithī′əsis\ [CYSTO- + LITHIASIS] The presence of one or more stones within the urinary bladder. Bladder stones may originate from a stone which has developed in the upper urinary tract and passed down the ureter into the bladder. They may also develop in the presence of a foreign body, such as a catheter tip or suture, within the bladder lumen, with or without concurrent presence of infection.

**cystolithotomy** \-lithät′əmē\ [CYSTO- + LITHOTOMY] CYSTOLITHECTOMY.

**cystoma** \sistō′mə\ [CYST- + -OMA] A cystic tumor. **colloid ovarian c.** MUCINOUS CYSTADENOMA OF THE OVARY. **simple c.** A cystic tumor containing a liquid or semisolid material.

**cystomatous** \sistäm′ətəs\ Pertaining to or resembling a cystoma.

**cystometer** \sistäm′ətər\ [CYSTO- + -METER] A device that measures urinary bladder pressure and capacity, used in the study and diagnostic evaluation of bladder function.

**cystometrogram** \-met′rəgram\ The tracing, recording intravesical pressure, that is obtained by cystometrography. Also *cystometric curve.*

**cystometry** \sistäm′ətrē\ Measurement of intravesical pressure and bladder capacity by means of a cystometer. Adj. cystometric.

**cystoparalysis** \-pəral′isis\ [CYSTO- + PARALYSIS] CYSTOPLEGIA.

**cystopexy** \sis′təpek′sē\ [CYSTO- + -PEXY] Surgical fixation of the bladder to the abdominal wall in treating cystocele or stress incontinence. Also *vesicofixation.*

**cystophotography** \sis′təfōtäg′rəfē\ The making of intravesical photographs through the cystoscope.

**cystophthisis** \sistäf′thisis\ [CYSTO- + PHTHISIS] Tuberculosis of the urinary bladder.

**cystoplegia** \-plē′jə\ [CYSTO- + -PLEGIA] Paralysis of the urinary bladder. Also *cystoparalysis.*

**cystoproctostomy** \-präktäs′təmē\ [CYSTO- + PROCTO- + -STOMY] Surgical creation of an opening between the urinary bladder and the rectum. Also *cystorectostomy, vesicorectostomy.*

**cystoprostatectomy** \-präs′tātek′təmē\ [CYSTO- + PROSTATECTOMY] Surgical removal of the urinary bladder and the prostate.

**cystoptosis** \sis′täptō′sis, sis′tətō′sis\ [CYSTO- + PTOSIS] Prolapse of a portion of the bladder mucosa into the urethra.

**cystorectocele** \-rek′təsēl\ [CYSTO- + RECTOCELE] A bulging of the bladder and rectum into the vagina as a result of weakening of the vaginal wall.

**cystorectostomy** \-rektäs′təmē\ CYSTOPROCTOSTOMY.

**cystorrhagia** \-rā′jə\ [CYSTO- + -RRHAGIA] Hemorrhage from the urinary bladder. Also *cystirrhagia.*

**cystorrhaphy** \sistôr′əfē\ [CYSTO- + -RRHAPHY] Suturing of the urinary bladder.

**cystosarcoma** \-särkō′mə\ **1** See under CYSTOSARCOMA PHYLLODES. **2** A sarcoma with cysts. **c. phyllodes** A tumor of the breast with a foliated structure composed of a mass of loose connective tissue containing duct epithelium. Such a tumor may reach a very large size but it rarely metastasizes. It has features of a fibroadenoma but greater connective-tissue cellularity. Also *Brodie's tumor, phyllodes tumor, cystadenoma phyllodes, cystadenosarcoma, fibrosarcoma phyllodes, giant mammary myxoma, cystofibroma papillare, mixed tumor of the breast.*

**cystoschisis** \sistäs′kisis\ EXSTROPHY OF THE BLADDER.

**cystoscope** \sis′təskōp\ [CYSTO- + -SCOPE] A metallic tube equipped with a lighting system, used for examination of the bladder interior, ureteral catheterization, and certain intravesical operations.

**cystoscopic** \-skäp′ik\ Pertaining to cystoscopy.

**cystoscopy** \sistäs′kəpē\ [CYSTO- + -SCOPY] Visual examination of the bladder interior with the cystoscope.

**cystospasm** \sis′təspazm\ [CYSTO- + SPASM] A spasmodic contraction of the urinary bladder.

**cystostomy** \sistäs′təmē\ [CYSTO- + -STOMY] Surgical creation of an opening into the urinary bladder. Also *vesicostomy.* **tubeless c.** The surgical creation of a tract between the urinary bladder and the skin of the lower abdomen wherein the tract is lined by bladder mucosa and skin. The lining prevents the tract from healing closed, thus eliminating the need for a catheter.

**cystotomy** \sistät′əmē\ [CYSTO- + -TOMY] Surgical incision into the bladder. Also *vesicotomy.* **suprapubic c.**

A surgical operation which creates an opening in the bladder through an incision in the abdominal wall made just above the pubic bone. The operation may be used for placement of a tube for urinary drainage, removal of a bladder stone, ureteral catheterization, or to provide direct access to the interior of the bladder for evaluation and treatment of a lesion within the bladder. Also *epicystotomy, Franco's operation.*

**cystoureteritis** \-yoorē'tərī'tis\ [CYSTO- + URETER + -ITIS] Inflammation of the ureters and the bladder.

**cystoureterocele** \-yoorē'tərōsēl'\ [CYSTO- + URETERO- + -CELE[1]] Protrusion of the bladder and ureter or ureters into the vagina.

**cystourethritis** \-yoo'rēthrī'tis\ [CYSTO- + URETHRITIS] Inflammation involving the bladder and the urethra.

**cystourethrocele** \-yoorē'thrəsēl'\ [CYSTO- + URETHRO- + -CELE[1]] Protrusion of the bladder and urethra into the vagina.

**cystourethrography** \-yur'ēthräg'rəfē\ [CYSTO- + URETHROGRAPHY] Radiographic study of the urinary bladder and urethra after their lumina have been filled with contrast medium. **micturating c.** VOIDING CYSTOURETHROGRAPHY. **retrograde c.** Cystourethrography in which the contrast medium is injected into the external urethral orifice. **voiding c.** Cystourethrography done while the patient is voiding urine which has been opacified by intravenous urography or more commonly by the instillation of contrast medium into the bladder via a urethral catheter or sometimes by direct percutaneous injection. Also *micturating cystourethrography.*

**cystourethroscope** \-yoorē'thrəskōp'\ [CYSTO- + URETHRO- + -SCOPE] An instrument for examining the interior of the bladder and the posterior urethra.

**cystous** \sis'təs\ CYSTIC.

**Cyt** Symbol for cytosine.

**cyt-** \sīt-\ CYTO-.

**cytarabine** $C_9H_{13}N_3O_5$. 4-Amino-1-$\beta$-D-arabinofuranosyl-2(1*H*)-pyrimidinone. A synthetic nucleoside that is an analogue of cytidine. It has antiviral activity against herpes infections and antineoplastic activity in the treatment of acute granulocytic leukemia and other types of acute leukemias.

**cytaster** \sī'tastər\ [CYT- + ASTER] Any of the asterlike figures containing a centriole, located in the cytoplasm near the nucleus, and involved in mitosis or meiosis.

**-cyte** \-sīt\ [Gk *kytos* hollow vessel, container] A combining form meaning cell.

**cythemolysis** \sī'thēmäl'isis, sī'tēm-\ HEMOLYSIS.

**cytidine** $N^1$-Ribosylcytosine, the nucleoside formed by linking C-1 of ribose to N-1 of cytosine. Also *ribofuranosylcytosine.* Symbol: Cyd

**cytidine diphosphate** Cytidine 5′-diphosphate. A nucleotide that is important mainly for its compounds, in which the terminal phosphate group is glycosylated or esterified (written CDP-X). Such compounds are donors of the X—$PO_2^-$— group, leaving CMP. Abbr. CDP

**cytidine diphosphate choline** Cyd(5′)—$PO_2^-$-—O—$PO_2^-$—O—$CH_2$—$CH_2$—$N^+Me_3$. The biologic donor of phosphocholine groups, as to a diacylglycerol to form phosphatidylcholine and leave CMP. Also *CDPcholine.*

**cytidine diphosphate ethanolamine** Cyd(5′)—*P*—O—*P*—O—$CH_2$—$CH_2$—$NH_2$. The biologic donor of *o*-phosphoethanolamine groups, as to a diacylglycerol to form phosphatidylethanolamine and leave CMP.

**cytidine monophosphate** **1** Cytidine 5′-phosphate. This compound is metabolically important because it is formed when cytidine diphosphate compounds act as donors. It is reused by conversion into CDP by cytidylate kinase, and thence to CTP. **2** Cytidine 2′- and 3′-phosphates, formed by alkaline hydrolysis of RNA.

**cytidine triphosphate** Cytidine 5′-triphosphate. It is made in the course of pyrimidine biosynthesis by amination of uridine triphosphate at the 4-position of the pyrimidine ring. This amination is achieved directly by interaction with ammonia in the bacteria, but with glutamine as amino donor in animals. Cytidine triphosphate reacts with phosphocholine with displacement of pyrophosphate to form CDPcholine, and other cytidine diphosphate compounds are similarly made. Symbol: CTP

**cytidylic acid** Any cytidine phosphate, usually cytidine 5′-phosphate, a nucleotide whose residues occur in RNA.

**cytisine** $C_{11}H_{14}ON_2$. A poisonous alkaloid found in the seeds of *Laburnum anagyroides* and *Cytisus laburnum.* Similar in effect to nicotine, it causes ganglionic blockage. Also *ulexine, laburinine.*

**cytisism** \sit'isizm\ The toxicity and symptoms resulting from the ingestion of seeds from the tree *Cytisus laburnum.* The characteristic symptoms include burning of the upper respiratory passages, diarrhea, thirst, vomiting, irregular pulse and prostration, aphasia, visual disturbances, and unconsciousness. Death may follow, due to respiratory paralysis.

**cyto-** \sī'tə-\ [Gk *kytos* a hollow vessel, container] A combining form meaning cell. Also *cyt-, kyto-.*

**cytoarchitecture** \-är'kətek'chər\ The arrangement or pattern of cells in a tissue or organ.

**cytobiology** \-bī·äl'əjē\ CYTOLOGY.

**cytoblast** \sī'təblast\ [CYTO- + -BLAST] An undifferentiated embryonic cell.

**cytocentrum** \-sen'trəm\ [CYTO- + CENTRUM] CENTROSOME.

**cytochalasin B** A fungal alkaloid that interferes with the assembly of actin filaments, and hence with the shape and movement of many eukaryotic cells.

**cytochemistry** \-kem'istrē\ The study of the chemical composition or the chemical activity of the cell. Adj. cytochemical.

**cytochrome** \sī'təkrōm\ [CYTO- + Gk *chrōm(a)* color] One of a number of heme-containing respiratory electron carriers, found especially in association with plasma membranes of aerobic bacteria and with the membranes of mitochondria of eukaryotes. They contain iron either in reduced form, Fe(II) or in oxidized form Fe(III). These forms are readily interconverted, but only one type of cytochrome (the cytochrome a component of cytochrome oxidase) can be oxidized by molecular oxygen. The Fe(II) forms show sharp absorption bands in the green (near 550 nm). The porphyrin group may be covalently bound to the protein by thioether linkage. The protein often binds the iron by coordination with histidine and methionine residues. At least five cytochromes (designated b, c, $c_1$, a, and $a_3$) have been found in mitochondrial inner membranes. Still others are found in plant, fungi, and bacteria.

**cytochrome a** A protein component of cytochrome oxidase, containing a heme A prosthetic group and characterized by its absorption spectrum. It accepts electrons from cytochrome c and transfers them to the cytochrome $a_3$ component.

**cytochrome $a_3$** A protein component of cytochrome oxidase, containing a heme A prosthetic group and characterized by its absorption spectrum. It is the terminal cytochrome in mitochondrial respiration, accepting electrons from the cytochrome a component and transferring them to molecular oxygen to form water.

**cytochrome b** A protein containing a heme prosthetic group, generally an integral membrane protein. It receives electrons from coenzyme Q and passes them to cytochrome c during mitochondria electron transport.

**cytochrome c** An iron-containing hemoprotein which acts as an electron transfer agent in oxidation-reduction reactions. It has a molecular weight of 13 000. Structurally it is a protein with a heme prosthetic group that has reacted with cysteine residues of the protein. It contains one atom of iron per molecule (0.43%) which is easily reduced by mild reducing agents such as dehydrogenase systems and which is oxidized by cytochrome oxidase. More than half of the amino acids in the protein moiety are arranged in an identical sequence in all species measured. The degree of difference in the primary structure of cytochrome c between species has been related to the degree of phylogenetic relationship between them. Man and rhesus monkeys differ in just one residue but fish and yeast differ in 48.

**cytochrome oxidase** A copper-containing heme protein (EC 1.9.3.1) responsible for the oxidation of cytochrome c using dioxygen. The sensitivity of cytochrome oxidase to cyanide accounts for the toxicity of cyanide. Also *cytochrome c oxidase*.

**cytochrome P-450** One of several heme proteins mostly associated with the microsomal electron-transport system of animal liver. They are involved in many hydroxylations by molecular oxygen, including hydroxylations of steroids and of foreign compounds such as drugs. The overall reaction involves oxidation of NADH or NADPH concomitant with substrate hydroxylation. Cytochrome P-450 is named from the intense absorption band at 450 nm of the complex with carbon monoxide of its Fe(II) form. Also *heme-thiolate protein*.

**cytocidal** \-sī′dəl\ Causing destruction or death of cells.

**cytocide** \sī′təsīd\ [CYTO- + -CIDE] Any agent which kills cells.

**cytocinesis** \-sinē′sis\ CYTOKINESIS.

**cytoclasis** \sītäk′ləsis\ [CYTO- + -CLASIS] Dissolution of a cell or cells.

**cytoclastic** \-klas′tik\ Pertaining to cytoclasis.

**cytode** \sī′tōd\ [CYT- + Gk *-ōdē(s),* suffix denoting like] A protoplasmic mass without a nucleus.

**cytodiagnosis** \-dī′agnō′sis\ Diagnosis of disease, particularly neoplasia, utilizing the microscopic examination of exfoliated cells. Also *cytoscopy*.

**cytodieresis** \-dī·er′əsis\ [CYTO- + Gk *diairesis* a dividing] CYTOKINESIS.

**cytodifferentiation** \-dif′ərenshē·ā′shən\ The progressive diversification of cells and tissues which occurs in the embryo, such as, for example, that seen in the differentiation of the primordial germ cells into spermatozoa and ova.

**cytogene** \sī′təjēn\ [CYTO- + GENE] PLASMAGENE.

**cytogenesis** \-jen′əsis\ [CYTO- + GENESIS] Cell origin and development. Also *cytogeny*. Adj. cytogenic.

**cytogeneticist** \-jənet′isist\ A specialist who uses cytologic techniques in the study of genetics, with a concentration on chromosomes.

**cytogenetics** \-jənet′iks\ The study of the physical constituents of heredity. Derived from both genetics and cytology, this field concentrates on the study of chromosomes, particularly their structure, replication, and recombination. **clinical c.** A branch of genetics that concerns the correlation of chromosome structure with alterations in the phenotype of the organism.

**cytogenic** \-jen′ik\ Pertaining to cell origin and development.

**cytogeny** \sitäj′ənē\ CYTOGENESIS.

**cytohistogenesis** \-his′təjen′əsis\ The development of structural features, such as the cytoskeleton, within cells.

**cytohistology** \-histäl′əjē\ *Obs.* CYTOLOGY.

**cytohyaloplasm** \-hī′əlōplazm′\ HYALOPLASM.

**cytoid** \sī′toid\ [CYT- + -OID] Resembling a cell.

**cyto-inhibition** \-in′hibish′ən\ The inhibiting effect of phagocytic cells on chemotherapeutic agents, as when phagocytization of certain bacteria or viruses protects them from the action of these agents.

**cytokinesis** \-kīnē′sis\ [CYTO- + Gk *kinēsis* a moving, motion] The process of division or segmentation of the cytoplasm of the cell, generally following nuclear division (karyokinesis). Also *cytodieresis, cellular fission*. Also *cytocinesis*.

**cytokinin** \-kī′nin\ One of several plant hormones that promote cell division, such as triacanthine.

**cytolemma** \-lem′ə\ PLASMA MEMBRANE.

**cytolist** \sī′təlist\ CYTOLYSIN.

**cytologist** \sītäl′əjist\ A biologist who studies cytology.

**cytology** \sītäl′əjē\ [CYTO- + -LOGY] The branch of biology concerned with the study of cells, including their anatomy, chemistry, pathology, and physiology. Also *cell biology, cytobiology, cytohistology* (obs.). Adj. cytologic. **exfoliative c.** A diagnostic method based on the microscopic examination of exfoliated cells. **nuclear c.** KARYOLOGY.

**cytolymph** \sī′təlimf\ HYALOPLASM.

**cytolysate** \sītäl′isāt\ The liquid component released from a cell when the cell membrane is ruptured. **blood c.** HEMOLYSATE.

**cytolysin** \sītäl′isin\ A substance that has the ability to destroy cell membranes. Also *cytolist*.

**cytolysis** \sītäl′isis\ [CYTO- + LYSIS] The process of degradation and disintegration of dead cells. **immune c.** Cell killing by damage to the plasma membrane, brought about by complement or lymphocytes (K cells) or myeloid effector cells in the presence of antibody, or alternatively, by specific lymphocytes.

**cytolysome** \sītäl′isōm\ LYSOSOME.

**cytolysosome** \-lī′sōsōm\ AUTOPHAGOSOME.

**cytolytic** \-lit′ik\ Capable of causing cell lysis.

**cytomegalic** \-məgal′ik\ Pertaining to or causing great enlargement of cells, usually also of their nuclei, as in the great enlargement of the epithelial cells of salivary glands caused by the cytomegalovirus.

**cytomegalovirus** \-meg′əlōvī′rəs\ [CYTO- + MEGALO- + VIRUS] Any of a group of herpes viruses which infect humans, mice, and other mammals and which differ in certain physical and chemical properties from other herpes viruses. Cytomegalovirus infection in humans is protean in its manifestations, including congenital disease in infants, a mononucleosis syndrome in normal adults, and hepatitis, pneumonia, gastrointestinal disease, or retinitis in immunocompromised adults. Also *salivary gland virus* (outmoded). See also CYTOMEGALIC INCLUSION DISEASE.

**cytomegaly** \-meg′əlē\ [CYTO- + -MEGALY] A pathologic enlargement of a cell or cells, so that the mass is much larger than normal.

**cytomembrane** \-mem′brān\ PLASMA MEMBRANE.

**cytometaplasia** \-met′əplā′zhə\ [CYTO- + METAPLASIA] A change in the structure of a cell.

**cytometer** \sītäm′ətər\ [CYTO- + -METER] A device for counting cells, as a hemocytometer. **eyepiece c.** A device that is incorporated into a microscope eyepiece to facilitate the counting of blood cells. **stage c.** A device that is used on a microscope stage to facilitate the counting of blood cells.

**cytometry** \sītäm′ətrē\ [CYTO- + -METRY] The enumeration of cells, especially of blood but also of other body fluids. **flow c.** A technique for measuring and characterizing particles, usually cells, suspended in fluid. The cells flow individually through an aperture, where they are exposed to light or electric current. Cell properties are determined by their effect on electrical transmission or on reflecting or absorbing light or fluorescence. Large numbers of cells are examined very rapidly and the results are analyzed by computer.

**cytomicrosome** \-mī′krəsōm\ MICROSOME.

**cytomorphology** \-môrfäl′əjē\ [CYTO- + MORPHOLOGY] The study of cell structure.

**cytomorphosis** \-môrfō′sis\ [CYTO- + Gk *morphōsis* formation] The structural changes occurring in a cell during its life.

**cytonecrosis** \-nəkrō′sis\ The morphologic changes developing in a cell after it has died.

**cytopathic** \-path′ik\ [CYTO- + PATH- + -IC] Injurious to cells or pertaining to cell injury; especially, denoting the damage caused by intracellular replication of viruses. Also *cytopathologic.*

**cytopathogenesis** \-path′əjen′əsis\ The mechanism by which injurious agents damage cells.

**cytopathogenetic** \-path′əjənet′ik\ Pertaining to cytopathogenesis. Also *cytopathogenic.*

**cytopathogenic** \-path′əjen′ik\ **1** Causing or tending to cause damage to cells. **2** CYTOPATHOGENETIC.

**cytopathologic** \-path′əläj′ik\ **1** Pertaining to cytopathology. **2** CYTOPATHIC.

**cytopathology** \-pathäl′əjē\ A subspecialty of anatomic pathology devoted to the study and diagnosis of diseases by means of the microscopic examination of smears of exfoliated cells. Such cells include those of the uterine cervix, the bronchial mucosa, and the epithelium of the urinary tract.

**cytopenia** \-pē′nē·ə\ [CYTO- + -PENIA] An abnormal decrease in numbers of cells, especially in the blood or bone marrow.

**cytophagocytosis** \-fag′əsītō′sis\ The ingestion of one cell by another, as seen in macrophages, unicellular parasites, and malignant cells. Also *cytophagy.*

**cytophagy** \sītäf′əjē\ CYTOPHAGOCYTOSIS.

**cytophil** \sī′təfil\ [CYTO- + -PHIL] A substance that has a tendency to bind onto cell surfaces. Adj. cytophilic.

**cytophotometer** \-fōtäm′ətər\ A photometer designed to measure the amount of light transmitted through specific small areas of a cell.

**cytophotometry** \-fōtäm′ətrē\ The measurement of the transmission of monochromatic light through various areas of the cell in order to localize specific organic substances. Adj. cytophotometric.

**cytophylaxis** \-fīlak′sis\ Any of the cellular defensive systems that serve to protect against attack by injurious agents, particularly infective organisms. Adj. cytophylactic.

**cytophysics** \-fiz′iks\ The physics of cell structure and function.

**cytophysiology** \-fiz′ē·äl′əjē\ The study of the functioning of living cells and their organelles. Also *cellular physiology.*

**cytopigment** \-pig′mənt\ Pigment contained within a cell.

**cytopipette** \-pipet′\ An elongated glass or plastic cylinder used, with a suction bulb, to aspirate fluid, especially vaginal fluid, for cytologic examination.

**cytoplasm** \sī′təplazm\ [CYTO- + -PLASM] The protoplasm of the cell which is outside of the nucleus. Adj. cytoplasmic.

**cytopreparation** \-rep′ərā′shən\ A preparation of isolated cells that is obtained from solid tissue, spread over the surface of a microscope slide, and stained for microscopic examination.

**cytoreticulum** \-retik′yələm\ [CYTO- + RETICULUM] The network of threadlike fibers within the cytoplasm of a cell. Also *cell network.*

**cytoscopy** \sītäs′kəpē\ [CYTO- + -SCOPY] CYTODIAGNOSIS.

**cytosiderin** \-sid′ərin\ An intracellular iron-containing pigment.

**cytosine** 4-Amino-2-hydroxypyrimidine. It exists predominantly as the tautomer 4-amino-1,2-dihydro-2-oxopyrimidine. It is one of the four bases found in DNA, where it is ribosylated on N-1 to form the nucleoside cytidine.

**cytosine arabinoside** The 2-epimer of cytidine. It is used in the treatment of leukemia. It is metabolized to form the nucleoside triphosphate, which inhibits DNA synthesis.

**cytosine deoxyriboside** A nucleoside that is composed of the pyrimidine base cytosine and the pentose deoxyribose. It is one of the four nucleosides present in DNA and the one which most often undergoes methylation *in vivo.* It base pairs with guanine deoxyriboside.

**cytoskeleton** \-skel′ətən\ The network of structural proteins on the interior of a cell that determines its characteristic shape, flexibility, and motility. In most cells the cytoskeleton is composed of microtubules, intermediate filaments, and microfilaments, some of which may traverse the cell. Actin and various fibrillar proteins are major components of the cytoskeleton.

**cytosmear** \sī′təsmir\ A thin layer of cells spread on the surface of a microscope slide for staining and examination, often for diagnostic purposes. Such cells may be collected by scraping a mucosal surface. Also *cytologic smear.*

**cytosol** \sī′təsôl\ HYALOPLASM.

**cytosome** \sī′təsōm\ [CYTO- + Gk *sōm(a)* body] The cell body excluding the nucleus.

**cytostatic** \-stat′ik\ Capable of inhibiting the growth and multiplication of cells, particularly neoplastic cells.

**cytosteatonecrosis** \-stē′ätōnekrō′sis\ [CYTO- + STEATO- + NECROSIS] SUBCUTANEOUS FAT NECROSIS.

**cytostome** \sī′təstōm\ [CYTO- + Gk *stom(a)* mouth] An opening in certain protozoa through which food is taken in.

**cytostromatic** \-strōmat′ik\ Pertaining to the stroma in a cell.

**cytotaxis** \-tak′sis\ The phenomenon of attracting or repelling cells; the movement of living cells in response to a stimulant. Also *cytotaxia.*

**cytotechnologist** \-teknäl′əjist\ A person who is trained in techniques used in the preparation of cells for microscopic examination and observation.

**cytotherapy** \-ther′əpē\ **1** The administration of embryonic animal cells for therapeutic purposes. **2** The administration of cytotoxic serum for therapeutic purposes.

**cytotoxic** \-täk′sik\ Having the effect of poisoning or destroying cells, as a drug or infective organism. Cytotoxic drugs are often used in chemotherapy of cancer.

**cytotoxicity** \-täksis′itē\ The property by which a substance is cytotoxic; the power to destroy cells.

**cytotoxin** \-täk′sin\ A cell poison that is either formed by an infective organism or administered as a drug, as in cancer chemotherapy.

**cytotropal** \sītät′rəpəl\ CYTOTROPIC.

**cytotrophoblast** \-träf′əblast\ A layer of trophoblastic cells (Langhans cells) with relatively pale-staining cytoplasm, which forms the inner trophoblastic layer of the placental chorionic villi during early pregnancy. Also *Langhans layer.*

**cytotropic** \-träp′ik\ [CYTO- + -TROPIC[1]] **1** Attracted to or moving toward cells. **2** Describing a property of certain classes of antibody that are able, without first complexing with antigen, to bind through their Fc region to cell receptors. For defs. 1 and 2 also *cytotropal.*

**cytozoic** \-zō′ik\ [CYTO- + *zo(o)* + -IC] Living intracellularly: said especially of certain parasitic protozoa.

**cytozoon** \-zō′ən\ [CYTO- + Gk *zōon* living being, animal] (*pl.* cytozoa) An intracellular protozoan parasite.

**cyturia** \sitoo′rē·ə\ [CYT- + -URIA] The presence of cells in the urine.

**Czapek** [Friedrich Johann Franz *Czapek,* Czech botanist, 1868–1921] Czapek-Dox solution. See under CZAPEK-DOX AGAR.

**Czerny** [Vincenz *Czerny,* German surgeon, 1842–1916] **1** See under SUTURE. **2** Czerny-Lembert suture. See under SUTURE.

# D

**D** **1** Symbol for deuterium. **2** Symbol for aspartic acid. **3** diopter. **4** duration. **5** dorsal.

**2,4-D** 2,4-dichlorophenoxyacetic acid.

**d** **1** Symbol for deci-: used with SI units. **2** Symbol for the unit, day.

**d.** **1** *dosis* (L, dose). **2** *detur* (L, let it be given). **3** *dexter* (L, right).

**D-** A prefix denoting a certain configuration of atoms around a chiral carbon atom. The enantiomeric configuration is designated L-.

**Da** Symbol for dalton.

**Daae** [Anders *Daae,* Norwegian physician, 1838–1910] Daae's disease, Daae-Finsen disease. See under EPIDEMIC PLEURODYNIA.

**Dabney** [William Cecil *Dabney,* U.S. physician, 1849–1894] Dabney's grip. See under EPIDEMIC PLEURODYNIA.

**dacarbazine** $C_6H_{10}N_6O$. 5-(3,3-Dimethyl-1-triazenyl)-1*H*-imidazole-4-carboxamide. An antineoplastic agent that is used to treat metastatic malignant melanoma, lymphomas (including Hodgkin's disease), and neuroblastomas. It is administered by intravenous injection.

**DaCosta** [Jacob Mendes *DaCosta,* U.S. physician, 1833–1900] Da Costa syndrome. See under NEUROCIRCULATORY ASTHENIA.

**dacry-** \dak′rə-\ DACRYO-.

**dacryadenitis** \-adənī′tis\ DACRYOADENITIS.

**dacryagogic** \-əgäj′ik\ DACRYOGENIC.

**dacryagogue** \dak′rē·əgäg′\ [DACRY- + -AGOGUE] A stimulant of tear formation.

**dacryo-** \dak′rē·ō-\ [Gk *dakry* or *dakryon* a tear] A combining form meaning (1) tears; (2) pertaining to the lacrimal apparatus. Also *dacry-.*

**dacryoadenectomy** \-ad′ənek′təmē\ [DACRYO- + ADEN- + -ECTOMY] Excision of a lacrimal gland.

**dacryoadenitis** \-ad′ənī′tis\ [DACRYO- + ADEN- + -ITIS] Inflammation of the lacrimal gland. Also *dacryadenitis.*

**dacryocanaliculitis** \-kan′əlik′yəlī′tis\ Inflammation of the lacrimal sac and lacrimal canaliculi (passages between the punctum and the sac).

**dacryocele** \dak′rē·əsēl′\ DACRYOCYSTOCELE.

**dacryocyst** \dak′rē·əsist′\ [DACRYO- + CYST] SACCUS LACRIMALIS.

**dacryocystalgia** \-sistal′jə\ [DACRYOCYST + -ALGIA] Pain in a lacrimal sac.

**dacryocystectomy** \-sistek′təmē\ [DACRYOCYST + -ECTOMY] Surgical removal of the lacrimal sac.

**dacryocystitis** \-sistī′tis\ [DACRYOCYST + -ITIS] Inflammation of the lacrimal sac.

**dacryocystitome** \-sis′tətōm\ DACRYOCYSTOTOME.

**dacryocysto-** A combining form meaning lacrimal sac.

**dacryocystocele** \-sis′təsēl\ A pathologic enlargement of the lacrimal sac usually due to occlusion of the nasolacrimal duct and retention of mucoid secretions. Also *dacryocele.*

**dacryocystography** \-sistäg′rəfē\ [DACRYOCYSTO- + -GRAPHY] Radiographic examination of the lacrimal sac after its opacification by an instilled contrast medium.

**dacryocystorhinostomy** \-sis′tôrīnäs′təmē\ [DACRYOCYSTO- + RHINO- + -STOMY] A surgically created opening between the lacrimal sac and the nasal cavity. Also *dacryocystorhinotomy, dacryorhinocystotomy, canaliculorhinostomy* (outmoded).

**dacryocystostomy** \-sistäst′əmē\ [DACRYOCYSTO- + -STOMY] A surgical opening into the lacrimal sac.

**dacryocystotome** \-sis′tətōm\ [DACRYOCYSTO- + -TOME] A knife designed for incising the lacrimal sac. Also *dacryocystitome.*

**dacryocystotomy** \-sistät′əmē\ [DACRYOCYSTO- + -TOMY] An incision into the lacrimal sac. Also *Ammon's operation.*

**dacryocyte** \dak′rē·əsīt\ An abnormally shaped erythrocyte that resembles a teardrop. Dacryocytes are characteristically found in blood films from persons with pernicious anemia or disorders that cause extramedullary hematopoiesis. Also *teardrop cell, tailed red cell.*

**dacryogenic** \-jen′ik\ [DACRYO- + -GENIC] Stimulating the production of tears. Also *dacryagogic.*

**dacryohemorrhea** \-hem′ôrē′ə\ [DACRYO- + HEMO- + -RRHEA] Hemorrhagic discharge from the lacrimal sac.

**dacryoid** \dak′rē·oid\ [DACRY- + -OID] Similar in appearance to a tear.

**dacryolith** \dak′rē·əlith′\ [DACRYO- + -LITH] A calcific deposit within the lacrimal drainage system, usually a consequence of fungus infection. Also *lacrimal calculus.*

**dacryolithiasis** \-lithī′əsis\ The condition characterized by the presence of calculi within the lacrimal drainage system.

**dacryoma** \dak′rē·ō′mə\ [DACRY- + -OMA] A lacrimal neoplasm or cyst.

**dacryopyorrhea** \-pī′ôrē′ə\ Purulent discharge from the lacrimal sac.

**dacryopyosis** \-pī·ō′sis\ Purulent inflammation of the lacrimal drainage system.

**dacryorhinocystotomy** \-rī′nōsistät′əmē\ DACRYOCYSTORHINOSTOMY.

**dacryorrhea** \-rē′ə\ [DACRYO- + -RRHEA] A pathologic, excessive discharge of tears.

**dacryosolenitis** \-sō′lenī′tis\ Inflammation of a duct of the lacrimal gland.

**dacryostenosis** \-stenō′sis\ Obstruction of the lacrimal drainage system.

**dactinomycin** ACTINOMYCIN D.

**dactyl** \dak′təl\ [Gk *daktyl(os)* finger] A finger or toe; a digit. Also *dactylus.*

**dactyl-** \dak′təl-\ DACTYLO-.

**dactylalgia** \dak′təlal′jə\ [DACTYL- + -ALGIA] Pain in a finger. Also *dactylodynia.*

**dactyledema** \dak′təlēdē′mə\ [DACTYL- + EDEMA] Swelling of a finger.

**dactylic** \daktil′ik\ Belonging to a digit.

**dactylitis** \dak′tilī′tis\ [DACTYL- + -ITIS] Inflammation or infection of a finger. **d. strumosa** DACTYLITIS TUBERCULOSA. **d. tuberculosa** Inflammation of the digits due to tuberculosis. Also *dactylitis strumosa.*

**dactylo-** \dak′təlō-\ [Gk *daktylos* finger] A combining form meaning (1) finger; (2) finger or toe; digit. Also *dactyl-.*

**dactylocampsodynia** \-kamp′sōdin′ē·ə\ [DACTYLO- + Gk *kampsodyn(os)* bent with pain + -IA] Painful flexion of the fingers.

**dactylodynia** \-din′e·ə\ [DACTYL- + -ODYNIA] DACTYLALGIA.

**dactylodystrophy** \-dis′trəfē\ A wasting of the fingers, which is seen in certain collagen diseases such as scleroderma.

**dactylogram** \dak′təlōgram′\ [DACTYLO- + -GRAM] FINGERPRINT.

**dactylography** \dak′təläg′rəfē\ [DACTYLO- + -GRAPHY] The study of fingerprints.

**dactylogryposis** \-grīpō′sis\ The developmental or acquired contracture or distortion of one or more digits.

**dactyloid** \dak′təloid\ [DACTYL- + -OID] Having the appearance of a finger.

**dactylolysis** \dak′təläl′isis\ [DACTYLO- + -LYSIS] Dissolution of the bone of a finger. **d. spontanea** AINHUM.

**dactylomegaly** \-meg′əlē\ [DACTYLO- + -MEGALY] MACRODACTYLY.

**dactyloscopy** \dak′təläs′kəpē\ [DACTYLO- + -SCOPY] The use of fingerprint impressions for purposes of identification.

**dactylose** \dak′təlōs\ [DACTYL- + -OSE[1]] Possessing fingerlike processes. Also *dactylous.*

**dactylospasm** \dak′təlōspazm′\ [DACTYLO- + SPASM] Vascular spasm of a finger, as in Raynaud's phenomenon.

**dactylosymphysis** \-sim′fisis\ SYNDACTYLY.

**dactylous** \dak′tələs\ DACTYLOSE.

**dactylus** \dak′tələs\ DACTYL.

**daisy** An informal term for MALARIAL ROSETTE.

**Dakin** [Henry Drysdale *Dakin,* English-born U.S. chemist, 1880–1952] Modified Dakin solution. See under SOLUTION.

**Dale** [Sir Henry Hallett *Dale,* English physiologist, 1875–1968] **1** Schultz-Dale technique. See under SCHULTZ-DALE REACTION. **2** Dale-Feldberg law. See under LAW.

**Dalrymple** [John *Dalrymple,* Scottish surgeon and oculist, 1803–1852] Dalrymple's disease. See under CYCLOKERATITIS.

**Dalton** [John *Dalton,* English chemist, 1766–1844] See under LAW.

**dalton** \dôl′tən\ [after John *Dalton,* 1766–1844, English chemist] A unit of mass equal to one-twelfth of the mass of an atom of isotope 12 of carbon, about $1.6598 \times 10^{-24}$ g; atomic mass unit. It is widely used in biochemistry. Symbol: Da

**dam** [Middle English] Something that blocks the passage of a fluid. **rubber d.** A thin sheet of rubber used to isolate one or more teeth from the environment of the mouth. For each tooth one makes a circular hole which is enlarged by stretching it over the crown of the tooth. When in position the circumference of the hole fits tightly around the neck of the tooth.

**damage / radiation d.** Damage to an organism, its organs, or its cells by exposure to ionizing radiation. The extent of damage and its repair depend upon the total dose and the kind of radiation used.

**damages / compensatory d.** In medical malpractice, the monetary sum determined by the court and awarded to a negligently injured party to compensate only for the financial loss suffered as a result of the injury. **punitive d.** A pecuniary award in a judicial proceeding, which is over and above the value assigned to compensate actual injury, loss, or detriment suffered by a plaintiff. Punitive damages are awarded because the wrong committed is reckless, oppressive, or malicious in nature. They are a form of punishment and deterrent.

**Dameshek** [William *Dameshek,* Russian-born U.S. physician and hematologist, 1900–1969] Estren-Dameshek syndrome. See under SYNDROME.

**damping** **1** Reduction of the amplitude of oscillations in a resonant system by dissipation of stored energy. Fluid in the lung causes damping of its normal resonant sound. **2** Resistive or mechanical loading of a system to progressively diminish the amplitude of oscillation. Used in a piezoelectric transducer to reduce the duration of its emitted pulse, as in echography.

**Dana** [Charles Loomis *Dana,* U.S. physician, 1852–1935] **1** Dana's operation. See under POSTERIOR RHIZOTOMY. **2** Putnam-Dana syndrome. See under SUBACUTE COMBINED DEGENERATION OF THE SPINAL CORD.

**Danbolt** [Niels Christian *Danbolt,* Swedish physician, born 1900] Danbolt-Closs syndrome. See under ACRODERMATITIS ENTEROPATHICA.

**Dance** [Jean Baptiste Hippolyte *Dance,* French physician, 1797–1832] See under SIGN.

**dance** Excessive arterial pulsation, as seen within an arteriovenous angioma or in any arteries when the pulse pressure is high, as in aortic regurgitation. **brachial d.** The lateral movement of a tortuous brachial artery with each pulsation, caused by arterial tortuosity and rigidity which are due to Monckeberg's arteriosclerosis. **hilar d.** Vigorous pulsation of the hilar arteries seen on fluoroscopy, characteristic of atrial septal defect. Also *hilus dance.* **St. Vitus d.** SYDENHAM'S CHOREA.

**dander** \dan′dər\ [origin unknown] Heterogeneous particles shed from the surface of the skin of various animals, as of cats and dogs, and commonly a cause of allergic reactions in atopic individuals. Dander consists of microorganisms, desquamated epithelial cells, fragments of hair, and sebaceous material.

**dandruff** [earlier *dander,* origin unknown + dialectal *hurf* scab, from Scandinavian, akin to Old Norse *hrufa* scab, crust] *Popular* PITYRIASIS CAPITIS.

**Dandy** [Walter Edward *Dandy,* U.S. surgeon, 1886–1946] Dandy-Walker deformity. See under DANDY-WALKER SYNDROME.

**Dane** [D. S. *Dane,* British virologist, flourished 20th century] See under PARTICLE.

**Danforth** [William Clark *Danforth,* U.S. obstetrician, 1878–1949] See under SIGN.

**Danielssen** [Daniel Cornelius *Danielssen,* Norwegian physician, 1815–1894] Danielssen-Boeck disease. See under SARCOIDOSIS.

**DANS** 1-Dimethylaminonaphthalene-5 sulfonyl chloride. A flurorochrome which combines with proteins and is used in immunofluorescent studies.

**dansyl** \dan′sil\ The group 5-(dimethylamino)naphthalene-1-sulfonyl. Dansyl chloride is used to add dansyl groups to the amino groups of peptides and proteins. Acid hydrolysis of the derivative thus formed gives the dansylamino acid of the residue that had been N-terminal. The fluorescence of dansylamino acids helps to identify them. Symbol: DNS

**danthron** $C_{14}H_8O_4$. 1,8-Dihydroxy-9,10-anthracenedione. It is a free anthrone, not a glycoside, as are the natural anthraquinone cathartics. It is used more commonly in veterinary medicine than in clinical practice.

**Danysz** [Jean *Danysz*, Polish pathologist, 1860–1928] See under VACCINE.

**dapsone** \dap′sōn\ $C_{12}H_{12}N_2O_2S$. 4,4′-Sulfonyldianiline, a drug used in the treatment of leprosy, and in dermatitis herpetiformis, in which disease the response to this drug is virtually diagnostic. It is also used in erythema elevatum diutinum, subcorneal pustular dermatosis, and occasionally in resistant acne.

**Darier** [Jean Ferdinand *Darier*, French dermatologist, 1856–1938] **1** See under SIGN. **2** Darier-Roussy sarcoid. See under SARCOID. **3** Darier's disease. See under KERATOSIS FOLLICULARIS. **4** Darier's disease. See under PSEUDOXANTHOMA ELASTICUM. **5** Darier's disease. See under ERYTHEMA ANNULARE CENTRIFUGUM. **6** Darier's disease. See under BENIGN FAMILIAL PEMPHIGUS.

**Darkschewitsch** [Liveri O. *Darkschewitsch*, Russian neurologist, 1858–1925] **1** Darkschewitsch's ganglion. See under NUCLEUS OF DARKSCHEWITSCH. **2** Fibers of Darkschewitsch. See under FIBER.

**Darling** [Samuel Taylor *Darling*, U.S. pathologist, 1872–1925] Darling's disease. See under HISTOPLASMOSIS.

**darmbrand** \därm′brunt\ [German *Darm* intestine + *Brand* a burning] A severe, hemorrhagic, necrotizing jejunitis with bloody diarrhea, shock, and abdominal pain, associated with significant mortality especially in children, recognized in Germany and other parts of Europe following World War II. It is now known to be the same condition as pigbel, caused by the toxin *Clostridium perfringens*. *Outmoded.*

**Darrow** [Daniel Cady *Darrow*, U.S. pediatrician, born 1895] See under SOLUTION.

**dartoid** \där′toid\ Having the characteristics of musculus dartos; exhibiting slow, involuntary contractions like a dartos muscle. Also *dartoic*.

**dartos** \där′təs\ [Gk (from *derein* to flay) flayed, stripped] MUSCULUS DARTOS. **d. muliebris** Nonstriated muscle fibers that are intermixed with a considerable amount of areolar and adipose tissue deep to the skin of the labia majora. It is analagous to the musculus dartos in the scrotum, which is much better developed and formed into a definite muscle layer.

**Darwin** [Charles Robert *Darwin*, English naturalist, 1809–1882] **1** Darwinian selection. See under NATURAL SELECTION. **2** See under REFLEX. **3** Darwinian fitness. See under FITNESS. **4** Darwinian tubercle. See under TUBERCULUM AURICULAE.

**darwinism** \där′winizm\ [after Charles Robert *Darwin*, English naturalist, 1809–1882] The evolutionary theory proposed by Charles Darwin in 1859 that all living things have evolved from earlier life forms in accordance with the principle of natural selection.

***Dasyprocta*** \das′ipräk′tə\ A genus of South American rodents, the agoutis, that serve as a reservoir host of *Trypanosoma cruzi*.

**DAT** **1** direct antiglobulin test. **2** A chemotherapy regimen that includes doxorubicin, cytosine arabinoside, and 6-thioguanine.

**data** (*sing.* datum) Facts or information used as a basis for analysis and for drawing conclusions, or for computer processing.

**database** \dā′təbās′\ The total data on one or more related subjects, such as a collection of data files stored in a computer containing all clinical laboratory results. Also *data base*.

**dating** / **carbon d.** The determination of the age of biologic materials by calculating the degree of radioactive decay of carbon 14.

**datum** \dā′təm\ [L (substantive from *datum*, neut. sing. of *datus*, past part. of *dare* to give, offer), a given fact] Singular of DATA.

**daturism** Poisoning by the alkaloids contained in *Datura stramonium* and other *Datura* species, primarily hyoscyamine and scopolamine.

**Daubenton** [Louis J. M. *Daubenton*, French physician, 1716–1800] See under PLANE, ANGLE.

**daughter** **1** Any nuclide that is an immediate product of the radioactive decay of another nuclide (the parent). **2** See under DAUGHTER CELL.

**daunorubicin** $C_{27}H_{29}NO_{10}$. An antibiotic substance with antineoplastic properties isolated from *Streptomyces peucetius*. It is used in the treatment of acute lymphocytic and acute granulocytic leukemia. Also *daunomycin*.

***Davainea madagascariensis*** *RAILLIETINA MADAGASCARIENSIS.*

**Davenport** [Harold Alvin *Davenport*, U.S. anatomist, born 1895] Davenport stain. See under DAVENPORT'S ALCOHOLIC SILVER NITRATE METHOD.

**Davidsohn** [Hermann *Davidsohn*, German physician, 1842–1911] See under SIGN.

**Davidsohn** [Israel *Davidsohn*, U.S. physician, born 1895] Davidsohn's differential test. See under PAUL-BUNNELL-DAVIDSOHN TEST.

**Davis** [John Staige *Davis*, U.S. surgeon, 1872–1946] **1** See under GAG. **2** Davis graft. See under PINCH GRAFT.

**Dawson** [James Robertson *Dawson*, U.S. pathologist, born 1908] Dawson's encephalitis. See under SUBACUTE SCLEROSING PANENCEPHALITIS.

**Day** [Richard Lawrence *Day*, U.S. pediatrician, born 1905] Riley-Day syndrome. See under FAMILIAL DYSAUTONOMIA.

**D and C** dilatation and curettage.

**dc** direct current.

**DCF** direct centrifugal flotation (method).

**d.d.** *detur ad* (L, let it be given to, a direction used in prescription writing).

**DDS** Doctor of Dental Surgery.

**DDSc** Doctor of Dental Science.

**DDT** DICHLORODIPHENYLTRICHLOROETHANE.

**D and E** dilatation and evacuation.

**de-** \dē-, də-\ [L *de* down, down from, away, after (in time) and from L *de-* from L *dis-*. See DIS-[1]] A prefix meaning (1) down; (2) away, take away; (3) completely; (4) reversal of, opposite of.

**DEACE** diethylaminochloroethane.

**deacylase** Any enzyme that removes an acyl group from a substance by hydrolysis.

**dead** **1** Having ceased to live; lifeless. • Criteria necessary for declaring an individual dead vary among different jurisdictions. In the United States a Uniform Determination of Death Act has been proposed (July 1981) that defines the criteria necessarily present for an individual to be declared dead. See under DEATH. In addition, an individual who has been missing for a prolonged time can legally be declared dead. The time criterion for this legal declaration of death varies depending upon the circumstances under which an individual is missing and varies among different jurisdictions. **2** Devoid of feeling; numb.

**DEAE-cellulose** DIETHYLAMINOETHYL CELLULOSE.

**deaf** [Old English *dēaf*, akin to Gk *typhlos* blind] **1** Partially or completely without hearing. **2** Pertaining to or denoting deafness.

**deafferentate** \dē·af′ərəntāt′\ To subject to deafferentation; remove or interrupt the afferent, or sensory, impulses of.

**deafferentation** \dē·af′ərəntā′shən\ The removal or interruption of afferent or sensory impulses by the destruction of sense organs, afferent pathways, and/or sensory relay nuclei.

**deaf-mute** DEAF MUTE.

**deaf-mutism** DEAF MUTISM. **endemic d.** Hearing loss and mutism in children that is usually associated with defective thyroid hormone biosynthesis and hypothyroidism and not with endemic goiter.

**deafness** Any degree of impaired hearing, from minimal to profound. Also *hearing loss.* **acoustic trauma d.** NOISE-INDUCED HEARING LOSS. **Bing-Siebenmann type genetic d.** A type of congenital deafness associated with hypoplasia of both cochlear and vestibular parts of the membranous inner ear. There are sometimes abnormalities of the central nervous system also. **central d.** Any hearing loss the cause of which is sited central to the cochlea and auditory nerve. **cerebral d.** CORTICAL DEAFNESS. **cochlear d.** Sensorineural deafness due to causes within the cochlea such as Menière's disease or hair-cell damage. **conductive d.** Hearing loss the cause of which is located in the external ear canal or middle-ear structures. Also *conduction deafness.* **congenital d.** Hearing loss present at birth or arising in the perinatal period. **cortical d.** Inability to perceive or to appreciate and interpret the meaning of sounds, especially speech, due to lesions of the auditory temporal cortex. Also *cerebral deafness.* **familial d.** Hearing loss which affects one or more members of several generations. It is not due to acquired causes such as industrial noise or suppuration in the middle-ear cleft, and it appears in a similar form in each family member affected. **familial perceptive d.** HEREDODEGENERATIVE DEAFNESS. **genetic d.** Deafness due to the inheritance of defective genes. The majority of such individuals are born deaf but a proportion become deaf later in life as in cases of heredodegenerative deafness and otosclerosis. **heredodegenerative d.** A hereditary sensorineural hearing loss that is either genetic or acquired *in utero.* It is of late onset, as late as the fifth decade, but then it becomes progressive. A number of disparate conditions are involved, including the Alport syndrome and congenital syphilis. Also *familial perceptive deafness.* **high frequency d.** Deafness involving particularly the perception of high-frequency sounds. **hysterical d.** NONORGANIC HEARING LOSS. **immune complex associated d.** AUTOIMMUNE SENSORINEURAL HEARING LOSS. **Mondini-Alexander type genetic d.** A type of congenital genetic deafness, associated with the Mondini malformation. Also *Mondini type genetic deafness.* **musical d.** AMUSIA. **nerve d.** Deafness due to a lesion of the cochlear nerve. • An outmoded term in technical usage, but still current in popular usage, where it applies to all varieties of sensorineural deafness. **neural d.** SENSORINEURAL HEARING LOSS. **noise-induced d.** NOISE-INDUCED HEARING LOSS. **organic d.** Hearing loss arising from ascertainable or presumed organic changes in the ear or its central connections. **ototoxic d.** OTOTOXIC HEARING LOSS. **perceptive d.** *Outmoded* SENSORINEURAL HEARING LOSS. **postlingual d.** Hearing loss developing after the subject has learned to speak. **prelingual d.** Severe hearing loss, usually sensorineural, occurring in childhood or infancy before the subject has learned to speak. The distinction from postlingual deafness is important because it is easier to maintain speech after it has been acquired than to acquire speech if there is little or no hearing. **retrocochlear d.** Sensorineural deafness due to causes central to the cochlea, such as lesions of the acoustic nerve, or disease involving the central connections of the cochlea within the brainstem. **Scheibe type genetic d.** The most common type of congenital genetic deafness, associated with the Scheibe lesion. **senile d.** *Incorrect* PRESBYCUSIS. **sensorineural d.** SENSORINEURAL HEARING LOSS. **syphilitic d.** Hearing loss arising as a result of syphilis. It may present as a slow, progressive, sensorineural loss, becoming profound in the later stages, or it may be congenital from maternal transmission, though the deafness is rarely present at birth. **tone d.** AMUSIA. **toxic d.** *Older term* OTOTOXIC HEARING LOSS. **transmission d.** CONDUCTIVE HEARING LOSS. **traumatic d.** Hearing loss caused by damage to middle-ear or inner-ear structures resulting from direct injury or head injury or as the result of a loud noise or blast. **vascular d.** Hearing loss arising from diminished blood supply to the inner ear. **word d.** A form of receptive aphasia limited to the inability to understand and interpret the meaning of words which are heard. Also *auditory imperception.*

**deamino-oxytocin** \dē·am′ənō-äk′sitō′sin\ An analogue of oxytocin. Lacking the C-9 amino group, it is more potent than oxytocin in stimulating contraction of the uterus at term and in promoting the ejection of milk.

**deanol acetamidobenzoate** $C_{13}H_{20}N_2O_4$. 4-(Acetylamino)benzoic acid compounded with 2-(dimethylamino)-ethanol (1:1). A salt form of dimethylaminoethanol, a precursor of choline, that is believed to be converted to acetylcholine in the brain. It has been used to treat hyperactive states and is classified also as an antidepressant agent. It is given orally.

**deaquation** \dē·äkwā′shən\ DEHYDRATION.

**dearg. pil.** *deargentur pilulae* (L, let the pills be silvered).

**death** [Old English *dēath,* akin to German *Tod* death] Cessation of life, generally considered to ensue in the absence of spontaneous breathing or heartbeat. In a society of high technology, however, absence of discernible brain function has sometimes been substituted for the above criteria. • In the United States a presidential commission voted in 1981 that a Uniform Determination of Death Act be adopted by all states, an action endorsed by the American Medical Association and American Bar Association. The Act reads: "An individual who has sustained either (1) irreversible cessation of circulatory and respiratory functions, or (2) irreversible cessation of all functions of the entire brain, including the brain stem, is dead. A determination of death must be made in accordance with accepted medical standards." **apparent d.** Cessation of vital physiologic functions, particularly cardiac and respiratory activity, which produces a state simulating actual death, but from which recovery is possible through the use of resuscitative efforts. **associated d.** A woman's death associated with but not directly attributed to a complication of pregnancy, confinement, or the puerperium, as a death from chronic valvular disease of a woman far advanced in pregnancy. Compare MATERNAL DEATH. **black d.** *Popular* BLACK PLAGUE. **brain d.** The termination of brain function, as evidenced by loss of all reflexes and electrical activity of the brain; irreversible coma. • As determined by the Harvard criteria, established 1968, brain death must meet the following criteria: (1) unreceptivity and unresponsiveness, i.e., no response even to painful stimuli such as hard pinching; (2) no movements after observation by a physician for an hour continuously, and no breathing after three minutes off a respirator; (3) no reflexes, including brainstem reflexes; pupils are fixed and dilated; (4) a "flat" electroencephalogram, considered of great "confirmatory value" if technically adequate; (5) all of these tests repeated at least 24 hours later with no change; (6) two conditions must be excluded: hypothermia and central nervous system depression by drugs such as barbiturates. —Report of the Ad Hoc Committee of the Harvard Medical School to Examine the Definition of Brain Death, *Journal of the American Medical Association* 205:337, 1968. **cot d.** A British term for SUDDEN INFANT DEATH SYNDROME. **crib d.** SUDDEN INFANT DEATH SYNDROME. **direct maternal d.** Death of a mother from obstetric complications during the antepartum, intrapartum, or postpartum stage of pregnancy, including any events resulting from attempts to treat or manage such complications. **early fetal d.** Intrauterine death occurring during the first 20 weeks of gestation. **fetal d.** INTRAUTERINE DEATH. **functional d.** Extensive and irreversible damage to the central nervous system with respiration and circulatory function maintained artificially. **genetic d.** In genetics and evolutionary biology, the failure of any organism to reproduce, whether through premature death, through infertility, or by choice. The individual's genotype is thus lost from the gene pool. **indirect maternal d.** Death of a mother during the antepartum, intrapartum, or postpartum stage of pregnancy due to aggravation of pre-existing disease or new nonobstetrical disease by the physiologic changes associated with the pregnancy. **infant d.** Death occurring under the age of one year. **instantaneous d.** Accidental death occurring immediately or within a very short time, usually 10–20 minutes following the accident. In negligence law, the determination that death was instantaneous excludes from consideration claims of pain and suffering in suits brought by survivors. Compare SUDDEN DEATH. **intermediate fetal d.** Intrauterine death occurring after 20 but not more than 28 weeks of gestation. **intrauterine d.** The death *in utero* of the complete products of conception, irrespective of the length of gestation. Also *fetal death*. **late fetal d.** Intrauterine death occurring after 28 weeks of gestation. **maternal d.** The death of a woman as a complication of pregnancy, confinement, or the puerperium. Compare ASSOCIATED DEATH. **neonatal d.** Death of a newborn during the first 28 days of life. Neonatal death is sometimes designated as early when it occurs during the first seven days, and late when it occurs between the seventh and 29th day of life. **nonmaternal d.** The death of a pregnant woman due to incidental or accidental causes totally unrelated to the pregnancy. **perinatal d.** Fetal or neonatal death, especially death occurring during the period from a few weeks before birth to four weeks after birth. **somatic d.** The death of the entire organism, as opposed to death of a part of an organ or an extremity. **sudden d.** Unexpected death due to any cause and occurring within a short time period following the cause. Death may be immediate but usually occurs within hours to a few days. Compare INSTANTANEOUS DEATH. **thymineless d.** Death of a cell caused by lack of thymine. It is not clear why nondividing cells need thymine, but inhibition of thymidylate biosynthesis eventually kills cells. Tumor cells are particularly vulnerable, because of the requirement for TTP in DNA formation, so thymidylate synthesis is a target in some forms of cancer chemotherapy. **violent d.** Unnatural death caused or accelerated by external, usually extreme or intense, physical forces.

**death-cap** The deadly poisonous fungus *Amanita phalloides.* Also *death-cup.*

**deaur. pil.** *deaurentur pilulae* (L, let the pills be gilded).

**debility** \dibil′itē\ [L *debil(itas)* (from *debil(is)* needy, disabled + *-itas* -ITY) neediness, infirmity] Weakness; loss of strength.

**debouch** \diboosh′\ [French *débouch(er)* (from *dé-* DE- + *bouche* mouth, from L *bucca* mouth) to flow from a smaller to a larger passage] To open or empty into a passage or canal.

**débouchement** \dābooshmäN′, diboosh′mənt\ The emptying or opening of one canal or passage into another, or the point at which one canal opens into another.

**Debré** [Robert *Debré,* French physician, born 1882] **1** Kocher-Debré-Semelaigne syndrome. See under DEBRÉ-SEMELAIGNE SYNDROME. **2** De Toni-Debré-Fanconi syndrome, Debré-de Toni-Fanconi syndrome. See under FANCONI SYNDROME.

**débride** \dābrēd′\ To excise by débridement.

**débridement** \dābrēdmäN′\ [French, from *débrider* to unbridle] The removal of nonviable tissue. It is usually done mechanically, but in some cases chemicals or enzymes are used. **enzymatic d.** Removal of nonviable tissue and foreign material by the use of vegetable enzymes that lyse nonliving tissue and spare living tissue. **major d.** A débridement of such magnitude that it is best accomplished in an operating theater with the use of an anesthetic. **minor d.** A wound cleansing that is brief enough or painless enough that it can generally be performed without an anesthetic or the need for an operating theater. **surgical d.** Mechanical removal of dead or infected tissue and foreign material from a wound or from diseased tissue. **tangential d.** TANGENTIAL EXCISION.

**debris** \dəbrē′\ [French *débris* (from Old French *desbrisier* to break apart, from *des-* down, away + *brisier* to break) rubble, rubbish, accumulated fragments] A useless accumulation of miscellaneous particles; waste in the form of fragments. **dermal d.** The accumulated serum, medication, and bits of necrotic dermis that form during the course of healing of a partial thickness burn. **d. of Malassez** RESTS OF MALASSEZ.

**debt / oxygen d.** The additional oxygen consumption above resting values that occurs at the end of a short period of intense work. It is the amount of oxygen required to restore the energy stores that were utilized anaerobically during the period of work. Also *oxygen deficit.*

**dec.** *decanta* (L, pour off: a direction used in pharmacy).

**deca-** \dek′ə-\ [Gk *deka* ten] A combining form denoting $10^1$, ten: used with SI units A seldom used form. Also *deka-*. Symbol: da

**decalcification** \dē′kalsifikā′shən\ The loss or removal of calcium salts from bones or teeth.

**decamethonium bromide** $C_{16}H_{38}Br_2N_2$. *N,N,N,-N′,N′,N′*-Hexamethyl-1,10-decanediaminium dibromide. A bis-trimethylammonium compound containing a 10-carbon atom bridge between the nitrogen atoms. It is an effective muscle relaxant drug of the depolarizing type, but is much more stable than succinylcholine.

**decannulation** \dēkan′yəlā′shən\ **1** The removal of an indwelling cannula. **2** The removal of a tracheostomy tube when it is no longer needed or as the first step in changing the tube. Also *detubation.*

**decapitate** \dēkap′itāt\ [Late L *decapitat(us),* past part. of *decapitare* to behead, from L *de* from + *caput,* gen. *capitis,* head] In experimental neurophysiology, designating a preparation in which the neuraxis is severed at the foramen magnum. The head is not necessarily removed.

**decapitation** \dēkap'itā'shən\ [*decapitat(e)* + -ION] Removal of the fetal head to facilitate delivery, a procedure that is obsolete among humans but is at times necessary in veterinary practice.

**decapsulation** \dēkap's$^y$əlā'shən\ [DE- + *capsul(e)* + -ATION] Removal of a capsule, usually a renal capsule (nephrocapsulectomy).

**decarboxylase** Any of a great variety of enzymes that catalyze the reaction R—COOH → R—H + $CO_2$. Those that act on amino acids usually contain pyridoxal phosphate.

**decarboxylation** \dē'kärbäk'silā'shən\ A reaction of the type R—COOH → R—H + $CO_2$, in which a carboxyl group is lost by a substance and carbon dioxide is produced, as in the reaction in which histidine yields histamine. **oxidative d.** The oxidation of a substance associated with the loss of a carboxyl group as carbon dioxide. The oxidation may be associated with an electron acceptor as nicotinamide adenine dinucleotide. An example is the reaction of pyruvate with pyruvate dehydrogenase $NAD^+$ and coenzyme A.

**decay** [Old French *decair* (from Vulgar L *decadere* to fall down or off, from L *de-* off, from + *cadere* to fall) to fall into ruin] **1** To decompose; rot. **2** To decline in health, strength, or vitality. **3** The process of decaying. **4** In radioactive materials, the spontaneous emission of charged particles from an unstable nucleus. **branching d.** The radioactive disintegration of a nuclide that has more than one mode of decay, each with its own type of emitted radiation. **dental d.** DENTAL CARIES. **free induction d.** The signal that emanates after a radio-frequency pulse has excited the nuclear spin system to resonance. The signal is termed "free" because the atomic nuclei precess freely without applying radio frequency. **isomeric level d.** ISOMERIC TRANSITION. **radioactive d.** A spontaneous change in a nucleus to a lower energy state, with the emission of energy in the form of photons or particles. Also *radioactive disintegration, spontaneous disintegration.*

**deceleration** \dēsel'ərā'shən\ **1** A decrease in velocity. Also *negative acceleration.* **2** The rate at which velocity decreases.

**decentered** \dēsen'tərd\ Positioned off axis: said of a lens.

**decentration** \dē'sentrā'shən\ [L *de-* away from, apart + *centr(um)* center + -ATION] Displacement of a lens system from perfect axial alignment.

**decerebellation** \dēser'əbelā'shən\ **1** Absence of cerebellar function. **2** The destruction of the cerebellum.

**decerebrate** \dēser'əbrāt\ **1** To remove higher cerebral function from, as by experimental transection of the neuraxis through the midbrain. Also *decerebrize.* **2** Denoting an absence of the cerebrum or of cerebral activity. Also *acerebral.*

**decerebration** \dēser'əbrā'shən\ [DE- + CEREBR- + -ATION] **1** The experimental procedure of rendering an animal behaviorally free of influence from the forebrain, either by destroying the forebrain or by isolating lower centers. **2** Absence of cerebral function, often the result of a tumor or other lesion of the midbrain and characterized principally by extreme extensor spasticity of all extremities.

**decerebrize** \dēser'əbrīz\ DECEREBRATE.

**dechlorurant** \dēklôr'yərənt\ An agent that decreases urinary chloride content.

**decholesterolization** \dē'kōles'tərôlīzā'shən\ Selective removal of cholesterol. Also *decholesterinization* (seldom used).

**deci-** \des'ə-\ [L *decem* ten] A combining form denoting $10^{-1}$, one tenth: used with SI units. Symbol: d

**decibel** \des'əbəl\ [DECI- + BEL] A unit of power ratio equal to 0.1 bel. Symbol: dB **d. A** A logarithmic unit of sound pressure or power, weighted by a function "A" which reduces the response to low and very high frequency sound in order to simulate the response of the human ear and give an indication of acceptability, or of loudness, or annoyance potential. When conditions of noise measurement are "A-weighted," a reference sound pressure of 20 micropascals ($20 \times 10^{-6}$ pascal) is used for sound pressure level, and a reference sound power of 1 picowatt ($10^{-12}$ watt) for sound power level. Symbol: dBA, dB(A)

**decidua** \disid'yoo·ə\ [L, short for *membrana decidua* deciduous membrane. See DECIDUOUS.] The thick endometrial lining of the uterus in pregnant mammals, all or part of which is shed with the placenta at or shortly after birth of the fetus. Also *caduca.* **d. basalis** The maternal part of the placenta directly underlying the chorionic sac at the site of implantation. Initially it is about 6 mm thick. It is penetrated to its deeper part by the cytotrophoblast, and increases in thickness as a result of growth in size and length of the villi of the chorion frondosum, and consequent expansion of the intervillous space. Only in the pathologic state termed "placenta accreta" does the cytotrophoblast penetrate the decidual plate to invade the underlying myometrium. Also *basal decidua.* **d. capsularis** The portion of the decidua directly overlying the chorionic sac and facing the uterine lumen which separates it from the decidua parietalis. By about 3½ months most of the decidua capsularis has atrophied allowing the chorion laeve to make direct contact with the epithelium of the decidua parietalis. It completely disappears by about 4½ months in all regions except at the placental margin. Also *capsular decidua.* **d. compacta** The surface and most compact zone of decidua. **ectopic d.** The occurrence of a decidual reaction outside of the endometrial cavity. **d. marginalis** The junction of the decidua basalis, decidua parietalis, and decidua capsularis. **d. parietalis** The portion of the endometrium which after implantation in man lines the uterus other than where the blastocyst is embedded. As the chorionic sac enlarges, the decidua capsularis thins out and degenerates and the chorion laeve fuses with the decidua parietalis. Also *parietal decidua.* **d. polyposa** Hyperplasia of the decidua leading to polyplike projections on the surface of the decidua. **d. spongiosa** The middle and spongy zone of the decidua, consisting of glands and numerous small blood vessels. **d. subchorialis** The decidual component of the thickening at the margin of a placenta.

**deciduitis** \disij'oo·ī'tis\ [*decidu(a)* + -ITIS] Inflammation or infection of the uterine decidua.

**deciduoma** \disij'oo·ō'mə\ [*decidu(a)* + -OMA] An intrauterine accumulation of decidual cells. **d. malignum** CHORIOCARCINOMA.

**deciduomatosis** \disij'oo·ōmətō'sis\ [DECIDUOMA + *t* + -OSIS ] The presence of decidua in the nonpregnant state.

**deciduosarcoma** \disij'oo·ōsärkō'mə\ [*decidu(a)* + *o* + SARCOMA] CHORIOCARCINOMA.

**deciduous** \disid'yoo·əs\ [L *deciduus* (from *decidere* to fall off, be shed, from *cadere* to fall) tending to be shed] Destined to be shed and replaced, as *deciduous teeth.*

**decision** A determination or judgment, as of a court. **Brawner d.** See under AMERICAN LAW INSTITUTE FORMULATION. **Durham d.** DURHAM RULE.

**declination** \dek'linā'shən\ [L *declinatio* (from *declinatus* past part. of *declinare* to turn away, vary) a turning aside] Ocular rotation away from the vertical in either direction.

**declive** \dēklīv'\ [L (from *declivis* sloping downward, from *clivus* a slope) a downslope, declivity] [NA] The vermian portion of the middle lobe of the cerebellum, between the fissura prima and the postlunate fissure, the culmen monticuli and folium vermis. It is continuous laterally with the lobulus simplex. Also *declivis, clivus monticuli, lobulus clivi.*

**decoagulant** 1 An agent that decreases the concentration of coagulation components in the blood. 2 ANTICOAGULANT.

**decoct.** *decoctum* (L, a decoction).

**decoction** [L *decoctio* (from DE- + L *coctus,* past part. of *coquere* to cook) a cooking down] 1 The process of boiling. 2 A medicinal or other drug preparation obtained by boiling. **Zimmermann's d.** A decoction consisting of rhubarb, potassium bitartrate, water, barley, and syrup, employed as a cathartic.

**decoctum** A decoction. **d. acaciae corticis** A decoction constituting a 6% aqueous extract of the bark from *Acacia arabica* or *A. decurrens.* It has been used in gargles and as an astringent. **d. aloes compositum** A decoction constituting a 1% aqueous extract of aloes and myrrh containing potassium carbonate, licorice, and compound tincture of cardamon. It was used as a purgative.

**decombustion** \dē′kəmbus′chən\ The removal of oxygen from a substance, as by strong heat in the presence of charcoal.

**decompensation** \dē′kämpənsā′shən\ 1 The absence of compensatory adjustments. 2 Following a lesion of the nervous system, the reappearance of the original functional deficits after a period during which they had disappeared due to compensation by other structures. Damage to a second brain structure usually triggers the decompensation. **Bekhterev d.** Appearance of nystagmus and other vestibular signs, directed to the side of damage to the vestibular apparatus or nerve, in an animal in which contralateral vestibular function had previously been abolished and in which compensation for those vestibular signs had taken place. Also *Bekhterev compensation.* **corneal d.** Failure of the corneal endothelium to perform its dehydrating function, with the result that the cornea becomes edematous.

**decomplementation** \dēkäm′pləmentā′shən\ The inactivation of complement in serum by any of a variety of agents.

**decomposition** Putrefaction of organic material. **d. of movements** ASYNERGY.

**decompression** \dē′kəmpresh′ən\ 1 The slow reduction of pressure on persons working in caissons or as deep-sea divers to prevent the onset of decompression sickness. 2 The reduction of atmospheric pressure on people who ascend to great heights. 3 Any operation to relieve pressure within a closed cavity or space, as the relief of intracranial pressure by removal of a portion of the cranium. **cardiac d.** A reduction of blood volume within the heart. **cerebral d.** Reduction of pressure in or on the brain. This is accomplished by a variety of measures, such as ventricular or cerebrospinal fluid drainage, systemic administration of chemicals to reduce the water content of the brain, and surgical removal of part of the brain, but principally by removal of part of the skull and incision of the dura mater to permit expansion of the brain. **d. of heart** Pericardiotomy with evacuation of a clot. Also *decompression of pericardium.* **intestinal d.** A procedure in which an obstructed bowel is either bypassed or exteriorized, as in a colostomy or ileostomy. It is performed to decrease intraluminal pressure, prevent perforation, and reestablish the fecal stream. It may occur spontaneously, opening into the free peritoneal cavity or into another hollow viscus. **Naffziger orbital d.** Surgical removal of the roof and lateral walls of the orbit to release intraorbital pressure, as for thyroid exophthalmos. **nerve d.** Reduction of pressure on a nerve to permit return of function, as by incision of the perineurium in the presence of an intraneural neuroma, or excision or deflection of tissue or strictures compressing a nerve. **d. of pericardium** DECOMPRESSION OF HEART. **d. of rectum** A surgical procedure in which excessive pressure in the rectum, resulting from distal obstruction, is relieved by bypass, division, or resection of the obstructive element. **d. of spinal cord** Reduction of pressure on the spinal cord, as by removal of spinous processes and laminae of the vertebrae where the spinal cord is compressed by extradural tissue, and opening of the dura mater also where compression is due to intradural disease. **suboccipital d.** Reduction of pressure on the cerebellum and structures in the posterior fossa by craniectomy of the occipital bone, sometimes with upper cervical laminectomy and incision of the dura mater. **subtemporal d.** Reduction of intracranial pressure by removal of cranial tissue beneath the temporal muscle and stellate incision of the dura mater to permit herniation of the temporal lobe. The operation was once employed in cases where increased intracranial pressure could not be attacked directly. Also *Cushing's operation.* **trigeminal d.** Reduction of pressure on the ganglion and root of the trigeminal nerve. This may be achieved by incision of the overlying dura and division of the superior petrosal sinus (Taarnhøj's operation). Another form of decompression employs separation of blood vessels, particularly the superior cerebellar artery from the root of the nerve near its juncture with the pons.

**decondensation** \dē′kändənsā′shən\ 1 Any process that results in transition of native chromatin to a more extended form in which core particles are separated by linker DNA in electron micrographs, creating the so-called beads-on-a-string configuration. 2 The process of chromosomes becoming more disperse during the cell cycle, in particular in moving from M to $G_1$ phases. Functionally, it is a requirement for transcription.

**deconditioning** \dē′kəndish′əning\ 1 The removal of a conditioned response. 2 Altered cardiovascular function associated with diuresis and reduced blood volume following prolonged periods of weightlessness.

**decongestant** \dē′kənjes′tənt\ An agent which reduces congestion, particularly nose drops intended to diminish congestion of the nasal lining.

**decontamination** \dē′kəntam′inā′shən\ [DE- + CONTAMINATION] The removal, reduction, or inactivation of a contaminant from a surface, structure, environment, an inanimate object including clothing, or a person, usually with the object of rendering the contaminated area or object safe or usable.

**decorticate** \dēkôr′tikāt\ [See DECORTICATION.] 1 To remove the cortex from (the cerebrum or cerebellum, or other organ such as the kidney). 2 Having had the cortex removed.

**decortication** \di′kôrtikā′shən\ [L *decorticatio* (from DE- + CORTEX + L *-atio* -ATION) a removing of the bark or rind] 1 A procedure in which a naturally occurring or pathologic outer layer of an organ or cavity is removed. It often is used in a pleural excision to allow entrapped lung tissue to expand, or in the removal of the renal capsule. 2 The degenerative loss of the cortical or outer layer of an organ or of a cavity lining. 3 Necrosis or destruction of the cerebral cortex with preserved brainstem function; the decorticate state. 4 The experimental procedure of removing or rendering nonfunctional the cerebral cortex. For defs. 1–4 also *excortication.* **arterial d.** A sympathectomy performed by removing periadventitial tissue containing sympathetic nerves near the arterial wall. **chemical d.** Removal of the cortical portion of an organ or structure by means of a chemical agent or by enzymatic digestion, rather than by surgical means. Also *enzymatic decortication.* **d. of lung** Surgical excision of the visceral pleura to permit the lung to expand. **renal d.** The removal of a renal capsule.

**decrement** \dek′rəmənt\ [L *decrement(um)* (from *decre(scere)* to decrease + *-mentum* -MENT) a decreasing in value] **1** Decrease or loss. **2** The amount of decrease or loss. **3** The abatement of symptoms of a disease.

**decrudescence** \dē′kroodes′əns\ [DE- + L *crudescens,* pres. part. of *crudescere* (from *crud(us)* rough, crude + *-escere,* inf. form denoting becoming) to become fierce or savage] A lessening of the intensity of symptoms; decrement.

**decub.** *decubitus* (L, lying down).

**decubation** \dē′kyoobā′shən\ [DE- + L *cubatio* (from *cubatus,* adaptation of *cubitus,* past part. of *cubare* to recline) a reclining] The final stage in the course of an infectious disease, from the disappearance of the symptoms to complete recovery and the absence of infecting organisms.

**decubital** \dikyoo′bitəl\ Of or relating to decubitus.

**decubitus** \dikyoo′bitəs\ [New L (from *decubitus,* past part. of L *decumbere* to be down), a lying down] **1** The position of a person lying down: often qualified by an indication of the part of the body resting on a surface, as *dorsal decubitus* (lying on the back). **2** A decubitus ulcer; bedsore. **d. acutus** A bedsore (decubitus ulcer) developing acutely in a hemiplegic patient on the affected side. **chronic d.** BEDSORE. **d. chronicus** BEDSORE. **dorsal d.** The position of a person lying on the back; a supine position. **lateral d.** In radiology, an examination with the patient lying on the side with the film in a vertical position and the radiation beam horizontal. **ventral d.** The position of a person lying on the abdomen; a prone position.

**decussate** \dēkus′āt\ **1** To cross, or pass at an angle from one side to the other, as fascicles, tracts, or pathways. **2** Crossing, as in the shape of an X.

**decussatio** \di′kusā′shō\ [L (from *decussis* an X mark, the numeral ten, a ten-*as* coin, from *dec(em)* ten + *assis* or *as,* a unit of weight and currency) an intersection of two lines] (*pl.* decussationes) DECUSSATION. **d. brachii conjunctivi** DECUSSATIO PEDUNCULORUM CEREBELLARIUM SUPERIORUM. **d. lemniscorum** A large, interwoven crossing of nerve fiber bundles (internal arcuate fibers) passing ventrorostrally from origins in the gracile and cuneate nuclei to form the medial lemnisci of the opposite side. The decussation lies dorsal to the pyramids and ventral to the central gray matter. Also *decussatio sensoria, sensory decussation, decussation of lemnisci.* **d. lemniscorum medialium** [NA] The crossing over the midline from one side of the brainstem to the other of the internal arcuate fibers derived from neurons having their cell bodies in the nucleus gracilis and nucleus cuneatus. It occurs ventral to the gray matter surrounding the central canal in a region just dorsal to the pyramids in the medulla oblongata. Also *decussation of medial lemniscus.* **d. motoria** DECUSSATIO PYRAMIDUM. **d. nervorum trochlearium** [NA] The complete crossing made by the trochlear nerves in the superior medullary velum. Also *decussation of trochlear nerves.* **d. pedunculorum cerebellarium superiorum** [NA] A crossing of the superior cerebellar peduncles that takes place ventral to the central gray matter in the midbrain. Also *decussation of superior cerebellar peduncles, decussation of the brachia conjunctiva, decussatio brachii conjunctivi.* **d. pyramidum** [NA] A massive, interwoven crossing of descending pyramidal fibers along the ventral aspect of the lower medulla oblongata. In humans, about three quarters of the fibers in the pyramids cross. Also *decussation of pyramids, pyramidal decussation, motor decussation, decussatio motoria.* **d. sensoria** DECUSSATIO LEMNISCORUM. **d. supraoptica dorsalis** DORSAL SUPRAOPTIC COMMISSURE. **d. supraoptica ventralis** VENTRAL SUPRAOPTIC COMMISSURE. **decussationes tegmenti** [NA] Two prominent decussations in the midbrain ventral to the central gray in the midbrain. The dorsal one consists of fascicles from the tectum and superior colliculus. The ventral one is formed by rubrospinal and rubroreticular fibers. Also *tegmental decussations, fountain decussations, decussationes tegmentorum, decussations of tegmentum.* **d. tegmenti dorsalis** DECUSSATION OF TECTOSPINAL TRACTS. **d. tegmenti ventralis** DECUSSATION OF RUBROSPINAL TRACTS. **decussationes tegmentorum** DECUSSATIONES TEGMENTI.

**decussation** \di′kusā′shən\ [L *decussatio.* See DECUSSATIO.] A midline crossing in the form of an X made by nerve or connective tissue fibers or fascicles. Also *decussatio.* **anterior hypothalamic d.** DORSAL SUPRAOPTIC COMMISSURE. **d. of the brachia conjunctiva** DECUSSATIO PEDUNCULORUM CEREBELLARIUM SUPERIORUM. **dorsal tegmental d.** DECUSSATION OF TECTOSPINAL TRACTS. **Forel's d.** DECUSSATION OF RUBROSPINAL TRACTS. • It is distinct from Forel's commissure (the supramamillary decussation). **fountain d.'s** DECUSSATIONES TEGMENTI. **fountain d. of Meynert** DECUSSATION OF TECTOSPINAL TRACTS. **Held's d.** The crossing of a small bundle of fibers arising in the ventral cochlear nucleus. After passing over the inferior cerebellar peduncle, the fibers swerve ventromedially as the acoustic striae cross the midline ventral to the medial longitudinal fasciculus and join the lateral lemniscus of the opposite side. The axons are smaller than those of the trapezoid body. **inferior hypothalamic d.** VENTRAL SUPRAOPTIC COMMISSURE. **d. of lemnisci** DECUSSATIO LEMNISCORUM. **d. of medial lemniscus** DECUSSATIO LEMNISCORUM MEDIALIUM. **motor d.** DECUSSATIO PYRAMIDUM. **optic d.** CHIASMA OPTICUM. **posterior hypothalamic d.** SUPRAMAMILLARY DECUSSATION. **pyramidal d.** DECUSSATIO PYRAMIDUM. **d. of pyramids** DECUSSATIO PYRAMIDUM. **d. of rubrospinal tracts** The crossing of rubrospinal fibers from one side of the midbrain to the other on their way from the red nucleus to the spinal cord. After arising from neurons in the red nucleus, the rubrospinal fibers cross immediately in the tegmental decussation ventral to the site of crossing of the tectospinal fibers. Rubrospinal fibers constitute the major part of this more ventrally located tegmental decussation. Also *ventral tegmental decussation, decussatio tegmenti ventralis, Forel's decussation.* See also DECUSSATIONES TEGMENTI. **sensory d.** DECUSSATIO LEMNISCORUM. **d. of superior cerebellar peduncles** DECUSSATIO PEDUNCULORUM CEREBELLARIUM SUPERIORUM. **superior hypothalamic d.** DORSAL SUPRAOPTIC COMMISSURE. **superior supraoptic d.** DORSAL SUPRAOPTIC COMMISSURE. **suprachiasmatic d.** VENTRAL SUPRAOPTIC COMMISSURE. **supramamillary d.** The midline crossing made by a small bundle of nerve fibers that passes from the globus pallidus to the contralateral subthalamic nucleus and adjacent midbrain reticular formation. It lies dorsal to the mamillary bodies. Also *posterior hypothalamic decussation, Forel's commissure.* **d. of tectospinal tracts** The crossing from one side of the midbrain to the other of fibers that form the tectospinal tract. These fibers originate in the superior colliculi, cross in the median raphe as the dorsal tegmental decussation, located just ventral to the oculomotor nucleus, and descend on the opposite side as the tectospinal tract. Also *dorsal tegmental decussation, decussatio tegmenti dorsalis, fountain decussation of Meynert*. See also DECUSSATIONES TEGMENTI. **tegmental d.'s** DECUSSATIONES TEGMENTI. **d.'s of tegmentum** DECUSSATIONES TEGMENTI. **d. of trochlear nerves** DECUSSATIO NERVORUM TROCHLEARIUM. **ventral supraoptic d.** VENTRAL SUPRAOPTIC COMMISSURE. **ventral tegmental d.** DECUSSATION OF RUBROSPINAL TRACTS.

**decussationes** \dēkus′āshō′nēz\ Plural of DECUSSATIO.

**dedifferentiation** \dēdif′əren′shē·ā′shən\ ANAPLASIA.

**deductible** \diduk′təbəl\ An amount of loss or expense for health care services that must be incurred by an insured individual before an insurer will assume liability for all or part of the remaining expenses. The level of deductibles are defined by the provisions of a health insurance plan.

**de-efferentation** \dē-ef′ərentā′shən\ [DE- + EFFERENT + -ATION] Motor denervation.

**deep** 1 Located beneath the surface. 2 Lying behind other structures.

**Deetjen** [Hermann *Deetjen*, German physician, 1867–1915] Deetjen's body. See under PLATELET.

**def** DEF INDEX.

**defatigation** \dē′fatigā′shən\ Muscle or nervous tissue fatigue.

**defaunate** \dēfô′nāt\ [DE- + *faun(a)* + -ATE] To eliminate animal or protozoan pests or parasites from (an infested area or an infected host).

**defecation** \def′əkā′shən\ [Late L *defaecatio* (from L *defaecare* to cleanse from the dregs, to clear, from *de-* from + *faex*, gen. *faecis*, the dregs of wine, sediment) a cleansing of impurities] The evacuation of fecal material from the rectum via the anus. Also *laxation, cacation, diachoresis*.

**defect** 1 A structural or functional abnormality, particularly one of developmental origin. 2 Any imperfection or failing. **acquired d.** An anatomic defect or loss or impairment of function not due to congenital factors but to trauma, infection, neoplastic change, or effects of the environment. Some defects may be described as prenatally acquired rather than congenital, such as those of the rubella syndrome. **aorticopulmonary septal d.** AORTICOPULMONARY WINDOW. **aortic septal d.** AORTICOPULMONARY WINDOW. **aortopulmonary d.** AORTICOPULMONARY WINDOW. **atrial septal d.** A persisting abnormal communication between the cardiac atria owing to the failure of any of the embryonic atrial septal structures to form and unite with other septal structures, or to be properly disposed. In humans, a failure of closure or fusion of the septum secundum results in an ostium secundum defect, and the failure of closure or fusion of the septum primum and endocardial cushions results in an ostium primum defect. A patent foramen ovale can also result in a functional atrial septal defect. Also *interatrial septal defect*. **atriventricular septal d.** A defect at the site of the normal atrioventricular septal structures which, potentially, permits a communication between all four chambers. It is always associated with a common atriventricular junction guarded by what is effectively a common valve, although the valve may be separated into distinct right- and left-sided orifices. **birth d.** CONGENITAL DEFECT. **complete type endocardial cushion d.** An atrioventricular septal defect with a common atrioventricular valve. It usually permits both interatrial and interventricular shunting. **congenital d.** Any structural or functional abnormality present at birth and thought to be of developmental origin. Also *birth defect*. **congenital ectodermal d.** Any of a heterogeneous group of developmental abnormalities characterized by the absence or abnormality of one or more ectodermal components, such as sweat glands, hair, nails, or teeth. The most common forms are hidrotic ectodermal dysplasia, an autosomal dominant condition, and anhidrotic ectodermal dysplasia, an X-linked condition. Also *ectodermal dysplasia, congenital ectodermal dysplasia*. **congenital pericardial d.** Congenital absence or other abnormality of part or all of the pericardium, commonly associated with other forms of congenital heart disease. **congenital reading d.** DEVELOPMENTAL DYSLEXIA. **cortical d.** A radiographic finding of a lucent zone in the cortex that is asymptomatic and benign. Also *subperiosteal cortical defect*. **dehalogenase d.** IODOTYROSINE DEIODINASE DEFECT. **developmental d.** Any deviation in embryonic, fetal, or postnatal development that results in a persistent abnormality in the structure or function of the individual. **endocardial cushion d.** A defect involving the failure of fusion or of ultimate disposition of embryonic atrioventricular cushions. It results in a persistent atrioventricular canal, or if of a lesser degree, in deficient leaflets of the mitral and tricuspid valves. **fibrous cortical d.** A common radiographic abnormality of the long bones in children consisting of an oval transparency in the cortex of the metaphysis and signifying an area of bone which has undergone necrosis and has been replaced by fibrous tissue. Large defects may cause pathological fracture. Spontaneous reconstitution of bone occurs in two to five years. **filling d.** Any abnormality of the gastrointestinal tract that becomes evident radiologically by failure of a contrast medium to fill some part of the tract, suggesting obstruction by foreign material or a tumor. **galactokinase d.** GALACTOSEMIA. **genetic d. of folate metabolism** Any of a group of rare autosomal recessive disorders characterized by onset early in life of seizures, mental retardation, and megaloblastic anemia. Included among these disorders is congenital folate malabsorption of unknown cause, dihydrofolate reductase deficiency, formiminotransferase deficiency, 5,10-methylene tetrahydrofolate reductase deficiency, and tetrahydrofolate methyltransferase deficiency. **3$\beta$-hydroxysteroid dehydrogenase d.** A rare form of congenital adrenocortical hyperplasia defined by a metabolic (enzymatic) block in the earliest stage of the biosynthetic pathway of cortisol. It occurs in the step between pregnenolone and progesterone. It is characterized by the presence of urinary steroids predominantly having the 3$\beta$-hydroxy-5-pregnene configuration, incomplete masculinization of the genital tract in affected males, a salt-losing syndrome, and early death. Also *3$\beta$-hydroxysteroid dehydrogenase deficiency*. **interatrial septal d.** ATRIAL SEPTAL DEFECT. **iodide transport d.** Familial goiter owing to absent or limited entry of iodide into the thyroid, despite raised concentrations of plasma thyrotropin, accompanied by a parallel abnormality in iodide transport by the salivary glands. **iodotyrosine coupling d.** Congenital goiter associated with a large, hyperactive thyroid gland but with low concentrations of thyroid hormone in plasma, raised concentrations of plasma iodotyrosines, and hypothyroidism. The defect is assumed to lie in the coupling of iodotyrosines to form iodothyronines. **iodotyrosine deiodinase d.** A familial enzymatic deficiency of the thyroid characterized by goiter, hypothyroidism, familial occurrence, and failure to deiodinate monoiodotyrosine or diiodotyrosine. Normal hormone synthesis is restored by administration of iodide. Also *dehalogenase defect*. **limb reduction d.** MEROMELIA. **luteal phase d.** Failure or inadequacy of the luteal (postovulatory or secretory) phase of the human menstrual cycle; the anatomic concomitant, in the uterine endometrium, of the anovulatory menstrual cycle. Such a defect may interfere with ability of a pregnancy to be maintained due to concomitant inadequate levels of progesterone. Also *luteal phase deficiency*. **metaphyseal fibrous d.** NONOSSIFYING FIBROMA. **neural-tube d.** Any developmental disorder, such as spina bifida, in an organ of the central nervous system which was derived from the embryonic neural tube. Neural-tube defects are usually caused by the failure of the neural tube to close in one or more of its segments. **obstructive ventilatory d.** A condition of the lung resulting in abnormal slowing of air flow, as detected by spirography. Compare RESTRICTIVE VENTILATORY DEFECT. **organification d.** The most common defect in thyroid hormone biosynthesis, characterized by thyroid enlargement, varying degrees of hypothyroidism, and sometimes deafness (Pendred syndrome). The biochemical abnormalities are absence of thyroidal iodide peroxidase or abnormality of thyroglobulin synthesis. **ostium primum d.** A deficiency of the atrioventricular septum which permits interatrial shunting. It is an "endocardial cushion defect" which is usually classified as an atrial septal defect, and it is often associated with other defects of atrioventricular canal embryogenesis. **ostium secundum d.** A defect of the atrial septum within the confines of the oval fossa. It is by far the commonest type of atrial septal defect. **partial type endocardial cushion d.** An atrioventricular septal defect with separate right and left atrioventricular orifices permitting only interatrial shunting. See also OSTIUM PRIMUM DEFECT. **polytopic field d.** A pattern of anomalies that result from the disturbance of a single developmental field, such as a malformation, deformation, or disruption sequence. **restrictive ventilatory d.** A condition of the lung resulting in reduced vital capacity without slowing of air flow, as detected by spirography. Compare OBSTRUCTIVE VENTILATORY DEFECT. **salt-losing d.** Any of several forms of congenital adrenocortical hyperplasia characterized by deficient biosynthesis of aldosterone in which renal sodium and water loss with consequent vasomotor collapse are the dominant clinical features. **serum iodoprotein d.** Congenital or familial goiter and hypothyroidism, probably owing to inadequate production of thyroglobulin in the thyroid. **subcortical d.** A bone lesion occurring on the inner surface of the cortex. **subperiosteal cortical d.** CORTICAL DEFECT. **ventricular septal d.** A communication between the ventricular chambers, usually resulting from a congenital malformation. It can also be due to ischemic heart disease or trauma, or be iatrogenic.

**defeminization** \dēfem′inīzā′shən\ [DE- + FEMINIZATION] Loss of estrogen effect upon the female secondary sex characters, as from surgical or natural menopause or a masculinizing ovarian or adrenal cortical tumor.

**defence** *Brit.* DEFENSE.

**defender / ear d.** HEARING PROTECTOR.

**defense** [French *défense* (from L *defensus*, past part. of *defendere* to ward off, defend) defense] **1** The act, process, or method by which the body or any of its systems or constituents protects itself in order to preserve health or homeostasis. **2** See under DEFENSE MECHANISM. **insanity d.** A plea, in a court of law, of not guilty of, or not fully responsible for, a criminal act by reason of mental illness. **muscular d.** GUARDING. **ur d.** See under UR-DEFENSE.

**deferens** \def′ərənz\ [L (gen. *deferentis*) pres. part. of *deferre* to carry away] **1** Conveying away; efferent. Also *deferent*. **2** Denoting the ductus deferens.

**deferent** \def′ərənt\ DEFERENS.

**deferentectomy** \def′ərentek′təmē\ [DEFERENT + -ECTOMY] VASECTOMY.

**deferential** \def′əren′shəl\ Pertaining to the ductus deferens.

**deferentitis** \def′ərentī′tis\ [DEFERENT + -ITIS] Inflammation of the ductus deferens.

**defervescence** \def′ərves′əns\ The lessening or subsiding of a fever.

**defervescent** \def′ərves′ənt\ **1** Of, causing, or characterized by defervescence, or the reduction of fever. **2** An agent that reduces a fever.

**defibrillation** \dēfib′rilā′shən\ [DE- + FIBRILLATION] The termination of atrial or ventricular fibrillation, usually by direct-current shock.

**defibrillator** \dēfib′rilā′tər\ An apparatus for administering electrical shock to terminate atrial or ventricular fibrillation or other arrhythmias. An external defibrillator is applied to the chest wall, and an internal defibrillator is applied directly to the heart.

**defibrinated** \dēfi′brinā′tid\ Freed of fibrinogen: said of blood or plasma.

# deficiency

**deficiency** \difish′ənsē\ [L *deficiens*, gen. *deficient(is)* pres. part. of *deficere* to be wanting, to fail + -Y] A lack or insufficiency. **acid-maltase d.** GLYCOGEN STORAGE DISEASE II. **adenosine deaminase d.** An enzyme deficiency inherited as an autosomal recessive, often associated with the combined immunodeficiency syndrome in children. **amylo-1,6-glucosidase d.** GLYCOGEN STORAGE DISEASE III. **amylo-(1,4-1,6)-transglucosidase d.** GLYCOGEN STORAGE DISEASE IV.. **$\alpha_1$-antitrypsin d.** **1** Any decrease in the functional activity, usually in plasma, of $\alpha_1$-antitrypsin. The deficiency may be acquired or be caused by a gene-determined protein abnormality. **2** A disorder of dominant heredity that is characterized by precocious pulmonary emphysema, hepatic cirrhosis, and pancreatic cysts of variable severity. It is associated with decreased plasma $\alpha_1$-antitrypsin activity. Affected individuals may be heterozygous for codominant alleles that individually are associated with intermediate deficiency, or homozygous for an allele associated with marked deficiency. Also *antitrypsin deficiency*. **apolipoprotein C-II d.** See under FAMILIAL HYPERLIPOPROTEINEMIA TYPE I. **argininosuccinic acid synthetase d.** One of the less rare autosomal recessive disorders of the urea cycle, in which a deficiency of the enzyme, orginosuccinic acid synthetase, inhibits the pathway of conversion of citrulline to arginine. Arginosuccinic acid, the precursor of arginine, accumulates in the blood, urine, and cerebrospinal fluid. Arginine, which is distal to the enzyme block, is at a low serum level. Hyperaminoacidemia results, with postprandial ammonemia. Clinical effects appear soon after birth in severe cases, with lethargy, tachypnea, hyperammonemia, respiratory distress, seizures, and coma. Later in infancy the manifestations are failure to thrive, developmental delay, seizures, hepatomegaly, and brittle hair. Later in childhood, mental defects, convulsions, cerebellar disorder, and cranial nerve palsies are seen. Also *argininosuccinase deficiency*. **brancher d.** GLYCOGEN STORAGE DISEASE IV.. **$C_1$ esterase inhibitor d.** HEREDITARY ANGIOEDEMA. **carnitine d.** A metabolic disorder usually of autosomal recessive inheritance which presents in two forms. In one the abnormality is virtually limited to skeletal muscle, giving rise to slowly progressive weakness particularly of proximal limb muscles, and muscle biopsy reveals substantial storage of neutral lipid, especially within Type I fibers. In the second variety, systemic carnitine deficiency, the muscular changes are associated with signs of hepatic dysfunction and severe metabolic acidosis, and the prognosis is much poorer. **carnitine palmityl transferase d.** A disorder of autosomal recessive inheritance in which there is a deficiency of carnitine palmityl transferase in skeletal muscle giving rise to episodes of muscle pain precipitated by exertion and often accompanied by myoglobinuria. **cerebroside sulfatase d.** METACHROMATIC LEUKODYSTROPHY. **complement d.** An absolute or partial deficiency of one or more of the constituents of the complement system. It can occur as a result of either disease, resulting in depletion or inactivation, or a hereditary failure to synthesize or to activate specific components. **congenital intrinsic factor d.** A hereditary disorder of autosomal recessive transmission. Homozygotes do not secrete intrinsic factor in gastric juice, and consequently they develop megaloblastic anemia, neuropathies, and other features of pernicious anemia within the first few years of life. **congenital lactase d.** Lack or inadequate supply of the enzyme lactase, normally produced in the cells of the brush border of the intestinal villi. Production of other enzymes may be normal. The disaccharide lactose of milk cannot be reduced to the monosaccharides glucose and galactose and passes unabsorbed to the colon, where its fermentation causes gaseous distension, acid diarrhea, and failure to thrive in infants. Siblings may be affected. Inheritance is probably recessive. **congenital myeloperoxidase d.** A disorder of autosomal recessive inheritance, characterized by recurrent pyogenic infections and absence of peroxidase activity in neutrophils. Also *Alius-Grignaschi anomaly.* **congenital transcobalamin II d.** A disorder, probably hereditary, in which a lack of plasma transcobalamin II prevents cells of all tissues from taking up cobalamin from plasma. Manifestations are convulsions, mental retardation, and megaloblastic anemia, beginning in early infancy. **cystathionine $\beta$-synthase d.** HOMOCYSTINURIA. **debrancher d.** GLYCOGEN STORAGE DISEASE III. **disaccharidase d.** See under DISACCHARIDE INTOLERANCE. **factor V d.** An autosomally inherited hemorrhagic disease resulting from a deficiency of plasma coagulation factor V. Also *parahemophilia, Owren's disease.* **factor VII d.** An autosomally recessive inherited reduction in clotting factor VII to less than 10% of normal activity, resulting in a bleeding tendency of marked variability, from mild epistaxis to severity mimicking classical hemophilia. Heterozygotes have no bleeding problems. Also *hereditary hypoproconvertinemia.* **factor IX d.** HEMOPHILIA B. **factor X d.** An autosomally inherited deficiency of plasma coagulation factor X. The deficiency results in a bleeding tendency. Also *Stuart-Prower factor deficiency.* **factor XII d.** An autosomally inherited deficiency of factor XII. Although *in vitro* coagulation is seriously impaired, there is no bleeding tendency. Also *Hageman's disease* (seldom used), *Hageman trait.* **factor XIII d.** An autosomally inherited hemorrhagic disease resulting from a deficiency of plasma coagulation factor XIII. **familial aldosterone d.** A rare, autosomal recessive inborn error of steroid metabolism that results in decreased synthesis of the hormone aldosterone. The clinical manifestations, obvious in infancy, include growth retardation, dehydration, failure to thrive, and intermittent fever. **familial high density lipoprotein d.** HIGH DENSITY LIPOPROTEIN DEFICIENCY. **folic acid d.** Reduction in the level of serum folate due either to dietary deficiency, malabsorption, or the effect of anticonvulsant drugs such as phenytoin. The neurologic effects of such a deficiency remain in dispute but dementia and/or polyneuropathy have been attributed to this cause. Megaloblastic anemia is the most consistent manifestation. **fructokinase d.** HEREDITARY FRUCTOSE INTOLERANCE. **$\alpha$-galactosidase d.** ANGIOKERATOMA CORPORIS DIFFUSUM. **glucocerebrosidase d.** 1 Any reduction in functional activity of glucocerebrosidase, an enzyme involved in glycosphingolipid catabolism. 2 GAUCHER'S DISEASE. **glucose-6-phosphatase d.** GLYCOGEN STORAGE DISEASE I. **glucose-6-phosphate dehydrogenase d.** A heterogeneous, X-linked recessive deficiency of the enzyme catalyzing the first step in glycolysis. A large number of rare variants and several polymorphic ones have been found, not all of which produce either deficient enzyme activity or clinical effect. The deficiency is the basis of favism, a sensitivity to primaquine, some other drug-induced hemolytic anemias, and chronic nonspherocytic hemolytic anemia. One polymorphic variant associated with the deficiency occurs in Blacks and another in Mediterranean populations. The locus for G6PD is located near the telomere of the long arm of the X chromosome, closely linked to factor VIII (hemophilia A) and to color blindness of the deutan and protan series. **$\alpha$-1,4-glucosidase d.** GLYCOGEN STORAGE DISEASE II. **glutathione synthetase d.** A deficiency or reduction in activity of the cellular enzyme glutathione synthetase. Two forms of hereditary deficiency of this enzyme are recognized: a deficiency of erythrocyte glutathione reductase alone, which is associated with mild hemolytic anemia and low concentration of glutathione in erythrocytes, and a deficiency of this enzyme in all cells, which is associated with neurologic degeneration, excretion of pyroglutamic acid in the urine, and mild hemolytic anemia. **heme synthetase d.** ERYTHROPOIETIC PROTOPORPHYRIA. **hepatic phosphorylase d.** GLYCOGEN STORAGE DISEASE VI. **hepatic phosphorylase kinase d.** GLYCOGEN STORAGE DISEASE VIII.. **HGPRTase d.** LESCH-NYHAN SYNDROME. **high density lipoprotein d.** A relative deficiency of high density lipoprotein (HDL). It is found in several hereditary defects of lipoprotein metabolism, including analphalipoproteinemia, the combined deficiency of apolipoproteins A-I and C-III, and heterozygosity or homozygosity for an apolipoprotein A-I deficiency. Also *familial high density lipoprotein deficiency.* **11$\beta$-hydroxylase d.** An uncommon form of congenital adrenocortical hyperplasia in which virilism and hypertension are the dominant clinical features. Plasma cortisol values are low and those of 11-deoxycorticosterone are raised. **17-hydroxylase d.** A rare form of congenital adrenocortical hyperplasia, characterized by insufficient secretion of sex hormones, cortisol, and aldosterone, but excessive production of corticosterone and 11-deoxycorticosterone. The clinical manifestations are hypogonadism and hypertension. **20-hydroxylase d.** An extremely rare and lethal form of congenital adrenocortical hyperplasia in which the adrenal cortices are massively enlarged and loaded with cholesterol and biosynthesis of adrenocortical steroid is severely impaired. Feminization occurs in both male and female neonates. **21-hydroxylase d.** The commonest form of congenital adrenocortical hyperplasia, in which a defect in the adrenocortical enzyme 21-hydroxylase causes deficient adrenocortical biosynthesis of cortisol and excessive production of adrenal androgens. See also CONGENITAL ADRENOCORTICAL HYPERPLASIA. **3$\beta$-hy-**

**droxysteroid dehydrogenase d.** 3β-HYDROXYSTEROID DEHYDROGENASE DEFECT. **hypoxanthine-guanine phosphoribosyltransferase d.** HYPOXANTHINE PHOSPHORIBOSYLTRANSFERASE DEFICIENCY. **hypoxanthine phosphoribosyltransferase d.** Hyperuricemia and uricolithiasis that results from a diminished activity of hypoxanthine-guanine phosphoribosyltransferase. The enzyme (symbolized HGPRT or HPRT) is encoded by a locus at Xq27, closely linked to α-galactosidase and glucose-6-phosphate dehydrogenase. The most severe genetic variant of this condition is the Lesch-Nyhan syndrome; less severe forms may present with gout. Also *hypoxanthine-guanine phosphoribosyltransferase deficiency, X-linked hyperuricemia.* **immunologic d.** IMMUNODEFICIENCY. **iron d.** A condition in which the quantity of iron in the body is less than normal, as reflected in absence of hemosiderin in bone marrow, lower than normal serum ferritin concentration, and, when severe, by low serum iron concentration, erythrocytic microcytosis and hypochromia, and anemia. Also *sideropenia, hypoferrism.* See also IRON DEFICIENCY ANEMIA. **iron d. in infancy** Anemia resulting from insufficiency of iron in an infant's diet. Milk contains practically no iron, but the period of milk dependency from birth to mixed feeding is normally bridged by the iron stores in the liver, acquired through the mother during fetal life. Premature babies have much smaller iron stores and therefore become deficient early. They will invariably be anemic during the first year of life or longer unless given oral iron supplements from the early weeks onward. **lactase d.** The relative or complete absence of the enzyme lactase, normally present in the brush border of small bowel epithelium and necessary for the digestion of the disaccharide lactose, the principal sugar in milk. Also *alactasia.* **lecithin-cholesterol acyl transferase d.** An autosomal recessive syndrome resulting from an inability to esterify cholesterol. The serum total cholesterol is elevated, and cholesterol accumulates in foam cells in the bone marrow, cornea, and glomeruli. Hemolytic anemia and renal failure are the important clinical consequences. This rare, genetically heterogeneous condition of worldwide occurrence was first described by Norum and Gjone in Norway in 1967. Also *LCAT deficiency, Norum's disease.* **lipoprotein lipase d.** See under FAMILIAL HYPERLIPOPROTEINEMIA TYPE I. **luteal phase d.** LUTEAL PHASE DEFECT. **mental d.** MENTAL RETARDATION. **muscle phosphofructokinase d.** GLYCOGEN STORAGE DISEASE VII.. **muscle phosphorylase d.** GLYCOGEN STORAGE DISEASE V. **phosphoglucomutase d.** A rare form of glycogen storage disease involving skeletal muscle and giving rise to a slowly progressive proximal myopathy. The condition has been attributed to a recessively inherited deficiency of the enzyme phosphoglucomutase. **phytanic acid oxidase d.** REFSUM'S DISEASE. **plasma thromboplastin antecedent d.** HEMOPHILIA C. **pseudocholinesterase d.** An autosomal recessive phenotype resulting in reduced serum cholinesterase activity. No clinical consequences are apparent unless a muscle relaxant, such as suxamethonium, is administered. Inability to metabolize the drug causes prolonged apnea. Also *suxamethonium sensitivity, postanesthesia apnea.* **pyridoxine d.** A deficiency of the enzyme pyridoxine, the chief constituent of vitamin $B_6$. In clinical practice the deficiency is most often secondary to the administration of drugs such as isoniazid, which inhibit the effects of the vitamin. It may also be due to malabsorption or to diet, as when it was omitted accidentally from manufactured baby food. In early infancy, pyridoxine deficiency may cause convulsions, in adult life, sensorimotor polyneuropathy. **pyruvate kinase d.** Chronic hemolytic anemia due to deficiency of erythrocyte pyruvate kinase. It is of autosomal recessive inheritance and is characterized by splenomegaly, frequently by cholelithiasis, and occasionally by stillbirth or failure to thrive. **riboflavin d.** A deficiency characterized by impaired cell oxidation which results in the clinical manifestations of angular stomatitis, cheilosis, glossitis, nasolabial seborrhea, invasion of the cornea by capillary blood vessels, lachrymation, and photophobia. It is diagnosed by measuring the activity of the enzyme erythrocyte glutathione reductase with and without flavin adenine dinucleotide added *in vitro.* An activation coefficient of over 1.20 with added flavin adenine dinucleotide indicates riboflavin deficiency. Also *hyporiboflavinosis.* **secondary lactase d.** A defect in the production of the enzyme lactase (which reduces lactose to galactose and glucose) resulting from damage to the intestinal mucosa, where it is normally produced in the brush border cells of the villi. Villous atrophy occurs in celiac disease and in various forms of enteritis. Unabsorbed lactose ferments in the colon, causing gaseous distension, loose acid stools, and failure of infants to thrive. Recovery of the villi on a strict gluten-free diet, or after recovery from enteritis, takes at least six weeks. Lactase secretion ceases in some adults for whom milk is not a regular food. **sphingomyelinase d.** Either type A or B of Niemann-Pick disease. **Stuart-Prower factor d.** FACTOR X DEFICIENCY. **thymus-dependent d.** THYMUS-DEPENDENT IMMUNODEFICIENCY. **thymus-independent d.** THYMUS-DEPENDENT IMMUNODEFICIENCY. **transferrin d.** ATRANSFERRINEMIA. **tryptophan d.** A deficiency of the amino acid tryptophan, seen in the diets of individuals who consume maize as a main source of protein. After prolonged exposure to such a diet, pellagra, a niacin deficiency disease, will be contracted unless niacin supplements are given. Because 60 mg of tryptophan are equivalent to 1 mg of niacin, tryptophan may be used to alleviate pellagra. Tryptophan can be converted into niacin, thus it serves as a substitute for a considerable portion of the niacin in the diet. **vitamin d.** A lack of a specific vitamin due to an inadequate dietary intake or to impaired absorption, as in malabsorption syndromes. Each vitamin deficiency leads to a given deficiency disease such as scurvy (vitamin C), rickets (vitamin D) and megaloblastic anemia (vitamin $B_{12}$). **vitamin A d.** A vitamin deficiency that leads to night blindness, xerophthalmia, keratomalacia, blindness, follicular keratosis, and stunting of growth. It is prevalent in hot, dry climates and results from a long-term diet deficient in dairy products and vegetables. Occasionally, it results from faulty absorption when diseases of the alimentary tract are present. Owing to the large store in the liver this takes many months of severe illness. Intercurrent infections and other diseases which restrict the dietary intake may precipitate clinical manifestations of retinol deficiency in patients whose normal diet contains small amounts of the vitamin. It is diagnosed by the presence of poor dark adaptation and low blood levels of retinol ($<200$ μg/l) and carotenoids ($<800$ μg/l). The level of carotenoids reflects the recent dietary intake of the precursor. **vitamin $B_6$ d.** See under PYRIDOXINE DEFICIENCY. **vitamin $B_{12}$ d.** A condition in which the amount of cobalamin (or vitamin $B_{12}$) in the body is less than normal, as reflected in low serum vitamin $B_{12}$ concentration and by erythrocytic macrocytosis, anemia, megaloblastic maturation of erythrocyte precursors in bone marrow, progressive neuropathies, neurosis, and psychosis. **vitamin E d.** A deficiency in vitamin E which in rats leads to increased oxidation of polyunsaturated fatty acids occurring chiefly in the muscles. This causes a higher oxygen uptake and the appearance of creatine and pentose sugar in the urine. Muscles weaken as a result of fatty degeneration and fibrosis in a manner that resembles muscular dystrophy in man, but no evidence is available to indicate that it is the same. Vitamin E deficiency affects reproduction as female rats become pregnant but the fetuses die *in utero* and males become sterile due to degeneration of the sperm-producing cells. When this deficiency is associated with protein deficiency, liver necrosis occurs. In humans, although vitamin E is probably necessary for normal metabolism, deficiency is rare. Some premature infants are born with an inadequate reserve of the vitamin and develop hemolytic anemia that is treatable with iron, folic acid, and tocopherol. Severe vitamin E deficiency also occurs in abetalipoproteinemia due to an inability to absorb vitamin E arising from a lack of $\beta$-lipoprotein. **vitamin K d.** An insufficient amount of vitamin K in the body, as reflected in bleeding due to reduction in synthesis of vitamin-K-dependent coagulation factors VII, IX, and X and prothrombin. The usual cause of vitamin K deficiency is impairment of intestinal absorption of this lipid-soluble vitamin as a result of biliary tract obstruction or abnormality of intestinal epithelium in sprue syndromes. **xanthine oxidase d.** 1 XANTHINURIA. 2 An autosomal recessive defect in the production or function in molybdenum cofactor. A xanthine oxidase deficiency, which results secondarily, can cause such clinical features as retardation and ectopia lentis when present concomitantly with deficient activity of sulfate oxidase. **X-linked mental d.** Any of a number of conditions causing mental retardation usually in association with one or more abnormalities, inherited as an X-linked recessive trait and occurring predominantly in males. Fragile X syndrome is the most common of these disorders. **xylitol dehydrogenase d.** PENTOSURIA. **L-xylulose reductase d.** PENTOSURIA.

**deficit** \def′isit\ [L, third person sing., pres. indicative active of *deficere* to be wanting, to fail] 1 An insufficient supply or quantity. 2 The amount by which a quantity is deficient; the difference between what is available and what is needed. **base d.** The negative value of base excess in the blood as titrated with strong base of pH 7.4 at a $P_{CO_2}$ of 40 mm Hg at 37°C, expressed in meq/liter. Also *alkali deficit.* **oxygen d.** 1 A deficiency in oxygen content or oxygen supply; hypoxemia or hypoxia. 2 OXYGEN DEBT. **pulse d.** The difference between the heart rate as measured at the apex and the arterial pulse rate, resulting from insufficient stroke volume in some beats to produce a pulse wave. It is a feature of atrial fibrillation. **reversible ischemic neurologic d.** A transient neurologic deficit that is characterized usually by motor, sensory, or ocular symptoms that last longer than 24 hours but clear completely within 72 hours. It is thus intermediate between a transient ischemic attack and a completed stroke.

**definitive** \difin′itiv\ Having all of the final or adult features although growth may not necessarily have finished: used especially of an organ or structure in the process of embryonic development.

**deflection** \diflek′shən\ [Late L *deflexio* (from L *deflexus,* past part. of *deflectere* to bend or turn aside) a bending or turning aside] In electroencephalography, any movement from the baseline of the recorded trace, caused by a change in electrical potential. **atrial d.** The deflection in the electrocardiogram caused by the passage of an electrical impulse through the atria. **His bundle d.** The deflection in the electrocardiogram caused by the passage of an electrical impulse through the bundle of His (fasciculus artrioventricularis). It is usually recorded from an intracardiac electrode. **intrinsic d.** The rapid decline from peak positivity to maximum negativity in a record of surface electric charges that occurs in a muscle during the passage of an action potential. **QRS d.** See under QRS COMPLEX.

**defloration** \def′lôrā′shən\ [Late L *defloratio* (from *defloratus,* past part. of *deflorare* to deprive of virginity, from L *de-* from + *flos,* gen. *floris,* flower) a depriving of virginity] Rupture of the hymen which may occur during the first sexual intercourse. It can also occur during the course of digital vaginal examination, masturbation, or through the use of vaginal tampons.

**defluvium** \difloo′vē·əm\ [L (from *defluere* to fall off or out, cease flowing, perish, decay), a falling off, falling out] **postpartum d.** Hair loss by a mother following delivery. Also *postpartum alopecia.* **d. unguium** ONYCHOMADESIS.

**defluxion** \difluk′shən\ [Late L *defluxio* (from *defluere* to flow down or out, from *fluere* to flow) a downflow, outflow] An abundant discharge.

**deformation** \dē′fôrmā′shən\ [L *deformatio* (from *deformare* to disfigure, from *de-* DIS- + *formare* to form) disfigurement, deformation] 1 The process of changing shape. 2 A defect in form, shape, or position of an organ, part of an organ, or part of a body that is caused by abnormal mechanical forces; a deformity. 3 DEFORMATION SEQUENCE.

**deformity** [L *deformitas* (from *deform(is)* misshapen + *-itas* -ITY) deformity, ugliness] A structural or functional deficiency or deviation. It is often of developmental origin but it may be acquired. **Arnold-Chiari d.** A congenital compression deformity of the cerebellum, medulla, and pons, characterized by herniation of the cerebellar tonsils and the distal portion of the medulla oblongata through the foramen magnum into the spinal canal. The fourth ventricle is compressed and firm adhesions occupy the cisterna magna. Although the presence of internal hydrocephalus would suggest that intracranial pressure pushes lower brain parts into the foramen, the frequently associated spina bifida (with or without meningocele or meningomyelocele) and attenuation of the spinal cord indicate that traction may play a role. Also *cerebellomedullary malformation syndrome.* **boutonnière d.** A finger deformity in which the proximal interphalangeal joint is flexed and the terminal interphalangeal joint extends. It is caused by damage to the central slip of the extensor tendon to the middle phalanx. Also *buttonhole deformity.* **cloverleaf d.** An alteration of the normal contour of the lumen of the duodenal bulb as seen radiologically, caused by focal scarring resulting in multiple outpouches having as their base a central area of fibrosis. **coup de sabre d.** The facial deformity resulting from facial hemiatrophy. The spontaneous loss of subcutaneous tissue gives the appearance of a saber wound. **Dandy-Walker d.** DANDY-WALKER SYNDROME. **dishface d.** FACIES SCAPHOIDEA. **equinus d.** TALIPES EQUINUS. **Erlenmeyer flask d.** A failure of bone remodeling characterized by a persistent metaphyseal widening that extends down into the diaphysis, resulting in a bone shape that resembles an Erlenmeyer flask. It is found in such bone dysplasias as onycho-osteodysplasia. **gun stock d.** CUBITUS VARUS. **Haglund's d.** ACHILLES BURSITIS. **hitchhiker's thumb d.** A hand deformity characteristic of diastrophic dwarfism in which the thumb is set at right angles to the axis of the other digits in the plane of the palm. **Ilfeld-Holder d.** A winging of the scapula with consequent reduced abduction of the upper limb. **intrinsic minus d.** A deformity of the fingers at the metacarpophalangeal joints that is characteristic of paralysis or weakening of the intrinsic musculature. **intrinsic plus**

**d.** A characteristic hyperextension deformity of the fingers at the metacarpophalangeal joints that occurs when the interossei muscles are contracted and foreshortened. **J-sella d.** The J-shaped appearance of the sella turcica on a lateral skull x ray that is characteristic of the mucopolysaccharidoses. **lobster-claw d.** A congenital cleft of one or more hands or feet due to the absence of the third or middle digit, and sometimes the second and fourth digits, with the result that the hand or foot bears some resemblance to the claw of a lobster. It is usually transmitted by autosomal dominant inheritance. Also *lobster claw hand.* See also CLEFT HAND, CLEFT FOOT. **Madelung's d.** A subluxation of the distal radioulnar joint secondary to abnormal growth and curvature of the distal radius marked by posterior bowing. Also *radius curvus, carpus curvus, Madelung syndrome.* **mermaid d.** SIRENOMELIA. **parachute d.** An anomaly of an atrioventricular valve whereby all the chordae insert into one papillary muscle, either because the papillary muscles are fused together or because one papillary muscle group is absent. It usually affects the mitral valve. **pinched tip d.** Extreme narrowing of the nasal tip as a result of injudicious surgery. Also *pinched nasal tip.* **polly-beak d.** A hooklike deformity of the nasal tip, usually as the result of lupus vulgaris with scarring and distortion of the columella nasi. **pseudolobster-claw d.** An incomplete lobster-claw deformity in which the middle or third digit is only partially suppressed. **recurvatum d.** A hyperextension deformity that is particularly common in the knee. **reduction d.** Any shortening or absence of any limb or parts thereof. **riding breeches d.** An accumulation of fat beneath the skin of the lateral aspect of the human thigh. It usually occurs in women and is amenable to cosmetic surgery. Also *trochanteric lipodystrophy.* **rocker-bottom d.** ROCKER-BOTTOM FLATFOOT. **round back d.** KYPHOSIS. **saddle d. of the nose** See under SADDLE NOSE. **seal-fin d.** Ulnar deviation of the fingers, as is seen in rheumatoid arthritis. **silver fork d.** The deformity resulting from a Colles fracture, so named because the relationship between the forearm and the wrist assumes the shape of a dinner fork. Also *Velpeau's deformity.* **simian d.** A deformity of the nose wherein the tip is raised and retracted and the anterior nares open forwards as in many of the apes. Most cases result from destruction of the front part of the nasal septum and contraction of scar tissue. **Sprengel's d.** The retention after birth of the elevated position of the scapulae in terms of vertebral levels, as is seen in the fetus. A definite cause has not been established. **swan-neck d.** A deformity of the fingers marked by hyperextension of the interphalangeal joint and flexion of the terminal interphalangeal joint. It is caused by overactivity or the contracture of the intrinsic muscles of the hand. **torsional d.** A limb or long bone deformity caused by abnormal rotation. **ulnar drift d.** See under ULNAR DRIFT. **Velpeau's d.** SILVER FORK DEFORMITY. **Volkmann's d.** A congenital dislocation at the tibiotarsal joint. **whistling d.** An unfavorable result following the repair of congenital cleft lip in which the incomplete approximation of muscle and mucosa result in a slight gap in the lip. This gap gives the patient the appearance of constantly whistling.

**deganglionate** \dēgang′glē·ōnāt′\ [L *de* away + GANGLION + -ATE] **1** To remove the ganglia of the somatic or the vegetative nervous system. **2** Having had the ganglia removed.

**degeneracy** \dijen′ərəsē\ The process of degenerating or the state of being degenerate.

**degenerate** \dijen′ərāt\ **1** To become worse or lose integrity; break down or deteriorate. **2** Characterized by degeneration.

# degeneration

**degeneration** \dijen′ərā′shən\ [Late L *degeneratio* (from L *degenerare* to decline from the standard of one's kind, from *de-* off, down from + *genus,* gen. *generis* a kind, race, origin) deterioration, debasement] **1** The process of becoming worse, or the condition resulting from such a process; deterioration. **2** A physical alteration in a cell, tissue, or organ, or in any organized structure, consisting of a breaking down into a disorganized or less organized state. **adipose d.** FATTY DEGENERATION. **albuminoid d.** CLOUDY SWELLING. **ascending d.** Wallerian degeneration affecting axons whose nerve cell bodies are located in the distal parts of the nervous system, such as nerve root ganglia. The degeneration progresses towards the spinal cord and brain. **atheromatous d.** Degenerative changes in arterial walls with formation of atheromas. **axonal d.** The changes occurring in neurons when their axons are cut or damaged. These consist of swelling, peripheral displacement of the nucleus, and chromatolysis. Also *Nissl's degeneration, retrograde degeneration, primary degeneration of Nissl.* **ballooning d.** A form of cell injury characterized by diffuse swelling of the cell, with a clear appearance of the cytoplasm due to increased water content. It may progress to cell death. Although nonspecific, this change is characteristic of viral infections such as viral hepatitis. **Best's macular d.** VITELLIFORM MACULAR DEGENERATION. **Canavan spongy d.** VAN BOGAERT'S FAMILIAL AXONAL SPONGY DEGENERATION. **carneous d.** RED DEGENERATION. **central d. of the corpus callosum** MARCHIAFAVA-BIGNAMI SYNDROME **cerebellar d.** Degeneration of specific parts or of the entire cerebellar cortex and/or cerebellar nuclei, comprising a group of disorders. Some of these are hereditary ataxias, others are of toxic or metabolic origin, and others of unknown cause. Ataxia is usually the most prominent of the various neurologic manifestations. **cerebellar d. of late onset** PRIMARY PROGRESSIVE CEREBELLAR DEGENERATION. **cerebellofugal d.** DYSSYNERGIA CEREBELLARIS MYOCLONICA. **cerebromacular d.** Any of a group of cerebral lipidoses, most of which give rise to progressive dementia, epilepsy, and spastic paralysis and in some of which a cherry-red spot is seen at the macula in the optic fundus. *Obs.* Also *cerebroretinal degeneration.* **cheesy d.** CASEOUS NECROSIS. **cloudy-swelling d.** See under CLOUDY SWELLING. **corticostriatonigral d.** A degenerative disorder of autosomal dominant inheritance affecting cells in the putamen and globus pallidus and giving rise to severe akinesia and rigidity with little or no tremor. The clinical picture resembles that of idiopathic parkinsonism but dementia is common. **corticostriatospinal d.** A progressive degenerative disease of the brain in which features of parkinsonism are associated with spastic paralysis of the limbs and sometimes with amyotrophy due to degeneration of anterior horn cells in the spinal cord. The etiology is unknown though in some cases there is evidence of dominant inheritance. Also *corticostriatospinal atrophy.* **cystic d.** A form of degeneration associated with formation of cystic structures. **cystic d. of adventitia** An uncommon pathologic disintegration of the outer part of arteries, usually the femoral or popliteal segments. The formation of cysts filled with a mucinous material may partially or completely occlude the arterial lumen. **descending d.** Wallerian degeneration affecting axons whose nerve cell bodies are located in the proximal parts of the central nervous system such as the motor cortex. **disciform macular d.** A roughly rounded or oval elevated deterioration of the center of the retina. Also *Kuhnt-Junius degeneration, Kuhnt-Junius disease.* **Doyne honeycomb d. of retina** A central retinal deterioration characterized by mulitple, closely packed drusen, somewhat resembling a honeycomb. Also *Doyne's familial colloid degeneration, familial colloid degeneration, Doyne's familial honeycombed choroiditis, giant drusen of macula, choroiditis guttata senilis, guttate choroidopathy, Tay's choroiditis.* **dystrophic d.** Degeneration due to an inadequate diet. **elastoid d.** Amyloid degeneration of the elastic tissue of arteries. **familial colloid d.** DOYNE HONEYCOMB DEGENERATION OF RETINA. **fascicular d.** Atrophy of bundles of muscle fibers occurring in diseases of the lower motor neuron such as motor neuron disease or amyotrophic lateral sclerosis. **fatty d.** The accumulation of fat-filled vacuoles in the parenchymal cells of an organ. Also *lipophanerosis, adipose degeneration.* **fibrinous d.** FIBRINOID NECROSIS. **fibroid d.** 1 Degeneration within fibrous tissue. 2 Involution or infarction of uterine myomata. **fibrous d.** Dissolution of tissue followed by scar formation. **floccular d.** CLOUDY SWELLING. **Gombault's d.** HEREDITARY HYPERTROPHIC INTERSTITIAL NEUROPATHY. **granular d.** CLOUDY SWELLING. **granulovacuolar d.** Vacuolation and granular change occurring in the cytoplasm of nerve cells in the hippocampus. It is an early histologic manifestation of Alzheimer's disease. **hematohyaloid d.** A stage of resolution of a thrombus, characterized by a glassy appearance due to homogeneous mixing of constituent erythrocytes and platelets. **hepatolenticular d.** WILSON'S DISEASE. **heredomacular d.** MACULAR DEGENERATION. **Holmes d.** PRIMARY PROGRESSIVE CEREBELLAR DEGENERATION. **hyaline d.** A nonspecific change of cells and tissues characterized by the replacement of normal structures by an amorphous, eosinophilic, and homogeneous material. It may be seen in fibrotic connective tissues, sclerotic glomeruli and, principally, in the arteriolar walls of old, hypertensive, and diabetic individuals. Also *vitreous degeneration.* **hydropic d.** A type of reversible degenerative change in which injured cells absorb water and swell, with characteristic appearance of small clear vacuoles, presumed to be distended, sequestered segments of endoplasmic reticulum. Denoting a moderately severe form of cellular injury, this type of change is seen most commonly in renal tubular cells in hypokalemia, and in hepatic or myocardial cells in certain other conditions. Also *vacuolar degeneration.* **infantile macular d.** VITELLIFORM MACULAR DEGENERATION. **infantile spongy d.** CANAVAN'S DISEASE. **juvenile macular d.** A genetic deterioration of the central retina with onset in the second decade of life. **Kuhnt-Junius d.** DISCIFORM MACULAR DEGENERATION. **late juvenile cerebromacular d.** ADULT CEROID-LIPOFUSCINOSIS. **lattice d. of the retina** A circumferential, peripheral deterioration of the retina resulting from vitreous traction. In advanced stages the retinal arterioles crossing the lesion resemble a lattice of white lines. This condition may be a precursor of detachment of the retina because it tends to lead to the formation of retinal holes. **lenticular d.** WILSON'S DISEASE. **lipoidal d.** A lipoidal accumulation in damaged tissue. **liquefaction d.** The degeneration and vacuolization of basal cells that is often seen in inflammatory disorders of the skin. **macular d.** Any genetically determined disorder of the eye which gives rise to progressive degeneration of the retina and choroid, such as retinitis pigmentosa. Also *heredomacular degeneration, tapetoretinal degeneration.* **Mönckeberg's d.** MÖNCKEBERG SCLEROSIS. **mucinous d.** A change in connective tissues due to the accumulation of mucoid, glycosaminoglycan-rich material. It is frequently not a true degeneration but rather a nonspecific reaction to injury. Also *mucous degeneration.* **mucoid d.** MYXOMATOUS DEGENERATION. **mucoid medial d.** CYSTIC MEDIAL NECROSIS. **mucous d.** MUCINOUS DEGENERATION. **multisystem d.** SHY-DRAGER SYNDROME. **myxomatous d.** A change in the texture of connective tissue in which there is a gelatinous consistency due to an increase in glycosaminoglycans. It is, for example, the characteristic change of mitral valve prolapse. Also *mucoid degeneration, mucoid softening.* **neurosomatic d.** Diffuse brain damage occurring as a consequence of frequent, severe or continuous epileptic seizures and of the cerebral anoxia which may accompany such events. The clinical manifestations include dementia, spasticity, and features resembling parkinsonism. **Nissl's d.** AXONAL DEGENERATION. **olivopontocerebellar d.** A progressive degenerative disease of autosomal dominant inheritance in which there is degeneration of the inferior olives and of the cerebellar cortex and dentatorubral system. The principal clinical features are static tremor, cerebellar ataxia, spastic paralysis of the limbs and progressive dementia. Also *Dejerine-Thomas atrophy.* **pallidal d.** Degeneration of the basal ganglia, particularly involving the globus pallidus. **paraneoplastic subacute cerebellar d.** PARANEOPLASTIC CEREBELLAR ATROPHY. **parenchymatous d.** CLOUDY SWELLING. **pigmentary d. of the globus pallidus** HALLERVORDEN-SPATZ DISEASE. **polychromatophilic d.** 1 BASOPHILIC STIPPLING OF ERYTHROCYTES. 2 A state in which erythrocytes stain with mixed areas of blue and pink cytoplasm. **polypoid d.** The appearance of a mucous membrane having polyplike formations due to the presence of severe edema. **polypoid d. of the vocal cords** REINKE EDEMA. **primary progressive cerebellar d.** A familial type of cerebellar degeneration presenting in the adult with slowly progressive ataxia, nystagmus, and tremor of the head and limbs. The disease affects the cerebellar cortex and the inferior olivary nucleus. Some authorities maintain that this degeneration represents a stage of development in olivopontocerebellar atrophy, another of the conditions in the hereditary ataxia group. Others take the view that it represents an independent entity. Also *cerebellar degeneration of late onset, Holmes degeneration, Holmes type cerebellar ataxia, Holmes ataxia.* **progressive lenticular d.** WILSON'S DISEASE. **progressive multisystem d.** SHY-DRAGER SYNDROME. **progressive pyramidopallidal d.** A progressive degenerative disorder, sometimes familial, giving features of extrapyramidal disease resembling those of parkinsonism and signs of bilateral corticospinal (pyramidal) tract involvement. *Imprecise.* **red d.** Hemorrhagic softening occurring in large neoplasms, particularly leiomyomas during pregnancy. The change is probably ischemic in nature, and usually undergoes cystic transformation. Also *carneous degeneration.* **retrograde d.** AXONAL DEGENERATION. **secondary d.** 1 WALLERIAN DEGENERATION. 2 Degeneration in any tract or pathway in the nervous system as a result of a primary lesion elsewhere. **senile disciform d.** A macular disorder resulting from invasion of the subretinal space by choroidal vessels and connective tissue via a break in the lamina vitrea. The etiology is a genetically determined aging process. Also *senile macular exudative choroiditis.* **spinocerebellar d. complicating carcinoma** PARANEOPLASTIC CEREBELLAR ATROPHY. **spongy d. of central nervous system** CANAVAN'S DISEASE. **spongy d. of white matter** CANAVAN'S DISEASE. **Stock's pigmentary d.** Retinal pigmentation and atrophy, as seen in Spielmeyer-Vogt disease. Also *Spielmeyer-Stock disease.* **striatonigral d.** SHY-DRAGER SYNDROME. **subacute combined d. of the spinal cord** The neurologic manifestations of vitamin $B_{12}$ deficiency, whether due to primary dietary insufficiency as in vegans or to malabsorption as in addisonian pernicious anemia. The manifestations of subacute combined degeneration of the spinal cord include symptoms and signs of sensory neuropathy and of posterior column and corticospinal tract dysfunction. Optic atrophy rarely occurs. Subacute combined degeneration of the brain can result in confusion and even dementia, reversible with treatment. If vitamin $B_{12}$ is given early, recovery may ultimately be complete. Also *combined sclerosis, combined system disease, Putnam-Dana syndrome, neuroanemic syndrome* (outmoded), *anemic myelitis* (incorrect), *posterolateral syndrome, combined subacute spinal sclerosis.* **system d.** In neurology, any disease selectively affecting, in a diffuse manner, one or more classes of nerve cells, such as the anterior horn cells, or fiber pathways, such as the spinocerebellar tracts. **tapetoretinal d.** MACULAR DEGENERATION. **traumatic d.** Any degenerative change in cells, tissues or organs produced by physical injury. **turbid-swelling d.** CLOUDY SWELLING. **Türck's d.** Ascending or descending degeneration in tracts of the spinal cord secondary to a primary lesion in the brain or brainstem (descending degeneration) or in, for example, the posterior nerve roots (ascending degeneration). **uratic d.** The changes that occur in tissues associated with the deposition of urates. *Seldom used.* **vacuolar d.** HYDROPIC DEGENERATION. **van Bogaert's familial axonal spongy d.** An infantile hereditary degenerative disease, probably metabolic, and due to cerebral edema resulting from mitochondrial dysfunction. It particularly affects Jews, and gives rise to severe mental retardation and generalized hypotonia, followed by involuntary movements, progressive optic atrophy and megalencephaly, with death usually before the age of two years. Also *Canavan's diffuse sclerosis, Canavan spongy degeneration, Canavan-van Bogaert-Bertrand disease.* **Virchow's d.** *Obs.* AMYLOIDOSIS. **vitelliform macular d.** A dominantly inherited disorder of the retinal pigment epithelium in which a conspicuous optic-disk-sized, discrete, yellow coloration of the macula appears in early life. Disproportionately good vision usually persists for many years. Also *infantile macular degeneration, Best disease, vitelliform degeneration of Best, vitelliform macular dystrophy, vitelliruptive macular degeneration, Best's macular degeneration.* **vitreous d.** *Obs.* HYALINE DEGENERATION. **wallerian d.** Degeneration and disintegration of an axon and secondarily of its myelin sheath distal to a lesion dividing it. Also *secondary degeneration.* **Wilson's d.** WILSON'S DISEASE. **Zenker's d.** HYALINE NECROSIS.

**degenerative** \dijen′ərətiv\ Relating to the process of degeneration.

**degerm** \dējurm′\ [DE- + GERM] To disinfect or sterilize.

**degloving** [L *de-* taking away + English *gloving,* from Old English *glōf* + -ING] The exposure of bone intraorally in preparation for an implant.

**deglut.** *deglutiatur* (L, let it be swallowed).

**deglutible** Able to be swallowed, as a pill or tablet of reasonable size.

**deglutition** \dē′glootish′ən\ [New L *deglutitio,* noun from L *degluttire* to gulp down, from *de-* down + *gluttire* to swallow (akin to *gula* throat, gullet)] SWALLOW.

**degradable** \digrād′əbəl\ Unstable and reducible to a simpler chemical form over a relatively short period of time.

**degranulation** \dēgran′yəlā′shən\ The process of shedding granules from cell cytoplasm to the exterior.

**degree** [Old French *degré* (from Vulgar L *degradus,* lit., a step down, from L *gradus* a step) a step, rank, degree] **1** A unit of angular measurement equal to $\pi/180$ radian; 1/360 of a complete revolution. **2** A unit on any of several scales of measurement, especially of temperature measurement. Symbol: ° **d. absolute** KELVIN. **d. Celsius** The unit of temperature of the Celsius scale. Also *degree centigrade* (older term). Symbol: °C **d. Fahrenheit** The unit of temperature of the Fahrenheit scale. Symbol: °F **d.'s of freedom** The number of the values in a given system that might be assigned arbitrarily. For example, given the mean of a sample of $N$ observations, deviations from the mean for $N-1$ of them could assume arbitrary values, but the deviation of the $N$th observation would have been determined. Hence the sample variance has $N-1$ degrees of freedom. In a contingency table with $m$ rows and $n$ columns there are $(m-1)(n-1)$ degrees of freedom. Thus a fourfold table has only one degree of freedom. This concept is of fundamental importance because most of the statistical distributions from which tests of significance are derived involve some function of the number of degrees of freedom. Abbr. *df* **d. Kelvin** *Outmoded* KELVIN.

**degustation** \dē′gustā′shən\ [L *degustatio* (from *degustare* to taste, have a bite or sip of, from *gustare* to taste) the act of tasting] The process of tasting. Also *gustation.*

**dehematize** \dēhem′ətīz\ To remove all blood from.

**dehemoglobinize** \dē′heməglō′binīz\ To remove all hemoglobin from (erythrocytes).

**dehiscence** \dihis′əns\ [New L *dehiscentia,* from L *dehiscere* to split open, develop a gap or hiatus, from *hiscere* to form a hiatus, from *hiare* to be open, gape] The formation of an opening along a seam; a split. **d. of alveolar process** The absence of bone on the buccal or the lingual surface of a tooth root. In this area the gingiva is attached directly to the cementum. Also *root dehiscence.* **Killian's d.** An interval between the oblique fibers of the thryopharyngeal component of the inferior constrictor muscle of pharynx and the horizontal cricopharyngeal fibers. It was once held responsible for the occurrence of pharyngeal diverticulum, but present-day opinion does not support this concept. **root d.** DEHISCENCE OF ALVEOLAR PROCESS. **d. of uterus** Occult separation of the uterine scar from a previous cesarean section.

**dehydrant** \dēhī′drənt\ An agent or drug that increases loss of body water, usually by increasing urinary output.

**dehydratase** Any enzyme that catalyzes the elimination of water from its substrate, such as serine dehydratase, which by such elimination forms 2-aminoacrylic acid from serine, and then spontaneously decomposes to pyruvate and ammonia.

**dehydrate** \dēhī′drāt\ [See DEHYDRATION.] To remove water from a substance or organism.

**dehydration** \dē′hīdrā′shən\ [DE- + HYDR- + -ATION] **1** The reduction or complete loss of water content. Also *exsiccosis, anhydration.* **2** The process of removing water from a substance. Also *deaquation.* **hypernatremic d.** A condition of water loss in the body that is not accompanied by a compensating sodium loss, thus creating an increased concentration of sodium salts in the blood. **vol-**

**untary d.** 1 A state of reduced water content in the body resulting from an intentionally inadequate water intake. 2 The process of reducing the water content of the body by intentionally limiting water intake.

**dehydro-** \dēhī′drō-\ [DE + HYDRO] 1 A combining form denoting the removal of a hydrogen atom from a molecule. 2 A combining form denoting the removal of two hydrogen atoms from adjacent atoms, as in the conversion of —$CH_2$—$CH_2$— into —CH═CH—.

**5,6-dehydroandrosterone** METHANDRIOL.

**dehydroascorbic acid** The oxidation product of ascorbic acid in which the —C(OH)═C(OH)— group is oxidized to —CO—CO—. Although it is reducible to ascorbic acid, it is unstable and breaks down irreversibly at neutral pH.

**7-dehydrocholesterol** A precursor of vitamin D that is widely distributed in animal fats, such as the oily secretions of mammalian skin and the oil of the preen gland in birds. Irradiation of this compound in the skin converts it to cholecalciferol.

**dehydrocholic acid** $C_{24}H_{34}O_5$. 3,7,12-Triketocholanic acid. It is an oxidation product of cholic acid, a derivative of bile salts. It stimulates the secretion of bile and is used when bile formation is deficient.

**dehydroemetine** A therapeutic agent used, usually in conjunction with other agents such as diiodohydroxyquinoline and chloroquine, in the treatment of amebic colitis and amebic liver abscess. It has largely been replaced by metronidazole and tinidazole.

**dehydroemetine resinate** An emetine derivative which is administered orally and is an effective agent against leishmaniasis.

**dehydroepiandrosterone** 3α-Hydroxyandrost-5-en-17-one. An androgen having a 3β-hydroxyl instead of the 3α-hydroxyl commonly found in reduced androgens. It is found in human urine, being especially abundant in cases of virilizing adrenocortical tumor. It is quantitatively the major androgenic hormone of the adrenal cortex, secreted at a rate of 1–10 mg per day in normal adult humans. Also *dehydroisoandrosterone* (seldom used).

**dehydroepiandrosterone sulfate** The sulfate of dehydroepiandrosterone, with which it is readily interconvertible. It is independently synthesized in the adrenal cortex to form a quantitatively major portion of the adrenal androgen. The secretion rate is 5 to 25 milligrams per day.

**dehydrogenase** Any enzyme that catalyzes the removal of a pair of hydrogen atoms from a molecule. Also *hydrogenlyase* (outmoded).

**dehydrogenate** \dē′hīdräj′ənāt\ To remove hydrogen, usually two hydrogen atoms, from a molecule.

**dehydroisoandrosterone** *Seldom used* DEHYDROEPIANDROSTERONE.

**deiteral** \dī′tərəl\ Denoting the Deiters nucleus (nucleus vestibularis lateralis).

**Deiters** [Otto Friedrich Karl *Deiters*, German anatomist, 1834–1863] 1 Deiters tract. See under TRACTUS VESTIBULOSPINALIS. 2 Deiters process. See under AXON. 3 Nucleus of Deiters. See under NUCLEUS VESTIBULARIS LATERALIS. 4 Deiters terminal frame. See under FRAME. 5 Deiters cell, phalangeal cell of Deiters. See under ASTROCYTE. 6 Deiter's cell, phalangeal cell of Deiters. See under EPITHELIOCYTUS PHALANGEUS EXTERNUS. 7 Deiters phalanges. See under PHALANX.

**déjà fait** \dāzhä fā′\ [French *déjà* already + *fait*, past part. of *faire* to do] Paramnesia in which subjects feel that what they are doing for the first time they have already done at some previous time.

**déjà vécu** \dāzhä′ vākʏ′, -kʸoo′\ [French *déjà* already + *vécu*, past part. of *vivre* to live] A powerful sense of recall of an experience one has lived through before, which may occur in temporal lobe epilepsy.

**déjà vu** \dāzhä vʏ′, vʸoo′\ [French *déjà* already + *vu*, past part. of *voir* to see] A form of paramnesia in which the subject has the intense feeling or conviction that a visual experience, as of a person or scene, has occurred before and is thus part of his memory, when in fact it has not occurred before. It is reported frequently in dreams, in association with neurotic depersonalization disorders, and in cerebral disorders such as temporal lobe epilepsy.

**dejecta** \dijek′tə\ [L, neut. pl. of *dejectus*, past part. of *dejicere* to cast down] Expelled feces; excrement.

**dejection** \dijek′shən\ [L *dejectio* (from *dejectus*, past part. of *dejicere* to cast down) a casting down or out] The lowered mood tone or feeling of sadness that is part of the clinical syndrome of depression. • Some writers use *dejection* to refer to depression itself.

**Dejerine** [Joseph Jules *Dejerine*, Swiss-born French neurologist, 1849–1917] 1 Dejerine's anterior bulbar syndrome, Dejerine's interolivary syndrome. See under MEDIAN MEDULLARY SYNDROME. 2 Klumpke-Dejerine paralysis. See under DEJERINE-KLUMPKE SYNDROME. 3 Dejerine-Lichtheim phenomenon. See under LICHTHEIM SIGN. 4 See under SIGN, SYNDROME. 5 Landouzy-Dejerine atrophy, Landouzy-Dejerine myopathy, Dejerine-Landouzy dystrophy, Landouzy-Dejerine dystrophy. See under FACIOSCAPULOHUMERAL MUSCULAR DYSTROPHY. 6 Verger-Dejerine syndrome. See under DEJERINE SYNDROME. 7 Dejerine-Thomas atrophy. See under OLIVOPONTOCEREBELLAR DEGENERATION. 8 Dejerine-Roussy syndrome, Roussy-Dejerine syndrome. See under THALAMIC SYNDROME. 9 Dejerine-Sottas syndrome, Dejerine disease. See under HEREDITARY HYPERTROPHIC INTERSTITIAL NEUROPATHY.

**deka-** \dek′ə-\ DECA-.

**de Kleijn** [Adrianus Paulus Huibertus Antonie *de Kleijn*, Dutch otorhinolaryngologist, flourished early 20th century] Magnus and de Kleijn neck reflex. See under REFLEX.

**Delafield** [Francis *Delafield*, U.S. pathologist, 1841–1915] See under FLUID.

**delamination** \dē′lamənā′shən\ [DE- + *lamin(a)* + -ATION] 1 A process in which a defined cellular layer is isolated from a cellular mass lacking obvious organization, such as the delamination of primary endoblast from the embryonic disk of mammals. 2 A process resulting from the division of one cellular layer into two layers, or by separation of two cellular layers by a newly formed cavity or by the extension of a preexisting cavity. Thus gastrulation in coelenterates consists of a delamination of the single-layered blastula into two distinct cellular layers, separated by the coelom.

**Delaney Clause** A part of the United States Food, Drug and Cosmetic Act that stipulates that no food additive is permitted that is considered unsafe. The clause states that a substance is unsafe "if it is found to induce cancer when ingested by man or animal, or if it is found, after tests which are appropriate for the evaluation of the safety of food additives, to induce cancer in man or animal . . ."

**de Lange** [Cornelia Catharina *de Lange*, Dutch physician, 1871–1950] Cornelia de Lange syndrome. See under DE LANGE SYNDROME.

**delay** / **conduction d.** The time elapsing between the initiation of a propagated impulse and its arrival at a distant point. The impulse may be an electrical impulse, passing along an axon, nerve, muscle fiber, cortical surface, etc., or a mechanical disturbance such as the pulse beat.

**intraventricular conduction d.** Delay in the passage of the depolarizing current through the ventricles. **pulse d.** The delay in leg pulses, relative to the radial pulse, characteristic of coarctation of the aorta. **synaptic d.** The time required for a nerve impulse to traverse a synapse.

**del Castillo** [E. B. *del Castillo,* Argentinian physician, flourished 20th century] **1** Argonz-del Castillo syndrome. See under SYNDROME. **2** Ahumada-del Castillo syndrome. See under SYNDROME. **3** Del Castillo syndrome. See under SERTOLI-CELL-ONLY SYNDROME.

**DeLee** [Joseph B. *DeLee,* U.S. obstetrician, 1869–1942] **1** See under FORCEPS, MANEUVER. **2** DeLee-Hillis obstetric stethoscope. See under STETHOSCOPE.

**deletion** \dilē′shən\ **1** In cytogenetics, a visible structural change in a chromosome caused by a loss of DNA and associated protein. The deletion can be at the end of the chromosome (terminal deletion) or internal (intercalary deletion). **2** In molecular biology, any loss, through mutation or rearrangement, of nucleotides from DNA in prokaryotic or eukaryotic chromosomes. The extent of the loss ranges from a single nucleotide to long stretches of DNA visible at the cytologic level. For defs. 1 and 2 also *chromosome deletion.* **intercalary d.** A loss of chromosome substance anywhere between the telomeres. **terminal d.** The loss of any amount of chromosome substance and one telomere. In reality, some telomere-specific DNA sequences persist to terminate the deleted chromosome.

**delimitation** \dēlim′itā′shən\ The determination of extent, as that to which a disease has affected a tissue or organ.

**delinquency** \diling′kwənsē\ [Late L *delinquentia* (from *delinquere* to fail, fall short, from *linquere* to leave, quit, forsake) failure in duty] Behavior by a juvenile that violates criminal law. Were it to occur in an adult, the same behavior would be labeled a crime punishable by law.

**delipidation** \dēlip′idā′shən\ [DE- + LIPID + -ATION] The removal of lipid from a specimen, usually by extraction with a solvent. This is often a stage in preparing material for microscopic examination.

**deliquescent** \del′əkwes′ənt\ [L *deliquescens,* gen. *deliquescentis,* pres. part. of *deliquescere* to melt away, dissipate, from *de-* away + *liquescere* to become liquid] Of a solid, taking up water vapor from the air to such an extent that it dissolves in this water and hence becomes liquid.

**délire oneirique** \dālir′ ônerēk′\ SOMNAMBULISM.

**deliria** \dilir′ē·ə\ Plural of DELIRIUM.

**deliriant** **1** Having the capacity to produce a state of delerium. **2** A deliriant drug or agent.

**delirifacient** **1** An agent that produces delirium. **2** Possessing the capability to produce delirium.

**delirium** \dilir′ē·əm\ [L (from *delirare* to rave, be out of one's mind, lit., to deviate from the furrow, from *de-* away + *lira* the ridge between furrows) frenzy, raving] (*pl.* deliriums, deliria) An organic brain syndrome characterized by clouding of consciousness, difficulty in sustaining attention, impaired orientation and memory, and perceptual disturbances leading to hallucinations. The subject feels confused and thoughts are fragmented and disjointed, often with an overlay of restlessness and excitement. **alcohol abstinence d.** DELIRIUM TREMENS. **alcoholic d.** Delirium associated with alcohol ingestion, as in the delirious form of alcohol intoxication, or in the case of alcohol withdrawal in a person who is physiologically dependent upon it (delirium tremens). **alcohol withdrawal d.** DELIRIUM TREMENS. **Bell's d.** DELIRIOUS MANIA. **collapse d.** DELIRIOUS MANIA. **d. cordis** ATRIAL FIBRILLATION. **febrile d.** Delirium occurring in association with fever, however caused. **d. grandiosum** DELUSION OF GRANDEUR. **d. grave** DELIRIOUS MANIA. **oneiric d.** SOMNAMBULISM. **organic d.** Delirium resulting from any organic disorder of the brain, including head injury, meningitis and encephalitis, or from toxic confusional states. **senile d.** *Imprecise* SENILE DEMENTIA. **specific febrile d.** Febrile delirium occurring in any specific infective illness. **traumatic d.** A state of confusion and acute hallucinosis following severe mechanical or thermal trauma. Although sometimes a postconcussive state, it often occurs without a head injury. **d. tremens** Delirium due to withdrawal of alcohol from a person who has become physiologically dependent on it. Characteristic symptoms are dysarthria, ataxia, disorientation, memory impairment, vivid hallucinations, and often delusion of persecution. The delirium is often secondary to intercurrent infection or injury. Also *alcohol withdrawal delirium, alcohol abstinence delirium, potomania* (obs.), *tremor potatorum.* See also ALCOHOL WITHDRAWAL SYNDROME.

**delitescence** \del′ites′əns\ [L *delitescens,* pres. part. of *delitescere* (from *de-* down, under + *latere* to lie low or hidden) to lie hidden] **1** The sudden disappearance of a tumor, a cutaneous lesion, or the signs and symptoms of a disease. **2** A latent or incubation period of a pathogen.

**deliver** [Old French *delivrer* to free, from L *de-* from + *liberare* to free] **1** To remove or expel with or without assistance (all or some of the products of a pregnancy). **2** To remove (a cataract).

**delivery** [Anglo-French *délivrée* a freeing, delivery. See deliver.] The process of giving birth. **abdominal d.** Delivery of an infant by cesarean section. **breech d.** Vaginal delivery of an infant in the breech presentation. **forceps d.** Vaginal delivery of an infant in the vertex presentation through the use of forceps applied to the infant's head. **high forceps d.** Vaginal delivery of an infant with the use of forceps applied to the infant's head before engagement has taken place. This procedure is no longer recommended in obstetrics. **low forceps d.** Vaginal delivery of an infant in the vertex presentation through application of forceps to the infant's head after the head has reached the perineal floor and the sagittal suture is in the anteroposterior diameter of the maternal outlet. Also *outlet forceps delivery.* **midforceps d.** Vaginal delivery of an infant in the vertex presentation through application of forceps to the infant's head after engagement but before the criteria for low forceps are met. **outlet forceps d.** LOW FORCEPS DELIVERY. **postmature d.** Delivery of an infant after a gestation longer than 42 weeks. **postmortem d.** Delivery of an infant after death of the mother. **premature d.** Delivery of an infant of premature size and prematurely in the gestation period. **spontaneous d.** Vaginal delivery of the products of conception without mechanical assistance. **vaginal d.** Delivery of an infant via the mother's lower reproductive tract.

**dell** [Middle English *dele, delle,* akin to Old English *dæl* valley] A small depression of the nail.

**delle** \del′ē\ [German *Delle* dent, depression] The central clear area of a stained erythrocyte.

**dellen** \del′ən\ [Dutch, pl. of *delle* low ground, a pit] Small, shallow depressions in Descemet's membrane resulting from degenerative changes in the corneal endothelium. Also *Fuchs dimples.*

**delta** **1** The name of the fourth letter of the Greek alphabet. Symbol: δ, Δ **2** A triangular space or surface. **d. fornicis** *Obs.* COMMISSURA FORNICIS. **Galton's d.** The triangular pattern of lines near the lower section of a fingerprint, a characteristic of loop pattern fingerprints in which the pattern area is surrounded by two diverging epidermal ridges (type lines). The ridge point nearest the type line divergence is Galton's delta. **d. mesoscapulae** The smooth, triangular area on the spine of the scapula at its junction with the medial margin, over which the tendon of the lower part of the trapezius muscle passes to its insertion just beyond.

**deltoid** \del′toid\ [Gk *deltoeidēs* (from *delt(a)* the letter Δ + *-eidēs* -like, -OID) delta-shaped, triangular] **1** Having the shape or outline of a triangle. **2** MUSCULUS DELTOIDEUS.

**deltopectoral** \del′təpek′tərəl\ Pertaining to the deltoid and pectoralis major muscles.

**delusion** [noun from L *deludere* (from *ludere* to play) to dupe, deceive] A false belief that is firmly maintained even when contradicted by social reality and even though it is not shared or validated by others of the same culture or environment. **autochthonous d.** A primary delusion that arises as an immediate experience within the subject and reflects a disturbance in symbolic meaning rather than a disturbance of perception, apperception, or intellect. **erotomaniacal d.** EROTOMANIA. **d. of grandeur** A delusion that one possesses wealth, beauty, or charm, or some combination of attributes that one believes is irresistible to the rest of humanity. Also *delirium grandiosum, expansive delusion, folie des grandeurs.* **d. of influence** The delusion that one is being affected or controlled by outside forces over which one has no control. **messianic d.** A delusion of grandeur consisting of the conviction that one is a messiah or God, i.e. the prophet chosen to save the world or lead people out of their present misery. **mood-incongruent d.** A delusional idea that is not in accord with the prevailing feeling tone or emotion of the subject, such as a delusion of omnipotence accompanied by fears of annihilation. **nihilistic d.** The delusion that the world, the self, or parts of either are nonexistent. A nihilistic delusion that occurs in some severely depressed patients is the conviction that their brain has rotted away. **d. of persecution** A delusion in which the subject believes that others are plotting against him by threatening him with disgrace, bodily harm, or control over his actions and thoughts. Also *persecutory delusion.* **primary d.** A delusion that arises as an immediate experience without reference to external events. It appears *de novo* rather than as a *post hoc* rationalization of something that has happened. **d. of reference** IDEA OF REFERENCE. **secondary d.** A delusion that is developed as a way of rationalizing a change that the patient perceives in himself or the outside world. A patient in hospital develops nausea and soon thereafter expresses the belief that his mother is trying to poison him, because the book she gave him a a week earlier "must" have contained a poison that upset his stomach. **self-referential d.** IDEA OF REFERENCE. **shared d.** A delusion that develops simultaneously in two or more people closely associated with one another. When the number of people involved is two, the condition is called folie à deux, when three are involved, folie à trois, etc. Also *collective insanity, communicated insanity, imposed insanity, induced insanity, psychosis of association, folie communiquée, folie imitative, folie imposée, folie induite, association neurosis, induced psychosis.* **somatic d.** A delusion of change in or dysfunction of one or more body parts or organ systems. **systematized d.** A delusion that is organized into a coherent plan that within itself maintains logic, order, and consistency, even though the logic is based upon a false initial assumption.

***Demansia*** \dēman′sē·ə\ [irreg. from Van *Diemen's* Land (now Tasmania), named for Anton van Diemen, Dutch merchant and administrator, 1593–1645 + -IA] An Australian genus of venomous snakes of the family Elapidae; the brown snakes.

**demarcation** \dē′märkā′shən\ The formation of distinct boundaries between tissues or structures. **surface d.** LINE OF DEMARCATION.

**demasculinization** \dēmas′kyəlinīzā′shən\ Reduction or loss of qualities normally characteristic of the male, as distinguished from acquisition of the characteristics of a female (feminization).

**demeclocycline** $C_{21}H_{21}ClN_2O_8$. 7-Chloro-6-demethyltetracycline. A broad-spectrum tetracycline antibiotic that inhibits bacterial protein synthesis in both Gram-positive and Gram-negative bacteria. It is given orally. Also *demethylchlortetracycline* (outmoded).

**dementia** \dimen′shə\ [L (from *demens*, gen. *dementis*, out of one's mind, from DE- + L *mens*, gen. *mentis*, mind), madness] A state in which there is a significant loss of intellectual capacity and cognitive functioning leading to impairment in social or occupational functioning, or both. It is believed that there is an organic disturbance in brain functioning which is not ordinarily wholly reversible. Also *athymia* (obs.), *aphrenia* (obs.). **alcoholic d.** KORSAKOFF PSYCHOSIS. **Alzheimer's d.** ALZHEIMER'S DISEASE. **arteriosclerotic d.** MULTI-INFARCT DEMENTIA. **boxers' d.** BOXERS' ENCEPHALOPATHY. **catatonic d.** CATATONIC SCHIZOPHRENIA. **chronic d.** *Seldom used* SCHIZOPHRENIA. **dialysis d.** A syndrome that develops in patients who have been on chronic hemodialysis for three to six years, characterized by intermittent speech dyspraxia followed by progressive myoclonus, tremors, personality changes, seizures, and psychosis, ending in dementia and death. Aluminum has been incriminated as an etiologic agent. Also *dialysis encephalopathy.* **hebephrenic d.** *Older term* HEBEPHRENIC SCHIZOPHRENIA. **d. infantilis** A pervasive developmental disorder or disintegrative psychosis of childhood with onset after an initial two or three year period of seemingly normal development. Symptoms include loss of social skills and speech and severe disturbances in emotions, behavior, and relationships, often accompanied by hyperactivity, stereotypy, and intellectual impairment. Also *Heller's disease.* **multi-infarct d.** Cerebral arteriosclerosis in which there are repeated infarcts within the brain causing enough brain tissue damage to produce dementia. It is characterized by abrupt onset and a fluctuating course of deterioration in memory, abstract thinking, judgment, impulse control, and character organization, in addition to focal neurologic signs. Also *arteriosclerotic dementia, arteriosclerotic brain disorder, vascular dementia.* **myxedematous d.** MYXEDEMA MADNESS. **paralytic d.** GENERAL PARESIS. **d. paranoides** *Outmoded* PARANOID SCHIZOPHRENIA. **paretic d.** GENERAL PARESIS. **post-traumatic d.** Dementia due to brain damage consequent upon severe head injury. **d. praecocissima** A pervasive developmental disorder of childhood, beginning often as early as the fourth year, characterized by stereotypies, posturing, echolalia, and marked intellectual deterioration. **d. praecox** *Older term* SCHIZOPHRENIA. **presenile d.** Any of a group of neurogenic degenerative diseases that have their onset before the age of the senium although their course resembles that of senile dementia. Pathologically, presenile and senile dementia are indistinguishable. At the present time the group includes Pick's disease, Alzheimer's disease, Huntington's disease, Wilson's disease, Parkinson-dementia complex, progressive supranuclear palsy, some forms of spinocerebellar degenerative disease, and Hallervorden-Spatz disease. Also *dementia praesenilis, presenile sclerosis.* **senile d.** A progressive, chronic dementia with onset in the senium. It is characterized by a steady deterioration in intellectual capacities, psychomotor abilities, including writing and speech, and sphincter control. Pathologic changes in the brain include neuronal loss and generalized atrophy and the appearance of new structural elements including senile plaques, granulovacuolar degeneration, and intraneural neurofibrillary tangle. Also *senile delirium* (imprecise), *geriopsychosis, degenerative insanity* (obs.), *senile insanity, senile psychosis.* **subcortical d.** *Seldom used* TARDIVE DYSMENTIA. **vascular d.** MULTI-INFARCT DEMENTIA.

**Demerol** A proprietary name for meperidine hydrochloride.

**demethylation** \dēmeth′ilā′shən\ The operation of removing a methyl group from a molecule, usually replacing it by hydrogen, or removing a positive charge as well.

**demethylchlortetracycline** *Outmoded* DEMECLOCYCLINE.

**demi-** \dem′ē-\ [French *demi* (from L *dimidius* half) half] A prefix meaning half.

**demifacet** \dem′ēfasət\ [DEMI- + FACET] One half, or part, of a plane articular surface, usually present on two adjacent bones that articulate with a third bone, such as some costal facets on the bodies of adjacent thoracic vertebrae. **inferior d. for head of rib** FOVEA COSTALIS INFERIOR. **superior d. for head of rib** FOVEA COSTALIS SUPERIOR.

**demigauntlet** \dem′əgôntlət\ DEMIGAUNTLET BANDAGE.

**demilune** \dem′əl$^y$oon\ [French *demi-lune* (from DEMI- + *lune* moon) a half-moon-shaped structure] **1** A crescent-shaped cell, as one of the serous cells of the submandibular salivary gland. **2** MALARIAL CRESCENT. **d. of Giannuzzi** A group of serous cells that are arranged in a crescent or demilune at the periphery of a mucous acinus in the submandibular salivary gland. Also *Giannuzzi's body, semilunar body, crescent of Giannuzzi.*

**demineralization** \dēmin′ərəlīzā′shən\ A decrease in the mineral content of a tissue. The term is used primarily to indicate calcium depletion of bone in such conditions as osteoporosis and osteomalacia.

**demodectic** \dem′ōdek′tik\ Pertaining to or caused by mites of the genus *Demodex.*.

***Demodex*** \dem′ōdeks\ [New L, from Gk *dēmó(s)* fat + *dēx* a worm] A genus of follicle mites in the family Demodicidae. They are usually found in the hair follicles and sebaceous glands of mammals, including man, and are causal agents of demodectic mange. ***D. folliculorum*** The follicular or hair follicle mite of man, parasitizing the hair follicles of eyelids, nose, and facial areas. Most persons infected are asymptomatic. Rates of infection for older persons run as high as 100 percent ranging down to about 20 percent in persons 10 to 20 years of age. Also *Acarus folliculorum, Simonea folliculorum.*

**demodiciasis** \dem′ōdisī′əsis\ DEMODICOSIS.

**Demodicidae** \dem′ōdis′idē\ [New L, from *Demodex,* gen. *Demodicis,* type genus + -IDAE] A family of minute mites (order Acarina) that parasitize the skin of man and other mammals, many of them living much of their life cycle within hair follicles. These mites are 0.1 to 0.4 mm long and have a striated abdomen with 4 pairs of stubby, five-segment legs.

**demodicosis** \dem′ōdikō′sis\ [*Demodic(is),* gen. of *DEMODEX,* + -OSIS] Infestation of the human pilosebaceous follicles with mites of the genus *Demodex.* Also *demodiciosis, demodiciasis.*

**demodulation** \dē′mädyəlā′shən\ The process of recovering the original modulating wave, as the audio waves, from the modulated carrier wave, as a radio-frequency wave.

**demographic** \dem′əgraf′ik\ Pertaining to demography.

**demography** \dimäg′rəfē\ [Gk *dēmo(s)* the people + -GRAPHY] The study of the structure, evolution, and specific characteristics of human populations, principally in quantitative terms.

**De Morgan** [Campbell *de Morgan,* English physician, 1811–1876] De Morgan spot, Campbell de Morgan spot. See under CHERRY ANGIOMA.

**demorphinization** \dēmôr′finīzā′shən\ The gradual removal of morphine or the substitution of less addictive or nonaddictive drugs as a means of overcoming morphine dependence.

**Demours** [Pierre *Demours,* French ophthalmologist, 1702–1795] Demours membrane.

**demulcent** [L *demulcens,* gen. *demulcentis,* pres. part. of *demulcere,* also *mulcere,* to soothe, smooth, caress] An agent that creates a protective effect on mucous membranes and relieves irritation. Demulcents are generally suspensions of gums or proteins that coat the surface of the mucous membranes.

**de Musset** [Alfred *de Musset,* French poet, 1810–1857] See under SIGN.

**demyelinate** \dēmī′əlināt′\ To destroy, damage, or remove the myelin sheath of (nerve fibers). Also *demyelinize.*

**demyelination** \dēmī′əlinā′shən\ The pathologic destruction and loss of the myelin sheath of nerve fibers. Also *demyelinization, myelinolysis.*

**demyelinize** \dēmī′əlinīz′\ DEMYELINATE.

**denarcotize** \dēnär′kətīz\ To deprive (a subject) of narcotics during treatment of addiction.

**denaturation** \dēnach′ərā′shən\ **1** An alteration of a substance, usually ethanol, to render it unfit for consumption. **2** An alteration of a substance without change in its covalent structure. This applies to substances whose molecules can have a specific folding, usually proteins and nucleic acids.

**dendr-** DENDRO-.

***Dendraspis*** \dendras′pis\ A genus of highly venomous snakes of the family Elapidae, including *D. polylapis* the black mamba. Species occur in central and southern Africa.

**dendraxon** \dendrak′sän\ A short axon or dendrite which branches close to its point of origin from the soma of its parent nerve cell.

**dendric** \den′drik\ DENDRITIC.

**dendriform** \den′drifôrm\ Branching like the limbs of a tree, as a *dendriform process.* Also *dendroid.*

**dendrite** \den′drīt\ [DENDR- + -ITE] A protoplasmic, usually branching process of a neuron. Typically, the multiple dendrites of a neuron conduct propagated impulses toward the cell body, whereas a single axon conducts impulses away from the cell body. However, the dendrites in some neurons exert effects on the cell body excitability primarily through (nonpropagated) electrotonic spread. Also *dendritum, dendron* (seldom used), *neurodendron, neurodendrite.* Adj. dendritic, dendric. **apical d.** A prominent dendrite that arises from the apex of a neuron, i.e., on the opposite side of the neuron from the axon hillock. The term is chiefly applicable to neurons in a polarly oriented layer, such as the pyramidal cells of the cortex. Also *dendritum apicale.* **basal d.** A dendrite that arises from a neuron elsewhere than at its apex. Also *dendritum basale.*

**dendritic** \dendrit′ik\ **1** Of or relating to the dendrite of a neuron. Also *dendric.* **2** Branching like a tree; arborescent.

**dendritum** \dendrī′təm\ [New L] DENDRITE. **d. apicale** APICAL DENDRITE. **d. basale** BASAL DENDRITE.

**dendro-** [Gk *dendron* a tree] A combining form denoting a tree or a branching structure. Also *dendr-*.

**dendrodendritic** \den′drōdendrit′ik\ Pertaining to a synaptic relationship in which the telodendria of one neuron end on dendrites of a second neuron.

**dendroid** \den′droid\ DENDRIFORM.

**dendron** \den′drän\ [Gk, tree] *Seldom used* DENDRITE.

**denervation** \dē′nurvā′shən\ Removal or loss of the nerve supply to an organ, a muscle, or any other part of the body.

**dengue** \deng′gē\ [prob. from pidgin Swahili *dinga*, from Swahili *kidinga pepo* or *kidingapopo* dengue fever, from obsol. Swahili *kidinga* fever; assimilated to Spanish *dengue* affectation, fussiness] An endemic and epidemic infectious disease of tropical and subtropical regions which is caused by a flavivirus (family Togaviridae), and is transmitted by mosquitoes of the subgenus *Stegomyia*, genus *Aedes*, especially *A. aegypti*. There are four distinct serotypes of the virus. An incubation period of three to six days is followed by an abrupt onset of symptoms. The disease, often diphasic, is characterized by a fever that may conform to a typical saddleback temperature curve. A rash appears on about the fifth day, and patients experience muscle and joint pain, and sometimes prolonged weakness and debility. Also *breakbone fever, bouquet fever, dandy fever, knokkelkoorts, dengue fever, stiffneck fever*. **hemorrhagic d.** DENGUE HEMORRHAGIC FEVER.

**denial** \dinī′əl\ A primitive psychological defense consisting of negation or disavowal of unpleasant reality. Also *avoidance*.

**denidation** \den′idā′shən\ [DE- + NIDATION] The sloughing and expulsion of endometrial tissue during the process of menstruation.

**Denis Brown** [*Denis Brown*, English surgeon, flourished 20th century] See under SPLINT, OPERATION.

***Denisonia*** \den′isō′nē·ə\ A genus of highly venomous snakes of the family Elapidae, including *D. superba*, the copperhead of Australia, Tasmania, and the Solomon Islands.

**denitrogenation** \dēnī′trōjənā′shən\ NITROGEN DESATURATION.

**Denker** [Alfred *Denker*, German otorhinolaryngologist, born 1863] See under OPERATION.

**Denny-Brown** [Derek Ernest *Denny-Brown*, New Zealand-born physician active in England and the United States, 1901–1981] Denny-Brown syndrome. See under DENNY-BROWN SENSORY NEUROPATHY.

**Denonvilliers** [Charles Pierre *Denonvilliers*, French surgeon, 1808–1872] Denonvilliers aponeurosis, Denonvilliers fascia, Denonvilliers ligament. See under SEPTUM RECTOVESICALE.

**dens** \denz\ [L (gen. *dentis*), tooth] (*pl.* dentes) **1** [NA] TOOTH. **2** A structure suggestive of a tooth. **dentes acustici** [NA] Toothlike elevations produced by a series of furrows intersecting at right angles to each other on the upper surface and free edge of the vestibular lip of the limbus laminae spiralis of the cochlear duct. They are covered by a layer of squamous epithelium. Also *auditory teeth of Huschke, hair teeth* (outmoded), *Corti's teeth, Corti's auditory teeth*. **dentes acuti** *Outmoded* DENTES INCISIVI. **dentes angulares** DENTES CANINI. **d. axis** [NA] The odontoid process of the second cervical vertebra. Also *dens epistrophei, odontoid apophysis, tooth of axis* (outmoded), *tooth of epistropheus* (outmoded), *odontoid bone, odontoid process of axis*. **dentes canini** [NA] The teeth that are the third in each quadrant starting from the midline; the canines. They have the longest roots of all the teeth and conical crowns, each terminating in a point that is gradually worn down by physiologic attrition. Also *dentes angulares*. **d. deciduus** (*pl.* dentes decidui) [NA] DECIDUOUS TOOTH. **d. epistrophei** DENS AXIS. **dentes incisivi** [NA] The four most anterior teeth in each jaw; incisors. Also *dentes acuti* (outmoded). **d. invaginatus** A tooth, usually an upper lateral incisor, with a deep invagination from the lingual surface. Thus the pulp chamber is filled with a tooth-shaped structure which has enamel as its inner layer. Also *dens in dente, invagination of enamel, dilated odontoma, gestant odontoma, dilated composite odontoma*. **dentes molares** [NA] The most posterior teeth in each jaw, two per quadrant in the human deciduous dentition, and three per quadrant in the permanent dentition; molars. **dentes premolares** [NA] The eight bicuspid teeth, two in each segment, located immediately in front of the dentes molares and behind the dentes canini. **d. sapientiae** THIRD MOLAR. **d. serotinus** THIRD MOLAR.

**densitometer** \den′sitäm′ətər\ A photoelectric device for the measurement of optical density, such as the blackness of an area in a photographic film. **film d.** A densitometer designed to measure the optical density in a photographic film after it has been exposed to light or to radiation.

**densitometry** \den′sitäm′ətrē\ [*densit(y)* + *o* + -METRY] Measurement of transmitted or reflected rays, used to calculate the density of a material or the intensity of light-affecting properties.

**density** [French *densité* (from L *densitas* thickness, from *densus* thick) weight relative to volume] Quantity per unit volume or per unit area. • When used without qualification, *density* refers to mass per unit volume (symbol ρ). **absolute d.** The mass of a substance per unit volume. **background d.** In radiology, the film blackening resulting from factors other than the radiation which passed through the irradiated object. **buoyant d.** The density of medium in which a given substance has a sedimentation coefficient of zero, because its molecules have the same effective density as the medium. Substances, such as nucleic acids of different base composition or of different isotopic composition, may be separated according to their buoyant density by centrifugation in a density gradient. **count information d.** The number of counts recorded per square centimeter in a scan or radionuclide image. Image content and quality are directly dependent on the count information density. Also *count density, scan information density*. **flux d.** The number of particles or photons passing per second through a square centimeter normal to the direction of flow; flux per square centimeter. **optical d.** ABSORBANCE. **relative d.** The ratio of the density of a substance to the density of a standard substance under specified conditions. For liquids and solids, the standard substance is usually water, often at 4°C although other temperatures may be specified. For gases, the standard may sometimes be the same gas under standard conditions of temperature and pressure. Also *specific gravity*. **scan information d.** COUNT INFORMATION DENSITY. **superhelix d.** The linking difference divided by the relaxed linking number. It determines transitions in DNA molecular structure, such as between B DNA and Z DNA. Symbol: σ

**densography** \denság′rəfē\ The measurement of film density by use of a densitometer.

**dent-** \dent-\ DENTI-.

**denta-** \den′tə-\ DENTI-.

**dental** [L *dens* (gen. *dentis*) tooth + -AL] **1** Of or relating to a tooth or teeth. **2** Relating to dentistry.

**dentate** \den′tāt\ [L *dentatus* (from *dens,* gen. *dentis* tooth) toothed] Possessing teeth or toothlike projections. Also *toothed.*

**dentatorubral** \den′tətōroo′brəl\ Designating fibers that arise in the dentate nucleus and project to the red nucleus.

**dentatothalamic** \den′tətōthalam′ik\ Pertaining to a projection from the dentate nucleus of the cerebellum that passes to the nucleus ventralis lateralis and, to a lesser extent, to the nucleus ventralis thalami anterior of the contralateral thalamus.

**dentatum** \dentā′təm\ [short for *corpus dentatum*] NUCLEUS DENTATUS CEREBELLI.

**dentes** \den′tēz\ Plural of DENS.

**denti-** \den′tə-\ [L *dens* (genitive *dentis*) tooth] A combining form meaning tooth, dental. Also *dent-, denta-, dento-.*

**denticle** \den′tikl\ [L *denticulus* (dim. of *dens* tooth) little tooth] A small calcified body found in the dental pulp. It is composed of dentin. Also *pulp stone.* **attached d.** A denticle attached to the wall of the pulp chamber. Also *adherent denticle.* **embedded d.** INTERSTITIAL DENTICLE. **false d.** A denticle having an amorphous structure not resembling dentin. **interstitial d.** A calcified body within a tooth, surrounded completely by dentin. Also *embedded denticle.*

**denticulation** \dentik′yəlā′shən\ One of the small, pointed projections of the denticulate ligament of the spinal cord extending across the subarachnoid space to the dura.

**dentifrice** \den′tifris\ [Middle English, from L *dentifricium* (from *dens,* gen. *dentis,* tooth + *fricare* to rub, polish) tooth powder] A preparation used for cleaning teeth, usually in the form of a paste or powder.

**dentigerous** \dentij′ərəs\ [DENTI- + *-ger* (from L *gerere* to carry, bear) suffix denoting carrying, bearing + -OUS] Bearing or containing a tooth or teeth.

**dentin** \den′tin\ [DENT- + -IN] The calcified tissue which forms the main part of the tooth. It is not cellular, as bone is, but is permeated throughout by tubules which contain the odontoblast processes and through which pain stimuli are conveyed. It is harder than bone but less hard than enamel. Also *dentinum.* Also *dentine* (British spelling). **adventitious d.** SECONDARY DENTIN. **hereditary opalescent d.** DENTINOGENESIS IMPERFECTA. **hypoplastic d.** Incompletely calcified dentin with many interglobular spaces. **irregular d.** See under SECONDARY DENTIN. **mantle d.** The first formed dentin, adjacent to the enamel or to the cementum. **opalescent d.** DENTINOGENESIS IMPERFECTA. **peritubular d.** The more highly mineralized layer lining the mature dentinal tubule. **reparative d.** A form of secondary dentin produced by severe pulp irritation. It may contain cellular inclusions but has no tubular pattern. **sclerotic d.** Dentin in which the tubules have been filled with calcified material in response to some prolonged stimulus. It is limited to the part of the dentin containing the tubules whose outer ends are stimulated. The affected area is relatively radiopaque but optically translucent. Also *transparent dentin, dentinal sclerosis.* **secondary d.** Additional dentin laid down on the pulpal side of normal dentin in response to a prolonged stimulus, such as caries, and giving some protection to the pulp. It may be tubular or nontubular; if the latter, it is called irregular dentin. Also *adventitious dentin.* **transparent d.** SCLEROTIC DENTIN.

**dentine** \den′tēn\ The British spelling of DENTIN.

**dentinoblast** \den′tinōblast′\ ODONTOBLAST.

**dentinoblastoma** \den′tinōblastō′mə\ [DENTIN + *o* + BLASTOMA] DENTINOMA.

**dentinogenesis** \den′tinōjen′əsis\ [DENTIN + *o* + GENESIS] The process of forming dentin, carried out by odontoblasts at the surface of the pulp. **d. imperfecta** A hereditary condition in which the formation of dentin is defective, and premature calcification of pulp chambers and root canals takes place. The enamel is transparent and the teeth take on a brown or opalescent appearance. Also *hereditary opalescent dentin, opalescent dentin, odontogenesis imperfecta, dentin dysplasia.*

**dentinoid** \den′tinoid\ [DENTIN + -OID] PREDENTIN.

**dentinoma** \den′tinō′mə\ [DENTIN + -OMA] A very rare benign jaw tumor of odontogenic epithelium and immature connective tissue, which forms dysplastic dentin. Also *dentinoblastoma, dentoma, dentinoid tumor.*

**dentinum** \den′tinəm\ DENTIN.

**dentist** [French *dentiste* (from DENT- + *-iste* -IST) a dentist] A person qualified to practice dentistry. Also *odontologist.*

**dentistry** \den′tistrē\ The art and science of preventing and treating dental and periodontal diseases and of providing restorations and prostheses. Also *odontology.* **conservative d.** The British term for OPERATIVE DENTISTRY. **forensic d.** Dental science applied to problems of law. It is concerned chiefly with dental identification of dead bodies, comparison and analysis of bite marks in criminal cases, interpretation and evaluation of criminally related traumatic injury of the oral tissues, and evaluation of alleged dental malpractice and negligence. Also *forensic odontology, dental jurisprudence.* **four-handed d.** A technique of operative dentistry in which the dentist's assistant passes instruments and performs manipulative tasks as required. **operative d.** Dentistry concerned principally with restorations, crowns and fixed bridges. Also *conservative dentistry* (British usage). **preventive d.** Dentistry concerned with the primary prevention of caries and periodontal diseases, particularly in public health fields. **prosthetic d.** Dentistry with the provision of prostheses. **restorative d.** Operative dentistry, periodontics, and prosthetic dentistry taken together.

**dentition** \dentish′ən\ [L *dentitio* (from *dentire* to grow teeth, teethe) dentition, teething] **1** The number, kinds, and arrangement of teeth in any animal. The dentition of a mammal can be described by a dental formula. **2** Teething or the eruption of teeth. **deciduous d.** Dentition of a young mammal, subsequently shed and replaced by permanent teeth. Also *primary dentition.* **mixed d.** Dentition of a child between the ages of six and twelve years, when the permanent teeth serially replace and add to the deciduous dentition. Also *transitional dentition.* **permanent d.** The adult dentition of thirty-two teeth, consisting in each quadrant of two incisors, one canine, two bicuspids, and three molars, in that order from the midline. Also *secondary dentition.* **predeciduous d.** Cornified structures in the mouth present before eruption of the deciduous teeth. **primary d.** DECIDUOUS DENTITION. **secondary d.** PERMANENT DENTITION. **transitional d.** MIXED DENTITION.

**dento-** \den′tō-\ DENTI-.

**dentoform** \den′tōfôrm\ [DENTO- + *form*] A representation of the teeth and jaws, used as a teaching aid.

**dentoliva** \-lī′və\ [DENT- + L *oliva* olive] *Obs.* NUCLEUS OLIVARIS.

**dentoma** \dentō′mə\ [DENT- + -OMA] DENTINOMA.

**dentulous** \den′tyələs\ [back formation from EDENTULOUS toothless] Having natural teeth. Compare EDENTULOUS.

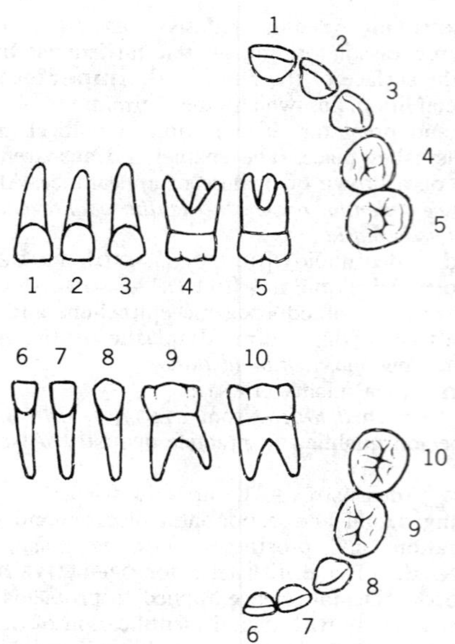


**Deciduous dentition** (1,6) Central incisor; (2,7) lateral incisor; (3,8) canine; (4,9) first molar; (5,10) second molar.

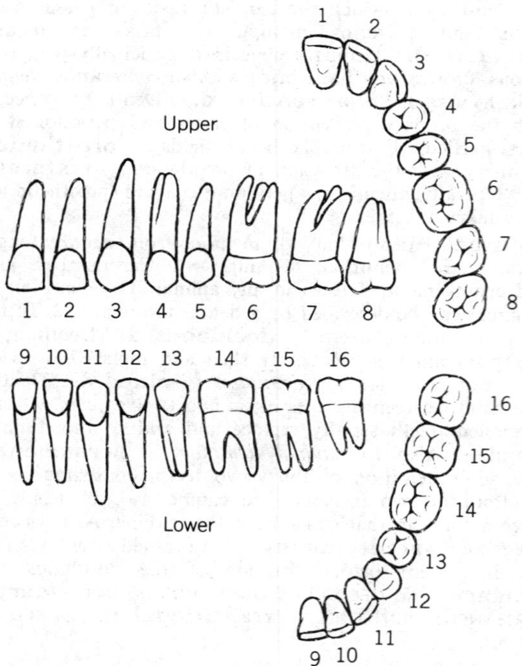


**Permanent dentition** (1,9) Central incisor; (2,10) lateral incisor; (3,11) canine; (4,12) first bicuspid; (5,13) second bicuspid; (6,14) first molar; (7,15) second molar; (8,16) third molar.

**denture** \den′chər\ [French (from L *dens* tooth), dentition, a set of (natural) teeth] A removable prosthesis replacing natural teeth and associated tissues. Also *dental plate* (older term). **complete d.** A denture replacing all the teeth in one jaw. Third molars are not usually placed on a denture. Also *full denture.* **duplicate d.** **1** An exact replica of a denture for use as a spare denture. **2** A denture that copies the original in appearance but is so constructed as to compensate for ridge resorption. **Every d.** A removable upper partial denture similar to the spoon denture, with extensions to contact the palatal aspects of one molar tooth on each side of the jaw. It is therefore tissue-borne. **fixed partial d.** BRIDGE. **full d.** COMPLETE DENTURE. **immediate d.** A denture fitted immediately after the removal of the teeth which it replaces. Also *immediate-insertion denture.* **implant d.** A denture, usually a complete denture, supported by one or more implants. **overlay d.** A denture, all or part of which covers the occlusal surfaces of natural teeth. Compare OVERDENTURE. **partial d.** A denture replacing some but not all of the teeth in a jaw. It may be fixed or removable. **permanent d.** A definitive denture, which is not a temporary, treatment, or transitional denture. The term *permanent* is used in a relative sense because, especially in the case of complete dentures, the tissues change shape with the passage of time. **skeleton d.** A removable, partial metal denture of which the base is constructed of connectors and bars to cover as little as possible of the mucosa. **spoon d.** A removable partial denture replacing one or a few upper anterior teeth. It has a base which covers most of the hard palate but does not have any clasps or touch the natural teeth except at the proximal surfaces adjacent to the replacement teeth. It is, therefore, a tissue-borne denture. **temporary d.** A denture worn for a short period, particularly soon after extractions, when there is rapid ridge resorption. **tooth-borne partial d.** A removable partial denture deriving its vertical support entirely from the natural teeth. **transitional d.** A removable partial denture to which additional teeth are added as more natural teeth are lost. **trial d.** A device used at a stage in the making of a denture in which artificial teeth are mounted with wax on a baseplate so that the shade and arrangement can be checked and altered if necessary.

**denturism** \den′chərizm\ A movement to legalize denturists with an emphasis on independent practice. ⟨"Denturism can be defined as a movement of dental-laboratory technicians who are seeking to be licensed independently from other dental-care practitioners, so that the dental-laboratory technician can directly serve the public." —*New England Journal of Medicine,* 16 Nov. 1978, 1131.⟩

**denturist** \den′chərist\ A dental laboratory technician licensed to supply dentures directly to the public. A term used chiefly in the U.S., Canada, and the United Kingdom.

**Denucé** [Maurice *Denucé,* French surgeon, 1859–1924] Denucé's ligament, quadrate ligament of Denucé. See under LIGAMENTUM QUADRATUM.

**denudation** \den″yoodā′shən\ The removal of epithelium by trauma, disease, or surgical excision.

**deontology** \dē′äntäl′əjē\ [Gk *deon,* gen. *deontos,* what is right or proper + -LOGY] The study of professional duties and courtesies.

**deorsumduction** \dē·ôr′sumduk′shən\ [L *deorsum* downward + DUCTION] INFRADUCTION.

**deorsumversion** \dē·ôr′sumvur′zhən\ [L *deorsum* downward + VERSION] INFRAVERSION.

**deoxy-** \dē·äk′sē-\ [DE + OXY-[1]] **1** A combining form applied to a group or compound from which an oxygen atom has been removed. **2** A prefix frequently used to designate the replacement of a hydroxyl group by a hydrogen atom. For defs. 1 and 2 also *desoxy-* (outmoded).

**deoxycholic acid** 3α,12α-Dihydroxy-5β-cholanic acid. A mammalian bile acid, found largely conjugated with taurine and glycine.

**11-deoxycorticosterone** $C_{21}H_{30}O_3$. 21-Hydroxypregn-4-ene-3,20-dione. An adrenocortical steroid with slight aldosteronelike activity, but little glucocorticoid activity. Because of this it was used medically before the discovery of aldosterone. It is secreted excessively in rare forms of congenital adrenocortical hyperplasia associated with hypertension. Also *Reichstein's compound Q* (older term). See also 17-HYDROXYLASE DEFICIENCY.

**deoxycorticosterone acetate** $C_{23}H_{32}O_4$. 21-Acetyloxypregn-4-ene-3,20-dione, the acetate ester of deoxycortisone. It is used for the same purposes as deoxycorticosterone and is given subcutaneously in depot form, or in tablets for buccal administration. Also *desoxycorticosterone acetate, deoxycortone.*

**deoxycorticosterone pivalate** $C_{26}H_{38}O_4$. The pivalate ester analogue of deoxycorticosterone. It is used for the same purposes as the acetate ester and it is given by intramuscular injection. Also *deoxycorticosterone trimethylacetate.*

**deoxycorticosterone trimethylacetate** DEOXYCORTICOSTERONE PIVALATE.

**deoxycortone** DEOXYCORTICOSTERONE ACETATE.

**deoxygenate** \dē·äk′səjənāt′\ To remove dioxygen: used of solutions, which may have dissolved oxygen removed from them by boiling or by subjecting to diminished pressure, or of substances that can combine with dioxygen, such as hemoglobin.

**deoxyhemoglobin** REDUCED HEMOGLOBIN.

**deoxynucleoside** \dē·äk′sēnʸoo′klē·əsīd\ A compound with a purine or pyrimidine base that is covalently linked through a ring nitrogen to the $C_1$ of deoxyribose.

**deoxypentosenucleic acid** DEOXYRIBONUCLEIC ACID.

**deoxyribonuclease** \-rī′bōnʸoo′klē·ās\ Any enzyme that hydrolyzes DNA. Also *DNAase, DNase, dornase* (obs.). **d. I** An enzyme (EC 3.1.21.1) that hydrolyzes oligonucleotides and DNA, with expulsion of the 3′-oxygen of one residue from the phosphorus atom of the next, so that the phosphate group is left on the 5′-oxygen in the products. It is obtained from the pancreas, and acts preferentially on double stranded DNA. **d. II** An enzyme (EC 3.1.22.1) that hydrolyzes oligonucleotides and DNA, with expulsion of the 5′-oxygen of a residue from its phosphorus atom, so that the phosphate group remains on the 3′-oxygen of the adjacent residue in the products. It is obtained from the pancreas, and acts preferentially on doubly stranded DNA.

**deoxyribonucleic acid** Any of numerous polymers of deoxyribonucleotides, which form the primary genetic material. The molecular weight is in the range of $10^6$–$10^9$. The molecule is generally composed of two linear unbranched strands arranged as a double helix. The nucleotides are composed of nitrogenous bases (purines or pyrimidines), the sugar deoxyribose, and phosphate. The bases are adenine, guanine, thymine, and cytosine. The molecule encodes the genetic information, with three adjacent nucleotides providing the information needed to add one amino acid to a polypeptide chain. See also entries under DNA. Also *desoxyribonucleic acid, chromonucleic acid, deoxypentosenucleic acid, desoxyribose nucleic acid, thymonucleic acid* (older term), *genetic material.* Abbr. DNA

**dep.** *depuratus* (L, purified).

**Depage** [Antoine *Depage,* Belgian surgeon, 1862–1925] See under POSITION.

**Department of Health and Human Services** The federal agency in the United States that is responsible for the administration of most health care programs; successor to the Department of Health, Education, and Welfare.

**depatterning** \dēpat′ərning\ The process of breaking up an existing pattern of thought, as in regressive electroshock therapy done to interrupt the pathologic patterns of neuronal interconnections in the hopes that as they realign themselves the interconnections will assume a more normal pattern.

**depend** **1** To rely on; need in order to function. **2** To be attached above with some freedom of motion; hang.

**dependence** DEPENDENCY.

**dependency** A psychologic and/or physiologic need for a person, an object, a substance, or a situation. Also *dependence.* **drug d.** Physiologic and psychological dependence upon a pharmacologic agent, as evidenced by tolerance of the drug by the body, the need for markedly increased amounts of the substance in order to achieve the desired effect, and by withdrawal symptoms when the substance is discontinued or reduced in amount. **psychological d.** The experience of an overpowering urge to continue the use of a drug to relieve tension once use has begun. This psychological reliance on the use of a particular substance may be distinguished from addiction, indicated by signs of physiologic withdrawal if the substance is discontinued. • The more general term *drug abuse* is increasingly employed to denote excessive use whether the need to continue the drug is of physiologic or psychological origin. **pyridoxine d.** A genetic disorder of infants characterized by seizures that cannot be controlled with anticonvulsants but can be prevented with large doses of pyridoxine. Some sufferers have intrauterine convulsions and others tonic-clonic seizures progressing to status epilepticus soon after parturition. Severe mental retardation occurs if it is not treated early with large doses of pyridoxine (5–25 mg per day). The defect is believed to be due to a poor affinity for pyridoxal phosphate of the pyridoxal-dependent enzyme glutamic acid decarboxylase. It has an autosomal recessive mode of inheritance, and is variable in its intensity of expression and time of first appearance. See also PYRIDOXINE DEFICIENCY.

**depersonalization** \dēpur′sənəlīzā′shən\ A nonspecific syndrome characterized by feelings of loss of one's personal identity and by feelings of being different, strange, or unreal. Depersonalization may appear in depression, dissociative disorders of a hysterical nature, schizophrenia, drug-induced toxic states, temporal lobe epilepsy, and states of fatigue. Also *dispersonalization, depersonalization syndrome.* **prolonged epileptic d.** DREAMY STATE.

**de Pezzer** [O. *de Pezzer,* French physician, flourished late 19th century] See under CATHETER.

**depilate** \dep′ilāt\ EPILATE.

**depilation** \dep′ilā′shən\ EPILATION.

**depilatory** \depil′ətôr′ē\ [L *depilat(us),* past part. of *depilare* (from *de-* from + *pil(us)* hair) to pull off the hair + -ORY] **1** Any agent used to remove or destroy hair. **2** Capable of removing or destroying hair. For defs. 1 and 2 also *epilatory.*

**deplete** \diplēt′\ To use up; empty.

**depletion** \diplē′shən\ [L *depletus* (past part. of *deplere* to empty out, from DE- + L *plere* to fill) emptied out] The act or process of depleting, as a body cavity of a fluid; the emptying, exhaustion, or reduction of a quantity or substance or of the strength of a power. **plasma d.** PLASMAPHERESIS.

**depolarization** \dēpō′lərīzā′shən\ [DE- + POLARIZATION] The process by which the resting potential of nerve or muscle is reversed, leading to increased excitation and eliciting a propagated impulse if of sufficient magnitude.

**depolarize** \dēpō′lərīz\ [DE- + POLARIZE] To reduce the negative potential across a cell membrane.

**depolarizer** \dēpō′lərīzər\ A chemical agent or substance that reduces or eliminates electrical polarization of an excitable membrane.

**Depo-Provera** A proprietary name for medroxyprogesterone acetate

**deportation** \dē′pôrtā′shən\ The breaking away of trophoblast cells from the placenta and their conveyance into the maternal circulation and thence to maternal organs such as the lungs. This is a relatively common occurrence in human pregnancy.

**deposit** [L *depositus* (past part. of *deponere* to put down, entrust, deposit) entrusted, deposited] The accumulation of a substance such as amyloid or hemosiderin in a tissue or organ. **active d.** The solid radioactive products resulting from the disintegration of a radioactive gas. **bismuth d.** A deposit of bismuth in the gingival tissues, causing the appearance of a blue-black line near the gingival margin. Also *bismuth line, bismuth stomatitis.* **dense d.'s** Very intense, electron-dense intramembranous deposits, characteristic of type II mesangiocapillary glomerulonephritis. **glomerular d.'s** Extracellular aggregations of substances not normally found in the glomerulus. The deposits usually contain proteins, especially immunoglobulins, fibrinogen, and complement, but may also be made up of or contain lipids, DNA, or metals such as silver, calcium, and iron. **hyaline d.** A glomerular deposit containing eosinophilic, homogeneous, smooth-appearing material. Lipid but little or no fibrin may be present. **mesangial d.** A deposit within the glomerular mesangial matrix or between the matrix and mesangial cell cytoplasm. **para-amyloid d.** A deposit in the renal interstitium or vessel walls of an acidophilic material that looks like amyloid but does not have the staining or electron-microscopic characteristics of amyloid. **renal amyloid d.** A deposit of amyloid material either in the glomeruli, blood vessels, or the interstitium, especially of the medulla. See also RENAL AMYLOIDOSIS. **subendothelial d.** A deposit located between the glomerular basement membrane and the endothelium. The deposit density may be greater, less, or the same as that of the basement membrane. **subepithelial d.** A deposit located on the outer or epithelial side of the glomerular basement membrane. The epithelial cell foot processes often surround the deposit and may appear to be fused. The deposits may be irregular in shape or may be a well-formed hump, as in immune complex renal disease.

**deposition** \dep′əzish′ən\ [L *depositio* (from *depositus,* past part. of *deponere* to put down, entrust, deposit) a depositing] **1** The act of depositing. **2** The accumulation of organic or inorganic debris. **urate d.** Accumulations of urates or uric acid in tissues, including joints, kidneys, and subcutaneous tissues.

**depot** [French *dépôt* (from L *depositum*) a deposit, store, depot] A particular tissue, organ, or general body compartment in which a drug or other agent has accumulated and is stored. **fat d.** A region of the body in which fat is stored.

**depressant** \dipres′ənt\ [*depress* + *-ant,* agentive suffix. See also DEPRESSION.] **1** Causing a reduction in activity, as of the central nervous system. **2** An agent that causes a reduction in activity. **cardiac d.** An agent which reduces myocardial contractility.

**depression** [L *depressio* (from *depressus,* past part. of *deprimere* to press or weight down) a pressing or weighing down] **1** A place or site pressed down or sunken below a surrounding surface, or the condition characterizing it. **2** A reduction in quantity or extent. **3** A psychiatric syndrome characterized by a lowering of mood tone, expressed as feelings of painful dejection with dimunition in self-esteem, difficulty in thinking, and psychomotor retardation or agitation. In addition, there may be disturbances in sleep, appetite, and weight and ideas of death or suicide. Also *melancholia, depressive reaction* (imprecise). **4** A reduction in the amplitude of an electroencephalographic recording. **agitated d.** **1** A clinical depression in which psychomotor agitation, rather than psychomotor retardation, is the prominent manifestation. **2** INVOLUTIONAL MELANCHOLIA. **anaclitic d.** A state of apparent depression that characterizes infants separated from their mothers for prolonged periods. It is marked by listlessness, immobility, expressionlessness, loss of appetite, and weight loss. **endogenous d.** A depression that arises *de novo,* independent of events that would appear adequate to justify or warrant it. • Some authors use the phrase in a purely descriptive manner to indicate that no clear-cut precipitants for the present episode can be elicited. Others use it to mean nonreactive, and therefore with a relatively poor prognosis in comparison with reactive depression. Others use it to indicate a depression accompanied by vegetative signs resulting in insomnia, weight loss, reduced libido, and, often, psychotic symptoms such as mood-incongruent delusions. In the last sense, endogenous depression is often considered to be organic in nature and based upon some defect in neurohormonal metabolism. Also *melancholia.* **freezing point d.** The effect of dissolved solutes on the freezing point of pure water, used to measure osmolality. One osmol dissolved in one kilogram depresses the freezing point 1.86°C. Serum and urine osmolality, usually determined in clinical settings by measuring freezing point depression in a suitably calibrated refrigerated bath, is expressed in mOsm/kg. **involutional d.** INVOLUTIONAL MELANCHOLIA. **Leão spreading d.** A phenomenon noted in the electrocorticogram in which depression of normal cortical rhythms spreads outward from the point of stimulation when certain areas of the exposed brain are stimulated. Also *spreading depression.* **neurotic d.** NEUROTIC DEPRESSIVE DISORDER. **pacchionian d.'s** FOVEOLAE GRANULARES. **precordial d.** FOSSA EPIGASTRICA. **psychotic d.** Any major depressive episode with gross impairment in reality testing. This may be an endogenous depression, a depression with a poor prognosis, a depression presumed to be primarily biologic in origin, a depression with a marked suicidal accompaniment or mood-incongruent features, or any combination of the foregoing. **pterygoid d.** FOVEA PTERYGOIDEA MANDIBULAE. **radial d.** FOSSA RADIALIS HUMERI. **reactive d.** A depression precipitated by an external event or situation, such as loss of a significant object. • In some classificatory schemes, reactive is used simply to mean occurring as a reaction. In others, it is used more specifically to indicate a depression of nonpsychotic or neurotic degree, of psychologic rather than biologic origin, or a depression with good prognosis. Also *situational depression, reactive depressive psychosis.* **retarded d.** A major depressive disorder with psychomotor retardation as a prominent symptom. **situational d.** REACTIVE DEPRESSION. **spreading d.** LEÃO SPREADING DEPRESSION. **supratrochlear d.** A shallow, transverse concavity just above the patellar surface at the lower end of the femur. **unipolar d.** A major affective disorder consisting of depressive episodes but without history or evidence of manic episodes. Also *unipolar psychosis.*

**depressomotor** \dipres′ōmō′tər\ **1** Of or relating to the lessening of movement. **2** DEPRESSOR.

**depressor** \dipres′ər\ **1** An agent that depresses by bringing about a reduction in activity. Also *depressomotor.*

2 Something that presses a structure in a downward direction: used of muscles and instruments. **d. anguli oris** MUSCULUS DEPRESSOR ANGULI ORIS. **d. epiglottidis** Those fibers of the thyroepiglottic muscle that depress the epiglottis, modifying the inlet of the larynx. **d. labii inferioris** MUSCULUS DEPRESSOR LABII INFERIORIS. **tongue d.** A flat instrument for pressing the tongue down against the floor of the mouth to facilitate examination of the mouth and throat or to maintain the airway in the unconscious or anesthetized subject. Also *tongue spatula.*

**deprivation** \dep′rivā′shən\ A condition or process within an organism evoked by the removal of something needed or desired either physiologically, such as food, or psychologically, such as the stimulation provided by contact with other human beings. In behavioral research with animal subjects, the degree of food or water deprivation is often manipulated to provide an operationally defined level of drive. **emotional d.** A lack of the usual kind and degree of psychologic support provided by interpersonal and environmental relationships. When this deprivation occurs in infancy or childhood and is sustained for any appreciable length of time, it interferes with the development of object relations and personality and may be associated with anaclitic depression and developmental disorders. **psychosocial d.** A level of psychological stimulation and social interaction below that which is necessary for normal mental development during the earliest years of life. **sensory d.** A condition, occurring either naturally or as an experimental manipulation, in which the normal or usual range of sensory stimulation impinging on an individual is markedly reduced, to a level below that required for normal central nervous system functioning. For example, a person is placed in a darkened, soundproofed, isolation chamber wearing cuffs or gloves to limit tactile experience. The restlessness, emotional upset, and sometimes delusional behavior that can be evoked by these restrictions underscores the human need for a certain measure of stimulus change in order to maintain normal functioning. Also *sensory isolation.* **thought d.** BLOCKING OF THOUGHT.

**deproteinization** \dēprō′tēnīzā′shən\ The removal of proteins, often a stage in treatment of a tissue extract in order to analyze its content of a substance of small molecular mass.

**depsipeptide** A peptide having some —NH— groups replaced by —O—. It is thus formed from both $\alpha$-amino acids and $\alpha$ hydroxy acids in amide and ester linkage. Several antibiotics are depsipeptides. An example is the cyclic depsipeptide valinomycin, which is an ionophore for potassium ions.

**depth** 1 Distance inward or downward. 2 Distance between a nearer and a farther point in an observer's line of sight or along the axis of any aiming or focusing system. **focal d.** The range of clear vision on either side of focus.

**depulization** \dē′pyoolīzā′shən\ [DE- + L *pul(ex)* a flea + *-iz(e)* + -ATION] The elimination of fleas from infested hosts or habitats. • The term has been used chiefly in antiplague work.

**depurant** \dep′yərənt\ DEPURATIVE.

**depurative** \dep′yərā′tiv\ [Late L *depurat(us),* past part. of *depurare* to purify, from L *de-* from + *purare* to purify, from *purus* pure, clean + -IVE] 1 Capable of purifying. Also *pellant.* 2 Any substance that purifies. Also *depurant.*

**depurination** \dēpyoo′rinā′shən\ The removal of purines from DNA, a process accomplished by acid treatment. The process of hydrolysis favors purines over pyrimidines, and DNA over RNA.

**de Quervain** [Fritz *de Quervain,* Swiss physician, 1868–1940] 1 Quervain's disease, Quervain syndrome. See under SYNDROME. 2 De Quervain's thyroiditis. See under SUBACUTE THYROIDITIS.

**der-** \der-\ [Gk *derē* neck] A combining form denoting the neck.

**derangement** \dirānj′mənt\ A defective configuration or the loss of a previously attained level of organization or functioning.

**Dercum** [Francis Xavier *Dercum,* U.S. neurologist, 1856–1931] Dercum's disease. See under NEUROLIPOMATOSIS DOLOROSA.

**derealization** \dē′rē·əlīzā′shən\ [DE- + REAL + *-iz(e)* + -ATION] The feeling that some or all of the external world has changed and is no longer familiar or real. It is reported most frequently in dissociative disorders of a hysterical nature, temporal lobe epilepsy, and schizophrenia.

**dereism** \dē′rē·izm\ [L *de-* from, away + *re,* ablative of *res* thing, reality + -ISM] Thinking and other mental activities that ignore reality and actual experience, such as occurs in a delusion. Dereism is often seen in schizophrenics. Also *derism.*

**derencephaly** \der′ənsef′əlē\ [DER- + ENCEPHAL- + -Y] The failure of closure in the cephalic and cervical regions of the neural tube, accompanied by erosion of the exposed neural tissues.

**derepression** \dē′ripresh′ən\ Preferential synthesis of an enzyme by removal or inactivation of a repressor that prevents expression of the appropriate genes.

**derism** \dē′rizm\ DEREISM.

**derivative** A substance derived from another by some specific modification of its molecule, usually by substitution or addition reactions. The derivative may be made in order to identify the original compound, or to protect some parts of the molecule when others react. **purified protein d.** Purified protein derivative of tuberculin. See under TUBERCULIN. **tricyclic d.** Any of the metabolites or chemical analogues of the tricyclic antidepressant drugs. Desipramine and nortriptyline, for example, are demethylated metabolites of tertiary tricyclics.

**derm-** \durm-\ DERMATO-.

**-derm** \-durm\ [Gk *derma* skin] A combining form denoting (1) a layer; (2) skin or integument.

**derma** \dur′mə\ [Gk, skin] DERMIS.

**derma-** \dur′mə-\ DERMATO-.

**-derma** \-durmə\ [Gk *derma* skin] A combining form meaning a kind of skin or a condition of the skin. • Some authorities have in the past differentiated *-dermia* from *-derma,* applying *poikilodermia,* for example, to a disease entity and *poikiloderma* to a symptom. The distinction is now no longer acceptable and there is a growing tendency to apply the form *-derma* in all contexts.

**dermabrader** \dur′məbrā′dər\ [DERM- + English *abrader* an agent used for abrading] 1 An instrument, often a rotating burr, that is used to perform dermabrasion. 2 The operator of such an instrument.

**dermabrasion** \-brā′zhən\ [DERM- + ABRASION] The surgical removal of irregularities of the skin, as scarring and embedded foreign materials. The skin is smoothed out by removing superficial layers of the skin with a dermatome or any of a variety of abrading devices, such as a rapidly turning wire brush or gritty paper or cloth. The remaining epithelium is then allowed to recover spontaneously. Also *planing.*

**dermacarrier** \-kar′ē·ər\ [DERMA + CARRIER] The part of a device that conveys a skin graft in the process of making a tanner mesh. It consists of a rigid, rectangular, plastic plate containing parallel grooves. Slits are cut between the grooves by a spiral blade positioned above the dermacarrier.

***Dermacentor*** \dur′məsen′tər\ [DERMA- + Gk *kentōr* a goader, stinger] A genus of ornate, moderate- to large-sized, hard ticks (family Ixodidae) with eyes and festoons. Some 31 species are known, most of which are three-host ticks, though a few one-host species are known. Immature stages usually feed on rodents, lagomorphs, and insectivores, while older stages feed on larger mammals. They are serious pests of herbivores in some areas and are also vectors of rickettsial and viral pathogens. ***D. andersoni*** The Rocky Mountain wood tick, a widely distributed, abundant pest in western North America, which serves as a vector of Rocky Mountain spotted fever, Colorado tick fever, and tularemia, and can also cause tick paralysis. Hosts include horses, cattle, sheep, deer, elk, antelope, grizzly bear, and coyotes. Larvae and nymphs feed on small mammals, chiefly rodents and rabbits. All three stages may feed on intermediate-sized animals, such as porcupines or jack rabbits. Also *Dermacentor venustus.* ***D. marginatus*** A species that serves as a vector of Russian spring-summer encephalitis virus, tick-borne encephalitis virus, as a reservoir of Omsk hemorrhagic fever virus in the USSR, as a possible vector of Crimean-Congo hemorrhagic fever virus and of *Babesia canis,* which causes canine babesiosis. ***D. occidentalis*** The Pacific Coast tick, a common species on the West Coast of the United States that parasitizes all domestic herbivores, deer, dogs, and man. It has been found infected in California and Oregon with Colorado tick fever virus. Other agents involving this species as a possible vector include Rocky Mountain spotted fever. ***D. variabilis*** The American dog tick, a species common in the eastern United States. It is the principal vector of Rocky Mountain spotted fever virus in the central and eastern United States, transmits tularemia, and may cause canine paralysis. ***D. venustus*** *DERMACENTOR ANDERSONI.*

***Dermacentroxenus*** \dur′məsen′träksē′nəs\ [DERMA- + Gk *kentro(n)* a prickle, sting + *xenos* a guest, host, stranger] A subgenus of *Rickettsia,* comprising an important group of pathogens carried by hard ticks, including *R. (D.) akari, R. (D.) australis, R. (D.) conorii, R. (D.) rickettsii, R. (D.) siberica,* and *R. (D.) tsutsugamushi.*. ***D. akari*** *RICKETTSIA AKARI.* ***D. australis*** *RICKETTSIA AUSTRALIS.* ***D. conori*** *RICKETTSIA CONORII.* ***D. orientalis*** *RICKETTSIA TSUTSUGAMUSHI.* ***D. rickettsi*** *RICKETTSIA RICKETTSII.*

**dermachalasis** \-kal′əsis\ [DERMA- + Gk *chalasis* (from *chalan* to make slack or loose) a slackening] CUTIS LAXA.

**dermal** \dur′məl\ [DERM- + -AL] **1** Pertaining to the skin. Also *dermic.* **2** Of or relating to the dermis. For defs. 1 and 2 also *dermatic.*

**dermalgia** \durmal′jə\ [DERM- + -ALGIA] Cutaneous pain occurring as a result of disease or dysfunction of the central or peripheral nervous system, as in tabes dorsalis or polyneuropathy. Also *dermatalgia.*

**dermamyiasis** \-mīyī′əsis\ DERMATOMYIASIS.

***Dermanyssus gallinae*** \-nis′əs galē′nē\ The chicken mite, a worldwide pest of chickens and other birds. Occasionally attacking humans, it causes an eruption and itching, particularly following sensitization.

**dermat-** \dur′mət-\ DERMATO-.

**dermatalgia** \-tal′jə\ DERMALGIA.

**dermatan sulfate** A polymer occurring in connective tissue and containing alternate residues of *N*-acetylgalactosamine-4-sulfate and L-iduronic acid. It thus differs from chondroitin-4-sulfate only in the configuration of the hexuronic acid moieties; and L-iduronic acid differs from D-glucuronic acid only in configuration at C-5. The linkage is [GalNAc4-$SO_3^-$($\beta$1-4)L-IdoA($\alpha$1-3)$]_n$. Also *chondroitin sulfate B.*

**dermatic** \dərmat′ik\ DERMAL.

**dermatitides** \dur′mətit′idēz\ Plural of DERMATITIS.

# dermatitis

**dermatitis** \dur′mətī′tis\ [DERMAT- + -ITIS] Any inflammatory skin disease. • The terms *dermatitis* and *eczema* are now regarded by most dermatologists as synonymous; however, some reserve eczema for use in describing a skin disease brought on by exposure to a substance in the workplace. **actinic d.** Dermatitis provoked by exposure to sunlight. Also *solar dermatitis, actinodermatitis.* **allergic contact d.** An acute inflammatory condition of the skin following topical exposure to an allergen to which the subject shows delayed hypersensitivity. **ancylostome d.** CUTANEOUS ANCYLOSTOMIASIS. **d. artefacta** Dermatitis that is wholly self-inflicted, either accidentally or deliberately. Also *autophytic dermatitis, dermatitis autophytica.* **ashy d.** ERYTHEMA DYSCHROMICUM PERSTANS. **atopic d.** ATOPIC ECZEMA. **autosensitization d.** SECONDARY SPREAD. **bathers' d.** Any form of irritable eruption related to contact with water. **berloque d.** A photosensitivity reaction following exposure to perfume containing a psoralen, usually bergamot oil. Also *perfume dermatitis.* **d. blastomycotica** CUTANEOUS BLASTOMYCOSIS. **carcinomatous d.** An inflammatory alteration of the skin due to an underlying carcinoma. **caterpillar d.** A form of allergic dermatitis resulting from contact with caterpillars that have urticarious hairs or spines, such as the larvae of the brown-tail moth, flannel moth, Io moth, or tussock moth. Also *caterpillar rash, moth dermatitis.* **cercarial d.** SCHISTOSOME DERMATITIS. **chemical d.** Inflammation of the skin caused by contact with or exposure to a chemical agent, and resulting in either allergic contact dermatitis or primary irritant dermatitis. The lesions are usually localized initially at the sites of exposure. **chronic superficial scaly d.** A chronic eczematous condition of unknown cause, characterized by round or oval erythematous scaly patches, often with fingerlike extensions, that occur on the trunk and limbs. **d. congelationis** FROSTBITE. **contact d.** An inflammation of the skin that is induced by external contact with substances that damage the skin by direct chemical action or through an immunological mechanism. Also *contact dermatosis.* **cumulative insult d.** Dermatitis caused by repeated exposure to a weak irritant such as a detergent. **diaper d.** Any eruption occurring in the skin that is usually covered by a diaper. It is often induced by prolonged contact with urine or feces. *Imprecise.* Also *napkin area dermatitis, Jacquet's dermatitis, dermatitis glutealis, napkin psoriasis* (imprecise). **dried fruit d.** A dermatitis caused by handling dried fruits infested with the dried fruit mite, *Carpoglyphus lactis,* of the family Carpoglyphidae. **eczematoid d.** ECZEMA. **epidemic exfoliative d.** TOXIC EPIDERMAL NECROLYSIS.

**dermato-** \dur′mətō-\ [Gk *derma* (genitive *dermatos*) skin] A combining form meaning skin, dermal. Also *derm-, derma-, dermo-, dermat-.*

**dermatoarthritis** \-arthrī′tis\ Any form of arthritis with a consistently associated rash, such as psoriatic arthritis. **lipid d.** Any of several illnesses, such as xanthoma and arthritis, which have simultaneously lipid abnormalities with cutaneous manifestations. Also *lipoid dermatoarthritis.*

***Dermatobia hominis*** \dur′mətō′bē·ə häm′inis\ The South American human botfly, commonly called tórsalo or berne. The adult fly resembles a bluebottle fly with brown wings. The larvae are parasitic in the skin of man, all domestic animals, monkeys, and some birds. It is an economically important cattle pest in Central and South America, causing heavy losses of milk, meat, and hides. Children are frequently attacked in these regions. The female fly does not deposit her eggs directly, but captures a bloodsucking insect (or tick) and deposits her eggs on its legs or body which then serves as a transport mechanism. The transported eggs hatch on contact with the host and release botfly larvae when the transport arthropod takes its blood meal. The larvae invade the skin, causing local warblelike lesions and swellings in which the larvae develop over a period of about six weeks. The mature larva then drops to the soil, enters it, and pupates. The life cycle usually requires three to four months.

**dermatobiasis** \-bī′əsis\ Infestation with *Dermatobia;* dermatobial myiasis.

**dermatodysplasia** \-displā′zhə\ [DERMATO- + DYSPLASIA] A developmental malformation of the skin.

**dermatofibroma** \-fībrō′mə\ [DERMATO- + FIBROMA] A benign nonencapsulated dermal lesion composed of a mixture of histiocytes and fibroblasts with varying amounts of collagen and thin-walled blood vessels. Also *reticulohistiocytoma, sclerosing hemangioma, histiocytoma* (not recommended), *histiocytoma cutis, reticulohistiocytic granuloma* (older term), *sclerosing angioma* (incorrect), *xanthofibroma thecocellulare* (obs.). **d. protuberans** DERMATOFIBROSARCOMA PROTUBERANS.

**dermatofibrosarcoma** \-fī′brəsärkō′mə\ A fibrosarcoma of low malignancy that arises in the skin. **progressive recurrent d.** A lesion of the dermal connective tissue that is characterized by the presence of atypical fibroblasts and a tendency to local recurrence. **d. protuberans** A fibrosarcoma of the skin which grows as a protruding nodular mass. The cells do not show great pleomorphism and are typically arranged in a cartwheel pattern. It is less malignant than the usual fibrosarcoma. Also *dermatofibroma protuberans.*

**dermatofibrosis** \-fībrō′sis\ A circumscribed dense fibrosis of the dermis. **disseminated lenticular d.** A syndrome characterized by multiple collagenomas evident mainly on the trunk and by the presence of osteopoikilosis. Also *Buschke-Ollendorff syndrome, dermatofibrosis lenticularis disseminata, familial cutaneous collagenoma.*

**dermatoglyphics** \-glif′iks\ [DERMATO- + Gk *glyph(ein)* to engrave, carve, scratch down + -ICS] **1** The epidermal ridge patterns of the volar skin surfaces of the fingers and toes and the palms and soles including single ridges and all of their configurational arrangements, but excluding flexion creases and other secondary foldings. **2** The anatomic study of the patterns of ridged skin as it relates to other scientific disciplines, particularly genetics, anthropology, and criminalistics. For defs. 1 and 2 also *dermoglyphics.*

**dermatographia** \-graf′ē·ə\ [DERMATO- + -GRAPH + -IA] DERMOGRAPHIA. **black d.** The discoloration of the skin by metal that appears after rubbing with a blunt point. It is most evident when the skin is covered with powder. **white d.** A white line on the skin, attributed either to small vessel constriction or to edema. It is part of the physiologic response to rubbing of the skin and is accentuated especially in atopic dermatitis.

**dermatographism** \dur′mətäg′rəfizm\ DERMOGRAPHISM.

**dermatoid** \dur′mətoid\ DERMOID.

**dermatologist** \dur′mətäl′əjist\ [*dermatolog(y)-* + -IST] A specialist in diseases of the skin.

**dermatology** \dur′mətäl′əjē\ [DERMATO- + -LOGY] The scientific study of diseases of the skin.

**dermatolysis palpebrarum** \dur′mətäl′isis pal′pəbrä′rəm\ Involvement of the eyelid skin in destructive cutaneous disease.

**dermatome** \dur′mətōm′\ [DERMA- + -TOME] **1** An area of skin innervated by a single dorsal spinal nerve root. In the thoracic region, the regular arrangement of the dermatomes in bands or girdles is reminiscent of the primary metameric segmentation. The regions supplied by the nerve roots overlap each other considerably so that division of a single root rarely gives any evident sensory loss. Elsewhere the dermatomes are less regularly arranged, largely because of the development of the limbs. Individual dermatomes are designated by the number of the nerve root (cervical, dorsal, lumbar, or sacral) which carries sensation from it. Also *dermatomic area, segmental area, rhizomere.* **2** That part of the embryonic mesenchyme beneath the epidermis, destined to form the dermis more or less in the dorsolateral region. It is derived from the external portion of the somite. Also *cutis plate, skin plate, dermatotome.* • Although the usual spelling is *dermatome,* some embryologists prefer the

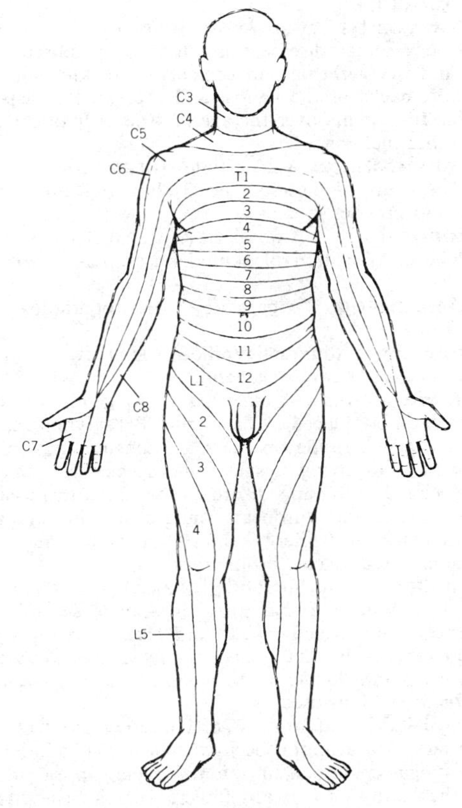


**Dermatomes**

spelling *dermotome* and consider that *dermatome* should be restricted to the cutaneous territories innervated by the segmental nerves. **3** A surgical instrument for obtaining (harvesting) partial thickness skin grafts. **Brown air-driven d.** A dermatome which incorporates adjustable guards for varying the width and thickness of the graft, and which has a replaceable reciprocating blade which is powered by a compressed air turbine. **drum d.** A manually operated dermatome in the shape of a half drum. Adhesive is applied to the surface of the drum, either in the form of glue or a special tape. The drum is then rolled across the surface of the skin, which it picks up while a guided knife attached to the drum cuts a split-thickness skin graft. It is available in a variety of sizes and styles. The Padgett and Reese dermatomes operate on the drum principle. **Padgett d.** An adjustable dermatome suitable for excising split-thickness or full-thickness grafts. **Reese d.** A dermatome designed for harvesting split-thickness grafts in the range of 0.20 to 0.86 mm.

**dermatomegaly** \-meg′əlē\ [DERMATO- + -MEGALY] Excessive folding of thickened skin which may occur as a developmental defect and may complicate acquired disorders such as acromegaly.

**dermatomycid** \-mī′sid\ DERMATOPHYTID.

**dermatomycin** \-mī′sin\ A fungal antigen substance which has the capacity to induce antibody formation in the human or animal host.

**dermatomyiasis** \-mīyī′əsis\ [DERMATO- + MYIASIS] Skin infestation with fly maggots developing in dermal lesions. Also *dermamyiasis.*

**dermatomyoma** \-mī·ō′mə\ [DERMATO- + MYOMA] LEIOMYOMA CUTIS.

**dermatomyositis** \-mī′əsī′tis\ [DERMATO- + MYOSITIS] A collagen vascular disease characterized by muscle inflammation and by erythema and edema of the skin, notably on the eyelids, backs of the hands, and the extensor aspects of the limbs. In patients over the age of 40 it is frequently associated with a malignancy.

**dermatoneurology** \-n$^y$urăl′əjē\ [DERMATO- + NEUROLOGY] The study of diseases and dysfunction affecting both the skin and nervous system.

**dermatonosology** \-nōsăl′əjē\ [DERMATO- + NOSOLOGY] The classification of skin diseases. Also *dermonosology.*

**dermatopathology** \-pathăl′əjē\ Histopathology of the skin.

**dermatopathy** \dur′mətăp′əthē\ [DERMATO- + -PATHY] Any skin disease. Also *dermopathy.*

***Dermatophagoides*** \-fagoi′dēz\ A genus of sarcoptiform mites, now placed in the family Pyroglyphidae. Members of the genus reside on the skin, consuming skin scales and detritus, not living tissues. One species, *D. saitoi,* has been associated with lung disorders. Several others, such as *D. pteronyssinus,* the European house-dust mite, are associated with house dust allergy. Infestation of humans may be accompanied by a severe chronic dermatitis.

**dermatophyte** \dur′mətōfīt′\ [DERMATO- + Gk *phyt(on)* a plant, tree, thing that has grown] Any of several species of imperfect fungi which invade and cause infections of the skin, hair, and nails. The genera involved are *Microsporum, Trichophyton,* and *Epidermophyton..* Also *dermophyte, cutaneous fungus* (seldom used).

**dermatophytid** \dur′mətăf′ətid\ [*dermatophyt(e)* + -ID²] A secondary skin eruption occurring in individuals having a primary fungal epidermal infection. Vesicles appear most often on the hands or between fingers and is believed to be caused by systemic antigens and skin-sensitizing antibodies. Also *dermatomycid, mycid* (obs.). Also *dermatophytide.*

**dermatophytosis** \-fītō′sis\ [*dermatophyt(e)* + -OSIS] A fungal infection of keratinized tissue, epidermis, hair, or nails, caused by one of several dermatophytes. Also *dermophytosis.* **d. interdigitale** TINEA INTERDIGITALIS.

**dermatoplastic** \-plas′tik\ Of or relating to dermatoplasty.

**dermatoplasty** \dur′mətōplas′tē\ [DERMATO- + -PLASTY] A plastic operation performed to replace injured skin. Also *dermoplasty.* **Thompson's d.** A treatment for lymphedema that includes the wide excision of involved skin and subcutaneous tissue with installation of buried dermal flaps, the latter deemed useful in increasing lymphatic drainage from the limb.

**dermatopolyneuritis** \-păl′ēn$^y$urī′tis\ [DERMATO- + POLYNEURITIS] PINK DISEASE.

**dermatosclerosis** \-sklerō′sis\ Fibrosis of the skin, as in sclerodactyly and progressive systemic sclerosis.

**dermatoses** \dur′mətō′sēz\ Plural of DERMATOSIS.

**dermatosis** \dur′mətō′sis\ [DERMAT- + -OSIS] Any disease of the skin. **acute febrile neutrophilic d.** An acute eruption of tender, dull red plaques and nodules accompanied by fever, and characterized histologically by intense focal infiltration of the dermis by polymorphonuclear leukocytes. It is often followed by the eventual development of reticulosis and impairment of the immune response mechanism. Also *Sweet syndrome.* **Bowen's precancerous d.** BOWEN'S DISEASE. **cholinogenic d.** CHOLINERGIC URTICARIA. **chronic bullous d. of childhood** An acute bullous disorder of children characterized by areas of erythema and blistering often around the genitals, lower abdomen, and buttocks. Bullae are formed at the dermo-epidermal junction beneath an intact epidermis and IgA can be found in this site. Spontaneous remission appears to occur within three to four years. **chronic hemosideric d.** Any skin disease accompanied by accumulation of hemosidirin in the dermis, including stasis dermatitis and Schamberg's disease (progressive pigmented purpuric dermatosis). **contact d.** CONTACT DERMATITIS. **industrial d.** OCCUPATIONAL DERMATITIS. **lichenoid d.** Any skin disease in which the lesions resemble those of lichen planus. **menstrual d.** A skin disease that recurs during or immediately before each menstrual period. **occupational d.** OCCUPATIONAL DERMATITIS. **d. papulosa nigra** A condition, thought to be related to seborrheic keratosis, that is found in Negroes and characterized by multiple papular lesions on the cheeks. Also *dermatitis papulosa nigra.* **pigmentary d.** Any skin disease showing increased or abnormal pigmentation. • The term is most often used to describe pigmented purpuric eruptions. **precancerous d.** BOWEN'S DISEASE. **progressive pigmented purpuric d.** A chronic dermatosis, usually of unknown etiology, due to a capillaritis and characterized by erythema, purpura, and hemosiderin staining. Also *Schamberg's disease, progressive pigmentary dermatosis, Schamberg's dermatosis.* **radiation d.** RADIATION DERMATITIS. **Schamberg's d.** PROGRESSIVE PIGMENTED PURPURIC DERMATOSIS. **seborrheic d.** SEBORRHEIC DERMATITIS. **subcorneal pustular d.** A chronic, benign, relapsing, pustular eruption in which the histology shows a subcorneal bulla containing polymorphonuclear leucocytes. The condition responds to treatment with dapsone. Also *Sneddon-Wilkinson disease.*

**dermatosome** \dur′mətōsōm′\ [DERMATO- + Gk *sōm(a)* body] A thickened region along a spindle fiber near the equatorial plate, during mitotic division.

**dermatosyphilis** \-sif′ilis\ Generalized syphilis manifesting itself in the skin. It is characteristic of secondary rather than late syphilis.

**dermatotome** \dur′mətōtōm′\ DERMATOME.

**dermatotropic** \-träp′ik\ [DERMATO- + -TROPIC[2]] Having an attraction or affinity for the skin: said chiefly of microorganisms. Also *dermotropic*.

**dermatozoiasis** \-zō·ī′əsis\ [*dermatozo(on)* + -IASIS] DERMATOZOONOSIS.

**dermatozoon** \-zō′än\ [DERMATO- + Gk *zōon* living being, animal] (*pl.* dermatozoa) An animal parasite that lives in or damages the skin.

**dermatozoonosis** \-zō′ənō′sis\ [DERMATOZOON + -OSIS] An eruption or skin disease caused by an animal parasite. Also *dermatozoiasis*.

**dermatropic** [DERMA- + -TROPIC[1]] Having an affinity for skin tissue.

**dermenchysis** \dermen′kisis\ [DERM- + Gk *enchysis* (from *enchein* to pour in, fill) a pouring in] The administration of medication beneath the skin, as by hypodermic injection.

**-dermia** \-dur′mē·ə\ [DERM- + -IA] A combining form denoting a condition of the skin. ● See note at -DERMA.

**dermic** \dur′mik\ DERMAL.

**dermis** \dur′mis\ [New L, back-formation from Gk *-dermis* as in *epidermis*] [NA] The connective tissue layer of the skin that lies deep to the epidermis and comprises a thin papillary layer and a deeper thick, dense reticular layer that merges into the tela subcutanea. The dermis contains plexuses of blood and lymphatic vessels, nerve fibers, sensory nerve endings, some fat, hair follicles, sebaceous glands, ducts of sweat glands, and smooth muscle fibers. It is tough and highly elastic, containing a high proportion of collagen and elastin fibers. It is very thick in the soles of the feet and palms of the hands. Also *corium, cutis vera, derma.* **reticular d.** The deep part of the dermis in which the collagen fibrils tend to form a network.

**dermo-** \dur′mō-\ DERMATO-.

**dermoactinomycosis** \-ak′tinōmīkō′sis\ Actinomycosis involving the skin and occurring in association with actinomycotic infection of deeper structures.

**dermoblast** \dur′mōblast\ [DERMO- + -BLAST] A precursor cell that arises from the lateral or somatic layer of the somites and gives rise to the cells of the dermis of the skin.

**dermocyma** \-sī′mə\ [DERMO- + Gk *kyma* the fetus in the womb, anything swollen] Unequal conjoined twins in which the smaller or parasitic member is covered by or imbedded within the skin of the host or larger member.

**dermogenesis** \-jen′əsis\ [DERMO- + GENESIS] The formation of the dermis or corium from the mesenchyme, probably derived from the dermatome. Fibrillae appear at the 30 mm stage in human embryos. Later they develop into collagenous and elastic fibers. At about 60 mm primitive papillae are present in the dermis.

**dermoglyphics** \-glif′iks\ DERMATOGLYPHICS.

**dermographia** \-graf′ē·ə\ [DERMO- + -GRAPH + -IA] The marking of the skin, usually in red, white, or black wheals. It is most often seen after rubbing the skin firmly with a blunted point. Also *dermatographia*.

**dermographism** \dərmäg′rəfizm\ [DERMO- + GRAPH- + -ISM] A tendency to readily show dermographia. Also *dermatographism, Ebbecke's reaction, factitious urticaria.*

**dermohygrometer** \-hīgräm′ətər\ An instrument for measuring skin resistance and thus determining the moisture of the skin surface, as in palmar sweating.

**dermoid** \dur′moid\ [DERM- + -OID] **1** Having features similar to the skin. Also *dermatoid.* **2** DERMOID CYST. **implantation d.** A cyst arising from ectodermal or epidermal cells that have been displaced, usually by injury, into deeper tissues. See also SEQUESTRATION CYST. **inclusion d.** DERMOID CYST. **intracranial d.** A dermoid cyst arising in the intracranial cavity. **intramedullary d.** A dermoid cyst arising within the substance of the spinal cord. **thyroid d.** A cyst within the thyroid gland, believed to originate from remnants of the thyroglossal duct. **tubal d.** A dermoid cyst arising in the uterine tube.

**dermolipoma** \-lipō′mə\ [DERMO- + LIPOMA] A tumorlike malformative mass of fibroadipose tissue beneath the conjunctiva.

**dermometer** \dərmäm′ətər\ [DERMO- + -METER] An instrument used to measure the resistance of the skin to the passage of direct electric current.

**dermomycosis** \-mīkō′sis\ [DERMO- + MYCOSIS] TINEA.

**dermomyotome** \-mī′ətōm\ [DERMO- + MYO- + -TOME] Cells of the dorsolateral part of each embryonic somite which form the muscle plate, or myotome, and the skin plate, or dermatome. Also *dermomyotome plate.* Adj. dermomyotomic, dermomuscular.

**dermoneurotropic** \-n[y]ur′əträp′ik\ Showing an affinity for both skin and neural tissue.

**dermonosology** \-nōsäl′əjē\ DERMATONOSOLOGY.

**dermopathy** \dərmäp′əthē\ DERMATOPATHY. **diabetic d.** A dermatosis occurring in association with diabetic microangiopathy. The initial lesion—an oval, dull red papule with some vesiculation—is usually found on the anterior surface of the legs and thighs. It leaves a small, sometimes pigmented, depressed scar on the shins.

**dermophyma venereum** \-fī′mə vəner′ē·əm\ A nodular lesion of the skin that is caused by a venereal, usually syphilitic, disease.

**dermophyte** \dur′mōfīt\ DERMATOPHYTE.

**dermophytosis** \-fītō′sis\ DERMATOPHYTOSIS.

**dermoplasty** \dur′mōplas′tē\ DERMATOPLASTY.

**dermoreaction** \-rē·ak′shən\ CUTANEOUS REACTION.

**dermorrhagia** \-rā′jē·ə\ HEMATIDROSIS.

**dermosynovitis** \-sin′ōvī′tis\ [DERMO- + SYNOVITIS] The simultaneous inflammation of the tendon or synovium and its overlying skin.

**dermotome** \dur′mōtōm\ See under DERMATOME.

**dermotoxin** \-täk′sin\ A toxin formed by certain staphylococci that induces necrosis when injected into the skin.

**dermotropic** \-träp′ik\ DERMATOTROPIC.

**dero-** \der′ō-\ DER-.

**DES** diethylstilbestrol.

**De Sanctis** [Carlo *De Sanctis,* Italian psychiatrist, born 1888] De Sanctis-Cacchione syndrome. See under SYNDROME.

**desaturation** The chemical transformation of a saturated compound into an unsaturated compound. **nitrogen d.** The reduction of nitrogen in body tissues by breathing gases that do not contain nitrogen, as in treating decompression sickness by having the patient inhale oxygen at low pressure. Also *denitrogenation.*

**Desault** [Pierre Joseph *Desault,* French surgeon 1744–1795] Desault's apparatus. See under BANDAGE.

**Descemet** [Jean *Descemet,* French physician 1732–1810] Descemet's membrane. See under LAMINA LIMITANS POSTERIOR CORNEAE.

**descemetitis** \des′əmetī′tis\ [*Descemet('s membrane)* + -ITIS] Inflammation of the innermost elastic layer of the cornea (Descemet's membrane).

**descemetocele** \des′əmet′ōsēl\ [*Descemet('s membrane)* + *o* + -CELE[1]] An outward bulging of the innermost elastic layer of the cornea (Descemet's membrane) that occurs when the stroma of the cornea is absent. Also *keratocele,* *keratodermatocele.*

**descendens** \dēsen′dənz\ [L (pres. part. of *descendere* to go down), descending] Denoting a structure or part that is directed downward; descending. **d. cervicalis** RADIX INFERIOR ANSAE CERVICALIS.

**descensus** \disen′səs\ [L, a descent] A moving downward; a descent or falling. **d. testis** DESCENT OF TESTIS. **d. uteri** PROLAPSE OF UTERUS. **d. ventriculi** GASTROPTOSIS.

**descent** 1 A downward movement or progression. 2 The process by which the human fetus progresses from the inlet to the outlet of the maternal pelvis during labor. **d. of testis** The change in position of the testis from its embryonic site on the posterior body wall into the scrotum during late fetal life in some mammalian species including primates. In man, the testes usually reach the scrotum by the end of the eighth month of fetal life but may remain undescended, either in the inguinal canal or within the abdomen. Descent is brought about through relative growth, the guidance of the gubernaculum, and hormonal influences. Failure of descent adversely affects spermatogenesis in man, but intra-abdominal retention of the testes is characteristic of elephants and cetaceans with no loss of reproductive ability. Many mammals, such as rodents, exhibit descent of testis only during the breeding season. When not reproductively active these mammals withdraw the testes to an inguinal position. Also *descensus testis.* **x d.** The downward deflection on an atrial or venous pulse tracing that follows the a wave. **y d.** The downward deflection on an atrial or venous pulse tracing from the peak of the v wave to the trough of the y. It is slow in cases of stenosis of the atrioventricular valves, and rapid when there is rapid ventricular filling as in regurgitant lesions.

**desensitization** \dēsen′sitīzā′shən\ The reduction or eradication of hypersensitive reaction to an antigen, as by repeated exposure to the antigen, leading to the formation of blocking antibodies. **anaphylactic d.** The transient desensitization of an individual to a specific antigen which may follow an anaphylactic reaction to that antigen.

**desensitize** \dēsen′sitīz\ 1 To subject to desensitization to an antigen. 2 To produce sensory denervation of.

**deserpidine** $C_{32}H_{38}N_2O_8$. 17α-Methoxy-18β-[(3,4,5-trimethylbenzoyl)oxy]-3β,20α-yohimban-16β-carboxylic acid methyl ester. An ester alkaloid obtained from the roots of *Rauwolfia canescens.* Its actions and uses are like those of reserpine. It is given orally as a sedative in acute anxiety states and in chronic psychoses.

**desexualize** \dēsek′shoo·əlīz\ To remove or decrease the sexual attractiveness of.

**desiccant** \des′ikənt\ [L *desiccans,* gen. *desiccantis* (pres. part. of *desiccare* to dry, drain, from *siccus* dry) drying, draining] 1 Causing dryness. Also *desiccative.* 2 A drying agent. For defs. 1 and 2 also *exsiccant.*

**desiccation** \des′ikā′shən\ The removal of moisture.

**desiccative** \des′ikā′tiv\ DESICCANT.

**desipramine hydrochloride** $C_{18}H_{23}ClN_2$. 10,11-Dihydro-*N*-methyl-5*H*-dibenz[*b,f*]azepine-5-propanamine hydrochloride. The monomethyl metabolite of imipramine that is also used as an antidepressant drug. Its properties are similar to those of imipramine, and it is given orally, usually as the hydrochloride salt.

**-desis** \-dē′sis, -dəsis\ [Gk *desis* a binding] A combining form meaning binding.

**Desjardins** [Abel *Desjardins,* French surgeon, flourished early 20th century] See under POINT.

**deslanoside** The deacetyl analogue of lanatoside C, prepared by alkaline degradation of lanaticide C. It is given intravenously for rapid digitalization of patients requiring a cardiac medication of this type.

**desm-** \dezm-\ DESMO-.

**desmectasis** \desmek′təsis\ [DESM- + ECTASIS] The hyperextension or stretching of a ligament.

**desmiognathus** \des′mē·ōnath′əs\ [Gk *desmio(s)* binding (adj.) + *gnathos* jaw, esp. the lower jaw] The parasitic member of epignathic twins represented by a head attached to the lower jaw or associated neck of the host. Also *dicephalus parasiticus.*

**desmitis** \desmī′tis\ [DESM- + -ITIS] An inflammation of a ligament.

**desmo-** \dez′mō-\ [Gk *desmos* band, bond, ligament] A combining form meaning bond or ligament. Also *desm-.*

**desmocranium** \-krā′nē·əm\ [DESMO- + CRANIUM] The embryonic mesodermal mass which becomes the primitive blastemal stage of the developing skull.

**desmocytoma** \-sītō′mə\ [DESMO- + CYT- + -OMA] FIBROMA.

**desmogenous** \desmäj′ənəs\ [DESMO- + -GENOUS] Deriving from a ligament or ligaments.

**desmohemoblast** \-hem′əblast\ MESENCHYME.

**desmoid** \des′moid\ [DESM- + -OID] 1 Consisting of scar tissue. 2 FIBROMATOSIS.

**desmology** \desmäl′əjē\ [DESMO- + -LOGY] The branch of anatomy dealing with the study of ligaments.

**desmoma** \desmō′mə\ DESMOID TUMOR.

**desmon** \des′män\ AMBOCEPTOR.

**desmopathy** \desmäp′əthē\ [DESMO- + -PATHY] A disease affecting a ligament.

**desmopexia** \-pek′sē·ə\ [DESMO- + *-pex(y)* + -IA] A uterine suspension operation in which the proximal round ligaments are attached to the anterior abdominal wall.

**desmoplasia** \-plā′zhə\ [DESMO- + -PLASIA] The formation of fibrous tissue: usually applied to carcinomas that incite a fibrogenic reaction in the surrounding stroma.

**desmoplastic** \-plas′tik\ Characterized by the development of fibrous tissue, adhesions, or scars.

**desmorrhexis** \-rek′sis\ [DESMO- + -RRHEXIS] A ligamentous rupture.

**desmosine** An amino acid with four amino and four carboxyl groups. It is formed in the protein elastin from four lysine residues with their side chains joined by oxidative cross-linking to form a substituted pyridine ring, so that it holds four polypeptide chains in a radial array. Elastin, unlike many other fibrous proteins, can thus undergo two-way stretch.

**desmosome** \des′mōsōm\ [DESMO- + Gk *sōma* body] A specialized contact site between adjacent cells seen particularly in epithelial tissues. Electron microscopy shows that there is a condensation of cytoplasmic filaments on either side, a widening of the intercellular gap, and some filamentous material within the gap. In light microscopy this site has been characterized as cross-bridges, intercellular bridges, or prickles. Also *macula adherens.*

**desmotomy** \desmät′əmē\ [DESMO- + -TOMY] The surgical division of a ligament.

**desoximetasone** $C_{22}H_{29}FO_4$. 9-Fluoro-11β,21-dihydroxy-16α-methylpregna-1,4-diene-3,20-dione, a corticosteroidal agent with anti-inflammatory and antipruritic activity. It is used topically for dermatologic conditions that respond to steroid therapy.

**desoxy-** \desäk′sē-\ *Outmoded* DEOXY-.

**desoxycorticosterone acetate** DEOXYCORTICOSTERONE ACETATE.

**Desoxyn** A proprietary name for methamphetamine hydrochloride.

**desoxyribonucleic acid** DEOXYRIBONUCLEIC ACID.
**desoxyribose nucleic acid** DEOXYRIBONUCLEIC ACID.
**desquamate** \des′kwəmāt\ [L *desquamare* (from *de-* off + *squama* fish scale) to scale or peel off] To shed or peel off in scales.
**desquamation** \des′kwəmā′shən\ [See DESQUAMATE.] The shedding of the outer layer, as of scales. Also *exfoliation*. **lamellar d. of the newborn** The desquamation in the newborn of the collodionlike scales that are characteristic of lamellar ichthyosis.
**desquamative** \des′kwəmā′tiv, deskwam′ətiv\ Inducing or resulting from desquamation. Also *exfoliative*.
**dessertspoon** A unit of capacity representing 10 milliliters. *Popular*. Symbol: dsp
**dest.** 1 *destilla* (L, distil). 2 *destillatus* (L, distilled).
**destil.** *destilla* (L, distil).
**2-desvinyl-2-formyl chlorophyll a** CHLOROPHYLL D.
**desynapsis** \dē′sinap′sis\ [DE- + SYNAPSIS] The premature separation of homologues during diplotene or diakinesis of the first meiotic division. It results in reduced chiasmata and, potentially, abnormal segregation and aneuploidy. Also *asynapsis*.
**desynchronization** \dēsing′krənīzā′shən\ 1 A phenomenon, usually resulting from disease, in which the electroencephalographically recorded wave forms from the two hemispheres do not occur in a synchronous manner. Normally the electrical activity of the brain is of roughly comparable amplitude and frequency over the two hemispheres and the wave forms recorded occur synchronously on opposite sides. 2 An electroencephalographic pattern of low amplitude and high frequency usually identified with periods of alertness during wakefulness or with REM periods during sleep; an activated electroencephalogram.
**det.** *detur* (L, let it be given).
**detachment** 1 A separation of anatomic parts or structures, as of a layer of the eye. 2 Separation of affect from the idea to which it was originally attached as a way of denying or defending against the idea. 3 Withdrawal from a situation, in the infant often manifested in drowsiness and sleep as a reaction to anxiety. **epiphyseal d.** SLIPPED EPIPHYSIS. **exudative retinal d.** Retinal detachment due to accumulation of fluid (probably a transudate) between the pigment epithelium and the neuroepithelium of the retina, secondary to severe hypertension, usually due to chronic renal failure. **retinal d.** The separation of the rods and cones from the pigment epithelium of the retina, leading to blindness unless repaired by emergency surgery. The condition is characterized by progressive loss of visual field over a variable period, usually days or weeks, often preceded by a sudden shower of hundreds of sootlike floating particles in the field of vision, a sensation caused by intravitreal hemorrhage from a tear of the retina. Also *amotio retinae, ablatio retinae, sublatio retinae*. **rhegmatogenous retinal d.** A retinal detachment resulting from a hole or tear in the retina, through which fluid vitreous humor can enter the subretinal space.
**detector** Any instrument used to note, and usually to quantify, the presence of a material under analysis. Chemical or physical signals may be recorded, such as changes in wave transmission, in gas pressure, in number of particles present, in pH, or in substrate concentration. **activation d.** ACTIVATION FOIL. **alpha wave d.** A circuit that uses a selective filter to detect the 8 to 13-Hz alpha waves from the electroencephalogram for use in biofeedback. **Doppler fetal heart d.** A device that transmits ultrasound through the abdominal wall to the fetal heart. Reflected ultrasound has a Doppler frequency shift that is proportional to heart motion. An acoustic output indicates heart rate. **flame ionization d.** A device that analyzes a gas or vapor by measuring the change in conductivity produced by the gas or vapor in a standard flame, usually hydrogen. **lie d.** *Popular* POLYGRAPH. **nonparalyzable d.** A radiation detector in which a pulse that impinges while the detection system is responding to a previous pulse is not counted but does not restart the recovery process. If every pulse restarted the recovery process, the detector might be paralyzed, since the detector is disabled during the recovery process. This system improves resolving time. **photocell d.** A photosensitive device that responds to changes in incident radiation by changing its current-voltage characteristics. **radiation d.** Any device designed for the detection of ionizing radiation. **scintillation d.** A radiation detector using a scintillating material that generates a minute flash of light each time an incident photon or particle imparts energy to it. Many kinds of crystals do this, sodium iodide being favored in medical work. There are also liquid and plastic scintillators. The detector commonly includes shielding, including collimation if required, and a photomultiplier tube that responds to the flash of light and generates an electrical pulse for each scintillation. This tube may be so designed that the pulse height indicates the energy deposited in the scintillator, thus making pulse-height spectrometry possible. **self-quenching d.** A gas-filled detector that can be operated in the Geiger-Müller region without requiring external electronic help to arrest each ion avalanche. During manufacture a small percentage of a suitable organic vapor or a halogen gas is introduced, with the result that each avalanche is stopped as soon as the output pulse is delivered. **smoke d.** A device, usually electronic, that activates a warning buzzer when exposed to the particulate matter in smoke. These inexpensive devices, when properly installed in homes and other buildings, can dramatically decrease burns and deaths from fires by providing an early warning. **sterility d.** Any of several devices used to demonstrate the efficiency of autoclaving. Common indicators are temperature-sensitive papers or liquids, or an aliquot of viable spores whose subsequent growth is prevented by exposure to a temperature of the desired level. **thermoluminescent d.** A dosimeter consisting of a crystalline structure of various configurations that can be inserted into a body or other material before irradiation. After the exposure the dosimeter is removed and heated, and its luminescence is a measure of the absorbed radiation. **threshold d.** An element or nuclide which will not be made radioactive by neutron capture until the neutron energy exceeds a threshold value characteristic of that element or nuclide.
**detergent** \ditur′jənt\ [L *detergens*, gen. *detergentis* (pres. part. of *detergere* to wipe off, cleanse, from *tergere* to rub, wipe) cleaning, wiping off] An amphipathic molecule such as a long-chain hydrocarbon, terminated at one end by a polar group, often charged. The charged polar group is highly soluble in water whereas the hydrocarbon does not readily enter the aqueous environment. Detergents allow fats to be suspended in water and thus act as cleaning agents. Also *wetting agent*. **anionic d.** A detergent whose molecule carries a negative charge, e.g. dodecyl sulfate, $CH_3—[CH_2]_{11}—O—SO_3^-$. **cationic d.** A detergent in which the polar part of the molecule carries a positive charge. An example is hexadecyltrimethylammonium as one of its salts.
**deterioration** \ditir′ē·ôrā′shən\ [noun from L *deteriorare* (from L *deterior* inferior) to worsen] 1 The process of becoming worse. 2 In psychiatry, progressive impairment in

mental functioning without the implication of irreversibility. **d. of affect** EMOTIONAL DETERIORATION. **emotional d.** Inability to maintain constant or appropriate affective contact with the environment, with resultant emotional blunting, apathy, and indifference to people and surroundings. Also *deterioration of affect.* **schizophrenic d.** Impairment of intellectual, affective, or social functioning as a result of schizophrenia. The term was once used to refer to a persisting core of symptoms that prevented return to fully normal status in every schizophrenic. Others have used the term for the disabilities of the chronic, intractable schizophrenic who does not respond to treatment. **simple senile d.** Senile dementia that is not complicated by delirium, delusions, or depression.

**determinant** \ditur′minənt\ [L *determinans,* gen. *determinantis,* pres. part. of *determinare* to limit, determine] Something that determines the nature or outcome of an occurrence; a determining factor. **antigenic d.** The small portion of an antigen that combines with a specific antibody. A single antigen molecule may carry several different antigenic determinants. Also *determinant, marker, epitope.* **germ-cell d.** A cytoplasmic body in the ovum which passes into the oocyte during gametogenesis. Also *oosome.* **hidden d.** INACCESSIBLE DETERMINANT. **inaccessible d.** An antigenic determinant on a complex antigen that is not accessible to antibody unless the molecule is unfolded or a covering group or molecule is removed. Also *hidden determinant, cryptodeterminant.* **resistance d.** The portion of a resistance plasmid that carries the resistance genes.

**determination** A conclusion or decision, especially one reached after deliberation, as of the nature of a disease or of the cause of death. **embryonic d.** The stage at which an embryonic tissue loses its ability to develop in several directions; it is, in a tissue sense, equivalent to differentiation in a cell. How the fate of a developing tissue is irrevocably fixed or determined is one of the fundamental problems of embryology. It implies the reception of instructions in chemical form (evocator) by regions having the potency to respond in an undeviating manner. **prior d.** The requirement imposed by a third party, usually an insurer, that a provider must justify the need for a particular service for a patient before actually providing care, except that payment may be made when prior authorization is not sought provided that it would have been approved as needed.

**determinism** \ditur′mənizm\ The philosophic doctrine that all natural phenomena, including human behavior, are the necessary consequences of antecedent causes.

**det. in dup.** *detur in duplo* (L, let twice as much be given). It is used in prescription writing.

**de Toni** [Giovanni *de Toni,* Italian pediatrician, born 1895] De Toni-Fanconi syndrome, de Toni-Debré-Fanconi syndrome, Debré-de Toni-Fanconi syndrome. See under FANCONI SYNDROME.

**detoxicate** \dētäk′sikāt\ DETOXIFY.

**detoxification** \dētäk′sifikā′shən\ **1** The inactivation of the toxic properties of substances in the body by enzymatic action, or by the administration of antidotes, producing less toxic or more easily excreted compounds. **2** The recovery, or the process of bringing about the recovery, of a patient from a state of dependence on alcohol or other drug. For defs. 1 and 2 also *detoxication, disintoxication.* **metabolic d.** A process by which the body converts toxic substances into biologically inactive materials.

**detoxify** \dētäk′səfī\ **1** To inactivate (a poison); to reduce or neutralize the toxic properties of (a substance). **2** To remove a toxic substance from (the body, an organ, or a system). **3** To effect the recovery of (a patient) from a state of dependence on alcohol or other drug. For defs. 1, 2, and 3 also *detoxicate.*

**detritus** \ditrī′təs\ [L, past part. of *deterere* to consume by wearing, wear out] Any residue of organic material, as that remaining after spontaneous sloughing or débridement; organic debris.

**detrusor** \ditroo′sər\ [New L (from L *detrus(us),* past part. of *detrudere* to thrust down by force + *-or* -OR)] A muscle whose contraction results in a pushing down or out. **d. urinae** MUSCULUS DETRUSOR VESICAE. **d. vesicae** MUSCULUS DETRUSOR VESICAE.

**d. et s.** *detur et signetur* (L, let it be given and labeled). It is used in prescription writing.

**detubation** \dē′tʸoobā′shən\ DECANNULATION.

**detuberculization** \dē′tʸUbur′kyəlīzā′shən\ The process of removing all tuberculous infections from persons or from a community.

**detumescence** \dē′tʸəmes′əns\ The subsidence of swelling or tumescence.

**deut-** \doot-\ DEUTERO-.

**deutan** \dʸoo′tan\ [*deut(er)* + *an,* from *an(omaly)* or *an(opia)*] A person suffering from green blindness, either deuteranomaly or deuteranopia.

**deuter-** \doo′tər-\ DEUTERO-.

**deuteranomaly** \dʸoo′tərənäm′əlē\ [DEUTER- + ANOMALY] A partial form of deuteranopia, in which the individual has a reduced ability to perceive green. Adj. deuteranomalous.

**deuteranope** \dʸoo′tərənōp′\ A person with deuteranopia.

**deuteranopia** \dʸoo′tərənō′pē·ə\ [DEUTER- + ANOPIA] A form of red-green color blindness in which the eye is insensitive to green color. Also *deuteranopsia.* Adj. deuteranopic.

**deuterate** To combine with or treat with deuterium. Also *deuterize.*

**deuteration** The insertion of deuterium into a molecule.

**deuterion** \dʸootir′ē·än\ DEUTERON.

**deuteripara** \dʸoo′tərip′ərə\ [DEUTER- + *i* + -PARA] SECUNDIPARA.

**deuterium** \dʸootir′ē·əm\ An isotope of hydrogen, mass number 2. Also *heavy hydrogen, deuterohydrogen, hydrogen 2.* Symbol: D, $^{2}H$

**deuterium oxide** $^{2}H_2O$. Water in which the hydrogen component consists of deuterium. Also *heavy water.*

**deuterize** DEUTERATE.

**deutero-** \doo′tərō-\ [Gk *deuteros* (adjective) second] A combining form meaning second, secondary. Also *deuto-, deut-, deuter-.*

**deuterohemophilia** \-hē′məfil′yə\ *Outmoded* HEMOPHILIA B.

**deuterohydrogen** \-hī′drəjən\ DEUTERIUM.

**Deuteromycetes** \-mīsē′tēz\ [DEUTERO- + -MYCETES] The form-class of fungi which have no demonstrable sexual stage of reproduction; the imperfect fungi. Many members of this group are causal agents of animal and plant diseases. Also *Fungi Imperfecti.*

**deuteron** \dʸoo′tərän\ The nucleus of deuterium, containing one proton and one neutron. Also *deuterion.*

**deuteropathy** \dʸoo′tərāp′əthē\ A disease secondary to another.

**deuteroplasm** \dʸoo′tərōplazm\ DEUTOPLASM.

**deuto-** \dʸoo′tō-\ DEUTERO-.

**deutoplasm** \dʸoo′təplazm\ [DEUTO- + -PLASM] The nutrient and other nonliving material in the cytoplasm of an ovum. Also *deuteroplasm.* See also VITELLUS.

**deutoplasmolysis** \-plazmäl′isis\ [DEUTOPLASM + *o* + LYSIS] Dissolution, destruction, and disintegration of deutoplasm for the nutrition of the developing ovum.

**devasation** \dē′vasā′shən\ DEVASCULARIZATION. **senile cortical d.** The diminution or loss of blood supply to the cerebral cortex in the aged as a result of atherosclerosis.

**devascularization** \dēvas′kyəler′īzā′shən\ Obstruction or obliteration of the blood vessels supplying an organ or tissue, resulting in loss of its blood supply. Also *devasation.*

**development** The processes by which a cell, an anatomic element, an organ, or a living individual increases in weight and volume at the same time as its form undergoes characteristic changes, as *embryonic development, larval development.* If there is an increase in volume only it is usually described as growth. **abnormal d.** Development of a cell, tissue, or entire embryo in a fashion which is contrary to the usually recognized form. Depending on the extent of the anomaly so produced, this may not be compatible with viability of the individual, or may result in a reduced life expectancy. • Current usage includes abnormality of function as well as of structure. **mosaic d.** Formation of an embryo in which discrete regions develop independently in a fixed and unalterable way as portions of a mosaic whole. Compare REGULATIVE DEVELOPMENT. **postnatal d.** MATURATION-DEVELOPMENT. **prenatal d.** Biologic maturation during fetal life, in the process of which structures, organs, and physiologic systems reach functional maturity by the time of birth, with the exception of the central nervous system, the reproductive organs, and the liver in a few respects. Psychological development, apparently dormant in prenatal life, must be proceeding because the fetus receives sensory impressions constantly. **psychomotor d.** The control of movement progressively achieved by infants and children in response to their psychologic needs and awareness of their surroundings. Precocious development, as measured by tests, does not predict intelligence with certainity. See also PSYCHOMOTOR RETARDATION. **psychosexual d.** Development of the different stages involving the maturation of the psyche. In psychoanalytic psychology, the stages of development reflect the development of object relationships (genital-psychical development), the vicissitudes of the libidinal and aggressive drives in relation to reality (libidinal development), and the development of mechanisms to accomplish the foregoing. **regulative d.** Embryonic development in which the growth of organs and tissues is determined through the action of inductors produced by surrounding parts. Compare MOSAIC DEVELOPMENT.

**developmental** \divel′əpmen′təl\ Of or relating to the period of time between conception and maturity at puberty or adulthood.

**Deventer** [Hendrik van *Deventer,* Dutch obstetrician, 1651–1724] See under PELVIS.

**Devergie** [Marie Guillaume Alphonse *Devergie,* French dermatologist, 1798–1879] **1** PUITS DE DEVERGIE. See under PUITS DE DEVERGIE. **2** See under ATTITUDE.

**deviance** \dē′vē·əns\ [See DEVIANT.] The state of differing significantly from a norm, as in behavior.

**deviant** \dē′vē·ənt\ [Late L *devians,* gen. *deviantis,* pres. part. of *deviare* to be erratic, stray. See DEVIATION.] **1** Diverging from the norm; abnormal. **2** An individual whose behavior differs from what is considered normal for that particular society.

**deviation** \dē′vē·ā′shən\ [Med L *deviatio* (from Late L *deviare* to stray, be deviant, from *devius* wandering, erratic, from *de-* off, away + *via* a way, road) divergence from a path or norm] **1** A turning aside or variation from a course or from a norm. **2** An instance of such an action or condition, as an abnormality or variation. **animal d.** The attracting of mosquitoes from human beings by proximity of animals serving as an alternate blood source. **axis d.** Deviation of the mean frontal axis of the QRS complex to the left or to the right of normal. **complement d.** The inhibition of complement-mediated hemolysis resulting from a condition of antibody excess. Also *Neisser-Wechsberg phenomenon.* **conjugate d. of the eyes** Parallel and usually symmetrical deviation of both eyes, usually to one side, much less often upwards or downwards. In a comatose patient this sign usually implies a massive destructive lesion, usually vascular, of the ipsilateral frontal lobe (the frontal eye-field), but an irritative lesion may, by contrast, cause deviation of the eyes, and often also of the head, to the contralateral side (an adversive attack). Also *ocular conjugate deviation.* **latent d.** A strabismic deviation usually masked by binocular fusion, but demonstrable when binocularity is blocked, as by occlusion of one eye. **manifest d.** A strabismic deviation spontaneously present under the usual conditions of binocular usage. Also *loxophthalmus.* **ocular conjugate d.** CONJUGATE DEVIATION OF THE EYES. **primary d.** The amount of strabismic deviation present when the individual is observing an object with the eye that is usually preferred in normal use. **secondary d.** The amount of strabismic deviation present when the individual is observing an object with the eye that is not usually preferred in normal use. **skew d.** Deviation of one eyeball downwards and inwards when compared with the other, which looks upwards and outwards. This sign is a rare manifestation of pontine lesions. Also *Hertwig-Magendie phenomenon, Hertwig-Magendie sign, Magendie sign, Magendie-Hertwig sign, seesaw strabismus, Magendie symptom, Hertwig-Magendie syndrome.* **squint d.** STRABISMIC DEVIATION. **standard d.** The square root of the variance. It is the measure of dispersion most often used in statistics. Abbr. SD **strabismic d.** The angular misalignment of the visual axes occurring in an individual with strabismus. Also *squint deviation.* **Vulpian's conjugate d.** ADVERSIVE ATTACK.

**Devic** [M. Eugene *Devic,* French physician, died 1930] Devic's disease. See under NEUROMYELITIS OPTICA.

**device** / **central-bearing d.** A tracing device that provides a central bearing point between upper and lower occlusal rims, contacting a plate attached to one of the rims. **contraceptive d.** A mechanical means of preventing conception, as a condom, diaphragm, or intrauterine device. **intrauterine d.** A plastic or metallic device worn in the uterus to prevent conception. Intrauterine devices are variously shaped but all approximate the size of the nonpregnant endometrial cavity, in which they are implanted and from which they can be removed, usually by a physician, when pregnancy is desired or because of complications, such as bleeding, that may occur. **medical d.** Any item or piece of equipment used in health care, excluding drugs. Specific legal definitions may specify which items are subject to governmental regulation as medical devices. **static imaging d.** GAMMA CAMERA.

**devitalize** \dēvī′təlīz\ To deprive of life or vitality, as by removing the pulp from a tooth.

**devolution** \dev′əloo′shən\ [Late L *devolutio* (from L *devolvere* to roll or fall down) corruption] **1** Systematic changes in phenotype toward less complexity, more simplistic development, or, perhaps, less selective advantage. Compare EVOLUTION. **2** *Seldom used* CATABOLISM.

**devolutive** \dev′əloo′tiv\ **1** Characterized by devolution. **2** Pertaining to or characterized by mental or neurologic impairment that specifically involves traits or functions of a most highly developed and complex nature, particularly those most recently acquired through evolution.

**Dewar** [James *Dewar,* Scottish chemist, 1842–1923] Dewar flask. See under VACUUM FLASK.

**dexamethasone** \dek'səmeth'əsōn\ $C_{22}H_{29}FO_5$. 9α-Fluoro-11β,17α,21-trihydroxy-16α-methyl-pregn-1,4-diene-3,20-dione. A synthetic analogue of the adrenocortical steroid, cortisol. It is used in the treatment of inflammatory, allergic, and neoplastic diseases.

**dexamethasone acetate** The acetate ester of dexamethasone. It is used for sustained activity by injection into lesions or soft tissues.

**dexamethasone sodium phosphate** $C_{22}H_{28}FNa_2O_8P$. The sodium phosphate ester analogue of dexamethasone. It is given intravenously, intramuscularly, or intra-articularly, or is topically applied, and it has the same properties as the parent compound.

**dexchlorpheniramine maleate** $C_{16}H_{19}ClN_2 \cdot C_4H_4O_4$. *d*-2-[*p*-Chloro-α-(2-dimethylaminoethyl)benzyl]pyridine maleate. The maleate salt of the dextrorotatory isomer of chlorpheniramine. Its use as an antihistaminic agent is identical to that of chlorpheniramine.

**Dexedrine** A proprietary name for dexamphetamine sulfate.

**dexter** \dek'stər\ [L, right, on the right side] Denoting the right side of a part, organ, structure, or the body.

**dextr-** \dekstr-\ DEXTRO-.

**dextrad** \deks'trad\ [DEXTR- + -AD] Toward the right side.

**dextral** \deks'trəl\ **1** Situated on the right side. **2** Right-handed.

**dextran** A polymer of glucose formed by bacteria from sucrose, usually α1,6-linked.

**dextran sulfate** The sulfuric acid ester of dextran. It is a charged polymer having anticoagulant and cholesterol-lowering properties. It has been found *in vitro* to inhibit the binding of human immunodeficiency virus to T lymphocytes and to inhibit viral replication. Its use clinically for HIV infection has not yet been established. It is administered intravenously and orally.

**dextriferron** A sterile complex of ferric hydroxide with partly hydrolyzed dextrin in water that contains about 20 mg of iron per ml. The solution can be injected slowly to provide iron when oral administration is not possible or practical.

**dextrin** The product of partial hydrolysis of starch or glycogen, consisting of a mixture of oligosaccharides and polysaccharides of glucose residues. **limit d.** A core produced from a natural, branched polysaccharide, usually glycogen or amylopectin, by exhaustive treatment with a degradative enzyme, such as exoamylase or phosphorylase, that removes units from nonreducing ends but cannot pass branch points. All exterior chains are therefore truncated, but none is removed. It therefore represents the limit of action of such enzymes.

**dextro-** \dek'strō-\ [L *dexter* (feminine *dextra*) right, on the right] **1** A combining form meaning right, to or on the right. **2** In stereochemistry, a combining form designating the dextrorotatory enantiomer of a substance. Compare LEVO-. Symbol: (+)

**dextrocardia** \-kär'dē·ə\ [DEXTRO- + -CARDIA] A malposition of the heart to the right rather than the left of the mediastinum. In most cases, the heart is simply displaced to the right of the midline and may be associated with situs inversus of other thoracic or abdominal viscera. **isolated d.** An abnormal position of the heart such that the cardiac mass is primarily within the right hemithorax but the atrial chambers are arranged in the usual way and the remaining thoracic organs are in their expected positions. Some authorities also insist that the apex points to the right, whereas others would make the definition irrespective of apex orientation. See also DEXTROVERSION OF THE HEART. **mirror-image d.** Dextrocardia occurring in situs inversus, in which a right-sided heart is the usual case. **secondary d.** The situation in which a normally structured heart occupies the right side of the chest as the consequence of extracardiac disease.

**dextrocerebral** \-ser'əbrəl\ Involving the right cerebral hemisphere.

**dextrocular** \deksträk'yələr\ [DEXTR- + OCULAR] Having the right eye dominant.

**dextroduction** \-duk'shən\ [DEXTRO- + DUCTION] A monocular movement to the right side.

**dextrogastria** \-gas'trē·ə\ [DEXTRO- + GASTR- + -IA] An anomaly in which the stomach is located in the right of the abdomen, usually associated with dextrocardia.

**dextrogyration** \-jīrā'shən\ DEXTROTORSION.

**dextromethorphan hydrobromide** $C_{18}H_{26}BrNO$. The dextrorotatory isomer of methorphan as the hydrobromide salt. It is used in syrups and tablets as an antitussive agent.

**dextroposition** \-pəzish'ən\ The condition in which a structure or organ, as the heart, normally found on the left side of the body is displaced to the right side. It is often indicative but not pathognomonic of situs inversus.

**dextrorotatory** \-rō'tətôr'ē\ Capable of rotating the plane of polarized light clockwise, when viewed toward the light source. Compare LEVOROTATORY. Symbol: *d*-, (+)

**dextrose** [DEXTR- + -OSE[2]] *Outmoded* GLUCOSE. • This name was originally given because, in contrast with fructose, it is dextrorotatory.

**dextrose monohydrate** $C_6H_{12}O_6 \cdot H_2O$. D-Glucose monohydrate; pure glucose. Also *medicinal glucose.*

**Dextrostix** A reagent paper strip impregnated with glucose oxidase, peroxidase, and a chromogen that is used to measure glucose concentrations in body fluids. Color change, proportional to glucose concentration, can be estimated visually by comparison with colored standards or with a reflectance meter. A proprietary name.

**dextrotorsion** \-tôr'shən\ [DEXTRO- + TORSION] A cyclodeviation in which the rotation of the eye is such as to turn the top of the eye to the right side of the individual. Also *dextrogyration.*

**dextroversion** \-vur'zhən\ [DEXTRO- + VERSION] **1** A turning or rotation to the right: used especially of the eyes. **2** An abnormal rotation or orientation to the right. **d. of the heart** An abnormal position of the heart such that the cardiac mass is mostly in the right chest and the apex points to the right, but with the usual arrangement of the atrial chambers and the other thoracic viscera. See also DEXTROCARDIA.

**DFDT** $C_{14}H_9Cl_3F_2$. Difluorodiphenyltricholoroethane, an insecticidal compound.

**DFP** diisopropyl fluorophosphate.

**DHL** diffuse histiocytic lymphoma.

**DI** diabetes insipidus.

**di-**[1] \di-, dī-\ DIS-[1].

**di-**[2] \dī-, di-\ [Gk *dis* (akin to Gk *dyo* two) twice, double] **1** A prefix meaning twice, double. **2** In organic chemistry, a prefix indicating doubling, or twice the usual amount, of a radical. Also *dis-*[2].

**di-**[3] \dī-, di-\ DIA-.

**dia-** \dī'ə-\ [Gk *dia* (as prefix *di-* before vowels) through]

A prefix meaning (1) through, between, across, apart; (2) completely. Also *di-*[3].

**diabetes** \dī′əbē′tēz\ [Gk *diabētēs* (from *diabainein* to pass through, from DIA- + *bainein* to step, walk, go) siphon, diabetes] Any of several conditions characterized by excessive output of urine (polyuria), as diabetes mellitus and diabetes insipidus. Adj. diabetic. • *Diabetes* is often used as a short form for diabetes mellitus. **adult-onset d.** MATURITY-ONSET DIABETES. **alloxan d.** Diabetes mellitus induced experimentally in animals by administration of alloxan which selectively destroys the beta cells of the islets of Langerhans. **asymptomatic d.** Measurable hyperglycemia and glucose intolerance without sufficient glycosuria to cause excessive excretion of urine (polyuria). **brittle d.** Diabetes mellitus in which the hyperglycemia is difficult to control. It is marked by abrupt and inexplicable swings between ketoacidosis and hypoglycemia. **bronze d.** Bronze pigmentation of the skin, diabetes mellitus, and bone and joint abnormalities as common manifestations of hemochromatosis. **chemical d.** LATENT DIABETES. **class A d.** Diabetes that is evident during pregnancy only and is revealed only by an abnormal glucose tolerance test. Also *gestational diabetes, pregnancy diabetes.* **congenital lipoatrophic d.** SEIP SYNDROME. **gestational d.** CLASS A DIABETES. **glucophosphatemic d.** An incomplete form of the de Toni-Fanconi syndrome, characterized by association of renal glycosuria and osteoporosis with bone pain and fractures, decreased serum in organic phosphorus, and increased serum alkaline phosphatose. It results from defective reabsorption of glucose and phosphorus by renal tube cells. Also *osteoporosis with renal diabetes.* **d. insipidus** A disease characterized by the output of large amounts of dilute urine (hyposthenuria), unquenchable thirst, and the incessant drinking of water (polydipsia). It occurs as a result of deficient secretion of vasopressin by the neurohypophysial unit. Its causes are idiopathic, or due to granuloma, tumor, or basilar skull fracture. It is sometimes difficult to distinguish from psychogenic polydipsia. Abbr. DI **insulin-dependent d. mellitus** Severe diabetes mellitus with onset usually in childhood or adolescence, associated with little or no endogenous insulin production, a genetic factor, and probably, abnormal immune mechanisms. Also *type-1 diabetes.* Compare NON-INSULIN-DEPENDENT DIABETES MELLITUS. Abbr. IDDM • This term has been recommended as applying to juvenile diabetes and brittle diabetes **juvenile d.** Diabetes mellitus affecting infants, children, and adolescents, persisting into adult life. It is thought to be a disease distinct from maturity-onset diabetes, having peculiar genetic characteristics and a strong familial tendency. It is characterized by severe insulinopenia and a strong propensity to the early development of microvascular and macrovascular degenerative complications. **latent d.** Asymptomatic diabetes mellitus which can sometimes be diagnosed by fasting hyperglycemia and always by postprandial hyperglycemia and a diabetic glucose tolerance curve. Also *chemical diabetes, masked diabetes, subclinical diabetes, pseudodiabetes.* Compare OVERT DIABETES. **lipoatrophic d.** A disease of children characterized by atrophy of subcutaneous and body fat, hyperlipemia, hepatomegaly, and insulin-resistant diabetes mellitus with much reduced binding of insulin to insulin receptors. It is invariably fatal. It has been postulated as a disorder of hypophysiotropic hormones owing to defective hypothalamic dopamine-$\beta$-hydroxylase. **masked d.** *Outmoded* LATENT DIABETES. **maturity-onset d.** Diabetes mellitus with onset after age 40 in overweight people. It is often asymptomatic, and compared to juvenile diabetes is characterized by a lesser degree of insulinopenia and less likelihood of ketoacidosis. It is often controllable with diet alone or with oral hypoglycemic agents, but can result in the development of microvascular and macrovascular complications. Also *obesity-associated diabetes, adult-onset diabetes.* **d. mellitus** A common disease of glucose homeostasis owing to actual or functional insulinopenia, characterized classically by polydipsia, polyuria, wasting, and death from ketoacidosis. The central defect, not yet understood, is related to inability of cells to take up and oxidize glucose, with ensuing hyperglycemia, glycosuria, polyuria, disordered catabolism of fats with ketosis, dehydration, and a shortened lifespan resulting chiefly from microvascular and macrovascular complications. Diabetes mellitus is a familial disease but its mode of inheritance is unknown. **metahypophysial d.** YOUNG'S DIABETES. **nephrogenic d. insipidus** A condition characterized by marked polyuria and polydipsia, due to congenital or acquired lesions of the renal collecting tubules, sometimes from reaction to lithium and demeclocycline which renders them insensitive to vasopressin. The urine is hypotonic. Also *water-losing nephritis, renal diabetes insipidus, vasopressin-resistant diabetes insipidus.* **neurogenic d.** Diabetes mellitus resulting from lesions in or disorders of the brain, usually involving the floor of the fourth ventricle or the hypothalamus. **non-insulin-dependent d. mellitus** Diabetes mellitus of adult onset, usually after age 40, associated with somewhat reduced, normal, or above-normal insulin production, a degree of genetic predisposition, and most often with exogenous obesity. Compare INSULIN-DEPENDENT DIABETES MELLITUS. Abbr. NIDDM • This term has been recommended as applying to maturity-onset diabetes. **obesity-associated d.** MATURITY-ONSET DIABETES. **overt d.** Diabetes mellitus with symptoms, as polyuria and polydipsia. Compare LATENT DIABETES. **pancreatic d.** Diabetes mellitus due to loss of pancreatic tissue, for example from chronic pancreatitis with atrophy or fibrosis, carcinoma of the pancreas, or pancreatectomy. **phlorhizin d.** Experimental diabetes mellitus produced by administration of the plant glucoside, phlorhizin. It poisons the renal tubule, glucose is not reabsorbed, gluconeogenesis increases, glycogen stores are depleted, fatty acid oxidation rises, and ketosis ensues. The syndrome produced is more akin to starvation and dehydration than to true diabetes mellitus. **phosphate d.** *Obs.* X-LINKED HYPOPHOSPHATEMIA. **piqûre d.** PUNCTURE DIABETES. **pregnancy d.** CLASS A DIABETES. **puncture d.** Glucosuria that results in experimental animals following a puncture wound to the brainstem made through the floor of the fourth ventricle. The mechanism of this phenomenon is unknown. Also *piqûre diabetes.* **renal d.** A benign hereditary condition, transmitted as a mendelian dominant, characterized by glycosuria without hyperglycemia, due to impaired reabsorption of glucose by the proximal renal tubules. In type A the maximum ability of the tubules to reabsorb glucose is reduced. In type B the maximum ability of the tubules to reabsorb glucose is normal overall, but is reduced in some nephrons. **renal amino acid d.** FANCONI SYNDROME. **renal d. insipidus** NEPHROGENIC DIABETES INSIPIDUS. **secondary d.** Diabetes mellitus owing to some definable cause, as pancreatic disease, hemochromatosis with pancreatic destruction, acromegaly, or Cushing syndrome. **starvation d.** Glucose intolerance associated with prolonged starvation. Administration of a glucose load is followed by hyperglycemia and glucosuria due to impaired pancreatic secretion of insulin and a reduced capacity of the liver to form glycogen. **steroid d.** Glucose intolerance induced by excessive doses of adrenal corticosteroids or in association with endogenous hypercortisolism (Cushing syndrome). It is characterized by a moderate requirement for insulin, resistance to ketoacidosis, and a relatively low rate of microvascular and macrovascular complication. **subclinical d.** LATENT DIABETES. **thiazide d.** Glucose intolerance produced by the administration of derivatives of benzene disulfonamide, such as hydrochlorothiazide. The mechanism is not established but may be related to diuretic-induced hypokalemia. **type-1 d.** INSULIN-DEPENDENT DIABETES MELLITUS. **vasopressin-resistant d. insipidus** NEPHROGENIC DIABETES INSIPIDUS. **Young's d.** Glucose intolerance induced experimentally in animals by protracted administration of pituitary extract specifically growth hormone. Also *metahypophysial diabetes.*

**diabetic** \dī′əbet′ik\ [*diabet(es)* + -IC] **1** Of, relating to, or affected by diabetes, especially diabetes mellitus. **2** One affected by diabetes, especially diabetes mellitus.

**diabetogenic** \dī′əbē′tōjen′ik\ [*diabet(es)* + *o* + -GENIC] Causing diabetes. Also *diabetogenetic.*

**diacetyl-*N*-allylnormorphine** DIACETYNALORPHINE.

**diacetyldapsone** ACEDAPSONE.

**diacetylmorphine** HEROIN.

**diacetyltannic acid** ACETANNIN.

**diacetynalorphine** A structural and functional analogue of nalorphine, with greater potency. It is used primarily in the treatment of morphine poisoning and addiction. Also *diacetyl-N-allylnormorphine.*

**diachoresis** \dī′əkôrē′sis\ DEFECATION.

**diaclasis** \dī·ak′ləsis\ OSTEOCLASIS.

**diaclast** \dī′əklast\ [DIA- + -CLAST] An instrument used to perforate the fetal skull for a craniectomy.

**diacrinous** \dī·ak′rinəs\ [DIA- + Gk *krin(ein)* to separate + -OUS] Of or relating to secretion of a glandular product as a homogeneous fluid rather than in the form of globules or granules. Compare PTYOCRINOUS.

**diacrisis** \dī·ak′risis\ [Gk *diakrisis* (from *diakrinein* to distinguish, discriminate, from DIA- + *krinein* to separate, choose) determination, decision] DIAGNOSIS.

**diacritic** \dī′əkrit′ik\ DIAGNOSTIC.

**diacylglycerol** Glycerol acylated on two of its hydroxyl groups, usually 1,2. Diacylglycerols are intermediates in the biosynthesis of fats (triacylglycerols) and of phospholipids. Also *diglyceride.*

**diadermic** \dī′ədur′mik\ PERCUTANEOUS.

**diadochocinesia** \dī·ad′əkōsīnē′zhə \ DIADOCHOKINESIA.

**diadochokinesia** \dī·ad′əkōkīnē′zhə \ [Gk *diadoch(ē)* succession, relay, taking turns + *kinēs(is)* movement + -IA] The ability to perform rapid, repetitive, coordinated movements such as repeated supination and pronation of a hand and forearm; the rapid performance of opposite motor behaviors. Also *diadochocinesia, diadochokinesis.* Adj. diadochokinetic, diadochocinetic.

**diagnose** \dī′agnōs\ [back-formation from DIAGNOSIS] To determine the nature or identity of (a disease), as by an analysis of signs and symptoms.

**diagnosis** \dī′əgnō′sis\ [Gk *diagnōsis* (from *diagignōskein* to distinguish, discriminate, diagnose, from *dia-* apart, between + root of *gnōsis* knowledge, recognition) discernment, means of distinguishing or resolving, diagnosis] (*pl.* diagnoses) **1** A determination of the nature or identity of a disease, typically based on an analysis of signs and symptoms, the patient's medical history, and often on the results of laboratory tests. Also *diacrisis.* **2** The art or process of making such a determination. **d. by exclusion** Identification of a patient's disease by eliminating all other known possibilities. Also *exognosis.* **clinical d.** The use of a subject's history, a physical examination, and laboratory findings to establish a diagnosis. **cytologic d.** Diagnosis arrived at by the microscopic study of exfoliated cells. **differential d.** **1** The process of making a diagnosis by comparing and analyzing the similarities and differences between the signs, symptoms, and other findings associated particularly with two or more diseases sharing certain characteristics. By this means, similar conditions are systematically eliminated from consideration. **2** A diagnosis made on this basis. Also *differentiation.* **direct d.** Rapid diagnosis made possible by the demonstration of characteristic morphologic lesions. **d. ex juvantibus** The identification of disease made on the basis of the patient's response to treatment. **laboratory d.** The use of laboratory findings to establish a diagnosis without reference to the subject's history or physical findings. **pathologic d.** Diagnosis arrived at by the observation of gross and microscopic findings affecting an organ or tissue. **physical d.** Diagnosis made on the basis of information gained by physical examination of the patient. **quick-section d.** A diagnosis that is derived from the examination of a frozen or cryostat section of diseased tissue. This method is used particularly during the course of a surgical operation when the surgeon requires guidance before proceding further.

**diagnostic** \dī′agnäs′tik\ [Gk *diagnōstikos* able to distinguish, pertaining to diagnosis] **1** Of, for, or relating to diagnosis. **2** Contributing to or useful in the process of reaching a diagnosis. For defs. 1 and 2 also *diacritic.*

**diagnostician** \dī′agnästish′ən\ **1** A practitioner considered with respect to the ability to make accurate diagnoses, as *a good diagnostician.* **2** An expert or specialist in diagnosis.

**diagnostics** \dī′agnäs′tiks\ The medical science concerned with diagnosis.

**diagram** \dī′əgram\ A plan or outline that graphically represents the structure of an object or illustrates relationships. **Berkow d.** A diagram of the body surface that uses the Berkow scale for estimating the extent of a burn. It is used to calculate the size of a burn as a percentage of total body surface. **burn d.** Any of several diagrams of the body surface, dividing it into percentages used to calculate the size of a burn in terms of percentage of total body surface. **vector d.** A diagram, based on the scalar electrocardiogram, demonstrating the magnitude, sense, and direction of the electromotor forces of the heart throughout a cardiac cycle.

**diagrammatic** \dī′əgrəmat′ik\ Based on or consisting of a diagram.

**diagraph** \dī′əgraf\ [DIA- + -GRAPH] An instrument used to record the outline of one or more parts of the body.

**diakinesis** \dī′əkīnē′sis\ [DIA- + KINESIS] The last phase of prophase I of meiosis, in which chromosome contraction reaches its maximum and the tetrad form can be observed. Chromosomes show two types of coiling, referred to as major and minor coils. During diakinesis the nucleolus disappears and the nuclear envelope is disrupted.

**Diakiogiannis** [*Diakiogiannis,* Greek physician, flourished 20th century] See under SIGN.

**dial** / **astigmatic d.** A pattern of evenly spaced radial lines used to detect the presence of an astigmatic refractive error by the difference of blackness seen in the meridian of astigmatic error.

**dialysance** \dī·al′isəns\ [*dialys(is)* + -ANCE] The rate of removal of a substance per unit of difference in the concentrations of the substance in blood and in the bath fluid of the artificial kidney.

**dialysate** \dī·al′isāt\ [*dialys(is)* + -ATE] The artificial kidney bath fluid during or after dialysis. Comparing substance concentration in the post-procedure dialysate with its concentration in the blood indicates the rate of removal of that substance.

**dialysis** \dī·al′isis\ [Gk (from *dialy(ein)* to separate, break up, from *dia-* apart, asunder + *lyein* to loosen, undo) separation, dissolution] **1** A technique to separate solute molecules of different sizes by diffusion of the smaller molecules through a semipermeable membrane into a solvent with a low or zero concentration of the solutes. It is used particularly to separate crystalloids, which pass freely across membranes of suitable pore size, from colloids, which remain confined. **2** A separation, avulsion, or disinsertion, as of the retina (dialysis retinae) or of the iris (iridodialysis). **acute d.** Dialysis performed over a limited period of time, usually less than six weeks, for an episode of acute renal failure. **chronic d.** MAINTENANCE DIALYSIS. **continuous ambulatory peritoneal d.** A form of maintenance dialysis in which dialysate remains continuously within the peritoneal cavity, with exchange of dialysate through a Tenckhoff catheter every four to eight hours, usually every six hours, seven days per week. The exchanges are performed manually, using two collapsible plastic bags, each containing one liter of dialysate. No equipment is required and the patient may remain ambulatory between exchanges. **continuous cycling peritoneal d.** A system of peritoneal dialysis for chronic renal failure therapy which utilizes automated intermittent peritoneal dialysis equipment to make several exchanges each night while the patient sleeps. During the day the patient allows 2 liters of peritoneal dialysate to dwell in the peritoneal cavity from a plastic bag as used in continuous ambulatory peritoneal dialysis. **cross d.** The simultaneous passage of blood of two individuals through a dialyzer, their blood being separated by a membrane. Toxic substances are removed from the recipient's blood while essential substances are transferred from the donor's to the recipient's blood. Cross dialysis is rarely used clinically but may be useful for experimental purposes. **equilibrium d.** A technique for measuring the extent of hapten binding to antibody. By having the antibody within a semipermeable membrane through which the hapten can diffuse, it is possible to measure at equilibrium the free concentration of hapten (outside the dialysis bag) and the bound concentration (the difference between the concentration outside and inside). From such measurements, antibody affinity and valence can be determined. **intermittent d.** Hemodialysis or peritoneal dialysis performed on an interrupte or irregular schedule. The schedule may be adjusted to the needs of the patient, and usually calls for dialysis once every one to four weeks. Compare PERIODIC DIALYSIS. **kidney d.** The removal of molecules of one or more substances from the blood of uremic or poisoned patients by passive diffusion through a semipermeable membrane into a dialysate with a concentration of the particular substance less than that in the blood. **maintenance d.** Hemodialysis or periotoneal dialysis performed on an intermittent or periodic basis and required for life or until renal transplantation. Also *chronic dialysis.* **periodic d.** Hemodialysis or peritoneal dialysis performed on a regular schedule, usually three times per week. Compare INTERMITTENT DIALYSIS. **peritoneal d.** A technique to remove molecules of one or more substances from the blood of uremic or poisoned patients by passive diffusion through the peritoneal membrane into fluid which is placed for several hours in the peritoneal cavity and then drawn off. The procedure usually is repeated after two hours. Also *peritoneal ultrafiltration.* **d. retinae** A circumferential tearing of the retina very near the ora serrata, leaving only a very narrow fringe of peripheral retina attached at the ora. Also *dialysis of the retina, disinsertion of the retina, retinodialysis.* **single-needle d.** Hemodialysis performed with a single intravenous catheter. This differs from the usual performance of hemodialysis, in which two separate needles are inserted, one supplying blood to the dialyzer and the other returning it to the patient. Single-needle dialysis may be performed with a needle that has a single lumen which is used with a device that reverses the flow so that blood is alternately aspirated and returned through the single needle. It may also be performed through a catheter with a double lumen, which permits continuous inflow and outflow of blood through each lumen.

**dialyzed** \dī′əlīzd\ Separated by unequal diffusion through a semipermeable membrane.

**dialyzer** \dī′əlīzər\ An apparatus for performing dialysis. **coil d.** A dialyzer in which the dialysis membrane is wrapped in a circular manner around a central point. The flow of blood and dialysate through the dialyzer are so arranged that totally separate compartments for blood and dialysate are created within the dialyzer, separated by the dialysis membrane which is supported by a plastic mesh. **hollow-fiber d.** A cylindrical hemodialyzer containing up to 22 000 longitudinally arranged hollow fiber capillary tubes. The dialyzer is so constructed that separate blood and dialysate compartments are maintained within the dialyzer. Blood enters and exits through either end of the device and courses through the lumens of the hollow fibers, while dialysate circulates past the external surface of the fibers. **parallel-flow d.** A hemodialyzer in which sheets of dialysis membrane are placed in the device to form parallel layers so that blood and dialysate circulate in separate compartments. Also *parallel-plate dialyzer.*

**diameter** \dī·am′ətər\ [Gk *diametros* (from *dia-* through, across + *metron* measure) diagonal, diametrical, diameter] In anatomy, a straight line, or chord, joining opposite points on the circumference of a spherical, or almost spherical, structure, part, or opening, and passing through its center. Dimensions are measured along such a line. **anterior sagittal d.** The distance between the inferior margin of the symphysis pubis and the midpoint of the transverse diameter of the pelvic outlet. **anteroposterior d.** The distance between points located on the anterior and posterior aspects of the body. **Baudelocque's d.** EXTERNAL CONJUGATE. **biparietal d.** The distance between the most prominent parts of the parietal bones. Also *posterotransverse diameter, parietal diameter.* **bisacromial d.** The distance between the outermost portions of the shoulders. **bisiliac d.** The widest distance between the iliac crests. **bispinous d.** The distance between the ischial spines. Also *interspinous diameter.* **bitemporal d.** The distance between the most prominent parts of the temporal bone. Also *temporal diameter.* **cervicobregmatic d.** The distance between the anterior fontanelle and the junction of the neck and skull. **coccygeopubic d.** The distance between the end of the coccyx and the inferior edge of the symphysis pubis. **d. conjugata** [NA] The anteroposterior diameter of the inlet, or superior aperture, of the pelvis, measured between the midpoints of the sacral promontory and the upper margin of the symphysis pubis. Also *conjugata, conjugate, true conjugate, true conjugate diameter, conjugate axis, conjugate of the inlet, anatomic conjugate, conjugata vera, internal conjugate.* **conjugate d.** Anteroposterior distances between specified points referable to the inlet of the pelvis. Also *conjugate axis* (outmoded). **craniometric d.** A line connecting skull landmarks of the same name, such as the biparietal diameter drawn between the prominent portions of the parietal bones located on each side of the skull. **diagonal conjugate d.** DIAGONAL CONJUGATE. **external conjugate d.** EXTERNAL CONJUGATE. **extracanthic d.** The distance between the lateral palpebral angles of the two eyes. **frontomental d.** The distance between the most prominent midpoint part of the frontal bone and the chin. **fronto-occipital d.** OCCIPITOFRONTAL DIAMETER. **intercanthic d.** The horizontal distance between the lateral and medial angles of the palpebral aperture. **intercristal d.** The distance between the midpoints of the crests of the ilium. **interspinous d.** BISPINOUS DIAMETER. **intertrochanteric d.** The distance between the trochanters of the femur. **left oblique d.** An oblique diameter of the pelvis which includes the sacroiliac articulation of the left side of the pelvis. **mean corpuscular d.** The mean diameter of erythrocytes in blood. **mento-occipital d.** OCCIPITOMENTAL DIAMETER. **mentoparietal d.** The distance between the chin and the top of the posterior skull or vertex. **d. obliqua pelvis** [NA] A measurement taken obliquely across the superior pelvic aperture, or pelvic inlet, from one iliopubic, or iliopectineal, eminence to the opposite sacroiliac joint. Also *oblique diameter.* **obstetric conjugate d.** OBSTETRIC CONJUGATE. **occipitofrontal d.** The distance between the most prominent midpoint parts of the frontal and occipital bones. Also *fronto-occipital diameter.* **occipitomental d.** The distance between the chin and the most prominent midpoint part of the occiput bone. Also *mento-occipital diameter.* **parietal d.** BIPARIETAL DIAMETER. **posterior sagittal d.** The distance from the tip of the sacrum to a right-angled intersection with a line drawn between the ischial tuberosities. **posterotransverse d.** BIPARIETAL DIAMETER. **pubotuberous d.** The perpendicular distance from the ischial tuberosity to the superior aspect of the symphysis pubis. **right oblique d.** An oblique diameter of the pelvis which includes the sacroiliac articulation of the right side of the pelvis. **sacropubic d.** The distance between the end of the sacrum and the inferior aspect of the symphysis pubis. **suboccipitobregmatic d.** The distance between the anterior fontanelle and the midpoint of the base of the occiput bone. **suboccipitofrontal d.** The distance between the most prominent midpoint part of the frontal bone and the base of the occiput bone. **suprasubparietal d.** The distance between a point just above a parietal eminence to a point just below the opposite parietal eminence. **temporal d.** BITEMPORAL DIAMETER. **d. transversa pelvis** [NA] The maximum transverse dimension of the superior pelvic aperture, measured between corresponding points on opposite sides of the pelvic brim. Also *transverse diameter of pelvis, transverse diameter of pelvic inlet.* **transverse d. of pelvic inlet** DIAMETER TRANSVERSA PELVIS. **transverse d. of pelvic outlet** The distance between the ischial tuberosities, measured between the lower borders of their medial surfaces. **transverse d. of pelvis** DIAMETER TRANSVERSA PELVIS. **true conjugate d.** DIAMETER CONJUGATA.

**diamine** A chemical compound containing two amino groups.

**diamine oxidase** Any of the copper-containing amine oxidases (EC 1.4.3.6). Members of this group oxidize several primary amines, monoamines as well as diamines.

**diaminodiphenyl sulfone** A synthetic chemotherapeutic agent used in the treatment of leprosy. Abbr. DAPS

**2,6-diaminopimelic acid** HOOC—CH($NH_2$)—[$CH_2$]$_3$—CH($NH_2$)—COOH. It is a component of many bacterial peptidoglycans, and is involved in cross-linking as the *meso-* or LL- compound. It is also an intermediate in lysine biosynthesis in green plants and bacteria (the diaminopimelate pathway).

**diaminopyrimidine** Any of a group of compounds (2,4-diaminopyrimidines) that includes a number of antimalarials.

**Diamond** [Louis Klein *Diamond,* U.S. physician, born 1902] Diamond-Blackfan syndrome. See under DIAMOND-BLACKFAN ANEMIA.

**diamorphine** HEROIN.

**diamthazole dihydrochloride** $C_{15}H_{25}Cl_2N_3OS$. 6-(2-Diethylaminoethoxy)-2-dimethylaminobenzothiazole dihydrochloride, an antifungal medication used in the treatment of infections from *Trichophyton, Microsporum,* and *Candida.* It is used topically in the form of an ointment, tincture, or dusting powder to treat such conditions as athlete's foot, ringworm of the nails, and tinea capitis.

**dianion** \dī-an′ī′ăn\ An anion carrying two negative charges, e.g. succinate, and $SO_4^{2-}$.

**diantebrachia** \dī′antēbrā′kē-ə\ [DI-[2] + ANTE- + L *brachia,* pl. of *brachium* arm] A congenital defect of the upper limb in which the forearm and varying degrees of the more distal segments appear to be duplicated.

**diapause** \dī′əpôz\ [DIA- + *pause*] EMBRYONIC DIAPAUSE. **embryonic d.** Any pause occurring in the process of embryonic development, or any delay or slowing down of embryonic development over a limited period. Also *diapause.* See also DELAYED IMPLANTATION.

**diapedesis** \dī′əpedē′sis\ [Gk *diapēdēsis* (from *dia-* through + *pēd(an)* to leap + *-ēsis* -ESIS) a leaping through or across] Passage through intact vessel walls of the formed elements of the blood. Also *diapedesia.* Adj. diapedetic.

**diaphoretic** \dī′əfôret′ik\ [Gk *diaphorētikos* (from *diaphorein* to disperse, cause to evaporate) promoting perspiration] **1** SUDORIFIC. **2** An agent capable of inducing sweating.

**diaphragm** \dī′əfram\ [Gk *diaphragma.* See DIAPHRAGMA.] **1** DIAPHRAGMA. **2** A contraceptive device used by women. See under CONTRACEPTIVE DIAPHRAGM. **3** A device with an adjustable opening through which the amount of light admitted can be controlled, as in a camera or microscope. **Akerlund d.** An adjustable lead diaphragm used in roentgenography to limit the radiation beam size to a circle of variable diameter. **Bucky d.** A grid, containing a series of thin lead strips, which moves between the patient and the film during a radiographic exposure. It is used to reduce the amount of scattered radiation reaching the film. Also *Bucky-Potter diaphragm, Potter-Bucky diaphragm, Bucky grid, Potter-Bucky grid.* **compression d.** A device used to apply external pressure to the part of the body being studied by fluoroscopy or roentgenography. **condensing d.** A variable aperture, situated in the condenser of a light microscope, that is capable of sharpening the image by eliminating peripheral light rays. **contraceptive d.** A contraceptive device, usually made of latex rubber, which is placed against the uterine cervix to block the passage of spermatozoa and to hold spermicidal cream or jelly. Contraceptive diaphragms are usually fitted by a physician but are applied by the woman herself prior to sexual intercourse and not worn otherwise. Also *vaginal diaphragm.* **filtration slit d. of glomerulus** FILTRATION SLIT MEMBRANE OF GLOMERULUS. **graduating d.** A glass disk that is accurately marked and placed within the eyepiece of a microscope in order to estimate the size of objects viewed in the microscope. Also *eyepiece graticule.*

**iris d.** A variable aperture in an optical system that can be opened and closed while always retaining a circular shape similar to the iris of the eye. **d. of mouth** MUSCULUS MYLOHYOIDEUS. **oral d.** MUSCULUS MYLOHYOIDEUS. **pelvic d.** DIAPHRAGMA PELVIS. **Potter-Bucky d.** BUCKY DIAPHRAGM. **respiratory d.** DIAPHRAGMA. **secondary d.** DIAPHRAGMA UROGENITALE. **d. of sella turcica** DIAPHRAGMA SELLAE. **thoracoabdominal d.** DIAPHRAGMA. **urogenital d.** DIAPHRAGMA UROGENITALE. **vaginal d.** CONTRACEPTIVE DIAPHRAGM.

**diaphragma** \dī′əfrag′mə\ [Gk (from *dia-* between, apart + *phragma* a fence, barrier, from *phrassein* to fence) a partition, midriff, diaphragm] **1** A thin tissue serving as a partition between adjacent spaces or regions. **2** [NA] The dome-shaped musculofibrous partition between the thoracic and abdominal cavities. It arises in three parts (sternal, costal, and lumbar) that ascend and are inserted into a central tendon that lies immediately below the pericardium. It is the principal muscle of respiration and assists the abdominal muscles in all acts of expulsion involving increased intra-abdominal pressure. In it are openings for the esophagus, aorta, and inferior vena cava. Also *midriff, diaphragmatic muscle, respiratory diaphragm, thoracoabdominal diaphragm, phren, interseptum.* For defs. 1 and 2 also *diaphragm.* **d. pelvis** [NA] The hammocklike part of the floor of the pelvic cavity, composed of the levator ani and coccygeus muscles of both sides meeting in the median plane, as well as the superior and inferior fascia of the pelvic diaphragm that invest these muscles. It supports the pelvic viscera, and is pierced by the anal canal, the urethra, and the vagina. Also *pelvic diaphragm.* **d. sellae** [NA] A tough, horizontal fold of dura mater that extends from the margins of the hypophysial fossa of the sphenoid bone, forming a roof for the sella turcica and separating the hypophysis from the optic chiasma and the base of the brain. The center of the fold is pierced by the infundibulum. Also *diaphragm of sella turcica, tentorium of hypophysis, pituitary folds.* **d. urogenitale** A triangular fibromuscular membrane spanning the ischiopubic rami superficial to the pelvic diaphragm and comprising the perineal membrane, the sphincter urethrae, and the deep transverse perineal muscles. The membrane is pierced by the urethra and a number of vessels, nerves, and ducts in both sexes, as well as the vagina in the female. Also *urogenital diaphragm, secondary diaphragm, Camper's ligament, fascia of urogenital trigone.*

**diaphragmata** \dī′əfrag′mətə\ Plural of DIAPHRAGMA.

**diaphragmatic** \dī′əfragmat′ik\ Of or pertaining to the diaphragm. Also *phrenic.*

**diaphyseal** \dī′əfiz′ē·əl\ Related to or associated with the shaft of a long bone. Also *diaphysary, diaphysial.*

**diaphysectomy** \dī′əfizek′təmē\ Surgical excision of all or part of a diaphysis.

**diaphyses** \dī·af′isēz\ Plural of DIAPHYSIS.

**diaphysial** \dī′əfiz′ē·əl\ DIAPHYSEAL.

**diaphysis** \dī·af′isis\ [Gk (from *diaphyesthai* to grow through or between, from *dia-* between + *phyesthai* to grow) growth through or between parts] [NA] The body, or shaft, of a long bone that ossifies from a primary center, in contrast to the extremities, or epiphyses, which ossify from secondary centers. It comprises a thick cylinder of compact bone surrounding a large medullary cavity.

**diaphysitis** \dī′əfizī′tis\ An inflammation of the diaphysis.

**diaplex** \dī′əpleks\ PLEXUS CHOROIDEUS VENTRICULI TERTII.

**diaplexus** \dī′əplek′səs\ *Outmoded* PLEXUS CHOROIDEUS VENTRICULI TERTII.

**diapnoic** \dī′apnō′ik\ [Gk *dia-* through + *pno(ē)* breath, vapor, exhalation + -IC] Of or relating to insensible sweating.

**diapophysis** \dī′əpäf′isis\ PROCESSUS ARTICULARIS SUPERIOR VERTEBRAE.

**diarrhea** \dī′ərē′ə\ [Gk *diarrhoia* (from DIA- + Gk *rheein* to flow) a flowing through, diarrhea] Abnormal fecal discharge characterized by frequent and/or watery stool. **choleraic d.** Acute, watery, choleralike diarrhea which may result in circulatory collapse. **climatic d.** Diarrhea due to climatic factors, often exposure to cold. **dientamoeba d.** Mild, chronic diarrhea due to infection with *Dientamoeba fragilis,* an ameba generally but not universally considered a pathogen in man. **epidemic d. in children** INFANTILE GASTROENTERITIS. **membranous d.** PSEUDOMEMBRANOUS COLITIS. **mucous d.** Diarrhea in which there is an increased quantity of mucus present. When accompanied by cramping abdominal pain, it may be a form of the irritable bowel syndrome. Also *mucomembranous diarrhea, enteromyxorrhea.* **osmotic d.** Diarrhea caused by an excess of osmotically active, nonabsorbable particles in the gut contents. **parenteral d.** Diarrhea resulting from extraintestinal disease. **serous d.** The passing of frequent watery stools. Stool electrolytes account for almost all the osmolality of the stool water. The diarrhea persists with fasting. Also *watery diarrhea.* **summer d.** *Outmoded* INFANTILE GASTROENTERITIS. **travelers' d.** An acute, infectious gastroenteritis usually caused by enterotoxigenic *Escherichia coli,* but also often related to infection with other organisms, such as *Shigella, Salmonella,* Rotavirus, and *Giardia lamblia.* It has an acute onset following exposure to contaminated drinking water or food, but it is self-limiting after two or three days. **virus d.** Diarrhea caused by a virus, such as rotavirus or Norwalk agent. **watery d.** SEROUS DIARRHEA.

**diarrheal** \dī′ərē′əl\ Of or relating to diarrhea. Also *diarrheic.*

**diarrhoea** *Brit.* DIARRHEA.

**diarthric** \dī·är′thrik\ [DI-[2] + ARTHR- + -IC] Pertaining to or affecting two joints; biarticular. Also *diarticular.*

**diarthrodial** \dī′ärthrō′dē·əl\ Pertaining to a synovial joint, formerly called a diarthrosis.

**diarthroses** \dī′ärthrō′sēz\ Plural of DIARTHROSIS.

**diarthrosis** \dī′ärthrō′sis\ [Gk *diarthrōsis* (from *di(a)-* through, apart + *arthrōsis* jointing, articulation) a movable articulation] ARTICULATIO SYNOVIALIS. **planiform d.** ARTICULATIO PLANA. **d. rotatoria** ARTICULATIO TROCHOIDEA.

**diarticular** \dī′ärtik′yələr\ DIARTHRIC.

**diascopy** \dī·as′kəpē\ [DIA- + -SCOPY] An examination of a skin lesion in which the blood is temporarily excluded from the lesion by application of firm pressure on the area of study using a slide of glass or other transparent material. Excluding the blood from the area facilitates the detection of cellular and other deposits in the dermis. Also *vitropressure.*

**diastase** [French (from Gk *diastasis* separation; see DIASTASIS) a substance that brings about a separation (hydrolysis) of starch; the first known digestive enzyme] An amylase, or mixture of amylases.

**diastasemia** \dī′əstəsē′mē·ə\ HYPERAMYLASEMIA.

**diastasis** \dī·as′təsis\ [Gk (from *diista(nai)* to set apart, from *di(a)-* + *(h)istanai* to stand, set) separation, parting, interval] **1** A separation, either imposed or not, between components of a structure or a process. **2** A separation of adjacent bones that do not articulate with each other as a result of damage to soft tissue structures. Such separations are seen along the shafts of the radius and ulna or the tibia and fibula. Also *divarication* (obs.). **d. cordis** DIASTOLE.

**diastema** \dīʹəstēʹmə\ [Gk *diastēma* an interval] (*pl.* diastemata) **1** Any abnormal cleft, space, or opening in or between parts. **2** A naturally occurring space between teeth in the same arch, as in a horse. **3** In man, an abnormally wide space between two teeth, usually the upper central incisors.

**diastemata** \dīʹəstemʹətə\ Plural of DIASTEMA.

**diastematocrania** \dīʹəstemʹətōkrāʹnē·ə\ [DIASTEMA + *-to-* + *cran(io)-* + -IA] A sagittal fissure between cranial bones persisting beyond the time of usual closure.

**diastematomyelia** \dīʹəstemʹətōmī·ēʹlyə\ [DIASTEMA + *-to-* + MYEL- + -IA] A longitudinal cleft or fissure in the spinal cord which may be either complete or localized at one or more vertebral levels. The cleft is often occupied by a bony or fibrocartilagenous spur or septum. Also *diastomyelia, diplomyelia.*

**diastematopyelia** \dīʹəstemʹətōpī·ēʹlyə\ [DIASTEMA + *-to-* + PYEL- + -IA] A congenital separation of the pelvic bones. It may involve the absence or cleft of the sacrum.

**diaster** \dīʹastər\ AMPHIASTER.

**diastereoisomer** \dīʹastirʹē·ō·īʹsōmirʹ\ Any stereoisomer that is not an enantiomer. The molecules therefore differ in some way other than being mirror images. They may do so by *cis-trans* isomerism at a double bond, or by having two chiral parts, one identical and one enantiomeric between the two molecules. Glucose and galactose, for example, are diastereoisomers, being enantiomeric at C-4, and identical, but chiral, in the rest of the molecule.

**diastole** \dī·asʹtəlē\ [Gk *diastolē* (from *diastellein* to expand, separate, from *dia-* apart + *stellein* to send, put) dilatation] The period of atrial and ventricular myocardial relaxation in the cardiac cycle. Also *diastasis cordis.* Compare SYSTOLE. **atrial d.** The period of myocardial relaxation in the atria during the cardiac cycle. Also *auricular diastole.* **end d.** The terminal part of diastole, immediately prior to the onset of systole. **ventricular d.** The period of myocardial relaxation in the ventricles during the cardiac cycle.

**diastolic** \dīʹəstälʹik\ Of or relating to diastole.

**diastomyelia** \dī·asʹtōmī·ēʹlyə\ DIASTEMATOMYELIA.

**diathermocoagulation** \dīʹəthurʹmōkō·agʹyəlāʹshən\ Surgical diathermy to coagulate tissue; electrocoagulation.

**diathermy** \dīʹəthurʹmē\ [DIA- + Gk *thermē* heat] Deep heating of body parts by conversion of energy from high-frequency electric current, electromagnetic wave energy, or ultrasound. It is a common adjunct to physical therapy, either to promote relaxation of muscles in spasm or of ligaments around a joint as a preparation for massage or exercise. Surgical diathermy utilizes high-frequency current at destructive levels to cause coagulation or desiccation. Also *endothermy, diathermic therapy.* **conventional d.** Diathermy that utilizes high-frequency currents ranging from 500 000 to 1 500 000 Hz and wavelengths between 100 and 600 meters. **long-wave d.** Diathermy using high-frequency currents with wavelengths between 100 and 300 meters. **microwave d.** Diathermy by microwave. A commonly used apparatus emits waves of 122 mm at a frequency of 2450 MHz. **pulsed d.** DUPLEX THERAPY. **short-wave d.** Diathermy utilizing wavelengths between 30 and 3 meters and frequencies between 10 and 100 MHz. This is the range of diathermy most commonly used for medical purposes. **ultrashort-wave d.** Diathermy using wavelengths shorter than 10 meters.

**diathesis** \dī·athʹəsis\ [Gk (from *diatithenai* to set out, arrange, dispose, from *dia-* through, throughout + *tithenai* to place, put) arrangement, disposition, constitution] An inborn tendency to develop certain diseases or other abnormal conditions; a constitutional susceptibility or predisposition. Adj. diathetic. **allergic d.** The genetically based susceptibility to develop immediate hypersensitivity to a variety of common environmental allergens. **asthenic d.** A predisposition to physical weakness. **explosive d.** EPILEPTOID PERSONALITY DISORDER. **exudative d.** The atopic state that predisposes one to eczema, asthma, and allergic rhinitis. **fibroplastic d.** The tendency to form scar tissue. **gouty d.** A predisposition to develop gout. **hemorrhagic d.** Any tendency to bleed. **lipogenic d.** A predisposition to obesity. **ossifying d.** A tendency to develop bone tissue. **spasmodic d.** SPASMOPHILIA. **thromboasthenic d.** GLANZMANN'S DISEASE. **traumatophilic d.** Proneness to accidents or to exposing oneself to physically or psychologically dangerous situations. **uric acid d.** A tendency to develop excess uric acid in the blood and tissues, leading to gout attacks or tophus deposits.

**diathetic** \dīʹəthetʹik\ Relating or attributed to a diathesis.

**diatomite** \dīʹətōmītʹ\ DIATOMACEOUS EARTH.

**diatoric** \dīʹətôrʹik\ [Gk *diator(os)* pierced + -IC] Pertaining to porcelain teeth which are attached to the base by means of perforations in the teeth as opposed to attachment by metal pins.

**diatrizoate sodium** $C_{11}H_8I_3N_2NaO_4$. The sodium salt of diatrizoic acid. It is used as an injectable radiopaque contrast medium for visualization of the biliary, urinary, and other systems.

**diatrizoic acid** $C_{11}H_9I_3N_2O_4$. 3,5-Diacetamido-2,4,6-triiodobenzoic acid, an acid used most commonly in the form of sodium or methylglucamine salts as a water-soluble contrast medium for intravascular administration, as in intravenous urography and angiography.

**diauxie** \dī·ôkʹsē\ [French, from DI-[2] + AUX- + *-ie* -Y] A two-step growth process on a mixture of nutrients, in which a microorganism exhausts a preferred compound before it is able to induce the enzymes required for the utilization of a second compound. This phenomenon has led to key studies on gene regulation, involving the induction of β-galactosidase and its catabolite repression by glucose. Adj. diauxic.

**diazepam** $C_{16}H_{13}ClN_2O$. 7-Chloro-1,3-dihydro-1-methyl-5-phenyl-2*H*-1,4-benzodiazepin-2-one, a commonly used pharmacologic agent with muscle relaxant, anticonvulsant, and tranquilizing properties. It is given orally or parenterally.

**diazo-** [DI-[2] + *azo(te)*] A combining form designating the presence in a molecule of the group —N=N—.

**diazomethane** $CH_2{=}N^+{=}N^-$. A yellow, explosive gas, which is easily liquefied. It is used, usually as its solution in diethyl ether, in chemical syntheses, especially for making methyl esters from acids and diazoketones from acid chlorides. It is highly toxic. Being a powerful methylating agent and so able to methylate nucleic acid, it is also carcinogenic and mutagenic.

**diazone** \dīʹəzōn\ [DIA- + ZONE] Dark bands seen in cross-sections of tooth enamel, formed by layers of enamel prisms.

**diazoxide** $C_8H_7ClN_2O_2S$. 7-Chloro-3-methyl-2*H*-1,2,4-benzothiadiazine 1,1-dioxide, a pharmacologic agent most commonly used in the emergency control of severe hypertension. It is also used as an oral medication to raise the level of the blood sugar.

**Dibenamine** A proprietary name for *N,N*-dibenzyl-*β*-chlorethylamine hydrochloride.
**dibenzothiazine** PHENOTHIAZINE.
***N,N*-dibenzyl-*β*-chlorethylamine hydrochloride** $C_{16}H_{18}ClN{\cdot}HCl$. An alpha-adrenergic blocking agent that has been used to treat some types of peripheral vascular disease and to diagnose pheochromocytoma. It is given orally or intravenously.
***N,N'*-dibenzylethylenediamine penicillin** BENZATHINE PENICILLIN G.
**diblastula** \dīblas′tyələ\ [DI-[2] + BLASTULA] A blastula in which both ectoderm and endoderm can be distinguished. Adj. diblastic.
**dibothriocephaliasis** \dībäth′rē·ōsef′əlī′əsis\ DIPHYLLOBOTHRIASIS.
***Dibothriocephalus*** \dībäth′rē·ōsef′ələs\ *DIPHYLLOBOTHRIUM.* ***D. latus*** *DIPHYLLOBOTHRIUM LATUM*
**dibromothymolsulfonphthalein** BROMOTHYMOL BLUE.
**dibucaine hydrochloride** An injectable topical anesthetic consisting of a quinoline derivative and having a long-lasting effect. Also *dibucaine.*
**dibutoline sulfate** $C_{30}H_{66}N_4O_8S$. Dibutylurethan of dimethylethyl-*β*-hydroxyethylammonium sulfate, an anticholinergic agent used as an antispasmodic.
**dibutyryl cyclic AMP** A derivative of cAMP which is less polar than cAMP but retains the biologic activity. This molecule can cross the cell membrane and inhibit cell division or suppress growth of certain tumor cells.
**DIC** disseminated intravascular coagulation.
**dicelous** \dīsē′ləs\ **1** Having two cavities. **2** Concave at both ends or on both sides. Also *dicoelous.*
**dicentric** \dīsen′trik\ Pertaining to a chromosome that has two centromeres.
**dicephalus** \dīsef′ələs\ [DI-[2] + -CEPHALUS] A conjoined twin with two heads. Also *bicephalus, diplocephalus, cephalodidymus.* **d. diauchenos** A dicephalus with two predominantly or completely separate necks. **d. dipus dibrachius** A dicephalus with an essentially normal body possessing only two arms and two legs. **d. dipus tetrabrachius** A dicephalus possessing two legs and four arms, signifying incomplete union in the thoracic part of the trunk. **d. dipus tribrachius** A dicephalus with two legs and three arms, signifying incomplete union in the pectoral and shoulder regions. **d. monauchenos** MONAUCHENOS. **d. parasiticus** DESMIOGNATHUS. **d. tripus tribrachius** A dicephalus with three legs and three arms.
**dicephaly** \dīsef′əlē\ [DI-[2] + CEPHAL- + -Y] The state of having two heads and a single body.
**dicheilia** \dīkī′lyə\ [DI-[2] + CHEIL- + -IA ] The condition of having a lip with an abnormal transverse fold which causes it to appear to be doubled.
**dicheiria** \dīkī′rē·ə\ [DI-[2] + CHEIR- + -IA ] POLYDACTYLY.
**dichloralphenazone** $C_{15}H_{18}Cl_6N_2O_5$. A derivative of chloral that generates chloral hydrate in the body. Administered orally, it is an effective hypnotic and sedative.
**dichlorisone** $C_{21}H_{26}Cl_2O_4$. 9,11*β*-Dichloro-17,21-dihydroxypregna-1,4-diene-3,20-dione, a glucocorticoid medication that is used particularly to treat skin allergic reactions and pruritic conditions that respond to steroid treatment. It is applied topically.
**dichloroacetic acid** $Cl_2CH—COOH$. A colorless, corrosive liquid, of sharp taste, solidifying at -4°C and boiling at 194°C. It is very soluble in water, ethanol and ether, and is a fairly strong acid (p*K* 1.3). It is used as a synthetic reagent in the preparation of organic thiosulfates and various medicaments. It irritates skin and mucous membranes.
**dichlorodiphenyltrichloroethane** $(ClC_6N_4)_2CH$-$CCl_3$. A persistent fat-soluble biocide which has been used against a wide variety of insects. It is a nonspecific poison and although banned in many parts of the world, its use continues. Also *DDT.*
**dichloronitrobenzene** 1-Chloro-24-dinitrobenzene, a compound used for studying contact or delayed hypersensitivity. A sensitizing dose is placed on one forearm and later the test dose is applied to the opposite forearm. Also *chlorodinitrobenzene, dinitrochlorobenzene.* Abbr. DCNB
**2,4-dichlorophenoxyacetic acid** $C_8H_6Cl_2O_3$. A white powder used as an herbicide, a component of Agent Orange. Its properties are similar to those of 2,4-trichlorophenoxyacetic acid, but it is less toxic. Abbr. 2,4-D
**dichloroxylenol** $C_8H_8Cl_2O$. 2,4-Dichloro-3,5-xylenol. An effective bacteriostatic agent structurally and functionally related to parachlorometaxylenol. It is highly effective against *Staphylococcus aureus.*
**dichlorphenamide** A carbonic anhydrase inhibitor which reduces intraocular pressure by reducing the formation of aqueous humor.
**dichogamous** \dīkäg′əməs\ [Gk *dich(a)* in two, asunder + GAM- + -OUS] Having two types of gametes which mature at different times, preventing self-fertilization. Compare HOMOGAMOUS.
**dichorionic** \dī′kôrē·än′ik\ [DI-[2] + CHORION + -IC] Possessing two separate chorions, as in *dichorionic twins.* Also *dichorial.*
**dichotomy** \dīkät′əmē\ [Gk *dichotomi(a)* (from *dich(a)* in two, asunder + *o* + *tom(os)* a cutting, from *temnein* to cut) a cutting in two parts] A division into two parts, especially opposing parts.
**dichroic** Exhibiting dichroism.
**dichroism** \dī′krō·izm\ [Gk *dichro(os)* two-colored + -ISM] The property of a substance to absorb left and right circularly polarized light to different extents. It is used to obtain information about the environment of a chromophore, because it is shown only by chiral chromophores or by chromophores in chiral environments. Also *circular dichroism.*
**dichromasy** \dīkrō′məsē\ DICHROMATOPSIA.
**dichromat** \dī′krōmat\ An individual with dichromatopsia.
**dichromatopsia** \dīkrō′mətäp′sē·ə\ [DI-[2] + CHROMAT- + -OPSIA] Color blindness in which the entire spectrum of colors is seen as various proportions of only two primary colors. Also *dichromasy, dichromism, dichromatism.* Adj. dichromatic, dichromic.
**Dick** [George Frederick *Dick,* U.S. physician and bacteriologist, 1881–1967] **1** Dick's method, Dick reaction. See under TEST. **2** Dick test toxin. See under ERYTHROGENIC TOXIN.
**Dick** [Gladys Henry *Dick,* U.S. bacteriologist, 1881–1963] **1** Dick's method, Dick reaction. See under TEST. **2** Dick test toxin. See under ERYTHROGENIC TOXIN.
**dicloxacillin** $C_{19}H_{17}Cl_2N_3O_5S$. A semisynthetic, penicillinase-resistant penicillin used, as the sodium salt, to treat infections, especially those caused by penicillin-resistant, Gram-positive organisms.
**dicloxacillin sodium** $C_{19}H_{16}Cl_2N_3NaO_5S{\cdot}H_2O$. 6-[3-(2,6-Dichlorophenyl)-5-methyl-4-isoxazole-carboxamido]penicillanic acid sodium. A semisynthetic antibiotic with penicillinase-resistant qualities. It is used in the treatment of infections caused by certain strains of staphylococci. It is given orally.

**dicoelous** \dīsē′ləs\ DICELOUS.

**dicoria** \dīkôr′ē·ə\ DIPLOCORIA.

**dicoumarol** \dīkoo′mərôl\ DICUMAROL.

**dicrotic** \dīkrät′ik\ [Gk *dikrot(os)* (from *dis* twice + *krotein* to beat, hammer) double-beating + -IC] **1** Characterized by having two waves: said of a pulse. Compare MONOCROTIC, TRICROTIC. **2** Being the second of two (waves): said of the pulse wave following the dicrotic notch.

**dictionary / genetic code d.** GENETIC CODE.

**dictyokinesis** \dik′tē·ōkīnē′sis\ The division of dictysomes and their distribution to two daughter cells during cell division.

**dictyoma** \dik′tē·ō′mə\ [Gk *dikty(on)* a net (retina) + -OMA] MEDULLOEPITHELIOMA.

**dictyosome** \dik′tē·ōsōm′\ [Gk *dictyo(n)* a net + *sōm(a)* body] A stack of cisternae forming a part of the Golgi apparatus. Golgi configurations in higher plants are often very complex, having many (even hundreds) of well-developed dictysomes in the Golgi apparatus. Also *Golgi body*.

**dictyotene** \dik′tē·ōtēn′\ A stage of oogenesis that interrupts prophase of the first meiotic division. No further crossing over occurs and the chromosomes disperse somewhat. In human females, this stage begins in the seventh month of fetal life and persists until the oogonial cell begins ovulation, an interval that may be as long as 50 years.

**dicumarol** \dīkoo′mərôl\ 3,3′-Methylene-bis(4-hydroxycoumarin). An anticoagulant derivative of coumarin that inhibits prothrombin synthesis in the liver. It is responsible for bleeding in animals ingesting spoiled sweet clover. Also *bishydroxycoumarin, melilotoxin*. Also *dicoumarol*.

**dicyclohexylcarbodiimide** $C_6H_{11}$—N═C═N—$C_6H_{11}$. The carbodiimide most used as a chemical reagent, as for peptide and polynucleotide synthesis. After acting as a condensing agent, between a carboxylic acid and an amine for example, it forms *N,N′*-dicyclohexylurea, which, being insoluble in most solvents, is easily removed. Dicyclohexylcarbodiimide reacts with carboxyl groups to activate them, and this is the basis of its reaction with a component of the $H^+$-transporting ATP synthase of mitochondria.

**didactylism** \dīdak′təlizm\ [DIDACTYL + -ISM] The state of having two digits on a hand or a foot.

**didelphia** \dīdel′fē·ə\ [DI-[2] + Gk *delph(ys)* uterus + -IA] A congenital condition in which the uterus consists of two predominantly separate, roughly parallel bodies. A uterus with this condition is commonly called a double uterus.

**dideoxyhexose** \dī′dē·äk′sēhek′sōs\ A group of unusual sugars characteristic of the lipopolysaccharide of various groups of salmonella: abequose, colitose, paratose, and tyvelose.

**didermal** \dīdur′məl\ [DI- + DERMAL] In embryology, characterized by having two germ layers, usually ectoderm and endoderm.

**didymitis** \did′imī′tis\ [Gk *didym(os)* double, a twin, testicle + -ITIS] ORCHITIS.

**didymous** \did′əməs\ [Gk *didym(os)* twin + -OUS] Having features indicative of conjoined twinning.

**-didymus** \-did′əməs\ [Gk *didymos* (from *dyo* two) double, twin] A combining form denoting conjoined twins. • In reference to twins united at a specified region of the body, this combining form is outmoded and being replaced by -PAGUS. See also CONJOINED TWINS.

**die[1]** \dī\ [Middle English *dien*, from Old Norse *deyja* to die] To suffer death. See under DEATH.

**die[2]** \dī\ [Old French *de* a die, prob. from L *datum* (neut. sing. of *datus*, past part. of *dare* to give) a thing given] A positive replica of a prepared tooth in metal or cement for the purpose of making a wax pattern on it for a cast restoration. **amalgam d.** A die prepared by condensing dental amalgam in a composition impression of a prepared tooth. **plated d.** A stone die with a metal surface obtained by electroplating the mold before casting the plaster. **stone d.** A die made of specially hard plaster of Paris.

**dieb. alt.** *diebus alternis* (L, on alternate days). It is used in prescription writing.

**dieb. tert.** *diebus tertiis* (L, every third day). It is used in prescription writing.

**diecious** \dī·ē′shəs\ [DI-[2] + Gk *oikia* a dwelling + -OUS] Denoting those taxa in which individuals are sexually distinct. Also *dioecious*.

**dieldrin** \dī·el′drin\ $C_{12}H_8Cl_6O$. A chlorinated hydrocarbon pesticide with long-lasting properties. It is used to control mosquitoes, ticks, sandflies, and other agricultural and forest pests. It is one of the more toxic members of its group, causing dizziness, nausea, and vomiting. In more serious cases convulsive seizures and coma may follow.

**dielectric** \dī′ilek′trik\ The insulating medium such as plastic, ceramic, or air between two plates of a capacitor.

**dielectrolysis** \dī′ilekträl′isis\ ELECTROPHORESIS.

**diembryony** \dī·em′brē·ənē\ [DI-[2] + Gk *embryon* embryo + -Y] Formation of two embryos from the same egg.

**diencephalic** \dī′ensəfal′ik\ Pertaining to or involving the diencephalon.

**diencephalohypophysial** \dī′ensef′əlōhī′pōfiz′ē·əl\ Pertaining to or connecting the diencephalon and hypophysis.

**diencephalon** \dī′ensef′əlän\ [DI-[3] + ENCEPHALON] [NA] The basal portion of the embryonic prosencephalon from which the hypothalamus, thalamus, and epithalamus are derived. Also *between-brain* (obs.), *thalamic brain* (obs.), *interbrain, thalamencephalon* (obs.).

**-diene** [DI-[2] + -ENE] See under -ENE.

***Dientamoeba fragilis*** \dī′entəmē′bə fraj′ilis\ A small flagellate, usually binucleated, which parasitizes humans and some other primates. It is mildly pathogenic or nonpathogenic, sometimes causing mild diarrhea or colicky distress. The life cycle is unknown but presumed to be by the fairly resistant trophozoites since no cysts have been found. Suggestions of transmission by pinworm eggs or other transport mechanisms have also been made. Though flagella are lacking, the organism is a flagellate, similar to *Histomonas* and, like the latter, probably related to the trichomonads, possibly in the family Monocercomonadidae.

**dieresis** \dī·er′əsis\ [Late L *diaeresis* (from Gk *diairesis* a dividing, division, from *dia-* through + *(h)airein* to take, seize) a division] A surgical procedure in which normally united body parts are divided by an incision.

**diesterase** Any enzyme that catalyzes the hydrolysis of a diester, usually a diester of phosphoric acid, and hence of general formula R—O—$PO_2^-$—O—R′. Such phosphodiesterases are involved in the hydrolysis of internucleotide bonds in nucleic acids and in the hydrolytic opening of cyclic nucleotides.

**diestrus** \dī·es′trəs\ [DI-[3] + ESTRUS] An interval of sexual inactivity between two periods of estrus. Also *diestrum*.

**diet** \dī′ət\ [L *diaeta* (from Gk *diaita* a way of living, life) diet, food] **1** The customary food intake of an individual or group of individuals over a given period of time. **2** A plan or method for consuming nutrients in order to meet certain specifications. **acid-ash d.** A diet designed to acidify the urine. It consists of foods that are acidic, such as meat, fish, eggs, and cereals and it contains little in the way of fruit, vegetables, cheese, and milk which are all alkali-producing foods. It is often prescribed as a prophylactic measure for patients with a tendency toward contracting particular types of urolithiasis. **alkali-ash d.** A diet that is alkaline in its composition. Such a diet is rich in fruit, vegetables, and milk, which are all alkaline foods. It contains minimal amounts of meat, fish, eggs, and cereals which tend to be acidic. **antiketogenic d.** A diet that is low in fat and high in carbohydrate, designed to prevent the formation of ketone bodies. **balanced d.** A diet that contains all the essential nutrients in sufficient quantities to provide for the daily needs of the body without increasing or decreasing body stores of nutrients. On such a diet a person would maintain body weight. **basal d.** A diet that provides just enough energy to meet the demands of basal metabolism. **basic d.** A diet that contains a considerable amount of alkaline ash. It is used to treat patients with certain types of urinary calculus. **bland d.** A diet intended to avoid foods that either irritate the gastrointestinal system or stimulate excess gastric-juice secretion. Such a regimen has been prescribed as suitable for patients with peptic ulcers, gastritis, irritable bowel syndrome, and certain other gastrointestinal disorders. However, no proof exists of the benefit of a bland diet compared to a regular diet in any of these conditions. **convalescent d.** A food regimen for one who is recovering from illness; a light diet. **elimination d.** A diet used to detect the cause of a food allergy. The foods commonly leading to an allergy are eliminated separately and in turn until the offending substance is identified. Diagnosis using elimination diets takes a long time, and such diets should only be used where the food sensitivity is very debilitating. Also *provocative diet.* **gluten-free d.** A diet used in the treatment of nontropical sprue (celiac disease) that excludes all gluten, which is found in wheat, rye, barley, oats, and similar grains. **gout d.** LOW PURINE DIET. **high calorie d.** A diet that provides more calories than needed to maintain body weight, often 3000–3500 calories per day. Underweight and convalescent patients would be given such a regimen. **high protein d.** A diet that contains large amounts of foods with high protein content such as meat, fish, poultry, nuts, legumes, and dairy products. Such diets contain about 20% of the total calories as protein and are prescribed for patients who are convalescing, patients with nephrotic syndrome, and patients suffering from hypoalbuminemia. **high sodium d.** A diet rich in sodium, chiefly in the form of sodium chloride (substantially more than ten grams a day). Such a diet is used mainly in treating Addison's disease, the salt-losing form of congenital adrenocortical hyperplasia, and salt-wasting nephropathy. **ketogenic d.** A diet which has been used to produce ketosis in order to control petit mal and grand mal epilepsy in children. Ketosis is induced by restriction of carbohydrate and protein with the majority of calories provided by fat. Since the diet is difficult to adhere to, it is reserved for those poorly controlled by multiple anticonvulsant drugs. It is now rarely used. **light d.** A fairly bland and easily digestible mixed diet that contains 100–120 g protein and is adequate in other nutrients. It is prescribed for convalescent medical and surgical patients. **low calorie d.** A diet that provides less energy than is required to meet the energy demands of the body and so leads to weight loss, usually a diet consisting of 1000 calories per day or less. Such diets are designed to contain all the essential nutrients in the correct proportions in order to ensure that only body fat is lost. They are usually prescribed for obese patients. **low fat d.** A diet that contains limited amounts of fat and is prescribed for obese individuals, those suffering from malabsorption states, and those with atherosclerosis. Such a diet contains no more than 20% of the dietary calories as fat. **low purine d.** A therapeutic diet used in the treatment of gout. It eliminates meat, fish, and poultry, and emphasizes dairy products, eggs, and vegetable proteins. Also *gout diet.* **low salt d.** A diet restricting sodium chloride intake. Such diets fall into three categories: mild (less than 2 g of salt per day), moderate (less than 1 g per day), and strict (less than 0.5 g per day). They are often prescribed for patients with hypertension or edema. Also *low sodium diet.* **macrobiotic d.** A diet consisting of grains and unprocessed foods. **obesity d.** REDUCING DIET. **provocative d.** ELIMINATION DIET. **rachitic d.** Any diet, usually one devoid of vitamin D and low in calcium, that leads to contraction of rickets. When given such a diet, an experimental animal will develop the deficiency disease, provided it is kept away from ultraviolet light. **reducing d.** A diet low in calories but containing all other essential nutrients in adequate quantities. It is designed to cause the loss of body weight, especially body fat. Also *obesity diet.* **salt free d.** A low-salt diet in which the patient does not add sodium chloride to his food. The only sodium chloride in the diet is that which occurs naturally in the foods. **Sippy d.** A diet for treatment (Sippy treatment or method) of peptic ulcer, no longer in use, consisting of large quantities of milk and cream administered on a careful schedule for 28 days. **smooth d.** A diet that contains very little that can act as a mechanical irritant in the gastrointestinal tract; a diet with a low content of roughage. **subsistence d.** A diet that contains all the essential nutrients in just adequate quantities (minimum dietary allowances) to sustain life.

**dietary** \dī′əter′ē\ Pertaining to or provided by a diet.

**dietetic** \dī′ətet′ik\ **1** Of or relating to diet or to dietetics. **2** Produced or adapted for use in particular types of diet: said of food products.

**dietetics** \dī′ətet′iks\ [Gk *diaitētik(ē),* fem. of *diaitētikos* pertaining to a way of living, + *s*] The study of the use of diet to maintain health and combat disease.

**diethylaminoethyl cellulose** Cellulose that has been treated in alkali with $Cl—CH_2—CH_2—NEt_2$, and hence bears $—CH_2—CH_2—NEt_2$ groups on some of its oxygen atoms. These groups are protonated below about pH 9, so that the material is an ion exchanger and is much used for the chromatography of proteins. Also *DEAE-cellulose.*

**diethylcarbamazine citrate** $C_{10}H_{21}N_3O{\cdot}C_6H_8O_7$. *N,N*-Diethyl-4-methyl-1-piperazinecarboxamide citrate. It is an effective antifilarial agent that is given orally.

**diethyl ether** $C_2H_5—O—C_2H_5$. A flammable, volatile liquid used for general inhalation anesthesia. It produces all stages of surgical anesthesia. Also *ether.*

**diethylpropion hydrochloride** $C_{13}H_{19}NO{\cdot}HCl$. 2-(Diethylamino)-1-phenyl-1-propanone hydrochloride. An adrenergic agent having a structural similarity to amphetamine and the amphetamine analogues. It is used mainly as an anorexic agent and is given orally.

**diethylstilbestrol** \dī·eth′əlstilbes′trôl\ $C_{18}H_{20}O_2$. A synthetic preparation possessing estrogenic properties. It is several times more effective than natural estrogens and may be given orally. Also *stilbestrol.* See also DES SYNDROME. Abbr. DES

**diethylstilbestrol diphosphate** A phosphate ester form of diethylstilbestrol. It is used for the same purposes and has the same properties as the parent drug. It is administered either orally or by intravenous injection.

**diethylstilboestrol** *Brit.* DIETHYLSTILBESTROL.

**diethyltoluamide** A colorless or yellowish liquid effective as an insect repellent.

**dietician** \dī′ətish′ən\ An expert in dietetics; a specialist in planning meals or diets.
**Dietl** [Jozef *Dietl,* Polish physician, 1804–1878] See under CRISIS.
**dietotherapy** \dī′ətōther′əpē\ DIET THERAPY.
**Dieulafoy** [Georges *Dieulafoy,* French physician, 1839–1911] See under ASPIRATOR, DISEASE.
**diff** difference.
**difference** / **alveolar-arterial oxygen d.** The difference between the tension of oxygen in the lung alveoli and that in the arterial blood. **cation-anion d.** ANION GAP. **interaural intensity d.** The small difference in the intensity of sound in one ear as compared with the other when the source of sound is not equidistant from both. This is considered an important phenomenon in the localization of sound. **interaural time d.** The difference in time at which an acoustic signal reaches one ear and then the other. Experimental manipulation of this parameter in the zero to three millisecond range results in a shift of the apparent location of the sound source. **just-noticeable d.** DIFFERENCE THRESHOLD. **linking d.** The difference between the number of superhelical turns present in a piece or region of DNA in a given configuration and the number of turns when the same molecule is relaxed. It is, in effect, the difference between the linking number and the relaxed linking number. Symbol: ↑
**differential** \dif′əren′shəl\ Relating to or exhibiting a difference. **nursing d.** Payment differential added to reimbursement to health care providers, usually inpatient facilities, to compensate for higher than average nursing costs attributable to one population group such as the elderly.
**differentiate** \dif′əren′shē·āt\ To increase in complexity and organization, as cells, tissues, organs, and structure during development.
**differentiated** \dif′əren′shē·ā′tid\ Exhibiting an increase in complexity and organization so that a final specialized condition has occurred: used especially of a cell, tissue, or organ during development.
**differentiation** \dif′əren′shē·ā′shən\ **1** The appearance of different characteristics in cells which were originally similar. It is a normal process in the course of embryogenesis by which the various tissues are formed (histogenesis) and also organs (organogenesis). Undifferentiated cells have the potential to become any of several different cell types, whereas differentiated cells are already committed to one cell type. **2** The transformation of general structures and of potential functions into specialized structures and functions. **3** DIFFERENTIAL DIAGNOSIS. **4** The removal of excess stain in order to give selective and clearly defined staining patterns. **dependent d.** Differentiation brought about by a stimulus acting from outside the cells or tissues, thus causing them to be determined in a way that would not otherwise have occurred. Once the stimulus has acted, however, the power of self-differentiation may be acquired. Also *correlative differentiation.* **functional d.** Differentiation that has reached the stage at which the cell or tissue starts to exhibit a specialized function. **invisible d.** The changes in a cell or group of cells resulting from chemodifferentiation, which determines their fate but without visible manifestation. **response d.** In operant conditioning, the learned differential response that comes to be made to only one stimulus among other possible stimuli as the result of positively reinforcing its occurrence, and of not rewarding or reinforcing responses made to similar, but incorrect, stimuli. **self d.** Differentiation resulting from internally generated instructions that seal the fates of the cells concerned so that they themselves differentiate along an undeviating path. **sexual d.** The process by which an embryo acquires the morphologic characteristics of its sex. At the start of development in vertebrates each embryo possesses a double assortment of genital ducts, the müllerian ducts with female potentialities and the wolffian ducts with male potentialities. Depending on the genetic sex of the embryo, one of these assortments will disappear and the genital organs will differentiate in a male or in a female direction. This differentiation is dependent on special fetal hormonal influences possibly secreted by the sex glands of the embryo.
**diffraction** \difrak′shən\ [L *diffractio* (from *diffractus,* past part. of *diffringere* to break in pieces, from DIS- + L *frangere* to break) a breaking in pieces, shattering] The modification in propagation of a wave, especially change in direction, as a result of passage by an obstacle or a heterogeneity in a medium. **x-ray d.** A technique in which the diffraction of x rays is measured as a beam of x rays focused upon molecules or crystals, providing precise information about the interatomic organization of the molecule with a resolution of about 1.5Å. Each chemical or element produces its characteristic diffraction pattern and can be identified by comparison of the pattern produced by an unknown with a standard pattern. Also *x-ray crystallography.*
**diffusate** \dif′yəsāt\ [*diffus(e)* + -ATE] After dialysis, the fraction consisting of material that has passed through the dialysis membrane and hence contains substances of relatively low molecular size.
**diffuse** \difyoos′\ [L *diffus(us),* past part. of *diffundere* to pour out or scatter, spread, disperse] Distributed broadly, and sometimes thereby diminished in intensity; spread out rather than concentrated.
**diffusible** \difyoo′zibəl\ Having the power to diffuse, usually in the context of having a low enough molecular size to diffuse through a specified membrane.
**diffusion** \difyoo′zhən\ [L *diffusio* (from *diffusus,* past part. of *diffundere* to scatter, spread, cheer) a scattering, spreading, cheering] The process whereby a substance is transported along a concentration gradient by the random movement of molecules. **alveolar capillary d.** An exchange of gas across the alveolocapillary membrane which comprises the alveolar epithelium, the interstitial space, and the capillary endothelium. **double d.** See under DOUBLE DIFFUSION TEST. **exchange d.** Movement by diffusion across a membrane, where a carrier is necessary, the carrier moving a molecule or ion into a cell at the same time it is carrying another ion or molecule out of the cell. **facilitated d.** Movement of molecules or ions across the plasma membrane, assisted by a carrier and driven by a diffusion gradient. The carrier improves the permeability of the membrane without altering the direction of movement. **free d.** The diffusion of one substance through another in the absence of an intervening membrane. **gel d.** See under GEL DIFFUSION TEST. **impeded d.** Diffusion that is restrained by an intervening membrane.
**dig.** *digeratur* (L, let it be digested).
**digallic acid** The substance formed by acylation of one molecule of gallic acid, on its O-3 atom, with another. It is found in many plant tannins, such as those of tea.
**digametic** \dī′gəmet′ik\ Capable of producing two types of gametes differing with respect to sex chromosomes. Human males are digametic, producing sperms that bear X or Y chromosomes; heterogametic.
**digastric** \dīgas′trik\ [DI-$^2$ + GASTR- + -IC ] Having two bellies, usually with reference to two fleshy parts of a muscle joined end to end by a tendon. Also *biventral, biventer.*
**Digenea** \dījē′nē·ə\ [DI-$^2$ + Gk *genea* birth, race, genera-

tion] A subclass (or order in some classifications) of parasitic flatworms of the class Trematoda, characterized by a life cycle involving a mollusk as first intermediate host, followed in most cases (excepting schistosomes) by a second intermediate transport host, then followed by the definitive or final host, a vertebrate. It includes all of the common flukes of man and other mammals.

**digenesis** \dījen′əsis\ [DI-[2] + GENESIS] Alternation of reproductive methods in different generations, as seen in the asexual cycle of trematodes in the mollusk intermediate host followed by the sexual cycle in the vertebrate host. Also *digenism.*

**digenetic** \dī′jənet′ik\ **1** Characterized by or referring to digenesis. **2** Pertaining to trematode worms of the subclass Digenea.

**digenic** \dījen′ik\ Characterized by or pertaining to digenesis.

**digenism** \dī′jənizm\ [DI-[2] + -GEN + -ISM] DIGENESIS.

**DiGeorge** [Angelo Mario *DiGeorge,* U.S. pediatrician, born 1921] See under SYNDROME.

**digest** [L *digestus,* past part. of *digerere* (from *di(s)-,* prefix indicating separation or dispersal, + *gerere* to carry, carry on, perform) to disseminate, distribute (as nutrients in the body)] **1** To break down (ingested food) into constituents from which nutrients can be absorbed. **2** To disintegrate (a substance) into simpler constituents by subjecting (that substance) to chemical action. **3** To soften (a substance) by moistening and heating. **meat d.** A culture medium prepared by enzymatic digestion of various kinds of meat. It is rich in amino acids and is widely used for cultivating fastidious pathogenic bacteria.

**digestant** \dījes′tənt\ **1** Effecting or promoting digestion. **2** An agent that promotes or stimulates digestion.

**digestion** \dījes′chən\ [L *digestio* (from *digerere* to distribute; see DIGEST) the distribution of nutrients in the body, secondary digestion (as distinguished from *concoctio* digestion in the alimentary tract)] **1** The process by which ingested food is broken down into smaller and simpler molecules suitable for absorption from the intestine. The process of digestion involves the action of gastric acid, bile, and enzymes secreted by the gastrointestinal mucosa and the pancreas. **2** The disintegration of a substance into simpler constituents by subjecting it to chemical action. **biliary d.** That component of gastrointestinal digestion in which bile is involved. **gastric d.** **1** The component of gastrointestinal digestion that takes place within the lumen of the stomach. **2** Digestion by gastric juice. **gastrointestinal d.** The process of converting food within the lumen of the gut into substances that can be absorbed and assimilated. **intestinal d.** The phase of gastrointestinal digestion that takes place within the lumen of the intestine. **pancreatic d.** **1** The phase of gastrointestinal digestion that involves the action of pancreatic juice. **2** Digestion by pancreatic juice. **primary d.** Digestion that takes place in the alimentary tract. **secondary d.** The series of metabolic processes whereby substances absorbed from the intestine are converted into nutrients that can be utilized or stored by the cells of the body. **tryptic d.** Digestion by trypsin; trypsinization.

**digestive** **1** Of or relating to digestion. **2** An agent that promotes digestion; a digestant.

**digit** \dij′it\ [L *digitus.* See DIGITUS.] **1** DIGITUS. **2** A single-character numeral. **binary d.** A character used to represent one of the two digits, either 0 or 1, in the binary number system. **sausage d.'s** Swollen digits, in which the swelling involves not only the joint capsule but the extra-articular areas, commonly seen in psoriatic arthritis.

**digital** \dij′ətəl\ **1** Pertaining to, resembling, or using a digit or digits. **2** Resembling an impression made by a finger. **3** Pertaining to data in the form of discrete states as contrasted to analog data in the form of continuously variable physical quantities.

**digitalgia paresthetica** Pain, paresthesiae, and numbness restricted to the distribution of a single digital nerve.

**digitalin** One of the main cardiotonic glycosides found in foxglove. It is a glycoside of the cardenolide 16-hydroxydigitoxygenin, as is gitoxin.

**digitalis** The dried leaf of *Digitalis purpurea,* the purple foxglove. It contains the glycosides digitoxin, gitoxin, and gitalin, which have the effect upon the heart of strengthening the force of contraction by a direct effect on the myocardium, and slowing the conduction in the auriculoventricular bundle, which prevents irregularities in the ventricular rhythm. It has been used in the treatment of congestive heart failure and accompanying edema. Poisoning can occur from an overdose of medication or from eating parts of the plant. Vomiting, diarrhea, headache, convulsions, and death may result. Commercial dried leaf preparations are standardized by biological assay. **powdered d.** A powdered preparation of digitalis leaf, standardized to produce a reliable uniformity of response. Also *prepared digitalis.*

**digitalization** \dij′itəlīzā′shən\ The administration of digitalis or one of its associated compounds in a dosage which achieves an optimal effect.

**digitaloid** Related to digitalis or resembling digitalis in its effects.

**digitate** \dij′itāt\ **1** Possessing several fingerlike processes or impressions. **2** Arranged like the fingers of the hand.

**digitation** \dij′itā′shən\ [English *digitat(e)* (from L *digitat(us)* having fingers or toes) + -ION] A fingerlike process, especially with reference to muscle attachments, such as those of musculus serratus anterior.

**digiti** \dij′itī\ Plural of DIGITUS.

**digitize** \dij′itīz\ **1** To convert analog signals into digital form. **2** To express an analog measurement in digital form.

**digitofibular** \dij′itōfib′yələr\ Pertaining to the lateral, or fibular, side of the toes.

**digitogenin** One of the sapogenins. One of its glycosides is digitonin.

**digitometatarsal** \dij′itōmet′ətär′səl\ Pertaining to the toes and the metatarsus.

**digitonide** A complex formed from digitonin and another compound, often a 3$\beta$-hydroxysteroid. It is used for precipitating and purifying the latter.

**digitonin** A saponin found in the foxglove. It consists of digitogenin glycosylated by a branched pentasaccharide. It is used in chemistry to precipitate 3$\beta$-hydroxysteroids as digitonides.

**digitoplantar** \dij′itōplan′tər\ Pertaining to the toes and the sole of the foot.

**digitoradial** \dij′itōrā′dē·əl\ Pertaining to the lateral, or radial, side of the fingers.

**digitotibial** \dij′itōtib′ē·əl\ Pertaining to the medial, or tibial, side of the toes.

**digitoulnar** \dij′itō·ul′nər\ Pertaining to the medial, or ulnar, side of the fingers.

**digitoxicity** \dig′itäksis′itē\ DIGITALIS TOXICITY.

**digitoxigenin** One of the cardenolides. It is released from digitoxin, the active principle of digitalis, by hydrolysis of the glycoside bonds.

**digitoxin** $C_{41}H_{64}O_{13}$. The major cardiotonic glycoside of digitalis. It consists of digitoxigenin and digitoxose, and its actions are similar to those of digitalis leaf preparations. It can be administered orally, intramuscularly, or intravenously.

**digitus** \dij′itəs\ [L, a finger, toe] A finger or toe. Also *digit.* **d. I** 1 HALLUX. 2 POLLEX. **d. II** 1 DIGITUS SECUNDUS. 2 INDEX. **d. III** 1 DIGITUS TERTIUS. 2 DIGITUS MEDIUS. **d. IV** 1 DIGITUS QUARTUS. 2 DIGITUS ANNULARIS. **d. V** DIGITUS MINIMUS. **d. annularis** [NA] The fourth, or ring, finger of the hand. Also *digitus quartus, digitus IV, ring finger.* **d. demonstrativus** INDEX. **d. extensus** Retraction or backward displacement of a finger. **d. malleus** MALLET FINGER. **digiti manus** [NA] The digits of the hand; the fingers. **d. medius** [NA] The middle, or third, finger. Also *digitus III, digitus tertius, middle finger.* **d. minimus** 1 [NA] The fifth, or little, finger. 2 [NA] The fifth, or smallest toe. Also *little toe.* For defs. 1 and 2 also *digitus quintus, digitus V.* **d. mortuus** WHITE FINGER. **digiti pedis** [NA] The digits of the foot; the toes. **d. postminimus** Any manifestation of a small supernumerary digit on the medial side of a fifth digit on a hand or foot. It may resemble a normal digit or consist of only a fleshy tab. **d. primus** 1 HALLUX. 2 POLLEX. **d. quartus** 1 [NA] The fourth digit of the foot. Also *digitus IV.* 2 DIGITUS ANNULARIS. **d. quintus** DIGITUS MINIMUS. **d. recellens** TRIGGER FINGER. **d. secundus** 1 [NA] The second digit, or toe, of the foot. Also *digitus II.* 2 INDEX. **d. tertius** 1 [NA] The third digit, or toe, of the foot. Also *digitus III.* 2 DIGITUS MEDIUS.

**diglossia** \dīgläs′ē·ə\ [DI-[2] + GLOSS- + -IA] BIFID TONGUE.

**diglossus** \dīgläs′əs\ [Gk *diglōssos* double-tongued] An individual with a bifid tongue.

**diglyceride** DIACYLGLYCEROL.

**dignathus** \dīnath′əs, dig·nā′thəs\ [DI-[2] + Gk *gnathos* the jaw, esp. the lower jaw] 1 An individual with cleft of the mandible. 2 A malformed fetus or newborn with a double lower jaw.

**digoxin** $C_{41}H_{64}O_{14}$. An important cardiotonic glycoside obtained from *Digitalis lanata* and occurring as colorless, odorless crystals or as a white or almost white powder with a bitter taste. It has the same actions as digitalis, and can be given orally, intramuscularly, or intravenously.

**Di Guglielmo** [Giovanni *Di Guglielmo,* Italian physician, 1886–1961] Di Guglielmo syndrome, Di Guglielmo disease. See under ERYTHROLEUKEMIA.

**diheteroxenic** \dīhet′ərōzen′ik\ [DI-[2] + *heteroxen(ous)* + -IC] Requiring two intermediate hosts: a characteristic of certain parasites.

**diheterozygote** \dīhet′ərōzī′gōt\ DOUBLE HETEROZYGOTE.

**dihybrid** \dīhī′brid\ DOUBLE HETEROZYGOTE.

**dihydrocodeine** $C_{18}H_{23}NO_3$. 6-Hydroxy-3-methoxy-*N*-methyl-4,5-epoxymorphinan. A narcotic analgesic, intermediate in activity between codeine and morphine and also used as an antitussive agent. It is generally administered as the bitartrate.

**dihydrocortisol** \dīhī′drōkôr′təsôl\ A more polar metabolic product of cortisol, having the double bond between C-4 and C-5 reduced, an intermediate step in hepatic cortisol metabolism in which the steroid is ultimately converted to tetrahydrocortisol, tetrahydrocortisone, and other polar products, which are excreted in the urine as glucuronides.

**dihydrocortisone** \dīhī′drōkôr′təsōn\ A $C_{21}$ metabolic product of cortisone having the double bond between C-4 and C-5 reduced, being an intermediate step in the hepatic pathway by which cortisol is degraded to more polar steroids, which are excreted in the urine as glucuronides.

**22,23-dihydroercalciol** VITAMIN $D_4$.

**dihydroergotamine** $C_{33}H_{37}N_5O_5$. A semisynthetic alkaloid produced from the ergot alkaloid ergotamine. It is used as an active adrenergic blocking agent in treating migraine headache.

**dihydrofolate reductase** An enzyme (EC 1.5.1.3) that catalyzes the conversion of dihydrofolate into tetrahydrofolate, using NADPH as hydrogen donor. Since dihydrofolate is produced in thymidylate biosynthesis for DNA formation, this enzyme is particularly necessary in rapidly proliferating tissue, such as some tumors, and its inhibitors are used in cancer chemotherapy.

**dihydrofolic acid** Any of the folic acids in which the pyrazine ring is in the dihydro form. To function as an acceptor of formyl, hydroxymethyl, etc., groups, this ring must be in the tetrahydro form, but transfer of a one-carbon moiety to form the 5-methyl group of thymidylate for DNA synthesis leaves the carrier in the dihydro form. It requires reduction, by dihydrofolate reductase, before it can function again.

**dihydrofolliculin** \dīhī′drōfälik′yəlin\ *Older term* ESTRADIOL.

**dihydrolipoamide acetyltransferase** The component (EC 2.3.1.12) of the pyruvate dehydrogenase complex that catalyzes reaction of a 1-hydroxyethyl group attached to thiamine diphosphate of another component of the complex to form *S*-acetyldihydrolipoyl groups. It also catalyzes transfer of acetyl groups between its own dihidrolipoyl groups and coenzyme A. Also *dihydrolipoyl transacetylase.*

**dihydrolipoamide dehydrogenase** A flavoprotein component (EC 1.6.4.3) of the 2-oxoacid dehydrogenase complexes. It acts on the dihydrolipoyl groups present as substituents on lysine residues of another component of the complex, after the acyl group derived by decarboxylation of the substrate has been transferred from them to coenzyme A, and it thus prepares these groups for a further round of reductive acylation. By removing the hydrogen atoms from the two thiol groups, it forms a 6,8-disulfide bond in a five-membered ring, and $NAD^+$is concurrently reduced to NADH. Also *dihydrolipoate dehydrogenase, lipoamide reductase.*

**dihydrolipoic acid** HS—$CH_2$—$CH_2$—CH(SH)—$[CH_2]_4$—COOH. 6,8-Dimercaptooctanoic acid, the reduced form of lipoic acid.

**dihydrolipoyl transacetylase** DIHYDROLIPOAMIDE ACETYLTRANSFERASE.

**dihydrostreptomycin** \dīhī′drōstrep′təmī′sin\ A derivative of streptomycin, no longer used because of its marked ototoxicity.

**dihydrotachysterol** $C_{28}H_{46}O$. 9,10-Secoergostra-5,7,22-trien-3$\beta$-ol, a reduced form of tachysterol that is used to raise calcium levels in the blood in conditions such as tetany. It is administered orally.

**dihydrotestosterone** \dīhī′drōtestäs′terōn\ A $C_{19}$ androgenic hormone formed through the action of the enzyme 5$\alpha$-reductase from testosterone in tissues, particularly those of the secondary sex organs. It is a potent androgen and may be the essential or intimate androgen which is the biologically active form of testosterone except in muscle and bone.

**dihydrouridine** \dīhī′drōyoor′idin\ A nucleoside found in tRNA and not present in mRNA, formed by a modification of uridine. It is a rare base.

**dihydroxyacetone** $CH_2OH$—CO—$CH_2OH$. A highly reactive ketone that normally exists as a dimer when pure, and is largely hydrated in water. It is the simplest ketose. Its phosphate is an intermediate in glycolysis. Also *glycerone.*

**dihydroxyacetone phosphate** HO—$CH_2$—CO—$CH_2$—O—$PO_3H_2$. An intermediate in glycolysis, in the utilization of glycerol, and in some other metabolic pathways. It is a substrate of the enzyme aldolase. Also *phosphodihydroxyacetone.*

**dihydroxyaluminum aminoacetate** $C_2H_6AlNO_4 \cdot xH_2O$. A basic aluminum salt of glycine occurring as a white powder. It is used as a gastric antacid in the form of tablets or as a magma. Also *aluminum aminoacetate, aluminum glycinate.*

**dihydroxyaluminum sodium carbonate** $CH_2AlNaO_5$. An aluminum salt of sodium carbonate that is used as an antacid.

**1,25-dihydroxycholecalciferol** The most active form known of vitamin D. It is a metabolic product, elaborated in the kidney, of 25-hydroxycholecalciferol. It is 300–1000 times more potent than cholecalciferol and stimulates the absorption of dietary calcium through the intestinal wall. Also *calcitriol.*

**dihydroxyestrin** *Older term* ESTRADIOL.

**3,4-dihydroxyphenylalanine** A systematic name for dopa.

**dihydroxyphenylpyruvic acid** A metabolite of dopa, formed by transamination.

**dihysteria** \dī′histir′ē·ə\ UTERUS DIDELPHYS.

**diiodohydroxyquin** $C_9H_5I_2NO$. 5,7-Diiodo-8-quinolinol. A therapeutic agent used, usually in conjunction with other agents such as chloroquine, tetracycline, or emetine, in the treatment of amebic colitis and amebic liver abscess. Gastrointestinal irritation and headaches are troublesome side-effects. It has largely been replaced by metronidazole and tinidazole. Also *iodoquinol.*

**diiodomethane** METHYLENE IODIDE.

**diiodophenylaminopropionic acid** DIIODOTYROSINE.

**diiodosalicylic acid** $C_7H_4I_2O_3$. 2-Hydroxy-3,5-diiodobenzoic acid. A colorless or slightly yellow, crystalline powder, used as a source of iodine, and in animal feeds to promote growth.

**diiodotyrosine** 2-Amino-3-(3,5-diiodo4-hydroxyphenyl)propionic acid. An intrathyroidal precursor of thyroxine and triiodothyronine. It is thought to be synthesized through the iodination of monoiodotyrosine. It is released into the circulation in excessive concentrations in certain cases of goitrous cretinism with inborn errors of thyroid hormone biosynthesis. Also *di-iodophenylaminoproprionic acid, iodogorgoic acid* (seldom used in the U.S.). Abbr. DIT

**diisopropyl fluorophosphate** $(Me_2CH—)_2P(=O)F$. A compound used as a long-acting cholinesterase inactivator in the treatment of glaucoma, and also to inhibit serine proteinases. It binds to their active centers and there phosphorylates the serine residue that is transiently acylated during the action of the enzyme. It is highly toxic because of its action on cholinergic nerves. Also *isoflurophate, diisopropyl phosphorofluoridate.* Abbr. DFP

**diisopropyl phosphorofluoridate** DIISOPROPYL FLUOROPHOSPHATE.

**diketopiperazine** The cyclic dipeptide formed from glycine or, by substitution of its methylene groups, any cyclic dipeptide.

**diktyoma** \dik′tē·ō′mə\ [Gk *diktyo(n)* a net (representing *retina*) + -OMA] MEDULLOEPITHELIOMA.

**dikwakwadi** \dik′wəkwä′dē\ A South African Bantu word for FAVUS.

**dil.** *dilue* (L, dilute or dissolve).

**dilaceration** \dī′lasərā′shən\ An abrupt bend of a tooth root caused by injury during formation.

**dilatancy** \dīlā′tənsē\ The property of certain gels, such as cytoplasm, of becoming solid when placed under pressure, i.e., of having viscosity increase as pressure increases.

**dilatation** \dil′ətā′shən\ [Late L *dilatatio* (from *dilatare* to extend, dilate, from *di(s)-* apart + L *latus* wide, large) expansion] **1** An enlargement or stretching of something beyond its normal size or extent, as an organ or vessel. **2** The condition of being dilated; an enlarged or distended state. For defs. 1 and 2 also *dilation.* **balloon d.** BALLOON ANGIOPLASTY. **d. of cervix** The opening up or stretching open of the uterine cervix. This may occur spontaneously, as in labor or spontaneous abortion, or may be brought about by medication or instruments. **d. and curettage** See under DILATATION AND CURETTAGE. **d. of the heart** Enlargement of the chambers of the heart. Also *cardiectasis.* **intraluminal d.** A technique to relieve arterial or venous stenoses by passage of dilating devices of metal or plastic, or inflatable balloons, through the arterial occlusions. **post-stenotic d.** Dilatation of a vessel or chamber of the heart distal to an area of stenosis. It is most commonly seen in association with valvular aortic or pulmonary stenosis. **supradiaphragmatic esophageal d.** PHRENIC AMPULLA.

**dilatation and curettage** \dil′ətā′shən\ Surgical dilatation of the cervix and curettage of the uterus for the diagnosis and treatment of pathologic conditions of the uterus and to terminate a pregnancy. Abbr. D and C

**dilatation and evacuation** \dil′ətā′shən\ A modification of the suction curettage method of abortion in which pregnancies in the second trimester are terminated by means of aspiration cannulae and forceps for removal of the products of conception. Abbr. D and E

**dilatator** \dil′ətā′tər\ DILATOR.

**dilate** \dī′lāt\ [L *dilat(are)* (from *dis-* apart + *latus* wide, large) to dilate, extend] To make or become wider or larger; expand in size or dimensions.

**dilation** \dīlā′shən\ **1** The act or action of dilating. **2** DILATATION.

**dilator** \dī′lātər\ **1** Something acting to dilate: said especially of certain muscles that widen, enlarge, or open parts, specifically blood vessels, canals, cavities, and orifices. **2** An agent inducing the dilatation of a structure or part, as the pupil or blood vessels. **3** A surgical instrument used to dilate an opening, cavity, or lumen. For defs. 1, 2, and 3 also *dilatator.* **Hegar's d.'s** Tapered, graduated metal dilators used for dilating the uterine cervix. **Kollmann's d.** An expandable device used to dilate the urethra. **laryngeal d.** Any of various instruments for dilating the narrowed laryngeal lumen in cases of laryngeal stenosis. **Mixter d.** A combined dilator, probe, and cannula made of metal and with a syringe fitting, used for common bile duct exploration. **Mosher d.** **1** An inflatable rubber bag on a flexible catheter, with an inflation system, used for treatment of esophageal achalasia by dilatation and divulsion. **2** A laryngeal cannula/dilator for use in upper airway obstruction. **Negus hydrostatic d.** A modification of the Tucker dilatable bag designed to be passed over a fine bougie introduced into the esophagus as a guide. **Plummer's d.** A pneumatically inflated esophageal dilator. **Starck d.** An expandable rubber-covered metal frame used to dilate the cardioesophageal junction in cardiospasm. **tracheal d.** An instrument for dilating the track through the soft tissues of the neck, in cases of tracheostomy, prior to introducing the tracheostomy tube or, in an emergency, if the tube is obstructed, to maintain the airway until another is introduced. **Tubbs d.** An instrument with separating blades that is used to dilate a stenosed mitral valve. It is passed through the wall of the left ventricle and directed into the valve orifice.

**diloxanide furoate** $C_{14}H_{11}Cl_2NO_4$. 4-(*N*-Methyl-2,2-dichloroacetamido)phenyl 2-furoate, a white crystalline powder that is used alone or in combination with other drugs to treat intestinal amebiasis.

**diluc.** *diluculo* (L, at daybreak).

**diluent** \dil′yoo·ənt\ The substance with which another is diluted.

**dilut.** *dilutus* (L, diluted).

**dilute** \diloot′, dī′loot\ [L *dilutus,* past part. of *diluere* (from *di(s)-* apart, away + *-luere,* combining stem of *lavare* to wash) to wash away, dissolve, dilute] **1** To lower the concentration of a substance, usually one in solution, by adding solvent. **2** Having a low concentration.

**dilution** [See DILUTE.] The process of decreasing the concentration of a solution by addition of water or another suitable solvent. **doubling d.** A serial dilution in which each aliquot is added to an equal volume of diluent. The concentration in each specimen is one half that of the preceding specimen. **isotope d.** Determination of the amount of a substance in a sample by adding to it a known amount of the same substance, isotopically labeled to an accurately known extent. The substance is then reisolated from the mixture. Its degree of isotopic labeling reflects the dilution of the added specimen by the material previously present. The advantage is that the method is independent of any losses during isolation. Isotope dilution can be applied to the determination of the volume of body compartments by administering a known quantity of isotope that will diffuse uniformly into the compartment being tested. The concentration of isotope in a specimen obtained after diffusion is complete permits calculation of the volume in which the isotope is diluted. **serial d.** A technique that dilutes an added material by a consistent factor in each of a series of tubes of diluent. **triple isotope d.** A technique for measuring three body compartments (vascular space, extracellular space, and total body water). Radionuclides with differing emitted radiations are labeled onto molecules that distribute selectively to the three compartments. After equilibration they can then be simultaneously measured.

**dim.** *dimidius* (L, one half).

***Dimastigamoeba*** \dimas′tigəmē′bə\ [DI-$^2$ + Gk *mastix,* gen. *mastigos,* a whip + AMOEBA] *NAEGLERIA.*

**dimefox** \dīmef′äks\ $C_4H_{12}FN_2OP$. Bis-(dimethylamino)-fluorophosphine oxide. A liquid with a fishy odor, prepared by fluorination of bis(dimethylamido)-phosphoryl chloride. It is a highly toxic cholinesterase inhibitor, used as a systemic insecticide.

**dimelia** \dīmē′lyə\ [DI-$^2$ + MEL-$^1$ + -IA] The duplication of all or a substantial part of a limb.

**dimenhydrinate** $C_{23}H_{28}ClN_5O_3$. 8-Chloro-3,7-dihydro-1,3-dimethyl-1*H*-purine-2,6-dione compounded with 2-(diphenylmethoxy)-*N,N*-dimethyl-ethanamine (1:1). An antihistaminic drug used primarily to prevent motion sickness and vomiting in pregnancy.

**dimension** [L *dimensio* (from *dimensus,* past part. of *dimetiri* to measure) a measuring] **1** An aspect of the spatial extent of an object, as length, width, or height. **2** Any of a small set of physical quantities regarded as fundamental measures in the sense that any physical quantity can be expressed as a product of powers of members of the set. The choice of members of the set, and even the number of members, is somewhat arbitrary, but mass, length, and time are often regarded as members of the set.

**dimer** \dī′mər\ [DI-$^2$ + Gk *mer(os)* a part] A compound resulting from the combination of two like molecules, in a strict sense without loss of atoms. Thus the dimer has twice the molecular weight of the single units (monomers). Adj. dimeric. **UV-induced d.** THYMINE DIMER. See under THYMINE.

**dimercaprol** $C_3H_8OS_2$. 2,3-Dimercaptopropanol. A colorless liquid with an unpleasant, mercaptan odor. It is a chelating agent developed as an antidote for lewisite, a war gas. As such, it acts by its affinity for the metal arsenic, which combines with it rather than with the SH groups of cell protein, forming a stable, nontoxic compound. It is also used as an antidote for poisoning by other metals, such as mercury, antimony, nickel, chromium, and bismuth, although it is relatively ineffective against lead. Also *antilewisite, British antilewisite.*

**dimethicone** A silicone oil used in protective creams and ointments as a barrier against industrial skin irritants and against the effects of ammonia in urine, as in infants and bed-ridden patients.

**dimethisoquin hydrochloride** $C_{17}H_{24}N_2O{\cdot}HCl$. 3-Butyl-1-[2-(dimethylamino)ethoxy]isoquinoline hydrochloride. A surface anesthetic agent used topically for the relief of itching, irritation, and mild sunburn.

**dimethisterone** $C_{23}H_{32}O_2$. 17$\alpha$-Hydroxy-6$\beta$-methyl-17-(1-propynyl)androst-4-en-3-one. A progestational agent effective when given orally. It is also used in combination with ethinyl estradiol as an oral contraceptive agent, and has been used to treat amenorrhea.

**dimethoxanate hydrochloride** $C_{19}H_{22}N_2O_3S{\cdot}HCl$. 10*H*-Phenothiazine-10-carboxylic acid 2-[2-(dimethylamino)ethoxy]ethyl ester hydrochloride, an agent with local anesthetic properties and value as an antitussive medication. It is given orally.

**dimethoxyphenyl penicillin sodium** METHICILLIN SODIUM.

**dimethylamine** $(CH_3)_2NH$. A colorless gas used in tanning, rubber, and soap industries. It occurs in decomposing nitrogenous matter, especially fish. At low concentrations in the air, it is readily recognized by a fishy odor. At high concentrations, it is difficult to distinguish from ammonia. It causes irritation of the nose and throat followed by coughing, sneezing, constriction of the larynx, difficulty in breathing, and pulmonary congestion and edema.

**5,6-dimethylbenzimidazole** $C_9H_{10}N_2$. Benzimidazole with two methyl substituents of the benzene ring. It is found, combined with ribose 5-phosphate as a nucleotide analogue, in vitamin $B_{12}$.

**dimethylmorphine** THEBAINE.

**dimethylnitrosamine** $C_2H_6N_2O$. A chemical used in industry as a solvent. It is formed by the interaction of nitrite with primary and secondary amines and by the action of nitrate-producing bacteria. It has been found in trace amounts in tobacco smoke condensates, in cured meat products, and in smoked and salted fish. It produces severe liver damage in the form of centrilobular necrosis in man and animals and is carcinogenic in animals.

**dimethylphenylpiperazinium** An experimental drug which has the effect of stimulating autonomic ganglia. Abbr. DMPP

**dimethyl phthalate** Phthalic acid esterified with methanol on both its carboxyl groups. It is often applied to the skin as an insect repellent.

**dimethyl sulfoxide** $Me_2SO$. A polar aprotic solvent, also used as a chemical reagent. It penetrates the skin and may carry solutes with it. Abbr. DMSO

**dimethyltubocurarine iodide** METOCURINE IODIDE.

**dimetria** \dīmē′trē·ə\ [DI-[2] + METR- + -IA] Any of several degrees of duplication of the uterine body or lumen. See also UTERUS DIDELPHYS, UTERUS BICORNIS.

**Dimitri** [Vincente *Dimitri,* Austrian-born Argentinian neurologist, 1885–1955] Dimitri's disease, Weber-Dimitri disease, Sturge-Weber-Dimitri disease. See under STURGE-WEBER SYNDROME.

**Dimmer** [Friedrich *Dimmer,* Austrian ophthalmologist, 1855–1926] Dimmer's keratitis. See under KERATITIS NUMMULARIS.

**dimorphism** \dīmôr′fizm\ [DI-[2] + MORPH- + -ISM] The condition of existing in two more or less distinct structural forms, each form possessing characteristic anatomical and other features. Adj. dimorphic. **physical d.** The property of a single compound existing in two different crystalline forms. **sexual d.** Exhibition within a species of anatomic, morphologic, endocrinologic, and behavioral differences between the male and female forms, whether haploid or diploid.

**dimorphobiotic** \dīmôr′fōbī·ät′ik\ [DI-[2] + MORPHO- + BIOTIC] Characterized by a regular alternation of parasitic and nonparasitic phases, as in the life cycle of gordian or horsehair worms (phylum Nematomorpha).

**dimoxyline phosphate** DIOXYLINE PHOSPHATE.

**dimple** A small depression of the skin. **anal d.** A cutaneous depression at the normal site of the anal orifice, seen in newborn infants with anal atresia. **Fuchs d.'s** DELLEN. **postanal d.** FOVEOLA COCCYGEA. **sacrococcygeal d.** A depression in the skin over the sacrococcygeal region, devoid of hair follicles and present at birth. Also *sacral bald spot.*

**dinitroaminophenol** PICRAMIC ACID.

**dinitrochlorobenzene** DICHLORONITROBENZENE.

**dinitro-*o*-cresol** $CH_3C_6H_2(NO_2)_2OH$. A compound used as a pesticide and fungicide. It is a homologue of dinitrophenol, but much more toxic. Mild poisoning causes lassitude, headache, and night sweats with weight loss. Acute poisoning is characterized by dyspnea and painful constriction of the chest. Its potentially lethal effects are due to interference with temperature regulation. Abbr. DNOC

**dinitrogen** $N_2$. The element nitrogen in its diatomic molecular form, in distinction from occurrence as free atoms or in combination with other elements.

**dinitrogen monoxide** NITROUS OXIDE.

**2,4-dinitrophenol** A compound frequently used an an uncoupler between oxidation and phosphorylation by mitochondria. It appears to act by discharging the gradient of hydrogen ions across the membrane, because both its protonated and deprotonated forms can pass through biologic membranes. It has a p$K$ of 4 and gives a yellow, quinonoid anion. It was once used as a slimming agent but is highly toxic and should not be consumed.

**Dinoflagellata** \dī′nōflaj′əlā′tə\ DINOFLAGELLIDA.

**dinoflagellate** \dī′nōflaj′əlāt\ [See DINOFLAGELLIDA.] A member of the order Dinoflagellida.

**Dinoflagellida** \dī′nōflajel′idə\ [Gk *dino(s)* a whirl, whirling + *flagell(um)* + *-ida,* suffix designating a taxonomic order] An order of protozoans of the phylum Sarcomastigophorea, marked by two heterodynamic flagella, complex cellulosic plates, and a unique nucleus with chromosomes of non-protein-complexed DNA. It includes aquatic microorganisms that are important in the food chain, such as *Ceratium, Gymnodinium,* and *Prorocentrum.* It also includes *Gonyaulax,* which is responsible for the red tide appearing periodically in marine waters and highly toxic to fish and other organisms. Also *Dinoflagellata.*

**d. in p. aeq.** *divide in partes aequales* (L, divide into equal parts): a direction used in prescription writing.

**dinucleotide** A substance formed by the linkage of two nucleotide molecules, either by ester combination between the phosphate group of one and a sugar hydroxyl group of the other, forming a phosphodiester link, or by combination of the two phospho groups to form a residue of diphosphoric acid. The first form may be a fragment of a nucleic acid molecule. Many coenzymes are dinucleotides of the second kind.

***Dioctophyma renale*** The largest of the nematodes; the giant kidney worm. It is found in dogs, foxes, wolves, and mink, but also reported in pigs, cattle, horses, and, rarely, in humans. Bright red in color and 35 cm (males) to over 100 cm (females) in length, these worms are usually found in the kidney but sometimes in the peritoneal cavity. It gradually destroys the kidney and may cause death of the host. The life cycle is via infected oligochaete worms and possibly one or several transport hosts. Also *Eustrongylus gigas, Eustrongylus visceralis, Strongylus gigas, Strongylus renalis.*

**diode** \dī′ōd\ [Gk *diodos* (from *di(a)* through + *(h)odos* way) a passage] A vacuum-tube or semiconducting device that permits the passage of current in one direction only and is used as a rectifier. **light-emitting d.** An electronic component that emits light when current passes through it. The common red type provides the readout for pocket calculators, but green and yellow types exist.

**Diodrast** A proprietary name for iodopyracet.

**dioecious** \dī·ē′shəs\ DIECIOUS.

**Diogenes** [*Diogenes,* Greek philosopher, 412–323 B.C.] See under SYNDROME.

**diopter** \dī·äp′tər\ [Gk *dioptēr* or *dioptra* (from *di(a)-* through, across + *-opt-* sight + *-t(ē)r,* instrumental suffix) any of several kinds of optical instrument; as a measure of lens power, back-formation from *dioptric*] A measure of the power of a lens, equal to the reciprocal of its focal length in meters. A converging lens is taken as positive, a diverging lens as negative. Also *dioptre, dioptry.* Abbr. D **prism d.** A unit used in measuring the deviating power of a prism. This power in prism diopters is 100 times the tangent of the angle of deviation of a ray of light. One prism diopter equals a deviation of one centimeter at one meter.

**dioptometry** \dī′äptäm′ətrē\ [DI-[3] + OPTO- + -METRY] Measurement of the refractive error of an eye by an optical device capable of determining the vergence of light rays.

**dioptre** \dī·äp′tər\ *Brit.* DIOPTER.

**dioptric** \dī·äp′trik\ [Gk *dioptrik(os)* (from *dioptr(a)* an instrument for taking levels and altitudes + *-ikos* -IC) pertaining to a diopter] Relating to the refraction of light by transmission, especially to the refractive strength of a lens as measured in diopters.

**dioptrics** \dī·äp′triks\ [DIOPTRIC + *s*] The science of the refraction of light by transmission.

**dioptry** \dī′äptrē\ DIOPTER.

**diovulatory** \dī·äv′yələtôr′ē\ [DI-[2] + OVULATORY] Discharging two ova from the ovary during a menstrual cycle.

**dioxin** \dī·äk′sin\ 2,3,7,8-Tetrachlorodibenzo-*p*-dioxin. A toxic chlorinated hydrocarbon formed at incineration sites at high temperatures from chlorine and hydrocarbon raw materials. It is also present as a contaminant in the preparation of 2,4,5-T, a well-known and widely used herbicide. Dioxin is a potent mutagen, teratogen, and carcinogen in laboratory animals. Evidence of adverse effects in man is largely from exposure in the workplace, causing chloracne, peripheral neuropathy, enlargement of the liver, and enzyme induction. There is no reliable evidence that dioxin is carcinogenic, teratogenic, or mutagenic in humans.

**dioxygenase** Any enzyme that catalyzes the oxidation

of a substrate by molecular oxygen (dioxygen) with the incorporation of both atoms of the oxygen into the substrate. Most dioxygenases that have been characterized contain iron and some also contain copper. An example is the enzyme that converts homogentisate into 4-maleylacetoacetate in the catabolism of tyrosine. This enzyme appears also to require ascorbic acid for optimal activity.

**dioxyline phosphate** $C_{22}H_{25}NO_4{\cdot}H_3PO_4$. 1-(4-Ethoxy-3-methoxybenzyl)-6,7-dimethoxy-3-methylesoquinoline dihydrogen phosphate, a synthetic agent like papaverine with similar pharmacologic properties. It is used as a vasodilator to reduce vascular spasm in conditions such as myocardial infarction, peripheral vascular diseases, and angina pectoris. It is given orally. Also *dimoxyline phosphate.*

**dipeptidase** Any enzyme that catalyzes the hydrolysis of a dipeptide to amino acids.

**dipeptide** A substance whose molecules consist of two amino-acid residues joined in peptide (amide) linkage. When the bond is between C-1 of one residue and N-2 of another, as it usually is, the dipeptide has the structure $NH_3^+$—CHR—CO—NH—CHR′—$COO^-$. Dipeptides are formed in the digestion of proteins.

***Dipetalonema*** \dīpet′əlōnē′mə\ [Gk *di-* twice + *petalo(n)* a leaf + *nēma* thread, tissue] A genus of filarial worms in the family Onchocercidae consisting of about 50 species. Adult worms live in connective tissue, membranes, or visceral surfaces and produce unsheathed microfilariae in blood or tissues. Several human parasites formerly classified as *Dipetalonema (D. perstans, D. streptocerca)* are now considered species of *Mansonella.*

**diphallia** \dīfal′yə\ [DI-[2] + PHALL- + -IA ] The partial or complete duplication of the penis in either the transverse or sagittal plane. Also *cleft penis.*

**diphasic** \dīfā′zik\ Occurring in or including two phases.

**diphebuzol** PHENYLBUTAZONE.

**diphemanil methylsulfate** $C_{21}H_{27}NO_4S$. 4-(Diphenylmethylene)-1,1-dimethylpiperidinium methylsulfate, a quaternary ammonium compound with pronounced anticholinergic activity. It is used to treat peptic ulcers and gastric hypermotility and hyperacidity, and it is employed to relieve pylorospasm. It is given orally.

**diphenadione** $C_{23}H_{16}O_3$. 2-(Diphenylacetyl)-*H*-indene-1,3(2*H*)-dione. An anticoagulant of the indanedione type. It is administered orally.

**diphenhydramine hydrochloride** $C_{17}H_{22}ClNO$. 2-Diphenylmethoxy-*N,N*-dimethylethanamine hydrochloride. An antihistaminic drug used for the treatment of allergic disorders. It can be given orally, intramuscularly, and intravenously. It is also used to prevent motion sickness. Also *benzhydramine hydrochloride.*

**diphenylaminearsine chloride** $NH(C_6H_4)_2AsCl$. A war gas that causes profuse watery nasal discharge, severe pain in the nose, sinuses, and chest, and coughing, sneezing, depression, and weakness. Also *adamsite.*

**diphenylchlorarsine** $(C_6H_5)_2AsCl$. A sternutator. It causes violent sneezing, coughing, headache, and retrosternal pain. Also *sneezing gas.*

**diphenylhydantoin** PHENYTOIN.

**diphenylhydantoin sodium** PHENYTOIN SODIUM.

**diphenylpyraline hydrochloride** $C_{19}H_{24}ClNO$. 4-(Diphenylmethoxy)-1-methylpiperidine hydrochloride, an antihistaminic agent of relatively short duration of action and less sedation than the phenothiazines. It is given orally for allergic conditions.

**diphosgene** \dīfäs′jēn\ $ClCOOCCl_3$. A gas which produces severe choking, lung irritation, and pulmonary edema. It was used in World War I as a poison gas. Also *perchloromethylformate, trichloromethylchloroformate.*

**diphosphate** Any anion, salt, or ester of diphosphoric acid, $(HO—)_2P(=O)—O—P(=O)(—OH)_2$. This substance is formed in many biologic reactions, such as nucleic acid synthesis, which are effectively rendered irreversible by the subsequent hydrolysis of the diphosphate formed. Also *pyrophosphate.* • The symbol $PP_i$ is used for salts of the uncombined acid, and the symbol *P—O—P* (shortened to *PP*) may be used for them whether free or combined.

**diphosphopyridine nucleotide** *Obs.* NICOTINAMIDE ADENINE DINUCLEOTIDE. Symbol: DPN

**diphthamide** \dif′thəmīd\ A modified histidine residue in eukaryotic protein elongation factor $EF_2$, which can be ADP-ribosylated by enzymatic action of diphtheria toxin.

**diphtheria** \difthir′ē·ə\ [French *dipht(h)érie*, from earlier *diphthérite* (from Gk *diphtheritis* clad in leather, from *diphther(a)* a piece of leather + *-itis*, fem. adjectival suffix) membranous inflammation, diphtheria] An acute infection caused by virulent strains of the *Corynebacterium diphtheriae,* commonly of the fauces but also of the larynx, trachea, nose, conjunctiva, vagina, and wounds of the skin. The local lesion is characteristic, and consists of a dense whitish gray membrane, made up of necrotic tissue, fibrin, and bacteria. When present in the larynx and trachea, this may produce asphyxia. The gravity of the infection is related not only to its locality but also to the production of an exotoxin which diffuses widely and threatens the subjects with the complications of myocarditis and cranial and peripheral neuritis. Past pandemics have been responsible for widespread mortality and morbidity, and although the disease has almost disappeared in many parts of the world, it remains endemic and still epidemic in many underprivileged areas. The widespread use of preventive immunization has contributed greatly to its declining incidence, and its treatment with penicillin to its diminished mortality. Antitoxin remains essential, however, to neutralize the toxin. Also *diphtheritis, morbus strangulatorius.* Adj. diphtherial, diphtheritic. **cutaneous d.** Infection of the skin by *Corynebacterium diphtheriae,* usually resulting in ulcerations with raised edges. The bacillus may also infect surgical wounds and chronic skin lesions or ulcers. **faucial d.** Diphtheria as it affects the fauces, the usual site of the disease. Appearing first on the tonsils, the characteristic membrane spreads frequently onto the soft palate and uvula. **d. gravis** Diphtheria caused by the *gravis* strain of *Corynebacterium diphtheriae* and therefore, if not promptly treated with antitoxin, likely to be complicated by myocarditis or peripheral neuritis. **laryngeal d.** Diphtheria as it affects the larynx. Diphtheria, first appearing on the tonsils, spreads to involve the larynx in about one case in four. This introduces a new element of special gravity, inasmuch as the characteristic membrane, spreading on to the vocal cords, obstructs the laryngeal airway and threatens the patient with asphyxia, often demanding urgent intubation or tracheostomy. In children, it produces hoarseness and a crouplike cough. Also *diphtheritic laryngitis, diphtheritic croup, pseudomembranous croup* (older term). **malignant d.** A fulminating form of diphtheria, described during the great outbreaks of the nineteenth century. Stiffness, headache, vomiting, petechial hemorrhages, and epistaxis were among the features which usually preceded collapse and a fatal outcome. **nasal d.** Rhinitis, usually unilateral, caused by *Corynebacterium diphtheriae,* occurring either as a primary infection or spreading to the nose from the fauces. It is usually an acute disease with the general features of diphtheria, but a chronic form, running a benign course with spontaneous recovery, occurs rarely. **pharyngeal d.** Diphtheria involving the pharynx or fauces, the usual site.

Also *Bretonneau's disease, Bretonneau's angina, angina diphtheritica.* **scarlatinal d.** Diphtheria occurring in conjunction with scarlet fever. **septic d.** Severe diphtheria where the classical symptoms and signs are altered by superinfection with pyogenic organisms, particularly *Streptococcus pyogenes.* **surgical d.** Diphtheria acquired by infection of a surgical wound. See also WOUND DIPHTHERIA. **wound d.** *Corynebacterium diphtheriae* infection of wounds, sores, or cuts. A pseudomembrane may form over a wound's surface.

**diphtherial** \difthir′ē·əl\ Pertaining to diphtheria or marked by its presence.

**diphtheric** \difthir′ik\ DIPHTHERITIC.

**diphtherin** \dif′thirin\ A diphtheria antigen used in skin testing.

**diphtheritic** \dif′thirit′ik\ Pertaining to or resembling diphtheria. Also *diphtheric.*

**diphtheritis** \dif′thirī′tis\ DIPHTHERIA.

**diphtheroid** \dif′thiroid\ **1** Similar to diphtheria or to the diphtheria bacillus. **2** Any corynebacterium other than *Corynebacterium diphtheriae.*

**diphtherotoxin** \dif′thirōtäk′sin\ DIPHTHERIA TOXIN.

**diphthong** \dif′thäng\ [Gk *diphthong(os)* (from *di(s)* twice + *phthongos* the voice, from *phthengesthai* to utter a sound) diphthong] A pair of vowel sounds uttered in rapid squence and perceived as one within a single syllable, as the vowel sound of *might* (aɪ).

**diphthongia** \difthän′jē·ə\ DIPLOPHONIA.

**diphyllobothriasis** \dīfil′ōbäthrī′əsis\ Infection with or the disease caused by the broad fish tapeworm of man, *Diphyllobothrium latum.* Human infection is acquired by ingestion of raw or undercooked fish infected with the plerocercoid larvae. In rare instances, a form of microcytic anemia may develop through differential absorption of vitamin $B_{12}$. Also *fish-tapeworm disease, dibothriocephaliasis.*

***Diphyllobothrium*** \dīfil′ōbäth′rē·əm\ [DI-[2] + PHYLLO- + BOTHRIUM] A genus of large tapeworms of the family Diphyllobothriidae, order Pseudophyllidea. Various fishes, such as trout and salmon are the adult hosts and copepods are the intermediate hosts. The larvae of some species can cause serious damage to the adult host during their migratory phase. Only *D. latum* is of widespread medical importance. The others reported from humans are of doubtful taxonomic validity. Also *Dibothriocephalus.* ***D. latum*** The broad fish tapeworm, common in humans and other fish-eating mammals in northern Europe, Japan, other parts of Asia, and in the north central United States. It can grow to 10 meters or more in length, with several thousand segments which usually are broader than long. The scolex is characterized by two sucking grooves, known as bothria, rather than the round suckers characteristic of cyclophyllidean tapeworms. Man acquires the infection through ingestion of raw or undercooked fresh-water fish that are infected from copepods that eat the motile larvae hatched from eggs passed into water by the infected final host. Also *Dibothriocephalus latus.* ***D. mansoni*** *SPIROMETRA MANSONI.* ***D. mansonoides*** *SPIROMETRA MANSONOIDES.*

**diphyodont** \dif′ē·ōdänt′\ [DI-[2] + Gk *phy(ein)* to produce, make to grow + -ODONT] Having two successive sets of dentitions, one deciduous and one permanent, as in man and most other mammalian species.

**dipl-** \dipl-\ DIPLO-.

**diplacusis** \dip′ləkoo′sis\ [DIPL- + -ACUSIS] The sensation of hearing two tones following the exhibition of a single tone. The sounds may be heard in one or both ears. The phenomenon is associated with cochlear dysfunction. Also *double hearing.* **binaural d.** Diplacusis in which the tone is heard differently in each ear. **disharmonic d.** Binaural diplacusis in which the subject hears a difference in the pitch of a note played in each ear. Also *double disharmonic hearing.* **monaural d.** A form of diplacusis in which the subject hears two tones in one ear when only one tone has been emitted.

**diplastic** \dīplas′tik\ [DI-[2] + PLASTIC] Capable of differentiating along either of two possible developmental pathways: said of a cell or tissue.

**diplegia** \dīplē′jə\ [DI-[2] + -PLEGIA] Any homonymous bilateral paralysis, such as double hemiplegia, paralysis of the upper or lower limbs (paraplegia), or bilateral facial paralysis (facial diplegia). The term is most often used in cases of spastic cerebral palsy with spastic weakness of all four limbs which affects the lower limbs more severely, such as Little's disease. Adj. diplegic. **atonic d.** FÖRSTER'S DIPLEGIA. **atonic-astatic d.** FÖRSTER'S DIPLEGIA. **cerebellar d.** Cerebral palsy in which symptoms and signs of cerebellar dysfunction predominate. **cerebral d.** SPASTIC DIPLEGIA. **congenital facial d.** MÖBIUS SYNDROME. **facial d.** Bilateral facial paralysis. Also *bifacial paralysis.* **flaccid d.** FÖRSTER'S DIPLEGIA. **Förster's d.** Infantile hypotonic cerebral paralysis, rarely inherited and much more often attributable to perinatal brain damage, occasionally to kernicterus. This condition may be accompanied by bilateral degeneration of the corpus striatum, of the cerebral cortex and corticospinal tracts, and also of the cerebellum. The main symptoms are hypotonia or atonia, either generalized or restricted to certain muscle groups, an increased range of passive joint movements, pendular tendon reflexes, postural abnormalities, ataxia, and often severe mental retardation. Also *atonia-astasia, infantile cerebrocerebellar diplegia, Förster's disease, Förster atonic-astatic syndrome, Förster syndrome, atonic-astasic encephalopathy, flaccid diplegia, hypotonic cerebral palsy, hypotonic diplegia, atonic diplegia, atonic-astatic diplegia.* **hypotonic d.** FÖRSTER'S DIPLEGIA. **infantile cerebral d.** LITTLE'S DISEASE. **infantile cerebrocerebellar d.** FÖRSTER'S DIPLEGIA. **masticatory d.** Bilateral paralysis of the motor division of the trigeminal nerve, giving rise to paralysis of lateral jaw movements involving the external pterygoid muscles and those of biting and chewing (involving the masseter and temporal muscles), with consequent dropping of the lower jaw. **spastic d.** Spastic weakness of the limbs, often affecting the legs more than the arms, present from birth and resulting from perinatal brain damage. It is one of the commonest forms of cerebral palsy. There may also be dysarthria, and when the child walks it is often with a scissors gait due to adductor spasm. Also *Little's disease, cerebral diplegia, tonic diplegia, cerebral spastic infantile paralysis, tabes spasmodica.* **tonic d.** SPASTIC DIPLEGIA.

**diplegic** \dīplē′jik\ Pertaining to or having diplegia.

**diplo-** \dip′lō-\ [Gk *diploos* (from *di-* two, twice + *pl(o)-*, root meaning fold; akin to L *duplex* folded over, double, and to English *twofold*) double] **1** A combining form meaning double, dual, twin. **2** A combining form meaning diploid. For defs. 1 and 2 also *dipl-*. Compare HAPLO-.

**diplobacillus** \-bəsil′əs\ (*pl.* diplobacilli) A type of bacillus found in cultures predominantly in pairs, usually end-to-end.

**diploblastic** \-blas′tik\ [DIPLO- + -BLAST + -IC] Formed from two embryonic germ layers.

**diplocardia** \-kär′dē·ə\ [DIPLO- + -CARDIA] A deepening of the cardiac fissures between the right and left chambers so as to suggest that the heart is divided into two lateral halves.

**diplocephalus** \-sef′ələs\ DICEPHALUS.
**diplocheiria** \-kir′ē·ə\ POLYDACTYLY.
**diplococci** \-käk′sī\ Plural of DIPLOCOCCUS.
**diplococcus** \-käk′əs\ (*pl.* diplococci) A type of coccus found in cultures predominantly in pairs. They are spherical or oval except where flattened at the region of contact.
***Diplococcus pneumoniae*** \-käk′əs noomō′ni·ē\ *Outmoded* STREPTOCOCCUS PNEUMONIAE.
**diplocoria** \-kôr′ē·ə\ [DIPLO- + *cor(e)*- + -IA] The presence of two pupils in one eye or irregularities of the pupil that suggest a doubled condition. Also *dicoria*.
**diploë** \dip′lō·ē\ [Gk *diploē* a fold, doubling, tissue between two layers or plates] [NA] The internal layer of trabecular bone that lies between the inner and outer tables of compact bone of the cranium and consists of cancellous tissue containing red bone marrow and large veins.
**diploetic** \-et′ik\ DIPLOIC.
**diplogenesis** \-jen′əsis\ [DIPLO- + GENESIS] The process or mechanism by which an embryo or part thereof is induced to become doubled.
**diploic** \diplō′ik\ Of or relating to the diploë. Also *diploetic*.
**diploid** \dip′loid\ [DIPL- + -OID] **1** Possessing two complete sets of homologous chromosomes. Compare HAPLOID. **2** An individual or cell that has two complete sets of homologous chromosomes. The somatic cells and the progenitors of the germ cells in eukaryotes are usually diploids.
**diploidy** \dip′loidē\ The condition of being diploid.
**diplokaryon** \-kar′ē·än\ A cell nucleus with twice the diploid number of chromosomes.
**diplomate** \dip′lōmāt\ **1** An individual who has a diploma. **2** A board certified physician. A usage occurring only in the U.S. • In Canada the equivalent of a diplomate (def. 2) is a Fellow of the Royal College. There is no exact equivalent of the word in this sense in the United Kingdom, where diplomas are granted by the royal colleges and by other organizations, or in Japan, where physicians are certified by the Ministry of Health.
**diplomyelia** \-mī·ē′lyə\ DIASTEMATOMYELIA.
**diplopagus** \dipläp′əgəs\ [DIPLO- + -PAGUS] Conjoined twins, especially when there is a relatively circumscribed union of the two, although one or more visceral organs may be shared.
**diplophase** \dip′lōfāz\ DIPLOTENE.
**diplophonia** \-fō′nē·ə\ [DIPLO- + PHON- + -IA] A quality of voice resulting from excitation of the vocal tract air column by vestibular fold activity as well as by the laryngeal folds. The resulting two fundamental laryngeal frequencies give a double-toned effect. This effect is seen in certain forms of dysphonia. Also *diphthongia*.
**diplopia** \diplō′pē·ə\ [DIPL- + -OPIA] The seeing of a single object as double, usually resulting from misalignment of the two eyes, but sometimes due to optical faults such as variations of density and consequently of refractive index within the crystalline lens. Also *double vision, visus duplicatus*. **binocular d.** Diplopia resulting from faulty alignment of the two eyes, which causes a different space projection of the two ocular images of the same object. This is the most common form of diplopia. **crossed d.** Diplopia in which the image seen by each eye is on the side opposite from the eye that sees the image. Also *heteronymous diplopia*. **direct d.** UNCROSSED DIPLOPIA. **facial fracture d.** Diplopia as a consequence of fractures of the facial bones that form the floor of the orbit. **heteronymous d.** CROSSED DIPLOPIA. **homonymous d.** UNCROSSED DIPLOPIA. **horizontal d.** Diplopia in which the two images appear side by side. **incongruous d.** PARADOXICAL DIPLOPIA. **intranasal tumor d.** Diplopia occurring when intranasal or paranasal tumors invade the orbit and displace the eye. **monocular d.** A ghostlike doubling of the image seen by one eye, due to dioptric imperfections within the crystalline lens. **paradoxical d.** A false localization of a diplopia image due to abnormal subjective orientation of the retina (anomalous retinal correspondence). Also *incongruous diplopia*. **physiologic d.** The normal visual reduplication of all objects seen at a distance other than at the point of fixation. This is normally ignored, although it can readily be observed by holding two fingers in front of the eyes, one at six inches, the other at one foot away. If one looks at either finger, the other will be seen as double. **uncrossed d.** Diplopia in which the image seen by each eye is on the same side as the eye that sees the image. Also *simple diplopia, direct diplopia, homonymous diplopia, temporal diplopia*. **vertical d.** Double vision in which one image is above the other.
**diplopodia** \-pō′dē·ə\ DIPODIA. • The term has been used erroneously as a synonym for polydactyly of the foot.
**diplosome** \dip′lōsōm\ [DIPLO- + Gk *sōm(a)* body] A pair of centrioles involved in spindle organization. They occur as orthogonal pairs close by the nuclear membrane and they separate to the spindle poles during karyokinesis. Also *paired allosome*.
**diplosomia** \-sō′mē·ə\ [DIPLO- + Gk *sōm(a)* body + -IA] A condition in equal conjoined twins involving the duplication of the trunk with limited fusion of parts. *Imprecise*.
**diplotene** \dip′lōtēn\ [DIPLO- + Gk *tain(ia)* a band, fillet] The fourth stage of the meiotic prophase. The paired, homologous chromosomes begin to separate but remain joined at the chiasmata. Also *diplophase*.
**diploteratology** \-ter′ətäl′əjē\ A subdivision of teratology concerned with the manifestations of conjoined twinning.
**Dipluridae** \diplʊr′idē\ A family of mygalomorph spiders of the suborder Orthognatha; the funnel-web spiders. Some members of the genera *Atrax* and *Trechona* have a bite that is dangerous to humans. See also *ATRAX*.
**dipodia** \dīpō′dē·ə\ [DI-[2] + POD- + -IA] **1** Any of various degrees of duplication of a foot. Also *diplopodia*. **2** In conjoined twins, the presence of two feet regardless of the degree of fusion elsewhere. **3** In sirenomelus, the presence of two feet or recognizable parts thereof.
**dipolar** \dīpō′lər\ BIPOLAR.
**dipole** \dī′pōl\ Two equal and opposite electrical charges or magnetic poles separated by a finite distance, regarded as a single entity.
**diprosopus** \dipräs′əpəs\ [Gk *diprosōpos* (from *di-* two + *prosōpon* face, from PROS- + Gk *ōps* eye) two-faced] Conjoined twins with two separate and generally complete faces regardless of the degree of fusion elsewhere. There is usually only one body. **d. parasiticus** Unequal conjoined twins in which the parasitic member is represented only by a small, poorly developed face.
**-dipsia** \-dip′sē·ə\ [Gk *dips(a)* thirst + -IA] A combining form indicating conditions associated with thirst or the ingestion of fluids.
**dipsogen** [Gk *dips(a)* thirst + *o* + -GEN] An agent that induces thirst.
**dipsogenic** Producing thirst.
**dipsomania** \dip′sōmā′nē·ə\ [Gk *dips(a)* thirst + *o* + -MANIA] **1** The pathologic use of alcohol. Also *potomania*. **2** ALCOHOLISM. **3** PERIODIC DRINKING BOUTS.
**dipstick** \dip′stik\ [English *dip* + *stick*] A chemically treated cellulose strip used to detect the presence of a given substance in urine.

**Diptera** \dip′tərə\ [Gk, neut. pl. of *dipteros* (from *di-* two + *ptera* wings) two-winged] A large order of holometabolous insects characterized by a single pair of membranous wings, the second pair being generally represented by halteres or balancing organs. The order is divided into three suborders, about 140 families, and about 100 000 species of flies, midges, gnats, and mosquitoes. It includes many of the most important pests and parasites of humans and domestic animals and vectors of human and animal diseases.

**dipteran** \dip′tərən\ **1** Belonging to or characteristic of the insect order Diptera. Also *dipterous.* **2** A member of the order Diptera.

**dipterous** \dip′tərəs\ [See DIPTERA.] **1** Having two wings: said primarily of certain insects. **2** DIPTERAN.

**dipygus** \dīpī′gəs\ [Gk *di(s)* + *pyg(ē)* rump, buttocks + *-us,* noun suffix] DUPLICITAS POSTERIOR. **d. parasiticus** Unequal conjoined twins in which the parasitic member is represented by a small or rudimentary pelvis and lower extremities attached to the pelvis or rump of the host member.

***Dipylidium caninum*** The most common tapeworm of dogs, also frequently found in cats. The larvae develop in dog fleas (*Ctenocephalides canis*), in lice (*Trichodectes canis*), and in the flea *Pulex irritans,* any of which can serve as intermediate hosts if the cysticercoids are ingested when the dog nips and swallows the infected pest insect. Man is occasionally infected through contact with dogs and dog fleas. Also *Taenia elliptica.*

**dipyridamole** A pyrimidine derivative that relaxes smooth muscle and inhibits platelet aggregation. It has been used in the treatment of angina pectoris and for prevention of intravascular coagulation.

**dipyrone** $C_{13}H_{18}N_3NaO_5S$. [(2,3-Dihydro-1,5-dimethyl-3-oxo-2-phenyl-1*H*-pyrazol-4-yl)methylamino]methanesulfonic acid sodium salt monohydrate, an effective antipyretic and analgesic of the pyrazole class. It is seldom used now because of the occasional but severe-to-fatal agranulocytosis associated with the use of these analgesics.

**Dirac** [Paul Adrien Maurice *Dirac,* English physicist, 1902–1984] Fermi-Dirac statistics. See under STATISTICS.

**direct** **1** Without an intervening medium or process; immediate. **2** Carried out on a tooth in the mouth as opposed to on a die made from an impression of the tooth. **3** Of or relating to the material used in or a stage in a direct procedure, as *direct wax pattern.*

**direction** / **pelvic d.** A line denoting the axis of the pelvic canal.

**directive** \direk′tiv\ Active or authoritarian: used especially of forms of psychotherapy that use exhortation or coercive methods rather than interpretative, analytic approaches.

**director** That which directs or channels movement or flow along a particular path. **grooved d.** A grooved metal probe used to control the direction and depth of surgical incisions.

***Dirofilaria*** \dī′rōfiler′ē·ə\ [L *dirus* terrible, ominous + *filaria*] A genus of filarial worms (family Dirofilariidae, superfamily Onchocercoidea). Most of the 31 species described are found in various mammals. Some human infections have been reported though these infections are usually self-limiting and aborted without complete development of the worm, as seen with "coin" lesions in the lung caused by *D. immitis.* Other species reported from humans (probably abnormal parasites of man, and probably identical to *D. immitis*) include *D. magalhaesi,* from the left ventricle of a Brazilian child, and *D. louisianensis,* from the inferior vena cava of an elderly woman. ***D. immitis*** The dog heartworm, a species found principally in the right ventricle and pulmonary arteries of dogs, wolves, and foxes. A cosmopolitan parasite, it is the source of an extract used as a nonspecific antigen in the diagnosis of human filariasis and in other serological tests. Human cases have been reported an a number of occasions, often identified as a pulmonary coin lesion. Also *Filaria immitis.* ***D. repens*** A species occurring in subcutaneous connective tissue of dogs, cats, wild carnivores, and man in Europe, Africa, and Asia. It causes local dermatitis, alopecia, and pruritus.

**dir. prop.** *directione propria* (L, with proper direction): used in prescription writing.

**dis-**[1] \dis-\ [L *dis-* prefix denoting separation or division, apart] A prefix meaning (1) reverse, opposite of; (2) not, un-; (3) away, apart, scattered. Also *di-*[1].

**dis-**[2] \dis-\ DI-[2].

**disability** A limitation or handicap in a person's ability to function normally in certain kinds of work, learning, or other necessary activity, to the extent that the person might be considered needful of some kind of benefit, exemption, compensation, special training, or the like because of such limitation. The extent of a disability, identified by a percentage, is often specified for qualifying for a specified legal benefit or service. Disability of 100 percent is equivalent to total disability. Impaired physical or mental health, injury, and congenital deformity are common causes of disability. **developmental d.** A failure to achieve some norm of expected behavioral competence during infancy, childhood, or adolescence. **learning d.** Any of those difficulties experienced by a child of normal intelligence in mastering one or more of the basic cognitive skills, i.e., speaking, reading, writing, or calculation, in the absence of any evident sensory or psychological disorder or cultural disadvantage: usually used in the plural. **major d.** A disability producing permanent and severe incapacity. In many countries persons with major disabilities are entitled to special benefits, such as prostheses, personal or attendance allowances, tax rebates, advantageous facilities in public transport, and special access to buildings.

**disable** **1** To produce permanent physical impairment with resulting loss of function of the impaired part of the body and with decreased or lost capacity to earn a living. **2** In criminal law, to intentionally produce bodily injury or harm which results in permanent or nonpermanent physical impairment.

**disaccharidase** Any enzyme that degrades lactose, sucrose, and any other disaccharide.

**disaccharide** A substance formed by the glycosylation of one sugar molecule by another. The disaccharide may be reducing, i.e., the glycosylated sugar residue may have a free anomeric carbon (as in lactose), or nonreducing, because the anomeric carbon atoms of the two components are joined to the same oxygen atom (as in sucrose).

**disarticulation** \dis′ärtik′yəlā′shən\ The amputation of a part through a joint. Also *exarticulation.* **knee d.** THROUGH-KNEE AMPUTATION.

**disassimilate** \dis′əsim′ilāt\ DISSIMILATE.

**disassociation** \dis′asō′sē·ā′shən\ DISSOCIATION.

**disazo-** DIAZO-.

**disc** **1** DISK. **2** DISCUS.

**disc-** \disk-\ DISCO-.

**discal** \dis′kəl\ Pertaining to intervertebral disk.

**discectomy** \disek′təmē\ DISKECTOMY.

**discharge** **1** The excretion or elimination of a substance, as from a body orifice or wound. **2** A substance so excreted. **3** An action potential from a nerve cell or group of nerve cells which can be amplified and recorded on an oscilloscope or similar equipment. **4** The sudden appearance in an electroencephalogram of a waveform which stands out clearly from the background activity, chiefly because of its increased voltage. **5** To administratively terminate the care of (a patient in an inpatient health care facility). **6** The act or process of discharging (a patient) or (of a patient's) being discharged. **conductive d.** The release of electrostatic charge from one conductor to another at a lower potential through a conducting material. **convective d.** The movement of charged particles away from a body charged to a sufficiently high voltage. Also *electric wind, effluve.* **critical epileptic d.** An electroencephalographic epileptic discharge which is associated with a clinical attack in an epileptic patient. Such paroxysms usually take the form of rhythmic spikes, spike-waves, sharp waves, and, less often, slow waves. Their distribution is general, bilateral, synchronous, and symmetrical over the whole scalp in generalized epilepsy; they may be general but of greater amplitude over one half of the scalp in unilateral epilepsy; they may be restricted to a localized area of the scalp in certain types of partial epilepsy; or they may be diffuse but of variable amplitude in different areas in some other types of partial epilepsy. **delta d.** DELTA WAVE. **diencephalic autonomic d.** Activity in the autonomic nervous system resulting from an activation of neurons in the hypothalamus. **disruptive d.** The sudden passage of current through an insulator as a result of breakdown of the material under electrostatic stress. **electroencephalographic epileptic d.** A wave or group of waves in the EEG indicating epileptic discharge. The discharge appears and disappears abruptly, and can be distinguished from the background activity in the EEG record by its frequency, shape, and amplitude. The usual appearance is of waves of such large amplitude and short duration that they appear as spikes or sharp waves, or as slow waves which constitute, with associated spikes, spike-wave complexes. **epileptic d.** A neuronal discharge reflecting the simultaneous activation of multiple cerebral neurons. Also *hypersynchronous neuronal discharge.* **focal epileptic d.** An electroencephalographic epileptic discharge, consistently confined to one part of the scalp. This is usually an interseizure epileptic discharge such as those which characterize most types of partial epilepsy. It is rare to find a critical epileptic discharge which remains localized to one particular area, even during a focal seizure. **generalized epileptic d.** An electroencephalographic epileptic discharge occurring in or between attacks and involving the entire scalp, and in which the components (spikes, spike-waves, or slow waves) are distributed bilaterally, synchronously, and symmetrically. **hypersynchronous neuronal d.** **1** EPILEPTIC DISCHARGE. **2** See under NEURONAL DISCHARGE. **myotonic d.** The bizarre, high-frequency discharge which is evoked in electromyography by movement of the recording electrode within skeletal muscle in patients with myotonia and which gives rise to a strident sound of variable pitch compared to that associated with dive bombers (the divebomber note). **nervous d.** Any spread of neuronal excitation with accompanying electrical activity, evoked by stimulation of neurons, whether physiological or experimental. Also *neural discharge.* **neuronal d.** A group of electrical potentials which reflect the activation of one or of several neurons. When numerous neurons fire off simultaneously, this is often called a *hypersynchronous neuronal discharge,* which for practical purposes is identical to epileptic discharge. **polysynaptic reflex d.** The motoneuron impulse discharge induced by an afferent fiber volley entering the dorsal horn to excite internuncial neurons that in turn excite the motoneuron pool. It is usually induced by excitation of cutaneous or slowly-conducting muscle afferent fibers. **pseudomyotonic d.** A bizarre, high-frequency discharge which may be recorded in the electromyogram with a concentric needle electrode and which resembles myotonic discharge except that the electrical activity begins and ends abruptly and does not wax and wane. It can be seen in a variety of neuromuscular diseases.

**dischronation** \dis′krōnā′shən\ [DIS[1] + CHRON- + -ATION] Alteration in the subject's biologic rhythms or biologic clock.

**disci** \dis′ī, dis′kī\ Plural of DISCUS.

**disci-** \dis′ē-\ DISCO-.

**disciform** \dis′ifôrm\ Disk-shaped. Also *diskiform.*

**discission** \disish′ən\ [L *discissio* (from *discissus,* past part. of *discindere* to tear apart, sever, from *dis-* apart + *scindere* to cut, tear) a tearing apart] A surgical cutting, as of a membrane such as the lens capsule. **d. of cataract** A surgical cutting of the lens capsule. **d. of the lens** An incision into the lens capsule to permit removal or spontaneous absorption of a cataract. **posterior d.** A surgical cutting of opacities of the posterior capsule of the lens, which may form after extracapsular cataract extraction.

**discitis** \disī′tis, diskī′tis\ DISKITIS.

**disclination** \dis′klinā′shən\ EXTORSION.

**disclosing** \disklō′zing\ The act of making dental plaque visible on the teeth by staining it with dyes like erythrocin.

**disclusion** \diskloo′zhən\ [L *disclusio* (from *discludere* to separate) a disjunction] **1** An opening of the jaw with no occlusal contacts. **2** The separation of occlusal contacts of groups of teeth.

**disco-** \dis′kō-\ [L *discus,* from Gk *diskos* a quoit, discus, disk] A combining form meaning disk, having the form of a disk. Also *disko-, disc-, disk-, disci-, diski-.*

**discoblastula** \-blas′tyələ\ A blastula resulting from meroblastic or discoidal cleavage in a megalecithal ovum. Adj. discoblastic.

**discogastrula** \-gas′troolə\ [DISCO- + GASTRULA] A gastrula produced from a blastula derived by meroblastic cleavage from a megalecithal ovum.

**discogenic** \-jen′ik\ [DISCO- + -GENIC] Caused by or stemming from an intervertebral disk. Also *discogenetic.*

**discography** \diskäg′rəfē\ DISKOGRAPHY.

**discoid** \dis′koid\ [DISC- + -OID] Roughly disk-shaped or characterized by disk-shaped lesions.

**discoidectomy** \dis′koidek′təmē\ DISKECTOMY.

**disconnection** \dis′kənek′shən\ **portoazygos d.** A nonshunt operation utilizing transection and reanastomosis of the proximal stomach, later accompanied in addition by extensive extragastric vascular ligature.

**discontinuity** \dis′käntənyoo′itē\ **ossicular d.** Interruption in the continuity of the chain of middle-ear ossicles, often as the result of destruction of the articular end of the long process of the incus in chronic otitis media with cholesteatoma. Trauma, both accidental and surgical, accounts for a number of cases, with dislocation of the incus as a relatively common lesion.

**discopathy** \diskäp′əthē\ DISKOPATHY.

**discoplacenta** \-pləsen′tə\ A placenta which is discoid in shape.

**discoplasm** \dis′kōplazm\ ERYTHROCYTE GHOST.

**discordance** \diskôr′dəns\ **1** In genetics, the occurrence of different phenotypes for a given genetically determined character in twins. **2** The occurrence of different phenotypes with respect to a given character among individuals or groups of individuals being examined. **3** An inappropriate or abnormal connection between segments of the heart. **atrioventricular d.** Any congenital defect in which the atria of the heart are connected to the wrong ventricles. **ventriculoarterial d.** Any congenital defect in which an artery arises from the wrong ventricle of the heart. See also TRANSPOSITION OF THE GREAT ARTERIES.

**discostroma** \-strō′mə\ ERYTHROCYTE GHOST.

**discotomy** \diskät′əmē\ [DISCO- + -TOMY] The surgical incision through the annulus fibrosus into the central areas of a disk.

**discrete** \diskrēt′\ [L *discretus* (from *discernere* to separate, distinguish, from *dis-* apart + *cernere* to sift, examine) separated, distinguished] Separate; individually distinct; not continuous or confluent.

**discrimination** \diskrim′ənā′shən\ The ability to recognize qualitative or quantitative differences between two or more sensory stimuli, often leading to differential reactions based upon the detection of such differences. **pitch d.** **1** The ability to perceive small increments of change in the frequency of a pure tone stimulus. **2** The perception of pitch change, as of intonation or in music. For defs. 1 and 2 also *tonal discrimination.* **speech d.** The ability to identify words and the component sounds of words: used especially in reference to the test results displayed by a speech audiogram. **tactile d.** The capability that an individual possesses to discern differences in the sense of touch, thus allowing the subject to distinguish fine touch, texture and other delicate and variable stimuli applied to the skin. **tonal d.** PITCH DISCRIMINATION. **two-point d.** **1** The ability to distinguish between two blunt points applied simultaneously to an area of skin. **2** The threshold distance at which two points can first be distinguished as being different from a single point on the skin. For defs. 1 and 2 also *two-point sensibility.*

**discriminator** \diskrim′ənā′tər\ PULSE-HEIGHT DISCRIMINATOR. **pulse-height d.** An electronic circuit that rejects all pulses whose height falls below a selected threshold value. Pulse heights above the threshold produce a pulse at the output. Also *discriminator.*

**discus** \dis′kəs\ [L, from Gk *diskos* a quoit, discus, disk-shaped object] (*pl.* disci) A circular, platelike structure. Also *disk, disc.* **d. articularis** [NA] A ring or plate of fibrocartilage or dense fibrous tissue, attached at its periphery to the fibrous capsule and extending into certain joint cavities, either partially or completely separating the opposed bony articular surfaces. If complete, the joint cavity is divided into two parts, both structurally and functionally, often permitting translation movements. Although such disks permit a better fit between the articular surfaces, their functions are not proven. Also *articular disk, interarticular disk, intra-articular disk, interarticular fibrocartilage, intra-articular fibrocartilage, interarticular cartilage, fibroplate.* **d. articularis articulationis acromioclavicularis** [NA] A pad of fibrocartilage often found within the acromioclavicular joint. Usually incomplete, it is located in the upper part of the joint attached to the fibrous capsule. Also *articular disk of acromioclavicular articulation, acromioclavicular disk, Weitbrecht's cartilage.* **d. articularis articulationis radioulnaris distalis** [NA] A triangular disk of fibrocartilage that connects the lower ends of the radius and the ulna, its broad apex attached to the angle between the base of the styloid process and the inferior surface of the head of the ulna, and its thin base attached to the margin separating the ulnar notch from the carpal articular surface of the radius. Also *articular disk of distal radioulnar articulation, triquetral cartilage, triquetrous cartilage, triangular disk of wrist, articular disk of wrist.* **d. articularis articulationis sternoclavicularis** [NA] A rounded plate of fibrocartilage attached to the upper margin of the sternal end of the clavicle, to the first costal cartilage and, by the rest of its circumference, to the fibrous capsule. It divides the joint cavity into two, movement between the clavicle and the disk being more extensive than that between the disk and the costal cartilage. Also *articular disk of sternoclavicular articulation, sternoclavicular disk, sternoclavicular fibrocartilage.* **d. articularis articulationis temporomandibularis** [NA] An oval plate of fibrous tissue that completely divides the temporomandibular joint so that the upper surface of the disk is concavo-convex and the inferior surface concave. Also *articular disk of temporomandibular joint, meniscus of temporomandibular joint, mandibular disk.* **d. interpubicus** [NA] A plate of fibrocartilage that is firmly adherent to the hyaline cartilage covering the medial surface of each pubic bone in the symphysis pubis. Also *interpubic disk, fibrocartilaginous interpubic lamina.* **disci intervertebrales** [NA] Plates of fibrocartilage interposed between the bodies of adjacent vertebrae from the axis to the sacrum, binding them firmly together. They are adherent to the hyaline cartilage on the upper and lower surfaces of the vertebral bodies, and are attached to the anterior and posterior longitudinal ligaments. The disks vary in thickness both within a disk and in different parts of the vertebral column. They are avascular, except for their periphery. Each disk consists of an outer, laminated part, annulus fibrosus, and an inner, pulpy core, nucleus pulposus. Also *intervertebral disks, fibrocartilagines intervertebrales, intervertebral cartilages, intervertebral fibrocartilages.* **d. nervi optici** [NA] A clearcut, whitish, circular spot visible on the fundus of the eye, medial to the fovea centralis. It marks the point of initial myelination of the retinal efferent fibers and their entry into the optic nerve. No rods and cones cover the area, so that functionally it is detectable as a blind spot. Also *optic papilla, papilla nervi optici* (outmoded), *papilla, head of optic nerve, optic disk.* **d. oophorus** CUMULUS OOPHORUS.

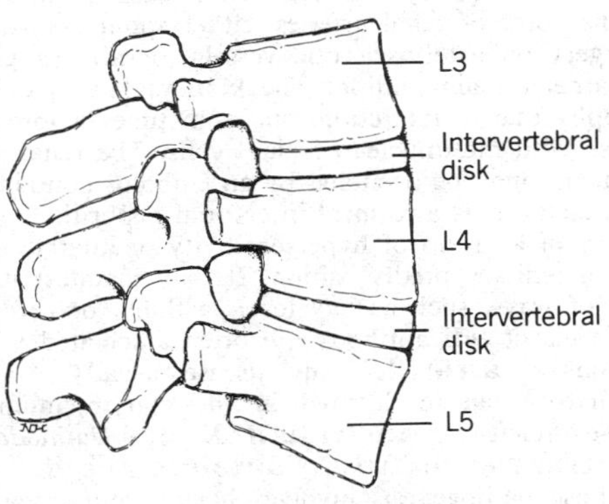

**Intervertebral disks**

**discuss** [L and Late L *discuss(us)*, past part. of *discutere*: in L to shatter, beat down, break up, in Late L to examine, discuss; from L *dis-* apart + *quatere* to shake violently] To cause to be dispersed or absorbed.

**discussive** DISCUTIENT.

**discutient** **1** Causing the dispersal or disappearance of a pathologic condition, such as a tumor. **2** A discutient agent. For defs. 1 and 2 also *discussive.*

# disease

**disease** [Old French *desaise* (from *des-* DIS-[1] + *aise* comfort, convenience, from L *adjacens* nearby, at hand) discomfort, illness] A condition which alters or interferes with the normal state of an organism and is usually characterized by the abnormal functioning of one or more of the host's systems, parts, or organs. It may be due to an unknown cause or may result from an inherent metabolic or structural deficiency, including congenital and hereditary defects and degenerative processes, or from such factors as stress, noxious stimuli, toxic agents, injury, or infection. A given disease is often manifested by a characteristic set of signs and symptoms, although a host organism can be asymptomatic while having microscopic, serologic, or immunologic evidence of disease. • *Disease* is usually distinguished from *injury*, the disruption of an organism's integrity, especially by an external agent, and often from *syndrome*, a complex of features descriptive of a disorder, especially a particular combination of phenotypic manifestations. See also note at SYNDROME. For particular disease entities not found under *disease*, see also under SYNDROME. **Acosta's d.** MOUNTAIN SICKNESS. **acute demyelinating d.** Any acute disease of the nervous system in which the predominant pathologic feature is demyelination. In the central nervous system, acute multiple sclerosis and postinfective encephalomyelitis are the most common; in the peripheral nervous system, the Guillain-Barré syndrome. **Adams d.** ADAMS-STOKES SYNDROME. **Adams-Stokes d.** ADAMS-STOKES SYNDROME. **Addison's d.** A chronic, wasting disease produced by gradual destruction of the adrenal cortex, most commonly due to an autoimmune process, less commonly caused by tuberculosis. If due to an autoimmune process, antibodies to adrenocortical cells are found in the patient's serum. It is characterized by weight loss, asthenia, prostration in the presence of minor illness, and acute exacerbations marked by high fever and shock. Patients are emaciated and in some cases the skin is a bronze color. The chemical lesions are cortisol and aldosterone deficiency with renal sodium loss. The disease can be successfully treated with cortisol and a synthetic mineralocorticoid. A form of the disease, which is inherited as an X-linked recessive trait, can occur in association with leukodystrophy. Also *primary adrenocortical insufficiency, primary adrenocortical failure, adrenocortical insufficiency, chronic adrenocortical insufficiency, adrenal tuberculosis* (older term). **adenocystic d.** CYSTIC MASTOPATHY. **adult celiac d.** Nontropical sprue in adults. Also *Gee-Thaysen disease.* **Albers-Schönberg d.** OSTEOPETROSIS. **Albert's d.** ACHILLES BURSITIS. **Albright's d.** A condition, affecting children and young adults, characterized by polyostotic fibrous dysplasia, unilateral patches of excessive cutaneous pigmentation, endocrine abnormalities, and unusually precocious puberty in females. Also *Albright syndrome, Albright-McCune-Sternberg syndrome, McCune-Albright syndrome.* **Alexander's d.** A rare variety of infantile leukodystrophy giving rise to severe mental retardation, paralysis and megalencephaly. Pathologically, there are eosinophilic hyaline bodies (Rosenthal fibers) distributed randomly throughout the cerebral white matter. Also *dysmyelinogenic leukodystrophy.* **allogeneic d.** A form of graft-versus-host disease produced by giving allogeneic lymphocytes to immunosuppressed animals. Also *homologous disease.* **Almeida's d.** SOUTH AMERICAN BLASTOMYCOSIS. **Alpers d.** ALPERS SYNDROME. **alpha heavy-chain d.** A lymphomalike disorder associated with an abnormal immunoglobulin IgA fragment. The condition occurs most commonly in persons from North Africa and Middle Eastern countries. It is characterized by diarrhea, steatorrhea, weight loss, and positive tests for malabsorption. There is marked lymphocytic and plasmacytic infiltration of the small intestine, often lymphomatous polyps of the stomach or intestines, and hypogammaglobulinemia. The Fab fragment of $\alpha$ heavy chains is secreted in large amounts in intestinal fluid and can also be demonstrated in blood or urine following concentration. **altitude d.** ALTITUDE SICKNESS. **alveolar hydatid d.** A disease caused by the larval form of *Echinococcus multilocularis* resulting in a multiloculate hydatid usually in the liver which produces a ramifying, continuously growing structure, not enclosed in a sheath as is the uniloculate hydatid of *E. granulosus.* The hepatic damage resembles a hepatoma and death is the usual result. **Alzheimer's d.** A form of degenerative brain disease resulting in progressive mental deterioration with disorientation, memory disturbance, and confusion, and leading to progressive dementia often accompanied by dysphasia and/or apraxia. The condition may also give rise ultimately to spastic weakness and paralysis of the limbs, epilepsy, and other variable neurologic signs. It usually runs a slow progressive course of five to ten years. It is marked morphologically by atrophy of the gyri and dilatation of the ventricles and, histologically, by atrophy and eventual loss of neurons, particularly in the outer cortical layer, with thick, strongly argyrophilic filaments (neurofibrillary tangles) in the neurons, by glial cell proliferation, by the presence of frequent senile plaques comprising amorphous argyrophilic deposits, and by granulovacuolar degeneration of hippocampal neurons. Also *Alzheimer's dementia, Alzheimer sclerosis.* • When the condition begins before the age of 65 years it is usually called *presenile dementia,* after that age *senile dementia.* **amyloid d.** AMYLOIDOSIS. **Anders d.** ADIPOSIS TUBEROSA SIMPLEX. **Andersen's d.** GLYCOGEN STORAGE DISEASE IV. **Anderson-Fabry d.** ANGIOKERATOMA CORPORIS DIFFUSUM. **Andrews d.** PUSTULOSIS PALMARIS ET PLANTARIS. **aortoiliac occlusive d.** Obstruction of the abdominal aorta, usually the consequence of a combination of atherosclerosis and thrombosis. Also *occlusive disease.* **Apert's d.** ACROCEPHALOSYNDACTYLY TYPE I. **Aran-Duchenne d.** PROGRESSIVE MUSCULAR ATROPHY. **Armenian d.** FAMILIAL MEDITERRANEAN FEVER. **Armstrong's d.** LYMPHOCYTIC CHORIOMENINGITIS. **atheroembolic renal d.** Acute or chronic renal failure caused by dislodgment of atheromatous emboli from the aorta or renal arteries, either spontaneously, or after surgery on arteriosclerotic vessels, or after angiography with catheter manipulation. The kidneys have patchy areas of atrophy due to infarction, and sometimes a foreign body response with multinucleated giant cells. The renal artery or its branches may be occluded by an embolus containing cholesterol clefts. It is a form of interstitial nephritis. **atopic d.** Any of a group of hypersensitivity or allergic disorders with a hereditary predisposition. It may manifest itself in a variety of ways, such as hay fever, asthma, or eczema. Elevated levels of IgE antibody are often associated with these conditions. **attic d.** Any disease, usually of a chronic inflammatory nature, located in the epitympanum of the middle-ear cleft. **Australian X d.** *Outmoded* MURRAY VALLEY ENCEPHALITIS. **autoimmune d.** Any disease whose pathogenesis involves host immune reactions to autoantigens. Autoantibodies to cell receptors may produce disease by agonist activity (as the antibody to thyrotrophin receptors in thyrotoxicosis) or by antagonist activity (as the antibody to acetylcholine receptors in myasthenia gravis). Immune complexes of non-organ-specific autoantigens and autoantibodies can give rise to glomerulonephritis and vasculitis, as occurs in systemic lupus erythematosus. Organ-specific autoantibodies may cause the destruction of the relevant cells if the antigens occur on cell or basement membranes. Thus autoantibodies to thyroid cells, adrenal cells, and the parietal cells of the stomach are implicated, respectively, in Hashimoto's disease, Addison's disease, and pernicious anemia. Autoantibodies to basement membrane give rise to the Goodpasture syndrome. Cellular immune reactions against autoantigens can be seen in experimental allergic encephalomyelitis and are believed to be similarly responsible for some forms of human encephalomyelitis. **autoimmune hemolytic d.** AUTOIMMUNE HEMOLYTIC ANEMIA. **autologous immune complex d.** A disease produced by complexes of the host's autologous antigens with autoantibodies formed to them. **Ayerza's d.** A form of cyanotic disease resulting from primary pulmonary hypertension or atherosclerosis with plexiform lesions of the arterioles, leading to polycythemia and hepatosplenomegaly. At one time attributed to syphilis, it is now thought to be due to a variety of disorders. Also *Ayerza syndrome.* **Baastrup's d.** KISSING SPINES. **Ballet's d.** EXTERNAL OPHTHALMOPLEGIA. **Ballingall's d.** MYCETOMA. **Baló's d.** A variety of cerebral diffuse sclerosis in which demyelination in the cerebral white matter occurs in concentric circles. It is probably not a specific disease entity but simply an unusual distribution of pathologic changes which may occur in cerebral multiple sclerosis or Schilder's disease. Also *concentric periaxial leukoencephalitis, Baló syndrome, Baló's concentric encephalitis, Baló's concentric sclerosis, encephalitis periaxialis concentrica, Greenfield's disease.* **Bamberger's d.** INFANTILE MASSIVE SPASM. **Bamberger-Marie d.** HYPERTROPHIC PULMONARY OSTEOARTHROPATHY. **Banti's d.** Splenomegaly and anemia secondary to portal hypertension. Also *Klemperer's disease.* **Barclay-Baron d.** VALLECULAR DYSPHAGIA. **Barcoo d.** VELDT SORE. **Barlow's d.** INFANTILE SCURVY. **Bassen-Kornzweig d.** ABETALIPOPROTEINEMIA. **Bateman's d.** 1 MOLLUSCUM CONTAGIOSUM. 2 A condition marked by the presence of both erythema nodosum and erythema multiforme. **Batten's d.** JUVENILE CEROID-LIPOFUSCINOSIS. **bauxite workers' d.** BAUXITE PNEUMOCONIOSIS. **Bayle's d.** GENERAL PARESIS. **Bazin's d.** ERYTHEMA INDURATUM. **Beard's d.** NEURASTHENIA. **beetle d.** SCARABIASIS. **Begbie's d.** *Rare* GRAVES DISEASE. **Béguez César d.** CHÉDIAK-HIGASHI ANOMALY. **Behçet's d.** BEHÇET SYNDROME. **Behr's d.** A hereditary macular degeneration occurring in adolescents or young adults. **Beigel's d.** WHITE PIEDRA. **Bennett's d.** LEUKEMIA. **Benson's d.** ASTEROID HYALOSIS. **Berger's d.** MESANGIAL IGA/IGG GLOMERULONEPHRITIS **Berlin's d.** A transient macular edema resulting from ocular contusion. **Bernhardt's d.** MERALGIA PARESTHETICA. **Besnier-Boeck d.** SARCOIDOSIS. **Besnier-Boeck-Schaumann d.** SARCOIDOSIS. **Best d.** VITELLIFORM MACULAR DEGENERATION. **Bielschowsky's d.** LATE INFANTILE CEROID-LIPOFUSCINOSIS. **Bielschowsky-Jansky d.** LATE INFANTILE CEROID-LIPOFUSCINOSIS. **Biermer's d.** PERNICIOUS ANEMIA. **big spleen d.** TROPICAL SPLENOMEGALY SYNDROME. **Bilderbeck's d.** PINK DISEASE. **Billroth's d.** TRAUMATIC MENINGOCELE. **Binswanger's d.** Progressive subcortical demyelination of the brain thought to be due to vascular insufficiency and giving rise to progressive dementia. The existence of this as a disease entity is in doubt. Also *chronic subcortical encephalitis, Binswanger's encephalitis, progressive subcortical encephalopathy, progressive subcortical gliosis, subcortical arteriosclerotic encephalopathy.* **bird-breeders' d.** A form of extrinsic allergic alveolitis occurring among bird breeders. It is caused by the inhalation of antigens contained in pigeon, parrot, and budgerigar droppings. Also *bird-breeders' lung, bird-fanciers' lung.* **bleeders' d.** HEMOPHILIA. **blinding d.** ONCHOCERCIASIS. **Bloodgood's d.** CYSTIC MASTOPATHY. **Blount's d.** OSTEOCHONDROSIS DEFORMANS TIBIAE. **Blumenthal's d.** ERYTHROLEUKEMIA. **Bodechtel-Guttmann d.** SUBACUTE SCLEROSING PANENCEPHALITIS. **Boeck's d.** SARCOIDOSIS. **Bornholm d.** EPIDEMIC PLEURODYNIA. • Named after *Bornholm* Island, Denmark **Boston exanthem d.** BOSTON EXANTHEM. **Bouillaud's d.** RHEUMATIC HEART DISEASE. **Bourneville's d.** TUBEROUS SCLEROSIS. **Bourneville-Brissaud d.** TUBEROUS SCLEROSIS. **Bourneville-Crouzon d.** TUBEROUS SCLEROSIS. **Bouveret's d.** PAROXYSMAL TACHYCARDIA. **Bowen's d.** A carcinoma in situ of the skin. Also *Bowen's precancerous dermatosis, precancerous dermatitis, precancerous dermatosis.* **Bowen's d. of the penis** An erythroplastic condition of the penis manifested by circumscribed, papular, velvety lesions with central atrophy. **brancher glycogen storage d.** GLYCOGEN STORAGE DISEASE IV. **brass-founders' d.** METAL-FUME FEVER. **braziers' d.** METAL-FUME FEVER. **Breda's d.** 1 MUCOCUTANEOUS LEISHMANIASIS. 2 *Outmoded* YAWS. **Bretonneau's d.** PHARYNGEAL DIPHTHERIA. **Breutsch's d.** SYDENHAM'S CHOREA. **bridegrooms' d.** Thrombosis affecting the pampiniform plexus. **Bright's d.** Any form of nephritis, particularly when glomerular in nature, characterized by proteinuria, hematuria, edema, hypertension, or nitrogen retention. *Outmoded.* **Brill's d.** A mild recrudescent typhus fever caused by reactivation of *Rickettsia prowazekii* retained from an infection early in life. It is seen principally in elderly persons who immigrated to the United States from Eastern Europe. Also *Brill-Zinsser disease, recrudescent typhus, sporadic typhus, benign typhus.* **Brill-Symmers d.** NODULAR LYMPHOMA. **Brill-Zinsser d.** BRILL'S DISEASE. **broad-beta d.** FAMILIAL HYPERLIPOPROTEINEMIA TYPE III. **Brodie's d.** Chronic synovitis secondary to infection, with boggy degeneration of the periarticular tissues. Also *Brodie's knee.* **Brown-Séquard d.** BROWN-SÉQUARD SYNDROME. **Brown-Symmers d.** ACUTE INFANTILE ENCEPHALOPATHY. **Brushfield-Wyatt d.** *Rare* STURGE-WEBER SYNDROME. **Bruton's d.** INFANTILE SEX-LINKED HYPOGAMMAGLOBULINEMIA. **Budd's d.** *Obs.* BUDD-CHIARI SYNDROME. **Budd-Chiari d.** BUDD-CHIARI SYNDROME. **Buerger's d.** THROMBOANGIITIS OBLITERANS. **Buschke's d.** CRYPTOCOCCOSIS. **Busquet's d.** Osteoperiostitis of the metatarsal bones that leads to exostoses on the dorsum of the foot. **Busse-Buschke d.** CRYPTOCOCCOSIS. **Byler's d.** A form of liver cirrhosis due to episodic bile stasis as a result of a fault in bile salt metabolism. Death occurs in the second to eighth year. It is of autosomal recessive inheritance and has been described in a large kinship of Amish people. Also *familial intrahepatic cholestasis.* **Caffey's d.** INFANTILE HYPEROSTOSIS. **caisson d.** DECOMPRESSION SICKNESS. **Calvé's d.** VERTEBRA PLANA. **Calvé-Perthes d.** PERTHES DISEASE. **Camurati-Engelmann d.** PROGRESSIVE DIAPHYSEAL DYSPLASIA. **Cana-**

**van's d.** A rare form of infantile cerebral leukodystrophy of autosomal recessive inheritance giving rise to severe mental retardation, spastic paralysis, blindness and death usually by 18 months of age. Pathologically, there are megalencephaly and widespread demyelination of cerebral white matter giving a diffuse spongy appearance. Also *infantile spongy degeneration, spongy degeneration of central nervous system, spongiform leukodystrophy, van Bogaert-Bertrand disease.* **Canavan-van Bogaert-Bertrand d.** VAN BOGAERT'S FAMILIAL AXONAL SPONGY DEGENERATION. **candle wax d.** MELORHEOSTOSIS. **Cannon's d.** ORAL FAMILIAL WHITE FOLDED DYSPLASIA. **carcinoid heart d.** Heart disease secondary to carcinoid. See also CARCINOID SYNDROME. **Caroli's d.** A congenital condition characterized by cystic dilatation of the intrahepatic bile ducts. Consequent bile stasis may result in cholangitis, cholelithiasis, or liver abscess. Also *congenital cystic disease of the liver.* **Carrión's d.** BARTONELLOSIS. **Castellani's d.** BRONCHOSPIROCHETOSIS. **cat-bite d.** CAT-BITE FEVER. **cat-scratch d.** A mild, self-limited infectious disease characterized by fever, regional lymphadenitis, and, occasionally, meningoencephalitis. The disease is usually transmitted by the scratch or bite of a cat. A small, pleomorphic bacillus has been implicated as the causative agent. Also *cat-scratch fever, cat-claw disease, nonbacterial regional lymphadenitis, benign lymphoreticulosis, benign reticulosis, benign inoculation reticulosis, cat-bite fever* (incorrect), *regional lymphadenitis* (imprecise and outmoded). **Cazenave's d.** 1 *Obs.* LUPUS ERYTHEMATOSUS. 2 PEMPHIGUS FOLIACEUS. **celiac d.** A malabsorption disease caused by sensitivity to gluten-containing foods, mainly wheat, and marked clinically by large, bulky, fat-containing stools, abdominal distention, and wasting. Removal of gluten from the diet is curative. Wheat and related grains (rye, barley, oats) must be strictly avoided. Although the condition usually presents within the first two years of life, it may occur at any age. Jejunal biopsy reveals flattening of the intestinal villi and provides a diagnostic test. Also *nontropical sprue, gluten enteropathy, idiopathic steatorrhea, celiac syndrome, celiac sprue, Thaysen's disease.* **central core d. of muscle** A relatively benign and nonprogressive form of congenital myopathy in which the majority of the muscle fibers show nonfunctioning central cores. It sometimes occurs sporadically, and is sometimes apparently of autosomal dominant inheritance. **ceroid storage d.** SYNDROME OF SEA-BLUE HISTIOCYTE. **Chagas d.** A disease caused by *Trypanosoma cruzi* and spread by the bite of blood-sucking, cone-nosed reduviid bugs of the subfamily Triatominae, such as *Triatoma infestans, Rhodnius prolixus, Panstrongylus megistus,* and *P. infestans,* which live in the thatched roofs of rural houses. It is found in Central and South America, especially Brazil. Reservoir hosts include dogs and cats, rodents, opossums, and species of armadillos. In humans, primary infection produces a local lesion (chagoma) usually on the face. Lymphatic and hematogenous spread of the trypanosomes follows. Trypanosomes enter cells, where they assume an amastigote form and multiply. Pseudocysts may form. Unilateral edema of the eyelid and face (Romana sign) may occur. The long-term features of the disease include damage to the myocardium and the myenteric plexuses of the gastrointestinal tract with subsequent megaesophagus and megacolon. Involvement of the central nervous system also occurs. Goiter may be a complication. In children, the disease is usually acute and frequently fatal, but in adults it pursues a chronic course. Treatment is with nifurtimox. Also *South American trypanosomiasis, Chagas-Cruz disease, American trypanosomiasis, Brazilian trypanosomiasis, Cruz trypanosomiasis, trypanosomiasis cruzi, barbeiro fever, schizotrypanosis, schizotrypanosomiasis.* **Chagas d. of the esophagus** TROPICAL CARDIOSPASM. **Chandler's d.** Aseptic necrosis of the femoral head. It is often seen as a complication of chronic alcoholism. **Charcot's d.** 1 OPHTHALMOPLEGIC MIGRAINE. 2 TABETIC ARTHROPATHY. **Charcot-Marie-Tooth d.** A genetically determined syndrome, usually of dominant inheritance, but due to an autosomal recessive gene in some families and in rare cases to an X-linked recessive gene. Sporadic cases occur. It usually begins in childhood with progressive wasting of leg muscles below the knee with footdrop and pes cavus, and later the small muscles of the hands and those of the forearms are usually involved. Wasting does not usually spread proximally above the knees and elbows, and vibration sense is usually impaired or lost at the ankles. In some cases there are associated features of other conditions of the hereditary ataxia group including optic atrophy and scoliosis and sometimes Argyll Robertson pupils are found. Recent work has shown that there are at least three varieties of this disease, one due to a demyelinating hypertrophic neuropathy related to Dejerine-Sottas disease, another due to axonal degeneration (the neuronal sensorimotor type), and a third due to anterior horn cell disease (the neuronal motor form), related to the spinal muscular atrophies. The condition usually runs a benign course and breeds true in individual families. Also *peroneal muscular atrophy, juvenile distal atrophic paralysis, Charcot-Marie-Tooth-Hoffmann syndrome, hereditary sensorimotor neuropathy types I-III, Charcot-Marie atrophy, peroneal atrophy, Tooth disease, Charcot-Marie-Tooth atrophy, Marie-Tooth disease, Tooth's atrophy, Charcot disease.* **Charlouis d.** *Outmoded* YAWS. **Chédiak-Higashi d.** CHÉDIAK-HIGASHI ANOMALY. **Chester's d.** Xanthomatosis of the long bones, which leads to pathologic fractures. **Chiari's d.** BUDD-CHIARI SYNDROME. **Chiari-Frommel d.** CHIARI-FROMMEL SYNDROME. **chignon d.** PIEDRA. **Christensen-Krabbe d.** KRABBE'S DISEASE. **Christian's d.** 1 HAND-SCHÜLLER-CHRISTIAN DISEASE. 2 RELAPSING FEBRILE NONSUPPURATIVE PANNICULITIS. **Christian-Weber d.** RELAPSING FEBRILE NONSUPPURATIVE PANNICULITIS. **Christmas d.** HEMOPHILIA B. **chronic granulomatous d.** An immunological disorder due to a metabolic fault in the intracellular bactericidal function of leukocytes. Patients may die of infection by organisms of quite low virulence. Infections starting in skin, the middle ear, or lung parenchyma are associated with chronic lymphadenopathy, hepatosplenomegaly, local granulomas, and draining sinuses. There is hypergammaglobulinemia. The disease becomes manifest in males in early childhood and is usually fatal in the first five to ten years of life. It is inherited as an X-linked recessive trait. Also *chronic familial granulomatosis, chronic X-linked granulomatosis.* **chronic hypertensive d. of pregnancy** A form of blood pressure elevation whereby the condition either antedates the pregnancy or is discovered prior to the twentieth week of pregnancy. **chronic obstructive pulmonary d.** A category of diseases that cause chronic limitation of air flow in the lungs, such as emphysema and chronic bronchitis. Abbr. COPD **chronic rheumatic heart d.** The long-term consequence of healed acute rheumatic myocarditis and endocarditis, characterized by stenosis and/or regurgitation of cardiac valves with an accompanying myocardial disorder. **Coats d.** EXUDATIVE RETINITIS. **Cogan's d.** COGAN SYNDROME. **cold hemolytic antibody d.** A hemolytic syndrome in which hemolytic anemia is associated with red cell agglutination that is induced by antibodies active below 37°C (cold agglutinins). It is usually characterized by mild anemia and Raynaud's phenomenon. Also *cold hemagglutinin disease.* Abbr. CHAD **collagen d.** Any of a wide variety of diseases characterized by widespread pathologic changes in connective tissue. Hypersensitivity or autoimmunity may play an important role in their pathogenesis. They are generally characterized by arthritis and diverse abnormalities of the skin and viscera. Among the many collagen diseases are systemic lupus erythematosus, progressive systemic sclerosis, dermatomyositis, rheumatoid arthritis, and polyarteritis. Also *collagenosis.* **combined immunodeficiency d.** SEVERE COMBINED IMMUNODEFICIENCY. **communicable d.** CONTAGIOUS DISEASE. **complicating d.** A disease that constitutes a complication of another disease. **Concato's d.** Polyserositis with effusions in the pericardium, pleura, and peritoneum. **congenital d.** 1 Any disease manifest or known to have been present at birth, particularly one of developmental or genetic origin. 2 Any disease that is genetically determined, whether or not manifest or diagnosed until after birth. **congenital cystic d. of the liver** CAROLI'S DISEASE. **congenital heart d.** Any malformation of the heart present at birth. It may be apparent at birth or become apparent later, or after recognition cease to be apparent in later childhood. The incidence is about 5–6 per 1000 among live births. Some forms are not compatible with extrauterine life. Anomalous communications between the right heart (serving the pulmonary circulation) and the left heart (serving the systemic circulation) allow the blood to be shunted from one side to the other according to the pressures in various chambers or vessels. The individual details of malformation determine the clinical picture, whether cyanotic or acyanotic, as well as the degree of handicap and the prognosis. Nearly all malformations are now amenable to surgery, with expectation of total correction in some and improvement in many. Congenital heart disease is commonly associated with other developmental defects and syndromes. Abbr. CHD **congenital Minamata d.** A neurologic disease resembling cerebral palsy that is seen in infants born to women who consumed food contaminated with mercury during the pregnancy. The mother does not always display postpartum signs of Minamata disease, thus indicating that the fetus is more susceptible to mercury posioning than the adult. **Conradi's d.** See under CHONDRODYSPLASIA PUNCTATA. **constitutional d.** A disease resulting from an inherent feature, as an inborn error of metabolism, as distinguished from an acquired disease, as by fortuitous infection. **contagious d.** A disease communicated between hosts either directly or indirectly. Also *communicable disease.* **convulsive tic d.** GILLES DE LA TOURETTE SYNDROME. **copper storage d.** WILSON'S DISEASE. **Corbus d.** GANGRENOUS BALANITIS. **Cori's d.** GLYCOGEN STORAGE DISEASE III. **Corrigan's d.** AORTIC REGURGITATION. **Corvisart's d.** 1 HYPERTROPHIC CARDIOMYOPATHY. 2 Tetralogy of Fallot with right aortic arch. **Cotugno's d.** SCIATICA. **Creutzfeldt-Jakob d.** A progressive degenerative brain disease of middle and late life, due to infection by a transmissible agent, believed to be a prion and characterized by a very long incubation period. In the typical case, the manifestations are rapidly progressive dementia with myoclonus and with typical periodic discharges in the electroencephalogram. The brain shows typical spongiform degeneration. In other cases the course is subacute with parkinsonian features, spasticity, and amyotrophy in addition to dementia. The condition is generally fatal in from six months to two years. Also *Jakob-Creutzfeldt disease, Jakob's disease, Jakob spastic pseudosclerosis, Creutzfeldt-Jakob syndrome, Creutzfeldt-Jakob presenile encephalopathy, Jones-Nevin syndrome, spongiform encephalopathy, striocortical syndrome.* **Crigler-Najjar d.** CRIGLER-NAJJAR SYNDROME. **Crohn's d.** A chronic inflammatory bowel disease involving the small intestine (most commonly the terminal ileum), the colon, or both, and characterized pathologically by transmural inflammation, deep linear ulceration, and often granulomas. Also *regional enteritis.* **Crouzon's d.** CRANIOFACIAL DYSOSTOSIS. **Cushing's d.** The pituitary-dependent form of Cushing syndrome, whether or not there is an adenoma of the adenohypophysis. See under CUSHING SYNDROME. Also *Cushing's basophilism.* **cyanotic heart d.** Heart disease complicated by cyanosis. Also *maladie bleue, blue disease* (outmoded, popular). **cystic d. of breast** CYSTIC MASTOPATHY. **cysticercus d.** CYSTICERCOSIS. **cystine storage d.** CYSTINOSIS. **cytomegalic inclusion d.** Systemic disease due to infection with cytomegalovirus. Of worldwide distribution, the disease may be congenital or acquired and is frequently asymptomatic. The virus may be transmitted transplacentally or acquired by sexual contact, blood transfusion, or transplantation of an infected organ. Symptomatic congenital infection may be characterized by hepatosplenomegaly, jaundice, purpura, microcephaly, cerebral calcifications, and chorioretinitis. Permanent psychomotor damage may result, with 75% of symptomatic infants having central nervous system sequelae in later years. Infection acquired after birth is usually benign but may produce respiratory symptoms with pneumonia, paroxysmal cough, petechial rash, hepatosplenomegaly, chorioretinitis, and gastric ulcerations. The virus can also cause a mononucleosis difficult to distinguish from Epstein-Barr virus mononucleosis. Renal transplant recipients on immunosuppressive therapy and persons with acquired immune deficiency syndrome (AIDS) are susceptible to acquisition of the virus or its reactivation. Also *cytomegalovirus disease.* **Daae's d.** EPIDEMIC PLEURODYNIA. **Daae-Finsen d.** EPIDEMIC PLEURODYNIA. **Dalrymple's d.** CYCLOKERATITIS. **Danielssen-Boeck d.** SARCOIDOSIS. **Darier's d.** 1 KERATOSIS FOLLICULARIS. 2 PSEUDOXANTHOMA ELASTICUM. 3 ERYTHEMA ANNULARE CENTRIFUGUM. 4 BENIGN FAMILIAL PEMPHIGUS. **Darling's d.** HISTOPLASMOSIS. **debrancher glycogen storage d.** GLYCOGEN STORAGE DISEASE III. **decompression d.** DECOMPRESSION SICKNESS. **deer-fly d.** TULAREMIA. **deficiency d.** A condition arising from the deficiency of an essential nutrient either through a lack of dietary intake of the nutrient or due to an inability to metabolize the nutrient. Examples of such diseases include beriberi, kwashiorkor, rickets, pellagra, and xerophthalmia. Also *deprivation disease.* **degenerative joint d.** OSTEOARTHRITIS. **degenerative joint d. of the lumbar spine** 1 Osteoarthritis of the zygapophyseal joints of the lumbar spine. 2 Degenerative disk disease of the lumbar spine. *Imprecise.* **Dejerine d.** HEREDITARY HYPERTROPHIC INTERSTITIAL NEUROPATHY. **demyelinating d.** Any disease of the central or peripheral nervous system in which demyelination is the predominant pathologic change. In the central nervous system, multiple sclerosis is the commonest demyelinating disease. **dense deposit d.** MEMBRANOPROLIFERATIVE GLOMERULONEPHRITIS. **deprivation d.** DEFICIENCY DISEASE. **de Quervain's d.** DE QUERVAIN SYNDROME. **Dercum's d.** NEUROLIPOMATOSIS DOLOROSA. **Devic's d.** NEUROMYELITIS OPTICA. **diatomite d.** DIATOMACEOUS EARTH PNEUMOCONIOSIS. **Dieulafoy's d.** Superficial ulceration of the gastric mucosa occurring over arterioles, leading to gastrointestinal bleeding. The cause of the ulceration, which occurs in otherwise healthy individuals, is unknown. **Di Guglielmo's d.** ERYTHROLEUKEMIA. **Dimitri's d.** STURGE-WEBER SYNDROME. **disappearing bone d.** A condition marked by a hemangiomatous lesion that gives rise to massive bone resorption. The bone seems to disappear when seen on a radiograph. **Döhle d.** SYPHILITIC AORTITIS. **Duchenne's d.** 1 DUCHENNE TYPE MUSCULAR DYSTROPHY. 2 MOTOR NEURON DISEASE. 3 TABES DORSALIS. **Dukes d.** EXANTHEM SUBITUM. **Dupré's d.** *Obs.* MENINGISM. **Dupuytren's d. of the foot** PLANTAR FIBROMATOSIS. **Duroziez d.** Congenital mitral stenosis, a rare condition usually associated with other anomalies such as aortic atresia. **Dutton's d.** AFRICAN TICK FEVER. **dynamic d.** FUNCTIONAL DISEASE. **Eales d.** A focal proliferation of new-formed blood vessels upon the retinal surface, invading the vitreous cavity. The etiology is unknown and the diagnosis does not include somewhat similar neovascularization associated with sickle-cell retinopathy, diabetic retinopathy, or retinopathy of prematurity. All of these disorders are variants of retinal vaso-occlusive disease. **Ebola virus d.** A severe and often fatal hemorrhagic fever caused by the Ebola virus and characterized by fever, nausea, vomiting, diarrhea, pharyngitis, dyspnea, cough, chest pain, prostration, and, after about five days, a morbilliform or vesicular rash, hepatitis, encephalitis, and disseminated intravascular coagulation. The case-fatality ratio is 50–70 percent, with death occurring 4–10 days after onset. Hitherto unknown, the disease occurred as an epidemic in Zaire and the Sudan in 1976–1977, with high mortality. The vector is unknown. The mode of transmission may be person-to-person. Ebola virus is closely related to but serologically distinct from Marburg virus. These two viruses are distinct from all others. Also *African hemorrhagic fever.* **Economo's d.** ENCEPHALITIS LETHARGICA. **Eddowes d.** LOBSTEIN SYNDROME. **Ehlers-Danlos d.** EHLERS-DANLOS SYNDROME. **Eisenmenger d.** EISENMENGER SYNDROME. **end-stage renal d.** Irreversible chronic renal failure that requires hemodialysis or transplantation for survival of the patient. *Popular.* **Engelmann's d.** PROGRESSIVE DIAPHYSEAL DYSPLASIA. **Engel-Recklinghausen d.** OSTEITIS FIBROSA CYSTICA. **English d.** RICKETS. **Engman's d.** INFECTIVE DERMATITIS. **eosinophilic collagen d.** An illness of uncertain classification characterized by fever, myalgia, arthralgia, and eosinophilia. It may be related to eosinophilic fasciitis or other hypereosinophilic syndromes. **eosinophilic endomyocardial d.** LÖFFLER'S ENDOCARDITIS. **epidemic hemorrhagic d.** EPIDEMIC HEMORRHAGIC FEVER. **Erb's d.** MUSCULAR DYSTROPHY. **Erb-Charcot d.** SYPHILITIC SPASTIC PARAPLEGIA. **Erb-Goldflam d.** MYASTHENIA GRAVIS. **Erb-Landouzy d.** MUSCULAR DYSTROPHY. **Eulenburg's d.** PARAMYOTONIA CONGENITA. **euthyroid Graves d.** A disorder of thyroid function in which the clinical and laboratory signs of hyperthyroidism are lacking but the thyroid gland is unresponsive to thyrotropin and to suppression by exogenous thyroid hormone, and the eyes show the typical features of thyrotoxic ophthalmopathy. **extramammary Paget's d.** See under PAGET'S DISEASE OF THE SKIN. **Fabry's d.** ANGIOKERATOMA CORPORIS DIFFUSUM. **Fahr's d.** A condition characterized morphologically by a protein deposit which undergoes secondary calcification in the walls of the blood vessels and adjacent parenchyma of the basal ganglia and dentate nuclei. The onset is in adolescence or middle age, and it usually gives rise to pyramidal, extrapyramidal, and cerebellar signs, reduced intelligence, and epileptic seizures, but it can sometimes be asymptomatic. Radiography shows that there are rounded, linear, or radiate shadows in the central nuclei, always bilateral. Calcification of the basal ganglia may sometimes occur in hypoparathyroidism. Recent work suggests that Fahr's disease is not a specific disease entity but a syndrome of multiple etiology. **familial hypophosphatemic bone d.** A heterogeneous condition of autosomal inheritance that is characterized by nonrachitic skeletal changes, a mild form of short stature and leg bowing, normal plasma calcium, and hypophosphatemia. Also *familial hypophosphatemic osteomalacia.* **Fanconi's d.** 1 FANCONI SYNDROME. 2 FANCONI'S ANEMIA. **Farber's d.** LIPOGRANULOMATOSIS. **fat-deficiency d.** A disease that manifests itself in rats and other animals by a failure to grow and by an eczematous dermatitis. The condition is due to a deficiency of the essential fatty acid, linoleic acid. Humans require just one gram per day, and it is rare to find a case of this disorder in human beings. Occasionally, it occurs in adults who have had a large portion of their small intestine removed but have not received total parenteral nutrition that includes lipids. The disease may occur in infants fed on low fat diets based on skimmed milk. Growth failure due to the disease has never been reported but eczema has been seen in both adults and children. **Fazio-Londe d.** INFANTILE PROGRESSIVE BULBAR PALSY. **Fc fragment d.** HEAVY CHAIN DISEASE. **Fede's d.** FRENAL ULCER. **Fenwick's d.** ATROPHIC GASTRITIS. **fibrocystic d.** 1 Any condition characterized by a combination of fibrosis and epithelial hyperplasia with cyst formation and occurring in a glandular tissue. It most typically affects the breast. 2 CYSTIC MASTOPATHY. **fibrocystic d. of bone** OSTEITIS FIBROSA CYSTICA. **fibrocystic d. of breast** CYSTIC MASTOPATHY. **fibrocystic d. of the pancreas** CYSTIC FIBROSIS. **fibromuscular d.** Nonatherosclerotic lesions of the renal artery or its primary branches, affecting the intima, media, elastica, or adventia, and often resulting in renovascular hypertension. Intimal fibroplasia is characterized by segmental circumferential fibrous tissue, usually in children or young adults in whom the elastica may be broken, resulting in a dissecting aneurysm. Fibromuscular hyperplasia (or dysplasia) represents various abnormalities in the intima, media, elastica, or adventia of the renal arterial wall, usually a localized overgrowth of the smooth muscle of the media. The involved artery may be tortuous, appear "corrugated" radiographically, and often is stenotic, causing renovascular hypertension. The lesion usually occurs in women 30–50 years of age, is often bilateral, and may be corrected surgically. Medial fibroplasia is often complicated by microaneurysms which produce a "string-of-beads" appearance on renal arteriography. Medial fibroplasia usually occurs in women 30–50 years of age and is often bilateral. Subadvential fibroplasia affects women 20–40 years of age and is characterized by marked stenosis due to dense collagen in the outer media, usually on the right. Also *fibromuscular hypertrophy.* **Fiedler's d.** ICTERIC LEPTOSPIROSIS. **fifth d.** ERYTHEMA INFECTIOSUM. **Filatov's d.** INFECTIOUS MONONUCLEOSIS. **Filatov-Dukes d.** EXANTHEM SUBITUM. **fish-skin d.** ICHTHYOSIS. **fish-tapeworm d.** DIPHYLLOBOTHRIASIS. **Flatau's d.** SCHILDER'S DISEASE. **Flatau-Schilder d.** SCHILDER'S DISEASE. **flax-dressers' d.** BYSSINOSIS. **flecked retina d.** Any of a variety of conditions accompanied by the appearance of multiple, small, light-colored spots in the fundus, including retinitis punctata albescens, fundus flavimaculatus, Kandori's fleck retina, and drusen. **Fleischner's d.** Osteochondritis of the proximal interphalangeal joints of the hands. **floating beta d.**

FAMILIAL HYPERLIPOPROTEINEMIA TYPE III. **focal d.** A disease that is limited to one or more specific sites. **Foix-Alajouanine d.** SUBACUTE NECROTIC MYELITIS. **Fölling's d.** *Outmoded* PHENYLKETONURIA. **foot-and-mouth d.** An acute, highly contagious, rhinoviral infection of wild and domestic animals, especially those with cloven hooves, which produces fever and a vesicular eruption on the lips, buccal cavity, pharynx, legs, feet, and sometimes, udders and teats. Man is occasionally infected and develops fever, malaise, headache, and vesiculation of the mouth, palms, and soles. Also *hoof-and-mouth disease, contagious aphthae, epizootic aphthae, aphthae epizooticae, malignant aphthae, aphthosa, aphthous fever, eczema epizootica.* **foot process d.** LIPOID NEPHROSIS. **Forbes d.** GLYCOGEN STORAGE DISEASE III. **Fordyce d.** FORDYCE SPOTS. **Förster's d.** 1 FÖRSTER'S DIPLEGIA. 2 AREOLAR CENTRAL CHOROIDITIS. **Fournier's d.** Fulminating gangrene of the external genitalia. Also *Fournier's gangrene.* **fourth d.** EXANTHEM SUBITUM. **Fox-Fordyce d.** A characteristic eruption of skin-colored papules, notably in the axillae, at the site of the apocrine gland ducts. It is comparable to miliaria of the eccrine sweat glands. Also *lichen axillaris.* **fracture d.** POST-TRAUMATIC OSTEOPOROSIS. **Francis d.** TULAREMIA. **Franklin's d.** GAMMA HEAVY-CHAIN DISEASE. **Frei's d.** LYMPHOGRANULOMA VENEREUM. **Freiberg's d.** KÖHLER SECOND DISEASE. **Friedländer's d.** ENDARTERITIS OBLITERANS. **Friedmann's d.** NARCOLEPSY. **Friedreich's d.** 1 A form of progressive hereditary ataxia of autosomal recessive inheritance beginning in childhood and giving rise to cerebellar ataxia, areflexia, extensor plantar responses, pes cavus, scoliosis, and variable amyotrophy. Less constant associations include cardiomyopathy and diabetes mellitus. Also *Friedreich's ataxia, Friedreich's tabes, hereditary spinal sclerosis.* 2 PARAMYOCLONUS MULTIPLEX. **Frommel's d.** CHIARI-FROMMEL SYNDROME. **functional d.** A disease in which functional impairment is unaccompanied by any ascertainable organic lesion. Also *dynamic disease.* **fusospirochetal d.** FUSOSPIROCHETOSIS. **Gaisböck's d.** STRESS ERYTHROCYTOSIS. **gamma heavy-chain d.** A lymphomalike disorder associated with an abnormal immunoglobulin IgG fragment in blood or urine. The condition is characterized by an atypical lymphocytic infiltration of lymph nodes, liver, and spleen that may simulate Hodgkin's disease, lymphosarcoma, or myeloma, and an abnormal protein in serum or urine that consists of the Fc fragment of IgG heavy chains. Also *Franklin's disease.* **Gamna's d.** SIDEROTIC SPLENOMEGALY. **Gamstorp's d.** PERIODIC PARALYSIS II. **Gandy-Gamna d.** SIDEROTIC SPLENOMEGALY. **Gandy-Nanta d.** SIDEROTIC SPLENOMEGALY. **garapata d.** Relapsing fever transmitted by ticks. • A term derived from the Spanish word *garrapatas,* tick. **Garré's d.** NONSUPPURATIVE OSTEOMYELITIS. **Gastaut's d.** LENNOX-GASTAUT SYNDROME. **Gaucher's d.** A group of inborn errors of glycosphingolipid (GSL) metabolism associated with deficiency of glucocerebrosidase. Type I, the most common variant, is characterized by deposition of GSL that is principally visceral and not neuronal. Hepatosplenomegaly, anemia, and bone erosions may be noted first in infancy or in late adulthood. In type II, infants develop both hepatosplenomegaly and severe neurologic deterioration, usually dying by age one year. In type III, the rarest variant, signs of visceral and neuronal GSL accumulation develop in childhood or early adulthood. All three forms are inherited as autosomal recessives. Also *glucocerebrosidase deficiency, glucocerebrosidosis.* **Gayet's d.** WERNICKE'S DISEASE. **Gee's d.** INFANTILE CELIAC DISEASE. **Gee-Herter-Heubner d.** INFANTILE CELIAC DISEASE. **Gee-Thaysen d.** ADULT CELIAC DISEASE. **genetic d.** HEREDITARY DISORDER. **Gerhardt's d.** ERYTHROMELALGIA. **Gerlier's d.** VESTIBULAR NEURONITIS. **Gibert's d.** PITYRIASIS ROSEA. **Gilbert's d.** GILBERT SYNDROME. **Gilchrist's d.** BLASTOMYCOSIS. **Gilles de la Tourette's d.** GILLES DE LA TOURETTE SYNDROME. **Glanzmann's d.** An autosomally inherited hemorrhagic disease with unique abnormalities of platelet function. Also *thrombasthenia, Glanzmann's thrombasthenia, thromboasthenic diathesis, thrombocytasthenia.* **glassblowers' d.** HEAT-RAY CATARACT. **Glisson's d.** RICKETS. **glomerular d.** GLOMERULOPATHY. **glomerular epithelial cell d.** LIPOID NEPHROSIS. **glycogen storage d.** A group of rare, autosomal recessive inborn errors of glycogen metabolism. Each type, designated by a Roman numeral, is due to a deficiency of a specific enzyme involved in glycogen catabolism, and is characterized by deposition of either abnormal quantities of glycogen, metabolic intermediates, or both in various organs. Also *glycogenosis.* **glycogen storage d. I** A disorder in which a deficiency of glucose-6-phosphatase prevents normal catabolism of glycogen and results in the massive deposition of structurally normal glycogen in tissues, particularly the liver. Its clinical effects are hypoglycemia, gout, growth retardation, and death before adulthood. Treatment consists of frequent feedings to prevent hypoglycemia. Also *von Gierke's disease, hepatorenal glycogen storage disease, glucose-6-phosphatase deficiency.* **glycogen storage d. II** A disorder caused by a deficiency of $\alpha$-1,4-glucosidase (acid maltase). It prevents the normal catabolism of glycogen and results in an accumulation of structurally normal glycogen in tissues, particularly the heart and the central nervous system. The clinical effects begin in infancy and include severe hypotonia, motor and mental retardation, and heart failure leading to early death. Also *Pompe's disease, $\alpha$-1,4-glucosidase deficiency, acid-maltase deficiency, glycogenosis type II.* **glycogen storage d. III** A disorder in which a deficiency of amylo-1,6-glucosidase results in the failure to completely catabolize glycogen and the accumulation of glycogen with short outer chains in the liver, heart, and skeletal muscle. The clinical features include growth retardation, hepatomegaly, and hypoglycemia. Also *debrancher deficiency, Cori's disease, Forbes disease, glycogenosis type III, amylo-1,6-glucosidase deficiency, debrancher glycogen storage disease.* **glycogen storage d. IV** A disorder in which a deficiency of amylo-(1,4-1,6)-transglucosidase results in an accumulation of abnormal glycogen in the skeletal muscle and liver. The clinical features include cirrhosis, portal hypertension, and death in childhood from hepatic failure. Also *Andersen's disease, brancher deficiency, amylopectinosis, brancher deficiency glycogenosis, brancher glycogen storage disease, amylo-(1,4-1,6)-transglucosidase deficiency.* **glycogen storage d. V** A disorder due to a deficiency of muscle phosphorylase. Affected individuals are normal at rest and during mild exercise. Fatigue appears soon after commencing anerobic exercise, attended usually by painful muscle cramps and, occasionally, by myoglobinuria which has caused renal failure in some. Also *McArdle's disease, muscle phosphorylase deficiency, glycogenosis type V, myophosphorylase deficiency glycogenosis, familial paroxysmal rhabdomyolysis.* **glycogen storage d. VI** A disorder that is probably due to a deficiency of hepatic phosphorylase activity. It may be heterogeneous. The clinical course is similar to but milder than glycogen storage disease I. Also *Hers disease, hepatic phosphorylase deficiency, hepatophosphorylase de-*

*ficiency glycogenosis, glycogenosis type VI.* **glycogen storage d. VII** A disorder due to deficiency of muscle phosphofructokinase. The clinical features are identical to glycogen storage disease V. Also *muscle phosphofructokinase deficiency, Tarui's disease.* **glycogen storage d. VIII** An X-linked disorder due to deficiency of the kinase which activates phosphorylase. Affected individuals are often asymptomatic but have hepatomegaly, increased liver glycogen, and diminished activity of hepatic phosphorylase B. Also *hepatic phosphorylase kinase deficiency.* **Goldflam's d.** MYASTHENIA GRAVIS. **Goldflam-Erb d.** MYASTHENIA GRAVIS. **Goldstein's d.** HEREDITARY HEMORRHAGIC TELANGIECTASIA. **Gowers d.** VASOVAGAL ATTACK. **Graefe's d.** PROGRESSIVE OPHTHALMOPLEGIA. **graft-versus-host d.** A disease caused by the transfer into an immunologically deficient host of allogeneic immunocompetent cells which, not being rejected, mount a reaction against the host's histocompatibility antigens. In experimental animals, it produces wasting disease (runt disease). In man, graft-versus-host disease involves principally the skin, the alimentary tract, and the liver, though other organs may be affected as well. Symptoms may include a morbilliform rash, severe diarrhea and abdominal pain, and jaundice. Graft-versus-host disease has been the major factor limiting the use of allogeneic bone marrow transplantation in man. However, progress in the ability to deplete native T cells from grafts with monoclonal antibodies carries the promise of overcoming the problem. Also *graft-versus-host reaction, GVH disease, GVH reaction, transplantation disease* (rare). Abbr. GVHD **Graves d.** Hyperthyroidism due to diffuse toxic goiter, probably of autoimmune origin, occurring most often in young women. It is characterized by weight loss, nervousness, disturbances of sleep, excessive heat intolerance and sweating, exophthalmos, fine tremor, swelling of the anterior neck, and tachycardia with raised metabolic rate and increased plasma concentration of the thyroid hormones. A self-limited disease, it can be treated pharmacologically, surgically, or with radioiodine. Also *Begbie's disease* (rare), *thyrotoxic cachexia* (obs.), *exophthalmic cachexia, Parry's disease* (chiefly British), *hyperthroidism* (ambiguous), *morbus basedowii, struma basedowificata.* **Greenfield's d.** BALÓ'S DISEASE. **green monkey d.** MARBURG VIRUS DISEASE. **Grisel's d.** NASOPHARYNGEAL TORTICOLLIS. **guinea worm d.** DRACONTIASIS. **GVH d.** GRAFT-VERSUS-HOST DISEASE. **Habermann's d.** PITYRIASIS LICHENOIDES. **Haff d.** Epidemic myoglobinuria occurring principally in fishermen and attributed to arsine contamination of coastal waters. • The term is derived from Königsberg *Haff,* a lagoon connected to the Baltic Sea and the site of such epidemics. **Hageman's d.** *Seldom used* FACTOR XII DEFICIENCY. **Haglund's d.** ACHILLES BURSITIS. **Hailey-Hailey d.** BENIGN FAMILIAL PEMPHIGUS. **Hallervorden-Spatz d.** A rare familial disease of autosomal recessive inheritance, starting usually during the first year of life with progressive stiffness which first affects the legs, then the arms and the facial muscles, the muscles of the mouth and of the pharynx. Subsequently athetoid movements and dementia are noted. Death usually occurs in the third year. There is progressive pigmentary degeneration of the globus pallidus and substantia nigra. There is now considerable controversy as to whe ther this is a single disease entity or a syndrome of multiple etiology. Also *pigmentary degeneration of the globus pallidus, status dysmyelinisatus, status dysmyelinatus, Hallervorden-Spatz syndrome.* **Hamman's d.** Spontaneous interstitial emphysema of the lung. Also *Hamman syndrome.* **Hamman-Rich d.** HAMMAN-RICH SYNDROME. **Hammond's d.** DOUBLE ATHETOSIS. **Hand's d.** HAND-SCHÜLLER-CHRISTIAN DISEASE. **hand-foot-and-mouth d.** An infectious disease usually seen in children and characterized by vesicular eruptions on the hands and feet and in the oropharynx. Sore throat and mouth and a low-grade fever also occur. It is caused principally by coxsackieviruses. **Hand-Schüller-Christian d.** Chronic multiple histiocytosis of bone, characterized by onset in childhood of destructive bone lesions, especially of the skull, loss of teeth, chronically draining ears, and diabetes insipidus that results from involvement of the sella turcica. Also *Hand's disease, Christian's disease, Schüller's disease, Schüller-Christian disease, normocholesteremic xanthomatosis, lipid granulomatosis, xanthomatosis generalisata ossium, chronic idiopathic xanthomatosis, Christian syndrome, Hand-Schüller-Christian syndrome, Hand syndrome, Schüller syndrome, Schüller-Christian syndrome.* **Hanot's d.** PRIMARY BILIARY CIRRHOSIS. **Hansen's d.** LEPROSY. **Harada's d.** HARADA SYNDROME. **hard-metal d.** A pneumoconiosis caused by exposure to the dust of hard metal manufactured from tungsten and carbon, with cobalt, the suspected agent of the disease, as a binder. It is characterized by respiratory distress towards the end of the work day. X rays show scattered nodular shadows. In severe cases there may be interstitial fibrosis of the lungs. **Hartnup's d.** A rare genetic disorder of tubular amino acid reabsorption of some monoamine monocarboxylic amino acids (excluding glycine, proline, and hydroxyproline). This disorder is associated with an increased requirement for nicotinamide, manifested by a pellagralike rash, cerebellar ataxia, diarrhea, and psychosis. Nicotinamide is a specific therapy. **Hashimoto's d.** A chronic, autoimmune disease of the thyroid, commoner in women, which presents as thyroid gland enlargement or hypothyroidism. The gland is densely infiltrated with lymphocytes and its substance ultimately destroyed, leading to myxedema. It sometimes occurs in association with other autoimmune diseases and occasionally as part of the course of Graves disease. Also *Hashimoto's thyroiditis, lymphocytic thyroiditis, struma lymphomatosa, Hashimoto struma, autoimmune thyroiditis, chronic lymphadenoid thyroiditis, chronic lymphocytic thyroiditis, chronic thyroiditis, lymphoid thyroiditis, lymphadenoid goiter, struma lymphatica* (seldom used). **heart d.** Any disorder affecting the endocardium, myocardium, pericardium, or coronary arteries. **heavy chain d.** A monoclonal gammopathy in which there is secretion of incomplete immunoglobulin heavy chains, not combined with any light chains. Deletions in the heavy chain constant region genes are responsible. Heavy chain disease of IgA ($\alpha$-chain disease), IgG ($\gamma$-chain disease), and IgM ($\mu$-chain disease) are all known. $\alpha$-chain disease is associated with an intestinal lymphoma and is found particularly in North Africa. $\gamma$-chain disease is associated with a lymphoma particularly affecting the pharyngeal ring. $\mu$-chain disease is often associated with chronic lymphocytic leukemia. Also *Fc fragment disease.* See also ALPHA HEAVY-CHAIN DISEASE, GAMMA HEAVY-CHAIN DISEASE. **Heberden's d.** Osteoarthritis of the hands. **Heerfordt's d.** HEERFORDT SYNDROME. **Heine-Medin d.** ACUTE ANTERIOR POLIOMYELITIS. **Heller's d.** DEMENTIA INFANTILIS. **Heller-Döhle d.** SYPHILITIC AORTITIS. **hemoglobin C d.** HOMOZYGOUS HEMOGLOBIN C. **hemoglobin C-thalassemia d.** HEMOGLOBIN C-$\beta$-THALASSEMIA. **hemoglobin D d.** HOMOZYGOUS HEMOGLOBIN D. **hemoglobin E d.** *Incorrect* HOMOZYGOUS HEMOGLOBIN E. **hemoglobin H d.** A thalassemia of moderate severity due to the inheritance of a gene for $\alpha$-thalassemia-1 from one parent and of a gene for $\alpha$-thalassemia-2 from the other parent, so that only one α-globin gene is functional. This results in marked reduction in α-globin chain formation and an excess of β-globin chains. The excess β-globin chains form a tetramer, $\beta_4$, or hemoglobin H, which usually comprises 5–15% of the total hemoglobin. The disorder is characterized by moderate anemia (venous hemoglobin concentration about 9 g/dl), mild hemolytic jaundice, and splenomegaly. **hemoglobin S-C d.** A serious sickling disorder due to inheritance of a gene for hemoglobin S from one parent and a gene for hemoglobin C from the other. The condition has all the features of homozygous hemoglobin S disease, but usually is somewhat milder. Also *sickle cell-hemoglobin C disease.* **hemoglobin S-D d.** A severe sickling disorder that results from inheritance of a gene for hemoglobin S from one parent and a gene for hemoglobin D-Punjab from the other. The disorder typically has all the features of homozygous hemoglobin S disease. Also *sickle cell-hemoglobin D disease.* **hemoglobin S-O-Arab d.** A severe sickling disorder that results from inheritance of a gene for hemoglobin S from one parent and a gene for hemoglobin O-Arab from the other. The disorder typically has all the features of homozygous hemoglobin S disease. The condition has often been mistaken for hemoglobin S-C disease because hemoglobins C and O-Arab have similar electrophoretic mobility. **hemolytic d. of the newborn** Any hemolytic disorder that is present at or shortly follows birth, as evidenced by anemia, jaundice, and greater than normal serum bilirubin concentration. Also *erythroleukoblastosis.* **hemorrhagic d. of the newborn** An exaggeration of the physiologic coagulation change that normally occurs during the first week of life. It reflects a deficiency of vitamin K. Also *hemophilia neonatorum* (incorrect), *morbus maculosus neonatorum.* **hemp-workers' d.** BYSSINOSIS. **Henneberg's d.** PSEUDOBULBAR PARALYSIS. **Henoch's d.** HENOCH-SCHÖNLEIN PURPURA. **hepatolenticular d.** WILSON'S DISEASE. **hepatorenal glycogen storage d.** GLYCOGEN STORAGE DISEASE I. **hereditary d.** HEREDITARY DISORDER. **Hers d.** GLYCOGEN STORAGE DISEASE VI. **Herter's d.** INFANTILE CELIAC DISEASE. **Herter-Heubner d.** INFANTILE CELIAC DISEASE. **hidebound d.** SCLERODERMA. **Hildenbrand's d.** TYPHUS. **Hirschsprung's d.** CONGENITAL MEGACOLON. **His-Werner d.** TRENCH FEVER. **Hodgkin's d.** A malignant neoplasm principally affecting lymph nodes and spleen, characterized by altered architecture of tissues and infiltration by lymphocytes, monocytes, plasma cells, eosinophils, fibroblasts, and Reed-Sternberg cells. Several histologic classifications have been made of Hodgkin's disease. One widely used is: lymphocyte predominance, mixed lymphocytic-histiocytic, nodular sclerosing, lymphocyte depleted. Also *lymphogranulomatosis, Reed-Hodgkin disease, Sternberg's disease, multiple lymphadenoma, lymphogranuloma malignum, malignant lymphogranulomatosis, granulomatous lymphoma, glandular sarcoma.* **Hodgkin's d. of lung** Involvement of the lung by Hodgkin's disease, either as the only manifestation or as one among others. **Hoffa's d.** A proliferation of the fat pad often with calcification, following injury to the knee joint. Also *Hoffa-Kastert disease.* **homologous d.** ALLOGENEIC DISEASE. **homozygous hemoglobin S d.** A severe and usually lethal disorder that results from inheritance of a gene for hemoglobin S from both parents. The disorder is characterized by pain crises affecting fingers, toes, joints or abdomen, pallor, jaundice, poorly healing ankle ulcers, aseptic necrosis of bones, and progressive renal impairment. Sickled erythrocytes, thin crescentic forms, can be demonstrated in blood treated with reducing agents or dilute formaldehyde. Also *sickle cell anemia.* **hoof-and-mouth d.** FOOT-AND-MOUTH DISEASE. **hookworm d.** The disease caused in various animals and man by hookworms, characterized usually by anemia but in severe infestations also causing ulceration and hemorrhage in the small intestine where the adult worms are attached to the mucosa. Common hookworms in dogs and cats are *Ancylostoma* spp. and *Uncinaria;* in cattle and sheep, *Bunostomum* spp.; and in man, *Ancylostoma* and *Necator.*. See also ANCYLOSTOMIASIS, NECATORIASIS. **Hünermann's d.** See under CHONDRODYSPLASIA PUNCTATA. **Hunt's d.** 1 JUVENILE PARALYSIS AGITANS. 2 DYSSYNERGIA CEREBELLARIS MYOCLONICA. **Huntington's d.** A chronic, dominantly inherited condition attributable to degeneration of the cerebral cortex and corpus striatum, especially the caudate nucleus. The onset is insidious, usually between 40 and 50 years of age, and is marked by choreic movements. These movements which are relatively slow in character, often showing some affinity with athetosis, may initially disappear when voluntary movements are made. Ultimately they cause a grotesque gait and severe dysarthria. This condition often gives rise initially to disorders of character and behavior such as irritability, impulsiveness, violence, fugue, sexual aberrations, even suicide. Eventually, patients suffer from chronic fatigue, apathy, poor memory, and progressive dementia. In those rare cases in which the condition begins in childhood or adolescence, it usually presents as the rigid form, with rigidity of extrapyramidal type in the limbs and trunk. Occasionally in cases showing the more usual onset in adult life dementia develops before the chorea. In the advanced stages pneumoencephalography may demonstrate atrophy of the caudate nucleus. The gene responsible for the disease lies on chromosome 4. Also *Huntington's chorea, chorea-athetosis-agitans syndrome* (obs.), *hereditary chorea, degenerative chorea, chronic chorea, chronic progressive hereditary chorea.* **Hurst's d.** ACUTE HEMORRHAGIC LEUKOENCEPHALITIS. **Hutchinson's d.** HUTCHINSON SUMMER PRURIGO. **Hutchinson-Boeck d.** SARCOIDOSIS. **hyaline membrane d.** RESPIRATORY DISTRESS SYNDROME OF NEWBORN. **hydatid d.** ECHINOCOCCOSIS. **hydatid d. of lung** Infection of the lung by *Echinococcus granulosus.* **hydroxyapatite d.** Acute painful arthritis or periarthritis associated with deposition of hydroxyapatite crystals in the involved area. Calcific tendinitis is an example. **hypertensive heart d.** Heart disease resulting from raised arterial pressure. **hypertensive renal d.** Disorder of renal structure or function as a result of sustained, systemic, arterial hypertension. **hypertensive vascular d.** Atherosclerosis of large arteries and thickening of arteriolar walls with narrowing of arteriolar lumens secondary to sustained hypertension. Involvement of vessels of the heart, brain, and kidneys are of greatest clinical importance and can cause myocardial failure or ischemia, cerebral thrombosis or hemorrhage, and renal failure respectively. **Icelandic d.** BENIGN MYALGIC ENCEPHALOMYELITIS. **I-cell d.** MUCOLIPIDOSIS II. **idiopathic d.** A disease that arises from unknown causes. • See note at IDIOPATHIC. **immune complex d.** Any of a group of numerous inflammatory conditions whose pathogenesis involves the deposition of immune complexes in tissue with fixation of complement and recruitment of polymorphonuclear leukocytes. There are two main types of immune complex disease: those where complexes are formed locally (as in the Arthus reaction), and those where complexes localize in tissue from the circulation (as in serum sickness). **infantile amaurotic familial d.** *Obs.* TAY-SACHS DISEASE. **infantile celiac d.** A condition in the first few weeks of infancy characterized by failure to thrive, bowel distension from lactose fermentation, loose stools, sometimes vomiting, and, when a jejunal biopsy is possible, villous atrophy of the mucosa. It results from feeding wheat germ-containing foods to an infant with gluten sensitivity. It is curable by administering a strict gluten-free diet. Also *Gee's disease, Gee-Herter-Heubner disease, Gee-Herter-Heubner syndrome, Herter-Heubner disease, Herter's disease, Herter's infantilism, celiac infantilism, intestinal infantilism.* **infectious d.** Disease caused by microbial agents or parasites. **inflammatory bowel d.** A category of diseases of unknown etiology characterized by chronic inflammation of the gastrointestinal tract. The major specific examples are ulcerative colitis and Crohn's disease. **inherited d.** HEREDITARY DISORDER. **iron storage d.** HEMOCHROMATOSIS. **irritable bowel d.** IRRITABLE BOWEL SYNDROME. **ischemic heart d.** Heart disease resulting from inadequate coronary blood flow. **itai-itai d.** A disease resulting from high cadmium intake and characterized by renal tubular proteinuria, impaired vitamin D metabolism, myalgia, and lumbar pain. Reported in Fuchu, Japan, in multiparous women over the age of 50, it results from industrial contamination of food, especially rice, and water. It can lead to osteomalacia with multiple fractures and a slow painful death. The precise etiology is obscure. Also *ouch-ouch disease.* **Itsenko's d.** A term used in the USSR for CUSHING SYNDROME. **Jaffe's d.** See under FIBROUS DYSPLASIA. **Jaffe-Lichtenstein d.** See under FIBROUS DYSPLASIA. **Jakob's d.** CREUTZFELDT-JAKOB DISEASE. **Jakob-Creutzfeldt d.** CREUTZFELDT-JAKOB DISEASE. **Jaksch d.** VON JAKSCH ANEMIA. **Janet's d.** PSYCHASTHENIA. **Jansen's d.** A hereditary form of metaphyseal dysplasia. **Jansky-Bielschowsky d.** LATE JUVENILE CEROID-LIPOFUSCINOSIS. **Jensen's d.** Retinochoroiditis juxtapapillaris sufficiently severe to damage the overlying nerve fibers with a consequential visual-field defect, typical of damage to the nerve fiber bundle. **Jessner-Kanof d.** LYMPHOCYTIC INFILTRATION OF SKIN. **Joseph's d.** ENCEPHALOPATHY WITH PROLINEMIA. **jumper d. of Maine** JUMPING FRENCHMEN OF MAINE. **jumping d.** CHOREOMANIA. **juvenile Paget's d.** HYPERPHOSPHATASIA. **Kahlbaum's d.** CATATONIC STUPOR. **Kalischer's d.** STURGE-WEBER SYNDROME. **Kaposi's d.** KAPOSI SARCOMA. **Katayama d.** KATAYAMA SYNDROME. **Kawasaki d.** KAWASAKI SYNDROME. **Kayser's d.** WILSON'S DISEASE. **kedani d.** SCRUB TYPHUS. **Kienböck's d.** Osteochondrosis of the carpal lunate bone. It may follow repeated trauma to the wrist joint. Also *lunatomalacia.* **kinky hair d.** MENKES SYNDROME. **Kinnier Wilson d.** WILSON'S DISEASE. **kissing d.** *Popular* INFECTIOUS MONONUCLEOSIS. • It was formerly believed that kissing was a major mode of transmission of the infection. **Klemperer's d.** BANTI'S DISEASE. **knight's d.** Infection of perianal abrasions such as those acquired by horseback riders from the chafing of the saddle. **Köhler's d.** Osteochondrosis of the navicular bone, often seen in adolescence. Also *epiphysitis juvenilis, osteochondritis of the tarsal navicular, os naviculare pedis retardatum, tarsal scaphoiditis.* **Köhler-Pellegrini-Stieda d.** PELLEGRINI-STIEDA DISEASE. **Köhler second d.** A thickening of the second metatarsal with osteochondrosis of the second metatarsal head, which gives rise to pain on standing and walking. Also *Freiberg's disease, Freiberg's infraction.* **König's d.** OSTEOCHONDRITIS DISSECANS. **Korsakoff's d.** KORSAKOFF PSYCHOSIS. **Kostmann's d.** 1 FANCONI'S ANEMIA. 2 CONGENITAL NEUTROPENIA. **Kozhevnikov's d.** CONTINUOUS PARTIAL EPILEPSY. **Krabbe's d.** 1 An infantile form of hereditary cerebral leukodystrophy, with onset at the age of four to six months, giving rise to progressive spastic weakness of the limbs, dementia, and sometimes hyperkinesia and tonic fits, and disturbances of ocular movement, leading to death within a few years. Sometimes there are also cerebellar signs, such as dysarthria, choreoathetoid movements, and difficulty in swallowing, the cerebrospinal fluid protein content is raised, and there may be clinical or electrophysiological evidence of polyneuropathy. The specific pathologic change is the presence in the white matter of the degenerating brain and peripheral nerves of large multinucleate cells (globoid cells). Also *Christensen-Krabbe disease, Krabbe type diffuse sclerosis, acute diffuse familial infantile cerebral sclerosis, Krabbe's leukodystrophy, globoid leukodystrophy, globoid cell leukodystrophy, Christensen-Krabbe progressive infantile cerebral poliodystrophy.* 2 CONGENITAL GENERALIZED MUSCULAR HYPOPLASIA. **Kufs d.** ADULT CEROID-LIPOFUSCINOSIS. **Kugelberg-Welander d.** JUVENILE FAMILIAL MUSCULAR ATROPHY. **Kuhnt-Junius d.** DISCIFORM MACULAR DEGENERATION. **Kümmell's d.** A complex of symptoms that develop following a compression fracture of a vertebra and are characterized by pain in the spine, intercostal neuralgia, kyphosis, and mild weakness of the lower limbs. Also *Kümmell-Verneuil disease, Kümmell spondylitis, spondylomalacia traumatica, traumatic spondylopathy, post-traumatic spondylitis.* **Kussmaul's d.** POLYARTERITIS NODOSA. **Kussmaul-Maier d.** POLYARTERITIS NODOSA. **Kwok's d.** CHINESE RESTAURANT SYNDROME. **laboratory d.** Any disease that does not occur naturally and is induced experimentally in a laboratory animal. **Laennec's d.** LAENNEC CIRRHOSIS. **Lafora's d.** PROGRESSIVE MYOCLONIC EPILEPSY. **Lafora body d.** PROGRESSIVE MYOCLONIC EPILEPSY. **Lancereaux-Mathieu d.** ICTERIC LEPTOSPIROSIS. **Landouzy's d.** ICTERIC LEPTOSPIROSIS. **Landry's d.** LANDRY'S PARALYSIS. **Lane's d.** ERYTHEMA PALMARE HEREDITARIUM. **Larrey-Weil d.** ICTERIC LEPTOSPIROSIS. **Larsen-Johansson d.** Osteochondrosis of the distal pole of the patella. Also *Larsen's disease, Sinding-Larsen-Johansson disease.* **Lauber's d.** FUNDUS ALBIPUNCTATUS. **Leber's d.** A hereditary bilateral optic atrophy affecting otherwise healthy young males. **Lederer's d.** LEDERER'S ANEMIA. **Legal's d.** GLOSSOPHARYNGEAL NEURALGIA. **Legg's d.** PERTHES DISEASE. **Legg-Calvé-Perthes d.** PERTHES DISEASE. **legionnaire's d.** An infectious disease caused by *Legionella pneumophila* and frequently characterized by severe pneumonia. First recognized after the occurrence of small, localized epidemics with a high mortality, it is now known to occur also, and not infrequently, in a less severe form. **Leigh's d.** SUBACUTE NECROTIZING ENCEPHALOPATHY. **Leiner's d.** A rare disorder of infancy, characterized by erythroderma, diarrhea, and recurrent infection. It is probably the result of an inherited defect of the complement system. **Lemierre's d.** A rare form of bacterial tonsillitis and pharyngitis caused by *Fusobacterium septicum* which may result in thrombophlebitis of the jugular vein with septic pulmonary embolus. **Lenegre's d.** Complete heart block due to primary degeneration of the atrioventricular conducting tissue. **Leri's d.** MELORHEOSTOSIS. **Leriche's d.** POST-TRAUMATIC OSTEOPOROSIS. **Letterer-Siwe d.** An acute generalized histiocytosis characterized by onset in infancy of fever, lymphadenopathy, enlargement of liver and spleen, eczematoid erythematous rash, anemia, and death. Also *systemic aleukemic reticuloendotheliosis* (obs.), *nonlipid histiocytosis.* **Lev's d.** Complete heart block resulting from sclerosis of the cardiac skeleton. **Lewandowsky-Lutz d.** EPIDERMODYSPLASIA VERRUCIFORMIS. **Leyden's d.** A form of cyclical vomiting. Episodes of nausea and vomiting occur at regular intervals of weeks to months and last hours to days, the intervals being symptom-free. **Libman-Sacks d.** LIBMAN-SACKS ENDOCARDITIS. **Lignac's d.** CYSTINOSIS. **lipid storage d.** LIPIDOSIS. **Lipschütz d.** A simple acute ulcer of the vulva, which may appear singly or in clusters. **Little's d.** 1 The commonest form of cerebral palsy, usually presenting with spastic diplegia and generally attributable to perinatal brain damage. There is marked difficulty in walking, with a typical "scissors" gait, but many other features of cerebral palsy such as choreoathetoid movements, dysarthria, and sometimes also epileptic fits and mental retardation occur in some cases. The spastic weakness is usually much more severe in the lower than in the upper limbs, but all four limbs may sometimes be equally involved. Also *infantile cerebral diplegia, congenital spasmodic limb stiffness, infantile spastic paralysis.* 2 SPASTIC DIPLEGIA. **Lobo's d.** LOBOMYCOSIS. **Lobstein's d.** LOBSTEIN SYNDROME. **local d.** A disease confined to one organ or part, as distinguished from systemic disease. **Löffler's d.** 1 LÖFFLER'S ENDOCARDITIS. 2 LÖFFLER SYNDROME. **Louis-Bar d.** ATAXIA-TELANGIECTASIA. **Lowe's d.** OCULOCEREBRORENAL SYNDROME. **Luft's d.** A form of myopathy associated with mitochondrial dysfunction and a severe hypermetabolic state not due to hyperthyroidism. **lung fluke d.** PARAGONIMIASIS. **Lutembacher's d.** LUTEMBACHER SYNDROME. **Lutz-Splendore-Almeida d.** SOUTH AMERICAN BLASTOMYCOSIS. **Lyell's d.** TOXIC EPIDERMAL NECROLYSIS. **Lyme d.** An epidemic inflammatory disease that often begins with a characteristic skin lesion called erythema chronicum migrans accompanied by headache, stiff neck, fever, and malaise and that weeks or months later manifests itself as migratory polyarthritis, intermittent oligoarthritis, chronic arthritis of the knees, chronic meningoencephalitis, cranial or peripheral neuropathy, migratory musculoskeletal pain, or cardiac abnormalities. First identified in Lyme, Connecticut, in 1975, the disease has subsequently been found to occur in at least fourteen states of the United States and in Europe and Australia. A penicillin-sensitive infectious agent transmitted by ticks of the *Ixodes* genus has long been suspected as the cause. Evidence published in 1983 and 1984 indicates that the causative agent is a spirochete, *Borrelia burgdorferi,* isolated from the gut of *Ixodes dammini* ticks in areas known to be endemic foci of Lyme disease and from the blood, skin, and cerebrospinal fluid of patients with the disease. Also *Lyme arthritis.* **lymphoproliferative d.** A neoplastic or systemic tumorlike proliferation of lymphocytes, as in lymphoid leukemia, malignantlymphomas, or in Waldenström's macroglobulinemia. Also *lymphoproliferative syndrome.* **lysosomal storage d.'s** Any of a large number of pathologic conditions characterized by either a deficiency of a function of a lysosome, the accumulation of a metabolic intermediate to excess in lysosomes, or, usually, both. Examples are the mucopolysaccharidoses, the sphingolipidoses, and mucolipidoses II and III. **Mackenzie's d.** X DISEASE. **Madelung's d.** DIFFUSE SYMMETRICAL LIPOMAS OF THE NECK. **Majocchi's d.** PURPURA ANNULARIS TELANGIECTODES. **malabsorption d.'s** See under MALABSORPTION SYNDROME. **mammary Paget's d.** A lesion of the nipple in which large, mucin-containing cells are in the epidermis. It is almost always associated with an underlying intraduct breast carcinoma. Also *Paget's disease of the nipple.* **Manson's d.** SCHISTOSOMIASIS MANSONI. **maple bark d.** A form of allergic alveolitis in workers who strip maple bark, and due to inhalation of spores of *Cryptostroma corticale* fungus which grows under the bark; cryptostromosis. **maple syrup urine d.** An inborn error of amino acid metabolism characterized by mental and motor retardation, episodes of metabolic acidosis associated with poor feeding, and urine that smells like maple syrup. The catabolism of leucine, isoleucine, and valine is blocked by a deficiency of branched-chain keto-acid decarboxylase. The condition, inherited as an autosomal recessive trait, can be effectively treated by a diet low in these amino acids and by pharmacologic doses of thiamine. Also *branched chain ketoaciduria, ketoaminoacidemia, maple sugar urine disease.* **marble bone d.** OSTEOPETROSIS. **Marburg virus d.** A severe and often fatal hemorrhagic fever caused by the Marburg virus and characterized by headache, high fever, nausea, vomiting, diarrhea, a maculopapular rash, hemorrhagic phenomena, and renal failure. The disease was first reported in 1967 in Marburg and Frankfurt, West Germany, and in Belgrade, Yugoslavia. The source of human infection proved to be African green or velvet monkeys (*Cercopithecus aethiops*) imported from Uganda for laboratory experiments. Additional cases occurred in southern Africa in 1975. The vector is unknown. Person-to-person spread is suspected. The virus is closely related to but serologically distinct from the Ebola virus. These two viruses are distinct from all others. Also *Marburg disease, green monkey disease.* **Marchiafava's d.** MARCHIAFAVA-BIGNAMI SYNDROME. **Marchiafava-Bignami d.** MARCHIAFAVA-BIGNAMI SYNDROME. **Marie-Bamberger d.** HYPERTROPHIC PULMONARY OSTEOARTHROPATHY. **Marie-Strümpell d.** 1 ANKYLOSING SPONDYLITIS. 2 ACUTE INFANTILE HEMIPLEGIA. **Marie-Tooth d.** CHARCOT-MARIE-TOOTH DISEASE. **Marion's d.** Congenital stenosis of the bladder neck with hypertrophy of the smooth muscle. The disease manifests itself in the child by recurrent febrile urinary infections, dysuria, incomplete urinary retention, and pseudoenuresis, and if not treated, will result in hydronephrosis and progressive renal failure. An acquired form may appear in the adult (neoforming disease of the bladder neck). Also *rigid induration of the bladder neck, congenital hypertrophy of the bladder neck, posterior stenosis of the urethra.* **Maroteaux-Lamy d.** MUCOPOLYSACCHARIDOSIS VI. **Martin's d.** Periosteal arthritis of the foot that is often seen in long-distance walkers. **mast cell d.** MASTOCYTOSIS. **Mathieu's d.** ICTERIC LEPTOSPIROSIS. **McArdle's d.** GLYCOGEN STORAGE DISEASE V. **μ-chain d.** See under HEAVY CHAIN DISEASE. **Medin's d.** ACUTE ANTERIOR POLIOMYELITIS. **Mediterranean d.** β-THALASSEMIA. **medullary cystic d.** A congenital or genetic nephropathy, characterized by the onset of polyuria and nocturia in childhood or early adolescence, followed by gradual development of anemia and uremia. Renal salt wastage, hyponatremia, and acidosis with hyperchloremia are common features. In children, retarded growth and renal osteodystrophy are usual. Tapetoretinal degeneration or retinitis pigmentosa may be present in a few patients. The disease usually is transmitted as an autosomal dominant trait. If the transmission is autosomal recessive, the disease is called familial juvenile nephronophthisis. Also *nephronophthisis.* **Ménétrier's d.** A condition characterized by gastric mucosal hypertrophy resulting in large rugae covering part or all of the stomach. Histologic findings typically include glandular hypertrophy with chief, parietal, and mucus-secreting cells lining elongated glands. This condition is frequently associated with hypoabuminemia due to excessive gastric protein loss. Also *hypertrophic gastropathy, hypertrophic gastritis, giant hypertrophic gastritis.* **Menière's d.** A disease of the inner ear which is usually progressive and characterized by the symptom triad of episodic vertigo, fluctuating hearing impairment, and tinnitus. Increased endolymphatic pressure produces distension of the membranous labyrinth. Many kinds of treatment, both medical and surgical, have been tried, although often without sustained success. Also *Menière syndrome, endolymphatic hydrops, labyrinthine hydrops* (incorrect). **Menkes d.** MENKES SYNDROME. **Merzbacher-Pelizaeus d.** PELIZAEUS-MERZBACHER DISEASE. **mesangial IgA/IgG d.** MESANGIAL IGA/-IGG GLOMERULONEPHRITIS. **Meyenburg's d.** RELAPSING POLYCHONDRITIS. **Meyer-Betz d.** FAMILIAL MYOGLOBINURIA. **Miana d.** MIANEH FEVER. **Mianeh d.** MIANEH FEVER. **microcystic d.** A form of the congenital nephrotic syndrome characterized by dilatation of the tubules and glomeruli by true cysts. The clinical manifestations begin in infancy or early childhood and include, in addition to the nephrotic syndrome, progressive renal failure, uremia, anemia, and renal osteodystrophy, with death usually before age two. **microdrepanocytic d.** HEMOGLOBIN S-β-THALASSEMIA. **milk alkali d.** MILK-ALKALI SYNDROME. **milk-borne d.'s** Diseases in which the pathogenic organism is commonly transmitted in milk. Among these diseases are cholera, dysentery, brucellosis, scarlet fever, tuberculosis, salmonellosis, and typhoid. **Miller's d.** OSTEOMALACIA. **Milroy's d.** HEREDITARY LYMPHEDEMA TYPE I. **Minamata d.** A severe neurologic disorder that occurred in the 1950s among those inhabitants of Minamata, Japan, who had consumed considerable quantities of seafood heavily contaminated with alkyl mercury compounds. The disease was characterized by peripheral neuropathy, ataxia, dysarthria, and loss of peripheral vision. The neurologic and mental disabilities were permanent and many cases resulted in death. **minimal change d.** LIPOID NEPHROSIS. **minimal lesion d.** LIPOID NEPHROSIS. **Mitchell's d.** ERYTHROMELALGIA. **mixed connective tissue d.** A rheumatic illness characterized by combined features of systemic lupus erythematosus and scleroderma (including pleurisy, Raynaud's phenomenon, and sclerodactyly) and defined by the presence of very high titer antibody to ribonucleoprotein in the absence of antibody to double-stranded DNA or Sm antigen. There is controversy whether mixed connective tissue disease represents a specific illness or a stage in the evolution of lupus or scleroderma. **mixed cryoglobulin d.** An illness characterized primarily by the presence of cryoglobulins containing two or more immunoglobulins, such as IgG and IgM, but often characterized also by cutaneous vasculitis, arthralgia, and nephritis. **Möbius d.** OPHTHALMOPLEGIC MIGRAINE. **Mondor's d.** Thrombophlebitis affecting the subcutaneous course of the thoracoepigastric vein of the breast and chest wall. **Monge's d.** MOUNTAIN SICKNESS. **Morgagni's d.** HYPEROSTOSIS FRONTALIS INTERNA. **Morquio's d.** MUCOPOLYSACCHARIDOSIS IV. **Mortimer's d.** SARCOIDOSIS. **Morvan's d.** MORVAN SYNDROME. **Moschcowitz d.** THROMBOTIC THROMBOCYTOPENIC PURPURA. **motor neuron d.** A progressive degenerative disease of unknown cause involving upper and lower motor neurons and giving rise to a combination of symptoms and signs due to upper and lower motor neuron dysfunction and usually ending in death within a few years of onset. Also *motor system disease, Duchenne's disease.* • When the bulbar muscles are predominantly involved the condition is usually called *progressive bulbar palsy,* when it begins with muscular weakness and wasting in the limb muscles it is called *progressive muscular atrophy,* and when the upper motor neurons are affected first with little atrophy of muscles it is called *amyotrophic lateral sclerosis.* In the United States, *amyotrophic lateral sclerosis* is often used to identify the disease as a whole. **Mouchet's d.** Osteochondrosis affecting the talus. **mountain d.** MOUNTAIN SICKNESS. **moyamoya d.** A cerebral vascular disease first reported in Japanese children in which there is occlusion of the major cerebral arteries so that the brain appears to be supplied with blood by a rete mirabile like that of lower animals. Chorea, symptoms of cerebral ischemia, and subarachnoid hemorrhage are among the clinical manifestations. **Mozer's d.** Myelosclerosis in an adult. **Mucha's d.** PITYRIASIS LICHENOIDES. **Mucha-Habermann d.** PITYRIASIS LICHENOIDES. **mule-spinners' d.** MINERAL OIL CANCER. **Münchmeyer's d.** FIBRODYSPLASIA OSSIFICANS PROGRESSIVA. **Murray Valley d.** MURRAY VALLEY ENCEPHALITIS. **mushroom workers' d.** An extrinsic alveolitis that occurs among workers who prepare mushroom beds from moldy compost, and due to inhalation of the spores of microorganisms growing in the compost such as *Micropolyspora faeni* and *Thermoactinomyces vulgaris* or of the mushrooms themselves. Also *mushroom pickers' disease, mushroom workers' lung.* **neuropathic joint d.** Joint destruction with microfractures occurring in subjects with neurologic sensory defects involving the affected joints, such as occurs in tabes dorsalis, syringomyelia, and diabetic neuropathy. **Nicolas-Favre d.** LYMPHOGRANULOMA VENEREUM. **Niemann-Pick d.** An autosomal recessive inborn error of sphingomyelin metabolism, characterized by hepatosplenomegaly, physical and mental retardation, and neurologic deterioration with onset by six months and death by age three years in the severe infantile form (type A). At least six overlapping clinical forms exist, labelled A to F, including adult-onset and non-neuronal types. The basic defect of types A and B is in the enzyme sphingomyelinase resulting in the accumulation of sphingomyelin in the nervous system. Also *sphingomyelin lipidosis, sphingomyelinosis.* **nil d.** LIPOID NEPHROSIS. **Nonne-Milroy d.** HEREDITARY LYMPHEDEMA TYPE I. **Norrie's d.** An X-linked recessive disorder of uncertain pathogenesis characterized by blindness, sensorineural deafness, and mental retardation. The eyes show retinal masses (pseudoglioma); hyperplasia of retinal, ciliary, and iris pigment epithelia; precocious cataracts; and phthisis bulbi. **Norum's d.** LECITHIN-CHOLESTEROL ACYL TRANSFERASE DEFICIENCY. **oasthouse urine d.** A rare congenital disorder of infancy in which defective renal and intestinal transport leads to increased urinary phenylpyruvic acid, tyrosine, and methionine. The urine has an odor similar to that of an oasthouse, dried celery, or burnt sugar. Clinical features include white hair, hyperpnea, convulsions, and mental retardation. The disorder probably is transmitted as an autosomal recessive. Also *methionine malabsorption syndrome.* **obstructive d.** A disease of the airways which causes an obstructive ventilatory defect. **occlusive d.** AORTOILIAC OCCLUSIVE DISEASE. **occupational d.** Any disease which is identified as being caused by the circumstances of an occupation or to which persons following a particular occupation are prone. The cause may be a physical agent, as in radiation dermatitis; a chemical agent, as in contact dermatitis or pneumoconiosis, where the effects are local, or in lead poisoning, where the effects are systemic; or a biologic agent, as in industrial anthrax, where the infecting organism may be accidently inoculated or inhaled. Other work factors, particularly psychosocial factors, may be etiologically important in common disorders such as hypertension, peptic ulcer, or mental illness. **Oguchi's d.** A rare stationary disorder of dark adaptation in which an anomalous photopigment becomes ophthalmoscopically visible after dark adaptation (Mizuo's phenomenon). **Ohara's d.** TULAREMIA. **Ollier's d.** UNILATERAL CHONDRODYSPLASIA. **ophthalmic Graves d.** EXOPHTHALMIC OPHTHALMOPLEGIA. **Opitz d.** THROMBOPHLEBITIC SPLENOMEGALY. **Oppenheim's d.** MYATONIA CONGENITA. **organic d.** A disease involving structural changes in organs or tissues. **oriental lung fluke d.** PARAGONIMIASIS. **Ormond's d.** IDIOPATHIC RETROPERITONEAL FIBROSIS. **Osgood-Schlatter d.** Osteochondrosis of the tibial tubercle. It is often seen following repeated trauma. Also *apophysitis tibialis adolescentium, Schlatter sprain, Schlatter's disease, rugby knee.* **Osler's d.** 1 POLYCYTHEMIA VERA. 2 HEREDITARY HEMORRHAGIC TELANGIECTASIA. **Osler-Vaquez d.** POLYCYTHEMIA VERA. **Osler-Weber-Rendu d.** HEREDITARY HEMORRHAGIC TELANGIECTASIA. **Otto's d.** PROTRUSIO ACETABULI. **ouch-ouch d.** ITAI-ITAI DISEASE. **Owren's d.** FACTOR V DEFICIENCY. **Paas d.** A familial complex of skeletal deformities that include unilateral or bilateral coxa valga, scoliosis, shortened phalanges, and spondylitis deformans of the lumbar vertebrae. **Paget's d.** OSTEITIS DEFORMANS. **Paget's d. of bone** OSTEITIS DEFORMANS. **Paget's d. of the nipple** MAMMARY PAGET'S DISEASE. **Paget's d. of the skin** A condition marked by a lesion in which large cells, singly or in small groups, infiltrate the epidermis. They typically contain mucus and do not invade the dermis. It is most frequently found in the nipple (mammary Paget's disease), and is associated with a carcinoma of the breast. Extramammary Paget's disease usually occurs in the anogenital region and may be associated with an underlying carcinoma. **Panner's d.** Osteochondrosis of the capitulum humeri. **Parkinson's d.** A disorder attributable to degeneration of the corpus striatum and the substantia nigra, associated with a reduced concentration of dopamine in the affected areas. The condition occurs in two principal forms. One is the idiopathic form or paralysis agitans, which usually develops in middle or late life with static tremor of the limbs, increasing plastic rigidity of the limbs and trunk, and akinesia or bradykinesia. The face is often masklike, there is a progressive stoop, the voice becomes slow and monotonous, the gait slow and shuffling, and there may be associated autonomic disturbances, such as excessive salivation and sweating. The other is the postencephalitic variety (postencephalitic parkinsonism), developing as a sequel of encephalitis lethargica, which shows similar manifestations but in which oculogyric crises and dementia are also frequent. See also entries under PARKINSONISM. Also *parkinsonism, spasmus agitans, tremor artuum, rigor tremens* (outmoded), *Parkinson syndrome, parkinsonian syndrome.* **parrot d.** PSITTACOSIS. **Parrot's d.** 1 ACHONDROPLASIA. 2 SYPHILITIC PSEUDOPARALYSIS. **Parry's d.** A term used chiefly in Great Britain for GRAVES DISEASE. **Payr's d.** SPLENIC FLEXURE SYNDROME. **Pelizaeus-Merzbacher d.** An early infantile form of progressive familial cerebral leukodystrophy. Its onset is a few months after birth, with head tremor, nystagmus, and athetoid movements, followed by ataxia, intention tremor, bradylalia, and progressive spastic paralysis of the limbs and trunk, with exaggerated tendon reflexes, extensor plantar responses, and abolition of the abdominal reflexes. Optic atrophy is sometimes seen. Mental development is relatively unimpaired until the late stages. Pathologically there is diffuse degeneration of the white matter of the brain and brainstem. No abnormal storage of lipid has yet been identified, and the cause is unknown. Also *familial centrolobular sclerosis, familial centrolobar sclerosis, Merzbacher-Pelizaeus disease, Pelizaeus-Merzbacher sclerosis, Pelizaeus-Merzbacher type diffuse sclerosis, aplasia axialis extracorticalis congenita.* **Pellegrini-Stieda d.** Post-traumatic ossification of the medial collateral ligament of the knee. Also *Köhler-Pellegrini-Stieda disease, Stieda disease, Pellegrini's disease.* **pelvic inflammatory d.** SALPINGO-OOPHORITIS. **periodic d.** Any disease marked by the regular recurrence of symptoms or attacks. **periodontal d.** Any disease affecting the periodontium, particularly chronic gingivitis and ensuing chronic periodontitis, which are endemic throughout the world. Also *parodontopathy.* **Perrin-Ferraton d.** SNAPPING HIP. **Perthes d.** Osteochondrosis of the proximal femoral epiphysis seen in young children. Also *Legg-Calvé-Perthes disease, Calvé-Perthes disease, Legg's disease, Waldenström's disease, osteochondritis deformans juvenilis, pseudocoxalgia.* **pestilential d.** Any of the five diseases (cholera, plague, smallpox, yellow fever, and typhus) which had given rise to major epidemics in the past and which had been and were still, up to the middle of the twentieth century, subject to defined quarantine procedures. Subsequently and until 1969, these diseases, together with relapsing fever, were referred to as quarantinable diseases. **Peyronie's d.** Sclerosis of the corpora cavernosa, of obscure origin and characterized by the presence in the erectile tissue of several hard nodules which provoke during erection a painful curve of the penis. Also *fibrous cavernitis, van Buren's disease, sclerosis of the corpora cavernosa, plastic induration of penis.* **Pfeiffer's d.** INFECTIOUS MONONUCLEOSIS. **Pick's d.** A form of presenile dementia caused by localized cerebral cortical atrophy of unknown origin, confined particularly to the frontal and temporal lobes. The condition, which may be familial, usually produces a relatively rapid change in personality, sometimes inappropriateness of affect and later a progressive dementia, often accompanied by dysphasia and by extrapyramidal features resembling those of parkinsonism. The histologic and ultrastructural appearances in the brain differ in several respects from those of the much commoner Alzheimer's disease. Also *Pick syndrome, Pick's gyral atrophy, Pick's convolutional atrophy, lobar sclerosis, lobar atrophy, atrophic sclerosis, circumscribed atrophy of the brain.* **pink d.** A severe and protracted illness of young children, chiefly of the teething age, characterized by cold, pink, sweaty extremities, hypotonia, tachycardia, hypotension, anorexia, and insomnia. Sudden death has been recorded. The cause is chronic poisoning with mercury in topical medicaments or teething powders. Also *acrodynia, dermatopolyneuritis, erythredema polyneuropathy, Bilderbeck's disease, Swift's disease, Swift-Feer disease, Selter's disease, vegetative neurosis, acrodynic erythema.* **plaster-of-Paris d.** Disuse atrophy of a limb encased in a plaster-of-Paris cast. **Plummer's d.** TOXIC NODULAR GOITER. **pneumatic hammer d.** VIBRATION DISEASE. **policeman's d.** TARSALGIA. **polycystic d. of the lung** Any of several diseases characterized by development of multiple cysts in the lung. *Outmoded.* **polycystic renal d.** A hereditary disease in which cysts distort the renal parenchyma, eventually causing enlargement of both kidneys, progressive renal failure, and uremia. **polycystic renal d., adult type** A form of polycystic renal disease transmitted as an autosomal dominant of high penetrance which increases with age. Although probably present at birth, the cysts enlarge so slowly that clinically there may be no symptoms until late middle age, when signs of hypertension, lumbar or abdominal pain, and renal failure appear. Many involved nephrons appear to retain some functional capacity and to contribute to urine formation. The kidneys become palpable before renal function begins to decline. On occasion the condition may be a chance finding during radiographic examination or at autopsy. The disease may be associated with cysts of the liver, pancreas, and spleen, and with aneurysms of the cerebral arteries. Death most commonly results from renal failure or complications of vascular disease, renal infection, or renal carcinoma. **polycystic renal d., childhood type** A form of polycystic renal disease transmitted as an autosomal recessive. The number of cysts and renal enlargement is less than in the infantile type. Intravenous urography may suggest medullary sponge kidney. Renal failure is inconstant, but chronic renal infection is common. **polycystic renal d., infantile type** A form of polycystic renal disease transmitted as an autosomal recessive. The distal tubules and collecting ducts are dilated, and result in very large kidneys which may cause dystocia. At birth the kidneys do not function, and oliguric renal failure supervenes rapidly. Death usually occurs in the perinatal period, although a few patients survive until adolescence. **Pompe's d.** GLYCOGEN STORAGE DISEASE II. **Poncet's d.** Inflammatory joint effusion accompanying advanced tuberculosis elsewhere in the body. Also *Poncet's rheumatism.* **Posada-Wernicke d.** COCCIDIOIDOMYCOSIS. **Pott's d.** TUBERCULOUS SPONDYLITIS. **Preiser's d.** Post-traumatic osteoporosis of the scaphoid bone of the wrist. **pseudo-Hurler's d.** MUCOLIPIDOSIS III. **pseudo-Pott's d.** Angular kyphosis attributable to a cause other than a tuberculous one. **psychosomatic d.** PSYCHOSOMATIC DISORDER. **pulmonary heart d.** Right-sided heart disease secondary to disorders of the lungs or pulmonary circulation. It may be acute, as in massive pulmonary embolism, or chronic, usually as a result of chronic obstructive airways disease. **pulseless d.** TAKAYASU'S ARTERITIS. **Purtscher's d.** Traumatic retinopathy, characterized by fundus hemorrhage, edema, and mechanical disruption. **Pyle's d.** METAPHYSEAL DYSPLASIA. **Quervain's d.** DE QUERVAIN SYNDROME. **rat-bite d.** RAT-BITE FEVER. **ray-fungus d.** ACTINOMYCOSIS. **Raynaud's d.** Raynaud's phenomenon, occurring as a primary or idiopathic disorder and marked by hyperreactive but otherwise normal vessels. Symptoms generally regress with time. **Recklinghausen's d.** See under NEUROFIBROMATOSIS. **Recklinghausen-Appelbaum d.** HEMOCHROMATOSIS. **Recklinghausen's d. of bone** OSTEITIS FIBROSA CYSTICA. **Reed-Hodgkin d.** HODGKIN'S DISEASE. **Refsum's d.** An autosomal recessive defect in catabolism of a branched-chain fatty acid, phytanic acid. Clinical features include a progressive pigmentary retinopathy with blindness, polyneuritis and cerebellar ataxia. Because humans do not synthesize phytanic acid, dietary manipulation to restrict intake of this fatty acid ameliorates but does not completely reverse the phenotype. The basic defect involves deficient activity of the first enzyme in the catabolic chain, one which catalyzes an alpha-oxidation. Also *phytanic acid oxidase deficiency.* **Reiter's d.** REITER SYNDROME. **renal arterial d.** Atherosclerosis or fibromuscular dysplasia of the main renal arteries or their branches. If the lesion sufficiently narrows the arterial lumen, hypertension may result. See also RENOVASCULAR HYPERTENSION. **Rendu-Osler-Weber d.** HEREDITARY HEMORRHAGIC TELANGIECTASIA. **restrictive d.** A disease of the lungs or chest which impairs lung inflation, thus leading to reduced total lung capacity and vital capacity. **rheumatic heart d.** Disease of the endocardium, myocardium, or pericardium as a consequence of rheumatic fever. Also *Bouillaud's disease, rheumatism of the heart.* **rheumatoid d.** Rheumatoid arthritis, especially its systemic manifestations. **rheumatoid lung d.** Any of several forms of lung disease found in association with rheumatoid arthritis, most commonly pulmonary fibrosis but also including rheumatoid nodules in the lung, the Caplan syndrome, and rheumatoid pleural effusions. **Ribbing's d.** 1 PROGRESSIVE DIAPHYSEAL DYSPLASIA. 2 A hereditary disorder of the skeleton marked by fragmented development of the long bone epiphyses, which may later form intra-articular loose bodies. **rice d.** BERIBERI. **Riedel's d.** RIEDEL STRUMA. **Riga-Fede d.** FRENAL ULCER. **Ritter's d.** PHYSIOLOGIC JAUNDICE. **Robles d.** ONCHOCERCIASIS. **Roger's d.** A small ventricular septal defect which causes no significant hemodynamic burden. Also *maladie de Roger.* See also ROGER'S MURMUR. **Rokitansky's d.** ACUTE YELLOW ATROPHY OF THE LIVER. **Romberg's d.** ROMBERG'S PROGRESSIVE FACIAL HEMIATROPHY. **Rossbach's d.** HYPERCHLORHYDRIA. **Rot's d.** MERALGIA PARESTHETICA. **Roth's d.** MERALGIA PARESTHETICA. **Royal Free d.** A form of benign myalgic encephalomyelitis which occurred in epidemic form in the nursing and other staff of the Royal Free Hospital in London in the 1950s. **Runeberg's d.** PERNICIOUS ANEMIA. **runt d.** A clinical syndrome in experimental animals which is a result of severe immunodeficiency produced by experimental manipulation. It is characterized by failure to thrive due to chronic infection. The condition was originally observed in neonatal mice subjected to experimental thymectomy. It is analogous to severe combined immunodeficiency seen in humans. Also *wasting disease* (outmoded), *runting disease, runting syndrome, neonatal thymectomy syndrome.* **runting d.** RUNT DISEASE. **Ruysch d.** CONGENITAL MEGACOLON. **sacroiliac d.** A pathologic process involving the sacroiliac joint. It once was believed to suggest tuberculosis, but is now more likely to be attributable to inflammatory sacroileitis. **salmon d.** SALMON POISONING. **Sander's d.** EPIDEMIC KERATOCONJUNCTIVITIS. **Sandhoff's d.** A form of cerebromacular degeneration similar to Tay-Sachs disease but which occurs in non-Jewish children and in which there is accumulation of both ganglioside $GM_2$ and globoside due to deficiency of both hexosaminidase A and B. **sandworm d.** CUTANEOUS LARVA MIGRANS. **Sanfilippo d.** A variety of gargoylism due to the abnormal storage of mucopolysaccharide in cerebral neurons. It resembles Hurler's disease except that the manifestations of central nervous system involvement are severe but the other somatic manifestations are mild. **San Joaquin Valley d.** COCCIDIOIDOMYCOSIS. **Schamberg's d.** PROGRESSIVE PIGMENTED PURPURIC DERMATOSIS. **Schaumann's d.** SARCOIDOSIS. **Scheuermann's d.** SCHEUERMANN'S KYPHOSIS. **Schilder's d.** A heritable progressive diffuse sclerosis of the cerebral white matter occurring in childhood between the ages of five and twelve years and giving rise to progressive visual deterioration, dementia, and spastic paralysis. There is massive demyelination of the posterior part of the cerebral hemispheres with sparing of the arcuate fibers. In some families there is an association with Addison's disease. Also *Flatau-Schilder disease, Schilder syndrome, cerebral centrolobar sclerosis.* **Schimmelbusch d.** CYSTIC MASTOPATHY. **Schlatter's d.** OSGOOD-SCHLATTER DISEASE. **Scholz d.** METACHROMATIC LEUKODYSTROPHY. **Scholz-Greenfield d.** METACHROMATIC LEUKODYSTROPHY. **Schönlein's d.** HENOCH-SCHÖNLEIN PURPURA. **Schönlein-Henoch d.** HENOCH-SCHÖNLEIN PURPURA. **Schottmüller's d.** PARATYPHOID FEVER. **Schül-**

**ler's d.** 1 HAND-SCHÜLLER-CHRISTIAN DISEASE. 2 *Seldom used* OSTEOPOROSIS CIRCUMSCRIPTA CRANII. **Schüller-Christian d.** HAND-SCHÜLLER-CHRISTIAN DISEASE. **Schultz d.** AGRANULOCYTOSIS. **sclerocystic d. of the ovary** POLYCYSTIC OVARY. **scleroderma heart d.** Heart disease due to progressive systemic sclerosis, usually consisting of pericarditis, pulmonary hypertension, arrhythmia, or cardiomyopathy. **Seitelberger's d.** INFANTILE NEUROAXONAL DYSTROPHY. **Selter's d.** PINK DISEASE. **septic d.** A disease resulting from infection by pyogenic microorganisms that have disseminated through the bloodstream. **serum d.** SERUM SICKNESS. **Sever's d.** A spurious radiographic diagnosis of fragmentation of the calcaneal epiphysis based on what is probably a normal variant. Also *calcaneal osteochondritis.* **severe combined immunodeficiency d.** SEVERE COMBINED IMMUNODEFICIENCY. **sexually transmitted d.** Any of a wide range of infectious diseases which are transmitted frequently but not necessarily exclusively by sexual contact, including not only the traditional venereal diseases such as syphilis and gonorrhea, but also hepatitis, group B streptococcal infection, *Chlamydia trachomatis* infection, nongonococcal urethritis, vaginitis, pubic lice, scabies, condyloma acuminatum, molluscum contagiosum, and viral illnesses such as herpes, cytomegalovirus, and acquired immune deficiency syndrome (AIDS). Abbr. STD **Sézary's d.** SÉZARY SYNDROME. **Shaver's d.** BAUXITE PNEUMOCONIOSIS. **shimamushi d.** SCRUB TYPHUS. **sickle cell d.** SICKLE CELL ANEMIA. **sickle cell-hemoglobin C d.** HEMOGLOBIN S-C DISEASE. **sickle cell-hemoglobin D d.** HEMOGLOBIN S-D DISEASE. **silk-stocking d.** ERYTHROCYANOSIS. **silo-fillers' d.** An occupational disease due to exposure to nitrogen oxides produced in silos. It may take the form of eye or upper airway irritation with cough and dyspnea. There is a delayed stage due to bronchiolitis and pulmonary edema with cyanosis and severe dyspnea. Also *silo workers' asthma.* **Simmonds d.** PANHYPOPITUITARISM. **Sinding-Larsen-Johansson d.** LARSEN-JOHANSSON DISEASE. **sixth d.** EXANTHEMA SUBITUM. **sixth venereal d.** *Obs.* LYMPHOGRANULOMA VENEREUM. **skinbound d.** SCLERODERMA. **sleeping d.** NARCOLEPSY. **small vessel d.** In diabetics, atherosclerotic involvement of metatarsal and digital arteries of the lower extremity as well as the generalized intimal and basement membrane thickening of arterioles and capillaries. Both findings are unusual in nondiabetics. **Sneddon-Wilkinson d.** SUBCORNEAL PUSTULAR DERMATOSIS. **social d.** *Popular* VENEREAL DISEASE. **Spielmeyer-Vogt d.** JUVENILE CEROID-LIPOFUSCINOSIS. **St. Aignon's d.** *Outmoded* FAVUS. **St. Anthony's d.** CHOREA. **Stanton's d.** MELIOIDOSIS. **Stargardt's d.** The commonest form of juvenile macular degeneration. **Steinert's d.** DYSTROPHIA MYOTONICA. **Sternberg's d.** HODGKIN'S DISEASE. **Stevens-Johnson d.** STEVENS-JOHNSON SYNDROME. **Sticker's d.** ERYTHEMA INFECTIOSUM. **Stieda's d.** PELLEGRINI-STIEDA DISEASE. **Still's d.** A form of juvenile rheumatoid arthritis characterized by high fever, rash, and polyarthritis. As originally described, splenomegaly and lymphadenopathy may also be present. **St. Modestus d.** CHOREA. **Stokes-Adams d.** ADAMS-STOKES SYNDROME. **storage d.** Any of a large number of pathologic conditions characterized by the accumulation of metabolic intermediates in cells. It is usually caused by a heritable enzyme deficiency or transport defect, and the accumulation of substances such as lipids and carbohydrates results in malfunction of organs in which the storage is greatest. Also *thesaurosis* (outmoded), *thesaurismosis* (outmoded). **Strachan's d.** STRACHAN-SCOTT SYNDROME. **structural d.** A pathologic process resulting in morphologic alterations recognizable by gross or microscopic examination. **Strümpell's d.** ACUTE INFANTILE HEMIPLEGIA. **Strümpell-Leichtenstern d.** ACUTE INFANTILE HEMIPLEGIA. **Strümpell-Marie d.** 1 ANKYLOSING SPONDYLITIS. 2 ACUTE INFANTILE HEMIPLEGIA. **Stühmer's d.** BALANITIS XEROTICA OBLITERANS. **Sturge's d.** STURGE-WEBER SYNDROME. **Sturge-Weber d.** STURGE-WEBER SYNDROME. **Sturge-Weber-Dimitri d.** STURGE-WEBER SYNDROME. **Sudeck's d.** POST-TRAUMATIC OSTEOPOROSIS. **Sutton's d.** PERIADENITIS MUCOSA NECROTICA RECURRENS. **Swediaur's d.** ACHILLES BURSITIS. **Swift's d.** PINK DISEASE. **Swift-Feer d.** PINK DISEASE. **swineherds' d.** Leptospirosis among farmers and persons handling livestock, especially swine that are carriers of the pathogen. The infection is usually acquired through scratches and abrasions in the skin, by contamination from the urine of infected animals. **Sylvest's d.** EPIDEMIC PLEURODYNIA. **Symmers d.** NODULAR LYMPHOMA. **systemic d.** A disease that affects the body as a whole rather than a single organ or part. **Takahara's d.** ACATALASIA. **Takayasu's d.** TAKAYASU'S ARTERITIS. **Tangier d.** ANALPHALIPOPROTEINEMIA. **tarabagan d.** Human plague derived from fleas of the tarabagan (Mongolian marmot). **Tarui's d.** GLYCOGEN STORAGE DISEASE VII. **Taussig-Bing d.** TAUSSIG-BING MALFORMATION. **Tay-Sachs d.** A rare and severe form of lipidosis of the nervous system due to a deficiency of the liposomal enzyme hexosaminidase A, causing accumulation and deposition of gangiosides $GM_2$ in brain cells, cerebellum, and axons of nerves. The onset is 4–6 months of age, with arrest, then decline of psychomotor development, irritability, hyperacusis, progressing to spasticity, convulsions, and decerebrate rigidity and death by the age of 3 years. A cherry red spot visible in the fundus oculi, due to degeneration of the retinal nerve fibers allowing the vascular chorion to show through at the macular area, is a diagnostic feature. It is of recessive inheritance and is particularly common in Ashkenazi Jews. Heterozygote screening and prenatal diagnosis have resulted in decreased incidence of the disease. Also *$GM_2$ gangliosidosis, infantile amaurotic familial disease* (obs.), *infantile amaurotic familial idiocy* (obs.). **Thaysen's d.** CELIAC DISEASE. **thick leg d.** OSTEOPETROTIC LYMPHOMATOSIS. **Thiemann's d.** Familial osteochondrosis of the phalangeal epiphyses. It occurs in childhood and gives rise to interphalangeal joint deformity. Also *familial osteoarthropathy of fingers.* **Thomsen's d.** MYOTONIA CONGENITA. **thyrocardiac d.** THYROTOXIC HEART DISEASE. **thyrotoxic heart d.** Heart disease due to hyperthyroidism. Also *thyrocardiac disease.* **Tietze's d.** COSTOCHONDRITIS. **Tommaselli's d.** Quinine poisoning, characterized by hematuria and pyrexia. Also *Tommaselli syndrome.* **Tooth d.** CHARCOT-MARIE-TOOTH DISEASE. **Tornwaldt's d.** TORNWALDT'S BURSITIS. **Tourette's d.** GILLES DE LA TOURETTE SYNDROME. **transplantation d.** *Rare* GRAFT-VERSUS-HOST DISEASE. **Trevor's d.** DYSPLASIA EPIPHYSIALIS HEMIMELICA. **Trinidad d.** PARALYSSA. **tropical d.** 1 Any disease common in tropical countries. The vast majority of tropical diseases have little or nothing to do with high ambient temperature but are associated with poor socioeconomic conditions. Most diseases which are prevalent today in tropical countries, especially water-borne bacterial infections, were world-wide a century ago. They have, for the most part, been eliminated except in poor or underdeveloped tropical countries where there may be severe food shortages, poor nutrition, and insufficient medical care. 2 A disease which can be contracted only in a hot climate because the responsible organism or its vector can exist only in such a climate. **tsutsugamushi d.** SCRUB TYPHUS. **tunnel d.** 1 MINERS' ANEMIA. 2 DECOMPRESSION SICKNESS. **Underwood's d.** SCLEREMA NEONATORUM. **unilateral multicystic d.** A congenital disorder in which cysts of varying size almost completely occupy one kidney. Remnants of atrophic nephrons or dilated tubules may persist. The condition usually is discovered by palpating a unilateral flank mass in an infant. **unilocular hydatid d.** A disease caused by a fluid-filled, unilocular hydatid cyst of *Echinococcus granulosus,* which has a germinative inner lining from which numerous scoleces and daughter colonies (brood capsules) are budded off. The cyst is lined with an enclosing laminated sheath which keeps the unilocular form. Hydatid disease usually affects the liver, but many other organs can be the site of growth of the hydatids. See also ECHINOCOCCOSIS, *ECHINOCOCCUS GRANULOSUS.* **Unna's d.** SEBORRHEIC DERMATITIS. **Unverricht's d.** PROGRESSIVE MYOCLONIC EPILEPSY. **Urbach-Oppenheim d.** NECROBIOSIS LIPOIDICA. **Urbach-Wiethe d.** LIPOID PROTEINOSIS. **uremic medullary cystic d.** A defect of the distal renal tubules resulting in an impaired concentration ability of the kidney, reported variously as a recessive or dominant trait affecting children or adults. Pathologically, the kidneys are contracted and show a widespread distribution of small cysts, most of which are situated in the medulla close to the junction with the cortex. There is glomerulosclerosis and interstitial fibrosis. Clinically, the onset is insidious with polyuria, anemia, salt wasting, impaired growth, and renal osteodystrophy. It progresses slowly to renal failure, usually during childhood or early adult life. It may be associated with retinal dystrophy. **vagrants' d.** Generalized dark pigmentation and skin hardening resulting from chronic infestation with body lice (pediculosis). Also *vagabonds' pigmentation, vagabonds' disease, morbus vagabondus, morbus errorum, parasitic melanoderma.* **valvular d.** Disease affecting one or more of the cardiac valves. **van Bogaert-Bertrand d.** CANAVAN'S DISEASE. **van Bogaert-Nyssen-Peiffer d.** METACHROMATIC LEUKODYSTROPHY. **van Buchem's d.** SCLEROSTEOSIS. **van Buren's d.** PEYRONIE'S DISEASE. **Vaquez d.** POLYCYTHEMIA VERA. **Vaquez-Osler d.** POLYCYTHEMIA VERA. **venereal d.** Any sexually transmitted disease, as syphilis, gonorrhea, chancroid, or lymphogranuloma venereum. Also *social disease* (popular). See also SEXUALLY TRANSMITTED DISEASE. • The legal definition of *venereal disease* varies from country to country **veno-occlusive d. of the liver** Obliteration of small hepatic vein radicles, sometimes associated with portal hypertension and progressing to cirrhosis. It may be due to any of a number of factors including intake of certain herbal teas in Jamaica. See also RETRORSINE. **Verneuil's d.** Bursitis due to tertiary syphilis. **Verse d.** INTERVERTEBRAL CALCINOSIS. **vibration d.** Raynaud's disease found in workers using vibrating tools such as power hammers. The stress of continued exposure to vibration causes injury to fingers (vibration-induced white fingers) and hands (dead hand). There may be bone changes, muscular weakness, and ulnar or median nerve degeneration. Also *vibration disorder, pneumatic hammer disease, traumatic vasospastic syndrome.* **Vidal's d.** LICHEN SIMPLEX. **Vincent's d.** 1 VINCENT'S ANGINA. 2 NECROTIZING ULCERATIVE GINGIVITIS. **Virchow's d.** LEONTIASIS OSSIUM. **Vogt's d.** DOUBLE ATHETOSIS. **Vogt-Spielmeyer d.** JUVENILE CEROID-LIPOFUSCINOSIS. **von Economo's d.** ENCEPHALITIS LETHARGICA. **von Gierke's d.** GLYCOGEN STORAGE DISEASE I. **von Recklinghausen's d.** See under NEUROFIBROMATOSIS. **von Willebrand's d.** Any of a heterogeneous group of autosomally inherited bleeding diseases resulting from a deficiency or abnormality of the Willebrand factor moiety of the plasma coagulation factor VIII complex. Clinical features include prolonged bleeding time, reduced platelet adhesiveness, and mucous membrane hemorrhage. Homozygotes have a more severe hemostatic abnormality than heterozygotes. Also *Willebrand syndrome.* **Voorhoeve's d.** OSTEOPATHIA STRIATA. **Vrolik's d.** OSTEOGENESIS IMPERFECTA CONGENITA. **Wagner's d.** COLLOID MILIUM. **Waldenström's d.** PERTHES DISEASE. **Wartenberg's d.** CHEIRALGIA PARESTHETICA. **Wassilieff's d.** ICTERIC LEPTOSPIROSIS. **wasting d.** 1 Any of various chronic diseases involving progressive deterioration, as pulmonary tuberculosis An outmoded, popular term. 2 *Outmoded* RUNT DISEASE. **Weber's d.** STURGE-WEBER SYNDROME. **Weber-Christian d.** RELAPSING FEBRILE NONSUPPURATIVE PANNICULITIS. **Weber-Dimitri d.** STURGE-WEBER SYNDROME. **Wegner's d.** Syphilitic pseudoparalysis marked by epiphyseal separation. Also *syphilitic osteochondritis.* **Weil's d.** ICTERIC LEPTOSPIROSIS. **Weir Mitchell's d.** ERYTHROMELALGIA. **Werdnig-Hoffmann d.** A disorder resulting from degeneration of the anterior horn cells in infancy and due to an autosomal recessive trait. It begins either *in utero* or in the first six months of life, and causes progressive flaccid paralysis with bilateral muscular atrophy which usually initially affects the muscles of the pelvic and shoulder girdles, ultimately affecting the entire musculature. The bulbar and respiratory muscles are soon involved and respiratory infection usually causes death within the first two years of life. Electromyography gives evidence of active progressive denervation of skeletal muscles, and muscle biopsy reveals isolated areas of atrophy of neurogenic type. Most cases previously diagnosed as myatonia congenita because of severe weakness and hypotonia present at birth proved to be suffering from Werdnig-Hoffmann disease. Also *acute infantile spinal muscular atrophy, Werdnig-Hoffmann syndrome, progressive spinal muscular atrophy of infancy, Hoffman's atrophy, Werdnig-Hoffmann paralysis, Hoffmann-Werdnig syndrome, Werdnig-Hoffman atrophy.* **Werner-His d.** TRENCH FEVER. **Werner Schultz d.** AGRANULOCYTOSIS. **Wernicke's d.** A manifestation of vitamin $B_1$ deficiency, occurring most often in alcoholic subjects but also resulting sometimes from malnutrition, or occurring as a sequel to gastrectomy, in which there is gliosis, capillary proliferation, and sometimes hemorrhage in the periaqueductal gray matter of the midbrain and in the mammillary bodies. The condition gives rise to nystagmus, paresis of ocular movement, and variable long tract signs. An associated polyneuropathy is often present and there is frequently an associated syndrome (Korsakoff psychosis) with difficulty in recording and retaining new impressions. Also *Wernicke's encephalopathy, Wernicke syndrome, encephalitis hemorrhagica superior, polio encephalitis acuta hemorrhagica, superior hemorrhagic polioencephalitis.* See also WERNICKE-KORSAKOFF PSYCHOSIS. **Westphal's d.** *Rare* PERIODIC PARALYSIS. **Wetherbee's d.** A form of familial spinal muscular atrophy due to degeneration of the anterior horns of the spinal cord, causing muscular atrophy and weakness, first in the distal portions of the lower limbs, later in the arms. The condition is closely related to juvenile familial muscular atrophy. **Whipple's d.** A systemic disease characterized by the infiltration of involved tissues with small bacilli and numerous large macrophages containing massive numbers of ingested small bacilli. Its manifestations may include intestinal malabsorption, fever, cutaneous hyperpigmentation, anemia, lymphadenopathy, arthralgia, arthritis, pleuritis, endocarditis, and central nervous system involvement. Also *intestinal lipodystrophy, lipophagic intestinal granulomatosis.* **whitespot d.** GUTTATE MORPHEA. **Whytt's d.** Tuberculous meningitis resulting in hydrocephalus. **Wilson's d.** A rare disease, inherited as an autosomal recessive trait and caused by a defect in copper metabolism that results in an excessive deposition of copper in the liver and other tissues. Eventually, the liver develops cirrhosis, the limbus of the cornea acquires a green/brown discoloration known as the Kayser-Fleischer ring, and degenerative changes appear in the basal ganglia of the brain. The serum copper level is normal or slightly low, serum ceruloplasmin levels are decreased, and there is a corresponding increase in albumin-bound copper. Associated clinical findings include involuntary movements, tremor, muscular rigidity, spastic contractures, psychic disturbances, dysphagia, and progressive cachexia. The progression of the disease and the development of liver and brain damage can be prevented by treatment with chelating agents such as penicillamine. Also *hepatolenticular degeneration, progressive lenticular degeneration, Wilson's degeneration, copper storage disease, Kinnier Wilson disease, Kayser's disease, familial hepatitis, Wilson syndrome.* **Winkelman's d.** JUVENILE PARALYSIS AGITANS. **Winkler's d.** CHRONIC NODULAR CHONDRODERMATITIS OF THE HELIX. **winter vomiting d.** An endemic or epidemic nonbacterial gastrointestinal infection caused by enteric viruses, specifically, Norwalklike and related agents. The disease commonly occurs in the winter months in temperate regions and is characterized by acute nausea, vomiting, and diarrhea of less than one to three days' duration. **Witkop-Von Sallmann d.** HEREDITARY BENIGN INTRAEPITHELIAL DYSKERATOSIS. **woolsorters' d.** INHALATION ANTHRAX. **x d.** A multisystem disease of unknown etiology characterized by gastrointestinal disturbance, dyspepsia, cold intolerance, and cardiorespiratory symptoms. Also *Mackenzie's disease.* **Zahorsky's d.** EXANTHEMA SUBITUM. **Ziehen-Oppenheim d.** DYSTONIA MUSCULORUM DEFORMANS.

**disengagement** \dis'engāj'mənt\ The liberating or extrication of the fetus from the lower birth canal as in a vaginal delivery.

**disequilibration** \disē'kwilibrā'shən\ Loss of the ability to maintain one's balance; instability.

**disequilibrium** \disē'kwilib'rē·əm\ **1** Any disturbance of equilibrium, whether physical or mental. **2** The manifestations or sensations of equilibratory disorder.

**disesthesia** \dis'esthē'zhə\ DYSESTHESIA.

**disfacilitation** \dis'fasil'itā'shən\ An inhibitory neural action that exerts its effect by removal or diminution of facilitation, as distinct from inhibition that can operate independently of excitatory effects.

**disgerminoma** \disjur'minō'mə\ DYSGERMINOMA.

**dish** A shallow, concave container made of glass or plastic and commonly employed in laboratory work such as microbial and tissue culture. **culture d.** PETRI DISH. **evaporating d.** A wide, shallow, concave vessel, usually made of glass or porcelain and used to evaporate substances by exposure to heat. **Petri d.** A shallow, circular dish with an overlapping cover, made of clear glass or plastic and used primarily for culture of microorganisms. Also *culture dish.*

**disharmony** / **maxillomandibular d.** Malposition of the maxilla with respect to the mandible. **occlusal d.** A lack of harmony between contacts of opposing occlusal surfaces of teeth and other tooth contacts during closed movements of the mandible.

**disinfect** \dis'infekt'\ To eliminate or inhibit the growth of pathogenic microorganisms.

**disinfectant** \dis'infek'tənt\ [*disinfect* + *-ant,* agentive suffix] An agent capable of eliminating or inhibiting pathogenic microorganisms, particularly one used on inert objects. **complete d.** An agent capable of eliminating both vegetative and spore forms of pathogenic microorganisms. **incomplete d.** A disinfectant that is incapable of killing spores although it is effective against vegetative cells.

**disinsertion** \dis'insur'shən\ The separation of a tendon from its bony insertion. **d. of the retina** DIALYSIS RETINAE.

**disintegrant** A substance included in tablets that causes them to disintegrate in the presence of moisture, dispersing the medicinal components. Also *disintegrator.*

**disintegration** \disin'təgrā'shən\ [DIS-[1] + INTEGRATION] Fragmentation or loss of cohesiveness and organization; the process of being broken up into parts or particles. **radioactive d.** RADIOACTIVE DECAY. **spontaneous d.** RADIOACTIVE DECAY.

**disintegrator** DISINTEGRANT.

**disintoxication** \dis'intäk'səkā'shən\ DETOXIFICATION.

**disjugate** \dis'joogāt\ [L *dis-* apart + *jugat(us),* past part. of *jugare* to fasten, bind, join] Not conjugate, as movements of the eye.

**disjunction** \disjungk'shən\ [DIS-[1] + JUNCTION] **1** The separation of paired chromosomes during anaphase of the first meiotic division. **2** The separation of sister chromatids during anaphase of the second meiotic division and of mitosis. **3** A separation of parts or structures normally joined. Also *dysjunction.* **craniofacial d.** See under LEFORT III FRACTURE.

**disjunctive** \disjungk'tiv\ **1** Of or pertaining to disjunction. **2** Not linked or in harmony, as binocular movements in which the eyes are not conjugate; disjugate.

# disk

**disk** [L *discus.* See DISCUS.] **1** DISCUS. **2** A flat, circular object, usually of slight breadth compared to its circular extent. Also *disc.* **A d.** A BAND. **abrasive d.** DENTAL DISK. **acromioclavicular d.** DISCUS ARTICULARIS ARTICULATIONIS ACROMIOCLAVICULARIS. **anangioid d.** An optic disk lacking or appearing to lack vasculature, a developmental defect. **anisotropic d.** A BAND. **anisotropous d.** A BAND. **articular d.** DISCUS ARTICULARIS. **articular d. of acromioclavicular articulation** DISCUS ARTICULARIS ARTICULATIONIS ACROMIOCLAVICULARIS. **articular d. of distal radioulnar articulation** DISCUS ARTICULARIS ARTICULATIONIS RADIOULNARIS DISTALIS. **articular d. of sternoclavicular articulation** DISCUS ARTICULARIS ARTICULATIONIS STERNOCLAVICULARIS. **articular d. of temporomandibular joint** DISCUS ARTICULARIS ARTICULATIONIS TEMPOROMANDIBULARIS. **articular d. of wrist** DISCUS ARTICULARIS ARTICULATIONIS RADIOULNARIS DISTALIS. **bilaminar embryonic d.** An embryonic disk in the early embryo when there is both an ectodermal and an endodermal layer present. **Bowman's d.** DISK OF STRIATED MUSCLE FIBERS. **choked d.** PAPILLEDEMA.

**ciliary d.** ORBICULUS CILIARIS. **cupped d.** An optic disk with abnormal excavation, most commonly produced by glaucomatous optic atrophy. **dental d.** A thin disk mounted on a mandrel, used in dentistry to cut, grind, or polish teeth. Abrasives of various types are embedded in the surfaces of the disk. Also *abrasive disk.* **ectodermal d.** The flattened, elongated plate of columnar ectodermal cells in the very early human embryo of about twelve days, having the amniotic cavity above and endoderm below. Also *ectodermal plate.* **embryonic d.** The first signs of an embryo in a cleaving ovum, seen as a thick plate of irregularly arranged cells within the formative or inner cell mass. Also *germinal disk.* **epiphyseal d.** CARTILAGO EPIPHYSIALIS. **equatorial d.** The mass of chromosomes, arranged as a disk, at the equator of a cell during the metaphase period of mitosis. Also *nuclear disk.* **floppy d.** A thin, flexible magnetic disk, about 5 inches in diameter, which is used for data and program storage in a small computer. Also *diskette.* **germinal d.** EMBRYONIC DISK. **hair d.** A richly innervated area of skin adjacent to a hair follicle. It consists of a thickened plaque of epithelial cells among which the unmyelinated terminals of a single axon ramify. Also *haarscheibe.* **herniated cervical d.** Rupture or protrusion of the nucleus pulposus in the cervical region, usually with radiculopathy. **herniated intervertebral d.** The protrusion of nucleus pulposus through disruption of the confining anulus fibrosus. Commonly the herniation causes compression and irritation of adjacent nerve roots and spinal cord. **herniated lumbar d.** Protrusion or herniation of the nucleus pulposus of the lumbar vertebral area, with or without radiculopathy. **I d.** I BAND. **interarticular d.** DISCUS ARTICULARIS. **intercalated d.** An irregular, densely staining layer at the interface where the end of one cardiac muscle abuts the next. It contains a series of desmosomes for attachment and specialized areas of close contact to facilitate the spread of excitation from one cell to the next. **intermediate d.** Z BAND. **interpubic d.** DISCUS INTERPUBICUS. **intervertebral d.'s** DISCI INTERVERTEBRALES. **intra-articular d.** 1 DISCUS ARTICULARIS. 2 MENISCUS ARTICULARIS. **isotropic d.** I BAND. **J d.** I BAND. **M d.** M BAND. **mandibular d.** DISCUS ARTICULARIS ARTICULATIONIS TEMPOROMANDIBULARIS. **Merkel's d.** MENISCUS TACTUS. **Miller d.** A microscope eyepiece graticule that is used for calculating the percentage of reticulocytes present in a blood film. **Newton's d.** An apparatus that combines the spectral colors to produce the appearance of white by means of a rapidly rotating circular pattern. **nuclear d.** EQUATORIAL DISK. **optic d.** DISCUS NERVI OPTICI. **pinhole d.** An opaque disk with a small opening (about 1 mm), designed to be held in front of the eye to block all light except that admitted by the pinhole. The pinhole admits only axial rays of light, which are not refracted, thus neutralizing any refractive error without the use of corrective lenses, thus permitting measurement of visual acuity without the need for a refractive correction. **Placido's d.** A pattern of concentric rings used to evaluate corneal curvature. The reflection of the rings upon the cornea suffers characteristic distortions if the corneal curvature is imperfect. **protruded d.** INTERVERTEBRAL DISK PROTRUSION. **Q d.** A BAND. **Ranvier's tactile d.'s** The cup-shaped axon terminals located adjacent to Grandry's corpuscles. **Rekoss d.** An optical device in which two superimposed disks, each mounted with a series of lenses, may be rotated so as to present multiple combinations of dioptric powers. This principle is the basis for a number of clinical optical examining instruments. **ruptured d.** INTERVERTEBRAL DISK PROTRUSION. **ruptured intervertebral d.** INTERVERTEBRAL DISK PROTRUSION. **sarcous d.** DISK OF STRIATED MUSCLE FIBERS. **slipped d.** *Popular* INTERVERTEBRAL DISK PROTRUSION. **stenopaic d.** A narrow slit aperture mounted in an optical lens holder, used to evaluate astigmatism. **sternoclavicular d.** DISCUS ARTICULARIS ARTICULATIONIS STERNOCLAVICULARIS. **d. of striated muscle fibers** One of the bands, visible by microscopy, that traverse skeletal muscle fibers, such as the A band and I band. Also *Bowman's disk, sarcous disk.* **stroboscopic d.** A disk that is partially opaque and partially open, so that when it rotates it produces a rapidly and regularly interrupted transmission of light for use in eye examinations. **tactile d.** MENISCUS TACTUS. **thin d.** Z BAND. **transverse d.** A BAND. **triangular d. of wrist** DISCUS ARTICULARIS ARTICULATIONIS RADIOULNARIS DISTALIS. **Z d.** Z BAND.

**disk-** \disk-\ DISCO-.

**diskectomy** \diskek′təmē\ The surgical excision of all or part of an intervertebral disk. Also *discoidectomy.* Also *discectomy.*

**diskette** \disket′\ FLOPPY DISK.

**diski-** \dis′kē-\ DISCO-.

**diskiform** \dis′kifôrm\ DISCIFORM.

**diskitis** \diskī′tis\ An inflammation of an intervertebral disk. Also *discitis.*

**disko-** \dis′kō-\ DISCO-.

**diskography** \diskäg′rəfē\ [DISKO- + -GRAPHY] Radiographic demonstration of the intervertebral disk by means of injection of a radiopaque water-soluble substance directly into the disk. The shape and integrity of the nucleus pulposus and annulus fibrosus may be evaluated. Also *nucleography.* Also *discography.*

**diskopathy** \diskäp′əthē\ [DISKO- + -PATHY] A disease of an intervertebral disk. Also *discopathy.*

**dislocate** \dis′lōkāt\ [See DISLOCATION.] To displace one or more bones of a joint from the normal position.

**dislocatio** \dis′lōkā′shō\ [L, dislocation. See DISLOCATION.] DISLOCATION. **d. erecta** A subglenoid dislocation of the shoulder joint whereby the humerus is held in a vertical position. Also *luxatio erecta.*

**dislocation** \dis′lōkā′shən\ [Med L *dislocatio* (from L *dis-* not + *locatio* a placing, from *locatus,* past part. of *locare* to place) dislocation] The displacement of one bone with respect to another through a joint. Also *luxatio, dislocatio, luxation.* **anterior d.** A dislocation in which the distal surface of a joint becomes displaced anteriorly. **anterior shoulder d.** A dislocation at the shoulder joint in which the head of the humerus displaces anteriorly out of the glenoid fossa. It is the most common shoulder dislocation. **d. of articular processes** The separation of two bones by displacement of a joint, as is seen in the spine. **Bell's d.** A traumatic dislocation of the atlantoaxial joint. **Bell-Dally d.** The spontaneous dislocation of the atlas without predisposing trauma. **Bennett's d.** A dislocation of the trapeziometacarpal joint of the thumb. **central d.** Injury of the hip joint whereby the femoral head is displaced through the floor of the acetabulum into the pelvis. **closed d.** A dislocation without a communicating wound. Also *simple dislocation.* **complete d.** A dislocation marked by a complete separation of the joint surfaces. **complicated d.** A dislocation with associated injuries to structures in the vicinity of the injured joint. **compound d.** OPEN DISLOCATION. **congenital d.**

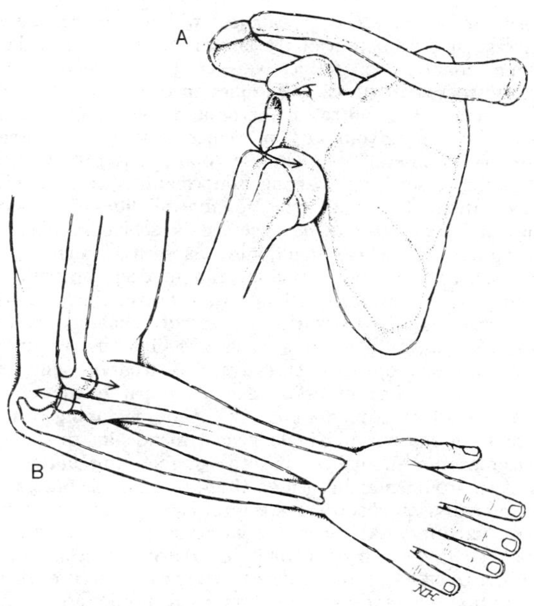


**Dislocations** (A) Subglenoid dislocation of shoulder; (B) dislocation of elbow.

**of the hip** The condition of the hip joint in which the head of the femur in a newborn infant easily slips backwards out of the acetabulum owing to its shape and the laxity of the ligaments. It is detectable at birth by the Ortolani sign, and is then curable by serial splintage. It may escape detection, however, until the second year of life when extensive and stressful orthopedic procedures are necessary to avert a lifelong limp. It is bilateral in 40 percent of cases and is seven times more frequent in girls than boys. Dominant inheritance occurs in some families in Italy and Yugoslavia. **consecutive d.** A dislocation in which the involved bone has changed its location subsequent to its position after the initial injury. **fracture d.** See under FRACTURE-DISLOCATION. **frank d.** A joint dislocation that is clinically apparent, as seen in a superficial joint such as the knee. **gamekeepers' d.** A dislocation of the metacarpophalangeal joint of the thumb. **habitual d.** A dislocation that recurs after reduction and often becomes a habit or volitional. **incomplete d.** SUBLUXATION. **incudomallear d.** Dislocation of the incus from the malleus. It is a rare occurrence which may result in cases of severe head injury or as an accident in the course of simple mastoidectomy. In either case, it is likely to be associated with incudostapedial dislocation or subluxation. **incudostapedial d.** Dislocation of the incus from the stapes. It is the most common of the traumatic disruptions of the ossicular chain. Severe head injury and, occasionally, surgical accident are responsible. **intrauterine d.** A joint dislocation of the fetus *in utero.* **Kienböck's d.** An isolated dislocation of the lunate bone of the wrist. **Lisfranc's d.** A dislocation of the forefoot across the tarsometatarsal joints. It is usually associated with fracture of one or more of the metatarsals. **Monteggia's d.** MONTEGGIA FRACTURE-DISLOCATION. **Nélaton's d.** A dislocation of the ankle in which the distal ends of the tibia and fibula are separated and the talus rides between them. **obturator d.** An inferior dislocation of the hip in which the femoral head rests in the obturator foramen. **old d.** A long-standing dislocation where secondary changes have taken place, with cartilage degeneration and fibrous scarring of the joint capsule and ligaments. **open d.** A dislocation complicated by a wound that communicates with the exterior. Also *compound dislocation.* **paralytic d.** A dislocation caused by the absence of muscle activity in paralytic conditions. **partial d.** SUBLUXATION. **pathologic d.** A joint dislocation seen as a complication of another disease such as paralysis, collagen disease, synovitis, or other generalized diseases. **perilunate d.** A dislocation of the entire carpus around the lunate bone, which remains attached to the radius. **posterior d.** A dislocation where the distal component lies posterior to the proximal joint surface. **posterior shoulder d.** An infrequent and sometimes undiagnosed shoulder dislocation whereby the humeral head lies posterior to the glenoid fossa. **recent d.** A dislocation in which insufficient time has passed for the development of secondary changes of inflammation and soft tissue scarring. **recurrent d.** A joint dislocation that recurs after the initial episode, often with minimal trauma. **sciatic d.** A posterior dislocation of the hip in which the femoral head damages the sciatic nerve. **simple d.** CLOSED DISLOCATION. **Smith's d.** A hyperextension injury of the foot with posterior displacement of the metatarsals and medial cuneiform bones. **subclavicular d.** A dislocation of the shoulder joint whereby the femoral head passes anteromedially to lie in the subclavicular region of the anterior chest wall. **subcoracoid d.** A dislocation of the shoulder whereby the humeral head lies anterosuperiorly beneath the coracoid process. **subglenoid d.** A shoulder dislocation in which the humeral head lies beneath the glenoid fossa. **unifacet d.** A vertebral dislocation in which one of the posterior facet joints is moved from its normal position. It is seen most commonly in the cervical spine. **unreduced d.** A dislocation in which the involved joint surfaces remain out of place. **vertebral d.** A dislocation that involves one or more of the intervertebral joints. It is often associated with a fracture. **voluntary d.** A dislocation that can be performed at will with relatively little pain.

**dismemberment** \dismem′bərmənt\ The removal of a limb or limbs.

**dismutation** \dis′myootā′shən\ A reaction in which atoms or electrons are transferred between two identical molecules, or parts of a molecule, to form different products. An example is the reaction of two triose phosphate molecules to form 3-phosphoglycerate and glycerol phosphate by the oxidation of one triose phosphate and the reduction of the other.

**disodium cromoglycate** $C_{23}H_{14}Na_2O_{11}$. A drug used prophylactically to treat those subject to allergic asthma and other allergic conditions, including allergic rhinitis. Its action is not fully understood, but it is associated with the stabilization of the activity of sensitized mast cells.

**disodium edetate** $C_{10}H_{14}N_2Na_2O_8$. (Ethylenedinitrilo)-tetraacetic acid disodium salt. A metal chelating agent used in the treatment of lead poisoning and hypercalcemia. Also *EDTA disodium, edetic acid disodium salt, edathamil disodium.*

**disome** \dī′sōm\ [DI-[2] + *(chromo)some*] **1** A chromosome set that consists of individually paired chromosomes. This is the normal situation in humans. **2** A chromosome set that exists as a pair of homologues.

**disomic** \dīsō′mik\ **1** Characterized by disomy.

2 Pertaining to a chromosome that exists in the cell as a pair of homologues.

**disomy** \dī′sōmē\ [*disom(e)* + -Y] The state of a chromosome set that consists of paired homologues. This is the usual state in humans and other diploid organisms.

**disopyramide** $C_{21}H_{29}N_3O$. α-[2-[Bis(1-methylethyl)-amino]-ethyl]-α-phenyl-2-pyridineacetamide. A drug that depresses the heart and is used as an antiarrhythmic agent. The phosphate salt has the same pharmacologic action, and can be given orally.

**disorder** [DIS-[1] + ORDER] A condition characterized by abnormal or disturbed function which may or may not be related to an identifiable structural cause or effect. **affective d.** Any disorder typified primarily by disturbances of mood, including the manic-depressive psychosis and the neurotic depressive disorder. **aggressive behavior d.** A group of conduct disturbances in children, characterized by physical violence against others or against property, or by thievery involving direct confrontation with a victim. **alcohol amnestic d.** KORSAKOFF PSYCHOSIS. **alcoholic brain d.'s** A group of brain disorders that are caused by or associated with alcoholism, including delirium tremens, pathologic intoxication, alcohol delirium, Wernicke-Korsakoff psychosis. **appetite d.** EATING DISORDER. **arteriosclerotic brain d.** MULTI-INFARCT DEMENTIA. **attention deficit d.** MINIMAL BRAIN DYSFUNCTION. **autonomic d.** Any disease or dysfunction of the autonomic nervous system. **behavior d.** Any of a group of childhood disorders that are manifested as abnormalities in personality development, including persisting undesirable traits or habits, antisocial behavior, neurotic traits that do not conform to any identifiable psychoneurotic pattern, or problems in school or vocational training. **bipolar d.** An affective disorder characterized by the occurrence of manic and depressive episodes, as in manic-depressive disorder. Bipolar disorders are often qualified by the most recent or most frequently recurring type of episode, as *manic* (or *depressed*) *bipolar disorder*. **brain d.** ORGANIC BRAIN SYNDROME. **cerebelloparenchymal d.** One of six autosomally inherited neurodegenerative disorders with variable age of onset, severity, and pathology that spare the pontine nuclei. **character d.** A disturbance in character consisting of any pattern of relating to the social environment that is so immutable as to limit effective functioning or satisfaction in interpersonal relationships. Such patterns are maladaptive because they are relatively inflexible and restrict the use of the subject's potentialities. Also *personality disorder, character neurosis*. **character impulse d.** IMPULSE DISORDER. **conduct d.** A type of behavior disorder characterized by repetitive and persistent antisocial activities. **consumptive thrombohemorrhagic d.** DISSEMINATED INTRAVASCULAR COAGULATION. **dissociative d.** In DSM-III, any of the syndromes whose central feature is sudden, temporary alteration in consciousness or identity. Included are multiple personality and depersonalization. **dysthymic d.** NEUROTIC DEPRESSIVE DISORDER. **eating d.** Any of a group of disorders involving abnormalities of appetite or food intake, or both, including anorexia nervosa, bulimia, pica, and rumination. Also *appetite disorder, dysorexia, parorexia*. **epileptoid personality d.** A character disorder typified by rigidity, seclusiveness, and a tendency toward irritability and overreaction to relatively innocuous stimuli which sometimes leads to acts of violence. Its cause is presumed to be based on organic cerebral dysfunction, as in brain trauma, temporal lobe epilepsy, or alchoholic encephalopathy. Also *epileptic personality disorder, explosive diathesis*. **equilibratory d.** Any disorder of the sense of balance, which may be caused by disease or dysfunction of the labyrinth, or of central labyrinthine connections. Subjective vertigo is usually present. **extrapyramidal d.** Malfunction of any motion believed to be under the control of the basal ganglia. Common manifestations are involuntary movements, such as chorea and tremor, or alteration in muscle tone. **gnostic d.'s** A group of disorders involving abnormalities of perception or recognition. This may refer to abnormalities of associative thinking such as may be observed in schizophrenia, to disturbances in cortical functioning as seen in some types of Broca's or syntactical aphasia, and to deep, epicritic sensation in contradistinction to protopathic sensation disturbances. **habit d.** A type of behavior disorder involving unfavorable habits, such as nail biting, thumb sucking, enuresis, open or excessive masturbation, and temper tantrums. **hereditary d.** Any pathologic condition whose etiology is predominantly genetic, including conditions due to mutations in single genes (mendelian disorders), to chromosome anomalies, and to collaborating mutant genes and environmental influences (multifactorial disorders). Fundamentally, all disorders are multifactorial and to some extent hereditary. Also *hereditary disease, genetic disease, inherited disease*. **hyperkinetic impulse d.** MINIMAL BRAIN DYSFUNCTION. **immunoproliferative d.** Any condition characterized by abnormal proliferation of lymphoid cells. Where the proliferating cell is a B lymphocyte, the disease may be accompanied by excessive and monoclonal immunoglobulin synthesis. **impulse d.** Any of a group of character disorders characterized by ego syntonicity, a pleasurable component, minimal distortion of the original id impulse, and some degree of lack of control. Included in this group are pathologic gambling, kleptomania, and pyromania. Also *character impulse disorder*. **isolated explosive d.** CATATHYMIC CRISIS. **LDL-receptor d.** FAMILIAL HYPERCHOLESTEROLEMIA. **manic-depressive d.** MANIC-DEPRESSIVE PSYCHOSIS. **mendelian d.** Any disorder resulting from autosomal recessive, autosomal dominant, or X-linked inheritance. **motility d.** An abnormality of movement, particularly the abnormal postures and gestures displayed in catatonic schizophrenia and in pervasive developmental disorders. **multifactorial d.** Any disorder resulting from a collaboration of mutant genes and environmental influences. **neurotic d.** NEUROSIS. **neurotic depressive d.** A disorder characterized by chronic or frequently recurring feelings of painful dejection or loss of interest or pleasure in usual activities, but not of sufficient degree to warrant a diagnosis as a major depressive episode. Also *dysthymic disorder, depressive neurosis, neurotic depression*. **organic behavior d.** Any organic brain syndrome exhibiting disordered behavior. **organic mental d.** ORGANIC BRAIN SYNDROME. **personality d.** CHARACTER DISORDER. **post-traumatic personality d.** Organic brain syndrome due to structural damage to the brain caused by head trauma. The clinical picture depends on the extent and location of the damage and consists usually of changes in usual behavior patterns or in the subject's characteristic style of relating to the environment. The postconcussional syndrome is one form of post-traumatic personality disorder. **post-traumatic stress d.** A disorder consisting of acute symptom formation in reaction to an earlier, overwhelming stress or trauma, as in combat neurosis. It may be characterized by recurrent thoughts or dreams of the stressful event, generally constricted responsiveness to the external environment except for exaggerated startle response, and sleep disturbances. Also *gross stress reaction, delayed stress* *syndrome.* **psychosomatic d.** A disorder with structural, physiologic, or other organic changes in one or more body systems, whose origin, at least in part, is related to emotional factors. Also *organ neurosis, psychophysiologic disorder, psychosomatic disease, visceral disorder, psychosomatic illness, psychosomatic reaction.* **schizoaffective d.** A disorder with elements of both an affective disorder and schizophrenia. As a result the clinician is unable to make a differential diagnosis between them. Some authorities use schizoaffective disorder to refer to episodes predominated by manic or melancholic features that occur in subjects with an underlying schizophrenic illness. **sleep d.** Any abnormality of the sleep-wake cycle, generally subdivided into four classes: (1) disorders of initiating and maintaining sleep (insomnia), such as sleep apnea and nocturnal myoclonus; (2) disorders of excessive somnolence, such as narcolepsy and Kleine-Levin syndrome; (3) disorders of the sleep-wake cycle, such as jet lag and work-shift syndromes; and (4) dysfunctions associated with sleep, sleep stages, or partial arousals (parasomnia), such as somnambulism, night terrors, nocturnal enuresis, nightmares, and sleep paralysis. **somatoform d.'s** A group of disorders in which the predominant symptoms resemble those of organic disorders even though no organic basis can be discovered. The group includes conversion and hypochondriasis. **stress d.** TRANSIENT SITUATIONAL PERSONALITY DISORDER. **thought d.** **1** Any abnormality in the process of thinking. **2** A disturbance seen in schizophrenia characterized by blocking of thought, thought deprivation, poverty of thought, or haphazard associations. For defs. 1 and 2 also *thinking disorder.* **Tourette's d.** GILLES DE LA TOURETTE SYNDROME **transient situational personality d.** A disorder consisting of acute symptom formation as a reaction to overwhelming stress or trauma with diminishment of symptoms when the stress is removed. Also *stress disorder, crisis reaction, acute situational reaction, adjustment reaction, stress reaction.* **vibration d.** VIBRATION DISEASE. **visceral d.** PSYCHOSOMATIC DISORDER. **XXX d.** A chromosomal disorder of phenotypic females with functioning ovaries. Subjects are affected by mental deficiency. **XXXX d.** A chromosomal disorder of phenotypic females with functioning ovaries and without identifying or characteristic anomalies. Subjects are affected by mental deficiency. **XXXXY d.** A chromosomal disorder of phenotypic males who are severely mentally deficient and have skeletal abnormalities and hypoplastic external genitalia. The condition is also characterized by sterility and androgen deficiency with associated anomalies, such as congenital heart disease, cleft palate, strabismus, microcephaly, and malformations of the face. Some diploid nuclei contain three chromatin bodies. **XXXY d.** A chromosomal disorder of phenotypic males marked by seminiferous tubule dysgenesis. It is similar to but more extreme than the Klinefelter syndrome (XXY disorder), characterized by mental deficiency, sterility, and hypoplastic external genitalia. **XXYY d.** A chromosomal disorder marked clinically by seminiferous tubule dysgenesis and by manifestations more extreme than those of the Klinefelter syndrome. It is associated with mental retardation, hypoplastic genitalia, tall stature and eunuchoid body proportions, unusual dermatoglyphic patterns, and peripheral vascular disease.

**disorganization** \dis'ôrgan'īzā'shən\ Profound structural alteration of an organ or tissue with associated impairment of function.

**disorientation** \disôr'ē·əntā'shən\ [DIS-[1] + ORIENTATION] Impaired understanding of temporal, spatial, or personal relationships suggestive of an underlying brain disorder. **right-left d.** An agnosic defect involving inability to distinguish between the right and left sides of the body and of the surroundings. It is one of the features of the Gerstmann syndrome.

**disparate** \dis'pərāt, dispar'it\ Not similar or comparable; different.

**disparity** \dispar'itē\ [Late L *disparitas,* from L *dis-* DIS-[1] + *paritas* parity, from *par* equal + *-itas* -ITY] **1** The condition of being disparate; lack of similarity. **2** A measure of the difference of two quantities.

**dispensary** \dispen'sərē\ **1** An outpatient facility or clinic, usually for treating primary care problems on a short-term basis; a facility that serves large, relatively healthy populations as in the military services. **2** A place, usually in a hospital or other institution, where medications can be obtained.

**dispensatory** A collection of information on sources, preparation, uses, and pharmacologic actions of official and nonofficial drugs used in the treatment of diseases. It is supplementary to a pharmacopeia or similar official treatise.

**Dispensatory of the United States of America** A collection of reports on both official and nonofficial drugs recognized in the United States Pharmacopeia, the British Pharmacopoeia, and other sources. It also includes drugs used in veterinary medicine.

**dispense** [L *dispensare* (from *dis-* DIS-[1] + *pensus,* past part. of *pendere* to weigh, pay) to weigh, pay, dispense, distribute] To compose and distribute (drugs) to patients, as in a pharmacy.

**dispermy** \dī'spurmē\ [DI- + SPERM + -Y] Penetration of two spermatozoa into one ovum.

**dispersal** \dispur'səl\ **flash d.** The prompt disintegration of a tablet or pill when placed on the tongue.

**dispersion** \dispur'shən\ [L *dispersio* (from *dispersus,* past part. of *dispergere* to scatter, from *dis-* apart + *spargere* to strew, throw about) dispersion] **1** The act or condition of scattering in different directions. **2** A more or less homogeneous distribution of particles of a substance in the body of another substance, used especially of a colloidal solution. **chromatic d.** **1** The variation of the speed of light in a medium with color, i.e., with wavelength. **2** The spreading of white light into a spectrum as a result of the different speeds of propagation of the different colors. **d. of light** **1** The spreading of white or other polychromatic light into its constituent colors, as by a prism or from chromatic aberration. **2** The quantitative variation of the refractive index of a substance with wavelength of light. **normal d.** NORMAL DISTRIBUTION. **optical rotatory d.** The dependence of optical rotation on wavelength. A change of sign of rotation occurs at the wavelength of maximal absorption of a chiral chromophore (the Cotton effect). Abbr. ORD

**dispersonalization** \dispur'sənalīzā'shən\ DEPERSONALIZATION.

**dispert** A dried, concentrated extract of a pharmacologically active plant or animal source, such as an endocrine gland.

***Dispholidus*** \disfäl'ədəs\ An African genus of venomous snakes of the family Colubridae. One species is *D. typus,* the boomslang.

**dispireme** \dīspī'rēm\ [DI-[2] + SPIREME] The telophase stage of mitosis, where the cytoplasm has divided, and the chromatin appears as a spiral, or coil, in each cytoplasmic mass. Also *dispira.*

**displacement** In psychiatry, an unconscious defense mechanism consisting of a shifting emotional charge or impulse from one object to another, or from one discharge pathway to another. **fetal d.** The shifting of a group of cells from their normal location during the process of fetal development. **fish-hook d.** A vertical orientation of the stomach so that the pylorus is directed upward and joins the duodenum at a sharper than usual angle when seen by radiography. This condition is associated with the tall, slender habitus. **mesial d.** MESIOVERSION. **Proetz d.** A method of treating chronic sinusitis with the object being the irrigation of the infected sinus by a noninvasive technique. The patient lies supine with the head low and the affected side of the nose is filled with a 0.5% ephedrine solution. Negative pressure is applied with a special syringe while the other side of the nose is kept closed by a finger and the nasopharynx by having the patient repeat "K-K-K." This draws pus from the sinuses and, when normal pressure is restored, admits the ephedrine solution in its place. Also *Proetz treatment.* **tissue d.** The change in position of a tissue due to pressure or mechanical forces.

**display** The presentation of graphic or alphanumeric information, as on a cathode-ray tube, or the manner of such presentation. **bistable d.** Ultrasound display in which all recorded spots have the same brightness. No gray-scale information is presented. **leading edge d.** Display of only the first portion of an ultrasonic echo from a tissue interface. This mode of display facilitates measurements between interfaces. **real-time d.** A display presented at essentially the same time the event occurs and distinguished from a delayed display presented after processing occurred. **refresh d.** A cathode-ray tube display with an image repetition rate high enough to prevent flickering.

**disposition** \dis′pəzish′ən\ [L *dispositio* (from *dispositus,* past part. of *disponere* to distribute) a placing in order] **1** Susceptibility, as to a disease. **2** Relatively enduring and consistent qualities of behavior that are characteristic of an individual and which allow a degree of prediction about what response is likely to be made when presented with specified stimulus situations.

**disproportion** / **borderline pelvic d.** A condition in which one or more of the pelvic diameters are shorter than normal, such that vaginal delivery of the fetal head may not be possible. **cephalopelvic d.** A condition whereby the size of the maternal pelvis is too small to allow vaginal delivery of the fetal head. **fiber type d.** A difference greater than 30 percent in fiber area or diameter between type I and type II muscle fibers. This abnormality has been identified in histochemically stained biopsy specimens from some infants and young children with benign congenital hypotonia or myopathy.

**disruption** \disrup′shən\ **1** The act or condition of being separated by force or burst asunder. **2** A defect in form, shape, or position of all or part of an organ or part of a body that is caused by interference with an intrinsically normal developmental process. **3** DISRUPTION SEQUENCE.

**disruptive** \disrup′tiv\ Leading to or causing disruption.

**Disse** [Joseph *Disse,* German anatomist, 1852–1912] Disse space. See under PERISINUSOIDAL SPACE.

**dissect** \disekt′\ [See DISSECTION.] To cut apart or separate the various tissues of the body so as to expose structures for the study of their organization.

**dissection** \disek′shən\ [L *dissectio* (from *dis-* apart + *sectio* a cutting, division, from *sectus,* past part. of *secare* to cut, cut off) a cutting apart] **1** The act of dissecting. **2** The appearance or state of a part or body after it has been dissected. **arterial d.** A pathological process characterized by the tearing of the intima of an artery, especially the aorta, and the migration of pulsatile blood flow into, within, and along the arterial wall, sometimes for great distances, as for example from the heart to the femoral artery along the aorta and iliac arteries. It is seen typically in young and middle-aged hypertensive subjects. The life-threatening complications associated with dissection relate to the occlusion of branch vessels (such as the carotid, coronary, mesenteric, or renal arteries) or to acute valvular insufficiency. Dissection of the aorta usually arises just above the aortic sinuses or beyond the left subclavian artery. Also *dissection, dissecting hematoma, dissecting aneurysm* (incorrect). **block d. of the neck** RADICAL NECK DISSECTION. **blunt d.** The separation of tissues along the naturally occurring tissue planes. **elective neck d.** PROPHYLACTIC NECK DISSECTION. **functional neck d.** An operation with the same aims as the radical neck dissection but which is designed to conserve certain functionally important structures, particularly the sternomastoid muscle and the accessory nerve. **partial neck d.** *En bloc* excision of the lymph nodes in a limited field of the neck, performed either for lymph node metastases or prophylactically. It is sometimes carried out during removal of the primary tumor. It is regarded as a controversial procedure. **radical neck d.** An operation designed to reverse a cancer of the head and neck and ablate the pathways or potential pathways of the lymphatic spread of the cancer. Usually, in order to assure the complete removal of the submandibular and cervical lymph nodes, the submandibular and sublingual salivary glands, the omohyoid and sternocleidomastoid muscles, and the deep jugular vein are removed along with the lymphatics. The operation may or may not be combined with that for removal of the primary tumor. Also *block dissection of the neck.* **prophylactic neck d.** Radical or partial neck dissection undertaken in the absence of demonstrable lymph node metastases. It is performed as a prophylactic measure in view of the liability of the diagnosed primary tumor to metastasize, sooner or later, to the regional lymph nodes in the neck. It is regarded as a controversial procedure. Also *elective neck dissection.* **sharp d.** A dissection performed by the incision of tissue. **suprahyoid neck d.** Partial neck dissection in which the whole lymph-bearing area between the hyoid bone and the mandible on one side or both, including the submandibular salivary glands, is removed *en bloc.*

**dissector** \disek′tər\ **1** One who dissects. **2** A surgical instrument used in dissection procedures.

**disseminated** \disem′inā′tid\ Widely spread throughout an organ, a system, or the whole body.

**dissepiment** \disep′imənt\ [L *dissaepimentum* (from *dis-* DIS-[1] + *saepire* to fence or hedge in + *-mentum* -MENT) a fencing or hedging in] A partition or septum.

**dissimilate** \disim′ilāt\ [DIS-[1] + *(as)similate.* See ASSIMILATION] To break down into components. Also *disassimilate.*

**dissociable** \disō′shē·əbəl\ Capable of dissociation.

**dissociation** \disō′sē·ā′shən\ [L *dissociatio* (from *dissociare* to separate, dissolve, from DIS-[1] + *sociare* to unite, associate with, from *socius* partner, companion) separation, incompatibility] **1** The separation, often reversible, of one molecule into two or more. **2** The separation or disengagement of one or more mental processes from the rest of the psychic apparatus, as in the separated states of consciousness in multiple personality and the amnesia of psychogenic fugue. For defs. 1 and 2 also *disassociation.* **albuminocytologic d. of cerebrospinal fluid** A pathologic increase in the total protein content of the cerebrospinal fluid with no increase in cells. This phenomenon is classically described as occurring in the Guillain-Barré syndrome but may also occur in spinal cord compression with a complete block, and in many other organic disorders of the spinal cord and brain. **atrial d.** Independent electrical activity of the two atria. **atrioventricular d.** Any disorder in which atria and ventricles are under the control of different pacemakers, as in complete heart block, or, more specifically, a disorder in which the atria are under a higher pacemaker and the ventricles under a lower one, even in the absence of organic atrioventricular block. Because the two pacemakers are initiating impulses almost synchronously, the territory of one is refractory to stimulation from the other. Sooner or later, the foci tend to fire asynchronously and the territory of the one may then be captured by the other (atrial or ventricular capture). Also *auriculoventricular dissociation, interference dissociation, dissociation by interference.* **d. by interference** ATRIOVENTRICULAR DISSOCIATION. **complete atrioventricular d.** COMPLETE HEART BLOCK. **electromechanical d.** Continuing electrical activity of the heart in the absence of mechanical cardiac function. Often a feature of cardiac rupture, it can also be caused by drugs. **interference d.** ATRIOVENTRICULAR DISSOCIATION. **longitudinal d.** Dissociation between the two atria or between the two ventricles, as opposed to atrioventricular dissociation. **Mobitz-type atrioventricular d.** MOBITZ BLOCK. **syringomyelic d.** Loss of the sense of pain and temperature, with preservation of tactile and deep sensibility, as seen in syringomyelia or syringobulbia. **tabetic d.** A type of dissociated sensory impairment seen particularly in tabes dorsalis in which deep sensibility, as pressure, deep pain, position, and joint sense, are selectively impaired, while superficial sensation, as of touch, cutaneous pain, and temperature, is intact.

**dissolution** \dis'əloo'shən\ [L *dissolutio*, from *dissolvere* to dissolve] The process of dissolving, or of breaking down.

**dissolve** \dizälv'\ [L *dissolvere* (from *dis-* apart, asunder + *solvere* to loosen, undo) to dismantle, disperse, dissolve] **1** Of a substance, to enter a liquid phase with the separation of its molecules or ions to form a solution. **2** To cause (a substance) to enter solution.

**dissonance** \dis'ənəns\ **cognitive d.** A psychological state in which incompatible beliefs, attitudes, knowledge, or other cognitions exist and are in conflict with each other, resulting in an uncomfortable state that motivates the individual to take action to reduce the dissonance. In theory, this can be accomplished by either adding consonant elements selectively or by reducing the importance or implications of the dissonant elements.

**dist.** *distilla* (L, distil).

**dist-** \dist-\ [L *distare* to be distant] A combining form meaning distal. Also *disti-, disto-.*

**distad** \dis'tad\ [DIST- + -AD] Towards a position away from center or away from a point of attachment; distally.

**distal** \dis'təl\ [*dist(ant)* + -AL] **1** Farthest or farther away from the beginning, the attached end, the center, or the midline. Compare PROXIMAL. **2** Farther or farthest away from the midline in the dental arch: used especially of the surface of a tooth. Compare MESIAL.

**distalis** \distā'lis\ [New L] Distal.

**distance** [L *distantia* (from *distans,* gen. *distantis,* pres. part. of *distare* to be at a distance, to differ) distance] The space between two points or places. **cone-surface d.** The distance from the end of a beam-defining cone to the surface of an object being radiographed. **focal d.** The distance between the primary focal point of a lens and the principal plane of the lens. **focal-skin d.** TARGET-SKIN DISTANCE. Abbr. FSD **half-intensity d.** The thickness of tissue required to halve the intensity of an ultrasonic beam. **interocclusal d.** The distance between the mandibular and maxillary occlusal surfaces in the rest position, usually measured by markings made on the face. Because the jaws do not open parallel to one another the distance varies from anterior to posterior. Also *interocclusal clearance, free-way space.* **interorbital d.** The distance between the bony orbits as measured from the angular process of one frontal bone to that of the other. **interpediculate d.** The distance between the pedicles of a vertebral body as measured on a frontal radiograph of the spine. **map d.** The distance between two gene loci on a chromosome which is measured in map units (centimorgans) and determined by the observed frequency of recombination. **object-film d.** The distance from the surface of an object being radiographed to the film, as measured along the central ray. **source-skin d.** TARGET-SKIN DISTANCE. Abbr. SSD **target-skin d.** The distance between the target in an x-ray tube and the skin of the patient being radiographed or treated with radiation. Also *focal-skin distance, source-skin distance.* Abbr. TSD **vertex d.** The distance of a spectacle lens from the cornea. This is of significance in the fitting of a strong lens, as in correction of aphakia, because the effective strength of a plus lens increases with distance, whereas the effective strength of a minus lens diminishes. **working d.** In a correctly focused compound microscope, the distance between the most distal lens of the objective lens system and the object being examined.

**distemper** \distem'pər\ [early modern English (from the verb *distemper* to derange the body's functions, from Med L *distemperare* to mix or temper disproportionately, e.g. the humors) an ailment, disorder] **1** Any of several infectious, primarily viral, diseases of domestic animals. **2** Any ailment or illness. An obsolete usage.

**distend** \distend'\ [L *distend(ere)* (from *dis-* apart + *tendere* to stretch) to extend, stretch out] To make or become larger, as a cyst or other enclosed part or organ, especially from internal pressure; expand or dilate.

**distensibility** \disten'səbil'itē\ The capability of distending.

**distension** \disten'shən\ [alteration of L *distentio* (from *distentus,* past part. of *distendere* to stretch out, extend) distension. See DISTEND.] The act of distending or the condition of being distended. Also *distention.*

**disti-** \dis'tē\ DIST-.

**distichiasis** \dis'tikī'əsis\ [Gk (from *distichos* in two rows, from *di-* two, double + *stichos* a row, line) growth of an extra row, as of eyelashes] The presence, usually genetic, of a double row of eyelashes, the abnormal row originating from hair bulbs located within the tarsal plate, thereby resulting in aberrant lashes arising from the posterior half of the eyelid margin. Also *distichia.*

**distillation** \dis'tilā'shən\ [L *destillatio, distillatio* (from *destillare* to drip, trickle down, from *de-* down + *stillare* to fall in drops, from *stilla* a drop) a dripping, trickling down, catarrh] The process of separating, purifying, or concentrating a volatile liquid by heating it to vaporization and then cooling the collected vapors to restore the liquid state. **cold d.** Distillation in which vaporization is achieved by lowering the atmospheric pressure in equilibrium with the liquid, rather than by raising the temperature. **destructive d.** Distillation in which vaporization is performed at a high temperature and low oxygen concentration. It results in the decomposition of complex compounds, often organic solids, into simpler volatile products. **dry d.** The destructive distillation of solids. **fractional d.** The separation of liquid components by exploiting their differences in boiling point and producing vapors at different temperatures so that the vapors are collected separately and condensed individually. **molecular d.** A method of purification of substances from crude sources, using very high vacuum and low temperature to condense the molecules that are thermolabile at higher temperatures. The process is used for separating fat-soluble vitamins, sterols, and certain hormones. **vacuum d.** Distillation into a low-pressure atmosphere in order to reduce the risk of decomposition by exposure to heat.

**disto-** \dis′tə-\ DIST-.

**distoceptor** \-sep′tər\ DISTANCE RECEPTOR.

**distoclusal** \-kloo′səl\ DISTO-OCCLUSAL.

**distoclusion** \-kloo′zhən\ [DISTO- + *(oc)clusion*] **1** The distal position of a lower tooth or teeth relative to the correct position in relation to the upper teeth. **2** Malrelation of dental arches, with the mandibular arch in a posterior position in relation to the maxillary arch. For defs. 1 and 2 also *disto-occlusion, distal occlusion, postnormal occlusion.* Compare MESIOCLUSION.

***Distoma*** \dis′tōmə\ [DI-[2] + Gk *stoma* mouth] A former genus of digenetic trematodes. Also *Distomum.* ***D. buski*** *Obs.* *FASCIOLOPSIS BUSKI* ***D. felineum*** *Obs.* *OPISTHORCHIS TENUICOLLIS.* ***D. haematobium*** *Obs.* *SCHISTOSOMA HAEMATOBIUM.* ***D. heterophyes*** *Obs.* *HETEROPHYES HETEROPHYES.* ***D. ringeri*** *Obs.* *PARAGONIMUS WESTERMANI.* ***D. westermani*** *Obs.* *PARAGONIMUS WESTERMANI.*

**distomiasis** \dis′tōmī′əsis\ [*Distom(a)* + -IASIS] The disease caused by trematodes (liver flukes). *Outmoded.*

***Distomum*** \dis′təməm\ *DISTOMA.*

**disto-occlusal** \-əkloo′səl\ **1** Pertaining to the distal and occlusal walls of a prepared cavity in a tooth. **2** Pertaining to the distal and occlusal surfaces of a restoration for a tooth. Also *distoclusal.* Abbr. DO

**disto-occlusion** \-əkloo′zhən\ DISTOCLUSION.

**distortion** \distôr′shən\ [L *distortio* (from *distortus,* past part. of *distorquere* to writhe, twist, distort, from *dis-* apart + *torquere* to turn, twist) distortion, writhing] In psychiatry, an unconscious defense mechanism in which thoughts are disguised so that they are not recognized as objectionable material and can thus gain expression which would otherwise be denied. **apperceptive d.** The interpretation of a percept on the basis of one's own motivations and experiences rather than on the basis of the objective appearance of the percept itself. Projective psychological tests generally present stimulus material of such ambiguity that the subject is forced to react idiosyncratically with his apperceptive distortions. **parataxic d.** A reaction of one person to another person that is based on a distorted evaluation. The distortion is a misinterpretation of the objectively verifiable significance of the object. In psychotherapy parataxic distortion is seen in transference.

**distoversion** \-vur′zhən\ [DISTO- + VERSION] The position of a tooth situated further from the median line than is normal.

**distractibility** \dis′traktəbil′itē\ An inability to maintain attention on one fixed object or incident. Attention shifts haphazardly in response to any stimulus that happens to occur no matter what its significance. Distractibility is frequent in manic episodes, and it is also a core element in hyperkinetic impulse disorder or minimal brain dysfunction.

**distraction** \distrak′shən\ **1** Mental disorder or derangement. • This usage is based on the fact that various kinds of mental illness interfere with the subject's ability to maintain fixed attention on one object. **2** The separation of joint surfaces beyond normal anatomical limits.

**distress** [Old French *destresse* (noun from L *distringere* to stretch apart, from *di(s)-* apart + *stringere* to bind, tighten) strain, stress, distress] **1** Physical or mental pain, suffering, or anxiety. **2** A dangerous condition requiring immediate intervention. **fetal d.** A clinical diagnosis suggesting possible anoxia of a fetus, an imprecise diagnosis usually based on changes in the fetal heart rate, the presence of meconium in the amniotic fluid, or abnormalities in biochemical parameters of pregnancy. The condition may be diagnosed antepartum or intrapartum. **idiopathic respiratory d. of newborn** RESPIRATORY DISTRESS SYNDROME OF NEWBORN.

**distribution** [L *distributio* (from *distribuere* to divide, distribute, from *dis-* denoting division + *tribuere* to give, yield, allot, from *tribus* tribe) distribution] **1** In statistics, the apportionment of an aggregate of data according to their numerical values or other attributes for the purpose of analysis or explication. **2** The pathway of or the area supplied by the branches of an artery or nerve. **3** The regional apportionment of certain tissues, such as fat or glands. **age d.** The distribution of a population or other specified group of persons by age. In official statistics, it is usual to tabulate by five-year or ten-year age groups, often with a finer breakdown for infancy (0 years) and early childhood (1–4 years). At the other extreme of the age range, an open-ended group (75 years and over or 85 years and over) is usually shown. **contagious d.** A frequency distribution compounded of two or more separate distributions. **continuous d.** The set of values on a continuous scale and between stated limits which a variable may assume. Theoretically the set is infinite, like the points on a line. In practice it is constrained only by the coarseness of the method of measurement involved in determining individual values. **discontinuous d.** In statistics, a distribution which is neither continuous nor discrete. **discrete d.** The set of values of a variable when the latter is constrained to take integral values only, as distinguished from a distribution when the possible values form a continuum. For example, the numbers of births per day in a hospital would form a discrete distribution whereas the birthweights would form a continuous distribution. **dose d.** In radiology, a chart showing the relative amounts of radiation dose absorbed by various parts of an irradiated object. **F d.** VARIANCE RATIO. **frequency d.** The arrangement of an aggregate of measurements according to the frequency with which they correspond to the values taken by one or more random variables. **gaussian d.** NORMAL DISTRIBUTION. **isodose d.** A chart or plan showing the relative dose within a patient or object from a beam of ionizing radiation, or from the combination of several beams of radiation. **Laplace-Gauss d.** NORMAL DISTRIBUTION. **marital status d.** The distribution of persons according to marital status, the usual categories being single, married, separated, and divorced, or of some object of interest according to the marital status of the subject, as the distribution of legal abortions according to the marital status of the woman. **negative binomial d.** A frequency distribution in which the relative frequencies are the successive terms of a binomial expression having a negative index. A classic example is provided by the frequency with which individuals in an occupational group sustain 0,1,2,3,...*n* accidents in a given time, such as one year. **normal d.** A continuous distribution in which the probability density associated with a random variable $x$ has as f($x$) the expression

$$\frac{1}{\sigma\sqrt{2\pi}}e^{-\frac{1}{2}\left(\frac{x-\mu}{\sigma}\right)^2}.$$

It is uniquely defined by the two parameters $\mu$ and $\sigma$, respectively the mean and the standard deviation of the distribution. The normal distribution is encountered whenever a random variable is subject to the influence of numerous causes of variability, the variation attributable to such factors being mutually independent and of the same order of magnitude. These conditions are often met with in nature; hence the important role of the normal distribution in the experimental sciences. The graphic form of the normal distribution, termed a *normal curve*, is characterized by the shape of a bell. Also *Laplace-Gauss distribution, gaussian distribution, normal dispersion.* **parity d.** The distribution of women by parity or of some object of interest (e.g., births, legal abortions, or pregnancies) according to the parity of the woman. **Pascal d.** NEGATIVE BINOMIAL DISTRIBUTION. **Poisson d.** A discrete distribution in which the probabilities associated with integral values of the random variable $x$ have the form $e^{-m}m^x/x!$ The distribution is uniquely determined by the value of the parameter $m$, which is the expectation or mean value predicted theoretically for the variable. The Poisson distribution can be regarded as the limit approached by the binomial distribution as the probability of the occurrence of a random event decreases. **saddle d.** Sensory innervation over the circumanal area and perineum; the distribution of the pudendal, perforating cutaneous, and coccygeal nerves. The uppermost, medial aspect of the thigh, the perineal branch of the posterior femoral cutaneous nerve, is sometimes included. **sampling d.** 1 The frequency distribution of a statistic, as predicted by theory. 2 The observed frequency distribution of values of a statistic in a set of samples. **skew d.** An asymmetric frequency distribution. If the distribution is unimodal and has a longer tail toward the upper range of values with the mean greater than the median, the distribution is said to be positively skewed. If the longer tail is towards the lower range the distribution is said to be negatively skewed. **standardized normal d.** A normal distribution having zero mean and unit standard deviation.

**districhiasis** \dis′trikī′əsis\ [DIS-[2] + TRICH- + -IASIS] The emergence of two hairs from one follicle.

**disturbance** [Old French *destorbance* (from L *disturbans,* pres. part. of *disturbare* to disperse, overthrow, from *dis-* apart + *turba* turmoil, a crowd, from Gk *tyrbē* disorder) disturbance] Any deviation or disruption of a normal state. **d.'s of affectivity** Abnormal, unexpected, or incomprehensible emotional reactions, including indifference, blunted or shallow emotionality, lack of adaptability, and disharmony or dissociation of mood from the idea it seems to accompany. Some authorities consider disturbances of affectivity one of the fundamental symptoms of the schizophrenias. **personality pattern d.** A group of character disorders, as defined in DSM-I, that included inadequate, schizoid, cyclothymic, and paranoid personalities. **personality trait d.** A group of character disorders, as defined in DSM-II, that included the emotionally unstable, the passive-aggressive, and the compulsive personalities. **sexual orientation d.** A disturbance in which there is dissatisfaction with, uncertainty about, or anxiety related to one's sexual preferences or behavior, such as is seen in ego-dystonic homosexuality.

**disulfide** —S—S—. The structure of two joined sulfur atoms or a substance that contains such atoms. See under DISULFIDE BOND.

**disulfiram** $C_{10}H_{20}N_2S_4$. Tetraethylthioperoxydicarbonic diamide. An antioxidant used therapeutically to create an aversion to alcohol. This agent inhibits the metabolism of acetaldehyde, an alcohol metabolite, and the accumulation of acetaldehyde produces disagreeable symptoms. Also *tetraethylthiuram disulfide.*

**disulfur dichloride** SULFUR MONOCHLORIDE.

**dithiazanine iodide** $C_{23}H_{23}IN_2S_2$. 3,3′-Diethylthiadicarbocyanine iodide. Green, crystalline powder, practically insoluble in water, very soluble in alcohol, but insoluble in ether. A toxic antihelmintic agent, formerly used against whipworms and threadworms.

**dithiol** A substance containing two thiol groups, such as dihydrolipoic acid. When thiol groups are close to each other, the substance has a high affinity for tervalent arsenic compounds and for many metal ions.

**dithionite** The ion $S_2O_4^{2-}$ or a salt containing it. It is a powerful reducing agent, easily oxidized to sulfite. It reduces methemoglobin to hemoglobin and reduces other Fe(III) compounds similarly. It reacts rapidly with oxygen to yield hydrogen peroxide, and more slowly with hydrogen peroxide to yield water. Also *hydrosulfite* (obs.), *hyposulfite* (outmoded).

**dithiothreitol** $CH_2SH$—CHOH—CHOH—$CH_2SH$. A compound used to reduce disulfide bonds in proteins. Because its oxidized form contains a six-membered ring, which is stable, the reaction has a favorable equilibrium constant. Also *Cleland's reagent.*

**dithranol** A British term for ANTHRALIN.

**Dittrich** [Franz *Dittrich,* German pathologist, 1815–1859] Buhl-Dittrich law. See under LAW.

**ditype** \dī′tīp\ See under NONPARENTAL DITYPE. **nonparental d.** One of the possible patterns of chromatid segregation at meiosis in which all of the chromatids are recombinant. For example, if two syntenic loci are both heterozygous, with the mutant alleles in cis configuration, then the nonparental ditype has the wild type allele at one locus and the mutant allele at the other locus on the same chromatid.

**diuresis** \dī′yUrē′sis\ [New L, from DI-[3] + -URESIS. See DIURETIC.] The excretion of unusually large quantities of urine. **alcohol d.** Diuresis that results from the presence of alcohol in the circulatory system. It is caused in part by inhibition of the release of antidiuretic hormones. **osmotic d.** Diuresis due to the presence of poorly absorbable solute in the nephron lumens, such as mannitol administered therapeutically, or excess amounts of glucose in diabetes mellitus. **water d.** Increased urine flow after water ingestion, believed to be the result of inhibition of antidiuretic hormone (vasopressin) secretion.

**diuretic** \dī′yUret′ik\ [Gk *diourētikos* (from *dioureisthai* to be passed in the urine, induce urination, from *di(a)-* through + *ourein* to urinate) diuretic] 1 Inducing a state of increased urine flow. 2 Any drug or factor that produces increased urine flow. Oral diuretics are widely used and are very effective. The thiazides inhibit sodium chloride reabsorption in the cortical diluting segment of the renal tubule, resulting in hypertonic urine. Ethacrynic acid and furosemide are very powerful diuretics and inhibit reabsorption throughout the nephron, especially that of chloride in the thick ascending limb of the loop of Henle. These two agents are effective in almost all cases and, in contrast to the thiazides, are effective in the presence of renal failure. Also *uragogue* (obs.). **cardiac d.** Any drug or factor, such as digitalis, that improves cardiac output in congestive heart failure sufficiently to increase renal blood flow and glomerular filtration, with resultant diuresis. **loop d.** A diuretic that acts especially on the thick ascending limb of the loop of Henle.

**diuria** \dīyoo′rē·ə\ [L *di(es)* day + -URIA] The increased frequency of urine flow while awake.

**diurnal** \dī·ur′nəl\ Pertaining to daytime, especially to a daytime period of animal activity. Compare NOCTURNAL.

**diurnule** A pill or other form of medication that contains a complete total daily dosage of a particular drug or agent.

**divalent** \dī′vālənt, dīvā′lənt\ BIVALENT.

**divarication** \dīver′ikā′shən\ *Obs.* DIASTASIS.

**divaricator** \dīver′ikā′tər\ [L *divaricat(us),* past part. of *divaricare* to cause to straddle, spread wide, splay + -OR] A static support used to maintain reduction of a congenitally dislocated hip.

**divergence** \divur′jəns, dī-\ [French (from L *divergens,* pres. part. of *divergere,* from *dis-* apart + *vergere* to turn), divergence] **1** A moving apart, usually of two paths, as of two light beams. **2** A moving apart of the two eyes in alignment in a horizontal plane. Also *negative convergence.* **beam d.** Outward spread of a beam in the far field.

**divergent** \dīvur′jənt\ [See DIVERGENCE.] Extending or moving in different directions.

**diversion** \divur′zhən\ [Late L *diversio* (from *diversus,* past part. of *divertere* to turn aside, digress) a changing course] A changed direction; deflection. **urinary d.** Surgical direction of urine flow outside of normal channels, as into the colon or an ileal conduit.

**diversity** \divur′sitē\ **combinatorial d.** The generation of many mRNA sequences from a few DNA sequences by rearranging, through somatic recombination, portions of a gene before transcription. It is the mechanism by which the variable regions of immunoglobulins are generated, resulting in antibodies specific for a wide range of antigens.

**diverticula** \dī′vərtik′yələ\ Plural of DIVERTICULUM.

**diverticular** \dī′vərtik′yələr\ Of or relating to diverticula or a diverticulum.

**diverticulectomy** \dī′vərtik′yəlek′təmē\ [*diverticul(um)* + -ECTOMY] The excision of a diverticulum.

**diverticulitis** \dī′vərtik′yəlī′tis\ [*diverticul(um)* + -ITIS] Inflammation of a diverticulum. It may be complicated by obstruction, bleeding, or perforation.

**diverticuloesophagostomy** \dī′vərtik′yəlō-ēsäf′əgäs′təmē\ An operation for the symptomatic relief of very large hypopharyngeal diverticula regarded as unsuitable for excision or Dohlman's operation. The lower end of the diverticulum is exposed in the chest and anastomosed to the esophagus end-to-side.

**diverticuloma** \dī′vərtik′yəlō′mə\ [*diverticul(um)* + -OMA] A mass or tumor in a diverticulum.

**diverticulopexy** \dī′vərtik′yəlōpek′sē \ [*diverticul(um)* + *o* + -PEXY] The surgical fixation of a diverticulum following its separation from subjacent tissue.

**diverticulosis** \dī′vərtik′yəlō′sis\ [*diverticul(um)* + -OSIS] The presence of multiple diverticula in a viscus, especially in the colon. Colonic diverticula are very commonly found in the middle-aged and elderly and are often asymptomatic. The lesions are acquired herniations of mucosa and submucosa through muscular layers of the colon wall. **d. of the gallbladder** ADENOMYOMATOSIS OF THE GALLBLADDER.

**diverticulum** \dī′vurtik′yələm\ [L (also *deverticulum*; from *divertere, devertere* to turn aside, from, respectively, *dis-* apart, *de* from, away + *vertere* to turn), a side way, bypath] (*pl.* diverticula) A localized sac or pouch formed in the wall of a hollow viscus and opening into its lumen. Common sites of origin include the ampulla of the ductus deferens, esophagus, intestines, and urinary bladder. **acquired d.** A diverticulum arising as a result of a pathological process weakening the wall of a hollow viscus. **acquired d. of the urinary bladder** A vesical diverticulum appearing at a point of decreased resistance to pressure, often resulting from urinary tract obstruction. **allantoic d.** The initial outgrowth from the endodermal embryonic hindgut, which later becomes the allantois. Also *allantoenteric diverticulum.* **diverticula ampullae ductus deferentis** [NA] Branched outpocketings of the mucous membrane into the adjacent muscular layer of the tortuous ampulla of the ductus deferens just before the latter narrows and joins the excretory duct of the seminal vesicle. **bladder d.** VESICAL DIVERTICULUM. **caliceal d.** An outward pouching of a renal calix. Cysts so formed usually cause no symptoms but may be complicated by stones and infections. Also *pyelocaliceal cyst, pyelogenic renal cyst.* **cervical d.** A diverticulum from the pharynx, representing persistence of an embryonic pharyngeal pouch, or from the skin on the side of the neck, representing persistence of an embryonic branchial groove. **congenital d.** A diverticulum of prenatal origin, usually resulting from abnormal persistence of an embryonic duct, tube, or other similar structure. **epiphrenic d.** A diverticulum originating just above the gastroesophageal junction. It usually protrudes toward the right side of the mediastinum. Also *supradiaphragmatic diverticulum.* **false d.** An intestinal diverticulum which passes through an established defect in the wall of the gut and therefore does not have a layer of muscle in its wall. **foregut d.** A cul-de-sac at the anterior extremity of the embryonic intestine, situated at the level of the dorsal surface of the cardiac recess. This arrangement lasts only until the pharyngeal membrane breaks down, towards the end of the third month, when the cephalic extremity of the intestine and the pharynx communicate directly with the amniotic cavity at the stomodeum. **Heister's d.** BULBUS SUPERIOR VENAE JUGULARIS. **hepatic d.** In an embryo, the endodermal diverticulum which arises close to the junction of the foregut and the yolk sac to give rise to the parenchymatous cells of the liver and the lining of the biliary apparatus (gallbladder, bile ducts). **hypopharyngeal d.** A circumscribed pouch of variable size created by herniation of the mucous membrane through a defect in the muscular coat at the junction of the pharynx and esophagus. Also *pharyngoesophageal diverticulum, Zenker's diverticulum, Zenker's pouch, pharyngocele.* **d. ilei** Any diverticulum from the ileum other than one associated with the embryonic yolk sac. **d. ilei verum** MECKEL'S DIVERTICULUM. **laryngeal d.** An unusual extension, in humans, of the saccule of the larynx, which is normally elongated in apes. **Meckel's d.** A vestige of the embryonic omphaloenteric duct. It may persist abnormally in the adult as a blind sac in the ileum, close to the ileocecal junction. Also *diverticulum ilei verum.* **Nuck's d.** A patent processus vaginalis peritonei in the female. **optic d.** Either of two bilateral diverticula which grow out from the inferolateral aspects of the diencephalon. The extremity of each diverticulum enlarges to form the optic vesicle, which becomes indented to form the optic cup. The cup becomes related to the developing lens placode at the ectodermal surface. The stalk of the diverticulum forms the basis of the future optic nerve. The optic cup, its layers derived from ectodermal nervous tissue, will give rise from the inner layer to the retina (pars optica retinae) and parts of the iris and of the ciliary body (pars optica caeca). The outer layer becomes the pigment layer of the retina. Also *optic evagination.* **pancreatic diverticula** A dorsal and a ventral endodermal diverticulum formed from the embryonic duodenum which will eventually fuse to form a single pancreas and its ducts. The ventral diverticulum gives rise to only the lower part of the head of the pancreas. **Pertik's d.** An occasional lateral extension of recessus pharyngeus. **pharyngeal d.** An outpocketing of the mucous membrane through the posterior wall of the pharynx between the thyropharyngeal and cricopharyngeal parts of the inferior constrictor muscle of the pharynx. **pharyngoesophageal d.** HYPOPHARYNGEAL DIVERTICULUM. **pineal d.** An embryonic evagination of the roof of the posterior part of the diencephalon (future third ventricle) which becomes the pineal gland. **pituitary d.** CRANIOPHARYNGEAL POUCH. **posterior pharyngeal d.** Either pharyngeal diverticulum or pharyngoesophageal diverticulum. **pulsion d.** A diverticulum resulting from herniation of the mucosa through a defect in the muscularis caused by high intraluminal pressures. Common sites for pulsion diverticula include the esophagus and the colon. Also *pressure diverticulum.* **pulsion d. of the esophagus** A fluid- or air-filled sac or pouch formed by hernial protrusion of the mucous membrane through the muscular coat of the esophagus or as a result of pressure within. It often results in the regurgitation of undigested food. **Rokitansky's d.** TRACTION DIVERTICULUM OF THE ESOPHAGUS. **supracondylar synovial diverticula** Hernial protrusions of the synovial membrane on the elbow joint occurring in the supracondylar region. **supradiaphragmatic d.** EPIPHRENIC DIVERTICULUM. **synovial d.** A hernial protrusion of synovial membrane through a joint capsule or tendon sheath. **thyroid d.** A midline downgrowth from the floor of the embryonic pharynx, just caudal to where the tuberculum impar will form, which becomes the thyroglossal duct and later most of the thyroid gland. **diverticula of trachea** Rare outpocketings of the mucous membrane of the trachea. Also *tracheal diverticula, tracheoaerocele* (rare). **traction d.** A diverticulum, usually in the esophagus, caused by external adhesive lesions that result in traction on the muscular coat and formation of the diverticulum. The traction is frequently caused by inflammatory lymph nodes in the mediastinum, usually tuberculous in nature. **traction d. of the esophagus** A localized distortion, angulation, or funnel-shaped bulging of the full thickness of the wall of the esophagus, caused by adhesions resulting from some external lesion near the midpoint of the esophagus. Also *Rokitansky's diverticulum.* **d. unci** In vertebrates, a recess of the temporal horn of the lateral ventricle formed by intrusion of the incus. **ureteric d.** URETERIC BUD. **d. of the utricle** A congenital anomaly in which midline fusion of the paramesonephric ducts produces a sac just behind the prostate. **vesical d.** A small pocket of vesical mucosa that penetrates the muscular coat of the bladder, most often seen in older people. Also *bladder diverticulum.* **Zenker's d.** HYPOPHARYNGEAL DIVERTICULUM.

**divicine** \dīvī′sin\ $C_4H_6N_4O_2$. A toxic pyrimidine base isolated from *Vicia sativa*, vetch. It may be the cause of lathyrism.

**divinyl ether** VINYL ETHER.

**division** [L *divisio* (from *dividere* to split, separate into parts, from *dis-* apart + root of *viduare* to deprive or bereave of, from *viduus* separated, widowed) a dividing, separation] **1** A separation into two or more parts. **2** A distinct part or branch of a larger structure, as of the brachial plexus. **cell d.** The division of a mother cell into two daughter cells. Cell division includes nuclear division (karyokinesis) and cytoplasmic division (cytokinesis). **craniosacral d.** SYSTEMA NERVOSUM AUTONOMICUM, PARS PARASYMPATHICA. **equational d.** Cell division in which the sister chromatids of a chromosome are separated. It is the second cell division in meiosis. **indirect nuclear d.** *Older term* MITOSIS. **maturation d.** One of the unequal meiotic divisions in oogenesis, from the germinal vesicle stage to the formation of a mature egg. **multiplicative d.** Division of a mother cell into more than two daughter cells. If the process follows fertilization, in which case division usually occurs in a cyst, the daughter cells are called sporozoites. If the division occurs without either prior fertilization of the mother cell or encystment, the daughter cells are called merozoites. **reduction d.** Cell division in which the homologous chromosomes pair, then later separate into the daughter cells. The daughter cells have only half the number of chromosomes as the parent cell. The first cell division in meiosis is a reduction division. **Remak's nuclear d.** AMITOSIS. **thoracicolumbar d.** SYSTEMA NERVOSUM AUTONOMICUM, PARS SYMPATHICA.

**Divry** [Paul *Divry,* Belgian physician, born 1889] Van Bogaert-Divry syndrome. See under SYNDROME.

**divulse** \divuls′\ [L *divuls(us),* past part. of *divellere* (from *di(s)-* apart + *vellere* to pluck, pull) to tear asunder] To separate by force; to rip asunder.

**divulsion** \divul′shən\ The act of pulling apart or separating.

**divulsor** \divul′sər\ [*divuls(e)* + -OR] An instrument used for dilatation of a cavity or canal.

**dizygotic** \dī′zīgät′ik\ [DI-$^2$ + ZYGOTIC] Formed from two separate zygotes, as fraternal or unlike twins.

**dizziness** A sensation of lightness in the head, of being dazed or giddy, as in the moments before fainting. Vertigo may cause dizziness but not all dizziness is vertigo.

**djenkolic acid** The amino acid formed by two molecules of cysteine linked sulfur-to-sulfur through a methylene group. It was first isolated in 1935 from the Djenkol bean. It is not a component of proteins.

**DL-** A prefix signifying a mixture of equal numbers of molecules of D- and L- enantiomers. Such a mixture behaves as a pure substance in its reactions with achiral reagents, since the two enantiomers have equal chances of entering such reactions.

***dl-*** An outmoded representation of DL-, from a time when it was not clear whether the letters implied configuration or optical rotation.

**D.M.D.** Doctor of Dental Medicine.

**DMF** [*d(ecayed)* + *m(issing)* + *f(illed)*] DMF INDEX.

**DMSO** dimethyl sulfoxide.

**DN** **1** dibucaine number. **2** dicrotic notch.

**Dn** decanem.

**DNA** deoxyribonucleic acid. **B D.** The usual form of double-chained DNA in which the helix is right-handed, the helical axis is in the center of the molecule, 2 grooves are present, and the pitch is 34. It is the classic, Watson-Crick double helix. Compare Z DNA. **complementary D.** **1** Any DNA chain complementary to a specified DNA sequence. **2** A DNA chain that is synthesized from, and is therefore complementary to, an RNA template using a reverse transcriptase. It is used in recombinant DNA technology for molecular cloning and for generating probes for hybridization studies. Also *copy DNA.* Abbr. cDNA **double-stranded D.** DNA in which two parallel, complementary polynucleotide chains are maintained in a double-helical conformation by the base pairing of nucleotides on opposite chains. Also *native DNA, duplex DNA.* Abbr. dsDNA **linker D.** In the nucleosome, the linear region of about 60 base pairs of DNA that separates each core particle. It is visible in electron micrographs of decondensed chromatin as the string portion of the "beads-on-a-string" appearance. **native D.** DOUBLE-STRANDED DNA. **rapidly reannealing D.** DNA that, on denaturation, rapidly reassumes the double-helical conformation. It usually has simple or highly repetitious nucleotide sequences and a

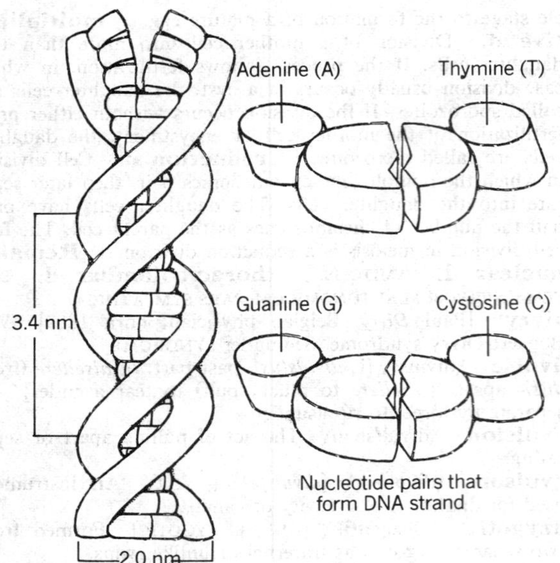


**DNA** (deoxyribonucleic acid)

relatively low cot value. Most types of satellite DNA are rapidly reannealing. Also *rapidly reassociating DNA*. **recombinant D.** DNA produced by molecular recombination *in vitro* of genetic material from two different sources. **repetitive D.** Any DNA sequence that is present in multiple copies in a given genome. It is characteristic of eukaryotic genomes, in which certain sequences are repeated in approximately $10^6$ copies, known as highly repetitive or simple-sequence DNA, and are found associated with constitutive heterochromatin and, to a lesser extent, are dispersed. Other sequences, called middle-repetitive DNA, are repeated $10^2$-$10^4$ times, and include certain structural genes for rRNA and histones. Compare SINGLE-COPY DNA. **satellite D.** Pieces of DNA that consist of many tandem repeats of some short sequence. These repeats may be identical or closely related to each other. Satellite DNA is often observed as a small peak separate from the peak of the main bulk of the DNA, when eukaryotic DNA is separated by buoyant density on centrifugation in a density gradient of cesium chloride. It rarely exceeds 5% of the DNA of the cell, and is often localized to heterochromatic regions of chromosomes, particularly centromeres. **single-copy D.** DNA sequences of eukaryotes that are found in one copy per genome. Most structural genes are part of this class. Also *unique DNA*. Compare REPETITIVE DNA. **single-stranded D.** A molecule of DNA with only one polynucleotide chain. A few of the bacterial viruses (0X174 and S13 *E. coli* viruses) have their genetic information on a single polynucleotide chain. During viral reproduction, the single polynucleotide strand (the + strand) acts as a template for the production of a complementary strand (the − strand), the + and − strands combine to form a double helix. **transferred D.** DNA, exogenous to a host cell's genome, that is introduced by a process such as transduction, microinjection, transfection, or transformation. Abbr. tDNA **unique D.** SINGLE-COPY DNA. **Z D.** A form of double-chained DNA in which the helix is left-handed, the helical axis is along the side of the molecule, and the pitch of the helix is 44.6. Also *Z form*. Compare B DNA.

**DNAase** DEOXYRIBONUCLEASE.

**DNA nucleotidyltransferase** The former official name of DNA POLYMERASE.

**DNA polymerase** An enzyme that makes DNA by adding deoxynucleoside 5′-phosphate residues to the 3′-hydroxyl of the previous residue with the expulsion of pyrophosphate from deoxynuocleoside triphosphates. Such enzymes may be DNA-directed, producing a sequence complementary to that of the directing DNA. These enzymes are involved in DNA replication and repair. On the other hand, they may be RNA-directed, in which case they are involved in the replication of certain RNA viruses. Also *DNA nucleotidyltransferase* (former official name). **RNA-directed D.** The enzyme (EC 2.7.7.49) that catalyzes synthesis of DNA from the four deoxynucleoside triphosphates, with release of pyrophosphate, using RNA as template. The enzyme is found in RNA-containing viruses, many of them oncogenic, whose replication requires the formation of complementary DNA in the animal host cell. It is widely used for synthesizing DNA for genetic engineering, using mRNA isolated from specialized cells as template, in order to obtain a specific gene.

**DNase** DEOXYRIBONUCLEASE.

**DNA topoisomerase** One of two enzymes (EC 5.99.1.2 and EC 5.99.1.3) that convert one topological isomer of DNA into another, with change in the degree of supercoiling. EC 5.99.1.2 catalyzes breaking of one strand, allowing relaxation of supercoiling, and rejoining. EC 5.99.1.3 is the ATP-hydrolyzing DNA topoisomerase, and it can produce less stable topological isomers.

**DNB** dinitrobenzene.

**DNCB** dinitrochlorobenzene (dichloronitrobenzene).

**DNFB** dinitrofluorobenzene (fluorodinitrobenzene).

**D.O.** Doctor of Osteopathy.

**DOA** dead on arrival (designating death prior to admission to a hospital).

**Doca** A proprietary name for desoxycorticosterone acetate.

***Dochmius duodenalis*** \däk′mē·əs doo′ōdənā′lis\ *ANCYLOSTOMA DUODENALE*.

**docimasy** \dō′simā′sē\ [Gk *dokimasia* (from *dokimos* tried, approved, from *dechesthai* to choose, approve) a proving, examination] The practice of using appropriate testing methods and techniques to document a claim or assertion made regarding the nature, quality, or quantity of a substance, such as a mineral or medication, or of a physiologic event. • The term was formerly used especially with reference to *pulmonary* and *intestinal docimasy*, in which the lungs and segments of doubly ligated intestinal tract of a dead newborn, particularly a suspected neonaticide, were placed in water. A finding that the organs floated was formerly considered absolute documentation that the neonate had been born alive and had breathed.

**doctor** [Middle English *doctour* (from L *doctor* a teacher, from *doc(ere)* to teach + *-tor*, agentive suffix) a teacher, master, scholar in any subject, including physick (medicine)] Any health care or medical science professional who holds a doctorate degree, as the degree of Medicinae Doctor, or Doctor of Medicine (M.D.). • *Doctor* is often used as a form of address prefixed to a name, in writing usually in its abbreviated form *Dr.* In the United Kingdom, a distinction is traditionally made between physicians and surgeons, the latter being addressed as *Mister* (*Mr.*). **barefoot d.** A medical auxiliary, especially in the rural areas of China, who is trained to diagnose and treat prevalent diseases, to dispense simple remedies, and to instruct in disease prevention and birth control. *Popular.* ⟨"The backbone of the early detection program are the paramedics, or barefoot doctors. . . . They screen large numbers of people for cancer in the rural communities and in the factories, as well as dispense herbal and modern medicines and birth control pills."—*Science News,* 25 Feb. 1978, 124.⟩

**doctrine** \däk′trin\ [L *doctrina* (from *doctor* a teacher) instruction] A set of principles or beliefs proffered for general acceptance. **Monro-Kellie d.** The principle of the constancy of intracranial blood volume. **d. of specific nerve energies** LAW OF SPECIFIC IRRITABILITY.

**dodeca-** \dō′dekə-\ [Gk *dōdeka* twelve] A combining form meaning twelve. Also *dodec-*.

**dodecadactylon** \-dak′təlän\ DUODENUM.

**dodecyl sulfate** The acid $CH_3$—$[CH_2]_{11}$—O—$SO_3H$, its anion, or any salt containing it. It is a commonly used anionic detergent. In a solution of the salt proteins show an electrophoretic mobility in a gel that depends on their molecular mass, but not on their original charge, which is swamped by the negative charge they acquire from adsorbing dodecyl sulfate anions. Determination of this mobility is used to find their molecular mass.

**Döderlein** [Albert Siegmund Gustav *Döderlein,* German obstetrician and gynecologist, 1860–1941] See under BACILLUS.

**DOE** dyspnea on exertion (exertional dyspnea).

**Doerfler** [Leo G. *Doerfler,* U.S. audiologist, born 1919] Doerfler-Stewart test. See under TEST.

**Dogiel** [Alexander Stanislavovic *Dogiel,* Russian histologist, 1852–1922] Dogiel's corpuscles. See under CORPUSCLE.

**Dogiel** [Jan *Dogiel,* Russian anatomist and physiologist, 1830–1905] See under ENDING.

**dogma** \dôg′mə\ **central d.** In biology, the scheme describing the interrelationships of the macromolecules that specify the transmission and translation of genetic information. It holds that both DNA and RNA can specify their own replication and can be transcribed one to the other, and that protein is translated from an RNA message.

**Döhle** [Paul *Döhle,* German pathologist, 1855–1928] **1** Döhle disease, Heller-Döhle disease. See under SYPHILITIC AORTITIS. **2** Döhle inclusion bodies. See under DÖHLE BODIES.

**Doisy** [Edward Adelbert *Doisy,* U.S. biochemist, born 1893] Allen-Doisy unit. See under MOUSE UNIT.

**dol** \dōl\ [L *dolor* ache, pain, grief] A subjective unit of pain intensity.

**Doléris** [Jacques-Amedee *Doléris,* French gynecologist, 1852–1938] See under OPERATION.

**dolicho-** \däl′əkō-\ [Gk *dolichos* long] A combining form meaning long. Also *dolich-*.

**dolichocephalic** \-səfal′ik\ Having a long, narrow head, with a cephalic index below 76. Also *dolichocephalous.*

**dolichocephalous** \-sef′ələs\ DOLICHOCEPHALIC.

**dolichocephaly** \-sef′əlē\ [DOLICHO- + CEPHAL- + -Y] Longness and narrowness of the head, with a cephalic index below 76.

**dolicho-mega-arteries** \-meg′ə-är′tərēs\ The suspected pathogenesis of arterial aneurysms, considered secondary to degeneration of the arterial media. The theory has gained popularity particularly in Europe.

**dolichomorphic** \-môr′fik\ Having an elongated, narrow body form. Also *longitypical.*

**dolichopellic** \-pel′ik\ DOLICHOPELVIC.

**dolichopelvic** \-pel′vik\ Having a long, narrow pelvis, with a pelvic index of 95 or above. Also *dolichopellic.*

**dolichostenomelia** \-stē′nōmē′lyə\ ARACHNODACTYLY.

**dolichuranic** \däl′ikyooran′ik\ Denoting a long narrow palate with a palatomaxillary index of less than 110.

**Döllinger** [Johann Ignaz J. *Döllinger,* German physician, 1770–1841] Döllinger's ring. See under SCHWALBE'S RING.

**dolor** \dō′lôr\ [L, pain, distress] Physical pain or mental anguish. **d. capitis** HEADACHE. **d. coxae** A pain in the hip.

**dolores** \dōlôr′ēz\ Plural of DOLOR.

**dolorimeter** \dō′lôrim′ətər\ [DOLOR + *i* + -METER] An instrument usually employing infrared radiation, for measuring the stimulus magnitude required for inducing pain.

**dolorimetry** \dō′lôrim′ətrē\ [DOLOR + *i* + -METRY] The measurement of subjective units of painful sensations.

**dolorogenic** \dōlôr′ōjen′ik\ [DOLOR + *o* + -GENIC] Pain-producing.

**domain** \dōmān′\ A region of a macromolecule with a certain structural or functional significance that distinguishes it from other regions of the same molecule. Domains of a protein molecule, for example, might be defined by secondary structure, such as an alpha-helix domain, or by binding properties, such as an antigen-binding domain. **immunoglobulin d.** A domain within an immunoglobulin. Immunoglobulins possess an obvious domain structure, with similar chain folding, some sequence homology, and similar disulfide bonds within domains.

**dome** / **pleural d.** CUPULA PLEURAE.

**dominance** \däm′ənəns\ **1** The state of being dominant. **2** In genetics, a property of the phenotype such that only one allele that determines the phenotype need be present in the genome, and that the action of this allele supersedes the action of the other allele present. Compare RECESSIVENESS. **cerebral d. 1** That state of organization of cerebral function in which one cerebral hemisphere, the dominant hemisphere, controls the functions of speech and of skilled cognition and execution. In right-handed persons, the left hemisphere is normally dominant. **2** The concept that all voluntary functions are controlled by the cerebral cortex. For defs. 1 and 2 also *laterality, lateral dominance.* **conditioned d.** A property of a phenotype such that, in certain conditions, inheritance is dominant, while in others it is recessive. In essence, the phenotype will be expressed when the determining allele is heterozygous in some situations and only when the allele is homozygous in other situations. **incomplete d.** The situation when the phenotype attributable to an allele, *A*, in the heterozygous diploid *Aa*, is intermediate to either homozygous genotype, *AA* or *aa*. Nearly all dominant human phenotypes have this characteristic. Also *partial dominance* (imprecise), *semidominance* (imprecise). **lateral d.** CEREBRAL DOMINANCE. **one-sided d.** Right or left handedness consequent upon cerebral dominance. **partial d.** *Imprecise* INCOMPLETE DOMINANCE. **reversed d. of the eyes** Dominance of the left eye in a right-handed person or vice versa.

**dominance-submission** \däm′ənəns-\ Denoting a continuum for rating or measuring the degree to which a given individual tends, in direct social relationships, either to control the behavior of others or to be dominated by others.

**dominant** \däm′ənənt\ [L *dominans* (pres. part. of *dominari* to reign, domineer, from *dominus* master, from *domus* a house) reigning, dominant] **1** Of or relating to a phenotype that is expressed when a particular allele is heterozygous as a result of the action of that allele. **2** Pertaining to the action of a heterozygous allele. **3** In mendelian genetics, of or relating to a phenotype that is invariant due to the action of a particular allele, whether that allele is homozygous or heterozygous. Compare RECESSIVE.

**domiphen bromide** $C_{22}H_{40}BrNO$. Dodecyldimethyl-2-phenoxyethylammonium bromide. An antiseptic agent employed therapeutically in the treatment of oral infections, such as sore throats. It is given in tablet or lozenge form.

**Donald** [Archibold *Donald,* English gynecologist, 1860–1937] Fothergill-Donald operation. See under MANCHESTER OPERATION.

**Donath** [Julius *Donath,* Austrian physician, 1870–1950] **1** Donath-Landsteiner cold autoantibody. See under DONATH-LANDSTEINER ANTIBODY. **2** See under PHENOMENON. **3** Donath's test. See under DONATH-LANDSTEINER TEST. **4** Donath-Landsteiner syndrome. See under PAROXYSMAL COLD HEMOGLOBINURIA.

**donda ndugu** \dôn′dä ndoo′goo\ [Swahili (from *donda* an ulcer, sore + *ndugu* a brother, sister, kinsman) lit., brother (i.e., chronic) ulcer] A disease that produces inflammation and edema of the legs, ultimately causing the involved skin to slough off. It is found in coastal areas of East Africa where the causative organisms are present in stagnant water.

**Donders** [Franz C. *Donders,* Dutch ophthalmologist, 1818–1889] See under SPACE, LAW, RING.

**donee** \dōnē′\ [*don(ate)* + *-ee* as in *employee*] One to whom something is given, especially the recipient of an organ graft; host.

**Don Juan** \dän wän′, dôn hwän′\ [after *Don Juan,* legendary Spanish seducer] A male sexual profligate, often with the implication that the erotomaniacal behavior is used as a defense against feelings of insecurity that the individual may have about his masculinity or against unconscious homosexual impulses.

**Donnan** [Frederick George *Donnan,* English chemist, 1870–1956] See under EQUILIBRIUM, EFFECT.

**donor** [*don(ate)* + -OR] **1** An individual organism from which a cell, tissue, or organ is removed for transplantation, either to another site on the same individual or to another individual. **2** In chemistry, the molecule (or ion, atom, etc.) that donates a specified entity, e.g., group, electron, etc., to another. **universal d.** An individual with group O blood type, so named because this blood can sometimes be given to individuals with other ABO blood types in emergency transfusions.

**Donovan** [Charles *Donovan,* Irish surgeon, 1863–1951] **1** Leishman-Donovan body. See under AMASTIGOTE. **2** Donovan bodies. See under BODY.

***Donovania granulomatis*** \dän′ōvā′nē·ə gran′yəlō′mətis\ *CALYMMATOBACTERIUM GRANULOMATIS.*

**donovanosis** \dän′əvənō′sis\ GRANULOMA INGUINALE.

**-dont** \-dänt\ -ODONT.

**dopa** \dō′pə\ 3,4-Dihydroxyphenylalanine. A substance formed from tyrosine and oxygen under the action of tyrosine 3-monooxygenase. It is an important intermediate in the formation of epinephrine and related catecholamines. It is catalytic in the oxidation of tyrosine to melanin by oxygen and monophenol monooxygenase. A synthetic form, levodopa, is used in the treatment of parkinsonism. Also *DOPA.*

**L-dopa** LEVODOPA.

**dopa decarboxylase** An enzyme (EC 4.1.1.28) that catalyzes the conversion of dopa into dopamine and carbon dioxide, a step in the biosynthesis of epinephrine.

**dopamine** \dō′pəmin\ 3,4-Dihydroxyphenethylamine. An intermediate in the biosynthesis of epinephrine. It is produced by decarboxylation of dopa and can be converted into norepinephrine by dopamine $\beta$-monooxygenase.

**dopamine hydroxylase** *Outmoded* DOPAMINE $\beta$-MONOOXYGENASE.

**dopamine $\beta$-monooxygenase** An enzyme (EC 1.14.17.1) that catalyzes the reaction of molecular oxygen with dopamine and ascorbate to yield norepinephrine and dehydroascorbate, thus hydroxylating the methylene group of dopamine that is attached to the benzene ring. Like other monooxygenases, it catalyzes the insertion into its substrate of only one oxygen atom from $O_2$. Also *dopamine hydroxylase* (outmoded).

**dopaminergic** \dō′pəminur′jik\ **1** Subject to activation by dopamine. **2** Of or relating to dopamine.

**dopa quinone** 4-(2-Amino-2-carboxyethyl)benzo-1,2-quinone. A substance formed from tyrosine via dopa by oxidizing the catechol grouping of dopa to its quinone. It is an intermediate in the formation of melanin. It is unstable because it contains both electrophilic and nucleophilic groups, and it polymerizes with the concomitant reduction of some of it to dopa.

**dope** A drug or agent administered for pleasure or to maintain an addiction, particularly a narcotic.

**Doppler** \däp′lər\ [Johann Christian *Doppler,* Austrian physicist and mathematician, 1803–1853] Relating to or utilizing the Doppler effect. **directional D.** Characterized by or pertaining to Doppler measurements in which information regarding motion toward or away from the transducer is preserved. **pulse D.** Characterized by or pertaining to Doppler imaging or flow detection in which pulsing is used to provide depth information.

**Doppler** [Johann Christian *Doppler,* Austrian physicist and mathematician, 1803–1853] **1** Doppler velocity signal, Doppler principle, Doppler phenomenon, Doppler shift. See under EFFECT. **2** Audio Doppler frequency. See under FREQUENCY. **3** Doppler flowmeter. See under FLOWMETER. **4** See under ULTRASOUND. **5** Laser Doppler velocimetry. See under VELOCIMETRY. **6** Doppler fetal heart detector. See under DETECTOR.

**Dorello** [Primo *Dorello,* Italian anatomist, born 1872] See under CANAL.

**dormant** \dôr′mənt\ [Middle French, pres. part. of *dormir* to sleep, from L *dormire* to sleep] Being in a state of suspended activity.

**dormifacient** HYPNOTIC.

**dornase** *Obs.* DEOXYRIBONUCLEASE. **pancreatic d.** A preparation of deoxyribonuclease from bovine pancreas. It is used in an aerosol to decrease the viscosity of pulmonary secretions and help clear the respiratory passages.

**Dorno** [Carl W. M. *Dorno,* Swiss climatologist, 1865–1942] Dorno's rays. See under RAY.

**Dorrance** [George Morris *Dorrance,* U.S. surgeon, 1877–1949] Dorrance operation. See under PALATAL PUSHBACK OPERATION.

**dors-** \dôrs-\ DORSO-.

**dorsa** \dôr′sə\ Plural of DORSUM.

**dorsad** \dôr′sad\ Toward the back or dorsal surface.

**dorsal** \dôr′səl\ [Med. L *dorsalis* (from L *dorsualis* situated on an animal's back, from *dorsum* back + *-alis* -AL) pertaining to the back] **1** Pertaining to the back of the body or to the dorsum of any part. **2** Relatively near the back or dorsum as compared with other structures or parts of the same kind nearer the front or belly side; in human anatomy, commonly equivalent to *posterior.* Compare VENTRAL.

**dorsalgia** \dôrsal′jə\ [DORS- + -ALGIA] A pain in the back. Also *dorsodynia, notalgia.*

**dorsalis** \dôrsā′lis\ [NA] Dorsal.

**dorsi-** \dôr′sə-\ DORSO-.

**dorsicumbent** \-kum′bənt\ SUPINE.

**dorsiduct** \dôr′sədukt\ To draw toward the back of the body or the dorsum of a part.

**dorsiflexion** \-flek′shən\ [DORSI- + FLEXION] Movement of the ankle in which the dorsum of the foot moves towards the anterior (cranial) aspect of the tibia or, in the forelimb of a quadruped, towards the radius. After dorsiflexion the foot or toes are said to be flexed upward away from the sole. Compare PLANTAR FLEXION.

**dorsiflexor** \-flek′sər\ A muscle that acts in dorsiflexion.

**dorsispinal** \-spī′nəl\ Pertaining to the back and the vertebral column.

**dorso-** \dôr′sō-\ [L *dorsum* back of a human or beast] A combining form meaning the back (of a body or part), dorsal. Also *dorsi-, dors-*.

**dorsoabdominal** \-abdäm′ənəl\ DORSOVENTRAL.

**dorsoanterior** \-antir′ē·ər\ [DORSO- + ANTERIOR] With the back of the fetus towards the front of the mother: said of an intrauterine position.

**dorsocephalad** \-sef′əlad\ Toward the back of the head.

**dorsodynia** \-din′ē·ə\ DORSALGIA.

**dorsoepitrochlearis** \-ep′iträk′lē·er′is\ LATISSIMOCONDYLARIS.

**dorsointerosseal** \-in′təräs′ē·əl\ Situated posteriorly between the metacarpal or the metatarsal bones. Also *dorsointerosseous.*

**dorsolateral** \-lat′ərəl\ Pertaining to the dorsal surface and the side of a part or the body. Also *laterodorsal.*

**dorsolumbar** \-lum′bər\ Pertaining to the back and the posterolateral region between the ribs and the iliac crest; lumbodorsal.

**dorsomedial** \-mē′dē·əl\ Situated at or near the medial side of the dorsal surface of an area.

**dorsomedian** \-mē′dē·ən\ Pertaining to, situated in, or denoting the median longitudinal line of the back.

**dorsomesial** \-mē′sē·əl\ Pertaining to the median longitudinal line of the back.

**dorsoposterior** \-pästir′ē·ər\ [DORSO- + POSTERIOR] With the back of the fetus towards the back of the mother: said of an intrauterine position.

**dorsoradial** \-rā′dē·əl\ Pertaining to or located on the radial side of the back of the forearm, hand, or fingers.

**dorsosacral** \-sā′krəl\ Pertaining to the back and the sacrum.

**dorsoventrad** \-ven′trad\ Extending in a direction from the dorsal to the ventral aspect.

**dorsoventral** \-ven′trəl\ **1** Pertaining to or extending between the back and the abdomen. **2** Directed from the back to the abdominal surface. For defs. 1 and 2 also *dorsoabdominal.*

**dorsum** \dôr′səm\ [L, the back of a human or animal] **1** The back. **2** An aspect of a body part, such as the back of the hand or the top of the foot, that is regarded as analagous to the back of the body. In reference to the anatomical position, the dorsum of most parts is either posterior or superior. **d. ilii** FACIES GLUTEA OSSIS ILII. **d. linguae** [NA] The superior and posterior surface of the body of the tongue, divided by a shallow median groove that extends posteriorly to the foramen cecum, which is at the apex of the sulcus terminalis separating the anterior from the posterior parts of the surface. The anterior part is covered by the lingual papillae, while the posterior surface is nodular due to the lingual tonsil in the submucosa. Also *dorsum of tongue.* **d. manus** [NA] The posterior aspect, or back, of the hand. **d. nasi** [NA] The rounded anterior border of the nose, extending from the root of nose to the apex, or tip. It is the junction of the sides of the nose, the uppermost part being the bridge. **d. pedis** [NA] The upper surface of the foot, the continuation of the front of the leg past the ankle joint. Also *regio dorsalis pedis.* **d. penis** The anterior surface of the flaccid penis or the posterosuperior surface of the erect penis. **d. of scapula** FACIES POSTERIOR SCAPULAE. **d. sellae** [NA] A quadrilateral plate of the body of the sphenoid bone projecting upward and forward to form the posterior surface of the sella turcica and ending superolaterally as the posterior clinoid process on each side. The sloping posterior surface, or clivus, is continuous inferiorly with the clivus of the occipital bone. Also *clinoid plate* (outmoded). **d. of testis** MARGO POSTERIOR TESTIS. **d. of tongue** DORSUM LINGUAE.

**dosage** [*dos(e)* + -AGE] The determination of the amount of a drug to be given. **gene d.** The number of copies of an allele, or of two similar alleles, in a genome. It is determined by ploidy, duplication, and deletion, and it is measured either indirectly, as by the amount of gene product, or directly, as by nucleic acid hybridization.

**dose** [Gk *dosis.* See DOSIS.] The amount given at one time of a therapeutic drug, diagnostic agent, or radioactivity. Also *dosis.* **absorbed d.** The energy imparted to a unit mass of tissue or other material by ionizing radiation, measured in grays or rads. Also *radiation absorbed dose, radiation dose.* **air d.** The radiation dose as measured in air, without scattering or backscattering material present. **booster d.** A second or subsequent dose of an immunizing agent, as a vaccine, usually given in attenuated form, to reinforce or restore the immunizing effect of the original dose. Also *booster.* **broken d.** REFRACTIVE DOSE. **central axis depth d.** The dose along the center of a beam of radiation entering a patient or object, expressed as a percentage of the maximum dose. **curative d.** The amount of any therapeutic agent required to produce a cure or correct a deficiency state of a particular nutritional component, such as a vitamin or mineral. Also *dosis efficax, dosis curativa.* **depth d.** The radiation dose delivered at a specified depth in a body or other material, usually expressed as a percentage of the maximum dose in the beam or of the surface dose. **divided d.** REFRACTIVE DOSE. **effective d.** The amount of a drug required to produce the therapeutic effect intended with its use. Abbr. ED **entrance d.** A radiation dose on the axis of a beam, at the surface of a phantom or patient, used in radiation therapy. **epilating d.** In radiotherapy, the dose required to produce primary loss of hair. **erythema d.** The dose of radiant energy sufficient to induce erythema, usually used in reference to ionizing radiation, ultraviolet light, or sunlight therapy. **exit d.** The absorbed dose from a beam of radiation at the surface of the patient or object where the beam emerges. **exposure d.** *Imprecise* EXPOSURE. ● The term is inaccurate because it is the dose that is absorbed. **fractional d.** REFRACTIVE DOSE. **fractionation d.** A method of irradiation in which the desired dose is administered in smaller portions, often daily, over an extended period. **genetically significant d.** A dose which results in the occurrence of genetic abnormalities in excess of those occurring naturally. It is usually applied to exposure to radiation. **immunizing d.** The amount of a given antigen which, upon administration, will elicit an immune response in the host. **initial d.** A first dose of a drug administered in an amount disproportionately large compared to the maintenance dose, in order to obtain therapeutic concentrations of the drug quickly. Also *loading dose, priming dose.* **integral d.** The total energy absorbed by a patient or an object exposed to radiation, equal to the product of the absorbed dose and the mass exposed to radiation. The units of integral dose are kilogram-rads and joules. Also *integral absorbed dose, volume dose* (incorrect) . **integral absorbed d.** INTEGRAL DOSE. **invariably lethal d.** $LD_{100}$. **$L_0$ d.** See under LIMES ZERO. **Lf d.** The quantity of diphtheria toxin or toxoid that flocculates most rapidly when mixed with one unit of antitoxin. The immunizing dose of toxoid is about 10 Lf. **limes nul d.** LIMES ZERO. **loading d.** INITIAL DOSE. **maintenance d.** **1** A dose that if given chronically will achieve the desired therapeutically effective concentrations after a time. **2** A dose designed to maintain stable function or condition rather than effect a cure or induce prophylaxis. **maximum d.** The largest amount of a drug that may safely be given to the average patient. **maximum permissible d.** The upper limit of permissible dose during a certain time period (e.g., a month) established by regulations. No harm is expected at this rate, but it should not be exceeded. **mean effective d.** MEDIAN EFFECTIVE DOSE. **mean lethal d.** MEDIAN LETHAL DOSE. **median effective d.** The amount of a material that induces the expected effect in 50 percent of susceptible subjects to whom it is administered. Also *mean effective dose.* Symbol: $ED_{50}$ **median infective d.** The quantity of pathogenic organisms that reliably causes infection to develop in 50 percent of susceptible subjects exposed to the organisms. Symbol: $ID_{50}$ **median lethal d.** The dose of biologically active material, usually a drug, a toxin, or a microorganism, that causes death in 50 percent of the exposed subjects. Also *mean lethal dose.* Symbol: $LD_{50}$ **minimal d.** The smallest amount of drug that can produce a physiologic effect in an adult. Also *minimum dose.* **minimal hemagglutinating d.** The smallest quantity of a hemagglutinating virus which will fully agglutinate a standard suspension of erythrocytes. A standard suspension of virus is often used to determine the amount of antibody to a given virus in a given serum. For example, the standard suspension of virus is added to each tube of a doubling dilution of serum. Erythrocytes are added to this mixture and agglutination indicates that dilution of serum in which virus has not been neutralized. **minimal hemolytic d.** The smallest quantity of complement which lyses a standard suspension of sensitized erythrocytes. Abbr. MHD **minimal infecting d.** The smallest amount of infective material regularly causing infection in 50 percent of a series of animals or cells. Symbol: $ID_{50}$ **minimal lethal d.** The lowest dose of a pathogenic organism or toxin that kills all of a group of test animals in a specified time. Abbr. MLD **minimal reacting d.** The smallest quantity of a toxic material that reliably produces a predetermined level of reaction in a susceptible subject. Abbr. MRD **minimum d.** MINIMAL DOSE. **minimum infective d.** The smallest quantity of an organism that is capable of producing infection in a susceptible host. **optimum d.** The dose of a drug required to produce the desired effects without causing any untoward symptoms or complications. Also *optimal dose.* **preventive d.** The smallest amount of a given nutrient, such as a vitamin, mineral, amino acid, or fatty acid, that will prevent the development of a deficiency disease caused by the absence of one of these nutrients from the diet. **priming d.** INITIAL DOSE. **radiation d.** ABSORBED DOSE. **radiation absorbed d.** ABSORBED DOSE. Abbr. rad **refractive d.** A fraction of a full dose given repeatedly at frequent intervals to add up to a full dose within a designated time. Also *broken dose, divided dose, fractional dose, dosis refracta.* **sensitizing d.** The quantity of antigenically active material capable of producing an immune response in a host who has had no previous contact with it. **skin d.** Absorbed radiation dose in the skin, resulting from ionization in the adjoining air together with backscattered photons from underlying tissues. **therapeutic d.** The quantity of a given vitamin prescribed for a person suffering from the consequences of a deficient amount of that vitamin. Usually the therapeutic dose is several times the recommended daily allowance. **threshold d.** The minimum absorbed dose of radiation capable of producing an observable effect. **threshold erythema d.** The smallest radiation absorbed dose that will produce appreciable reddening of the skin. **tissue d.** In radiology, the amount of radiation absorbed in a tissue or organ. **unit d.** A single dose of a drug provided in an individual labeled packet, container, or syringe. **volume d.** *Incorrect* INTEGRAL DOSE.

**dosimeter** \dōsim′ətər\ [*dosi(s)* + -METER] Any instrument used to measure the amount of radiation. Also *dosage meter.* **film d.** FILM BADGE. **integrating d.** A dosimeter giving the total charge delivered during an irradiation. **noise d.** An instrument used to record total noise exposure. It is worn by industrial workers exposed to high ambient noise levels. **pocket d.** POCKET CHAMBER.

**dosimetrist** \dōsim′ətrist\ **1** A person who performs dose measurements. **2** In radiation therapy, a person trained to make radiation measurements and also perform treatment-planning calculations.

**dosimetry** \dōsim′ətrē\ [*dosi(s)* + -METRY] In radiology, the science of the measurement of radiation doses, as from x rays or gamma rays. Adj. dosimetric. **photographic d.** The estimation of absorbed dose of radiation from the blackening of photographic film, as read on a densitometer. **thermoluminescent d.** The measurement of ionizing radiation by materials, such as lithium fluoride, which, after exposure to radiation, emit light when subsequently heated. Abbr. TLD

**dosis** [Gk *dosis* (from *didonai* to give) a giving, gift, dose] DOSE. **d. curativa** CURATIVE DOSE. **d. efficax** CURATIVE DOSE. **d. refracta** REFRACTIVE DOSE.

**dot** A small spot or mark, as a defect of a different color from the background against which it is observed. **Gunn's d.'s** Minute punctate reflections from the inner surface of the retina, occurring physiologically in the macular region of the eyes of healthy young people, perhaps due to dimpling of the surface by traction from Müller's fibers. **Maurer's d.'s** Irregular intraerythrocytic inclusions found in cells infected by malarial organisms and revealed when stained with the Leishman stain. Also *Maurer's clefts, Maurer spots, Maurer stippling, Christopher spots, Stephen spots.* **Mittendorf's d.** The mesodermal remnant of the anterior end of the hyaloid artery, located just behind the crystalline lens. It may persist as a congenital anomaly but it does not affect vision. **Schüffner's d.'s** SCHÜFFNER'S GRANULES. **Trantas d.'s** Whitish limbal deposits found in vernal conjunctivitis.

**double-blind** Characterized by concealment to both experimenter and subjects as to which subjects are exposed to the variable being tested and which are functioning as controls. Double-blind tests are designed to eliminate bias resulting from knowledge of the nature of the test. In a double-blind trial of a drug, for example, neither observer nor subject is aware of the subjects given the active material as distinguished from a placebo. Also *double-masked.*

**double-masked** DOUBLE-BLIND. ⟨"Besides photocoagulation, ETDRS will also use a double-masked trial protocol (ophthalmologists eschew the term 'double-blind') to compare long-term aspirin ingestion, 500 mg a day, with placebo" —*Medical World News,* 29 Oct. 1979, 62.⟩

**double-stranded** Having the two polynucleotide molecular chains wound round each other, with pairing between complementary bases which joins the two strands: said of DNA, or occasionally of RNA.

**douche** \doosh\ [French (from Italian *doccia* a water pipe, akin to *doccione* a water conduit, from L *ductio,* gen. *ductionis,* a means of conveying water, from *ducere* to convey) a douche, shower] **1** A jet or localized spray of liquid, gas, or vapor directed into a body cavity or onto a part. **2** A device for administering a douche. **air d.** A pressurized current of air introduced into a body cavity. **Scotch d.** TRANSITION DOUCHE. **transition d.** A douche using alternating hot and cold water streams. Also *Scotch douche.*

**Douglas** [Claude Gordon *Douglas,* English physiologist, 1882–1963] See under BAG.

**Douglas** [James *Douglas,* Scottish anatomist, 1675–1742] **1** Douglas septum. See under CLOACAL SEPTUM. **2** Douglas cul-de-sac, Douglas space, pouch of Douglas. See under EXCAVATIO RECTOUTERINA. **3** Lateral fold of Douglas. See under FOLD. **4** See under ABSCESS. **5** Douglas fold, Douglas ligament. See under PLICA RECTOUTERINA. **6** Douglas fold, line of Douglas, semicircular line of Douglas. See under LINEA ARCUATA VAGINAE MUSCULI RECTI ABDOMINIS.

**Douglas** [John C. *Douglas,* Irish obstetrician, 1777–1850] See under MECHANISM, METHOD.

**dowel** \dou′əl\ A metal post inserted into the root canal of a tooth to support an artificial crown. Also *post, pivot* (outmoded).

**Dowex** Ion exchange resins, both cation and anion exchangers. A proprietary name.

**Down** [John Langdon Haydon *Down,* English physician, 1828–1896] **1** See under SYNDROME. **2** Translocation Down syndrome. See under SYNDROME.

**down** [Old Norse *dúnn* soft feathers] LANUGO.

**Downey** [H. *Downey,* U.S. hematologist, 1877–1959] Downey cell. See under ATYPICAL LYMPHOCYTE.

**downgaze** INFRAVERSION.

**downstream** **1** In a chromosome, the nucleotide sequences 3′ to the end of the last exon of a gene. Compare UPSTREAM. **2** Designating any nucleotide sequence in a gene that is removed in the direction of transcription from a reference sequence. For example, the termination codon is downstream from the initiation codon.

**Dox** [Arthur Wayland *Dox,* U.S. chemist, born 1882] Czapek-Dox solution. See under CZAPEK-DOX AGAR.

**doxapram hydrochloride** $C_{24}H_{30}N_2O_2 \cdot HCl \cdot H_2O$. 1-Ethyl-4-[2-(morpholinyl)ethyl]-3,3-diphenyl-2-pyrrolidinone monohydrochloride monohydrate. A respiratory stimulant employed in the treatment of postanesthetic respiratory depression and distress. It is given intravenously.

**doxepin hydrochloride** $C_{19}H_{21}NO \cdot HCl$. 3-Dibenz[*b,e*]-oxepin-11(6*H*)ylidene-*N,N*-dimethyl- 1-propanamine hydrochloride. An antidepressant drug of the tricyclic class. It has both antidepressant and antianxiety properties.

**doxycycline** $C_{22}H_{24}N_2O_8$. α-6-Deoxy-5-hydroxytetracycline. A yellow, crystalline powder, soluble in water and alcohol, slightly soluble in chloroform and ether, and having a wide range of antibiotic activity against both Gram-positive and Gram-negative organisms. It is similar in its activity to tetracycline hydrochloride.

**doxycycline hyclate** DOXYCYCLINE HYDROCHLORIDE.

**doxycycline hydrochloride** $C_{22}H_{25}ClN_2O_8$. The hydrochloride salt of doxycycline. It has the same properties and uses as the parent drug. Also *doxycycline hyclate.*

**Doyen** [Eugene Louis *Doyen,* French surgeon, 1859–1916] See under OPERATION, CLAMP, GAG.

**Doyère** [Louis Michel François *Doyère,* French physiologist, 1811–1863] Doyère's hillock. See under MOTOR END-PLATE.

**Doyne** [Robert Walter *Doyne,* English ophthalmologist, 1857–1896] Doyne's familial colloid degeneration, Doyne's familial honeycombed choroiditis. See under DOYNE HONEYCOMB DEGENERATION OF RETINA.

**D.P.** Doctor of Pharmacy.

**d.p.** *directione propria* (L, with proper direction).

**DPN** diphosphopyridine nucleotide (nicotinamide adenine dinucleotide). This abbreviation has been replaced by NAD.

**DR** **1** reaction of degeneration. **2** diabetic retinopathy.

**Dr.** doctor (used as a title of address prefixed to a name). • See note at DOCTOR.

**drachm** \dram\ *Brit.* DRAM. **fluid d.** In Great Britain, a unit of capacity equal to 1/1280 (UK) gallon, 1/8 (UK) fluid ounce, or 3.551 63 milliliters. An obsolete unit. Also *fluid dram.* Symbol: fl dr

**dracontiasis** \drak′äntī′əsis\ [Gk *drakontiasis* (from *drakont(ion),* guinea worm, dim. of *drakōn* dragon) guinea worm disease] An infection with the filarial nematode worm *Dracunculus medinensis,* occurring in the Middle East, India, parts of South America, and tropical and northern Africa. The source of infection is drinking water containing water fleas (copepods, *Cyclops* spp.) carrying the infective larvae. Ingested larvae are freed by digestion, migrate to the body cavity and mature. The female, when gravid, migrates to subcutaneous tissues, usually feet and legs. She secretes an enzyme which produces a bullous lesion in which larvae are formed. The lesion bursts when the infected person enters a step-in-well to collect water, discharging a milky fluid containing numerous larvae. These in turn reinfect the water and are fed upon by water fleas to continue the cycle. Secondary infection of the worm-track causes cellulitis, periarticular fibrosis, and arthritis. Metronidazole and thiabendazole are of value therapeutically, but the ultimate solution is to eliminate *Cyclops* spp. from drinking water. Also *guinea worm disease, dracunculosis, dracunculiasis.*

**dracuncular** \drəkung′kyələr\ Referring to nematodes of the genus *Dracunculus..*

**dracunculiasis** \drəkung′kyəlī′əsis\ DRACONTIASIS.

**dracunculosis** \drəkung′kyəlō′sis\ DRACONTIASIS.

***Dracunculus*** \drəkung′kyələs\ A genus of nematodes (superfamily Dracunculoidea) distantly related to filarial worms. Adult females are up to one meter in length. The intermediate host is a freshwater copepod which ingests larvae that exit from a blister in the skin of the final host induced by the adult female worm. The adult parasitizes the subcutis of the host which includes mink, otters, dogs, raccoons, skunks, and man. ***D. medinensis*** The guinea worm, a nematode which may be as much as 120 cm long. The larvae are ingested by copepods (*Cyclops* spp.) which serve as intermediate hosts. Humans and various domestic animals, principally in the Middle East, Africa, and India, become infected by drinking water containing the copepods. Also *Filaria medinensis, Gordius medinensis, Vena medinensis.* See also DRACONTIASIS.

**draft** A dose of a liquid medicine; a potion. **black d.** COMPOUND MIXTURE OF SENNA.

**drag** The lower side of a dental flask. **solvent d.** The effect that net solvent flow through a membrane exerts on the passage of solute across the same membrane.

**dragée** [French (irreg. from L *tragemata,* from Gk *tragēmata* dried fruits or other sweets, from *trōgein* to nibble, munch, eat) a fruit confection, sugar-coated pill] A pill or tablet that is sugar-coated; a medicated candy or confection.

**Drager** [Glenn Albert *Drager,* U.S. neurologist, born 1917] Shy-Drager syndrome. See under SYNDROME.

**drain** [Old English *dreahnian* to strain out, dry, akin to English *dry*] An appliance or piece of material that acts as a channel for the escape of fluid from a cavity, or of pus and other matter from a wound or a focus of suppuration. **cigarette d.** A drain consisting of a gauze wick inside a rubber tube. Also *Penrose drain.* **quarantine d.** A surgically inserted drain that isolates the discharge from the environment. **stab wound d.** A surgical drain introduced into the primary drainage area via a cutaneous incision apart from the operative wound.

**drainage** The drawing off or outflow of fluids or of solid material contained in it, as from a cavity or a wound. **anomalous pulmonary venous d.** A developmental defect in which some or all of the venous blood from the lungs, normally discharged into the left cardiac atrium, is taken instead to the right atrium or to any of a number of systemic veins entering the right atrium. The embryologic error probably lies with the failure of the early venous evagination from the left atrium to form or to establish contact with the venous plexus surrounding the lung buds, thereby favoring retention of the early systemic drainage of the lungs. **closed pleural d.** Drainage of fluid or air from the pleural cavity by insertion through the chest wall of a tube, the other end of which does not permit entry of air into the chest. **dependent d.** Drainage from the lowest or dependent part. **open d.** Drainage of fluid from the lung or pleura by means of a tube that is not closed to entry of air at the other end. **postural d.** Drainage of the bronchial system by coughing while positioned in such a way that the drainage is facilitated by gravity. **Roux-Y d.**

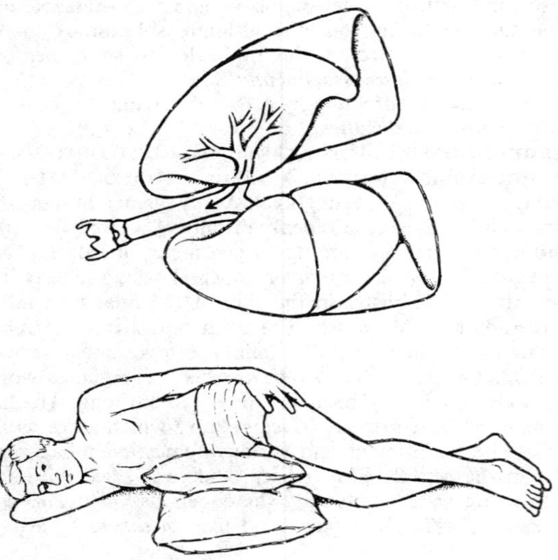

Postural drainage of left lung

The drainage of a structure by using a Roux-en-Y anastomosis. **suction d.** Drainage of a part using suction equipment attached to the drain. **tidal d.** Drainage of the urinary bladder by means of a device that alternately fills and empties the bladder. **ventriculoatrial d.** The shunting of ventricular fluid into the right atrium of the heart by means of a system that connects a ventricular catheter to a graded pressure valve and then to a catheter that passes subcutaneously to the internal jugular vein and down to the atrium. It is used to treat hydrocephalus. **Wangensteen d.** An obsolete method of drainage through an indwelling gastric or duodenal tube, produced by gentle continuous negative pressure created by a siphon.

**drain-tube** *Incorrect* VENTILATION TUBE. • The intention is not to drain the secretions but to ventilate the middle ear.

**dram** \dram\ [L *drachma,* from Gk *drachmē* a coin, an Attic unit of weight, related to *dragma* a handful] **1** An apothecaries' unit of mass or weight equal to 60 grains; 3.887 93 grams. **2** An avoirdupois unit of mass or weight equal to 1/16 ounce; 1.771 85 gram. Symbol: dr Also *apothecaries' dram.* Also *drachm* (British spelling). Symbol: dram **fluid d.** **1** A unit of capacity equal to 1/1024 (US) gallon; 1/8 (US) fluid ounce; 3.696 69 milliliters. Also *liquid dram.* Symbol: fl dr, liq dr **2** FLUID DRACHM.

**drapes** Sterilized sheets, commonly of waterproofed paper or linen, that are used to establish a sterile field at the site of an operative incision.

**draught** *Brit.* DRAFT.

**dream** [Old Norse *draumr* dream, assimilated in form to Old English *drēam* joy, music, noise] Images and/or thoughts mediated by the mind during sleep and often mimicking perception in the wakeful state. Dreams are experienced normally by humans and other animals. In a psychoanalytic framework, dreams consist of both manifest content and latent content. **wet d.** NOCTURNAL EMISSION.

**drepanocyte** \drep'ənōsīt'\ [Gk *drepan(ē)* a sickle + -CYTE] SICKLE CELL.

**Dresbach** [Melvin *Dresbach,* U.S. physician, 1874–1946] **1** Dresbach's anemia. See under SICKLE CELL ANEMIA. **2** Dresbach syndrome. See under HEREDITARY ELLIPTOCYTOSIS.

**dressing** An artificial wound cover; a bandage. See also entries under BANDAGE and GAUZE. **adhesive absorbent d.** A self-contained bandage with an absorbent gauze center and an adhesive coated cloth or plastic periphery. Also *adhesive bandage.* **biologic d.** A wound covering derived from living tissue, usually human skin, pig skin, or amnion. If such dressings adhere, they protect the wound from dessication and infection. **bolus d.** TIE-OVER DRESSING. **cement d.** **1** A temporary restoration in a tooth. **2** A protective cover for a wound after a surgical operation particularly after periodontal surgery. **cocoon d.** A piece of gauze affixed to the skin around a wound with an adhesive material such as collodion. The raised central portion gives the dressing the appearance of an insect's cocoon. **cross d.** TRANSVESTISM. **fixed d.** A plaster of Paris–impregnated dressing used for immobilization. **Lister's d.** A dressing made of gauze saturated with carbolic acid. It was the first antiseptic dressing used to pack open wounds. **occlusive d.** A dressing, generally bulky, designed to keep a wound from being exposed to air. **pressure d.** A dressing which exerts continuous pressure on the underlying tissues, usually to collapse empty spaces in which serum or blood might otherwise collect. The pressure is applied either by a bandage wrapped tightly around a part of the body or by elastic adhesive tape securely anchored to adjacent areas. **stent d.** A tie-over dressing in which the principal material is a thermoplastic dental wax made to conform accurately to the surface to be dressed. It is a thick, pliable material which becomes rigid when dry. It is typically used during the immediate postoperative period. Also *Stent's mass.* **tie-over d.** A dressing which is held in place by putting sutures with long ends in the tissues all around the dressing and then tying the long ends over the dressing. Also *bolus dressing.* **wet-to-dry d.** A moistened coarse gauze dressing applied to a wound and allowed to dry over several hours. Wound debris sticks to the dressing, and when the dressing is removed the wound is débrided. Such treatment is effective but painful.

**Dressler** [William *Dressler,* Polish-born U.S. physician, 1890–1969] Dressler syndrome. See under POST-MYOCARDIAL INFARCTION SYNDROME.

**Dreyer** [Georges *Dreyer,* English pathologist, 1873–1934] See under TEST.

**DRG** diagnosis-related group.

**drift** A gradual movement, as of a structure from an original or normal position, produced by environmental circumstances and often having the appearance of random movement. **antigenic d.** 1 The emergence of serologically novel strains of microbes or viruses to which the host population is not immune. 2 The lesser form of antigenic variation in influenza viruses, believed to be due to mutations, as distinguished from antigenic shift. **genetic d.** Any fluctuation in gene frequency in a given population due to random variation from generation to generation, randomly fluctuating selection pressures, or sampling error. The effects of genetic drift are more prominent the smaller the population studied and may lead to fixation or extinction of alleles regardless of an allele's adaptive value. Also *Sewall Wright effect, random genetic drift.* **mesial d.** The physiologic movement of teeth mesially that compensates for the loss of enamel caused by proximal abrasion. **radial d.** Deviation of the fingers to the radial (thumb) side of the hand, usually due to a chronic arthritis such as rheumatoid arthritis. **ulnar d.** Deviation of the fingers to the ulnar (little finger) side of the hand associated with chronic arthritis at the metacarpophalangeal joint. This is a characteristic deformity of rheumatoid arthritis.

**drifting** The slow horizontal movement of teeth within the bone. Bone is resorbed on the side toward which the tooth is drifting and is laid down on the opposite side. Drifting may be physiologic, as in mesial drift, or pathologic, when it is associated with periodontal pocketing. Also *tooth migration.*

**drill** An instrument for boring into or through bone or other hard substances. **cannulated d.** A drill containing a hole through its center. The hole is used to guide the drill over a trocar. **mirror d.** Practice in the voluntary suppression of facial tics in front of a mirror.

**drinker** / **problem d.** The drinker whose use of alcohol is undisciplined or inappropriate in regard to amount, time, occasion, locale, or behavioral effects. Any dependence on alcohol in this case is of a psychologic, rather than physiologic, nature. There is neither loss of control nor signs of progression to physiologic dependence, but alcohol is used to relieve body or mental pain and distress.

**drinking** / **binge d.** PERIODIC DRINKING BOUTS. **episodic excessive d.** Alcoholism, as defined in DSM-II, characterized by episodes of intoxication, with clearcut alteration in behavior or impairment of coordination or speech, occurring at least four times a year. **habitual excessive d.** Alcoholism, as defined in DSM-II, characterized by more than 12 episodes of intoxication a year. **periodic d.** PERIODIC DRINKING BOUTS.

**drip** / **intravenous d.** The slow instillation of fluid into a vein. Also *drip phleboclysis, slow phleboclysis.* **postnasal d.** The sensation or sometimes the objective evidence of secretions or inflammatory products dripping or running from the nasopharynx into the oropharynx.

**drive** An aroused condition of the organism based on the physiologic changes associated with either tissue needs, or of noxious stimulation, giving rise to behaviors that are directed toward the elimination of these conditions by removing the tissue need, or the source of noxious stimulation. Drive impels the subject into activity that will reduce the tension and restore the organism to its preexisting level of equilibrium or homeostasis. In the dual instinct theory of psychoanalysis, two drives are distinguished, the sexual or erotic and the aggressive or destructive. **acquired d.** A drive that is not innate for the species but results from experience or learning. Examples include drug addiction and the social motivation of "saving face." *Imprecise.* Also *learned drive, secondary drive.* **exploratory d.** The curiosity or stimulus-seeking drive hypothesized to account for those activities, manipulations, and locomotions of an organism which appear to derive not from any physiologic need but to be based rather in the need of the organism to investigate and to orient itself in respect to novel aspects of its environment. **learned d.** ACQUIRED DRIVE. **meiotic d.** Any process that results in a violation of Mendel's second law, with certain genes represented disproportionately in progeny independent of selective effects on individual alleles. It is often due to chromosome aberrations that interfere with normal meiosis and cause nonrandom assortment. **secondary d.** ACQUIRED DRIVE.

**driving** A phenomenon seen in the electroencephalogram in which cortical rhythms are seen to follow the frequency of a rhythmic and repetitive sensory stimulus. See also FOLLOWING.

**dRNA** DNA-like RNA.

**dromic** \drō′mik\ [back-formation from ANTIDROMIC] Pertaining to nerve impulses that course in a normal direction, such as from dendrite to cell body or from the cell body down the axon or from receptor to cell body.

**dromo-** \dräm′ō-\ [Gk *dromos* a course, a running] A combining form meaning a running or flow.

**dromograph** \dräm′ōgraf\ [DROMO- + -GRAPH] An instrument for measuring the speed of blood flow.

**dromostanolone propionate** $C_{23}H_{36}O_3$. 2α-Methyl-17β-(1-oxopropoxy)-5α-androstan-3-one, an anabolic, androgenic steroid that is used as an antineoplastic agent to provide symptomatic relief in cases of advanced metastatic breast cancer. It is given intramuscularly. Also *drostanolone propionate.*

**drop** [Old English *dropa,* akin to *drēopan* to drip] **1** A spherical globule of liquid that falls from a pipet or other similar dispenser when it discharges a minute mass of fluid. **2** The state of falling or dangling, as a structural member lacking tonus. **ankle d.** FOOTDROP. **capsular d.** A collection of hyalin in droplet form in the glomerular capsule, once thought to be specific for diabetic glomerulosclerosis but subsequently recognized occasionally in a variety of other glomerular lesions. **enamel d.** ENAMEL PEARL. **hanging d.** A drop of liquid held by surface tension to the undersurface of a slide or cover glass. It is used in microscopic examination of microorganisms. Also *hanging drop technique.* **lid d.** PTOSIS. **steel d.'s** Astyptic and astringent solution consisting of a 15% w/v ferric chloride and 22–24% w/v ethanol solution. **wrist d.** WRISTDROP.

**droperidol** $C_{22}H_{22}FN_3O_2$. 1-[1-[3-(4-Fluorobenzoyl)-propyl]-1,2,3,6-tetrahydro-4-pyridyl]-2-benzimidazolinone, a tranquilizing agent that is used for its antianxiety, sedative, and antiemetic effects prior to surgery. Its properties are similar to those of haloperidol. It is given orally or by intravenous or intramuscular injection.

**droplet** A liquid particle of very small mass capable of remaining in suspension in a gas. **Flügge's d.'s** The small droplets emitted during loud or forcible speaking and which may result in transmission of airborne infections. **hyaline d.** A refractile, acidophilic droplet, PAS-positive and silver methenamine positive, which may vary from less than a micron to several microns in diameter. One type contains lipofuscin, another protein. **lipid d.** A droplet composed of lipid in cell cytoplasm, often a renal tubular cell. By light microscopy, lipid droplets appear as vacuoles in paraffin-embedded sections, and by electron microscopy as droplets composed of black or gray osmiophilic material surrounded by a single membrane. Lipid droplets may result from absorption of excess lipids or from defective metabolism of lipids. **protein d.** A hyaline droplet composed of protein, located mainly in the proximal tubule cells, resulting from absorption from the tubular fluid of protein in amounts greater than that metabolizable by the tubule cells. By electron microscopy, protein droplets are homogeneous, electron-dense, and surrounded by a single membrane.

**dropper** A pipet or tube having a constricted tip and fitted with a bulb to dispense liquid medications as drops.

**drop phalangette** \fal′ənjet′\ A permanently flexed position of a distal phalanx of finger or toe, such as may occur in mallet finger.

**dropsy** \dräp′sē\ [Middle English *dropesie,* short for *ydropesie,* from L *hydropisis,* also *hydrops* (from Gk *hydrōps* dropsy, from *hydōr* water) dropsy] Edema or effusion. *Older term.* **abdominal d.** ASCITES. **d. of amnion** HYDRAMNIOS. **articular d.** HYDRARTHROSIS. **cardiac d.** Severe edema secondary to heart failure; cardiac edema. **d. of chest** HYDROTHORAX. **epidemic d.** A sudden onset of serous fluid formation in tissue spaces and serous cavities, especially prevalent in rice-eating populations. It is apparently caused by eating mustard oil, which contains argemone oil derived from *Argemone mexicana,* the prickly poppy, a contaminant of the mustard crop. It resembles wet beriberi, but there is no paralysis or anesthesia. There may be fever and generalized aching with an exanthem on the face, trunk, and limbs. Nodular eruptions and acute glaucoma are other manifestations. **famine d.** NUTRITIONAL EDEMA. **lymphatic d.** Edema occurring as the result of obstruction of lymphatic channels. *Obs.* **nutritional d.** NUTRITIONAL EDEMA. **d. of pericardium** PERICARDIAL EFFUSION. **peritoneal d.** ASCITES. **salpingian d.** HYDROSALPINX. **tubal d.** HYDROSALPINX. **wet d.** **1** WET BERIBERI. **2** NUTRITIONAL EDEMA.

**drostanolone propionate** DROMOSTANOLONE PROPIONATE.

**drowning** [English *drown,* from Middle English *drounen,* akin to Old Norse *drukna* to drown, and to Old English *druncnian* to become drunk, be drowned; + -ING] Death by asphyxiation resulting from aspiration of liquid into the respiratory tract, usually though not always due to submersion in water. **freshwater d.** Death resulting from aspiration of hypo-osmolar water. Large shifts of fluid and electrolytes may occur, resulting in hemodilution, hemolysis, circulatory overload, and hyponatremia. **saltwater d.** Death resulting from aspiration of hyperosmolar water. Large shifts of fluid and electrolytes may occur, resulting in hemoconcentration, pulmonary edema, hypernatremia, and heart failure. **secondary d.** Death of a victim who initially survived drowning that occurs as a result of the delayed effects of liquid aspiration on the lungs.

**drug** [Old French *drogue* (from an uncertain Teutonic root) a drug] **1** A medicinal chemical compound that is used for the treatment of diseases, for the prevention of pathologic states, or for the diagnosis of disease conditions in man and animals. **2** Any nonfood substance that is taken or administered in relatively small amounts to alter or control the subject's physical, mental, or emotional state. **3** To administer a drug, especially a narcotic, to (a subject). • Used in this sense, the term can imply excessive dosages that cause harm to the subject. **antagonistic d.** A drug that counteracts, neutralizes, or acts in the opposite way as another drug. **controlled d.** A drug whose distribution is regulated and monitored under governmental requirements. **crude d.** An unrefined, natural source of a therapeutic substance. **ethical d.** PRESCRIPTION DRUG. **investigational new d.** The designation for a new drug that is under study in the first clinical patients for its effects under carefully controlled conditions. Approval for such studies is obtained from the Food and Drug Administration, Bureau of Drugs, after a review of earlier, preclinical, animal studies. Proof of efficacy and safety is required to advance to new drug status. Abbr. IND **over-the-counter d.** A pharmaceutical which does not require a prescription to obtain, as determined by governmental authorities in each country. **prescription d.** A pharmaceutical which requires physician or other health-care provider approval to purchase and which must be obtained from a pharmacy or other authorized location. Governmental authorities determine who can prescribe drugs and where they may be sold. Also *ethical drug.* **proprietary d.** A drug or other medicinal agent protected by patent from being copied or produced by any party, except with the authorization of the patent holder.

**drug-fast** *Outmoded* DRUG-RESISTANT.

**druggist** One who prepares and dispenses drugs; pharmacist.

**drug-resistant** \-risis′tənt\ Able to grow in the presence of a concentration of an antimicrobial agent that inhibits or kills other related organisms. The term is used of mutants isolated in the laboratory, strains within a species found in nature, and sometimes entire species. Drug resistance may be due either to chromosomal mutations that alter the accessibility or the structure or amount of the component with which the drug interacts, or to added genes that code for an inactivating enzyme. Also *drug-fast* (outmoded).

**drum** [Dutch *trom* drum] MEMBRANA TYMPANI. **Bárány d.** A striped drum which can be rotated and used to induce optokinetic nystagmus. **blue d.** The appearance of the tympanic membrane in some cases of cholesterol granuloma. The brownish oily exudate present in the middle ear makes the tympanic membrane look as if it were slate blue.

**drumhead** MEMBRANA TYMPANI.

**drumstick** DRUMSTICK APPENDAGE.

**drunkenness** The state of being drunk; acute alcoholism. Also *ebriety.* **sleep d.** A condition in which there is a prolonged transition period from sleep to wakefulness characterized by confusion and, sometimes, irrational, impulsive, or even violent behavior. It seems to occur only in male adults.

**drusen** \droo′zən\ [German, pl. of *Druse* a druse, geode] **1** Multiple hyaline excrescences deposited upon the lamina vitrea of the ocular fundus as a result of degenerative changes. **2** Gliotic nodules occurring within the optic disk, sometimes a manifestation of tuberous sclerosis, but sometimes of no clinical significance and resulting in the appearance of pseudopapilledema. **giant d. of macula** DOYNE HONEYCOMB DEGENERATION OF RETINA.

**DS** desynchronized sleep.

**D.Sc.** Doctor of Science.

**dsDNA** double-stranded DNA.
**DSM-I** Diagnostic and Statistical Manual of Mental Disorders, 1st edition, 1952, authorized by the American Psychiatric Association.
**DSM-II** Diagnostic and Statistical Manual of Mental Disorders, 2nd edition, 1968 revision.
**DSM-III** Diagnostic and Statistical Manual of Mental Disorders, 3rd edition, 1980 revision. DSM-III conforms in general with ICD-9-CM, the 9th edition of the International Classification of Diseases modified for clinical use in the United States. It often provides greater detail than is possible in the ICD and includes more recent data than were incorporated in ICD-9. In addition, it provides descriptions of disease entities with inclusion and exclusion criteria, and it employs a multiaxial classificatory system. A revised edition, DSM-III R, was published in 1987.
**DT** 1 delirium tremens. 2 duration tetany. 3 double tachycardia.
**d.t.d.** *datur talis dosis* (L, give of such a dose).
**DTP** distal tingling on percussion (Tinel sign).
**DTR** deep tendon reflex.
**DTPA** diethylenetriaminepentaacetic acid.
**dualism** \d^y^oo′alizm\ Any doctrine or theory that asserts the existence of two distinct and independent substances, principles, or constituents, such as Descartes' theory, that the human person consists of mind and body, two entities independent of and irreducibly distinct from each other.
**Duane** [Alexander *Duane*, U.S. ophthalmologist, 1858–1926] Stilling-Turk-Duane syndrome. See under DUANE SYNDROME.
**duazomycin** An antibiotic agent with antineoplastic properties, obtained from *Streptomyces ambofaciens*. It has been used in combination with other antineoplastic drugs. Also *duazomycin A*.
**duazomycin C** *Outmoded* AMBOMYCIN.
**Dubin** [Isadore Nathan *Dubin*, U.S. pathologist, born 1913] Dubin-Johnson syndrome. See under SYNDROME.
**Du Bois** [Eugene Floyd *Du Bois*, U.S. physiologist, 1882–1959] 1 Aub-Dubois standards. See under DUBOIS STANDARD. 2 See under FORMULA.
**Dubois** [Paul Antoine *Dubois*, French obstetrician, 1795–1871] See under SIGN, ABSCESS.
**DuBois-Reymond** [Emil Heinrich *DuBois-Reymond*, German physiologist, 1818–1896] See under LAW.
**Dubovitz** [Victor *Dubovitz*, South African physician, born 1931] See under SYNDROME.
**Dubreuilh** [M. W. *Dubreuilh*, French dermatologist, flourished early 20th century] Precancerous melanosis of Dubreuilh. See under HUTCHINSON'S MELANOTIC FRECKLE.
**Duchenne** [Guillaume Benjamin Amand *Duchenne*, French physician, 1806–1875] 1 See under SIGN, SYNDROME. 2 Duchenne's paralysis, Duchenne-Erb paralysis, Erb-Duchenne paralysis. See under DUCHENNE-ERB SYNDROME. 3 Duchenne's paralysis, Duchenne's myopathy, Duchenne's progressive muscular dystrophy, Duchenne's disease. See under DUCHENNE TYPE MUSCULAR DYSTROPHY. 4 Duchenne syndrome, Aran-Duchenne disease. See under PROGRESSIVE MUSCULAR ATROPHY. 5 Duchenne syndrome. See under PROGRESSIVE BULBAR PALSY. 6 Aran-Duchenne amyotrophy, Aran-Duchenne muscular atrophy. See under PROGRESSIVE MUSCULAR ATROPHY. 7 Duchenne-Landouzy dystrophy. See under FACIOSCAPULOHUMERAL MUSCULAR DYSTROPHY. 8 Duchenne's disease. See under MOTOR NEURON DISEASE. 9 Duchenne's disease. See under TABES DORSALIS.
**Ducrey** [Augusto *Ducrey*, Italian dermatologist, 1860–1940] Ducrey's bacillus. See under *HAEMOPHILUS DUCREYI*.

# duct

**duct** [L *ductus* (from *ductus*, past part. of *ducere* to lead) a leading, drawing out, a line] DUCTUS. **aberrant d.'s** DUCTULI ABERRANTES. **accessory bile d.'s** 1 Minute aberrant ducts occasionally present in the triangular ligaments of the liver. Also *aberrant bile ducts*. 2 Aberrant segmental or area ducts which have an extrahepatic course. They usually drain the right half of the liver and terminate in a hepatic duct or in the gallbladder. Also *accessory hepatic ducts*. **accessory pancreatic d.** DUCTUS PANCREATICUS ACCESSORIUS. **adipose d.** SEBACEOUS DUCT. **allantoic d.** ALLANTOIC STALK. **alveolar d.'s** DUCTULI ALVEOLARES. **amniotic d.** A short diverticulum extending from the human amniotic cavity into a stalk of mesoderm which connects the amnion to the trophoblast. **anterior semicircular d.** DUCTUS SEMICIRCULARIS ANTERIOR. **d. of Arantius** DUCTUS VENOSUS. **Bartholin's d.** DUCTUS SUBLINGUALIS MAJOR. **Bellini's d.** 1 DUCTUS PAPILLARIS. 2 TUBULUS COLLIGENS RECTUS. **Bernard's d.** DUCTUS PANCREATICUS ACCESSORIUS. **bile d.** 1 Any duct carrying bile within and from the liver to the duodenum. Also *biliary duct*. 2 *Popular* DUCTUS CHOLEDOCHUS. **biliary d.** 1 BILE DUCT. 2 One of the ductuli biliferi. Also *biliferous duct*. **cervical d.** A passage leading from the exterior of the embryo into the transient cervical sinus. **choledochous d.** DUCTUS CHOLEDOCHUS. **cochlear d.** DUCTUS COCHLEARIS. **collecting d.** TUBULUS RENALIS COLLIGENS. **common bile d.** DUCTUS CHOLEDOCHUS. **common hepatic d.** DUCTUS HEPATICUS COMMUNIS. **common pharyngobranchial d.** The inner portion of the fourth pharyngeal pouch, which provides a common passage for the lateral portion of the fourth and the fifth pouch. **cowperian d.** DUCTUS GLANDULAE BULBOURETHRALIS. **craniopharyngeal d.** A duct which temporarily connects the adenohypophysis, following its differentiation from the distal end of the craniopharyngeal pouch (Rathke's pouch), to the stomatodeum. The duct subsequently becomes obliterated and disappears. **d. of Cuvier** COMMON CARDINAL VEIN. **cystic d.** DUCTUS CYSTICUS. **deferent d.** DUCTUS DEFERENS. **dorsal pancreatic d.** A duct of the embryonic dorsal pancreatic outgrowth or bud which will eventually drain the tail, body, and upper part of the head of the pancreas. **efferent d.** A duct that carries secretions away from a gland. **efferent d.'s of testis** DUCTULI EFFERENTES TESTIS. **ejaculatory d.** DUCTUS EJACULATORIUS. **endolymphatic d.** DUCTUS ENDOLYMPHATICUS. **d. of epididymis** DUCTUS EPIDIDYMIDIS. **epigenital d.'s** The five to twelve excretory tubules in the gonadal region of the male embryo, situated at the cranial pole and which persist after the regression of the mesonephros. The two first become isolated to constitute the ductuli aberrantes superiores. The others retain connection with the rete testis to form the vasa efferentia of the testis. Also *collecting tubules of the mesonephros*. **d. of epoöphoron** LONGITUDINAL DUCT OF EPOÖPHORON. **excretory d.'s** DUCTUS EXCRETORIUS. **excretory d. of bulbourethral gland** DUCTUS GLANDULAE BULBOURETHRALIS. **excretory d.'s of lacrimal gland** DUCTULI EXCRETORII GLANDULAE LACRIMALIS. **excretory d. of seminal vesicle** DUCTUS EXCRETORIUS VESICULAE SEMINALIS. **excretory d. of testis** DUCTUS DEFERENS. **extrahepatic bile d.'s** Excretory ducts that convey bile from the liver to the duodenum, including the right and left hepatic ducts, the common hepatic duct, the cystic duct, and the common bile duct. **frontonasal d.** The mucosa-lined bony channel draining the frontal sinus into the anterior end of either the middle nasal meatus of the infundibulum ethmoidale. Also *nasofrontal duct, infundibulum of frontal sinus.* **d. of gallbladder** DUCTUS CYSTICUS. **Gartner's d.** LONGITUDINAL DUCT OF EPOÖPHORON. **genital d.** GENITAL CANAL. **Hensen's d.** DUCTUS REUNIENS. **hepaticopancreatic d.** DUCTUS PANCREATICUS. **incisive d.** A duct in the hard palate between the primitive palate and the lateral palatine shelves from the maxillary processes. In man the duct becomes covered by mucous membrane, but in many mammals it remains open as an incisive canal. **intercalated d.** A thin branched tubule connected by either simple apposition or intercellular canaliculi to the secretory acini of a gland, such as a salivary gland. Several of such initial ducts drain into an intralobular duct. Also *intercalary duct.* **interlobar d.** A duct that drains two or more lobes of a gland or organ. **interlobular d.** 1 A duct formed by the union of two or more intralobular ducts. It unites with others to drain the lobules of a gland or an organ. 2 DUCTUS INTERLOBULARIS BILIFER. **interlobular bile d.** DUCTUS INTERLOBULARIS BILIFER. **lacrimal d.** A fine, angulated canal in each eyelid that commences at the punctum on the edge of the eyelid and runs medially to end in the lacrimal sac at the upper end of the nasolacrimal duct; canaliculus lacrimalis. **lacrimonasal d.** DUCTUS NASOLACRIMALIS. **lactiferous d.'s** DUCTUS LACTIFERI. **lateral semicircular d.** DUCTUS SEMICIRCULARIS LATERALIS. **left d. of caudate lobe** DUCTUS LOBI CAUDATI SINISTER. **left hepatic d.** DUCTUS HEPATICUS SINISTER. **left lymphatic d.** DUCTUS THORACICUS. **longitudinal d. of epoöphoron** A rudiment of the mesonephric duct which extends medially in the broad ligament of the uterus almost parallel to the outer part of the uterine tube. It may extend farther alongside the uterus to the level of the internal os, enter the uterine muscle and descend into the cervix uteri from where it continues downward in the lateral vaginal wall and ends near the hymen. Cysts may develop at any part of its course, particularly at the cranial end, as a cystic vesicular appendage. Also *duct of epoöphoron, Gartner's duct, ductus epoophori longitudinalis.* **Luschka's d.'s** LUSCHKA'S CRYPTS. **lymphatic d.'s** 1 Ductus lymphaticus dexter and ductus thoracicus. 2 VASA LYMPHATICA. **major sublingual d.** DUCTUS SUBLINGUALIS MAJOR. **mammary d.'s** DUCTUS LACTIFERI. **mesonephric d.** An embryonic duct which communicates between the pronephros and the cloaca. It is formed in association with rudiments of the pronephric kidney which are taken over to form the excretory duct by the mesonephros. It develops into various ducts of the reproductive system in the male, being represented by the epididymis, the vas deferens and the common ejaculatory duct, and into vestigial structures in the female. Also *wolffian duct.* **metanephric d.** The duct formed by the elongating stalk of the ureteric bud, or metanephric diverticulum, that grows out from the mesonephric duct towards the metanephrogenic mass of the embryo. The cephalic end of the duct develops into the renal pelvis, while the caudal end forms the ureter. **milk d.'s** DUCTUS LACTIFERI. **minor sublingual d.'s** DUCTUS SUBLINGUALES MINORES. **müllerian d.** PARAMESONEPHRIC DUCT. **nasal d.** DUCTUS NASOLACRIMALIS. **nasofrontal d.** FRONTONASAL DUCT. **nasolacrimal d.** DUCTUS NASOLACRIMALIS. **nephric d.** 1 PRONEPHRIC DUCT. 2 *Outmoded* URETER **ovarian d.** TUBA UTERINA. **pancreatic d.** DUCTUS PANCREATICUS. **papillary d.** 1 DUCTUS PAPILLARIS. 2 One of Bellini's tubules. **paragenital d.'s** Excretory tubules of the caudal region of the male embryo persisting after the regression of the mesonephros and which form the massa innominata or paradidymis. **paramesonephric d.** Either of a pair of ducts which first appear in embryos of about 10 mm crown-rump length as an invagination of the coelomic epithelium into the mesenchyme. In the male the greater part of each duct retrogresses early in embryonic life. In female mammals these ducts become specialized, the cranial parts become the uterine tubes, the intermediate parts fuse to a varying degree to form the uterus, while the caudal portions unite and contribute to the development of the upper part of the vagina. Also *müllerian duct.* **paraurethral d.'s** DUCTUS PARAURETHRALES. **parotid d.** DUCTUS PAROTIDEUS. **d. of Pecquet** DUCTUS THORACICUS. **perilymphatic d.** AQUEDUCTUS COCHLEAE. **periotic d.** AQUEDUCTUS COCHLEAE. **persistent craniopharyngeal d.** The remnant in postnatal life of the craniopharyngeal pouch along the embryonic course of its growth from the pharynx to the hypothalamus. The duct may persist in part as a cyst, a strand of glandular tissue, or a column of connective tissue between the nasopharynx and the anterior lobe of the pituitary gland. **persistent mesonephric d.** A congenital retention of all or parts of the embryonic mesonephric duct, occurring in females. Isolated segments may form retention cysts. In the male the mesonephric duct becomes the vas deferens. **persistent omphalomesenteric d.** Any postnatal residual remnant of the embryonic omphalomesenteric duct, or yolk stalk, between the ileum and the umbilicus. It may take the form in part of a patent duct lined with epithelium, a ligamentous strand, or a ligamentous strand containing one or more cysts. **persistent thyroglossal d.** Any postnatal residual remnant of the embryonic thyroglossal duct or thyroid diverticulum between the isthmus of the thyroid gland and the cecal foramen at the base of the tongue. Such a duct often consists in part of discrete nodules of thyroid tissue dispersed at intervals in a fibrous strand between the base of the tongue and the thyroid. **posterior semicircular d.** DUCTUS SEMICIRCULARIS POSTERIOR. **primary genital d.'s** The mesonephric and paramesonephric ducts. **pronephric d.** A longitudinal excretory embryonic duct of the pronephros, formed by union of the ends of the segmental pronephric tubules and draining into the cloaca of lower vertebrates. It was thought to be the precursor of the mesonephric duct, but it is now considered too vestigial in human embryos. **prostatic d.'s** DUCTULI PROSTATICI. **right d. of caudate lobe** DUCTUS LOBI CAUDATI DEXTER. **right hepatic d.** DUCTUS HEPATICUS DEXTER. **right lymphatic d.** DUCTUS LYMPHATICUS DEXTER. **right thoracic d.** DUCTUS LYMPHATICUS DEXTER. **d.'s of Rivinus** DUCTUS SUBLINGUALES MINORES. **sacculoutricular d.** DUCTUS UTRICULOSACCULARIS. **salivary d.'s** 1 The excretory ducts of salivary glands in and around the mouth that convey saliva to the oral cavity. 2 SECRETORY DUCTS. **d. of Santorini** DUCTUS PANCREATICUS ACCESSORIUS. **Schüller's d.'s** DUCTUS PARAURETHRALES. **sebaceous d.** The duct that connects the sebaceous gland to the hair follicle. Also *adipose duct.* **secretory d.'s** The tubules connected to secretory acini inside the smallest lobules of salivary glands, slightly larger than intercalated ducts, and leading into intralobular ducts. They have a striated epithelium. Also *striated ducts, salivary ducts.* **segmental d.** A pronephric or mesonephric duct. **semicircular d.'s** DUCTUS SEMI-

CIRCULARES. **seminal d.'s** Ducts conveying spermatozoa and seminal fluid to the exterior, namely, ductus deferens, ductus excretorius vesiculae seminalis, and ductus ejaculatorius. **d. of seminal vesicle** DUCTUS EXCRETORIUS VESICULAE SEMINALIS. **Skene's d.'s** DUCTUS PARAURETHRALES. **spermatic d.** DUCTUS DEFERENS. **d. of Steno** DUCTUS PAROTIDEUS. **Stensen's d.** DUCTUS PAROTIDEUS. **striated d.'s** SECRETORY DUCTS. **sublingual d.'s** Ductus sublingualis major and ductus sublinguales minores. **submandibular d.** DUCTUS SUBMANDIBULARIS. **submaxillary d. of Wharton** *Outmoded* DUCTUS SUBMANDIBULARIS. **superior semicircular d.** DUCTUS SEMICIRCULARIS ANTERIOR. **sweat d.** The portion of the sweat gland that conveys sweat from the sweat gland coil to the surface. Also *ductus sudoriferus.* **tear d.'s** The lacrimal passages, including the ducts of the lacrimal gland and the nasolacrimal duct.

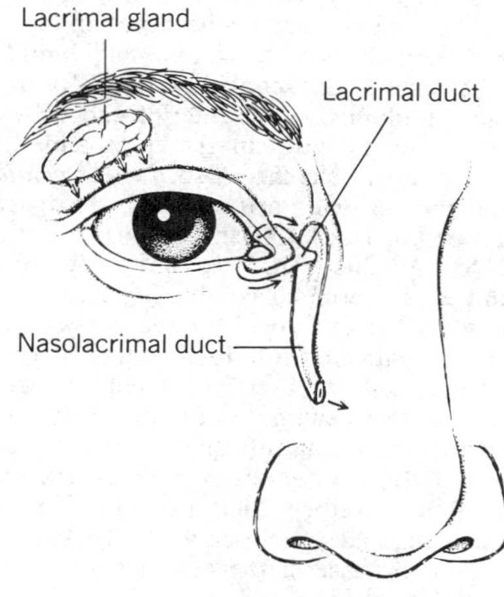


**Tear ducts**

**testicular d.** DUCTUS DEFERENS. **thoracic d.** DUCTUS THORACICUS. **thyrocervical d.** THYROPHARYNGEAL DUCT. **thyroglossal d.** A duct in the embryo extending between the thyroid gland and a small depression, the foramen cecum, on the posterior part of the tongue. In normal development it is completely reabsorbed, but it may persist in whole or in part. Fistulas and cysts may be found along the track of a persistent thyroglossal duct. **thyropharyngeal d.** A diverticulum or duct related to the fourth pharyngeal pouch in the embryo. It has been considered to provide tissue to the lateral lobe of the thyroid gland during development. Also *thyrocervical duct.* **utriculosaccular d.** DUCTUS UTRICULOSACCULARIS. **ventral pancreatic d.** A duct of the ventral pancreatic rudiment or bud which opens into the duodenum. It forms the proximal end of the definitive main pancreatic duct, and anastomoses with the dorsal pancreatic duct which contributes the distal part of the definitive duct. **vitelline d.** OMPHALOMESENTERIC CANAL. **Walther's d.'s** DUCTUS SUBLINGUALES MINORES. **Wharton's d.** DUCTUS SUBMANDIBULARIS. **d. of Wirsung** DUCTUS PANCREATICUS. **wolffian d.** MESONEPHRIC DUCT.

**ductal** \duk′təl\ Pertaining to a duct.

**ductile** \duk′til\ [L *ductilis* (from *ducere* to lead, pull, draw out) drawn along, ductile] Capable of being shaped or drawn out, as into the form of a wire: said of a substance, especially certain metals.

**ductility** \duktil′itē\ The property of being ductile.

**duction** \duk′shən\ [L *ductio* (from *ducere* to lead, convey, pull) conveyance, pulling] The movement of one eye in any direction, including abduction (outward), adduction (inward), supraduction (upward), or infraduction (downward). Compare VERGENCE.

**ductless** \dukt′lis\ Lacking an excretory duct: said of the endocrine glands (the glands of internal secretion) whose products are secreted directly into the bloodstream.

**ductular** \duk′tyələr\ Pertaining to a ductule.

**ductule** \dukt′yool\ DUCTULUS. **aberrant d.'s** DUCTULI ABERRANTES. **alveolar d.'s** DUCTULI ALVEOLARES. **biliary d.** **1** DUCTULUS BILIFER. **2** Any of the small ducts draining segments of the lobes of the liver. **cranial aberrant d.** DUCTULUS ABERRANS SUPERIOR. **efferent d.'s of testis** DUCTULI EFFERENTES TESTIS. **excretory d.'s of lacrimal gland** DUCTULI EXCRETORII GLANDULAE LACRIMALIS. **Haller's aberrant d.** DUCTULUS ABERRANS INFERIOR. **inferior aberrant d.** DUCTULUS ABERRANS INFERIOR. **d.'s of prostate gland** DUCTULI PROSTATICI. **superior aberrant d.** DUCTULUS ABERRANS SUPERIOR. **transverse d.'s of epoöphoron** Ten to fifteen short tubules, remnants of the tubules of the mesonephros, in the lateral part of the mesosalpinx, ending blindly towards the ovary while their other ends enter the longitudinal duct of the epoophoron. Also *ductuli transversi epoophori.*

**ductuli** \duk′tyəlī\ Plural of DUCTULUS.

**ductulus** \duk′tyələs\ [L (dim. of *ductus*; see DUCTUS) a small duct] **1** A very small duct. **2** One of the smallest initial branches of a duct that are either in contact with the acini of a gland or in an organ; tubule. For defs. 1 and 2 also *ductule.* **d. aberrans inferior** [NA] A coiled, blind tubule often connected to the inferior part of the ductus epididymidis or to the beginning of the ductus deferens. It is sometimes dilated distally, and occasionally not connected. Also *inferior aberrant ductule, caudal aberrant ductule, Haller's aberrant ductule.* **d. aberrans superior** **1** [NA] A long, blind tubule in the head of the epididymis, connected to the rete testis. **2** One, or sometimes more, of the most cranial tubules of the mesonephros, remaining as a blindly ending vestige in the adult epididymis. For defs. 1 and 2 also *superior aberrant ductule, cranial aberrant ductule, vasculum aberrans* (outmoded), *vas aberrans* (outmoded). **ductuli aberrantes** [NA] Embryonic mesonephric tubules that persist into adult life as blind epithelial tubules, the most cranial one or two forming the ductulus aberrans superior connected to the head of epididymis and rete testis, and a caudal tubule persisting as the ductulus aberrans inferior related to the tail of epididymis. Also *aberrant ductules, aberrant ducts.* **ductuli alveolares** [NA] Several tortuous, thin-walled tubes that extend from each respiratory bronchiole and then branch into the expanded atria leading into the alveolar saccules or sacs. Pulmonary alveoli pouch out sideways from the walls. Also *alveolar ducts, alveolar ductules.* **d. bilifer** Any of the smallest branches of the bile ducts, which are situated at the periphery of the hepatic lobules and connect the bile canaliculi with interlobular bile ducts. Also *biliary ductule, biliary canal.* **ductuli efferentes testis** [NA] Up to twenty tubules continuing from the rete testis at the superior part of the mediastinum testis and piercing the tunica albuginea testis to enter the head of the epididymis, where they end in the lobules. Also *efferent ductules of testis, efferent ducts of testis.* **ductuli excretorii glandulae lacrimalis** [NA] The excretory ducts of the lacrimal gland that open into the superior fornix of the conjunctival sac. Also *ductus lacrimales, excretory ductules of lacrimal gland, excretory ducts of lacrimal gland.* **ductuli prostatici** [NA] Ten to thirty excretory ducts draining the glandular substance of the prostate gland and ending in the floor of the prostatic sinus on each side of the urethral crest in the prostatic part of the urethra. Also *ductules of prostate gland, ductus prostatici, prostatic ducts.* **ductuli transversi epoophori** TRANSVERSE DUCTULES OF EPOÖPHORON.

**ductus** \duk′təs\ [L (from *ductus,* past part. of *ducere* to lead, conduct, convey, akin to English *tow*) conveyance, pulling, drawing out, a line] (*pl.* ductus) A tubular channel for conducting excretions, secretions, or any other fluid. Also *duct.* **d. aberrans** Either ductulus aberrans superior or ductulus aberrans inferior. **d. arteriosus** A canal derived in the embryo from part of the left sixth aortic arch artery, which is a continuation of the origin of the terminal branches of the pulmonary trunk. It anastomoses with the lower end of the arch of the aorta below the origin of the left subclavian artery (at the level of the aortic isthmus). In the fetus up until birth it drains the major part of the pulmonary output directly into the aorta. It normally closes down after birth, then atrophies over the next few weeks to form the fibrous ligamentum arteriosum. When it remains patent after birth it gives rise to a not uncommon clinical condition, patent or persistent ductus arteriosus. **d. arteriosus bilateralis** A persistence of both embryonic sixth aortic arches connecting the ventral and dorsal aortae in the embryo and the left ventricle descending aorta of the fetus and newborn. If both remain patent beyond early infancy, the trachea and esophagus may be constricted within a vascular ring. Also *double ductus arteriosus.* **d. choledochus** [NA] The large duct formed just below the porta hepatis by the union of the common hepatic and cystic ducts. Also *choledochous duct, common bile duct, choledochus, bile duct* (popular). **d. cochlearis** [NA] A triangular membranous duct winding within the outer wall of the two and three-quarter turns of the bony cochlea of the internal ear, its basal end connecting with the saccule by the ductus reuniens and its upper end reaching the apex of the cochlea, where it ends blindly at the cecum cupulare. Its posterior wall is the basilar membrane stretching between the osseous spiral lamina and the spiral ligament and separating the duct from the scala tympani. The anterior wall is the vestibular membrane separating the duct from the scala vestibuli, and the outer wall is the thickened endosteum lining the bony canal. The highly specialized cellular organ of hearing, the spiral organ, rests on the basilar membrane that conveys the peripheral processes of the ganglion cells of the cochlear nerve to the organ. It contains endolymph. Also *cochlear duct, membranous cochlea, scala media, Löwenberg's canal.* **d. cysticus** [NA] The short duct that extends from the neck of the gallbladder to its junction with the common hepatic duct to form the common bile duct at a variable distance from the porta hepatis. Also *cystic duct, duct of gallbladder.* **d. deferens** [NA] The continuation of the ductus epididymidis in the tail of the epididymis, ascending in the spermatic cord to traverse the inguinal canal and pass through the deep inguinal ring to enter the minor pelvis. It runs outside the parietal peritoneum to the posterior surface, or base, of the urinary bladder, where it crosses the ureter and turns down on the medial side of the seminal vesicle to join its duct and form the ejaculatory duct at the base of the prostate. Also *deferent duct, vas deferens* (outmoded)*, excretory duct of testis, spermatic duct, testicular duct.* **double d. arteriosus** DUCTUS ARTERIOSUS BILATERALIS. **d. ejaculatorius** [NA] A duct formed between the base of the urinary bladder and the base of the prostate by the union of the ductus deferens and the duct of the seminal vesicle. It passes anteroinferiorly through the prostate and along the side of the prostatic utricle to end on the colliculus seminalis on or within the slitlike orifice of the prostatic utricle. Also *ejaculatory duct.* **d. endolymphaticus** [NA] A membranous tube arising from the posterior part of the saccule and joined by the ductus utriculosaccularis before passing inferomedially along the aqueduct of the vestibule to end as a blind sac, saccus endolymphaticus, under the dura mater on the posterior surface of the petrous part of the temporal bone. Also *endolymphatic duct, aqueduct of vestibule.* **d. epididymidis** [NA] A fine tube commencing in the caput epididymidis and receiving the efferent ducts of the lobuli epididymidis posteriorly. It then becomes highly convoluted and forms the body and tail of the epididymis, at the inferior end of which it becomes uncoiled, and increases in thickness and diameter to continue as the ductus deferens. Also *duct of epididymis, canal of epididymis.* **d. epoophori longitudinalis** [NA] LONGITUDINAL DUCT OF EPOÖPHORON. **d. excretorius** [NA] A duct that is lined by nonsecretory epithelium and is the terminal conducting passage of a complex exocrine gland. It is formed by successive unions of intralobular, interlobular, and interlobar ducts. It conducts the secretion of gland cells to a free external or internal body surface. The duct epithelium varies and may occasionally modify the nature and concentration of the secretion. Also *excretory duct.* **d. excretorius vesiculae seminalis** [NA] The straight excretory duct that leaves the lower medial end of each seminal vesicle between the base of the urinary bladder and the base of the prostate to join the ductus deferens on its lateral side and form the ejaculatory duct. Also *excretory duct of seminal vesicle, duct of seminal vesicle.* **d. glandulae bulbourethralis** [NA] The long, thin duct of each bulbourethral gland that extends anteriorly outside the mucous membrane of the membranous part of the urethra and pierces the perineal membrane to traverse the bulb of the corpus spongiosum penis and open on the floor of the spongy part of the urethra. Also *excretory duct of bulbourethral gland, cowperian duct.* **d. hepaticus communis** [NA] The duct formed near the right end of the porta hepatis by the union of the left and right hepatic ducts. It then runs in the lesser omentum on the right side of the hepatic artery and in front of the portal vein to join the cystic duct and form the common bile duct at a variable distance from the porta hepatis. Also *common hepatic duct.* **d. hepaticus dexter** [NA] The duct formed at the right margin of the porta hepatis by the union of the biliary ductules from the anterior and posterior segments of the right lobe of the liver. It also receives a ductule from the caudate process and the right duct of the caudate lobe. It is about 1 cm long and joins the left hepatic duct to form the common hepatic duct. Also *right hepatic duct.* **d. hepaticus sinister** [NA] The duct formed in the porta hepatis by the union of the biliary ductules from the lateral and medial segments of the left lobe of the liver and from the quadrate lobe. It also receives the left duct of the caudate lobe. It joins the right hepatic duct to form the common hepatic duct. Also *left hepatic duct.* **d. interlobularis bilifer** The bile-carrying duct that forms part of the hepatic triad in the portal canal. It is connected to both the bilecanaliculi and the ductuli biliferi. Also *interlobular duct, interlobular biliary canal, interlobular bile duct.* **d. lacrimales** DUCTULI EXCRETORII GLANDULAE LACRIMALIS. **d. lactiferi** [NA] Terminal ducts of about 20 lobes of the mammary gland that traverse the breast tissue in a radial fashion to open separately on the surface of the papilla, or nipple. Deep to the areola each duct expands into a lactiferous sinus, which then narrows again at the base of the nipple. Also *lactiferous ducts, mammary ducts, milk ducts, galactophorous tubules, lactiferous tubules.* **d. lobi caudati dexter** [NA] The bile duct that drains the right half of the caudate lobe and the caudate process of the liver and terminates in the right hepatic duct. Also *right duct of caudate lobe.* **d. lobi caudati sinister** [NA] The bile ductule draining the left half of the caudate lobe of the liver and terminating in the left hepatic duct. Also *left duct of caudate lobe.* **d. lymphaticus dexter** [NA] A short lymphatic trunk situated along the medial margin of the right scalenus anterior muscle at the root of the neck, where it ends by opening into the junction of the internal jugular and right subclavian veins. It is usually formed by the right jugular, subclavian, and bronchomediastinal lymphatic trunks, any one of which may end separately in the right brachiocephalic vein. Also *right lymphatic duct, right thoracic duct.* **d. nasolacrimalis** [NA] A membranous tube within a bony canal extending from the lower end of the lacrimal sac to the anterior part of the inferior nasal meatus, where it opens. It is surrounded by an extensive venous plexus that forms an erectile tissue. Also *nasolacrimal duct, lacrimonasal duct, nasal duct.* **d. pancreaticus** [NA] The main excretory duct of the pancreas which runs in the glandular substance from the tip through the body and the head, receiving ducts from the lobules en route. It ends in the wall of the descending part of the duodenum by uniting with the common bile duct to form the ampulla hepatopancreatica. Occasionally it opens separately into the duodenum. Also *pancreatic duct, canal of Wirsung, duct of Wirsung, hepaticopancreatic duct.* **d. pancreaticus accessorius** [NA] An occasional additional excretory duct that drains the lower part of the head of the pancreas and runs upwards in front and to the right of the main pancreatic duct. It terminates at the minor duodenal papilla in the descending part of the duodenum. Also *accessory pancreatic duct, duct of Santorini, Bernard's duct.* **d. papillaris** One of the wide tubes that are formed by the union of the collecting or straight tubules from the medullary rays of the renal cortex. They terminate on the apex of the renal papilla forming the area cribrosa. Also *Bellini's duct, papillary duct.* **d. paraurethrales** [NA] Ducts draining some urethral glands on each side of the lower end of the female urethra and extending through the submucosa to end in small openings on the lateral edges of the external urethral orifice. Also *paraurethral ducts, Guérin's glands, Skene's ducts, Skene's glands, paraurethral glands, Schüllers glands, paraurethral tubules, Skene's tubules.* **d. parotideus** [NA] The excretory duct of the parotid gland, commencing at the union of two main branches in the anterior portion of the gland and extending horizontally forwards over the masseter muscle. At the muscle's anterior margin it turns sharply inward through the corpus adiposum buccae to pierce the buccinator muscle and open on a papilla in the mucous membrane of the cheek opposite the upper second molar tooth. Also *parotid duct, Stensen's canal, Stensen's duct, duct of Steno.* **patent d. arteriosus** The persistence of a functional lumen in the ductus arteriosus beyond the time of its usual occlusion by fibrous tissue during the first few weeks of postnatal life. The channel is derived from the sixth aortic arch, which in fetal life conveys right ventricular blood directly to the descending aorta and thus bypasses the pulmonary circulation. Also *persistent ductus arteriosus.* **d. perilymphaticus** AQUEDUCTUS COCHLEAE. **persistent d. arteriosus** PATENT DUCTUS ARTERIOSUS. **d. prostatici** DUCTULI PROSTATICI. **d. reuniens** [NA] A narrow, short membranous duct uniting the lower end of the cochlear duct, just beyond the cecum vestibulare, to the saccule. Also *canalis reuniens, Hensen's duct, Hensen's canal.* **right-sided d. arteriosus** A persistence of the right-sided embryonic sixth aortic arch as the fetal shunt between the pulmonary trunk and the descending aorta. Usually a right-sided duct is found instead of the left duct in the presence of other malformations, notably pulmonary atresia, but there may be bilateral ducts. Also *reversed ductus arteriosus.* **d. semicirculares** [NA] The anterior, lateral, and posterior semicircular ducts of the membranous labyrinth that occupy about one fourth of the diameter of the osseous semicircular canals of the internal ear. They are arranged approximately at right angles to each other. All the ducts contain endolymph, while perilymph separates them from the osseous canals. Also *semicircular ducts, membranous semicircular canals.* **d. semicircularis anterior** [NA] The membranous duct within the bony anterior semicircular canal that lies in the vertical plane and has its ampulla at the anterolateral end. Its medial end, or crus, joins that of the posterior semicircular duct to form the crus commune, which enters the utricle. Also *anterior semicircular duct, superior semicircular duct.* **d. semicircularis lateralis** [NA] The membranous duct within the bony lateral semicircular canal which lies in the horizontal plane and has its ampulla at the anterolateral end close to that of the anterior semicircular duct and the other end, or crus, opening into the utricle. Also *lateral semicircular duct.* **d. semicircularis posterior** [NA] The membranous duct within the bony posterior semicircular canal that lies in the vertical plane and has its ampulla at its inferior end, while its medial end, or crus, joins the medial end of the anterior semicircular duct to form the crus commune, which then joins the utricle. Also *posterior semicircular duct.* **d. sublinguales minores** [NA] Many short excretory ducts of the sublingual gland that open on tiny papillae on the summit of the plica sublingualis just superior to the gland. Also *minor sublingual ducts, ducts of Rivinus, canals of Rivinus, Walther's ducts, canals of Walther.* **d. sublingualis major** [NA] A single excretory duct that receives some ducts from the anterior part of the sublingual gland and opens adjacent to the submandibular duct on the caruncula sublingualis next to the frenulum of the tongue. Also *major sublingual duct, Bartholin's duct.* **d. submandibularis** [NA] A long, thin duct draining the submandibular salivary gland and emerging from the deep part of the gland to pass through its anterior part, where it receives additional small ducts. It terminates on the summit of the caruncula sublingualis next to the frenulum of the tongue on the floor of the mouth. Also *submandibular duct, submaxillary duct of Wharton* (outmoded), *Wharton's duct.* **d. sudoriferus** SWEAT DUCT. **d. thoracicus** [NA] The large lymphatic trunk which extends upwards from the upper end of the cisterna chyli opposite the upper lumbar vertebrae through the aortic orifice of the diaphragm and anterior to the thoracic vertebrae in the posterior mediastinum until it reaches the root of the neck on the left side of the esophagus where it arches upwards, forwards and then downwards to terminate in the junction of the left internal jugular and subclavian veins. It may terminate in either vein or break into branches which open into both veins. It drains most of the lymph of the body below the diaphragm and from the left half of the body above the diaphragm. Also *thoracic duct, left lymphatic duct, duct of Pecquet, van Hoorne's canal.* **d. utriculosaccularis** [NA] A narrow, membranous canal connecting the anteromedial part of the utricle to the ductus endolymphaticus just after it leaves the saccule. Also *utriculosaccular duct, utriculosaccular canal, sacculoutricular duct, sacculoutricular canal.* **d. venosus** A venous channel which, in the fetus, connects the left branch of the portal vein with the inferior vena cava and thus allows a proportion of blood returned from the placenta (via the umbilical vein which also joins the portal vein) to bypass the liver. Shortly after birth the channel constricts and then fibroses to leave the ligamentum venosum. Also *canal of Arantius, duct of Arantius.*

**Duddell** [Benedictus *Duddell,* English oculist, flourished 18th century] Duddell's membrane. See under LAMINA LIMITANS POSTERIOR CORNEAE.

**Duguet** [Jean Baptiste *Duguet,* French physician, born 1837] Bouveret-Duguet ulcer. See under ULCER.

**Duhot** [Robert *Duhot,* Belgian urologist and dermatologist, born 1867] See under LINE.

**Dührssen** [Alfred *Dührssen,* German obstetrician and gynecologist, 1862–1933] **1** See under OPERATION. **2** Dührssen's incisions. See under INCISION.

**duipara** \doo·ip′ərə\ [L *du(o)* two + *i* + PARA] SECUNDIPARA.

**Duke** [William Waddell *Duke,* U.S. pathologist, 1883–1945] Duke's method. See under DUKE BLEEDING TIME TEST.

**Dukes** [Clement *Dukes,* English physician, 1845–1925] Dukes disease, Filatov-Dukes disease. See under EXANTHEM SUBITUM.

**Dukes** [Cuthbert Esquire *Dukes,* English pathologist, 1890–1977] See under CLASSIFICATION.

**dulcin** A non-nutritive sweetening compound, moderately soluble in water. It is about 250 times sweeter than cane sugar, but is not used clinically because it causes liver tumors in rats. Also *phenetidinnurea.*

**dulcitol** GALACTITOL.

**dull** **1** Not sharp or bright. **2** Lacking resonance on percussion.

**dumas** \doo′mas\ A word used in Sri Lanka for FOOT YAWS.

**dumb** [Old English (from a Germanic word prob. originally meaning stupid; later, in somelanguages, inarticulate, speechless) mute] MUTE. • The colloquial American use of *dumb* to mean "stupid," which probably derives from the influence of German *dumm* "stupid," has rendered its use in the sense of "mute" unacceptable in many contexts.

**dumbbell / d.'s of Schäfer** Isolated matter found in striated muscle tissue.

**dumbness** The condition of being mute. **pure word d.** BROCA'S APHASIA.

**dummy** A term for PACIFIER used in Britain and New Zealand.

**Duncan** [James Matthews *Duncan,* Scottish gynecologist, 1826–1890] See under POSITION, MECHANISM.

**duodenal** \d$^{y}$oo′ōdē′nəl\ Pertaining to the duodenum.

**duodenectomy** \d$^{y}$oo′ōdenek′təmē\ [*duoden(um)* + -ECTOMY] The surgical removal of duodenal tissue.

**duodenitis** \d$^{y}$oo′ōdenī′tis\ Inflammation of the duodenum, either acute or chronic, most often involving the duodenal bulb. While it is sometimes associated with an increased risk of duodenal ulcer, many patients with radiographic or endoscopic evidence of duodenitis are asymptomatic.

**duodeno-** \d$^{y}$oo′ədē′nə-\ [L *duodeni* twelve. See DUODENUM.] A combining form denoting the duodenum.

**duodenocholecystostomy** \-kō′ləsistäs′təmē\ CHOLECYSTODUODENOSTOMY.

**duodenocholedochotomy** \-kō′lēdōkät′əmē\ [DUODENO- + CHOLEDOCHO- + -TOMY] The surgical incision of the common bile duct and the duodenum.

**duodenocystostomy** \-sistäs′təmē\ CHOLECYSTODUODENOSTOMY.

**duodenoduodenostomy** \-d$^{y}$oo′ədənäs′təmē\ The surgical anastomosis of the two portions of a divided duodenum.

**duodenoenterostomy** \-en′tərä s′təmē\ [DUODENO- + ENTERO- + -STOMY] A surgical anastomosis between the duodenum and another part of the small intestine.

**duodenography** \d$^{y}$oo′ədənäg′rəfē\ Roentgenography of the duodenum, especially after it has been filled with a contrast agent. **hypotonic d.** Radiologic examination of the duodenum by filling an atonic duodenum (made so by pharmacologic agents) with barium. By providing greater anatomic detail, it allows earlier detection of pancreatic or ampullary carcinomas, for example, than conventional barium x-ray studies.

**duodenoileostomy** \-il′ē·äs′təmē\ [DUODENO- + ILEO- + -STOMY] A surgical anastomosis between the duodenum and the ileum.

**duodenojejunostomy** \-jəjoonäs′təmē\ [DUODENO- + JEJUNO- + -STOMY] A surgical anastomosis between the duodenum and the jejunum.

**duodenolysis** \d$^{y}$oo′ədənäl′isis\ A surgical operation to release the duodenum from adhesions.

**duodenopancreatectomy** \-pan′krē·ətek′təmē\ [DUODENO- + PANCREAT- + -ECTOMY] The surgical excision of the duodenum in continuity with the pancreas.

**duodenoplasty** \d$^{y}$oo·ad′ənōplas′tē\ [DUODENO- + -PLASTY] Any restorative or reparative operation upon the duodenum.

**duodenorrhaphy** \d$^{y}$oo′ədənôr′əfē\ [DUODENO- + -RRHAPHY] The suturing of the duodenum. Also *duodenorraphia.*

**duodenoscope** \d$^{y}$oo·ad′ənōskōp′\ An instrument designed to allow direct inspection of the upper gastrointestinal tract as far as the proximal duodenum. It is usually flexible, using fiberoptic bundles for illumination and visualization.

**duodenoscopy** \d$^{y}$oo′ədənäs′kəpē\ Examination of the duodenum by means of an endoscope.

**duodenostomy** \d$^{y}$oo′ədənäs′təmē\ The creation of a stoma in the duodenum.

**duodenotomy** \d$^{y}$oo′ədənät′əmē\ [DUODENO- + -TOMY] A surgical incision of the duodenum.

**duodenum** \d$^{y}$oo′ədē′nəm\ [short for Med L *intestinum duodenum digitorum* intestine of twelve fingers' breadths, from *duodeni* a group of twelve (from *duodecim* twelve) + *digitorum* of fingers] [NA] The first and widest part of the small intestine. It commences at the pyloric ostium, forms a C-shaped curve encircling the head of the pancreas, and terminates at the duodenojejunal flexure by continuing as the jejunum. It has no mesentery, is only partly covered by peritoneum, and is mainly related posteriorly to the right kidney, inferior vena cava, and the abdominal aorta. It is subdivided into pars superior, or first part; pars descendens, or second part; pars horizontalis, or third part; and pars ascendens, or fourth part. Also *dodecadactylon.*

**duoparental** \d$^{y}$oo′ōpəren′təl\ BIPARENTAL.

**duovirus** \dʸoo′ōvī′rəs\ *Outmoded* ROTAVIRUS.

**Duplay** [Simon-Emmanuel *Duplay,* French surgeon, 1836–1924] Duplay syndrome. See under CALCIFIC TENDINITIS.

**duplication** [L *duplicatio* (from *duplicare* to fold over, bend double, from *duplex,* gen. *duplicis* folded over, double, from *du(o)-* two + *-plex* -fold) a doubling] The doubling or apparent doubling during development of a part, an entire organ, or a major region of the body which is not normally doubled. **chromosome d.** A chromosome aberration in which a cytologically distinct portion of a chromosome occurs in more than one location in the karyotype. Duplications may be intrachromosomal or interchromosomal. In the latter case, they would also be characterized as a translocation. **tandem d.** **1** The occurrence of identical nucleotide sequences or genes in the same orientation adjacent to one another on a chromosome. It is the usual organization of satellite and other highly repetitious eukaryotic DNA's and a potential mechanism for genetic evolution. Also *tandem repeat.* **2** A chromosome aberration in which a cytogenetically distinct region of a chromosome is present in at least two adjacent copies.

**duplicature** \doo′plikā′chər\ A folding or doubling, as of the peritoneum or any membrane.

**duplicitas** \dooplis′itas\ [Late L (from L *duplex* double; see DUPLICATION) doubling, duplicity] The doubling or apparent doubling of a part, an entire organ, or a major region of the body. • This term was commonly used to designate conjoined twins but increasingly is supplanted by the suffix *-pagus,* preceded by the name of the region or regions at which union occurs. **d. anterior** Equal conjoined twins with union confined to the lower half of the body, particularly the pelvis and lower extremities, but with doubling of the upper parts, particularly the head and neck and often the thorax. Also *duplicitas superior.* **d. asymmetros** Unequal conjoined twins, particularly those in which the parasitic member is represented only by a poorly developed duplicate of either the upper or the lower half of the body. Also *heteropagus.* **d. completa** Equal conjoined twins in which both members are fully developed except for a restricted area of union. **d. inferior** DUPLICITAS POSTERIOR. **d. posterior** Equal conjoined twins with union confined to the upper half of the body, particularly the head and neck and often the thorax, but with the pelvis and lower extremities separate and intact. Also *ileadelphus, pygodidymus, iliadelphus.* **d. superior** DUPLICITAS ANTERIOR.

**dupp** \dup\ An onomatopoeic term, used to represent the second heart sound on auscultation.

**Dupré** [Ernest Pierre *Dupré,* French physician, 1862–1921] Dupré's disease, Dupré syndrome. See under MENINGISM.

**Dupuy-Dutemps** [Louis *Dupuy-Dutemps,* French ophthalmologist, 1871–1946] **1** Dupuy-Dutemps sign. See under LEVATOR SIGN. **2** See under OPERATION. **3** Dutemps-Cestan sign, Dupuy-Dutemps and Cestan sign. See under CESTAN SIGN.

**Dupuytren** [Guillaume *Dupuytren,* French surgeon and anatomist, 1777–1835] **1** See under SUTURE, HYDROCELE, FRACTURE, SIGN. **2** Dupuytren's fascia. See under APONEUROSIS PALMARIS. **3** Dupuytren's disease of the foot. See under PLANTAR FIBROMATOSIS.

**dura** \dʸoo′rə\ [L *dura,* fem. of *durus* hard] DURA MATER.

**dural** \dʸoo′rəl\ Of or denoting the dura mater.

**dura mater** \dʸoo′rə mā′tər\ [Med L, lit., tough mother, from *dura* (fem. of *durus* hard, tough) + *mater,* lit. transl. of Arabic *'umm* mother, matrix, protective covering (as in *'umm ad-dimāgh* covering of the brain)] The outermost and toughest of the meninges of the brain and spinal cord. In the head, the dura mater is scarcely distinguishable from the periosteum of the cranium, but at spinal levels it is separated from the vertebrae and the covering ligaments by the epidural space. The smooth inner surface is cleanly separable from the arachnoid by a cleft or potential space, the subdural space. Also *pachymeninx, scleromeninx, dura.* Adj. dural, duramatral. **d. encephali** [NA] The dura mater covering the brain, including sleevelike projections about the optic nerve and several other cranial nerves. Also *dura mater of brain, cranial dura mater, theca cerebri* (obs.). **d. spinalis** [NA] The dura mater that envelops the spinal cord and cauda equina. Included are dural prolongations extending outward around the spinal roots, and the filum terminale externale. Also *dura mater of spinal cord, endorrhachis, theca vertebralis* (obs.).

**Durand** [Paul *Durand,* French physician active in Tunisia, born 1895] **1** See under VACCINE. **2** Durand and Giroud vaccine. See under VACCINE.

**Duran-Reynals** [Francisco *Duran-Reynals,* U.S. bacteriologist, 1899–1958] Duran-Reynals factor, Reynals factor. See under HYALURONIDASE.

**duraplasty** \dʸoo′rəplas′tē\ [*dura (mater)* + -PLASTY] The repair of the dura mater by suture or by replacement of defective tissue with a substitute.

**duration** A period of elapsed time. **pulse d.** The temporal length of a pulse of light, sound, electric current, radio waves, etc. Also *pulse length, pulse width.*

**dur. dolor.** *durante dolore* (L, while the pain lasts).

**Durham** [*Durham,* U.S. criminal, flourished 20th century] See under RULE.

**Durham** [Arthur Edward *Durham,* English surgeon, 1834–1895] See under TROCAR, TUBE.

**Duroziez** [Paul Louis *Duroziez,* French physician, 1826–1897] **1** See under DISEASE. **2** Duroziez's murmur, Duroziez sign. See under MURMUR.

**Dutton** [Joseph Everett *Dutton,* English physician, 1874–1905] **1** Dutton's relapsing fever, Dutton's disease. See under AFRICAN TICK FEVER. **2** See under SPIROCHETE.

**Duverney** [Joseph-Guichard *Duverney,* French anatomist, 1648–1730] **1** Duverney's gland. See under GLANDULA VESTIBULARIS MAJOR. **2** Duverney's fissure. See under INCISURAE CARTILAGINIS MEATUS ACUSTICI. **3** Duverney's muscle. See under PARS LACRIMALIS MUSCULI ORBICULARIS OCULI.

**DV** **1** dependent variable. **2** dilute volume.

**D.V.M.** Doctor of Veterinary Medicine.

**dwale** \dwāl\ BELLADONNA.

**dwarf** [Old English *dweorg, dweorh*] An undersized individual for whom there is no expectation of attaining a size in the range typical for persons of like age, race, and sex. Even with special therapeutic measures the likelihood of normal growth is limited. For different forms of dwarfism, see also under DWARFISM. Also *nanus, nanosomus.* **achondroplastic d.** A dwarf whose short stature stems from defective cartilaginous growth and development of the long bones and not from deficient secretion of hormones. Characteristically, the arms and legs are short, the head and trunk are of normal size, sexual development is normal, and there is no pituitary disease. Also *chrondrodystrophic dwarf.* **adrenal d.** A dwarf whose short stature is due to early closure of the osseous epiphyses in children with congenital adrenocortical hyperplasia and excessive secretion of adrenal androgens. **ateliotic d.** A hypophysial dwarf in whom pituitary gonadotropin secretion is preserved, with consequent normal development of primary and secondary sex characters and the capacity for sexual reproduction. Also *sexual* *dwarf, sexual ateliotic dwarf, primordial dwarf, idiopathic dwarf* (imprecise), *Seckel dwarf.* **chondrodystrophic d.** ACHONDROPLASTIC DWARF. **deformed d.** A dwarf who is of disproportionate short stature, with a discrepancy between the relative size of the limbs and the trunk. **hypophysial d.** A dwarf whose stature results from deficient or absent secretion of the growth hormone of the anterior pituitary. It is often associated with insufficiency of the pituitary tropic hormones, consequent failure of gonadal development, and severely diminished thyroid and adrenocortical function. The condition is sometimes familial and sometimes sporadic. Also *pituitary dwarf, hypopituitary dwarf, panhypopituitary dwarf, prepubertal dwarf, Lévi-Lorain dwarf, Paltauf's dwarf* (seldom used), *hyposomatotropic dwarf, Lorain-Lévi dwarf.* **hypoplastic d.** A dwarf having relatively normal proportions of limbs and trunk. **hyposomatotropic d.** HYPOPHYSIAL DWARF. **hypothyroid d.** A dwarf whose failure of linear growth is due to primary hypothyroidism in infancy, as in cretinism. **idiopathic d.** *Imprecise* ATELIOTIC DWARF. **Laron d.** A dwarf whose short stature is due to ineffectiveness of growth hormone action associated with normal plasma growth hormone concentrations, specifically to deficient somatomedin generation in response to growth hormone. **Lévi-Lorain d.** *Older term* HYPOPHYSIAL DWARF. **Lorain-Lévi d.** HYPOPHYSIAL DWARF. **micromelic d.** A dwarf with very small extremities. **Paltauf's d.** *Seldom used* HYPOPHYSIAL DWARF. **panhypopituitary d.** HYPOPHYSIAL DWARF. **phocomelic d.** An abnormally small person having the associated developmental malformation of phocomelia. **pituitary d.** HYPOPHYSIAL DWARF. **prepubertal d.** HYPOPHYSIAL DWARF. **primordial d.** ATELIOTIC DWARF. **rachitic d.** One who has been dwarfed as a result of rickets. Such an individual has a high, prominently bossed forehead, poorly developed teeth with thin pitted enamel, prominence of the sternum (pigeon chest), a transverse depression passing from the costal cartilages to the axillae which deepens with inspiration (Harrison sulcus), kyphosis or lordosis of the spine, enlargement of the lower ends of the femur and tibia, and fibular bowing of the long bones. **Russell d.** A child with features similar to those of the Silver-Russell syndrome, having in addition a degree of mental retardation and a propensity for ketotic hypoglycemia, but no skeletal asymmetries. **Seckel d.** ATELIOTIC DWARF. **senile d.** A dwarf whose failure of linear growth is due to progeria and not to an endocrine deficiency. **sexual d.** ATELIOTIC DWARF. **sexual ateliotic d.** ATELIOTIC DWARF.

**dwarfism** \dwôr′fizm\ [DWARF + -ISM] The condition of being a dwarf. For different forms of dwarfism, see also under DWARF. Also *nanism, nanosomia, nanosoma.* **acromelic d.** Dwarfism characterized by a marked shortening of the distal limbs. It is a feature of several osteochondrodysplasias, usually in association with shortening of other body segments. Also *acromelia.* **camptomelic d.** CAMPTOMELIC DYSPLASIA. **cardiac d.** Dwarfism secondary to a congenital cyanotic heart disease. **chondrodystrophic d.** See under CHONDRODYSTROPHY. **diabetic d.** Growth retardation associated with juvenile diabetes mellitus. **exostotic d.** Short stature associated with multiple hereditary exostoses. **hypophysial d.** Dwarfism resulting from deficient or absent secretion of the growth hormone of the anterior pituitary. Also *Lorain-Lévi syndrome, hypopituitary dwarfism, hypophysial infantilism* (older term), *idiopathic infantilism* (older term), *pituitary infantilism* (older term), *proportionate infantilism* (older term), *Lévi-Lorain infantilism* (outmoded), *Lorain's infantilism* (outmoded), *Lévi-Lorain type, Lorain type, prepubertal panhypopituitarism.* See also HYPOPHYSIAL DWARF. **hypopituitary d.** HYPOPHYSIAL DWARFISM. **mesomelic d.** Dwarfism associated with marked shortening of the forearms and lower legs; a feature of several osteochondrodysplasias. Also *mesomelia.* **micromelic d.** Disproportionate dwarfism characterized by small limbs, as is seen in achondroplasia. **myxedematous d.** THYROID DWARFISM. **pituitary d. I** An autosomal recessive syndrome of proportionate short stature due to a deficiency of growth hormone and the normal production and regulation of other anterior pituitary hormones. In some cases, it is due to a deletion of the human growth locus on chromosome 17. **pituitary d. III** Panhypopituitary dwarfism that occurs sporadically or is inherited as an autosomal recessive trait. The growth hormone and gonadotropins are deficient, as may be ACTH and TSH. Growth retardation is proportionate and is associated with a marked reduction in bone age. The condition is effectively treated by early growth hormone replacement. Also *Hanhart syndrome.* **polydystrophic d.** MUCOPOLYSACCHARIDOSIS III. **Pott's d.** A short stature caused by kyphosis of the spine secondary to vertebral destruction by tuberculosis. **pseudometatropic d.** SPONDYLOMETAEPIPHYSEAL DYSPLASIA. **psychosocial d.** Severe stunting of growth occurring as a sequela to the maternal deprivation syndrome. **renal d.** The retardation of growth during childhood by chronic renal failure, usually due to some congenital renal disorder. Renal rickets and renal osteodystrophy as well as a negative nitrogen balance and other less well understood nutritional deficiencies are important in the development of renal dwarfism. **rhizomelic d.** Dwarfism associated with marked shortening of the proximal limbs. It is a feature of several osteochondrodysplasias, including achondroplasia. Also *rhizomelia.* **thanatophoric d.** THANATOPHORIC DYSPLASIA. **thyroid d.** Dwarfism associated with cretinism. Also *myxedematous dwarfism.*

**Dy** Symbol for the element, dysprosium.

**dyad** \dī′ad\ [Gk *dyas,* gen. *dyados* (from *dyo* two) the number two, a pair] **1** The two cells that are produced by the first meiotic division. **2** Either of the two pairs of homologous chromatids, joined at the centromere, that result from disjunction of a tetrad during the first meiotic division.

**dyadic** \dī·ad′ik\ Of or pertaining to a dyad.

**dyaster** \dī′astər\ AMPHIASTER.

**dyclonine hydrochloride** $C_{18}H_{27}NO_2 \cdot HCl$. 1-(4-butoxyphenyl)-3-(1-piperidinyl)-1-propanone, an agent used as a topical local anesthetic to the skin and mucous membranes and to the conjunctiva. It also has bactericidal and fungicidal activity.

**dydrogesterone** $C_{21}H_{28}O_2$. (9β,10α)-Pregna-4,6-diene-3,20-dione. A white, crystalline powder that is a synthetic progestational compound. It is used in the diagnosis and subsequent treatment of primary amenorrhea and for the treatment of dysmenorrhea. It is also used in combination with estrogens in the treatment of menorrhagia. Also *isopregnenone.*

**dye** \dī\ [Old English *dēag*] A substance capable of binding to tissue components, which can subsequently be identified by the color imparted to them by the chromophore grouping on the dye molecules. **acidic d.** ACID STAIN. **azo d.** Any dyestuff in which the chromophore has an azo group. Widely used commercially, these dyes can be compounded as acid or basic dyes. **basic d.** BASIC STAIN. **fluorescein d.'s** FLUORESCEIN. **metachromatic d.** A dyestuff that causes tissue elements, notably sulfated polysaccharides, some sialic acid mucins, and ribonucleic acid, to assume a color different from that of the dye, usually one of a shorter wavelength. Also *metachromatic stain.* **vital d.** VITAL STAIN.

**Dyke** [Sidney Campbell *Dyke,* English physician, born 1886] Dyke-Young syndrome. See under SYNDROME.

**-dymus** \-dəməs\ [New L, back-formation from -DIDYMUS] A suffix denoting duplication or other supernumerary state, used in combination with a number root such as *tri-* or *tetra-*. ● In modern usage such terms to designate conjoined twins are being supplanted by the suffix *-pagus,* preceded by the name of the region or regions where union occurs.

**dynamic** \dīnam′ik\ [Gk *dynamikos* (from *dynamis* power, force) powerful, efficacious] **1** Pertaining to motion or to kinetic energy. **2** Characterized by activity or change. **3** Functional or processual. **4** Pertaining to motives, drives, or psychic forces.

**dynamics** \dīnam′iks\ [Gk *dynam(is)* strength, power + -ICS] The branch of physics that deals with the study of forces and motion. **group d.** The study of group formation and function and of the cause-and-effect relationships that can be identified among the interactions of members of the group. **topological d.** A field of mathematics that describes the way interconnected systems such as heart cells interact to yield irregularities such as arrhythmias.

**dynamo-** \dī′nəmō-\ [Gk *dynamis* power] A combining form meaning power, force, strength, or movement.

**dynamograph** \dīnam′əgraf\ [DYNAMO- + -GRAPH] An instrument for measuring and recording the strength of a muscle contraction.

**dynamometer** \dī′nəmäm′ətər\ [DYNAMO- + -METER] An instrument for measuring the energy resulting from the action of any mechanical force, as that exerted by muscle contraction.

**dynamopathic** \-path′ik\ Affecting function or the ability to move.

**dynamophoric** \-fôr′ik\ [DYNAMO- + *phor-* + -IC] Contributing to energy production.

**dynamoscope** \dīnam′ōskōp\ [DYNAMO- + -SCOPE] An instrument for observing functional activity usually taking place within the body.

**dyne** \dīn\ [French (from Gk *dyn(amis)* force), a unit of force in the cgs system] Special name for a unit of force in the CGS system, equal to the force which, acting on a mass of one gram, gives to it an acceleration of one centimeter per second squared; $10^{-5}$ newton. Symbol: dyn **d. -second per centimeter to the fifth power** A unit of vascular resistance to flow, 0.1 kilopascal second per liter. Symbol: $dyn{\cdot}s/cm^5$, $dyn{\cdot}s{\cdot}cm^{-5}$

**dynein** \dī′nēn\ A protein of eukaryotic cilia and flagella. It uses the hydrolysis of ATP to perform the mechanical work involved in the movement of these organelles.

**dyphylline** $C_{10}H_{14}N_4O_4$. 7-(2,3-Dihydroxypropyl)-3,7-dihydro-1,3-dimethyl-1*H*-purine-2,6-dione. A theophylline analogue with the properties of a peripheral vasodilator, a diuretic, a bronchodilator and a cardiac stimulant. It is used in the treatment of bronchial asthma as well as in bronchospasm secondary to chronic bronchitis and emphysema. Also *glyphylline, hyphylline.*

**dys-** \dis-\ [Gk, mis-, mal-, bad, faulty] A prefix meaning bad, defective, difficult, disordered, abnormal. Compare EU-.

**dysacousis** \dis′əkoo′sis\ DYSACUSIS.

**dysacusis** \dis′əkoo′sis\ [DYS- + -ACUSIS] A disorder characterized by a distortion in the quality of the sounds being heard, as of musical notes. It sometimes causes a sense of discomfort in the patient. Also *acoustic hyperesthesia, auditory hyperesthesia, auditory dysesthesia.* Also *dysacousis.*

**dysadaptation** \dis′adaptā′shən\ [DYS- + ADAPTATION] Inability of the eye to change its sensitivity to variations of intensity of light, as normally occurs spontaneously. Also *dysaptation.*

**dysaesthesia** *Brit.* DYSESTHESIA.

**dysallilognathia** \disal′ilōnā′thē·ə\ A growth abnormality resulting in a disproportion between the mandible and the maxilla.

**dysaphia** \disā′fē·ə\ [DYS- + Gk *(h)aph(ē)* a touching + -IA] Distortion or impairment of the sense of touch. Also *dyshaphia.* Adj. dyshaphic.

**dysaptation** \dis′aptā′shən\ DYSADAPTATION.

**dysarthria** \disär′thrē·ə\ [DYS- + ARTHR- + -IA ] A disorder of articulation due to a motor disturbance involving the upper or lower motor neurons, neuromuscular junctions, or skeletal muscles concerned in this process. **ataxic d.** CEREBELLAR DYSARTHRIA. **cerebellar d.** Dysarthria due to disease or dysfunction of the cerebellum. In its most clearly-defined form this gives rise to scanning speech with slurring and separation of the syllables. Also *ataxic dysarthria, ataxiophemia* (outmoded), *ataxophemia* (outmoded). **developmental d.** A developmental disorder of speech which may occur alone or in association with cerebral palsy. The affected children have particular difficulty in pronouncing consonants. **d. literalis** *Seldom used* STUTTERING. **spastic d.** The variety of dysarthria associated with spasticity of the muscles of articulation, as in some patients with cerebral palsy and in adults with progressive bulbar palsy, in which the sounds burst out in an explosive fashion. **d. syllabaris spasmodica** *Seldom used* STUTTERING.

**dysarthric** \disärth′rik\ Pertaining to or affected by dysarthria.

**dysarthrosis** \dis′ärthrō′sis\ [DYS- + ARTHR- + -OSIS ] **1** The malformation of one or more joints. **2** The development of a joint where none is normally present. **craniofacial d.** CRANIOFACIAL DYSOSTOSIS.

**dysautonomia** \dis′ôtənō′mē·ə\ [DYS- + Gk *autonomia* (from *autos* self + *nemein* to control) independence] Dysfunction of the autonomic nervous system. **familial d.** An autosomal recessive neurologic disorder, found predominantly in Ashkenazi Jews, that is characterized by a lack of tearing, emotional lability, increased sweating, corneal anesthesia, and erythematous blotching of the skin. The basic defect is unclear. Also *Riley-Day syndrome.*

**dysbarism** \dis′barizm\ [DYS- + BAR- + -ISM] A condition associated with exposure to very low or rapidly changing atmospheric pressure. Symptoms include pain in or near joints, giddiness, headache, numbness of limbs, chest pain, and shortness of breath. **altitude d.** AEROTITIS.

**dysbasia** \disbā′zhə\ [DYS- + Gk *bas(is)* a step + -IA] Difficulty in walking, including excessively fast steps (tachybasia), or very small steps (brachybasia). *Seldom used.* **d. lordotica progressiva** DYSTONIA MUSCULORUM DEFORMANS.

**dysbetalipoproteinemia** \disbā′təlip′əprō′tēnē′mē·ə\ FAMILIAL HYPERLIPOPROTEINEMIA TYPE III.

**dysbiosis** \dis′bī·ō′sis\ [DYS- + BIOSIS] Perturbation of the normal equilibrium of flora or fauna in a particular environment.

**dysbolism** \dis′bōlizm\ [DYS- + *(meta)bolism*] Any metabolic abnormality.

**dyscalculia** \dis′kəlkyoo′lē·ə\ [DYS- + L *calcul(are)* to compute + -IA] Impairment of the ability to calculate and to use numbers, resulting from a lesion of the dominant parietal lobe.

**dyscephalia** \dis′efā′lyə\ DYSCEPHALY.

**dyscephaly** \disef′əlē\ [DYS- + CEPHAL- + -Y] Any malformation of the head or face. Also *dyscephalia*.
**dyscheiria** \diskī′rē·ə\ [DYS- + Gk *cheir* the hand, hand and arm, arm + -IA] Inability to decide which side of the body has received a sensory stimulus. Also *dyschiria*.
**dyschezia** \diskē′zhə\ [DYS- + Gk *chez(ein)* to defecate + -IA] Difficult or painful defecation. Also *dyschesia*.
**dyschiasia** \dis′kī·ā′zhə\ [DYS- + Gk *chiaz(ein)* to make a cross, as an X + -IA] Difficulty in localizing sensory stimuli.
**dyschiria** \diskī′rē·ə\ DYSCHEIRIA.
**dyschondrogenesis** \dis′kändrōjen′əsis\ The defective development of cartilage.
**dyschondroplasia** \dis′kändrōplā′zhə\ [DYS- + CHONDROPLASIA] Any abnormality in cartilage formation and proliferation that persists into the metaphyseal and diaphyseal regions of the long bones. It may be unilateral or bilateral, and rarely it is confined to one bone, such as the pelvis. Dwarfism of individual bones may occur.
**dyschondrosteosis** \dis′kändräs′tē·ō′sis\ [DYS- + CHONDR- + OSTE- + -OSIS] A hereditary dyschondroplasia that gives rise to short stature, excessive ossification of the epiphyses, and broad diaphyses of the long bones. Joint stiffness is apparent in the hands and feet. Also *Léri's pleonosteosis, Léri-Weill syndrome*.
**dyschromatopsia** \dis′krōmətäp′sē·ə\ [DYS- + *chromat-* + -OPSIA] A faulty color discrimination resulting in incomplete color blindness.
**dyschromatosis** \dis′krōmətō′sis\ An abnormality of pigmentation.
**dyschronometria** \dis′kränōmē′trē·ə\ [DYS- + CHRONO- + METR- + -IA] An impairment of the initiation, speed, duration, and cessation of movements, resulting from cerebellar dysfunction.
**dyschronous** \dis′krənəs\ Lacking in synchrony; not synchronous.
**dyschylia** \diskī′lyə\ [DYS- + *chyl(e)* + -IA] Any disorder of the chyle or of its formation.
**dyscinesia** \dis′ īnē′zhə\ DYSKINESIA.
**dyscrasia** \diskrā′zhə\ [Gk *dyskrasia* (from DYS- + Gk *kras(is)* a mixing + -IA) bad temperament] Any abnormal condition of the body. **blood d.** Any abnormality of blood cells or bone marrow. Also *hemodyscrasia, hematodyscrasia*. **plasma cell d.** An abnormality of plasma cells, usually malignant, expressed as paraproteinemia or as multiple myeloma.
**dysdiadochokinesia** \dis′dī·ad′ōkōkīnē′zhə\ [DYS- + DIADOCHOKINESIA] Impairment of rapid repetitive pronation and supination of the open hand due to cerebellar dysfunction. Adj. dysdiadochokinetic.
**dysenteric** \dis′enter′ik\ Relating to or affected with dysentery.
**dysenteriform** \dis′enter′iform\ Resembling dysentery; dysenterylike.
**dysentery** \dis′enter′ē\ [Gk *dysenteria* (from DYS- + *enter(on)* bowel + -IA) dysentery] A condition characterized by difficult or painful bowel movements, usually related to inflammation or infection of the intestinal tract, with associated diarrhea, abdominal cramping and possibly the passage of mucus or blood with the stool. **amebic d.** Dysentery caused by infection by pathogenic amebas, usually *Entamoeba histolytica*, and characterized by diarrhea which may be severe, often with blood and mucus. Symptoms usually include abdominal pain and, when the rectum is involved, tenesmus. See also AMEBIASIS. **asylum d.** INSTITUTIONAL DYSENTERY. **bacillary d.** An infectious disease caused by bacteria of the *Shigella* species and characterized by bloody diarrhea. The disease is common in, but not restricted to, tropical regions. The worst case is usually that caused by *S. dysenteriae I*. Stool mucus, abdominal pain, tenesmus, and dehydration may also be present. Identical symptoms can, however, be produced by other bacteria. Also *Flexner's dysentery, Japanese dysentery, Shiga's dysentery*. **balantidial d.** Dysentery caused by the ciliate protozoan *Balantidium coli*. It is sometimes mistaken for amebic dysentery. **bilharzial d.** SCHISTOSOMAL DYSENTERY. **catarrhal d.** *Obs.* SPRUE. **ciliate d.** A dysentery caused by ciliate organisms such as the human and pig parasite *Balantidium coli*.. **flagellate d.** GIARDIASIS DYSENTERY. **Flexner's d.** BACILLARY DYSENTERY. **giardiasis d.** Dysentery caused by the parasitic protozoan flagellate *Giardia lamblia*.. Also *flagellate dysentery*. **helminthic d.** Dysentery caused by infection with intestinal worms. **institutional d.** Bacillary dysentery occurring in a closed community, as among patients in mental institutions. Also *asylum dysentery*. **Japanese d.** BACILLARY DYSENTERY. **malignant d.** A severe form of dysentery which may lead rapidly to death. **schistosomal d.** Dysentery associated with intestinal schistosomiasis caused by *Schistosoma mansoni*. Also *bilharzial dysentery*. **Shiga's d.** BACILLARY DYSENTERY. **Sonne d.** A usually mild form of bacillary dysentery caused by *Shigella sonnei*. It most commonly affects children living in temperate areas.
**dysequilibrium** \dis′ēkwəlib′rē·əm\ Any disturbance of the equilibrium in any physiologic system, but especially in the vestibular and related systems.
**dyserythropoiesis** \dis′irith′rōpoi·ē′sis\ [DYS- + ERYTHROPOIESIS] Abnormal formation of erythrocytes, often manifested by misshapen nuclei or binucleated or multinucleated erythrocyte precursors in bone marrow. Dyserythropoiesis is characteristic of pernicious anemia, some thalassemias, sideroblastic anemias, myeloproliferative disorders, erythroleukemia, and the congenital dyserythropoietic anemias. Also *dyshematopoiesis, dyshemopoiesis*.
**dyserythropoietic** \dis′irith′rōpoi·et′ik\ Characterized by dyserythropoiesis. Also *dyshematopoietic, dyshemopoietic*.
**dysesthesia** \dis′esthē′zhə\ [DYS- + -ESTHESIA] Abnormal spontaneous sensation, often with an unpleasant quality, including, for example, itching, pins and needles, burning, or sensations as of hot or cold water, or of an electric shock. These are symptoms of disease or dysfunction of sensory pathways but are not in themselves specific or diagnostic, although some types of dysesthesia may be of limited diagnostic value, such as burning sensations in the skin occurring as a result of lesions in the spinothalamic tract. Also *disesthesia*. Adj. dysesthetic. **auditory d.** DYSACUSIS.
**dysfibrinogenemia** \dis′fībrin′ōjənē′mē·ə\ An autosomally inherited condition marked by any of various abnormal fibrinogens in the plasma. These fibrinogens clot slowly, yet thrombosis is a more commonmanifestation. Each type of dysfibrinogenemia is named for the city in which the corresponding abnormal fibrinogen was discovered.
**dysfunction** \disfungk′shən\ [DYS- + FUNCTION] Any disordered or abnormal functioning, especially of an organ. **central auditory d.** Any form of hearing disorder other than the forms of hearing loss associated with conductive or sensorineural deafness. The effects are not usually related to alteration of hearing threshold but to problems in the accurate spatial localization of sound, or of its identification or recognition. Such disorders may affect the comprehension of spoken language, as in sensory aphasia. **constitutional hepatic d.** GILBERT SYNDROME. **hypertonic uterine d.** Abnormal uterine contractions

which tend to occur in the latent phase of labor, are painful and incoordinate, and which often can be corrected through the use of sedation. **hypotonic uterine d.** Abnormal uterine contractions during labor, characterized by low intensity, relative painlessness and occurrence in the active phase of labor. They can often be corrected through the use of oxytocic drugs. **minimal brain d.** A syndrome characterized in children by short attention span, impulsivity, excitability with extraordinary emotional reactions to ordinary disappointments, distractibility, irritability, and often motor hyperactivity. Ability to perform coordinated movements requiring high motor skills is impaired, as are balance and kinesthetic and epicritic sensibility. Developmental delay may be manifested in acquiring the skills of reading and writing, often associated with poor tolerance for frustration and sometimes aggravated by parental and educational pressures to perform normally or better. Also *attention deficit disorder, clumsy child syndrome, minimal cerebral dysfunction, dyssynchronous child syndrome, minimal brain dysfunction syndrome, hyperkinetic impulse disorder, neurophrenia* (seldom used), *minimal chronic brain syndrome, nonpsychotic organic brain syndrome.* **orgasmic d.** Psychosexual disorder characterized by delayed or absent orgasm or ejaculation despite an adequate sexual excitement phase. Inhibited male or female orgasm, ejaculatory impotence, and frigidity are all examples of orgasmic dysfunction. **papillary muscle d.** Disorder of the mitral valve apparatus resulting from disease of the papillary muscles. Usually the consequence of myocardial ischemia or infarction, it causes mitral regurgitation. Also *papillary muscle syndrome.*

**dysgalactia** \dis′gəlak′tē·ə\ [DYS- + GALACT- + -IA] Poor or inadequate milk production.

**dysgammaglobulinemia** \disgam′əgläb′yəlinē′mē·ə\ [DYS- + GAMMA GLOBULIN + -EMIA] An immunologic deficiency state characterized by selective deficiencies of one or more but not all classes of immunoglobulins. The result is an increased susceptibility to infectious diseases in which humoral immunity plays the major role. *Imprecise.* Also *dysimmunoglobulinemia.*

**dysgenesis** \disjen′əsis\ [DYS- + GENESIS] Any abnormality of development. • The term is often applied specifically to teratogenic abnormality, but is used more broadly as well of any deficiency in development **disseminated nodular d. of the frontal surface layer** MOREL-WILDI SYNDROME. **gonadal d.** 1 The deficient development of the ovaries or testes, particularly absence of the germinal elements. It is said to occur more frequently in female than in male subjects, but the apparent disparity is probably due to differentiation of the genitalia in a female direction regardless of gonadal gender when male humoral influences from the embryonic gonads are inadequate. Also *germinal aplasia* (rare). 2 *Imprecise* TURNER SYNDROME. **iridocorneal mesodermal d.** RIEGER SYNDROME. **Rieger's d.** RIEGER SYNDROME. **seminiferous tubule d.** The agenesis or marked deficiency of male germinal elements, usually characterized by extensive hyalinization of the seminiferous tubules. The body habitus tends to be eunuchoid, and a lowered level of androgen secretion may be present. This condition is typically seen in the Klinefelter syndrome.

**dysgenic** \disjen′ik\ [Gk *dysgen(ēs)* low-born + -IC] Relating to or tending to produce genetic deterioration in a population.

**dysgenics** \disjen′iks\ The study of genetic deterioration in populations.

**dysgerminoma** \dis′jərminō′mə\ [DYS- + L *germen*, gen. *germinis*, sprout, fetus, seed + -OMA] A malignant tumor of the ovary composed of large round cells with clear, glycogen-containing cytoplasm resembling primitive germ cells. It is the ovarian counterpart of the testicular seminoma. Also *ovarian seminoma.* Also *disgerminoma.*

**dysgeusia** \disgyoo′zhə, disjoo′sē·ə\ [DYS- + Gk *geus(is)* taste + -IA] Any perversion of taste perception.

**dysglobulinemia** \disgläb′yəlinē′mē·ə\ Abnormality of the globulins in the blood, as in incomplete immunoglobulin deficiencies or in conditions involving the presence of paraproteins.

**dysgnathia** \disnā′thē·ə\ [DYS- + GNATH- + -IA] Any developmental abnormality of the maxilla or mandible or both jaws.

**dysgonesis** \dis′gōnē′sis\ [DYS- + GON-[2] + -ESIS] Dysfunction of the reproductive organs.

**dysgonic** \disgän′ik\ [DYS- + GON-[2] + -IC] Growing slowly: used especially of strains of the tubercle bacillus. *Outmoded.*

**dysgrammataxia** \dis′gramətak′sē·ə\ [DYS- + Gk *gramma* that which is drawn or written + *tax(is)* an arranging + -IA] Difficulty in combining into an integrated whole the various symbols comprising a word or phrase.

**dysgrammatism** \disgram′ətizm\ AGRAMMATISM.

**dysgraphia** \disgraf′ē·ə\ [DYS- + GRAPH- + -IA] **1** In children, difficulty in learning to write. This difficulty may be an apraxia for writing movements or a form of expressive dysphasia involving the use of written symbols. **2** In adults, acquired difficulty in writing. It is of cerebral origin and less severe than total agraphia. Also *status dysgraphicus.* Adj. dysgraphic.

**dyshematopoiesis** \dis·hem′ətōpoi·ē′sis\ DYSERYTHROPOIESIS.

**dyshematopoietic** \dis·hem′ətōpoi·et′ik\ DYSERYTHROPOIETIC.

**dyshemopoiesis** \dis·hē′məpoi·ē′sis\ DYSERYTHROPOIESIS.

**dyshemopoietic** \dis·hē′məpoi·et′ik\ DYSERYTHROPOIETIC.

**dysimmunoglobulinemia** \disim′yənōgläb′yəlinē′mē·ə\ DYSGAMMAGLOBULINEMIA.

**dysjunction** \disjungk′shən\ DISJUNCTION.

**dyskaryosis** \diskar′ē·ō′sis\ [DYS- + *kary(o)-* + -OSIS] A state in which one or more cells contain abnormal nuclei and yet the cytoplasm shows normal differentiation.

**dyskaryotic** \disker′ē·ät′ik\ Of or relating to dyskaryosis.

**dyskeratoma** \disker′ətō′mə\ [DYS- + KERATOMA] A keratotic tumor. **warty d.** A cystic, tumorlike invagination of the epidermis, containing keratin and parakeratin with villouslike projections extending into the lumen. It usually occurs on the face, neck, or scalp. Also *isolated dyskeratosis follicularis.*

**dyskeratosis** \dis′kerətō′sis\ [DYS- + KERATOSIS] An abnormal and premature keratinization of epidermal cells. **d. congenita** A syndrome of cutaneous hyperpigmentation, nail dystrophy, leukoplakia, lacrimal duct atresia, deforming periarticular atrophic skin changes, and pancytopenia. The oral lesions appear in childhood, and other changes progress with age. X-linked recessive inheritance accounts for the overwhelming predominance of affected males, but genetic heterogeneity exists. The biochemical defect is unknown. Also *Zinsser-Cole-Engman syndrome.* **hereditary benign intraepithelial d.** An autosomal dominant condition that affects the oral mucosa and conjunctiva and results in a leukoplakia-like abnormality that is not premalignant and pterygia-like eye lesions. Also *Witkop-Von Sallman disease.* **isolated d. follicularis**

WARTY DYSKERATOMA.

**dyskinesia** \dis′kinē′zhə\ [Gk *dyskinēsia* (from DYS- + *kinēs(is)* motion + -IA) difficulty in moving] **1** Any abnormality of movement, such as incoordination, spasm, or irregular and ill-formed movements. **2** Any bizarre spontaneous movements such as the irregular and intermittent protrusion of the tongue and associated lip movements (facial dyskinesia) which may result from phenothiazines. Also *dyscinesia.* Adj. dyskinetic. **biliary d.** Functional abnormality of gallbladder and biliary tract contractions, causing postprandial right upper quadrant pain. **BLM d.** TARDIVE DYSKINESIA. **buccal-lingual-masticatory d.** TARDIVE DYSKINESIA. **facial d.** TARDIVE DYSKINESIA. **occupational d.** OCCUPATIONAL CRAMP. **orofacial d.** TARDIVE DYSKINESIA. **phenothiazine-induced d.** KULENKAMPFF-TARNOW SYNDROME. **tardive d.** Slow, rhythmic, sterotyped, repetitive, involuntary movements of the tongue, lips, and mouth, and sometimes also of the trunk and limbs, that appear as a complication of neuroleptic drug administration, usually after a year or more of treatment. Also *orofacial dyskinesia, dyskinesia tarda, facial dyskinesia, buccal-lingual-masticatory syndrome, BLM syndrome, buccal-lingual-masticatory dyskinesia, BLM dyskinesia.* **tracheobronchial d.** Impairment of the muscular action of the trachea and bronchi as a result of abnormalities of its fibrous and elastic tissue.

**dyskinetic** \dis′kinet′ik\ Pertaining to or affected by dyskinesia.

**dyslalia** \dislā′lyə\ [DYS- + -LALIA] **1** Difficulty in articulating because of an abnormality or lesion of the organs of phonation and articulation. **2** A benign developmental speech disorder characterized by multiple consonant substitutions. The condition, which usually becomes apparent between the ages of eighteen months and three years, carries an excellent prognosis. It is probably a mild and reversible form of developmental articulatory apraxia.

**dyslexia** \dislek′sē·ə\ [DYS- + Gk *lex(is)* word, discourse, from *legein* to speak, say, recite, read aloud + -IA] **1** Impairment of the ability to read. The condition may be developmental, being then a form of developmental receptive aphasia or word blindness, or it may be acquired, resulting from a lesion in the dominant parietal lobe. **2** Difficulty in identifying, understanding and reproducing written symbols. Adj. dyslexic. **congenital d.** DEVELOPMENTAL DYSLEXIA. **developmental d.** Abnormal difficulty in learning to read, in a person of normal intelligence. Also *evolutive dyslexia, congenital dyslexia, congenital reading defect, developmental alexia.*

**dyslipidosis** \dis′lipidō′sis\ Any disorder of fat metabolism. Also *dislipoidosis.*

**dysmature** \disməty̆oor′\ [DYS- + MATURE] Marked by inappropriately low birthweight for gestational age: said of an infant.

**dysmaturity** \dis′məty̆oo′ritē\ [DYS- + MATURITY] Failure of normal placental function appropriate to a particular stage in placental development. **pulmonary d.** WILSON-MIKITY SYNDROME.

**dysmegalopsia** \dis′megəläp′sē·ə\ [DYS- + *megal(o)-* + -OPSIA] DYSMETROPSIA.

**dysmelia** \dismē′lyə\ [DYS- + MEL[1] + -IA] Any malformation of a limb, especially meromelia.

**dysmenorrhea** \dis′menôrē′ə\ [DYS- + MENORRHEA] Painful menstruation; the colicky lower abdominal pain of ovulatory menstruation. Also *algomenorrhea, menstrual colic, menalgia, menorrhalgia, menstrual cramps, colica scortorum.* **acquired d.** Dysmenorrhea resulting from abnormalities of the vagina or pelvis, i.e., caused by lesions outside the uterus. **congestive d.** Painful menstruation supposed to be caused by undue congestion and vasodilatation of the pelvic organs of reproduction. Also *pelvic congestion syndrome.* **inflammatory d.** Dysmenorrhea resulting from inflammation of the female genital tract. **d. intermenstrualis** MITTELSCHMERZ. **membranous d.** Dysmenorrhea accompanied by the passage of membranous portions of the menstrual decidua. **primary d.** Dysmenorrhea which begins at menarche or a year or so later. **secondary d.** Painful menstruation beginning some time after menarche and usually due to some underlying pathologic condition. **ureteric d.** Painful ureteral spasm during menses. **vaginal d.** Dysmenorrhea resulting from a pathological condition of the vagina, such as an inflammation or tumor.

**dysmentia** \dismen′shə\ [DYS- + L *mens*, gen. *mentis,* mind + -IA] Pseudodementia or pseudoimbecility, based primarily on psychological factors. **tardive d.** A behavioral disorder associated with long-term neuroleptic drug treatment characterized by loquaciousness, speaking loudly, disconnected and often inappropriate thoughts, a generally euphoric mood with occasional bursts of hostility or petulance, and social withdrawal or autistic preoccupation broken by episodes of intrusive overactivity. Also *iatrogenic schizophrenia, tardive psychosis, subcortical dementia* (seldom used).

**dysmetria** \dismet′rē·ə\ [DYS- + Gk *metr(on)* measure + -IA] Inability, in the performance of a movement, to judge direction and distance, seen particularly when the patient attempts to touch his nose or the examiner's finger with his finger, or his knee with his heel. The movement, while generally in the right direction, either veers to the side of the target or overshoots (hypermetria). This sign is due to disease or dysfunction of the cerebellar hemisphere or of cerebellar tracts or connections. Unlike sensory ataxia caused by impairment of deep sensibility, it is not increased by closing the eyes. Adj. dysmetric. **ocular motor d.** Difficulty in fixating the eyes upon an object, so that they overshoot and then oscillate beyond and short of the target a few times before accurate fixation is achieved. It is a sign of cerebellar dysfunction.

**dysmetropsia** \dis′mətrap′sē·ə\ [DYS- + Gk *metr(on)* measure + -OPSIA] Inability to assess correctly the size of an object by looking at it. Also *dysmegalopsia.*

**dysmimia** \dismim′ē·ə\ [DYS- + Gk *mim(os)* an imitator, mime + -IA] Difficulty in expressing one's meaning by gestures or mimicry.

**dysmnesia** \disnē′zhə\ [DYS- + Gk *mnēs(is)* memory + -IA] **1** Impaired memory, particularly those disturbances in memory and thinking that precede the establishment of irreversible dementia. **2** DYSMNESIC SYNDROME.

**dysmorphia** \dismôr′fē·ə\ [Gk (from DYS- + *morph(ē)* form, shape + -IA) misshapenness] An abnormality of shape or size, usually of developmental origin.

**dysmorphogenesis** \dis′môrfōjen′əsis\ [*dysmorph(ia)* + GENESIS] TERATOGENESIS.

**dysmorphology** \dis′môrfäl′əjē\ [*dysmorph(ia)* + -LOGY] TERATOLOGY.

**dysmorphophobia** \dismôr′fəfō′bē·ə\ [*dysmorph(ia)* + -PHOBIA] Morbid fear of developing a physical deformity.

**dysmyelination** \dis′mī·əlinā′shən\ Disordered myelination in the central or peripheral nervous system.

**dysmyelopoietic** \dismī′əlōpoi·et′ik\ Characterized by disordered or abnormal myelopoiesis.

**dysnomia** \disnō′mē·ə\ [DYS- + Gk *(o)nom(a)* name + -IA] Partial nominal aphasia.

**dysodynia** \dis′ōdin′ē·ə\ [DYS- + -ODYNIA] Uterine contractions during labor that do not produce cervical dilatation or descent of the presenting fetal part.

**dysontogenesis** \dis′äntōjen′əsis\ [DYS- + ONTOGENESIS] Failure of proper development. Adj. dysontogenetic.

**dysorexia** \dis′ôrek′sē·ə\ [Gk (from DYS- + *orex(is)* yearning, appetite + -IA) a lack of appetite] EATING DISORDER.

**dysostosis** \dis′ästō′sis\ [DYS- + OSTOSIS] Defective bone formation, due to faulty ossification of fetal cartilages. **acrofacial d.** NAGER'S ACROFACIAL DYSOSTOSIS. **cleidocranial d.** CLEIDOCRANIAL DYSPLASIA. **craniofacial d.** An autosomal dominant inherited condition in which there is hypoplasia of the maxilla and a beaked nose. The eyes are widely separated, exophthalmic, and marked by a squint or strabismus. Also *maxillonasal dysostosis, craniofacial dysarthrosis, Crouzon's disease, Crouzon syndrome.* **d. enchondralis epiphysaria** DYSPLASIA EPIPHYSIALIS MULTIPLEX. **mandibulofacial d.** An autosomal dominant malformation syndrome characterized by antimongoloid slant of the eyes, eyelid coloboma, micrognathia, macrostomia, microtia, and hypoplastic zygomatic arches. Secondary hearing loss and mental retardation may result. Also *Treacher Collins syndrome, Treacher Collins-Franceschetti syndrome, mandibular dysostosis.* **maxillonasal d.** CRANIOFACIAL DYSOSTOSIS. **metaphyseal d.** A form of dysostosis in which the cartilage cells and trabeculae extend down into the metaphyses, failing to undergo normal endochondral ossification and remodelling. The metaphyseal areas of the long bones are expanded with thinned cortices. **d. multiplex** A nonspecific, generalized dysostosis that is defined radiologically and is characterized by short, broad tubular bones, anterior wedging and beaking of vertebrae, and scaphocephaly. It occurs in the mucopolysaccharidoses and mucolipidoses. **Nager's acrofacial d.** Mandibulofacial dysostosis with limb anomalies such as absence of the radius, hypoplastic thumbs, or radioulnar synostosis. Also *acrofacial dysostosis, Nager syndrome.* **nasomaxillary d.** A defect in the normal ossification or growth of the maxilla and the bones forming the nose, resulting in hypoplasia of the maxilla and hypotelorism. Also *Binder syndrome.* **orodigitofacial d.** OROFACIODIGITAL SYNDROME. **otomandibular d.** Hypoplasia of the mandible, the temporomandibular joint, and other structures derived from and associated with the embryonic first branchial arch.

**dyspareunia** \dis′pəroo′nē·ə\ [Gk *dyspareun(os)* (from DYS- + Gk *para* beside + *eunē* a bed, the marriage bed) ill-mated + -IA] Coitus associated with recurrent, persistent genital pain.

**dyspepsia** \dispep′sē·ə\ [Gk (from DYS- + *peps(is)* digestion + -IA) indigestion] Indigestion; an upset stomach. **functional d.** A functional disturbance of the upper gastrointestinal tract characterized by abdominal discomfort, bloating, and, to a variable degree, nausea.

**dyspeptic** \dispep′tik\ Characterized by or affected by dyspepsia.

**dysphagia** \disfā′jə\ [DYS- + Gk *phag(ein)* to eat + -IA] Difficulty in swallowing; a sensation of food sticking in the esophagus. Also *aphagopraxia, dysphagy.* **d. globosa** GLOBUS HYSTERICUS. **d. inflammatoria** Dysphagia caused by esophagitis. **d. lusoria** Dysphagia due to compression of the esophagus by an aberrant right subclavian artery. • The Latin adjective *lusoria* is derived from *lusus,* play, sport, referring here to a "sport of nature" or congenital anomaly. **d. paralytica** Dysphagia due to paralysis of the muscles of swallowing. **sideropenic d.** PLUMMER-VINSON SYNDROME. **d. spastica** Dysphagia due to spasticity of the muscles of swallowing. **tropical d.** TROPICAL CARDIOSPASM. **vallecular d.** A state in which a portion of food or, rarely, a foreign body becomes lodged in one or other of the epiglottic valleculae. Also *Barclay-Baron disease.*

**dysphagic** \disfā′jik\ Characterized by or affected by dysphagia.

**dysphagy** \dis′fəjē\ DYSPHAGIA.

**dysphasia** \disfā′zhə\ [DYS- + Gk *phas(is)* a speech, a saying + -IA] Impairment of the production or appreciation of speech, due to a cerebral lesion. It is a defect less severe than that of aphasia, although often the two terms are used interchangeably.

**dysphemia** \disfē′mē·ə\ *Seldom used* STUTTERING.

**dysphonia** \disfō′nē·ə\ [DYS- + PHON- + -IA] Abnormal phonation. Adj. dysphonic. **d. plicae ventricularis** An abnormal, low-pitched, rough vocalization, produced, not by the vocal cords, but by the ventricular bands. It often occurs when an attempt is made to disguise some underlying vocal cord disease. **spastic d.** Dysphonia due to paroxysms of glottic spasm, occurring mainly in those liable to overuse of the voice and in association with anxiety.

**dysphonic** \disfän′ik\ Pertaining to or affected by dysphonia.

**dysphylaxia** \dis′fīlak′sē·ə\ [DYS- + Gk *phylax(is)* a watching, guarding + -IA] Premature spontaneous arousal from sleep, such as early morning waking.

# dysplasia

**dysplasia** \displā′zhə\ [DYS- + -PLASIA] **1** Incomplete or aberrant development of a part, system, or region of the body. Compare APLASIA, AGENESIS, HYPOPLASIA. **2** Cellular atypia and architectural distortion considered to represent a potential for malignancy, i.e. a precancerous lesion. The term is used typically for epithelial tissues such as cervix, larynx, stomach, colon, and liver. Degrees of dysplasia are described as mild, moderate, and severe. **anhidrotic ectodermal d.** An X-linked condition that is more severe in hemizygous males, who exhibit an absence of sweat glands and teeth, hypotrichosis, and mild nail dystrophy. Heterozygous females show reduced or malformed teeth, mild hypohidrosis, and hypoplastic breasts. An autosomal dominant form may occur. Also *Christ-Siemens syndrome, Christ-Siemens-Touraine syndrome, hypohidrotic ectodermal dysplasia, anhydrotic ectodermal dysplasia.* **asphyxiating thoracic d.** ASPHYXIATING THORACIC DYSTROPHY. **atriodigital d.** HOLT-ORAM SYNDROME. **bronchopulmonary d.** A chronic respiratory disorder particularly liable to affect infants recovering from respiratory distress syndrome who have required high concentrations of oxygen and positive pressure pulmonary ventilation. It is due to epithelial lung damage followed by bronchiolar metaplasia and interstitial fibrosis. The respiratory distress continues instead of easing after seven to ten days. Full recovery may take up to 12 months. **camptomelic d.** A group of autosomal recessive, congenital skeletal dysplasias that are characterized by bowing and angulation of tubular bones, especially those of the limbs. Long-limb and two short-limb forms have been recognized, and, because of the XY gonadal dysgenesis in some phenotypic females, the condition affects more females than males. Many subjects die in infancy of respiratory complications. Also *camptomelic dwarfism, camptomelic syndrome.* **caudal d.** 1 A rare developmental agenesis of the sacrococcygeal segments of the vertebral column and spinal cord with consequent paralysis and sensory loss in lower limb muscles and often sphincter dysfunction, present from birth. 2 Any of various malformations, particularly of skeletal structures and especially of the pelvis and lower extremities. It is thought to be more frequent in the offspring of diabetic mothers than in the general population. Also *caudal dysplasia syndrome.* **d. of cervix** Dysplasia of the epithelium of the uterine cervix in which neoplastic cells occupy one to two thirds of the layering. **chondroectodermal d.** ELLIS-VAN CREVELD SYNDROME. **cleidocranial d.** An autosomal dominant osteochondrodysplasia characterized by moderate, proportionate short stature; narrow, drooping shoulders due to aplasia of the clavicles; delayed closure of the fontanels, and malerupted or supernumerary teeth. Also *osteodental dysplasia, cleidocranial dysostosis.* **congenital alveolar d.** Respiratory distress of unknown causation in the newborn. **congenital ectodermal d.** CONGENITAL ECTODERMAL DEFECT. **congenital d. of the hip** A condition found in children under five years of age in which the epiphysis is late in appearing and the roentgenogram has a mottled appearance. The epiphysis does not fragment and heals completely when relieved of bearing weight. **craniocarpotarsal d.** WHISTLING FACE–WINDMILL VANE HAND SYNDROME. **craniometaphyseal d. of Pyle** See under METAPHYSEAL DYSPLASIA. **craniotelencephalic d.** A form of craniostenosis caused by premature fusion of the coronal, metopic, and sagittal sutures, particularly affecting constriction or distortion of the anterior part of the cranial cavity. **dental d.** A developmental abnormality of the structure of a tooth, such as amelogenesis imperfecta of enamel and dentinogenesis imperfecta of dentin. **dentin d.** DENTINOGENESIS IMPERFECTA. **diaphyseal d.** PROGRESSIVE DIAPHYSEAL DYSPLASIA. **disseminated juvenile fibrous d. of the jaws** CHERUBISM. **ectodermal d.** 1 The maldevelopment of those tissues, such as skin, hair, and teeth, that are derived from embryonic ectoderm. 2 CONGENITAL ECTODERMAL DEFECT. **enamel d.** AMELOGENESIS IMPERFECTA. **encephalo-ophthalmic d.** The deficient or aberrant development of the eyes associated with abnormal organogenesis of the brain. **epiphyseal d.** METAPHYSEAL DYSPLASIA. **d. epiphysialis hemimelica** An overgrowth of the long bone epiphyses caused by an increase in the number of normally formed cartilage cells in the epiphyseal plate. It is seen most often in the distal femur or proximal tibia, but it may also occur in the talus in children. Adjacent joint movement may become limited. Also *epiphyseal hyperplasia, Trevor's disease, tarsomegaly.* **d. epiphysialis multiplex** A genetic disorder characterized by dwarfism in the form of slight, short limbs and short stubby digits in both the hands and feet. The epiphyseal centers of the limbs ossify irregularly in extent, timing, and shape, and enlarge without an increase in length. The condition is usually diagnosed in the young child at the onset of walking. It has been linked as an autosomal dominant characteristic. Also *multiple epiphyseal dysplasia, dysostosis enchondralis epiphysaria.* **extracranial fibromuscular d.** A nonarteriosclerotic occlusive condition of the cervical arteries, most commonly the carotid artery. It is characterized by alternating stenoses and dilatations and may be associated with occlusion, transient ischemic attacks, or stroke. **familial fibrous d. of the jaws** CHERUBISM. **fibromuscular d.** See under FIBROMUSCULAR DISEASE. **fibrous d.** An abnormality of the bone-forming mesenchyme marked by the replacement of the bony trabeculae by a stroma of fibrous tissue and even tissue to form a cyst or abnormal expansion of the bone. It can be found as a single lesion (monostotic fibrous dysplasia) or as multiple lesions, a condition known as polyostotic fibrous dysplasia, the Jaffe-Lichtenstein disease or syndrome, or Jaffe's disease. **fibrous d. of jaw** Fibrous dysplasia that occurs in the jaw alone or also in other bony sites. It usually leads to facial deformity. **hereditary bone d.** OSTEOCHONDRODYSPLASIA. **hereditary ectodermal d.** Any of the hereditary syndromes with primary abnormalities of tissues derived from the ectoderm. **hereditary renal-retinal d.** Any condition characterized by pigmentary retinopathy and progressive renal failure and associated with glomerular and vascular sclerosis and tubular atrophy. Clinical variability suggests that several forms exist, each heritable as an autosomal recessive trait. In no case has the basic defect been determined. **hidrotic ectodermal d.** An autosomal dominant syndrome characterized by total alopecia, severe nail dystrophy, scattered skin hyperpigmentation, normal teeth, and normal sweat and sebaceous gland function. It is less common than the anhidrotic form. Also *Clouston syndrome.* **hypohidrotic ectodermal d.** ANHIDROTIC ECTODERMAL DYSPLASIA. **d. linguofacialis** OROFACIODIGITAL SYNDROME. **mammary d.** CYSTIC MASTOPATHY. **metaphyseal d.** Dysplasia resulting from a failure of tubular remodeling just distal to the epiphyseal growth plate of long bones. This failure may leave the bones uniformly expanded and osteoporotic. When associated with overgrowth of the skull bones (leontiasis ossea), there may be cranial nerve involvement with blindness and hearing impairment, a condition called craniometaphyseal dysplasia of Pyle. The stature is normal. Also *epiphyseal dysplasia, Pyle's disease.* **monostotic fibrous d.** See under FIBROUS DYSPLASIA. **multiple epiphyseal d.** DYSPLASIA EPIPHYSIALIS MULTIPLEX. **nuclear d.** Impaired development of cranial nerve nuclei. It is one cause of the Möbius syndrome. **oculoauricular d.** OCULOAURICULOVERTEBRAL DYSPLASIA. **oculoauriculovertebral d.** A malformation syndrome characterized by facial asymmetry, frontal bossing, mandibular hypoplasia, epibulbar dermoids, preauricular appendages, ear malformations with conductive deafness, and vertebral anomalies. Most cases are sporadic and the recurrence risk in sibs is about 1%. Genetic heterogeneity is likely, and autosomal dominant inheritance does occur. Also *Goldenhar syndrome, oculovertebral syndrome, oculoauricular dysplasia.* **oculodentodigital d.** An autosomal dominant syndrome characterized by an abnormal facies that exhibits hypertelorism and a thin nose, eyes characterized by microphthalmia and pupillary membranes, abnormal enamel, soft tissue syndactyly, and skeletal dysplasia, with metaphyseal widening of the long bones. Also *ODD syndrome, oculodento-osseous syndrome.* **olfactory genital d.** KALLMANN SYNDROME. **oral familial white folded d.** An uncommon hereditary disease chiefly of the oral mucous membrane and sometimes of the mucosa of the nose, vagina, or rectum. It is often a congenital condition. The mucosa anywhere in the mouth may be affected, assuming a folded, spongy, opalescent appearance. Also *white folded gingivostomatosis, Cannon's disease, congenital oral leukokeratosis.* **osseous d.** The presence of a cementoma or exostosis, caused by the abnormal development of the cemental connective tissue cells surrounding the root of a tooth. **osteodental d.** CLEIDOCRANIAL DYSPLASIA. **polyostotic fibrous d.** See under FIBROUS DYSPLASIA. **progressive diaphyseal d.** A symmetrical, fusiform thickening of the mid-diaphyseal cortex, particularly of the femur, tibia, and fibula, although it can affect the flat bones as well with decreased hematopoiesid. Muscles become atrophied and weakened. It presents with varying severity early in childhood and may not be discovered until adulthood. It is frequently familial, but no definite inherited pattern has been established. Also *diaphyseal sclerosis, Camurati-Engelmann disease, Ribbing's disease, Engelmann's disease, diaphyseal dysplasia, osteopathia hyperostotica multiplex infantilis.* **pseudoachondroplastic d.** Any of several chondrodysplasias that are characterized by disproportionate short stature with a relatively normal trunk, the shortness usually not evident during infancy; a normal cranium and facies; and joint instability and deformity. Two autosomal dominant and an autosomal recessive form occur. Also *pseudoachondroplastic spondyloepiphyseal dysplasia, PAT-SED.* **renal d.** Disruption of any parts of the kidneys by persistence of fetal structures or mesonephric tissue, or both, either unilaterally or bilaterally. Dysplastic kidneys may be of any size or shape, and may or may not be cystic. **retinal d.** The absence or deficiency of neural elements in the retina with compensating excessive glial tissue. **skeletal d.** OSTEOCHONDRODYSPLASIA. **skeletodental d.** An abnormal development in the relationship of the maxilla to mandible, or to the base of the skull, along with an abnormal relationship of the teeth in opposing jaws. **spondyloepimetaphyseal d.** SPONDYLOMETAEPIPHYSEAL DYSPLASIA. **spondyloepiphyseal d.** Short trunk, short limb dwarfism that is caused by an ossification defect of epiphyseal growth in the vertebral column as well as the extremity growth plates, particularly those proximal ones in the vicinity of the shoulder and pelvic girdles. The condition has been described among family members with varying genetic types of inheritance, including autosomal dominant, recessive, and X-linked recessive. The dominant form may also be associated with ocular abnormalities as well as odontoid process hypoplasia. Although usually diagnosed in early childhood, it may become evident in a small-statured individual with the early onset of osteoarthrosis. **spondylometaepiphyseal d.** A skeletal dysplasia of unclear inheritance and basic defect that is characterized by abnormal facies, short limbs, clubfoot, kyphoscoliosis, and deafness due to recurrent otitis. Also *spondyloepimetaphyseal dysplasia, Strudwick syndrome, pseudometatropic dwarfism.* **thanatophoric d.** A severe chondrodysplasia that results in marked micromelia, abnormal facies, small thorax, disorganization of the central nervous system, and death within days of birth. Also *thanatophoric dwarfism.* **ventriculoradial d.** A skeletal syndrome in which absence of the radius or thumb or both is associated with a patent interventricular septum.

**dysplastic** \displas′tik\ Pertaining to or characterized by dysplasia.

**dyspnea** \dispnē′ə\ [L *dyspnoea,* from Gk *dyspnoia* (from DYS- + *pno(ē)* breath + -IA) difficulty in breathing] Shortness of breath; labored or difficult breathing; breathlessness. **cardiac d.** Dyspnea due to cardiac disease, most commonly occurring on exercise. **exertional d.** Dyspnea provoked by physical effort. **expiratory d.** Dyspnea more marked on breathing out, as in bronchial asthma. **inspiratory d.** Dyspnea more marked on breathing in, as in bilateral abductor paralysis of the larynx. **nocturnal d.** Dyspnea that occurs during sleep. **orthostatic d.** PLATYPNEA. **paroxysmal nocturnal d.** Dyspnea occurring in sudden episodes at night, usually due to acute left ventricular heart failure.

**dyspneic** \disp·nē′ik\ Relating to or affected by dyspnea.

**dyspnoea** \disp·nē′ə\ *Brit.* DYSPNEA.

**dyspoiesis** \dis′pō·ē′sis\ [DYS- + -POIESIS] A disorder of production, usually of cells such as hematopoietic cells.

**dyspoietic** \dis·′pō·et′ik\ Denoting any organ, tissue, or cell line that shows abnormal development.

**dysponderal** \dispän′dərəl\ [DYS- + L *pondus,* gen. *ponderis,* weight + -AL] Obese or underweight; not of ideal weight.

**dyspraxia** \disprak′sē·ə\ [Gk (from *dys-* DYS- + *prassein* to work, achieve) ill success] A disorder of movement, involving impairment of the ability to carry out a skilled activity in the absence of paralysis, ataxia, or any other abnormality of the primary motor pathways controlling movement. Like apraxia, which implies total loss rather than impairment of the particular skill, it may be developmental or acquired, resulting from a cerebral lesion. Adj. dyspraxic, dyspractic. • *Apraxia* and *dyspraxia* are often used interchangeably.

**dysprosium** \disprō′sē·əm\ Element number 66, having atomic weight 162.50. It is a rare earth metal of the lanthanide series. Symbol: Dy

**dysprosody** \disprās′ōdē\ [DYS- + PROSODY] Any abnormality of the cadence and pitch of speech.

**dysproteinemia** \disprō′tēnē′mē·ə\ Any disease associated with abnormal serum proteins. Qualitative or quantitative abnormalities may involve any serum protein, including lipoproteins.

**dysprothrombinemia** \dis′prōthrăm′binē′mē·ə\ [DYS- + PROTHROMBIN + -EMIA] A rare, autosomally inherited bleeding disease resulting from an abnormality of the prothrombin molecule.

**dysraphia** \disrā′fē·ə\ [DYS- + Gk *rhaph(ē)* a seam, suture + -IA] The absence of fusion or incomplete fusion of embryonic folds or other primordia, particularly in relation to the neural tube. Also *dysraphism.* **prosencephalic d.** Incomplete closure of the embryonic neural tube in the prosencephalic or forebrain region. **spinal d.** Incomplete closure of the embryonic neural tube in the spinal but not in the cephalic region of the neural axis.

**dysrhythmia** \disriTH′mē·ə\ [DYS- + Gk *rhythm(os)* rhythm + -IA] Disordered or abnormal rhythm. **cerebral d.** In electroencephalography, diffuse, complex, abnormal and disorganized electrical activity of cerebral origin. Some distinguish between slow dysrhythmia, in which theta or delta rhythm predominates, and rapid dysrhythmia, in which the predominant frequencies are greater than 14 Hz. *Seldom used.* **cortical d.** In electroencephalography, any disorganization of the normal rhythms that is believed to originate in the cerebral cortex. **paroxysmal cerebral d.** Episodic, recurrent, or paroxysmal discharges of abnormal electrical activity as shown in the electroencephalogram, often associated with epilepsy. **d. pneumophrasia** A disorder in which speech is interrupted by an abnormal pattern of breathing. **sinus d.** SINUS ARRHYTHMIA.

**dyssomatognosia** \disō′mətägnō′zhə\ [DYS- + SOMATO- + Gk *-gnōs(is)* knowledge + -IA] A subjective impression that all, or part of, the body has become deformed, for example that it has become smaller, or that a limb or part of a limb belongs to someone else; a form of agnosia for somatic sensation; a defect of the body image. Compare ASOMATOGNOSIA.

**dyssomnia** \disäm′nē·ə\ Any disorder of sleep or abnormal sleep pattern.

**dysspermia** \dispur′mē·ə\ [DYS- + SPERM + -IA] An abnormal condition of the spermatozoa.

**dysstasia** \distā′zhə\ [DYS- + *-stas(is)* + -IA] Difficulty in standing. Also *dystasia.* Adj. dysstatic. **hereditary**

**areflexic d.** ROUSSY-LÉVY SYNDROME.

**dysstatic** \distat′ik\ Pertaining to or affected by dysstasia.

**dyssynergia** \dis′inur′jē·ə\ [DYS- + Gk *synergia* (from SYN- + Gk *erg(on)* work + -IA) assistance, cooperation] ATAXIA. **d. cerebellaris myoclonica** A degenerative condition of autosomal recessive inheritance affecting chiefly the cerebellar dentate nuclei and the superior cerebellar peduncles. The condition, which has its onset in infancy, gives rise to epileptic seizures, myoclonus, and progressive cerebellar ataxia with severe dysarthria. Also *progressive cerebellar tremor, Ramsay Hunt syndrome, dyssynergia cerebellaris progressiva, dentate cerebellar ataxia, cerebellofugal degeneration ataxia, progressive cerebellar asynergy, cerebellofugal degeneration, Hunt's disease.*

**dyssynergy** \disin′ərjē\ [See DYSSYNERGIA.] ATAXIA.

**dystasia** \distā′zhə\ [*dy(s)-* + *-stas(is)* + -IA] DYSSTASIA.

**dystaxia** \distak′sē·ə\ [DYS- + *(a)taxia*] An attenuated form of ataxia. *Seldom used.*

**dystectia** \distek′shə\ [DYS- + L *tect(um)* a covering, roof + -IA] DYSRAPHIA.

**dysthymia** \disthīm′ē·ə\ [Gk (from DYS- + *thym(os)* temper, spirit + -IA) despondency] Depression, usually of less severity than psychotic depression or major depressive disorder.

**dystocia** \distō′shə\ [Gk *dystokia* (from DYS- + *tokos* childbirth) difficult delivery] Abnormally slow progress in labor due to ineffective uterine contractions, abnormality of fetal size or presentation, or abnormalities of the birth canal. These conditions may occur individually or in combination.

**dystonia** \distō′nē·ə\ [DYS- + Gk *ton(os)* tension + -IA] Any abnormality of muscle tone. Adj. dystonic. **attitudinal d.** Any of various symptomatic forms of torsion spasm or dystonia, secondary to infection such as epidemic encephalitis or to degenerative lesions such as hepatolenticular degeneration, in contrast to primary torsion spasm or dystonia musculorum deformans. **autonomic d.** Impaired excitability of the autonomic nervous system, which can be seen as sympathicotonia, as vagotonia, or as simultaneous hyperexcitability of both sympathetic and vagal nervous systems (amphotonia). **d. deformans progressiva** DYSTONIA MUSCULORUM DEFORMANS. **hypersympatheticotonic d.** SYMPATHETICOTONIA. **kinetic d.** Localized dystonic movements, often restricted to certain muscle groups in the head, trunk, or limbs. It is a localized form of torsion spasm or dystonia musculorum deformans, and may be symptomatic of a focal brain lesion or, like the generalized form, of unknown cause. **lenticular d.** Dystonia associated with a lesion of the lenticular nucleus. Also *dystonia lenticularis.* **d. musculorum deformans** A rare progressive disorder of the nervous system which sometimes occurs sporadically but is more often inherited. The principal tissue changes are in the basal ganglia but are very poorly defined. A severe form with autosomal recessive inheritance is seen particularly in Jews and begins in childhood or adolescence. A less severe dominantly inherited form of later onset has also been described. The condition usually begins with a gait disorder due to inversion and plantar flexion of one foot, but eventually there develop fixed alterations in posture with involuntary movements and rigidity involving especially the axial muscles of the head, neck and trunk, and walking becomes impossible. Also *torsion dystonia, torsion spasm, progressive torsion spasm, dystonia deformans progressiva, dysbasia lordotica progressiva, Ziehen-Oppenheim disease, tortipelvis.* **periodic d.** PAROXYSMAL KINESOGENIC CHOREOATHETOSIS. **torsion d.** DYSTONIA MUSCULORUM DEFORMANS.

**dystonic** \distän′ik\ Pertaining to or suffering from dystonia.

**dystopia** \distō′pē·ə\ [DYS- + Gk *top(os)* a place + -IA] ECTOPIA. **crossed d. of the kidney** A congenital anomaly in which, during embryonic life, one kidney crosses the midline to the other side. The abnormally placed kidney usually is small and below the normal kidney. The crossing kidney sometimes may be fused with its mate. The long, tortuous course of the blood vessels and ureter makes obstruction common. The diagnosis is made by intravenous pyelography. **simple renal d.** An abnormal position of one or both kidneys in a lumbar, iliac, or pelvic position. Pelvic kidneys often are fused. Also *simple renal ectopia.*

**dystrophia** \distrō′fē·ə\ [DYS- + Gk *troph(ē)* nourishment + -IA] DYSTROPHY. **d. adiposogenitalis** FRÖHLICH SYNDROME. **d. brevicollis** A condition manifested in features similar to the Fröhlich syndrome, accompanied by a foreshortening of the neck into the shoulders. It is not associated with congenital segmental defects of the cervical spine, as is seen in the Klippel-Feil syndrome. **d. mediana canaliformis** MEDIAN CANALIFORM DYSTROPHY OF THE NAIL. **d. myotonica** A dominantly inherited condition characterized by myotonia, often best demonstrated in the tongue and hand muscles, and associated with a progressive muscular dystrophy which involves particularly the facial muscles, the sternomastoids and the distal muscles of the limbs but not initially the small muscles of the hands and feet. Associated features include frontal baldness in the male, testicular atrophy, cataracts, cardiomyopathy, thickness of the skull vault, a small sella turcica, and abnormalities of the serum immunoglobulins. Infants suffering from the disease, almost invariably born to affected mothers rather than fathers, display developmental delay, generalized hypotonia, and sometimes mental retardation, and develop the more characteristic features of the disease in adolescence. Also *myotonia atrophica, myotonic myopathy, Steinert's disease, myotonic dystrophy, myotonic atrophy, myotonia dystrophica.* **d. unguis mediana canaliformis** MEDIAN CANALIFORM DYSTROPHY OF THE NAIL. **d. unguium** Any abnormality of the nails.

**dystrophic** \disträf′ik\ [DYS- + -TROPHIC] Pertaining to improper nutrition.

**dystrophoneurosis** \disträf′ōnʸŭrō′sis\ [DYS- + TROPHO- + NEUROSIS] Any disease of the nervous system that leads to malnutrition, such as anorexia nervosa, or that arises from malnutrition, such as the Wernicke-Korsakoff syndrome which is due to vitamin $B_1$ deficiency.

**dystrophy** \dis′trəfē\ [New L *dystrophia.* See DYSTROPHIA.] A degeneratve disorder of the structure or function of an organ due to improper nutrition. Such abnormalities include a wide variety of conditions, including neuromuscular disorders, and are often congenital. Also *dystrophia, paratrophy* (obs.). **adiposogenital d.** FRÖHLICH SYNDROME. **Albright's d.** ALBRIGHT'S HEREDITARY OSTEODYSTROPHY. **arthritic d.** Dystrophy, usually rheumatoid in type, with typical deformities of hands and feet as well as large joints. Because of disuse as well as the rheumatoid pathology, there is marked osteoporosis of bones. **asphyxiating thoracic d.** A generalized skeletal dysplasia that is inherited as an autosomal recessive trait and that causes respiratory distress and most often death in infancy. Its features include a small, nonexpansile thorax, short ribs, deformity of the pelvis and limb bones, and renal changes. Also *Jeune syndrome, thoracic-pelvic-phalangeal dystrophy, asphyxiating thoracic dysplasia.* **Becker type muscular d.** Muscular dystrophy due to an X-linked recessive gene and having a pattern of muscular involvement which resembles that of the Duchenne type but with later onset and a course more benign, with survival usually into middle life. **Biber-Haab-Dimmer d.** LATTICE DYSTROPHY OF THE CORNEA. **congenital muscular d.** Any of a group of conditions, sometimes sporadic and sometimes of autosomal recessive inheritance, giving rise to severe infantile hypotonia from birth and motor developmental delay, in which the changes in the muscles resemble those of other forms of muscular dystrophy. Severe, rapidly progressive and fatal varieties have been described, but in some cases the condition is relatively benign and nonprogressive. *Imprecise.* **corneal d.** A spontaneous degeneration of the cornea having a genetic basis. See also GRANULAR CORNEAL DYSTROPHY, MACULAR CORNEAL DYSTROPHY. **crystalline d. of the cornea** A familial degeneration of the cornea in which discrete deposits may be seen in the stroma with slit lamp or pathologic section. **Dejerine-Landouzy d.** FACIOSCAPULOHUMERAL MUSCULAR DYSTROPHY. **distal muscular d.** Muscular dystrophy beginning in the distal muscles of the arms and legs and gradually spreading proximally. Some cases are sporadic, but an autosomal dominant form is also seen, especially in Sweden. **Duchenne-Landouzy d.** FACIOSCAPULOHUMERAL MUSCULAR DYSTROPHY. **Duchenne's progressive muscular d.** DUCHENNE TYPE MUSCULAR DYSTROPHY. **Duchenne type muscular d.** The commonest and most severe form of muscular dystrophy, due to an X-linked recessive gene, and therefore manifest in males and transmitted by clinically unaffected carrier females. It usually begins with difficulty in walking, in rising from the floor and in climbing stairs at about the age of three years, causes confinement to a wheelchair by the age of 10 years, and results in death from respiratory infection or cardiac failure, due to an associated cardiomyopathy, by about the age of 20. In the early stages enlargement (pseudohypertrophy) of certain muscles, as calves and deltoids, is common. Later contractures and skeletal deformity are common. Also *Duchenne's progressive muscular dystrophy, Duchenne's myopathy, pseudohypertrophic muscular atrophy, Duchenne's disease, Duchenne's paralysis, pseudohypertrophic muscular dystrophy* (outmoded). **endothelial corneal d.** Degeneration of the posterior cellular layer of the cornea. **facioscapulohumeral muscular d.** A dominantly inherited form of muscular dystrophy, sometimes beginning in childhood but more often in adolescence or early adult life, resulting in facial muscular weakness with a typical pouting appearance of the lips, early selective atrophy of scapulohumeral muscles and early involvement of the anterior tibial and peroneal muscles in the legs. The condition shows marked variation in severity in different affected members of the same family but many cases run an exceptionally benign course with a normal life expectation. Also *Landouzy-Dejerine myopathy, Landouzy-Dejerine atrophy, facioscapulohumeral atrophy, Dejerine-Landouzy dystrophy, Duchenne-Landouzy dystrophy, Landouzy's dystrophy, Landouzy-Dejerine dystrophy.* **Fröhlich's adiposogenital d.** FRÖHLICH SYNDROME. **Fuchs d.** Degeneration of the corneal endothelium. **granular corneal d.** A genetic disorder characterized by degeneration of the cornea marked by the presence of grayish white granules within the stroma. It is autosomal dominant. Also *Groenouw type I corneal dystrophy.* **Groenouw type I corneal d.** GRANULAR CORNEAL DYSTROPHY. **Groenouw type II corneal d.** MACULAR CORNEAL DYSTROPHY. **gutter d. of cornea** A degeneration causing a loss of the surface thickness near the periphery of the cornea. **hypophysial d.** HYPOPITUITARISM. **infantile neuroaxonal d.** A rare, progressive recessively inherited form of neurodegenerative disease with neonatal onset. It is characterized by cerebellar cortical atrophy, internal hydrocephalus, spongy degeneration and lipid accumulation in the caudate and lenticular nuclei and globus pallidus, and axonal degeneration in the optic tracts and the posterior columns of the spinal cord. The clinical signs are arrest of mental and physical development marked by an inability to learn how to walk and talk, generalized hypotonia, arreflexia and later spasticity, contractures, hyperreflexia and ataxia, double incontinence, pendular nystagmus, amaurosis, vestibular defects, and deafness. Also *Seitelberger syndrome, neuroaxonal dystrophy, Seitelberger's disease, neuroaxonal proteid dystrophy, progressive neuroaxonal dystrophy, spastic amaurotic axonal idiocy* (obs.). **juvenile progressive muscular d.** LIMB-GIRDLE MUSCULAR DYSTROPHY. **Landouzy's d.** FACIOSCAPULOHUMERAL MUSCULAR DYSTROPHY. **Landouzy-Dejerine d.** FACIOSCAPULOHUMERAL MUSCULAR DYSTROPHY. **lattice d. of the cornea** A genetic degeneration of the cornea, in which opaque lines traverse the corneal stroma, fancifully compared to a lattice pattern. Also *Biber-Haab-Dimmer dystrophy.* **Leyden-Möbius d.** LIMB-GIRDLE MUSCULAR DYSTROPHY. **limb-girdle muscular d.** A form of muscular dystrophy, usually of autosomal recessive inheritance, which begins in adolescence or adult life and runs a relatively benign course. It may begin in either the shoulder girdle (scapulohumeral muscular dystrophy) or the pelvic girdle (pelvifemoral muscular dystrophy), spreading to the other muscle group after an interval that may be many years. Many cases so diagnosed in the past have proved to be spinal muscular atrophy or, in the pelvifemoral group, Becker type muscular dystrophy. Also *juvenile progressive muscular dystrophy, Simmerlin's dystrophy, Erb's palsy, Erb's paralysis, Leyden-Möbius dystrophy.* **macular corneal d.** A genetic disorder characterized by progressive degeneration of the cornea marked by the presence of gray, punctate opacities within the stroma. Onset is usually between 5–9 years of age. It is autosonal recessive. Also *Groenouw Type II corneal dystrophy.* **median canaliform d. of the nail** A split of the canal in the nail plate, usually just off-center, that starts at the cuticle and progresses to the free edge. Feathery cracks extend laterally from the split, giving the appearance of an inverted fir tree. Its cause is unknown. Also *median nail dystrophy, solenonychia, dystrophia unguis mediana canaliformis, dystrophia mediana canaliformis.* **muscular d.** Any of a group of genetically determined, primary degenerative myopathies of unknown etiology, characterized by various patterns of selective atrophy and weakness of the voluntary muscles, leading as a rule to progressive disability. In some types, certain muscles demonstrate, at least for a time, enlargement or pseudohypertrophy. The tendon reflexes are lost early in the affected muscles, and muscular contractures and skeletal deformity are common in the later stages. Various enzymes, as transaminases, aldolase, and creatine kinase, are increased in the blood serum, electromyography shows myopathic changes, and muscle biopsy demonstrates random variation in muscle size and shape, necrosis and phagocytosis of fibers, regenerative activity, and infiltration with fat and connective tissue in varying degree. Also *progressive muscular dystrophy, primary progressive myopathy, progressive atrophic myopathy, primary progressive amyotrophy, Erb-Landouzy disease, myodystrophia, myodystrophy, Erb's disease.* Abbr. MD **myotonic d.** DYSTROPHIA MYOTONICA. **neuroaxonal d.** INFANTILE NEUROAXONAL DYSTROPHY. **neuroaxonal proteid d.** INFANTILE NEUROAXONAL DYSTROPHY. **ocular muscular d.** Progressive muscular dystrophy involving the external ocular muscles. Some degree of involvement of the facial and limb muscles is also seen in most cases and the condition may be sporadic or of autosomal recessive or dominant inheritance. **oculocerebrorenal d.** OCULOCEREBRORENAL SYNDROME. **oculopharyngeal muscular d.** A muscular dystrophy which affects first the external ocular and pharyngeal muscles, giving rise to bilateral ptosis, impairment of ocular movement in all directions and dysphagia, followed by variable involvement of facial, trunk and limb muscles. It is usually of autosomal dominant inheritance and many affected families have proved to be of French-Canadian ancestry. Recent evidence suggests that morphologic changes in the mitochondria can usually be seen by electron microscopy in the affected muscles. **progressive muscular d.** MUSCULAR DYSTROPHY. **progressive neuroaxonal d.** INFANTILE NEUROAXONAL DYSTROPHY. **progressive tapetochoroidal d.** CHOROIDEREMIA. **pseudohypertrophic muscular d.** 1 Any of the forms of muscular dystrophy in which enlargement or pseudohypertrophy of muscle occurs. This is most often seen in the Duchenne and Becker types. Also *atrophia musculorum lipomatosa.* 2 *Outmoded* DUCHENNE TYPE MUSCULAR DYSTROPHY. **reflex sympathetic d.** 1 REFLEX DYSTROPHY OF THE UPPER EXTREMITY. 2 SYMPATHETIC DYSTROPHY. **reflex d. of the upper extremity** A painful swelling of the hand, usually but not invariably associated with pericapsulitis of the shoulder joint (a "frozen" shoulder). In long-lasting cases osteoporosis and atrophy of the bones of the hand may develop (Sudeck's atrophy). The condition is usually relieved by sympathectomy. Also *hand-shoulder syndrome, shoulder-hand syndrome, reflex sympathetic dystrophy.* **sex-linked muscular d.** X-LINKED MUSCULAR DYSTROPHY. **Simmerlin's d.** LIMB-GIRDLE MUSCULAR DYSTROPHY. **speckled d. of the cornea** A familial degeneration of the cornea in which irregular mottling of the cornea is visible upon biomicroscopic examination. **sympathetic d.** A poorly understood disease of the sympathetic nerves, occurring after sometimes trivial trauma to an extremity. The extremity becomes painful, swollen, erythematous, hyperesthetic, and sensitive to temperature fluctuations. The condition can be relieved by sympathetic denervation of the limb. Also *reflex sympathetic dystrophy.* **tapetochoroidal d.** CHOROIDEREMIA. **thoracic-pelvic-phalangeal d.** ASPHYXIATING THORACIC DYSTROPHY. **vitelliform macular d.** VITELLIFORM MACULAR DEGENERATION. **X-linked muscular d.** The Duchenne and Becker types of muscular dystrophy. Much rarer X-linked subvarieties have been described, and scapuloperoneal muscular dystrophy is rarely due to an X-linked gene. Also *sex-linked muscular dystrophy.*

**dysuria** \disyoo′rē·ə\ [Gk *dysouria* (from DYS- + *our(ein)* to urinate + -IA) difficulty in urinating] Painful or difficult urination, generally caused by lower urinary tract disease, such as cystitis, urethritis, urethral stricture, and prostatic disease. Also *dysuresia.* **spastic d.** Difficulty in urinating caused by bladder spasm.

**dysvitaminosis** \dis′vītəminō′sis\ [DYS- + VITAMIN + -OSIS] Any disease due to an intake of too little of a given vitamin (as beriberi, rickets, or pellagra) or too much of a given vitamin.

# E

**E** 1 Symbol for exa-: used with SI units. 2 Symbol for glutamic acid.

**E.** 1 emmetropia. 2 eye.

**$E_1$** A symbol for the first generation to appear after the exposure of a progenitor cell or a parental organism to some mutagen, often irradiation.

**$E_h$** The oxidation-reduction potential of a given solution or combination of reactants, calculated from the standard redox potential of the electron-donor and electron-receptor pair and the concentrations of donor and acceptor species actually present.

**e-** \e-, i-\ EX-[1].

**(*E*)-** [German *entgegen* opposite] A stereochemical prefix describing the placing of substituents about a double bond, e.g. C═C. Substituents are placed in a priority order based on atomic number of the nearest atom. If this atom is identical for two substituents, the atom with the substituent of highest priority takes priority. Supplementary rules define the order in more complex cases. If the double bond has the two substituents of highest priority on opposite sides it is designated (*E*)-, if the reverse, it is designated (*Z*)-.

**EA** 1 erythrocyte antibody 2 educational age.

**EAC** erythrocyte antibody complement.

**EACA** ϵ aminocaproic acid.

**ead.** *eadem* (L, the same).

**EAE** experimental allergic encephalomyelitis.

**EAHF** eczema, asthma, and hay fever. See under EAHF complex.

**Eales** [Henri *Eales,* English physician, 1852–1913] See under DISEASE.

**EAP** epiallopregnanolone.

**ear** [Old English *ēare* (akin to L *auris* and Gk *ous,* gen. *ōtos*)] 1 The organ of hearing; auris. 2 The auricula, or external ear. *Popular.* **artificial e.** ACOUSTIC COUPLER. **bat e.** LOP EAR. **Blainville e.'s** Asymmetrical auricles of the ear. **cat e.** An auricle of the ear folded downward upon itself. **cauliflower e.** A severe deformity of the auricle resulting from injury, often repeated injury, to the external ear. Also *prizefighter ear.* **cockleshell e.** A severe form of constricted ear in which the ear appears to be tubular in shape. **constricted e.** A variety of congenital deformity of the ear in which the helix appears to have been shortened, causing protrusion and cupping of the ear. **Darwin's e.** An auricle of the ear in which the superior border of the helix is not rolled over and has an angular contour suggestive of the ear of certain monkeys. **dead e.** The ear, so damaged by disease, drugs, or trauma, including surgical trauma, that all function, both hearing and vestibular, is destroyed. This is judged and demonstrated by the absence of audiometric and caloric responses. **external e.** AURIS EXTERNA. **glue e.** *Popular* SECRETORY OTITIS MEDIA. **inner e.** AURIS INTERNA. **internal e.** AURIS INTERNA. **lop e.** An auricle that lacks the usual degree of flaring and appears to emerge from the side of the head at a right angle. Also *bat ear.* **middle e.** AURIS MEDIA. **Morel e.** A congenitally abnormal auricle characterized by large size, reduced sharpness of the usual folds, grooves, and contours, and edges that tend to be thinner than usual. **Mozart e.** A congenitally abnormal auricle in which the crura of the antihelix and the helix are united so as to cause the upper part of the auricle to bulge outward. • The composer Wolfgang A. Mozart is said to have had this deformity. **outer e.** *Seldom used* AURIS EXTERNA. **prizefighter e.** CAULIFLOWER EAR. **satyr e.** A congenitally abnormal auricle in which the helix lacks the usual rolled contour and the tubercle is unusually prominent. **scroll e.** A congenitally abnormal auricle in which the posterior margin is rolled forward. **shell e.** An ear in which the helical fold is absent. **No. 1 Stahl e.** A congenitally abnormal auricle in which the helix and antihelix coalesce, tending to obliterate the fossa scaphoidea and the fossa ovalis cordis. **No. 2 Stahl e.** A congenitally abnormal auricle in which the antihelix has three instead of the usual two crura. **Wildermuth's e.** A congenitally abnormal auricle in which the helix is deficient or is rolled toward the head, rather than away from it. The antihelix thus forms the most prominent part of the external ear.

**earache** Pain in the ear, often of a prolonged nature. A variety of otalgia, earache may or may not be due to disease of the ear. Pain may be referred to the ear from disease in an adjacent site such as the teeth or pharynx.

**eardrum** MEMBRANA TYMPANI.

**earlobe** The soft, lowest part of the auricle of the ear, situated below the antitragus, devoid of cartilage and consisting of fatty and fibrous tissue; lobulus auriculae.

**earphone** The electroacoustical component of a headset, telephone, or hearing-aid receiver, by which electrical energy is converted into sound. **electrostatic e.** An earphone with an electrical charge between one electrode or backplate and the diaphragm which forms the other electrode. It is driven by the alternating voltage output of an amplifier.

**earpit** PREAURICULAR SINUS.

**earth** Soil; dirt. Also *terra.* **alkaline e.** **1** Any of the metallic elements beryllium, magnesium, calcium, strontium, barium, or radium. They are characterized by easy oxidation of the metal to the 2+ cation. **2** Any of the oxides of these metals. The original, but now outmoded usage. **diatomaceous e.** A compound containing 96 percent silica derived from the siliceous skeletons of aquatic plants. It is used as an abrasive or for polishing, filtering, or insulating. Heavy exposure can cause pneumoconiosis. Also *infusorial earth, siliceous earth, diatomite, kieselguhr.*

**earwax** CERUMEN.

**earwig** [Old English *erwicga,* from *ēare* ear + *wicga* insect, worm] A member of the insect order Dermaptera (*Foricula auricularia*), so named because of the popular notion that it could wriggle its way into the head through the ear. Although not infrequently, and in common with many other insects, it finds its way into the external auditory meatus, it is fortunately unable to proceed further and may be removed without difficulty.

**eating / binge e.** See under BULIMIA.

**Eaton**

**Eaton** [Monroe Davis *Eaton,* U.S. bacteriologist, born 1904] **1** See under AGENT. **2** Eaton agent pneumonia. See under MYCOPLASMAL PNEUMONIA.

**EB** elementary body.

***Eberthella*** \ē′bərthel′ə\ A former genus of enteric pathogens, especially *E. typhosa,* now absorbed into the larger genus *Salmonella.*

**Ebner** [Anton Gilbert Viktor *Ebner* von Rofenstein, Austrian physician and histologist, 1842–1925] **1** Ebner's glands. See under GLANDULA GUSTATORIA. **2** See under RETICULUM.

**ebriety** \ēbrī′ətē\ DRUNKENNESS.

**Ebstein** [Wilhelm *Ebstein* German internist, pathologist, and medical historian, 1836–1912] **1** Ebstein's malformation. See under ANOMALY. **2** Ebstein-like malformation of the mitral valve. See under MALFORMATION. **3** Armanni-Ebstein cells. See under CELL. **4** Armanni-Ebstein change. See under CHANGE. **5** Ebstein's lesion. See under ARMANNI-EBSTEIN LESION. **6** Murchison-Pel-Ebstein fever, Pel-Ebstein pyrexia, Pel-Ebstein symptom. See under PEL-EBSTEIN FEVER.

**ebullition** \eb′əlish′ən\ [Late L *ebullitio* (from *e(x)-* out + *bullire* to bubble, from *bulla* a bubble) a boiling or bubbling up] The act or process of boiling in which a liquid vaporizes rapidly, producing bubbles and turbulent movement.

**eburnation** \ē′bərnā′shən\ [L *eburn(us)* made of or pertaining to ivory + -ATION] **1** The thinning or absence of articular cartilage, as occurs in degenerative joint disease, such that the subchondral bone is exposed and lines parts of the articular cavity. With time, this bone becomes dense and acquires a polished appearance. Also *bone sclerosis.* **2** The polished, burnished appearance taken on by exposed dentin; dentin eburnation. See also SCLEROTIC DENTIN.

**eburneous** \ēbur′nē·əs\ [L *eburneus* made of or pertaining to ivory] Having the appearance of ivory.

**EBV** Epstein-Barr virus.

**EC** Initials used before a number to signify that this number is allotted in *Enzyme Nomenclature,* published for the International Union of Biochemistry (originally by the "Enzyme Commission" of the Union). The numbers that follow allot the enzyme to the class of reaction that it catalyzes.

**ec-** \ek-, ik-\ EX-[2].

**ecbolic** \ekbäl′ik\ [Gk *ekbol(ē)* (from *ekballein* to throw out, expel, from *ek-* out + *ballein* to throw) expulsion, throwing out + -IC] OXYTOCIC.

**ecbolium** An agent that causes contractions of the uterus and may cause abortion or induce parturition.

**ecbovirus** \ek′bōvī′rəs\ [from *e(nteric) c(ytopathogenic) b(ovine) o(rphan)* + VIRUS] Any of a group of nonpathogenic picornaviruses isolated from cattle. Also *ECBO virus.*

**eccentric** \eksen′trik\ **1** Deviating from a center or from a usual course. **2** Occurring or located away from a center or from a usual position or location.

**eccentrochondro-osteodystrophy** \eksen′trəkän′drō-äs′tē·ədis′trəfē\ MUCOPOLYSACCHARIDOSIS IV.

**ecchondroma** \ek′ändrō′mə\ OSTEOCHONDROMA.

**ecchondrosis** \ek′ändrō′sis\ [EC- + CHONDR- + -OSIS ] Multiple osteochondromas (ecchondromas).

**ecchondrotome** \ekän′drətōm\ [EC- + CHONDRO- + -TOME] An instrument for excising cartilage.

**ecchymosis** \ek′imō′sis\ [Gk *ekchymōsis* (from EK- + Gk *chymos* juice, from *cheein* to pour out, shed, spill) ecchymosis] (*pl.* ecchymoses) A discoloration of the skin caused by the extravasation of blood. **Roederer's e.** Areas of ecchymosis or petechiae on the pleural and pericardial surfaces of stillborn infants believed to be secondary to attempted respiration.

**eccrine** \ek′rin, ek′rīn\ [Gk *ekkrin(ein)* (from *ek-* out + *krinein* to separate) to separate out, excrete] **1** Of or relating to a secretion from the sweat gland that is produced without the loss of cell substance and gives rise to ordinary watery sweat. Compare APOCRINE. **2** EXOCRINE.

**ecdemic** \ekdem′ik\ [Gk *ekdēm(os)* away from home + -IC] Relating to a nonlocalized factor, as a disease caused by an imported factor or organism.

**ecdysis** \ek′disis\ [Gk *ekdysis* a shedding, putting off] The shedding of the outer layer of skin or of a shell. This process is common in many species of animals and insects, not only during development but also during the adult stage. **erythrocytic e.** ERYTHROCYTORRHEXIS.

**ECF** 1 eosinophil chemotactic factor. 2 extracellular fluid.

**ECG** electrocardiogram.

**echidnin** \əkid′nin\ The toxic principle in viper venom.

***Echidnophaga gallinacea*** \ek′idnäf′əgə gal′inā′sē·ə\ The sticktight flea, an important pest of poultry, occurring worldwide and known to attack humans. The adult fleas tend to form dense masses on the heads of chickens and in the ears of other domestic animals.

**echin-** \əkīn-, ek′in-\ ECHINO-.

**echinate** \ek′ināt\ [ECHIN- + -ATE] ECHINULATE.

**echino-** \əkī′nō-\ [Gk *echinos* hedgehog, urchin, prickly shell] A combining form meaning spiny, prickly. Also *echin-*.

**echinococcosis** \-käkō′sis\ [*Echinococc(us)* + -OSIS] A disease caused by the presence and growth of larval tapeworms or hydatids of the genus *Echinococcus*. The most common form is the unilocular hydatid cyst of *E. granulosus* which usually develops in the liver but may also develop in the lung, brain, kidney, spleen, the peritoneal cavity, or within the long bones, among other sites. The other type is the alveolar or multilocular hydatid cyst of *E. multilocularis*. The disease occurs wherever sheep and dogs live in close contact with man. Human infection is from food contaminated with dog feces, which contain larvae of the parasite. Also *hydatid disease, echinococciasis, hydatidosis*. **e. of the kidney** A hydatid cyst in the kidney parenchyma manifested by hematuria and loin pain.

**echinococcotomy** \-käkät′əmē\ [*Echinococc(us)* + -TOMY] The surgical removal of a hydatid cyst, usually from liver, peritoneum, lung, or brain tissue.

***Echinococcus*** \ekī′nōkäk′əs\ [ECHINO- + New L *coccus* (from Gk *kokkos* seed, berry, oak gall) a berrylike object or cyst] A genus of small cyclophyllidean tapeworms of the family Taeniidae. The adult worms, found in canids and other carnivores but not in humans, are extremely small, consisting of only two or three segments. Larvae form hydatid cysts in various herbivorous mammals and in humans. ***E. alveolaris*** *ECHINOCOCCUS MULTILOCULARIS*. ***E. granulosus*** A species in which the adult worm is found in dogs, wolves, and rarely, in cats. The larvae may develop in nearly all mammals including man. Larval forms produce slow-growing unilocular hydatid cysts usually in the liver but also in lungs, kidneys, and other organs. A dog-sheep cycle is common in sheep-raising areas, though a zoonotic cycle may also occur. Also *Taenia echinococcus*. ***E. multilocularis*** The alveohydatid tapeworm of foxes, coyotes, dogs, and cats. The larvae are found in microtine rodents, and, infrequently, in herbivores and man. The larvae produce multilocular or alveolar cysts in the liver which are usually fatal to the host. Also *Echinococcus alveolaris*.

**echinocyte** \əkī′nōsīt\ [ECHINO- + -CYTE] An erythrocyte with evenly distributed, uniform thorny membrane projections. It is seen in azotemia and in some erythrocyte enzyme deficiencies. Also *burr cell, burr erythrocyte, crenocyte, crenated erythrocyte*.

***Echinolaelaps*** \-lē′laps\ A genus of mites in the large family Laelaptidae. They are found on rodents and are common in stable litter. The bite, for humans, causes intense itching. Some species are vectors of parasitic sporozoans of the genus *Hepatozoon*. Also *Laelaps, Lelaps*.

**echinophthalmia** \əkī′näfthal′mē·ə\ [ECHIN- + OPHTHALMIA] MARGINAL BLEPHARITIS.

***Echinorhynchus*** \-ring′kəs\ [ECHINO- + Gk *rhynchos* a snout, beak] A genus of acanthocephalan worms that are parasitic in various fishes. ***E. gigas*** *MACRACANTHORHYNCHUS HIRUDINACEUS*. ***E. hominis*** *MACRACANTHORHYNCHUS HIRUDINACEUS*.

***Echinostoma*** \ek′inäs′tōmə\ A genus of parasitic trematodes of the family Echinostomatidae with a cosmopolitan distribution and a wide range of hosts and including several species that have been found in humans. They parasitize the small intestine and may cause enteritis. ***E. malayanum*** A species that is normally parasitic in swine, but which is also reported in humans in Southeast Asia. Human infection occurs through ingestion of metacercariae in freshwater snails. Also *Artyfechinostomum sufrartyfex*..

**echinulate** \əkin′yəlāt\ [Late L *echinul(us)*, dim. of L *echinus* sea urchin, prickly polycarp of a chestnut, from Gk *echinos* sea urchin, hedgehog + -ATE] Covered with very small spines or prickles; having spiny projections or outgrowths. Also *echinate*.

***Echis*** \ē′kis\ A genus of venomous snakes of the family Viperidae occurring in Africa and western Asia. Specimens are usually less than one meter in length. The genus includes *E. carinatus*, the carpet viper.

**echnothiophate iodide** $C_9H_{23}INO_3PS$. 2-[(Diethoxyphosphinyl)-thio]-*N,N,N*-trimethylethanaminium iodide. An organophosphate type of anticholinesterase compound. It is used for its cholingeric activity and long duration in the treatment of chronic glaucoma.

**echo** \ek′ō\ [L, from Gk *ēchō* an echo] 1 A repetition of sounds due to reflection by an obstacle. 2 Any repetition of a wave pattern by reflection, or by other process of reconstruction after a time delay. 3 Any imitative repetition. **cochlear e.** Stimulated acoustic emission in response to a transient stimulus, usually a click. In humans this response is delayed by 5–15 msec, and is clearly distinguishable from the stimulus. Also *Kemp echo*. **metallic e.** A metallic quality of heart sounds encountered in some patients with pneumothorax or pneumopericardium. **midline e.** The ultrasonic echo from midline intracranial structures. A displacement is regarded as indicative of an intracranial lesion, pressure from which has shifted the midline structures.

**echocardiogram** \-kär′dē·əgram′\ [ECHO + CARDIOGRAM] The display obtained by echocardiography, an ultrasound image of the heart.

**echocardiography** \ek′ōkär′dē·äg′rəfē\ [ECHO + CARDIOGRAPHY] The recording of an ultrasound image of the heart. A transducer, usually placed on the chest wall, is employed to transmit very high frequency waves that are reflected from tissue interfaces and to detect the reflected waves. Also *ultrasonic cardiography*. **cross-sectional e.** Echocardiography in which a moving image of the heart is obtained by mechanical or electronic scanning. In the former method, the beam is moved in an arc by a mechanical scanner, the transducer is oscillated, or a series of transducers is rotated. In the latter, a phased-array system of multiple ultrasonic elements is steered electronically. Also *real-time echocardiography, two-dimensional echocardiography*. **M-mode e.** Echocardiography in which the reflected sound waves are displayed on a graph in which the horizontal axis represents time and the vertical axis distance from the transducer. **real-time e.** CROSS-SECTIONAL ECHOCARDIOGRAPHY. **two-dimensional e.** CROSS-SECTIONAL ECHOCARDIOGRAPHY.

**echoencephalogram** \-ensef′əlōgram′\ [ECHO + ENCEPHALOGRAM] The trace recorded by echoencephalography. In the simple A-scan, echoes are produced by reflection of the ultrasound pulses from the inner and outer tables of the skull and from midline structures. By measuring the distance of the midline from the inner table of the skull when recordings are made from each side, it can be determined whether the midline is displaced. With more sophisticated equipment, the B-scan can give an indication of the cerebral ventricular outline and other useful information.

**echoencephalograph** \-ensef′əlōgraf′\ [ECHO + ENCEPHALOGRAPH] The instrument used for carrying out echoencephalography. The standard A-scan equipment consists of a device for emission of high-frequency ultrasound, which excites a transducer that converts reflected ultrasound into electrical oscillations; a circuit for detection and a circuit for amplification; a cathode-ray screen, which displays the electrical signals; and a camera, which records the display (the echoencephalogram). **midline e.** An echoencephalograph which measures the echo distance between each lateral surface of the skull and the midline structures of the brain. Any inequality indicates displacement of the midline structures. A midline echoencephalograph is performed by a computerized unit which calculates any degree of shift and displays it on a bar graph.

**echoencephalography** \-ensef′äläg′rəfē\ [ECHO + ENCEPHALOGRAPHY] A technique for examining the intracranial structures with the use of ultrasound. Space-occupying lesions may cause displacement of the echo which is reflected from midline structures in the brain. The transducer produces ultrasound pulses which are reflected when they encounter an obstacle. The transducer which is sensitive to reflected ultrasound, is placed on the temporoparietal region of the skull, against the top of the ear or near it. The reflected ultrasonic echoes are converted into an electrical signal which is seen on a cathode ray screen as vertical deflection of a horizontal baseline, the time interval between the starting and finishing signal indicating the position of the structure causing the echo. The electrical signal (the echoencephalogram) is recorded photographically. Also *neurosonology.*

**echogenic** \-jen′ik\ [ECHO + -GENIC] Producing echoes.

**echogenicity** \-jənis′itē\ [ECHOGENIC + -ITY] The echo-producing ability of a medium.

**echogram** \ek′ōgram\ ULTRASONOGRAM.

**echographia** \-graf′ē·ə\ [ECHO + -GRAPH + -IA ] Aphasia in which the patient cannot express his thoughts in writing but can copy a written or printed script.

**echography** \ekäg′rəfē\ ULTRASONOGRAPHY.

**echoing** \ek′ō·ing\ **thought e.** THOUGHT AUDITION.

**echokinesis** \-kinē′sis\ [ECHO + KINESIS] ECHOPRAXIA.

**echolalia** \-lā′lyə\ [ECHO + -LALIA] Spontaneous repetition of a meaningless phrase. Also *echophrasia, echo speech.*

**echomimia** \-mim′ē·ə\ [ECHO + Gk *mim(os)* an imitator + -IA] ECHOPRAXIA.

**echomotism** \-mō′tizm\ [ECHO + L *mot(us),* past part. of *movere* to move + -ISM] ECHOPRAXIA.

**echophrasia** \-frā′zhə\ [ECHO + Gk *phras(is)* speech + -IA] ECHOLALIA.

**echopraxia** \-prak′sē·ə\ [ECHO + Gk *prax(is)* a doing, acting + -IA] Pathologic imitation of another's actions, often compulsive or semiautomatic in nature. Also *echokinesis, echomimia, echomotism, hypermimia.*

**echoscope** \ek′ōskōp\ [ECHO + -SCOPE] ULTRASONOGRAPH.

**echovirus** \ek′ōvī′rəs\ [from *enteric cytopath(ogen)ic human orphan* + VIRUS] Any of a group of enteroviruses, constituting 31 serotypes and worldwide in distribution, which are a major cause of aseptic meningitis, a variety of exanthems and other febrile syndromes in humans. Echoviruses are a rare cause of epidemic pleurodynia. They may cause gastroenteritis and diarrhea. Also *ECHO virus.*

**Ecker** [Alexander *Ecker,* German anatomist, 1816–1887] Ecker's fissure. See under SULCUS OCCIPITALIS TRANSVERSUS.

**Ecker** [Enrique Eduardo *Ecker,* Dutch West Indian-born U.S. pathologist, born 1887] Rees and Ecker diluting fluid, Ecker's fluid. See under REES-ECKER SOLUTION.

**eclabium** \eklā′bē·əm\ [EC- + LABIUM] Eversion of the lip, as that due to the contraction of scar tissue.

**eclampsia** \iklamp′sē·ə\ [Gk *eklamps(is)* (from *ek-* out + *lampein* to shine) a flash, sudden development + -IA] The occurrence in a preeclamptic woman in the prepartum or postpartum of one or more convulsions that are not due to other cerebral conditions such as epilepsy or cerebral hemorrhage. Also *glomerular capillary endotheliosis.* Adj. eclamptic. **cerebral e.** Eclampsia with cerebral symptoms such as convulsions or coma. **e. nutans** *Obs.* INFANTILE MASSIVE SPASM. **puerperal e.** Eclampsia occurring in the puerperium. **superimposed e.** The development of eclampsia in a pregnant woman with preexisting chronic hypertensive or renal disease.

**eclampsism** \eklamp′sizm\ PREECLAMPSIA.

**eclamptogenic** \eklamp′təjen′ik\ Giving rise to eclampsia.

**eclipse** [Gk *ekleipsis* an eclipse] A stage in viral replication which occurs shortly after attachment and before the first appearance of new virions. During this stage, neither the original inoculum nor progeny virus is detectable. Also *eclipse period.*

**ecmnesia** \eknē′zhə\ [EC- + Gk *mnēs(is)* memory + -IA] Defective recent or short-term memory with retention of long-term memory.

**ecmovirus** \ek′mōvī′rəs\ [from *e(nteric) c(ytopathogenic) m(onkey) o(rphan)* + VIRUS] Any of a group of nonpathogenic picornaviruses isolated from monkey kidneys. Also *ECMO virus.*

**eco-** \ē′kō-, ek′ō-\ [Gk *oikos* house, household affairs or management] A combining form meaning (1) household; (2) environment, especially as it relates to the life of an organism or group of organisms. Also *oeco-, oiko-.*

**E.Coch.G.** electrocochleography.

***E. coli*** *Escherichia coli.*

**ecology** \ikäl′əjē\ [Gk *oikos* house, household + -LOGY] The study of the interrelationships between organisms and their environment. Also *bionomics.* **human e.** The science of ecology applied to human populations or groups.

**Economo** [Constantin Alexander von *Economo,* Austrian neurologist, 1876–1931] Economo's disease, von Economo's disease, Economo's encephalitis, von Economo's encephalitis. See under ENCEPHALITIS LETHARGICA.

**economy** \ikän′əmē\ [Gk *oikonomia* (from *oikos* house, household + *nom(os)* law, ordinance, usage + -IA) household management] **token e.** A technique of behavior therapy in which desired behavior, when it occurs, is rewarded by a concrete object, such as a token or scrip. The object may then be applied toward the purchase or acquisition of desired goods or services.

**ecoparasite** \-par′əsīt\ [ECO- + PARASITE] ECOSITE.

**écorché** \ākôrshā′\ [French, past part. of *écorcher* (from Late L *excorticare* to peel, from L *ex-* out + *cortex,* gen. *corticis,* rind, bark) to remove the skin] An anatomical presentation, either a painting, drawing, or manikin, of a human or animal without the skin, so as to reveal the muscles for study.

**ecosite** \ē′kōsīt\ [ECO- + *(para)site*] A microparasite to which the host is normally immune or well adapted. Also *oecosite, ecoparasite, oikosite.*

**ecotropic** \-träp′ik\ Of or pertaining to a virus that may either be integrated into the genome of a host cell as a provirus, or may propagate within those cells. Compare XENOTROPIC.

**ECS** electroconvulsive shock.

**ecsovirus** \ek′sōvī′rəs\ [from *e(nteric) c(ytopathogenic) s(wine) o(rphan)* + VIRUS] A picornavirus isolated from the intestine of swine that is cytopathogenic in tissue culture but causes no known disease. Also *ECSO virus*.

**ecstrophy** \ek′strəfē\ EXSTROPHY.

**ECT** electroconvulsive treatment (electroconvulsive therapy).

**ect-** \ekt-\ ECTO-.

**ectad** \ek′tad\ [ECT- + -AD] Directed outward; from the inside out.

**ectal** \ek′təl\ [ECT- + -AL] Outer or superficial; toward the outside of a part or the body.

**ectasia** \ektā′zhə\ [Gk *ektasis* (from EK- + Gk *tasis* a stretching, from *teinein* to stretch + -IA) a stretching out] The dilatation of a duct, vessel, or hollow viscus, usually resulting from obstruction to flow or intrinsic degenerative changes of the wall. Also *ectasis*. **corneal e.** KERATECTASIA. **diffuse arterial e.** CIRSOID ANEURYSM. **mammary duct e.** A chronic condition of the breast characterized by dilatation of the mammary ducts with inspissation of their secretions. Frequently this condition is part of fibrocystic disease of the breast and is associated with ductal and periductal chronic inflammation. **papillary e.** A circumscribed permanent dilatation of the dermal capillaries, as seen in angiokeratoma. **senile e.** Visibly dilated capillaries or venules seen in the elderly.

**ectasis** \ek′təsis\ [Gk *ektasis*. See ECTASIA.] ECTASIA.

**ectatic** \ektat′ik\ Of or relating to ectasia.

**ectethmoid** \ekteth′moid\ Either of the two labyrinths, or lateral masses, of the ethmoid bone.

**ecthyma** \ekthī′mə, ek′thimə\ [Gk *ekthyma* a pustule, pimple, breaking out] A heavily crusted pyogenic infection that leaves a scar. It is often seen on the legs and forearms of malnourished subjects. **e. gangrenosum** A necrotic and ulcerous skin lesion occurring in response to a focus of infection, as of *Pseudomonas aeruginosa*, often in malnourished children or in the newborn with impaired immune defenses. Instead of a healthy inflammatory response to infection, an ulcer deepens into a circular area of gangrene, beyond which is an intensely red flush. **e. syphiliticum** The ulcerated pustular skin lesions of syphilis. **e. vacciniform syphiloide** Ecthyma resembling that of tertiary syphilis.

**ecto-** \ek′tō-, ek′tə-\ [Gk *ektos* outside, without, out of] A prefix meaning outside, external, without. Also *ect-*.

**ectobiology** \-bī·äl′əjē\ The study of the properties, composition, specific enzymes, and binding sites of the cell surface.

**ectoblast** \ek′təblast\ [ECTO- + -BLAST] ECTODERM. **primary e.** A superficial layer of the early embryo, from which the chordamesoderm has not yet separated, and which invaginates from the primitive streak and from Hensen's node to give rise to the chordamesoderm.

**ectocardia** \-kär′dē·ə\ [ECTO- + -CARDIA] The developmental misplacement of the heart, especially in an external position.

**ectocondyle** \-kän′dīl\ The lateral condyle of a bone.

**ectocornea** \-kôr′nē·ə\ LAMINA LIMITANS ANTERIOR CORNEAE.

**ectocranial** \-krā′nē·əl\ Pertaining to the exterior of the skull. Also *exocranial*.

**ectocyst** \ek′təsist\ [ECTO- + CYST] The outer laminated membrane of a hydatid cyst or the outer portion of a dermoid cyst.

**ectoderm** \ek′tədurm′\ [ECTO- + -DERM] A superficial germ layer developing on the outside of the embryo. It differentiates into neuroblast and epiblast and will give rise, on the one hand, to the nervous system and elements of the special senses under the inductive influence of axial chordamesoderm, and on the other hand to the epidermis and its derivatives under the influence of the lateral mesoderm. Also *ectoblast*. Adj. ectodermal, ectodermic. **amniotic e.** The epithelial lining of the amniotic sac and covering of the umbilical cord, in continuity with the epiblastic layer of the fetus. Morphologically it is derived from ectoderm. At the end of gestation it appears as a simple cubical or squamous epithelium. **basal e.** The inner layer of fetal epidermis derived from ectoderm. It becomes the stratum germinativum of the basal layer of adult skin. **blastodermic e.** PRIMITIVE ECTODERM. **chorionic e.** TROPHOBLAST. **epithelial e.** That portion of the ectoderm of the early embryo which moves away from neurectoderm to give rise to epidermis and epidermal structures. Also *superficial ectoderm*. **extraembryonic e.** An ectodermal derivative which is situated outside the confines of the developing embryo. **neural e.** That part of the ectoderm of the embryonic disk which will give rise to the neural groove and the neural tube. **primitive e.** A thin layer of cells, probably trophoblastic in origin, which covers the embryonic inner cell mass. In man and some other mammals, this layer does not disappear and thus the inner cell mass cells are not exposed to the exterior. Also *blastodermic ectoderm, primary ectoderm, Rauber's layer*. **superficial e.** EPITHELIAL ECTODERM.

**ectodermal** \-dur′məl\ Pertaining to or consisting of ectoderm. Also *ectodermic*.

**ectodermatosis** \-dur′mətō′sis\ ECTODERMOSIS.

**ectodermic** \-dur′mik\ ECTODERMAL.

**ectodermoidal** \-dərmoi′dəl\ [ECTODERM + -OID + -AL] Resembling or in some way simulating ectoderm.

**ectodermosis** \-dərmō′sis\ [ECTODERM + -OSIS] Any developmental defect that involves ectodermal derivatives. Also *ectodermatosis*. **e. erosiva pluriorificialis** STEVENS-JOHNSON SYNDROME.

**ectoentad** \-en′tad\ From without inward.

**ectoenzyme** \-en′zīm\ Any enzyme occurring within the membrane of a cell whose active site is on the outer surface, so that it takes up substrate and releases product on the outside of the cell.

**ectogenic** \-jen′ik\ EXOGENOUS.

**ectogenous** \ektäj′ənəs\ **1** Capable of developing outside the host organism: said especially of parasitic microorganisms. Also *ectogenic*. **2** EXOGENOUS.

**ectoglia** \ektäg′lē·ə\ [ECTO- + GLIA] An external, marginal layer of the neural tube at an early stage in embryonic development.

**ectogony** \ektäg′ənē\ [ECTO- + -GONY] Any effect on the maternal organism brought about by the embryo or fetus during pregnancy.

**ectolecithal** \-les′ithəl\ [ECTO- + LECITHAL] Describing an ovum whose yolk is distributed primarily around its cortex.

**-ectome** \-ek′tōm\ [EC- + -TOME] A combining form denoting a surgical instrument used for excision.

**ectomeninx** \-mē′ningks\ [ECTO- + MENINX] A dense, mesenchymatous layer in the embryo, surrounding the central nervous system, which gives rise to the dura mater and contributes to the skull. Also *meninx primitiva*.

**ectomere** \ek′təmir\ [ECTO- + -MERE] Any one of the blastomeres which contribute to the formation of the ectoderm.

**ectomesenchyme** \-mes′ənkīm\ [ECTO- + MESENCHYME] Mesectoderm that has reached the stage of mesenchyme.

**ectomorph** \ek′təmôrf\ An individual who has the characteristics of ectomorphy.

**ectomorphic** \-môr′fik\ Characterized by ectomorphy.

**ectomorphy** \ek′təmôrfē\ A type of human body conformation in which the individual is tall, thin, and asthenic with long limbs and extremities, a narrow chest, and small breasts. Compare ENDOMORPHY, MESOMORPHY.

**-ectomy** \-ek′təmē\ [Gk *ektomē* (from *ek* out of, away from + *tomē* a cutting, a cutting off, a cut, from *temnein* to cut) a cutting out] A combining form meaning the surgical removal of (a part); excision.

**ectopagia** \-pā′jə\ [ECTO- + *-pag(us)* + -IA] The condition of equal conjoined twins united to one another laterally.

**ectoparasite** \-par′əsīt\ [ECTO- + PARASITE] A parasite that lives on and feeds on the surface of the body of its host.

**ectoparasiticide** \-par′əsit′əsīd\ [*ectoparasit(e)* + *i* + -CIDE] An agent destructive to ectoparasites.

**ectoparasitism** \-par′əsitizm\ The relationship of an ectoparasite to its host; infestation by ectoparasites.

**ectoperitoneal** \-per′itənē′əl\ Pertaining to the external, or parietal, surface of the peritoneum.

**ectophyte** \ek′təfīt\ [ECTO- + Gk *phyt(on)* a plant, tree] A plant symbiont living on the surface of its host.

**ectophytic** \-fit′ik\ **1** Pertaining to ectophytes or to the ectophyte-host relationship. **2** EXOPHYTIC.

**ectopia** \ektō′pē·ə\ [New L (from Gk *ektop(os)* out of place, displaced + -IA)] Abnormal developmental placement or exposure to the surface of any organ or part. Also *dystopia, heterotopia, heterotaxia.* Adj. ectopic. **e. cordis** A congenital exposure of the heart through or on the anterior thoracic wall. The sternum is either cleft or deficient and the pericardium is incomplete. **e. cordis abdominalis** The apparent abnormal placement of the heart inferiorly into the abdominal cavity. It occurs with the absence of or major deficiency in the diaphragm. **e. lentis** A displacement of the lens from the normal position by either developmental or mechanical causes. **e. pupillae congenita** An eccentric displacement of the pupil within the iris that occurs during prenatal development. **renal e.** DYSTOPIC KIDNEY. **simple renal e.** SIMPLE RENAL DYSTOPIA. **e. testis** ECTOPIC TESTIS. **e. vesicae** EXSTROPHY OF THE BLADDER. **visceral e.** The partial or complete exposure of major thoracic and abdominal viscera resulting from incomplete development of the ventral body wall.

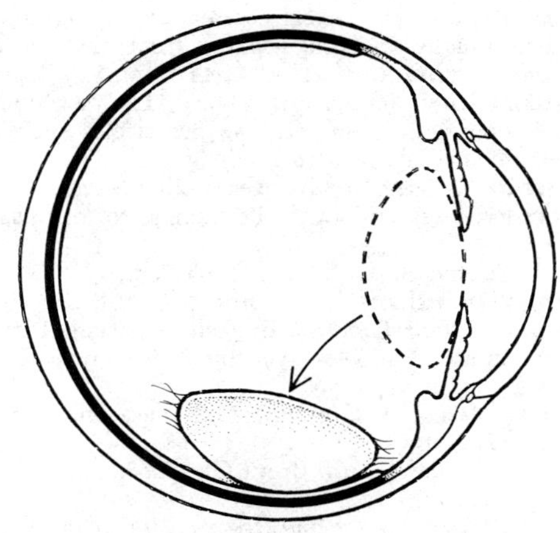
**Ectopia lentis**

**ectopic** \ektäp′ik\ [Gk *ektop(os)* (from *ek-* out + *topos* place) out of place + -IC] Out of place, outside the usual range of locations or relationships, or abnormally exposed to view.

**ectoplasm** \ek′təplazm\ [ECTO- + -PLASM] The thin layer of cytoplasm just inside of the cell membrane. It usually is dense and contains many microfilaments. Also *exoplasm.* Compare ENDOPLASM. Adj. ectoplasmatic.

**ectoplastic** \-plas′tik\ Describing a cell whose shape or morphology is established by the cell surface.

**ectoretina** \-ret′ənə\ RETINAL PIGMENT EPITHELIUM.

**ectosarc** \ek′təsärk\ PLASMA MEMBRANE.

**ectoskeleton** \-skel′ətən\ EXOSKELETON.

**ectosphere** \ek′təsfir\ [ECTO- + SPHERE] The outer layer or zone of a centrosome, seen at the poles of the spindle apparatus.

**ectosteal** \ektäs′tē·əl\ **1** Pertaining to or located on the external aspect of a bone. **2** Pertaining to ectostosis.

**ectostosis** \ek′tästō′sis\ [ECT- + OSTOSIS] Ossification commencing under the perichondrium or the periosteum.

**ectothermic** \-thur′mik\ POIKILOTHERMIC.

**ectothermy** \ek′təthurmē\ POIKILOTHERMY.

**ectothrix** \ek′təthriks\ [ECTO- + Gk *thrix* hair] **1** A form of hair invasion by a dermatophyte in which arthrospores develop on the surface of the infected hair shaft. **2** Those species of dermatophyte that produce arthrospores on the surface of the hair shaft, such as *Microsporum audouinii* and *Trichophyton mentagrophytes.*

**ectotoxemia** \-täksē′mē·ə\ [ECTO- + TOXEMIA] Toxemia due to any substance introduced into the body from an external source.

**ectotoxin** \-täk′sin\ EXOTOXIN.

**ectozoa** \-zō′ə\ Plural of ECTOZOON.

**ectozoic** \-zō′ik\ Of or pertaining to ectozoa. Also *ectozoal.*

**ectozoon** \-zō′ən\ [ECTO- + Gk *zōon* living being, animal] (*pl.* ectozoa) An animal organism living externally on another animal.

**ectro-** \ek′trə-\ [Gk *ektrōsis* miscarriage] A combining form denoting congenital absence, as of a part normally present.

**ectrocheiry** \-kī′rē\ ACHEIRIA.

**ectrochiry** \-kī′rē\ ACHEIRIA.

**ectrodactyly** \-dak′təlē\ [ECTRO- + DACTYL- + -Y ] The developmental absence of one or more digits (fingers or toes), with the total absence of all parts of a digital ray; that is, metacarpal or metatarsal parts and all phalanges. Also *oligodactyly, hypodactyly, adactyly.*

**ectromelia** \-mē′lyə\ [ECTRO- + MEL-[1] + -IA] AMELIA.

**ectromelic** \-mel′ik\ [ECTRO- + MEL[1] + -IC ] Affected by or pertaining to amelia.

**ectrometacarpia** \-met′əkär′pē·ə\ [ECTRO- + *metacarp(al)* + -IA] The developmental absence of one or more metacarpal bones.

**ectrometatarsia** \-met′ətär′sē·ə\ [ECTRO- + *metatars(al)* + -IA] A developmental absence of one or more metatarsal bones.

**ectropion** \ektrō′pē·än\ [Gk *ektropion* (from EK- + Gk *tropē* a turn, turning, from *trepein* to turn) a turning out or away] Eversion, especially of the margin of the eyelid, as due to relaxation of the supporting structures, paralysis of the orbicularis oculi muscle, or external cicatricial contraction. **cervical e.** Eversion of the cervix where the columnar epithelium has extended onto the portio vaginalis. **e. cicatriceum** The eversion of an eyelid margin caused by a scar in the lid itself or contracture of the surrounding skin. Also *cicatricial ectropion.* **flaccid e.** PARALYTIC ECTROPION. **mechanical e.** Ectropion of the eyelid due to posterior pressure, as from a mass. **paralytic e.** Ectropion of the lower eyelid due to paralysis of the facial muscles. Also *flaccid ectropion.* **e. of pigment layer** ECTROPION UVEAE. **senile e.** Malposition of the lower eyelid so that its margin is displaced away from contact with the eye, arising from the etiology of spontaneous relaxation of the supporting structures because of aging. Also *ectropion senilis.* **e. uveae** Displacement of the posterior pigment layer of the iris around the pupil edge, to lie upon the anterior surface of the iris. Also *ectropion of pigment layer.*

**ectropionize** \ektrō′pē·əniz\ [ECTROPION + -IZE] To turn inside out.

**ectropody** \ekträp′ədē\ [ECTRO- + POD- + -Y] APODIA.

**ectrosyndactyly** \-sindak′təlē\ [ECTRO- + SYNDACTYLY] The developmental absence of one or more digits and fusion of the remaining digits on the same hand or foot.

**ectylurea** $C_7H_{12}N_2O_2$. *N*-(2-Ethylisocrotonoyl)urea, a mild sedative that has been used to treat simple anxiety and tension.

**ectype** \ek′tīp\ [Gk *ektypos* (from *ek-* out + *typos* impression, cast, form) distinct, standing out] **1** An individual with an unusual physical or mental makeup or appearance. **2** ECTYPIA.

**ectypia** \ekti′pē·ə\ [*ectyp(e)* + -IA] A condition marked by an unusual physical or mental makeup. Also *ectype.*

**eczema** \ek′zimə\ [Gk *ekzema* (from EK- + Gk *zeein* to boil, seethe) anything thrown off or out by heat] An inflammatory skin reaction characterized histologically by spongiosis and clinically by a variety of features, including pruritus, erythema, clustered papules or vesicles, hyperkeratosis with scaling, exudation of serum, and crusting. Also *eczematoid dermatitis, eczematoid reaction.* See also DERMATITIS. **asteatotic e.** A form of eczema characterized by dry, fissured skin. Abnormal water loss as a result of decreased skin lipids is thought to play a part in the pathogenesis. The condition tends to affect elderly people, and it tends to worsen in winter. Also *dermatitis hiemalis, fissured eczema.* **atopic e.** The characteristic clinical type of eczema associated with atopy. It usually begins between the ages of two and six months, persists into childhood, and then tends to clear. The face is often the first area to be affected, and then the flexures. The intense pruritus often causes severe excoriation, and the skin may become lichenified. The unaffected skin is often dry. Also *infantile eczema, atopic dermatitis.* **autoallergic e.** An ill-defined condition which is proposed as a possible mechanism for the secondary spread of eczema. It has been suggested that a cytotoxic antibody directed against the epidermis may occur in the blood of some patients with active eczema. **bakers' e.** Occupational dermatitis of bakers, due to contact with flour, sugar, and food additives, and exacerbated by moisture. These substances can act as either primary irritants or as sensitizers. It may also be caused by a mite that infects grain, *Acarus siro (Tyrophagus farina).* **bullous e. of the legs** A form of eczema in which persistent blisters develop on the lower legs, usually in elderly subjects. In some, the condition appears to be a localized form of pemphigoid that develops in a subject with preexistent eczema. **dry e.** A form of nummular eczema in which the lesions are dry and slightly scaly and never obviously papulovesicular. The eruption persists for months without remission, yet causes the subject little discomfort. Also *eczema siccum.* **dyshidrotic e.** Pompholyx in which sweat retention is thought to play a causative role. **dyskeratotic e. of the hand** Eczema in which intensely irritable hyperkeratotic patches develop on the palms and palmar surfaces of the fingers. Painful fissures are common. The condition usually affects middle-aged or elderly men. **fissured e.** **1** Hyperkeratotic eczema in which cracks or fissures have developed. Also *eczema fissum, eczema rhagadiforme.* **2** ASTEATOTIC ECZEMA. **e. herpeticum** A serious, generalized vesicular eruption caused by a herpes simplex virus and complicating a pre-existing dermatologic condition, usually atopic eczematous dermatitis. In appearance, the eruption is indistinguishable from that of eczema vaccinatum. **e. hypertrophicum** LICHENIFICATION. **infantile e.** ATOPIC ECZEMA. **infective e.** INFECTIVE DERMATITIS. **intertriginous e.** Eczema affecting apposed skin surfaces. See also INTERTRIGO. **lichenoid e.** Eczema that has been lichenified from repeated rubbing and scratching. The affected area is thickened and the skin markings are increased. Around the edge of the plaque there may be small lichenoid papules. **e. marginatum** TINEA CRURIS. **e. medicamentosa** DRUG ERUPTION. **nipple e.** Dermatitis of the nipples. A biopsy may be required to distinguish this condition from the more serious mammary Paget's disease. **occupational e.** OCCUPATIONAL DERMATITIS. **e. parasiticum** An eczematous eruption secondary to parasitic infestation, notably to scabies and pediculosis. **phlyctenular e.** A rare eczema marked by small tense vesicles that are confined to the thenar eminence and wrist. The vesicles may be mistaken for pustules, though their minute structure is eczematous. **pustular e.** Eczema in which pustules develop as a result of a secondary bacterial infection that is usually staphylococcal in origin. Also *eczema pustulosum.* **e. rhagadiforme** FISSURED ECZEMA. **seborrheic e.** SEBORRHEIC DERMATITIS. **e. siccum** DRY ECZEMA. **stasis e.** A distinctive pattern of eczema due to chronic venous stasis of the legs, which usually exhibit obvious varicose veins or leashes of dilated venules. The eczema is often accompanied by brawny edema, diffuse brown pigmentation, and venous ulcerations of the affected area, typically the lower part of the leg. Also *stasis dermatitis, varicose eczema.* **e. vaccinatum** A vesicular eruption produced by the vaccinia virus, often seen as a complication of a topical eczematous dermatitis and in appearance usually indistinguishable from that of eczema herpeticum. **varicose e.** STASIS ECZEMA.

**eczematization** \ekzem′ətīzā′shən\ The development of eczema secondary to a pre-existing dermatosis such as scabies. This often results from scratching.

**eczematoid** \eksem′ətoid\ Resembling eczema.

**eczematous** \eksem′ətəs\ Pertaining to or resembling eczema.

**ED** **1** effective dose. **2** erythema dose.

**edathamil disodium** DISODIUM EDETATE.

**Eddowes** [Alfred *Eddowes,* English physician, 1850–1946] Eddowes disease, Eddowes syndrome. See under LOBSTEIN SYNDROME.

**Edebohls** [George *Edebohls,* U.S. surgeon, 1853–1908] See under POSITION.

**edeitis** \ē′dē·ī′tis\ [*ede(a)* (from Gk *aidoia* the genitals) the external genitals + -ITIS] VULVITIS.

**edema** \idē′mə\ [Gk *oidēma* (from *oidein* to swell) a swelling] The presence of excessive fluid in the tissue spaces.

Also *oedema* (British spelling). **alimentary e.** NUTRITIONAL EDEMA. **angioneurotic e.** A chronic, episodic, potentially fatal condition characterized by circumscribed areas of subcutaneous edema, abdominal pain, and laryngeal edema. In those cases attributed to a $C_1$ esterase inhibitor deficiency, the condition is referred to as hereditary angioedema. Also *angioedema, Quincke's edema, angioneuroedema.* **brain e.** CEREBRAL EDEMA. **brawny e.** Inflammatory lymph that tends to become organized. *Seldom used.* Also *plastic lymph.* **e. bullosum vesicae** The presence of intercellular fluid tissues on the mucous bladder wall. **Calabar e.** CALABAR SWELLINGS. **cardiac e.** Peripheral edema secondary to cardiac disease. It is a feature of right-sided heart failure, associated with high venous pressure and sodium retention. **cerebral e.** Diffuse or focal brain swelling due to an increase in intracellular but more particularly in extracellular fluid. Diffuse edema has many causes, some of known etiology, as in lead poisoning or hypertensive encephalopathy, but some of unknown cause, as benign intracranial hypertension. Localized edema may result from neoplasms, local injury, inflammation (cerebral abscess), infarction, and many other processes. Also *wet brain, encephaloedema, brain swelling, brain edema, cerebral congestion, coup de sang* (An imprecise and outmoded term). **dependent e.** Edema affecting predominantly the dependent parts of the body. **famine e.** NUTRITIONAL EDEMA. **gaseous e.** Edema with the presence of gas, as seen in clostridial infections. **gestational e.** Edema which occurs as a normal physiologic consequence of pregnancy. **e. glottidis** Edematous swelling of the glottic soft tissues. • This term was once commonly applied to cases now regarded as examples of subglottic edema. **hereditary e.** HEREDITARY ANGIOEDEMA. **hereditary angioneurotic e.** *Outmoded* HEREDITARY ANGIOEDEMA. **high-altitude pulmonary e.** An accumulation of fluid in the lungs resulting from rapidly reduced atmospheric pressure. **idiopathic e.** Edema occurring usually in women, not necessarily in consonance with the menstrual cycle. It is generally believed to be due not to hormonal abnormality, but to a "capillary leak" of serum protein leading to an unfavorable change in tissue osmotic pressure conducive to leakage of serum fluids into peripheral tissues. **inflammatory e.** The characteristic localized edema of acute inflammatory reactions. **insulin e.** Edema occurring locally at the site of insulin injection, perhaps of allergic origin. **interstitial e.** An accumulation of excess fluid in tissue whenever the extracellular fluid space is expanded, causing separation of the tissue's normal elements. If the edema persists in renal tissue, collagen and other elements of fibrosis may develop within a week or so. **lymphatic e.** LYMPHEDEMA. **menstrual e.** A generalized, peripheral edema occurring in the few days preceding and the first days of menstruation, when the menstrual cycles are normal. It is associated with ovulation and is usually absent when the cycles are anovulatory. The swelling affects the face, especially the periorbital region, the breasts, hands, and other areas. It is accompanied by increased venous pressure or by signs or symptoms of hepatic or renal dysfunction, more likely related to estrogen- or progesterone-conditioned changes in capillary permeability than to hormone-induced retention of sodium and water. **mucous e.** *Outmoded* MYXEDEMA. **nephritic e.** Edema associated with circulatory congestion secondary to acute renal failure and characterized by venous congestion, pulmonary congestion and gallop rhythm, and peripheral edema. Circulation time is rapid. See also ACUTE NEPHRITIC SYNDROME. **nonpitting e.** Edema associated with tissue induration so that the affected part cannot be pitted by finger pressure. Compare PITTING EDEMA. **nutritional e.** Edema caused by a prolonged dietary deficiency of protein, as occurs in kwashiorkor. The degree of edema is largely dependent on the level of albumin in the blood and hence to the amount of protein in the diet. Other factors, including salt and water in the diet, are also important. Although it occasionally involves the whole body, including the face, in most cases it is most marked in the lower limbs. Also *famine dropsy, wet dropsy, alimentary edema, famine edema, nutritional dropsy.* **passive e.** Edema resulting from venous or lymphatic engorgement. **pitting e.** Edema characterized by prolonged persistence of pits caused by finger pressure. It is usually seen in uncomplicated forms of edema such as those caused by congestive heart failure, hypoproteinemia, and vascular obstruction. Compare NONPITTING EDEMA. **placental e.** Accumulation of fluid in the placental villi causing them to become swollen with distended tips. **pulmonary e.** Accumulation of abnormally large amounts of watery fluid within the pulmonary alveoli. **purulent e.** Edema caused by an acute purulent inflammation. **Quincke's e.** ANGIONEUROTIC EDEMA. **Reinke e.** A common variety of chronic laryngitis consisting of bilateral symmetrical polypoid swelling of the whole length of the membranous part of the vocal cords. Also *polypoid degeneration of the vocal cords.* **renal e.** 1 Edema of the renal parenchyma. 2 Peripheral edema due to any renal disease. *Ambiguous.* **salt e.** An abnormal accumulation of fluid in the body tissues resulting from excessive dietary intake of sodium chloride. **solid e.** *Rare* MYXEDEMA. **subglottic e.** Edematous swelling of the loose submucosa of the lining of the elastic cone of the larynx. It is a feature of severe acute laryngitis and laryngotracheitis, particularly in children. More rarely it is a feature of various kinds of acute noninfective laryngitis in all age groups. Stridor and croupy cough are the main symptoms and respiratory obstruction an ever-present risk. **toxic e.** Edema caused by a poisonous or toxic substance. **tubular e.** Edema of renal tubule cells characterized by separation of endoplasmic reticulum, increase in size and number of vacuoles, swelling of mitochondria, decrease in number of ribosomes, and absence of organelles in the cytoplasm. These changes are the first to occur in acute cellular injury due to any cause and may be difficult to differentiate from postmortem effects. Cessation of blood flow leads to these changes within minutes. Also *tubular hydropic change, tubular cloudy swelling.* **turban e.** Pseudoedema of the epiglottis, so-called because of the turbanlike appearance of the swollen epiglottis on indirect laryngoscopy. It is one of the many manifestations of laryngeal tuberculosis. **wound e.** The increase in fluid content of tissues within and surrounding a wound, resulting from increased capillary permeability as a consequence of the mediators of inflammation.

**edematous** \ēdem′ətəs\ Affected by edema. Also *hydropic* (rare).

**edentate** \ēden′tāt\ [L *edentat(us),* past part. of *edentare* to deprive of teeth] Toothless.

**edentulous** \ēden′tyələs\ [L *edentulus* (from *e-*, *ex-* loss, lack of + *dens,* gen. *dent(is)* tooth + *-ulus* adj. suffix) toothless, having lost one's teeth] Without teeth. Compare DENTULOUS.

**edetate** An anion derived from ethylenediaminetetraacetic acid (EDTA).

**edetate calcium disodium** A mixture of the dihydrate and trihydrate of the calcium disodium salt of ethylenediaminetetraacetate. Also *sodium calcium edetate, calcium disodium versenate, calcium disodium edetate, calcium diso-*

*dium ethylenediaminetetraacetate.*

**edetate disodium** The disodium salt of ethylenediaminetetraacetate. It is used as a chelating agent, particularly for calcium and trace metals.

**edetate sodium** The sodium salt of ethylenediaminetetraacetic acid. It is used as a chelating agent for trace metals.

**edetate trisodium** The trisodium salt of ethylenediaminetetraacetate. It is used as a chelating agent.

**edetic acid** ETHYLENEDIAMINETETRAACETIC ACID.

**edetic acid disodium salt** DISODIUM EDETATE.

**edible** [Late L *edibilis* (from L *ed(ere)* to eat + *-ibilis* -IBLE) edible] Suitable for eating.

**Edinger** [Ludwig *Edinger*, German anatomist, 1855–1918] **1** Habenulodiencephalic tract of Edinger. See under TRACT. **2** See under LAW. **3** Edinger-Westphal nucleus, Edinger's nucleus. See under NUCLEUS OCULOMOTORIUS ACCESSORIUS.

**Edison** [Thomas Alva *Edison*, U.S. inventor, 1847–1931] See under EFFECT.

**editor** \ed′itər\ A specialized computer program that manipulates text data in a program to provide an easy way to insert new text or correct errors.

**EDR** electrodermal response (psychogalvanic response).

**edrophonium bromide** $C_{10}H_{16}BrNO$. *N*-Ethyl-3-hydroxy-*N,N*-dimethylbenzenaminium bromide, a short-acting anticholinesterase agent that has been used in a diagnostic test for myasthenia gravis. It is also employed as an antidote for excessive intake of curariform drugs and to treat a myasthenic crisis. It is given intramuscularly or intravenously.

**edrophonium chloride** $C_{10}H_{16}ClNO$. Ethyl(3-hydroxyphenyl)dimethylammoniumchloride, the chloride salt of edrophonium. Its properties and uses are the same as those of edrophonium bromide.

**EDTA** ethylenediaminetetraacetic acid.

**EDTA disodium** DISODIUM EDETATE.

**education / compensatory e.** HABILITATION.

**educator / health e.** A health care professional who provides instruction and guidance, in health care settings or elsewhere in the community, on how to maintain good health or how to cope with illness and to facilitate recovery.

**educt** **1** Any type of extract. **2** A drug or active agent extracted in a form unchanged from that present in a cruder therapeutic preparation.

**edulcorant** Serving as a sweetening agent.

**edulcorate** The process of sweetening; to make sweeter.

**Edwards** [John Hilton *Edwards*, English geneticist, born 1928] Edwards syndrome. See under TRISOMY 18 SYNDROME.

**Edwards** [M. L. *Edwards*, U.S. physician, flourished 20th century] Starr-Edwards prosthesis. See under PROSTHESIS.

***Edwardsiella*** \ed′wərdsyel′ə\ A group of motile, hydrogen-sulfide-producing, lactose-negative organisms that closely resemble *Salmonella* and occasionally cause disease in man. They are isolated commonly from reptiles.

**EEE** eastern equine encephalomyelitis.

**EEG** **1** electroencephalogram. **2** electroencephalography.

**EENT** eye, ear, nose, and throat. • This is a popular abbreviation which, to some extent, has been replaced by ENT (ear, nose, and throat) as the specialties of ophthalmology and otorhinolaryngology have grown apart.

**EF** elongation factor (in protein synthesis).

**ef-** \ef-, əf-\ EX-[1].

**effacement** \ifās′mənt\ [French (from L *ex-* from + French *face* face + *-ment* -MENT), an effacing] The thinning out of the uterine cervix prior to or during labor by the taking up of the uppermost muscular fibers in the vicinity of the internal os into the lower uterine segment.

# effect

**effect** [L *effectus* (from *effectus*, past part. of *efficere* to bring to pass, from *ef-* + L *facere* to do, make) an effect, result] A result of an action or agency; something caused. **accumulative e.** CUMULATIVE EFFECT. **additive e.** The combined effect of two or more agents that equals the sum of their separate effects. **adverse e.** An unintended, deleterious reaction occurring after administration of a substance at levels normally not intended to produce such an effect. **anachoretic e.** The collection or deposition of material at a particular site, such as binding of cadmium and zinc to metallothionein in the liver and kidney. **Anrep e.** Increased impedance to cardiac output. **Auger e.** An atomic process, which may occur as an alternative to characteristic x-ray emission, in which the energy released in the filling of an inner-shell vacancy is transferred to an outer-shell electron, which is then emitted from the atom. **Bainbridge e.** Acceleration of the heartbeat in response to a rise in pressure and distension. The effect is not a reflex, but is caused by a mechanical effect on the cardiac pacemaker fibers. Also *Bainbridge reflex.* **Bezold-Jarisch e.** BEZOLD REFLEX. **Bohr e.** The lowering of affinity of hemoglobin for oxygen evoked by carbon dioxide. This effect is due both to the lowering of pH and to the combination of carbon dioxide with amino groups, and assists the release of oxygen in the tissues. **cis-trans position e.** A condition that may arise in an organism both diploid for and carrying two mutations in a given gene or cistron. When the mutations occur on the same chromosome (cis position) the phenotype is wild type; when the mutations are on different chromosomes (trans position) the mutant phenotype emerges. Recombination can cause expression of the mutant phenotype through a shift of the mutations from cis to trans. See also COUPLING, REPULSION. **clasp-knife e.** CLASP-KNIFE RIGIDITY. **cohort e.** GENERATION EFFECT. **columella e.** The transmission of sound across the middle ear effected by a single ossicle, as in birds (the single ossicle being the columella), but in particular as produced in man by the type 3 tympanoplasty operation. **Compton e.** The interaction between a photon and an outer atomic electron which is loosely bound or free. The photon is deflected, losing some of its energy to the electron. See also COMPTON ELECTRON, COMPTON SCATTERING. **contrast e.** An intensification of the difference between two stimuli received in the same sense mode that results from presenting them closely in space or time. This awareness of difference is heightened particularly if the stimuli are of opposing quality, such as a sour taste immediately following a sweet one. **Cotton e.** A change of the sign of optical rotation of a specimen as the wavelength of observation is changed, this change occurring at the wavelength of an absorption band. It is said to be positive if the rotation is positive at wavelengths above the change of sign. This effect is shown by chiral chromophores, or by chromophores in chiral environments, such as pyridoxal phosphate (itself achiral) when enzyme-bound. **Crabtree e.** The suppression of aerobic oxidative processes in certain tissues upon the addition of glucose. Compare PASTEUR EFFECT. **crowding e.** **1** The growth-inhibiting or deleterious effect on individual organisms induced by excessive numbers; said, for example, of intestinal parasites, especially cestodes. **2** The effect on humans of high population density, marked by the inability to control the amount, rate, or quality of social interchange, hence usually experienced as a negative effect. **cumulative e.** The enhancement produced by the summation of repeated exposures or doses when the rate of intake exceeds the rate of elimination. Also *accumulative effect.* **cytopathic e.** A pathologic effect on cells, as that produced by virus infection. Often it consists of a rounding up of the infected cell and the development of increased refractility. **Deelman e.** The localization of a tumor to an area previously treated with a carcinogen and scarified. **Donnan e.** The influence on the distribution of diffusible charged particles on two sides of a membrane created by indiffusible charged particles restricted to one side. **Doppler e.** Difference between emitted and perceived frequency due to motion of source, reflector, or receiver of a wave. Also *Doppler shift, Doppler velocity signal, Doppler phenomenon, Doppler principle.* **Edison e.** The thermionic emission of charged particles from a hot filament. **electrophonic e.** *Seldom used* COCHLEAR MICROPHONICS. **electrotonic e.** The altered excitability of nerve or muscle caused by the direct spread of electrical current in tissue. It involves no generation of new current by action potentials. **Fahraeus-Lindqvist e.** The decrease in measured viscosity observed when a flow of blood or other liquid suspension of particles is measured in tubes of small diameter, usually below 0.5 mm. **field e.** The static, three-dimensional distribution of potentials dependent solely upon distance and electrical impedance of the tissue when surrounding a locus of hyperpolarization or hypopolarization. **founder e.** The occurrence of a restricted number of genotypes, or of a rare allele, in a population because of the contribution to the gene pool by a small number of founders. It is one mechanism for the occurrence of rare hereditary disorders, especially recessives, in populations that have existed in isolation, the other mechanism being mutation in an earlier generation. **gene dosage e.** In bacterial genetics, the proportionality of the synthesis of a product to the number of copies of its gene, for those genes that are not repressed. **generation e.** An observed difference, as in the incidence of a disease, among two or more generations due to differences in the environment to which each had been exposed. Also *cohort effect.* **glucose e.** The inhibition by glucose of the induction of microbial genes that specify early steps of catabolic pathways. This inhibition can be either by inducer exclusion, i.e. the prevention by glucose or its analogs of the initial penetration of a substrate into a cell, or by catabolite repression, i.e. the decreased expression of relevant genes in the presence of glucose. *Rare.* **graded e.** An effect, the intensity or severity of which is directly related to dosage. Compare QUANTAL EFFECT. **Haldane e.** The fact that oxygenation of hemoglobin lowers its affinity for carbon dioxide. It is the converse of the Bohr effect. **heel e.** The reduction in radiation received by the part of the film which is on the anode side of the x-ray tube, because of increased absorption of x rays which are emitted at an angle close to the target angle. **Hering e.** The generation of new impulses following the arrival of a synchronized potential at the artificial synapse formed at the cut end of a nerve. **hybrid e.** An animal or plant produced by parents of two different species or strains is thought to be biologically stronger and more resistant to diseases. **hyperchromic e.** The increase of absorbance at 260 nm of DNA when its ordered, double-stranded structure is lost, as on heating. **hypochromic e.** The phenomenon that the bases of DNA show a diminished absorbance at 260 nm in the ordered, double-stranded structure, in comparison with that of the compounds free in solution. **inductive e.** The effect of one group in a molecule on the reactivity of another when this effect is transmitted as a simple electrostatic effect through the molecule, rather than by stabilizing a different bond structure. **internal photoelectric e.** The ejection of an electron from the atom by a process in which emitted fluorescent photons interact with one of the orbital electrons and the energy exchange is sufficient to eject the electron. **inverse photoelectric e.** The emission of x rays or ultraviolet radiation from a surface bombarded with high-energy electrons. **isomorphic e.** The induction by trauma or nonspecific inflammation of specific changes in a disorder, such as psoriasis, lichen planus, or eczema, that is already present in a subject in active or latent form. Also *Köbner's phenomenon, isomorphous provocative reaction.* **isotope e.** The effect of atomic mass of the various isotopes of an element, on the chemical behavior of compounds that contain them. Although the isotopes are all chemically similar, isotopic substitution can affect rates of reaction and equilibrium constants. **Mierzejewski e.** The disproportionate development of gray and white matter in the brain, the gray being excessive. **muscarinic e.** The effect, exerted by acetylcholine as a peripheral parasympathetic humoral transmitter substance, that is mimicked by muscarine and antagonized by atropine. Compare NICOTINE EFFECT. **nicotine e.** The effect exerted by acetylcholine in ganglia of the autonomic nervous system or at the motor end-plate that is mimicked by nicotine. It is not antagonized by atropine, but may be antagonized by hexamethonium or curare. Also *nicotinic effect.* Compare MUSCARINIC EFFECT. **Orbeli e.** The phenomenon wherein the response of a fatigued nerve-muscle preparation can be enhanced by electrical sympathetic nerve stimulation. Also *Orbeli phenomenon.* **Pasteur e.** The effect of oxygen in lowering the rate of glycolysis, often manifested as a lowering of glucose uptake. It is the result of a metabolic control that comes into effect when the organism has enough ATP. Much less glucose is required to form a specified amount of ATP under aerobic conditions than under anaerobic ones, so oxygen has the effect of raising the ATP concentration. Also *Pasteur's reaction.* Compare CRABTREE EFFECT. **photoelectric e.** The interaction between a photon and one of the more firmly bound electrons in an atom. The photon disappears, imparting all of its energy to the electron, which is knocked out of the atom. The resulting orbital vacancy is filled in by electrons farther out, with the emission of a characteristic x ray. The interaction is most likely when the energy of the photon matches the binding energy of the electron. The effect is prominent, therefore, in materials with high proton numbers, as lead, tungsten, etc., which make good radiation shields. **piezoelectric e.** Generation of an electrical potential when certain crystalline materials are mechanically stressed, or conversely, the generation of a mechanical strain when an electric field is applied to such a crystalline material. **placebo e.** The effect produced by a simulated drug known to have no active ingredients. Knowledge of this inactivity is not given to the patient, but is available to the physician. Placebos are used to evaluate the psychological effects of giving medicine, as opposed to the real therapeutic effects of the therapeutic compound. **position e.** Any change in expression of a gene caused by altering its physical position with respect to the nucleotide sequences or to the genes which neighbor it. Two classes have been defined based on studies in eukaryotes other than primates: the cis-trans type and the variegated type. **Purkinje e.** The displacement towards the shorter wavelengths of sensitivity to brightness under conditions of scotopic, as compared to photopic, vision. It explains why blue colors appear relatively brighter in weak light and yellow hues appear relatively brighter in stronger light. Also *Purkinje phenomenon, Purkinje shift.* **quantal e.** An effect, such as death or the occurrence of a tumor, which either happens or does not happen, showing no gradation. Compare GRADED EFFECT. **relative biologic e.** RELATIVE BIOLOGIC EFFECTIVENESS. **second gas e.** An effect observed when a mixture of two anesthetic gases, such as nitrous oxide and oxygen, is breathed. The greater initial uptake from the alveoli of one of the gases (nitrous oxide) in pulmonary capillary blood will augment the inspiratory volume and increase the concentration and uptake of the second gas (oxygen). **side e.** SIDE-EFFECT. **Soret e.** The development of a concentration gradient in a tube of solution subjected to a prolonged temperature gradient. Also *Soret phenomenon.* **specific dynamic e.** SPECIFIC DYNAMIC ACTION. **Stiles-Crawford e.** The phenomenon in which light entering through the center of the pupil appears brighter than the same light when entering through a peripheral part of the pupil. **treppe e.** STAIRCASE PHENOMENON. **Tyndall e.** The rendering visible of a beam of light passing through a transparent medium containing suspended particles. Also *Tyndall phenomenon.* **variegated position e.** The emergence of a mutant phenotype in a diploid organism that is heterozygous for a mutant allele when the activity of the wild type allele is partially or totally repressed by a change in the chromosome, such as heterochromatization, in the region of the genetic locus. **Venturi e.** The fall in pressure and increase in speed of flow observed when a fluid travels through a constricted portion of a tube. **Vulpian's e.** The slow contraction of the denervated lingual muscles which may be evoked by stimulating the chorda tympani after division of the hypoglossal nerve. **Wever-Bray e.** COCHLEAR MICROPHONIC POTENTIAL. **Zeeman e.** The separation of a spectral line into two or more lines, having different polarization properties, by placement of the source in a strong magnetic field.

**effectiveness** \ifek′tivnis\ **1** The extent to which a drug or other agent achieves its intended therapeutic purpose. **2** The measure of the extent to which items of service, such as the number of treatments given, are successful in achieving defined goals of improving health or curing or controlling disease. **relative biologic e.** The ratio of the biologic effects produced by a given amount of ionizing radiation to those effects produced by an equal amount of radiation of a standard type, usually taken as 250 kV x rays. Also *relative biologic effect.*

**effector** \ifek′tər\ An organ that responds to nervous impulses either by movement (muscle, chromatophore), secretion (exocrine and endocrine glands), or release of an electrical discharge (electric organ), as of an electric eel. Also *effector organ.* **allosteric e.** A substance that affects the activity of an enzyme by binding to it at a site other than the substrate-binding site. The rates at which metabolic conversion occur are often controlled in response to the needs of the organism by such effectors.

**effemination** \ifem′ənā′shən\ FEMINIZATION.

**efferent** \ef′ərənt\ [L *efferens*, gen. *efferentis*, pres. part. of *efferre* (from *e(x)-* out, away + *ferre* to carry) to carry away] Conveying outward or away from the center, as nerve impulses, fluid such as blood or lymph, or information. Also *efferential.* Compare AFFERENT. **$\alpha$-e.** A motoneuron or its myelinated axon of large caliber exclusively innervating extrafusal muscle fibers. It contributes to the early $\alpha$-wave of an evoked ventral root neurogram. Also *$\alpha$-fiber.* **$\beta$-e.** A motoneuron or axon that supplies motor endplates to both extrafusal (skeletal) and intrafusal muscle fibers. Also *skeletofusimotor fiber, $\beta$-fiber, $\beta$ motor fiber.* **dynamic $\gamma$-e.** A fusimotor neuron whose activation enhances the phasic response of the primary ending of a muscle spindle to an abrupt change, i.e., in spindle length. The effect is thought to be due to contraction of the nuclear $bag_1$ intrafusal fibers. **$\gamma$-e.** A small motoneuron or its myelinated axon that innervates one or more of the intrafusal fibers in a muscle spindle but none of the extrafusal fibers. Such small axons contribute to the relatively late $\gamma$-wave in an evoked neurogram monitored from a ventral root. Most spindles receive two distinct types of $\gamma$-efferents, called dynamic and static $\gamma$-efferents. Also *$\gamma$-fiber, fusimotor fiber.* **general visceral e.** **1** Denoting the motor innervation of the heart, the smooth muscle, and glands of the viscera. **2** A general visceral efferent fiber. **somatic e.** **1** Denoting nerve fibers that transmit impulses to extra- and intrafusal fibers in muscle. **2** A somatic efferent fiber. **special visceral e.** **1** Denoting motor fibers innervating muscles of branchial arch origin, i.e., the muscles of mastication, and those of the face, middle ear, pharynx, larynx, and upper esophagus. The sternocleidomastoid and trapezius muscles are usually included. **2** A special visceral efferent fiber. **static $\gamma$-e.** A fusimotor neuron whose activation depresses the dynamic sensitivity of the primary ending and enhances static discharge of the secondary ending in response to steady stretch. **visceral e.** **1** Denoting autonomic nerve fibers that innervate the internal organs. **2** A visceral efferent fiber.

**efferential** \ef′əren′shəl\ EFFERENT.

**effervescent** [L *effervescens*, gen. *effervescentis*, pres. part. of *effervescere* (from *ef-* out + *fervescere* to begin to be hot or to boil, from *fervere* to burn, seethe, boil) to begin to boil] Rapidly producing gas in the form of small bubbles within a liquid.

**efficacy** \ef′əkəsē\ The effectiveness of a therapy, drug, or other intervention in the theoretical optimal state under ideal conditions.

**efficiency** [L *efficien(tia)* (from *efficiens*, pres. part. of *efficere* to effect) the power to effect] **1** The ratio of useful output of a dynamic system to the input, in terms of power, energy, quantity of electricity, etc. **2** In statistics, the degree of accuracy with which a sample statistic estimates the parameter of interest. **counting e.** INTRINSIC COUNTER EFFICIENCY. **detection e.** INTRINSIC COUNTER EFFICIENCY. **intrinsic counter e.** The ratio of the number of pulses actually counted to the number of particles reaching the detector in the same time. It is the product of the intrinsic detector efficiency and the window efficiency. Also *counting efficiency, detection efficiency.* **photopeak e.** PEAK-TO-TOTAL RATIO. **production e.** **1** The ratio of tissue formed to the energy intake by an organism. **2** Energy in the tissue formed divided by energy intake. **window e.** The ratio of the number of pulses passed by the electronic window of the pulse-height analyzer to the number delivered by the detector in the same time. It is not always identical to the peak-to-total ratio, since sometimes the window should not cover the whole total-absorption peak.

**effloresce** [L *effloresce(re)* (from *ef-* for *ex-* out, out of + *florescere* to begin to blossom, from *flos* a flower, blossom) to bloom, blossom] To lose water of crystallization or combined water when exposed to fairly dry air. The solid that effloresces thereby becomes covered with a powder of the dehydrated material.

**efflorescence** \ef′lôres′əns\ [French, a flowering. See EF-

FLORESCE.] **1** A skin eruption, particularly one that arises in relation to an infectious or other systemic disease. **2** The process or result of efflorescing chemically. Adj. efflorescent.

**efflorescent** Showing a tendency to effloresce.

**effluve** \ifloov′\ [French, from L *effluvium.* See EFFLUVIUM.] CONVECTIVE DISCHARGE.

**effluvia** \ifloo′vē·ə\ Plural of EFFLUVIUM.

**effluvium** \ifloo′vē·əm\ [L (from *effluere* to flow out, fall out, escape, from *ef-, ex-* out + *fluere* to flow) outflow, discharge] **1** A shedding of a surface body part such as hair. **2** An emanation or outflow, especially of noxious matter. **anagen e.** The diffuse loss of hair in the anagen phase of the hair cycle, as seen after the administration of cytotoxic drugs. **telogen e.** The diffuse loss of hair in the telogen phase of the hair cycle, as seen after a fever.

**effusion** \ifyoo′zhən\ [L *effusio* (from *effundere* to pour out, from *ef-* EX- + *fundere* to pour) a discharge, emission] The escape of fluid and its accumulation in tissues or a body cavity. **chylous e.** An effusion rich in lymph, usually resulting from obstruction of the thoracic duct. **middle-ear e.** **1** An effusion occurring in the middle ear. **2** SECRETORY OTITIS MEDIA. **pericardial e.** A collection of fluid within the pericardial space. Also *dropsy of pericardium.* **pleural e.** A collection of fluid within the pleural space. Also *pleurorrhea.* **subdural e.** The escape of cerebrospinal fluid from the subarachnoid into the subdural space.

**eg-** \eg-, əg-\ EN-.

**egest** \ējest′\ [L *egest(us),* past part. of *egerere* (from *e(x)-* out + *gerere* to bear, carry) to bring forth, discharge] To eliminate or discharge (waste or indigestible material) from the body: used most commonly of microorganisms and lower animals.

**egesta** \ējes′tə\ [L, neut. pl. of *egestus.* See EGEST.] Material that has been egested.

**egestion** \ējes′chən\ [L *egestio* (from *egestus,* past part. of *egerere* to cast forth) a voiding] The elimination or discharge of indigestible or unassimilable material that has been ingested.

**egg** [Old Norse *egg,* replacing Old English *æg,* akin to German *Ei,* L *ovum,* and Gk *ōion,* all meaning *egg*] The female gamete which may be fertilized by a male gamete in sexual reproduction; an ovum.

**Egger** [Fritz *Egger,* Swiss internist, 1863–1938] See under LINE.

**eglandulous** \ēglan′dyələs\ Lacking glands.

**ego** \ē′gō, eg′ō\ [L (akin to Gk *egō,* I), I] The part of the psychic apparatus that mediates between the self and the outside world. Its prime function is to perceive reality and to adapt to it. **body e.** The psychic representations of one's self and one's body, which form the core of the body image.

**ego-alien** \-ā′lyən\ EGO-DYSTONIC.

**egobronchophony** \-bränkäf′ənē\ EGOPHONY.

**ego-dystonic** \-distän′ik\ Referring to anything that is recognized as not being a part of the self and, in particular, anything that is unacceptable to the ego. Also *ego-alien.*

**egomania** \-mā′nē·ə\ [EGO + -MANIA] An exaggerated sense of one's importance and worth. Also *autophilia.*

**egophony** \ēgäf′ənē\ [Gk *aïx,* gen. *aïgos,* a goat + PHON- + -Y] A vocal sound likened to the bleating of a goat heard on auscultation of the chest over pleural effusion. Also *capriloquism, bronchoegophony, egobronchophony.*

**ego-strength** \ē′gō-strength′\ The extent to which the ego satisfactorily performs its functions of mediating between superego, id, and reality, and of integrating those functions with enough flexibility so that energy is preserved for creativity and other unforeseen demands on the ego.

**ego-syntonic** \-sintän′ik\ Consonant and compatible with, and acceptable to, the ego.

**EHBF** **1** estimated hepatic blood flow. **2** extrahepatic blood flow.

**Ehlers** [Edward L. *Ehlers,* Danish dermatologist, 1863–1937] Ehlers-Danlos syndrome. See under SYNDROME.

**Ehrenritter** [Johann *Ehrenritter,* Austrian anatomist, died 1790] Ehrenritter's ganglion. See under GANGLION SUPERIUS NERVI GLOSSOPHARYNGEI.

**Ehrlich** [P. *Ehrlich,* German ophthalmologist, flourished late 19th century] See under TUMOR.

**Ehrlich** [Paul *Ehrlich,* German bacteriologist, 1854–1915] **1** Ehrlich's aldehyde reagent. See under REAGENT. **2** Ehrlich's diazo reagent. See under DIAZO REAGENT. **3** Ehrlich's benzaldehyde reaction. See under EHRLICH'S TEST. **4** See under EHRLICH'S HEMATOXYLIN. **5** Ehrlich's hemoglobinemic bodies. See under HEINZ BODIES. **6** Ehrlich's triacid stain. See under EHRLICH'S TRIPLE STAIN. **7** Ehrlich side-chain theory, Ehrlich's theory, Ehrlich's postulate. See under SIDE CHAIN THEORY. **8** Ehrlich's neutral stain. See under STAIN. **9** Biermer-Ehrlich anemia. See under PERNICIOUS ANEMIA.

**Ehrlich 606** ARSPHENAMINE.

**Eichhorst** [Hermann Ludwig *Eichhorst,* Swiss physician, 1849–1921] See under ATROPHY.

**eiconometer** \ī′kōnäm′ətər\ EIKONOMETER.

**eicosa-** \īkō′sə-\ ICOSA-.

**eid-** \īd-\ EIDO-.

**eidetic** \īdet′ik\ [Gk *eidētikos* (from *eidos* form, shape) pertaining to form or shape] Characterized by or involving mental imagery that is so clear and detailed as to appear nearly hallucinatory and as if being perceived rather than being revived from memory.

**eido-** \ī′dō-\ [Gk *eidos* form, shape] A combining form meaning image. Also *eid-.*

**eidogen** \ī′dōjən\ [EIDO- + -GEN] A substance capable of modifying the development of an embryonic organ during its formation, and after its induction has occurred. See also INDUCTOR.

**EIEC** enteroinvasive *Escherichia coli.*

***Eikenella corrodens*** \ī′kənel′ə kôrō′dəns\ A species of facultative, Gram-negative, rod-shaped bacteria associated with periodontal disease.

**eikonometer** \ī′kōnäm′ətər\ [Gk *eikōn* image, semblance + *o* + -METER] A device for measuring differences in the perception of size by the two eyes. Also *eiconometer.*

**eiloid** \ī′loid\ [Gk *eil(ein)* to roll, twist tight + -OID] Having the appearance of a coil or roll.

***Eimeria*** [after Theodor Gustav Heinrich *Eimer,* German zoologist, 1843–1898] A genus of coccidian protozoan parasites (family Eimeriidae), many species of which are economically important as causes of coccidiosis, infecting domesticated birds and mammals as well as many wild vertebrates. The oocyst contains four sporocysts, each of which has two sporozoites. The disease agents are especially pathogenic in young animals crowded or penned under unsanitary conditions, as they become infected by ingesting oocysts in the feces of infected individuals. Some species have been found as pseudoparasites in the human intestine, where they are nonpathogenic.

**Einhorn** [Max *Einhorn,* Russian-born gastroenterologist, 1862–1953] Einhorn string test. See under STRING TEST.

**einsteinium** A synthetic transuranium element having atomic number 99. It was first identified in debris from a thermonuclear explosion. Twelve isotopes are known, having mass numbers ranging from 245 to 256. The longest lived, einsteinium 254, has a half-life of 276 days. Symbol: Es

**Einthoven** [Willem *Einthoven,* Dutch physiologist, 1860–1927] **1** See under TRIANGLE, LAW. **2** Einthoven galvanometer. See under STRING GALVANOMETER.

**Eisenmenger** [Victor *Eisenmenger,* German physician, 1864–1932] **1** Eisenmenger's tetralogy. See under COMPLEX. **2** Eisenmenger disease. See under SYNDROME.

**eisodic** \īsäd′ik\ AFFERENT.

**eiweissmilch** \ī′vīsmilsH′\ [German *Eiweiss* (from *Ei* egg + *weiss* white) egg white + *Milch* milk] Albumen milk, made from white of egg.

**ejaculate** \ijak′yəlāt\ [L *ejaculatus,* past part. of *ejaculari* (from *e(x)-* out + *jaculari* to hurl, from *jaculum* javelin, from *jacere* to throw) to shoot out] **1** To discharge or expel suddenly. **2** The semen expelled in one ejaculation. Also *ejaculum.*

**ejaculatio** \ijak′yəlā′shē·ō\ [New L] EJACULATION. **e. deficiens** Inadequate ejaculation. **e. praecox** PREMATURE EJACULATION. **e. retardata** The psychosexual dysfunction of persistent inappropriate delay in the ejaculation of semen during sexual activity. It is often classified as a form of sexual impotence. Also *inhibited male orgasm.*

**ejaculation** \ijak′yəlā′shən\ [*ejaculat(e)* + -ION] A discharge or sudden emission, especially of semen. Also *ejaculatio.* **premature e.** The psychosexual dysfunction of persistent inability to maintain reasonable control over the timing of the ejaculation of semen during sexual activity, such that the ejaculation occurs before it is intended. Also *ejaculatio praecox.* **e. of semen** The sudden expulsion from the urethra by the male of fluid containing secretions of the prostate, epididymus, seminal vesicles, and ductus deferens which include spermatozoa.

**ejaculator** \ijak′yəlā′tər\ A muscle involved in ejaculation.

**ejaculum** \ijak′yələm\ EJACULATE.

**ejecta** \ijek′tə\ [L (from *ejecta,* neut. pl. of *ejectus,* past part. of *ejicere* to cast out, expel), things cast out] Materials ejected from the body; excreted waste materials.

**ejection** \ijek′shən\ **milk e.** The forceful expulsion of milk from the nipple in response to suckling. See also LET-DOWN REFLEX.

**ejector** \ijek′tər\ A device used for expelling or ejecting a substance from a space. **saliva e.** **1** A suction device for removing excess saliva from the mouth during dental treatment; an aspirator using the venturi effect of a water jet. Also *dental pump, saliva pump.* **2** The interchangeable sterilizable mouthpiece for such a device; an aspirator tip.

**ejusd.** *ejusdem* (L, of the same).

**ek-** \ek-, ik-\ EX-[2].

**eka-** [Sanskrit *eka* one] A prefix used to designate a chemical element and its position in the periodic table prior to its discovery or naming: applied to the known element it is expected to follow.

**Ekbom** [Karl Axel *Ekbom,* Swedish neurologist, born 1907] Ekbom syndrome. See under RESTLESS LEGS SYNDROME.

**EKG** electrocardiogram.

**EKY** electrokymogram.

**el-** \el-, il-\ EN-.

**elaeo-** \ē′lē·ō-\ ELEO-.

**elaio-** \ē′lē·ō-\ ELEO-.

**elaioplast** \ilē′ōplast\ [ELAIO- + -PLAST] A large cell containing oil or fat which appears in areas of fat necrosis as a result of trauma.

**Elapidae** \ilap′idē\ A large family of venomous snakes containing some 181 species distributed in tropical and subtropical regions. Their fangs are fixed rigidly at the front of the upper jaw, and each anterior maxillary tooth is grooved or perforated. The venom is neurotoxic. The family includes cobras, kraits, coral snakes, mambas, and brown snakes. Adj. elapid.

***Elaps*** \ē′laps\ MICRURUS.

**elast-** \ilast-\ ELASTO-.

**elastance** \ilas′təns\ [ELAST- + -ANCE] The recoil pressure resulting from a unit change of volume of a hollow viscus; the reciprocal of compliance. Compare COMPLIANCE.

**elastase** A serine proteinase (EC 3.4.21.11) produced in the pancreas. It has a large sequence in common with trypsin, and it splits peptides on the C-terminal side of hydrophobic residues.

**elastic** [ELAST- + -IC] Tending to resume its initial shape after being stretched or bent. **intermaxillary e.** A small elastic band used to exert a force on a tooth or teeth taking its anchorage from the opposite jaw.

**elasticity** \ē′lastis′itē\ The quality or condition of being elastic. **physical e. of muscle** That property of a muscle by which it can yield to passive stretch. **physiologic e. of muscle** That property of a muscle by which it can alter its length in response to nervous stimulation. **total e. of muscle** The combined effects of physical elasticity and physiological elasticity on a muscle.

**elastin** An elastic protein found in artery walls. Its chains are cross-linked by the formation of desmosine and related residues from lysine residues in the separate chains.

**elasto-** \ilas′tō-\ [New L *elast(icus)* (from Gk *elastikos* driven on, set in motion, from *elaunein* to drive on, set in motion) propulsive, ductile] A combining form meaning elasticity, elastic. Also *elast-.*

**elastoblast** \ilas′tōblast\ [ELASTO- + -BLAST] A cell that is capable of forming elastic fibers.

**elastofibroma** \ilas′tōfībrō′mə\ [ELASTO- + FIBR- + -OMA] A benign tumor containing fibrous and elastic tissues. It usually occurs in the subscapular region in elderly people. **e. dorsi** A benign lesion with an elastin-filled core surrounded by a collagen matrix. It is most commonly seen in the subscapular area of elderly patients. **perforating e.** A benign dermal tumor composed of both elastic tissue and collagen, part of which is situated in the dermis.

**elastoid** \ilas′toid\ [ELAST- + -OID] A substance formed by hyaline degeneration of the elastic lamina of blood vessels sometimes noted in postpartum uteri.

**elastoidosis** \ilas′toidō′sis\ [ELAST- + -OID + -OSIS ] **nodular e.** NODULAR ELASTOSIS OF THE SKIN.

**elastoma** \il′astō′mə\ [ELAST- + -OMA] An abnormality in quality or quantity of either cutaneous collagen or elastic fibers in the dermis. **juvenile e.** A connective tissue nevus characterized by proliferation of abnormal elastic fibers in the dermis. **Miescher's e.** ELASTOSIS PERFORANS SERPIGINOSA.

**elastomer** \ilas′tōmir′\ A man-made material with elastic properties resembling those of rubber.

**elastometer** \ē′lastäm′ətər\ [ELASTO- + -METER] An instrument for measuring elasticity, as of tissue.

**elastosis** \ilastō′sis\ [ELAST- + -OSIS] Degeneration and fragmentation of elastic fibers. Adj. elastotic. **e. intrapapillare** ELASTOSIS PERFORANS SERPIGINOSA. **nodular e. of the skin** Chronic solar degenerative elastosis that gives rise to yellow, irregularly thickened skin, and comedones and follicular cysts, which are found most often around the orbits and on the cheeks. Also *Favre-Racouchot syndrome, nodular elastoidosis.* **e. perforans serpiginosa** Keratotic papules arranged in a ring or in a serpiginous form that arise from the skin, along with an excess of elastic tissue in the dermis. Also *Miescher's elastoma, elastosis intrapapillare, reactive perforating elastosis.* **senile e.** The degeneration of the elastic tissue of the dermis, due to old age. Also *elastosis senilis.*

**Elaut** [Leon Jozef Stephaan *Elaut,* Belgian anatomist, flourished 20th century] See under TRIANGLE.

**elbow** [Old English *elboga, elnboga,* from *eln* forearm (akin to L *ulna* forearm and Gk *ōlenē* forearm) + *boga* bow, bend] The joint between the arm and the forearm and the region immediately around it; cubitus. **baseball pitchers' e.** Premature osteoarthrosis of the radiohumeral joint. It can be caused by repeated trauma, as is seen in baseball pitching. **beat e.** Bursitis and/or subcutaneous cellulitis around the elbow. It occurs among miners and is due to prolonged external friction or pressure. Similar conditions occur in the hand and knee. **capped e.** OLECRANON BURSITIS. **golfers' e.** Inflammation of the medial epicondyle of the humerus. Also *elbow pain syndrome.* **little leaguers' e.** Osteochondrosis of the capitulum of the humerus which is often seen in children who take part in pitching sports, such as baseball. **miners' e.** OLECRANON BURSITIS. **pulled e.** Distal subluxation of the head of the radius. **students' e.** OLECRANON BURSITIS.

**elective** \ilek′tiv\ Optional or nonurgent, as in *elective surgery.*

**electricity** [*electr(o)-* + -IC + -ITY] The separation or movement of electrons and protons; either the separation of charges by friction (static electricity), or the movement of charges caused by magnetism and chemical batteries (current flow).

**electro-** \ilek′trō-\ [Gk *ēlektron* amber] A combining form meaning electricity, electric.

**electroacupuncture** \-ak′yəpungk′chər\ [ELECTRO- + ACUPUNCTURE] A procedure for relief of pain or spasticity consisting of electrical stimulation through a needle electrode, which usually is inserted into the vicinity of a nerve.

**electroanalgesia** \-an′aljē′sē·ə\ [ELECTRO- + ANALGESIA] Diminution of pain through stimulation with an electric current. It may involve stimulation of brain or spinal cord structures through indwelling electrodes, or stimulation of a peripheral nerve.

**electroanesthesia** \-an′esthē′zhə\ ELECTRICAL ANESTHESIA.

**electroaugmentation** \-ôg′məntā′shən\ Electrical pacing of the heart.

**electrobasograph** \-bā′sōgraf\ An apparatus for measuring the weight bearing period of limbs during walking.

**electrobiologic** \-bi′əläj′ik\ BIOELECTRIC.

**electrobioscopy** \-bī·äs′kəpē\ The recording of electrical activity in a tissue or organism in order to determine whether it is alive.

**electrocapillarity** \-kap′iler′itē\ The change in position of the interface between two liquids in a capillary tube when a voltage is applied across them. Also *electrocapillary action.*

**electrocardiogram** \-kär′dē·ōgram′\ [ELECTRO- + CARDIOGRAM] The graphic recording of the potentials of the heart detected on the surface of the body by electrocardiography. The most common electrocardiogram, called lead II, has as its principal components the P wave, the QRS complex, and the T wave. Abbr. ECG, EKG **bipolar e.** An electrocardiogram obtained by recording the difference in voltage between two electrodes at different sites on the body surface. **scalar e.** The usual electrocardiogram which plots voltage versus time, as distinguished from the vectorcardiogram, which plots voltage versus phase. **unipolar e.** An electrocardiogram which shows the potential de-

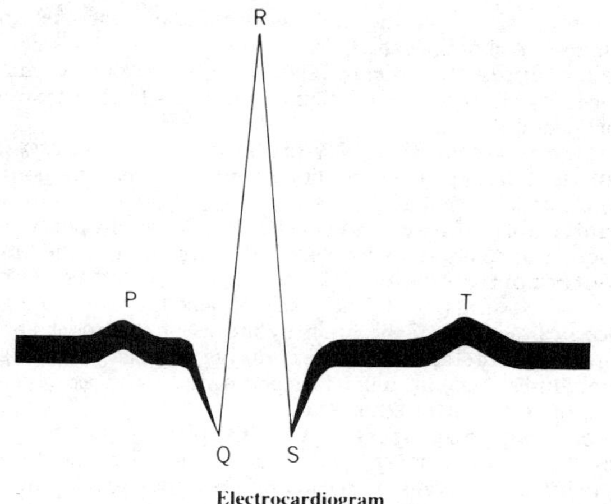

Electrocardiogram

tected by a single electrode. In practice, this is obtained by using an exploring electrode and a second electrode such as a Wilson central terminal which is assumed to have zero potential.

**electrocardiograph** [ELECTRO- + CARDIOGRAPH] An instrument used for making electrocardiograms. It contains a lead-switching network, a differential amplifier, and a strip-chart recorder to trace the electrocardiogram on paper output.

**electrocardiography** \-kär′dē·äg′rəfē\ [ELECTRO- + CARDIOGRAPHY] The recording and study of the electrical activity of the heart. **intrabronchial e.** The recording of an electrocardiogram with an exploring electrode in a bronchus. **intracardiac e.** The recording of electrocardiograms by means of electrodes within the cardiac cavities. **precordial e.** The recording of electrical activity from electrodes placed on the anterior chest wall.

**electrocatalysis** \-kətal′isis\ [ELECTRO- + CATALYSIS] The breaking down of a substance by electric stimulation.

**electrocauterization** \-kô′tərīzā′shən\ The establishment of hemostasis through the use of an electrocautery.

**electrocautery** \-kô′tərē\ [ELECTRO- + CAUTERY] The destruction or coagulation of tissue by the application of electric current, as to obtain hemostasis.

**electrocerebellogram** \-ser′əbel′əgram\ A record of the electrical activity displayed by the cerebellum. Using electrodes with suitably small contacts, it is distinguished by random, high-frequency activity.

**electrocision** \-sizh′ən\ [ELECTRO- + *(ex)cision*] The excision of tissue following the application of an electric current.

**electrocoagulation** \-kō·ag′yəlā′shən\ Coagulation by the heat of an electric spark created by a high-frequency alternating current applied across two terminals. Also *electric coagulation.*

**electrocochleogram** \-käk′lē·əgram′\ A graphic record of auditory threshold as measured by electrocochleography.

**electrocochleography** \-käk′lē·äg′rəfē\ [ELECTRO- + *cochle(a)* + *o* + -GRAPHY] The measurement of auditory threshold for rapid trains of clicks at specified intensities, determined by the changes noted in computer-averaged electrical potential, and detected by means of a fine transtympanic electrode placed in the middle-ear mucosa near the round window. Abbr. E.Coch.G.

**electrocoma** \-kō′mə\ [ELECTRO- + COMA] Coma induced by electrical stimulation of the brain for the treatment for mental illness.

**electrocontractility** \-kän′traktil′itē\ [ELECTRO- + CONTRACTILITY] Contractility of muscle fibers induced by an electrical stimulus.

**electroconvulsive** \-kənvul′siv\ Pertaining to the induction of convulsions by electrical stimulation of the brain.

**electrocorticogram** \-kôr′tikəgram′\ [ELECTRO- + CORTICO- + -GRAM] **1** The trace obtained by recording the electrical activity of the brain by means of electrodes applied directly to the cerebral cortex, during clinical neurosurgical procedures and in animal experiments. Also *corticogram.* **2** *Incorrect* DEPTH RECORDING.

**electrocorticography** \-kôr′tikäg′rəfē\ [ELECTRO- + CORTICO- + -GRAPHY] The technique of recording electrical activity of the brain by means of electrodes applied directly to the exposed cerebral cortex. Abbr. ECoG

**electrocortin** *Outmoded* ALDOSTERONE.

**electrocution** \-kyoo′shən\ [ELECTRO- + *(exe)cute* + -ION] Death resulting from the passage of electric current through the body. Death is usually caused by the induction of ventricular fibrillation or standstill.

**electrocystography** \-sistäg′rəfē\ [ELECTRO- + CYSTOGRAPHY] The recording of varying electrical currents in the urinary bladder.

**electrode** \ilek′trōd\ [ELECTR- + Gk *(h)odos* a way, path, road] An electrical conductor used to pass charge or current to or from a gas, solution, semiconductor, another metallic conductor, or tissue. **active e.** THERAPEUTIC ELECTRODE. **carbon dioxide e.** An electrode that determines the partial carbon dioxide pressure of a fluid specimen by measuring the pH change across a gas-permeable membrane separating the specimen from a bicarbonate buffer solution of known pH within the electrode. **central terminal e.** In unipolar electrocardiography, the exploring electrode connected to the Wilson central terminal. **Clark e.** A platinum wire electrode used in measuring arterial blood oxygen. When current of an appropriate voltage is applied, oxygen flows from the specimen through a gas-permeable membrane and is destroyed at the platinum surface. **dispersive e.** In electrosurgery, the large electrode usually placed on the buttocks or thigh to collect the current and return it to the electrosurgical unit. Also *return electrode, butt plate, safety plate, patient plate, silent electrode, indifferent electrode, fixed electrode.* **esophageal e.** An electrode placed in the esophagus to obtain electrocardiographic records from this region or used for electrical pacemaking. **fixed e.** **1** INDIFFERENT ELECTRODE. **2** DISPERSIVE ELECTRODE. **glass e.** An electrode for measuring the pH of a solution, based on the fact that a thin sheet of glass is permeable to hydrogen ions but not to other ions. The apparatus so called often contains both electrodes of a cell within it, i.e. a reference electrode as well as the glass electrode proper, and a salt bridge for connecting them, so that the potential produced by the cell depends on the pH of the solution in which the apparatus is immersed. **indifferent e.** **1** An electrode remote from the biopotential source and serving as a reference for the active electrode. **2** The Wilson central terminal used in unipolar electrocardiography for recording the precordial leads. For defs. 1 and 2 also *fixed electrode.* **3** DISPERSIVE ELECTRODE. **ion-selective e.** An electrode used for measurement of specific ions in body fluids. Selectivity may be achieved by use of appropriate buffer solutions, partially permeable membranes, or ion-exchange materials. **return e.** DISPERSIVE ELECTRODE. **reversible e.** An electrode such as the silver/silver chloride electrode in which the electrochemical reaction is reversible, which results in a low resistance to direct current. **silent e.** DISPERSIVE ELECTRODE. **therapeutic e.** An electrode filled with therapeutic agents. Also *active electrode.* **transcutaneous oxygen e.** A device that measures the oxygen tension in the skin without penetrating the tissues.

**electrodesiccation** \-des′ikā′shən\ Destruction of tissue with a needle-shaped electrode through which is passed high frequency currents.

**electrodiagnosis** \-di′əgnō′sis\ The diagnosis of disease or dysfunction of the central and peripheral nervous systems and voluntary muscles by any method utilizing electrical stimulation or recording electrical activity.

**electrodialysis** \-dī·al′isis\ Dialysis in an electric field, used to speed movement of large molecules.

**electrodialyzer** \-dī′əlīzər\ A dialyzer that rapidly removes electrolytes from colloids by applying an electric field across the semipermeable membrane.

**electroencephalogram** \-ensef′əlōgram′\ [ELECTRO- + ENCEPHALO- + -GRAM] The trace obtained when the electrical activity of the brain is recorded by means of electrodes placed upon the intact scalp. Abbr. EEG **isoelectric e.** An electroencephalogram in which no recognizable wave-

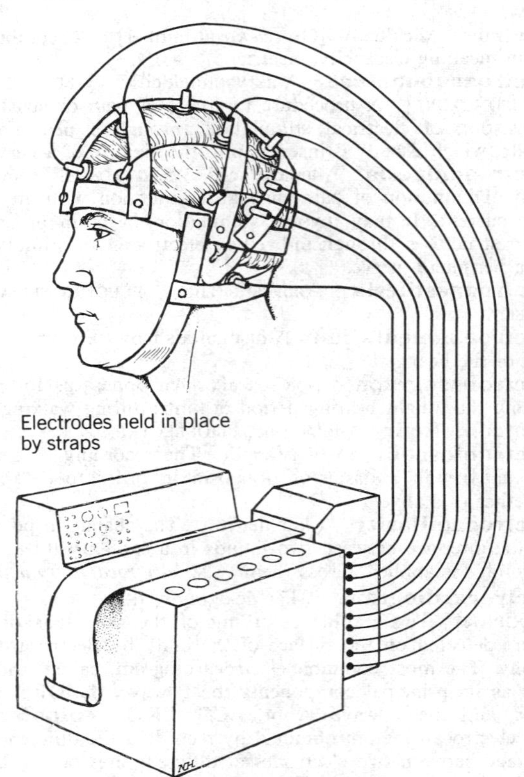


**Electroencephalography**

forms or deviations from the baseline of electrical activity can be discerned as arising from the brain. This is defined as the absence of potentials of more than 2 microvolts observed in a 30-minute recording using electrode pairs 10cm or more apart. This finding usually but not invariably indicates brain death. Also *flat electroencephalogram.*

**electroencephalograph** \-ensef′əlōgraf′\ [ELECTRO- + ENCEPHALO- + -GRAPH] An instrument which is used to amplify and record the electrical activity of the brain, either through the intact skull and scalp, or directly from the exposed cerebral cortex (electrocorticography). It is made up of a number of channels, each of which comprises an amplifying and recording instrument which records the electrical events beneath and between a pair of recording electrodes.

**electroencephalography** \-ensef′əläg′rəfē\ [ELECTRO- + ENCEPHALO- + -GRAPHY] A technique for recording the electrical activity of the brain, through the intact skull and scalp, using an electroencephalograph. It is of particular value in the investigation and diagnosis of epilepsy and may be helpful in localizing some intracranial lesions and in the diagnosis of various brain diseases. Abbr. EEG

**electroexcision** \-eksizh′ən\ Any excision of tissue performed by electrosurgical means. Also *electroresection.*

**electrogastrogram** \-gas′trəgram\ [ELECTRO- + GASTRO- + -GRAM] A record of the electrical activity of the stomach musculature.

**electrogenic** \-jen′ik\ [ELECTRO- + -GENIC] Denoting a process, such as the pumping of ions across a membrane, in which net charge is transferred, so that an electrical field is set up unless the charge can be dissipated by another process. The $Na^+/K^+$-transporting ATPase is electrogenic, as it pumps three sodium ions in one direction for each two potassium ions pumped in the other.

**electroglottography** \-glätäg′rəfē\ ELECTROLARYNGOGRAPHY.

**electrogoniometer** \-gän′ē·äm′ətər\ [ELECTRO- + GONIOMETER] An instrument used to measure positions of flexion and extension of a hinge joint.

**electrogram** \ilek′trōgram\ [ELECTRO- + -GRAM] A record of changes in electrical activity. Also *electrograph.*

**electrography** \ē′lektäg′rəfē\ [ELECTRO- + -GRAPHY] Any technique involving the recording of electrical potentials in resting tissues or organs, and of changes in these potentials during physiologic or pathologic activity. **His bundle e.** The recording of electrograms from the His bundle (atrioventricular bundle), usually by intravenous introduction of an electrode.

**electrogustometer** \-gustäm′ətər\ An apparatus for applying a direct electrical current to points on the tongue as a means of testing the sense of taste. The anode is applied to different points on the protruded tongue and the current necessary to produce an acid taste is noted.

**electrogustometry** \-gustäm′ətrē\ [ELECTRO- + GUSTOMETRY] Assessment of the integrity of the sense of taste using graded electrical stimuli applied to the lingual mucosa.

**electrohemostasis** \-hēmäs′təsis\ [ELECTRO- + HEMOSTASIS] The use of high-frequency electric currents to stop bleeding.

**electrohysterogram** \-his′tərōgram′\ [ELECTRO- + HYSTERO- + -GRAM] A record of the electrical activity of the uterine musculature.

**electroimmunoassay** \-im′yənō·as′ā\ ROCKET ELECTROPHORESIS.

**electroimmunodiffusion** \-im′yənōdifyoo′zhən\ [ELECTRO- + IMMUNODIFFUSION] The diffusion of antigen and antibody through an electric field, as in the Laurell rocket immunoelectrophoresis.

**electrokymograph** \-kī′mōgraf\ [ELECTRO- + KYMOGRAPH] An instrument that records changes in density of examined structures or organs, or motions of the borders of organs, by recording the changes in the transmission of a well-collimated, narrow beam of radiation.

**electrokymography** \-kīmäg′rəfē\ The study of motion of borders of organs by using an electrokymograph.

**electrolaryngogram** \-lering′gōgram\ The oscilloscopic record of vocal cord activity made by means of electrolaryngography. Also *laryngogram, glottogram.*

**electrolaryngograph** \-lering′gōgraf\ An instrument for recording the activity of the vocal cords during phonation and respiration. It consists of a pair of electrodes, one for application to either side of the neck adjacent to the larynx, a generator, amplifier, and oscilloscope. Also *laryngograph, glottograph.*

**electrolaryngography** \-ler′ing·gäg′rəfē\ The recording, using an electrolaryngograph, of the activity of the vocal cords from potentials arising in the laryngeal muscles during phonation and respiration. Also *laryngography, electroglottography, glottography.*

**electrolithotrity** \-lithät′ritē\ [ELECTRO- + LITHOTRITY] Disintegration of calculi by application of an electric current.

**electrolysis** [ELECTRO- + LYSIS] The chemical decomposition of a substance by the reactions that occur to its constituent ions at electrodes when an electric current is passed through the molten substance or, more usually, through a solution of the substance. Electrolysis is widely used to destroy hair follicles in the treatment of hirsutism. Also *galvanolysis.*

**electrolyte** \ilek′trəlīt\ [ELECTRO- + Gk *lytos* dissoluble] A substance that yields ions in solution so that its solutions conduct electricity.

**electrolyzer** \ilek′trəlīzər\ An instrument for removing fibromas or relieving urethral strictures by electrolysis.

**electromanometer** \-manäm′ətər\ [ELECTRO- + MANOMETER] An apparatus for measuring the pressure of gases or liquids that uses an electric signal as the indicator.

**electromanometry** \-manäm′ətrē\ The measurement of pressure, as of the cerebrospinal fluid during lumbar puncture, by electrical means.

**electrometer** \il′ekträm′ətər\ [ELECTRO- + -METER] An instrument for measuring the electrostatic potential difference between two conductors. It is typically used to measure the charge on a capacitor type of ionization chamber or the potential difference of a pH electrode.

**electrometrogram** \-met′rəgram\ [ELECTRO- + METRO- + -GRAM] An instrument that can record changes in the electrical potentials of uterine musculature.

**electromyogram** \-mī′əgram\ A record of the spiking electrical discharge of a muscle, motor unit, or muscle fiber generated in response to neural impulses or arising spontaneously.

**electromyography** \-mī·äg′rəfē\ [ELECTRO- + MYOGRAPHY] The recording of electrical activity associated with muscular activity, often used in clinical diagnosis of muscular disorders. **ureteral e.** The recording of varying electrical currents during contractions of the ureter.

**electron** \ilek′trän\ [*electr(o)-* + -ON] An elementary charged particle carrying unit negative charge of $1.6 \times 10^{-19}$ coulombs. Electrons form the outer parts of atoms, and are responsible for the bonding between them. Also *negatron.* **Auger e.** An electron emitted from an excited atom through the Auger effect. **Compton e.** The electron recoil resulting from the interaction of an x ray or gamma ray in the process known as the Compton effect.

**free e.** An electron in or beyond the outermost electron shells of an atom. It is unbound or very weakly bound. **secondary e.** An electron knocked out of its normal habitat by an incident photon or particle. Also *recoil electron.* **thermionic e.** An electron emitted by heating a substance. **valence e.** One or more of the electrons in an atom's outermost, incomplete electron shell. Such electrons are exchanged or shared in chemical reactions.

**electronarcosis** \-närkō′sis\ Narcosis created with use of electroconvulsive therapy in which the clonic phase is limited by continued electrical stimulation for several minutes. Also *galvanonarcosis.*

**electron-dense** \ilek′trän-dens′\ Characterized by being relatively opaque to the passage of the electron beam in an electron microscope. Such an object will appear as a dark area on the viewing screen and photographic print.

**electronegative** \-neg′ətiv\ Having the power to attract electrons, and thus likely to become negatively charged when combined with a less electronegative atom or group.

**electroneuromyography** \-n$^y$ur′ōmī·äg′rəfē\ [ELECTRO- + NEUROMYOGRAPHY] The recording of electrical activity of muscle induced by electric stimulation of nerve.

**electronic** \ē′lekträn′ik\ Of or pertaining to devices, circuits, and systems that use devices that control the flow of electrons, such as vacuum tubes and transistors.

**electron-microscopic** \ilek′trän-mī′krəskäp′ik\ Of or relating to electron microscopy.

**electronvolt** \ilek′trənvōlt′\ [ELECTRON + VOLT] A unit of energy used in particle physics equal to the kinetic energy acquired by an electron in passing through a potential difference of one volt in vacuum, a noncoherent unit used in conjunction with SI. Its experimentally obtained value is 1.602 19 $\times 10^{-19}$ joule. Symbol: eV

**electronystagmography** \-nis′tagmäg′rəfē\ The registering of eye movements in spontaneous and induced nystagmus, using either a bioelectric or a photoelectric technique. The bioelectric method records the changes in electrical potential produced by movements of the eye in the plane of two electrodes placed on either side of the eye or, if vertical nystagmus is to be measured, above and below the eye. Its important clinical application is the testing of vestibular function. Also *electro-oculography.* Abbr. ENG

**electrophile** \ilek′trəfīl\ [ELECTRO- + -PHILE] A chemical species with affinity for electrons and hence reactive with species rich in electrons.

**electrophoresis** \-fôrē′sis\ [ELECTRO- + -PHORESIS] The migration of charged particles in a solution under the influence of an applied electric current. Also *cataphoresis, dielectrolysis, electric chromatography.* **countercurrent e.** COUNTERIMMUNOELECTROPHORESIS. **disk e.** An electrophoretic technique that separates proteins by their physical interaction with the supporting medium as well as by electrophoretic mobility. Proteins migrate through layered gels of differing pore size and/or pH, forming discontinuous and concentrated disks of individual molecules within the gel layers. **gel e.** An electrophoretic technique in which the charged material migrates through an agar gel rather than upon a fluid-impregnated solid strip. **paper e.** An electrophoretic technique in which the charged materials migrate upon a paper strip impregnated with an electrolyte solution through which the electric current passes. **polyacrylamide gel e.** Electrophoretic techniques in which the supporting medium, polyacrylamide gel, serves as a molecular sieve so that separation occurs by size and shape of the protein molecules as well as by electrophoretic mobility. **rocket e.** A precipitin technique in which the preparation of antigen is moved by application of an electric current through a medium that contains evenly dispersed antibody. The rapid migration of antigen produces changing concentrations of antigen relative to the antibody, and precipitin lines form in a convex pattern likened to the shape of an ascending rocket. Also *electroimmunoassay.* **zone e.** The electrophoretic separation of migrating molecules in a conducting medium which is immobilized onto an inert supporting medium such as paper, cellulose acetate, or agar gel. Zone electrophoresis allows more manipulation of the separated proteins than moving-boundary electrophoresis.

**electrophoretic** \-fôret′ik\ Pertaining to or resulting from electrophoresis.

**electrophoretogram** \-fôret′əgram\ [*electrophoret(ic)* + *o* + -GRAM] **1** The pattern produced by fixing or staining the bands of protein that have been separated by electrophoresis on a supporting medium. **2** The densitometer tracing generated by analyzing a strip of electrophoretically separated proteins. For defs. 1 and 2 also *ionopherogram.*

**electrophotometer** \-fōtäm′ətər\ PHOTOELECTRIC COLORIMETER.

**electrophysiology** \-fiz′ē·äl′əjē\ [ELECTRO- + PHYSIOLOGY] **1** The study of the electric phenomena associated with the functions of living organisms. **2** The study of the function of living organisms by using electric and electronic techniques.

**electropneumograph** \-n$^y$oo′mōgraf\ An electrical apparatus that records respiratory movements.

**electropositive** \-päs′ətiv\ Tending to lose electrons.

**electroprosthesis** \-prästhē′sis\ [ELECTRO- + PROSTHESIS] A prosthetic device which delivers patterned electrical stimuli to a peripheral nerve or brain site for a functionally beneficial effect.

**electroradiometer** \-rā′dē·äm′ətər\ An electroscope of any of several designs suitable for the measurement of ionizing radiation arriving through the air. Typically, a microscopic, electrically conducting fiber (e.g., silvered quartz) is suspended in a chamber, close to and connected with an insulated wire support. An electrostatic charge is applied, and the like charges deflect the fiber away from the support, the movement being monitored with a microscope and scale. As the radiation of interest ionizes the enclosed gases, slow discharge occurs, and the fiber retreats toward its resting position, the rate of movement indicating the intensity of the radiation.

**electroresection** \-risek′shən\ [ELECTRO- + RESECTION] ELECTROEXCISION.

**electroretinogram** \-ret′ənōgram′\ [ELECTRO- + *retin(a)* + *o* + -GRAM] A recording of the electrical potentials evoked in the retina and ocular fundus in response to a visual stimulus. Abbr. ERG **E e.** An electroretinogram that exhibits excitatory characteristics derived from the rods. **I e.** An electroretinogram that exhibits inhibitory characteristics derived from the cones.

**electroretinography** \-ret′inäg′rəfē\ [ELECTRO- + RETINOGRAPHY] The measurement of the electric potentials of the light-stimulated eye by means of an electroretinograph.

**electroscission** \-sish′ən\ [ELECTRO- + SCISSION] The cutting of tissue by electrosurgical methods.

**electroscope** \ilek′trōskōp\ [ELECTRO- + -SCOPE] Any device for detecting or indicating the presence of an electrostatic charge.

**electrosection** \-sek′shən\ A surgical procedure that involves an electrosurgical incision.

**electroshock** \ilek′trōshäk\ See under ELECTROCONVULSIVE THERAPY.

**electrosome** \ilek′trōsōm\ [ELECTRO- + Gk *sōm(a)* body] MITOCHONDRION.

**electrospectrogram** \-spek′trōgram\ A record produced by electrospectrography.
**electrospectrography** \-spekträg′rəfē\ Automatic frequency analysis of the constituent wave forms of the electroencephalogram.
**electrospinogram** \-spī′nōgram\ A record of the electrical activity of the spinal cord.
**electrospinography** \-spīnäg′rəfē\ The process of recording and analyzing the electrical activity of the spinal cord.
**electrosurgery** \-sur′jərē\ The surgical use of electricity for cutting, desiccation, and coagulation, usually by applying radio-frequency current to a blade or wire loop.
**electrosyneresis** \-siner′əsis\ IMMUNOFILTRATION.
**electrotaxis** \-tak′sis\ [ELECTRO- + TAXIS] The movement of cells or organisms in response to electric current. It can be either negative, when movement is toward the anode, or positive, when movement is toward the cathode. Also *galvanotaxis.*
**electrotherapy** \-ther′əpē\ Any therapeutic use of electricity. Also *electrotherapeutics.*
**electrothrombosis** \-thrämbō′sis\ [ELECTRO- + THROMBOSIS] The production of a thrombus within a blood vessel by introducing an electric current to coagulate the blood.
**electrotome** \ilek′trōtōm\ [ELECTRO- + -TOME] Any electrosurgical cutting instrument.
**electrotomy** \ē′lekträt′əmē\ [ELECTRO- + -TOMY] Electroexcision in which an electric current of high frequency, high voltage, and low amperage is used so that no tissue coagulation occurs.
**electrotonic** \-tän′ik\ Of or related to electrotonus.
**electrotonus** \-tō′nəs\ [ELECTRO- + TONUS] **1** The state in which a tissue or organism is being subjected to a steady polarizing electrical current. **2** Alteration in excitability and conductivity of an excitable tissue, cell, or membrane in the vicinity of an electrode imposing a steady polarizing current.
**electrotrephine** \-trē′fīn\ An electrically operated trephine for perforating the skull.
**electrotropism** \ē′lekträt′rəpizm\ [ELECTRO- + TROPISM] The movement of a cell or organism in response to an electrical stimulus.
**electroureterogram** \-yoorē′tərōgram′\ [ELECTRO- + URETEROGRAM] The recording produced by ureteral electromyography.
**electroversion** \-vur′zhən\ The termination of an arrhythmia by countershock.
**electrovert** \ilek′trōvurt\ To terminate (an arrhythmia) by countershock.
**electuary** \ilek′choo·er′ē\ [Late L *electuarium* (irreg. from Gk *ekleikton* a medicine that melts in the mouth, from *ekleichein* to lick up, from *leichein* to lick) a candied medication, electuary] A medication prepared by combining a powdered drug with honey or syrup. Also *linctus, lincture.* **e. of senna** A syrup containing powdered senna leaf, tamarind, cassia pulp, prune, licorice extract, sucrose, and water. It is used as a laxative. Also *confection of senna.*
**eleidin** \elē′idin\ A substance related to keratin and found in the stratum lucidum of the epidermis.
**element** [L *elementum* (usu. in pl. *elementa* first principles, elements) an element] **1** A substance all of whose atoms have identical nuclear charge. **2** A simple or fundamental component of a more complex entity. **anatomic e.** Any primary morphologic unit, such as a cell or muscle fiber, that constitutes an organ or tissue. **formed e.'s** Erythrocytes, leukocytes, and platelets. **labile e.** A cell group that continues to divide during the life of the individual and retains the capacity for further differentiation. **tissue e.** A cell, connective tissue fiber, or other basic component from which tissues are constructed. Also *morphologic element.* **trace e.** A chemical element that is essential in minute amounts to an organism's metabolism. **transduced e.** Any fragment of nucleic acid that enters a host cell by the process of transduction. **transducer e.** One piece in an array of many transducers used, for example, in an ultrasonic scanner. **transition e.** An element that possesses, either in the elemental form or in an ionic form, a partly filled *d* or *f* shell of electrons. Such elements are metals, exhibit variable valence, and form some colored cations and some paramagnetic compounds. Transition elements represent a transition from strongly electropositive elements to noble metals. **transposable e.** Any piece of duplex DNA capable of moving from one location in a genome to another, as a transposon in bacteria. **transuranic e.** Any element of atomic number greater than 92. Also *transuranium element.*
**elementary** Of or relating to an element; essential, primary, or rudimentary.
**elemicin** \ēlem′isin\ $C_{12}H_{16}O_3$. A hallucinogenic substance present in the seeds and aril of *Myristica fragrans,* nutmeg.
**eleo-** \ē′lē·ō-\ [Gk *elaion* olive oil] A combining form denoting oil. Also *elaeo-, elaio-.*
**eleoma** \el′ē·ō′mə\ [*ele(o)-* + -OMA] A tumorlike lesion resulting from the injection of oil into tissue.
**elephantiasic** \el′əfan′tē·as′ik\ Relating to elephantiasis. Also *elephantiac.*
**elephantiasis** \el′əfantī′əsis\ [Gk (from *elephas,* gen. *elephant(os)* an elephant) elephantiasis] **1** A condition characterized by chronically edematous and thickened tissue, especially the tissues of the genitals and lower extremities, regardless of cause. **2** FILARIAL ELEPHANTIASIS. **e. chirurgica** Massive edema of the arm, especially lymphedema which develops as the result of interruption of axillary lymphatic channels following a radical mastectomy. **e. congenita angiomatosa** KLIPPEL-TRENAUNAY-WEBER SYNDROME. **congenital e.** HEREDITARY LYMPHEDEMA TYPE I. **filarial e.** A disease caused by filariasis and characterized by inflammation and obstruction of lymphatic channels with subsequent lymphatic edema of the limbs and/or other parts of the trunk or head. The edema leads to hypertrophy of the connective tissues and thickening and overgrowth of the malpighian layer of the skin. The legs and external genitalia are most frequently involved, and their appearance in advanced cases resembles that of an elephant's foreleg. The disease is irreversible when fully developed. It is caused by infection with the filarial nematodes *Wuchereria bancrofti* and *Brugia malayi.* The former is the causative organism in most tropical countries, especially Africa, and the latter is the causative organism in Asia and the Far East. Also *elephantiasis, mal de Cayenne, myelolymphangioma, pes febricitans, chyloderma.* **e. italica** PELLAGRA. **e. leishmaniana** The edema and hypertrophy of tissues caused by leishmaniasis, as distinguished from filarial elephantiasis. **e. neuromatosa** The appearance of elephantiasis due to numerous neurofibromas as in neurofibromatosis. **e. nostras** Gross lymphedema of a limb that is not attributable to an exotic cause. It may occur as a result of a developmental defect. **e. scroti** Chronic scrotal filarial elephantiasis; filarial chylocele. Also *lymphoscrotum.*
**elephantoid** \el′əfan′toid\ [*elephant* + -OID] Resembling elephantiasis.
**elevation** An eminence; a raised area. **tactile e.'s**

The cutaneous papillae, rich in sensory nerve endings, found on the skin of the palm and to a lesser extent on the sole of the foot. Also *toruli tactiles.* **tubal e.** TORUS TUBARIUS.

**elevator** [Late L (from *elevatus,* past part. of *elevare* to lift up, alleviate), one who or that which raises] **1** An instrument used to detach a membrane from the surface of bone, used in the manner of a scraper. **2** An instrument used to reposition a fractured and displaced bone. **3** See under DENTAL ELEVATOR. **Cushing periosteal e.** A periosteal elevator designed for use on the skull but now commonly employed in other branches of surgery as well. Also *Cushing elevator.* **dental e.** An instrument used for the removal of teeth or tooth roots. There are two basic types, the most common type having a fine single blade, straight or angled to the shaft, which is used principally with a wedging action, sometimes with rotation of the shaft. The blade is forced into and enlarges the periodontal ligament space. Right and left versions of angled dental elevators are mirror images of each other. The other type of dental elevator is a screw elevator. **Freer e.** An instrument for elevating the mucoperichondrium and mucoperiosteum from the underlying cartilage and bone in submucous resection of the nasal septum. **Lempert e.** LEMPERT RUGINE. **malar e.** A surgical instrument used for repositioning a fracture of the cheek bone. **palatal e.** PALATE RETRACTOR. **periosteal e.** A blunt, flat instrument used during surgery for the separation of periosteum from underlying bone. **Pierce e.** A double-ended dissector for use in a submucous resection operation. Blades are angled to the right and left. **e. of prostate** MUSCULUS LEVATOR PROSTATAE.

**eliminant** \əlim′ənənt\ An agent that promotes excretion, elimination, or evacuation of waste.

**elimination** [L *eliminatus,* past part. of *eliminare* to turn out of doors, from EX- + L *limen* threshold] **1** The excretion of waste products. **2** Any process of removal or exclusion. **immune e.** The removal of antigen from the bloodstream of immune individuals as a result of interaction with antibody followed by ingestion by phagocytes. Also *immune clearance.*

**ELISA** enzyme-linked immunosorbent assay.

**elixir** [Arabic *al-iksīr* (from Gk *xēros* dry, from *xērainein* to dry up) a medium through which a transformation is made] A clear, sweetened, hydroalcoholic solution for oral use containing flavoring substances and medicinal ingredients. **acetaminophen e.** An elixir containing 95 to 105 percent of the labeled amount of acetaminophen. The usual concentrations are 24, 30, and 100 mg per ml. It is used as an analgesic medication. **adjuvant e.** An elixir containing glycyrrhiza. Also *glycyrrhiza elixir.* **amobarbital e.** An elixir containing 95 to 105 percent of the labeled amount of amobarbital. The usual concentration is 22 mg in 5 ml of solution. It is used as a sedative. **e. anisi** A solution containing aniseed oil, fennel oil, bitter almond oil, alcohol, syrup, and water. It is used as a carminative agent. **aromatic e.** A hydroalcoholic solution of which 1000 ml contains orange oil 2.4 ml, lemon oil 0.6 ml, coriander oil 0.24 ml, anise oil 0.06 ml, syrup 375 ml, and talc 30 g. It is used as a vehicle for dispensing medications. Also *simple elixir.* **cascara e.** An elixir produced by percolating cascara, licorice, and light magnesium oxide with boiling water. The solvent is then evaporated and the remaining compound flavored with glycerin and a volatile oil, usually coriander oil since it is most effective in masking the bitterness of cascara. It is used as a purgative. **compound benzaldehyde e.** An aqueous solution containing benzaldehyde 500 μl, vanillin 1 g, orange flower water 150 ml, alcohol 50 ml, and simple syrup 400 ml in each 1000 ml of liquid. It is used as a vehicle for pharmaceutical preparations. **e. of diamorphine and terpin** A solution containing diamorphine hydrochloride, terpin hydrate, alcohol, glycerin, and wild cherry syrup. It is used in the treatment of coughs. **glycerinated gentian e.** A solution containing gentian and taraxacum fluid extracts, compound cardamom tincture, raspberry syrup, sweet orange peel tincture, phosphoric acid, ethyl acetate, glycerin, sucrose, and alcohol in purified water. It is used as a vehicle flavoring agent for medications. **glycyrrhiza e.** ADJUVANT ELIXIR. **high-alcoholic e.** An elixir containing compound orange spirit 4 ml, saccharin 3 g, glycerin 200 ml, and enough alcohol to yield 1000 ml of solution. **isoalcoholic e.** A solution prepared by mixing low-alcoholic and high-alcoholic elixir in proportions sufficient to yield the desired strength of alcohol. Isoalcoholic solutions are prepared to serve as vehicles for various medications that require solvents of different alcoholic strengths. **lactated pepsin e.** An aqueous solution containing a proteolytic enzyme from the glandular layer of the fresh stomach of the hog, lactic acid, glycerin, alcohol, orange oil, and amaranth solution. **low-alcoholic e.** An elixir containing compound orange spirit 10 ml, alcohol 100 ml, glycerin 200 ml, sucrose 320 g, and sufficient purified water to yield 1000 ml of solution. **e. of nux vomica** A solution containing nux vomica tincture, compound cardamom tincture, syrup, and chloroform water. **simple e.** AROMATIC ELIXIR. **sodium pentobarbital e.** An elixir containing sodium pentobarbital 4 g, glycerin 450 ml, alcohol 150 ml, orange oil 0.75 ml, caramel 2 g, simple syrup 150 ml, diluted hydrochloric acid 6 ml, and enough purified water to make 1000 ml of solution. It is used as a hypnotic medication. **terpin hydrate e.** An elixir containing a mixture of terpin hydrate, sweet orange peel tincture, benzaldehyde, glycerin, alcohol, and syrup in purified water. It is used as an expectorant. **terpin hydrate and codeine e.** A solution prepared from 2 g codeine and sufficient terpin hydrate elixir to yield 1000 ml. It is used as an expectorant. **e. valerianae et chloralis compositum** A solution containing potassium bromide, chloral hydrate, liquid extract of valerian, orange oil, lemon oil, coriander oil, aniseed oil, syrup, alcohol, and water. It is used as a sedative.

**-ella** \-el′ə, -ələ\ [L, dim. suffix] A suffix denoting little one.

**Elliot** [George Thomson *Elliot,* U.S. dermatologist, 1851–1935] See under SIGN.

**Elliot** [John Wheelock *Elliot,* U.S. surgeon, 1852–1925] See under POSITION.

**ellipsoid** \ilip′soid\ **1** Having the shape of an ellipse. **2** Any structure possessing a spindle shape, such as a sheathed artery.

**elliptocytary** \ilip′tōsī′tərē\ ELLIPTOCYTIC.

**elliptocyte** \ilip′tōsīt\ An elliptic erythrocyte. Also *ovalocyte, cameloid cell.*

**elliptocytic** \ilip′tōsit′ik\ Relating to or resulting from elliptocytes. Also *elliptocytotic, elliptocytary, ovalocytary.*

**elliptocytosis** \ilip′tōsītō′sis\ The presence of elliptocytes in blood. Also *ovalocytosis.* **hereditary e.** An autosomally inherited abnormality of the erythrocyte membrane, in which many erythrocytes are elliptic, accompanied at times by premature red cell destruction and anemia. Also *elliptocytic anemia, Dresbach syndrome, ovalocytary anemia.*

**elliptocytotic** \ilip′tōsītät′ik\ ELLIPTOCYTIC.

**Ellis** [Richard White Bernard *Ellis,* English physician, born 1902] Ellis-van Creveld syndrome. See under SYNDROME.

**Ellison** [Edwin Homer *Ellison,* U.S. surgeon, 1918–1970]

1 Zollinger-Ellison tumor. See under TUMOR. 2 Zollinger-Ellison syndrome. See under SYNDROME.

**Ellsworth** [Read McLane *Ellsworth*, U.S. physician, born 1899] Ellsworth-Howard test. See under TEST.

**elopement** [Anglo-French *aloper*, prob. from Middle English *aleapen, alepen* to leap, run away, from Old English *ahleapan* to run away, + -MENT] Escape or absence without permission from a psychiatric hospital.

**Elsberg** [Charles Albert *Elsberg*, U.S. surgeon, 1871–1948] See under TEST.

**Elschnig** [Anton Philipp *Elschnig*, Austrian ophthalmologist, 1863–1939] 1 Elschnig pearls. See under ELSCHNIG BODIES. 2 Koerber-Salus-Elschnig syndrome. See under AQUEDUCT OF SYLVIUS SYNDROME.

**Elsner** [Christoph Friedrich *Elsner*, German physician, 1749–1820] Elsner's asthma. See under ANGINA PECTORIS.

**eluate** \el′yoo·āt\ The material obtained by elution.

**eluent** \el′yoo·ənt\ A fluid medium used in obtaining material separated by elution.

**elute** \ēloot′\ To subject to elution.

**elution** \ēloo′shən\ [From L *elutus*, past part. of *eluere* to wash out, cleanse, rinse, from EX- + L *luere* (from Gk *lyein* to loosen) to wash] 1 The separation of one or more constituents from a biologic or physical complex, as, for example, detaching immunoglobulin from a cell surface or removing adsorbed materials from a chromatographic column. 2 The separation of solids from one another by washing or by suspension in media of differing density. For defs. 1 and 2 also *elutriation*. **affinity e.** The elution of a substance from a solid material to which it is adsorbed, when this is achieved by adding to the solution a ligand with which the substance has a natural affinity. Thus an enzyme may be eluted from an ion exchanger by its substrate if this substrate has the same charge as the exchanger. Highly specific elution can often be obtained, and hence high purification of enzymes. **gradient e.** The elution of adsorbed substances by a solution of gradually changing composition, designed to become a steadily more powerful eluting agent, e.g. of increasing salt strength if the substances are adsorbed by ion exchange. This method is used in the purification of proteins.

**elutriation** \ēloo′trē·ā′shən\ [L *elutriatus*, past part. of *elutriare* to wash out] 1 The separation of mixtures of particulate solids by suspending the particles in fluid and allowing sedimentation to occur according to differences in density. 2 ELUTION.

**elytro-** \el′ətrō-\ [Gk *elytron* sheath, covering] A combining form denoting the vagina.

**elytroceliotomy** \-sē′lē·ät′əmē\ [ELYTRO- + CELIO- + -TOMY] CULDOCENTESIS.

**elytroplasty** \el′ətrōplas′tē\ [ELYTRO- + -PLASTY] COLPOPLASTY.

**elytropolypus** \-päl′ipəs\ COLPOPOLYPUS.

**Elzholz** [Adolf *Elzholz*, Austrian psychiatrist, 1863–1925] Elzholz bodies. See under BODY.

**EM** emmetropia.

**em-** \em-, əm-\ EN-.

**emaciated** \imā′shē·ā′tid\ Characterized by emaciation.

**emaciation** \imā′shē·ā′shən\ [from L *emaciatus*, past part. of *emaciare* to make lean, from *e-* E- intensive + *macies* leanness, from *macer* lean] A condition characterized by the loss of excessive quantities of body tissues resulting in a loss of weight, which might occur as a result of starvation.

**emailloblast** \emī′lōblast, emā′lō-\ AMELOBLAST.

**emanation** \em′ənā′shən\ [Late L *emanatio* (from L *emanatus*, past part. of *emanare* to flow out, run out) a flowing out] Radon, thoron, and actinon considered as isotopes of a single element. Symbol: Em • *Radon, thoron*, and *actinon* are convenient and practical names. They indicate at once the series to which the nuclide belongs, and they distinguish radon, which is clinically usable, from the other two, which have only academic interest due to their short half-lives. From a logical standpoint however, the designations *emanation 222, emanation 220*, and *emanation 219*, respectively, are more suitable **radium e.** RADON.

**emancipation** \iman′sipā′shən\ Acquisition by an embryonic region of autonomy in its development.

**emasculation** \imas′kyəlā′shən\ [L *emascul(are)* (from *e(x)-* out, off + *masculus* male) to deprive of virility + -ATION] 1 Castration of the male. 2 Removal of the male external genitalia. 3 Deprivation of masculinity or virility.

***Embadomonas*** \em′bədäm′ənəs\ [Gk *embas*, gen. *embados*, a slipper + *monas* single, a unit] *RETORTAMONAS*

**embalm** [Middle English *embalmen*, from Middle French *embaumer* to embalm (from *en-* IN- + *basme* balm, from L *balsamum* balsam, balm)] To treat (a dead body) with chemical preservatives, pigments, and antiseptic agents to produce a lifelike appearance and to impede early postmortem putrefaction.

**Embden** [Gustav *Embden*, German biochemist, 1874–1933] 1 Embden-Meyerhof cycle. See under EMBDEN-MEYERHOF PATHWAY. 2 Embden ester. See under GLUCOSE 6-PHOSPHATE.

**embed** \embed′\ To permeate and surround a block of tissue with a substance that can harden sufficiently to support that tissue during the preparation of a histologic section. Also *imbed*.

**embolectomy** \em′bōlek′təmē\ [*embol(us)* + -ECTOMY] The removal of an embolus through an incision in a blood vessel.

**emboli** \em′bōlī\ Plural of EMBOLUS.

**embolic** \embäl′ik\ Pertaining to or resulting from an embolism.

**emboliform** \embäl′ifôrm\ Resembling an embolus.

**embolism** \em′bōlizm\ [*embol(us)* + -ISM] The obstruction of a vessel by solid or gaseous matter which has been transported through the bloodstream. **air e.** The obstruction of a vessel by bubbles of air, usually as a result of introduction into veins by trauma, surgery or the faulty intravenous administration of fluid. Also *aeroembolism, pneumathemia, pneumohemia, aeremia*. **amniotic fluid e.** An embolus consisting of amniotic fluid which is forced into the maternal vasculature by tumultuous contractions occurring near the end of the second stage of labor. The condition is associated with the abrupt onset of shock, dyspnea, and coagulopathy and frequently proceeds to death of the mother. Also *amniotic fluid infusion*. **bacterial e.** Obstruction of a vessel by a mass of bacteria. **bland e.** An uninfected thrombotic embolism. **bone marrow e.** Obstruction of a vessel by bone marrow, usually as a result of a fractured long bone. **capillary e.** Blocking of capillaries, usually by bacteria. **cerebral e.** The blockage of a cerebral artery or arteriole by an embolus transported from some point in the arterial circulation at a distance from the point of vascular occlusion. Thrombi in the heart or major arteries of the neck are the major sources of cerebral emboli. **coronary e.** Obstruction of a coronary artery by an embolus, usually derived from the vegetations of infective endocarditis or a thrombus from a prosthetic valve. **crossed e.** PARADOXICAL EMBOLISM. **fat e.** The obstruction of vessels by fat globules, usually as a consequence of fractures of long bones but also occur-

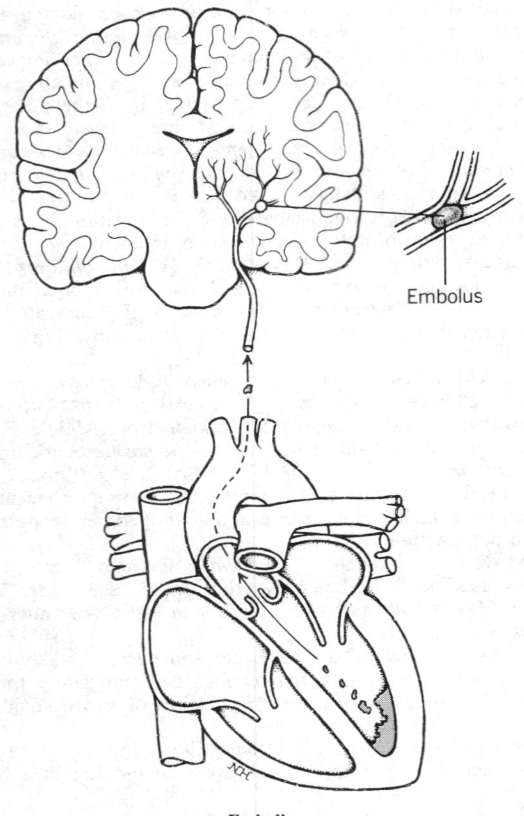

Embolism

ring in burns and in fatty degeneration of the liver. Also *oil embolism.* **hematogenous e.** Embolism due to blood clot. **infective e.** Obstruction of a vessel by infected material. Also *pyemic embolism.* **miliary e.** Multiple simultaneous emboli, as, for example, to many small arteries of the feet from an aortic aneurysm, or to several different peripheral arteries from a cardiac source. **oil e.** FAT EMBOLISM. **paradoxical e.** Embolism as the result of a clot which originates on the venous side of the circulation but embolizes to the arterial side because of a right-to-left shunt in the central circulation. This is usually through a patent foramen ovale but it can also occur through atrial or ventricular septal defects. Also *crossed embolism.* **pulmonary e.** Embolic occlusion of a major pulmonary artery or one or more of its branches. **pyemic e.** INFECTIVE EMBOLISM. **retinal e.** Embolic occlusion of the central artery of the retina. **saddle e.** Embolic occlusion of the bifurcation of the aorta and the common iliac arteries. **tumor e.** Embolic occlusion due to neoplastic tissue. **venous e.** Embolism arising from venous thrombosis.

**embolization** \em′bōlīzā′shən\ [*embol(us)* + *-iz(e)* + -ATION] The occlusion of a blood vessel or group of blood vessels, as in an arteriovenous anomaly, by a transported blood clot or any foreign material such as muscle, plastic beads, iron filings, inflated balloon, etc.

**embolotherapy** \em′bōlōther′əpē\ The therapeutic blocking of arteries by the installation of a small fragment of muscle, blood clot, or other material through a catheter. It is performed to correct problems of bleeding, a tumor, or an arteriovenous fistula.

**embolus** \em′bōləs\ [New L, from Gk *embolos* (from *emballein* to throw in, put in, from *em-* in + *ballein* to throw) a plug, stopper, wedge] (*pl.* emboli) **1** A thrombus formed within or a foreign material introduced into the vascular tree and carried by the bloodstream to a site where it lodges and obstructs further flow of blood. **2** NUCLEUS EMBOLIFORMIS CEREBELLI. **air e.** An air bubble or bubbles obstructing a vessel. See also AIR EMBOLISM. **cholesterol e.** An embolus containing cholesterol and usually derived from the breakdown of an atheromatous plaque in the wall of an artery. **fat e.** An embolus consisting of fat globules or oily material. Also *oil embolus.* See also FAT EMBOLISM. **pantaloon e.** SADDLE EMBOLUS. **platelet e.** An embolus made up of a clump of platelets, usually arising from a mural thrombus forming upon the surface of an atheromatous plaque. **pulmonary e.** A thrombus, usually stemming from deep venous thrombosis of the pelvis and thigh, that is passed into the pulmonary arterial circulation. Occasionally other materials, notably amniotic fluid, air bubbles, or foreign bodies, may embolize in the lungs. **renal cholesterol e.** Partial or complete obstruction of small intrarenal arteries by needle-shaped cholesterol crystals, sometimes resulting in renal infarcts. The embolus originates from an atheroma of the aorta or a main renal artery, usually following vascular surgery or angiography. **saddle e.** An embolus overriding the bifurcation of the aorta and blocking both iliac arteries. Also *riding embolus, straddling embolus, pantaloon embolus.*

**emboly** \em′bōlē\ [Gk *embolē* (from *en-* in + *ballein* to throw) a throwing in, entrance, insertion] The process of invagination of the blastula, which results in the formation of the gastrula.

**embouchement** \äNbooshmäN′\ [French (from *(s')emboucher(r)* to flow into, from *em-* EN- + *bouche* mouth, from L *bucca* mouth + French *-ment* -MENT), a flowing into] The opening of one blood vessel into another.

**embrasure** \embrā′zhər\ [French (from *ébraser* to enlarge progressively from the outside to the inside, as a fortification window), the opening for a door or window] A space, widening from within outwards, between two or more flat or curved surfaces. **interdental e.** The space between the proximal surfaces of two adjacent teeth and the outer surface of the interdental soft tissue. In health, the embrasure is shallow. In disease, it may be filled with enlarged gingiva or deepened by loss of gingiva. Also *interdental space.*

**embrocation** The application of a liquid medicinal material, usually a liniment, to the body surface. *Rare.*

**embry-** \em′brē-\ EMBRYO-.

**embryatrics** \em′brē·at′riks\ [EMBRY- + *-(i)atrics*] Any matter or topic related to or involving the investigation and treatment of an embryo and, by extension, of a fetus.

**embryectomy** \em′brē·ek′təmē\ [EMBRY- + -ECTOMY] The excision of an embryo, especially an extrauterine embryo.

**embryo** \em′brē·ō\ [Gk *embryon* (from EM- + Gk *bryein* to be full of, to swell) fruit of the womb before birth, an embryo] The juvenile stage of an animal when within an egg, enclosed in egg membranes, or inside the maternal organism. The life period of an embryo is usually considered to extend from the start of cleavage until escape from the enveloping egg membranes. In man an embryo, by convention, exists from cleavage until the eighth week of intrauterine life when

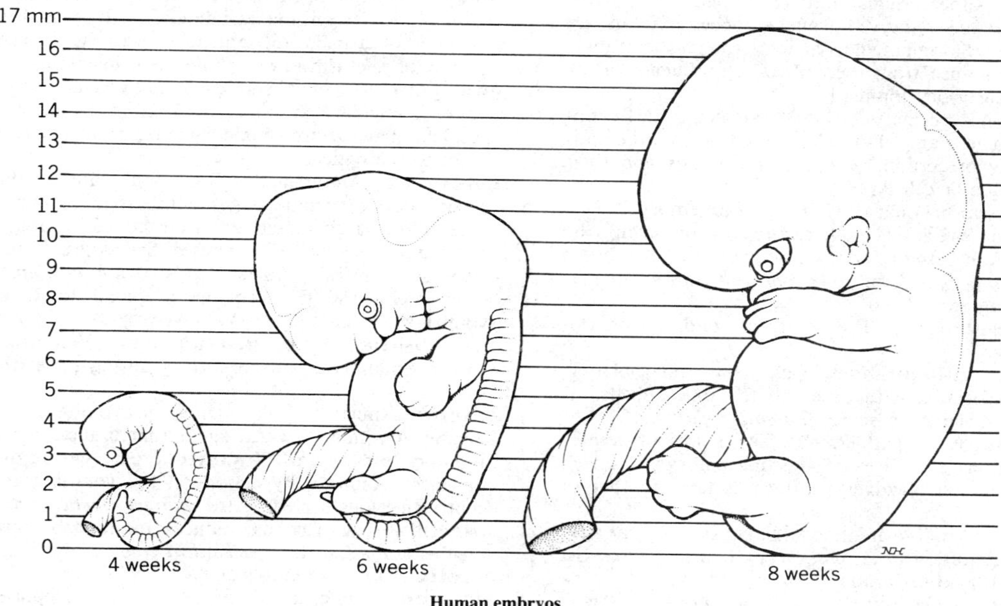


**Human embryos**

its form has virtually become established. Thereafter it is called a fetus. **hexacanth e.** The six-hooked tapeworm embryo (subclass Cestoda) that forms within the eggshell and, after hatching in an appropriate intermediate host, claws its way into its tissues to form the next larval stage, such as the cysticercus or cysticercoid. **presomite e.** The stage in the development of an embryo before any somites have appeared. **previllous e.** The stage in the development of an embryo before any villi have appeared on the chorion. **somite e.** The stage of embryonic development which starts with the appearance of the first somite and ends when somite formation has been completed.

**embryo-** \em′brē·ō-\ [Gk *embryon* embryo] A combining form meaning embryo. Also *embry-*.

**embryoblast** \em′brē·ōblast′\ [EMBRYO- + -BLAST] The portion of the ovum from which the embryo itself develops, with the exclusion of the extraembryonic structures.

**embryocardia** \-kär′dē·ə\ [EMBRYO- + -CARDIA] FETAL RHYTHM.

**embryocidal** \-sī′dəl\ Causing death of an embryo.

**embryoctony** \em′brē·äk′tənē\ [EMBRYO- + Gk *ktono(s)* a killing + -Y] Destruction of a living embryo or fetus by artificial means.

**embryogenesis** \-jen′əsis\ The development of an embryo, in animals from the initial fertilization of an egg. Principal events include cleavages; formation of germ layers, of somites and of branchial arches; histogenesis and organogenesis. Adj. embryogenic. • While *embryogenesis* really refers to the stage of constitution of the embryo proper, the term is often extended to cover the entire developmental process from egg to adult. **accelerated e.** TACHYGENESIS.

**embryogeny** \em′brē·äj′ənē\ [EMBRYO- + GEN- + -Y ] The origination of an embryo or its initial means of formation; the act or process of producing an embryo. Adj. embryogenic, embryogenetic.

**embryograph** \em′brē·ōgraf′\ [EMBRYO- + -GRAPH] An old-fashioned but still occasionally useful method of drawing outlines of sections of embryos using a camera lucida.

**embryologic** \-läj′ik\ Pertaining to embryology.

**embryologist** \em′brē·äl′əjist\ One who specializes in embryology.

**embryology** \em′brē·äl′əjē\ [EMBRYO + -LOGY] The study of the development of plant or animal organisms from a seed or an egg to the establishment of form and shape, but not necessarily to that of adult or definitive size. Modern embryology has advanced beyond descriptions of developmental stages of the individual and evolutionary history of tissues, organs, and parts to a realization of the importance of genetics, molecular biology and biochemistry, teratogens and abnormal development. Embryology now deals primarily with the complex interrelations of processes that bring about normal and abnormal development. **causal e.** A branch of embryology which considers the mechanisms involved in embryonic development. **chemical e.** The study of the chemistry of embryologic processes, including the biochemical analysis of eggs, embryos and their parts. **comparative e.** The study of the similarities and differences in the developmental processes exhibited by the various groups of organisms. **descriptive e.** The description of the successive phases exhibited by any organism during its development from an egg. The establishment of sound descriptive embryology has allowed the development of the modern experimental approach, which searches for an understanding of the control of embryologic processes. **experimental e.** The study of embryonic development under experimental and usually artificial conditions to determine the driving forces behind it.

**embryoma** \em′brē·ō′mə\ [EMBRY- + -OMA] **1** Any tumor containing embryonal-type tissues, such as a nephroblastoma or a retinoblastoma. **2** TERATOMA.

**embryomorphous** \-môr′fəs\ [EMBRYO- + -MORPHOUS] **1** Resembling an embryo in shape, form, or development.

2 Designating abnormal tissue elements which may develop in the gonads, or other organs, and which were at one time supposed to have been derived from a conception but are more likely to have originated from isolated, plastic embryonic tissue that escaped from the controlling influence of organizers during early development.

**embryonal** \em′brē·ənal\ 1 EMBRYONIC. 2 Resembling an embryonic stage of development; poorly differentiated: said chiefly of certain malignant neoplasms and their characteristic tissue or cell types.

**embryonate** \em′brē·ənāt′\ Containing an embryo.

**embryonic** \em′brē·än′ik\ Of, relating to, or having the characteristics of an embryo. Also *embryonal.*

**embryoniferous** \-nif′ərəs\ [Gk *embryon* embryo + *i* + -FEROUS] Bearing an embryo.

**embryony** \em′brē·ənē\ The ability or condition of producing an embryo.

**embryopathia rubeolaris** \-path′ē·ə roo′bē·ōler′is\ Embryopathy associated with or attributed to a rubella infection during pregnancy. Also *rubella embryopathy.*

**embryopathology** \-pathäl′əjē\ The study of teratogenic manifestations and diseases affecting embryos, as well as of the transmission of adverse influences from mother to embryo.

**embryopathy** \em′brē·äp′əthē\ [EMBRYO- + -PATHY] Any abnormal condition in an embryo or fetus. **rubella e.** EMBRYOPATHIA RUBEOLARIS.

**embryoplastic** \-plas′tik\ [EMBRYO + -PLAST + -IC ] Of or relating to embryo formation.

**embryotomy** \em′brē·ät′əmē\ [Gk *embryotomia* (from *embryo(n)* embryo, fetus + *tom-*, stem designating cutting, section + *-ia*, derivative noun suffix) the cutting apart of a fetus] The breaking apart or mechanical destruction of a fetus to allow vaginal delivery.

**embryotoxic** Producing or having the capacity to produce embryotoxicity.

**embryotoxicity** \-täksis′itē\ [EMBRYO- + TOXICITY] Any toxic effect observed in an embryo or later recognized as having begun in the embryonic period, that is either induced or inherent. The four commonly identified embryotoxic manifestations are death, growth retardation, malformation, and postnatal functional defect.

**embryotoxon** \-täk′sän\ [EMBRYO + Gk *toxon* a bow, arch] A mesodermal dysgenesis resulting in the presence of abnormal connective tissue remaining on the inner surface of the peripheral cornea. This appears as a faint white ring extending from the trabecular meshwork to the periphery of Descemet's membrane. **anterior e.** ARCUS JUVENILIS.

**embryotroph** \-träf\ [EMBRYO + Gk *troph(ē)* nourishment] A product of maternal origin derived from cellular destruction or from secretion of uterine glands, providing nutrition to the embryo from the start of or during its development. A hemophagous organ at the margin of the placenta in Carnivora performs such a role. A secretion from uterine glands (uterine milk) occurs in porcines and ruminants. Such embryotrophic substances are called paraplacental histotrophe. In contrast, those elements assuring respiration or nutrition for the embryo which pass through the chorionic villi are sometimes called hemotroph, as they are derived from maternal blood.

**embryotrophic** \-träf′ik\ [EMBRYO- + -TROPHIC] Pertaining to the nourishment of the embryo: usually applied to maternal tissues and substances that undergo degradation to be absorbed by embryonic elements.

**EMC** encephalomyocarditis.

**emedullate** \imed′yəlāt\ [E- + *medull(a)* + -ATE] To excise bone marrow.

**emeiocytosis** \imī′ōsītō′sis\ EXOCYTOSIS.

**emepronium bromide** A quarternary ammonium compound with antimuscarinic effects. It is used in the management of urinary incontinence, urgency, or excessive frequency of micturition due to detrusor instability.

**emergency** 1 A sudden or unexpected event which requires immediate attention. 2 In medicine, an illness or accident that requires immediate treatment to prevent further harm to the patient.

**emergent** \imur′jənt\ Becoming manifest through successive developmental stages until attaining final form: said especially of a characteristic or structural feature.

**emesia** \əmē′zhə\ [Gk, nausea. See EMESIS.] VOMITING.

**emesis** \em′əsis, əmē′sis\ [Gk (from *eme(ein)* to vomit, from prehistoric Gk root *weme-*, akin to L *vome(re)* to vomit) throwing up, emesis] VOMITING. **fecal e.** FECAL VOMITING. **e. gravidarum** Vomiting associated with pregnancy, usually occurring during the sixth to twelfth week.

**emetic** \imet′ik\ [Gk *emetikos* provoking emesis] 1 Inducing vomiting. 2 An agent that induces vomiting. Also *vomitory* (older term). **central e.** A drug or agent that produces vomiting by action on the vomiting center in the central nervous system. Also *indirect emetic, systemic emetic.* **direct e.** A drug that induces vomiting by acting directly on the stomach. Also *mechanical emetic.*

**emeticology** EMETOLOGY.

**emetine** \em′ətin\ $C_{29}H_{40}N_2O_4$. Methylcephaeline, an alkaloid obtained from ipecac or produced synthetically. It has been used to treat amebiasis and schistosomiasis.

**emetine hydrochloride** The hydrochloride of the emetic alkaloid $C_{29}H_{40}N_2O_4$, of ipecac, used in the treatment of acute amebiasis. It is formed from two molecules of dopamine and a monoterpene unit. The molecule contains five rings, the two from dopamine remaining aromatic.

**emetology** The science and study of factors affecting vomiting and the vomiting reflex. Also *emeticology.*

**EMF** 1 electromotive force. 2 erythrocyte maturation factor.

**EMG** electromyogram.

**EMI** electromagnetic interference.

**-emia** \-ē′mē·ə\ [New L *-aemia* (from Gk *-aimia*, from *(h)aim(a)* blood + -IA)] A combining form denoting a condition of the blood. Also *-hemia, -aemia* (British spelling).

**eminence** \em′inəns\ [L *eminentia.* See EMINENTIA.] EMINENTIA. **alveolar e.'s** JUGA ALVEOLARIA. **arcuate e.** EMINENTIA ARCUATA. **articular e. of temporal bone** TUBERCULUM ARTICULARE OSSIS TEMPORALIS. **bicipital e.** TUBEROSITAS RADII. **canine e.** A bulge on the surface of the maxilla, caused by the root of the canine tooth. **coccygeal e.** CORNU SACRALE. **collateral e. of lateral ventricle** EMINENTIA COLLATERALIS VENTRICULI LATERALIS. **collateral e. of Meckel** EMINENTIA COLLATERALIS VENTRICULI LATERALIS. **e. of concha** EMINENTIA CONCHAE. **cruciate e.** EMINENTIA CRUCIFORMIS. **cruciform e. of occipital bone** EMINENTIA CRUCIFORMIS. **deltoid e.** TUBEROSITAS DELTOIDEA HUMERI. **Doyère's e.** *Outmoded* MOTOR END-PLATE. **facial e.** COLLICULUS FACIALIS. **frontal e.** TUBER FRONTALE. **hypobranchial e.** A median elevation on the floor of the developing embryonic pharynx. It receives the ventral portions of the third, fourth, and later the second visceral arches (copula). The caudal part of the eminence forms the epiglottis and the ventral portion blends with the rudiment of the tongue to form its posterior or pharyngeal part. See also LINGUAL COPULA. **hypoglossal e.** TRIGONUM NERVI HYPOGLOSSI. **hypothenar e.**

HYPOTHENAR. **iliopectineal e.** EMINENTIA ILIOPUBICA. **iliopubic e.** EMINENTIA ILIOPUBICA. **intercondylar e. of tibia** EMINENTIA INTERCONDYLARIS. **intercondyloid e.** EMINENTIA INTERCONDYLARIS. **jugular e.** TUBERCULUM JUGULARE OSSIS OCCIPITALIS. **lateral e.'s of the tuber cinereum** A pair of slightly convex prominences visible on the ventral surface of the hypothalamus, one on each side, in the lateral tuber cinereum region. The lateral eminences of the tuber cinereum are located caudal to the optic chiasma and rostral to the mammillary bodies, and at the same level as the infundibulum, but lateral to it. **mamillary e.** CORPUS MAMILLARE. **medial e. of fourth ventricle** EMINENTIA MEDIALIS FOSSAE RHOMBOIDEAE. **medial e. of rhomboid fossa** EMINENTIA MEDIALIS FOSSAE RHOMBOIDEAE. **median e. of neurohypophysis** The tapering ring of nervous tissue joining the hypothalamus above with the infundibular stem below. Phylogenetically, developmentally, and in permeability characteristics it is more closely related to the neurohypophysis than the hypothalamus. Functionally, it influences the adenohypophysis through humoral transport over the hypophysioportal system, which originates in the eminence. Also *median eminence of hypothalamus, median eminence of tuber cinereum.* **median e. of hypothalamus** MEDIAN EMINENCE OF NEUROHYPOPHYSIS. **median e. of tuber cinereum** MEDIAN EMINENCE OF NEUROHYPOPHYSIS. **occipital e.** An embryonic ridge that develops into the bulb of the posterior, or occipital, horn of the lateral ventricle of the brain, deep to the parieto-occipital fissure. **olivary e.** OLIVA. **orbital e.** EMINENTIA ORBITALIS. **parietal e.** TUBER PARIETALE. **postchiasmatic e.** *Obs.* TUBER CINEREUM. **postinfundibular e.** A single swelling between the infundibulum and mammillary bodies. It lies over the infundibular (arcuate) nucleus. **pyramidal e.** EMINENTIA PYRAMIDALIS. **radial e. of wrist** EMINENTIA CARPI RADIALIS. **e. of scapha** EMINENTIA SCAPHAE. **e. of superior semicircular canal** EMINENTIA ARCUATA. **supracondylar e.** EPICONDYLUS. **terete e.** EMINENTIA MEDIALIS FOSSAE RHOMBOIDEAE. **thenar e.** THENAR. **e. of triangular fossa of auricle** EMINENTIA FOSSAE TRIANGULARIS AURICULAE. **trigeminal e.** EMINENTIA TRIGEMINA. **ulnar e. of wrist** EMINENTIA CARPI ULNARIS. **vagal e.** TRIGONUM NERVI VAGI.

**eminentia** \em′inen′shə\ [L (from *eminens,* gen. *eminentis,* pres. part. of *eminire* to stand out, jut out), a prominence, protuberance] A prominence, ridge, or projection; a raised area, usually on the surface of a bone. Also *eminence.* **e. abducentis** COLLICULUS FACIALIS. **e. acoustica** An elevated area in the lateral angle of the fourth ventricle. It overlies vestibular nuclei and is crossed by the auditory striae. *Obs.* **e. arcuata** [NA] An irregularly-rounded elevation on the upper, or anterior, surface of the petrous part of the temporal bone, located near its center posterolateral to a depression in the bony roof of the internal acoustic meatus and the cochlea. The elevation is produced by the arched anterior semicircular canal deep to it. Also *arcuate eminence, eminence of superior semicircular canal.* **e. carpi radialis** The proximal part of the lateral pillar of the carpal groove, formed by the tubercle of the scaphoid bone projecting anteriorly, and palpable as a rounded knob at the medial side of the proximal end of the thenar eminence just beyond the distal crease of the wrist. *Outmoded.* Also *radial eminence of wrist.* **e. carpi ulnaris** The proximal part of the medial pillar of the carpal groove, formed by the pisiform bone projecting anteriorly, and palpable in the medial part of the proximal end of the hypothenar eminence just beyond the distal crease of the wrist. *Outmoded.* Also *ulnar eminence of wrist.* **e. cinerea cuneiformis** TRIGONUM NERVI VAGI. **e. collateralis ventriculi lateralis** [NA] An elongate swelling in the inferior cornu of the lateral ventricle, running lateral and parallel to the hippocampus, and continuing posteriorly into the collateral trigone. It corresponds to the collateral fissure. Also *collateral eminence of lateral ventricle, collateral eminence of Meckel.* **e. conchae** [NA] The convex prominence on the cranial surface of the auricular cartilage corresponding to the depression of the concha on the lateral surface. Also *eminence of concha.* **e. cruciformis** [NA] The crosslike arrangement on the internal aspect of the squamous part of the occipital bone formed by a series of ridges, longitudinal and transverse, intersecting at the internal occipital protuberance. The median longitudinal ridges are those forming the groove for the superior sagittal sinus above the intersection and the internal occipital crest below, while horizontally and at right angles are the ridges forming the grooves for the right and left transverse sinuses. Also *cruciform eminence of occipital bone, cruciate eminence, occipital cross.* **e. facialis** COLLICULUS FACIALIS. **e. fossae triangularis auriculae** [NA] A small oval projection on the cranial surface of the auricular cartilage corresponding to the triangular fossa on the lateral surface. Also *eminence of triangular fossa of auricle.* **e. gracilis** TUBERCULUM NUCLEI GRACILIS. **e. hypoglossi** TRIGONUM NERVI HYPOGLOSSI. **e. iliopectinea** EMINENTIA ILIOPUBICA. **e. iliopubica** [NA] A rounded elevation forming the lateral boundary, or base, of the triangular pectineal surface of the superior ramus of the pubis, and located at the junction of the superior ramus with the body of the ilium. Also *iliopubic eminence, eminentia iliopectinea, iliopectineal eminence, iliopubic tuber, iliopubic tubercle, iliopectineal tubercle, iliopectineal crest of pubis.* **e. intercondylaris** [NA] A spinous prominence surmounted by the medial and lateral intercondylar tubercles, located on the proximal extremity of the tibia between the condylar articular surfaces on each side and between the anterior and posterior intercondylar areas anteroposteriorly. Also *spinous process of tibia, eminentia intercondyloidea, tubercle of tibia* (outmoded), *intercondylar process of tibia, intercondylar eminence of tibia.* **e. intercondyloidea** EMINENTIA INTERCONDYLARIS. **e. medialis fossae rhomboideae** [NA] A caudally tapering area and swelling in the floor of the fourth ventricle, bounded by the sulcus medianus and the sulcus limitans. Also *eminentia teres, terete eminence, medial eminence of rhomboid fossa, medial eminence of fourth ventricle.* **e. orbitalis** [NA] A small tubercle often present on the orbital surface of the zygomatic bone just below the frontozygomatic suture, providing attachment for the lacertus musculi recti lateralis bulbi. Also *orbital tubercle, lateral orbital tubercle, palpebral tubercle, Whitnall's tubercle, orbital eminence, lateral palpebral tubercle.* **e. pyramidalis** [NA] A small, hollow, conical bony projection behind the fenestra vestibuli and anterior to the vertical part of the facial canal on the posterior, or mastoid, wall of the middle ear. It contains the stapedius muscle. Also *pyramidal eminence, pyramid of tympanum.* **e. restiformis** A large prominence on the dorsolateral aspect of the medulla, formed by the inferior cerebellar peduncle as it curves dorsalward to reach the cerebellum. **e. scaphae** [NA] The long, rounded and arched cartilaginous elevation on the cranial surface of the auricle corresponding to the scapha, or scaphoid fossa, of the lateral surface. Also *eminence of scapha.* **e. symphysis** PROTUBERANTIA MENTALIS. **e. teres**

EMINENTIA MEDIALIS FOSSAE RHOMBOIDEAE. **e. trigemina** A slight, longitudinal prominence made along the dorsolateral aspect of the medulla by the spinal tract and the nucleus of the fifth cranial nerve. Also *trigeminal eminence, column of Rolando.* **e. vagi** 1 A slight, longitudinal elevation in the floor of the fourth ventricle overlying the dorsal nucleus of the vagus nerve. It is included within the trigonum vagi. 2 *Imprecise* TRIGONUM NERVI VAGI.

**emiocytosis** \em′ē·ōsītō′sis\ EXOCYTOSIS.

**emissaria** \em′iser′ē·ə\ Plural of EMISSARIUM.

**emissarium** \em′iser′ē·əm\ [L (from *emiss(us)*, past part. of *emittere* to send forth or out + *-arium* -ARY), a sluice, sink, watergate] (*pl.* emissaria) *Outmoded* VENA EMISSARIA.

**emissary** \em′iser′ē\ VENA EMISSARIA.

**emission** \imish′ən\ [L *emissio* (from *emittere* to send forth or out) a sending out, darting forth] 1 Something discharged or let out, as gaseous or particulate matter into the atmosphere. 2 A pathologic or physiologic discharge, usually a fluid, from the body. **cold e.** The emission of electrons from an unheated cathode by the use of a very strong electric field. Also *field emission.* **nasal e.** The escape of air from the nose during speech, as in the production of nasal consonants and vowels and, in a more marked degree, in cases of velopharyngeal insufficiency. Also *nasal escape.* **nocturnal e.** A discharge of semen during the period of sleep. Also *spermatorrhea dormientium, wet dream.*

**emissivity** \em′isiv′itē\ The ratio of the amount of radiant energy given off by a surface to that of a black surface at the same temperature.

**EMIT** enzyme-multiplied immunoassay technique.

**emittance** \imit′əns\ **luminous e.** *Outmoded* LUMEN PER SQUARE METER.

**emmenagogic** \imen′əgäj′ik\ Inducing menstruation.

**emmenagogue** \imen′əgäg\ [Gk *emmēna* (from *emmēnos* monthly, from EM- + Gk *mēn* a month) menses + -AGOGUE ] A substance which induces menstruation. **direct e.** A drug that initiates menstruation by acting directly on female reproductive organs. **indirect e.** A drug that starts menstruation by correcting a condition responsible for amenorrhea.

**emmenology** \em′ənäl′əjē\ [Gk *emmēn(os)* monthly + *o* + -LOGY] The study of menstruation and its disorders.

**Emmet** [Thomas Addis *Emmet,* U.S. gynecologist, 1828–1919] Emmet's operation. See under TRACHELORRHAPHY.

**emmetrope** \em′ətrōp\ [Gk *emmetr(os)* (from *en-* in + *metron* a measure) in measure + -OPE] A person with no refractive error of the eyes.

**emmetropia** \em′ətrō′pē·ə\ [Gk *emmetr(os)* in measure + -OPIA] The optical condition of an eye free of refractive error. Adj. emmetropic.

***Emmonsiella*** \em′ənsyel′ə\ The perfect state of the fungus *Histoplasma.*

**emodin** $C_{15}H_{10}O_5$. 1,3,8-Trihydroxy-6-methyl-9,10-anthracenedione. A constituent of rhubarb root, used as a cathartic. Also *frangulic acid.*

**emollient** [L *emolliens,* gen. *emollientis,* pres. part. of *emollire* to make soft or tender, from *e-* E- + *mollis* soft] 1 Softening or soothing. 2 Any agent that softens the skin and renders it more pliant. For defs. 1 and 2 also *malactic.*

**emotiomotor** \imō′shē·ōmō′tər\ Of or relating to motor activity that is influenced by emotion.

**emotion** [French (from L *emotus,* past part. of *emovere* to move out, stir up, agitate, dislocate, from *e-* E- + *movere* to move), agitation provoked by joy, fear, surprise and other conditions] A complex reaction by the whole organism, often to an abrupt shift in social circumstances, involving widespread bodily changes in visceral function, such as heartbeat, breathing, and glandular secretion, and characterized mentally by strong feelings, excitement, agitation, and turmoil. A distinctive feeling tone is associated with each of the principal emotions, such as fear or anger.

**emotiovascular** \imō′shē·ōvas′kyələr\ Of or relating to vascular changes resulting from emotion.

**e.m.p.** *ex modo prescripto* (L, after the manner prescribed; as directed).

**empasma** A dusting powder, used for external application to the skin.

**empathy** \em′pəthē\ [EM- + *-pathy* as in *sympathy*; transl. of German *Einfühlung* in(sight into others') feelings] The identification of oneself with another as a means of recognizing and comprehending the experience and attendant sensations, emotions, and thoughts of the other. Adj. empathic, empathetic.

**emperipolesis** \emper′ēpōlē′sis\ [EM- + PERIPOLESIS] The active movement of one cell through the cytoplasm of another cell, as neutrophils normally wander through the cytoplasm of megakaryocytes or, in tissue culture, through the cytoplasm of macrophages.

**emphysema** \em′fisē′mə\ [Gk *emphysēma* (from *emphysan* to inflate, from *em-* EN- + *physan* to blow, puff) inflation, swelling, tympanites] 1 Accumulation of air in connective tissue. 2 A condition in which there is dilatation of the pulmonary alveoli distal to the terminal bronchioles with destruction of their walls; pulmonary emphysema. **aging-lung e.** SENILE EMPHYSEMA. **atrophic e.** SENILE EMPHYSEMA. **bullous e.** Emphysema associated with bullae in the lung tissue. Also *cystic emphysema.* **centriacinar e.** Emphysema involving predominantly the central part of the pulmonary acinus. Also *centrilobular emphysema.* **chronic hypertrophic e.** HYPERTROPHIC EMPHYSEMA. **compensatory e.** Increased distension of healthy lung to compensate for loss of volume of another part of the lung. Also *compensating emphysema.* **cystic e.** BULLOUS EMPHYSEMA. **diffuse e.** PANACINAR EMPHYSEMA. **ectatic e.** PANACINAR EMPHYSEMA. **false e.** A deformity of the chest wall in which the anteroposterior diameter of the chest is abnormally large. It mimics the characteristic appearance of the chest in pulmonary emphysema. **familial e.** Emphysema that tends to occur in several members of a family. It is often associated with deficiency of $\alpha_1$-antitrypsin in the blood. **focal e.** Pulmonary emphysema occurring in separate foci rather than diffusely in the lung tissue. See also FOCAL DUST EMPHYSEMA. **focal dust e.** Focal emphysema usually occurring as a feature of coal workers' pneumoconiosis. Coal dust collects in foci up to 5 mm in diameter around small bronchioles. **hypertrophic e.** Emphysema characterized by large lungs. The enlargement is due to overinflation, however, and not to hypertrophy of tissues. Also *chronic hypertrophic emphysema.* **infantile lobar e.** Emphysema of a lobe of the lung in an infant, usually due to congenital abnormality of the lobar bronchus. **interstitial e.** Accumulation of air in the interstitial tissues of the lung. **intestinal e.** The presence of air or gas within the intestinal wall. **mediastinal e.** PNEUMOMEDIASTINUM. **obstructive e.** Overdistension of lung beyond a partial obstruction of its bronchus. **panacinar e.** Emphysema involving all parts of the pulmonary acinus. Also *panlobular emphysema, ectatic emphysema, vesicular emphysema, diffuse emphysema.* **paraseptal e.** Emphysema involving alveoli adjacent to interlobar septa. **pulmonary e.** A condition characterized by dilatation of the pulmonary alveoli and respiratory bronchioles with destruction of their walls. **senile e.** A condition of aging lungs due to normal atrophic changes which superficially resembles true emphysema. Also *atrophic emphysema, aging-lung emphysema, small-lunged emphysema.* **small-lunged e.** SENILE EMPHYSEMA. **subgaleal e.** The presence of air or gas beneath the galea aponeurotica. It is usually the result of an injury that lacerates or penetrates the scalp. Also *extracranial pneumatocele.* **traumatic e.** The presence of air in tissue planes where it is not normally found as a result of injury, generally to the lung. The air is commonly found in subcutaneous tissues or in the mediastinum. **vesicular e.** PANACINAR EMPHYSEMA.

**emphysematous** \em′fisem′ətəs\ Affected with or relating to emphysema.

**Empirin** Headache tablets containing acetylsalicylic acid, phenacetin, and caffeine. A proprietary name.

**emplastic** 1 Adhesive or gluelike: used of a substance, such as a plaster. 2 A medicinal agent that causes constipation.

**emplastration** The application of a plaster or a salve.

**emprosthotonos** \em′prästhät′ənəs\ [Gk (from *emprosth(en)* in front + *tonos* tension) drawn stiffly forward] A tetanic spasm of the trunk in which the body is acutely flexed so that the head and feet are brought together. Also *episthotonos.*

**empyema** \em′pī·ē′mə\ [Gk *empyēma* (from EM- + Gk *pyon* pus) an internal abscess] The accumulation of pus in a cavity, especially in the thoracic cavity. Adj. empyemic. **e. articuli** PYARTHROSIS. **e. benignum** Thoracic empyema occurring without fever or constitutional symptoms. Also *latent empyema.* **extradural e.** EXTRADURAL ABSCESS. **interlobar e.** A collection of pus located between lobes of the lung. **latent e.** EMPYEMA BENIGNUM. **loculated e.** The presence of multiple pus-filled cavities. **metapneumonic e.** Empyema that follows pneumonia. **e. necessitatis** Thoracic empyema in which the infectious process penetrates the chest wall, leading to the formation of a subcutaneous swelling or abscess which may rupture externally. **subdural e.** SUBDURAL ABSCESS. **thoracic e.** A collection of pus in the pleural cavity.

**EMS** emergency medical service.

**EMT** emergency medical technician.

**emul.** *emulsum* (L, emulsion).

**emulgent** Purifying by straining or extraction: used of a process.

**emulsification** \imul′sifikā′shən\ 1 The formation of an emulsion. 2 The dispersal of a bacterial colony in an aqueous medium. An outmoded usage.

**emulsion** \imul′shən\ [L *emulsio* (from E- + L *mulsus,* past part. of *mulgere* to milk, akin to Gk *amelgein* to milk) a milking or draining out] The dispersion of one insoluble liquid in another liquid. The liquid in smaller quantity (disperse phase) is in the form of particles suspended in the other (continuous phase). Examples are cream (fat in water) and butter (water in fat). An emulsifying agent is often needed at the interface to prevent coalescence of the droplets, as the use of protein in milk. **bacillary e.** A form of adjuvant in which the supernatant fluid of a suspension of pulverized tubercule bacilli is mixed with equal parts of glycerin. **benzyl benzoate e.** An aqueous suspension of benzylbenzoate that is used topically as a scabicide. **e. of cod-liver oil** An aqueous suspension of cod liver oil in water containing gum acacia, tragacanth, bitter almond oil, saccharin sodium, and chloroform. **e. of liquid paraffin with cascara** An emulsion containing mineral oil, cascara elixir, and water in a stable suspension. **e. of liquid paraffin and phenolphthalein** A mineral oil emulsion containing 0.34% phenolphthalein. **e. of peppermint** An mixture of oil of peppermint and water (1:10) and quillaia liquid extract, 0.25 ml per 100 ml. It is used as an aromatic carminative. **perlsucht bacillen e.** The original tuberculin prepared from cultures of bovine tubercle bacilli. Also *perlsucht tuberculin original, perlsucht tuberculin rest.* Abbr. PBE **water-in-oil e.** A dispersion of water droplets in a medium of vegetable or mineral oil, used as a suspending medium for injected antigens. Antigens suspended in water-in-oil emulsions usually have greater immunizing potency than those suspended in oil-in-water emulsions.

**emunctory** \imungk′tərē\ [L *emunct(us),* past part. of *emungere* to clear (the nose) of mucus (from *e-* out + *mucus* mucus) + -ORY] An organ of the body that serves to carry off body wastes.

**emylcamate** $C_7H_{15}NO_2$. A compound that has tranquilizing properties similar to those of meprobamate.

**en-** \en-, ən-\ [Gk *en* (as prefix *en-* assimilated to *g, k, ch, x* as *eg-,* to *l* as *el-,* to *b, m, p, ph, ps* as *em-,* sometimes to *r* as *er-*) in, at, on, within, near] A prefix meaning in, into. Also *eg-, em-, el-, er-.*

**enalapril** $C_{20}H_{28}N_2O_5$. 1-[*N*-[1-(Ethoxycarbonyl)-3-phenylpropyl]-L-alanyl]-L-proline. The prodrug form of an angiotensin converting enzyme inhibitor. It is administered orally as the maleate salt. Enalapril loses an ethyl ester group by hydrolysis to yield enalaprilat, the active inhibitor of angiotensin converting enzyme. Enalapril is used in the treatment of hypertension and congestive heart failure, and may occasionally cause headache.

**enamel** \inam′əl\ [Anglo-French *enameler* (from Old French *en-,* prefix meaning to apply, put on + *a(s)mal,* variant of *esmal* enamel, from Frankish *smalt,* akin to English *smelt*) to enamel] A highly mineralized tissue produced by epithelial cells, which forms a layer superficial to the dentin on the crowns of teeth. Also *enamelum, adamantine layer, stratum adamantinum, adamantine substance of tooth.* **gnarled e.** Enamel in which the prisms intertwine. **hereditary brown e.** AMELOGENESIS IMPERFECTA. **hypoplastic e.** Defective enamel produced by defective formation of matrix. The enamel may be very thin or pitted, or may consist of small nodules, but what enamel there is, is hard, of normal translucency, and is not specially liable to caries. The condition may be hereditary, congenital, as from syphilis, or dietary, as in fluorosis. **mottled e.** Enamel of normal thickness with irregular patches of white or brown or both. If only one or two teeth are affected, the cause is idiopathic or may be due to infection from a deciduous tooth during formation of the permanent tooth. If all the teeth are affected, the mottling is usually caused by fluorosis. Mottled enamel is not more liable to caries than normal enamel.

**enameloblast** \inam′əlōblast′\ AMELOBLAST.

**enamelogenesis** \inam′əlōjen′əsis\ [ENAMEL + *o* + GENESIS] AMELOGENESIS.

**enameloma** \inam′əlō′mə\ [ENAMEL + -OMA] ENAMEL PEARL.

**enamelum** \inam′ələm\ ENAMEL.

**enanthema** \en′ənthē′mə\ [EN- + *-anthema* as in EXANTHEMA] An eruption on a mucous membrane. Also *enanthem.* Adj. enanthematous.

**enantiomer** \enan′tē·əmər\ [Gk *enantio(s)* opposite, over against, reverse + *mer(os)* part] One of a pair of compounds that differ only in being mirror images of each other in molecular structure. Since all internal interactions are identical, their properties and reactions with achiral reagents are identical, hence they bear the same chemical name. They are distinguished from each other by chiral reagents, such as enzymes. Enantiomers have optical rotations equal in magnitude but opposite in sign. Also *optical isomer*.

**enantiopathia** \inan′tē·ōpath′ē·ə\ [Gk *enantio(s)* opposite + -PATHIA] **1** A condition in which the effects of each of two diseases tend to counteract the other disease. **2** A disease in such a relationship with another. Also *enantiopathy*.

**enarthrodial** \en′ärthrō′dē·əl\ Pertaining to an enarthrosis, or spheroidal articulation.

**enarthrosis** \en′ärthrō′sis\ [Gk *enarthrōsis* (from *en-* in + *arthrōsis* jointing, articulation) a ball-and-socket joint] ARTICULATIO SPHEROIDEA.

**encapsidate** \enkap′sidāt\ To enclose the nucleocapsid of a virus in a protein coat.

**encapsulated** Enclosed within a capsule.

**encapsulation** \enkap′sʸəlā′shən\ The process of enclosing or being enclosed within a capsule.

**encarditis** \en′kärdī′tis\ ENDOCARDITIS.

**encatarrhaphy** \en′kətär′əfē\ [EN- + CATA- + -RRHAPHY] The placing of a tissue or an organ in a pocket created by sewing the adjacent tissues together over the structure. Also *enkatarrhaphy*.

**-ence** \-əns\ [L *-entia* (from *-ens,* gen. *-entis,* pres. part. of verbs ending in *-ere* or *-ire* + -IA) noun suffix denoting action, process, quality, state, or amount] A noun suffix denoting action, state, or condition.

**enceinte** \änsent′\ [French, pregnant, from Late L *incincta* ungirt, without girdle] Pregnant.

**encephal-** \ensef′əl-\ ENCEPHALO-.

**encephalalgia** \ensef′əlal′jə\ [ENCEPHAL- + -ALGIA] Pain in the head; headache. Also *encephalodynia*.

**encéphale isolé** \änsāfāl′ ēzōlā′\ Denoting an animal preparation in which the neuraxis has been transected at the junction of the medulla oblongata and the spinal cord, and in which the brain is the subject of experimental interest. It results in a waking EEG pattern. Also *isolated brain*.

**encephalic** \en′sefal′ik\ Relating to the encephalon.

**encephalitic** \ensef′əlit′ik\ Pertaining to or suffering from encephalitis.

**encephalitides** \ensef′əlit′idēz\ Plural of ENCEPHALITIS.

# encephalitis

**encephalitis** \en′sefəlī′tis\ [Gk *enkephal(os)* (from EN- + Gk *kephalē* the head) the brain + -ITIS] (*pl.* encephalitides) Any inflammation of the substance of the brain, whether of viral, microbial, or parasitic origin. Adj. encephalitic. • When the process involves the entire central nervous system it is called *encephalomyelitis,* or, less often, *neuraxitis.* **e. A** ENCEPHALITIS LETHARGICA. **acute disseminated e.** ACUTE DISSEMINATED ENCEPHALOMYELITIS. **acute necrotic e.** A morphologic and clinical variety of viral encephalitis characterized by the abrupt onset of a severe febrile illness with early meningoencephalitic signs, especially rapid impairment of consciousness, and generalized epileptic fits, rapidly progressing to coma and death. The cerebrospinal fluid is usually clear, but sometimes bloodstained, and contains numerous cells, particularly lymphocytes, and a high protein count, although the glucose concentration is usually normal. Hyperpyrexia is common. Morphologically, the damage involves the rhinencephalon and insula (central lobe), and produces massive areas of swelling and inflammatory necrosis, particularly in the cortex of the temporal lobe, which is sometimes more severe unilaterally. In the affected area there is diffuse microglial hyperplasia. Acidophilic inclusions may be found in the neurons and glia of neighboring necrotic regions, and there may be other areas of inflammation at a distance, particularly in the brainstem and cerebellum. In most cases electron microscopy with fluorescent antibody staining reveals the presence of particles of herpes simplex virus, but it is possible that the herpes virus is not always the causative agent. The extent of the necrosis and of the hemorrhage suggests that allergic and circulatory factors also play a part. Some patients recover partially or completely if subjected to early surgical decompression, with diagnostic biopsy, combined with massive doses of steroids and antiviral agents. Also *acute necrotizing encephalitis.* **acute postinfectious e.** POSTINFECTIOUS ENCEPHALITIS. **American e.** ST. LOUIS ENCEPHALITIS. **arbovirus e.** Any type of encephalitis caused by one of the arboviruses, which have the ability to multiply in vertebrate and invertebrate tissues, as of blood-sucking arthropods which act as vectors. Different types of arbovirus encephalitis have in common various pathologic characteristics, including perivascular infiltration of mononuclear cells, distension of the Virchow-Robin spaces, neuronal damage, with satellitosis and neuronophagia, and the scattering at random of microglial foci in the brain and spinal cord. Viruses transmitted by arthropod vectors include those belonging to several different virus families; Bunyaviridae, Togaviridae, Reoviridae, Rhabdoviridae. Specific viruses differ according to their insect vector and their geographic distribution. Microbiologic diagnosis is carried out by isolation of the virus from the blood or cerebrospinal fluid during the first few days of the illness by intracerebral inoculation of suckling mice, and the virus can often be isolated from the brain after death. Immunoassay is carried out by neutralization or inhibition of red cell clumping in the presence of reference sera. Serodiagnosis may be achieved by complement fixation tests, red cell agglutination inhibition tests, or by virus neutralization tests. Also *arthropod-transmitted encephalitis.* **Australian X e.** *Outmoded* MURRAY VALLEY ENCEPHALITIS. **e. B** JAPANESE B ENCEPHALITIS. **Baló's concentric e.** BALÓ'S DISEASE. **benign myalgic e.** BENIGN MYALGIC ENCEPHALOMYELITIS. **Binswanger's e.** BINSWANGER'S DISEASE. **boutonneuse e.** A cerebral complication of boutonneuse fever, attacking various parts of the brain, such as the central grey nuclei, medulla oblongata, or pyramidal tracts and occurring either at the onset of the infection or at the start of convalescence. There may be neurologic sequelae, particularly hemiplegia. **e. C** ST. LOUIS ENCEPHALITIS. **Calabrian e.** CONDORELLI'S ENCEPHALITIS. **California e.** A usually mild meningoencephalitis caused by bungaviruses of the California group. First described in California in 1943, the disease has since been reported in the upper midwestern U.S. and in North Carolina. **Central European e.** See under TICK-BORNE ENCEPHALITIS. **cerebellar e.** An acute inflammatory process involving the cerebellum, either solely or predominantly, and usually attributable to a neurotropic virus. One specific form of this condition is acute cerebellar ataxia of infancy. Also *acute cerebellitis, parencephalitis.* **chronic subcortical e.** BINSWANGER'S DISEASE. **Condorelli's e.** A type of viral encephalitis similar to St. Louis encephalitis, endemic in Sicily, and marked morphologically by glial micronodular foci scattered throughout the cerebral cortex. Affected patients often become cachectic and may develop epilepsy. Also *Sicilian encephalitis, Calabrian encephalitis, Condorelli syndrome.* **Coxsackie e.**

Encephalitis due to one of the coxsackieviruses. **Dawson's e.** SUBACUTE SCLEROSING PANENCEPHALITIS. **diffuse sclerosing e.** SUBACUTE SCLEROSING PANENCEPHALITIS. **eastern equine e.** EASTERN EQUINE ENCEPHALOMYELITIS. **eastern North American e.** A type of equine encephalitis, predominating along the east coast of the United States from New Hampshire to Texas, and transmitted by various mosquitoes. **Economo's e.** ENCEPHALITIS LETHARGICA. **equine e.** A type of encephalitis caused by any of three arboviruses (eastern and western equine encephalitis, and Venezuelan equine encephalitis) all having in common the ability to damage, often permanently, the central nervous system of the horse and of man. Transmission of infection is accomplished by mosquitoes from animal reservoirs of the virus, usually wild birds. These types of encephalitis are very often fatal in horses and severe in man though not as frequently fatal. **hemorrhagic e.** Any acute encephalitis marked morphologically by hemorrhagic foci within the brain. This pathologic change is seen in many viral encephalitides, especially herpes simplex encephalitis, and in acute hemorrhagic leukoencephalitis. **hemorrhagic arsphenamine e.** Acute hemorrhagic leukoencephalitis or brain purpura following the administration of arsphenamine. **e. hemorrhagica superior** WERNICKE'S DISEASE. **herpesvirus e.** An acute encephalitis caused by a herpes simplex virus. The most common cause of the disease in adults is herpes simplex virus type 1 (HSV-1), while in neonates HSV-2 is most often implicated. Also *herpes encephalitis, herpes simplex encephalitis, herpetic encephalitis.* See also ACUTE NECROTIC ENCEPHALITIS. **Ilheus e.** A Brazilian mosquito-borne encephalitis caused by the Ilheus virus. **inclusion e.** SUBACUTE SCLEROSING PANENCEPHALITIS. **inclusion body e.** SUBACUTE SCLEROSING PANENCEPHALITIS. **infantile e.** Acute disseminated encephalomyelitis following an exanthematous infection occurring in childhood. **influenzal e.** Encephalitis occurring as a complication of influenza. **Japanese B e.** A type of epidemic encephalitis attributable to a flavivirus (group B togavirus), identified in Japan in 1924 but subsequently rediscovered in Malaysia and in India. Somnolence, epileptic fits, and acute psychosis are some of the symptoms noted during the course of this disease, which is transmitted by mosquitoes of the genus *Culex*, particularly *C. tritaeniorhynchus*, originally infecting various wild birds, especially herons. Also *encephalitis B, Russian autumnal encephalitis, summer encephalitis, Japanese encephalitis.* **lead e.** LEAD ENCEPHALOPATHY. **Leichtenstern's e.** ACUTE HEMORRHAGIC LEUKOENCEPHALITIS. **e. lethargica** An acute infection which occurred as an epidemic at the end of the First World War, but which is seen nowadays only sporadically, if at all. It may affect the entire neuraxis (neuraxitis) or only part of it, and is often accompanied by lesions of the central gray nuclei. The symptomatology may be very varied, but clinical diagnosis may be made by the presence of certain characteristic symptoms such as somnolence, reversal of the sleep rhythm, oculomotor paralysis, local or general myoclonus, hiccups, and psychic disturbances with psychomotor excitation, the latter being seen most frequently in children. The cerebrospinal fluid is normal or only slightly abnormal, sometimes with a raised glucose and a slightly raised protein content, but with little or no pleocytosis. This condition may result in complete recovery or it may be followed by serious sequelae such as postencephalitic parkinsonism, or be rapidly fatal in an acute phase. To date, the etiology is still unknown and no virus has been isolated, though typical Loewi bodies or inclusions may be found in the substantia nigra. Also *lethargic encephalitis, encephalitis A, von Economo's encephalitis, von Economo's disease, epidemic neuraxitis, polioencephalitis infectiva, talking sickness.* **limbic e.** Encephalitis involving one or both limbic lobes of the brain. Most such cases are due to the herpes simplex virus and are acute, but subacute or chronic encephalitis involving the limbic lobes has been described as a complication of carcinoma. **Mengo e.** A viral encephalitis and myocarditis occurring in Africa and due to the Mengo virus. **mumps e.** A manifestation of mumps virus infection, having a symptomatology more often that of a meningoencephalitis than of a pure encephalitis or of encephalomyelitis. It usually occurs five to seven days after the onset of infection, whether or not the latter includes parotitis. It can be differentiated from other forms of postinfectious encephalitis in that the mumps virus, which can be isolated from the cerebrospinal fluid, appears to be directly responsible. **Murray Valley e.** A viral encephalomyelitis which has occurred in epidemics in Australia since 1917. Most cases occurred in the Murray Valley of Australia. The disease is caused by a flavivirus (group B togavirus) and is transmitted to man by the *Culex annulirostris* mosquito. Also *Murray Valley disease, Australian X disease* (outmoded), *Australian X encephalitis* (outmoded), *X encephalitis* (outmoded). **otitic e.** Encephalitis spreading to the ipsilateral temporal lobe of the brain or to the cerebellum, stemming from an infection in the ear and usually occurring as a stage in the formation of a temporal lobe or cerebellar abscess. **e. periaxialis concentrica** BALÓ'S DISEASE. **e. periaxialis diffusa** See under SCHILDER'S DISEASE. **perivenous e.** ACUTE DISSEMINATED ENCEPHALOMYELITIS. **postexanthematous e.** POSTEXANTHEMATOUS ENCEPHALOMYELITIS. **postinfectious e.** POSTINFECTIOUS ENCEPHALOMYELITIS. **postvaccinal e.** POSTVACCINAL ENCEPHALOMYELITIS. **Powassan e.** A tick-borne viral encephalitis described in Canada in 1958, caused by a flavivirus. **purulent e.** Encephalitis attributable to the activity of pyogenic bacteria, and marked by the production of pus. This condition may be diffuse or localized (cerebral abscess), and indeed a phase of diffuse suppurative encephalitis in one cerebral or cerebellar hemisphere often precedes the development of an abscess. Also *pyogenic encephalitis, suppurative encephalitis.* **Russian autumnal e.** JAPANESE B ENCEPHALITIS. **Russian spring-summer e.** See under TICK-BORNE ENCEPHALITIS. **Schilder's e.** See under SCHILDER'S DISEASE. **Semliki Forest e.** A mosquito-borne viral encephalitis which occurs in western Uganda and is due to the Semliki Forest virus. It occurs also in west Africa. **Sicilian e.** CONDORELLI'S ENCEPHALITIS. **St. Louis e.** A type of encephalitis caused by a flavivirus (group B togavirus), usually occurring in epidemic form in the western and central regions of the United States, but also in Panama and Trinidad. It is transmitted by mosquitoes of the genus *Culex* which have themselves been infected by wild birds and which can transmit the disease to domestic animals and to man. Also *American encephalitis, encephalitis C.* **Strümpell-Leichtenstern e.** ACUTE HEMORRHAGIC LEUKOENCEPHALITIS. **subacute inclusion body e.** SUBACUTE SCLEROSING PANENCEPHALITIS. **summer e.** JAPANESE B ENCEPHALITIS. **suppurative e.** PURULENT ENCEPHALITIS. **tick-borne e.** Encephalitis occurring in Siberia and eastern and central Europe caused by a flavivirus (group B togavirus) and transmitted to man by ixodid ticks or via unpasteurized goat's milk. There are two antigenically distinguishable subtypes of the virus, one occurring in the eastern USSR and one in central Europe. The eastern subtype causes more severe disease, with headache, fever, nausea, vomiting, hyperesthesia, photophobia, and, in severe cases, convulsions, delirium, coma, paralysis, or involvement of bulbar centers and cervical spinal cord. Residual paralysis is common, and there is a 15–20% fatality rate. The central European subtype causes disease with a diphasic course and 0–5% mortality. An influenzalike illness is followed by an asymptomatic interval which is succeeded by abrupt onset of fever, headache, nausea, vomiting, and a benign meningoencephalitis. The eastern type, prevalent in the eastern provinces of the Soviet Union in spring and summer, is known as Russian spring-summer encephalitis, Far Eastern encephalitis, Far East Russian encephalitis, Russian endemic encephalitis, Russian tick-borne encephalitis, taiga tick meningoencephalitis, forest-spring encephalitis, vernal encephalitis, vernoestival encephalitis, woodcutters' encephalitis. The central European subtype is known as Central European encephalitis, Central European tick-borne encephalitis, biundulant meningoencephalitis, diphasic milk fever, Central European tick-borne fever, Czechoslovakian tick-borne encephalitis. **torula e.** Meningoencephalitis due to *Cryptococcus neoformans* (*Torula histolytica*). **toxoplasmic e.** Encephalitis in toxoplasmosis, a common effect of this disease, especially following intrauterine infection. **typhoid e.** Encephalitis or encephalopathy occurring in severe typhoid fever and considered to be caused by toxins released by the typhoid bacillus. Clinically it is characterized by circulatory collapse and stupor alternating with psychomotor agitation, acute delirium, or convulsions. Also *cerebrotyphus* (incorrect). **van Bogaert's e.** SUBACUTE SCLEROSING PANENCEPHALITIS. **varicella e.** Encephalitis accompanying or following varicella (chickenpox). **Venezuelan e.** VENEZUELAN EQUINE ENCEPHALOMYELITIS. **Venezuelan equine e.** VENEZUELAN EQUINE ENCEPHALOMYELITIS. **viral e.** Any type of encephalitis caused by a virus. There are two main types: encephalitis associated with the multiplication of various viruses, such as arbovirus, poliovirus, herpes virus, or mumps virus, in the nervous system; and encephalitis which occurs during the course of exanthemata of viral origin, such as vaccinia, measles, German measles, and chickenpox. In these infections it is still uncertain whether the virus multiplies in the nervous tissue, or whether, as is generally believed, the encephalitis is an allergic or hypersensitivity reaction of the same type as that which occurs in "experimental allergic encephalitis," which can be induced in animals by the injection of brain tissue with Freund's adjuvant. In encephalitis lethargica, another important variety of encephalitis, the causative agent has not been identified. **von Economo's e.** ENCEPHALITIS LETHARGICA. **western equine e.** WESTERN EQUINE ENCEPHALOMYELITIS. **West Nile e.** WEST NILE FEVER. **X e.** *Outmoded* MURRAY VALLEY ENCEPHALITIS.

**encephalitogen** \ensef'əlit'əjən\ [*encephalit(is)* + *o* + -GEN] Any agent which, when injected experimentally with adjuvant into an animal, induces encephalitis. Also *encephalogen.*

***Encephalitozoon*** \en'sefal'itōzō'ən\ [*encephalit(is)* + *o* + Gk *zōon* a living being, animal] A genus of microsporidian protozoans in the phylum Microspora, order Microsporida. They are parasitic in warm-blooded vertebrates and differ from members of the related genus *Nosema,* which chiefly parasitize invertebrates, by a peculiar double-nucleated condition.

**encephalization** \ensef'əlīzā'shən\ [ENCEPHAL- + *-iz(e)* + -ATION] The formation of the head or brain of an embryo.

**encephalo-** \ensef'əlō-\ [Gk *enkephalos* (from EN- + *kephalē* the head) the brain] A combining form denoting the brain. Also *encephal-.*

**encephalocele** \ensef'əlōsēl'\ [ENCEPHALO- + -CELE[1]] A herniation of the brain and meninges usually through a developmental defect in the skull and usually at one of the major sutures of the cranium, but not limited to these sites. A covering of skin or mucous membrane is initially present but may be ruptured as the herniation enlarges. Also *craniocele, cranium bifidum, encephalomeningocele, cephalocele, meningoencephalocele.* **orbital e.** An encephalocele with a herniation of the brain into or through the orbit.

**encephaloclastic** \-klas'tik\ [ENCEPHALO- + -CLAST + -IC] Describing or pertaining to the late effects of a lesion causing breakdown of brain substance.

**encephalocoele** \ensef'əlōsēl'\ **1** The entire cranial cavity. **2** The cerebral ventricles considered as a whole.

**encephalocystocele** \-sis'təsēl\ [ENCEPHALO- + CYSTO- + -CELE] HYDROENCEPHALOCELE.

**encephalocystomeningocele** \-sis'təmening'gōsēl\ [ENCEPHALO- + CYSTO- + MENINGOCELE] HYDROENCEPHALOCELE.

**encephalodynia** \-din'ē·ə\ [ENCEPHAL- + -ODYNIA] ENCEPHALALGIA.

**encephalodysplasia** \-displā'zhə\ [ENCEPHALO- + DYSPLASIA] Any developmental abnormality of the brain.

**encephaloedema** \ensef'əlidē'mə\ [ENCEPHAL- + OEDEMA] CEREBRAL EDEMA.

**encephalogen** \ensef'əlōjən\ ENCEPHALITOGEN.

**encephalogram** \ensef'əlōgram'\ [ENCEPHALO- + -GRAM] A record on film from a radiographic examination of the subarachnoid spaces and ventricular system after the injection of air or, less often, of opaque material into the subarachnoid space. This is usually done by means of spinal or suboccipital puncture into the subarachnoid space.

**encephalography** \ensef'əläg'rəfē\ [ENCEPHALO- + -GRAPHY] Roentgenography of the brain. **air e.** PNEUMOENCEPHALOGRAPHY. **fractional e.** A type of pneumoencephalography for the study of different portions of the intracranial subarachnoid spaces and ventricles. Increments of air or oxygen are injected into the subarachnoid space usually via spinal lumbar puncture. After each injection radiographs of the skull are made in different projections. **gamma e.** Scintigraphy used for examination of the brain, notable for the diagnosis of expansile neurosurgical lesions. The most common radiopharmaceutical used to be serum albumin labeled with radioactive iodine, or less commonly radioactive copper or arsenic. Radioactivity was measured at the surface of the skull. An area of increased activity indicated in general the presence of a tumor or other cause of blood brain barrier breakdown or increased capillary permeability. It has been largely superseded by imaging procedures, most commonly with 99m technetium pertechnetate. Also *cerebral gammography, gamma scan.* **positive contrast e.** Radiographic study of the subarachnoid spaces and ventricles of the brain after injection of a radiopaque contrast material into the cerebrospinal fluid.

**encephaloid** \ensef'əloid\ [ENCEPHAL- + -OID] Resembling the brain or brain tissue.

**encephalolith** \ensef'əlōlith'\ [ENCEPHALO- + -LITH] A calculus or concretion in the brain or ventricles.

**encephalomalacia** \-məlā'shə\ [ENCEPHALO- + MALACIA] A softening of any part of the brain from whatever cause. Also *cerebromalacia.* **periventricular e.** A form of cerebral softening in the white matter around the cerebral ventricles found in many infants with cerebral palsy.

**encephalomeningitis** \-men'injī'tis\ MENINGOENCEPHALITIS.

**encephalomeningocele** \-mening′gōsēl\ ENCEPHALOCELE.

**encephalomeningopathy** \-men′ing·gäp′əthē\ [ENCEPHALO- + MENINGO- + -PATHY] Any disease process involving the brain and the meninges.

**encephalomyelitis** \-mī·əlī′tis\ [ENCEPHALO- + MYEL- + -ITIS] Any disorder giving rise to inflammation of the brain and spinal cord. The condition is often of viral origin, but may be due to allergy or hypersensitivity. Also *myelencephalitis, myeloencephalitis.* **acute disseminated e.** Any acute or subacute disease of the brain and spinal cord complicating viral or other banal infections (e.g., measles, rubella, varicella, influenza) that do not normally affect the central nervous system or following prophylactic immunization against smallpox, rabies, influenza, or tetanus. It is not known whether the illness is due to direct invasion of the brain by the virus or to an allergic or hypersensitivity reaction. Measles and mumps viruses have been isolated from the brains of patients with acute disseminated encephalomyelitis. The symptomatology is varied and may include fever, headache, vomiting, drowsiness, depressed consciousness, coma, convulsions, behavioral disturbances, visual impairment, paralysis, and ataxia. Pathologically, the basic lesion is the presence in the brain of mononuclear cells around small veins, chiefly in the white matter. This is accompanied by perivascular demyelination. Mortality and the frequency of sequelae vary depending on the virus involved. Also *acute postinfectious encephalitis, acute disseminated encephalitis, perivenous encephalitis.* **benign myalgic e.** An epidemic disease reported from many different parts of the world and characterized by muscle pain, weakness, mood depressions, and sensory symptoms and often by severe fatigue lasting for several months. No causal agent has been identified. Some believe the condition to be due to a viral infection but the cerebrospinal fluid is invariably normal. Many epidemics have occurred in closed institutions such as nursing homes, convents, and schools and some believe the condition to be a form of mass hysteria. Also *myalgic asthenia, epidemic myalgic encephalomyelopathy, Icelandic disease, epidemic neuromyasthenia, benign myalgic encephalitis.* **eastern equine e.** A severe encephalomyelitis due to an alphavirus, the eastern equine encephalitis virus, and transmitted to horses and to man by infected mosquitoes, usually *Culiseta melanura.* The disease may be distributed worldwide, but it is seen primarily in the eastern United States and Canada. In man, illness begins abruptly, with headache, fever, chills, nausea, and vomiting, and infection progresses rapidly to the central nervous system, producing confusion, somnolence, and sometimes profound coma. Illness is usually more severe in children, and they seldom recover completely. The fatality rate is about 70 percent. Also *eastern equine encephalitis.* Abbr. EEE **experimental allergic e.** Acute disseminated encephalomyelitis experimentally produced in laboratory animals by injections of preparations of spinal cord or brain from infected animals. **Kelly's e.** ACUTE INFANTILE ENCEPHALOPATHY. **postexanthematous e.** Acute disseminated encephalomyelitis following an exanthem, such as measles. See under ACUTE DISSEMINATED ENCEPHALOMYELITIS. Also *postexanthematous encephalitis.* **postimmunization e.** POSTVACCINAL ENCEPHALOMYELITIS. **postinfectious e.** Acute disseminated encephalomyelitis occurring as a sequel to an infection such as influenza or mumps. See under ACUTE DISSEMINATED ENCEPHALOMYELITIS. Also *acute postinfectious encephalitis, postinfectious encephalitis, postinfection encephalomyelopathy.* **postvaccinal e.** Acute disseminated encephalomyelitis following prophylactic immunization or vaccination, as for influenza, tetanus, rabies, pertussis, or smallpox. See under ACUTE DISSEMINATED ENCEPHALOMYELITIS. Also *postvaccinal encephalopathy, postimmunization encephalomyelopathy, postvaccinal encephalitis.* **Venezuelan equine e.** An encephalomyelitis due to an alphavirus, the Venezuelan equine encephalitis virus, and transmitted to horses and man by mosquitoes of at least ten different genera. It is seen primarily in South and Central America, but many cases, including a large equine epidemic, have occurred in the southern United States, especially Texas. The disease in man may be a subclinical infection, a benign influenzalike illness, a fulminant systemic illness, or a severe febrile encephalomyelitis. Recovery is usually uneventful, although fulminant systemic disease may be rapidly fatal. Also *Venezuelan equine encephalitis, Venezuelan encephalitis.* Abbr. VEE **viral e.** Any type of encephalomyelitis attributable to a virus. Also *virus encephalomyelitis.* **western equine e.** An encephalomyelitis caused by an alphavirus, the western equine encephalitis virus, and transmitted to horses and to man by mosquitoes, usually *Culex tarsalis* and *Culiseta melanura.* It is seen primarily in the western regions of the United States, Canada, and Mexico. Symptoms resemble those of eastern equine encephalomyelitis, but the disease usually takes a less severe course and has a fatality rate of about 10 percent. Also *western equine encephalitis.* Abbr. WEE **zoster e.** Encephalomyelitis due to the varicella-zoster virus.

**encephalomyelocele** \-mī′əlōsēl\ [ENCEPHALO- + MYELO- + -CELE] A developmental defect in the occipital region of the skull and the upper cervical vertebrae through which brain tissue, the upper spinal cord, and associated meninges have herniated.

**encephalomyeloneuropathy** \-mī′əlōnʸUräp′əthē\ [ENCEPHALO- + MYELO- + NEUROPATHY] Any disease involving the brain, spinal cord, and peripheral nerves.

**encephalomyelopathy** \-mī′əläp′əthē\ [ENCEPHALO- + MYELO- + -PATHY] Any disease involving the brain and spinal cord. Also *encephalomyelosis, neuroencephalomyelopathy.* **epidemic myalgic e.** BENIGN MYALGIC ENCEPHALOMYELITIS. **Leigh's necrotizing e.** SUBACUTE NECROTIZING ENCEPHALOPATHY. **postinfection e.** POSTINFECTIOUS ENCEPHALOMYELITIS. **postvaccinal e.** POSTVACCINAL ENCEPHALOMYELITIS. **subacute necrotizing e.** SUBACUTE NECROTIZING ENCEPHALOPATHY.

**encephalomyeloradiculitis** \-mī′əlōrədik′yəlī′tis\ [ENCEPHALO- + MYELO- + RADICULITIS] Inflammation of the brain, spinal cord, and spinal roots.

**encephalomyeloradiculoneuritis** \-mī′əlōrədik′yəlōnʸUrī′tis\ [ENCEPHALO- + MYELO- + RADICULO- + NEURITIS] Inflammation of the brain, spinal cord, spinal roots, and peripheral nerves.

**encephalomyeloradiculopathy** \-mī′əlōrədik′yəläp′əthē\ [ENCEPHALO- + MYELO- + RADICULO- + -PATHY] Any disease involving the brain, spinal cord, and spinal roots.

**encephalomyelosis** \-mī′əlō′sis\ [ENCEPHALO- + MYELO- + -SIS] ENCEPHALOMYELOPATHY.

**encephalomyocarditis** \-mī′əkärdī′tis\ A syndrome of myocarditis with heart failure and meningoencephalitis in the neonate, resulting from infection with a coxsackievirus (group B, types 1–5). In severe cases, there is rapid progression to cyanosis and circulatory collapse, and in fatal cases there is usually disseminated viral infection with involvement of the central nervous system, liver, pancreas, or adrenal glands. Mortality is approximately 50 percent.

**encephalon** \ensef′əlän\ [New L, from Gk *enkephalon,* variant of *enkephalos* (from EN- + *kephalē* the head) that which is inside the head, brain] [NA] BRAIN.

**encephalopathia** \-path′ē·ə\ ENCEPHALOPATHY.

**encephalopathy** \ensef′əläp′əthē\ [ENCEPHALO- + -PATHY] 1 Any disease or degenerative condition of the brain. 2 An acute reaction of the brain to a variety of toxic or infective agents, without any actual inflammation such as occurs in encephalitis. Also *encephalopathia.* Adj. encephalopathic. **acute infantile e.** A hyperacute form of encephalopathy which attacks very young children. The onset is marked by fever, vomiting, irritability, and neck stiffness, and it is ultimately characterized by bulbar and cerebral disturbances, such as respiratory difficulty, strabismus, nystagmus, ptosis, facial paralysis, hemiplegia, generalized convulsions, and coma. It is often fatal within a few days. This appears to be a syndrome of multiple etiology, sometimes but not invariably due to viral infection. Also *Brown-Symmers disease, Kelly's encepyhalomyelitis, acute toxic encephalopathy.* **alcoholic e.** Any disturbance of brain function due to or associated with alcohol ingestion, including the short-term dysfunction associated with acute intoxication and longer lasting or irreversible organic changes such as those of the Wernicke-Korsakoff psychosis. **anoxic e.** POSTANOXIC ENCEPHALOPATHY. **arsenical e.** A rare, fatal complication, formerly seen during the course of treatment of syphilis with organic arsenical compounds. The condition usually started three days after the third injection, with a violent headache, which was rapidly followed by fever, convulsions, and delirium, and rapidly progressed to coma. **atonic-astasic e.** FÖRSTER'S DIPLEGIA. **biliary e.** HEPATIC ENCEPHALOPATHY. **bilirubin e.** KERNICTERUS. **boxers' e.** A state of multifocal softening in the cerebral cortex, subcortical white matter and basal ganglia, often associated with absence or cavitation of the septum pellucidum and with defects of memory and intellect, and clinical features resembling those of parkinsonism, occurring in professional boxers as a consequence of repeated cerebral trauma. Also *punch-drunk syndrome, Friedmann syndrome, Friedmann's complex, boxers' syndrome, traumatic encephalopathy of boxers, Friedmann's vasomotor syndrome, traumatic parkinsonism.* **callosal demyelinating e.** MARCHIAFAVA-BIGNAMI SYNDROME. **chronic traumatic e.** Any chronic encephalopathy resulting from a single major head injury or from repeated brain injury such as that occurring in professional boxers or steeplechase jockeys. **Creutzfeldt-Jakob presenile e.** CREUTZFELDT-JAKOB DISEASE. **cystic multilocular e.** A pathological change in the brain with multiple areas of softening and consequent cyst formation in the cerebral substance, believed to result from infarction due to arterial disease and found in some children with cerebral palsy. **dialysis e.** DIALYSIS DEMENTIA. **e. and fatty degeneration of viscera** REYE SYNDROME. **e. with formiminotransferase deficiency** A congenital metabolic disease of young children, marked by psychomotor retardation, hepatomegaly, muscle hypertonia, and urinary excretion of formiminoglutamic acid. **hepatic e.** A cerebral complication of cirrhosis of the liver or of portocaval anastomosis, related to a rise in blood ammonia levels because the diseased liver is unable to metabolize absorbed amino acids or because these enter the systemic circulation through anastomoses between the portal and systemic circulations. The condition is marked by symptoms ranging from mild irritability to coma and is often accompanied by flapping tremor of the outstretched hands (asterixis). The symptoms may either regress with treatment or may lead to irreversible hepatic coma. Also *biliary encephalopathy, coma hepaticum, hepatic coma, portocaval encephalopathy, portal-systemic encephalopathy, portosystemic encephalopathy, hepatocerebral syndrome.* **hypercalcemic e.** Drowsiness, confusion, or stupor resulting from hypercalcemia. **hypernatremic e.** Convulsions and impairment of consciousness resulting from hypernatremia occurring either in infancy as a result of excess salt intake or in adults as a result of hypothalamic lesions such as tumors. **hypertensive e.** Coma, convulsions, or transient manifestations of cerebral dysfunction resulting from a sudden severe rise in systemic blood pressure such as that which may occur in malignant hypertension, eclampsia, acute nephritis, or in pheochromocytoma. **hypoglycemic e.** Coma, convulsions, or transient manifestations of cerebral dysfunction, including disordered mentation, resulting from hypoglycemia, however produced. **hypoxic e.** A state of cerebral dysfunction due to oxygen deficiency. **infantile myoclonic e.** An encephalopathy of unknown cause beginning acutely in infancy but running a benign but protracted course with exacerbations and remissions and giving rise to opsoclonus, limb myoclonus and irritability. Also *dancing eye–dancing feet syndrome, subacute myoclonic encephalopathy.* **lead e.** A group of cerebral symptoms caused by lead poisoning and resulting in diffuse cerebral edema. The symptoms may include depression, insomnia, headache, convulsive attacks, transient blindness, aphasia, transient deafness, loss of consciousness, and coma. Also *lead encephalitis, saturnine encephalopathy.* **Leigh's e.** SUBACUTE NECROTIZING ENCEPHALOPATHY. **metabolic e.** Any encephalopathy consequent upon a generalized change in the metabolism of the brain or in its extracellular environment. Also *metabolic craniopathy.* **necrotizing e.** Any encephalopathy, such as some of toxic origin, in which there is necrosis of brain tissue. **palindromic e.** RECURRENT ENCEPHALOPATHY. **para-Wernicke e.** SUBACUTE NECROTIZING ENCEPHALOPATHY. **pertussis e.** Drowsiness, coma, and/or convulsions complicating pertussis. **portal-systemic e.** HEPATIC ENCEPHALOPATHY. **portocaval e.** HEPATIC ENCEPHALOPATHY. • This term is sometimes reserved for cases that may follow surgical portocaval anastomosis. **portosystemic e.** HEPATIC ENCEPHALOPATHY. **postanoxic e.** A state of progressive cerebral dysfunction following an interval of apparent recovery from a coma induced by oxygen deficiency. Also *anoxic encephalopathy.* **post-traumatic e.** A syndrome characterized by headache, giddiness, insomnia, irritability, loss of memory, and intolerance of alcohol, among other symptoms, occurring as a sequel of a single concussive head injury. Also *post-traumatic syndrome.* **postvaccinal e.** POSTVACCINAL ENCEPHALOMYELITIS. **progressive multifocal e.** PROGRESSIVE MULTIFOCAL LEUKOENCEPHALOPATHY. **progressive subcortical e.** BINSWANGER'S DISEASE. **progressive traumatic e.** A syndrome occurring after concussion, developing slowly and progressively, seen rarely in cases of severe brain injury or, more commonly, after repeated trauma in professional boxers or steeplechase jockeys. It is marked by incoordination of movement, tremor, dysarthria, parkinsonian features, and some degree of intellectual impairment. Boxers' encephalopathy is one variety of this syndrome. Also *traumatic progressive encephalopathy.* **e. with prolinemia** Encephalopathy attributable to a congenital metabolic defect involving heterocyclic amino acids, manifested as hyperprolinemia and excessive urinary excretion of proline, hydroxyproline, and glycine. The clinical signs are convulsions, a moderate degree of psychomotor retardation, muscle hypotonia, and hearing defects. Also *Joseph's disease, familial hyperprolinemia.* **recurrent e.** Any form of encephalopathy which shows a tendency to recur. Also *palindromic encepha-*

*lopathy.* **rheumatic e.** SYDENHAM'S CHOREA. **saturnine e.** LEAD ENCEPHALOPATHY. **spongiform e.** CREUTZFELDT-JAKOB DISEASE. **subacute myoclonic e.** INFANTILE MYOCLONIC ENCEPHALOPATHY. **subacute necrotizing e.** An autosomal recessive, degenerative neurologic disorder characterized by foci of necrosis, vascular proliferation, and gliosis in the brainstem and spinal cord. Symptoms include hyporeflexia, hypotonia, seizures, ophthalmoplegia, irregular breathing, and lactic acidosis. The histopathologic changes resemble those of Wernicke's encephalopathy. Abnormalities of thiamine and pyruvate metabolism occur, but the basic defect is not clear. It usually develops in infancy, where it is characterized by a failure to thrive, but milder cases of late onset have been described. Also *Leigh's disease, subacute necrotizing encephalomyelopathy, Leigh's necrotizing encephalomyelopathy, para-Wernicke encephalopathy, Leigh's encephalopathy.* **subcortical arteriosclerotic e.** BINSWANGER'S DISEASE. **toxic e.** Any encephalopathy resulting from the action of an exogenous or endogenous toxin. **traumatic e. of boxers** BOXERS' ENCEPHALOPATHY. **traumatic progressive e.** PROGRESSIVE TRAUMATIC ENCEPHALOPATHY. **e. with tyrosinuria** Encephalopathy of the newborn, attributable to an inherited defect of tyrosine metabolism, with hypertyrosinuria, giving rise clinically to severe generalized weakness, lack of psychomotor development, convulsions, and nystagmus. **uremic e.** AZOTEMIC ENCEPHALOSIS. **Wernicke's e.** WERNICKE'S DISEASE.

**encephalopuncture** \-pungk′chər\ The introduction of a needle or trochar into the brain.

**encephalorachidian** \-rəkid′ē·ən\ CEREBROSPINAL.

**encephaloradiculitis** \-rədik′yəlī′tis\ [ENCEPHALO- + RADICULITIS] Inflammation of the brain and spinal nerve roots.

**encephalorrhagia** \-rā′jə\ [ENCEPHALO- + -RRHAGIA] INTRACEREBRAL HEMORRHAGE.

**encephaloschisis** \ensef′əläs′kisis\ [ENCEPHALO- + -SCHISIS] Any defect in the closure of the neural tube in the region of the brain.

**encephalosis** \ensef′əlō′sis\ [ENCEPHAL- + -OSIS] Any form of organic disease or dysfunction of the brain. *Outmoded.* **azotemic e.** A neurologic syndrome which occurs in patients with raised blood nitrogen levels and which is marked by intellectual apathy and mental confusion, often with hallucinations, delirium, and bouts of agitation alternating with a state of collapse. Also *uremic encephalopathy.*

**encephalospinal** \-spī′nəl\ CEREBROSPINAL.

**encephalotome** \ensef′əlōtōm′\ [ENCEPHALO- + -TOME] An instrument for incising the brain.

**enchondral** \enkän′drəl\ INTRACARTILAGINOUS.

**enchondroma** \en′kändrō′mə\ [EN- + CHONDR- + -OMA] A benign cartilaginous growth within bone. Also *medullary chondroma, true chondroma, endochondroma.* **multiple e.'s** ENCHONDROMATOSIS. **multiple congenital e.'s** UNILATERAL CHONDRODYSPLASIA. **e. petrificum** OSTEOCHONDROMA.

**enchondromatosis** \enkän′drōmətō′sis\ [ENCHONDROMA + *t* + -OSIS] A condition characterized by multiple nests of cartilage cells which originate from the growth plate, but which do not become ossified. As growth continues the cartilage nests migrate into the bony metaphyses and cause thinning of the overlying cortex, which results in bone weakness. Also *skeletal enchondromatosis, enchondrosis, multiple enchondromas, genotypic chondrodysplasia.*

**enchondromatous** \en′kändräm′ətəs\ Pertaining to an enchondroma.

**enchondrosis** \en′kändrō′sis\ ENCHONDROMATOSIS.

**enclave** \en′klāv, äNkläv′\ [French (from Old French *enclave(r)* to enclose, from assumed Vulgar L *inclavare* to enclose, lock in, from L *in-* IN-[1] + *clavis* a key), a territory enclosed by another] A protected environment within an organ, tissue, or cell where external influences have either little or no effect.

**enclosure** An enclosed area or space. **Charnley e.** An ultraclean operating environment that is surrounded by nonporous material. The air that enters the enclosure is purified and frequently changed to prevent infection of exposed tissues during extended surgical procedures.

**encolpismus** \en′kälpiz′məs\ [New L, from Gk *enkolpismos* (from *kolpos* vagina) a vaginal douche or medication] A medicinal pessary inserted into the vagina.

**encopresis** \en′kōprē′sis\ [EN- + COPR- + -ESIS] Fecal incontinence not due to organic defect, but most commonly a result of faulty toilet training, mental retardation, or regression.

**encounter** A contact between a patient and a provider in which some health care is given. It is a measure used for record keeping or statistical purposes.

**encranius** \enkrā′nē·əs\ [New L, from Gk *en-* in + *krani(on)* the upper part of the head, the skull + *-us,* noun suffix] Unequal conjoined twins in which the parasitic member is partly or wholly included within the cranial cavity of the host.

**encysted** \ensis′tid\ Enclosed within a sac or cyst wall.

**encystment** \ensist′mənt\ The process of becoming encysted.

**end** / **C-terminal e.** C TERMINUS. **distal e.** In dental anatomy, the surface of a tooth that faces away from the midpoint of the dental arch. **N-terminal e.** N TERMINUS. **reducing e.** The end of a molecule of an oligosaccharide or polysaccharide that possesses a hydroxyl group on the anomeric carbon of the terminal residue. This residue is glycosylated by the second residue, but does not glycosylate another sugar. **sticky e.** The single-stranded end of double-stranded DNA that is produced by the action of a nuclease specific for a sequence that is identical with its complementary sequence. The single-stranded piece can therefore complement with, and so adhere to, the end of every other DNA fragment so produced, including the other end of the same fragment. **taste e.** TASTE ENDING.

**end-** \end-\ ENDO-.

**endadelphos** \end′ədel′fəs\ [END- + Gk *adelphos* brother, twin] Unequal conjoined twins in which the parasitic member is included within the body of the host.

**Endamoebidae** \end′əmē′bidē\ [*Endamoeb(a)* + -IDAE] A family of amebas that live in the digestive tracts of various animals. The genera, differentiated on the basis of nuclear structure, include *Endamoeba,* parasitic in invertebrates, and *Entamoeba, Iodamoeba,* and *Endolimax,* in vertebrates. Also *Entamoebidae.*

**endangiitis** \end′anjē·ī′tis\ [END- + ANGI- + -ITIS] Inflammation of the intima of a vessel; intimitis.

**endaortitis** \end′ā·ôrtī′tis\ [END- + AORTITIS] Inflammation of the intima of the aorta.

**endarterectomize** \end′ärtərek′təmīz\ [*endarterectom(y)* + -IZE] To remove an atherosclerotic occlusion or stenosis by dissecting the diseased intima and media from the underlying healthy adventitia.

**endarterectomy** \end′ärtərek′təmē\ [END- + *arter(i)-* + -ECTOMY] The excision of an atheromatous inner coat of an artery. **eversion e.** An endarterectomy in which an atherosclerotic artery is divided at its distal end and its more proximal atherosclerotic core is dissected free by cephalad eversion of the outer nondiseased part of the proximal artery. The core is then removed after the artery is divided a second time above the area of atherosclerotic involvement. The two sites of arterial division are then reanastomosed. **gas e.** An endarterectomy in which the dissection of the atherosclerotic plaque is carried out by high-pressure gas that is instilled into the vessel wall through a hand-held needle or cannula. **transaortic e.** An endarterectomy technique of renal or visceral artery orifices performed by opening the clamped aorta and removing the arterial plaque from within the aortic lumen.

**endarterial** \end′ärtir′ē·əl\ **1** Within an artery; intra-arterial. **2** Pertaining to the inner lining of an artery. For defs. 1 and 2 also *endoarterial.*

**endarteritis** \end′ärtərī′tis\ [END- + ARTERITIS] Inflammation of the intima of an artery. Also *endoarteritis.* **Heubner specific e.** SYPHILITIC CEREBRAL ENDARTERITIS. **e. obliterans** The narrowing of small arteries as a result of cellular proliferation of the intima. This is a nonspecific response to injury and it is seen, for example, in the vasa vasorum in syphilis of the aorta. Also *Friedländer's disease.* **spinal e.** Endarteritis of the arteries supplying the spinal cord. **syphilitic cerebral e.** Endarteritis due to syphilis affecting the arteries supplying the brain. Also *Heubner specific endarteritis.*

**endarterium** \end′ärtir′ē·əm\ The tunica interna of an artery.

**endarteropathy** \end′ärtəräp′əthē\ Any disorder involving the intima of arteries. **digital e.** Abnormality of the small digital arteries, associated with Raynaud's phenomenon. The latter is a vasospastic condition and so the involved vessels are morphologically normal. Only late in its course some degree of nonspecific intimal thickening may appear.

**endaural** \endôr′əl\ [END- + AURAL] Within the ear.

**endbrain** TELENCEPHALON.

**end-brush** TELODENDRON.

**end-bulb** **1** Any globose terminal of a sensory fiber in the skin, mucosa, fascial layers, etc. **2** The rounded terminal of a recurrent collateral of a dorsal root ganglion cell. It may contact either the cell body or the capsule. **3** END FOOT. **cylindrical e.** A tactile receptor of the conjunctiva having an elongated central axis cylinder, a lamellated sheath, and a capsule of connective tissue. It is a variety of the corpuscula tactus. **e. of Held** In the ventral cochlear nucleus as seen in a Golgi preparation, a small bulb with short rootlike processes at the end of a primary cochlear axon. It clasps the body of a secondary sensory neuron. **e.'s of Krause** CORPUSCULA BULBOIDEA.

**end-diastolic** \-dī′əstäl′ik\ Referring to the terminal part of diastole, immediately before the onset of systole.

**endemic** \endem′ik\ [Gk *endēm(os)* (from *en-* in + *dēmos* the people) native + -IC] Describing a disease which occurs persistently in an area or among a given population or group. Compare EPIDEMIC.

**endemicity** \en′dəmis′ətē\ The characteristic of being endemic.

**endepidermis** \end′epidur′mis\ EPITHELIUM.

**endergonic** \end′ərgän′ik\ Describing a reaction that proceeds with uptake of energy, often Gibbs energy. Compare EXERGONIC.

**end-flake** *Outmoded* MOTOR ENDPLATE.

**ending** / **annulospiral e.** PRIMARY ENDING. • Because the ending does not have an annulospiral configuration in the spindles of all species, the term primary ending is preferred. **ball-of-thread e.'s** RUFFINI'S CORPUSCLES. **basket e.'s** TERMINAISONS EN PANIER. **calyciform e.** A nerve synaptic terminal in the form of a cup or goblet. • The term was first used to describe auditory fiber terminals of the cochlear nuclei, but the form is also seen in other structures, such as a ciliary ganglion. **Dogiel e.** A nonencapsulated, arboriform ending in the intramuscular connective tissue of the mammalian abdominal and thoracic musculature. It is supplied by a thick, myelinated axon. **encapsulated nerve e.'s** CORPUSCULA NERVOSA TERMINALIA. **en plaque e.** TERMINAISON EN PLAQUE. **epilemmal e.'s** The major sensory endings in muscle. The term reflects the older view that terminals of sensory axons end on the surface of muscle fibers, whereas motor axons penetrate the sacrolemma. *Outmoded.* **free nerve e.** *Imprecise* CORPUSCULUM NERVOSUM ACAPSULATUM. **Golgi-Mazzoni e.'s** Encapsulated sensory nerve endings found in the skin and especially common in subcutaneous tissues of the fingers and toes, where they serve tactile sensibility. They are lamellated corpuscles of globular shape having relatively few lamellae and a large central core containing a profusely branching axon terminal. Also *Golgi-Mazzone corpuscles.* **grape e.'s** A motor axon terminal appearing as a fibrillar tangle with multiple, punctate synaptic contacts. Such endings are found in tonic skeletal muscles of lower vertebrates and on some fibers of mammalian extraocular muscles, and resemble the trail endings on intrafusal bag fibers. It was once held that they were terminals of sympathetic or parasympathetic fibers, but it is now thought that they are terminals of ordinary skeletomotor neurons innervating certain slow-contracting muscle fibers. Also *terminaisons en grappe, grapelike terminals.* **nerve e.** Any terminal structure of the axon, such as a synaptic ending, an afferent axon sense organ of deep and superficial somatic structures, or that portion of the axon containing synaptic vesicles. **nonencapsulated e.** FREE NERVE ENDING. **pain e.** NOCICEPTOR. **palisade e.** An eye-muscle sensory organ having a form appearing like a basket of branches embracing the end of a single muscle fiber. It may be a tension receptor for the type I muscle fibers found in eye muscles. **primary e.** The major sensory terminal in a muscle spindle, consisting of axonal branches that clasp or spiral around each of the intrafusal fibers at its midpoint. It is called primary by reason of its central position, its persistence when other sensory endings are absent, the large diameter of its axon, and because only one such afferent is found in a spindle. It senses static and dynamic changes in muscle length. Also *annulospiral ending.* Compare SECONDARY ENDING. **Ruffini's e.'s** RUFFINI'S CORPUSCLES. **secondary e.** A sensory axon terminal of spraylike, clasping, or spiraling configuration found on either side of the primary ending in a mammalian muscle spindle. There may be several such secondary wrappings and axons in a spindle, or it may lack them entirely. The ending is a slowly adapting sensor of muscle length. Compare PRIMARY ENDING. **spiral e.** A sensory ending of eye muscles consisting in its most typical form of a half dozen turns encircling a muscle fiber. It differs from a muscle spindle in having either no capsule or a feeble one, and no specialized motor supply. **spray e.'s** RUFFINI'S CORPUSCLES. **synaptic e.** A terminal portion of an axon, the site of impulse transmission, characterized morphologically by synaptic vesicles and membrane thickenings. **taste e.** The axon terminal innervating gustatory receptors of the tongue and oropharynx that respond to sapid molecular stimuli. Excitation elicits sensory reports of taste usually expressed as sweet, sour, bitter, or acid. Also *taste end.* **trail e.** A motor ending found on some intrafusal muscle fibers consisting of one or several naked filaments bearing multiple loci of cholinergic synaptic contact with the fiber: so called because it appears to trail or wander over the surface of the muscle fibers. **ultraterminal e.** A motor endplate at the end of an unmyelinated axon branch which has itself emerged from another motor endplate on the same or a neighboring muscle fiber. **unencapsulated e.** FREE NERVE ENDING.

**Endo** [Shigeru *Endo*, Japanese bacteriologist, active in Germany, 1869–1937] See under AGAR.

**endo-** \en′dō-\ [Gk *endon* within] A prefix meaning within, inside. Also *end-*. • In anatomy and embryology, the combining forms *endo-* and *ento-* are used interchangeably, as in *endoderm* and *entoderm*. In keeping with *Nomina Anatomica* 5th edition, 1980, this dictionary uses *endo-* as the preferred form for all anatomic and embryologic terms.

**endoabdominal** \-abdäm′ənəl\ Pertaining to the interior of the abdomen.

**endoamylase** Any amylase that hydrolyzes bonds remote from the nonreducing ends of starch molecules.

**endoaneurysmoplasty** \-an′yooriz′məplas′tē\ The repair, reconstruction, or obliteration of an aneurysm by suturing from within the sac.

**endoaneurysmorrhaphy** \-an′yoorizmôr′əfē\ The treatment of an aneurysm by suture ligation of inflow and outflow orifices from within the aneurysmal sac or by the insertion of a prosthetic graft into the aneurysmal sac from within.

**endoarterial** \-ärtir′ē·əl\ ENDARTERIAL.

**endoarteritis** \-är′təri′tis\ ENDARTERITIS.

**endobiotic** \-bī·ät′ik\ Living within the body of another organism.

**endoblast** \en′dōblast\ [ENDO- + -BLAST] An undifferentiated embryonic cell destined to become an endodermal cell, recognized by its position in an early embryo and by its cytochemical and cytoplasmic characteristics. Also *entoblast*. Adj. endoblastic.

**endocardial** 1 Pertaining to the endocardium. 2 Within the heart.

**endocardiography** \-kär′dē·äg′rəfē\ [ENDO- + CARDIOGRAPHY] Electrocardiography from an exploring electrode within the heart, for example to measure responses of the bundle of His during conduction studies.

**endocarditis** \-kärdī′tis\ [*endocard(ium)* + -ITIS] An inflammatory disorder of the endocardium, often involving the cardiac valves. Also *encarditis*. **abacterial thrombotic e.** NONBACTERIAL THROMBOTIC ENDOCARDITIS. **acute bacterial e.** Bacterial endocarditis of a fulminating type, usually caused by pyogenic bacteria, particularly the staphylococci. Also *septic endocarditis*. **atypical verrucous e.** LIBMAN-SACKS ENDOCARDITIS. **bacterial e.** Endocarditis as a result of bacterial infection. **e. benigna** LIBMAN-SACKS ENDOCARDITIS. **chronic e.** Chronic inflammatory change in the endocardium, especially affecting the valve cusps. **constrictive e.** LÖFFLER'S ENDOCARDITIS. **Coxsackie e.** Endocarditis resulting from infection by coxsackievirus. **gonococcal e.** Endocarditis due to gonococcal infection. **infective e.** Endocarditis, mainly of the cardiac valves, as a result of infection by microorganisms including bacteria, viruses, and fungi. Also *infectious endocarditis*. **e. lenta** SUBACUTE BACTERIAL ENDOCARDITIS. **Libman-Sacks e.** A nonbacterial verrucous endocarditis often associated with systemic lupus erythematosus. Also *atypical verrucous endocarditis, nonbacterial verrucous endocarditis, endocarditis benigna, Libman-Sacks disease, Libman-Sacks syndrome.* **Löffler's e.** Endocarditis accompanying the Löffler syndrome and characterized by thickening of the endocardium, eosinophilia, and the clinical picture of restrictive or obliterative cardiomyopathy. Also *Löffler's parietal fibroplastic endocarditis, constrictive endocarditis, eosinophilic endomyocardial disease, Löffler's disease.* **malignant e.** A rapidly progressive acute endocarditis; acute bacterial endocarditis. **marantic e.** NONBACTERIAL THROMBOTIC ENDOCARDITIS. **mural e.** Endocarditis affecting the walls of the cardiac chambers as opposed to the valvular structures. Also *parietal endocarditis*. **nonbacterial thrombotic e.** Endocarditis characterized by uninfected thrombotic vegetations, often associated with terminal illness such as cancer and prone to lead to sterile emboli. Also *abacterial thrombotic endocarditis, marantic endocarditis.* **nonbacterial verrucous e.** LIBMAN-SACKS ENDOCARDITIS. **parietal e.** MURAL ENDOCARDITIS. **pulmonic e.** Endocarditis affecting the pulmonic valve. **rheumatic e.** Endocarditis as a component of rheumatic fever or other rheumatic diseases. **rickettsial e.** Endocarditis caused by *Coxiella burnetii*, usually associated with other manifestations of chronic Q fever infection including hepatomegaly. **septic e.** ACUTE BACTERIAL ENDOCARDITIS. **subacute bacterial e.** Bacterial endocarditis which pursues a relatively slow course, being characterized by a low fever, anemia, and emboli and, in its most classical form, associated with progressive valvular disorder, splenomegaly, clubbing, and petechiae. Also *endocarditis lenta*. **ulcerative e.** Endocarditis in which there is a rapid ulceration of the affected structures, especially the valves. **valvular e.** Endocarditis affecting one or more of the cardiac valves. **verrucous e.** Endocarditis characterized by sterile wartlike aggregations of fibrin, platelets, and leukocytes on the free margins of the atrioventricular valves. It is usually part of a collagen vascular disease such as systemic lupus erythematosus. Also *verrucous carditis*. **verrucous nonbacterial e.** The occurrence of sterile nodules on the heart valve. The condition occurs in subjects with various noninfectious chronic illnesses, such as malignancies, systemic lupus erythematosus, and the like. **viridans e.** Endocarditis resulting from *Streptococcus viridans* infection.

**endocardium** \-kär′dē·əm\ [New L, from ENDO- + Gk *kardia* heart] [NA] The thin layer of endothelial cells resting on fibroelastic tissue that lines the chambers of the heart and is continuous with the endothelium of the large blood vessels. By folding on itself, it helps to form the valves of the heart.

**endocellular** \-sel′yələr\ INTRACELLULAR.

**endocervical** 1 Within the cervical canal. 2 Pertaining to the endometrium of the cervical canal.

**endocervicitis** \-sur′visī′tis\ [*endocervic(al)* + -ITIS] Inflammation of the cervical canal. Also *endotrachelitis*.

**endochondral** \-kän′drəl\ INTRACARTILAGINOUS.

**endochondroma** \-kändrō′mə\ ENCHONDROMA.

**endochrome** \en′dōkrōm\ A coloring matter or pigment within a cell.

**endochylema** \-kīlē′mə\ HYALOPLASM.

**endocommensal** \-kəmen′səl\ 1 Living and obtaining nourishment within the body of another organism without exhibiting a parasitic effect. 2 An endocommensal organism.

**endocorpuscular** \-kôrpus′kyələr\ INTRACORPUSCULAR.

**endocranial** \-krā′nē·əl\ Located within the skull.

**endocraniosis** \-krā′nē·ō′sis\ HYPEROSTOSIS FRONTALIS INTERNA.

**endocranium** \-krā′nē·əm\ [ENDO- + CRANIUM] The inner lining of the cranium, consisting of the outer (endosteal) layer of the dura mater adherent to the cranial bone.

**endocrine** \en′dəkrin, en′dəkrīn\ [ENDO- + Gk *krin(ein)* to separate] **1** Secreting into the bloodstream: said of a gland that delivers a substance into the circulation and that has an effect at a remote site. **2** Of or concerning secretion into the bloodstream of a chemical transmitter which has an effect at a remote site. Compare EXOCRINE.

**endocrinism** \endäk′rinizm\ [*endocrin(e)* + -ISM] ENDOCRINOPATHY.

**endocrinologist** \-krinäl′əjist\ A specialist in endocrinology.

**endocrinology** \-krinäl′əjē\ [*endocrin(e)* + *o* + -LOGY] The study of endocrine glands and of the chemistry, physiology, and pharmacology of hormones, of the functions of internal secretions upon the organism as a whole, and of disorders of endocrine function.

**endocrinopathy** \-krinäp′əthē\ [*endocrin(e)* + *o* + -PATHY] Any disorder of any endocrine gland. *Imprecise.* Also *endocrinism.*

**endocrinotherapy** \-krī′nōther′əpē\ HORMONOTHERAPY.

**endocyst** \en′dōsist\ [ENDO- + CYST] The germinative inner membrane of a hydatid cyst.

**endocystitis** \-sistī′tis\ [ENDO- + CYSTITIS] Inflammation of the mucous inner surface of the bladder.

**endocytize** \-sī′tīz\ To ingest by endocytosis. Also *endocytose.*

**endocytosis** \-sītō′sis\ [ENDO- + CYT- + -OSIS] The process whereby material is brought into the cytoplasm in a vesicle, the membrane of which is derived from the cell membrane. If the material includes a particle, the process is called phagocytosis. If only a fluid is contained in the vesicle, the process is called pinocytosis.

**endoderm** \en′dōdurm′\ [ENDO- + -DERM] The inner layer of the embryo, giving rise to the primitive intestine and the yolk sac. It forms the epithelium of the digestive tube. In its middle part, glands related to the gut, such as the liver and pancreas, are derived from it. In the foregut region, related to the pharynx, it contributes to the thyroid, the lungs, and through the branchial arches to the parathyroids and the thymus. In its posterior part, it gives rise ventrally to the allantois, while its terminal part forms the cloaca. In mammals the endoderm is isolated by division of the deep aspect of the embryonic mass, but its origin varies widely according to the zoological group and its type of gastrulation. Also *entoderm.* Adj. endodermal, endodermic. **primary e.** The first endodermal cells to appear. **primitive e.** The lining layer of the gastrula. It gives rise to the yolk sac and the gut epithelium. **yolk-sac e.** The lining of the yolk sac, made of endoderm.

**endodermoreaction** \-dur′mərē·ak′shən\ [ENDODERM + *o* + REACTION] TRAMBUSTI'S REACTION.

**endodiascope** \-dī′əskōp\ [ENDO- + DIA- + -SCOPE] An x-ray tube small enough to be placed inside a body cavity for the diagnostic or therapeutic use of the x rays.

**endodontia** \-dän′shə\ [END- + -ODONTIA] ENDODONTOLOGY.

**endodontics** \-dän′tiks\ The application of endodontology in practice.

**endodontist** \-dän′tist\ A dentist who specializes in endodontics.

**endodontium** \-dän′tē·əm\ DENTAL PULP.

**endodontology** \-däntäl′əjē\ [END- + ODONTO- + -LOGY] The study of diseases of the dental pulp and their sequelae. Also *endodontia.*

**endodural** \-d$^{y}$oo′rəl\ Within the dura mater; especially, denoting a potential cleft within the thickness of the spinal dura mater. Electrodes are sometimes implanted at this level.

**endodyogeny** \-dī·äj′ənē\ [ENDO- + Gk *dyo* two + -GEN + -Y] Reproduction by internal budding, as found among species of the genera *Toxoplasma, Besnoitia, Sarcocystis,* and *Frenkelia,* in which trophozoites form two organisms within a parent cell and are subsequently freed when the cell ruptures. See also SCHIZOGONY.

**endoectothrix** \-ek′təthriks\ An invasion of the hair by a dermatophyte, marked by the presence of fungal elements both within and on the surface of the hair shaft. • By convention, the terms *endothrix* and *ectothrix* are used to describe the location of arthrospores while ignoring the site of the mycelium. Most authorities now agree that no dermatophyte species forms arthrospores in both sites, and in all ectothrix infections there is mycelium within the hair shaft.

**endoelectrontherapy** \-ilek′tränther′əpē\ [ENDO- + ELECTRON + THERAPY] Radiation, with electrons, of tumors located within body cavities. A cone attached to the source of the electrons is placed into the orifice, sparing the surface tissues.

**endoenzyme** \-en′zīm\ **1** Any enzyme that acts within a cell. **2** Any enzyme that acts on links within chains of a macromolecule, as opposed to acting only on such links near unblocked ends of the chains.

**endogamy** \endäg′əmē\ [ENDO- + GAM- + -Y] **1** Reproductive union between eukaryotic organisms descended from a recent common ancestor. The parental cells share common genes although the genotypes need not be identical. **2** Mating or marriage within a tribe, clan, community, or other social group. To the extent that the group may be based on descent from fairly recent common ancestors, endogamy implies inbreeding. Compare EXOGAMY.

**endogenote** \-jē′nōt\ In genetic recombination, the chromosome of the recipient cell.

**endogenous** \endäj′ənəs\ [Gk *endogen(ēs)* (from *endo(n)* inside, domestic + *gen(os)* offspring) born in the house + -OUS] Originating within an organism, or resulting from causes within the organism.

**endogeny** \endäj′ənē\ [*endogen(ous)* + -Y] Development within an organism.

**endognathion** \-nā′thē·än\ [New L (from Gk *endo(n)* within + New L *gnathion,* irreg. from Gk *gnathos* jaw)] The medial segment of the human premaxilla, or incisive bone.

**endointoxication** \-intäk′səkā′shən\ Poisoning caused by toxic substances formed within the organism. Also *endogenic toxicosis.*

**endolaryngeal** \-lərin′jē·əl\ Within the larynx.

**endolemma** \-lem′ə\ *Outmoded* ENDONEURIUM.

***Endolimax*** \-lī′maks\ [ENDO- + L *limax* a slug, snail] A genus of small amebas (order Amoebida, superclass Rhizopoda) found in the intestine of humans and other animals, both vertebrate and invertebrate. Generally considered a commensal, it causes no known disease. It is characterized by a vesicular nucleus with a large, irregularly shaped endosome of chromatin granules. Transmission is through cysts.

**endolymph** \en′dōlimf\ ENDOLYMPHA.

**endolympha** \-lim′fə\ [ENDO- + LYMPHA] [NA] A secretion that fills the membranous labyrinth of the internal ear. It resembles intracellular fluid in its ionic composition, but its source and mode of production is uncertain. Its composition differs from perilymph. Also *endolymph, Scarpa's fluid* (outmoded), *liquor of Scarpa, otic fluid* (outmoded), *vitrina auris* (outmoded), *vitrina auditoria* (outmoded).

**endolymphangial** \-limfan′jē·əl\ **1** Within a lymph vessel. **2** Pertaining to the inner coat of a lymph vessel.

**endolymphangitis** \-lim′fanjī′tis\ Inflammation of the

inner coat of lymph vessels. **e. proliferans** A partial or complete lymphatic luminal obliteration that results from repeated subcutaneous inflammation which causes endothelial swelling. It has been suggested as a cause of lymphedema.

**endolymphatic** \-limfat′ik\ Pertaining to the endolymph.

**endolysin** \endäl′isin\ Bactericidal material present in extracts of host cells. **leukocytic e.** Any of a group of bactericidal substances extracted from polymorphonuclear leukocytes.

**endomeninges** \-mənin′jēz\ [ENDO- + *meninges*, pl. of MENINX] A layer of embryonic mesenchyme surrounding the neural tube and from which the pia mater and the arachnoid develop.

**endomesoderm** \-mes′ədurm\ Mesoderm derived from endoderm in the bilaminar embryonic disk.

**endometrectomy** \-mētrek′təmē\ [*endometr(ium)* + -ECTOMY] Surgical removal of the endometrium. This can be accomplished by utilizing caustic chemicals, or by curettage in the postabortal or puerperal period.

**endometrial** \-mē′trē·əl\ Pertaining to the endometrium or uterine cavity.

**endometrioma** \-mē′trē·ō′mə\ A hemorrhagic cyst resulting from endometriosis. The name is given to the larger of such cystic structures, particularly those measuring more than 8 cm in diameter. Also *Sampson cyst.*

**endometriosis** \-mē′trē·ō′sis\ [*endometri(um)* + -OSIS] The presence of functional endometrial glands or stroma or both in locations outside the uterus. In order of descending frequency, these ectopic sites include the ovaries, broad ligaments, rectovaginal septum, umbilicus, and laparotomy scars. The endometrial glands respond to hormonal stimuli, resulting in cyclic menstrual bleeding in the ectopic foci. Blood accumulates in cystic structures that are surrounded by inflammatory adhesions. Dysmenorrhea and pelvic pain are the main symptoms. Also *adenomyosis externa, adenomyosis of fallopian tube, endometrial implants, endometriosis externa.* **colonic e.** The presence of ectopic endometrium in the colon. It is frequently associated with smooth muscle hypertrophy and may result in intestinal obstruction. **cutaneous e.** The presence of ectopic endometrial tissue in the skin, usually in the vulvar area. **cystic e.** Endometriosis characterized by cystic accumulations of menstrual secretions. Larger cysts are called endometriomas. **e. externa** ENDOMETRIOSIS. **e. interna** ADENOMYOSIS. **interstitial e.** ENDOLYMPHATIC STROMAL MYOSIS. **ovarian e.** Endometriosis involving the ovary, usually characterized by the presence of blue cysts on the surface and adjacent peritoneum. In more advanced cases, large cysts filled with old menstrual blood are formed ("chocolate" cysts). Also *adenoma endometrioides ovarii.* **tubal e.** The presence of endometrial glands and stroma in the wall of the uterine tube. Also *adenomyosis tubae.* **e. uterina** ADENOMYOSIS.

**endometriotic** \-mē′trē·ät′ik\ Referring to or characterized by endometriosis.

**endometritis** \-mitrī′tis\ [*endometr(ium)* + -ITIS] Inflammation of the endometrium. **decidual e.** Inflammation or infection of the decidua during or just after pregnancy. **exfoliative e.** MEMBRANOUS ENDOMETRITIS. **membranous e.** Inflammation of the endometrium with formation of a pseudomembrane composed of cellular debris and a leukocytic inflammatory infiltrate. Also *exfoliative endometritis.* **puerperal e.** The postpartum occurrence of inflammation or infection of the endometrium. Also *lochometritis, lochiometritis.* **syncytial e.** An accentuation of the morphologic features of the placental site. The endometrium and myometrium are infiltrated by trophoblastic cells, with varying degrees of inflammation. The lesion is benign. Also *syncytioma.* **e. tuberosa papulosa** DECIDUAL CAST.

**endometrium** \-mē′trē·əm\ [New L, from ENDO- + Gk *mētra* the womb + new L *-ium*, noun suffix] TUNICA MUCOSA UTERI. **Swiss-cheese e.** CYSTIC-GLANDULAR HYPERPLASIA OF THE ENDOMETRIUM.

**endometrorrhagia** \-met′rôrā′jə\ METRORRHAGIA.

**endomitosis** \-mītō′sis\ (*pl.* endomitoses) A process in differentiating or differentiated somatic cells in which variable early stages of normal mitosis occur within the nucleus, including chromosome replication (endoreduplication), but the mitotic apparatus and metaphase plate do not form and the nucleus does not divide. If no obvious mitotic stages occur, then an increase in ploidy will be the only evidence, a process called masked endomitosis.

**endomixis** \-mik′sis\ [ENDO- + Gk *mixis* a mixing, sexual intercourse] SELF-FERTILIZATION.

**endomorph** \en′dōmôrf\ An individual who has the characteristics of endomorphy.

**endomorphic** \-môr′fik\ Characterized by endomorphy.

**endomorphy** \en′dōmôr′fē\ [ENDO- + MORPH- + -Y] A type of human body conformation in which there is relative predominance of soft tissues and viscera, resulting in a rounded body habitus. Compare ECTOMORPHY, MESOMORPHY.

**endomyelography** \-mī′əläg′rəfē\ [ENDO- + MYELOGRAPHY] Radiographic examination of the spinal intramedullary cavity, notably in syringomyelia, by means of injection of contrast material into it.

**endomyocardial** \-mī′əkär′dē·əl\ Pertaining to or affecting both endocardium and myocardium.

**endomyocarditis** \-mī′əkärdī′tis\ [ENDO- + MYOCARDITIS] Inflammation affecting both endocardium and myocardium.

**endomyometritis** \-mī′əmētrī′tis\ [ENDO- + MYOMETRITIS] Inflammation of the endometrium and myometrium which usually occurs after an abortion or term delivery, but which can on occasion occur at a time not associated with a recent pregnancy. Also *metroendometritis.*

**endomysium** \-mis′ē·əm\ [ENDO- + Gk *mys* muscle, mouse + L *-ium*, neut. sing. noun suffix] The connective tissue layer that surrounds an individual muscle fiber or cell. Also *internal perimysium.*

**endonephritis** \-nəfrī′tis\ [ENDO- + NEPHRITIS] *Outmoded* PYELITIS.

**endoneurial** \-nʸŭr′ē·əl\ Pertaining to the connective tissue and related cells of the endoneurium of the peripheral nerves.

**endoneuritis** \-nʸŭrī′tis\ [*endoneur(ium)* + -ITIS] Inflammation of the endoneurium.

**endoneurium** \-nʸŭr′ē·əm\ [ENDO- + NEUR- + L *-ium*, neut. sing. noun termination] The connective tissue surrounding individual peripheral nerve myelinated axons or the Schwann cells enveloping several unmyelinated axons. Also *Key-Retzius sheath, endoneurial sheath, epilemma* (outmoded), *endolemma* (outmoded).

**endoneurolysis** \-nʸŭräl′isis\ [ENDO- + NEUROLYSIS] HERSAGE.

**endonuclear** \-nʸoo′klē·ər\ Situated or occurring within the nucleus of a cell.

**endonuclease** Any of a class of hydrolytic enzymes which hydrolyze polynucleotide chains within the chains, i.e., not acting near their ends. One class of endonucleases (restriction endonucleases or restriction enzymes) have become important tools in recombinant DNA technology. Compare

EXONUCLEASE. **restriction e.** One of a class of species-specific microbial enzymes capable of degrading duplex DNA at specific nucleotide sequences. *In vivo,* host DNA is protected by modification of the recognition sequence. These enzymes have been widely applied in studying genetic organization and in recombinant DNA technology. Also *restriction enzyme.*

**endonucleolus** \-nʸooklē′ələs\ A small region in the nucleolus, usually centrally located, which is difficult to stain.

**endoparasital** \-par′əsī′təl\ ENDOPARASITIC.

**endoparasite** \-par′əsīt\ [ENDO- + PARASITE] A parasite that lives within its host. Various kinds of endoparasites characteristically occupy body cavities such as the digestive tract, tissues such as muscle, subcutaneous tissue, or blood, particular organs such as the liver, or the interior of cells.

**endoparasitic** \-par′əsit′ik\ **1** Living parasitically within the body of a host. **2** Of or pertaining to endoparasites. Also *endoparasital.*

**endoparasitism** \-par′əsitizm\ Internal parasitism; the relation of an endoparasite to its host.

**endopeptidase** Any peptidase that hydrolyzes bonds remote from the ends of the substrate molecules.

**endopericardial** \-per′ikär′dē·əl\ Pertaining to or affecting both endocardium and pericardium.

**endoperineuritis** \-per′inyʊrī′tis\ [ENDO- + PERINEURITIS] Inflammation of the endoneurium and perineurium.

**endoperoxide** A compound with an internally located peroxide (—O—O—) group. The intermediary in prostaglandin synthesis, prostaglandin G, has an endoperoxide group, attached to the cyclopentane ring, that is cleaved in the formation of physiologically active prostaglandins.

**endoperoxide isomerase** An enzyme involved in prostaglandin synthesis that splits the endoperoxide group (—O—O—) of prostaglandin $G_2$, resulting in hydroxyl and keto side groups at carbons 9 and 11.

**endophasia** \-fā′zhə\ [ENDO- + Gk *phas(is)* speech + -IA] A phenomenon in which an individual moves the lips and other organs of articulation as if intending to utter words but produces no sound.

**endophlebitis** \-fləbī′tis\ [ENDO- + PHLEBITIS] Inflammation of the intima of a vein. **e. hepatica obliterans** BUDD-CHIARI SYNDROME. **proliferative e.** PHLEBOSCLEROSIS.

**endophthalmitis** \en′däfthalmī′tis\ [END- + OPHTHALM- + -ITIS] Inflammation of the interior of the eye. **e. phacoanaphylactica** Intraocular inflammation due to a toxic response to the protein of the crystalline lens.

**endophthalmos** \en′däfthal′məs\ ENOPHTHALMOS.

**endophytic** \-fit′ik\ [ENDO- + Gk *phyt(os)* (from *phyein* to grow) grown, growing + -IC] Growing or progressing inward within the interior of an organ or other structure: said of certain tumors.

**endoplasm** \en′dōplazm\ [ENDO- + -PLASM] The inner portion of the cytoplasm, which generally contains granular material and is more fluid than the outer ectoplasm. The flow of endoplasm and physical change between endoplasm and ectoplasm are responsible for ameboid movement among the amebae. Also *entoplasm, endosarc, entosarc.*

**endoplasmic** Pertaining to or located in the endoplasm.

**endopolygeny** \-pəlij′ənē\ [ENDO- + POLY- + -GEN + -Y] Asexual reproduction characterized by the formation of more than two offspring within the parent cell. Two or more nuclear divisions occur prior to merozoite formation, as in the internal budding seen in *Toxoplasma gondii.*. See also SCHIZOGONY.

**endoradiosonde** \-rā′dē·ōsänd′\ [ENDO- + *radiosonde* (from *radio* + French *sonde* SOUND²) a radio tracing or sampling device] A swallowable pill miniature implantable instrument that measures physiologic variables such as pressure, temperature, and pH and transmits these by radiotelemetry to a receiver outside the body. Also *radio pill, telemetry capsule, radiotelemetry capsule.*

**endoradiotherapy** \-rā′dē·ōther′əpē\ Radiotherapy of internal organs by the insertion of a radioactive source into a body cavity, such as the rectum, vagina, trachea, esophagus, etc.

**endoreduplication** \-ridʸoop′likā′shən\ The process of chromosome replication occurring in endomitosis. See under ENDOMITOSIS.

**end-organ** \end′-ôrgən\ See under ORGAN.

**endorphin** \endôr′fin\ Any or all of the endogenous morphinelike substances isolated from the pituitary gland. Three components, $\alpha$, $\beta$, and $\gamma$, constitute peptide sequences of $\beta$-lipotropin.

**$\alpha$-endorphin** An endogenous opiatelike peptide, comprising the amino acid sequence 61 to 76 in the $\beta$-lipotropin molecule which is assumed to be the prohormone for the endorphins. It possesses analgesic and behavioral effects in animals, generally less potent than $\beta$-endorphin.

**$\beta$-endorphin** An opioid peptide elaborated in and secreted by cells of the basal hypothalamus and the intermediate and anterior lobes of the pituitary; the material is a single-chain peptide comprising amino acids 61-91 of the $\beta$-lipotropin molecule, has analgesic and behavioral effects in mammals, and appears to be secreted by the same pituitary cells and controlled by the same regulatory mechanisms as is pituitary corticotropin.

**$\gamma$-endorphin** An endogenous opiatelike peptide comprising the amino acid sequence 61-77 in the $\beta$-lipotropin molecule and having properties similar to those of $\beta$-endorphin but with lesser potency.

**endorrhachis** \-rā′kis\ [ENDO- + Gk *rhachis* the back, spine, backbone] DURA MATER SPINALIS.

**endosalpingitis** \-sal′pinjī′tis\ [ENDO- + SALPINGITIS] Inflammation of the epithelium of the oviduct.

**endosalpingoma** \-sal′ping·gō′mə\ [ENDO- + SALPING- + -OMA] Localized endometriosis of the oviduct.

**endosalpingosis** \-sal′ping·gō′sis\ [ENDO- + SALPING- + -OSIS] The presence of fallopian tube epithelium outside of the tube proper. Frequently, the tubal epithelium is located on the ovarian surface close to the fimbria. It may also follow surgical intervention such as hysterectomy.

**endosalpinx** \-sal′pingks\ [ENDO- + SALPINX] The mucosa of the oviduct (fallopian tube). It contains three types of cells (ciliated, nonciliated, and intercalary).

**endosarc** \en′dōsärk\ ENDOPLASM.

**endoscope** \en′dōskōp\ [ENDO- + -SCOPE] A device for visualizing the interior of a body cavity.

**endoscopic** \-skäp′ik\ Of, by, or relating to endoscopy.

**endoscopy** \endäs′kəpē\ Inspection of an internal cavity using an endoscope. **peroral e.** Endoscopy performed by way of the mouth, as in esophagoscopy. **transcolonic e.** Endoscopic examination of the colon through an opening in the colonic wall.

**endoskeleton** \-skel′ətən\ The internal supporting bony and cartilaginous framework of an animal; the vertebrate skeleton. Also *neuroskeleton.*

**endosmosis** \en′däzmō′sis\ [END- + OSMOSIS] Osmosis involving movement of a liquid into a cell or cavity. Compare EXOSMOSIS.

**endosome** \en′dōsōm\ [ENDO- + Gk *sōm(a)* body] A more or less central body in the vesicular nucleus of certain protozoa. It lacks DNA, as indicated by a negative Feulgen reaction. The endosome is characteristic of trypanosomes, parasitic amebas, and phytoflagellates. The chromatin, which is Feulgen-positive, is found between the nuclear membrane and the endosome.

**endospore** \en′dōspôr\ [ENDO- + SPORE] **1** BACTERIAL SPORE. **2** ENDOSPORIUM.

**endosporium** \-spôr′ē·əm\ [New L (from Gk *endo(n)* within + *spor(a)* seed + L *-ium*, neut. sing. noun suffix)] The inner layer of a spore envelope. Also *endospore*.

**endosteal** \endäs′tē·əl\ Of or relating to the endosteum.

**endosteohyperostosis** \endäs′tē·ōhī′pərästō′sis\ VAN BUCHEM SYNDROME.

**endosteum** \endäs′tē·əm\ [New L, from END- + Gk *osteon* bone] [NA] A vascular membrane composed of condensed areolar tissue lining the central medullary cavity and the connecting intratrabecular spaces in the ends of bones. It is both osteogenic and hemopoietic. Also *medullary membrane, perimyelis*.

**endotenon** \-ten′än\ [ENDO- + Gk *tenōn* sinew] A loose connective tissue framework between and around the main bundles of collagen fibers in a tendon. Also *endotendineum*.

**endothelial** \-thē′lē·əl\ Pertaining to or consisting of endothelium.

**endothelialization** \-thē′lē·əlīzā′shən\ **1** The repair of the endothelial surfaces of vessels. **2** The invasion of repair tissue by endothelial cells.

**endothelio-** \en′dōthē′lē·ō-\ [See ENDOTHELIUM.] A combining form denoting endothelium.

**endothelioid** \-thē′lē·oid\ Resembling endothelium.

**endothelioma** \-thē′lē·ō′mə\ [*endotheli(um)* + -OMA] Any tumor composed of vascular endothelial cells. • *Endothelioma* is usually used as a component of a more detailed term, as *hemangioendothelioma* or *lymphangioendothelioma*. The term has also been used for mesothelioma and Ewing sarcoma and is therefore ambiguous. **diffuse e.** EWING SARCOMA. **perithelial e.** HEMANGIOPERICYTOMA.

**endotheliosis** \-thē′lē·ō′sis\ [*endotheli(um)* + -OSIS] A state of endothelial excess. **glomerular capillary e.** ECLAMPSIA.

**endotheliotoxin** \-thē′lē·ōtäk′sin\ A toxin which catalyzes the endothelial cells of capillaries and small veins to produce severe hemorrhages.

**endothelium** \-thē′lē·əm\ [ENDO- + *(epi)thelium*] A single layer of squamous epithelial cells arranged on the surface of connective tissue that lines the heart, blood vascular, and lymphatic channels. It derives from flattened embryonic mesenchymal cells. **e. camerae anterioris bulbi** The layer of polygonal, squamous cells that covers the posterior surface of the posterior limiting lamina of the cornea and the anterior surface of the iris. It also lines the spaces of the iridocorneal angle. *Outmoded.* Also *endothelium of anterior chamber, epithelium posterius corneae, corneal endothelium, endothelium camerae anterioris oculi* (outmoded). **extraembryonic e.** Lining cells of blood vessels originating in structures outside the embryo, as of the vessels which develop in various parts of the placenta or its membranes. **vascular e.** A single layer of flattened cells that forms the innermost lining of the blood vascular system. This lining is able to function as a semipermeable structure in many capillary vessels. Also *endothelial tissue*.

**endothermic** \-thur′mik\ **1** HOMEOTHERMIC. **2** Proceeding with intake of heat.

**endothermy** \en′dōthur′mē\ **1** DIATHERMY. **2** HOMEOTHERMY.

**endothoracic** \-thôras′ik\ Within the thorax. Also *intrathoracic*.

**endothrix** \en′dōthriks\ [ENDO- + Gk *thrix* hair] **1** A form of hair invasion by a dermatophyte in which arthrospores develop within the hair shaft. **2** Those species of dermatophyte that produce arthrospores within the hair shaft, such as *Trichophyton tonsurans* and *Trichophyton violaceum*.

**endothyroidopexy** \-thīroi′dəpek′sē\ [ENDO- + THYROID + *o* + -PEXY] Surgical translocation of the thyroid gland from its normal site in front of the trachea to a pocket created in the side of the neck. Also *endothyropexy*.

**endotoxemia** \-täksē′mē·ə\ The presence in blood of endotoxin. Endotoxemia is commonly associated with severe hypotension that is usually fatal.

**endotoxic** \-täk′sik\ Relating to or possessing endotoxin.

**endotoxicosis** \-täk′sikō′sis\ Poisoning due to the presence of an endotoxin.

**endotoxin** \-täk′sin\ [ENDO- + TOXIN] The lipopolysaccharide of the outer membrane of Gram-negative bacteria, extractable from cells with trichloroacetic acid but not naturally released in quantity until cell lysis. The lipid A portion of the lipopolysaccharide is responsible for its toxic effects, which include leukopenia, thrombocytopenia, fever, and shock. Unlike the specific exotoxins, endotoxins from various organisms have similar pathogenic effects. Also *bacterial pyrogen*.

**endotoxoid** \-täk′soid\ A toxoid prepared from an endotoxin.

**endotracheal** Within or through the trachea.

**endotrachelitis** \-trā′kəlī′tis\ [ENDO- + TRACHEL- + -ITIS] ENDOCERVICITIS.

**endourethral** INTRAURETHRAL.

**endplate / motor e.** The expanded terminal of a motor axon in synaptic contact with a striated muscle fiber, together with the subneural apparatus of the muscle fiber. The transmission of the excitatory stimulus between the two cells is achieved by the release of acetylcholine from the nerve fiber. A palisadelike interdigitation of axon terminal with muscle plasmalemmal folds usually increases the area of synaptic contact.It occurs in various forms, such as plaque endings, grape endings, and trail endings. Also *myoneural junction, Doyère's eminence* (outmoded), *end-flake* (outmoded), *motorial end organ* (obs.), *neuromuscular junction, Doyère's hillock, myoceptor, terminal nerve-plate of Rouget* (obs.), *motor plate, tache motrice*.

**endyma** \en′dimə\ *Obs.* EPENDYMA.

**-ene** [L suffix *-enus*; Gk suffix *-enos*] A suffix used to indicate the presence of a double bond. It replaces the suffix *-ane* in the name of a hydrocarbon. It can have multiplicative prefixes attached to it, as *butadiene* from *butane*, and also locants, as *but-2-ene*. Some old chemical names, such as *acetylene*, end in *-ene* without carrying this meaning.

**enema** \en′əmə\ [Gk (from *enienai* to inject, send in, from EN- + *hienai* to send) injection, enema] Injection of a liquid per rectum, or the liquid to be injected. Also *clyster* (older term). **barium e.** The instillation of a barium sulfate suspension or emulsion into the rectum to fill the colon for roentgenographic examination of the large bowel. Also *contrast enema*. **double contrast e.** Instillation of air into the colon per rectum, either after partial filling of the large bowel with a barium sulfate emulsion or suspension or after evacuation of a barium enema. The distension of the bowel by the air after preliminary coating of the mucosa permits roentgenographic air-contrast examination of the colon. **high e.** An enema of any material inserted high into the colon, usually via a tube. **sedative e.** **1** A general sedative administered as an enema and containing paraldehyde, tribromoethanol, chloral, and bromide. **2** A local sedative to the gastrointestinal tract, given as an enema containing opium in starch or starch mucilage. **starch e.** A sedative enema of starch mucilage, consisting of starch thickened by heating in water. **starch-and-opium e.** A starch mucilage enema containing tincture of opium.

**energizer / psychic e.** A drug or agent that produces a heightened mood, increased emotional excitability or responsiveness. Representative drugs of this type are the tricyclic antidepressants, the monoamine oxidase inhibitors, as well as the amphetamines.

**energy** [Gk *energeia* (from EN- + Gk *ergon* work) an act, operation, energy] The amount of work that can be done by a system. **e. of activation** The energy that must be supplied to a system in order to initiate a reaction. For covalent bonds to be broken they must temporarily acquire extra energy, pushing the bonded atoms further apart. Once the reaction is activated it will proceed releasing energy. **atomic e.** *Popular* NUCLEAR ENERGY. **binding e.** The amount of energy which must be supplied to an electron to separate it from the nucleus. Its value depends on the atomic number and the orbit in which the electron is located. **disintegration e.** The total energy difference involved in a nuclear disintegration. **excitation e.** The energy difference between the excited state of an atom or molecule and the ground state. Thus it is the energy which must be supplied in order to excite the atom or molecule. **free e.** A system's maximum potential for doing useful work, either Gibbs energy, which applies to a system at constant temperature and constant pressure, or Helmholtz energy, which applies to systems at constant volume and constant temperature. Since constant temperature and pressure are biologic conditions, Gibbs energy is usually meant in biologic contexts. **Gibbs e.** A system's potential, dependent on composition, temperature, etc., for doing useful work at constant temperature and pressure. Under these conditions it tends to decrease in all spontaneous reactions. The change in Gibbs energy, symbolized $\Delta G$, is thus negative for reactions going towards equilibrium, zero for reactions at equilibrium, and positive for reactions being forced from equilibrium, as for an electric cell being charged. **kinetic e.** The component of energy possessed by a body in motion that results from its motion. **latent e.** POTENTIAL ENERGY. **nuclear e.** Energy released by the fission of the nuclei of heavy atoms, as in a nuclear reactor, or by the fusion of light elements to form heavier ones. Also *atomic energy* (popular). **phosphate bond e.** The Gibbs energy for the hydrolysis of a compound of formula $R—PO(OH)_2$ to R—H and $H_3PO_4$. It is a measure of how powerful a donor the first compound is of the phospho group. **e. of position** POTENTIAL ENERGY. **potential e.** The component of energy possessed by a body or system by virtue of its position in space or its configuration. Also *energy of position, latent energy*. **recoil e.** 1 The energy imparted to a target body by an incident body. 2 The energy imparted to the residual system in an atomic or nuclear decay process. **specific nerve e.** LAW OF SPECIFIC IRRITABILITY.

**energy-rich** Describing a bond whose hydrolysis is accompanied by a large fall in standard Gibbs energy, or a compound containing that kind of bond. Such compounds are good donors of the group joined by these bonds, because they are by definition good donors (at least in the sense of equilibrium position) of the groups to water. The term does not refer to bond energy in the physicochemical sense of the energy required to break the bond with formation of radicals or ions. Also *high-energy*.

**enervation** \en′ərvā′shən\ Nerve interruption or removal. *Outmoded.*

**enflagellation** \enflaj′əlā′shən\ Development of flagella.

**enflurane** \en′floorān\ $CHF_2—O—CF_2—CHClF$. A nonflammable, volatile general anesthetic in liquid form, consisting of a halogenated ether with a fluorene substitution. When administered, it results in a low metabolism rate and little cardiac arrhythmia.

**ENG** electronystagmography.

**engagement** The descent of the biparietal plane of the fetal skull to a level below that of the inlet of the maternal pelvis.

**engastrius** \engas′trē·əs\ [EN- + Gk *gastēr* the belly + L *-ius*, noun suffix] Unequal conjoined twins in which the parasitic member is incorporated within the abdominal cavity of the host.

**Engel** [Gerhard *Engel*, German physician, flourished mid-19th century] Engel-Recklinghausen disease. See under OSTEITIS FIBROSA CYSTICA.

**Engelmann** [Guido *Engelmann*, German surgeon, born 1876] Camurati-Engelmann disease, Engelmann's disease. See under PROGRESSIVE DIAPHYSEAL DYSPLASIA.

**engineering / biomedical e.** The application of the tools of mathematics and the physical sciences to biologic and medical problems. Also *bioengineering*. **genetic e.** 1 The deliberate alteration of the genome of an organism, as, for example, the isolation of a piece of the DNA of a different organism and incorporation of it into the genome to give the recipient desired characteristics. 2 Any process or combination of processes that bypass, wholly or in part, the usual reproductive cycle of a cell or an organism. It includes artificial insemination, *in vitro* fertilization, and prenatal diagnosis with termination of genetically abnormal fetuses. **human e.** The application of psychological principles to match the human operator, often of a machine, to the task to be performed. It includes a consideration of such factors as the complexity of the control system, the physical conditions of work, skills, and learning ability needed, operator comfort and fatigue, and the like.

**englobement** \englōb′mənt\ PHAGOCYTOSIS.

**Engman** [Martin Feeney *Engman*, U.S. dermatologist, 1869–1953] 1 Engman's disease. See under INFECTIVE DERMATITIS. 2 Zinser-Cole-Engman syndrome. See under DYSKERATOSIS CONGENITA.

**engorged** \engôrjd′\ So filled with fluid as to be swollen; distended.

**engorgement** \engôrj′mənt\ A complete filling with fluid. **breast e.** Distension of the female breasts until they become firm and nodular due to stasis in the venous and lymphatic system. This process is a normal accompaniment of lactation.

**engram** \en′gram\ [EN- + -GRAM] MEMORY TRACE.

**en grappe** \äN gräp′\ [French *en* in + *grappe* a cluster] Consisting of grapelike clusters, as fungal spores, especially the microconidia of certain dermatophytes. Compare EN THYRSE.

**enhancement** \enhans′mənt\ [Old French *enhalcier* (ultimately from L *altus* high) to heighten, increase] IMMUNOLOGIC ENHANCEMENT. **acoustic e.** Increased echo amplitude from reflectors that lie behind a weakly attenuating structure. Compare ACOUSTIC SHADOW. **contrast e.** An increase in the apparent difference between bright and dark regions on a recorded image, achieved by electronic or computer adjustment. **immunologic e.** 1 Increased growth and survival of allogenic organ or tumor transplants in a host which has antibody to the organ graft or tumor. Enhancement is attributed to the presence of antibodies to class 2 MHC antigens on potential antigen-presenting cells within the graft, thereby inhibiting effective antigen presentation. 2 Any of various means of augmenting immune response. For defs. 1 and 2 also *enhancement.*

**enhancer** \enhan′sər\ A nucleotide sequence that increases the transcription of a linked gene.

**enhexymal** HEXOBARBITAL.

**enkatarrhaphy** \en′kətär′əfē\ ENCATARRHAPHY.

**enkephalin** Either of two peptides, of sequence Tyr-Gly-Gly-Phe-Xaa, found in the nervous system, where Xaa is Met (in [Met]enkephalin) or Leu (in [Leu]enkephalin). They relieve pain and have many of the actions of morphine. [Leu] enkephalin is released from $\beta$-endorphin by proteolysis.

**enlargement** **1** The condition of being or becoming larger. **2** A large or thickened part of a structure. **cervical e.** INTUMESCENTIA CERVICALIS. **hereditary gingival e.** GINGIVAL FIBROMATOSIS. **idiopathic gingival e.** GINGIVAL FIBROMATOSIS. **lumbar e.** INTUMESCENTIA LUMBALIS.

**enol** \ē′nôl\ [-ENE + -OL] The tautomer of a carbonyl compound R—CO—CHR′R″ of formula R—C(OH)=CR′R″.

**enolase** An enzyme (EC 4.2.1.11) that catalyzes the elimination of water from 2-phosphoglycerate to yield phosphoenolpyruvate, and the reverse reaction. This is a step in the pathways of glycolysis and gluconeogenesis. The enzyme has an absolute requirement for $Mg^{2+}$ or $Mn^{2+}$ and is strongly inhibited by fluoride, particularly in the presence of phosphate.

**enolization** \ē′nōlīzā′shən\ The formation of an enol from a carbonyl compound.

**enophthalmos** \en′äfthal′məs\ [EN- + Gk *ophthalmos* the eye] Abnormal posterior displacement of the eye within the orbit. Also *enophthalmus, endophthalmos.*

**enorganic** \en′ôrgan′ik\ [EN- + ORGANIC] Describing a permanent and characteristic feature of an organism.

**enostosis** \en′ästō′sis\ [EN- + OST- + -OSIS] Abnormal bone formation in the medullary cavity of a bone. Also *entostosis.*

**enoxidase** \enäk′sidās\ An enzyme which causes oxidation of wine, rendering it less palatable.

**enoyl-ACP reductase** An enzyme that catalyzes the formation of a saturated *S*-acyl group on acyl carrier protein by transfer of hydrogens from NADPH + $H^+$ to the 2,3-double bond of an unsaturated group on the acyl carrier protein in the course of fatty acid biosynthesis in bacteria.

**enoyl-CoA hydratase** The enzyme (EC 4.2.1.17) that catalyzes the addition of the elements of water to a 2,3-*trans*-enoyl-CoA to yield a (3*S*)-3-hydroxyacyl-CoA. This is a reaction in the pathway of fatty-acid oxidation.

**en plaque** \äN plak′\ See under TERMINAISON EN PLAQUE.

**enrichment** The addition of nutrients, either to foods (as the addition of vitamin D to milk, vitamin C to fruit juices, iodide to table salt, and B vitamins to flour and rice) or to microbiologic culture media. Also *fortification.*

**ensiform** \en′sifôrm\ Sword-shaped; xiphoid.

**ensisternum** \en′sistur′nəm\ PROCESSUS XIPHOIDEUS.

**ensomphalus** \ensäm′fələs\ [Gk *en-* IN- + *sōm(a)* body + *(om)phalos* the navel] Equal conjoined twins that share no vital organs and are united minimally by superficial tissues in the abdominal or thoracic region.

**ENT** [*e(ar,) n(ose, and) t(hroat)* ] OTORHINOLARYNGOLOGY.

**ent-** \ent-\ ENTO-.

**entad** \en′tad\ [ENT- + -AD] Toward the inside; inward.

**ental** \en′təl\ Central; inner.

**entalação** \ēNtalasouN′\ [Portuguese (from *ental(ar)* to put in a tight spot, to splint, from *en-, em* in, into + *tal(a)* a splint + *-ação* -ATION) difficulty (swallowing), dysphagia] TROPICAL CARDIOSPASM.

**entamebiasis** \en′təmēbī′əsis\ ENTAMOEBIASIS.

***Entamoeba*** \ent′əmē′bə\ [ENT- + AMOEBA] A genus of amebas (order Amoebida, superclass Rhizopoda) most of which are parasitic in the intestine of mammals and birds. ***E. buccalis*** *ENTAMOEBA GINGIVALIS.* ***E. coli*** A large, nonpathogenic ameba found in the large intestine of humans. It is important mainly because of possible confusion with the pathogenic species *E. histolytica..* Also *Amoeba coli.* ***E. dispar*** *ENTAMOEBA HISTOLYTICA.* ***E. dysenteriae*** *ENTAMOEBA HISTOLYTICA.* ***E. gingivalis*** A species found in the mouth of humans, especially around the gums and in tartar on the teeth. Although frequently found in the presence of dental caries and gum disease, it is not thought to be a primary pathogen. It is also found in other primates, dogs, and cats. Also *Entamoeba buccalis, Amoeba buccalis, Amoeba dentalis.* ***E. hartmanni*** A nonpathogenic species found in the large intestine of humans, other primates, and dogs. It is frequently confused with *E. histolytica,* since it appears to be identical except for its smaller size. Once considered a small race of *E. histolytica,* it is now classed as a distinct species or strain. ***E. histolytica*** The only important pathogen of the genus, causing amebic dysentery in humans. It can cause ulceration of the walls of the large intestine and, transported by portal circulation, invade the liver and produce hepatic abscesses. Less frequently it spreads to other organs, including the lungs, brain, and skin. Also *Amoeba dysenteriae, Amoeba histolytica, Caudamoeba sinensis, Entamoeba dispar, Entamoeba dysenteriae, Entamoeba tetragena, Karyamoebina falcata.* ***E. moshkowskii*** A free-living saprophytic species found in sewage and municipal water supplies, but not an animal or human parasite. It is similar to *E. histolytica* and may cause diagnostic confusion if it is present in drinking water. ***E. tetragena*** *ENTAMOEBA HISTOLYTICA.*

**entamoebiasis** \en′təmēbī′əsis\ [*Entamoeb(a)* + -IASIS] Infection with amebas of the genus *Entamoeba,* especially *E. histolytica;* amebiasis. Also *entamebiasis.* **e. coli** The presence of *Entamoeba coli* in the colon. *Entamoeba coli* is a harmless protozoan frequently found as a commensal in the human colon throughout the world. Cysts and trophozoites should be distinguished from those of the pathogenic *E. histolytica.*

**Entamoebidae** \en′təmē′bidē\ ENDAMOEBIDAE.

**entepicondyle** \entep′ikän′dīl\ [ENT- + EPICONDYLE] *Outmoded* EPICONDYLUS MEDIALIS HUMERI.

**enter-** \enter-, en′tər-\ ENTERO-.

**enterectomy** \en′tərek′təmē\ [ENTER- + -ECTOMY] The surgical removal of all or part of the intestine.

**enteric** \enter′ik\ [Gk *enterikos* (from *enteron* intestine) intestinal] **1** Of or relating to the intestine, especially the small intestine. **2** Intended to be dissolved or digested in the intestine but not in the stomach: said especially of capsules and pill coatings that protect their contents from the action of gastric juice.

**enteric-coated** Designating tablets or pills protected by an external coating which prevents the release of the active contents until the medication has passed through the stomach and entered the small intestinal tract. It is used to avoid gastric irritation or destruction of the drug by the gastric acidity and digestion.

**entericoid** \enter′ikoid\ [*enteric (fever)* + -OID] Resembling typhoid fever.

**enterics** \enter′iks\ Enteric bacteria; any bacteria found in the intestinal tract, especially the Enterobacteriaceae.

**enteritis** \en′tərī′tis\ [ENTER- + -ITIS] Inflammation of the mucosa of the small intestine. Also *enteronitis.* **e. cystica chronica** Enteritis resulting in dilatation of intestinal glands. **diphtheritic e.** Enteritis resulting in a thick membrane simulating the pharyngeal membrane of diphtheria. ***Escherichia coli* e.** Acute gastrointestinal infection caused by Gram-negative motile rods which ferment lactose and glucose, usually with gas-formation. There are numerous serotypes, many of which produce heat-stable and heat-labile enterotoxins and others of which are direct intestinal pathogens. This is the main organism responsible for travelers' diarrhea, which is caused by an acute replacement of the colonic flora by a "foreign" serotype of *E. coli.* **mucomembranous e.** *Outmoded* IRRITABLE BOWEL SYNDROME. **mucous e.** *Outmoded* IRRITABLE BOWEL SYNDROME. **e. necroticans** Enteritis caused by *Clostridium perfringens,* resulting in mucosal necrosis. Also *necrotizing enteritis.* **necrotizing e.** 1 A condition of the intestine characterized by widespread necrosis involving mucosa alone or extending through all layers. It is usually a consequence of infarction of intestinal tissue secondary to vascular occlusion. 2 ENTERITIS NECROTICANS. **phlegmonous e.** A severe inflammatory condition of the small intestine characterized pathologically by marked infiltration with acute inflammatory cells. It most commonly complicates other intestinal disorders such as strangulated hernia or intestinal obstruction. **e. polyposa** Enteritis characterized by polypoid growths. **pseudomembranous e.** PSEUDOMEMBRANOUS COLITIS. **regional e.** CROHN'S DISEASE.

**entero-** \en′tərō-\ [Gk *enteron* (from *entos* within, inside) gut, bowel] A combining form denoting the intestines. Also *enter-*.

**enteroanastomosis** \-ənas′təmō′sis\ The surgical creation of an anastomosis between two parts of the intestine. Also *enteroenterostomy.*

**enteroapocleisis** \-ap′ōklī′sis\ ENTEROAPOKLEISIS.

**enteroapokleisis** \-ap′ōklī′sis\ [ENTERO- + Gk *apokleisis* (from *apo-* away, off + *kleisis* shutting, closure) a shutting out] The surgical exclusion of a segment of intestine from the normal fecal flow. Also *enteroapocleisis.*

***Enterobacter*** \-bak′tər\ A genus of microorganisms that form a neutral fermentation product, butanediol, and hence can grow heavily and form large quantities of gas. It is found primarily on plants, but some *Enterobacter* species are common opportunistic pathogens. ***E. aerogenes*** A lactose-positive enterobacterium whose butanediol fermentation yields neutral products, thus permitting heavier growth and gas production than the mixed-acid fermentation of *Escherichia.* The IMViC set of tests is used to distinguish *E. aerogenes* from *Escherichia coli* as an index of fecal contamination of water supplies. Also *Aerobacter aerogenes* (outmoded). ***E. agglomerans*** An enterobacterium frequently encountered as an opportunistic pathogen. ***E. alvei*** *HAFNIA ALVEI.* ***E. cloacae*** The *Enterobacter* species most often encountered in man, *E. aerogenes* being more frequent in soil and in plants. ***E. hafniae*** *HAFNIA ALVEI.*

**Enterobacteriaceae** \-baktir′ē·ā′si·ē\ [ENTERO- + BACTERI- + -ACEAE] A large family of Gram-negative, facultative, oxidase-negative, peritrichously flagellated or nonmotile rods with simple growth requirements; the enterobacteria. It includes genera that are primarily normal inhabitants or pathogens of the vertebrate intestinal tract (*Escherichia, Edwardsiella, Citrobacter, Salmonella, Shigella,* and *Hafnia*), pathogens for other organs (*Klebsiella* and *Yersinia*), or primarily inhabitants of soil or plants (*Enterobacter, Proteus, Serratia,* and *Erwinia*). Organisms intermediate between the type strains, by biochemical and serologic criteria, are often encountered.

**enterobacterium** \-baktir′ē·əm\ [ENTERO- + BACTERIUM] (*pl.* enterobacteria) Any microorganism of the family Enterobacteriaceae.

**enterobactin** \-bak′tin\ ENTEROCHELIN.

**enterobiasis** \-bī′əsis\ [*Enterob(ius)* + -IASIS] Infection with worms of the genus *Enterobius,* especially *E. vermicularis,* the pinworm that infects humans. Although most patients are asymptomatic, pruritus ani may be a prominent and distressing result of infection.

***Enterobius*** \en′tirō′bē·əs\ A genus of oxyurid nematodes found in the large intestine and cecum of primates. ***E. vermicularis*** A species of pinworm, or seatworm, occurring in humans. It is parasitic in the large intestine. Infection is common in children, sometimes causing perianal itching or general restlessness, but serious illness is rare. Also *Oxyuris vermicularis, Ascaris vermicularis.*

**enterocele** \en′tirōsēl′\ [Gk *enterokēlē* (from *entero(n)* intestine + *kēlē* hernia) hernia or rupture of an intestine] 1 An intestinal hernia. 2 POSTERIOR VAGINAL HERNIA.

**enterocentesis** \-sentē′sis\ [ENTERO- + -CENTESIS] The puncturing of the intestine by surgical means.

**enteroceptor** \-sep′tər\ [ENTERO- + *(re)ceptor*] An internal sense organ generally associated with viscera or visceroceptors but denoting any sense organ responsive to changes in internal milieu.

**enterochelin** \-kē′lin\ A cyclic trimer of 2,3-dihydroxybenzoylserine, formed by enteric bacteria, that chelates $Fe^{3+}$ and promotes its uptake. Also *enterobactin.*

**enterochirurgia** \-kīrur′jē·ə\ [ENTERO- + L *chirurgia* surgery] Any surgical procedure performed on the intestine.

**enterocholecystostomy** \-kō′ləsistäs′təmē\ CHOLECYSTENTEROANASTOMOSIS.

**enterocholecystotomy** \-kō′ləsistät′əmē\ CHOLECYSTOENTEROTOMY.

**enterocleisis** \-klī′sis\ [ENTERO- + -CLEISIS] Surgical closure of a defect in the intestinal wall. **omental e.** The closure of a defect in the intestine with a sutured fold of omentum.

**enteroclysis** \en′tiräk′lisis\ [ENTERO- + CLYSIS] A high colonic enema. Also *enteroclysm.*

**enterococcemia** \-käksē′mē·ə\ [*enterococc(us)* + -EMIA] A condition in which enterococci are present in the blood.

**enterococcus** \-käk′əs\ [ENTERO- + COCCUS] (*pl.* enterococci) An organism of the species *Streptococcus faecalis.*

**enterocoelic** \-sē′lik\ [ENTERO- + COEL- + -IC ] Designating an embryo in which the primitive segments are formed from a series of evaginations of the primitive intestine. Compare SCHIZOCOELIC.

**enterocolectomy** \-kōlek′təmē\ [ENTERO- + COLECTOMY] A surgical resection of the intestine, including parts of the ileum, cecum, and colon.

**enterocolic** \-kō′lik\ Of or relating to the small intestine and the colon.

**enterocolitis** \-kōlī′tis\ [ENTERO- + COLITIS] Inflammation involving the mucosa of both large and small intestine. Also *coloenteritis.* **antibiotic e.** Inflammation of the colonic mucosal lining associated with antibiotic use. **pseudomembranous e.** PSEUDOMEMBRANOUS COLITIS. **regional e.** Crohn's disease involving parts of the small intestine and colon.

**enterocolostomy** \-kōläs′təmē\ [ENTERO- + COLO- + -STOMY] The surgical formation of a communication between a segment of small intestine and the colon. It is usually formed following intestinal resection or to bypass an obstruction.

**enterocyst** \en′tirōsist′\ A fluid-filled sac within the peritoneal lining of the intestine.

**enterocystocele** \-sist′əsēl\ [ENTERO- + CYSTO- + -CELE] A hernia involving the urinary bladder and the intestine.

**enterocystoma** \-sistō′mə\ VITELLOINTESTINAL CYST.

**enterocyte** \en′tirōsīt′\ [ENTERO- + -CYTE] One of the cells that forms the lining epithelium of the intestine.

**enteroenteric** \-enter′ik\ Involving or relating two or more segments of the intestine; intestinointestinal. Also *enterointestinal.*

**enteroenterostomy** \-en′tərās′təmē\ [ENTERO- + ENTEROSTOMY] ENTEROANASTOMOSIS.

**enterogastritis** \-gastrī′tis\ [ENTERO- + GASTRITIS] Inflammation of the intestinal and stomach mucosa; gastroenteritis.

**enterogastrone** \-gas′trōn\ An intestinal hormone which inhibits gastric secretion and emptying. It is not certain whether this material is separate from cholecystokinin.

**enterogram** \en′tirōgram′\ [ENTERO- + -GRAM] A visual record of the motor activity of the intestine.

**enterohepatocele** \-hep′ətōsēl′\ [ENTERO- + HEPATO- + -CELE] A developmental umbilical hernia containing some liver and intestine. The abdominal wall is developmentally deficient or atrophic or both at the base of the hernial sac.

**enterohepatopexy** \-hep′ətōpek′sē\ [ENTERO- + HEPATO- + -PEXY] A surgical procedure in which the small intestine or the large intestine is anchored to the liver.

**enterohydrocele** \-hī′drəsēl\ A hydrocele containing a loop of intestine as well as peritoneal secretions.

**enteroidea** \en′təroi′dē·ə\ [New L, from *enter(ic)* + *-oidea,* taxonomic suffix used for broader categories] A category of febrile diseases caused by intestinal bacteria. It includes enteric fevers, caused by *Salmonella* species, and parenteric fevers, caused by bacteria other than *Salmonella.*

**enterointestinal** \-intes′tənəl\ ENTEROENTERIC.

**enteroinvasive** \-invā′siv\ Causing intestinal disease by invading mucosal cells: used of bacteria, especially *Shigella* and certain strains of *Escherichia coli.*

**enterolith** \en′tirōlith′\ [ENTERO- + -LITH] An intestinal calculus, especially one consisting of ingested material.

**enterolithiasis** \-lithī′əsis\ [ENTEROLITH + -IASIS] A condition which there are calculi (enteroliths) in the intestine.

**enterology** \en′tiräl′əjē\ [ENTERO- + -LOGY] The study of the intestine, its physiology, pathophysiology, and diseases.

**enterolysis** \en′tiräl′isis\ [ENTERO- + LYSIS] The surgical division of adhesions involving the intestine.

**enteromegaly** \-meg′əlē\ [ENTERO- + -MEGALY] Abnormal largeness of the intestine; megaloenteron.

**enteromenia** \-mē′nē·ə\ [ENTERO- + *men(o)-* + -IA] Cyclic bleeding into the small intestine at the time of menstruation from an implantation of endometriosis at that site.

**enteromerocele** \-mer′ōsēl\ [ENTERO- + MERO-$^2$ + -CELE$^1$] FEMORAL HERNIA.

**enteromycosis** \-mīkō′sis\ An intestinal infection with pathogenic fungi, most commonly *Candida.*

**enteromyiasis** \-mīyī′əsis\ INTESTINAL MYIASIS.

**enteromyxorrhea** \-mik′sôrē′ə\ MUCOUS DIARRHEA.

**enteron** \en′tərän\ [Gk (from *entos* within, inside) gut, intestine] **1** CANALIS ALIMENTARIUS. **2** INTESTINUM TENUE.

**enteronitis** \-nī′tis\ [ENTERON + -ITIS] ENTERITIS. **polytropous e.** *Older term* ACUTE INFECTIOUS GASTROENTERITIS.

**enteroparalysis** \-pəral′isis\ ENTEROPLEGIA.

**enteroparesis** \-pərē′sis\ A relaxation and dilatation of the intestine.

**enteropathogenic** \-path′əjen′ik\ Pathogenic for the intestine.

**enteropathy** \en′tiräp′əthē\ [ENTERO- + -PATHY] Disease of the intestines. **gluten e.** CELIAC DISEASE.

**enteropeptidase** An enzyme secreted by the intestine that hydrolyzes the bond between the Lys-6 and Ile-7 residues of trypsinogen and thus produces trypsin.

**enteropexy** \en′tirōpek′sē\ [ENTERO- + -PEXY] The surgical fixation of the intestine to itself or to the abdominal wall in order to prevent the formation of intestinal obstruction caused by adhesions. Also *enteropexia.*

**enteroplasty** \en′tirōplas′tē\ [ENTERO- + -PLASTY] Any plastic operation on the intestine, such as closure of a perforation or enlargement of a constricted area.

**enteroplegia** \-plē′jə\ [ENTERO- + -PLEGIA] Lack of intestinal motility, as in adynamic ileus. Also *enteroparalysis.*

**enteroplex** \en′tirōpleks′\ [ENTERO- + L *plex(us),* past part. of *plectere* to braid, plait] A surgical instrument used to unite two cut ends of intestine.

**enteroplexy** \en′tirōplek′sē\ [ENTEROPLEX + -Y] The surgical union of two divided ends of intestine in order to reestablish luminal continuity.

**enteroptosis** \en′tiräptō′sis\ [ENTERO- + -PTOSIS] Descent of the viscera on upright posture due largely to a laxity of mesenteric attachments. This ptosis is now believed to have no pathologic significance. Also *enteroptosia.*

**enteroptotic** \en′tiräptät′ik\ Relating to or characterized by enteroptosis.

**enteroptychia** \en′tirōtik′ē·ə\ [ENTERO- + Gk *ptyx,* gen. *ptychos,* a fold + *-ia* -IA] The surgical plication of intestine to prevent the formation of adhesions. Also *enteroptychy.*

**enterorrhaphy** \en′tirôr′əfē\ [ENTERO- + -RRHAPHY] The repair of the intestine with sutures. **circular e.** An anastomosis of two ends of divided intestine created by invaginating one end in the other and securing it with sutures.

**enterorrhexis** \-rek′sis\ [ENTERO- + -RRHEXIS] A rupture or perforation of the intestine.

**enteroscope** \en′tirōskōp′\ [ENTERO- + -SCOPE] An endoscope for examining the intestinal interior.

**enterosepsis** \-sep′sis\ Sepsis from intestinal bacterial origin.

**enterostasis** \-stā′sis\ [ENTERO- + STASIS] INTESTINAL STASIS.

**enterostenosis** \-stenō′sis\ [ENTERO- + STENOSIS] A narrowing in the intestinal lumen.

**enterostomal** \-stō′məl\ Of or relating to an enterostomy.

**enterostomy** \en′tiräs′təmē\ [ENTERO- + -STOMY] The creation of a stoma in the intestine to permit the expulsion of the intestinal contents. **gun-barrel e.** The creation of intestinal stomata through the abdominal wall such that the segments of intestine exit in a parallel fashion, as a double-barrel gun.

**enterotomy** \en′tirät′əmē\ [ENTERO- + -TOMY] An incision into the intestine.

**enterotoxemia** \-täksē′mē·ə\ Systemic toxemia due to absorption of toxic products produced by pathogenic gut flora.

**enterotoxigenic** \-täk′səjen′ik\ Pertaining to or producing substances toxic to intestinal tissue.

**enterotoxin** \-täk′sin\ Any bacterial exoprotein that causes increased exudation of fluid in the gastrointestinal tract. Heat-labile toxins are released by *Vibrio cholerae* and by certain strains of *Escherichia coli, Pseudomonas aeruginosa, Clostridium perfringens,* and *Clostridium difficile.* Some organisms also release a smaller, heat-stable toxin. The genes for enterotoxins are often carried on plasmids. See also LABILE TOXIN, STABLE TOXIN. **perfringens e.** A substance produced during sporulation by certain strains of *Clostridium perfringens* and a cause of acute food poisoning.

**enterotropic** \-träp′ik\ [ENTERO- + -TROPIC[1]] Having an effect on the intestine.

**enterotyphus** \-tī′fəs\ TYPHOID FEVER.

**enterouria** \-yoo′rē·ə\ ENTERURIA.

**enterovaginal** \-vaj′ənəl\ Pertaining to or connecting the intestine and the vagina.

**enterovesical** \-ves′ikəl\ Relating or connecting the intestine and the urinary bladder, as a fistula.

**enterovirus** \-vī′rəs\ [ENTERO- + VIRUS] Any picornavirus of the genus *Enterovirus,* which includes human polioviruses, coxsackie viruses, echoviruses, and more recently identified viruses that are assigned type numbers because of problems with the previous classification scheme.

**enterozoic** \-zō′ik\ Pertaining to or caused by an enterozoon.

**enterozoon** \-zō′än\ [ENTERO- + Gk *zōon* living being, animal] (*pl.* enterozoa) An animal organism which lives in the intestine.

**enteruria** \en′taroo′rēə\ [ENTER- + -URIA] The presence of fecal material in the urine, denoting a fistulous communication between the intestines and the urinary tract. Also *enterouria.*

**enthalpy** \en′thalpē\ [Gk *enthalp(ein)* to warm in, glow + -Y] A measure of the heat content of a system usually expressed with respect to some suitable reference state. Enthalpy equals the sum of the internal energy and the product of pressure and volume. Symbol: H

**enthlasis** \en′thləsis\ A comminuted depressed skull fracture.

**en thyrse** \äN tērs′\ [French *en* in, on + *thyrse* (from Gk *thyrs(os)* the stalk of an umbelliferous plant) a cluster of flowers in pyramidal form] Describing spores arranged singly along both sides of a hypha, as fungal spores, especially the microconidia of certain dermatophytes. Compare EN GRAPPE.

**ento-** \en′tə-\ [Gk *entos* in, within, inside] A prefix meaning within, inside. Also *ent-.* • See note at ENDO-.

**entoblast** \en′təblast\ [ENTO- + -BLAST] ENDOBLAST.

**entocele** \en′təsēl\ [ENTO- + -CELE[1]] A hernia within the abdomen.

**entochondrostosis** \-kän′drästō′sis\ Osteogenesis within cartilage.

**entochoroidea** \-kôroi′dē·ə\ COMPLEXUS BASALIS CHOROIDEAE.

**entocondyle** \-kän′dīl\ The medial condyle of any long bone. Adj. entocondylar.

**entocuneiform** \-kyoo′nē·ifôrm′\ OS CUNEIFORME MEDIALE.

**entocyte** \en′təsīt\ [ENTO- + -CYTE] The material contained within a cell; the totality of the components inside the plasmalemma.

**entoderm** \en′tədurm\ [ENTO- + -DERM] ENDODERM. **primitive e.** The lining layer of the gastrula, which gives rise to the yolk sac and the gut epithelium.

**entomere** \en′təmir\ A blastomere that will give rise to an endodermal cell.

**entomo-** \en′təmō-\ [Gk *entomon* (from *entemnein* to cut up, in reference to the insect's segmented body) insect] A combining form meaning insects.

**entomogenous** \-mäj′ənəs\ [ENTOMO- + -GENOUS] **1** Caused by or derived from insects. **2** Growing or developing in or on insects.

**entomologist** \-mäl′əjist\ A student of, or specialist in, the science of entomology.

**entomology** \-mäl′əjē\ [ENTOMO- + -LOGY] The scientific study of insects. Also *insectology.* **medical e.** The study of insects or, more broadly, of arthropods, that inflict harm, cause disease, or transmit infection to humans.

**entomophagous** \-mäf′əgəs\ [ENTOMO- + -PHAGOUS] Insect-eating; insectivorous.

***Entomophthora*** \-mäf′thərə\ [ENTOMO- + Gk *phthora* destruction, ruin, corruption] A genus of fungi noted for their parasitic habit on and in insects, as well as for causing entomophthoromycotic granules and nasal polyps in man.

**Entomophthorales** An order of insect-parasitizing fungi, a few of which are human pathogens, causative agents of entomophthoromycosis.

**entomophthoromycosis** \-mäf′thərəmikō′sis\ [*Entomophthor(ales)* + MYCOSIS] Any of several phycomycoses brought about by fungi of the genera *Basidiobolus* and *Conidiobolus.*

**Entomospira** \-mōspī′rə\ *BORRELIA.*

**ento-occipital** \-äksip′ətəl\ Located between the median plane of the skull and the occipital gyrus of a cerebral hemisphere.

**entopic** \entäp′ik\ [Gk *entop(os)* (from *en-* in + *topos* a place) in or of a place + -IC] Occurring in the normal place. Also *eutopic.*

**entoplasm** \en′təplazm\ ENDOPLASM.

**entoptic** \entäp′tik\ [ENT- + OPT- + -IC] Denoting visual phenomena of intraocular origin, such as traction or impact phosphenes caused by vitreous movements.

**entoptoscopy** \en′täptäs′kəpē\ [ENT- + OPTO- + -SCOPY] Evaluation of the transparency of the ocular media. Adj. entoptoscopic.

**entoretina** \-ret′ənə\ The neural retina, extending from the nuclei of the rods and cones to the nerve fiber layer. Also *Henle's nervous layer.*

**entorhinal** \-rī′nəl\ Pertaining to the region of the temporal lobe medial to the rhinal fissure; specifically of the cortical area of the parahippocampal gyrus (entorhinal area).

**entosarc** \en′təsärk\ ENDOPLASM.

**entostosis** \en′tästō′sis\ ENOSTOSIS.

**entotympanic** \-timpan′ik\ Within the tympanic cavity.

**entozoal** \-zō′əl\ Pertaining to animal organisms that live within other animals.

**entozoon** \-zō′ən\ [ENTO- + Gk *zōon* living being, animal] (*pl.* entozoa) An animal organism that lives within another animal.

**entrance** / **superior e. to glottis** ADITUS GLOTTIDIS SUPERIOR.

**entrapment** \entrap′mənt\ The partial or complete extrinsic compression of a vessel by surrounding muscle, tendon, or bone, particularly in an anatomic hiatus such as the adductor canal.

**entropion** \entrō′pē·än\ [EN- + *-tropion* as in ECTROPION] An inward turning or inversion of a part or edge, especially of the margin of the eyelid, as may occur with orbicularis oculi contraction upon a flaccid eyelidor from internal cicatricial contraction. **cicatricial e.** Inward turning of the eyelid due to the shrinkage of scar tissue. Also *entropion cicatriceum, contraction entropion.* **spastic e.** Inward turning of the eyelid due to contraction of the orbicularis oculi muscle. Also *spasmodic entropion, entropion spasticum.* **e. uveae** Entropion of the pigment margin of the pupil, as may occur in severe iridocyclitis with posterior synechiae.

**entropy** \en′trəpē\ [German *Entropie* (coined from EN-, taken as meaning *Inhalt* contents, + Gk *tropē* a turn, change) lit., transformation-content] A measure of the disorder of the molecules of a system.

**entypy** \en′tīpē\ [EN- + Gk *typ(os)* mold, form + -Y] A type of gastrulation in which the endoderm eventually comes to lie outside the ectoderm.

**enucleate** \inoo′klē·āt\ [E- + *nucle(o)-* + -ATE] **1** To remove as a structurally integral unit, as the eyeball or a tumor from a capsule. **2** To remove the nucleus from (a cell).

**enuresis** \en′yoorē′sis\ [New L, from Gk *enour(ein)* to urinate in (e.g. bed) + -ESIS] Incontinence of urine, with full bladder emptying, after the age at which bladder control should have been attained. Also *uracrasia, uracratia*. Adj. enuretic. **epileptic e.** ENURETIC EPILEPSY. **nocturnal e.** Enuresis occurring while asleep at night. It is due to a delay in maturation of the mechanism, partly cerebral, of inhibition of the infantile response of the bladder in sleep, so that complete emptying takes place into the bed. One in seven children is said to suffer from nocturnal enuresis. After continence has been learned a recurrence may signify stress or unhappiness in the child's life. Also *bedwetting*.

**envelope** [French *envelopper* (origin unknown) to cover] **1** A membrane or other thin structure that encloses something. **2** A lipid-containing material that is external to the nucleocapsid in many kinds of virus. It is usually derived from the host cell membrane. Also *peplos*. **basilar membrane e.** LAMINA BASILARIS DUCTUS COCHLEARIS. **cell e.** The layers that surround the contents of a bacterial cell, including the cytoplasmic membrane and the peptidoglycan wall, and often a capsule. Gram-negative bacteria also have an outer membrane outside the peptidoglycan. **egg e.'s** EGG MEMBRANES. **nuclear e.** A boundary between the nucleus and the cytoplasm of a eukaryotic cell, composed of two unit membranes separated by the perinuclear space. The outer surface of the nuclear envelope faces the cytoplasm and is often studded with ribosomes. The inner and outer membranes of the envelope are fused at intervals to form nuclear pores.

**envenom** \enven′əm\ To introduce venom into; to poison by injection or contact with venom.

**envenomation** \enven′əmā′shən\ Poisoning by venom, as from the bite or sting of certain arthropods, reptiles, and other animals.

**environment** [French *environ* around, about + -MENT] All of the physical, chemical, and biologic features that act on an organism at any one time. **controlled e.** A space surrounding a patient where air temperature, humidity, and flow can be regulated. The patient's bed is usually surrounded by a specially designed plastic curtain with provision for a laminar flow of air. Such devices are used to provide strict isolation for patients with compromised immune defenses. **external e.** The environment within which an organism lives and breathes. Also *milieu extérieur*. Compare INTERNAL ENVIRONMENT. **internal e.** The fluid within the body that surrounds and bathes the cells. Also *milieu intérieur*. Compare EXTERNAL ENVIRONMENT.

**envy** Desire for something that belongs to another. **penis e.** In psychoanalytic psychology, the female's desire for a penis. It is part of the castration complex.

**enzygotic** \en′zīgät′ik\ MONOZYGOTIC.

**enzymatic** \en′zīmat′ik\ Pertaining to or catalyzed by an enzyme. Also *enzymic*.

**enzyme** \en′zīm\ [German *Enzym* (from Late Gk *enzym(os)* leavened, from Gk *en-* IN-[1] + *zymē* a leaven) enzyme] Any biologic catalyst. Enzymes are present in all living matter. All prove to be proteins. Also *ferment* (obs.). See also EC. **adaptive e.** INDUCIBLE ENZYME. **collagenolytic e.** An enzyme with collagenase activity that is obtained from *Clostridium histolyticum*. It is used to a limited extent in the débridement of skin ulcers and burns by assisting in the healing process. **condensing e.** *Outmoded* CITRATE SYNTHASE. **constitutive e.** An enzyme formed without requiring an inducer. Many constitutive enzymes are repressible by the end product. Compare INDUCIBLE ENZYME. See also CONSTITUTIVE MUTATION. **debranching e.** Any enzyme that removes branching points during the degradation of a branched macromolecule, usually a polysaccharide. **débridement e.'s** Enzymes, such as streptokinase and streptodornase, that have been used to digest clotted blood and fibrinous or purulent exudates and to supplement surgical drainage and cleaning of an affected area. The use of enzymes for these purposes is most successful when draining sinuses and infected wounds and ulcers. **digestant e.'s** A combination of several enzymes with amylolytic, proteolytic, and lipolytic activities that compensate for a reduced function of similar enzymes of pancreatic origin. They contribute to digestion in the small intestine. The medication is generally formulated in capsules for release in the duodenum. **early e.** An enzyme produced by a cell as a result of infection by a virus and produced early in the course of multiplication of the virus. Such enzymes are usually specified by the nucleic acid sequence first introduced into the cell on infection. **fibrinolytic e.'s** Enzymes that engage in hydrolytic activity with fibrin. Examples include fibrinolysin bovine plasma and a similar enzyme from *Aspergillus oryzae*. They have been used alone or in combination with other lytic enzymes and antibiotics to assist in the resolution of fibrinous exudates. These agents have been applied topically in ointments. Limited success has been achieved in the use of fibrinolytic enzymes to recanalize occluded arteries by direct application. **inducible e.** An enzyme that is formed only in the presence of a specific inducer, usually its substrate or a chemical analogue thereof. Enzyme induction is now recognized as a special example of gene regulation. Also *adaptive enzyme*. Compare CONSTITUTIVE ENZYME. **late e.** An enzyme produced by a cell as a result of infection by a virus, and produced late in the course of multiplication of the virus. Such enzymes are often specified by the nucleic acid sequences last introduced into the cell on infection. **Lohmann's e.** CREATINE KINASE. **malic e.** MALATE DEHYDROGENASE (OXALOACETATE DECARBOXYLATING). **old yellow e.** A flavoprotein capable of catalyzing NADPH oxidation. It was originally thought to be part of a respiratory chain. **proteolytic e.** PROTEINASE. **regulatory e.** An enzyme subject to natural controls whose rate of action controls the rate of the metabolic pathway in which it participates. **repair e.** An enzyme whose function is to repair damaged nucleic acid, such as that damaged by photochemical reaction. **restriction e.** RESTRICTION ENDONUCLEASE. **Schardinger e.** XANTHINE OXIDASE. **serum e.** Any protein that is capable of enzymatic activity and that is found routinely or in pathologic states in the blood plasma.

**Enzyme Commission** See under EC.

**enzymic** ENZYMATIC.

**enzymology** \en′zīmäl′əjē\ [*enzym(e)* + *o* + -LOGY] The study of enzymes.

**enzymopathy** \en′zīmäp′əthē\ **1** Any abnormality of normal enzyme function. It usually stems from a genetic defect of protein synthesis, modification, or transport that reduces or abolishes activity of a specific enzyme. **2** INBORN ERROR OF METABOLISM.

**eosin** \ē′ōsin\ [Gk *ēōs* the dawn + -IN] A red synthetic xanthene dye that is used as a cytoplasmic counterstain to hematoxylin. Also *yellowish eosin, water-soluble eosin, eosin Y*. **e. Y** EOSIN.

**eosinoblast** \ē′ōsin′əblast\ A myeloblast which will mature into an eosinophil.

**eosinocyte** \ē′ōsin′əsīt\ EOSINOPHIL.

**eosinopenia** \ē′ōsin′əpē′nē·ə \ An abnormal decrease in the number of circulating eosinophilic leukocytes. Also *hypo-eosinophilia.* **hormonal e.** Eosinopenia due to humoral factors, most often excess adrenal cortical substances.

**eosinophil** \ē′ōsin′əfil\ [EOSIN + *o* + -PHIL] A cell or histologic structure that stains intensely with the acid dye eosin. Eosinophils of the anterior lobe of the pituitary gland are the source of growth hormone and prolactin. Eosinophils of the blood (eosinophilic leukocytes) are granulocytes that typically have two nuclear lobes and numerous large cytoplasmic granules that stain red-orange with Romanowsky dyes. Eosinophils play a role in hypersensitivity reactions. Also *acidophil, acidophilic cell, acidocyte, eosinocyte.*

**eosinophilia** \ē′ōsin′ōfil′yə\ **1** An abnormal increase in the number of circulating eosinophilic leukocytes. **2** The presence of increased eosinophil precursors in the bone marrow. **3** The property of staining intensely with eosin. **hereditary e.** A rare, autosomal dominant disorder characterized by mild eosinophilia. Also *familial eosinophilia.* **Löffler's e.** LÖFFLER SYNDROME. **pulmonary infiltration e.** Infiltration of the lungs by eosinophils, characteristic of the Löffler syndrome. **tropical pulmonary e.** A syndrome of wasting, cough, bronchospasm, and eosinophilia occurring in many tropical countries and attributed to nematode infection. Also *tropical eosinophilia, eosinophilic lung, Weingarten syndrome.*

**eosinophilic** \ē′ōsin′əfil′ik\ Having the property of staining with eosin: said of cells or histologic structures. Also *eosinophilous, eosinophilocytic.*

**eosinophilous** \ē′ōsinäf′ələs\ EOSINOPHILIC.

**eosin Y** EOSIN.

**ep-** \ep-, əp-\ EPI-.

**epactal** \epak′təl\ [Gk *epakt(os)* (from *epagein* to bring in, introduce, from *epi-* upon, to + *agein* to lead, bring) acquired, adventitious, intercalated] **1** Supernumerary. **2** Of or relating to the small bones found along the cranial sutures.

**eparterial** \ep′ärtir′ē·əl\ Situated on or above an artery. Compare HYPARTERIAL. • The term was first suggested and used with reference to the branches of bronchi as related to the pulmonary artery.

**epaxial** \epak′sē·əl\ Situated above or behind an axis, usually applied to the axis of the vertebral column or of a limb.

**ependyma** \epen′dimə\ [Gk *ependyma* (from EPI- + Gk *endyma* a garment, from *endyein* to put on) an upper garment] **1** The inner cellular layer of the embryonic neural tube. **2** [NA] The ciliated cell lining of the adult cerebral ventricles and the central canal of the spinal cord. For defs. 1 and 2 also *endyma* (obs.). Adj. ependymal.

**ependymitis** \ep′endimī′tis\ [*ependym(a)* + -ITIS] Inflammation of the ependyma.

**ependymoblast** \epen′dimōblast′\ [*ependym(a)* + *o* + -BLAST] Embryonic ependymal spongioblast.

**ependymoblastoma** \epen′dimōblastō′mə\ [*ependym(a)* + *o* + BLASTOMA] A malignant form of ependymoma showing anaplasia, invasive properties, and necrosis. It may resemble glioblastoma. It is not clear whether ependymoblastoma is an entity distinct from anaplastic ependymoma.

**ependymocyte** \epen′dimōsīt′\ [*ependym(a)* + *o* + -CYTE] A cell derived from the embryonic ependymal layer lining the central canal and ventricles, possessing a ciliated ventricular surface and zonula occludens junctions with adjacent cells of the same type. Compare TANACYTE.

**ependymoma** \epen′dimō′mə\ [*ependym(a)* + -OMA] A tumor composed of ependymal cells forming rosettes, canals, and perivascular pseudorosettes. Blepharoplasts may be demonstrated in the cytoplasm along the luminal margins. The tumor typically projects from an ependymal surface. The floor of the fourth ventricle, the region of the central canal of the spinal cord, the lateral, and third ventricle are common sites. Growth is usually slow. Also *ependymocytoma, ependymal glioma.* **anaplastic e.** The malignant counterpart of an ependymoma. Also *malignant ependymoma.* **myxopapillary e.** A tumor of the cauda equina composed of ependymal cells arranged in a papillary manner over cores of hyaline connective tissue. Mucin is in the tumor cells. **papillary e.** A rare form of ependymoma similar to choroid plexus papilloma.

**eph-** \ef-, if-\ EPI-.

**ephapse** \ef′aps\ [Gk *ephapsis* (from *ephaptein* to touch, border on) a touching] A site of contact between neurites, principally axons, where electrical interactions may occur in the absence of synaptic specialization. Adj. ephaptic.

**ephebiatrics** [Gk *ephēb(os)* (from *ep-* upon + *hēb(ē)* manhood, youth) arrived at puberty + -IATRICS] ADOLESCENT MEDICINE.

**ephedrine** $C_{10}H_{15}NO$. An adrenergic compound that is synthesized or extracted from species of *Ephedra*. Ephedrine is a sympathomimetic that produces effects similar to epinephrine in stimulating the myocardium and being a vasoconstrictor. It is also used as a bronchodilator.

**ephedrine sulfate** The sulfate salt of ephedrine. It has the same properties and uses as the parent compound, and it is administered orally, parenterally, and as an inhalant.

**Ephemeridae** \ef′əmer′idē\ [Gk *ephēmer(os)* (from *ep-* on, upon + *hēmera* a day) lasting a day, short-lived + -IDAE] A family in the insect order Ephemeroptera, the mayflies. The type genus, *Ephemera*, and others are associated with asthma due to sensitization from inhalation of cast skins and bits of dried materials from the large swarms of these abundant insects.

**epi-** \ep′i-, ep′ē-\ [Gk *epi* on, upon] **1** A prefix meaning (1) upon, above, over, outside; (2) near, next to, beside. Also *ep-, eph-.* **2** A prefix denoting a chemical substance obtained by means of an epimerization.

**epiallopreganolone** \-al′ōpregnan′əlōn\ A $C_{21}$ corticosteroid found in pregnancy urine and probably of fetal adrenal cortical origin. It appears to serve as a precursor in the biosynthesis of $C_{19}$ androgenic hormones.

**epiandrosterone** \-andräs′tərōn\ $C_{19}H_{30}O_2$. 3$\beta$-Hydroxy-5$\alpha$-androstan-17-one. An androgen excreted in the urine of both male and female. It is a less abundant metabolite of testosterone and androstenedione and a less potent androgen than its 3$\alpha$ isomer, androsterone. It is included in the measurement of urinary 17-ketosteroids. Also *isoandrosterone.*

**epiblast** \ep′iblast\ [EPI- + -BLAST] That part of the outermost (ectoderm) germ layer which gives rise to the skin and its derivatives. It results from the ectoblast dividing into neuroblast and epiblast. Adj. epiblastic.

**epiblepharon** \-blef′ərän\ [EPI- + BLEPHARON] A developmental, abnormal fold of skin that parallels the margin of either the upper or lower eyelid.

**epibranchial** \-brang′kē·əl\ Placed above or dorsal to the branchial arches or branchial grooves.

**epicanthic** \-kan′thik\ Pertaining to the epicanthus or plica palpebronasalis. Also *epicanthal, epicanthine.*

**epicanthus** \-kan′thəs\ [EPI- + CANTHUS] PLICA PALPEBRONASALIS. **e. inversus** A developmental crescentic fold of skin extending from the lower eyelid to the inner canthus. It is often associated with congenital blepharoptosis.

**epicarcinogen** \-kär′sənəjən\ [EPI- + CARCINOGEN] A substance that augments the action of a carcinogen.

**epicardia** \-kär′dē·ə\ [EPI- + CARDIA] The lowest portion of the esophagus, connecting with the upper stomach.

**epicardial** \-kär′dē·əl\ **1** Pertaining to the epicardia. **2** Pertaining to the epicardium.

**epicardiectomy** \-kär′dē·ek′təmē\ [*epicardi(um)* + -ECTOMY] Excision of the epicardium, usually associated with removal of the pericardium in patients with constrictive pericarditis.

**epicardium** \-kär′dē·əm\ LAMINA VISCERALIS PERICARDII.

**epicentral** \-sen′trəl\ Attached to a vertebral body (centrum).

**epichordal** \-kôr′dəl\ Situated dorsal to the notochord of embryos.

**epicillin** $C_{16}H_{21}N_3O_4S$. 6-[D-α-Amino-2-(1,4-cyclohexadien-1-yl)acetamido]-penicillanic acid. A bactericidal agent with a spectrum of activity similar to that of ampicillin. It is inactivated by penicillinase and there is cross-resistance with ampicillin.

**epicomus** \epik′əməs\ [EPI- + Gk *kom(ē)* the hair of the head + *-us*, L noun suffix] CRANIOPAGUS PARASITICUS.

**epicondyle** \ep′ikän′dīl, -dəl\ EPICONDYLUS. **external e. of femur** EPICONDYLUS LATERALIS OSSIS FEMORIS. **external e. of humerus** EPICONDYLUS LATERALIS HUMERI. **internal e. of femur** EPICONDYLUS MEDIALIS OSSIS FEMORIS. **internal e. of humerus** EPICONDYLUS MEDIALIS HUMERI. **lateral e. of femur** EPICONDYLUS LATERALIS OSSIS FEMORIS. **lateral e. of humerus** EPICONDYLUS LATERALIS HUMERI. **medial e. of femur** EPICONDYLUS MEDIALIS OSSIS FEMORIS. **medial e. of humerus** EPICONDYLUS MEDIALIS HUMERI.

**epicondyli** \-kän′dəlī\ Plural of EPICONDYLUS.

**epicondylitis** \ep′ikän′dilī′tis\ [*epicondyl(e)* + -ITIS] Inflammation or pain arising from an epicondyle. **lateral e.** An inflammation at the common extensor origin of the wrist extensor muscles at the elbow. It is commonly produced by repetitive power movements of the wrist and forearm, as in playing tennis. **medial e.** An inflammation of the flexor muscles of the forearm where they take origin from the medial epicondyle of the humerus. It is often seen in golfers.

**epicondylus** \ep′ikän′diləs\ [EPI- + CONDYLUS] A protuberance on a bone adjacent to, above, or upon a condyle. It usually serves as an attachment for ligaments and tendons. Also *epicondyle, supracondylar eminence.* **e. lateralis humeri** [NA] The blunt, rounded nonarticular part of the condyle of the humerus at the lower end of the lateral margin of humerus. On its anterolateral aspect is a facet for the origin of the superficial group of extensor muscles of the forearm, while posteriorly the anconeus muscle is attached. To its lower edge the radial collateral ligament of elbow joint is attached. It is palpable posteriorly. Also *lateral epicondyle of humerus, external epicondyle of humerus, external condyle of humerus, lateral condyle of humerus, radial condyle of humerus, condylus lateralis humeri, extensor condyle of humerus.* **e. lateralis ossis femoris** [NA] The short, prominent projection on the lateral aspect of the lateral condyle of the femur, serving as the attachment of the fibular collateral ligament of knee joint. A groove for the popliteus muscle separates the epicondyle from the articular margin inferiorly. Also *lateral epicondyle of femur, external epicondyle of femur.* **e. medialis humeri** [NA] The prominent subcutaneous, rounded projection on the medial side of the condyle of the humerus, the anterior surface giving origin to the superficial group of flexors of the forearm. The ulnar nerve is directly posterior to it. To its lower part areattached the anterior and posterior bands of the ulnar collateral ligament of the elbow joint. Also *medial epicondyle of humerus, internal epicondyle of humerus, condylus medialis humeri, flexor condyle of humerus, internal condyle of humerus, medial condyle of humerus, ulnar condyle of humerus, epitrochlea, entepicondyle* (outmoded). **e. medialis ossis femoris** [NA] The most prominent point on the medial aspect of the medial condyle of the femur, inferior and anterior to the projecting adductor tubercle and serving as the attachment of the tibial collateral ligament of knee joint. Also *medial epicondyle of femur, internal epicondyle of femur.*

**epicostal** \-käs′təl\ Situated above or on a rib.

**epicotyl** \-kät′il\ [EPI- + Gk *kotyl(ēdōn)* a cuplike hollow] The upper part of an embryo or seedling above the cotyledon or seed leaf.

**epicranium** \-krā′nē·əm\ The whole extent of the scalp, comprising skin, connective tissue, musculus epicranius, loose areolar tissue, and pericranium.

**epicrisis[1]** \ep′ikrī′sis\ [EPI- + *crisis*] A second crisis in the course of a disease.

**epicrisis[2]** \epik′rəsis\ [Gk *epikrisis* (from *epikrinein* to decide, adjudge) a judgment upon] A summation or analysis of a case of disease after its termination.

**epicritic** \-krit′ik\ [Gk *epikritik(os)* judgmental, from *epikrit(os),* verbal of *epikrinein* to give judgment upon + *-ikos* -IC] Pertaining to fine discrimination: said of cutaneous nerves and pathways subserving the tactile perception of small stimulus variations. • The term was devised by Sir Henry Head to characterize lemniscal system sensory function. Its usefulness has been controversial.

**epicystotomy** \-sistät′əmē\ [EPI- + CYSTOTOMY] SUPRAPUBIC CYSTOTOMY.

**epicyte** \ep′isīt\ [EPI- + -CYTE] **1** A plasma membrane surrounding an animal cell, especially a protozoan. **2** An epithelial cell.

**epidemic** \-dem′ik\ [adj. from early modern English *epidemy* an epidemic, from French *épidémie,* from Gk *epidēmia* a visit among the people, an epidemic, from *epidēmos* (from *epi* upon, among + *dēmos* people, inhabitants) sojourning among the people, prevalent, epidemic] **1** Having unusually high or significantly increased incidence in a given population and period of time: said of diseases, as in *cholera was epidemic here in 1832.* Compare ENDEMIC. **2** An unusual increase, not necessarily within a short time, in the number of cases of a transmissible disease previously existing only at an endemic level in a region or population, or the appearance of an unusual number of cases of a disease which was not recognized as being endemic in a region or population. • In modern usage, this term has been extended to apply to any considerable increase in illness whether or not transmissible, or to an increase in other events such as accidents, suicides, etc. **3** Pertaining to or characterized by epidemics.

**epidemiologic** \-dē′mē·əläj′ik\ Pertaining to epidemiology.

**epidemiology** \-dē′mē·äl′əjē\ [Gk *epidēmio(s)* (from *epi-on* + *dēmos* the people) among the people + -LOGY] **1** The study of the frequency, distribution, and causation of disease, both infectious and noninfectious, in a population, based upon the investigation of factors in the physical and social environment. Other biologic and social phenomena, apart from disease, that are subject to similar influences, may also be studied from an epidemiologic point of view, as in the epidemiology of accidents. **2** The study of epidemic disease. **clinical e.** Epidemiology based on observations made in clinical practice as distinguished from those made on the scale of populations.

**epiderm-** EPIDERMO-.

**epidermal** \-dur′məl\ Pertaining to the epidermis.

**epidermat-** EPIDERMO-.

**epidermatitis** \-dur′mətī′tis\ [EPIDERMAT- + -ITIS] Inflammation of the epidermis. *Seldom used.* Also *epidermitis.*

**epidermato-** EPIDERMO-.

**epidermatozoonosis** \-dur′mətōzō′ənō′sis\ EPIZOONOSIS.

**epidermicula** \-dərmik′yələ\ CUTICULAR LAYER.

**epidermidalization** \-dur′mədəlizā′shən\ The conversion of mucous epithelium into stratified epidermis.

**epidermides** \-dur′midēz\ Plural of EPIDERMIS.

**epidermis** \-dur′mis\ [Gk (from *epi-* EPI- + *derma* skin) the outer skin, epidermis] [NA] The outermost layers of the skin, of ectodermal origin and consisting of a basal layer, a prickle cell layer, a granular layer, a clear layer, and an outer horny layer. Also *tegumentary epithelium.*

**epidermitis** \-dərmī′tis\ [EPIDERM- + -ITIS] EPIDERMATITIS.

**epidermo-** [Gk *epidermis* outer skin] A combining form denoting the epidermis. Also *epiderm-, epidermat-, epidermato-.*

**epidermodysplasia** \-dur′mədisplā′zhə\ [EPIDERMO- + DYSPLASIA] The abnormal development of the epidermis. **e. verruciformis** An abnormality characterized by the early development of extensive virus warts, some of which may eventually undergo malignant change. It results from an inherited defect in the body's response to a human papovavirus. Also *Lewandowsky-Lutz disease.*

**epidermoid** \-dur′moid\ [EPIDERM- + -OID] Like or composed of epidermis. **cerebrospinal e.** An epidermoid cyst arising within the cranial cavity or spinal canal.

**epidermolysis** \ep′idərmäl′isis\ [EPIDERMO- + Gk *lysis* dissolution, loosing] The separation of keratinocytes, usually leading to blister formation. **e. bullosa** A group of disorders characterized by blistering of the skin and often the mucosae at sites of minor trauma. **e. bullosa dystrophica** DYSTROPHIC EPIDERMOLYSIS BULLOSA. **e. bullosa dystrophica (dominant)** A variant of epidermolysis bullosa in which blistering occurs after birth. It is usually relatively mild and rarely affects the mucous membranes. It is transmitted by an autosomal dominant gene. Also *hyperplastic epidermolysis bullosa* (outmoded). **e. bullosa dystrophica (recessive)** A variant of epidermolysis bullosa in which blisters occur at birth. The mouth and esophagus are usually involved. It is often severe, deformities occur, and it may be fatal. It is of autosomal recessive origin. The bullae occur under the basement membrane and electron microscopy shows diminished numbers of anchoring fibrils. Also *polydysplastic epidermolysis bullosa* (outmoded), *Hallopeau-Siemens syndrome.* **e. bullosa letalis** Epidermolysis bullosa marked by extensive blistering, with the cleft forming between the plasma membrane and basal lamina. Inherited through an autosomal recessive gene, it is often progressive and lethal, although mild forms exist among long-term survivors. Also *epidermolysis bullosa lethalis* (rare), *epidermolysis bullosa hereditaria letalis* (outmoded), *Herlitz syndrome.* **e. bullosa simplex** Epidermolysis bullosa in which blisters are formed within the basal cell layer of the epidermis on the hands, feet, trunk, and perioral area. It is of autosomal dominant inheritance. Also *simple epidermolysis bullosa.* **e. bullosa simplex of hands and feet** A variant of epidermolysis bullosa in which blisters occur on the hands and feet following minor trauma and heal without scarring. Clearage occurs between the suprabasal and granular layers of the epidermis. It is of autosomal dominant inheritance. Also *Weber-Cockayne epidermolysis bullosa* (rare). **dystrophic e. bullosa** A rare, severely disabling bullous disease, the inheritance of which is determined by an autosomal recessive gene. The bullae form in the upper dermis. Also *epidermolysis bullosa dystrophica, dysplastic epidermolysis bullosa.* **hyperplastic e. bullosa** *Outmoded* EPIDERMOLYSIS BULLOSA DYSTROPHICA (DOMINANT). **polydysplastic e. bullosa** *Outmoded* EPIDERMOLYSIS BULLOSA DYSTROPHICA (RECESSIVE). **simple e. bullosa** EPIDERMOLYSIS BULLOSA SIMPLEX. **Weber-Cockayne e. bullosa** *Rare* EPIDERMOLYSIS BULLOSA SYMPLEX OF HANDS AND FEET.

***Epidermophyton*** \ep′idərmäf′itän\ [EPIDERMO- + Gk *phyton* a tree, plant] A genus of fungi many of which have been implicated as causative agents of dermatophytosis. ***E. purpureum*** *TRICHOPHYTON RUBRUM.* ***E. rubrum*** *TRICHOPHYTON RUBRUM.*

**epidermophytosis** \-dur′məfītō′sis\ A dermatomycosis brought about by any of several dermatophytes, including species of *Epidermophyton.* **e. axillaris** TRICHOMYCOSIS AXILLARIS.

**epidermopoiesis** \-dur′məpoi·ē′sis\ [EPIDERMO- + -POIESIS] The formation of epidermis, whether in an embryo or in any organism at any stage in its existence.

**epidermosis** \-dərmō′sis\ Any disease of the epidermis. *Obs.* **aural e.** CHOLESTEATOMA.

**epididymectomy** \-did′əmek′təmē\ [*epididym(o)-* + -ECTOMY] Surgical excision of the epididymis, an operation usually performed for treatment of chronic epididymitis. Partial epididymectomy may be required in conjunction with excision of a spermatocele.

**epididymis** \-did′imis\ [Gk *epididymos* (from *epi-* upon + *didymos* testicle) outer membrane of the testicle] [NA] A crescentic cordlike structure applied to the posterior margin and overlapping the upper pole and lateral surface of the testis. The upper expanded part, or head, consists of 15–20 coiled tubules, or lobuli epididymidis. They join into a single convoluted duct, the ductus epididymidis, that passes through the body and tail where, at the lower pole of the testis, it turns upwards as the ductus deferens. It is connected to the testis by the efferent ductules at its head and by loose areolar tissue and the reflection of the two layers of the tunica vaginalis elsewhere. Also *parorchis* (outmoded).

**epididymitis** \-did′əmī′tis\ [*epididym(is)* + -ITIS] Inflammation of the epididymis. Acute epididymitis is characterized by an enlarged, indurated, exquisitely tender epididymis, with thickening and erythema of the overlying scrotal skin. All or part of the epididymis may be involved. Chronic epididymitis may be mildly symptomatic, manifested only by some induration and nodularity of the epididymis. The etiology is unclear, but may include bacterial infection, chemical irritation, or tuberculosis. **spermatogenic e.** Inflammation due to the presence of spermatozoa in the tissues of the epididymis.

**epididymo-** \ep′idid′əmō-\ [Gk *epi* on, upon + *didymo(s)* (from *dis* twice, double) a twin, testicle] A combining form denoting the epididymis.

**epididymodeferentectomy** \-did′əmōdef′ərentek′təmē\ [EPIDIDYMO- + *(ductus) deferens,* gen. *deferent(is)* + -ECTOMY] Surgical removal of the epididymis and the ductus deferens.

**epididymo-orchitis** \-did′əmō-ôrkī′tis\ [EPIDIDYMO- +

ORCHITIS] Inflammation of both the epididymis and testis. The condition, manifested by induration, swelling, and tenderness of both the epididymis and testis (the two organs often becoming confluent with one another) may mask an underlying testicular neoplasm.

**epididymotomy** \-did′əmät′əmē\ [EPIDIDYMO- + -TOMY] Incision into the epididymis.

**epididymovasectomy** \-did′əmōvazek′təmē\ [EPIDIDYMO- + VAS- + -ECTOMY] Surgical removal of the epididymis and part of the ductus deferens.

**epididymovasostomy** \-did′əmōvasäs′təmē\ [EPIDIDYMO- + VASOSTOMY] Surgical creation of an anastomosis of the epididymis with the ductus deferens. Also *vasoepididymostomy.*

**epidural** \-d$^y$oo′rəl\ [EPI- + DURAL] **1** Overlying the dura mater. **2** Filling the potential space between the dura and cranium, as in epidural hemorrhage. Also *extrameningeal.*

**epiduritis** \-d$^y$oorī′tis\ [EPI- + *dur(a mater)* + -ITIS] Inflammation of the surface of the spinal or cranial dura mater or in the space immediately outside it. *Seldom used.* **acute e.** ACUTE SPINAL PACHYMENINGITIS.

**epidurography** \-d$^y$ooräg′rəfē\ [EPI- + *dur(a mater)* + *o* + -GRAPHY] Radiographic visualization of the vertebral epidural space after injection of air or contrast material into the epidural space.

**epiestriol** \-es′tri·ôl\ Any of the epimers of estriol. Several are found in pregnancy urine and originating in the fetoplacental unit. They include 16-epiestriol ($16\beta,17\beta$); 16,17-epiestriol ($16\beta,17\alpha$); and 17-epiestriol ($16\alpha,17\alpha$).

**epigamous** \epig′əməs\ [EPI- + GAM- + -OUS] Taking place after fertilization of the ovum.

**epigastralgia** \-gastral′jə\ [*epigastr(ium)* + -ALGIA] Pain in the epigastric region of the abdomen.

**epigastric** \-gas′trik\ Of or pertaining to the epigastrium.

**epigastrium** \-gas′trē·əm\ [New L, from Gk *epigastrion* (from *epigastrios* over the belly, from *epi-* over + *gastēr* belly) the wall of the abdomen above the navel] REGIO EPIGASTRICA.

**epigastrius** \-gas′trē·əs\ Unequal conjoined twins in which the parasitic member is united with the host in the epigastric region. Also *epigastrius parasiticus.*

**epigastrocele** \-gas′trəsēl\ [*epigastr(ium)* + *o* + -CELE[1]] A hernia in the epigastrium.

**epigenesis** \-jen′əsis\ [EPI- + GENESIS] A theory which holds that all the first blastomeres produced by a fertilized egg have similar potentialities of development and consequently that the embryo is not preformed in the ovum but develops gradually by the successive formation of new parts. In fact each of first blastomeres of the sea urchin and of urodeles can, after isolation, form an entire larva. Modern embryology explains such occurrences in terms of activation of the genome. Adj. epigenetic.

**epiglottectomy** \-glätek′təmē\ [*epiglott(is)* + -ECTOMY] Excision of the suprahyoid portion of the epiglottis. It is usually performed for treatment of malignant disease and normally carried out by the anterior pharyngotomy route.

**epiglottis** \-glät′is\ [Gk *epiglōttis* (from *epi-* on + *glōtta* the tongue) the epiglottis] [NA] An unpaired, leaflike plate of elastic fibrocartilage situated behind the root of the tongue and the hyoid bone and in front of and overhanging the inlet of the larynx. Its tapered inferior part, or stalk, is attached by the thyroepiglottic ligament to the thyroid cartilage, while its rounded free end points upwards. The mucous membrane covering its anterior surface is reflected onto the pharyngeal part of the tongue, and that covering the posterior surface overlies the tuberculum epiglotticum and some pits containing mucous glands, while the mucous membrane attached to thc margins is reflected posteriorly as the aryepiglottic folds.

**epiglottitis** \-glätī′tis\ [*epiglott(is)* + -ITIS] **1** Inflammation of the epiglottis. **2** SUPRAGLOTTIC LARYNGITIS.

**epignathus** \-nā′thəs\ [EPI- + Gk *gnathos* the jaw, esp. the lower jaw] Unequal conjoined twins in which the parasitic member is attached to the host in the region of the lower jaw. Also *epignathus parasiticus.*

**epihyal** \-hī′əl\ **1** Pertaining to the upper portion of the ventral part of the hyoid arch. **2** Denoting a cartilage or bone occurring in the center of the stylohyoid ligament.

**epikeratomileusis** \-ker′ətōmiloo′sis\ [EPI- + KERATOMILEUSIS] A surgical technique of refractive keratoplasty in which a lathe-cut lens of donor cornea is sutured to the Bowman's membrane surface of the recipient cornea. The purpose of this procedure is the correction of refractive error.

**epilamellar** \-ləmel′ər\ Lying on and attached to the basement membrane.

**epilate** \ep′ilāt\ [E- + *pil(o)* + -ATE] To remove hair. Also *depilate.*

**epilation** \-lā′shən\ [French *épilation* (from *é-* E- + L *pil(us)* a hair + *-ation* -ATION) the act of removing hair] **1** The permanent removal of a hair, such as a misdirected cilium, including destruction of its bulb. **2** The destruction of hairs, often including their roots, by radiation or other diffuse injury. For defs. 1 and 2 also *depilation.*

**epilatory** \epil′ətôr′ē\ DEPILATORY.

**epilemma** \-lem′ə\ [EPI- + Gk *lemma* peel, husk, skin] *Outmoded* ENDONEURIUM.

**epilepsia** \ep′ilep′sē·ə\ [Late L, from Gk *epilēpsia* (from *epilambanein* to attack, seize, from *epi-*, intensifying prefix, + *lambanein* to grasp) a seizure, epileptic seizure] EPILEPSY. **e. arithmetica** A form of reflex epilepsy in which attacks are precipitated by attempting to carry out arithmetical calculations or to solve any mathematical problem. **e. gravior** MAJOR EPILEPSY. **e. major** MAJOR EPILEPSY. **e. minor** MINOR EPILEPSY. **e. mitis** PETIT MAL. **e. procursiva** PROCURSIVE EPILEPSY. **e. rotatoria** PROCURSIVE EPILEPSY. **e. tarda** SENILE EPILEPSY.

# epilepsy

**epilepsy** \ep′ilep′sē\ [Late L *epilepsia.* See EPILEPSIA.] A neurologic disorder characterized by the tendency to suffer recurrent seizures or fits, whether minor or major. The condition may be idiopathic due to no obvious cause or symptomatic, resulting from a focal cerebral lesion, from diffuse brain disease, or from some metabolic disturbance affecting cerebral function. Also *epilepsia.* • Some authorities reserved the term *epilepsy* in the past for the idiopathic disorder and classified seizures resulting from known organic disease as epileptiform, but this distinction is no longer tenable, especially since modern techniques of investigation, particularly the electroencephalogram and CAT scan, have shown that many attacks which would once have been classified as idiopathic are in fact symptomatic of unsuspected cerebral lesions. See also note at FIT. Adj. epileptic. **abdominal e.** Any attack of epilepsy in which abdominal symptoms constitute the aura or warning or a part of the attack. Also

*Moore syndrome.* **abortive e.** **1** SUBCLINICAL EPILEPSY. **2** EPILEPTIC AURA. **accelerative e.** PROCURSIVE EPILEPSY. **acousticogenic e.** REFLEX AUDITORY EPILEPSY. **acousticomotor e.** REFLEX AUDITORY EPILEPSY. **acquired e.** *Outmoded* SYMPTOMATIC EPILEPSY. **activated e.** Attacks of epilepsy induced by photic or pharmacological techniques of cerebral activation in order to study epileptic discharges recorded in the electroencephalogram. **adult e.** Epilepsy beginning in adult life. In fact, with the exception of idiopathic petit mal, any form of epilepsy may begin in this age group, although a significantly greater proportion of adults than children who develop epilepsy prove to be suffering from the symptomatic as distinct from the idiopathic variety. **adversive e.** Focal epilepsy in which there is turning of the head and eyes, and less often of the trunk, towards one side. This form of epilepsy is usually due to a contralateral frontal lobe lesion involving the frontal eye field (Brodmann's area 8). **affective e.** An attack of epilepsy in which affective symptoms, such as fear, anxiety, or depression, are common, and which usually results from focal epileptic discharge arising in one or other temporal lobe (temporal lobe or complex partial epilepsy). **akinetic e.** ATONIC EPILEPSY. **alcoholic e.** Epilepsy associated with the ingestion of alcohol, which in a patient suffering from idiopathic or symptomatic epilepsy may precipitate an attack. Sudden withdrawal of alcohol from a chronic alcoholic may also precipitate an attack. **alternating e.** Epilepsy in which the attacks are characterized by unilateral convulsive movements occurring successively on opposite sides of the body, either in successive attacks or less often in a single attack. Such phenomena may in rare cases result from a unilateral prerolandic epileptogenic focus, but more often their pathogenesis is obscure. **ambulatory e.** Epilepsy, usually of temporal lobe origin, in which the attacks give rise to automatism in the form of walking of which the patient is subsequently unaware when the attack is over. • When such attacks are prolonged so that the patient continues to walk in a dreamlike or trancelike state, the term *epileptic fugue* is sometimes used. **amygdaloid e.** An attack of epilepsy arising as a consequence of focal discharge originating in the amygdaloid nucleus. Rhythmic chewing and lip-smacking movements often occur in such an attack along with other variable manifestations dependent upon the extent to which the discharge spread throughout the temporal lobe. **aphasic e.** Focal epilepsy marked by attacks in which the patient, though conscious, is transiently aphasic. Such attacks result from focal epileptic discharge arising in either Broca's or Wernicke's area. **atonic e.** A form of epilepsy accompanied by loss of postural tone leading to collapse. In some episodes, which may be associated with a spike-wave rhythm of 3 Hz, the loss of tone is also rhythmical and, occurring simultaneously with the slow wave of each spike-wave complex, may induce collapse of the body in a series of jerks. In episodes which are electroencephalographically atypical, on the other hand, the loss of tone may be sudden and violent so that the patient falls heavily to the ground and may injure himself but does not convulse. Also *akinetic epilepsy, atonic "drop" epilepsy.* **audiogenic e.** REFLEX AUDITORY EPILEPSY. **audiosensory e.** REFLEX AUDITORY EPILEPSY. **auditory e.** A type of focal or partial epilepsy in which the attack is characterized usually by unformed, less often formed, auditory hallucinations or in which such phenomena constitute the aura of the attack. **auditory hallucinatory e.** A type of partial or temporal lobe epilepsy in which auditory hallucinations are prominent. These are either crude and unformed, arising as a consequence of abnormal discharge originating in the primary auditory cortex, or complex and formed (a recollection of remembered sounds such as speech, music, etc.) and are due to involvement of the auditory association areas. Sometimes the hallucination constitutes the first symptom, or aura, of the attack, sometimes it occurs during a more complex attack with other manifestations. **auditory illusional e.** A type of focal epilepsy in which attacks result from a neuronal discharge arising in the temporal cortex, and in which sounds in the patient's environment which he is capable of hearing become distorted, or louder or softer than in fact they are, or else their nature, meaning, and significance is misinterpreted. These attacks are to be distinguished from those of auditory hallucinatory epilepsy in which true auditory hallucinations occur without external auditory stimulation. **autonomic e.** Attacks of parietal, less often generalized, epilepsy, in which the manifestations are predominantly autonomic. So-called diencephalic epileptic attacks are thought to give rise to tachycardia, hypertension, pupillary dilatation, piloerection, profuse sweating, and disturbances of respiratory rhythm, but there is still some dispute as to whether diencephalic epilepsy can be separately identified. However it is clear that many forms of partial epilepsy due to discharge arising in the temporal lobe, cingulate gyrus, insular and peri-insular region consistently give autonomic manifestations including many of the above symptoms as well as salivation and epigastric and other abdominal sensations. These manifestations may be succeeded or accompanied by disordered consciousness and other manifestations of temporal lobe (partial complex) epilepsy and even by generalized convulsions, depending upon the extent and rapidity of spread of the epileptic discharge. An imprecise term. Also *visceral epilepsy, visceral aura, autonomic aura.* **Bravais-jacksonian e.** JACKSONIAN EPILEPSY. **catamenial e.** Epilepsy in which attacks arise in relation to the menstrual periods. Also *menstrual epilepsy, ovarioepilepsy.* **centrencephalic e.** Epilepsy consequent upon abnormal discharges presumed to arise in the reticular substance of the midbrain and thalamus, giving rise to bilaterally synchronous and symmetrical epileptic activity spreading to the cerebral cortex. This is the archetype of so-called idiopathic epilepsy. Petit mal accompanied by generalized 3 Hz spike-wave discharge is the most typical example, but some cases of idiopathic grand mal are still believed to be due to a similar mechanism. Also *central epilepsy, diencephalic epilepsy, mesodiencephalic epilepsy, midbrain epilepsy.* **chronic focal e.** CONTINUOUS PARTIAL EPILEPSY. **cingulate e.** A type of focal epilepsy in which the neuronal discharge or the lesion which causes the attack involves the cingulate gyrus of the cerebral cortex. The attacks are characterized by autonomic symptoms, such as sweating, palpitations, or tachycardia, and emotional symptoms, such as anxiety, and may be difficult to distinguish from panic attacks of psychogenic origin. **conditioned e.** Epilepsy in which attacks are precipitated by a conditioned reflex. There is little if any evidence to suggest that this form of epilepsy can be distinguished from the many specific varieties of reflex epilepsy. **contact e.** A rare form of reflex epilepsy in which attacks are precipitated by sudden, unexpected physical contact with a part of the patient's body or by other appropriate somatic sensory stimuli. Such attacks are rarely of the major or grand mal type. More common is myoclonus precipitated by a tap ("startle" epilepsy). In many such cases an auditory stimulus, such as a sudden noise, may have a similar effect. **continuous e.** STATUS EPILEPTICUS. **continuous partial e.** An attack of somatomotor epilepsy with persistent and continuous jerking movements involving that part of the body in which the jacksonian convulsions began. Also *Kozhevnikov syndrome, Kozhevnikov's disease, Kozhevnikov's epilepsy, chronic focal epilepsy, continuous epilepsy, focal status.* **contraversive e.** Adversive epilepsy in which the head, eyes, and sometimes the trunk turn to the side opposite to the causal frontal lobe lesion. **cortical e.** Focal epilepsy in which the attacks result, initially at least, from a neuronal discharge restricted to one part of the cerebral cortex. According to the area of the cortex involved, it is possible to differentiate adversive frontal epilepsy, supplementary motor area epilepsy, secondary sensory motor area epilepsy, and cingulate, frontal, insular, occipital, opercular, pararhinal, parietal, postrolandic, prerolandic, temporal, uncinate epilepsy, and other types. **cryptogenic e.** IDIOPATHIC EPILEPSY. **cyclical e.** Epilepsy in which attacks occur spontaneously, but not randomly, being separated by more or less regular and predictable intervals. In most cases they do not seem to be related to any apparent predisposing factor, and their periodicity, which is governed by some unknown biologic mechanism, is significant only when analyzed statistically. Less frequently, there is some obvious factor which may determine the periodicity, such as diurnal rhythms (sleep epilepsy or waking epilepsy) or the menstrual cycle (catamenial epilepsy). **diencephalic e.** CENTRENCEPHALIC EPILEPSY. **diencephalic autonomic e.** A syndrome marked by epileptic attacks caused by thalamic compression or invasion by a tumor. The attacks may be accompanied by peripheral vasodilatation, sweating, sialorrhea, tears, nystagmus, hypothermia, hypertension, and bradypnea, and are classified in the group of autonomic epilepsies. Also *Penfield syndrome.* **diurnal e.** Epilepsy in which the attacks occur during the day, when the patient is awake. Compare NOCTURNAL EPILEPSY. **dysmnesic e.** A type of focal epilepsy in which the attacks arise from a hypersynchronous neuronal discharge in the temporal lobe, and in which the fundamental and sometimes only feature is a greater or lesser degree of disturbance of memory. Usually classified as manifestations of dysmnesic epilepsy are ecmnesic hallucinations, epileptic panoramic vision (the "private cinema phenomenon"), and feelings of déjà-vu or, conversely, of detachment or depersonalization (jamais-vu). Also *paramnesic epilepsy, dysmnesic aura, paramnesic aura.* **enuretic e.** Incontinence of urine occurring as a consistent manifestation in minor attacks of epilepsy with brief impairment of consciousness. This is distinguished by some authorities from the incontinence which commonly occurs during an attack of major epilepsy, but it is doubtful whether this distinction is of any diagnostic value or validity. Also *epileptic enuresis.* **essential e.** IDIOPATHIC EPILEPSY. **familial e.** Epilepsy occurring in several members of the same family, usually because of a marked genetic predisposition. • When the predisposition is so powerful that it is the major if not the sole factor which causes epilepsy in different members of the family, this may be considered true hereditary epilepsy, which is always characterized by generalized epileptic attacks from the outset, often of the petit mal variety. When predisposition is less important and merely renders different members of the same family likely to suffer attacks due to various precipitating factors, the term *hereditary epilepsy* is no longer justified and the term *familial epilepsy* is more appropriate. **febrile e.** Childhood epilepsy in which the attacks are regularly precipitated by bouts of fever. **focal e.** Epilepsy in which the attacks are caused by a neuronal discharge arising in a localized area of one hemisphere, and usually characterized electroencephalographically by a localized discharge which can be recorded from that part of the scalp overlying the discharging cortical area. Clinically, these attacks have very variable manifestations, depending upon the function of the neurons involved in the discharge. They can be classified either by the presence of primary symptoms, including motor symptoms (somatomotor or jacksonian attacks, versive attacks, etc.), sensory symptoms (somatosensory, visual, or other attacks), and autonomic symptoms, such as epigastric attacks, or by the presence of complex symptomatology, including purely mental or emotional attacks (dysmnesic or ideatory attacks, etc.), attacks with psychosensory symptoms (illusional or hallucinatory), and attacks with psychomotor symptoms, such as automatism. Attacks of focal epilepsy can also be classified according to the region of origin. Also *local epilepsy, partial epilepsy, cerebral seizure.* **fortuitous e.** SPONTANEOUS EPILEPSY. **gaze e.** 1 An attack of epilepsy reflexly provoked by gazing at an object. 2 Any form of epilepsy in which conjugate ocular deviation occurs. Thus in petit mal the eyes may deviate upwards, while in versive or adversive epilepsy the eyes may deviate to the side opposite to the causal frontal lesion either in a tonic manner or in saccadic movements (oculoclonic epilepsy). An obsolete usage. **gelastic e.** Attacks of epilepsy in which uncontrollable laughter occurs before or during the attacks. **generalized e.** Epilepsy characterized by attacks which result from bilateral synchronous discharges arising centrally and spreading to involve both cerebral hemispheres, and which are usually accompanied by generalized and synchronous spike, sharp wave, slow wave, or spike-wave discharges in the EEG. The attacks may be minor as petit mal, or major (grand mal), atonic or akinetic, or less often myoclonic. The attacks may result from a disorder of function of unknown cause which begins in the upper midbrain and/or thalamus (primary generalized, or idiopathic epilepsy) or may be due to a focal discharge beginning in the cortex but spreading rapidly to the diencephalon and there evoking similar generalized discharges (secondary generalized epilepsy). **generalized flexion e.** INFANTILE MASSIVE SPASM. **grand mal e.** MAJOR EPILEPSY. **e. gravidarum** Epilepsy in which the attacks occur mainly or entirely when the patient is pregnant. This type of epilepsy is uncommon in that pregnancy more often reduces and may even suppress the attacks in many epileptic women. A somewhat different circumstance is the case of epilepsy resulting from severe toxemia of pregnancy (puerperal eclampsia). Also *pregnancy epilepsy.* **gustatory e.** 1 A type of focal or temporal lobe epilepsy in which one symptom is an abnormal, usually unpleasant taste in the mouth either constituting the aura of the attack or occurring during it. These attacks are the result of neuronal discharge arising in the specific cortical area of the temporal lobe which controls the sense of taste, or in the surrounding area of the brain. 2 A reflex epileptic attack thought to be precipitated by a powerful taste. The concept of reflex gustatory epileptic attacks has been questioned. **haut mal e.** MAJOR EPILEPSY. **hereditary e.** See under FAMILIAL EPILEPSY. **hysteriform e.** Temporal lobe or focal epilepsy with manifestations in the attacks which are sometimes reminiscent of hysteria. **ideational e.** A rare form of focal or partial epilepsy, resulting from discharge arising in the frontotemporal region, in which the patient experiences a compulsive recurring thought or idea which may have no substance in fact and is therefore delusional, or else it is an idea present in the patient's mind before the attack during which it becomes insistently persistent or recurrent. True delusions are very rarely epileptic. Often after the attack the patient remembers that he experienced an obsessive or compulsive thought during the episode but is unable to recall its content. **idiopathic e.** Epilepsy due to constitutional factors or of undetermined cause. Also *essential epilepsy, cryptogenic epilepsy, psychoepilepsy* (obs.). **illusional e.** A form of focal epilepsy usually resulting from discharge arising in the temporal region which causes attacks in which the patient experiences sensory illusions. Thus the patient, whose consciousness is usually retained, may see visual images which are distorted, being, for example, larger (macropsia) or smaller (micropsia) than normal. Alternatively the patient may experience an illusory interpretation of the meaning or significance of other sensory experiences. **induced e.** REFLEX EPILEPSY. **insular e.** Epilepsy in which the causative neuronal discharge arises in the insuloperi-insular region. The attacks often have complex manifestations, but principally affect the sense of taste (primary or complex, illusional or hallucinatory attacks) with accompanying autonomic symptoms, chiefly epigastric or abdominal. **jacksonian e.** Focal epilepsy resulting from localized cortical neuronal discharge arising usually in the motor cortex and demonstrating a march of manifestations as the discharge spreads to contiguous cortical areas. Also *Bravais-jacksonian epilepsy, localized epilepsy.* **kinesogenic e.** MOVEMENT-INDUCED EPILEPSY. **Kozhevnikov's e.** CONTINUOUS PARTIAL EPILEPSY. **larval e.** Epileptic discharges in the electroencephalogram which are not accompanied by any recognizable clinical manifestations. Also *latent epilepsy.* **latent e.** LARVAL EPILEPSY. **local e.** FOCAL EPILEPSY. **localized e.** JACKSONIAN EPILEPSY. **luminosensible e.** PHOTIC EPILEPSY. **major e.** Generalized epilepsy in which the attacks, usually lasting for about one minute, are characterized clinically by loss of consciousness and by convulsions which are first tonic, then clonic, and electroencephalographically by a rapid rhythm which becomes progressively slower and of greater amplitude during the tonic contraction, and which is rhythmically interrupted by slow waves during the clonic contraction. The attack always ends in stertorous coma lasting about five to ten minutes. Also *grand mal, mal comitial, falling sickness, epilepsia major, epilepsia gravior, haut mal epilepsy, grand mal epilepsy, haut mal.* **masked e.** Any of various symptoms, such as cyclical vomiting, occurring in patients not known to suffer overt attacks of epilepsy but once attributed incorrectly to subclinical epileptic activity, often on the basis of nonspecific EEG abnormalities. *Obs.* **masticatory e.** A type of oropharyngeal epilepsy in which the attacks are marked by rhythmic chewing movements and often by profuse salivation during the period of unconsciousness. **matutinal e.** MORNING EPILEPSY. **menstrual e.** CATAMENIAL EPILEPSY. **mental e.** PSYCHIC EPILEPSY. **mesodiencephalic e.** CENTRENCEPHALIC EPILEPSY. **metabolic e.** Epilepsy resulting from disturbances of cerebral metabolism. In adults major convulsions may occur as a consequence of many metabolic disturbances, including hypoxia, uremia, and drug withdrawals, and may depend at least in part upon a constitutional predisposition (low convulsive threshold). In neonates and young infants attacks resulting from metabolic disturbances are more common, and the causes include hypoglycemia, hypocalcemia, pyridoxine deficiency, and phenylketonuria. **midbrain e.** CENTRENCEPHALIC EPILEPSY. **minor e.** Any attack of epilepsy which does not give rise to major convulsions. Also *epilepsia minor.* • This is a somewhat imprecise term used by some to identify typical petit mal. Such attacks are a form of minor epilepsy, but not all minor epilepsy is petit mal. **minor focal e.** Jacksonian epilepsy in which the attacks are mild and of brief duration. Also *paraepilepsy.* **morning e.** Epilepsy in which the attacks occur usually or always in the morning, shortly after awakening. The attacks are usually major in type, and may be preceded or accompanied by myoclonus. Also *waking epilepsy, matutinal epilepsy.* **morpheic e.** NOCTURNAL EPILEPSY. **movement-induced e.** A rare type of reflex epilepsy, showing some affinities with "startle" epilepsy, in which attacks are precipitated by an abrupt movement, as when the patient rises suddenly from a chair. Some such attacks are of tonic epilepsy, very brief, and frequently unilateral in distribution. Their sudden onset causes change in posture, which has led to some confusion with brief episodes of paroxysmal kinesogenic choreoathetosis which is probably not an epileptic phenomenon. Also *kinesogenic epilepsy.* **musicogenic e.** Epilepsy in which the attacks, usually of the focal type and arising in the temporal lobe, are regularly induced by the sound of music. The precise mechanism by which these attacks of reflex epilepsy are precipitated is still unknown. It seems that in most cases it is the emotional overtones of the music rather than the actual sound which triggers the attack. Also *musicolepsy.* **myoclonic e.** Any form of epilepsy of which myoclonus is one manifestation. Brief myoclonic jerks occur occasionally in association with attacks of petit mal and may also occur particularly in the mornings in patients suffering from idiopathic major epilepsy but do not then accompany the major convulsions. The movements of prolonged jacksonian epilepsy (continuous partial epilepsy) may resemble myoclonus. The latter phenomenon is, however, a striking manifestation, along with major attacks, in progressive myoclonic epilepsy (Unverricht's disease) and can also be a manifestation of many diffuse degenerative brain diseases, such as cerebral lipidosis, subacute sclerosing panencephalitis, and Creutzfeldt-Jakob disease. . *Imprecise.* **myoclonic e. with Lafora bodies** PROGRESSIVE MYOCLONIC EPILEPSY. **nocturnal e.** Epilepsy in which the attacks occur chiefly or invariably at night while the patient is asleep. Also *sleep epilepsy, morpheic epilepsy.* Compare DIURNAL EPILEPSY. **occipital e.** Any form of epilepsy in which the neuronal discharge which causes the attacks arises in the occipital cortex. The attacks generally, but not invariably, give rise to crude or complex visual symptoms (illusions or hallucinations). **olfactory e.** 1 A type of focal epilepsy producing olfactory illusions or hallucinations, the smells evoked being usually unpleasant. The attacks result from a neuronal discharge arising in the specific olfactory cortex. 2 A form of reflex epilepsy which some authorities believe can be evoked by powerful odors, but the existence of which is denied by others. **opercular e.** A type of epilepsy in which the neuronal discharge which induces the attacks involves the walls of the sylvian fissure and the peri-insular region. These attacks often have a complex symptomatology, comprising hypersalivation with involuntary mastication and clouding of consciousness. **opisthotonic e.** Attacks of epilepsy or tonic fits in which opisthotonus occurs, usually implying brainstem dysfunction. **oral e.** OROPHARYNGEAL EPILEPSY. **oropharyngeal e.** A type of focal epilepsy in which the attacks result from a neuronal discharge arising in the insuloperi-insular or opercular region. Hypersalivation is a common manifestation, and is in rare cases the only symptom (salivatory epilepsy). In other cases, this is combined with rhythmic movements of the lips and tongue, with involuntary swallowing movements, or with masticatory movements (masticatory epilepsy). There may also be associated emotional, psychosensory, or psychomotor manifestations. Also *oral epilepsy, pharyngeal epilepsy.* **paramnesic e.** DYSMNESIC EPILEPSY. **partial e.** FOCAL EPILEPSY. **petit mal e.** PETIT MAL. **pharyngeal e.** OROPHARYNGEAL EPILEPSY. **photic e.** Attacks of epilepsy induced by any visual stimulus such as flashing light. Also *photogenic epilepsy, photosensory epilepsy, luminosensible epilepsy, visuosensory epilepsy.* See also REFLEX VISUAL EPILEPSY. **postcentral e.** PRIMARY SOMATOSENSORY EPILEPSY. **posthemiplegic e.** Epileptic attacks developing in a patient with hemiplegia, usually beginning focally in the paralyzed limbs. **postrolandic e.** PRIMARY SOMATOSENSORY EPILEPSY. **post-traumatic e.** Epilepsy following brain damage caused by a head injury. Post-traumatic epileptic attacks are often of the focal type but sometimes become generalized, and the manifestations are governed by the location of the cerebral lesion. Penetrating brain injuries or depressed skull fractures with injury to the underlying brain most often give rise to epilepsy, but most patients with post-traumatic epilepsy have suffered closed head injuries, which are much more frequent. In such cases the risk of post-traumatic epilepsy is roughly proportional to the severity of the injury, as assessed by the duration of post-traumatic amnesia. The fact that cerebral contusions following closed head injury often involve the temporal lobe explains why post-traumatic epilepsy is often of the temporal lobe type. Epilepsy more often follows relatively minor closed head injury in children than in adults. Those patients suffering epileptic attacks within one week of the head injury are more likely to develop late post-traumatic epilepsy in the subsequent weeks, months, and years. Also *traumatic epilepsy.* **pregnancy e.** EPILEPSY GRAVIDARUM. **primary auditory e.** Focal or partial epilepsy resulting from an epileptic discharge arising in the primary auditory area of the temporal cortex and giving rise to unformed auditory hallucinations (unidentifiable sounds). Also *primary auditory aura.* **primary gustatory e.** A type of focal epilepsy in which the attacks are the result of a hypersynchronous neuronal discharge arising in the insular, peri-insular or opercular cortex, the main or only symptoms of which are unpleasant taste sensations (parageusia) relating to three of the four primary taste modalities, particularly bitterness, and less frequently to sweetness and salinity. Also *gustatory aura.* **primary olfactory e.** A type of focal epilepsy in which attacks result from hypersynchronous neuronal discharge arising in the uncinate cortex, and which give rise, entirely or mainly, to spontaneous smell sensations (parosmia) which the patient is usually unable to identify, although they are usually classed as unpleasant. • When the olfactory sensation is succeeded by other epileptic manifestations, it is called an *olfactory aura.* **primary sensory e.** A type of focal epilepsy in which the basic feature, which is often the first and sometimes the only symptom, comprises spontaneous sensations involving somatosensory, visual, auditory, gustatory, olfactory, or vestibular mechanisms, and which is caused by a neuronal discharge arising in a specific sensory area of the brain. Primary sensory attacks should be differentiated from illusional and hallucinatory attacks which also involve the different senses but which are more complex. • When they are followed by other manifestations, particularly convulsions, these sensory symptoms are sometimes termed an "aura." **primary somatosensory e.** A type of focal epilepsy in which attacks are caused by a hypersynchronous neuronal discharge arising in the postrolandic area, and which give rise, wholly or partly, to spontaneous sensations (paresthesiae) which may be negative in nature, such as numbness, but are more often positive, such as prickling, tingling, or "pins and needles." Such paresthesiae affect the part of the body opposite to the cortical discharge and may spread by jacksonian march. The patient often remains conscious during these attacks, which may develop into somatomotor attacks as the motor cortex becomes involved. Also *sensory aura, somatosensory aura, postrolandic epilepsy, somesthetic epilepsy, postcentral epilepsy.* **primary visual e.** A type of focal epilepsy in which the attacks result from neuronal discharge arising in the occipital cortex, and which take the form, in whole or in part, of spontaneous visual sensations (paropsia) which may be negative in type (scotoma) or, more usually, positive (phosphenes or crude flashes of light), and which usually occupy the visual hemifield opposite to the hemisphere involved. Attacks of primary visual epilepsy can be distinguished from attacks of visual hallucinatory epilepsy. • When other epileptic manifestations follow, these sensations are called a *visual aura.* **procursive e.** Focal epilepsy, usually of the temporal lobe type, in which the attacks are characterized by brief confusional ambulatory automatism. The patient walks a short distance, usually forwards, colliding with obstacles in his way. Attacks of procursive epilepsy must be differentiated from confusional automatism occurring after epileptic attacks. These are more frequent and often longer-lasting, and the patient may walk aimlessly, even into dangerous situations and for comparatively long distances. Also *accelerative epilepsy, epilepsia rotatoria, epilepsia procursiva.* **progressive myoclonic e.** A progressive degenerative brain disorder of autosomal dominant inheritance characterized by severe myoclonus, major convulsions and progressive dementia and accompanied by the presence of Lafora bodies, due to the storage of abnormal mucopolysaccharide, in neurons of the cerebral cortex and especially of the dentate nuclei of the cerebellum. Also *Unverricht's disease, Lafora body disease, Lafora's disease, myoclonic epilepsy with Lafora bodies, Unverricht syndrome, Unverricht's myoclonia.* **psychic e.** A type of focal epilepsy in which the attacks result from a neuronal discharge arising in the temporal cortex, or, much more rarely, in the frontal lobe. These attacks produce complex mental and emotional symptoms and include ideational epilepsy, dysmnesic epilepsy and affective epilepsy. Also *psychic aura* (incorrect), *mental epilepsy.* **psychomotor e.** *Obs.* TEMPORAL LOBE EPILEPSY. **pubertal e.** Epilepsy beginning at or about puberty. Generalized (idiopathic) epilepsy, or partial attacks associated with temporal lobe damage resulting from birth trauma often begin at this age. Typical petit mal often disappears at puberty, but may be superseded by major (grand mal) attacks. **reflex e.** A type of epilepsy in which attacks are regularly induced by a single precipitating factor. Reflex epilepsies include self-induced epilepsy, as in the case of some children with petit mal who induce attacks by passing their fingers regularly in front of their eyes to produce flickering light, and attacks induced by many other sensory stimuli, such as in photic epilepsy, television epilepsy, reading epilepsy, musicogenic epilepsy, or movement-induced epilepsy. Also *induced epilepsy.* **reflex auditory e.** An unusual type of reflex epilepsy induced by a noise, which is usually short, loud, and unexpected. The attack may be short and resemble myoclonus, being accompanied by a burst of spikes and waves or of generalized multispike-waves in the EEG, but more often it is prolonged and then resembles an attack of tonic epilepsy with generalized desynchronization of the EEG. The fact that the noise which triggers off the attack is more effective when it is unexpected explains why such attacks are often classified as "startle" epilepsy. Also *acousticogenic epilepsy, acousticomotor epilepsy, audiogenic epilepsy, audiosensory epilepsy, sonosensory epilepsy, auditory epilepsy* (seldom used). **reflex autonomic e.** A type of reflex epilepsy once thought to be induced by visceral afferent impulses. Most such attacks including the so-called cardiac, laryngeal, ophthalmic, ovarian, and pleural varieties are, in fact, episodes of reflex syncope and not epilepsy, and the existence of this form of epilepsy, for instance after eating a heavy meal, is in considerable doubt. **reflex visual e.** A type of epilepsy in which most, or all, of the attacks are induced by visual sensory stimuli. This is by far the most common variety of reflex epilepsy. It can be subdivided according to the type of visual stimulus which precipitates the attack, as television epilepsy, photic epilepsy, visual exploration epilepsy, or self-induced epilepsy. In rare cases attacks may be precipitated by saccadic ocular movements or by gazing at an object which is bright or which demonstrates strong visual contrasts (gaze epilepsy or pattern-induced epilepsy) and even by reading. Not all individuals who show paroxysmal discharges in the EEG induced by photic stimulation (flickering light), nor even those in whom an occasional attack of epilepsy can be induced by such stimuli, are suffering from true reflex visual epilepsy, in the usual clinical meaning of the term. Also *visual epilepsy*. **secondary e.** SYMPTOMATIC EPILEPSY. **secondary generalized e.** A phenomenon in which a jacksonian epileptic discharge, arising from a cortical lesion, radiates to midline reticular substance and precipitates a generalized epileptic discharge which in turn causes a major convulsion. **seesaw e.** Alternating epilepsy in which unilateral convulsive movements occur now on one side of the body, now on the other. **self-induced e.** An unusual form of epilepsy induced by the patient at will. Usually this occurs in children with petit mal who have discovered an effective way of precipitating their attacks. These generally take the form of reflex visual epilepsy which is induced by the subject staring at the sun and passing his open fingers rapidly back and forward in front of his eyes. More rarely, the subject can induce attacks simply by closing his eyes, by staring fixedly at a bright object or by overbreathing. **senile e.** Epilepsy which occurs in the elderly. There is no etiological or other reason why this type of epilepsy should be separately identified. Although many cases result from cerebral infarction due to atherosclerosis, the causes are multiple. Also *epilepsia tarda, tardy epilepsy*. **sensory e.** **1** Any form of focal epilepsy in which the basic clinical feature consists of simple or complex sensory manifestations. These are often the first and sometimes the only symptom. They include attacks of primary sensory epilepsy, illusional and hallucinatory epilepsy, and other varieties. The attacks can be classified according to the sense involved in the neuronal discharge, which may be auditory, gustatory, olfactory, somatosensory, visual, or vestibular. **2** Any epileptic attack precipitated by a specific sensory stimulus. **serial e.** Frequent epileptic attacks with recovery of consciousness between the attacks. **somatomotor e.** A type of focal epilepsy in which the attacks are caused by a neuronal discharge arising in the prerolandic area of the cortex and which result in tonic or clonic convulsions of any part of the opposite side of the body, to which they may be restricted, or from whence they may be propagated to adjoining areas by jacksonian march. The patient is conscious during these attacks, which may, however, culminate in secondary generalized convulsions with loss of consciousness. **somatosensory reflex e.** A type of reflex epilepsy induced by exteroceptive somatic sensory afferent stimuli. This includes contact epilepsy (attacks induced by physical contact) and movement-induced epilepsy. There is some dispute as to whether it is the sensory stimulus or the associated startle or emotional shock which is the precipitant. **somesthetic e.** PRIMARY SOMATOSENSORY EPILEPSY. **somnambulistic e.** Attacks of epilepsy in which automatism, resembling the automatic behavior of sleepwalking, occurs. Also *somnambulic epilepsy*. **sonosensory e.** REFLEX AUDITORY EPILEPSY. **spontaneous e.** An isolated epileptic attack which occurs without any evident causal or precipitating factor. Also *fortuitous epilepsy*. **startle e.** A type of reflex epilepsy in which attacks are brought on by a short, sharp and unexpected stimulus, giving rise to a start of surprise. Such a stimulus is usually auditory, such as a slamming door, car horn, telephone, or bell; exteroceptive, such as an unexpected tap on a part of the body, but particularly on the head or shoulders; or proprioceptive, such as being jolted in a crowd, stumbling, or any sudden violent movement. The attacks usually take the form of tonic attacks with desynchronization of the EEG and, occasionally, massive myoclonus with spike-wave or multispike-wave discharges. In hemiplegic or hemiparetic subjects the tonic attacks induced by noise or movement are often unilateral, predominantly involving the paralyzed side. **subclinical e.** An epileptic attack accompanied by characteristic discharges in the EEG but with such slight clinical manifestations that it may go unnoticed. The confusion of so-called petit mal status is often so identified and may be recognized only through EEG recording. It is also believed that postepileptic (Todd's) paralysis may be due to continuing subclinical epileptic discharge following a clinically overt focal attack. Also *abortive epilepsy, subclinical absence, subclinical epileptic attack*. **symptomatic e.** Any form of epilepsy in which the attacks are symptomatic of an underlying brain disease, metabolic disturbance, or focal lesion. Also *acquired epilepsy* (outmoded), *secondary epilepsy*. **tardy e.** SENILE EPILEPSY. **television e.** A type of reflex visual epilepsy in which attacks regularly occur in light-sensitive subjects, when they are watching television. These attacks must be distinguished from syncope of emotional origin precipitated by the emotional content of the program. Diagnosis may be facilitated by the demonstration of light-sensitivity while an EEG is being recorded during intermittent photic stimulation. **temporal e.** TEMPORAL LOBE EPILEPSY. **temporal lobe e.** Any type of partial epilepsy in which the causative neuronal discharge involves all or part of the temporal lobe. The attacks include epilepsy with primary symptoms of the illusional, hallucinatory, auditory, olfactory, or gustatory type, as well as those with psychic, psychosensory, or psychomotor symptoms. Also *temporal epilepsy, psychomotor epilepsy, psychic equivalent*. **tonic e.** A type of generalized epilepsy in which the attacks, which are of brief duration (about 10 seconds), are characterized clinically by impaired consciousness and tonic spasm chiefly of the postural muscles, usually resulting in an opisthotonic position. Electroencephalographically, they show a rapid rhythm which progressively slows and becomes of greater amplitude. Tonic attacks are usually considered, both clinically and electroencephalographically, to be tonicoclonic attacks restricted to the initial tonic phase. They usually occur in children, particularly in the presence of diffuse brain damage. However, focal tonic attacks giving a transient fixed alteration in posture of a single limb without convulsive jerking also occur, sometimes in patients with multiple sclerosis. Tonic attacks must be distinguished from the similar transient opisthotonus which may be seen in patients with posterior fossa tumors. **tornado e.** Epilepsy with an aura of intense rotational vertigo. **traumatic e.** POST-TRAUMATIC EPILEPSY. **uncinate e.** A type of temporal lobe epilepsy in which the causative neuronal discharge arises in the anteromedial aspect of the temporal lobe, and in particular in the uncinate area of the hippocampal gyrus. These attacks usually cause simple or complex olfactory illusions or hallucinations, in isolation or combined with other symptoms, particularly impairment of consciousness and a dreamlike state. **unilateral e.** Epilepsy in which the convulsive movements are limited to or originate in the face, limbs, and/or trunk on one side of the body. The attacks may be tonic or tonicoclonic, and may sometimes spread to become generalized with loss of consciousness. The corresponding EEG discharge is usually limited, at least initially, to the opposite cerebral hemisphere. **versive e.** A type of focal epilepsy in which the attacks give rise to conjugate deviation of the eyes, head, and/or trunk either towards the side opposite to that in which the epileptic discharge arises (adversive or contraversive epilepsy), or, very rarely, towards the same side (ipsiversive epilepsy). These attacks can be classified as clonic conjugate deviation of the eyes (oculoclonic epilepsy), which often culminates in tonic deviation of the eyes, as a result of discharge of occipital neurons; tonic conjugate deviation of the eyes, arising from discharge of neurons in the frontal eye field; and tonic conjugate deviation of the head, eyes, and trunk as a result of neuronal discharge from the frontal, temporal, and/or supplementary motor areas. When twisting of the body makes the patient turn around once or twice, this is referred to as a gyratory or rotatory attack. **vertiginous e.** A rare type of focal epilepsy in which the attacks result from neuronal discharge arising from an as yet undetermined part of the temporal cortex, and which produces sensations of true rotatory vertigo. Attacks of vertiginous epilepsy must be differentiated from simple transitory impairment of consciousness which some patients refer to as "giddiness." Also *vertiginous aura, aura vertiginosa.* **visceral e.** AUTONOMIC EPILEPSY. **visual e.** **1** Any type of focal epilepsy in which spontaneous visual sensations occur as a consequence of neuronal discharge arising in the specific visual cortex or its surrounding areas. **2** REFLEX VISUAL EPILEPSY. **visual hallucinatory e.** A type of focal epilepsy resulting from neuronal discharge arising in the temporo-occipital cortex, during which the patient experiences visual hallucinations. If the attacks arise in the primary visual cortex (primary visual epilepsy) these hallucinations are crude and unformed, as flashes of light, but if they arise in the visual association areas, formed hallucinations may be experienced, including the vivid evocation of well-remembered scenes. Alternatively there may be distortion of visual images which look larger or smaller than normal. In rare cases the patient may see an image of himself outside his own body (autoscopy). Also *visual illusional epilepsy.* See also PRIMARY VISUAL EPILEPSY. **visuosensory e.** PHOTIC EPILEPSY. **vocal e.** A type of focal epilepsy in which the attacks, which usually result from a discharge arising in the inferior rolandic or supplementary motor area, take the form of continuous or rhythmically modulated repetition of a vowel. Also *epileptic vocalization, iterative vocalization.* **waking e.** MORNING EPILEPSY.

**epileptic** \-lep′tik\ [French *épileptique* (from Gk *epilēptikos* pertaining to a seizure) epileptic] **1** Of or relating to epilepsy. Also *comitial.* **2** A person who has epilepsy.

**epileptiform** \-lep′tifôrm\ Resembling epilepsy; having characteristics resembling those of epilepsy.

**epileptogenic** \-lep′təjen′ik\ Likely to cause or precipitate an epileptic attack. For example, cerebral tumor or atrophic scar may be epileptogenic, as may various drugs such as leptazol (pentylenetetrazol), if administered in large enough doses.

**epileptogenous** \-leptäj′ənəs\ Pertaining to a part of the brain in which an epileptic discharge originates.

**epileptoid** \-lep′toid\ Suggesting or resembling epilepsy.

**epileptologist** \-leptäl′əjist\ A doctor who specializes in the study and treatment of epilepsy.

**epileptology** \-leptäl′əjē\ That branch of medicine dealing with the study of epilepsy.

**epiloia** \-loi′ə\ TUBEROUS SCLEROSIS.

**epimastigote** \-mas′tigōt\ [EPI- + MASTIGOTE] A stage in the development of certain flagellate protozoa in which the flagellum arises from the kinetoplast just in front of the nucleus and emerges from the anterior of the organism, forming an undulating membrane. Also *crithidia* (outmoded), *crithidial stage* (outmoded).

**epimenorrhagia** \-men′ôrā′jə\ [EPI- + MENO- + -RRHAGIA] HYPERMENORRHEA.

**epimenorrhea** \-men′ôrē′ə\ [EPI- + MENORRHEA] HYPERMENORRHEA.

**epimer** \ep′imər\ One of two isomers that differ by inversion of configuration at one chiral center when this is not the only chiral center in the molecule. Thus inversion of the hydroxyl group on carbon 3 of a sterol leads to an episterol, the epimer of the first. A more restrictive definition in sugar chemistry limits the term *epimers* to sugars that differ only in the stereochemistry of the carbon atom next to the reducing carbon. Thus the epimer of glucose is mannose, and the epimer of ribulose is xylulose. If one adopts the wider definition one speaks of epimers for the glucose-galactose pair (which differ only on carbon 4) and of D-glucose as the 5-epimer of L-idose.

**epimerase** Any enzyme that catalyzes the interchange of two of the four different substituents at a chiral carbon atom in a compound that contains at least one other chiral center. Hence it catalyzes the conversion of a substrate into its epimer. If on the other hand the center at which the conversion occurs were the only chiral center in the molecule, the product would be the enantiomer of the substrate, and the enzyme would consequently be a racemase.

**epimerization** \ep′imər′īzā′shən\ A chemical reaction leading to the transformation of a chiral compound into its epimer.

**epimorphosis** \-môrfō′sis\ Regeneration of organized tissues or of a part of an organism at the site where the original was cut off or became separated. Adj. epimorphic.

**epimyocardium** \-mī′əkär′dē·əm\ [EPI- + MYOCARDIUM] MYOEPICARDIAL MANTLE.

**epimysium** \-mis′ē·əm\ [New L, from EPI- + Gk *mys* muscle] The connective tissue that surrounds a muscle belly. Also *perimysium externum, external perimysium.*

**epinephrectomy** \-nəfrek′təmē\ [*epinephr(os)* + -ECTOMY] *Outmoded* ADRENALECTOMY.

**epinephrine** \-nef′rin\ [*epinephr(os)* + -INE] 3,4-dihydroxy-$\alpha$-[(methylamino)methyl] benzyl alcohol, a sympathomimetic hormone synthesized by the adrenal medulla. It is released into the circulation in response to stress, splanchnic nerve stimulation, and hypoglycemia. The hormone acts upon both $\alpha$- and $\beta$-adrenergic receptors to raise peripheral vascular resistance, decrease peripheral blood flow, and induce tachycardia and glycogenolysis. The pharmaceutical preparation (levorotatory or *R*-isomer) is widely used in several compounds as a heart and blood pressure stimulant and as a bronchodilator in acute asthma. Also *adrenaline* (British usage), *chromaffin hormone* (older term), *sphygmogenin* (older term). **racemic e.** A mixture of the *d* and *l* forms of epinephrine. Ninety percent of the adrenergic activity is due to the *l*-isomer component. The racemic mixture arises by synthetic preparation of the compound.

**epinephrine bitartrate** $C_{13}H_{19}NO_9$. The bitartrate salt of epinephrine. It is used as a convenient form of L-epinephrine in ophthalmic solutions and in other preparations of sympathomimetic and vasoconstrictor medications, for its adrenergic properties.

**epinephroma** \-nəfrō′mə\ [EPI- + NEPHR- + -OMA] *Obs.* RENAL CELL CARCINOMA.

**epinephros** \-nef′räs\ [Gk *epi-* at, upon + *nephros* kidney] GLANDULA SUPRARENALIS.

**epineural** \-nʸŏŏr′əl\ [EPI- + NEURAL] Overlying the neural arch of a vertebra.

**epineurial** \-nʸŏŏr′ē·əl\ Denoting the epineurium of an entire peripheral nerve bundle.

**epineurium** \-nʸŏŏr′ē·əm\ [New L, from EPI- + Gk *neuron* sinew, nerve] [NA] The outer sheath of cellular and collagenous connective tissue covering a peripheral nerve. Adj. epineurial.

**epinosic** \-nō′sik\ [EPI- + Gk *nos(os)* illness, disease + -IC] Secondary to an illness, as in *epinosic gain.*

**epiorchium** \-ôr′kē·əm\ *Outmoded* LAMINA VISCERALIS TUNICAE VAGINALIS TESTIS.

**epipericardial** \-per′ikär′dē·əl\ Situated on or around the pericardium.

**epipharyngeal** \-fərin′jē·əl\ NASOPHARYNGEAL.

**epipharyngitis** \-far′ənjī′tis\ NASOPHARYNGITIS.

**epiphenomenon** \-fənäm′ənän\ An incidental event or symptom occurring as an accompaniment of a disease but not essentially or typically with it.

**epiphora** \epif′ərə\ [Gk (from *epipher(esthai)* to rush upon, impend, accumulate, from *epi-* upon + *pherein* to bear, carry) impact, eruption, flood of tears] An overflow of tears escaping from the conjunctival sac, as may occur with faulty function of the lacrimal drainage system or from excessive lacrimation. Also *stillicidium lacrimarum* (outmoded).

**epiphyseal** \-fiz′ē·əl\ Pertaining to or resembling an epiphysis. Also *epiphysial.*

**epiphysectomy** \-fizek′təmē\ [*epiphys(is)* + -ECTOMY] The surgical excision of a bony epiphysis.

**epiphyses** \epif′isēz\ Plural of EPIPHYSIS.

**epiphysial** \-fiz′ē·əl\ EPIPHYSEAL.

**epiphysiodesis** \-fiz′ē·ōdē′sis\ [*epiphysi(s)* + *o* + -DESIS] The premature bony fusion of a growth plate either caused by a pathologic disorder or following surgery to arrest longitudinal bone growth.

**epiphysioid** \-fiz′ē·oid\ Resembling epiphyses: said of the small bones of the hands and feet that develop from a center of ossification in a manner similar to those with epiphyses.

**epiphysiolisthesis** \-fiz′ē·ōlisthē′sis\ [*epiphysi(s)* + Gk *olisthēsis* slippage, dislocation] SLIPPED EPIPHYSIS.

**epiphysiolysis** \-fiz′ē·äl′isis\ The separation of an epiphysis from the end of a long bone. **distraction e.** A method of lengthening a long bone by distracting the epiphysis, separating it from the metaphysis by a fracture through the growth plate.

**epiphysis** \epif′isis\ [Gk (from EPI- + *physis* growth, from *phyein* to bring forth, make to grow) a growing upon, excrescence] The end of a long bone that develops from a secondary center of ossification. It is separated from the shaft of the bone by the growth plate, but in the adult it is fused to the shaft. Also *osteoepiphysis.* **capital e.** The epiphysis of the femoral head which articulates the acetabulum. **e. cerebri** CORPUS PINEALE. **slipped e.** The displacement of an epiphysis from the end of a long bone. Also *epiphysiolisthesis, epiphyseal detachment.* **slipped capital femoral e.** A condition most commonly seen in adolescence in which the upper femoral epiphysis becomes displaced by a fracture through or a weakness of the growth plate. **stippled e.** The abnormal appearance on radiography of the epiphyses in subjects with chondrodystrophia congenita punctata.

**epiphysitis** \-fisī′tis\ [*epiphys(is)* + -ITIS] An inflammation of an epiphysis. **e. juvenilis** KÖHLER'S DISEASE. **vertebral e.** SCHEUERMANN'S KYPHOSIS.

**epipial** \-pī′əl\ Overlying the pia mater.

**epiplo-** \əpip′lō-\ [Gk *epiploon* (from *epiplein* to sail upon, to float upon) caul of the entrails, omentum] A combining form denoting the omentum.

**epiploa** \epip′lō·ə\ Plural of EPIPLOON.

**epiplocele** \epip′lōsēl\ [Gk *epiplokēlē* (from *epiplo(on)* omentum + *kēlē* hernia) an omental hernia] A hernia containing omental tissue.

**epiploectomy** \epip′lō·ek′təmē\ [EPIPLO- + -ECTOMY] OMENTECTOMY.

**epiploic** \ep′iplō′ik\ [EPIPLO- + -IC] Pertaining to the omentum.

**epiploitis** \epip′lō·ī′tis\ [EPIPLO- + -ITIS] OMENTITIS. **Sherlock's e.** TUBEROUS SCLEROSIS.

**epiploon** \epip′lō·än\ [Gk *epiploon* the caul of the entrails, omentum] OMENTUM. **great e.** *Outmoded* OMENTUM MAJUS. **lesser e.** *Outmoded* OMENTUM MINUS.

**epiplopexia** \epip′lōpek′sē·ə\ OMENTOPEXY.

**epiplopexy** \epip′lōpek′sē\ [EPIPLO- + -PEXY] OMENTOPEXY.

**epiplorrhaphy** \ep′iplôr′əfē\ [EPIPLO- + -RRHAPHY] OMENTORRHAPHY.

**epipygus** \-pī′gəs\ [EPI- + Gk *pyg(ē)* the rump, buttocks + L *-us,* noun suffix] Unequal conjoined twins in which the parasitic member is united to the host at the sacral region or the buttocks. Also *epipygus parasiticus.* **e. parasiticus** EPIPYGUS.

**epipyramis** \-pir′əmis\ A supernumerary bone that is sometimes found in the wrist. Also *epitriquetrum.*

**epirotulian** \-rōtyoo′lē·ən\ Above the patella.

**episclera** \-sklir′ə\ The loose connective tissue framework just external to the scleral surface. Adj. episcleral.

**episcleral** \-sklir′əl\ [EPI- + SCLERAL] Referring to the tissues upon the surface of the ocular sclera.

**episcleritis** \-sklirī′tis\ [*episcler(a)* + -ITIS] An inflammation of the superficial sclera and immediately overlying connective tissue. **e. partialis fugax** A transient inflammation affecting only a portion of the visible anterior area of the scleral surface.

**episclerotitis** EPISCLERITIS.

**episio-** \əpiz′ē·ō\ [Gk *episeion* region of the pubes] A combining form denoting the vulva.

**episioperineoplasty** \əpiz′ē·ōper′inē′ōplas′tē\ A plastic reconstruction of the perineum in which an episiotomy is carried out.

**episioplasty** \əpiz′ē·ōplas′tē\ [EPISIO- + -PLASTY] A plastic reconstruction of an episiotomy scar.

**episiorrhaphy** \əpiz′ē·ôr′əfē\ [EPISIO- + -RRHAPHY] Repair of an episiotomy.

**episiotomy** \epiz′ē·ät′əmē\ [EPISIO- + -TOMY] An incision from the vagina towards the rectum utilized to facilitate vaginal delivery of a baby. **median e.** An episiotomy incision made in the midline directly towards the rectal opening. **mediolateral e.** An episiotomy incision made from the vagina towards the ischiorectal fossa in an effort to avoid possible entry into the rectum.

**episode** \ep′isōd\ [Gk *epeisodion* (neut. of *epeisodios* coming in beside, episodic, from EPI- + Gk *eis* into + *hodos* a way, path, road) an entrance, episode] An event that is in some way different or distinctive and therefore stands out from the normal course, as of an illness. Adj. episodic. **acute schizophrenic e.** The sudden appearance of grossly psychotic symptoms such as bizarre delusions, delusions of persecution accompanied by hallucinations, auditory hallucinations consisting of voices commenting on the subject's behavior or thoughts, or incoherence or other marked abnormality of associations. The episode may also take the form of a relapse in chronic schizophrenia. **psycholeptic e.** A sudden decrease in mental tension associated with the appearance or eruption of irrational unconscious elements into consciousness or with the development of conversion symptoms or other symptoms or syndromes. *Obs.* **psychomotor e.** A transient alteration in behavior or the state of consciousness coincident with abnormal electrical activity of the brain. These episodes are usually related to temporal lobe seizures.

**episome** \ep′isōm\ [EPI- + Gk *sōm(a)* body] Genetic material in a bacterium that can either replicate independently or be integrated into the chromosome and replicate with it. Examples include plasmids and the DNA of temperate bacteriophages.

**epispadias** \ep′ispā′dē·əs\ [EPI- + Gk *span* to draw out, pluck off, tear] A condition in which the urethra opens into a groove on the dorsal aspect of the penis. This malformation presents an embryologic enigma. **balanic e.** A condition in which the urethra opens on the dorsal aspect of the glans penis. Also *glandular epispadias.* **female e.** The presence of a fissure in the anterior wall of the female urethra. It is probably not homologous to epispadias as seen in the male. **glandular e.** BALANIC EPISPADIAS. **penopubic e.** Epispadias associated with faulty development of the pubic bones or with symphysis. This condition is regularly seen in cases of exstrophy of the bladder.

**epispastic** \-spas′tik\ [EPI- + SPASTIC] VESICANT.

**episplenitis** \-splēnī′tis\ Inflammation of the splenic capsule (tunica fibrosa lienis).

**epistasis** \əpis′təsis\ [Gk *epistasis* (from *epistanai,* Ionic Gk for *ephistanai*) a bringing to a stop, a standing upon, scum] **1** The suppression of the phenotypic expression of one gene by another gene. **2** The suppression of a secretion or excretion. **3** The surface film that forms on urine. For defs. 1, 2, and 3 also *epistasy.*

**epistatic** \-stat′ik\ Suppressing the phenotypic expression of another gene: said of a gene.

**epistaxis** \-stak′sis\ [EPI- + Gk *staxis* a dropping, dripping] Blood loss from within the nose, either from the anterior nares or into the nasopharynx and usually both. The many causes include neoplasm and trauma, but usually it occurs in the absence of any major or progressive disease, and the blood loss itself is the principal problem. Also *nosebleed, nose bleed, nasal hemorrhage.*

**episternal** \-stur′nəl\ Situated over or on the sternum.

**episthotonos** \ep′isthät′ənəs\ [erroneously formed by analogy with *opisthotonos.* See OPISTHOTONOS.] EMPROSTHOTONOS.

**epistropheus** \-strō′fē·əs\ [New L (from Gk *epistrophē* a turning about + New L *-us,* masc. noun suffix)] *Obs.* AXIS. Adj. epistrophic.

**episylvian** \-sil′vē·ən\ [EPI- + SYLVIAN] The frontal and parietal portions of the cerebrum lying above the lateral sulcus.

**epitarsus** \-tär′səs\ [EPI- + TARSUS] A developmental defect of the eyelids, in which folds of conjunctiva from the cul-de-sac are adherent to the tarsal conjunctiva.

**epitendineum** \-tendin′ē·əm\ Condensed areolar connective tissue ensheathing a tendon and containing collagen and elastic fibers. It is continuous with connective tissue both surrounding it and between the tendon fascicles. Also *epitenon.*

**epitenon** \-tē′nän\ EPITENDINEUM.

**epithalamic** \-thalam′ik\ **1** Of or denoting the epithalamus. **2** Derived from the embryonic epithalamus (dorsal thalamic plate). **3** Situated above the thalamus.

**epithalamus** \-thal′əməs\ [EPI- + THALAMUS] [NA] The embryonic dorsal plate of the diencephalon that gives rise to the habenular, paraventricular, and pretectal nuclei and the corpus pineale. Adj. epithalamic.

**epithelia** \-thē′lyə\ Plural of EPITHELIUM.

**epithelial** \-thē′lē·əl\ [*epitheli(um)* + -AL] Of or relating to epithelium.

**epithelialization** \-thē′lē·əlīzā′shən\ The stage in wound healing at which epithelial cells bridge the underlying surface to close the wound.

**epithelialize** \-thē′lē·əlīz\ To cover with epithelial cells. Also *epithelize.*

**epitheliitis** \-thē′lē·ī′tis\ [*epitheli(um)* + -ITIS] An inflammation of the epithelium. Also *epithelitis.*

**epithelio-** \ep′ithē′lē·ō-\ [New L *epithelium* (from Gk *epi* on + *thēlē* nipple) epithelium] A combining form denoting epithelium.

**epitheliocytus** \-sī′təs\ A cell that forms part of the covering or lining of a surface of the body; epithelial cell. **e. basalis gustatorius** One of the three major cell types that comprise a taste bud. It is situated in a basal position and is probably a stem or blastemal cell capable of giving rise to all the major cell types by mitosis. Also *basal cell of taste bud.* **e. phalangeus externus** One of the cells that form three rows serving as supports for both the three rows of outer hair cells and the nerve endings at the base of the hair cells of the spiral organ. An additional row is added in each of the second and third coils of the cochlea. The prism-shaped cell body is characterized by a microtubule-containing fibrillar bundle that runs through its axis, starting from hemidesmosomes on the basal cell membrane and extending to the surface alongside a hair cell where it expands into a flat plate, or phalanx. Where the body begins to taper into a thin process its protoplasm expands and forms an excavation to lodge the base of the hair cell it supports. Also *outer phalangeal cell, Deiters cell, phalangeal cell of Deiters.* **e. phalangeus internus** One of the cells forming a single row on the inner surface of the inner pillars of the spiral organ (of Corti). The cell bodies have a nucleus near their bases. The latter are situated in the space between the bases of the inner pillars and the foramina nervosa on the basilar membrane. Each body contains a fine bundle of tonofibrils and ends at the surface in a small cuticular plate. They support the inner hair cells. Also *inner phalangeal cell.* **e. pilosus columnaris** EPITHELIOCYTUS SENSORIUS PILOSUS EXTERNUS. **e. sensorius gustatorius** One of the three major cell types that comprise a taste bud. It is situated between the supporting, or sustentacular, cells. Between 4 and 20 are present in each taste bud. Each is slender and long with a central nucleus and a short taste hair, or microvillus, on the free surface that projects into the lumen of the taste bud. Each forms a modified synaptic contact with terminal branches of the afferent gustatory nerves. Also *taste receptor cell, neuroepithelial taste cell.* **e. sensorius pilosus externus** One of the hair cells that form three rows between the outer pillars and the outer phalangeal cells of the spiral organ (of Corti). Additional rows are added in each of the second and upper coils of the cochlea. It is columnar-shaped, with a rounded lower end that contains the nucleus. The base fits into a recess of a supporting phalangeal cell. On the free surface are about 100 stereocilia without kinocilia that are longer than those of the inner hair cells and fit in the holes of the reticular membrane by short, bristlelike outgrowths. It is one of the neuroepithelial receptors stimulated by sound waves. Also *outer hair cell, epitheliocytosus pilosus columnaris.* **e. sensorius pilosus internus** One of the hair cells that form a single row between the inner pillars of the spiral organ (of Corti) on the one side and the inner phalangeal and the border cells on the other. It is piriform-shaped with its nucleus in its expanded base that rests in a hollowed recess of a supporting phalangeal cell. The slender free surface has about 50 stereocilia lacking kinocilia that fit in the holes of the reticular membrane by short bristlelike outgrowths. It is one of the neuroepithelial receptors stimulated by sound waves. Also *inner hair cell, epitheliocytus sensorius pilosus piriformis.* **e. sensorius pilosus piriformis** EPITHELIOCYTUS SENSORIUS PILOSUS INTERNUS. **e. sustentans gustatorius** One of the three major cell types that comprise a taste bud. It is spindle-shaped, and several are arranged like staves of a barrel around a pitlike cavity leading to the porus gustatorius. Microvilli are located at the apex of each cell. The cells wrap around and support the sensory, or receptor, cells and contain dense bodies of a secretory nature. Also *incasing cell* (outmoded), *supporting cell of taste bud, sustentacular cell of taste bud.*

**epitheliofibril** \-fī′bril\ TONOFIBRIL.

**epitheliogenetic** \-jənet′ik\ [EPITHELIO- + GENETIC] Resulting from epithelial proliferation.

**epitheliogenic** \-jen′ik\ [EPITHELIO- + -GENIC] Forming epithelium.

**epithelioid** [*epitheli(um)* + -OID] **1** Resembling epithelium or epithelial cells. **2** Characterized by epithelioid cells: said of certain tumors.

**epitheliolysis** \ep′ithē′lē·äl′isis\ The destruction of epithelium.

**epitheliolytic** \-lit′ik\ [EPITHELIO- + LYTIC] Causing the destruction of epithelium.

**epithelioma** \ep′ithē′lē·ō′mə\ [*epitheli(o)-* + -OMA] **1** CARCINOMA. **2** Any of several kinds of benign epithelial tumor. **e. adenoides cysticum** TRICHOEPITHELIOMA. • This term is used especially for the multiple and inherited form. **basal cell e.** BASAL CELL CARCINOMA. **basisquamous e.** BASOSQUAMOUS CARCINOMA. **benign calcifying e.** PILOMATRIXOMA. **calcified e.** PILOMATRIXOMA. **chorionic e.** CHORIOCARCINOMA. **e. cuniculatum** CARCINOMA CUNICULATUM. **Ferguson-Smith type e.** SELF-HEALING SQUAMOUS EPITHELIOMA. **glandular e.** *Obs.* ADENOCARCINOMA. **intraepidermal e.** CARCINOMA IN SITU. **Malherbe's e.** PILOMATRIXOMA. **e. molluscum** Epithelioma marked by self-healing tumors on the face that resemble molluscum contagiosum. **morpheic e.** MORPHEA TYPE BASAL CELL CARCINOMA. **pigmented basal-cell e.** A basal cell carcinoma containing melanin. **pseudocystic e.** A tumor derived from epithelium containing dilated spaces that are not lined with epithelium as in a true cyst. **self-healing squamous e.** A genetically determined condition characterized by the appearance of crops of craggy, nodular lesions that resolve spontaneously and heal with scarring. Also *Ferguson-Smith type epithelioma.* **squamous cell e.** SQUAMOUS CELL CARCINOMA.

**epitheliomatosis** \-mətō′sis\ [EPITHELIOMA + *t* + -OSIS] CARCINOMATOSIS.

**epitheliomatous** \ep′ithē′lē·äm′ətəs\ [EPITHELIOMA + *t* + -OUS] Referring to a carcinoma, as in *pseudoepitheliomatous hyperplasia.*

**epitheliosis** \ep′ithē′lē·ō′sis\ [EPITHELI- + -OSIS] A proliferation of conjunctival epithelium.

**epitheliotropic** \-träp′ik\ [EPITHELIO- + -TROPIC[1]] Characterized by an affinity for epithelial cells.

**epithelitis** \ep′ithēlī′tis\ EPITHELIITIS.

**epithelium** \ep′ithē′lē·əm\ [New L (from EPI- + Gk *thēlē* the nipple + New L *-ium,* noun suffix)] [NA] The cellular covering of the skin and mucous membranes. Also *endepidermis.* **anterior e. of cornea** EPITHELIUM ANTERIUS CORNEAE. **e. anterius corneae** [NA] The five layers of cells that cover the anterior surface of the cornea and become continuous with the conjunctival epithelium over the sclera at the sclerocorneal junction. The superficial flattened squamous cells do not usually become keratinized. Most of the cells are prickle cells, and the epithelium is extremely sensitive, containing many free nerve endings and having a great capacity for regeneration. Also *anterior epithelium of cornea, corneal epithelium* (outmoded). **ciliated e.** **1** Epithelium bearing cilia on its surface. **2** CILIAL RETINA. **coelomic e.** The lining of any coelomic cavity. It is derived from somatic and splanchnic mesoderm with the line of junction marking the subdivision into a parietal and a visceral layer. The primitive coelom is at first lined by cuboidal mesodermal cells. Later they flatten to form the mesothelium. **columnar e.** Epithelium consisting of columnar

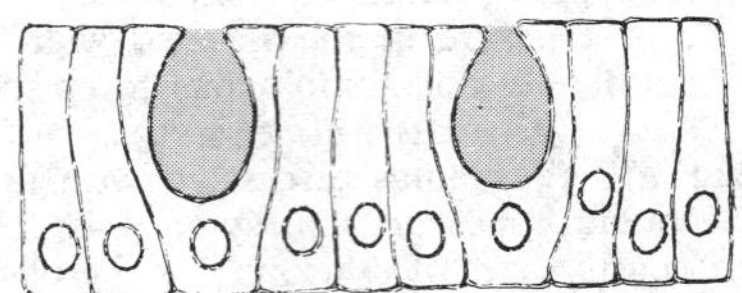

Columnar epithelium of intestines

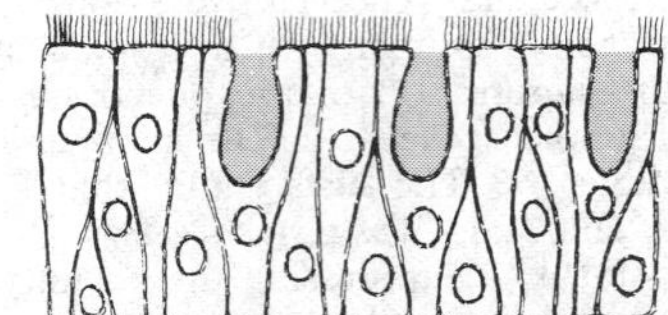

Pseudostratified ciliated columnar epithelium

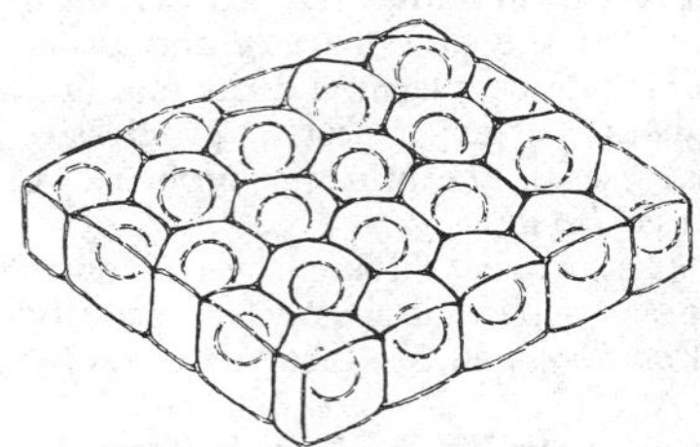

Simple cuboidal epithelium

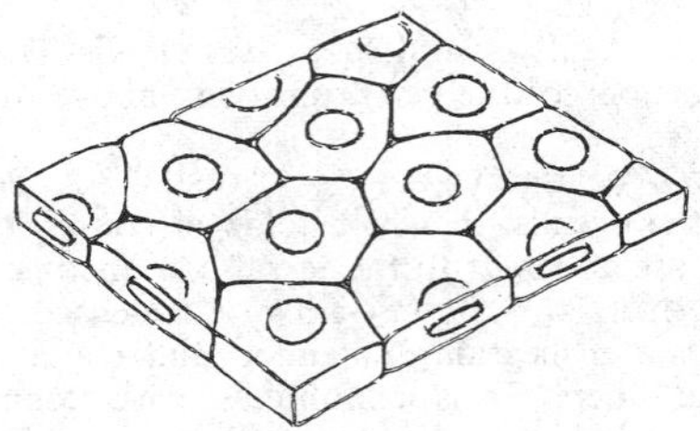

Squamous epithelium

**Types of epithelium**

cells. **corneal e.** *Outmoded* EPITHELIUM ANTERIUS CORNEAE. **crevicular e.** SULCULAR EPITHELIUM. **cuboidal e.** Epithelium consisting of cells of cuboidal shape. **dental e.** ENAMEL EPITHELIUM. **e. ductus semicircularis** The squamous epithelium lining each semicircular duct, similar to that lining the utricle and saccule of the internal ear. *Outmoded.* **enamel e.** The basal cell layer of the epithelial enamel organ. Also *dental epithelium.* **external enamel e.** OUTER ENAMEL EPITHELIUM. **follicular e.** A layer of cells that lines a follicle. **germinal e.** That part of the coelomic epithelium which covers the developing gonad and which gives rise to ingrowths of cords of cells by its proliferation. Early in development the cords are invaded by germ cells (gonocytes) which will become spermatogonia or oogonia while the cord cells give rise to their enveloping cells (either Sertoli cells or follicular membrana granulosa cells). Also *Waldeyer's layer.* **gingival e.** The stratified squamous epithelium of the gingiva. **glandular e.** Epithelium containing glandular cells. **inner enamel e.** The basal epithelial cells forming the inner layer or pulpal surface of the enamel organ. **junctional e.** The epithelial collar that provides the epithelial attachment to the tooth surface. It is continuous with but structurally distinct from the sulcular epithelium. **laminated e.** STRATIFIED EPITHELIUM. **e. of lens** EPITHELIUM LENTIS. **e. lentis** [NA] The layer of transparent, flattened hexagonal cells covering the anterior surface of the lens of the eye. Towards the equator the cells become columnar and arranged in meridional rows, gradually becoming transformed to lens fibers and forming the nuclear or transition zone. Also *epithelium of lens, subcapsular epithelium.* **mesenchymal e.** The epithelial lining of the subdural and subarachnoid spaces and the fluid-filled cavities of the eye and inner ear. **mucous e.** An epithelium containing cells that secrete mucus, as seen in the respiratory tract and gastric mucosa. **muscle e.** MYOEPITHELIUM. **myxopleomorphic e.** PLEOMORPHIC ADENOMA. **nerve e.** 1 The epithelial cells of the ependymal layer of the embryo that give rise to neuroblasts and the spongioblasts that form astrocytes and oligodendrocytes. 2 The sensory epithelium of the optic and otic placodes. Also *neurepithelium, neuroepithelium.* **olfactory e.** A pseudostratified sensory epithelium lining the roof of the nasal cavity containing olfactory cells and supporting cells. **oral e.** The epithelium of the oral mucosa. **outer enamel e.** The basal epithelial cells forming the outer layer of the enamel organ. Also *external enamel epithelium.* **pavement e.** Epithelium consisting of a single layer of flat cells. **pigmented e.** Epithelium that comprises pigment-bearing cells. Also *pigmentary epithelium.* **e. pigmentosum partis ciliaris retinae** [NA] The deeper of the two layers of ciliary epithelium which covers the inner surface of the ciliary body. It consists of cuboidal or columnar cells loaded with pigment granules and is continuous posteriorly with the pigmented layer of the pars optica retinae at the ora serrata, while anteriorly it continues on to the posterior surface of the iris. It is firmly united to the superficial, nonpigmented layer of epithelium by an intervening basement membrane. In addition, the deeper layer is united to the ciliary stroma by its own basement membrane which extends posteriorly into the basal lamina (Bruch's membrane) of the choroid. Also *epithelium pigmentosum corporis ciliaris, pigmented layer of ciliary body, pigmented layer of ciliary part of retina, stratum pigmenti corporis ciliaris* (outmoded). **e. posterius corneae** ENDOTHELIUM CAMERAE ANTERIORIS BULBI. **e. posterius pigmentosum partis iridicae retinae** [NA] The posterior, heavily pigmented layer of cuboidal cells that lines the posterior surface of the iris. The cells are held together by junctional complexes and are separated from the posterior chamber of the eye by the fine internal limiting membrane. The layer is continuous posteriorly with the nonpigmented layer of the pars ciliaris retinae, whereas deep or anterior to it is another, less pigmented layer of cuboidal cells which is continuous with the pigmented layer of the pars ciliaris retinae. Also *pigmented layer of iris, stratum pigmenti iridis* (outmoded). **protective e.** Epithelium that provides protection: said of the epidermis. **pseudostratified e.** Epithelium in which the cell nuclei are arranged at different levels, although all the cells are attached to the basement membrane. **pyramidal e.** 1 A layer of transitional epithelium that covers a pyramid of the kidney. 2 An epithelial layer composed of cells that have a pyramidal shape. **reduced enamel e.** The residual epithelium of the enamel organ that covers the enamel surface of a tooth following amelogenesis. **respiratory e.** The pseudostratified columnar ciliated epithelium with goblet cells lining the conducting air passages of the respiratory tract, namely, the nasal cavity, nasopharynx, larynx, trachea, and principal bronchi. **retinal pigment e.** The outermost layer of the retina, composed of a single layer of cuboidal cells that contain melanin pigment. Also *ectoretina.* **seminiferous e.** The lining of the seminiferous tubules, comprising Sertoli cells, spermatogonia, spermatocytes, and spermatids. **sensory e.** The neurepithelial cells that give rise to the neural structures of the optic and otic placodes. Also *sense epithelium.* **simple e.** Epithelium consisting of a single layer of cells. **squamous e.** Epithelium consisting of flattened cells. Also *tabular epithelium.* **stratified e.** Epithelium consisting of more than one layer of cells. Also *laminated epithelium.* **stratified ciliated columnar e.** A multilayered epithelium, the surface layer being composed of tall cells bearing cilia. Most of the respiratory tract is lined by epithelium of this type. **stratified squamous e.** A multilayered epithelium, the surface layer of which consists of flattened cells that may or may not be cornified. **subcapsular e.** 1 The epithelial lining of the outer capsule of sensory and autonomic ganglia. 2 The epithelial lining of any capsular structure. 3 EPITHELIUM LENTIS. **sulcular e.** The epithelium lining the outer wall of the gingival sulcus, extending from the gingival margin to the junctional epithelium. Also *crevicular epithelium, sulcal epithelium.* **e. superficiale ovarii** [NA] The layer derived from the embryonic germinal epithelium, comprising simple cuboidal or columnar cells in infancy and flattened cells in adults, which covers the free surface of the ovary. Deep to it is the tunica albuginea. Also *Waldeyer's layer.* **surface e.** One or more layers of specialized cells that cover the body surfaces and line the internal cavities. It performs a generally protective function, preventing dehydration and loss of body substances, but it may be locally adapted for either absorption or secretion. **tabular e.** SQUAMOUS EPITHELIUM. **tegumentary e.** EPIDERMIS. **tessellated e.** Epithelium composed of flattened, interdigitating cells. **transitional e.** Epithelium present in the mucous membrane of excretory passages of the urinary tract, capable of modifying the arrangement of its constituent cells according to the degree of distention of the bladder, and yet remaining impervious to the urine within the lumen of the urinary tract. **visceral e.** A single layer of flattened mesothelial cells that covers the various organs lying within the coelomic cavities. Together with the parietal epithelium it forms a continuous lining for the pleural, pericardial, and peritoneal cavities.

**epithelization** \ep′ithē′līzā′shən\ EPITHELIALIZATION.
**epithelize** \ep′ithē′līz\ EPITHELIALIZE.
**epithet** \ep′əthet\ [Gk *epithet(os)* (from *epitithenai* to put or place on or by) added or attached to] In scientific nomenclature, any of those parts of a genus name that serve to identify the species or variety within the genus: often qualified by the taxonomic classification so identified, as *specific epithet.*
**epitope** \ep′itōp\ [EPI- + Gk *top(os)* a place] ANTIGENIC DETERMINANT.
**epitrichium** \-trik′ē·əm\ [EPI- + TRICH- + L *-ium,* noun suffix] A superficial large-celled layer which temporarily covers the fetal skin and its primitive hairs. It either breaks up in pieces or else in some forms is sloughed en masse before or at birth. Also *dome cells.*
**epitriquetrum** \-trīkwē′trəm\ EPIPYRAMIS.
**epitrochlea** \-träk′lē·ə\ EPICONDYLUS MEDIALIS HUMERI.
**epitrochlear** \-träk′lē·ər\ Pertaining to the epitrochlea.
**epitrochleitis** \-träk′lē·ī′tis\ An inflammation about the epitrochlear region of the humerus. It is associated with disease of the epitrochlear lymph node.
**epituberculosis** \-t^yubur′kyəlō′sis\ A benign pulmonary condition which appears as a dense, homogenous shadow in the roentgenogram and which occurs in tuberculin-positive individuals, usually infants and children. There may be accompanying fever and nonproductive cough. There is gradual, complete clearing of the lesion. The condition may be due to atelectasis secondary to bronchial compression by tuberculous lymph nodes.
**epitympanic** \-timpan′ik\ Situated above the tympanic cavity.
**epitympanum** \-tim′pənəm\ RECESSUS EPITYMPANICUS.
**epitype** \ep′itīp\ [EPI- + *type*] A group of similar epitopes.
**epizoa** \-zō′ə\ Plural of EPIZOON.
**epizoic** \-zō′ik\ Living on the surface of an animal.
**epizoon** \-zō′än\ [EPI- + Gk *zōon* living being, animal] (*pl.* epizoa) An animal organism that lives on the surface of a host animal; an ectozoon.
**epizoonosis** \-zō′ənō′sis\ A disease caused by an animal parasite in or on the skin. Also *epidermatozoonosis.*
**Epon** A plastic substance used to embed specimens for ultrastructural study. A proprietary name.
**eponychium** \ep′ōnik′ē·əm\ [New L, from EP- + Gk *onyx,* gen. *onychos* nail] (*pl.* eponychia) **1** [NA] A fold of epidermis which overlaps the base of the nail; cuticle. **2** A cutaneous elevation near the end of an embryonic finger or toe marking the place of origin of a nail. For defs. 1 and 2 also *epionychium.*
**eponym** \ep′ənim\ [Gk *eponym(os)* (from *ep(i)-* upon + *onym(a),* Aeolian Gk for Attic *onoma* a name) named after, giving one's name to; as substantive, a surname] **1** A person whose name has been used in a term and from which the term is or may be derived, as Albert Einstein in *einsteinium* or James Clerk Maxwell in *maxwell.* **2** A term derived or thought to be derived from the name of a person, as *Parkinson's disease* or *Gram-negative.* Adj. eponymous, eponymic.
**eponymous** \epän′əməs\ Formed from or resembling an eponym; especially, named after a person, as *eponymous term.* Also *eponymic.*
**epoophorectomy** \ep′ō·äf′ôrek′təmē \ [*epoöphor(on)* + -ECTOMY ] The surgical excision of the epoöphoron.
**epoöphoron** \ep′ō·äf′ôrän\ [EP- + OOPHORON] [NA] The remains of the cranial portions of the mesonephros and the mesonephric duct that persist into adult life, respectively, as a longitudinal duct (of Gartner) closed at both ends, and several ductuli transversi that open into the longitudinal duct. They are located between the layers of the mesosalpinx near the ovary where the longitudinal duct is parallel to the uterine tube. Also *corpus pampiniforme, pampiniform body, Rosenmüller's body, Rosenmüller's organ, parovarium, proövarium.*
**epoprostenol** \ep′ōpräs′tənôl\ PROSTAGLANDIN $I_2$.
**epoxy-** [EP- + OXY-[1]] A combining form signifying the replacement of one hydrogen atom on each of two adjacent carbon atoms by an oxygen atom which therefore bridges them to form a three-membered ring. The compound formed is known as an epoxide.
**epoxymethamine bromide** METHSCOPOLAMINE BROMIDE.
**EPR** electrophrenic respiration.
**EPS** exophthalmos-producing substance.
**EPSP** excitatory postsynaptic potential. **aggregate E.** The EPSP produced in a neuron by the population of axons that synapse on the neuron from one peripheral source, e.g., the depolarization of a motoneuron resulting from stimulation of the nerve to the homonymous muscle.
**Epstein** [Alois *Epstein,* Czech pediatrician, 1849–1918] Epstein's pearls. See under PEARL.
**Epstein** [Emil *Epstein,* Austrian biochemist, flourished 20th century] Van Bogaert-Scherer-Epstein syndrome. See under CEREBROTENDINOUS XANTHOMATOSIS.
**Epstein** [Michael Anthony *Epstein,* English physician, born 1921] Epstein-Barr virus. See under VIRUS.
**epulides** Plural of EPULIS.
**epulis** \epyoo′lis\ [Gk *epoulis* (from EPI- + Gk *oulon* a gum; mostly in pl. *oula* the gums) a gumboil] A localized swelling of the gingiva, sessile or pedunculated in form. It may be inflammatory in origin or a true tumor. **congenital e. of newborn** A pedunculated hamartoma of the tissues of the gum of newborn infants, almost exclusively females. It is usually found in the region of the upper central incisors. **fibrous e.** A fibrosed granulomatous epulis. **giant cell e.** PERIPHERAL GIANT CELL REPARATIVE GRANULOMA. **granulomatous e.** An epulis consisting of granulation tissue caused by chronic irritation. **pigmented e.** MELANOTIC NEUROECTODERMAL TUMOR. **e. of pregnancy** A focal, highly vascularized epulis which bleeds readily if traumatized, occurring during pregnancy but regressing following delivery. It is of inflammatory origin associated with irritation around a tooth.
**epulofibroma** \ep′yəlōfībrō′mə\ [*epul(is)* + *o* + FIBROMA] A fibroma of the gingiva.
**epulosis** \ep′yəlō′sis\ [Gk *epoulōsis* a scarring over, healing] *Seldom used* CICATRIZATION.
**epulotic** \ep′yəlät′ik\ Concerning or causing epulosis (cicitrization).
**eq** equivalent
**equalization** \ē′kwəlīzā′shən\ The process of making equal or uniform. **pressure e.** The correction of alternobaric abnormalities in the middle ears or paranasal sinuses to avoid or treat barotrauma. This correction usually occurs physiologically but may call for such measures as the introduction of ventilation tubes and nasal decongestion.
**equation** \ikwā′zhən\ [L *aequatio* (from *aequatus,* past part. of *aequare* to make equal) an equaling, equalizing] A statement expressing the equality of two quantities. **alveolar gas e.** An equation which relates the tension of oxygen in the alveoli to the tension of oxygen in inspired air, the tension of carbon dioxide in the alveoli, and the respiratory exchange ratio. **Arrhenius e.** The equation $k = A\ \exp(-E_a/RT)$, which relates $k$, the rate constant for a chemical reaction, to $T$, the absolute temperature, where $R$ is

the gas constant, and where $E_a$, the energy of activation, and $A$ are parameters characteristic of the reaction. **Ayala's e.** AYALA'S QUOTIENT. **Bohr's e.** An equation for calculating the ratio of dead space to tidal volume based on the expired and arterial $CO_2$ concentrations:

$$\frac{\text{dead space volume}}{\text{tidal volume}} = \frac{\text{arterial } CO_2 - \text{expired } CO_2}{\text{arterial } CO_2}.$$

**Gompertz e.** A mathematical equation stating that the probability of death in humans doubles every eight years after age 35. **Henderson-Hasselbalch e.** The equation pH = p$K$ + log([base]/[acid]), which relates the pH of a solution to the p$K$ of any dissociating species in it and to the concentrations of the protonated and unprotonated forms of that species, i.e. the concentrations of an acid and its conjugate base. **Hill e.** An equation used to express the fractional saturation of a molecule with a ligand as a function of ligand concentration, e.g., the saturation of hemoglobin with oxygen. The empirical equation is: $y/1-y=ks^n$, where $y$ = degree of saturation, $s$ = concentration of free ligand, and $n$ = Hill coefficient, which cannot exceed the number of binding sites. $k$ = a proportionality constant. **Larmor e.** An equation used in nuclear magnetic resonance calculations: $\omega_o=\gamma H_o$, where $\omega_o$ is the Larmor frequency, $\gamma$ is the gyromagnetic ratio, and $H_o$ is the strength of the magnetic field. **Lineweaver-Burk e.** LINEWEAVER-BURK PLOT. **Michaelis-Menten e.** The equation $v = V{\cdot}s/(s + K)$, which expresses the way in which the rate, $v$, of an enzyme-catalyzed reaction varies with the concentration, $s$, of free substrate. It contains two empirical constants: $V$, the limiting velocity (sometimes written as $V_{max}$), and $K_m$, the Michaelis constant. Also *Michaelis equation.* **Nernst e.** A formula that expresses the relationship between the electric potential between two compartments and relative concentrations of an ion in the two compartments when the system is in equilibrium:

$$E = \frac{RT}{zF} \ln \frac{[C_1]}{[C_2]},$$

where $E$ is the equilibrium potential in mV, $R$ is the universal gas constant, $T$ is the absolute temperature, $z$ is the ionic charge of the ion, $F$ is Faraday's constant, and $C_1$ and $C_2$ are the respective concentrations of the ion in the two compartments. **Poiseuille's e.** POISEUILLE'S LAW. **Ussing e.** An equation which predicts whether movement of an ion across a membrane involves active transport. If no active transport is involved, then the ratio of external to internal concentrations multiplied by exponential $zEF/RT$, where $z$ is the charge of the ion, $E$ the potential difference across the membrane, $F$ the Faraday constant, $R$ the gas constant, and $T$ the absolute temperature. **van't Hoff e.** An equation which relates the osmotic pressure exerted by a solution to the concentration of the solute: $\pi=CRT$, where $\pi$ equals the osmotic pressure, $C$ equals the molar concentration of the solute, $R$ = the gas constant 0.082 liter atmospheres per degree per mole, and $T$ equals the absolute temperature.

**equator** [Late L *aequator* (from L *aequatus*, past part. of *aequare* to make equal, + *-or* -OR) an equalizer] In anatomy, an imaginary line encircling a spherical organ midway between its two poles, dividing the surface into two approximately equal parts. **e. bulbi oculi** [NA] An imaginary line encircling the eyeball midway between the anterior and posterior poles. Also *equator of eyeball.* **e. of cell** An imaginary line encircling a cell which is equidistant from each pole, as a line around an egg between the animal pole and the vegetal pole. **e. of crystalline lens** EQUATOR LENTIS. **e. of eyeball** EQUATOR BULBI OCULI. **e. lentis** [NA] The marginal circumference of the lens of the eye, situated midway between the anterior and posterior poles of the lens. Also *equator of lens, equator of crystalline lens.*

**equi-** \ē′kwi-, ē′kwē-\ [ L *aequus* level, equal, smooth, similar, just] A combining form meaning equal, equally.

**equiaxial** \-ak′sē·əl\ Possessing axes of equal length.

**equicaloric** \-kəlôr′ik\ [EQUI- + CALORIC] Having the same caloric value. Also *isocaloric.*

**equil** equilibration

**equilibration** \-librā′shən\ Adjustment to bring into equilibrium. **occlusal e.** Adjustment of the occlusal surfaces of teeth in order to produce balanced occlusion or harmonious cuspal relationships.

**equilibrium** [L *aequilibrium* (from *aequus* level, equal + *libr(a)* scales, a balance + *-ium,* noun suffix) equality of weight] **1** A state in which a chemical is proceeding equally rapidly in the forward and reverse directions. **2** A state in which chemical or physical forces are equal and opposite. **acid-base e.** ACID-BASE BALANCE. **body e.** ENERGY BALANCE. **calorie e.** ENERGY BALANCE. **carbon e.** CARBON BALANCE. **Donnan e.** The equilibrium of small ions between a solution containing charged macromolecules and one without them, as across a membrane permeable to small but not to large ions. **dynamic e.** A state of equilibrium, with emphasis on the fact that individual reactions are rapid even though they balance out in net effect. **fluid e.** WATER BALANCE. **genetic e.** In a randomly mating population, a state in which the frequencies of the alleles of a given gene or genotype remain constant through successive generations and conform to the Hardy-Weinberg law. Mutation, drift, selection, and migration are the most important factors that tend to disrupt genetic equilibrium. Also *genotypic equilibrium.* **Hardy-Weinberg e.** The situation in a randomly breeding population in which gene frequencies are in accordance with the predictions of the Hardy-Weinberg law. **homeostatic e.** HOMEOSTASIS. **metabolic e.** METABOLIC BALANCE. **mutational e.** **1** A state of balance between the elimination of mutant alleles because of negative fitness and the addition of mutant alleles by new mutation. **2** With respect to neutral mutations, the situation of balance between mutation and drift, such that any individual selected at random in a population will be homozygous at a given locus. **3** In a freely breeding population, a balance between positive and negative mutations such that net selective pressure is zero. **nitrogen e.** NITROGEN BALANCE. **protein e.** PROTEIN BALANCE. **radioactive e.** The condition established in a radioactive preparation including one or more members of radioactive series when the disintegration rates of the successive members of the series become equal. The overall disintegration rate of the preparation is then constant, at least on a time scale that is short compared with the longest half-life involved. **secular e.** Equilibrium between the members of a radioactive series, when the parent is a radionuclide with a half-life much longer than the half-lives of the daughter products. **transient e.** The equilibrium between parent and daughter radionuclides when they are confined together and both have rather short half-lives. The quantity of the daughter builds up until its disintegration rate is equal to that of the parent, as in the conversion from molybdenum 99 to technetium 99m. Compare SECULAR EQUILIBRIUM. **water e.** WATER BALANCE.

**equinocavus** \ikwī′nōkā′vəs\ [*equin(us)* + L *cavus* concave] TALIPES CAVUS.

**equinovalgus** \ikwī'nōval'gəs\ [*equin(us)* + VALGUS] TALIPES EQUINOVALGUS.

**equinovarus** \ikwī'nōver'əs\ [*equin(us)* + VARUS] TALIPES EQUINOVARUS.

**equinus** \ikwī'nəs\ [L, equine] Like or suggestive of a horse: applied especially to human foot deformities that prevent normal plantigrade weight-bearing. See also TALIPES EQUINUS.

**equipotential** \-pōten'shəl\ In embryonic cells or tissues, having the developmental capability of progressing in similar ways and to a similar extent. Thus the cells of a very early two-cell embryo each have the power of developing into an individual organism.

**equipotentiality** \-pōten'shē·al'itē\ The hypothesized ability of intact regions of the cerebral cortex to assume the functions of damaged parts of the cortex well enough to permit functional performance in learning tasks of a general kind.

**equitoxic** \-täk'sik\ Of equal toxicity.

**equivalence** \ikwiv'ələns\ **1** The proportionate concentrations of any two materials such that they combine with or displace one another maximally. **2** The concentrations of antigen and antibody that produce optimum formation of immune complexes.

**equivalent** \ikwiv'ələnt\ [French *équivalent* (from L *aequus* level, equal + *valens*, gen. *valentis*, strong) having equal force] **1** The weight in grams of an element that combines with or displaces one gram of hydrogen. **2** The weight of substance contained in one liter of normal solution. **3** Having the same valence. *Outmoded.* **caloric e. of oxygen** The amount of energy produced in the body per liter of oxygen taken in. The value is a function of the composition of the food being utilized (fuel value). **calorie e.** The number of calories contained in a given quantity of food. **concrete e.** The thickness of concrete that has the same shielding properties, for a given kind of radiation, as the substance of interest (e.g., earth). **dose e.** Absorbed dose multiplied by a quality factor whose function is to make allowance for the different biological effectiveness of various kinds of radiation, as related to linear energy transfer. Such a factor converts rads to rems. **genetic lethal e.** LETHAL EQUIVALENT. **gram e.** EQUIVALENT WEIGHT. **isodynamic e.** The quantity of food that is equivalent to a fixed quantity of another food in the energy it gives. Since fat gives 9.3 calories per gram and carbohydrate 4.1 calories per gram, 4.1 grams of fat is the isodynamic equivalent of 9.3 grams of carbohydrate. **lead e.** The thickness of lead that has the same shielding properties, for a given kind of radiation, as the substance of interest (e.g., brick). **lethal e.** A genetic measure of the deleterious genes carried in a heterozygous state by an individual organism: that is, genes that, when homozygous, result in reduced fitness. An individual who is heterozygous for five genes, each of which, if homozygous, reduces fitness by 20%, is said to have one lethal equivalent. Also *genetic lethal equivalent, lethal equivalent value.* **maximum permissible dose e.** The maximum permissible absorbed dose, adjusted for the kind of radiation and for the parts or extent of the body exposed. **nitrogen e.** The equivalent by weight in nitrogen of protein catabolized by the body. One gram of nitrogen is equal to 6.25 grams of protein catabolized by the body. This equivalent is used in the measurement of protein breakdown by analysis of the nitrogen excreted in the urine. **psychic e.** TEMPORAL LOBE EPILEPSY. **toxic e.** A measure of toxicity expressed as the amount of a substance per kilogram of body weight required to kill a test animal. **ventilation e.** The ratio of ventilatory volume to oxygen consumption.

**ER** **1** emergency room. **2** external resistance. **3** evoked response (evoked potential).

**Er** Symbol for the element, erbium.

**er** endoplasmic reticulum.

**er-** \er-, ir-\ EN-.

**-er** \-ər\ [Germanic *-ar(jaz)*, from L *-arius*, agentive suffix] A suffix denoting a person or thing that performs a specified action.

**ERA** electric response audiometry.

**eradication** \irad'ikā'shən\ [Late L *eradicatio* (from L *eradicare* to pull up by the root, from *ex* out + *radix*, gen. *radicis*, root) an uprooting] Total elimination, as of an endemic disease or of the vector of such disease.

**Erb** [Wilhelm Heinrich *Erb*, German neurologist, 1840–1921] **1** Erb's paraplegia, Erb spastic paraplegia, Erb syphilitic spinal paralysis, Erb-Charcot disease, Erb's paralysis, Erb's palsy. See under SYPHILITIC SPASTIC PARAPLEGIA. **2** Duchenne-Erb paralysis, Erb-Duchenne paralysis, Erb's paralysis, Erb's palsy. See under DUCHENNE-ERB SYNDROME. **3** See under REACTION, SIGN, PHENOMENON, POINT. **4** Erb sclerosis. See under PRIMARY LATERAL SCLEROSIS. **5** Erb syndrome, Erb-Goldflam syndrome, Erb-Oppenheim-Goldflam syndrome, Erb-Goldflam disease, Goldflam-Erb disease. See under MYASTHENIA GRAVIS. **6** Erb's paralysis, Erb's palsy. See under LIMB-GIRDLE MUSCULAR DYSTROPHY. **7** Erb-Landouzy disease, Erb's disease. See under MUSCULAR DYSTROPHY.

**Erben** [Siegmund *Erben*, Austrian neurologist, born 1863] Erben's phenomenon, Erben sign. See under REFLEX.

**ERBF** effective renal blood flow.

**Erc** erythrocyte.

**ercalciol** \urkal'sē·ôl\ ERGOCALCIFEROL.

**Erdheim** [Jakob *Erdheim*, Austrian physician, 1874–1937] Erdheim syndrome, Erdheim's cystic medial necrosis. See under CYSTIC MEDIAL NECROSIS.

**erectile** \irek'tīl\ **1** Capable of being placed upright. **2** Capable of becoming tumescent or turgid.

**erection** The engorgement with blood, stiffening, and elevation of erectile tissue, especially of the penis.

**erector** \irek'tər\ [L *erectus*, past part. of *erigere* to set up, lift up + -OR] A structure, such as a muscle, that causes a part either to stand up or out, to be held up or out, or to become erect. Also *arrector*.

**erethetical** \er'əthet'ikəl\ ERETHISMIC.

**erethism** \er'ithizm\ [Gk *erethisma* a stirring up, exciting] **1** A state of excessive irritability and of heightened and intense emotional reactivity and lability. **2** A mental disturbance characterized by emotional irritability, shyness, and depression occurring in chronic inorganic mercury poisoning. *Older term.* Also *hydrargyromania*. **sexual e.** An unusually strong reaction to sexual stimulation, as in nymphomania, or satyriasis. *Older term.*

**erethismic** \er'əthiz'mik\ **1** Pertaining to or precipitating erethism. Also *erethetical, erethistic.* **2** A person suffering from erethism.

**erethisophrenia** \er'əthiz'ōfrē'nē·ə \ [Gk *erethis-*, stem of *erethizein* to stir up, anger, excite + -PHRENIA] *Outmoded* MANIC-DEPRESSIVE PSYCHOSIS.

**erethistic** \er'əthis'tik\ ERETHISMIC.

**ereuth-** \irooth-\ ERYTHRO-.

**ERG** electroretinogram.

**erg** \urg\ [Gk *erg(on)* work] Special name for the derived unit of work in the CGS system, the work done when the point of application of a force of one dyne is displaced through a distance of one centimeter in the direction of the force; $10^{-7}$ joule. Symbol: erg

**ergasia** \urgā′zhə\ [Gk *ergasia* work] **1** The total psychobiologic activity of an individual. **2** A potential for work.

**ergastic** \urgas′tik\ Of or relating to ergasia.

**ergastoplasm** \urgas′təplazm\ ENDOPLASMIC RETICULUM. • This term may be used when considering the staining properties of this cytoplasm, i.e., its affinity for basic stains such as pyronine and methylene blue, whereas *granular endoplasmic reticulum* is defined in terms of structure as revealed by electron microscopy.

**ergo-** \ur′gō-\ [Gk *ergon* work] A combining form meaning work.

**ergocalciferol** \-kalsif′ərôl\ A form of vitamin D that is made by irradiating ergosterol with ultraviolet light. Irradiation gives rise to a number of compounds, some toxic, of which only ergocalciferol has significant antirachitic properties. It is widely used in clinical medicine. It is rarely found in plant and animal tissues except in certain fish-liver oils. It differs from cholecalciferol by possessing a methyl group on C-24 and a 22(23) double bond. Also *vitamin $D_2$, activated ergosterol, irradiated ergosterol, viosterol, ercalciol.*

**ergoesthesiograph** \-esthē′zē·əgraf\ ERGOMETER.

**ergogenesis** \-jen′əsis\ [ERGO- + GENESIS] The process of developing energy necessary to function.

**ergograph** \ur′gōgraf\ [ERGO- + -GRAPH] ERGOMETER. **Mosso's e.** An ergometer for studying finger flexion.

**ergometer** \urgäm′ətər\ [ERGO- + -METER] An instrument for recording the amount of work done during muscular activity. Also *ergograph, ergoesthesiograph.* Adj. ergometric. **bicycle e.** A stationary bicycle system used to measure the amount of energy expended while performing a cycling movement.

**ergometrine** ERGONOVINE.

**ergometry** \urgäm′ətrē\ [ERGO- + -METRY] The process of recording the amount of work performed during muscular activity.

**ergonomics** \ur′gənäm′iks\ [ERGO- + *(eco)nomics*] The study and design of work situations, taking into account the anatomic, physiologic, and psychological variabilities of the people who will work within the given environment.

**ergonovine** $C_{19}H_{23}N_3O_2$. An alkaloid either produced synthetically or obtained from ergot. It is a direct muscle stimulant and has been used as an oxytocic to produce strong, rhythmic contractions of the uterus and also to treat migraine headache. Also *ergometrine, ergostetrine, ergotocine.*

**ergonovine maleate** $C_{23}H_{27}N_3O_6$. 9,10-Didehydro-*N*-(2-hydroxy-1-methylethyl)-6-methylergoline-8$\beta$(S)-carboxamide maleate, the maleate salt of ergonovine. It is used as an oxytocic agent and for the preventive treatment of migraine headaches. It can be given orally, intramuscularly, or intravenously.

**ergosome** \ur′gəsōm\ POLYRIBOSOME.

**ergostat** \ur′gəstat\ [ERGO- + -STAT] An apparatus for exercising muscles.

**ergosterol** A sterol of fungal cell membranes. It differs from cholesterol in possessing two extra double bonds, at C-7 and C-22, and an extra methyl group on C-24. Some polyene antibiotics have selectivity for yeasts rather than mammalian cells because of slightly higher affinity for ergosterol than for the cholesterol of animal membranes. When exposed to ultraviolet light, ergosterol gives rise to several related substances, of which ergocalciferol (vitamin $D_2$) is the only one with antirachitic properties. Some of the other substances created are toxic. **activated e.** ERGOCALCIFEROL. **irradiated e.** ERGOCALCIFEROL.

**ergostetrine** ERGONOVINE.

**ergot** \er′gät, ur′gät\ **1** A fungus, *Claviceps purpurea,* growing as a parasite on grains of rye. Ingestion of ergot may cause vomiting, diarrhea, and peripheral circulatory changes leading to gangrene. **2** A similar parasite of other cereals and grasses. **hydrogenated e. alkaloids** Semistynthetic derivatives of ergot alkaloids that are prepared by catalytic hydrogenation of the natural alkaloids to saturate the D ring of lysergic acid.

**ergotamine** \urgät′əmēn\ One of several alkaloids produced by *Claviceps purpurea* (ergot), containing, in part, lysergic acid. Several medicinal uses are made of this fungal by-product.

**ergotamine tartrate** $C_{70}H_{76}N_{10}O_{16}$. 12′-Hydroxy-2′-methyl-5′$\alpha$-(phenylmethyl)ergotaman-3′,6′,18-trione tartrate, an ergot alkaloid with vasoconstrictor properties. It has been used in the prevention of migraine headaches. Absorption from oral doses is variable, but subcutaneous or intramuscular injection is more reliable and the effects take place more quickly.

**ergotherapy** \-ther′əpē\ The therapeutic use of physical effort.

**ergothioneine** 3-(2-Mercaptoimidazol-4-yl-2-(trimethylammonio) propionic acid. A substance derived from histidine by substitution of a mercapto group on C-2 of the imidazole ring and three methylations of the ammonio group. It occurs in erythrocytes. Also *thioneine.*

**ergotinin** \urgät′inin\ An alkaloid isolated from the ergot fungus, *Claviceps purpurea,* which is known to cause a toxic action.

**ergotism** \ur′gətizm\ [ERGOT + -ISM] Poisoning caused by ingestion of grain contaminated with ergot, *Claviceps purpurea,* or by chronic excessive use of the drug. The signs and symptoms of poisoning are ataxia, tremors, convulsions, stimulation of the uterus, and severe vasoconstriction in the extremities leading to gangrene if allowed to persist.

**ergotocine** ERGONOVINE.

**ergotoxine** \-täk′sin\ A 1:1:1 mixture of ergocornine, ergocristine, and ergocryptine obtained from ergot (*Claviceps purpurea*). It has marked stimulating effects on smooth muscle of the uterus and blood vessels.

**eriodictyon** A fluidextract or syrup derived from the dried leaf of *Eriodictyon californicum.* It is used as an expectorant and to mask the taste of bitter drugs.

**erisiphake** \eris′ifāk\ ERYSIPHAKE.

***Eristalis tenax*** \er′istā′lis tē′naks\ The drone fly, a species of syrphid fly that resembles a drone bee. The fly lays its eggs on liquid manure or excrement. The larvae, so-called rat-tail maggots, can cause enteric pseudomyiasis in humans. Fecal contamination with these larvae doubtless occurs, but passage of the actual worms in human stools, especially of children, has also been authenticated. These cases are pseudoparasitic in that no prolonged parasitic period of intestinal myiasis is involved, although a few cases of intestinal disturbances in children over a period of weeks have been reported.

**Erlenmeyer** [Richard August Carl Emil *Erlenmeyer,* German chemist, 1825–1909] **1** See under FLASK. **2** Erlenmeyer flask deformity. See under DEFORMITY.

**Ernst** [Paul *Ernst,* Swiss pathologist, 1859–1937] Babès-Ernst corpuscles, Babès-Ernst granules. See under BABÈS-ERNST BODIES.

**erogenous** \iräj′ənəs\ [Gk *erō(s)* love + -GENOUS] **1** Libidinal or erotic. **2** Capable of erotic arousal.

**eros** \ir′äs, er′əs\ [Gk *erōs* love, desire] SEXUAL INSTINCT.

**erosio** \erō′sē·ō\ [L (from *erosus,* past part. of *erodere* to gnaw off or away, consume), erosion] EROSION. **e. interdigitalis blastomycetica** Interdigital infection with *Candida albicans.* The likelihood of the infection is increased by frequent exposure of the hands to water and by limitation of finger mobility, as by arthritis. Also *erosio interdigitalis saccharomycetica.*

**erosion** [L *erosio.* See EROSIO.] 1 The process of wearing away, as in the formation of a superficial ulcer or the loss of dental tissue resulting from the effects of abrasion. 2 A superficial ulcer. Also *erosio.* **cervical e.** The alteration of the epithelium on a portion of the uterine cervix as a result of ulceration by infection. **dental e.** The loss of tooth substance, particularly enamel, by the acid action of food such as citrus fruits, gastric regurgitation, or industrial fumes such as those found in an electric battery factory or battery servicing department. Erosion occurs at nonocclusal surfaces and the tissue loss may be further increased by dental abrasion. Dental erosion may also be of mechanical origin caused by abrasive dusts in granules or by the practice of craftsmen of holding nails in the mouth.

**erosive** \irō′siv\ Characterized by or producing erosion.

**erotic** \irät′ik\ [Gk *erōtikos* (from *erōs,* gen. *erōtos* love, passion) of or caused by love] Possessing libidinal qualities; sexually stimulating.

**erotico-** \irät′əkō-\ EROTO-.

**eroticomania** \irät′əkōmā′nē·ə\ EROTOMANIA.

**eroto-** \irō′tə-, irät′ə-\ [Gk *erōs,* gen. *erōtos* love, desire] A combining form meaning sexual desire. Also *erotico-.*

**erotogenic** \irät′əjen′ik\ [EROTO- + -GENIC] Originating from or giving rise to libidinal energies.

**erotomania** \irät′əmā′nē·ə\ [EROTO- + -MANIA] 1 A delusion that one is loved by another. Also *eroticomania, erotomaniacal delusion, amorous paranoia.* 2 Obsessive sexual activity or preoccupation.

**ERPF** effective renal plasma flow.

**errhine** \er′īn\ [Gk *errhin(on)* (from *er-* in + *rhis,* gen. *rhinos,* nose) sternutatory medicine] Any drug serving as a nasal irritant thus increasing discharge of nasal fluid.

**error** [L, a wandering about] 1 The difference between the measured, observed, or calculated value and the true value. 2 A deviation or defect in structure or function, as *inborn error of metabolism.* **absolute e.** The difference between an observed value and the real value of that being observed. **biased e.** An error which distorts a statistical result in a systematic way, unlike random errors, whose distortions tend to cancel each other out. **copy e.** Any mutation that arises during DNA replication from a failure to insert nucleotides complementary to those in the parent DNA chain. **experimental e.** In statistics, the random variation shown in measurements repeated under the same conditions. The precision with which experimental error can be measured depends on the statistical properties of the experimental design. **inborn e. of metabolism** 1 Any abnormality of a metabolic process that is due to a gene-determined defect. Most result from deficient activity of a specific enzyme, are inherited as autosomal or X-linked recessives, and cause some clinical effect. The phenotype can be detected at birth (or *in utero*) if the metabolic block is assayed biochemically, although pathologic consequences may be either delayed until later life or may be benign. Also *enzymopathy.* 2 The concept, originated by A. E. Garrod in 1902, that biochemical disturbances of physiology originate in heritable defects in enzyme function. **sampling e.** That part of the difference between a population value and an estimate thereof, derived from a random sample, which is due to the fact that only a sample of values is observed, as distinct from errors due to imperfect selection, bias in response or estimation, or errors in observation and recording. Sampling error, itself a random variable, is inversely proportional to the square root of the size of the sample. **standard e.** The positive square root of the variance of a a set of observations or of a function of the set. The standard error of the mean of a set of observations is equal to the standard deviation of the observations divided by the square root of their number. Abbr. SE **type I e.** The error of rejecting a statistical hypothesis when it should have been accepted, that is, when it is true. **type II e.** The error of accepting a statistical hypothesis when it should have been rejected, that is, when it is false.

**eructation** \ē′ruktā′shən\ [L *eructatio* (from *eructare* to belch up, spew out, from *ructus* a belch) belching, disgorgement] The explosive oral expulsion of gas from the stomach; belching; a belch. **nervous e.** A neurosis characterized by repeated belching.

**erugation** \er′oogā′shən\ [E- + *rug(a)* + -ATION] RHYTIDECTOMY.

**eruption** \irup′shən\ [L *eruptio* (from *eruptus,* past part. of *erumpere* to break open, cause to burst forth) a breaking open, bursting forth] 1 The process of breaking out with a skin rash. 2 A visible rash or other cutaneous disruption. 3 See under ERUPTION OF TEETH. **active e.** The movement of a tooth from its germinative position into the oral cavity. **butterfly e.** A rash on the nose and cheeks in a distribution that resembles the shape of a butterfly. It is suggestive of but not pathognomonic of lupus erythematosus. Also *butterfly, butterfly patch, butterfly rash.* **clinical e.** The penetration of a tooth through the mucosa and into the oral cavity. **continuous e.** Tooth eruption which occurs throughout life because of the continuous production of dental tissues. **creeping e.** CUTANEOUS LARVA MIGRANS. **delayed e.** 1 A general delay in the eruption of the deciduous or permanent teeth. It may be associated with defective development of the skeleton, as in rickets, or with local obstacles, as in hereditary gingival fibromatosis. 2 A delay in the eruption of individual teeth, caused by lack of space, the retention of a deciduous tooth, or the presence of a dentigerous cyst. **demodectic e.** Demodectic acariasis occurring in humans. **drug e.** Dermatitis caused by a drug or medicine, whether administered systemically or topically. Also *drug rash, dermatitis medicamentosa, eczema medicamentosa, medicinal rash.* **fixed e.** An eruption recurring at the identical site or sites. **Kaposi's varicelliform e.** Either eczema herpeticum or eczema vaccinatum. Also *pustulosis vacciniformis acuta.* **morbilliform e.** An eruption that resembles the rash of measles. **partial e.** A state of incomplete eruption of a tooth made more or less permanent by an obstructive condition such as impaction. **passive e.** The physiologic retraction of the gingiva after a newly erupted tooth has met its opponent, giving the appearance of further movement of the tooth relative to the bone. **polymorphous light e.** A variable acquired light sensitivity eruption, characterized by the development of plaques or papules on light-exposed skin. Also *polymorphous photodermatitis.* **sandworm e.** CUTANEOUS LARVA MIGRANS. **serum e.** The urticarial eruption that forms a characteristic feature of serum sickness. **summer e.** MILIARIA. **surgical e.** The eruption of a tooth facilitated by the removal of overlying bone or other obstacle such as a supernumerary tooth or dentigerous cyst. It is sometimes necessary to apply traction to the unerupted tooth. **e. of teeth** 1 Piercing of the integuments of the gums by the crowns or cutting edges of the teeth as they develop. Eruption follows an orderly sequence, beginning with the two lower central incisors at the age of about six months and continuing until the full set of 20, the deciduous, first dentition, or milk teeth, is complete at about 30 months. At the age of about seven years the eruption of the second or permanent dentition and shedding of the milk teeth, starting with the lower first molar (six years), takes place until a full set of 32 teeth is present by the end of adolescence. There are many exceptions to the speed and orderliness of the sequence of eruption and occasionally one or more teeth remain permanently unerupted. 2 The movement of teeth towards the occlusal plane. **total e.** The complete eruption of a tooth including passive eruption. **vaccinal e.** Any eruption that is induced by vaccination against smallpox.

**ERV** expiratory reserve volume.

**-ery** \-erē\ [Middle English *-erie,* from Old French] A suffix meaning practice, trade. Also *-ry.*

**erysipelas** \er′isip′ələs\ [Gk, prob. akin to *erythros* red and *pella* skin] An acute skin infection by hemolytic streptococci, principally group A, characterized by a well-demarcated, spreading, erythematous inflammation, most commonly on the face, accompanied by pain and fever. Also *St. Anthony's fire.* **e. bullosum** Erysipelas complicated by the formation of bullae. **gangrenous e.** Erysipelas in which areas of necrosis occur. **hemorrhagic e.** Erysipelas accompanied by ecchymoses. **e. migrans** Erysipelas involving multiple sites successively. It may clear quickly in one part of the body only to appear in another part. Also *migratory erysipelas, wandering erysipelas.* **wandering e.** ERYSIPELAS MIGRANS.

**erysipeloid** \er′isip′əloid\ 1 Resembling or acting like erysipelas. 2 An infection, usually cutaneous, caused by *Erysipelothrix rhusiopathiae.* Also *erysipeloid of Rosenbach.*

***Erysipelothrix rhusiopathiae*** \er′isip′əlōthriks′ roo′sē·ōpath′i·ē\ A Gram-positive, nonsporulating, aerobic to microaerophilic bacillus, similar to *Listeria* in structure and in its wide distribution in nature. It occurs primarily in food handlers, entering the human skin through abrasions and causing erysipeloid. Also *Erysipelothrix insidiosa.*

**erysiphake** \eris′ifāk\ [Gk *erysi(s)* a dragging, drawing + *phak(os)* a lentil] A small suction cup for grasping the lens during a cataract extraction. Also *erisiphake.*

**eryth-** \irith-\ ERYTHRO-.

**erythema** \er′ithē′mə\ [Gk *erythēma* (from *erythainein* to redden, from *erythros* red) redness on the skin] An increased redness of the skin that is caused by capillary dilatation. **acrodynic e.** PINK DISEASE. **acute infectious e.** An acute infectious exanthematous fever, believed to be of viral origin, that is characterized by a confluent facial rash and a less profuse maculopapular eruption of the trunk and limbs. **e. annulare centrifugum** A symptomatic annular erythema characterized by the development of rings that increase in size, usually on the trunk. **e. a pudore** A mottled erythema of the neck and chest. It may accompany emotional blushing. **e. arthriticum epidemicum** HAVERHILL FEVER. **e. caloricum** Erythema induced by exposure to heat or light. **e. chronicum migrans** A centrifugal annular erythema of the skin which is the characteristic initial lesion of Lyme disease. It is caused by a newly recognized, penicillin-sensitive, *Treponema*-like spirochete residing in the gut of *Amblyomma americanum* and *Ixodes dammani* ticks, the arthropod vectors of Lyme disease. **circinate syphilitic e.** Erythema composed of the macular lesions of syphilis, which form as circles or parts of circles and which may coalesce. It is often associated with a relapse of syphilis following inadequate treatment with heavy metals. Also *neurosyphilid.* **cold e.** A hypersensitivity reaction to cold stimuli characterized by local vasodilatation. It appears to be hereditary and is thought to be produced by local serotonin release. **diaper e.** The inflammatory changes induced in parts of the area covered by a diaper and caused by chemical irritation and microbial activity. **e. dyschromicum perstans** A dermatosis of unknown origin in which grayish plaques on the trunk, limbs, and face present macules of hypomelanosis or hypermelanosis. **e. endemicum** PELLAGRA. **e. induratum** A chronic nodular vasculitis as seen in the calves in young women. Tuberculosis is one of several possible causes. **e. infectiosum** A mild systemic illness accompanied by a very distinctive rash, occasionally occurring in epidemic form mainly in children. The rash begins as an erythema on the cheeks, having the appearance of a slapped cheek. It subsequently invades the trunk, extremities, palms, and soles in a maculopapular form, which may be itchy and leave a reticular pattern as it fades. Mean duration is 11 days. The cause is unknown. Also *fifth disease, megalerythema, Sticker's disease.* **Jacquet's e.** Diaper dermatitis in which eroded and ulcerated papules are a conspicuous feature. Also *papuloerosive erythema.* **e. marginatum** ERYTHEMA MARGINATUM RHEUMATICUM. **e. marginatum rheumaticum** An eruption of rings or segments of rings, usually on the trunk, that is seen in about 10 percent of subjects with rheumatic fever. **e. multiforme** A distinctive reaction of the skin and mucous membranes that is characterized by the more or less symmetrical development of edematous papules, plaques, or bullae, predominantly on the extensor aspects of the extremities and on the buccolabial mucous membranes. It can be precipitated by various microbial agents, by drugs, or by other diseases. **e. multiforme bullosum** STEVENS-JOHNSON SYNDROME. **e. necroticans** 1 LUCIO PHENOMENON. 2 A rare necrotizing skin reaction complicating lepromatous leprosy. **e. neonatorum** A common benign and macular erythema evident in early infancy. **e. nodosum** An acute, self-limiting eruption of inflammatory nodules on the lower legs, and, less often, on the thighs and arms, often accompanied by an acute arthritis of the ankles. It may be produced by microbial agents, by drugs, or by other diseases. **e. nodosum leprosum** The dermatological component of the immune complex reaction that may complicate lepromatous leprosy. It is characterized by transient erythematous lesions which occasionally become vesicular or bullous. Abbr. ENL. **e. nodosum syphiliticum** SYPHILITIC ERYTHEMA NODOSUM. **e. nuchae** STORK BITE. **nummular e.** TINEA CIRCINATA. **palmar e.** A redness of the palms that occurs in pregnancy or in the presence of certain systemic diseases, notably those of the liver. **e. palmare hereditarium** Diffuse palmar eythema of early onset, apparently an isolated autosomal dominant trait. Also *Lane's disease.* **papuloerosive e.** JACQUET'S ERYTHEMA. **e. papulosum** An eruption of papules on a background of erythema. **pellagroid e.** Erythema resembling that which occurs in pellagra. Similar in appearance to severe sunburn, it is symmetrical over the parts of the body exposed to sunlight, especially the backs of the hands, the wrists, arms, face, and neck. **rheumatic e.** ERYTHEMA MARGINATUM RHEUMATICUM. **e. subitum** EXANTHEM SUBITUM. **syphilitic e. nodosum** A nodular syphilid of the skin of the shins or arms. Also *erythema nodosum syphiliticum.* **e. toxicum** A generalized erythema caused by a drug or other chemical substance or a bacterial toxin. **e. urticans** *Seldom used* URTICARIA.

**erythematous** \er′ithem′ətəs\ Affected by or characterized by erythema.

**erythr-** \irithr-\ ERYTHRO-.

**erythralgia** \er′ithral′jə\ ERYTHROMELALGIA.

**erythrasma** \er′ithraz′mə\ [ERYTHR- + Gk *-asma,* noun termination] A common, mild, chronic infection of the skin by *Corynebacterium minutissimum.*

**erythremia** \er′ithrē′mē·ə\ [ERYTHR- + -EMIA] **1** ERYTHROCYTOSIS. **2** POLYCYTHEMIA VERA. **acute e.** ERYTHROLEUKEMIA. **chronic e.** POLYCYTHEMIA VERA. **high-altitude e.** A greater than normal erythrocyte count, hemoglobin concentration, and hematocrit of blood, which is adaptive to the lower oxygen tension of air at high altitudes. This phenomenon occurs in persons living at moderate elevations, as in the Alps or the Rocky Mountains, and is quite marked in persons residing at extreme elevations, as in the Andes or Himalayas.

**erythritol** $CH_2OH—CHOH—CHOH—CH_2OH$. The $C_4$-sugar alcohol formed by reduction of erythrose. It is achiral, since its two chiral centers are mirror images of each other. It is found in the fetal fluids and placenta of cattle and several other animals, but not in man. It stimulates the growth of *Brucella,* and hence may account for the unusual viscerotropism of this organism.

**erythrityl tetranitrate** $C_4H_6N_4O_{12}$. 1,2,3,4-Butanetetrol tetranitrate, an orally effective nitrate that is often formulated in sustained release forms. It is used to treat and reduce the incidence of attacks of angina pectoris. Also *trinitrol.*

**erythro-** \irith′rō-\ [Gk *erythros* red] A combining form meaning (1) red; (2) erythrocyte. Also *ereuth-, eryth-, erythr-.*

**erythroblast** \irith′rōblast′\ [ERYTHRO- + -BLAST] Any nucleated cell that is a precursor of erythrocytes, including all cells of the normoblastic and megaloblastic series of erythrocytic maturation. Also *erythrocytoblast.* **acidophilic e.** ORTHOCHROMATIC NORMOBLAST. **basophilic e.** BASOPHILIC NORMOBLAST. **early e.** BASOPHILIC NORMOBLAST. **eosinophilic e.** ORTHOCHROMATIC NORMOBLAST. **intermediate e.** POLYCHROMATOPHILIC NORMOBLAST. **late e.** ORTHOCHROMATIC NORMOBLAST. **orthochromatic e.** ORTHOCHROMATIC NORMOBLAST. **oxyphilic e.** ORTHOCHROMATIC NORMOBLAST. **polychromatophilic e.** POLYCHROMATOPHILIC NORMOBLAST.

**erythroblastemia** \-blastē′mē·ə\ ERYTHROBLASTOSIS.

**erythroblastic** \-blas′tik\ NORMOBLASTIC.

**erythroblastoma** \-blastō′mə\ A soft-tissue mass composed of erythroblasts. Such masses may occur in patients with severe anemias, and may cause compression of the brain, spinal cord, or other vital structures. Also *extramedullary hematopoietic tumor.*

**erythroblastomatosis** \-blas′tōmətō′sis\ The presence of numerous erythroblastomas in different tissues or organs.

**erythroblastopenia** \-blas′tōpē′nē·ə\ Diminution or absence of erythrocyte precursors in bone marrow. **idiopathic transitory e.** An anemia of childhood due to temporary suppression of erythropoiesis, usually following a viral or bacterial infection. Besides the anemia, there is reticulocytopenia and nearly complete absence of normoblasts in bone marrow. The cause is unknown. Recovery is spontaneous within a few weeks. Also *transitory erythroblastopenia of childhood.*

**erythroblastosis** \-blastō′sis\ [ERYTHROBLAST + -OSIS] The presence of nucleated erythrocyte precursors in circulating blood. Also *erythroblastemia.* **e. fetalis** Severe hemolytic disease of the newborn, typically accompanied by the presence of numerous nucleated erythrocyte precursors in the blood and high concentration of bilirubin in serum. Formerly, incompatibility of Rh antigens of fetal and maternal blood was the principal cause. Also *erythroblastosis neonatorum, icterus gravis neonatorum.*

**erythroblastotic** \-blastät′ik\ Pertaining to, characterized by, or resulting from erythroblastosis.

**erythrocatalysis** \-kətal′isis\ ERYTHROPHAGOCYTOSIS.

**erythrochromia** \-krō′mē·ə\ [ERYTHRO- + CHROM- + -IA] A red appearance of the cerebrospinal fluid, attributable to the presence of red blood cells.

**erythrocuprein** SUPEROXIDE DISMUTASE.

**erythrocyanosis** \-sī′ənō′sis\ [ERYTHRO- + CYANOSIS] A disorder characterized by swelling and blueness of the legs. It occurs chiefly in young women and seems to result from vascular spasm associated with inadequate protection. Also *erythrocyanosis supramalleolaris, silk-stocking disease.* **e. frigida** A benign condition of the skin of the lower extremities characterized by sluggish cutaneous circulation that results in a bluish red discoloration. **e. supramalleolaris** ERYTHROCYANOSIS.

**erythrocyte** \irith′rōsīt′\ [ERYTHRO- + -CYTE] An anucleate cell, normally the most common formed element in circulating blood, filled with hemoglobin and shaped as a biconcave disk. Also *red cell, red blood cell, red corpuscle, red blood corpuscle.* **basophilic e.** An erythrocyte with affinity for basic dyes, usually a young cell with residual cytoplasmic ribosomal RNA. **burr e.** ECHINOCYTE. **crenated e.** ECHINOCYTE. **dichromatic e.** POLYCHROMATOPHILIC ERYTHROCYTE. **orthochromatic e.** An erythrocyte whose cytoplasm exhibits solely acidophilic staining. **polychromatophilic e.** An erythrocyte which, when stained, displays both basophilia and eosinophilia of varying intensity in different parts of its cytoplasm. Also *polychromatic erythrocyte, dichromatic erythrocyte.* **reticulated e.** RETICULOCYTE. **target e.** A red blood cell that resembles a target or "bull's eye" on microscopic examination. Electron microscopy indicates that target erythrocytes are bell-shaped. The deformity in shape is due to a relative redundancy of erythrocyte membrane for the size of the cell. Also *Mexican hat cell, target cell.*

**erythrocyte transketolase** A thiamin-dependent enzyme used to assess a person's thiamin status. The enzyme is measured in red blood cells in the presence and absence of added thiamin pyrophosphate. If the enzyme activity increases by more than 25 percent in the presence of excess thiamin pyrophosphate, it indicates thiamin deficiency.

**erythrocythemia** \-sīthē′mē·ə\ ERYTHROCYTOSIS.

**erythrocytic** \-sit′ik\ Of or relating to erythrocytes.

**erythrocytoblast** \-sī′təblast\ ERYTHROBLAST.

**erythrocytolysin** \-sītäl′isin\ HEMOLYSIN.

**erythrocytolysis** \-sītäl′isis\ HEMOLYSIS.

**erythrocytometer** \-sītäm′ətər\ A device used in the enumeration of erythrocytes. Also *erythrometer.*

**erythrocytometry** \-sītäm′ətrē\ The enumeration of erythrocytes in a blood specimen or other body fluid. Also *erythrometry.*

**erythrocyto-opsonin** \-sī′tō-äp′sənin\ HEMOLYSIN.

**erythrocytopenia** \-sī′təpē′nē·ə\ A decrease in the number or concentration of erythrocytes; anemia. Also *erythropenia.*

**erythrocytophagy** \-sītäf′əjē\ ERYTHROPHAGOCYTOSIS.

**erythrocytopoiesis** \-sī′təpoi·ē′sis\ ERYTHROPOIESIS.

**erythrocytorrhexis** \-sī′tôrek′sis\ [*erythrocyt(e)* + -RRHEXIS ] A degenerative alteration in the appearance of erythrocytes, characterized by the extrusion of filaments of erythrocyte membrane (myelin figures). This occurs in blood that has been incubated for a few days *in vitro* or *in vivo* following extensive burns or in some hemolytic disorders. Also *microspherulation, erythrocytic ecdysis.*

**erythrocytosis** \-sītō′sis\ [*erythrocyt(e)* + -OSIS] A greater than normal number of erythrocytes in the blood;

polycythemia. Also *erythrocythemia, erythremia, hypercythemia, hypererythrocythemia.* **anoxemic e.** COMPENSATORY POLYCYTHEMIA. **renal e.** Increased production of erythrocytes in certain renal diseases, such as polycystic renal disease, presumbably due to increased secretion of erythropoietin by the kidney. **stress e.** A condition in which the hematocrit, erythrocyte count, or hemoglobin concentration of venous blood exceeds normal limits as a consequence of less than normal plasma volume rather than being due to increased numbers of erythrocytes. The spurious " erythrocytosis" was once believed to occur mostly in tense, obese middle-aged males. It is probably not a single entity. Also *stress polycythemia, polycythemia hypertonica, Gaisböck syndrome, Gaisböck's disease, pseudopolycythemia.*

**erythrocyturia** \-sītʸoo′rē·ə\ [*erythrocyt(e)* + -URIA] HEMATURIA.

**erythroderma** \-dur′mə\ [ERYTHRO- + -DERMA] Extensive, often universal, persistent erythema of the skin. It is usually associated with exfoliation. Also *generalized exfoliative dermatitis.* **bullous ichthyosiform e.** An autosomal dominant generalized skin disorder of congenital or perinatal onset that is characterized by epidermal erosions, skin infection, and abnormal arrangement of tonofibrils. Also *bullous erythroderma ichthyosiformis congenita of Brocq, bullous ichthyosiform hyperkeratosis.* **congenital ichthyosiform e.** SJÖGREN-LARSSON SYNDROME. **desquamative e.** EXFOLIATIVE ERYTHRODERMA. **exfoliative e.** Extensive and persistent erythema associated with exfoliation. Also *desquamative erythroderma.* **ichthyosiform e.** SJÖGREN-LARSSON SYNDROME. **e. ichthyosiforme congenitum** SJÖGREN-LARSSON SYNDROME. **leukemic e.** A generalized red rash, often pruritic, that may occur in chronic lymphocytic leukemia or the Sézary syndrome as a result of cutaneous infiltration by the leukemic cells. **lymphoblastic e.** Any generalized erythroderma with cutaneous infiltration of immature lymphocytes, such as the Sézary syndrome. *Obs.* **e. psoriaticum** Erythroderma arising from or based on psoriasis. **resistant maculopapular scaly e.** PARAPSORIASIS EN PLAQUES.

**erythrogenesis** \-jen′əsis\ ERYTHROPOIESIS. **e. imperfecta** FANCONI'S ANEMIA.

**erythrogenic** \-jen′ik\ **1** Causing a red color or a red skin rash. **2** Causing the formation of erythrocytes. Seldom used in this sense.

**erythroid** \er′ithroid, irith′roid\ Pertaining to erythrocytes and erythrocyte precursors.

**erythrokatalysis** \-kətal′isis\ [ERYTHRO- + Gk *katalysis* (from KATA + LYSIS) a dissolving] ERYTHROPHAGOCYTOSIS.

**erythrokeratoderma** \-ker′ətōdur′mə\ [ERYTHRO- + KERATODERMA] Hyperkeratosis in the presence of erythema. It is seen in several hereditary disorders of keratinization. Also *erythrokeratodermia.* **progressive symmetrical verrucous e.** A genetically determined syndrome in which plaques of erythrokeratoderma develop on the extremities from infancy to puberty, sparing the palms and soles. Also *Gottron syndrome.*

**erythrokinetics** \-kinet′iks\ **1** The rate of formation and destruction of erythrocytes. **2** The length of time an erythrocyte remains in the blood before it is removed and destroyed.

**erythroleukemia** \-lookē′mē·ə\ A malignant proliferation of erythrocyte precursors, characterized by anemia, abnormal erythrocyte precursors in blood films, and a marked increase in erythrocyte precursors in bone marrow, most of which are morphologically bizarre. Myeloblasts may also be increased, especially in late stages. Also *Di Guglielmo's disease, acute erythremia, Blumenthal's disease, Di Guglielmo syndrome.*

**erythroleukoblastosis** \-loo′kəblastō′sis\ HEMOLYTIC DISEASE OF THE NEWBORN.

**erythrolysin** \er′ithräl′isin\ HEMOLYSIN.

**erythrolysis** \er′ithräl′isis\ HEMOLYSIS.

**erythromelalgia** \-melal′jə\ [ERYTHRO- + MEL-[1] + -ALGIA] A syndrome in which a painful burning sensation in one or more extremities is associated with conspicuous erythema and a raised skin temperature. Also *terminal neuritis* (outmoded), *erythralgia, Gerhardt's disease, Mitchell's disease, Weir Mitchell's disease.*

**erythrometer** \er′ithräm′ətər\ ERYTHROCYTOMETER.

**erythrometry** \er′ithräm′ətrē\ ERYTHROCYTOMETRY.

**erythromycin** $C_{37}H_{67}NO_{13}$. A naturally occurring macrolide antibiotic produced by *Streptomyces erythreus.* It is effective against a wide spectrum of Gram-positive and Gram-negative bacteria, and it is highly effective against *Mycoplasma pneumoniae.* It is used in treating patients who have shown an allergic reaction toward penicillin and against organisms resistant to penicillin medications. It is given orally, topically, and parenterally, and it is formulated in a variety of salts for more favorable pharmacokinetic properties of the medication. **e. B** BERYTHROMYCIN.

**erythromycin estolate** $C_{40}H_{71}NO_{14}{\cdot}C_{12}H_{26}O_4S$. The lauryl sulfate ester form of erythromycin. It is given orally for the same indications as the parent drug. Also *erythromycin propionate lauryl sulfate.*

**erythromycin ethylcarbonate** $C_{40}H_{71}NO_{15}$. The ethylcarbonate salt of erythromycin. It is used by oral administration for the same indications as the parent drug.

**erythromycin ethylsuccinate** $C_{43}H_{75}NO_{16}$. The ethylsuccinate salt form of erythromycin. It is given orally or intramuscularly for the same indications as the parent drug.

**erythromycin gluceptate** $C_{37}H_{67}NO_{13}{\cdot}C_7H_{14}O_8$. The gluceptate (glucoheptonate) salt form of erythromycin. It is given intravenously for the same indications as the parent drug.

**erythromycin lactobionate** $C_{37}H_{67}NO_{13}{\cdot}C_{12}H_{22}O_{12}$. The lactobionate (lactobiono-δ-lactone) salt form of erythromycin. It is used for the same indications as the parent drug. It is given intravenously.

**erythromycin propionate** $C_{40}H_{71}NO_{14}$. The propionate salt form of erythromycin. It is used by oral administration for the same indications as the parent drug.

**erythromycin propionate lauryl sulfate** ERYTHROMYCIN ESTOLATE.

**erythromycin stearate** $C_{37}H_{67}NO_{13}{\cdot}C_{18}H_{36}O_2$. The stearate salt form of erythromycin. It is given orally, and used for the same indications as the parent drug.

**erythron** \irith′rän\ All of the erythrocytes as well as their precursors, in both blood and bone marrow, taken as a whole.

**erythroparasite** \-par′əsīt\ Any organism that parasitizes erythrocytes.

**erythropenia** \-pē′nē·ə\ ERYTHROCYTOPENIA.

**erythrophage** \irith′rōfāj\ ERYTHROPHAGOCYTE.

**erythrophagia** \-fā′jə\ ERYTHROPHAGOCYTOSIS.

**erythrophagocyte** \-fag′əsīt\ Any cell that engulfs and destroys erythrocytes. Also *erythrophage, hematophage, hemophage, hematophagocyte, hemophagocyte.*

**erythrophagocytosis** \-fag′əsītō′sis\ The engulfment and destruction of erythrocytes by phagocytes. Also *erythrocytophagy, erythrophagy, erythrophagia, erythrocatalysis, erythrokatalysis, hemophagocytosis.*

**erythrophagous** \er′ithräf′əgəs\ Pertaining to or characterized by erythrophagocytosis.

**erythrophagy** \er′ithräf′əjē\ ERYTHROPHAGOCYTOSIS.

**erythrophobia** \-fō′bē·ə\ [ERYTHRO- + -PHOBIA] Pathologic fear of red, of blood, or of blushing.

**erythrophore** \irith′rōfôr\ A chromatophore which has a red-brown color and is insoluble in alcohol. Also *allophore*.

**erythroplasia** \-plā′zhə\ [ERYTHRO- + -PLASIA] A condition in which painless erythematous lesions occur in areas covered by squamous epithelium, such as a mucous membrane. **e. of Queyrat** A rare, intraepidermal squamous cell carcinoma presenting as a sharply marginated, flat plaque on the glans penis. **Zoon's e.** A nonmalignant condition affecting the glans penis (plasma cell balanitis) or the vulva (plasma cell vulvitis), in which small erythematous papular lesions are seen on mucosal and cutaneous surfaces. It is characterized histologically by plasma cell infiltration of the dermis, epidermal atrophy, and spongiosis.

**erythropoiesis** \-poi·ē′sis\ [ERYTHRO- + -POIESIS] The formation of erythrocytes. Also *erythrogenesis, erythrocytopoiesis*. Adj. erythropoietic.

**erythropoietin** \-poi′ətin\ A protein with MW of approximately 46 000, synthesized mainly in the kidney, which directly stimulates erythropoiesis in bone marrow.

**erythropsia** \er′ithräp′sē·ə\ [ERYTHR- + -OPSIA] A color vision fault in which red is abnormally prominent, occurring most commonly following prolonged exposure of a aphakic eye to bright light.

**erythropyknosis** \-pik·nō′sis\ The alteration in erythrocytes caused by malarial parasites, resulting in the so-called brassy bodies.

**erythrosarcoma** \-särkō′mə\ ERYTHROBLASTIC MYELOSARCOMA.

**erythrose** One of the two isomeric aldose tetroses (the other being threose) of the formula CHO—CHOH—CHOH—$CH_2OH$. Erythrose on oxidation to tartaric acid gives the meso compound. Its 4-phosphate is an intermediate in the pentose-phosphate pathway and in photosynthesis. It can be derived from fructose 6-phosphate and a $C_2$-acceptor (an aldose) by the action of transketolase, and from sedoheptulose 7-phosphate and a $C_3$-acceptor by the action of transaldolase.

**erythrosin** The sodium or potassium salt of iodeosin. It is soluble in water or alcohol and is used as a biologic stain and an artificial food color.

**erythrosis** \er′ithrō′sis\ [ERYTHR- + -OSIS] A reddish or ruddy color of the skin occurring in polycythemia. **e. of Bechterew** An often familial disorder, intermediate between acrocyanosis and erythromelalgia, that is characterized by redness and swelling of the hands, feet, nose, and ears. It begins in childhood and runs a chronic progressive course.

**Es** Symbol for the element, einsteinium.

**escape** The emergence of a lower cardiac pacemaker from the usual suppression by a higher one. If the sinuatrial discharge rate slows or a conduction defect occurs, an ectopic impulse may arise because of escape of pacemaker in the atrioventricular junctional tissue or ventricular tissue, which then controls ventricular activity. **atrioventricular e.** ATRIOVENTRICULAR JUNCTIONAL ESCAPE. **atrioventricular junctional e.** The emergence of a pacemaker in the atrioventricular junctional tissue. It escapes from the control of the sinuatrial node when discharge from the latter becomes abnormally slow. Also *atrioventricular escape, nodal escape, vagal escape*. **nasal e.** NASAL EMISSION. **nodal e.** ATRIOVENTRICULAR JUNCTIONAL ESCAPE. **vagal e.** ATRIOVENTRICULAR JUNCTIONAL ESCAPE. **ventricular e.** An ectopic beat arising from a ventricular pacemaker which has escaped from control from higher centers.

**-escence** \-es′əns\ [See -ESCENT.] A suffix meaning the action or becoming or the state of being.

**-escent** \-es′ənt\ [L *-escens*, gen. *-escentis*, pres. participial ending of verbs whose infinitives end in *-escere*] A suffix meaning beginning to be, becoming.

**eschar** \es′kär\ [Gk *eschara* hearth, fireplace, scab. See also SCAR.] A slough produced by a caustic or corrosive substance. **burn e.** The nonviable skin debris, composed of devitalized dermis and coagulum, on the surface of a full thickness or deep dermal burn. It should be distinguished from the crusts that form on a superficial burn as a result of coagulated plasma.

**escharotic** \es′kärät′ik\ [Gk *escharōtikos* tending to cause an eschar] **1** Caustic; corrosive. **2** A chemical agent with caustic or corrosive properties.

**escharotomy** \es′kärät′əmē\ [ESCHAR + *o* + -TOMY] A procedure involving incisions made through a burn eschar to relieve pressure underneath. It is frequently needed in cases of full thickness circumferential burns of the extremities or of the chest.

**Escherich** [Theodor *Escherich*, German physician, 1857–1911] See under TEST, SIGN.

***Escherichia coli*** \esh′ərik′ē·ə kō′lī \ [after Theodor *Escherich* (German physician, 1857–1911) + L *coli* of the colon] A species of enterobacteria that can ferment lactose by the mixed acid fermentation and releases dihydrogen from the resulting formic acid. Citrate is not utilized. It is the major facultative anaerobe of the gut flora. Some strains are invasive or toxigenic, the enterotoxins (LT and ST) being coded by plasmids. It is also a major cause of urinary tract infections and of neonatal meningitis. Many serologic types have been distinguished.

**eseptate** \ēsep′tāt\ Without a septum or septa.

**eserine** \es′ərin\ PHYSOSTIGMINE.

**ESF** erythropoietic stimulating factor.

**-esis** \-ē′sis\ [Gk stem vowel *-ē-* + noun-forming suffix *-sis*] A suffix usually denoting a process, as in *diapedesis*.

**Esmarch** [Johann Friedrich August von *Esmarch*, German surgeon, 1823–1908] See under TOURNIQUET.

**eso-** \es′ō-, ē′sō-\ [Gk *esō* within] A prefix meaning inner, within, or inward.

**esodeviation** \ē′sōdēv′ē·ā′shən\ [ESO- + DEVIATION] A misalignment of one eye into an abnormally convergent position.

**esodic** \ēsäd′ik\ AFFERENT.

**esophagalgia** \esäf′əgal′jə\ [*esophag(o)-* + -ALGIA] Pain in the esophagus. Also *esophagodynia*.

**esophageal** \esäf′əjē′əl, ē′sōfā′jē·əl\ Pertaining to the esophagus.

**esophagectasia** \esäf′əjektā′zhə\ [*esophag(o)-* + ECTASIA] Enlargement or dilatation of the esophagus. Also *esophagectasis, esophagoectasis*.

**esophagectasis** \esäf′əjek′təsis\ ESOPHAGECTASIA.

**esophagectomy** \esäf′əjek′təmē\ [*esophag(o)-* + -ECTOMY] The surgical excision of the greater part of the esophagus, especially for the cure or palliation of carcinoma of the esophagus or of the esophagus and cardia. It is followed by gastric or colonic replacement.

**esophagismus** \esäf′əjiz′məs\ Muscular spasm of the esophagus; esophagospasm. Also *esophagism*.

**esophagitis** \esäf′əjī′tis\ [*esophag(o)-* + -ITIS] Inflammation of the esophagus. **acute corrosive e.** Inflammation of the esophagus due to ingestion of strong chemicals. Substances most commonly ingested or swallowed are strong acids such as sulfuric or nitric acid, alkalis such as sodium hydroxide or potash, oxalic acid, iodine, bichloride of mercury, arsenic, silver nitrate, and phenol. **chronic hy-**

**perkeratotic e.** Chronic inflammation of the esophagus with hyperkeratinization due to iron deficiency. **peptic e.** Esophagitis caused by acid reflex from the stomach. Also *reflux esophagitis.* **reflux e.** PEPTIC ESOPHAGITIS. **thrush e.** Esophagitis caused by the thrush fungus (*Candida* spp.).

**esophago-** \esäf′əgō-\ [Gk *oisophágos* (from *ois-*, stem of *pherein* to carry + *phagein* to eat) esophagus] A combining form denoting the esophagus. Also *oesophago-* (British spelling).

**esophagocardiomyotomy** \-kär′dē·ōmī·ät′əmē\ CARDIOMYOTOMY.

**esophagocele** \esäf′əgōsēl′\ [ESOPHAGO- + -CELE[1]] An abnormal protrusion of mucosa and submucosa through the muscular layer of the esophagus.

**esophagocologastrostomy** \-kō′ləgasträs′təmē\ [ESOPHAGO- + COLO- + GASTRO- + -STOMY] The surgical interposition of a segment of colon following esophageal resection to recreate continuity of the esophagus with the stomach.

**esophagoduodenostomy** \-d$^y$oo′ōdenäs′təmē\ A surgical anastomosis between the esophagus and the duodenum. Such a procedure usually follows a removal or bypass of the stomach.

**esophagodynia** \-din′ē·ə\ [*esophag(o)-* + -ODYNIA] ESOPHAGALGIA.

**esophagoectasis** \-ek′təsis\ ESOPHAGECTASIA.

**esophagoenterostomy** \-en′təräs′təmē\ [ESOPHAGO- + ENTERO- + -STOMY] A surgical anastomosis of the esophagus and a segment of intestine.

**esophagoesophagostomy** \-esäf′əgas′təmē\ A surgical anastomosis of two formerly separated segments of esophagus.

**esophagofundopexy** \-fun′dōpek′sē\ [ESOPHAGO- + *fund(us)* + *o* + -PEXY] The surgical fixation of the esophagus to the fundus of the stomach. It is often performed to prevent reflux of the gastric contents into the esophagus.

**esophagogastrectomy** \-gastrek′təmē\ [ESOPHAGO- + GASTRECTOMY] The surgical removal of part of the esophagus and adjacent stomach tissue.

**esophagogastric** \-gas′trik\ Relating to both esophagus and stomach.

**esophagogastroanastomosis** \-gas′trō-ənas′təmō′sis\ GASTROESOPHAGOSTOMY.

**esophagogastromyotomy** \-gas′trōmī·ät′əmē\ An incision through the muscles of the esophagus and stomach.

**esophagogastroplasty** \-gas′trəplas′tē\ Plastic repair of the junction of the esophagus and stomach. Also *cardioplasty.*

**esophagogastroscopy** \-gasträs′kəpē\ [ESOPHAGO- + GASTROSCOPY] Examination of the esophagus and stomach with an endoscope.

**esophagogastrostomy** \-gasträs′təmē\ GASTROESOPHAGOSTOMY.

**esophagogram** \esäf′əgōgram′\ A roentgenogram obtained during esophagography.

**esophagography** \esäf′əgäg′rəfē\ [ESOPHAGO- + -GRAPHY] Roentgenography of the esophagus while or immediately after the patient swallows a positive contrast medium such as barium sulfate suspended in water.

**esophagohiatal** \-hī·ā′təl\ Relating to the esophageal hiatus, or to the esophagus and the esophageal hiatus.

**esophagojejunogastrostomosis** \-jəjoo′nōgasträs′tōmō′sis\ [ESOPHAGO- + JEJUNO- + GASTRO- + *(ana)-stomosis*] The surgical interposition of a segment of jejunum between the esophagus and the stomach to preserve alimentary continuity. Also *gastrojejunoesophagostomy, esophagojejunogastrostomy.*

**esophagojejunogastrostomy** \-jəjoo′nōgasträs′təmē\ ESOPHAGOJEJUNOGASTROSTOMOSIS.

**esophagojejunoplasty** \-jəjoo′nōplas′tē\ [ESOPHAGO- + JEJUNO- + -PLASTY] The surgical repair of a defect in the esophagus by using a segment of jejunum.

**esophagojejunostomy** \-jəjoonäs′təmē\ [ESOPHAGO- + JEJUNO- + -STOMY] The surgical creation of a communication between the esophagus and the jejunum.

**esophagolaryngectomy** \-lar′injek′təmē\ An inaccurate term for ESOPHAGOPHARYNGOLARYNGECTOMY.

**esophagology** \esäf′əgäl′əjē\ [ESOPHAGO- + -LOGY] The study of the esophagus and its diseases.

**esophagomyotomy** \-mī·ät′əmē\ CARDIOMYOTOMY. **Heller e.** CARDIOMYOTOMY.

**esophagopharyngolaryngectomy** \-fəring′gōlar′injek′təmē\ Excision of the larynx in continuity with the laryngopharynx and esophagus as a preliminary to the restoration of swallowing by visceral transposition via the posterior mediastinum. The operation is indicated for certain malignant tumors of the cervical esophagus and hypopharynx. Also *esophagolaryngectomy* (inaccurate).

**esophagoplasty** \esäf′əgōplas′tē\ Plastic repair or complete reconstruction of the esophagus.

**esophagoplication** \-plīkā′shən\ [ESOPHAGO- + PLICATION] The reduction in size of the lumen of a segment of the esophagus or of an esophageal pouch by the creation and suturing of vertical folds.

**esophagoscope** \esäf′əgōskōp\ [ESOPHAGO- + -SCOPE] Any of various instruments for the endoscopic examination of the esophagus. **Negus e.** A rigid endoscope that is modified with a slot near its distal end. When inserted into the esophagus of a subject with bleeding esophageal varices,

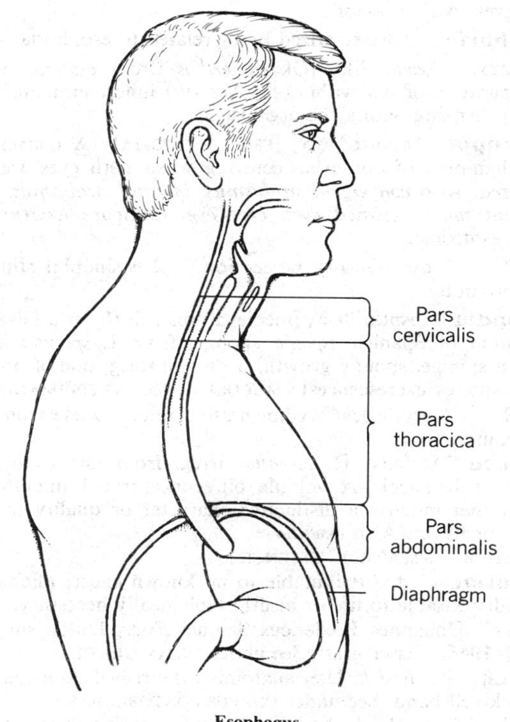


Esophagus

each varix can be trapped within the slot for injection sclerotherapy.

**esophagoscopy** \esäf′əgäs′kəpē\ Visualization of the esophagus with an esophagoscope.

**esophagospasm** \esäf′əgōspazm′\ Spasm of the esophageal walls. See also DIFFUSE ESOPHAGEAL SPASM.

**esophagostenosis** \-stenō′sis\ [ESOPHAGO- + STENOSIS] Abnormal narrowing of the esophagus.

**esophagostoma** \esäf′əgäs′təmə\ [ESOPHAGO- + STOMA] The external opening of a surgically created communication between the skin and the esophagus.

**esophagostomy** \esäf′əgäs′təmē\ [ESOPHAGO- + -STOMY] The surgical creation of a stoma into the esophagus.

**esophagotomy** \esäf′əgät′əmē\ [ESOPHAGO- + -TOMY] An incision into the esophagus.

**esophagotracheal** \-trā′kē·əl\ Relating or connecting the esophagus and the trachea.

**esophagus** \esäf′əgəs\ [Gk *oisophagos* (from *ois*-, fut. stem of *pherein* to carry + *phagein* to eat) esophagus] (*pl.* esophagi) [NA] The vertical muscular tube that connects the pharynx to the stomach. It extends from the lower margin of the cricoid cartilage opposite the sixth cervical vertebra to the level of the eleventh thoracic vertebra. It is constricted at its commencement, behind the arch of the aorta, behind the left principal bronchus, and where it pierces the diaphragm. It is divided into pars cervicalis, pars thoracica, and pars abdominalis. **Barrett's e.** Glandular metaplasia of the esophageal mucosa. It is considered a sequel to chronic reflux esophagitis and a lesion with a risk for the development of adenocarcinoma of the esophagus.

**esophoria** \es′ōfôr′ē·ə\ [ESO- + -PHORIA] A convergent misalignment of one eye which occurs when binocular fusion is prevented, as by covering the eye, but not when both eyes are uncovered; a latent tendency to convergent deviation of the eyes. Adj. esophoric.

**esophoric** Characterized by or related to esophoria.

**esoteric** \es′əter′ik\ [Gk *esōterikos* (from *esōteros* inner, comparative of *esō* within + *-ikos* -IC) inner, intimate, esoteric] Arising within the organism.

**esotropia** \es′ōtrō′pē·ə\ [ESO- + TROPIA] A convergent misalignment of one eye, occurring when both eyes are uncovered. Also *convergent strabismus, internal strabismus, convergent squint, crossed eyes, cross-eye*. Compare EXOTROPIA. Adj. esotropic.

**ESP** 1 extrasensory perception. 2 eosinophil stimulator promoter.

**espundia** \espUn′dē·ə\ [medieval Spanish (from a false latinization of Spanish *esponja* sponge, from L *spongia*, from Gk, a sponge, spongy growth) a disease (orig. one of horses) with spongy excrescences] MUCOCUTANEOUS LEISHMANIASIS.

**ESR** 1 erythrocyte sedimentation rate. 2 electron spin resonance.

**essence** \es′əns\ [L *essentia* (irreg. from *esse* to be) essence, substance] A volatile oil, concentrated tincture, or spirit that imparts a distinctive character or quality to perfume or flavor. Also *essentia*.

**essentia** \esen′shə\ ESSENCE.

**essential** 1 Attributable to no known cause; idiopathic. 2 Indispensable to life or health: biologically necessary.

**Esser** [Johannes Fredericus Samuel *Esser*, Dutch surgeon, 1877–1946] Esser graft. See under INLAY GRAFT.

**Essick** [C. *Essick*, U.S. anatomist, flourished 20th century] Essick cell band. See under CORPUS PONTOBULBARE.

**EST** electroshock therapy (electroconvulsive therapy).

**ester** \es′tər\ [German coinage, prob. from *Es(sigä)ther* acetic ether, i.e., ethyl acetate] A compound derived from an acid by replacing an acidic hydroxyl group with an alkoxyl group. If the acid is a carboxylic acid, R—COOH, its ester has the structure R—CO—O—R′. Biologically important esters include nucleic acids (esters of phosphoric acid) and fats. **Cori e.** *Older term* GLUCOSE 1-PHOSPHATE. **Embden e.** *Obs.* GLUCOSE 6-PHOSPHATE. **Robison e.** *Obs.* GLUCOSE 6-PHOSPHATE.

**esterase** Any enzyme that catalyzes the hydrolysis of an ester.

**esterify** \ester′ifī\ To convert an acid into its ester.

**Estes** [William Lawrence *Estes*, Jr., U.S. surgeon, 1885–1940] See under OPERATION.

**esthematology** \esthē′mətäl′əjē\ [Gk *aisthēma*, gen. *aisthēmato(s)* perception, sense + -LOGY] The study of the senses and of the organs and structures which subserve them.

**esthesia** \esthē′zhə\ [Gk *aisthēs(is)* perception by the senses, esp. by feeling + -IA] Ability to perceive a sensation: sensibility: often used in combination. Adj. esthesic.

**esthesio-** \esthē′zē·ō-\ [Gk *aisthēsis* perception by the senses, especially by feeling] A combining form meaning sensation, sensory perception. Also *aesthesio-* (British spelling).

**esthesioblast** \esthē′zē·ōblast′\ [ESTHESIO- + -BLAST] GANGLIOBLAST.

**esthesiogen** \esthē′zē·əjən\ An agent capable of inducing a sensation.

**esthesiography** \esthē′zē·äg′rəfē\ ESTHESIOMETRY.

**esthesiology** \esthē′zē·äl′əjē\ [ESTHESIO- + -LOGY] The science or study of the senses.

**esthesiometry** \esthē′zē·äm′ətrē\ [ESTHESIO- + -METRY] 1 The study or description of sensory mechanisms. 2 The determination of areas of sensation on the skin. For defs. 1 and 2 also *esthesiography*.

**esthesioneurocytoma** \-n$^y$Ur′əsītō′mə\ *Rare* OLFACTORY NEUROCYTOMA.

**esthesioneuroepithelioma** \-n$^y$Ur′ō·ep′ithē′lē·ō′mə\ NEUROEPITHELIOMA.

**esthesiophysiology** \-fiz′ē·äl′əjē\ The physiology of the senses; sensory physiology.

**esthetic** \esthet′ik\ 1 Of or relating to sensation; esthesic. 2 Having to do with qualities of appearance or attractiveness, especially when compared to the normal range of such qualities. For defs. 1 and 2 also *aesthetic*.

**estimation** [L *aestimatio* (from *aestimatus*, past part. of *aestimare* to value, appreciate) a valuing, price] In statistics, a technique for establishing the value of a parameter on the basis of a sample of observations. If the observations are taken from a random sample, the precision of the resulting estimate of the parameter can be given an exact expression. **magnitude e.** A method of psychophysical ratio scaling in which an observer makes direct numerical estimates of subjective stimulus magnitudes. A standard stimulus is first presented and the subject told that the sensation it produces has a given numerical value, such as 100. Alternatively, the arbitrarily chosen value may be assigned by the observer himself. Other comparison stimuli are then presented and the observer is asked to assign a number to the sensation relative to the standard stimulus. The data obtained from several observers may then be pooled to construct a ratio scale of subjective magnitude, using the geometric mean. **numerical e.** A calculation of the estimated date of an expectant mother's confinement by counting 296 days from a single episode of fruitful coitus.

**estival** \es′tivəl\ Occurring in or relating to summer.

**estivation** \es′tivā′shən\ [L *aestiv(are)* (from *aestivus* pertaining to summer, from *aestas* summer) to spend the summer + -ATION] A regular period of dormant inactivity occurring during seasons of drought. It occurs in lungfish, some snails, many reptiles and insects, and some small mammals. Also *summer torpor.* Compare HIBERNATION.

**estivoautumnal** \es′tivō·ôtum′nəl\ [*estiv(al)* + *autumnal*] Pertaining to or occurring in the summer and autumn.

**Estlander** [Jakob August *Estlander,* Finnish surgeon, 1831–1881] **1** See under FLAP. **2** Abbé-Estlander operation. See under OPERATION.

**estradiol** \es′trədī′ôl, estrā′dē·ôl\ $C_{18}H_{24}O_2$. Estra-1,3,5(10)triene-3,17β-diol. The most potent estrogenic hormone in humans, synthesized and secreted by the ovarian follicle, the fetoplacental unit, and perhaps by the adrenal cortex, and found together with many metabolites in the plasma and urine of mammals, particularly during gestation. The hormone exists in two forms, 17α and 12β, of which the latter is the more potent. Biologic functions are to induce estrus and to promote the growth of the endometrium and the maturation of the other female secondary sex characters. Pharmaceutical preparations and derivatives are widely used to treat estrogen deficiency and as components of antiovulatory contraceptive agents. Also *dihydrofolliculin* (older term), *dihydroxyestrin* (older term).

**β-estradiol** See under ESTRADIOL.

**estradiol benzoate** The benzoate derivative of estradiol. It is a form of estrogenic medication that is given parenterally. Also *benzogynestryl, benzestrofol, hydroxyestrin benzoate.*

**estradiol cypionate** $C_{26}H_{36}O_3$. Estradiol 17β-cyclopentanepropionate. A product obtained from estradiol 3,17β-dicyclopentane propionate and potassium carbonate. It is a lipid-soluble form of estradiol used for estrogenic hormone therapy.

**estradiol dipropionate** The dipropionate ester form of estradiol. It is used as an estrogenic medication because of its slow rate of absorption and long period of activity.

**estradiol enanthate** The 17-heptanoate ester of estradiol. It is given intramuscularly.

**estradiol undecylate** The 17-undecanoate ester of estradiol. It is used as an intramuscularly injected preparation of estradiol.

**estradiol valerate** The 17-valerate ester of estradiol. It is used as an intramuscularly injected form of estradiol.

**estrane** $C_{18}H_{30}$. The parent hydrocarbon of the estrogens. It contains the steroid ring system without any side chains except the methyl group at the C/D ring junction.

**Estren** [Solomon *Estren,* Russian-born U.S. physician, born 1918] Estren-Dameshek syndrome. See under SYNDROME.

**estrenol** \es′trənôl\ $C_{18}H_{24}O$. 1,3,5(10)-Estratriene-3-ol. An estrogenic steroid. *Rare.*

**estriasis** \estrī′əsis\ OESTRIASIS.

**estrin** \es′trin\ *Older term* ESTROGEN.

**estrinization** \es′trinīzā′shən\ The biologic change resulting from the presence of estrogenic substances in the circulation.

**estriol** \es′trē·ôl\ $C_{18}H_{24}O_3$. Estra-1,3,5(10)-triene-3β,16α,17β-triol. An abundant but relatively weak estrogen found in mammalian urine, especially during pregnancy. It is a major metabolic product of estradiol and estrone. Also *trihydroxyestrin.*

**estrogen** \es′trəjən\ [*estr(us)* + -GEN] Any of a class of $C_{18}$ steroid hormones synthesized and secreted by the ovarian follicle, the fetoplacental unit, the testis, and perhaps by the adrenal cortex. The biologic properties include induction of estrus in the adult female, of growth and maturation of the female secondary sex characters, and preparation of the endometrium in conjuction with progesterone for implantation of the fertilized ovum and the support of pregnancy. Estrogens are excreted mainly in the urine as sulfates and glucuronides of many metabolites, as estriol, estetrol, hydroxylated estrones, estradiols, and many others. Pharmaceutical uses include treatment of ovarian deficiency, the symptoms of menopause, metastatic cancers of the prostate and breast, and osteoporosis, as well as the inhibition of lactation. Estrogens are also widely used as components of oral contraceptive agents. Also *estrogenic hormone, estrin* (older term), *hysterythrine* (outmoded), *theelol* (older term). **conjugated e.'s** The sodium salts of the estrogenic compounds, primarily estrone and equilin, that are present as sulfate ester conjugates in pregnant mare urine. These sulfate conjugated estrogens are effective orally because of sulfatases that release the principal estrogens. Also *conjugated estrogen hormones.* **esterified e.'s** The mixed sodium salts of estrogenic esters, primarily of estrone, that are present in pregnant mare urine. They are used for oral estrogenic therapy. **e. glucuronides** A major and varied group of estrogen metabolites, synthesized mostly in the liver and excreted in the urine. They are not used therapeutically.

**estrogenic** \es′trəjen′ik\ Of or relating to estrogen, or producing the biologic effects of estrogen.

**estrone** One of the main metabolites of estradiol. It is found in urine. It differs from estradiol in having C-17 oxidized from CHOH to CO.

**estrone sulfate** The sulfate ester of estrone and a metabolite of estrone. It is used pharmaceutically in tablet form or in aqueous or oily suspension to treat conditions where estrogenic therapy is indicated.

**estrous** \es′trəs\ **1** Pertaining to estrus, the period of intense sexual activity and mating in lower animals, especially the female of the species. **2** Pertaining to the changes in the genitalia produced by the administration of estrogenic substances.

**estruation** \es′troo·ā′shən\ ESTRUS.

**estrus** \es′trəs\ [L *oestrus,* from Gk *oistros* gadfly, sting, agony, frenzy] The period of receptivity to mating which occurs immediately prior to ovulation in most mammals other than humans. Also *oestrus* (British spelling), *estruation, estrum, heat.* Adj. estrous, estrual.

**Et** Symbol for the ethyl group, $CH_3$—$CH_2$—.

**état** \ātä′\ [French (from Old French *estat,* from L *status* position, standing) state, status] A state or condition. **é. criblé** STATUS CRIBROSUS. **é. dysmelinique** Any state of disordered or abnormal myelination. **é. lacunaire** A lacunar state of the brain resulting from multifocal infarction. **é. marbré** The abnormal marbled appearance of the corpus striatum described in neuropathologic specimens in some patients with cerebral palsy. Also *marble state, status marmoratus.* **é. vermoulu** A condition of the cerebral cortex in some cases of advanced arteriosclerosis, in which the surface of the brain appears "worm-eaten" by ulceration.

**etch** / **acid e.** A technique for increasing the retention of plastic fillings in enamel. An organic acid which may be 30–50% phosphoric acid is applied to render the enamel surface more porous.

**ETEC** enterotoxic *Escherichia coli* (strains which produce an extracellular exotoxin).

**ethacrynic acid** $C_{13}H_{12}Cl_2O_4$. [2,3-Dichloro-4-(2-methylene-1-oxobutyl)phenoxy]acetic acid, a potent diuretic agent of the high-ceiling group. It inhibits the reabsorption of sodium and chloride in the ascending loop of Henle. It is administered orally, and a sodium salt form is available for intravenous use.

**ethambutol hydrochloride** $C_{10}H_{25}ClN_2O_2$. *d-N,N'*-bis(1-hydromethylpropyl)ethylenediamine hydrochloride, a compound used as an antibacterial agent, particularly against tuberculosis. A dihydrochloride salt of the same substance is also used for the same purposes.

**ethamivan** $C_{12}H_{17}NO_3$. *N,N*-Diethylvanillamide, a respiratory stimulant. It affects the respiratory system centrally and has been used in cases of respiratory depression. It is administered orally or by parenteral injection.

**ethamoxytriphetol** An antiestrogen which itself lacks estrogenic properties and which opposes some but not all the peripheral actions of natural and synthetic estrogens.

**ethanal** See under ACETALDEHYDE.

**ethanoic acid** Systematic name for acetic acid.

**ethanol** $CH_3—CH_2OH$. A colorless liquid of density 0.789. It has a pleasant smell, is inflammable, and is miscible with water (azeotrope of 96% ethanol commercially available) and with ether, chloroform, and methanol. Because of its solvent power it is used for various extractions. A 70% solution is used as an antiseptic. It is used in histologic techniques as a dehydrating agent and, undiluted, as a fixative. It is formed by fermentation of sugars. Its immediate source is the reduction by NADH of acetaldehyde formed by decarboxylation of pyruvate. In reverse, ethanol can be used by cells after oxidation by $NAD^+$, in the presence of alcohol dehydrogenase, into acetaldehyde, itself oxidized in the presence of aldehyde dehydrogenase into acetic acid or acetyl-CoA. Because of its lipid solubility it alters lipoprotein membranes of cells and of mitochondria. It is toxic to hepatic cells and nervous cells. Also *alcohol, ethyl alcohol* (outmoded).

**ethanolamine** The trivial name for 2-AMINOETHANOL.

**ethanolism** \eth′ənôlizm\ Habitual excessive consumption of ethanol; alcoholism.

**ethanoyl** ACETYL.

**ethaverine hydrochloride** $C_{24}H_{30}ClNO_4$. 6,7-Diethoxy-1-(3,4-diethoxybenzyl)-isoquinoline hydrochloride. The substance is used as an antispasmodic agent. Also *ethylpapaverine hydrochloride.*

**ethchlorvynol** $C_7H_9ClO$. 1-Chloro-3-ethyl-1-penten-4-yn-3-ol. A colorless or yellow viscous liquid with sedative and hypnotic properties. It is administered orally.

**ethene** The systematic name for ethylene.

**ethenesulfonic acid homopolymer sodium salt** LYAPOLATE SODIUM.

**ethenyl** The systematic name for vinyl.

**ether** \ē′thər\ [New L *aether* (from L, from Gk *aithēr* the heavens, sky, air) a subtle gas] **1** A compound of general formula R—O—R′ where R and R′ are alkyl or phenyl radicals. **2** DIETHYL ETHER.

**etherization** \ē′thərīzā′shən\ The production of general anesthesia using diethyl ether.

**ethical** \eth′ikəl\ **1** Of or relating to ethics. **2** In accordance with the principles of professional ethics. **3** Permitted to be sold or distributed only with a physician's prescription: said of a drug.

**ethics** \eth′iks\ [Gk *ēthikē* (from *ēthikos* moral, from *ēthos* custom, usage, character) moral philosophy] A set of principles of right conduct, such as those governing the actions of an individual or a professional group, or the philosophy underlying such principles. Adj. ethical. **medical e.** The ethical principles that govern professional conduct in medicine.

**ethinamate** $C_9H_{13}NO_2$. 1-Ethynylcyclohexanol carbamate, a carbamic acid ester with rapid onset but of brief hypnotic activity. It is used to induce sleep and is given orally.

**ethinyl** ETHYNYL.

**Ethiodol** A preparation of iodine combined with fatty esters of poppyseed oil. It is used as a roentgenographic contrast medium, as in lymphangiography. A proprietary name.

**ethionamide** 2-Ethyl thioisonicotinamide. A yellow powder used with other drugs to treat tuberculosis.

**Ethiopian** \ē′thē·ō′pē·ən\ **1** Pertaining to the peoples of Africa and constituting one of the five races of man defined by Blumenbach in 1795 according to head characteristics. **2** An individual of this race. **3** Pertaining to the biogeographic region that includes Africa, southern Arabia, and some islands in the Indian Ocean.

**ethisterone** $C_{21}H_{28}O_2$. 17$\beta$-hydroxy-17$\alpha$-pregn-4-en-20-yn-3-one, a progestin and a synthetic steroid that is used chiefly as a component of oral contraceptive drugs. Also *ethynyl testosterone, pregneninolone.*

**ethmo-** \eth′mō-\ [Gk *ēthmos* sieve] A combining form denoting the ethmoid bone.

**ethmofrontal** ETHMOIDOFRONTAL.

**ethmoid** \eth′moid\ [Gk *ēthmoeidēs* (from *ēthmos* a strainer, sieve) perforated, sievelike] **1** Sievelike; cribriform. **2** OS ETHMOIDALE.

**ethmoidal** \ethmoi′dəl\ Pertaining to or adjacent to the ethmoid bone.

**ethmoidectomy** \eth′moidek′təmē\ [ETHMOID + -ECTOMY] The exenteration of the ethmoidal air cells in cases of ethmoiditis often at the same time as the removal of nasal polyps. The operation may be performed by the intranasal, external, or transantral routes. **transantral e.** Ethmoidectomy performed through the maxillary sinus. Also *transmaxillary ethmoidectomy, Horgan's operation.*

**ethmoiditis** \eth′moidī′tis\ [ETHMOID + -ITIS] ETHMOIDAL SINUSITIS.

**ethmoidofrontal** Pertaining to the ethmoid bone and the frontal bone. Also *ethmofrontal.*

**ethmoidolacrimal** Pertaining to the ethmoid bone and the lacrimal bone. Also *ethmolacrimal.*

**ethmoidomaxillary** Pertaining to the ethmoid bone and the maxilla. Also *ethmomaxillary.*

**ethmoidonasal** Pertaining to the ethmoid bone and the nasal bone. Also *ethmonasal.*

**ethmoidopalatal** Pertaining to the ethmoid bone and the bony palate. Also *ethmopalatal.*

**ethmoidopalatine** Pertaining to the ethmoid bone and the palatine bones.

**ethmoidosphenoid** Pertaining to the ethmoid bone and the sphenoid bone. Also *ethmosphenoid.*

**ethmoidovomerine** Pertaining to the ethmoid bone and the vomer.

**ethmolacrimal** ETHMOIDOLACRIMAL.

**ethmomaxillary** ETHMOIDOMAXILLARY.

**ethmonasal** ETHMOIDONASAL.

**ethmopalatal** ETHMOIDOPALATAL.

**ethmosphenoid** ETHMOIDOSPHENOID.

**ethmoturbinal** \eth′mōtur′binəl\ **1** The superior or middle nasal concha. **2** Having to do with one of these conchae.

**ethnic** \eth′nik\ [Gk *ethnikos* (from *ethnos* a nation, people) national, of a people] Designating the physical and cultural traits that distinguish members of one society or larger human group from members of other such groups.

**ethnobiology** \eth′nōbī·äl′əjē\ **1** The biological study of human races. **2** The study of ethnic groups as they are affected by the biological factors in their environment.

**ethnography** \ethnäg′rəfē\ **1** The description and classification of human racial groups. An outmoded usage. **2** The descriptive study of ethnic groups, or of a particular ethnic group.

**ethnologic** \eth′nōläj′ik\ Pertaining to ethnology.

**ethnology** \ethnäl′əjē\ [Gk *ethno(s)* a nation, people + -LOGY] **1** The study of the human races, their origins, relationships, and characteristics. **2** The anthropological study of ethnic groups.

**ethnopsychiatry** \-sīkī·′ətrē\ [Gk *ethno(s)* a nation, people, race + English *psychiatry*] The study of the effects of culture on psychiatric disorders and their manifestations. Also *comparative psychiatry, cross-cultural psychiatry.*

**ethocaine** PROCAINE HYDROCHLORIDE.

**ethoheptazine** $C_{16}H_{23}NO_2$. 4-Carbethoxy-1-methyl-4-phenylazacycloheptane, a compound that is used clinically as an analgesic for mild to moderate pain. It is usually given orally as the citrate salt.

**ethology** \ethäl′əjē\ [Gk *ētho(s)* custom, manners, habits of man, also of animals + -LOGY] The study of animal behavior under natural conditions or in a laboratory where natural conditions have been simulated.

**ethopropazine hydrochloride** $C_{19}H_{25}ClN_2S$. *N,N*-Diethyl-$\alpha$-methyl-10*H*-phenothiazine-10-ethanamine hydrochloride, a phenothiazine derivative with anticholinergic activity. It is used in the treatment of parkinsonism and extrapyramidal symptoms from other phenothiazines. It is given orally. Also *isothiazine hydrochloride.*

**ethosuximide** $C_7H_{11}NO_2$. 3-Ethyl-3-methyl-2,5-pyrrolidinedione, an anticonvulsant drug that is preferred for treatment of petit mal epilepsy. It is effective in myoclonic spasms, but it is not usually so for temporal lobe seizures or generalized tonic-clonic seizures. It is given orally.

**ethotoin** $C_{11}H_{12}N_2O_2$. 3-Ethyl-5-phenyl-2,4-imidazoledinedione, an anticonvulsant agent with a structure similar to that of phenytoin. It is less effective than phenytoin and is usually used in combination with other anticonvulsant drugs such as phenobarbital or phenytoin for the treatment of grand mal epilepsy. It is given orally.

**ethoxazene hydrochloride** $C_{14}H_{17}ClN_4O$. 4-[(4-Ethoxyphenyl)azo]-1,3-benzenediamine hydrochloride, a reddish powder which is insoluble in water. It is used as a local analgesic for pain from urinary tract infections, and it is given orally.

**ethoxy-** [*eth(yl)* + OXY-[1]] A combining form denoting the presence of an ethoxy ($C_2H_5$—O—) group in a molecule.

**ethoxzolamide** $C_9H_{10}N_2O_3S_2$. 6-Ethoxy-2-benzothiazolesulfonamide, a carbonic anhydrase inhibitor that is used to reduce intraocular pressure in the treatment of glaucoma. It is administered orally.

**ethyl** \eth′il\ [*eth(er)* + -YL] The group $CH_3$—$CH_2$—, derived from ethane.

**ethyl alcohol** *Outmoded* ETHANOL.

**ethyl aminobenzoate** $C_9H_{11}NO_2$. *p*-Aminobenzoic acid ethyl ester, a surface local anesthetic agent that is used to treat pain or irritation of the skin and mucous membranes. It is applied as a cream, solution, or ointment, or ingested in lozenges.

**ethylation** \eth′ilā′shən\ The process of substituting hydrogen by ethyl groups.

**ethyl biscoumacetate** $C_{22}H_{16}O_8$. 4-Hydroxy-$\alpha$-(4-hydroxy-2-oxo-2*H*-1-benzopyran-3-yl)-2-oxo-2*H*-1-benzopyran-3-acetic acid ethyl ester, a synthetic anticoagulant that is effective orally.

**ethyl chloride** $C_2H_5Cl$ A volatile liquid used as a local anesthetic on the skin and mucous membrane by virtue of its refrigerant properties. It was also used up to about 1950 as a general anesthetic for the extraction of teeth.

**ethylenediaminetetraacetic acid** (HOOC—$CH_2$—$)_2$-N—$CH_2$—$CH_2$—N(—$CH_2$—COOH$)_2$. A chelating agent with high affinity for many kinds of metal ions that possess two or more positive charges, such as magnesium. The formula shown is conventional, in that the nitrogen atoms become protonated more easily than the carboxylate groups. This agent is also useful in separating cells or removing them from glass surfaces in tissue cultures. The sodium salt is used as a water softener and to stabilize solutions of various compounds. Also *versene, ethylenedinitrilotetraacetic acid, edetic acid.* Abbr. EDTA

**ethylene dibromide** $C_2H_4Br_2$. 1,2-Dibromoethane, a heavy liquid with a chloroformlike odor, used as a fumigant for the protection of stored foodstuffs against insects, rodents, and nematodes. It has been shown to be carcinogenic in experimental animals, and limits on its use on foodstuffs have been established in the United States by the Environmental Protection Agency, with some states setting lower limits, although its carcinogenicity in humans has not been established. Abbr. EDB

**ethylenedinitrilotetraacetic acid** ETHYLENEDIAMINETETRAACETIC ACID.

**ethylene oxide** $C_2H_4O$. A gaseous cyclic compound, an epoxide, that alkylates $NH_2$ and OH groups, in much the same way as formaldehyde. It is widely used for chemical disinfection.

**ethyl eosin** The ethyl ester of eosin, which renders it alcohol-soluble.

**ethyl green** BRILLIANT GREEN.

**ethyl hydrocupreine** An antibacterial agent which is relatively specific for the pneumococcus, *Streptococcus pneumoniae.* It is used in disk testing to confirm the identity of *S. pneumoniae* in clinical laboratories.

**ethyl iodophenylundecylate** IOPHENDYLATE.

**ethylmalonyl-adipicaciduria** \eth′əlmal′əniladip′ikas′idʸoo′rē·ə\ GLUTARIC ACIDURIA TYPE IIB.

**ethyl mercaptan** $CH_3$—$CH_2$—SH. A volatile, easily oxidized liquid with an unpleasant smell. It is used as an additive to natural and refrigerant gases to serve as a warning agent for gas leaks.

**ethylnorepinephrine hydrochloride** $C_{10}H_{16}ClNO_3$. 4-(2-Amino-1-hydroxylbutyl)-1,2-benzenediol hydrochloride, the hydrochloride salt of ethylnorepinephrine. It is usually administered subcutaneously or intramuscularly to relieve bronchial asthma by bronchodilatation.

**ethylpapaverine hydrochloride** ETHAVERINE HYDROCHLORIDE.

**ethynyl** The —C≡CH radical in organic compounds. Also *ethinyl.*

**ethynyl estradiol** 17$\alpha$-Ethynyl-1,3,5 (10)-estratriene-3,17-$\beta$-diol. A semisynthetic analogue of 17$\beta$-estradiol. It is an extremely potent estrogenic agent, which is given orally.

**ethynyl testosterone** ETHISTERONE.

**etidocaine hydrochloride** $C_{17}H_{29}ClN_2O$. *N*-(2,6-Dimethylphenyl)-2-(ethylpropylamino)-butanamide hydrochloride, the hydrochloride salt of etidocaine. It is used as a local anasthetic and is characterized by rapid onset of effects and long duration of action.

**etio-** \ē′tē·ō-\ [Gk *aitia* cause] A combining form meaning cause. Also *aetio-* (British spelling).

**etiocholane** *Obs.* ANDROSTANE.

**etiocholanolone** 3$\alpha$-Hydroxy-5$\beta$-androstan-17-one, a weakly androgenic 17-ketosteroid, quantitatively a major metabolite, along with androsterone, of testosterone, androstenedione, and dehydroepiandrosterone.

**etiolation** \-lā′shən\ [French *étiol(er)* to cause yellowing in green plants left in darkness + -ATION] **1** A blanched condition in green plants that is caused by a lack of light or by disease. **2** A pallor of the skin resulting from light deprivation.

**etiologic** \-läj′ik\ Of or relating to etiology.

**etiology** \ē′tē·äl′əjē\ [Med L *aetiologia* (from Gk *aitiologia* a giving proof or cause, from *aitia* cause, origin + *log(os)* a telling) a stating of causation] **1** The systematic study of the causes of disease. **2** The cause or causes of a particular disease.

**etiopathic** \-path′ik\ Pertaining to the pathogenesis of a disease.

**etiotropic** \-träp′ik\ [ETIO- + -TROPIC[1]] Directed against the cause of a disease: said of a treatment or medication. Compare NOSOTROPIC.

**etrotomy** \ēträt′əmē\ [Gk *ētro(n)* the belly + -TOMY] A hypogastric incision; suprapubic incision.

**Eu** Symbol for the element, europium.

**eu-** \yoo-\ [Gk *eu* (adverb) well] A prefix meaning (1) good, well, normal; (2) true, typical. Compare DYS-.

**euangiotic** \yoo′anjē·ät′ik\ [EU- + ANGIO- + *t* + -IC] Containing a normal supply of blood vessels.

***Eubacterium*** \yoo′baktir′ē·əm\ A genus of Gram-positive, rod-shaped, obligate anaerobes that differ from clostridia in that they do not form spores. Many species have been isolated from human lesions or feces, as well as from soil or spoiled food. Their pathogenicity is uncertain.

**eubolism** \yoo′bōlizm\ [EU- + *(meta)bolism*] The presence of a normal metabolism.

**β-eucaine** $C_{15}H_{21}NO_2$. 2,2,6-Trimethyl-4-piperidinol benzoate. A local anesthetic agent with properties like those of cocaine. Also *benzamine hydrdochloride.*

**eucalyptol** $C_{10}H_{18}O$. The anhydride of methane-1,8-diol, obtained from eucalyptus oil. It is a component of the oils of eucalyptus, cardamom, canella, sage, rosemary, lavender, ginger, and wormseed. It has a camphorlike odor and a pungent, spicy taste and has both irritant and antiseptic properties. It is used as a flavoring agent and an ingredient in medicines to treat upper respiratory diseases. Also *cajeputol, cineole.*

**eucapnia** \yookap′nē·ə\ NORMOCAPNIA.

**eucaryote** \yookar′ē·ōt\ EUKARYOTE.

**Eucestoda** \yoo′sestō′də\ [EU- + CESTODA] CESTODA.

**euchlorhydria** \yoo′klôrhī′drē·ə\ [EU- + CHLORHYDRIA] A state marked by a normal concentration of hydrochloric acid in gastric juice.

**euchromatic** \yoo′krōmat′ik\ Relating to or characteristic of euchromatin.

**euchromatin** \yookrō′mətin\ Chromatin that becomes uncoiled, or diffuse, during interphase. It appears as stained bands in polytene chromosomes, whereas it appears less densely stained in most chromosomes. It contains little highly repetitious DNA, is actively transcribed, and is associated with relatively more nonhistone protein than is heterochromatin. Compare HETEROCHROMATIN.

**euchromatopsy** \yookrō′mətäp′sē·ə\ [EU- + CHROMAT- + -OPSY] The condition of normal color vision.

**euchromosome** \yookrō′məsōm\ *Obs.* AUTOSOME.

**eucodeine** $C_{18}H_{21}O_3N{\cdot}(BrCH_3)$. Codeine methyl bromide. An analogue of codeine which is also used as a sedative.

**eudiometer** \yoo′dē·äm′ətər\ [Gk *eudi(a)* fair weather + *o* + -METER] An instrument used in the volumetric analysis of gases and, in particular, pollutants in the air.

**eudipsia** \yoodip′sē·ə\ [EU- + -DIPSIA] Normal thirst.

**euergasia** \yoo′urgā′zhə\ [EU- + ERGASIA] A normal psychobiologic state. *Seldom used.* Also *orthergasia, euergasis.*

**Euflagellata** \yooflaj′əlā′tə\ A former name for MASTIGOPHORA.

**eugenetics** \yoo′jənet′iks\ EUGENICS.

**eugenicist** \yoojen′isist\ One who studies, investigates, practices, or advocates eugenic theory or implementation. Also *eugenist.*

**eugenics** \yoojen′iks\ [Gk *eugen(ēs)* (from EU- + Gk *genos* race, descent) well-born, of noble race + -ICS] The alteration of certain phenotypic traits through selective breeding. It is applied especially to the alteration of traits in humans in order to improve the species. Also *eugenetics.* **negative e.** The process of altering phenotypic traits in a species by discouraging or preventing reproduction by members with less desirable traits. **positive e.** The process of altering phenotypic traits in a species by encouraging or requiring reproduction by members who have desirable traits.

**eugenism** \yoo′jənizm\ The belief or philosophy that the human species can be improved through selective breeding.

**eugenist** \yoojen′ist\ EUGENICIST.

**eugenol** $C_{10}H_{12}O_2$. A phenol that occurs in volatile oils, including those of clove and allspice. It is a dental obtundent and has been used as an antiseptic in endodontic treatments. Mixed into a paste with zinc oxide, it is used as a temporary filling, an impression material, and as a surgical pack following periodontal surgery. It is also used in perfumery as a substitute for clove oil.

**euglobulin** In an obsolescent classification, a protein that is a globulin in that it is precipitated by half-saturated ammonium sulfate, and further is insoluble in water but soluble in dilute salt solutions. Most blood immunoglobulins are euglobulins.

**euglycemia** \yoo′glīsē′mē·ə\ [EU- + GLYCEMIA] A normal concentration of glucose in the blood, plasma, or serum.

**eugnosia** \yoonō′sē·ə\ [EU- + Gk *gnōs(is)* knowledge + -IA] The ability to synthesize sensory stimuli into perceptual experience.

**eugnostic** \yoonäs′tik\ [EU- + Gk *gnōstikos* (from *gnōsis* knowledge) concerning knowledge] Pertaining to the normal perception of sensory stimuli.

**eukaryote** \yookar′ē·ōt\ [EU- + *kary(o)-* + Gk *-ōtē(s)*, suffix denoting native, inhabitant] An organism with cells having a well-defined nucleus enclosed by a nuclear envelope, multiple chromosomes, and a mitotic cycle. Also *eucaryote.* Compare PROKARYOTE. Adj. eukaryotic, eucaryotic.

**eukinesia** \yoo′kīnē′zhə\ Possessing the normal ability to perform motor function. Also *eukinesis.*

**eulaminate** \yoolam′ināt\ [EU- + *lamin(a)* + -ATE] Possessing the normal six layers: used of certain areas of the cerebral cortex.

**Eulenburg** [Albert *Eulenburg,* German neurologist, 1840–1917] Eulenburg's disease. See under PARAMYOTONIA CONGENITA.

**eumenorrhea** \yoo′menôrē′ə\ [EU- + MENORRHEA] Normal menstruation.

**eumorphics** \yoomôr′fiks\ The branch of orthopedics that deals with the correction of deformity and return to normal form.

**eumorphism** \yoomôr′fizm\ [EU- + MORPH- + -ISM ] The maintaining of a normal shape by a cell.

**eumycetoma** \yoomī′sētō′mə\ [EU- + MYCETOMA] A tumorlike mass composed of fungal hyphae, as in *Madurella mycetomatis* and *M. grisea* infections.

**eunuch** \yoo′nək\ [Gk *eunouch(os)* (from *eun(ē)* a bed + *ech(ein)* to have, hold) guardian of the bed] A man or boy whose testes have been ablated or destroyed by disease, especially a male castrated before puberty so that secondary sex characters never develop and the bodily proportions remain typical of the prepubertal state or of eunuchoidism. **fertile e.** Eunuchoidism due to deficient secretion of luteinizing hormone and subnormal testosterone production, but with evidence of normal follicle-stimulating hormone function, FSH levels being normal and spermatogenesis variably present. Treatment can be successfully carried out with human chorionic gonadotropin or an androgen.

**eunuchism** \yoo′nəkizm\ [EUNUCH + -ISM] The state of being a eunuch. **pituitary e.** Eunuchism related to aleydigism resulting from failure of anterior pituitary luteinizing hormone to stimulate the Leydig (testosterone-producing) cells of the testis. *Older term.*

**eunuchoid** \yoo′nəkoid\ [EUNUCH + -OID] 1 Resembling a eunuch; having the bodily proportions and the androgen deficiency characteristic of eunuchoidism. 2 A genetic male with gonadal dysgenesis.

**eunuchoidism** \yoo′nəkoid′izm\ [EUNUCH + -OID + -ISM] Relative deficiency of androgenic hormone in the male, with underdevelopment of the male secondary sex characters and typical bodily proportions, the arm span and pubis-to-floor measurement exceeding that of pubis-to-crown by more than five centimeters. These abnormal proportions are due to delayed osseous epiphysial closure resulting from delayed puberty, testicular hypoplasia, or subnormal androgen production from any cause. **female e.** Eunuchoid bodily proportions and underdevelopment of the female secondary sex characters in adolescent girls or women due to estrogen deficiency from any cause before and at the time of expected puberty. **hypergonadotropic e.** Hypogonadism, eunuchoid bodily proportions, and varying degrees of underdevelopment of the male secondary sex characters in men. The level of pituitary gonadotropic hormones in the blood is elevated owing to the deficiency of androgenic hormones from the testis which normally repress gonadotropin secretion. The condition is seen in the Klinefelter syndrome (semniferous tubule dysgenesis), XYY syndrome, Sertoli-cell-only syndrome, and adult semniferous tubule failure of several types, including sometimes the male climacteric. **hypogonadotropic e.** Eunuchoid bodily proportions, subnormal production of androgen, and relative failure of secondary sex characters to develop owing to primary deficiency of the secretion of anterior pituitary gonadotropin. Also *pituitary eunuchoidism.*

**euonymin** A cathartic obtained by the extraction and distillation of bark from the tree *Euonymus atropurpureus.* The extract is combined with one-fourth its weight of calcium phosphate to keep it in powder form as a final product.

**euparal** \yoo′pəral\ A mixture of eucalyptol and paraldehyde, with camphor and phenyl salicylate, that is used as a mounting medium for histologic preparations.

**eupatheoscope** \yoopath′ē·ōskōp′\ [Gk *eupathē(s)* comfortable + *o* + -SCOPE] An instrument used indoors to measure the combined effects of air temperature, air movement, and radiation, and thus quantify the degree of environmental warmth experienced by the human body.

**eupatorin** $C_{18}H_{16}O_7$. 3′,5-Dihydroxy-4′,6,7-trimethoxyflavone. An active agent derived from *Eupatorium perfoliatum.* It is used as an emetic medication.

**eupepsia** \yoopep′sē·ə\ [EU- + *-pepsia* as in *dyspepsia*] The condition of normal digestion.

**eupeptic** \yoopep′tik\ [*eupep(sia)* + *t* + -IC] Referring to or promoting good digestion.

**euphenics** \yoofē′niks\ Any improvement in the phenotype of an organism through planned manipulation, such as medical treatment.

**euphoriant** \yoofôr′ē·ənt\ ANTIDEPRESSANT.

**euplasia** \yooplā′zhə\ [EU- + -PLASIA] A balanced or normal rate of cellular proliferation.

**euplastic** \yooplas′tik\ [EU- + -PLAST + -IC] Pertaining to normal growth or healing, both in embryos and in tissue repair.

**euploid** \yoo′ploid\ [EU- + -PLOID] 1 Pertaining to a cell or organism whose chromosome constitution is a whole-number multiple of the haploid set, such as diploid or triploid. 2 Such a cell or organism. Compare ANEUPLOID.

**euploidy** \yooploi′dē\ [EUPLOID + -Y] The state of a cell or organism having a chromosome constitution that a is whole-number multiple of the haploid set. Also *euploid state.* Compare ANEUPLOIDY.

**eupnea** \yoop·nē′ə\ [Gk *eupnoia* (from EU- + *pno(ē)* breath + -IA) easy breathing] Normal breathing, in contradistinction to difficult breathing (dyspnea), abnormally rapid or deep breathing (hyperpnea), abnormally slow breathing (bradypnea), and the like. Adj. eupneic.

**eupraxia** \yooprak′sē·ə\ [Gk (from EU- + *praxis* action) successful action, good conduct] An ability to perform normally skilled and coordinated movements.

**eurodontia** \yoo′rōdän′shə\ [Gk *eur(ōs)* mold, decay + -ODONTIA] *Obs.* DENTAL CARIES.

**European Pharmacopeia** A pharmacopeia produced under the auspices of the Council of Europe (Partial Agreement) and published in English and French versions. It has legal force in those countries that have ratified the European Pharmacopeia Convention superseding the corresponding national pharmacopeias.

**europium** \yoorō′pē·əm\ Element number 63, having atomic weight 151.96. It is the most reactive element in the lanthanide series and one of the rarest. There are 17 isotopes known, two of them stable. Symbol: Eu

**eury-** \yoo′ri-, yoo′rē-\ [Gk *eurys* wide] A combining form meaning wide.

**eurymeric** \-mer′ik\ In osteometry, denoting an upper femur that is circular in cross section.

**euryopia** \-ō′pē·ə\ [EURY- + -OPIA] A normal variant of facial topography in which the interorbital distance is increased but not to the degree to suggest teratic or pathologic associations, as in hypertelorism.

***Euscorpius italicus*** \yooskôr′pē·əs ital′ikəs\ A species of scorpion of Europe and North Africa; the black scorpion.

**Eustachi** [Bartolomeo *Eustachi,* Italian physician, surgeon, and anatomist, 1524–1574] 1 Eustachian tube, eustachian canal. See under TUBA AUDITIVA. 2 Eustachian valve. See under VALVULA VENAE CAVAE INFERIORIS.

**eusthenia** \yoosthē′nē·ə\ [EU- + STHEN- + -IA] A state of normal strength.

**eutectic** \yootek′tik\ [Gk *eutēkt(os)* (from *eu-* well + *tēktos* verbal adj. of *tēkein* to melt) easily melted or dissolved + -IC] 1 Having the lowest possible melting point: said especially of a mixture whose melting point is lower than that of any of its individual constituents. 2 Having a fixed melting point: used of a mixture, often an alloy.

**euthanasia** \yoo′thənā′zhə\ [Gk (from *eu-* well + *-thanasia,* combining form from *thanatos* death), easy death] The act or practice of deliberately but painlessly killing, or allowing to die, a person suffering the stress attending the approach of death from an incurable illness or suffering intractable pain, with or without that person's consent or expressed desire. Active, or positive, euthanasia, popularly known as mercy killing, involves actions that serve to cause or hasten death, such as administering an overdose of a drug. Passive, or negative, euthanasia consists in withholding medical treatment that might prolong life. **passive e.**

The act of hastening the death of an incurable, terminally ill, and usually comatose patient by withholding or withdrawing life-support systems. The practice is legally acceptable providing consulting physicians agree in writing that the situation is hopeless and prior consent for the act has been obtained from next of kin. Also *orthothanasia.*

**euthenics** \yoothen′iks\ [Gk *euthēn(ēs)* flourishing + -ICS] The discipline that seeks to improve human welfare by modifying the environment.

**euthermic** \yoothur′mik\ [EU- + THERM- + -IC] **1** Of or relating to a state of warmth. **2** Possessing a normal temperature.

**euthyroid** \yoothī′roid\ [EU- + THYROID] Having a normally functioning thyroid gland and normal thyroid hormone.

**euthyscope** \yoo′thiskōp\ [Gk *euthy(s)* straight, direct + -SCOPE] A modified ophthalmoscope used to treat amblyopic eccentric fixation by dazzling the retina surrounding the central portion of the macula, thereby rendering the periphery less sensitive than the suppressed fovea, which is kept within a disk of shadow during the dazzling illumination.

**eutopic** \yootäp′ik\ ENTOPIC.

***Eutrombicula alfreddugesi*** \yoo′trämbik′yələ al′frədəjē′sī\ *TROMBICULA ALFREDDUGESI.*

**eV** Symbol for the unit, electronvolt.

**evacuant** **1** Promoting evacuation or expulsion. **2** A drug or agent that allows for the expulsion of some material from an organ or organ system, particularly the gastrointestinal tract: a purgative.

**evacuate** \ivak′yoo·āt\ [L *evacuat(us),* past part. of *evacuare* (from *e-* out + *vacuus* empty) to empty out] To discharge or cause to be discharged from the body, especially the contents of the bowels.

**evacuation** \ivak′yoo·ā′shən\ [Late L *evacuatio* (from L *evacuatus,* past part. of *evacuare* to empty out) an emptying out] Removal of material, or an emptying, especially of the bowel.

**evagination** \ivaj′ənā′shən\ [L *evaginatus,* past part. of *evaginare* (from *e-* out + *vagina* sheath) to unsheathe] An outpouching of the wall of a tissue or part. **optic e.** OPTIC DIVERTICULUM.

**evanescent** \ev′ənes′ənt\ Existing briefly before becoming nonfunctional or disappearing.

**Evans** [Herbert Meleon *Evans,* U.S. anatomist and embryologist, 1882–1971] See under BLUE.

**Evans** [Robert Sherman *Evans,* U.S. physician, born 1912] See under SYNDROME.

**evenomation** \iven′ōmā′shən\ [E- + VENOM + -ATION ] Removal or neutralization of venom in a victim of envenomation.

**event** / **ionizing e.** Any interaction that generates an ion or groups of ions. **positron annihilation e.** The interaction of an incident positron with an electron, resulting in the conversion of the mass energy (and any kinetic energy) of both into radiation. Also *annihilation reaction.* **scattering e.** SCATTERING COLLISION.

**eventration** \ē′ventrā′shən\ [French *éventration* (from E- + L *venter,* gen. *ventris,* the belly + *-ation* -ATION) act of disemboweling] The protrusion of abdominal viscera, particularly the intestines, through an open abdominal wall. **congenital e. of the diaphragm** An abnormal upward protrusion of a part of the diaphragm. The diaphragm is thin and atrophic and covers variable displaced abdominal viscera. The eventration usually occurs on the left side. **diaphragmatic e.** Cephalad displacement of a part of the diaphragm by the abdominal viscera, usually resulting from phrenic nerve paralysis or from congenital muscular deficiency in the diaphragm. **umbilical e.** The herniation of a major portion of the abdominal viscera through an enlarged umbilical opening, the usual constriction of the umbilical cord where it joins the embryonic abdominal wall having failed to occur. The condition is secondary to persistence of the midgut hernia of embryonic life or the result of subsequent hypoplasia of the abdominal wall, or both.

**eversion** \ivur′zhən\ [L *eversio* (from *evertere* to turn out; see EVERT) a turning out, expulsion] A turning outwards or turning inside out.

**evert** \ivurt\ [L *evertere* (from *e(x)-* out + *vertere* to turn) to turn inside out or upside down] **1** To turn outward, as of the foot. **2** To turn inside out, as of the eyelid.

**evertor** \ivur′tər\ A muscle that turns a part, such as the foot, outward.

**évidement** \āvēdmäɴ′\ [French (from *évider* to hollow out, from *vide* empty) a hollowing out, exenteration] The surgical removal of diseased tissue from a cavity or organ.

**evidence** [L *evidentia* (from *evidens,* gen. *evidentis,* visible + -IA) visibility, clarity] All of the testimony, documents, displays, objects, and material substances presented to a court of law for the purpose of proving or disproving an alleged fact. **circumstantial e.** Those proven or accepted facts presented as evidence in a judicial proceeding, which are not based on actual observation or direct knowledge but which tend to establish the contested fact by inference. Also *indirect evidence.* **expert e.** EXPERT TESTIMONY. **indirect e.** CIRCUMSTANTIAL EVIDENCE. **physical e.** That evidence which is physically real or demonstrative, as opposed to verbal, and which can be seen and examined by jurors, such as the murder weapon used in a homicide. **trace e.** Physical evidence of small, usually microscopic size, which is recovered from a crime scene, or found on the body or clothing of a victim or assailant, or found on an object involved in a crime, such as blood and seminal stains, hairs and fibers, fingerprints, glass fragments, paint chips, and soil samples. Such evidence is used to establish a connection between the crime and its perpetrator or victim.

**eviration** \ē′virā′shən\ [L *evir(are)* (from *e(x)-* out + *vir* man) to emasculate + -ATION] FEMINIZATION.

**eviscerate** \ivis′ərāt\ [L *eviscerare* (from *e(x)-* out + *viscera* inner parts) to disembowel] **1** To remove viscera or a viscus from the body. **2** To extrude by injury or surgical intervention, as the intestines.

**evisceration** \ivis′ərā′shən\ [L *eviscer(are)* to disembowel + -ATION. See EVISCERATE.] **1** The surgical removal of viscera or a viscus. **2** The loss or removal of abdominal viscera; disemboweling. **3** The removal of the contents of the eye with retention of the sclera.

**evisceroneurotomy** \ivis′ərōnʸʊrät′əmē\ Evisceration of the eye combined with cutting of the optic nerve or removal of a portion of the nerve.

**evocation** \ev′ōkā′shən\ [L *evocatio* (from *evocare* to call out or forth) a calling out or forth, eliciting] The induction of the morphogenetic potential of a particular tissue during embryogenesis by the action of a single chemical substance, the evocator.

**evocator** \ev′ōkā′tər\ **1** Any chemical substance which has the property of evoking latent potentialities for development in a region in an embryo. An evocator provides a morphogenetic stimulus. Also *morphogenetic hormone, inducing agent.* **2** INDUCTOR.

**evolution** \ev′əloo′shən\ [L *evolutio* (from *evolutus,* past part. of *evolvere* to roll out, unroll) an unrolling, opening] The irreversible process of gradual change in successive generations, tending toward increased complexity and differentiation of structure and function, and occurring by the accumulation of genetic mutations over time. Compare DEVOLUTION. **convergent e.** The independent development of similar character states in two or more phylogenetic lineages even though they receive from the common ancestor neither the adaptations involved nor the characteristics that channel the development of those adaptations. This usually occurs as a response to similar environmental pressures. Convergence often occurs due to similarity of function, such as the evolution of wings in the ancestors of birds, bats, and flies. • See note at PARALLEL EVOLUTION. **parallel e.** The independent development of a similar character state in lineages that inherit the potential for the development of such a character state from a common ancestor, but do not directly inherit the similar character state. • As it is generally not possible to determine whether such a potential was present in the common ancestor, *parallel evolution* is most often used interchangeably with *convergent evolution*. Convergent evolution occurs when descendants resemble each other more than their ancestors did with respect to a given characteristic. Parallel evolution occurs when lineages have changed in similar ways, so that the descendants are as similar to each other as their ancestors were.

**evulsio** \ivul′sē·ō\ [L (from *evulsus*, past part. of *evellere* to tear or pull out, remove), a tearing or pulling out, removing] EVULSION. **e. nervi optici** Mechanical rupture of the optic nerve from the sclera.

**evulsion** \ivul′shən\ [L *evulsio*. See EVULSIO.] Extraction by force. Also *evulsio*.

**Ewart** [William *Ewart*, English physician, 1848–1929] See under SIGN, PROCEDURE.

**Ewing** [James *Ewing*, U.S. pathologist, 1866–1943] Ewing's tumor. See under SARCOMA.

**ex-**[1] \eks-\ [L *ex* (as prefix *ex-* before vowels or consonants, *e-* before consonants except *f-*, *ef-* before *f*) out of, from] A prefix meaning (1) out of, from, away from; (2) lacking, being without; (3) thoroughly. Also *e-*,*ef-*.

**ex-**[2] \eks-\ [Gk *ex-* (as prefix *ek-* before vowels) from out of, away, from] A prefix meaning out of, from. Also *ek-*, *ec-*.

**exa-** \ek′sə-\ A combining form denoting $10^{18}$: used with SI units. Symbol: E

**exacerbation** \igzas′ərbā′shən\ [Late L *exacerbatio* (from L *exacerbatus*, past part. of *exacerbare* to exasperate, from *ex-* out + *acerbus* harsh, bitter, from *acer* sharp) exasperation, intensification] An increase in the severity of a disease or its manifestations.

**examination** [L *examinatio* (from *examinare* to weigh, balance, scrutinize, from *examen* a balance, weight, control, from *exigere* to exact, require, from *ex-* out + *agere* to drive, do, act) a weighing, scrutiny] An inspection or investigation, often to establish a diagnosis or to assess the condition of a patient undergoing treatment. **air-contrast e.** Roentgenography of a hollow viscus, such as the colon, after coating the lining or mucosa of its lumen with a radiopaque contrast medium, such as barium sulfate, and then distending the lumen with air. **gastrointestinal e.** An x-ray examination of the gastrointestinal tract using barium or other radiologic contrast medium. Examination of the upper gastrointestinal tract usually follows the oral administration of barium meal. The lower tract is examined by barium enema. Also *gastrointestinal study*.

**examinee** \igzam′ənē\ A person being examined; the subject of an examination.

**examiner** A person conducting an examination. **medical e.** 1 An appointed medical officer with training or expertise in forensic pathology who is empowered to investigate certain categories of death which are defined by law. Medical examiners are charged with responsibilities virtually identical to those of elected coroners, whom they have replaced in many states, counties, and municipalities in the United States. 2 A physician who practices as an employee of private or public enterprise and whose services are specified by the employer. The examination of prospective purchasers of life insurance is one such service.

**exanimation** \igzan′əmā′shən\ [L *exanimatio* (from *exanimatus*, past part. of *exanimare* to deprive of breath, terrify, kill, from *ex-* from + *anima* breath) a depriving of breath, terror] 1 Coma. 2 Death.

**exanthem** \eksan′thəm\ [Gk *exanthēma* (from *exanthein* to bloom, flower, break out, from *anthos* flower) eruption, efflorescence] 1 A rash that develops as a cutaneous manifestation of an infectious disease. 2 A rash that arises from a sensitivity to a drug. For defs. 1 and 2 also *exanthema*. **Boston e.** An acute febrile exanthematous illness caused by echovirus 16 and probably other enterovirus types. The rash generally appears shortly after the fever subsides and consists of salmon-pink macules with indistinct borders. The eruption predominates over the face and upper part of the chest but frequently extends to the extremities. The rash subsides after a few days, and recovery is always uneventful. Also *Boston exanthem disease*. **e. subitum** An acute illness of young children, probably due to a virus, occurring sporadically and rarely in epidemics, and characterized by high fever terminating in an abrupt return to normal temperature on the fourth day. Within 48 hours after the disappearance of fever, a bright pink macular rash resembling measles appears on the trunk and neck, but unlike measles, it practically spares the face. Adenopathy in the cervical and posterior auricular regions is often present. Also *roseola infantum, fourth disease, parascarlatina, Dukes disease, Filatov-Dukes disease, Zahorsky's disease, sixth disease, erythema subitum, roseola infantilis*.

**exanthema** \eks′anthē′mə\ EXANTHEM.

**exanthemata** \eks′ənthē′mətə\ Plural of EXANTHEMA.

**exanthrope** \ek′santhrōp\ [EX-[2] + Gk *anthrōp(os)* man] An etiologic factor or agent situated outside the body in which it causes disease.

**exarticulation** \eks′ärtik′yəlā′shən\ DISARTICULATION.

**excarnation** \eks′kärnā′shən\ [Late L *excarnatus*, past part. of *excarnare* (from L *ex-* out + *caro*, gen. *carnis*, flesh) to strip of flesh] The removal of soft tissue from an anatomic specimen to show underlying osteoarticular structures.

**excavatio** \eks′kəvā′shē·ō\ [L (from *excavare* to hollow out, from EX- + L *cavus* hollow, concave) a scooping or hollowing out] A cavity, a pouchlike space, or recess. Also *excavation*. **e. disci** [NA] The slight depression in the central part of the optic disk where the optic nerve pierces the retina. Also *optic cup, physiologic cup, excavation of optic disk, physiologic excavation*. **e. rectouterina** [NA] A deep pouch formed by the reflection of peritoneum from the anterior surface of the rectum onto the posterior fornix of the vagina and the posterior, or intestinal, surface of the uterus. The pouch contains the terminal coils of the ileum and the sigmoid colon. Also *rectouterine excavation, Douglas cul-de-sac, pouch of Douglas, Douglas space, rectouterine pouch, rectovaginal pouch*. **e. rectovesicalis** [NA] The portion of the peritoneal cavity between the upper two thirds of the rectum and the superior surface of the urinary bladder in the male. Also *rectovesical excavation, rectovesical pouch*. **e. vesicouterina** [NA] The shallow pouch formed by the reflection of peritoneum from the anterior, or vesical, surface of the uterus at the level of the isthmus onto the superior surface of the urinary bladder. Also *vesicouterine* *excavation, uterovesical pouch, vesicouterine pouch, cavum vesicouterinum.*

**excavation** \eks′kəvā′shən\ [L *excavatio.* See EXCAVATIO.] **1** EXCAVATIO. **2** The process or act of hollowing out a space or cavity. **e. of optic disk** EXCAVATIO DISCI. **physiologic e.** EXCAVATIO DISCI. **rectouterine e.** EXCAVATIO RECTOUTERINA. **rectovesical e.** EXCAVATIO RECTOVESICALIS. **vesicouterine e.** EXCAVATIO VESICOUTERINA.

**excavationes** \eks′kəvā′shē·ō′nēz\ Plural of EXCAVATIO.

**excavator** \eks′kəvā′tər\ [L *excavat(us)* (past part. of *excavare* to excavate, from *ex-* out + *cavare* to make hollow) + -OR] A surgical instrument, often in the form of a scoop, used for hollowing out tissue. **dental e.** A hand instrument, usually with a spoon-shaped tip, used to scrape or lift carious dentin from a tooth. There is a large variety of tip sizes and angulations.

**excernent** \eksur′nənt\ [L *excernens,* gen. *excernentis,* pres. part. of *excernere* to separate] **1** Capable of bringing about expulsion. **2** An agent used to bring about expulsion.

**excess** / **antibody e.** In an antigen-antibody precipitation, the region in which increasing amounts of antibody (with a fixed amount of antigen) yield no further amounts of precipitate and where free antibody remains in the supernatant. Compare ANTIGEN EXCESS. **antigen e.** In an antigen-antibody reaction, the addition of sufficient antigen to saturate the antibody and leave uncombined antigen in solution. Because the antigen-antibody complexes do not form large cross-linked aggregates under these conditions, they are soluble. Compare ANTIBODY EXCESS. **base e.** Blood base concentration in mEq/l as measured by titration with strong acid at 37°C to pH 7.4 at a carbon dioxide partial pressure of 40 mm Hg.

**exchange** / **ion e.** The reversible exchange of ions in solution with ions of similar charge attached to an insoluble material. **sister chromatid e.** A recombination, detectable cytologically using fluorescent markers of newly replicated DNA, between sister chromatids. It occurs in the meiotic tetrad or in the duplicated mitotic chromosome. Also *mitotic recombination, intrachromosomal recombination.*

**exchangeable** Denoting a pool of a substance within which an added quantity of the substance will be distributed after a relatively short interval. The pool of exchangeable material is commonly measured by isotope dilution.

**exchanger** \iks·chān′jər\ A device for transferring substances or properties. **anion e.** One of two types of synthetic resin with the property of liberating certain ions in exchange for others from the medium. Anion exchangers in the hydroxide form are used to treat gastric hyperacidity. They have the advantage in comparison with alkaline medicaments of not disturbing the acid-base balance. The acid bound in the stomach is released in the intestine. Anion exchangers are used in chemical isolations, including amino-acid analysis of protein hydrolysates, and in softening and purifying water. **cation e.** A solid containing negatively charged groups. It can exchange the cations that are counter ions for these groups with a solution, e.g. it can take up calcium ions in exchange for hydrogen ions. Cation exchangers in the hydrogen form were once used to treat cardiac or renal edema, but they are less efficient than modern diuretics and resulted in metabolic disturbances. Cation exchangers are used in chemical isolations including amino-acid analysis of protein hydrolysates, and in softening and purifying water. Proteins, in particular, may be separated by differential binding to such exchangers. They bind by their positive charges, and their affinity can be modulated by altering their charges, via the pH of the medium, and by altering the concentration of competing cations in the solution. **heat e.** Any device that promotes rapid heat transfer beween two flowing media, such as that used for cooling or warming blood in extracorporeal circulation. **ion e.** An anion or cation exchanger.

**excipient** \eksip′ē·ənt\ [L *excipiens,* gen. *excipientis,* pres. part. of *excipere* (from *ex-* out + *capere* to catch, take) to take out, take up, absorb] A pharmacologically inactive substance which is combined with a drug to confer a suitable physical form to the mixture and facilitate the administration of the drug.

**excise** \eksīz′\ [L *excis(us),* past part. of *excidere* (from *ex-* out + *caedere* to cut) to cut out or off] To remove by cutting.

**excision** \eksizh′ən\ [L *excisio* (from *excisus,* past part. of *excidere* to cut out or off) a cutting out or off] The removal by cutting of tissue, a structure, or an organ. Also *exsection.* **fascial e.** An excision of a full thickness burn and the subcutaneous fat down to the investing muscle fascia. Also *formal excision.* **multiple partial e.'s** A method of excising large skin lesions. A portion of the lesion is excised and the resulting defect is closed. After a waiting period lasting from weeks to months, which allows relaxation of the surrounding tissues, an additional portion of the lesion is excised. The process is repeated until the lesion has been completely excised. Also *Ferris Smith technique.* **narrow e.** The complete operative removal of a lesion with slim margins. **primary e.** Surgical removal of a burn prior to spontaneous separation of the eschar. **sequential e.** TANGENTIAL EXCISION. **tangential e.** The excision of any lesion through a plane which is tangential to the surface from which it originates. The defect may be allowed to re-epithelialize spontaneously, but in the case of skin, it may be overgrafted. Also *sequential excision, tangential débridement.* **wide e.** The complete operative removal of a lesion with broad margins.

**excitability** \eksī′təbil′itē\ [L *excit(are)* to rouse forth, arouse + -ABILITY] The property of being excited by and reacting to a stimulus. Also *irritability.* **direct e.** The excitability of muscle to an electrical stimulus applied directly to its surface. **exteroceptive e.** Susceptibility to respond to a physical change external to the organism. **indirect e.** Excitability of muscle to an electrical stimulus of the nerve. **proprioceptive e.** Susceptibility to physical changes inducing nerve impulse activity within the organism. **rhythmic e.** The tendency of neurons to respond repetitively to a single, often sustained, stimulus. **seismogenic e.** The tendency or susceptibility to respond to a repetitive mechanical stimulus. Also *vibratory sensitivity.* **subliminal e.** The susceptibility of nerve and muscle to stimuli below the threshold for impulse generation and muscle contraction.

**excitation** \ek′sītā′shən\ [L *excitatio* (from *excitare* to disturb, provoke, rouse, from *citare* to call, summon) arousal, liveliness] **1** The stimulation of a nerve cell or muscle fiber causing a response, such as a membrane depolarization. **2** The condition of being excited. **3** The addition of energy to a system or to a molecule, converting it from a ground state to an excited state. The energy may move an electron from its orbital to an outer orbital having a higher energy level. **anomalous atrioventricular e.** WOLFF-PARKINSON-WHITE SYNDROME. **catatonic e.** CATATONIC EXCITEMENT. **direct e.** Induction of contraction in a muscle through electrodes resting on its surface. Both activation of the muscle fibers themselves and indirect activation of them through intramuscular nerve trunks can be involved, but stimulation of the muscle fibers is usually intended. **ephaptic e.** The direct transfer of a nervous impulse from one axon to another, either across an intact axonal membrane or where demyelinated axons come into physical contact with one another.

**excitatory** \iksī′tətôr′ē\ 1 Susceptible to excitation or able to excite. Also *excitative, irritative* (obs.). 2 Demonstrating or marked by excitation.

**excitement** [L *excitare* to rouse forth, arouse + -MENT] A state marked by agitation, hyperactivity, or hyperirritability. **anniversary e.** An episode of agitation that recurs on specific calendar days which are significant to the patient. It is most commonly seen in schizophrenic patients. **catatonic e.** A state of excitement seen in some forms of catatonic schizophrenia. Such a state is manifested in hyperkinesia, stereotypy, mannerisms, automatism, and impulsivity. Also *catatonic excitation.* **psychomotor e.** A state of mental excitement and physical overactivity, as seen in patients with delirium.

**exclave** \eks′klāv\ [EX- + *-clave* as in *enclave*, from L *clav(is)* key] Part of an organ displaced to an ectopic site, thereby constituting an accessory organ. Exclaves of thyroid, thymus, spleen, and pancreas are not uncommon.

**exclusion** \iksklōō′zhən\ 1 The act or condition of being kept apart or shut out. 2 An operation in which an organ is divided or a portion of an organ is detached but not removed.

**exconjugant** \ikskän′jəgənt\ A ciliate protozoan at the stage following separation after sexual conjugation and before mitotic division has begun.

**excoriation** \ikskôr′ē·ā′shən\ [Med L *excoriatio* (from L *excoriatus*, past part. of *excoriare* to flay, strip off the skin, from *ex-* out + *corium* hide, skin, bark) a stripping off of skin] A superficial loss of substance, as may be produced on the skin by scratching. **neurotic e.** A self-inflicted excoriation, usually on the face, back, or shoulders of a subject under stress.

**excortication** \ekskôr′təkā′shən\ DECORTICATION.

**excrement** \eks′krəmənt\ [L *excrement(um)* (from *excernere* to separate out; see EXCRETE) refuse, excrement]

**excrementitious** \eks′krəmentish′əs\ Relating to or characteristic of excrement.

**excrescence** \ekskres′əns\ [L *excrescentia* (from *excrescens*, gen. *excrescentis*, pres. part. of *excrescere* to grow out, fungate, from *ex-* out + *crescere* to grow) outgrowths] A projection of abnormal tissue from a surface such as the skin, a mucosa, or a heart valve. **fungating e.** A fungal infection of the umbilical cord at the point of separation. Also *fungous excrescence.* **Lambl's e.'s** Small warty or polypoid excrescences occurring on cardiac valves. They may result from organization of thrombi or myxoid degeneration.

**excreta** \ekskrē′tə\ [L, neut. pl. of *excretus*, past part. of *excernere* to separate, sift out] Materials excreted from the body, such as feces and urine.

**excrete** \ekskrēt′\ [L *excret(us)*, past part. of *excernere* (from *ex-* out + *cernere* to sift) to separate out, sift out] To separate out and eliminate (waste products) from the body.

**excreter** \ekskrē′tər\ [*excret(e)* + -ER] A carrier who excretes pathogenic organisms in the urine or feces.

**excretion** \ekskrē′shən\ [Vulgar L *excretio* a separating of waste matter. See EXCRETE.] The separating out and elimination of the waste products of digestion and metabolism. **fractional e.** The fraction of a substance filtered at the glomerulus that appears in the urine, calculated from the clearance of the substance divided by the glomerular filtration rate. **renal tubular e.** The net transfer of solute by the renal tubular cells to the tubular lumen. **renal tubular hydrogen e.** The net transfer of hydrogen ions by the renal tubular cells to the tubular lumen, calculated from the sum of ammonium ions and titratable acid excreted in urine.

**excursion** [L *excursio* (from *excurrere* to run out, hasten forth, from EX- + L *currere* to run) a sortie, expedition] The movement or deviation of an object or substance, usually implying the possibility of return to the original position or state, as a movement of the mandible away from the rest position. **lateral e.** Excursion of the mandible to the right or left until the mandibular buccal cusps are level with those of the maxillary teeth. **respiratory e.** The amount of movement (of chest wall or diaphragm) during breathing.

**excyclodeviation** \eksī′klōdē′vē·ā′shən\ [EX-[2] + CYCLO- + DEVIATION] Torsional displacement of an eye on its anteroposterior axis, so that its upper (12 o'clock) part is rotated outward in the direction of the temple. Also *negative torsion, lateral torsion.*

**excyclophoria** \eksī′klōfôr′ē·ə\ [EX-[2] + CYCLO- + PHORIA] A latent extorsion of the eyes with respect to each other.

**excyclotropia** \eksī′klōtrō′pē·ə\ [EX-[2] + CYCLO- + TROPIA] A manifest extorsion of the eyes with respect to each other.

**excyst** \eksist′\ [EX-[2] + CYST] To emerge, or be released, from a cyst. See also EXCYSTATION.

**excystation** \ek′sistā′shən\ [EXCYST + -ATION] Emergence from a cyst, as occurs after parasitic protozoa with cystic stages are ingested by the final host. Also *excystment.*

**exelcymosis** \ek′selsīmō′sis\ EXTRACTION.

**exencephalocele** \ek′sensef′əlōsēl′\ A herniation of brain tissue and an enclosing sac of meninges through a defect in the skull.

**exencephaly** \ek′sensef′əlē\ [EX-[2] + ENCEPHAL- + -Y] Herniation of or in situ exposure of the brain owing to deficient development of the skull. There is usually no meningeal covering over the exposed brain tissue which consequently undergoes extensive erosion during the fetal period. The reduced mass of blood vessels and residual nervous tissue typically seen in anencephaly is the end result of prolonged intrauterine erosion of an exencephalic brain. Such erosion of brain tissue does not occur in animals with short gestation periods.

**exenteration** \eksen′tərā′shən\ [L *exenter(are)*, from Gk *exenterizein* (from *ex(o)-* out + *enteron* bowel) to disembowel + -ATION] 1 Removal of the contents of a body cavity, as of the pelvis; evisceration. 2 The removal of the eye along with the associated structures within the orbit. **anterior pelvic e.** The in-continuity excision of the lower ureters, bladder, uterus, vagina, adnexa, pelvic peritoneum, and lymph nodes, used for treatment of carcinoma of the cervix extending into the bladder. Usually the remaining parts of the ureters are reimplanted in a segment of intestinal conduit. **pelvic e.** TOTAL PELVIC EXENTERATION. **posterior pelvic e.** An in-continuity surgical excision of the pelvic colon, uterus, vagina, and adnexa, leaving the lower urinary tract intact. **total pelvic e.** 1 The exenteration of all the pelvic organs including the pelvic lymph nodes and the entire pelvic peritoneum. 2 The in-continuity removal of the lower ureters, bladder, uterus, adnexa, vagina, rectum, pelvic peritoneum, and lymph nodes, used for treatment of carcinoma of the cervix which extends to the bladder and rectum or for severe infection of the pelvic organs. Also *pelvic exenteration, Brunschwig's operation.*

**exenteritis** \eksen′tərī′tis\ Inflammation of the outermost layers of the intestinal tract.

**exercise** [French *exercice,* from L *exercitium* (from *exercere* to exercise, utilize, from *ex-* out + *arcere* to confine, contain, from *arca* a box, chest) exercise, training] Repetitive or systematically varied activity that in appropriate circumstances has, or is intended to have, a cumulative or long-range effect of improving, maintaining, or restoring health or skill, or that is used for diagnosis or testing. **active assisted e.** Exercise done voluntarily by an individual with assistance from another individual. **active resistive e.** Exercise done voluntarily by an individual with resistance applied by another individual. **Fournier's e.'s** A series of movements designed to reveal incipient ataxia, as they show up clumsiness, incoordination, and hesitant movements. **Frenkel's e.'s** Muscle exercises recommended for the treatment of ataxia. Also *Frenkel's treatment.* **graduated resistance e.** PROGRESSIVE RESISTIVE EXERCISE. **isokinetic e.** Exercise in which the motion of a joint is carried out at a constant speed, as regulated by an appropriate device. See also ISOKINETIC CONTRACTION. **isometric e.** Exercise in which there is active, voluntary contraction of muscles without producing motion of the joints to which they are attached. Also *static exercise, muscle-setting exercise.* See also ISOMETRIC CONTRACTION. **isotonic e.** Exercise in which there is active, voluntary contraction of muscles producing motion of the joints to which they are attached. See also ISOTONIC CONTRACTION. **muscle-setting e.** ISOMETRIC EXERCISE. **neuromuscular facilitation e.** An exercise used to enhance contraction or relaxation of muscles. **passive e.** Exercise in which a patient's body part is moved by another individual or external force, without contraction of the patient's muscles. **progressive assistive e.** A modification of the progressive resistive exercise technique utilized when the patient's muscle strength is inadequate to overcome the force of gravity. Assistance is provided to remove the effect of gravity either by the therapist or through use of a suspension device, pulleys, or a powder board. **progressive resistive e.** A course of active resistive exercise in which resistance or weight is progressively increased. Also *progressive resistance exercise, graduated resistance exercise.* **static e.** ISOMETRIC EXERCISE.

**exeresis** \ekser′əsis\ [New L, from Gk *exairesis* a removal] The surgical excision of a part.

**exergonic** \ek′sərgän′ik\ Describing a process accompanied by a loss (output) of energy, often of a specified form such as Gibbs energy. Also *exoergic, exoenergetic.* Compare ENDERGONIC.

**exfetation** \eks′fētā′shən\ [EX-[1] + FETATION] ECTOPIC PREGNANCY.

**exflagellation** \eksflaj′əlā′shən\ [EX- + *flagell(um)* + -ATION] The emergence of flagellalike microgametes, as occurs in the stomach of anopheline malaria mosquitoes a few moments after taking a blood meal from an infected human host.

**exfoliate** \eksfō′lē·āt\ [See EXFOLIATION.] To remove or slough off (as epithelial cells) from an exposed layer.

**exfoliatin** \eksfō′lē·ətin\ A plasmid-coded protein that is produced by some strains of *Staphylococcus aureus* and that cleaves desmosomes in the stratum granulosum of the epidermis, thus causing various forms of exfoliative skin disease. Also *epidermolytic toxin.*

**exfoliation** \eksfō′lē·ā′shən\ [Med L *exfoliatio* (from *exfoliare* to strip leaves from, from *ex-* out, off + *folia* leaves) a stripping off of leaves] **1** Removal or sloughing from an exposed layer, as of epithelial cells. **2** DESQUAMATION.

**exfoliative** **1** Pertaining to or done by exfoliation. **2** DESQUAMATIVE.

**exhalant** \eks·hā′lənt\ Something that is exhaled.

**exhale** [L *exhal(are)* (from *ex-* out + *halare* to breathe) to exhale] To breathe out; expire.

**exhaustion** \igzôs′chən\ [L *exhaust(us),* past part. of *exhaurire* (from *ex-* out + *haurire* to draw, scoop up) to drain, empty out + -ION] **1** The depletion of energy stores resulting in muscle fatigue to the point where physical activity cannot be performed. **2** The depletion or extraction of the active ingredients of a substance. **anhidrotic heat e.** HEATSTROKE. **cold e.** A condition characterized by drowsiness, fatigue, and eventually loss of consciousness resulting from exposure to cold or failure to adapt to lowered environmental temperature, a consequence of accidental hypothermia. **heat e.** A circulatory disorder resulting from prolonged exposure to a hot environment. Excessive perspiration results in extracellular and plasma volume depletion, causing symptoms of dizziness, headache, fatigue, and drowsiness. It is a less severe form of heatstroke and is distinguished from heatstroke by a normal body temperature. Also *heat syncope, ignisation, heat prostration.*

**exhib.** *exhibeatur* (L, let it be given).

**exhibition** [L *exhibitio* (from *exhibere* to produce, present, provide, from *ex-* out + *habere* to have) production, appearance, provision] The administration of a drug or remedy.

**exhibitionism** \ek′səbish′ənizm\ The practice by a male of exposing his genitals in the presence of strangers, usually females and often children, to achieve sexual gratification; a type of paraphilia.

**exhilarant** \egzil′ərənt\ **1** Enlivening; exhilarating. **2** An agent that enlivens or exhilarates.

**exhumation** \eks′hyoomā′shən\ [from Med L *exhumatus,* past part. of *exhumare,* from L *ex-* from out of + *humus* earth, soil] The removal of a body, previously buried, from the earth. Exhumation may be performed for many reasons, such as the need to establish that a previously unrecognized injury or illness existed. In the United States and Great Britain, legal authorization is required before an exhumation can be carried out.

**exitus** \ek′sitəs\ [L (from *exitus,* past part. of *exire* to go out), a going out, termination] **1** Exit; outlet. **2** Death.

**Exner** [Sigmund *Exner,* Austrian physiologist, 1846–1926] **1** Call-Exner body. See under BODY. **2** Exner's plexus. See under MOLECULAR PLEXUS.

**exo-** \ek′sō-\ [Gk *exō* without, on the outside] A prefix meaning outside, external.

**exoamylase** Any amylase that hydrolyzes starch by splitting sugar molecules from the ends (outsides) of chains.

**exocardial** \-kär′dē·əl\ **1** Located or formed outside the heart. **2** Pertaining to ectocardia; ectocardial.

**exoccipital** \ek′säksip′itəl\ *[ex(o)-* + *occipit(o)-* + -AL] Each of two identical and symmetric bony (cartilaginous) pieces which constitute in a fetus the lateral masses of the occiput.

**exochorion** \-kôr′ē·än\ [EXO- + CHORION] The part of the chorion which develops from embryonic ectoderm.

**exocoelom** \-sē′ləm\ [EXO- + COELOM] EXTRAEMBRYONIC COELOM.

**exocranial** \-krā′nē·əl\ ECTOCRANIAL.

**exocrine** \ek′sōkrin\ [EXO- + Gk *krin(ein)* to separate] Secreting in the direction of the body surface, usually through a duct. Also *eccrine.* Compare ENDOCRINE.

**exocytosis** \-sītō′sis\ [EXO- + CYT- + -OSIS] A mechanism for transport of substances out of a cell by enclosure in the plasma membrane followed by expulsion from the cell.

Also *reverse pinocytosis, emiocytosis, emeiocytosis.*

**exodeviation** \-dē'vē·ā'shən\ [EXO- + DEVIATION] A misalignment of the eye into an abnormally divergent position; latent or manifest outward separation of the visual axes of the two eyes.

**exodontia** \-dän'shə\ [EX-$^2$ + -ODONTIA] The study of the deliberate removal of teeth as a part of dental treatment.

**exoenergetic** \-en'ərjet'ik\ EXERGONIC.

**exoenzyme** \-en'zīm\ **1** Any enzyme that is oriented in a cell surface so that it acts on substrates outside the cell. **2** Any enzyme that acts on the external ends of chains of a macromolecule and willnot act on similar links within those chains.

**exoergic** \-ur'jik\ EXERGONIC.

**exoerythrocytic** \-irith'rəsit'ik\ [EXO- + *erythrocyt(e)* + -IC] External to erythrocytes: Usually said of the asexual developmental stages of malarial parasites occurring for example, in parenchymal cells in the liver. Also *metaerythrocytic.*

**exogamy** \eksäg'əmē\ [EXO- + GAM- + -Y] **1** Reproductive union between eukaryotic organisms that are not descended from a recent common ancestor or which are genotypically less similar than the average of random pairings. **2** Mating or marriage between members of different tribes, clans, communities, or other social groups. To the extent that the groups differ in their ancestry, exogamy implies outbreeding. Compare ENDOGAMY.

**exogastrulation** \-gas'trəlā'shən\ [EXO- + GASTRULATION] Abnormal development in which there has been interference with the normal processes of gastrulation causing evagination of the primitive gut to the exterior. Also *extrogastrulation.*

**exogenetic** \-jənet'ik\ EXOGENOUS.

**exogenous** \eksäj'ənəs\ [EXO- + -GENOUS] **1** Produced or otherwise originating outside the organism. Also *exogenetic.* **2** Growing outward; exophytic. For defs. 1 and 2 also *exogenic, ectogenous, ectogenic.*

**exognathion** \ek'sägnā'thē·än\ The maxilla, excluding the endognathion and mesognathion.

**exognosis** \ek'sägnō'sis\ DIAGNOSIS BY EXCLUSION.

**exohormone** \-hôr'mōn\ PHEROMONE.

**exometer** \eksäm'ətər\ An apparatus, no longer used, to measure the ability of x rays to produce fluorescence.

**exomphalos** \eksäm'fələs\ [EX-$^2$ + Gk *omphalos* navel] OMPHALOCELE.

**exon** \ek'sän\ [*ex(o)-* + -ON] In genetics, a subregion of a gene of higher organisms that codes for some portion of the processed mRNA which, in turn, is translated into protein. Also *coding sequence.* Compare INTRON.

**exonuclease** \-n$^y$oo'klē·ās\ Any of a class of hydrolytic enzymes which remove one of the terminal nucleotides from a polynucleotide chain. Compare ENDONUCLEASE.

**5'-exonuclease** PHOSPHODIESTERASE I.

**exopathic** \-path'ik\ Being or relating to exopathy; produced by a pathogen arising outside the host: said of a disease.

**exopathy** \eksäp'əthē\ [EXO- + -PATHY] A disease of an organism produced by a pathogen arising outside the host.

**exopeptidase** Any enzyme that hydrolyzes a protein or peptide by splitting amino acids or, rarely, dipeptides from the ends of the substrate molecules.

**exophoria** \-fôr'ē·ə\ [EXO- + PHORIA] Latent outward separation of the visual axes of the two eyes. Adj. exophoric.

**exophthalmic** \ek'säfthal'mik\ Relating to or characterized by exophthalmos.

**exophthalmometer** \ek'säfthalmäm'ətər\ A device for measuring the anteroposterior position of the eye within the orbit. The reference points are usually the apex of the cornea and the lateral orbital rim. Also *protometer, proptometer, ophthalmostat, ophthalmostatometer, orthometer.*

**exophthalmometry** \ek'säfthalmäm'ətrē\ [*exophthalmo(s)* + -METRY] The measurement of the anteroposterior position of the eye within the orbit, corresponding to the distance in millimeters between the corneal apex and the lateral orbital rim.

**exophthalmos** \ek'säfthal'məs\ [Gk (from *ex(o)-* out + *ophthalmos* eye) having eyes that bulge out] An abnormally forward, protuberant position of the eye within the orbit. Also *proptosis, ophthalmocele* (rare), *ophthalmoptosis, protopsis* (rare), *exorbitism* (rare), *exophthalmus* (rare). **endocrine e.** Exophthalmos related to dysfunction of an endocrine gland such as the thyroid in hyperthyroidism. **malignant e.** Thyrotoxic exophthalmos of sufficient severity to damage the health and function of the eye and adnexa, as proptosis of the globe, ulceration of the cornea, paralysis of the extraocular muscles and impairment or loss of vision. **pulsating e.** Forward displacement of the eye within its socket, varying in amount synchronously with the arterial pulse. The pulsation is transmitted from the brain through a defect in the bony orbit. **thyrotoxic e.** Exophthalmos associated with Graves disease. In the benign form there is an illusion of apparent forward displacement of the eye owing to widening of the palpebral fissures, as a result of the synergistic actions of excessive thyroid hormone and catecholamines. True exophthalmos results from mucopolysaccharide accumulation in the retro-orbital space with consequent proptosis of the globe, and may progress to malignant exophthalmos. **thyrotropic e.** A forward displacement of the eyes found in various forms of Graves disease and attributed to the thyrotropic hormone of the pituitary rather than to thyroid hormone. Also *hyperophthalmopathic syndrome.*

**exophthalmus** \ek'säfthal'məs\ *Rare* EXOPHTHALMOS.

**exophyte** \ek'sōfīt\ A parasite that lives on the exterior of its plant host.

**exophytic** \-fit'ik\ **1** Of or relating to an exophyte. **2** Characterized by a proliferation on the surface or outer epithelium of an organ or structure in which the growth originated. Also *ectophytic.*

**exoplasm** \ek'sōplazm\ ECTOPLASM.

**exorbitism** \eksôr'bitizm\ *Rare* EXOPHTHALMOS.

**exoresis** \ek'sôrē'sis\ AVULSION.

**exosepsis** \-sep'sis\ [EXO- + SEPSIS] Septic poisoning the source of which is external to the body.

**exoskeleton** \-skel'ətən\ **1** A more or less rigid integument of an animal body, such as the chitinous or calcareous external skeleton of various invertebrates, especially arthropods, which gives support and often a shape to the animal. Growth occurs only as the exoskeleton is shed and replaced. **2** In vertebrates, the portions of the integument, such as hair, nails, and teeth, produced by the epidermis. For defs. 1 and 2 also *ectoskeleton.*

**exosmosis** \ek'säzmō'sis\ [EX-$^2$ + OSMOSIS] Osmosis involving movement of a liquid out of a cell or cavity. Compare ENDOSMOSIS.

**exosomesthesia** \-sō'mesthē'zhə\ [EXO- + Gk *sōm(a)* the body + ESTHESIA] An illusional sensory experience seen in some patients with parietal lobe lesions in which the patient locates a sensory stimulus which has actually been applied to the surface of the body at some point in extrapersonal space.

**exosplenopexy** \-splē'nəpek'sē\ [EXO- + SPLENO- + -PEXY] The surgical fixation of the spleen within the wound or outside of the body.

**exostectomy** \ek′sästek′təmē\ The surgical removal of an exostosis. Also *exostosectomy.*

**exostosis** \ek′sästō′sis\ [Gk *exostōsis* (from EX-[2] + *ost(eon)* bone + -OSIS) a bony outgrowth] (*pl.* exostoses) A benign bony protuberance that grows from the surface of a bone in response to inflammation or repeated trauma. Adj. exostotic. **e. bursata** A cartilage-capped exostosis that arises near a joint. Over it lies an adventitial bursa. **e. cartilaginea** An exostosis with a large cartilage cap that originates from the peripheral area of the growth plate. **cartilaginous e.** OSTEOCHONDROMA. **dental e.** A calcified growth on the root of a tooth. **hereditary multiple exostoses** A hereditary disorder of bone development whereby exostoses develop from the peripheral regions of the growth plates and become inclined away from the epiphysis. Also *multiple cartilaginous exostoses, multiple exostoses, osteomatosis.* See also OSTEOCHONDROMA. **ivory e.** A smooth, flattened bony protuberance that consists of compact bone. It is seen most often on the skull. **multiple exostoses** HEREDITARY MULTIPLE EXOSTOSES. **multiple cartilaginous exostoses** HEREDITARY MULTIPLE EXOSTOSES. **osteocartilaginous e.** OSTEOCHONDROMA.

**exostotic** \ek′sästät′ik\ Of or relating to an exostosis.

**exoteric** \-ter′ik\ Arising or developing outside the organism; external.

**exothermal** **1** EXOTHERMIC. **2** POIKILOTHERMIC.

**exothermic** \-thur′mik\ **1** Denoting a reaction that gives out heat, i.e. a reaction of negative enthalpy. **2** POIKILOTHERMIC.

**exothymopexy** \-thī′məpek′sē\ The removal of the thymus gland from its normal site and suturing of it to the underside of the sternum.

**exothyroidopexy** \-thīroi′dōpek′sē\ EXOTHYROPEXY.

**exothyropexia** \-thī′rōpek′sē·ə\ EXOTHYROPEXY.

**exothyropexy** \-thī′rōpek′sē\ [EXO- + THYRO- + -PEXY ] The surgical removal and fixation of thyroid tissue to the skin surface in order to permit shrinkage or dessication. Also *exothyroidopexy, exothyropexia.*

**exotic** \igzät′ik\ [L *exoticus* (from Gk *exōtikos* foreign, from *exō* on the outside) from a strange country] Describing something not originating in the place where it is found, as a disease the cause of which lies outside the region in which the case or cases have occurred and which does not usually affect the population of the region.

**exotoxic** \-täk′sik\ Of or relating to an exotoxin.

**exotoxin** \-täk′sin\ Any extracellular toxin formed by bacteria. Toxin-forming bacteria include the botulinum, diphtheria, and tetanus bacilli and one species of shigella. The exotoxins are neurotoxins, appear to be proteins, are denatured by heat, and, with the exception of the botulinum toxin, are destroyed by proteolytic enzymes. Treatment with formaldehyde destroys their toxic qualities but not their antigenic properties. Crystalline type A botulinum toxin is the most potent of all poisonous substances, with a median lethal dose of $4.5 \times 10^{-9}$ mg in the mouse. Also *ectotoxin.*

**exotropia** \-trō′pē·ə\ [EXO- + TROPIA] A manifest lateral misalignment of the visual axes of the two eyes; divergent misalignment of the eyes. Also *divergent strabismus, external strabismus, divergent squint, walleye, wall eye.* Compare ESOTROPIA. Adj. exotropic.

**expander** A substance used to expand such as a substance used to increase the volume of blood or plasma. Also *extender.* **plasma volume e.** A sterile liquid whose composition makes it suitable for intravenous use. It may be a colloid or crystalloid material. It may be derived from normal human plasma. The substance functions to increase circulating intravascular fluid volume. Also *plasma substitute.*

**expansion** [Late L *expansio* (from L *expansus,* past part. of *expandere* to stretch out, extend) a stretching out, spreading] **1** An increase in size or volume. **2** A measure of such an increase; the increment by which a quantity has increased. **3** A broadened part of an anatomic structure. **aliform e.** A wing-shaped expansion of a structure, as the greater and lesser wings of the sphenoid bone. **dorsal digital e.** EXTENSOR EXPANSION. **extensor e.** The triangular aponeurotic flattening of each tendon of the extensor digitorum muscle, joined by tendinous fibers from the interossei and a lumbrical muscle over the dorsum of the metacarpophalangeal joint and the base of the proximal phalanx. It is adherent to the joint capsule and sends some fibers anteriorly for attachment to the palmar aponeurosis and the base of the proximal phalanx. Distally the expansion separates into a central and two lateral bands that insert into the bases of the middle and distal phalanges respectively. The tendons of the extensor digitorum longus muscle of the lower limb have similar expansions. Also *extensor aponeurosis, dorsal digital expansion.* **fibrous e.'s of eye muscles** Fibrous bands that extend from the tubular sheaths of the orbital muscles to the adjacent walls of the orbital cavity, tending to limit the actions of the muscles. **hygroscopic e.** Expansion, caused by excess water, of a plaster of Paris and water mixture as it sets. **setting e.** Expansion that takes place during the setting of materials such as plaster of Paris, dental amalgam, and acrylic resin. **thermal e.** An increase in size caused by an increase in temperature. **wax e.** In dentistry, the expansion of a wax pattern during investment with a heated investing material. Expansion of the pattern or of the mold after wax removal is necessary to compensate for contraction of the cast metal as it cools.

**expectancy** The probability of the occurrence of an eventuality specified in advance. **life e.** EXPECTATION OF LIFE.

**expectant** Awaiting the birth of a child.

**expectation** / **e. of life** The average number of years of life stated by a life table as remaining to each person or other animal of a specified age, given the age-specific death rates on which the table is based. Also *life expectancy.* **e. of life at birth** MEAN LENGTH OF LIFE.

**expectorant** \ekspek′tərənt\ [L *expectorans,* gen. *expectorantis,* pres. part. of *expectorare* to drive from the breast, expectorate (from EX- + L *pectus,* gen. *pectoris* breast)] **1** Promoting the ejection of sputum from the air passages. Also *apophlegmatic.* **2** An agent which increases or promotes expectoration.

**expectorate** \ekspek′tərāt\ [See EXPECTORANT.] To expel matter from the respiratory tract through the mouth.

**expectoration** \ekspek′tərā′shən\ [See EXPECTORANT.] The act of expelling material from the respiratory tract through the mouth. **rusty e.** The expectoration of rust-colored sputum, usually due to altered blood.

**expel** To drive out by force, as a fetus by the force of uterine contractions.

**expellent** A drug or agent used for expelling worms or other parasites from the alimentary canal.

**expense** / **ancillary e.'s** Costs for health care services such as radiology, laboratory, and drug services but excluding hospital room and board and professional services such as those of a physician or other health professional personnel.

**experiment** [L *experimentum* (from *experiri* to try, test, learn from experience, akin to *peritus* expert) test, trial, experience] **1** A procedure performed to test a hypothesis, confirm a fact, or demonstrate a principle. **2** To perform an experiment. **bulbocapnine e.** A demonstration in which animals are injected with bulbocapnine to increase muscle tone while the animal is at rest. The effect of the bulbocapnine is negated by voluntary movement. **control e.** An experiment or study that employs a standard (or control) against which the effects observed in a different group or subject to whom the variable being tested has been exposed can be compared. See also CONTROL. **crossover e.** An experiment or study in which each of two matched groups alternately serves as control and experimental group. See also CROSS-OVER. **defect e.** A method of ascertaining the effect on development of destroying a region or part of an embryo, sometimes employed in fate mapping studies. **double-blind e.** An experiment or study characterized by concealment to both experimenter and subjects as to which subjects are exposed to the variable being tested and which are functioning as controls. See also DOUBLE-BLIND. **Küss e.** A demonstration of the impermeability of the bladder to opiate drugs in which opiates are placed directly into the bladder but do not produce opiate poisoning in the body. **Mariotte's e.** A demonstration of the blind spot in the visual field. With one eye covered, the subject fixes the other eye on a cross that has been marked on a card, which also bears a large spot. The card is moved to and from the face to illustrate that at a certain point the image of the spot will be lost. **Müller's e.** A demonstration of the effect on the arterial pulse that occurs when making a forced inspiratory effort with the glottis closed. Also *Müller's maneuver.* Compare VALSALVA MANEUVER. **Nussbaum's e.** The demonstration of the function of renal tubules in animals such as frogs. The renal arteries are ligated to cut off the blood supply to the glomeruli. **O'Beirne's e.** The simulation of a strangulated hernia by injection of air or fluid into a loop of intestine that has been passed through a hole in a piece of paper or cardboard. **Scheiner's e.** The demonstration of the focusing ability of the eye by looking at an object, usually a pin, through two appropriately positioned pinholes in a card. If the object is in focus, only one image is observed; if not, more than one image is seen. **Stensen's e.** A demonstration of the importance of the abdominal aorta to the blood supply of the lumbar region of the spinal cord. Experimental compression of the abdominal aorta alters the functional integrity of the lower spinal cord and this results in paralysis of the hindquarters in animals. **Toynbee's e.** An experiment to demonstrate the effect on the air pressure in the tympanic cavity of swallowing with both the nose and mouth closed. • Joseph Toynbee, the pioneer London otologist, 1815–1866, was the first specialist in this field to base his practice on the painstaking study of pathologic material. **Valsalva's e.** VALSALVA MANEUVER.

**expert** / **medical e.** A physician, nurse, or other medical practitioner who is qualified to provide expert evidence and who testifies as an expert witness in his professional capacity in a legal proceeding. Opinions of medical experts are allowed into evidence but are restricted to the realm of medical certainty. The expert is not allowed to express opinions that should be formulated by the jury. **medicolegal e.** An individual with education, training, and experience in forensic medicine. In the capacity of expert witness, a medicolegal expert can give an opinion in a court of law on the basis of the evidence presented to him or on the basis of factual material he has gathered.

**expiration** \eks′pərā′shən\ [L *ex(s)piratio* (from *ex(s)pirare* to exhale; see EXPIRE) exhalation] **1** The act or process of breathing out; in humans, the expulsion of air from lungs as part of the process of respiration. **2** Death.

**expire** [Old French *expirer,* from L *ex(s)pirare* (from *ex-* out + *spirare* to breathe) to breathe out, breathe one's last] **1** To breathe out as part of the process of respiration. **2** To die.

**explant** \eksplant′\ [EX-[2] + *(im)plant*] **1** To transfer (viable tissue) from a living organism to an artificial medium, as for laboratory culture. **2** Tissue that has been explanted for laboratory culture. **cellular e.** TISSUE CULTURE.

**explode** [L *explode(re)* to drive out by clapping. See EXPLOSION.] **1** To cause to release energy suddenly, usually with a loud report. **2** To burst violently as a result of pressure from within; undergo explosion. **3** To increase rapidly and suddenly; multiply in number, as the incidence of disease.

**exploration** [L *exploratio* (from *exploratus,* past part. of *explorare* to spy out, examine, explore) a spying, searching] Investigation or examination of a part or organ of the body for diagnostic purposes by touch, instrument, or operation.

**exploratory** \iksplôr′ətôr′ē\ Designating a diagnostic procedure, especially surgery, to investigate or examine a part or organ of the body.

**explorer** PROBE.

**explosion** [L *explosio* (from *explosus,* past part. of *explodere* to drive out by clapping, from EX- + L *plodere,* for *plaudere,* to clap, applaud, from Gk *platagein* to clap the hands loudly) a driving out by clapping] **1** A sudden release of energy, usually accompanied by a loud report. **2** A sudden and rapid increase, as of the incidence of disease in an epidemic.

**explosive** [L *explos(us),* past part. of *explodere* to drive out by clapping + -IVE. See EXPLOSION.] A material that, when detonated, expands instantaneously with destructive force.

**exponent** \ikspō′nənt\ A superscript placed to the right of a mathematical expression and designating the power to which the mathematical quantity is to be raised. Adj. exponential.

**exposure** [EX- + French *poser* to place, put, from L *positus,* past part. of *ponere* to place, put] In radiology and radiation protection, the amount of x- or gamma radiation at some point, as determined by the amount of ionization produced in air at that point. The unit of exposure is the roentgen. Also *air exposure, exposure dose* (imprecise). **air e.** EXPOSURE. **double e.** A radiograph obtained by two separate exposures of an area on the same film. **pulp e.** The creation of continuity between the dental pulp and a carious cavity or the oral cavity. It may be carious, accidental, or caused by fracture of the tooth.

**express** To extract or force out by pressing or squeezing.

**expression** [French *expression* (from L *expressus,* past part. of *exprimere* to press out, force out, from EX- + L *premere* to press) a pressing out, manner of expressing] The act of expressing; extraction or expulsion by pressure or by squeezing out. **manual e. of placenta** The act of squeezing or exerting pressure on the uterus to facilitate expulsion of the placenta after delivery of a baby.

**expressive** Of or relating to expression, as speech.

**expressivity** \eks′presiv′itē\ The extent to which a phenotype, primarily determined by a gene, appears in a given individual. Measured in quantitative or qualitative terms, the expression of a gene depends on numerous factors including age, sex, environment, and the action of other genes.

**expulsion** \ikspul′shən\ [L *expulsio* (from *expulsus,* past part. of *expellere* to drive out or away) expulsion] The act or process of forcing out or driving out. **spontaneous e. of placenta** Vaginal delivery of the placenta without the use of traction or abdominal pressure.

**expulsive** \ikspul′siv\ Tending to force out or drive out.

**exsanguinate** \eksang′gwənāt\ [L *exsanguinat(us)* (from *ex-* EX-[1] + *sanguis*, gen. *sanguinis*, blood + *-atus* -ATE) without blood] **1** To drain of blood. **2** Deprived of blood; bloodless.

**exsanguination** \eksang′gwənā′shən\ [See EXSANGUINATE.] Hemorrhage within a body cavity or externally in quantities sufficient to cause death.

**exsanguine** \eksang′gwin\ Bloodless.

**exsect** \eksekt′\ [L *exsect(us)*, past part. of *exsectare* (from *ex-* out + *sectare* to cut) to cut out] EXCISE.

**exsection** \eksek′shən\ [EXSECT + -ION] EXCISION.

**exsiccant** \ek′sikənt\ [L *exsiccans*, gen. *exsiccantis*, pres. part. of *exsiccare* to dry up] DESICCANT.

**exsiccate** [L *exsiccat(us)*, past part. of *exsiccare* (from *ex-* from + *siccus* dry) to dry up] DESICCATE.

**exsiccosis** \ek′sikō′sis\ [*exsicc(ate)* + -OSIS] DEHYDRATION.

**exsorption** \eksôrp′shən\ [L *exsorptus*, past part. of *exsorbere* to swallow, absorb, drain juice from] The movement of substances from within outward, as from the blood into the intestinal lumen or out of cells.

**exstrophy** \ek′strōfē\ [Gk *ekstroph(ē)* (from *ekstrephein* to turn inside out, from *ek-* out + *strephein* to turn, twist) eversion, dislocation + -Y] A congenital anomaly in which a hollow organ has its wall everted, thus establishing a communication with the exterior. Also *extrophy* (mispelling), *ecstrophy*. **e. of the bladder** A congenital anomaly of the urinary bladder characterized by absence of the anterior wall of the bladder and overlying abdominal wall, with eversion of the posterior bladder wall so that urine from the ureteral orifices drains to the exterior. Associated anomalies include epispadias and, rarely, carcinoma may develop. Also *extroversion of the bladder, hernia of the bladder, ectopia vesicae, schistocystis, cystoschisis.*

**ext.** *extractum* (L, extract).

**extend** To straighten a limb or other body part at a joint. Compare FLEX.

**extender** **1** A substance added to another to dilute or modify it or to increase its volume. **2** EXPANDER. **artificial plasma e.** Plasma volume expander which is synthetic in nature and is not derived from fractionation of normal human plasma. **dental e.** A term sometimes used in the U.S. for DENTAL ASSISTANT. **physician e.** PHYSICIAN ASSISTANT.

**extension** [L *extensus*, past part. of *extendere* to stretch out, extend] **1** The straightening of a limb. **2** The lengthening of a structure by axial traction. **Buck's e.** A method of applying longitudinal traction to one or both lower limbs. Adhesive tape, applied to the limb, is attached to a cord which is connected to weights and passed over a pulley. The foot of the bed is elevated so that the body acts as a counterweight. Also *Buck's traction.* **nail e.** SKELETAL TRACTION. **e. for prevention** The enlargement of a carious cavity at the margins beyond that required to remove the caries. The object is to place the cavity margin in a situation not conducive to the formation of further caries. This is achieved by including all fissures in the cavity and by extending proximal parts of the cavity margin so that they are easily cleaned with a toothbrush or are subgingival. **ridge e.** The increasing of the area of an edentulous ridge by surgically deepening the adjacent sulcus or sulci. Also *Kazanjian's procedure.* **skeletal e.** SKELETAL TRACTION. **Steinmann's e.** Skeletal traction in which a transfixing pin is placed into the os calcis for fractures of the tibia or into the tibial tubercle for fractures of the femur. The traction force is applied through weights and pulleys that are attached to the pin. **tectoseptal e.** The contribution of maxillary mesoderm to the formation of the nasal septum in the embryo. The primitive septum is formed from the deep portion of the frontonasal process and receives this mesodermal extension as it grows downwards and backwards towards the palatal processes to become the definitive nasal septum.

**extensor** \iksten′sər\ **1** A muscle that causes the movable part on one side of a joint either to move away from the other side or to move with the other side to approach a straight line. **2** A muscle that causes the movable part of a joint in the upper limb or the hip joint to move posteriorly or dorsally. **3** A muscle that causes the movable part of the knee, ankle, or toe joints to move anteriorly. Compare FLEXOR. **e. carpi radialis accessorius** A variant of the radial extensors of the wrist that usually arises as a slip of one or both muscles and is inserted onto the base of the metacarpal or the proximal phalanx of the thumb, the abductor pollicis brevis, or an adjacent structure. **e. carpi radialis intermedius** A variant of the radial extensors of the wrist that has an origin similar to that of the extensor carpi radialis accessorius but is inserted into the base of either the second or third metacarpal bone, or both. **long radial e. of wrist** MUSCULUS EXTENSOR CARPI RADIALIS LONGUS. **ulnar e. of wrist** MUSCULUS EXTENSOR CARPI ULNARIS.

**exterior** Of or on the outside.

**exteriorize** \ikstir′ē·ərīz\ To expose so as to make part of an exterior surface, as an organ or bodily structure, for the purpose of observation and study, promoting healing, or treatment.

**extern** \ek′stərn\ [French *externe* (from L *externus* outside) a nonresident student] A health professions student who is receiving training in a health care facility under a specific type of program for field training.

**external** \ikstur′nəl\ **1** Of or situated on the outside or on an outer surface. **2** EXTERNUS.

**externalia** \ek′stərnā′lē·ə\ The external genitalia. *Outmoded.*

**externalization** \ikstur′nəlīzā′shən\ [*external* + *-iz(e)* + -ATION] The process by which the young child comes gradually to differentiate between the self and not-self.

**externalize** \ikstur′nəlīz\ To project or turn an internal conflict onto the external world.

**externus** \ikstur′nəs\ [L, outward, external] **1** On, near, or relating to the outside of the body, an organ or part; away from the center of a cavity or on its exterior. Also *external.* **2** An outmoded and incorrect term for LATERALIS.

**extero-** \ek′stərō-\ [L *exter* on the outside, without] A prefix meaning outside, outer.

**exteroceptive** \-sep′tiv\ [EXTERO- + *(re)ceptive*] Denoting receptor sensitivity to external environmental changes capable of exciting the skin.

**exteroceptor** \-sep′tər\ [EXTERO- + *(re)ceptor*] A sensory receptor that responds to stimuli generated in the external environment, such as the pain, touch, and pressure receptors in the skin and the visual and auditory receptors. Compare ENTEROCEPTOR.

**extinction** [L *ex(s)tinctio* (from *ex(s)tinguere* to extinguish, quench, wipe out, from *ex-*, intensifying prefix + *stinguere* to quench) extinction, annihilation] **1** In classical or operant conditioning, the progressive weakening of a conditioned response and the decreased likelihood of its appearance as a result of omission of the reward or reinforcement. **2** INATTENTION PHENOMENON. **3** The disappearance or extermination of a species. **4** In genetics, the loss of a given allele from a population.

**extinguish** In classical or operant conditioning, to subject to the process of extinction: said of a response.

**extirpate** \ek′stərpāt\ [L *ex(s)tirpare* (from *ex-* out + *stirps* trunk, root) to pull up by the trunk or root] To excise completely, as an organ or a pathologic process; remove in its entirety.

**extirpation** \ek′stərpā′shən\ [L *ex(s)tirpatio* an uprooting. See EXTIRPATE.] The excision of an entire organ or of a pathologic process. **pulp e.** PULP REMOVAL.

**extorsion** \ekstôr′shən\ [EX-[1] + TORSION] Rotary movement of an eye in the upper part of the vertical meridian in a lateral direction. Also *disclination*.

**extortor** \ekstôr′tər\ **1** An ocular muscle that produces extorsion of the eye, namely, the inferior oblique muscle when the eye is abducted, and the inferior rectus muscle when it is adducted. **2** A lateral rotator.

**extra-** \ek′strə-\ [L *extra* (from *exter* on the outside, without) on the outside, without, in addition] A prefix meaning outside, beyond, in addition.

**extra-adrenal** \-ədrē′nəl\ Situated on or external to the suprarenal, or adrenal, gland.

**extra-amniotic** \-am′nē·ät′ik\ Occurring outside the amniotic cavity.

**extra-articular** \-ärtik′yələr\ Describing or pertaining to structures about but not within the joints, such as tendons, bursae, and other bone and/or muscle structures. Also *extracapsular*.

**extrabronchial** \-bräng′kē·əl\ Situated outside or independently of the bronchi.

**extracapsular** \-kap′s$^y$ələr\ **1** Pertaining to the space outside a capsule. **2** EXTRA-ARTICULAR.

**extracardiac** \-kär′dē·ak\ [EXTRA- + CARDIAC] Occurring or originating outside the heart. Also *extracardial*.

**extracartilaginous** \-kär′təlaj′ənəs\ Beyond the cartilage: used especially of a surgical incision about the ear designed to avoid cutting through the cartilages of the ear.

**extracellular** \-sel′yələr\ External to cells; occurring or functioning outside of cells.

**extracerebral** \-ser′əbrəl\ On the outside of or beyond the cerebral surface.

**extrachromosomal** \-krō′məsō′məl\ Pertaining to any cellular process that occurs away from the chromosomes or to a structure that is separate from the chromosome.

**extracorporeal** Of or situated on the outside of the body. Also *extracorporal*.

**extracorpuscular** \-kôrpus′kyələr\ Situated or occurring outside a cell, especially outside an erythrocyte.

**extracorticospinal** \-kôr′təkōspī′nəl\ EXTRAPYRAMIDAL.

**extract** [L *extractus*, past part. of *extrahere* to draw out, drag out, from EX- + L *trahere* to draw, draw away] **1** To remove, as a concentrate, by the action of a solvent. **2** A concentrated drug preparation of vegetable or animal origin obtained by removal of the active constituent with an appropriate solvent, evaporation of all or nearly all of the solvent, and adjustment of the remaining mass or powder to a prescribed standard. Extracts can be obtained in three forms: semiliquid or syrupy consistency, pilular or solid, and a dry powder. Also *extractum*. **3** To remove by force or pressure. **alcoholic e.** A solid extract product obtained by extraction of the alcohol-soluble elements of a drug source, followed by evaporation of the alcohol. **allergenic e.** An extract containing a substance, usually a protein, from a source such as food, bacteria, pollen, or any substance a person may be sensitive to. These extracts are used for diagnosis or desensitization therapy in conditions of hypersensitivity to the particular substance. **alum precipitated poison ivy e.** An extract used to counteract rhus dermatitis due to poison ivy, *Toxicodendron radicans*. It is a pyridine extract of poison ivy designed to be slowly absorbed. **animal e.** An extract prepared from constituents of animal origin. **beef e.** An extract prepared through the concentration of beef broth and used in compounding certain prescriptions. Also *extractum carnis*. **Buchner e.** An extract of yeast that is cell-free but able to catalyze fermentative reactions. **chondrus e.** A tan powder obtained from the dried seaweed *Chondrus crispus*. It is used as a protective agent externally and internally. Also *Irish moss extract*. **compound e.** An extract containing more than one active agent. **dry e.** POWDERED EXTRACT. **equivalent e.** A fluid extract possessing, weight for weight, the same strength as the original drug. **euphorbia liquid e.** An extract obtained by percolation of the dried plant *Euphorbia hirta* with 45 percent alcohol. The plant contains not less than 16 percent extractable material. The extract is used as a constituent of cough medicines and for preparations to treat asthma. **fluid e.** FLUIDEXTRACT. **glycyrrhiza e.** A brown powder made from the rhizome and foots of plants of the *Glycyrrhiza* species. The extract is used as a flavoring agent. Also *licorice root extract*. **henbane e.** HYOSCYAMUS EXTRACT. **hydroalcoholic e.** A solid extract prepared by extracting the soluble constituents of a drug with alcohol and water, followed by evaporation. **hyoscyamus e.** An extract in pilular or powdered form containing 155 mg of hyoscyamus alkaloids, primarily hyoscyamine and hyoscine, in each 100 g. It was formerly used as an anticholinergic agent. Also *henbane extract*. **Irish moss e.** CHONDRUS EXTRACT. **licorice root e.** GLYCYRRHIZA EXTRACT. **liquid e.** FLUIDEXTRACT. **liquid liver e.** LIVER SOLUTION. **liver e.** A slightly hygroscopic brown powder that is derived from mammalian livers and is used to promote hematopoiesis. Also *extractum hepatis*. **e. of male fern** ASPIDIUM OLEORESIN. **malt e.** A sweet, viscous, light brown liquid or powder obtained by extracting the partially and artificially germinated grain of barley. The extract contains dextrin, maltose, glucose, and amylolytic enzymes. It is used as a nutritive and emulsifying agent. **meat e.** A preparation obtained by boiling meat and concentrating the broth. It is rich in cofactors and is used to enrich bacterial culture media. **nux vomica e.** A powder derived from nux vomica containing 7–7.75 g of strychnine in each 100 g of powder. Although used in the past, strychnine preparations are without any therapeutic value, and may cause fatal poisoning. Also *extractum nucis vomicae*. **ox bile e.** A brownish to greenish yellow powder or granular preparation from the fresh bile of the ox. The extract contains at least 45% cholic acid, and possesses a characteristic odor and bitter taste. It is used as a choleretic medication. Also *powdered oxgall extract, extractum fellis bovis, ox gall*. **parathyroid e.** PARATHYROID INJECTION. **pilular e.** An extract prepared in the form of a thick paste using liquid glucose, malt extract, or glycerin as the diluent. Also *solid extract*. **placental e.** An extract containing globulins derived from human placenta. It is used to immunize children against measles. **poison ivy e.** An extract made from the fresh leaves of poison ivy, *Toxicodendron radicans*. It is used in the prevention of rhus dermatitis due to poison ivy by providing an agent effective in desensitizing an individual. **poison oak e.** An extract made from the fresh leaves of poison oak, *Toxicodendron diversilobum*. It is used in the prevention of rhus dermatitis due to poison oak by providing an agent capable of desensitizing an individual. **pollen e.** A preparation made from the pollen of specific plants to be used in the diagnosis and treatment of inhalant allergies to those plants. **powdered e.** A dry powder extract prepared using starch, sucrose, lactose, powdered glycyrrhiza, magnesium carbonate, magnesium oxide, or calcium phosphate as a diluent. Also *dry extract.* **powdered oxgall e.** OX BILE EXTRACT. **protein e.** An extract of a substance consisting of only the protein portion, to which a sensitivity is suspected. It may be utilized for either diagnosis or desensitization. **pure glycyrrhiza e.** An extract made from the rizome and the roots of varieties of *Glycyrrhiza glabra.* It is used in the compounding of aromatic cascara sagrada fluid extract. Also *pure licorice root extract.* **semiliquid e.** An extract that has been evaporated to a syrupy consistency. **soft e.** An extract that has the consistency of honey. These preparations are awkward to work with and are seldom used. **solid e.** PILULAR EXTRACT. **yeast e.** A powder extract prepared from a water-soluble, peptonelike derivative of yeast cells.

**extractant** \ikstrak′tənt\ An agent used to extract a substance, as from a mixture or tissue.

**extraction** \ikstrak′shən\ [L *extractio* (from *extractus,* past part. of *extrahere* to draw out or away) an extracting] **1** The act or process of extracting, as by surgical intervention. **2** The deliberate removal of a tooth as a part of dental treatment. For defs. 1 and 2 also *exelcymosis.* **3** The preparation of a pharmaceutical extract. **breech e.** Traction on an infant presenting as a breech in order to facilitate vaginal delivery. **intracapsular e.** Cataract extraction within an intact lens capsule. **menstrual e.** A procedure intended to produce abortion and carried out usually within the first six weeks from the first day of the last menstrual period, using a suction device to aspirate the contents of the uterine cavity. **partial breech e.** Extraction of an infant in the breech presentation after the forces of labor have allowed delivery to the level of the umbilicus. **phenol water e.** A method which employs phenol ($C_6H_5OH$) in water to extract lipids or proteins from bacteria. It is useful in the extraction and purification of lipopolysaccharides from Gram-negative bacteria. **serial e.** The planned extraction of deciduous and permanent teeth during the period of the mixed dentition. It is a form of interceptive orthodontic treatment in cases of overcrowding where it is seen that the extraction of a permanent tooth will be necessary at some stage of treatment. By the premature removal of a tooth to precede the eruption of an adjacent tooth, normal arch alignment can be achieved without the use of orthodontic appliances. **total breech e.** Extraction of the entire infant in the breech presentation without benefit of partial delivery by the forces of labor. **vacuum e.** Extraction of an infant from the birth canal utilizing a cuplike suction device applied to the fetal head which facilitates traction on the infant.

**extractor** \ikstrak′tər\ [EXTRACT + -OR] An instrument used for extraction of tissue or a foreign body.

**extractum** [L (from *extractum,* neut. of *extractus,* past part. of *extrahere* to draw out, drag out), an extract] EXTRACT. **e. carnis** BEEF EXTRACT. **e. fellis bovis** OX BILE EXTRACT. **e. hepatis** LIVER EXTRACT. **e. nucis vomicae** NUX VOMICA EXTRACT.

**extracystic** \-sis′tik\ Situated outside or beyond the urinary bladder or gallbladder.

**extradural** \-d^y^oo′rəl\ External to the dura mater.

**extraembryonic** \-em′brē·än′ik\ [EXTRA- + EMBRYONIC] Describing a part that does not become a constituent part of the embryo proper: used especially of the fetal membranes and structure outside the body stalk.

**extraepiphyseal** \-ep′ifiz′ē·əl\ Not attached or related to the epiphysis.

**extrafusal** \-fyoo′zəl\ [EXTRA- + L *fus(us)* a spindle + -AL] Denoting the tissue in a muscle exclusive of its spindles. • The term is used when a distinction is to be made between components contained within the muscle spindle capsule and other elements in the muscle.

**extramastoiditis** \-mas′toidī′tis\ An inflammation localized to the external surface of the mastoid process and surrounding soft tissues.

**extramedullary** \-med′yəler′ē\ External to the spinal cord.

**extrameningeal** \-menin′jē·əl\ EPIDURAL.

**extraneous** \ikstrā′nē·əs\ Arising, occurring, or belonging outside an organism.

**extraneural** \-n^y^ʊr′əl\ Affecting, involving, or pertaining to tissues other than neural tissue; not neural.

**extranuclear** \-n^y^oo′klē·ər\ [EXTRA- + NUCLEAR] Located or occurring outside of the nucleus, as in the cytoplasm.

**extraocular** \-äk′yələr\ [EXTRA- + OCULAR] Designating a location near to the eye but not within the eyeball.

**extraperineal** \-per′inē′əl\ Pertaining to the area around the perineum.

**extraphysiologic** \-fiz′ē·öläj′ik\ Pertaining to phenomena outside the normal physiologic processes, hence pathologic.

**extraplacental** \-pləsen′təl\ **1** Occurring outside the placenta. **2** Not dependent upon the placenta.

**extrapleural** \-plʊr′əl\ Outside the parietal pleura.

**extrapolation** \ikstrap′əlā′shən\ [EXTRA- + *(inter)polate,* from L *interpolatus,* past part. of *interpolare* to polish, furbish, give new form, + -ION] The projection or extension of directly established knowledge to an area not presently open to observation, as the calculation, on the basis of known data, of values obtaining outside the range of direct measurement or of the known data.

**extrapyramidal** \-piram′ədəl\ **1** Situated outside the corticospinal (pyramidal) tract. Also *extracorticospinal.* **2** Pertaining to the basal ganglia, red nucleus, vestibular nuclei, and reticular formation and their descending connections which modulate background activity for the motor system.

**extrarenal** \-rē′nəl\ Located outside the kidney.

**extrasensory** \-sen′sərē\ [EXTRA- + SENSORY] Not mediated by any of the known senses: used especially of an individual's claimed awareness of some external event or object.

**extraspinal** \-spī′nəl\ Of mechanisms, not involving the spinal cord.

**extrastriate** \-strī′āt\ Denoting cortical areas that mediate visual functions but do not have the characteristic cytoarchitecture of the striate visual cortex.

**extrasystole** \-sis′təlē\ [EXTRA- + SYSTOLE] A cardiac depolarization originating outside the sinuatrial node. Also *premature systole.* **atrial e.** Extrasystole arising in the atrium but not from the sinuatrial node. Also *auricular extrasystole.* **atrioventricular junctional e.** Extrasystole arising in the atrioventricular junctional tissue. Also *atrioventricular extrasystole, auriculoventricular extrasystole, A-V extrasystole, junctional extrasystole, nodal extrasystole, A-V nodal extrasystole.* **auricular e.** ATRIAL EXTRASYSTOLE. **auriculoventricular e.** ATRIOVENTRICULAR JUNCTIONAL EXTRASYSTOLE. **A-V e.** ATRIOVENTRICULAR JUNCTIONAL EXTRASYSTOLE. **A-V nodal e.** ATRIOVENTRICULAR JUNCTIONAL EXTRASYSTOLE. **infra-**

**nodal e.** VENTRICULAR EXTRASYSTOLE. **interpolated e.** An extrasystole which is interposed between two normal beats and fails to affect their time relationship. **junctional e.** ATRIOVENTRICULAR JUNCTIONAL EXTRASYSTOLE. **nodal e.** ATRIOVENTRICULAR JUNCTIONAL EXTRASYSTOLE. **return e.** An echo beat in which the impulse deriving from a ventricular extrasystole ascends towards the atrium and then returns to reactivate the ventricle. **supraventricular e.** Extrasystole deriving from above the ventricle. **ventricular e.** Extrasystole arising in the ventricles. Also *infranodal extrasystole.*

**extratubal** \-tʸoo′bəl\ Outside a tube, especially the eustachian or fallopian tubes.

**extratympanic** \-timpan′ik\ Immediately outside of the tympanic cavity.

**extrauterine** \-yoo′tərin\ [EXTRA- + UTERINE] **1** Occurring outside the uterus. **2** Not dependent upon the uterus.

**extravaginal** \-vaj′ənəl\ [EXTRA- + VAGINAL] **1** Occurring outside the vagina. **2** Not dependent upon the vagina.

**extravasate** \ikstrav′əsāt\ [EXTRA- + VAS + -ATE] To leak fluid or blood outside the confines of the vessel that is expected to contain it.

**extravasation** \ikstrav′əsā′shən\ [*extravasat(e)* + -ION] **1** The leakage of blood or fluid outside of the vessel that was expected to contain it. **2** The blood or fluid found in the tissues following such leakage. **pyelosinus e.** Extravasation of radiopaque contrast material from the renal collecting system during retrograde pyelography, usually the result of increased urinary pressure secondary to urinary obstruction. It is occasionally seen in the course of intravenous urography.

**extravascular** \-vas′kyələr\ [EXTRA- + VASCULAR] Outside the blood vessels.

**extraversion** \-vur′zhən\ EXTROVERSION.

**extravert** \ek′strəvurt\ EXTROVERT.

**extremital** \ikstrem′ətəl\ Pertaining to or located at an extremity; distal.

**extremitas** \ikstrem′itäs\ [L (from *extremus,* superl. of *exter* or *exterus* outer, external + *-itas,* -ITY), an end or extremity of a thing, the exterior] **1** The distal or peripheral portion of a limb or any elongated structure or organ. **2** An upper or lower limb; membrum. **3** A hand or foot. For defs. 1, 2, and 3 also *extremity.* **e. acromialis claviculae** [NA] The flattened lateral end of the clavicle that has an inferolaterally directed oval facet for articulation with the medial surface of the acromion in the acromioclavicular articulation. Also *acromial extremity of clavicle.* **e. anterior splenis** [NA] The wide, flattened anterior end of the spleen which is directed anteroinferiorly and connects the upper and lower margins. It is related to the left colic flexure and the phrenicocolic ligament. Also *anterior extremity of spleen, tail of spleen* (outmoded). **e. inferior 1** *Outmoded* MEMBRUM INFERIUS. **2** The lower end of an organ, as of the kidney and testis. **e. inferior renis** [NA] The rounded lower end of the kidney, which is usually smaller, thinner, and further from the median plane than the upper extremity. Also *inferior extremity of kidney, inferior pole of kidney.* **e. inferior testis** [NA] The rounded, smooth lower end of the testis, which is directed posteromedially and attached to the tail of the epididymis by areolar tissue and a reflection of the tunica vaginalis. Also *inferior extremity of testis, inferior pole of testis, caudal pole of testis.* **e. posterior splenis** [NA] The rounded, blunt posterior end of the spleen, narrower than the anterior end and directed posterosuperiorly toward the vertebral column. Also *posterior extremity of spleen.* **e. sternalis claviculae** [NA] The expanded medial end of the clavicle, having an irregular triangular articular surface directed slightly inferomedially to articulate with the clavicular notch of the manubrium sterni through an articular disk. The articular surface extends onto the inferior surface of the clavicle to articulate with the first costal cartilage. Its circumference is roughened to provide attachment for the capsule and ligaments of the joint, and the superior margin also has the articular disk attached to it. Also *sternal extremity of clavicle.* **e. superior 1** *Outmoded* MEMBRUM SUPERIUS. **2** The upper end of an organ, as of the kidney or testis. **e. superior renis** [NA] The rounded upper end of the kidney, which is usually larger, thicker, and nearer the median plane than the lower extremity. It is related to the suprarenal gland. Also *superior extremity of kidney, upper pole of kidney.* **e. superior testis** [NA] The convex, smooth upper end of the testis. It is directed anterolaterally and connected directly with the head of the epididymis by the efferent ductules of the testis. The visceral layer of tunica vaginalis covers part of it before being reflected on to the head of the epididymis. Also *superior extremity of testis, upper pole of testis, cranial pole of testis.* **e. tubaria ovarii** [NA] The larger, rounded superior end of the ovary, having the ovarian fimbria of the uterine tube and the suspensory ligament of the ovary attached to it. It usually lies close to the external iliac vein. Also *tubal extremity of ovary.* **e. uterina ovarii** [NA] The lower end of the ovary, narrower than the tubal extremity and directed towards the uterus, to the lateral angle of which it is attached by the ligament of the ovary. Also *uterine extremity of ovary, pelvic extremity of ovary.*

**extremitates** \ikstrem′itā′tēz\ Plural of EXTREMITAS.

**extremity** \ikstrem′itē\ [L *extremitas.* See EXTREMITAS.] EXTREMITAS. **acromial e. of clavicle** EXTREMITAS ACROMIALIS CLAVICULAE. **anterior e. of spleen** EXTREMITAS ANTERIOR SPLENIS. **cartilaginous e. of rib** CARTILAGO COSTALIS. **fimbriated e. of fallopian tube** FIMBRIA OVARICA. **inferior e.** MEMBRUM INFERIUS. **inferior e. of kidney** EXTREMITAS INFERIOR RENIS. **inferior e. of testis** EXTREMITAS INFERIOR TESTIS. **lower e.** MEMBRUM INFERIUS. **pelvic e. of ovary** EXTREMITAS UTERINA OVARII. **posterior e. of spleen** EXTREMITAS POSTERIOR SPLENIS. **proximal e. of phalanx of finger** BASIS PHALANGIS DIGITORUM MANUS. **proximal e. of phalanx of toe** BASIS PHALANGIS DIGITORUM PEDIS. **sternal e. of clavicle** EXTREMITAS STERNALIS CLAVICULAE. **superior e.** MEMBRUM SUPERIUS. **superior e. of kidney** EXTREMITAS SUPERIOR RENIS. **superior e. of testis** EXTREMITAS SUPERIOR TESTIS. **tubal e. of ovary** EXTREMITAS TUBARIA OVARII. **upper e.** MEMBRUM SUPERIUS. **uterine e. of ovary** EXTREMITAS UTERINA OVARII.

**extrinsic** \ikstrin′sik\ [L *extrinsecus* (from *exter* outer + *-im,* adv. suffix, + *secus* alongside; ending *-ec(us)* assimilated in English to -IC) from outside, externally] **1** Originating from outside the organism; exogenous. **2** Not an internal or integral part of the organ served: said of anatomic structures. Compare INTRINSIC.

**extro-** \ek′strō-\ [by analogy to INTRO-] A prefix meaning outer or outward.

**extrogastrulation** \-gas′trəlā′shən\ EXOGASTRULATION.

**extrophy** A misspelling of EXSTROPHY.

**extroversion** \-vur′zhən\ **1** A personality trait that orients one toward external events, other people, and social interactions rather than toward inner feelings or thoughts.

2 Eversion of a hollow organ. For defs. 1 and 2 also *extraversion*. **e. of the bladder** EXSTROPHY OF THE BLADDER.

**extrovert** \ek′strəvurt\ [EXTRO- + L *vert(ere)* to turn] One whose personality exhibits the characteristics of extroversion. Also *extravert*.

**extrusion** \ikstroo′zhən\ [Med L *extrusio* (from L *extrusus*, past part. of *extrudere* to drive or thrust out, exclude) a driving or thrusting out] 1 The action of pushing or forcing out. 2 The condition resulting from the action of pushing or forcing out, as of a displaced part or organ. **e. of tooth** 1 The slight temporary displacement of a tooth toward the occlusal plane, without damaging the main fiber bundles, by acute apical periodontitis. 2 The permanent displacement of a tooth with its supporting structures toward the occlusal plane when the antagonistic teeth are absent; overeruption. For defs. 1 and 2 also *extrudoclusion*.

**extubate** \ikst$^y$oo′bāt, ek′st$^y$əbāt\ To remove a tube from.

**extubation** \eks′t$^y$oobā′shən\ The withdrawal of a tube, as from an organ or orifice.

**exuberant** \igzoo′bərənt\ Plentiful or superabundant in production; displaying profuse proliferation.

**exudate** \ek′soodāt, eks′yoodāt\ [L *exudat(us), exsudatus*, past part. of *exudare, exsudare* to sweat out, discharge by sweating, from *ex-* EX-[1] + *sudor* sweat] An extravascular fluid characteristic of the inflammatory reaction, containing a high protein level, cells and cellular debris and having a specific gravity above 1.020. It accumulates in tissues or is deposited on surfaces such as the pleura. **catarrhal e.** A mucus-rich exudate associated with inflammation of a mucosal membrane. **cotton wool e.'s** COTTON WOOL PATCHES. **fibrinous e.** An exudate rich in fibrin, as seen in rheumatic pericarditis and the early stages of pneumococcal pneumonia. **gingival e.** GINGIVAL FLUID. **hemorrhagic e.** An exudate containing many red blood cells as a result of rupture of vessels or diapedesis of erythrocytes. Also *sanguineous exudate*. **inflammatory e.** An exudate containing variable amounts of fibrin, plasma proteins, and inflammatory cells. **purulent e.** An exudate composed mainly of pus. It is characteristically caused by bacteria such as staphylococci, pneumococci, and gonococci. **sanguineous e.** HEMORRHAGIC EXUDATE. **serofibrinous e.** A serous exudate with added fibrin. In general, it indicates the existence of a more severe type of injury than that resulting in a simple serous exudate, since large fibrinogen molecules have leaked out of the blood vessels. **serous e.** An exudate having a composition similar to that of the blood serum. It is derived from either the blood or the secretion of mesothelial cells. A good example is the skin blister caused by a burn. Serous exudates are characteristic of the early stages of acute inflammation.

**exudation** \eks′yoodā′shən\ [Late L *exudatio, exsudatio*. See EXUDATE.] The escape of intravascular contents, including fluids and cells, into the tissues, due to an increase in vascular permeability caused by an inflammatory reaction to injury.

**exude** \igzood′\ [L *exud(are), exsudare*. See EXUDATE.] To ooze from blood vessels into the surrounding tissues, usually in association with inflammation.

**exutory** \iksyoo′tərē\ [L *exut(us)*, past part. of *exuere* to strip off, draw out, remove + -ORY] Drawing up or off; promoting draining.

**eye** [Old English *ēage*, akin to German *Auge* eye] 1 The visual apparatus; oculus. 2 The general area of the eye, including the lids. *Popular*. **black e.** A discoloration of the eyelids, conjunctiva, and periorbital tissues caused by hemorrhage into the tissues following trauma or operation. **blear e.** A poorly defined term for a minor inflammation or irritation of the eye and eyelids, perhaps with the connotation of an etiology of debauchery or poor hygiene. *Popular*. **compound e.** The multifaceted eye of arthropods, chiefly found in insects. **crossed e.'s** ESOTROPIA. **cyclopean e.** CYCLOPIA. **exciting e.** The originally injured eye in sympathetic ophthalmia. Also *primary eye*. **fixating e.** The eye used for observing the object of regard under the given conditions of binocular vision. **hare's e.** LAGOPHTHALMOS. **lazy e.** SUPPRESSION AMBLYOPIA. **pink e.** ACUTE CONTAGIOUS CONJUNCTIVITIS. **primary e.** EXCITING EYE. **secondary e.** The uninjured eye suffering from sympathetic ophthalmia. **shipyard e.** EPIDEMIC KERATOCONJUNCTIVITIS. **Snellen's reform e.** A rather large, hollow, artificial eye used to compensate for the loss of orbital volume caused by ocular enucleation. **wall e.** EXOTROPIA.

**eyeball** BULBUS OCULI.

**eyebrow** 1 Either of the two raised arches of skin, with short, thick hairs, that overlie the supraorbital margins; supercilium. 2 The hairs of each of these arches; supercilia. Adj. superciliary.

**eyecup** A container with an oval opening that can be fitted snugly against the skin around the eye to bathe it with medicated liquid when the face is turned upward and the eyelid opened. This is an unsanitary device, the use of which should be discouraged. Also *eye cup*.

**eyeglass** [*eye* + *glass*] A spectacle lens.

**eyeglasses** Optical lenses mounted before the eyes to correct for refractive error or for protective purposes. Also *spectacles, ocular prosthesis* (outmoded).

**eyeground** FUNDUS OCULI.

**eyelash** One of the short, thick hairs that is attached along the free edge of the eyelids; cilium.

**eyelid** Either the palpebra inferior or palpebra superior. Also *lid*. **lower e.** PALPEBRA INFERIOR. **upper e.** PALPEBRA SUPERIOR.

**eyepiece** The lens or lens system of a compound microscope or telescope that magnifies and transmits to the eye of the viewer the image originating in the objective lens system. Also *ocular*. **comparison e.** A system of ocular lenses that transmits in a single field side-by-side images from two different objective systems. **compensating e.** Ocular lenses that are used in a compound microscope to compensate for the spherical and chromatic aberration of the objective lens system. **demonstration e.** A system of prisms and mirrors that transmits the image from a single objective system to two or more ocular systems. It permits the simultaneous viewing of a single specimen by several observers. **huygenian e.** An uncorrected optical system of two planoconvex lenses used as an ocular for compound microscopes. Both convex surfaces face toward the objective. Also *Huygen's ocular*. **widefield e.** A system of ocular lenses in which additional lenses are used to raise the eyepoint and widen the in-focus viewing field. Also *wide-field ocular*.

**eyespot** A light-sensitive pigmented spot or chromatophore in some unicellular organisms and invertebrates. Also *ocellus*.

**eyestrain** [*eye* + *strain*] Ocular discomfort attributed to use of the eyes. *Popular*.

# F

**F** 1 Symbol for the unit, farad. 2 Chemical symbol for the element, fluorine. 3 Symbol for phenylalanine. 4 Symbol for variance ratio.

**F.** 1 Fahrenheit (scale). 2 visual field. 3 French (catheter size). See under FRENCH SCALE. 4 formula.

**$F_1$** A symbol used in genetics for the hybrid progeny resulting from the first mating of two organisms that differ by at least one phenotypic trait; the first filial generation.

**$F_2$** A symbol used in genetics for the progeny resulting from the mating of two members of the first filial generation; the second filial generation.

**°F** Symbol for the unit, degree Fahrenheit.

**f** 1 Symbol for femto-: used with SI units. 2 frequency.

**FA** 1 fluorescent antibody (fluorescein-labeled antibody). 2 femoral artery. 3 Fanconi's anemia. 4 fluorescent assay.

**Fab** [from *Fragment, antigen-binding*] See under FAB FRAGMENT.

**fabella** \fəbel′ə\ [L *fab(a)* a bean + *-ella*, diminishing suffix] A small sesamoid of bone or fibrocartilage frequently occurring in the lateral head of the gastrocnemius muscle.

**Faber** [Knud Helge *Faber*, Danish physician, 1862–1956] Faber's anemia, Faber syndrome. See under IRON DEFICIENCY ANEMIA.

**fabism** \fā′bizm\ FAVISM.

**fabrication** \fab′rəkā′shən\ 1 CONFABULATION. 2 Conscious and willful distortion of the truth; lying.

**Fabricius** [Girolamo *Fabricius* ab Aquapendente, Italian anatomist and embryologist, 1533–1619] See under BURSA.

**Fabry** [Johannes *Fabry*, German physician, 1860–1930] Fabry's disease, Fabry syndrome. See under ANGIOKERATOMA CORPORIS DIFFUSUM.

**face** [French (from L *facies* shape, form, face), face] The front, or anterior, aspect of the head from the top of the forehead to the point of the chin; facies. **bony f.** FACIES OSSEA CRANII. **cushingoid f.** MOON FACE. **hatchet f.** MYOPATHIC FACIES. **hippocratic f.** FACIES HIPPOCRATICA. **masklike f.** The expressionless, unblinking facial appearance typical of parkinsonism. Also *mask face, Parkinson's facies.* **moon f.** The round face characteristic of Cushing syndrome, with prominent fatty deposits in the temporal fossae and the cheeks. Also *cushingoid face, cushingoid facies, moon facies.*

**face-bow** A device attached to the teeth or occlusal rims for recording the position of the hinge axis and transferring it to an articulator. **adjustable axis f.** A face-bow with condyle rods adjustable in the vertical plane. Also *kinematic face-bow.*

**face-lift** A plastic operation to eliminate or greatly decrease wrinkles and sagging of the soft tissues covering the face and neck, thus producing a more youthful appearance. Also *melocervicoplasty, face-lift operation.*

**facet** \fas′ət\ [French *facette* (dim. of *face* face) a little face] A small, smooth, flat surface, often rounded, on a hard structure, such as bone. **acromial f.** FACIES ARTICULARIS ACROMIALIS CLAVICULAE. **anterior articular f. of axis** FACIES ARTICULARIS ANTERIOR AXIS. **anterior articular f. of talus** FACIES ARTICULARIS CALCANEA ANTERIOR TALI. **anterior calcaneal f.** 1 FACIES ARTICULARIS CALCANEA ANTERIOR TALI. 2 FACIES ARTICULARIS TALARIS ANTERIOR CALCANEI. **anterior costal f.** FACIES ARTICULARIS TUBERCULI COSTAE. **articular f.** A small, smooth surface located on a bone at the site of articulation with another structure and covered with articular cartilage. **articular f. of anterior arch of atlas** FOVEA DENTIS ATLANTIS. **articular f.'s for rib cartilages** INCISURAE COSTALES STERNI. **auricular f. of sacrum** FACIES AURICULARIS OSSIS SACRI. **circular articular f. of atlas** FOVEA DENTIS ATLANTIS. **clavicular f.** INCISURA CLAVICULARIS STERNI. **costal f.'s of sternum** INCISURAE COSTALES STERNI. **costal f. of transverse process** FOVEA COSTALIS PROCESSUS TRANSVERSUS. **fibular articular f. of tibia** FACIES ARTICULARIS FIBULARIS TIBIAE. **inferior articular f. of atlas** FACIES ARTICULARIS INFERIOR ATLANTIS. **inferior costal f.** FACIES ARTICULARIS TUBERCULI COSTAE. **lateral malleolar f. of talus** FACIES MALLEOLARIS LATERALIS TALI. **lateral f.'s of sternum** INCISURAE COSTALES STERNI. **Lenoir's f.** A narrow articular facet on the medial edge of the patella for the lateral margin of the medial condyle of the femur in extreme flexion. **locked f.'s of spine** A dislocation of the zygapophyseal joints, with complete overlapping of the joint surfaces. It most commonly occurs in the cervical spine. **medial malleolar f. of talus** FACIES MALLEOLARIS MEDIALIS TALI. **middle articular f. of talus** FACIES ARTICULARIS CALCANEA MEDIA TALI. **posterior articular f. of talus** FACIES ARTICULARIS CALCANEA POSTERIOR TALI. **posterior costal f.** FACIES ARTICULARIS CAPITIS COSTAE. **posterior medial f. of calcaneus** FACIES ARTICULARIS TALARIS MEDIA CALCANEI. **squatting f.** An adventitious articular facet found on the anterior aspect of the lower end of the tibia, with a reciprocal facet on the neck of the talus. It is found in individuals who habitually adopt a squatting position. **sternal articular f. of clavicle** FACIES ARTICULARIS STERNALIS CLAVICULAE. **superior articular f. of atlas** FACIES ARTICULARIS SUPERIOR ATLANTIS. **superior costal f.** FACIES ARTICULARIS CAPITIS COSTAE. **superior costal f. of vertebra** FOVEA COSTALIS SUPERIOR. **f. for tubercle of rib** FOVEA COSTALIS PROCESSUS TRANSVERSUS. **wear f.** A flattened polished surface of a tooth produced by grinding contact between occluding surfaces.

**facetectomy** \fas′ətek′təmē\ [FACET + -ECTOMY] Excision of an articular facet.

# facies

**facies** \fā′shi·ēz\ [L, shape, form, face] (*pl.* facies) 1 [NA] The face. 2 [NA] A surface of a structure, organ, or part of the body. 3 A facial expression. **acromegalic f.** The enlarged face characteristic of acromegaly, with increased length (due chiefly to lengthening of the maxilla), prominent frontal bosses, prominent zygomas, prognathism, increased size of the nose and ears, and an overall aspect of increased mass. **adenoid f.** The facial expression often observed in children with nasal obstruction resulting from adenoid hypertrophy and characterized by mouth breathing and a vacant, dull expression. **f. anterior antebrachii** REGIO ANTEBRACHIALIS ANTERIOR. **f. anterior brachii** REGIO BRACHIALIS ANTERIOR. **f. anterior corneae** [NA] The broad, elliptical, outer surface of the cornea which is covered by epithelium and faces the eyelids. Also *anterior surface of cornea.* **f. anterior cruris** REGIO CRURALIS ANTERIOR. **f. anterior dentium premolarium et molarium** The mesially directed surface of premolar and molar teeth. **f. anterior femoris** REGIO FEMORALIS ANTERIOR. **f. anterior glandulae suprarenalis** [NA] The anterior, or ventral, surface of the adrenal gland, that of the right being in contact with the inferior vena cava and the bare area of the liver, while that of the left is related to the stomach through the omental bursa, and to the pancreas and splenic artery directly. Also *anterior surface of suprarenal gland.* **f. anterior iridis** [NA] The outer surface of the iris which faces the cornea, forms part of the posterior wall of the anterior chamber of the eye, and extends from the pupillary border to its junction with the ciliary body. It comprises the annulus iridis major and annulus iridis minor and presents delicate, sinuous radiations caused by blood vessels shining through it. It is covered by the endothelium of the anterior chamber in infancy. Also *anterior surface of iris, anterior limiting layer of iris.* **f. anterior lateralis humeri** [NA] The anterolateral surface of the humerus, extending between the anterior and lateral margins. **f. anterior lentis** [NA] The outer surface of the lens which faces the anterior chamber of the eye and is in contact with the pupillary margin of the iris. It is covered by a single layer of epithelium which is bounded by the capsule. Also *anterior surface of lens.* **f. anterior maxillae** [NA] The surface of the body of maxilla that is directed anterolaterally. Its medial margin forms the nasal notch, which ends anteroinferiorly in the anterior nasal spine, and laterally it is separated from the infratemporal surface by the zygomatic process. Superiorly, the infraorbital margin separates it from the orbital surface, and just below the margin is the infraorbital foramen. **f. anterior medialis humeri** [NA] The anteromedial surface of the humerus, situated between the anterior and medial margins. Its upper third forms the floor of the intertubercular sulcus where the latissimus dorsi muscle is inserted, while near its middle the coracobrachialis muscle is inserted, and the rest of the surface provides partial origin for the brachialis muscle. Also *anteromedial surface of humerus.* **f. anterior palpebrarum** [NA] The outer surface of the eyelids, which is formed by skin and meets the posterior surface at the free margin of each eyelid. There the thin skin is continuous with the palpebral conjunctiva. Also *anterior surface of eyelids.* **f. anterior pancreatis** [NA] The slightly concave surface of the pancreas that lies between the anterior and superior margins and faces anterosuperiorly to come into contact with the posteroinferior surface of the stomach through the omental bursa. Also *anterior surface of pancreas.* **f. anterior partis petrosae ossis temporalis** [NA] The somewhat triangular anterior, or superior, surface of the petrous part of the temporal bone that forms part of the floor of the middle cranial fossa. Posterior to its apex, its major features include the trigeminal impression, grooves for the greater and the lesser petrosal nerves, the arcuate eminence, and the roof of the tympanic cavity. **f. anterior patellae** [NA] The convex anterior surface of the patella, marked by longitudinal striations and foramina of nutrient vessels, over which fibers of the common tendon of the quadriceps femoris muscle are prolonged into the ligamentum patellae. It is separated from the skin by a bursa. **f. anterior prostatae** [NA] The convex anterior surface that extends from the base to the apex of the prostate and lies behind the pubic symphysis from which it is separated by the prostatic and vesical venous plexuses and some fat and areolar tissue. **f. anterior radii** [NA] The anterior surface of the radius, situated between the anterior and the interosseous margins and providing attachment on the proximal two-thirds for the origin of the flexor pollicis longus muscle, and in the distal third for the insertion of the pronator quadratus muscle. The nutrient foramen is just below the proximal third. **f. anterior renis** [NA] The convex surface of the kidney that faces anterolaterally and has different relations to organs and vessels on the two sides. On the right side it is covered by peritoneum where it is related to the liver and coils of small intestine, but is bare against the suprarenal gland, descending part of the duodenum, and right colic flexure. On the left side, it is covered by peritoneum where it is related to the stomach, spleen, jejunum, and left colic flexure, but it is bare in relation to the body of the pancreas, the splenic vessels, and left suprarenal gland. Also *anterior surface of kidney.* **f. anterior ulnae** [NA] The anterior surface of the ulna, situated between the anterior and the interosseous margins and grooved in its proximal three-fourths for the origin of the flexor digitorum profundus muscle, while distally it is narrow and convex for the origin of the pronator quadratus muscle. The nutrient foramen is just below the proximal third. **f. anterolateralis cartilaginis arytenoideae** [NA] The convex, irregular anterolateral surface of the arytenoid cartilage, crossed sinuously from the apex to the vocal process by the arcuate crest, separating the fovea triangularis above from the fovea oblongata below. **f. articulares inferiores vertebrarum** The oval, concave surfaces on the inferior articular processes of the vertebrae that are directed inferiorly, anteriorly and, often, medially. **f. articulares superiores vertebrarum** The flat surfaces on the superior articular processes of the vertebrae that are directed superiorly, posteriorly, and laterally in a plane slightly anterior to that of the inferior articular surfaces. **f. articularis acromialis** [NA] The small, oval articular surface on the medial border of the acromion of scapula for the acromial articular surface of the clavicle. **f. articularis acromialis claviculae** [NA] The smooth, oval articular surface at the lateral end of the clavicle, directed laterally and downward for the articular surface of the acromion. Also *acromial articular surface of clavicle, acromial facet.* **f. articularis anterior axis** [NA] The small, oval facet on the anterior surface of the dens of the axis vertebra for articulation with the fovea dentis on the posterior surface of the anterior arch of atlas. Also *anterior articular facet of axis, anterior articular process of axis.* **f. articularis arytenoidea cartilaginis cricoideae** [NA] An oval, convex articular facet on each superolateral aspect of the posterior surface at the upper border of the cricoid cartilage that articulates with the base of the arytenoid cartilage. **f. articularis calcanea anterior tali** [NA] A small, oval articular facet on the plantar aspect of the head of talus that rests on the plantar calcaneonavicular ligament and on the anterior articular surface on the upper aspect of the calcaneus. Also *anterior calcaneal facet, anterior articular facet of talus.* **f. articularis calcanea media tali** The elongated, convex middle calcaneal facet on the inferomedial aspect of the articular head of talus that articulates with the sustentaculum tali of the calcaneus. Also *middle articular facet of talus.* **f. articularis calcanea posterior tali** [NA] The concave, oblong articular surface set transversely across the inferior surface of the body of talus for articulation with a corresponding articular surface on the superior surface of the calcaneus in the subtalar joint. Also *posterior articular facet of talus.* **f. articularis capitis costae** [NA] The articular surface on the head of a rib that is divided by a crest into two convex facets that articulate with the bodies of two adjacent vertebrae. The articular surfaces of the heads of the first, tenth, eleventh, and twelfth ribs are usually not divided. Also *posterior costal facet, superior costal facet.* **f. articularis capitis fibulae** [NA] The circular articular surface on the medial side of the head of fibula that is directed anterosuperiorly for the lateral condyle of the tibia in the tibiofibular joint. **f. articularis carpi radii** [NA] The concave, quadrilateral articular surface at the distal extremity of the radius, divided by a small vertical ridge so that the medial quadrangular portion articulates with the lunate bone and the lateral triangular portion articulates with the scaphoid bone. Also *carpal articular surface of radius.* **f. articularis cartilaginis arytenoideae** [NA] A small articular surface on the concave base of the arytenoid cartilage for articulation with a facet on the superolateral aspect of the posterior surface of the cricoid cartilage. **f. articularis cuboidea calcanei** [NA] The concavoconvex, quadrangular anterior surface of the calcaneus that articulates with the cuboid bone to form the calcaneocuboid joint. Also *cuboid articular surface of calcaneus.* **f. articularis fibularis tibiae** [NA] The flat, circular articular surface on the posterolateral aspect of the lateral condyle of tibia, directed posteroinferiorly for the head of the fibula to form the tibiofibular joint. Also *fibular articular facet of tibia.* **f. articularis inferior atlantis** The circular and slightly hollowed surface on the inferior aspect of the lateral mass of the atlas, facing medially and downward to articulate with a similar superior articular facet on the axis in the lateral atlantoaxial joint. Also *inferior articular fovea of atlas, fovea articularis inferior atlantis, inferior articular facet of atlas, inferior articular fossa of atlas, inferior articular pit of atlas.* **f. articularis inferior tibiae** [NA] The smooth, quadrangular surface, wider in front than behind and concave anteroposteriorly, on the inferior aspect of the distal extremity of the tibia, and articulating with the body of the talus. Medially it is continuous with the malleolar articular surface. Also *inferior articular surface of tibia.* **f. articularis malleoli fibulae** [NA] The anterosuperior part of the medial surface of the lateral malleolus of fibula, triangular-shaped and convex and articulating with the lateral side of the talus. Also *lateral malleolar fovea of fibula, fovea of lateral malleolus.* **f. articularis malleoli tibiae** [NA] The smooth lateral surface of the medial malleolus of tibia that articulates with the medial side of the talus. It is continuous with the inferior articular surface of tibia. **f. articularis navicularis tali** [NA] The oval and convex anterior part of the large articular surface on the head of the talus, for articulation with the navicular bone. **f. articularis ossis temporalis** [NA] The anterior, articular portion of the mandibular fossa, oval and deeply concave and formed by the squamous part of temporal bone, extending anteriorly onto the articular tubercle and articulating with the articular disk of the temporomandibular joint. **f. articularis ossium** Any articular surface of a bone; a joint surface. **f. articularis patellae** [NA] The upper part of the posterior surface of the patella, divided by a vertical ridge into two angulated surfaces, both of which articulate with the respective condyles of the femur. **f. articularis posterior axis** [NA] A smooth, grooved surface on the posterior aspect of the dens of axis that abuts against the transverse ligament of the atlas. **f. articularis sternalis claviculae** [NA] The somewhat triangular surface on the sternal end of the clavicle, directed inferomedially to articulate with the clavicular notch of the manubrium sterni through the interposed articular disk attached to the superior margin of the surface. Also *sternal articular facet of clavicle.* **f. articularis superior atlantis** [NA] The elongated, bean-shaped, concave articular facet on the superior surface of each lateral mass of the atlas for articulation with a corresponding convex occipital condyle in the atlanto-occipital joint on each side. Also *fovea articularis superior atlantis, superior articular pit of atlas, superior articular surface of atlas, superior articular facet of atlas, superior articular fossa of atlas, condyloid fossa of atlas, superior articular sinus of atlas* (outmoded). **f. articularis superior tibiae** [NA] The expanded, oval articular surface on the proximal extremity of the tibia, subdivided by a median nonarticular intercondylar area into medial and lateral articular surfaces for the condyles of the femur. Also *condyloid surface of tibia, superior articular surface of tibia.* **f. articularis talaris anterior calcanei** [NA] The most anterior of the three articular surfaces on the superior aspect of the calcaneus that articulate with three corresponding facets on the overlying talus. Also *anterior talar articular surface of calcaneus, anterior calcaneal facet.* **f. articularis talaris media calcanei** [NA] The middle facet of the three articular surfaces on the superior aspect of the calcaneus. It is larger than the anterior facet, behind which it is located on the sustentaculum tali. Also *middle talar articular surface of calcaneus, posterior medial facet of calcaneus.* **f. articularis talaris posterior calcanei** [NA] The most posterior of the three articular surfaces on the superior aspect of the calcaneus. Large and oval, it is located in the center of the superior surface. Also *posterior talar articular surface of calcaneus.* **f. articularis thyroidea cartilaginis cricoideae** [NA] A circular articular facet facing posterolaterally on the cricoid cartilage, at the junction of the arch with the lamina, for articulation with the inferior horn of the thyroid cartilage on each side. **f. articularis tuberculi costae** [NA] A small, raised, oval facet on the medial portion of the tubercle of a rib for articulation with the transverse process of the numerically corresponding vertebra. Also *anterior costal facet, inferior costal facet.* **f. auricularis ossis ilii** [NA] The rough, ear-shaped surface at the anteroinferior end of the sacropelvic surface of the ilium that articulates with the auricular surface of the sacrum in the sacroiliac joint. Also *auricular facet of iliac bone.* **f. auricularis ossis sacri** [NA] The ear-shaped articular surface on the upper part of the lateral surface of the lateral portion of the sacrum that articulates with the auricular surface of the ilium in the sacroiliac joint. Also *lateral articular surface of sacral bone* (outmoded), *auricular plane of sacral bone, auricular facet of sacrum.* **f. bovina** A cowlike facial appearance owing to orbital hypertelorism. It is seen in cases of the Crouzon syndrome. **f. cerebralis alae majoris** [NA] The concave inner surface of the greater wing of the sphenoid bone, forming part of the middle cranial fossa and supporting the anterior part of the temporal lobe of cerebrum. Among the numerous foramina piercing it are the foramen rotundum, foramen ovale, and foramen spinosum. **f. cerebralis partis squamosae ossis temporalis** [NA] The concave internal surface of the squamous part of the temporal bone, its depressions corresponding to the convolutions of the temporal lobe and its grooves being formed by branches of the middle meningeal vessels. **f. colica splenis** [NA] The flattened impression on the lateral extremity of the visceral surface of the spleen which is related to the left colic flexure and phrenicocolic ligament. Also *colic impression of spleen, colic surface of spleen.* **f. convexa cerebri** FACIES SUPEROLATERALIS CEREBRI. **f. costalis pulmonis** [NA] The convex outer surface of each lung. It corresponds to the inner surface of the thoracic wall and is in contact with the costal pleura. Also *costal surface of lung.* **f. costalis scapulae** [NA] The triangular concave surface of the scapula that faces anteromedially toward the thorax and forms the subscapular fossa, the surface of which is ridged for the attachment of tendinous intersections of the subscapularis muscle. Near the medial margin is a longitudinal ridge for attachment of the serratus anterior muscle. Also *anterior surface of scapula, costal surface of scapula.* **cushingoid f.** MOON FACE. **f. diaphragmatica cordis** [NA] The inferior surface of the heart, separated from the sternocostal surface by the right margin and resting on the central tendon and part of the left muscular portion of the diaphragm, from which it is separated by the pericardium. Also *diaphragmatic surface of heart.* **f. diaphragmatica hepatis** [NA] The extensive convex surface of the liver, which is related to the diaphragm and is divided into anterior, posterior, right, and superior parts. Also *diaphragmatic surface of liver.* **f. diaphragmatica pulmonis** [NA] The concave, semilunar inferior surface of each lung which rests on the diaphragm and is separated from it by pleura. Also *diaphragmatic surface of lung.* **f. diaphragmatica splenis** [NA] The convex, and largest, surface of the spleen. It is directed superiorly and posterolaterally to the left and is related to the inferior surface of the diaphragm that separates it from the left pleura and lung and the ninth through eleventh ribs. Also *diaphragmatic surface of spleen.* **f. digitales dorsales manus** [NA] The posterior, or dorsal, surfaces of the fingers. **f. digitales ventrales manus** [NA] The anterior, or palmar, surfaces of the fingers. **f. dolorosa** The drawn appearance of the face of an individual suffering pain. **f. dorsales digitorum pedis** The superior, or dorsal, surfaces of the toes. **f. dorsalis ossis sacri** [NA] The triangular and markedly convex posterior surface of the sacrum, ridged by the median, intermediate, and lateral sacral crests, perforated by four dorsal sacral foramina on either side, and providing origin for the erector spinae and multifidus muscles. Also *posterior surface of sacrum.* **f. dorsalis radii** FACIES POSTERIOR RADII. **f. dorsalis ulnae** FACIES POSTERIOR ULNAE. **f. externa ossis frontalis** [NA] The convex, smooth outer surface of the frontal bone, marked by the frontal eminence on each side, and occasionally by a remnant of the frontal, or metopic, suture centrally. **f. externa ossis parietalis** [NA] The convex, smooth outer surface of the parietal bone, crossed transversely below the center by the superior and the inferior temporal lines, above which is the bulge of the parietal eminence. **f. gastrica splenis** [NA] The broad and deeply concave area on the visceral surface of the spleen. It is directed anterosuperiorly and medially and is related to the posterior surface of the stomach through the greater sac of the peritoneum. Near its lower margin is the fissure for the hilum of the spleen. Also *gastric surface of spleen, gastric impression of spleen.* **f. glutea ossis ilii** [NA] The outer surface of the ala of ilium, convex anteriorly and concave posteriorly, divided into four areas by posterior, inferior, and anterior gluteal lines, the upper three areas being for attachments of the gluteus maximus, medius, and minimus muscles. Also *dorsum ilii.* **f. hepatica** The drawn facial expression and appearance of a person with a chronic disorder of the liver, usually characterized as sunken eyes and cheeks, a sallow complexion with dilated capillaries, and spider angiomata. **f. hippocratica** A facial appearance associated with impending death. It is characterized by dull, sunken eyes; hollow temples and cheeks; and drooping lower jaw. Also *hippocratic face.* **Hutchinson's f.** The appearance of congenital syphilis, including frontal bony prominence, sunken bridge of the nose, and deformed peg-shaped incisor teeth. **f. inferior cerebri** The basal surface of the cerebrum. Also *basis encephali, basis cerebri, base of brain.* **f. inferior hemispherii cerebelli** The inferior surface of the cerebellar hemispheres in the posterior cranial fossa. **f. inferior hemispherii cerebri** The basal cerebral surfaces lying upon the anterior and middle cranial fossae and the tentorium cerebelli. Also *base of cerebrum.* **f. inferior linguae** [NA] The inferior surface of the freely mobile body of the tongue that faces the floor of the mouth. It is covered by thin, smooth mucous membrane that forms the frenulum in the midline, on each side of which the lingual vein produces an elevation between it and the plica fimbriata. **f. inferior pancreatis** [NA] The narrow surface of the body of the pancreas which faces inferiorly and is covered with peritoneum of the posteroinferior layer of the transverse mesocolon. It is related to the duodenojejunal flexure, jejunum, and left colic flexure. Also *inferior surface of pancreas.* **f. inferior partis petrosae ossis temporalis** [NA] The inferior surface of the petrous part of the temporal bone, forming an irregular section of the external surface of the base of skull, the main features of which are, anteroposteriorly, the circular opening of the carotid canal, the deep depression of the jugular fossa, the styloid process, and the stylomastoid foramen. **f. inferolateralis prostatae** [NA] The convex inferolateral surface on each side of the prostate, related to the superior surface of the levator ani muscle, from which it is separated by the fibrous tissue forming the prostatic sheath and containing the prostatic plexus of veins. **f. infratemporalis maxillae** [NA] The convex surface of the maxilla facing laterally and posteriorly and forming the anterior wall of the infratemporal fossa. Also *infratemporal surface of maxilla.* **f. interlobaris pulmonis** [NA] The surface of each lobe of the lung which faces either the oblique or the horizontal fissure. Also *interlobar surface of lung.* **f. interna ossis frontalis** [NA] The concave internal surface of the frontal bone, divided in the midline by the longitudinal groove of superior sagittal sinus, below which is the frontal crest terminating at the foramen cecum. Also *inner table of frontal bone* (outmoded), *frontal fossa.* **f. interna ossis parietalis** [NA] The concave internal surface of the parietal bone, having light digitate impressions and marked vascular grooves produced by the middle meningeal vessels. Along the superior margin is part of the groove of the superior sagittal sinus, adjacent to which are pits for arachnoid granulations. **f. intestinalis uteri** [NA] The convex posterior surface of the uterus adjacent to the intestine. **f. lateralis brachii** The outer, or lateral, surface of the arm between the acromial angle and the elbow joint. **f. lateralis cruris** The outer, or lateral, surface of the leg extending from the knee joint to the lateral malleolus. **f. lateralis femoris** The outer, or lateral, surface of the thigh, flattened due to the presence of the iliotibial tract. **f. lateralis fibulae** [NA] The surface between the anterior and the posterior margins of the fibula. **f. lateralis ossis zygomatici** [NA] The convex outer surface of the zygomatic bone on which is located the zygomaticofacial foramen and which provides for the origin of both zygomatic muscles. **f. lateralis radii** [NA] The convex outer surface of the radius on which the supinator muscle is inserted proximally and the pronator teres muscle near the middle. **f. lateralis testis** [NA] The convex, smooth lateral surface of the testis situated between the anterior and posterior borders and invested by the visceral layer of tunica vaginalis. Near the upper pole the appendix testis may be attached. **f. lateralis tibiae** [NA] The lateral surface of the tibia lying between the anterior and the interosseous margins and providing attachment on its proximal two thirds for the tibialis anterior muscle. Also *external border of tibia.* **leonine f.** The nodulation, thickening, and fissuring of facial skin in lepromatous leprosy that imparts a lionlike appearance. Also *leontiasis* (obs.), *facies leontina, facies leprosa.* **f. lunata acetabuli** [NA] The horseshoe-shaped articular portion of the acetabulum, deficient inferiorly and on which the femur articulates in the hip joint. Also *articular surface of acetabulum.* **f. malleolaris lateralis tali** [NA] The lateral surface of the body of the talus, having a large triangular facet for articulation with the lateral malleolus and terminating inferiorly in the lateral process. Also *lateral malleolar facet of talus.* **f. malleolaris medialis tali** [NA] The medial surface of the body of the talus, the upper part of which has a horizontal, comma-shaped surface covered with cartilage, continuous with the superior surface, for articulation with the medial malleolus of tibia, while the lower part has numerous vascular foramina and gives attachment to deep fibers of the medial collateral ligament of the ankle joint. Also *medial malleolar facet of talus.* **Marshall Hall's f.** The facies seen in hydrocephalus, characterized by broadening of the forehead with increased prominence of the frontal bones, giving the face a triangular appearance. **f. maxillaris alae majoris** [NA] A small area on the anteroinferior aspect of the greater wing of the sphenoid bone, located at the base of the lateral lamina of the pterygoid process and forming part of the posterior wall of the pterygopalatine fossa, where it is perforated by the foramen rotundum. **f. maxillaris laminae perpendicularis ossis palatini** [NA] The irregular lateral surface of the perpendicular plate of the palatine bone, divided by a vertical groove that superiorly forms the medial wall of the pterygopalatine fossa and inferiorly becomes the greater palatine sulcus, which is converted into a canal by a similar groove on the nasal surface of the maxilla articulating with it. **f. mediales digitorum manus** The medial surfaces of the fingers along which digital vessels and nerves course. Also *ulnar margins of fingers.* **f. mediales digitorum pedis** The medial surfaces of the toes along which digital vessels and nerves course. **f. medialis brachii** The inner, or medial, surface of the arm from the apex of the axilla to the elbow joint. **f. medialis cartilaginis arytenoideae** [NA] The narrow, flat medial surface of each arytenoid cartilage, covered by mucous membrane and lying parallel to each other, forming the intercartilaginous part of the rima glottidis between their lower margins. **f. medialis cerebri** The median surface of the cerebral cortex facing the midline of the sagittal sulcus and underlying the falx cerebri. **f. medialis cruris** The inner, or medial, surface of the leg between the knee and the ankle joints. **f. medialis femoris** The inner, or medial, surface of the thigh. **f. medialis fibulae** [NA] The surface of the fibula between the anterior and interosseous margins, very narrow proximally but broad distally, providing origin for the extensor digitorum longus, peroneus tertius, and extensor hallucis longus muscles. **f. medialis ovarii** [NA] The rounded medial surface of the ovary, largely overlapped by the fimbriated end of the uterine tube and the mesosalpinx and partly related to a loop of intestine. **f. medialis testis** [NA] The convex, smooth medial surface of the testis, invested by the visceral layer of the tunica vaginalis and situated between the anterior and posterior borders of the testis. It faces the opposite testis but is also directed anteriorly and inferiorly to some degree. **f. medialis tibiae** [NA] The medial surface of tibia, lying between the medial and anterior margins and receiving the tendons of insertion of the sartorius, gracilis, and semitendinosus muscles on its broad proximal end. **f. medialis ulnae** [NA] The smooth, rounded medial surface of the ulna that gives attachment to part of the origin of the flexor digitorum profundus muscle on the proximal two-thirds. Distally it is subcutaneous. **f. mediastinalis pulmonis** [NA] The medial concave surface of each lung, related to the mediastinum and containing the hilum of the lung. Also *mediastinal surface of lung, medial surface of lung.* **mitral f.** The highly colored, slightly cyanotic flush over the malar region in patients with long-standing mitral stenosis. Also *mitrotricuspid facies.* **mitrotricuspid f.** MITRAL FACIES. **moon f.** MOON FACE. **myasthenic f.** The facial appearance in myasthenia gravis, characterized usually by bilateral ptosis, drooping and expressionless facial muscles, and, when the patient smiles, a typical myasthenic grimace. **myopathic f.** Any of the facial appearances seen in myopathy. The two most characteristic abnormalities of facial appearance are seen in facioscapulohumeral muscular dystrophy, where the affected individual cannot close the eyes and there is a pouting appearance of the lips (tapir mouth), and in dystrophia myotonica, in which there is hollowing of the temporal fossae, bilateral ptosis and a lugubrious expression. Also *hatchet face.* **myxedematous f.** The appearance of the face associated with myxedema, showing a yellowish pallor and puffiness, particularly around the eyes, and producing a general impression of lethargy and sluggishness. **f. nasalis laminae horizontalis ossis palatini** [NA] The smooth, concave upper surface of the horizontal plate of the palatine bone that forms the posterior part of the floor of the nasal cavity. **f. nasalis laminae perpendicularis ossis palatini** [NA] The medial surface of the perpendicular plate of the palatine bone that presents the ethmoidal and conchal crests separating three depressions that form part of the walls of the superior, middle, and inferior meatus of the nose. Also *facies nasalis partis perpendicularis ossis palatini.* **f. nasalis maxillae** [NA] The nasal surface of the maxilla that helps to form the lateral wall of the nasal cavity. Posterior to it is a large, irregular gap, or hiatus, leading into the maxillary sinus, just anterior to which is the downward sloping lacrimal groove. More anteriorly on the smooth surface is the conchal crest, above which is the wall of the atrium of the middle meatus, while below is the inferior meatus. **f. nasalis partis perpendicularis ossis palatini** FACIES NASALIS LAMINAE PERPENDICULARIS OSSIS PALATINI. **f. orbitalis alae majoris** [NA] The quadrilateral anteromedial surface of the greater wing of the sphenoid bone that forms the posterior part of the lateral wall of the orbit. Also *facies orbitalis alae magnae, orbital border of sphenoid bone, orbital surface of sphenoid bone.* **f. orbitalis maxillae** [NA] A triangular surface of the maxilla that forms most of the floor of the orbit, which is traversed by the infraorbital groove and canal. **f. orbitalis ossis frontalis** [NA] The concave, smooth orbital surface of the frontal bone forming most of the roof of the orbital cavity, its anterior edge being the supraorbital margin, just posterior to which on the lateral side is the fossa for the lacrimal gland, while the trochlear fovea, or spine, is on the medial side. Also *orbital fossa.* **f. orbitalis ossis zygomatici** [NA] The concave orbital surface of the zygomatic bone that takes part in the formation of the lateral wall of the orbit, on which are located the zygomatico-orbital foramina. **f. ossea cranii** The bony skeleton of the face. Also *bony face.* **f. palatina laminae horizontalis ossis palatini** [NA] The inferior surface of the horizontal plate of the palatine bone, forming the posterior one-fourth of the hard palate with the corresponding surface of the opposite bone, their medial borders meeting at the median palatine suture. Also *facies palatina partis horizontalis ossis palatini* (outmoded). **paralytic f.** The facial appearance resulting from unilateral or bilateral paralysis of the facial muscles. When unilateral, the eye on the affected side cannot be closed and the affected corner of the mouth droops in comparison with the other side. **Parkinson's f.** MASKLIKE FACE. **f. patellaris femoris** [NA] The trochlear surface between and continuous with the articular surfaces of the condyles of the femur anteriorly, for articulation with the patella. Also *trochlea of femur* (outmoded). **f. pelvica ossis sacri** [NA] The concave anterior surface of the sacrum, directed anteroinferiorly and forming part of the posterior wall of the pelvic cavity. Four central transverse ridges indicate the lines of fusion between the five sacral vertebrae, at the extremities of which are four pelvic sacral foramina on each side. The bars of bone between these foramina represent costal elements fused to the vertebrae. Also *anterior surface of sacrum.* **f. plantares digitorum pedis** The inferior, or plantar, surfaces of the toes. **f. poplitea femoris** [NA] The triangular area at the lower end of the posterior surface of the femoral shaft, located between the medial and lateral supracondylar lines that come together at the apex of this area as the linea aspera. This surface forms the upper part of the floor of the popliteal fossa, a pad of fat separating it from the popliteal artery. Also *planum popliteum femoris, popliteal triangle of femur.* **f. posterior antebrachii** REGIO ANTEBRACHIALIS POSTERIOR. **f. posterior brachii** REGIO BRACHIALIS POSTERIOR. **f. posterior cartilaginis arytenoideae** [NA] The concave, triangular posterior surface of the arytenoid cartilage, covered by the transverse arytenoid muscle. **f. posterior corneae** [NA] The posterior surface of the cornea which faces the anterior chamber of the eye and is lined by the posterior limiting lamina and the endothelium of the anterior chamber. At its periphery it meets the iris at the iridocorneal angle. Also *posterior surface of cornea.* **f. posterior cruris** REGIO CRURALIS POSTERIOR. **f. posterior femoris** REGIO FEMORALIS POSTERIOR. **f. posterior fibulae** [NA] The large surface between the interosseous and posterior margins of the fibula, divided longitudinally into two in its upper two-thirds by the medial crest for the attachment of an intermuscular septum that separates the tibialis posterior muscle arising on its medial side and the soleus and flexor hallucis longus muscles from its posterior side. **f. posterior glandulae suprarenalis** [NA] The surface of the suprarenal gland which is directed posteromedially and is related to the diaphragm on each side. Also *posterior surface of suprarenal gland.* **f. posterior humeri** [NA] The dorsal surface of the humerus lying between the lateral and medial margins, divided into two by the oblique, shallow groove of the radial nerve that runs from superomedial to inferolateral across the middle third. **f. posterior iridis** [NA] The surface of the iris which forms the anterior wall of the posterior chamber of the eye and rests against the anterior surface of the lens near the pupil. It is covered with a double layer of heavily pigmented epithelium, or the iridial portion of the retina, the outer, or anterior, layer of which becomes differentiated into smooth muscles, namely, the sphincter pupillae and the dilator pupillae. Also *posterior surface of iris.* **f. posterior lentis** [NA] The posterior surface of the lens which rests in the hyaloid fossa of the vitreous body. At its periphery some of the zonular fibers are attached. Also *posterior surface of lens.* **f. posterior palpebrarum** [NA] The internal surface of the eyelids which faces the eyeball and is covered by the conjunctiva. At its free margin, where it is continuous with the anterior surface of each eyelid, are the openings of the tarsal glands which are embedded in the tarsal plate deep to the conjunctiva. Also *posterior surface of eyelids.* **f. posterior pancreatis** [NA] The flattened posterior surface of the body of the pancreas. It has no peritoneal covering and is related posteriorly to the aorta and origin of the superior mesenteric artery, the left suprarenal gland, left kidney, and renal vein. Also *posterior surface of pancreas.* **f. posterior partis petrosae ossis temporalis** [NA] The surface of the petrous part of the temporal bone, forming the anterior part of the posterior cranial fossa. **f. posterior prostatae** [NA] The convex posterior surface of the prostate separated from the lower part of the rectum by the prostatic sheath and the rectovesical septum. **f. posterior radii** [NA] The posterior surface of the radius lying between the interosseous and the posterior margins, the upper part of which gives origin to the abductor pollicis longus muscle proximally and the extensor pollicis brevis distally, while the lower part is only covered by the extensor pollicis longus and brevis muscles. Also *facies dorsalis radii.* **f. posterior renis** [NA] The surface of the kidney which faces posteromedially, is devoid of peritoneum, and is related to the posterior abdominal wall. Also *posterior surface of kidney.* **f. posterior scapulae** [NA] The convex posterior surface of the scapula, divided by the somewhat horizontal spine of scapula into a small supraspinous fossa for the supraspinatus muscle and a larger infraspinous fossa for the infraspinatus muscle. Also *dorsal surface of scapula, posterior surface of scapula, dorsum of scapula.* **f. posterior tibiae** [NA] The posterior surface of the tibia lying between the interosseous and medial margins. **f. posterior ulnae** [NA] The posterior surface of the ulna lying between the interosseous and the posterior margins. Also *facies dorsalis ulnae.* **Potter f.** A combination of facial features consisting of orbital hypertelorism, low-set ears, receding chin, and a flat nose, characteristically seen in a newborn infant with bilateral renal agenesis or other severe renal malformations. **f. pulmonalis cordis** [NA] The convex left surface of the heart, formed mainly by the left ventricle and partly by the left atrium and producing the cardiac impression on the medial surface of the left lung. Also *pulmonary surface of heart, left border of heart* (outmoded), *left margin of heart* (outmoded). **f. renalis glandulae suprarenalis** [NA] The concave inferolateral surface of each suprarenal gland which lies against the superior extremity of its corresponding kidney. Also *renal surface of suprarenal gland, basis glandulae suprarenalis, inferior margin of suprarenal gland.* **f. renalis splenis** [NA] The slightly concave area on the lower part of the visceral surface of the spleen which rests posteromedially against the superolateral part of the rounded anterior surface of the left kidney and, occasionally, the adjacent suprarenal gland. Also *renal surface of spleen, facies renalis lienis.* **f. sacropelvica ossis ilii** [NA] The posterior part of the medial aspect of the ilium, located behind and below the iliac fossa. It is subdivided into three areas posteroanteriorly: the iliac tuberosity, a rough area just below the posterior part of the iliac crest mainly for the attachment of the interosseous and dorsal sacroiliac ligaments; the auricular surface;

and the pelvic surface, lying between the inferior margin of the auricular surface and the superior margin of the greater sciatic notch and forming part of the wall of pelvis minor. Also *sacropelvic surface of ilium.* **f. scaphoidea** A face that appears concave in profile, due to a protruding forehead, depressed nose and upper jaw, and a prominent chin. Also *dishface deformity.* **f. sternocostalis cordis** [NA] The anterior surface of the heart, facing anterosuperiorly and to the left and formed partly by the right atrium above and to the right and mainly by the ventricles, two-thirds by the right and one-third by the left. Also *sternocostal surface of heart.* **f. superior hemispherii cerebelli** The rostral, superior face of the cerebellum, consisting essentially of those portions rostral to the horizontal cerebellar fissure. **f. superior trochleae tali** [NA] The broad upper surface of the talus, widest anteriorly, convex anteroposteriorly, and concave from side to side, that articulates with the inferior articular surface of the tibia in the ankle joint. Also *superior surface of talus.* **f. superolateralis cerebri** [NA] The outer convex surface of the cerebral hemispheres underlying the calvaria. Also *facies convexa cerebri.* **f. symphysialis** [NA] The elongated, oval medial surface of the body of the pubis that articulates with the opposite pubis in the symphysis pubis. Also *symphysial surface of pubis.* **tabetic f.** Bilateral ptosis with compensatory wrinkling of the forehead seen in some cases of advanced tabes dorsalis. **f. temporalis alae magnae** FACIES TEMPORALIS ALAE MAJORIS. **f. temporalis alae majoris** [NA] The convex outer, or lateral, surface of the greater wing of the sphenoid bone, divided by the horizontal infratemporal crest into a large upper part, a portion of the temporal fossa, and a small lower part, a portion of the wall of the infratemporal fossa. • Some textbooks refer to the upper part as the temporal surface, and to the lower part as the infratemporal surface of the greater wing of sphenoid bone. **f. temporalis ossis frontalis** [NA] A small concave area posterior to the temporal line on the lateral aspect of the frontal bone that helps to form the wall of the temporal fossa. Also *temporal surface of frontal bone.* **f. temporalis ossis zygomatici** [NA] A small concave area facing posteromedially on the zygomatic bone, the posterior part of which extends upwards on the frontal process to form the anterior boundary of the temporal fossa. A backward extension on the medial part of the temporal process helps to form the lateral wall of the infratemporal fossa. The surface has a foramen for the zygomaticotemporal nerve. **f. temporalis partis squamosae** [NA] The large, convex anterior portion of the outer surface of the squamous part of the temporal bone that participates in the posterior part of the wall of the temporal fossa. **typhoid f.** The facial appearance characteristic of typhoid fever, marked by moderate flushing, lustrous and sunken eyes, a vacant, apathetic expression, and ashen color. Also *facies typhosa.* **f. urethralis penis** [NA] The inferior surface of the penis, in apposition with the scrotum and opposite to the dorsal aspect of the penis. **f. vesicalis uteri** [NA] The normally flattened anterior surface of the body of the uterus, in apposition with the urinary bladder from which it is separated by the vesicouterine excavation, or peritoneal pouch. **f. visceralis hepatis** [NA] The surface of the liver that faces inferiorly and posteriorly and is covered by peritoneum, except over the fossa for the gallbladder, at the porta hepatis, and in the fissure for ligamentum teres. It is divided into the right, left, and quadrate lobes, which are closely related to adjacent abdominal organs, such as the right kidney, stomach, transverse colon, gallbladder, and duodenum. Also *visceral surface of liver, inferior surface of liver.* **f. visceralis splenis** [NA] The medial surface of the spleen. It faces the abdominal organs and is divided into facies colica, facies gastrica, and facies renalis, which are related to the left colic flexure, the stomach, and the left kidney, respectively. The hilum of the spleen is situated on the gastric surface. Also *visceral surface of spleen.*

**facilitation** \fəsil′itā′shən\ [*facilit(y)* + -ATION] The neural process of enhancing or promoting synaptic events or reflex actions whereby the sum of separate inputs is additive. **associative f.** That process by which one association, already established, makes it easier to form another association to one of its elements. Thus, having already established an association between moon and June, an association between moon and spoon (or June and spoon) would be facilitated. **proprioceptive neuromuscular f.** The use of proprioceptive stimuli and reflex patterns to enhance contraction or relaxation of muscles. **f. of reflexes** REINFORCEMENT OF REFLEXES. **Wedensky's f.** The additive effect of an appropriately timed sequence of electric shocks, resulting in greater amplitude of muscle contraction than with a single shock of the same strength.

**facilitatory** \fəsil′ətətôr′ē\ Producing or promoting facilitation.

**facility** \fəsil′itē\ [L *facilitas* (from *facilis* easy to do, easy, from *facere* to make, do + *-itas* -ITY) readiness, easiness] A physical plant, along with its equipment and supplies, in which services are provided. **extended care f.** An inpatient health care facility providing skilled nursing and related services for long-term stays not appropriate to community hospitals. **intermediate care f.** A health care facility that provides inpatient care that is less complex or sophisticated than that of a general or community hospital or a skilled nursing facility but which is required by patients needing long-term institutionalization because of their mental or physical condition. **skilled nursing f.** An inpatient health care facility which provides care for patients that do not require the services of a community hospital but do require nursing care due to injury, disability, or mental health problems.

**facing** The visible tooth-colored part of a combined metal/nonmetal crown or unit of a prosthesis.

**facio-** \fā′shē·ō-\ [L *facies* face] A combining form denoting the face.

**facioplegia** \fā′shē·ōplē′jə\ FACIAL PARALYSIS.

**factitious** \faktish′əs\ Not occurring naturally; artificial or contrived.

# factor

**factor** [L (from *fact(us)*, past part. of *facere* to make, do + *-or* -OR), a maker, doer] **1** Any agent or element which helps to produce a result, as in an enzyme reaction, blood coagulation, or hormonal change. **2** A determinant of a mendelian character; a gene. An outmoded usage. **f. I** FIBRINOGEN. • The I in this term represents the roman numeral for 1, not the letter I. **f. II** PROTHROMBIN. **f. III** *Rare* THROMBOPLASTIN. **f. IV** The calcium present in plasma. *Seldom used.* **f. V** The coagulation factor that, when activated, is the cofactor of factor Xa in the formation of prothrombinase. Also *labile factor* (obs.), *proaccelerin, accelerator globulin, cofactor V, accelerator factor.* **f. VI** The original designation for activated factor V (accelerin). This term is no longer applied to any coagulation factor. **f. VII** A plasma coagulation factor intermediate in the clotting cascade. It dominates the "extrinsic" coagulation pathway. Also *stable factor, proconvertin, serum prothrombin conversion accelerator* (outmoded), *kappa factor, cothromboplastin.* **f. VIII** A plasma coagulation factor whose inherited deficiency is responsible for classic hemophilia (lack of factor VIII: C) or von Willebrand's disease (lack of factor VIII R: Ag). It is deficient in acute disseminated intravascular coagulation. Also *antihemophilic factor, antihemophilic factor A, hemophilic factor A, platelet cofactor I, thromboplastic plasma component, antihemophilic globulin* (original term). **f. VIII:c** The coagulant moiety of the factor VIII complex, having a molecular weight of about 250 000. This is primarily deficient in classic hemophilia. **f. VIII:CAg** The plasma protein that normally has factor VIII:C coagulant activity. Patients with or without hemophilia who develop anti-factor VIII antibodies do so against factor VIII:-CAg. **f. VIIIR:Ag** The noncoagulatnt portion of factor VIIIR:Ag, which is necessary for platelets to adhere to damaged endothelium. This accounts for the long bleeding time in patients with von Willebrand's disease, who have a deficiency of this factor. This factor must also be present in adequate amounts in order for the antibiotic ristocetin to clump platelets. Also *Willebrand factor, transhemophilin, ristocetin cofactor, ristocetin factor, factor VIII T.* **f. VIII T** FACTOR VIIIR:AG. **f. IX** A plasma coagulation factor that may be deficient on an inherited basis (hemophilia B), or an acquired basis (vitamin K deficiency). Also *plasma thromboplastin component, Christmas factor, platelet cofactor II, autoprothrombin II, antihemophilic factor B, hemophilic factor B.* **f. X** A vitamin K-dependent plasma coagulation factor. When activated (factor Xa) it combines with activated factor V (factor Va) plus calcium and phospholipid to form the prothrombinase complex. Also *Stuart factor, Prower factor, Stuart-Prower factor, autoprothrombin I.* **f. XI** A plasma coagulation factor that forms the bridge between the activation factors, such as factor XII, and the hemophilic factors, factors IX and VIII. Deficiency of factor XI causes a bleeding tendency. Also *plasma thromboplastin antecedent, antihemophilic factor C, hemophilic factor C.* **f. XII** One of the activation factors initiating the intrinsic coagulation pathway. There is no bleeding diathesis when this factor is deficient. Also *Hageman factor, glass factor.* **f. XIII** An enzyme of blood plasma that cross-links strands of fibrin monomers, thus creating a mesh of polymerized fibrin and stabilizing the blood clot. Also *fibrin stabilizing factor, fibrinase, fibrinoligase, Laki-Lorand factor.* **accelerator f.** FACTOR V. **activated clotting f.'s** Products with clotting activity generated from the inactive plasma clotting proteins during the coagulation process. The inactive proteins have been assigned Roman numerals, and the active products have an *a* appended. Thus proaccelerin is factor V and accelerin is factor Va. **activation f.** Any of three plasma coagulation factors that, when activated, initiate the intrinsic clotting cascade. They are factor XII, prekallikrein (Fletcher factor), and high-molecular weight kininogen (Fitzgerald factor). Bleeding does not result from deficiencies of these factors. Also *contact activation factor.* **amplification f.** The ratio of output voltage to input voltage in the operation of an electronic or other amplifier, or one of its components. In a pulse amplifier this factor is equal to the voltage at the peak of an output pulse divided by that at the peak of the corresponding input pulse. **animal protein f.** VITAMIN $B_{12}$. **antiacrodynia f.** VITAMIN $B_6$. **antialopecia f.** INOSITOL. **antianemia f.** VITAMIN $B_{12}$. **antiberiberi f.** THIAMIN. **anti-black-tongue f.** NIACIN. **anticanities f.** PANTOTHENIC ACID. **antidermatitis f. of chicks** PANTOTHENIC ACID. **antidermatitis f. of rats** VITAMIN $B_6$. **anti-egg-white f.** BIOTIN. **antihemophilic f.** FACTOR VIII. **antihemophilic f. A** FACTOR VIII. **antihemophilic f. B** FACTOR IX. **antihemophilic f. C** FACTOR XI. **antihemorrhagic f.** VITAMIN K. **antineuritic f.** THIAMIN. **antipellagra f.** NIACIN. **antirachitic f.** VITAMIN D. **antiscorbutic f.** VITAMIN C. **antisterility f.** VITAMIN E. **antixerophthalmia f.** VITAMIN A. **atrial natriuretic f.** A heart atrial extract which produces marked natriuresis and diuresis when injected into rats. A synthetic form has been produced. **f. B** The component of the alternative complement pathway that is the homolog of C2 in the classical pathway. It is the zymogen of a complex serine protease. Factor B complexes with C3b in the presence of magnesium ions and is then cleaved by factor D to give rise to two products, Ba and C3b,Bb, the latter being the C3-converting enzyme of the alternative complement pathway. **backscatter f.** The ratio of the exposure or of the absorbed dose at a point on the surface of a patient or phantom to the exposure or absorbed dose due to primary photons only. **Bittner milk f.** MOUSE MAMMARY TUMOR VIRUS. **buildup f.** In a beam of high energy x rays or gamma rays the ratio of the peak absorbed dose to the surface absorbed dose. **calibration f.** A multiplier applied to the numerical reading of an instrument to convert a quantity with one physical dimension to a more informative one, for example counts per second to millicuries of radioactivity. **CAMP f.** A product of group B streptococci, seen when streptococci are grown on a blood agar plate near a hemolytic strain of *Staphylococcus aureus.* The factor enlarges the zone of $\beta$-hemolysis that surrounds the streaked colonies of *S. aureus.* **Castle's f.** INTRINSIC FACTOR. **chick antipellagra f.** PANTOTHENIC ACID. **chick growth f.** STREPTOGENIN. **chick growth f. S** STREPTOGENIN. **Christmas f.** FACTOR IX. **clearing f.** LIPOPROTEIN LIPASE. **clumping f.** Surface-bound coagulase of *Staphylococcus aureus,* which causes clumping in plasma by reaction with fibrinogen. **C3 nephritic f.** An autoantibody present in the plasma of some patients with membranoproliferative glomerulonephritis who have low plasma complement activity. The autoantibody has specificity for the C3b,Bb complex of the alternative pathway of complement activation, and it stabilizes the system for enzymatic cleavage of C3 to C3a and C3b. **coagulation f.'s** Any of the plasma proteins in the coagulation cascade plus calcium and thromboplastin. **conglutinogen-activating f.** FACTOR I. **contact activation f.** ACTIVATION FACTOR. **cord f.** 6,6′-Dimycolyl trehalose, a component of the cell envelope of *Mycobacterium tuberculosis* that promotes virulence and serpentine growth. **coupling f.'s** Substances which allow, or restore, mitochondrial oxidation to bring about phosphorylation so that adenosine triphosphate can again be produced, especially in mitochondria in which these processes have been uncoupled. **cow manure f.** VITAMIN $B_{12}$. **f. D** A serine protease of molecular weight 25 000 daltons which occurs in fully active form in plasma and is an essential component of the alternative pathway of complement activation. It cleaves Fb when this protein is bound to C3b. **decapacitation f.** A factor that prevents capacitation of spermatozoa, such that the ability of spermatozoa to fertilize an ovum is impaired. **decay accelerating f.** An erythrocyte membrane protein which functions as a control protein of the complement system. It accelerates the decomposition of $\overline{C4b,2b}$, the C3-converting enzyme of the classical pathway, into its components. Decay accelerating factor is absent on the abnormal erythrocytes of patients with paroxysmal nocturnal hemoglobinuria. **depolarization f.** The process of decreasing the membrane potential of a cell by any course in which the absolute potential value becomes less negative. **Duran-Reynals f.** **duty f.** Pulse duration multiplied by pulse repetition frequency. For example, in ultrasonography the pulse duration of 1 μs and a pulse repetition frequency of 2000 pulses/s yields a low duty factor of 0.002. **elongation f.** One of several cytoplasmic proteins that function cyclically during each addition of an amino acid in polypeptide chain elongation. In bacteria EFTu complexes with aminoacyl-tRNA and GTP to form a ternary complex that binds to the ribosome in the recognition step. EFTu·GDP is released and then interacts with EFTs, which leads to replacement of the GDP by GTP. EFG, complexed with GTP, participates in the translocation step in chain elongation, and it is released after hydrolysis of the GTP. In eukaryotic systems similar factors are called EF-1 and EF-2. **eluate f.** VITAMIN $B_6$. **eosinophil chemotactic f.** A lymphokine that, when activated by immune complexes, attracts blood eosinophils to sites of inflammation. **epidermal growth f.** A protein substance, extracted from submaxillary glands of male mice, which when administered to immature mice induces more rapid eyelid opening, eruption of teeth, and growth of epidermal structures. Larger doses may inhibit these processes. **essential food f.'s** Substances that are required by the body to sustain life but which cannot be synthesized by the body and so must be supplied exogenously by the diet. Such substances include linoleic acid, the vitamins and minerals, and the essential amino acids, specifically tryptophan, phenylalanine, lysine, threonine, valine, methionine, leucine, and isoleucine. Histidine is an essential amino acid during childhood. **extrinsic f.** VITAMIN $B_{12}$. **F f.** A particular plasmid that codes efficiently for transfer of itself, and also of the bacterial chromosome, by conjugation. This plasmid is the one with which bacterial conjugation was discovered in *Escherichia coli*. It is unusually efficient because it lacks a gene, present in most conjugative plasmids, that represses the transfer operon. Also *F plasmid, F agent, fertility factor*. **fertility f.** 1 F FACTOR. 2 Any conjugative plasmid. **fibrin stabilizing f.** FACTOR XIII. **filtrate f.** PANTOTHENIC ACID. **Fletcher f.** The original term for PREKALLIKREIN. • *Fletcher* was the name of the family in which an inherited deficiency of this factor was discovered. **F-prime f.** An F factor that has incorporated specific host genes and thus mediates their high-frequency transfer by conjugation. **Fy f.** The gene responsible for expressing the red cell phenotype Fy(a-b-) which is commonly found in blacks and rarely in whites. The Fy factor is so named because it is part of the Du*ffy* blood group. **G f.** G FACTOR OF SPEARMAN. **general f.** G FACTOR OF SPEARMAN. **glass f.** FACTOR XII. **growth f.** 1 Any factor essential to skeletal or somatic growth, such as vitamin D, minerals, or the growth hormone. 2 A substance that is required for or that enhances growth of a particular microbe. Most growth factors are nutrients utilized by the cell, but some, as albumin or starch, are protective, acting by binding toxic compounds, especially soap, in the medium. **growth hormone inhibitory f.** SOMATOSTATIN. **G f. of Spearman** A unitary factor said to underlie performance scores earned on virtually all tests of mental ability and to contribute to and be responsible for the tendency for all cognitive measures to be positively related. Individuals are held to possess this general factor of mental ability in varying amounts, and it is to this ability to reason, to perceive relationships, and to educe correlates from them that reference is made when speaking of the individual's intelligence. Also *G component, general ability, general factor, G factor*. **f. H** 1 BIOTIN. 2 One of the control proteins of the complement system. Factor H binds to C3b and allows its cleavage by factor I. **Hageman f.** FACTOR XII. **hemophilic f. A** FACTOR VIII. **hemophilic f. B** FACTOR IX. **hemophilic f. C** FACTOR XI. **H f. of Lewis** The substances liberated into the skin after rubbing with a blunt instrument as part of the triple response of Lewis. It was presumed by Lewis, probably correctly, to be histamine with or without other pharmacologically active substances. **human f. IX complex** A fraction prepared from the supernatant plasma after precipitating human antihemophilic globulin. It is a concentrated mixture of coagulation factors II, VII, IX, and X, and it is used to treat bleeding episodes in patients with hemophilia B. **f. I** One of the control proteins of the complement system. It is a serine protease occurring in fully active form in plasma which cleaves C3b to iC3b. This reaction is of central importance in the control of the alternative complement pathway. Factor I will also cleave iC3b to C3c and C3dg; and C4b to C4c and C4d. All factor I cleavage requires the substrate to be bound to a substrate modifying protein. Also *C3b inactivator, conglutinogen-activating factor*. • The *I* in this term represents the letter I, not the roman numeral. **IgG rheumatoid f.** Immunoglobulin G with antibody activity against the Fc portion of a normal immunoglobulin G molecule. **IgM rheumatoid f.** The classic rheumatoid factor, consisting of an immunoglobulin M molecule with antibody activity directed against the Fc portion of a normal immunoglobulin G molecule. **initiation f.** One of several protein factors that participate in the initiation step in protein synthesis and then are released from the ribosome as it moves on into chain elongation. Bacteria have three initiation factors (IF-1, IF-2, IF-3). Eukaryotic cells have a larger number. **insulin-antagonizing f.** Any nonhormonal insulin antagonist, such as a fatty acid. **intermediate lobe inhibiting f.** MELANOCYTE STIMULATING HORMONE INHIBITORY HORMONE. **intrinsic f.** A glycoprotein of molecular weight in the order of 50 000 which is produced by normal gastric parietal cells. It dimerizes when it combines with vitamin $B_{12}$ to give a complex consisting of two molecules of intrinsic factor and two molecules of vitamin $B_{12}$. In this form $B_{12}$ is permitted to enter ileal mucosal cells. Deficiency of intrinsic factor impairs the absorption of $B_{12}$. This is common in old people. Also *Castle's factor*. **kappa f.** 1 A large, complex particle composed of DNA, RNA, and protein, occurring in the cytoplasm of certain strains of paramecia. Strains having kappa particles produce toxic materials which kill sensitive strains of paramecia. 2 FACTOR VII. **labile f.** *Obs.* FACTOR V. **lactogenic f.** *Outmoded* PROLACTIN. **Laki-Lorand f.** FACTOR XIII. **LE f.** ANTINUCLEAR ANTIBODY. **LE cell f.** ANTINUCLEAR ANTIBODY. **letdown f.** *Outmoded* PROLACTIN. **lethal f.** LETHAL ALLELE. **leukocyte migration inhibition f.** A lymphokine that inhibits migration of polymorphonuclear leukocytes. **leukopenic f.** A hypothetical substance postulated to occur in inflammatory conditions as a result of cell death, and causing reduction in number of blood leukocytes. Endotoxin, derived from bacterial cell walls, is a well-defined leukopenic factor. **liver f.** A factor in liver that was found to cause remissions of pernicious anemia. Its purified form is vitamin $B_{12}$. **liver filtrate f.** PANTOTHENIC ACID. **LLD f.** VITAMIN $B_{12}$. **lupus erythematosus f.** ANTINUCLEAR ANTIBODY. **lu-**

**teinizing hormone releasing f.** GONADOTROPIN RELEASING HORMONE. Abbr. LHRF, LRF **lymph node permeability f.** A substance derived from extracts of lymph nodes having the capacity to increase the permeability of vessels. Abbr. LNPF **lymphocyte-activating f.** INTERLEUKIN-1. **lymphocytosis-promoting f.** A protein product of *Bordetella pertussis* that stimulates lymphocyte production and may be responsible for other toxic effects. **macrophage-activating f.** A lymphokine that enhances phagocytic, bactericidal, and tumoricidal activities of macrophages. **macrophage chemotactic f.** A lymphokine that stimulates migration of macrophages. **macrophage migration inhibition f.** MIGRATION INHIBITION FACTOR. **maturation f.** Any substance, real or hypothetical, which can cause differentiation or maturation of a cell. **melanocyte inhibiting f.** MELATONIN. **melanocyte stimulating hormone release inhibiting f.** MELANOCYTE STIMULATING HORMONE INHIBITORY HORMONE. **migration inhibition f.** A protein of approximately 70 000 daltons released from sensitized lymphocytes and which inhibits the mobility of macrophages. Also *macrophage migration inhibition factor.* Abbr. MIF **milk f.** MOUSE MAMMARY TUMOR VIRUS. **mitogenic f.** A substance that stimulates transformation, DNA synthesis, and mitosis in immunocompetent lymphocytes. **modifying f.** MODIFYING GENE. **mouse antialopecia f.** INOSITOL. **mouse mammary tumor f.** MOUSE MAMMARY TUMOR VIRUS. **müllerian regression f.** A protein hormone secreted by the Sertoli cells of the fetal testis. The hormone induces the normal involution of the embryonic müllerian duct structures in the male. Also *müllerian duct inhibiting factor.* **multiple f.'s** Two or more genetic loci, the individual actions of which cannot be separated from their cooperative action in producing a recognizable character. **nerve growth f.** A specific protein which causes cells of embryonic spinal ganglia to send out axons. Snake venom and submaxillary salivary glands of mice contain very potent nerve growth factors. **neutrophil chemotactic f.** A lymphokine that stimulates migration of neutrophils. **osteoclast activating f.** A lymphokine that stimulates osteoclasts thus causing resorption of bone. **Passovoy f.** A coagulation activation factor that acts near factor XI in the coagulation cascade. **plasma thromboplastin f.** Any intrinsic coagulation plasma factor that promotes acceleration of the conversion of prothrombin to thrombin. Three such factors are recognized: factors VIII, IX, and XI. **platelet f.** Any of several substances that are primarily located within platelets or on their surface membranes and that contribute to coagulation by affecting platelet aggregation, adhesion, or retraction, or accelerate conversion of prothrombin to thrombin. Adsorbed substances are not considered platelet factors. Seven platelet factors are recognized. • Whereas coagulation factors are assigned Roman numerals, platelet factors are assigned Arabic numerals 1–7. **platelet activating f.** Acetyl glyceryl ether phosphorylcholine, a substance released by neutrophils, monocytes, mast cells, and basophils that causes platelets to aggregate and release $\beta$-thromboglobulin, 5-hydroxytryptamine, and platelet factor 4. **platelet derived growth f.** A heat-stable protein having a molecular weight of 13 000, which is contained in the $\alpha$-granules of platelets. It stimulates proliferation of smooth-muscle cells in tissue culture. Abbr. PDGF **Prower f.** FACTOR X. **quality f.** A number which relates the relative biologic effect of different types of radiation and is used in the field of radiation protection. The International Commission on Radiological Protection has assigned the quality factor values of from 1 to 20, depending on the linear energy transfer, defined in terms of the collision stopping power. Multiplying the absorbed dose in rads by the quality factor gives the dose in rems. Symbol: Q **R f.** Any of a large group of plasmids characterized by the presence of genes that cause resistance to various antimicrobial agents, mostly by coding for enzymes that inactivate the agent. Factors are classified in terms of incompatibility group or in terms of their pattern of resistance genes. Also *resistance factor, R plasmid.* See also FERTILITY INHIBITION. **rat acrodynia f.** PYRIDOXINE. **reducing f.** VITAMIN C. **resistance f.** R FACTOR. **resistance transfer f.** The part of a resistance plasmid, sometimes found alone, that codes for its own replication and machinery of conjugation. Combined with R-determinants, which code for enzymes that inactivate various antimicrobial agents, it becomes a resistance factor (R factor). Abbr. RTF **Reynals f.** HYALURONIDASE. **Rh f.** RH ANTIGEN. **Rhesus f.** RH ANTIGEN. **rheumatoid f.** An immunoglobulin, usually pentameric IgM but sometimes monomeric IgM or IgG, that is defined by its reactivity with the Fc portion of IgG. Rheumatoid factor is commonly present in the serum of patients with rheumatoid arthritis. **f. rho** The transcription termination factor, which promotes release of RNA polymerase from DNA. Its deficiency in mutants results in suppression of operon polarity. **risk f.** In epidemiology, an attribute or circumstance associated with an enhanced risk of developing or of dying from a specific disease. **ristocetin f.** FACTOR VIIIR:AG. **f. S** BIOTIN. **secretor f.** **1** A genetically-determined agent responsible for the secretion in body fluids of water-soluble A, B, or H substances, corresponding to the ABO type of the individual. Individuals who inherit the factor are secretors, those lacking it are nonsecretors. **2** SECRETOR. **sex f.** CONJUGATIVE PLASMID. **sigma f.** One of the subunits of bacterial DNA-directed RNA polymerase. It binds to the rest of the enzyme and enables it to bind to a promoter site in DNA while diminishing its affinity for the rest of the DNA. The sigma factor functions only during the initiation of a new RNA chain, after which it is released and recycled to another RNA polymerase. **skin f.** BIOTIN. **skin reactive f.** A lymphokine that causes local cutaneous inflammatory reactions. **somatotropin-releasing f.** GROWTH HORMONE RELEASING HORMONE. **specific macrophage arming f.** A lymphokine that causes macrophages to be cytotoxic for tumor cells. **spreading f.** HYALURONIDASE. **stable f.** FACTOR VII. **Stuart f.** FACTOR X. **Stuart-Prower f.** FACTOR X. **sulfation f.** *Outmoded* SOMATOMEDIN. **T-cell growth f.** INTERLEUKIN-2. **T-cell replacing f.** A lymphokine that augments antiheterologous erythrocyte plaque-forming cell responses. **termination f.** TERMINATION SEQUENCE. **thyroid stimulating hormone releasing f.** THYROTROPIN RELEASING HORMONE. Abbr. TSH-RF **thyrotoxic complement-fixation f.** One of several abnormal proteins found in the serum of patients with Graves disease. Its presence provides support for an autoimmune basis of this type of hyperthyroidism. **tissue plasminogen f.** TISSUE PLASMINOGEN ACTIVATOR. **transfer f.** **1** An activity found in the dialysate of leukocyte extracts from subjects who show delayed hypersensitivity to an antigen which is claimed to confer, when injected into other human subjects who are believed not to have encountered the antigen concerned, the specific delayed hypersensitivity to that antigen. **2** Single breath carbon monoxide diffusing capacity per unit lung volume. A British term. • Transfer factor is calculated and expressed in the American literature as the carbon monoxide diffusing capacity (DCO) divided by the calculated alveolar volume at which the test is performed (D/V). **transfer f. II** TRANSLOCASE. **transforming f.** A fragment of bacterial DNA which is capable of being integrated into the genome of a recipient bacterium. The term applies especially to type transformation in the pneumococcus, which was the initial observation of this phenomenon. **transmethylation f.** CHOLINE. **transmission f.** The ratio of the radiation intensity behind a protective barrier or other material to the radiation intensity at the surface. **tumor-angiogenesis f.** A substance produced by cancer cells which stimulates nearby blood vessels to grow into the tumor. **tumor cell migration inhibition f.** A lymphokine that inhibits migration of tumor cells. **tumor necrosis f.** A naturally occurring substance that causes necrosis of tumor cells. **f. V** NICOTINAMIDE ADENINE DINUCLEOTIDE. • The *V* in this term represents the letter V, not the roman numeral. **vascular permeability f.** A lymphokine that increases vascular permeability and induces inflammatory reactions. **vascular tissue f.** TISSUE PLASMINOGEN ACTIVATOR. **virulence f.** 1 Any genetic variable that affects virulence of a microbe or virus. 2 Any feature whose elimination may have a large effect, such as formation of a capsule, of a toxin, or of a surface molecule required for adherence. Also *aggressin* (obs.). **f. W** BIOTIN. **Willebrand f.** FACTOR VIIIR:AG. **Y f.** PYRIDOXINE. **yeast eluate f.** PYRIDOXINE. **yeast filtrate f.** PANTOTHENIC ACID.

**factorial** \faktôr′ē·əl\ For any given positive integer *n*: the product, written *n*!, of the first *n* positive integers. Thus, factorial 4, or 4!, is equal to $4 \times 3 \times 2 \times 1$, or 24. By convention, $0! = 1$.

**facultative** \fak′əltā′tiv\ 1 Able to live under more than one set of conditions, as in the case of certain organisms which can adapt to either a parasitic or nonparasitic existence, or which can grow either anaerobically or aerobically. Compare OBLIGATE. 2 Characterized by the capacity to operate or function in adapting to particular circumstances, as homosexuality in response to conditions where it is accepted and no heterosexual object is available, as in prisons.

**FAD** flavin adenine dinucleotide.

**faecalith** \fē′kəlith\ *Brit.* FECALITH.

**faeces** \fē′sēz\ *Brit.* FECES.

**faex** [L (gen. *faecis*), the dregs or lees of a liquid, esp. wine, brine of pickles] 1 A sediment or other material at the bottom of a solution. 2 YEAST.

**Faget** [Jean Charles *Faget*, French physician, 1818–1884] Faget sign. See under FAGET'S LAW.

**Fahr** [Theodor *Fahr*, German neurologist, 1877–1945] See under DISEASE.

**Fahraeus** [Robin Sanno *Fahraeus*, Swedish pathologist and anatomist, 1888–1968] 1 Fahraeus-Lindqvist effect. See under EFFECT. 2 Fahraeus reaction, Fahraeus test. See under ERYTHROCYTE SEDIMENTATION.

**Fahrenheit** [Daniel Gabriel *Fahrenheit*, German-Dutch physicist, 1689–1736] 1 Degree Fahrenheit. See under DEGREE. 2 See under THERMOMETER.

**fail-safe** Describing a circuit or system that fails in a way that prevents harm or destruction. An example of a fail-safe device is a mechanism on an anesthesia machine which will automatically shut off the delivery of nitrous oxide to a patient whenever the oxygen supply falls below a safe level.

**failure** [French *faillir* (inf. used as noun; from L *fallere* to deceive) to make a default; a failing] A condition or instance of not functioning or not functioning adequately. **acute anuric renal f.** Acute renal failure with no urine output. This is rare, but is most likely to develop in complete urinary obstruction, acute glomerulonephritis, bilateral cortical necrosis, and vascular disorders. **acute oliguric renal f.** Sudden renal excretory failure characterized by oliguria of less than 400 ml per 24 hours and rapidly increasing azotemia. Correctable causes include urinary tract obstruction, decreased renal blood flow and glomerular filtration rate associated with decreased extracellular and intravascular volumes, and transient hypotension. The most common cause of acute renal failure is hypotension after trauma, burns, or surgical shock. Other causes include nephrotoxins, acute glomerular diseases, acute interstitial disease, acute intravascular hemolysis, and acute renal vascular disorders such as embolus, thrombosis, vasculitis, and bilateral cortical necrosis. In approximately half of the cases the etiology is difficult to establish. **acute polyuric renal f.** Acute renal failure characterized by urinary output greater than 1 liter per 24 hours. This is most common in acute renal failure due to drugs and anesthetic agents. **acute renal f.** Sudden decrease of kidney function usually manifested by oliguria or rarely anuria. **backward heart f.** Heart failure attributable to a rise in filling pressure of the heart and a consequent rise in venous pressure: a mechanism proposed as the major cause of the manifestations of congestive heart failure. Compare FORWARD HEART FAILURE. **biventricular f.** Cardiac failure involving both right and left ventricles. **congestive heart f.** Heart failure manifested by congestion of the lungs if the left ventricle is involved, or by peripheral venous engorgement, hepatomegaly, and edema if the right ventricle has failed. Abbr. CHF **forward heart f.** Heart failure attributable to low cardiac output. It is proposed that the manifestations of congestive heart failure, such as pulmonary edema, hepatomegaly, and peripheral edema, are the consequence of low cardiac output and therefore of inadequate renal blood flow, leading to retention of sodium and water. Compare BACKWARD HEART FAILURE. **heart f.** Inability of the heart to meet the circulatory needs of the body, or meeting those needs only at the expense of excessively high venous pressures. Also *cardiac insufficiency*. **hepatic f.** A syndrome that results from massive necrosis of liver cells and marked by the inability of the liver to perform such synthetic and metabolic functions as bilirubin metabolism or synthesis of coagulation factors II, V, VII, IX, and X. It is manifested by progressive jaundice, fluid retention, hypoglycemia, and encephalopathy, and has a very high mortality rate. **high output heart f.** Failure of the heart to meet the needs of the body in spite of a higher than normal cardiac output, as seen in thyrotoxicosis, anemia, beriberi, and Paget's disease. **high output renal f.** Acute renal failure characterized by the kidney's inability to concentrate urine, thus producing normal or supranormal volumes of urine. Because urine output is normal or increased, the condition may be misdiagnosed. Recovery can be expected if the condition is diagnosed and treated. **kidney f.** RENAL FAILURE. **left-sided heart f.** Heart failure in which the manifestations are related to failure of the left ventricle or high pressure in the left atrium. Also *left heart failure*. **liver f.** See under HEPATIC FAILURE. **low output heart f.** Cardiac failure in which inadequate cardiac output is a major feature. **peripheral circulatory f.** Failure of the circulation as a consequence of inadequate peripheral vascular function. See also SHOCK. **prerenal f.** Renal failure due to decreased renal blood flow and glomerular filtration rate, associated with shock, volume depletion, congestive heart failure, or renal artery obstruction. Except for the last, prerenal failure is readily reversible by appropriate therapy. **primary adrenocortical f.** ADDISON'S DISEASE. **pump f.** Cardiac failure as a result of inadequate pumping function of the heart. **renal f.** Acute or chronic decrease in renal function associated with uremic symptoms, due to any cause. Lesser degrees of renal function impairment usually are termed renal insufficiency. Also *kidney failure.* **respiratory f.** Failure of the respiratory system to maintain normal tensions of oxygen or carbon dioxide in the arterial blood. **right-sided heart f.** Heart failure due to failure of the right ventricle or an excessively high pressure in the right atrium. Also *right heart failure.* **secondary adrenocortical f.** SECONDARY ADRENOCORTICAL INSUFFICIENCY. **secondary glandular f.** Deficiency of a hormone secreted by a particular gland owing to absence of stimulation by the hormone of another gland. Secondary hypogonadism, for example, results from anterior pituitary gonadotropin insufficiency. **template f.** A failure of the template of DNA or RNA to be correctly replicated, transcribed, or translated, thus interfering with a cell's ability to synthesize functional proteins, considered as one explanation of cellular aging.

**faint** [Middle English *feint,* from Old French *feint,* past part. of *feindre* to fain, dissimulate, from L *fingere* to touch] SYNCOPE.

**fainting** A sudden loss of consciousness due to transient global diminution of cerebral blood flow.

**Fajersztajn** [J. *Fajersztajn,* Austrian neurologist, flourished late 19th–early 20th centuries] Fajersztajn's test. See under FAJERSZTAJN'S CROSSED SCIATIC SIGN.

**falces** \fal′sēz\ Plural of FALX.

**falcial** \fal′shəl\ Pertaining to a falx.

**Fallopio** [Gabriele *Fallopio* (*Fallopius*), Italian anatomist, 1523–1562] **1** Foramen of Fallopio. See under HIATUS CANALIS NERVI PETROSI MAJORIS. **2** Aqueduct of Fallopius, fallopian aqueduct, fallopian canal, canalis facialis fallopii. See under CANALIS FACIALIS. **3** Fallopian tube. See under TUBA UTERINA.

**Fallot** [Étienne Louis Arthur *Fallot,* French physician, 1850–1911] **1** See under PENTALOGY, TRILOGY. **2** Fallot syndrome, Fallot's tetrad. See under TETRALOGY.

**fallout** Fine radioactive dust or other material projected into the atmosphere by a nuclear explosion and later resettling to earth.

**Falls** [Harold Francis *Falls,* U.S. opththalmologist and geneticist, born 1909] Rundles-Falls syndrome. See under HEREDITARY SIDEROBLASTIC ANEMIA.

**falx** \falks\ [L (gen. *falcis*), a scythe, sickle] (*pl.* falces) **1** A sickle-shaped structure or tissue. **2** Either the falx cerebri or the falx cerebelli. **aponeurotic f.** FALX INGUINALIS. **f. aponeurotica** FALX INGUINALIS. **f. cerebelli** [NA] A fold of dura mater lying in the midsagittal plane, separating the two cerebellar hemispheres. Also *falciform process of cerebellum.* **f. cerebri** [NA] A midline fold of dura mater situated superiorly in the midsagittal plane that separates the two cerebral hemispheres. Also *falciform process of cerebrum.* **f. inguinalis** [NA] The conjoint tendon of the transverse and internal oblique muscles of the abdomen, arching over the spermatic cord in the male and the round ligament of the uterus in the female and descending behind the superficial inguinal ring to its insertion on the crest and the pecten of the pubis, while it fuses medially with the anterior lamina of the rectus sheath. Occasionally the lateral fibers are continuous with the interfoveolar ligament. Also *conjoint tendon, conjoined tendon, tendo conjunctivus, inguinal falx, aponeurotic falx, falx aponeurotica.*

**familial** \fəmil′yəl\ **1** Of or pertaining to the family. **2** Affecting more members of a family than would be predicted on the basis of mere chance.

**family** [L *familia* (from *famulus* a household slave) the slaves, or the whole household, of one master] **1** A social group, especially a human social group, comprising parents and their offspring and sometimes other relatives. **2** A biological taxonomic group ranking above the genus and below the order. **extended f.** A group related by blood or marriage, extending over three or more generations, and including collateral relatives, their spouses, and offspring to an extent varying according to custom and mores in different cultures. **form-f.** See under FORM. **Jukes f.** A pseudonymous family descended from five sisters from New York State that was studied by the sociologist and penal reformer R.L. Dugdale in the 1870s. Many family members were described as criminals, paupers, or feeble-minded. Dugdale, who assigned the pseudonym Jukes to the family, ascribed these defects to such environmental influences as malnutrition, illiteracy, and congenital infections. Later authors distorted the data and ignored Dugdale's conclusions by promulgating genetic causes for the so-called defects. The Jukes family became a prototype for hereditarians seeking negative eugenic solutions to societal problems. **Kallikak f.** A pseudonymous family from New Jersey sired by a Revolutionary War soldier and studied by H.H. Goodard in 1912. In one branch of the family, descended from an illegitimate son, more than one quarter of the relatives were described as feeble-minded, illegitimate, prostitutes, or alcoholics. The legitimate branch contained relatives described as intelligent and respectable. The study was cited by hereditarians in support of negative eugenic solutions to societal problems, particularly low intelligence. **nuclear f.** A family unit comprising the father, mother, and their unmarried children.

**fan** [Old English *fann,* from L *vannus* a winnowing fan] **macular f.** A fanlike or stellate area of lipoidal deposits in the macula area of the retina occurring as a consequence of severe papilledema or as a result of other abnormal vascular permeability. Also *macular star.*

**Fanconi** [Guido *Fanconi,* Swiss pediatrician, born 1892] **1** Wissler-Fanconi syndrome. See under SYNDROME. **2** Fanconi's pancytopenia, Fanconi syndrome, Fanconi's disease. See under FANCONI'S ANEMIA. **3** De Toni-Fanconi syndrome, de Toni-Debré-Fanconi syndrome, Debré-de Toni-Fanconi syndrome, Fanconi's disease. See under FANCONI SYNDROME. **4** Lignac-Fanconi syndrome. See under CYSTINOSIS.

**fango** \fan′gō\ See under FANGO THERAPY.

***Fannia*** \fan′ē·ə\ A genus of flies of the family Muscidae. The larvae of some species cause myiasis and pseudomyiasis in humans. ***F. canicularis*** The lesser housefly. It is largely black with yellow markings on the sides of the abdomen, and is more slender than the common housefly. It is thought to cause intestinal myiasis in Europe, though feces may actually be contaminated in the environment. ***F. scalaris*** The latrine fly, larger than *F. canicularis* and differentiated from it by having two rather than three stripes on the adult thorax. It lays its eggs on human and animal excrement more frequently than on decaying vegetable material.

**fanning** The spreading movement of the second to the fifth toes seen on eliciting the plantar reflex in patients with an extensor plantar response (Babinski's sign).

**Fansidar** An antimicrobial agent consisting of a fixed combination of pyrimethamine and sulfadiazine and effective in the prevention of chloroquine-resistant malaria. A proprietary name.

**fantascope** \fan′təskōp\ [Gk *phanta(sma)* an image presented to the mind + -SCOPE] RETINOSCOPE.
**fantasy** A group of symbols synthesized into a unified story by the secondary process of the ego; an imagining. Also *phantasia*.
**Farabeuf** [Louis Hubert *Farabeuf*, French surgeon, 1841–1910] See under TRIANGLE.
**farad** \far′ad\ [after Michael *Faraday*, English chemist and physicist, 1791–1867] The special name for the SI derived unit of capacitance, the capacitance of a capacitor between the plates of which there appears a difference of electric potential of one volt when it is charged by a quantity of electricity of one coulomb; 1 farad = 1 coulomb/1 volt. Symbol: F
**Faraday** [Michael *Faraday*, English chemist and physicist, 1791–1867] See under CAGE, CONSTANT.
**faradic** \fərad′ik\ Of or relating to the asymmetric alternating current used in faradism.
**faradism** \far′ədizm\ The therapeutic application of faradic current used principally for the stimulation of muscles and nerves. Also *faradization*.
**faradize** \far′ədīz\ To subject to, or to treat with, a faradic current; to treat by faradism.
**faradocontractility** \far′ədōkän′traktil′itē \ [FARAD + *o* + *contractility*] The ability of muscle to respond to an alternating electric current.
**faradomuscular** \far′ədōmus′kyələr\ Denoting the effect of an alternating current in exciting muscle.
**Farber** [Sidney *Farber*, U.S. pathologist, 1903–1973] **1** See under TEST. **2** Farber's disease. See under LIPOGRANULOMATOSIS.
**farnesol** $C_{15}H_{25}OH$. 3,7,11-trimethyldodeca-2,6,10-trien-1-ol. A terpene alcohol with *trans* configuration of the 2 and 6 double bonds and containing three isoprene units. It occurs in plants. Its diphosphate (pyrophosphate) is an intermediate in the biosynthesis of sterols and many terpenes.
**farnesyl pyrophosphate** The ester of diphosphoric acid with farnesol. It is formed by elimination of diphosphate from a molecule of dimethylallyl pyrophosphate and two molecules of isopentenyl pyrophosphate. It is an intermediate in the biosynthesis of sterols, via squalene, and of various terpenes.
**farnoquinone** *Obs.* MENAQUINONE.
**Farr** [William *Farr*, English medical statistician, 1807–1883] See under LAW.
**Farre** [Arthur *Farre*, English obstetrician and gynecologist, 1811–1887] Farre's white line. See under LINE.
**Farre** [John Richard *Farre*, English physician, 1775–1862] Farre's tubercles. See under TUBERCLE.
**farsighted** [*far* + *sighted* (having sight)] HYPEROPIC.
**farsightedness** HYPEROPIA.
**fasc.** *fasciculus* (L, bundle).

# fascia

**fascia** \fash′ē·ə\ [L (akin to *fascis* a bundle) a band, strip, wrapping] (*pl.* fasciae) A layer or sheet of connective tissue composed mainly either of loose areolar tissue or compactly arranged collagen fibers and found subcutaneously investing or separating muscles and various structures and organs of the body. It may be a simple, single sheet or complex and multilayered, and is usually divided into superficial fascia, immediately beneath the skin, and deep fascia. **alar f. of pharynx** A sheet of fascia extending medially from the carotid sheath to the pharyngeal part of the buccopharyngeal fascia, fusing with it along the posterior median line of the pharynx from the base of the skull to the level of the seventh cervical vertebra and also attaching to the transverse processes of the cervical vertebrae. **f. antebrachii** [NA] The deep fascia of the forearm investing the muscles and sending septa between them. It is firmly attached to the posterior margin of ulna and the posterior surface of olecranon, and is continuous proximally with brachial fascia and distally with deep fascia of the hand. It is strengthened by transverse, longitudinal, and oblique fibers attached to certain bony parts and to tendons, especially at the wrist where it is thickened to form the extensor retinaculum posteriorly and the palmar carpal ligament and the flexor retinaculum anteriorly. **f. axillaris** [NA] A dome-shaped fibrous membrane that stretches across the base of the pyramidal-shaped axilla between the lower borders of the pectoralis major and latissimus dorsi muscles, continuous laterally with the brachial fascia and medially with fascia over the serratus anterior muscle. Because the clavipectoral fascia is attached to it by the suspensory ligament of axilla, the axillary fascia is raised during elevation of the arm, producing the hollowing of the armpit. Also *axillary fascia*. **bicipital f.** APONEUROSIS MUSCULI BICIPITIS BRACHII. **f. brachii** [NA] The deep fascia investing the muscles of the arm, continuous proximally with the axillary fascia and that of the muscles of the shoulder, and distally with the antebrachial fascia. It is anchored to the distal half of the humerus by the medial and lateral intermuscular septa, to the epicondyles, and to the posterior surface of olecranon. It is pierced by nerves and vessels, the largest being the basilic vein. Also *brachial fascia*. **f. buccopharyngealis** [NA] The thin layer of fibrous tissue surrounding the constrictor muscles of the pharynx, extending anteriorly to cover the buccinator muscle and blending superiorly with the pharyngobasilar fascia. Inferiorly it extends forwards to blend with the pretracheal fascia and the sheath of the thyroid gland. **Buck's f.** FASCIA PENIS PROFUNDA. **bulbar f.** VAGINA BULBI. **f. of Camper** The superficial, or fatty, layer of the superficial fascia of the lower third of the anterior abdominal wall, becoming continuous over the inguinal ligament with the superficial fascia of the thigh, while more centrally it extends into the penis as its superficial fascia, while in the female it continues into the labia majora. In the penis it loses its fat and continues into the scrotum, where it develops a few dartos muscle fibers. Occasionally it fuses with the deep layer (Scarpa's fascia) in the penis and scrotum. **f. cervicalis** [NA] The deep fascia investing the neck and extending around and between muscles, vessels, and viscera as fibrous sheets and sheaths. Deep to the superficial fascia and platysma, it roofs the anterior triangle of the neck, surrounds the sternocleidomastoid muscle, roofs the posterior triangle, encloses the trapezius muscle, and becomes continuous with the ligamentum nuchae. Superiorly it is attached to the inferior margin of mandible, ascending to form the masseteric fascia and parotid fascia before attaching to, among others, the zygoma, the mastoid process, and the superior nuchal line. Inferiorly it attaches to the clavicle and the manubrium sterni. More deeply in the neck, it forms the pretracheal fascia, prevertebral fascia, stylomandibular ligament, and the carotid sheath. Also *cervical fascia, fascia of neck*. **cervical visceral f.** LAMINA PRETRACHEALIS FASCIAE CERVICALIS. **f. cinerea** GYRUS FASCIOLARIS. **f. clavipectoralis** [NA] A strong sheet of connective tissue between the subclavius and pectoralis minor muscles, deep to the pectoralis major and attached to the first rib medially and the coracoid process of scapula laterally, the latter part often being designated the costocoracoid ligament, or membrane. Superiorly it splits around the subclavius to attach to the clavicle, and inferiorly it splits around the pectoralis minor to rejoin below it and continue inferiorly to fuse with the axillary fascia. The fascia above pectoralis minor is pierced by lymphatics, the cephalic vein, the lateral pectoral nerve, and thoracoacromial vessels. Also *clavicoracoaxillary aponeurosis, costocoracoid membrane.* **f. clitoridis** [NA] The dense fibrous tissue surrounding the body of the clitoris and continuous with the suspensory ligament. The fascia is not as clearly demarcated as that of the penis. Also *fascia of clitoris.* **Colles f.** FASCIA PERINEI SUPERFICIALIS. **f. cremasterica** A sheet of loosely arranged fasciculi of the cremaster muscle joined together by loose connective tissue, extending from the superficial inguinal ring down the spermatic cord to the testis and lying between the external and the internal spermatic fasciae. Also *cremasteric fascia, Scarpa sheath.* **f. cribrosa** [NA] The deep layer of superficial fascia that covers the saphenous opening in the fascia lata femoris, continuous with the margins of the opening and with the femoral sheath and pierced by the great saphenous vein, branches of the femoral artery, and lymph vessels. These perforations create a sievelike appearance. Also *cribriform lamina* (outmoded), *cribriform membrane.* **f. cruris** [NA] The investing deep fascia of the leg, continuous with the fascia lata and attached superiorly to the patella, ligamentum patellae, condyles of tibia, and head of fibula, and inferiorly to the malleoli and the back of the calcaneus. It is adherent to periosteum on the subcutaneous medial surface of the tibia, and from its deep surface arise muscles, the anterior and posterior crural intermuscular septa, and the deep transverse fascia of the leg. Around the ankle it is reinforced to form the superior and inferior extensor retinacula, the flexor retinaculum, and the peroneal retinacula. Also *crural fascia, crural aponeurosis, fascia of leg.* **Cruveilhier's f.** FASCIA PERINEI SUPERFICIALIS. **dartos f. of scrotum** TUNICA DARTOS. **deep f.** Compact connective tissue sheets that invest muscles and form intermuscular septa between them, become thickened around joints to form retinacula over tendons, vessels and nerves, ensheath certain vessels or nerves, fuse with periosteum over bone, or form osseofibrous channels or fibrous sheaths over tendons, and may invest certain organs and glands. **deep f. of back** FASCIA THORACOLUMBALIS. **deep cervical f.** FASCIA NUCHAE. **deep f. of penis** FASCIA PENIS PROFUNDA. **Denonvilliers f.** SEPTUM RECTOVESICALE. **f. dentata hippocampi** GYRUS DENTATUS. **dentate f.** GYRUS DENTATUS. **Dupuytren's f.** APONEUROSIS PALMARIS. **f. diaphragmatis pelvis inferior** [NA] The thin layer of fascia that lines the inferior surface of the levator ani and coccygeus muscles on each side, as well as the medial wall of the ischiorectal fossa. Also *superficial perineal aponeurosis, inferior layer of pelvic diaphragm.* **f. diaphragmatis pelvis superior** [NA] The fascia lining the superior, or pelvic, surface of the levator ani and coccygeus muscles on each side, blending medially with the visceral pelvic fascia. Also *aponeurosis of superior surface of levator ani muscle, superior perineal aponeurosis, superior layer of pelvic diaphragm.* **f. diaphragmatis urogenitalis inferior** MEMBRANA PERINEI. **f. diaphragmatis urogenitalis superior** The layer of superficial fascia that was once believed to separate the sphincter urethrae muscle from the prostate gland. It is now known that this layer does not,in fact, exist. Also *deep layer of triangular ligament, deep layer of urogenital diaphragm.* **dorsal f. of foot** FASCIA DORSALIS PEDIS. **dorsal f. of hand** FASCIA DORSALIS MANUS. **f. dorsalis manus** [NA] The deep fascia on the back of the hand, continuous with the antebrachial fascia and split around the extensor tendons on the hand, fusing with the tendons on the back of the fingers. Also *dorsal fascia of hand.* **f. dorsalis pedis** [NA] A thin fascial membrane continuous with fascia cruris at the inferior extensor retinaculum and extending to the dorsum of the toes where it forms fibrous sheaths for the extensor tendons. Also *dorsal fascia of foot.* **endoabdominal f.** FASCIA TRANSVERSALIS. **f. endopelvina** The areolar connective tissue between and investing the pelvic viscera, continuous with extraperitoneal tissue and condensed in places into membranes, ligaments and folds, such as the uterosacral, lateral cervical, uterovesicular, pubovesical, and puboprostatic ligaments. Also *endopelvic fascia.* **f. endothoracica** [NA] The thin layer of loose connective tissue that lines the internal surface of the thoracic cavity, lying outside the parietal pleura and fusing with the periosteum of the ribs and sternum. Also *endothoracic fascia.* **external cervical f.** LAMINA SUPERFICIALIS FASCIAE CERVICALIS. **external spermatic f.** FASCIA SPERMATICA EXTERNA. **f. extraperitonealis** [NA] The layer of fascia external to the parietal peritoneum and deep to the abdominal and pelvic walls. It varies in quantity and may contain fat in different areas, such as around the kidney. In some areas, such as behind the linea alba, it may be dense, causing the peritoneum to adhere to the wall. In others it may be very loose, permitting organs to distend it. Also *extraperitoneal fascia.* **fibroareolar f.** TELA SUBCUTANEA. **Gerota's f.** FASCIA RENALIS. **gluteal f.** Fascia lata that descends as a dense layer from the iliac crest over the gluteus medius muscle to the upper margin of the gluteus maximus muscle. There it splits into two layers, one superficial to the gluteus maximus and one deep to it. At the lower border of the muscle they reunite. **f. of Godman** The prolongation of the pretracheal fascia into the superior mediastinum. **hypogastric f.** FASCIA PELVIS. **hypothenar f.** The thin medial part of the palmar aponeurosis that covers the hypothenar muscles and becomes continuous medially with the fascia on the dorsum of the hand and laterally with the central part of the aponeurosis. **iliac f.** 1 FASCIA ILIACA. 2 ARCUS ILIOPECTINEUS. **f. iliaca** [NA] The fascia covering the psoas and iliacus muscles. It is especially thick in the inguinal region, where it is firmly adherent to the internal aspect of the inguinal ligament and the transversalis fascia lateral to the femoral vessels, and forms the arcus iliopectineus. Also *iliac fascia.* • In some texts, the iliac and psoas portions are described separately as the iliac fascia and psoas fascia. **iliopectineal f.** ARCUS ILIOPECTINEUS. **f. of insertion** APONEUROSIS OF INSERTION. **internal spermatic f.** FASCIA SPERMATICA INTERNA. **investing f.** APONEUROSIS OF INVESTMENT. **lacrimal f.** The thick anterior layer of the periorbita that extends from the lacrimal crest of the maxilla to the crest of the lacrimal bone, forming the roof of the fossa for the lacrimal sac and separating the sac from the medial palpebral ligament anteriorly and from the lacrimal part of musculus orbicularis oculi posteriorly. **f. lata femoris** [NA] The deep fascia investing the hip and thigh regions, thin medially and posteriorly and thick and strong laterally, where it forms the iliotibial tract. It provides intermuscular septa in the gluteal region as well as the medial, lateral, and posterior septa in the thigh where they are anchored to the linea aspera and separate the extensor, adductor, and flexor groups of muscles. Also *femoral aponeurosis.* **f. of leg** FASCIA CRURIS. **lumbar f.** FASCIA THORACOLUMBALIS. **lumbo-**

**dorsal f.** FASCIA THORACOLUMBALIS. **f. lunata** The deep fascia lining and arching over the ischioanal fossa and comprising the inferior fascia of pelvic diaphragm and either the obturator fascia below the arcus tendineus musculus levator ani or an upward extension of the sheath of pudendal canal. The latter blends with the inferior fascia and attaches to the falciform process of sacrotuberous ligament. **f. masseterica** [NA] A layer of deep cervical fascia that spreads upwards from the inferior and posterior margins of the mandible to cover and attach to the masseter muscle, while superficially it forms the parotid fascia investing the gland. Also *masseteric fascia.* • Some texts consider it to be an extension of the parotid fascia. **middle f. of pharynx** *Outmoded* FASCIA PHARYNGOBASILARIS. **fasciae musculares bulbi** [NA] Tubular fibrous sheaths of the bulbar muscles which thicken and fuse with the vagina bulbi where it is pierced by each of the muscles. Proximally they thin out and fuse with the perimysium and may form expansions such as the medial and lateral check ligaments. Also *muscular fasciae of eye, fasciae musculares oculi.* (outmoded). **fasciae musculares oculi** *Outmoded* FASCIAE MUSCULARES BULBI. **muscular fasciae of eye** FASCIAE MUSCULARES BULBI. **f. of nape** FASCIA NUCHAE. **f. of neck** FASCIA CERVICALIS. **f. nuchae** [NA] The investing fascial layer of the deep muscles at the back of the neck, including a series of membranes attached to it that surround groups of deep muscles. Also *nuchal fascia, fascia of nape, deep cervical fascia.* **f. obturatoria** [NA] That part of the parietal pelvic fascia that covers the internal surface of the obturator internus muscle. Also *obturator fascia.* **fasciae orbitales** [NA] The tissues connecting and supporting the various contents of the orbit, including the periorbita, septum orbitale, fasciae musculares, vagina bulbi, and corpus adiposum orbitae. Also *orbital fasciae.* **palmar f.** APONEUROSIS PALMARIS. **palpebral f.** SEPTUM ORBITALE. **parietal pelvic f.** FASCIA PELVIS PARIETALIS. **parietal f. of pelvis** FASCIA PELVIS PARIETALIS. **f. parotidea** [NA] An extension, forward of the investing layer of the deep cervical fascia, from the anterior border of the sternocleidomastoid muscle that splits and invests the parotid gland. The superficial part then extends anteriorly to form the masseteric fascia and attach to the zygomatic arch, while the deep layer fuses with the fascia of the posterior belly of the digastric muscle, attaches to the styloid process, and forms the stylomandibular ligament. Also *parotid fascia.* **f. parotideomasseterica** Fascia parotidea and fascia masseterica together. **f. pectinea** An extension of the iliac fascia behind the femoral vessels, attaching to the pecten pubis where it is continuous with the deep layer of fascia lata that forms the inferomedial margin of the saphenous opening and turns upwards and laterally behind the femoral vessels and in front of the pectineus muscle to attach to the pecten pubis. Also *Cowper's ligament, pubic fascia, pectineal fascia.* **f. pectoralis** [NA] The thin membrane that invests the pectoralis major muscle, continuous at its lower border with the axillary fascia and attached medially to the sternum and superiorly to the clavicle. Also *pectoral fascia.* **pelvic f.** FASCIA PELVIS. **f. pelvis** [NA] The overall fascial sheaths of the pelvis, comprising the parietal pelvic fascia, visceral pelvic fascia, and endopelvic fascia. Also *pelvic fascia, hypogastric fascia.* **f. pelvis parietalis** [NA] The fascia lining the inner walls of the pelvis, including the muscles passing from the pelvic cavity to the gluteal region, namely, obturator internus and piriformis, as well as the muscles of the pelvic diaphragm on both superior and inferior aspects. Also *parietal layer of pelvic fascia, parietal fascia of pelvis, parietal pelvic fascia, parietal part of pelvic fascia.* **f. pelvis visceralis** [NA] The fascia that surrounds the various organs and vessels of the pelvis, comprising the endopelvic fascia of specific viscera and the fascia associated with the pelvic peritoneum. Also *visceral pelvic fascia, visceral fascia of pelvis, visceral layer of pelvic fascia, visceral part of pelvic fascia.* **f. penis profunda** [NA] The condensed deep layer of the superficial fascia of the penis, continuous proximally and superiorly with the membranous layer of the superficial fascia of the anterior abdominal wall, and inferiorly with the tunica dartos of the scrotum and the membranous layer in the urogenital triangle where it encloses the crura and the bulb of penis and is joined to the perineal membrane and the perineal body. Also *deep fascia of penis, fascia penis, Buck's fascia.* **f. penis superficialis** [NA] The subcutaneous loose areolar tissue surrounding the penis, devoid of fat and continuous proximally and superiorly with the fatty layer of the superficial fascia of the anterior abdominal wall, and inferiorly with the tunica dartos of the scrotum. Also *superficial fascia of penis.* **f. perinei superficialis** [NA] The superficial fascia of the perineum, separated into a superficial, fatty layer and a deeper, membranous layer continuous with similar layers on the anterior abdominal wall. The fatty layer becomes the superficial fascia of the penis and the tunica dartos in the scrotum. The membranous layer forms the deep fascia of the penis and is continuous with the tunica dartos in the scrotum, whereas in the urogenital triangle it is attached to the margins of the ischiopubic rami over the crura of the penis as far posteriorly as the ischial tuberosities. The arrangement is modified in the female to accommodate the vagina. Also *superficial fascia of perineum, Colles fascia, Cruveilhier's fascia, superficial perineal fascia, anoscrotal fascia* (outmoded), *fascia superficialis perinei* (outmoded). • *Nomina Anatomica* does not distinguish between the fatty and membranous layers. Strictly, though, Colles fascia designates the membranous layer, and Cruveilhier's fascia the fatty layer. **perirenal f.** FASCIA RENALIS. **f. pharyngobasilaris** [NA] The fibrous layer of the wall of the pharynx situated between the mucous and muscular layers, thick superiorly where it is attached to the base of the skull and adjacent structures where the pharyngeal muscle fibers are absent and becoming thinner as it descends. It is supported posteriorly by the pharyngeal raphe, which provides attachment for the pharyngeal constrictor muscles. Also *pharyngobasilar fascia, pharyngobasilar aponeurosis, pharyngeal aponeurosis, pharyngobasilar coat, pharyngobasilar tunic, pharyngeal tunic, pharyngobasilar membrane.* **f. phrenicopleuralis** [NA] A flimsy layer of endothoracic fascia that binds the diaphragmatic pleura to the superior surface of the diaphragm. Also *phrenicopleural fascia.* **plantar f.** APONEUROSIS PLANTARIS. **popliteal f.** An extension of fascia cruris over the popliteal fossa where it is strengthenedby transverse fibers and pierced by the small saphenous vein. **pretracheal f.** LAMINA PRETRACHEALIS FASCIAE CERVICALIS. **prevertebral f.** LAMINA PREVERTEBRALIS FASCIAE CERVICALIS. **f. prevertebralis** LAMINA PREVERTEBRALIS FASCIAE CERVICALIS. **f. prostatae** Visceral fascia of the pelvis that ensheathes the prostate gland and its capsule, continuous anteriorly with the puboprostatic ligaments and inferiorly with the fascia on the deep aspects of the transversus perinei profundus and the sphincter urethrae muscles. Also *fascia of prostate, sheath of prostate.* **psoas f.** The fascia covering the psoas muscle. Also *fascia psoatis.* **pubic f.** FASCIA PECTINEA. **f. of quadratus lumborum muscle** See under FASCIA THORACOLUMBALIS. **rectovaginal f.** SEPTUM RECTOVAGINALE. **rectovesical f.** SEPTUM RECTOVESICALE.

**renal f.** FASCIA RENALIS. **f. renalis** [NA] A sheath of condensed fibroareolar tissue that surrounds the kidney and perirenal fat. It is connected to the fibrous capsule of the kidney by fibrous bands that pierce the perirenal fat. It consists of an anterior and a posterior layer, which are fused at the lateral margin of the kidney. Also *renal fascia, perirenal fascia, Gerota's fascia, fibrous sheath of kidney.* **Richet's f.** A fold of subperitoneal fascia surrounding the ligamentum teres hepatis as it pierces the fibers of the transversus abdominis muscle. **scalene f.** MEMBRANA SUPRAPLEURALIS. **Scarpa's f.** The deep or membranous layer of the superficial fascia in the lower part of the anterior abdominal wall. Inferiorly it is attached to the fascia lata in a straight line lateral to the pubic tubercles, whereas between them it is continuous with the membranous layer of the superficial fascia of the perineum. **semilunar f.** APONEUROSIS MUSCULI BICIPITIS BRACHII. **Sibson's f.** MEMBRANA SUPRAPLEURALIS. **f. spermatica externa** [NA] A tubulosaccular sheath that forms the outermost covering layer of the spermatic cord and testis. It is composed of fibrous tissue that extends down from the margins of the superficial inguinal ring in the aponeurosis of the external oblique muscle of the abdomen and the overlying fascia. Also *external spermatic fascia.* **f. spermatica interna** [NA] A tubulosaccular sheath forming the innermost covering layer of the spermatic cord and testis and being a prolongation of the transversalis fascia at the deep inguinal ring, thereby surrounding the structures passing through the ring and along the inguinal canal. Also *internal spermatic fascia.* **subcutaneous f.** TELA SUBCUTANEA. **subperitoneal f.** 1 FASCIA EXTRAPERITONEALIS. 2 TELA SUBSEROSA PERITONEI. **f. subperitonealis** FASCIA EXTRAPERITONEALIS. **f. subscapularis** The thin membranous layer attached to the total circumference of the subscapular fossa of the scapula, and providing origin from its deep surface to some fibers of the subscapularis muscle. Also *subscapular aponeurosis.* **superficial f.** TELA SUBCUTANEA. **superficial f. of penis** FASCIA PENIS SUPERFICIALIS. **f. superficialis perinei** *Outmoded* FASCIA PERINEI SUPERFICIALIS. **superficial perineal f.** FASCIA PERINEI SUPERFICIALIS. **superficial f. of perineum** FASCIA PERINEI SUPERFICIALIS. **superior f. of urogenital f.** See under SPATIUM PERINEI PROFUNDUM. **f. of Tarin** GYRUS DENTATUS. **f. tarini** GYRUS DENTATUS. **f. temporalis** [NA] A fibrous sheet covering the temporalis muscle and attached superiorly to the superior temporal line of the parietal bone and the temporal line of the frontal bone. Inferiorly it splits into two layers, the more superficial of which is attached to the lateral border and the deep one to the medial border of the zygomatic arch. Between the layers is some fat and small nerves and vessels. Also *temporal fascia, temporal aponeurosis.* **f. of Tenon** VAGINA BULBI. **thenar f.** The thin fibrous lateral part of the palmar aponeurosis that covers the thenar muscles and is continuous laterally with the fascia on the dorsum of the hand and medially with the central portion of the aponeurosis. **f. thoracolumbalis** [NA] The fascia covering the deep muscles of the back of the trunk and continuous superiorly with the nuchal fascia. In the thoracic region it separates the vertebral extensors from the more superficial muscles to the shoulder girdle and upper limb, and is attached laterally to the angles of the ribs and medially to the spines of vertebrae. In the lumbar region there are three layers of fascia that fuse lateral to the quadratus lumborum muscle into a common lamella from which arise parts of transversus abdominis and internal oblique muscles. The posterior layer covers the erector spinae muscle and is attached to the spines of lumbar and sacral vertebrae and their supraspinous ligaments, while the origin of the latissimus dorsi muscle blends with it to form the lumbar aponeurosis. The middle layer, between the erector spinae and quadratus lumborum, is attached to the tips of the transverse processes of lumbar vertebrae, while the anterior layer anterior to the quadratus lumborum is attached medially to the anterior surfaces of those transverse processes and inferiorly to the iliac crest and iliolumbar ligament. The anterior layer blends with the fascia transversalis and psoas fascia. Also *thoracolumbar fascia, lumbodorsal fascia, deep fascia of back, lumbar aponeurosis, lumbar fascia.* **tibial f.** *Outmoded* FASCIA CRURIS. **f. of Toldt** 1 The subperitoneal fascial layer posterior to the ascending colon (the right fascia of Toldt) and the descending colon (the left fascia of Toldt). It results from the fusion of the parietal peritoneum with the peritoneum covering corresponding parts of the colon or, when present, their mesocolon. 2 A fixation of fascial layers behind the body of the pancreas that is continuous with the fascia of Treitz. **f. transversalis** [NA] The layer of connective tissue between the extensive internal surface of the transversus abdominis muscle and the subperitoneal fascia, the right and left sides fusing behind the linea alba. It is continuous superiorly with the diaphragmatic fascia, posteriorly with the anterior layer of the thoracolumbar and psoas fasciae, while inferiorly it is attached to the iliac crest and the posterior edge of the inguinal ligament, where it is continuous with the iliac fascia. It is also attached to pecten pubis behind the conjoint tendon, helping to form the pectineal ligament. It forms the anterior wall of the femoral sheath. Also *transverse fascia, endoabdominal fascia.* **f. of Treitz** A layer of fascia that is situated behind the head of the pancreas and separates it from structures on the posterior abdominal wall, namely the right crus of the diaphragm, abdominal aorta, inferior vena cava, and right renal vein. **triangular f. of abdomen** LIGAMENTUM REFLEXUM. **triangular f. of Quain** LIGAMENTUM REFLEXUM. **Tyrrell's f.** SEPTUM RECTOVESICALE. **umbilicovesical f.** The deeper layer of the transversalis fascia and its continuation along the anterior surface of the bladder that forms the dorsal boundary of the retropubic space. *Outmoded.* Also *umbilical prevesical fascia.* **f. of urogenital trigone** DIAPHRAGMA UROGENITALE. **visceral pelvic f.** FASCIA PELVIS VISCERALIS. **visceral f. of pelvis** FASCIA PELVIS VISCERALIS. **volar f.** APONEUROSIS PALMARIS.

**fasciae** \fash′i·ē\ Plural of FASCIA.

**fascial** \fash′ē·əl\ Pertaining to a fascia.

**fascicle** \fas′ikl\ [L *fasciculus,* dim. of *fascis* a bundle of wood, rods, twigs, reeds, or straws] 1 A group of nerve fibers coursing in the same direction and often subserving a similar function. 2 FASCICULUS. **gracile f.** FASCICULUS GRACILIS MEDULLAE SPINALIS. **longitudinal f.'s of cruciform ligament** FASCICULI LONGITUDINALES LIGAMENTI CRUCIFORMIS ATLANTIS.

**fascicular** \fəsik′yələr\ 1 Pertaining to a fasciculus. 2 FASCICULATED.

**fasciculated** \fəsik′yəlā′tid\ Arranged in clusters or bundles. Also *fascicular.*

**fasciculation** \fəsik′yəlā′shən\ [*fascicul(us)* + -ATION] Spontaneous contraction of bundles of skeletal muscle fibers resulting in a localized twitching or flickering which can be seen under the skin or a mucous membrane but does not produce movement at a joint. Compare FIBRILLATION. Also *muscular tremor.* **benign f.** Fasciculation usually in the calf muscles or first interosseous space, less often in other muscles, which is benign and of no pathologic significance. Benign coarse fasciculation is a prominent feature of one form of myokymia.

**fasciculi** \fəsik′yəlī\ Plural of FASCICULUS.

**fasciculitis** \fəsik′yəli′tis\ [*fascicul(us)* + -ITIS] Inflammation limited to a few fascicles, usually of a nerve. **f. optica** *Outmoded* OPTIC NEURITIS.

# fasciculus

**fasciculus** \fəsik′yələs\ [L (dim. of *fascis* a bundle, packet), a little bundle or packet] (*pl.* fasciculi) A bundle of muscle, nerve, or connective tissue fibers. Also *fascicle.* **f. aberrans of Monakow** TRACTUS RUBROSPINALIS. **f. anterior proprius flechsigi** The fasciculi proprii, intersegmental axons, bordering the gray matter of the spinal ventral horn running in the anterior funiculus. **anterior pyramidal f.** TRACTUS CORTICOSPINALIS VENTRALIS. **f. anterolateralis superficialis Gowersi** TRACTUS SPINOCEREBELLARIS VENTRALIS. **f. arcuatus** FASCICULUS LONGITUDINALIS SUPERIOR CEREBRI. **f. atrioventricularis** [NA] A slender bundle of cardiac muscle fibers specially differentiated to conduct impulses for the contraction of cardiac muscle. It commences at the atrioventricular node in the lower part of the interatrial septum and passes subendocardially through the right trigonum fibrosum to reach the interventricular septum, ventral to which it divides into a right and a left crus, or limb. Each passes down either side of the septum to branch out to the walls of the ventricles. Also *atrioventricular bundle, A-V bundle, Kent's bundle, bundle of His, Kent-His bundle, bundle of Stanley Kent, His band, Gaskell's bridge* (outmoded), *ventriculonector, atrioventricular band.* **f. of Burdach** FASCICULUS CUNEATUS BURDACHI. **calcarine f.** A short bundle of association fibers lying beneath the calcarine sulcus and reciprocally connecting the upper and lower banks. **central tegmental f.** TRACTUS TEGMENTALIS CENTRALIS. **cerebellospinal f.** *Imprecise* TRACTUS SPINOCEREBELLARIS DORSALIS. **f. cerebellospinalis** *Imprecise* TRACTUS SPINOCEREBELLARIS DORSALIS. **f. cerebrospinalis anterior** TRACTUS CORTICOSPINALIS VENTRALIS. **f. cerebrospinalis lateralis** TRACTUS CORTICOSPINALIS LATERALIS. **f. circumolivaris pyramidalis** A bundle of axons coursing from the surface of the medullary pyramid, over the inferior olivary protuberance, and into the pons. **crossed pyramidal f.** TRACTUS CORTICOSPINALIS LATERALIS. **cuneate f. of Burdach** FASCICULUS CUNEATUS BURDACHI. **cuneate f. of medulla oblongata** FASCICULUS CUNEATUS MEDULLAE OBLONGATAE. **cuneate f. of spinal cord** FASCICULUS CUNEATUS MEDULLAE SPINALIS. **f. cuneatus burdachi** The fasciculus cuneatus medullae spinalis, along with its rostral continuation, the fasciculus cuneatus medullae oblongatae. Also *fasciculus cuneatus, cuneate fasciculus of Burdach, fasciculus of Burdach, Burdach's tract, column of Burdach.* **f. cuneatus medullae oblongatae** [NA] The rostral continuation of the cuneate fasciculus of the spinal cord, overlying the cuneate nucleus of the medulla oblongata. Also *cuneate fasciculus of medulla oblongata, funiculus cuneatus medullae oblongatae* (outmoded), *funiculus cuneatus Burdachi* (outmoded), *cuneate funiculus.* **f. cuneatus medullae spinalis** [NA] The axonal bundle forming the lateral portion of the posterior (dorsal) column and constituting the largest demarcated fascicle of myelinated fibers in the spinal cord. It is composed chiefly of large ascending axons arising from spinal ganglion cells of the cervical and upper thoracic levels that terminate in the cuneate nucleus (Burdach's nucleus) of the medulla oblongata. It also contains ascending axons from neurons of the spinal dorsal horn and a few descending interfascicular axons. Also *cuneate fasciculus of spinal cord.* **direct pyramidal f.** TRACTUS CORTICOSPINALIS VENTRALIS. **dorsal longitudinal f.** FASCICULUS LONGITUDINALIS DORSALIS. **dorsolateral f.** TRACTUS DORSOLATERALIS. **f. dorsolateralis** TRACTUS DORSOLATERALIS. **extrapyramidal motor f.** An outmoded and imprecise term for TRACTUS RUBROSPINALIS. **fastigiobulbar f.** An efferent bundle of cerebellar fibers emerging from the fastigial nucleus via the uncinate fasciculus (of Russell) arching around the superior cerebellar peduncle. Fibers from the rostral fastigial nucleus are uncrossed, sweep ventromedially, and terminate in the vestibular nuclei and dorsomedial parts of the pontine and medullary reticular formation. The larger, crossed component arises from the caudal fastigial nucleus and terminates in the medullary lateral reticular nucleus and perihypoglossal nucleus. **Flechsig's fasciculi** FASCICULI PROPRII. **f. of Foville** STRIA TERMINALIS. **f. of Goll** FASCICULUS GRACILIS MEDULLAE SPINALIS. **f. of Gowers** TRACTUS SPINOCEREBELLARIS VENTRALIS. **f. gracilis** 1 FASCICULUS GRACILIS MEDULLAE SPINALIS. 2 FASCICULUS GRACILIS MEDULLAE OBLONGATAE. **f. gracilis Golli** FASCICULUS GRACILIS MEDULLAE SPINALIS. **f. gracilis medullae oblongatae** [NA] The rostral continuation of the spinal fasciculus gracilis medullae spinalis, overlying and penetrating the nucleus gracilis in the medulla oblongata. Also *fasciculus gracilis, funiculus gracilis* (outmoded), *funiculus gracilis medullae oblongatae, posterior pyramid of medulla oblongata.* **f. gracilis medullae spinalis** [NA] A slender axonal bundle forming the medial segment of the posterior (dorsal) column. It is composed largely of long ascending axons from spinal ganglion cells of the lower thoracic, lumbar, and sacral levels of the spinal cord that terminate in the gracile nucleus of the medulla oblongata. It also contains ascending axons from posterior horn neurons, and a sector of interfascicular axons. Also *fasciculus gracilis, gracile fascicle, fasciculus gracilis Golli, fasciculus of Goll, column of Goll, tract of Goll.* **gyral f.** The subcortical association fibers running between gyri of the cerebral cortex. **inferior longitudinal f. of cerebrum** FASCICULUS LONGITUDINALIS INFERIOR CEREBRI. **f. interfascicularis** [NA] The descending axonal branches of the medial division of the spinal nerve dorsal roots situated between the fasciculi gracilis and cuneatus of the cervical and thoracic spinal cord. It also contains some descending axons from the dorsal horn. Also *comma tract of Schultze, bundle of Schultze* (obs.), *fasciculus semilunaris, interfascicular fasciculus, comma tract, Schultze's tract, semilunar tract.* **lateral cerebrospinal f.** TRACTUS CORTICOSPINALIS LATERALIS. **f. lateralis plexus brachialis** [NA] A major component of the brachial plexus formed proximally by the joining of anterior divisions of the superior and middle trunks, in its course giving rise to the lateral pectoral nerve, and splitting distally into a lateral component of the median nerve and the musculocutaneous nerve. It carries axons of $C_{4-7}$ segmental levels. Also *lateral cord of brachial plexus.* **f. lateralis proprius flechsigi** The fasciculi proprii, intersegmental axons, bordering the lateral ventral horn of the spinal cord in the lateral funiculus. **lateral pyramidal f.** TRACTUS CORTICOSPINALIS LATERALIS. **f. lenticularis** The bundle of fibers emerging from the globus pallidus of the lenticular nucleus, continuing below the zona incerta in the dorsal part of the ansa lenticularis, and entering the H field of Forel to form the fasciculus thalamicus. Also *field $H_2$ of Forel.* See also H FIELDS OF FOREL. **longitudinal fasciculi of cruciform ligament** FASCICULI LONGITUDINALES LIGAMENTI CRUCIFORMIS ATLANTIS. **fasciculi longitudinales** Collectively, the several longitudinal fiber tracts of the central nervous system. **fasciculi longitudinales ligamenti cruciformis atlantis** [NA] Thick, longitudinal bundles of ligamentous fibers that extend from the anterior margin of the foramen magnum to the posterior surface of the body of the axis vertebra. In between, they blend with the transverse ligament of the atlas, forming the cruciform ligament. Also *longitudinal fasciculi of cruciform ligament, longitudinal fascicles of cruciform ligament.* **fasciculi longitudinales pontis** The axonal bundles in the ventral pons arising from the cerebral cortex and constituting the corticonuclear and corticopontine components of the pyramidal tract. Also *fasciculi longitudinales pyramidales pontis.* **f. longitudinalis dorsalis** [NA] A small bundle of axons consisting principally of descending axons from the medial and periventricular hypothalamus to the mesencephalic central gray and the dorsal tegmental nucleus. Also *dorsal longitudinal fasciculus, Schütz bundle, tract of Schütz, periventricular tract, periependymal tract.* **f. longitudinalis inferior cerebri** [NA] The grossly delimited large myelinated bundle of association fibers coursing along the inferior horn of the lateral ventricle, reciprocally connecting the temporal and occipital lobes and including most of the geniculocalcarine tract. Also *inferior longitudinal fasciculus of cerebrum, inferior longitudinal bundle.* **f. longitudinalis medialis** [NA] A prominent myelinated bundle, close tothe midline and below the central gray matter, extending from the upper mesencephalon to the upper cervical levels of the spinal cord. It consists largely of axons from the vestibular nuclei ascending to the abducens, trochlear, and oculomotor nuclei and descending to motoneurons innervating the neck musculature. Also *medial longitudinal fasciculus, posterior longitudinal fasciculus, medial longitudinal bundle, posterior longitudinal bundle.* **f. longitudinalis medialis medullae oblongatae** [NA] The portion of the fasciculus longitudinalis medialis within the medulla oblongata, coursing rostrally from the vestibular nuclei and caudally to motoneurons of the accessory nerve. **f. longitudinalis medialis pontis** The portion of the fasciculus longitudinalis medialis within the pons, chiefly innervating the motor nuclei of extraocular muscles. Also *fasciculus teres* (outmoded). **f. longitudinalis superior cerebri** [NA] The poorly demarcated, longitudinally directed, lateral bundle of cortical association fibers reciprocally connecting the frontal, temporal, parietal, and occipital lobes. Also *fasciculus arcuatus, superior longitudinal fasciculus of cerebrum, superior longitudinal bundle.* **maculary f.** A bundle of fibers in the optic nerve, derived from ganglion cells that radiate from the macula lutea of the retina. **mamillotegmental f.** The tract connecting the mamillary nuclei of the hypothalamus with the dorsal and ventral tegmental nuclei (of Gudden). **f. mamillothalamicus** [NA] The myelinated axon bundle extending between the hypothalamic mamillary nuclei and the anterior nuclei of the thalamus. Also *fasciculus of Vicq d'Azyr, fasciculus thalamomamillaris, mamillothalamic fasciculus, thalamomamillary bundle, bundle of Vicq d'Azyr, tractus mamillothalamicus, tract of Vicq d'Azyr, mamillothalamic tract.* **f. medialis plexus brachialis** [NA] In the brachial plexus, a cord formed by the anterior division of the inferior trunk ($C_8$ and $T_1$). It gives rise to the medial pectoral, medial brachial, and medial antebrachial cutaneous nerves, and as terminal branches, the ulnar nerve and the medial root of the median nerve. Also *medial cord of brachial plexus.* **f. medialis telencephali** MEDIAL FOREBRAIN BUNDLE. **medial longitudinal f.** FASCICULUS LONGITUDINALIS MEDIALIS. **median triangular f.** FASCICULUS TRIANGULARIS. **Meynert's f.** FASCICULUS RETROFLEXUS. **Monakow's f.** TRACTUS RUBROSPINALIS. **f. obliquus crucis cerebri** A fiber bundle passing from the lateral part of the cerebral peduncle obliquely backward and medialward across the peduncle to enter the interpeduncular fossa at the pontine gray and tegmentum. **f. obliquus pontis** An indistinct bundle of fibers on the ventral pontine surface running obliquely lateral and caudal from the anteromedial portion of the pons. **f. occipitofrontalis inferior** The deep part of the fasciculus uncinatus, connecting the cortex of the frontal and occipital lobes. Also *inferior occipitofrontal bundle.* **f. occipitofrontalis superior** A bundle of association fibers connecting frontal and occipital gyri coursing within the fasciculus subcallosus. **occipitothalamic f.** *Seldom used* RADIATIO OPTICA. **oval f.** FASCICULUS SEPTOMARGINALIS. **f. pedunculomamillaris** An ascending axonal bundle arising in the midbrain dorsal and ventral tegmental nuclei that projects mainly upon the lateral mamillary nucleus, with some fibers ascending in the medial forebrain bundle. **perpendicular f.** A vertical bundle of cortical association fibers interconnecting regions of the temporal, parietal, and occipital lobes. **fasciculi pontis longitudinales** The numerous bundles of myelinated, principally descending fibers running in the rostrocaudal axis of the pons. Also *longitudinal fibers of pons.* **posterior longitudinal f.** FASCICULUS LONGITUDINALIS MEDIALIS. **posterior longitudinal f. of medulla oblongata** The portion of the fasciculus longitudinalis dorsalis within the medulla oblongata. **f. posterior plexus brachialis** [NA] The posterior nerve cord of the brachial plexus. It is formed by posterior divisions of the superior, middle, and inferior trunks of $C_5$ through $C_8$ or $T_1$, giving rise to the subscapular, thoracodorsal, axillary, and radial nerves. Also *posterior cord of brachial plexus.* **f. precommissuralis** Interhemispheric axons rostral to the anterior commissure of the cerebrum. **prerubral f.** STRIORUBRAL TRACT. **fasciculi proprii** Intersegmental ascending and descending axonal bundles of the spinal cord lying superficial to the gray matter of the anterior, lateral, and posterior funiculi. Also *Flechsig's fasciculi, ground bundles of Flechsig, proprius bundles of spinal cord, proper fasciculi of cord, basis bundles* (outmoded), *fundamental bundles* (obs.), *spinospinal tracts, lateral intersegmental tract.* **fasciculi pyramidales medullae oblongatae** FIBRAE PYRAMIDALES MEDULLAE OBLONGATAE. **f. pyramidalis anterior** TRACTUS CORTICOSPINALIS VENTRALIS. **f. pyramidalis lateralis** TRACTUS CORTICOSPINALIS LATERALIS. **f. retroflexus** [NA] A myelinated bundle of nerve fibers which have their neuronal cell bodies in the habenular nuclei of the epithalamus and which terminate in the ipsilateral interpeduncular nucleus of the mesencephalon. It is the largest efferent pathway from the habenula, and in its course it passes through the rostromedial part of the red nucleus. Also *tractus habenulointerpeduncularis, habenulointerpeduncular tract, Meynert's tract, Meynert's bundle, Meynert's fasciculus, habenulopeduncular tract* (incorrect), *fibers of Meynert.* **f. of Rolando** The elevated portion of the fasciculus cuneatus, overlying the bulge of the nucleus cuneatus in the medulla oblongata. Also *funiculus of Rolando.* **f. rotundus** *Seldom used* TRACTUS SOLITARIUS. **f. semilunaris** FASCICULUS INTERFASCICULARIS. **f. septomarginalis** [NA] The myelinated, descending axons in the lumbar dorsal column near the posterior septum that in the sacral cord form a superficial, median triangular zone, the fasciculus triangularis. Also *septomarginal fasciculus, oval bundle of Flechsig, oval area of Flechsig, septomarginal tract, tract of Bruce and Muir, Bruce's tract, Hoche's tract, oval fasciculus.* **solitary f.** TRACTUS SOLITARIUS. **f. subcallosus** A thin bundle of axons on the ventricular surface of the angle formed by the corpus callosum and the internal capsule. It is thought to contain fibers extending from the frontal motor cortex to the caudate nucleus, and cortical association fibers connecting the frontal, temporal, and occipital lobes. There is ambiguity about whether it includes the tapetum of the corpus callosum and the fasciculus occipitofrontalis superior. Also *subcallosal bundle, subcallosal fasciculus.* **f. sulcomarginalis** [NA] A lamina of descending dorsal root fibers running in the anteromedial funiculus of the spinal cord along the margin of the anterior fissure. Also *sulcomarginal fasciculus, sulcomarginal tract.* **superior longitudinal f. of cerebrum** FASCICULUS LONGITUDINALIS SUPERIOR CEREBRI. **f. teres** *Outmoded* FASCICULUS LONGITUDINALIS MEDIALIS PONTIS. **f. thalamicus** [NA] The myelinated bundle of axons entering the rostral portion of the thalamic ventral nuclear group dorsal to the zona incerta via the H field of Forel. These axons originate primarily in the globus pallidus and the dentate and red nuclei, course through the fasciculus lenticularis (field $H_2$), and terminate principally in the rostral nuclei of the ventral thalamic nuclear group. Also *field $H_1$ of Forel, thalamic fasciculus.* See also H FIELDS OF FOREL. **f. thalamomamillaris** FASCICULUS MAMILLOTHALAMICUS. **transverse fasciculi of palmar aponeurosis** FASCICULI TRANSVERSI APONEUROSIS PALMARIS. **transverse fasciculi of plantar aponeurosis** FASCICULI TRANSVERSI APONEUROSIS PLANTARIS. **fasciculi transversi aponeurosis palmaris** [NA] The transverse fibers on the deep aspect of the palmar aponeurosis that thicken to form strong ligamentous bands in the webs of the fingers, closing the gaps between the more superficial longitudinal bands to the fingers. Also *transverse fasciculi of palmar aponeurosis, transverse bundles of palmar aponeurosis.* **fasciculi transversi aponeurosis plantaris** [NA] Well-marked transverse bundles of fibers that close the gaps between the longitudinal digital bands of the plantar aponeurosis at the webs of the toes. Also *transverse fasciculi of plantar aponeurosis.* **f. triangularis** A group of descending fibers in the dorsal columns of the lumbosacral spinal cord that consists in large part of intersegmental connections. Also *median triangular fasciculus, triangular fasciculus, Gombault-Philippe triangle, tract of Philippe-Gombault, triangular tract of Philippe-Gombault, median root zone.* **f. of Türck** TRACTUS CORTICOSPINALIS VENTRALIS. **f. uncinatus** [NA] A bundle of frontotemporal association fibers extending between the orbitofrontal region to the uncus and parahippocampal gyrus. Also *uncinate fasciculus, unciform fasciculus, uncinate bundle.* **uncrossed pyramidal f.** TRACTUS CORTICOSPINALIS VENTRALIS. **f. ventrolateralis superficialis** TRACTUS SPINOCEREBELLARIS VENTRALIS. **f. of Vicq d'Azyr** FASCICULUS MAMILLOTHALAMICUS.

**fasciectomy** \fas′ē·ek′təmē\ [*fasci(a)* + -ECTOMY] Excision of a fascia, such as the fascia lata.

**fasciitis** \fas′ē·ī′tis\ [*fasci(a)* + -ITIS] Inflammation of a fascia. Also *fascitis, fibrofascitis.* **eosinophilic f.** Fasciitis of unknown cause, usually chronic, accompanied by marked increase in blood eosinophils. **necrotizing f.** A rapidly advancing soft-tissue infection that moves along fascial planes causing disruption of the fascial blood supply. It is usually caused by a synergistic infection of two bacterial species and can be fatal if not surgically treated. **nodular f.** A benign soft tissue growth typically developing rapidly in the upper extremities, trunk, or neck of young adults. It can be easily confused with a sarcoma because of its infiltrative margins and rapid growth in relation to a fascia. Microscopically, it consists of a reactive proliferation of myofibrasts in a loose, myxoid matrix. Also *pseudosarcomatous fibromatosis, subcutaneous pseudosarcomatous fibromatosis.* **perirenal f.** IDIOPATHIC RETROPERITONEAL FIBROSIS. **proliferative f.** A benign soft tissue growth very similar to nodular fasciitis, from which it can be differentiated by the presence of large, basophilic cells resembling rhabdomyoblasts, or ganglion cells. It tends to affect patients older than 45 and involves the skeletal muscles of the shoulder, thorax, and thigh. **pseudosarcomatous f.** A benign but rapidly progressive fibroblastic growth extending from superficial fascia into subcutaneous fat or muscle. High cellularity and mitotic activity simulate sarcoma.

***Fasciola*** \fəsē′ōlə\ [L (dim. of *fascia.* See FASCIA.) a little band] A genus of large digenetic flukes of the class Trematoda. They are parasitic in the liver of herbivorous animals and, infrequently, of humans. ***F. gigantica*** The giant liver fluke, a trematode found primarily in herbivores and occasionally in humans in Africa, Asia, Australasia, and Hawaii. It is similar in appearance to *F. hepatica* but larger and without an apical cone. Human infection is usually acquired by eating raw watercress contaminated by sheep feces. Adult flukes inhabit bile ducts which become distended and thick-walled. Sheep are more susceptible than cattle to the damaging effects of migration of flukes through the liver parenchyma. Severe anemia and death can occur. Praziquantel is the treatment of choice. ***F. hepatica*** The sheep liver fluke, a common trematode found in sheep, cattle, goats, horses, other animals including, though rarely, humans. Various species of snails of the genus *Lymnaea* serve as first intermediate hosts. The cercariae leave the snail, encyst on vegetation, and are ingested by the final host. In heavy infections extensive damage to the liver by migrating immature flukes causes severe hemorrhage, anemia, and even death. Adult flukes inhabit the bile ducts which become greatly thickened, fibrosed, and distended. ***F. heterophyes*** *HETEROPHYES HETEROPHYES*

**fasciola** \fəsē′ələ\ [See *FASCIOLA.*] A small strip or band of nerve fibers. **f. cinerea cinguli** GYRUS FASCIOLARIS. **f. dentata** GYRUS DENTATUS.

**fasciolae** \fəsē′əlē\ Plural of FASCIOLA.

**fasciolar** \fəsē′ələr\ **1** Denoting the gyrus fasciolaris. **2** Pertaining to a fasciola.

**fascioliasis** \fas′ē·əlī′əsis\ Infection with flukes of the genus *Fasciola,* especially *F. hepatica.*

**Fasciolidae** \fas′ē·äl′idē\ [*Fasciol(a)* + -IDAE] A family of large, leaf-shaped distomous digenetic flukes that are parasitic in mammals. It includes the genera *Fasciola, Fascioloides,* and *Fasciolopsis,* which can infect animals and humans.

**fasciolopsiasis** \fas′ē·ōläpsī′əsis\ Infection with flukes of the genus *Fasciolopsis.*

***Fasciolopsis*** \fas′ē·ōläp′sis\ [*Fasciol(a)* + -OPSIS] A genus of large flukes in the family Fasciolidae. Besides *F. buski,* it contains *F. fuelleborni,* which has been found in humans in India and Egypt, and *F. rathouisi,* found in humans in China. ***F. buski*** A species found in the small intestine of humans, pigs, and other mammals in eastern and southeastern Asia. In heavy infections, the flukes cause nausea, diarrhea, and malabsorption. Intermediate hosts include the snail genera *Planorbis* and *Segmentina,* which release cercariae that develop into the infective metacercariae on water chestnuts and other aquatic vegetation. Also *Distoma buski* (obs.).

**fasciorrhaphy** \fash′ē·ôr′əfē\ [*fasci(a)* + *o* + -RRHAPHY] An operation involving suturing of a fascia or of an aponeurosis. Also *aponeurorrhaphy.*

**fasciotomy** \fash′ē·ät′əmē\ [*fasci(a)* + *o* + -TOMY] Incision in the fascia that invests muscles, usually performed to release pressure on the invested muscles, nerves, and blood vessels, especially in the forearm or calf.

**fascitis** \fəsī′tis\ FASCIITIS.

**fast**[1] [Old English *fæst,* akin to German *fest* firm, fast] **1** Securely fastened; immobilized. **2** Resistant to dissolution or decolorization.

**fast**[2] **1** To abstain from food, usually for a set period or on a set schedule. **2** A period of abstention from food.

**fast-glycolytic** \-glī′kōlit′ik\ Denoting the fast-contracting, glycolysis-dependent, fatigue-susceptible type of motor unit or muscle fiber.

**fastidious** \fastid′ē·əs\ In microorganisms, having complex growth requirements.

**fastigial** \fastij′ē·əl\ Denoting the nucleus fastigii or fibers emanating from it.

**fastigiobulbar** \fastij′ē·əbul′bər\ Denoting nerve fibers from the cerebellar fastigial nucleus to the pons.

**fastigium** \fastij′ē·əm\ [L (from *fastus* elevation), roof, slope] The peak of the roof of the fourth ventricle of the brain, formed by the angle of union between the superior medullary velum and the nodulus cerebelli.

**fast-oxidative-glycolytic** \-äk′sidā′tiv-glī′kōlit′ik\ Denoting motor units or muscle fibers that are fast-contracting, fatigue-resistant, and capable of utilizing both oxidative and glycolytic pathways for the energy used in contraction.

**fat** [Old English *fætt* (noun, adj.)] Any of class of naturally occurring neutral organic compounds formed by ester bonds between three fatty acid molecules and one molecule of glycerol. They are insoluble in water, soluble in ether, and combustible. Fats are distinguished from oils in that fats are solid at 20°C and lower temperatures. Fats are rich in energy (9.3 kcal/g) and are stored in cells and tissues. **body f.** That portion of the body that consists of fat. It represents about 14% of the body weight of a man of ideal body composition and about 28% of a woman. However, the ratio of body fat to body weight varies widely among normal subjects. **bound f.** In a cell, a lipid component that is not demonstrable with conventional fat stains. Also *masked fat.* **brown f.** INTERSCAPULAR GLAND. **chyle f.** An emulsion of fat within the lymphatic system. **depot f.** Body stores of triglyceride fat. Usually found in limited areas, such as the abdominal wall, it constitutes the main energy reserve. **masked f.** BOUND FAT. **molecular f.** Intracellular fat within numerous minute vacuoles. **neutral f.** A fat composed entirely of triglyceride esters, containing no free fatty acids. **wool f.** LANOLIN. **yellow f.** The usual type of adipose tissue, as distinguished from the brown fat characteristic of the interscapular gland.

**fatal** \fā′təl\ [L *fatalis* (from *fatum* fate, a prophetic utterance, from *fari* to speak, utter) fatal, fateful] Causing death.

**fatality** \fātal′ətē\ **1** A death, especially one resulting from a specific disease, trauma, or other misfortune. **2** In medical statistics, the probability of an illness proving fatal, expressed as a percentage; fatality rate. **case f.** FATALITY RATE.

**fate** The ultimate state of development normally achieved by any embryonic cell or region of an early embryo. See also FATE MAP. **potential f.** Collectively, the possible fates of a cell or group of cells or of a part or even whole region of an embryo. The prospective fate is chosen from among the possible fates. Also *prospective potency.* **prospective f.** The development normally achieved by a part or region of an embryo, assuming no external interference is involved to modify the normal course of events. Also *prospective significance.*

**fatigability** \fat′əgəbil′itē\ The condition of being subject to fatigue; tendency to tire or become exhausted.

**fatigue** [French (from L *fatigare* to weary, tire), weariness] A state of weariness of mind and body following prolonged or excessive exertion or prolonged sensory stimulation. It results in loss of capacity to respond to stimulation. **auditory f.** Decreased response to a steady state tone or noise. The subject perceives the sound as diminishing in loudness. **flying f.** JET LAG. **industrial f.** Fatigue caused by prolonged or excessive work and exacerbated by monotony or by exposure to extreme conditions, as of heat and cold. It may lead to lowered output, mistakes, and accidents. **stance f.** A state of weariness or exhaustion produced by prolonged standing. **stimulation f.** A rise in the threshold of response to electrical stimulation in a nerve or nerve fiber as a result of prior repetitive stimulation.

**fatty** Composed of, resembling, or associated with fat: used particularly of chemical compounds whose molecules contain long chains of methylene groups. Thus fatty alcohols are long-chain alcohols, derivable by reduction of fatty acids.

**fatty acid** Any acid of formula $CH_3$—$[CH_2]_n$—COOH. Such acids occur in biologic material, particularly as esters in fats and phospholipids. **essential f.** Any of the interconvertible polyunsaturated fatty acids required in the diet and not made in mammals, such as linoleic acid. **free f.'s** Fatty acids that are not esterified, e.g. as fat or as phospholipid. Thus the albumin-bound fatty acid of the blood is included, since its binding to albumin is noncovalent. **nonesterified f.** A fatty acid in free form, in contrast with acyl groups in fats. It may, however, be noncovalently bound to a protein, as to serum albumin. **polyunsaturated f.'s** Monobasic aliphatic acids containing only carbon, hydrogen, and oxygen. They are made up of an alkyl radical attached to the carboxyl group and have more than one double bond. They fall into several groups: linoleic series with two double bonds between carbon atoms 9 and 10 and 12 and 13 (Δ 9 and 12) and general formula $C_nH2_n$—COOH, linolenic series with three double bonds (Δ 9, 12, and 15) and general formula $C_nH_{2n-5}$ COOH, fatty acids with four double bonds (Δ 5, 8, 11, and 14), such as arachidonic acid, and general formula $C_nH_{2n-7}$ COOH, and those with five double bonds such as clupanodonic acid. Good sources are certain vegetable oils such as peanut, cottonseed, corn, sunflower, and safflower. They have a blood cholesterol lowering effect but increase the requirement for vitamin E.

**fatty-acid synthase complex** The enzyme complex responsible for the biosynthesis of fatty acid from acetyl-CoA, malonyl-CoA, and NADPH. It has several active centers, on which condensation and reduction reactions occur.

**fauces** \fô′sēz\ [L, the gullet, pharynx, throat, a narrow passage, mouth] [NA] The narrowed space and surrounding structures between the oral cavity and the pharynx. It includes the isthmus and arches of the fauces, as well as the tonsillar fossa and the palatine tonsil. Also *throat.* Adj. faucial.

**fauna** \fô′nə\ [after Late L *Fauna* sister or wife of Faunus a nature god; adopted by Linnaeus as a parallel to Flora] The composite animal community of a given area, period, or habitat.

**fauntail** \fôn′tāl\ A tuft of long, fine hair in the lumbosacral region that usually overlies a defect, as that in diastematomyelia.
**Faust** [Ernest Carroll *Faust,* U.S. parasitologist, flourished 20th century] See under METHOD.
**faute de mieux** \fōt də myœ′\ [French, (for) lack of better] A situation in which a same-sex partner is acceptable because there is no opposite-sex partner. Such situations often occur in prisons or military installations.
**faveolar** \fāvē′ələr\ Pertaining or belonging to a faveolus.
**faveolate** \fāvē′əlāt\ [*faveol(us)* + -ATE] Having a pitted surface.
**faveoli** \fāvē′əlī\ Plural of FAVEOLUS.
**faveolus** \fāvē′ələs\ [New L, dim. of L *favus* honeycomb] **1** A small depression or pit. **2** ALVEOLUS.
**favic** \fā′vik\ Having the character of favus. • The term is usually applied to a fungal mycelium that grows in a branched pattern, such as *Trichophyton schoenleinii,* the cause of favus.
**favid** \fā′vid\ [*fav(us)* + -ID[2]] A dermatophytid reaction provoked by an infection (favus) due to *Trichophyton schoenleinii.* Also *favide.*
**favism** \fā′vizm\ Severe hemolytic anemia that follows ingestion of fava beans in some persons with glucose-6-phosphate dehydrogenase deficiency (Mediterranean variant). Also *Baghdad spring anemia* (seldom used), *fabism.*
**Favre** [Maurice Jules *Favre,* French physician, 1876–1954] **1** Favre-Racouchot syndrome. See under NODULAR ELASTOSIS OF THE SKIN. **2** Gamna-Favre bodies. See under MIYAGAWA BODIES.
**favus** \fā′vəs\ [L, honeycomb] A disease of the hair follicle which results in a cup-shaped crust (scutula). If the crust is removed, an oozing, red lesion will be exposed. In most instances the agent of this disease is *Trichophyton schoenleinii..* Also *St. Aignon's disease.* **f. circinatus** An oozing crusty type of ringworm in which the lesion is considerably larger and generally circular.
**faxen-psychosis** \fak′sən-\ [German *Faxen* buffoonery + PSYCHOSIS] BUFFOONERY PSYCHOSIS.
**Fazio** [E. *Fazio,* Italian physician, 1849–1902] **1** Fazio-Londe atrophy. See under ATROPHY. **2** Fazio-Londe syndrome, Fazio-Londe disease. See under INFANTILE PROGRESSIVE BULBAR PALSY.
**Fc** See under FC FRAGMENT.
**FCA** Freund's complete adjuvant.
**F-Cortef** A proprietary name for fludrocortisone
**FD** **1** focal distance. **2** fatal dose (lethal dose).
**Fd** See under FD FRAGMENT.
**FDA** Food and Drug Administration.
**FD & C** Federal Food, Drug and Cosmetic: used to designate approved food colorings, such as coal-tar colors.
**FDNB** fluoro-2,4-dinitrobenzene.
**F-duction** \-duk′shən\ A gene transfer from a donor bacterium to a recipient in which a piece of donor DNA is incorporated into the F plasmid and is transferred by conjugation. The modified plasmid is called F′ (F-prime). Also *sexduction.*
**Fe** Symbol for the element, iron.
**fear** [Old English *fær* peril, sudden attack, akin to German *(Ge)fahr* danger] A strong, primitive emotional reaction to a specific danger that exists or is perceived, characterized subjectively by feelings of unpleasantness and agitation, and behaviorally by postures and movements to bring about escape or concealment. Fear responses are dependent on the action of diencephalic centers in the brain, and are accompanied by widespread physiologic changes in the body mediated by the sympathetic nervous system, such as sweating or a rapid heartbeat.
**Feather** [Norman *Feather,* English physicist, born 1904] See under ANALYSIS.
**feature** Any characteristic element, as of a structure, condition, or appearance.
**feb. dur.** *febre durante* (L, while the fever lasts).
**febricide** \feb′risīd\ ANTIPYRETIC.
**febricity** \febris′itē\ The condition of having a fever.
**febrifacient** \feb′rifā′shənt\ **1** Fever-producing. **2** A febrifacient agent.
**febrifugal** \febrif′yəgəl\ ANTIPYRETIC.
**febrifuge** \feb′rifyooj\ ANTIPYRETIC.
**febrile** \feb′rəl, fē′brəl, feb′rīl\ [Med L *febril(is)* (from L *febris* fever) pertaining to fever] Of or characterized by fever. Also *pyretic, pyrexial.*
**febris** \fē′bris\ [L (popularly but prob. erroneously supposed to be akin to L *fervere* to boil, be boiling hot) a fever] Fever. **f. entericoides** PARENTERIC FEVER. **f. melitensis** MALTA FEVER. **f. recurrens** RELAPSING FEVER. **f. rubra** SCARLET FEVER. **f. undulans** UNDULANT FEVER. See under BRUCELLOSIS.
**fecal** \fē′kəl\ Of or relating to feces.
**fecalith** \fē′kəlith\ A solid mass of fecal material found in the colon or identified as a radiopaque object on an abdominal radiograph; a fecal calculus. Also *coprolith, stercolith.*
**fecaloid** \fē′kəloid\ Bearing a resemblance to feces.
**fecaloma** \fē′kəlō′mə\ [FECAL + -OMA] STERCOROMA.
**fecaluria** \fē′kəloo′rē·ə\ [FECAL + -URIA] The presence of feces in the urine, associated with a fistula between the colon or rectum and the bladder.
**feces** \fē′sēz\ [L *faeces,* pl. of *faex* dregs, lees] The excreta expelled from the anus, consisting of undigested material, bacteria, mucosal cells, and mucus.
**Fechner** [Gustav Theodor *Fechner,* German psychologist, 1801–1887] **1** See under FRACTION, LAW. **2** Weber-Fechner law. See under LAW.
**fecundate** \fē′kəndāt\ [L *fecundat(us),* past part. of *fecundare* (from *fecundus* fruitful, fertile) to fertilize, make fruitful] To fertilize; to make fertile.
**fecundation** \fē′kəndā′shən\ [L *fecundatus,* past part. of *fecundare* (akin to *fetus*) to make fertile or fruitful] FERTILIZATION. **artificial f.** ARTIFICIAL INSEMINATION.
**fecundity** \fēkun′ditē\ [L *fecunditas* (from *fecundus* fruitful, fertile) fruitfulness, fertility] In demography, the ability to conceive; reproductive potential as distinguished from reproductive performance (fertility).
**Fede** [Francesco *Fede,* Italian physician, 1832–1913] Fede's disease, Riga-Fede disease. See under FRENAL ULCER.
**Federici** [Cesare *Federici,* Italian physician, 1832–1892] See under SIGN.
**fee / f. for service** A method of charging or paying for health care services whereby the provider bills or is reimbursed a defined amount for each service.
**feeblemindedness** *Older term* MENTAL RETARDATION.
**feedback** In a system, the return of a fraction of the output to the input for use in regulation. **alpha f.** A type of relaxation training in which the subject receives information about his electroencephalogram and learns under what conditions alpha waves, characteristic of relaxed and peaceful wakefulness, are produced. **delayed auditory f.** Interference with a subject's hearing of his own speech, typically by using special headphones that impose a delay of 200 to 300 milliseconds on the transmission of the sound. In the ordinary person such a delay produces marked distortion in speech, while in some schizophrenic patients the delay has

remarkably little effect on speech patterns. Abbr. DAF **negative f.** A process in which the output of a system acts upon the input to decrease its action. For example, increased circulating hormone causes decreased hormone production. **positive f.** A process in which the output of a system acts upon the input to reinforce its action. For example, placing a microphone near a loudspeaker reinforces the undesirable sustained oscillations in a public-address system.

**feeding** The process of taking or giving food. **artificial f.** The feeding of an infant by any means other than suckling at the breast. **breast f.** The nourishment of an infant by the act of suckling; the obtaining of breast milk by sucking at the mother's breast. The infant controls its own intake which reduces the possibility of overfeeding. The composition of the milk is normally such as to satisfy completely the infant's nutrient needs. **demand f.** Giving nourishment to a child when he signals he is hungry, typically by crying, rather than feeding according to a rigidly imposed schedule. **drip f.** INTRAVENOUS FEEDING. **intravenous f.** The intravenous administration of five or ten percent glucose solutions with electrolytes and vitamins. Because of the inability to provide sufficient calories to meet the needs of undernourished or hypermetabolic patients and to provide the patient with adequate amino acids, it can only be used for a short period. Long-term intravenous feeding requires total parenteral feeding or hyperalimentation which provides the patient with all the essential nutrients. Also *drip feeding, drip treatment.* **nasal f.** The taking in of food through a tube inserted into the stomach via the nose. **sham f.** 1 An experimental procedure in which food is chewed and swallowed but is then diverted to the exterior by way of an esophageal fistula in order to prevent it from entering the stomach. 2 An experiment in which food is chewed but is expectorated rather than swallowed. **tube f.** The supplying of nutrients through a tube placed in the stomach by way of the nostril, pharynx, and esophagus or through a tube inserted into the stomach or jejunum at operation. Gastrostomy and jejunostomy feedings are only used when it is not possible to pass an intragastric tube or when there is gross disease of the stomach, respectively. Feeds are usually presented every four hours in a volume of 250 ml followed by 50 ml of water to rinse the tube. Distasteful medicines may also be administered through a tube.

**feeling** 1 Any conscious state containing some elements not obviously referable to the immediate environment. 2 The subjective aspect of affective or emotional experience; an awareness of one's mood or of a particular emotional reaction. **f.'s of estrangement** A sense of being apart from people and outer reality because external objects seem unfamiliar or unreal. Feelings of estrangement are frequent in dissociative states and certain types of schizophrenia and affective disorders. Such feelings may take the form of nihilistic delusions. Also *feelings of unreality.*

**Feer** [Walther Emil *Feer,* Swiss pediatrician, 1864–1955] Swift-Feer disease. See under PINK DISEASE.

**feet** Plural of FOOT.

**Fegeler** [Ferdinand *Fegeler,* German dermatologist, flourished 20th century] See under SYNDROME.

**Fehleisen** [Friedrich *Fehleisen,* German-born U.S. physician, 1854–1924] Fehleisen streptococcus. See under *STREPTOCOCCUS PYOGENES.*

**Fehling** [Hermann Christian von *Fehling,* German chemist, 1812–1885] Fehling's test. See under FEHLING SOLUTION.

**Feichtiger** [H. *Feichtiger,* German physician, flourished mid-20th century] Ullrich-Feichtiger syndrome. See under SYNDROME.

**Feil** [Andre *Feil,* French physician, born 1884] **1** Klippel-Feil sign. See under SIGN. **2** Klippel-Feil syndrome. See under SYNDROME. **3** Klippel-Feil malformation. See under MALFORMATION.

**Feiss** [Henry O. *Feiss,* U.S. orthopedic surgeon, flourished 20th century] See under LINE.

**fel** \fel\ BILE.

**Feldberg** [Wilhelm Siegmund *Feldberg,* German-born British physiologist, born 1900] Dale-Feldberg law. See under LAW.

**Feldman** [Harry Alfred *Feldman,* U.S. epidemiologist, born 1914] Sabin-Feldman dye test. See under TEST.

**Felix** [Arthur *Felix,* Czech bacteriologist, 1887–1956] **1** Felix-Weil reaction, Weil-Felix reaction. See under WEIL-FELIX TEST. **2** See under VACCINE.

**Felix** [Jules *Felix,* French physician, 1838–1912] Felix Vi serum. See under SERUM.

**fellatio** \fəlā′shō, fəlā′shē·ō\ [New L, from L *fellare* to suck] Oral stimulation of the penis.

**felon** \fel′ən\ [Old French (prob. from L *fel* bile, bitterness, perh. assimilated to Old French *fel, felon* traitorous, treacherous) an ulcer, abscess] A suppurating abscess or infection of the distal phalanx of the finger. **bone f.** A felon involving subperiosteal bone and causing necrosis. **deep f.** A felon located deep within a structure such as the bone cortex or subcutaneous tissue. **subcutaneous f.** A felon that involves tissues below the skin surface. **subcuticular f.** A felon that arises between the dermis and the epidermis. Also *subepithelial felon, superficial felon.* **subperiosteal f.** A felon involving the periosteum. **thecal f.** A felon involving a synovial sheath. Also *thecal whitlow.*

**felony** \fel′ənē\ [See FELON.] A very serious crime defined by legal statute and most commonly punished by imprisonment in a penitentiary. Adj. felonious.

**feltwork** Any layer of densely interwoven nerve fibers. **Kaes f.** BEKHTEREV'S LAYER.

**Felty** [Augustus Roi *Felty,* U.S. physician, born 1895] See under SYNDROME.

**female** [Middle English, altered by the influence of *male* from Old French *femelle* female, from L *femella,* dim. of *femina* a female, woman] **1** Of or pertaining to the sex that in animals produces ova and brings forth young. **2** An individual of the female sex, as a woman. **genetic f.** **1** A human possessing a normal female karyotype, 46,XX. **2** In any species, an individual possessing the karyotype that is usually present in the female. **3** A female pseudohermaphrodite in which the karyotype is 46,XX. The gonads are ovaries, a uterus is present, and the external genitalia are virilized or ambiguous. *Outmoded.*

**feminine** [Old French *feminin* feminine, from L *femininus* female, from *femin(a)* a woman] Of or relating to the female sex; having the qualities characteristic of women.

**femininity** \fem′ənin′itē\ The state of being feminine; possession of the normal characteristics of women.

**feminism** \fem′ənizm\ *Older term* FEMINIZATION. **mammary f.** *Seldom used* GYNECOMASTIA.

**feminization** \fem′ənīzā′shən\ **1** The development in the male of secondary sex characters of a female, as regression of masculine body hair and assumption of feminine body contour. Also *effemination, eviration, feminism* (older term). **2** Normal development of secondary sex characters in the female. **testicular f.** A condition that prevents both embryologic and postnatal androgen-dependent development. It is due to a defective or absent cellular androgen receptor, the genetic locus for which is on the X chromosome. The phenotype in the affected hemizygote includes the absence of the ovaries, uterus, and tubes; inguinal or abdominal testes; a vagina and female external genitalia; female habitus and breast development; the absence of virilization; and a 46,XY karyotype. A similar phenotype occurs in numerous forms of male pseudohermaphroditism, including incomplete testicular feminization in which clitoromegaly at birth and mild virilization at puberty occur. Also *testicular feminization syndrome, Morris syndrome* (seldom used), *androgen insensitivity syndrome*.

**feminize** \fem′ənīz\ 1 To induce the development of female secondary sex characters in the female. 2 To promote the development of female secondary sex characters in the male.

**femora** \fem′ərə\ Plural of FEMUR.

**femoral** \fem′ərəl\ Pertaining or belonging to the femur or the thigh.

**femorocele** \fem′ərəsēl′\ [*femor(al)* + *o* + -CELE[1]] FEMORAL HERNIA.

**femto-** \fem′tō-\ [Danish *femten* fifteen] A combining form denoting $10^{-15}$: used with SI units. Symbol: f

**femur** \fē′mər\ [L, the thigh] (*pl.* femora) 1 [NA] The long bone of the thigh, extending from the hip joint to the knee joint; the proximal bone in the hindlimb of vertebrates. Also *thigh bone, femoral bone.* 2 [NA] The thigh; regio femoralis.

**fenbencillin** PHENBENICILLIN.

**fenestra** \fənes′trə\ [L a window] (*pl.* fenestrae) 1 In anatomy, an opening between two chambers or spaces, usually in the wall between them; a window. 2 Any opening resembling a window, as in some plaster casts, surgical drapes, or surgical instruments. **f. choledocha** The opening into the duodenum made by the common bile duct and the pancreatic duct. **f. cochleae** [NA] A small, rounded, recessed opening in the medial wall of the tympanic cavity, located behind and below the fenestra vestibuli, under cover of the projecting edge of the promontory and communicating with scala tympani of the cochlea from which it is separated by the secondary tympanic membrane. Also *fenestra of cochlea, round window, fenestra rotunda* (outmoded), *cochlear window, porta labyrinthi* (outmoded). **f. ovalis** *Outmoded* FENESTRA VESTIBULI. **f. rotunda** *Outmoded* FENESTRA COCHLEAE. **f. vestibuli** [NA] A small oval opening located posterosuperior to the promontory on the medial wall of the tympanic cavity and communicating with the vestibule of the internal ear. It has the base of the stapes covering it and fixed by the annular ligament to its margin. Also *oval window, fenestra ovalis* (outmoded), *vestibular window.*

**fenestrae** \fines′trē\ Plural of FENESTRA.

**fenestrate** \fen′əstrāt\ To create one or more openings in (tissue).

**fenestrated** \fen′əstrā′tid\ Perforated by one or more openings, as tissue.

**fenestration** \fen′əstrā′shən\ [*fenestr(a)* + -ATION] 1 FENESTRATION OPERATION. 2 The establishment of a fistulous opening (fenestra) usually to bypass some obstruction. **f. of alveolar process** A circumscribed opening in the alveolar bone over the root of a tooth. If the opening is not circumscribed it is called a dehiscence. **aortopulmonary f.** AORTICOPULMONARY WINDOW.

**fenoprofen calcium** $C_{30}H_{26}CaO_6 \cdot 2H_2O$. $\alpha$-Methyl-3-phenoxybenzeneacetic acid calcium dihydrate. It is used as an analgesic and anti-inflammatory agent.

**fentanyl** $C_{22}H_{28}N_2O$. *N*-Phenyl-*N*-[1-(2-phenylethyl)-4-piperidinyl]propanamide, a narcotic analgesic with actions that resemble those of morphine. It is used therapeutically for the same purposes as morphine and has the same addicting potential. It is given intravenously or intramuscularly.

**fentanyl citrate** $C_{28}H_{36}N_2O_8$. *N*-Phenyl-*N*-[1-(2-phenylethyl)-4-piperidinyl]-propanamide citrate, a potent analgesic that is related to the synthetic phenylpiperidine derivatives. Its effects are like those of morphine, but its duration of action is shorter than meperidine or morphine. It is administered parenterally, and chronic use can lead to addiction.

**Fenwick** [Edwin Hurry *Fenwick*, English physician, 1856–1944] Fenwick-Hunner ulcer. See under HUNNER'S ULCER.

**Fenwick** [Samuel *Fenwick*, English physician, 1821–1902] Fenwick's disease. See under ATROPHIC GASTRITIS.

**-fer** \-fər\ [L *ferre* to bear] A combining form meaning one that bears.

**fer-de-lance** \fer′dəlänˢ′, -lans′\ [French, spearhead] The venomous snake *Bothrops atrox*.

**Féréol** [Louis Henri Felix *Féréol*, French physician, 1825–1891] Féréol's nodes. See under RHEUMATIC NODULES.

**Ferguson-Smith** [John *Ferguson-Smith*, English dermatologist, flourished 20th century] Ferguson-Smith type epithelioma. See under SELF-HEALING SQUAMOUS EPITHELIOMA.

**Fergusson** [Sir William *Fergusson*, Scottish surgeon, 1808–1877] Fergusson's incision. See under WEBER-FERGUSSON INCISION.

**ferment** \fur′mənt\ [French (from L *fermentum* for *fervimentum* leaven, yeast, from *fervere* to be boiling hot, ferment) agent causing fermentation] 1 *Obs.* ENZYME. 2 To undergo or bring about fermentation. **fibrin f.** *Obs.* THROMBIN. **glycolytic f.** Any enzyme involved in the digestion of glucose or other simple sugars.

**fermentation** \fur′məntā′shən\ [FERMENT + -ATION] The anaerobic catabolism of organic substances by organisms, usually microorganisms. In contrast to respiration, the final electron acceptors for the oxidation of organic substrates are also organic. Reduced end-products thus accumulate. Also *zymosis, zymolysis, zymohydrolysis.* **acetone-butanol f.** *n*-BUTANOL FERMENTATION. **alcoholic f.** The breakdown of sugars to ethanol and carbon dioxide as performed by yeast. **amino acid f.** Any of a variety of fermentations, prominent in putrefaction and in cheese manufacture, that oxidize one amino acid and reduce another. **butanediol f.** A fermentation that yields, via the glycolytic pathway, the nonacidic products butanediol and its oxidation product, acetoin. It is characteristic of *Enterobacter* species and is used to differentiate this genus from coliforms. Also *butylene glycol fermentation.* ***n*-butanol f.** A bacterial fermentation (e.g., in clostridia and bacteroides) that yields principally *n*-butyric acid, acetone, and *n*-butanol ($CH_3CH_2CH_2CH_2OH$), via head-to-tail condensation of two acetyl groups. Also *butyric fermentation, acetone-butanol fermentation.* **butylene glycol f.** BUTANEDIOL FERMENTATION. **butyric f.** *n*-BUTANOL FERMENTATION. **formic f.** MIXED ACID FERMENTATION. **heterolactic f.** A fermentation in which C atoms 4,5,6 of hexose are converted to lactic acid and atoms 1,2,3 to carbon dioxide and acetic acid (or alcohol). **mixed acid f.** A fermentation, characteristic of *Escherichia coli* and many other Enterobacteriaceae, that yields primarily acetic acid and formic acid which is often converted to $H_2$ and $CO_2$. In this fermentation, the acetic acid is formed via acetyl CoA, which can generate ATP, thus yielding more energy per mole of sugar than the lactic or the ethanolic fermentation. Also *formic fermentation.* **propionic f.** The process of breakdown of sugars by bacteria, especially *Propionibacterium*, in which propionic acid is produced, together with some acetic acid and either succinic acid or carbon dioxide. In Swiss cheese, these organisms use the lactic acid formed by other organisms as carbon source, converting it to propionic and acetic acids with the liberation of carbon dioxide. The propionic acid contributes to the flavor while the carbon dioxide is responsible for the holes in the cheese. **stormy milk f.** Fermentation that involves clotting with entrapment of gas bubbles in a milk-containing medium. It is characteristic of the clostridia of gas gangrene.

**Fermi** [Claudio *Fermi,* Italian physician, born 1862] See under VACCINE.

**Fermi** [Enrico *Fermi,* Italian-born U.S. physicist, 1901–1954] Fermi-Dirac statistics. See under STATISTICS.

**fermium** \fur′mē·əm\ A synthetic radioactive element of the actinide series, having atomic number 100. Fermium 257, discovered in 1954, is produced by neutron bombardment of plutonium. Ten isotopes are known. Fermium 257 has the longest half-life, 80 days. Symbol: Fm

**ferning** \fur′ning\ CERVICAL MUCUS ARBORIZATION.

**-ferous** \-fərəs\ [L *ferre* to bear] A combining form meaning bearing, producing.

**Ferrata** [Adolfo *Ferrata,* Italian physician, 1880–1946] Ferrata cell. See under HEMOHISTIOBLAST.

**ferrate** An anion with irons as the central atom, such as hexacyanoferrate(III), i.e. $Fe(CN)_6^{3-}$.

**Ferraton** [Louis *Ferraton,* French surgeon, born 1860] Perrin-Ferraton disease. See under SNAPPING HIP.

**ferredoxin** Any of a class of iron-sulfur compounds found in photosynthetic and anaerobic bacteria and photosynthetic plants, where they serve as electron carriers with very low redox potentials.

**Ferrein** [Antoine *Ferrein,* French surgeon and anatomist, 1693–1769] **1** Ferrein's cord. See under PLICA VOCALIS. **2** Ferrein's ligament. See under LIGAMENTUM LATERALE ARTICULATIONIS TEMPOROMANDIBULARIS. **3** Ferrein's canal. See under RIVUS LACRIMALIS. **4** Ferrein's tubules. See under TUBULE. **5** Pyramid of Ferrein. See under PARS RADIATA LOBULI CORTICALIS RENIS. **6** Ferrein's vasa aberrantia. See under VAS. **7** See under FORAMEN.

**ferri-** \fer′ē-\ [L *ferrum* iron] A combining form denoting iron, especially iron(III).

**ferric** \fer′ik\ [L *ferr(um)* iron + -IC] Denoting compounds containing iron in the Fe(III) state.

**ferric ammonium citrate** IRON AND AMMONIUM CITRATE.

**ferric ammonium sulfate** IRON AND AMMONIUM SULFATE.

**ferric citrate** A mixture of ferric iron and citric acid in an indefinitely defined composition. It is in the form of solid red transparent scales or a brown powder which is soluble in water. It is used as a source of iron to treat iron-deficiency anemia. Also *iron citrate.*

**ferric glycerophosphate** $C_9H_{21}Fe_2O_{18}P_3$. Solid orange-to-yellow transparent scales or powder which are soluble in water. It is used as a hematinic agent. Also *iron glycerophosphate.*

**ferric hydroxide with magnesium oxide** $Fe_2O_3{\cdot}3H_2O$. Ferric hydroxide, mixed with a suspension of magnesium oxide. It has been alleged to be an antidote for arsenic poisoning.

**ferric hypophosphite** $FeH_6O_6P_3$. A white or gray-white powder which is soluble in water. It has been used as a hematinic agent. Also *iron hypophosphite.*

**ferric pyrophosphate** $Fe_4O_{21}P_6$. A bioavailable form of iron that is used as a hematinic.

**ferric sodium edetate** Ferric monosodium ethylenediaminetetracetate, a chelated preparation of iron(III) used in the treatment of iron deficiency anemia.

**ferricyanide** The ion $Fe(CN)_6^{3-}$, and salts that contain it. It is a mild oxidizing agent, and is systematically and increasingly called hexacyanoferrate(III).

**ferriheme** HEME.

**ferrihemochrome** Any respiratory pigment containing iron(III).

**ferrihemoglobin** METHEMOGLOBIN.

**ferriporphyrin** Any porphyrin containing iron(III).

**ferriprotoporphyrin** Any protoporphyrin containing iron(III).

**Ferris Smith** [*Ferris Smith,* U.S. otolaryngologist, born 1884] Ferris Smith technique. See under MULTIPLE PARTIAL EXCISIONS.

**ferritin** A protein constituting a storage form of iron in liver and other tissues. It consists of an outer shell of 24 molecules of a protein of mass 18.5 kDa, surrounding a crystalline region of iron(III), largely as its hydroxide, which may be filled to a variable extent. When completely filled, the ferritin contains 23% iron. This gives it high electron density, a property used in the technique of ferritin labeling.

**ferro-** \fer′ō-\ [L *ferrum* iron] A combining form denoting iron, especially iron(II).

**ferrochelatase** The enzyme (EC 4.99.1.1) responsible for heme synthesis by catalyzing the reaction of protoporphyrin with iron(II) to yield heme with displacement of two hydrogen ions. This is a step in the biosynthesis of hemoglobin. Also *heme synthetase.*

**ferrocholinate** $C_{11}H_{24}FeNO_{11}$. A mixture of equal molar concentrations of choline dihydrogen citrate and ferric hydroxide or ferrous carbonate. It is used as a hematinic agent. Also *iron choline citrate.*

**ferrocyanide** The ion $Fe(CN)_6^{4-}$, and salts that contain it. It is a mild reducing agent, and is systematically and increasingly called hexacyanoferrate(II).

**ferroelectric** \fer′ō·ilek′trik\ Denoting crystalline materials in which an external electric field can create a permanent electric polarization, much as an external magnetic field creates a permanent magnet.

**ferrography** \feräg′rəfē\ [FERRO- + -GRAPHY] A method of treating a sample of synovial fluid with a solution rich in magnetic ions and exposing it to a magnetic field which sorts out breakdown products by size and structure.

**ferrokinetics** \fer′ōkinet′iks\ The changes undergone by elemental iron in the body in the course of its absorption, distribution, metabolism, and excretion.

**ferrotherapy** Treatment with iron or iron compounds.

**ferrous** \fer′əs\ [L *ferr(um)* iron + -OUS] Denoting compounds containing iron, particularly in the Fe(II) state.

**ferrous fumarate** $C_4H_2FeO_4$. A bioavailable powder of iron used as a hematinic agent. It is prepared by mixing ferrous sulfate and sodium fumarate.

**ferrous gluconate** $C_{12}H_{22}FeO_{14}$. A bioavailable form of iron that is used as a hematinic and as a food coloring and flavoring agent. Also *iron gluconate.*

**ferrous iodide** $FeI_2{\cdot}5H_2O$. A deliquescent compound of iron used in tonic syrups. Also *iron iodide.*

**ferrous lactate** $(CH_3CHOHCOO)_2Fe{\cdot}3H_2O$. A compound of iron used in the treatment of iron deficiency anemia. Also *iron lactate.*

**ferrous sulfate** $FeSO_4{\cdot}7H_2O$. Bluish green crystals or granules that are a very commonly used form of iron in medical tonics and for the treatment of iron deficiency anemia. Also *copperas, green vitriol, iron protosulfate, iron sulfate.*

**ferruginous** \feroo′jənəs\ Containing iron.

**Ferry** [Erwin Sidney *Ferry,* U.S. physicist, 1868–1956] Ferry-Porter law. See under LAW.

**fertility** [L *fertilitas* (from *fertilis* fruitful, fertile, from *ferre* to bear) fruitfulness] **1** The condition of being fertile; capacity to conceive and bear offspring. Also *uberty* (seldom used). **2** In demography, reproductive performance as distinguished from reproductive capacity or fecundity. **3** The influence of births on population change. **effective f.** REPRODUCTION PROBABILITY.

**fertilization** [L *fertilis* fruitful, fertile + -IZE + -ATION] The process of union of a sperm and an ovum in order to form a zygote in either animals or plants. In man, fertilization takes place usually in the outer third of the uterine tube shortly after ovulation. One spermatozoon penetrates the zona pellucida of the ovum and then enters the ovum itself to form the male pronucleus. This soon joins the female pronucleus of the ovum to provide the nucleus of the zygote with the diploid number of chromosomes. The process of fertilization is the normal means of stimulation of development of a single-celled ovum into an individual of a particular species. See also PARTHENOGENESIS. **cross f.** The fertilization of a gamete of one organism by a gamete from another organism, as distinguished from self-fertilization.

**fertilizin** \fur′təlīzin\ A substance associated with the plasma membrane of the ovum of some species, which is capable of agglutinating and binding spermatozoa of the same species to the ovum. In the sea urchin, it has been characterized as a glycoprotein with a molecular weight in the region of 300 000.

**ferv.** *fervens* (L, boiling).

**fester** \fes′tər\ [Middle English *fester, festre,* from Middle French *festre* sore, from L *fistula* a pipe, reed, ulcer] **1** A suppurating ulcer. **2** To become inflamed and suppurate superficially.

**festination** \fes′tinā′shən\ [L *festinatio* (from *festinare* to hurry) a hurrying] FESTINATING GAIT. Adj. festinant.

**festoon** \festoon′\ [French *feston* (from Italian *festone* festoon, from *festa* a holyday feast, from Vulgar L *festa* feast) a garland] **1** One of the segments found on the posterior submarginal border of the dorsum of certain hard ticks, consisting of rectangular divisions separated by grooves in the edge of the dorsum. **2** GINGIVAL FESTOON. **gingival f.** **1** The curved shape of the gingival margin. **2** A simulation of this in a prosthesis. **3** A thickening and rounding of the gingival margin caused by inflammation. Also *festoon.*

**fetal** \fē′təl\ [*fet(us)* + -AL] Of or relating to a fetus. For humans, the fetal stage of intrauterine development extends from the ninth week of pregnancy until term.

**fetalism** \fē′təlizm\ Persistence of a fetal character into postnatal life, as may occur in the vascular system.

**fetation** [*fet(us)* + -ATION] Fetal growth and development taking place inside the uterus.

**feti-** \fē′tē-\ FETO-.

**feticide** \fē′tisīd\ [FETI- + -CIDE] The killing or destruction of a fetus, usually by artificial means.

**fetish** \fet′ish\ [French *fétiche* (from Portuguese *feitiço* a charm, from L *facticius,* artificial) an object venerated as an idol] A body part or material thing, associated with the love object, whose presence is necessary for the subject's sexual excitement. The fetish may totally replace the need for the love object itself.

**fetishism** \fet′ishizm\ A paraphilia consisting of the preferred or obligatory use of an object (fetish) in order to achieve sexual excitement.

**feto-** \fē′tō-\ [L *fetus.* See FETUS.] A combining form meaning fetus, fetal. Also *feti-, foeti-, foeto-.*

**fetoamniotic** \fē′tō·am′nē·ät′ik\ Relating to both the fetus and the amnion.

**fetoglobulin** \fē′tōgläb′yəlin\ FETOPROTEIN.

**fetologist** \fētäl′əjist\ A specialist in fetology.

**fetology** \fētäl′əjē\ [FETO- + -LOGY] The scientific study of the fetus. • The study of the fetus is often considered to be part of embryology, but *fetology* is still used when a distinction is necessary between study of the embryo and study of the fetus.

**fetomaternal** \fē′tōmətur′nəl\ Pertaining to the relationship between the fetus and the mother.

**fetometry** \fētäm′ətrē\ [FETO- + -METRY] Measurement of the fetus. The term usually applies to skull diameters. **roentgen f.** The measurement of fetal head size by roentgenographic methods.

**fetopathy** \fētäp′əthē\ [FETO- + -PATHY] Any morbid state or condition in a fetus *in utero,* or, by extension, in a newborn infant. It may be of developmental, infectious, inflammatory, or traumatic origin.

**fetoplacental** \fē′tōplasen′təl\ Pertaining to the relationship between the fetus and placenta.

**fetoprotein** \fē′tōprō′tēn\ One of a number of proteins found in fetal blood. $\alpha$-fetoprotein is the fetal equivalent of albumin. It is produced in adults by hepatomas and certain teratomas for which its presence is a marker. $\alpha$-fetoprotein is immunosuppressive and may play some part in the immunosuppression associated with tumors that secrete it. $\beta$- and $\gamma$-fetoproteins are associated with various neoplasms in the adult. Also *fetoglobulin.*

**fetor** \fē′tər\ [L *foetor* foul smell, stench] A strong, offensive smell or stench. **f. ex ore** *Rare* FETOR ORIS. **f. hepaticus** A unique sweet, musty smell of the breath which may occur in patients with severe hepatocellular disease. Its exact cause it not known. Also *liver breath.* **f. oris** Foul breath. The cause may be apparent, such as disease within the mouth (dental caries, severe ulcerative stomatitis, ulceromembranous pharyngitis etc.) or the nose (ozena, malignant disease etc.) but frequently defies diagnosis. Also *halitosis, fetor ex ore* (rare).

**fetoscope** \fē′təskōp\ [FETO- + -SCOPE] **1** An instrument utilized to detect and measure the fetal heartbeat. **2** An instrument utilized to visualize a fetus through transabdominal insertion of the device into the amniotic cavity.

**fetoscopy** \fētäs′kəpē\ [FETO- + -SCOPY] The direct visualization of a fetus using a fetoscope.

**fetotoxic** \fē′tōtäk′sik\ [FETO- + TOXIC] **1** Characteristic of an agent that is toxic to the fetus; that is, to the conceptus after completion of organogenesis. **2** Descriptive of toxic effects on the conceptus at any time during intrauterine life. These effects are not limited to lethality but also may include malformation and intrauterine growth retardation. Compare EMBRYOTOXIC.

**fetus** \fē′təs\ [L (from the adj. *fetus,* fem. *feta* pregnant, akin to *fecundus* fertile) parturition, offspring, unborn offspring] The unborn child or offspring while still in the uterus during the later part of gestation and after the time of appearance of the major systems and parts during the embryonic period. A fetus displays the beginnings of adult features of the species and the fetal period is principally one of growth. A human embryo becomes a fetus at about the end of the eighth week after fertilization. **f. acardius** A fetus or newborn infant lacking a heart. **calcified f.** LITHOPEDION. **f. compressus** FETUS PAPYRACEUS. **harlequin f.** A fetus or newborn, often premature, infant with the most severe form of ichthyosis vulgaris. The keratin layer of the skin is so thickened as to interfere with vital functions. The multidirectional cracks in the skin produce a harlequin pattern of diamond-shaped, grayish brown plaques. In addition, the face, hands, and feet may be malformed. The condition is transmitted as a recessive trait and is incompatible with survival for more than a few hours or days. **mummified f.** LITHOPEDION. **paper-doll f.** FETUS PAPYRACEUS. **papyraceous f.** FETUS PAPYRACEUS. **f. papyraceus** The remains of a dead twin which during intrauterine development died and was pressed flat against the uterine wall by the living twin. Also *fetus compressus, paper-doll fetus, papyraceous fetus.* **retroperitoneal f. in fetu** A conjoined twin situated outside the peritoneum, usually on the posterior abdominal wall, of the host fetus. Although retroperitoneal, it is covered by an amniotic sac and protrudes forward into the peritoneal cavity of the host. The parasitic twin may contain organs and limbs with some vertical axis symmetry, and it is removable with good prognosis during infancy of the host.

**Feulgen** [Robert Joachim *Feulgen,* German biochemist, 1884–1955] Feulgen procedure, Feulgen's test, Feulgen reaction. See under METHOD.

**Feulgen-positive** \foil′gen-\ [after Robert *Feulgen,* German biochemist, 1884–1955 + *positive*] Describing any cytologic structure that stains as a result of the Feulgen method: used especially in reference to DNA.

**FEV** forced expired volume.

# fever

**fever** [Old English *fēfor,* from L *febris.* See FEBRIS.] **1** An increase of body temperature above normal. Also *pyrexia.* **2** Any state of ill health in which an elevated body temperature is a primary symptom. **abortus f.** Brucellosis in humans caused by *Brucella abortus.* It is generally contracted from cattle or cow's milk. **adynamic f.** Low-grade fever in patients who are generally weak or asthenic. An imprecise and outmoded term. Also *asthenic fever.* **African hemorrhagic f.** EBOLA VIRUS DISEASE. **African tick f.** A tick-borne endemic relapsing fever caused by the spirochete *Borrelia duttoni,* transmitted by *Ornithodoros moubata.* Also *Dutton's relapsing fever, Dutton's disease.* **f. and ague** *Obs.* MALARIA. **Andaman A f.** Leptospirosis caused by a strain of *Leptospira icterohaemorrhagiae* first isolated in the Andaman Islands. **aphthous f.** FOOT-AND-MOUTH DISEASE. **apyretic typhoid f.** A form of typhoid fever in which the temperature remains nearly normal. **Argentinian hemorrhagic f.** An acute, severe disease caused by the Junín virus, an arenavirus contracted from the urine of infected rodents, and marked by fever, chills, lymphadenopathy, headache, myalgia, leukopenia, shock, hemorrhagic, neurologic manifestations, and renal involvement. Also *Junín fever, South American hemorrhagic fever.* **artificial f.** INDUCED FEVER. **aseptic f.** Fever that accompanies an aseptic wound and that is brought on by the absorption of noninfected but injured tissue. **Assam f.** KALA-AZAR. **auric f.** A toxic reaction to gold, characterized by dermatitis which is expressed as erythema, urticaria, or rash. Temporary nephritis with albuminuria may sometimes occur. Blood dyscrasias such as leukopenia, agranulocytosis, and thrombopenia have also been reported. **Australian Q f.** Q FEVER. **Australian tick f.** NORTH QUEENSLAND TICK TYPHUS. **autumn f.** **1** NANUKAYAMI. **2** SEVEN-DAY FEVER. **Bangkok hemorrhagic f.** DENGUE HEMORRHAGIC FEVER. **barbeiro f.** CHAGAS DISEASE. **biduotertian f.** Tertian malaria in which paroxysms of fever are nearly continuous resulting from infection by two broods of parasites, with merozoite release occurring on alternate days. **bilious f.** A febrile illness characterized by bilious vomiting. *Obs.* **black f.** KALA-AZAR. **blackwater f.** An acute intravascular hemolysis associated with falciparum malaria. The urine becomes dark brown or black. It may occur as a single crisis in which more than half the circulating erythrocytes are hemolyzed intravenously, or repeated smaller crises may occur. The disease is frequently fatal. It occurs mainly among foreigners in malarial countries, who have previously had attacks of falciparum malaria inadequately treated by quinine. Quinine often precipitates an attack, but its etiologic role is still unclear. The disease is quite unusual where newer synthetic antimalarial drugs are used. Also *hemolytic malaria, melanuric fever.* **Bolivian hemorrhagic f.** Hemorrhagic fever caused by the Machupo virus (an arenavirus), clinically similar to Argentinian hemorrhagic fever, with involvement of hematopoietic, cardiovascular, renal, clotting, and central nervous systems. There is 10–20 percent mortality. Also *South American hemorrhagic fever.* **bouquet f.** DENGUE. **boutonneuse f.** A tick-borne disease caused by *Rickettsia conorii,* widespread in the Mediterranean, Africa, and India. It is characterized by an initial necrotic skin lesion (tache noire), headache, muscle pain, and a skin rash covering the entire body, including palms of hands and soles of feet. Also *African tick typhus, Mediterranean fever, Marseilles fever, Mediterranean tick fever, South African tick-bite fever, fièvre boutonneuse.* **brass-founders' f.** METAL-FUME FEVER. **Brazilian spotted f.** ROCKY MOUNTAIN SPOTTED FEVER. **breakbone f.** DENGUE. **Brisbane f.** Q FEVER. **Bullis f.** A mild disease characterized by fever, leukopenia, postorbital and occipital headache, and lymphadenitis. It is thought to be caused by a species of *Rickettsia* and transmitted by the Lone Star tick (*Amblyomma americanum*). Also *Texas tick fever, Lone Star fever.* • It was given its name following an epidemic originating at Camp Bullis, Texas, in 1942. **burdwan f.** KALA-AZAR. **Bushy Creek f.** FORT BRAGG FEVER. **Bwamba f.** A mild, febrile disease of viral origin which resembles yellow fever and occurs in central Africa, particularly Uganda. There are many strains of the virus, which is transmitted by *Anopheles gambiae.* Headache and backache are the main symptoms, which usually subside in 5–7 days. • The name is derived from *Bwamba* forest in the western province of Uganda. **cachectic f.** KALA-AZAR. **cachexial f.** KALA-AZAR. **canefield f.** Leptospirosis occurring among canefield workers, caused principally by *Leptospira interrogans* serovar *australis.* **carbuncular f.** ANTHRAX. **cat f.** FELINE VIRAL ENTERITIS. **cat-bite f.** **1** An infectious disease caused by *Pasteurella multocida* and spread to humans by the bite of a cat. An abscess forms at the site of injury. Also *cat-bite disease.* **2** *Incorrect* CAT-SCRATCH DISEASE. **cat-scratch f.** CAT-SCRATCH DISEASE. **Central Asian hemorrhagic f.** A tick-borne hemorrhagic fever due to the Congo virus (a togavirus) and reported in Kazakhstan and Uzbekistan. It is thought to be transmitted by the tick *Hyalomma anatolicum.* **cerebrospinal f.** CEREBROSPINAL MENINGITIS. **Charcot's f.** INTERMITTENT HEPATIC FEVER. **Charcot's intermittent f.** INTERMITTENT HEPATIC FEVER. **chikungunya f.** CHIKUNGUNYA. **childbed f.** *Older term* PUERPERAL FEVER. **Colombian tick f.** ROCKY MOUNTAIN SPOTTED FEVER. **Colorado tick f.** A febrile illness of man caused by an orbivirus (Colorado tick fever virus) and transmitted by *Dermacentor andersoni* ticks from small rodents. The disease occurs only in the region where the tick resides, i.e. in the Rocky Mountains and westward, with the majority of cases reported in Colorado. The signs and symptoms are nearly identical to those of Rocky Mountain spotted fever, although there is usually no rash. Developing 3–6 days after the infecting tick bite, the disease is characterized by high fever (biphasic in 50% of cases), chills, myalgia, severe headache, nausea and vomiting, ocular and abdominal pain, and, in a majority of cases, leukopenia. The virus is erythrocyte-associated and persists in the blood for two weeks to two months after onset of illness. Also *Colorado fever, mountain tick fever.* **Crimean hemorrhagic f.** A hemorrhagic fever caused by a virus of the Crimean-Congo group of the Bunyaviridae and transmitted principally by the tick *Hyalomma marginatum,* which occurs in the Crimea and the lower Don and Volga river valleys. **cyclic f.** A fever that recurs regularly. **Cyprus f.** MALTA FEVER. **dandy f.** DENGUE. **deer-fly f.** TULAREMIA. **dehydration f.** Rise of body temperature in the newborn on the second to fifth day of life, when the combination of a high room temperature and low fluid intake reduces the insensible evaporation from the lungs and heat loss in the breath. Also *inanition fever, exsiccation fever.* **dengue f.** DENGUE. **dengue hemorrhagic f.** A form of dengue characterized by hemorrhagic manifestations. It often occurs in epidemics in large urban centers in Asia, and is associated with a substantial mortality rate (50 percent or more), especially in children. Thrombocytopenia, concurrent hemoconcentration, and circulatory failure (dengue hemorrhagic shock syndrome), probably mediated by immunopathologic mechanisms, are important features of the disease. Intensive care with fluid replacement, blood transfusion, and administration of corticosteroids plays a part in management. Also *hemorrhagic dengue, Bangkok hemorrhagic fever, Philippine hemorrhagic fever, Thai hemorrhagic fever.* **digestive f.** *Obs.* DIETARY INDUCED THERMOGENESIS. **diphasic milk f.** The central European subtype of tick-borne encephalitis. See under TICK-BORNE ENCEPHALITIS. **drug f.** An elevated body temperature brought about by the administration of a drug. These reactions are not uncommon from vaccines, some antibiotics, and antineoplastic agents. Usually the effect is over when medication is stopped. **Dumdum f.** KALA-AZAR. **Dutton's relapsing f.** AFRICAN TICK FEVER. **endemic relapsing f.** See under RELAPSING FEVER. **enteric f.** A febrile illness caused by bacteria of the genus *Salmonella*; typhoid fever or paratyphoid fever. **entericoid f.** PARENTERIC FEVER. **ephemeral f.** Any fever of brief duration. **epidemic hemorrhagic f.** An acute infectious disease seen in northeastern Asia, caused by the Hantaan virus and transmitted by field rodents. The disease is characterized by fever, purpura, vascular damage, renal failure, prostration, and shock. Also *epidemic hemorrhagic disease, Far Eastern hemorrhagic fever, Korean hemorrhagic fever, Songo fever, epidemic nephrosonephritis, nephrosonephritis* (rare). **estivo-autumnal f.** ESTIVOAUTUMNAL MALARIA. **etiocholanolone f.** An episodic fever due to periodic elevations of plasma 5$\beta$-androstane (etiocholanolone). **exsiccation f.** DEHYDRATION FEVER. **familial Mediterranean f.** A hereditary disease found in persons of Mediterranean origin, consisting of episodic fever, arthritis, serositis, and sometimes complicated by amyloidosis. Also *Armenian disease, familial paroxysmal peritonitis.* **famine f.** TYPHUS. **Far Eastern hemorrhagic f.** EPIDEMIC HEMORRHAGIC FEVER. **fatigue f.** A fever that follows violent and/or prolonged exercise. **Fort Bragg f.** Leptospirosis, presumably due to *Leptospira autumnalis,* characterized by fever and a pretibial rash. Also *Bushy Creek fever, pretibial fever.* **foundrymen's f.** METAL-FUME FEVER. **Gambian f.** An irregular, recurrent, febrile condition lasting from one to four days, with from two to five days between relapses, and characterized by rapid pulse and breathing, and enlargement of the spleen. It is caused by the presence of *Trypanosoma gambiense,* the agent of Gambian trypanosomiasis, in the bloodstream. **glandular f.** INFECTIOUS MONONUCLEOSIS. **Guáitara f.** OROYA FEVER. **Hankow f.** Schistosomiasis due to *Schistosoma japonicum.* **harvest f.** A type of leptospirosis characterized by conjunctivitis, vomiting, diarrhea, abdominal pains, stupor, and fever. Occurring principally among field workers during harvest, it is caused by *Leptospira interrogans* serovar *grippotyphosa.* **Hasami f.** Mild leptospirosis caused by *Leptospira autumnalis* or a similar leptospiral agent and occurring in Japan, especially in the Hasami district of Nagasaki Prefecture. **Haverhill f.** An illness characterized by fever, chills, an erythematous eruption, headache, and arthritis. One causative agent is *Streptobacillus moniliformis,* which has been recovered from raw milk believed to be contaminated by rats. First identified in Haverhill, Massachusetts in 1926, it occurs in epidemics and in isolated cases. Also *streptobacillary fever, erythema arthriticum epidemicum.* See also RAT-BITE FEVER. **hay f.** Allergic rhinitis due to pollen hypersensitivity and therefore seasonal. In the United States, ragweed pollen is the usual allergen and August and September the season, whereas in the United Kingdom, grass pollens are most often incriminated and the season runs from the end of May until the middle of July. Also *seasonal nasal allergy, summer catarrh* (rare), *autumnal catarrh, Bostock's catarrh* (obs.). **hematuric bilious f.** *Plasmodium falciparum* malaria associated with hematuria. *Rare.* **hemoglobinuric f.** BLACKWATER FEVER. **hemorrhagic f.** A category of infectious diseases of diverse viral origin characterized generally by fever, myalgia, headache, capillaritis, and hemorrhagic manifestations often followed by focal inflammation and necrosis. The mortality rate among those suffering from these fevers ranges from 10 to 50 percent. Hemorrhagic fevers include Argentinian hemorrhagic fever, Bolivian hemorrhagic fever, Crimean hemorrhagic fever, African hemorrhagic fever, Omsk hemorrhagic fever, Kyasanur forest disease, Ebola virus disease, Marburg disease, yellow fever, hemorrhagic dengue, and epidemic hemorrhagic fever. **herpetic f.** Infection of the mucous membranes of the mouth and lips and surrounding skin with herpes simplex virus, usually herpes simplex virus type 1, associated with fever, chills, and, occasionally, sore throat. **Herxheimer's f.** HERXHEIMER REACTION. **hospital f.** EPIDEMIC LOUSE-BORNE TYPHUS. **icterohemorrhagic f.** ICTERIC LEPTOSPIROSIS. **Ilheus f.** A febrile disease, sometimes with encephalitis, of eastern Brazil and other parts of South and Central America, caused by the Ilheus virus (a flavivirus). **inanition f.** DEHYDRATION FEVER. **induced f.** Fever caused deliberately by procedures such as the application of heat or the administration of a pyrogen. Also *artificial fever.* **intermittent f.** Any fever characterized by recurrent episodes of elevated temperature occurring between periods of normal temperature. **intermittent hepatic f.** An intermittent fever, usually septic or hectic, caused by episodes of biliary tract infection and obstruction as a result of gallstones. Also *Charcot's fever, Charcot's intermittent fever.* **Jaccoud's dissociated f.** Meningitis and fever in association with a slow and irregular pulse. It was originally observed in cases of tuberculous meningitis. *Obs.* **Japanese flood f.** SCRUB TYPHUS. **jungle yellow f.** Yellow fever endemic among primates in African and Central and South American forests which is occasionally transmitted to humans by infected treetop-breeding mosquitoes, usually of the genus *Aedes,* but *Haemogogus* and *Sabethes* may also be responsible. Also *sylvan yellow fever.* **Junín f.** ARGENTINIAN HEMORRHAGIC FEVER. **kedani f.** SCRUB TYPHUS. **Kenya f.** KENYA TYPHUS. **Kew Gardens f.** RICKETTSIALPOX. **Kew Gardens spotted f.** RICKETTSIALPOX. **Kinkian f.** SCHISTOSOMIASIS JAPONICA. **Kinkiang f.** SCHISTOSOMIASIS JAPONICA. **Korean hemorrhagic f.** EPIDEMIC HEMORRHAGIC FEVER. **Kyoto f.** A kind of nanukayami or seven-day fever seen in the vicinity of Kyoto, Japan. **Lassa f.** A highly communicable, hemorrhagic fever caused by the Lassa virus (an arenavirus) and occurring principally in west Africa, where it is endemic or hyperendemic. It has also been reported from Zimbabwe and South Africa. Rodents (especially *Mastomys natalensis*) constitute the only known reservoir of infection, and the disease is spread from person to person by multiple routes. It ranges in severity from a mild infection to a fatal multisystem illness and is characterized by fever, diarrhea, myalgia, severe pharyngitis, headache, epigastric and chest pain, vomiting, and cough. In fatal cases, hypovolemia, hypotension, pleural effusion, ascites, and pulmonary edema may develop. Virologic studies and a complement fixation test are of value in diagnosis. Hospital outbreaks have produced the highest mortality rates. Strict isolation is essential. Ribavirin when administered intravenously appears to be a promising treatment. Injection of human convalescent serum has been used for therapy, but its efficacy is not known. **lemming f.** In man an infectious disease in Norway, thought to be attributable to contamination of drinking water by the excreta and drowned bodies of lemmings infected with *Francisella tularensis.* **leprotic f.** The fever which characterizes the early stage of leprosy and is a part of the lepra reaction. **Lone Star f.** BULLIS FEVER. **louse-borne relapsing f.** A spirochetal disease, spread by lice, characterized by alternating fevers and apyrexial episodes. It is caused by *Borrelia recurrentis.* Distibution is widespread in Africa, Asia, and South America. **macular f.** **1** Any febrile disease characterized by a macular cutaneous eruption. **2** *Obs.* TYPHUS. **malarial f.** MALARIA. **malignant tertian f.** FALCIPARUM MALARIA. **Malta f.** Brucellosis in humans caused by *Brucella melitensis.* It is common on Mediterranean islands and coastal areas but is also widely distributed elsewhere. Also *febris melitensis, melitensis, Cyprus fever, Mediterranean phthisis, Mediterranean fever.* **Marseilles f.** BOUTONNEUSE FEVER. **marsh f.** MALARIA. **Mediterranean f.** **1** MALTA FEVER. **2** BOUTONNEUSE FEVER. **Mediterranean tick f.** BOUTONNEUSE FEVER. **Mediterranean yellow f.** *Outmoded* ICTERIC LEPTOSPIROSIS. **melanuric f.** BLACKWATER FEVER. **metabolic f.** A fever caused by a disturbance of the heat-regulating mechanism of the body, a condition seen in some metabolic disorders. It may be associated with dehydration or an electrolyte imbalance. **metal-fume f.** A condition caused by exposure to zinc fumes in the smelting of zinc ores, in galvanizing or welding, in cutting galvanized iron, etc. Inhaled zinc oxide destroys cells in lung alveoli, producing proteins which are absorbed and cause malaise, shivering, fever, and muscular pains. Recovery is almost always complete within 24 hours. Metal fumes other than zinc may also cause this condition. Also *brass-founders' ague, spelter-workers' ague, welders' ague, zinc-smelters' ague, brass chill, braziers' chill, spelters' chill, zinc chill, brass-founders' fever, foundrymen's fever, spelters' fever, zinc-fume fever.* **Meuse f.** TRENCH FEVER. **Mexican spotted f.** ROCKY MOUNTAIN SPOTTED FEVER. **Mianeh f.** A form of relapsing fever present in Iran and other parts of the Middle East. It is caused by *Borrelia persica* and commonly characterized by eye complications and jaundice. Though spread by a tick, it is considered clinically distinct from the classical tick-borne and louse-borne relapsing fevers. There may be a high death rate. Also *Persian relapsing fever, Miana disease, Mianeh disease.* Also *Miana fever.* **milk f.** Fever occurring in women during the immediate postpartum period and associated with the onset of lactation. *Seldom used.* **miniature scarlet f.** A rare reaction following immunization with a scarlet fever prophylactic containing a toxin of *Streptococcus pyogenes* and characterized by a generalized scarlatiniform rash, malaise, nausea, and vomiting. **mite f.** SCRUB TYPHUS. **monoleptic f.** Any fever which is continuous, in contrast to one which occurs in two or more paroxysms (polyleptic). **Mossman f.** A febrile disease occurring in sugar cane cutters in Australia. It was formerly thought to be caused by *Leptospira australis* but is probably a rickettsial infection, perhaps a form of scrub typhus. ● The name is derived from the *Mossman* district of north Queensland, Australia. **mountain tick f.** COLORADO TICK FEVER. **mud f.** Leptospirosis caused by *Leptospira interrogans* serovar *grippotyphosa,* occurring principally among workers in flooded fields or other muddy workplaces. See also HARVEST FEVER. **Murchison-Pel-Ebstein f.** PEL-EBSTEIN FEVER. **nanukayami f.** NANUKAYAMI. **neurogenic f.** Pyrexia occurring in disorders of the central nervous system, not due to infection but to a disturbance of brain centers responsible for temperature control. **north Queensland tick f.** NORTH QUEENSLAND TICK TYPHUS. **Omsk hemorrhagic f.** A hemorrhagic fever occurring seasonally or epidemically in southwestern Siberia and caused by a tick-borne flavivirus. The disease is characterized by fever, headache, bronchopneumonia, hemorrhagic and encephalitic manifestations, and, rarely, shock. **O'nyong-nyong f.** An acute epidemic disease that occurs in Uganda and Kenya, caused by a mosquito-borne alphavirus and characterized by fever, lymphadenitis, arthritis, and rash. An epidemic affecting 5 million people occurred in northern Uganda in 1959. **Oroya f.** The acute, febrile phase of bartonellosis. Also *Guáitara fever.* See also BARTONELLOSIS. ● A severe epidemic occurred among laborers in 1870 during construction of the railway between Lima and La Oroya, a mining center in the high Andes. **Pahvant Valley f.** TULAREMIA. **paludal f.** MALARIA. **pappataci f.** SANDFLY FEVER. ● *Pappataci* is the Italian word for sandfly. **paramalta f.** Any febrile illness resembling Malta fever but not caused by *Brucella melitensis.* Also *paramelitensis fever, paraundulant fever.* **paratyphoid f.** Enteric fever caused by *Salmonella* serotypes other than *S. typhi,* especially *S. paratyphi, S. schottmuelleri* (formerly *S. paratyphi* B), and *S. hirschfeldii* (formerly *S. paratyphi* C). The clinical features of the disease are essentially identical with those of typhoid fever, but paratyphoid fever is usually a milder illness than typhoid. Also *Schottmüller's disease, paratyphoid.* **paraundulant f.** PARAMALTA FEVER. **parenteric f.** A febrile illness which has the characteristics of typhoid or paratyphoid fever but which is not caused by *Salmonella* organisms. Also *entericoid fever, febris entericoides.* **parrot f.** PSITTACOSIS. **Pel-Ebstein f.** Recurrent episodes of fever that persist for several days, separated by afebrile intervals that last for several days to a few weeks. Pel-Ebstein fever is a manifestation of Hodgkin's disease. Also *Murchison-Pel-Ebstein fever, Pell-Ebstein pyrexia, Pel-Ebstein symptom.* **periodic f.** **1** Recurrent episodes of fever interspersed with periods of wellness. It is a feature of several syndromes, including familial Mediterranean fever, an autosomal recessive trait. **2** A specific, rare autosomal dominant condition of idiopathic fever in otherwise well individuals. **Persian relapsing f.** MIANEH FEVER. **petechial f.** CEREBROSPINAL MENINGITIS. **pharyngoconjunctival f.** An epidemic, febrile illness caused primarily by adenovirus types 3, 4, 7, 14, and 21 and usually affecting school-age children. It is characterized by fever, pharyngitis resembling that seen in streptococcal infections, and, in about 35–50% of cases, conjunctivitis. Accompanying symptoms may include myalgia, headache, chills, and dizziness. **Philippine hemorrhagic f.** DENGUE HEMORRHAGIC FEVER. **phlebotomus f.** SANDFLY FEVER. **polyleptic f.** RELAPSING FEVER. **polymer fume f.** A disorder with symptoms similar to those of metal-fume fever, caused by exposure to fumes emitted during the burning of polymers such as Teflon or paratetrafluoroethylene. **Pomona f.** Leptospirosis caused by *Leptospira pomona* and occurring mostly in hogs and cattle. The disease is spread to humans by contact with the urine of an infected animal, usually through scratches or abrasions of the skin. In adult animals infection is often asymptomatic but young animals may become acutely ill with jaundice, hemolytic anemia, and hemoglobinuria. Late abortions and neonatal deaths may also occur. **pretibial f.** FORT BRAGG FEVER. **puerperal f.** Endometritis, often associated with septicemia, following childbirth or abortion. The infection is usually due to streptococci but occasionally is caused by *Mycoplasma hominis* or *Ureaplasma urealyticum.* In the preantibiotic era this disease was associated with a high death rate. Also *childbed fever* (older term), *puerperal sepsis, puerperal septicemia.* **pythogenic f.** TYPHOID FEVER. **Q f.** A globally distributed infectious disease caused by the rickettsia *Coxiella burnetii* and first observed in Brisbane, Australia. It is usually transmitted to man from cattle, sheep, and goats when aerosolized particles containing the infectious agent are inhaled. Manifestations include fever, headache, myalgia, and pneumonia. The disease is most prevalent in areas where cattle, sheep, and goats are raised. Also *Australian Q fever, Brisbane fever.* • The disease was designated Q fever in the original report in 1937 "until further knowledge should allow a better name." Though further knowledge was soon forthcoming, the nonce designation has prevailed. **quartan f.** MALARIAE MALARIA. **Queensland coastal f.** SCRUB TYPHUS. **Queensland tick f.** NORTH QUEENSLAND TICK TYPHUS. **quintan f.** TRENCH FEVER. **quintana f.** TRENCH FEVER. **quotidian f.** Fever recurring daily, as in some types of malaria. **rabbit f.** TULAREMIA. **rat-bite f.** A febrile infectious disease acquired through the bite of a rat or other rodent or, rarely, through ingestion of contaminated milk. There are two forms of the disease: sodoku (spirillary fever), caused by *Spirillum minor* and occurring most often in Japan, and Haverhill fever (streptobacillary fever), caused by *Streptobacillus moniliformis* and occurring most commonly in the United States. Fever, chills, localized lymphangitis and lymphadenitis, and a characteristic rash are seen in both forms of the disease. Half of the cases of Haverhill fever also exhibit a nonsuppurative migrating polyarthritis. Also *rat-bite disease, morbus morsus muris.* **recurrent f.** RELAPSING FEVER. **relapsing f.** One of a group of acute febrile diseases occurring worldwide and caused by arthropod-borne spirochetes of the genus *Borrelia.* Epidemic relapsing fever is caused by *V. recurrentis,* has a person-to-person cycle, and is transmitted by the human body louse. Endemic relapsing fever is caused by various *Borrelia* species and is transmitted by ticks of the genus *Ornithodoros.* The disease is characterized by alternating febrile and afebrile episodes, each lasting two to nine days, with recurrence and abatement of symptoms. A petechial rash, conjunctival infection and hepatosplenomegaly may be present. Diagnosis is made from blood films. Tetracycline, and less frequently, erythromycin are used in treatment. Herxheimer reactions are common. Mortality rates of up to 70 percent have been reported in untreated patients, but with adequate treatment mortality may be reduced to 5 percent. Also *febris recurrens, polyleptic fever, recurrent fever, typhinia.* **remittent f.** Fever in which the temperature fluctuates significantly in the course of a day but is still above normal at its lowest point. **rheumatic f.** An acute, self-limited, febrile disease occurring as a sequela to a group A streptococcal pharyngeal infection and affecting children and young adults. The disease is characterized by fever and nonsuppurative inflammation of the heart, joints, subcutaneous tissue, and central nervous system. Myocardial and valvular damage may result, particularly if there are recurrent attacks of the disease. Also *inflammatory rheumatism, polyarthritis rheumatica acuta.* **rice-field f.** Leptospirosis contracted by rice-field workers. **Rift Valley f.** An acute, infectious, febrile disease caused by a bunyavirus and transmitted by *Culex* and *Aedes* mosquitoes and by contact with infected tissues. The incubation period is 3–6 days. It occurs in eastern, western, and southern Africa and in Egypt. It affects man as well as sheep, cattle, goats, camels, antelope, and rodents. Hepatic necrosis is a consistent finding. In severe cases there is encephalitis, retinitis, and hemorrhagic fever. A vaccine is available. Mortality from the disease is approximately 10–15 percent. Also *enzootic hepatitis.* **river f. of Japan** SCRUB TYPHUS. **Rocky Mountain spotted f.** An acute, febrile illness caused by *Rickettsia rickettsii* and transmitted by various ticks, the usual vectors in the United States being *Amblyomma americanum, Dermacentor variabilis,* and *Dermacentor andersoni.* Sudden onset of fever, headache, and myalgia occur within a few days of the infective tick bite and a characteristic macular, petechial rash appears first on the extremities and spreads centripetally. Widely distributed in the western hemisphere, the disease is known by a variety of regional names. Also *spotted fever, Brazilian spotted fever, Colombian tick fever, Tobia fever* (Colombian), *Mexican spotted fever, São Paulo fever, São Paulo typhus, fiebre manchada, Colorado fever.* **Russian headache f.** Fever and headache associated with tick-borne flaviviruses, such as Omsk hemorrhagic fever virus and tick-borne encephalitis viruses. **Sakushu f.** A type of seven-day epidemic fever, probably leptospiral, occurring in the autumn in Japan, especially in Okayama Prefecture. **sandfly f.** A febrile illness caused by a bunyavirus transmitted by the sandfly *Phlebotomus papatasii.* The disease occurs endemically in the Mediterranean region, the Middle East, and central Asia, and sporadically elsewhere. It is characterized by a three-day fever, headache, conjunctivitis, leukopenia, and malaise. Also *phlebotomus fever, pappataci fever.* **San Joaquin f.** COCCIDIOIDOMYCOSIS. **São Paulo f.** ROCKY MOUNTAIN SPOTTED FEVER. **scarlet f.** An acute, contagious illness which results from infection, usually of the pharynx, with group A $\beta$-hemolytic streptococci which elaborate erythrogenic toxin. The disease most commonly affects the pharynx but may follow streptococcal infections of wounds or the birth canal. It is characterized by fever, acute exudative pharyngitis, tonsilitis (or endometritis in the case of puerperal infection), a red enanthem, and a scarlet red exanthem which is followed by extensive desquamation. In the antibiotic era, severe forms of the disease are rarely seen. Certain other bacteria, for example staphylococci, may occasionally produce erythrogenic toxins and so give rise to a syndrome resembling scarlet fever. Also *scarlatina.* **septic f.** Elevation of body temperature, commonly to 40°C or more, due to the presence of bacteria or bacterial toxins in blood. **seven-day f.** 1 NANUKAYAMI. 2 Any of various forms of anicteric leptospirosis or similar diseases occurring in Japan, such as Hasami fever or Sakushu fever. 3 A denguelike fever occurring in India at the end of summer. For defs 1, 2, and 3 also *autumn fever.* • The term is imprecise and may apply to diverse febrile illnesses including dengue **shinbone f.** TRENCH FEVER. **ship f.** EPIDEMIC LOUSE-BORNE TYPHUS. **slime f.** MUD FEVER. **snail f.** SCHISTOSOMIASIS. **solar f.** 1 DENGUE. 2 SUNSTROKE. **South African tick-bite f.** BOUTONNEUSE FEVER. **South American hemorrhagic f.** 1 ARGENTINIAN HEMORRHAGIC FEVER. 2 BOLIVIAN HEMORRHAGIC FEVER. **spelters' f.** METAL-FUME FEVER. **spirillar f.** SODOKU. **spirillary f.** SODOKU. **spirillum f.** SODOKU. **splenic f.** ANTHRAX. **spotted f.** 1 ROCKY MOUNTAIN SPOTTED FEVER. 2 Any of various other tick-borne rickettsioses characterized by cutaneous eruptions, such as boutonneuse fever, north Queensland tick typhus, or Siberian tick typhus. **stiffneck f.** 1 DENGUE. 2 CEREBROSPINAL MENINGITIS. **streptobacillary f.** HAVERHILL FEVER. **sulfonamide f.** A toxic reaction to sulfonamides. The symptoms include fever, anemia, leukopenia, dermatitis, and nephritis, the last being due to the precipitation of crystals in the collecting tubules of the kidney. **sweat f.** MILIARIA. **sylvan yellow f.** JUNGLE YELLOW FEVER. **tetanoid f.** CEREBROSPINAL MENINGITIS. **Texas tick f.** BULLIS FEVER. **Thai hemorrhagic f.** DENGUE HEMORRHAGIC FEVER. **therapeutic f.** The induced fever used in fever therapy. **thermic f.** HEATSTROKE. **thirst f.** A fever associated with dehydration. **tick-borne relapsing f.** A spirochetal disease, spread by ticks, characterized by alternating fevers and apyrexial episodes. It is caused by several species of *Borrelia,* especially *B. duttoni.* Distribution is widespread in Africa, Asia, the Middle East, and central and South America. **Tobia f.** A Colombian term for ROCKY MOUNTAIN SPOTTED FEVER. **trench f.** A louse-borne relapsing fever caused by *Rochalimaea quintana* (formerly *Rickettsia quintana*). The disease was epidemic in Europe during the First World War. It is characterized by paroxysms of fever, chills, headache, myalgia (especially of the back and legs), and a rash on the trunk. Also *quintan fever, Meuse fever, shinbone fever, Volhynia fever, Wolhynia fever, His-Werner disease, Werner-His disease, quintana fever.* **trypanosome f.** TRYPANOSOMIASIS. **tsutsugamushi f.** SCRUB TYPHUS. **typhoid f.** An acute, febrile illness caused by *Salmonella typhi* and usually acquired as a result of ingesting contaminated water or food. The disease may occur in epidemic form and is characterized by headache, chills, myalgia, diarrhea, bacteremia, abdominal distention, and splenomegaly. Characteristic rose-colored spots appear in the early stages of some cases. In severe cases prostration, intestinal perforation, and hemorrhage may occur. A vaccine is available. Also *enterotyphus, pythogenic fever, typhoid.* **typhus f.** TYPHUS. **undulant f.** Brucellosis in humans. Also *Bruce's septicemia, febris undulans.* **urban f.** A form of tropical typhus, usually flea-borne, occurring in urban areas. **urban yellow f.** The classical or urban cycle of human yellow fever transmitted by *Aedes aegypti.* **urinary f.** A fever caused by a urinary tract infection. **urticarial f.** SCHISTOSOMIASIS JAPONICA. **uveoparotid f.** HEERFORDT SYNDROME. **vaccinal f.** Fever occurring subsequent to vaccination. **valley f.** COCCIDIOIDOMYCOSIS. **Volhynia f.** TRENCH FEVER. **West Nile f.** A mild fever resembling dengue, caused by a group B arbovirus which has antigenic similarities to the Japanese B, Murray B Valley, and St. Louis encephalitis viruses. The natural reservoir probably exists in birds. It is spread by many species of *Culex* mosquitoes, some *Anopheles,* and one *Mansonia* species. It is also spread by ticks, such as *Argas hermanni* in Egypt, or several *Ornithodoros* species in the USSR. The virus has been isolated in Africa, India, the USSR, and the Middle East. Also *West Nile encephalitis.* **Whitmore's f.** MELIOIDOSIS. **Wolhynia f.** TRENCH FEVER. **wound f.** A fever resulting from a bacterial infection within a wound. **Yangtze Valley f.** SCHISTOSOMIASIS JAPONICA. **yellow f.** An infectious disease caused by a flavivirus of the togavirus family, transmitted between humans by the *Aedes aegypti* mosquito (urban yellow fever) and from animals to humans by various species of mosquitoes (jungle or sylvan yellow fever). The disease is endemic in tropical areas of Central and South America and Africa. The reservoir of infection may be in man (urban cycle) or in animals (sylvan or jungle cycle), especially primates. The disease is characterized by jaundice, fever, chills, headache, gastrointestinal hemorrhage, and albuminuria. In fatal cases, liver histology establishes the diagnosis. Control of the disease depends on destruction of the vector. Vaccines are available. The attenuated 17D strain is given subcutaneously and renders excellent protection for ten years. There is no specific treatment for the disease. Also *yellow jack* (popular), *amarillic typhus* (outmoded). **Zika f.** An acute degenerative disease of the central nervous system, involving especially the hippocampus, which occurs in Africa and Malaysia. The presentation and clinical picture resemble dengue. It is caused by a flavivirus first isolated from monkeys and from the mosquito *Aedes africanus,* which appears to be the insect vector, in the Zika forest of Uganda. **zinc-fume f.** METAL-FUME FEVER.

**FF** filtration fraction.

**FFT** flicker fusion threshold.

**FGT** female genital tract.

**f.h.** *fiat haustus* (L, let a draught be made).

**FIA** Freund's incomplete adjuvant.

**fiat** Let there be made, as used in prescription writing.

# fiber

**fiber** [L *fibra.* See FIBRA.] FIBRA. **Ia f.** PRIMARY AFFERENT. **Ib f.** GROUP IB FIBER. **A f.'s** All peripheral myelinated axons, originally defined as the "A" elevation of the compound action potential, thus constituting the fastest conducting nerve fibers. Each subdivision, α–δ, can be further defined in terms of sensory and motor functional categories as well as axonal diameter. **α-f.** α-EFFERENT. **accelerator f.** A sympathetic nerve fiber that, when stimulated, increases the heart rate. Also *augmentor fiber, accelerating fiber, cardiac accelerator fiber.* **accessory f.** A fiber of the ciliary zonule that is not attached to the lens capsule directly. Also *auxiliary fiber.* **adrenergic f.'s**

Sympathetic nerve fibers for which norepinephrine or epinephrine serve as synaptic transmitter. **afferent f.** A nerve fiber conducting towards a nucleus or center. Also *centripetal fiber, sensory fiber.* **anterior external arcuate f.'s** FIBRAE ARCUATAE EXTERNAE VENTRALES. **archiform f.'s** FIBRAE INTERCRURALES. **arcuate f.'s** 1 Collectively, the various fascicles of arcuate fibers in the brainstem, including the fibrae arcuatae internae, fibrae arcuatae externae ventrales, and fibrae arcuatae externae dorsales. 2 FIBRAE ARCUATAE CEREBRI. **arcuate f.'s of cerebrum** FIBRAE ARCUATAE CEREBRI. **argentaffin f.** A nerve fiber that can be stained by silver solutions without the addition of an external reducing agent. Also *argentophil fiber, argentophilic fiber.* **argyrophilic f.** A nerve fiber that can be stained by silver solutions only in the presence of an external reducing agent. **association f.'s** The nerve fibers connecting different regions of the cerebral cortex within the same hemisphere. They consist of short association fibers that curve beneath each sulcus, connecting adjacent gyri, and long association fibers that interconnect different lobes. **augmentor f.** ACCELERATOR FIBER. **auxiliary f.** ACCESSORY FIBER. **B f.'s** Myelinated nerve fibers of up to 3 μm diameter and conduction rates of up to 15 m/s. They occur primarily in autonomic nerves as preganglionic fibers. **β-f.** β-EFFERENT. **Bergmann's f.'s** Glial processes of specialized astrocytes (Bergmann cells) in the molecular layer of the cerebellar cortex that extend through that layer to the pia. **Berneheimer's f.'s** A band of nerve fibers extending from the dorsal optic tract to the subthalamic nucleus (nucleus of Luys), unconfirmed in experimental studies of the optic tract axonal trajectory. **β motor f.** β-EFFERENT. **f.'s of Bogrov** Nerve fibers that pass from the optic tract to the thalamus. **bone f.'s** Collagen fibers that connect a tendon, ligament, fascia, or periosteum to underlying bone. Also *Sharpey's fibers.* **Brücke's f.'s** FIBRAE MERIDIONALES MUSCULI CILIARIS. **bulbospiral f.'s** A group of cardiac muscle fibers that run a spiral course in the walls of the atria and ventricles of the heart. **Burdach's f.'s** Axons of the fasciculus cuneatus medullae oblongatae (column of Burdach) terminating in the nucleus cuneatus (nucleus of Burdach's column). **C f.'s** Unmyelinated, slowly-conducting axons of the peripheral nervous system, usually found in small bundles ensheathed by a single Schwann cell. They constitute the majority of autonomic axons, and also innervate a variety of deep and cutaneous sense organs including nociceptors, thermoreceptors, and sensitive mechanoreceptors. **capsular f.'s** Nerve fibers of the cerebral internal capsule. *Imprecise.* **cardiac accelerator f.** ACCELERATOR FIBER. **cardiac depressor f.** A cholinergic nerve fiber that supplies the heart and causes a fall in cardiac output and a drop in blood pressure. **cardiac pressor f.** A sympathetic nerve fiber that supplies the heart and, when stimulated, causes an increase in cardiac output and a rise in blood pressure. **centripetal f.** AFFERENT FIBER. **cerebrospinal f.'s** FIBRAE CORTICOSPINALES. **chief f.'s** Those fibers of the ciliary zonule that are attached to the lens capsule. They are supported by accessory fibers which are attached to them at various angles. *Outmoded.* Also *principal fibers, main fibers, white fibers.* **cholinergic f.** An axon that releases the neurotransmitter acetylcholine at its synaptic terminals. **chromatic f.** A threadlike fiber or chromatin observed in the early mitotic nucleus. **chromosomal f.** CHROMOSOMAL SPINDLE FIBER. **chromosomal spindle f.** A fiber which is visible microscopically during prometaphase to telophase of cell division and which extends from the centrosome to the centromere (actually the kinetochore) of each chromosome. The structure of the spindle and the composition of the fibers vary among organisms, but all contain microtubules and help orchestrate segregation of daughter chromosomes. Also *chromosomal fiber, traction fiber, chromosomal microtubule, half-spindle fiber, kinetochore microtubule.* **cilioequatorial f.'s** Those fibers of the ciliary zonule that are attached to the equator of the lens. *Outmoded.* **cilioposterocapsular f.'s** The fine curved fibers of the ciliary zonule that are attached to the posterior surface of the lens capsule. *Outmoded.* **circular f.'s of ciliary muscle** FIBRAE CIRCULARES MUSCULI CILIARIS. **climbing f.'s of cerebellum** Myelinated axons emanating from the inferior olivary complex and extending through the cerebellar granular layer, where they climb along the extensive tree of Purkinje neuron dendrites, contacting the smooth dendritic branches and forming powerful excitatory synapses. Collaterals also contact cerebellar stellate, basket, and Golgi cells. **collagen f.** The predominant type of connective tissue fiber, synthesized from tropocollagen subunits by fibroblasts. The individual fibers have a characteristic periodicity of 64 nm when examined by electron microscopy. **collateral f.'s of Winslow** *Outmoded* FIBRAE INTERCRURALES. **commissural f.'s** 1 Nerve fibers that cross the midline to connect symmetric, homotopic zones of the cerebral cortex via the corpus callosum and anterior commissure. 2 Nerve fibers that cross the midline to connect symmetric zones throughout the brain and spinal cord. **cone f.'s** The fibers that extend from either side of the retinal cone bodies or cells. Stout, smooth inner fibers that resemble axons descend from the bodies of all cones to the middle zone of the outer plexiform layer, where they end in the club-shaped cone pedicles. Their lengths and course vary according to the region of the retina. The short, outer fibers extend from the cell body in the outer fovea and resemble dendrites physiologically. **conjunctival f.'s** Nerve fibers from the trigeminal nerve that supply the conjunctival membrane. The opthalmic division deals with the upper half and the maxillary branch with the lower half. **continuous f.** CONTINUOUS SPINDLE FIBER. **continuous spindle f.** A fiber visible microscopically during prometaphase to telophase of cell division which extends between the two poles of the spindle apparatus and which does not terminate at a chromosome kinetochore. Also *continuous fiber, interzonal fiber.* **corticobulbar f.'s** FIBRAE CORTICONUCLEARES. **corticofugal f.** An axon that emanates from a neuron cell body within the cerebral or cerebellar cortex and enters the underlying white matter. **corticonuclear f.'s** FIBRAE CORTICONUCLEARES. **corticopetal f.** An axon entering the cerebral or cerebellar cortex from the underlying white matter and terminating in the cortical neuropil. **corticopontine f.'s** FIBRAE CORTICOPONTINAE. **corticorubral f.'s** The sparse nerve fibers arising in the cerebral cortex and descending in the internal capsule to the region of the red nucleus. **corticospinal f.'s** FIBRAE CORTICOSPINALES. **corticostriate f.'s** Corticofugal fibers that are derived in large numbers from neurons in nearly all regions of the cerebral cortex and that project to the striatum (caudate nucleus and putamen). Some corticostriate fibers project to the ipsilateral striatum, while others cross in the corpus callosum and project to the contralateral striatum. **corticothalamic f.'s** FIBRAE CORTICOTHALAMICAE. **dark f.** TYPE I MUSCLE FIBER. **f.'s of Darkschewitsch** Nerve fibers derived from neurons in the nucleus of Darkschewitsch that course in the posterior commissure but whose precise terminations are not well known. **daugh-**

**ter f.** One of the muscle fibers formed by the splitting of a single parent fiber. **dentinal f.** *Obs.* ODONTOBLASTIC PROCESS. **dentinogenic f.'s** KORFF'S FIBERS. **dietary f.** The structural parts of plant foods such as fruits, vegetables, grains, nuts, and beans. It includes the coatings, such as the bran around brown rice or whole wheat, and the networks throughout a plant, as in celery, carrots, and sweet potatoes. Fiber is that part of ingested plant material which is not broken down and digested in the human gastrointestinal tract. A low fiber dietary intake is thought to be associated with constipation, diverticulitis, colon cancer, gallbladder disease, and appendicitis. **Dieters f.'s** STILLING'S FIBERS. **dorsal arcuate f.'s** FIBRAE ARCUATAE EXTERNAE DORSALES. **dorsal external arcuate f.'s** FIBRAE ARCUATAE EXTERNAE DORSALES. **efferent f.** An axon emanating from a neural center containing its neuron cell body. • The term is largely used to denote motor pathways. **elastic f.'s** Connective tissue fibers that display considerable flexibility. They branch and rejoin freely, forming a network and imparting a yellowish tinge to the tissue when present in quantity. They are found in the skin, the walls of larger blood vessels, and the ligamenta flava of the neck. Also *yellow fibers.* **external arcuate f.'s** FIBRAE ARCUATAE EXTERNAE. **extrafusal muscle f.** Any skeletal muscle fiber other than the modified intrafusal fibers within muscle spindles. **fastigioperiventricular f.'s** Fascicles arising in the fastigial nucleus which leave the anterior cerebellar peduncle to enter the periventricular gray and the dorsal nucleus of the raphe. **flocculo-oculomotor f.'s of Wallenberg-Klimoff** Fascicles passing from the cerebellar flocculus to the oculomotor nuclei. **frontopontine f.'s** TRACTUS FRONTOPONTINUS. **fusimotor f.** γ-EFFERENT. **γ-f.** γ-EFFERENT. **giant f.** GIANT AXON. **gingival f.** A collagen fiber which is an intrinsic component of the gingiva or which enters it from adjacent structures. **Goll's f.'s** Nerve fibers extending from the nucleus gracilis (nucleus of Goll's column) to the cerebellar vermal cortex. **f.'s of Gratiolet** RADIATIO OPTICA. **Gratiolet's radiating f.'s** RADIATIO OPTICA. **gray f.'s** FIBERS OF REMAK. **group I f.** One of the largest sensory fibers in cutaneous or muscle nerves, having a diameter of 12–22 μm and a conduction rate of 72–130 m/s. They supply the primary endings of muscle spindles, tendon organs, and to a lesser degree other mechanoreceptors. **group Ia f.** PRIMARY AFFERENT. **group Ib f.** **1** A large, myelinated axon leading from the sensory terminal in a tendon organ. **2** Such an axon, along with the sensory terminal itself. Also *Ib afferent, Ib fiber, tendon organ afferent.* **group II f.** In mammalian nerves, a myelinated fiber of intermediate diameter, i.e., of 6–12 μm, with variation according to species. It may arise in one of several types of sensory receptors, as in the secondary ending of a muscle spindle. **group III f.** One of the smallest, unmyelinated sensory fibers in cutaneous and muscle nerves, having a diameter of 1–7 μm and a conduction rate of 6–30 m/s. They supply nociceptive, blood-vessel, and hair-follicle receptors. **half-spindle f.** CHROMOSOMAL SPINDLE FIBER. **Herxheimer's f.'s** HERXHEIMER SPIRALS. **IF f.** INTRAFUSAL MUSCLE FIBER. **impulse-conducting f.** PURKINJE'S FIBER. **inhibitory f.'s** Axons whose synaptic action on neuron somata, dendrites, and axons suppresses membrane excitatory events to produce a reduction in membrane potential change and/or the rate of impulse discharge. **interciliary f.'s** The short fibers of the ciliary zonule that are located between the ciliary processes and join the longer fibers so as to serve as supports. *Outmoded.* **intercolumnar f.'s** FIBRAE INTERCRURALES. **intercrural f.'s** FIBRAE INTERCRURALES. **internal arcuate f.'s** FIBRAE ARCUATAE INTERNAE. **internuncial f.'s** Axons connecting neurons, especially neurons intrinsic to the same nuclear group or cortical field. **interzonal f.** CONTINUOUS SPINDLE FIBER. **intrafusal f.** INTRAFUSAL MUSCLE FIBER. **intrafusal muscle f.** One of the specialized muscle fibers in a muscle spindle. In mammals, three distinct types of fibers are distinguished within each spindle by their ultrastructural, histochemical, and contractile characteristics. They are all striated, and have a concentration (or bag) of nuclei at their mid-length. They receive innervation from dynamic fusimotor fibers and are responsible for the dynamic component in stretch sensitivity of the spindle primary ending. Also *intrafusal fiber, IF fiber, intrafusal bag fiber.* **isotropic f.** I BAND. **Korff's f.'s** Channels between odontoblasts which occur during the initial formation of dentin and which resemble corkscrew-shaped fibers when stained with silver. Also *dentinogenic fibers.* **Kühne's f.** MUSCLE SPINDLE. **lattice f.'s** Fibers, such as collagen fibers, arranged in the form of a lattice, as determined by light or electron microscopy. **Lenhossek's f.'s** STILLING'S FIBERS. **f.'s of lens** FIBRAE LENTIS. **light f.'s** Fibers which do not take a histopathologic stain deeply. **longitudinal f.'s of pons** FASCICULI PONTIS LONGITUDINALES. **main f.'s** CHIEF FIBERS. **mantle f.** CHROMOSOMAL SPINDLE FIBER. **Mauthner's f.** One of several types of giant nerve fibers found in the central nervous system of lower vertebrate and invertebrate forms. The Mauthner fibers are derived from a pair of Mauthner neuron cell bodies located in the lower brainstem, one on each side of the midline, in many species of fish and amphibians. Dendrites extend from the Mauthner neuron cell body laterally and ventrally and receive impulses from vestibular, acoustic, cerebellar and trigeminal sources, while the Mauthner fibers cross the midline and descend to the caudal end of the spinal cord, providing a fast-conducting pathway to motoneurons that supply the tail muscles. The Mauthner fiber is an essential part of a reflex mechanism that allows these animals a rapid motor reaction to vibratory and other startling stimuli. **medullated f.'s** MYELINATED FIBERS. **meridional f.'s of ciliary muscle** FIBRAE MERIDIONALES MUSCULI CILIARIS. **f.'s of Meynert** FASCICULUS RETROFLEXUS. **Monakow's f.'s** TRACTUS RUBROSPINALIS. **mossy f.** Myelinated afferent axons to the cerebellar cortex terminating broadly in the granular layer, where they form numerous complex glomerular synaptic arrangements. **motor f.** An efferent axon, arising from a motoneuron in the anterior horn of the spinal cord or a motor nucleus in the brain stem, that innervates several skeletal muscle fibers, constituting a motor unit. **Müller's f.'s** Complex supporting neuroglial elements with oval nuclei and cell bodies in the middle zone of the inner nuclear layer from which long vertical processes extend radially through most of the thickness of the retina between the two limiting membranes and form the internal limiting membrane. Dendritic processes spread horizontally into the plexiform layers and form a network around the bodies of cells in the nuclear and ganglion cell layers. The cell bodies of the radial fibers have recesses and projections which fit around and support bodies of the neighboring nerve cells. Also *sustentacular fibers, retinal gliocytes.* **muscle f.** The single unit of an intact muscle, composed of one or more muscle cells. Also *myofiber* (seldom used). **myelinated f.'s** Axons whitish in appearance due to their covering of myelin. These fibers correspond to the A group of the compound action potential, denoting the fastest impulse-conducting elements. Also *medullated fibers.* **naked f.** An unencapsulated sensory nerve ending that lacks either a myelin sheath or Schwann cell covering. **nerve f.** 1 AXON. 2 The axon with its Schwann sheath, which forms myelin around some axons; the individual unit of a nerve trunk, subdivided into myelinated and unmyelinated fibers. **neuroglial f.** A fibrillar structure in the cytoplasm of a neuroglial cell. **non-**

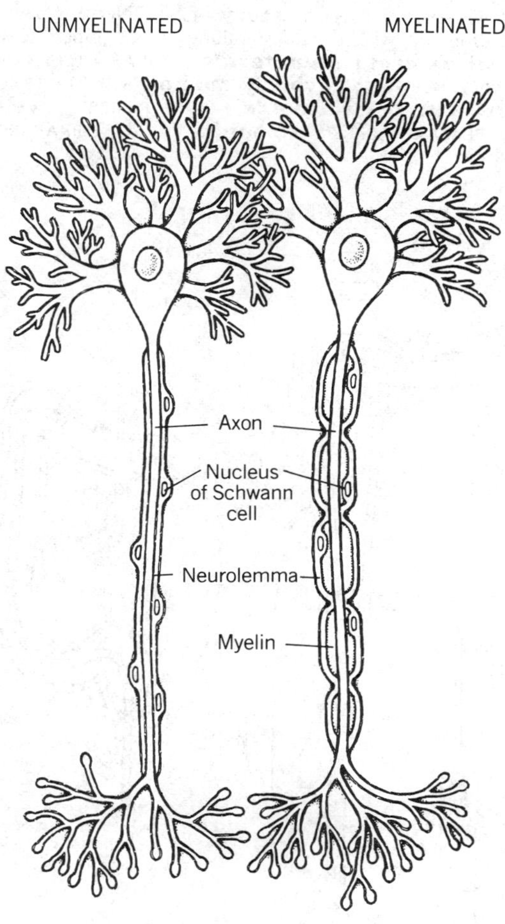


**Nerve fibers**

**medullated f.'s** UNMYELINATED FIBERS. **nuclear bag f.** An intrafusal fiber distinguished by relatively large size and a cluster of as many as 100 nuclei at the midlength. Two types, $bag_1$ and $bag_2$, differing markedly in histochemical, ultrastructural, and contractile characteristics, are usually present in a mammalian muscle spindle. **nuclear chain muscle f.** An intrafusal fiber in mammalian muscle spindles characterized by a chain of nuclei at midlength, extremely fast contraction, and innervation by static fusimotor fibers. **oblique f.'s of stomach** FIBRAE OBLIQUAE GASTRICAE. **olfactory f.'s** NERVI OLFACTORII. **olivocerebellar f.'s** TRACTUS OLIVOCEREBELLARIS. **orbiculoanterocapsular f.'s** Those fibers of the ciliary zonule that extend to the capsule on the posterior surface of the lens and lie close to the vitreous body. *Outmoded.* **orbiculociliary f.'s** Fibers of the ciliary zonule that extend between and beyond the ciliary processes to become continuous with the basement membranes of the superficial layer of epithelial cells over the orbiculus ciliaris. *Outmoded.* **orbiculoposterocapsular f.'s** Long fibers of the ciliary zonule that are continuous with the vitreous membrane. *Outmoded.* **osteocollagenous f.'s** Collagen fibers that develop in osteoid and become part of the bone matrix. **osteogenetic f.'s** The collagen fibers within osteoid around which bone mineralization occurs. Also *osteogenic fibers.* **pale muscle f.** TYPE II MUSCLE FIBER. **pallidohypothalamic f.'s** Efferent axons that arise in the globus pallidus and project to the ventromedial nucleus of the hypothalamus. **pallidothalamic f.'s** See under LENTICULOTHALAMIC TRACT. **palliopontine f.** TRACTUS CORTICOPONTINUS. **parent f.** A muscle fiber which, through longitudinal division (splitting), gives rise to two or more separate fibers. **perforating f.'s** A connective tissue collagen fiber that passes through the cortex of a bone. **periventricular f.'s** FIBRAE PERIVENTRICULARES. **pilomotor f.'s** The unmyelinated nerve fibers supplying the arrector muscles of the hair follicles. **postcommissural f.'s** Axons of the descending column of the fornix that course behind the anterior commissure and terminate in the mamillary nuclei of the hypothalamus. **posterior arcuate f.'s** FIBRAE ARCUATAE EXTERNAE DORSALES. **postganglionic f.'s** Peripheral nerve axons that emanate from sympathetic and parasympathetic ganglia and innervate viscera, glands, and smooth muscle. **precollagenous f.'s** *Obs.* RETICULAR FIBERS. **precommissural f.'s** Axons in the descending column of the fornix that course rostral to the anterior commissure and terminate in the septal nuclei. **preganglionic f.'s** Autonomic axons in peripheral nerves that emanate from cell bodies within the spinal cord or brain stem and terminate in peripheral sympathetic and parasympathetic ganglia. **pressor f.** A sympathetic nerve fiber that causes vasoconstriction and a corresponding rise in blood pressure. **principal f.'s** 1 CHIEF FIBERS. 2 Collagen fibers in the periodontal ligament, attaching the root of a tooth to the bone of the socket. Arranged in bundles, they follow a wavy course and can be grouped as oblique, apical, horizontal, crestal, and transseptal fibers. **projection f.'s** Axons which emanate from a circumscribed neuronal aggregate and which can be traced to a specific distant structure, such as the thalamocortical projection fibers. Also *projection tract.* **Prussak's f.'s** Connective tissue fibers connecting the apex of the lateral process of the malleus with the margins of the tympanic notch bounding the flaccid part of the tympanic membrane. **Purkinje's f.** One of the cardiac muscle cells that are modified for rapid conduction of the excitatory impulse from the atrioventricular node to the ventricular muscle. Also *impulse-conducting fiber.* **pyramidal f.'s of medulla oblongata** FIBRAE PYRAMIDALES MEDULLAE OBLONGATAE. **radiating f.'s of anterior chondrosternal ligaments** LIGAMENTA STERNOCOSTALIA RADIATA. **radicular f.'s** FILA RADICULARIA NERVORUM SPINALIUM. **ragged-red muscle f.'s** The disorganized type I muscle fibers seen in histochemically stained sections in cases of mitochondrial myopathy. **Rasmussen's nerve f.'s** OLIVOCOCHLEAR BUNDLE OF RASMUSSEN. **red muscle f.** TYPE I MUSCLE FIBER. **Reissner's f.** The highly refractile rod extending along the central canal of the spinal cord in primitive vertebrates, believed to be involved in neurosecretory function. In Amphioxus, it originates in the infundibular organ. • It was first described in the cord of Petromyzon by Ernst Reissner in 1860. **f.'s of Remak** Unmyelinated postganglionic axons of the sympathetic nervous system. Also *gray fibers.* **reticular f.'s** Small, connective-tissue fibers identifiable with a silver stain. Also *precollagenous fibers* (obs.). **reticuloreticular f.'s** RETICULORETICULAR TRACT. **ring f.'s** RINGBINDEN. **Ritter's f.** One of a number of fibers lying between the rods and cones of the retina. It was believed to be an optic nerve fiber, but now it is considered to be an artifact. **rod f.'s** Smooth protoplasmic threads of uniform thickness and varying length that connect the rod processes to the cell bodies in the retina. Physiologically, the outer fibers resemble dendrites while the inner fibers resemble axons. **Rolando's f.'s** FIBRAE ARCUATAE EXTERNAE. **Rosenthal f.'s** Eosinophilic masses found in the cytoplasm of astrocytes. They are elongated, carrot-shaped, dense, and homogeneous, and show positive PTAH staining. Associated with advanced, long-standing gliosis, they are seen in such conditions as Alexander's disease, syringomyelia, and juvenile pilocytic astrocytoma. **Sappey's f.'s** Smooth muscle fibers in the medial and lateral check ligaments of the eyeball. **Schroeder's f.'s** STILLING'S FIBERS. **secretomotoric f.'s** Postganglionic, parasympathetic axons the electrical stimulation of which results in secretory activity, such as that elicited by the vasodilator fibers to the submandibular salivary gland. Also *secretomotor nerves, secretory nerves, secretory fibers.* **sensory f.** AFFERENT FIBER. **Sharpey's f.'s** BONE FIBERS. **short association f.'s** Nerve fibers connecting adjacent gyri in the cerebral cortex. **skeletofusimotor f.** $\beta$-EFFERENT. **spinal parasympathetic f.'s** Neurons homologous to parasympathetic fibers which were thought to synapse in the dorsal root ganglia with secondary neurons that innervated skeletal muscle fibers. • The hypothesis has been discredited, and the term is of historical interest only. **spindle f.** Any of the microtubules which form the spindle shaped structure between the poles during mitosis and meiosis, especially those extending from pole to pole (continuous spindle fibers), or those which extend from the centrosome to the centromere (chromosomal spindle fibers). **Stilling's f.'s** Axonal bundles of the formatio reticularis medullae oblongatae. Also *Lenhossek's fibers, Dieters fibers, Schroeder's fibers.* **striated muscle f.** A muscle cell in which the actin and myosin filaments are arranged in a structured pattern. Microscopy reveals a series of transverse bands or stripes across the length of the cells. Such striations can be seen in both cardiac muscle and skeletal muscle. Also *rhabdium* (obs.). **sustentacular f.'s** MÜLLER'S FIBERS. **T f.** An axon that branches at right angles, giving rise to two separate axons extending in opposite directions. This form is typical of axonal bifurcations in sensory ganglion cells. **thalamocortical f.'s** FIBRAE CORTICOTHALAMICAE. **thalamostriate f.'s** THALAMOSTRIATE RADIATION. **Tomes f.** ODONTOBLASTIC PROCESS. **traction f.** CHROMOSOMAL SPINDLE FIBER. **transverse f.'s of pons** FIBRAE PONTIS TRANSVERSAE. **type I muscle f.** A skeletal muscle fiber that is predominantly concerned with slow, tonic contractions. Such fibers contain abundant myoglobin, mitochondria, and oxidative enzymes, yet lack phosphatase enzymes. Also *red muscle fiber, dark fiber.* **type II muscle f.** A skeletal muscle fiber that is predominantly concerned with rapid contractions. Such fibers contain abundant glycogen and phosphatase enzymes but are relatively lacking in mitochondria and oxidative enzymes. Also *pale muscle fiber.* **ultraterminal f.** The final unmyelinated branch of a myelinated axon before it expands to form a synaptic enlargement, such as the motor endplate. **unmyelinated f.'s** Axons lacking a myelin sheath. In peripheral nerves, they are surrounded by Schwann cytoplasm, with several axons per Schwann cell. In the central nervous system, they form bundles lacking a glial sheath. Also *nonmedullated fibers, unmyelinated axons.* **varicose f.'s** Axons displaying variations in diameter along their length in the form of bulges or varicosities. They are often a consequence of postmortem changes. **vasoconstrictor f.'s** Nerve fibers the stimulation of which causes constriction of blood vessels. **vasodilatory f.'s** Nerve fibers the stimulation of which causes dilatation of blood vessels. **ventral external arcuate f.'s** FIBRAE ARCUATAE EXTERNAE VENTRALES. **von Monakow's f.'s** TRACTUS RUBROSPINALIS. **white f.'s** CHIEF FIBERS. **yellow f.'s** ELASTIC FIBERS. **zonular f.'s** FIBRAE ZONULARES.

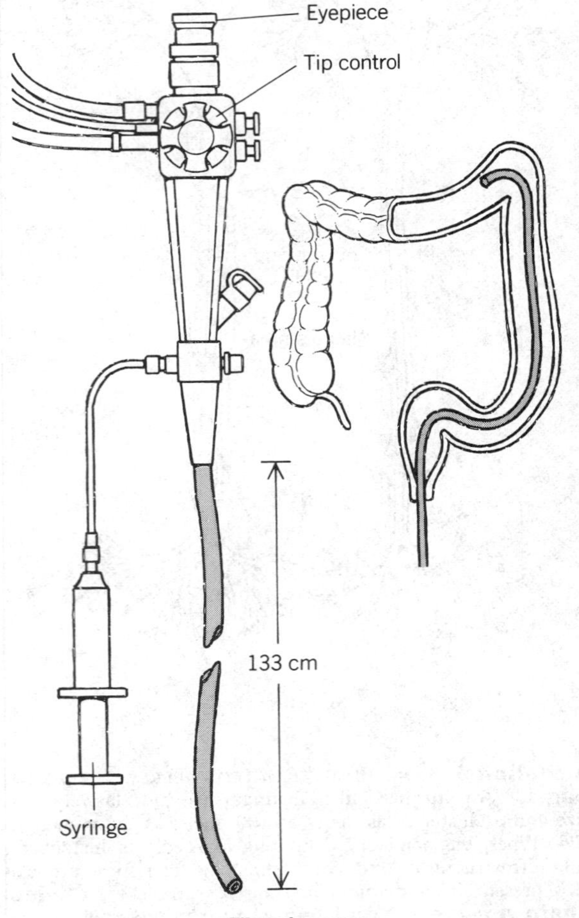


**Fibercolonoscope**

**fibercolonoscope** \-kōlän′əskōp\ [FIBER + COLONOSCOPE] An instrument for examining the colon that utilizes fiberoptics.

**fibergastroscope** \-gas′trəskōp\ [FIBER + GASTRO-

SCOPE] An instrument for examining the stomach that utilizes fiberoptics. Also *gastric fiberscope.*

**fiberglass** \fī′bərglas\ Glass spun in thin fibrous form. It is increasingly used in industry to replace asbestos as an insulating material. It can cause skin irritation, and it possibly affects the respiratory tract. Unlike asbestos exposure, there is no definite evidence that workers exposed to fiberglass risk lung cancer or mesothelioma.

**fiberoptics** \-äp′tiks\ [FIBER + OPTICS] A bundle of parallel thin transparent glass or plastic fibers individually clad with material having a lower index of refraction. The fibers transmit light by total internal reflection. A fiberoptic endoscope bends around corners and transmits images from internal organs to the exterior.

**fiberscope** \fī′bərskōp\ [FIBER + -SCOPE] A flexible instrument used for internal examination that utilizes fiberoptic bundles. Also *fibrescope.* **gastric f.** FIBERGASTROSCOPE.

**fibr-** \fībr-, fibr-\ FIBRO-.

**fibra** \fī′brə\ [L, a ridge between fissures, blade of grass, rootlet] (*pl.* fibrae) A long, threadlike strand of nerve, muscle, or connective tissue. Also *fiber.* **fibrae annulares** Either pars annularis vaginae fibrosae digitorum manus or pars annularis vaginae fibrosae digitorum pedis. **fibrae arcuatae cerebri** [NA] Short arc-shaped bundles of association fibers running through the white matter underlying the cerebral cortex, connecting adjacent gyri. Also *fibrae propriae, arcuate fibers of cerebrum, arcuate fibers.* **fibrae arcuatae externae** Axons that arise from the arcuate nuclei of the medullary pyramid and run laterally on the surface of the medulla oblongata into the inferior cerebellar peduncle. Also *external arcuate fibers, Rolando's fibers.* **fibrae arcuatae externae anteriores** FIBRAE ARCUATAE EXTERNAE VENTRALES. **fibrae arcuatae externae dorsales** [NA] Fascicles of fibers arising in the accessory cuneate nucleus that enter the cerebellum by way of the inferior cerebellar peduncle on the same side. They comprise the fibers in the cuneocerebellar pathway, and transmit afferent proprioceptive impulses from the cervical spinal segments that serve the upper limb. The fibers course to the medulla by way of the fasciculus cuneatus. Also *fibrae arcuatae externae posteriores, posterior arcuate fibers, dorsal arcuate fibers, dorsal external arcuate fibers.* **fibrae arcuatae externae posteriores** FIBRAE ARCUATAE EXTERNAE DORSALES. **fibrae arcuatae externae ventrales** [NA] Fascicles of fibers that arise in the arcuate nuclei located in the ventromedial aspect of the medulla oblongata. Emerging from the ventral median fissure, these fibers course laterally, dorsally, and superiorly over the surface of the medulla to reach the posterior spinocerebellar tract, which they accompany to the cerebellum by way of the inferior cerebellar peduncle. Also *anterior external arcuate fibers, fibrae arcuatae externae anteriores, ventral external arcuate fibers.* **fibrae arcuatae internae** [NA] Axons that arise in the nuclei gracilis and cuneatus and course in a lateroventral arc to form the midline decussation of the medial lemniscus, which terminates principally in the ventral nuclear group of the thalamus. Also *internal arcuate fibers.* **fibrae cerebello-olivares** TRACTUS OLIVOCEREBELLARIS. **fibrae circulares musculi ciliaris** [NA] A sphincteric band of muscle fibers of the ciliary muscle situated internal to the meridional fibers near the base of the iris and close to the periphery of the lens. Also *circular fibers of ciliary muscle, Müller's muscle, Rouget's muscle.* **fibrae corticonucleares** [NA] Axons arising broadly from the cerebral cortex, and in primates principally from the precentral gyrus, that join corticospinal (pyramidal tract) axons in their course through the internal capsule and cerebral peduncles, and then disperse to innervate various somatic motor nuclei of the midbrain, pons, and medulla oblongata. Also *corticobulbar fibers, corticonuclear fibers.* **fibrae corticopontinae** [NA] Axons that arise in the cerebral cortexand descend in the internal capsule and cerebral peduncles together with axons destined to form the pyramidal tracts, but which terminate in various nuclei of the pons. Also *corticopontine fibers.* **fibrae corticoreticulares** [NA] Axons that arise from the cerebral cortex and descend together with corticospinal fibers to terminate on neurons of the pontine and medullary reticular formation. **fibrae corticospinales** [NA] Corticospinal axons arising broadly from the cerebral cortex, and in primates principally from the precentral gyrus. These axons descend through the internal capsule, cerebral peduncles, mesencephalon, and pons, and enter the medullary pyramids before descending into the white matter of the spinal cord. Also *corticospinal fibers, cerebrospinal fibers.* **fibrae corticothalamicae** [NA] Large numbers of corticofugal nerve fibers, derived from neuronal cell bodies located in specific regions of the cerebral cortex, that project to the several thalamic nuclei. Also *corticothalamic fibers, thalamocortical fibers.* **fibrae intercrurales** [NA] Arched transverse fibers of the aponeurosis of the external oblique muscle of the abdomen that pass upward and toward the midline, reinforcing the junction of the crura at the apex of the superficial inguinal ring. Also *intercrural fibers, collateral fibers of Winslow* (outmoded), *intercolumnar fibers, archiform fibers.* **fibrae lentis** [NA] Elongated bands of curved fibers that constitute the substance of the lens of the eye. Young fibers close to the surface have nuclei and narrow serrated edges which interdigitate, forming concentric laminae, while the ends of the fibers meet at the sutures. Older fibers in the dense inner portion of the lens lose their nuclei. The fibers extend from the sutures on the anterior surface to those on the posterior surface, but they do not extend from pole to pole. Also *fibers of lens.* **fibrae meridionales musculi ciliaris** [NA] The outermost fibers of the ciliary muscle which run posteriorly in a longitudinal direction from the pectinate ligament into the stroma of the choroid. There many of them end by branching. Also *meridional fibers of ciliary muscle, fibrae meridionales brueckei* (outmoded), *Brücke's fibers.* **fibrae obliquae gastricae** [NA] The oblique muscle fibers that form the innermost layer of the tunica muscularis of the stomach, being internal to the circular layer. Also *fibrae obliquae ventriculi, oblique fibers of stomach, Gavard's muscle.* **fibrae periventriculares** [NA] Axons within the central gray matter surrounding the third and fourth ventricles and cerebral aqueduct that are believed to originate in the hypothalamus and terminate in the thalamus, midbrain tectum, pontine and medullary reticular formation, and raphe nuclei. A partially myelinated bundle is segregated ventromedially, forming the dorsal longitudinal fasciculus (of Schütz), which runs in the subependymal portion of the central gray, terminating partly on surrounding neurons and partly on the dorsal tegmental nucleus. Also *periventricular fibers.* **fibrae pontis profundae** The deep internal axons of the fibrae pontis transversae. **fibrae pontis superficiales** The more superficial axons of the fibrae pontis transversae. **fibrae pontis transversae** [NA] Axons that arise in the pontine nuclei and course laterally in the ventral pons, where most cross the midline to form the middle cerebellar peduncles. Also *transverse fibers of pons.* **fibrae propriae** FIBRAE ARCUATAE CEREBRI. **fibrae pyramidales medullae oblongatae** Axons within the pyramidal tract surrounding the midline at the base of the medulla oblongata. Also *pyramidal fibers of medulla oblongata, fasciculi pyramidales medullae oblongatae.* **fibrae zonulares** [NA] Fine, elastic filaments that arise from the surface of the epithelium of the ciliary body as far back as the ora serrata and especially from the corona ciliaris and extend to the equatorial region of the lens of the eye. Through their attachments, the ciliary muscle produces changes in the curvature of the lens during accommodation. Collectively they form the zonula ciliaris. Also *zonular fibers.*

**fibrae** \fī′brē\ Plural of FIBRA.

**fibration** \fībrā′shən\ [FIBR- + -ATION] **1** The organizational pattern of a fibrous structure. **2** The process of forming fibers.

**fibre** \fī′bər\ *Brit.* FIBER.

**fibremia** \fībrē′mē·ə\ FIBRINEMIA.

**fibrescope** \fī′bərskōp\ FIBERSCOPE.

**fibril** \fī′bril\ [New L *fibrilla* (dim. of FIBRA) a little fiber] A small fiber or a component of a fiber. Also *fibrilla, microfibril.* **Alzheimer f.** INTRANEURAL FIBRILLARY TANGLE. **axial f.'s** The organs of locomotion in spirochetes, arising near each terminus of the helical protoplasmic cylinder and each extending between that body and the outer envelope. **border f.'s** BRUSH BORDER. **cytoplasmic f.'s** Fine filaments within the cytoplasm of cells, including thin filaments of actin, various intermediate filaments, and thick filaments of myosin. **dentinal f.** A collagen fiber of the matrix of dentin. *Outmoded.* **fibroglia f.'s** FIBROGLIA. **muscle f.** MYOFIBRIL. **nerve f.** NEUROFIBRIL. **young collagen f.'s** Fine collagen fibers that form at the surface of fibroblasts as a result of the condensation of tropocollagen molecules secreted by the cells.

**fibrilla** \fībril′ə\ (*pl.* fibrillae) FIBRIL.

**fibrillar** \fī′brilər\ Characteristic of or resembling a fibril. Also *fibrillary.*

**fibrillate** \fī′brilāt\ [See FIBRILLATION.] To undergo a spontaneous and uncoordinated twitching of individual muscle fibers.

**fibrillated** \fī′brilā′tid\ Composed of fibrils. Also *fibrillate.*

**fibrillation** \fī′brilā′shən\ [*fibrill(a)* + -ATION] Spontaneous contraction of single muscle fibers which can be recorded electromyographically and which is usually a manifestation of denervation, with wallerian degeneration of at least some motor axons. It initially appears three weeks after division of the motor nerve fibers and may persist for as long as the active process of denervation continues. Fibrillation cannot be observed through the skin but may in rare cases be visible in the tongue. Also *fibrillary contraction.* Compare FASCICULATION. **atrial f.** An arrhythmia, characterized by total disorganization of atrial electrical activity, in which multiple wavelets course in a chaotic fashion across the atrium. Impulses are conducted in a random fashion to the ventricles causing ventricular activity which is quite irregular and usually fast. Also *delirium cordis.* **ventricular f.** An arrhythmia characterized by totally disorganized ventricular electrical activity, associated with a clinical picture of cardiac arrest. Abbr. VF

**fibrillogenesis** \fībril′ōjen′əsis\ [*fibrill(a)* + *o* + GENESIS] The formation of fibrils.

**fibrillolysis** \fī′briläl′isis\ The process of destruction and degradation of fibrils.

**fibrin** [*fibr(a)* + -IN] The protein responsible for the formation of a blood clot. It is formed from plasma fibrinogen following removal of anionic peptides by the proteolytic plasma enzyme thrombin. **stroma f.** Fibrin presumed to have arisen from the stroma of blood cells.

**fibrinase** \fī′brinās\ FACTOR XIII.

**fibrinemia** \fī′brinē′mē·ə\ The presence of fibrin in the blood. Also *fibremia.*

**fibrinocellular** \fī′brinōsel′yələr\ Consisting of cells within a fibrin network.

**fibrinogen** \fībrin′əjən\ The precursor of fibrin in clot formation. It is a plasma glycoprotein of about 340 000 daltons, consisting of three pairs of subunits (designated $\alpha$, $\beta$, and $\gamma$). Thrombin induces clotting by the conversion of fibrinogen to fibrin monomer. The monomers then polymerize to form a clot. Also *factor I.* • The variant listed above refers to the roman numeral for 1, not the letter. **human f.** A preparation of fibrinogen obtained from human blood and given therapeutically for the treatment of hypofibrinogenemia.

**fibrinogenesis** \fī′brinōjen′əsis\ The formation of fibrin.

**fibrinogenolysis** \fī′brinōjenäl′isis\ The destruction of fibrinogen by action of an enzyme such as plasmin.

**fibrinogenopenia** \fī′brinōjen′ōpē′nē·ə\ HYPOFIBRINOGENEMIA. Adj. fibrinogenopenic.

**fibrinoid** \fī′brinoid\ [FIBRIN + -OID] Homogeneous, eosinophilic, acellular material resembling fibrin, typically seen in the wall of blood vessels when there is increased endothelial permeability, as in necrotizing vasculitis. **canalized f.** Fibrinoid material with a canalized structure, found on the chorionic plate in late pregnancy. See also LANGHANS STRIA. **placental f.** The fibrin and fibrinoid material which, from early in normal human pregnancy, is found between maternal and fetal tissues and is also related to syncytial villi. This material may prevent escape of placental transplantation antigens to the mother.

**fibrinoligase** \fī′brinäl′igās\ FACTOR XIII.

**fibrinolysis** \fī′brinäl′isis\ The digestion of fibrin, usually by action of an enzyme such as plasmin that is normally present in plasma or by a bacterial enzyme such as streptokinase. Fibrinolysis is usually accompanied by fibrinogenolysis.

**fibrinolytic** \fī′brinōlit′ik\ Of, relating to, or producing fibrinolysis.

**fibrinopeptide** One of the peptides released by thrombin from the N terminus of two of the three chains of fibrinogen to produce fibrin. Each has several negative charges.

**fibrinopurulent** \fī′brinōpyʊr′′ələnt\ Composed of fibrin and pus, as the exudate typically seen in the early stages of the acute inflammatory response, when exudation predominates over suppuration.

**fibrinous** \fī′brinəs\ Like or related to fibrin.

**fibrinuria** \fī′brinoo′rē·ə\ [*fibrin(ogen)* + -URIA] Excretion of fibrinogen or its products in the urine. This is an indication of glomerular damage, usually severe.

**fibro-** \fī′brō-\ [L *fibra* fiber] A combining form meaning fiber, fibrous tissue. Also *fibr-.*

**fibroadenoma** \-ad′ənō′mə\ [FIBRO- + ADENOMA] A benign tumor containing proliferating glandular and stromal components. It is typically found in the female breast. Also *adenoma fibrosum.* **intracanalicular f.** A fibroadenoma of the breast in which the proliferating stroma compresses, elongates, and distorts the glandular elements. **pericanalicular f.** A fibroadenoma of the breast in which the stromal component proliferates in a relatively regular manner around the glandular elements, leading to less distortion than in the intracanalicular form. Also *periacinar fibroadenoma.*

**fibroangioma** \-an′jē·ō′mə\ [FIBRO- + ANGIOMA] An angioma containing much fibrous tissue. • *Sclerosing hemangioma* is more commonly used when a vascular tumor appears to be undergoing involution and fibrosis.

**fibroblast** \fī′brōblast\ [FIBRO- + -BLAST] **1** A connective-tissue cell, usually large and spindle-shaped, with an oval, pale-staining nucleus, and cytoplasmic processes at the ends. The cell functions in the production of fibers and amorphous ground substance. **2** An undifferentiated connective tissue cell which differentiates into chondroblasts, collagenoblasts, and osteoblasts. For defs. 1 and 2 also *inocyte, phorocyte, phoroblast.* **contractile f.** MYOFIBROBLAST.

**fibroblastoma** \-blastō′mə\ [FIBRO- + BLASTOMA] **1** *Outmoded* FIBROMA. **2** *Outmoded* FIBROSARCOMA.

**fibrocalcific** \-kalsif′ik\ Formed largely from connective tissue fibers and impregnated with calcium salts.

**fibrocartilage** \-kär′tilij\ [FIBRO- + CARTILAGE] FIBROCARTILAGO. **f. of the auricle** CARTILAGO AURICULAE. **basal f.** BASILAR CARTILAGE. **basilar f.** SYNCHONDROSIS SPHENO-OCCIPITALIS. **circumferential f.** Fibrocartilage that surrounds a joint. **connecting f.** Fibrocartilage joining two bones as in a synchondrosis. Also *spongy fibrocartilage.* **cotyloid f.** LABRUM ACETABULARE. **elastic f.** Fibrocartilage in which the connective tissue fibers are primarily of the yellow elastic type. Also *yellow fibrocartilage, yellow cartilage, reticular cartilage, elastic cartilage.* **external semilunar f.** MENISCUS LATERALIS ARTICULATIONIS GENUS. **glenoid f.** That part of the fibrocartilaginous palmar and plantar ligaments that is attached to the bases of the proximal phalanges of the digits, providing grooves for the passage of the flexor tendons. Their deep surfaces form parts of the articular facets for the heads of the metacarpal and metatarsal bones, and they are lined by synovial membrane. In the thumb and great toe the grooves articulate with sesamoid bones. *Outmoded.* **interarticular f.** DISCUS ARTICULARIS. **internal semilunar f.** MENISCUS MEDIALIS ARTICULATIONIS GENUS. **intervertebral f.'s** DISCI INTERVERTEBRALES. **intra-articular f.** DISCUS ARTICULARIS. **spongy f.** CONNECTING FIBROCARTILAGE. **sternoclavicular f.** DISCUS ARTICULARIS ARTICULATIONIS STERNOCLAVICULARIS. **stratiform f.** Fibrocartilage found outside the joint spaces in and around tendon sheaths. **white f.** A fibrocartilage in which the connective tissue fibers are primarily of the collagenous type. **yellow f.** ELASTIC FIBROCARTILAGE.

**fibrocartilagines** \-kär′tilaj′inēz\ Plural of FIBROCARTILAGO.

**fibrocartilaginous** \-kär′tilaj′inəs\ Pertaining to or composed of fibrocartilage.

**fibrocartilago** \-kär′tilā′go\ [FIBRO- + CARTILAGO] Cartilage in which the matrix of the chondrocytes, or cartilage cells, consists mainly of bundles of dense white fibrous tissue, or collagen. Transitional between cartilage and connective tissue, it combines toughness with elasticity, and occurs in such tissues as intervertebral and articular disks, labrum acetabulare, and labrum glenoidale. Also *fibrocartilage.* **f. basalis** BASILAR CARTILAGE. **fibrocartilagines intervertebrales** DISCI INTERVERTEBRALES.

**fibrocavitary** \-kav′iter′ē\ A lesion comprised of abscess cavities surrounded by dense fibrosis, characteristic of chronic pulmonary tuberculosis.

**fibrocellular** \-sel′yələr\ Formed largely from connective tissue fibers and cells, with a minimum of intercellular matrix.

**fibrocementoma** \-sē′mentō′mə\ [FIBRO- + CEMENTOMA] CEMENTIFYING FIBROMA.

**fibrochondritis** \-kändrī′tis\ Inflammation of fibrocartilage.

**fibrocongestive** \-känjes′tiv\ Characteristic of the diffuse atrophy and fibrosis in an organ subject to chronic vascular congestion, as in congestive splenomegaly.

**fibrocystic** \-sis′tik\ Containing fibrous and cystic components.

**fibrocyte** \fī′brōsīt\ [FIBRO- + -CYTE] A mature connective-tissue cell. The cytoplasm is less abundant and less basophilic than the cytoplasm of a fibroblast.

**fibrodysplasia** \-displā′zhə\ **1** Dysplasia of fibrous connective tissue. **2** FIBRODYSPLASIA OSSIFICANS PROGRESSIVA. **f. ossificans progressiva** The progressive deposition of heterotopic bone in connective tissue throughout the body, especially in skeletal muscle, tendons, and ligaments. It results in calcified subcutaneous masses, immobility, and death from respiratory compromise. Congenital hallux valgus should arouse suspicion of this disorder. While an autosomal dominant trait, most cases are sporadic and reproduction is markedly limited by the condition. Also *fibrodysplasia ossificans multiplex progressiva, fibrodysplasia, myositis ossificans progressiva, Münchmeyer's disease, Münchmeyer syndrome.* **renal artery f.** An occlusive condition of the renal arteries, characterized pathologically by exuberant ingrowth of smooth muscle cells and fibroblasts. The condition is characterized by multiple stenoses with interspersed aneurysmal dilatations and may cause renovascular hypertension or diminished renal function.

**fibroelastosis** \-il′astō′sis\ [FIBRO- + ELASTOSIS] A form of scar tissue in which there is deposition of elastic as well as fibrous tissue. It is commonly seen in the endocardium, among other sites. **f. cordis** ENDOMYOCARDIAL FIBROELASTOSIS. **endocardial f.** A disorder characterized by thickening of the endocardium with the presence of elastic and collagenous fibers. Primary endocardial fibroelastosis occurs as a lone feature, particularly involving the left ventricle. Secondary fibroelastosis occurs in association with disorders in which the left ventricle is dilated, such as ventricular septal defect or persistent ductus arteriosus. Also *subendocardial sclerosis.* **endomyocardial f.** Congenital thickening of the ventricular mural endocardium with subendocardial changes in the myocardium, mainly evidenced by excessive amounts of fibrous and elastic tissue. Cardiac valves are usually thickened and may be malformed. Some studies suggest a viral etiology. Also *fibroelastosis cordis.*

**fibroendothelioma** [FIBRO- + ENDOTHELIOMA] A tumor with fibrous and endothelial components.

**fibroepithelioma** [FIBRO- + EPITHELIOMA] A tumor with fibrous and epithelial components. **premalignant f.** A skin tumor in which cords of basal cells surround islands of fibrous stroma. It is considered to be a form of basal cell carcinoma. Also *premalignant fibroepithelial tumor.*

**fibrofascitis** \-fəsī′tis\ [FIBRO- + *fasc(ia)* + -ITIS] FASCIITIS.

**fibrogenesis** \-jen′əsis\ The process of synthesizing collagen reticulin or elastic fibers. **f. imperfecta ossium** A rare disorder of bone, caused by a defect in the collagen, that is characterized by multiple fractures and osteoporosis. It resembles osteogenesis imperfecta, but it usually presents in adult life.

**fibroglia** \fībräg′lē·ə\ [FIBRO- + GLIA] Fine connective tissue fibrils attached to the external aspect of a fibroblast after the secretion of tropocollagen molecules by the cell. Also *fibroglia fibrils.*

**fibroid** \fī′broid\ [FIBR- + -OID] LEIOMYOMA.

**fibroidectomy** \fī′broidek′təmē\ [FIBROID + -ECTOMY] The surgical excision of a dense fibrous mass or masses, especially a uterine fibromyoma or leiomyoma. Also *fibromectomy.*

**fibrokeratoma** \-ker′ətō′mə\ A benign keratotic outgrowth, usually from the region of a finger joint. It is probably a response to trauma.

**fibrolaminar** \-lam′inər\ Formed from layers of connective tissue fibers.

**fibroleiomyoma** \-lī′ōmī·ō′mə\ [FIBRO- + LEIOMYOMA] A leiomyoma with a prominent fibrous component.

**fibrolipoma** \-lipō′mə\ [FIBRO- + LIPOMA] A lipoma containing mature fibrous tissue. It is most common in the skin, where it is usually pedunculated. Also *fibroma molle, soft fibroma, lipofibroma, lipoma fibrosum.*

**fibroma** \fībrō′mə\ [FIBR- + -OMA] A benign tumor composed of fibroblasts forming collagen. It can occur in a variety of tissues. Also *fibroblastoma* (outmoded), *fibroplastic tumor, fibrous tumor, desmocytoma.* **ameloblastic f.** A benign jaw tumor with odontogenic epithelium embedded in cellular mesodermal tissue that resembles dental papilla but without odontoblasts. It usually occurs in the mandible of children. **calcified f.** A fibroma containing calcifications. **cementifying f.** A jaw tumor containing cellular fibrous tissue with small basophilic masses of cementumlike tissue. It usually occurs in the mandible of adults. Also *fibrocementoma.* **chondromyxoid f.** A benign tumor characterized by lobulated areas of spindle-shaped or stellate cells with abundant myxoid or chondroid intercellular material, separated by zones of more cellular tissue rich in spindle-shaped or rounded cells with a varying number of multinucleated giant cells of different sizes. Large pleomorphic cells may be present and can result in confusion with chondrosarcoma. This type of lesion is usually situated in the metaphyseal region of a long bone, particularly the upper tibia, and produces an expansion of part of the cortex. Lesions of the tarsal and metatarsal bones are not infrequent. The patients are adolescents or young adults, and males and females are affected in equal numbers. **f. cutis** A fibroma in the skin. **cystic f.** A fibroma containing cysts. **f. durum** A fibroma made firm by the presence of dense mature collagen. Also *hard fibroma.* **endoneural f.** NEUROFIBROMA. **hard f.** FIBROMA DURUM. **irritation f.** An overgrowth of fibrous tissue at the margin of a denture which has been abrading the mucosa for a long time. It is not a true tumor. **f. molle** FIBROLIPOMA. **myxoid f.** FIBROMYXOMA. **nonossifying f.** A lesion of growing children in the metaphyseal regions of long bones, in which bone is replaced by fibrous tissue containing giant cells, hemosiderin, and lipid-laden histiocytes. Also *metaphyseal fibrous defect, nonosteogenic fibroma.* **odontogenic f.** A fibroma occurring in the jaws and containing strands or islands of epithelial cells. Also *fibrous odontoma.* **ossifying f.** An encapsulated neoplasm, mainly of the jaws, that consists of fibrous tissue containing varying amounts of metaplastic bone and mineralized masses that have rounded outlines and few entrapped cells. Although the lesional tissue may be indistinguishable from fibrous dysplasia, it is an encapsulated growth that behaves as a benign neoplasm. Also *fibro-osteoma, osteofibroma.* **parasitic f.** A leiomyoma which detaches from the uterus, finds a new growth site on the peritoneum, and acquires an alternate blood supply. **periapical f.** A fibroma occurring adjacent to the apex of a vital tooth. In some cases it develops into a cementoma. **periungual f.** A fibrous nodule that develops beneath the nail folds in cases of tuberous sclerosis. It is a pathognomic feature of the disease. Also *Koenen's tumor.* **recurrent digital f.** One of a group of disorders of connective tissue in which flesh-colored nodules form on the extensor aspects of the terminal phalanges of the fingers and toes in infants. There is a tendency to recurrence. Spontaneous regression occurs in two to three years. There is abundant normal collagen in the lesions and spindle-shaped cells containing small round intracytoplasmic bodies. The cause is unknown. Also *digital fibromatosis, infantile digital fibromatosis.* **senile f.** CUTANEOUS FIBROUS POLYP. **soft f.** FIBROLIPOMA. **submucous f.** A fibroma developing beneath a mucous membrane and usually projecting into the overlying lumen. **f. of the testis** A benign growth of the testicular tunica which may occur as a solitary, large ovoid tumor or as multiple nodules. Calcification may occur. On palpation, it resembles a bunch of grapes. **f. xanthoma** FIBROUS HISTIOCYTOMA.

**fibromatosis** \-mətō′sis\ [FIBROMA + *t* + -OSIS] A group of tumorlike lesions of fibrous tissue, characterized by active proliferation, and including keloid, nodular fasciitis, palmar, penile, plantar, abdominal, and aggressive fibromatoses, and fibromatosis colli. **aggressive f.** A locally invasive tumorlike proliferation of fibrous tissue. **f. colli** A fibrous proliferation in the sternocleidomastoid muscle, typically occurring in children. It can be bilateral. Contraction of the affected muscle may lead to torticollis. **digital f.** RECURRENT DIGITAL FIBROMA. **gingival f.** A fibrous enlargement of the gingiva, which may be idiopathic or hereditary. The deciduous and permanent dentition may be affected, eruption delayed or prevented and teeth displaced. Another type develops in the posterior regions of the jaws, with eruption of the permanent molar teeth. Also *hereditary gingival enlargement, idiopathic gingival enlargement.* **infantile digital f.** RECURRENT DIGITAL FIBROMA. **palmar f.** Fibromatosis originating in the palmar aponeuroses and leading to Dupuytren's contracture. **plantar f.** Fibromatosis originating in the plantar aponeuroses and leading to progressive contracture of the toes. **pseudosarcomatous f.** NODULAR FASCIITIS. **subcutaneous pseudosarcomatous f.** NODULAR FASCIITIS.

**fibromatous** \fībrō′mətəs\ Relating to or characterized by fibromas.

**fibromectomy** \-mek′təmē\ FIBROIDECTOMY.

**fibromyoma** \-mī·ō′mə\ [FIBRO- + MYOMA] LEIOMYOMA. **f. uteri** LEIOMYOMA UTERI.

**fibromyomectomy** \-mī′ōmek′təmē\ [*fibromyom(a)* + -ECTOMY] The surgical excision of a dense fibromuscular mass or masses.

**fibromyositis** \-mī·ōsī′tis\ Nonspecific inflammation and fibrous replacement of skeletal muscle.

**fibromyotomy** \-mī·ät′əmē\ [*fibromyo(ma)* + -TOMY] A surgical procedure in which an incision is made into one or more fibromuscular masses.

**fibromyxolipoma** \-mik′sōlipō′mə\ MYXOLIPOMA.

**fibromyxoma** \-miksō′mə\ [FIBRO- + MYX- + -OMA] A tumor composed of fibrous and myxomatous tissue. Also *myxofibroma, myxoid fibroma.*

**fibromyxosarcoma** \-mik′sōsärkō′mə\ A sarcoma composed of fibrous and myxomatous elements.

**fibronectin** A protein of the extracellular matrix. It assists cells, especially fibroblasts, to adhere to each other. Fibroblasts derived from tumors produce less fibronectin than do normal ones.

**fibroneuroma** \-nʸurō′mə\ [FIBRO- + NEUROMA] A benign neoplasm occurring in a peripheral nerve and containing both fibrous and neural elements.

**fibroneurosarcoma** \-nʸur′ōsärkō′mə\ [FIBRO- + NEURO- + SARCOMA] **1** A malignant neoplasm occurring in a peripheral nerve and containing both fibrous and neural elements. **2** MALIGNANT SCHWANNOMA.

**fibronuclear** \-noo′klē·ər\ Composed of nucleated fibers.

**fibro-odontoma** \-ō′däntō′mə\ [FIBRO- + ODONTOMA] AMELOBLASTIC FIBRO-ODONTOMA. **ameloblastic f.** A tumor resembling an ameloblastic fibroma but containing dentin and enamel. Also *ameloblastic odontoma, fibro-odontoma.*

**fibro-osteoma** \-äs′tē·ō′mə\ [FIBRO- + OSTEOMA] OSSIFYING FIBROMA.

**fibropapilloma** \-pap′ilō′mə\ A papilloma with a prominent fibrous tissue component. • The term is poor as it emphasizes the stroma but does not describe the epithelial component, as transitional or squamous, of what is basically an epithelial tumor.

**fibroplasia** \-plā′zhə\ [FIBRO- + -PLASIA] The formation of fibrous tissue. **intimal f.** A form of fibromuscular disease of the renal arteries characterized by stenosis related to segmental circumferential fibrous changes in the internal elastic membrane, usually in children and young adults. The condition can be unilateral or bilateral. If the elastic is disrupted, dissecting aneurysms may develop. Hypertension is a common complication, which may be corrected by vascular surgery or nephrectomy. **medial f.** A form of fibromuscular disease of the renal arteries, usually bilateral, characterized by fibrous hyperplasia of the media with microaneurysms which produce a "string-of-beads" appearance on an arteriogram. The condition usually occurs in women from 30 to 50 years of age, and is complicated by hypertension. It may be corrected by surgery. **myointimal f.** A thickening of a damaged vessel's inner lining that follows an episode of trauma, such as vascular surgery. The thickening is brought about by the exuberant ingrowth of fibroblasts and smooth muscle cells. See under FIBROMUSCULAR DISEASE. **retrolental f.** The end stage of oxygen-induced retinopathy of prematurity, in which the detached retina and a mass of fibrovascular tissue lie just behind the lens. Also *Terry syndrome.* **subadventitial f.** A form of fibromuscular disease of the renal arteries, characterized by deposition of collagen in the outer media, usually in women from 20 to 40 years of age. The renal artery, especially on the right, usually is severely stenosed with resultant hypertension, which can be corrected surgically.

**fibroplate** \-plāt\ DISCUS ARTICULARIS.

**fibroreticulate** \-retik′yəlit\ Pertaining to or comprising a network of fibers.

**fibrosarcoma** \-särkō′mə\ [FIBRO- + SARCOMA] A malignant tumor of fibroblastic cells. The histologic appearance is chiefly of interlacing, densely cellular fascicles of spindle cells, often forming a herringbone pattern. Reticulin fibers are closely related to the tumor cells. Collagen production is a constant feature. No other form of cellular differentiation should be present. Mitoses are usually frequent. Pleomorphism may be marked. Metastasis is chiefly by the bloodstream. Also *fibroblastoma* (outmoded). **ameloblastic f.** A malignant odontogenic neoplasm similar to the ameloblastic fibroma but in which the stromal component shows the features of a sarcoma. Also *ameloblastic sarcoma.* **f. of the nerve sheath** MALIGNANT SCHWANNOMA. **odontogenic f.** A very rare fibrosarcoma arising from odontogenic tissue. **f. phyllodes** CYSTOSARCOMA PHYLLODES. **renal f.** An uncommon malignant tumor which arises from the renal capsule. Growth may be rapid, although many such tumors are encapsulated.

**fibrosclerosis** \-sklerō′sis\ Advanced fibrosis where most fibroblasts have been replaced by dense collagen. **multifocal f.** Sclerosis occurring in multiple areas, as in retroperitoneal fibrosis.

**fibrose** \fī′brōs\ To form fibrous tissue; to scar.

**fibroserous** \-sir′əs\ Pertaining to a structure composed of fibrous tissue elements and having a serous surface.

**fibrosis** \fībrō′sis\ [FIBR- + -OSIS] The deposition of collagen, usually in the form of a scar but also in the interstitium, surrounding parenchymal cells. It occurs in the healing stage of inflammation when restoration of normal anatomic integrity is not possible. **bauxite pulmonary f.** BAUXITE PNEUMOCONIOSIS. **condensation f.** The apparent focal increase in fibrous tissue in an organ due to the necrosis and resorption of parenchyma and subsequent approximation of the surviving stroma. **congenital hepatic f.** An idiopathic congenital fibrosis of the liver, usually accompanied by bile ductular proliferation within the fibrotic bands. Also *congenital hepatic cirrhosis.* **cystic f.** An autosomal recessive disorder characterized by a decreased pancreatic exocrine function that leads to maldigestion, decreased mucociliary transport with chronic sinopulmonary infections, and abnormal sweat gland function which causes high electrolyte concentrations. It is usually diagnosed in infancy on account of meconium ileus or failure to thrive, or in early childhood because of pulmonary infections. Mild variants may escape detection until adulthood. The effects of the disorder include sterility, deafness, and intraocular damage. The worst effects are seen in the bronchial tree, where the infected, viscid secretions cannot be eliminated and chronic bronchopneumonia leads to death in childhood, adolescence, or early adult life. Survival has been extended through aggressive treatment until the third decade on average. It is the most common lethal condition in Caucasian children, with a heterozygote frequency of 1 in 40. Also *cystic fibrosis of pancreas, mucoviscidosis, fibrocystic disease of pancreas, congenital pancreatic steatorrhea* (older term). **cystic f. of pancreas** CYSTIC FIBROSIS. **diffuse interstitial pulmonary f.** Widespread accumulation of fibrous tissue in alveolar walls and interstitial tissues of the lungs. Also *interstitial pneumonia, cirrhosis of the lung* (obs.), *pulmonary cirrhosis.* **endomyocardial f.** A form of restrictive cardiomyopathy characterized by pronounced thickening of the endocardium and adjacent myocardium by dense fibrous tissue. The fibrosis involves the ventricles and sometimes extends to the atrioventricular valves, particularly the mitral valve. The condition is endemic in Africa and its etiology is unknown. Also *endocardial fibrosis, subendocardial sclerosis.* **glomerular f.** The presence of collagen in the glomerular mesangial region, segmental scars, or in fibrous crescents. Small deposits of collagen can be seen only on electron microscopy, but larger amounts are demonstrable on light microscopy. **hepatic f.** Fibrosis in the liver, usually the result of previous inflammation and a necessary component of hepatic cirrhosis. **idiopathic retroperitoneal f.** Fibrosis of the peritoneal tissue, resulting at times in compression of the great vessels and the ureters. Also *retroperitoneal fibrosis, periureteritis plastica, Ormond's disease, perirenal fasciitis.* **mediastinal f.** Fibrosis occurring within the mediastinum and often compressing the mediastinal structures. Also *fibrous mediastinitis, indurative mediastinitis.* **neoplastic f.** PROLIFERATIVE FIBROSIS. **panmural f. of the bladder** CHRONIC INTERSTITIAL CYSTITIS. **periureteric f.** Retroperitoneal fibrosis causing ureteric obstruction. **pipestem f.** SYMMERS PIPESTEM FIBROSIS. **pleural f.** The presence of abnormal amounts of fibrous tissue in the pleura. **postfibrinous f.** Organization and fibrosis of a fibrinous exudate. **progressive massive f.** An advanced form of pneumoconiosis in which simple pneumoconiosis progresses to form one or more masses of fibrous tissue intermingled with dust, usually located in the upper part of the lung. Its cause is unknown, but it is probably related to dust burden and possibly to an immunologic process. It occurs in coal miners and has been described as a complication of other pneumoconioses. Also *complicated pneumoconiosis, collagenous pneumoconiosis.* **proliferative f.** Excessive production of fibrous elements that continues after the stimulus has ceased. Also *neoplastic fibrosis.* **pulmonary f.** The accumulation of abnormal quantities of fibrous tissue in the lung. **renal f.** The presence of collagen anywhere in the kidney, involving glomeruli or the interstitium of the cortex, medulla, or capsule. Fibrosis of the renal cortex can occur in almost any renal disease, but is especially common in nephrosclerosis, chronic glomerulonephritis, and interstitial nephritis. **retroperitoneal f.** IDIOPATHIC RETROPERITONEAL FIBROSIS. **root sleeve f.** Fibrosis of the dural covering of the spinal nerves and/or nerve roots as they pass through the intervertebral foramina. **Symmers pipestem f.** Periportal and perilobular fibrosis of the liver in schistosomiasis, occurring in response to trapped embolic eggs and egg products of schistosomes, especially *Schistosoma mansoni.* This condition results in characteristic, grossly observable accumulations of white fibrotic tissue. Also *pipestem fibrosis, Symmers fibrosis.*

**fibrositis** \-sī′tis\ [New L *fibros(us)* (from L *fibr(a)* fiber, filament + *-osus* -OSE) fibrous + -ITIS] A condition of uncertain cause characterized by diffuse myalgia, sometimes with trigger points. Some authorities feel this is a psychological illness, others regard it as physiologic. Also *intramuscular fibrositis, rheumatoid myositis.* **traumatic f.** A nonspecific inflammation of fibrous tissue caused by single or multiple traumatic episodes, resulting in painful, tender areas and joint motion limitations or muscle weakness.

**fibrosplenomegaly** \-splē′nōmeg′əlē\ Splenomegaly with fibrosis. **congestive f.** CHRONIC CONGESTIVE SPLENOMEGALY.

**fibrothorax** \-thôr′aks\ Fibrosis of the pleural space, often causing adhesion of the pleural surfaces, seen as opacified hemithorax on chest radiograph. Thick, nonexpansile fibrous tissue may lead to restriction of lung motion. Also *pachypleuritis.*

**fibrotic** \fībrät′ik\ Characterized by fibrosis.

**fibrous** \fī′brəs\ Characterized by, composed of, or resembling fibers.

**fibrovascular** \-vas′kyələr\ Formed primarily from connective tissue fibers with a good supply of blood vessels.

**fibroxanthoma** \-zanthō′mə\ [FIBRO- + XANTHOMA] FIBROUS HISTIOCYTOMA.

**fibula** \fib′yələ\ [L (from *fi(gere)* to fasten, fix + *-bula,* instrumental suffix) a clasp, buckle, brace, pin] [NA] The slender lateral, or outer, bone of the leg, articulating with the tibia superiorly and taking part in the ankle joint inferiorly. It is less important than the tibia as a weightbearing bone. Also *fibular bone, perone, canna minor* (outmoded), *paracnemis* (outmoded), *paracnemidion* (outmoded).

**fibular** \fib′yələr\ Pertaining or belonging to the fibula. Also *peroneal, fibularis.*

**fibulation** \fib′yəlā′shən\ INFIBULATION.

**-fic** \-fik\ [L *-ficus* (from *facere* to do, make + *-us,* adj. or noun ending), causative suffix] A combining form meaning making or causing.

**-fication** \-fikā′shən\ [-FIC + -ATION] A suffix denoting the process of making.

**Fick** [Adolf Eugen *Fick,* German physician, 1829–1901] **1** See under METHOD. **2** Fick formula. See under PRINCIPLE.

**ficosis** \fīkō′sis\ [L *fic(us)* a fig + -OSIS] SYCOSIS.

**Fiedler** [Carl Ludwig Alfred *Fiedler,* German physician, 1835–1921] **1** Fiedler's myocarditis. See under ACUTE ISOLATED MYOCARDITIS. **2** Fiedler's disease. See under ICTERIC LEPTOSPIROSIS.

**field** **1** An area or surface that can be seen or defined, as in function or extent. **2** In microscopy, the area which can be viewed at one time with a particular lens system. **3** The space surrounding a charged particle or other force-creating body, throughout which the force is effective. **adversive f.** Any region of the cerebral cortex which upon stimulation causes turning of the head and eyes and sometimes of the body toward the opposite side. **auditory f.** The primary auditory receptive area of the cerebral cortex. **binocular f.** The area that can be seen with both eyes simultaneously. This excludes the 30° temporal monocular field of each eye. **centrocecal area of f.** See under AREA. **Cohnheim's f.'s** Myofibrillar areas seen in cross-section of muscle fiber. **developmental f.** MORPHOGENETIC FIELD. **electromagnetic f.** **1** The field by means of which electrically charged bodies interact. **2** A region in which there exist electric and/or magnetic fields. **electrostatic f.** The region surrounding a charged body or particle throughout which another charged body will experience a force of attraction or repulsion. **far f.** **1** That region of the field where the angular field distribution is independent of distance. **2** In ultrasound, the region of the sound beam beyond the distance $r^2/\lambda$ where r is the radius of the transducer and $\lambda$ is the wavelength. It is the region of the sound beam in which the beam diameter increases as the distance from the transducer increases. Also *Fraunhofer zone, far zone.* **f. of fixation** The extent of excursion, measured in degrees, of which the eye is capable in the various directions of gaze. **Flechsig's f.** MYELINOGENETIC FIELD. **Forel's f.** H FIELDS OF FOREL. **frontal eye f.** The region of the cerebral cortex of the frontal lobe, corresponding approximately to area 8 of Brodmann, from which adversive (nonconjugate) eye movements can be elicited by electrical stimulation. Also *eye area, frontal adversive field.* **H f.'s of Forel** An H-shaped configuration of myelinated fibers as seen on coronal section of the prerubral portion of the cerebrum. It is comprised of a ventral stratum of incoming fibers from the lenticular nucleus (fasciculus lenticularis) and a dorsal layer of emergent fibers (fasciculus thalamicus), which together embrace the zona incerta and merge medially as the ansa lenticularis. Also *area Foreli, Forel's field.* **f. $H_1$ of Forel** FASCICULUS THALAMICUS. **f. $H_2$ of Forel** FASCICULUS LENTICULARIS. **high-power f.** The portion of a microscope slide visible under a high-power objective lens. It is the basis for quantifying discrete objects. **individuation f.** A localized region within a developing embryo which is influenced by the presence of a single modifying substance or organizer. The organizer has the ability to rearrange the regional structure of both itself and the adjacent tissue so that they form part of an integrated embryo. **low-power f.** The portion of a microscope slide seen when a low-magnification objective lens system is used. It serves as a unit of areal measure for calculating the concentration of discrete objects. **magnetic f.** A condition in a region of space in the neighborhood of a magnet or of an electric current, characterized by the existence of a torque on a test magnet. **morphogenetic f.** The region of an embryo which is generally larger than its main derivatives, out of which definite structures, such as organs, normally develop. Also *developmental field.* **myelinogenetic f.** Any fiber pathways or tracts in the central or peripheral nervous system in which the process of myelination is taking place or about to take place. Also *Flechsig's field.* **near f.** 1 That region of the field between the antenna and the far field. 2 In ultrasound, the region of the beam within a distance of $r^2/\lambda$ where r is the radius of the transducer and λ is the wavelength. It is the region of a beam in which the beam diameter decreases as the distance from the transducer increases. Also *Fresnel zone, near zone.* **occipital eye f.** The cerebral cortex surrounding the calcarine fissure, including striate (area 17) and peristriate fields (areas 18 and 19), the electrical stimulation of which elicits conjugate eye movements towards the opposite side. **perceptual f.** The totality of all aspects of the external world of which the individual is aware at a given moment. The sensory field, created by sense organ reactivity to actual objects in the outer world, interacts with the mental set of the individual and with the effects of prior experience so that what is perceived is an active process and not a mere registration of stimuli reaching the sense organs. **prefrontal eye f.** FRONTAL EYE FIELD. **primary nail f.** The earliest sign of the development of the nail as a flattened plate on the terminal phalanx of a finger or toe. **receptive f.** 1 The area of skin or deeper structures capable upon adequate stimulation of exciting a discharge in a sensory axon, nerve, root, or rootlet. It represents the extent of ramification of the axons. 2 SENSITIVE AREA. **subicular f.'s** The cytoarchitectonically defined cortex of the hippocampal gyrus, lateral to the hippocampus proper and medial to the rhinal fissure. It is sometimes subdivided into subiculum, presubiculum, and prosubiculum and is often considered a part of the hippocampus distinct from the CA fields. **surplus f.** The remaining portion of the visual field on the side of an incomplete hemianopsia. **tactile f.** An area concerned with touch sensation within which it is not possible to distinguish two stimuli applied simultaneously. **visual f.** The area that is visible to an eye at a given position. Also *field of vision.* **Wernicke's f.** 1 The myelinated fibers traversing the lateral posterior and pulvinar nuclei of the thalamus. 2 The cortical field comprising Wernicke's area in the posterior superior temporal gyrus, including the supramarginal and angular gyri. This area is believed to be a speech center.

**field-dependent** Characterizing those persons whose interpretation of events occurring within their perceptual field is strongly governed by cues supplied by the surrounding frame of reference. Such individuals, when attempting to adjust to a true vertical a luminous rod viewed in a darkened room, are more influenced by the position of a surrounding luminous square which is also slightly tilted than are field-independent subjects, who reposition the rod in a way less influenced by the immediate embedding context.

**Fielding** [George Hunsley *Fielding,* English anatomist and ophthalmologist, 1801–1871] Fielding's membrane. See under TAPETUM.

**Fiessinger** [Noel *Fiessinger,* French physician, 1881–1946] 1 Fiessinger-Leroy-Reiter syndrome. See under REITER SYNDROME. 2 Fiessinger-Rendu syndrome. See under STEVENS-JOHNSON SYNDROME.

**fièvre** \fē·ev′r\ [French, fever] Fever. **f. boutonneuse** BOUTONNEUSE FEVER.

**FIGLU** formiminoglutamic acid.

**figure** [L *figura* (akin to *fingere* to shape, mold, fashion) a form, shape, figure] 1 A shape or outline. 2 An amount or a number representing it. 3 A person taken to be representative of a type or role. **achromatic f.** MITOTIC APPARATUS. **chromatic f.** The pattern formed by the chromosomes during mitosis or meiosis. Also *nuclear figure.* **fortification f.** TEICHOPSIA. **mitotic f.** MITOTIC APPARATUS. **myelin f.** A lysosome that contains a laminated structure composed of incompletely digested cytoplasmic membranes. **nuclear f.** CHROMATIC FIGURE. **Stifel's f.** A white spot upon a dark background, intended for demonstration of the physiologic blind spot.

**fila** \fī′lə\ Plural of FILUM.

**filament** \fil′əmənt\ [L *filamentum* (from *filare* to spin, from *filum* a thread + *-mentum* -MENT) a small thread] A long, threadlike structure. Also *filamentum.* **acrosomal f.** A thin, stiff filament projecting from the head of the spermatozoon, formed by elongation of a central part of the acrosome. It plays a part in penetration of the ovum at fertilization. **actin f.** One of the smaller of the two types of myofilament that can be demonstrated in skeletal muscle by electron microscopy. They are attached at one end to the Z band and the other ends interdigitate with the myosin filaments. **axial f.** AXONEME. **intermediate f.** One of the fibrous components of the cytoskeleton of a cell. Such filaments are approximately 10 nm in diameter and are intermediate in size between microfilaments and the large filaments such as myosin. **linin f.** The threadlike achromatic material which forms a network in the nucleus of a cell. The chromatin appears as granules along the filaments. **root f.'s of spinal nerves** FILA RADICULARIA NERVORUM SPINALIUM. **spermatic f.** A short segment at the end of the tail of a spermatozoon, characterized by lack of a sheath and with irregular arrangement and extent of the axial fibrile. **terminal f.** FILUM TERMINALE. **terminal f. of spinal dura mater** FILUM DURAE MATRIS SPINALIS.

**filamenta** \fil′əmen′tə\ Plural of FILAMENTUM.

**filamentation** \fil′əmentā′shən\ [FILAMENT + -ATION] A shape change manifested by bacilli growing in adverse conditions, as in the presence of antibodies or antibiotics, wherein normal, short, rod-shaped forms change to elongated threadlike forms. Also *thread reaction.*

**filamentous** \fil′əmen′təs\ Forming or consisting of filaments.

**filamentum** \fil′əmen′təm\ FILAMENT.

***Filaria*** \filer′ē·ə\ [See FILARIA.] A genus of secernentean (phasmidian) nematodes of the superfamily Filarioidea, family Filariidae. The genus formerly included all of the filarial worms with microfilariae, but these have been assigned to

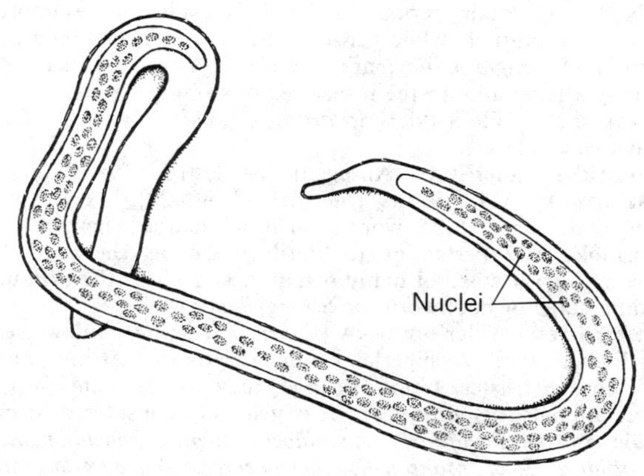


**Filaria** (microfilaria of *Wuchereria bancrofti*)

families such as Onchocercidae, Dirofilariidae, and Dipetolonematidae in the superfamily Onchocercoidea. Only a few species, chiefly mustelid parasites, remain as true members of the genus, the related cattle filariae being assigned to the genus *Parafilaria*. ***F. bancrofti*** WUCHERERIA BANCROFTI. ***F. demarquayi*** MANSONELLA OZZARDI. ***F. diurna*** LOA LOA. ***F. immitis*** DIROFILARIA IMMITIS. ***F. juncea*** MANSONELLA OZZARDI. ***F. loa*** LOA LOA. ***F. malaya*** BRUGIA MALAYI. ***F. medinensis*** DRACUNCULUS MEDINENSIS. ***F. nocturna*** WUCHERERIA BANCROFTI. ***F. ozzardi*** MANSONELLA OZZARDI. ***F. streptocerca*** MANSONELLA STREPTOCERCA. ***F. volvulus*** ONCHOCERCA VOLVULUS.

**filaria** \filer′ē·ə\ [L *filum* thread + -ARIA] (*pl.* filariae) Any nematode in the suborder Filarina (including the superfamilies Filarioidea and Onchocercoidea) but especially any onchocercid nematode that has microfilariae parasitic in the blood or tissues of the host. **Bancroft's f.** A filarial nematode of the species *Wuchereria bancrofti*. **Brug's f.** A filarial nematode of the species *Brugia malayi*.

**filariae** \filer′i·ē\ Plural of FILARIA.

**filarial** \filer′ē·əl\ Of or pertaining to filariae.

**filariasis** \fil′ərī′əsis\ [*Filar(ia)* + -IASIS] Infection with filarial nematode worms, common in many tropical and subtropical regions, especially west Africa, India, southeast Asia, and South America. Adult worms live in the lymphatics, skin, connective tissue, or serous membranes, producing live embryos (microfilariae). *Wuchereria bancrofti* and *Brugia malayi* are associated with lymphatic obstruction, which may result in elephantiasis and chyluria. *Onchocerca volvulus* causes river blindness, rashes, and subcutaneous nodules. *Loa loa* is responsible for Calabar swellings. *Dracunculus medinensis* (the guinea worm) causes dracontiasis. Other species are less pathogenic. Inflammation and lymphatic obstruction may continue after the death of the worms. **Bancroft's f.** Infection with *Wuchereria bancrofti*. Also *bancroftian filariasis, bancroftiasis*. **Brug's f.** MALAYAN FILARIASIS. **Malayan f.** A filarial infection caused by *Brugia malayi* and transmitted by *Mansonia* and *Anopheles* mosquitoes. The disease occurs in Malaysia, Borneo, Indonesia, India, and much of southeast Asia. It is characterized by lymphatic obstruction and lymphangitis as occur in *Wuchereria bancrofti* infections. The swelling, however, is usually more distal and is usually confined to the arms below the elbows and to the legs below the knees. Also *filariasis malayi, Brug's filariasis*. **Ozzard's f.** Infection with *Mansonella ozzardi* filariae. **periodic f.** Filariasis in which microfilariae are found in the bloodstream only during certain periods in the daily cycle. For example, *Loa loa* is diurnal, while certain strains of *Wuchereria bancrofti* and *Brugia malayi* are nocturnal. This periodicity is usually attributable to the insect vector's biting habits.

**filaricidal** \filer′isī′dəl\ [*filari(a)* + *-cid(e)* + -AL] Destructive to filariae.

**filaricide** \filer′isīd\ An agent that destroys filariae.

**filariform** \filer′ifôrm\ [*filari(a)* + -FORM] **1** Resembling small nematode worms such as filariae; hairlike or threadlike. **2** Pertaining to filariform larvae, the third or infective larval stage of many nematodes, such as the skin-invading stage of hookworm or *Strongyloides* larvae.

**Filarioidea** \filer′ē·oi′dē·ə\ [*Filari(a)* + *-oidea*, suffix used for higher taxa] A superfamily of nematodes that are parasitic in the tissues, blood, or body cavities of many vertebrate animals including man. It is generally considered to include *Filaria, Parafilaria, Acanthocheilonema, Dipetalonema, Dirofilaria, Loa, Mansonella, Onchocerca, Wuchereria,* and *Brugia*. In some classifications, the superfamily Filarioidea includes only the family Filariidae with only the genera *Filaria* and *Parafilaria* of medical or veterinary interest, while the other genera (possessing microfilariae) are placed in a separate superfamily, Onchocercoidea, in the family Onchocercidae.

**filarious** \filer′ē·əs\ **1** Pertaining to or due to filariae. **2** Infected with filariae.

**Filatov** [Nils Feodorovich *Filatov*, Russian pediatrician, 1847–1902] **1** Filatov-Dukes disease. See under EXANTHEM SUBITUM. **2** Filatov's disease. See under INFECTIOUS MONONUCLEOSIS.

**Filatov** [Vladimir Petrovich *Filatov*, Russian ophthalmologist, 1875–1956] **1** Filatov flap. See under TUBED FLAP. **2** Filatov-Gillies tubed pedicle. See under PEDICLE.

**Fildes** [Paul Gordon *Fildes*, English bacteriologist, born 1882] See under LAW.

**file** [Old English *fīl, fēol* ] Any of various instruments having a hard, ridged surface that can be applied abrasively to another surface to cut, smooth, or polish it. **root canal f.** A fine tapering wire with a fine-pitch thread, used to scrape the sides of root canals. It is held in the fingers and used with a push-pull action.

**filial** \fil′ē·əl\ Pertaining to offspring with respect to the parental generation.

**filiform** \fil′ifôrm\ Having the form of a filament; threadlike.

**filigree** \fil′igrē′\ An open arrangement of fine silver or stainless steel wire.

**fillet** \fil′it\ **1** LEMNISCUS. **2** To surgically remove a bone so that only soft tissue remains, such as removing a phalanx in order to correct the deformity in a toe.

**filling** **1** The act of putting into a prepared cavity or root canal a material that acts as a substitute for the lost tooth substance. **2** The finished restoration produced by filling. **complex f.** COMPOUND FILLING. **composite f.** A filling made with a mixture of a setting resin and siliceous particles. **compound f.** A filling which involves more than one surface of a tooth, such as a mesio-occlusal filling. Also *complex filling*. **direct f.** A filling created by placing a plastic material into the cavity, where it sets. **indirect f.** A filling created by taking an impression and making a model of the prepared cavity. The restoration is then prepared to fit the model, usually in cast gold, and is subsequently cemented into the prepared cavity. **postresection f.** A root canal filling placed after an apicoectomy, usually from the apical end of the root canal. Also *retrograde filling, retrofilling, retrograde amalgam*. **retrograde f.** POSTRESECTION FILLING.

**film** [Middle English *filme*, from Old English *filmen, fylmen* membrane, akin to Gk *pelma* sole of the foot or shoe and to Old English *fell* skin] **1** A thin coating or layer. **2** A roll or sheet of material coated with an emulsion to render it light-sensitive or sensitive to other forms of radiant energy for producing photographs, roentgenograms, or other visual records. **baseline f.** A roentgenogram which is used as a reference for comparison with subsequent similar roentgenograms of the same area. **bite-wing f.** BITE-WING RADIOGRAPH. **fibrin f.** A substitute membrane made of human fibrin, usually used to repair defects in the dura. **nonscreen f.** Radiographic film intended for use without intensifying screens. **occlusal f.** OCCLUSAL RADIOGRAPH. **panoramic x-ray f.** PANORAMIC RADIOGRAPH. **periapical f.** PERIAPICAL RADIOGRAPH. **port f.** A roentgenogram, usually made with the radiation source for treatment, to demonstrate the size, shape, and location of the area being treated. **precorneal f.** The tear film upon the corneal surface. **preliminary f.**

SCOUT FILM. **scout f.** A plain film taken prior to radiologic examination with contrast medium, such as in intravenous urography or barium enema. Also *preliminary film, survey radiograph.* **spot f.** A rapid-exposure roentgenogram taken during fluoroscopy. **stripping f.** A film, used for autoradiography, having a sensitive photographic emulsion which can be stripped from a prepared matrix, the emulsion being applied directly to the section of the radionuclide-containing specimen for exposure and later developed. **x-ray f.** A very thin flexible transparent sheet of plastic, e.g., cellulose acetate, coated on one side or both sides with a radiant-energy sensitive emulsion, used in radiology. The term is used for both nonexposed and exposed film.

**filopod** \fil′əpäd\ FILOPODIUM.

**filopodia** \fī′ləpō′dē·ə\ Plural of FILOPODIUM.

**filopodium** \fī′ləpō′dē·əm\ [*fil(um)* + *o* + *(pseudo)-podium*] (*pl.* filopodia) A slender, hyaline pseudopodium largely composed of ectoplasm that is seen in certain free-living amebas. The pseudopodia often anastomose, fuse locally, and form thin sheets of cytoplasm. Also *filopod.*

**filter** [French *filtre* (from Italian *filtro* a filter, from Late Med L *filtrum* a filter, from Germanic *filt(iz)* felt) a filter] **1** A device that traps particles suspended in a fluid (liquid or gas) that is passed through it. **2** A device or material through which a mixture of penetrating radiations can pass, but which selectively absorbs some components (usually those with lower energy, or longer wavelength) more than others, thus "purifying" the transmitted beam. **band-pass f.** A component of an electronic amplifying system, designed to pass a desired range of frequencies while attenuating undesired noise above and below this range. This improves the signal-to-noise ratio. **band-stop f.** A filter that rejects a band of frequencies and passes higher and lower frequencies. **barrier f.** A filter used in fluorescence microscopy to protect the eye of the viewer from exposure to light of the wavelengths that excite the fluorochrome. **excitation f.** A filter used in fluorescence microscopy that restricts the light reaching the specimen to only those wavelengths capable of exciting the fluorochrome. **Greenfield f.** A caval interruption device that is designed to be inserted transvenously, either through the jugular or femoral route, into the inferior vena cava. There it remains permanently to block thrombi from embolizing to the central pulmonary circulation. **high-pass f.** A component of an electronic amplifying system designed to pass desired high frequencies while attenuating undesired noise below a selected cutoff frequency. This improves the signal-to-noise ratio. **low-pass f.** A component of an electronic amplifying system, designed to pass desired low frequencies while attenuating all undesired noise above a selected cutoff frequency. This improves the signal-to-noise ratio. **membrane f.** A filter of graded porosity, usually made of nitrocellulose. It may be used to sterilize media, to prepare culture filtrates, and to enumerate bacteria in dilute suspensions, as in water bacteriology, by collection on the filter followed by its incubation in contact with the surface of a solid medium. **notch f.** A filter that rejects a narrow band of frequencies and passes higher and lower frequencies. **Thoraeus f.** A filter consisting primarily of tin, usually about 0.44 mm, backed by 0.25 mm Cu and 1.0 mm Al, used to harden the beam in high-voltage radiation therapy. **ultraviolet f.** A filter that only transmits light rays of the ultraviolet range. It is used in microscopy, spectrophotometry, photography, and in the excitation of fluorescence. **umbrella f.** A filter in the shape of an umbrella placed in the inferior vena cava to prevent pulmonary embolism. **wedge f.** A filter of graduated thickness, used to cause a progressive decrease in the dose rate across a radiation beam. **Wood's f.** A glass that contains 9 percent nickel oxide and only transmits light that exceeds 365 nm. It is used in the Wood's lamp with ultraviolet light.

**filterable** \fil′tərəbl\ Small enough in particle size to pass through a filter of a given pore size. Also *filtrable.*

**filtrable** \fil′trəbl\ FILTERABLE.

**filtrate** \fil′trāt\ That portion of a solution that passes through a filter. **bacterial f.** The filtrate from a bacterial culture which has been passed through a filter fine enough to retain the bacterial cells. **Folin's protein-free f.** A preparation of blood serum from which proteins have been removed by precipitation with sodium tungstate and sulfuric acid, with the resulting chocolate brown semisolid material removed by filtration through filter paper. **glomerular f.** The ultrafiltrate of plasma formed across the glomerular capillary wall. All diffusible solutes of plasma appear in the glomerular filtrate in the same concentration as in plasma, corrected for Donnan's equilibrium.

**filtration** \filtrā′shən\ **1** Separation of particulate matter from solution by passage through a filter. **2** Sterilization of fluids by passage through a membrane or other filter with fine enough pores to retain all bacteria. **3** The interposition of a radiation-absorbing material that allows only a selective range of wavelengths to pass through. **gel f.** See under GEL FILTRATION CHROMATOGRAPHY. **glomerular f.** The ultrafiltration of solutes from the blood across the glomerular capillary basement into the Bowman space.

**filtrum** \fil′trəm\ PHILTRUM. **Merkel's f.** FILTRUM VENTRICULI. **f. ventriculi** A shallow, vertical furrow between the corniculate cartilage and the cuneiform cartilage in the posterior part of the aryepiglottic fold. Inferiorly it is continuous with the sinus of the larynx. . *Outmoded.* Also *Merkel's fossa, Merkel's filtrum.*

**filum** \fī′ləm\ [L (perhaps akin to *fibra* rootlet or to *funis* rope) a thread, string, filament] (*pl.* fila) A threadlike structure. **fila anastomotica nervi acustici** The nerve filaments extending between the seventh and eighth nerve roots. **f. durae matris spinalis** [NA] The slender, connective-tissue continuation of the filum terminale of the spinal cord, forming the coccygeal ligament, which fuses with the posterior periosteal surface of the coccyx. Also *filum of spinal dura mater, terminal filament of spinal dura mater.* **fila olfactoria** NERVI OLFACTORII. **fila radicularia nervorum spinalium** [NA] The threadlike filaments of the dispersed axonal bundles of the dorsal and ventral roots of the spinal cord. Also *root filaments of spinal nerves, fila radicularia, radicular fibers.* **f. of spinal dura mater** FILUM DURAE MATRIS SPINALIS. **f. terminale** The slender, threadlike prolongation of the conus medullaris of the spinal cord. It extends downward to the fundus of the dural sac at the level of the second sacral vertebra, where it penetrates the dura and fuses with the filum of the dura mater to form the coccygeal ligament, which in turn fuses with the periosteum of the posterior surface of the coccyx. The rostral portion contains a prolongation of the central canal, but this is composed mostly of pial connective tissue. Also *terminal filament.*

**fimbria** \fim′brē·ə\ [L, a fringe, thread, fiber] (*pl.* fimbriae) **1** A fringelike structure; a fringed border or edge. **2** Collectively, the very fine filamentous projections from the surface of cells or bacteria. The individual filaments usually have a diameter of 0.01 μm or less and a length of 1–2 μm. Also *fringe, lacinia* (outmoded). **fimbriae of fallopian tube** FIMBRIAE TUBAE UTERINAE. **f. hippocampi** [NA] A narrow band of fibrous white matter (myelinated axons), which form the fornix, situated on the medial ventricular surface of the hippocampus. Also *fimbria of hippocampus, corpus fimbriatum hippocampi.* **f. ovarica** [NA] The longest and most grooved of the fimbriae tubae uterinae, lying along the free border of the mesosalpinx as far as the tubal end of the ovary. Also *fimbriated extremity of fallopian tube, ovarian fimbria, infundibulo-ovarian ligament.* **fimbriae of tongue** PLICA FIMBRIATA. **fimbriae tubae uterinae** [NA] A number of irregular, fingerlike processes extending from the circumference of the expanded abdominal end, or infundibulum, of the uterine tube. They are lined by a mucous membrane thrown into longitudinal folds continuous with those in the infundibulum. Also *fimbriae of uterine tube, fimbriae of fallopian tube.*

**fimbrial** \fim′brē·əl\ Pertaining to a fimbria.

**fimbriation** \fim′brē·ā′shən\ **1** The process of forming fimbriae. **2** The condition of having fimbriae or a fringed border.

**fimbriectomy** \fim′brē-ek′təmē\ [*fimbri(a)* + -ECTOMY] Amputation of the fimbria of the fallopian tube for purposes of sterilization.

**fimbriocele** \fim′brē-əsēl′\ [*fimbri(a)* + *o* + -CELE[1]] A vaginal herniation of the fimbriae of the oviduct.

**fimbriodentate** \fim′brē-əden′tāt\ Denoting the fimbria of the fornix and the underlying dentate gyrus from which it is separated by a groove (fimbriodentate sulcus).

**fimbrioplasty** \fim′brē-əplas′tē\ [*fimbri(a)* + *o* + -PLASTY] The surgical freeing of the fimbria of an ovarian tube when obstruction is present.

**Finckh** [Johann *Finckh*, German psychiatrist, born 1873] Finckh's test. See under PROVERBS TEST.

**finder** A microscope slide that has been marked out in numbered squares in order to facilitate the locating of a given point on the slide.

**finger** [Old English] Any one of the five digits of the hand. **baseball f.** MALLET FINGER. **clubbed f.** A bulbous enlargement of the terminal segment of the finger. It is seen in infants and children with various diseases of the thoracic organs, particularly with certain congenital heart diseases, or it may be inherited. There is no constant osseous change in the terminal phalanx, but the surrounding fibrous tissue proliferates excessively. Also *drumstick finger.* **dead f.** WHITE FINGER. **drop f.** MALLET FINGER. **drumstick f.** CLUBBED FINGER. **first f.** POLLEX. **hammer f.** MALLET FINGER. **index f.** INDEX. **lock f.** A finger with bony or fibrous ankylosis. **mallet f.** A flexion deformity of the terminal phalanx of the finger provoked by striking the dorsum of the finger tip. It is caused by the complete or partial rupture of the extensor tendon to the terminal phalanx or by the avulsion of its bony insertion. It can be passively, but not actively, corrected. Also *baseball finger, drop finger, hammer finger, digitus malleus.* **middle f.** DIGITUS MEDIUS. **ring f.** DIGITUS ANNULARIS. **snapping f.** TRIGGER FINGER. **spade f.'s** The thickened, square-tipped fingers of acromegaly, due mainly to an increase in soft tissue. **spider f.** ARACHNODACTYLY. **spring f.** **1** TRIGGER FINGER. **2** A finger that resists the extremes of flexion or extension. **stuck f.** TRIGGER FINGER. **trigger f.** A deformity of the finger in which the digit becomes stuck in flexion at the proximal interphalangeal joint. The condition is due to entrapment of the flexor tendon at the entrance of the fibrous flexor sheath. Also *stuck finger, snapping finger, spring finger, digitus recellens.* **vibration-induced white f.'s** See under VIBRATION DISEASE. **washerwoman's f.'s** Shriveled fingers caused by extreme dehydration, as seen in the terminal stages of cholera. **waxy f.** Cyanotic mottling and numbness of the fingers due to impaired circulation, as seen in the Raynaud syndrome. **webbed f.'s** A slight degree of syndactyly in which adjacent fingers are joined by a fold of skin of greater distal extent than is usually seen. There is no union of fibrous or osseous elements. Also *palmature.* **white f.** A condition characterized by numbness and blanching of the fingers, especially in workers who use vibrating hand tools such as pneumatic hammers and chain saws in cold environments. It constitutes an occupational variant of the Raynaud syndrome. Also *dead finger, digitus mortuus.*

**fingerdrop** One of the results of radial (musculospiral) nerve paralysis characterized by inability to extend the fingers at the metacarpophalangeal joints. It is often associated with wristdrop and other evidences of radial nerve paralysis depending on the level of the nerve lesion.

**fingerprint** **1** The transferred impression of the dermatoglyphic pattern of the distal phalangeal volar surface of a finger or thumb, formed by intentional or chance contact of the distal phalanx with a surface that will retain the impression. Also *dactylogram.* **2** The result of an analytic technique capable of distinguishing between or separating similar compounds, such as the final position on a chromatographic plate of individual peptides from a mixture of peptides subjected to two-dimensional paper chromatography. **chance f.'s** Fingerprints left unintentionally when contact of ridged skin is made with a surface that retains the dermatoglyphic pattern, such as fingerprints on a polished surface where the deposited perspiration and oily skin secretions leave ridge impressions. Also *trace fingerprints.* **latent f.'s** Chance fingerprints which are invisible or barely visible. Enhancement techniques, such as dusting the suspected surface with powder or exposing it to iodine fumes, are required to detect their presence. **record f.'s** Fingerprints made by applying ink or other suitable staining material to the volar surfaces of the distal phalanges and rolling each fingertip across an assigned space on a white card or paper. They are used for identification and comparison purposes. **trace f.'s** CHANCE FINGERPRINTS.

**Finkeldey** [Wilhelm *Finkeldey*, German pathologist, flourished 20th century] Warthin-Finkeldey cell. See under CELL.

**Finney** [John Miller Turpin *Finney*, U.S. surgeon, 1863–1942] Finney's operation. See under PYLOROPLASTY.

**Finochietto** [Enrique *Finochietto*, Argentinian surgeon, 1881–1948] See under STIRRUP.

**Finsen** [Jon Constant *Finsen*, Icelandic physician, born 1826] Daae-Finsen disease. See under DISEASE.

**Finsen** [Niels Ryberg *Finsen*, Danish physician, 1860–1904] See under LAMP.

**Finzi** [Neville Samuel *Finzi*, English radiotherapist, born 1881] Finzi-Harmer operation. See under OPERATION.

**fire** [Old English *fȳr*; akin to Gk *pyr* fire] **Saint Anthony's f.** ERGOTISM

**firedamp** [FIRE + early modern English *damp* (prob. from medieval Dutch or Low German) vapor, gas, fumes] A colorless, odorless gas, composed mainly of methane (more than 60%), nitrogen, and carbon dioxide, that occurs naturally in coal mines. Although it has no physiologic action on its own it creates a hazard as a simple asphyxiant. It is inflammable and gives rise to the risk of explosion in mines.

**first aid** See under AID.

**Fisher** [Miller *Fisher*, U.S. physician, born 1910] Miller Fisher syndrome. See under FISHER SYNDROME.

**Fisher** [Ronald Aylmer *Fisher*, English statistician and geneticist, 1890–1962] Fisher's exact test of probability. See under TEST.

**fishing** In laboratory usage, the picking of single colonies from a culture with a needle or toothpick.

**Fiske** [Cyrus Hartwell *Fiske*, U.S. biochemist, born 1890] Fiske and Subbarow method. See under METHOD.

**fission** \fish′ən\ [L *fissio* (from *fissus*, past part. of *findere* to cleave, cut) a cleaving, dividing] The act of splitting or breaking apart, as an atomic nucleus or the nucleus of a cell. **binary f.** Asexual reproduction by the splitting of a cell by nuclear division (karyokinesis) followed by cytoplasmic separation (cytokinesis) to form two new cells of equal size, a common method of reproduction of various protists. **bud f.** GEMMATION. **cellular f.** CYTOKINESIS. **multiple f.** A series of nuclear divisions followed by the division of the body of the cell into an equal number of parts, each with a daughter nucleus, as is seen in the asexual reproduction of sporozoa (schizogony), or the result of sexual fusion (sporogomy). A specialized form of multiple fission is called endopolygeny, in which daughter cells form within their cell membranes in the cytoplasm of the mother cell rather than at the periphery. Compare SIMPLE FISSION. **nuclear f.** The splitting of a heavy nucleus into two roughly equal parts, with the release of large amounts of energy. A few naturally occurring nuclides undergo spontaneous fission, but ordinarily fission will not occur unless the nucleus can absorb external neutrons or gamma photons, thus causing instability. Fission of a given nuclide leads to any of a variety of pairs of daughter nuclides rather than just a prespecified pair. **simple f.** The division of the cell nucleus followed by division of the body of the cell into two equal parts; binary fission. Compare MULTIPLE FISSION.

**fissula** \fis′yələ\ [Late L, dim. of L *fissum* cleft, fissure] A small cleft or fissure. **f. ante fenestram** An oblique, slitlike space through the lateral wall of the internal ear that is filled with a strip of connective tissue extending from the vestibule immediately in front of the fenestra vestibuli to the mucoperiosteum of the tympanic cavity near the processus cochleariformis. It is considered to be an appendage of the perilymphatic labyrinth. Also *Cozzolino's zone.*

**fissura** \fisyoo′rə\ [Late L (from *fiss(us)*, past part. of *findere* to cleave, cut + *-ura* -URE), fissure, cleft, groove] (*pl.* fissurae) A furrow, groove, or cleft, especially a deep fold separating gyri in the cerebral cortex; sulcus. Also *fissure.* • Though close in meaning, *fissura* usually denotes a deeper, and *sulcus* a more shallow furrow. **f. antitragohelicina** [NA] A deep notch in the auricular cartilage separating the cauda helicis posteriorly from the antitragus anteriorly. Also *antitragohelicine fissure, posterior fissure of auricle.* **f. calcarina** SULCUS CALCARINUS. **fissurae cerebelli** [NA] Major grooves separating the corpus cerebelli into lobes and lobules. **f. cerebri lateralis Sylvii** SULCUS LATERALIS CEREBRI. **f. choroidea** The linear evagination of the choroid plexus along the walls of the lateral ventricles. Also *Schwalbe's fissure.* **f. collateralis** SULCUS COLLATERALIS. **f. dentata** SULCUS HIPPOCAMPI. **f. hippocampi** SULCUS HIPPOCAMPI. **f. horizontalis cerebelli** [NA] The horizontal fissure separating the ansiform lobule of the hemispheres into the rostral crus I (superior semilunar lobule) and caudal crus II (inferior semilunar lobule). Medially, it separates the folium vermis from the tuber vermis. Also *sulcus horizontalis cerebelli, great horizontal fissure, horizontal fissure of cerebellum.* **f. horizontalis pulmonis dextri** [NA] A short, deep horizontal cleft that extends from the anterior margin of the right lung to the hilum, where it meets the oblique fissure and separates the superior from the middle lobe. Also *horizontal fissure of right lung.* **f. in ano** ANAL FISSURE. **f. ligamenti teretis** [NA] A fissure of variable depth on the visceral surface of the liver. It extends from a notch on the inferior margin to the left extremity of the porta hepatis, where it meets the fissure for ligamentum venosum. It separates the quadrate lobe from the left lobe and lodges the ligamentum teres of the liver. Also *fissure for ligamentum teres, fissure of round ligament, umbilical fissure* (outmoded), *fossa for ligamentum teres.* **f. ligamenti venosi** [NA] A deep groove on the posterior part of the diaphragmatic surface of the liver that separates the caudate lobe from the left lobe and contains the two layers of the lesser omentum. Inferiorly it reaches the left extremity of the porta hepatis, where it meets the fissure for ligamentum teres. Also *fissure for ligamentum venosum.* **f. longitudinalis cerebri** [NA] The largest and deepest cerebral fissure, separating the two cerebral hemispheres. Also *superior longitudinal sulcus, longitudinal fissure, longitudinal fissure of cerebrum, intercerebral fissure.* **f. mediana anterior** FISSURA MEDIANA ANTERIOR MEDULLAE SPINALIS. **f. mediana anterior medullae oblongatae** [NA] The continuation of the median fissure of the ventral spinal cord into the medulla oblongata, where it becomes more shallow. Also *anterior median fissure of medulla oblongata, fissura mediana ventralis medullae oblongatae.* **f. mediana anterior medullae spinalis** [NA] The deep midline fissure parting the ventral spinal cord throughout its length. Also *fissura mediana anterior, sulcus medianus, anterior median fissure of spinal cord, anteromedian groove of spinal cord, Haller's line* (obs.), *sulcus ventralis medullae spinalis.* **f. mediana posterior medullae oblongatae** SULCUS MEDIANUS POSTERIOR MEDULLAE OBLONGATAE. **f. mediana ventralis medullae oblongatae** [NA] FISSURA MEDIANA ANTERIOR MEDULLAE OBLONGATAE. **f. obliqua pulmonis** [NA] A long, deep cleft that extends from the costal to the mediastinal surface of each lung and from a point below the apex on the posterior margin obliquely through the hilum to the inferior margin close to its junction with the anterior margin. It separates the superior and inferior lobes in the left lung and the inferior lobe from the superior and middle lobes in the right lung. Also *oblique fissure of lung.* **f. orbitalis inferior** [NA] The cleft at the apex of the orbit between the lateral and inferior walls. It is bounded laterally and posteriorly by the inferior margin of the orbital surface of the greater wing of the sphenoid bone, and anteriorly and medially by the orbital process of the palatine bone and the posterior margin of the orbital surface of the maxilla. It serves as a communication between the orbit and the pterygopalatine fossa medially and the infratemporal fossa laterally. Through it pass the maxillary nerve, the infraorbital vessels, and connections between the ophthalmic veins and the pterygoid venous plexus. Also *inferior orbital fissure.* **f. orbitalis superior** [NA] An oblique, narrow cleft at the apex of the orbit between the lateral wall and roof. Its long axis is directed medially, posteriorly, and inferiorly. It lies between the greater and lesser wings of the sphenoid bone and connects the orbit with the middle cranial fossa. It transmits numerous structures including the ophthalmic, oculomotor, trochlear, and abducent nerves and the ophthalmic veins. Also *superior orbital fissure, superior sphenoidal fissure* (outmoded), *sphenoidal fissure* (outmoded). **f. parieto-occipitalis** SULCUS PARIETO-OCCIPITALIS. **f. petro-occipitalis** [NA] A cranial fissure extending caudally from the foramen lacerum between the basioccipital and the posterior and inferior borders of the petrous portion of the temporal bone. Also *occipital fissure, petrobasilar fissure, petro-occipital fissure.* **f. petrosquamosa** A superficial cranial fissure following the line of fusion of the petrous and squamous portions of the temporal bone. Also *petrosquamous fissure, petrosquamous suture.* **f. petrotympanica**

[NA] The medial part of the tympanosquamous fissure in the mandibular fossa of the temporal bone, situated between the inferiorly projecting anterolateral edge of the tegmen tympani and the tympanic part of the temporal bone. It transmits the chorda tympani from the tympanic cavity, the anterior tympanic branch of the maxillary artery, and part of the anterior ligament of the malleus. In the tympanic cavity the fissure opens just above the flaccid part of the tympanic membrane and contains the anterior process of the malleus. Also *petrotympanic fissure, glaserian fissure, tympanic fissure, tympanosquamous fissure.* **f. posterolateralis cerebelli** The first fissure to appear in the development of the cerebellum, separating the corpus cerebelli from the flocculonodular lobe. Also *floccular fissure.* **f. prima cerebelli** [NA] The primary cerebellar fissure, separating the anterior from the posterior lobe. It extends laterally into the hemispheres from behind the culmen, separating the culmen and declive medially and the posterior and superior semilunar lobules laterally. Also *superior anterior fissure, primary fissure.* **f. pterygoidea** INCISURA PTERYGOIDEA. **f. pterygomaxillaris** [NA] The V-shaped cleft between the back of the maxilla and the pterygoid process of the sphenoid bone through which the infratemporal fossa communicates medially with the pterygopalatine fossa, giving passage to the maxillary nerve and the terminal part of the maxillary artery. Also *pterygomaxillary fissure, pterygopalatine fissure.* **f. secunda cerebelli** [NA] A fissure, located on the anterior surface of the cerebellum, that separates the pyramis and uvula portions of the cerebellar vermis. Also *secondary fissure.* **f. spheno-occipitalis** The fissure filled with cartilage in the synchondrosis spheno-occipitalis before it is ossified. Also *spheno-occipital fissure, basilar fissure, occipitosphenoidal fissure.* **f. sphenopetrosa** [NA] The slit between the petrous part of the temporal bone and the lateral portion of the posterior margin of the greater wing of sphenoid, just medial to the sphenoidal spine. The fissure is filled with fibrocartilage, forming a synchondrosis. Also *angular fissure, petrosphenoidal fissure, sphenopetrosal fissure.* **f. transversa cerebelli** The transverse indentation between the nodulus and the cerebellar peduncles. Also *transverse fissure of cerebellum.* **f. transversa cerebri** [NA] The cleft separating the corpus callosum and fornix from the underlying diencephalon rostrally and the cerebellum caudally, where the fissure is occupied by the tentorium cerebelli. The fissure contains a double layer of pia, the lower portion of which forms the invaginated tela choroidea of the third ventricle. Also *fissure of Bichat, cerebral fissure of Bichat, great fissure of cerebrum, great transverse fissure of cerebrum, transverse fissure of cerebrum.* **f. tympanomastoidea** [NA] A slit usually located on the inferior aspect of the skull lateral to the base of the styloid process and between the tympanic part and the mastoid process of the temporal bone. Opening into the fissure is the mastoid canaliculus. Also *tympanomastoid fissure, petromastoid fissure, auricular fissure of temporal bone.* **f. tympanosquamosa** [NA] A transverse fissure between the tympanic and the squamous parts of the temporal bone, observed externally in the mandibular fossa. It is relatively wide in the infant but in the adult narrows to a slit into which the anterolateral edge of the tegmen tympani turns downward, dividing the medial part of the fissure into the petrosquamous fissure anteriorly and the petrotympanic fissure posteriorly. Also *tympanosquamous fissure, squamotympanic fissure, anterior tympanosquamous fissure.*

**fissurae** \fisyoo′rē\ Plural of FISSURA.

**fissural** \fish′ʊrəl\ Pertaining to a fissure.

**fissuration** \fish′ʊrā′shən\ [*fissur(e)* + -ATION] The formation of furrows or fissures, especially in the cerebral and cerebellar cortices during the development of gyri and folia respectively.

# fissure

**fissure** \fish′ər\ [L *fissura.* See FISSURA.] FISSURA. **Ammon's f.** HIPPOCAMPAL FISSURE. **amygdaline f.** A variable groove near the cerebral temporal pole extending toward the uncus. **anal f.** A mucosal tear of the anus. Also *fissura in ano, Allingham's ulcer.* **angular f.** FISSURA SPHENOPETROSA. **anterior median f. of medulla oblongata** FISSURA MEDIANA ANTERIOR MEDULLAE OBLONGATAE. **anterior median f. of spinal cord** FISSURA MEDIANA ANTERIOR MEDULLAE SPINALIS. **anterior paracentral f.** A transverse fissure in the frontal lobe motor cerebral cortex approximately parallel to the sulcus centralis and forming the rostral limit of the precentral gyrus. **anterior tympanosquamous f.** FISSURA TYMPANOSQUAMOSA. **antitragohelicine f.** FISSURA ANTITRAGOHELICINA. **ape f.** *Obs.* SULCUS LUNATUS. **f. of aqueduct of vestibule** APERTURA EXTERNA AQUEDUCTUS VESTIBULI. **arciform f.** HIPPOCAMPAL FISSURE. **auricular f. of temporal bone** FISSURA TYMPANOMASTOIDEA. **basal f.** DECIDUAL FISSURE. **basilar f.** FISSURA SPHENO-OCCIPITALIS. **basisylvian f.** In the human brain, the portion of the sulcus lateralis cerebri (sylvian fissure) extending down from the temporal lobe toward the orbital surface of the frontal lobe. **f. of Bichat** FISSURA TRANSVERSA CEREBRI. **branchial f.'s** BRANCHIAL CLEFTS. **Broca's f.** Branches of the sulcus lateralis cerebri of the inferior frontal lobule associated with Broca's motor speech area on the left hemisphere of humans. **Burdach's f.** The hidden circumferential cleft that separates the insula from the operculum. **calcarine f.** SULCUS CALCARINUS. **callosal f.** SULCUS CORPORIS CALLOSI. **callosomarginal f.** SULCUS CINGULI. **central f.** SULCUS CENTRALIS CEREBRI. **cerebral f.'s** SULCI CEREBRI. **cerebral f. of Bichat** FISSURA TRANSVERSA CEREBRI. **f.'s of cerebrum** SULCI CEREBRI. **cervical f.** An epithelially lined opening on the side of the neck that is a persistent remnant of one of the embryonic branchial grooves. It may be the external termination of either a sinus tract or a fistula connecting with the pharynx. **choroid f.** A fissure present in the brain of the human embryo from the third month. It arches upwards and backwards from the interventricular foramen on the medial aspect of the telencephalon. It marks the invagination of the medial wall of the developing hemisphere by vascular tissue which will constitute the choroid plexus of the lateral ventricle. Also *fetal fissure.* **choroidal f. of eye** A cleft on the inferior aspect of the embryonic optic vesicle continuing on to the optic stalk, resulting from the original invagination of the optic vesicle also involving its under side. The tips of the cleft close during the seventh week in human development. Also *optic fissure, fetal fissure of optic cup.* **Clevenger's f.** SULCUS TEMPORALIS INFERIOR. **collateral f.** SULCUS COLLATERALIS. **decidual f.** A space or cleft developing in the decidua basalis toward the end of pregnancy. Also *basal fissure.* **dentate f.** SULCUS HIPPOCAMPI. **f. of ductus venosus** A fissure on the inferior aspect of the developing liver. The depression becomes deeper as the liver grows and is the fissure of the ductus venosus. When the ductus venosus closes after birth and becomes a fibrous remnant it lies in a deep cleft lying between the left lobe and the caudate lobe of the liver then called the fissure for ligamentum venosum. Also *fissure of the venous ligament.* **Duverney's f.'s** INCISURAE CARTILAGINIS MEATUS ACUSTICI. **Ecker's f.** SULCUS OCCIPITALIS TRANSVERSUS. **entorbital f.** An inconstant sulcus on the base of the human frontal lobe lying between the orbital and olfactory sulci. **fetal f.** CHOROID FISSURE. **fetal f. of optic cup** CHOROIDAL FISSURE OF EYE. **floccular f.** FISSURA POSTEROLATERALIS CEREBELLI. **genitovesical f.** A groove between the genital cord and the bladder of the fetus which in the female becomes the excavation between the uterus and the bladder. **glaserian f.** FISSURA PETROTYMPANICA. **f. of glottis** RIMA GLOTTIDIS. **great f. of cerebrum** FISSURA TRANSVERSA CEREBRI. **great horizontal f.** FISSURA HORIZONTALIS CEREBELLI. **great transverse f. of cerebrum** FISSURA TRANSVERSA CEREBRI. **hippocampal f.** 1 In a human embryo of about two months, a longitudinal fissure with an inferior concavity extending from the interventricular foramen to the temporal lobe. Also *Ammon's fissure, arciform fissure.* 2 SULCUS HIPPOCAMPI. **f. of hippocampus** SULCUS HIPPOCAMPI. **horizontal f. of cerebellum** FISSURA HORIZONTALIS CEREBELLI. **horizontal f. of right lung** FISSURA HORIZONTALIS PULMONIS DEXTRI. **inferior orbital f.** FISSURA ORBITALIS INFERIOR. **inferofrontal f.** SULCUS FRONTALIS INFERIOR. **intercerebral f.** FISSURA LONGITUDINALIS CEREBRI. **intercotyledonary f.'s** Fissures or grooves which separate the cotyledons on the maternal aspect of the placenta. **interparietal f.** SULCUS INTRAPARIETALIS. **intratonsillar f.** FOSSA SUPRATONSILLARIS. **lateral cerebral f.** SULCUS LATERALIS CEREBRI. **lateral f. of cerebrum** SULCUS LATERALIS CEREBRI. **f. for ligamentum teres** FISSURA LIGAMENTI TERETIS. **f. for ligamentum venosum** FISSURA LIGAMENTI VENOSI. **linguogingival f.** A fissure on the lingual surface of an upper incisor tooth extending from the lingual fossa towards the root. **longitudinal f.** FISSURA LONGITUDINALIS CEREBRI. **longitudinal f. of cerebellum** VALLECULA CEREBELLI. **longitudinal f. of cerebrum** FISSURA LONGITUDINALIS CEREBRI. **f. of Monro** SULCUS HYPOTHALAMICUS. **oblique f. of lung** FISSURA OBLIQUA PULMONIS. **occipital f.** FISSURA PETROOCCIPITALIS. **occipitosphenoidal f.** FISSURA SPHENOOCCIPITALIS. **optic f.** CHOROIDAL FISSURE OF EYE. **oral f.** RIMA ORIS. **f. of palpebrae** RIMA PALPEBRARUM. **palpebral f.** RIMA PALPEBRARUM. **Pansch's f.** SULCUS INTRAPARIETALIS. **parafloccular f.** The indentation between the flocculus and paraflocculus of the cerebellum. **parieto-occipital f.** SULCUS PARIETO-OCCIPITALIS. **parietosphenoid f.** INCISURA PARIETALIS OSSIS TEMPORALIS. **petrobasilar f.** FISSURA PETRO-OCCIPITALIS. **petromastoid f.** FISSURA TYMPANOMASTOIDEA. **petro-occipital f.** FISSURA PETRO-OCCIPITALIS. **petrosphenoidal f.** FISSURA SPHENOPETROSA. **petrosquamous f.** FISSURA PETROSQUAMOSA. **petrotympanic f.** FISSURA PETROTYMPANICA. **portal f.** PORTA HEPATIS. **postcentral f.** SULCUS POSTCENTRALIS. **posterior f. of auricle** FISSURA ANTITRAGOHELICINA. **posterior median f. of medulla oblongata** SULCUS MEDIANUS POSTERIOR MEDULLAE OBLONGATAE. **posterior median f. of spinal cord** SULCUS MEDIANUS POSTERIOR MEDULLAE SPINALIS. **posterolateral f.** SULCUS POSTEROLATERALIS CEREBELLI. **postlingual f.** The superior, transverse cerebellar fissure separating the lingula from the lobus centralis. **postlunate f.** The superior, transverse cerebellar fissure between the lunate and ansiform lobule. **postpyramidal f.** The fissure separating the cerebellar pyramis from the tuber vermis. **precentral f.** SULCUS PRECENTRALIS. **precuneal f.** A variable fissure in the rostral cuneus of the cerebrum. **prepyramidal f.** The fissure separating the cerebellar pyramis and uvula. **presylvian f.** The rostral continuation of the sulcus lateralis cerebri. **primary f.** FISSURA PRIMA CEREBELLI. **pterygoid f.** INCISURA PTERYGOIDEA. **pterygomaxillary f.** FISSURA PTERYGOMAXILLARIS. **pterygopalatine f.** FISSURA PTERYGOMAXILLARIS. **pterygopalatine f. of palatine bone** SULCUS PALATINUS MAJOR OSSIS PALATINI. **pudendal f.** RIMA PUDENDI. **retrotonsillar f.** A deep fissure on the inferior surface of the cerebellar hemisphere anterior to the biventral lobule and posterior to the tonsil of the cerebellum. It is continuous with the anterior part of the sulcus valleculae, which also bounds the tonsil. **rhinal f.** 1 The sulcus or fissure which demarcates the olfactory cortex or rhinencephalon from adjacent regions of the cerebral surface. In the human brain it lies lateral to the uncus. Also *rhinal sulcus.* 2 SULCUS RHINALIS. **f. of Rolando** SULCUS CENTRALIS CEREBRI. **f. of round ligament** FISSURA LIGAMENTI TERETIS. **sagittal portal f.** An intrahepatic plane that extends through the fossa for the gallbladder to the left side of the fossa for the inferior vena cava. It divides the liver into right and left functional lobes, according to the distribution of the right and left hepatic vessels and bile ducts. It passes along the course of the intermediate hepatic vein. **sagittal f. of liver** FOSSA SAGITTALIS SINISTRA HEPATIS. **Santorini's f.'s** INCISURAE CARTILAGINIS MEATUS ACUSTICI. **Schwalbe's f.** FISSURA CHOROIDEA. **sclerotomic f.** Loosening of cells which occurs transitorily to subdivide each sclerotomic segment into a cranial and a caudal half around the notochord and which becomes incorporated in the perichordal disk. **secondary f.** FISSURA SECUNDA CEREBELLI. **simian f.** *Obs.* SULCUS LUNATUS. **sphenoidal f.** *Outmoded* FISSURA ORBITALIS SUPERIOR. **spheno-occipital f.** FISSURA SPHENO-OCCIPITALIS. **sphenopetrosal f.** FISSURA SPHENOPETROSA. **squamotympanic f.** FISSURA TYMPANOSQUAMOSA. **subfrontal f.** SULCUS FRONTALIS INFERIOR. **subsylvian f.** 1 The posterior branch of the sulcus lateralis cerebri. 2 A variable posterolateral fissure on the base of the frontal lobe. *Obs.* **subtemporal f.** A variable fissure in the inferior temporal gyrus. **superficial petrosal f.** HIATUS CANALIS NERVI PETROSI MAJORIS. **superior anterior f.** FISSURA PRIMA CEREBELLI. **superior orbital f.** FISSURA ORBITALIS SUPERIOR. **superior sphenoidal f.** *Outmoded* FISSURA ORBITALIS SUPERIOR. **supertemporal f.** SULCUS TEMPORALIS SUPERIOR. **sylvian f.** SULCUS LATERALIS CEREBRI. **f. of Sylvius** SULCUS LATERALIS CEREBRI. **transtemporal f.** A variable, short, transverse fissure on the lateral temporal lobe. **transverse f.** PORTA HEPATIS. **transverse f. of cerebellum** FISSURA TRANSVERSA CEREBELLI. **transverse f. of cerebrum** FISSURA TRANSVERSA CEREBRI. **transverse occipital f.** SULCUS OCCIPITALIS TRANSVERSUS. **tympanic f.** FISSURA PETROTYMPANICA. **tympanomastoid f.** FISSURA TYMPANOMASTOIDEA. **tympanosquamous f.** 1 FISSURA TYMPANOSQUAMOSA. 2 *Outmoded* FISSURA PETROTYMPANICA. **urogenital f.** RIMA PUDENDI. **vestibular f. of the cochlea** A slitlike gap between the free edge of the projecting osseous spiral lamina and the tip of the secondary spiral lamina that projects inwards from the outer wall of the lower part of the first turn of the bony cochlea. **f. of the vestibule** RIMA VESTIBULI. **zygal f.** An H-shaped configuration produced by a transverse fissure linking two parallel cerebral fissures. **zygomaticosphenoid f.** SUTURA SPHENOZYGOMATICA.

# fistula

**fistula** \fis′tyoolə\ [L, a pipe, conduit, tube, fistula] (*pl.* fistulas, fistulae) An abnormal communication between two normally unconnected structures, body cavities, or the surface of the body. **abdominal f.** A communicating tract between an abdominal organ and the external surface of the abdomen. **alveolar f.** ALVEOLAR SINUS. **anal f.** A fistula with one end opening onto the mucosal epithelium of the anus or nearby skin. Also *perirectal fistula.* **aortocaval f.** A communication that develops between the aorta and the inferior vena cava, usually between the infrarenal aorta and vena cava because of an aortic aneurysm. It may occasionally occur as a result of penetrating abdominal trauma. **aortoduodenal f.** See under AORTOENTERIC FISTULA. **aortoenteric f.** A communication that develops between the aorta and the gastrointestinal tract. It is most common between the proximal suture line of an aortic prosthesis and the nearby duodenum (referred to as an aortoduodenal fistula), forming as a consequence of a pseudoaneurysm at the suture line. It may rarely develop primarily between an aortic aneurysm and the overlying bowel. **arteriovenous f.** An abnormal communication between an artery and a vein, allowing shunting of blood from the arterial system. It may either result from trauma or be congenital. **f. auris congenita** PREAURICULAR SINUS. **f. bimucosa** An abnormal passage both ends of which open on mucosal surfaces. **blind f.** An abnormal passage arising on an internal organ or the skin and ending in a cul-de-sac. Also *incomplete fistula.* **branchial f.** An abnormal passage representing persistence of the embryonic branchial system of arches, grooves, and pouches. The position of the fistula depends upon which of the four arches and associated grooves and pouches have persisted. In all instances the embryonic pharynx or one of its derivatives communicates with the exterior through a persistent external groove or fissure on the side of the face or neck. Also *cervicoaural fistula.* **Brescia-Cimino f.** RADIOCEPHALIC FISTULA. **bronchobiliary f.** A fistula between a bronchus and intrahepatic bile ducts. It may be a complication of trauma or hepatic abscesses with transdiaphragmatic extension into the chest. **bronchoesophageal f.** An abnormal communication between a bronchus and the esophagus allowing aspiration of esophageal contents into the lungs. This type of fistula may occur in association with an erosive tumor involving either of these structures. Also *esophagobronchial fistula.* **bronchopleural f.** An abnormal communication between a bronchus and the pleural cavity. Also *pleurobronchial fistula.* **caroticocavernous f.** A rupture of the intracavernous portion of the internal carotid artery, allowing arterial blood to pass directly into the venous sinus. It usually results either from trauma or from aneurysmal rupture. Also *carotid-cavernous fistula.* **cerebrospinal fluid f.** A fistula, caused by injury or disease or complicating surgical procedures on the ear, nose or paranasal sinuses, by which cerebrospinal fluid escapes from the ear or nose or, having passed via the nasopharynx, is swallowed. **cervical f.** A branchial fistula representing abnormal persistence of the epithelial tissues of the second, third, or fourth embryonic branchial arch, which connects the pharynx with the exterior. The external opening is on the side of the neck, as opposed to being on the face anterior to the auricle. **cervicoaural f.** BRANCHIAL FISTULA. **cholecystoduodenal f.** A communication between the gallbladder and the duodenum resulting from chronic irritation and inflammation of the gallbladder and adjacent duodenal wall, a complication of severe cholecystitis. Large gallstones may pass through the fistula into the duodenum and be carried distally where they may cause intestinal obstruction. This condition may be diagnosed by radiographic evidence of intrabiliary air. **chylous f.** A fistula resulting in an external leakage of chyle as a result of injury to the abdominal lymphatics, especially the cisterna magna. **complete f.** A pathological communication between two sites, one end of which may open to a mucosal or cutaneous surface. **congenital preauricular f.** PREAURICULAR SINUS. **congenital urethrorectal f.** A congenital anomaly resulting from incomplete separation of the rectum from the posterior urethral segment of the bladder, permitting passage of urine through the rectum and feces through the urethra. Also *congenital rectourethral fistula.* **craniosinus f.** A fistula between the subarachnoid space of the brain and one of the paranasal sinuses, allowing the flow of cerebrospinal fluid into the nose. **dental f.** A fistula between the apical region of a tooth and the gingival mucosa which may drain pus from an apical abscess. Also *gingival fistula.* **enterocutaneous f.** A fistula between the small or large intestine and the abdominal skin. **enterovaginal f.** A fistula between the vagina and an adjacent portion of intestine, usually the rectum. **enterovesical f.** A fistula between the urinary bladder and an adherent portion of intestine. **esophagobronchial f.** BRONCHOESOPHAGEAL FISTULA. **esophagotracheal f.** TRACHEOESOPHAGEAL FISTULA. **external f.** A fistula between an internal organ and the skin, generally accompanied by inflammation and drainage to the outside. **fecal f.** A fistula between the lumen of the distal intestine and the abdominal skin which discharges feces to the outside. This type of fistula can be a sequel of any process that results in intestinal perforation, such as diverticulitis, regional enteritis, carcinoma, radiation damage, or the passage of a foreign body. Also *intestinal fistula, stercoral fistula.* **frontal sinus f.** A fistula in the fronto-orbital region leading into the frontal sinus. It occasionally persists at the site of drainage of frontal sinus suppuration or of frontal sinus mucocele. It can occur, though rarely, as the result of trauma or of surgical excision. **gastric f.** An abnormal passage through the abdominal wall communicating the lumen of the stomach with the outside. A surgically created passage (gastrostomy) is often created for feeding purposes. **gastrocolic f.** A fistula between the stomach and the colon. It is usually a complication of gastric surgery for peptic ulcer, or it may result from neoplastic invasion. **gastrojejunal f.** An abnormal communication between the stomach and the jejunum. It may develop as a complication of marginal ulcer following surgery for peptic ulcer. **gingival f.** DENTAL FISTULA. **horseshoe f.** An anal fistula forming a semicircular tract communicating at both extremities with the surface of the perianal skin. **f. in ano** A fistulous tract in close proximity to the anus that opens to the surface of the skin and may communicate with the rectum. **incomplete f.** BLIND FISTULA. **internal f.** A fistula between two internal, generally hollow, organs. **intestinal f.** FECAL FISTULA. **lacrimal f.** An abnormal communication between the lacrimal duct or sac and the external skin of the periorbital area. **lacteal f.** A fistula between a lactiferous duct and the periareolar skin of the breast. **f. of lip** A very rare hereditary defect at the margin of the lower lip, consisting of a small pit 5–25 mm long. It is usually bilateral and is associated with other deformities, such as clefts. **lymphatic f.** An abnormal communication with a lymphatic vessel allowing drainage of lymph out of the lymphatic system. This type of fistula is often congenital and found in the neck. **Mann-Bollman f.** An artificial communication produced surgically for experimental purposes: a segment of intestine is isolated, the proximal end is sutured to the abdominal wall and the distal end is anastomosed side to side to the proximal jejunum or duodenum. Due to intrinsic peristalsis, there is minimal leakage through the abdominal wall, and food as well as other substances can be administered directly through the abdominal orifice. **mediastinobronchial f.** A fistula between a bronchus and the mediastinal cavity. It may be a complication of lung resection in which the bronchial stump leaks into the mediastinum. **mucus f.** DRY COLOSTOMY. **oroantral f.** An abnormal communicating passage between the maxillary sinus and the oral cavity, occurring most commonly in the region of the first or second molar teeth following surgical manipulation of that area or infection of the maxillary sinus. **oronasal f.** A fistula between the interior of the mouth and the nose, usually through the hard palate. The causes include neoplastic and granulomatous ulceration and certain surgical procedures, sometimes for the relief of such diseases. Rarely, accidental trauma may be responsible. **parietal f.** An abnormal passage through the abdominal or thoracic wall that either ends blindly or communicates with some external structure. **perilymph f.** A fistula between the periotic compartment of the inner ear and the middle ear, permitting the escape of perilymph into the tympanic cavity. It occurs usually in the oval window region as a complication of stapedectomy. **perirectal f.** ANAL FISTULA. **pharyngeal f.** An abnormal, often congenital passage communicating the pharynx with the skin of the neck. **pilonidal sinus f.** A sinus tract developed in the subcutaneous tissues of the intergluteal fold that opens to the outside at a point located from four to five cm posterior to the anus. Seen most commonly among young white males with straight black hair, this lesion is a giant cell foreign body reaction to inverted hairs that lodge in the dermis in skin folds subject to irritation and inflammation. These sinuses frequently become infected, causing chronic suppuration and requiring surgical removal. Also *pilonidal fistula.* **pleurobronchial f.** BRONCHOPLEURAL FISTULA. **pleurocutaneous f.** A communication between the pleural cavity and the skin. **preauricular f.** PREAURICULAR SINUS. **radiocephalic f.** An anastomosis of the radial artery and cephalic vein at the wrist. It is usually created to bring about the development of large venous channels in the forearm of subjects who require vascular access for hemodialysis. Also *Brescia-Cimino fistula.* **rectovaginal f.** An abnormal communication between the rectum and vagina often resulting in serious infections of the vaginal mucosa ascending to the cervix. **rectovesical f.** An abnormal communication between the urinary bladder and the rectum often resulting from tumor invasion. It causes severe cystitis and the presence of gas and feces in the urine. **salivary f.** An abnormal communication from a salivary duct allowing drainage of saliva to the outside or into the oral cavity through a newly formed passage. **spermatic f.** A fistula communicating with either the seminal ducts or the testicular parenchyma. **stercoral f.** FECAL FISTULA. **submental f.** A form of salivary fistula connecting a salivary duct with a cutaneous opening below the chin. **Thiry's f.** An artificially produced isolation of a segment of intestine for the purpose of collecting intestinal juice for experimental use. The procedure generally involves isolation of a loop of intestine, attachment of one end to the abdominal wall for drainage, and occlusion of the other end. Also *Thiry-Vella fistula.* **thoracic f.** A fistula through the thoracic wall that communicates with the pulmonary parenchyma or a loculated portion of the pleural cavity. **tracheoesophageal f.** A communication between the esophagus and trachea. It is a life-threatening condition that can be either congenital or acquired. As a congenital condition it occurs almost always in association with congenital esophageal atresia, and in acquired cases it is usually a complication of esophageal carcinoma, the result of the misuse of cuffed tracheostomy tubes, or, rarely, due to the presence of impacted esophageal foreign bodies. Also *esophagotracheal fistula.* **umbilical f.** A fistula between the intestine and umbilicus resulting from patency of the vitello-intestinal duct after birth. When the umbilical cord is cut, an open intestinal fistula is formed. Intestinal obstruction resulting from evagination and prolapse of intestinal loops through the fistula is a serious and life-threatening complication. **urachal f.** An abnormal communication between the urachus and other internal structures, most commonly the rectum. Rarely, the fistula is between the urachus and the bladder, resulting in escape of urine through the umbilicus. **ureterocervical f.** An abnormal communication between the cervix and the ureter. **urinary f.** An abnormal communication of the urinary tract with other internal structures allowing drainage of urine from the system and predisposing to ascending urinary tract infections. **uterovesical f.** An abnormal communication between the uterus and the urinary bladder. **Vella's f.** An isolated loop of intestine, both ends of which are exteri-

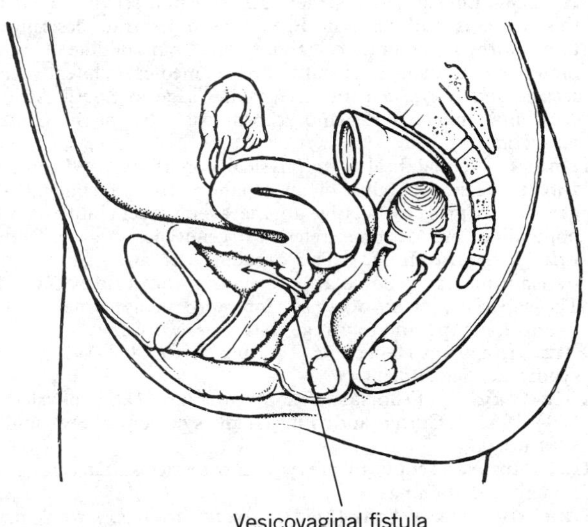

orized through the abdominal wall. It is used to study intestinal secretions. **vesical f.** Any abnormal communication of the urinary bladder with other structures. **vesicoabdominal f.** A fistula between the urinary bladder and the abdominal skin. **vesicocolonic f.** An abnormal communication between the urinary bladder and the colon. **vesicointestinal f.** An abnormal communication between the urinary bladder and the intestine. **vesicorectal f.** An abnormal communication between the urinary bladder and the rectum. **vesicoumbilical f.** A fistulous connection between the urinary bladder and the umbilicus, representing persistence of the embryonic continuity between the cloaca and the allantois. The fistula courses through the urachus and allows urine to escape at the umbilicus. **vesicovaginal f.** An abnormal communication between the urinary bladder and the vagina, often resulting from erosion by advanced carcinoma of the cervix. **vitelline f.** A persistence of the embryonic vitelline duct between the terminal ileum and the umbilicus, allowing fecal material to escape at the umbilicus.

**fistulae** \fis′tyəlē\ Plural of FISTULA.

**fistulation** \fis′tyəlā′shən\ FISTULIZATION.

**fistulatome** \fis′tyələtōm′\ [FISTULA + -TOME] A surgical instrument used to incise a fistula.

**fistulectomy** \fis′tyəlek′təmē\ [*fistul(a)* + -ECTOMY] A surgical procedure in which a fistula or extra-anatomic communication is removed. Also *syringectomy.*

**fistulization** \fis′tyəlīzā′shən\ The formation of an abnormal communication between two structures, one of which is usually a hollow organ or cavity. Also *fistulation.*

**fistulize** \fis′tyəlīze\ **1** To make (a fistula) surgically. **2** To develop a fistula, as by a disease process.

**fistuloenterostomy** \fis′tyəlō·en′təräs′təmē\ [*fistul(a)* + ENTERO- + -STOMY] A surgical operation for repair of a biliary or pancreatic fistula, in which a permanent connection is established between the fistula and the small intestine and the abnormal opening is closed.

**fistulography** \fis′tyəläg′rəfē\ Radiographic examination of a fistulous tract after injecting it with an opaque contrast medium through its external orifice.

**fistulotomy** \fis′tyəlät′əmē\ [*fistul(a)* + *o* + -TOMY] A surgical incision into a fistula. Also *syringotomy.*

**fistulous** \fis′tyələs\ Pertaining to the presence of a fistula.

**fit** [Old English *fitt* a strife] An epileptic seizure. • *Fit* in this sense is still used in Britain as a neutral, descriptive term without pejorative connotation, but in the United States and Canada it is outmoded in medical contexts, and *seizure* and *convulsion* are preferred. Usage in South Africa, Australia, and New Zealand accords with that of the United Kingdom.

**fitness** Good health or physical condition. **darwinian f.** The capability of an organism for transmitting its genome to progeny relative to the average capability of the population or to some reference genotype. Also *adaptive value.* **genetic f.** The capability of an organism for transmitting its genome to progeny. **reproductive f.** The capability of an organism for reproducing, usually relative to the population average. Also *survival value.*

**Fitz** [Reginald Heber *Fitz,* U.S. physician 1843–1913] Fitz syndrome. See under LAW.

**Fitz-Hugh** [Thomas *Fitz-Hugh,* Jr., U.S. physician, 1894–1963] Curtis and Fitz-Hugh syndrome. See under SYNDROME.

**fix** In microscopy, to preserve and render suitable for sectioning and staining.

**fixation** \fiksā′shən\ [Med L *fixatio* (from L *fix(us),* past part. of *figere* to fix, fasten, affix + *-atio* -ATION) an act of fixing or fixating] **1** The act of directing vision at a given point. **2** Persistence of libidinal or aggressive cathexis at an infantile level to a greater than usual degree, thereby constituting a focus for subsequent regression and expression of neurotic conflicts. Also *psychic inertia.* **3** In genetics, the attainment of a given allele of a gene frequency of 1.0, either by drift or by selection. Also *fixing.* **4** In chemistry, the formation of a stable compound. **5** The preservation of tissue for microscopic analysis, usually by immersion in a substance, as alcohol, that quickly kills and hardens it. **6** The act of immobilizing fragments of fractured bone, as with pins or screws. **arch bar f.** A method of holding the upper teeth firmly in occlusion with the lower teeth, used in the treatment of fractures of the jaws. Narrow strips of malleable metal, having small hooks attached at intervals, are wired to the outside of each dental arch, and the hooks of the upper arch bar are connected to those of the lower with rubber bands or wires. **binocular f.** Simultaneous observation of the object of regard by foveas of both eyes. **complement f.** The removal of components of complement from serum by reaction with immune complexes, antibody-coated cells or bacteria, or other material that activates complement. Also *Bordet and Gengou reaction, complement fixation reaction.* See also COMPLEMENT FIXATION TEST. **external pin f.** A method of securing the fractured parts of the mandible using metal pins which penetrate the skin and underlying tissues and are fixed into the bone. The outer ends are linked together with metal bars. **intermaxillary f.** MAXILLOMANDIBULAR FIXATION. **internal f.** The maintenance of a fracture reduction by the application of bone plates, screws, pins, wires, or any other means involving a surgical implant. **intramedullary f.** A method of maintaining fracture reduction and stabilization in a long bone in which a metal rod is inserted in the medullary canal of the bone across the fracture site. **intraosseous f.** A method of securing the fractured parts of the mandible or maxilla by means of wires, pins, plates, or screws, which are covered by the tissues after being put in place. **maxillomandibular f.** The fixing of the normal jaws together by means of wires as a treatment for obesity. Also *intermaxillary fixation.* **nitrogen f.** One of the phases of the nitrogen cycle in nature in which molecular nitrogen, $N_2$, is transformed into nitrates and ammonia. This fixation may be chemical, biologic, or electrical. The chemical process involves transformation into ammonia, followed by conversion of this into ammonium sulfate, urea, cyanamide, and nitrate. The biologic process occurs only in prokaryotes. It is rapid in certain blue-green bacteria (cyanobacteria) and in *Rhizobium* and *Azobacter* species, but it also occurs in many other species, including *Klebsiella.* The electrical process occurs in thunderstorms when ammonium nitrate is synthesized and is found dissolved in rain water. **postural f.** A method of correcting a bone or joint deformity by the use of slings and splints. **reflex ocular f.** The normal mechanism whereby the eyes fix upon and follow a moving object. **skeletal f.** The immobilization of a part or joint in which metal wires or pins are placed directly through bone and are then attached to external traction devices.

**fixative** \fik′sətiv\ [Med L *fixat(io)* fixation + -IVE] A chemical agent used in the preparation of a histologic specimen to maintain the essential structure of its constituent elements. Various substances are used for this, such as formaldehyde, which cross-links proteins and renders them insoluble. **Bouin's f.** BOUIN'S FLUID. **denture f.** DENTURE ADHESIVE. **glutaraldehyde f.** **1** A fixative used in specimen preparation for electron microscopy, consisting of a 4% solution of glutaraldehyde dissolved in phosphate or cacodylate buffer together with calcium chloride. It is the best general fixative for this purpose, and does not simultaneously stain the tissue. **2** A fixative used in preparation and sterilization of heterograft or allograft cardiac valves. **Helly's f.** HELLY'S FLUID. **lanthanum permanganate f.** A fixative solution used in electron microscopy in which lanthanum and potassium permanganate clearly demonstrate the cell membranes but preserve less well such intracytoplasmic structures as ribosomes. **Palade's f.** A fixative solution, suitable for electron microscopy, that contains osmium tetroxide dissolved in veronal acetate buffer. **paraformaldehyde f.** A fixative solution for use in electron microscopy that contains methanol-free formaldehyde and provides a high standard of tissue preservation. **potassium permanganate f.** A fixative solution for electron microscopy that is based on potassium permanganate. **Rhodin's f.** An isotonic solution for electron microscopy that contains osmium tetroxide dissolved in veronal acetate buffer. **Schaudinn's f.** A solution containing mercuric chloride, alcohol, and acetic acid, used to fix smears for cytologic examination. **Zenker's f.** ZENKER'S FLUID. **Zenker-formol f.** HELLY'S FLUID.

**fixing** FIXATION.

**fl.** fluid.

**flaccidity** \flaksid′itē\ The property of being soft and relaxed.

**Flack** [Martin William *Flack*, English physiologist, 1882–1931] Flack's node, Keith-Flack node, sinuatrial node of Keith and Flack. See under NODUS SINUATRIALIS.

**flagella** \fləjel′ə\ Plural of FLAGELLUM.

**flagellar** \fləjel′ər\ Pertaining to a flagellum or to organisms possessing flagella.

**flagellate** \flaj′əlāt\ [*flagell(um)* + -ATE] **1** Having one or more flagella. **2** An organism having one or more flagella, especially a protozoan of the subphylum Mastigophora. **3** To whip; to subject to flagellation.

**flagellated** \flaj′əlā′tid\ Having one or more flagella.

**flagellation** \flaj′əlā′shən\ **1** The whipping or beating of another or oneself as a means of sexual gratification. **2** The formation or arrangement of flagella.

**flagelliform** \fləjel′ifôrm\ Shaped like a flagellum.

**flagellin** A protein of molecular mass 53 kDa. It is the constituent of the helical filament of a bacterial flagellum.

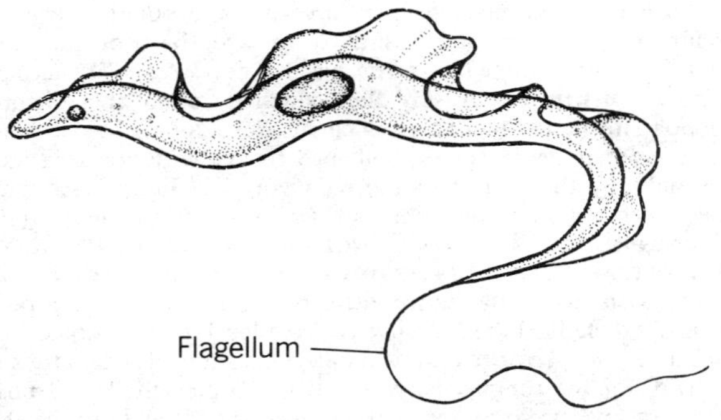

**Flagellum of Mastigophora**

**flagellum** \fləjel′əm\ [L (dim. of *flagrum*, a whip, scourge) a whip, lash, tentacle] (*pl.* flagella) **1** In protozoa, a locomotor organelle found in all Mastigophora and in intermediate forms of certain amebas and sporozoans. It is the definitive structure of flagellates. It is a filamentous cytoplasmic projection with a central axial filament or axoneme composed of a central and nine peripheral fibrils. The flagellum arises from a basal body. **2** In bacteria, a filament consisting of a helical chain of molecules of a single protein (flagellin) attached by a hooklike sheath to a basal body embedded in the wall and membrane. Locomotion is caused by rotation.

**flail** \flāl\ Capable of abnormal mobility, as of a joint, or paradoxical mobility, as of the chest wall following injury.

**flame** [French *flamme* (from L *flamma* flame, blaze) a flame] **1** The gaseous material that results from a rapid chemical reaction between a combustible material and oxygen or other oxidizing agent, usually in the form of an ascending cone that gives off energy as heat and light. **2** To expose noncombustible material to a flame for purposes of heat sterilization. **3** To expose combustible material to a flame for purposes of photometric analysis. **capillary f.** STORK BITE.

**flange** \flanj\ [Possibly from Old French *flangir* to bend, turn] A projecting edge, especially one providing guidance or serving as a means of attachment. **denture f.** The part of a denture base that extends into the vestibule of the mouth or into the alveololingual sulcus.

**flank** [Middle English *flanke*, from Old French *flanc* flank, from Germanic presumed *hlanka* flank, hip] The side of the trunk between the lowest rib and the iliac crest; latus.

# flap

**flap** [Middle English *flappe*] **1** In reconstructive surgery, one to several associated tissue layers dissected and transferred to a nearby site with an intact blood supply, or separated and transplanted to a distant site, with revascularization through anastomoses of recipient and donor arteries and veins. Also *surgical flap*. **2** PEDICLE GRAFT. **3** ASTERIXIS. **Abbe f.** A cross-lip flap, usually for reconstructing the upper lip. The triangular flap from the central part of the donor lip is rotated through 180 degrees as a small pedicle and sutured into the defect in the other lip. Also *Abbe lip flap*. **advancement f.** SLIDING FLAP. **axial f.** A pedicled skin flap which has its blood supplied entirely by a known artery and vein which are in the pedicle and which traverse the flap. Also *arterialized flap, arterial flap, axial pattern flap*. **axilloabdominal f.** THORACOEPIGASTRIC FLAP. **bilobed f.** A pedicle graft consisting of a larger tongue and a smaller tongue of tissue, both based on a single stem and the whole somewhat V-shaped. After surgical excision of a lesion not far from the larger tongue, the latter is rotated into the defect to cover it, while the smaller tongue is rotated into the donor defect from the larger tongue. The donor defect from the smaller tongue is closed by undermining the edges and bringing them together with sutures. Also *Zimany's bilobed flap*. **bipedicle f.** A flap devised with a soft tissue attachment at either end, thereby enhancing the vascular supply. Such flaps rarely die but they cannot be moved as far as a single pedicle flap. Also *double pedicle flap, bridge flap*. **Björk f.** A rectangular flap from the anterior tracheal wall, hinged downwards and stitched to the lower lip of the skin incision so as to facilitate the introduction of the tube in tracheostomy. **bone f.** A reflected plate of the cranium hinging on attached temporal muscle. Also *osteoplastic flap.* **bridge f.**

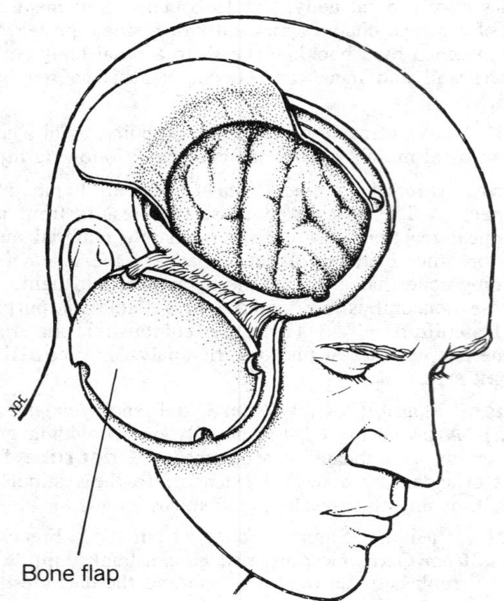


BIPEDICLE FLAP. **buccal f.** A flap from the mucosa of the internal surface of the cheek used to cover defects after ablative surgery in the oral and pharyngeal regions. Also *cheek flap.* **cellulocutaneous f.** SKIN FLAP. **cervical f.** Any flap fashioned from the tissues of the neck. **cheek f.** BUCCAL FLAP. **composite f.** Any flap, other than a skin flap, containing a considerable quantity of two or more tissues, as an osteocutaneous flap or a myocutaneous flap. Also *compound flap.* **coronal f.** A flap created to obtain surgical exposure of the bones of the naso-orbital region without leaving facial scars. A skin incision is made transversely in the scalp in the area of the coronal suture, and the flap of scalp and forehead tissues are reflected forward and downward. At the completion of the operation the flap is returned to its original position. **cross-finger f.** A flap that is fashioned from the tissues of one finger and transferred to an adjacent finger. **cross-leg f.** A flap raised on one leg and transferred to the other. Such flaps require several weeks of immobilization while the new blood supply becomes established. **cross-lip f.** A flap for repairing a defect in one lip raised from the other and rotated across the mouth on a pedicle containing the coronary (labial) blood vessels. The pedicle is divided after three weeks, by which time the flap can be expected to have acquired an adequate blood supply from the receiving lip. **delayed f.** A pedicled skin flap which is prepared before transfer by a series of operation at intervals of seven or more days so as to divest the flap of a portion of its normal blood supply and augment the blood supply coming through the pedicle. The procedure is used most frequently in the preparation of random flaps. **deltopectoral f.** An axial flap taken from the skin and subcutaneous tissues of the anterior chest wall and the front of the shoulder. Its blood supply comes from the internal mammary artery. **direct f.** A skin flap which is elevated from its donor area and applied to the recipient area in the same operation, without any intervening procedure. Also *immediate transfer flap.* **dorsalis pedis f.** An axial flap receiving its blood supply from the dorsalis pedis artery, and fashioned from the skin and subcutaneous tissue on the top of the foot. **double pedicle f.** BIPEDICLE FLAP. **eave f.** A method of deepening the helical sulcus of the ear. The lateral superior skin of the ear is elevated as a broad flap based at the superior free border of the ear. The under surface is then skin-grafted, and the overall effect resembles the eaves of a roof. **Estlander f.** A cross-lip flap for repairing a defect in the lateral part of one lip with a flap raised from the vermilion border of the other and rotated so that the pedicle becomes the new commissure. **fan f.** Any fan-shaped flap. **Filatov f.** TUBED FLAP. **forehead f.** A flap of forehead skin and subcutaneous tissue based on the superficial temporal artery, used in plastic reconstruction within the mouth or of the lateral wall of the oropharynx. Also *temporal flap.* **free f.** A skin flap or composite flap having no continuous pedicle or tether between the donor and recipient sites. After being completely elevated, as an island flap, on a long stalk of its nourishing artery and vein(s), the base of the stalk is severed and the flap is transferred to the distant recipient site, where it is revascularized by anastomosing its artery and vein(s) to comparable isolated vessels in the new site. Also *microvascular free graft.* **free bone f.** A segment of cranium, unattached to muscle, removed in surgical exposure of the brain and replaced as the wound is closed. • Its designation as a flap is a misnomer. **French f.** SLIDING FLAP. **Gillies f.** TUBED FLAP. **groin f.** An axial flap fashioned from tissues centered over the inguinal crease and receiving its blood supply from branches of the femoral artery and vein. **hinge f.** TURNOVER FLAP. **immediate transfer f.** DIRECT FLAP. **Indian f.** A skin flap from the forehead used for partial or total reconstruction of the nose. • This flap was described about 900 B. C. in the Sushruta Samhitá of ancient India. Many modifications have been developed since that time. **intercalated f.** One of two adjacent flaps which can be transposed, as in a Z-plasty. **island f.** A flap, usually a skin flap, which is completely raised so that it remains attached to the donor area only by the long pedicle of its nourishing artery and vein(s). In order to be transferred to another site, a subcutaneous tunnel is created between the donor and recipient sites. The flap is put through the tunnel, keeping the nourishing vessels intact. **Italian f.** A pedicled skin flap from the arm, used for partial or total reconstruction of the nose. After the arm flap is raised on its pedicle, the forearm is brought over the scalp, the head is rotated slightly toward the arm, and the flap is sutured in place in the nasal defect. Also *Tagliacozzi flap.* **jump f.** A skin flap which is raised at a distant donor site and attached to a carrier, usually the wrist, and later, sometimes in stages, detached from the donor area and brought by the carrier to the recipient site. Jump flaps may be tubed or may be kept flat as in an open jump flap. **Langenbeck f.** VON LANGENBECK'S BIPEDICLED MUCOPERIOSTEAL FLAP **latissimus dorsi muscle f.** A flap consisting of the entire latissimus dorsi muscle or a portion thereof. Its blood supply is provided by the thoracodorsal artery. **lingual f.** A flap consisting of a lengthwise portion of the tongue, between 20 to 40 percent, based posteriorly and used to reconstruct defects of the floor of the mouth and alveolus as well as buccal defects following ablative surgery. Also *tongue flap*. **liver f.** Asterixis in hepatic encephalopathy. **local f.** A flap having its donor area contiguous or very near to the recipient site. **Millard island f.** A method of lengthening the palate wherein a mucoperiosteal island flap from the anterior palate, receiving its blood supply from the greater palatine artery, is inserted, with the mucosa on the nasal side, between the hard and soft palates. **mucomuscular f.** A flap incorporating muscle and the overlying mucous membrane. **mucoperiosteal f.** A flap of mucous membrane with underlying periosteum taken from bone of the hard palate. **muscle f.** A pedicle graft consisting entirely of muscle. **myocutaneous f.** A flap consisting of a muscle, usually in its entirety, together with all the overlying tissue, including the skin. Also *musculocutaneous flap*. **nasolabial f.** A flap fashioned from the tissues in the vicinity of the nasolabial fold. **neurovascular f.** An axial flap with its sensory nerves retained intact. **osteoplastic f.** BONE FLAP. **pectoral muscle f.** A flap consisting of the entire pectoralis muscle or a portion thereof. Its major blood supply is from branches of the thoracoacromial artery and vein. **pericoronal f.** Gingiva overlying but not attached to the crown of a partially erupted tooth. **pharyngeal f.** 1 A flap raised from the posterior pharyngeal wall, as in a palatopharyngoplasty. 2 Any flap from the pharynx. **random f.** A skin flap with its blood supply coming from a number of small and unidentified vessels, often running in various directions, rather than from a single and known main artery with its accompanying veins. Also *random pattern flap*. **rope f.** TUBED FLAP. **rotation f.** A local flap for which the tissue is advanced into its new position by rotating the tissue about an axis in the center of the flap. **sandwich f.** A flap consisting of two flaps placed back to back. **scalping f.** A flap consisting of a temporarily elevated scalp which is used as a carrier for the forehead or small segments of the hair-bearing scalp that are utilized in the reconstruction of the nose or eyebrows. When its use as a carrier is complete, it is returned to its original position. **skin f.** A flap consisting of the entire thickness of the skin plus part or all of the subjacent subcutaneous fat. Also *cellocutaneous flap*. **sliding f.** A skin flap designed and elevated adjacent to a defect and then, taking advantage of the stretchability of the skin, pulled over the defect and sutured in place. This flap is usually applicable only to small defects. Also *advancement flap, French flap*. **split thickness f.** In periodontal surgery, a flap of epithelium and connective tissue which does not include the periosteum. **subcutaneous pedicle f.** TUNNEL FLAP. **surgical f.** FLAP. **Tagliacozzi f.** ITALIAN FLAP. **temporal f.** FOREHEAD FLAP. **tensor fasciae latae muscle f.** A flap consisting of the entire tensor fascia latae muscle or a portion thereof. Its vascular pedicle is the lateral circumflex femoral artery. **thoracoabdominal f.** A flap fashioned from the tissues of both the abdominal and chest walls. **thoracoepigastric f.** A flap, usually superiorly based, that is fashioned from the combined tissues of the lateral chest wall and the anterior abdominal wall. Also *axilloabdominal flap*. **tongue f.** 1 LINGUAL FLAP. 2 Any flap fashioned from the tongue. **transposition f.** A flap that is moved at an angle in order to reach the recipient site. The movement is around a vertical axis located in the base of the flap. **trapdoor f.** A flap, roughly square in shape and left attached on one border, that consists of an elevated segment of skin and subcutaneous tissue. It is created to obtain surgical exposure and is returned to its original position after completion of the operation. **tubed f.** A flap created by making two long, parallel cuts through the skin and subcutaneous tissue, undermining the area between the incisions, then suturing the two skin edges of the flap together, with the epidermis facing outward, to make a rope, or tube, of the skin and subcutaneous tissue. Also *tube flap, tubed pedicle flap, Filatov flap, Gillies flap, rope flap*. **tunnel f.** A long, rectangular, skin flap in which the pedicle is denuded of all contiguous epidermis, and the flap is then passed through a subcutaneous tunnel to the recipient site so that the denuded pedicle lies in the tunnel and the skin-covered portion emerges on the other side to cover the original defect. Also *subcutaneous pedicle flap*. **turnover f.** A flap in which the axis of rotation lies along the length of its base, thus causing the surface of the flap to be inverted and to lie adjacent to its original position. It is a type often used as a lining flap. Also *hinge flap*. **von Langenbeck's bipedicled mucoperiosteal f.** A flap used in closure of a complete cleft of the palate, consisting of the entire thickness of oral mucosa and periosteum on one side of the hard palate from front to back. The anterior pedicle contains the incisive artery and vein and the posterior pedicle contains the major palatine artery and vein. Also *Langenbeck flap*. **V-Y f.** A V-shaped flap that is elongated to cover a greater area of tissue. The flap, which is at first triangular, is undermined and then pulled so that the area is then sutured in the shape of a Y. **Z-f.** A flap consisting of two triangular flaps formed from a Z-shaped incision that has been made through the skin and subcutaneous tissues. The two flaps are rotated and then interchanged, which serves to rotate the axis of tension, originally along the central limb of a the Z-shaped incision, by 90 percent. **Zimany's bilobed f.** BILOBED FLAP.

**flare** [Middle English *fleare*] 1 The visible reflection of light from the aqueous or vitreous humors made turbid by a pathologic amount of protein present because of breakdown of the blood-aqueous barrier. Flare is recognized by biomicroscopic observation of the path of a sharply focused beam of light. 2 The eccentric deposition of soot, unburned powder, and metal shavings and thermal burning of the skin on one side of a short-range, gunshot entrance wound. Also *flip*. **f. of the nostrils** ALAE NASI.

**flash** [Middle English *flaschen*] The flange of surplus material surrounding a dental cast which is made in a two-part mold. It prevents complete closure of the flask.

**flashblindness** See under BLINDNESS.

**flask** [French *flasque* (from Late L *flasca* or *flasco* a keg, bottle; perh. from Germanic; possibly from alter. of L *vasculum* a small vessel) a bottle or flask] 1 A narrow-mouthed, usually glass container, often with a rounded or expanded lower portion, that is used for storage and manipulation of fluids. 2 A metal box or cylinder that is used to contain investment material when making a mold, as for a denture. **Carrel f.** A flask used in tissue culture. The elongated neck may be slanted from the vertical at any angle from a slight deviation to a right angle. **casting f.** A flask for use with refractory investment in casting with molten metal. Also *casting ring*. **Dewar f.** VACUUM FLASK. **Erlenmeyer f.** A glass laboratory flask with a broad base, cone-shaped body, and a relatively short neck. **vacuum f.** A double-walled glass container, often with silvered surfaces. An evacuated space between the two walls provides thermal insulation between the contents of the flask and the environment. Also *Dewar flask*. **volumetric f.** A flask with a relatively large body and a slender, elongated neck marked to denote a precise quantity of liquid that the container holds.

**flat** 1 Lacking irregularities or curvature: said of a surface, or of a line on a graph. 2 Lacking resonance: said of auscultatory sounds. 3 Somewhat lower than a standard or intended pitch: said of musical tones.

**Flatau** [Edward *Flatau*, Polish neurologist, 1869–1932] 1 See under LAW. 2 Flatau's disease, Flatau-Schilder disease. See under SCHILDER'S DISEASE.

**flatfoot** TALIPES PLANUS. **rocker-bottom f.** A congenitally malformed foot in which a congenital dislocation of the talonavicular joint results in a convex contour to the sole. It may be associated with the chromosomal defect of autosomal trisomy, especially of 13–15 and 18. Also *rocker-bottom foot, congenital convex club foot, convex foot, rocker-bottom deformity.* **spastic f.** A painful variety of flatfoot which is believed to result from spasm of the peroneal muscles with consequent partial eversion of the foot. Also *spasmodic talipes planus, talipes spasmodicus.* **static f.** The stabilized, fixed loss of the normal longitudinal arch of the foot.

**flattening** In psychiatry, the leveling, impoverishment, or dulling of emotional reactivity.

**flatulence** \flach′ələns\ [French, irreg. from L *flatus*, past part. of *flare* to blow, breathe] The presence of an excessive amount of gas in the stomach or intestine.

**flatus** \flā′təs\ [L, substantive from *flatus*, past part. of *flare* to blow, breathe] 1 Gas generated in the stomach or the intestinal tract. 2 Gas expelled from the intestinal tract. **f. vaginalis** Audible expulsion of gas from the vagina.

**flatworm** Any worm belonging to the phylum Platyhelminthes.

**flav-** \flāv-\ FLAVO-.

**flavacidin** AMYLPENICILLIN SODIUM.

**flavianic acid** $C_{10}H_6N_2O_8S$. A naphthol derivative used to precipitate arginine and histidine in protein hydrolysis. As the sodium or potassium salt, it is used in tissue stains.

**flavicin** AMYLPENICILLIN SODIUM.

**flavin** \flā′vin\ [FLAV- + -IN] Any of a few compounds that contain the tricyclic nucleus dimethylisoalloxazine, which consists of dimethylbenzene fused to a pterin ring. In its oxidized, quinonoid form it is yellow. Most natural flavins are combined forms of riboflavin.

**flavin adenine dinucleotide** A prosthetic group of many oxidizing enzymes, which can exist in oxidized or reduced forms. It consists of a diphosphate residue, esterified with adenosine on one phosphorus and riboflavin on the other.

**flavin mononucleotide** Riboflavin 5′-phosphate, the prosthetic group of some enzymes. Also *isoalloxazine mononucleotide, riboflavin phosphate, riboflavin mononucleotide, vitamin $B_2$ phosphate.*

**flavivirus** \flā′vivī′rəs\ [L *flav(us)* yellow (as in yellow fever) + VIRUS] Any of a large group of RNA viruses (formerly group B arboviruses) belonging to the genus *Flavivirus*, family Togaviridae. These viruses produce a variety of febrile systemic syndromes and meningoencephalitis in humans.

**flavo-** \flā′vō-\ [L *flavus* yellow] A combining form meaning yellow. Also *flav-*.

***Flavobacterium*** \-baktir′ē·əm\ [FLAVO- + BACTERIUM] A genus of Gram-negative, mostly nonmotile bacilli, found in nature, that form yellow to red pigmented colonies, and that ferment so slowly that they are often mistaken for nonfermenters (especially for pseudomonads). *F. meningosepticum* often causes serious illness in the newborn.

**flavoprotein** A yellow protein containing a flavin as prosthetic group.

**flavor** \flā′vər\ 1 A distinctive taste. The olfactory sense as well as the gustatory sense contributes to the sensation of flavor. 2 To impart a flavor to; especially, in pharmacology, to disguise the taste of by admixing additives: used of medicines taken orally.

**flavoxate hydrochloride** $C_{24}H_{26}ClNO_4$. 3-Methyl-4-oxo-2-phenyl-4*H*-1-benzopyran-8-carboxylic acid 2-piperidinoethyl ester hydrochloride, an anticholinergic drug with local anesthetic and analgesic properties. It is also capable of relaxing smooth muscles. it is administered orally for urinary tract pain and discomfort from inflammation of the bladder and urinary tract components.

**flay** \flā\ To tear away strips of skin and subcutaneous tissues by repetitive blows, as in whipping.

**fld.** fluid.

**flea** [Old English *flēah*, akin to L *pulex* flea and Gk *psylla* flea] A dorsoventrally flattened, wingless, ectoparasitic insect of the order Siphonaptera equipped with an extraordinarily developed jumping third pair of legs, mouth parts adapted for sucking blood, smooth body segments with posteriorly directed ctenoid or comblike hairs, and extremely complex genitalia. Some 1500 species are known ectoparasites of warmblooded animals, particularly rodents. Many

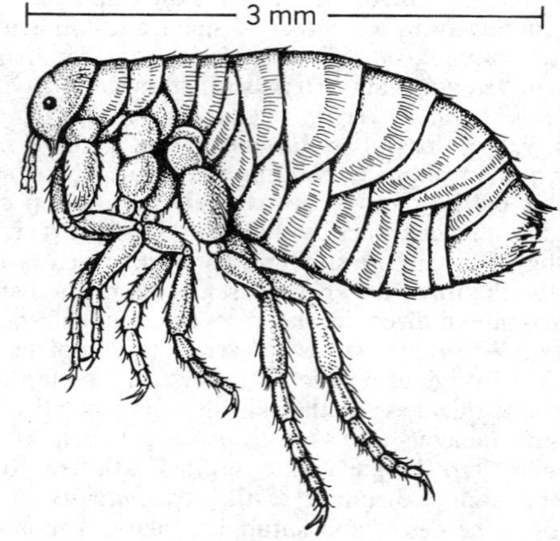


**Human flea** (*Pulex irritans*)

species attack man and are carriers of a number of diseases such as plague and typhus, and many species are intermediate hosts of helminths of birds and mammals. **burrowing f.** A flea of the species *Tunga penetrans*; a chigoe. **cat f.** A flea of the species *Ctenocephalides felis*. **chigger f.** CHIGOE. **chigoe f.** CHIGOE. **common f.** HUMAN FLEA. **dog f.** A flea of the species *Ctenocephalides canis*. **human f.** A flea of the species *Pulex irritans*. Also *common flea*. **jigger f.** CHIGOE. **oriental rat f.** A flea of the species *Xenopsylla cheopis*. **rat f.** Any of several species of fleas found as ectoparasites of rats, some of which are involved in transmission of plague, including *Xenopsylla cheopis, X. brasiliensis*, and *X. astia*. **sand f.** CHIGOE. **sticktight f.** A flea of the species *Echidnophaga gallinacea*. **water f.** Popular COPEPOD.

**Flechsig** [Paul Emil *Flechsig*, German neurologist, 1847–1929] 1 Ground bundles of Flechsig. See under BUNDLE. 2 Flechsig's fasciculi. See under FASCICULI PROPRII.

3 Flechsig's tract. See under TRACTUS SPINOCEREBELLARIS DORSALIS. 4 Flechsig's myelogenetic law. See under MYELOGENETIC LAW. 5 Oval area of Flechsig, oval bundle of Flechsig. See under FASCICULUS SEPTOMARGINALIS. 6 Fasciculus anterior proprius flechsigi, fasciculus lateralis proprius flechsigi. See under FASCICULUS. 7 Flechsig's field. See under MYELINOGENETIC FIELD.

**fleece** A neural fiber network.

**Fleischer** [Richard *Fleischer,* German physician, 1848–1909] 1 Fleischer-Strümpell ring. See under FLEISCHER KERATOCONUS RING. 2 Kayser-Fleischer ring. See under RING. 3 See under VORTEX.

**Fleischmann** [Gottfried *Fleischmann,* German anatomist, 1777–1853] Fleischmann's bursa. See under BURSA SUBLINGUALIS.

**Fleischner** [Felix *Fleischner,* German-born U.S. radiologist and physician, born 1893] 1 See under LINE. 2 See under DISEASE.

**Flemming** [Walther *Flemming,* German anatomist, 1843–1905] 1 Flemming center. See under GERMINAL CENTER. 2 Flemming's liquid, Flemming solution. See under FLEMMING'S FIXING FLUID.

**flesh** [Old English *flæsc;* akin to German *Fleisch* flesh] 1 The muscular tissues of the body. 2 The soft outer tissues of the animal body, including the muscles. **goose f.** Skin in which piloerection has taken place as a reaction to cold or emotion. Also *cutis anserina, gooseflesh, goose bumps.* **live f.** MYOKYMIA. **proud f.** 1 GRANULATION TISSUE. 2 Exuberant granulation tissue that has overgrown the boundaries and contours of the wound where it was formed.

**flex** To bend a limb or other body part at a joint. Compare EXTEND.

**flexibilitas** \flek'sibil'itas\ FLEXIBILITY. **f. cerea** A characteristic of catalepsy in which the patient allows bending of the limbs or body into a particular posture or attitude which is maintained for inordinate periods of time. Also *waxy flexibility.*

**flexibility** The property of being flexible. Also *flexibilitas.* **waxy f.** FLEXIBILITAS CEREA.

**flexible** Capable of bending without breaking. Also *flexile.*

**flexion** \flek'shən\ [L *flexio* (from *flexus,* past part. of *flectere* to bend, turn) a bending, winding] The movement of parts of the body, usually around an axis which is transverse or obliquely transverse. It usually results in a diminution of the angle between two ventral surfaces. **lateral f.** The act of bending to the right or left. **mass f.** A general contraction of flexor musculature, such as occurs when a mass reflex is triggered in the chronic spinal patient. **plantar f.** Movement of the ankle and tarsal joints in which the dorsum of the foot moves away from the anterior (cranial) aspect of the tibia or, in the forelimb of a quadruped, from the radius. After plantar flexion the foot or toes are said to be extended downward in the direction of the sole. Also *plantiflexion.* Compare DORSIFLEXION. **posterior f.** The approximation of the two sides of a joint posteriorly. *Outmoded.* • The term is sometimes incorrectly used by clinicians when referring to movements of the vertebral column as extension or hyperextension is taking place. **universal f.** Flexion of the fetal parts onto the body as a normal process during labor.

**Flexner** [Simon *Flexner,* U.S. pathologist, 1863–1946] 1 See under SERUM. 2 Flexner's dysentery. See under BACILLARY DYSENTERY. 3 Flexner-Jobling carcinosarcoma. See under CARCINOSARCOMA.

**flexor** \flek'sər\ [New L, from L *flex(us),* past part. of *flectere* to bend + *-or* -OR] A muscle that produces an approximation of the movable part on one side of a joint to the fixed side to a varying degree. In general, the approximation results in a forward movement of the movable part except in the lower limb, where, in the case of the knee, ankle, and toe joints, it produces a posterior movement of the movable part. Compare EXTENSOR.

**flexura** \flekshoo'rə\ [L (from *flexus,* past part. of *flectere* to bend, bow, turn) a bending, winding, turning] An angulation or bend, usually in a structure or organ. Also *flexure.* **f. coli dextra** [NA] The bend between the terminal part of the ascending colon and the beginning of the transverse colon. It is situated below the right lobe of the liver and anterior to the inferolateral part of the anterior surface of the right kidney. Also *right flexure of colon, right colic flexure, hepatic flexure of colon.* **f. coli sinistra** [NA] The acute bend between the termination of the transverse colon and the commencement of the descending colon. It is situated in the left hypochondriac region, inferior to the lateral extremity of the spleen and tail of the pancreas and anterior to the left kidney. It is attached to the diaphragm by the phrenicocolic ligament. Also *left flexure of colon, left colic flexure, splenic flexure of colon.* **f. duodeni inferior** [NA] The bend between the descending part and the horizontal part of the duodenum. It is situated at the right side of the lower border of the third lumbar vertebra and of the inferior vena cava. Also *inferior flexure of duodenum, inferior angle of duodenum.* **f. duodeni superior** [NA] The acute bend between the superior part and the descending part of the duodenum, which is usually located below the neck of the gallbladder. Also *superior flexure of duodenum, superior angle of duodenum.* **f. duodenojejunalis** [NA] The sharp bend between the end of the ascending part of the duodenum and the commencement of the jejunum, which is situated at the level of the upper border of the second lumbar vertebra. It is fixed posteriorly by the suspensory muscle of the duodenum and is related to the body of the pancreas superiorly and the transverse colon and mesocolon anteriorly. Also *duodenojejunal flexure, duodenojejunal angle.* **f. perinealis recti** [NA] The sharp backward bend of the terminal part of the rectum at the anorectal junction. Also *perineal flexure of rectum.* **f. sacralis recti** [NA] The anteroposterior curvature of the upper part of the rectum. It has its concavity directed anteriorly. Also *sacral flexure of rectum.*

**flexurae** \flekshoo'rē\ Plural of FLEXURA.

**flexure** \flek'shər\ FLEXURA. **basicranial f.** PONTINE FLEXURE. **caudal f.** The ventral curvature which develops at the hind end of an embryo and ends in the tail. Also *sacral flexure.* **cephalic f.** In the embryo, a flexure (concave below) on the inferior aspect of the cranial extremity of the closed neural tube at the level of the midbrain. Also *mesencephalic flexure, head bend.* **cervical f.** An encephalic flexure of the embryo, the first to appear, at the junction of the rhombencephalon and the spinal cord. Also *nuchal flexure, neck bend.* **dorsal f.** The curvature that develops ventrally in the thoracic region of the developing embryo. **duodenojejunal f.** FLEXURA DUODENOJEJUNALIS. **encephalic f.** Any of three flexures that appear in the developing neural tube as a result of unequal growth of its different parts. Two are concave ventrally (cephalic and cervical flexures), one is convex ventrally (pontine). **hepatic f. of colon** FLEXURA COLI DEXTRA. **inferior f. of duodenum** FLEXURA DUODENI INFERIOR. **left colic f.** FLEXURA COLI SINISTRA. **lumbar f.** The anteriorly convex curvature of the lumbar region of the vertebral column. **mesencephalic f.** CE-

PHALIC FLEXURE. **nuchal f.** CERVICAL FLEXURE. **perineal f.** Ventral curvature in the embryo where the back sweeps round to the perineum. **perineal f. of rectum** FLEXURA PERINEALIS RECTI. **pontine f.** An encephalic flexure of the embryo which develops in the rhombencephalon between the metencephalon and the myelencephalon. Also *basicranial flexure.* **right colic f.** FLEXURA COLI DEXTRA. **right f. of colon** FLEXURA COLI DEXTRA. **sacral f.** CAUDAL FLEXURE. **sacral f. of rectum** FLEXURA SACRALIS RECTI. **sigmoid f. of colon** *Outmoded* COLON SIGMOIDEUM. **splenic f. of colon** FLEXURA COLI SINISTRA. **superior f. of duodenum** FLEXURA DUODENI SUPERIOR.

**flicker** [Old English *flicorian* to move the wings] The quality of visual sensation produced by a rapid and regular intermittance of a stimulus within the visual field.

**flight / f. of ideas** Rapid speech with the speaker switching from one topic to another, as in manic states. Also *topical flight.* **f. into disease** The conversion of a mental conflict into physical symptoms, as seen in neurotic disorders. **topical f.** FLIGHT OF IDEAS.

**Flint** [Austin *Flint,* U.S. physician, 1812–1886] Flint's murmur. See under AUSTIN FLINT MURMUR.

**Flint** [Austin *Flint,* Jr., U.S. physiologist, 1836–1915] Flint's arcade. See under ARTERIAE ARCUATAE RENIS.

**flip** FLARE.

**floaters** \flō′tərs\ Apparent visual opacities perceived as drifting in suspension in front of the eye. This is due to the presence of opacities in the posterior portion of the vitreous humor, a position from which a shadow can be cast upon the retina. Floaters may represent benign embryologic remnants or acquired pathologic changes within the vitreous humor.

**floating** 1 Unattached; free or partly free, as the lowest two pairs of ribs, whose anterior ends are not connected to the cartilages above. 2 Being or capable of being displaced from its normal position, as a kidney.

**floc** \fläk\ [L *floc(cus)* a lock or pile of wool] The fluffy, woolly, or lumpy precipitates that result when an antigen and antibody unite in a flocculation reaction. *Popular.*

**floccillation** \fläk′silā′shən\ [L *flocc(us)* a tuft of cotton + *-ill(us),* masc. diminishing suffix + English -ATION] CARPHOLOGY.

**floccular** \fläk′yələr\ [*floccul(us)* + -AR] 1 Of or relating to the fluffy, woolly or lumpy precipitates that develop after some antigen-antibody reactions. 2 Pertaining to the flocculus of the cerebellum.

**flocculation** \fläk′yəlā′shən\ [*floccul(e)* + -ATION] The formation of fluffy, woolly, or lumpy precipitates following the combination of an antibody with colloidally suspended particulate antigens. This immunologic reaction is often performed to detect bacterial antibodies.

**flocculent** \fläk′yələnt\ 1 Precipitated from a fluid as fluffy lumps. 2 Growing in loose aggregates in a liquid medium, as bacteria.

**flocculi** Plural of FLOCCULUS.

**flocculus** \fläk′yələs\ [Late L (dim. of L *floccus* a lock or pile of wool), a small lock or pile of wool] (*pl.* flocculi) [NA] A downward-hanging, semidetached lobule at the lower extremity of each cerebellar hemisphere, continuous with the nodulus of the vermis. Also *nucleus nervi pneumogastrici* (obs.), *floccular process.* **accessory f.** The small, lateral, lobular extension of the cerebellar flocculus. Also *paraflocculus, secondary flocculus, flocculus secondarii.*

**Flood** [Valentine *Flood,* Irish surgeon, 1800–1847] See under LIGAMENT.

**flooding** Prolonged exposure of the phobic subject to the very object or situation he fears, as a form of therapy.

**floor** [Old English *flor,* akin to L *planus* level, flat] The inferior, or lowest, surface of any cavity or hollow organ; the surface joining the lowest parts of the walls of any space, area, or organ. **jugular f. of tympanic cavity** PARIES JUGULARIS CAVITATIS TYMPANICAE. **f. of orbit** PARIES INFERIOR ORBITAE.

**flora** \flôr′ə\ [L *Flora* goddess of flowers.] 1 The plants of a particular geographical area or period of time. 2 The total microbial population of a localized region, as of the intestinal tract or the skin. **intestinal f.** The highly mixed bacterial population in the feces. The intestinal contents are anaerobic, and the facultative organisms that can grow on aerobic plates, consisting largely of Enterobacteriaceae, are in fact usually greatly outnumbered by obligate anaerobes (bacteroids). **oral f.** The microorganisms normally resident in the oral cavity.

**Florence** [Albert *Florence,* French physician, 1851–1927] See under REACTION.

**florid** \flôr′id\ [L *florid(us)* (from *flos,* gen. *floris,* a flower) flowery, blooming, bright-colored] 1 Bright red, as a skin lesion. 2 Fully represented or developed, as the symptoms of a disease.

**flow** [Old English *flōwan* (akin to L *pluere* to rain but unrelated to L *fluere* to flow) to flow] 1 The movement of a fluid or the course of such movement. 2 A measure of the quantity or rate of the movement of a fluid, as of blood through the vessels or of air in inspiration into the lungs. **axoplasmic f.** The physiologic movement of protein molecules along an axon. Fast and slow rates of flow have been described and studied using radioactively labeled substances. **cerebral blood f.** The volume of blood that passes through vessels of the brain in a given period, usually measured between the carotid artery and jugular vein. **effective pulmonary blood f.** Pulmonary blood flow available for gas exchange. **effective renal blood f.** Blood flow calculated by dividing the effective renal plasma flow by unity minus the hematocrit ratio. **effective renal plasma f.** The plasma flow that perfuses the renal parenchyma, approximately 90 percent of total renal plasma flow. The remaining 10 percent is presumed to perfuse the supporting tissues of the kidney. It is measured by the clearance method, using agents such as *p*-amino hippurate (PAH) at such low plasma concentrations that all of the agent is removed during one passage through the kidney. **gene f.** The transfer of genes between distinct populations of the same species through mating. It may influence allele frequency and evolution. Also *gene spread.* **laminar f.** 1 A directional flow of air in a controlled environment with the use of fan and filter, used to decrease contamination by airborne bacteria. 2 A type of flow by liquids in tubes in which successive cylindrical layers of fluid move with decreasing velocity as one proceeds from the axis of flow to the wall of the tube. Cohesive forces between the wall and the liquid limit the movement of an infinitesimally thin layer of fluid at the periphery but the movement of inner layers of fluid upon one another is related to the viscosity of the fluid. **maximal midexpiratory f.** The greatest flow of air generated during the midpart of a forced exhalation. **peak expiratory f.** The greatest flow rate attained during a forced exhalation: a measure of airway obstruction. **renal blood f.** TOTAL RENAL BLOOD FLOW. Abbr. RBF **total renal blood f.** Blood flow to the entire kidney. Also *renal blood flow.*

**Flower** [Sir William Henry *Flower,* English surgeon and anatomist, 1831–1899] 1 Flower's bone. See under EPIPTERIC BONE. 2 Flower's index. See under DENTAL INDEX.

**flowers** [variant of Middle English *flour(es)*, from Old French, from L *flos*, gen. *floris* flower, flowering, growth or deposit on a surface, fine powder] The form of a drug or chemical obtained by sublimation.

**flowmeter** \flō′mē′tər\ An instrument for measuring the rate at which a volume of liquids or gases is moving within a closed hydraulic system. Examples include instruments which measure rate of blood flow within arteries and veins, and rate of gas flow within the airways. Also *stromuhr.* **Doppler f.** A blood flowmeter that continuously transmits ultrasound into a vessel. Reflected ultrasound has a Doppler frequency shift that is proportional to blood cell velocity. An acoustic output provides information on blood velocity, while a recorder indicates blood flow averaged across the cross-section. Also *continuous wave Doppler flowmeter.* **dry f.** A flowmeter which measures gas flow quantitatively. A bobbin is placed in a tapered tube attached to the source of gas, and as the gas is released the bobbin will rise. **electromagnetic f.** A device measuring blood flow based upon the voltage created by blood moving through a magnetic field. **pulsed Doppler f.** A blood flowmeter that transmits pulses of ultrasound into the vessel. Reflected ultrasound has a Doppler frequency shift that is proportional to blood cell velocity. It displays velocity versus radial position as it changes with time.

**floxuridine** $C_9H_{11}FN_2O_5$. 2′-Deoxy-5-fluorouridine. An antineoplastic drug that is an analogue of fluorouracil. It is used in the treatment of carcinomas and is given by intra-arterial infusion. Abbr. FUDR

**flu** \floo\ *Popular* INFLUENZA. **intestinal f.** A viral infection of the gastrointestinal tract usually resulting in emesis or diarrhea.

**flucrylate** $C_7H_6F_3NO_2$. 2,2,2-Trifluoro-1-methylethyl-2-cyanoacrylate. A tissue adhesive used in surgical procedures.

**flucytosine** $C_4H_4FN_3O$. 5-Fluorocytosine. An antifungal agent employed in the treatment of serious fungal infections from *Candida* and *Cryptococcus* organisms.

**fludrocortisone** $C_{23}H_{31}FO_6$. 21-(Acetyloxy)-9α-fluoro-11β17α-dihydroxy-pregn-4-ene-3,20-dione. A synthetic corticosteroid possessing both glucocorticoid and mineralcorticoid activities. It is used as a replacement therapy in mineralcorticoid insufficiency and in congenital adrenocortical hyperplasia. Also *fluohydrisone, fluohydrocortisone.*

**fludrocortisone acetate** $C_{23}H_{31}FO_6$ The acetate ester form of fluorocortisone. It is used as an anti-inflammatory drug, with uses and actions like those of hydrocortisone and deoxycortisone.

**fluence** \floo′əns, flʏ·äns′\ INTEGRAL NEUTRON FLUX. **energy f.** In radiation dosimetry, the sum of the energies of all the particles which enter a sphere of unit cross-sectional area.

**flufenamic acid** $C_{14}H_{10}F_3NO_2$. 3′-Trifluoromethyldiphenylamine-2-carboxylic acid. It is used as an anti-inflammatory agent and as an analgesic.

**flügelplatte** \flē′gəlplät′ə, flʏ′-\ [German *Flügel* a wing, fin, blade + *Platte* plate] ALAR LAMINA.

**fluid** [French *fluide* (from L *fluidus* flowing, fluid, from *fluere* to flow) fluid (adj.)] **1** Capable of flowing, as a liquid or gas. **2** A fluid substance; a liquid or gas. **Altmann's f.** A fixative solution, comprising potassium dichromate and osmium tetroxide, that is used for the demonstration of all cytologic structures except chromosomes. Also *Altmann's liquid.* **amniotic f.** The fluid that accumulates in the amnion, in human embryos from the twelfth day. It increases in quantity until it surrounds the embryo and then the fetus, except at the point of attachment of the umbilical cord. The amount decreases slightly after the seventh month in human pregnancy and about one liter is present at term. Initially it resembles blood plasma in composition but it becomes diluted as pregnancy advances, presumably due to the addition of fetal urine. The fluid probably derives mostly from the fetal membranes and the fetus, but maternal factors may play a part. It contains desquamated fetal epithelial cells and may also in some mammals contain shed lanugo and partially calcified, precociously erupted, deciduous teeth. The fluid may be drawn off by the procedure of amniocentesis. Also *liquor amnii, aqua amnii, waters* (older term). **ascitic f.** The serous fluid found in the peritoneal cavity in ascites. It is usually composed of water, proteins in a concentration of 1 to 2 g/100 ml, and other solutes found in the plasma. **Bouin's f.** A solution of picric acid, formaldehyde, and acetic acid used as a fixative for detailed nuclear study and the preservation of glycogen. In recent years it has been used extensively for renal biopsy material. Also *Bouin's fixative, Bouin solution.* **cerebrospinal f.** LIQUOR CEREBROSPINALIS. Abbr. CSF. **crevicular f.** GINGIVAL FLUID. **decalcifying f.** Any solution that removes calcium from tissues and leaves organic constituents intact for sectioning. **Delafield's f.** A fixative solution that contains osmic acid, chromic acid, acetic acid, and alcohol. It is suitable for delicate histologic material. **Ecker's f.** REES-ECKER SOLUTION. **extracellular f.** Any fluid not contained within the cell membrane, such as plasma, interstitial fluid, and joint fluid, and fluid within body cavities or pleural or pericardial spaces. **extravascular f.** Any fluid not contained within the vascular system, generally excluding intracellular fluid but including interstitial fluid and fluid within body cavities. **Flemming's fixing f.** A widely used cytological fixative, containing osmium tetroxide, chromic acid, and glacial acetic acid. Also *Flemming's liquid, Flemming solution.* **follicular f.** The fluid which surrounds the maturing oocyte within the ovarian follicle and which is partially exuded with the oocyte at ovulation. Its origin is not clearly understood and primary, secondary and tertiary types of fluid have been described which vary in consistency and viscosity as the follicle enlarges. Also *liquor folliculi.* **formol-Müller f.** ORTH SOLUTION. **Gendre's f.** A histologic fixative containing picric acid, acetic acid, and formaldehyde. It is excellent for the preservation of glycogen. **gingival f.** A flow of clear fluid, not pus, from the gingival sulcus or periodontal pocket. It contains a large number of substances derived from the subgingival plaque, the gingival tissues, and the interaction between these two. It also contains large numbers of polymorphonuclear leukocytes. In perfect gingival health there is no flow. In chronic gingivitis and chronic periodontitis the rate of flow varies with the degree of inflammation, and the measurement of the flow is used in periodontal research as an indication of the degree of inflammation present. Also *crevicular fluid, gingival exudate.* **Helly's f.** A fixative solution comprising mercuric chloride, potassium dichromate, and formaldehyde with the addition of sodium sulfate for osmotic purposes. It is an excellent cytoplasmic fixative that is used particularly for delicate tissues and in situations where cytoplasmic details are important. Also *Helly's fixative, Zenker-formol fixative.* **interstitial f.** Body fluid contained within the spaces between cells, excluding intracellular fluid, intravascular fluid, and fluid contained within body cavities. Also *tissue fluid, intercellular lymph, tissue lymph* (outmoded). **intracellular f.** Fluid contained within a cell. **intraocular f.** HUMOR AQUOSUS. **labyrinthine f.** *Outmoded* PERILYMPHA. **non-newtonian f.** A fluid whose viscosity changes with the gradient of rate of flow. Solutions of fibrous macromolecules are examples, the alignment of the molecules with the flow diminishing the viscosity. **otic f.** *Outmoded* ENDOLYMPHA. **pericardial f.** The small amount of fluid in the pericardial cavity that facilitates movement of the heart within the pericardium. Also *liquor pericardii, aqua pericardii, pericardial serum.* **Rees and Ecker diluting f.** REES-ECKER SOLUTION. **saline f.** SALINE. **Scarpa's f.** *Outmoded* ENDOLYMPHA. **seminal f.** SEMEN. **serous f.** A clear, watery fluid produced within the body, especially in body cavities or in sterile abscesses. Also *serofluid.* **synovial f.** SYNOVIA. **Thoma's f.** A strong decalcifying solution composed of nitric acid in alcohol. Also *Thoma's liquid.* **tissue f.** INTERSTITIAL FLUID. **transcellular f.** That part of the extracellular fluid volume that is derived from the intracellular volume by active transport across cell membranes. **ventricular f.** The cerebrospinal fluid that is found within the ventricles of the brain. **Zenker's f.** A fixative solution that contains mercuric chloride, potassium dichromate, and glacial acetic acid. It provides for excellent preservation of cell cytoplasm. Also *Zenker's fixative, Zenker solution.*

**fluidextract** A liquid preparation of a drug dissolved in alcohol in a concentration such that one milliliter of the solution contains the extracted material from one gram of the drug source. Also *fluidextractum, liquid extract.* Also *fluid extract.*

**fluidglycerates** Preparations that contain 50 percent glycerin by volume with no alcohol in the formulation. Such a preparation is made equivalent to a fluidextract, as 1 ml of solution contains the material extracted from 1 g of the crude drug.

**fluidism** \floo′idizm\ HUMORALISM.

**fluidounce** \floo′idouns′\ See under FLUID OUNCE.

**fluidrachm** \floo′idram′\ See under FLUID DRACHM.

**fluidram** See under FLUID DRAM.

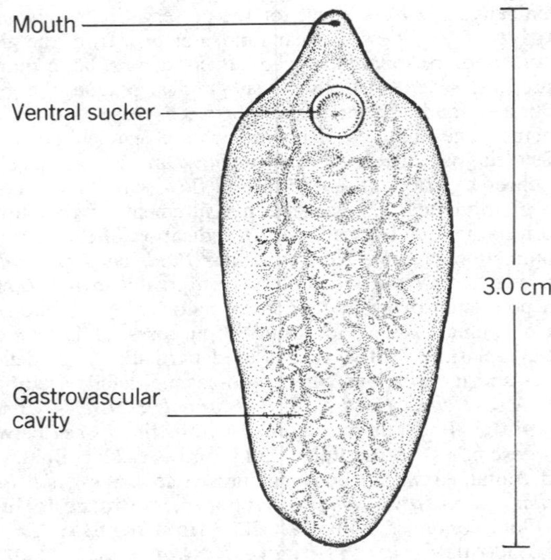


**Liver fluke** (*Fasciola hepatica*)

**fluke** \flook\ [Old English *flōc* a flatfish, flounder] A parasitic flatworm of the class Trematoda; a trematode. There are over 4000 species of flatworms of the class Trematoda. Also *fluke worm.* **blood f.** A trematode worm that inhabits blood vessels of vertebrates; a member of the family Schistomatidae (superfamily Schistosomatoidea). **bronchial f.** A fluke of the species *Paragonimus westermani.*. **cat liver f.** A fluke of the species *Opisthorchis tenuicollis.* **Chinese liver f.** A fluke of the species *Clonorchis sinensis.* Also *oriental fluke.* **digenetic f.** **1** A member of the trematode order (or subclass in other systems) Digenea. **2** A fluke having two stages of reproduction, asexual in the larval form and sexual in the adult form. **liver f.** Any of various trematode worms that infect the liver and biliary system of their definitive host. Examples are *Fasciola hepatica, Clonorchis sinensis, Opisthorchis* spp., and *Dicrocoelium* spp. **lung f.** A trematode worm that parasitizes the lung of its host, such as *Haematoloechus* of frogs or *Paragonimus westermani* of humans. **oriental f.** CHINESE LIVER FLUKE. **sheep liver f.** A fluke of the species *Fasciola hepatica.*

**flukicide** \floo′kisīd\ [*fluk(e)* + *i* + -CIDE] A substance used to kill parasitic flukes.

**flumen** \floo′mən\ [L (from *fluere* to flow) a river, stream] (*pl.* flumina) A stream. **flumina pilorum** Groups of hair growing in the skin so as to produce hair tracts that slope in a common direction in specific regions, such as the hairs on the extensor surface of the forearms that are directed ulnarward. Also *hair streams.*

**flumethasone** $C_{22}H_{28}F_2O_5$. 6α,9α-Difluoro-11β,17α,21-trihydroxy-16α-methylpregna-1,4-diene-3,20-dione. A synthetic glucocorticoid used primarily as a topical anti-inflammatory drug to treat skin conditions that respond to steroid therapy. It is usually given as the acetate or pivalate ester.

**flumethasone pivalate** $C_{27}H_{36}F_2O_6$. The pivalate (dimethylpropionate) ester through the C-21 position of the steroid. It has the same uses and properties as the parent drug.

**flumina** \floo′minə\ Plural of FLUMEN.

**flunarizine hydrochloride** $C_{26}H_{28}Cl_2F_2N_2$. 1-Cinnamyl-4-(di-*p*-fluorobenzhydryl)piperazine. The dihydrochloride salt form of flunarizine, used as a vasodilator.

**fluo-** \floo′ə-\ FLUOR-.

**fluocinoline acetonide** $C_{24}H_{30}F_2O_6$. 6α,9α-Difluoro-11β,21-dihydroxy-16α,17α-isopropylidenedioxypregna-1,4-diene-3,20-dione. A synthetic glucocorticoid. It is used topically as an anti-inflammatory drug to treat dermatologic conditions that respond to steroid therapy.

**fluocinonide** $C_{26}H_{32}F_2O_7$. The 21-acetate ester of fluocinolone acetonide. It has the same anti-inflammatory and antipruritic properties as the parent drug and is used topically for steroid-responsive dermatoses.

**fluohydrisone** FLUDROCORTISONE.

**fluohydrocortisone** FLUDROCORTISONE.

**fluor** \floo′ôr\ [L (from *fluere* to flow), a flow, flux. See also FLUOR-.] **1** One of a class of solids that has the property of fluorescence, useful for detector construction. **2** A flow or flux. An outmoded usage. **f. albus** LEUKORRHEA. **plastic f.** A synthetic material that has the characteristic of emitting a flash of light as the result of an ionizing event within it.

**fluor-** \floo′ər-, flôr-\ [early modern English *fluor* (from L, a flow, flux) a mineral used as a flux in smelting] A combining form denoting (1) fluorine; (2) fluorescence. Also *fluo-, fluori-, fluoro-.*

**fluorapatite** \floorap′ətīt\ $Ca_{10}(PO_4)_6F_2$. The form of apatite in which fluorite ions replace the commoner hydroxide ions, the inorganic portion of bone made up largely of calcium phosphate or hydroxyapatite. Fluorapatite is formed in tooth enamel in the developmental and maturing stages and continues to be added to the enamel surface but at a declining rate as the tooth ages, ceasing when the tooth is completely mineralized. Fluorapatite serves to harden bone and makes teeth more resistant to caries.

**fluorecin** LEUCOFLUORESCEIN.

**fluorescein** \floores′ē·in\ $C_{20}H_{12}O_5$. An orange-red crystalline compound that produces a green fluorescence in an alkaline solution. As the isothiocyanate derivative it can be coupled to proteins, especially immunoglobulins, for use in immunofluorescence techniques. In a dilute solution as the sodium compound, it is used to detect ophthalmic lesions and to evaluate blood circulation. Also *fluorescein dyes.*

**fluorescence** \floo′əres′əns\ [*fluor(spar)* native calcium fluoride (in which the phenomenon was observed) + *-escence* as in opalescence] **1** Photoluminescence in which the initial state of the radiative transition is a singlet state. **2** Any photoluminescence in which the emission ceases within a fraction of a second upon cessation of the stimulating radiation. *Imprecise.* Compare PHOSPHORESCENCE. **natural f.** AUTOFLUORESCENCE. **nonspecific f.** Fluorescence spontaneously present in a preparation, not resulting from an attachment of a fluorochrome-labeled specific antibody or reagent. **x-ray f.** Emission of characteristic x rays from an atom as a result of the absorption of higher energy radiation.

**fluori-** \floo′ərē-, flôr′ē-\ FLUOR-.

**fluoridation** \-idā′shən\ Adjustment of the fluoride level in a water supply by the addition or injection of a substance which will provide sufficient fluoride ions for the desired concentration to be attained for dental health and in particular, the reduction of caries. In temperate climates, the optimum level is approximately one part per million of fluoride ion.

**fluoride** \floo′ərīd\ $F^-$. The anion formed from fluorine, or a salt containing it. **topical f.** An agent containing fluoride for application to the teeth to increase resistance to caries. It may be in the form of a solution, gel, paste, varnish, or mouthwash.

**fluoridization** \-idīzā′shən\ **1** The addition of fluoride to foods or drinks, other than by means of the public water supply. **2** The topical applications of fluoride solution to the teeth.

**fluorine** \floo′rēn\ Element number 9, having atomic weight 18.9984. Fluorine is a member of the halogen family and it is the most electronegative and reactive of all elements, forming compounds even with the usually inert gases krypton, xenon, and radon. The valence is 1. In elemental form it is a pale yellow, corrosive gas. Both the gas and its compounds are very toxic. In trace amounts, however, it is possibly a constituent of teeth and bones, and it is known to be an essential factor in the growth of rats. Soluble fluoride is often introduced into drinking water supplies in order to increase the resistance to caries of developing teeth. Fluorine 19 is the sole stable isotope occurring in nature. Symbol: F

**fluoro-** \floo′ərō-, flôr′ō-\ FLUOR-.

**fluorocarbon** One of a group of hydrocarbons in which some or all of the hydrogen has been substituted by fluorine. It is characterized by a low boiling point and chemical inertness, and it is used as a refrigerant fluid and in fire extinguishers and aerosol sprays. Also *fluorinated hydrocarbon.*

**fluorochrome** \floo′rōkrōm\ A fluorescent substance used to impart fluorescence to a cell, tissue, or type of molecule in the tissue.

**fluorochroming** \floo′rōkrō′ming\ The attachment of a fluorescent compound to a protein, usually as a marker for an immunoglobulin.

**fluorocitric acid** HOOC—CHF—C(OH)(COOH)—$CH_2$—COOH. One of the diastereoisomers of this compound is highly toxic because it inhibits aconitase and blocks the citric acid cycle. This diastereoisomer is formed, by a process that has been termed "lethal synthesis," from fluoroacetyl-CoA and oxaloacetate by citrate synthase.

**9α-fluorocortisol** A synthetic corticosteroid. The fluorine substitution is made because it inhibits activity little but inhibits catabolism more and so prolongs the activity of the compound.

**fluorography** \flooräg′rəfē\ [FLUORO- + -GRAPHY] PHOTOFLUOROGRAPHY. **digital f.** Fluorography in which the x-ray images are digitized so that they may be computer processed for contrast enhancement. See also DIGITAL SUBTRACTION ANGIOGRAPHY.

**fluorometholone** $C_{22}H_{29}FO_4$. 9α-Fluoro-11β,17α-dihydroxy-6α-methyl-1,4-pregnadiene-3,20-dione. A glucocorticoid agent possessing anti-inflammatory activity. It may be applied topically to the skin in the form of a cream.

***p*-fluorophenylalanine** An analogue of phenylalanine which can be incorporated into proteins in its place. The products formed may still be functional, but they are often less stable than the natural proteins.

**fluorophosphate** Phosphorofluoridate. Any of the anions and esters of $(HO)_2P(F){=}O$. Simple dialkyl fluorophosphates, $(RO)_2P(F){=}O$, are powerful inhibitors of cholinesterase and of serine proteinases. The nucleophilic group of each of these enzymes, which normally attacks the carbonyl group of the substrate, becomes phosphorylated by displacing fluoride from the inhibitor.

**fluororoentgenography** \-rent′genäg′rəfē\ PHOTOFLUOROGRAPHY.

**fluoroscope** \floo′rəskōp\ [FLUORO- + -SCOPE] Any apparatus which contains a fluorescent screen that absorbs x rays and produces a visible image which continuously shows the passage of x ray through an object. All modern fluoroscopes use some form of image amplifier, and most display the image on a television monitor.

**fluoroscopic** Relating to fluoroscopy or use of the fluoroscope.

**fluoroscopy** \flooräs′kəpē\ Examination by a fluoroscope.

**fluorosis** \floorō′sis\ [FLUOR- + -OSIS] The long-term effects of the ingestion of excessive amounts of dietary fluoride. These may include chronic endemic dental fluorosis (mottled enamel) and osteosclerosis.

**fluorouracil** $C_4H_3FN_2O_2$. 5-Fluoro-2,4(1*H*,3*H*)-pyrimidinedione. A fluoro-substituted pyrimidine used as an antimetabolite by its conversion *in vivo* to the deoxynucleotide, a compound that inhibits thymidylate synthetase and inhibits DNA synthesis. It is used as an antineoplastic drug against colorectal carcinoma and some other types of cancer. It is administered intravenously. It is also used topically for the treatment of multiple actinic keratoses of the skin.

**fluoxymesterone** $C_{20}H_{29}FO_3$. 9-α-fluoro-11β, 17β-hydroxy-17α-methylandrost-4-en-3-one. A white, crystalline powder, practically insoluble in water but soluble in alcohol. It is used for the same conditions as methyltestosterone, and is also given to cancer patients as an anabolic steroid.

**fluphenazine dihydrochloride** $C_{22}H_{28}Cl_2F_3N_3OS$. 4-[3-[2-(Trifluoromethyl)-10*H*-phenothiazin-10-yl]propyl]-1-piperazineethanol dihydrochloride. A piperazine phenothiazine derivative with the ability to prevent nausea from toxins, radiation treatment, and cytotoxic drugs. It is ineffective against motion sickness. It is also used as an antipsychotic tranquilizer. It is administered orally or intramuscularly.

**fluprednisolone** $C_{21}H_{27}FO_5$. A fluoridated prednisolone analogue with glucocorticoid and anti-inflammatory properties. Flupredisolone and its valerate salt are used for the management of allergic and arthritic disorders.

**flurandrenolide** $C_{24}H_{33}FO_6$. 6α-fluoro-11β,21-dihydroxy-16α,17-[(1-methylethylidene)bis-(oxy)]pregn-4-ene-3,20-dione. A synthetic glucocorticoid with anti-inflammatory actions. It is used in dermatologic conditions that respond to these agents. It also has antipruritic and vasoconstrictive properties.

**flurazepam hydrochloride** $C_{21}H_{25}Cl_3FN_3O$. C-Chloro-1-[2-(diethylamino)ethyl]-5-(*o*-fluorophenyl)-1,3-dihydro-2*H*-1,4-benzodiazepin-2-one dihydrochloride. It is used as a sedative and hypnotic and given orally.

**fluroxene** \flooräk′sēn\ $CH_2{=}CH{-}O{-}CH_2{-}CF_3$. A slightly flammable, volatile liquid with a pungent odor, that is used as a general anesthetic. *Obs.*

**flush** **1** A reddening of tissue caused by vasodilatation. **2** To wash out or cleanse with a brisk flow of liquid, usually water. **atropine f.** A reaction characterized by reddening and dryness of the skin over the face and neck regions. This is observed when atropine is given in overdose amounts. **carcinoid f.** The episodic flush, thought to be hormonally induced by vasoactive kinins or serotonin, occurring in patients with carcinoid syndrome. **flamingo f.** SCHWARTZE SIGN. **harlequin f.** HARLEQUIN COLOR CHANGE. **hectic f.** The heightening of facial coloring associated with a rise in body temperature. **histamine f.** A flushing of the face and upper trunk as a result of the sudden release of histamine from drugs or from the mast cells in some forms of mastocytosis. **limbal f.** Hyperemia in the circumcorneal region, of importance because it usually indicates presence of a severe inflammation of the anterior portion of the eye. **malar f.** A flush over the cheek bones. **menopausal f.** Intermittent flushing and sweating due to vasodilatation accompanying estrogen withdrawal in the menopause.

**fluspirilene** $C_{29}H_{31}F_2N_3O$. 8-[4,4-Bis(*p*-fluorophenyl)-butyl]-1-phenyl-1,3,8-triazaspiro[4,5]-decan-4-one. An antipsychotic agent occurring as a white crystalline solid. It is administered orally.

**flutter** A rapid vibrating or pulsating activity. **atrial f.** An arrhythmia in which atrial activation is occurring in a regular fashion at a rate between 260 and 320 per minute. It is probably the result of a reentrant circuit. Usually only a proportion of atrial impulses are conducted to the ventricles, most commonly as a 2:1 block with a ventricular rate of 130 to 160 per minute. **impure f.** An arrhythmia in which there appears at times to be organized atrial flutter while at other times it more closely resembles atrial fibrillation. **ventricular f.** A form of ventricular tachycardia in which the ventricular rate is much faster than usual (in the neighborhood of 300 per minute), and which often degenerates into ventricular fibrillation.

**flutter-fibrillation** \-fī′brilā′shən\ An arrhythmia which varies in appearance between atrial flutter and atrial fibrillation.

**flux** \fluks\ [L *fluxus* (from *fluxus,* past part. of *fluere* to flow) a flow, flowing] **1** An excessive discharge of fluid. **2** The movement of any vector quantity through an area, per unit time. Also *fluxion.* **integral neutron f.** The product of the flux of neutrons and the time, usually expressed in neutrons per square centimeter. Also *fluence.* **luminous f.** The rate of flow of radiant energy, expressed in lumens. **neutron f.** The intensity of a neutron beam, expressed as the number of neutrons per second crossing a unit area.

**fluxion** \fluk′shən\ FLUX.

**fly** [Old English *flēoge, flȳge*] Any winged insect of the order Diptera other than those called gnats, midges, or mosquitoes. The term is also used in the names of certain non-dipteran insects such as caddis flies. **black f.** BLACKFLY. **blow f.** BLOWFLY. **bluebottle f.** A fly of a metallic blue color in the genus *Calliphora.* **bot f.** BOTFLY. **caddis f.** An insect of the order Trichoptera, whose freshwater aquatic larvae construct a characteristic tube, or caddis, from which the head or legs can emerge for feeding or movement. The adults have membranous wings covered with hairs which, when shed, produce allergic symptoms in sensitized persons. **cheese f.** A fly of the species *Piophila casei.* **deer f.** Any of various tabanid flies of the genus *Chrysops,* especially *C. discalis.* **eye f.** A fly which hovers around or attacks the eye, such as *Siphunculina funicola.* See also *HIPPELATES.* **filth f.** A fly, such as *Musca domestica,* that feeds or breeds on garbage, feces, or the like. **flesh f.** Any of various kinds of fly whose larvae feed on the living or necrotic flesh of vertebrates or cause myiasis, such as screwworm flies of the genera *Cochliomyia, Sarcophaga,* and *Wohlfahrtia* and blowflies of the genus *Calliphora.* **fruit f.** **1** A fly of the family Drosophilidae, such as *Drosophila melanogaster.* Also *vinegar fly, pomace fly.* **2** A fly of the family Trypetidae (Tephritidae), such as *Ceratitis capitata,* the Mediterranean fruit fly. **gad f.** See under GADFLY. **horse f.** HORSEFLY. **house f.** HOUSEFLY. **hover f.** A fly of the family Syrphidae, such as *Helophilus* or *Eristalis.* **latrine f.** A fly of the species *Fannia scalaris.* **louse f.** A bloodsucking ectoparasitic fly of the family Hippoboscidae, especially one of the genus *Hippobosca.* **mangrove f.** An African fly of the genus *Chrysops,* such as *C. dimidiata* or *C. silacea.* Also *mango fly.* **pomace f.** FRUIT FLY. **sand f.** SANDFLY. **screwworm f.** Any of various calliphorid or sarcophagid flies. See also SCREWWORM. **Spanish f.** **1** A blister beetle of the species *Cantharis vesicatoria.* **2** *Popular* CANTHARIDES. **stable f.** A fly of the genus *Stomoxys,* especially one of the species *S. calcitrans.* **tsetse f.** An African fly of the genus *Glossina,* which includes the vectors of African trypoanosomiasis. Also *tsetse, tzetze.* **vinegar f.** FRUIT FLY.

**f.m.** *fiat mistura* (L, have a mixture made).

**Fm** Symbol for the element, fermium.

**FMG** foreign medical graduate.

**FMN** flavin mononucleotide.

**foam** / **fibrin f.** Fibrin derived from fractionation of human blood. It was formerly applied to bleeding surfaces to control oozing of blood, but its use is now obsolete.

**focal** \fō′kəl\ Relating to or constituting a focus.

**foci** \fō′sī\ Plural of FOCUS.

**focimeter** \fōsim′ətər\ A device for measuring the dioptric strength of a lens.

**focus** \fō′kəs\ [L, hearth, fireplace] (*pl.* foci) **1** The point at which rays of parallel light, heat, or sound intersect after reflection from a mirror or refraction from a lens. Also *focal point.* **2** The source or central area, as of an infection or other pathologic process. **Assmann f.** A localized inflammatory lesion, usually in the subapical region of the lung, which is an early phase of pulmonary tuberculosis. Also *Assman's tuberculous infiltrate.* **conjugate f.** Each of two points in an optical system such that each is the image point of the other regarded as object point. **epileptic f.** **1** The totality of the neural tissue involved in a focal epileptic discharge. When the discharge spreads and ultimately becomes generalized, the term denotes that site in the brain from which the discharge originated. 2 In electroencephalography, localized spike or sharp wave discharges occurring between attacks in an epileptic patient. For defs. 1 and 2 also *epileptogenic focus.* **Ghon f.** GHON TUBERCLE. **negative f.** 1 The location of a virtual image in an optical system. 2 A focus on the same side of the lens as the object. **principal foci** The location at which an optical system brings parallel light to a point. **real f.** The location at which an optical system places a convergent image. **spike f.** A recurring spike discharge in the electroencephalogram usually indicative of a focus of epileptic discharge in the underlying brain. **virtual f.** The location at which an optical system places a divergent image. Also *point of dispersion.*

**focusing** \fō′kəsing\ **dynamic f.** Electronically changing the focal distance of a receiving transducer array so that it equals the distance to the propagating transmitted pulse. **electronic f.** Focusing an ultrasonic beam by electronic phasing of electrical pulses applied to the elements of a linear phased transducer array. **isoelectric f.** An electrophoretic technique in which migrating proteins are additionally characterized according to their isoelectric point. A pH gradient is established in the support medium and proteins migrate until they reach the pH zone that equals the isoelectric point of the individual molecule.

**Foerster** [Otfrid *Foerster,* Polish neurosurgeon, 1873–1941] See under SIGN.

**foeti-** \fē′tē-\ FETO-.

**foeto-** \fē′tō-\ FETO-.

**foetor** \fē′tər\ *Brit.* FETOR.

**foetus** \fē′təs\ *Brit.* FETUS.

**fog** 1 A colloid system in which the dispersion medium is a gas and the dispersed particles are liquid. 2 A suspension of very small moisture droplets in the air. • By international meteorological agreement, the term *fog* is used scientifically when the horizontal visibility at the earth's surface is less than 1 km, while *haze* and *mist* describe lesser degrees of visual impairment. **mental f.** CLOUDING OF CONSCIOUSNESS.

**Fogarty** [Thomas J. *Fogarty,* U.S. thoracic surgeon, born 1934] See under CATHETER.

**fogging** The deliberate blurring of distance vision used as a technique for preventing unconscious accommodation when testing for refractive error by placing an excessively convex lens before the eye of a hypermetrope or an excessively concave lens before the eye of a myope.

**foil** [French *feuille* (from L *folium* a leaf) leaf] A very thin pliable sheet of metal. In dental usage foil often refers to gold foil or even a gold foil restoration. **activation f.** A material used to measure a neutron flux or flux density by means of the radioactivity induced due to neutron capture in the foil. Also *activation detector.* **gold f.** An exceedingly thin foil of gold. If the gold is pure and is kept clean, the foil has the property of cold-welding to itself under pressure. It is used for dental restorations by adding small rolled-up pieces one at a time with considerable pressure. Also *fibrous gold.* **platinum f.** Foil of pure platinum used as a foundation for making porcelain full crowns because of its high melting point.

**Foix** [Charles *Foix,* French neurologist, 1882–1927] **1** Foix paramedian syndrome. See under MEDIAN MEDULLARY SYNDROME. **2** Marie-Foix sign. See under SIGN. **3** Foix-Alajouanine syndrome, Foix-Alajouanine disease. See under SUBACUTE NECROTIC MYELITIS.

**folate** Any of the various ionized forms of folic acid.

# fold

**fold** 1 An edge or margin produced by doubling a layer of a tissue or a structure over on itself. 2 A ridge formed by a flexure in a tissue or organ; plica. **alar f.'s** PLICAE ALARES. **amniotic f.** Extraembryonic ectoderm with mesoderm that gives rise in many vertebrates to the amnion by folding together over the early embryo and fusing at junctions, thus closing off the amniotic cavity. The amnion of human embryos is not formed in this way but is the result of cavitation between the embryonic disk and the cytotrophoblast. **anterior mallear f. of tympanic membrane** PLICA MALLEARIS ANTERIOR MEMBRANAE TYMPANI. **aryepiglottic f.** PLICA ARYEPIGLOTTICA. **arytenoepiglottidean f.** PLICA ARYEPIGLOTTICA. **avascular f. of Treves** PLICA ILEOCAECALIS. **axillary f.'s** Plica axillaris anterior and plica axillaris posterior. **Brachet's mesolateral f.** MESOLATERAL FOLD. **bulboventricular f.** A fold or pleat in the developing heart tube between the bulbus cordis and the ventricle. It either atrophies or is absorbed as the proximal part of the bulbus is incorporated into the right ventricle. **caudal genital f.** An elevation on the posterior abdominal wall of an embryo, extending caudally from the caudal pole of the gonad and containing the upper portion of the gubernaculum. **caval f.** A ridge raised on the posterior abdominal wall of an embryo by the inferior vena cava where it passes to the posterior aspect of the liver. **cecal f.'s** PLICAE CAECALES. **cholecystoduodenocolic f.** CYSTICODUODENAL LIGAMENT. **ciliary f.'s** PLICAE CILIARES. **circular f.'s** PLICAE CIRCULARES. **conjunctival f.** PALPEBRAL FOLD. **costocolic f.** LIGAMENTUM PHRENICOCOLICUM. **cranial genital f.** A ridge raised by connective tissue on the posterior abdominal wall of an embryo, stretching cranially from the upper pole of the gonad. It involutes to become the diaphragmatic ligament. **cutaneous f.'s of anus** Skin corrugations at the lower margin of the anal canal which are probably produced by the corrugator cutis ani muscle. **Douglas f.** 1 PLICA RECTOUTERINA. 2 LINEA ARCUATA VAGINAE MUSCULI RECTI ABDOMINIS. **duodenojejunal f.** PLICA DUODENALIS SUPERIOR. **duodenomesocolic f.** PLICA DUODENALIS INFERIOR. **epicanthic f.** PLICA PALPEBRONASALIS. **epigastric f.** PLICA UMBILICALIS LATERALIS. **falciform f. of fascia lata** MARGO FALCIFORMIS HIATUS SAPHENUS. **false vocal f.** PLICA VESTIBULARIS. **fimbriated f.** PLICA FIMBRIATA. **gastric f.'s** PLICAE GASTRICAE. **gastropancreatic f.** PLICA GASTROPANCREATICA. **gastropancreatic f.'s of Huschke** The plica gastropancreatica and the plica hepatopancreatica. **genital f.** Either of a pair of posterior prolongations of mesoderm from the primitive streak, which skirt each side of the cloacal membrane to raise the surface ectoderm into folds extending from the genital tubercle. The folds give rise primarily to the labia minora. **gluteal f.** SULCUS GLUTEALIS. **Guérin's f.** VALVULA FOSSAE NAVICULARIS. **Hasner's f.** PLICA LACRIMALIS. **head and tail f.'s** A tucking under of the front and back of the embryonic disk so that the embryo is folded up ventrally along its longitudinal axis. This phenomenon, which in man occurs about the 21st day after fertilization, happens at the start of neurulation and marks the beginning of the processes which gradually delimit the embryo from its adnexa to which up until then it had been intimately related. **Heister's f.** PLICA SPIRALIS. **Hensing's f.** LIGAMENTUM PHRENICOCOLICUM. **hepatopancreatic f.** PLICA HEPATOPANCREATICA. **horizontal f.'s of rectum** PLICAE TRANSVERSALES RECTI. **ileocecal f.** PLICA ILEOCAECALIS. **iliopubic f. of Thompson** A transverse band of thickened connective tissue that runs parallel to the inguinal ligament, reinforcing its posterior margin from close to the anterior superior iliac spine to the pubic tubercle. It is considered to be thickened transversalis fascia that is joined by the recurved aponeurotic fibers of the external oblique muscle. It is also attached to the fascia iliaca laterally and to Henle's ligament medially. **incudal f.** PLICA INCUDIS. **inferior duodenal f.** PLICA DUODENALIS INFERIOR. **infrapatellar synovial f.** PLICA SYNOVIALIS INFRAPATELLARIS. **interarytenoid f.** PLICA INTERARYTENOIDEA. **interureteric f.** PLICA INTERURETERICA. **iridial f.'s** PLICAE IRIDIS. **junctional f.** A ridge of cytoplasm of a muscle cell between the secondary clefts produced by infolding of the sarcolemma at a myoneural junction. **Kerckring's f.'s of small intestine** PLICAE CIRCULARES. **Kohlrausch f.'s** PLICAE TRANSVERSALES RECTI. **lacrimal f.** PLICA LACRIMALIS. **f.'s of large intestine** PLICAE SEMILUNARES COLI. **f. of laryngeal nerve** In the laryngopharynx, the elevated fold of mucous membrane overlying the internal branch of the superior laryngeal nerve. **lateral f.** A fold at both the right and left sides of a young embryo which gradually constricts and cuts off the yolk sac. **lateral f. of Douglas** Either the plica rectouterina or the sacrogenital fold. **lateral glossoepiglottic f.** PLICA GLOSSOEPIGLOTTICA LATERALIS. **lateral nasal f.** An elevation on the outer side of the nasal placode in the embryo. It gives rise to much of the ala or wing of the nostril. **lateral umbilical f.** PLICA UMBILICALIS LATERALIS. **f. of the left vena cava** PLICA VENAE CAVAE SINISTRAE. **longitudinal f. of duodenum** PLICA LONGITUDINALIS DUODENI. **mammary f.** The lower fold marking the line of attachment of the breast to the anterior chest wall. **medial nasal f.** An elevation on the medial side of each nasal placode in the embryo, which will, with its neighbor, give rise to the fleshy part of the nasal septum. Also *globular process.* **medial umbilical f.** PLICA UMBILICALIS MEDIALIS. **median glossoepiglottic f.** PLICA GLOSSOEPIGLOTTICA MEDIANA. **median umbilical f.** PLICA UMBILICALIS MEDIANA. **medullary f.** NEURAL FOLD. **mesolateral f.** The right layer of the dorsal mesentery of the embryonic foregut that becomes isolated by the formation of the upper recess of the lesser sac, or vestibule, and forms the caval mesentery in which the upper segment of the inferior vena cava develops. Also *Brachet's mesolateral fold.* **middle glossoepiglottic f.** PLICA GLOSSOEPIGLOTTICA MEDIANA. **middle umbilical f.** PLICA UMBILICALIS MEDIANA. **mucolabial f.** The arched fold of mucous membrane extending from the gums to the inner surface of each lip. In the median plane it forms a raised fold, the frenulum. **mucous f.'s of rectum** COLUMNAE ANALES. **nasal f.** The medial and lateral elevated edges of the two olfactory pits in the embryo which contribute to the formation of the edges of the primitive anterior nares. **nasolabial f.** SULCUS NASOLABIALIS. **nasopharyngeal f.** PLICA SALPINGOPALATINA. **Nélaton's f.** The most prominent of the transverse mucosal folds within the rectum. It is located at the junction of the middle and lower thirds. Also *Nélaton sphincter.* **neural f.** One of the two edges of the neural groove which rise high, fold over, and fuse to form the neural tube. Also *medullary fold, neural ridge.* **opercular f.** A fold of connective tissue adhering the palatine tonsil to the palatoglossal arch. **palmate f.'s** PLICAE PALMATAE. **palpebral f.** Either fornix conjunctivae inferior or fornix conjunctivae superior. Also *conjunctival fold.* **palpebronasal f.** PLICA PALPEBRONASALIS. **pancreaticogastric f.** PLICA GASTROPANCREATICA. **paraduodenal f.** PLICA PARADUODENALIS. **parietoperitoneal f.** A fold of fetal peritoneum stretching from the left side of the ascending colon to the parietal peritoneum on the right. **patellar synovial f.** PLICA SYNOVIALIS INFRAPATELLARIS. **Pawlik's f.'s** The proximal part of the columna rugarum anterior and its rugae vaginales, related to the trigone of the bladder anteriorly. **pituitary f.'s** DIAPHRAGMA SELLAE. **pleuroperitoneal f.** A fold of parietal (somatopleuric) mesoderm semilunar in shape, which contributes, together with the septum transversum, to the formation of the diaphragm and its crura. **posterior mallear f. of tympanic membrane** PLICA MALLEARIS POSTERIOR MEMBRANAE TYMPANI. **primitive f.** One of the ridges flanking the primitive groove that extends axially along the surface of the primitive streak. **rectal f.'s** PLICAE TRANSVERSALES RECTI. **rectouterine f.** PLICA RECTOUTERINA. **rectovaginal f.** A peritoneal fold that extends from the back of the posterior fornix of the vagina to the front of the rectum and forms the bottom of the rectouterine pouch. Also *posterior ligament of uterus.* **rectovesical f.** SACROGENITAL FOLD. **Rindfleisch f.'s** Crescentic folds in the serous pericardium around the ascending aorta. **sacrogenital f.** A peritoneal fold that extends from the posterior surface of the urinary bladder to the sides of the rectum and the front of the sacrum, bounding the rectovesical pouch in the male. It corresponds in part with the rectouterine fold in the female. Also *rectovesical fold, posterior false ligaments of bladder.* **salpingopalatine f.** PLICA SALPINGOPALATINA. **salpingopharyngeal f.** PLICA SALPINGOPHARYNGEA. **f.'s of scrotum** Transverse ridges of skin, both parallel and irregular, that extend laterally from the median raphe across the anterior and lateral surfaces of the scrotum. They are produced by the dartos muscle, the fibers of which are at right angles to the ridges. **semilunar f.'s of colon** PLICAE SEMILUNARES COLI. **semilunar f. of conjunctiva** PLICA SEMILUNARIS CONJUNCTIVAE. **semilunar f. of transversalis fascia** LIGAMENTUM INTERFOVEOLARE. **sigmoid f.'s of colon** PLICAE SEMILUNARES COLI. **spiral f.** PLICA SPIRALIS. **spiral f. of cystic duct** PLICA SPIRALIS. **stapedial f.** PLICA STAPEDIS. **sublingual f.** PLICA SUBLINGUALIS. **superior duodenal f.** PLICA DUODENALIS SUPERIOR. **synovial f.** PLICA SYNOVIALIS. **tail f.** See under HEAD AND TAIL FOLDS. **transverse palatine f.'s** PLICAE PALATINAE TRANSVERSAE. **transverse f.'s of rectum** PLICAE TRANSVERSALES RECTI. **transverse vesical f.** PLICA VESICALIS TRANSVERSA. **Treves f.** 1 PLICA ILEOCAECALIS. 2 PLICA CAECALIS VASCULARIS. **triangular f.** PLICA TRIANGULARIS. **triangular f. of His** PLICA TRIANGULARIS. **tubal f.'s of uterine tube** PLICAE TUBARIAE TUBAE UTERINAE. **f. of the urachus** PLICA UMBILICALIS MEDIANA. **urethral f.** UROGENITAL RIDGE. **urogenital f.** UROGENITAL RIDGE. **uterosacral f.** PLICA RECTOUTERINA. **vaginal f.'s** RUGAE VAGINALES. **vascular f. of cecum** PLICA CAECALIS VASCULARIS. **Vater's f.** A prominent, hoodlike fold of mucous membrane that is situated proximal to the greater duodenal papilla and at the lower extremity of the plica longitudinalis in the descending part of the duodenum. **vestibular f.** PLICA VESTIBULARIS. **villous f.'s of stomach** PLICAE VILLOSAE GASTRICAE. **vocal f.** PLICA VOCALIS.

**Foley** [Frederic Eugene Basil *Foley,* U.S. urologist, 1891–1966] **1** Foley Y-type ureteropelvioplasty. See under FOLEY Y-PLASTY. **2** See under CATHETER.

**folia** \fō′lyə\ Plural of FOLIUM.

**folic acid** Any of a number of compounds including pteroic acid and its conjugates with one or more molecules of glutamic acid. The glutamic residues are joined by acylation of the amino group of one by the γ-carboxyl of the next. Folic acid is a vitamin, since it is required in the form of tetrahydrofolate, produced by enzymic reduction, for carrying various one-carbon groups in metabolism. Deficiency leads to megaloblastic anemia.

**folie** \fōlē′\ [French (from L *follis* a leather ball, balloon), madness] **1** Acquired insanity. **2** Any psychologic abnormality. **f. à deux** The simultaneous appearance of psychosis in two persons closely associated with one another. Also *double insanity, simultaneous delusion.* See also SHARED DELUSION. **f. communiquée** SHARED DELUSION. **f. des grandeurs** DELUSION OF GRANDEUR. **f. du doute** An obsessive-compulsive neurosis characterized by repeated checking to see if a mistake was made or to be sure something was done properly. Also *doubting mania, checking compulsion, folie raisonnante, doubting insanity.* **f. imitative** SHARED DELUSION. **f. imposée** SHARED DELUSION. **f. induite** SHARED DELUSION. **f. raisonnante** FOLIE DU DOUTE.

**Folin** [Otto *Folin,* Swedish-born U.S. biochemist, 1867–1934] **1** Folin and Wu test. See under TEST. **2** Folin's protein-free filtrate. See under FILTRATE. **3** Folin and Svedberg method. See under METHOD.

**folinic acid** $C_{20}H_{23}N_7O_7$. 5-Formyl-5,6,7,8 tetra-hydropteroyl-L-glutamic acid. An active form of folic acid used in the treatment of megaloblastic anemia resulting from folic acid deficiency, as opposed to that arising from vitamin $B_{12}$ deficiency. It is also used in other forms of folic acid deficiency, such as that arising from the chronic administration of folic acid antagonists. Also *leucovorin.*

**folium** \fō′lē·əm\ [L (akin to Gk *phyllon* a leaf), a leaf] (*pl.* folia) [NA] A leaflike structure or part, as those in the cerebellum. **f. cacuminis** *Obs.* FOLIUM VERMIS. **folia cerebelli** [NA] The extensive, parallel leaflike structures formed by the folds of cerebellar cortex. Also *folia of cerebellum.* **folia of cerebellum** FOLIA CEREBELLI. **f. vermis** [NA] The small superior portion of the cerebellar vermis lying between the tuber vermis and the declive. Also *folium cacuminis.*

**Folli** [Cecilio Folli (*Folius*), Italian anatomist, 1615–1660] Process of Folius. See under PROCESSUS ANTERIOR MALLEI.

**follicle** \fäl′ikl\ [L *folliculus.* See FOLLICULUS.] A small, saclike depression. Also *folliculus.* Adj. follicular. **aggregated f.'s** FOLLICULI LYMPHATICI AGGREGATI. **aggregated lymphatic f.'s of Peyer** PEYER'S PATCHES. **anovular ovarian f.** CORPUS ATRETICUM. **atretic f.** CORPUS ATRETICUM. **atretic ovarian f.** CORPUS ATRETICUM. **closed f.** A completely closed sac or pouch. **dental f. 1** A mesenchymal condensation surrounding a tooth germ. **2** A fibrous envelope surrounding the crown of a tooth prior to its eruption through the oral mucosa. Also *odontotheca.* **gastric f.** GLANDULA GASTRICA PROPRIA. **germinal f.** GERMINAL CENTER. **graafian f.** VESICULAR OVARIAN FOLLICLE. **hair f.** The tube of epidermal cells at the base of which the hair matrix forms the hair shaft. Also *folliculus pili.* **intestinal f.'s** GLANDULAE INTESTINALES. **laryngeal lymphatic f.'s** NODULI LYMPHATICI AGGREGATI CAVITATIS LARYNGIS. **Lieberkühn's f.'s** GLANDULAE INTESTINALES. **lingual f.'s** FOLLICULI LINGUALES. **lymphatic f.** NODULUS LYMPHATICUS. **lymphatic f.'s of tongue** FOLLICULI LINGUALES. **Montgomery's f.'s** MONTGOMERY'S GLANDS. **nabothian f.'s** NABOTHIAN CYSTS. **nasal mucous f.'s** *Outmoded* GLANDULAE NASALES. **ovarian f.** The egg-containing, fluid-filled sphere that develops in the ovary and ruptures at ovulation to liberate the ovum. It is also an endocrine gland, producing estrogens and giving rise after ovulation to a corpus luteum. It appears first as a primordial follicle with the oocyte surrounded by a single layer of flattened follicular cells, then by a single layer of cuboidal or columnar cells (and called a primary follicle). Follicles mature at intervals depending on the type of reproductive pattern in response to the follicle-stimulating hormone (FSH)

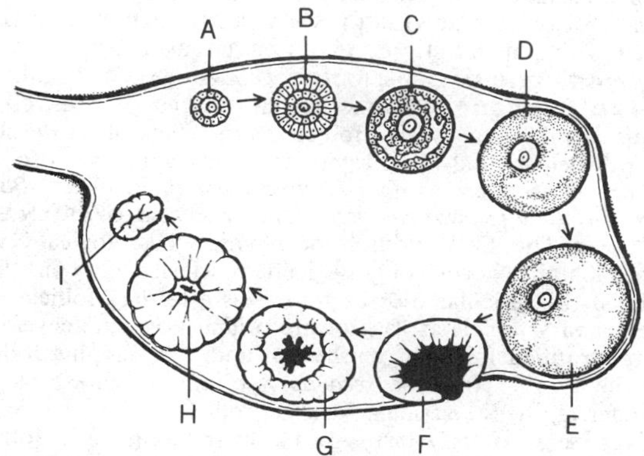


**Ovarian follicle** (A) Primary follicle; (B) double-layered follicle; (C) follicle at beginning of antrum formation; (D) follicle approaching maturity; (E) mature follicle; (F) corpus hemorrhagicum; (G) young corpus luteum; (H) corpus luteum; (I) corpus albicans.

from the anterior lobe of the pituitary. The epithelial covering becomes a many-layered membrana granulosa and a second outer covering is added, the theca interna. An antrum usually forms in the granulosa layer and fluid, liquor folliculi, accumulates as the follicle enlarges. The oocyte, usually a secondary oocyte by the stage of antrum formation, is surrounded by granulosa cells forming the corona radiata and is mounted eccentrically on the follicle wall on the cumulus oophorous. This stage is sometimes called a secondary or vesicular or graafian follicle. Only about 300 follicles mature and rupture at ovulation during a woman's reproductive life. The others degenerate at various stages of maturation by the process of follicular atresia. **pilosebaceous f.** An invagination of the epidermis that extends down to the hair root sheath and communicates with a sebaceous gland. **polyovular ovarian f.** A follicle containing more than one oocyte. The condition has been reported in many mammalian types, including humans, but apart from some marsupials it is thought that polyovular follicles become atretic and do not give rise to multiple births. **primary f.** A lymphoid follicle that has not received an antigenic stimulus. **primary ovarian f.** An ovarian follicle at an early stage in its development succeeding that of the primordial follicle when the oocyte is surrounded by a single layer of cuboidal or columnar follicle cells. Also *folliculus ovaricus primarius.* **primordial ovarian f.** The earliest and smallest type of ovarian follicle, consisting of an oogonium or oocyte surrounded by a single layer of follicle cells. It is formed by the time of birth or just afterwards in most mammals by division of oogonia. Some 400 000 are present in each human ovary at birth. The number falls rapidly, due to atresia, to about half at puberty and none remains a few years after the menopause. Also *folliculus ovaricus primordialis.* **sebaceous f.** A pilosebaceous unit in which the sebaceous gland is prominent. **secondary f.** 1 VESICULAR OVARIAN FOLLICLE. 2 An ovarian follicle at the stage of its development when it is enveloped by a stratified follicular epithelium and a developing follicular theca. Also *folliculus ovaricus secundarius.* • See note at VESICULAR OVARIAN FOLLICLE. 3 A follicle which has developed a germinal center following antigenic stimulation. **solitary f.** A single rounded collection of lymphoid cells within a tissue or organ. **splenic lymph f.'s** FOLLICULI LYMPHATICI SPLENICI. **tertiary f.** VESICULAR OVARIAN FOLLICLE. • See note at VESICULAR OVARIAN FOLLICLE. **thyroid f.** FOLLICULUS GLANDULAE THYROIDEAE. **f. of thyroid gland** FOLLICULUS GLANDULAE THYROIDEAE. **f.'s of tongue** FOLLICULI LINGUALES. **vesicular ovarian f.** An ovarian follicle at the stage of its development when a fluid-filled cavity (antrum) appears. Also *secondary follicle, tertiary follicle, graafian follicle, ovisac, Baer's vesicle, folliculus ovaricus vesiculosus.* See also OVARIAN FOLLICLE. • The Fifth Edition of Nomina Histologica (1983, based on the world congress held in Mexico City in 1980) defined the vesicular ovarian follicle as a tertiary follicle, and a secondary follicle as "a growing primary ovocyte enveloped by a stratified follicular epithelium and a developing follicular theca . . ." However, *secondary follicle* is well established as referring to the vesicular ovarian follicle.

**follicular** \fōlik′yələr\ 1 Of or relating to a follicle. 2 Characterized by or consisting of follicles.

**folliculi** \fōlik′yəlī\ Plural of FOLLICULUS.

**folliculitis** \fōlik′yəlī′tis\ [*follicul(us)* + -ITIS] Inflammation of one or more follicles. **f. abscedens et suffodiens** A burrowing, suppurating folliculitis of the scalp. **f. cruris atrophicans** Pustular folliculitis that leads to cicatricial alopecia of the lower leg. It occurs predominantly in males and in tropical climates. **f. decalvans** Folliculitis that results in alopecia. **f. decalvans cryptococcica** A scarring folliculitis of the scalp caused by a yeast species. **Gram-negative f.** A pustular or papular inflammation of the hair follicles due to infection with Gram-negative bacteria such as *Proteus.* This is a rare complication of the antibiotic treatment of acne vulgaris. **industrial f.** OIL ACNE. **keloidal f.** KELOID ACNE. **f. nares perforans** Inflammation of a hair follicle in the nasal vestibule, that progresses to abscess formation, the abscess discharging eventually through the skin adjacent to the nasolabial or nasobuccal sulcus. **oil f.** OIL ACNE. **f. ulerythematosa reticulata** VERMICULATE ATROPHODERMA OF THE CHEEKS.

**folliculoma** \fōlik′yəlō′mə\ [*follicul(us)* + -OMA] GRANULOSA CELL TUMOR. **f. lipidique** A Sertoli cell tumor in which the tumor cells are distended with lipid.

**folliculus** \fōlik′yələs\ [L (dim. of *follis* a leather bag, esp. a pair of bellows), a little sack or bag] (*pl.* folliculi) 1 FOLLICLE. 2 A spherical collection of cells which may contain a cavity. **f. glandulae thyroideae** [NA] Any of the rounded, hollow cellular units that form the lobules of each lobe of the thyroid gland and consist of an outer layer of epithelial cells of varying size surrounding a space containing jelly-like colloid. Between the units is highly vascular connective tissue, as well as nerve fibers and lymphatics. The shape of the follicle cells vary with the activity of the gland, their secretions being hormones. Also *thyroid follicle, follicle of thyroid gland.* **folliculi linguales** [NA] Nodules of lymphoid tissue in the submucous layer of the pharyngeal part of the tongue that produce a number of bulgings on the surface and are collectively termed the lingual tonsil. Also *lingual follicles, follicles of tongue, lymphatic follicles of tongue.* **folliculi lymphatici aggregati** A group of lymphatic follicles. Also *aggregate nodule, aggregated follicles, Peyer's glands.* See also PEYER'S PATCHES. **folliculi lymphatici laryngei** NODULI LYMPHATICI AGGREGATI CAVITATIS LARYNGIS. **folliculi lymphatici splenici** [NA] Nodular localized enlargements of the sheaths of lymphatic tissue that surround the small arteriolar branches of the splenic arteries as far as their divisions into capillaries and form the white pulp of the spleen. Also *malpighian bodies of spleen, malpighian corpuscles of spleen, malpighian glands, splenic lymph follicles, splenic lymph nodules, malpighian nodules, splenic corpuscles.* **f. lymphaticus** NODULUS LYMPHATICUS. **f. ovaricus primarius** PRIMARY OVARIAN FOLLICLE. **f. ovaricus primordialis** PRIMORDIAL OVARIAN FOLLICLE. **f. ovaricus secundarius** SECONDARY FOLLICLE. • See note at VESICULAR OVARIAN FOLLICLE. **f. ovaricus vesiculosus** VESICULAR OVARIAN FOLLICLE. **f. pili** [NA] HAIR FOLLICLE.

**Fölling** [Ivar Asbjorn *Fölling,* Norwegian physician, born 1888] Fölling's disease. See under PHENYLKETONURIA.

**following** In electroencephalography, a phenomenon in which repeated sensory stimuli, such as photic stimulation, cause cortical response patterns characterized by one response wave for each stimulus. This is sometimes described as "driving" the brain waves, so that the alpha rhythm varies in frequency according to the frequency of the stimulus or at a frequency that represents a harmonic of the latter.

**follow-up** 1 Done or administered to a patient subsequent to the initial diagnosis or treatment, as *follow-up care.* 2 A follow-up measure or treatment.

**Foltz** [Jean Charles Eugene *Foltz,* French ophthalmologist, 1822–1876] Valvule of Foltz. See under VALVE.

**fomentation** \fō′məntā′shən\ [Late L *fomentatio* (from *fomentare* to foment, from *fomentum* poultice, from L *fovere* to warm) application of a poultice] 1 The use of hot, moist applications, especially to ease pain or reduce inflammation. 2 The hot, moist substance or material used in fomentation, such as a poultice.

**fomes** \fō′mēz\ [L (akin to *fovere* to warm, keep warm, foster), tinder] (*pl.* fomites) Any nonpathogenic substance or inanimate object other than food that is capable of harboring or transmitting pathogenic microorganisms. Also *fomite.*

**fomite** \fō′mīt\ [back-formation from plural *fomites*] FOMES.

**fomites** \fō′mitēz\ Plural of FOMES.

**fons pulsatilis** \fänz pulsat′ilis\ ANTERIOR FONTANEL.

**fontactoscope** \fäntak′təskōp\ [L *fons,* gen. *fontis,* spring + Gk *act(is)* a ray, beam + *o* + -SCOPE] An electroscope designed for measuring the radioactivity of water and gases.

**Fontan** [François *Fontan,* French thoracic surgeon, born 1929] See under OPERATION.

**Fontana** [Arturo *Fontana,* Italian dermatologist, 1873–1950] See under STAIN.

**Fontana** [Felice *Fontana,* Italian neurologist, 1730–1805] 1 Fontana's markings. See under MARKING. 2 Fontana spaces. See under SPATIA ANGULI IRIDOCORNEALIS.

**fontanel** \fän′tənel′\ [French *fontanelle* (dim. of *fontaine* fountain, basin of a fountain, from Late L *fontana*, from L *fons*, gen. *fontis* a spring) lit., a small fountain basin] FONTICULUS. **anterior f.** The fontanel located at the junction of the coronal, frontal, and sagittal sutures of a fetal or newborn skull. Also *fonticulus quadrangularis, bregmatic fontanel, quadrangular fontanel, frontal fontanel, fonticulus frontalis major, fonticulus major, fonticulus anterior, fons pulsatilis, bregmatic space* (outmoded). **anterolateral f.** SPHENOIDAL FONTANEL. **bregmatic f.** ANTERIOR FONTANEL. **Casser's f.** MASTOID FONTANEL. **cranial f.'s** FONTICULI CRANII. **frontal f.** ANTERIOR FONTANEL. **Gerdy's f.** SAGITTAL FONTANEL. **lateral f.'s** Fonticulus sphenoidalis and fonticulus mastoideus. **mastoid f.** The fontanel located at the junction of the lambdoidal, occipitomastoid, and parietomastoid sutures of a fetal or newborn skull. Also *fonticulus mastoideus, Casser's fontanel, posterolateral fontanel, posterotemporal fontanel.* **occipital f.** The fontanel located at the junction of the lambdoidal and sagittal sutures of the fetal or newborn skull. Also *posterior fontanel, triangular fontanel, fonticulus minor, fonticulus occipitalis, fonticulus posterior, fonticulus triangularis.* **posterior f.** OCCIPITAL FONTANEL. **posterolateral f.** MASTOID FONTANEL. **posterotemporal f.** MASTOID FONTANEL. **quadrangular f.** ANTERIOR FONTANEL. **sagittal f.** A fontanel that occasionally occurs along the sagittal suture in a fetal or newborn skull. Also *Gerdy's fontanel.* **sphenoidal f.** A fontanel located at the articulations of the parietal, frontal, sphenoidal, and temporal bones in the fetal or newborn skull. Also *anterolateral fontanel, fonticulus sphenoidalis.* **supraoccipital f.** The membranous area in front of the cartilaginous precursor of the supraoccipital bone in the fetus. **triangular f.** OCCIPITAL FONTANEL.

**fontanelle** \fän′tənel′\ FONTICULUS.

**fonticuli** \fäntik′yəlī\ Plural of FONTICULUS.

**fonticulus** \fäntik′yələs\ [L (dim. of *fons*, gen. *fontis*, a spring, fountain), a little spring; used as a latinization of French *fontanelle*. See FONTANEL.] An unossified area of the fibrous membrane that forms the fetal cranial vault before ossification begins, usually present for varying periods up to two years after birth, depending on the site. There are six main areas, one at each angle of the parietal bones, those in the median plane fusing into two areas. The membrane consists of the periosteum externally and the dura mater internally. Also *fontanel, fontanelle.* See also FONTICULI CRANII. **f. anterior** ANTERIOR FONTANEL. **fonticuli cranii** [NA] The unossified areas, occupied by membrane, in the developing human skull, found principally at the angles of the parietal bone, comprising the fonticulus anterior, fonticulus posterior, fonticulus sphenoidalis, and fonticulus mastoideus. Also *cranial fontanels.* **f. frontalis major** ANTERIOR FONTANEL. **f. major** ANTERIOR FONTANEL. **f. mastoideus** MASTOID FONTANEL. **f. minor** OCCIPITAL FONTANEL. **f. occipitalis** OCCIPITAL FONTANEL. **f. posterior** OCCIPITAL FONTANEL. **f. quadrangularis** ANTERIOR FONTANEL. **f. sphenoidalis** SPHENOIDAL FONTANEL. **f. triangularis** OCCIPITAL FONTANEL.

**food** [Old English *fōda*, akin to L *pascere* to feed and *pabulum* food] Any substance that can be used by the body to provide some essential nutrient and/or energy.

**foot** [Old English *fōt*, akin to L *pes*, gen. *pedis*, foot and to Gk *pous*, gen. *podos*, foot] (*pl.* feet) **1** A unit of length equal to 1/3 yard; 0.3048 meter exactly. Symbol: ft **2** The distal end of the lower limb; pes. **athlete's f.** *Popular* TINEA PEDIS. **bifid f.** CLEFT FOOT. **broad f.** A broadening of the distal foot that is caused by the separation of the metatarsal heads and collapse of the transverse arch. Also *metatarsus latus, talipes transversoplanus, splay foot, spread foot.* **burning feet** A form of nutritional sensory polyneuropathy of uncertain cause, but probably due to vitamin B deficiency, giving a severe burning sensation in the feet. Also *hot feet, ignipedites.* **cavus f.** A foot with a high longitudinal arch. **Charcot's f.** A deformity of the foot resulting from arthropathy, consequent to neurologic lesions of tabes dorsalis. **claw f.** A foot deformity characterized by a high longitudinal arch, abnormal flexion of the interphalangeal joints, and hyperextension of the toes at the metatarsophalangeal joints. Also *gampsodactyly.* **cleft f.** A developmental defect in which one or more of the three central digits are absent, as in lobster-claw deformity, or abnormally aligned with respect to other digits, so that the usual interdigital space extends into the metatarsal region. Also *bifid foot, split foot.* See also LOBSTER-CLAW DEFORMITY. **club f.** TALIPES. **congenital convex club f.** ROCKER-BOTTOM FLATFOOT. **convex f.** ROCKER-BOTTOM FLATFOOT. **dancers' f.** Traumatic inflammation of the second and third metatarsal heads. The condition is quite painful and is usually associated with dancing. **drop f.** FOOTDROP. **end f.** The terminal expansion of an axon at the site of synaptic contact on the soma or dendrite of a neuron. Also *bouton terminal, axon terminal, terminal button, synaptic button, synaptic knob, endbulb, neuropodium.* **end feet of Held** Distinctive, large terminal expansions of cochlear nerve synapses. • When first described, it was believed that neurofibrils extended across these contacts. **equinus club f.** TALIPES EQUINOVARUS. **flat f.** Talipes planus. See also entries under FLATFOOT. **Friedreich's club f.** Pes cavus and other foot deformities occurring in Friedreich's disease. **fungus f.** MADURA FOOT. **hollow f.** TALIPES CAVUS. **hot feet** BURNING FEET. **f. lambert** A unit of luminance equal to the luminance of a uniform diffuser emitting one lumen per square foot, equal to 3.426 25 nit, 3.426 25 candela per square meter. Symbol: ft La **Madura f.** Mycetoma of the foot caused by *Actinomadura madurae* (formerly *Streptomyces madurae)* and found in India, northern Africa, Cyprus, and South America. Entry of the organism follows trauma. Multiple sinuses ultimately develop. Antifungal agents are sometimes effective, but amputation is frequently necessary. Also *fungus foot.* See also MYCETOMA. **paralytic club f.** Pes cavus developing as a consequence of lower motor neuron paralysis of the long flexor and extensor muscles of the leg and of the intrinsic muscles of the foot. **rocker-bottom f.** ROCKER-BOTTOM FLATFOOT. **root f.** One of the fine digitations on the lower aspect of the basal cells of the epidermis. **SACH f.** An artificial ankle-foot component of a prosthesis, shaped like a human foot, with a solid, nonmovable articulation to the prosthetic shank and including a cushion heel that absorbs the impact of heel strike. • SACH is an acronym formed from *single axis cushion heel.* **septic f.** Ischemic necrosis of the skin appendages of the foot that extends into the deep tissues along fascial planes. It is usually seen in diabetics and often requires emergency treatment by guillotine amputation. **splay f.** BROAD FOOT. **split f.** CLEFT FOOT. **spread f.** BROAD FOOT. **stump f.** TALIPES. **sucker f.** The terminal expansion of an astrocytic (glial) process on the basal lamina of a small blood vessel in the central nervous system. Also *vascular footplate, sucker process.* **tip f.** TALIPES EQUINUS. **trench f.** The painful, vascular response of the feet to prolonged exposure to damp and cold, aggravated by physical inactivity.

Such conditions were experienced by many soldiers in trench warfare in World War I. Signs include swelling and inflammation and, in the most severe cases, gangrene. Also *water-bite.* **valgus club f.** TALIPES EQUINOVALGUS. **varus club f.** TALIPES EQUINOVARUS. **weak f.** A precursory stage of flatfoot.

**footdrop** Plantar flexion of the foot caused by paralysis or paresis of the muscles of the anterior compartment of the leg, making it impossible to dorsiflex the foot and leading to a high-stepping gait. Also *drop foot, ankle drop.*

**foot-engine** A treadle-operated dental drilling machine.

**foot lambert** \lam′bərt\ See under FOOT.

**footplate** 1 BASIS STAPEDIS. 2 PEDICEL. **vascular f.** SUCKER FOOT.

**footprint** The impression of the dermatoglyphic pattern, flexion creases, and secondary folds of the sole of the foot and the plantar aspects of the toes, made by applying ink to these surfaces and pressing them on paper. Footprints, like palmprints, are used chiefly as supplemental records for identification of newborn infants, and rarely in cases of criminal identification.

**forage** \fôr′ij\ [French, a drilling, piercing] A surgical procedure involving a V-shaped incision of the prostate to treat hypertrophy and obstruction.

# foramen

**foramen** \fôrā′mən\ [L (from *forare* to bore, pierce), a hole, opening] (*pl.* foramina) An opening, perforation, or hole into or through a structure or tissue, particularly a bone. **accessory f.** A foramen on the root of a tooth which opens into the root canal or pulp chamber in addition to the apical foramen. **foramina alveolaria maxillae** Openings on the infratemporal surface of the maxilla which transmit the posterior superior alveolar nerves and vessels. Also *posterior superior alveolar foramina.* **anterior condyloid f.** CANALIS HYPOGLOSSI. **anterior ethmoidal f.** FORAMEN ETHMOIDALE ANTERIUS. **anterior sacral foramina** FORAMINA SACRALIA ANTERIORA. **aortic f.** HIATUS AORTICUS. **apical f. of tooth** An opening at or near the apex of the root of a tooth through which vessels and nerves enter and leave the pulp. **arachnoid f.** APERTURA MEDIANA VENTRICULI QUARTI. **Bichat's f.** *Obs.* CISTERNA VENAE MAGNAE CEREBRI. **f. bursae omentalis majoris** An opening produced by the encroachment of the left gastropancreatic fold of the left gastric artery and the right gastropancreatic fold of the hepatic artery on the omental bursa so that it is divided into a superior and an inferior recess that communicate through the opening in the constriction. Also *foramen of omental bursa.* **f. caecum** A blind foramen; an incomplete perforation. Also *foramen cecum.* **f. caecum linguae** [NA] A prominent median pit at the apex of the sulcus terminalis that separates the dorsum of the tongue into anterior and posterior parts. The pit is the site of the upper end of the thyroid diverticulum in the embryo. Also *foramen cecum of tongue, morgagnian foramen.* **f. caecum ossis frontalis** [NA] An opening produced between the notch in the frontal crest and the notched base of the crista galli at the frontoethmoidal suture. Rarely, an emissary vein passes through it to connect the superior sagittal sinus with the nasal veins. Also *cecal foramen.* **caroticoclinoid f.** An occasional foramen produced by a bar of bone bridging the gap between the anterior and the middle clinoid processes of the sphenoid bone. It provides passage for the internal carotid artery when it leaves the cavernous sinus at the end of the carotid sulcus. **caroticotympanic foramina** CANALICULI CAROTICOTYMPANICI. **cecal f.** FORAMEN CAECUM OSSIS FRONTALIS. **f. cecum** FORAMEN CAECUM. **f. cecum of tongue** FORAMEN CAECUM LINGUAE. **conjugate f.** A foramen produced by apposing notches at the junction of two bones, such as foramen caecum ossis frontalis. **f. costotransversarium** A gap occupied by the costotransverse ligament between the posterior surface of the neck of a rib and the anterior aspect of the transverse process and pedicle of the corresponding vertebra. Also *costotransverse foramen.* **cotyloid f.** The opening formed deep to the transverse ligament as it spans the acetabular notch, giving passage to vessels and a nerve to the hip joint. **cribroethmoid f.** FORAMEN ETHMOIDALE ANTERIUS. **f. diaphragmatis sellae** The small opening in the diaphragma sellae covering the sella turcica that accommodates the stalk of the pituitary gland extending from the base of the hypothalamus. Also *foramen of Pacchioni, pacchionian foramen.* **emissary f.** Any foramen in the skull through which an emissary vein passes, providing communication between dural venous sinuses and veins outside the skull. **esophageal f.** HIATUS ESOPHAGEUS. **ethmoidal foramina** FORAMINA ETHMOIDALIA. **f. ethmoidale anterius** [NA] An opening near the anterior end of the frontoethmoidal suture at the junction of the superior and medial walls of the orbit that transmits the anterior ethmoidal nerve and vessels. Also *anterior ethmoidal foramen.* **f. ethmoidale posterius** [NA] An opening near the posterior end of the frontoethmoidal suture at the junction of the superior and medial walls of the orbit that transmits the posterior ethmoidal nerve and vessels. Also *posterior ethmoidal foramen.* **foramina ethmoidalia** [NA] The foramen ethmoidale anterius and the foramen ethmoidale posterius considered together. Also *ethmoidal foramina, orbital canals, ethmoidal canals.* **external auditory f.** MEATUS ACUSTICUS EXTERNUS. **f. of Fallopio** HIATUS CANALIS NERVI PETROSI MAJORIS. **Ferrein's f.** HIATUS CANALIS NERVI PETROSI MAJORIS. **f. frontale** [NA] An occasional foramen, present in about 50 percent of humans, that is located on the supraorbital margin of the frontal bone just medial to the supraorbital notch or foramen. It transmits the supratrochlear artery and the medial branch of the supraorbital nerve and is formed by a small bar of bone bridging over the incisura frontalis. Also *frontal foramen, medial frontal foramen.* **Galen's f.** The orifice of the anterior cardiac vein in the right atrium draining blood from the front of the right ventricle. **great f.** FORAMEN MAGNUM. **greater ischiadic f.** FORAMEN ISCHIADICUM MAJUS. **greater palatine f.** FORAMEN PALATINUM MAJUS. **great occipital f.** FORAMEN MAGNUM. **hemal f.** An opening limited by the hemal arch. Also *visceral foramen.* **Hyrtl's f.** PORUS CROTAPHITICOBUCCINATORIUS. **f. incisivum** [NA] One of the lower openings of the four incisive canals that lead from the floor of the nasal cavity into the incisive fossa lying immediately behind the incisor teeth anteriorly in the median plane of the hard palate and transmitting the nasopalatine nerves. Also *incisive foramen, anterior palatine canal.* **inferior occipital f.** FORAMEN MAGNUM. **f. infraorbitale** [NA] The anterior opening of the infraorbital canal situated on the anterior surface of the body of the maxilla just below the inferior margin of the orbital opening and above the canine fossa. It transmits the infraorbital nerve and vessels. Also *infraorbital* *foramen.* **innominate f.** A very small opening occasionally located posteromedial to foramen ovale in the greater wing of the sphenoid bone through which the small, or lesser, petrosal nerve may leave the skull to pass on to the otic ganglion. **interatrial f. secundum** OSTIUM SECUNDUM. **internal auditory f.** PORUS ACUSTICUS INTERNUS. **f. interventriculare** [NA] The opening between one lateral ventricle and the third ventricle. It lies between the column of the fornix and the anterior end of the thalamus. Also *foramen of Monro, foramen interventriculare Monroi, interventricular foramen, interventricular opening.* **f. intervertebrale** [NA] The passage formed by the apposition of the vertebral notches of two adjacent vertebrae, transmitting a spinal nerve and vessels. Also *intervertebral foramen.* **foramina intervertebralia ossis sacri** [NA] Four forked channels through which the four pairs of both pelvic and dorsal sacral foramina communicate with the sacral canal through its lateral wall. Also *intervertebral foramina of sacrum, intersacral canals.* **f. ischiadicum majus** [NA] The large aperture of the greater sciatic notch of hip bone spanned by the sacrotuberous ligament and separated from the lesser sciatic foramen by the sacrospinous ligament. Passing through it are the piriformis muscle separating the superior gluteal vessels and nerves above it from the inferior gluteal vessels and nerves, internal pudendal vessels, and pudendal, sciatic, and other nerves below it. Also *greater ischiadic foramen.* **f. ischiadicum minus** [NA] The small aperture of the lesser sciatic notch of hip bone spanned by the sacrotuberous ligament and separated from the greater sciatic foramen by the sacrospinous ligament. The bony surface is covered by cartilage over which pass the tendon of the obturator internus muscle and its nerve, while the internal pudendal vessels and pudendal nerve re-enter the pelvis through it from the greater sciatic foramen. Also *lesser ischiadic foramen.* **f. jugulare** [NA] An irregularly rounded and deep orifice on the base of the skull, usually larger on the right side, located at the posterior end of the petro-occipital suture and formed anteriorly by the jugular fossa of the petrous part of the temporal bone apposing, posteriorly, the jugular notch on the jugular process lateral to the condyle of the occipital bone. It is partially divided by the processus intrajugularis, lateral to which is the sigmoid sinus, while medial to it are, anteroposteriorly, the inferior petrosal sinus, the glossopharyngeal, vagus, and accessory nerves, and the internal jugular vein. The foramen is posterior to foramen caroticum externum and medial to the base of the styloid process. Also *jugular foramen.* **f. lacerum** [NA] An opening with a serrated margin located at the base of the skull between the basilar part of the occipital bone, the junction of the body and greater wing of the sphenoid bone, and the apex of the petrous part of temporal bone. It is normally closed inferiorly by fibrocartilage on which the internal carotid artery rests as the artery leaves the foramen caroticum internum and bends upwards to the cavernous sinus. Also *middle lacerate foramen.* **foramina of Lannelongue** The largest of the foramina venarum minimarum. **lateral f.** An opening on the side of the root of a tooth which leads into the root canal. **lateral incisive f.** The most lateral of several openings of the incisive canals into the incisive fossa posterior to the upper incisor teeth. It conducts the nasopalatine nerve and the terminal branch of the greater palatine artery. **lesser ischiadic f.** FORAMEN ISCHIADICUM MINUS. **lesser palatine foramina** FORAMINA PALATINA MINORA. **f. magnum** [NA] The largest cranial foramen, the midline opening of the occipital bones through which emerges the medulla oblongata extending caudally into the vertebral canal. Also *great foramen, occipital foramen, inferior occipital foramen, foramen occipitale magnum, great occipital foramen.* **mandibular f.** An opening on the medial surface of the ascending ramus of the mandible which transmits the inferior alveolar nerve and vessels. Also *foramen mandibulae, foramen mandibulare, posterior maxillary foramen.* **f. mastoideum** [NA] A small opening behind the mastoid process of the temporal bone, near or on the occipitomastoid suture, for transmission of an emissary vein from the sigmoid sinus and a branch of the occipital artery to the dura mater. Its location is very variable. Also *mastoid foramen.* **maxillary f.** HIATUS MAXILLARIS. **medial frontal f.** FORAMEN FRONTALE. **median incisive f.** One of two incisive foramina occasionally present and opening on the anterior and posterior walls of the incisive fossa of the bony palate. **mental f.** An opening on the lateral surface of the mandible adjacent to the premolar teeth which transmits the mental nerve and vessels. **middle lacerate f.** *Outmoded* FORAMEN LACERUM. **f. of Monro** FORAMEN INTERVENTRICULARE. **Morgagni's f.** The occasional deficiency between the costal and sternal origins of the respiratory diaphragm, filled on each side with areolar tissue and transmitting the superior epigastric vessels and lymphatic vessels. Also *pleuroperitoneal foramen, trigonum sternocostale* (outmoded), *Larrey space, sternocostal triangle, Larrey's cleft.* **morgagnian f.** FORAMEN CAECUM LINGUAE. **nasal foramina** Small openings on the external, or facial, surface of the nasal bone for transmission of tributaries of the angular vein. Also *foramina nasalia* (outmoded). **foramina nervosa limbus laminae spiralis osseae** [NA] Numerous openings on the tympanic lip of the limbus laminae spiralis osseae of the cochlear labyrinth for the transmission of the branches of the cochlear nerve to the spiral organ. Also *habenula perforata.* **nutrient f.** An aperture, perforation, or passage through the cortex of the bone that carries the blood vessels to the medullary space. Also *foramen nutricium.* **f. obturatum** [NA] A large, irregularly oval opening bounded above and laterally by the acetabulum and acetabular notch, anteromedially and posterolaterally by the pubis and ischium respectively, and anteroinferiorly by the ischiopubic ramus. Attached to its circumference is a fibrous membrane, except superiorly at the obturator canal. Also *obturator foramen.* **occipital f.** FORAMEN MAGNUM. **f. occipitale magnum** FORAMEN MAGNUM. **olfactory f.** One of numerous foramina arranged in rows on the lamina cribrosa of the ethmoid bone through which pass filaments of the olfactory nerve. **f. of omental bursa** FORAMEN BURSAE OMENTALIS MAJORIS. **f. omentale** [NA] A short peritoneal canal between the omental bursa and the greater sac of abdominal peritoneum. It is bounded anteriorly by the right margin of the lesser omentum, inferiorly by the superior part of the duodenum, posteriorly by the inferior vena cava, and superiorly by the caudate process of liver. It is located just to the right of the midline. Also *hiatus of Winslow, opening of omental bursa, opening to lesser sac of peritonium, epiploic orifice.* **optic f. of sclera** The opening in the lamina cribrosa sclerae that gives passage to the central retinal artery and vein. Also *porus opticus.* **optic f. of sphenoid bone** CANALIS OPTICUS. **f. opticum ossis sphenoidalis** *Outmoded* CANALIS OPTICUS. **f. ovale** A valved communication between the right atrium and left atrium in the fetal heart. It is usually an obliquely elongated cleft bounded by the upper edge of the persisting part of the septum primum and by the lower edge of the septum secundum. The part of the septum primum that overlaps the cleft is called the valve of the foramen ovale. The foramen serves to direct oxygenated blood from the fetal inferior vena to the left atrium. It is obliterated shortly after birth in most individuals because increase in pressure in the left atrium closes the valve and fusion leaves a depression on the right side of the interatrial wall, called the fossa ovalis, lying inside the arched edge, or annulus ovalis, of the septum secundum. Not infrequently fusion is incomplete but the opening is small and possibly still valvular so that function is unimpaired. In a minority the opening remains unclosed in postnatal life and constitutes a patent foramen ovale. Also *Botallo's foramen* (obs.). See also OSTIUM PRIMUM, OSTIUM SECUNDUM. **f. ovale alae majoris** [NA] A large oval foramen near the middle of the posterior margin of the greater wing of the sphenoid bone between foramen rotundum anteriorly and foramen spinosum posterolaterally, transmitting the mandibular nerve to the infratemporal fossa along with the accessory meningeal artery and, occasionally, the lesser petrosal nerve. Also *oval foramen of sphenoid bone.* **f. ovale cordis** OSTIUM SECUNDUM. **f. ovale of Pacchioni** *Outmoded* INCISURA TENTORII. **oval f. of fetus** OSTIUM SECUNDUM. **oval f. of sphenoid bone** FORAMEN OVALE ALAE MAJORIS. **f. of Pacchioni** FORAMEN DIAPHRAGMATIS SELLAE. **pacchionian f.** FORAMEN DIAPHRAGMATIS SELLAE. **foramina palatina minora** [NA] Two or more small openings piercing the pyramidal process of the palatine bone in each posterolateral angle of the bony palate behind the greater palatine foramina and transmitting the lesser palatine nerves and vessels from their canals. Also *lesser palatine foramina.* **foramina of palatine tonsil** FOSSULAE TONSILLARES TONSILLAE PALATINAE. **f. palatinum majus** [NA] The lower orifice of the greater palatine canal that opens on the posterolateral part of the bony palate just behind the palatomaxillary suture and transmits the greater palatine nerve and vessels. Also *greater palatine foramen.* **foramina papillaria renis** [NA] The numerous openings of the papillary ducts of Bellini on the summit of a renal papilla, forming the area cribrosa and discharging the urine into the minor calices. Also *papillary foramina of kidney.* **f. parietale** [NA] A small, round opening, occasionally absent on one or both sides, adjacent to the sagittal margin of the parietal bone near lambda and transmitting an emissary vein from the superior sagittal sinus. **patent f. ovale** The valvelike aperture in the interatrial septum which remains patent in some 25 percent of adults, as a result of failed fusion of the embryonic septum secundum in such manner as to close the foramen of the septum primum. Also *acleistocardia.* **pleuroperitoneal f.** 1 MORGAGNI'S FORAMEN. 2 *Incorrect* HIATUS PLEUROPERITONEALIS. **posterior condyloid f.** CANALIS CONDYLARIS. **posterior ethmoidal f.** FORAMEN ETHMOIDALE POSTERIUS. **posterior maxillary f.** MANDIBULAR FORAMEN. **posterior sacral foramina** FORAMINA SACRALIA POSTERIORA. **posterior superior alveolar foramina** FORAMINA ALVEOLARIA MAXILLAE. **primary interventricular f.** CHANNEL OF HALLER. **f. primum** OSTIUM PRIMUM. **f. processus transversi** [NA] A rounded opening that pierces the transverse process of the cervical vertebrae, through the upper six of which it transmits the vertebral artery, vein, and plexus of sympathetic nerves. Also *transverse foramen.* **pterygoalar f.** PORUS CROTAPHITICOBUCCINATORIUS. **f. rotundum ossis sphenoidalis** [NA] A circular opening in the anteromedial part of the greater wing of the sphenoid bone, anterior to foramen ovale and inferomedial to the superior orbital fissure and conducting the maxillary nerve to the pterygopalatine fossa. Also *superior maxillary canal.*

**foramina sacralia anteriora** [NA] Four pairs of large openings located at the ends of the transverse lines on the anterior, or pelvic, surface of the sacrum that are linked by the intervertebral foramina to the sacral canal, from which they transmit the ventral rami of the first four sacral nerves, arteries, and veins. Also *anterior sacral foramina.* **foramina sacralia posteriora** [NA] Four paired large openings on the posterior surface of the sacrum located between the intermediate sacral crest and articular tubercles medially, and the lateral sacral crest and transverse tubercles laterally. The intervertebral foramina link them with the sacral canal, from which they transmit dorsal rami of the first four sacral nerves, arteries, and veins. Also *posterior sacral foramina.* **f. of saphenous vein** HIATUS SAPHENUS. **f. secundum** OSTIUM SECUNDUM. **f. singulare** [NA] An isolated foramen below and behind the inferior vestibular area, on the vertical plate of the fundus of the internal acoustic meatus. It transmits the nerve to the ampulla of the posterior semicircular duct of the internal ear. **foramina of smallest veins of heart** FORAMINA VENARUM MINIMARUM CORDIS. **f. sphenopalatinum** [NA] The foramen in the upper part of the medial wall of the pterygopalatine fossa, formed by the orbital process of the perpendicular plate of the palatine bone anteriorly, its sphenoidal process posteriorly and the body of the sphenoid bone above. Through it the fossa communicates with the nasal cavity posterior to the superior meatus, and transmits the nasopalatine and superior nasal nerves and the sphenopalatine vessels. Also *sphenopalatine foramen.* **f. spinosum** [NA] A small, circular opening in the posterior angle of the greater wing of the sphenoid bone, situated posterolateral to the foramen ovale and anteromedial to the spine of the sphenoid on the infratemporal surface. It transmits the middle meningeal artery and the meningeal branch of the mandibular nerve to the middle cranial fossa. Also *spinous foramen.* **f. stylomastoideum** [NA] An opening between the root of the styloid process and the anterior end of the mastoid notch on the inferior surface of the petrous part of the temporal bone. It is the external opening of the facial canal and transmits the facial nerve, the stylomastoid branch of the posterior auricular artery and, occasionally, the auricular branch of the vagus nerve. **f. supraorbitale** [NA] The foramen at the junction of the medial and intermediate thirds of the supraorbital margin which is formed by bone or fibrous tissue bridging over the incisura supraorbitalis. It transmits the supraorbital nerve and vessels and has an opening in its floor for a diploic vein. Also *supraorbital foramen.* **f. of Tarin** *Outmoded* HIATUS CANALIS NERVI PETROSI MAJORIS. **f. thyroideum** [NA] An occasional opening in the upper part of the lamina of the thyroid cartilage transmitting the superior laryngeal vessels and resulting from the incomplete fusion of the fourth and fifth branchial cartilages. Also *thyroid foramen.* **tonsillar foramina** Either fossulae tonsillares tonsillae palatinae or fossulae tonsillares tonsillae pharyngeae. **transverse f.** FORAMEN PROCESSUS TRANSVERSI. **transverse accessory f.** A small foramen frequently present in the transverse process of the sixth cervical vertebra, posterior to and smaller than the foramen processus transversi. It may transmit a vein and it is seldom present in other cervical vertebrae. **f. venae cavae** [NA] The highest of the three major openings in the respiratory diaphragm, situated at the junction of the right leaf with the middle part of its tendon and transmitting the inferior vena cava and some branches of the right phrenic nerve. Also *vena caval foramen, vena caval hiatus, opening for vena cava, opening of inferior vena cava.* **foramina venarum minimarum cordis** [NA] The minute orifices of the venae cardiacae minimae opening on the internal surface of the walls, especially the septal and right lateral, of the right atrium. Also *foramina of smallest veins of heart, pores of Vieussens, foraminula of Lannelongue.* **f. vertebrale** [NA] The large space behind the body of a vertebra, bounded posteriorly and laterally by the vertebral arch, varying in shape in different parts of the vertebral column and containing mostly the spinal cord, meninges and associated vessels. Also *spinal aperture, vertebral foramen.* **visceral f.** HEMAL FORAMEN. **Weitbrecht's f.** An opening, variable in size and occurrence, in the fibrous capsule of the shoulder joint, situated between the superior and middle glenohumeral ligaments, through which the bursa under the tendon of the subscapularis muscle communicates with the joint cavity. Also *foramen ovale of Weitbrecht.* **f. zygomaticofaciale** [NA] The opening near the orbital margin on the lateral surface of the zygomatic bone for the zygomaticofacial nerve and vessels. Also *zygomaticofacial foramen, zygomaticofacial canal.* **f. zygomatico-orbitale** [NA] Either of two openings on the orbital surface of the zygomatic bone leading to two canals that terminate in the zygomaticofacial foramen and the zygomaticotemporal foramen. Also *zygomatico-orbital foramen.* **f. zygomaticotemporale** [NA] The opening on the temporal surface and near the base of the frontal process of the zygomatic bone for transmission of the zygomaticotemporal nerve and branch of lacrimal artery. Also *zygomaticotemporal foramen, zygomaticotemporal canal.*

**foramina** \fôram′inə\ Plural of FORAMEN.

**foraminal** \fôram′inəl\ Pertaining to a foramen.

**foraminotomy** \fôr′aminät′əmē\ [*foramin(is),* gen. of L *foramen* a hole, opening + *o* + -TOMY] Enlargement of an aperture in the skull or the vertebra for passage of a nerve.

**foraminulate** \fôr′amin′yəlit\ Possessing a foraminulum or foraminula. Also *foraminulous, foraminulose.*

**foraminulose** \fôr′amin′yəlōs\ FORAMINULATE.

**foraminulous** \fôr′amin′yələs\ FORAMINULATE.

**foraminulum** \fôr′amin′yələm\ A very small foramen. **foraminula of Lannelongue** *Outmoded* FORAMINA VENARUM MINIMARUM CORDIS.

**foration** \fôrā′shən\ [L *forat(us),* past part. of *forare* to bore, pierce + -ION] TREPHINING.

**Forbes** [A. P. *Forbes,* U.S. physician, flourished mid-20th century] Forbes-Albright syndrome. See under SYNDROME.

**Forbes** [Gilbert Burnett *Forbes,* U.S. pediatrician, born 1915] Forbes disease. See under GLYCOGEN STORAGE DISEASE III.

**force** [French (from Vulgar L *fortia* strength, from L *fortis* strong) power, strength] That influence which produces or tends to produce acceleration of a body. **catabiotic f.** The energy derived from the metabolism of food. **catabolic f.** Energy obtained from the conversion of complex substances to simpler compounds in living cells. **chewing f.** MASTICATORY FORCE. **electromotive f.** The relative potential between two dissimilar electrodes in the same electrolyte. Abbr. EMF **field f.'s** Hypothetical forces which are thought to play a part in the individuation process during early embryonic development by means of which organizers influence adjacent cells and tissues. See also INDIVIDUATION FIELD. **masticatory f.** The force exerted by the muscles of mastication. Also *chewing force, biting strength.* **occlusal f.** The force applied to teeth by opposing teeth or interposed food. Also *biting pressure, occlusal pressure.* **radiation f.** The force exerted on a body by radiation incident on it. **f. of recoil of the lung** The force with which the lung, because of its inherent elasticity, tends to retract and lose volume when not held in contact with the thoracic wall. **shearing f.** The stress existing between the bony skeleton and the skin overlying it when a patient, sitting propped up in bed, slides down and the skin continues to adhere to the surface with which it is in contact, i.e., the mattress. The stress causes disruption of blood vessels and body tissues and it predisposes the patient to the formation of a decubitus ulcer. **van der Waals f.'s** Relatively weak forces of attraction between all molecules, due to interaction of oscillating electrical dipoles, even in molecules with no permanent dipoles. They were recognized from the equations of van der Waals for representing the deviation of behavior of actual gases from the ideal gas laws.

# forceps

**forceps** \fôr′seps\ [L (from *for(mus)* hot + *-ceps,* from *capere* to hold, seize) a pair of tongs, pincers] **1** A surgical instrument that is used for grasping tissues or surgical materials. It may resemble scissors, with a locking mechanism at the handles to maintain a desired position, or it may look like tweezers. **2** An anatomic structure with a forcipate or pincerlike shape. Adj. forcipate, forcipal. **Adams f.** A powerful forceps with flattened oval-shaped blades for gripping the nasal septum in the Adams operation. **adenoid f.** Forceps with cupped or fenestrated blades for removing the adenoids or adenoid remnants left behind after the use of an adenoid curette or adenotome, or for excising a sample of a postnasal tumor as a biopsy specimen. **Allis f.** A tissue forceps with fine-toothed, incurved jaws, widely used in several branches of surgery. **f. anterior** FORCEPS MINOR. **Asch f.** A forceps for centralizing the displaced nasal septum in cases of fracture of the nose. The forceps are applied to the interior of the nose with one blade on either side of the septum. **axis-traction f.** Obstetrical forceps designed to exert traction in an axis corresponding to that of the lower maternal birth canal. **Bailey-Williamson f.** A modified version of the Elliot obstetrical forceps with fenestrated blades and with lengthened shanks which accentuate their cephalic curve. **Ballenger's f.** Curved, locking forceps which are a modification of volsella forceps, used in seizing the tonsil in tonsillectomy. **Barton f.** An obstetrical forceps utilized to exert traction on a fetal head in the occiput transverse position. It consists of a hinged anterior blade and a rigid posterior blade. **bayonet f.** Forceps shaped like a bayonet, commonly used in the treatment and surgery of the nose and ear. The object of the design is to prevent the fingers holding the forceps from obscuring a view of the tips of the forceps. **bone f.** Forceps with sharp curved beaks, meeting edge-to-edge, used for the removal of bone. **bone-cutting f.** Plierlike forceps that are used to cut bone or cartilage. **bone-nibbling f.** Forceps used to remove small sections of bone or cartilage. Also *gouge forceps.* **Brenner f.** A type of obstetrical forceps utilized in breech presentations. **bulldog f.** A small spring forceps, the jaws usually covered with rubber tubing, used for occluding blood vessels. **capsule f.** A surgical instrument for grasping the lens capsule during cataract extraction. **cartilage f.** Forceps used to extract cartilage in a surgical procedure. **chalazion f.** A surgical instrument for securing the everted eyelid during incision and curettage of a retention cyst of the meibomian gland. It is also used during removal of lesions from the lip or cheek. **Chamberlen f.** A forerunner of modern obstetrical forceps developed by four generations of English physicians, the Chamberlens, between 1600 and 1728. Their instrument was one of the first designed to save not only the mother's life but the infant's life as well. **clamp f.** Locking forceps that are used to compress arteries, the pedicle of a tumor, and the like. **f. of corpus callosum** The forceps minor and forceps major of the corpus callosum. **crocodile f.** Any of a variety of forceps having elongated jaws with only the upper jaw being hinged. Light-weight forceps of this kind are commonly used in modern otologic surgery. **DeLee f.** An obstetrical forceps similar to Simpson's forceps but consisting of longer shanks and modified handles. **dental extracting f.** Forceps with curved beaks shaped to fit the roots of teeth. There is a large variety of design, often named after the tooth which the design fits, such as upper right molar forceps. Also *dental forceps, extracting forceps.* **depilatory f.** EPILATING FORCEPS. **dissecting f.** Forceps used to separate and delineate tissues and organs. Also *dissection forceps.* **double-action f.** A surgical scissorlike instrument that is constructed with two joints or hinges between the blades and handles. It is used for applying pressure to compress or divide tissues. **dural f.** A two-bladed surgical instrument having small teeth. It is used for grasping the dura mater. **Elliot f.** Obstetrical forceps consisting of a rounded cephalic curve with fenestrated blades and overlapping of the shanks. **epilating f.** An instrument used to pluck hair. Also *depilatory forceps.* **extracting f.** DENTAL EXTRACTING FORCEPS. **failed f.** The unsuccessful application of obstetrical forceps, usually due to cephalopelvic disproportion, incomplete cervical dilatation, or malposition of the fetal head. **fixation f.** Tweezerlike forceps with serrated tips that are used to stabilize tissues during operative procedures. Also *rat-tooth forceps.* **Foster-Ballenger f.** A punch forceps with flattened blades, one fenestrated to receive the other, for cutting out portions of the septal cartilage in submucous resection of the nasal septum. **galea f.** WILLETT FORCEPS. **Garrison's f.** LUIKART FORCEPS. **Good f.** An obstetrical forceps similar to Simpson's forceps. **gouge f.** BONE-NIBBLING FORCEPS. **Haig Ferguson f.** An obstetrical forceps similar in design to Simpson's forceps. **Hawks-Dennen f.** A modified version of Simpson's obstetrical forceps with the shanks bent backwards to form an exaggerated perineal curve in order to facilitate axis traction. **high f.** The application of obstetrical forceps to an unengaged fetal head, an application very rarely if ever utilized by modern-day obstetricians. Also *inlet forceps.* **inlet f.** HIGH FORCEPS. **insertion f.** POINT FORCEPS. **Jansen f.** **1** A cranked punch forceps designed for operations on the sphenoidal sinus. **2** A bayonet-shaped rongeur used in mastoid surgery. **Kerrison f.** A tympanic rongeur designed to minimize the risk of injury to the facial nerve during mastoid surgery. **Kielland f.** An obstetrical forceps primarily utilized for rotation with narrow, separated handles, a sliding lock, overlapping shanks, and a bayonet appearance of the blades and shanks due to a reversed pelvic curve. **Kocher's f.** Forceps with teethlike projections for holding tissue during surgery or for compressing bleeding tissue. **lion-jawed f.** Strong, long-handled, serrated forceps that are used to hold large pieces or shafts of bone. **lock f.** POINT FORCEPS. **low f.** The application of obstetrical forceps after the fetal head has reached the perineal floor and with the sagittal suture in the anteroposterior diameter of the maternal outlet. Also *outlet forceps.* **Luc's f.** A stout forceps, with angled blades and cupped or, more often, fenestrated jaws of different shapes and sizes. They are widely used in nasal surgery, particularly in turbinectomy and for removing nasal polyps. **Luikart f.** An obstetrical forceps similar to the Tucker-McLean forceps with overlapping shanks with a sliding lock, handles similar to those on the Kielland forceps, and blades with an incomplete fenestration (pseudofenestration) on the cephalic side of the blades. Also *Garrison's forceps.* **f. major** [NA] The interhemispheric fibers of the occipital cerebral cortex extending through the splenium of the corpus callosum. Also *forceps posterior.* **McKenzie f.** Forceps designed for the application of neurosurgical clips. **mid f.** The application of obstetrical forceps after engagement of the fetal head but prior to meeting the criteria for low forceps. Also *median forceps, mid-plane forceps.* **f. minor** [NA] The interhemispheric fibers of the frontal cerebral cortex extending through the genu of the corpus callosum and coursing forward. Also *forceps anterior.* **mosquito f.** Small delicate forceps for holding tissue. **Negus ligature f.** An artery forceps with backward curving tips designed for use in tonsillectomy to facilitate the tying of ligatures around bleeding points in the tonsil bed. Also *Negus tonsil artery forceps.* **nonfenestrated f.** Obstetrical forceps in which the blades consist of solid metal without a window or fenestration. **obstetrical f.** An instrument usually consisting of two blades, each connected to a handle by a shank and utilized to exert traction on a fetal head or to rotate the fetal head in order to facilitate vaginal delivery. **Ostrom f.** A backward cutting punch forceps designed for enlarging the antrostome forwards in in-

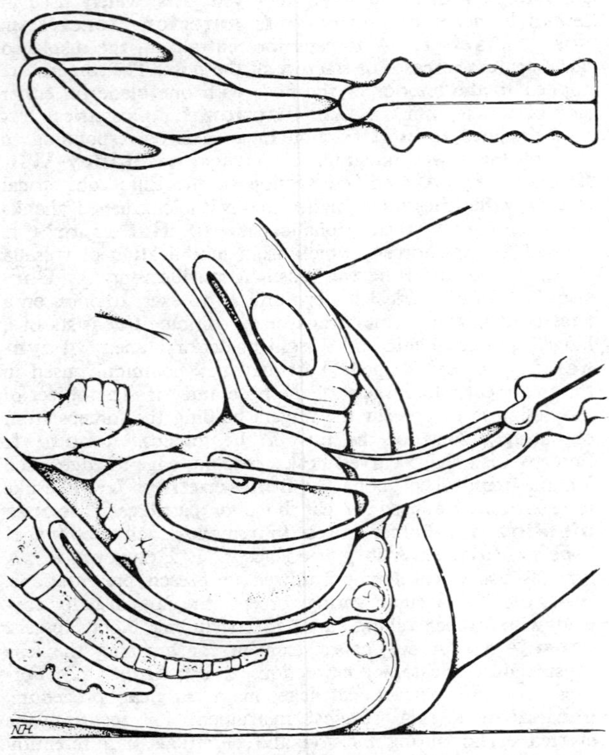


**Obstetrical forceps**

tranasal antrostomy. **outlet f.** LOW FORCEPS. **ovum f.** A surgical forceps having blades with oval tips designed for removing tissue from the uterus following an incomplete abortion or at the time of a dilatation and curettage in search of an endometrial polyp. **Piper f.** An obstetrical forceps with long shanks and a perineal curve. It is designed to be applied to an aftercoming head in order to facilitate the vaginal delivery of an infant in the breech presentation. **placenta f.** A forceps usually consisting of fenestrated blades which are passed transcervically in order to grasp and extract placental tissue still lying within the uterine cavity. **point f.** Fine forceps, with serrated or longitudinally grooved beaks, used for inserting points such as gutta-percha points into root canals. The beaks can be locked in the closed position. Also *lock forceps, insertion forceps.* **f. posterior** FORCEPS MAJOR. **punch f.** A forceps used to punch out a small sample of tissue for biopsy. **rat-tooth f.** FIXATION FORCEPS. **rib-cutting f.** Forceps designed to divide ribs. **rongeur f.** Bone cutting forceps that combine a rongeur-type cutting head with forceps handle and have a double fulcrum lever action to enhance mechanical power. They are used to remove small fragments of bone during an exposure procedure. **root-splitting f.** Dental forceps with cutting blades for separating the roots of multirooted teeth. **rubber dam clamp f.** Forceps with curved, ball-ended beaks, used for holding and opening rubber dam clamps. The beaks can be locked in the open position. Also *clamp holder, rubber dam clamp holder.* **sequestrum f.** Plierlike forceps with strong serrated locking teeth that are used to remove fragments of dead bone. **Simpson's f.** An obstetrical forceps consisting of a long, tapered cephalic curve with fenestrated blades and parallel separated shanks. **sinus f.** A forceps designed with narrow, tapered blades, used to gain entrance to or enlarge an abscess. **speculum f.** Long-handled forceps designed to be used through a speculum. **sponge-holding f.** SPONGE HOLDER. **spring f.** Lightweight forceps with two opposable blades separated by spring tension. **suture f.** NEEDLE HOLDER. **tenaculum f.** Forceps having two blades, both of which have a sharp hook, used for grasping and stabilizing tissues. **thumb f.** TISSUE FORCEPS. **tissue f.** Forceps having two fine-toothed blades, designed for gentle, nontraumatic manipulation of tissues. Also *thumb forceps.* **torsion f.** Forceps utilizing torsion or twisting to stop hemorrhaging of an artery. **towel f.** TOWEL CLIP. **tubular f.** Long, slender forceps designed to be used through a speculum or a very limited incision. **Tucker-McLean f.** A modified version of the Elliot obstetrical forceps with either semifenestrated or nonfenestrated blades and with lengthened shanks which accentuate their cephalic curve. **uterine f.** A long, slender, curved instrument with blunted serrations, used to remove tissue or insert packing in the uterus. **volsella f.** A long forceps with sharp teeth on the end, used in some gynecologic procedures to grasp tissues and apply torsion or traction. Also *vulsella, volsella.* **Walsham f.** A forceps for correcting lateral deviation of the fractured nose. With one blade inside the nose and the other, surrounded by a piece of rubber tubing, outside, the fractured nasal bones are disimpacted and repositioned. **Willett f.** An instrument formerly utilized to control hemorrhage from a placenta previa. A T-shaped clamp is attached transcervically to the fetal scalp and a 1–2 pound weight is applied to the clamp via a pulley in order to compress the low-lying placenta. It may also be of use in assisting the delivery of a dead fetus. Also *Willett's clamp, galea forceps.*

**Forchheimer** [Frederick *Forchheimer,* U.S. physician, 1853–1913] Forchheimer spots. See under SPOT.

**forcipate** Shaped like forceps. Also *forcipal.*

**forcipressure** \fôr′sipresh′ər\ A technique for arresting hemorrhage by compressing the artery with the forceps.

**Fordyce** [John Addison *Fordyce,* U.S. dermatologist, 1858–1925] **1** Fox-Fordyce disease. See under DISEASE. **2** Fordyce disease, Fordyce granules. See under FORDYCE SPOTS.

**forearm** ANTEBRACHIUM.

**forebrain** [*fore* + *brain*] PROSENCEPHALON.

**forefinger** INDEX.

**forefoot** **1** An anterior foot of a quadruped. **2** The distal or anterior part of the human foot: used most often with respect to the fitting of shoes, prostheses, or the like.

**foregilding** \fôr′gilding\ The impregnation of fresh nerve fibers with gold chloride solution. The process is particularly suitable for the demonstration of nerve endings.

**foregut** The anterior portion of the embryonic intestine from which the pharynx, esophagus and stomach, and the proximal part of the duodenum and its derivatives will develop.

**forehead** The region of the face between the eyebrows and the hairline; frons. **bony f.** FRONS CRANII.

**foreign** [Old French *forain,* from Late L *foranus* foreign, on the outside, from L *foras* out of doors, from Old L *fora* door] In immunology, deriving from a source other than the subject's own tissues (self); being or relating to nonself.

**Forel** [Auguste Henri *Forel,* Swiss neurologist, 1848–1931] **1** Forel's decussation. See under DECUSSATION OF RUBROSPINAL TRACTS. **2** Area Foreli, Forel's field. See under H FIELDS OF FOREL. **3** Forel's commissure. See under SUPRAMAMILLARY DECUSSATION. **4** Field $H_1$ of Forel. See under FASCICULUS THALAMICUS. **5** Field $H_2$ of Forel. See under FASCICULUS LENTICULARIS.

**foreleg** **1** An anterior limb of a quadruped. **2** The distal part of the human leg, near the ankle: used most often with respect to the fitting of prostheses or the like.

**foremilk** COLOSTRUM.

**forensic** \fəren′sik\ [L *forens(is)* pertaining to a forum where justice was publicly administered + -IC] Pertaining to or concerned with courts of justice or public debate.

**foreplay** The sexual activity which immediately precedes intromission and intercourse.

**foreseeability of harm** \fôrsē′əbil′itē\ The ability to foresee or predict that a negligent act or the negligent failure to act would introduce a risk of injury or damage that would not otherwise have existed. In malpractice cases where negligence is charged, it must be proven that a reasonably prudent person would have been able to predict that a negligent act or omission would, in all probability, have resulted in injury or damage, and the injuries or damages can be directly related to the negligent act or omission.

**foreskin** \fôr′skin\ PREPUTIUM PENIS. **hooded f.** The appearance of the prepuce in hypospadias, when the prepuce only partially covers the glans penis.

**forespore** \fôr′spôr\ A region of increased refractility seen with the light microscope in bacteria beginning to form a spore. At this stage the electron microscope shows an invaginated double layer of cytoplasmic membrane surrounding a chromosome and associated cytoplasm.

**forewaters** [*fore* + *waters*] The portion of the amniotic membranes and the contained fluid which lies between the fetal head and the opening of the uterine cervix.

**fork** / **replication f.** The region in a DNA molecule where replication occurs. Before the fork there is one fiber of double-stranded parental DNA, and at the fork the two strands separate, each being copied and soon possessing a newly synthesized complementary strand. Also *growing point.* **tuning f.** A two-pronged instrument resembling a long U with a short stem attached to its base. For clinical purposes the stem has a disk-shaped foot. When the fork is tapped against a firm surface the prongs vibrate virtually at a single characteristic frequency depending on the length and mass of the fork. The tuning fork has been of immense historic and practical importance in the development of tests of hearing for different tones and in facilitating the diagnosis between conductive and sensorineural hearing loss. Low frequency tuning forks are also used in neurologic diagnosis to assess the subject's vibration sense.

**form** 1 Shape or configuration of an object or body. 2 When prefixed to a taxon, as in *form-genus* or *form-class,* denoting a grouping of organisms that lack a sexual reproductive stage: used especially in classifying the imperfect fungi. **accolé f.** A surface adherent form of *Plasmodium falciparum* in which the early stage trophozoite (ring form) appears to cling to the outside of the human red cell. Also *appliqué form, appliqué.* **replicative f.** The double-stranded form of viral DNA capable of replicating in a host cell. Many viruses of single-stranded nucleic acid direct the synthesis of a complementary strand to produce such a replicative form, which then multiplies in the cell. **resistance f.** That factor in the determination of the shape of a prepared tooth cavity which takes into account the need to support the restoration against occlusal forces. **retention f.** That factor in the determination of the shape of a prepared tooth cavity which takes into account the need for the restoration to be retained in the cavity. **trypanosomal f.** *Outmoded* TRYPOMASTIGOTE. **wax f.** WAX PATTERN. **Z f.** Z DNA.

**-form** \-fôrm\ [L *forma* form, shape] A combining form meaning having the form or appearance of.

**formal** FORMALDEHYDE SOLUTION.

**formaldehyde** \fôrmal′dəhīd\ H—CHO. Methanal. It is a highly reactive aldehyde, largely hydrated in water and easily reversibly polymerized. It is somewhat toxic and can be used to fix and preserve animal tissues.

**formalin** *Outmoded* FORMALDEHYDE SOLUTION.

**formant** \fôr′mənt\ [L *formans,* gen. *formantis,* pres. part. of *formare* to form] A restricted band of relatively high acoustic energy in comparison with other harmonics or overtones. Its center frequency and the total number of formants depend on the characteristics of the resonating chamber related to the primary sound source. It is of particular importance in the acoustic phonetics of speech. The shape of the supraglottic part of the vocal tract is capable of considerable variation, with direct effects on its performance as a series of linked resonators, most clearly seen in the production of vowels.

**formatio** \fôrmā′shō\ [L (from *formare* to form, shape) a forming, shaping] [NA] Any structure having a definite shape. Also *formation.* **f. hippocampalis** HIPPOCAMPAL FORMATION. **f. reticularis** [NA] Diffusely organized neural tissue consisting characteristically of a meshwork of both large and small neuronal cell bodies and their dendrites, axons, and branching collaterals found in the gray matter of the spinal cord, the central core region of the medulla oblongata, pons, and midbrain, and extending rostrally into the medial thalamus and hypothalamus. They exert profound effects upon all sensory and motor systems as well as the rest-activity cycle, i.e., sleep and wakefulness. Also *reticular formation, reticular substance, substantia reticularis, reticular system.* **f. reticularis medullae oblongatae** [NA] The diffuse, poorly circumscribed cell groups and fiber tracts of the medulla oblongata, interspersed among the main nuclei and tracts. Also *medullary reticular formation, reticular formation of medulla oblongata.* **f. reticularis medullae spinalis** [NA] The medial, intermediate portion of thespinal gray matter, consisting of scattered cell groups and fiber tracts. Also *reticular formation of spinal cord.* **f. reticularis mesencephali** [NA] The midbrain reticular formation, interposed between the substantia nigra and the periaqueductal gray matter. Also *formatio reticularis pedunculi cerebri, reticular formation of mesencephalon.* **f. reticularis pedunculi cerebri** FORMATIO RETICULARIS MESENCEPHALI. **f. reticularis pontis** [NA] The nuclei and tracts located principally in the tegmentum of the pons, including the central tegmental reticular nucleus (nucleus dissipata), the superior central pontine tegmental nucleus (associated with the pneumotaxic center), and the medial and lateral ventral tegmental nuclei. Also *reticular formation of pons.*

**formation** [L *formatio.* See FORMATIO.] 1 The process of forming or developing. 2 The result of such a process; something formed. 3 FORMATIO. **Ammon's f.** HIPPOCAMPUS. • The term is named after *Ammon,* the ram-headed deity of ancient Egypt. **chiasma f.** The process during meiosis of chromosomal crossing over in which pairs of homologous chromosomes physically join at chiasmata. **endochondral bone f.** ENDOCHONDRAL OSSIFICATION. **hippocampal f.** The fascia dentata, fornix, hippocampus, and subicular fields. *Imprecise.* Also *formatio hippocampalis, gyrus hippocampi* (imprecise). **intracartilaginous bone f.** ENDOCHONDRAL OSTEOGENESIS. **intramembranous bone f.** The process of creating the structure of bone directly through osteoblastic activity in a noncartilaginous matrix. **medullary reticular f.** FORMATIO RETICULARIS MEDULLAE OBLONGATAE. **palisade f.** Cells arranged with their long axis in a parallel manner to give a picket fence effect. This formation typically occurs in neurilemmomas. A similar appearance can be seen around areas of necrosis in glioblastomas. **reaction f.** An unconscious defense mechanism of the ego consisting of denying the presence of unacceptable infantile urges and therefore altering one's character and one's way of relating to the external world. **reticular f.** FORMATIO RETICULARIS. **reticular f. of medulla oblongata** FORMATIO RETICULARIS MEDULLAE OBLONGATAE. **reticular f. of mesencephalon** FORMATIO RETICULARIS MESENCEPHALI. **reticular f. of pons** FORMATIO RETICULARIS PONTIS. **reticular f. of spinal cord** FORMATIO RETICULARIS MEDULLAE SPINALIS. **rouleaux f.** The arrangement of erythrocytes in overlapping fashion, suggesting a stack of coins. **white reticular f.** SUBSTANTIA RETICULARIS ALBA MEDULLAE OBLONGATAE.

**formationes** \fôr′māshō′nēz\ Plural of FORMATIO.

**formative** \fôr′mətiv\ Having to do with the shaping or molding of the final product of any developmental process.

**forme fruste** \fôrm froost, frʏst\ (*pl.* formes frustes) An incomplete or abortive form of a disease or anomaly.

**forme tardive** \fôrm tärdiv′\ Late-appearing manifestations of a disease with variable age of onset and which is normally seen at a younger age. For example, epiloia (tuberose sclerosis) may present no serious symptoms until late in life.

**form-genus** \fôrm-jē′nəs\ See under FORM.

**formic** \fôr′mik\ [L *formic(a)* an ant] 1 Of or relating to ants. 2 Relating to or derived from formic acid.

**formic acid** H—COOH. A weak acid (p$K$ 3.7), that is colorless, corrosive, and harmful to the skin. It has the distinctive smell of ants, which secrete it. It is used as a reducing agent, and is miscible with water, alcohol, and ether. It can be formed from the metabolism of many biochemical compounds, such as serine or glycine, or by the oxidation of "one-carbon compounds," such as formaldehyde or methanol, which may be free or combined with tetrahydrofolic acid. However, the metabolically active forms are $N^{10}$- and $N^5$- formyl tetrahydrofolic acids, which are intermediates in the biosynthesis of purines.

**formicant** \fôr′mikənt\ Describing or producing formication.

**formication** \fôr′mikā′shən\ [L *formic(a)* an ant + -ATION] A sensation of insects creeping in or under one or more areas of the skin. It is most commonly reported in drug and alcohol abusers. Also *crawling, Magnan sign, Magnan symptom.*

**formiciasis** \fôr′misī′əsis\ [*formic (acid)* + -IASIS] Formic acid poisoning from ant bites.

**formimino** The group HN═CH—. This group is transferred to tetrahydrofolate during the catabolism of histidine.

***N*-formiminoglutamate** HN═CH—NH—CH(COOH)—$CH_2$—$CH_2$—COOH. The substance whose formula is shown and its ionized forms. It is an intermediate in the catabolism of histidine.

**formiminonoglutamic acid** HN═CH—NH—CH(COOH)—$CH_2$—$CH_2$—COOH. An intermediate in the breakdown of histidine, it transfers its formimino group to tetrahydrofolate.

**formiminoglutamicaciduria** \fôrmim′inōglootam′ikas′idoo′rē·ə\ The excessive urinary excretion of formiminoglutamic acid. It occurs in two distinct autosomal recessive inborn errors of metabolism: cyclodeaminase deficiency, in which patients are severely mentally retarded with cerebral cortical atrophy, and formiminotransferase deficiency, in which patients have variable but mild neurologic abnormalities.

**formiminoglycine** $H_2N^+$═CH—NH—$CH_2$—$COO^-$. A substance found as a metabolite in the breakdown of purines. It yields glycine by transferring its $H_2N^+$═CH— group to tetrahydrofolate.

**formiminotetrahydrofolate** Tetrahydrofolate substituted on N-5 with the formimino group. It is derived from formiminoglutamate in histidine breakdown or from formiminoglycine in purine breakdown. It is metabolized to liberate ammonia with formation of 5,10 methenyltetrahydrofolate.

**formiminotransferase** Any enzyme that transfers the formimino group. Also *transformiminase.*

**forminitrazole** $C_4H_3N_3O_3S$. A bacteriostatic agent that is used in the treatment of trichomoniasis vaginitis.

**formol saline** A widely used general purpose fixative solution that contains 10 percent formaldehyde in physiologic saline.

**formol sublimate** A compound fixative composed of mercuric chloride and formaldehyde. It is a swift histological fixative that enhances subsequent staining.

**formula** [L (dim. of *forma* form, shape), a rule, form, order, condition] **1** A designation of the structure or composition of a chemical that uses symbols and signs to identify the structural characteristics. **2** The ingredients and directions that are to be combined for the preparation of a medicinal drug or application. **3** An algebraic or symbolic expression of a rule or concept. **Arneth's f.** The proportions of segmented neutrophils, when classified by number of nuclear lobes. Also *Arneth's count.* **Bazett f.** A formula for correcting the Q-T interval for the effects of rate (where RR is the time interval in seconds between successive R waves): $QTc = \frac{QT}{\sqrt{RR}}$. **Casper's f.** A formula used in forensic medicine: the amount of putrefaction occurring in one week in a body exposed to air equals that amount occurring in two weeks in a body in water or the amount occurring in eight weeks in a body in soil. Putrefaction is assumed to occur at a set rate. The formula is used as a rule of thumb to assess the time of death in decaying or decomposing bodies. However, it is a useful approximation only in temperate climates. **dental f.** A concise representation of the number of incisors, canines, premolars, and molars in the dentition of a particular animal. **Du Bois f.** A formula that relates the surface area of the body to the body weight and height: $O = W^{0.425} \times H^{0.725} \times 71.84$, where O = surface area in $cm^2$, W = weight in kg, and H = height in cm. **extemporaneous f.** A prescription for a medicinal preparation that must be prepared just before being dispensed and not taken from stock or off the shelf. **Fick f.** See under FICK PRINCIPLE. **Gorlin f.** A formula for calculating the area of a cardiac valve orifice: Valve area = blood flow ÷ K × 44.5 × $\sqrt{P1-P2}$, (where valve area is in square centimeters, blood flow is in mm/sec during the time of valve opening, K is an empirical constant, and P1 and P2 are the mean pressures in mmHg on either side of the valve during the time it is open). **Hamilton-Stewart f.** A formula for calculating cardiac output following the rapid injection of an indicator substance: F = *i*/CT (where *F* = blood flow in liters/min; *i*, the injected substance in mg; *C*, the average concentration of the injected substance during the primary curve; and *T*, the duration of the primary curve, i.e., the curve in which there is no recirculation of the injected substance). **official f.** An approved and accepted formula that has been recognized and designated by a pharmacopeia or similar authoritative group. **Poisson-Pearson f.** A formula for the percentage error in calculating the endemic index of malaria for a population given the spleen rate estimated from a sample and the size of the population under 15 years:

$$\frac{200}{n}\sqrt{\frac{2(n-x)}{n}}\sqrt{1-\frac{(n-1)}{(N-1)}},$$

where $n$ is the size of the sample, $x$ the number with enlarged spleens, $N$ the size of the child population, and $x/n$ is the estimated spleen rate. **Rollier's f.** A formula used to increase progressively the ultraviolet dosage being applied to the body, to prevent excessive use of ultraviolet radiation. **vertebral f.** A numerical representation of the number of vertebrae usually found in the cervical, thoracic, lumbar, sacral, and coccygeal regions, namely, C 7, T 12, L 5, S 5, Co (or Cd) 4 = 33, for humans. **Vierordt-Meeh f.** A formula that relates the surface area of the body to the body weight and height: $O = mP^{2/3}$, where O = surface area, m = height, and P = weight.

**formulary** \fôr′myəler′ē\ **1** A listing of drugs, usually by generic name, and usually including all drugs available through a pharmacy or health care plan. **2** A published collection of formulas used in compounding drugs. See also NATIONAL FORMULARY.

**formulation** \fôr′myəlā′shən\ **ALI f.** AMERICAN LAW INSTITUTE FORMULATION. **American Law Institute f.** "A person is not responsible for criminal conduct if at the time of such conduct as a result of mental disease or defect he lacks substantial capacity either to appreciate the wrongfulness of his conduct or to conform his conduct to the requirements of law." It was first adopted in

1966 by the Second Circuit U.S. Court of Appeals based on the case of the United States vs Brawner. Also *American Law Institute rule, ALI formulation.*

**formyl** \fôr′mil\ The group H—CO—; the acyl group derived from formic acid.

**formylation** \fôr′milā′shən\ The process of replacing a hydrogen atom by the formyl group.

***N*-formylmethionine** HCO—NH—CH(COOH)—$[CH_2]_2$—S—$CH_3$. The acylated amino acid with which bacterial protein synthesis starts. It is produced as formylmethionyl-tRNA by formylation of one of the two forms of methionyl-tRNA, and is transferred on the ribosome onto the second residue of the protein being synthesized, releasing its tRNA.

**formyltetrahydrofolate** Tetrahydrofolate formylated on N-5 or N-10. Each of these compounds is an intermediate in some biologic formylations. They can be derived by oxidation of methylenetetrahydrofolate as well as by direct formylation.

**fornical** \fôr′nikl\ Pertaining or belonging to a fornix.

**fornicate** \fôr′nikit\ Arched or vaulted; shaped like a fornix.

**fornix** \fôr′niks\ [L, a furnacelike ceiling, an arch, vault] **1** Any archlike structure, or the concave recess produced by such a structure. **2** FORNIX CEREBRI. **anterior f.** PARS ANTERIOR FORNICIS VAGINAE. **f. cerebri** [NA] Large, paired myelinated tracts that emerge from the hippocampus, arch and fuse beneath the corpus callosum, and descend in separate columns to the septal region (precommissural fornix) and mamillary bodies (postcommissural fornix). It contains mainly efferent fibers arising from the subiculum and hippocampus, but numerous other afferent and efferent connections have been described. Also *fornix of cerebrum, cerebral fornix, psalis* (outmoded), *cerebral trigone, trigonum cerebrale, fornix.* **f. of conjunctiva** Either the fornix conjunctivae superior or the fornix conjunctivae inferior. **f. conjunctivae inferior** [NA] The line of reflection of the conjunctiva from the inner surface of the lower eyelid to the eyeball. Also *inferior conjunctival fornix.* **f. conjunctivae superior** [NA] The line of reflection of the conjunctiva from the inner surface of the upper eyelid to the eyeball. The excretory ductules of the lacrimal gland open into its lateral part. Also *superior conjunctival fornix.* **f. gastricus** FUNDUS GASTRICUS. **inferior conjunctival f.** FORNIX CONJUNCTIVAE INFERIOR. **f. of lacrimal sac** FORNIX SACCI LACRIMALIS. **lateral f.** PARS LATERALIS FORNICIS VAGINAE. **f. longus** The portion of the fornix cerebri bundle emerging from the hippocampus in its longitudinal course above the diencephalon, before forming the descending columns. **f. pharyngis** [NA] The arched roof and adjacent posterior wall of the nasopharynx that is attached to the inferior surface of the basilar part of the occipital bone and the adjoining body of the sphenoid bone and related anteriorly to the nasal choanae. Its mucous membrane contains the pharyngeal tonsil. Also *fornix of pharynx, vault of pharynx.* **posterior f.** PARS POSTERIOR FORNICIS VAGINAE. **f. sacci lacrimalis** [NA] The dome-shaped upper junction of the lateral and medial walls of the lacrimal sac which is situated above the level of the opening of the lacrimal canaliculi. Also *fornix of lacrimal sac.* **f. of the stomach** FUNDUS GASTRICUS. **superior conjunctival f.** FORNIX CONJUNCTIVAE SUPERIOR. **f. vaginae** [NA] The arched recess surrounding the vaginal portion of the uterine cervix at the upper end of the vagina. The continuous space is divided into pars anterior, pars lateralis, and pars posterior in relation to the walls of the vagina. Also *fundus of vagina.* **f. ventricularis** FUNDUS GASTRICUS.

**Foroblique** A telescopic lens used especially in cystoscopes A trade name.

**Forssman** [John *Forssman,* Swedish pathologist, 1868–1947] **1** See under ANTIBODY, SHOCK. **2** Forssman's lipoid. See under ANTIGEN.

**Förster** [Carl Friedrich Richard *Förster,* German ophthalmologist, 1825–1902] **1** Förster's choroiditis, Förster's disease. See under AREOLAR CENTRAL CHOROIDITIS. **2** Förster's disease. See under DIPLEGIA.

**fortification** \fôr′təfikā′shən\ ENRICHMENT.

**FORTRAN** [*for(mula) tran(slation)*] A high-level scientific programming language designed for problems expressed in algebraic notation.

**fosfomycin** \fäs′fōmī′sin\ PHOSPHONOMYCIN.

**Foshay** [Lee *Foshay,* U.S. bacteriologist, 1896–1961] Foshay serum. See under ANTITULARENSE SERUM.

# fossa

**fossa** \fäs′ə\ [L (from fem. of *fossus,* past part. of *fodere* to dig), a ditch, trench] (*pl.* fossae) A trenchlike depression, hollow area, or recess. **f. acetabuli** [NA] The rough nonarticular portion above the acetabular notch forming the floor of the acetabulum. Also *acetabular fossa.* **adipose fossae** Spaces in the subcutaneous areolar tissue in the breast that contain varying amounts of fat, producing the contour of the breast. **anterior cranial f.** FOSSA CRANII ANTERIOR. **anterior intercondylar f. of tibia** AREA INTERCONDYLARIS ANTERIOR TIBIAE. **f. anthelicis** [NA] The curved, vertical groove on the cranial surface of the auricular cartilage corresponding to the anthelix on the lateral surface. Also *fossa of anthelix.* **articular f. for odontoid process of axis** FOVEA DENTIS ATLANTIS. **f. axillaris** The pyramidal fossa between the upper part of the medial side of the arm and the lateral side of the upper thorax. It provides passage for the brachial plexus and axillary vessels between the upper limb and the neck and trunk, and it contains lymph nodes, fat, and connective tissue. Also *maschale, axilla, axillary space, axillary fossa, armpit, arm pit, axil.* **canine f.** A shallow depression on the anterolateral surface of the maxilla, above and lateral to the canine eminence, which gives origin to the levator anguli oris muscle. Also *fossa canina, maxillary fossa, suborbital fossa.* **cerebral f.** Any of the following: (1) fossa cranii anterior; (2) fossa cranii media; (3) fossa cranii posterior. **f. cerebri lateralis Sylvii** FOSSA LATERALIS CEREBRI. **f. condylaris** The depression behind each occipital condyle that receives the posterior margin of the superior facet of the atlas when the head is extended. Also *condylar fossa.* **condyloid f. of atlas** FACIES ARTICULARIS SUPERIOR ATLANTIS. **f. coronoidea humeri** [NA] An oval pit situated anteriorly and proximal to the trochlea of the humerus into which the coronoid process of ulna fits during flexion of the elbow joint. Also *coronoid fossa of humerus, coronoid fossa, anterior supratrochlear fovea, fovea of coronoid process, greater anterior fovea of humerus, supratrochlear fovea of humerus.* **cranial f.** Either fossa cranii anterior, fossa cranii media, or fossa cranii posterior. **f. cranii anterior** [NA] The anterior of the three subdivisions of the internal cranial base, depressed to fit the rounded lower aspect of the frontal lobes of the cerebrum, and limited in front and on the sides by the frontal bone. Also *anterior cranial fossa.* **f. cranii media** [NA] The irregular depression in the middle of the internal surface of the base of the cranium, situated at a lower level than the anterior fossa and consisting of a central and two lateral portions. On each side it lodges the temporal lobe of the cerebrum while in the center the hypophysis cerebri is contained. Also *middle cranial fossa.* **f. cranii posterior** [NA] The posterior, largest, and deepest depression of the internal surface of the irregular base of the cranium, bounded anteriorly by the dorsum sellae of the sphenoid bone, laterally by the superior margin of the petrous part of the temporal bone and the mastoid angle of the parietal bone, and posteriorly by the squamous part of the occipital bone below the transverse sinuses. The floor is constituted by the occipital bone, which supports the cerebellum posteriorly and the pons and medulla oblongata anteriorly. Also *posterior cranial fossa.* **Cruveilhier's f.** FOSSA SCAPHOIDEA OSSIS SPHENOIDALIS. **f. cubitalis** [NA] A triangular hollow in front of the elbow joint between the pronator teres muscle medially, the brachioradialis muscle laterally, and a base formed by an imaginary line between the humeral epicondyles. Also *cubital fossa, chelidon, triangle of elbow, antecubital space.* **digastric f.** 1 FOSSA DIGASTRICA. 2 INCISURA MASTOIDEA OSSIS TEMPORALIS. **f. digastrica** [NA] A small rough pit on the base of the mandible on each side of the midline for the attachment of the anterior belly of the digastric muscle. Also *digastric fossa, digastric fovea, digastric impression.* **duodenal f.** Either recessus duodenalis inferior or recessus duodenalis superior. **duodenojejunal f.** 1 RECESSUS DUODENALIS SUPERIOR. 2 A deep peritoneal recess which is situated between the duodenojejunal junction and the root of the transverse mesocolon on the left of the abdominal aorta and below the pancreas. It lies behind a peritoneal fold formed by the left colic artery. Also *mesocolic recess.* **epigastric f.** 1 FOSSA EPIGASTRICA. 2 FOSSA SUPRAVESICALIS. **f. epigastrica** A small depression on the anterior abdominal wall which is situated just below the xiphoid process in the epigastric region. Also *epigastric fossa, precordial depression.* **ethmoid f.** A groove on the cribriform plate of the ethmoid bone on each side of the crista galli occupied by the olfactory bulb and pierced by numerous foramina for filaments of the olfactory nerve. Also *olfactory fossa, olfactory groove.* **femoral f.** A small depression in the parietal peritoneum overlying the annulus femoralis and separated from the lower end of the lateral inguinal fossa by the medial end of the inguinal ligament. Also *crural fovea, femoral fovea, hiatus femoralis.* **frontal f.** FACIES INTERNA OSSIS FRONTALIS. **f. of gallbladder** FOSSA VESICAE BILIARIS. **f. of gasserian ganglion** *Outmoded* IMPRESSIO TRIGEMINALIS OSSIS TEMPORALIS. **f. glandulae lacrimalis** [NA] A rounded, shallow depression situated on the anterolateral part of the orbital surface of the frontal bone and medial to the zygomatic process of the frontal bone. In it the orbital part of the lacrimal gland is lodged. Also *fossa of lacrimal gland.* **glenoid f.** CAVITAS GLENOIDALIS. **glenoid f. of scapula** CAVITAS GLENOIDALIS. **glossoepiglottic f.** VALLECULA EPIGLOTTICA. **greater f. of Scarpa** TRIGONUM FEMORALE. **greater supraclavicular f.** TRIGONUM OMOCLAVICULARE. **Gruber's f.** GRUBER'S CUL-DE-SAC. **Gruber-Landzert f.** 1 RECESSUS PARADUODENALIS. 2 A superior duodenal recess that extends behind the duodenojejunal flexure. **Hartmann's f.** RECESSUS ILEOCECALIS INFERIOR. **f. of head of femur** FOVEA CAPITIS OSSIS FEMORIS. **f. hyaloidea** [NA] A deep concavity on the front of the vitreous body against which the posterior surface of the lens fits. Also *hyaloid fossa.* **f. hypophysialis** [NA] The deep hollow in the center of the sella turcica of the sphenoid bone occupied by the hypophysis cerebri. The floor is perforated by foramina for blood vessels. Also *hypophysial fossa, pituitary fossa.* **ileocolic f.** RECESSUS ILEOCECALIS SUPERIOR. **f. iliaca** [NA] The hollow anterior and superior part of the medial surface of the ilium, anterior to the sacropelvic surface and bounded above by the iliac crest and below by the arcuate line. It provides attachment for the iliacus muscle. Also *iliac fossa.* **f. iliopectinea** The deep groove between the psoas major and iliacus muscles laterally and the pectineus and adductor longus muscles medially, in which the femoral vessels lie proximally in the femoral triangle. Also *iliopectineal fossa, iliopectineal trigone.* **f. incisiva** [NA] A funnel-shaped depression that is situated in the median plane of the bony palate just behind the incisor teeth. It contains the lower openings of the two lateral incisive canals in its lateral walls, one on each side, extending from the nasal cavity and providing passage for the nasopalatine nerves and the termination of the greater palatine arteries. In addition, the median anterior and posterior incisive foramina may be present and open in the depression in the midline, the left nasopalatine nerve then passing through the anterior foramen and the right nasopalatine nerve passing through the posterior foramen. Also *incisive fossa.* **incisive f. of maxilla** A small depression on the anterior surface of the maxilla above the lateral incisor tooth that gives origin to the depressor septi muscle. Also *myrtiform fossa, prenasal fossa.* **f. incudis** [NA] A small depression in the posteroinferior part of the epitympanic recess in which the short process of the incus is lodged, attached by ligamentous fibers. Also *incudal fossa.* **f. of incus** FOSSA INCUDIS. **inferior articular f. of atlas** FACIES ARTICULARIS INFERIOR ATLANTIS. **inferior costal f.** FOVEA COSTALIS INFERIOR. **inferior duodenal f.** RECESSUS DUODENALIS INFERIOR. **inferior duodenojejunal f.** An occasional peritoneal recess that is situated in the duodenojejunal flexure and is limited anteriorly by a peritoneal fold extending from the ascending portion of the duodenum to the origin of the jejunum. It is open inferiorly and to the left. **inferior ileocecal f.** RECESSUS ILEOCECALIS INFERIOR. **inferior f. of omental sac** RECESSUS INFERIOR OMENTALIS. **f. infraclavicularis** [NA] The triangular depression below the clavicle and between the superior border of the pectoralis major muscle and the anterior border of the deltoid muscle, containing the cephalic vein and the deltoid branch of the thoracoacromial artery. Also *infraclavicular fossa, infraclavicular region, infraclavicular triangle, regio infraclavicularis* (outmoded), *Mohrenheim's space.* **infraduodenal f.** An occasional small peritoneal recess situated just below the horizontal part of the duodenum. **f. infraspinata** [NA] The large triangular area formed by the inferior surface of the spine of the scapula and the posterior surface of the scapula below it. Most of the area is occupied by the origin of the infraspinatus muscle. Also *infraspinous fossa, infraspinous region.* **f. infratemporalis** [NA] An irregular space below and medial to the zygomatic arch, bounded anteriorly by the posterolateral, or infratemporal, surface of the maxilla, superiorly by the infratemporal surface of the greater wing of the sphenoid bone and a part of the squamous temporal bone, and medially by the lateral pterygoid lamina. Laterally it is only partly bounded by the ramus of the mandible, while behind and below it is open. Its roof is pierced by the foramen ovale and foramen spinosum in the greater wing of the sphenoid bone. The anterior and medial walls are united inferiorly but separated superiorly by the pterygomaxillary fissure, through which it communicates with the pterygopalatine fossa. It also communicates superiorly with the temporal fossa through the gap medial to the zygomatic arch, and anteriorly with the orbit through the inferior orbital fissure. Also *infratemporal fossa.* **f. inguinalis lateralis** [NA] The depression in the parietal peritoneum that is lateral to the lateral umbilical fold formed by the inferior epigastric vessels on the inner surface of the anterior abdominal wall. The fossa is related to the deep inguinal ring inferiorly and corresponds to the saccus vaginalis in the embryo. Also *lateral inguinal fossa, fovea inguinalis lateralis, lateral inguinal fovea, external inguinal fovea.* **f. inguinalis medialis** [NA] The depression in the parietal peritoneum that lies between the lateral umbilical fold formed by inferior epigastric vessels and the medial umbilical fold formed by the obliterated umbilical artery on the inner surface of the anterior abdominal wall. Also *medial inguinal fossa, fovea inguinalis medialis, internal inguinal fovea, medial inguinal fovea, middle inguinal fovea.* **f. intercondylaris femoris** [NA] A deep notch separating the projecting cartilage-covered condyles of the femur posteriorly and providing attachment for the anterior and posterior cruciate ligaments of the knee joint on the opposed surfaces of the condyles and for the infrapatellar synovial fold anteriorly, while posteriorly the intercondylar line separates the notch from the popliteal surface of the femur. Also *intercondylar fossa of femur, intercondylar notch of femur, intercondylar notch.* **f. intercruralis** FOSSA INTERPEDUNCULARIS. **f. interpeduncularis** [NA] The midline depression between the cerebral peduncles, the site of the interpeduncular cistern. Also *interpeduncular fossa, fossa intercruralis, interpeduncular space, interpeduncular trigone, trigonum interpedunculare, interpeduncular recess.* **intersigmoid f.** RECESSUS INTERSIGMOIDEUS. **intrabulbar f.** The dilated segment of the spongiose part of the male urethra in the bulb of the penis just beyond the perineal membrane. **f. ischioanalis** [NA] The wedge-shaped space that is bounded medially by the inferior fascia of the pelvic diaphragm and the sphincter ani externus, laterally by the inner aspect of the ischial tuberosity and the obturator fascia, posteriorly by the sacrotuberous ligament and lower part of the gluteus maximus muscle, and anteriorly by the perineal membrane. The floor or base is formed by the skin of the perineum while the apex is roofed over by fascia arching between the medial and lateral walls. The space is filled by a pad of fat traversed by vessels and nerves, while the pudendal canal is situated along the lateral wall. Also *ischioanal fossa, ischiorectal excavation.* **Jobert's f.** A furrow formed between the distal part of the adductor magnus muscle anteriorly and the sartorius and gracilis muscles posteriorly when the knee is flexed and the thigh is rotated laterally. **f. of Jonnesco** 1 RECESSUS DUODENALIS SUPERIOR. 2 A peritoneal recess between the superior and the inferior duodenal folds on the left of the duodenojejunal flexure. **jugular f.** FOSSA SUPRACLAVICULARIS MINOR. **f. jugularis ossis temporalis** [NA] A deep, rounded depression behind the external opening of the carotid canal on the inferior aspect of the posterior portion of the petrous part of the temporal bone. It forms the anterior and lateral part of the wall of the jugular foramen and lodges the superior bulb of the internal jugular vein. The roof separates it from the tympanic cavity and in its lateral wall is the mastoid canaliculus. Also *jugular fossa of temporal bone.* **f. of lacrimal gland** FOSSA GLANDULAE LACRIMALIS. **f. of lacrimal sac** FOSSA SACCI LACRIMALIS. **Landzert's f.** RECESSUS PARADUODENALIS. **lateral f. of brain** FOSSA LATERALIS CEREBRI. **lateral f. of cerebrum** FOSSA LATERALIS CEREBRI. **lateral inguinal f.** FOSSA INGUINALIS LATERALIS. **f. lateralis cerebri** [NA] A slight depression that appears at the beginning of the fourth fetal month in the lateral surface of the cerebrum anterior and superior to the temporal pole. As the cortical lobes develop, the lateral cerebral fossa becomes submerged and overlapped by the opercula of the frontal, parietal, and temporal lobes. Its floor becomes the insula, and it opens toward the anterior perforated substance at the base of the cerebrum. Also *vallecula sylvii, vallecula fossa sylvii, vallecula cerebri lateralis, sylvian fossa, fossa of Sylvius, lateral fossa of cerebrum, fossa occipitalis cerebralis* (obs.), *fossa cerebri lateralis Sylvii, fossa lateralis cerebri, lateral fossa of brain.* **f. of lateral malleolus** FOSSA MALLEOLI LATERALIS. **lateral pharyngeal f.** RECESSUS PHARYNGEUS. **lateral f. of preputial space** Either of two shallow fossae that extend laterally from the frenulum preputii penis in the preputial space along the collum glandis penis. **f. of lateral pterygoid muscle** FOVEA PTERYGOIDEA MANDIBULAE. **lesser supraclavicular f.** FOSSA SUPRACLAVICULARIS MINOR. **f. for ligamentum teres** FISSURA LIGAMENTI TERETIS. **longitudinal fossae of right liver** FOSSAE SAGITTALES DEXTRAE HEPATIS. **Luschka's f.** RECESSUS ILEOCECALIS SUPERIOR. **f. malleoli lateralis** [NA] An oval depression at the lower end of the fibula behind the malleolar articular surface for the talus, pierced by many vascular foramina and attaching the posterior tibiofibular and posterior talofibular ligaments. Also *fossa of lateral malleolus.* **f. mandibularis** [NA] The deep, oval concavity, with its long axis directed posteromedially, at the root of the zygomatic process on the inferior surface of the squamous part of the temporal bone, for articulation with the mandibular condyle through the articular disk. The small nonarticular posterior wall of the fossa is formed by the temporal part of the temporal bone, anterior to which is the squamotympanic fissue. Also *mandibular fossa.* **mastoid f. of temporal bone** FOVEOLA SUPRAMEATICA. **maxillary f.** CANINE FOSSA. **medial inguinal f.** FOSSA INGUINALIS MEDIALIS. **Merkel's f.** FILTRUM VENTRICULI. **mesentericoparietal f.** An occasional peritoneal recess that is situated below the horizontal part of the duodenum and invaginates the adjacent base of the mesentery to the right. The large orifice is covered anteriorly by a fold of peritoneum formed by the superior mesenteric artery. It is more common in fetuses than in adults. Also *Waldeyer's fossa.* **middle cranial f.** FOSSA CRANII MEDIA. **myrtiform f.** INCISIVE FOSSA OF MAXILLA. **f. navicularis urethrae** [NA] A dilated portion of the male urethra, flattened from side to side, within the glans penis. In its dorsal wall is a pitlike recess, lacuna magna. Also *navicular fossa of male urethra, crypt of Morgagni, fovea of Morgagni.* **navicular f. of male urethra** FOSSA NAVICULARIS URETHRAE. **occipital f.** Any of the four depressions on the internal surface of the squamous part of the occipital bone that are separated by the grooves for the transverse sinuses, extending laterally from the internal occipital protuberance, and by the sulcus of superior sagittal sinus and internal occipital crest, extending superiorly and inferiorly, respectively, from the protuberance. The upper two lodge the poles of the occipital lobes of the cerebrum while the lower two lodge the hemispheres of the cerebellum. **f. occipitalis cerebralis** *Obs.* FOSSA LATERALIS CEREBRI. **occlusal f.** An irregular rounded depression on the occlusal surface of a tooth. **f. olecrani** [NA] A deep oval depression on the posterior aspect of the condyle of the humerus above the trochlea, into which the tip of the olecranon process of ulna fits during extension of the elbow. Its floor is thin and may be perforated. Also *olecranon fossa.* **olfactory f.** ETHMOID FOSSA. **orbital f.** FACIES ORBITALIS OSSIS FRONTALIS. **oval f. of heart** FOSSA OVALIS CORDIS. **f. ovalis** 1 FOSSA OVALIS CORDIS. 2 HIATUS SAPHENUS. **f. ovalis cordis** [NA] An oval depression bounded by the prominent limbus fossae ovalis on the lower part of the interatrial septum in the right atrium, situated to the left of and above the opening of the inferior vena cava. Its floor represents the septum primum of the fetal heart. Also *oval fossa of heart, fossa ovalis.* **oval f. of thigh** HIATUS SAPHENUS. **f. ovarica** [NA] A peritoneum-lined depression occupied by the ovary on the lateral wall of the pelvis, bounded anteriorly by the obliterated umbilical artery, posteriorly by the internal iliac artery and the ureter, superiorly by the external iliac vessels, and inferiorly by the obturator vessels and nerve. Also *ovarian fossa.* **fossae of Pacchioni** FOVEOLAE GRANULARES. **paraduodenal f.** RECESSUS PARADUODENALIS. **pararectal f.** A peritoneal recess that is situated on either side of the upper part of the rectum and varies in size with the fullness of the rectum. It contains the sigmoid colon on the left and the lower part of the ileum on the right. **f. paravesicalis** [NA] A peritoneal depression on each side of the urinary bladder that is bounded medially by the lateral margin of the superior vesical surface and laterally by a raised fold of peritoneum covering the ductus deferens in the male and the round ligament of the uterus in the female. The degree of distension of the bladder determines the size and depth of the fossa. When the bladder is empty the fossa is crossed by the transverse vesical fold, when present. Posteriorly the fossa is separated from the pararectal fossa by peritoneal ridges formed by the internal iliac vessels and ureter as well as, in the female, the broad ligament of the uterus. Also *paravesical fossa, paracystic pouch, paravesical pouch.* **petrosal f.** FOSSULA PETROSA. **f. for petrosal ganglion** *Outmoded* FOSSULA PETROSA. **piriform f.** RECESSUS PIRIFORMIS. **pituitary f.** FOSSA HYPOPHYSIALIS. **f. poplitea** [NA] A diamond-shaped area behind the knee joint, bounded superiorly by the semitendinosus and semimembranosus muscles medially and the biceps femoris muscle laterally, while inferiorly the medial wall is the medial head of the gastrocnemius and the lateral wall is the lateral head of the gastrocnemius and plantaris muscles. The floor is formed by the popliteal surface of femur, the oblique posterior ligament of knee joint, and the popliteus muscle and its fascia. The roof is the popliteal fascia pierced by the small saphenous vein. During flexion of the knee the boundaries and the hollow between them become obvious. Also *popliteal fossa, popliteal cavity, popliteal space, poples, ham.* **postauditory f.** FOVEOLA SUPRAMEATICA. **posterior cranial f.** FOSSA CRANII POSTERIOR. **posterior intercondylar f. of tibia** AREA INTERCONDYLARIS POSTERIOR TIBIAE. **prenasal f.** INCISIVE FOSSA OF MAXILLA. **f. pterygoidea ossis sphenoidalis** [NA] The deep, elongated space separating the medial and lateral pterygoid laminae, open posteriorly and closed anteriorly by the fusion of the laminae and containing the medial pterygoid and tensor veli palatini muscles. Also *pterygoid fossa of sphenoid bone.* **pterygoid f. of sphenoid bone** FOSSA PTERYGOIDEA OSSIS SPHENOIDALIS. **f. pterygopalatina** [NA] A small pyramidal space bounded anteriorly by the superomedial portion of the posterior surface of the maxilla, posteriorly by the root of the pterygoid process and the adjacent part of the greater wing of the sphenoid bone, medially by the upper portion of the perpendicular plate of the palatine bone, and laterally communicating with the infratemporal fossa through the pterygomaxillary fissure. Inferiorly the anterior and posterior walls meet at the opening of the greater palatine canal. The space also communicates anteriorly with the orbit through the inferior orbital fissure, and medially with the nasal cavity through the sphenopalatine foramen. The major contents comprise the maxillary nerve and vessels and the pterygopalatine ganglion and their branches. Also *pterygopalatine fossa.* **radial f.** 1 FOSSA RADIALIS HUMERI. 2 *Outmoded* AREA NERVI FACIALIS. **f. radialis humeri** [NA] A small, shallow hollow lateral to the coronoid fossa and above the capitulum of the condyle of humerus into which the rim of the head of the radius fits during full flexion of the elbow joint. Also *radial fossa of humerus, radial depression, fovea for head of radius, lesser anterior fovea of humerus, radial fossa.* **retrocecal f.** RECESSUS RETROCAECALIS. **retrocolic f.** A variant of recessus retrocecalis in which there is incomplete fusion of the ascending colon with the parietal peritoneum, allowing a peritoneal recess to extend between the ascending colon and the posterior abdominal wall. It may contain the vermiform appendix. **retroduodenal f.** RECESSUS RETRODUODENALIS. **f. rhomboidea** [NA] The diamond-shaped floor of the fourth ventricle forming the roof of the medulla oblongata and caudal pons. Also *rhomboid fossa.* **Rosenmüller's f.** RECESSUS PHARYNGEUS. **f. sacci lacrimalis** [NA] The vertical depression on the anteromedial wall of the orbit that contains the lacrimal sac and its fascia and is formed by the lacrimal sulcus of the lacrimal bone and the frontal process of the maxilla. It is limited posteriorly by the posterior lacrimal crest. Also *lacrimal groove, fossa of lacrimal sac.* **fossae sagittales dextrae hepatis** The longitudinal grooves on the visceral surface of the right lobe of the liver that are formed by the fossa vesicae biliaris and sulcus venae cavae. *Outmoded.* Also *longitudinal fossae of right liver.* **f. sagittalis sinistra hepatis** A longitudinal groove on the visceral surface of the left lobe of the liver which is formed by fissura ligamenti teretis anteriorly and fissura ligamenti venosi posteriorly. *Outmoded.* Also *sagittal fissure of liver.* **scaphoid f.** 1 *Outmoded* SCAPHA. 2 *Outmoded* FOSSA TRIANGULARIS AURICULAE. **f. scaphoidea** 1 *Outmoded* SCAPHA. 2 *Outmoded* FOSSA SCAPHOIDEA OSSIS SPHENOIDALIS. **f. scaphoidea ossis sphenoidalis** [NA] A small, oval depression formed by the splitting of the upper end of the posterior margin of the medial pterygoid plate, lying at the upper end of the pterygoid fossa and providing attachment for part of the tensor veli palatini muscle. Also *scaphoid fossa of sphenoid bone, fossa scaphoidea* (outmoded), *scaphoid fossa* (outmoded), *Cruveilhier's fossa.* **semilunar f. of ulna** INCISURA TROCHLEARIS ULNAE. **sigmoid f.** SULCUS SINUS TRANSVERSI. **sigmoid f. of temporal bone** SULCUS SINUS SIGMOIDEI OSSIS TEMPORALIS. **sigmoid f. of ulna** INCISURA TROCHLEARIS ULNAE. **f. subarcuata ossis temporalis** [NA] An irregular pit just below the superior petrosal sinus and posterosuperior to the internal acoustic meatus, situated on the posterior surface of the petrous part of the temporal bone and containing a small vein and a fold of dura mater. In fetal life the pit is large, containing the cerebellar flocculus and extending under the anterior semicircular canal. Also *subarcuate fossa of temporal bone, subarcuate hiatus.* **f. subinguinalis** The shallow depression that overlies the base of the femoral triangle just below the groin. **sublingual f.** FOVEA SUBLINGUALIS. **submandibular f.** FOVEA SUBMANDIBULARIS. **suborbital f.** CANINE FOSSA. **subpyramidal f.** An insignificant depression below the pyramid and behind the fenestra cochleae on the posteromedial wall of the middle ear. **f. subscapularis** [NA] The major, central portion of the concave costal surface of the scapula, providing origin for the subscapularis muscle and ridged for attachment of tendinous intersections. Also *subscapular fossa.* **subsigmoid f.** An occasional peritoneal space between the root of the sigmoid mesocolon and the mesocolon of the descending colon when the latter is present. **superior articular f. of atlas** FACIES ARTICULARIS SUPERIOR ATLANTIS. **superior costal f.** FOVEA COSTALIS SUPERIOR. **superior duodenal f.** RECESSUS DUODENALIS SUPERIOR. **superior ileocecal f.** RECESSUS ILEOCECALIS SUPERIOR. **superior f. of omental sac** RECESSUS SUPERIOR OMENTALIS. **superior retroduodenal f.** A rare variant of recessus retroduodenalis in which the pocket is situated behind the duodenojejunal flexure. **supinator f.** A small triangular hollow distal to the radial notch of the ulna and between the diverging proximal ends of the interosseous margin. The anterior part of the hollow receives the radial tuberosity during pronation, while the posterior part and the supinator crest posterior to it provide origin to part of the supinator muscle. **f. supraclavicularis minor** [NA] A small triangular space above and behind the clavicle between the sternal and the clavicular heads of origin of the sternocleidomastoid muscle. The area is roofed over by external cervical fascia. Also *lesser supraclavicular fossa, jugular fossa.* **supracondyloid f.** An insignificant groove between the adductor tubercle and the medial epicondyle of the femur, for part of the origin of medial head of gastrocnemius muscle. **supramastoid f.** FOVEOLA SUPRAMEATICA. **f. supraspinata** [NA] The hollow formed by the superior surface of the spine of scapula and the posterior surface of scapula above it, the medial two thirds of which provides origin for the supraspinatus muscle. It is about one fourth the area of the infraspinous fossa. Also *supraspinous fossa, supraspinous region.* **suprasternal f.** SUPRASTERNAL SPACE. **supratonsillar f.** FOSSA SUPRATONSILLARIS. **f. supratonsillaris** 1 [NA] A space above the palatine tonsil, especially obvious in the adult when the tonsil is diminished in size. 2 A horizontal semilunar cleft in the upper part of the palatine tonsil. Also *intratonsillar cleft* (outmoded), *intratonsillar fissure.* For defs. 1 and 2 also *supratonsillar fossa, supratonsillar recess.* **f. supravesicalis** [NA] The depression in the parietal peritoneum between the median umbilical fold formed by the urachus and the medial umbilical fold formed by the obliterated umbilical artery on the internal surface of the anterior abdominal wall. The fossa is particularly obvious when the urinary bladder is empty. Also *supravesical fossa, supravesical fovea, epigastric fossa.* **sylvian f.** 1 FOSSA LATERALIS CEREBRI. 2 SULCUS LATERALIS CEREBRI. **f. of Sylvius** 1 FOSSA LATERALIS CEREBRI. 2 SULCUS LATERALIS CEREBRI. **f. temporalis** [NA] The space on the lateral side of the cranium bounded superiorly and posteriorly by the temporal line, laterally by the zygomatic arch, and anteriorly by the temporal surface of the zygomatic bone, while inferiorly it is continuous with the infratemporal fossa deep to the zygomatic arch. It is occupied by the temporalis muscle, which is attached to its floor. Also *temporal fossa.* **tibiofemoral f.** A space palpable on each side of the apex of the patella between the femoral and tibial condyles, especially when the knee is flexed. **f. tonsillaris** [NA] A triangular depression lodging the palatine tonsil between the palatoglossal and palatopharyngeal arches. Also *tonsillar fossa, tonsillar sinus.* **transverse costal f.** FOVEA COSTALIS PROCESSUS TRANSVERSUS. **f. of Treitz** RECESSUS DUODENALIS INFERIOR. **f. triangularis auriculae** [NA] A small triangular depression lying between the two diverging crura of the anthelix at its upper end. Also *triangular fossa of auricle, scaphoid fossa* (outmoded). **f. trochanterica** [NA] A deep pit on the concave medial surface of the curved posterosuperior part of the greater trochanter of femur into which the obturator externus muscle is inserted. Also *trochanteric fossa.* **trochlear f.** FOVEA TROCHLEARIS. **f. vesicae biliaris** [NA] A shallow oval impression for the gallbladder on the visceral surface of the right lobe of the liver. It extends from the inferior margin of the liver to the right end of the porta hepatis and lies on the right of the quadrate lobe. It is usually not covered by peritoneum. Also *fossa of gallbladder, fossa vesicae felleae, vallecula ovata* (outmoded). **f. vesicae felleae** FOSSA VESICAE BILIARIS. **vestibular f.** FOSSA VESTIBULI VAGINAE. **f. vestibuli vaginae** [NA] A portion of the vestibule that forms a shallow depression between the frenulum of the labia minora and the vaginal orfice. Also *vestibular fossa, fossa of vestibule of vagina.* **Waldeyer's f.** 1 MESENTERICOPARIETAL FOSSA. 2 Duodenal fossa; either recessus duodenalis superior or recessus duodenalis inferior.

**fossae** \fäs′ē\ Plural of FOSSA.

**fossette** \fäset′\ A small pit or depression; fossula.

**fossula** \fäs′yələ\ [L (dim. of *fossa* a ditch, trench), a small ditch or trench] A small pit or depression. **f. fenestrae cochleae** [NA] The deep hollow posteroinferior to the promontory at the bottom of which is the fenestra cochleae in the medial wall of the middle ear. Also *fossula of cochlear window.* **f. fenestrae vestibuli** [NA] A depression situated posterosuperior to the promontory at the bottom of which is the fenestra vestibuli in the medial wall of the middle ear. Also *fossula of vestibular window.* **inferior costal f.** FOVEA COSTALIS INFERIOR. **f. petrosa** [NA] A small notch located on the inferior surface of the petrous portion of the temporal bone, located between the jugular fossa and the external orifice of the carotid canal. It lodges the inferior (or petrous) ganglion of the glossopharyngeal nerve, and nearby is located the canaliculus tympanicus through which courses the tympanic branch of the glossopharyngeal nerve on its way to the middle ear. Also *petrous fossula, vallecula for petrosal ganglion, receptaculum ganglii petrosi, petrosal fossula, petrosal fossa, fossula of petrous ganglion, fossa for petrosal ganglion* (outmoded). **f. post fenestram** An inconstant evagination of the connective tissue of the perilymphatic space into a hollow in the lateral wall of the internal ear immediately behind the vestibular window and between the latter and the nonampullated end of the lateral semicircular canal. **superior costal f.** FOVEA COSTALIS SUPERIOR. **fossulae tonsillares tonsillae palatinae** [NA] The pitlike openings of the deep, tubular tonsillar crypts on the medial surface of the palatine tonsil. Also *tonsillar fossulae of palatine tonsil, foramina of palatine tonsil, crypts of palatine tonsil.* **fossulae tonsillares tonsillae pharyngealis** [NA] The surface openings of the cleftlike invaginations of diffuse lymphoid tissue in the pharyngeal tonsil. Also *tonsillar fossulae of pharyngeal tonsil, fossulae tonsillares tonsillae pharyngeae, crypts of pharyngeal tonsil, sulci of pharyngeal tonsil.* **f. of vestibular window** FOSSULA FENESTRAE VESTIBULI.

**fossulae** \fäs′yəlē\ Plural of FOSSULA.

**fossulate** \fäs′yəlāt\ Having a small fossa or groove.

**Foster Kennedy** [Robert *Foster Kennedy,* U.S. neurologist, 1884–1952] See under SYNDROME.

**Fothergill** [William Edward *Fothergill,* English gynecologist, 1865–1926] 1 See under OPERATION. 2 Manchester-Fothergill operation, Fothergill-Donald operation. See under MANCHESTER OPERATION.

**Fouchet** [André *Fouchet,* French chemist and physician, born 1894] See under REAGENT.

**foudroyant** \foodroi′ənt, foodrô·äyäN′\ FULMINANT.

**fouling** \fou′ling\ In forensic medicine, the solid, black, circular zone of deposited soot surrounding the edges of skin or clothing caused by the passage of a projectile, as by the near contact or penetration of a bullet.

**foundation** The combination of tooth substance and restorative material such as cement, gold, or amalgam, made when the tooth substance itself is insufficient to make a satisfactory support for a full crown. **denture f.** STRESS-BEARING AREA. **medical f.** An organization of physicians, in the United States primarily, usually sponsored by a local medical society which is involved in certain activities such as peer review and sponsorship or operation of prepaid health care plans. Also *foundation for medical care.*

**fourchette** \foorshet′\ [French (dim. of *fourche* pitchfork, from L *furca* fork), fork, fork-shaped object] FRENULUM LABIORUM PUDENDI.

**Fourier** [Jean Baptiste Joseph *Fourier,* French mathematician, 1768–1830] See under ANALYSIS.

**Fourneau 190** [after Ernest François Auguste *Fourneau,* French chemist, 1872–1949] ACETARSOL.

**Fourneau 309** [after E. F. A. *Fourneau*] SURAMIN.

**Fourneau 933** [after E. F. A. *Fourneau*] PIPEROXAN HYDROCHLORIDE.

**Fournier** [Jean Alfred *Fournier,* French dermatologist, 1832–1914] **1** Fournier's gangrene. See under FOURNIER'S DISEASE. **2** Fournier's exercises. See under EXERCISE. **3** See under SIGN. **4** Fournier sign. See under SABER SHIN.

**fovea** \fō′vē·ə\ [L, a pit, pitfall] (*pl.* foveae) **1** A small fossa, pit, or depression. **2** FOVEA CENTRALIS RETINAE. **anterior supratrochlear f.** FOSSA CORONOIDEA HUMERI. **f. articularis capitis radii** [NA] A shallow, circular depression on the proximal end of the head of the radius for articulation with the capitulum of the humerus. Also *fovea of little head of radius.* **f. articularis inferior atlantis** FACIES ARTICULARIS INFERIOR ATLANTIS. **f. articularis superior atlantis** FACIES ARTICULARIS SUPERIOR ATLANTIS. **articular foveae for rib cartilages** INCISURAE COSTALES STERNI. **f. capitis ossis femoris** [NA] A small pit just posteroinferior to the middle of the head of the femur, not covered by cartilage and providing attachment for the ligament of head of femur. Also *fovea of head of femur, fossa of head of femur.* **f. cardiaca** INCISURA CARDIACA PULMONIS SINISTRI. **caudal f.** FOVEA INFERIOR. **f. centralis retinae** [NA] The conical central depression in the macula retinae where the retina is very thin so that rays of light have free passage to the layer of photoreceptors, mostly cones. This is the area of most distinct vision to which the visual axis is directed. Also *central fovea of retina, fovea centralis, fovea.* **f. of coronoid process** FOSSA CORONOIDEA HUMERI. **f. costalis inferior** [NA] A hollowed articular facet near the inferior margin of the vertebral body and anterior to the vertebral notch of most thoracic vertebrae for articulation with the head of a rib. Also *inferior costal fovea, inferior costal fossa, inferior costal fossula, inferior costal pit, inferior demifacet for head of rib.* **f. costalis processus transversus** [NA] A small hollow pit on the anterolateral surface of the transverse processes of most thoracic vertebrae for articulation with the tubercle of a rib to form a costotransverse joint. Also *costal pit of transverse process, transverse costal fovea, transverse costal fossa, costal facet of transverse process, facet for tubercle of rib.* **f. costalis superior** [NA] A hollowed articular facet, usually larger than the inferior fovea, located near the superior margin of the vertebral body anterior to the base of the pedicle of most thoracic vertebrae for articulation with the head of a rib. Also *superior costal fovea, superior costal facet of vertebra, superior costal fossa, superior costal fossula, superior demifacet for head of rib.* **costal foveae of sternum** INCISURAE COSTALES STERNI. **cranial f.** FOVEA SUPERIOR. **crural f.** FEMORAL FOSSA. **f. dentis atlantis** [NA] A rounded, concave facet on the posterior surface of the anterior arch of the atlas for articulation with the dens of the axis in the median atlantoaxial joint. Also *dental fovea of atlas, circular articular facet of atlas, articular fossa for odontoid process of axis, articular facet of anterior arch of atlas.* **digastric f.** FOSSA DIGASTRICA. **external inguinal f.** FOSSA INGUINALIS LATERALIS. **femoral f.** FEMORAL FOSSA. **f. of fourth ventricle** FOVEA INFERIOR. **foveae of fourth ventricle** The fovea inferior and the fovea superior. **greater anterior f. of humerus** FOSSA CORONOIDEA HUMERI. **f. of head of femur** FOVEA CAPITIS OSSIS FEMORIS. **f. for head of radius** FOSSA RADIALIS HUMERI. **f. inferior** A small indentation of the sulcus limitans in the floor of the fourth ventricle at the caudal end of the striae medullares. Also *inferior fovea of floor of fourth ventricle, fovea of fourth ventricle, caudal fovea.* **inferior articular f. of atlas** FACIES ARTICULARIS INFERIOR ATLANTIS. **inferior costal f.** FOVEA COSTALIS INFERIOR. **inferior f. of floor of fourth ventricle** FOVEA INFERIOR. **f. inguinalis lateralis** FOSSA INGUINALIS LATERALIS. **f. inguinalis medialis** FOSSA INGUINALIS MEDIALIS. **internal inguinal f.** FOSSA INGUINALIS MEDIALIS. **lateral inguinal f.** FOSSA INGUINALIS LATERALIS. **lateral malleolar f. of fibula** FACIES ARTICULARIS MALLEOLI FIBULAE. **f. of lateral malleolus** FACIES ARTICULARIS MALLEOLI FIBULAE. **lesser anterior f. of humerus** FOSSA RADIALIS HUMERI. **f. of little head of radius** FOVEA ARTICULARIS CAPITIS RADII. **medial inguinal f.** FOSSA INGUINALIS MEDIALIS. **middle inguinal f.** FOSSA INGUINALIS MEDIALIS. **f. of Morgagni** FOSSA NAVICULARIS URETHRAE. **f. nuchae** A depression in the midline of the back of the neck just below the external occipital protuberance. **f. oblonga cartilaginis arytenoideae** [NA] An oblong depression below the lower part of the arcuate crest on the anterolateral surface of the arytenoid cartilage that provides attachment for the vocalis and lateral cricoarytenoid muscles. Also *oblong fovea of arytenoid cartilage, oblong pit of arytenoid cartilage.* **f. pterygoidea mandibulae** [NA] The rough depression on the anteromedial aspect of the neck of the condylar process of the mandible for the attachment of lateral pterygoid muscle. Also *pterygoid fovea, pterygoid depression, pterygoid pit, fossa of lateral pterygoid muscle.* **f. sublingualis** [NA] A smooth triangular depression above the anterior end of the mylohyoid line, posterolateral to the mental spine of the mandible and lodging the sublingual salivary gland. Also *sublingual fossa, sublingual fovea.* **f. submandibularis** [NA] An elongated shallow depression below the middle portion of the mylohyoid line and muscle on the inner surface of the body of the mandible which lodges the submandibular salivary gland and some submandibular lymph nodes. Also *submandibular fossa, submandibular fovea.* **f. superior** A small indentation of the sulcus limitans in the fourth ventricle at the rostral end of the striae medullares. Also *superior fovea of sulcus limitans, cranial fovea.* **superior costal f.** FOVEA COSTALIS SUPERIOR. **superior f. of sulcus limitans** FOVEA SUPERIOR. **supratrochlear f. of humerus** FOSSA CORONOIDEA HUMERI. **supravesical f.** FOSSA SUPRAVESICALIS. **f.**

**of talus** SULCUS TALI. **transverse costal f.** FOVEA COSTALIS PROCESSUS TRANSVERSUS. **f. triangularis cartilaginis arytenoideae** [NA] A triangular depression above the lower part of the arcuate crest on the anterolateral surface of the arytenoid cartilage that provides attachment for the vestibular ligament and lodges some mucous glands. Also *triangular pit of arytenoid cartilage, triangular foveola.* **f. trigemini** A small depression in the rostral floor of the fourth ventricle lying anterolateral to the facial colliculus and overlying the motor and main sensory trigeminal nuclei. **f. trochlearis** [NA] A small, shallow depression at the anteromedial angle of the roof of the orbital cavity just behind the medial end of the supraorbital margin for the attachment of the fibrocartilaginous trochlea of the superior oblique muscle. It is often occupied by the trochlear spine. Also *trochlear fovea, trochlear fossa.*

**foveate** \fō′vē·āt\ Having foveae; pitted.

**foveation** \fō′vē·ā′shən\ Pitting, as of the skin.

**foveola** \fōvē′ōlə\ [New L (dim. of FOVEA), a very small pit] (*pl.* foveolae) **1** A small pit, fossa, or depression. **2** ALVEOLUS. **f. coccygea** [NA] A shallow dimple often present in the skin over the coccyx. It marks the point at which the embryonic neural tube made a caudal contact with the ectoderm. The dimple is created by a bundle of white fibrous tissue that extends from the tip of the last coccygeal vertebra to the skin. Also *coccygeal foveola, postanal dimple, postanal pit.* **foveolae gastricae** [NA] Slitlike furrows on the surface of the mucous membrane of the stomach into the bottoms of which the gastric glands open. Because of their large number, the mucosa has a honeycomb appearance. Also *gastric pits, gastric pits of Frey.* **foveolae granulares** [NA] A number of irregular depressions that are on the inner surface of the parietal bones on each side of the sagittal sulcus and are occupied by the arachnoid granulations. They increase in size and number with advancing age. Also *granular foveolae, pacchionian depressions, meningeal impression, fossae of Pacchioni.* **f. suprameatica** [NA] A small pit that marks the center of the suprameatal triangle and is situated below the supramastoid crest and behind the suprameatal spine at the junction of the superior and posterior margins of the external acoustic meatus. Also *mastoid fossa of temporal bone, postauditory fossa, supramastoid fossa.* **triangular f.** FOVEA TRIANGULARIS CARTILAGINIS ARYTENOIDEAE.

**foveolae** \fōvē′ōlē\ Plural of FOVEOLA.

**foveolar** \fōvē′ōlər\ Pertaining to a foveola.

**foveolate** \fōvē′ōlāt\ Displaying foveolae.

**Foville** [Achille-Louis *Foville,* French physician, 1799–1878] **1** Fasciculus of Foville. See under STRIA TERMINALIS. **2** Foville superior syndrome, Foville's median syndrome. See under FOVILLE'S PEDUNCULAR SYNDROME.

**Fowler** [George Ryerson *Fowler,* U.S. surgeon, 1848–1906] See under POSITION.

**Fowler** [Thomas *Fowler,* English physician, 1736–1801] Fowler solution. See under POTASSIUM ARSENITE SOLUTION.

**Fox** [George Henry *Fox,* U.S. dermatologist, 1846–1937] Fox-Fordyce disease. See under DISEASE.

**foxglove** [Old English *foxes* fox's + *glōfa* glove] Any of various plants of the genus *Digitalis.* **Austrian f.** *DIGITALIS LANTANA* LEAF. **woolly f.** *DIGITALIS LANTANA* LEAF.

**FP** Symbol for properdin.

**f.p.** **1** freezing point. **2** *fiat potio* (L, let a potion be made).

**f. pil.** *fiant pilulae* (L, let pills be made).

**fPt** fasting patient.

**FR** **1** flocculation reaction. **2** fixed ratio.

**Fr** Symbol for the element, francium.

**fract. dos.** *fracta dosi* (L, in divided doses).

**fraction** [Late L *fractio* (from L *frangere* to break) a breaking into portions] A portion of a mixture obtained by a separation technique, as by centrifugation, distillation, or precipitation, and representing a discrete constituent of the mixture. **absorbed f.** The fraction of energy, radiated by an embedded radionuclide, that is absorbed within a specified volume of a living body or other absorbing mass. **blood plasma f.** HUMAN PLASMA PROTEIN FRACTION. **dried human plasma protein f.** Plasma protein fraction from which all water has been removed by dehydration or lyophilization. Also *dried human plasma, blood-plasma powder.* **ejection f.** An index of the heart pumping function. It equals the proportion of total blood volume that is expelled from the heart with each heartbeat. **Fechner f.** A measure of contrast sensitivity of the eye, $dB/B$, where $B$ is the brightness of a large field of view and $dB$ the difference of brightness which is just distinguishable on a small area within that field. **filtration f.** The ratio of glomerular filtration rate to effective renal plasma flow. This represents the amount of effective renal plasma flow filtered at the glomerulus. In disease, the filtration fraction reflects relative change in effective renal plasma flow and glomerular filtration rate, being increased when the afferent glomerular arterioles are relatively constricted, as in hypertension and congestive heart failure, or decreased in glomerular diseases, as in acute glomerulonephritis and the nephrotic syndrome. **human plasma protein f.** Plasma pooled from several donors to which certain preservatives and salts are added so that it is isotonic and iso-oncotic with normal human plasma. The product is heat-treated at 60°C for 10 hours to eliminate viable hepatitis virus particles. Also *blood plasma fraction, plasma fraction, pooled plasma.* **microsome f.** A membrane-rich fraction obtained as the components of a tissue homogenate are separated with an ultracentrifuge. Most of the membranes are formed from Golgi complexes or from endoplasmic reticulum. **mole f.** The amount of substance of a component ($x$) divided by the amount of substance of the mixture (all components of the system), expressed in mol/mol. Also *substance fraction.* Abbr. molfr. Symbol: $x_x$ **plasma f.** HUMAN PLASMA PROTEIN FRACTION. **plasma protein f.** A sterile solution of selected plasma proteins obtained from the pooled plasma of adult blood donors. The preparation contains 4.5 to 5.5 g of protein per 100 ml, with albumin representing 83 to 90 percent of the protein; the rest is largely alpha and beta globulins. It is used for its oncotic properties, much the same as albumin solutions. **recombination f.** RECOMBINATION FREQUENCY. **sampling f.** SAMPLING RATIO. **soluble f.** The cell cytoplasm in distinction from the organelles, such as mitochondria, that are suspended in it. **substance f.** MOLE FRACTION. **volume f.** Of a component of a system, the volume of the component divided by the volume of the system, expressed in l/l or $m^3/m^3$.

**fractional** \frak′shənəl\ Constituting a fraction; partial.

**fractionate** \frak′shənāt\ **1** To separate constituent materials into discrete portions or categories. **2** To divide a quantity of radiation or other therapeutic intervention so as to administer small portions at timed intervals.

**fractionation** \frak′shənā′shən\ [FRACTION + -ATION] **1** Separation of a mixture according to differences among the constituents in regard to some property, such as boiling point or solubility. **2** In radiation therapy, the use of small doses of radiation given at intervals. Also *dose fractionation, fractionated treatment, fractionated radiation.*

**cell f.** A method used to separate various cellular components. The tissue or cells are homogenized and the homogenate is centrifuged to separate the particles on the basis of density and/or sedimentation velocity. **Cohn f.** The separation of plasma proteins by treatment of plasma with cold mixtures of water and ethanol in varying proportions. By this technique major plasma proteins are obtained in the following fractions: fibrinogen in fraction I, beta and gamma globulins in fractions II and III, alpha globulin in fraction IV, and albumen in fraction V. Also *cold ethanol fractionation.* **dose f.** FRACTIONATION.

**fractography** \fraktäg′rəfē\ An examination, by light or electron microscopy, of fractured surfaces such as cells and membranes.

# fracture

**fracture** \frak′chər\ [L *fractura* (from *fract(us),* past part. of *frangere* to break, shatter + *-ura* -URE) a breaking] **1** A break in the continuity of a structure such as bone, cartilage, or metal. **2** A discontinuity in the mechanical strength of a structure. **3** To cause to have a break in continuity. **abduction f.** A fracture in which the distal part is displaced away from the midline. **adduction f.** A fracture in which the distal part is displaced towards the midline. **apophyseal f.** The avulsion of a small fragment of an apophysis or epiphyseal center. It is most often seen in growing children. **articular f.** INTRA-ARTICULAR FRACTURE. **atrophic f.** A fracture of an atrophic bone, occurring spontaneously or as a result of minimal trauma. **avulsion f.** A bone fracture that is caused by the pulling away of a tendon, muscle, ligament, or joint capsule from the bone while taking with it a fragment of the bone. **Barton's f.** A fracture-dislocation of the radius at the wrist joint. **basal skull f.** A fracture, usually linear, through the bony floor of the skull. It may be clinically manifested by rhinorrhea, collection of blood on the deep side of the tympanic membrane, otorrhea, or the Battle sign. **basocervical f.** A basal neck fracture of the femur at the junction with the trochanteric line. **bending f.** GREENSTICK FRACTURE. **Bennett's f.** A fracture-dislocation of the base of the first metacarpal bone that involves the carpo-metacarpal joint. **birth f.** Fracture of a fetal bone which occurs during the process of delivery. **blow-out f.** A fracture through the floor of the orbit caused by a blow on the eye with a sudden increase in pressure of the orbital contents. Part of the orbital contents may become trapped in the fracture site, particularly the inferior rectus or inferior oblique muscles, resulting in diplopia on upward gaze. **boxers' f.** A fracture through the neck of a metacarpal bone. It is usually seen on the first or fifth metacarpal and is marked by anterior displacement. **bucket-handle f.** BUCKET-HANDLE TEAR. **bumper f.** A comminuted, often bilateral, fracture of the upper tibia and fibula, caused by a motor vehicle striking a pedestrian, with the point of impact being immediately below the knee of the pedestrian. Also *fender fracture, bumper injury.* **bursting f.** An expansile comminuted fracture that usually occurs in the distal phalanx. Also *tuft fracture.* **butterfly f.** A comminuted fracture characterized by one large central fragment and two smaller adjacent fragments. **chip f.** The separation of a small sheared-off fragment of bone adjacent to a joint space. **chisel f.** The displacement of a fragment of the radial head. **cleavage f.** A fracture of the lower end of the humerus that involves the cartilage and bone of the capitulum. **closed f.** A fracture in which the overlying soft tissue and skin remain intact. Also *subcutaneous fracture.* **Colles f.** A fracture in which the lower end of the radius is displaced backwards and upwards to produce the silver-fork deformity. Avulsion of the ulnar styloid process usually takes place as well. Also *silver-fork fracture.* **comminuted f.** A fracture that results in numerous fragments. **complete f.** A fracture in which the bone is completely broken across. **complicated f.** A fracture accompanied by adjacent tissue or organ damage. **compound f.** A fracture in continuity with the external environment through divided skin or mucous membrane. Also *open fracture.* **compound skull f.** Fracture of the skull accompanied by laceration of the overlying scalp. **compression f.** A fracture of the calcaneus or a vertebral body that is usually produced by vertical forces associated with a fall from a height. **condylar f.** A fracture through a condyle, usually that at the lower end of the humerus or femur. **congenital f.** INTRAUTERINE FRACTURE. **contrecoup f.** A linear fracture of the skull occurring on the side of the head opposite the direct blow. **cortical f.** LINEAR FRACTURE. **cough f.** A fracture, usually of the middle ribs, produced by excessive coughing. **craniofacial dysjunction f.** LEFORT III FRACTURE. **crush f.** A fracture, usually produced by a blunt force, that results in multiple, depressed fragments. **dentate f.** A fracture in which the oppos-

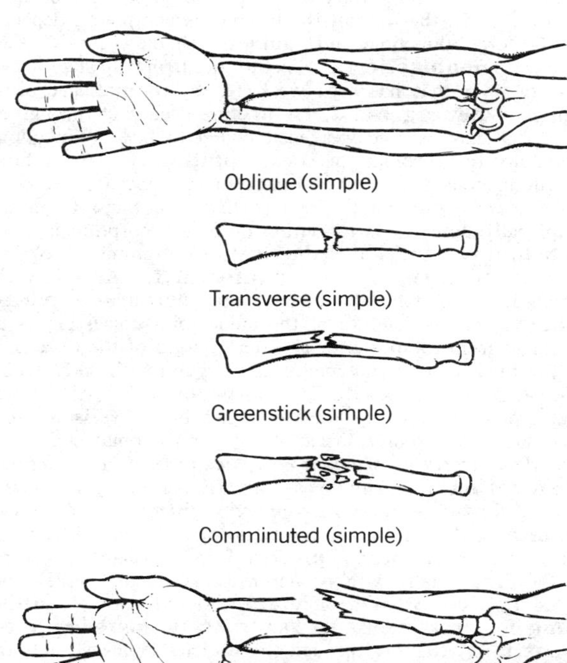

**Bone fractures**

ing fragment surfaces are serrated and fit into each other. **depressed skull f.** Fracture of the skull with inward displacement of fragments of bone. Also *derby hat fracture, ping-pong fracture, depressed fracture.* **diastatic skull f.** Fracture of the skull resulting in separation of bone fragments. **direct f.** A fracture that occurs at the point of injury. **dislocation f.** See under FRACTURE-DISLOCATION. **displaced f.** A fracture in which the fragments are separated and are not in alignment. **double f.** A fracture at two points on the same bone. Also *segmental fracture.* **Dupuytren's f.** A fracture of the lower fibula complicated by a dislocation of the ankle joint. **Duverney's f.** A fracture of the ilium that is directed from the anterior superior iliac spine. **endocrine f.** A pathologic fracture through weakened bone produced by an endocrine disorder such as hyperparathyroidism or thyrotoxicosis. **f. en rave** A transverse fracture of, but not across, a cortex surface. **epiphyseal f.** The traumatic separation of the epiphyseal plate of a long bone, with or without a fracture involving the adjacent bone. **extracapsular f.** A fracture in a bone that is adjacent to a joint but outside the attachment of the capsule. It is usually seen in the humerus or femur. **fatigue f.** A fracture that occurs usually in the short bones of the foot when exposed to repeated or undue loading, such as in marching. **fender f.** BUMPER FRACTURE. **fissure f.** LINEAR FRACTURE. **freeze f.** A procedure for preparing materials for observation with an electron microscope, in which materials are rapidly frozen and then fractured. The fracture of the ice occurs along natural structures, such as the membranes of cellular organelles, so that their structure can be revealed by electron microscopy of the fractured surface. **Galeazzi's f.** A fracture of the lower end of the radius accompanied by dislocation of the ulna at the wrist. **Gosselin's f.** A v-shaped fracture of the lower end of the tibia that involves the ankle joint. **greenstick f.** An incomplete fracture, usually seen in children, in which only the convex side of the cortex is broken with bending of the bone. Also *willow fracture, hickory-stick fracture, bending fracture.* **Guérin's f.** LEFORT I FRACTURE. **hairline f.** A small fracture of bone without displacement. Also *microfracture.* **heat f.'s** Artifactual fractures of the long bones and skull, found in burned bodies, occurring post mortem from heat. The fracture lines tend to be curved, and in the skull, they often radiate laterally from a common point located near the vertex. **hickory-stick f.** GREENSTICK FRACTURE. **horizontal maxillary f.** LEFORT I FRACTURE. **idiopathic f.** A pathologic break in a weakened bone without a known cause. **impacted f.** A fracture in which the fragments are driven into each other with a resulting reestablishment of some stability. **incomplete f.** A break or rupture of bone that does not involved the total bone segment or length. Also *infracture, infraction.* **indirect f.** A fracture, usually of the skull, that occurs at a site away from the traumatic force. **inflammatory f.** A pathologic fracture of a bone that occurs through a lesion caused by osteitis or osteomyelitis. **intertrochanteric f.** A fracture between the two trochanters of the upper femur. **intra-articular f.** A fracture through a joint surface. Also *articular fracture, intracapsular fracture.* **intraperiosteal f.** A fracture through the cortex that does not rupture the periosteum. **intrauterine f.** A fracture of a fetal bone when the fetus is within the uterus. It is usually traumatic in origin. Also *congenital fracture.* **joint f.** A fracture within the joint capsule. **lead pipe f.** A crack, seen in young bones, in one cortex with bulging of the opposite cortex. **LeFort f.** A fracture of the skull involving any or all of the maxillary, nasal, zygomatic, or orbital bones. Also *midfacial fracture.* **LeFort I f.** A midfacial fracture involving the maxilla. Also *horizontal maxillary fracture, transverse maxillary fracture, Guérin's fracture.* **LeFort II f.** A midfacial fracture in which the main fracture lines meet at the nasion. Also *pyramidal fracture.* **LeFort III f.** A fracture in which the facial bones are separated from the cranium. Also *craniofacial dysjunction fracture, transverse facial fracture.* **linear f.** A fracture extending down along the length of the bone. Also *fissure fracture, cortical fracture.* **Lisfranc's f.** Multiple fractures across the midtarsal bones and the bases of the metatarsal bones. **longitudinal f.** A fracture in the long axis of a long bone. **loose f.** A fracture in which the bone ends are freely mobile and not in contact. **malar f.** Fracture of the lateral part of the central third of the facial skeleton caused by a direct blow to the malar bone resulting usually in flattening of the cheek, epistaxis, gross swelling and bruising of the lower eyelid and, often, double vision. **mallet f.** The avulsion of a dorsal fragment of the epiphysis of the terminal phalanx of the finger. **march f.** STRESS FRACTURE. **midfacial f.** LEFORT FRACTURE. **Monteggia's f.** MONTEGGIA FRACTURE-DISLOCATION. **Moore's f.** A fracture of the distal half of the radial shaft together with dislocation of the ulnar head and entrapment of the styloid process by the wrist ligaments. **multiple f.** More than one fracture occurring in the same bone without communication between fracture points. **nasal f.** Fracture of the bony nasal skeleton, commonly of the nasal bones alone but, in more severe cases, of the frontal processes of the maxillae also. The cartilaginous septum is frequently involved. The degree of deformity, extent of comminution, severity of epistaxis, and whether or not the fracture is compound depend on the force, direction, and nature of the blow causing the injury. **neoplastic f.** Fracture occurring through a region of bone that has been weakened by the presence of a tumor. **neurogenic f.** A fracture occurring through a bone that has become weakened owing to lack of function secondary to neurologic disease. **oblique f.** A fracture of a long bone that runs obliquely to the long axis. **occult f.** A symptomatic fracture that is not visible radiographically until callus formation or bone resorption is seen more than two weeks after the onset of symptoms. **open f.** COMPOUND FRACTURE. **panfacial f.** An injury in which all of the facial bones have been fractured. **paratrooper f.** A fracture of the ankle joint consisting of a fragment from the posterior articular margin of the tibia and of the medial or lateral malleolus. **parry f.** MONTEGGIA FRACTURE-DISLOCATION. **pathologic f.** A fracture that occurs through any bone weakened by a preexisting disease such as a tumor, osteoporosis, or osteomalacia. Also *secondary fracture, spontaneous fracture, trophic fracture.* **perforating f.** Any open fracture caused by a missile passing through a bone. Also *puncture fracture.* **pertrochanteric f.** A fracture of the proximal femur involving the greater trochanter. **pillion f.** A T-shaped fracture of the distal femur with posterior displacement of the condyles. It is caused by a blow to the flexed knee. **ping-pong f.** DEPRESSED SKULL FRACTURE. **posterior element f.** A fracture through the pedicles or facet joints of the vertebrae. **Pott's f.** A fracture, usually oblique, of the lateral malleolus of the fibula, with an avulsion transverse fracture of the tibial medial malleolus. The hindfoot is outwardly displaced at the mortice of the ankle joint. **pressure f.** A resorption and fracturing of bone due to an adjacent tumor. **puncture f.** PERFORATING FRAC-

TURE. **pyramidal f.** LEFORT II FRACTURE. **reverse Colles f.** A fracture of the lower end of the radius in which the radial fragment is displaced anteriorly. It is usually caused by a direct blow to the dorsal aspect of the radius. **secondary f.** PATHOLOGIC FRACTURE. **segmental f.** DOUBLE FRACTURE. **shaft f.** A fracture through or across the shaft of a long bone. **Shepherd's f.** An avulsion or shear fracture of the posterior process of the talus. **silver-fork f.** COLLES FRACTURE. **simple f.** A closed fracture without significant soft tissue injury or displacement. **simple skull f.** A fracture of the skull that is linear and closed. **skull f.** A break in the continuity of the skull caused by trauma. **spiral f.** A fracture of a long bone that is spiral or helical in outline and is due to torsional force. Also *torsion fracture*. **splintered f.** A comminuted fracture in which the numerous fragments are thin and sharp. **spontaneous f.** PATHOLOGIC FRACTURE. **sprain f.** An avulsion fracture of a small piece of bone or cartilage with its attached ligament or tendon by a sudden force. Also *strain fracture*. **sprinters' f.** The avulsion of the anterior superior or inferior iliac spine of the ilium due to excessive muscle pull. **stellate f.** A fracture resulting from a central impact of force, with the fracture lines radiating outward. **strain f.** SPRAIN FRACTURE. **stress f.** A fracture that results from repetitive strong forces in the shafts of weight-bearing long bones adjacent to muscle attachments, such as the tibia or fibula. It is often seen in runners or ballet dancers. Also *march fracture*. **subcapital f.** A fracture at the junction of the head and neck of the femur. **subcutaneous f.** CLOSED FRACTURE. **subperiosteal f.** A cortical crack without displacement or irregularity, suggesting that the periosteum is still intact. **subtrochanteric f.** A transverse fracture at the junction of the femoral shaft and the lesser trochanter. **supracondylar f.** A fracture above the lines of the condyles in either the humerus or the femur. **surgical neck f.** A fracture line through the surgical neck of the humerus. **temporal bone f.** Fracture of the skull involving the temporal bone. Eighty percent of such fractures involve the long axis of the petrous portion of the bone and are likely to be accompanied by bleeding into the tympanic cavity or bleeding from the ear together with impaired hearing of the conduction type. Transverse fractures of the petrous portion are likely to involve the inner ear, resulting in irreversible sensorineural deafness. This is a common injury, particularly in road accidents. **tibial plateau f.** A fracture through one or both tibial plateaus, usually with downward or oblique displacement. **torsion f.** SPIRAL FRACTURE. **transcervical f.** An intracapsular fracture through the neck of the femur. **transverse f.** A fracture across the longitudinal axis of the bone. **transverse facial f.** LEFORT III FRACTURE **transverse maxillary f.** LEFORT I FRACTURE. **trimalleolar f.** A fracture through both lateral and medial malleoli of the ankle joint as well as the posterior process of the tibia. **trophic f.** PATHOLOGIC FRACTURE. **tuft f.** BURSTING FRACTURE. **ununited f.** A fracture in which the callus fails to unite the bone ends, resulting in abnormal mobility, i.e., a false joint. **vertebra plana f.** A fracture through the plate of a vertebral body. **willow f.** GREENSTICK FRACTURE.

**fracture-dislocation** \frak′chər-dis′lōkā′shən\ A fracture or fractures associated with instability and disruption of articulating surfaces making up a joint. **Monteggia f.** A displaced fracture of the upper end of the ulnar shaft with dislocation of the radial head. Also *Monteggia's fracture, parry fracture, Monteggia's dislocation*. **posterior f.** A fracture-dislocation, usually of the hip joint, in which the posterior margin has been sheared off by the dislocating femoral head. It can also be seen at the elbow joint, where the anterior margin of the ulnar coronoid process is sheared off by the humerus.

**fradicin** A substance with antibiotic activity against some fungi. It is isolated from *Streptomyces fradiae*.

**fragilitas** \frəjil′itas\ [L (from *fragil(is)* fragile, from *frangere* to break, shatter + *-itas* -ITY), frailty, weakness] FRAGILITY.

**fragility** [L *fragilitas*. See FRAGILITAS.] The likelihood of being damaged or destroyed. Also *fragilitas*. **f. of blood** ERYTHROCYTE FRAGILITY. **capillary f.** Excessive liability of the capillaries to rupture, as in purpura. **erythrocyte f.** The pattern of susceptibility of erythrocytes to hemolysis, when subjected to graduated hypotonic saline solutions. Also *fragility of blood*. **mechanical f.** The ease with which erythrocytes are disrupted by shear stress. **osmotic f.** The susceptibility of erythrocytes to lyse in hypotonic solutions of sodium chloride. Erythrocytes of normal blood exhibit very little lysis in NaCl solution of 0.5 g/dl concentration, whereas blood that contains spherocytes lyse at this or higher salt concentration. A test for osmotic fragility is used in the diagnosis of hereditary spherocytosis.

**fragilocyte** \frəjil′əsīt\ SPHEROCYTE.

**fragilocytosis** \frəjil′ōsītō′sis\ SPHEROCYTOSIS.

**fragment** \frag′mənt\ [L *fragmentum* (from *frang(ere)* to break + *-mentum* -MENT) a piece broken off] **1** A part detached or broken off. **2** One of the parts of an antibody molecule obtained by treatment with a proteinase. The two main fragments are Fab and Fc. Fab contains the antigen-binding site and comprises the complete light chain and about half the heavy chain of the immunoglobulin molecule. Fc comprises half the heavy chain and can be crystallized, since Fc molecules from different antibodies have identical structures. **f. A** The smaller of the two fragments into which diphtheria toxin is split by various proteases. It is the enzymatically active moiety of the toxin and the part that enters the host cell. **f. B** The larger of the two fragments of diphtheria toxin, which functions in binding the toxin to a host cell receptor. **Fab f.** A fragment of the immunoglobulin molecule obtained following papain hydrolysis of the molecule. The Fab moiety has an approximate molecular mass of 45 000 daltons and consists of one light chain linked to the N-terminal portion of the contiguous heavy chain. Two Fab fragments are obtained from the hydrolysis of one 7 S immunoglobulin and each fragment contains one antibody combining site. **$F(ab')_2$ f.** The major fragment of immunoglobulins obtained after pepsin digestion of the molecule. It has a molecular weight of 90 000 daltons and retains the two antibody combining sites but does not have the major Fc fragment. It is a useful tool in immunologic research, since it will not bind specifically to Fc receptor present on the surface of many tissue cells. **Fc f.** A fragment of the immunoglobulin molecule which has a molecular weight of 45 000 daltons and is obtained following papain digestion of the molecule. Unlike papain digestion of immunoglobulins, this fragment contains no antibody combining sites but does retain its site for complement fixation and for binding to Fc receptors in tissues. **Fc′ f.** The smaller molecular weight material following papain digestion of immunoglobulin molecules. It consists of a dimer of the C-terminal half of the two Fc fragments and has a molecular weight of 24 000 daltons. It has no antibody combining activity. **Fd f.** The heavy chain fragment of the immunoglobulin molecule obtained after papain digestion. It contains both the constant and variable region of the heavy chain molecule. The variable region of the heavy chain is involved in the antibody combining site of immunoglobulins. Also *Fd piece.* **fission f.** Any daughter nuclide produced by a fission event. There are two daughters per fission, and they are not necessarily alike. The mass numbers from the fission of uranium 235, for example, range from 72 to a little over 160. Most fragments are radioactive. The amounts of each produced vary widely. **one-carbon f.** Any of the formyl, formimino, hydroxymethyl, and methyl groups, and their equivalents, carried on tetrahydrofolate and metabolically interconvertible. They are used in various biosyntheses, as that of purines. **papain f.** Any of the various fragments of the immunoglobulin molecule obtained after papain digestion of the immunoglobulin. **Spengler's f.'s** Small, spherical bodies found in the sputum of patients with pulmonary tuberculosis.

**frambesia** [New L *framboesia,* from French *framboise* raspberry; so called from the typical appearance of the secondary lesions] YAWS. **f. tropica** YAWS.

**frambesioma** [*frambesi(a)* + -OMA] MOTHER YAW.

**framboesia** [See FRAMBESIA.] YAWS.

**frame** / **Balkan f.** A frame consisting of overhead bars attached to a hospital-type bed to which can be attached suspension slings, traction units, and weight-resisted pulley systems. Also *Balkan splint.* **Deiters terminal f.** A platelike expansion at the free end of each of the phalangeal processes of the outer phalangeal cells of Deiters that ends on the reticular lamina and connects the cells of Deiters to the hair cells and the supporting cells of Hensen at the outer side of the spiral organ of Corti. *Outmoded.* **occluding f.** A simple type of nonhinged articulator. **rubber dam f.** A wire frame for holding a rubber dam in a stretched state while teeth are isolated from the mouth. **Stryker f.** A rigid stretcher-type frame used to rotate a patient without active or passive motion of the patient's trunk and limbs. **suture f.** A rectangular, metal frame designed for attachment to a mouth gag, sometimes used in operations for the repair of cleft palate. It is provided with a means for retaining in an orderly way the long ends of a number of sutures until the surgeon is ready to cut them short. **trial f.** A spectacle frame designed to hold interchangeable optical lenses during an examination for refractive error. **unidentified reading f.** A nucleotide sequence, bounded by an initiation codon and a termination codon, that does not encode any known protein. Abbr. URF

**frame shift** See under FRAME-SHIFT MUTATION.

**framework** The metal part of a partial denture. Also *skeleton of partial denture.* **scleral f.** The part of the iridocorneal angle adjacent to the sclera. **uveal f.** RETICULUM TRABECULARE SCLERAE.

**Franceschetti** [Adolphe *Franceschetti,* Swiss ophthalmologist, born 1896] Treacher Collins-Franceschetti syndrome. See under MANDIBULOFACIAL DYSOSTOSIS.

**Francis** [Edward *Francis,* U.S. bacteriologist, 1872–1957] Francis disease. See under TULAREMIA.

***Francisella tularensis*** \fran'sisel'ə too'lərən'sis\ A very small, nonmobile, unencapsulated, aerobic, Gram-negative bacillus which causes tularemia. It has complex growth requirements, including a high concentration of a sulfhydryl compound, and it grows slowly and forms minute colonies. The organism is an intracellular parasite. It is transmitted to humans from rabbits and other wild animals by the deer fly, ticks, contact with animals, and ingestion of meat, the manifestations depending largely on the site of entry. The organism is dangerous in the laboratory. It can penetrate unbroken skin and a very small dose is infectious. Also *Pasteurella tularensis* (former name).

**francium** \fran'sē·əm\ A radioactive element having atomic number 87. Its position in the periodic table identifies it as the heaviest of the alkali metals. About 20 very short-lived isotopes have been made synthetically. The only naturally occurring isotope is a decay product of actinium having mass number 223. No weighable amount has been isolated. It decays by emitting alpha particles and electrons and has a half-life of 22 minutes. Symbol: Fr

**Franco** [Pierre *Franco,* French surgeon, 1500–1561] Franco's operation. See under SUPRAPUBIC CYSTOTOMY.

**François** [Jules *François,* Belgian ophthalmologist, flourished mid-20th century] Hallermann-Streiff-François syndrome. See under HALLERMANN-STREIFF SYNDROME.

**frangulic acid** EMODIN.

**Frank** [Otto *Frank,* German physiologist, 1865–1944] **1** Frank-Starling curve. See under STARLING'S CURVE. **2** Frank-Starling mechanism. See under MECHANISM.

**Frank** [Rudolf *Frank,* Austrian surgeon, 1862–1913] Ssabanejew-Frank operation. See under FRANK'S OPERATION.

**Fränkel** [Henri *Fränkel,* French ophthalmologist, born 1864] Bordier-Fränkel sign. See under SIGN.

**Frankenhäuser** [Ferdinand *Frankenhäuser,* German gynecologist, 1832–1894] Frankenhäuser's ganglion. See under CERVICAL GANGLION OF UTERUS.

**Franklin** [Edward Claus *Franklin,* German-born U.S. physician, born 1928] Franklin's disease. See under GAMMA HEAVY-CHAIN DISEASE.

**Fraser** [G. R. *Fraser,* British geneticist, flourished 20th century] Fraser syndrome. See under CRYPTOPHTHALMIA-SYNDACTYLY SYNDROME.

**fraternal** \frətur'nəl\ [Med L *fraternalis* (from L *fraternus* of brothers, from *frater* brother) pertaining to brothers] **1** Having a brotherly or sibling relationship. **2** Derived from separately fertilized ova: said of twins.

**fratricide** \fra'trisīd\ [L *frater,* gen. *fratris,* brother + -CIDE] **1** The killing of one's own brother or sister. **2** One who commits fratricide.

**Fraunhofer** [Joseph *Fraunhofer,* German physicist, 1787–1826] Fraunhofer zone. See under FAR FIELD.

**Frazier** [Charles Harrison *Frazier,* U.S. surgeon, 1870–1936] Frazier-Spiller operation. See under OPERATION.

**FRC** functional residual capacity.

**freckle** [Middle English *frekel, frakel,* from the Scandinavian] A light brown pigmented macule that develops on light-exposed skin in a genetically predisposed subject. Also *sunspot, macula solaris, lentigo aestiva.* **Hutchinson's melanotic f.** A pigmented lesion of the malar region of the face containing abnormal melanocytes in the epidermis. The lesion can become a malignant melanoma. Also *precancerous melanosis of Dubreuilh, lentigo maligna, Hutchinson's malignant lentigo, malignant lentigo.*

**Fredet** [Pierre *Fredet,* French surgeon, 1870–1946] Fredet-Ramstedt operation. See under PYLOROMYOTOMY.

**free-living** **1** Not parasitic; not metabolically dependent on another living organism. **2** Nonsessile; not permanently attached; motile.

**Freeman** [E. A. *Freeman,* English physician, flourished mid-20th century] Freeman-Sheldon syndrome. See under WHISTLING FACE-WINDMILL VANE HAND SYNDROME.

**Freer** [Otto Tiger *Freer,* U.S. surgeon, 1857–1932] See under ELEVATOR.

**freeze** / **frame f.** Display of a single frame of a real-time sequence, as in ultrasound, to allow close examination of specific features of the image.

**freeze-drying** LYOPHILIZATION.

**freeze-etching** A method of forming a stable replica of

a small particle for examination in an electron microscope. The particle is frozen in a block of ice, partially etched by warming, and subsequently coated with a shadowing technique to form the stable replica.

**freeze-substitution** A freezing technique that is used to facilitate the impregnation of embedding media into tissues prior to electron microscopy.

**Frei** [Wilhelm Siegmund *Frei,* German dermatologist, 1885–1943] Frei's disease. See under LYMPHOGRANULOMA VENEREUM.

**Freiberg** [Albert Henry *Freiberg,* U.S. surgeon, 1869–1940] Freiberg's disease, Freiberg's infraction. See under KÖHLER SECOND DISEASE.

**Frejka** [Bedrich *Frejka,* Czech physician, born 1890] Frejka pillow. See under FREJKA PILLOW SPLINT.

**fremitus** \frem′itəs\ [L (from *fremere* to growl, mutter) a murmuring, roaring] A palpable vibration. **tactile f.** A fremitus felt on palpation, especially of the chest. **vocal f.** The fremitus felt on palpation of the chest during phonation. Abbr. VF

**frena** \frē′nə\ Plural of FRENUM.

**frenal** \frē′nəl\ Pertaining to a frenum.

**frenectomy** \frēnek′təmē\ [*fren(um)* + -ECTOMY] A surgical procedure in which a frenum is excised.

**Frenkel** [Heinrich S. *Frenkel*-Heiden, German neurologist, 1860–1931] **1** Frenkel's treatment. See under FRENKEL'S EXERCISES. **2** See under SYMPTOM. **3** Frenkel's movements. See under MOVEMENT.

**frenoplasty** \frē′nōplas′tē\ [*fren(um)* + *o* + -PLASTY] A plastic operation on a frenulum.

**frenotomy** \frēnät′əmē\ [*fren(um)* + *o* + -TOMY] The surgical cutting of a frenum, usually of the lingual frenum for the correction of ankyloglossia.

**frenula** \fren′yələ\ Plural of FRENULUM.

**frenulum** \fren′yələm\ [Late L (dim. of L *frenum* a bridle, bit, reins), a small bridle] (*pl.* frenula) A fold of mucous membrane or other tissue that prevents, controls, or limits the movements of an organ or part to which it is attached; a small frenum. **f. of anterior medullary velum** FRENULUM VELI MEDULLARIS SUPERIOR. **f. cerebelli** FRENULUM VELI MEDULLARIS SUPERIOR. **f. clitoridis** [NA] The small fold on the under-surface of the clitoris formed by the lower division of the anterior ends of the labia minora meeting under and uniting with the clitoris. Also *frenulum of clitoris.* **f. of duodenal papilla** A variable fold of mucous membrane that extends downward from the lower margin of the papilla duodeni major and is a continuation of the plica longitudinalis duodeni. **f. of Giacomini** GIACOMINI'S BAND. **f. of ileocecal valve** FRENULUM VALVAE ILEALIS. **f. of ileocolic valve** FRENULUM VALVAE ILEALIS. **f. labii inferioris** [NA] The small raised fold of mucous membrane connecting the inner surface of the lower lip with the lower gum in the median plane. Also *frenulum of inferior lip.* **f. labii superioris** [NA] The prominent raised fold of mucous membrane connecting the inner surface of the upper lip with the upper gum in the median plane. Also *frenulum of superior lip.* **f. labiorum pudendi** [NA] The fold of skin joining the posterior ends of the labia minora across the midline and anterior to the posterior commissure. Also *frenulum of pudendal labia, frenulum pudendi, fourchette, frenum of labia.* **f. linguae** [NA] The raised median, vertical fold of mucous membrane connecting the inferior surface of the tongue to the floor of the mouth. Also *frenulum of tongue, frenum of tongue, lingual frenum, glossodesmus* (seldom used). **f. linguae cerebelli** VINCULA LINGULAE CEREBELLI. **f. of Macdowel** An aponeurotic sheet spreading across the bicipital groove of the humerus from the tendon of insertion of the pectoralis major muscle. Also *Macdowel's frenum.* **f. of Morgagni** FRENULUM VALVAE ILEALIS. **f. preputii penis** [NA] A small median fold of skin on the urethral surface of the penis extending from the deep surface of the prepuce to the glans penis just behind the external urethral orifice. Also *frenulum of prepuce of penis.* **f. of pudendal labia** FRENULUM LABIORUM PUDENDI. **f. pudendi** FRENULUM LABIORUM PUDENDI. **f. of superior lip** FRENULUM LABII SUPERIORIS. **f. of superior medullary velum** FRENULUM VELI MEDULLARIS SUPERIOR. **f. synoviale** Any one of the vincula tendinum. **f. of tongue** FRENULUM LINGUAE. **f. valvae ilealis** A ridge that is formed by the fused lips of the ileocecal valve. It runs laterally and downwards, demarcating the cecum from the ascending colon. Also *frenulum of ileocecal valve, frenulum of ileocolic valve, frenulum valvae ileocecalis, frenula valvulae coli, frenulum of Morgagni, frenum of Morgagni, frenum of valve of colon.* **f. veli medullaris superior** [NA] A band running from the rostral end of the superior medullary velum to the longitudinal groove between the inferior colliculi. Also *frenulum of superior medullary velum, frenulum of anterior medullary velum, frenulum veli medullaris anterioris, frenulum cerebelli.*

**frenum** \frē′nəm\ [L *frenum* a bridle, bit, reins] (*pl.* frenums, frena) A body structure that serves to restrain or check movement. Also *bridle.* **buccal f.** A fold of mucosa stretching from the cheek to the alveolar process in the canine region. **f. of labia** FRENULUM LABIORUM PUDENDI. **labial f.** A fold of mucosa stretching from the lip to the alveolar process between the central incisor teeth. **lingual f.** FRENULUM LINGUAE. **Macdowel's f.** FRENULUM OF MACDOWEL. **f. of Morgagni** FRENULUM VALVAE ILEALIS. **f. of tongue** FRENULUM LINGUAE. **f. of valve of colon** FRENULUM VALVAE ILEALIS.

**frenzy** \fren′zē\ [Old French *frenesie* from Med L *phrenesia* madness, from L *phrenesis* frenzy, madness, from Gk *phrenitis* (from *phrēn* the mind + *-itis* -ITIS) delirium of fever, frenzy] Delirium induced by meningitis or by other acute cerebral conditions. *Outmoded.*

**frequency** \frē′kwənsē\ [L *frequentia* (from *frequens* repeated), frequency] **1** In statistics, the number of occurrences of a given event or the number of observations falling within a given class. Also *absolute frequency.* **2** The number of complete variations (cycles) of an electromagnetic or acoustic wave occurring in one second. **audio f.** Sonic frequency in the audible range: between about 20 and 20 000 Hz for humans. **audio Doppler f.** Doppler shift presented as audible sound. **center f.** The dominant frequency present in an ultrasound pulse. **critical flicker fusion f.** The slowest rate of stroboscopic presentation of a light at which the illumination is perceived as a constant and unvarying light. Also *fusion frequency.* **cutoff f.** The frequency of a system identified with the transition between those frequencies that pass through the system and those that are attenuated, and where the attenuation is 3 dB. **dominant f.** In the electroencephalogram, the frequency, usually that of the alpha rhythm, which dominates the record. **fusion f.** CRITICAL FLICKER FUSION FREQUENCY. **gene f.** In a defined population, the frequency of a specific allele at a given genetic locus. **high f.** **1** A frequency that is high in comparison to a given standard such as the pitch frequency of middle C. **2** A radio frequency in the range of 3 to 30 megahertz. **Larmor f.** The frequency of precession of a rotator whose angular momentum is associated with a magnetic moment (as in the case of an electron or nucleus) when subjected to a magnetic field. See also LARMOR EQUATION. **mutant f.** The proportion of a particular mutant in a population. It depends not only on mutation rate but on the accumulation of the progeny of mutants arising in the culture. **nearest neighbor f.** With reference to nucleic acids of a given organism, usually DNA, the relative frequency with which two nucleotides are adjacent. **projection f.** The proportion of neurons in a circumscribed nucleus synaptically contacted by a given or average fiber projecting onto the nucleus, e.g., the percentage of motoneurons in a muscle's motor pool with which a primary spindle afferent makes contact. **recombination f.** **1** The frequency of genetic recombination between two given syntenic loci. It is determined by dividing the number of individuals in a given sibship in whom recombination occurred by the total number of individuals. For loci sufficiently closely linked that multiple crossovers are infrequent, the recombination frequency is a measure of map distance. **2** The frequency of transfer of a bacterial gene from a donor to a recipient. **3** The frequency of crossover between two genetic markers in a merozygote. **4** The frequency of recombination between markers in two viral genomes infecting the same cell. For defs. 1, 2, 3, and 4 also *recombination fraction*. Abbr. RF **rectified radio f.** A radio frequency signal which has been converted from alternating to direct current form. **relative f.** In statistics, a frequency expressed as a proportion of the total number of events or of some other totality. **respiratory f.** The rate of breathing, measured usually by the number of breaths per minute. Also *ventilatory frequency*. **subsonic f.** A frequency below the audible range. **ultrasonic f.** Frequency of vibration above the audible range, especially in the range of 1 to 10 MHz. **ventilatory f.** RESPIRATORY FREQUENCY.

**Fresnel** [Augustin Jean *Fresnel*, French physicist, 1788–1827] Fresnel zone. See under NEAR FIELD.

**fretum** \frē′təm\ [L, a place of passage, strait, channel] In anatomy, a constriction, narrowing, or channel.

**freudian** \froi′dē·ən\ [after Sigmund *Freud*, Austrian neurologist and psychiatrist, 1856–1939 + *-ian*, suffix denoting pertaining to] **1** Relating to concepts proposed by Freud in the development of his theories of psychoanalytic psychology and technique. **2** See under PSYCHOANALYSIS.

**Freund** [Jules Thomas *Freund*, U.S. immunologist, 1890–1960] **1** See under ADJUVANT. **2** Freund's incomplete adjuvant. See under ADJUVANT. **3** Freund's complete adjuvant. See under ADJUVANT.

**Freund** [Wilhelm Alexander *Freund*, German surgeon, 1833–1918] See under ANOMALY.

**Frey** [Heinrich *Frey*, Swiss histologist, born 1822] Gastric pits of Frey. See under FOVEOLAE GASTRICAE.

**Frey** [Lucie *Frey*, Polish physician, 1852–1932] Frey-Baillarger syndrome, Frey syndrome. See under AURICULOTEMPORAL SYNDROME.

**Frey** [Maximilian Ruppert Franz von *Frey*, Austrian-born German physician, 1852–1932] Frey's hairs. See under HAIR.

**Freyer** [Peter Johnston *Freyer*, English surgeon, 1851–1921] See under OPERATION.

**FRF** follicle releasing factor.

**Fricke** [Johann Karl Georg *Fricke*, German surgeon, 1790–1841] See under BANDAGE.

**Friderichsen** [Carl *Friderichsen*, Danish pediatrician, born 1886] Waterhouse-Friderichsen syndrome. See under SYNDROME.

**Friedländer** [Karl *Friedländer*, German physician, 1847–1887] **1** Friedländer's bacillus. See under *KLEBSIELLA PNEUMONIAE*. **2** Friedländer's disease. See under ENDARTERITIS OBLITERANS. **3** Friedländer's pneumonia. See under *KLEBSIELLA* PNEUMONIA.

**Friedman** [Emanuel A. *Friedman*, U.S. physician, born 1926] See under CURVE.

**Friedman** [Maurice Harold *Friedman*, U.S. physician, born 1903] Friedman-Lapham test, Friedman test. See under FRIEDMAN TEST.

**Friedmann** [Max *Friedmann*, German neurologist, 1858–1925] **1** Friedmann's complex, Friedmann syndrome, Friedmann's vasomotor syndrome. See under BOXERS' ENCEPHALOPATHY. **2** Friedmann's disease. See under NARCOLEPSY.

**Friedreich** [Nikolaus *Friedreich*, German physician, 1826–1882] **1** See under FOOT, SIGN. **2** Friedreich's ataxia, Friedreich's tabes. See under FRIEDREICH'S DISEASE.

**Friend** [Charlotte *Friend*, U.S. microbiologist, born 1921] See under VIRUS.

**frigidity** \frijid′itē\ [Late L *frigiditas* (from L *frigid(us)* cold + *-itas* -ITY) frigidity] Emotional coldness; unresponsiveness. **sexual f.** Female psychosexual dysfunction that may reflect inhibited sexual desire, sexual excitement, or orgasm, or any combination thereof. The end result is failure to achieve orgasm through coitus. Also *sexual anesthesia*.

**frigolabile** \frig′ōlā′bīl\ [L *frig(us)* cold (noun) + *o* + LABILE] Readily damaged by cold.

**frigostabile** \frig′ōstā′bīl\ FRIGOSTABLE.

**frigostable** \frig′ōstā′bl\ [L *frig(us)* cold (noun) + *o* + *stabil(is)* stable] Resistant to cold. Also *frigostabile*.

**frigotherapy** \frig′ōther′əpē\ CRYOTHERAPY.

**frill** \fril\ [possibly from Flemish *frul* frill, edge] The posterior iris pigment of neuroectodermal origin that is visible as a thin brown edge of the pupil. **iris f.** IRIS COLLARETTE.

**fringe** [Old French *frenge* (from alter. of L *fimbria*. See FIMBRIA.) a fringe, border] FIMBRIA. **subliminal f.** A region within a neuron pool from which no discharge of impulses takes place during weak stimulation of one or other of two afferent nerves but from which discharge of impulses does occur if the afferent nerves are stimulated simultaneously.

**Fröhlich** [Alfred *Fröhlich*, Austrian-born pharmacologist active in the United States, 1871–1953] Babinski-Fröhlich syndrome, Fröhlich's adiposogenital dystrophy. See under FRÖHLICH SYNDROME.

**Froin** [Georges *Froin*, French physician, born 1874] Nonne-Froin syndrome, Lépine-Froin syndrome. See under FROIN SYNDROME.

**Froment** [Jules *Froment*, French physician, 1878–1946] **1** Froment's paper sign. See under NEWSPAPER SIGN. **2** See under SIGN. **3** Froment sign. See under ROGER'S COUNTER SIGN.

**Frommann** [Carl *Frommann*, German anatomist, 1831–1892] Frommann's lines. See under STRIATIONS OF FROMMANN.

**Frommel** [Richard Julius Ernst *Frommel*, German gynecologist, 1854–1912] Frommel's disease, Chiari-Frommel disease, Frommel-Chiari syndrome. See under CHIARI-FROMMEL SYNDROME.

**frondose** \fràn′dōs\ [L *frondos(us)* (from *frons*, gen. *frondis*, leaf of a tree, branch or tree with leaves + *-osus* -OSE[1]) leafy] Bearing leaflike, tufted, or villous structures.

**frons** \fränz\ [L, the brow, forehead] The region of the face between the eyebrows and the hairline; forehead. Also *brow*. **f. cranii** [NA] The external surface of the fron-

tal bone corresponding to the forehead. Also *bony forehead, frons of cranium.*
**front** / **wave f.** A continuous surface at which all vibratory motion has the same phase at a given instant.
**frontad** \frun′tad\ [*front(o)-* + -AD] Toward the front or the frontal aspect.
**frontal** \frun′təl\ **1** Pertaining to the forehead or the frontal bone. **2** Pertaining to the coronal or frontal plane. **3** Pertaining to the front or frontal aspect.
**frontalis** \fruntā′lis\ [New L] Frontal.
**frontipetal** \fruntip′ətl\ [L *frons,* gen. *frontis,* brow, forepart + -PETAL] Directed towards the front.
**fronto-** \frun′tō-\ [L *frons-,* gen. *front(is)* forehead] A combining form meaning front, frontal, or frontal bone.
**frontocerebellar** \-ser′əbel′ər\ Denoting fiber tracts from the frontal cerebral cortex extending through the pons to the cerebellum. Also *frontopontocerebellar.*
**frontoethmoidectomy** \-eth′moidek′təmē\ EXTERNAL FRONTOETHMOIDECTOMY. **external f.** An operation intended for the relief of chronic frontal sinusitis either alone or with ethmoidal disease, particularly when there are nasal polyps. A curved skin incision (Howarth's incision) is made medial to the inner canthus of the eye and the frontal sinus opened through its floor. The ethmoidal air cells are broken into through the medial wall of the orbit and exenterated, providing a pathway to drain the frontal sinus into the nose beneath the middle concha. There are many modifications known by the names of their advocates. Also *frontoethmoidectomy.*
**frontomalar** \-mā′lər\ FRONTOZYGOMATIC.
**frontomaxillary** \-mak′siler′ē\ Pertaining to the frontal bone and the maxilla.
**frontomental** \-men′təl\ Pertaining to the forehead or frontal bone and the chin.
**frontonasal** \-nā′zəl\ Pertaining to the frontal and nasal bones or to the frontal sinus and nasal cavity. Also *nasofrontal.*
**fronto-occipital** \-äksip′ətl\ Pertaining to the frontal and occipital bones or to the forehead and the occiput.
**fronto-orbital** \-ôr′bitəl\ Pertaining to the frontal bone and the orbital cavity.
**frontoparietal** \-pərī′ətəl\ PARIETOFRONTAL.
**frontopontine** \-pän′tīn\ Denoting the tractus frontopontinus (Arnold's bundle).
**frontopontocerebellar** \-pän′tōser′əbel′ər\ FRONTOCEREBELLAR.
**frontotemporal** \-tem′pərəl\ Pertaining to the frontal and the temporal bones. Also *temporofrontal.*
**frontozygomatic** -zī′gəmat′ik Pertaining to the frontal and zygomatic bones. Also *frontomalar.*
**Froriep** [August Friedrich von *Froriep,* German anatomist, 1849–1917] See under GANGLION.
**Frost** [William Adams *Frost,* English ophthalmologist, 1853–1935] See under SUTURE.
**frost** / **uremic f.** Fine, white, crystalline powder on the skin of patients with uremia, secondary to increased urea excreted with sweat which has then evaporated.
**frostbite** Tissue destruction resulting from exposure to low environmental temperature. The extent of damage is difficult to determine on first inspection. **deep f.** Tissue destruction extending beyond the skin and involving subcutaneous tissues, muscle, and/or bone. Also *third degree frostbite.* **superficial f.** Frostbite confined to the skin. **third degree f.** DEEP FROSTBITE.
**froth** \fräth\ **f. of drowning** The abundant white, occasionally blood-tinged, foamy liquid that exudes from the nose and mouth of drowning victims. The fluid is an admixture of mucus, proteins, and inhaled water. The finding of this frothy fluid in corpses recovered from water is a strong indication of drowning death.
**frottage** \frôtäzh′\ [French (from *frott(er)* to rub, from L *fricare* to rub) rubbing, friction] The obtaining of sexual gratification by rubbing against the sexual object.
**fructi-** FRUCTO-.
**fructivorous** \fruktiv′ərəs\ Existing on a diet composed of fruit. Also *frugivorous.*
**fructo-** [L *fructus* fruit] A combining form denoting relationship to fructose, as in *phosphofructokinase.* Also *fructi-.*
**fructofuranose** Fructose in its furanose form; a hemiacetal formed between its carbonyl group and O-5. This is only a minor form in solution, where the more stable 6-membered ring is favored, but occurs if O-6 is substituted (as in fructose 6-phosphate), and it predominates also in glycosides of fructose, such as sucrose.
**fructokinase** The enzyme (EC 2.7.1.4) that catalyzes the reaction of fructose with ATP to form ADP and fructose 1-phosphate. In animals, this is one of the ways in which fructose derived from the digestion of sucrose can enter metabolism. It is also a route for the assimilation of fructose by microorganisms.
**fructopyranose** Fructose in its pyranose form; a hemiacetal formed between its carbonyl group and O-6. This form predominates in solution. The alternative fructofuranose form is commoner in glycosidically linked fructose.
**fructose** \fruk′tōs, frʊk′-\ [L *fruct(us)* fruit + -OSE[2]] $CH_2OH—[CHOH]_3—CO—CH_2OH$. A 6-carbon ketose sugar with the same configuration at its chiral atoms as that of glucose. It exists mainly in the pyranose form when uncombined. Its main occurrences are in combination as sucrose, and as phosphates, which are intermediates in several pathways of carbohydrate metabolism. It is the most rapidly absorbed simple sugar and is sweeter than sucrose. Also *levulose* (outmoded).
**fructose-bisphosphatase** The enzyme (EC 3.1.3.11) that catalyzes the hydrolysis of fructose 1,6-bisphosphate to fructose 6-phosphate and orthophosphate. It is allosterically controlled, being inhibited by AMP and activated by citrate. The progress of glycolysis depends on its being inactive, whereas gluconeogenesis requires its activity.
**fructose 1,6-bisphosphate** Fructose carrying phosphate groups on O-1 and O-6. It is an intermediate in glycolysis, being formed from ATP and fructose 6-phosphate under the influence of phosphofructokinase, and also in gluconeogenesis, being formed by aldol condensation of triose phosphates. Also *fructose 1,6-diphosphate.*
**fructose 2,6-bisphosphate** The glycoside formed between fructose 6-phosphate and phosphoric acid. It stimulates phosphofructokinase and inhibits fructose-bisphosphatase, thereby stimulating glycolysis. In liver, its concentration falls in response to stimulation by glucagon.
**fructose-bisphosphate aldolase** The enzyme (EC 4.1.2.13) of the glycolytic pathway that catalyzes the interconversion of fructose 1,6-bisphosphate with glyceraldehyde 3-phosphate and glycerone phosphate (dihydroxyacetone phosphate), often simply known as aldolase. It is highly specific for glycerone phosphate, but catalyzes its condensation with a variety of aldehydes. Also *aldolase.*
**fructose 1,6-diphosphate** FRUCTOSE 1,6-BISPHOSPHATE.
**fructosemia** \fruk′təsē′mē·ə\ The presence of fructose in blood. Also *levulosemia.*
**fructose 1-phosphate** The product of fructokinase. It is an intermediate in the catabolism of fructose. A specific aldolase converts it in the liver into glyceraldehyde and dihydroxyacetone phosphate.

**fructose 6-phosphate** An intermediate in glycolysis. It is formed by the isomerization of glucose 6-phosphate and is a substrate for phosphofructokinase, which converts it into fructose 1,6-bisphosphate. It can also be formed, especially in adipose tissue, by phosphorylation of fructose with hexokinase.

**fructosidase** Any enzyme capable of liberating fructose, possibly substituted by other sugars, from glycoside linkage by hydrolysis.

**fructoside** Any compound containing fructose in glycosidic linkage, such as sucrose, which is $\beta$-D-fructofuranosyl-(2′1)-$\alpha$-D-glucopyranoside.

**fructosuria** \fruk′təsoo′rē·ə\ The excretion of fructose in the urine. **benign f.** A rare, asymptomatic, metabolic defect, apparently confined to Jewish people, in which an excess blood fructose level after meals is associated with fructosuria. The condition probably is due to a deficiency of hepatic fructokinase. Also *essential fructosuria.* **essential f.** BENIGN FRUCTOSURIA.

**fructosyl** The group formed by removing the 2-hydroxyl group from the furanose or, occasionally, pyranose form of fructose.

**frugivorous** \froojiv′ərəs\ FRUCTIVOROUS.

**fruitarian** \frooter′ē·ən\ [FRUIT + *-arian* as in *vegetarian*] One who lives on a diet consisting mainly of fruit.

**fruitarianism** \frooter′ē·ənizm\ [FRUITARIAN + -ISM] The consumption of a diet composed chiefly of fruit.

**frust.** *frustillatum* (L, in small pieces).

**FSH** follicle stimulating hormone.

**FSHRH** follicle stimulating hormone releasing hormone.

**ft.** *fiat* (L, let it be made).

**FTI** free thyroxine index.

**ft. mas. div. in pil.** *fiat massa dividenda in pilulae* (L, let a mass be made, to be divided into pills).

**ft. pulv.** *fiat pulvis* (L, let a powder be made).

**Fuchs** [Ernst *Fuchs*, Austrian ophthalmologist, 1851–1930] **1** See under SIGN, COLOBOMA, DYSTROPHY. **2** Fuchs syndrome. See under HETEROCHROMIC CYCLITIS. **3** Crypts of Fuchs. See under CRYPTS OF IRIS. **4** Fuchs dimples. See under DELLEN.

**fuchsin** \fook′sin\ [after Leonhard *Fuchs*, German physician and botanist, 1501–1566 + -IN] Any of several dyes or stains that impart a red or purple color. They may be either acid or basic. **acid f.** A synthetic acid dye that is the sulfonated derivative of basic fuchsin. It is used in the van Gieson and Masson trichrome connective tissue stains. Also *acid fuchsin stain, rubin.* **basic f.** A biologic stain that is a mixture of pararosanilin, rosanilin, and magenta II. It is a powerful dye used in the Ziehl-Neelsen technique and is the main constituent of Schiff's reagent. Also *aniline red, basic rubin, basic fuchsin stain, magenta, diamond fuchsin.* **diamond f.** BASIC FUCHSIN.

**fuchsinophil** \fooksin′əfil\ Denoting the affinity of a tissue structure for acidic or basic fuchsin. Also *fuchsinophilic, fuchsinophilous.*

**fucose** L-Fucose (6-deoxy-L-galactose). A substance that occurs widely in the carbohydrates of glycoproteins. It is produced as its GDP derivative from GDP-D-mannose by a series of reactions in which C-6 is deoxygenated and the centers at C-3 and C-5 are epimerized. D-Fucose is used experimentally as a noncatabolizable analogue of galactose.

**fucoside** A glycoside of fucose.

**fucosidosis** \fyoo′kōsidō′sis\ Either of two types of an autosomal recessive inborn error of glycoprotein degradation due to deficiency of the enzyme $\alpha$-fucosidase. The two major clinical variants share mild coarsening of the facies, hepatosplenomegaly, mental retardation, and vacuolated lymphocytes. Type I is of infantile onset with frequent seizures. Type II is of childhood onset and causes the development of tortuous conjunctival vessels and angiokeratoma.

**FUDR** floxuridine.

**Fuerbringer** [Paul Walther *Fuerbringer*, German physician, 1849–1930] See under LAW.

**-fuge** \-fyooj\ [L *fugare* to put to flight] A combining form designating an agent that expels or rids of.

**fugu** \foo′goo\ The Japanese name for PUFFER.

**fugue** \fyoog\ [French (from Italian *fuga* flight, fugue in music, from L *fuga* a fleeing, flight, desire to escape, akin to Gk *phygē* flight), a fugue in music, escape] A condition in which the subject takes leave of his usual activities and wanders about. Typically the individual suffers from amnesia for the period he is absent from his usual activities. **epileptic f.** Prolonged epileptic automatjsm, lasting for several hours, and in rare cases for days, and occurring during a postepileptic confusional state, usually in cases of temporal lobe epilepsy.

**fulgurant** \ful′gyərənt\ Piercing; intense. Also *fulgurating.*

**fulgurate** \ful′gyərāt\ To destroy (tissue) with a sparking electrode.

**fulgurating** \ful′gyərāting\ **1** FULGURANT. **2** Of or relating to fulguration.

**fulguration** \ful′gyərā′shən\ [L *fulguratio* (from *fulguratus*, past part. of *fulgurare* to send lightning flashes, from *fulgur* lightning) a lightning flash] A method of destroying tissue using a sparking, movable electrode.

**fulgurize** \ful′gyərīz\ To treat (necrotic tissue) by fulguration.

**Fülleborn** [Friedrich *Fülleborn*, German parasitologist, 1866–1933] See under METHOD.

**Fuller** [Eugene *Fuller*, U.S. urologist, 1858–1930] See under OPERATION.

**fulminant** \ful′mənənt\ [L *fulminans*, gen. *fulminantis*, pres. part. of *fulminare* to fulminate, strike with lightning] Sudden and severe, as the onset of an illness; hyperacute. Also *fulminating, foudroyant.*

**fulminating** \ful′mənāting\ FULMINANT.

**fumarase** The original name for FUMARATE HYDRATASE. • The name was changed because the ending *-ase* applied to the name of a substrate normally implies that the enzyme hydrolyzes that substrate. Fumarase catalyzes the reversible hydration of fumarate to malate.

**fumarate hydratase** The enzyme (EC 4.2.1.2) that catalyzes the readily reversible *trans* addition of water to fumarate to form (*S*)-malate. This is a step in the citric acid cycle.

**fumaric acid** HOOC—CH═CH—COOH. The isomer of butenedioic acid with *trans* configuration. It is an intermediate in the citric acid cyle, being made from succinic acid by dehydrogenation, and being converted into malic acid by addition of the elements of water.

**fumarylacetoacetic acid** (2*E*)-4,6-Dioxooct-2-endioic acid. An intermediate in the catabolism of phenylalanine and tyrosine, in which it is formed by isomerization of maleylacetoacetic acid and is hydrolyzed to form fumaric and acetoacetic acids.

**fume** [L *fum(are)* (from *fumus* smoke, fume) to emit smoke or fumes] **1** A noxious and usually odorous gaseous emanation. **2** To give out fumes.

**fumigacin** *Outmoded* HELVOLIC ACID.

**fumigant** \fyoo′məgənt\ [L *fumigans*, gen. *fumigantis*, pres. part. of *fumigare* to smoke, from *fumus* smoke] A gas or aerosol used for disinfecting rooms or materials.

**functio** \fungk′shō\ FUNCTION. **f. laesa** A loss of function.

**function** [L *functio* (from *functus,* past part. of *fungi* to do, execute) a doing, executing] **1** The action or office performed by an organ, part, or substance of the body. Also *functio.* **2** The characteristic action of a compound due to its composition or structure. **arousal f.** The capacity that a sensory stimulus possesses to induce a state of vigilance, awareness, or readiness in the cerebral cortex; the induction of an activated electroencephalogram by a sensory stimulus. **carnotic f.** The relationship between the amount of heat lost and the quantity of work performed as a result of the heat expended. Also *Carnot's function.* **discriminant f.** An algebraic expression embodying a linear combination of variables that contribute to differentiating or discriminating two or more conditions or categories. **ego f.** The work of the ego in perceiving reality, mediating between it and the person and adapting the person to reality. Its tasks include perception, self-awareness, motor control, defense mechanisms, replacement of the primary process of the id with the secondary process, memory, affects, thinking, thought synthesis, and creativity. **group f.** The harmonious contacts of a group of teeth with their antagonists. **isomeric f.** The sensory, motor, or reflexive function of an isolated segment of the spinal cord. **life table f.** See under LIFE TABLE. **linear f.** A function of the general form $y=a+bx$ where $a$ and $b$ are constants. The graph of $y$ against $x$ is a straight line with slope$=b$ and intercept$=a$. **line-spread f.** A plot of count rate against the position of a thin "line" source of radioactivity as it is moved, at right angles to the line, across the field of vision of a collimated detector. The line source is oriented at right angles to the detector's axis, and the distance from the detector is kept constant throughout a given pass. This distance must be specified, since the spread is a function of the distance. **logistic f.** A function expressing the relationship between two variables, $x$ and $y$, that has the general form:

$$y = \frac{k}{1+e^{a+bx}},$$

where $a$ and $b$ are parameters and $e$ is the exponential constant (= 2.71828 ...). The growth (or decline) in populations may be represented at least aproximately by the logistic function, with $x$ as time and $y$ as size. With suitable parameters a logistic function may also express the risk of disease ($y$) according to the level ($x$) of a risk factor. **multiple logistic f.** A function used in the statistical analysis of the results of epidemiologic investigations to assess the relative contribution of several independent variables to the outcome under study. An example would be the influence of blood pressure, serum cholesterol, and smoking, separately, on the occurrence of coronary heart disease.

**functional** \fungk′shənəl\ **1** Of or relation to a function; specifically, serving to contribute to the operation of a bodily function. **2** Having no known organic cause, as *functional disorder.*

**funda** \fun′də\ [L, a sling] A four-tailed bandage used in a slinglike fashion, as, for example, to support and limit the motion of the mandible.

**fundal** \fun′dl\ Of or pertaining to a fundus.

**fundament** [L *fundament(um)* (from *funda(re)* to lay a foundation (from *fundus* bottom) + *-mentum* -MENT) a foundation] **1** In anatomy, the anus and surrounding region; the buttocks. **2** The base of a part or structure. **3** A structure when it first begins to develop its shape or form.

**fundectomy** \fundek′təmē\ FUNDUSECTOMY.

**fundi** \fun′dī\ Plural of FUNDUS.

**fundic** \fun′dik\ Pertaining to a fundus.

**fundiform** \fun′difôrm\ Having a slinglike configuration.

**fundoplasty** \fun′dəplas′tē\ [*fund(us)* + *o* + -PLASTY] GASTROESOPHAGOPLASTY.

**fundoplication** \fun′dəplikā′shən\ Plication of the fundus of the stomach around the lower esophagus, a surgical treatment for gastroesophageal reflux.

**fundoscopy** \fundäs′kəpē\ [*fund(us)* + *o* + -SCOPY] *Imprecise* OPHTHALMOSCOPY.

**fundus** \fun′dəs\ [L, the bottom or base of a thing] The deepest part of an organ, or a part opposite the main opening to or from a hollow organ. **f. albipunctatus** A genetic disease of the retinal pigment epithelium, characterized by the appearance of multiple, small, discrete, pale, rounded discolorations of this layer. It is generally benign. Also *Lauber's disease.* **f. of eye** FUNDUS OCULI. **f. flavimaculatus** A genetic disease of the retinal pigment epithelium, characterized by the appearance of multiple, small, elongated, pale discolorations of this layer. It often is associated with a juvenile macular degeneration. **f. of gallbladder** FUNDUS VESICAE BILIARIS. **f. gastricus** [NA] The dome-shaped part of the stomach which is situated above and to the left of the cardiac orifice and is usually distended with gas. Also *fundus of stomach, fundus ventriculi, fornix gastricus, fornix ventricularis, fornix of stomach.* • In radiologic anatomy, the term *fornix gastricus* is more common than *fundus gastricus.* **f. of internal acoustic meatus** FUNDUS MEATUS ACUSTICI INTERNI. **leopard f.** TESSELATED FUNDUS. **f. meatus acustici interni** [NA] The lateral end or bottom of the internal acoustic meatus, formed by a vertical plate of bone which separates it from the internal ear and is divided by the transverse crest. Above the crest the facial nerve area is anterior to the superior vestibular area, while below the crest the tractus spiralis foraminosus is anterior to the inferior vestibular area and the foramen singulare. Also *fundus of internal acoustic meatus.* **f. oculi** The posterior part of the interior of the eye as viewed on ophthalmoscopy. It comprises the optic part of the retina and parts of the choroid and sclera. Also *fundus of eye, eyeground.* **f. of stomach** FUNDUS GASTRICUS. **tesselated f.** The mottled appearance of the fundus of the eye when a moderate amount of choroidal melanin contrasts with the reddish choroidal vessels, a normal variant of the fundus pattern. Also *tigroid fundus, leopard fundus, tigroid retina, leopard retina.* **tigroid f.** TESSELATED FUNDUS. **f. of urinary bladder** FUNDUS VESICAE URINARIAE. **f. uteri** [NA] The domelike upper part of the body of the uterus that lies above the plane through the points of attachment of the uterine tubes. It is covered with peritoneum continuous with that on the anterior and posterior surfaces. Also *fundus of uterus.* **f. of vagina** FORNIX VAGINAE. **f. ventriculi** FUNDUS GASTRICUS. **f. vesicae biliaris** [NA] The rounded, dilated end of the gallbladder that usually extends downwards and forwards beyond the inferior margin of the liver to come into contact with the anterior abdominal wall at the point where the ninth costal cartilage meets the right lateral line. It is covered by peritoneum. Also *fundus of gallbladder.* **f. vesicae urinariae** [NA] The triangular base of the urinary bladder, directed posteriorly and inferiorly. In males it is separated from the rectum by the rectovesical pouch of peritoneum superiorly and by the seminal vesicles, deferent ducts, and rectovesical fascia inferiorly. In females it is related to the cervix uteri and the upper part of the anterior wall of the vagina. The internal aspect of the fundus constitutes the trigonum vesicae. Also *fundus of urinary bladder, infundibulum of urinary bladder, base of bladder.*

**funduscope** \fun′dəskōp\ [*fundu(s)* + -SCOPE] *Imprecise* OPHTHALMOSCOPE.

**funduscopy** \fundus′kəpē\ [*fundu(s)* + -SCOPY] *Imprecise* OPHTHALMOSCOPY.

**fundusectomy** \fun′dəsek′təmē\ [FUNDUS + -ECTOMY] **1** A surgical removal of the base of or a broad part of an organ. Also *fundectomy.* **2** The surgical removal of the fundus of the stomach.

**fungal** \fung′gəl\ Of, pertaining to, charactistic of, or caused by a fungus. Also *fungous.*

**fungating** \fung′gāting\ Descriptive of a lesion that, by virtue of its proliferative capacity, protrudes from its site of origin as a spongy growth.

**fungemia** \funjē′mē·ə\ MYCETHEMIA.

**fungi** \fun′jī\ Plural of FUNGUS.

**fungicidal** \fun′jisī′dəl\ Destructive of or deleterious to fungi.

**fungicide** \fun′jisīd\ [*fung(us)* + -CIDE] Any agent used to kill or inhibit fungi.

**fungicidin** *Outmoded* NYSTATIN.

**Fungi Imperfecti** \fun′jī im′pərfek′tī\ DEUTEROMYCETES.

**fungimycin** An antifungal antibiotic agent obtained from *Streptomyces coelicolor* var. *aminophilus.* It is an amorphous yellow solid that is practically insoluble in water. It is an aromatic antibiotic and it contains an amino-sugar, perosamine. Also *perimycin.*

**fungistat** \fun′jistat\ [*fung(us)* + -STAT] Any agent that inhibits fungal growth without killing the fungus. Also *mycostat.*

**fungistatic** \fun′jistat′ik\ Inhibiting the growth of a fungus or fungi.

**fungitoxicity** The attribute of having a destructive effect on fungi.

**fungoid** \fung′goid\ Resembling or having characteristics of a fungus. Also *fungous, mycetoid, mycoid.*

**fungosity** \fungäs′itē\ A fungus or funguslike growth.

**fungous** \fung′gəs\ **1** FUNGOID. **2** FUNGAL.

**funguria** \fung·goo′rē·ə\ The presence of a fungus in the urine.

**fungus** \fung′gəs\ [L (prob. akin to Gk *spongos, sphongos* a sponge), a mushroom, fungus, mildew] (*pl.* fungi) Any of a large group of achlorophyllous, spore-bearing eukaryotes having either a typically walled thallus with absorptive nutrition or an unwalled thallus with saprophytic nutrition. **beefsteak f.** The fungus *Gyromitra esculenta* (sometimes classified as *Helvella esculenta*). It is generally believed that eastern North American forms of the fungus contain varying amounts of monomethylhydrazine. This fungus can cause gastrointestinal upsets, and some instances of death have been recorded. Also *lorchel.* **biphasic fungi** False yeasts, such as *Candida,* which are able to grow by budding to typical ovoid yeast cells or develop in a mycelial form. **f. of the brain** A morbid, granulating protrusion of brain tissue through an opening in the skull. Also *cerebral fungus, fungus cerebri.* **f. cerebri** FUNGUS OF THE BRAIN. **cutaneous f.** *Seldom used* DERMATOPHYTE. **dimorphic f.** Any fungus that is capable of responding to environmental conditions by growing a different form for each substrate, such as a filamentous form on or in a solid substrate, and a yeastlike form in liquid media. **fission f.** *Obs.* BACTERIUM. • This is a literal translation of *schizomycete.* **foot f.** See under MYCETOMA. **imperfect f.** Any member of the form-class Deuteromyces; a fungus having no known sexual stage of reproduction. **kefir f.** A mixture of yeasts and bacteria used to produce kefir milk, a fermented milk popular in the Balkans. **perfect f.** Any fungus whose sexual and asexual methods of reproduction are known. **ray f.** *Outmoded* ACTINOMYCETE. **thrush f.** *CANDIDA ALBICANS.* **umbilical f.** GRANULOMA OF THE UMBILICUS. **yeastlike f.** Any fungus which lacks the sexual means of reproduction and which is also diphasic, one form resembling ovoid yeast cells and the other form being hyphal.

**funic** \fyoo′nik\ **1** Pertaining to a funis. **2** Pertaining to the umbilical cord. For defs. 1 and 2 also *funicular.*

**funicle** \fyoo′nikl\ FUNICULUS.

**funicular** \fyoonik′yələr\ **1** Pertaining to any funiculus. **2** FUNIC.

**funiculate** \fyoonik′yəlit\ Possessing or forming a funiculus.

**funiculi** \fyoonik′yəlī\ Plural of FUNICULUS.

**funiculitis** \fyoonik′yəlī′tis\ [*funicul(us)* + -ITIS] **1** Inflammation of the spermatic cord. Also *corditis.* **2** Inflammation of a spinal nerve or of a nerve fiber tract within the spinal canal. **filarial f.** Lymphatic filariasis caused by *Wuchereria bancrofti* or *Brugia malayi* with secondary involvement of the spermatic cord.

**funiculopexy** \fyoonik′yəlōpek′sē\ [*funicul(us)* + *o* + -PEXY] Surgical correction of undescended testes by suturing the spermatic cord to surrounding tissue.

**funiculus** \fyoonik′yələs\ [L (dim. of *funis* a rope, cord), a thin rope] [NA] A small cordlike or bandlike structure, as of nerve fibers. Also *funicle.* **f. anterior medullae spinalis** [NA] The white matter of the spinal cord lying between the anterior median fissure and the ventral root entry zone and containing longitudinal ascending and descending tracts. Also *ventral funiculus, funiculus ventralis, anterior funiculus of spinal cord, columna ventralis medullae spinalis.* **cuneate f.** FASCICULUS CUNEATUS MEDULLAE OBLONGATAE. **f. cuneatus Burdachi** *Outmoded* FASCICULUS CUNEATUS MEDULLAE OBLONGATAE. **f. cuneatus lateralis** The longitudinal tract of the medulla oblongata that is lateral to the cuneate funiculus and demarcated laterally by the rootlets of the spinal accessory nerve. It contains afferent fibers from the upper cervical dorsal roots to the external cuneate nucleus, and some fibers of the dorsolateral tract of the spinal cord. **f. cuneatus medullae oblongatae** *Outmoded* FASCICULUS CUNEATUS MEDULLAE OBLONGATAE. **dorsal f.** FUNICULUS POSTERIOR MEDULLAE SPINALIS. **f. dorsalis** FUNICULUS POSTERIOR MEDULLAE SPINALIS. **f. gracilis** *Outmoded* FASCICULUS GRACILIS MEDULLAE OBLONGATAE. **f. gracilis medullae oblongatae** *Obs.* FASCICULUS GRACILIS MEDULLAE OBLONGATAE. **hepatic f.** *Outmoded* DUCTUS CHOLEDOCHUS. **hepatic f. of Rauber** ARTERIA HEPATICA PROPRIA. **f. lateralis medullae oblongatae** [NA] The medullary continuation of the lateral funiculus of the spinal cord, consisting principally of the anterolateral and spinocerebellar tracts. Also *lateral funiculus of medulla oblongata.* **f. lateralis medullae spinalis** [NA] The white matter of the spinal cord lateral to the dorsal and ventral horns, especially the ascending tracts. Also *lateral funiculus of spinal cord, anterolateral column, columna lateralis medullae spinalis.* **lateral f. of medulla oblongata** FUNICULUS LATERALIS MEDULLAE OBLONGATAE. **lateral f. of spinal cord** FUNICULUS LATERALIS MEDULLAE SPINALIS. **ligamentous f.** LIGAMENTUM COLLATERALE CARPI ULNARE. **funiculi medullae spinalis** Longitudinally oriented segments of the white matter of the spinal cord. Dorsal, lateral, and ventral funiculi are recognized.

Also *funiculi of spinal cord.* **f. posterior medullae spinalis** [NA] The longitudinal white matter between the posterior median sulcus and the dorsal root entry zone, consisting principally of myelinated ascending axons including a large component derived from spinal ganglion cells, most of which terminate in the cuneate and gracile nuclei of the medulla oblongata. It consists of two main components, the medial (gracile) and lateral (cuneate) fasciculi. Also *dorsal funiculus, funiculus dorsalis, posterior funiculus of spinal cord, columna dorsalis medullae spinalis.* **f. of Rolando** FASCICULUS OF ROLANDO. **f. separans** [NA] The oblique ridge on the caudal floor of the fourth ventricle of the medulla oblongata that separates the area postrema and the vagal trigone. **f. solitarius** TRACTUS SOLITARIUS. **f. spermaticus** [NA] The rounded cord extending from the deep inguinal ring and suspending the testis in the scrotum. It is composed of the testicular, cremasteric, and deferential arteries, the testicular veins and pampiniform plexus, lymph vessels, nerves, and the ductus deferens, which in their course through the inguinal canal become surrounded by the internal spermatic fascia, the cremasteric fascia, and the external spermatic fascia that extend down into the wall of the scrotum. Also *spermatic cord, chorda spermatica* (outmoded), *testicular cord.* **funiculi of spinal cord** FUNICULI MEDULLAE SPINALIS. **f. teres** The median eminence of the floor of the fourth ventricle of the medulla. *Obs.* **ventral f.** FUNICULUS ANTERIOR MEDULLAE SPINALIS. **f. ventralis** FUNICULUS ANTERIOR MEDULLAE SPINALIS.

**funis** \fyoo′nis\ [L, a rope, cord] **1** Any ropelike structure. **2** UMBILICAL CORD. **f. argenteus** *Obs.* MEDULLA SPINALIS. • The term derives from the spinal cord's fancied resemblance to a silver rope.

**funnel** \fun′əl\ [Provençal *fonilh* (from L *fundibulum*, variant of *infundibulum* a funnel, from *fundere* to pour) a funnel] **1** A device used to transfer or filter liquids that has a wide upper orifice and tapers, often in conical shape, to a narrow neck through which effluent flows in a controllable fashion. **2** An infundibulum. **muscular f.** The area bounded by the four rectus muscles of the eyeball. It resembles a funnel in shape. *Outmoded.* **pial f.** The adventitial sheath surrounding blood vessels leaving and entering the central nervous system, forming a funnel-shaped channel, the Virchow-Robin space, containing cerebrospinal fluid.

**FUO** fever of undetermined origin.

**Furacin** A proprietary name for nitrofurazone.

**furan** The heterocyclic compound whose molecule consists of a ring of four —CH= groups and an oxygen atom.

**furanose** A sugar in the 5-membered ring form produced by reaction of the 5-hydroxyl group with the aldehyde group in an aldose, or of the 6-hydroxyl group with the 2-carbonyl group in a ulose.

**furanoside** Any glycoside in which the sugar is in its furanose form, i.e. as a five-membered ring. Nucleosides are in the furanoside form, and fructosyl groups, as in sucrose, are usually furanosides.

**furazolidone** $C_8H_7N_3O_5$. 3-[[(5-Nitro-2-furanyl)methylene]amino]-2-oxazolidinone. An antibacterial and antiprotozoal agent that is used as both a topical anti-infective and as an oral antibacterial drug. It is specific for many Gram-negative enteric bacterial species. It is used in the treatment of diarrhea, enteritis, and, often with nifuroxime, candidal, bacterial, and trichomonal forms of vaginitis.

**furazolium** $C_9H_7N_3O_3S$. 6,7-Dihydro-3-(5-nitro-2-furanyl)-5*H*-imidazo[2,1-*b*]thiazolium. An antibacterial agent. It is also prepared as the tartrate and chloride salts.

**furazolium chloride** $C_9H_8ClN_3O_3S$. 6,7-Dihydro-3-(5-nitro-2-furanyl)-5*H*-imidazo[2,1-*b*]thiazol-4-ium chloride. An antibacterial agent.

**furazosin** \fyooraz′əsin\ PRAZOSIN.

**furca** \fur′kə\ [L, a fork] In anatomy, a fork, usually referring to a two-pronged fork.

**furcal** \fur′kəl\ Forklike; forked or branched. Also *furcate.*

**furcate** \fur′kāt\ FURCAL.

**furcation** \furkā′shən\ [Med L *furcatio* (from *furcare* to branch, from L *furca* a two-pronged fork) a branching, forking] A region of a multirooted tooth where the individual roots leave the common root stock.

**furcula** \fur′kyələ\ [L, dim. of FURCA] A forked ridge, like an inverted U, in the ventral wall of the primitive pharynx. The groove contained between the ridges of the furcula is continued downwards on the ventral wall of the foregut as the laryngotracheal groove from which the lower part of the larynx, trachea, bronchial tree, and lungs will eventually develop.

**furfur** [L, bran, scales on head, face, skin] A dry, branlike scale, such as that of pityriasis capitis.

**furfuraceous** Resembling furfur; scaling.

**furocoumarin** \fyoor′ōkoo′mərin\ PSORALEN.

**furor** \fyoo′rər\ [L (from *furere* to rage, rave), madness, raving, frenzy] Rage; agitation; frenzy.

**furosemide** $C_{12}H_{11}ClN_2O_5S$. 5-(Aminosulfonyl)-4-chloro-2-[(2-furanylmethyl)amino]benzoic acid, a diuretic that inhibits chloride and sodium reabsorption in the ascending loop of Henle. It is used to treat hypertension and to relieve edema that stems from cardiac, hepatic, or renal disease. It is given orally, but parenteral administration may be employed. Also *fursemide.*

**furrow** \fur′ō\ [Old English *furh*] A groove or v-shaped hollow; a sulcus. **atrioventricular f.** SULCUS CORONARIUS CORDIS. **digital f.** The flexure line on the anterior, or palmar, surface of any finger opposite the interphalangeal or metacarpophalangeal joints. **division f.** One of the ringlike indentations on an animal cell during cytokinesis, due to infolding of the plasma membrane. The cytoplasm beneath the division furrow contains a dense ring of microfilaments (the contractile ring) encircling the cell like a purse string. **genital f.** The groove on the caudal surface of the genital tubercle of the two month old fetus, which becomes the primary urethral groove. Also *genital groove.* **gluteal f.** CRENA ANI. **mentolabial f.** SULCUS MENTOLABIALIS. **nympholabial f.** The groove separating the labium majus and labium minus. **primitive f.** A longitudinal groove on the outer surface of the primitive streak. **Schmorl's f.** A variable linear depression across the surface of the apex of the lung thought to be secondary to developmental variation of the first rib. Some observers believe the associated pulmonary tissue to be more than normally susceptible to tuberculosis. **scleral f.** SULCUS SCLERAE. **Sibson's f.** The hollow between the lower border of the pectoralis major muscle and the thoracic wall. Also *Sibson's groove.* **skin f.'s** SULCI CUTIS.

**fursemide** FUROSEMIDE.

**Furst** [William *Furst*, U.S. physician, flourished mid-20th century] Ostrum-Furst syndrome. See under KLIPPEL-FEIL SYNDROME.

**Furth** [Jacob *Furth*, Hungarian-born pathologist active in the U.S., born 1896] See under TUMOR.

**furuncle** \fyoor′ungkl\ [L *furunculus* (dim. of *fur* a thief) a petty thief, a sap-stealing shoot or twig, a bump left where the twig has been pruned, a boil] A deep staphylococcal folliculitis. Also *furunculus, boil* (popular).

**furuncular** \fyoorung′kyələr\ FURUNCULOUS.

**furunculosis** \fyoorung′kyəlō′sis\ [*furuncul(us)* + -OSIS]

A condition marked by the presence of furuncles.

**furunculous** \fyoorung′kyələs\ Pertaining to a furuncle. Also *furuncular*.

**furunculus** \fyoorung′kyələs\ FURUNCLE.

**fury / alcoholic f.** PATHOLOGIC INTOXICATION.

***Fusarium*** \fyooser′ē·əm\ [New L, from L *fusus* a spindle] A form-genus of imperfect fungi, some of which are agents of mycotic keratitis.

**fuscin** \fus′in\ [L *fusc(us)* dark, dusky + -IN] The melanin pigment of the retinal pigment epithelium.

**fusicellular** \fyoo′sisel′yələr\ Composed of spindle-shaped cells. Also *fusocellular*.

**fusidic acid** $C_{16}H_{30}O_6$. A fermentation product derived from the fungus *Fusidium coccineum* and employed as an antibiotic.

**fusiform** \fyoo′sifôrm\ [L *fus(us)* spindle + *i* + -FORM] Shaped like a spindle; pointed at both ends.

**fusimotor** \fyoo′simō′tər\ **1** Denoting specificially the γ-efferent nerve fibers which innervate the intrafusal fibers of muscle spindles, in distinction to skeletofusimotor and skeletomotor fibers. **2** Denoting any motor innervation of intrafusal fibers. **3** Denoting the contractile activity of intrafusal fibers.

**fusion** \fyoo′zhən\ [L *fusio* (from *fusus*, past part. of *fundere* to pour) a pouring out] **1** Perception of a flickering light as a single, uninterrupted stimulus once the critical flicker frequency is reached. **2** The formation of an ankylosis. **3** Union of two adjacent tooth germs along their whole length or partially. This may result in a large abnormally-shaped tooth or two teeth united at crown or root level. In true fusion the dentin is confluent. Deciduous, permanent, or supernumerary teeth may be involved. **binocular f.** The cortical synthesis of the visual impulses of the same image from both eyes to form an integrated perceptual sensation. **cell f.** The merging of two cells to form one cell. When cells are grown *in vitro* the incidence of fusion is greatly increased by the presence of deactivated Sendai virus, which, by adhering strongly to cell surfaces holds cells together and thus increases the opportunity for fusion. **centric f.** A chromosome rearrangement in which the centromeres of two homologous or nonhomologous chromosomes fuse. It usually involves two acrocentric chromosomes with generation of a metacentric or submetacentric chromosome and a fragment that is composed of the satellites of the original chromosomes. The fragment is usually lost during the next mitosis. **diaphyseal-epiphyseal f.** The operative arrest of growth in the length of a bone by fusing the diaphysis and epiphysis. It is used in treating discrepancies in leg length. **flicker f.** The ability of the visual system to perceive a rapid alternation of light and dark as a steady and uniform illumination. This normally occurs when the alternation occurs more rapidly than at 50 Hz. **nuclear f.** The coalescence of two light atomic nuclei to form a single heavier one. Some of the combined mass disappears, being converted into energy. Because of repulsion between the two positively charged nuclei, strong forces must be present to drive them together. In thermonuclear fusion this is provided by exceedingly high thermal energy. **renal f.** FUSED KIDNEY. **spinal f.** The union of two or more vertebrae, congenitally as a result of infection, or due to a surgical operation designed to abolish motion between vertebrae. Also *vertebral fusion*.

***Fusobacterium*** \fyoo′sōbaktir′ē·əm\ [*fus(us)* + *o* + BACTERIUM] A genus of Gram-negative anaerobic rods with tapered ends, often found in human cavities and in abscesses. They differ morphologically from the genus *Bacteroides* (both being in the family Bacteroidaceae), and also in forming butyric acid as a major fermentation product. ***F. fusiformis*** The type species of *Fusobacterium*. It is a probable cause of Vincent's angina. Also *Fusobacterium nucleatum, Fusobacterium plautivincenti, Bacteroides fusiformis* (older term), *Bacillus fusiformis* (obs.), *Vincent's bacillus*.

**fusocellular** \fyoo′sōsel′yələr\ FUSICELLULAR.

**fusospirochetal** \fyoo′sōspī′rōkē′təl\ Pertaining to the association of *Fusobacterium* species and spirochetes in mixed infections.

**fusospirochetosis** \fyoo′sōspī′rōkētō′sis\ Infection with *Fusobacterium* species and spirochetes, involving most commonly the throat, mouth, and gums. These organisms may also be implicated in lung abscesses, vulvovaginitis, and balanitis. Also *fusospirochetal disease, fusospirillosis*. See also VINCENT'S ANGINA, NECROTIZING ULCERATIVE GINGIVITIS.

**fusus** \fyoo′səs\ [L, a spindle] (*pl.* fusi.) A minute, spindle-shaped object or part. **cortical fusi** The spindle-shaped air spaces in the cortex of the hair shaft. **fracture fusi** Clefts between the fibrils of the hair cortex which are produced by trauma. **f. neuromuscularis** MUSCLE SPINDLE. **f. neurotendineus** TENDON ORGAN.

**-fy** \-fī\ [from Old French *-fier*, suffix denoting to make, from L *-ficare*, from *facere* to make, do] A suffix meaning to make or form into.

# G

**G** **1** Symbol for giga-: used with SI units. **2** Symbol for glycine. **3** Symbol for guanosine. **4** gravitational constant. **5** gonidial (colony).

**$G_1$** A phase of the interphase stage of the cell cycle that precedes DNA synthesis (S phase).

**$G_2$** A phase of the interphase stage of the cell cycle that follows DNA synthesis (S phase) and precedes mitosis.

**g** Symbol for the unit, gram.

**g.** gravity.

**γ** The third letter of the Greek alphabet, gamma.

**GA** glutaric aciduria.
**Ga** Symbol for the element gallium.

**GABA** γ-aminobutyric acid.

**gadfly** \gad′flī\ Any of various biting, blood-sucking flies of the genus *Tabanus* or of the genus *Hypoderma,* such as the heel fly and ox-warble fly, which cause myiasis in cattle, deer, horses, and occasionally in man.

**gadolinium** A rare-earth metal having atomic number 64 and atomic weight 157.25. Seven isotopes occur naturally, six of them stable and the seventh, of 0.2% natural abundance, having a half-life of $1.1 \times 10^{14}$ years. Ten other unstable isotopes have been described. Symbol: Gd

**Gaffky** [Georg Theodor August *Gaffky,* German bacteriologist, 1850–1918] Gaffky table. See under SCALE.

**gag** [Middle English *gaggen* to strangle, of imitative origin] **1** An instrument for forcing open or holding open the mouth of the unconscious patient, particularly when under general anesthesia, and often designed to facilitate surgical access to the mouth, pharynx, and larynx. **2** To strain involuntarily to vomit; retch. **Davis g.** An instrument combining an incisor gag and tongue depressor, with the latter incorporating an anesthetic tube. It is used extensively in peroral surgery, particularly dissection tonsillectomy. The chief advantage lies in the manner of use. The gag is introduced and supported with the patient's head hyperextended and the shoulders raised, thereby reducing the risk of the inhalation of blood, which gravitates away from the lower air passages towards the nasopharynx. **Doyen g.** A widely used variety of incisor gag. **incisor g.** A mouth gag designed to act by application between the incisor teeth. **Mason g.** A widely used variety of molar gag. **molar g.** A mouth gag designed to act by application between the molar teeth.

**gage** \gāj\ GAUGE.

**gain** An increase in signal voltage or power from input to output in an electronic amplifier or system. **antigen g.** The appearance in cells of new antigenic determinants which were not normally present or expressed in the parent cell. **end g.** PARANOSIC GAIN. **epinosic g.** Those advantages, of a secondary nature, that may be derived from an illness or its symptoms, such as the attentiveness and overprotection showered on an invalid by family members. Also *secondary gain.* **near g.** Electronic amplification of echoes returning from structures close to the ultrasound transducer. **paranosic g.** The fundamental gain derived from an illness, such as the avoidance of anxiety in neurosis. Also *primary gain, paranosis, end gain.* **secondary g.** EPINOSIC GAIN. **swept g.** Compensation for the effects of attenuation by increasing gain with time from when a pulse was emitted by an ultrasound imaging system. Also *attenuation compensation, electronic distance compensation, time gain compensation.*

**Gairdner** [Sir William Tennant *Gairdner,* Scottish physician, 1824–1907] Gairdner's coin test. See under COIN SOUND.

**Gaisböck** [Felix *Gaisböck,* Austrian internist, 1868–1955] Gaisböck's disease, Gaisböck syndrome. See under STRESS ERYTHROCYTOSIS.

**gait** \gāt\ The way in which an individual walks. **antalgic g.** A form of gait in which the patient uses a cane, crutch, or other means to avoid painful weight-bearing. **ataxic g.** An unsteady gait, due as a rule either to cerebellar ataxia or to sensory ataxia. Also *staggering gait.* **cerebellar g.** A staggering, swaying, and unstable gait, like that of intoxication, seen in cases of bilateral or central cerebellar lesions. In truncal ataxia due to midbrain cerebellar lesions, the patient walks on a broad base and has difficulty in stopping and in turning. When the cerebellar syndrome is unilateral, there is a tendency to deviate to the affected side. **drag-to g.** A gait in which the patient drags an impaired lower limb towards the advanced crutch. **drunken g.** The ataxic gait seen in intoxication with alcohol or other drugs, such as barbiturates. Also *staggering gait, reeling gait.* **duck g.** MYOPATHIC GAIT. **equine g.** STEPPAGE GAIT. **festinating g.** A type of gait characteristic of some extrapyramidal syndromes and particularly of parkinsonism. It consists of involuntary acceleration of the gait, in which very small steps are taken (marche à petits pas), with the body leaning forward, as if chasing its center of gravity. Also *festination.* **footdrop g.** STEPPAGE GAIT. **four-point g.** A sequential gait pattern alternating a crutch or cane with placement of the opposite foot: right crutch, left foot, left crutch, right foot. **gluteal g.** The gait produced by paralysis of the gluteus medius muscle and characterized by marked tilting of the pelvis and trunk towards the affected side with every other step. This type of gait is seen particularly in patients with congenital hip dislocation. Also *Trendelenburg gait.* **gluteus maximus g.** A lurching backward movement of the trunk in order to place the center of gravity over the supporting limb, commonly used when there is weakness of the gluteus maximus on the side of that limb. **gluteus medius g.** A compensatory shifting of the trunk laterally, to the weakened gluteus medius side, in order to place the center of gravity closer to the supporting limb. **heel-toe g.** A normal walking pattern in which the heel strikes first and then the toes push off the surface. **hemiplegic g.** The gait of a patient with hemiplegia. The affected arm and hand are held flexed across the front of the trunk and there is extensor spasticity with circumduction of the affected leg. **myopathic g.** A type of gait in which the patient rolls from side to side in walking, with accentuation of the lumbar lordosis, as is seen in myopathy and in other neuromuscular disorders that cause weakness of the pelvic girdle musculature. Also *duck gait, waddling gait.* **paraparetic g.** The spastic gait seen in patients with spastic weakness of the lower limbs. **Petren g.** MARCHE À PETITS PAS. **reeling g.** DRUNKEN GAIT. **scissor g.** The type of spastic gait seen in patients with Little's disease in which with each step one leg crosses over in front of the other. Also *scissoring, cross-legged progression.* **skaters' g.** Walking accomplished with abrupt flinging movements of the arms and legs and with repeated flexion and extension of the trunk, as seen in some patients with Huntington's disease. **spastic g.** The gait which results from spasticity. When both lower limbs are spastic, the patient walks stiffly, scraping the feet along the ground. With severe spasticity, as in cerebral diplegia, the legs may cross each other alternately while walking ("scissors"). In hemiplegia there may be circumduction or dragging of the affected leg. **spastic equinus g.** A gait characterized by spastic and incoordinated movements of the lower limbs, with weight borne primarily on the forefoot since the ankles are plantar flexed. There is often associated adduction and internal rotation of the hips causing the knees and feet to turn inward. **staggering g.** **1** ATAXIC GAIT. **2** DRUNKEN GAIT. **stamping g.** TABETIC GAIT. **star g.** See under BABINSKI-WEILL TEST. **steppage g.** A gait in which the advancing foot is lifted high and the toes barely clear the ground or drag along the floor. It is due to paralysis of the anterior tibial muscles as in polyneuropathy and peroneal nerve injuries. Also *footdrop gait, equine gait.* **swaying g.** The ataxic gait of cerebellar ataxia. **swing-through g.** A gait in which both crutches are advanced to the same point and then the patient lifts both feet off the ground, swinging and landing ahead of the crutches. **swing-to g.** A gait in which both crutches are advanced and the patient then swings both limbs so that the feet are advanced the same distance as the crutches. **tabetic g.** A gait due to sensory ataxia in tabes dorsalis, in which steps are taken on a wide base with slapping of the feet heavily on descent. Often the subject watches his feet as he walks so that he will know where they are. Tabetic gait is due to posterior column disease with consequent loss of proprioception. Also *stamping gait.* **tandem g.** Heel-to-toe walking, used in neurology as a test for the presence of ataxia. **three-point g.** A gait pattern in which both crutches and the impaired lower limb are advanced together and then the uninvolved lower limb is advanced by itself. **Todd's g.** HELICOPODIA. **Trendelenburg g.** GLUTEAL GAIT. **two-point g.** A gait in which a crutch or cane is advanced together with the opposite lower limb. **waddling g.** MYOPATHIC GAIT.

**galact-** \gəlakt-, gal′akt-\ GALACTO-.

**galactagogin** \gəlak′təgäg′in\ HUMAN PLACENTAL LACTOGEN.

**galactagogue** \gəlak′təgäg\ [GALACT- + -AGOGUE] Any agent that promotes the flow of breast milk. Also *galactogogue, lactogogue.*

**galactemia** \gal′əktē′mē·ə\ The presence of milk in the blood.

**galactic** \gəlak′tik\ [Gk *galaktik(os)* (from *gala,* gen. *galaktos,* milk + *-ikos* -IC) pertaining to milk, milky] Of, pertaining to, denoting, or characteristic of breast milk.

**galactin** \gəlak′tin\ *Outmoded* PROLACTIN.

**galactitol** The achiral alcohol formed by reducing the —CHO group of galactose to —$CH_2$OH. It is formed in a type of galactosemia associated with a lack of galactokinase, and its accumulation leads to cataract formation in the eye. It is found in manna and other plant products. Also *dulcitol.*

**galacto-** \gəlak′tō-\ [Gk *gala,* gen. *galaktos* milk] A combining form meaning (1) milk; (2) milky, milklike; (3) galactose. Also *galact-.*

**galactocele** \gəlak′təsēl\ [GALACTO- + -CELE[2]] A mammary gland cyst containing milk, presumably caused by duct obstruction. Also *lactocele, lacteal cyst, milk cyst, lacteal tumor, galactoma.*

**galactocerebroside** A cerebroside whose hexose sugar is galactose, i.e. an *O*-galactosyl-*N*-acylsphingoid. Such compounds are the main cerebrosides of brain and myelin.

**galactography** \gal′əktäg′rəfē\ [GALACTO- + -GRAPHY] Radiographic examination of the mammary ducts after the injection of a radiopaque medium into them.

**galactokinase** The enzyme (EC 2.7.1.6) that catalyzes the phosphorylation of galactose to yield galactose 1-phosphate at the expense of ATP. This reaction enables galactose formed by digestion of lactose to be metabolized.

**galactolipid** Any lipid containing galactose residues. Many glycolipids of cell surfaces do so, with galactose linked either directly to a ceramide or through glucose. Galactolipids are found in the myelin sheath of nerves and in the brain.

**galactoma** \gal′əktō′mə\ [GALACT- + -OMA] GALACTOCELE.

**galactopexy** \gəlak′təpek′sē\ The incorporation of galactose into tissues.

**galactophlebitis** \-flebī′tis\ [GALACTO- + PHLEBITIS] PHLEGMASIA ALBA DOLENS.

**galactophorous** \gal′əktäf′ərəs\ LACTIFEROUS.

**galactopoiesis** \-poi·ē′sis\ LACTOGENESIS.

**galactopoietic** \-poi·et′ik\ LACTOGENIC.

**galactorrhea** \-rē′ə\ [GALACTO- + -RRHEA] Excessive or persistent flow of milk from the breasts due to a pathologic condition of either sex unrelated to the puerperium. Also *lactorrhea.*

**galactosamine** 2-Amino-2-deoxygalactose. A substance found widely as a constituent of glycoproteins. Its *N*-acetylated residues occur in chondroitin.

**galactose** A 6-carbon aldose sugar, differing from glucose in its configuration at C-4. It is a constituent of lactose, which is hydrolyzed by $\beta$-galactosidase to galactose and glucose. Galactose can subsequently give rise to glucose by an epimerization at C-4, but this involves the prior formation of UDP-galactose which then forms UDP-glucose.

**galactosemia** \-sē′mē·ə\ [*galactos(e)* + -EMIA] A metabolic defect in the conversion of galactose, a monosaccharide derived from lactose in milk, to glucose, due to a deficiency of galactose-1-phosphate uridyltransferase, which is one of four enzymes involved. The process takes place in the liver and in red cells in which an accumulation of galactose-1-phosphate is found and is suspected of being the toxic substance giving rise to clinical symptoms including the principal tetrad of hepatomegaly, cataracts, marasmus, and mental retardation. Galactosuria and amino-aciduria may result from possible renal damage. All these symptoms, except brain damage, may regress completely if the subject is placed on a galactose-free diet. Brain damage can be prevented by early diagnosis by demonstration of excess galactose-1-phosphate in the infant's red cells. In a family with a previously affected child, subsequent children should be tested for a galactokinase deficiency in the red cells of cord blood and given lactose-free milk until the result is known. The condition isinherited as an autosomal recessive trait. Also *galactokinase defect, congenital galactosemia in infants, hereditary galactose intolerance.*

**galactose-1-phosphate uridylyltransferase** The enzyme (EC 2.7.7.10) that transfers a uridylyl group from UDP-glucose onto the phosphate group of galactose 1-phosphate to form UDP-galactose and glucose 1-phosphate. The step is involved in lactose synthesis and in the metabolism of galactose derived from lactose. Also *phosphogalactose uridylyltransferase.*

**galactosidase** Any enzyme hydrolyzing galactosides. Thus $\beta$-galactosidases hydrolyze lactose. Study of the synthesis by bacteria of $\beta$-galatosidase and other enzymes concerned in lactose metabolism has revealed simultaneous control of transcription of related genes. Deficiency of various isomers results in the $GM_1$ gangliosidoses and in mucopolysaccharidosis IVB.

**galactoside** A compound containing a galactose residue whose aldehyde group is bound as an acetal with the hydroxyl group on C-5 or C-4 and with another alcohol.

**galactoside acetylase** An enzyme which transfers an acetyl group from acetylcoenzyme A to $\beta$-galactoses. The duction is under control of the Lac operon in *Escherichia coli.*

**galactoside permease** A membrane protein which is responsible for allowing galactoside to enter the cytoplasm. Production of this protein is controlled by the Lac operon in *Escherichia coli.*.

**galactosis** \gal′əktō′sis\ [GALACT- + -OSIS] LACTATION.

**galactosuria** \-soo′rē·ə\ [*galactos(e)* + -URIA] The excretion of galactose in the urine. This occurs only when the diet contains galactose.

**galactosyl** The group formed by removal of the hydroxyl group from C-1 of a ring (hemiacetal) form of galactose.

**galactotoxin** \-täk′sin\ A toxic substance of unknown composition found in decomposed milk. Also *galactotoxicon.*

**galacturia** \gal′əktoo′rē·ə\ [GALACT- + -URIA] *Obs.* CHYLURIA.

**Galant** [Ivan Borisovich *Galant,* Russian psychiatrist, born 1893] See under REFLEX.

**galea** \gā′lē·ə\ [L, a helmet] A structure shaped like a helmet. **g. aponeurotica** [NA] The fibrous membrane that not only joins the six component parts of the epicranius muscle to each other but is also anchored posteriorly to the external occipital protuberance and supreme nuchal line, anteriorly to the skin near the eyebrows, and laterally to muscles of the ear and to the zygomatic arch, thereby covering the calvaria deep to the superficial fascia of the scalp. Also *epicranial aponeurosis, galea, aponeurosis of occipitofrontal muscle, tendinous part of epicranius muscle.*

**Galeati** [Domenico Gusmano *Galeati,* Italian physician, 1686–1775] Galeati's glands. See under GLANDULAE INTESTINALES.

**Galeazzi** [Riccardo *Galeazzi,* Italian orthopedic surgeon, 1866–1952] See under FRACTURE.

**Galen** [Claudius *Galen,* Greek physician active in Rome, c. 130–200 A.D.] **1** See under FORAMEN. **2** Galen's ventricle. See under VENTRICULUS LARYNGIS. **3** Galen's veins. See under VENAE CARDIACAE ANTERIORES. **4** Galen's veins. See under VEIN. **5** Ansa of Galen, Galen's nerve, Galen's anastomosis. See under RAMUS COMMUNICANS NERVI LARYNGEI SUPERIORIS CUM NERVO LARYNGEO INFERIORE. **6** Great vein of Galen. See under VENA MAGNA CEREBRI.

**Galeotti** [Gino *Galeotti,* Italian bacteriologist, born 1867] Lustig-Galeotti vaccine. See under VACCINE.

**gall** \gôl\ [Old English *gealla* (akin to Old English *geolu* yellow) ] BILE. **ox g.** OX BILE EXTRACT.

**gallacetophenone** $C_8H_8O_4$. 2′,3′,4′-Trihydroxyacetophenone. A phenolic compound which is used as an antiseptic for external use only.

**gallamine triethiodide** $C_{30}H_{60}I_3N_3O_3$. 2,2′,2″-[1,2,3-Benzenetriyltris(oxy)]tris(*N,N,N*-triethylethanaminium] triiodide. A synthetic muscle relaxant that inhibits neurotransmission at the myoneural junction. It is given intravenously during surgical procedures, or for endoscopic or intubation operations. It may produce respiratory paralysis that requires artificial respiration. Its actions are reversed by neostigmine. Also *benzcurine iodide.*

**gallbladder** VESICA BILIARIS. **mobile g.** A gallbladder that is not attached to the ventral surface of the liver but is freely movable on the cystic duct or is restrained only by a ligamentous attachment. **phrygian cap g.** See under PHRYGIAN CAP. **sandpaper g.** Cholesterolosis of the gallbladder. **strawberry g.** The appearance of the gallbladder affected by cholesterolosis, in which a strawberrylike appearance develops due to the infiltration of cholesterol into the mucosa, with accompanying inflammation.

**Galli Mainini** [Carlos *Galli Mainini,* Argentinian physician, 1879–1943] Galli Mainini test. See under MALE FROG TEST.

**gallium** \gal′ē·əm\ A rare metallic element having atomic number 31 and atomic weight 69.737. It has a low melting point (29.78°C) and can exist as a liquid at room temperature. Two stable isotopes occur in nature and 12 unstable isotopes are known. Valences are 2 and 3. Gallium of-

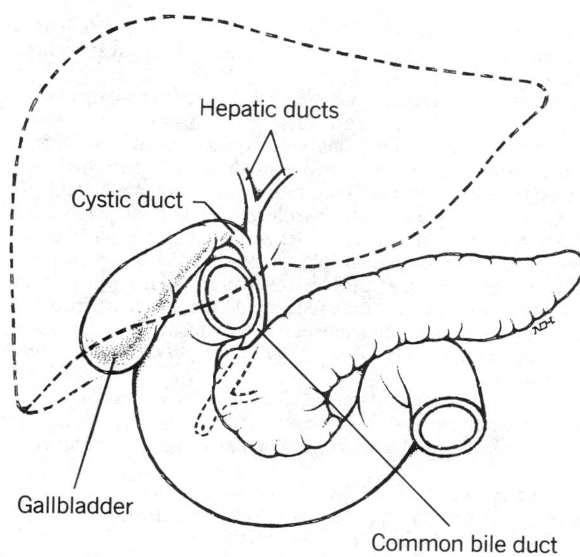


Gallbladder

ten accumulates in tumors and inflammatory processes. Symbol: Ga

**gallium 67** A radioactive isotope of gallium that decays by orbital electron capture. The half-life is 78.26 hours. Symbol: $^{67}$Ga

**gallium 68** A radioactive isotope of gallium that decays by positron emission and orbital electron capture. The half-life is 68.2 minutes. Symbol: $^{68}$Ga

**gallocyanin** A synthetic blue dye that is used together with chrome alum as a mordant to stain both DNA and RNA within cells.

**gallop** \gal′əp\ See under GALLOP RHYTHM. **atrial g.** The atrial component of a gallop rhythm. **$S_3$ g.** Gallop rhythm due to the presence of a third heart sound; ventricular gallop. **systolic g.** Gallop rhythm due to an extra sound during systole. **ventricular g.** Gallop rhythm due to ventricular filling; $S_3$ gallop.

**gallotannic acid** TANNIC ACID.

**gallstone** A concretion formed primarily of cholesterol, bile pigments, or a mixture of the two, found in the gallbladder or the biliary tree. Also *biliary calculus, cholelith.*

**Galton** [Francis *Galton,* English anthropologist, 1822–1911] **1** Galton system of classification of fingerprints. See under SYSTEM. **2** See under DELTA, WHISTLE. **3** Galton's law of regression. See under LAW.

**galvanic** \galvan′ik\ Pertaining to galvanism.

**galvanism** \gal′vənizm\ [after Luigi *Galvani,* Italian physician and physicist, 1737–1798 + -ISM] **1** Direct current electricity as that from a chemical battery. **2** GALVANO THERAPY. **dental g.** The formation of a painful electric current in the teeth by the presence of two dissimilar metals in the saliva, which acts as an electrolyte. An amalgam restoration in intermittent contact with a gold restoration may cause this effect.

**galvano-** \gal′vənō-\ [after Luigi *Galvani,* Italian physician and physicist, 1737-1798] A combining form designating galvanism or galvanic current.

**galvanocautery** \-kô′tərē\ ELECTRIC CAUTERY.

**galvanogustometer** \-gustäm′ətər\ An instrument for testing taste sensation by applying an electrical stimulus to the lingual mucosa.
**galvanoionization** \-ī′ənīzā′shən\ IONTOPHORESIS.
**galvanolysis** ELECTROLYSIS.
**galvanometer** \gal′vənäm′ətər\ [GALVANO- + -METER] An instrument for measuring a small electric current flowing through a wire or coil that moves in a magnetic field. The output is observed as the needle movement on a meter, deflection of a light beam, or deflection of a pen such as that on an electrocardiograph recorder. Also *rheometer.* **string g.** A thin thread of silvered quartz or platinum stretched in a strong magnetic field. An arc lamp projected the optically magnified movements to form the first electrocardiograph in 1901. Also *Einthoven's galvanometer, thread galvanometer.*
**galvanonarcosis** \-närkō′sis\ ELECTRONARCOSIS.
**galvanosurgery** \-sur′jərē\ [GALVANO- + SURGERY] The surgical use of an electric current to cut or cauterize tissue.
**galvanotaxis** \-tak′sis\ ELECTROTAXIS.
**galvanotherapy** \-ther′əpē\ The therapeutic use of galvanic electric currents. Also *galvanism.*
**galvanotonus** \-tō′nəs\ Muscular contraction induced by direct current. **nonpermanent g.** Nonsustained muscular contraction induced by direct current. **permanent g.** Sustained muscular contraction in response to direct current.
**gam-** \gam-\ GAMO-.
**gambir** \gam′bir\ CATECHU.
**gamblegram** \gam′bəlgram\ A bar graph representation of the electrolyte composition of body fluids in normal and diseased states.
**gamete** \gam′ēt\ [Gk *gametēs* a husband, *gametē* a wife, from *gamos* marriage] A mature cell with a haploid chromosome set that participates in sexual reproduction. Two gametes of opposite sex (in humans, the male sperm and the female ovum) fuse to form a diploid zygote.
**gametic** \gəmet′ik\ Referring to or of parallel function to a gamete.
**gameticidal** \gam′ətosī′dəl\ GAMETOCIDAL.
**gameticide** \gəmē′tisīd\ GAMETOCIDE.
**gameto-** \gam′ətō-\ [Gk *gametē* wife, *gametēs* husband] A combining form meaning gamete.
**gametoblast** \-blast\ [GAMETO- + -BLAST] *Obs.* SPOROZOITE.
**gametocidal** \gam′ətəsī′dəl\ [GAMETO- + *cid(e)* + -AL] Destructive to gametes or gametocytes. Also *gameticidal.*
**gametocide** \-sīd\ [GAMETO- + -CIDE] An agent that kills gametes or gametocytes. Also *gameticide.*
**gametocyte** \gəmē′təsīt\ [GAMETO- + -CYTE] A cell able to produce one or more sexual (haploid) progeny, the male or female gametes which undergo fusion to complete the sexual phase of reproduction. A great many types of such cells are found in both plants and animals, and many examples can be found among the sporozoan protozoa. Also *gamont.*
**gametocytemia** \gəmē′təsītē′mē·ə\ [*gametocyt(e)* + -EMIA] The presence of gametocytes, as, for example, of protozoan parasites, in the blood of the host.
**gametogenesis** \-jen′əsis\ The process of formation and maturation of gametes.
**gametogenic** \-jen′ik\ **1** Of or relating to gametogenesis. **2** Capable of gametogenesis.
**gametogony** \gam′ətäg′ənē\ [GAMETO- + -GONY] The gamete-producing stage in the sexual reproductive cycle, as in many protozoa, including *Plasmodium* species. In the latter, gametocytes are produced in the human blood stream. After ingestion by the mosquito vector, the gametes are released, leading to zygote formation, followed by growth of the oocyst from the zygote (ookinete) and production of great numbers of sporozoites. Also *gametogonia, gamogony.*
**gametoid** \gam′ətoid\ Resembling gametes; having characteristics of reproductive cells.
**gametophagia** \-fā′jə\ [GAMETO- + -PHAGIA] The elimination of the male or female element during conjugation of unicellular organisms. Also *gamophagia.*
**gametotropic** \-träp′ik\ [GAMETO- + -TROPIC[1]] Attracted to gametes; having an affinity for gametes.
**gamma** \gam′ə\ [third letter of the Gk alphabet] **1** The name of the third letter of the Greek alphabet. **2** A gamma ray or photon. **3** A unit of magnetic field strength equal to $10^{-5}$ oersted; 0.795 775 × $10^{-3}$ ampere per meter. An obsolete unit. Symbol: $\gamma$ **4** An obsolete, informal term for MICROGRAM.
**gammacism** \gam′əsizm\ A defect of speech, occurring mostly in younger children, in which the sounds represented by *g* and *k* are not articulated, being replaced by other sounds, usually that represented by *d*. It results in the "baby talk" of young children.
**Gammacorten** A proprietary name for dexamethasone.
**gamma-emitter** \gam′ə-\ Any nuclide that emits gamma photons.
**gamma globulin** See under GLOBULIN.
**gammaglobulinopathy** \gam′əgläb′yəlinäp′əthē\ GAMMOPATHY.
**gammexane** \gamek′sān\ LINDANE.
**gammography** \gamäg′rəfē\ Imaging by means of gamma radiation; scintigraphy. *Rare.* **cerebral g.** GAMMA ENCEPHALOGRAPHY.
**gammopathy** \gamäp′əthē\ [*gamm(a globulin)* + *o* + -PATHY] Any quantitative or qualitative abnormality of plasma immunoglobulins, such as agammaglobulinemia, hyperglobulinemia, and the monoclonal hypergammaglobulinemia associated with multiple myeloma. Also *immunoglobulinopathy, gammaglobulinopathy.* **benign monoclonal g.** MONOCLONAL GAMMOPATHY OF UNDETERMINED SIGNIFICANCE. **biclonal g.** A condition in which serum contains abnormal globulins that are derived from two separate clones of abnormally proliferating B lymphocytes. **monoclonal g.** An immunoproliferative disorder characterized by the abnormal proliferation of a single clone of lymphoid cells, which results in an excess of one specific class of immunoglobulins. Diseases in this category include multiple myeloma, macroglobulinemia, and heavy chain disease. **monoclonal g. of undetermined significance** A greater than normal serum concentration of immunoglobulin of type IgG or IgM, represented as a homogeneous single band on serum protein electrophoresis, of either kappa or lambda light chain type, but not both, in a patient who is otherwise well and without other evidence of myeloma. The monoclonal protein is usually less than 2.0 g/l. Plasma cells may be slightly increased in bone marrow, but they are not immature or myeloma cells. Bone lesions are absent. The condition is usually very indolent, but approximately 15% of patients ultimately develop myeloma or Waldenström's macroglobulinemia. Also *benign monoclonal gammopathy.*
**Gamna** [Carlo *Gamna*, Italian physician, 1886–1950] **1** Gamna-Favre bodies. See under MIYAGAWA BODIES. **2** Gamna nodules, Gandy-Gamna nodules. See under GAMNA-GANDY BODIES. **3** Gandy-Gamna spleen, Gamna's disease. See under SIDEROTIC SPLENOMEGALY.
**gamo-** \gam′ō-\ [Gk *gamos* marriage] A combining form

meaning (1) united, joined; (2) sexually united. Also *gam-*.

**gamogenesis** \gam′əjen′əsis\ SEXUAL REPRODUCTION.

**gamogony** \gamäg′ənē\ GAMETOGONY.

**gamont** \gam′änt\ GAMETOCYTE.

**gamophagia** \gam′əfā′jə\ [GAMO- + -PHAGIA] GAMETOPHAGIA.

**Gamper** [E. *Gamper,* Austrian neurologist, 1887–1938] See under REFLEX.

**gampsodactyly** \gamp′sōdak′təlē\ [Gk *gampso(s)* curved, having curved talons + DACTYL- + -Y] CLAW FOOT.

**Gamstorp** [Ingrid *Gamstorp,* Swedish pediatrician, flourished mid-20th century] Gamstorp's disease. See under PERIODIC PARALYSIS II.

**Gandy** [Charles *Gandy,* French physician, born 1872] **1** Gandy-Gamna nodules. See under GAMNA-GANDY BODIES. **2** Gandy-Nanta disease, Gandy-Gamna disease, Gandy-Gamna spleen. See under SIDEROTIC SPLENOMEGALY.

**gangli-** \gang′glē-\ GANGLIO-.

**ganglia** \gang′glē·ə\ Plural of GANGLION.

**ganglial** \gang′glē·əl\ GANGLIONIC.

**gangliectomy** \gang′glē·ek′təmē\ GANGLIONECTOMY.

**gangliitis** \gang·glē·ī′tis\ GANGLIONITIS.

**ganglio-** \gang′glē·ō-\ [Gk *ganglion* swelling, knot] A combining form meaning ganglion. Also *gangli-*.

**ganglioblast** \gang′glē·əblast′\ [GANGLIO- + -BLAST] One of the immature cells, similar to neuroblasts, which differentiate into the principal cells of nerve ganglia. Also *esthesioblast.*

**gangliocyte** \gang′glē·əsīt′\ [GANGLIO- + -CYTE] GANGLION CELL.

**gangliocytoma** \-sītō′mə\ [*gangliocyt(e)* + -OMA] A tumor of ganglion cells. Non-neoplastic glial elements may be present.

**ganglioglioma** \-glī·ō′mə\ [GANGLIO- + GLIOMA] A tumor of ganglion cells and neoplastic glial cells. Also *glioneuroma, ganglionic glioma, neuroastrocytoma, neuroglioma ganglionare.*

**ganglioglioneuroma** \-glī′ōn$^y$Urō′mə\ [GANGLIO- + GLIO- + NEUROMA] A tumor of ganglion cells, glial cells, and nerve fibers.

**gangliolytic** \-lit′ik\ **1** GANGLIOPLEGIC. **2** Denoting a substance capable of destroying ganglion cells.

# ganglion

**ganglion** \gang′glē·än\ [Gk *ganglion* a knot, swelling] (*pl.* ganglia, ganglions) **1** [NA] An aggregation of neuron cell bodies in the peripheral nervous system, such as the sensory root ganglia and the autonomic ganglia. Also *neuroganglion, nerve ganglion.* **2** A knot or mass of connective or nerve tissue, or a cystic swelling containing jellylike fluid rich in mucopolysaccharides, arising from the synovium of a tendon on the dorsum of the wrist or foot, or within a semilunar cartilage of a knee. Also *peritendinitis serosa.* **accessory ganglia** GANGLIA INTERMEDIA. **acoustic g.** **1** A ganglion mass differentiated in the embryo from the cranial neural crest lying between the rhombencephalon and the developing labyrinth. It is formed from the caudal part of the larger acousticofacial ganglion and divides into two parts, the cochlear (spiral) ganglion and the vestibular ganglion. Also *vestibulocochlear ganglion.* **2** GANGLION SPIRALE COCHLEAE. **acousticofacial g.** An embryonic ganglion-mass arising from neural crest cells and initially common to the seventh and eighth cranial nerves. At the 7 mm stage in man (end of the fourth week) the cranial portion of the ganglion-mass separates to become the geniculate ganglion of the facial nerve. The caudal portion becomes the acoustic (vestibulocochlear) ganglion which divides into two parts, the vestibular and the cochlear (spiral) ganglia. **Andersch g.** GANGLION INFERIUS NERVI GLOSSOPHARYNGEI. **ganglia aorticorenalia** [NA] The semidetached inferior extension of the ganglia of the celiac plexus. Also *aorticorenal ganglion, nephrolumbar ganglia* (obs.). **Arnold's g.** **1** GANGLION OTICUM. **2** GLOMUS CAROTICUM. **auditory g.** GANGLION SPIRALE COCHLEAE. **Auerbach's g.** Any of the small aggregates of parasympathetic ganglion cells of the myenteric plexus (Auerbach's plexus). Also *Auerbach's node.* **auricular g.** *Seldom used* GANGLION OTICUM. **autonomic ganglia** Any of the visceral ganglia associated with the sympathetic or parasympathetic nervous system. **azygous g.** GANGLION IMPAR. **basal ganglia** The nuclear masses of gray matter in the cerebrum, comprising the corpus striatum (caudate, putamen, and globus pallidus) and the amygdaloid complex, sometimes including the claustrum and septal nuclei. Also *basal nuclei.* **Bezold's g.** A linear aggregation of parasympathetic ganglion cells in the interatrial septum. **Bidder's ganglia** VENTRICULAR GANGLIA. **Blandin's g.** GANGLION SUBMANDIBULARE. **Bochdalek's g.** A ganglionlike structure containing no ganglion cells and located on the superior alveolar nerve. Also *ganglion bochdalekii.* • The structure was described by the Czech anatomist V.A. Bochdalek in 1855, and is believed to be the plexus dentalis superior. **Bock's g.** INFERIOR CAROTID GANGLION. **Böttcher's g.** GANGLION SPIRALE COCHLEAE. **cardiac ganglia** GANGLIA CARDIACA. **ganglia cardiaca** [NA] Parasympathetic ganglia of the cardiac plexus lying between the aortic arch and the bifurcation of the pulmonary artery. Also *cardiac ganglia, Wrisberg's ganglion.* **carotid g.** **1** GLOMUS CAROTICUM. **2** INFERIOR CAROTID GANGLION. **ganglia celiaca** [NA] A pair of large sympathetic prevertebral ganglia within the diaphragmatic celiac plexus located on the upper part of the abdominal aorta. They innervate the stomach, spleen, liver, gallbladder, and the small and large intestines. Also *celiac ganglia, solar ganglia.* **cerebrospinal ganglia** The ganglia associated with the afferent cranial and spinal nerve roots, containing the cell bodies of sensory neurons. They differ from other ganglia in lacking dendrites and synapses on their cell bodies. **g. cervicale inferius** A portion of the ganglion cervicothoracicum (stellate ganglion). Also *inferior cervical ganglion.* **g. cervicale medium** [NA] The small middle cervical sympathetic ganglion at about the level of the cricoid cartilage. Its postganglionic axons innervate the cervical region, upper extremity, and heart. Also *inferior thyroid ganglion, middle cervical ganglion.* **g. cervicale superius** [NA] The largest and most rostral ganglion of the sympathetic trunk, lying anterior to the second and third cervical vertebrae between the internal carotid artery and the internal jugular vein. Also *superior cervical ganglion.* **cervical g. of uterus** A parasympathetic ganglion near the uterine cervix. Also *Lee's ganglion, Frankenhäuser's ganglion, cervicouterine ganglion.* **g. cervicothoracicum** [NA] The sympathetic ganglion at the seventh cervical level, usually partially fused with the first thoracic ganglion. Its postganglionic axons innervate the heart, upper extremity, neck, and head. Also *cervicothoracic* *ganglion, stellate ganglion.* **cervicouterine g.** CERVICAL GANGLION OF UTERUS. **g. ciliare** [NA] A small parasympathetic ganglion lying in the posterior orbit between the optic nerve and external rectus muscle. Its postganglionic axons innervate the ciliary muscle and the pupillary sphincter. Also *lenticular ganglion* (obs.), *Schacher's ganglion* (seldom used), *ciliary ganglion, ophthalmic ganglion, optic ganglion, orbital ganglion.* **ciliary g.** GANGLION CILIARE. **Cloquet's g.** A ganglion of the nasopalatine nerve, the existence of which has been questioned. **coccygeal g.** GANGLION IMPAR. **collateral g.** Any of the sympathetic ganglia of the mesenteric plexus surrounding the abdominal aorta and its major branches. **compound g.** A cystic swelling of a tendon sheath that is constricted by a ligament around the sheath. **Corti's g.** GANGLION SPIRALE COCHLEAE. **Darkschewitsch's g.** *Obs.* NUCLEUS OF DARKSCHEWITSCH. **diaphragmatic ganglia** GANGLIA PHRENICA. **diffuse g.** A swelling, usually on the dorsum of the hand or wrist, composed of tendon sheath, synovium, and synovial fluid. **dorsal root g.** GANGLION SPINALE. **g. of duct of Botallo** NODUS LIGAMENTIS ARTERIOSI. **Ehrenritter's g.** GANGLION SUPERIUS NERVI GLOSSOPHARYNGEI. **g. extracraniale** GANGLION INFERIUS NERVI GLOSSOPHARYNGEI. **g. of facial nerve** GANGLION GENICULI. **false g.** An enlargement of a peripheral nerve not containing ganglion cells. **Frankenhäuser's g.** CERVICAL GANGLION OF UTERUS. **Froriep's g.** A transient embryonic dorsal root ganglion related to the metencephalon and probably to the structures of the fourth occipital somite. **Gasser's g.** GANGLION TRIGEMINALE. **gasserian g.** GANGLION TRIGEMINALE. **g. geniculi** [NA] The intracranial sensory ganglion of the facial nerve root associated with the nervus intermedius gustatory receptors of the anterior two thirds of the tongue. Also *ganglion of facial nerve, geniculate ganglion.* **g. of habenulae** The habenular nuclear complex of the thalamus, derived from the embryonic epithalamus. **hepatic g.** An autonomic ganglion located near the hepatic artery. **Huber's g.** A cerebrospinal ganglion sometimes found at the $C_1$ level. There is usually no sensory ganglion at this level in man and other higher mammals. *Obs.* **hypogastric ganglia** *Imprecise* GANGLIA PELVINA. **hypoglossal g.** A ganglion associated with sensory fibers of the twelfth cranial nerve. The ganglion is present at one stage of embryonic development but regresses and is rarely seen in the adult. **g. impar** [NA] The unpaired, most caudal ganglion of the sympathetic trunk, lying in front of the coccyx. Also *coccygeal ganglion, Walther's ganglion, azygous ganglion.* **inferior carotid g.** A small ganglion on the ventral surface of the internal carotid artery in the cavernous sinus. Also *Bock's ganglion, Laumonier's ganglion, Schmiedel's ganglion, carotid ganglion.* **inferior cervical g.** GANGLION CERVICALE INFERIUS. **inferior g. of glossopharyngeal nerve** GANGLION INFERIUS NERVI GLOSSOPHARYNGEI. **inferior jugular g.** GANGLION INFERIUS NERVI GLOSSOPHARYNGEI. **inferior mesenteric g.** GANGLION MESENTERICUM INFERIUS. **inferior petrosal g.** GANGLION INFERIUS NERVI GLOSSOPHARYNGEI. **inferior thyroid g.** GANGLION CERVICALE MEDIUM. **inferior vagal g.** GANGLION INFERIUS NERVI VAGI. **inferior g. of vagus** GANGLION INFERIUS NERVI VAGI. **g. inferius nervi glossopharyngei** The lower of the two sensory ganglia on the glossopharyngeal nerve at the site of its entrance into the jugular foramen. Also *ganglion petrosum, petrous ganglion, petrosal ganglion, ganglion extracraniale, Andersch ganglion, inferior ganglion of glossopharyngeal nerve, inferior jugular ganglion, inferior petrosal ganglion, lower ganglion of glossopharyngeal nerve.* **g. inferius nervi vagi** The large inferior sensory ganglion of the vagus located below the jugular foramen at the level of the first and second cervical vertebrae. Also *nodose ganglion, ganglion nodosum, inferior vagal ganglion, inferior ganglion of vagus, lower ganglion of vagus nerve.* **intercarotid g.** *Outmoded* GLOMUS CAROTICUM. **intercrural g.** NUCLEUS INTERPEDUNCULARIS. **ganglia intermedia** Small aggregates of sympathetic ganglion cells on the rami communicantes in the cervical, lower thoracic, and upper lumbar levels of the spinal cord. Also *accessory ganglia, intermediate ganglia.* **intermediary g.** *Outmoded* GANGLION VERTEBRALE. **intermediate ganglia** GANGLIA INTERMEDIA. **interpeduncular g.** NUCLEUS INTERPEDUNCULARIS. **g. intervertebrale** GANGLION SPINALE. **intracranial g.** GANGLION SUPERIUS NERVI GLOSSOPHARYNGEI. **g. isthmi** *Obs.* NUCLEUS INTERPEDUNCULARIS. **g. jugulare nervi vagi** GANGLION SUPERIUS NERVI VAGI. **jugular g. of glossopharyngeal nerve** GANGLION SUPERIUS NERVI GLOSSOPHARYNGEI. **jugular g. of vagus nerve** GANGLION SUPERIUS NERVI VAGI. **Küttner's g.** A constant, large lymph node, belonging to the superior deep cervical group, that lies on the internal jugular vein at the point where it is crossed by the posterior belly of the digastric muscle, to which a large number of marginal lymphatic vessels of the tongue converge. **Langley's g.** A collection of ganglion cells found in the hilus of the submandibular gland of most mammals. **Laumonier's g.** INFERIOR CAROTID GANGLION. **Lee's g.** CERVICAL GANGLION OF UTERUS. **lenticular g.** *Obs.* GANGLION CILIARE. **lesser g. of Meckel** GANGLION SUBMANDIBULARE. **lingual g.** *Obs.* GANGLION SUBMANDIBULARE. **Lobstein's g.** GANGLION SPLANCHNICUM. **Loetwig's g.** BULBUS CORDIS. **lower g. of glossopharyngeal nerve** GANGLION INFERIUS NERVI GLOSSOPHARYNGEI. **lower g. of vagus nerve** GANGLION INFERIUS NERVI VAGI. **Ludwig's g.** A small parasympathetic ganglion of the cardiac interatrial plexus innervating the right atrium. **ganglia lumbalia** [NA] The four or five pairs of lumbar sympathetic ganglia on the border of the psoas muscles. Also *lumbar ganglia.* **Luschka's g.** GLOMUS COCCYGEUM. **maxillary g.** *Outmoded* GANGLION SUBMANDIBULARE. **Meckel's g.** GANGLION PTERYGOPALATINUM. **Meissner's g.** The numerous aggregates of parasympathetic ganglion cells in the submucosal plexus (of Meissner). **g. mesentericum inferius** [NA] The inferior ganglion of the sympathetic prevertebral chain in the inferior mesenteric plexus, innervating the descending and sigmoid colon. Also *inferior mesenteric ganglion.* **g. mesentericum superius** [NA] One or more paired sympathetic ganglia forming part of the celiac ganglion at the origin of the superior mesenteric artery. Also *superior mesenteric ganglion.* **middle cervical g.** GANGLION CERVICALE MEDIUM. **g. of Müller** GANGLION SUPERIUS NERVI GLOSSOPHARYNGEI. **nasal g.** GANGLION PTERYGOPALATINUM. **nephrolumbar ganglia** *Obs.* GANGLIA AORTICORENALIA. **nerve g.** GANGLION. **g. nervi splanchnici** GANGLION SPLANCHNICUM. **nodose g.** GANGLION INFERIUS NERVI VAGI. **g. nodosum** GANGLION INFERIUS NERVI VAGI. **olfactory g.** BULBUS OLFACTORIUS. **ophthalmic g.** GANGLION CILIARE. **optic g.** GANGLION CILIARE. **orbital g.** GANGLION CILIARE. **g. oticum** [NA] A parasympathetic ganglion, located below the foramen ovale medial to the mandibular nerve, that innervates the parotid gland and receives preganglionic fibers from the glossopharyngeal nerve via the lesser petrosal nerve. Also *otic ganglion, auricular ganglion* (seldom used), *Arnold's ganglion, splanchnic ganglion of Arnold, otoganglion* (seldom used). **parasympathetic ganglia** The peripheral postganglionic, cholinergic ganglia innervated by preganglionic neurons of the brainstem and middle (second to fourth) sacral segments of the spinal cord. **paravertebral g.** One of the ganglia of the thoracolumbar sympathetic trunk. **pelvic ganglia** GANGLIA PELVINA. **ganglia pelvina** [NA] The parasympathetic and sympathetic ganglia within the pelvic plexus of both sides. Also *pelvic ganglia, hypogastric ganglia* (imprecise). **periosteal g.** A ganglion cyst occurring in a subperiosteal location. **petrosal g.** GANGLION INFERIUS NERVI GLOSSOPHARYNGEI. **g. petrosum** GANGLION INFERIUS NERVI GLOSSOPHARYNGEI. **petrous g.** GANGLION INFERIUS NERVI GLOSSOPHARYNGEI. **ganglia phrenica** [NA] The small aggregates of sympathetic ganglion cells of the phrenic plexus adjacent to the celiac plexus. Also *diaphragmatic ganglia, phrenic ganglia.* **ganglia plexuum autonomicorum** [NA] Aggregates of ganglion cells of autonomic plexuses such as the sympathetic celiac and inferior mesenteric ganglia, along with the parasympathetic ganglia of the myenteric plexus. Also *ganglia of sympathetic plexuses.* **ganglia plexuum sympathicorum** Aggregates of sympathetic postganglionic neurons lying in plexuses of autonomic fibers. **posterior root g.** GANGLION SPINALE. **prevertebral ganglia** The irregular aggregates of sympathetic ganglia lying anterior to the vertebral column in the mesenteric plexuses of the thorax and abdomen surrounding the abdominal aorta and its main visceral branches. **prostatic g.** A ganglion of the prostatic plexus lying on the prostate gland. **pterygopalatine g.** GANGLION PTERYGOPALATINUM. **g. pterygopalatinum** [NA] The small parasympathetic ganglion in the upper pterygopalatine fossa. Its preganglionic innervation is via the greater petrosal nerve, and its postganglionic axons innervate the lacrimal, palatine, and nasal glands. Also *sphenopalatine ganglion, ganglion sphenopalatinum, Meckel's ganglion, nasal ganglion, pterygopalatine ganglion.* **Remak's g.** 1 SINOATRIAL GANGLION. 2 A sympathetic ganglion on the inferior vena cava at the diaphragm. 3 A ganglion of the gastric plexus. **ganglia renalia** [NA] Small, scattered, sympathetic ganglia in the renal plexus. Also *renal ganglia.* **g. retinae** The outer portion of the internal nuclear layer of the retina, containing bipolar, horizontal, and amacrine cells. **Ribes g.** The most rostral sympathetic ganglion on the anterior communicating artery of the brain. It is rarely seen. **ganglia sacralia** [NA] The three or four ganglia of the sacralpart of the sympathetic trunk. Also *sacral ganglia.* **Scarpa's g.** GANGLION VESTIBULARE. **Schacher's g.** *Seldom used* GANGLION CILIARE. **Schmiedel's g.** INFERIOR CAROTID GANGLION. **semilunar g.** 1 GANGLION TRIGEMINALE. 2 Either of the ganglia celiaca. **g. semilunare gasseri** GANGLION TRIGEMINALE. **sensory g.** GANGLION SPINALE. **sinoatrial g.** A sympathetic ganglion in the cardiac sinoatrial wall near the superior vena cava. Also *Remak's ganglion.* **sinus g.** A small collection of parasympathetic neurons found near the point of entrance of the coronary sinus into the right atrium. *Seldom used.* **solar ganglia** *Outmoded* GANGLIA CELIACA. **sphenopalatine g.** GANGLION PTERYGOPALATINUM. **g. sphenopalatinum** GANGLION PTERYGOPALATINUM. **spinal g.** GANGLION SPINALE. **g. spinale** [NA] The sensory ganglion of each spinal dorsal root, containing neuron cell bodies whose peripheral neurites form or contact so-

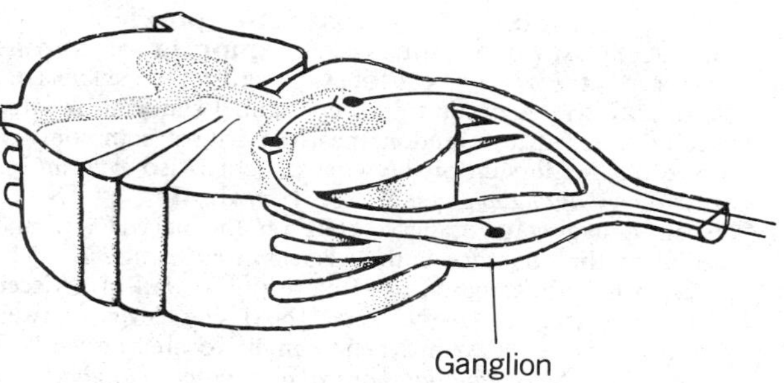


**Spinal (dorsal root) ganglion**

matosensory end organs in the skin, deep tissue, and viscera. Also *dorsal root ganglion, posterior root ganglion, sensory ganglion, spinal ganglion, ganglion intervertebrale.* **g. spirale cochleae** [NA] The olongate, spiral ganglion of the cochlear division of the eighth nerve within the temporal bone modiolus. Its peripheral axons terminate in the spiral organ (of Corti), and its central root ends in the brainstem cochlear nuclear complex. Also *auditory ganglion, acoustic ganglion, Corti's ganglion, spiral ganglion, spiral ganglion of cochlear nerve, ganglion spirale nervi cochleae, ganglion spirale partis cochlearis nervi octavi, Böttcher's ganglion.* **splanchnic g.** GANGLION SPLANCHNICUM. **splanchnic g. of Arnold** GANGLION OTICUM. **g. splanchnicum** [NA] The variable small sympathetic ganglion on the greater splanchnic nerve at the $T_{12}$ vertebral level innervating portions of the gastrointestinal tract. Also *splanchnic ganglion, splanchnic ganglion of Lobstein, ganglion nervi splanchnici, Lobstein's ganglion.* **stellate g.** GANGLION CERVICOTHORACICUM. **g. sublinguale** A ganglion constituted by some parasympathetic nerve cells which are occasionally found on fibers running distally from the submandibular ganglion to the lingual nerve. It is believed to be distributed to the sublingual salivary gland but its function is not yet clearly understood. Also *sublingual ganglion of Blandin.* **g. submandibulare** [NA] A small parasympathetic ganglion on the lingual nerve above the submandibular gland. It controls salivary secretion of the submandibular and sublingual glands, receiving preganglionic fibers via the chorda tympani of the facial nerve. Also *submandibular ganglion, ganglion submaxillare, Blandin's ganglion, lesser ganglion of Meckel, lingual ganglion, maxillary ganglion.* **superior carotid g.** A sympathetic ganglion of the upper internal carotid plexus. **superior cervical g.** GANGLION CERVICALE SUPERIUS. **superior g. of glossopharyngeal nerve** GANGLION SUPERIUS NERVI GLOSSOPHARYNGEI. **superior mesenteric g.** GANGLION MESENTERICUM SUPERIUS. **superior g. of vagus nerve** GANGLION SUPERIUS NERVI VAGI. **g. superius nervi glossopharyngei** [NA] The upper of the two sensory ganglia on the glossopharyngeal nerve in the jugular foramen. Also *superior ganglion of glossopharyngeal nerve, Ehrenritter's ganglion, intracranial ganglion, ganglion superius, ganglion of Müller, jugular ganglion of glossopharyngeal nerve.* **g. superius nervi vagi** [NA] The small sensory ganglion on the vagus nerve in the jugular foramen. Its peripheral processes extend into the vagus, meningeal, and auricular nerves. Also *jugular ganglion of vagus nerve, superior ganglion of vagus nerve, ganglion jugulare nervi vagi.* **suprarenal g.** A small sympathetic ganglion of the celiac portion of the prevertebral plexus supplying the adrenal gland. **ganglia of sympathetic plexuses** GANGLIA PLEXUUM AUTONOMICORUM. **ganglia of sympathetic trunk** GANGLIA TRUNCI SYMPATHICI. **synovial g.** A cystic tumor containing synovial-like fluid, usually attached to a tendon sheath and most commonly observed on the dorsum of the wrist or foot. Also *synovial cyst, myxoid cyst, ganglion cyst.* **g. terminale** **1** [NA] A dispersed aggregate of nerve cells on the nervus terminalis medial to the olfactory bulb. Also *terminal ganglion.* **2** A parasympathetic ganglion in or close to the wall of a visceral organ. **ganglia thoracica** [NA] The eleven or twelve paired paravertebral sympathetic ganglia located at the heads of the ribs. Also *ganglia thoracalia, thoracic ganglia.* **g. trigeminale** [NA] A large sensory ganglion on the portio major of the trigeminal nerve, containing segments for the ophthalmic, maxillary, and mandibular nerves. It lies on the anterior slope of the petrous pyramid and is partially surrounded by an extension of the subarachnoid space (cavum trigeminale). Also *semilunar ganglion, ganglion semilunare gasseri, Gasser's ganglion, gasserian ganglion, trigeminal ganglion, ganglion of trigeminal nerve.* **Troisier's g.** An enlarged supraclavicular lymph node associated with a mediastinal tumor. **ganglia trunci sympathici** [NA] The ganglia of the sympathetic trunk extending from the superior cervical ganglion caudally to the ganglion impar. Also *ganglia of sympathetic trunk.* **g. tympanicum** [NA] A ganglion on the tympanic branch of the glossopharyngeal nerve in the petrous portion of the temporal bone. Also *tympanic ganglion.* **Valentin's g.** **1** A ganglion on the superior alveolar nerve. Also *tympanic ganglion of Valentin.* **2** An enlargement on the tympanic branch of the glossopharyngeal nerve. **ventricular ganglia** Aggregates of parasympathetic ganglion cells in the inferior portion in the interatrial septum of the heart. Also *Bidder's ganglia.* **g. vertebrale** [NA] A small, variable sympathetic ganglion between the middle cervical ganglion and the cervicothoracic ganglion. Its postganglionic fibers are distributed in the brachial plexus and in the vertebral nerve and plexus. Also *vertebral ganglion, intermediary ganglion* (outmoded). **g. vestibulare** [NA] The sensory ganglion of the vestibular portion of the eighth nerve, located in the internal auditory meatus. It innervates the sensory epithelium of the saccule, utricle, and semicircular canal, and its central processes terminate in the medullary vestibular nuclei. Also *vestibular ganglion, Scarpa's ganglion, vestibular end organ* (outmoded). **vestibulocochlear g.** ACOUSTIC GANGLION. **Walther's g.** GANGLION IMPAR. **Wrisberg's g.** GANGLIA CARDIACA. • This ganglion should not be confused with the geniculate ganglion associated with the nervus intermedius (nerve of Wrisberg).

**ganglionated** \gang′glē·ənā′tid\ Denoting structures, especially visceral ones, containing ganglia.

**ganglionectomy** \-nek′təmē\ [GANGLION + -ECTOMY] Excision of a ganglion. Also *gangliectomy.*

**ganglioneuroblastoma** \-nʸUr′əblastō′mə\ A tumor of varying degrees of malignancy composed of a mixture of neuroblasts and ganglion cells in various stages of differentiation. As in neuroblastoma, the majority occur along the thoracolumbar sympathetic chain or in the adrenal gland. They are most common in children under five years of age. In rare cases maturation into a ganglioneuroma occurs. Increased catecholamine levels may be observed. Also *gangliosympathicoblastoma.*

**ganglioneurofibroma** \-nʸUr′əfībrō′mə\ A neurofibroma with ganglion cells. Also *ganglionic neuroma.* **melanogenic g.** A ganglioneurofibroma containing melanin.

**ganglioneuroma** \-nʸUrō′mə\ [GANGLIO- + NEUROMA] A benign tumor composed of mature ganglion cells associated with well-differentiated neurofibromatous elements. Also *neurofibroma gangliocellulare, neurofibroma ganglionare, ganglionic neuroma, neuroma verum, neuroganglioma.* **dumbbell g.** HOURGLASS TUMOR. **hourglass g.** HOURGLASS TUMOR.

**ganglioneuromatosis** \-nʸUr′əmatō′sis\ Multiple widespread ganglioneuromas.

**ganglionic** \gang′glē·än′ik\ Pertaining to a ganglion. Also *ganglial.*

**ganglionitis** \-nī′tis\ [GANGLION + -ITIS] Nonspecific inflammation of an autonomic ganglion. Also *gangliitis.* **acute posterior g.** HERPES ZOSTER. **gasserian g.** HERPES OPHTHALMICUS.

**ganglionoplegic** \gang′glē·än′əplē′jik\ GANGLIOPLEGIC.

**ganglionostomy** \-näs′təmē\ [GANGLION + *o* + -STOMY] A surgical procedure that creates an opening into a cystic lesion on a tendon sheath, particularly on the dorsum of the wrist.

**ganglioplegic** \-plē′jik\ A chemical substance that blocks conduction in autonomic ganglia. Also *gangliolytic, ganglionoplegic.*

**ganglioside** [GANGLI- + *-os(e)*[2] + -IDE[1]] Any glycolipid consisting of a ceramide glycosylated with an oligosaccharide that contains at least one residue of sialic acid. Such glycolipids are important components of cell membranes. **g. GM$_1$** A ganglioside consisting of ceramide glycosylated by a particular oligosaccharide. This oligosaccharide contains five residues: one of glucose, two of galactose, one of *N*-acetylgalactosamine, and one of *N*-acetylneuraminic acid. **g. GM$_2$** A ganglioside related to ganglioside GM$_1$ by lacking a terminal galactose residue.

**gangliosidoses** \-sīdō′sēz\ Plural of GANGLIOSIDOSIS.

**gangliosidosis** \-sīdō′sis\ Any of the several inborn errors of ganglioside metabolism that cause an accumulation of gangliosides in nervous tissue, primarily in lysosomes. They are due in all but one case to a deficit of a catabolic enzyme. One synthetic defect is known. Also *ganglioside lipidosis.* **general g.** GM$_1$ GANGLIOSIDOSIS. **GM$_1$ g.** Any of several inborn errors of ganglioside GM$_1$ catabolism. All are autosomal recessive, result in neuronal and somatic accumulation of GM$_1$ gangliosides, and are associated with GM$_1$ $\beta$-galactosidase deficiency. Several distinct, and apparently allelic, disorders are known, which have widely variable phenotypes and ages of onset. The most severe begins in early infancy and causes severe skeletal changes and rapid neurologic deterioration. Also *general gangliosidosis, neurovisceral lipidosis.* **GM$_2$ g.** TAY-SACHS DISEASE.

**gangliosympathectomy** \-sim′pəthek′təmē\ Ganglionectomy of sympathetic ganglia.

**gangliosympathicoblastoma** \-simpath′əkōblastō′mə\ GANGLIONEUROBLASTOMA.

**Gangolphe** [Louis *Gangolphe,* French surgeon, 1858–1920] See under SIGN.

**gangosa** \gang·gō′sə\ [Spanish, from *gangoso* speaking with a nasal twang; of onomatopoeic origin] A form of treponematosis, tertiary yaws. Ulceration occurs in the nasal and palatal structures and nasopharynx, which it ultimately destroys. It is found in any region in which yaws is endemic, particularly Africa, South America, southeast Asia, and the Pacific. Also *rhinopharyngitis mutilans, ogo, kaninloma.*

**gangrene** \gang′grēn\ [L *gangraena* , from Gk *gangraina* (akin to *grainein* to gnaw) gangrene] A form of coagulative necrosis principally due to ischemia that is modified by the liquefactive action of bacteria and polymorphonuclear leukocytes. **chemical g.** Tissue necrosis resulting from the application or injection of various chemical agents. It is seen with extravasation of vasoactive drugs and, in drug abusers, from the inadvertent intra-arterial injection of intravenous preparations. **circumscribed g.** Gangrene that is demarcated from the surrounding viable tissue by an inflammatory rim. **cold g.** DRY GANGRENE. **cutaneous g.** Necrosis of the skin. **decubital g.** BEDSORE. **diabetic g.** Gangrene due to peripheral vascular insufficiency associated with diabetes mellitus. It most commonly affects the toes or feet, rarely the fingers. **disseminated cutaneous g.** GANGRENOUS DERMATITIS OF INFANTS. **dry g.** A type of gangrene where coagulative necrosis predominates, resulting in mummification of the affected tissue. The liquefactive action of bacteria and leukocytes is minimal or absent. Also *cold gangrene.* **embolic g.** Gangrene due to embolic occlusion of the arterial supply of a tissue. **emphysematous g.** GAS GANGRENE. **epidemic g.** Gangrene resulting from ergotism, which formerly occurred in epidemics caused by local consumption of contaminated grain. **Fournier's g.** FOURNIER'S DISEASE. **gas g.** Gangrene characterized by a fulminant, painful, and severely toxic infection, typically in a wound, by any of several species of the anaerobic bacterium *Clostridium,* especially *C. welchii,* with putrefaction of tissue and the formation of gas. Surgery is the usual treatment. Also *progressive emphysematous necrosis, emphysematous gangrene.* **hospital g.** BEDSORE. **hot g.** INFLAMMATORY GANGRENE. **humid g.** WET GANGRENE. **inflammatory g.** Gangrene that develops as a complication of inflammation. Also *hot gangrene.* **ischemic g.** A condition of one or more digits or the skin of the distal foot in far-advanced arterial insufficiency, where actual tissue necrosis has occurred. In dry gangrene the dead tissue has simply mummified, while in wet gangrene, secondary infection has occurred, threatening the more proximal limb. **Meleney synergistic g.** PROGRESSIVE POSTOPERATIVE GANGRENE. **moist g.** WET GANGRENE. **oral g.** CANCRUM ORIS. **presenile spontaneous g.** Gangrene due to thromboangiitis obliterans. **pressure g.** BEDSORE. **primary g.** Gangrene occurring in a tissue not previously inflamed. **progressive g.** Gangrene lacking demarcation from healthy tissue and which continues to expand. **progressive bacterial synergistic g.** A superficial, spreading infection, often following surgery, due to synergistic multiplication of microaerophilic streptococci and *Staphylococcus aureus* and resulting in destruction of tissue. **progressive postoperative g.** Cutaneous gangrene caused by a microaerophilic streptococcus in a rare complication of an abdominal surgical wound. Also *Meleney synergistic gangrene.* **secondary g.** Gangrene developing within an inflammatory focus. **senile g.** A form of dry gangrene of the lower extremities seen in the elderly and resulting from advanced occlusive atherosclerosis. **static g.** Gangrene resulting from severe venous stasis. Also *venous gangrene.* **thrombotic g.** Gangrene as a consequence of arterial thrombosis. **traumatic g.** Gangrene resulting from traumatic injury that interferes with the blood supply to the affected region. **trophic g.** Gangrene developing in part of an extremity which has been deprived of sensory innervation and in which trophic changes have occurred. **venous g.** STATIC GANGRENE. **wet g.** A form of gangrene in which the necrotic tissues are soft, edematous, and inflamed. It is commonly the result of bacterial infection. Also *moist gangrene, humid gangrene.*

**gangrenous** \gang′grənəs\ Pertaining to or characterized by gangrene.

**ganja** \gän′jä\ MARIHUANA.

**ganoblast** \gan′ōblast\ AMELOBLAST.

**Ganong** [William Francis *Ganong,* U.S. physiologist, born 1924] Lown-Ganong-Levine syndrome. See under SHORT PR SYNDROME.

**Ganser** [Sigbert Joseph Maria *Ganser,* German psychiatrist, 1853–1931] **1** Ganser state, Ganser symptom. See under GANSER SYNDROME. **2** Commissure of Ganser. See under DORSAL SUPRAOPTIC COMMISSURE.

**Gant** [Frederick James *Gant,* English surgeon, 1825–1905] See under LINE.

**gantry** \gan′trē\ The cylindrical opening located at or near the center of an imaging scanner into which the subject is placed.

**Ganz** [William *Ganz,* U.S. cardiologist,born 1919] Swan-Ganz catheter. See under CATHETER.

**gap** / **air-bone g.** The difference between the impaired air-conduction auditory threshold and the better or normal bone-conduction threshold. It is indicative of middle-ear pathology. **anion g.** The excess of unmeasured anions over unmeasured cations, comprising the negative charges contributed by phosphates, sulfates, and other metabolites. It is approximated by subtracting the sum of chloride and bicarbonate anions from the sum of sodium and potassium cations. The normal range of 12 to 18 mEq/liter is exceeded in ketoacidosis, severe alcohol toxicity, lactic acidosis, renal failure, and in many toxic ingestions. Also *cation-anion difference.* **auscultatory g.** A period of silence, in the measurement of blood pressure by sphygmomanometry, following the initial period of sounds as the pressure falls in the manometer. It is mainly encountered in hypertension and aortic stenosis. Also *silent gap.* **Bochdalek's g.** PLEUROPERICARDIAL HIATUS. **chromatid g.** In cytogenetics, a region of a chromatid which is euchromatic and which, presumably because of less compact packing of chromatin, does not stain in usual cytologic preparations but which is more extensive than an unstained band. A gap does not disrupt the continuity of the chromatid. Gaps on human karyotypes are termed marker sites, markers, or fragile sites. **silent g.** AUSCULTATORY GAP.

**Gardner** [Eldon John *Gardner,* U.S. geneticist, born 1909] Fitzgerald-Gardner syndrome. See under GARDNER SYNDROME.

**garg.** *gargarismus* (L, gargle).

**gargalanesthesia** \gär′gəlan′esthē′zhə\ Absence of sensibility for tickle.

**gargalesthesia** \gär′glesthē′zhə\ [Gk *gargal(os)* a tickling, itching + ESTHESIA] The sense of tickle. Adj. gargalesthetic.

**gargle** [Middle French *gargouiller* to gurgle, of onomatopoeic origin] **1** To rinse the throat by agitating fluid there with the head back, the soft palate being caused to vibrate against the back of the tongue by a controlled expiration. **2** A preparation, usually medicated, with which to rinse the throat.

**gargoylism** \gär′goilizm\ [English *gargoyl(e)* (from Old French *gargouille* throat, waterspout, gargoyle) + -ISM] *Outmoded* MUCOPOLYSACCHARIDOSIS IH. **X-linked recessive g.** *Outmoded* MUCOPOLYSACCHARIDOSIS II.

**Garland** [Hugh *Garland,* English neurologist, flourished mid-20th century] Marinesco-Garland syndrome, Marinesco-Sjögren-Garland syndrome. See under MARINESCO-SJÖGREN SYNDROME.

**garment** / **elastic g.** Any of several specially measured and fitted elastic bandages used to provide constant pressure over a healed burn in hopes of reducing hypertrophic scarring.

**Garré** [Karl *Garré,* Swiss surgeon and bacteriologist,

1857–1928] Garré's disease, Garré's osteitis. See under NONSUPPURATIVE OSTEOMYELITIS.

**garrot** \gar′ət, gərōt′\ [French (from the Germanic), a tourniquet] SPANISH WINDLASS.

**Gartner** [Hermann Treschow *Gartner*, Danish anatomist, 1785–1827] **1** See under CYST. **2** Gartner's duct. See under LONGITUDINAL DUCT OF EPOÖPHORON.

**gas** [a term invented by Jean-Baptiste van Helmont, Belgian chemist, 1577–1644; suggested by Gk *chaos* chaos, space] A substance in the state of matter in which its molecules are widely dispersed and spend only a small fraction of time in strong interaction with each other (collision). **alveolar g.** Air that has been subjected to gas exchange with pulmonary blood through the epithelium of the lung alveoli. Also *alveolar air.* **blood g.** Gas dissolved in blood. **carrier g.** A gas, usually oxygen with or without nitrous oxide, used as a conveyor of liquid anesthetics that have been vaporized for inhalation. **choking g.** SUFFOCATING GAS. **hemolytic g.** ARSINE. **inert g.** Any gas unreactive under specified experimental conditions, sometimes nitrogen, but usually one of the noble gases, as these are particularly inert. **lacrimator g.** TEAR GAS. **laughing g.** NITROUS OXIDE. **marsh g.** See under METHANE. **nerve g.** Any of a group of organophosphate compounds which interfere with the central, peripheral, and parasympathetic nervous systems by inhibiting cholinesterase. **premixed g.** A fixed combination of gases, as oxygen and nitrous oxide, in compressed gas cylinders, used for analgesia or general anesthesia. **sewer g.** The mixture of gases and vapors formed in a sewer as a result of the decomposition of organic matter in the sewage. If not properly vented, toxic amounts of hydrogen sulfide may accumulate. **sneezing g.** DIPHENYLCHLORARSINE. **suffocating g.** A war gas which causes extreme damage to the lungs and respiratory tract. Also *choking gas.* **sweet g.** CARBON MONOXIDE. **tear g.** A volatile fluid that is dispersed in the air to induce tearing and irritation of the eyes as a means of temporarily disabling a person or controlling a crowd. Also *lacrimator, lacrimator gas.* **war g.** A chemical warfare agent, either a true gas or a finely dispersed liquid or solid, which produces a toxic or strongly irritant effect. On the basis of physiologic action there are five classes of war gas: lacrimators, lung irritants, sternutators, systemic poisons, and vesicants.

**gaseous** \gas′ē·əs, gash′əs\ Of the nature of gas.

**Gaskell** [Walter Holbrook *Gaskell*, English physiologist, 1847–1914] Gaskell's bridge. See under FASCICULUS ATRIOVENTRICULARIS.

**gasometry** \gasäm′ətrē\ The measurement of gas volume, either as constituents of a gaseous mixture or as the product evolved in an analytic reaction.

**gasp** [Middle English *gaspen* to gasp, from Old Norse *geispa* to yawn] A short, sharp inspiration of air.

**Gasser** [Johann Ludwig *Gasser*, Austrian anatomist, 1723–1765] **1** Gasserian syndrome. See under GASSERIAN GANGLION SYNDROME. **2** Ganglion semilunare Gasseri, Gasser's ganglion. See under GANGLION TRIGEMINALE.

**gasserectomy** \gas′ərek′təmē\ [*gasser(ian ganglion)* + -ECTOMY] Excision of the gasserian ganglion of the trigeminal nerve.

**Gastaut** [Henri Jean-Pascal *Gastaut*, French biologist, born 1915] Gastaut's disease. See under LENNOX-GASTAUT SYNDROME.

**gaster** \gas′tər\ [Gk *gastēr* belly] [NA] The most dilated part of the digestive tube, situated in the upper part of the abdominal cavity and extending from the cardiac orifice at the termination of the esophagus to the pyloric orifice that opens into the duodenum. It presents two borders, namely, the greater and lesser curvatures; and two surfaces, namely, anterosuperior and posteroinferior; and its body separates the fundus at the proximal end from the pyloric antrum distally. Also *ventriculus, stomach.*

**gaster-** \gas′tər-\ GASTERO-.

**-gaster** \-gastər\ [Gk *gastēr* belly] A combining form meaning (1) stomach or digestive tract; (2) belly, abdomen.

**gastero-** \gas′tərō-\ [Gk *gastēr* belly] A combining form meaning stomach or digestive tract. Also *gaster-*.

***Gasterophilus intestinalis*** \gas′təräf′iləs intes′tənal′is\ A species of horse botfly which deposits its eggs on hairs mainly of a horse's shoulders and forelegs. Human infection also occurs, producing a form of cutaneous larva migrans. The newly hatched larvae penetrate human skin and produce visible, tortuous dermal burrows. These larvae, about 1–2 mm long, do not develop beyond the first stage and usually can easily be surgically removed from the skin. In the horse the larval bots attach to the cardiac part of the gastric mucosa but even large numbers of them are well tolerated.

**gastr-** \gastr-\ GASTRO-.

**gastralgia** \gastral′jə\ [GASTR- + -ALGIA] STOMACHACHE.

**gastramine** BETAZOLE HYDROCHLORIDE.

**gastrectomy** \gastrek′təmē\ [GASTR- + -ECTOMY] A surgical procedure in which all or part of the stomach is removed. **antecolic g.** A surgical procedure in which all or part of the stomach is removed and the loop of jejunum that bears the efferent loop is sutured anterior to the transverse colon. **physiologic g.** A procedure in which gastric function is arrested either chemically, neurologically, or by means of a limited resection.

**gastric** \gas′trik\ [GASTR- + -IC] Affecting, originating in, or relating to the stomach.

**gastrin** \gas′trin\ [GASTR- + -IN] A gastrointestinal hormone, the most powerful known stimulant of gastric acid secretion. It is located in G cells of the gastric antrum and proximal duodenum, less abundantly in the small and large intestinal mucosa and in delta cells of the islets of Langerhans. Gastrin release is stimulated after eating, vagus nerve activation, or insulin hypoglycemia and is secreted excessively in the Zollinger-Ellison syndrome. Also *gastric secretin.*

**gastrinoma** \gas′trinō′mə\ [GASTRIN + -OMA] An endocrine tumor which produces gastrin. It occurs most frequently in the pancreas, less often in the duodenum, and rarely in the stomach. It morphologically resembles the carcinoid or the islet cell tumor. It may be malignant. Gastrin overproduction can lead to the Zollinger-Ellison syndrome. Also *G-cell tumor, G-cell carcinoid.*

**gastritic** \gastrit′ik\ Affected by or relating to gastritis.

**gastritis** \gastrī′tis\ [GASTR- + -ITIS] Inflammation of the mucosal lining of the stomach. **antral g.** Gastritis primarily affecting the gastric antrum. **atrophic g.** Idiopathic, chronic gastritis characterized by diffuse atrophy of the mucosa, loss of the normal rugal folds, and diminished or absent production of gastric acid and intrinsic factor, which may lead to pernicious anemia. It is also associated with an increased risk of gastric cancer. Also *Fenwick's disease.* **catarrhal g.** Inflammation and hypertrophy of the mucosal lining of the stomach associated with secretion of excessive quantities of mucus and gastric juices. **corrosive g.** Acute necrotizing destructive gastritis following ingestion of highly concentrated acid or alkaline agents. Also *chemical gastritis.* **erosive g.** Gastritis with erosions or ulcerations of the gastric mucosa. Also *exfoliative gastritis.* **giant hypertrophic g.** MÉNÉTRIER'S DISEASE.

**granulomatous g.** Gastritis characterized by the presence of a granulomatous mucosal infiltrate such as may occur in patients with tuberculosis, sarcoidosis, or regional enteritis. **hypertrophic g.** MÉNÉTRIER'S DISEASE. **phlegmonous g.** SUPPURATIVE GASTRITIS. **pseudomembranous g.** Inflammation of the stomach characterized by formation of a pseudomembrane over the gastric mucosa. **radiation g.** Gastritis from exposure to radiation, usually x-ray irradiation. **suppurative g.** Severe inflammation of the stomach caused by transmural purulent infection of the gastric wall. Also *phlegmonous gastritis.* **toxic g.** Gastritis secondary to drug, toxin, or corrosive injury. **uremic g.** Inflammation of the stomach occurring in association with renal failure and characterized by a variety of pathologic findings, varying from mucosal petechiae to superficial ulceration and submucosal hemorrhage, and by clinical symptoms such as anorexia, nausea, and vomiting.

**gastro-** \gas′trō-\ [Gk *gastēr* belly] A combining form denoting (1) stomach; (2) belly, abdomen. Also *gastr-*.

**gastroacephalus** \-əsef′ələs\ [GASTRO- + Gk *a-* priv. + -CEPHALUS] Unequal conjoined twins in which an acephalic parasite is attached at the abdomen of the host.

**gastroanastomosis** \-ənas′tōmō′sis\ [GASTRO- + ANASTOMOSIS] GASTROGASTROSTOMY.

**gastrocamera** \-kam′ərə\ [GASTRO- + CAMERA] A small photographic instrument which may be passed into the stomach to record the state of the gastric mucosa. It is now largely replaced by fiberoptic endoscopes.

**gastrocele** \gas′trəsēl\ [GASTRO- + -CELE[1]] A hernia involving a part of the stomach.

**gastrocnemius** \gas′trəkē′m\ [New L (from Gk *gastroknēmē* the calf, from *gast(ē)r* belly + *knēmē* leg, shank) pertaining to the calf] MUSCULUS GASTROCNEMIUS.

**gastrocoele** \gas′trəsēl\ [GASTRO- + -COELE] ARCHENTERON.

**gastrocolic** \-käl′ik\ Relating to or connecting the stomach and the colon.

**gastrocolostomy** \-kōläs′təmē\ [GASTRO- + COLO- + -STOMY] The surgical creation of an opening between the colon and the stomach. Such an opening may rarely occur spontaneously after trauma, inflammation, or formation of a neoplasm.

**gastrocolotomy** \-kōlät′əmē\ [GASTRO- + COLO- + -TOMY] A surgical procedure in which an incision is made into the stomach and colon.

**gastrodisciasis** \-disī′əsis\ [*Gastrodisc(us)* + -IASIS] Infection with *Gastrodiscoides hominis,* a trematode that inhabits the cecum and the colon of cynomolgus monkeys, pigs, and man in India, Asia, and the Philippines. It is characterized by mild, mucoid diarrhea.

***Gastrodiscoides*** \-diskoi′dēz\ [alter. of *Gastrodiscus*] A genus of amphistome trematodes parasitic in the intestine of humans and other mammals. The species *Gastrodiscoides hominis* (formerly called *Gastrodiscus hominis* and *Amphistomum hominis*) has been reported to occur in humans, rodents, and certain primates in southeast Asia, India, and the Philippines. It is a cone-shaped, fleshy, pink worm typical of the family Paramphistomatidae (though it is sometimes placed in a separate family, Gastrodiscidae). The planorbid snail *Helicorbus coenosus* has served in India as an experimental intermediate host. Transmission to humans is presumed to be via metacercariae encysted on aquatic plants.

***Gastrodiscus hominis*** \-dis′kəs häm′ənis\ See under *GASTRODISCOIDES.*

**gastroduodenal** \-d^yoo′ədē′nəl\ Relating to or connecting the stomach and the duodenum.

**gastroduodenectomy** \-d^yoo′ədənek′təmē\ [GASTRO- + DUODEN- + -ECTOMY] A surgical procedure in which a part or all of the duodenum and stomach are removed.

**gastroduodenitis** \-d^yoo′ədənī′tis\ [GASTRO- + DUODEN- + -ITIS] Inflammation of the stomach and duodenum, often peptic in origin.

**gastroduodenoenterostomy** \-d^yoo′ədē′nō·en′təräs′təmē\ [GASTRO- + DUODENOENTEROSTOMY] A surgical procedure that creates an opening between the stomach, the duodenum, and the small bowel following a resection or bypass procedure. Usually created surgically, it may rarely result from a spontaneous traumatic, neoplastic, or inflammatory process.

**gastroduodenoscopy** \-d^yoo′ədənäs′kəpē\ [GASTRO- + DUODENO- + -SCOPY] Examination of the interior of the stomach and duodenum by means of a gastroscope.

**gastroduodenostomy** \-d^yoo′ədənäs′təmē\ [GASTRO- + DUODENO- + -STOMY ] A surgical procedure involving a resection or bypass that creates an opening between the stomach and the duodenum. It may occur spontaneously after trauma, neoplasm, or inflammatory disease, but this is rare.

**gastrodynia** \-din′yə\ [GASTR- + -ODYNIA] STOMACHACHE.

**gastroenteric** \-enter′ik\ Pertaining to or connecting the stomach and small intestine.

**gastroenteritis** \-en′tərī′tis\ [GASTRO- + ENTERITIS] A syndrome characterized by gastrointestinal symptoms, including nausea and vomiting, diarrhea, and abdominal discomfort, and usually viral, bacterial, or parasitic in origin. There may or may not be inflammation of the intestinal tract. **acute infectious g.** Acute inflammation of the stomach and small intestine due to viral or bacterial infection. **eosinophilic g.** A form of gastroenteritis with eosinophilia of the peripheral blood, eosinophilic infiltration of the lamina propria of the stomach and small intestine, and varying amounts of abdominal pain, diarrhea, and malabsorption. **infantile g.** A form of gastroenteritis common in children in the first two or three years of life, and characterized by acute vomiting and diarrhea leading to dehydration. There is a high mortality rate among victims, particularly in communities with a low socioeconomic standard. The infecting agent may be bacterial or viral. Also *summer diarrhea* (outmoded), *cholera infantum, epidemic diarrhea in children.*

**gastroenteroanastomosis** \-en′tərō·ənas′təmō′sis\ [GASTRO- + ENTERO- + ANASTOMOSIS] GASTROENTEROSTOMY.

**gastroenterocolitis** \-en′tərōkōlī′tis\ [GASTRO- + ENTEROCOLITIS] Inflammation of the stomach, the small intestine, and the colon.

**gastroenterocolostomy** \-en′tərōkōläs′təmē\ [GASTRO- + ENTEROCOLOSTOMY] A surgical procedure involving a bypass or resection that creates an opening between the stomach, the small bowel, and the large bowel. Rarely, it may occur spontaneously after trauma, neoplasm, or inflammatory disease.

**gastroenterologic** Of or pertaining to gastroenterology.

**gastroenterologist** \-en′təräl′əjist\ A specialist in gastroenterology.

**gastroenterology** \-en′təräl′əjē\ [GASTRO- + ENTERO- + -LOGY] The branch of medicine dealing with the function and disorders of the stomach, small and large intestines, esophagus, pancreas, liver, and biliary tract.

**gastroenteropathy** \-en′təräp′əthē\ [GASTRO- + ENTEROPATHY] Any disorder of the stomach or small or large bowel.

**gastroenteroplasty** \-en′tərōplas′tē\ Any plastic operation involving the stomach and an adjacent segment of small intestine.

**gastroenterostomy** \-en′tərăs′təmē\ [GASTRO- + ENTERO- + -STOMY] A surgical procedure involving a resection or bypass that creates an opening between the stomach and the small bowel. Although it may occur spontaneously after trauma, neoplasm formation, or inflammation, such cases are rare. Also *gastroenteroanastomosis, gastronesteostomy.* **Roux en Y g.** A surgical procedure involving a bypass or resection, using a defunctionalized Y-shaped jejunal limb to create a connection between the stomach and the small bowel. Also *Roux's gastroenterostomy, Roux-Y gastrojejunostomy.*

**gastroenterotomy** \-en′tərăt′əmē\ [GASTRO- + ENTERO- + -TOMY] A surgical incision into the stomach and the small bowel.

**gastroepiploic** \-ep′iplō′ik\ [GASTRO- + EPIPLOIC] Pertaining to the stomach and the greater omentum.

**gastroesophageal** \-ēsăf′əjē′əl\ Pertaining to the stomach and the esophagus.

**gastroesophagitis** \-ēsăf′əjī′tis\ [GASTRO- + ESOPHAG- + -ITIS] Inflammation, usually peptic in origin, of the stomach and the esophagus.

**gastroesophagoplasty** \-ēsăf′əgōplas′tē\ [GASTRO- + ESOPHAGO- + -PLASTY] Any plastic operation on the lower end of the esophagus and the cardiac end of the stomach, usually for the relief of stricture or reflux esophagitis. Also *fundoplasty.* See also FUNDOPLICATION.

**gastroesophagostomy** \-ēsăf′əgăs′təmē\ A surgical procedure, involving a resection or bypass, that creates an opening between the stomach and the esophagus. It may result from trauma, neoplasm, or inflammation, but this is rare. Also *esophagogastrostomy, esophagogastroanastomosis.*

**gastrofiberscope** \-fī′bərskōp\ FIBEROPTIC GASTROSCOPE.

**gastrogastrostomy** \-gasträs′təmē\ [GASTRO- + GASTRO- + -STOMY] A surgical procedure involving a partial gastric resection or biopsy, creating an opening between two parts of the stomach. Also *gastroanastomosis.*

**gastrogavage** \-gaväzh′\ [GASTRO- + GAVAGE] Feeding via nasogastric intubation.

**gastrogenic** \-jen′ik\ Originating in the stomach.

**gastrograph** \gas′trəgraf\ [GASTRO- + -GRAPH] An instrument for recording gastric motility. Also *gastrokinesograph.*

**gastrohydrorrhea** \-hī′drôrē′ə\ Gastric hypersecretion.

**gastroileitis** \-il′ē·ī′tis\ [GASTRO- + ILEITIS] Inflammation of the stomach and the ileum.

**gastroileostomy** \-il′ē·äs′təmē\ A surgical anastomosis of the stomach to the ileum. Such a connection, which has no therapeutic use and causes death from malnutrition, has occasionally been made erroneously in place of a gastrojejunostomy.

**gastrointestinal** \-intes′tənəl\ Relating to the stomach and the intestines.

**gastrojejunoesophagostomy** \-jəjoo′nō·ēsäf′əgäs′təmē\ ESOPHAGOJEJUNOGASTROSTOMOSIS.

**gastrojejunostomy** \-jəjoonäs′təmē\ A surgical anastomosis creating a direct connection between the stomach and the jejunum. **Roux-Y g.** ROUX EN Y GASTROENTEROSTOMY.

**gastrokinesograph** \-kīnē′sōgraf\ GASTROGRAPH.

**gastrolavage** \-ləväzh′\ [GASTRO- + LAVAGE] Irrigation of the stomach via a nasogastric tube.

**gastrolienal** \-lī′ənəl\ Relating to or connecting the stomach and the spleen; gastrosplenic.

**gastrolithiasis** \-lithī′əsis\ [GASTRO- + LITHIASIS] A condition characterized by the tendency to form gastric calculi.

**gastrology** \gasträl′əjē\ [GASTRO- + -LOGY] That branch of medical science devoted to the study of the stomach and its diseases.

**gastrolysis** \gasträl′isis\ [GASTRO- + LYSIS] A surgical procedure in which the adhesions that surround the stomach are lysed in preparation for a gastric resection or to expose perigastric structures.

**gastromalacia** \-məlā′shə\ A softening of the gastric wall usually involving the mucosa and submucosa, commonly an incidental autopsy finding indicating advanced autolysis.

**gastromelus** \gasträm′ələs\ [GASTRO- + Gk *melos* limb] Unequal conjoined twins in which the parasitic member is represented by a supernumerary limb attached to the abdomen of the host.

**gastromenia** \-mē′nē·ə\ [GASTRO- + *men(o)-* + -IA] Gastric hemorrhage as a form of vicarious menstruation or possibly secondary to endometriosis of the gastrointestinal tract.

**gastromycosis** \-mīkō′sis\ Any fungal disease involving the stomach, as gastritis occurring in disseminated histoplasmosis or mucormycosis, or *Candida* infection of the stomach occurring in immunocompromised hosts.

**gastromyotomy** \-mi·ät′əmē\ [GASTRO- + MYOTOMY] A surgical incision into the stomach wall down to but not through the mucosa.

**gastronesteostomy** \-nes′tē·äs′təmē\ GASTROENTEROSTOMY.

**gastro-oesophagostomy** \-ēsäf′əgäs′təmē\ *Brit.* GASTROESOPHAGOSTOMY.

**gastro-omental** \-ōmen′təl\ Pertaining to the stomach and omentum.

**gastropagus** \gasträp′əgəs\ [GASTRO- + -PAGUS] Equal conjoined twins united at the abdominal region. **g. parasiticus** Unequal conjoined twins in which the parasite is attached to the abdomen of the host.

**gastroparalysis** \-pəral′isis\ [GASTRO- + PARALYSIS] Loss of smooth muscle function in the stomach; gastroparesis.

**gastroparesis** \-pərē′sis\ An incomplete gastric paralysis, seen especially in diabetic acidosis or coma. *Seldom used.* Also *gastroplegia.*

**gastropathy** \gasträp′əthē\ [GASTRO- + -PATHY] A pathologic condition of the stomach; a disease of the stomach. **hypertrophic g.** MÉNÉTRIER'S DISEASE.

**gastropexy** \gas′trəpek′sē\ [GASTRO- + -PEXY] A surgical procedure in which the stomach is fixed or resuspended to change the axis or relative position of the gastroesophageal junction.

**gastrophore** \gas′trəfôr\ [GASTRO- + -PHORE] A surgical device designed to support the stomach during operative procedures involving that organ.

**gastroplasty** \gas′trəplas′tē\ [GASTRO- + -PLASTY] Any plastic operation on the stomach.

**gastroplegia** \-plē′jə\ GASTROPARESIS.

**gastroplication** \-plikā′shən\ [GASTRO- + PLICATION] A surgical procedure in which a fold is created in a redundant gastric wall in order to reduce its size. Also *gastroptyxis, stomach reefing.*

**gastroptosis** \gas′träptō′sis\ [GASTRO- + -PTOSIS] Downward displacement of the stomach. Also *ventroptosis, descensus ventriculi.*

**gastroptyxis** \gas′trōtik′sis\ [GASTRO- + Gk *ptyxis* a fold] GASTROPLICATION.

**gastropylorectomy** \-pī′lôrek′təmē\ [GASTRO- + PYLO-

RECTOMY] A surgical procedure in which the pylorus and part of the stomach proximal to the pylorus are resected.

**gastrorrhagia** \-rā′jə\ [GASTRO- + -RRHAGIA] Hemorrhage from the mucosal surface of the stomach.

**gastrorrhaphy** \gastrôr′əfē\ Closure of an incision into or laceration of the stomach.

**gastrorrhea** \-rē′ə\ [GASTRO- + -RRHEA] Excessive secretion of gastric juice or of mucus by the stomach.

**gastrorrhexis** \-rek′sis\ [GASTRO- + -RRHEXIS] Gastric rupture.

**gastroschisis** \gasträs′kisis\ [GASTRO- + Gk *schisis* a cleaving, division] Failure of closure of the embryonic anterior abdominal wall at the midventral line. The viscera may protrude with or without a complete or partial covering of a membrane, variably comprised of modified skin, peritoneum, and muscle aponeuroses. The abdominal wall may be left in a deficient state. When the thorax is involved, the condition is called thoracogastroschisis.

**gastroscope** \gas′trəskōp\ [GASTRO- + -SCOPE] An instrument used to visualize the mucosal surface of the stomach. **fiberoptic g.** An endoscope made with flexible synthetic fibers permitting observation of the stomach. Also *gastrofiberscope.*

**gastroscopy** \gasträs′kəpē\ [GASTRO- + -SCOPY] Inspection of the inner surface of the stomach with an endoscope.

**gastrospasm** \gas′trəspazm\ Spasm of the walls of the stomach.

**gastrostenosis** \-stinō′sis\ [GASTRO- + STENOSIS] A narrowing of the stomach lumen.

**gastrostomy** \gasträs′təmē\ [GASTRO- + -STOMY] A surgical procedure creating an opening into the stomach from the abdominal wall for drainage or feeding purposes. Also *gastrostomosis.* **Beck's g.** A surgical procedure creating an opening between the skin and the stomach, utilizing a tube created from the greater curvature of the gastric wall. Also *Beck's method.* **Stamm g.** A surgical procedure for gastric decompression and/or feeding, in which a mushroom catheter is inserted through two concentric purse-string sutures into the stomach. The anterior gastric wall is then tacked securely to the peritoneal surface of the anterior abdominal wall.

**gastrosuccorrhea** \-suk′ôrē′ə\ [GASTRO- + SUCCORRHEA] Excessive secretion of gastric juice.

**gastrothoracopagus** \-thôr′əkäp′əgəs\ THORACOGASTROPAGUS.

**gastrotomy** \gasträt′əmē\ [GASTRO- + -TOMY] A surgical procedure in which one or more incisions are made into the stomach.

**gastrotonometer** \-tōnäm′ətər\ [GASTRO- + TONOMETER] An apparatus used to measure intragastric pressure.

**gastrotonometry** \-tōnäm′ətrē\ [GASTRO- + TONOMETRY] The measurement of intragastric pressure.

**gastrotoxin** \-täk′sin\ Any toxic substance that exerts an adverse effect on the stomach.

**gastrotropic** \-träp′ik\ [GASTRO- + -TROPIC[1]] Having an effect upon the stomach.

**gastrula** \gas′troolə\ [New L (dim. of *gaster* stomach) primitive gut stage] A stage in embryonic development, following that of the blastula, during which there appears for the first time, as the result of morphogenetic movements, several layers (two or three, depending on the animal group) representing the primary germ layers of ectoderm, mesoderm, and endoderm. This process of formation (gastrulation) establishes the anteroposterior axis of the body in the embryo.

**gastrulation** \gas′troolā′shən\ [*gastrul(a)* + -ATION] The process by which the blastula is developed to the gastrula, a folding of a portion of the blastula on to the opposed part. It is during this part of embryonic development that the segmental ovum generally obtains three primary germ layers. The mechanics of gastrulation differ among animal groups.

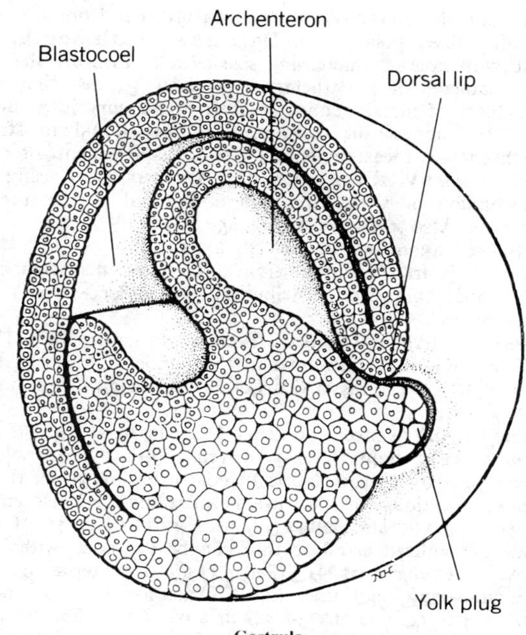


Gastrula

**gate** [Old English *geat, gæt* a gate, opening] **1** A combinational logic circuit whose output is determined by the states of its inputs. **2** The control electrode in a field-effect transistor. **3** An interval of time during which an electronic circuit is operative and can pass data. **AND g.** A combinational logic circuit that gives a high, or 1, output only if all inputs are high.

**gating** \gā′ting\ **1** The process of selecting those portions of a wave that lie between certain times or amplitudes. **2** The process by which sodium channels become opened during the electrical activity of a neuron.

**gatism** \gā′tizm, gätism′\ [French *gâtisme* (from *gâter* to spoil, ruin, from L *vastare* to lay waste) a physical or mental deterioration] Bladder and rectal incontinence.

**Gaucher** [Philippe Charles Ernst *Gaucher,* French physician, 1854–1918] **1** Gaucher lipid. See under CEREBROSIDE. **2** See under CELL. **3** See under GAUCHER'S DISEASE.

**gauge** \gāj\ [French *jauge* (from the Germanic) gauge] **1** Any of various instruments used to measure a physical quantity, either directly or by converting one physical quantity into another giving an observable output, as a blood-pressure gauge. **2** Any arbitrarily chosen range of sizes, as of wires, generally referred to by numbers. **3** A specific size within such a range of sizes, as a 16-gauge hypodermic needle. For defs. 1, 2, and 3 also *gage.* **beta ray g.** An instrument using a source of beta radiation and a radiation detector to measure the thickness of a material, such as plastic foil, by detecting the transmission of the beta rays through it. **bite g.** A device used in prosthodontics to determine the rest position, by measurement from the nose or other fixed point. Also *bitegauge*. **catheter g.** A plate with holes of increasing size used to measure the outside diameter of a catheter. **strain g.** A thin wire transducer of metal, semiconductor, or mercury in a rubber tube. Its increase in resistance is proportional to strain, which enables measurement of stress, displacement, or pressure. **x-ray thickness g.** An instrument using the transmission of x rays through a material to measure its thickness. Also *x-ray emission gauge*.

**gauntlet** \gônt′lit\ GAUNTLET BANDAGE.

**Gauss** [Carl Friedrich *Gauss*, German mathematician, 1777–1855] Gaussian distribution. See under NORMAL DISTRIBUTION.

**Gaussel** [Amans *Gaussel*, French physician, 1871–1937] **1** Grasset-Gaussel phenomenon. See under GRASSET'S PHENOMENON. **2** Grasset-Gaussel-Hoover sign. See under SIGN.

**gauze** \gôz\ [sixteenth-century English, from *Gaza*, Palestine, where a light, loosely woven fabric was made] A woven, usually cotton, fabric of coarse or fine mesh that is treated in various ways for use as a dressing. See also entries under BANDAGE and DRESSING. **absorbable g.** Gauze made of oxidized cellulose that can be degraded within the body. **absorbent g.** Gauze made of material that will take up serum and other liquid exudation from a wound. **antiseptic g.** Gauze to which any of a number of antimicrobial agents have been added. Common among these are dyes, iodinated compounds, and sulfonamides. **fine mesh g.** A narrow woven, single-layer cotton dressing. The small interstices do not allow much adherence of the dressing to the serum and wound exudate. As a result there is less trauma to the wound or fresh graft when the dressing is removed. **petrolatum g.** Gauze impregnated with petrolatum to exclude air from the wound and thus prevent drying. **ribbon g.** Gauze made in a long thin strip and used to pack a deep wound so as to keep the edges apart and allow healing from the interior outward. **tullegras g.** TULLE GRAS.

**gavage** \gaväzh′\ [French (from *gaver* to force-feed (animals), from Picard French *gav(e)* throat) a gorging, force-feeding] Alimentation via a tube placed into the stomach.

**Gavard** [Hyacinthe *Gavard*, French anatomist, 1753–1802] Gavard's muscle. See under FIBRAE OBLIQUAE GASTRICAE.

**Gay-Lussac** [Joseph Louis *Gay-Lussac*, French chemist and physicist, 1778–1850] Gay-Lussac law. See under LAW.

**gaze** **1** To direct the eyes persistently. **2** The act of gazing; a stable and persistent direction of the eyes. **conjugate g.** Simultaneous movement of both eyes into a position of use.

**GBM** glomerular basement membrane.

**G + C** Guanine paired with cytosine, as in DNA. See also BASE RATIO.

**Gd** Symbol for the element, gadolinium.

**GDH** **1** glucose dehydrogenase. **2** glutamate dehydrogenase. **3** glycerol-3-phosphate dehydrogenase. • Because of its various meanings this abbreviation is best avoided.

**GDP** guanosine diphosphate.

**Ge** Symbol for the element, germanium.

**Gee** [Samuel Jones *Gee*, English physician, 1839–1911] **1** Gee's disease, Gee-Herter-Heubner disease, Gee-Herter-Heubner syndrome. See under INFANTILE CELIAC DISEASE. **2** Gee-Thaysen disease. See under ADULT CELIAC DISEASE.

**gegenhalten** \gā′gənhul′tən\ [German *gegen* against, counter + *halten* to hold, stop] Uneven resistance to passive movement of the limbs. Superficially it resembles in some cases the lead-pipe or cogwheel rigidity of parkinsonism and may be noted in some stuporous or demented patients. Also *paratonia*.

**Geigel** [Richard *Geigel*, German physician, 1859–1930] See under REFLEX.

**Geiger** [Hans Wilhelm *Geiger*, German physicist, 1882–1945] **1** Geiger-Müller counter. See under COUNTER. **2** Geiger-Nuttall law. See under LAW. **3** Geiger-Müller survey meter. See under METER. **4** See under REGION, PLATEAU, THRESHOLD. **5** Geiger-Müller tube. See under TUBE.

**gel** \jel\ [short for GELATIN] A phase that is largely liquid but incapable of flow because it is held rigid by molecular chains, usually cross-linked, that pass through it.

**gelatin** \jel′ətin\ [French *gélatine* (from L *gelatus*, past part. of *gelare* to cause to freeze) gelatin] A soluble protein obtained by boiling collagen with water, during which process the collagen is partly degraded. **g. compound phenolized** A preparation with a gelatin base containing zinc oxide, glycerin, water, and phenol. It is used in bandages that are applied to the skin for the treatment of ulcers and burns. **formalin g.** Gelatin that has been treated with an enteric coating to render it insoluble. Capsules or coverings for pills from such material are protected from the acidity of the stomach and remain intact until they reach the alkaline conditions of the small intestine. **medicated g.** A gelatin base that contains medicinally active agents. It is most often applied topically. **zinc g.** A medicinal preparation that is composed of 15 percent zinc oxide, gelatin, water, and glycerin. It is applied topically and serves as a protective coating.

**gelatinosa** Gelatinous: said of portions of the nervous system.

**gelatinous** \jəlat′ənəs\ **1** Having a gelatinlike consistency that varies with moisture conditions: often used of a layer or part of a fungus. **2** Pertaining to or resembling gelatin; jellylike.

**gelation** \jəlā′shən\ [GEL + -ATION] The process of gel formation.

**Gélineau** [Jean Baptiste Edouard *Gélineau*, French neurologist, born 1859] Gélineau syndrome. See under NARCOLEPSY.

**Gellé** [Marie Ernest *Gellé*, French otologist, 1834–1923] See under TEST.

**gel. quav.** *gelatina quavis* (L, in any kind of jelly).

**gelsemism** \jel′səmizm\ [*Gelsem(ium)* + -ISM] Poisoning caused by the ingestion of the Carolina or yellow jessamine, *Gelsemium sempervirens*. The symptoms are muscular weakness, excessive perspiration, and respiratory depression.

**geminate** \jem′ənit\ [L *geminat(us)*, past part. of *geminare* to double] Occurring in pairs. Also *geminous*.

**gemination** \jem′ənā′shən\ [L *geminatio* (from *geminatus*, past part. of *geminare* to double, be double) a doubling] The union of two teeth. **false g.** The joining together of two normal teeth by an overgrowth of cementum.

**geminous** \jem′ənəs\ GEMINATE.

**gemistocyte** \jemis′təsīt\ [Gk *gemisto(s)* laden, full + -CYTE] PROTOPLASMIC ASTROCYTE.

**gemistocytic** \jəmis′tōsit′ik\ Describing, pertaining to, or consisting of gemistocytes: used especially of certain astrocytomas.

**gemistocytoma** \jəmis′təsītō′mə\ GEMISTOCYTIC ASTROCYTOMA.

**gemmation** \jəmā′shən\ [L *gemmat(us)*, past part. of *gemmare* to put forth buds or gems + -ION] Asexual cell reproduction in which part of the cell body organizes as a separate growth on the surface or within the parent body, and then differentiates as a new individual. Also *bud fission*.

**gen-** \jen-\ GENO-.

**-gen** \-jən\ [Gk *gennan* to beget, produce, create] A combining form meaning (1) something that produces or evokes (a specified substance or reaction); (2) something produced.

**gena** \jē′nə\ [L (akin to Gk *genys* chin and English *chin*) cheek] BUCCA.

**genal** \jē′nəl\ BUCCAL.

**gender** \jen′dər\ [Middle English *gendre,* from Old French *genre* kind, from L *genus* , gen. *generis* class, kind] Sex; a categorical differentiation of organisms based on sex.

**gene** \jēn\ [German *Gen* (shortened from earlier *Pangen* pangene, coined from *pangenesis,* Darwin's then prevalent theory of generation; see PANGENESIS) a hereditary factor] A segment of DNA (or RNA in certain viruses) that codes for a specific polypeptide or RNA molecule. See also CISTRON. **allelic g.** ALLELE. **amorphic g.** An allele that produces either no product or a nonfunctional product. The effect on phenotype is not predictable, can vary from none to extreme, and depends on the action of the companion allele in diploid organisms, among many factors. Also *amorph.* **antimutator g.** A gene whose mutation can decrease the spontaneous mutation rate. **autosomal g.** Any gene located on an autosomal chromosome. **complementary g.'s** Two or more genetic loci that interact, generally through their products, with the resulting phenotype being distinct from those of any of the loci acting independently. Also *reciprocal genes.* **control g.** REGULATOR GENE. **cumulative g.** POLYGENE. **cytoplasmic g.** Any gene that ordinarily exists on nucleic acid in the cytoplasm, especially one on mitochondrial or chloroplast chromosomes. **dominant g.** An allele that directs the production or appearance of a mendelian dominant phenotype, regardless of whether the allele is heterozygous or homozygous. Also *dominant allele.* **hemizygous g.** Any gene present in but one copy in a cell or organism that is diploid or polyploid: used especially of genes on either sex chromosome in the heterogametic sex. **histocompatibility g.** A gene determining the specificity of tissue antigenicity and therefore the compatibility of donor and recipient in transplantation. **holandric g.** **1** A gene that occurs only in the male of a species. *Popular.* **2** Y-LINKED GENE. **hologynic g.'s** **1** Genes that determine traits limited to females. *Popular.* **2** In humans, genes that determine X-linked dominant traits lethal *in utero* to hemizygous males or autosomal traits limited to females. **3** In certain species in which the female is the heterogametic sex, genes linked to the female-determining sex chromosome, such as the W chromosome. **homeotic g.** A mutant gene whose effect on phenotype is homeosis. Such genes, when not mutated, are thought to have roles in developmental processes. **Ir g.** **1** A gene specifying an immune response function. **2** A gene in the major histocompatibility complex of the mouse. **jumping g.** TRANSPOSABLE GENE. **leaky g.** HYPOMORPH. **lethal g.** LETHAL ALLELE. **major g.** Any gene whose effect on the phenotype is evident, regardless of how this effect is modulated by the rest of the genotype. **marker g.** Any gene that determines a distinct phenotype and can therefore be used in experimental genetics. **mimic g.** **1** An allele that results in a phenotype similar to that of a distinct genetic locus. **2** An allele that causes a genocopy or genetic mimic. **modifying g.** A gene that affects the phenotypic expression of another genetic locus. The interaction may enhance, reduce, or suppress the action of the modified locus. Also *modifying factor, modifier, modification allele.* **mutant g.** Any allele distinct in structure or function from the wild-type allele because of mutation at that genetic locus. **mutator g.** A gene whose mutation can increase the spontaneous mutation rate. In bacteria several mechanisms, affecting DNA repair or the accuracy of DNA replication, have been identified. **nonstructural g.** A genetic locus whose function is other than to determine the amino acid sequence of a polypeptide chain. Compare STRUCTURAL GENE. **operator g.** See under OPERATOR LOCUS. **g. pool** See under POOL. **recessive g.** In diploid organisms, an allele that, when homozygous, directs the production or appearance of a mendelian recessive phenotype. Also *recessive allele.* **reciprocal g.'s** COMPLEMENTARY GENES. **regulator g.** A genetic locus that regulates expression of one or more other genes. Also *control gene, regulator.* **repressor g.** A regulator gene that directs the synthesis of a regulator protein, usually a repressor. **resistance g.** Any locus that encodes a product, process, or trait capable of rendering a cell or organism less susceptible to, usually, a specific deleterious agent. An example would be a gene encoding penicillinase that results in resistance of a bacterium to penicillin. **restorer g.** A gene that reverses the changes brought about by cytoplasmically induced sterility. Restorer genes have been isolated for use as fertility agents in plant genetics. **Rh g.'s** Genes that encode the rhesus blood group antigens. They are located on the distal short arm of chromosome 1. **sex-influenced g.** A genetic locus that determines a sex-influenced phenotype. It may be either linked to a sex chromosome or autosomal. *Popular.* Also *sex-conditioned gene.* **sex-limited g.** A genetic locus, whether autosomal or linked to a sex chromosome, that determines a sex-limited phenotype. *Popular.* **sex-linked g.** **1** A genetic locus located on a sex chromosome. **2** *Imprecise* X-LINKED GENE. **silent g.** SILENT ALLELE. **split g.** A gene which consists of at least two coding sequences, separated by introns. Most genes of higher organisms are split, whereas bacterial and viral genes are rarely split. **structural g.** A genetic locus that determines the amino acid sequence of a polypeptide. The gene coding for RNA molecules such as transfer RNAs or ribosomal RNAs are considered by some to be structural genes also. Compare NONSTRUCTURAL GENE. **sublethal g.** SUBLETHAL ALLELE. **suppressor g.** A gene capable of blocking or otherwise modifying the effect of a mutation in a separate locus. **switch g.** In developmental genetics, a regulator gene that determines the developmental sequence of an organism. **syntenic g.'s** Genes located on the same chromosome. **taster g.** PTC LOCUS. **transposable g.** A transposon that contains a coding sequence. Also *jumping gene* (popular). **tRNA g.** A gene that codes for a transfer RNA molecule. **uninducible g.** A gene which is present as a part of the genome, but which is not transcribed even in the presence of an inducer. **wild-type g.** An allele that, when heterozygous, specifies a dominant wild-type phenotype or, when homozygous, specifies either a recessive or a dominant wild-type phenotype. **X-linked g.** A genetic locus on the X chromosome in any species. Also *sex-linked gene* (imprecise). **Y-linked g.** A genetic locus on the Y chromosome in any species. Also *holandric gene.*

**geneogenous** \jē′nē·äj′ənəs\ CONGENITAL.

**genera** \jen′ərə\ Plural of GENUS[1].

**generalize** \jen′ərəlīz\ To progress from local to general: said of a disease.

**generation** [French *génération* (from L *generatio,* from *generare* to beget, produce, from *genus;* see GENUS) generation] **1** Reproduction. **2** One complete cycle from parents to offspring in the life of sexually reproducing organisms. **3** The group of individuals descended from a given ancestor in the same number of parent-offspring cycles.

4 In demography, a group of persons born during a given period, usually a calendar year. 5 In demography, the offspring of a group of persons born during a calendar year. **asexual g.** ASEXUAL REPRODUCTION. **direct g.** ASEXUAL REPRODUCTION. **first filial g.** All offspring resulting from the sexual reproduction of two individuals. Symbol: $F_1$ **nonsexual g.** ASEXUAL REPRODUCTION. **parental g.** 1 All individuals in a population of approximately the same age as a designated set of parents. *Popular.* 2 In genetics, all sibs and first cousins of a particular set of parents. 3 In experimental genetics, the original two individuals in a breeding experiment, the mating of which produced the first filial generation. Symbol: $P_1$ **second filial g.** All offspring produced by the sexual reproduction of two individuals who were members of the first filial generation. Symbol: $F_2$ **sexual g.** SEXUAL REPRODUCTION. **spontaneous g.** The theory that living organisms are created from nonliving matter. Also *abiogenesis, autogenesis, archegony* (seldom used). **virgin g.** PARTHENOGENESIS.

**generative** \jen′ərətiv\ [L *generat(us),* past part. of *generare* to beget, produce + -IVE] Pertaining to the reproductive process.

**generator** [L, a begetter, producer] 1 Anything that produces a particular form of matter or energy. 2 A device that produces electricity by conversion from other forms of energy, such as mechanical, nuclear, or chemical energy. **asynchronous pulse g.** A pulse generator which is unaffected by cardiac electrical activity and generates pulses at a fixed rate. Also *fixed-rate pulse generator.* **atrial synchronous pulse g.** A pulse generator which is triggered by normal atrial activity to stimulate the ventricle. Also *atrial triggered pulse generator.* **demand pulse g.** VENTRICULAR INHIBITED PULSE GENERATOR. **electrostatic g.** An apparatus for producing a high voltage by the separation of electric charges. Also *static machine.* **fixed-rate pulse g.** ASYNCHRONOUS PULSE GENERATOR. **pattern g.** The neuronal circuitry directly involved in the production of a stereotyped form of motor activity of complex, usually repetitive pattern, such as ambulation, swimming, or chewing. The pattern generator is at once the total of distinctive interneuronal connections and the activity channeled through them which results in the pattern behavior. **pulse g.** An electronic device that generates sharp pulses, usually of very short duration and either regular or random in timing. **radionuclide g.** A device that contains a relatively long-lived parent radionuclide fixed to an ion exchange column from which a daughter radionuclide may be eluted. • In nuclear medicine, this is commonly termed a "cow," because it is "milked" from time to time. **standby pulse g.** VENTRICULAR INHIBITED PULSE GENERATOR. **supervoltage g.** An apparatus for producing voltages greater than one million volts, for use in x-ray therapy. **technetium-99m g.** A radionuclide generator that produces the daughter nuclide, technetium 99m, from the parent, molybdenum 99. **Van de Graaff g.** An apparatus for producing a high voltage, typically several million volts, by means of a fast-moving belt stretched between two pulleys. Electric charges are sprayed onto the belt at one pulley and taken off at the other. Also *Van de Graaff machine.* **ventricular inhibited pulse g.** A pulse generator whose activity is inhibited by intrinsic ventricular activity. Also *demand pulse generator, standby pulse generator.* **ventricular triggered pulse g.** A pulse generator which delivers its impulse synchronously with natural ventricular activity unless this fails, in which case it provides a pacemaking impulse. Also *ventricular synchronous pulse generator.*

**generic** \jəner′ik\ 1 Of or relating to a genus. 2 Nonproprietary, as a drug that can be substituted for a proprietary brand in a prescription.

**genesis** \jen′əsis\ [Gk (from root of *gignesthai* to become, be, be born) origin, source, birth, race, descent] The process of being formed; origin; beginning: often used in combination, as in *spermatogenesis.*

**gene-splicing** \jēn′-splī′sing\ The *in vitro* manipulation of DNA or RNA to achieve rearrangement of an organism's genes; molecular recombination. The introduction of a foreign nucleotide sequence into a specific location in the host genome, as in bacterial recombination.

**genetic** \jənet′ik\ 1 Of or pertaining to genesis or origins. 2 Of or relating to the study of genetics. 3 Referring to or pertaining to anything controlled or defined by genes. Also *genic.* 4 HERITABLE.

**geneticist** \jənet′əsist\ One who specializes in the acquisition and application of knowledge about heredity and genetic processes.

**genetics** \jənet′iks\ That branch of the life sciences that deals with the structure and function of genes; the expression of genes in individuals, families, and populations; and the causes and extent of genetic variation. **behavioral g.** A subfield of psychology concerned with investigating the influence of heredity on behavior. It combines the methods of psychology and genetics to inquire into the influence of heredity and environment on behavior, and especially into the nature of their interactions. **biochemical g.** That amalgamation of the sciences of biochemistry and genetics that focuses on the expression of normal and mutant genes in individuals and populations, usually at the level of enzymes and other proteins. **clinical g.** That branch of medicine involved with the diagnosis and treatment of human disorders caused, at least in part, by abnormal genes or chromosomes in patients and their families. **developmental g.** The study of the genetic and epigenetic control and modulation of organismal development. **human g.** That branch of genetics concerned with humans. Included are clinical genetics, medical genetics, and the study of the genetic foundations of human phenotypic variation. **medical g.** That branch of medicine concerned with clinical genetics as well as the discovery, nosology, epidemiology, and pathogenesis of hereditary disorders. **microbial g.** The branch of genetics concerned with microorganisms, especially bacteria, viruses, and phage. **molecular g.** The branch of genetics that focuses on the molecular structure of nucleic acids, the molecular organization of genetic information, and the processes through which this information is expressed. **population g.** The branch of genetics that focuses on gene and allele frequencies and their interactions in populations, as well as the forces and processes that alter gene frequencies. **statistical g.** The branch of genetics concerned with the analysis of data or the elaboration of genetic theory in quantitative terms according to the precepts of statistics.

**Gengou** [Octave *Gengou,* Belgian bacteriologist, 1875–1957] 1 Bordet-Gengou agar. See under AGAR. 2 Bordet-Gengou bacillus. See under *BORDETELLA PERTUSSIS.* 3 Bordet and Gengou reaction. See under COMPLEMENT FIXATION.

**genial** \jēn′yəl\ [Gk *genei(on)* chin, jaw, cheek + -AL] Pertaining to the chin. Also *genian.*

**genic** \jē′nik, jen′ik\ GENETIC.

**-genic** \-jen′ik\ [-GEN + -IC] A combining form meaning producing, creating.

**genicula** \jənik′yələ\ Plural of GENICULUM.

**genicular** \jənik′yələr\ Of or pertaining to the knee, or genus.

**geniculate** \jənik′yəlit\ [*genicul(um)* + -ATE] Resembling or shaped like a knee in a flexed position; bent sharply.

**geniculocalcarine** \jənik′yəlōkal′kərīn\ Denoting the visual radiation fibers projecting from the lateral geniculate body to the calcarine portion of the visual cortex.

**geniculotemporal** \jənik′yəlōtem′pərəl\ Denoting the visual radiation fibers emanating from the lateral geniculate body and coursing around the temporal horn of the lateral ventricle en route to the visual cortex.

**geniculum** \jenik′yələm\ [L (dim. of *genu* the knee) a small knee, knob, knot] **1** A small acute bend or angulation, resembling a knee, in a structure or organ. **2** A kneelike or knotlike structure. **g. canalis facialis** [NA] The sharp, posteriorly directed bend in the lateral part of the facial canal above the vestibular part of the internal ear and in the petrous part of the temporal bone where the canal runs from the internal acoustic meatus. The canal is dilated at this bend, where it lodges the geniculate ganglion. Also *genu of facial canal, little knee of facial canal, geniculum of facial canal.* **g. nervi facialis** [NA] The portion of the facial nerve root within the facial canal that bends sharply posteriorly at the site of the geniculate ganglion. Also *external genu of facial nerve, genu of facial nerve* (imprecise), *geniculum of facial nerve.* Compare GENU NERVI FACIALIS.

**genio-** \jē′nē·ō-\ [Gk *geneion* chin, jaw, cheek] A combining form meaning (1) chin; (2) cheek. Also *geny-*.

**geniocheiloplasty** \-kī′ləplas′tē\ [GENIO- + CHEILOPLASTY] Any plastic operation on the lower lip and chin. Also *genycheiloplasty, genychiloplasty.*

**genioglossus** \-gläs′əs\ MUSCULUS GENIOGLOSSUS.

**geniohyoglossus** \-hī′ōgläs′əs\ MUSCULUS GENIOGLOSSUS.

**geniohyoid** \-hī′oid\ **1** Pertaining to the chin and the hyoid bone. **2** Denoting the musculus geniohyoideus.

**genioplasty** \jē′nē-ōplas′tē\ [GENIO- + -PLASTY] Any plastic surgical procedure on the chin, usually one designed to enlarge, reduce, or change the shape of the chin. Also *genyplasty.*

**genital** \jen′itəl\ [L *genitalis (from genitus,* past part. of *gignere* to create, produce, beget, bear) generative, procreative] Of or relating to the reproductive organs (the genitals), or to reproduction.

**genitalia** \jen′itā′lyə\ [L (neut. pl. of *genitalis* generative; see GENITAL) the genitals] The organs of reproduction in both males and females, usually used in reference to external genitals. Also *genitals, reproductive organs.* **ambiguous external g.** External genitalia not conforming clearly to either the male or female pattern. Causes include chromosome defects, metabolic errors of hormone synthesis, and anatomical malformations. **external g.** The organa genitalia masculina externa and the organa genitalia feminina externa. **indifferent g.** The embryonic genital organs before differentiation into the organs peculiar to either sex.

**genitals** \jen′itəlz\ GENITALIA.

**genito-** \jen′itō-\ [L *genitus* (past participle of *gignere* to beget, produce) begotten, produced] A combining form meaning genital.

**genitoinfectious** \-infek′shəs\ VENEREAL.

**genitoplasty** \jen′itōplas′tē\ [GENITO- + -PLASTY] Any plastic operation on the genitalia.

**genitourinary** \-yoo′riner′ē\ UROGENITAL.

**Gennari** [Francesco *Gennari,* Italian anatomist, 1750–1795] Line of Gennari, stripe of Gennari, Gennari's layer, stria of Gennari. See under BAND.

**geno-** \jen′ə-\ [Gk *gennan* to beget, produce, bring forth] A combining form meaning (1) genetic, gene; (2) genital; (3) genus, race, nation. Also *gen-*.

**genocopy** \jen′əkäpē\ An individual whose phenotype is similar to or indistinguishable from another individual of different genotype. Also *genetic mimic, isophene.*

**genome** \jē′nōm\ [German *Genom,* from GEN- + *-om* -OME; influenced by the (unrelated) ending of *chromosome*] **1** The total genetic information present in a cell. **2** In diploid cells, the genetic information contained in one chromosome set. **3** The genetic information contained in a haploid gamete of a diploid organism.

**genomic** \jənō′mik\ **1** Of or pertaining to the genome. **2** In molecular genetics, referring to DNA purified from and representative of the nuclear DNA.

**genotype** \jen′ətīp\ **1** The total genetic information in a somatic cell, or the total potential genetic information in a germ cell or an organism. **2** The genetic constitution at one or several loci in a given cell or organism.

**genotypic** \jen′ətip′ik\ Of or relating to a genotype.

**-genous** \-jənəs\ [-GEN + -OUS] A combining form meaning (1) producing; (2) produced by.

**gentamicin** \jen′təmī′sin\ A broad-spectrum, aminocyclitol antibiotic elaborated by *Micromonospora purpurea* and *M. echinospora.* It inhibits bacterial protein synthesis and is active against many Gram-negative and Gram-positive bacteria, particularly *Pseudomonas aeruginosa.* The sulfate salt is used. The major side effect is that this drug is ototoxic and may cause irreversible damage. Also *gentamycin.*

**gentian** \jen′shən\ A drug prepared from dried, fermented rhizomes and roots of *Gentiana lutea* of the Gentianaceae family. It has been used as a bitter tonic to stimulate gastric secretion and improve the appetite. Also *bitter root.*

**gentiavern** \jen′shəvurn\ GENTIAN VIOLET.

**gentrogenin** BOTOGENIN.

**genu** \jē′noo\ [L (akin to Gk *gony* knee and *gōnia* corner, angle) the knee] (*pl.* genua) **1** GENUS[2]. **2** Any of various angulated or curved anatomic structures suggestive of a bent knee. **g. capsulae internae** [NA] The angular bend formed by the anterior and posterior limbs of the internal capsule. Also *genu of internal capsule, knee of internal capsule.* **g. corporis callosi** [NA] The ventrally directed, kneelike bend at the rostrum of the corpus callosum. Also *genu of corpus callosum.* **external g. of facial nerve** GENICULUM NERVI FACIALIS. **g. extrorsum** GENU VARUM. **g. of facial canal** GENICULUM CANALIS FACIALIS. **g. of facial nerve** **1** GENU NERVI FACIALIS. **2** *Imprecise* GENICULUM NERVI FACIALIS. **g. impressum** A deformity of the knees in which the knee is bent to one side with abnormal positioning of the patella upwards and to that side. **g. of internal capsule** GENU CAPSULAE INTERNAE. **internal g. of facial nerve** GENU NERVI FACIALIS. **g. internum radicis nervi facialis** GENU NERVI FACIALIS. **g. introrsum** GENU VALGUM. **g. nervi facialis** [NA] The bend in the motor fibers of the facial nerve at the point where they arch over the abducens nucleus, resulting in an elevation of the floor of the fourth ventricle (the facial colliculus), before coursing ventrally to emerge from the brainstem. Also *internal genu of facial nerve, genu of facial nerve, genu internum radicis nervi facialis.* Compare GENICULUM NERVI FACIALIS. **g. recurvatum** A congenital hyperextension at the knee joint, giving a forward concavity of the lower extremity when fully extended. Also *back knee.* **g. valgum** A congenital curvature of the lower extremity so that the knees are abnormally approximated and the ankles abnormally divergent. Also *genu introrsum, knock-knee, tragopodia, tibia valga.* **g. varum** A congenital curvature of the lower extremities that results in the knees being abnormally divergent and the ankles abnormally approximated. Also *bowleg, genu extrorsum, tibia vara, bandy leg.*

**genua** \jen′ʸoo·ə\ 1 Plural of GENU. 2 Plural of GENUS[2].

**genual** \jen′ʸoo·əl\ Pertaining to or resembling a genu, or knee; genicular.

**genus[1]** \jē′nəs\ [L (from root of *(gi)gnere* to bring into being; akin to Gk *genos* race, stock, kind) origin, stock, race, kind] (*pl.* genera) A taxonomic group ranking below a family and including one or more species.

**genus[2]** \jē′nəs, jen′əs\ [L, variant of *genu* knee] (*pl.* genua) [NA] The region of the knee joint, comprising the regio genus anterior, regio genus posterior, and the fossa poplitea; the knee. Also *genu.*

**geny-** \jen′ē-\ [Gk *genys* chin] GENIO-.

**genyantrum** \jen′ē·an′trəm\ *Outmoded* SINUS MAXILLARIS.

**genycheiloplasty** \jen′ēkī′lōplas′tē\ GENIOCHEILOPLASTY.

**genychiloplasty** \jen′ēkī′lōplas′tē\ GENIOCHEILOPLASTY.

**genyplasty** \jen′ēplas′tē\ GENIOPLASTY.

**geo-** \jē′ō-\ [Gk *gē* the earth, land] A combining form meaning earth, soil.

**geode** \jē′ōd\ [from its similarity to a stone geode] In anatomy, an enlarged lymphatic space or the dilatation occurring where several lymphatic capillaries join together. *Outmoded.*

**geomedicine** \jē′ōmed′əsən\ [*geo(graphic)* + MEDICINE] The branch of medicine concerned with the influence of environmental, climatic, and topographic conditions on health and the prevalence of disease in different parts of the world. Also *nosochthonography* (seldom used), *nosogeography* (seldom used).

**geometry** \jē·äm′ətrē\ In nuclear medicine, any of the various arrangements between a radioactive source and a detector that affect the accuracy of counting or measurement. Also *counting geometry.* **good g.** A physical relationship between a radioactive source and a detector that is favorable to the quantitative counting of the source. Two factors are usually involved: the necessity to minimize the fraction of the emitted radiation that misses the detector entirely, and the necessity to minimize the effects of scattered radiation. The latter is often beyond the experimenter's control, as when the source is buried in a patient.

**geotrichosis** \jē′ōtrikō′sis\ Infection due to the fungus *Geotrichum candidum.* It affects humans, with lesions developing in the mouth and in the digestive and respiratory systems.

**ger-** \jer′-\ GERO-.

**geraniol** $Me_2C{=}CH{-}CH_2{-}CH_2{-}C(Me){=}CH{-}CH_2OH$. An alcohol found in plant oils in the *trans* configuration. Its molecule contains two isoprene units. Its ester with diphosphoric acid (geranyl pyrophosphate) is an important metabolic intermediate.

**geranyl pyrophosphate** The ester of geraniol and diphosphoric acid. It is an intermediate in the synthesis of steroids and terpenes, being formed from isopentenyl pyrophosphate and dimethylallyl pyrophosphate. It reacts with a further molecule of isopentenyl pyrophosphate to form farnesyl pyrophosphate.

**Gerdy** [Pierre Nicholas, *Gerdy,* French surgeon, 1797–1856] 1 Gerdy's fontanel. See under SAGITTAL FONTANEL. 2 Gerdy's ligament. See under SUSPENSORY LIGAMENT OF AXILLA.

**gereology** \jer′ē·äl′əjē\ GERONTOLOGY.

**Gerhardt** [Carl Jakob Christian Adolph *Gerhardt,* German physician, 1833–1902] Gerhardt's disease. See under ERYTHROMELALGIA.

**geriatric** \jer′ē·at′rik\ [GER- + -IATRIC] 1 Pertaining to geriatrics. 2 Pertaining to old age.

**geriatrician** \jer′ē·ətrish′ən\ A physician who specializes in the practice of geriatric medicine. Also *geriatrist.*

**geriatrics** \jer′ē·at′riks\ [GER- + -IATRICS] *Popular* GERIATRIC MEDICINE. **dental g.** GERODONTICS.

**geriatrist** \jer′ē·at′rist\ GERIATRICIAN.

**geriodontics** \jer′ē·ədän′tiks\ GERODONTICS.

**geriopsychosis** \jer′ē·əsīkō′sis\ SENILE DEMENTIA.

**Gerlach** [Andreas Christian *Gerlach,* German veterinary surgeon, 1811–1877] Gerlach's valvula. See under LIGAMENTUM PECTINATUM ANGULI IRIDOCORNEALIS.

**Gerlach** [Joseph von *Gerlach,* German anatomist, 1820–1896] 1 See under VALVE. 2 Gerlach's annular tendon, annular ring of Gerlach. See under ANNULUS FIBROCARTILAGINEUS MEMBRANAE TYMPANI. 3 Gerlach's tonsil. See under TONSILLA TUBARIA.

**Gerlier** [Felix *Gerlier,* Swiss physician, 1840–1914] 1 Gerlier's disease. See under VESTIBULAR NEURONITIS. 2 Gerlier syndrome. See under DISEASE. 3 Gerlier syndrome. See under PALLIDAL SYNDROME.

**germ** \jurm\ [French *germe* (from L *germen,* gen. *germinis,* sprout, bud, from root of L *gignere* to generate) a rudiment or embryonic form, source; the "germ" of a disease: a pathogen] 1 The portion of an ovum which divides to give rise to the embryo, the rest of the ovum (including the yolk) being responsible for providing nourishment. 2 A rudiment or primordium; an embryonic precursor, as *tooth germ, germ layer.* 3 Constituting the reproductive or genetic material of an organism, as *germ cell, germ plasm.* 4 A microorganism capable of causing a disease. **dental g.** TOOTH GERM. **enamel g.** An epithelial bud which develops at an early stage of tooth formation. **tooth g.** An embryonic precursor or dental organ of a tooth which develops at intervals along the dental lamina in the shape of a cap of ectoderm with mesenchyme on its inner aspect, forming the dental papilla which will become the dentine and the pulp. The dental organ soon becomes bell-shaped (the bell stage) and four cell layers develop: an external dental epithelium, a stellate reticulum, a stratum intermedium, and an internal dental epithelium. The latter becomes folded to determine the crown pattern of the tooth, and its cells, now called ameloblasts, lay down the enamel. Odontoblasts develop from the superficial cells of the dental papilla and lay down predentin which is the precursor of dentin. Also *dental germ.*

**germanium** \jərmā′nē·əm\ A metallic element having atomic number 32 and atomic weight 72.59. Five stable natural isotopes are known and 12 radioactive isotopes have been identified. Valences are 2 and 4. Elemental germanium is a brittle, crystalline solid with a metallic luster. The element is a semiconductor and is important in the manufacture of electronic and optical instruments. Symbol: Ge

**germ-free** \jurm′-frē\ AXENIC.

**germicidal** \jur′məsī′dəl\ [*germicid(e)* + -AL] Able to destroy microorganisms.

**germicide** \jur′məsīd\ [GERM + *i* + -CIDE] An agent capable of destroying microorganisms.

**germinal** \jur′mənəl\ [L *germen,* gen. *germinis,* a bud, seed + -AL] Of or relating to a germ cell or to germination.

**germination** \jur′mənā′shən\ [L *germinatio* (from *germinatus,* past part. of *germinare* to sprout, put forth) a sprouting, budding] The initiation of growth by a bud, seed, spore, or other structure.

**germinative** \jur′minətiv\ 1 Of or relating to a germ cell. 2 Pertaining to the process of germination.

**germinoblast** \jur′mənōblast′\ 1 LARGE NONCLEAVED FOLLICULAR CENTER CELL. 2 SMALL NONCLEAVED FOLLICULAR CENTER CELL.

**germinocyte** \jur′mənōsīt′\ 1 LARGE CLEAVED FOLLICULAR CENTER CELL. 2 SMALL CLEAVED FOLLICULAR CENTER CELL.

**germinoma** \jur′mənō′mə\ [L *germen*, gen. *germinis*, a bud, sprout + -OMA] A malignant tumor composed of large, primitive, round cells resembling germ cells. It occurs in the pineal region, mediastinum, and retroperitoneum. It is histologically indistinguishable from testicular seminoma and ovarian dysgerminoma. **pineal g.** A germinoma of the pineal region. It is indistinguishable from the testicular seminoma or ovarian dysgerminoma. Geminomas are the most frequent tumor of the pineal region.

**gero-** \jer′ō-\ [Gk *gerōn* (genitive *gerontos*) old man] A combining form meaning old age, relating to old people. Also *geronto-, geront-, ger-.*

**geroderma** \jer′ōdur′mə\ [GERO- + -DERMA] Atrophy of the skin, as that seen in old age. Also *gerodermia.* **g. osteodysplastica** A hereditary disorder, transmitted as an autosomal recessive trait and usually seen in women, that is characterized by dystrophy of the skin and genitalia, osteoporosis, and prominent bony trabeculae which are visible radiographically.

**gerodermia** \jer′ōdur′mē·ə\ GERODERMA.

**gerodontics** \jer′ōdän′tiks\ [GER- + odont- + -ICS] The practice of dentistry aimed at treating old people. Also *dental geriatrics, geriodontics, gerodontia.*

**geromorphism** [GERO- + MORPH- + ISM] Bodily characteristics of old age in the young; premature senility.

**geront-** \jeränt-\ GERO-.

**geronto-** \jerän′tō-, jer′äntō-\ GERO-.

**gerontologist** \jer′əntäl′əjist\ One who specializes in gerontology.

**gerontology** \jer′əntäl′əjē\ [GERONTO- + -LOGY] 1 The study of aging as a biologic, sociological, and psychological process. Also *gereology, nostology* (obs.). 2 Clinical gerontology; geriatric medicine.

**gerontopia** \jer′əntō′pē·ə\ [GERONT- + -OPIA] SECOND SIGHT.

**gerontotherapy** \-ther′əpē\ [GERONTO- + THERAPY] *Seldom used* GERIATRIC MEDICINE.

**gerontotoxon** \-täk′sän\ [GERONTO- + Gk *toxon* a bow] ARCUS SENILIS.

**gerontoxon** \jer′əntäk′sän\ [Gk *gerōn* old man + *toxon* a bow] ARCUS SENILIS.

**geropsychiatry** \jer′ōsīkī′ətrē\ [GERO- + PSYCHIATRY] PSYCHOGERIATRICS.

**Gerota** [Dimitru *Gerota,* Rumanian surgeon, 1867–1939] 1 Gerota's fascia. See under FASCIA RENALIS. 2 See under METHOD.

**Gersh** [Isidore *Gersh,* U.S. histologist, born 1907] Altmann-Gersh method. See under METHOD.

**Gerstmann** [Josef *Gerstmann,* Austrian neurologist, 1887–1969] See under SYNDROME.

**gerüstmark** \gərʏst′märk, gərist′-\ [German *Gerüst* scaffold + *Mark* marrow, pith] The presence in scurvy of connective tissue within the bone marrow.

**Gesell** [Arnold Lucius *Gesell,* U.S. psychologist, 1880–1961] Gesell developmental scales. See under SCALE.

**gestagen** \jes′təjən\ PROGESTOGEN.

**gestalt** \gəshtält′, gəstôlt′\ [German (old past part. of *stellen* to place, set up, arrange) form, shape, figure] (*pl.* gestalten) A perceptual configuration organized in such a way as to lend it properties that exceed the summation of its component parts; a pattern, a figure, or a perceptually integrated whole.

**gestaltism** \gəshtäl′tizm\ GESTALT PSYCHOLOGY.

**gestation** \jestā′shən\ [L *gestatio* (from *gestare* to carry, from *gerere* to produce, bear, carry) a bearing, carrying in the womb] The duration of the embryo in the uterus, from fertilization of the ovum until delivery; the period of normal pregnancy.

**GFR** glomerular filtration rate.

**GH** growth hormone.

**GHIH** growth hormone inhibiting hormone.

**Ghon** [Anton *Ghon,* Czech pathologist, 1866–1936] 1 Ghon focus, Ghon's primary lesion. See under GHON TUBERCLE. 2 Ghon complex. See under PRIMARY COMPLEX.

**ghost** The faint and barely perceivable remains of some object, especially of an erythrocyte. Also *shadow, phantom.* **erythrocyte g.** The hemoglobin-free erythrocyte membrane, usually obtained by lysing erythrocytes with hypotonic solutions. Also *ghost corpuscle, phantom corpuscle, shadow corpuscle, discoplasm, blood ghost, erythrocyte stroma, discostroma, ghost cell, phantom cell, shadow cell.*

**GHRH** growth hormone releasing hormone.

**GHRIH** growth hormone release inhibiting hormone.

**GI** gastrointestinal.

**Giacomini** [Carlo *Giacomini,* Italian anatomist, 1841–1898] Frenulum of Giacomini. See under BAND.

**Giannuzzi** [Giuseppe *Giannuzzi,* Italian physiologist, 1839–1876] 1 Giannuzzi's body, crescent of Giannuzzi. See under DEMILUNE OF GIANNUZZI. 2 Cell of Giannuzzi. See under DEMILUNE CELL.

**Gianotti** [Ferdinando *Gianotti,* Italian dermatologist, born 1920] Gianotti-Crosti syndrome. See under INFANTILE PAPULAR ACRODERMATITIS.

**giant** 1 A person or creature of great size. 2 MEGASOME.

**giantism** \jī′əntizm\ [GIANT + -ISM] GIGANTISM.

***Giardia*** \jē·är′dē·ə\ [after Alfred *Giard,* French biologist, 1846–1908 + -IA] A genus of parasitic flagellates (order Diplomonadida, class Zoomastigophorea) found in the small intestine of many mammals, including humans. The question of which species besides *G. lamblia* may be responsible for human giardiasis remains unresolved. Also *Lamblia.* ***G. intestinalis*** *GIARDIA LAMBLIA* ***G. lamblia*** The common intestinal flagellate of humans, an abundant, cosmopolitan parasite, and probably the most common protozoan human parasite in the United States. It is spread by drinking water contaminated with human feces or feces of infected animals, such as rodents and possibly domesticated animals. Also *Giardia intestinalis, Lamblia intestinalis.*

**giardiasis** \jē′ärdī′əsis\ [*Giard(ia)* + -IASIS] 1 Infection with protozoa of the genus *Giardia.* 2 Specifically, human infection with *Giardia lamblia*; lambliasis. Heavy infection may cause protracted diarrhea with symptoms suggestive of malabsorption. Light infections are usually asymptomatic but are probably capable of causing disease if the host's resistance falls. Some human infections have been shown to be derived from animals via mountain streams and other sources, but most are transmitted by human sewage in public water supplies.

**gibber** \gib′ər\ [L, hump] A humplike or pouchlike enlargement or projection. **g. inferior thalami** NUCLEUS POSTERIOR THALAMI. **g. ulnae** *Outmoded* OLECRANON.

**Gibbs** [Josiah Willard *Gibbs,* U.S. physicist, 1839–1903]

See under ENERGY.

**gibbus** \gib′əs\ [L, a hump, hunch] An angulation of the spine due to anterior collapse of the disk space and vertebral bodies. It is usually caused by an abscess, especially a tuberculous abscess.

**Gibert** [Camille Melchior *Gibert,* French dermatologist, 1797–1866] Gibert's disease, Gibert's pityriasis. See under PITYRIASIS ROSEA.

**Gibson** [George Alexander *Gibson,* Scottish physician, 1854–1913] See under MURMUR.

**Gibson** [Stanley *Gibson,* U.S. pediatrician, born 1883] Potts-Smith-Gibson operation. See under POTTS OPERATION.

**Giemsa** [Berthold Gustav Carl *Giemsa,* German chemotherapeutist, 1867–1948] See under METHOD, STAIN.

**Gierke** [Hans Paul Bernard *Gierke,* German anatomist, 1847–1886] Gierke cells. See under CELL.

**Gifford** [Harold *Gifford,* U.S. ophthalmologist, 1858–1929] **1** Gifford's reflex, Gifford-Galassi reflex. See under WESTPHAL-PILTZ REFLEX. **2** See under OPERATION.

**giga-** \jī′gə-\ [Gk *gigas* a giant] A combining form denoting $10^9$: used with SI units. Symbol: G

**gigabecquerel** \-bek′ərəl\ [GIGA- + BECQUEREL] A unit of activity of a radionuclide equal to $10^9$ becquerel. Symbol: GBq

**gigantism** \jī′gantizm\ [*gigant(o)-* + -ISM] **1** The state or quality of having excessively large stature; abnormally large size. **2** PITUITARY GIGANTISM. **acromegalic g.** Gigantism combined with changes in osseous and soft tissues characteristic of acromegaly in patients who because of an adenohypophysial tumor, began secreting growth hormone excessively before puberty and before epiphysial closure, the hormonal excess persisting into adult life. Also *acromegalogigantism.* **cerebral g.** SOTOS SYNDROME. **constitutional g.** Excessively large stature with normal body proportions and without demonstrable endocrine or other somatic dysfunction; gigantism attributed to genetic factors. Also *normal gigantism, primordial gigantism* (rare). **digital g.** MACRODACTYLY. **fetal g.** A size or weight in excess of the usual range in a fetus or newborn infant, often seen in the offspring of diabetic mothers or other conditions predisposing to postmaturity. **hyperpituitary g.** PITUITARY GIGANTISM. **hypothalamic g.** Gigantism associated with excessive release of growth hormone by the adenohypophysis, presumably owing to failure or deficiency of hypothalamic somatostatin (growth hormone inhibiting hormone). **normal g.** CONSTITUTIONAL GIGANTISM. **pituitary g.** Gigantism owing to excessive secretion of growth hormone by an adenohypophysial tumor or hypoplasia of the adenohypophysial alpha cells. Also *hyperpituitary gigantism, Launois syndrome, gigantism.* • When used without qualification, *gigantism* usually refers to pituitary gigantism. **primordial g.** *Rare* CONSTITUTIONAL GIGANTISM. **total lipodystrophy and acromegaloid g.** See under SEIP SYNDROME.

**giganto-** \jīgan′tə-\ [Gk *gigas* (genitive *gigantos*) a giant] A combining form meaning great in size, enormously large.

***Gigantobilharzia*** \-bilhär′zē·ə\ A genus of schistosome blood flukes (family Schistosomatidae) infecting birds. Some have been implicated in human cercarial dermatitis, or swimmer's itch.

**gigantomastia** \-mas′tē·ə\ [GIGANTO- + MAST- + -IA] Excessive growth of the breasts.

***Gigantorhynchus hirudinaceus*** \-ring′kəs hiroo′dinā′sē·əs\ *MACRACANTHORHYNCHUS HIRUDINACEUS.*

**gigantosoma** \-sō′mə\ [GIGANTO- + Gk *sōma* body] *Older term* GIGANTISM.

**Gilbert** [Augustin-Nicholas *Gilbert,* French physician, 1858–1927] **1** See under SYNDROME. **2** Gilbert-Behçet syndrome. See under BEHÇET SYNDROME.

**Gilchrist** [Thomas Caspar *Gilchrist,* U.S. physician, 1862–1927] Gilchrist's mycosis, Gilchrist's disease. See under BLASTOMYCOSIS.

**gilding** \gil′ding\ The application of gold salts or of a thin layer of gold to biologic material, especially fixed nerve tissue.

**Gilford** [Hastings *Gilford,* English physician, 1861–1941] Hutchinson-Gilford syndrome. See under PROGERIA.

**Gill** [Arthur Bruce *Gill,* U.S. orthopedic surgeon, 1876–1965] See under OPERATION.

**Gilles de la Tourette** [Georges Edouard Albert Brutus *Gilles de la Tourette,* French physician, 1859–1904] Gilles de la Tourette's disease, Tourette's disease, Tourette's disorder, Tourette syndrome. See under SYNDROME.

**Gillette** [Eugene Paulin *Gillette,* French surgeon, 1836–1886] Gillette suspensory ligament. See under TENDO CRICOESOPHAGEUS.

**Gilliam** [David Tod *Gilliam,* U.S. gynecologist, 1844–1923] See under OPERATION.

**Gillies** [Harold Delf *Gillies,* New Zealand surgeon, 1882–1960] **1** Gillies flap. See under TUBED FLAP. See under FLAP. **2** Filatov-Gillies tubed pedicle. See under PEDICLE.

**Gimbernat** [Antonio de *Gimbernat,* Spanish surgeon and anatomist, 1734–1816] **1** Gimbernat's ligament, lacunar ligament of Gimbernat. See under LIGAMENTUM LACUNARE. **2** Reflex ligament of Gimbernat. See under LIGAMENTUM REFLEXUM.

**gingiva** \jin′jivə, jinjī′və\ [L, the gum of the mouth] (*pl.* gingivae) A combination of epithelial and connective tissues that surrounds and is attached to the tooth and alveolar bone and extends to the mucogingival junction; the gum. On the palatal side it is a rim of tissue that merges with the masticatory mucosa of the hard palate. Also *oula* (outmoded), *ula* (outmoded). **areolar g.** The loose areolar connective tissue overlying part of the alveolar process. This is no longer considered to be part of the gingiva. *Outmoded.* **attached g.** The major portion of the gingiva, which is firmly bound down to the underlying bone and tooth. Also *gingival zone* (outmoded). **cleft g.** GINGIVAL CLEFT. **free g.** The collar of gingival tissue surrounding the gingival sulcus. This sulcus may be absent in the healthy state. *Outmoded.*

**gingivae** \jinjī′vē\ Plural of GINGIVA.

**gingival** \jinjī′vəl\ Of or relating to the gingivae.

**gingivectomy** \jin′jīvek′təmē\ [*gingiv(a)* + -ECTOMY] The elimination of a gingival or periodontal pocket by excision. The bevel of raw tissue left is then covered by a surgical pack for 7–10 days while re-epithelialization is occurring. In a reverse-bevel gingivectomy, the initial incision is directed towards the apices of the roots and the gingiva remaining is sutured interdentally to bring the raw surfaces into contact with the teeth.

**gingivitis** \jin′jivī′tis\ [*gingiv(o)-* + -ITIS] Any inflammatory condition of the gingivae, regardless of the etiology. **acute necrotizing g.** NECROTIZING ULCERATIVE GINGIVITIS. **acute ulcerative g.** NECROTIZING ULCERATIVE GINGIVITIS.. Abbr. AUG **bismuth g.** Chronic gingivitis modified by the systemic influence of a bismuth compound in a medicine. A dark bluish line in the gingiva is related to plaque stagnation areas. **chronic desquamative g.** Uncommon plaque-associated gingivitis in which the oral gingival epithelium becomes extremely thin as a result of cellular desquamation and the gingiva bright red and sharply demarcated from the normal tissue. This lesion is not to be confused with erosive lichen planus, benign mucous membrane pemphigoid, pemphigus, or foreign-body reactions. Also *desquamative gingivitis.* **diphenylhydantoin g.** A plaque-associated gingivitis showing marked hyperplasia caused by the systemic action of an anticoagulant drug diphenylhydantoin sodium (phenytoin sodium in British usage) used in treating epilepsy. Also *Dilantin gingival hyperplasia* (used especially in the U.S.). **eruptive g.** Gingivitis around erupting teeth. Mild trauma may produce false pockets allowing increased stagnation areas for plaque accumulation. With further eruption, these areas are reduced. **g. gravidarum** PREGNANCY GINGIVITIS. **hormonal g.** A plaque-associated gingivitis modified and aggravated by sex steroids released during phases of the menstrual cycle or pregnancy or administered in the form of contraceptives. The disease may present as a hyperplastic lesion called a pregnancy tumor (epulis). Hormonal imbalance may also be a factor in the hyperplastic gingivitis of puberty. **hyperplastic g.** Chronically enlarged and inflamed gingival tissues. The gingivitis is plaque-associated but may have been modified by systemic factors, such as pregnancy or ingestion of Dilantin sodium. **marginal g.** Gingivitis limited to the gingival margins and the interdental col. **necrotizing ulcerative g.** A disease involving necrosis and ulceration of the surface of the gingiva with underlying inflammation. It begins in an area of gingiva in contact with plaque, often interdental, and results in the clinically pathognomonic "punched-out" papilla. The plaque is characterized by a complex flora with relative proliferation of fusiform bacilli and spirochetes. The spirochetes penetrate the apparently still vital gingival tissues. The disease is associated with a typical fetor oris. Also *acute ulcerative gingivitis, acute necrotizing gingivitis, ulceromembranous gingivitis, Vincent's disease, trench mouth, Vincent stomatitis, fusospirochetal stomatitis.* Abbr. NUG **pregnancy g.** A plaque-associated gingivitis that has been exacerbated by pregnancy. It is sometimes considered a form of hormonal gingivitis. It may be hemorrhagic and hyperplastic in type. Also *gingivitis gravidarum.* **puberty g.** Hyperplastic, plaque-associated chronic gingivitis in children of pubertal age or in adolescents. It is assumed to be a form of hormonal gingivitis. **scorbutic g.** Hemorrhagic gingivitis associated with vitamin C deficiency. **ulceromembranous g.** NECROTIZING ULCERATIVE GINGIVITIS.

**gingivo-** \jin′jivō-\ [L *gingiva* the gum] A combining form denoting the gingivae.

**gingivoplasty** \jin′jivōplas′tē\ [GINGIVO- + -PLASTY] A surgical procedure to improve the contours of the gingiva and facilitate plaque control.

**gingivostomatitis** \jin′jivōstō′mətī′tis\ Inflammation of the gingivae and the mucosa of the oral cavity. **herpetic g.** HERPETIC STOMATITIS. **necrotizing ulcerative g.** The extension of necrotizing ulcerative gingivitis to involve adjacent oral mucosa. The tonsillar region may be involved (Vincent's angina), and extensive gangrene may occur (cancrum oris). **primary herpetic g.** An infection of the mouth by the herpes simplex virus, occurring usually in the first five years of life, rarely in adults. The characteristic vesicular lesions of the gingivae, but also of the tongue and lips, quickly give way to small painful ulcers. Fever and local lymphadenopathy are the rule. **white folded g.** WHITE SPONGE NEVUS.

**gingivostomatosis** \-stō′mətō′sis\ **white folded g.** WHITE SPONGE NEVUS.

**ginglyform** \jin′glifôrm\ GINGLYMOID.

**ginglymoarthrodial** \jin′glimō′ärthrō′dē·əl\ Pertaining to a joint with elements of both hinge and plane joints.

**ginglymoid** \jin′glimoid\ Pertaining to or resembling a ginglymus, or hinge joint. Also *ginglyform.*

**ginglymus** \jin′gliməs\ [New L, from Gk *ginglymos* hinge] [NA] A uniaxial synovial joint in which movement is generally limited to to-and-fro movements in one plane, like a door on a hinge. Typically, the joint has powerful collateral ligaments tending to contain the movements, such as in the humeroulnar joint. Also *hinge joint, ginglymoid joint, hinge articulation.* **helicoid g.** ARTICULATIO TROCHOIDEA. **lateral g.** ARTICULATIO TROCHOIDEA.

**Giordano** [Davide *Giordano,* Italian surgeon, 1864–1954] Giordano sphincter. See under MUSCULUS SPHINCTER DUCTUS CHOLEDOCHI.

**Girard** [Alfred Conrad *Girard,* Swiss-born U.S. surgeon, 1841–1914] **1** See under TREATMENT. **2** Girard's method. See under TREATMENT.

**girdle** An encircling structure or area; cingulum. **hip g.** CINGULUM MEMBRI INFERIORIS. **Hitzig's g.** A girdle of sensory loss around the trunk, situated at breast level, and corresponding to the region innervated by the third, fourth, fifth, and sixth dorsal nerves. This is sometimes an early manifestation of tabes dorsalis. **g. of inferior extremity** CINGULUM MEMBRI INFERIORIS. **limb g.** Either cingulum membri inferioris or cingulum membri superioris. **limbal g. of Vogt** A narrow fenestrated white crescent situated in the very superficial layers of the peripheral cornea in the nasal and temporal interpalpebral space. It is a benign, asymptomatic change of no significance. Also *limbus girdle.* **limbus g.** LIMBAL GIRDLE OF VOGT. **Neptune's g.** A wet pack worn around the abdomen. **pectoral g.** CINGULUM MEMBRI SUPERIORIS. **pelvic g.** CINGULUM MEMBRI INFERIORIS. **shoulder g.** CINGULUM MEMBRI SUPERIORIS. **g. of superior extremity** CINGULUM MEMBRI SUPERIORIS. **thoracic g.** CINGULUM MEMBRI SUPERIORIS. **upper limb g.** CINGULUM MEMBRI SUPERIORIS.

**Girdner** [John Harvey *Girdner,* U.S. physician, 1856–1933] Girdner's probe. See under ELECTRIC PROBE.

**githagism** \gith′əjizm\ [*(Agrostemma) githag(o)* + -ISM] Poisoning by seeds of corn cockle, *Agrostemma githago.* They contain the toxic substances agrostemmic acid and githagin, a glucoside. Corn cockle is a common weed whose seed is often found mixed in wheat. When ingested, it causes irritation of the digestive tract, vomiting, nausea, diarrhea, depressed respiration, and vertigo. Also *corn cockle poisoning.*

**Gitterfasern** \git′ərfä′zərn\ [German *Gitter* lattice, trellis + *Fasern,* pl. of *Faser* thread, fiber] The reticular fibers of the dermis.

**GIX** A proprietary name for DFDT.

**Gjessing** [Leiv Rolvssoen *Gjessing,* Norwegian physician, born 1918] See under SYNDROME.

**gl.** *glandula* (L, gland).

**glabella** \gləbel′ə\ [New L (substantive from fem. of *glabellus,* dim. of L *glaber* bare, smooth) a small hairless spot] [NA] A craniometric point situated in the midline of the frontal bone at the most prominent point between the medial ends of the superciliary arches. Also *metopic point, intercilium.*

**glabrous** \glā′brəs\ [L *glaber,* gen. *glabris,* bald, bare + -OUS] Smooth: used especially in reference to a surface that lacks terminal hair but is not strictly hairless.

**gladiolic acid** $C_{11}H_{10}O_5$. 2,3-Diformyl-6-methoxy-5-methylbenzoic acid, a naturally occurring antibiotic substance from *Penicillium gladioli.* It also has antifungal properties.

**gladiolus** \glədī′ələs, glad′i·ō′ləs\ [L, a small sword, from *gladius* a sword] CORPUS STERNI.

**gladiomanubrial** \glad′ē·ōmənoo′brē·əl\ Pertaining to the gladiolus and the manubrium of the sternum.

**glairy** \gler′ē\ Resembling glair, as in texture; viscid; glutinous.

# gland

**gland** [French *glande,* from Old French *glandre* a gland, esp. a swollen gland or lymph node, from L *glandula.* See GLANDULA.] **1** An organized group of epithelial cells, either tightly clustered or scattered, that produces a secretion or an excretion for discharge; glandula. **2** A lymph node, glomus, follicle, or other glandlike structure that has no glandular function. *Outmoded.* **accessory adrenal g.'s** GLANDULAE SUPRARENALES ACCESSORIAE. **accessory lacrimal g.'s** GLANDULAE LACRIMALES ACCESSORIAE. **accessory mammary g.'s 1** SUPERNUMERARY MAMMAE. **2** *Outmoded* MONTGOMERY'S GLANDS. **accessory parotid g.** GLANDULA PAROTIDEA ACCESSORIA. **accessory salivary g.'s** GLANDULAE SALIVARIAE MINORES. **accessory suprarenal g.'s** GLANDULAE SUPRARENALES ACCESSORIAE. **accessory thyroid g.'s** Small remnants of thyroid tissue, residua of embryogenesis, along the course of the thyroglossal duct and in the thorax. Also *suprahyoid glands, glandulae thyroideae accessoriae.* **acid g.** GLANDULA GASTRICA PROPRIA. **acinar g.** ACINOUS GLAND. **acinotubular g.** A gland made up of both tubules and acini. Also *tubuloacinar gland.* **acinous g.** A gland that is formed of cells arranged in small clusters which often encompass central lumens. Also *alveolar gland, acinar gland.* **adrenal g.** GLANDULA SUPRARENALIS. **Albarrán's g.'s** SUBCERVICAL GLANDS OF ALBARRÁN. **albuminous g.** Any gland that secretes a notably proteinaceous substance. **alveolar g.** ACINOUS GLAND. **anterior lingual g.** GLANDULA LINGUALIS ANTERIOR. **anterior lingual g. of Blandin and Nuhn** GLANDULA LINGUALIS ANTERIOR. **aortic g.'s** CORPORA PARA-AORTICA. **apical g. of tongue** GLANDULA LINGUALIS ANTERIOR. **apocrine g.** A gland whose secretory discharge contains a part (the apex) of the secreting cell, as in certain sweat glands. **apocrine sweat g.** A gland that opens into the hair follicle via a duct above the sebaceous duct. Such glands are small and inactive during childhood but enlarge at puberty. They are usually confined to the axillary and anogenital skin and to the areolae of the breasts. **areolar g.'s** MONTGOMERY'S GLANDS. **arterial g.** A small aggregation of arteriovenous anastomoses or vascular tissue, such as the glomus coccygeum. *Outmoded.* **arytenoid g.** GLANDULA ARYTENOIDEA. **atrabiliary g.** *Outmoded* GLANDULA SUPRARENALIS. **axillary g.'s** NODI LYMPHATICI AXILLARES. **Bartholin's g.** GLAN-

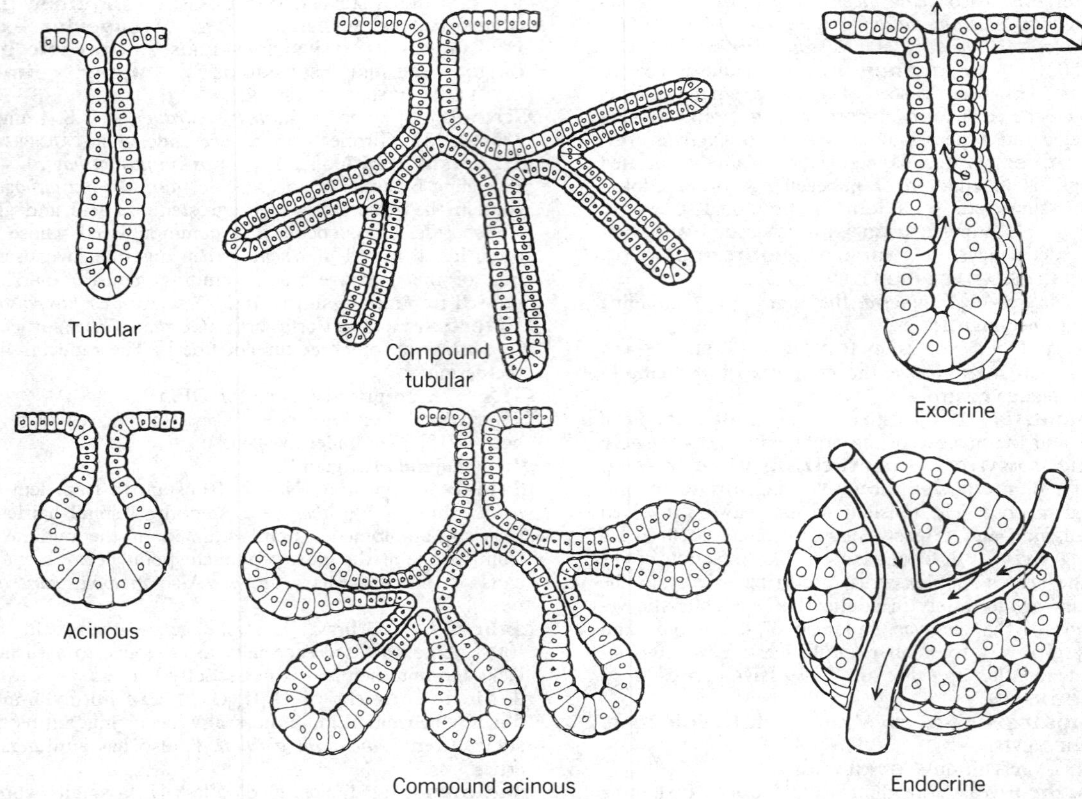


**Glands**

DULA VESTIBULARIS MAJOR. **Bauhin's g.'s** GLANDULA LINGUALIS ANTERIOR. **Baumgarten's g.'s** Convoluted tubular glands that are situated near the fornices in the medial part of the palpebral conjunctiva and open on the surface of the conjunctiva. Also *Henle's glands.* **g.'s of biliary mucosa** GLANDULAE MUCOSAE BILIOSAE. **Blandin's g.** GLANDULA LINGUALIS ANTERIOR. **Blandin and Nuhn g.** GLANDULA LINGUALIS ANTERIOR. **Boerhaave's g.'s** SWEAT GLANDS. **Bonnot's g.** INTERSCAPULAR GLAND. **Bowman's g.** GLANDULA OLFACTORIA. **brachial g.'s** NODI LYMPHATICI BRACHIALES. **bronchial g.'s** GLANDULAE BRONCHIALES. **Bruch's g.'s** Lymphatic follicles situated in the conjunctiva of the lower eyelid chiefly near the medial palpebral commissure. **Brunner's g.'s** GLANDULAE DUODENALES. **buccal g.'s** GLANDULAE BUCCALES. **bulbocavernous g.** GLANDULA BULBOURETHRALIS. **bulbourethral g.** GLANDULA BULBOURETHRALIS. **carotid g.** GLOMUS CAROTICUM. **g.'s of the caruncle** The sebaceous and sweat glands within the lacrimal caruncle. **celiac g.'s** NODI LYMPHATICI COELIACI. **ceruminous g.'s** The wax-forming glands of the external ear, located in the external portions of the external auditory meatus. Also *glandulae ceruminosae.* **cervical g.'s of uterus** GLANDULAE CERVICALES UTERI. **cheek g.'s** GLANDULAE BUCCALES. **choroid g.** PLEXUS CHOROIDEUS. **Ciaccio's g.'s** GLANDULAE LACRIMALES ACCESSORIAE. **ciliary g.'s** GLANDULAE CILIARES PALPEBRARUM. **Cloquet's g.** CLOQUET'S NODE. **Cobelli's g.** GLANDULA CARDIACA ESOPHAGI. **coil g.** CONVOLUTED GLAND. **compound g.** Any exocrine gland comprising multiple units whose ducts unite to form ductules and ducts of progressively larger size. The salivary glands and the pancreas are glands of this kind. **conjunctival g.'s** GLANDULAE CONJUNCTIVALES. **convoluted g.** A tubular gland of the skin, as a sweat gland, whose secretory, proximal end is coiled like a glomerulus. Also *coil gland.* **Cowper's g.** GLANDULA BULBOURETHRALIS. **ductless g.'s** ENDOCRINE GLANDS. **duodenal g.'s** GLANDULAE DUODENALES. **Duverney's g.** GLANDULA VESTIBULARIS MAJOR. **Ebner's g.'s** GLANDULA GUSTATORIA. **eccrine g.** Any of the more numerous type of sweat glands, whose cells do not form part of its secretary discharge, thus distinguishing them from apocrine glands; a merocrine gland. **Eglis g.'s** Small mucous glands in the renal pelvis. **endocrine g.'s** Glands that secrete gland-specific molecules, or hormones, directly into the bloodstream. The hormones influence body functions generally and at remote anatomic sites. Endocrine glands include the pituitary gland, the thyroid, parathyroids, adrenals, gonads, pancreatic islets, and specialized cells of the gastrointestinal tract and the lung. The status of the pineal and the thymus as endocrine glands is controversial. Also *ductless glands, glandulae endocrinae, glandulae sine ductibus.* **endoepithelial g.** INTRAEPITHELIAL GLAND. **endometrial g.'s** GLANDULAE UTERINAE. **epithelial g.** A mass of glandular cells within an epithelium. **esophageal g.'s** GLANDULAE ESOPHAGEAE. **esophageal g. proper** GLANDULA ESOPHAGEA PROPRIA. **excretory g.** A gland excreting the products of metabolism from the system, as the sweat glands. **exocrine g.** A gland which secretes its product to an internal or external surface through a duct or system of ducts, as the sweat glands or salivary glands. **extraparotid lymph g.'s** Nodi lymphatici parotidei superficiales. *Outmoded.* See under NODI LYMPHATICI PAROTIDEI SUPERFICIALES. **Fraenkel's g.'s** Minute laryngeal glands situated just below the vocal

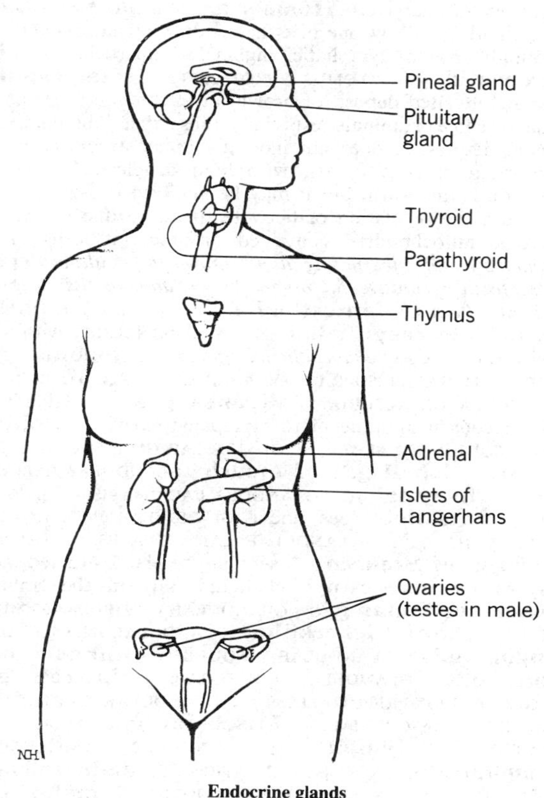


**Endocrine glands**

folds. **fundic g.** GLANDULA GASTRICA PROPRIA. **fundus g.** GLANDULA GASTRICA PROPRIA. **Galeati's g.'s** GLANDULAE INTESTINALES. **gastric g.'s** The several groups and types of glands secreting the gastric juice, including glandula cardiaca, glandula gastrica propria, and glandula pylorica. They contain zymogenic, oxyntic, and mucous cells. **gastric g. proper** GLANDULA GASTRICA PROPRIA. **gastroepiploic g.'s** The nodi lymphatici gastrici dextri and nodi lymphatici gastrici sinistri. **genal g.'s** GLANDULAE BUCCALES. **gingival g.'s** SERRES GLANDS. **glomerate g.'s** GLOMIFORM GLANDS. **glomiform g.'s** Arteriovenous shunts in the skin. Also *glomerate glands, glandulae glomiformes, glomus bodies.* • The term is inaccurate, since the bodies referred to are not glands. **greater vestibular g.** GLANDULA VESTIBULARIS MAJOR. **Guérin's g.'s** **1** DUCTUS PARAURETHRALES. **2** GLANDULAE URETHRALES URETHRAE FEMININAE. **gustatory g.** GLANDULA GUSTATORIA. **g.'s of Haller** GLANDULAE PREPUTIALES. **haversian g.'s** Villi synoviales or adipose tissue that is covered by a synovial lining in the joints. **hematopoietic g.'s** Those organs or glands that contribute to blood formation in fetal or postnatal life, including the thymus, liver, spleen, lymph glands, and bone marrow. *Seldom used.* **hemolymph g.'s** HE-

MOLYMPH NODE. **Henle's g.'s** BAUMGARTEN'S GLANDS. **heterocrine g.** GLANDULA SEROMUCOSA. **hibernating g.** INTERSCAPULAR GLAND. **holocrine g.** An exocrine gland whose secreting cells form part of its secretory discharge. **Home's g.** SUBTRIGONAL GLAND. **inguinal g.** Any one of either nodi lymphatici inguinales profundi or nodi lymphatici inguinales superficiales. **intercarotid g.** GLOMUS CAROTICUM. **interscapular g.** A lobulated deposit of brown fat in the interscapular region of some mammals, especially those that hibernate, and human fetuses. It does not have glandular structure, and is comprised of cells gorged with lipid droplets. Its specific function is unknown, but it may be involved in heat production and the regulation of body temperature due to the numerous mitochondria contained in the fat cells. Also *Bonnot's gland, hibernating gland, brown fat, multilocular adipose tissue, primitive fat organ, brown adipose tissue, textus adiposus fuscus.* **intestinal g.'s** GLANDULAE INTESTINALES. **intraepithelial g.** A gland located within an epithelium. Also *endoepithelial gland.* **jugular g.'s** NODI LYMPHATICI SUPRACLAVICULARES. **Kölliker's g.** GLANDULA OLFACTORIA. **Krause g.'s** 1 Glands in the mucous membrane of the tympanic cavity. 2 GLANDULAE CONJUNCTIVALES. 3 GLANDULAE LACRIMALES ACCESSORIAE. **labial g.'s of mouth** GLANDULAE LABIALES ORIS. **lacrimal g.** GLANDULA LACRIMALIS. **g.'s of large intestine** See under GLANDULAE INTESTINALES. **laryngeal g.'s** GLANDULAE LARYNGEALES. **lateral nasal g. of Stensen** A serous-type gland situated laterally in the nasal cavity but found only in the embryo. **lesser vestibular g.'s** GLANDULAE VESTIBULARES MINORES. **g.'s of Lieberkühn** GLANDULAE INTESTINALES. **lingual g.'s** GLANDULAE LINGUALES. **lingual mucous g.'s** GLANDULAE LINGUALES. **Littre's g.'s** 1 GLANDULAE PREPUTIALES. 2 GLANDULAE URETHRALES URETHRAE MASCULINAE. **Luschka's g.** GLOMUS COCCYGEUM. **lymph g.** NODUS LYMPHATICUS. **lymphatic g.** NODUS LYMPHATICUS. **main salivary g.'s** GLANDULAE SALIVARIAE MAJORES. **malar g.'s** GLANDULAE BUCCALES. **malpighian g.'s** FOLLICULI LYMPHATICI SPLENICI. **mammary g.** GLANDULA MAMMARIA. **marrow-lymph g.** A lymph gland that is largely composed of hematopoietic cells, and that serves as a site of blood formation, as normally occurs in embryonic and fetal life. *Rare.* **master g.** *Popular* PITUITARY GLAND. **meibomian g.'s** GLANDULAE TARSALES. **merocrine g.** An exocrine gland whose cells do not form part of its secretory discharge, as the commonest form of human sweat gland. **mesenteric g.'s** NODI LYMPHATICI MESENTERICI. **mesocolic g.'s** NODI LYMPHATICI MESOCOLICI. **metrial g.** A collection of cellular elements concerned with the nutrition of the embryo. It comprises giant cells of the maternal part of the placenta, the myometrial gland, and hypertrophied epithelial cells. **minor salivary g.'s** GLANDULAE SALIVARIAE MINORES. **mixed g.** GLANDULA SEROMUCOSA. **molar g.'s** GLANDULAE MOLARES. **Moll's g.'s** GLANDULAE CILIARES PALPEBRARUM. **Montgomery's g.'s** The enlarged sebaceous glands seen on the areola of the nipple during pregnancy. Also *glandulae areolares, glandulae sebaceae mammae, areolar gland, Montgomery's follicles.* **Morgagni's g.'s** GLANDULAE URETHRALES URETHRAE MASCULINAE. **g.'s of mouth** GLANDULAE ORIS. **mucilaginous g.'s** SYNOVIAL VILLI. **muciparous g.** GLANDULA MUCOSA. **mucous g.** GLANDULA MUCOSA. **mucous g.'s of auditory tube** GLANDULAE TUBARIAE. **mucous g.'s of duodenum** GLANDULAE DUODENALES. **mucous g.'s of eustachian tube** GLANDULAE TUBARIAE. **mucous g. of the urethra** A mucous gland that lies in the connective tissue around the penile part of the male urethra. **myometrial g.** A collection of cells which respond to steroids and are diffusely distributed during pregnancy in the myometrium of rabbits and some rodents. The myometrial gland has been considered a possible source of a hormone. **nabothian g.'s** NABOTHIAN CYSTS. **nasal g.'s** GLANDULAE NASALES. **Nuhn's g.** GLANDULA LINGUALIS ANTERIOR. **odoriferous g.'s of prepuce** GLANDULAE PREPUTIALES. **oil g.'s** SEBACEOUS GLANDS. **olfactory g.** GLANDULA OLFACTORIA. **oxyntic g.** GLANDULA GASTRICA PROPRIA. **pacchionian g.'s** GRANULATIONES ARACHNOIDEALES. **palatine g.'s** GLANDULAE PALATINAE. **palpebral g.'s** GLANDULAE TARSALES. **pancreaticosplenic g.'s** Nodi lymphatici pancreatici and nodi lymphatici splenici considered together. **parafrenal g.'s** Preputial glands that open alongside the frenulum of the prepuce. **parathyroid g.'s** Yellow bodies that occur in pairs behind or in the substance of the thyroid gland. They arise embryologically from the branchial clefts, In humans they usually comprise two superior and two inferior glands. Composed of chief cells and oxyphil cells, they secrete parathyroid hormone, the principal endocrine regulator of calcium and phosphorus and of the metabolism of bone. Also *glandulae parathyroideae, Sandström's bodies.* **paraurethral g.'s** 1 DUCTUS PARAURETHRALES. 2 GLANDULAE URETHRALES URETHRAE FEMININAE. **parotid g.** GLANDULA PAROTIDEA. **pectoral g.'s** NODI LYMPHATICI AXILLARES. **peptic g.** GLANDULA GASTRICA PROPRIA. **perspiratory g.'s** SWEAT GLANDS. **Peyer's g.'s** FOLLICULI LYMPHATICI AGGREGATI. **pharyngeal g.'s** GLANDULAE PHARYNGEAE. **pharyngeal pituitary g.** A group of adenohypophysial cells embedded in small clusters in the sphenoid bone, richly innervated but with a blood supply lacking in hypothalamic hypophysiotropic hormones. It may play a role in the secretion of anterior pituitary hormone. **Philip's g.'s** Lymph nodes situated in the anterior tr iangle of the neck close to the sternoclavicular joint. They become enlarged in children suffering from pulmonary tuberculosis, by extension from a primary focus in the apex of the lung, via the bronchial and hilar lymph nodes. **pilar g.'s** Sebaceous glands opening into hair follicles. **pineal g.** CORPUS PINEALE. **pituitary g.** An unpaired, ovoid body that lies below the hypothalamus in the pituitary fossa of the sella turcica; the hypophysis. In humans it weighs 400–900 mg. It is attached to the tuber cinereum by a stalk containing the hypothalamic-hypophysial portal venous system (which conveys to the pituitary the hypothalamic hypophysiotropic hormones) and the supraopticoneurohypophysial neurosecretory tract (which acts as a conduit for the neurohypophysial peptides oxytocin and vasopressin and their carrier proteins). The gland consists of two main lobes. The anterior lobe, the adenohypophysis, arises in embryogenesis from the ectodermal roof of the stomatodeum. It has three constituent parts, the pars distalis, or main body of the adenohypophysis; the pars intermedia, which is not a separate entity in man; and the pars tuberalis, which forms a tenuous cell layer on the outer surface of the pituitary stalk. The posterior lobe, the neurohypophysis, arises in embryogenesis from an outpouching of the hypothalamic floor, and includes the pars posterior, the infundibular stem, and the median eminence. Regulated by the hypothalamic releasing hormones, the adenohypophysis periodically secretes growth hormone, prolactin, thyrotropin, adrenocorticotropin, gonadotropin, and lipotropin. These hormones exert a major regulatory influence through other endocrine glands upon growth, development, maturation, and reproduction. Acted upon by many stimuli, the chief being the osmolarity of the plasma, the supraoptic nuclei secrete vasopressin, which is ultimately released from the neurohypophysis. The neurohypophysis also releases oxytocin at parturition, but the physiologic role of this hormone in man is not fully understood. Also *glandula pituitaria, hypophysis cerebri, pituitary body, master gland* (popular), *glandula basilaris, pituitarium.* **Poirier's g.** A lymph node located in the base of the broad ligament of the uterus where the uterine artery crosses medially over the ureter. **preputial g.'s** GLANDULAE PREPUTIALES. **principal lacrimal g.** PARS ORBITALIS GLANDULAE LACRIMALIS. **prostate g.** PROSTATA. **puberty g.'s** Leydig interstitial cells in the testis and lutein cells in the ovary. **pyloric g.** GLANDULA PYLORICA. **racemose g.'s** Exocrine glands that have a ramifying duct system and attached cluster of acini. **retromolar g.'s** GLANDULAE MOLARES. **Rivinus g.** GLANDULA SUBLINGUALIS. **Rosenmüller's g.** 1 CLOQUET'S NODE. 2 PARS PALPEBRALIS GLANDULAE LACRIMALIS. **saccular g.** An exocrine gland that is composed of one or more sacs lined with secretory cells. **salivary g.** One of either glandulae salivariae majores or glandulae salivariae minores. **Schüller's g.'s** 1 Diverticula of the ductus epoophori longitudinalis. 2 DUCTUS PARAURETHRALES. **sebaceous g.'s** Small lobulated glands in the dermis that produce sebum by a process of holocrine secretion. Most sebaceous glands open via the sebaceous duct into a hair follicle, but in a few sites, such as the female genitalia, the glands open directly onto the skin surface. Also *oil glands, glandulae sebaceae.* **sebaceous g.'s of eyelids** GLANDULAE SEBACEAE PALPEBRARUM. **sentinel g.** An enlarged regional lymph node calling attention to a nearby disease process, usually inflammatory in nature. It often refers to an enlarged lymph node adjacent to an ulcer of the stomach. **seromucous g.** GLANDULA SEROMUCOSA. **serous g.** An exocrine gland that secretes a wheylike or watery fluid that contains proteins such as lysozymes and digestive enzymes. The nuclei of the cells are spherical and placed near the base of the cell and the apical cytoplasm contains zymogen granules. Also *glandula serosa.* **Serres g.'s** Aggregations of epithelial cells situated in the gingival mucosa of the newborn infant. Also *gingival glands.* **sexual g.** The testis or ovary. **g.'s of Shambaugh** The specialized stratified columnar epithelium of the stria vascularis on the outer wall of the cochlear duct that some investigators believe secretes endolymph. *Imprecise.* **Sigmund's g.'s** NODI LYMPHATICI CUBITALES. **simple g.** An exocrine gland that is drained by a duct without branches. **Skene's g.'s** GLANDULAE URETHRALES URETHRAE FEMININAE. **g.'s of small intestine** See under GLANDULAE INTESTINALES. **splenolymph g.** A hemal node that contains tissue resembling that of the spleen. **Stahr's g.** One of the nodi lymphatici faciales, situated adjacent to the facial artery as it crosses the base of the mandible. **subauricular g.'s** NODI LYMPHATICI MASTOIDEI. **subcervical g.'s of Albarrán** Submucosal glands of the prostatic part of the urethra that are situated just distal to the neck of the urinary bladder where the subtrigonal glands are located. Some consider these glands to be true mucous glands. It is believed by some authorities that hyperplasia of the glands produces the so-called middle lobe hypertrophy of the prostate. Also *Albarrán's glands, Albarrán's tubules.* **sublingual g.** GLANDULA SUBLINGUALIS. **submandibular g.** GLANDULA SUBMANDIBULARIS. **subtrigonal g.** 1 One of several epithelial outgrowths of the urethra during development of the glandular tissue of the prostate which are situated beneath the mucous membrane near the apex of the trigone of the urinary bladder and constitute part of the middle lobe of the prostate, especially when they undergo hyperplasia. They lie deep to and form the uvula vesicae. Also *Home's gland, Home's lobe.* 2 GLANDULA TRIGONI VESICAE. **sudoriferous g.'s** SWEAT GLANDS. **sudoriparous g.'s** SWEAT GLANDS. **suprahyoid g.'s** ACCESSORY THYROID GLANDS. **suprahyoid accessory thyroid g.** GLANDULA THYROIDEA ACCESSORIA SUPRAHYOIDEA. **suprarenal g.** GLANDULA SUPRARENALIS. **Suzanne's g.** A mucous gland situated in the mucous membrane of the floor of the mouth near the midline. **sweat g.'s** Glands in the skin that produce sweat. Also *glandulae sudoriferae, sudoriferous glands, perspiratory glands, Boerhaave's glands, sudoriparous glands.* See also APOCRINE SWEAT GLAND, ECCRINE GLAND. **synovial g.'s** SYNOVIAL VILLI. **target g.** A gland whose function is affected by an external influence, as the thyroid gland, gonads, or the adrenal cortex by an anterior pituitary hormone. **tarsal g.'s** GLANDULAE TARSALES. **Theile's g.'s** LUSCHKA'S CRYPTS. **thymus g.** THYMUS. **thyroid g.** A highly vascular endocrine gland weighing 10 to 60 g in the human adult, located in the front of the neck and closely apposed to the upper part of the trachea, and consisting of two lobes joined in front by an isthmus. It arises embryologically from the pharyngeal floor. The gland is ultimately concerned with nutrition, having the capacity to concentrate iodine and forming the thyroid hormones, thyroxine and triiodothyronine, which play a major part in regulating metabolic rate, rate of cellular oxygen consumption, normal growth, and orderly somatic and mental development. It consists of follicles 200 μm in diameter, among which are interspersed parafollicular cells that secrete thyrocalcitonin, which is important in calcium metabolism. Also *glandula thyroidea, thyroidea, thyroid body* (outmoded). **Tiedemann's g.** GLANDULA VESTIBULARIS MAJOR. **g.'s of tongue** GLANDULAE LINGUALES. **tracheal g.'s** GLANDULAE TRACHEALES. **trachoma g.'s** Follicular enlargements of the conjunctiva due to infection with *Chlamydia trachomatis.* **tubular g.** An exocrine gland whose component cells are arranged in the form of tube about a central lumen. **tubuloacinar g.** ACINOTUBULAR GLAND. **tympanic g.** A minute ganglionic mass situated on the tympanic nerve in its canaliculus. **g.'s of Tyson** GLANDULAE PREPUTIALES. **unicellular g.** A single cell that secretes directly onto a surface, as the goblet cells that line the large bowel mucosa. **urethral g.'s of female urethra** GLANDULAE URETHRALES URETHRAE FEMININAE. **urethral g.'s of male urethra** GLANDULAE URETHRALES URETHRAE MASCULINAE. **uterine g.'s** GLANDULAE UTERINAE. **utricular g.'s** GLANDULAE UTERINAE. **vesical g.'s** 1 Mucous follicles in the mucous membrane of the urinary bladder, especially near the neck. 2 GLANDULA TRIGONI VESICAE. **vestibular g.'s** Glandula vestibularis major and glandulae vestibulares minores. **Virchow's g.** SENTINEL NODE. **Waldeyer's g.'s** Small sweat glands in the skin of the attached margin of the eyelid, especially the lower. **Wasmann's g.** GLANDULA GASTRICA PROPRIA. **Weber's g.'s** Lingual mucous glands situated in the posterior part of the tongue at its margins. **Wepfer's g.'s** GLANDULAE DUODENALES. **Willis g.** CORPUS ALBICANS. **g.'s of Wolfring** GLANDULAE LACRIMALES ACCESSORIAE. **g.'s of Zeis** GLANDULAE SEBACEAE PALPEBRARUM. **Zuckerkandl's**

**g.** An occasional accessory thyroid gland situated left of center on the front of the hyoid bone.
**glanders** \glan′dərz\ [Old French *glandres* (from L *glandulae* glands) swollen glands, esp. in the neck] A serious, often fatal, infectious disease of horses, mules, and donkeys caused by *Pseudomonas mallei* and characterized by ulcerous nodules in the upper respiratory tract, lungs, and skin. When the lymphatic system is affected, with formation of nodules and abscesses (farcy buds), the disease is known as farcy. In the chronic form, large stellate scars in the mucosa of the nasal septum are characteristic. Formerly distributed worldwide, it has been eliminated or controlled in many countries, including the United States. Man and many other animals species are susceptible to infection. Human infection acquired from an infected animal or another human case, can be a chronic suppurative infection or acute, being localized and suppurative, pulmonary, or septicemic. The septicemic form is always fatal.
**glandes** \glan′dēz\ Plural of GLANS.

## glandula

**glandula** \glan′dyələ\ [L (dim. of *glans*, gen. *glandis*, an acorn) a gland or lymph node, esp. of the neck] (*pl.* glandulae) An organized group of epithelial cells, either tightly clustered or scattered, that produces a secretion or an excretion for discharge; gland. Either it may discharge directly onto a surface or via a duct (exocrine gland) or it may discharge into the blood and lymph streams (endocrine gland). The classification of glands is based either on structure or the nature and composition of the secretions. Also *glandule*. **glandulae areolares** MONTGOMERY'S GLANDS. **g. arytenoidea** One of several laryngeal glands located in the triangular fovea of the arytenoid cartilage and around the cuneiform cartilage in the free edge of the aryepiglottic fold. Also *arytenoid gland*. **g. atrabiliaris** GLANDULA SUPRARENALIS. **g. basilaris** PITUITARY GLAND. **glandulae bronchiales** [NA] Mixed mucoserous and mucous glands situated in the submucosa of the bronchi. Their ducts penetrate the more superficial layers to open on the surface of the mucous membrane. Also *bronchial glands*. **glandulae buccales** [NA] Small mucous glands situated between the mucous membrane of the cheek and the buccinator muscle. Also *buccal gland, genal glands, cheek glands, malar glands*. **g. bulbourethralis** [NA] A small, rounded, lobulated gland situated on each side of the membranous urethra just superior to the perineal membrane and the bulb of the penis and surrounded by the sphincter urethrae. The lobules are invested with fibrous tissue and comprise acini of columnar epithelium. Its excretory duct pierces the perineal membrane and opens on the floor of the spongy part of the urethra. It is homologous to the greater vestibular gland in the female. Also *bulbourethral gland, Cowper's gland, anteprostate, antiprostate, bulbocavernous gland*. **g. cardiaca esophagi** Any of the small compound tubuloalveolar glands that are situated at the extremities of the esophagus. One group is at a level between the cricoid cartilage and the fifth tracheal cartilage and a lower group is near the cardiac orifice of the stomach. The glands are limited to the lamina propria mucosae, and their large ducts open on the tip of a papilla. They vary considerably or may be absent entirely. Also *Cobelli's gland*. **g. cardiaca gastrica** One of a small number of simple and compound tubular glands that are situated in a narrow ring-shaped area near the cardiac orifice of the stomach. Mucus-secreting cells are common, whereas zymogenic and oxyntic cells are scarce. They closely resemble the superficial mucosal glands in the esophagus adjacent to the cardiac orifice. **glandulae ceruminosae** CERUMINOUS GLANDS. **glandulae cervicales uteri** [NA] Extensively branched large glands situated in the mucosa of the cervical canal of the uterus and lined with a tall columnar epithelium that secretes a clear, alkaline mucus. Also *cervical glands of uterus*. **glandulae ciliares palpebrarum** [NA] A number of large, modified sweat glands that form several rows near the free margin of each eyelid and open either into or near the follicles of the eyelashes. The nature of their secretion is uncertain. Also *ciliary glands, Moll's glands*. **glandulae conjunctivales** [NA] Groups of mucus-secreting goblet cells that are either scattered throughout the epithelium of the conjunctiva or are lining irregular invaginations of the epithelium, especially where it is reduced to two cell layers at the upper edge of the tarsus. Also *conjunctival glands, Krause glands*. **g. cutis** A gland of the skin. **glandulae duodenales** [NA] Mucous tubuloalveolar glands that are situated in the submucosa of the duodenum, most extensively in the superior part and diminishing in number towards the jejunum. Their excretory ducts pierce the muscularis mucosae and open into the intestinal glands. Also *duodenal glands, Brunner's glands, Wepfer's glands, cryptae mucosae duodeni, mucous crypts of duodenum, mucous glands of duodenum*. **glandulae endocrinae** [NA] ENDOCRINE GLANDS. **g. epiglottica** One of several mucous glands located in little pits on both surfaces of the epiglottis. **glandulae esophageae** The glandula esophagea propria and glandula cardiaca esophagi considered together. Also *esophageal glands*. **g. esophagea propria** One of the small compound glands with branched tubuloalveolar secretory portions that contain only mucous glands and are situated in the submucosa of the middle two thirds of the esophagus. Their long, dilated main ducts pierce the lamina muscularis mucosae to open on the mucosal surface. Also *esophageal gland proper*. **g. gastrica propria** One of the main gastric glands that are situated in the mucosa of the body and fundus of the stomach and open into the bottom of the gastric pits. Some are compound racemose while others are simple tubular glands and they contain highly differentiated cells including chief or zymogenic cells, oxyntic or parietal cells, argentaffin cells, mucous neck cells and undifferentiated cells. Also *gastric gland proper, fundic gland, fundus gland, Wasmann's gland, gastric follicle, oxyntic gland, acid gland, peptic gland*. **glandulae glomiformes** GLOMIFORM GLANDS. **g. gustatoria** [NA] One of the specialized racemose serous or albuminous glands located in the muscle tissue of the tongue near the taste buds, the ducts of which open mostly into the sulci surrounding the vallate papillae. Also *gustatory gland, Ebner's gland*. **g. intercarotica** GLOMUS CAROTICUM. **glandulae intestinales** [NA] Numerous tubular glands in the mucous membrane of the small and large intestine. They are simple tubular structures or crypts, set at right angles to the surface, that extend deeply through the thickness of the mucosa to the muscularis mucosae. In the small intestine they open by small round apertures between the bases of the villi, the epithelium of which continues into the glands and contains large zymogenic cells of Paneth at the bottom of the crypts. Scattered in their epithelium are argentaffin cells. In the large intestine their epithelium contains more goblet cells than are seen in the small intestine and there are no Paneth cells. Also *intestinal glands, glands of Lieberkühn,* *crypts of Lieberkühn, Lieberkühn's follicles, intestinal follicles, Galeati's glands.* **glandulae labiales oris** [NA] Small, rounded mucous glands, situated between the mucous membrane of the lips and the orbicularis oris muscle, the ducts of which open into the vestibule of the mouth. Also *labial glands of mouth.* **glandulae lacrimales accessoriae** [NA] Small tear-secreting glands that are situated near and in the conjunctival fornices, being more numerous in the upper eyelid than the lower. Also *accessory lacrimal glands, Krause glands, glands of Wolfring, Ciaccio's glands.* **g. lacrimalis** [NA] The large tear-secreting gland that is situated in the anterolateral part of the orbital cavity above the lateral angle of the eye. There its fine excretory ducts open into the superior conjunctival fornix. Its anterior margin lies against the orbital septum. It is imperfectly divided into two unequal parts by the tendinous expansion of the levator palpebrae superioris muscle, namely the pars orbitalis and pars palpebralis. It is a compound tubuloalveolar gland comprising many small lobules. Also *lacrimal gland.* **glandulae laryngeales** [NA] Mucous glands situated in the mucous membrane of the larynx, designated according to their location glandula epiglottica, glandula arytenoidea, glandula ventriculi laryngis, and glandula sacculi laryngis, as well as in the infraglottic cavity. They were formerly designated simply as anterior, middle, and posterior groups. Also *laryngeal glands.* **glandulae linguales** [NA] Mucous and serous glands located in the mucous membrane of the tongue. The mucous glands (glandula lingualis apicalis and glandula radicis linguae) are numerous in the posterior part but are also found along the margins and at the tip. The racemose serous glands are located near taste buds, their ducts opening into the sulci of the vallate papillae. Also *lingual glands, lingual mucous glands, glands of tongue.* **g. lingualis anterior** [NA] One of a pair of mixed, though chiefly mucous, glands situated on the inferior surface of the apex of the tongue, on either side of the midline adjacent to the frenulum. Also *anterior lingual gland, anterior lingual gland of Blandin and Nuhn, apical gland of tongue, Bauhin's gland, Blandin's gland, Blandin and Nuhn gland, Nuhn's gland.* **g. mammaria** [NA] The glandular element, or parenchyma, of the mamma, or breast, which undergoes growth and development after puberty in the female but remains rudimentary in the male. It is situated in the superficial fascia on each side of the front of the thorax, being separated from the ribs by the pectoral and thoracic muscles. It comprises about 15 to 20 lobes composed of lobules formed by acini and surrounded by areolar tissue, blood vessels, and lymphatics. The lobules are drained by ducts that join together so that each lobe has a single lactiferous duct opening on the surface of the nipple, or papilla. The lobes and ducts are distributed in a radial fashion around the nipple. The lobules and lobes are held together by connective tissue and surrounded by varying amounts of fat, giving the mamma its contour. The glandular structure varies with age, pregnancy, and lactation and secretes milk when functioning. Also *mammary gland.* **glandulae molares** [NA] Several of the larger buccal glands situated external to the buccinator muscle and around the entrance of the parotid duct in the cheek. Their ducts pierce the buccinator and open into the oral cavity opposite the upper third molar tooth. Also *molar glands, retromolar glands.* **g. mucosa** A unicellular or multicellular gland containing mucous or goblet cells that usually have small, dark nuclei flattened against the basal plasma membrane of the cell and a clear cytoplasm containing pale droplets of mucigen, a protein-polysaccharide complex. Mucigen leaves the cell to form mucin, the basic constituent of mucus. Also *mucous gland, muciparous gland, cryptae mucosae.* **glandulae mucosae biliosae** [NA] Numerous lobulated mucous glands situated in the mucous membrane of the neck of the gallbladder and groups of tubuloalveolar glands distributed throughout the mucosa of the larger bile ducts. Also *glands of biliary mucosa.* **glandulae nasales** [NA] Groups of serous and mucous glands situated deep to the basal lamina of the respiratory epithelium of the nasal cavity. Also *nasal glands, nasal mucous follicles* (outmoded). **g. olfactoria** One of the several branched tubuloalveolar glands deep to the olfactory epithelium of the nasal mucous membrane, on the surface of which their narrow, short ducts open. Also *olfactory gland, Bowman's gland, Kölliker's gland.* **glandulae oris** [NA] Glandulae salivariae majores and glandulae salivariae minores. Also *glands of mouth.* **glandulae palatinae** [NA] Numerous mucous glands situated between the periosteum and the mucous membrane of the posterior half of the bony palate and beneath and in the mucous membrane of both surfaces of the soft palate, especially on the inferior surface and around the uvula. Those on the superior surface are mixed glands. Also *palatine glands.* **glandulae parathyroideae** PARATHYROID GLANDS. **g. parotidea** [NA] The largest of the main salivary glands, shaped like an inverted three-sided pyramid and situated below and anterior to the external acoustic meatus in the gap between the mandible and the sternocleidomastoid muscle. Superiorly it reaches the zygomatic arch and inferiorly extends beyond the angle of the mandible. It is divided into a pars superficialis and a pars profunda by the branches of the facial nerve, the superficial part extending forward over the masseter muscle and ending in the parotid duct, while the deep portion extends medially to the styloid process behind the mandible. Its investing capsule is derived from the deep cervical fascia. Within the substance of the gland are the external carotid artery and its terminal branches as well as the retromandibular vein and its tributaries and termination. Its lobules contain only serous alveoli. Also *parotid gland, glandula parotis, parotid.* **g. parotidea accessoria** [NA] The most anterior portion of the superficial part of the parotid gland, either fully or partially detached, situated between the zygomatic arch above and the parotid duct below. It is present in about 30 percent of individuals and its duct joins the parotid duct. Also *accessory parotid gland, glandula parotis accessoria, accessory part of parotid gland.* **g. parotis** GLANDULA PAROTIDEA. **g. parotis accessoria** GLANDULA PAROTIDEA ACCESSORIA. **glandulae pharyngeae** [NA] Mucous glands situated beneath the mucous membrane of the pharynx and especially numerous in the nasopharynx around the orifices of the auditory tubes. Also *pharyngeal glands.* **g. pituitaria** PITUITARY GLAND. **glandulae preputiales** [NA] A few modified sebaceous glands situated on the corona and the neck of the glans penis that secrete smegma. Also *preputial glands, Littre's crypts, Littre's glands, Haller's crypts, glands of Haller, glands of Tyson, crypts of Tyson.* **g. pylorica** One of the simple, branched tubular glands that are situated in the pyloric part of the stomach. Each comprises a few short convoluted tubules opening into the gastric pits which extend deep into the mucous membrane. The epithelial cells are mainly of the mucous type with some oxyntic cells. They may also produce gastrin. Also *pyloric gland.* **g. sacculi laryngis** One of several laryngeal glands located in the saccule of the larynx. **glandulae salivariae majores** [NA] The three pairs of main salivary glands, the ducts of which carry their secretions into the oral cavity to assist the process of digestion. They are the glandula parotidea, glandula sublingualis, and glandula submandibularis. Also *main salivary glands.* **glandulae salivariae minores** [NA] Numerous small glands in the mucous membrane of the tongue, lips, cheeks and palate that produce either mucous or serous secretions or both so as to assist the process of digestion in the oral cavity. Also *minor salivary glands, accessory salivary glands.* **glandulae sebaceae** SEBACEOUS GLANDS. **glandulae sebaceae mammae** MONTGOMERY'S GLANDS. **glandulae sebaceae palpebrarum** [NA] Small sebaceous glands that are situated in the eyelids and open into the follicles of the eyelashes. In addition, they are also associated with the sparse, downy hairs on the skin of the eyelids. Also *sebaceous glands of eyelids, glands of Zeis.* **g. seromucosa** [NA] A mixed exocrine gland containing either mucous and serous secretory units or acini with both mucous and serous cells. In various glands one or other type of cell may predominate, affecting the constitution of the secretion produced. Also *seromucous gland, mixed gland, heterocrine gland.* **g. serosa** SEROUS GLAND. **glandulae sine ductibus** ENDOCRINE GLANDS. **g. sublingualis** [NA] The smallest of the three main salivary glands situated in the floor of the mouth deep to the mucous membrane on each side of the lateral surface of the tongue, resting on the mylohyoid muscle and lying along the medial surface of the anterior part of the corpus mandibulae above the mylohyoid line. Also *sublingual gland, Rivinus gland.* **g. submandibularis** [NA] One of the three main salivary glands, part of which is superficial to the posterior part of the mylohyoid muscle, and part deep to the muscle. It is ovoid in shape and variable in size, situated deep to the posterior part of the corpus mandibulae and extending downward into the digastric triangle of the neck. It is crossed superficially by the facial vein, while the facial artery grooves the posterosuperior part of the gland and then emerges between its lateral surface and the mandible. Its long excretory duct crosses the hyoglossus muscle and lingual nerve to open in the floor of the mouth, one on each side of the base of the frenulum of the tongue. Also *submandibular gland.* **glandulae sudoriferae** SWEAT GLANDS. **glandulae suprarenales accessoriae** [NA] Isolated, encapsulated nodules of either cortical tissue only (cortical bodies) or medullary and cortical tissue of the suprarenal gland. They may be located either in areolar tissue near the main gland and the celiac axis or in or near the kidney, along the ureter, in or near the ovaries, in the broad ligament of the uterus, in the spermatic cord, or in the caput epididymidis. Also *accessory suprarenal glands, accessory adrenal capsules, accessory adrenal glands.* **g. suprarenalis** A paired endocrine gland that is pyramidal in shape on the right and crescentic on the left, flattened anteroposteriorly, and situated on the anterosuperior aspect of each kidney. It is retroperitoneal, enclosed in the renal fascia, and composed of a mesodermal cortex and an ectodermal medulla. The embryologically fused cortex forms the greater part of the gland and comprises three layers, the zona glomerulosa, zona fasiculata, and zona reticularis, which contain no chromaffin tissue and secrete lipids. The cortex, essential to life, is regulated by two hormones. One, adenohypophysial adrenocorticotropin, maintains the glandular structure and stimulates the secretion of more than thirty $C_{21}$ corticosteroids such as cortisol, adrenal androgens, progestins, and perhaps estrogens. The second, renin-angiotensin, controls aldosterone secretion. The medulla secretes epinephrine and norepinephrine. Its irregular chromaffin cells form either rounded masses or short cords surrounded by venules and blood capillaries. The medulla can be extirpated without lethality. Also *adrenal gland, suprarenal gland, atrabiliary gland* (outmoded), *paranephros* (outmoded), *adrenal body, suprarenal body, adrenal capsule, epinephros, renicapsule* (outmoded), *glandula atrabiliaris, suprarene* (outmoded). **glandulae tarsales** [NA] A row of about 30 modified sebaceous glands embedded transversely in a groove in the tarsus of each eyelid. They have lobulated terminal alveolar portions which are connected by short lateral branching ducts to long central excretory ducts. The long ducts are lined with stratified squamous epithelium and open on the inner free margins of the eyelids. Their oily secretion forms a barrier for the tears so that they do not overflow on to the cheeks. Also *tarsal glands, meibomian glands, palpebral glands.* **g. thyroidea** [NA] THYROID GLAND. **g. thyroidea accessoria suprahyoidea** A small, isolated nodule of thyroid tissue occasionally located in the midline above the hyoid bone. Also *suprahyoid accessory thyroid gland.* **glandulae thyroideae accessoriae** [NA] ACCESSORY THYROID GLANDS. **glandulae tracheales** Small tubuloacinous, mixed mucous glands situated mostly in the submucosa between the cartilaginous rings and on the posterior wall of the trachea. Their short ducts pierce the elastic fibers of the lamina propria to open on the inner surface of the trachea. Also *tracheal glands.* **g. trigoni vesicae** One of the glands in the mucous membrane near the internal urethral opening in the urinary bladder, considered by some authorities to be true mucous glands. Pathological enlargement may produce urinary obstruction. Also *vesical gland, subtrigonal gland.* **glandulae tubariae** [NA] Mucous glands of the auditory tube that are located, associated with lymph nodules, in the loose, thick mucosa of the cartilaginous portion, particularly near the pharynx. Also *mucous glands of auditory tube, mucous glands of eustachian tube.* **glandulae urethrales urethrae femininae** [NA] A number of small mucous glands situated in the mucous membrane of the female urethra and opening separately on its surface. A group of glands on each side of the distal end of the urethra occasionally open into the paraurethral duct. Also *urethral glands of female urethra, paraurethral glands, Skene's glands, Guerin's glands, cryptae urethrae muliebris.* **glandulae urethrales urethrae masculinae** [NA] Numerous small glands and follicles situated in the submucosa of the proximal two-thirds of the spongy part of the male urethra that open in the grooves between the longitudinal folds of the urethra. Also *urethral glands of male urethra, Littre's glands, crypts of Littre, Morgagni's glands.* **glandulae uterinae** [NA] Tubular glands found within the inner layer of the uterine wall. These glands undergo cyclical changes in the reproductive phase of life that constitute the menstrual cycle. Also *uterine glands, endometrial glands, utricular glands.* **g. ventriculi laryngis** One of several laryngeal glands located on the vestibular fold and in the ventricle of the larynx. **glandulae vestibulares minores** [NA] Numerous small mucous glands that open on the surface of the vestibule between the external urethral orifice and the vaginal orifice. Also *lesser vestibular glands.* **g. vestibularis major** [NA] A small, oval tubuloalveolar gland situated on each side of the vaginal orifice contiguous with and medial to the posterior end of the bulb of the vestibule, its duct opening between the labium minus and the vaginal orifice. It is homologous to the bulbourethral gland in the male. Also *greater vestibular gland, Bartholin's gland, Duverney's gland, Tiedemann's gland.*

**glandulae** \glan′dyəlē\ Plural of GLANDULA.

**glandular** \glan′dyələr\ Of, resembling, or having the characteristics of a gland.

**glandule** \glan′dyool\ GLANDULA.

**glans** \glanz\ [L, acorn] An acorn-shaped, rounded body

or mass of tissue, specifically the glans penis and glans clitoridis. **g. clitoridis** [NA] The small, rounded free end of the body of the clitoris, composed of erectile tissue and covered by a highly sensitive epithelium. Overhanging it superiorly is the prepuce and inferiorly the frenulum is attached to it. It is homologous to the glans penis in the male. Also *glans of clitoris.* **g. of clitoris** GLANS CLITORIDIS. **g. penis** [NA] The conical expansion of the corpus spongiosum at the distal extremity of the penis. Its proximal end, or base, forms the corona glandis projecting over the distal ends of the corpora cavernosa, which are attached in its proximal concavity. The spongy urethra pierces it and opens on its distal end. The thin skin of the penis attaches around its neck and extends over it as a double fold forming the prepuce. Also *head of penis.*

**Glanzmann** [Eduard *Glanzmann,* Swiss physician, 1887–1959] Glanzmann's thrombasthenia. See under GLANZMANN'S DISEASE.

**glare** An irritating sensation accompanying visual perception of very bright light, either direct or reflected. It can sharply reduce perception of one's normal field of vision.

**glass** [Old English *glæs,* akin to Old English *glær* amber and Old English *geolu* yellow] A hard, brittle, usually transparent substance formed by fusing sand with various oxides. See also GLASSES. **cover g.** A thin disk or oblong of glass placed upon material to be examined microscopically. It is often used with a sealing material to provide permanent protection. Also *coverslip.* Also *coverglass.* **holvi g.** VITA GLASS. **lithium g.** A lithium-containing glass used for x-ray tubes which produce photons of very low voltage, such as grenz ray tubes. **object g.** OBJECTIVE. **optical g.** Any type of fine quality glass with uniform refracting properties, suitable for the manufacture of lenses. **quartz g.** A glass composed of the mineral, quartz, which has the property of transmitting ultraviolet rays. **vita g.** Glass containing a high percentage of quartz and especially transparent to ultraviolet light. Also *holvi glass, vitaglass.* **watch g.** A shallow concave glass vessel that is similar in shape and appearance to the crystal of a large pocket watch. It is used for evaporating small quantities of fluid or containing reagents whose interaction is to be viewed with the naked eye. **Wood's g.** A nickel oxide filter glass used with ultraviolet light to remove the visible radiation so that any weak fluorescence may be seen. It is used to detect ringworm infection of the scalp. See also WOOD'S LIGHT.

**glasses** Eyeglasses; optical spectacles. **bifocal g.** Eyeglasses for the correction of presbyopia in which the left and right lenses are each divided into two separate segments with different focal distances, the upper portions for distant vision and the lower portions for near vision. Also *bifocals.* **Frenzel g.** A pair of shielded glasses fitted with +20 diopter biconvex lenses and enclosed with a source of illumination for use in the investigation of nystagmus and in caloric testing, so as to abolish optic fixation and facilitate observation of the subject's eyes. **hyperbolic g.** Lenses designed with an exaggerated anterior convexity. **trifocal g.** Eyeglasses in which the left and right lenses are divided into three separate segments with different focal distances, the upper portions for seeing at infinity, the middle portions for seeing at arm's length, and the lower portions for near vision.

**glasspox** \glas′päks\ *Obs.* ALASTRIM.

**Glauber** [Johann Rudolph *Glauber,* German chemist, 1604–1670] See under SALT.

**glaucoma** \glôkō′mə\ [Gk *glaukōma* (from *glauk(os)* gleaming, bluish green, gray) cataract, glaucoma (not clearly distinguished until modern times)] An increase of intraocular pressure sufficient to damage the structure or function of the eye. Also *choroiditis serosa, green cataract* (obs.), *oculus caesius.* Adj. glaucomatous. **acute congestive g.** Increased intraocular pressure to an angle-closure mechanism, as that of angle-closure glaucoma or narrow-angle glaucoma. **air-block g.** Increased intraocular pressure due to interference with aqueous flow caused by a bubble of gas within the anterior chamber. **angle-closure g.** Glaucoma due to obstruction of aqueous outflow by occlusion of the trabecular meshwork from mechanical contact with the peripheral iris. Also *closed-angle glaucoma.* **angle-recession g.** A post-traumatic increase in intraocular pressure associated with a circumferential rupture of the portion of the ciliary body between the scleral spur and the iris base. Such an injury widens the angle of the anterior chamber. **aphakic g.** Increased intraocular pressure occurring in an eye without its crystalline lens. **apoplectic g.** In-

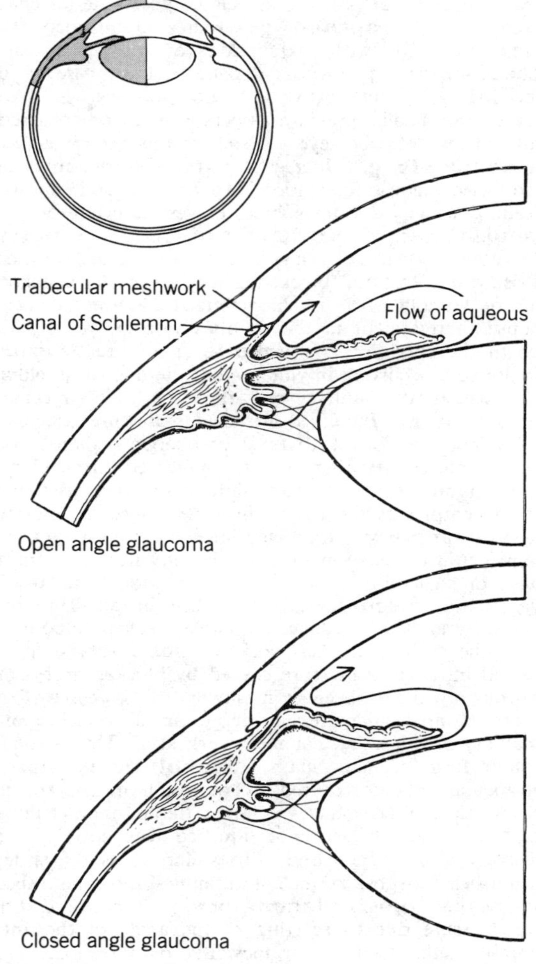

**Glaucoma**

creased intraocular pressure associated with anterior chamber hemorrhage. **capsular g.** Increased intraocular pressure associated with exfoliation of the lens capsule. **closed-angle g.** ANGLE-CLOSURE GLAUCOMA. **congenital g.** BUPHTHALMOS. **congestive g.** An increased intraocular pressure associated with obvious redness and edema of the eye. Also *incompensated glaucoma.* **hemorrhagic g.** Increased intraocular pressure associated with neovascularization of the iris and intraocular bleeding, usually due to diabetes or venous occlusion. **incompensated g.** CONGESTIVE GLAUCOMA. **infantile g.** BUPHTHALMOS. **inverse g.** Increased intraocular pressure due to pupil block mechanisms, as by a dislocated lens or vitreous. This is characterized by a paradoxical response to treatment in that miotics worsen and mydriatics benefit the condition. **juvenile g.** Increased intraocular pressure occurring in young adult life due to developmental structural faults of the outflow mechanism. **lenticular g.** Increased intraocular pressure secondary to faulty lens position or to toxic or allergic responses of the cortex lentis. **malignant g.** Increased intraocular pressure resulting from a forward shift of the vitreous structure, which compresses the iris against the trabecular meshwork. **narrow-angle g.** Increased intraocular pressure resulting from forward displacement of the iris towards the cornea because of structural reasons in the anterior segment of the eye. **neovascular g.** Increased intraocular pressure caused by growth of connective tissue and new blood vessels upon the trabecular meshwork. **obstructive g.** Increased intraocular pressure caused by blocked access of the aqueous to the trabecular meshwork. **open-angle g.** Increased intraocular pressure due to an inherent loss of permeability of the trabecular meshwork itself. This is the commonest form of glaucoma. **phakolytic g.** Increased intraocular pressure caused by occlusion of the trabecular meshwork of macrophages entering the anterior chamber in response to the presence of liquefied lens cortex. **pigmentary g.** Increased intraocular pressure associated with a heavy deposit of melanin granules upon the trabecular meshwork. **postinflammatory g.** Increased intraocular pressure due to scarring of the angle of the anterior chamber subsequent to iridocyclitis or infection. **primary g.** Spontaneously occurring inherited glaucoma, the more common form of glaucoma, either open-angle or closed-angle. **pseudoexfoliative capsular g.** Increased intraocular pressure associated with the shedding of lens capsular material. **secondary g.** Increased intraocular pressure due to ocular disease rather than to an inherited tendency to glaucoma. **vitreous-block g.** Increased intraocular pressure due to occlusion of the pupil by the vitreous humor, usually occurring in aphakic eyes.

**glaucomatous** \glôkō′mətəs\ Of or pertaining to glaucoma; associated with increased intraocular pressure.

**GLC** gas-liquid chromatography.

**Glc** Symbol for glucose.

**GlcA** 1 Symbol for glucuronic acid. 2 Symbol for gluconic acid.

**GlcN** A symbol for glucosamine (systematically 2-amino-2-deoxyglucose).

**GlcNAc** Symbol for *N*-acetylglucosamine.

**GlcUA** Symbol for glucuronic acid. • The preferred symbol is GlcA.

**gleet** \glēt\ [Middle English *glet, glette* (from L *glittus* sticky) slime] 1 Chronic gonococcal urethritis. 2 The slight mucous discharge seen in the chronic stage of gonococcal urethritis.

**Glenn** [William Wallace Lumpkin *Glenn*, U.S. cardiovascular surgeon, born 1914] See under OPERATION.

**glenohumeral** \glē′nōhyoo′mərəl\ Pertaining to the glenoid cavity of the scapula and the humerus.

**glenoid** \glē′noid\ [Gk *glēnoeidēs* (from *glēnē* a shallow socket) socketlike] Pertaining, belonging to, or resembling the glenoid cavity of the scapula.

**GLI** gastrointestinal glucagonlike immunoreactivity.

**glia** \glī′ə, glē′ə\ [Gk *glia,* also *gloia* glue] NEUROGLIA. **cytoplasmic g.** Glial cells, usually astrocytes, containing abundant perikaryal cytoplasm. **g. of Fañanás** CELLS OF FAÑANÁS. **fibrillary g.** Astrocytes possessing numerous silver-impregnated fibrils consisting of bundles of microfilaments. They are often prominent in zones of neural degeneration in which astrocytic processes proliferate.

**gliacyte** \glī′əsīt\ [GLIA + -CYTE] A neuroglial cell body. Also *gliocyte, gliocytus.*

**glial** \glī′əl\ Of or pertaining to neuroglia.

**glide** / **mandibular g.** Lateral or protrusive movement of the mandible with teeth or other occluding surfaces in contact. Also *gliding movement of the mandible.* **occlusal g.** An eccentric movement of the mandible during closure caused by a deflective occlusal contact.

**glio-** \glī′ō-, glē′ō-\ [Gk *glia* or *gloia* glue] A combining form meaning (1) glue, gluelike; (2) gliomatous.

**glioblast** \glī′əblast\ SPONGIOBLAST.

**glioblastoma** \-blastō′mə\ [GLIO- + BLASTOMA] A highly malignant brain tumor composed of glial tissue. It contains poorly differentiated cells and areas of necrosis, pseudopalisading, vascular endothelial proliferation, hemorrhage, and invasive growth. It usually occurs in the cerebral hemispheres of adults. Also *glioblastoma multiforme, spongioblastoma multiforme.* **giant cell g.** A glioblastoma with a predominance of bizarre, multinucleated giant cells. Also *monstrocellular sarcoma, magnocellular glioblastoma.* **magnocellular g.** GIANT CELL GLIOBLASTOMA. **g. multiforme** GLIOBLASTOMA.

**gliocyte** \glī′əsīt\ GLIACYTE. **retinal g.'s** MÜLLER'S FIBERS.

**gliocytoma** \-sītō′mə\ GLIOMA.

**gliocytus** \-sī′təs\ GLIACYTE. **g. radiatus** CELLS OF FAÑANÁS.

**gliofibrilla** \-fībril′ə\ One of the cytoplasmic filaments within a glial cell. These filaments are primarily composed of glial fibrillary acid protein.

**gliofibrillary** \-fī′briler′ē\ Pertaining to the silver-impregnated fibrils of neuroglial cells, consisting chiefly of microfilaments of astrocytic cytoplasmic processes.

**gliofibrosarcoma** \-fī′brōsärkō′mə\ [GLIO- + FIBROSARCOMA] A glioblastoma with a fibrosarcomatous component.

**gliogenous** \glī·äj′ənəs\ Derived from or pertaining to glial cells. *Obs.*

**glioma** \glī·ō′mə\ [*gli(o)-* + -OMA] A tumor of glial cells, such as astrocytoma, glioblastoma, or oligodendroglioma. Also *gliocytoma, neurogliocytoma, neuroglioma, neurospongioma.* Adj. gliomatous. **astrocytic g.** ASTROCYTOMA. **g. endophytum** A glioma of the inner part of the retina. It may enter into the vitreous space. **ependymal g.** EPENDYMOMA. **g. exophytum** A glioma of the outer part of the retina. It may enter into the choroid. **extramedullary g.** HETEROTOPIC GLIOMA. **ganglionic g.** GANGLIOGLIOMA. **heterotopic g.** A glioma formed outside the central nervous system. Also *extramedullary glioma.* **malignant peripheral g.** MALIGNANT SCHWANNOMA. **mixed g.** A glioma with more than one cell type. Most commonly it is an oligoastrocytoma. **nasal g.** *Incorrect* NASAL GLIAL HETEROTOPIA. **optic g.** A glioma arising from the optic nerve. **peripheral**

**g.** *Outmoded* NEURILEMMOMA. **g. retinae** A glioma arising from the retina. **g. sarcomatosum** A glioblastoma with a sarcomatous component.

**gliomatosis** \-mətō′sis\ Diffuse gliomatous change. **g. cerebri** A rare disease in which there is diffuse involvement of the cerebral hemispheres by neoplastic glial cells. Also *astrocytomatosis cerebri, oligodendrogliomatosis cerebri.*

**gliomatous** \glī·äm′ətəs\ Characteristic of a glioma.

**glioneuroma** \-n$^y$urō′mə\ [GLIO- + NEUROMA] GANGLIOGLIOMA.

**gliophagia** \-fā′jə\ [GLIO- + -PHAGIA] The condition in which neuroglial cells are phagocytosed by other cells.

**gliopil** \glī′əpil\ [GLIO- + Gk *pil(os)* wool or hair wrought into felt] The matrix of glial cell processes, consisting principally of astrocytes.

**gliosarcoma** \-särkō′mə\ **1** A malignant glioma. **2** A mixed glioblastoma and sarcoma.

**gliosis** \glī·ō′sis\ [*gli(o)-* + -OSIS] Proliferation of astrocytes in response to disease or injury. It is one means of scar formation in the central nervous system. Also *astrogliosis.* **diffuse g.** Gliosis occurring diffusely throughout the central nervous system. **hypertrophic nodular g.** Severe diffuse but patchy gliosis producing general as well as nodular enlargement of the cerebral hemispheres. This condition is seen particularly in tuberous sclerosis. **progressive subcortical g.** BINSWANGER'S DISEASE.

**gliosome** \glī′əsōm\ [GLIO- + -SOME] A cytoplasmic organelle or inclusion seen in neuroglial cells by light microscopy. They are probably mostly mitochondria but may also include liposomes and lysosomes.

**Glisson** [Francis *Glisson*, English anatomist, physiologist, and pathologist, 1597–1677] **1** See under CIRRHOSIS, SLING. **2** Glisson's capsule. See under CAPSULA FIBROSA PERIVASCULARIS. **3** Glisson's capsule. See under TUNICA FIBROSA HEPATIS. **4** Glisson's disease. See under RICKETS.

**glissonitis** \glis′ənī′tis\ [*Glisson('s) capsule* + -ITIS] PERIHEPATITIS.

**Gln** Symbol for glutamine.

**global** \glō′bəl\ **1** Of or relating to a globe, as the eye. **2** Of or involving the entire world. **3** Considered in its entirety; with attention to the broadest view of the situation.

**globe** [L *globus.* See GLOBUS.] A spherical mass, as the eye; globus.

**globefish** \glōb′fish\ PUFFER.

**globi** \glō′bī\ Plural of GLOBUS.

**globin** [*glob(us)* + -IN] The protein of hemoglobin after removal of heme.

**globoid** \glō′boid\ Having a shape similar to that of a sphere.

**globose** \glō′bōs\ Having the shape of a globe; globular.

**globoside** A compound, usually a glycosphingolipid, containing Gal($\alpha$1-4)Gal($\beta$1-4)Glc(globotriaose) or GalNAc($\beta$1-3)Gal($\alpha$1-4)Gal($\beta$1-4)Glc(globotetraose) as its oligosaccharide.

**globular** \gläb′yələr\ **1** Characterized by a spherical shape. **2** Consisting of globules.

**globule** \gläb′yəl\ [French (from L *globulus,* dim. of *globus* a ball, sphere), a very small spherical body] **1** Any small spheroidal particle. Also *globulus.* **2** A blood cell or corpuscle; especially, an erythrocyte. An obsolete usage. **dentin g.'s** Small spherical bodies of mineralized matrix seen in regions of dentin in which mineralization is incomplete. **Morgagni's g.'s** Fluid droplets within a cataractous lens.

**globuli** \gläb′yəlī\ Plural of GLOBULUS.

**globulin** \gläb′yəlin\ [*globul(e)* + -IN] A category of protein, comprising those that are soluble in dilute salt solutions and are precipitated by half saturation with ammonium sulfate, in distinction from the albumins, which require complete saturation to precipitate them. Typical globulins were once considered to be insoluble in water in the absence of salt, but the globulins have since been subdivided into the euglobulins, which possess this property, and the pseudoglobulins, which dissolve even in the absence of salt. **accelerator g.** FACTOR V. Abbr. AcG **alpha g.** Any of the globulins of plasma which have the greatest electrophoretic mobility of the globulins in neutral or alkaline solutions. **antihemophilic g.** The original term for FACTOR VIII. Abbr. AHG **antihuman g.** An antibody directed against human globulin: usually applied to the antibodies against human immunoglobulins used to detect incomplete antibodies to erythrocytes by the antiglobulin (Coombs) test. **antilymphocyte g.** An antibody directed against lymphocyte surface antigens. Such antibodies are produced by immunization of experimental animals with heterologous lymphocytes and are used as immunosuppressive agents, for example in organ transplantation. Antilymphocyte antibodies may also occur spontaneously in the presence of disease states such as systemic lupus erythematosus. Abbr. ALG **Bence Jones g.** BENCE JONES PROTEIN. **beta g.** Any of the globulins of blood plasma characterized by electrophoretic mobility intermediate between those of alpha (fast) and gamma (slow). **beta-1A g.** Immunoelectrophoretic designation of the major C3 conversion product found in serum after complement activation. It corresponds to the fragment properly called iC3b, but has also been used as an alternative name for the later C3 breakdown product C3c, which is difficult to distinguish from iC3b on immunoelectrophoresis. Native C3 (immunoelectrophoretic designation $\eta$1C globulin) has a slower mobility. **beta-2A g.** *Obs.* IMMUNOGLOBULIN A. **beta-1C g.** *Obs.* C3. **beta-1E g.** *Obs.* C4. **beta-1F g.** *Obs.* C5. **beta-2M g.** *Obs.* IMMUNOGLOBULIN M. **corticosteroid-binding g.** An alpha globulin that binds and transports biologically active, unconjugated cortisol in plasma. Also *transcortin, corticosteroid-binding protein.* **D antigen immune g.** The globulin fraction of human serum directed against the D antigens of the rhesus blood group system. It is now given within 36 hours of the birth of an Rh+ child to an Rh− mother to prevent isoimmunization of the mother. **gamma g.** **1** A group of plasma proteins characterized by very slow electrophorectic mobility in alkaline buffers. Most antibodies are gamma globulins and gamma globulins are thus usually identified with immunoglobulins. **2** IMMUNOGLOBULIN. **gamma-A g.** *Obs.* IMMUNOGLOBULIN A. **gamma-D g.** *Obs.* IMMUNOGLOBULIN D. **gamma-E g.** *Obs.* IMMUNOGLOBULIN E. **gamma-G g.** *Obs.* IMMUNOGLOBULIN G. **gamma-M g.** *Obs.* IMMUNOGLOBULIN M. **human gamma g.** **1** The fraction of human serum that migrates most anodically on electrophoresis. **2** IMMUNOGLOBULIN G. **human rabies immune g.** A preparation of human immunoglobulin based on pooled plasma from individuals who had been recently vaccinated against rabies. It is used with rabies vaccine for protection in people bitten by rabid animals or those who have been in contact with saliva from an animal suspected of being rabid. **immune g.** IMMUNOGLOBULIN. **measles immune g.** A sterile preparation from pooled human plasma of people convalescent from or immunized against measles, which contains 90% gamma globulin and 10–18 g of protein per 100 ml. It is used to prevent or modify measles in susceptible people previously exposed to a measles infection, within 6 days of that exposure. **pertussis immune g.** A sterile preparation of immunoglobulins of pooled plasma from adult human donors who previously were immunized with pertussis vaccine. It contains glycine as a stabilizing agent and some suitable preservative. It is used to confer passive protection against whooping cough to individuals exposed to that disease. **$\mathbf{rh_O}$(D) immune g.** A sterile globulin solution prepared from human blood plasma containing immunoglobulins to the erythrocyte factor $Rh_o$(D). Intramuscular injection is used to prevent production of $Rh_o$(D) antibodies in $Rh_o$(D)-negative mothers following birth or miscarriage of an $Rh_o$(D)-positive baby or fetus, avoiding erythroblastosis fetalis in a subsequent pregnancy if the child is $Rh_o$(D)-positive. **T g.** A large immunoglobulin band seen in the electrophoresis of horse serum following hyperimmunization. It is postulated to be a subclass of IgG. **tetanus immune g.** A sterile gamma globulin solution used in the prophylaxis and treatment of tetanus. It is prepared from the blood plasma of normal adult human subjects who have been immunized with tetanus toxoid. **thyroxine-binding g.** A serum globulin having a mass of about 60 000 daltons, moving electrophoretically between $\alpha_1$- and $\alpha_2$-globulin, which at one major binding site binds thyroxine and, less readily, triiodothyronine and acts as their carrier protein in the circulation. Serum concentration of the globulin is raised during pregnancy and estrogen administration, lowered when testosterone is given, and is deficient in one or more genetic disorders. Also *thyroid-binding globulin* (imprecise). Abbr. TBG **vitamin D-binding g.** A protein synthesized in the liver, migrating in the $\alpha 2$ globulin band on electrophoresis. It binds both natural D vitamins and the metabolically active hydroxylated forms. Several phenotypic variants can be identified, but no association has been found between protein variants and pathophysiologic conditions. Levels decline in severe hepatocellular diseases. Also *Gc protein.*

**globulinuria** \gläb′yəlinoo′rē·ə\ [GLOBULIN + -URIA] The excretion of serum globulins in the urine, an indication of nonselective proteinuria resulting from severe glomerular damage.

**globulolysis** \gläb′yəläl′isis\ HEMOLYSIS.

**globulolytic** \gläb′yəlōlit′ik\ HEMOLYTIC.

**globulus** \gläb′yələs\ (*pl.* globuli) GLOBULE. **globuli ossei** Rounded areas of bone tissue found with in the lacunae of calcified cartilage.

**globulysis** \glōbyoo′lisis\ HEMOLYSIS.

**globus** \glō′bəs\ [L, ball, sphere, globe] (*pl.* globi) **1** A spherical mass. **2** A lump or swelling. **3** In leprology, a macrophage swollen by its content of leprosy bacilli, as seen in lepromatous leprosy. **g. abdominalis** A subjective sensation as if there were a lump in the abdomen. **g. hystericus** The sensation of a lump in the throat that is not due to organic pathology. It may appear as the single symptom of conversion hysteria, or it may constitute a significant part of an anxiety disorder or of anorexia nervosa. **g. pallidus** The smaller, medial portion of the lentiform nucleus, which is divided by the lamina medullaris medialis into a lateral or external part and a medial or internal part. The globus pallidus is separated from the more laterally located putamen by the lamina medullaris lateralis. Afferent fibers reach the globus pallidus from the putamen, subthalamic nucleus, substantia nigra, thalamus, and cerebral cortex, while efferent fibers from the globus pallidus course to the nucleus ventralis anterior of the thalamus and the subthalamic nucleus in the diencephalon, the substantia nigra and red nucleus in the midbrain, and the reticular formation and inferior olivary nucleus in the lower brainstem. Also *pallidus, paleostriatum.* Adj. pallidal, paleostriatal.

**glomangioma** \glōman′jē·ō′mə\ [*glom(us)* + ANGIOMA] GLOMUS TUMOR.

**glomangiosis** \glōman′jē·ō′sis\ The occurrence of multiple arteriovenular anastomoses in a tissue or organ. **pulmonary g.** Arteriovenular anastomoses occurring in severe pulmonary hypertension.

**glome** \glōm\ GLOMUS.

**glomectomy** \glōmek′təmē\ [*glom(us)* + -ECTOMY] Excision of a glomus, especially the glomus caroticum.

**glomera** \gläm′ərə\ Plural of GLOMUS.

**glomerular** \glōmer′yələr\ Of or relating to a glomerulus.

**glomeruli** \glōmer′yəlī\ Plural of GLOMERULUS.

**glomerulitis** \glōmer′yəlī′tis\ [*glomerul(us)* + -ITIS] Inflammation of renal glomeruli with endothelial cell proliferation and often with infiltration by leukocytes. It may occur in a variety of diseases. ● *Glomerulitis* usually denotes a relatively mild inflammation of the glomeruli, but is a nonspecific term. **focal g.** Glomerulitis involving only some glomeruli, usually less than half the glomeruli. **segmental g.** Glomerulitis involving only a single tuft or portion of a tuft rather than the entire glomerulus, typically seen in lupus erythematosus.

**glomerulonephritis** \glōmer′yəlōnefrī′tis\ [*glomerul(us)* + *o* + NEPHRITIS] Any glomerular disease characterized by acute, subacute, or chronic inflammation. Also *glomerular nephritis.* ● This term has been inappropriately used at times to designate noninflammatory lesions, as in *membranous glomerulonephritis.* **acute g.** ACUTE DIFFUSE GLOMERULONEPHRITIS. **acute benign hemorrhagic g.** A syndrome of transient hematuria and proteinuria following any type of infection, rarely accompanied by hypertension, edema, or more than mild renal functional impairment. This syndrome also may represent mild poststreptococcal acute glomerulonephritis. Renal biopsy may reveal the underlying lesion to be a mild, diffuse, acute, proliferative glomerulonephritis or focal glomerulitis. When the syndrome is recurrent, it usually is associated with mesangial IgG/IgA glomerulonephritis. **acute diffuse g.** An acute inflammatory process involving glomeruli, characterized by endothelial and mesangial proliferation, and often leukocytic infiltration. Deposition of soluble antigen-antibody complexes is the most common pathogenesis, especially after pharyngeal or skin infections due to nephritogenic strains of group A hemolytic streptococci, bacterial endocarditis, and other infections. Acute glomerulonephritis also may follow minor infections, or be associated with systemic diseases such as Henoch-Schönlein purpura, systemic lupus erythematosus, the Goodpasture syndrome, and periarteritis nodosa. Clinically the disease may be characterized by the acute nephritic syndrome, or may be so mild that it can be detected only by serial urinalysis. Also *acute nephritis, acute glomerulonephritis, acute hemorrhagic nephritis.* **acute nonpoststreptococcal g.** A form of acute benign hemorrhagic glomerulonephritis, not caused by group A hemolytic streptoccal infection. It sometimes occurs in epidemics and is presumably of viral etiology. Complete recovery is the rule. **acute poststreptococcal g.** POSTSTREPTOCOCCAL ACUTE GLOMERULONEPHRITIS. **antiglomerular basement membrane antibody g.** GOODPASTURE SYNDROME. **autoimmune g.** An experimental glomerular disease, produced in sheep by injection of a glomerular basement membrane preparation plus Freund's adjuvant, and presumably due to autoantibodies against the glomerular basement membrane. Also *Steblay nephritis.* **chronic g.** Any chronic renal disease of glomerular origin. A few instances follow acute glomerulonephritis that fails to heal, but most begin with asymptomatic proteinuria, the nephrotic syndrome, hypertension, slowly developing chronic renal failure, or uremic symptoms. Even if an accurate pathologic diagnosis is established by renal biopsy, the etiology rarely is known. **circulating immune-complex g.** Any of a group of glomerular diseases characterized by deposition of circulating antigen-antibody complexes along the glomerular capillary basement membrane in an irregular, granular pattern as revealed by immunofluorescent microscopy and by electron microscopy. The glomerular lesions may be proliferative, exudative, or both. Circulating immune-complex glomerulonephritis includes glomerulonephritis associated with group A hemolytic streptococcal infections, subacute bacterial endocarditis, malaria, lupus erythematosus, periarteritis, and other conditions. Also *immune-complex glomerulonephritis.* **congenital chronic g.** CONGENITAL GLOMERULOSCLEROSIS. **crescentic g.** EXTRACAPILLARY GLOMERULONEPHRITIS. **diffuse lupus g.** A renal complication of systemic lupus erythematosus in which all glomeruli are involved, with proliferative or membranous changes. See also DIFFUSE PROLIFERATIVE GLOMERULONEPHRITIS. **diffuse proliferative g.** A form of glomerulonephritis that may occur during the course of systemic lupus erythematosus, characterized by proteinuria, hematuria, cylinduria, and renal functional impairment. **extracapillary g.** Extracapillary proliferation of epithelial cells (crescents) lining Bowman's space. Crescents may occur in a variety of glomerular diseases including poststreptococcal acute glomerulonephritis and idiopathic rapidly progressive glomerulonephritis, or may occur as part of systemic disorders such as the Goodpasture syndrome, glomerulonephritis associated with bacterial endocarditis, polyarteritis, Henoch-Schönlein purpura, systemic lupus erythematosus, and essential mixed cryoglobulinemia. Involvement of more than 50 percent of the glomeruli is usually associated with the clinical syndrome of rapidly progressive glomerulonephritis. Also *crescentic glomerulonephritis, extracapillary acute proliferative glomerulonephritis.* **extracapillary acute proliferative g.** EXTRACAPILLARY GLOMERULONEPHRITIS. **focal g.** Proliferation in some but not all glomeruli. Leukocytes, fibrin, and necrosis also may be present in the lesions. Such lesions occur in systemic diseases such as polyarteritis, systemic lupus erythematosus, subacute bacterial endocarditis, and Schönlein-Henoch purpura. Other cases are associated with recurrent hematuria, asymptomatic proteinuria, or the nephrotic syndrome. **focal embolic g.** A condition characterized by proliferative, focal, and sometimes necrotizing glomerular lesions, usually associated with subacute bacterial endocarditis due to a variety of organisms but especially to *Streptococcus viridans* or staphylococci. Also *focal proliferative glomerulonephritis, embolic nephritis, focal embolic nephritis, Löhlein's nephritis.* **focal necrotizing g.** Necrosis of some or parts of some glomeruli, as evidenced by nuclear fragmentation and debris. Total necrosis of glomeruli results form occlusion of their blood supply. **focal proliferative g.** FOCAL EMBOLIC GLOMERULONEPHRITIS. **focal sclerosing g.** FOCAL GLOMERULOSCLEROSIS. **hypocomplementemic g.** MEMBRANOPROLIFERATIVE GLOMERULONEPHRITIS. **immune-complex g.** CIRCULATING IMMUNE-COMPLEX GLOMERULONEPHRITIS. **membranoproliferative g.** A form of chronic glomerulonephritis characterized by mesangial cell proliferation, increased mesangial matrix, and thickened glomerular capillary walls. The thickened capillary wall results from interposition of mesangial matrix and cell cytoplasm between the glomerular basement membrane and the endothelium. Two types of membranoproliferative glomerulonephritis are distinguished by electron microscopy. Type 1 is characterized by electron-dense deposits between the endothelium and the glomerular basement membrane, and type 2 by very electron-dense deposits within the basement membrane. By immunofluorescent technique C3, properdin, and to a lesser extent C3 activator are distributed as granular deposits along the capillary wall. IgG and IgM are present in approximately half the cases. The disease, which may occur at any age, is often associated with the nephrotic syndrome and is accompanied by slowly progressive renal failure over five to ten years. Spontaneous remissions sometimes occur. Type 2 is sometimes associated with partial lipodystrophy. Also *mesangiocapillary glomerulonephritis, dense deposit disease, hypocomplementemic glomerulonephritis.* **membranous g.** A disease characterized by heavy proteinuria and often by the nephrotic syndrome. Progressive renal failure is usual, but spontaneous remissions may occur in approximately 20 percent of the cases. Histologically, diffuse membranous lesions are characterized by protein deposits initially on the epithelial side of the glomerular capillary membrane. Basement membrane material subsequently separates the deposits, forming spikes and thickening of the membrane. The deposits contain gamma globulin and complement ($C_3$) in a granular distribution. Also *membranous glomerulopathy, membranous nephropathy.* **mesangial IgA/IgG g.** A glomerulonephritis characterized by diffuse enlargement and hypercellularity of the mesangial regions which on immunofluorescent stain contain large amounts of IgA and some IgG in most instances. Clinical features include recurrent hematuria, usually associated with respiratory infections, and persistent proteinuria only rarely great enough to result in the nephrotic syndrome. Renal failure may develop after several years and is slowly progressive. Also *Berger's disease, mesangial IgA/IgG disease, mesangial IgA/IgG nephropathy, mesangial nephropathy, mesangial proliferative glomerulonephritis.* **mesangiocapillary g.** MEMBRANOPROLIFERATIVE GLOMERULONEPHRITIS. **postinfectious acute g.** Acute glomerulonephritis following an infection. Some instances may represent a nonspecific response to infection characterized by a focal glomerulitis and asymptomatic urine abnormalities, while others may be related to circulating immune complexes as in poststreptococcal acute glomerulonephritis. **poststreptococcal acute g.** A disorder, most common in childhood, characterized by sudden onset of proteinuria, hematuria, and cylindruria, often associated with hypertension, renal function impairment, and circulatory congestion in varying combinations. It begins 5 to 28 days after infection with a nephritogenic strain of group A hemolytic streptococci. The severity may vary from asymptomatic urine abnormalities to acute oliguric renal failure. The healing rate is high, especially in children. However, chronic glomerulonephritis follows some severe instances, usually in adults. The glomeruli are diffusely involved with endothelial cell proliferation and infiltration with polymorphonuclear leukocytes. In severe instances crescents and adhesions between the glomerular tufts and Bowman's capsule are present. By immunofluorescent techniques, IgG, complement (usually C3, sometimes C4), and properdin are deposited in a granular pattern along the epithelial side of the glomerular basement membrane. By electron microscopy characteristic electron-dense "humps" are observed up to six weeks after onset along the epithelial side of the glomerular capillary basement membrane. The latent period, glomerular deposits, and the presence of serum cryoglobulins and reduced serum complement suggest that the disorder is associated with circulating immune complexes. Also *acute poststreptoccal glomerulonephritis, poststreptococcal* *nephritis.* **proliferative g.** Any lesion characterized by proliferation of glomerular, epithelial, endothelial, or mesangial cells. **rapidly progressive g.** A syndrome characterized histologically by diffuse extracapillary proliferation with crescent formation, and clinically by rapidly progressive renal insufficiency, which leads to end-stage renal disease in weeks or months. The syndrome can be associated with poststreptococcal acute glomerulonephritis, mesangiocapillary glomerulonephritis, malignant hypertension, the Goodpasture syndrome, and idiopathic rapidly progressive glomerulonephritis. In the latter case, immunofluorescent study reveals deposition in a linear fashion of IgG along glomerular capillary basement membranes can be demonstrated in association with antiglomerular basement membrane antibodies in the serum. The glomerular lesions are identical to those of the Goodpasture syndrome. Also *subacute glomerulonephritis* (outmoded), *subacute nephritis.* **segmental g.** Glomerulonephritis limited to segments of some or all glomeruli. It is a form of focal glomerulonephritis. **subacute g.** *Outmoded* RAPIDLY PROGRESSIVE GLOMERULONEPHRITIS.

**glomerulopathy** \glōmer′yəläp′əthē\ [*glomerul(us)* + *o* + -PATHY] Any lesion that involves the glomeruli. **diabetic g.** Any renal complication of diabetes mellitus involving glomeruli and including diffuse or nodular diabetic glomerulosclerosis. **membranous g.** MEMBRANOUS GLOMERULONEPHRITIS. **minimum change g.** LIPOID NEPHROSIS.

**glomerulosclerosis** \glōmer′yəlōsklerō′sis\ [*glomerul(us)* + *o* + SCLEROSIS] Replacement of all or part of some or all glomeruli by collagen, mesangial matrix, or fibrillar material. This condition may be diffuse or focal and may follow proliferative glomerular lesions, or may be associated with vascular lesions, diabetes, or some instances of idiopathic nephrotic syndrome. Also *glomerular sclerosis.* **congenital g.** Small and scarred glomeruli in the renal cortex of infants. If extensive, tubular atrophy and interstitial fibrosis may lead to renal failure during the first year of life. The cause is unknown. Also *congenital chronic glomerulonephritis.* **diabetic g.** A common and serious complication of diabetes mellitus, characterized by diffuse but irregular thickening of the glomerular capillary basement membrane and mesangial areas. Accumulations of strongly acidophilic and PAS-positive mesangial matrix form nodules of varying size in the centers of peripheral capillary loops. Nodules may occur in association with diffuse glomerular changes. Both types of lesions may be associated with hyaline deposits ("exudative droplets"). Arteriolosclerosis involving both the afferent and efferent glomerular arterioles is characteristic of diabetes mellitus. Diabetic glomerulosclerosis is part of a generalized microangiopathy that involves arterioles of many organs, including the retina, and is characterized by proteinuria, microscopic hematuria, progressive renal failure, and sometimes the nephrotic syndrome. Also *intercapillary glomerulosclerosis, nodular glomerulosclerosis, Kimmelstiel-Wilson syndrome.* **diffuse g.** Sclerosis of all or almost all glomeruli. **focal g.** **1** Sclerosis of some but not all glomeruli. **2** A renal disease characterized by the nephrotic syndrome and hyaline foci in some glomeruli, at first involving only the juxtamedullary glomeruli. Microscopic hematuria is common, and hypertension and chronic renal failure develop within a few years. Remissions are rare, whether spontaneous or treatment-induced. The etiology is unknown. Although many features, including diffuse smudging of epithelial foot processes on electron microscopy, are similar to lipoid nephrosis, focal glomerulosclerosis probably is a separate entity. Also *congenital nephrosclerosis, focal sclerosing glomerulonephritis.* **intercapillary g.** DIABETIC GLOMERULOSCLEROSIS. **nodular g.** DIABETIC GLOMERULOSCLEROSIS.

**glomerulus** \glōmer′yələs\ [New L, dim. of L *glomus* a ball of thread] (*pl.* glomeruli) **1** A knot or tuft of convoluted capillary blood vessels or nerve fibers. **2** [NA] In the renal cortex and columns, a tufted network of anastomosing capillaries derived from an afferent arteriole (arteriola

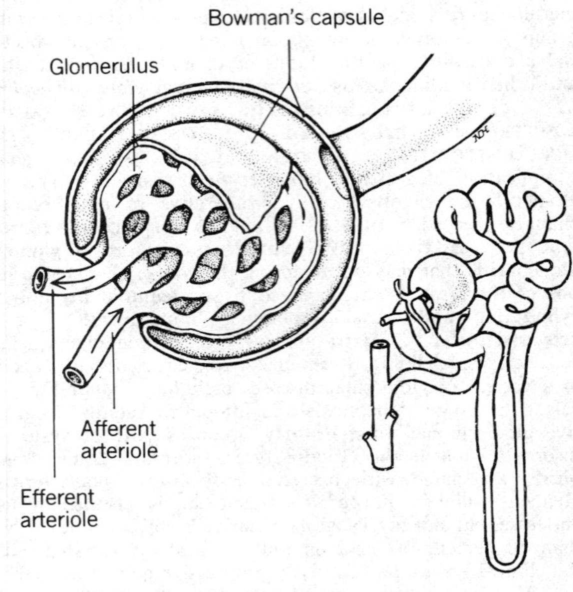


**Glomerulus**

glomerularis afferense) and ending in an efferent arteriole (arteriola glomerularis efferens) which enter and leave at the vascular pole of a renal corpuscle. It is held together by loose connective tissue and surrounded by the glomerular capsule (capsula glomeruli). **glomeruli arteriosi cochleae** [NA] The capillary network formed by the ramification of the cochlear branch of the labyrinthine artery in the lamina spiralis and basilar membrane of the cochlea. **caudal arterial glomeruli** GLOMUS COCCYGEUM. **g. of mesonephros** One of the excretory units of the mesonephros which may be functional for a short time in the embryo. Each lies medial to the mesonephric duct and is supplied by a lateral branch from the aorta. **nonencapsulated nerve g.** A spherical terminal cluster of nerve fibers associated with an internal organ and lacking a specialized corpuscular surrounding structure. **olfactory g.** One of a series of rounded areas of neuropil containing complex axodendritic and dendrodendritic synapses between olfactory afferent nerve fibers and the apical dendrites of the mitral and tufted cells and the dendrites of periglomerular cells in the glomerular layer of the main and accessory olfactory bulbs. **g. of pronephros** An arterial tuft covered by a thin epithelium which projects into the coelom in lower vertebrates having a functional pronephros. Waste is excreted into the coelom and removed through segmentally arranged nephrostomes to the pronephric duct.

**glomus** \glō′məs\ [L (gen. *glomeris*), a clue, skein, ball of thread] (*pl.* glomera) [NA] A neurovascular body, generally ball-shaped, containing richly innervated small arterioles. Also *vascular gland, glome.* Adj. glomic. **glomera aortica** CORPORA PARA-AORTICA. **g. caroticum** [NA] A small, oval neurovascular body situated at the bifurcation of each common carotid artery, containing chemoreceptors that monitor blood gas concentration and aid in the regulation of respiration by means of central connections via the glossopharyngeal nerve. Also *carotid glomus, glomus caroti-deum, carorid body, carotid gland, intercarotid gland, glandula intercarotica, Arnold's ganglion, carotid ganglion, intercarotid ganglion* (outmoded), *nodulus intercaroticus* (outmoded). **g. choroideum** [NA] The enlarged body of choroid plexus in the lateral ventricle at the junction of the main body with the inferior horn. Also *choroid glomus.* **g. coccygeum** [NA] A small, irregularly rounded mass in front of the apex of the coccyx and at the termination of the median sacral vessels that communicate with it by efferent and afferent vessels. It is composed of a large central nodule surrounded by smaller nodules each of which is composed of spherical or polyhedral epithelial cells surrounding a sinusoidal capillary that takes part in a complex arrangement of arteriolovenular anastomoses. The cells are considered to be shortened muscle cells of the tunica media of vessels adjacent to the dilated capillaries. Its functions are not clearly understood. Similar masses are found anterior to the caudal vertebrae of many other mammals. Also *coccygeal glomus, Luschka's body, Luschka's ganglion, Luschka's gland, corpus coccygeum, coccygeal vascular plexus, coccygeal arterial glomeruli* (outmoded). **digital g.** A structure that provides a short circuit of blood directly from arterioles to venules in the dermis of the fingers and toes as well as the palms and soles, face, and ears. Also *cutaneous glomus, neuromyoarterial glomus.* **g. intravagale** One of a number of small bodies, similar in structure to that of the carotid body, situated near the arch of the aorta, ductus arteriosus, and right subclavian artery, supplied by branches of the vagus nerve and considered to contain chemoreceptor endings. *Outmoded.* **g. jugulare** A microscopic neurovascular specialization in the adventitia of the jugular bulb. **neuromyoarterial g.** DIGITAL GLOMUS.

**gloss-** \gläs-\ GLOSSO-.

**glossa** \gläs′ə\ [Gk *glōssa* the tongue] LINGUA.

**glossal** \gläs′əl\ Pertaining to the tongue; lingual.

**glossalgia** \gläsal′jə\ GLOSSODYNIA.

**glossectomy** \gläsek′təmē\ [GLOSS- + -ECTOMY] Surgical removal of the tongue.

***Glossina*** \gläsī′nə\ A genus of African muscoid flies, the tsetse flies, which are vectors of the various trypanosomes that cause African trypanosomiasis of humans and domestic animals. Both sexes feed exclusively and avidly on the blood of vertebrates. Twenty-two species have been described. The feeding and breeding habits of these flies, in the so-called tsetse belts or fly belts, determine the distribution of the various trypanosomes they carry. Of particular adaptive importance in the survival of these flies is their pupiparous habit, the female fly possessing "milk glands" which enable a single larva to pass through its first three larval instars within the female, protected from external conditions and predation. The larvae are deposited on loose soil, into which they burrow by peristaltic movements. The integument quickly hardens to form a puparium within which the fourth larval and the pupal stage develop. ***G. morsitans*** A savanna-inhabitating species that transmits *Trypanosoma brucei* , the agent of nagana in central Africa and *T. (brucei) rhodesiense,* the cause of Rhodesian, or east African, human sleeping sickness. ***G. pallidipes*** The chief vector of the trypanosome that causes nagana, the rapidly fatal trypanosomiasis of cattle. It also transmits *Trypanosoma rhodesiense,* the agent of human east African sleeping sickness. ***G. palpalis*** A species of tsetse fly that transmits *Trypanosoma gambiense,* an agent of Gambian, or west African, sleeping sickness. The illness is associated with riverine vegetation and villages located along water courses, in keeping with the local distribution patterns of the vector fly.

**glossitis** \gläsī′tis\ [GLOSS- + -ITIS] Inflammation, usually superficial, of the tongue. **atrophic g.** HUNTER'S GLOSSITIS. **benign migratory g.** GEOGRAPHIC TONGUE. **chronic superficial g.** Red, swollen, and painful tongue, which may be smooth in its entirety or in patches, associated with many systemic diseases, including pernicious anemia, neural disturbances, and vitamin B deficiency. It is due to tissue atrophy. Also *Moeller's glossitis.* **Clarke-Fournier g.** INTERSTITIAL SCLEROUS GLOSSITIS. **cortical superficial sclerotic g.** Chronic superficial glossitis characterized by red or whitish plaques and both superficial induration and atrophic furrows, an appearance seen in a number of varieties of chronic glossitis, for instance the hobnail tongue of tertiary syphilis. **deep sclerotic g.** INTERSTITIAL SCLEROUS GLOSSITIS. **exfoliative g.** GEOGRAPHIC TONGUE. **Fournier's g.** INTERSTITIAL SCLEROUS GLOSSITIS. **gummatous g.** Chronic, diffuse, interstitial glossitis caused by syphilis. Also *gummatory glossitis* (rare). **Hunter's g.** Glossitis associated with pernicious anemia, in which the tongue is smooth and red. Also *atrophic glossitis.* **interstitial sclerous g.** Glossitis associated with tertiary syphilis, in which there are nodules, lobulation, and induration. Also *Clark-Fournier glossitis, Fournier's glossitis, deep sclerotic glossitis.* **median rhomboid g.** A rare congenital anomaly characterized by a smooth, oval, red patch in the midline of the dorsum of the tongue immediately anterior to the circumvallate papillae, due to the persistence of the tuberculum impar on the surface of the tongue. **g. migrans** GEOGRAPHIC TONGUE. **Moeller's g.** CHRONIC SUPERFICIAL GLOSSITIS. **monilial g.** Thrush affecting the tongue. **syphilitic g.** Inflammation of the tongue due to syphilis. Although lesions of the tongue may occur in primary and secondary syphilis, the term is usually preserved for the hobnail tongue of the late disease. One-third of such lesions progress to carcinoma of the tongue. **ulceromembranous g.** Ulceration of the tongue associated with the formation of membranes, as seen in granulocytopenia and necrotizing ulcerative gingivitis.

**glosso-** \gläs′ō-\ [Gk *glōssa* or *glōtta* tongue] A combining form meaning (1) the tongue; (2) speech, language. Also *gloss-, glotto-.*

**glossodesmus** \-dez′məs\ *Seldom used* FRENULUM LINGUAE.

**glossodynamometer** \-dī′nəmäm′ətər\ An instrument for measuring the strength of the muscles of the tongue.

**glossodynia** \-din′yə\ [GLOSS- + -ODYNIA] **1** Pain in the tongue. **2** Paresthesia marked by a burning sensation of the tongue. A wide variety of causes have been proposed but frequently no cause can be found. For defs. 1 and 2 also *glossalgia* (seldom used). **g. exfoliativa** Painful, bald, beefy tongue, seen in certain deficiency diseases. Many varieties of glossitis, such as Hunter's glossitis, are characterized as such.

**glossograph** \gläs′əgraf\ [GLOSSO- + -GRAPH] An instrument for recording movements of the tongue during speech.

**glossohyal** \-hī′əl\ HYOGLOSSAL.

**glossohyoidal** \-hī·oi′dəl\ HYOGLOSSAL.

**glossology** \gläsäl′əjē\ [GLOSSO- + -LOGY] The study of the tongue and the conditions affecting it.
**glossolysis** \gläsäl′isis\ [GLOSSO- + LYSIS] GLOSSOPLEGIA.
**glossomantia** \-man′tē·ə\ [GLOSSO- + Gk *manteia* a prophesying, power of divination] A prognosis of a disease on the basis of the appearance of the tongue.
**glossopexy** \gläs′əpek′sē\ [GLOSSO- + -PEXY] The attachment of the tongue to the lower lip to prevent asphyxia in the Pierre Robin syndrome.
**glossopharyngeal** \-fərin′jē·əl\ Pertaining to the tongue and the pharynx.
**glossopharyngeus** \-fərin′jē·əs\ **1** PARS GLOSSOPHARYNGEA MUSCULI CONSTRICTORIS PHARYNGIS SUPERIORIS. **2** NERVUS GLOSSOPHARYNGEUS.
**glossoplasty** \gläs′əplas′tē\ [GLOSSO- + -PLASTY] A plastic operation performed on the tongue.
**glossoplegia** \-plē′jə\ [GLOSSO- + -PLEGIA] Paralysis of the tongue. This is usually unilateral, caused by damage to the hypoglossal nerve, and it brings about deviation of the tongue towards the affected side on protrusion. Also *glossolysis.*
**glossoptosis** \gläs′äptō′sis\ The prolapse backwards and downwards of the abnormally small tongue characteristic of the Pierre Robin syndrome.
**glottal** \glät′l\ Of or relating to the glottis. Also *glottic, glottidean.*
**glottides** \glät′idēz\ Plural of GLOTTIS.
**glottis** \glät′is\ [Gk *glōttis* (from *glōtta,* Attic form of *glōssa* tongue, reed of a pipe) mouthpiece of a pipe, mouth of the windpipe] [NA] The vocal apparatus of the larynx, composed of the two vocal folds and the intermembranous part of the rima glottidis between them. **false g.** RIMA VESTIBULI. **intercartilaginous g.** PARS INTERCARTILAGINEA RIMAE GLOTTIDIS. **respiratory g.** PARS INTERCARTILAGINEA RIMAE GLOTTIDIS. **true g.** RIMA GLOTTIDIS.
**glotto-** \glät′ō-\ GLOSSO-.
**glottogram** \glät′əgram\ [GLOTTO- + -GRAM] ELECTROLARYNGOGRAM.
**glottograph** \glät′əgraf\ ELECTROLARYNGOGRAPH.
**glottography** \glätäg′rəfē\ ELECTROLARYNGOGRAPHY.
**glow / cathode g.** The incandescence appearing at the surface of the cathode of a discharge tube. Also *negative glow.*
**Glu** Symbol for glutamic acid.
**gluc-** \glook-\ GLUCO-.
**glucagon** \gloo′kəgän\ [GLUC- + Gk *agōn* (pres. part. of *agein* to bring, bring on) bringing on, eliciting] A 29-residue peptide hormone secreted by the $\alpha$-cells of the pancreatic islets of Langerhans and released in response to hypoglycemia, amino-acid administration, dietary protein, and pituitary growth hormone. Its effects generally oppose those of insulin, stimulating liver cells to release glucose from stored glycogen through its activation of adenylate cyclase in the cell membrane, thus raising the intracellular concentration of cyclic AMP (adenosine 3′,5′-cyclic phosphate). The hormone appears to exert subtle effects in concert with insulin upon glucose homeostasis, and it probably plays a part in the pathogenesis of diabetes mellitus.
**glucagon hydrochloride** A pharmaceutical preparation of glucagon. It has found limited clinical use in the experimental treatment of some cases of heart failure and in diagnostic tests of hypoglycemic disorders.
**glucagonoma** \gloo′kəgänō′mə\ [GLUCAGON + -OMA] An islet cell tumor of the alpha cells of the pancreas which secretes glucagon. It can occur clinically with diabetes mellitus, and may be malignant. Also *alpha cell tumor.*
**gluci-** \gloo′sē-\ GLUCO-.
**Gluck** [Themistokles *Gluck,* German surgeon, born 1853] See under INCISION.
**gluco-** \gloo′kō-\ [Gk *gleukos* (akin to *glykys* sweet) sweetness] A combining form denoting glucose. Also *gluc-, gluci-.*
**glucocerebrosidosis** \-ser′əbrōsīdō′sis\ GAUCHER'S DISEASE.
**glucocorticoid** A $C_{21}$ adrenocortical steroid hormone which stimulates gluconeogenesis, chiefly in the liver, and opposes the hypoglycemic action of insulin. In man the major natural glucocorticoid is cortisol. In rats and mice, it is corticosterone. All the semisynthetic hormones used to treat allergic and inflammatory diseases are glucocorticoids. Also *glucosteroid, S. hormone* (older term), *glucocorticosteroid.*
**glucogenesis** The formation of glucose from the dissolution of glycogen.
**glucohemia** \-hē′mē·ə\ GLYCEMIA.
**glucokinase** The enzyme (EC 2.7.1.2) that catalyzes the reaction of glucose and ATP to yield glucose 6-phosphate and ADP, and has a greater specificity for glucose than does hexokinase. This enzyme has not been found in mammals, but the term is sometimes applied to the liver isoenzyme of hexokinase, because its affinity for glucose and fructose is lowered in comparison with the muscle isoenzymes, so that it may appear inactive with fructose at the concentrations used for assay. This isoenzyme is not easily saturated with glucose ($K_m$ 10mM, compared with 0.1 mM for muscle isoenzymes), and so the rate of reaction it catalyzes increases with the blood sugar concentration. It also differs in not being inhibited by glucose 6-phosphate.
**Glucomannan** A fiber extracted from konjac tubers and marketed as a slimming aid. It swells when mixed with fluid in the stomach, thus giving the feeling of satiety. A proprietary name.
**gluconate** The anion derived from gluconic acid, a salt containing it, or more rarely an ester.
**gluconeogenesis** \-nē′ōjen′əsis\ [GLUCO- + NEO- + GENESIS] The formation of glucose or glucose residues of glycogen, from noncarbohydrate sources, especially from amino acids derived from proteins. Thus alanine yields pyruvate by transamination, and much but not all of the subsequent pathway is the reverse of glycolysis.
**gluconic acid** The acid formed by oxidation of C-1 of glucose to form a carboxyl group. The oxidation of glucose by glucose oxidase, an enzyme found in molds, produces its lactone together with hydrogen peroxide.
**gluconolactone** A lactone derived from gluconic acid, usually the 1,4- or the 1,5-lactone. 6-Phosphoglucono-1,5-lactone is the initial product of glucose-6-phosphate dehydrogenase, and glucono-1,5-lactone is likewise the initial product of glucose oxidase. In each case dehydrogenation of the —O—CHOH— group in the ring forms —O—CO—.
**glucopenia** \-pē′nē·ə\ [*gluc(ose)* + -PENIA] A condition marked by a lower-than-normal concentration of glucose in the blood and tissues.
**glucophylline** THEOPHYLLINE METHYLGLUCAMINE.
**glucopyranose** Glucose in its pyranose form. This form greatly predominates for free glucose, in which pyranose, furanose and chain forms equilibrate, and in natural glucosides and polysaccharides, where they do not.
**glucosamine** 2-Amino-2-deoxyglucose, an important component of many polysaccharides, usually acetylated on its amino group. Such polysaccharides occur, for example, in bacterial call walls. Cell membrane glycoproteins also contain glucosamine in the oligosaccharides attached to their outer portions. Symbol: GlcN

**glucosaminephosphate isomerase** The enzyme (EC 5.3.1.10) that catalyzes the interconversion of glucosamine 6-phosphate and water with fructose 6-phosphate and ammonia. It is so named because the first product is presumed to be the imine of fructose 6-phosphate and ammonia formed by isomerization of glucosamine phosphate. It provides a pathway for the breakdown of glucosamine. Another enzyme, present in liver and some molds, glucosaminephosphate isomerase (glutamine-forming) (EC 5.3.1.19), catalyzes a similar reaction in which glutamate replaces water, and the products are therefore fructose 6-phosphate and glutamine.

**glucose** \gloo′kōs\ [French (irreg. from Gk *gleukos*, must, sweet new wine, akin to *glykys* sweet), the sugar of grapes, of potato flour] The sugar present in blood. It is the most stable aldohexose because in its predominant pyranose form C-6 and all hydroxyl groups are equatorial substituents of the ring. It occurs widely in combined form, usually esterified with orthophosphoric acid, in metabolic pathways. Also *starch sugar.* **liquid g.** A colorless, odorless, viscous syrup consisting of dextrose, maltose, dextrins, and water, prepared by the incomplete acid hydrolysis of starch. Also *corn syrup.* **medicinal g.** DEXTROSE MONOHYDRATE.

**glucose oxidase** An enzyme (EC 1.1.3.4) that catalyzes the oxidation of glucose to gluconolactone, which in turn hydrolyzes spontaneously to gluconic acid with the concomitant reduction of oxygen to hydrogen peroxide. It is not found in mammals and it is usually derived from molds. Many methods for determining glucose concentration depend on measurement of the hydrogen peroxide that it forms. This enzyme was originally isolated from the mold *Penicillium notatum* and was mistakenly thought to be an antibiotic because of the antibacterial action of the hydrogen peroxide. Also *notatin* (obs.), *penicillin B* (obs.).

**glucose-6-phosphatase** The enzyme (EC 3.1.3.9) that hydrolyzes glucose 6-phosphate to glucose and orthophosphate. It occurs in liver and enables liver cells to regulate blood glucose concentration. Elaborate mechanisms exist for controlling its activity.

**glucose 1-phosphate** An important metabolic intermediate, interconvertible with glucose 6-phosphate. It is on the route of glycogen synthesis as well as being the direct product of glycogen breakdown by phosphorylase. Unlike glucose 6-phosphate, it is a glycoside. Also *Cori ester* (older term).

**glucose 6-phosphate** An important metabolic intermediate, it is the product of phosphorylation of glucose by hexokinase, glucokinase, or, in all anaerobic bacteria, phosphotransferase. It may be oxidized by glucose-6-phosphate dehydrogenase, interconverted with glucose 1-phosphate on the route to or from glycogen, or interconverted with fructose 6-phosphate in the glycolytic pathway. Also *Embden ester* (obs.), *Robison ester* (obs.).

**glucose-6-phosphate dehydrogenase** The enzyme (EC 1.1.1.49) that catalyzes the conversion of glucose 6-phosphate into 6-phosphogluconolactone with concomitant reduction of $NADP^+$ to NADPH. This is the first step of the oxidative pentose phosphate pathway. The NADPH formed is used for reductions in fatty acid synthesis, etc.

**glucose-phosphate isomerase** The enzyme (EC 5.3.1.9) that catalyzes the interconversion of glucose 6-phosphate and fructose 6-phosphate, an early step of glycolysis. Also *oxoisomerase* (outmoded), *phosphohexoisomerase.*

**glucose-1-phosphate phosphodismutase** An enzyme (EC 2.7.1.41) which catalyzes the conversion of two molecules of D-glucose 1-phosphate into D-glucose and D-glucose 1,6-bisphosphate.

**glucose-1-phosphate uridylyltransferase** The enzyme (EC 2.7.7.9) that catalyzes the transfer of a uridylyl group from UTP onto glucose 1-phosphate to form UDPglucose and diphosphate. It is important in the formation of glycogen, because UDPglucose is the donor of glucosyl groups for the biosynthesis of glycogen and of some other polysaccharides.

**glucosidase** Any enzyme, such as an amylase, that catalyzes the hydrolysis of a glucoside.

**glucoside** A compound in which the hydroxyl group on C-1 of a ring form of glucose is substituted, i.e. the potential aldehyde group is combined as an acetal with two alcoholic hydroxyl groups, one of them already in the glucose molecule on C-4 or C-5, the other from another molecule. Polysaccharides of glucose are glucosides.

**glucosinolate progoitrin** A natural inhibitor of the synthesis of thyroxine, found in brassica seeds and in lesser amounts in their leaves and roots. This substance is inactive until converted to the active goitrin 5-vinyloxazolidine-2-thione by the enzyme thioglucosidase. This enzyme is destroyed by cooking, thus preventing the production of the goitrogen.

**glucosteroid** GLUCOCORTICOID.

**glucosulfone sodium** $C_{24}H_{34}N_2Na_2O_{18}S_3$. 1,1′-[Sulfonylbis(4,1-phenyleneimino)]bis[1-deoxy-1-sulfo-D-glucitol] disodium salt. An antibacterial agent with leprostatic action. It is used as an injectable solution.

**glucosuria** \-soo′rē·ə\ GLYCOSURIA.

**glucosyl** The group formed from a ring form of glucose by removing the hydroxyl group on C-1.

**glucuronate** The anion derived from glucuronic acid.

**glucuronic acid** The substance formed from glucose by oxidizing C-6 from —$CH_2$OH to —COOH. It occurs in polysaccharides, and many substances are excreted in the urine in the form of glycosides of glucuronic acid.

**glucuronidase** Any enzyme that hydrolyzes the glycoside bond formed between glucuronic acid and an alcohol. The best known is β-glucuronidase (EC 3.2.1.31), which has little specificity for the alcohol, but more specific enzymes are also known. It is used in the chemical analysis of urine, as for steroid hormones, to release metabolites that are combined as glucuronides.

**glucuronide** A glycoside of glucuronic acid. Many substances such as steroid metabolites are converted into their glucuronides to solublize them for excretion.

**glue** / **plasma g.** PLASMA CLOT.

**glutamate** **1** A negatively charged ion derived from glutamic acid. It may bear a net charge of −1 or −2 according to pH. A glutamate residue in a protein is the deprotonated form of a glutamic residue, i.e. the form that occurs at neutral pH. **2** An ester of glutamic acid.

**glutamate decarboxylase** The enzyme (EC 4.1.1.15) that catalyzes the decarboxylation of glutamic acid. The product is 4-aminobutyrate, which is important as a neurotransmitter, especially in arthropods. Also *glutamic decarboxylase.*

**glutamate dehydrogenase** An enzyme that catalyzes the reaction: glutamate + $NAD(P)^+ \rightleftharpoons$ 2-oxoglutarate + $NH_4^+$ + NAD(P)H. It is probably responsible for both the biosynthesis and the catabolism of glutamate, and hence indirectly, via transamination, of other amino acids.

**glutamate oxaloacetate transaminase** A previous name for ASPARTATE AMINOTRANSFERASE. Abbr. GOT

**glutamate pyruvate transaminase** ALANINE AMINOTRANSFERASE.

**glutamic acid** HOOC—$CH_2$—$CH_2$—$CH(NH_2)$—COOH. An amino acid central to the metabolism of other amino acids, especially because it can reversibly transfer its nitrogen to many 2-oxoacids to form a new amino acid and 2-oxoglutarate. It can also form 2-oxoglutarate and ammonia with concomitant reduction of $NAD^+$ (or $NADP^+$), and the reverse of this reaction is a route of its biosythesis. Its conversion into glutamine allows some storage of ammonia. In microorganisms its formation from glutamine and 2-oxoglutarate, in which the amide nitrogen is transferred, is a key step in a major route of assimilation of ammonia nitrogen. Also *aminoglutaric acid.*

**glutamic acid hydrochloride** $C_5H_9NO_4{\cdot}HCl$. A dicarboxylic amino acid which has been used as an acidifying agent in cases of achlorhydria and hypochlorhydria, and as an antiepileptic agent.

**glutamic decarboxylase** GLUTAMATE DECARBOXYLASE.

**glutamic semialdehyde** $HCO{-}[CH_2]_2{-}CH(NH_3^+){-}COO^-$. An intermediate in the metabolism of glutamate, from which it can be formed by reduction of γ-glutamyl phosphate, in turn formed from glutamate and ATP. It is on the pathway of conversion of glutamate into proline, and on the pathways of glutamate formation from ornithine and proline.

**glutaminase** The enzyme (EC 3.5.1.2) that catalyzes the hydrolysis of glutamine to form glutamate and ammonia.

**glutamine** $H_2N{-}CO{-}CH_2{-}CH_2{-}CH(NH_2){-}COOH$. An amide of glutamic acid. It is also one of the 20 amino acids incorporated into proteins. Many animal cells require it, although the whole organism can make it via glutamate. It is made by glutamine synthase, by a reaction that enables ammonia to be stored. Symbol: Gln

**glutamine synthase** The enzyme (EC 6.3.1.2) that catalyzes the reaction: glutamate + $NH_3$ + ATP ⇌ glutamine + ADP + orthophosphate. This enables ammonia to be stored. In bacteria this reaction is a key step in the assimilation of ammonia. In addition, glutamine is an intermediate in many biosyntheses, including those of amino acids, purines and pyrimidines, and the enzyme is subject to elaborate control mechanisms.

**glutaminyl** The group $H_2N{-}CO{-}CH_2{-}CH_2{-}CH(NH_2){-}CO{-}$, derived from glutamine.

**glutamyl** The group $HOOC{-}CH_2{-}CH_2{-}CH(NH_2){-}CO{-}$, derived from glutamic acid.

**γ-glutamyl** The group $HOOC{-}CH(NH_2){-}CH_2{-}CH_2{-}CO{-}$, derived from glutamic acid. It occurs in glutathione.

**γ-glutamyl transpeptidase** An enzyme that catalyzes the transfer of glutamyl groups among peptides or amino acids. It is derived primarily from the liver, although renal and pancreatic cells contain substantial quantities. Serum levels are markedly elevated in obstructive liver disease and hepatocellular carcinoma, and moderately elevated with liver cell damage. It is usually measured as an indirect index of ethanol ingestion, because hepatocellular levels increase temporarily after stimulation by alcohol, barbiturates, and phenytoins. Also *γ-glutamyl transferase.*

**glutaraldehyde** $OCH[CH_2]_3$ CHO. A chemical having a molecular mass of 100 daltons, commonly used as a fixative in preservation of tissue for electron microscopy. Also *1,5-pentanediol.*

**glutaredoxin** A small protein, of molecular mass about 12 kDa, containing one disulfide bond. Its reduced form can function as the reductant for converting ribonucleotides into 2′-deoxyribonucleotides for DNA synthesis, and its oxidized form can be reduced by glutathione.

**glutaryl-CoA synthetase** An enzyme (EC 6.2.1.6) that catalyzes the conversion of glutarate, adenosine triphosphate, and coenzyme A into adenosine diphosphate, orthophosphate, and glutaryl-CoA.

**glutathione** The peptide γ-glutamylcysteinylglycine. In animals, it supplies reducing power to keep hemoglobin in its Fe(II) state despite spontaneous oxidation. It can also reduce ribonucleoside diphosphates to 2′-deoxyribonucleoside diphosphates. Its oxidized form, the dimeric disulfide, is reconverted into the thiol form by glutathione reductase.

**glutathione reductase** A flavoprotein enzyme (EC 1.6.4.2) that catalyzes the reduction of oxidized glutathione using NADPH or NADH as hydrogen donor.

**gluteal** \gloo′tē·əl\ [*glute(us)* + -AL] Pertaining to the buttocks or to one of their component structures.

**gluten** \gloo′tən\ [L, glue] The part of the wheat seed consisting of protein. It causes intestinal inflammation to those who have celiac disease.

**glutenin** One of the main components of gluten.

**gluteofemoral** \gloo′tē·ōfem′ərəl\ **1** Pertaining to the buttock and the thigh. **2** Pertaining to a gluteal muscle and the thigh or the femoral bone.

**glutethimide** $C_{13}H_{15}NO_2$. 2-Ethyl-2-phenylglutarimide. A piperidinedione derivative that is used as a sedative and hypnotic. It is general central nervous system depressant, and it is used in the treatment of insomnia and as preoperative medication for its sedative properties. It is given orally.

**gluteus** [New L (from Gk *gloutos* a buttock) pertaining to the buttocks] Denoting any of the gluteal muscles: musculus gluteus maximus, medius, or minimus.

**glutinous** \gloo′tənəs\ Gluelike; gummy; sticky.

**glutitis** \glootī′tis\ [Gk *glout(os)* the rump, bottom + -ITIS] An inflammation of the muscles of the buttocks.

**Glx** A symbol for a residue that may be glutamic acid, or glutamine, or 5-oxoproline, or 4-carboxyglutamic acid. Any method of locating the residue in a protein or peptide that uses acid hydrolysis converts all the last three into glutamic acid, and hence cannot distinguish between these four residues.

**Gly** Symbol for glycine.

**glyc-** \glīk-\ GLYCO-.

**glycemia** \glīsē′mē·ə\ [GLYC- + -EMIA] The presence of glucose in the blood. Also *glycohemia, glucohemia, glycosemia.*

**glyceraldehyde** $CH_2OH{-}CHOH{-}CHO$. The simplest chiral sugar. Its dextrorotatory form, D-glyceraldehyde, was taken as the standard of D configuration for sugars. It is the *R* compound. Also *glyceric aldehyde* (obs.), *glycerose* (obs.), *glyceral.*

**glyceraldehyde 3-phosphate** $CHO{-}CHOH{-}CH_2{-}O{-}PO_3H_2$. A three-carbon intermediate in glycolysis, formed when fructose 1,6-bisphosphate is cleaved under the influence of aldolase. It is interconvertible with the other triose phosphate produced with it, dihydroxyacetone phosphate. Also *3-phosphoglyceraldehyde.*

**glyceraldehyde-3-phosphate dehydrogenase** Any of the enzymes (EC 1.2.1.9, 1.2.1.12, and 1.2.1.13) that catalyze the oxidation of glyceraldehyde 3-phosphate to form either 3-phosphoglycerate with concomitant reduction of $NADP^+$, or, with uptake of orthosphosphate and concomitant reduction of $NAD^+$or $NADP^+$, 3-phosphoglyceroyl phosphate. The term when unqualified refers to the enzyme (EC 1.2.1.12) that uses $NAD^+$as hydrogen acceptor and forms 3-phosphoglyceroyl phosphate. This enzyme catalyzes an important step in the glycolytic pathway. The enzyme reacts with substrate through the thiol group of a cysteine residue, so that if the enzyme is portrayed as E—SH and the substrate as R—CHO, the hemithioacetal E—S—CHOH—R is formed and is then dehydrogenated to form an acyl enzyme, which can transfer the acyl group to orthophosphate to complete the reaction. The 3-phosphoglyceroyl phosphate formed can phosphorylate ADP to form ATP. The mammalian enzyme is a tetramer of four identical polypeptide chains, each of about 330 residues.

**glyceric acid** $CH_2OH—CHOH—COOH$. A compound that is an intermediate in the metabolism of glycolate by bacteria and plants, but whose phosphates are biologically more important as glycolytic intermediates. Its 2,3-bisphosphate regulates the affinity of hemoglobin for oxygen. Symbol: Gri

**glyceric aldehyde** *Obs.* GLYCERALDEHYDE.

**glyceride** A compound of glycerol.

**glycerin** \glis′ərin\ [French *glycérine* (from Gk *glyker(os)* sweet + -INE) glycerin] GLYCEROL. **g. of alum** A solution of potassium sulfate in water and glycerol. It is used as a topical astringent. **g. of boric acid** A thick, yellow, liquid prepared by dissolving boric acid in glycerol at 140–150°C. The product contains 31% w/w of boric acid. The weak bacteriostatic and fungistatic powers of boric acid, and the possible absorption of boric acid through abraded and broken skin areas, limit the usefulness of this medication. Also *boroglycerin glycerite.* **compound g. of thymol** A liquid mixture containing thymol, volatile oils, menthol, and glycerol. It has been used as a mouthwash. **g. of ichthammol** A preparation containing 10% ichthammol in glycerin w/w which has been used as ear drops for external ear inflammatory conditions. **g. of lead subacetate** A solution of lead subacetate ($C_4H_{10}O_8Pb_3$) in glycerin and water to a concentration of 1.48 g per ml. It has been used externally as an astringent solution for sprains and bruises. **g. of pepsin** A suspension of pepsin in water and glycerin with hydrochloric acid as a vehicle. It is used to administer pepsin to patients with a deficiency of this proteolytic enzyme. **phenol g.** A solution of phenol in glycerin, 16% w/w. It is further diluted with glycerin for use as a local treatment for mouth ulcers or tonsillitis. Dilute preparations in glycerin are also used as ear drops. **starch g.** A mixture of starch, glycerin, and water. It is a translucent jelly, and has been used as a protective ointment or coating on inflamed skin. Also *starch glycerite.*

**glycerinated** Treated with glycerol: used especially of muscle fibers extracted with glycerol to remove small molecules and leave the system of actin and myosin, to which substrates and effectors can be added.

**glycerine** GLYCEROL.

**glycerite** A solution or mixture of medicines with glycerol as the main solvent. Also *glyceritum.* **boroglycerin g.** GLYCERIN OF BORIC ACID. **starch g.** STARCH GLYCERIN.

**glyceritum** GLYCERITE.

**glycerol** ($CH_2OH$ CHOH $CH_2OH$). Trihydroxyproprane, a clear, colorless, syrupy liquid obtained from the hydrolysis of neutral fats. It is used as a solvent, an emollient, and a suppository. Also *glycerin, glycerine.*

**glycerol kinase** The enzyme (EC 2.7.1.30) that catalyzes the conversion of glycerol into *sn*-glycerol 3-phosphate by transfer of a phospho group from ATP with concomitant formation of ADP.

**glycerol phosphate** An ester of glycerol with phosphoric acid. The natural glycerol phosphate, formed by glycerol kinase from glycerol and ATP, or by glycerol-3-phosphate dehydrogenase by reduction of glycerone phosphate, is the *R* compound. It is known as *sn*-glycerol 3-phosphate, the prefix *sn* indicating stereospecific numbering in which the pro-*S* hydroxymethyl group is numbered 1. Glycerol phosphate is an intermediate in the metabolism of glycerol derived from fats. Also *glycerophosphate.*

**glycerol-phosphate dehydrogenase** Any enzyme that dehydrogenates glycerol phosphate. The commonest of such enzymes (EC 1.1.1.8) uses $NAD^+$ as hydrogen acceptor, and its activity provides a means of reoxidizing NADH when glycolysis is accelerating, and the concentration of pyruvate (in plants acetaldehyde) is low, because glycerone phosphate can act as the oxidant. It may also allow glycerol phosphate derived from glycerol to enter the glycolytic pathway, although in bacteria this oxidation is effected by a glycerol-phosphate dehydrogenase (EC 1.1.99.5) that uses a flavin as immediate hydrogen acceptor.

**glycerone** DIHYDROXYACETONE. Symbol: Grn

**glycerophosphate** GLYCEROL PHOSPHATE.

**glycinamide ribonucleotide** A substance whose molecule is composed of a ribose phosphate with the amide nitrogen of glycinamide linked to C-1 of the ribose. It is an intermediate in purine biosynthesis. Also *N-(5-phosphoribosyl)glycineamide.*

**glycinate** The anion, or occasionally an ester, derived from glycine.

**glycine** \glī′sēn\ [Gk *glyk(ys)* sweet + -INE] $NH_2$-$CH_2COOH$. α-Amino acetic acid. The simplest of the amino acids and a common constituent of proteins.

**glycine amidinotransferase** The enzyme (EC 2.1.4.1) that catalyzes the transfer of the amidino group —C(=NH)—$NH_2$ from arginine to glycine with the formation of ornithine and guanidinoacetate, a step in the biosynthesis of creatine.

**glycinemia** \glī′sinē′mē·ə\ HYPERGLYCINEMIA.

**glycinol** 2-AMINOETHANOL.

**glycinuria** \glī′sinoo′rē·ə\ [*glycin(e)* + -URIA] Excretion of excess amounts of glycine in the urine. Also *hyperglycinuria.* **de Vries type renal g.** Excess excretion of glycine in the urine, often associated with nephrolithiasis and hypophosphatemic rickets. It is inherited as a dominant trait. **hereditary g.** A rare condition, genetically transmitted as a dominant, characterized by hyperglycinuria with normoglycinemia due to decreased renal tubular reabsorption of glycine.

***Glyciphagus*** \glīsif′əgəs\ *GLYCYPHAGUS.*

**glyco-** \glī′kō-\ [Gk *glykys* sweet] A combining form meaning (1) sugar or any saccharide; (2) glycine. Also *glyc-.*

**glycobiarsol** $C_8H_9AsBiNO_6$. A pentavalent arsenical which also contains bismuth. It is used as an amebicidal drug in treating intestinal infections.

**glycocalyx** \-kā′liks\ A thin layer of acid polysaccharides, particularly sialic acid, adherent to the outer surface of many cells. It may be the site of intense enzyme activity and also contains the surface antigens of the cell. Also *fuzzy coat.*

**glycocholic acid** The conjugate of cholic acid with glycine, containing an amide bond between the carboxyl group of cholic acid and the amino group of glycine. It is present in mammalian bile.

**glycogen** \glī′kəjən\ [GLYCO- + -GEN] A storage polysaccharide, found in mammalian liver and muscle, and in microorganisms. It conists of glucose residues joined by $\alpha$1-4 links, with branches formed by occasional $\alpha$1-6 links.

**glycogenesis** 1 The formation or elaboration of glycogen. 2 The production of glucose. *Older term.*

**glycogenic** \-jen′ik\ [GLYCO- + -GENIC] Capable of forming carbohydrate: said of substances that can act as precursors of glycogen.

**glycogenolysis** \-jənäl′isis\ The process of glycogen breakdown.

**glycogenolytic** \-jen′əlit′ik\ Capable of causing glycogen breakdown.

**glycogenosis** \-jenō′sis\ [GLYCOGEN + -OSIS] GLYCOGEN STORAGE DISEASE. **brancher deficiency g.** GLYCOGEN STORAGE DISEASE IV. **hepatophosphorylase deficiency g.** GLYCOGEN STORAGE DISEASE VI. **myophosphorylase deficiency g.** GLYCOGEN STORAGE DISEASE V. **g. type II** GLYCOGEN STORAGE DISEASE II. **g. type III** GLYCOGEN STORAGE DISEASE III. **g. type V** GLYCOGEN STORAGE DISEASE V. **g. type VI** GLYCOGEN STORAGE DISEASE VI.

**glycogen phosphorylase** The phosphorylase (EC 2.4.1.1) that acts on glycogen, catalyzing its reaction with orthophosphate to form glucose 1-phosphate.

**glycogen synthase** The enzyme (EC 2.4.1.11) responsible for the synthesis of glycogen. It acts by transferring glucosyl groups from UDPglucose onto the O-4 atom of the terminal residue of an existing glycogen chain. This enzyme is phosphorylated by the cAMP-dependent protein kinase. In its phosphorylated form it is inactive except in the presence of glucose 6-phosphate. This control allows glycogen synthesis to be shut off when glycogen breakdown is enhanced in response to hormones such as epinephrine. Also *UDPG-glycogen transglucosidase* (outmoded).

**glycogeusia** \-joo′sē·ə\ [GLYCO- + Gk *geus(is)* taste + -IA] A spontaneous sensation of a sweet taste in the mouth.

**glycohemia** \-hē′mē·ə\ GLYCEMIA.

**glycolic acid** HO—$CH_2$—COOH. 2-Hydroxyacetic acid.

**glycolipid** \-lip′id\ Any lipid which contains a carbohydrate group. **blood group A g.** A ANTIGEN. **blood group B g.** B ANTIGEN.

**glycolysis** \glīkäl′isis\ [GLYCO- + LYSIS] The breakdown of carbohydrate, such as glycogen, to a simpler compound, such as pyruvate. This process does not require oxygen, but in order to regenerate $NAD^+$used during glycolysis, the end-product has also to serve as a hydrogen acceptor. A variety of substances, such as lactate, ethanol and carbon dioxide, succinate, and propionate are thus formed. This overall sequence forms the basis of many industrially important fermentations. Adj. glycolytic.

**glycolytic** Concerned with glycolysis, as an enzyme catalyzing one of the steps of glycolysis.

**glyconeogenesis** \-nē′ōjen′əsis\ The formation of glycogen or other carbohydrate from noncarbohydrate sources, such as lactic acid or some amino acids derived from the breakdown of protein.

**glycopenia** \-pē′nē·ə\ [GLYCO- + -PENIA] A condition marked by a lower-than-normal concentration of sugar in the blood and tissues.

**glycopeptide** A compound of a peptide and a carbohydrate. Such compounds are formed by the partial hydrolysis of glycoproteins.

**glycopexia** \-pek′sē·ə\ The incorporation of sugars into tissues. Also *glycopexis.*

**glycophorin A** One of the major proteins of the erythrocyte cytoskeleton. It is a glycoprotein that contains 131 amino acids. Glycophorin spans the lipid bilayer of the membrane, with its carbohydrate-rich region on the exterior surface, its hydrophobic region with the lipid bilayer, and its interior C terminus attached to spectrin. Glycophorin is the MNSs blood group surface antigen. It is believed to constitute the anion channel.

**glycoprotein** A conjugated protein containing one or more carbohydrate residues. The glycoproteins are important components of the plasma membrane, as well as of mucin and chondroitin.

**glycoregulation** \-reg′yəlā′shən\ The control of the processes associated with the metabolism of sugar.

**glycorrhachia** \-rā′kē·ə\ [GLYCO- + -RRHACHIA] An abnormally high sugar content in the cerebrospinal fluid.

**glycosaminoglycan** A polysaccharide that contains amino sugars or monosaccharides in which one of the —OH groups is replaced with an —$NH_2$ group. They occur either alone or in combination with proteins. Also *mucopolysaccharide.*

**glycosemia** \-sē′mē·ə\ GLYCEMIA.

**glycosidase** Any enzyme that catalyzes the hydrolysis of a glycoside.

**glycoside** Any substance consisting of an alcohol with the hydrogen of its hydroxyl group replaced by a glycosyl group. The alcohol can be released from it by acid hydrolysis, and is known as the aglycone. **cardiac g.** Any of the glycosides of a cardenolide. They are found in plants and possess cardiotonic action.

***N*-glycoside** A substance containing a glycosylated nitrogen atom, it is analogous with a glycoside but with nitrogen in place of oxygen. Nucleosides are *N*-glycosides.

**glycostasis** \-stā′sis\ The maintenance of a constant sugar concentration in the body.

**glycosuria** \-s^y oo′rē·ə\ [*glycos(e)* (obsol. variant of GLUCOSE) + -URIA] Excretion of abnormal amounts of glucose in urine. Normal persons may excrete up to 200 mg/24 hours of glucose and other sugars, and other substances with reducing activity, notably ascorbic acid. Glycosuria results either from excessively high plasma glucose levels or from reduced renal capacity to reabsorb glucose from normal plasma ultrafiltrate. Also *glucosuria.* Adj. glycosuric. **alimentary g.** Glycosuria secondary to excess dietary sugar intake. **artificial g.** The presence in the urine of sugar added inadvertently or else deliberately and surreptitiously by the patient. Also *factitious glycosuria.* **benign g.** RENAL GLYCOSURIA. **diabetic g.** Excessive excretion of glucose in the urine secondary to the hyperglycemia of diabetes mellitus. **factitious g.** ARTIFICIAL GLYCOSURIA. **hyperglycemic g.** Glycosuria due to hyperglycemia, as in diabetes mellitus or rapid intravenous injection of glucose. **nondiabetic g.** Glycosuria due to any cause other than diabetes mellitus including renal and alimentary glycosuria. **phlorizin g.** Glycosuria produced in experimental animals by injection of phlorizin. The phlorizin decreases or abolishes renal tubular reabsorption of glucose. **pituitary g.** **1** Glycosuria associated with the hyperglycemia of acromegaly due to excessive growth hormone. *Older term.* **2** Glycosuria accompanying the hypercortisolism that occurs in the pituitary-dependent form of the Cushing syndrome. **renal g.** **1** The benign, usually asymptomatic presence of glucose in the urine when the blood glucose is normal, due to defective reabsorption of glucose by the proximal convoluted tubules. Familial renal glycosuria may be inherited as an autosomal recessive trait. **2** Glycosuria in the presence of normal blood glucose, due to defective reabsorption of glucose by diseased renal tubules, which may be part of the Fanconi syndrome, chronic renal failure, or due to effects on the renal tubules of toxins or poisons, such as the heavy metals, phlorizin, and carbon monoxide. Also *benign glycosuria.*

**glycosuric acid** HOMOGENTISIC ACID.

**glycosyl** The group formed from a sugar, oligosaccharide, or polysaccharide by removal of its anomeric hydroxyl group.

**glycosylation** \-səlā′shən\ **1** Substitution with a glycosyl group. **2** The formation, by nonenzymatic means, of an irreversible bond between glucose and the N-terminal valine of the hemoglobin $\beta$ chain to form a detectable, electrophoretically fast-moving hemoglobin, hemoglobin $A_{1c}$, the level of which rises in association with the raised blood glucose concentration in uncontrolled or poorly controlled diabetes mellitus.

**glycosyltransferase** Any of the enzymes that transfer glycosyl groups, including enzymes responsible for the synthesis of polysaccharides and those responsible for their phosphorolysis. Enzymes that hydrolyze polysaccharides are not so classed, although they transfer glycosyl groups onto water.

**glycotropic** \-träp′ik\ Acting upon or influenced by the concentration of sugar.

***Glycyphagus*** \glīsif′əgəs\ A genus of mites that infest stored food products and induce dermatitis among grocers and other food handlers. The reaction may be caused by the bites directly or may be a contact allergy. Also *Glyciphagus.*

**glycyrrhiza** \glis′ərī′zə\ [Gk *glykyrrhiza* (from *glyky(s)* sweet + *rhiza* root) licorice] The dried roots of *Glycyrrhiza glabra,* used in extracts and syrups as a demulcent, expectorant, and flavoring vehicle for drugs. Also *licorice, licorice root, liquorice, sweet root.*

**glycyrrhizic acid** $C_{42}H_{62}O_{16}$. A glycoside found in licorice root.

**glyoxalin** *Outmoded* IMIDAZOLE.

**glyoxylate** An anion, salt, or ester of glyoxylic acid.

**glyoxylic acid** CHO—COOH. 2-Oxoacetic acid. An intermediate in the glyoxylate pathway, by which plants and microorganisms, but not higher animals, can convert fat into carbohydrate. The aldehyde group is hydrated both in solution and in the solid form.

**glyoxysome** \glī·äk′sisōm\ [*glyoxy(late)* + -SOME] An organelle in the cells of plants and of some eukaryotic microorganisms that contains the enzymes necessary to catalyze the glyoxylate cycle.

**glyphylline** DYPHYLLINE.

**Glytheonate** A proprietary name for theophylline sodium glycinate.

**Gm** See under GM ALLOTYPE.

**gm** Symbol for the unit, gram. An incorrect symbol.

**GMP** guanosine monophosphate.

**gnat** \nat\ [Old English *gnætt*] Any of various small dipteran insects, especially pestiferous ones, such as blackflies, biting midges, or sandflies. • The term *gnat* also includes mosquitoes in British and South African usage, but not in U.S. usage. **buffalo g.** BLACKFLY. **eye g.** A fly of the genus *Hippelates,* especially *H. pusio.*

**gnath-** \nath-\ GNATHO-.

**gnathic** \nā′thik, nath′ik\ [GNATH- + -IC] Pertaining to the cheek or jaw, or to the alveolar process.

**gnathion** \nā′thē·än\ [New L, irreg. from Gk *gnathos* the jaw, esp. the lower jaw] A point on the surface of the mandible in the sagittal plane midway between the most anterior and the most inferior points on the chin.

**gnatho-** \nath′ō-\ [Gk *gnathos* jaw, especially lower jaw] A combining form denoting the jaw. Also *gnath-.*

**gnathocephalus** \-sef′ələs\ [GNATHO- + -CEPHALUS] A malformed embryo, fetus, or neonate lacking most of the head above the mandibular arch or the lower jaw.

**gnathodynamometer** \-dī′nəmäm′ətər\ [GNATHO- + DYNAMOMETER] An instrument for measuring forces exerted by the teeth. Also *occlusometer.*

**gnathology** \nāthäl′əjē\ [GNATHO- + -LOGY] The study of the forces exerted by the teeth, especially during mastication.

**gnathopalatoschisis** \-pal′ətäs′kisis\ [GNATHO- + PALATO- + -SCHISIS] A facial cleft in which the prepalate or premaxilla as well as the palate is cleft. In the usual cleft of jaw and palate, the cleft passes to either or both sides of the premaxilla.

**gnathoplasty** \nā′thəplas′tē\ [GNATHO- + -PLASTY] Any plastic operation on either jaw.

**gnathoplegia** \-plē′jə\ [GNATHO- + -PLEGIA] Paralysis of the muscles of the cheek.

**gnathoschisis** \nāthäs′kisis\ [GNATHO- + -SCHISIS] A cleft of the jaw, usually of the maxilla, thus the usual cleft of lip and jaw. Rarely the mandible and lower lip may show midline hypoplasia of sufficient degree to constitute a developmental defect.

***Gnathostoma*** \nathäs′təmə\ [GNATHO- + Gk *stoma* the mouth] A genus of some 19 species of spiruroid nematodes (family Gnathostomatidae) parasitic in the stomach wall of cats, dogs, other predatory mammals, and occasionally humans. Members of the genus have heads with rows of cuticular spines, and multiple-host aquatic life cycles, involving copepods and a varied assortment of aquatic second intermediate hosts. They may also use a series of transport or paratenic hosts, leading to the final, carnivorous, mammalian host. In humans, they have been associated with a cutaneous larva migrans, especially in southeastern Asia.

**gnathostomiasis** \-stōmī′əsis\ [*Gnathostom(a)* + -IASIS] Infection with *Gnathostoma,* especially *G. spinigerum.* The larvae may affect the skin and subcutaneous tissues, and the adult worms sometimes cause intestinal infections.

**gnotobiology** \nō′tōbī·äl′əjē\ [Gk *gnōto(s)* known + BIOLOGY] The maintenance of laboratory animals all of whose microbiologic commensals are known, or which have been reared as germ-free. Also *gnotobiotics.*

**gnotophoric** \nō′tōfôr′ik\ Harboring a known flora and fauna on the body.

**GnRH** gonadotropin releasing hormone.

**goal** **1** Any target for behavior or incentive for action. **2** In experimental usage, an end result, specified in advance by the experimenter, the accomplishment of which completes a behavioral sequence.

**godet** \gōdet′, gōdā′\ [French, a drinking cup without foot or handle] SCUTULUM.

**Godman** [John Davidson *Godman,* U.S. anatomist, 1794–1830] See under FASCIA.

**Goeckerman** [William Henry *Goeckerman,* U.S. dermatologist, 1884–1954] See under TREATMENT.

**Goethe** [Johann Wolfgang von *Goethe,* German writer, statesman, and scientist, 1749–1832] **1** See under BONE. **2** Goethe's bone. See under OS INCISIVUM.

**Gofman** [Moses *Gofman,* German physician, born 1897] See under TEST.

**goiter** \goi′tər\ [French *goitre* (from L *guttur* the throat) goiter] Any diffuse or nodular enlargement or swelling of the thyroid gland, often visible as a prominence in the lower anterior neck. Also *struma, thyromegaly.* Adj. goitrous, strumous. **aberrant g.** Goiter affecting an ectopic or supernumerary thyroid gland, usually in the anterior and superior mediastinum. **adenomatous g.** NODULAR GOITER. **Basedow's g.** A diffuse nontoxic goiter that becomes toxic or hyperfunctional after iodine administration. **cabbage g.** Diet-induced goiter caused by the goitrogenic substances contained in cabbage and related plants. **colloid g.** A diffuse enlargement of the thyroid gland caused by greatly distended, colloid-filled follicles. This is the typical form of endemic goiter seen in areas of iodine deficiency. Also *follicular goiter, parenchymatous goiter, struma colloides, struma parenchymatosa, adenoma gelatinosum.* **congenital g.** Goiter present in the neonate or due to heritable deficiency of one of several enzymes involved in the biosynthesis of thyroid hormone. There is subnormal thyroid hor-

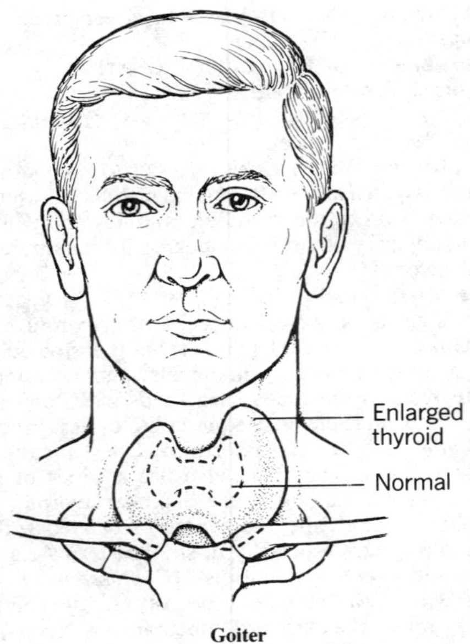


Goiter

mone secretion, excessive pituitary secretion of thyrotropin, and consequent hypertrophy of the thyroid gland. **diving g.** A goiter, located at the level of the sternal notch, that is freely movable and thus may change its location from above to below the sternal notch. Also *wandering goiter.* **endemic g.** Goiter occurring in parts of the world where the iodine content of the diet is low, as in the Alps, the Andes, the Himalayas, and the Great Lakes region of North America. In some areas dietary goitrogens may also be operative, as in Africa and South America. Also *nontoxic diffuse goiter.* **exophthalmic g.** Goiter associated with proptosis of the eyeballs, as seen in Graves disease. **familial g.** **1** Goiter associated with heritable inborn errors of thyroid hormone biosynthesis. Also *familial goitrous hypothyroidism.* **2** Goiter afflicting extended families in a region where goiter is endemic. An imprecise usage. **familial g. with deaf-mutism** Nerve-deafness associated with familial goiter which is inherited as an autosomal recessive defect. The basic thyroid defect may be a partial failure of the incorporation of iodide into organic hormones. The subjects are euthyroid. Also *Pendred syndrome.* **follicular g.** COLLOID GOITER. **intrathoracic g.** A form of goiter that extends into the thoracic cavity, usually the superior and anterior mediastinum in proximity to the thymus or thymic remnant. Also *plunging goiter, struma endothoracica.* **lingual g.** A mass of ectopic thyroid tissue lying at the base of the tongue in the region from which the embryonic thyroglossal duct arose. Also *struma lingualis, struma baseos linguae.* **lymphadenoid g.** HASHIMOTO'S DISEASE. **myxedematous g.** Any goiter associated with severe hypothyroidism, congenital or acquired. **nodular g.** The usual form of goiter, in which the enlarged gland has a nodular pattern due to the development of multiple, discrete foci of hyperplasia with interstitial fibrosis and sometimes calcification. Also *adenomatous goiter.* **nontoxic g.** Any goiter not associated with hyperthyroidism or thyrotoxicosis. There are two types, diffuse (endemic goiter) and nodular (nontoxic nodular goiter). **parenchymatous g.** COLLOID GOITER. **plunging g.** INTRATHORACIC GOITER. **simple g.** Goiter with normal thyroid function. **substernal g.** Goiter affecting primarily the isthmus, with downward extension into the substernal region. Also *substernal struma, retrosternal struma.* **thoracic g.** An enlargement of accessory or ectopic thyroid tissue in the superior mediastinum. Thryoid tissue, either coextensive with or separate from the normally located thyroid gland, may develop in the upper thorax in association with the thymus. It tends to become goitrous under conditions similar to those affecting thyroid tissue generally, as in dietary iodine lack. **toxic g.** Goiter associated with hyperthyroidism and thyrotoxicosis. There are two types, diffuse (toxic diffuse goiter) and nodular (toxic nodular goiter). **toxic diffuse g.** Diffuse, generalized enlargement of the thyroid, accompanied by hyperthyroidism and thyrotoxicosis and often with exophthalmos. **toxic nodular g.** Nodular goiter, more often single than multiple, accompanied by hyperthyroidism and thyrotoxicosis and not usually associated with exophthalmos. Also *Plummer's disease.* **wandering g.** DIVING GOITER.

**goitre** \goiʹtər\ *Brit.* GOITER.

**goitrogen** \goiʹtrəjən\ [*goit(e)r* + *o* + -GEN] Any goiter-producing substance, as contained in peanuts, turnips and rutabagas, thiourea and its derivatives, thionamides, aminoheterocyclic compounds, substituted phenols, thicyanate and perchlorate ions.

**goitrogenic** \goiˈtrəjenʹik\ Tending to produce goiter. Also *goitrogenous.*

**gold** Element number 79, having atomic weight 196.9665. It is a soft, heavy (specific gravity, 19.32), malleable and ductile yellow metal that does not tarnish in air. The sole stable isotope, gold 197, is found free and also combined in the lithosphere and is present in sea water in concentrations as high as 2 mg/ton. Eighteen radioactive isotopes are known. Gold is used in dentistry and in some pharmaceuticals. Symbol: Au **fibrous g.** GOLD FOIL. See under FOIL. **inlay g.** An alloy of which the principal ingredient is gold, used in cast restorations. **radioactive g.** Any of the 25 radioactive isotopes of gold, ranging in atomic mass from 185 to 203 and having half-lives from 0.44 millisecond to 183 days. Also *radiogold.*

**gold 198** A radioactive isotope of gold, emitting beta and gamma radiation. In years past, it was used in a colloid preparation for liver imaging but has been replaced by technetium 99m agents. Intracavitary injection of a colloidal preparation of gold 198 has been used for treatment of peritoneal and pleural effusions. Interstitial implantation of gold 198 seeds or wires is used in tumor therapy. Physical half-life is 2.7 days. Symbol: $^{198}$Au

**Goldberger** [Joseph *Goldberger,* U.S. physician, 1874–1929] Anderson and Goldberger test. See under TEST.

**Goldblatt** [Harry *Goldblatt,* U.S. pathologist, 1891–1977] **1** See under KIDNEY. **2** Goldblatt phenomenon. See under HYPERTENSION.

**Golden** [William Wolfe *Golden,* U.S. physician, 1866–1929] See under SIGN.

**Goldenhar** [Maurice *Goldenhar,* Swiss physician, flourished mid-20th century] Goldenhar syndrome. See under OCULOAURICULOVERTEBRAL DYSPLASIA.

**Goldflam** [Samuel Valfovish *Goldflam,* Polish neurologist, 1852–1932] Hoppe-Goldflam syndrome, Erb-Goldflam syndrome, Erb-Oppenheim-Goldflam syndrome, Goldflam's disease, Goldflam-Erb disease, Erb-Goldflam disease. See under MYASTHENIA GRAVIS.

**gold sodium thiomalate** AUROTHIOMALATE DISODIUM.

**Goldstein** [Hyman Isaac *Goldstein,* U.S. physician, 1887–1954] **1** See under HEMATEMESIS, HEMOPTYSIS, SIGN. **2** Goldstein's disease. See under HEREDITARY HEMORRHAGIC TELANGIECTASIA.

**Goldstein** [Kurt *Goldstein,* German-born U.S. psychologist, 1878–1965] **1** Goldstein syndrome, Goldstein-Reichmann syndrome. See under ACQUIRED CEREBELLAR SYNDROME. **2** See under CLASSIFICATION. **3** Weigl-Goldstein-Scheerer test. See under TEST.

**gold thioglucose** An insoluble colloidal gold compound, used in the treatment of rheumatoid arthritis.

**gold thiomalate** A soluble gold compound, used in the treatment of rheumatoid arthritis.

**gold toning** The optimal step in the silver impregnation techniques for reticulin, fungi, and axons, using gold chloride to provide a completely permanent preparation with a neutral black color of high density. Also *aftergilding.*

**Golé** [L. *Golé,* French physician, flourished 20th century] Touraine-Solente-Golé syndrome. See under PACHYDERMOPERIOSTOSIS.

**Golgi** [Camillo *Golgi,* Italian histologist, 1843–1926] **1** Golgi type I neurons. See under NEURON. **2** Golgi type II neurons. See under NEURON. **3** See under METHOD. **4** Cox modification of Golgi's corrosive sublimate method. See under METHOD. **5** Golgi complex. See under APPARATUS. **6** Golgi body. See under DICTYOSOME. **7** Golgi-Mazzoni corpuscles. See under GOLGI-MAZZONI ENDINGS. **8** Golgi cisternae. See under CISTERNA. **9** Holmgren-Golgi canals. See under ENDOPLASMIC RETICULUM. **10** Golgi cells. See under GOLGI TYPE I NEURON, GOLGI TYPE II NEURON. **11** See under THEORY.

**Goll** [Friedrich *Goll,* Swiss anatomist, 1829–1903] **1** Goll's fibers. See under FIBER. **2** Nucleus of Goll's column. See under NUCLEUS GRACILIS. **3** Column of Goll, fasciculus gracilis Golli, fasciculus of Goll. See under FASCICULUS GRACILIS MEDULLAE SPINALIS. **4** Tract of Goll. See under COLUMNA POSTEROMEDIANA.

**Goltz** [Robert William *Goltz,* U.S. physician, born 1923] Goltz syndrome. See under FOCAL DERMAL HYPOPLASIA.

**Gombault** [François Alexis Albert *Gombault,* French neurologist, 1844–1904] **1** Tract of Philippe-Gombault, triangular tract of Philippe-Gombault, Gombault-Philippe triangle. See under FASCICULUS TRIANGULARIS. **2** Gombault's degeneration. See under HEREDITARY HYPERTROPHIC INTERSTITIAL NEUROPATHY.

**gomitoli** \gōmit′ōlē\ [Italian, pl. of *gomitolo* a coil or ball of thread] A network of specialized capillaries in the hypothalamic-hypophysial portal venous system of the infundibular stalk that envelops the terminal anteriolar branches of the superior hypophyseal arteries and empties into the hypophysial portal veins. It is often associated with the pathogenesis of the Sheehan syndrome.

**Gomori** [George *Gomori,* Hungarian-born U.S. pathologist, 1904–1957] Gomori stain. See under METHOD.

**Gompertz** [Benjamin *Gompertz,* English mathematician, 1779–1865] **1** See under EQUATION, LAW. **2** Gompertz curve. See under GROWTH CURVE.

**gomphosis** \gämfō′sis\ [Gk *gomphōsis* (from *gomphos* a bolt, peg) a bolting together, peg articulation] [NA] A type of fibrous joint in which the roots of teeth are fixed in sockets in the mandible and the maxilla by the periodontal ligament. Also *peg-and-socket joint, socket joint of tooth, clavation, incuneation, peg-and-socket suture.*

**gon-**[1] \gän-\ GONY-.

**gon-**[2] \gän-\ GONO-.

**gonacratia** \gän′əkrā′shə\ [GON-[2] + Gk *akrateia* (early form of *akrasia*) incontinence] SPERMATORRHEA.

**gonad** \gän′ad, gō′nad\ [Gk *gon(ē)* generation, generative organ + *-ad* as in *monad* (a unit, one of a pair or set)] A structure capable of producing a gamete; testis or ovary. Adj. gonadal. **indifferent g.** An undifferentiated gonad in the embryo, which has not acquired the characteristics of an ovary or a testis. **primitive g.** An often undifferentiated anlage in an early embryo, destined to become either a testis or an ovary. **streak g.** An undeveloped gonadal structure located in the broad ligament in close proximity to the fallopian tube. It is characteristically seen in individuals with Turner syndrome, with XO genotype, in which the phenotypic development is female. It is composed of whorled connective tissue stroma with no germinal or secretory cells. The etiology is unclear, as mice with an XO genotype possess morphologically normal ovaries and may have definite, if limited, fertility.

**gonadectomy** \gän′ədek′təmē\ [GONAD + -ECTOMY] The surgical removal of one or both gonads.

**gonadoblastoma** \gän′ədōblastō′mə\ An ovarian or testicular tumor composed of large germ cells similar to those of seminoma and dysgerminoma and small cells resembling immature Sertoli and granulosa cells. The stroma may contain Leydig cells. The tumor almost always arises in those with dysgenetic gonads. Most subjects are phenotypic females who have a Y chromosome. Also *dysgenetic gonadoma.*

**gonadocentric** \gän′ədōsen′trik\ Focused on the genitals, as in adolescent and adult sexuality when genital primacy is attained.

**gonadogenesis** \gän′ədōjen′əsis\ [GONAD + *o* + GENESIS ] Embryonic development of the ovaries or testes according to the sex of the individual.

**gonadoma** \gän′ədō′mə\ [GONAD + -OMA] A tumor of a gonad. **dysgenetic g.** GONADOBLASTOMA.

**gonadotrope** \gän′ədōtrōp′\ A gonadotropin-secreting cell of the anterior pituitary. Also *gonadotroph.*

**gonadotrophic** \gän′ədōträf′ik\ GONADOTROPIC.

**gonadotrophin** \gän′ədōträf′in\ GONADOTROPIN. **luteotrophic g.** *Outmoded* PROLACTIN.

**gonadotropic** \gän′ədōträp′ik\ Acting to stimulate the gonads: used especially of the hormones of the adenohypophysis and the placenta which regulate the structure, function, and development of the gonads. Also *gonadotrophic.*

**gonadotropin** \gän′ədōtrō′pin\ [GONAD + *o* + *trop(ic)* + -IN] Any hormone acting to stimulate the gonads, regulate their development, structure, or hormone-secreting functions, or contribute to gametogenesis, as the follicle-stimulating hormone or luteinizing hormone of the pituitary and the chorionic gonadotropin secreted by the placenta. Also *gonadotrophin, gonadotropic hormone.* **chorionic g.** The gonadotropin synthesized and secreted by the placenta. The hormone is a glycopeptide having an $\alpha$ subunit virtually identical to those of luteinizing hormone and thyroid-stimulating hormone and a specific $\beta$ subunit responsible for its gonadotropic activity. Its actions resemble those of luteinizing hormone. Presence of this hormone in urine in early pregnancy is the basis for most pregnancy tests. Human chorionic gonadotropin maintains the secretory integrity of the corpus luteum of pregnancy. The urinary preparation is used pharmaceutically to treat cryptorchidism and to induce ovulation in anovulatory women. The hormone is secreted in excess in hydatidiform mole, choriocarcinoma, and certain tumors of the testis. Chorionic gonadotropin from the urine of pregnant women and pregnant mares' serum is used in the treatment of hypogonadism. Also *anterior-pituitary-like* *substance.* Abbr. CG **equine g.** PREGNANT MARE SERUM GONADOTROPIN. **human chorionic g.** See under CHORIONIC GONADOTROPIN. Abbr. HCG **human menopausal g.** The gonadotropin isolated and concentrated from the urine of postmenopausal women. The pharmaceutical preparation is used to stimulate ovulation in infertile women. **pituitary g.** A gonadotropin secreted by the pituitary, as distinguished from chorionic gonadotropin; follicle-stimulating hormone or luteinizing hormone. **pregnant mare serum g.** A gonadotropin obtained from the serum of pregnant mares. It has a molecular weight of about 53 000 and contains a high concentration of carbohydrate and sialic acid. Also *equine gonadotropin.* Abbr. PMSG

**gonaduct** \gän′ədukt\ Oviduct or seminal duct.

**gonangiectomy** \gän′anjē·ek′təmē\ [GON-[2] + ANGI- + -ECTOMY] VASECTOMY.

**gonarthrosis** \gän′ärthrō′sis\ Arthritis of the knee.

**gonarthrotomy** \gän′ärthrät′əmē\ An operative opening into the knee.

**gonecyst** [Gk *gonē* seed + CYST] *Obs.* VESICULA SEMINALIS.

**gonecystitis** \gän′əsistī′tis\ [GONECYST + -ITIS] Inflammation of the seminal vesicles.

**gonecystolith** \gän′əsis′təlith\ [GONECYST + *o* + -LITH] A calculus or mass in a seminal vesicle.

**goneitis** \gän′ē·ī′tis\ GONITIS.

***Gongylonema pulchrum*** \gän′jilōnē′mə pul′krəm\ A cosmopolitan species of gullet worm found in the esophageal mucosa and rumen of wild and domestic ruminants, and also in bears, pigs, and humans. It is transmitted by coprophagous beetles. Human infections are usually caused by immature worms.

**gonia** \gō′nē·ə\ Plural of GONION.

**gonial** \gō′nē·əl\ Pertaining to the gonion.

**gonidium** \gōnid′ē·əm\ [GON-[2] + -IDIUM] (*pl.* gonidia) One of the motile reproductive cells of certain nitrogen-fixing bacteria. Adj. gonidial.

**gonio-** \gō′nē·ō-\ [Gk *gōnia* corner, angle] A combining form meaning angle.

**goniolens** \gō′nē·ōlens′\ [GONIO- + LENS] A contact lens that modifies the corneal refraction of light so as to permit observation of the details of the peripheral angle of the anterior chamber, evaluation of which is particularly important in glaucoma.

**gonioma** \gän′ē·ō′mə\ [GON-[2] + *i* + -OMA] A tumor of germ cells.

**goniometer** \gän′ē·äm′ətər\ [GONIO- + -METER] An instrument used to measure angles. In medicine, it is often used to test the range of flexion/extension in joints.

**gonion** \gō′nē·än\ [New L, irreg. from Gk *gōnia* corner, angle] A craniometric point situated at the apex of the angle of the mandible formed by the body and the ramus.

**goniophotography** \-fōtäg′rəfē\ The technique of obtaining pictures of the angle of the anterior chamber of the eye.

**gonioprism** \gō′nē·ōprizm′\ **Allen g.** A four-sided contact lens used for microscopic viewing of the internal aspect of the peripheral circumference of the anterior chamber of the eye.

**goniopuncture** \-pungk′chər\ [GONIO- + PUNCTURE] Perforation from within the trabecular meshwork and scleral structures to create a fistula leading from the anterior chamber to the subconjunctival space, particularly useful in the management of congenital glaucoma.

**gonioscope** \gō′nē·ōskōp′\ [GONIO- + -SCOPE] A device for viewing the anterior chamber angle of the eye *in vivo.*

**gonioscopy** \gō′nē·äs′kəpē\ Examination of the anterior chamber angle of the eye by means of a gonioscope.

**goniosynechia** \-sinek′ē·ə\ [GONIO- + SYNECHIA] Adhesion between the peripheral iris and the trabecular meshwork.

**goniotomy** \gō′nē·ät′əmē\ [GONIO- — -TOMY] A wide incision of the trabecular meshwork, performed by approaching from within the eye via a puncture entering the opposite limbal area, useful in management of congenital glaucoma. Also *Barkan's operation.*

**gonitis** \gōnī′tis\ [Gk *gon(y)* knee + -ITIS] An inflammation of the knee. Also *goneitis.* **g. tuberculosa** A tuberculous inflammation of the knee.

**gono-** \gän′ə-\ [Gk *gonē* seed] A combining form meaning seed, semen. Also *gon-*[2].

**gonocele** \gän′əsēl\ [GONO- + -CELE[1]] A cystic distention of the spermatic cord.

**gonocide** \gän′əsīd\ GONOCOCCOCIDE.

**gonococcal** \-käk′əl\ Pertaining to or caused by gonococci (*Neisseria gonorrheae).*

**gonococcemia** \-käksē′mē·ə\ [*gonococc(us)* + -EMIA] The presence of gonococci in the bloodstream.

**gonococci** \-käk′sī\ Plural of GONOCOCCUS.

**gonococcocide** \-käk′əsīd\ [*gonococc(us)* + *o* + -CIDE] A substance capable of killing the *Neisseria gonorrhoeae.* Also *gonococcide, gonocide.* Adj. gonococcocidal.

**gonococcus** \-käk′əs\ [*gono(rrhea)* + COCCUS] (*pl.* gonococci) An organism of the species *Neisseria gonorrhoeae.*

**gonocyte** \gän′əsīt\ [GONO- + -CYTE] **1** GERM CELL. **2** A secondary oocyte or secondary spermatocyte. **primordial g.** ARCHIGONOCYTE.

**gonocytoma** \-sītō′mə\ [*gonocyt(e)* + -OMA] A tumor of germ cells.

**gonoducts** \gän′ədukts\ [GONO- + *ducts,* pl. of DUCT] The mesonephric and paramesonephric ducts considered together.

**gonomery** \gänäm′ərē\ [GONO- + *-mer(e)* + -Y] A condition in which paternal and maternal chromosomes remain in separate groups and do not completely fuse.

**gonorrhea** \gän′ərē′ə\ [Late L *gonorrhoea,* from Gk *gonorroia* (from *gono(s)* seed + *rhoia* a flow) leakage of semen (an ancient misnomer)] Infection of the genitourinary organs and more rarely of the rectum, pharynx, or conjunctiva caused by *Neisseria gonorrhoeae.* The disease, detectable three to five days after sexual contact with an infected partner, is usually characterized by a purulent urethral discharge in men. Symptoms are less prominent in women. Complications include salpingitis, chronic pelvic inflammatory disease with sterility, and hematogenous dissemination producing arthritis and rash. Also *blenorrhagia, clap* (popular).

**gonorrhoea** \gän′ôrē′ə\ *Brit.* GONORRHEA.

**gonoscheocele** \gänäs′kē·ōsēl′\ [GON-[2] + OSCHEO- + -CELE[1]] Testicular swelling due to excessive seminal fluid.

**gonotoxemia** \-täksē′mē·ə\ A toxic state caused by the presence in blood of substances derived from *Neisseria gonorrhoeae.*

**gony-** \gän′ē-\ [Gk *gony* knee] A combining form denoting the knee. Also *gon-.*

**-gony** \-gənē\ [Gk *gonos* or *gonē* (from root of *gignesthai* to be, become, be born) that which is begotten, offspring] A combining form denoting reproduction.

**gonyalgia** \-al′jə\ [GONY- + -ALGIA] Pain in the knee. **g. paresthetica** Pain and paresthesia occurring in the distribution of the infrapatellar branch of the saphenous nerve.

***Gonyaulax*** \-ô′leks\ A genus of marine dinoflagellates (order Dinoflagellida, class Phytomastigophorea) known to cause paralytic shellfish poisoning. These protozoans can synthesize and secrete a toxin that is often fatal to humans who eat filter-feeding shellfish (mussels, clams, oysters, scallops) that have filtered out the flagellates from the water. The flagellates are not destroyed by the shellfish but continue to produce their toxin in an unusual form of protective symbiosis.

**gonycampsis** \-kamp′sis\ An abnormal curvature of the knee.

**gonyoncus** \-äng′kəs\ A tumorous swelling of the knee.

**Good** [R. A. *Good,* U.S. pediatrician, born 1922] Good syndrome. See under IMMUNODEFICIENCY WITH THYMOMA.

**Goodell** [William *Goodell,* U. S. gynecologist, 1829–1894] Goodell's law. See under SIGN.

**Goormaghtigh** [Norbert *Goormaghtigh,* Belgian physicist, 1890–1960] **1** Apparatus of Goormaghtigh. See under JUXTAGLOMERULAR APPARATUS. **2** Goormaghtigh cells. See under JUXTAGLOMERULAR CELLS.

**gooseflesh** GOOSE FLESH. See under FLESH.

**Gopalan** [C. *Gopalan,* Indian biochemist, flourished 20th century] Gopalan syndrome. See under BURNING FEET SYNDROME.

***Gordius*** \gôr′dē·əs\ A genus of the phylum Nematomorpha (or Gordiacea), the horsehair snakes, or horsehair worms. Adults are free-living, elongate, rather stiff-bodied aschelminths related to the nematodes. The larval forms undergo nearly all of their growth and development in the body cavity of an insect or other arthropod host. The fully developed larva leaves its host, usually killing it in the process, only when the host is in or near water. ***G. aquaticus*** A species sometimes found as a pseudoparasite in the human intestinal tract following ingestion of infected insects or drinking water containing infective larvae. ***G. medinensis*** *DRACUNCULUS MEDINENSIS* ***G. robustus*** A species found as a pseudoparasite in human intestines and reported also in periorbital tissues and the urinary tract, probably as a result of ingesting water containing infective larvae.

**Gordon** [Alfred *Gordon,* U.S. neurologist, 1874–1953] **1** Gordon's test, Gordon sign. See under REFLEX. **2** See under SIGN.

**Gorlin** [Richard *Gorlin,* U.S. cardiologist, born 1926] See under FORMULA.

**Gorlin** [Robert James *Gorlin,* U.S. oral pathologist, born 1923] Gorlin syndrome. See under BASAL CELL NEVUS SYNDROME.

**Gosselin** [Leon Athanase *Gosselin,* French surgeon, 1815–1887] See under FRACTURE.

**gossypol** $C_{30}H_{30}O_8$. A sesquiterpene phenol that is a toxic principle found in cottonseed meal and cottonseed cake. It has been used in China as a male antifertility agent.

**GOT** glutamate oxaloacetate transaminase (aspartate aminotransferase).

**Göthlin** [Gustaf *Göthlin,* Swedish physiologist, 1874–1949] See under TEST.

**Gottlieb** [Bernhard *Gottlieb,* Austrian dentist, 1885–1950] Gottlieb's cuticle. See under PRIMARY CUTICLE.

**Gottron** [Heinrich Adolf *Gottron,* German dermatologist, born 1890] **1** See under SIGN. **2** Gottron syndrome. See under PROGRESSIVE SYMMETRICAL VERRUCOUS ERYTHROKERATODERMA.

**Gottstein** [Jacob *Gottstein,* German otologist, 1832–1895] Gottstein's basal process. See under PROCESS.

**gouge** [Middle English *gowge,* from Old French *gouge,* from Vulgar L *gubia* for late L *gulbia* a hollow chisel] A chisel-like surgical instrument with a handle and a blade that is U-shaped in cross section. It is designed to facilitate bone and cartilage removal. **Kelley g.** A surgical instrument with a handle and sharp blade designed to harvest a free graft of cartilage.

**Gougerot** [Henri *Gougerot,* French physician, 1881–1955] **1** See under TRIAD. **2** Gougerot-Carteaud syndrome. See under CONFLUENT AND RETICULATE PAPILLOMATOSIS.

**goundou** \goon′doo\ [French, from a West African language] A nasal osteoblastic periostitis, a sequel to yaws. It is characterized by purulent nasal discharge, headache, and painless symmetric nasal swellings. Orbital invasion and visual impairment may develop at a later stage. The condition occurs in West and Central Africa and in South America. A similar disease is found in the larger apes. Also *anákhré, henpue.*

**gout** \gout\ [French *goutte* (from L *gutta* a drop) a drop, dripping, gout; the disease was attributed to a defluxion or dripping of morbid humors into a joint] Acute or chronic arthritis due to the presence of monosodium urate crystals in polymorphonuclear leukocytes within the joint space or as tophi. Also *uratic arthritis, gouty arthritis, uarthritis, urarthritis.* **latent g.** A condition, usually hyperuricemia, predisposing one to an attack of gout. Also *masked gout.* **lead g.** Gout associated with lead poisoning, specifically lead nephropathy. Also *saturnine gout.* **masked g.** LATENT GOUT. **oxalic g.** Musculoskeletal pain associated with oxalosis. **primary g.** Gout occurring spontaneously and not induced by lead poisoning, myeloproliferative disease, or other states. **rheumatic g.** *Imprecise* POLYMYALGIA RHEUMATICA. **saturnine g.** LEAD GOUT. **secondary g.** Gout associated with hyperuricemia of nongenetic origin, such as a myeloproliferative disorder or diuretic therapy. **tophaceous g.** Chronic gout associated with deposits of monosodium urate (tophi) either subcutaneously or in or near joints.

**gouty** [GOUT + -Y] Pertaining to or having gout.

**government / patient g.** A situation, in a therapeutic community, in which the patients participate in the administration of their ward or unit in the hospital.

**Gowers** [Sir William Richard *Gowers,* English neurologist, 1845–1915] **1** Gowers disease, Gowers syndrome. See under VASOVAGAL ATTACK. **2** Panatrophy of Gowers. See under PANATROPHY. **3** See under SIGN. **4** Fasciculus of Gowers, Gowers tract. See under TRACTUS SPINOCEREBELLARIS VENTRALIS.

**GP** **1** general practitioner. **2** general paresis.

**G6PD** glucose-6-phosphate dehydrogenase.

**GPI** gingival periodontal index.

**gracile** \gras′il\ [French (from L *gracilis* tall, slender), slender] Slender or lightly built.

**gracilothalamic** \gras′əlōthəlam′ik\ Denoting the projection from one gracile nucleus to the opposite nucleus ventralis posterolateralis of the thalamus.

**grad.** *gradatim* (L, by degrees).

**g·rad** Symbol for the unit, gram-rad.

**gradatim** \gradā′təm\ Gradually.

**Gradenigo** [Giuseppe *Gradenigo,* Italian otorhinolaryngologist, 1859–1926] Gradenigo-Lannois syndrome. See under GRADENIGO SYNDROME.

**gradient** \grā′dyənt\ [L *gradiens,* gen. *gradientis,* pres. part. of *gradi* to step] The rate of change of pressure, oxygen tension, or other variable as a function of distance, time, or other continuously changing influence. **g. of approach** The changing strength of the attractiveness of a positive goal as it is approached, growing stronger as it is neared and marked by a measurable increase in effort. **atrioventricular g.** The difference, during diastole, between atrial and ventricular pressures. **g. of avoidance**

The relative decrease in the attractiveness of a negative goal as it is neared; marked by a tendency to draw away from it. **axial g.** The rate of change of a variable with position along an axis. **concentration g.** The changing concentration of solute in solvent before equilibrium is reached, reflecting the effect of mass or solubility on dispersal in a confined system. **mitral g.** The pressure difference across the mitral valve during diastole. **proton g.** A higher concentration of protons on one side of the inner mitochondrial membrane as compared to the other side. The establishment of this gradient by transport stores free energy and the free energy of this gradient then drives the phosphorylation reaction. The proton gradient is essential to the chemiosmotic hypothesis. **systolic g.** The pressure difference across a semilunar valve during systole. **ventricular g.** The net difference in electrical activity between the algebraic sum of the area enclosed within the QRS complex and that within the T wave of the electrocardiogram.

**graduate** [Med L *graduat(us)*, past part. of *graduare* (from L *gradus* a step, degree) to graduate] A container, usually cylindrical and with a pouring lip, that is marked off in units of fluid volume and is used to contain, measure, and pour liquids.

**graduated** Marked with a scale by which measurements can be taken.

**Graefe** [Albrecht Friedrich Wilhelm Ernst von *Graefe*, German ophthalmologist, 1828–1870] **1** See under OPERATION, TEST. **2** Von Graefe sign, Graefe sign. See under EYELID LAG. **3** Graefe's disease. See under PROGRESSIVE OPHTHALMOPLEGIA.

**Graefenberg** [Ernst *Graefenberg*, German gynecologist, active in the U.S., 1881–1957] See under RING.

# graft

**graft** [Middle English *graffe*, from French *greffe* (from L *graphium* an iron pen or stylus) a branch or bud inserted into another plant] **1** Tissue, living or preserved, that is transferred from one location to another on the same organism or from one organism to another. • In strict usage, the term *graft* means a free graft. **2** To transfer such tissue. **3** The operation of transferring such tissue. **activated g.** A graft in which a nerve and blood supply have devel-

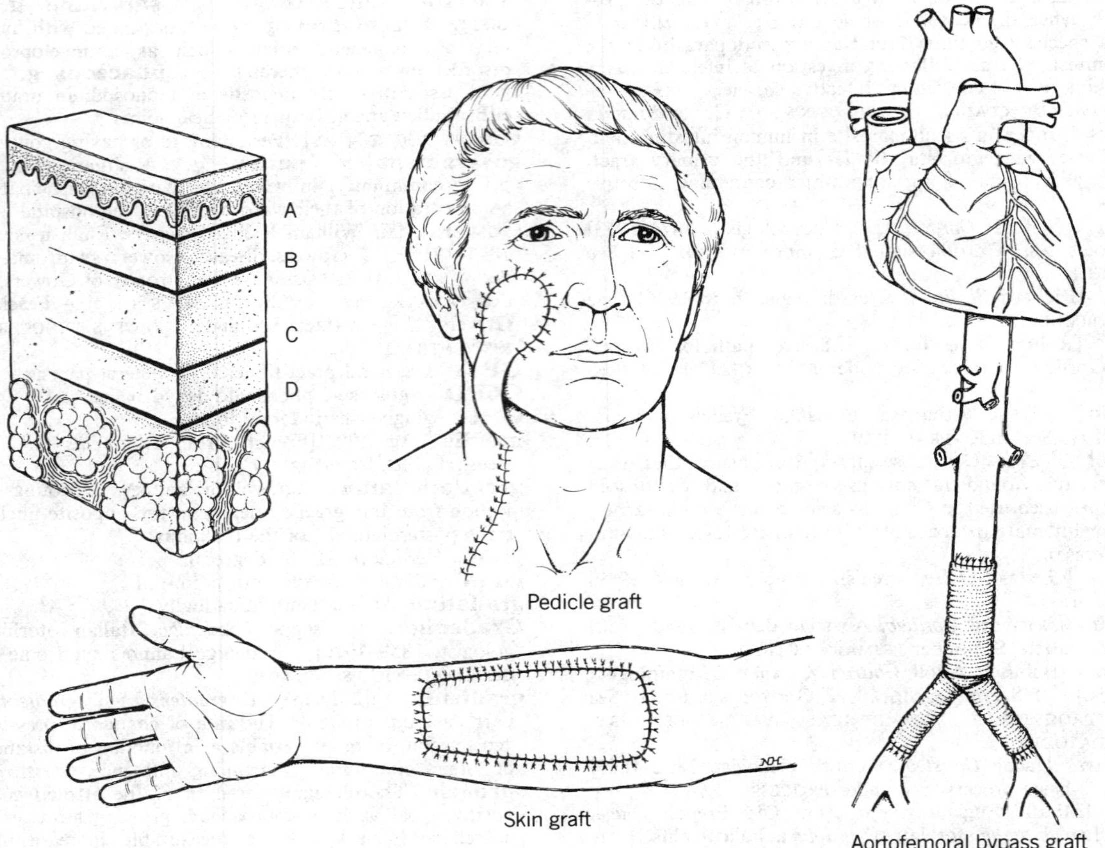


**Grafts** (A, B, C) Split-thickness grafts; (D) full-thickness graft.

oped. **allogeneic g.** ALLOGRAFT. **alloplast g.** A graft of an inert material. **animal g.** A graft from an animal to a human being. Also *zoograft.* **anorganic bone g.** KIEL BONE GRAFT. **aortofemoral bypass g.** A conduit, usually composed of prosthetic material, that joins the aorta to the common femoral arteries in cases of aortoiliac occlusive disease. Such grafts are usually constructed to connect both common femoral arteries and thus have the configuration of an inverted Y. **aortorenal bypass g.** A conduit of autogenous vein or artery or of prosthetic material that links the aorta to the renal artery beyond a point of stenosis or occlusion. It is usually designed to correct inadequate arterial blood flow to a kidney. **autodermic g.** A skin autograft. *Older term.* Also *autoepidermic graft.* **autogenous g.** A graft from another part of the same individual, such as the implantation of bone marrow from the iliac crest to the mandible. **autologous g.** *Older term* AUTOGRAFT. **axillofemoral bypass g.** An extra-anatomic bypass in which the axillary artery is used as the source for blood flow through a graft, usually of prosthetic material, to the common femoral artery. It is often used to bypass the site of aortoiliac occlusive disease in subjects who might not tolerate a direct surgical attack upon the aorta. Also *axillobifemoral bypass graft.* **Blair-Brown g.** SPLIT-SKIN GRAFT. **brephoplastic g.** BREPHOPLASTY. **bridge g.** INTERPOSITION GRAFT. **cable g.** A graft in which several small-caliber nerves are used to form a cable to bridge a gap in nerve anastomosis. **cantilever g.** A graft of bone, cartilage, or alloplastic material which is secured to the nasal bones or the frontal bone, and extends downward to support the tip of the nose. **chondrocutaneous g.** A graft consisting of contiguous skin and cartilage, usually obtained from the ear. **composite g.** Any graft, contiguous in nature, consisting of tissues of more than one type. **crossover bypass g.** An extra-anatomic vascular reconstruction, usually between the femoral vessels in both groins, performed to bypass unilateral iliac vessel occlusion. **cutis g.** DERMAL GRAFT. **Davis g.** PINCH GRAFT. **delayed g.** **1** A skin graft which is elevated and then sutured back onto its donor area, where it remains for a time before being transferred. **2** A split-skin graft which is applied to a surgically created raw surface one or more days after the excision which resulted in this recipient area. **derma-fat-fascia g.** A free graft consisting of dermis and the attached subjacent subcutaneous fat and fascia. Such a graft is sometimes inserted subcutaneously in a depressed area to fill out the contour. **dermal g.** A free graft consisting of part or all of the thickness of the dermis without any attached epidermis or subcutaneous fat. Also *cutis graft, dermic graft, dermis graft.* **dermis-fat g.** A graft consisting of dermis and contiguous fat. Also *dermis-fat composite graft.* **diced cartilage g.'s** Cartilage grafts, usually from the human rib, cut into many small pieces. Such grafts were once used by molding the pieces into the shape desired. **epidermic g.** A very thin split-skin graft consisting of the epidermis but less than the usual amount of dermis. An old-fashioned misnomer. **Esser g.** INLAY GRAFT. **extracranial-intracranial bypass g.** The anastomosis of a branch of the external carotid artery, such as the superficial temporal artery, with an intracranial artery, such as the middle cerebral artery or one of its branches, in order to revascularize the intracranial artery. It is usually performed to relieve atherosclerotic stenoses or occlusions of the intracranial carotid artery. Such a procedure may also be performed using autogenous vein bypass grafts from the common or external carotid artery. **fascia g.** A free graft of fascia. Such a graft is sometimes used in ribbon form as a strong suture, sometimes as a pad of several thicknesses in a subcutaneous pocket to fill out defects of contour, and sometimes for other purposes. **fascia-fat g.** A graft consisting of fascia and contiguous fat. **fascicular g.** A nerve graft in which each fascicle is sutured to a corresponding fascicle in the recipient nerve. **femoral-femoral g.** The connection of both common femoral arteries by a graft of autogenous or prosthetic material, usually in order to bypass a unilateral iliac artery stenosis or occlusion. **femoral-tibial bypass g.** A conduit, either autogenous vein or prosthetic material, that joins the common femoral artery at the groin and one of the tibial arteries below the popliteal trifurcation. **free g.** A graft completely detached from the donor area and transferred to the recipient area without the use of vascular anastomoses. **free gingival g.** A graft of masticatory mucosa which is completely detached from its donor site and used to extend the area of attached gingiva. **full-thickness g.** A skin graft containing all the elements of the skin (epidermis and dermis) but none of the subcutaneous tissue. Such a graft will produce better cosmetic and functional results than a split-thickness graft, but its survival rate is more tenuous and the donor site must be grafted or surgically closed. Also *Krause-Wolfe graft, Wolfe-Krause graft, Wolfe's graft.* **heterodermic g.** A xenograft of skin. *Older term.* **heterogenous g.** XENOGRAFT. **heterologous g.** *Older term* XENOGRAFT. **heteroplastic g.** *Older term* XENOGRAFT. **heterotopic g.** A graft of an organ or tissue to a site where it is not normally found. Also *heterotopic transplantation.* **homogenous g.** ALLOGRAFT. **homologous g.** *Older term* ALLOGRAFT. **homoplastic g.** *Older term* ALLOGRAFT. **ileal g.** A graft consisting of a portion of the ileum. **iliac g.** A bone graft utilizing the ilium, especially the crest of the ilium, as the donor site. **inlay g.** A split-skin graft which is wrapped, raw side out, around a mold, usually of stent dressing, and buried just under the skin or mucosa. After the graft has taken, the overlying cover is cut through down to the mold, which is removed. The graft may remain as a pocket or trench, or it may gradually flatten to produce more laxity in the area. Also *Esser graft, skin graft inlay, epithelial inlay.* **interposition g.** Tissue or prosthetic material used to bridge a gap, as to replace a missing segment of artery or reconstitute a missing segment of nerve. Also *bridge graft.* **isogeneic g.** ISOGRAFT. **isologous g.** ISOGRAFT. **isoplastic g.** ISOGRAFT. **Kiel bone g.** A preserved, dry, deproteinized bone graft from a young calf, intended for use in human patients. It was once thought that these grafts were nonantigenic and would stimulate the growth of new bone, but the results were often disappointing and they are seldom used today. Also *anorganic bone graft, Kiel graft.* **Krause-Wolfe g.** FULL-THICKNESS GRAFT. **mesh g.** A split-skin graft containing multiple small slits, usually cut by machine. When tension is applied, these slits open out into spaces and the area of the graft increases. **mesocaval H g.** A mesocaval shunt constructed to relieve portal hypertension. It is most often composed of a short segment of prosthetic material and connects the superior mesenteric vein and the inferior vena cava. Also *Drapanas shunt.* **microvascular free g.** FREE FLAP. **nerve g.** The interposition of a human or animal nerve segment to bridge a gap between the ends of a divided nerve. **Ollier-Thiersch g.** A thin split-skin graft cut with an old-fashioned straight razor or similar blade. Also *thin-split graft, Thiersch graft, Ollier graft, razor graft, Thiersch operation.* **onlay g.** Any graft, of any tissue, that is applied by laying it on a flat or convex surface. Also *onlay, outlay.* **orthotopic g.** A graft of an organ or tissue to a site where the tissue is normally found. Also *orthotopic transplantation, homotopic transplantation.* **panel g.** The construction of a large-caliber venous conduit by longitudinally incising a vein, then laterally suturing segments of the opened vein to form a panel. **parathyroid g.** A procedure sometimes done experimentally after removal of more than one parathyroid for hyperparathyroidism in which a small piece of the patient's own parathyroid is implanted subcutaneously in order to provide for continued secretion of parathyroid hormone. **patch g.** A graft of autologous tissue or inert prosthetic material used to enlarge the lumen of tubular structures. It is used primarily in surgery on blood vessels, ureters, or bile ducts. **pedicle g.** A full-thickness graft, or a graft including subcutaneous tissues or even deeper tissues, in which the blood supply is retained, either by leaving the tissue permanently or temporarily attached to its site of origin, or by anastomosing blood vessels within the tissue to blood vessels at the recipient site. Also *flap.* **pedicled bone g.** An autograft consisting of bone, usually covered with surrounding soft tissue and transferred on a pedicle of soft tissue containing the nutrient vessels to the bone so that the bone graft remains continuously alive. **periosteal g.** A graft of periosteum, the purpose of which is to produce bone in the recipient area. **pinch g.** A skin graft obtained by pinching up a small bit of skin with a thumb forceps and cutting it off with a knife or scissors. When many of these are placed on a wound, the epithelial cells from the edges coalesce to heal over the recipient bed. **preserved bone g.** A bone graft preserved by physical or chemical means or both for a considerable period of time between removal and use. Usually these are bone homografts removed from a human patient shortly after death and preserved in a bone bank in a hospital or other institution. **prosthetic vascular g.** Any of a variety of artificial blood vessel substitutes. The earliest grafts were composed of metal, but these have been superseded by Dacron, polytetrafluoroethylene, and, most recently, silicone rubber, polycarbons, and other new materials. **razor g.** OLLIER-THIERSCH GRAFT. **Reverdin g.** A full-thickness graft produced by elevating a cone of skin on the point of a straight needle and cutting off the top portion of this cone. A number of these grafts are placed at intervals of about one centimeter on a raw recipient site. The separate pieces will fuse and form one whole graft. Also *Reverdin's method, seed graft, Reverdin's operation.* **seed g.** REVERDIN GRAFT. **sequential g.** A conduit that uses a bypass graft already in place as a blood flow source to other more distal arteries. It is commonly used in coronary artery bypass grafting and occasionally in tibial vessel reconstruction. Also *snake graft.* **sheet g.** A skin transplant removed from the donor site with a dermatome and placed on the recipient site as a single piece without alteration. **skin g.** A piece of skin, partial-thickness or full-thickness, completely removed from one part of the body and transferred to a raw area on another part of the same body (autograft), or transferred from one individual to another of the same species (allograft), or transferred from one individual to another of a different species (xenograft). The transfer is done without surgical vascular anastomoses. **snake g.** SEQUENTIAL GRAFT. **splenorenal bypass g.** An anastomosis of the splenic artery, which is disconnected from the spleen and dissected from its bed, to the renal artery beyond a point of stenosis or occlusion. **split-rib g.** A bone graft utilizing a rib or ribs that have been split along their long axes. Such a graft is useful in reconstructing the skull or facial bones. **split-skin g.** A free graft of skin consisting of the entire thickness of the epidermis and part of the thickness of the dermis. The donor site regenerates skin from the remnant of dermis left on it. Such a graft can be cut in large sheets to repair large raw areas. Also *Blair-Brown graft.* **split-thickness g.** A graft of oral mucosa or skin utilizing only a portion of the thickness available at the donor site. Compare FULL-THICKNESS GRAFT. **stent g.** A skin graft held in place with a tie-over dressing. • Formerly, the term was used only when the material in the dressing was dental wax (stent dressing), but now it is used regardless of the material. **syngeneic g.** ISOGRAFT. **Thiersch g.** OLLIER-THIERSCH GRAFT. **thin-split g.** OLLIER-THIERSCH GRAFT. **vascular g.** A segment of artery, vein, or prosthetic conduit that is used to bypass or replace a diseased vessel. **vein g.** A graft utilizing an intact segment of vein as a means of bypassing a blocked arterial segment or of replacing an arterial segment that is missing. **Wolfe's g.** FULL-THICKNESS GRAFT. **Wolfe-Krause g.** FULL-THICKNESS GRAFT. **xenogeneic g.** XENOGRAFT.

**grafting** / **interfascicular nerve g.** The technique of placing individual grafts between each of the fascicles of a severed nerve to bridge the gap. Also *fascicular nerve grafting.* **mesh g.** A method of expanding a skin transplant by running it through a special device that cuts multiple slits in the sheet of skin. Depending on the length of the slits, the graft can be expanded in ratios of up to twelve to one to cover larger areas than the original sheet.

**Graham** [Evarts Ambrose *Graham,* U.S. surgeon, 1883–1957] Graham's test. See under CHOLECYSTOGRAPHY.

**Graham** [Thomas *Graham,* Scottish chemist, 1805–1869] See under LAW.

**grain** [Old French *grein* a seed, a grain, from L *granum* a seed; and Old French *grainne* seed or grain in general, from L *grana,* pl. of L *granum*] A unit of mass or weight equal to 1/7000 pound; 64.798 $91 \times 10^{-6}$ kilogram, 64.798 91 milligrams. The grain is the same in avoirdupois, apothecaries', and troy weight. Symbol: gr

**grains** Dyskeratotic, parakeratotic cells present in the epidermis in cases of keratosis follicularis.

**Gram** [Hans Christian Joachim *Gram,* Danish physician, 1853–1938] Gram's method. See under GRAM STAIN.

**gram** [French *gramme,* from Gk *gramma* that which is drawn or written, a small weight] A unit of mass or weight equal to 0.001 kilogram; 15.43 grains, or 0.035 27 ounce. Symbol: g

**-gram** \-gram\ [Gk *gramma* that which is drawn or written, a letter, a small weight] A combining form meaning a record, something written.

**Gram-amphophilic** \-am′fəfil′ik\ Staining positively in part and negatively in part with the Gram stain.

**gram-atom** The quantity of an element having a mass in grams numerically equal to the atomic weight. One gram-atom contains the Avogadro number of atoms. Also *gram-atomic weight, g atom.*

**gram-calorie** 15°C CALORIE. Symbol: g-cal.

**gramicidin** A cyclic decapeptide antibiotic formed by *Bacillus brevis.* Its molecule consists of the sequence D-Phe-L-Pro-L-Val-L-Orn-L-Leu occurring twice. Peptide bond formation in its biosynthesis is accomplished by transfer of aminoacyl groups from their thioesters formed with thiol groups in the enzyme complex that makes it. It enters biologic membranes and renders them permeable to cations including $Na^+$ and $K^+$.

**Gram-negative** [after Hans Christian Joachim *Gram,*

Danish physician, 1853–1938] Decolorized by alcohol or acetone when stained with the Gram stain. Gram-negative bacteria have an inner (cytoplasmic) membrane, a very thin murein wall, often only a single peptidoglycan layer, and a surrounding, adherent outer membrane. • The lower-case form *gram-negative* is often preferred in the United States.

**Gram-positive** [after Hans Christian Joachim *Gram*, Danish physician, 1853–1938] Not decolorized by alcohol or acetone when stained with the Gram stain. Gram-positive bacteria have a multilayered murein wall and no outer membrane. • The lower-case form *gram-positive* is often preferred in the United States.

**gram-rad** \gram′-rad\ A unit of absorbed dose of ionizing radiation, equal to 100 ergs; $10^{-5}$ joule. Symbol: g·rad

**gram-roentgen** \gram′-rent′gen\ In radiology, formerly the unit of integral dose, defined as the real energy conversion when one roentgen is delivered to one gram of air (83.7 ergs). This unit has been superseded by the gram-rad (100 ergs) and the kilogram-gray (1 joule).

**grand mal** \gräN mäl′\ [French *grand* great + *mal* sickness] MAJOR EPILEPSY. • This term was once used to identify any convulsive epileptic attack with major manifestations, as opposed to petit mal.

**Granger** [Amedee *Granger*, U.S. radiologist, 1879–1939] See under LINE.

**granular** \gran′yələr\ Having a texture like grains of sand or salt. Also *granulose, granuliform.*

**granulate** \gran′yəlāt\ **1** To undergo granulation; to form granulation tissue. **2** Composed of or covered with granules; granular.

**granulatio** \gran′yəlā′shō\ [Late L *granul(um)* (dim. of *granum* a grain ) a little grain + *-atio* -ATION] A granular, collagenous body. **granulationes arachnoideales** [NA] The numerous bulbous protrusions of the arachnoid extending chiefly into the sagittal sinus and venous lacunae, and constituting the main site of cerebrospinal fluid reabsorption into venous blood. Similar, less numerous arachnoid granulations are found in the transverse sinus and elsewhere. Those to either side of the sagittal sinus become calcified with increasing age, are visible with the naked eye, and often indent the calvaria. Also *pacchionian bodies, pacchionian glands, pacchionian granulations, arachnoidal granulations, granulationes arachnoideales Pacchioni, granulationes cerebrales, granulationes pacchioni, meningeal granules, arachnoid villi.*

**granulation** \gran′yəlā′shən\ [L *granulatio.* See GRANULATIO.] The formation of a tissue composed of capillaries, fibroblasts, and inflammatory cells. It is characteristic of wounds healing by second intention. **arachnoidal g.'s** GRANULATIONES ARACHNOIDEALES. **exuberant g.'s** The overproduction of granulation tissue associated with a healing wound. **hypertrophic g.** The process by which granulation tissue in a chronic wound, if unimpeded by wound closure, may become exuberant and rise above the edges of the wound. **pacchionian g.'s** GRANULATIONES ARACHNOIDEALES. **pyroninophlic g.'s** Cytoplasmic granules, which are composed of RNA, that have a particular affinity for the histologic stain pyronin. **Reilly g.'s** Alder-Reilly bodies. See under ALDER-REILLY ANOMALY. **Virchow's g.'s** Focal areas of glial proliferation in the ependymal and subependymal area around the lateral cerebral ventricles found in patients with general paresis.

**granulationes** \gran′yəlāshō′nēz\ Plural of GRANULATIO.

**granule** \gran′yəl\ [Late L *granulum* (dim. of *granum* a grain, akin to English *corn*) a little grain] **1** A small mass or particle, as a beadlike mass of tissue. **2** Any small sugar-coated or gelatin-coated pill containing a minute dose of a drug. **acrosomal g.** A large granule formed by fusion of proacrosomal granules during spermiogenesis and enclosed within a large acrosomal vesicle. It spreads out over the nuclear membrane, flattens, and forms a cap over the nucleus in man, bull, and ram, but the form is more complicated in rodents and other mammals. **alpha g.'s** **1** Platelet granules that contain mostly platelet-derived growth factor, and also platelet factor 4, fibrinogen, β thromboglobulin, and thrombin-sensitive protein. **2** Granules of the alpha cells of the islets of the pancreas, presumed to be the source of glucagon. **3** Granules of the pituitary gland. **Altmann's g.** MITOCHONDRION. **amphophil g.'s** Granules in the cytoplasm of cells that take up both acidophilic and basophilic dyes. **azurophil g.** A granule, approximately 0.1 μm in diameter, that is commonly found in the cytoplasm of normal lymphocytes, especially natural killer lymphocytes, and that stains red or violet with azure dyes. Also *kappa granule.* **Babès-Ernst g.'s** BABÈS-ERNST BODIES. **basal g.** BASAL BODY. **basophil g.'s** Cytoplasmic granules that stain with basic dyes. **Bensley specific g.'s** Granules in the cytoplasm of any of the cells of the pancreatic islets of Langerhans. **beta g.'s** Secretory or presecretory granules in the cytoplasm of the beta cells of the pancreatic islets, which contain insulin and C-peptide, and in the various beta cells or basophilic cells of the anterior pituitary, containing adrenocorticotropin, β-lipotropin, endorphins, and in other cells, the gonadotropins. **Bollinger's g.'s** Small yellowish granular masses seen in the cutaneous lesions of botryomycosis, composed of heterogeneous aggregates of Gram-positive cocci, generally staphylococci. **Bütschli g.'s** Enlargements or swellings located along the fibers of the mitotic spindle in an ovum. **chromophobe g.'s** Cytoplasmic granules that fail to stain with either acid or basic dyes, usually as a consequence of a relationship to secretory inactivity in the cells of the anterior lobe of the hypophysis. **cone g.** The nucleus of a cone cell in the external nuclear lamina of the retina. **cortical g.'s** Subcortically located round or elliptical membrane-bound bodies, usually 0.5 μm–0.8 μm in diameter, found in animal oocytes. These are particularly visible just before fertilization. Following sperm fusion with the egg's vitelline membrane their contents (largely mucopolysaccharides) are released into the perivitelline space (cortical reaction). This consequently modifies the properties both of the vitellus and zona pellucida (zona reaction) so that additional sperm penetration is inhibited. The cortical granules are probably derived from the coalescence of tiny vesicles produced by the Golgi apparatus. **cytoplasmic g.** A granule in the cytoplasm of a cell. **delta g.'s** Cytoplasmic granules in delta cells of the pancreatic islets. **dense core g.** NEUROSECRETORY GRANULE. **eosinophil g.'s** Cytoplasmic granules with a particular affinity for acidic dyes; especially, granules that are present in the cytoplasm of a class of polymorphonuclear leukocytes. These granules are relatively large, approximately 0.5 to 1.0 micron, round, numerous, and stain red to red-orange with Romanowsky dyes. They release a protein (eosinophil basic protein) that is toxic on contact to bacteria or living cells. **Fordyce g.'s** FORDYCE SPOTS. **fuchsinophil g.'s** Cytoplasmic granules that stain preferentially with acid or basic fuchsin. **glycogen g.'s** Small particles of glycogen that can be identified within the cytoplasm of cells by electron microscopy. The granules vary between 15 nm and 45 nm in diameter. **Heinz g.'s** HEINZ BODIES. **interstitial g.** A fine eosinophilic particle within cell cytoplasm. It corresponds to a mitochondrion in electron microscopy. **Isaac's g.'s** RETICULAR SUBSTANCE. **juxtaglomerular g.'s** Granules in cells of the juxtaglomerular apparatus which represent secretion or storage of renin. **kappa g.** AZUROPHIL GRANULE. **keratohyaline g.** Cytoplasmic material that is identifiable by light microscopy within the cells of the granular layer of the epidermis. It is considered to be the precursor of keratin. **Langerhans cell g.** A tennis racket-shaped cytoplasmic inclusion within a Langerhans cell of the epidermis, which is considered to be specific to this cell type. **lipofuscin g.** A form of hyaline droplet containing lipofuscin and reflecting cellular damage. Lipofuscin granules are yellow-brown in unstained section and appear on electron microscopy as vacuoles filled with granular and membranous material. An estimate of the age of an animal can often be made based on the number of lipofuscin granules. **mast-cell g.** A metachromatic particle within the cytoplasm of a mast cell. Heparin sulfate, histamine, and serotonin have been identified within such granules. **melanin g.** MELANOSOME. **meningeal g.'s** GRANULATIONES ARACHNOIDEALES. **mucinogen g.'s** Cytoplasmic granules that are visible in mucous secretory cells. **mucous g.** A cytoplasmic vesicle that contains mucin. **neurosecretory g.** A small intracytoplasmic vesicle that contains an electron-dense aggregate of neurosecretory material such as oxytocin, vasopressin, or norepinephrine. Also *dense core granule, neurosecretory sphere.* **neutrophil g.'s** Minute granules, generally less than 0.1 μm in diameter, that are numerous in the cytoplasm of a class of polymorphonuclear leukocytes, and that stain a pale rose color with Romanowsky dyes. The granules are lysosomes that contain peroxidases and esterases. **Nissl g.'s** NISSL SUBSTANCE. **Palade g.** RIBOSOME. **Paschen's g.'s** GUARNIERI BODIES. **pigment g.'s** Colored or pigmented granules in a cell, generally cytoplasmic granules. **polar g.'s** VOLUTIN GRANULES. **proacrosomal g.'s** The granular precursors of the acrosome situated inside the acroblast during spermiogenesis. Several of the cisternae in the Golgi complex accumulate these protein granules which fuse to form a single acrosomal granule containing much carbohydrate. **prosecretion g.'s** Cytoplasmic granules containing materials that will be secreted from the cell. **rod g.** The nucleus of a rod cell in the external nuclear lamina of the retina. **Schüffner's g.'s** Numerous minute reddish granules that stipple erythrocytes infected with *Plasmodium vivax* or *P. ovale,* when stained with a Romanowsky dye. Such granules do not appear in erythrocytes infected with *P. malariae* or *P. falciparum.* Also *Schüffner's dots, Schüffner stippling, malarial stippling.* **secondary g.** SPECIFIC GRANULE. **secretory g.** SECRETORY VACUOLE. **seminal g.'s** Very small granular masses formed in seminal fluid. **specific g.** The smaller type of lysosome that is found in the cytoplasm of mature neutrophil polymorphs and that contains alkaline phosphatase, collagenase, and aminopeptidase. Also *secondary granule.* **sulfur g.'s** Characteristic yellow granular bodies found in the exudate of actinomycotic lesions. **tannophil g.'s** Cytoplasmic granules that are readily identified after mordanting with tannic acid. **toxic g.'s** Small, basophilic, intracytoplasmic granules found in leukocytes, at one time believed to be related to infections. They probably represent aberrantly developed lysosomes. **volutin g.'s** Metachromatic particles consisting of free nucleic acids stored in granular form in the cytoplasm of certain microorganisms such as coccidia and trypanosomes, protozoa that undergo rapid nuclear division and require substantial quantities of nucleic acids. Also *polar granules.* **yolk g.'s** Nutritive, nonliving material made of fatty and albuminous substance synthesized by the cytoplasm of most animal ova in the form of only a few or of many granules. The amount present enables the classification of egg types. **zymogen g.'s** Granules in the cytoplasm of enzyme-secreting cells such as those of the salivary glands or pancreas. The granules contain the zymogenic material.

**granuliform** \gran′yəlifôrm′\ GRANULAR.

**granulo-** \-gran′yəlō-\ [Late L *granulum.* See GRANULE.] A combining form meaning granule, granular, or granulation.

**granuloblast** \gran′yələblast′\ A precursor granular cell giving rise to any adult blood cell containing granules, such as the various types of leukocyte.

**granulocytapheresis** \-sī′təferē′sis\ Leukapheresis for the collection specifically of granulocytes.

**granulocyte** \gran′yəlōsīt′\ [GRANULO- + -CYTE] A leukocyte that characteristically contains many granules in its cytoplasm. Included among granulocytes are neutrophils, eosinophils, basophils, and the precursors of these cells. Also *granular leukocyte.* **heterophil g.** NEUTROPHIL. **neutrophil g.** NEUTROPHIL. **polymorphonuclear g.** SEGMENTED NEUTROPHIL.

**granulocytopenia** \-sī′təpē′nē·ə\ An abnormally decreased number of granulocytes in the blood. Also *granulopenia, hypogranulocytosis.*

**granulocytopoiesis** \-sī′təpoi·ē′sis\ GRANULOPOIESIS.

**granulocytopoietic** \-sī′təpoi·et′ik\ GRANULOPOIETIC.

**granulocytosis** \-sītō′sis\ Increased numbers of granulocytes in blood or tissue.

**granuloma** \gran′yəlō′mə\ [*granul(e)* + -OMA] (*pl.* granulomas, granulomata) **1** A chronic inflammatory lesion characterized by an accumulation of macrophages which have undergone epithelioid transformation, with or without lymphocytes and multinuclear giant cells, into a discrete granule. **2** A chronic inflammatory lesion which forms microscopic or macroscopic nodules in response to multiple infectious, immunologic, neoplastic, or foreign body challenges. For defs. 1 and 2 also *granulation tumor.* **adjuvant g.** An inflammatory lesion that forms at the site of injection of adjuvants, particularly complete Freund's adjuvant. **alum g.** A small inflammatory lesion that occurs at the injection site of aluminum adjuvant. **amebic g.** A rare form of colonic amebiasis characterized by a tumorlike induration of the wall due to exuberant granulation tissue. **g. annulare** A benign skin disorder of unknown origin characterized clinically by small dermal nodules that sometimes appear in annular configuration, and histologically by a histiocytic and granulomatous response to focal necrobiosis of collagen. **apical g.** PERIAPICAL GRANULOMA. **aquarium g.** FISH TANK GRANULOMA. **benign g. of thyroid** A chronic inflammatory disease of the thyroid, which enlarges and eventually becomes very firm. **beryllium g.** The characteristic lesion of berylliosis, consisting of a usually non-caseating granuloma with multinucleated giant cells. It is most frequently seen in the lung, but the skin, liver, and spleen may also be involved. ***Candida* g.** **1** One of the granulomatous, crusted nodules of the scalp, face, mucous membranes, and fingers occurring in chronic, generalized candidiasis in association with impaired immune response. Also *candidal granuloma, Monilia granuloma.* **2** Any granuloma seen in tissues infected by *Candida* oranisms. **central giant cell reparative g.** A giant cell reparative granuloma occurring in one of the bones of the jaw. **cholesterol g.** A chronic granulomatous inflammatory disease involving both the tympanic and mastoid segments of the middle-ear cleft and regarded as a late stage in the progress of chronic exudative otitis media. The granulations are typified by cholesterol crystals and foreign-body giant cells. A brownish glairy exudate filling the tympanic cavity and mastoid air cells gives a characteristic bluish appearance when viewed through the tympanic membrane. **chronic g.** PERIAPICAL GRANULOMA. **coccidioidal g.** COCCIDIOIDOMA. **g. contagiosum** GRANULOMA INGUINALE. **dental g.** PERIAPICAL GRANULOMA. **eosinophilic g.** 1 A circumscribed, cystic lesion of bone most often seen in children and adolescents, consisting of histiocytes and eosinophils. See also HISTIOCYTOSIS. 2 The eosinophilic intestinal wall mass resulting from infection with the roundworm *Anisakis marina.* **eosinophilic g. of the skin** The least severe form of histiocytosis, characterized by papular lesions and ulcerated plaques. Histologically the granulomatous lesions contain many eosinophils as well as histiocytes. **favic g.** A chronic granulomatous ringworm infection due to *Trichophyton schoenleinii.* **fish tank g.** A chronic, ulcerative skin lesion, usually on the forearm, caused by *Mycobacterium marinum* infection. It is the same as swimming pool granuloma, but is generally seen in persons who keep fish as a hobby and generally acquired in the process of cleaning a fish tank or aquarium. Also *aquarium granuloma.* **g. fissuratum** A chronic inflammatory response of the skin to repeated localized trauma, as is seen in the transversely ridged soft red nodule that forms on the skin because of the pressure of the earpiece of spectacles. Also *fissured angioma.* **foreign body g.** A granuloma caused by the aspiration, injection, or inoculation of foreign matter. The granuloma is usually noncaseating, and the foreign body is often visible within it. **g. fungoides** MYCOSIS FUNGOIDES. **giant cell reparative g.** A benign tumorlike lesion arising as an abnormal reaction to injury and containing numerous multinuclear giant cells. It occurs in the gingiva or in the bones of the jaw. **g. gluteale infantum** Dull red granulomatous nodules in the diaper area of infants. Topical corticosteroids favor this development in which *Candida albicans* is believed to play a part. **g. inguinale** A chronic, ulcerogranulomatous venereal disease of the skin and mucous membranes caused by the Gram-negative bacillus *Calymmatobacterium granulomatis* (formerly *Donovania granulomatis* or Donovan's bodies). It is characterized by ulcerating skin lesions on the genitalia which contain macrophages packed with Donovan bodies. Rectovaginal fistula is a common complication. The disease is most commonly seen in tropical and subtropical areas and is especially common in Papua New Guinea. Also *donovanosis, granuloma contagiosum, granuloma pudendi, venereal granuloma.* **intubation g.** Laryngeal granuloma occurring at the site of minor injury caused by laryngeal intubation, usually during general anesthesia. The principal site is somewhere on the vocal cords, usually over the vocal processes of the arytenoid cartilages. **iodide g.** A follicular skin rash, one of many types of cutaneous reaction caused by the intake of iodides in sensitized individuals. **lethal midline g.** A rare, progressive disease of unknown etiology, characterized by local erosive destruction of the paranasal sinuses, palate, and nose, with later extention to the orbits and other facial structures. The process involves nonspecific acute or chronic inflammation resulting in necrosis of soft tissue, bone, and cartilage with or without the formation of granulomas. Also *midline granuloma, malignant granuloma of the face.* **lipoid g.** A granuloma characterized by lipid-containing foamy histiocytes. It may be caused by excessive amounts of endogenous or exogenous lipid. **lipophagic g.** A granuloma occurring when subcutaneous fat undergoes necrosis, usually as a result of traumatic injury. This lesion is characterized by a central focus of necrotic, oily debris surrounded by lipid-laden macrophages, proliferating fibroblasts, and granulation tissue. **Majocchi's g.** An uncommon chronic infection of the hair follicles of the lower leg caused by a ringworm species, typically *Trichophyton rubrum.* It usually arises by extension of primary tinea pedis. Also *hypertrophic ringworm, trichophytic granuloma, tinea profunda.* **malignant g. of the face** LETHAL MIDLINE GRANULOMA. **midline g.** LETHAL MIDLINE GRANULOMA. ***Monilia* g.** *CANDIDA* GRANULOMA. **paracoccidioidal g.** SOUTH AMERICAN BLASTOMYCOSIS. **periapical g.** Granuloma occurring adjacent to the apex of a nonvital tooth. Also *apical granuloma, chronic granuloma, dental granuloma.* **peripheral giant cell reparative g.** A giant cell reparative granuloma occurring on the gingiva. Also *giant cell epulis.* **plasma cell g.** A granulomatous inflammatory response in which plasma cells predominate. At times it is not a true granuloma, but rather a nonspecific chronic inflammatory infiltrate largely composed of mature plasma cells. **g. of the prostate** A chronic inflammatory process of the prostate probably caused by partial obstruction of the larger ducts followed by chronic inflammation and the formation of granulomatous nodules. **g. pudendi** GRANULOMA INGUINALE. **pyogenic g.** An exophytic red nodule occurring primarily in the skin and oral mucosa and composed of proliferated capillaries in an edematous stroma containing inflammatory cells. Undoubtedly benign, this lesion is believed by some to be an exaggerated response to minor trauma, i.e., exuberant granulation tissue. Others classify it as a polypoid form of capillary hemangioma. Also *septic granuloma, granulation tumor.* **reticulohistiocytic g.** *Older term* DERMATOFIBROMA. **rheumatic g.'s** Granulomas and/or subcutaneous nodules appearing in various parts of the body in certain types of inflammatory rheumatic disease, such as rheumatoid arthritis and rheumatic fever. **septic g.** PYOGENIC GRANULOMA. **swimming pool g.** A chronic skin infection caused by *Mycobacterium marinum* and acquired in nonchlorinated swimming pools or lakes. **g. telangiectaticum** A granuloma composed of dilated small blood vessels. **trichophytic g.** MAJOCCHI'S GRANULOMA. **umbilical g.** Granulation tissue that forms on the umbilical cord stump of newborn infants. **g. of the umbilicus** A small mass of granulation tissue formed at the site of separation of the umbilical cord, which the dermal epithelium cannot cover and which gives rise to a discharge of thin pus from the navel. It is curable by judicious application of silver nitrate. Also *umbilical fungus.* **venereal g.** GRANULOMA INGUINALE. **Wegener's g.** See under WEGENER'S GRANULOMATOSIS.

**granulomatosis** \-mətō′sis\ [GRANULOMA + *t* + -OSIS ] A condition or disease characterized by multiple granulomas. **beryllium g.** A granulomatous condition of the lung resembling sarcoidosis and resulting from exposure to beryllium. **chronic familial g.** CHRONIC GRANULOMATOUS DISEASE. **chronic X-linked g.** CHRONIC GRANULOMATOUS DISEASE. **lipid g.** HAND-SCHÜLLER-CHRISTIAN DISEASE. **lipophagic intestinal g.** WHIPPLE'S DISEASE. **lymphomatoid g.** A rare disease characterized by vasculitis and lymphoid infiltrates in nodules within the lung, subcutaneous tissue, and brain. **necrotizing respiratory g.** Wegener's granulomatosis in the respiratory tract. **reticuloendothelial g.** HISTIOCYTOSIS. **Wegener's g.** An illness of unknown cause characterized by necrotizing sinusitis, other oral and ocular infiltrative granulomas, necrotizing pneumonia with nodules, systemic vasculitis, and glomerulonephritis. The disease occurs in two forms, limited Wegener's granulomatosis, which does not involve the kidneys, and generalized Wegener's granulomatosis, in which the kidneys are involved. Also *Wegener syndrome.*

**granulomatous** \gran′yəläm′ətəs\ [GRANULOMA + *t* + -OUS] Describing or pertaining to a form of subacute inflammation in which there is exuberant proliferation of inflammatory cells and reactive fibrous or glial tissue.

**granulomere** \gran′yələmir′\ The central portion of a blood platelet as seen on a stained blood smear, characterized by purplish granules. Compare HYALOMERE.

**granulopenia** \-pē′nē·ə\ GRANULOCYTOPENIA.

**granulopexy** \gran′yələpek′sē\ Fixation of granules.

**granuloplasm** \gran′yələplazm′\ **1** The portion of the cytoplasm which contains granules. **2** The more centrally located cytoplasm of amebas and certain other unicellular organisms.

**granuloplastic** \-plas′tik\ Having the capacity to form granules.

**granulopoiesis** \-poi·ē′sis\ The normal maturation and release of granulocytes by the bone marrow. Also *granulocytopoiesis.*

**granulopoietic** \-poi·et′ik\ Pertaining to or stimulating granulopoiesis. Also *granulocytopoietic.*

**granulose** \gran′yəlōs\ GRANULAR.

**granulovacuolar** \-vak′yoo·ō′lər\ Characterized by the presence of both granules and vacuoles in the cytoplasm, as seen in neurons in Alzheimer's disease.

**graph-** \graf-\ GRAPHO-.

**-graph** \-graf\ [Gk *graphein* to write, draw, record] A combining form meaning (1) an instrument that writes or records; (2) a record, something written.

**grapho-** \graf′ō-\ [Gk *graphein* to write, draw, record] A combining form meaning writing, a record. Also *graph-.*

**graphology** \grafäl′əjē\ [GRAPHO- + -LOGY] The analysis of handwriting for the purpose of assessing or predicting personality type and character traits. Also *graphopathology.* **forensic g.** The comparative analysis of handwriting samples and handwritten documents in order to determine the authenticity of questioned documents.

**graphomotor** \-mō′tər\ [GRAPHO- + MOTOR] Describing, pertaining to, or affecting the movements used in writing.

**graphopathology** \-pathäl′əjē\ GRAPHOLOGY.

**graphospasm** \graf′əspazm\ [GRAPHO- + SPASM] WRITERS' CRAMP.

**-graphy** \-grəfē\ [Gk *graphein* to write, draw, record] A combining form meaning (1) writing, a record; (2) a manner or means of writing or recording.

**GRAS** [from *generally regarded as safe*] Designating a list of food additives that were introduced before the Delaney Law was passed in 1958. They are assumed to be safe and there are no restrictions on their use. Any substance on the list found to be unsafe is immediately banned and removed from the list.

**grasping / forced g.** GRASP REFLEX.

**Grasset** [Joseph *Grasset,* French physician, 1849–1918] **1** Grasset's law. See under LANDOUZY-GRASSET LAW. **2** Grasset-Gaussel phenomenon, Grasset-Bychowski sign, Grasset sign. See under GRASSET'S PHENOMENON. **3** Grasset-Gaussel-Hoover sign. See under SIGN.

**graticule** \grat′ikyool\ [French (alteration of L *craticula* latticework, dim. of *cratis* a wicker frame or basket), a grid] A grid, usually of plastic, for measurement of quantities displayed on the cathode-ray tube of an oscilloscope. **eyepiece g.** GRADUATING DIAPHRAGM.

**grating** A perforated frame or latticework. **diffraction g.** A device that consists of closely ruled, parallel, equidistant lines on a transparent or polished plate. It is used to produce spectra of transmitted or reflected light, through interference of the waves diffracted by the individual rulings.

**Gratiolet** [Louis Pierre *Gratiolet,* French anatomist and physiologist, 1815–1865] **1** Peduncular ansa of Gratiolet. See under ANSA PEDUNCULARIS. **2** Fibers of Gratiolet, radiation of Gratiolet, radiatio occipitothalamica Gratioleti, Gratiolet's radiating fibers. See under RADIATIO OPTICA.

**grattage** \grätäzh′\ [French, a scratching] The removal of surface scale by gentle scraping. The technique is used in the diagnostic examination of suspected psoriasis.

**gravel** [Middle English, from Old French *gravelle,* dim. of *grave* coarse or pebbly sand] Granular urinary-tract concretions, smaller than calculi and ordinarily the size of pinheads, which can be passed through the urethra without discomfort.

**Graves** [Robert James *Graves,* Irish physician, 1796–1863] **1** See under DISEASE. **2** Euthyroid Graves disease. See under DISEASE. **3** Graves scapula. See under SCAPHOID SCAPULA.

**gravid** \grav′id\ Pregnant.

**gravida** \grav′idə\ [L (from *gravis* heavy) pregnant] A pregnant woman. A numerical designation is often used following the term to denote the total number of pregnancies the woman has experienced including the current one. For example, a woman who has had one prior pregnancy and is currently pregnant is designated *gravida 2.*

**gravidity** \grəvid′itē\ PREGNANCY.

**gravimeter** \grəvim′ətər\ An apparatus for measuring specific gravity. Also *gravitometer.*

**gravimetric** \grav′imet′rik\ [L *gravi(s)* weighty + *metric(us)* pertaining to measuring] Of or relating to measurement by weight.

**gravistatic** \grav′istat′tik\ Relating to the accumulation of body fluids or sedimentary material in dependent parts from the effects of gravity.

**gravitation** \grav′itā′shən\ The force of attraction between any two bodies. Also *gravity.* See also NEWTON'S LAW OF GRAVITATION.

**gravitometer** \grav′itäm′ətər\ GRAVIMETER.

**gravity** \grav′itē\ [L *gravitas* (from *grav(is)* weighty + *-itas* -ITY) weightiness] GRAVITATION. • Physicists tend to use *gravity* to mean the force exerted on an object near the surface of a celestial body, such as the Earth or the moon, and to use *gravitation* for the general phenomenon, but for most purposes they can be used interchangeably. **specific g.** RELATIVE DENSITY. **standard g.** STANDARD ACCELERATION OF FREE FALL.

**Grawitz** [Paul Albert *Grawitz,* German pathologist, 1850–1932] **1** Grawitz tumor. See under RENAL CELL CARCINOMA. **2** See under CACHEXIA.

**Gray** [Joseph Alexander *Gray,* Australian physician, 1884–1966] Bragg-Gray principle. See under PRINCIPLE.

**gray¹** [after Louis Harold *Gray,* British radiologist, 1905–1965] Special name for the SI derived unit of absorbed dose in the field of ionizing radiation, equal to one joule per kilogram. The absorbed dose is the mean energy imparted by ionizing radiation to matter per unit of mass of irradiated material at the place of interest. Symbol: Gy **g. per second** The SI derived unit of radiation absorbed dose rate. 1 gray per second = 100 rad per second. Symbol: Gy/s, $Gy{\cdot}s^{-1}$

**gray²** SUBSTANTIA GRISEA. **central g.** SUBSTANTIA GRISEA CENTRALIS CEREBRI. **periaqueductal g.** SUB-

STANTIA GRISEA CENTRALIS CEREBRI.

**gray-out** Mild, short-lived, or partial loss of consciousness, most commonly due to temporary anoxemia.

**green** 1 A color of the visible spectrum falling between blue and yellow. 2 A substance, usually a stain or dye, that is green in appearance, or that produces a cytochemical reaction resulting in green staining. For chemical names including *green,* see under the chemical name. **acid g.** LIGHT GREEN S F YELLOWISH. **brilliant g.** A basic arylmethane synthetic dye used sometimes as a stain for bacteria, spirochetes, fungi, and yeasts. It is used more frequently as a constituent of bacteriologic media, as in the brilliant green bile medium for the identification of *Escherichia coli.* Also *ethyl green, new solid green.* **diamond g.** MALACHITE GREEN. **fast g.** A dye that is closely related to light green chemically and has been used as an alternative to it in staining techniques where greater permanency is required. **fast acid g. N** LIGHT GREEN S F YELLOWISH. **fast g. FCF** A dye that substitutes for light green SF yellowish but that has superior resistance to fading. It is used in various staining techniques involving bacteria, collagen fibers, and plant histology. **Hoffman g.** IODINE GREEN. **light g. N** MALACHITE GREEN. **light g. S F yellowish** A synthetic acid dye derived from brilliant green. It is used as a stain for microorganisms and for collagen fibers in Masson's trichrome modification of the Mallory aniline blue method. Also *acid green, fast acid green N.* **malachite g.** A diaminotriphenylmethane dye variously used as a counterstain, as a vital stain, as an indicator at both pH 0.0–2.0 and 11.6–14.0 ranges, and as a constituent in Löwenstein-Jensen agar for mycobacteria. It has also been used as an antiseptic and antimycotic agent. Also *diamond green, solid green O, Victoria green, light green N.* **new solid g.** BRILLIANT GREEN. **solid g. O** MALACHITE GREEN. **Victoria g.** MALACHITE GREEN.

**Greenfield** [Joseph Godwin *Greenfield,* English neuropathologist, 1844–1958] 1 Greenfield's disease. See under BALÓ'S DISEASE. 2 Greenfield syndrome, Scholz-Greenfield disease. See under METACHROMATIC LEUKODYSTROPHY.

**Greenwood** [Major *Greenwood,* English physician, born 1880] Greenwood-Yule method. See under METHOD.

**Greig** [David Middleton *Greig,* Scottish scientist, 1864–1936] Greig syndrome. See under ORBITAL HYPERTELORISM.

**Greither** [Aloys *Greither,* German dermatologist, born 1913] See under SYNDROME.

**Greppi** [Encrico *Greppi,* Italian hematologist, born 1896] Microelliptopoikilocytic anemia of Rietti, Greppi, and Micheli. See under ANEMIA.

**Grey Turner** See under TURNER.

**gribouillist** \grēbooyist′\ [French *gribouill(e)* a foolish, naive, disorganized person + -IST] One who accentuates the most unattractive aspects of old age, particularly in a way intended to promote guilt among other people.

**grid** [short for *gridiron*] In radiology, a series of very thin lead strips separated by spacers which are transparent to x rays. The strips are set on edge, parallel to the beam axis, and reduce the amount of scattered x rays reaching the film. **Amsler g.** A checkerboardlike pattern of lines used as a background for the subjective drawing of visual field defects. **baby g.** Any of various growth charts of weight and length of babies. **Bucky g.** BUCKY DIAPHRAGM. **fixed g.** STATIONARY GRID. **focused g.** A radiographic grid in which the lead strips are angled slightly so that they focus on a line at a specified distance, which determines the optimal placement of the x-ray tube. **moving g.** A radiographic grid which moves during the x-ray exposure, in order to blur out the shadows caused by the lead strips. **parallel g.** A radiographic grid in which the lead strips are parallel to each other in their longitudinal axis. **Potter-Bucky g.** BUCKY DIAPHRAGM. **stationary g.** A radiographic grid that does not move during the x-ray exposure. Also *fixed grid.* **Thoms g.** A grid used in pelvimetry to allow direct measurement from the radiograph of pelvic diameters. **Wetzel g.** Formerly, a growth chart of heights and weights for children according to age. A second measurement of the child after a sufficient interval, when plotted on the grid, gave the growth trend of that child, whether accelerating, slowing, arrested, catching up, or normal.

**Gridley** [Mary F. *Gridley,* U.S. medical technologist, 1908–1954] See under STAIN.

**Griffith** [Frederick *Griffith,* English bacteriologist, died 1941] See under CLASSIFICATION.

**grinding** / **night g.** BRUXISM. **selective g.** Alteration of the occlusal surfaces of the teeth by grinding away points or areas of contact. Also *spot grinding.*

**grinding-in** A method of adjusting the occlusal surfaces of the teeth by moving the jaws (or the equivalents thereof on an articulator) relative to one another with an abrasive paste in between the upper and lower occlusal surfaces. Also *milling-in.*

**grip** *Older term* INFLUENZA. • In this sense, the French spelling *grippe* is more usual. **Dabney's g.** EPIDEMIC PLEURODYNIA. **devil's g.** EPIDEMIC PLEURODYNIA.

**grippe** \grip\ [French (from *gripper* to seize, from Low German *gripan* to clutch, seize), an epidemic catarrh, influenza] *Older term* INFLUENZA.

**grisein** An antibiotic produced by strains of *Streptomyces griseus.* It is an amorphous red powder containing ferric iron. Acid hydrolysis yields 3-methyluracil and at least two amino acids. It is active against some Gram-positive and Gram-negative bacteria and certain fungi.

**Grisel** [P. *Grisel,* French physician, flourished early 20th century] Grisel's disease. See under NASOPHARYNGEAL TORTICOLLIS.

**griseofulvin** $C_{17}H_{17}ClO_6$. A naturally occurring antibiotic derived from *Penicillium griseofulvum.* It is used in the treatment of fungal infections of the skin. It is given orally.

**Grisolle** [Augustin *Grisolle,* French physician, 1811–1869] See under SIGN.

**gristle** \gris′əl\ CARTILAGE.

**Gritti** [Rocco *Gritti,* Italian surgeon, 1828–1920] 1 Gritti's operation. See under GRITTI'S AMPUTATION. 2 Gritti-Stokes amputation. See under AMPUTATION.

**Grocco** [Pietro *Grocco,* Italian physician, 1856–1916] See under SIGN.

**Groenouw** [Arthur *Groenouw,* German ophthalmologist, 1862–1945] 1 Groenouw type I corneal dystrophy. See under GRANULAR CORNEAL DYSTROPHY. 2 Groenouw type II corneal dystrophy. See under MACULAR CORNEAL DYSTROPHY.

**groin** \groin\ [early modern English rendering of *grine,* also *grinde,* from Middle English *grynde,* from Old English *grynde* abyss] The curved linear groove forming the junction between the anterior abdominal wall and the front of the thigh lateral to the perineal area. Also *inguen.*

**grommet** \gräm′it\ [obsolete French *gromette* (now *gourmette*) a bridle chain for curbing animals] *Popular* VENTILATION TUBE.

**Grönblad** [Esther Elisabeth *Grönblad,* Swedish ophthalmologist, born 1898] Grönblad-Strandberg syndrome. See under PSEUDOXANTHOMA ELASTICUM.

# groove

**groove** [Middle English *grofe,* from Middle Dutch *groeve* a furrow, ditch] A linear depression or furrow found on the surfaces of teeth, bones, and other anatomical structures. **alveolobuccal g.** The curved groove at the uppermost and lowermost margins of the vestibule of the mouth that is formed by the mucous membrane reflected from the gums to the cheeks and lips. Also *alveolobuccal sulcus, gingivobuccal sulcus.* **alveololabial g.** The groove that develops in the embryo between the lips and the jaws. It is a deepening of the labiodental lamina. Also *alveolabial sulcus, gingivobuccal groove, gingivolabial sulcus.* **alveololingual g.** A groove that develops in the embryo between the tongue and the lower jaw. Also *alveololingual sulcus.* **anterior auricular g.** INCISURA ANTERIOR AURIS. **anterior interventricular g.** SULCUS INTERVENTRICULARIS ANTERIOR. **anterior paramedian g. of spinal cord** SULCUS INTERMEDIUS ANTERIOR MEDULLAE SPINALIS. **anterolateral g. of medulla oblongata** SULCUS LATERALIS ANTERIOR MEDULLAE OBLONGATAE. **anterolateral g. of spinal cord** SULCUS LATERALIS ANTERIOR MEDULLAE SPINALIS. **anteromedian g. of spinal cord** FISSURA MEDIANA ANTERIOR MEDULLAE SPINALIS. **arterial g.'s** SULCI ARTERIOSI. **atrioventricular g.** SULCUS CORONARIUS CORDIS. **auriculoventricular g.** SULCUS CORONARIUS CORDIS. **basilar g.** SULCUS BASILARIS PONTIS. **bicipital g. of humerus** SULCUS INTERTUBERCULARIS HUMERI. **Blessig's g.** The future ora serrata of the retina, seen in the developing eye as a groove between the nervous part of the retina and its ciliary part. **branchial g.** A furrow on the outside of an embryo, lying between two branchial arches and having its floor made of ectoderm. Also *visceral groove.* **carotid g. of sphenoid bone** SULCUS CAROTICUS OSSIS SPHENOIDALIS. **cavernous g. of sphenoid bone** SULCUS CAROTICUS OSSIS SPHENOIDALIS. **cerebral g.** The cerebral portion of the neural groove. **chiasmatic g.** SULCUS PRECHIASMATICUS. **costal g.** SULCUS COSTAE. **deltopectoral g.** The curved vertical groove between the anterior margin of the deltoid muscle and the clavicular part of the pectoralis major muscle in which the cephalic vein and deltoid branch of the thoracoacromial artery are situated. It is continuous superiorly with the fossa infraclavicularis. **developmental g.** A groove on the surface of an anatomical structure such as a tooth or a bone, which is an intrinsically determined feature of its shape. Also *developmental line.* **digastric g.** INCISURA MASTOIDEA OSSIS TEMPORALIS. **duodenopyloric g.** PYLORIC CONSTRICTION. **ethmoidal g.** SULCUS ETHMOIDALIS OSSIS NASALIS. **g. for eustachian tube** SULCUS TUBAE AUDITIVAE. **g. for facial artery on mandible** A groove on the base of the mandible that is immediately anterior to the angle and is traversed by the facial artery. **free gingival g.** A groove on the surface of the gingiva at the junction between the free and attached gingiva. **genital g.** GENITAL FURROW. **g. of great superficial petrosal nerve** SULCUS NERVI PETROSI MAJORIS. **hamular g.** SULCUS HAMULI PTERYGOIDEI. **Harrison's g.** A horizontal indentation of the ribs making up the chest wall opposite the attachment of the diaphragm, produced by softening of the bones in rachitic children. Also *Harrison sulcus.* **g. of helix** SCAPHA. **inferior dental g.** The inferior dental (mandibular) canal during development in the embryo. At first it is not closed over by bone on its medial (lingual) aspect. **infraorbital g. of maxilla** SULCUS INFRAORBITALIS MAXILLAE. **interatrial g.** A slight sulcus extending between the left sides of the superior and inferior venae cavae on the external dorsal surface of the heart, indicating the division between the right and left atria and usually only visible if the heart is somewhat distended. Also *interatrial sulcus.* **interdental g.** A vertical furrow on the surface of the interdental papilla. **interosseous g. of calcaneus** SULCUS CALCANEI. **intertubercular g. of humerus** SULCUS INTERTUBERCULARIS HUMERI. **labial g.** A thin ectodermal formation in the embryo which, after delamination, forms the gingivolabial furrow (alveololabial sulcus). From its internal part the dental lamina originates. **lacrimal g.** FOSSA SACCI LACRIMALIS. **g. of lacrimal bone** SULCUS LACRIMALIS OSSIS LACRIMALIS. **laryngotracheal g.** A ventrally placed gutter at the caudal end of the primitive pharyngeal floor in an embryo, marking the site of early development of the larynx and trachea. **lateral bicipital g.** SULCUS BICIPITALIS LATERALIS. **lateral g. of occipital bone** SULCUS SINUS TRANSVERSI. **lateral phallic g.** A groove on each side of the developing penis in the embryo, separating it from the future scrotum. **g. of Lucas** STRIA SPINOSA. **mastoid g.** INCISURA MASTOIDEA OSSIS TEMPORALIS. **medial bicipital g.** SULCUS BICIPITALIS MEDIALIS. **medullary g.** NEURAL GROOVE. **meningeal g.'s** Sulci arteriosi and sulci venosi. **g. for middle temporal artery** SULCUS ARTERIAE TEMPORALIS MEDIAE. **musculospiral g.** SULCUS NERVI RADIALIS. **mylohyoid g.** SULCUS MYLOHYOIDEUS MANDIBULAE. **nail g.** SULCUS MATRICIS UNGUIS. **nasal g.** SULCUS ETHMOIDALIS OSSIS NASALIS. **g. for nasal nerve** SULCUS ETHMOIDALIS OSSIS NASALIS. **nasolabial g.** SULCUS NASOLABIALIS. **nasolacrimal g.** An elongated thickening that forms from ectoderm medial to the nasomaxillary groove and sinks below the surface, becomes canalized, and gives rise to the nasolacrimal duct. **nasomaxillary g.** The groove formed at the line of union of the maxillary and lateral nasal processes during the development of the cheek. **naso-optic g.** ORBITONASAL CLEFT. **nasopalatine g.** A narrow, deep channel running anteroinferiorly on each lateral surface of the vomer, lodging the nasopalatine nerve and vessels. **nasopharyngeal g.** A shallow sulcus on the lateral nasal wall extending from the body of the sphenoid bone to the junction of the hard and soft palates and separating the nasal fossa posteriorly from the nasopharynx. **neural g.** A groove, formed in an early temporary stage in the development of the central nervous system, situated in the middle of the embryo in front of Hensen's node. It follows the neural plate stage and is formed by sinking in of the neural plate to give rise to a midline groove. The margins of the groove fold over and meet centrally, at first in its middle portion, to begin the formation of the neural tube containing the neural canal. Also *medullary groove.* **nuchal g.** The vertical median furrow of the nape of the neck. **nutrient artery g.** A linear translucency produced on a radiograph of a bone by the canal of a nutrient artery. **obturator g.** SULCUS OBTURATORIUS OSSIS PUBIS. **g. for occipital artery** SULCUS ARTERIAE OCCIPITALIS. **olfactory g.** 1 SULCUS OLFACTORIUS NASI. 2 ETHMOID FOSSA. **optic g.** SULCUS PRECHIASMATICUS. **palatine g.'s of maxilla** SULCI PALATINI MAXILLAE. **palatine g. of palatine bone** SULCUS PALATINUS MAJOR OSSIS PALATINI. **pala-**

**tomaxillary g. of palatine bone** SULCUS PALATINUS MAJOR OSSIS PALATINI. **palatovaginal g.** SULCUS PALATOVAGINALIS. **paracolic g.'s** SULCI PARACOLICI. **pharyngeal g.** A groove delineating adjacent pharyngeal or branchial arches. Pharyngeal grooves are of two varieties, endodermal and ectodermal. Endodermal grooves are found in the foregut and extend laterally to form pouches. Ectodermal grooves lie opposite the endodermal pouches. **pharyngotympanic g.** SULCUS TUBAE AUDITIVAE. **popliteal g.** A deep, smooth sulcus below and behind the lateral epicondyle of the femur, the anterior portion of which gives attachment to the tendon of the popliteus muscle, while the posterior part receives the tendon in full flexion of the knee joint. **posterior auricular g.** SULCUS AURICULAE POSTERIOR. **posterior interventricular g.** SULCUS INTERVENTRICULARIS POSTERIOR. **posterior paramedian g. of spinal cord** SULCUS INTERMEDIUS POSTERIOR MEDULLAE SPINALIS. **posterolateral g. of spinal cord** SULCUS LATERALIS POSTERIOR MEDULLAE SPINALIS. **preauricular g. of ilium** PREAURICULAR SULCUS. **preputiolabial g.** A depression separating the two genital folds in female embryos. Also *urogenital groove.* **primary labial g.** LABIAL LAMINA. **primary urethral g.** A median groove that develops along the caudal surface of the embryonic phallus. It is in contact with the lower margin of the urethral plate and its raised margins are the genital folds. The groove deepens and eventually becomes the greater part of the spongy urethra. Also *urethral groove.* **primitive g.** PRIMITIVE STREAK. **primitive dental g.** DENTAL LAMINA. **radial g.** SULCUS NERVI RADIALIS. **g. for radial nerve** SULCUS NERVI RADIALIS. **rhombic g.** One of the grooves between the segments or neuromeres of the rhombencephalon. **sagittal g.** SULCUS SINUS SAGITTALIS SUPERIORIS. **second branchial g.** The U.S. term for HYOBRANCHIAL CLEFT. **Sibson's g.** SIBSON'S FURROW. **sigmoid g. of temporal bone** SULCUS SINUS SIGMOIDEI OSSIS TEMPORALIS. **g. of small superficial petrosal nerve** SULCUS NERVI PETROSI MINORIS. **sphenobasilar g.** The shallow depression on the superior surface of the basiocciput and the dorsum sellae of the sphenoid bone to which the ventral surface of the pons is related. **spiral g.** SULCUS NERVI RADIALIS. **g. of subclavius muscle** A transverse groove in the middle third of the inferior surface of the clavicle for the proximal attachment of the subclavius muscle. The clavipectoral fascia is attached to the anterior and posterior margins of the groove. A nutrient foramen is located in the lateral end of the groove. **subcostal g.** SULCUS COSTAE. **g. for superior longitudinal sinus** SULCUS SINUS SAGITTALIS SUPERIORIS. **tracheobronchial g.** A median groove that appears in the floor of the embryonic pharynx and is rapidly converted into a tubular outgrowth parallel to the foregut. It is the primordium of the larynx, trachea, bronchi, and lungs. Also *laryngotracheal groove.* **trigeminal g.** The earliest indication in the embryo of the formation of the ganglion of the trigeminal nerve. **tympanic g.** SULCUS TYMPANICUS OSSIS TEMPORALIS. **ulnar g.** SULCUS NERVI ULNARIS. **g. of ulnar nerve** SULCUS NERVI ULNARIS. **urethral g.** PRIMARY URETHRAL GROOVE. **urogenital g.** PREPUTIOLABIAL GROOVE. **venous g.'s** SULCI VENOSI. **Verga's lacrimal g.** A furrow occasionally found in the lateral wall of the inferior meatus of the nose, extending downward just below the opening of the nasolacrimal duct. **vertebral g.** A marked hollow on each side of the spinous processes of the vertebral column, posterior to the laminae and the transverse processes and occupied by the deep muscles of the back. **visceral g.** BRANCHIAL GROOVE.

**Gross** [Ludwik *Gross*, Polish-born U.S. physician, born 1904] See under LEUKEMIA.

**gross** Visible to the naked eye; macroscopic.

**ground** **1** A point in an electric circuit used as a common reference for measuring voltages. **2** The connection between an electric circuit and the earth. **3** A backdrop or setting on which something else, the figure, is displayed or superimposed; background. Difficulty in differentiating the figure from the ground is characteristic of some organic mental disorders.

**group** **1** A set or class. **2** An assemblage. **3** A number of mutually bonded atoms in a molecule, forming an identifiable part of that molecule. **A g.** In human cytogenetics, the largest metacentric chromosomes, numbers 1, 2, and 3. **alkalescens-dispar g.** A group of nonpathogenic Enterobacteriaceae, classified formerly with *Shigella* (because they do not form gas) but now with *Escherichia coli.* **Arizona g.** A group of microorganisms sometimes classified as *Salmonella arizonae.* They are very similar to *Salmonella* biochemically and in pathogenesis, but often lactose-positive. Reptiles seem to be the natural reservoir. **B g.** In human cytogenetics, the largest submetacentric chromosomes, numbers 4 and 5. **Bethesda-Ballerup g.** A group of enteric bacteria, closely related metabolically and antigenically to *Escherichia coli* and now included in *Citrobacter.* **blood g.** See under BLOODGROUP. **C g.** In human cytogenetics, the submetacentric chromosomes intermediate in length to those in the B and E groups, namely numbers 6 through 12 and the X. **California g.** A group of eleven serologically related mosquito-borne bunyaviruses found in the United States, Europe, and Africa. Five viruses of the group are associated with human illness ranging from mild fever to encephalitis. **closed g.** A therapy group to which no new patients are admitted once the series of sessions has begun. **compatibility g.** INCOMPATIBILITY GROUP. **continuous g.** OPEN GROUP. **control g.** A group used as a control in an experiment or study (control experiment). See under CONTROL. Compare EXPERIMENTAL GROUP. **D g.** In human cytogenetics, the largest acrocentric chromosomes, numbers 13, 14, and 15. **diagnosis-related g.** In the United States, a group of conditions for which health-care treatment has been received and charges are to be assessed, considered to be related by diagnoses, with the object of establishing in a prospective manner a specific, reimbursable fee or range of fees for an episode of care for each such group. Thus, all diagnoses within a group are reimbursed at the same rate, regardless of length-of-stay in an inpatient facility, the severity of illness, or the specific services provided. This system was initiated primarily for prospective payment of inpatient care under the Medicare program. Abbr. DRG • In Japan, a similar payment system was instituted in 1983 specifically for the care of those over 70 years of age. In the United Kingdom, no comparable system exists, although the concept is reflected in the term *performance indicator,* broadly applied to various hospital services, including administrative services as well as patient management. **E g.** In human cytogenetics, the smallest of the submetacentric chromosomes, numbers 16, 17, and 18. **encounter g.** A therapy group in which there is an emphasis on intensive face-to-face interaction, the encouraging of interpersonal confrontation and self-disclosure, and a striving to modify behavior on the basis of increased awareness of self and of how others react to one's self. The encounter group is an outgrowth of sensitivity training. Also *T-group, sensitivity training group.* **experimental g.** The group in a control experiment that is exposed to the variable under study. Compare CONTROL GROUP. **F g.** In human cytogenetics, the smallest of the metacentric chromosomes, numbers 19 and 20. **G g.** In human cytogenetics, the smallest acrocentric chromosomes, numbers 21 and 22, and the Y. **incompatibility g.** A group of plasmids with the same specificity in the system regulating their copy number. As a result, a cell infected with two plasmids of the same group will soon yield progeny lines that contain one or the other. This feature is a fundamental criterion for classifying plasmids. Also *compatibility group.* **leukocyte g.** White cells typed by antigenic determinants and generally recognized by their reactivity with corresponding antibodies by agglutination, cytotoxicity, or fluorescence. **linkage g.** Two or more genes found by family, biochemical, or cytogenetic studies to be linked. Such genes do not segregate independently, in apparent violation of Mendel's second law. All genes of a given linkage group are syntenic, but all syntenic loci are not necessarily linked in the genetic sense and may show independent assortment through crossing over. **marathon g.** A type of encounter group that meets for long stretches of time, sometimes for as long as 48 or 72 hours without interruption except for short sleep periods and toilet breaks. **open g.** A therapy group that accepts new participants at any time. Also *continuous group.* **prosthetic g.** A group in a protein molecule not composed of amino-acid residues. The flavin of a flavoprotein is an example. The prosthetic group of an enzyme often plays a part in the reaction it catalyzes. It differs from a coenzyme in being more tightly bound so that it remains with the enzyme when this is isolated. **reporter g.** A group in a molecule, often inserted artificially, that is capable of providing information about the parts of the molecule around it. It possesses some measurable characteristic, such as absorbance, fluorescence, or nuclear magnetic resonance signal, whose nature is responsive to changes in its environment. Such groups in proteins have been used to indicate conformation changes or the binding of ligands. **sensitivity training g.** ENCOUNTER GROUP. **ventral thalamic g.** The several nuclei lying ventrolateral to the internal medullary lamina, constituting the thalamic centers for somatosensory and motor integration.

**grouping / blood g.** Typing of blood cell antigenic determinants by their specific reactivity with corresponding antibodies and generally determined *in vitro* by cell agglutination. (For specific blood groups, see under BLOOD GROUP.).

**growth** 1 The process by which an organism increases in size as part of its normal development. 2 Any increase in size of an organism or part. 3 A tumor. 4 An increase in the number of units making up a whole, as, for example, population growth, or growth of a tissue or organ by cellular multiplication. **absolute g.** An actual increase in size, in whole or in part. **accretionary g.** Any growth process involving an increase in the amount of intercellular, nonliving substances. **allometric g.** The growth of a part of the body as an exponential function of the growth of the body as a whole. **appositional g.** A growth process which occurs by increase at the edges or on the outside of a structure, thus adding new material or tissue at the periphery. **auxetic g.** AUXESIS. **confluent g.** The growth of animal cells to form a sheet in which the cells are brought into intimate contact. Normally this results in cessation of DNA synthesis and of further growth (contact inhibition), but many types of cancer cell continue to grow. **differential g.** The difference in growth rates as exhibited by the several parts of a structure or an organism. **histiotypic g.** Profuse uncontrolled growth of cells. **interstitial g.** Growth occurring inside a structure or organ by increase in number and size of the elements or components contained within them. **multiplicative g.** Growth which results from an increase in number of cells. **new g.** NEOPLASM.

**Gruber** [Maximilian Franz Maria von *Gruber,* Austrian bacteriologist, 1853–1927] Gruber-Widal reaction, Gruber's reaction, Gruber-Widal test. See under WIDAL TEST.

**Gruber** [Wenzel Leopold *Gruber,* Russian anatomist, 1814–1890] **1** Gruber's fossa, sac of Gruber. See under GRUBER'S CUL-DE-SAC. **2** Gruber-Landzert fossa. See under RECESSUS PARADUODENALIS. **3** Gruber-Landzert fossa. See under FOSSA.

**grumous** \groo′məs\ [L *grum(us)* a mound, heap + -OUS] Describing a semisolid material containing small, lumpy concretions: often used of the gross appearance of the contents of advanced atheromatous plaques. Also *grumose.*

**grundplatte** \grUnt′plät′ə\ [German *Grund* ground, bottom, base + *Platte* a board, slab, plate] BASAL LAMINA.

**Grünwald** [Ludwig *Grünwald,* German rhinologist, born 1863] May-Grünwald stain. See under STAIN.

**Grütz** [Otto *Grütz,* German dermatologist, born 1886] Bürger-Grütz syndrome. See under FAMILIAL HYPERLIPOPROTEINEMIA TYPE I.

**gryochrome** \grī′ōkrōm\ Designating any nerve cell or neuronal perikaryon containing stainable granules in its cytoplasm, such as the anterior horn cells of the spinal cord.

**gryphosis** \grīfō′sis\ ONYCHOGRYPOSIS.

**gryposis** \grīpō′sis\ [Gk *gryp(os)* curved, esp. hook-nosed + -OSIS] ONYCHOGRYPOSIS. **g. penis** CHORDEE. **g. unguium** ONYCHOGRYPOSIS.

**GSH** Symbol for reduced glutathione.

**GSR** galvanic skin response (psychogalvanic response).

**GSSG** Symbol for oxidized glutathione.

**gt.** *gutta* (L, drop).

**GTO** Golgi tendon organ (tendon organ).

**GTP** guanosine triphosphate.

**gtt.** *guttae* (L, drops).

**GU** **1** genitourinary. **2** gastric ulcer.

**Gua** Symbol for guanine.

**guaiacol** \gwī′əkôl\ $C_7H_8O_2$. 2-Methoxyphenol, a phenolic compound of creosote produced primarily by destructive distillation of beechwood. It has antiseptic, disinfectant, deodorant, expectorant, and mucolytic properties. It may be synthesized from catechol and may be used to synthesize vanillin. Also *catechol methyl ether, methylcatechol.*

**guaiacol carbonate** $C_{15}H_{14}O_5$. Carbonic acid bis(2-methoxyphenyl)ester, a white, crystalline powder used as an expectorant medication.

**guaiacum resin** A resin obtained from the wood of certain *Guaiacum* species. It has mild laxative and diuretic actions and it has been used to treat rheumatism. The resin is also used in a test for occult blood in feces that also employs acetic acid and hydrogen peroxide.

**guaifenesin** $C_{10}H_{14}O_4$. 3-(2-Methoxyphenoxy)-1,2-propanediol, a compound that is believed to reduce the viscosity of sputum. It is used as an expectorant in cough medicine.

**guanazolo** AZAGUANINE.

**guanethidine sulfate** $C_{20}H_{46}N_8O_4S$. 2-(1′-Azacyclooctyl)ethylguanidine sulfate, a compound that is used in the management of moderate to severe hypertension, and for hypertension secondary to renal disease, amyloidosis, and renal artery stenosis. It is given orally.

**guanidine** $(NH_2)_2C{=}NH$. A strong base (p*K* 13.6), which forms a highly symmetrical cation. Strong solutions of its hydrochloride are used to denature and dissolve proteins.

**guanidine phosphate** 1 A salt between guanidine and phosphoric acid. 2 *Incorrect* PHOSPHOGUANIDINE.

**guanidino** The group $NH_2—C(=NH)—NH—$, derived from guanidine. It is strongly basic and is an important feature of the arginine molecule.

**guanidinoacetic acid** $NH_2—C(=NH_2^+)—NH—CH_2—COO^-$. An intermediate in the biosynthesis of creatine, it is formed by transfer of an amidino group from arginine onto glycine by glycine amidinotransferase.

**γ-guanidinobutyramide** $H_2N—C(=NH)—NH—[CH_2]_3—CO—NH_2$. A compound related in structure to both arginine and γ-aminobutyric acid, found to lower urea and influence autonomic neuropathy in diabetes.

**guanidinosuccinic acid** A complex of guanidine and succinic acid, having a molecular weight of approximately 158, that accumulates in the blood of uremic patients and inhibits platelet aggregation. The hemorrhagic diathesis of uremia has been attributed to this substance.

**guanine** \gwä′nēn\ [*guan(o)* from Spanish, from Quechua *huanu* dung) bird droppings, fertilizer + -INE] One of the two purines found in all nucleic acids; 2-amino-6-hydroxypurine and its tautomers, predominantly 2-amino-6-oxo-1,6-dihydropurine. Its nucleotides are important in a number of biologic processes, such as the decarboxylation of oxaloacetate, the oxidation of 2-oxoglutarate, and, in bacteria, the integration of the biosynthesis of proteins and nucleic acids.

**guanine deoxyriboside** A nucleoside, composed of the purine base guanine and the pentose deoxyribose. It is one of the four nucleosides present in DNA, and it base-pairs with cytosine deoxyriboside.

**guanophores** \gwän′ōfôrs\ [*guan(ine)* + *o* + -PHORE] Epidermal cells, found in some poikilotherms, which contain granules rich in guanine. The granules give the animal a metallic luster, usually gold or silver.

**guanosine** The nucleoside formed by condensation of guanine and ribose. It is a constituent of nucleic acids and of many biologically important nucleotides. Also *ribofuranosylguanine.*

**guanosine diphosphate** The nucleotide formed by esterification of O-5′ of guanosine with diphosphoric (pyrophosphoric) acid. Symbol: GDP

**guanosine triphosphate** The nucleotide formed by esterification of O-5′ of guanosine with triphosphoric acid. It is the precursor of guanosine-phosphate residues in RNA, and also acts as an intermediate in biologically important energy-transfer and biosynthetic processes. Symbol: GTP

**guanyl** *Obs.* AMIDINO.

**guanylate cyclase** The enzyme (EC 4.6.1.2) responsible for the breakdown of GTP into cGMP and diphosphate. Guanylate cyclase is an important metabolic regulator in bacteria and in higher cells. Some enterotoxins act by activating this enzyme. Also *guanyl cyclase, guanylyl cyclase.*

**guanylic acid** A guanosine phosphate, usually guanosine 5′-phosphate. Its residues occur in RNA and in several nucleotides.

**guanyloribonuclease** RIBONUCLEASE $T_1$.

**guanylyl cyclase** GUANYLATE CYCLASE.

**guanylyl methylene diphosphonate** The anhydride between GMP and methylenebis(phosphonic acid), i.e., the analogue of GTP in which the oxygen atom between P-β and P-γ is replaced by $CH_2$. It is a competitive inhibitor of guanosine triphosphate reactions in protein synthesis.

**guard** A device that protects or shields. **bite g.** A removable appliance that covers the occlusal surfaces of the teeth in one jaw. It is used to protect teeth from occlusal stress and in the treatment of temporomandibular joint pain. Also *occlusal overlay appliance.* **mouth g.** A device for protecting the teeth from injury during sporting activities. It covers the teeth occlusally, labially, and buccally, and extends into the labial and buccal vestibules. It is made in one piece of resilient material, such as rubber, on casts of the teeth and gums. **night g.** A bite guard worn only during sleep.

**guarding** A reflex or voluntary reaction of a subject during physical examination that firmly contracts the abdominal wall, thereby making deep palpation difficult. It is usually associated with an underlying inflammatory process. Also *muscular defense.*

**Guarnieri** [Giuseppe *Guarnieri,* Italian pathologist, 1856–1918] Guarnieri's corpuscles, Guarnieri's inclusions. See under GUARNIERI BODIES.

**gubernaculum** \gʸoo′bərnak′yələm\ [L (from *guberna(re)* to steer, govern, from Gk *kybernan* to steer, govern) a steering oar, rudder] A fibrous cord directing the course of a structure attached to it during development. **g. dentis** An epithelial tract that for some time attaches the apex of unerupted deciduous and permanent teeth to the gum epithelium. It is a remnant of the dental lamina and eventually disappears completely. **g. testis** A fibromuscular cord which, in the male embryo, connects the lower pole of the wolffian body (mesonephros) to the part of the inguinal peritoneum that sends out, through the abdominal wall, a diverticulum called the processus vaginalis. The gubernaculum is crossed on its ventral aspect by the urogenital cord. The gubernaculum then becomes adherent to the lower pole of the testis, as it starts to descend and connects it through the cord and the processus vaginalis to the coverings of the genital swelling. There is thus formed a pathway for the descent of the testis: intra-abdominal within the inguinal fold of peritoneum, then intraparietal within the bulk of the abdominal muscles (internal oblique and transversus where the inguinal canal will form), and finally extra-abdominal within the scrotum. The testis normally descends along this pathway to reach the scrotum where it projects into the distal end of the processus vaginalis which later becomes the tunica vaginalis testis. The gubernaculum in adult males contributes to the fascial coverings of the testis and spermatic cord. In adult females the homologous structure is retained as the round ligament of the uterus and the ligament of the ovary.

**Gubler** [Adolphe Marie *Gubler,* French physician, 1821–1879] 1 See under SIGN, TUMOR. 2 Gubler's hemiplegia, Gubler's paralysis, Millard-Gubler paralysis, Gubler-Millard paralysis. See under MILLARD-GUBLER SYNDROME.

**Gudden** [Johann Bernhard Aloys von *Gudden,* German psychiatrist, 1824–1886] 1 See under LAW. 2 Tegmental nuclei of Gudden. See under NUCLEI TEGMENTI MESENCEPHALICI. 3 Commissura inferior guddeni. See under GUDDEN'S COMMISSURE.

**Guedel** [Arthur Ernest *Guedel,* U.S. anesthesiologist, 1883–1956] Guedel stages of general anesthesia. See under STAGE.

**Guenther** [Carl Oskar *Guenther,* German physician, 1854–1929] See under STAIN.

**Guérin** [Alphonse François Marie *Guérin,* French surgeon, 1816–1895] 1 Guérin's glands. See under DUCTUS PARAURETHRALES. 2 Guérin's glands. See under GLANDULAE URETHRALES URETHRAE FEMININAE. 3 Guérin's fold, valvule of Guérin, Guérin's valve. See under VALVULA FOSSAE NAVICULARIS. 4 Guérin's fracture. See under LEFORT I FRACTURE. 5 Guérin sinus. See under LACUNA MAGNA.

**Guérin** [Camille *Guérin,* French bacteriologist, 1872–1961]

Calmette-Guérin bacillus. See under BACILLUS.

**guidance** 1 Counseling and supportive psychotherapy that encourages the subject to set specific goals and to avoid anxiety-provoking situations. 2 The act or process of guiding. **child g.** Measures taken to enhance familial and social supports available during a child's developmental years as a means of preventing or minimizing the chances of the development of mental illness. **contact g.** The condition in which the direction of growth of a cellular process or the direction of cellular movement is dependent upon the contour of the solid substratum with which the cell is in physical contact. The influence of nonuniform surfaces on cell growth or movement is seen during embryogenesis or in tissue culture.

**guide** 1 A device that directs the course of something else, as by preceding it or confining its motion, or that indicates by pointing. 2 To serve as a guide for. **anterior g.** INCISAL GUIDE. **condylar g.** That part of an articulator which controls the path of the simulated condyle. **incisal g.** That part of an articulator which simulates the natural incisal guidance angle. Also *anterior guide.* **light g.** Fiberoptics used for illumination only and not for transmitting images. **mold g.** A series of samples, photographs, or diagrams showing the various shapes and sizes of artificial teeth available from a manufacturer.

**guideline** 1 A line used as a guide or indicator. 2 A statement or rule that serves to guide conduct in accordance with policy. **clasp g.** SURVEY LINE.

**Guidi** [Guido *Guidi* (Vidius), Italian-born anatomist active in France, 1500–1569] Canal of Guidi, canalis pterygoideus Vidii. See under CANALIS PTERYGOIDEUS.

**Guillain** [Georges *Guillain,* French neurologist, 1876–1961] 1 Barré-Guillain syndrome, Guillain-Barré polyneuritis, Guillain-Barré-Strohl syndrome, Landry-Guillain-Barré syndrome. See under GUILLAIN-BARRÉ SYNDROME. 2 Guillain-Barré reflex. See under SOLE-TAP REFLEX.

**guillotine** \gil′ətēn\ [French, originally a machine for beheading with a sharp blade sliding down vertical guides, after Joseph Ignace *Guillotin,* French physician, 1738–1814] A sharp surgical instrument designed to excise the tonsils or the uvula. **tonsil g.** One of a family of instruments for performing tonsillectomy, all descended from the Physick tonsillotome. Modern instruments do not cut off the tonsils, as the name suggests, but enucleate them. Also *tonsillotome* (obs.).

**guinea pig** \gin′ē\ A rodent of the genus *Cavia* used extensively in biologic research.

**gula** \gul′ə, goo′lə\ GULLET.

**gulf** / **Lecat's g.** A dilatation of the lumen of the bulb of the urethra just beyond the membranous portion where the ducts of the bulbourethral glands open.

**gullet** \gul′it\ [Middle English *golet,* from Middle French *goulet,* dim. of Old French *gole, goule* throat, from L *gula* gullet, windpipe, neck] The hollow muscular canal extending from the mouth to the stomach, comprising the pharynx and the esophagus. Also *gula.*

**gum**[1] [Old French *gomme* (from L *gummi,* also *cummi,* from Gk *kommi,* from Egyptian *qemai* acacia gum) gum, resin] A diverse group of complex carbohydrate derivatives that are amorphous, translucent, and water-soluble, and that are produced by plants following mechanical injury. **acacia g.** ACACIA. **g. arabic** ACACIA. **g. benjamin** BENZOIN. **g. benzoin** BENZOIN. **g. dragon** GUM TRAGACANTH. **g. guaiac** A resin obtained from the heartwood of *Guiacum officinale* and *Guiacum sanctum.* It is a hard, glossy, reddish brown substance that takes on a green color on long exposure to the air. It has a balsamic odor and a slightly acrid taste. The powder made from the resin is yellow-brown becoming olive-brown on exposure to air. It dissolves incompletely but readily in alcohol, ether, chloroform, and alkalis, and dissolves slightly in carbon disulfide and benzene. It is used as a preservative or antioxidant in foods. **Indian g.** STERCULIA GUM. **g. juniper** SANDARAC. **karaya g.** STERCULIA GUM. **Kordofan g.** ACACIA. **g. opium** OPIUM. **g. senegal** ACACIA. **sterculia g.** An exudate obtained from several species of *Sterculia,* the most important being *S. urens.* It is used as a bulk cathartic. Also *Bassora gum, karaya gum, Indian gum, ghatti gum, karaya, Indian tragacanth.* **g. tragacanth** The gummy exudate obtained from several species of *Astragalus,* the most important commercially being *A. gummifer.* It is used pharmaceutically as an emulsifying agent, adhesive, and emollient. Also *gum dragon, tragacanth, mucilago tragacanthae.*

**gum**[2] [Old English *gōma* (akin to German *Gaumen* palate and to Gk *chaunos* gaping) palate, in pl., jaws] The gingiva or the mucosa covering edentulous ridges; usually used in the plural. **blue g.** The appearance of gingiva with a lead line.

**gumboil** \gum′boil\ [GUM[2] + BOIL] See under ALVEOLAR ABSCESS.

**gumma** \gum′ə\ [New L (from L *gummi* gum) a gummy or rubbery lesion] (*pl.* gummas, gummata) The characteristic but inconstant lesion of tertiary syphilis. It may be solitary or multiple, range from microscopic to several centimeters in diameter, and is most commonly found in the liver, testis, bone, skin, and mucosal areas. Gummas have a rubbery consistency and are often surrounded by a fibrous capsule. Microscopically, the center consists of necrotic debris with faint outlines of preexisting structures. Epithelioid cells, occasional multinucleated giant cells, and plasma cells surround the necrotic center. Gummas are clinically important because of local tissue destruction. The large ones must be differentiated from neoplasms. Therapy shrinks the gumma, which becomes a fibrotic scar. Also *gummy tumor.* **tuberculous g.** A granulomatous nodule of tuberculous origin. Also *scrofuloderma gummosa, scrofulous gumma.*

**gummata** \gum′ətə\ Plural of GUMMA.

**gummatous** \gum′ətəs\ Having the gross appearance of a gumma.

**Gunn** See under MARCUS GUNN.

**Gunn** [Moses *Gunn,* U.S. surgeon, 1822–1887] See under LAW.

**Gunning** [Thomas Brian *Gunning,* U.S. dentist, 1813–1889] See under SPLINT.

**Günz** [Justus *Günz,* German anatomist, 1714–1789] See under LIGAMENT.

**Günzberg** [Alfred *Günzberg,* German physician, born 1861] See under SIGN.

**Guo** Symbol for guanosine.

**gurney** \gur′nē\ [orig. *Gurney,* the name of a taxicab company, later applied jocularly to horse-drawn patrol wagons and police ambulances and subsequently to wheeled stretchers] A wheeled stretcher or cart for the transport of patients, usually within a hospital.

**gustation** \gustā′shən\ DEGUSTATION.

**gustatory** \gus′tətôr′ē\ [L *gustat(us),* past part. of *gustare* to taste + -ORY] Having to do with the sense of taste.

**gustometry** \gustäm′ətrē\ [L *gust(us)* a tasting + *o* + -METRY] The measurement of taste thresholds either by applying the appropriate stimulus (salt, sweet, sour, or bitter) to the dorsum of the tongue or by the technique of electrogustometry.

**gut** [Old English *guttas* (pl.) viscera, akin to *geotan* to pour] **1** The digestive or alimentary tract, or a part of it; in embryology, the foregut, midgut or hindgut. **2** INTESTINE. **3** Surgical suture material, such as catgut, originally made of animal intestines. **blind g.** CAECUM. **postanal g.** The extension tailwards of the posterior part of the embryonic intestine (the hindgut) beyond the cloacal membrane. It becomes obliterated and disappears early in development. Also *tailgut.* **primitive g.** ARCHENTERON. **ribbon g.** A broad band of animal intestine that has been heated and processed and is used to reinforce surgical suture lines where the natural tissues are weakened. **silkworm g.** A strand of treated and processed suture material drawn from a silkworm. It is fairly stiff and nonabsorbable. **surgical g.** CATGUT.

**Guthrie** [George James *Guthrie,* English surgeon, 1785–1856] Guthrie's muscle. See under MUSCULUS SPHINCTER URETHRAE.

**Guthrie** [Robert *Guthrie,* U.S. pediatrician and microbiologist, born 1916] See under TEST.

**Gutmann** [Carl *Gutmann,* German physician, born 1872] Michaelis-Gutmann bodies. See under BODY.

**gutta** [L, a drop, a small quantity] (*pl.* guttae.) A drop. **guttae ophthalmicae** HASSALL-HENLE BODIES. **g. serena** *Obs.* AMAUROSIS.

**gutta-percha** \gut′əpur′chə\ [Malay *getah* gum + *percha* the tree yielding the juice] A thermoplastic material made from the latex of certain sapotaceous trees which has been used as a temporary filling in dentistry.

**guttat.** *guttatim* (L, drop by drop).

**guttate** \gut′āt\ Denoting a lesion of the skin having the shape of a drop.

**gutter** **1** A shallow furrow. **2** One of the sulci paracolici. **paracolic g.'s** SULCI PARACOLICI. **pleuroperitoneal g.'s** Paired gutters between somatopleure and splanchnopleure which at one stage constitute the posterior parts on each side of the primitive coelomic cavity (becoming closed off as the coelomic duct). Each pleuroperitoneal communication is subsequently obliterated, between the fifth and eighth weeks of gestation, by the formation of a pleuroperitoneal membrane and by the enlargement of neighboring organs such as the liver on the right and the suprarenal gland on the left. **synaptic g.** SYNAPTIC TROUGH.

**guttering** \gut′əring\ An operation in which the surface of a bone is grooved deeply.

**Guttmann** [E. *Guttmann,* German physician, flourished 20th century] Bodechtel-Guttmann disease. See under SUBACUTE SCLEROSING PANENCEPHALITIS.

**gutt. quibusd.** *guttis quibusdam* (L, with a few drops).

**guttur** \gut′oor, gut′ər\ [L, the throat] The throat.

**guttural** \gut′ərəl\ [L *guttur* the throat + -AL] **1** Concerned with or relating to the throat. **2** The quality of an individual's speech and of certain spoken languages in which there is a greater proportion of sounds produced with the posterior part of the tongue in the velar or pharyngeal regions of the vocal tract.

**Guye** [Ambroise Arnold Guillaume *Guye,* Dutch laryngologist, 1839–1904] Guye sign. See under GUYE'S APROSEXIA.

**Guyon** [Jean Casimir Felix *Guyon,* French surgeon, 1831–1920] Guyon's operation. See under AMPUTATION.

**GVH** graft-versus-host (reaction).

**GVHD** graft-versus-host disease.

**Gy** Symbol for the unit, gray.

**gymnastics** \jimnas′tiks\ **ocular g.** Exercises consisting of movement of the eyes into various positions. **Swedish g.** A system of exercises developed by a Swedish fencing master in 1813, originally for use in the military but later proposed as a means of attaining physical fitness for the general population. It involves detailed directions classifying starting positions and specific degrees of activity, and regulating dosage and progress. As a result of royal backing and the founding of the Central Institute of Gymnastics in Stockholm, this program, to which massage was added, became known as Swedish gymnastics and massage. Also *Swedish movement, Ling's method, lingism.*

**gymno-** \jim′nə-\ [Gk *gymnos* naked, lightly clad] A combining form meaning naked, bare, exposed.

***Gymnothorax*** \jim′nōthôr′aks\ A genus of marine eels of the family Muraenidae; the moray eels. They occur on tropical reefs and have caused cases of poisoning when eaten.

**gyn-** \jīn-\ GYNECO-.

**gynaeco-** \jī′nəkō-\ *Brit.* GYNECO-.

**gynaecology** *Brit.* GYNECOLOGY.

**gynaecomastia** *Brit.* GYNECOMASTIA.

***Gynaecophorus*** \gī′nəkäf′ərəs\ A former name for *SCHISTOSOMA.*

**gynandria** \jinan′drē·ə\ *Imprecise* HERMAPHRODITISM.

**gynandroblastoma** \jinan′drəblastō′mə\ [GYN- + ANDRO- + BLASTOMA] A very rare ovarian tumor in which collections of granulosa cells with typical Call-Exner bodies coexist with hollow tubules lined by Sertoli cells. Used morphologically, the term does not imply a specific type of hormone production.

**gynandroid** \jinan′droid\ [GYN- + ANDROID] FEMALE PSEUDOHERMAPHRODITE.

**gynandromorph** \jinan′drəmôrf\ [GYN- + ANDRO- + -MORPH] An individual having both male and female external genitalia and/or secondary sexual features.

**gynandromorphism** \jinan′drəmôr′fizm\ [GYN- + ANDRO- + MORPH- + -ISM] HERMAPHRODITISM.

**gynandromorphous** \jinan′drəmôr′fəs\ Possessing both male and female anatomic characteristics. Also *hermaphroditic.*

**gynatresia** \jin′ətrē′zhə\ [GYN- + ATRESIA] An occlusion of any part of the female genital tract, particularly an occlusion of the vagina by a residual urogenital membrane.

**gyne-** \jī′nə-\ GYNECO-.

**gynec-** \jī′nək-\ GYNECO-.

**gyneco-** \jī′nəkō-, jin′əkō-, gī′nəkō-\ [Gk *gynē* (genitive *gynaikos*) a woman] A combining form meaning woman or female. Also *gyn-, gyne-, gyno-, gynaeco-* (British spelling).

**gynecography** \jin′əkäg′rəfē\ [GYNECO- + -GRAPHY] Radiography of the female genital organs using air or other gas injected intraperitoneally as a contrast medium. Also *gynography.*

**gynecoid** \jin′əkoid\ [GYNEC- + -OID] Pertaining to or resembling women.

**gynecologist** \gī′nəkäl′əjist\ A physician who specializes in gynecology.

**gynecology** \gī′nəkäl′əjē\ [GYNECO- + -LOGY] The branch of medicine which devotes itself to the care and prevention of genital tract disorders in women and which for the most part is not concerned with pregnancy. Gynecology is also associated with public-health functions, and includes family planning, preconception counseling, genetic counseling, and sexual therapy. Also *gyniatry.* Adj. gynecologic, gynecological.

**gynecomania** \-mā′nē·ə\ [GYNECO- + -MANIA] SATYRIASIS.

**gynecomastia** \-mas′tē·ə\ [GYNECO- + MAST- + -IA] Enlargement of the male breast, occurring sometimes in mild form as a normal phenomenon of male puberty, and as a sequela of various pathologic conditions, such as the Klinefelter syndrome, or hepatic cirrhosis, or thyrotoxicosis. The bulk of the overgrowth is fibrous, regardless of cause. Galactorrhea occurs uncommonly. Also *mammary feminism* (older term).

**gynecophoral** \-fôr′əl\ [GYNECO- + PHOR- + -AL] See under GYNECOPHORIC CANAL.

**gynephilia** \ji′nəfil′yə\ [GYNE- + -PHILIA] SATYRIASIS.

**gyneplasty** \jī′nəplas′tē\ GYNOPLASTY.

**gyniatry** \jin′ē·at′rē\ [GYN- + -IATRY] GYNECOLOGY.

**gyno-** \jī′nə-\ GYNECO-.

**gynogenesis** \jī′nəjen′əsis\ [GYNO- + GENESIS] Development of an embryo from an egg that has been stimulated by a male gamete, but where the spermatozoon does not contribute any genetic material to the conceptus.

**gynography** \jinäg′rəfē\ GYNECOGRAPHY.

**gynoid** \jī′noid\ GYNECOID.

**gynomerogon** \jin′əmer′əgän\ [GYNO- + MERO-$^1$ + Gk *gon(os)* offspring, procreation] An organism derived from an ovum possessing solely a female pronucleus and thus with maternal chromosomes only. Also *gynomerogone.*

**gynomerogony** \jin′əmeräg′ənē\ [GYNO- + MERO-$^1$ + -GONY] Development of the part of a fertilized ovum having only the female pronucleus with its maternal chromosomes.

**gynoplasty** \jī′nəplas′tē\ [GYNO- + -PLASTY] Reconstructive surgery of the female reproductive organs. Also *gyneplasty.*

**gyr-** \jīr-\ GYRO-.

**gyral** \jī′rəl\ Pertaining to a gyrus.

**gyrase** \jī′rās\ A name for the ATP-hydrolyzing DNA topoisomerase (EC 5.99.1.3), the enzyme that unwinds the DNA helix, introducing a region of positive supercoiling into the duplex ahead of the replication fork. Also *helicase.*

**gyrate** \jī′rāt\ Twisted or coiled; convoluted.

**gyre** \jī′r\ *Obs.* GYRUS.

**gyrectomy** \jīrek′təmē\ [GYR- + -ECTOMY] Excision of a convolution, or gyrus, of the cerebrum.

**gyrencephalic** \jīren′səfal′ik\ [GYR- + ENCEPHAL- + -IC] Denoting the presence of convolutions in the cerebral cortex.

**gyri** \jī′rī\ Plural of GYRUS.

**gyro-** \jī′rə-\ [Gk *gyros* ring, circle] A combining form meaning (1) ring, ringlike; (2) rotating, rotatory. Also *gyr-.*

**gyromele** \jī′rəmēl\ [GYRO- + Gk *mēlē* a probe] A flexible rod passed through a stomach tube and rotated with any of several attachments affixed to the end. It was formerly used for stomach cleansing or other treatment and for taking specimens for culture.

## gyrus

**gyrus** \jī′rəs\ [L (from Gk *gyros* a ring, circle), a circle, circuit, ring] (*pl.* gyri) An elevation of the cerebral cortex resulting from the infolding of adjacent sulci or fissures; convolution. Also *gyre* (obs.). **g. angularis** [NA] The gyrus of the inferior parietal lobule formed by the caudal union of the superior and middle temporal gyri. Also *angular gyrus.* **gyri annectentes** The small gyri (convolutions) within the sulcal depths formed by inconstant, small indentations or furrows. Also *annectant gyri, transitional gyri, transitional convolutions.* **anterior central g.** GYRUS PRECENTRALIS. **ascending frontal g.** GYRUS PRECENTRALIS. **ascending parietal g.** GYRUS POSTCENTRALIS. **gyri breves insulae** [NA] The short, rostral gyri on the insular surface, within the lateral sulcus. Also *preinsular gyri, short gyri of insula, gyri operti* (obs.). **Broca's g.** BROCA'S MOTOR SPEECH AREA. **callosal g.** GYRUS CINGULI. **g. callosus** GYRUS CINGULI. **g. centralis anterior** GYRUS PRECENTRALIS. **g. centralis posterior** GYRUS POSTCENTRALIS. **g. cinguli** [NA] The convolution on the medial surface of the cerebrum surrounding the corpus callosum, consisting of a transitional cortex (principally Brodmann's areas 24 and 23) and the retrosplenial fields. Also *callosal convolution, mesocortex, limbic cortex, gyrus callosus, callosal gyrus, rhinencephalic arch, cingulum hemispherii, cingulate gyrus, cingulate cortex.* **g. cunei** CUNEUS. **cuneolingual gyri** The gyri on the medial surface of the human cerebral hemisphere surrounding the calcarine sulcus and containing portions of the visual areas. **deep gyri** GYRI PROFUNDI CEREBRI. **deep transitional g.** The central, transverse zone of cortex in the fetal human cerebrum that forms the buried portion of the sulcus centralis in later development. **g. dentatus** [NA] The innermost cortex of the hippocampal gyrus capping the hippocampal fissure. It consists of a zonal lamina, a densely packed granular layer, and a loose pyramidal or polymorphic layer bounded on its ventricular surface by a myelinated tract, the alveus hippocampi. Also *fascia dentata hippocampi, dentate gyrus, dentate band, dentate fascia, fascia of Tarin, fascia tarini, fasciola dentata.* **g. descendens** POSTERIOR OCCIPITAL GYRUS. **g. epicallosus** INDUSIUM GRISEUM. **external orbital g.** GYRUS ORBITALIS LATERALIS. **g. fasciolaris** [NA] The band of cortex surrounding the splenium of the corpus callosum, contiguous with the underlying induseum griseum rostrally and with the hippocampal formation ventrocaudally. Also *fasciola cinerea cinguli, fascia cinerea, splenial gyrus.* **g. fornicatus** LIMBIC LOBE. **g. frontalis inferior** [NA] The inferior convolution below the inferior frontal sulcus of the anthropoid cerebral cortex, divided into triangular, orbital, and opercular sectors by branches of the lateral sulcus. Also *Broca's convolution, inferior frontal gyrus, Broca's region.* **g. frontalis medialis** [NA] A convolution on the medial surface of the frontal lobe, lying above the sulcus cinguli and extending dorsally to meet the superior frontal gyrus. Also *medial frontal gyrus, gyrus marginalis, marginal gyrus of Turner.* **g. frontalis medius** [NA] The middle convolution of the frontal lobe, extending rostrally from the precentral gyrus and bordered by the superior and inferior frontal sulci. Also *middle frontal gyrus.* **g. frontalis superior** [NA] A frontal lobe convolution extending forward from the precentral gyrus above the sulcus frontalis superior. Also *superior frontal gyrus.* **g. fusiformis** A convolution on the ventral surface of the temporal lobe, bounded laterally by the inferior temporal gyrus and limited medially by the collateral and rhinal sulci. It comprises medial and lateral lobules, the gyri occipitotemporalis medialis and lateralis. Also *fusiform gyrus, fusiform lobule.* **g. geniculi** GYRUS SUBCALLOSUS. **Heschl's gyri** The obliquely oriented transverse temporal gyri lying on the temporal operculum of the lateral sulcus. They are the site of the primary auditory cortex (Brodmann's area 41 and probably a portion of area 42). Also *Heschl's convolutions.* **hippocampal g.** 1 GYRUS HIPPOCAMPI. 2 *Imprecise* GYRUS PARAHIPPOCAMPALIS. **g. hippocampi** 1 [NA] The hippocampal cortical fields (of Ammon's horn), sometimes including the fascia dentata and the subiculum. Also *hippocampal gyrus.* 2 *Imprecise* HIPPOCAMPAL FORMATION. **inferior frontal g.** GYRUS FRONTALIS INFERIOR. **inferior occipital g.** The more ventral of the two gyri on the lateral surface of the occipital lobe, limited anteriorly by the occipital lateral sulcus. **inferior temporal g.** GYRUS TEMPORALIS INFERIOR.

**g. infracalcarinus** GYRUS LINGUALIS. **gyri insulae** [NA] The gyri forming the surface of the insula, deep within the lateral sulcus, comprising the gyrus longus insulae and the gyri breves insulae. **internal orbital g.** GYRUS ORBITALIS MEDIALIS. **g. intralimbicus** The caudal bulge of the uncus at its junction with the hippocampus. **lateral occipital gyri** The two gyri (superior and inferior) on the lateral surface of the occipital lobe, delimited by the lateral occipital sulcus. **lateral occipitotemporal g.** GYRUS OCCIPITOTEMPORALIS LATERALIS. **g. limbicus** LIMBIC LOBE. **g. lingualis** [NA] A rostrally oriented, tongue-shaped gyrus on the medial and ventral surfaces of the occipital and temporal lobes, separated from the cuneus by the calcarine sulcus and from the fusiform gyrus by the collateral sulcus. It is the site of contralateral, upper quadrant visual field representation. Also *gyrus infracalcarinus, lingual gyrus.* **g. longus insulae** [NA] The largest and most caudal of the longitudinally oriented gyri of the insula. It lies within the lateral sulcus. Also *long gyrus of insula.* **g. marginalis** GYRUS FRONTALIS MEDIALIS. **marginal g. of Turner** GYRUS FRONTALIS MEDIALIS. **medial frontal g.** GYRUS FRONTALIS MEDIALIS. **medial occipitotemporal g.** GYRUS OCCIPITOTEMPORALIS MEDIALIS. **middle frontal g.** GYRUS FRONTALIS MEDIUS. **middle temporal g.** GYRUS TEMPORALIS MEDIUS. **g. occipitotemporalis lateralis** [NA] The lateral portion of the fusiform gyrus. It is continuous with the inferior temporal gyrus laterally and is separated from the medial portion of the fusiform gyrus by the occipitotemporal sulcus. Also *lateral occipitotemporal gyrus, occipitotemporal convolution.* **g. occipitotemporalis medialis** [NA] The medial portion of the fusiform gyrus. It lies on the ventral surface of the temporal lobe and extends between the collateral sulcus and the occipitotemporal sulcus. Also *medial occipitotemporal gyrus.* **gyri operti** *Obs.* GYRI BREVES INSULAE. **gyri orbitales** [NA] The several irregular convolutions on the basal surface of the frontal lobe overlying the orbit and lateral to the olfactory sulcus. Also *orbital gyri.* **g. orbitalis lateralis** The most lateral of the contiguous convoluted orbital gyri on the base of the human frontal lobe. Also *external orbital gyrus.* **g. orbitalis medialis** The most medial of the contiguous convoluted orbital gyri on the base of the human frontal lobe cortex. Also *internal orbital gyrus.* **g. paracentralis** A convolution on the medial surface of the cerebral hemisphere continuous with the precentral and postcentral gyri at the termination of the central sulcus, bounded ventrally by the cingulate sulcus. It is the site of sensory and motor representation of the lower extremities and of a separate, supplementary representation of the entire body (called the supplementary motor cortex). Also *paracentral gyrus.* **g. parahippocampalis** [NA] A convolution on the ventral and medial surface of the temporal lobe, lying between the hippocampal sulcus medially and the collateral (rhinal) sulcus laterally. It contains the subicular and entorhinal cortical fields. Also *parahippocampal gyrus, hippocampal gyrus* (imprecise). **parahippocaudal g.** The cerebral cortex between the rhinal fissure marking the neocortical boundary and the hippocampal fissure marking the site of contact with the hippocampus proper. **parasplenial g.** A convolution on the medial surface of the carnivore brain adjacent to the splenium. It is bordered superiorly by the parasplenial sulcus, and inferiorly by the corpus callosum. **paraterminal g.** GYRUS SUBCALLOSUS. **g. paraterminalis** [NA] GYRUS SUBCALLOSUS. **g. postcentralis** [NA] The rostral convolution of the parietal lobe, lying behind the central sulcus and anterior to the postcentral sulcus. It is the primary area of somatosensory cortex, corresponding approximately to Brodmann's areas 3, 1, and 2. Also *posterior central gyrus, postrolandic gyrus, ascending parietal gyrus, gyrus centralis posterior, postcentral gyrus.* **posterior occipital g.** The inferior portion of the gyrus occipitalis lateralis. Also *gyrus descendens.* **postrolandic g.** GYRUS POSTCENTRALIS. **precentral g.** GYRUS PRECENTRALIS. **g. precentralis** [NA] The caudal convolution of the frontal lobe anterior to the central sulcus. It is the thickest cortical area, the principal site of origin of the corticospinal tract, and the principal motor area, corresponding approximately to Brodmann's area 4 and a portion of area 6. Also *anterior central gyrus, precentral gyrus, prerolandic gyrus, ascending frontal gyrus, gyrus centralis anterior.* **preinsular gyri** GYRI BREVES INSULAE. **prerolandic g.** GYRUS PRECENTRALIS. **gyri profundi cerebri** Gyri of cerebral cortex, formed within the depths of sulci, that reach the surface. Also *deep gyri.* **quadrate g.** *Seldom used* PRECUNEUS. **g. rectus** [NA] The medial convolution on the orbital surface of the frontal lobe, bordered laterally by the olfactory sulcus. Also *straight gyrus.* **retrosplenial g.** The posterior continuation of the cingulate gyrus, extending behind the splenium of the corpus callosum. See also RETROSPLENIAL CORTEX. **g. of Retzius** **1** GYRUS INTRALIMBICUS. **2** LIMEN INSULAE. **g. rolandicus** A rarely found gyrus of the human cerebral cortex in the anomalous condition in which two central sulci are present. **short gyri of insula** GYRI BREVES INSULAE. **splenial g.** GYRUS FASCIOLARIS. **straight g.** GYRUS RECTUS. **subcalcarine g.** The gyrus forming the inferior lip of the calcarine sulcus. **g. subcallosus** [NA] A thin, paramedian gyrus rostral and ventral to the genu of the corpus callosum. Also *gyrus paraterminalis, Zuckerkandl's convolution, subcallosal gyrus, gyrus geniculi, external marginal arc of Zuckerkandl, area paraterminalis, septal area, paraterminal gyrus, corpus paraterminalis, pedunculus corporis callosi* (obs.). **superior frontal g.** GYRUS FRONTALIS SUPERIOR. **superior occipital g.** The uppermost of the gyri on the lateral surface of the occipital lobe, lying above the lateral occipital sulcus. **superior temporal g.** GYRUS TEMPORALIS SUPERIOR. **g. supracallosus** The thin horizontal band lying between the cingulate gyrus and the corpus callosum containing the indusium griseum (hippocampal rudiment). Also *supracallosal gyrus.* **g. supramarginalis** [NA] The convolution of the inferior portion of the parietal lobe surrounding the caudal end of the lateral sulcus and continuous anteriorly with the superior temporal gyrus. Also *supramarginal gyrus.* **gyri temporales transversi** [NA] The transverse convolutions of the superior temporal gyrus lying within the lateral sulcus. It is the site of the primary auditory cortex. The anterior transverse temporal gyrus is called Heschl's gyrus or convolution. Also *transverse temporal gyri.* **g. temporalis inferior** [NA] The longitudinal inferolateral gyrus of the temporal lobe, below the inferior temporal sulcus and continuous caudally with the lateral occipitotemporal gyrus. Also *inferior temporal gyrus.* **g. temporalis medius** [NA] The middle longitudinal gyrus of the temporal lobe, bounded by the superior and inferior temporal sulci. Also *second temporal convolution, middle temporal gyrus.* **g. temporalis superior** [NA] The horizontal, dorsal sulcus of the temporal lobe lying above the superior temporal sulcus and below the lateral sulcus, merging caudally with the supramarginal gyrus. Also *first temporal convolution, superior temporal gyrus.* **transitional gyri** GYRI ANNECTENTES. **transverse gyri of Heschl** AUDITORY CORTEX. **transverse temporal gyri** GYRI TEMPORA-

LES TRANSVERSI. **uncinate g.** UNCUS. **g. uncinatus** UNCUS.

**Gy/s** Symbol for the unit, gray per second.
**Gy·s$^{-1}$** Symbol for the unit, gray per second.

# H

**H** 1 Symbol for the element, hydrogen. 2 Symbol for histidine.
**$^2$H** Symbol for deuterium.
**$^3$H** Symbol for tritium.
**h** 1 Symbol for hecto-: used with SI units. 2 Symbol for the unit, hour.
***H*** 1 Symbol for the quantity, magnetic field strength, expressed in amperes per meter. 2 Symbol for the quantity, magnetization, expressed in amperes per meter.
**Haab** [Otto *Haab,* Swiss ophthalmologist, 1850–1931] 1 See under REFLEX. 2 Biber-Haab-Dimmer dystrophy. See under LATTICE DYSTROPHY OF THE CORNEA.
**Haagensen** [Cushman Davis *Haagensen,* U.S. surgeon, born 1900] See under TEST.
**haarscheibe** \här′shībə\ [German *Haar* + *Scheibe* disk] HAIR DISK.
**Habel** [Karl *Habel,* U.S. virologist, born 1908] See under METHOD.
**habena** \həbē′nə\ [L (from *habere* to have, hold), a thong, strap] Any straplike fibrous structure, resembling a bridle; frenum.
**habenula** \həben′yələ\ [dim. of *habena.* See HABENA.] (*pl.* habenulae) 1 A small, straplike fibrous structure; frenulum. 2 [NA] A caudal, dorsal thalamic nuclear group derived from the embryonic epithalamus bordering the third ventricle. Its association with the overlying pineal gland is evident in some species. The habenular complex consists of a medial nucleus with neurosecretory cells, and a lateral nucleus from which the main efferent tract, the habenulointerpeduncular tract, arises. Also *habenula conarii, habenular body.* **h. conarii** HABENULA. **h. perforata** FORAMINA NERVOSA LIMBUS LAMINAE SPIRALIS OSSEAE. **h. urethralis** Either of the two whitish lines extending from the external urethral orifice to the glans clitoridis in young females, considered by some to be related to the two slender bands of erectile tissue connecting the anterior ends of the bulbs of the vestibule to the glans. *Outmoded.*
**habenular** \həben′yələr\ Denoting the habenula.
**Haber** [Henry *Haber,* English dermatologist, flourished mid-20th century] See under SYNDROME.
**Habermann** [Rudolf *Habermann,* German dermatologist, 1884–1941] Habermann's disease, Mucha-Habermann disease, Mucha-Habermann syndrome. See under PITYRIASIS LICHENOIDES.
**habilitation** \həbil′itā′shən\ [Med L *habilitatio* (from Late L *habilitatus,* past part. of *habilitare* to make suitable) a making suitable or fit] Training given to develop skills not previously possessed, as in compensation for early-acquired handicaps or congenital defects. Also *compensatory education.*
**habit** [L *habitus.* See HABITUS.] 1 A learned response, practiced often enough to have become relatively permanent and virtually automatic, requiring very little conscious attention for an efficient execution. Habitual responses are notable for their invariance and ease of evocation. 2 A habitus or diathesis. **position h.** The tendency for an experimental subject to go to a specific place in the test apparatus, or to select one side consistently in making a discrimination response. **tongue h.** Habitual malposition of the tongue, as in the forward malposition of lisping.
**habituation** \həbich′oo·ā′shən\ [Med L *habituatio* (from Late L *habituare* to bring into a bodily condition, from L *habitus* condition, habit) habituation] 1 The process of gradual adaptation to a stimulus or an environment. 2 The development of a habit of using, or psychological dependence on, a nonaddictive or potentially addictive substance. See also ADDICTION.
**habitus** \hab′itəs\ [L (from *habitus,* past. part. of *habere* to have, hold), habit, condition, fashion, state of health, attire] 1 Physical appearance; physique or attitude. 2 The physical appearance of one who is particularly subject to a specific disease or condition. **h. phthisicus** A general bodily appearance, characterized by pallor, thinness, and limited muscular and osseous development, formerly thought to indicate a predisposition to tuberculosis.
**habu** \hä′boo\ The highly venomous snake *Trimeresurus flavoviridis,* found on the Ryukyu Islands.
**hachement** \äshmäN′\ [French (from *hache(r)* to cut into small pieces + *-ment* -MENT), a cutting into small pieces] A form of massage in which the therapist uses chopping or hacking strokes to improve circulation and muscle tone.
**HACS** hyperactive child syndrome.
**Hadfield** [Geoffrey *Hadfield,* English pathologist, born 1889] Hadfield-Clarke syndrome. See under CLARKE-HADFIELD SYNDROME.
***Hadrurus*** \hadroo′rəs\ A genus of scorpions characterized by having many setae on the stinger. The most common species is *H. arizonensis,* the large hairy scorpion, found in the southwestern United States. It has a very painful sting but there is very little systemic reaction to it.
**Haeckel** [Ernst Heinrich *Haeckel,* German biologist, 1834–1919] Haeckel's law, Müller-Haeckel law. See under RECAPITULATION THEORY.
**haem** \hēm\ *Brit.* HEME.
**haem-** \hēm-, hem-\ *Brit.* HEM-. See under HEMO-.
***Haemadipsa*** \hē′mədip′sə\ [HAEM- + *a* + Gk *dipsa* thirst] A genus of terrestrial leeches of the family Gnathobdellidae, found in the Far East and South America, especially in tropical forests. The leeches, 2–3 cm long when not engorged, are found on leaves and under stones in damp places and quickly drop onto or attach to human or animal skin, adhere with their posterior sucker, lacerate a wound that bleeds freely, and engorge large amounts of blood, usually exceeding their body weight and more than doubling their volume.
***Haemagogus*** \hē′məgō′gəs\ A genus of tree-hole-breeding treetop mosquitoes, many species of which are vectors of jungle yellow fever in Central and South America. They are closely related to *Aedes,* with brilliantly metallic colors. Some of the important species in the transmission of jungle yellow fever, such as *H. spegazzinii falco* and *H. splendens,* have become adapted to breeding in waterfilled hollows, tree stumps, cut bamboo stalks, or even old tires and water tanks

at the forest fringe.

**haemangioma** *Brit.* HEMANGIOMA.

***Haemaphysalis*** \hē′məfī′səlis\ [HAEM- + *a* + Gk *physalis* a bladder, bubble] A genus of mostly small inornate ticks characterized by a lack of eyes, the presence of festoons, and a distinctive basis capituli. The sexes are usually similar. The larvae and nymphs parasitize small mammals and birds, and the adults are found on larger animals and some birds. Among the approximately 150 species described, several are medically important as vectors of infectious agents, particularly viruses. ***H. cinnabarina*** A species, found principally in the drier regions of British Columbia, containing strains which can cause tick paralysis, or ascending paraplegia, in humans and various animals. ***H. concinna*** A vector of *Rickettsia sibirica,* the agent of Siberian tick typhus. It is also a vector of a form of Russian spring-summer encephalitis virus found in China and the eastern USSR. ***H. leporispalustris*** The rabbit tick, widely distributed in the western hemisphere. It is a vector of Colorado tick fever virus, rickettsias including the agent of Rocky Mountain spotted fever, and *Francisella tularensis,* the agent of tularemia. It is medically important only in maintaining infection in wild animal reservoir hosts. ***H. spinigera*** A species that transmits Kyasanur Forest disease among tropical forest workers in India.

**haemato-** \hē′mətō-\ *Brit.* HEMATO-. See under HEMO-.

***Haematobia*** \hē′mətō′bē·ə\ A genus of muscid flies, including highly irritating and economically costly horn flies such as *H. irritans* and *H. minuta.*

**haematocrit** \hēmat′əkrit\ *Brit.* HEMATOCRIT.

**haematology** \hē′mətäl′əjē\ *Brit.* HEMATOLOGY.

**haematoma** *Brit.* HEMATOMA.

***Haematopinus suis*** \hē′mətōpī′nəs soo′is\ A large (5–6 mm) louse of swine, the so-called blue louse or common pig louse. It is the only louse infesting pigs and it is cosmopolitan in distribution. It is a serious pest of hogs and also feeds readily on humans.

***Haematosiphon*** \hē′mətōsī′fən\ A genus of bedbugs similar to *Cimex,* but with longer legs and an unusually elongated sucking proboscis and beak. ***H. inodorus*** The poultry bug or Mexican chicken bug; a bedbug that attacks chickens, owls, eagles, and condors in southwestern United States and Mexico. It rarely attacks humans though it may be severe among poultry handlers.

**haematuria** \hē′mətʸoo′rē·ə\ *Brit.* HEMATURIA.

***Haementeria*** \hē′menter′ē·ə\ A genus of leeches in the family Rhynchobdellidae. It includes *H. officinalis,* the medicinal leech of South and Central America. Also *Hementaria.*

**-haemia** \-hē′mē·ə\ *Brit.* -HEMIA.

**haemo-** \hē′mō-\ *Brit.* HEMO-.

**haemodialysis** \-dī·al′isis\ *Brit.* HEMODIALYSIS.

**haemoglobin** \hē′məglō′bin, hē′məglō′bin\ *Brit.* HEMOGLOBIN.

**haemoglobinuria** \-glō′binoo′rē·ə\ *Brit.* HEMOGLOBINURIA.

**haemolysis** \hēmäl′isis\ *Brit.* HEMOLYSIS.

**haemolytic** \-lit′ik\ *Brit.* HEMOLYTIC.

**haemophilia** *Brit.* HEMOPHILIA.

***Haemophilus*** \hēmäf′iləs\ [HAEMO- + Gk *philos* beloved, loving] A genus of small, Gram-negative, nonmotile facultatively anaerobic coccobacilli with complex growth requirements provided by blood. These requirements include the heat-stable factor X (hemin) and the heat-labile factor V (nicotinamide adenine dinucleotide). They are generally grown on chocolate agar, in which mild heating has released the factors and destroyed an inhibitor of factor V. Growth is often enhanced by elevated carbon dioxide concentrations. The major species is *H. influenzae.* Also *Hemophilus.* ***H. aegyptius*** A species, very similar to *H. influenzae,* that produces purulent conjunctivitis. Also *Koch-Weeks bacillus.* ***H. ducreyi*** A hemophilus that causes chancroid. Also *Ducrey's bacillus.* ***H. haemolyticus*** A nonpathogenic hemophilus often present in the upper respiratory tract. It forms β-hemolytic colonies, especially with rabbit blood, that are easily mistaken for those of *Streptococcus pyogenes.* ***H. influenzae*** A hemophilus found normally in the human nasopharynx; the influenza bacillus. Strains with polysaccharide capsules, of six types (designated *a* to *f*), may cause disease. Type *b* is the most frequent. The organism is the commonest cause of meningitis in children. It also causes sinusitis, otitis media, pneumonia, arthritis, and a fulminating epiglottitis and obstructive laryngitis. The organism was once considered, mistakenly, the cause of pandemic influenza. Also *Pfeiffer's bacillus.* ***H. parainfluenzae*** An organism closely related to *H. influenzae,* often found as a commensal in the human respiratory tract.

**haemorrhage** \hem′ərij\ *Brit.* HEMORRHAGE.

**haemorrhoids** \hem′əroidz\ *Brit.* HEMORRHOIDS.

**haemosiderosis** \-sid′ərō′sis\ *Brit.* HEMOSIDEROSIS.

**Haemosporidia** \hē′mōspôrid′ē·ə\ [pl. of HAEMOSPORIDIUM.] A former order of sporozoans in the class Telosporidia, equivalent to the present suborder Haemosporina in the order Eucoccidiida, class Sporozoea. Many of the most important pathogens of humans, domestic animals, and birds are included, notably the malarial parasites of the genus *Plasmodium* and various bird pathogens included in the genus *Leucocytozoon..* Also *Hemosporidia.*

**haemosporidian** \hē′mōspôrid′ē·ən\ **1** Pertaining to or belonging to the former sporozoan order Haemosporidia (now replaced by the suborder Haemosporina). **2** A member of the Haemosporidia (Haemosporina).

**haemosporidium** \hē′mōspôrid′ē·əm\ [HAEMO- + SPOR- + -IDIUM] (*pl.* haemosporidia) Any of the sporozoan blood parasites formerly classified as members of the order Haemosporidia and now as members of the suborder Haemosporina. Also *hemosporidium, hematosporidium.*

**Haemosporina** \hē′mōspôr′inə\ A suborder of sporozoans in the order Eucoccidiida, equivalent to the former order Haemosporidia. It includes the genera *Haemoproteus, Hepatocystis, Leucocytozoon,* and *Plasmodium..*

**haemostasis** \hēmäs′təsis, hē′mōstā′sis\ *Brit.* HEMOSTASIS.

**haemostatic** \-stat′ik\ *Brit.* HEMOSTATIC.

**haemothorax** \-thôr′aks\ *Brit.* HEMOTHORAX.

**haemozoin** \-zō′in\ *Brit.* HEMOZOIN.

**Haenel** [Heinrich G. *Haenel,* German neurologist, 1874–1942] Haenel's variant. See under SYMPTOM.

**Haffkine** [Waldemar Mordecai Wolff *Haffkine,* Russian bacteriologist, 1860–1930] See under VACCINE.

***Hafnia alvei*** \haf′nē·ə alvē′ī\ An enterobacterium found in feces and in nature. It is an opportunistic pathogen. Also *Enterobacter hafniae, Enterobacter alvei.*

**hafnium** Element number 72, having atomic weight 178.49. It is found combined in minerals containing zirconium, which it resembles chemically. One of its six natural isotopes, hafnium 74, is radioactive, having a half-life of $2 \times 10^{15}$ years and emitting alpha particles. Many additional radioactive isotopes have been identified, with mass numbers ranging from 168 to 183 and half-lives from 5 seconds to $9 \times 10^{6}$ years. The metal absorbs neutrons and is used to make control rods for nuclear reactors. Symbol: Hf

**Hagedorn** [Werner *Hagedorn,* German surgeon, 1831–1894] See under NEEDLE.

**Haglund** [Sims Emil Patrik *Haglund*, Swedish physician, 1870–1937] Haglund's disease, Haglund's deformity. See under ACHILLES BURSITIS.

**hahnemannism** \hä′nəmənizʹm\ [after Samuel C. F. *Hahnemann*, German physician, 1755–1843 + -ISM] HOMEOPATHY.

**Haidinger** [Wilhelm Karl von *Haidinger*, Austrian mineralogist, 1795–1871] Haidinger's brushes. See under BRUSH.

**Haig Ferguson** [James *Haig Ferguson*, Scottish obstetrician, born 1862] See under FORCEPS.

**Hailey** [Hugh E. *Hailey*, U.S. dermatologist, born 1909] Hailey-Hailey disease. See under BENIGN FAMILIAL PEMPHIGUS.

**Hailey** [William Howard *Hailey*, U.S. dermatologist, 1898–1967] Hailey-Hailey disease. See under BENIGN FAMILIAL PEMPHIGUS.

**hair** [Old English *hær*] A keratinized threadlike skin appendage consisting of cornified epidermal cells that is formed in specialized follicles and is a characteristic feature of mammals; pilus. **auditory h.'s** The stereocilia and kinocilia of each cellula sensoria pilosa located on the inner surface of the utricle, saccule, and semicircular ducts and in the auditory portion of the inner ear. The cells communicate with afferent vestibular fibers. *Imprecise.* **bamboo h.** TRICHORRHEXIS INVAGINATA. **bayonet h.** A structural defect of the hair shaft in which the shaft tapers to a fine point above a spindle-shaped thickening of the cortex immediately below the tip of the hair. The origin of the defect is uncertain. **beaded h.** Hair characterized by regular elliptical nodes separated by internodes. It is a shaft defect characteristic of monilethrix. Also *moniliform hair.* **burrowing h.** A hair that fails to emerge from the follicle and grows into its wall. **club h.** A hair in the telogen phase of the hair cycle. It is the state in which it is shed in all physiologic and in some pathologic circumstances. Also *resting hair.* **exclamation point h.** A broken hair shaft of normal caliber and 5–10 mm in length, tapering to an atrophic or shrunken bulb or to a more or less normal club. Such hairs are characteristic of the periphery of extending patches of alopecia areata. **Frey's h.'s** A device composed of stiff hairs mounted at right angles to the end of a wooden handle. It is used to measure skin touch sensitivity. The hairs are graded in tensile strength and can be flexed according to the degree of pressure exerted, thus enabling the examiner to measure sensory tactile acuity. **gustatory h.'s** The hairlike protrusions of taste cells, consisting of microvilli. Also *taste hairs.* **ingrown h.** The penetration of the surface epidermis or the wall of a follicle by the tip of a tightly coiled hair. It commonly occurs on the neck, when the resulting inflammatory changes give rise to pseudofolliculitis. **moniliform h.** BEADED HAIR. **pubic h.** The terminal hair of the mons pubis. **resting h.** CLUB HAIR. **ringed h.** A hereditary defect of the hair shaft in which light bands on the shaft mark areas containing an increased number of air spaces within the cortex. Also *thrix annulata.* **sensory h.'s** The hairlike cilia, stereocilia, and microvilli of the sensory cells of the olfactory epithelium, the hair cells of the organ of Corti, the ampullary crests and the maculae of the utricle and saccule, and the cells of the taste buds. **stellate h.** A hair that shows terminal splitting, the divergent parts of the hair assuming a starlike pattern. **stinging h.'s** Rigid, glandular hairlike structures found on certain plants and urticating insects, such as the tussock moths, browntail moths, and other caterpillars that secrete an irritating or acrid fluid at the base of the stinging hair or spine. **taste h.'s** GUSTATORY HAIRS. **terminal h.** The long, strong hair of the scalp, eyebrows, eyelashes, male beard, axillae, and pubic region of the adult human.

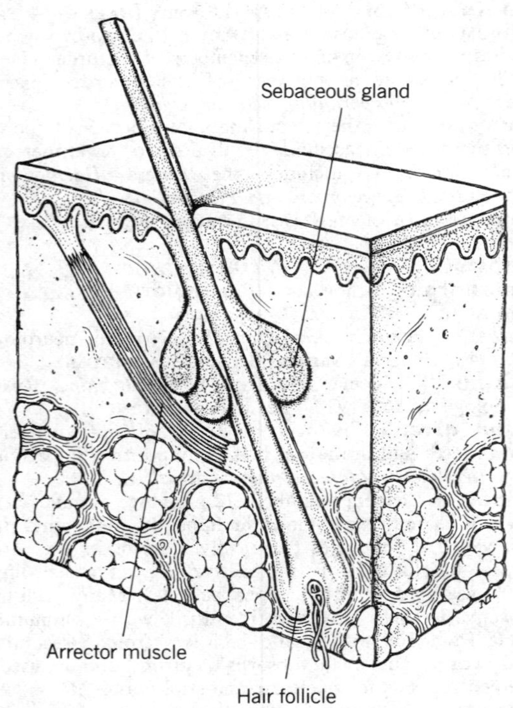


**Hair**

**hairball** TRICHOBEZOAR.

**haircast** A trichobezoar which has filled and acquired the shape of a segment of the alimentary canal, usually the stomach.

**hairworm** [HAIR + WORM] **1** A nematode worm of the genus *Trichostrongylus.*. **2** A nematode worm of the genus *Capillaria.*. **3** HORSEHAIR WORM.

**Hajek** [M. *Hajek*, Austrian otolaryngologist, 1861–1941] See under OPERATION.

**Halban** [Josef Van *Halban*, Austrian gynecologist, 1870–1937] See under SIGN.

**halcinonide** $C_{24}H_{32}ClFO_5$. 21-Chloro-9α-fluoro-11β-hydroxy-16α,17α-isopropylidenedioxypregn-4-ene-3,20-dione, a synthetic steroidal agent that is used topically as an anti-inflammatory medication.

**Haldane** [John Burdon Sanderson *Haldane*, Scottish geneticist, 1892–1964] See under LAW.

**Haldane** [John Scott *Haldane*, Scottish physiologist, 1860–1936] **1** Haldane's chamber. See under HALDANE APPARATUS. **2** Haldane-Priestley sampling. See under SAMPLING. **3** See under EFFECT.

**half-cycle** Half of a sequential movement or period.

**half-layer** HALF-VALUE LAYER.

**half-life** **1** See under RADIOACTIVE HALF-LIFE. **2** The time taken for the concentration of a substance to fall to half its initial value. This time is independent of the initial concentration in many processes, as for example in radioactive decay, and approximately so for others, as in the elimination of many foreign substances from the body. **antibody h.** A measurement of the mean lifetime of antibodies after synthesis, most often referring to the time required to eliminate 50 percent of a known quantity of immunoglobulin from the circulation. **effective h.** The time required for half of the original amount of a constituent to disappear from a biological or other system, whether because of radioactive decay or any other process such as diffusion or chemical change. Symbol: $t^1/_2$ **physical h.** RADIOACTIVE HALF-LIFE. **radioactive h.** The time required for the radioactivity of a sample of a radionuclide to decrease to half of its initial value, and thus the time when half of its atoms have disintegrated. The half-life of a radionuclide is a physical constant which is equal to 0.693 divided by the disintegration constant. Also *physical half-life.* Symbol: $T^1/_2$

**half-moon** A crescent-shaped structure or marking; a lunula or demilune. **red h.** The suffused lunula characteristic of cardiac failure.

**half-thickness** HALF-VALUE LAYER.

**half-time** The time after which half remains of the amount originally present of a given substance. This time will be constant for any substance being destroyed by a first-order reaction, e.g. radioactive decay. See also HALF-LIFE.

**halide** Any of the ions, or the salts that contain them, derived from a halogen atom by addition of an electron.

**halisteresis** \həlis′tərē′sis\ [Gk *hals,* gen. *hal(os)* salt + *i* + *sterēsis* (from *sterein* to deprive) lack, deprivation] *Obs.* OSTEOMALACIA. **h. cerea** A waxlike softening of bone.

**halitosis** \hal′itō′sis\ [L *halit(us)* breath, exhalation + -OSIS] FETOR ORIS.

**halitus** \hal′itəs\ [L, breath, vapor, exhalation] Breath; exhalation. **h. saturninus** LEAD BREATH.

**Hallé** [Adrien Joseph Marie Noel *Hallé,* French physician, 1859–1947] See under POINT.

**Haller** [Albrecht von *Haller,* Swiss physiologist, 1708–1777] **1** See under CHANNEL, ANSA. **2** Haller's line. See under FISSURA MEDIANA ANTERIOR MEDULLAE SPINALIS. **3** Lateral lumbocostal arch of Haller. See under LIGAMENTUM ARCUATUM LATERALE. **4** Haller's arches. See under ARCH. **5** Haller's crypts. See under GLANDULAE PREPUTIALES. **6** Medial lumbocostal arch of Haller. See under LIGAMENTUM ARCUATUM MEDIALE. **7** Venous ring of Haller. See under PLEXUS VENOSUS AREOLARIS. **8** Haller's cones. See under LOBULI EPIDIDYMIDIS. **9** Haller's layer, Haller's membrane. See under LAMINA VASCULOSA CHOROIDEAE. **10** Haller's aberrant ductule. See under DUCTULUS ABERRANS INFERIOR.

**Hallervorden** [Julius *Hallervorden,* German neurologist, 1882–1965] Hallervorden-Spatz syndrome. See under HALLERVORDEN-SPATZ DISEASE.

**hallex** \hal′eks\ HALLUX.

**Hallgren** [Bertil *Hallgren,* Swedish geneticist, flourished mid-20th century] See under SYNDROME.

**Hallopeau** [François Henri *Hallopeau,* French dermatologist, 1842–1919] **1** Hallopeau's acrodermatitis. See under ACRODERMATITIS CONTINUA. **2** Hallopeau-Siemens syndrome. See under EPIDERMOLYSIS BULLOSA DYSTROPHICA (RECESSIVE).

**halluces** \hal′yəsēz\ Plural of HALLUX.

**hallucination** \həloo′sinā′shən\ [L *hallucinatio* or *alucinatio* (from *hallucinari* or *alucinari* to daydream, dote, from Gk *alyein* to wander in the mind, be ill at ease) idle dream, delusion] A false sensory perception unrelated to any external stimulus, such as hearing voices when one is alone in a forest, or seeing people coming out of the fireplace when one is in an empty room. **autoscopic h.** AUTOSCOPY. **blank h.** A hallucination in which there is a disorder of one's sense of equilibrium and space. It may be typified by the rhythmic approaching and receding of objects. Also *Isakower phenomenon, dream screen, abstract perception.* **epileptic h.** A somatosensory, visual, or auditory hallucination, occurring either as one manifestation or as the entire evidence of an attack of epilepsy, and usually resulting from neuronal discharge arising in the sensory association areas. Epileptic hallucinations can be differentiated from epileptic illusions and from attacks of primary sensory epilepsy. Also *hallucinatory aura* (incorrect). **hypnagogic h.** A hallucination, usually visual, that occurs during the transitional phase from being awake to sleeping. **hypnopompic h.** A hallucination, usually visual, that occurs in the half-awake state between sleeping and full arousal. **lilliputian h.** MICROPSIA. **microptic h.** MICROPSIA. **h. of perception** An auditory hallucination involving a voice whose origin is outside the body of the subject. **psychomotor h.** A hallucination that parts of one's body are being transferred to different regions of the body. **stump h.** PHANTOM LIMB.

**hallucinatory** \həloo′sinətôr′ē\ Pertaining to or characterized by hallucinations.

**hallucinogen** \həloo′sinəjən, hal′yəsin′əjən\ A drug that is capable of producing hallucinations, such as mescaline or LSD. Also *psychotomimetic, psychotogen.*

**hallucinogenic** \həloo′sinəjen′ik\ Giving rise to hallucinations. Also *psychotogenic, psychotomimetic.*

**hallucinosis** \həloo′sinō′sis\ [*hallucin(ation)* + -OSIS] The occurrence of hallucinations, usually visual or auditory, without disorientation or intellectual impairment. Adj. hallucinotic. **acute alcoholic h.** An acute hallucinatory state occurring in a clear intellectual state and without other features of delirium, sometimes observed in alcoholics following an unusual excess of alcohol intake or, less commonly, as a part of alcohol withdrawal. Most often the hallucinations are auditory and derogatory or critical in content, and sometimes they are accompanied by paranoid delusions of a persecutory nature.

**hallucinotic** \həloo′sinät′ik\ Characterized by hallucinosis; causing or subject to hallucinations.

**hallux** \hal′uks\ [L, the big toe] [NA] The big toe; the first digit of the foot. Also *pollex pedis, hallex, great toe, digitus primus, digitus I.* **h. dolorosa** A painful condition of the big toe that is seen in flatfoot deformity. **h. flexus** A hammer toe deformity characterized by acute flexion of the interphalangeal joint. Also *hallux malleus.* **h. malleus** HALLUX FLEXUS. **h. rigidus** A painful limitation of motion in the metatarsophalangeal joint of the big toe in flexion. Also *stiff toe.* **h. valgus** A displacement of the big toe away from the midline at the metatarsophalangeal joint. When the joint is covered with an adventitious bursa, it is called a bunion. **h. varus** A displacement of the big toe towards the midline and away from the other toes.

**halmatogenesis** \hal′mətōjen′əsis\ [Gk *halma* a leap, jump, + GENESIS] SALTATORY VARIATION.

**halo** \hā′lō\ [L (from Gk *halōs* a threshing floor, the disk of the sun or moon), a halo, circle around the sun or moon] **1** A circumferential scattering of light around its focus or origin. **2** A type of cranial skeletal traction used to immobilize the neck or keep pressure off the scalp. **anemic h.** A pale area surrounding a skin lesion. **glaucomatous h.** A rainbow-colored ring seen around lights when the cornea is edematous due to increased intraocular pressure. Also *halo glaucomatosus.* **peripapillary senile h.** CIRCUMPAPILLARY CHORIORETINAL ATROPHY. **h. sat-**

**urninus** LEAD LINE. **senile h.** CIRCUMPAPILLARY CHORIORETINAL ATROPHY.

**halo-** \hal′ō\ [Gk *hals,* gen. *halos* (akin to L *sal* salt) salt] **1** A combining form designating a salt. **2** A combining form designating replacement of a hydrogen atom by an atom of any halogen.

**halodermia** \-dur′mē·ə\ [*halo(gen)* + DERM- + -IA] A skin condition caused by exposure to certain halogens, such as bromine, chlorine, and iodine, either by inhalation, ingestion, or skin absorption.

**halogen** [HALO- + -GEN] An element of group VII of the periodic table, including fluorine, chlorine, bromine, iodine, and astatine. All form stable anions on addition of an electron to an atom of the element.

**halogenation** \hal′əjənā′shən\ The chemical reaction of adding halogen to a molecule. This may be by an addition of the element to a double bond, or it may be by a substitution reaction. Such reactions are common in organic synthesis. Tyrosine is halogenated to form diiodotyrosine in the biosynthesis of thyroxin.

**halometer** \hālām′ətər\ A device for measuring the scattering of light to the side of the object or focus.

**halometry** \hālām′ətrē\ [HALO + -METRY] Measurement of the scattering of light to the side of the object or focus by a halometer.

**haloperidol** $C_{21}H_{23}ClFNO_2$. A neuroleptic drug of the butyrophenone class.

**halosteresis** \həläs′tərē′sis\ OSTEOMALACIA.

**halothane** \hal′ōthān\ $CHBrCl—CF_3$. Bromochlorotrifluoroethane. A nonflammable general anesthetic which occurs in liquid form but which can be converted into a vapor for inhalation. It consists of a halogenated trifluoride amide and will produce all stages of general anesthesia.

**Halsted** [William Stewart *Halsted,* U.S. surgeon, 1852–1922] **1** Halsted radical mastectomy, Halsted's operation. See under RADICAL MASTECTOMY. **2** See under SUTURE, OPERATION.

**halzoun** \hal′zoon\ [Arabic *ḥalzūn* snail] An acute parasitic pharyngitis causing respiratory distress or blockage, nasal and lacrimal discharges, episodic sneezing and coughing, hemolysis, dyspnea, dysphonia, dysphagia, and frontal headache, associated with the eating of raw liver or other viscera of sheep, goat, camel, or ox infected with *Fasciola hepatica.* It is prevalent in parts of the Near and Middle East, north Africa, and south Asia. Nymphs of the pentastome worm *Linguatula serrata* have also been recovered from the nasal passages and throats of a number of persons suffering from this syndrome in Lebanon. Other trematodes have also been held responsible for it.

**Ham** [Thomas Hale *Ham,* U.S. physician, born 1905] See under TEST.

**ham** [Old English *hamm,* akin to Gk *knēmē* the leg, shank] **1** FOSSA POPLITEA. **2** The buttock and the back of the thigh, or the back of the thigh below the buttock.

**hamamelis** \ham′əmē′lis\ The dried leaves of *Hamamelis virginiana,* which have been used as an astringent. An extract made from them has been used in making suppositories and in treating hemorrhoids. Also *witch hazel.*

**hamartochondromatosis** \ham′ärtōkän′drōmətō′sis\ [*hamarto(ma)* + CHONDROMATOSIS] Multiple cartilaginous hamartomas.

**hamartoma** \ham′ärtō′mə\ [Gk *hamart(ia),* also *hamart(ēma)* a failure, error, sin + -OMA] A benign tumor or tumorlike lesion composed of one or more tissues normal to the organ but abnormally mixed and overgrown. For example, a hamartoma of the lung may contain a mixture of cartilage, connective tissue, and bronchial epithelium. Compare CHORISTOMA. **chondromatous h.** CHONDROMA OF LUNG. **fetal h.** MESOBLASTIC NEPHROMA. **leiomyomatous h.** MESOBLASTIC NEPHROMA. **neuromuscular h.** A tumorlike lesion containing differentiated skeletal muscle admixed with nerves. It is multinodular, separated by fibrous tissue bands, and associated with major nerves. It typically occurs in infancy. Also *benign Triton tumor.* **renal h.** RENAL ANGIOMYOLIPOMA. **temporal h.** A malformation of developmental origin situated in the temporal lobe of the brain.

**hamartomatous** \ham′ärtäm′ətəs\ Of the nature of or resembling a hamartoma.

**hamate** \hā′māt\ [L *hamatus* (from *hamus* a hook, barb) hooked, hooklike] **1** OS HAMATUM. **2** Hook-shaped at the tip. Also *hamose.*

**hamatum** \həmā′təm\ OS HAMATUM.

**Hamberger** [Georg Erhard *Hamberger,* German physician, 1697–1755] See under SCHEMA.

**Hamburger** [Franz *Hamburger,* German physician, born 1874] See under TEST.

**Hamburger** [Hartog Jakob *Hamburger,* Dutch physiologist, 1859–1924] Hamburger phenomenon, shift of Hamburger.

**Hamilton** [David James *Hamilton,* Scottish pathologist, 1849–1909] See under METHOD.

**Hamilton** [Frank Hastings *Hamilton,* U.S. surgeon, 1813–1886] See under PSEUDOPHLEGMON.

**Hamman** [Louis *Hamman,* U.S. physician, 1877–1946] **1** Hamman syndrome. See under DISEASE. **2** Hamman-Rich disease. See under HAMMAN-RICH SYNDROME.

**hammer** MALLEUS.

**Hammerschlag** [Albert *Hammerschlag,* Austrian physician, 1863–1935] See under METHOD, TEST.

**hammock** / **pelvic h.** A suspensory support for a fractured pelvis.

**Hammond** [William Alexander *Hammond,* U.S. neurologist, 1823–1900] Hammond syndrome, Hammond's disease. See under DOUBLE ATHETOSIS.

**hamose** \hā′mōs\ HAMATE.

**Hampton** [Aubrey Otis *Hampton,* U.S. radiologist, 1900–1955] See under MANEUVER.

**hamstring** \ham′string\ [early modern English HAM + *string* tendon] **1** See under HAMSTRING TENDON. **2** See under HAMSTRING MUSCLE. **lateral h.** The tendon of insertion of the biceps femoris muscle. Also *outer hamstring.* **medial h.'s** The tendons of insertion of the semimembranosus and semitendinosus muscles. Also *inner hamstrings.*

**hamular** \ham′yələr\ Hook-shaped; unciform.

**hamulate** \ham′yəlit\ Shaped like or possessing a small hook. Also *hamulose.*

**hamulus** \ham′yələs\ [L (dim. of *hamus* a hook, thorn), a little hook] A small, hooklike structure. **h. of ethmoid bone** PROCESSUS UNCINATUS OSSIS ETHMOIDALIS. **frontal h.** ALA CRISTAE GALLI. **h. of hamate bone** HAMULUS OSSIS HAMATI. **h. lacrimalis** [NA] The hooklike process, situated at the lower end of the vertical posterior lacrimal crest on the orbital surface of the lacrimal bone, that turns anteriorly to articulate with the orbital surface of the maxilla, forming the upper bony opening of the nasolacrimal canal. Also *lacrimal hamulus, hamular process of lacrimal bone.* **h. laminae spiralis** [NA] The hooklike termination of the osseous spiral lamina at its apex after it has wound around the modiolus of the cochlea. Also *rostrum of spiral lamina* (outmoded). **h. ossis hamati** [NA] The hooklike projection, flattened from side to side, on the palmar surface of the hamate bone to which the flexor retinaculum, pisohamate ligament, and two hypothenar muscles are attached. Also *hamulus of hamate bone, hook of hamate bone.* **h. pterygoideus** [NA] The narrow, curved, fingerlike projection from the inferior end of the medial pterygoid plate of the sphenoid bone on the lateral side of which there is a groove for the tendon of the tensor veli palatini muscle that hooks around it to the soft palate. Also *pterygoid hamulus, hamular process of sphenoid bone.* **trochlear h.** SPINA TROCHLEARIS.

**hamycin** A polyene, antifungal antibiotic obtained from *Streptomyces pimprina.* It is very similar to trichomycin and candicidin. Also *primamycin.*

**Hand** [Alfred *Hand,* Jr., U.S. pediatrician, 1868–1949] Hand-Schüller-Christian syndrome, Hand syndrome. See under HAND-SCHÜLLER-CHRISTIAN DISEASE.

**hand** The extremity of the upper limb distal to the forearm; manus. **accoucheur's h.** The position of the hand in tetany, as in hypocalcemia of hypoparathyroidism, the hand being flexed at the wrist, the fingers flexed at the metacarpophalangeal joints but extended at the interphangeal joints, with the thumb tightly flexed over and into the palm. Also *obstetrician's hand.* **ape h.** A developmental defect in which the thumb extends almost at right angles to the longitudinal axis of the hand, resembling the nonapposed position of the thumb of the great apes. **apostolic h.** PREACHER'S HAND. **beat h.** Cellulitis of the hand occurring among miners and caused by friction and pressure. **benediction h.** PREACHER'S HAND. **Charcot's h.** PREACHER'S HAND. **claw h.** A hand which superficially resembles a claw and which usually results from an ulnar nerve lesion or from some other process causing diffuse atrophy and weakness of the interosseous and lumbrical muscles. The digits are hyperextended at the metacarpophalangeal joints, and flexed at the interphalangeal joints. Also *clawhand, griffin-claw hand, griffin claw.* **cleft h.** 1 LOBSTER CLAW HAND. 2 A congenital defect in which separation between any two adjacent fingers extends into the metacarpal region. More often than not, this defect involves lobster-claw deformity, with the partial or total absence of one or more of the middle digits. Also *split hand.* See also LOBSTER-CLAW DEFORMITY. **dead h.** See under VIBRATION DISEASE. **drop h.** WRISTDROP. **fakir's h.** A hand with fingers maximally and firmly flexed into the palm. This is almost invariably due to hysterical contracture, much less often to organic contracture. *Older term.* **flipper h.** 1 A hand that lacks spontaneous motion due to destruction of most of the wrist and interphalangeal joints by inflammatory arthritis. 2 A hand affected by a severe form of syndactyly. **griffin-claw h.** CLAW HAND. **Krukenberg's h.** KRUKENBERG'S ARM. **lobster claw h.** 1 An attitude of the hand, sometimes seen in syringomyelia, in which the thumb is held away from the index finger, which is semiflexed, giving a pincerlike appearance. The three other fingers are strongly flexed. Also *cleft hand.* 2 LOBSTER-CLAW DEFORMITY. **mitten h.** Multiple syndactyl deformities of the fingers. **obstetrician's h.** ACCOUCHEUR'S HAND. **opera-glass h.** A hand in which the joints are severely damaged by inflammatory arthritis resulting in telescoped fingers. **phantom h.** A sensation, following amputation, as if the hand were still present. See under PHANTOM LIMB. **preacher's h.** A position of the hand marked by flexion of the two terminal phalanges of all the fingers and extension of the first, with extension of the hand at the wrist. This may be caused by paralysis of the ulnar and median nerves, precluding any action antagonistic to that of the long extensor muscles or by a lesion of the first thoracic spinal nerve or inner cord of the brachial plexus. Often the flexion of the little and ring fingers is more striking than that of the others. Also *Charcot's hand, benediction hand, apostolic hand.* **split h.** CLEFT HAND. **succulent h.** A hand that is swollen and plump, with dimpling over the knuckles. It is sometimes caused by edema resulting from immobility and dependency but more often due to brawny swelling and induration of the soft tissues. It is most often seen in syringomyelia but can develop in other conditions such as shoulder-hand syndrome or reflex dystrophy of the upper extremity. It has been attributed at least in part to the effects of loss of pain and temperature sensation and repeated minor trauma. **trench h.** Frostbite of the hand, resulting in a loss of soft tissue and skin, which produces stiffness and atrophy. **trident h.** The hand characteristically seen in achondroplasia in which all digits tend to be of equal length, with fingers somewhat splayed at the first interphalangeal joint.

**handicap** [obsolete English, a game in which forfeits were drawn from a cap, alteration of *hand in cap*] A physical or mental limitation, which may be correctable, in the ability to function normally.

**handicapped** Limited in a physical or mental capacity, such that the ability to function normally is impaired. Legal definitions in some jurisdictions have been determined to fix standards of eligibility for specific programs and services. **perceptually h.** Having limitations of activity and ability related to sensory difficulties, frequently, resulting from birth defects or subsequent injury or illness.

**handle** / **h. of malleus** MANUBRIUM MALLEI.

**Handley** [William Sampson *Handley,* English surgeon, 1872–1962] Handley's method. See under LYMPHANGIOPLASTY.

**handpiece** 1 A device, held in the hand, that holds the bur and either transmits rotational power from a dental engine to the bur or has within it a small engine. 2 A similar device for producing vibratory movements of a tip, which replaces the bur.

**handprint** 1 The patterned impression of the epidermal ridges and skin creases of the fingers, thumb, and palm, made by chance contact of an individual's hand with a surface capable of retaining the impression. 2 The impression made by applying ink or some other substance to the hand and pressing the hand on paper or another suitable medium. Handprints of newborns are often made for the purpose of identification, and occasionally they are required for biologic investigations and in cases of disputed paternity.

**handshaking** The exchange of a certain sequence of control signals by two communication devices such as modems to synchronize transmission of data.

**Hanfmann** [Eugenia *Hanfmann,* U.S. psychologist, flourished 20th century] Hanfmann-Kasanin test. See under TEST.

**hanging** Subjecting to asphyxial injury or death by ligature strangulation in which the weight of the victim's suspended body produces the force to tighten the ligature. Death results from compression of the upper airway and cervical blood vessels, except in a judicial hanging in which the sudden snap of the laterally placed knot when the victim is dropped is designed to fracture the upper cervical vertebrae and cause transection of the spinal cord.

**hangnail** [alteration of *agnail* (from Old English *angnægl* a corn, from *ang(e)* pain (akin to English *anger*) + Old English *nægl* a metal nail) a sore around a toenail or fingernail] A hard spicule at the edge of the nail. It is common among nail biters.

**Hanhart** [Ernst *Hanhart,* Swiss internist, flourished mid-20th century] 1 Hanhart syndrome. See under PITUITARY DWARFISM III. 2 Hanhart syndrome. See under AGLOSSIA-ADACTYLIA SYNDROME.

**Hanlon** [C. Rollins *Hanlon,* U.S. surgeon, born 1915] Blalock-Hanlon operation. See under OPERATION.

**Hannover** [Adolph *Hannover,* Danish anatomist, 1814–1894] Hannover's canal. See under SPATIUM ZONULARE.

**Hanot** [Victor Charles *Hanot,* French physician, 1844–1896] Hanot cirrhosis, Hanot's disease, Hanot syndrome. See under PRIMARY BILIARY CIRRHOSIS.

**Hansen** [Gerhard Henrik Armauer *Hansen,* Norwegian bacteriologist, 1841–1912] **1** Hansen's disease. See under LEPROSY. **2** Hansen's bacillus. See under LEPROSY BACILLUS.

**hanseniasis** \han′səni′əsis\ [after Gerhard Henrik Armauer *Hansen,* Norwegian bacteriologist and physician, 1841–1912 + -IASIS] *Rare* LEPROSY.

***Hansenula anomala*** \hansen′yələ ənäm′ələ\ A nonpathogenic species of yeast fungus sometimes found as normal flora of the throat and digestive tract of humans.

**haphalgesia** \haf′aljē′zē·ə\ [Gk *haph(ē)* a touching, sense of touch + ALGESIA] Cutaneous pain caused by the faintest contact, occurring in hysterical states and in diseases such as tabes. Also *aphalgesia.*

**hapl-** \hapl-\ HAPLO-.

**haplo-** \hap′lə-\ [Gk *haplo(os)* (from *ha-* one, single, + *plo-* fold; akin to L *simplex* single-layered) single, simple] **1** A combining form meaning single or simple. **2** A combining form meaning haploid. For defs. 1 and 2 also *hapl-.* Compare DIPLO-.

**haplodiploidy** \-dip′loidē\ [HAPLO- + DIPLOIDY] A state in which males develop from unfertilized ova and are haploid, and females develop from fertilized ova and are diploid, as in honeybees. Compare HAPLOID-DIPLOID MOSAICISM.

**haploid** \hap′loid\ [HAPL- + -OID] **1** Having a chromosome complement composed either of a single chromosome (as in bacteria and viruses) or multiple nonhomologous chromosomes (as in the gametes of eukaryotes). In humans, the haploid number of chromosomes is 23, and it is the normal situation in ova and sperm. Also *monoploid.* Compare DIPLOID. **2** A cell or organism having such a chromosome complement. Also *haplont.*

**haploidy** \hap′loidē\ The condition of having a single set of nonhomologous chromosomes. Also *haploid state.*

**haplomycosis** \-mīkō′sis\ ADIASPIROMYCOSIS.

**haplont** \hap′länt\ HAPLOID.

**haploscope** \hap′ləskōp\ [HAPLO- + -SCOPE] A device presenting a separate picture to each eye. Adj. haploscopic. **mirror h.** A device that uses mirrors in order to show a different view to each eye, used in the study of binocular vision and in treatment of its disorders.

**haplosporangin** \-spôran′jin\ An antigen prepared from the fungus *Chrysosporium parva* and used in serologic testing for coccidioidomycosis.

**haplotype** \hap′lətīp\ **1** In linked genes, the alleles contributed from one or the other parent. **2** A linear combination of specific linked alleles or nucleotide sequences, such as restriction enzyme site polymorphisms, that are inherited in coupling (as the alleles of the Rh locus) and may be subject to linkage disequilibrium (as the alleles of the major histocompatibility complex).

**hapt-** \hapt-\ HAPTO-.

**hapte-** \hap′tə-\ HAPTO-.

**hapten** \hap′tən\ [German, from HAPT- + *-en* -IN or -INE] A substance that is unable to induce antibody formation but that can react with antibody: applied especially to organic chemicals of low molecular weight. To raise antibodies to haptens it is necessary to couple them to an immunogenic "carrier" molecule which can recruit a helper T cell response. Also *partial antigen, incomplete antigen, proantigen.* Also *haptin, haptene.* Adj. haptenic.

**hapto-** \hap′tə-\ [Gk *haptein* to touch, handle, fasten to or on, perceive] A combining form meaning (1) touching; (2) binding. Also *hapt-, hapte-.*

**haptoglobin** \-glō′bin\ [HAPTO- + *(hemo)globin*] An $\alpha_2$ globulin, normally present in plasma, that specifically binds hemoglobin released from erythrocytes lysed within the circulating blood.

**haptophore** \hap′təfôr\ [HAPTO- + -PHORE] In Ehrlich's side chain theory of the nature of antibodies, the group that gave the antibody its specific activity. It thus corresponds to the antigen-binding site. *Obs.* Adj. haptophorous, haptophoric.

**Harada** [Einosuke *Harada,* Japanese surgeon, 1892–1947] Harada's disease. See under SYNDROME.

**hardening** The process of making or becoming firm. **h. of the arteries** ARTERIOSCLEROSIS.

**hardness** The property of a solid that characterizes its resistance to scratching or indentation. **indentation h.** The measure of a material's resistance to being dented by a standard load applied to a measured surface area.

**Hardy** [Godfrey Harold *Hardy,* English mathematician, 1877–1947] **1** Hardy-Weinberg law. See under LAW. **2** Hardy-Weinberg equilibrium. See under EQUILIBRIUM.

**Hare** [Edward Selleck *Hare,* English physician, 1812–1838] Hare syndrome. See under PANCOAST SYNDROME.

**harelip** [HARE + LIP] CLEFT LIP. **bilateral h.** A harelip with the upper lip cleft on both sides of the philtrum and premaxilla. Also *double harelip.* **lateral h.** A harelip consisting of a unilateral cleft of the upper lip on one side or the other of the philtrum and premaxilla, with or without an associated cleft of the maxilla. Also *unilateral harelip.* **median h.** A harelip consisting of a cleft of the upper lip and maxilla at the midline. It results from failed development of the embryonic medial nasal processes. It is analogous to the midline cleft normally seen in a hare. **unilateral h.** LATERAL HARELIP.

**harmaline** \här′məlin\ $C_{13}H_{14}ON_2$. A cardioactive alkaloid obtained from the seeds and roots of *Peganum harmala.*

**Harmer** [William Douglas *Harmer,* English otolaryngologist, born 1873] Finzi-Harmer operation. See under OPERATION.

**harmine** \här′min\ $C_{13}H_{12}N_2O$. A $\beta$-carboline alkaloid found in a variety of plants, including *Peganum harmala* and *Banisteria caapi.* A central nervous system stimulant and inhibitor of monoamine oxidase, it is used to treat paralysis agitans. Its sedative and depressive effect is usually more pronounced than its hallucinogenic effect.

**harmonic** \härmän′ik\ A sinusoidal component of a periodic wave having a frequency that is an integral multiple of the fundamental frequency. Twice the fundamental frequency is the second harmonic.

**harmony** / **occlusal h.** A dental occlusion compatible with complete health of teeth, periodontium, temporomandibular joints, and neuromuscular mechanisms.

**harness** / **shoulder h.** A restraint attached to the frame of a motor vehicle, passing diagonally from behind a shoulder and fastening next to the opposite hip of a seated passenger or the driver. It prevents forward motion of the upper torso during sudden deceleration and is more effective in preventing injury than a lap belt alone.

**harpoon** An elongated, thin, barbed surgical instrument designed to obtain a small sample of tissue for diagnostic testing.

**Harris** [Franklin I. *Harris,* U.S. surgeon, born 1895] See under TUBE.

**Harris** [Henry Albert *Harris*, English anatomist, 1886–1968] Harris line. See under GROWTH ARREST LINE.
**Harris** [Henry Fauntleroy *Harris*, U.S. physician, 1867–1926] See under HEMATOXYLIN.
**Harris** [James Arthur *Harris*, U.S. scientist, born 1880] Harris and Benedict standard. See under STANDARD.
**Harrison** [Edward *Harrison*, English physician, 1766–1838] Harrison sulcus. See under GROOVE.
**Harrison** [Harold Edward *Harrison*, U.S. physician, born 1908] See under TEST.
**Harrison Antinarcotic Act** An act regulating the importation, sale, and use of all substances defined in the act as narcotics. It was originally passed by the U.S. Congress in 1914, and amended several times subsequently.
**Harrower** [Henry Robert *Harrower*, U.S. physician, born 1883] See under HYPOTHESIS.
**harrowing** \har′ō·ing\ [Middle English *harwe*, prob. akin to Gk *keirein* to clip, cut out, hew off, + -ING] HERSAGE.
**Hartel** [Fritz *Hartel*, German surgeon, flourished early 20th century] See under TREATMENT, METHOD.
**Hartley** [Frank *Hartley*, U.S. surgeon, 1857–1913] Hartley-Krause operation. See under OPERATION.
**Hartman** [Le Roy Leo *Hartman*, U.S. dentist, 1893–1951] See under SOLUTION.
**Hartmann** [Arthus *Hartmann*, German laryngologist, 1849–1931] See under SPECULUM.
**Hartmann** [Henri *Hartmann*, French surgeon, 1860–1952] **1** Hartmann's critical point. See under POINT OF SUDECK. **2** See under POUCH.
**Hartmann** [Robert *Hartmann*, German anatomist, 1831–1893] Hartmann's fossa. See under RECESSUS ILEOCECALIS INFERIOR.
***Hartmannella*** \härt′manel′ə\ A genus of amebas (order Amoebida) normally free-living, although some species are facultative parasites in the respiratory passages and central nervous system of mammals, including humans.
**Hartnup** [Edward *Hartnup*, English hospital patient of 20th century] See under SYNDROME.
**harvest** To obtain (tissue or an organ) from a donor for use in another site in the same subject or as a transplant into another subject.
**Hashimoto** [Hakaru *Hashimoto*, Japanese surgeon, 1881–1934] Hashimoto struma, Hashimoto's thyroiditis. See under HASHIMOTO'S DISEASE.
**hashish** \hash′ish, hashēsh′\ [Arabic *ḥashīsh* grass, hay, dried hemp, hashish] A resin obtained from the Indian hemp plant, *Cannabis sativa*, smoked or ingested for its intoxicating qualities.
**Hasner** [Joseph Ritter von Artha *Hasner*, Czech physician, 1819–1892] Hasner's fold, Hasner's valve. See under PLICA LACRIMALIS.
**Hassall** [Arthur Hill *Hassall*, English physician, 1817–1894] **1** Virchow-Hassall body, Hassall's body. See under HASSALL'S CORPUSCLE. **2** Hassall-Henle warts. See under HASSALL-HENLE BODIES.
**Hasselbalch** [Karl Albert *Hasselbalch*, Danish biochemist and physician, 1874–1962] Henderson-Hasselbalch equation. See under EQUATION.
**Hata** [Sahachiro *Hata*, Japanese physician, 1873–1938] See under PHENOMENON.
**hatchet** A manual dental instrument, the tip of which is a very small, angled chisel. Also *enamel hatchet*.
**Haudek** [Martin *Haudek*, Austrian roentgenologist, 1880–1931] Haudek sign. See under NICHE.
**haunch** \hônch\ The hips and buttocks considered as a single unit.
**haust.** *haustus* (L, a draft).
**haustra** \hôs′trə\ **1** Plural of HAUSTRUM. **2** HAUSTRA COLI.
**haustral** \hôs′trəl\ **1** Pertaining to a haustrum. **2** Of or relating to the haustra coli.
**haustrations** \hôstrā′shəns\ HAUSTRA COLI.
**haustrum** \hôs′trəm\ [L (from *haur(ire)* to draw or scoop up + *-trum*, instrumental suffix) a scoop of a waterwheel] (*pl.* haustra) Any one of the pouches, or sacculations, in the wall of the colon. **cecal haustra** Haustra coli located on the cecum. **haustra coli** [NA] The sacculations of the colon that are formed because of the shortness of the taeniae coli relative to the circular muscle coat and the length of the large intestine. The number and distribution of the sacculations are modified according to the physiologic status of the colon, and they disappear in the vicinity of the rectum. In the newborn and infants they are fewer and shallower than in adults. Also *haustra of colon, haustrations, haustra, colic sacculations, colic haustra*.
**haustus** [L (from *haurire* to draw forth or out, drink off), a drawing, drinking, draft] **1** A potion. **2** A measure of a liquid drug or medicinal preparation. **h. niger** COMPOUND MIXTURE OF SENNA.
**haut mal** \ō mäl′\ [French *haut* high + *mal* sickness] MAJOR EPILEPSY.
**HAV** HEPATITIS A VIRUS.
**Haven** [Hale *Haven*, U.S. neurologist, born 1902] Haven syndrome. See under SCALENUS ANTERIOR SYNDROME.
***Haverhillia multiformis*** \hā′vərhil′ē·ə mul′tifôr′mis\ *STREPTOBACILLUS MONILIFORMIS*.
**Hawes** [Sir Richard Brunel *Hawes*, English physician, flourished 20th century] Hawes-Pallister-Landor syndrome. See under STRACHAN-SCOTT SYNDROME.
**Hayem** [Georges *Hayem*, French physician, 1841–1933] **1** See under SOLUTION. **2** Hayem's elementary corpuscle. See under PLATELET. **3** Hayem's hematoblast. See under HEMOCYTOBLAST.
**hay fever** See under FEVER.
**Hayflick** [Leonard *Hayflick*, U.S. microbiologist, born 1928] See under PHENOMENON.
**hayrake** HAYRAKE SPLINT.
**hazard** [Middle English, from Old French *hazard* a dice game, from Arabic *az-zahr* the dice, dice game] **1** A circumstance or agent that increases the probability of loss or damage. **2** The chance that injury will result from exposure to a substance under specified conditions of use.
**Hb** hemoglobin (or hemoglobin concentration).
**$HB_cAg$** hepatitis B core antigen.
**HBeAg** hepatitis B e antigen.
**$HB_sAg$** hepatitis B surface antigen.
**$HbO_2$** oxyhemoglobin (oxygenated hemoglobin).
**HBV** hepatitis B virus.
**HCG** Human chorionic gonadotropin.
**HCT** hematocrit.
**$HD_{50}$** [from *hemolyzing dose*] The amount of complement which will cause hemolysis of 50 percent of a population of sensitized red blood cells.
**h.d.** *hora decubitus* (L, at bedtime).
**HDL** high-density lipoprotein.
**HDN** hemolytic disease of the newborn.
**H and E** hematoxylin and eosin stain.
**He** Symbol for the element, helium.
**Head** [Sir Henry *Head*, English neurologist, 1861–1940] **1** See under CLASSIFICATION. **2** Head-Holmes syndrome. See under SYNDROME.
**head** [Old English *hēafod*, akin to L *caput* head] **1** The upper extremity of the human body; caput. It comprises the

cranium and the face. **2** The proximal or superior extremity of any organ or structure. **articular h.** The cartilage-covered rounded extremity of a bone that articulates with another bone. **h. of astragalus** CAPUT TALI. **box h.** The characteristically flattened head which results from rickets. **h. of condyloid process of mandible** CAPUT MANDIBULAE. **coronoid h. of pronator teres muscle** CAPUT ULNARE MUSCULI PRONATORIS TERETIS. **drum h.** MEMBRANA TYMPANI. **engaged h.** A fetal head which as the presenting part has descended to a level such that the biparietal plane of the fetal head is below that of the pelvic inlet. **h. of epididymis** CAPUT EPIDIDYMIDIS. **h. of femur** CAPUT OSSIS FEMORIS. **h. of fibula** CAPUT FIBULAE. **floating h.** A condition in which the fetal head as the presenting part lies well above the plane of the pelvic inlet. **hourglass h.** A head having a transverse depression on the skull at the coronal suture. It can be a manifestation of congenital syphilis. **humeral h. of flexor carpi ulnaris muscle** CAPUT HUMERALE MUSCULI FLEXORIS CARPI ULNARIS. **humeral h. of flexor digitorum sublimis muscle** CAPUT HUMEROULNARE MUSCULI FLEXORIS DIGITORUM SUPERFICIALIS. **humeral h. of pronator teres muscle** CAPUT HUMERALE MUSCULI PRONATORIS TERETIS. **humeroulnar h. of flexor digitorum superficialis** CAPUT HUMEROULNARE MUSCULI FLEXORIS DIGITORUM SUPERFICIALIS. **h. of humerus** CAPUT HUMERI. **lateral h. of gastrocnemius muscle** CAPUT LATERALE MUSCULI GASTROCNEMII. **lateral h. of triceps brachii muscle** CAPUT LATERALE MUSCULI TRICIPITIS BRACHII. **lateral h. of triceps muscle** CAPUT LATERALE MUSCULI TRICIPITIS BRACHII. **little h. of humerus** CAPITULUM HUMERI. **long h. of biceps brachii muscle** CAPUT LONGUM MUSCULI BICIPITIS BRACHII. **long h. of biceps femoris muscle** CAPUT LONGUM MUSCULI BICIPITIS FEMORIS. **long h. of triceps brachii muscle** CAPUT LONGUM MUSCULI TRICIPITIS BRACHII. **long h. of triceps muscle** CAPUT LONGUM MUSCULI TRICIPITIS BRACHII. **h. of malleus** CAPUT MALLEI. **h. of mandible** **1** CAPUT MANDIBULAE. **2** PROCESSUS CONDYLARIS MANDIBULAE. **medial h. of biceps brachii muscle** CAPUT BREVE MUSCULI BICIPITIS BRACHII. **medial h. of gastrocnemius muscle** CAPUT MEDIALE MUSCULI GASTROCNEMII. **medial h. of triceps brachii muscle** CAPUT MEDIALE MUSCULI TRICIPITIS BRACHII. **medial h. of triceps muscle** CAPUT MEDIALE MUSCULI TRICIPITIS BRACHII. **h. of metacarpal bone** CAPUT METACARPALIS. **h. of metatarsal bone** CAPUT METATARSALE. **h. of muscle** CAPUT MUSCULI. **oblique h. of adductor hallucis muscle** CAPUT OBLIQUUM MUSCULI ADDUCTORIS HALLUCIS. **oblique h. of adductor pollicis muscle** CAPUT OBLIQUUM MUSCULI ADDUCTORIS POLLICIS. **h. of optic nerve** DISCUS NERVI OPTICI. **overriding h.** An unengaged fetal head which as the presenting part lies over the symphysis pubis. **h. of pancreas** CAPUT PANCREATIS. **h. of penis** GLANS PENIS. **h. of phalanx of fingers** CAPUT PHALANGIS DIGITORUM MANUS. **h. of phalanx of toes** CAPUT PHALANGIS DIGITORUM PEDIS. **radial h. of flexor digitorum superficialis muscle** CAPUT RADIALE MUSCULI FLEXORIS DIGITORUM SUPERFICIALIS. **h. of radius** CAPUT RADII. **h. of rib** CAPUT COSTAE. **short h. of biceps brachii muscle** CAPUT BREVE MUSCULI BICIPITIS BRACHII. **short h. of biceps femoris muscle** CAPUT BREVE MUSCULI BICIPITIS FEMORIS. **h. of spermatozoon** The ovoid head of a male germ cell or spermatozoon. It is somewhat pear-shaped in man because the tip is flattened. It is nearly 4 μm long and consists of a nucleus enclosed by a nuclear membrane with its front half covered by a two-layered cap (the acrosome). **h. of stapes** CAPUT STAPEDIS. **h. of talus** CAPUT TALI. **h. of thigh bone** CAPUT OSSIS FEMORIS. **tower h.** OXYCEPHALY. **transverse h. of adductor hallucis muscle** CAPUT TRANSVERSUM MUSCULI ADDUCTORIS HALLUCIS. **transverse h. of adductor pollicis muscle** CAPUT TRANSVERSUM MUSCULI ADDUCTORIS POLLICIS. **h. of ulna** CAPUT ULNAE. **ulnar h. of flexor carpi ulnaris muscle** CAPUT ULNARE MUSCULI FLEXORIS CARPI ULNARIS. **ulnar h. of pronator teres muscle** CAPUT ULNARE MUSCULI PRONATORIS TERETIS. **white h.** FAVUS.

**headache** [Old English *hēafod æce*] Pain in the head. Also *angina capitis, dolor capitis.* **bilious h.** MIGRAINE HEADACHE. **blind h.** MIGRAINE HEADACHE. **cluster h.** MIGRAINOUS NEURALGIA. **congestive h.** Headache resulting either from vascular dilatation or from raised intracranial pressure. An imprecise and outmoded term. **cough h.** A syndrome in which attacks of severe headache are precipitated by coughing. This may be a benign syndrome for which no cause is discovered but cough headache sometimes occurs in patients with raised intracranial pressure. **drainage h.** LUMBAR PUNCTURE HEADACHE. **dynamite h.** Headache due to the hypotensive effects of the nitroglycerin component of dynamite. It is accompanied by arterial dilatation, increased heart rate, and a reduced blood pressure. Workers usually acclimatize rapidly to this hypotensive action. Headache is a common symptom on first exposure and on Monday mornings after loss of acclimatization. Also *nitroglycerin headache.* **fibrositic h.** A headache involving the occipital region of the skull. There is often pain and tenderness associated with the presence of small nodules in the scalp. It is often evoked by atmospheric cold. **histamine h.** MIGRAINOUS NEURALGIA. **Horton's vascular h.** MIGRAINOUS NEURALGIA. **jolt h.** Headache induced by sudden head movement. **lumbar puncture h.** Headache due to reduced intracranial pressure after lumbar puncture resulting from leakage of cerebrospinal fluid through the hole in the dura mater left by the exploring needle. Also *drainage headache, postspinal headache, puncture headache, spinal headache, spinal-fluid loss headache.* **meningeal h.** Headache due to inflammation or irritation of the meninges, usually accompanied by neck stiffness. **migraine h.** The typical paroxysmal throbbing headache occurring in attacks of migraine. Also *bilious headache, blind headache, sick headache.* **neuralgic h.** Any headache involving the head and neck in which pain radiates or shoots along the course of a sensory nerve or is sharp, intermittent, and transient in character. **nitroglycerin h.** DYNAMITE HEADACHE. **organic h.** Any headache due to physical as distinct from mental disease. **paraplegic h.** Transient pressor headache occurring in paraplegic patients in whom a sudden sharp rise in systemic blood pressure may be reflexly induced by stimuli originating below the level of the spinal cord lesion, such as distension of the bladder or rectum. **postconcussional h.** Recurrent headache following a closed head injury giving rise to concussion. This headache usually declines in frequency and severity with the passage of time and ultimately resolves. **postspinal h.** LUMBAR PUNCTURE HEADACHE. **pressor h.** Headache due to transient or persistent arterial hypotension or to pharmacologic pressor agents. **puncture h.** LUMBAR PUNCTURE HEADACHE. **pyrexial h.** Headache developing in the context of fever. **reflex h.** A form of headache resulting from a disease or abnormality outside the brain. Also *symptomatic headache.* **sick h.** MIGRAINE HEADACHE. **spinal h.** LUMBAR PUNCTURE HEADACHE. **spinal-fluid loss h.** LUMBAR PUNCTURE HEADACHE. **symptomatic h.** REFLEX HEADACHE. **toxic h.** A headache resulting from systemic poisoning. **traction h.** Headache resulting from traction upon pain-sensitive intracranial or extracranial structures such as the dura mater, arteries, veins, and muscles. **traumatic h.** Headache following head injury. **vacuum h.** Frontal headache apparently due to obstruction of the ostia of the anterior group of paranasal sinuses. The obstruction is said to be caused by swelling of the mucosa beneath the middle nasal concha leading to absorption of air in the sinuses and the establishment of a partial vacuum. **vascular h.** A headache resulting from disease or dysfunction of extracranial or intracranial arteries. **vasomotor h.** Headache resulting from constriction or, alternatively, from vasodilatation, of extracranial or intracranial arteries.

**headcap** A cap-shaped device, fitting closely to the skull and used in occipital anchorage.

**headgear** The headcap or neck device used as the base for external anchorage in orthodontic treatment.

**headgut** FOREGUT.

**headlight** An electric light incorporated into a head mirror worn on a headband, enabling the wearer, as a surgeon, to observe deeply situated structures under good illumination while leaving his hands free.

**head-nodding** SPASMUS NUTANS.

**head wrapping** A method once used to treat hydrocephalus by constricting the infant's head in tight bandages. *Obs.*

**Heaf** [Frederick R. G. *Heaf,* English physician, born 1894] See under TEST.

**heal** [Middle English *helen,* from Old English *hælan*] **1** To make or become whole or well. **2** To bring about the recovery of (a lesion).

**healing** [Old English *hælan*] The act of making or the process of becoming whole or healthy; restoration to health. **h. by first intention** The normal, uncomplicated healing of a wound. It is seen in small, smooth lacerations and sutured surgical wounds when continuity is reestablished without infection or granulation tissue. Also *primary adhesion, primary union, immediate union.* **h. by second intention** A type of healing of a surface wound, usually large and irregular or infected, which is characterized by development of granulation tissue from the depth and margins of the wound. Eventually, the epithelium grows over and covers the defect. It often results in a prominent scar. Also *secondary adhesion, healing by granulation.* **faith h.** Treatment of disease through prayer, often invoking faith in God's power to heal or in the healing power of faith itself. **mental h.** PSYCHOTHERAPY.

**health** [Old English *hælth* (from *hāl* whole)] **1** A state of well-being of an organism or part of one, characterized by normal function and unattended by disease. • *Health* is defined in the constitution of the World Health Organization as "a state of complete physical, mental, and social well-being and not merely the absence of disease and infirmity." **2** The relative condition of an individual, either physiologic or psychologic, as in *ill health.* **occupational h.** A professional discipline designed to promote and protect the health of workers by identifying and controlling health hazards in the workplace. Occupational health comprises mainly occupational medicine and occupational hygiene but also includes ergonomics and occupational psychology. **public h.** **1** Services designed to promote the health of populations, especially those provided on a community rather than individual basis. **2** The publicly organized system through which members of the health professions and others work to reduce morbidity and mortality. **3** The health status of a population as measured by morbidity and mortality indices and other relevant information.

**hearing** A primary sensory and perceptual function. Extremely small rapidly recurring variations of air pressure originating from a sound source often some distance away are converted first into vibrations of the tympanic membrane and ossicular chain, so matching variations in air pressure to variations in fluid pressure within the inner ear, and subsequently initiating neural activity through the organ of Corti. Hearing does not only refer to middle-ear or end-organ activity but includes all that takes place from the periphery to the higher auditory and related centers until the sound enters consciousness and is located and identified. **double h.** DIPLACUSIS. **double disharmonic h.** DISHARMONIC DIPLACUSIS. **residual h.** The hearing remaining available to an individual with a hearing loss. In audiometric terms this lies between the sometimes greatly increased auditory threshold and the upper limit of hearing when discomfort is experienced on exposure to very loud sounds.

**hearing aid** See under AID.

**hearing loss** See under LOSS.

**heart** [Old English *heorte,* akin to L *cor,* gen. *cordis,* heart, and Gk *kardia* heart] The hollow, chambered organ that serves as the muscular pump for the circulation of the blood; cor. **addisonian h.** The small, ptotic heart of untreated Addison's disease. At necropsy, there is a characteristic brown degeneration of myocardium, now rarely encountered since most patients are treated. **amyloid h.** A heart infiltrated by amyloid, as is usually the case in senile amyloidosis. **armored h.** Chronic adhesive pericarditis

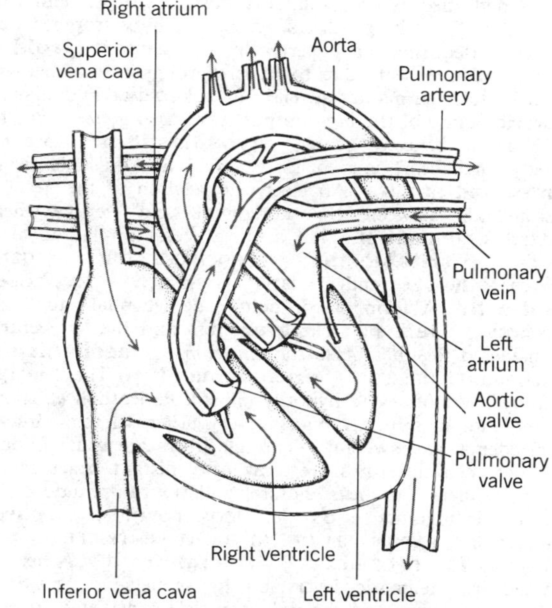


**Cross-section of heart** (showing circulation)

with calcification. Also *panzerherz.* **artificial h.** Any of various extracorporeal or intracorporeal circulatory devices used as a substitute for the heart or a part of it. An implanted device consisting of two separate ventricles for perfusion of both systemic and pulmonary circulations, as the Jarvik heart, is powered by an external air-driven system. Also *mechanical heart.* **athlete's h.** Hypertrophy of the heart due to athletic activity. It is not thought that this type of hypertrophy is ever pathologic. Also *athletic heart.* **atrophic h.** CARDIAC ATROPHY. **beer h.** BEER-DRINKER'S CARDIOMYOPATHY. **beriberi h.** The enlarged heart and associated cardiac disorders resulting from thiamin deficiency. The heart becomes enlarged with the right side becoming very prominent. The pulmonary second sound is accentuated. Tachycardia occurs at the slightest physical exertion, and heart failure of the right side, precipitated by physiologic stress, is the end result. **boat-shaped h.** The shape of the heart seen radiologically, suggestive of a boat, in some cases of aortic regurgitation as a result of combined dilatation and hypertrophy. **booster h.** AUXILIARY VENTRICLE. **bovine h.** COR BOVINUM. **drop h.** A condition in which the heart appears long and thin, usually in tall asthenic individuals but also occurring in conditions where the diaphragm is unusually low, as in asthma or emphysema. Also *hanging heart, pendulous heart, suspended heart, cardioptosis, cardioptosia.* **extracorporeal h.** An artificial heart device located outside the body as in a heart-lung machine. **fatty h.** A non-specific accumulation of fat within the myocardium, usually the consequence either of chronic mild hypoxia as seen in anemia, or ischemia associated with coronary atherosclerosis. Other causes include toxic injury, myocarditis, and cardiomyopathy. The microscopic distribution of fat tends to be in the form of small cytoplasmic droplets. Also *steatosis cordis, adipositas cordis.* **flask-shaped h.** The radiological appearance of the heart in pericardial effusion. **goiter h.** HYPERTHYROID HEART. **hairy h.** PERICARDITIS VILLOSA. **hanging h.** DROP HEART. **horizontal h.** The electrical position of the heart in which the QRS deflection is predominantly positive in aVL and negative in aVF. **hypertensive h.** A hypertrophied heart as a consequence of hypertension. **hyperthyroid h.** An overactive heart due to hyperthyroidism and characterized by tachycardia and a tendency to atrial arrhythmias and cardiac failure of the high output type. Also *goiter heart, thyroid heart, thyrotoxic heart.* **hypoplastic h.** An abnormally small heart as seen, for example, in Addison's disease. **intermediate h.** An electrical position of the heart intermediate between the horizontal and vertical heart. **intracorporeal h.** An artificial heart implanted in the body. **irritable h.** NEUROCIRCULATORY ASTHENIA. **Jarvik h.** See under ARTIFICIAL HEART. **kyphoscoliotic h.** A form of cor pulmonale secondary to kyphoscoliosis. **left h.** The left atrium and the left ventricle considered together. Also *cor sinistrum.* **mechanical h.** ARTIFICIAL HEART. **myxedema h.** The enlarged, flabby heart of severe hypothyroidism. Pericardial effusion is sometimes present. Coronary artery atherosclerosis, interstitial edema, and swelling of muscle fibers are usual findings. Clinical characteristics are slow rate, distant heart sounds, some tendency to heart failure, and low amplitude on the electrocardiogram. **ox h.** COR BOVINUM. **parchment h.** HYPOPLASIA OF THE RIGHT VENTRICLE. **pendulous h.** DROP HEART. **rheumatic h.** A heart affected by rheumatic fever and its sequelae. **right h.** The right atrium and the right ventricle considered together. Also *cor dextrum, cor venosum* (outmoded). **sabot h.** COEUR EN SABOT. **scleroderma h.** The structural and functional changes seen in the heart in progressive systemic sclerosis. These changes are nonspecific and include interstitial myocardial fibrosis, thickening of small vessels, and possibly vasospasm. **semihorizontal h.** The electrical position of the heart when it is between the horizontal and intermediate positions, with a QRS axis of approximately 0°. **semivertical h.** The electrical position of the heart when it is situated between the intermediate and vertical positions with an electrical axis of approximately 60°. **soldier's h.** NEUROCIRCULATORY ASTHENIA. **stony h.** ISCHEMIC CONTRACTURE OF THE LEFT VENTRICLE. **suspended h.** DROP HEART. **tabby cat h.** The appearance of heart muscle affected by pale areas of fatty degeneration; tigering. Also *tiger heart, tiger lily heart.* **three-chambered h.** COR TRILOCULARE. **thrush breast h.** Patchy fatty change of the myocardium that appears streaked due to alternating lipid-laden and normal myofibers. **thyroid h.** HYPERTHYROID HEART. **thyrotoxic h.** HYPERTHYROID HEART. **tiger h.** TABBY CAT HEART. **tiger lily h.** TABBY CAT HEART. **Traube's h.** Heart disease as a consequence of renal disease. **triatrial h.** COR TRIATRIUM. **trilocular h.** COR TRILOCULARE. **vertical h.** The electrical position of the heart in which there is a dominant R wave in aVF and an S wave and negative T wave in aVL, the electrical axis of the QRS being approximately +90°. **wooden shoe h.** COEUR EN SABOT.

**heartbeat** A contraction of the heart; a complete cardiac cycle. Also *ictus cordis.*

**heartburn** [early modern English *hart-burne,* translation of Gk *kardialgia.* See CARDIALGIA.] A substernal burning sensation usually due to the reflux of gastric acid into the esophagus. Also *pyrosis, phagopyrosis, brash, cardialgia.*

**heartworm** A filarial worm of the species *Dirofilaria immitis.*

**heat** 1 A form of energy that is caused by motion of molecules. 2 A sensation resulting from exposure of the body to high temperatures. 3 ESTRUS. **animal h.** The heat resulting from biologic processes in living animals. **blood h.** BODY TEMPERATURE. **h. of compression** The heat produced by simple compression of a body or substance. **conductive h.** The heat transmitted from a body of higher temperature to one of lower temperature by flow of heat through a material body. **conversive h.** The heat produced from the absorption of radiation. **dry h.** The heat of a moistureless environment. **h. of fusion** The heat required to convert a substance from a solid to a liquid state without a temperature change. **latent h.** The heat lost or gained by a body or system undergoing a change in state but without a change in temperature. **prickly h.** MILIARIA RUBRA. **radiant h.** Heat transferred from one point to another without an intervening conductive medium, such as heat from the sun or a heating lamp; a form of electromagnetic radiation. **sensible h.** The heat that produces an elevation in temperature in a body that absorbs it. **specific h.** The amount of heat required to change the temperature of a known mass of a substance 1°C divided by the amount of heat required to change the temperature of an equal mass of water by the same number of degrees. The specific heat of water is 1.0. **h. of vaporization** The heat required to convert a substance from a liquid to a gaseous state without a temperature change.

**Heath** [Christopher *Heath,* English surgeon, 1835–1905] See under OPERATION.

**heating** / **conductive h.** Transfer of heat by direct

contact with a warm object such as a hot pack or hot water bottle. **convective h.** Application of heat by means of an intermediary fluid substance such as warmed air or water. **conversive h.** Application of heat by conversion of energy from a form other than heat, as in diathermy or ultrasound therapy. **radiant h.** Application of heat radiating directly as electromagnetic waves, either luminous or nonluminous, and from a natural source such as the sun or from special devices such as a heat lamp or other radiator. **reflex h.** Heating of one portion of the body by reflex vasodilation secondary to heat application at a distance. **ultrasonic h.** Heating by absorption of ultrasound.

**heat-labile** Having the property of being destroyed by a rise in temperature. This property is often used in biochemistry as evidence that a process involves the action of proteins, often enzymes.

**heatstroke** [HEAT + STROKE] A condition caused by environmental temperatures too high for the body's compensatory mechanism. It is characterized by dry skin, high body temperature, nausea, headache, thirst, and confusion. If untreated, it can lead to coma and death. Also *heat apoplexy, thermoplegia, thermic fever, heat hyperpyrexia, heat pyrexia, anhidrotic heat exhaustion.*

**heave** / **parasternal h.** Palpable elevation of the ribs adjacent to the sternum with heartbeat, usually due to enlargement of the right ventricle.

**hebdom.** *hebdomada* (L, a week).

**hebephrenia** \hē′bəfrē′nē·ə\ [Gk *hēbē* manhood, freshness of youth, time just before manhood + -PHRENIA] A subtype of schizophrenia characterized by marked disorganization of speech and behavior, inappropriate affect, and unsystematized and bizarre delusions that are often concerned with ideas of omnipotence, sex change, cosmic identification, and rebirth.

**hebephrenic** \hē′bəfren′ik\ Having the characteristics of hebephrenia.

**Heberden** [William *Heberden*, Sr., English physician, 1710–1801] **1** Heberden's arthropathy, Heberden sign. See under HEBERDEN'S NODES. **2** Heberden's rheumatism. See under OSTEOARTHRITIS.

**heboid** \hē′boid\ Having characteristics similar to hebephrenia. *Outmoded.*

**heboidophrenia** \hēboi′dəfrē′nē·ə\ [HEBOID + *o* + -PHRENIA] *Outmoded* SIMPLE SCHIZOPHRENIA.

**Hecht** [Victor *Hecht*, Austrian pathologist, flourished early 20th century] Hecht's pneumonia. See under GIANT CELL PNEUMONIA.

**Hecker** [Karl von *Hecker*, German obstetrician, 1827–1882] See under LAW.

**hectic** \hek′tik\ [Gk *hektikos* (from *hexis* a habit, condition) habitual, recurrent, hectic] Characterized by wide swings in temperature which recur daily: said of a fever or of a condition involving such a fever.

**hecto-** \hek′tə-\ [Gk *hekaton* hundred] A combining form denoting $10^2$, one hundred: used with SI units. Symbol: h

**Hedinger** [Christoph Ernst *Hedinger*, Swiss pathologist, born 1917] Hedinger syndrome. See under CARCINOID SYNDROME.

**hedrocele** \hed′rōsēl\ [Gk *hedr(a)* the fundament + *o* + -CELE[2]] RECTAL PROLAPSE.

**heel** **1** The distal end of a part. **2** The rounded protuberance forming the posterior end of the foot; calx. **anterior h.** A bar of leather placed behind the weight-bearing line of the metatarsal heads on the sole of a shoe. It is designed to redistribute the weight-bearing forces of the foot. **black h.** Bluish black specks occurring just above the hyperkeratotic edge of the heel, due to rupture of superficial capillaries and accumulation of blood in the dermis and epidermis. It usually occurs in athletic adolescent girls. Also *talon noir, basketball heels.* **cracked h.'s** Hyperkeratotic heels marked by fissures. **painful h.** Pain or local tenderness on the plantar surface of the heel when bearing weight. Also *calcodynia.* **prominent h.** A painful swelling around the posterior aspect of the os calcis at the attachment of the Achilles tendon. **Thomas h.** A 4.7 mm rise of leather that is placed along the inner side of the shoe heel and extended forward onto the longitudinal arch area. It is used as an additional support and to force the foot into a more inverted position to correct flatfoot deformities.

**HEENT** head, eyes, ears, nose, throat.

**Heerfordt** [Christian Frederik *Heerfordt*, Danish oculist, born 1871] Heerfordt's disease. See under SYNDROME.

**Hefke** [H. W. *Hefke*, U.S. radiologist, born 1871] Hefke-Turner sign. See under OBTURATOR SIGN.

**Hegar** [Alfred *Hegar*, German gynecologist, 1830–1914] **1** Hegar's dilators. See under DILATOR. **2** See under SIGN.

**Hegglin** [Robert Marquand *Hegglin*, Swiss internist, born 1907] Hegglin's anomaly. See under MAY-HEGGLIN ANOMALY.

**Heidenhain** [Rudolf Peter Heinrich *Heidenhain*, German physiologist, 1834–1897] **1** See under POUCH. **2** Heidenhain's iron hematoxylin stain. See under HEIDENHAIN'S IRON HEMATOXYLIN.

**height** A distance or a corresponding measurement from the lowest part to the top of an object or part. **h. of contour** The points of greatest convexity of a tooth, relative to a more or less vertical reference line through the crown. The height of contour may change when the reference line is inclined to different angles. Also *surveyed height of contour.* **cusp h.** The average height of the cusps of a tooth measured perpendicularly from the central fossa. **sitting h.** The height of the vertex of a child above a table he is sitting on, when the external auditory meatus and the lower edge of the orbit are in a horizontal plane, (the Frankfort plane), the back is held straight with no sagging or rounding, and the weight is taken by the ischial tuberosities on the table, to ensure which the thighs should be kept just clear of the surface of the table by placing the feet on a stool of suitable height. Also *sitting vertex height.* **sitting vertex h.** SITTING HEIGHT. **standing h.** A measurement of a child's height taken with the child standing upright against a wall or fixed ruler. It is the distance between the horizontal plane of the vertex, when the external auditory meatus and the lower edge of the orbit are in a horizontal plane (the Frankfort plane) and the floor. The heels of the subject must be together, knees straight, and buttocks and upper back touching the measuring rod or wall. **surveyed h. of contour** HEIGHT OF CONTOUR.

**Heimlich** [Henry Jay *Heimlich*, U.S. surgeon, born 1920] See under MANEUVER.

**Heineke** [Walter Hermann *Heineke*, German surgeon, 1834–1901] **1** See under OPERATION. **2** Heineke-Mikulicz operation. See under HEINEKE-MIKULICZ PYLOROPLASTY.

**Heinz** [Robert *Heinz*, German pathologist, 1865–1924] **1** Heinz body test. See under TEST. **2** Heinz granules. See under HEINZ BODIES. **3** Heinz-body anemia. See under ANEMIA. **4** Heinz-body anemia, congenital Heinz-body anemia. See under UNSTABLE HEMOGLOBIN HEMOLYTIC ANEMIA.

**Heister** [Lorenz *Heister*, German anatomist, 1683–1758] **1** Heister's fold, valvula spiralis heisteri, spiral valve of Heister, Heister's valve. See under PLICA SPIRALIS. **2** Heister's diverticulum. See under BULBUS SUPERIOR VENAE JUGULARIS.

**helcoid** \hel′koid\ [Gk *helko(s)* a sore, ulcer + -OID] Resembling an ulcer.

**helcology** \helkäl′əjē\ [Gk *helko(s)* a sore, ulcer + -LOGY] The study of ulcers.

**helcosis** \helkō′sis\ [Gk *helkōsis* (from *helkoun* to ulcerate, from *helkos* a sore, ulcer) ulceration] ULCERATION.

**Held** [Hans *Held*, German anatomist, 1866–1942] **1** End feet of Held. See under FOOT. **2** Striae of Held. See under STRIAE MEDULLARES VENTRICULI QUARTI. **3** End-bulb of Held. See under END-BULB. **4** See under DECUSSATION. **5** His-Held space. See under PERIVASCULAR SPACE.

**heli-** \hē′lē-\ HELIO-.

**helianthin** \hē′lē·an′thin\ METHYL ORANGE.

**heliation** \hē′lē·ā′shən\ HELIOTHERAPY.

**helic-** \hel′ik-\ HELICO-.

**helical** \hel′ikl\ Referring to or having the shape of a helix.

**helicase** \hel′ikās\ GYRASE.

**helices** \hel′isēz\ Plural of HELIX.

**helico-** \hel′ikō-\ [Gk *helix* (genitive *helikos*) coil, spiral, whirl] A combining form meaning (1) helical, spiral; (2) pertaining to a scala or cochlea. Also *helic-*.

**helicopodia** \-pō′dē·ə\ [HELICO- + -POD + -IA] A sweeping type of gait observed in spastic hemiplegia, resulting from the inability of the leg to be moved forward without describing an arc, the radius of which is external to the body, with the foot scraping the ground. This is due to a combination of extensor spasticity, causing difficulty in flexing the knee, together with spastic footdrop. Also *Todd's gait*. Adj. helicopod.

**helicotrema** \-trē′mə\ [HELICO- + Gk *trēma* an aperture, perforation] [NA] The narrow opening connecting the scala tympani to the scala vestibuli at the apex of the modiolus of the cochlea where the cochlear duct ends. It is bounded by the hamulus of the spiral lamina. Also *Breschet's hiatus, Scarpa's hiatus.*

**helio-** \hē′lē·ō-\ [Gk *hēlios* the sun] A combining form denoting the sun or sunlight. Also *heli-*.

**heliosis** \hē′lē·ō′sis\ [Gk *hēliōsis* (from *hēliousthai* to be exposed to the sun, sunburnt, sun-struck, from *hēlios* the sun) exposure to the sun] SUNSTROKE.

**heliotherapy** \-ther′əpē\ The use of the sun's rays for therapeutic purposes. Also *heliation, solar therapy, solar treatment.*

**helium** \hē′lē·əm\ Element number 2, having atomic weight 4.0026. It is a chemically inert gas, the second most abundant element (after hydrogen) in the universe, though it is present in the earth's atmosphere in a concentration of only about five parts per million. It tends to escape from the earth, but it is constantly replenished as a radioactive decay product, since alpha particles, emitted from many of the natural radioactive minerals, are the nuclei of helium atoms. Natural helium consists of two stable isotopes, helium 3 (comprising only about 0.00013%) and helium 4 (virtually 100%). The boiling point of helium is close to absolute zero, and the liquid displays unique properties that are of great interest in physics research. Being much less soluble in blood than nitrogen, helium is used in place of nitrogen in artificial atmospheres for divers, caisson workers, and the like. Symbol: He

**helix** \hē′liks\ [Gk (akin to L *volvere* to roll and English *whelk*) a spiral, coil] (*pl.* helices, helixes) **1** A circular pattern in which each successive loop is a constant distance from the last, in the manner of a spring, and every point of the pattern is equidistant from its central axis, such that any two lines drawn through corresponding points of successive loops would be parallel. Adj. helical. **2** [NA] The prominent curved outer rim of the auricle of the external ear. It is separated from the anthelix by the scapha. **alpha h.** One of the regular arrangements of amino-acid residues in proteins. It is a helix of 3.6 residues per turn, with each carbonyl group hydrogen-bonded to the fourth NH group towards the C terminus of the chain. Many proteins have regions of such helix, with side chains pointing out from the helix axis. Also *Pauling-Corey helix.* **double h.** The molecular arrangement of double-stranded DNA. Each of the two polynucleotide chains forms a right-handed coil. Bases of the nucleotides project toward the axis of the helix. The chains are complementary with the C-5′ end of one chain pairing with the C-3′ end of the second chain. The coil makes one turn each 3.4 nm, with 10 nucleotides per turn. The polynucleotide chains are held together by hydrogen bonds between bases, adenine bonding to thymine and cytosine to guanine. Also *Watson-Crick helix, twin helix.* **Pauling-Corey h.** ALPHA HELIX. **twin h.** DOUBLE HELIX. **Watson-Crick h.** DOUBLE HELIX.

**Hellendall** [Hugo *Hellendall*, German gynecologist, born 1872] Hellendall's sign. See under CULLEN SIGN.

**Heller** [Arnold Ludwig Gotthilf *Heller*, German pathologist, 1840–1913] **1** Heller-Döhle disease. See under SYPHILITIC AORTITIS. **2** See under PLEXUS.

**Heller** [Ernst *Heller*, German surgeon, 1877–1964] Heller's operation, Heller esophagomyotomy. See under CARDIOMYOTOMY.

**Heller** [Theodor O. *Heller*, German neuropsychiatrist, born 1869] Heller's disease. See under DEMENTIA INFANTILIS.

**Hellin** [Dyonizy *Hellin*, Polish pathologist, 1867–1935] See under LAW.

**Helly** [Konrad *Helly*, Swiss pathologist, born 1875] Helly's fixative. See under FLUID.

**Helmholtz** [Hermann Ludwig Ferdinand von *Helmholtz*, German physicist and physiologist, 1821–1894] **1** Young-Helmholtz theory. See under HELMHOLTZ THEORY OF COLOR VISION. **2** See under LIGAMENT. **3** Helmholtz theory of hearing. See under THEORY.

**helminth** \hel′minth\ [Gk *helmins*, gen. *helminthos*, a worm] A parasitic worm, especially a cestode, trematode, or nematode parasite of vertebrates.

**helminthagogue** \helmin′thəgäg\ ANTHELMINTIC.

**helminthemesis** \hel′minthem′əsis\ [HELMINTH + EMESIS] The vomiting of intestinal worms.

**helminthiasis** \hel′minthī′əsis\ [Gk *helmins*, gen. *helminthos*, a worm + -IASIS] Any infection with helminths. **cutaneous h.** CUTANEOUS LARVA MIGRANS.

**helminthic** \helmin′thik\ HELMINTIC.

**helminthicide** \helmin′thisīd\ [HELMINTH + *i* + -CIDE] A compound lethal to helminths; an anthelmintic.

**helminthism** \hel′minthizm\ [HELMINTH + -ISM] The presence of worms; helminthiasis.

**helminthoid** \helmin′thoid\ Resembling a worm; wormlike.

**helminthology** \hel′minthäl′əjē\ [HELMINTH + *o* + -LOGY] The scientific study of parasitic worms. Also *scolecology.*

**helmintic** \helmin′tik\ [*helmint(h)* + -IC] Relating to or infected with parasitic worms or helminths. Also *helminthic, helminthous.*

**helo-** \hē′lō-\ [Gk *hēlos* nail, wart, callus, corn] A combining form meaning (1) nail or callus; (2) wart, warty.

***Heloderma*** \-dur′mə\ A genus of poisonous lizards of the family Helodermatidae, containing two extant species, *H.*

*suspectum*, the gila monster, and *H. horridum*, the Mexican beaded lizard. They are found in the southwestern United States and Mexico, and are the only lizards known to be poisonous.

**heloderma** \-dur′mə\ [HELO- + -DERMA] A warty or nodulated condition of the skin. *Obs.*

**heloma** \hēlō′mə\ [*hel(o)*- + -OMA] CORN.

***Helophilus*** \hēläf′ələs\ A genus of flies (family Syrphidae) known as hover flies. The larvae (rat-tail maggots) may cause myiasis in nasal cavities or intestines of man or domestic animals. See also RAT-TAIL MAGGOT.

**helplessness** / **learned h.** The condition of passivity or apathy that can be created by subjecting an experimental animal to unavoidable noxious stimulation, such as electric shock. Because humans faced with stressful and uncontrollable events may also exhibit apathy which can then generalize to other situations, this animal model has been proposed as a key for understanding states of depression.

**helvellic acid** $C_{12}H_{20}O_7$. An extremely toxic hemolytic constituent of the fungus *Helvella infula*.

**Helvetius** [Johannis Claudius Adrian *Helvetius*, French anatomist, born 1685] Ligaments of Helvetius. See under LIGAMENTA PYLORI.

**helvolic acid** $C_{33}H_{44}O_8$. An antibiotic chemical derived from cultures of *Aspergillus fumigatus*. Also *fumigacin* (outmoded).

**Helweg** [Hans Kristian Saxtorph *Helweg*, Danish physician, 1847–1901] **1** Bundle of Helweg. See under BUNDLE. **2** Helweg's tract. See under TRACTUS OLIVOSPINALIS.

**hem-** \hēm-, hem-\ HEMO-.

**hema-** \hē′mə-, hem′ə-\ HEMO-.

**hemachromatosis** \-krō′mətō′sis\ HEMOCHROMATOSIS.

**hemachrome** \hē′məkrōm\ HEMOCHROME.

**hemachrosis** \-krō′sis\ Abnormally increased redness of the blood, as seen in carbon monoxide poisoning or in the presence of cyanhemoglobin.

**hemacyte** \hē′məsīt\ HEMOCYTE.

**hemacytometer** \-sītäm′ətər\ HEMOCYTOMETER.

**hemacytopoiesis** \-sī′təpoi·ē′sis\ HEMATOPOIESIS.

**hemadsorbent** \hē′madsôr′bənt\ **1** Causing or characterized by hemadsorption. **2** A substance causing hemadsorption.

**hemadsorption** \hē′madsôrp′shən\ [HEM- + ADSORPTION] **1** The adherence of red cells to mammalian cells or viruses whose surfaces possess receptors. **2** A technique in which antiglobulin antibodies are coupled to erythrocytes and used to detect antibodies bound on tissue cells. **mixed h.** MIXED ANTIGLOBULIN REACTION.

**hemadynometry** \-dīnäm′ətrē\ HEMOMANOMETRY.

**hemafacient** \-fā′shənt\ Promoting hematopoiesis.

**hemagglutination** \-gloo′tinā′shən\ [HEM- + AGGLUTINATION] Agglutination of erythrocytes, induced by antibody to erythrocyte antigens or to antigens adsorbed on their surface, or by other hemagglutinins. Also *hemoagglutination*. **passive h.** Passive agglutination in which red blood cells are the indicator particles to which an antigen has been adsorbed. **viral h.** Agglutination of erythrocytes brought about by a virus, such as the mumps virus or an influenza virus.

**hemagglutinin** \-gloo′tinin\ A substance capable of causing agglutination of erythrocytes: used especially of the surface components of myxoviruses and paramyxoviruses that have this activity, but also applicable to antierythrocyte antibodies. Also *hemoagglutinin*. **cold h.** An erythrocyte-agglutinating antibody, usually of anti-I specificity and IgM class, which is active only at temperatures below 37°C. This reflects the low affinity of the antibodies. Cold hemagglutinins are found in man following infections with *Mycoplasma pneumoniae*, but more usually as a result of a lymphoproliferative process. In this case they are monoclonal. **warm h.** An erythrocyte-agglutinating antibody which is active at normal body temperature (37°C). These antibodies are usually characterized by high affinity and are often IgG.

**hemagogic** \-gäj′ik\ Any substance which stimulates flow of blood.

**hemagonium** \-gō′nē·əm\ HEMOCYTOBLAST.

**hemal** \hē′mal\ **1** Of, pertaining to, or characteristic of blood or blood vessels. **2** Designating the area ventral to the spine, which contains the heart and great vessels.

**hemalum** \hēmā′ləm\ ALUM HEMATOXYLIN. **Mayer's h.** An alum hematoxylin solution containing sodium iodate as an oxidant. It is often used where acid-alcohol differentiation would be inappropriate. Also *Mayer solution*.

**hemanalysis** \hē′mənal′isis\ Examination or analysis of the blood.

**hemangiectasia** \hē′manjē·ektā′zhə\ ANGIECTASIA.

**hemangio-** \hēman′jē·ō-, həman′jē·ō-\ [HEM- + ANGIO-] A combining form denoting blood vessels.

**hemangioblast** \hēman′jē·ōblast′\ [HEMANGIO- + -BLAST] One of the precursor cells which give rise in an embryo to both blood cells and blood vessels.

**hemangioblastoma** \-blastō′mə\ [HEMANGIOBLAST + -OMA] A vascular tumor of the central nervous system composed of capillary type blood vessels separated by stromal cells. Histologically it resembles the hemangioblastic meningioma, but it arises mainly in the cerebellum, medulla, or spinal cord. It may be part of von Hippel-Lindau syndrome. Also *angioblastoma*. **h. retinae** ANGIOMATOSIS RETINAE.

**hemangioendothelioma** \-en′dothē′lē·ō′mə\ [HEMANGIO- + ENDOTHELIOMA] A tumor of blood vessels, mainly capillaries, with prominent endothelial cells. It may occur in benign or malignant forms. **benign h.** ANGIOENDOTHELIOMA. **infantile h.** A hemangioendothelioma of infants, typically in the liver. It may be locally aggressive and replace large portions of the organ. **malignant h.** ANGIOSARCOMA. **h. tuberosum multiplex** Multiple vascular nodules caused by hyperplasia of the endothelium of dermal blood vessels.

**hemangiofibroma** \-fībrō′mə\ ANGIOFIBROMA.

**hemangiogliomatosis retinae** \-glī′ōmətō′sis ret′inē\ ANGIOMATOSIS RETINAE.

**hemangiolymphangioma** \-lim′fanjē·ō′mə\ HEMOLYMPHANGIOMA.

**hemangioma** \hēman′jē·ō′mə\ [HEM- + ANGIOMA] A benign lesion composed of proliferated blood vessels. It may occur in various forms, such as capillary, venous, or cavernous, and is subtyped accordingly. In many of the lesions of this group, the distinction between malformations and neoplasms is difficult and in some cases unresolved. • *Angioma* is often used synonymously but can also apply to lymphangioma. **capillary h.** A nevoid vascular defect consisting of a dense cluster of capillaries of various size separated by a sparse network of reticular tissue. The endothelial cells making up the walls of the capillaries are large and tend to protrude into the lumina so as to reduce the internal diameter. Also *hemangioma congenitale, hemangioma simplex, capillary angioma, capillary nevus*. **cavernous h.** A hemangioma composed of large channels lined by a single layer of endothelial cells. Also *cavernoma, cavernous angioma*. **cirsoid h.** RACEMOSE HEMANGIOMA. **h. congenitale** CAPILLARY HEMANGIOMA. **h. hypertrophicum cutis** ANGIOMA CUTIS. **h. of the kidney** RENAL HEMANGI-

OMA. **multiple hemorrhagic h. of Kaposi** KAPOSI SARCOMA. **h. planum extensum** A large cutaneous hemangioma which is not noticeably elevated above the general level of the skin. **racemose h.** A lesion resembling a malformation composed of tortuous, thick-walled blood vessels of the venous and arterial type. Also *cirsoid hemangioma.* **renal h.** A hemangioma usually arising in the medulla. Intermittent hematuria is the most common symptom, often associated with renal colic due to clots in the ureter. Differential diagnosis includes malignant tumors and calculi. When the diagnosis is not clear nephrectomy is indicated. Also *hemangioma of the kidney.* **sclerosing h.** DERMATOFIBROMA. **h. simplex** CAPILLARY HEMANGIOMA. **venous h.** A hemangioma composed of irregular medium-to-large-sized vessels, predominantly of the venous type. **verrucous keratotic h.** A lesion in which the epidermis shows verruciform projections with dilated capillaries in close apposition to the basal layer and simulating angiokeratoma, but with vascular changes extending into the underlying dermis and subcutis, usually in the form of a capillary angioma. Also *verrucous hemangioma.*

**hemangiomatosis** \-mətō′sis\ [HEM- + ANGIOMATOSIS] Regional or diffuse proliferation of capillaries or thin-walled vascular structures with or without a congenital arteriovenous fistula. Sometimes this lesion is accompanied by overgrowth of fat and/or bone. Also *angiomatosis.* **h. retinae** ANGIOMATOSIS RETINAE. **systemic h.** A condition involving one or more organs or tissues which is characterized by multicentric or diffuse hemangiomatous lesions. Rendu-Osler-Weber disease, Sturge-Weber disease, the Mafucci syndrome, the Bourneville syndrome, and von Hippel-Lindau syndrome are forms of systemic hemangiomato sis.

**hemangiomyolipoma** \-mī′əlipō′mə\ ANGIOMYOLIPOMA.

**hemangiopericyte** \-per′isīt\ PERICYTE.

**hemangiopericytoma** \-per′isītō′mə\ [HEMANGIO- + *pericyt(e)* + -OMA] A vascular tumor in which the pericytic cells of vessel walls proliferate. Microscopically the tumor cells surround vascular channels which are lined by a single layer of endothelial cells. The tumor may be benign or malignant. Also *perithelioma, perithelial endothelioma, periangioma, pericytoma.* **renal h.** JUXTAGLOMERULAR CELL TUMOR.

**hemangiosarcoma** \-särkō′mə\ ANGIOSARCOMA.

**hemaphein** \-fē′in\ A derivative of hemoglobin that imparts a brown color to serum or urine. Adj. hemapheic.

**hemapheresis** \-fer′əsis\ [HEM- + APHERESIS.] The process of separating freshly drawn blood into various constituents, retaining the desired portions, and returning the remaining portions to the donor. Erythrocytes are virtually always one of the components returned. Components retained may be plasma, leukocytes, or platelets, or some combination of these. The restoration of erythrocytes and replacement of lost fluids prevent the donor from experiencing untoward effects from repeated donations, so the process can be repeated more than once, at intervals as short as 48 hours. Also *apheresis, pheresis* (widely used but incorrect).

**hemapoiesis** \-poi·ē′sis\ HEMATOPOIESIS.

**hemapoietic** \-poi·et′ik\ HEMATOPOIETIC.

**hemapophysis** \-päf′isis\ [HEM- + APOPHYSIS] The anterior segment of the hemal arch. A costal cartilage can be regarded as an apophysis of the hemal spine.

**hemarthrosis** \hem′ärthrō′sis\ A hemorrhage into a joint. Also *hemarthros.*

**hemat-** \hē′mət-, hem′ət-\ HEMO-.

**hematal** \hē′mətəl, hem′ətəl\ [HEMAT- + -AL] Relating to blood or blood vessels; hemal.

**hematemesis** \-tem′əsis\ [HEMAT- + EMESIS] The vomiting of blood, which may be clearly recognizable as such or may be in an altered state as dark-colored or blackish material. **Goldstein's h.** Hematemesis resulting from bleeding telangiectases in the gastric mucosa.

**hemathermal** \-thur′məl\ [HEMA- + THERMAL] HOMEOTHERMIC.

**hemathermous** \-thur′məs\ HOMEOTHERMIC.

**hemathidrosis** \hē′matidrō′sis\ HEMATIDROSIS.

**hemathorax** \-thôr′aks\ HEMOTHORAX.

**hematic** \hēmat′ik\ [Gk *haimatikos* (from *haima* blood) sanguineous, of blood] Pertaining to blood.

**hematid** \hem′ətid\ [HEMAT- + -ID[2]] A skin eruption due to hypersensitivity to a component of blood.

**hematidrosis** \hē′matidrō′sis\ [HEMAT- + *(h)idrosis*] The perspiring of blood-tinged sweat. Also *hemathidrosis, hematohidrosis, dermorrhagia, sudor cruentus* (obs.), *sudor sanguineus* (obs.), *bloody sweat.*

**hematimeter** \-tim′ətər\ HEMOCYTOMETER.

**hematin** \hē′mətin, hem′ətin\ [HEMAT- + -IN] A complex of porphyrin and hydroxide ion with iron(III). It may be isolated from hemoglobin as the dimer formed by dehydration, in which the two iron atoms are linked by an oxygen bridge. **acid h.** A brown pigment released from hemoglobin upon treatment with hydrochloric acid. It is apparently identical with heme.

**hematinemia** \-tinē′mē·ə\ The presence of heme in blood, usually bound to hemopexin.

**hematinic** \-tin′ik\ Any substance that promotes blood formation, such as iron, vitamin $B_{12}$, or folic acid. Also *hematinogen, hematonic.*

**hematinometer** \-tinäm′ətər\ HEMOGLOBINOMETER.

**hemato-** \hē′mətō-, hem′ətō-\ HEMO-.

**hematobia** \hē′mətō′bē·ə\ Plural of HEMATOBIUM.

**hematobilia** \-bil′yə\ [HEMATO- + *bil(i)-* + -IA] The presence of blood within the biliary system. Also *hemobilia.*

**hematobium** \hē′mətō′bē·əm\ [HEMATO- + New L *-bium,* neut. of *-bius,* combining form from Gk *bios* life] (*pl.* hematobia) Any microorganism, particularly an animal form or hematozoon, which is parasitic in the blood.

**hematoblast** \hē′mətōblast′\ HEMOCYTOBLAST. **Hayem's h.** HEMOCYTOBLAST.

**hematoblastosis** \-blastō′sis\ HEMOBLASTOSIS.

**hematocele** \hē′mətōsēl′\ [HEMATO- + -CELE[1]] A collection of extravasated blood in a cavity or part, often forming a tumorlike or cystlike swelling, especially in the tunica vaginalis testis. **parametric h.** RECTOUTERINE HEMATOCELE. **pelvic h.** A collection of effused blood within the peritoneal cavity; usually, a rectouterine hematocele. **pudendal h.** A hematocele in a labium of the pudenda. **rectouterine h.** A collection of blood in the rectouterine excavation (pouch of Douglas). Also *parametric hematocele.* **scrotal h.** A hematocele of the scrotum, either in the subcutaneous tissue or within the cavity of the tunica vaginalis. **vaginal h.** A hematocele of the tunica vaginalis testis.

**hematocelia** \-sē′lē·ə\ HEMATOCOELIA.

**hematochezia** \-kē′zē·ə\ [HEMATO- + Gk *chez(ein)* to defecate + -IA] The passage of bright red, easily identifiable blood from the anus, usually a sign of fresh bleeding distal to the ileocecal valve. Also *hemochezia.* Compare MELENA.

**hematochlorin** \-klôr′in\ A green hemoglobin degradation product obtained from placentas. It may be a mixture of verdohemoglobin and related pigments.

**hematochromatosis** \-krō′mətō′sis\ HEMOCHROMATOSIS.

**hematochylocele** \-kī′ləsēl\ A localized collection of both blood and chyle, as seen in the tunica vaginalis of the testis in filariasis.

**hematocoelia** \-sē′lē·ə\ [HEMATO- + COEL- + -IA ] Bleeding into the peritoneal cavity. Also *hematocelia.*

**hematocolpometra** \-käl′pəmē′trə\ [HEMATO- + COLPO- + Gk *mētra* uterus] A collection of blood in the uterus and vagina, usually because of an imperforate hymen or vaginal atresia.

**hematocolpos** \-käl′pəs\ [HEMATO- + Gk *kolpos* womb, vagina] Retention of blood in the vagina usually because of an imperforate hymen. Also *hematokolpos, retained menstruation.*

**hematocrit** \hēmat′ōkrit\ [HEMATO- + Gk *krit(ēs)* a discerner, judge, arbiter] **1** The proportion of erythrocytes in blood, as determined by centrifugation of anticoagulated blood and the calculation:

$$100 \times \frac{\text{volume of packed erythrocytes}}{\text{volume of specimen}}.$$

Also *packed cell volume.* **2** With some automated particle counters, the product 0.1 × mean corpuscular volume × erythrocyte count. **3** Originally, the centrifuge used to determine the ratio of the volume of packed erythrocytes per unit volume of blood. An obsolete usage. For defs. 1, 2, and 3 also *hematokrit* (German spelling). **whole body h.** The volume of erythrocytes (×100) per unit volume of blood for all the blood in circulation. Usually this is determined by measuring, for example with radiolabeled albumen, the plasma volume and the total erythrocyte volume of blood, and then calculating:

$$\text{whole body hematocrit} = \frac{100 \times \text{total erythrocyte volume}}{\text{plasma volume} + \text{total erythrocyte volume}}.$$

**Wintrobe's h.** **1** The proportion of packed erythrocytes in a column of blood following centrifugation for 30 minutes at relative centrifugal force 2260. **2** A graduated glass tube, 10 cm in length with a uniform internal diameter, used for making this measurement.

**hematocyst** \hēmat′ōsist′\ **1** A cyst that contains blood. **2** The presence of blood in the urinary bladder. For defs. 1 and 2 also *hematocystis.*

**hematocyte** \hēmat′ōsīt′\ HEMOCYTE.

**hematocytoblast** \-sī′tōblast\ HEMOCYTOBLAST.

**hematocytolysis** \-sītäl′isis\ HEMOLYSIS.

**hematocytometer** \-sītäm′ətər\ HEMOCYTOMETER.

**hematocytopenia** \-sī′təpē′nē·ə\ A less than normal number of cells in blood, as in erythrocytopenia, leukopenia, neutropenia, lymphocytopenia, thrombocytopenia, and pancytopenia.

**hematocytosis** \-sītō′sis\ POLYCYTHEMIA.

**hematodyscrasia** \-diskrā′zhə\ BLOOD DYSCRASIA.

**hematodystrophy** \-dis′trəfē\ NUTRITIONAL ANEMIA.

**hematoencephalic** \-en′səfal′ik\ Pertaining to a suffusion of blood in the intracranial cavity.

**hematogenesis** \-jen′əsis\ HEMATOPOIESIS.

**hematogenous** \hē′mətäj′ənəs\ [HEMATO- + -GENOUS] Arising from the blood or disseminated by the bloodstream. Also *hematogenic* (rare).

**hematogone** \hē′mətōgōn′\ [HEMATO- + Gk *gonē* seed, stock, progenitor] A lymphocytelike cell, normally present in bone marrow, that is approximately 7 $\mu$m in diameter, has very condensed nuclear chromatin without nucleoli, and contains very little cytoplasm. The relationship of hematogones to other blood cells is unclear. They have been considered to be the common hematopoietic stem cells. Also *lymphoid hemoblast of Pappenheim, myelogone.*

**hematohidrosis** \-hidrō′sis\ HEMATIDROSIS.

**hematohistioblast** \-his′tē·əblast′\ HEMOHISTIOBLAST.

**hematoidin** \hē′mətoi′din\ An iron-free derivative of hemoglobin that resembles bilirubin.

**hematokolpos** \-käl′pəs\ HEMATOCOLPOS.

**hematokrit** The German spelling of HEMATOCRIT. • This spelling occasionally appears in English-language texts.

**hematologist** \hē′mətäl′əjist\ A medical scientist specializing in hematology.

**hematology** \hē′mətäl′əjē\ [HEMATO- + -LOGY] The science of blood and blood-forming tissues, including disorders thereof. Also *hemology.*

**hematolymphangioma** \-lim′fanjē·ō′mə\ HEMOLYMPHANGIOMA.

**hematolysis** \hē′mətäl′isis\ HEMOLYSIS.

**hematolytic** \-lit′ik\ HEMOLYTIC.

**hematoma** \-tō′mə\ [HEMAT- + -OMA] A localized accumulation of blood in a tissue or space. It is usually composed of clotted blood in various stages of organization depending on the length of time it is present. Among the most common causes are trauma, erosion of a blood vessel by pathologic processes such as cancer or abscess, and disorders of blood coagulation. **aneurysmal h.** FALSE ANEURYSM. **h. auris** A condition usually resulting from injury to the external ear in which blood is extravasated between the perichondrium and the cartilage, producing a characteristic unsightly swelling of the pinna. Boxers and rugby football players are particularly at risk. Cases of spontaneous hematoma have sometimes been reported. Failure to evacuate the hematoma promptly may lead to cauliflower ear. **cystic h.** A hematoma which, in the the process of organization, has developed a wall and whose contents have undergone liquefaction. **dissecting h.** ARTERIAL DISSECTION. **epidural h.** A collection of blood external to the dura, usually found within the skull following fracture. Also *extradural hematoma.* **intracerebral h.** An accumulation of blood within the substance of the brain, a common cause of death, dependent on the size and location of the accumulation. **intramural h.** A hematoma located in the wall of a hollow organ. **nasal septum h.** Hematoma located beneath the mucoperichondrium and mucoperiosteum of the nasal septum. It can occur either

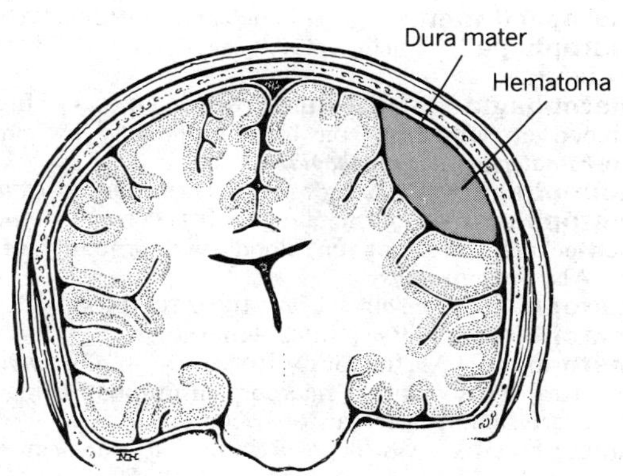


**Subdural hematoma** (showing frontal section of brain)

postoperatively, for instance following submucous resection of the septum, or as a result of accidental trauma. The latter is particularly liable to infection with the formation of a nasal septum abscess. **perinephric h.** A collection of blood anywhere around the kidney, caused by trauma, surgery, or rupture of a blood vessel. **puerperal h.** A hematoma that occurs during the postpartum period. **retroperitoneal h.** Hemorrhage into the retroperitoneal or perirenal areas caused by injury, including a renal biopsy. It may produce severe pain, hematuria, and swelling. **subchorial tuberous h. of the placenta** TUBEROUS MOLE. **subdural h.** A collection of blood between the dura and arachnoid. Intracranially, the hematoma usually comes from torn veins near the longitudinal venous sinus. Also *hemorrhagic internal pachymeningitis* (obs.). **subungual h.** A localized collection of blood beneath a digital nail. **tuberous subchorial h.** TUBEROUS MOLE.

**hematomanometer** \-manäm′ətər\ SPHYGMOMANOMETER.

**hematomediastinum** \-mē′dē·asti′nəm\ HEMOMEDIASTINUM.

**hematometakinesis** \-met′əkīnē′sis\ [HEMATO- + Gk *metakinēsis* (from *meta-* change, trans- + *kinēsis* movement) shift, dislocation] The redistribution of blood from one part of the body to another. Also *borrowing-lending hemodynamic phenomenon, hemometakinesia, hemometakinesis.*

**hematometer** \hem′ətäm′ətər\ HEMOGLOBINOMETER.

**hematometra** \-mē′trə\ [HEMATO- + Gk *mētra* the uterus] An accumulation of blood in the uterus usually due to obstruction either at the level of the uterine cervix or occasionally due to an imperforate hymen. Also *hemometra.*

**hematomole** \hē′mətōmōl′\ [HEMATO- + MOLE[2]] TUBEROUS MOLE.

**hematomphalocele** \hē′mətämfal′əsēl\ The presence of frank blood within an omphalocele.

**hematomphalus** \hē′mətäm′fələs\ [HEMAT- + Gk *omphalos* the navel] CULLEN SIGN.

**hematomyelia** \-mī·ē′lē·ə\ [HEMATO- + MYEL- + -IA] Hemorrhage within the spinal cord occurring spontaneously or as a result of trauma. Also *hematorrhachis interna.*

**hematomyelopore** \-mī′əlōpôr′\ [HEMATO- + MYELO- + PORE] Posthemorrhagic cavitation or softening of the spinal cord.

**hematonic** \hē′mətän′ik\ HEMATINIC.

**hematopathology** \-pathäl′əjē\ The pathology of blood and of blood-forming and lymphoid tissues.

**hematopedesis** \-pədē′sis\ HEMODIAPEDESIS.

**hematopericardium** \-per′ikär′dē·əm\ HEMOPERICARDIUM.

**hematoperitoneum** \-per′itənē′əm\ HEMOPERITONEUM.

**hematophage** \hē′mətōfāj′, hem′ətōfāj′\ ERYTHROPHAGOCYTE.

**hematophagia** \-fā′jə\ [HEMATO- + -PHAGIA] Ingestion of blood or subsistence on blood, especially by parasites. Also *hematophagy, hemophagia.*

**hematophagocyte** \-fag′əsīt\ ERYTHROPHAGOCYTE.

**hematophagous** \hē′mətäf′əgəs\ [HEMATO- + -PHAGOUS] Bloodsucking; subsisting on blood: said primarily of parasites. Also *sanguivorous.*

**hematophagy** \hē′mətäf′əjē\ HEMATOPHAGIA.

**hematophilia** \-fil′yə\ HEMOPHILIA.

**hematophyte** \hē′mətōfīt′\ [HEMATO- + Gk *phyt(on)* a plant, tree] Any plantlike microorganism found living in the blood, for example, a fungus or bacterium.

**hematophytic** \-fit′ik\ Relating to or caused by hematophytes.

**hematopiesis** \-pī·ē′sis\ [HEMATO- + Gk *piesis* a pressing, squeezing] *Outmoded* BLOOD PRESSURE.

**hematoplasmopathy** \-plazmäp′əthē\ HEMOPLASMOPATHY.

**hematoplast** \hem′ətōplast′\ HEMOCYTOBLAST.

**hematoplastic** \-plas′tik\ HEMATOPOIETIC.

**hematopoiesis** \-poi·ē′sis\ [HEMATO- + -POIESIS] The growth and maturation of the formed elements of the blood. Also *hemapoiesis, hemacytopoiesis, hematogenesis, hemogenesis, hemocytogenesis, hemocytopoiesis, hemopoiesis, sanguification* (rare), *sanguinification* (rare). Adj. hematopoietic. **extramedullary h.** The production of formed elements of the blood in tissues outside of the bone marrow.

**hematopoietic** \-poi·et′ik\ [Gk *haimatopoiētikos* blood-making] **1** Relating to hematopoiesis. Also *hemapoietic, hemogenic, hematoplastic, hemopoietic, hemopoiesic, sanguinopoietic.* **2** Any agent that promotes hematopoiesis.

**hematoporphyria** \-pôrfir′ē·ə\ *Obs.* PORPHYRIA.

**hematoporphyrin** \-pôr′firin\ A porphyrin two of whose pyrrole rings have methyl and 1-hydroxyethyl substituents, and two have methyl and 2-carboxyethyl substituents. Hematoporphyrins are not found in nature, but can be prepared from the protoporphyrin of hemoglobin by addition of the elements of water to its vinyl groups.

**hematoporphyrinemia** \-pôr′firinē′mē·ə\ The presence of hematoporphyrin in plasma or serum. *Seldom used.*

**hematoporphyrinism** \-pôr′firinizm′\ A clinical syndrome of hematoporphyrinemia and cutaneous sensitivity to sunlight.

**hematoporphyrinuria** \-pôr′firinoo′rē·ə\ The excretion of hematoporphyrin, a degradation product of hemoglobin, in the urine.

**hematorrhachis** \-rā′kis\ [HEMATO- + Gk *rhachis* the back, spine, backbone] The effusion of blood into the spinal canal. Also *hemorrhachis.* **h. externa** The effusion of blood into the spinal canal, sparing the spinal cord itself. Also *intramedullary hemorrhage.* **h. interna** HEMATOMYELIA.

**hematosalpinx** \-sal′pingks\ [HEMATO- + Gk *salpinx* a tube] An accumulation of blood in a fallopian tube often in association with a tubal ectopic pregnancy. Also *hemosalpinx.*

**hematosarcoma** \-särkō′mə\ *Rare* LYMPHOMA.

**hematoscheocele** \hē′mətäs′kē·əsēl′\ [HEMAT- + OSCHEO- + -CELE[1]] An accumulation of blood in the scrotum.

**hematosepsis** \-sep′sis\ SEPTICEMIA.

**hematospermatocele** \-spur′mətōsēl′\ A spermatocele that contains blood.

**hematospermia** \-spur′mē·ə\ HEMOSPERMIA.

**hematosporidium** \-spôrid′ē·əm\ HAEMOSPORIDIUM.

**hematostatic** \-stat′ik\ **1** Characterized by or resulting from stagnation of the blood. **2** HEMOSTATIC.

**hematotherapy** \-ther′əpē\ HEMOTHERAPY.

**hematothermal** \-thur′məl\ [HEMATO- + THERMAL] HOMEOTHERMIC.

**hematothorax** \-thôr′aks\ HEMOTHORAX.

**hematotoxic** \-täk′sik\ HEMOTOXIC.

**hematotoxin** \-täk′sin\ Any substance that damages blood or blood cells or blood-forming organs.

**hematotropic** \-träp′ik\ HEMOTROPIC.

**hematotympanum** \-tim′pənəm\ HEMOTYMPANUM.

**hematoxic** \-täk′sik\ HEMOTOXIC.

**hematoxylin** \-täk′silin\ An extract from the heartwood of the tree *Haematoxylon campechianum* that is extensively used as a stain for nuclear chromatin. Hematoxylin itself is colorless and needs to be oxidized to the dye hematein, either by natural oxidation by exposure to light and air or by chemical oxidation using sodium iodate or mercuric oxide. Hematein on its own has a poor affinity for tissue and requires a mordant which is usually a salt of a heavy metal. **Ehrlich's h.** An alum hematoxylin that naturally oxidizes to its active form, hematin, over a period of about two months. Also *Ehrlich's acid hematoxylin.* **Harris h.** An alum hematoxylin in which mercuric oxide is used as an oxidant. It provides particularly clear nuclear staining. **Heidenhain's iron h.** A form of iron hematoxylin in which ferric ammonium sulfate is used as a combined oxidizing agent and mordant on tissue specimens, staining nuclei a deep purple. Also *Heidenhain's iron hematoxylin stain.* **Weigert's iron h.** A nuclear stain using alcoholic hematoxylin and ferric chloride. It is the standard iron hematoxylin solution used for staining nuclei. Also *Weigert solution, Weigert's iron hematoxylin stain.*

**hematozoa** \-zō′ə\ Plural of HEMATOZOON.

**hematozoic** \-zō′ik\ [HEMATO- + *zo(o)-* + -IC] Parasitic in the blood of vertebrates: said principally of protozoa. Also *hemozoic.*

**hematozoon** \-zō′ən\ [HEMATO- + Gk *zōon* living being, animal] (*pl.* hematozoa) A protozoon that is parasitic in the blood of vertebrates. Also *hemozoon.*

**hematrophe** \hē′mətrōf\ HEMOTROPH.

**hematuria** \-t$^y$oo′rē·ə\ [HEMAT- + -URIA] Excretion of urine containing blood, either gross (visible) or microscopic (seen only by microscopic examination). The source of bleeding may be the kidney, ureter, bladder, urethra, or prostate. Also *erythrocyturia.* **Egyptian h.** SCHISTOSOMIASIS HAEMATOBIA. **endemic h.** SCHISTOSOMIASIS HAEMATOBIA. **essential h.** Hematuria of unknown cause. **false h.** Red blood cells in the urine from sources other than the urinary tract, as in contamination from feces or vaginal secretions. **hereditary h.** HEREDITARY NEPHRITIS. **initial h.** Hematuria only at the beginning of urination, a sign of a urethral lesion. **recurrent h.** A form of glomerulonephritis characterized by recurrent gross or microscopic hematuria in association with infections. Edema, hypertension, and renal functional impairment are uncommon. The most common histologic finding is focal glomerulonephritis, sometimes with IgA deposition in the mesangium. The prognosis usually is excellent. **renal h.** Red blood cells in the urine due to lesions in the kidneys rather than other urinary tract sources. Red blood cell casts signify glomerular origin of hematuria. **terminal h.** Hematuria at the end of micturition, reflecting a hemorrhagic lesion in the posterior urethra or base of the bladder. **total h.** Hematuria throughout micturition, reflecting a hemorrhagic lesion in the kidneys or ureter. **urethral h.** The passing of blood in the urine due to a urethral hemorrhage. **vesical h.** Blood in the urine from a hemorrhage in the bladder.

**heme** \hēm\ [contraction of HEMATIN] Any iron-porphyrin coordination complex. Porphyrins bind iron(II) and iron(III) very tightly. Also *oxyhematin, oxyheme, oxyhemochromogen, ferriheme.*

***Hementaria*** \hē′menter′ē·ə\ *HAEMENTARIA.*

**hemeralope** \hem′əralōp′\ An individual with hemeralopia.

**hemeralopia** \hem′ərəlō′pē·ə\ [Gk *hēmeralōp(s)* (from *hēmer(a)* the day, daylight + *al(aos)* blind + *ōps* the eye) blind by day + -IA] Inability to see well in bright illumination. Also *day blindness.* • This term is commonly used incorrectly to designate night blindness (nyctalopia).

***Hemerocampa leukostigma*** \hem′ərōkam′pə loo′kōstig′mə\ The white-marked tussock moth, whose larvae bear urticating venomous white hairs that can cause a severe dermatitis.

**hemi-** \hem′ē-\ [Gk *hēmi-* (akin to L *semi-*) half] A prefix meaning (1) half or partial; (2) pertaining to one lateral half of the body or a part; unilateral.

**-hemia** \-hē′mē·ə\ -EMIA.

**hemiacardius** \-əkär′dē·əs\ [HEMI- + ACARDIUS] Conjoined twins in which circulation of both is effected partially or wholly by the heart of only one member.

**hemiacetal** **1** A compound containing the grouping —C(OH)(OR)—. It is formed reversibly by combination of the carbonyl group —CO— with the alcohol R—OH. A second molecule of alcohol could convert it into the acetal —$C(OR)_2$—, which would not revert so easily to the free carbonyl compound. The ring forms of sugars are hemiacetals, formed by combination of a carbonyl group with a hydroxyl group within the same molecule. **2** Such a substance having the carbonyl group contributed only by an aldehyde rather than by a ketone. In the latter case, the term *hemiketal* was once used. An obsolete usage.

**hemiachromatopsia** \-ak′rōmətäp′sē·ə\ [HEMI- + ACHROMATOPSIA] Faulty color perception in a portion of the visual field, due to neurologic disease rather than to the inherited forms of color blindness. Also *hemichromatopsia, color hemianopia.*

**hemiagenesis** \-əjen′əsis\ Agenesis of only one of a pair of organs or unilateral agenesis of an organ normally displaying prominent bilaterality, such as the cerebrum or the cerebellum of the brain.

**hemiageusia** \-əjoo′zē·ə\ [HEMI- + AGEUSIA] Lack or partial loss of the sense of taste on one side of the tongue. Also *hemiageustia.*

**hemiagnosia** \-əgnō′zhə\ [HEMI- + AGNOSIA] Agnosia restricted to half of the body, with regard to the sense of touch, or to half the visual field of each eye, with regard to visual perception. **h. for pain** Hemiasomatognosia giving rise to lack of reaction to painful stimuli restricted to one half of the body.

**hemialbumin** \-albyoo′min\ A polypeptide sometimes found in the urine of patients with osteomalacia or diphtheria. *Outmoded.* Also *hemialbumose.*

**hemianalgesia** \-an′əljē′zē·ə\ Analgesia on one side of the body.

**hemianencephaly** \-an′ənsef′əlē\ Anencephaly affecting one side or primarily one side of the brain and related cranial structures.

**hemianesthesia** \-an′esthē′zhə\ [HEMI- + ANESTHESIA] Loss of sensation on one side of the body. **alternate h.** Loss of feeling on one side of the face due to a lesion of the trigeminal nucleus or tract which also involves ascending sensory pathways resulting in loss of sensation over the contralateral trunk and limbs. The most typical picture is that seen in the Wallenberg syndrome. **bulbar h.** Loss of sensation on one half of the body due to a contralateral brainstem lesion, sometimes associated with hemiplegia, such as that occurring in the paramedian syndrome and in the syndromes of Schmidt and Avellis, in Jackson's lateral bulbar syndrome, and in the Wallenberg syndrome. **cerebral h.** Hemianesthesia resulting from a cerebral lesion. **crossed h.** Hemianesthesia due to a contralateral lesion in the central nervous system. Also *hemianesthesia cruciata.* **peduncular h.** Hemianesthesia due to a lesion of the opposite cerebral peduncle. This may involve all forms of sensation or may affect only pain and temperature sense, touch, or deep sensibility, depending upon the situation and extent of the lesion. Sometimes there is an associated hemiplegia on the side of the impaired sensation and/or a third nerve palsy with signs of cerebellar dysfunction on the side of the lesion.

**hemianopia** \-anō'pyə\ [HEMI- + ANOPIA] Inability to see in half of the visual field. Also *hemianopsia.* Adj. hemianopic. **altitudinal h.** The loss of the upper or lower half of the field of vision. **bilateral h.** BINOCULAR HEMIANOPIA. **binasal h.** Loss of the medial half of the visual field in both eyes. **binocular h.** Loss of half of the visual field in both eyes. Also *bilateral hemianopia.* **bitemporal h.** Loss of the lateral half of the field of vision in both eyes. **color h.** HEMIACHROMATOPSIA. **congruous h.** A loss of part or all of half of the visual field that has exactly identical borders in both eyes. **crossed h.** Loss of opposite vertical halves of the visual fields in the two eyes, top loss on one side, bottom on the other. **heteronymous h.** Loss of different (crossed) halves of the visual field for each eye, as loss of the right field in one eye and of the left field in the other. **homonymous h.** Loss of the same (uncrossed) halves of the visual field for each eye, as loss of the right field for each eye. **incongruous h.** Losses of half of the visual field that are of different extent in each eye. **nasal h.** Loss of all or part of the medial half of the visual field. **quadrantic h.** Loss of all or part of a fourth of the visual field, bounded by the vertical and horizontal midlines. **relative h.** Loss of all or part of half of the visual field that is demonstrable only when the test objects are simultaneously presented on both sides of the visual field. **temporal h.** Loss of all or part of the lateral half of the visual field. **true h.** Loss of vision of half of the visual field, affecting both eyes, and limited to one side of the vertical midline, as would result from a visual pathway lesion at or posterior to the optic chiasm.

**hemianopic** \-anō'pik\ Characterized by or relating to hemianopia; being unable to see in all or part of half of the visual field. Also *hemianoptic.*

**hemianopsia** \-anäp'sē·ə\ HEMIANOPIA. Adj. hemianoptic.

**hemianosmia** \-anäz'mē·ə\ Anosmia affecting only one side of the nose.

**hemiasomatognosia** \-əsō'mətägnō'zhə\ [HEMI- + ASOMATOGNOSIA] Inability to appreciate and interpret somatic sensation upon one side of the body.

**hemiatonia** \-ətō'nē·ə\ Unilateral muscular atonia (flaccid paralysis) or hypotonia.

**hemiatrophy** \-at'rōfē\ [HEMI- + ATROPHY] Atrophy of tissues involving one side of the body or one half of a structure, organ, or part. Also *hemihypoplasia.* **facial h.** ROMBERG'S PROGRESSIVE FACIAL HEMIATROPHY. **progressive lingual h.** A progressive, unilateral paralysis of the tongue, accompanied by atrophy. **Romberg's progressive facial h.** A rare condition characterized by unilateral facial atrophy, involving especially the subcutaneous tissues. The condition, of unknown cause, occurs more frequently in women, first appears in adolescence, and is slowly progressive. Also *Romberg's disease, facial trophoneurosis, Parry-Romberg syndrome, facial hemiatrophy, trophoneurosis of Romberg.*

**hemiballismus** \-baliz'məs\ [HEMI- + Gk *ballismos* a throwing oneself about] A syndrome, usually of sudden onset, in elderly patients, giving rise to violent, writhing, involuntary movements, often of wide excursion, and confined to one half of the body. The movements are continuous and often exhausting but cease during sleep. It results from cerebral vascular disease and is usually due to infarction of one subthalamic nucleus (corpus Luysii) or of the pathway connecting this nucleus to the midbrain. The condition was often fatal in the past, due to exhaustion, but can now sometimes be controlled by phenothiazine drugs or abolished by stereotaxic surgery. Milder forms of the condition may be identified as hemichorea. Also *syndrome of the corpus Luysii, subthalamic syndrome, hemiballism, body of Luys syndrome.*

**hemic** \hem'ik\ Related to blood or blood flow.

**hemicardia** \-kär'dē·ə\ [HEMI- + -CARDIA] A developmentally defective heart with only two chambers, a single atrium and a single ventricle. These chambers have structural features common to the respective right and left chambers, therefore efforts to identify them with the normal right and left chambers are meaningless. Also *cor biloculare.*

**hemicardius** \-kär'dē·əs\ An embryo, fetus, or neonate with hemicardia, that is only half of the usual four-chambered heart.

**hemicellulose** Any of several alkali-soluble polysaccharides found in the walls of plant cells. They include polymers of xylose, mannose, L-arabinose, glucuronic acid, and galacturonic acid.

**hemicentrum** \-sen'trəm\ [HEMI- + CENTRUM] Either of the two lateral halves of a body of a vertebra.

**hemicephalalgia** \-sef'əlal'jə\ [HEMI- + CEPHALALGIA] HEMICRANIA.

**hemicephaly** \-sef'əlē\ [HEMI- + CEPHAL- + -Y] Agenesis or partial agenesis of the cerebral hemispheres. The basal ganglia may be present to a variable degree but the brainstem and cerebellum tend to be normally formed.

**hemicerebrum** \-ser'əbrəm\ The cerebral hemisphere of one side. Also *hemiencephalon.*

**hemichorea** \-kôrē'ə\ Chorea in which the choreic movements affect only one half of the body. Also *hemiplegic chorea, hemilateral chorea, chorea dimidiata, unilateral chorea, one-sided chorea.* **paralytic h.** Hemichorea giving such a degree of weakness and hypotonia in the affected limbs that hemiplegia is simulated. **posthemiplegic h.** Hemichorea developing as a sequel of hemiplegia. **preparalytic h.** A condition in which choreiform movements in the affected limbs precede the development of hemiplegia.

**hemichromatopsia** \-krō'mətäp'sē·ə\ HEMIACHROMATOPSIA.

**hemicolectomy** \-kōlek'təmē\ [HEMI- + COLECTOMY] The surgical removal of approximately half of the large bowel. **left h.** The surgical removal of the large bowel from the midtransverse colon to the rectum. **right h.** The surgical removal of a few distal centimeters of the small bowel and the large bowel from the cecum to the midtransverse colon.

**hemicorporectomy** \-kôr'pôrek'təmē\ The surgical removal of the lower half of the body, including all of the pelvic contents and the pelvic bones.

**hemicrania** \-krā'nē·ə\ [Gk *hēmikrania* (from HEMI- + *kranion* skull, head + -IA) a headache on one side] **1** Pain or neuralgia on one side of the head. Also *hemicephalalgia.* **2** MIGRAINE.

**hemicraniectomy** \-krā'nē·ek'təmē\ [HEMI- + CRANIECTOMY] Removal of one side of the cranium, as for extensive decompression of the brain. Also *hemicraniotomy.*

**hemicraniosis** \-krā'nē·ō'sis\ An enlargement of one side of the cranium and/or face.

**hemicraniotomy** \-krā'nē·ät'əmē\ [HEMI- + CRANIOTOMY] HEMICRANIECTOMY.

**hemidesmosome** \-dez'mōsōm\ An attachment point between an epidermal cell and the underlying basement membrane, seen by electron microscopy to correspond to one-half of a desmosome.

**hemidiaphoresis** \-dī'əfôrē'sis\ [HEMI- + Gk *diaphorēsis* evaporation, perspiration] HEMIHYPERHIDROSIS.

**hemidiaphragm** \-dī′əfram\ One half of the diaphragm (right or left).
**hemidrosis** \-drō′sis\ HEMIHIDROSIS.
**hemidysesthesia** \-dis′esthē′zhə\ Spontaneous abnormal sensation occurring over one half of the body.
**hemiectromelia** \-ek′trəmē′lyə\ [HEMI + ECTROMELIA] A reduction deformity of the limbs on one side of the body.
**hemiencephalon** \-ensef′əlän\ HEMICEREBRUM.
**hemifacial** \-fā′shəl\ [HEMI- + FACIAL] Describing, pertaining to, or affecting one side of the face only.
**hemigastrectomy** \-gastrek′təmē\ The surgical removal of approximately half of the stomach.
**hemigeusia** \-joo′zē·ə\ [HEMI- + Gk *geus(is)* taste + -IA] Taste sensation on one side of the tongue only.
**hemigigantism** \-jī′gantizm\ Extreme hypertrophy of a lateral half of the body or of one or more parts on one side of the body.
**hemiglossitis** \-gläsī′tis\ Glossitis confined to one side of the tongue.
**hemiglossoplegia** \-gläs′əplē′jə\ [HEMI- + GLOSSOPLEGIA] Paralysis of one side of the tongue.
**hemignathia** \-nā′thē·ə\ [HEMI- + GNATH- + -IA] Defective development of the mandibular region on one side.
**hemihepatectomy** \-hep′ətek′təmē\ The surgical removal of approximately half of the liver.
**hemihidrosis** \-hidrō′sis\ [HEMI- + HIDROSIS] Sweating confined to one side of the body. Also *hemidrosis.*
**hemihydranencephaly** \-hī′dranənsef′əlē\ Hydranencephaly affecting only one side of the head.
**hemihypalgesia** \-hī′paljē′zē·ə\ A reduction in pain sensibility on one half of the body.
**hemihyperesthesia** \-hī′pəresthē′zhe\ [HEMI- + HYPERESTHESIA] An apparent heightening of acuteness of perception of touch on one side of the body.
**hemihyperhidrosis** \-hī′pərhidrō′sis\ [HEMI- + HYPERHIDROSIS ] Excessive sweating on one side of the body. Also *hemidiaphoresis, hyperhidrosis unilateralis.*
**hemihyperplasia** \-hī′pərplā′zhə\ Hyperplasia of tissues on one side of the body or on one side of an organ or part.
**hemihypertrophy** \-hīpur′trəfē\ Hypertrophy of tissues, organs, or parts on one side of the body.
**hemihypesthesia** \-hī′pesthē′zhə\ [HEMI- + HYP- + -ESTHESIA] Impairment of the sense of touch over one half of the body. Also *hemihypoesthesia.*
**hemihypoesthesia** HEMIHYPESTHESIA.
**hemihypogeusia** \-hī′pōjoo′zē·ə\ [HEMI- + HYPOGEUSIA] Reduced perception of taste on one side of the tongue.
**hemihypoplasia** \-hī′pōplā′zhə\ [HEMI- + HYPOPLASIA] HEMIATROPHY.
**hemihypothermia** \-hī′pōthur′mē·ə\ A condition in which the temperature upon one side of the body is lower than on the other.
**hemikaryon** \-kar′ē·än\ The nucleus of a cell which contains the haploid number of chromosomes.
**hemilaminectomy** \-lam′inek′təmē\ Excision of a vertebral lamina on one side. Also *hemilaminotomy.*
**hemilaryngectomy** \-lar′injek′təmē\ [HEMI- + LARYNGECTOMY] An operation to remove half the larynx for malignant disease localized strictly within the part removed. See also HEMILARYNX. **horizontal h.** Hemilaryngectomy in which the part of the larynx removed is that situated above the level of the vocal folds, including the hyoid bone, epiglottis, and ventricular bands. Also *supraglottic laryngectomy.* **vertical h.** A partial laryngectomy in which the greater part of the hemilarynx situated to one side of the anteroposterior midline vertical plane is removed.
**hemilarynx** \-lar′ingks\ Half the larynx; particularly a half that is surgically removed. It can be either the half to one side of the midline vertical plane through the laryngeal eminence or the half above the horizontal plane transecting the larynx immediately above the true vocal cords.
**hemilateral** \-lat′ərəl\ Pertaining to or involving the outer half of one side.
**hemimacrocephaly** \-mak′rəsef′əlē\ [HEMI- + MACROCEPHALY] Hemihypertrophy affecting the head.
**hemimacroglossia** \-mak′rəgläs′ē·ə\ Enlargement of the tongue confined to one side.
**hemimandible** \-man′dibl\ Either half of the mandible situated on one side or the other of the midline vertical plane passing through the symphysis menti.
**hemimandibulectomy** \-mandib′yəlek′təmē\ Surgical excision of half the mandible, from close to the symphysis menti to, and including, the mandibular condyle. It is undertaken chiefly for the removal of various tumors confined to this part. Reconstruction may make use of a bone graft or of a metal implant splint.
**hemimandibuloglossectomy** \-mandib′yəlōgläsek′təmē\ Hemimandibulectomy combined with excision of part of the tongue. It is undertaken for malignant disease involving both mandible and tongue. Reconstruction presents formidable problems.
**hemimelia** \-mē′lyə\ [HEMI- + MEL-[1] + -IA ] A developmental defect involving major reduction in the distal portion of a limb. It is one of the conditions that can result when a pregnant woman takes thalidomide. Compare PHOCOMELIA. **axial h.** The agenesis of one of the distal long bones of a limb. **transverse h.** The natural developmental amputation of a limb at the elbow or wrist in an upper extremity or at the knee or ankle in a lower extremity.
**hemimetabolous** \-mətab′ələs\ [HEMI- + Gk *metabol(os)* changeable + -OUS] Characterized by gradual or simple metamorphosis, involving a series of preadult nymphal stages: said primarily of insects. Compare HOLOMETABOLOUS.
**hemiparalysis** \-pəral′isis\ [HEMI- + PARALYSIS] HEMIPLEGIA.
**hemiparaplegia** \-per′əplē′jə\ [HEMI- + PARAPLEGIA] Paralysis of one side of the lower half of the body. • This usage is incorrect as *paraplegia* by definition means paralysis of both lower limbs.
**hemiparesis** \-pərē′sis\ [HEMI- + PARESIS] Slight or incomplete motor weakness affecting one side of the body.
**hemiparesthesia** \-per′esthē′zhə\ [HEMI- + PARESTHESIA] Paresthesia restricted to one half of the body.
**hemiparkinsonism** \-pär′kinsənizm′\ [HEMI- + PARKINSONISM] Parkinsonism in which the abnormal physical signs are restricted to one half of the body.
**hemipelvectomy** \-pelvek′təmē\ The surgical removal of half of the bony pelvis.
**hemipelvis** \-pel′vis\ Either of the two lateral halves of a pelvis.
**hemipelvisectomy** \-pel′visek′təmē\ HINDQUARTER AMPUTATION.
**hemiphalangectomy** \-fal′anjek′təmē\ An excision of part of a digit.
**hemiplegia** \-plē′jə\ [HEMI- + -PLEGIA] Paralysis of one half of the body. The paralysis may be total, involving face, limbs, and trunk, or partial (hemiparesis). Bilateral hemiplegia may occur, giving a clinical picture which is difficult to distinguish from quadriplegia. Also *hemiparalysis, semiplegia.* Adj. hemiplegic. **acute infantile h.** An acute cerebral disorder affecting infants and children up to about two years, characterized by hemiplegia, lateralized seizures, and severe neurologic residual defects. Fever and coma are com-

mon. The etiology is manifold and includes thrombosis of the internal carotid artery and cortical thrombophlebitis secondary to severe dehydration. Also *Marie-Strümpell disease, polioencephalitis of Marie-Strümpell, hemiconvulsive-hemiplegic syndrome, Strümpell's disease, Strümpell-Leichtenstern disease, H.H.E. syndrome, Strümpell-Marie disease.* **h. alternans hypoglossica** MEDIAN MEDULLARY SYNDROME. **alternate h.** CROSSED HEMIPLEGIA. **alternating oculomotor h.** WEBER SYNDROME. **ascending h.** Hemiplegia in which paralysis begins in the foot and leg and spreads upwards to the trunk and upper limb. **Avellis h.** AVELLIS PARALYSIS. **bulbar h.** Any type of hemiplegia caused by damage to the medulla oblongata. **capsular h.** Hemiplegia resulting from a lesion of the contralateral internal capsule. **cerebellar h.** Severe unilateral ataxia due to a lesion of the ipsilateral cerebellum or of cerebellar pathways in the brainstem on the same side. Strictly, although the affected limbs may be grossly ataxic and also weak, this is not a true hemiplegia. **cerebral h.** Hemiplegia due to any cerebral lesion. **collateral h.** Hemiplegia occurring on the same side as the cerebral lesion. This may be due, among other causes, to pressure upon the contralateral crus cerebri against the free edge of the tentorium cerebelli, produced by a space-occupying lesion. **congenital h.** Hemiplegia present at birth and attributable to impaired cerebral development or to birth trauma. A form of cerebral palsy, it is rarely discernible before the age of two or three months. **contralateral h.** The usual form of hemiplegia, occurring on the side opposite to the cerebral lesion. **crossed h.** Hemiplegia due to a contralateral brainstem lesion which may have produced signs of cranial nerve dysfunction or cerebellar signs on the side of the lesion (the side opposite to the hemiplegia). Also *hemiplegia cruciata, alternate hemiplegia, stauroplegia.* **facial h.** Unilateral facial paralysis. Also *hemiprosoplegia.* **faciobrachial h.** Paralysis of one side of the face and of the arm on the same side. **faciolingual h.** Paralysis of one side of the face and of half the tongue on the same side. **flaccid h.** Hemiplegia with atonia or severe hypotonia and absent or depressed tendon reflexes in the affected limbs. This may be an initial manifestation of an acute lesion, such as an infarct, in the opposite cerebral hemisphere, seen in the phase of "shock", in which case spasticity often develops subsequently in the affected limbs. But when there is extensive involvement of the parietal sensory cortex as well as motor cortex, flaccidity may persist in the paralyzed limbs. **functional h.** HYSTERICAL HEMIPLEGIA. **Gubler's h.** MILLARD-GUBLER SYNDROME. **hysterical h.** Hemiplegia due to subconscious mental motivation and not to any physical cause, usually developing as a means of escape from a stressful situation. Often there is also total loss of all forms of sensation in the affected limbs. Also *functional hemiplegia.* **infantile h.** Hemiplegia which may be present from birth, normally due to perinatal brain damage, or which develops during infancy. It may develop acutely and is often associated with seizures occurring at the onset. It is usually due to infarction resulting from arterial or, less often, cerebral venous occlusion, but may in rare cases be due to encephalitis or encephalopathy. A hemiplegia developing gradually in infancy or early childhood may be a manifestation of the Sturge-Weber syndrome. **organic h.** Any form of hemiplegia due to a physical lesion of the nervous system. **peduncular h.** Hemiplegia due to a lesion of the contralateral cerebral peduncle. **pontine h.** Hemiplegia due to a contralateral pontine lesion. In most cases, this is associated with signs of cranial nerve or cerebellar dysfunction on the side of the lesion. **puerperal h.** Hemiplegia due to cerebral vascular disease developing in the puerperium. **spastic h.** Hemiplegia with spasticity, as distinct from flaccidity, of the affected limbs. **spinal h.** Hemiplegia resulting from a unilateral lesion of the pyramidal (corticospinal) tract in the spinal cord. The face is spared. Depending upon the extent of the lesion, sensory pathways may also be affected. **superior alternate h.** WEBER SYNDROME

**hemiplegic** \-plē′jik\ Pertaining to hemiplegia.

**hemiprosoplegia** \-präs′əplē′jə\ [HEMI- + *proso(p)-* + -PLEGIA] FACIAL HEMIPLEGIA.

**hemiprostatectomy** \-präs′tətek′təmē\ [HEMI- + PROSTATECTOMY] The surgical removal of one of the lateral halves of the prostate.

**Hemiptera** \hemip′tərə\ [HEMI- + Gk *ptera* (pl. of *pteron* feather) feathers, wings] An order of hemimetabolous insects, the true bugs, which includes many species of varied habits and structures, but all equipped with piercing and sucking mouthparts. A few are of medical importance, being adapted for bloodsucking, enabling them to be disease vectors. The triatomine or cone-nosed bugs serve to transmit the flagellate *Trypanosoma cruzi,* the agent of Chagas disease. *Cimex lectularius,* the common bedbug, is a member of the order. Though a notorious pest and bloodsucker, it appears not to serve as an efficient vector of human parasites.

**hemipterous** \hemip′tərəs\ Of or belonging to the order Hemiptera.

**hemisacralization** \-sā′krəlizā′shən\ The unilateral fusion of the transverse process of the fifth lumbar vertebra to the wing of the sacrum.

**hemisection** A longitudinal section in the median plane. **h. of the spinal cord** A longitudinal incision dividing the spinal cord in the midline.

**hemiseptum** **1** Half of a septum. **2** HEMISEPTUM CEREBRI. **h. cerebri** The septum pellucidum of one side of the telencephalon. Also *hemiseptum.*

**hemisotonic** \hēmī′sōtän′ik\ [HEM- + ISOTONIC] Having the same osmolarity as the blood.

**hemispasm** \hem′ēspazm\ [HEMI- + SPASM] Unilateral spasm. **facial h.** Spasmodic unilateral contraction of facial muscles, usually due to an irritative lesion of the facial nerve in its canal, less often to a lesion of the facial nucleus in the brainstem. This is a not infrequent sequel of facial paralysis (Bell's palsy). Also *clonic facial spasm, facial myoclonus, facial myospasm.* **glossolabial h.** Unilateral recurrent contraction of tongue and lip muscles, which may extend to the orbicularis oculi or be associated with blepharospasm. This may be hysterical, but similar manifestations can occur in facial dyskinesia due to phenothiazine drugs.

**hemisphere** \hem′isfir\ [L *hemisphaerium.* See HEMISPHERIUM.] HEMISPHERIUM. **animal h.** In a cleaving telolecithal ovum, the hemisphere where the yolk material does not accumulate. Compare VEGETAL HEMISPHERE. **cerebellar h.** HEMISPHERIUM CEREBELLI. **cerebral h.** HEMISPHERIUM CEREBRI. **dominant h.** The cerebral hemisphere which controls speech and executive and cognitive skills. This is almost invariably the left hemisphere in right-handed individuals. In the left-handed, it is usually the right, but sometimes it may be the left. Also *talking hemisphere.* **nondominant h.** The cerebral hemisphere other than the dominant one, such that ablation results in a less severe deficit. Also *mute hemisphere.* **talking h.** DOMINANT HEMISPHERE. **vegetal h.** The hemisphere of a cleaving ovum of the telolecithal type where the yolk becomes concentrated. Compare ANIMAL HEMISPHERE.

**hemispherectomy** \-sfirek′təmē\ [*hemispher(e)* + -ECTOMY] Excision or extensive resection of one cerebral hemisphere.

**hemispheria** \-sfir′ē·ə\ Plural of HEMISPHERIUM.

**hemispherium** \-sfir′ē·əm\ [L *hemisphaerium* (from Gk *hēmisphairion* a small hemisphere, from *hēmi-* half + *sphairion* a little ball or sphere) hemisphere] Half of a spherical structure or organ such as the cerebrum or cerebellum. Also *hemisphere*. **h. bulbi urethrae** Each lateral half of the bulbus penis (occasionally called bulbus urethrae), on each side of the commencement of the spongy part of the urethra. **h. cerebelli** [NA] The cerebellar hemisphere of one side, lateral to the midline vermis and consisting of the lobuli centralis, quadrangularis, simplex, semilunaris, biventer, and tonsil. Also *cerebellar hemisphere*. **h. cerebri** [NA] The largest mass of the brain on either side, derived from the embryonic telencephalon and consisting principally of the cerebral cortex and the underlying basal ganglia and their associated fiber systems. Also *cerebral hemisphere*.

**hemisyndrome** \-sin′drōm\ [HEMI- + SYNDROME] Any syndrome in which the symptoms and signs of disease or dysfunction are confined to one side of the body.

**hemiterpene** A terpene formed from a single isoprene unit and of formula $C_5H_8$.

**hemithermoanesthesia** \-thur′mə·an′esthē′zhə\ [HEMI- + THERMO- + ANESTHESIA] Loss or impairment of temperature sensation on one side of the body.

**hemithorax** \-thôr′aks\ One of the two lateral halves of the chest.

**hemitoxin** \-täk′sin\ A toxin that has half of its original toxicity.

**hemitremor** \hem′ētrem′ər\ [HEMI- + TREMOR] Tremor on only one side of the body.

**hemivertebra** \-vur′təbrə\ A failure in the development of a lateral half, or major part thereof, of a vertebra. It is usually accompanied by agenesis of the rib ordinarily associated with the missing vertebral part.

**hemizygote** \-zī′gōt\ A cell, tissue, organism, or sex having but one copy of a specific gene, genes, chromosome segment, or entire chromosome in its otherwise diploid genome. The human male is a hemizygote with reference to the X and Y chromosomes.

**hemizygous** \-zī′gəs\ **1** Of or pertaining to a specific gene, group of genes, chromosome segment, or entire chromosome that is present only once in an otherwise diploid genome. **2** Referring to a cell, tissue, organism, or sex that is in some way a hemizygote. The heterogametic sex of a species is hemizygous for genes on both sex chromosomes. For defs. 1 and 2 also *hemizygotic*.

**hemlock** \hem′läk\ [Old English *hemlic*, prob. from Finno-Ugrian, akin to Finnish *humala* hop plant] A plant of the species *Conium maculatum*; poison hemlock.

**hemo-** \hē′mō-\ [Gk *haima* (genitive *haimatos*) blood] A combining form meaning blood. Also *haemo-* (British spelling), *hem-, hema-, haem-* (British spelling), *hemat-, hemato-, haemato-* (British spelling).

**hemoagglutination** \-əgloo′tinā′shən\ HEMAGGLUTINATION.

**hemoagglutinin** \-əgloo′tinin\ HEMAGGLUTININ.

**hemobilia** \-bil′yə\ HEMATOBILIA.

**hemoblast** \hē′mōblast\ HEMOCYTOBLAST. **lymphoid h. of Pappenheim** HEMATOGONE.

**hemoblastosis** \-blastō′sis\ Any neoplastic disorder of the hematopoietic system, such as leukemias of all types, malignant lymphomas, myeloma, polycythemia vera, and essential thrombocythemia. *Rare*. Also *hematoblastosis, hemolymphadenosis, hemomyelosis*.

**hemocatheresis** \-kəther′əsis\ *Seldom used* HEMOLYSIS.

**hemocele** \hē′mōsēl\ HEMOCOEL.

**hemochezia** \-kē′zē·ə\ HEMATOCHEZIA.

**hemocholecyst** \-ko′ləsist\ A hollow structure, usually the gallbladder, containing both blood and bile and resulting from nontraumatic hemorrhage.

**hemocholecystitis** \-kō′ləsistī′tis\ [HEMO- + CHOLECYSTITIS] Inflammation of the gallbladder accompanied by bleeding into the gallbladder.

**hemochorial** \-kôr′ē·əl\ [HEMO- + *chori(on)* + -AL] Pertaining to a type of placentation containing only trophoblast, connective tissue, and endothelium, occurring in lower rodents, bats, and anthropoids. The endothelium of uterine vessels is lost and blood circulates in channels in the fetal syncytium.

**hemochromatosis** \-krō′mətō′sis\ [HEMO- + CHROMATOSIS] A chronic, progressive disease of unclear pathogenesis that is associated with iron overload and iron deposition in many tissues. The idiopathic form is an autosomal recessive condition. A similar phenotype, hemosiderosis, can result from multiple transfusions or a diet very high in iron. Clinical sequelae include a bronze hue to the skin, hepatic failure with cirrhosis, diabetes, heart failure, pituitary insufficiency, and arthropathy. Also *hemachromatosis, hematochromatosis, Recklinghausen-Applebaum disease, iron storage disease*. **exogenous h.** Hemochromatosis caused by an excess of iron taken into the body, as through repeated blood transfusions or prolonged and excessive ingestion of iron.

**hemochrome** \hē′mōkrōm\ Any oxygen-carrying pigment of blood. The hemochrome of vertebrates is hemoglobin. A variety of hemochromes occur in invertebrate species, such as hemocyanin, erythrocruorin, chlorocruorin, and hemoerythrin. Also *hemachrome*.

**hemochromogen** \-krō′məjən\ Any substance that contains heme in combination with protein or other constituents. **hemoglobin h.** Denatured hemoglobin.

**hemochromometer** \-krōmäm′ətər\ HEMOGLOBINOMETER.

**hemochromometry** \-krōmäm′ətrē\ HEMOGLOBINOMETRY.

**hemoclip** \hē′mōklip\ [HEMO- + *clip*] A malleable metal clip used to occlude small vessels during a surgical operation or to mark structures for radiographic study or postoperative irradiation.

**hemocoagulin** \-kō·ag′yəlin\ A substance in the venom of certain snakes, especially vipers, that induces the clotting of blood.

**hemocoel** \hē′mōsēl\ [HEMO- + *coel(om)*] **1** A body cavity in which blood circulates freely without being confined to vessels, as in arthropods. **2** In vertebrates, the part of the coelomic body cavity involved in the development of the heart. For defs. 1 and 2 also *hemocoelom, hemocele*.

**hemoconcentration** \-kän′səntrā′shən\ A relative increase in the proportion of cellular components of blood due to reduction in the fluid component. Hemoconcentration may result from dehydration, from severe or extensive burns, or transiently in an extremity from prolonged application of a tourniquet prior to drawing a blood specimen.

**hemocrine** \hē′məkrin\ [HEMO- + *-crine* as in *endocrine*] Capable of producing a hormonal influence in the blood.

**hemoculture** \hē′mōkul′chər\ Culture of the blood to isolate microbial agents, usually bacteria.

**hemocyanin** \-sī′ənin\ An oxygen-carrying, copper-containing blood pigment found in arthopods and mollusks. It is often used as an experimental antigen in immunologic studies.

**hemocyte** \hē′mōsīt\ [HEMO- + -CYTE] Any formed element of the blood. Also *hematocyte*. Also *hemacyte*.

**hemocytoblast** \-sī′təblast\ [*hemocyt(e)* + *o* + -BLAST] The totipotential precursor of mesenchymal origin, probably of lymphoid appearance, which can develop into any of the formed blood elements. It is the keystone of the monophyletic theory of hematopoiesis. Also *hematoblast, Hayem's hematoblast, hematocytoblast, hematoplast, hemoblast, hemagonium, lymphoidocyte*.

**hemocytoblastoma** \-sī′təblastō′mə\ LEUKEMIA.

**hemocytocatheresis** \-sī′təkəther′əsis\ HEMOLYSIS.

**hemocytogenesis** \-sī′təjen′əsis\ HEMATOPOIESIS.

**hemocytolytic** \-sī′təlit′ik\ HEMOLYTIC.

**hemocytometer** \-sītäm′ətər\ A device used in the microscopic enumeration of blood cells. It consists of a thin glass tablet on which are scored grids of precise dimensions, so that when a 0.1 mm thick film of diluted blood is placed above the grids, the number of cells in a volume of blood may be determined by microscopic examination. Also *counting chamber, hemacytometer, hematocytometer, hematimeter, Zappert's chamber*.

**hemocytophagia** \-sī′təfā′jə\ The ingestion of blood cells by phagocytes.

**hemocytophagic** \-sī′təfā′jik\ **1** Relating to hemocytophagia. **2** Capable of ingesting blood cells: used of phagocytes.

**hemocytopoiesis** \-sī′təpō·ē′sis\ HEMATOPOIESIS.

**hemodiafiltration** \-dī′əfiltrā′shən\ SIMULTANEOUS HEMODIALYSIS AND HEMOFILTRATION. See under HEMOFILTRATION.

**hemodialysis** \-dī·al′isis\ [HEMO- + DIALYSIS] A process by which certain molecules are removed from circulating blood of uremic patients by diffusion through a semipermeable membrane. Access to blood is achieved through an external arteriovenous shunt, or more commonly, an arteriovenous fistula produced surgically. **sequential ultrafiltration-h.** A process by which fluid, electrolytes, and substances of relatively small molecular weight are removed from whole blood by convective transport through a conventional hemodialysis membrane combined with ultrafiltration. The ultrafiltration may be performed before or after the hemodialysis. **simultaneous h. and hemofiltration** See under HEMOFILTRATION.

**hemodialyzer** \-dī′əlī′zər\ An apparatus by which hemodialysis may be carried out, blood being separated by a semipermeable membrane from a solution of such composition as to cause diffusion of certain unwanted molecules out of the blood. A variety of different hemodialysis machines and semipermeable membranes are available. Treatments are given two or three times weekly in endstage renal disease, with repeated access to the vascular system usually through an internal, surgically produced arteriovenous shunt. Also *artificial kidney* (popular). **ultrafiltration h.** A hemodialyzer in which fluid pressure causes filtration of a protein-free fluid out of the blood, used in the management of fluid overload in the presence of acute or chronic renal failure, or in intractable congestive heart failure.

**hemodiapedesis** \-dī′əpədē′sis\ The passage of red cells through capillary walls into the tissues. Also *hematopedesis*.

**hemodilution** \-diloo′shən\ The reduction of hematocrit, or the lowering of hemoglobin or erythrocyte concentration of blood, resulting from augmentation of plasma volume.

**hemodromography** \-drōmäg′rəfē\ [HEMO- + DROMO- + -GRAPHY] The procedure of recording blood flow velocity. Also *hemodromometry*.

**hemodromometry** \-drōmäm′ətrē\ HEMODROMOGRAPHY.

**hemodynamics** \-dīnam′iks\ The science concerned with the study of blood circulation. Also *hemohydraulics*.

**hemodynamometry** \-dī′nəmäm′ətrē\ HEMOMANOMETRY.

**hemodyscrasia** \-diskrā′zhə\ BLOOD DYSCRASIA.

**hemoendothelial** \-en′dəthē′lē·əl\ Describing a type of placentation in which maternal blood comes in contact with the endothelium of the placenta, occurring in rats, guinea pigs, and rabbits. The endothelium alone, of fetal vessels, separates fetal blood from the maternal blood sinuses. See also HEMOENDOTHELIAL PLACENTA.

**hemofiltration** \-filtrā′shən\ [HEMO- + FILTRATION] An extracorporeal process by which the fluid and solute composition of blood and body fluids can be corrected by a

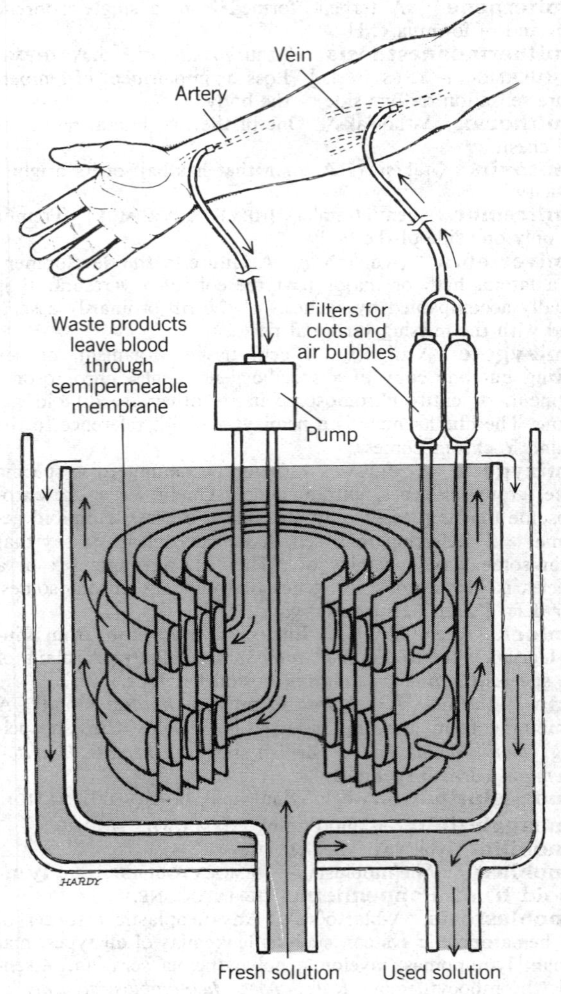


**Hemodialysis**

combination of ultrafiltration and convective solute loss and dilution with physiologic saline solution. Dilution may occur before or after the ultrafiltration. This treatment requires an apparatus similar to a hemodialyzer. The membrane has a high ultrafiltration capability. Usually rates of blood flow of 250–350 ml/min are required to maintain ultrafiltration rates in the range of 50–150 ml/min. The process removes 25–30 liters of ultrafiltrate during a period of five or six hours. During therapy, simultaneous reinfusion of a physiologic saline solution is required. Equipment which can balance fluid removal and replacement, preventing marked intravascular shifts, is necessary for the performance of hemofiltration. Although the technique is less efficient than hemodialysis for removing substances of small molecular weight, such as urea nitrogen and creatinine, it has the advantage of efficient removal of excess fluid without cardiovascular instability. The technique also allows for the removal of substances of larger molecular weight. Increased protein loss could mean retrogression if repeated therapy is necessary. **simultaneous hemodialysis and h.** A system of extracorporeal treatment which utilizes convective and diffusive transport simultaneously. Membranes must have high permeability for fluid and be satisfactory for hemodialysis, such as polyacrylonitrile or cellulose acetate. The patient may be simultaneously hemodialyzed while up to 100 ml of ultrafiltrate is removed each minute. A replacement solution is reinfused at the rate of 60–90 ml/min. The combined and additive effectiveness of diffusion and convective transport results in a reduction of treatment time. Also, the combined therapy results in a lower incidence of cardiovascular instability during treatment. Also *hemodiafiltration.*

**hemoflagellate** \-flaj′əlāt\ [HEMO- + FLAGELLATE] Any flagellate protozoan of the family Trypanosomatidae that is parasitic in the blood. Found in many species of birds and animals, including man, hemoflagellates include the genera *Trypanosoma* and *Leishmania,* which contain species that are important human and animal pathogens, causing a wide spectrum of diseases.

**hemofuscin** \-fyoo′sin\ A yellow-brown nonferrous pigment present in the tissues in hemochromatosis.

**hemogenesis** \-jen′əsis\ HEMATOPOIESIS.

**hemogenic** \-jen′ik\ HEMATOPOIETIC.

**hemoglobin** \hē′məglō′bin, hē′məglō′bin\ [HEMO- + GLOBIN (for GLOBULIN)] A heme protein of approximately 64 000 MW that transports oxygen and carbon dioxide and constitutes approximately 99% of the protein content of mammalian erythrocytes. It also occurs in other animal phyla and in plants, as in root nodules of legumes (leghemoglobin). Hemoglobin is a tetramer of four subunits, each consisting of a globin chain of amino acids and a heme group. **h. A** The predominant form of human hemoglobin, the molecule of which consists of two $\alpha$ and two $\beta$ chains. **h. $A_2$** A normally present component of hemoglobin that is a tetramer of $\alpha$ and $\delta$ globin chains, i.e. $\alpha_2\delta_2$. Hemoglobin $A_2$ normally makes up 1.5–3% of the hemoglobin in adults or children of age greater than six months. An elevated proportion of hemoglobin $A_2$ is usually indicative of $\beta$-thalassemia trait. **h. $A_{ic}$** A minor form of hemoglobin in normal blood. It contains carbohydrate linked to the N-terminal valine of the $\beta$ chains, probably in the form of the Amadori rearrangement product of glucosylated protein, i.e. the furanose form of fructose in which O-1 is replaced by the amino group of the valine residue. Its concentration is raised in diabetes. See also GLYCOSYLATED HEMOGLOBIN. **abnormal h.** Any hemoglobin found in only a minority of individuals. Such hemoglobins often contain a single change in amino-acid sequence. **h. Bart's** A hemoglobin variant that is a tetramer of $\gamma$ chains ($\gamma_4$) and which, when present in blood, is evidence of $\alpha$-thalassemia. **h. C** An abnormal human hemoglobin in which lysine occurs instead of glutamate at position 6 of the beta chain, i.e. $\beta$6(A2)Glu→Lys. This is due to a mutation at the beta locus, allelic to the mutation for hemoglobin S. The presence of hemoglobin C causes a mild hemolytic anemia in the heterozygote and a more severe disorder when homozygous. Hemoglobin C is common in West Africa and among a small proportion of black Americans. **h. Constant Spring** A hemoglobin variant in which the $\alpha$ chain is extended by addition of 31 amino acids to the C-terminal end as a result of mutation of a nonsense (termination) codon of DNA. When present in blood, it usually comprises 1–3% of the total hemoglobin, and has the effect of a mild $\alpha$-thalassemia trait. Although described from the village of Constant Spring, Jamaica, hemoglobin Constant Spring is found only in Asians. It is a common hemoglobin variant in Chinese and in Southeast Asians. **h. D** Any of a group of hemoglobin variants due to amino acid substitutions in the $\beta$-globin chain that confer abnormal electrophoretic mobility. The most common of these is hemoglobin D-Punjab (or hemoglobin D-Los Angeles), which differs from normal adult hemoglobin A by having glutamine rather than glutamic acid as the 121st amino acid of the $\beta$-globin chain, i.e. $\beta$121(GH4)Glu→Gln. **h. E** A hemoglobin variant that differs from the normal hemoglobin A by having lysine rather than glutamic acid as the 26th amino acid of the $\beta$-globin chain, i.e. $\beta$26(B8) Glu→Lys. Hemoglobin E is very common in persons of Southeast Asian ancestry. **h. F** The predominant hemoglobin of fetal life. It is a tetramer of $\alpha$ and $\gamma$ globin chains, $\alpha_2\gamma_2$, and has a higher affinity for oxygen than does adult hemoglobin. At birth, hemoglobin F is 50–70% of the total hemoglobin, but the proportion of hemoglobin F declines rapidly. In adults and children of age greater than one year, hemoglobin F normally is not more than 1% of total hemoglobin. Elevated proportions of hemoglobin F occur in thalassemias and other chronic anemias. Also *fetal hemoglobin.* **fast h.'s** Those variant hemoglobins that, upon electrophoresis at pH 8.6–9.0, run ahead of the normal hemoglobin A. They are more negatively charged than hemoglobin A. Glycosylated hemoglobin is the fast hemoglobin component that is in the first fraction eluted from certain ion-exchange resin chromatography columns. **fetal h.** HEMOGLOBIN F. **h. G** Any of several hemoglobin variants that exhibit mobility identical with, or just slightly greater than hemoglobin S upon electrophoresis in alkaline media. The most commonly encountered is hemoglobin G-Philadelphia [$\alpha$68(E17)Asn→Lys], a hemoglobin variant that is found commonly in the blood of black people. Other G-hemoglobins are rare. **glycosylated h.** Any complex of hemoglobin with glucose or related monosaccharides, in which the monosaccharide binds to the N-terminal end of the $\beta$ globin chain. Among glycosylated hemoglobins are hemoglobin $A_{IC}$, a complex of hemoglobin A with glucose; $A_{Ia1}$, a complex of hemoglobin A with fructose diphosphate; and $A_{Ia2}$, a complex of hemoglobin A with glucose 6-phosphate. **h. Gower** Either of two human hemoglobins normally present in blood during the first three months of embryonic life. They contain the prefetal globin chains $\zeta$ (a prefetal $\alpha$ chain) and $\epsilon$ (a prefetal non-$\alpha$ chain). Hemoglobin Gower-1 is $\zeta_2\epsilon_2$ and hemoglobin Gower-2 is $\alpha_2\epsilon_2$. • The term is never used without specifying it as Gower-1 or Gower-2. **h. H** A hemoglobin variant that is a tetramer of $\beta$-globin chains, ($\beta_4$). Hemoglobin H is an expression of $\alpha$-thalassemia. Rarely it occurs as an epiphenomenon of erythroleukemia. **homozygous h. C** A disorder that results from inheritance of a gene for hemoglobin C from both parents. The condition is associated with mild anemia, erythrocytic hypochromia, and numerous target erythrocytes. Also *called hemoglobin C disease.* **homozygous h. D** A minor disorder that results from inheritance of a gene for hemoglobin D from both parents. Homozygous hemoglobin D-Punjab has been associated with mild erythrocytic microcytosis. It is very rare except in northwest India. Also *hemoglobin D disease.* **homozygous h. E** A minor condition due to inheritance of a gene for hemoglobin E from both parents. The condition is associated with moderate erythrocytic microcytosis and hypochromia, and occasionally with minimal anemia. Also *hemoglobin E disease* (incorrect). **h. J** Any of several hemoglobin variants that exhibit more rapid anodal mobility than hemoglobin A upon electrophoresis in alkaline media. In such media, the position of hemoglobin J is as far ahead of (anodal to) hemoglobin A as hemoglobin S is behind (cathodal to)hemoglobin A. Hemoglobins J-Baltimore [$\beta$15(A12)Gly$\rightarrow$Asp] and J-Oxford [$\alpha$15(A13)Gly$\rightarrow$Asp] are found occasionally in blood specimens of blacks and Caucasians respectively. All other J-hemoglobins are very rare. **h. K** Any of three hemoglobin variants, with amino acid substitutions in the $\beta$ chain, that exhibit slightly faster anodal mobility than hemoglobin A, but less than hemoglobin J, upon electrophoresis in alkaline media. Of the three K-hemoglobins, (K-Woolwich, K-Ibadan, and K-Cameroon), all were reported in blood specimens from black persons, and all appear to be quite rare. **h. Köln** An unstable hemoglobin variant that causes continual mild hemolytic anemia, jaundice, and splenomegaly. Although rare, it is the unstable hemoglobin most commonly encountered in people of north European origin. Hemoglobin Köln is $\beta$98(FG5) Val$\rightarrow$Met. **h. Lepore** An abnormal human hemoglobin in which two normal $\alpha$ chains pair with two abnormal globin chains, the latter being 146 amino acids long and composed of the N-terminal portion of normal $\delta$-globin chains and the C-terminal portion of normal $\beta$-globin chains. It is thought to arise from unequal recombination between the closely linked delta and beta globin genes. • This hemoglobin is named for the family in which the variant was first discovered. **h. M** Any of a group of hemoglobin variants in which the heme iron of one pair of globin chains is in the Fe(III) state because of an amino acid substitution. **mean corpuscular h.** The average amount of hemoglobin per erythrocyte in a sample of blood, expressed in picograms. It is calculated by dividing hemoglobin (in grams per liter) by erythrocyte count. Also *blood quotient.* Abbr. MCH, MCHg **h. N** Any of three hemoglobin variants, with amino acid substitutions in the $\beta$ chain, that exhibit a slightly more rapid anodal mobility than hemoglobin J upon electrophoresis in alkaline media. Hemoglobin N-Baltimore [$\beta$95(FG2)Lys$\rightarrow$Glu] is found occasionally in blood specimens of black persons. The other N-hemoglobins are very rare. **h. O** Any of three hemoglobin variants that exhibit mobility identical with that of hemoglobin C upon electrophoresis in alkaline media. The most commonly encountered is hemoglobin O-Arab [$\beta$121(GH4)Glu$\rightarrow$Lys], a hemoglobin variant that is found occasionally in the blood of black people or of Bulgarians. **oxidized h.** 1 METHEMOGLOBIN. 2 OXYHEMOGLOBIN. • Because of the ambiguity of this term, it is best avoided. **reduced h.** The deoxygenated form of hemoglobin. Also *deoxyhemoglobin.* **h. S** An abnormal human hemoglobin due to the presence of a valine residue instead of glutamate at position 6 of the $\beta$-globin chain, i.e. $\beta$6(A2)Glu$\rightarrow$Val. This mutation results in a conformational alteration in the hemoglobin molecule when deoxygenation occurs, with the result that the erythocyte assumes a "sickle" shape. When both alleles at the beta locus have this mutation, sickle cell disease results. Heterozygosity for the mutant allele and the normal allele results in sickle cell trait. Hemoglobin S occurs in approximately 8% of black people in North America. Also *sickle hemoglobin.* Abbr. HbS **sickle h.** HEMOGLOBIN S. **slow h.'s** Hemoglobin variants which, on electrophoresis at pH 8.6–9.0, migrate more slowly toward the anode than does the normal hemoglobin A. The reason for their slow electrophoretic mobility is that they contain more positively charged amino acids than does hemoglobin A. **unstable h.** A hemoglobin variant that precipitates more readily than does normal adult hemoglobin A upon mild heating or chemical or mechanical stress. **h. Zürich** An unstable hemoglobin variant that predisposes a person having it to hemolytic anemia when sulfonamides are ingested. Hemoglobin Zürich is $\beta$63(E7) His$\rightarrow$Arg. The condition is very rare.

**hemoglobinemia** \\-glō'binē'mē·ə\\ [HEMOGLOBIN + -EMIA] A greater than normal concentration of hemoglobin in plasma. Also *hyperhemoglobinemia.*

**hemoglobinometer** \\-glō'binäm'ətər\\ An instrument for determining hemoglobin concentration of blood, plasma, or other fluids. Also *hematinometer, hematometer, hemochromoneter, hemometer.*

**hemoglobinometry** \\-glō'binäm'ətrē\\ The determination of hemoglobin concentration of blood, plasma, or other fluids. Also *hemochromometry, hemometry.*

**hemoglobinopathy** \\-glō'binäp'əthē\\ Any abnormality of the hemoglobin molecule, whether inherited or acquired, quantitative or qualitative, including unbalanced globin chain production, amino acid substitutions, deletions, and additions within globin chains, and abnormalities of the heme group. Most hemoglobinopathies do not result in clinical disease.

**hemoglobinuria** \\-glō'binoo'rē·ə\\ [HEMOGLOBIN + -URIA] The presence of free hemoglobin or its derivatives in urine, whenever its concentration in plasma exceeds the maximum saturation of plasma haptoglobin. The urine is dark brown in color. Hemoglobinuria should be differentiated from lysis of erythrocytes during hematuria by dilute or alkaline urine. Hemoglobinuria may result from toxins, some infections, incompatible blood transfusions, extensive burns, excessive physical exertion, and as a feature of paroxysmal nocturnal hypoglobinuria, or paroxysmal cold hemoglobinuria. Sudden hemoglobinuria may be a primary cause of or a contributing factor to acute renal failure. Also *methemoglobinuria.* **intermittent h.** Recurrent attacks of hemoglobinuria characteristic of paroxysmal nocturnal hemoglobinuria or paroxysmal cold hemoglobinuria. **malarial h.** BLACKWATER FEVER. **march h.** An episodic form of hemolysis, caused by unusually intense or prolonged physical activity (such as running or marching) sufficient to cause mechanical injury to circulating erythrocytes. **paroxysmal cold h.** A rare disorder characterized by acute severe hemolytic anemia following exposure to cold. There is usually hemoglobinuria, and a serum test for Donath-Landsteiner antibody is positive. Also *Donath-Landsteiner syndrome.* **paroxysmal nocturnal h.** A rare disorder, reflecting acquired erythrocyte hypersensitivity to the lytic effect of complement, that is manifested by intravascular hemolysis, hemoglobinuria, hemosiderinuria, positive Ham test, Crosby test, and sucrose lysis test, and is often accompanied by other cytopenias. Also *Marchiafava-Micheli syndrome* (rare). • The name implies increased nocturnal hemolysis, because the first morning urine is most concentrated and pigments from hemolysis more noticeable. In fact, hemolysis is not greater at night.

**hemoglobinuric** \-glō'binoo'rik\ Of or pertaining to hemoglobinuria.

**hemogram** \hē'mōgram\ COMPLETE BLOOD COUNT.

**hemohistioblast** \-his'tē·əblast'\ [HEMO- + HISTIOBLAST] A mesenchymal progenitor capable of differentiating into any normal cellular element of blood. Also *hematohistioblast, Ferrata cell.*

**hemohydraulics** \-hīdrôl'iks\ HEMODYNAMICS.

**hemokinesis** \-kīnē'sis\ The movement of blood.

**hemokinetic** \-kinet'ik\ Pertaining to blood flow.

**hemology** \hēmäl'əjē\ HEMATOLOGY.

**hemolymph** \hē'mōlimf\ **1** The circulating body fluids, including blood and lymph, taken as a whole. **2** A type of body fluid in certain invertebrates, analogous to both blood and lymph. It may be found free in the body cavity, or in restricted parts of the coelom, or within the vascular bed, as in insects.

**hemolymphadenosis** \-limfad'ənō'sis\ HEMOBLASTOSIS.

**hemolymphangioma** \-limfan'jē·ō'mə\ [HEMO- + LYMPHANGIOMA] A tumor composed of blood vessels and lymphatics. Also *hematolymphangioma, hemangiolymphangioma.*

**hemolymphocytotoxin** \-lim'fəsī'tətäk'sin\ A factor found in the hemolymph of invertebrates which has the ability to kill mammalian cells. Such factors are quite frequent but seem to have no close relationship to the antibodies or complement components found in vertebrates.

**hemolysate** \hēmäl'isāt\ [*hemolys(is)* + -ATE] The fluid that is formed upon lysis of blood cells. Also *blood cytolysate.*

**hemolysin** \hēmäl'isin\ [*hemolys(is)* + -IN] An antibody capable of inducing red cell destruction in the presence of complement. Also *erythrolysin, erythrocytolysin, erythrocyto-opsonin.* **α-h.** The most common of the four cytolytic toxins produced by *Staphylococcus aureus.* It lyses rabbit but not human erythrocytes. When injected into experimental animals it causes aggregation and lysis of platelets of man and rabbits, and causes local necrosis of skin and tissue. **β-h.** One of the four cytolytic toxins produced by *Staphylococcus aureus,* found most often in bovine strains and in about 20 percent of human strains. A hot-cold lysin, it lyses sheep, beef, and human erythrocytes only when incubation at 37°C is followed by refrigeration. **γ-h.** One of the four cytolytic toxins produced by *Staphylococcus aureus.* It consists of two components that synergistically induce hemolysis of rabbit, sheep, and human erythrocytes. Its action is inhibited by sulfated polymers, including agar. **δ-h.** One of the four cytolytic toxins produced by *Staphylococcus aureus.* It has a broad range of lytic and cytotoxic activity, but serum phospholipids inhibit its action and it therefore may not exert an effect *in vivo.* **acid h.** A hemolytic antibody with a pH optimum below 7.0. **bacterial h.** Any hemolysin produced by bacteria. **cold h.** DONATH-LANDSTEINER ANTIBODY. **immune h.** A hemolytic antibody produced in the host animal or individual after immunizing exposure to blood cells carrying the antigen for which the antibody is specific. It may be a human antibody against an alloantigen or an antibody raised in animals against a heterogenous antigen. **natural h.** A naturally occurring antibody capable of inducing red cell destruction in the presence of complement. **specific h.** Antibody capable of inducing red cell destruction by its specific reactivity with the corresponding antigen on the red cell surface and complement fixation.

**hemolysis** \hēmäl'isis\ [HEMO- + LYSIS] The destruction or dissolution of erythrocytes. Also *erythrocytolysis, erythrolysis, cythemolysis, globulysis, globulolysis, hemocatheresis* (seldom used), *hematocytolysis, hemolyzation* (seldom used), *hematolysis, hemocytocatheresis, hemoclastic reaction.* Adj. hemolytic. **α h.** The partial decomposition of hemoglobin characteristic of certain strains of streptococci and pneumococci. It appears as a greenish color surrounding a bacterial colony in blood agar. Also *viridans hemolysis.* **β h.** Hemolysis in which a transparent area is apparent surrounding a colony of certain pathogenic bacteria in blood agar. **contact h.** Accelerated destruction of erythrocytes as a result of mechanical stress during or following contact with a foreign surface. **immune h.** The lysis by complement of antibody-sensitized erythrocytes. **osmotic h.** Disruption of erythrocytes, and loss of their cytosol, as a consequence of swelling and bursting in hypotonic solution. **passive h.** Hemolysis occurring in the presence of complement and antibody directed to an antigen adsorbed or chemically coupled onto the surface of erythrocytes. It is used as a test for antibodies to various antigens that can be bound to erythrocytes. **siderogenous h.** Any condition in which accelerated destruction of blood (hemolysis) is associated with increased body iron stores, as in thalassemia major. **viridans h.** α HEMOLYSIS.

**hemolytic** \-lit'ik\ Relating to, characterized by, or producing hemolysis. Also *hematolytic, hyperhemolytic, hemocytolytic, globulolytic.*

**hemolyzable** \-lī'zəbl\ Subject to hemolysis.

**hemolyze** \hē'mōlīz\ To subject to or undergo hemolysis. Also *lake.*

**hemomanometry** \-mənäm'ətrē\ The process of blood pressure measurement. Also *hemodynamometry, hemadynometry.*

**hemomediastinum** \-mē'dē·astī'nəm\ A hematoma in the mediastinum. Also *hematomediastinum.*

**hemometakinesia** \-met'əkinē'zhə\ HEMATOMETAKINESIS.

**hemometakinesis** \-met'əkinē'sis\ HEMATOMETAKINESIS.

**hemometer** \hēmäm'ətər\ HEMOGLOBINOMETER.

**hemometra** \-mē'trə\ HEMATOMETRA.

**hemometry** \hēmäm'ətrē\ HEMOGLOBINOMETRY.

**hemomyelosis** \-mī'əlō'sis\ HEMOBLASTOSIS.

**hemonormoblast** \-nôr'məblast\ NORMOBLAST.

**hemopathology** \-pathäl'əjē\ **1** Disease of the blood or blood-forming organs or lymphatic tissues. **2** The study, especially by histologic technique, of diseases of the blood or blood-forming organs or lymphatic tissues.

**hemopathy** \hēmäp'əthē\ [HEMO- + -PATHY] Any disease primarily involving the blood or blood-forming organs. Adj. hemopathic.

**hemoperfusion** \-pərfyoo'zhən\ [HEMO- + PERFUSION] The removal of substances from blood by passage through a column containing a substance over the surface of which the blood passes and comes into contact before leaving the column and returning to the patient. In contradistinction to hemodialysis, there is no semipermeable dialysis membrane and no dialysate. Blood comes directly into contact with the sorbent contained within the column, or the sorbent may be coated with a material preventing direct contact between the blood and the active ingredient of the column, if such contact would be detrimental, as by damaging or trapping formed elements of the blood, or by permitting embolization of the active ingredient of the column into the blood. A variety of substances may be used as the active ingredient in the column over which blood is perfused. Selection of the active ingredient is determined by its affinity for the substance or substances whose removal from blood is desired. **charcoal h.** Hemoperfusion performed through a column containing charcoal, usually activated charcoal. **resin h.** Hemoperfusion performed through a column containing a resin as absorbent. A large variety of resins are available.

**hemopericardium** \-per′ikär′dē·əm\ Blood in the pericardial space. Also *hematopericardium.*

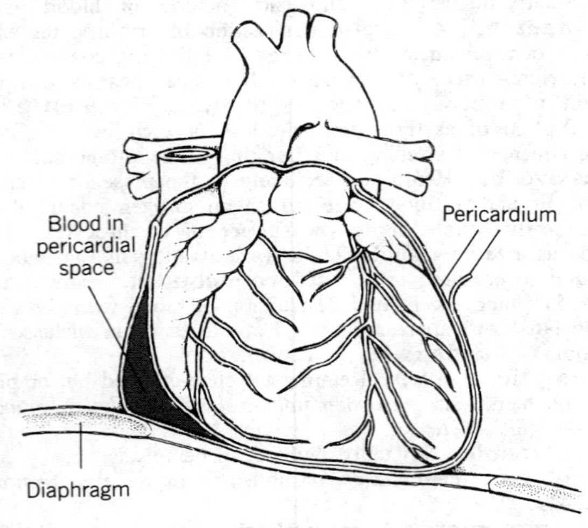


**Hemopericardium**

**hemoperitoneum** \-per′itōnē′·əm\ The presence of frank blood within the peritoneal cavity. Also *hematoperitoneum.*

**hemopexin** \-pek′sin\ [HEMO- + Gk *pēx(is)* fixation, binding + -IN] A plasma beta-globulin, produced by the liver, that binds heme when heme appears in plasma. The heme-hemopexin complex is removed from plasma by macrophages.

**hemophage** \hē′mōfāj\ ERYTHROPHAGOCYTE.

**hemophagia** \-fā′jə\ [HEMO- + -PHAGIA] HEMATOPHAGIA.

**hemophagocyte** \-fag′əsīt\ ERYTHROPHAGOCYTE.

**hemophagocytosis** \-fag′əsītō′sis\ ERYTHROPHAGOCYTOSIS.

**hemophil** \hē′mōfil\ [HEMO- + -PHIL] **1** Any of the microorganisms which culture most successfully on media containing blood. **2** Any organism which prefers, or thrives on, blood.

**hemophilia** \-fil′yə\ [HEMO- + -PHILIA] A serious inherited hemorrhagic disease. Hemophilias A and B are X-linked while factor XI deficiency (hemophilia C) is autosomal. Also *bleeders' disease, thromboplastinopenia* (obs.), *hematophilia.* Adj. hemophilic. **h. A** An X-linked recessive disorder of blood coagulation due to deficiency of the coagulation moiety of factor VIII. The gene for factor VIII is located near the telomere of the long arm of the X chromosome, closely linked to the gene encoding glucose-6-phosphate dehydrogenase. Morbidity and mortality can be improved considerably by infusion of concentrates of human coagulation factors enriched for factor VIII. Also *classical hemophilia.* See also VON WILLEBRAND'S DISEASE. **h. B** An X-linked hereditary bleeding disease caused by a deficiency of factor IX. Also *factor IX deficiency, Christmas disease, deuterohemophilia* (outmoded). **h. C** An autosomally inherited bleeding disease resulting from a deficiency of factor XI. Also *Rosenthal syndrome, plasma thromboplastin antecedent deficiency.* **classical h.** HEMOPHILIA A. **h. neonatorum** *Incorrect* HEMORRHAGIC DISEASE OF THE NEWBORN. **vascular h.** The association of a prolonged bleeding time with a reduction of plasmatic factor VIII. Most, if not all, patients with vascular hemophilia have von Willebrand's disease.

**hemophiliac** \-fil′ē·ak\ A person or animal with hemophilia.

**hemophilic** \-fil′ik\ Relating to hemophilia or hemophiliacs.

**hemophilioid** \-fil′ē·oid\ Describing any bleeding tendency, usually of unknown origin, resembling one or another hemophilia.

***Hemophilus*** \hēmäf′ələs\ *HAEMOPHILUS.* • Although not officially correct, this spelling is preferred by many microbiologists in the United States.

**hemophilus** \hēmäf′ələs\ Any microorganism of the genus *Haemophilus.*

**hemophoresis** \-fôrē′sis\ [HEMO- + -PHORESIS] The movement of blood.

**hemophthisis** \hēmäf′thisis, hē′mäfthis′is\ Anemia due to impaired formation of erythrocytes.

**hemoplasmopathy** \-plazmäp′əthē\ Any disease characterized by quantitative or qualitative disturbance of plasma proteins. Also *hematoplasmopathy.*

**hemoplastic** \-plas′tik\ Relating to the growth and maturation of formed elements of the blood.

**hemopleura** \-plŏŏr′ə\ HEMOTHORAX.

**hemopneumopericardium** \-n$^y$oo′mōper′ikär′dē·əm\ The presence of both blood and gas in the pericardial space.

**hemopneumothorax** \-n$^y$oo′mōthôr′aks\ The presence of blood and air in the pleural cavity.

**hemopoiesic** \-poi·ē′sik\ HEMATOPOIETIC.

**hemopoiesis** \-poi·ē′sis\ HEMATOPOIESIS.

**hemopoietic** \-poi·et′ik\ HEMATOPOIETIC.

**hemoposia** \-pō′zhə\ [Gk *haimoposia* (from *haima* blood + *posis* drinking, a drink) the drinking of blood] The drinking of blood, as by vampire bats, insects, or other metazoan parasites, or by humans for nutrition, therapy, or ritual purposes.

**hemoprotein** Any protein containing a heme group, such as hemoglobin or cytochrome c.

**hemoprotozoa** \-prō′tōzō′ə\ (*sing.* hemoprotozoon) Protozoan parasites that circulate in the bloodstream during some stage in their development, for example, plasmodia and trypanosomes.

**hemoptysic** \hē′mäptī′sik\ Relating to or characterized by hemoptysis. Also *hemoptoic, hemoptic.*

**hemoptysis** \hēmäp′tisis\ [HEMO- + Gk *ptysis* a spitting] The expectoration of blood. **endemic h.** PARAGONIMIASIS. **Goldstein's h.** Hemoptysis due to telangiectasia of the tracheobronchial tree. **oriental h.** PARAGONIMIASIS. **parasitic h.** PARAGONIMIASIS. **vicarious h.** The coughing up of blood at the time of menstruation, usually caused by endometriosis of the lung or bronchial passages.

**hemorepellant** \-ripel′ənt\ **1** Resistant to wetting by blood: said of a surface or substance. **2** A hemorepellant surface or substance.

**hemorheology** \hem′ôrē·äl′əjē\ [HEMO- + RHEOLOGY] The study of the effect of blood flow on the constituents of the blood, especially the cellular components, and upon the vessel walls. Also *hemorrheology.* Adj. hemorheologic.

**hemorrhachis** \hēmôr′əkis\ HEMATORRHACHIS.

**hemorrhage** \hem′ərij\ [Gk *haimorragia* (from *haima*

blood + *-rragia*, from *rheg(nynai)* to burst forth + -IA) profuse bleeding, hemorrhage] **1** The escape of blood from blood vessels. Such bleeding continues until external pressure exceeds that within the blood vessel. **2** An accumulation of extravasated blood. See also PETECHIA, PURPURA, ECCHYMOSIS, HEMATOMA. **accidental antepartum h.** ABRUPTIO PLACENTAE. **arterial h.** Hemorrhage from a ruptured artery. **capillary h.** Hemorrhage from damaged capillary vessels. **capsular h.** Cerebral hemorrhage occurring in the internal capsule. **capsuloganglionic h.** Cerebral hemorrhage involving the internal capsule and basal ganglia. **cerebellar h.** Hemorrhage arising in or extending into the cerebellum. **cerebral h.** Hemorrhage occurring in one cerebral hemisphere or, less often, in both. The many causes include arteriosclerosis, hypertension, aneurysm, angioma, cerebral tumor, head injury, arteritis, and blood diseases. Also *ictus sanguinis.* **concealed h.** Hemorrhage that is not apparent on the surface. **critical h.** Hemorrhage that threatens either life or the function of the organ into which the bleeding occurs. **epidural h.** EXTRADURAL HEMORRHAGE. **external h.** Blood escaping through a wound in the skin. Unless issuing from deep-seated blood vessels, it can usually be controlled by direct pressure. **extradural h.** Hemorrhage occurring between the dura mater and the skull, usually caused by head injury with skull fracture and division of the middle meningeal artery or one of its branches. Also *epidural hemorrhage.* **fetomaternal h.** Leakage of fetal blood cells into the maternal circulation. This usually occurs at the time of placental separation. **fibrinolytic h.** Hemorrhage due to a disorder of the fibrinolytic system. **flame-shaped h.'s** Bleeding into the nerve fiber layer of the retina, recognizable by its linear configuration. Also *flame spots.* **glomerular h.** The presence of blood in the glomerular capsular space. This is a feature of glomerulonephritis. **internal h.** Bleeding that is confined within the body cavity. It is usually not readily apparent on physical examination, but may be suspected from systemic reactions to blood loss. **intracerebral h.** Hemorrhage arising within the cerebrum. Also *encephalorrhagia.* **intracranial h.** Hemorrhage occurring anywhere within the cranial cavity. **intradural h.** SUBDURAL HEMORRHAGE. **intramedullary h.** HEMATOMYELIA. **intrapartum h.** The occurrence of hemorrhage usually due to abruptio placentae or placenta previa during labor. **intraventricular h.** Hemorrhage arising within the cerebral ventricles. **massive h.** Hemorrhage severe enough to cause shock. In otherwise healthy individuals this amounts to 15 to 20 percent of the blood volume, or about 1.2 liters in a person weighing 70 kg. **meningeal h.** SUBARACHNOID HEMORRHAGE. **nasal h.** EPISTAXIS. **neonatal subdural h.** Subdural hemorrhage occurring in neonates. **parenchymatous h.** Hemorrhage into the parenchyma of an organ. **petechial h.** Punctate hemorrhage under the skin, producing petechiae. **pontine h.** Hemorrhage arising in or extending into the pons. **postpartum h.** The occurrence of hemorrhage during the postpartum period. The most frequent causes are uterine atony, retained placental tissue, or an unrecognized laceration of the birth canal. **primary h.** **1** Hemorrhage immediately following injury. **2** SPONTANEOUS HEMORRHAGE. **pulmonary h. in newborn** Hemorrhage into the pulmonary alveoli, and to a lesser degree into the interstitial tissue of the lung, a complication of the respiratory distress syndrome, pneumonia, or severe anoxia, and a common autopsy finding in neonatal deaths from varied causes. Symptoms are respiratory distress and oozing of frothy blood from nose and mouth, with death ensuing in 48 hours. **punctate h.** Hemorrhage at minute points in the skin or other organs. **recurring h.** Recurrent episodes of capillary hemorrhage. **renal h.** Hemorrhage from or into a kidney. *Imprecise.* **secondary h.** **1** Hemorrhage that is delayed following injury. It usually occurs when a vessel is damaged but is able to withstand the internal pressure for a time. It also occurs when an expanding hematoma finally ruptures the capsule of an organ such as the liver, spleen, or kidney. **2** Bleeding that is delayed following surgery. It may be caused by slippage of a ligature by or elevation of the patient's blood pressure enough to overcome pressure external to the blood vessel. **slit h.** A linear extension of intracerebral hemorrhage usually found in the white matter, separating fiber bundles or tracts. **splinter h.** A linear hemorrhage found at the base of or under the nail bed. It is diagnostically important in bacterial endocarditis, microembolic disease, and some forms of vasculitis. It may also occur as a result of minor trauma to the fingers. **spontaneous h.** Hemorrhage occurring without evident provocation. Also *primary hemorrhage.* **subarachnoid h.** Hemorrhage occurring in the subarachnoid space. The many causes include intracranial aneurysm, angioma, head injury, neoplasia, and blood disease. Also *meningeal hemorrhage.* **subconjunctival h.** Hemorrhage beneath the conjunctiva, arising spontaneously or resulting from trauma. **subdural h.** Hemorrhage occurring in the subdural space, between the dura and the arachnoid. This usually results from head injury with rupture of veins which traverse the space, and it can be acute, subacute, or chronic. In rare cases it results from blood or liver disease or occurs as a complication of anticoagulant therapy. Also *intradural hemorrhage.* **subgaleal h.** Hemorrhage arising beneath the galea aponeurotica. **subhyaloid h.** Hemorrhage occurring between the retina and the hyaloid membrane of the eye which separates the retina from the vitreous. It is usually brick-red in color, extending outwards from the optic disk and is diagnostic of subarachnoid hemorrhage. **venous h.** Loss of blood from a vein.

**hemorrhagic** \hem′əraj′ik\ Causing, resulting from, or characterized by hemorrhage.

**hemorrhagin** \hem′ərā′jin\ A toxic substance present in certain venoms and plant seeds, such as snake venom and castor beans (*Ricinus communis*). It causes extensive destruction of the endothelial cells in blood vessels.

**hemorrheology** \hem′ôrē·äl′əjē\ HEMORHEOLOGY. Adj. hemorrheologic.

**hemorrhoid** \hem′əroid\ [Gk *haimorrois,* pl. *haimorroides* (from *haim(a)* blood + *rhoē* a flow) tending to bleed, veins that tend to bleed, piles] A varicosity of one of the veins comprising the hemorrhoidal venous plexus (plexus venosus rectalis). **combined h.** MIXED HEMORRHOID. **external h.** A hemorrhoid below the pectinate line, covered by anal skin, and involving only the inferior venous plexus. Also *cutaneous hemorrhoid.* **internal h.** A hemorrhoid above the pectinate line, covered by mucous membrane, and involving the superior venous plexus. **mixed h.** A hemorrhoid extending above and below the pectinate line, usually representing a connection between the superior and inferior rectal venous plexuses. Also *combined hemorrhoid, mucocutaneous hemorrhoid.* **prolapsed h.** An internal hemorrhoid which protrudes from the anus. **strangulated h.** A prolapsed internal hemorrhoid which has been cut off from its blood supply. **thrombosed h.** A strangulated hemorrhoid which, because of compromised blood flow, has become thrombosed. The hemorrhoid becomes hard, tender, and nonreducible and results in perianal pain.

**hemorrhoidal** \hem′əroi′dəl\ **1** Of or relating to hemorrhoids. **2** Rectal: designating arteries, veins, and nerves of the rectum.

**hemorrhoidectomy** \hem′əroidek′təmē\ [HEMORRHOID + -ECTOMY] Surgical excision or removal of hemorrhoids.

**hemorrhoidolysis** \hem′əroidäl′isis\ The destruction of hemorrhoids by means other than direct surgical removal, as by diathermy or chemical treatment.

**hemorrhoids** \hem′əroidz\ A condition in which there are varicosities in veins of the hemorrhoidal plexus, often associated with hematochezia, pruritus ani, or anorectal pain. Although often associated with constipation, its cause is not known. Also *piles.*

**hemosalpinx** \-sal′pingks\ HEMATOSALPINX.

**hemosarcoma** \-särkō′mə\ *Obs.* LEUKEMIA.

**hemosiderin** [HEMO- + *sider(o)-* + -IN] An iron-rich protein found in the liver and some other organs. It is probably a form of ferritin.

**hemosiderosis** \-sid′ərō′sis\ [*hemosider(in)* + -OSIS] The deposition of iron within tissues, either diffusely or focally, not associated with injury or fibrosis of the affected organs. **hepatic h.** Deposition of large quantities of iron in hepatic tissue, generally seen within sinusoidal Kupffer cells and not resulting in hepatic cirrhosis or fibrosis. **nutritional h.** The presence of excess iron in the body arising from an excessive dietary intake and demonstrated by the presence of hemosiderin in the tissues. When slight overloading occurs, the iron is deposited in the liver's parenchymal cells but no clinical manifestations are apparent. With increasing iron intake, the Kupffer cells become loaded and eventually their portals contract. This may result in fibrosis and be a contributing cause to cirrhosis. Alcoholics who drink inexpensive wines rich in iron (10–350 mg/l) are especially subject to the condition. Hemosiderosis is also common among those peoples who traditionally cook in iron pots. Also *nutritional siderosis.* **pulmonary h.** The presence of hemosiderin-laden macrophages within alveoli and interstitium of the lung. In addition to an idiopathic form occurring in children and young adults, it may result from severe left-sided heart failure and the Goodpasture syndrome. **transfusional h.** Chronic iron overload that results from repeated blood transfusions.

**hemospermia** \-spur′mē·ə\ [HEMO- + SPERM + -IA ] The occurrence of blood in the semen. Also *hematospermia.*

**hemosporidium** \-spôrid′ē·əm\ HAEMOSPORIDIUM.

**hemosporine** \-spôr′in\ [HEMO- + *spor(e)* + -INE] **1** Pertaining or belonging to the suborder Haemosporina of the sporozoan order Eucoccidiida; haemosporidian. **2** A sporozoan blood parasite belonging to the suborder Haemosporina; a haemosporidium.

**hemostasis** \hēmäs′təsis, hē′mōstā′sis\ [Gk *haimostasis* (from *haima* blood + *(hi)sta(nai)* to stand, stop + *-sis* derivative noun suffix) a styptic] The arrest of hemorrhage. Also *hemostasia.*

**hemostat** \hē′mōstat\ [HEMO- + Gk *-statēs* -stopping, -stopper] A device or material designed to occlude or compress tissues or vessels in order to control bleeding, as during surgery or following trauma. Also *angioclast* (obs.).

**hemostatic** \-stat′ik\ [late Gk *haimostatikos* styptic] **1** Tending to cause hemostasis. Also *hematostatic.* **2** An agent that causes hemostasis. For defs 1 and 2 also *hemostyptic.* **capillary h.** An agent which arrests capillary hemorrhage.

**hemostyptic** \-stip′tik\ HEMOSTATIC.

**hemotherapy** \-ther′əpē\ The administration of blood or such blood components as packed erythrocytes, platelets, leukocytes, plasma, or serum. Also *hematotherapy, hemotherapeutics* (rare).

**hemothorax** \-thôr′aks\ A collection of blood within the pleural cavity. It may be either internal or external to the pleura but not within the mediastinum. Also *hematothorax, hemathorax, hemopleura.*

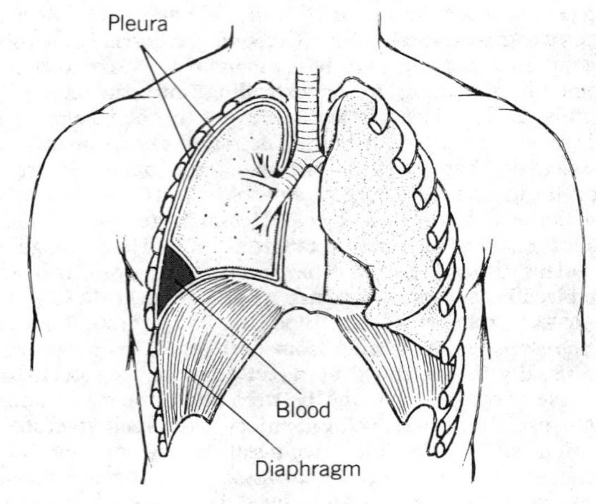


**Hemothorax**

**hemotoxic** \-täk′sik\ Having the property of damaging blood cells. Also *hematotoxic, hematoxic.*

**hemotoxicity** \-täksis′itē\ Injury to blood or blood-forming tissues by drugs, chemicals, or other substances.

**hemotoxin** \-täk′sin\ Any substance that is injurious to blood cells, causing them to be destroyed or removed from circulation at a greater than normal rate.

**hemotroph** \hē′mōträf\ [HEMO- + Gk *troph(ē)* nourishment] The nutrients supplied to an embryo by maternal blood either as carried by the bloodstream or from blood cells. Also *hemotrophe.* Adj. hemotrophic.

**hemotropic** \-träp′ik\ **1** Having an affinity for blood or blood cells. **2** Influencing phagocytic cells to migrate toward blood. For defs. 1 and 2 also *hematotropic.*

**hemotympanum** \-tim′pənəm\ Hemorrhage into the tympanic cavity. It often occurs after head injury and indicates a skull fracture involving the middle ear. Also *hematotympanum.*

**hemozoic** \-zō′ik\ HEMATOZOIC.

**hemozoin** \-zō′in\ The pigment product of malarial breakdown of hemoglobin in the infected red blood cell.

**hemozoon** \-zō′ən\ HEMATOZOON.

**hemp** [Old English *hænep*, akin to Gk *kannabis* hemp] CANNABIS. • The word *hemp* is applied chiefly to varieties of cannabis that are cultivated for their fiber. The word also enters into the names of various other plants or their products that are similar in some respect, such as *Manila hemp, Canada hemp.* **American h.** CANNABIS. **Indian h.** **1** CANNABIS. **2** A plant of the species *Apocynum cannabinum*; Canada hemp. • This ambiguous term is derived either by reference to India, where much cannabis has been grown, or to North American Indians, who have used *A. cannabinum* in various ways.

**HEMPAS** hereditary erythroblastic multinuclearity

with positive acid serum test. See under CONGENITAL DYSERYTHROPOIETIC ANEMIA.

**Henderson** [Lawrence Joseph *Henderson,* U.S. biochemist, 1878–1942] Henderson-Hasselbalch equation. See under EQUATION.

***Hendersonula*** A genus of black or grey molds found on vegetation in tropical regions of Africa, India, and the West Indies. It is capable of causing skin and nail disease in man in a form that closely resembles *Trichophyton rubrum* ringworm. The usual species are *Hendersonula toruloidea* and *Scytalidium hyalinum.*

**hendersonulosis** \hen′dərsän′yəlō′sis\ An infection of the skin or nails with the saprophytic mold *Hendersonula toruloidea.*

**Henke** [Wilhelm *Henke,* German anatomist, 1834–1896] **1** Henke's triangle, Henke's trigone. See under TRIGONUM INGUINALE. **2** Henke space. See under SPATIUM RETROPHARYNGEUM.

**Henle** [Friedrich Gustav Jacob *Henle,* German anatomist and pathologist, 1809–1885] **1** See under LIGAMENT, BAND. **2** Henle's reaction. See under CHROMAFFIN REACTION. **3** See under LAYER. **4** Henle's nervous layer. See under ENTORETINA. **5** Henle's elastic membrane. See under EXTERNAL ELASTIC LAMINA. **6** Henle's ansa, Henle's canal. See under LOOP OF HENLE. **7** Hassall-Henle warts. See under HASSALL-HENLE BODIES. **8** Henle's membrane. See under COMPLEXUS BASALIS CHOROIDEAE. **9** Henle's glands. See under GLAND. **10** Henle's ampulla. See under AMPULLA DUCTUS DEFERENTIS. **11** Crural canal of Henle. See under CANALIS ADDUCTORIUS. **12** Lumbocostal ligament of Henle. See under LIGAMENTUM LUMBOCOSTALE. **13** Henle's fiber layer. See under LAYER. **14** Inferior ligament of neck of rib of Henle. See under LIGAMENTUM COSTOTRANSVERSARIUM. **15** Henle's tubules. See under TUBULE. **16** Spine of Henle. See under SPINA SUPRAMEATUM. **17** Muscle of Henle. See under MUSCULUS AURICULARIS ANTERIOR. **18** Henle's fenestrated membrane. See under MEMBRANE. **19** Thick limb of the loop of Henle. See under THICK ASCENDING LIMB. **20** Thin limb of the loop of Henle. See under LIMB.

**Henneberg** [Richard *Henneberg,* German physician, born 1868] **1** Henneberg's disease. See under PSEUDOBULBAR PARALYSIS. **2** Scholz-Bielschowsky-Henneberg diffuse cerebral sclerosis. See under METACHROMATIC LEUKODYSTROPHY.

**Henoch** [Eduard Heinrich *Henoch,* German pediatrician, 1820–1910] **1** Schönlein-Henoch purpura nephritis. See under NEPHRITIS. **2** Schönlein-Henoch disease, Henoch's disease, Henoch's purpura, Schönlein-Henoch purpura, Schönlein-Henoch syndrome, Henoch-Schönlein syndrome. See under HENOCH-SCHÖNLEIN PURPURA.

**henogenesis** \hen′ōjen′əsis\ ONTOGENY.

**henpue** \henpoo′yē\ [West African] GOUNDOU.

**Henry** [Sir Edward Richard *Henry,* English goverment official, 1850–1931] Henry system of classification of fingerprints. See under SYSTEM.

**Henry** [William *Henry,* English chemist, 1775–1836] See under LAW.

**henry** \hen′rē\ [after Joseph *Henry,* US physicist, 1797–1878] (*pl.* henrys, henries) The SI derived unit of inductance; the inductance of a closed circuit in which an electromotive force of one volt is produced when the electric current in the circuit varies uniformly at the rate of one ampere per second; 1 henry = 1 volt × 1 second / 1 ampere. Symbol: H

**Henseleit** [Kurt *Henseleit,* German biochemist, born 1907] Krebs-Henseleit cycle. See under UREA CYCLE.

**Hensen** [Viktor *Hensen,* German physiologist, 1835–1924] **1** See under NODE, KNOT, STRIPE. **2** Hensen's plane. See under H BAND. **3** Hensen's canal. See under DUCTUS REUNIENS. **4** Hensen cells. See under CELL. **5** Hensen's duct. See under DUCTUS REUNIENS.

**Hensing** [Friedrich W. *Hensing,* German anatomist, 1719–1745] Hensing's fold, Hensing's ligament. See under LIGAMENTUM PHRENICOCOLICUM.

**hepar** \hē′pär\ [New L (gen. *hepatis*), from Gk *hēpar,* gen. *hēpatos* (akin to L *iecur* liver) the liver] [NA] A wedge-shaped, reddish brown gland that is situated in the upper right portion of the abdominal cavity immediately beneath the diaphragm; liver. It is the largest organ in the body and weighs an average of 1500 g in adults. Its diaphragmatic surface is in contact with the diaphragm and adjacent body walls, and its visceral surface is related to abdominal organs. It is divided into right and left lobes, and on its visceral surface its caudate and quadrate lobes are demarcated by various fissures and the porta hepatis. The internal substance is divided into segments on the basis of the ramification of the bile ducts and the hepatic vessels. It is almost totally invested by peritoneum, on the inner aspect of which is a connective tissue capsule. It has a dual blood supply from the hepatic artery and the portal vein and drains through multiple hepatic veins into the inferior vena cava. For information on the physiologic function of the organ, see LIVER. **h. adiposum** FATTY LIVER. **h. lobatum** The grossly misshapen and scarred liver that develops after congenital syphilis. It is characterized by multiple lobes of variable size separated by deep fissures resulting from the scars of healed syphilitic gummas.

**heparan sulfate** A polysaccharide derived from a sequence of alternating residues of D-glucuronic acid and *N*-acetylglucosamine by partial deacetylation and sulfation of amino groups. As the process proceeds, inversion at C-5 of the D-glucuronic residues forms L-iduronic residues, which also become sulfated at O-2, and the glucosamine residues are sulfated at O-6. As these processes advance, the heparan sulfate becomes heparin.

**heparin** \hep′ərin\ [HEPAR + -IN] A polysaccharide, consisting typically of alternate residues of L-iduronic acid 2-sulfate and 2-deoxy-2-sulfoaminoglucose 6-sulfate. The processes that form it from heparan sulfate may, however, not be complete, so less sulfated residues and glucuronic residues may be present. Its anticoagulant properties are probably due to its binding to thrombin and antithrombin in plasma and assisting their combination. It may also affect lipid metabolism by binding lipoprotein lipase to cell surfaces.

**heparinase** *Outmoded* HEPARIN LYASE.

**heparinemia** \hep′ərinē′mē·ə\ Active heparin circulating in the blood. Normally, negligible amounts are found in the blood, and demonstrable amounts reflect a very rare state in man unless exogenous heparin has been administered.

**heparinize** \hep′ərinīz′\ To administer heparin in order to achieve some degree of anticoagulation.

**heparin lyase** The enzyme (EC 4.2.2.7) that degrades heparin by an elimination reaction in which a hexosamine residue is liberated as a new reducing end by cleavage of the oxygen it glycosylates from a glucuronate residue, with the introduction of a 4,5-double bond in the latter. Also *heparinase* (outmoded).

**heparitinuria** \hep′ərit′inoo′rē·ə\ The presence of heparan sulfate in the urine, as may occur in mucopolysaccharidoses, notably the Hurler syndrome.

**hepat-** \hepat-\ HEPATO-.

**hepatalgia** \hep′ətal′jə\ Pain in the liver, most often related to capsular distension.

**hepatauxe** \hep′ətôk′sē\ [HEPAT- + Gk *auxē* growth, increase] HEPATOMEGALY.

**hepatectomy** \hep′ətek′təmē\ [HEPAT- + -ECTOMY] The surgical removal of all or a part of the liver.

**hepatic** \həpat′ik\ [Gk *hēpatik(os)* (from *hēpar*, gen. *hēpatos*, the liver + *-ikos* -IC) pertaining to the liver] Of or relating to the liver.

**hepatico-** \həpat′əkō-\ [See HEPATIC.] A combining form meaning (1) hepatic; (2) hepatic bile duct.

**hepaticocholangiojejunostomy** \-kōlan′jē·ōjē′joo-näs′təmē\ [HEPATICO- + CHOLANGIO- + JEJUNO- + -STOMY] The surgical creation of an opening between the common hepatic bile duct and a proximal loop of small intestine in order to bypass obstructed or damaged distal biliary ducts. It may also involve a second communication with another bile duct.

**hepaticocholedochostomy** \-kōled′ōkäs′təmē\ [HEPATICO- + CHOLEDOCHO- + -STOMY] The surgical creation of an opening between the common hepatic duct and the common bile duct.

**hepaticodochotomy** \-dōkät′əmē\ [HEPATICO- + *(chole)docho-* + -TOMY] A surgical procedure in which an incision is made into the hepatic and common bile ducts.

**hepaticoduodenostomy** \-doo′ədēnäs′təmē\ A surgically created opening between the common hepatic duct and the duodenum. It is performed to alleviate damage to or an obstruction of the distal biliary tree.

**hepaticoenterostomy** \-en′təräs′təmē\ The surgical creation of an opening between a hepatic bile duct and the small bowel. It is usually performed to bypass the distal biliary tree after resection, because of an obstruction, or because of trauma.

**hepaticogastrostomy** \-gasträs′təmē\ A surgical procedure creating an opening between a hepatic bile duct and the stomach.

**hepaticojejunostomy** \-jē′joonäs′təmē\ The surgical creation of an opening between a hepatic bile duct and the proximal small intestine. It is frequently performed following biliary duct resection or for damage or obstruction of the distal biliary tree.

***Hepaticola*** \hep′ətik′ələ\ *CAPILLARIA.*

**hepaticoliasis** \-lī′əsis\ CAPILLARIASIS.

**hepaticolithotomy** \-lithät′əmē\ [HEPATICO- + LITHOTOMY] A surgical procedure in which an incision is made into a hepatic bile duct for the purpose of stone removal.

**hepaticolithotripsy** \-lith′ətrip′sē\ A surgical procedure in which hepatic duct stones are crushed to facilitate their passage or removal.

**hepaticostomy** \həpat′əkäs′təmē\ [HEPATICO- + -STOMY] A surgical procedure in which an incision is made into a hepatic bile duct to permit drainage, usually through a tube.

**hepaticotomy** \həpat′əkät′əmē\ [HEPATICO- + -TOMY] A surgical incision into a hepatic bile duct.

**hepatitic** \hep′ətit′ik\ Of or relating to hepatitis.

**hepatitides** \hep′ətit′idēz\ Plural of HEPATITIS.

**hepatitis** \hepətī′tis\ [HEPAT- + -ITIS] **1** Inflammation of the liver, involving alteration of hepatocytes, either degenerative or necrotic. **2** Any of various diseases characterized primarily by liver inflammation. **h. A** An acute illness of global distribution caused by hepatitis virus A, a picornavirus. After an incubation period of two to six weeks, the disease begins with fever, nonspecific gastrointestinal symptoms, and malaise. Subsequently, hepatosplenomegaly, jaundice, dark urine, and pruritis usually develop, with convalescence marked by persistent malaise, fatigue, and slight liver function abnormalities. The disease is usually acquired by oral consumption of contaminated material or by close person-to-person contact, especially via the fecal-oral route. It is rarely transmitted by blood transfusion. Hepatitis A occurs most frequently in children and young adults. Also *infectious hepatitis, viral hepatitis type A, epidemic hepatitis, epidemic catarrhal jaundice.* **active chronic h.** See under CHRONIC ACTIVE HEPATITIS. **amebic h.** Invasion of the liver by trophozoites of *Entamoeba histolytica.* **anicteric h.** An inflammatory process in the liver not accompanied by jaundice. **h. B** Inflammation of the liver caused by hepatitis B virus. The infectious agent may circulate in the blood for long periods of time (months or years) and is characteristically transmitted by parenteral, percutaneous, or permucosal inoculation of even minute amounts of blood, blood products, or bodily secretions. The disease may be acute or chronic, symptomatic or asymptomatic. Also *viral hepatitis type B, homologous serum hepatitis, human serum jaundice, homologous serum jaundice.* **cholestatic h.** An inflammatory process in the liver accompanied by manifestations of cholestasis. Also *cholangiolitic hepatitis.* **chronic active h.** A chronic inflammatory disease of the liver characterized by progressive destruction of the hepatic lobule, progressing to scarring and cirrhosis. Known etiologies are hepatitis virus, drugs, and certain autoimmune phenomena. The morphologic lesion of chronic active hepatitis can also be seen as part of the spectra of Wilson's disease and primary biliary cirrhosis. Also *chronic aggressive hepatitis, subacute hepatitis, relapsing epidemic jaundice* (outmoded). **chronic interstitial h.** CIRRHOSIS OF THE LIVER. **chronic persistent h.** A chronic hepatitis manifested histologically by an infiltrate of inflammatory cells in the portal areas without disruption of the limiting plate, with minimal piecemeal necrosis and without fibrosis. Known causative agents include hepatitis B virus and a virus of non-A, non-B hepatitis. Clinical manifestations include mild fatigue and malaise, but most patients are asymptomatic. **delta agent h.** Infection with delta agent, an RNA virus, occurring as a coinfection with hepatitis B or as a superinfection in a hepatitis B carrier and manifested as a fulminant, acute, or chronic exacerbation of hepatitis B infection. The agent is transmissible person-to-person via percutaneous or permucosal exposure to infected blood, serous fluid, or bodily secretions, but the presence in the host of hepatitis B surface antigen (HBsAg) is necessary for its replication. There is an unusually high incidence of cirrhosis in persons with chronic hepatitis due to delta agent superinfection. Delta agent infection probably occurs worldwide and is endemic in Italy. Incidence in the United States is low except among users of intravenous drugs. Also *delta hepatitis.* **enzootic h.** RIFT VALLEY FEVER. **epidemic h.** HEPATITIS A. **h. externa** PERIHEPATITIS. **familial h.** WILSON'S DISEASE. **fulminant h.** A rare form of hepatitis which rapidly develops massive liver damage characterized by acute yellow atrophy, commonly ending in coma and death. In most cases it is the result of viral or toxic liver injury. **giant cell h.** A histologic pattern of liver damage where multinucleate giant cells are conspicuous. It occurs particularly in newborn infants as a response to a variety of noxious agents. **homologous serum h.** HEPATITIS B. **infectious h.** HEPATITIS A. **ischemic h.** Inflammatory change in the liver, most prominent in the centrolobular zone, caused by acute hepatic ischemia and characterized by dramatic elevations of serum transaminase concentrations. **long-incubation h.** SERUM HEPATITIS. **lupoid h.** Chronic active hepatitis characterized by LE cells in the circulating blood. Despite the immunologic abnormalities, the illness is not thought to be related to systemic lupus erythematosus. Also *plasma cell* *hepatitis.* **neonatal h.** A giant cell hepatitis of unknown cause although possibly due to maternal-infant transmission of hepatitis B. It is one of the main causes of an obstructive type of jaundice in the newborn infant. Recovery is sometimes complete, but the condition may develop into hepatic cirrhosis. **non-A, non-B h.** Hepatitis in humans apparently caused by an as-yet uncharacterized retrovirus or retroviruslike agent. Diagnosis continues to depend on serological exclusion of hepatitis A and B viruses, cytomegalovirus, and Epstein-Barr virus. The clinical picture is indistinguishable from that produced by hepatitis B virus, it may be acquired by transfusion of blood and blood products, and infection may lead to chronic active or chronic persistent hepatitis. **plasma cell h.** LUPOID HEPATITIS. **post-transfusion h.** Hepatitis occurring following a blood transfusion. The vast majority of cases are caused by either hepatitis B or non-A, non-B virus. Also *transfusion hepatitis.* **serum h.** Viral hepatitis transmitted parenterally (by contaminated needles or the administration of infective blood products) or by oral ingestion of contaminated material. This general category of hepatitis is now usually specified according to the types of virus responsible: either hapatitis B, non-A, or non-B hepatitis, or delta agent hepatitis. Also *long-incubation hepatitis, syringe jaundice, transfusion jaundice.* **subacute h.** CHRONIC ACTIVE HEPATITIS. **toxic h.** Hepatitis caused by the administration of or exposure to a toxic compound. Also *toxipathic hepatitis.* **toxipathic h.** TOXIC HEPATITIS. **transfusion h.** POST-TRANSFUSION HEPATITIS. **viral h.** Any inflammation of the liver caused by a virus, including hepatitis A, hepatitis B, non-A, non-B hepatitis, delta agent hepatitis, and hepatitis due to Epstein-Barr virus, cytomegalovirus, or yellow fever virus. The clinical manifestations range from asymptomatic to fulminant disease resulting in coma and early death. Common symptoms are malaise, weakness, and nausea, and icterus occurs in approximately 25% of cases. Recovery is usually complete, but chronic hepatitis may occur after hepatitis B, non-A, non-B hepatitis, or delta agent hepatitis. **viral h. type A** HEPATITIS A. **viral h. type B** HEPATITIS B.

**hepatization** \hep′ətīzā′shən\ The transformation of a loose tissue into a dense, homogenous mass with the texture and consistency of liver. It usually denotes the conversion of normal lung to the consolidated inflammatory infiltrate of lobar pneumonia. **gray h.** The gross appearance of the second stage in the evolution of lobar pneumonia in which the lung parenchyma is firm rather than spongy, and has a grayish discoloration. This color is due to the degradation of leukocytes, red blood cells, and fibrin that fill the alveoli. **red h.** Hepatization in which the affected portion of lung is firm and red as a result of hyperemia and extravasation of blood in the early stages of pneumonia.

**hepatized** \hep′ətīzd\ Denoting an organ or structure that has been altered by disease so as to have the consistency of liver.

**hepato-** \hep′ətō-\ [Gk *hēpar*, gen. *hēpatos* liver] A combining form denoting the liver. Also *hepat-*.

**hepatobiliary** \-bil′i·er′ē\ Pertaining to the liver and biliary system.

**hepatoblast** \hep′ətōblast′\ [HEPATO- + -BLAST] The precursor in the fetus of the parenchymatous hepatic cell of the liver.

**hepatoblastoma** \-blastō′mə\ [HEPATOBLAST + -OMA] A malignant tumor of the liver, composed of cells resembling embryonal and fetal hepatic parenchyma with or without mesenchymal elements, such as cartilage and bone. It occurs mainly in early childhood and is not associated with cirrhosis. Also *embryonal mixed tumor.*

**hepatocarcinoma** \-kär′sinō′mə\ HEPATOCELLULAR CARCINOMA.

**hepatocele** \hep′ətōsēl′\ [HEPATO- + -CELE[1]] A herniation of part of the liver.

**hepatocellular** \-sel′yələr\ Pertaining to liver cells.

**hepatocerebral** \-ser′əbrəl\ [HEPATO- + CEREBRAL] Describing, pertaining to, or affecting the liver and brain.

**hepatocholangeitis** \-kōlan′jē·ī′tis\ HEPATOCHOLANGITIS.

**hepatocholangioduodenostomy** \-kōlan′jē·ōdoo′ədēnäs′təmē\ [HEPATO- + CHOLANGIO- + DUODENO- + -STOMY] A surgical procedure creating an opening between the hepatic biliary tree and the duodenum in order to treat distal biliary tract disease.

**hepatocholangioenterostomy** \-kōlan′jē·ō·en′təräs′təmē\ The surgical formation of an opening between the hepatic bile ducts and the small bowel in order to treat distal biliary tract disease.

**hepatocholangiogastrostomy** \-kōlan′jē·ōgasträs′təmē\ A surgical procedure that creates an opening between the hepatic ducts and the stomach. It is performed to bypass diseased areas of the distal biliary tract.

**hepatocholangiojejunostomy** \-kōlan′jē·ōjē′joonäs′təmē\ The surgical creation of an opening between the hepatic ducts and the proximal part of the small bowel. It is performed to bypass a diseased biliary tract.

**hepatocholangiostomy** \-kōlan′jē·äs′təmē\ A surgical procedure creating an opening between the hepatic ducts and the skin, usually through a tube, for the purpose of drainage.

**hepatocholangitis** \-kō′lanjī′tis\ [HEPATO- + *cholang(io)-* + -ITIS] Inflammation of the liver and biliary ducts. Also *hepatocholangeitis.*

**hepatocirrhosis** \-sirō′sis\ CIRRHOSIS OF THE LIVER.

**hepatocolic** \-käl′ik\ Referring to the liver and the colon.

**hepatocystic** \-sis′tik\ Referring to the liver and the gallbladder. Also *hepatovesicular.*

**hepatocyte** \hep′ətōsīt′\ LIVER CELL.

**hepatoduodenal** \-doo′ədē′nəl\ Referring to the liver and duodenum.

**hepatoduodenostomy** \-doo′ədēnäs′təmē\ A surgical procedure creating an opening between the liver and the duodenum for the purpose of bile drainage.

**hepatodystrophy** \-dis′trəfē\ ACUTE YELLOW ATROPHY OF THE LIVER.

**hepatoenteric** \-enter′ik\ Referring to the liver and intestine.

**hepatoenterostomy** \-en′təräs′təmē\ A surgical procedure creating an opening between the liver and small bowel for the purpose of biliary decompression and drainage.

**hepatogastric** \-gas′trik\ Referring to the liver and stomach.

**hepatogenous** \hep′ətäj′ənəs\ Originating in or from the liver. Also *hepatogenic.*

**hepatogram** \hep′ətōgram′\ A radiograph of the liver. **emission h.** LIVER SCAN. **isotope h.** *Incorrect* LIVER SCAN. **radionuclide h.** LIVER SCAN.

**hepatography** \hep′ətäg′rəfē\ [HEPATO- + -GRAPHY] Radiography of the liver usually after the injection of a contrast agent into the hepatic artery or retrogradely into hepatic veins. The liver can also be made radiopaque as a result of picking up special contrast agents, such as thorotrast or iodinated fat preparations, by the reticuloendothelial system. This method has experimental use only.

**hepatohemia** \-hē′mē·ə\ [HEPATO- + HEM- + -IA] Congestion of the sinusoids of the liver.

**hepatoid** \hep′ətoid\ Resembling the liver or liver tissue.
**hepatojugular** \-jug′yələr\ Referring to the liver and jugular vein, as in *hepatojuglar reflux*.
**hepatolenticular** \-lentik′yələr\ Involving the liver and the lenticular nucleus, as in *hepatolenticular degeneration*.
**hepatolienal** \-lī′ənəl\ [HEPATO- + LIEN- + -AL] Referring to the liver and the spleen; hepatosplenic.
**hepatolienography** \-lī′ənäg′rəfē\ HEPATOSPLENOGRAPHY.
**hepatolienomegaly** \-lī′ənōmeg′əlē\ HEPATOSPLENOMEGALY.
**hepatolith** \hep′ətōlith′\ A calculus in an intrahepatic bile duct.
**hepatolithectomy** \-lithek′təmē\ [HEPATOLITH + -ECTOMY] The surgical removal of one or more stones from the liver.
**hepatolithiasis** \-lithī′əsis\ A pathologic condition characterized by the presence of calculi within the intrahepatic bile ducts.
**hepatologist** A specialist in hepatology.
**hepatology** \hep′ətäl′əjē\ [HEPATO- + -LOGY] The study of the liver and its diseases.
**hepatoma** \hep′ətō′mə\ [HEPAT- + -OMA] **1** A primary tumor of the liver parenchymal cells. **2** HEPATOCELLULAR CARCINOMA. **3** A benign or malignant experimental tumor of liver parenchymal cells. **malignant h.** HEPATOCELLULAR CARCINOMA.
**hepatomalacia** \-məlā′shə\ A condition marked by the softening of the liver.
**hepatomegalia** \-məgā′lyə\ HEPATOMEGALY. **h. glycogenica** GLYCOGENIC HEPATOMEGALY.
**hepatomegaly** \-meg′əlē\ [HEPATO- + -MEGALY] Enlargement of the liver. Also *hepatomegalia, hepatauxe*. **glycogenic h.** Enlargement of the liver caused by a glycogen storage disease. Also *hepatomegalia glycogenica*.
**hepatonephritis** \-nəfrī′tis\ Simultaneous inflammation of the liver and kidneys, as in leptospirosis.
**hepatopathic** \-path′ik\ Causing or relating to liver disease.
**hepatopathy** \hep′ətäp′əthē\ [HEPATO- + -PATHY] Disease of the liver.
**hepatoperitonitis** \-per′itōnī′tis\ Inflammation of the hepatic peritoneum.
**hepatopexy** \hep′ətōpek′sē\ [HEPATO- + -PEXY] A surgical procedure in which the liver is resuspended to prevent ptosis.
**hepatophlebitis** \-fləbī′tis\ Inflammation of veins in the liver.
**hepatophlebography** \-fləbäg′rəfē\ Radiologic visualization of the hepatic venous outflow tracts.
**hepatoportal** \-pôr′təl\ Relating to the portal venous system of the liver.
**hepatoptosis** \hep′ətōtō′sis\ Ptosis of the liver.
**hepatorenal** \-rē′nəl\ Relating to the liver and kidneys.
**hepatorrhagia** \hep′ətôrā′jə\ [HEPATO- + -RRHAGIA] Bleeding from the liver.
**hepatorrhaphy** \hep′ətôr′əfē\ [HEPATO- + -RRHAPHY] A surgical procedure in which sutures are placed in the liver substance either for repair of a defect or for fixation.
**hepatorrhexia** \hep′ətôrek′sē·ə\ [HEPATO- + *-rrhex(is)* + -IA] Rupture of the liver.
**hepatosplenic** \-splē′nik\ Relating to or connecting the liver and the spleen; hepatolienal.
**hepatosplenitis** \-splēnī′tis\ Inflammation of the liver and the spleen.
**hepatosplenography** \-splēnäg′rəfē\ [HEPATO- + SPLENO- + -GRAPHY] Radiography of the liver and spleen, usually after opacification of these organs by injecting contrast medium into feeding vessels, such as the celiac axis, or by intravenous administration of radiopaque preparations which are picked up by the cells of the reticuloendothelial system. Also *hepatolienography*.
**hepatosplenomegaly** \-splē′nəmeg′əlē\ Simultaneous enlargement of the liver and spleen. Also *hepatolienomegaly, splenohepatomegaly*.
**hepatosplenopathy** \-splēnäp′əthē\ A disorder of the liver and the spleen.
**hepatostomy** \hep′ətäs′təmē\ [HEPATO- + -STOMY] A surgical procedure creating an opening between the liver and the skin, usually through a tube, in order to establish drainage.
**hepatotomy** \hep′ətät′əmē\ [HEPATO- + -TOMY] A surgical incision into the liver.
**hepatotoxic** \-täk′sik\ Toxic to the liver.
**hepatotoxicity** \-täksis′itē\ Toxicity with respect to the liver; the property of being toxic to the liver.
**hepatotoxin** \-täk′sin\ [HEPATO- + TOXIN] A drug, chemical, or other substance toxic to the liver.
**hepatotropic** \-träp′ik\ Having an affinity for the liver; specifically affecting the liver.
**hepatovesicular** \-vesik′yələr\ HEPATOCYSTIC.
**HEPES** *N*-2-hydroxyethylpiperazine-*N′*-propanesulfonic acid. It is used as a buffer, all of whose forms are impermeable to biologic membranes due to the presence of the sulfo group. The p*K* values of piperazine are greatly depressed in this compound, and the p*K* of 7.5 normally used is that between its zwitterionic and anionic forms.
**hept-** \hept-\ HEPTA-.
**hepta-** \hep′tə-\ [Gk *hepta* seven] A combining form meaning seven.
**heptabarbital** $C_{13}H_{18}N_2O_3$. 5-(1-Cyclohepten-1-yl)-5-ethylbarbituric acid, a barbiturate with sedative and hypnotic properties. It is a short-acting agent, is given orally, and may lead to habituation or addiction.
**heptylpenicillin** PENICILLIN K.
**herb** \urb, hurb\ [L *herba* a small plant, herb, grass] A prepared drug that consists of plants or plant parts.
**Herbert** [Herbert *Herbert*, English ophthalmic surgeon, 1865–1942] **1** See under OPERATION. **2** Herbert's pits. See under PIT.
**herbivore** \hur′bəvôr′\ [New L *herbivorus* (from L *herb(a)* grass, herb + *vorare* to eat, devour) feeding on grass and herbs] An animal that is a member of the second trophic level in the food chain and that feeds primarily on vegetation.
**herbivorous** [See HERBIVORE.] Characterized by a plant-eating diet.
**hereditary** \həred′iter′ē\ Transmitted or transmissable from parent to child through the genes. Also *inborn*.
**heredity** [L *hereditas* (from *heres* an heir) inheritance] **1** The genetic endowment an offspring receives from the parents. **2** The transmission of genetic information from parents to offspring. **autosomal h.** AUTOSOMAL INHERITANCE. **dominant h.** DOMINANT INHERITANCE. **X-linked h.** X-LINKED INHERITANCE.
**heredo-** \her′ədō-\ [L *heres* (genitive *heredis*) heir] A combining form meaning heredity, hereditary.
**heredoataxia** \-ətak′sē·ə\ Any of the group of hereditary ataxias.
**heredodegeneration** \-dējen′ərā′shən\ Any hereditary degeneration of the nervous system. **spinocerebellar h.** Any of a group of hereditary ataxias including Friedreich's disease, Marie's cerebellar ataxia, the Roussy-Lévy syndrome, olivopontocerebellar degeneration, and many

other inherited degenerative diseases of the nervous system.

**heredosyphilis** \-sif′əlis\ CONGENITAL SYPHILIS.

**heredosyphilitic** \-sif′əlit′ik\ Of or relating to congenital syphilis.

***Herellea*** \herel′ē·ə\ A former genus of aerobic, Gram-negative diplobacilli, now included in *Acinetobacter*.

**herelleosis** \herel′ē·ō′sis\ An infection caused by bacteria of the genus *Herellea*.

**Hering** [Heinrich Ewald *Hering*, German physiologist, 1866–1948] **1** See under EFFECT. **2** Hering's nerve. See under RAMUS SINUS CAROTICI NERVI GLOSSOPHARYNGEI. **3** Hering-Breuer reflex. See under REFLEX.

**Hering** [Karl Ewald Constantin *Hering*, German physiologist, 1834–1918] **1** See under TEST, THEORY. **2** Canal of Hering. See under CHOLANGIOLE.

**heritability** \her′itəbil′itē\ Any measure of capability of being inherited. **broad sense h.** The proportion of the phenotypic variance that is due to genetic factors. It can be calculated from the analysis of twins:

$$H = \frac{V_{DZ} - V_{MZ}}{V_{DZ}},$$

where $H$ is broad sense heritability and $V_{DZ}$ and $V_{MZ}$ are the means of the squares of the differences between members of dizygotic and monozygotic twin pairs, respectively.

$$H' = \frac{r_{MZ} - r_{DZ}}{1 - r_{DZ}},$$

where $r_{DZ}$ and $r_{MZ}$ are the intraclass correlations for dizygotic and monozygotic twin pairs. $H$ and $H'$ are approximately equal provided the total variance for dizygotic twins does not differ too greatly from that for monozygotic twins. **narrow sense h.** The proportion of the phenotypic variance that is due to additive genetic variation.

$$h^2 = \frac{V_A}{V_A + V_D + V_E},$$

where $h^2$ is narrow sense heritability, $V_A$ is the additive genetic variance, $V_D$ is the dominance variance, and $V_E$ is the environmental variance.

**heritable** \her′itəbl\ **1** Capable of being inherited. **2** Referring to a phenotype determined by a gene. For defs. 1 and 2 also *genetic*.

**heritage** **1** All characteristics passed from one generation to the next, irrespective of genetic considerations. *Popular.* **2** All characteristics, due in part to genes, that are transmitted from one generation to the next.

**Herlitz** [Carl Gillis *Herlitz*, Swedish pediatrician, born 1902] Herlitz syndrome. See under EPIDERMOLYSIS BULLOSA LETALIS.

**Hermansky** [F. *Hermansky*, Czech internist, flourished 20th century] Hermansky-Pudlak syndrome. See under SYNDROME.

**hermaphrodism** \hərmaf′rōdizm\ HERMAPHRODITISM.

**hermaphrodite** \hərmaf′rōdīt\ [after *Hermaphroditos*, mythological son of *Hermes* (Mercury) and *Aphrodite* (Venus)] An individual with some anatomic attributes of both sexes. **true h.** A person who has both ovarian and testicular tissue and a highly variable clinical syndrome ranging from external genitalia which simulate normal male or female structures through any degree of ambiguity. Gonads are of three types: testis on one side, ovary on the other; ovotestes on each side; ovotestis on one side, testis or ovary on the other. Internal genitalia are variable. Chromosomal constitution is normal male or female or XX/XY chimerism or XY/XXY mosaicism. Also *true intersex*.

**hermaphroditic** \hərmaf′rōdit′ik\ GYNANDROMORPHOUS.

**hermaphroditism** \hərmaf′rōdīt′izm\ [*hermaphrodit(e)* + -ISM] The condition of having both male and female anatomic characteristics. Also *hermaphrodism, hermaphroditismus, gynadromorphism, gynandria* (imprecise). **bilateral h.** True hermaphroditism in which ovarian and testicular tissue is present on both sides. **lateral h.** True hermaphroditism in which an ovary is present on one side and a testis on the other, without admixture of gonadal tissue. **ovotesticular h.** TRUE HERMAPHRODITISM. **protandrous h.** The condition in a hermaphroditic organism in which the male reproductive organs develop earlier than the female organs. **protogynous h.** Hermaphroditism in which the female reproductive organs develop earlier than the male organs. **synchronous h.** Hermaphroditism in which female and male generative functions occur concurrently, or sometimes alternately. **transverse h.** Pseudohermaphroditism in which the gonads are characteristic of one sex and the external genitalia are characteristic of the other. **true h.** The condition of being a true hermaphrodite. Also *hermaphroditismus verus*. **unilateral h.** The presence of both ovarian and testicular tissue on one side of the body and of either an ovary or a testis on the other side.

**hermaphroditismus** \hərmaf′rōdītiz′məs\ [See HERMAPHRODITISM.] HERMAPHRODITISM. **h. verus** TRUE HERMAPHRODITISM.

**hermetic** \hərmet′ik\ Sealed by fusion to ensure a very low rate of gas or water-vapor leakage.

**hernia** \hur′nē·ə\ [L, hernia, rupture] Protrusion of an organ or tissue through an abnormal opening. Also *rupture* (popular). **annular h.** INDIRECT INGUINAL HERNIA. **Birkett's h.** A hernia of the stratum synoviale through the stratum fibrosum of a joint capsule. Also *synovial hernia*. **h. of the bladder** EXSTROPHY OF THE BLADDER. **h. of the brain** Protrusion of the brain through a defect in the skull, the falx cerebri, or the tentorium cerebelli, or through anatomical openings such as the incisura of the tentorium or the foramen magnum. Also *cerebral hernia*. **h. of the broad ligament of the uterus** A protrusion of a loop of intestine into the substance of the broad ligament of the uterus. Also *broad-ligament hernia*. **cerebral h.** HERNIA OF THE BRAIN. **Cloquet's h.** PECTINEAL HERNIA. **complete h.** A hernia which has passed entirely through the orifice: applied especially to an indirect inguinal hernia that has passed into the scrotum or the labium majus. **Cooper's h.** RETROPERITONEAL HERNIA. **crural h.** FEMORAL HERNIA. **diaphragmatic h.** A hernia of abdominal viscera into the thorax at any of several areas of the diaphragm, most commonly in one of the less supported areas such as the pleuroperitoneal membrane, Morgagni's foramen, or the esophageal hiatus. It may also occur at other points owing to congenital underdevelopment of the usual muscular and tendinous supports. In the newborn, it most commonly occurs through the pleuroperitoneal canal (foramen of Bochdalek). **direct inguinal h.** An inguinal hernia which leaves the abdomen between the inferior epigastric artery and the rectus muscle. Also *direct hernia, internal hernia*. **exomphalos h.** OMPHALOCELE. **femoral h.** A hernia of intestine into the femoral canal. Also *femorocele, enteromerocele, crural hernia*. **funicular h.** A hernia involving either the spermatic or the umbilical cord. **gastroesophageal h.** A hiatal hernia involving a portion of stomach and esophagus. **hiatal h.** Hernia through the diaphragmatic hiatus, usually of a portion of the stomach and lower esophagus. It may be a sliding hernia or a paraesophageal hernia. Also *hiatus hernia, parahiatal diaphragmatic hernia.* **incarcerated h.** A hernia which cannot be reduced. Also *irreducible hernia.* **incisional h.** A hernia occurring at the site of a surgical incision, usually in the abdomen. **incomplete h.** A hernia which has not passed entirely through the orifice. **indirect inguinal h.** An inguinal hernia in which the internal orifice is the deep inguinal

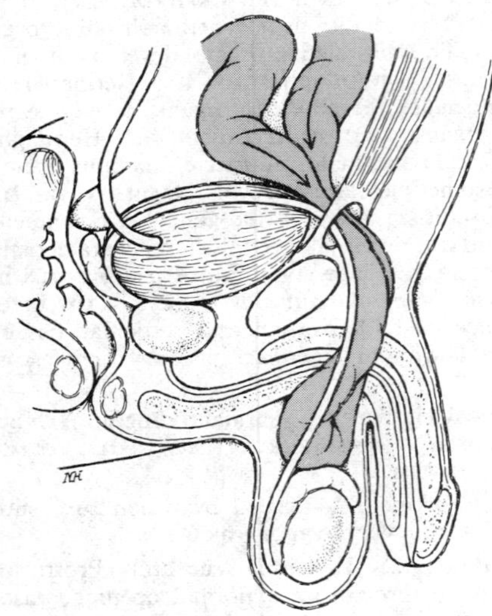

Indirect inguinal hernia

ring. Also *indirect hernia, annular hernia, oblique hernia.* **infantile h.** A congenital inguinal hernia. **inguinal h.** Hernia into the inguinal canal. See also DIRECT INGUINAL HERNIA, INDIRECT INGUINAL HERNIA. **inguinofemoral h.** Hernia into both the inguinal and the femoral canal. **internal h.** 1 A hernia not involving the abdominal wall. 2 DIRECT INGUINAL HERNIA. **irreducible h.** INCARCERATED HERNIA. **Laugier's h.** A femoral hernia passing through the lacunar ligament. **h. of the lung** Protrusion of the lung through a defect in the chest wall or diaphragm. Also *pneumatocele, pneumocele, pneumonocele.* **h. of the nucleus pulposus** INTERVERTEBRAL DISK PROTRUSION. **oblique h.** INDIRECT INGUINAL HERNIA. **obturator h.** A hernia through the obturator canal. **paraesophageal h.** A form of hiatal hernia in which the gastroesophageal junction remains in its infradiaphragmatic position and the fundus and body of the stomach herniate into the thorax. **parahiatal diaphragmatic h.** HIATAL HERNIA. **para-umbilical h.** Protrusion of an infant's viscera, through a weakness in the rectus fascia just above the umbilical scar. This hernia, which is uncommon, has no tendency to disappear spontaneously. **pectineal h.** A femoral hernia that enters the femoral canal and perforates the pectineus fascia rather than the fascia cribosa, simulating an obturator hernia. Also *pectineal crural hernia, Cloquet's hernia.* **posterior vaginal h.** Downward displacement of the pouch of Douglas (excavatio rectouterina). Also *enterocele.* **pudendal h.** Hernia in the pudendum via the levator muscle. **pulsion h.** Hernia produced by a sudden force such as an increase in intra-abdominal pressure. **rectal h.** Hernia of a loop of small intestine into the wall of the rectum. **rectovaginal h.** RECTOCELE. **reducible h.** Hernia in which the protruding portion of bowel may be manipulated back into its normal position. **retroperitoneal h.** Hernia of intestine into the retroperitoneum, usually in the region of the retroperitoneal duodenum. Also *Cooper's hernia.* **sciatic h.** Hernia through the greater sciatic foramen. Also *ischiocele.* **scrotal h.** An inguinal hernia that extends into the scrotum. Also *orchiocele, oscheocele, scrotocele.* **sliding h.** A hernia either of the cecum or of the sigmoid colon into the parietal peritoneum. **strangulated h.** An incarcerated hernia which may become ischemic and gangrenous. **synovial h.** BIRKETT'S HERNIA. **tentorial h.** TENTORIAL HERNIATION. **tonsillar h.** TONSILLAR HERNIATION. **transmesenteric h.** A herniation of a loop or larger segment of intestine through a defect of a mesentery, which is often of developmental origin. **h. of the tunica albuginea** A minute hernia in which seminiferous epithelium penetrates through the tunica albuginea of the testis. **umbilical h.** A protrusion of a segment of the gastrointestinal tract and/or the great omentum through a defect in the abdominal wall at the umbilicus, the herniated mass being circumscribed and covered by normal skin. It is almost universal in children in tropical countries, sometimes to a late age, but it is a self-curing condition. Compare OMPHALOCELE. **ventral h.** The herniation of peritoneal contents through the abdominal wall, often associated with a defect resulting from an incompletely closed surgical incision. Also *laparocele.*

**hernial** \hur′nē·əl\ Of or referring to a hernia.

**herniated** \hur′nē·ā′tid\ Having undergone herniation; protruding through a hernial opening.

**herniation** \hur′nē·ā′shən\ The formation of a hernia; rupture. **caudal transtentorial h.** Herniation of the brain caudally through the hiatus of the tentorium. **cingulate h.** Hernia of the cingulate gyrus beneath the falx cerebri. **disk h.** The protrusion of nucleus pulposus material through the annulus fibrosus of an intervertebral disk. Also *intervertebral disk herniation.* **foraminal h.** Herniation through an anatomic opening, usually of the cerebellar tonsils through the foramen magnum or the rostral displacement of the cerebral peduncles through the tentorial incisura. **intervertebral disk h.** DISK HERNIATION. **h. of nucleus pulposus** A protrusion of the nucleus pulposus of the intervertebral disk through a tear in the anulus fibrosus. **rostral transtentorial h.** Partial protrusion of the temporal lobe through the incisura of the tentorium, the result of supratentorial pressure at birth. **subfalcial h.** Herniation of the medial aspects of a cerebral hemisphere beneath the inferior edge of the falx cerebri. **tentorial h.** Herniation of the brain through the tentorial hiatus, usually involving the inferomedial portion of one or both temporal lobes (the uncus), due to supratentorial pressure. Also *tentorial hernia, uncal herniation.* **tonsillar h.** Herniation of one or both cerebellar tonsils through the foramen magnum due to intracranial pressure. Also *tonsillar hernia.* **transtentorial h.** Herniation of the brain through the tentorial hiatus. **uncal h.** TENTORIAL HERNIATION.

**hernio-** \hur′nē·ō-\ [L *hernia* rupture] A combining form meaning hernia.

**hernioenterotomy** \-en′tərät′əmē\ [HERNIO- + ENTEROTOMY] A surgical procedure that combines a hernia repair with an incision into the small bowel.

**herniolaparotomy** \-lap′ərät′əmē\ [HERNIO- + LAPA-

ROTOMY] A surgical procedure in which an incision into the abdominal cavity is combined with a hernia repair.

**herniology** \hur′nē·äl′əjē\ [HERNIO- + -LOGY] The study of hernias.

**hernioplasty** \hur′nē·əplas′tē\ [HERNIO- + -PLASTY] Any surgical procedure for repairing a hernia. **Cooper's ligament h.** MCVAY'S OPERATION.

**herniopuncture** \hur′nē·əpungk′chər\ [HERNIO- + PUNCTURE] A surgical procedure in which a hole is made in a hernia sac.

**herniorrhaphy** \hur′nē·ôr′əfē\ [HERNIO- + -RRHAPHY] A sutural procedure designed to repair a hernia.

**herniotomy** \hur′nē·ät′əmē\ [HERNIO- + -TOMY] Any surgical procedure that involves an incision into a hernia, usually to effect a repair. Also *celotomy, kelotomy.*

**heroic** \hirō′ik\ Involving extreme risk to a patient but resorted to in an effort to save life: said of a procedure.

**heroin** \her′əwin\ [German, from Gk *herō(s)* a hero (supposedly from the exalted feelings the drug can produce) + -IN] $C_{21}H_{23}O_5N$. A derivative of morphine that is formed by acetylation. It produces intense euphoria and excitation, and its use is likely to result in dependence and addiction. Also *diamorphine, diacetylmorphine, acetomorphine.*

**herpangina** \hurp′anjī′nə\ [*herp(es)* + ANGINA] An infectious disease caused by group A coxsackieviruses and characterized by fever, dysplasia, severe sore throat, anorexia, malaise, and typical gray-white vesicles in the tonsillar region. The disease occurs most frequently in children under seven years of age. Also *benign croupous angina, pharyngitis herpetica.*

**herpes** \hur′pēz\ [Gk *herpēs* (from *herpein* to creep, crawl, akin to L *serpere* to creep, crawl) herpes zoster] **1** Either of two diseases caused by a herpesvirus and characterized by a vesicular eruption: herpes simplex or herpes zoster. • When not followed by *zoster* or by *virus,* the word *herpes* now usually refers specifically to herpes simplex. **2** Any of various serpiginous skin diseases. An obsolete usage. **buccal h.** Herpes simplex appearing on the buccal mucous membrane. **h. digitalis** Herpes simplex that involves one or more fingers or toes. **h. disseminatus** The presence of scattered varicelliform vesicles in a subject with herpes zoster. **h. facialis** Herpes simplex on the face. **h. febrilis** Herpes simplex manifested as a fever blister (cold sore) or accompanying fever. See also HERPES LABIALIS. **h. generalisatus** Herpes zoster occurring as a generalized vesicular eruption, usually in the presence of an immune defect. **genital h.** Genital infection with *Herpesvirus hominis,* the herpes simplex virus (HSV), usually HSV-2. Most often transmitted by sexual contact and affecting both males and females, the infection is characterized clinically by itching, hyperemia, and the formation of closely grouped vesicles filled with clear fluid at the site of the infection. These rupture and develop into superficial ulcerations which heal after several weeks but recur in most patients and become active and infective again. Primary infection is frequently associated with systemic manifestations such as fever, malaise, anorexia, and bilateral inguinal lymphadenopathy. Also *herpes genitalis, herpes progenitalis.* **h. gestationis** A rare disease characterized by an itchy erythematous eruption which later blisters. Clinically it resembles pemphigoid but occurs only in late pregnancy and the puerperium. It recurs in successive pregnancies and can be reactivated by the oral contraceptive. Histologically there are foci of epidermal basal cell necrosis over the tips of dermal papillae and subepidermal blister formation. Patients have an IgG (herpes gestationis factor) circulating which fixes complement to the basement membrane zone. Symptomatic treatment is often sufficient although occasionally corticosteroids may be necessary to control blistering. Also *dermatitis gestationis.* **h. labialis** Herpes simplex manifested as an acute vesicular eruption on the lip or lips; a labial cold sore. The infection is usually acquired in childhood, and exacerbations may occur throughout life, especially during febrile illnesses such as pneumonia and malaria. Also *labial herpes.* **lingual h.** Herpes simplex on the tongue. **menstrual h.** Herpes simplex recurring in the premenstrual or menstrual phase of the menstrual cycle. **h. mentalis** Herpex simplex below the chin. **nasal h.** An eruption on or in the nose due either to the herpes simplex virus or to the virus of herpes zoster. **nasal h. simplex** The characteristic eruption around the anterior nares caused by the herpes simplex virus. In many individuals such sores are liable to recur whenever the patient has a cold or is overexposed to the sun, as the virus resides in the cells of the skin and becomes active in response to local irritation. **nasal h. zoster** A painful vesicular eruption which may occur on the skin of the external nose, in the nasal vestibule or, rarely, within the nasal cavity, due to herpes zoster of the maxillary division of the trigeminal nerve. Postherpetic pain may persist after the eruption has healed. The diagnosis may be more apparent if vesicles appear elsewhere in the distribution of the second division of the affected nerve, for instance on the ipsilateral cheek, but not across the midline. **neuralgic h.** Genital herpes marked by painful straining of the bladder and rectum. **ocular h.** Infection of any part of the eye with either herpes simplex or herpes zoster virus. **h. ophthalmicus** Herpes zoster involving the trigeminal ganglion and giving rise to pain and vesiculation in the distribution of the first division of the trigeminus, often including the cornea. Also *herpes zoster ophthalmicus, zoster ophthalmicus, zona ophthalmica, gasserian ganglionitis.* **orofacial h. simplex** An eruption around the mouth or nose or, less often, elsewhere on the face, due to infection with the virus of herpes simplex. **h. praeputialis** Genital herpes affecting the prepuce. **h. progenitalis** GENITAL HERPES. **h. pyaemicus** PUSTULAR PSORIASIS. **recurrent h.** HERPES SIMPLEX RECURRENS. **h. simplex** A disease caused by infection with *Herpesvirus hominis* (herpes simplex virus), types 1 and 2, usually characterized by vesicles 3–6 mm in diameter developing around the lips or nostrils (usually type 1) or in the genital area (usually type 2). Infection may also involve the eye, the brain, or the meninges. The principal mode of spread is direct contact, usually by means of infected secretions. Once acquired, infection may be recurrent, and recurrences may be precipitated by physical illness or emotional stress. Neonatal infection may occur in offspring of mothers with active cervical herpes. **h. simplex recurrens** Herpes simplex that tends to recur at or near the same site. Also *herpes recurrens, recurrent herpes.* **traumatic h.** Herpes simplex developing at the site of recent trauma, as may occur in wrestling and other body-contact sports. **h. zoster** An acute viral disease resulting from the activation of a latent herpesvirus (varicella-zoster virus) and characterized by inflammation of sensory ganglia, radicular neuralgic pain, and the usually unilateral eruption of groups of varicellalike vesicular lesions in a dermatomic distribution. Vesicles at sites distant from the primary infection occur in 2–5% of cases and more often in immunocompromised persons. The frequency of disseminated infection increases with age and with immunosuppression. Also *shingles, zoster, zona, zona ignea* (older term), *zona serpiginosa, acute posterior ganglionitis.* **h. zoster auricularis** A painful eruption of vesicles in the concha of the ear or elsewhere in or around the ear, due to infection with the virus of herpes zoster. Some cases are complicated by facial paralysis, deafness, and vertigo. Postherpetic neuralgia may occur particularly in the elderly. Also *zoster auricularis, herpes zoster oticus, zoster oticus.* See also RAMSAY HUNT SYNDROME. **h. zoster ophthalmicus** HERPES OPHTHALMICUS. **h. zoster oticus** HERPES ZOSTER AURICULARIS. **h. zoster varicellosus** Disseminated herpes zoster characterized by a varicelliform eruption.

***Herpesvirus*** \hur′pēzvī′rəs\ A generic designation comprising various herpes viruses, including herpes simplex viruses, varicella-zoster virus, and Epstein-Barr virus. ***H. hominis*** A genus-species designation for herpes simplex virus. ***H. papio*** A herpesvirus of baboons which is related to Epstein-Barr virus of humans. ***H. simiae*** A genus-species designation for herpes B virus. ***H. suis*** A genus-species designation for pseudorabies virus.

**herpesvirus** \hur′pēzvī′rəs\ **1** A virus belonging to the genus *Herpesvirus.* **2** Any herpes virus; a virus belonging to the family Herpetoviridae. **h. B** HERPES B VIRUS. **h. simian B** HERPES B VIRUS.

**herpetic** \hərpet′ik\ [Gk *herpēs,* gen. *herpēt(os)* shingles + -IC] **1** Pertaining to herpes. **2** Of or relating to the herpesviruses.

**Herpetoviridae** \hur′pətōvir′idē\ [*herpet(ic)* + *vir(us)* + -IDAE] A family of large, enveloped, DNA-containing viruses. Those causing human disease belong to two genera: *Herpesvirus,* which includes herpes simplex virus, varicella-zoster virus, and Epstein-Barr virus, and *Cytomegalovirus,* which includes the agent of cytomegalic inclusion disease.

**Herrick** [James Bryan *Herrick,* U.S. physician, 1861–1954] Herrick's anemia. See under SICKLE CELL ANEMIA.

**hersage** \ersäzh′\ [French (from L *irpex* or *hirpex* a harrow), a harrowing] The separation of fibers of a scarred nerve. Also *combing, harrowing, endoneurolysis.*

**Herter** [Christian Archibald *Herter,* U.S. physician, 1865–1910] Herter's disease, Herter-Heubner disease, Gee-Herter-Heubner syndrome, Herter's infantilism. See under INFANTILE CELIAC DISEASE.

**Hertig** [Arthur T. *Hertig,* U.S. pathologist, born 1904] Hertig-Rock ova. See under OVUM.

**Hertwig** [Richard Carl Wilhelm Theodor von *Hertwig,* German zoologist, 1850–1937] Hertwig-Magendie phenomenon, Magendie-Hertwig sign, Hertwig-Magendie sign, Hertwig-Magendie syndrome. See under SKEW DEVIATION.

**Hertwig** [Wilhelm August Oskar *Hertwig,* German physiologist, 1849–1922] See under SHEATH.

**hertz** \hurts\ [after Heinrich Rudolph *Hertz,* German physicist, 1857–1894] (*pl.* hertz) Special name for the SI derived unit of frequency, the frequency of a periodic phenomenon having a periodic time of one second; one cycle per second. Symbol: Hz

**Herxheimer** [Karl *Herxheimer,* German dermatologist, 1861–1944] **1** Jarisch-Herxheimer reaction, Herxheimer's fever. See under HERXHEIMER REACTION. **2** Herxheimer's fibers. See under HERXHEIMER SPIRALS.

**Heschl** [Richard L. *Heschl,* Austrian pathologist, 1824–1881] Transverse gyri of Heschl. See under AUDITORY CORTEX.

**Hess** [Alfred Fabian *Hess,* U.S. physician, 1875–1933] Hess capillary test. See under TEST.

**Hess** [Walter Rudolf *Hess,* Swiss physiologist, 1881–1973] Trophotropic zone of Hess. See under ZONE.

**Hesselbach** [Franz Kaspar *Hesselbach,* German surgeon, 1759–1816] **1** Hesselbach's ligament. See under LIGAMENTUM INTERFOVEOLARE. **2** Hesselbach's triangle. See under TRIGONUM INGUINALE.

**heter-** \het′ər-\ HETERO-.

**heterauxesis** \het′ərôkzē′sis\ [HETER- + AUXESIS] The disproportionate growth of a part in relation to another part of the same organism.

**heterecious** \het′ərē′shəs\ [HETER- + *oiki(a)* a dwelling + -OUS] Requiring more than one host to complete the life cycle: a characteristic of many parasites. Also *heteroecious, metecious, metoecious, heteroxenous, metoxenous.* Compare AUTECIOUS.

**heterecism** \het′ərē′sizm\ [HETER- + *oik(ia)* a dwelling + -ISM] A life cycle pattern, characteristic of many parasites, in which more than one host is required for the organism to complete its life cycle. Also *heteroxeny, metoxeny, metaxeny.* Also *heteroecism.*

**heterergic** \het′ərur′jik\ [HETER- + *erg(o)-* + -IC] Capable of producing varying pharmacologic effects: said of drugs or pharmaceutical agents.

**hetero-** \het′ərō-\ [Gk *heteros* (adjective) other, one of two] **1** A combining form meaning other, different. **2** In organic chemistry, a combining form specifically meaning containing elements other than carbon. Also *heter-.* Compare HOMO-.

**heteroagglutinin** \-əgloo′tinin\ An antibody that agglutinates xenogeneic erythrocytes. Also *heterohemoagglutinin.*

**heteroallele** \-əlēl′\ In diploid cells, a mutant allele whose paired allele on the homologous chromosome also carries a mutation but in a different codon.

**heteroallelic** \-əlē′lik\ Pertaining to mutant alleles that differ from the wild type because of mutations in different codons.

**heteroatom** An atom other than carbon, especially such an atom in a chain of carbon atoms.

**heteroauxin** \-ôk′sin\ *Obs.* INDOLE-3-ACETIC ACID. • This name was given when it was thought to be only one of the auxins, and that other substances were the main plant growth hormones.

***Heterobilharzia americana*** \-bilhär′zē·ə əmer′ikän′ə\ A species of schistosome found in mesenteric veins of the lynx and other mammals. The cercariae may cause a dermatitis common among oil workers in Louisiana.

**heteroblastic** \-blas′tik\ [HETERO- + *blast(o)-* + -IC] Derived from different kinds of precursor or from various embryonic cell types.

**heterocaryon** \-kar′ē·än\ HETEROKARYON.

**heterocephalus** \-sef′ələs\ [HETERO- + -CEPHALUS] Conjoined twins with heads of unequal size.

**heterochiral** \-kī′rəl\ [HETERO- + CHIR- + -AL] Relating to the other hand.

**heterochromatin** \-krō′mətin\ Regions of chromosomes characterized by condensation during interphase, late replication of DNA, transcriptional inactivity, and enrichment for highly repititious DNA. Compare EUCHROMATIN. **constitutive h.** Heterochromatin such as that at the centromere which is relatively invariant in an organism, regardless of cell type, state of differentiation, or transcriptional acitivity of the cell or of the surrounding euchromatin. **facultative h.** Heterochromatin that may become euchromatin, depending on the cell type, developmental stage, or sex. The inactive X chromosome in mammalian females is largely facultative heterochromatin. **paracentric h.** Heterochromatin that surrounds the centromere of a chromosome.

**heterochromia** \-krō′mē·ə\ [HETERO- + CHROM- + -IA] The presence of more than one color where uniformity of color is normal. Also *heterochromatosis.* **binocular h.** Variations in the color of the iris affecting both eyes, with or without associated pigmentation defects elsewhere in the body. **monocular h.** Loss of part of the melanin pigmentation of one iris.

**heterochromosome** \-krō′məsōm\ ALLOSOME.

**heterochronia** \-krō′nē·ə\ [Gk *heterochron(os)* (from HETERO- + *chronos* time) belonging to different times + -IA] The development of tissues, organs, or other parts of an organism out of normal temporal sequence.

**heterocladic** \-klad′ik\ [HETERO- + Gk *klad(os)* a branch + -IC] Relating to or characterized by anastomosis between branches of different arterial trunks.

**heterocrisis** \-krī′sis\ A crisis marked by unusual symptoms or occurring at an unusual time.

**heterocycle** A closed chain (ring) in an organic molecule in which at least one of the ring atoms is replaced by an atom other than carbon, such as O, N, S, P, Se, As, and B. Heterocyclic compounds are extremely numerous, and some, like pyrroles, furans, oxazines, thiazines, pyrimidines, and purines, play important parts in biologic chemistry and the dyestuffs industry.

**heterocyclic** [HETERO- + CYCLIC] Designating a compound whose molecule contains a ring of atoms of which one or more is not carbon.

**heterocytotropic** \-sī′tətrăp′ik\ [HETERO- + CYTO- + -TROPIC[1]] Having an affinity for cells of another species.

**heterodont** \het′ərōdänt′\ [*heter(o)-* + -ODONT] Denoting a dentition in which the teeth are specialized into different types, such as the incisors, canines, premolars, and molars of mammals.

**heteroduplex** \-doo′pleks\ **1** Any double-stranded nucleic acid, either totally or partially base paired, in which the two strands are derived from different sources, such as different species. **2** A completely or partially base paired nucleic acid in which one strand is DNA and the other is RNA.

**heteroecious** \-ē′shəs\ HETERECIOUS.

**heteroecism** \-ē′sizm\ HETERECISM.

**heterofermentative** \-fərmen′tətiv\ Carrying out heterolactic fermentation. Also *heterolactic.* Compare HOMOFERMENTATIVE.

**heterogamete** \-gam′ēt\ Any gamete that differs in structure or size from the one that is usually joined in fertilization with it, as in the human ovum and sperm.

**heterogametic** \-gəmet′ik\ **1** Referring to or characterized by the production of different kinds of gametes, usually in reference to the sex chromosome present. In humans, males are heterogametic. **2** Referring to or characterized by the production of gametes that differ in size or structure. Humans are heterogametic in this regard.

**heterogamy** \het′ərăg′əmē\ [HETERO- + *gam(o)-* + -Y] **1** A mating preference for individuals of unlike characteristics. **2** The reproduction of plants by indirect pollination. Compare HOMOGAMY.

**heterogeneic** \-jənē′ik\ HETEROGENIC.

**heterogeneity** \-jənē′itē\ GENETIC HETEROGENEITY. **genetic h.** The occurrence of different mutations, either at a single locus or at distinct loci, that determine the same phenotype. Also *heterogenicity, heterogeneity.*

**heterogeneous** \-jē′nē·əs\ HETEROGENIC.

**heterogenesis** \-jen′əsis\ Origination or development by asexual multiplication, sport, or bud variation.

**heterogenic** \-jen′ik\ Characterized by heterogeneity. Also *heterogenetic, heterogeneous, heterogenous, heterogeneic.*

**heterogenicity** \-jənis′itē\ GENETIC HETEROGENEITY.

**heterogenote** \-jē′nōt\ A bacterium which is heterozygous for a region of a chromosome owing to the presence of an F-prime factor or a transducing phage.

**heterogenous** \het′əräj′ənəs\ HETEROGENIC.

**heterogeusia** \-joo′zē·ə\ [HETERO- + Gk *geus(is)* taste + -IA] A variety of dysgeusia characterized by a persistent, consistent change in the taste of all food and drink, for example everything may taste sweet.

**heterogonic** \-gän′ik\ [HETERO- + GON-[2] + -IC] Characterizing an alternative cycle in which larvae, under appropriate circumstances, develop into free-living male and female adults instead of developing directly into the infective parasitic form. Alternative heterogonic and homogonic cycles are seen in rhabditoid nematode worms. See also *STRONGYLOIDES.*

**heterograft** \het′ərōgraft′\ XENOGRAFT. **bovine h.** A prosthetic vascular graft composed of preserved calf carotid artery.

**heterohemagglutinin** \-hem′əgloo′tinin\ HETEROAGGLUTININ.

**heterohemolysin** \-hēmäl′isin\ An antibody occurring naturally or raised by immunization which is effective in producing a complement-mediated lysis of xenogeneic erythrocytes.

**heteroinoculation** \-inäk′yəlā′shən\ [HETERO- + INOCULATION] Inoculation of one individual with a microorganism from another.

**heterointoxication** \-intäk′sikā′shən\ Poisoning resulting from the introduction of an exogenous substance into the body. Also *heterotoxis.*

**heterokaryon** \-kar′ē·än\ A cell that contains two or more genetically different nuclei in a common cytoplasm, as somatic cell hybrids, or cells of some ascomycetes or basidiomycetes. Also *heterocaryon.* Compare HOMOKARYON.

**heterokeratoplasty** \-ker′ətōplas′tē\ [HETERO- + KERATOPLASTY] The transplantation of a cornea to an individual of a different species of animal.

**heterokinesia** \-kīnē′zhə\ [HETERO- + KINESIA] Difficulty in performing a movement, due to the fact that one limb is moved spontaneously when one attempts to move the other (allokinesia or mirror movement), or that a movement contrary to the one desired is made.

**heterolactic** \-lak′tik\ HETEROFERMENTATIVE.

**heterolateral** \-lat′rəl\ CONTRALATERAL.

**heterolecithal** \-les′ithəl\ [HETERO- + LECITH- + -AL] Describing an ovum in which yolk substances are unequally distributed.

**heterologous** \het′əräl′əgəs\ [HETERO- + *-logous* as in HOMOLOGOUS] **1** Different: said of a graft between divergent species. Also *xenogenic, xenogeneic, heterospecific.* **2** Noncorresponding, as two nonhomologous chromosomes, or an antigen and an antibody that do not interact. Compare HOMOLOGOUS.

**heterolysosome** \-lī′səsōm\ [HETERO- + LYSOSOME] A membrane-limited organelle in the cytoplasm of the cell which is formed by fusion of a phagosome and a lysosome.

**heterometric** \-met′rik\ [HETERO- + Gk *metr(on)* measure + -IC] Concerning changes in dimension.

**heterometropia** \-mətrō′pē·ə\ [HETERO- + Gk *metr(on)* measure + -OPIA] A difference in the refractive errors of the two eyes.

**heteromorphic** \-môr′fik\ HETEROMORPHOUS.

**heteromorphosis** \-môrfō′sis\ The regeneration of a structure, part, or organ different from that lost or removed.

**heteromorphous** \-môr′fəs\ [Gk *heteromorphos* (from HETERO- + *morphē* form) of different forms] **1** Departing from the norm in shape or structure. **2** Exhibiting variation in form: anisomorphous. For defs. 1 and 2 also *heteromorphic.*

**heteronymous** \het′ərän′əməs\ [Gk *heterōnymos* (from

HETERO- + *onyma* name) having a different name] **1** Corresponding to the opposite side, as an image on the right projected from the left eye; crossed. **2** Of or relating to another muscle: said of the response in one muscle, motoneuron, or nerve upon stimulation of the nerve to a second muscle, which is usually a synergist. Compare HOMONYMOUS.

**heteropagus** \het′əräp′əgəs\ [HETERO- + -PAGUS] DUPLICITAS ASYMMETROS.

**heterophany** \het′əräf′ənē\ [Gk *heterophan(ēs)* (from HETERO- + *-phanēs* -appearing, from *phainesthai* to appear) diverse in appearance + -Y] Variation in the manifestations of a certain disease or condition.

**heterophil** \het′ərōfil′\ [HETERO- + -PHIL] Having the property of reacting or combining with more than one substance, as an antiserum that reacts with both human and sheep erythrocytes or a cell that is stainable by both acidic and basic dyes.

**heterophonia** \-fō′nē·ə\ [HETERO- + PHON- + -IA ] Disordered voice production resulting from inflammatory, structural, neurologic, or psychogenic factors. Also *heterophony.*

**heterophoria** \-fôr′ē·ə\ [HETERO- + -PHORIA] A latent tendency to misalignment of the eyes in any direction, recognizable only when fusion is interrupted, as by covering one eye. Adj. heterophoric.

**heterophydiasis** \-fīdī′əsis\ HETEROPHYIASIS.

***Heterophyes*** \het′əräf′i·ēz\ A genus of small fish-borne trematodes of the family Heterophyidae, parasitic in the small intestine of humans, dogs, cats, other mammals, and fish-eating birds. Infection of the final host occurs through ingestion of raw or undercooked infected fish, which are in turn infected from cercariae from infected first intermediate snail hosts. Also *Cotylogonimus.* ***H. heterophyes*** A species parasitic in the cecum and small intestine of man and other fish-eating mammals; the Egyptian or small intestinal fluke. It is widely distributed in Egypt and the Far East. Also *Distoma heterophyes* (obs.), *Fasciola heterophyes, Mesogonimus heterophyes.* ***H. katsuradai*** A species of trematode, smaller in size than *H. heterophyes,* which occurs in Japan. Infections resulting from ingestion of raw, smoked, pickled, or undercooked fresh- or brackish-water fish are common.

**heterophyiasis** \-fī·ī′əsis\ [*Heterophy(es)* + -IASIS] Infection with flukes of the genus *Heterophyes.*. Also *heterophydiasis.*

**Heterophyidae** \-fī′idē\ [*Heterophy(es)* + -IDAE] A family of small trematodes which are freshwater-fish-borne parasites of fish-eating birds, humans, and other mammals. It includes the genus *Heterophyes,* species of which are common human parasites. Some members of the family are thought to cause blockage of coronary vessels by the extremely small eggs of the parasites that enter the submucosa and the mesenteric circulation. These cases, reported chiefly in the Philippines, involved bird heterophyids not well adapted to humans.

**heteroplasia** \-plā′zhə\ [HETERO- + -PLASIA] **1** The development of cells or tissues of a distinctive type in a location where they do not normally occur. Also *alloplasia.* **2** An abnormal position, termination, or origin of an organ or part that is otherwise normal, as an ectopic termination of the ureter.

**heteroplasm** \het′ərōplazm′\ [HETERO- + -PLASM] A tissue found in an abnormal location.

**heteroplastic** \-plas′tik\ Exhibiting heteroplasia; ectopic.

**heteroplastid** \-plas′tid\ XENOGRAFT.

**heteroplasty** \het′ərōplas′tē\ [HETERO- + -PLASTY] *Obs.* HETEROTRANSPLANTATION.

**heteroploidy** \het′ərōploi′dē\ [HETERO- + -PLOID + -Y ] The condition of a cell or an individual organism that has a number of chromosomes different from the usual haploid or diploid complement, as the states of aneuploidy and polyploidy.

***Heteropoda venatoria*** \het′əräp′ədə ven′ətôr′ē·ə\ A large spider, confused with tarantulas, often found in shipments of tropical fruit, particularly bananas. The bite of this spider is painful but not serious.

**heteropsychology** \-sīkäl′əjē\ ABNORMAL PSYCHOLOGY.

**Heteroptera** \het′əräp′tərə\ [HETERO- + Gk *ptera* feathers, wings (pl. of *pteron* feather)] A suborder of bugs in the order Hemiptera. Most possess two pairs of wings, one coriaceous or horny, the other membranous. The medically important families Reduviidae and Cimicidae are included in the suborder.

**heterosexual** \-sek′shoo·əl\ **1** Characterized by heterosexuality. **2** A heterosexual individual.

**heterosexuality** \-sek′shoo·al′itē\ [HETERO- + SEXUALITY] Sexuality directed toward the opposite sex.

**heterosmia** \het′əräz′mē·ə\ [HETER- + *osm(o)-*[2] + -IA] A disorder of the sense of smell in which the odor perceived is at variance with the stimulus producing it.

**heterosome** \het′ərōsōm′\ *Rare* SEX CHROMOSOME.

**heterospecific** \-spəsif′ik\ HETEROLOGOUS.

**heterotaxia** \-tak′sē·ə\ ECTOPIA.

**heterotherapy** \-ther′əpē\ Treatment directed at the chief symptoms of a disorder.

**heterothermic** \-thur′mik\ POIKILOTHERMIC.

**heterothermy** \-thur′mē\ POIKILOTHERMY.

**heterotonia** \-tō′nē·ə\ A condition characterized by variations in muscle tone.

**heterotopia** \-tō′pē·ə\ [HETERO- + Gk *top(os)* place + -IA] ECTOPIA. **nasal glial h.** A tumorlike mass of mature glial tissue occurring intranasally or at the base of the nose. Astrocytes may simulate nerve cells. Also *nasal glioma* (incorrect). **neuronal h.** A pathologic state in which neurons are found in parts of the brain (as in the white matter) where they are not normally present.

**heterotopic** \-täp′ik\ Describing or relating to heterotopia.

**heterotoxic** \-täk′sik\ Producing toxic effects in individuals of a different species from the originating individual. Compare HOMEOTOXIC.

**heterotoxin** \-täk′sin\ [HETERO- + TOXIN] A toxin which produces adverse effects in individuals of a different species from the originating individual.

**heterotoxis** \-täk′sis\ HETEROINTOXICATION.

**heterotransplant** \-trans′plant\ XENOGRAFT.

**heterotransplantation** \-trans′plantā′shən\ An operation involving the transplantation of tissue or an organ from an unrelated species (xenograft) to replace lost or damaged tissue. Also *heteroplasty* (obs.), *xenoplasty.*

**heterotroph** \het′ərəträf′\ [HETERO- + Gk *troph(ē)* nourishment] An organism unable to synthesize nutrients from inorganic compounds and therefore dependent on complex organic molecules from external sources for growth. Also *metatroph.* Compare AUTOTROPH.

**heterotrophic** \-träf′ik\ **1** Of or relating to a heterotroph. **2** Denoting the mode of nutrition characterizing heterotrophs; requiring complex organic molecules as sources of carbon and other nutrients. For defs 1 and 2 also *metatrophic.*

**heterotropia** \-trō′pē·ə\ [HETERO- + TROPIA] STRABISMUS.

**heterotropy** \het′ərät′rəpē\ STRABISMUS.
**heterotype** \het′ərōtīp′\ A representative of a population whose characters are widely divergent from the mean for that population. Compare HOMOTYPE.
**heterovaccine** \-vak′sēn\ A vaccine manufactured from a microorganism different from the causative agent of the disease for which the vaccine is used.
**heteroxenous** \het′əräk′sənəs\ [HETERO- + *xen(o)-* + -OUS] HETERECIOUS.
**heteroxeny** \het′əräk′sənē\ [HETERO- + *xen(o)-* + -Y] HETERECISM.
**heterozygosis** \-zīgō′sis\ The union of gametes of unlike genetic constitution to form a zygote.
**heterozygosity** \-zīgäs′itē\ A condition of a diploid or polyploid organism in which different alleles are found at one or more loci.
**heterozygote** \-zī′gōt\ An individual having different alleles at one or more genetic loci in homologous chromosome segments. This situation provides a much greater potential store of genetic diversity than is possible in a population of homozygotes with identical alleles at these loci. **compound h.** GENETIC COMPOUND. **double h.** A cell or organism that is heterozygous at two separate genetic loci. In experimental genetics, it is usually the offspring of parents who were homozygous for different alleles at two loci. Also *dihybrid, diheterozygote.* **inversion h.** A cell or organism that contains an inverted region of chromosome or detectable DNA sequence at one allele at one or more loci.
**heterozygous** \-zī′gəs\ [Gk *heterozyg(os)* (from HETERO- + *zygon* a yoke) unevenly yoked, not a matched pair + -OUS] Characterized by different alleles at a given locus: used especially of diploid or polyploid cells or organisms. Also *heterozygotic.* Compare HOMOZYGOUS.
**Heublein** [Arthur Carl *Heublein*, U.S. radiologist, 1879–1932] See under METHOD.
**Heubner** [Johann Otto Leonhard *Heubner*, German pediatrician, 1843–1926] **1** Heubner's specific endarteritis. See under SYPHILITIC CEREBRAL ENDARTERITIS. **2** Herter-Heubner disease, Gee-Herter-Heubner disease, Gee-Herter-Heubner syndrome. See under INFANTILE CELIAC DISEASE. **3** See under ARTERY.
**Heuser** [Chester *Heuser*, U.S. embryologist, 1885–1965] Heuser's membrane. See under EXOCOELOMIC MEMBRANE.
**hex-** \heks-\ HEXA-.
**hexa-** \hek′sə-\ [Gk *hex* six] A combining form meaning six. Also *hex-*.
**hexacanth** \hek′səkanth\ [HEX- + -ACANTH] ONCOSPHERE.
**hexachlorane** HEXACHLOROCYCLOHEXANE.
**hexachlorobenzene** $C_6Cl_6$. A white crystalline solid used as a fungicidal dressing on seed grains. It is not known to cause poisoning to workers manufacturing it or using it in the field. Poisoning has occurred among persons who have eaten wheat treated with this fungicide.
**hexachlorocyclohexane** $C_6H_6Cl_6$. A halogenated hydrocarbon that is an effective agent in the treatment of scabies and pediculosis. It is used in creams, ointments, and shampoos. The gamma isomer is lindane, which is used as an insecticide. Poisoning may occur from ingestion or prolonged inhalation. Also *hexachlorane, benzene hexachloride.*
**hexachlorophane** HEXACHLOROPHENE.
**hexachlorophene** $C_{13}H_6Cl_6O_2$. 2,2′-Methylenebis-[3,4,6-trichlorophenol]. A mild detergent that is used as a topical antiseptic agent and as a component of some soaps and scrubbing preparations. It is contraindicated for burn or skin dressings, the skin of infants, or other situations in which absorption of the chemical might occur and lead to toxic reactions. Also *compound G-11, hexachlorophane.*
**hexachromic** \-krō′mik\ [HEXA- + CHROM- + -IC] Descriptive of the ability to perceive six of the major spectral hues, the faulty discrimination usually being in the short wavelength end of the visible spectrum.
**hexadimethrine bromide** $(C_{13}H_{30}Br_2N_2)_X$. *N,N,N′,N′*-Tetramethyl-1,6-hexanediamine polymer with 1,3-dibromopropane. A polymer with basic properties that has the capacity to combine with and neutralize the effects of heparin and prevent its anticoagulant action.
**hexamethonium** $(CH_3)_3N^+—[CH_2]_6—N^+(CH_3)_3$. A ganglion-blocking agent, available as its chloride or bromide, used for the treatment of hypertension.
**hexamethylenaminesalicylsulfonic acid** METHENAMINE.
**hexamethyl violet** CRYSTAL VIOLET.
**hexamine** METHENAMINE.
**hexamine hippurate** METHENAMINE HIPPURATE.
**hexamine mandelate** METHENAMINE MANDELATE.
**hexane** $CH_3—[CH_2]_4—CH_3$. The saturated hydrocarbon whose molecules have unbranched chains of six carbon atoms.
**hexanoic acid** $CH_3—[CH_2]_4—COOH$. One of the lower fatty acids. Its residues occur in milk fat. Also *caproic acid* (outmoded).
**hexavaccine** \-vak′sēn\ A vaccine composed of six different antigens.
**hexavitamin** A combination of vitamins containing six components: Vitamins A, C, and D, and thiamine hydrochloride, riboflavin, and nicotinamide. It is formed into a tablet or capsule for oral administration.
**hexaxial** \heksak′sē·əl\ Having or pertaining to six axes, as in the hexaxial reference system, used for determining the electrical axis of the heart.
**hexenmilch** \hek′sənmilsh, -milsH\ [German, witches' milk] WITCH'S MILK.
**hexestrol** \hek′səstrôl\ $C_{18}H_{22}O_2$. 4,4′-(1,2-Diethyl-1,2-ethanediyl)bisphenol, a synthetic derivative of diethylstilbestrol, used orally and parenterally in substitutive and pharmacologic estrogen therapy.
**hexetidine** $C_{21}H_{45}N_3$. 1,3-Bis(2-ethylhexyl)hexahydro-5-methyl-5-pyrimidinamine. An oil used as a 0.1% solution in mouth and throat infections. The agent has antibacterial and antiprotozoal activity, and it is effective against *Candida* infections as well as mixed bacterial infections.
**hexobarbital** $C_{12}H_{16}N_2O_3$. 5-(1-Cyclohexen-1-yl)-1,5-dimethylbarbituric acid, a barbiturate used therapeutically as a sedative and short-acting hypnotic. It is given orally. Also *enhexymal, methexenyl.*
**hexocyclium methylsulfate** $C_{21}H_{36}N_2O_5S$. 4-(β-Cyclohexyl-β-hydroxy-β-phenethyl)-1,1-dimethylpiperazinium methylsulfate. A quarternary anticholinergic agent that is used to decrease gastric motility and gastric secretory activity. In larger doses it is also used to produce parasympathetic blockade. It is given orally.
**hexokinase** The enzyme (EC 2.7.1.1) that catalyzes the transfer of a phosphate group from ATP to glucose to yield glucose 6-phosphate. Most of its forms, such as those of muscle, have a low Michaelis constant for glucose and are normally saturated by it. The main liver isoenzyme, however, has a Michaelis constant comparable with the glucose concentration in the blood, and therefore phosphorylates more glucose when this concentration is raised.
**hexonate** The anion or salt of a hexonic acid, i.e. the acid formed by oxidation of C-1 of an aldohexose to yield a carboxyl group.

**hexonic acid** The acid formed by oxidation of C-1 of an aldohexose to yield a carboxyl group.

**hexosamine** The derivative of an aldohexose in which one hydroxyl group, normally on C-2, is replaced by an amino group.

**hexosaminidase** Any enzyme that catalyzes the hydrolysis of glycosides formed by hexosamines or *N*-acylated hexosamines. The removal of *N*-acetylglucosamine and *N*-acetylgalactosamine residues from glycolipids is a function of hexosaminidases. **h. A** The more negatively charged (pI = 5) of two hexosaminidases found in tissues. It catalyzes the hydrolytic cleavage of *N*-acetylglucosamine residues from glycolipids. If the enzyme is absent as in Tay-Sachs disease, a ganglioside accumulates. **h. B** The less negatively charged of two hexosaminidases found in tissues. It has an isoelectric point of 7. Unlike hexosaminidase A, it is not deficient in Tay-Sachs disease.

**hexose** [HEX- + -OSE[2]] A sugar whose molecule consists of a chain of six carbon atoms, such as glucose or fructose.

**hexosephosphoric esters** Phosphate esters of hexose sugars. They are important intermediates in carbohydrate metabolism.

**hexylcaine hydrochloride** $C_{16}H_{24}ClNO_2$. 1-(Cyclohexylamino)-2-propanol benzoate (ester) hydrochloride, a local anesthetic used primarily for topical anesthesia of intact membranes of the respiratory tract, the upper gastrointestinal tract, and the urinary tract.

**hexylresorcinol** $C_{12}H_{18}O_2$. 4-Hexyl-1,3-benzenediol, an antiseptic used in a solution which usually contains glycerin in water, as a wash, or for application to topical wounds or membranes. It is also administered internally as an antihelminthic against roundworms and hookworms.

**Hey** [William *Hey*, English surgeon, 1736–1819] Hey's ligament. See under MARGO FALCIFORMIS HIATUS SAPHENUS.

**Heyer** [W. T. *Heyer*, U.S. scientist, born 1902] Pudenz-Heyer valve. See under VALVE.

**Heyman** [James *Heyman*, Swedish gynecologist, born 1882] See under TECHNIQUE.

**Heymans** [Corneille Jean François *Heymans*, Belgian physiologist, 1892–1968] See under LAW.

**Hf** Symbol for the element, hafnium.

**Hfr** Denoting a strain of *Escherichia coli* capable of high-frequency gene transfer to a recipient because its F plasmid has integrated into the host chromosome. The site of integration determines the locus of entry of the chromosome.

**HFT** high-frequency transduction (denoting certain strains of bacteriophage).

**Hft** high-frequency transduction (denoting certain strains of bacteriophage).

**Hg** Symbol for the element, mercury.

**Hgb** hemoglobin.

**HGH** human growth hormone.

**HGPRT** hypoxanthine-guanine-phosphoribosyl transferase.

**hiatal** \hī·ā′tl\ Of or referring to a hiatus, especially the esophageal hiatus of the diaphragm.

**hiation** \hī·ā′shən\ [L *hiat(us)*, past part. of *hiare* to gape, yawn + -ION] YAWNING.

**hiatopexy** \hī·at′ōpek′sē\ [L *hiat(us)* an opening, a gaping + *o* + -PEXY] A surgical procedure to repair a space, gap, or widened opening, usually employing suture plication. Also *hiatopexia.*

**hiatus** \hī·ā′təs\ [L (from *hiare* to gape, stand open) an opening, gap] Any large opening, gap, or cleft; a foramen. **h. aorticus** [NA] The osseoaponeurotic opening in, or behind, the diaphragm, bounded by the median arcuate ligament anteriorly, the right and left crura of the diaphragm on either side, and the lower border of the body of twelfth thoracic vertebra posteriorly, transmitting the aorta, the thoracic duct and, occasionally, the azygos vein. Also *aortic opening, aortic foramen, aortic hiatus, aortic opening in diaphragm, aortic orifice.* **Breschet's h.** HELICOTREMA. **buccal h.** A cleft at the angle of the mouth in the embryo, which, if it persists, gives rise to macrostomia. Also *transverse facial cleft.* **h. of canal for greater petrosal nerve** HIATUS CANALIS NERVI PETROSI MAJORIS. **h. canalis nervi petrosi majoris** [NA] The opening in the anterior petrous portion of the temporal bone that leads to the facial canal and contains the greater petrosal nerve and a branch of the middle meningeal artery. Also *hiatus of canal for greater petrosal nerve, hiatus canalis facialis, hiatus of facial canal, hiatus for greater superficial petrosal nerve, superficial petrosal fissure, foramen of Fallopio, hiatus of Fallopius, hiatus of fallopian canal, hiatus fallopii, false hiatus of fallopian canal, spurious aperture of facial canal* (outmoded), *foramen of Tarin* (outmoded), *Ferrein's foramen.* **h. canalis nervi petrosi minoris** [NA] The small lateral opening in the petrous portion of the temporal bone through which the lesser petrosal nerve passes. Also *hiatus of canal for lesser petrosal nerve, opening for lesser superficial petrosal nerve, opening for smaller superficial petrosal nerve.* **h. esophageus** [NA] The oval opening formed by the separation of the medial muscular fibers of the right crus of the diaphragm at the level of the tenth thoracic vertebra, transmitting the esophagus, the anterior and posterior vagal trunks, and esophageal branches of the left gastric vessels. Also *esophageal hiatus, esophageal foramen, esophageal opening in diaphragm.* **h. of facial canal** HIATUS CANALIS NERVI PETROSI MAJORIS. **h. of fallopian canal** HIATUS CANALIS NERVI PETROSI MAJORIS. **h. fallopii** HIATUS CANALIS NERVI PETROSI MAJORIS. **h. of Fallopius** HIATUS CANALIS NERVI PETROSI MAJORIS. **false h. of fallopian canal** HIATUS CANALIS NERVI PETROSI MAJORIS. **h. femoralis** FEMORAL FOSSA. **h. for greater superficial petrosal nerve** HIATUS CANALIS NERVI PETROSI MAJORIS. **h. leukemicus** A maturation gap in the granulocytic series that is often seen in acute granulocytic leukemia. For example, there may be myeloblasts, progranulocytes, and mature neutrophils, without any cells of the normally intermediate stages of maturation. **h. maxillaris** [NA] The large, irregular aperture opening into the maxillary sinus on the posterosuperior aspect of the nasal surface of the maxilla, partly closed by the perpendicular plate of palatine bone, the maxillary process of inferior nasal concha, the uncinate process of ethmoid, and part of the lacrimal bone. Also *maxillary hiatus, maxillary foramen, ostium maxillare, orifice of maxillary sinus.* **neural h.** An opening in the neural tube of early embryos during the closure process which eventually results in a complete neural tube with anterior and posterior neuropores. **pleuropericardial h.** An opening by which the early pericardial cavity communicates with each pleural canal. Subsequently each hiatus is closed off by the corresponding pleuropericardial fold, and contributes to the definitive diaphragm. If not closed, each opening is a potential site of a diaphragmatic hernia. Also *pleuroperitoneal sinus.* **h. sacralis** [NA] An inverted U-shaped opening at the apex of the dorsal surface of the sacrum, produced by the failure of the laminae of the fifth, and often the fourth, sacral vertebra to meet in the midline. This opening into the sacral canal is roofed over by the superficial dorsal sacrococcygeal ligament. Also *sacral hiatus, inferior opening of sacral canal.* **h. saphenus** [NA] The opening in the fascia lata of the thigh just below and lateral to the pubic tubercle, closed by the cribriform fascia through which pass the great saphenous vein to join the femoral vein, as well as small arteries, veins, and lymphatics. Also *saphenous hiatus, saphenous opening, oval fossa of thigh, fossa ovalis, foramen of saphenous vein.* **Scarpa's h.** HELICOTREMA. **h. of Schwalbe** The gap between the obturator fascia and the origin of the levator ani muscle when the latter occasionally arises by a tendinous sling attached only to bone anteriorly and posteriorly. The gap is a potential communication between the pelvic cavity and the ischioanal fossa. **h. semilunaris** [NA] A curved, long and narrow fissure between the free, posterior border of the uncinate process of the ethmoid bone inferiorly and the rounded ethmoidal bulla superiorly. It is continuous anteriorly with the ethmoidal infundibulum in the lateral wall of the middle meatus of the nasal cavity, and often receives the opening of the maxillary sinus. Also *semilunar hiatus, semilunar opening of ethmoid bone.* **subarcuate h.** FOSSA SUBARCUATA OSSIS TEMPORALIS. **h. tendineus** [NA] The large osseoaponeurotic opening in the tendon of the adductor magnus muscle at the medial supracondylar line about the junction of the middle and lower thirds of the thigh through which the femoral vessels pass from the adductor canal into the popliteal fossa. Also *tendinous opening, opening in adductor magnus muscle.* **tentorial h.** INCISURA TENTORII. **h. totalis sacralis** A gap extending along the whole dorsal wall of the sacral canal due to failure of the laminae to meet in the midline. **vena caval h.** FORAMEN VENAE CAVAE. **h. of Winslow** FORAMEN OMENTALE.

**hibernation** \hī'bərnā'shən\ [L *hibernatus,* past part. of *hibernare* (akin to *hiems* winter) to winter] A period of dormant inactivity, marked by hypothermia, that occurs in winter among many rodents, bats, and some large carnivores, such as the bear. Also *winter torpor.* Compare ESTIVATION. **artificial h.** A drug-induced state of narcosis and reduced metabolic activity resembling the natural state of hibernation exhibited by certain animal species.

**hibernoma** \hī'bərnō'mə\ [L *hibern(us)* pertaining to winter + -OMA; so called because the tumor suggests a fad pad of some hibernating animals] A benign, lobulated and encapsulated tumor made up of granular or vacuolated, round, acidophilic cells having the appearance of brown fat. It usually involves the shoulder and neck region of young adults. Also *fetal fat cell lipoma, brown fat tumor.*

**hiccough** \hik'up\ HICCUP.

**hiccup** \hik'up\ [earlier *hikop,* of imitative origin] **1** An involuntary, spasmodic diaphragmatic contraction interrupted by a sudden closure of the glottis which results in a characteristic sound. Also *singultus, singultation, spasmolygmus.* Also *hiccough.* **2** To produce a hiccup or hiccups. **epidemic h.** An uncommon disorder, thought to be a monosymptomatic manifestation of encephalitis lethargica, in which strong recurrent diaphragmatic contractions occur and are often accompanied by glottal spasm, possibly for several hours or even for days. Also *diaphragmatic myoclonus.*

**Hicks** See under BRAXTON HICKS.

**hidebound** \hīd'bound\ Adhering tightly to the subcutaneous tissues, as of the skin in scleroderma.

**hidr-** \hidr-, hīdr-\ HIDRO-.

**hidradenitis** \hī'dradənī'tis\ [HIDR- + ADENITIS] An inflammation of the sweat glands. It most often affects the apocrine sweat glands. Also *hydradenitis.* **h. axillaris** Hidradenitis suppurativa of the axillary region. **h. suppurativa** A chronic infective disorder that involves apocrine gland follicles of the axilla and anogenital region producing indolent discharging sinuses. Some cases are associated with acne conglobata. Also *apocrine acne.*

**hidradenoma** \hidrad'ənō'mə\ [HIDR- + ADENOMA] A sweat gland adenoma. Also *hidroadenoma.* Also *hydradenoma.* **clear cell h.** ECCRINE ACROSPIROMA. **eruptive h.** SYRINGOMA. **h. eruptivum** SYRINGOMA. **papillary h.** A benign sweat gland tumor composed of papillae arranged in a lacelike pattern with superficial apocrine-type cells. It occurs in women in the anogenital region. Also *papilliferous hidradenoma, apocrine adenoma.*

**hidro-** \hid'rō-, hī'drō-\ [Gk *hidrōs* sweat] A combining form denoting sweat or sweat glands. Also *hidr-.*

**hidroa** \hidrō'ə\ [Gk *hidrōa* (from *hidrōs* sweat) heat rash] **1** Any skin condition occurring with associated abnormal sweating. *Seldom used.* **2** HYDROA.

**hidroadenoma** \-ad'ənō'mə\ HIDRADENOMA.

**hidrocystoma** \-sistō'mə\ A benign sweat gland tumor with single or multiple cysts that are lined by apocrine cells and occasional papillary structures. Also *hydrocystadenoma.* Also *hydrocystoma.*

**hidrorrhea** \hid'rôrē'ə\ HYPERHIDROSIS.

**hidroschesis** \hidräs'kəsis\ HYPOHIDROSIS.

**hidrosis** [Gk *hidrōsis* (from *hidrōs* sweat) sweating, perspiration] HYPERHIDROSIS.

**hidrotic** \hidrät'ik\ Of, relating to, or inducing sweating or increased sweating; sudorific or hyperhydrotic.

**hierarchy** \hī'rärkē\ **anxiety h.** The ranking of stimuli or situations to which a phobic patient responds with anxiety, ranging from those least fear-provoking to those most anxiety-provoking. This gradual series can then be used to gradually reduce crippling anxiety-laden responses by means of behavior modification techniques, such as systematic desensitization.

**hieric** \hī·er'ik\ [Gk *hier(os)* sacred, sacral + -IC] SACRAL.

**hierolisthesis** \hī'ərōlisthē'sis\ [Gk *hier(on osteon)* the sacrum + *olisthēsis* slippage, dislocation, from *olisthein* to slip] A displacement of the sacrum which results in an abnormal angulation at the lumbosacral junction.

**Higashi** [Ototaka *Higashi,* Japanese physician, flourished mid-20th century] Chédiak-Higashi disease, Chédiak-Steinbrinck-Higashi anomaly. See under CHÉDIAK-HIGASHI ANOMALY.

**high-energy** ENERGY-RICH.

**Highmore** [Nathaniel *Highmore,* English anatomist, 1613–1685] **1** Antrum of Highmore. See under SINUS MAXILLARIS. **2** Body of Highmore. See under MEDIASTINUM TESTIS.

**high-risk** **1** More liable to develop a disease or sustain an injury than others in the population at large or in some other defined group. ⟨"babies classified as 'high risk' have distinctly different cry patterns from 'normals.' High risk was determined by the prevalence among mothers during pregnancy of factors such as toxemia, narrow birth canal, infection and poor nutrition. . . . many high risk babies displayed these traits: Took longer to respond to the cry stimulus [;] sustained their cry for less time but took an average of 11 seconds longer to start crying after being snapped with a rubber band; had a pitch twice as high as normals." —*Science News,* 19 Nov. 1983, 327.⟩ **2** More hazardous for the patient than an alternative procedure. **3** Having a poor prognosis.

**high-spin** Denoting the state of a transition metal ion in which the electrons have as few paired spins as possible and are therefore spread among different orbitals. This state is energetically favored when different orbitals differ little in energy, usually because no strong interactions with electrons of ligands are provided in particular directions. This form of iron(II) is just favored in hemoglobin, and the iron in its high-spin state is larger than in its low-spin state and is further out of the plane of the porphyrin, whereas the low-spin state is favored in oxyhemoglobin.

**high-spinal** \-spī′nəl\ With reference to spinal preparations, denoting the highest cervical levels of the spinal cord, above the outflow of the phrenic nerve.

**hila** \hī′lə\ Plural of HILUM.

**Hildenbrand** [Johann Valentin Edler von *Hildenbrand*, Austrian physician, 1763–1818] Hildenbrand's disease. See under TYPHUS.

**hili** \hī′lī\ Plural of HILUS.

**hilifuge** \hī′lifyooj\ [*hil(um)* + *i* + -FUGE] Extending in a radiating pattern from a hilum, especially that of the lung: said of the configuration of a density seen on a chest radiograph, as in pulmonary edema.

**Hill** [Archibald Vivian *Hill*, English physiologist, 1886–1977] See under COEFFICIENT, EQUATION.

**Hill** [Robin *Hill*, English chemist, flourished early 20th century] See under REACTION.

**Hillis** [David S. *Hillis*, U.S. obstetrician and gynecologist, 1873–1942] **1** DeLee-Hillis obstetric stethoscope. See under STETHOSCOPE. **2** Müller-Hillis maneuver. See under MANEUVER.

**hillock** \hil′ək\ A small prominence or elevated part. **anal h.** ANAL TUBERCLE. **auricular h.'s** EAR HILLOCKS. **axon h.** The conical portion of the axon as it emerges from a neuron soma, distinguished by a relative paucity of Nissl bodies and a specialized plasmalemma. It is believed to be the site of initiation of the conducted action potential. Also *nerve hillock*. **Doyère's h.** MOTOR ENDPLATE. **ear h.'s** Small mounds on the side of the head of an embryo which are destined to form the external ear. Also *auricular hillocks*. **facial h.** COLLICULUS FACIALIS. **nerve h.** AXON HILLOCK. **seminal h.** COLLICULUS SEMINALIS.

**Hilton** [John *Hilton*, English surgeon, 1804–1878] **1** See under LAW. **2** Hilton's white line. See under LINE. **3** Hilton sac. See under SACCULUS LARYNGIS. **4** Hilton's muscle. See under MUSCULUS ARYEPIGLOTTICUS.

**hilum** \hī′ləm\ [L, a minute thing, a trifle; supposed orig. meaning: the "eye" of a bean, where it was attached to the pod] A small gap or hollow in an organ where vessels, nerves, and ducts enter or leave it. Also *hilus* (outmoded). Adj. hilar. **h. of caudal olivary nucleus** HILUM NUCLEI OLIVARIS CAUDALIS. **h. glandulae suprarenalis** A short groove for the passage of the corresponding suprarenal vein, which is situated on the anterior surface of each suprarenal gland. Also *hilum of suprarenal gland*. **h. of inferior olivary nucleus** HILUM NUCLEI OLIVARIS CAUDALIS. **h. of kidney** HILUM RENALE. **h. lienis** *Outmoded* HILUM SPLENICUM. **h. of lung** HILUM PULMONIS. **h. nodi lymphatici** A depression on one side of a lymph node through which the efferent lymph vessel emerges and its blood vessels enter and leave. Dense fibrous tissue extends from it into the medulla. Also *hilum of lymph node*. **h. nuclei dentati** [NA] The axonal core of the dentate nucleus of the cerebellum, giving rise to fibers of the superior cerebellar peduncle. **h. nuclei olivaris caudalis** The medial axonal core of the inferior olivary nucleus of the medulla oblongata. Also *hilum of olivary nucleus, hilum of inferior olivary nucleus, hilum of caudal olivary nucleus*. **h. ovarii** [NA] A slit in the mesovarian border of the ovary through which its arteries, veins, and lymphatics enter or leave. Also *hilum of ovary*. **h. pulmonis** [NA] The depression on the mediastinal surface of each lung through which the structures of the root of the lung enter or leave the lung. Also *hilum of lung, pulmonary hilum*. **renal h.** HILUM RENALE. **h. renale** [NA] A deep vertical fissure in the medial margin of each kidney that contains the renal artery, vein, and nerves and the renal pelvis. The vein usually lies anterior to the artery and the pelvis is often posterior to both. Also *hilum of kidney, porta renis, renal hilum*. **h. splenicum** [NA] A fissure in the lower part of the gastric surface of the spleen for the passage of the splenic vessels and nerves. Also *hilum of spleen, hilum lienis* (outmoded). **h. of suprarenal gland** HILUM GLANDULAE SUPRARENALIS.

**hilus** \hī′ləs\ *Outmoded* HILUM.

**hinchazón** \in′chäzôn′\ [Spanish, swelling (referring to the edema of wet beriberi)] A Cuban term for BERIBERI.

**hindbrain** \hīnd′-\ RHOMBENCEPHALON.

**hindfoot** \hīnd′-\ The foot structure posterior to the midtarsal joint.

**hindgut** \hīnd′gut\ [*hind* + GUT] The posterior segment of the embryonic intestine, precursor of the sigmoid colon and the rectum. It is extended by the cloaca, the partitioning of which separates the anal canal from the urogenital sinus. It is temporarily extended in the tail bud by a diverticulum, the postanal gut, which usually disappears before the end of the fifth week in human development.

**hind-kidney** \hīnd′-\ METANEPHROS.

**hindwater** \hīnd′-\ [*hind* + *water*] That portion of the amniotic fluid that lies behind the presenting fetal part.

**hinge-bow** \hinj′-bō\ A face-bow used in locating the external projection of the hinge axis on the face.

**hip** [Old English *hype* (prob. from a root meaning to bend, akin to L *cubitum* elbow and *cubare* to recline) the hip] **1** ARTICULATIO COXAE. **2** The lateral bulge of the body below the waist and lateral to the hip joint. **snapping h.** The crepitus and associated audible snapping noise that occurs when the fascia lata tendon rides over an enlarged posterior margin of the greater trochanter of the femur. Also *Perrin-Ferraton disease*.

***Hippelates*** \hip′əlā′tēz\ A genus of acalyptrate flies of the western hemisphere (family Chloropidae, order Diptera) known as eye gnats. Attracted to eye secretions and fluids of man and animals, some species are believed to transmit conjunctivitis, bovine mastitis, and yaws. ***H. flavipes*** A tropical species thought to be involved in mechanical transmission of yaws in Haiti and Jamaica. ***H. pusio*** The black-bodied, shining eye gnat of California and Florida. Also found in other southern states, it is a mechanical vector of a form of epidemic conjunctivitis and a particularly troublesome pest.

**hippo-** \hip′ō-, hip′ə-\ [Gk *hippos* horse] A combining form meaning horse.

***Hippobosca*** \-bäs′kə\ A genus of primarily Old World louse flies of the family Hippoboscidae, ectoparasitic on mammals and ostriches. Species reported to attack humans include *H. equina, H. variegata, H. camelina,* and *H. longipennis*.

**hippocampus** \-kam′pəs\ [New L (from Gk *hippokampos* seahorse, from *hippos* horse + *kampos* sea monster), a seahorse] [NA] An infolded region of the cerebral cortex forming an arched elevation in the floor of the lateral ventricle bordering the choroid fissure. It is composed of two sectors: Ammon's horn, or hippocampus proper, and the dentate gyrus, both of which together are sometimes called the hippocampal formation. The laminar structure constitutes a unique form of allocortex, with white matter (the alveus) on the surface. The main afferent connections derive from the entorhinal cortex of the parahippocampal gyrus. It gives rise to a large efferent bundle, the fornix, partially originating in the subiculum and projecting to the mamillary nuclei, septal nuclei, and anterior nuclei of the thalamus. Also *hippocampus major, cornu Ammonis, horn of Ammon, pes hippocampi major.* Adj. hippocampal.

**Hippocrates** \hipäk′rətēz\ **1** A physician of ancient Greece (460 B.C.–377 B.C.), customarily described as the "Father of Medicine" in recognition of his contribution to the scientific foundation of medicine through his and his followers' writings and practice. His name is also associated with the fundamental principles of medical ethics through the Hippocratic Oath, an ancient oath of uncertain origin still sworn by new physicians. **2** Cord of Hippocrates. See under TENDO CALCANEUS. **3** Hippocratic maneuver. See under MANEUVER.

**hippocratic** \-krat′ik\ Associated with or attributed to Hippocrates.

**Hippuran** A proprietary name for iodohippurate sodium

**hippuric acid** $C_6H_5—CO—NH—CH_2—COOH$. *N*-Benzoylglycine, the form in which benzoic acid is mainly excreted in the urine.

**hippus** \hip′əs\ [New L, from Gk *hippos* a horse, an eye ailment causing winking] A spasmodic alternation of large and small pupil size occurring spontaneously or associated with light or accommodation reflexes. Also *pupillary athetosis, bounding pupil.*

**hirci** \hur′sī\ [See HIRCUS.] (*sing.* hircus) [NA] Axillary hair.

**hircus** \hur′kəs\ [L, he-goat, goatlike smell, smell of the armpits] (*pl.* hirci) An axillary hair.

**Hirschberg** [Julius *Hirschberg*, German ophthalmologist, 1843–1925] Hirschberg's test for strabismus. See under TEST.

**Hirschberg** [Leonard Keene *Hirschberg*, U.S. physician, born 1877] Hirschberg's reflex. See under ADDUCTOR REFLEX OF FOOT.

**Hirschfeld** [Isador *Hirschfeld*, U.S. dentist, 1881–1965] **1** See under METHOD. **2** Hirschfeld's canals. See under INTERDENTAL CANALS.

**Hirschsprung** [Harald *Hirschsprung*, Danish pediatrician, 1830–1916] Hirschsprung's disease. See under CONGENITAL MEGACOLON.

**hirsute** \hur′soot\ [L *hirsutus* hairy, shaggy] Characterized by hirsutism.

**hirsuties** \hərsoo′shi·ēz\ . HIRSUTISM. **h. papillaris penis** HIRSUTOID PAPILLOMAS OF THE PENIS.

**hirsutism** \hur′sootizm\ [*hirsut(e)* + -ISM] The growth of hair in women in the male sexual pattern, either in part or wholly. Also *trichosis hirsuties, hirsuties.* Compare HYPERTRICHOSIS. **constitutional h.** Hirsutism in women due to hereditary factors and not to excessive androgen secretion. Also *idiopathic hirsutism.*

**hirudicide** \hiroo′disīd\ [L *hirudo*, gen. *hirudi(nis)* leech + -CIDE] An agent that destroys leeches.

**hirudin** \hiroo′din\ A substance secreted by the salivary glands of leeches. It acts as an antithrombin, preventing the coagulation of blood.

**Hirudinea** \hir′oodin′ē·ə\ [L *hirudo*, gen. *hirudinis* a leech + *-ea* (neut. pl. of *-eus* English *-eous*), suffix denoting a class] The leeches, a class of worms of the phylum Annelida that includes the genera *Haementeria, Helobdella, Hirudo, Hirudinaria, Haemadipsa, Haemopis, Limnatis, Macrobdella,* and *Pontobdella,* characterized by an extremely branched alimentary system for food storage, flat, segmented bodies, and a sucker at the posterior and often the anterior end. Most feed on the tissues of soft-bodied invertebrates, such as snails, but a number take the blood and exudates of vertebrates. Fish are frequently attacked, as are amphibians and other aquatic organisms. Human infestation often occurs while bathing or drinking hastily from contaminated pools. The worms enter rapidly and attach deep within the nostrils, pharynx, throat, ears, urethra, or vagina. The land leeches of the Far East (*Haemadipsa*) and South America, especially in humid or tropical rainforests, are notorious for mass attacks on horses, cattle or humans, often causing death.

**hirudiniasis** \hiroo′dinī′əsis\ [L *hirudo*, gen. *hirudin(is)* a leech + -IASIS] A condition caused by an attack by leeches, generally resulting in blockage of channels such as the urethra, or bleeding caused by a temporary attachment in the nares, pharynx, or ears. **external h.** Hirudiniasis resulting from attachment of aquatic or land leeches to the skin, resulting in blood loss, possible secondary infection, and transmission of parasites. **internal h.** Hirudiniasis resulting from accidental ingestion through drinking, or invasion of the mouth, nose, pharynx, larynx or genitalia.

**hirudinization** \hiroo′dinīzā′shən\ The injection of hirudin in order to prevent coagulation of blood.

**hirudinize** \hiroo′dinīz\ To render (blood) incoagulable by the addition of hirudin. This may be *in vitro* or done by the leech (*Hirudo*) during blood sucking.

***Hirudo*** \hiroo′dō\ [L, a leech, bloodsucker] A genus of leeches (family Gnathobdellidae, class Hirudinea), used traditionally for blood-letting or hirudinization. Also *Iatrobdella, Sanguisuga.* ***H. japonica*** The medicinal leech used for therapy in Japan. ***H. javanica*** A species found in Java and Burma, reported to cause internal hirudiniasis. ***H. medicinalis*** The medicinal leech, formerly a species of great importance in medicine as a therapeutic agent for hemorrhoids and many other conditions, and still in use by some local practitioners, especially in the Orient. Aquatic leeches serve as intermediate hosts for trypanosomes and sporozoan parasites of fish, amphibians, and turtles.

**His** [Wilhelm *His*, Jr., Swiss-born anatomist active in Germany, 1863–1934] **1** See under ELECTROGRAPHY. **2** His-Werner disease, Werner-His disease. See under TRENCH FEVER. **3** Kent-His bundle, His band, bundle of His. See under FASCICULUS ATRIOVENTRICULARIS. **4** Bifurcation of bundle of His. See under BIFURCATION. **5** His-Tawara node. See under NODUS ATRIOVENTRICULARIS. **6** Trunk of bundle of His. See under TRUNCUS FASCICULI ATRIOVENTRICULARIS. **7** His spindle. See under AORTIC SPINDLE.

**His** [Wilhelm *His*, Sr., Swiss-born anatomist active in Germany, 1831–1904] **1** See under RULE. **2** Isthmus of His. See under ISTHMUS RHOMBENCEPHALI. **3** His perivascular space, His-Held space. See under PERIVASCULAR SPACE. **4** His tubercle. See under TUBERCULUM AURICULAE.

**His** Symbol for histidine.

**Hiss** [Philip Hanson *Hiss*, U.S. bacteriologist, 1868–1913] Hiss capsule stain. See under STAIN.

**hist-** \hist-\ HISTO-.

**histaminase** A copper-containing amine oxidase. *Outmoded.* • This term is misleading because it suggests that the reaction is a hydrolysis rather than an oxidation.

**histamine** \his′təmin\ [*hist(idine)* + AMINE] Imidazolylethylamine. The substance formed by decarboxylation of histidine. It is released from mast cells during the allergic response. It stimulates the contraction of smooth muscle and increases vascular permeability.

**histamine acid phosphate** HISTAMINE PHOSPHATE.

**histamine dihydrochloride** $C_5H_9N_3{\cdot}2HCl$. A compound with the same general properties and actions as histamine.

**histamine-fast** Not responsive to histamine.

**histaminemia** \histam′inē′mē·ə\ The presence of histamine in the blood.

**histamine phosphate** $C_5H_9N_3{\cdot}2H_3PO_4$. The diphosphate salt of histamine, which is used as a diagnostic tool for the study of gastric secretions and in the treatment of some allergic conditions. Also *histamine acid phosphate*.

**histidase** *Outmoded* HISTIDINE AMMONIA-LYASE.

**histidinase** *Outmoded* HISTIDINE AMMONIA-LYASE.

**histidine** \his′tidin\ One of the amino acids incorporated into proteins. Its molecule consists of alanine substituted on C-3 by imidazole (at C-4 of the imidazole). The imidazole ring is weakly basic, so histidine residues in proteins are partly, but not overwhelmingly, protonated at neutral pH. They are involved in the catalytic mechanism of several enzymes.

**histidine ammonia-lyase** The enzyme (EC 4.3.1.3) that catalyzes the interconversion of histidine with ammonia and urocanate, the *trans* isomer of 3-(imidazol-4-yl)propenoic acid. This is a step in the catabolism of histidine. Also *histidase* (outmoded), *histidinase* (outmoded).

**histidine decarboxylase** The enzyme (EC 4.1.1.22) that catalyzes the conversion of histidine into histamine and carbon dioxide.

**histidinemia** \his′tidinē′mē·ə\ A rare inborn error of amino acid metabolism characterized by an elevated level of plasma histidine, excessive urinary excretion of histidine and imidazole metabolites, mental retardation, and defective speech. It is caused by a deficiency of histidine $\alpha$-deaminase that is inherited as an autosomal recessive trait.

**histidinuria** \his′tidinoo′rē·ə\ The excessive urinary excretion of histidine. The condition is a feature of histidinemia.

**histio-** \his′tē·ō-\ [Gk *histion* web, cloth, sheet] A combining form denoting tissue, especially connective tissue.

**histioblast** [HISTIO- + -BLAST] A histiocyte precursor.

**histiocyte** \his′tē·əsīt′\ [HISTIO- + -CYTE] A connective-tissue macrophage. Also *histocyte, reticulum cell, reticuloendothelial cell, reticular cell.* **cardiac h.** A multinucleate cell found in the inflammatory nodules of rheumatic carditis. Such cells may represent a fusion of macrophages or alternatively a damaged and degenerating cardiac muscle cell. Also *Anichkov cell, Anichkov's myocyte.* **sea-blue h.** A histiocyte that contains an excess of ceroid pigment within the cytoplasm.

**histiocytoma** \-sītō′mə\ [*histiocyt(e)* + -OMA] **1** DERMATOFIBROMA. **2** Any of various tumors characterized by a predominance of histiocytes. • The use of this term without qualification is not recommended, because of the possible confusion of dermatofibroma with (benign or malignant) fibrous histiocytoma. **h. cutis** DERMATOFIBROMA. **fibrous h.** A benign tumor of histiocytes and fibroblasts which typically grow in a storiform pattern. Lipid-laden macrophages, as foam cells and giant cells, are also present. It is most commonly found in the dermis. Also *fibroxanthoma, lipoid histiocytoma, fibroma xanthoma, xanthofibroma.* See also MALIGNANT FIBROUS HISTIOCYTOMA. **juvenile h.** JUVENILE XANTHOMA. **lipoid h.** FIBROUS HISTIOCYTOMA. **malignant fibrous h.** The malignant counterpart of a fibrous histiocytoma. Also *malignant fibroxanthoma, xanthosarcoma.*

**histiocytosis** \-sītō′sis\ [*histiocyt(e)* + -OSIS] Any of several disorders in which there is proliferation of histiocytes without any known underlying cause, such as infection, or disorder of lipid metabolism. Histiocytosis may be solitary or multiple, and may be restricted to bone or may be generalized. It is seen in eosinophilic granuloma, Hand-Schüller-Christian disease, and Letterer-Siwe disease, but although these disorders may be neoplastic in nature they are to be distinguished from malignant histiocytosis, which is a separate entity. Also *histocytosis, histiocytosis X, reticuloendothelial granulomatosis.* **malignant h.** A rapidly progressive neoplastic proliferation of histiocytes, especially those of bone marrow, liver, and spleen. The disorder is characterized by fever, enlargement of spleen and liver, pancytopenia, and infiltration of bone marrow by large, bizarre histiocytes that typically exhibit much erythrophagocytosis. Also *histiocytic medullary reticulosis, bony reticulosis.* **nonlipid h.** LETTERER-SIWE DISEASE. **pulmonary h.** An uncommon condition of unknown cause characterized by proliferation of histiocytes and granulomas in the lungs, often with subsequent fibrosis. **sinus h.** A nonspecific, benign reactive change of lymph nodes characterized by proliferation of histiocytes within peripheral and medullary sinuses. It may be seen in lymph nodes draining certain carcinomas. **h. X** HISTIOCYTOSIS.

**histiogenic** \-jen′ik\ HISTOGENOUS.

**histioma** \his′tē·ō′mə\ [*histi(o)-* + -OMA] *Obs.* NEOPLASM.

**histiotrophe** \his′tē·ətrōf′\ HISTOTROPH.

**histo-** \his′tō-\ [Gk *histos* loom, web of loom, warp] A combining form denoting (1) tissue; (2) a web or network. Also *hist-*.

**histoautoradiography** \-ô′tōrā′dē·äg′rəfē\ The process or technique of producing autoradiographs from histologic sections of tissue.

**histoblast** \his′təblast\ [HISTO- + -BLAST] One of the precursor cells that give rise to the tissues of the body, usually in the embryo and fetus but also later in life.

**histochemistry** The chemistry of tissues, especially in the sense of the characterization of the distribution of specific chemical compounds within cells. Also *histologic chemistry*.

**histochemotherapy** CHEMOTHERAPY.

**histocompatibility** \-kəmpat′əbil′itē\ A compatibility between the genotypes of donor and host such that a graft generally will not be rejected. Genetically determined alloantigens, present on the surface of nucleated cells of many tissues and easily detected on blood leukocytes, determine histocompatibility. The best studied antigens are those of the H-2 histocompatibility system in mice and the HLA histocompatibility system in man.

**histocompatible** \-kəmpat′əbəl\ Marked by histocompatibility; not likely to induce an immune response leading to rejection: said especially of a tissue graft or organ transplant.

**histocyte** \his′təsīt\ HISTIOCYTE.

**histocytosis** \-sītō′sis\ HISTIOCYTOSIS.

**histodifferentiation** \-dif′əren′shē·ā′shən\ The development of the characteristics peculiar to a particular tissue type from less organized groups of cells.

**histofluorescence** \-flôres′əns\ Fluorescence produced in tissue by the administration of some substance, such as one that had been previously irradiated.

**histogenesis** \-jen′əsis\ [HISTO- + GENESIS] The creation and development of tissues arising from undifferentiated embryonic cells. Also *histogeny, morphologic synthesis.* Adj. histogenetic.

**histogenous** \histäj′ənəs\ Of or relating to histogenesis. Also *histiogenic*.

**histogeny** \histäj′ənē\ HISTOGENESIS.

**histogram** \his′təgram\ [HISTO- + -GRAM] A graphic representation of a frequency distribution by means of a set of rectangles, the base of each representing a class-interval and the area being proportional to the frequency of that class.

**histoincompatibility** \-in′kəmpat′əbil′itē\ An incompatibility between the genotypes of donor and host such that a graft will almost invariably be rejected.

**histoincompatible** \-in'kəmpat'əbəl\ Marked by histoincompatibility; likely to induce an immune response leading to rejection: said especially of a tissue graft or organ transplant.

**histologist** \histäl'əjist\ A specialist in histology. Also *microanatomist.*

**histology** \histäl'əjē\ [HISTO- + -LOGY] An integral subspecialty of anatomy wherein the tissues and cells of an organism's structures are treated with special chemicals and studied with the light microscope. Also *microscopic anatomy, micranatomy, microanatomy, microhistology, histomorphology, histologic anatomy, minute anatomy.* Adj. histologic. **pathologic h.** HISTOPATHOLOGY. **topographic h.** The study of cell and tissue specialization according to the anatomic site in which they occur.

**histolysis** \histäl'isis\ Dissolution of tissue. Also *physiolysis.* Adj. histolytic.

**histoma** \histō'mə\ [HIST- + -OMA] *Obs.* NEOPLASM.

**histomorphology** \-môrfäl'əjē\ HISTOLOGY.

**histone** One of the strongly basic proteins usually associated with DNA in eukaryotic nuclei. There are five main types, and they show very little variation in sequence from one species to another.

**histonuria** \-noo'rē·ə\ [*histon(e)* + -URIA] The presence of histone in the urine, associated with dissolution of cells, as occurs in leukemias and in febrile and wasting illnesses.

**histopathogenesis** \-path'əjen'əsis\ Abnormal embryonic development of cells or tissues; abnormal histogenesis.

**histopathology** \-pathäl'əjē\ [HISTO- + PATHOLOGY] The study of the structural alterations of cells and tissues caused by disease.

**histophysiology** \-fiz'ē·äl'əjē\ The relationship between the microscopic structure and the function of living things.

***Histoplasma*** \-plaz'mə\ [HISTO- + PLASMA] A genus of dimorphic fungi that includes the agent of histoplasmosis, *Histoplasma capsulatum.* The perfect state is *Emmonsiella.*

**histoplasmin** \-plaz'min\ A sterile liquid preparation containing soluble antigenic material that is derived from cultures of *Histoplasma capsulatum.* It is injected intradermally as a skin test for the presence of cell-mediated immunity to *H. capsulatum* .

**histoplasmoma** \-plazmō'mə\ [*Histoplasm(a)* + -OMA] A tissue response to *Histoplasma capsulatum* consisting of a small tumorlike nodule, often located in the lung or in a lymph node. The nodule may contain calcifications in a caseous center or concentric rings of calcification.

**histoplasmosis** \-plazmō'sis\ A systemic fungal disease contracted by inhalation of spores of *Histoplasma capsulatum.* It may vary in severity from an asymptomatic infection to an acute influenzalike respiratory illness to a progressive disseminated disease, usually fatal if untreated, marked by hepatosplenomegaly, lymphadenopathy, fever, and organ or system involvement such as endocarditis or hypoadrenalism. The disease may also occur as a chronic cavitary pulmonary infection. Healing lesions frequently undergo calcification. Histoplasmosis occurs worldwide but is endemic in some areas, such as the Ohio and lower Mississippi river valleys of the south central United States. Also *Darling's disease.* **African h.** A systemic fungal disease reported in Africa (especially west Africa) and caused by *Histoplasma duboisii,* which although producing a separate disease is identical in culture to *H. capsulatum.* There are characteristic cutaneous nodules, papules, or ulcers, bony lesions, and lymphadenopathy with liquefaction necrosis. The portal of entry is thought to be respiratory. Diagnosis is from biopsy or smears from skin or bone lesions.

**historadiography** \-rā'dē·äg'rəfē\ Microradiography of tissue sections.

**history / case h.** A recording of information relating to a particular case, as in medicine, social work, or the like. **medical h.** A recording, often in written form as part of the medical record, of a patient's prior medical and health care status, illnesses, treatments, and problems.

**histospectroscopy** \-spekträs'kəpē\ The application of spectroscopy to tissue sections.

**histotome** \his'tətōm\ [HISTO- + -TOME] MICROTOME.

**histotoxic** \-täk'sik\ Toxic to or destructive of tissue: used especially in reference to infection by bacteria such as *Clostridium perfringens,* which form tissue-destroying enzymes.

**histotroph** \his'təträf\ [HISTO- + Gk *trophē* nourishment] The nutrients supplied to the mammalian embryo from the maternal tissues as distinct from that derived from the maternal blood and bloodstream, which is called hemotroph. Also *histiotrophe.* Adj. histotrophic, histiotrophic.

**histotropic** \-träp'ik\ [HISTO- + -TROPIC[1]] Having an affinity for tissue cells: said of certain chemicals, stains, and parasites.

**histozoic** \-zō'ik\ [HISTO- + *zo(o)-* + -IC] Living within host tissues: used especially of protozoan parasites.

**Hitzig** [Eduard *Hitzig,* German neurologist and psychiatrist, 1838–1907] See under GIRDLE, SYNDROME.

**HIV** human immunodeficiency virus.

**hives** [Scots dialect] URTICARIA.

**Hl** **1** latent hyperopia. **2** half-life. **3** hearing loss.

**HLA** **1** human leukocyte antigen. **2** human leukocyte, locus A. • *HL-A* or *HLA* referred originally to locus A, but subsequently various loci have been identified and are designated as *HLA-A, HLA-B, HLA-C,* and *HLA-D.*

**HL-A** human leukocyte, locus A. See under HLA.

**Hm** manifest hyperopia.

**HMG** human menopausal gonadotropin.

**HMO** health maintenance organization.

**hnRNA** heterogeneous nuclear RNA.

**Ho** Symbol for the element, holmium.

**hoarse** [Middle English *hors,* from Old Norse *hārs,* superseding Old English *hās* hoarse] **1** Husky, croaking, rough: said of the sound of the voice. **2** Suffering from such a change of voice.

**hoarseness** The condition of being hoarse.

**Hoboken** [Nicolaas *Hoboken,* Dutch anatomist and physician, 1632–1678] Hoboken's valves, valvulae Hobokenii. See under VALVE.

**Hoche** [Alfred Erich *Hoche,* German psychiatrist, 1865–1945] Hoche's tract. See under FASCICULUS SEPTOMARGINALIS.

**Hochsinger** [Karl *Hochsinger,* Austrian pediatrician, born 1860] See under PHENOMENON, SIGN.

**Hodge** [Hugh Lenox *Hodge,* U.S. gynecologist, 1796–1873] **1** See under PESSARY, MANEUVER. **2** Hodge's planes. See under PLANE.

**Hodgen** [John Thompson *Hodgen,* U.S. surgeon, 1826–1882] Hodgen's apparatus. See under SPLINT.

**Hodgkin** [Alan Lloyd *Hodgkin,* British physiologist, born 1914] See under CYCLE.

**Hodgkin** [Thomas *Hodgkin,* English physician, 1798–1866] **1** Reed-Hodgkin disease. See under HODGKIN'S DISEASE. **2** Hodgkin's disease of lung. See under DISEASE. **3** Hodgkin cells. See under STERNBERG-REED CELLS. **4** Non-Hodgkin's lymphoma. See under LYMPHOMA.

**hodograph** \hō'dōgraf\ An instrument that records the movements of locomotion.

**hodology** [Gk *hodo(s)* path, road, way + -LOGY] The

scientific study of tracts or pathways in the central nervous system.

**Hoehne** [Ottomar *Hoehne,* German gynecologist, 1871–1932] See under SIGN.

**Hoeppli** [Reinhard J. C. *Hoeppli,* German parasitologist, born 1893] See under PHENOMENON.

**hof** \hōf\ [German *Hof* courtyard] A pale or lucent area in the cytoplasm of cells stained with Romanowsky stains (such as the Wright stain), corresponding to the Golgi zone. A hof is characteristically seen in plasma cells and osteoblasts, toward the center of the cell from the eccentrically located nuclei. **nuclear h.** A deep nuclear indentation that is often situated opposite the Golgi apparatus. Also *nuclear pocket.*

**Hofbauer** [J. Isfred Isidore *Hofbauer,* U.S. gynecologist, 1878–1961] Hofbauer cells. See under CELL.

**Hoffa** [Albert *Hoffa,* German surgeon, 1859–1907] **1** Hoffa's operation, Hoffa-Lorenz operation. See under LORENZ OPERATION. **2** Hoffa-Kastert disease. See under HOFFA'S DISEASE.

**Hoffmann** [Johann *Hoffmann,* German neurologist, 1857–1919] **1** See under REFLEX, SYNDROME, SIGN, PHENOMENON. **2** Werdnig-Hoffmann paralysis, Hoffmann's atrophy, Werdnig-Hoffmann atrophy, Hoffmann-Werdnig syndrome, Werdnig-Hoffmann syndrome. See under WERDNIG-HOFFMANN DISEASE.

**Hofmann** [Georg von *Hofmann* Wellenhof, Austrian bacteriologist, 1843–1890] Hofmann's bacillus. See under *CORYNEBACTERIUM PSEUDODIPHTHERITICUM.*

**Hofmeister** [Franz von *Hofmeister,* German surgeon, 1867–1926] See under OPERATION.

**Hoguet** [Joseph Pierre *Hoguet,* U.S. surgeon, 1882–1946] See under MANEUVER.

**Hoke** [Michael *Hoke,* U.S. surgeon, 1872–1944] See under OPERATION.

**hol-** \häl-\ HOLO-.

**holandric** \hälan′drik\ Pertaining to traits, usually heritable ones, that only occur in the males of a species.

**hold / inspiratory h.** A device used to delay the onset of expiration during mechanical ventilation.

**Holden** [Luther *Holden,* English anatomist, 1815–1905] See under LINE.

**holder / broach h.** A manual dental instrument with a chuck for holding broaches securely during endodontic treatment. **clamp h.** RUBBER DAM CLAMP FORCEPS. **needle h.** A surgical device somewhat resembling scissors that is designed to hold a needle near the points of the blades and thus facilitate the placement of surgical sutures. Also *suture forceps.* **rubber dam h.** A device for holding a rubber dam in place. It may be a wire frame with lugs on which the rubber is stretched, or an arrangement of clips attached to elastics that encircle the head. **rubber dam clamp h.** RUBBER DAM CLAMP FORCEPS. **sponge h.** A surgical instrument with two blades and two handles that is designed to hold small absorbent pads. It is used for blunt dissection and hemostasis. Also *sponge-holding forceps.*

**holdfast** An organ found on certain parasites used for adherence, such as the scolex of tapeworms, highly modified for sucking and attachment to the intestinal wall of a vertebrate host, or the special basal structure by which Trichomycetes fungi attach to their insect hosts.

**hole / burr h.** An opening in the skull made with a burr.

**Holger Nielsen** [*Holger Nielsen,* Danish army officer, 1866–1955] Holger Nielsen method. See under COPENHAGEN METHOD.

**holiday / drug h.** A period during which maintenance drugs used in the treatment or suppression of mental illnesses, are discontinued, to assess the level of activity of the underlying disorder and to prevent or minimize undesirable side effects.

**holistic** \hōlis′tik\ [HOL- + -IST + -IC] Pertaining to or considering the whole rather than just individual parts or aspects. See also HOLISTIC MEDICINE.

**Holl** [Moritz *Holl,* Austrian surgeon, 1852–1920] See under LIGAMENT.

**Hollander** [Franklin *Hollander,* U.S. physiologist, 1899–1966] See under TEST.

**Hollenhorst** [Robert William *Hollenhorst,* U.S. ophthalmologist, born 1913] Hollenhorst bodies. See under PLAQUE.

**hollow** In anatomy, a depression or concavity in a surface. **Sebileau's h.** A depression on the floor of the mouth between the sublingual fold and the inferior surface of the tongue. *Outmoded.*

**hollow-back** LORDOSIS.

**Holmes** [Eric Gordon *Holmes,* English neurologist, born 1897] Stewart-Holmes sign. See under SIGN.

**Holmes** [Gordon Morgan *Holmes,* English neurologist, 1876–1965] **1** Holmes-Adie syndrome. See under ADIE SYNDROME. **2** Holmes phenomenon, Holmes-Stewart phenomenon, Holmes sign. See under HOLMES REBOUND PHENOMENON. **3** Holmes ataxia, Holmes type cerebellar ataxia, Holmes degeneration, Holmes familial cerebellar degeneration. See under PRIMARY PROGRESSIVE CEREBELLAR DEGENERATION. **4** Head-Holmes syndrome. See under SYNDROME.

**Holmes** [Timothy *Holmes,* English surgeon, 1825–1907] See under OPERATION.

**Holmgren** [Alarik Frithiof *Holmgren,* Swedish physiologist, 1831–1897] See under TEST.

**Holmgren** [Emil Algot *Holmgren,* Swedish histologist, 1866–1922] Holmgren-Golgi canals. See under ENDOPLASMIC RETICULUM.

**holmium** Element number 67, having atomic weight 164.93. Holmium is a somewhat toxic rare-earth metal. One stable isotope occurs in nature and many synthetic radioisotopes have been identified. Symbol: Ho

**holo-** \häl′ə-, hō′lə-\ [Gk *holos* whole, complete] A combining form meaning whole, complete, integral, undivided. Also *hol-.*

**holoacardius** \-əkär′de·əs\ [HOLO- + ACARDIUS] A monozygotic twin that lacks a heart and depends for circulation of blood upon the heart of the more nearly normal twin via the placenta and umbilical cord.

**holoanencephaly** \-an′ənsef′əlē\ [HOLO- + ANENCEPHALY] The total absence of the brain and cranium.

**holoblast** \häl′əblast\ [HOLO- + -BLAST] An early embryo in which cleavage is total. Adj. holoblastic.

**holoblastic** \-blas′tik\ [HOLO- + -BLAST + -IC] See under HOLOBLASTIC CLEAVAGE.

**holocephaly** \-sef′əlē\ [HOLO- + CEPHAL- + -Y] A condition in which the head is normal in the presence of demonstrable malformation elsewhere in the body.

**holocortex** \-kôr′teks\ [HOLO- + CORTEX] The cerebral cortex, conceived as formed by a continuous and contiguous migration. It includes the isocortex, cingulate region, and Ammon's formation.

**holocrine** \häl′əkrin\ [HOLO- + Gk *krin(ein)* to separate] Denoting or characterized by secretion in which the secreting cells form part of the secretory product. Compare MEROCRINE.

**holodiastolic** \-dī′astäl′ik\ Occupying the whole of diastole.

**holoendemic** \-endem′ik\ [HOLO- + ENDEMIC] HYPERENDEMIC.
**holoenzyme** \-en′zīm\ An enzyme including its removable prosthetic group, in distinction from the apoenzyme formed when the prosthetic group is removed.
**hologamy** \hōläg′əmē\ A characteristic by which the gametes of an organism are indistinguishable from somatic cells. Reproduction involves the fusion of two gametes, as is seen in unicellular organisms.
**hologastroschisis** \-gasträs′kisis\ [HOLO- + GASTRO- + -SCHISIS] A developmental defect in the body wall caused by the failure of the anterior (or ventral, in quadrupeds) abdominal wall to close about the umbilicus. It represents an extreme degree of omphalocele.
**hologram** \hō′ləgram\ [HOLO- + -GRAM] An interference pattern recorded on photographic film by using a split beam of coherent light. When the film is illuminated from behind by coherent light, the viewer sees a three-dimensional image.
**holography** \hōläg′rəfē\ [HOLO- + -GRAPHY] The process of recording or viewing a hologram. **acoustic h.** An imaging technique whereby a diffraction pattern is first generated from the original object and an image is subsequently reconstructed by coherent radiation.
**hologynic** \-jin′ik\ Pertaining to traits, usually heritable ones, that occur in the females of a species.
**holometabolous** \-mətab′ələs\ [HOLO- + Gk *metabol(os)* changeable + -OUS] Characterized by complete metamorphosis, with fully distinct larval, pupal, and imago stages: said of insects. Compare HEMIMETABOLOUS.
**holonephros** \-nef′rəs\ [HOLO- + Gk *nephros* kidney] All of the embryonic renal tubular systems considered as an all-embracing, continuous series. Also *segmental organ.* • There are anatomic and other attributes to indicate resemblances between the tubules of the pronephros, mesonephros, and metanephros, and so the term *holonephros* would include all three of these tubular excretory systems.
**holophytic** \-fit′ik\ Capable of manufacturing food from inorganic sources, like a green plant: said of certain protozoa.
**holoplexia** \-plek′sē·ə\ [HOLO- + Gk *plēx(is)* (from *plēssein* to strike) a stroke + -IA] GENERAL PARESIS.
**holoprosencephaly** \-präs′ənsef′əlē\ The failure of the embryonic prosencephalon, or forebrain, to differentiate into two cerebral hemispheres and the diencephalon. It is seen in severe degrees of cyclopia. **familial alobar h.** The autosomal recessive inheritance of malformations of the cranium (orbital hypotelorism), the face (median cleft lip and palate), and the brain (absence of the corpus callosum and/or a single ventricle).
**holorachischisis** \-rākis′kisis\ RACHISCHISIS TOTALIS.
**holoschisis** \hōläs′kisis, häl′əskī′sis\ [HOLO- + -SCHISIS] AMITOSIS.
**holosymphysis** \-sim′fisis\ A complete continuity: said of bones.
**holosystolic** \-sistäl′ik\ Occupying the whole of systole; pansystolic.
**holotelencephaly** \-tel′ənsef′əlē\ [HOLO- + *telencephal(on)* + -Y] The persistence of a single cerebral lobe and a single cerebral ventricle because of the failure of the embryonic telencephalon to differentiate into two hemispheres. It is seen in arrhinencephaly and severe degrees of cyclopia.
***Holothyrus*** \-thī′rəs\ A genus of mites parasitic in poultry and other domestic animals. A species from Mauritius, *H. coccinella* has poisoned ducks, geese, and chickens that ingested it. In humans this species may cause a painful swelling of the tongue and throat.
**holotopy** \hōlät′əpē\ The position of a part or an organ with respect to the whole body or organism.
**holotrichous** \hōlät′rikəs\ [HOLO- + TRICH- + -OUS ] Having cilia of approximately equal length over the entire body surface: said of microorganisms.
**holozoic** \-zō′ik\ Concerning the ingestion and metabolism of food in a manner common to most animals, involving heterotrophic nutrition, in which the energy source or food is derived directly from the cells or cell products of other organisms, as distinguished from saprozoic organisms.
**Holt** [Mary Clayton *Holt,* English pediatrician, flourished 20th century] Holt-Oram syndrome. See under SYNDROME.
**Holth** [Soren *Holth,* Norwegian ophthalmologist, 1863–1937] See under OPERATION.
**Holzknecht** [Guido *Holzknecht,* Austrian roentgenologist, 1872–1931] Lambert-Holzknecht law. See under LAW.
**homalocephalus** \häm′əlōsef′ələs\ An individual possessing a flat head.
**homalography** \häm′əläg′rəfē\ [Gk *homalo(s)* level, in the same plane + -GRAPHY] The study of the structural organization of a body by plane sections of parts or regions, or by drawings of such sections.
***Homalomyia*** \häm′əlōmī′yə\ A genus of flies of which the larvae may cause accidental intestinal myiasis in animals or humans.
**Homans** [John *Homans,* U.S. surgeon, 1877–1954] See under SIGN.
**homatropine** $C_{16}H_{21}NO_3$. An alkaloid medication made by combining in ester form tropine and mandelic acid. It is used as an antispasmodic because of its anticholinergic action as a parasympathetic blocking agent like atropine. Its salts are used as mydriatics.
**homatropine hydrobromide** $C_{16}H_{21}NO_3 \cdot HBr$. A white, crystalline powder that is used as a cycloplegic and mydratic agent. It is given topically in the conjunctiva.
**homatropine methylbromide** $C_{17}H_{24}BrNO_3$. The methylbromide salt of homatropine, which has the same properties as the parent drug. It is a parasympatholytic agent and used in the treatment of spasms in the gastrointestinal tract. It is given orally.
**homaxial** \hōmak′sē·əl\ Possessing axes of equal length, as in a sphere.
**Home** [Sir Everard *Home,* English surgeon, 1756–1832] Home's lobe, Home's gland. See under SUBTRIGONAL GLAND.
**home** / **nursing h.** A health care institution which provides various levels of long-term care for people who usually have medical disabilities or limitations in activity or mobility. • The term is used in this sense in many countries (except Japan), but in some (such as the United Kingdom and South Africa) it may apply also to some institutions providing short-term acute care. **residential h.** A residence provided for any of various groups requiring special care, such as the old or the handicapped. Such a home typically provides room and board and limited personal assistance in a group or family setting within the community.
**homecious** \hōmē′shəs\ AUTECIOUS.
**homeo-** \hō′mē·ə-\ [Gk *homoios* like, resembling] A combining form meaning like, similar, same. Also *homoeo-* (variant British spelling), *homoio-*.
**homeograft** \hō′mē·əgraft′\ ALLOGRAFT.
**homeometric** \-met′rik\ Maintaining like size.
**homeomorphous** \-môr′fəs\ [Gk *homoiomorphos* having the same form] Of like form and shape.
**homeopath** \hō′mē·əpath′\ A practitioner of homeopathy.
**homeopathy** \hō′mē·äp′əthē\ [HOMEO- + -PATHY] A

system of medicine in which the treatment of disease depends upon the administration of minute doses of drugs that would in larger doses produce symptoms of the disease being treated. Homeopathy was originally propounded by Samuel C. F. Hahnemann (1755–1843), a German physician. Also *hahnemannism*. Compare ALLOPATHY. Adj. homeopathic.

**homeoplasia** \-plā′zhə\ [HOMEO- + -PLASIA] The growth of new tissue similar to the tissue present in the region. Also *homoioplasia*.

**homeorrhesis** \hō′mē·ôrē′sis\ [HOMEO- + *-rrhe(a)* + -SIS] The continuation of a biological process along an unchanged course that remains unaffected by potentially diverting influences.

**homeosis** \hō′mē·ō′sis\ [Gk *homoiōsis* (from *homoios* similar) assimilation, establishment of a resemblance] A change or substitution in one structure or organ of the body to or by a related or homologous structure from another body segment. Adj. homeotic.

**homeostasis** \-stā′sis\ [HOMEO- + -STASIS] **1** The relative stability of the internal environment of a normal organism which is preserved through feedback mechanisms despite the presence of influences capable of causing profound changes. For example, when oxygen level decreases, sensors cause respiration to increase to preserve a level within a limited variability consistent with normal functioning. Also *homeostatic equilibrium*. **2** Those processes considered collectively by which homeostasis is maintained by normal organisms. For defs. 1 and 2 also *homoiostasis*. **genetic h.** In a breeding population, the combination of forces and processes that stabilize the genotype. **immunologic h.** The immunologic condition of a normal animal, in which an immune response is produced by the introduction of foreign antigens but not by the animal's own antigens.

**homeotherapy** \-ther′əpē\ Therapy or prevention of a disease using a material similar to, but not identical with, the pathogenic agent of that disease. See also HOMEOPATHY.

**homeotherm** \hō′mē·əthurm′\ [Gk *homoiothermos* (from *homoio(s)* similar + *thermē* heat) equally warm] An animal that can maintain a more or less constant body temperature by metabolic activity and by modifications that carefully regulate the rate of heat exchange with the environment. Also *homotherm, warm-blooded animal*.

**homeothermic** \-thur′mik\ Exhibiting or characterized by homeothermy. Also *homeothermal, hemathermal, hematothermal, hemathermous, homoiothermal, homoiothermic, homothermal, homothermic, endothermic, warm-blooded*.

**homeothermy** \-thur′mē\ [HOMEO- + THERM- + -Y] The maintenance of a constant body temperature independent of ambient temperatures. Homeothermy is typical only of birds and mammals. Also *endothermy*.

**homeotoxic** \-täk′sik\ Producing toxic effects in individuals of the same species as the originating individual; characteristic of or pertaining to a homeotoxin. Also *isotoxic*. Compare HETEROTOXIC.

**homeotoxin** \-täk′sin\ A toxin from an individual which is toxic to other individuals of the same species. Also *isotoxin*. Also *homoeotoxin, homoiotoxin*.

**homeotransplant** \-trans′plant\ ALLOGRAFT.

**homeotransplantation** \-trans′plantā′shən\ ALLOTRANSPLANTATION.

**homeotypic** \-tip′ik\ Pertaining to or resembling the normal or usual cell type: used especially of products of the second meiotic division of the male germ cells.

**homergic** \hōmur′jik\ [*hom(o)-* + *erg(o)-* + -IC] Characterizing drugs or pharmacologic agents that produce the same type of pharmacologic effects, even though they may not accomplish this by the same mechanism or by the same receptors.

**homicide** \häm′isīd\ [L *homicid(ium)* (from *homo*, gen. *homi(nis)* a human being + *caedere* to kill) homicide] **1** The killing of a human being by the act, by omission, or by negligence under circumstances which may be justifiable, excusable, or felonious. **2** One who commits homicide.

**hominid** \häm′ənid\ **1** Belonging to the primate family Hominidae. **2** A member of the primate family Hominidae.

**Hominidae** \hämin′idē\ The primate family comprising humans and the ancestral and collateral forms most closely related to them. There is only one extant genus, *Homo*, but numerous earlier forms are known from the fossil record. Some zoologists include the anthropoid apes in this family.

***Homo*** \hō′mō\ [L, a human being, man] A genus of the family Hominidae of which *H. sapiens* is the only living species. Extinct species such as *H. habilis* and *H. erectus* are known from fossil remains, as are *H. neanderthalensis* and others which are now often considered subspecies of *H. sapiens*. ***H. heidelbergensis*** See under HEIDELBERG MAN. ***H. neanderthalensis*** A fossil human species represented by the type specimen from La Chapelle-aux-Saints, France. Many other examples are known from Europe and the Middle East. The skeleton of this species is typically of short stature and robust structure, with large joints and a large cranial capacity. The face is large and projects forward from heavy brow ridges. Sites yielding Neandertal remains are mostly dated to between 50 000 and 100 000 years before the present. Some authorities regard Neandertal man as belonging to the species *Homo sapiens*, designating it as the subspecies *H. sapiens neanderthalensis*. ***H. sapiens*** The species that includes all the living races of mankind. It is characterized by striding, upright bipedalism, brain size in the order of 1350 $cm^3$, and an orthognathic face with a chin. These characters, as well as several others, serve to distinguish modern human anatomy from that of other species such as *H. habilis* and *H. erectus*. Early examples of *H. sapiens* are known from Swanscombe, England and Omo, Ethiopia, dated to between 100 000 and 250 000 years before the present. Some authorities recognize fossil subspecies such as *H. sapiens neanderthalensis, H. sapiens rhodesiensis, H. sapiens steinheimensis*, and others.

**homo-** \hō′mō-, häm′ə-\ [Gk *homos* one and the same] **1** A combining form meaning same, alike. **2** In organic chemistry, a combining form indicating the addition of a methylene group to a compound. Compare HETERO-.

**homoblastic** \-blas′tik\ Derived from one particular type of tissue.

**homocladic** \-klad′ik\ [HOMO- + Gk *klad(os)* a branch + -IC] Relating to or characterized by anastomosis between small branches of the same artery.

**homocysteine** $HS{-}CH_2{-}CH_2{-}CH(NH_3^+){-}COO^-$. An amino acid not incorporated into proteins but important as an intermediate in the metabolism of cysteine and methionine. In the breakdown of methionine it reacts with serine to form cystathionine, and it can alternatively by methylated to yield methionine. Symbol: Hcy

**homocysteine methyltransferase** **1** The enzyme (EC 2.1.1.10) present in plants and microorganisms that is responsible for the methylation of homocysteine to yield methionine. It uses *S*-adenosylmethionine or *S*-methylmethionine as methyl donor. **2** The cobamide-containing enzyme that uses methyltetrahydrofolate as methyl donor.

**homocystine** \-sis′tin\ $[S{\cdot}CH_2{\cdot}CH_2{\cdot}CH(NH_2)COOH]_2$. A substance made by the demethylation of methionine. It provides a source of sulfur for the body and is homologous to cystine.

**homocystinemia** \-sis′tinē′mē·ə\ The presence of homocystine in blood, a rare finding in patients with homocystinuria.

**homocystinuria** \-sis′tinoo′rē·ə\ **1** The abnormal excretion of homocysteine or homocystine in the urine. It is usually due to one of several inborn errors of transsulfuration, but it can also be caused by drugs or bacterial contamination of the urine. **2** A clinical condition caused by a deficiency of cystathionine β-synthase. The condition is of widely variable severity and is characterized by overgrowth of tubular bones, osteoporosis, ectopia lentis, thrombosis, and mental retardation. In one of at least two biochemical (and perhaps allelic) variants, the administration of pyridoxine increases enzyme activity, corrects biochemical abnormalities, and reduces the likelihood of further clinical deterioration. Also *cystathionine β-synthase deficiency*.

**homocytotropic** \-sī′tətrāp′ik\ [HOMO- + CYTOTROPIC] Capable of binding to cells of the same animal species: said of antibodies.

**homodromous** \hōmäd′rəməs\ [Gk *homodromos* (from HOMO- + *dromos* course) running on the same course] Moving in the same direction, or directing activity toward the same end.

**homodynamic** Of or relating to drugs or pharmacological agents that interact specifically with the same receptor and thus produce the same type of pharmacological response.

**homodynamy** \-dī′nəmē\ Similarity in structure and development of parts or organs arranged in series along the main axis of the body. Also *metameric homology, serial homology*.

**homoecious** \hōmē′shəs\ AUTECIOUS.

**homoeo-** \hō′mē·ə-\ *Brit.* HOMEO-.

**homoeopathy** *Brit.* HOMEOPATHY.

**homoeosis** *Brit.* HOMEOSIS.

**homoeostasis** *Brit.* HOMEOSTASIS.

**homoeotoxin** \hō′mē·ətäk′sin\ HOMEOTOXIN.

**homofermentative** \-fərmen′tətiv\ Carrying out homolactic fermentation. Also *homolactic*. Compare HETEROFERMENTATIVE.

**homogametic** \-gəmet′ik\ **1** Referring to or characterized by the production of the same kinds of gametes, usually in reference to the sex chromosome present. In humans, females are homogametic. **2** Referring to or characterized by the production of gametes that are of the same size or structure.

**homogamous** \hōmäg′əməs\ Having male and female sex organs functional at the same time. Compare DICHOGAMOUS.

**homogamy** \hōmäg′əmē\ A mating preference between organisms that share certain aspects of phenotype or are of similar genotype. It is a contributing factor to assortative mating. Compare HETEROGAMY.

**homogenate** \hōmäj′ənāt\ [HOMO- + -GEN + -ATE] Material that has been reduced to a uniform consistency by homogenization.

**homogeneity** \-jənē′itē\ The property of having all its parts the same. Of chemical substances it signifies purity, because all the molecules are identical.

**homogeneization** \-jē′nē·īzā′shən\ HOMOGENIZATION.

**homogeneous** \-jē′nē·əs\ Possessing homogeneity.

**homogenization** \hōmäj′ənīzā′shən\ The process whereby material is reduced to a uniform consistency. Also *homogeneization*.

**homogenize** \hōmäj′ənīz\ To reduce to uniform consistency or composition; to render homogeneous.

**homogenous** \hōmäj′ənəs\ [HOMO- + -GENOUS] Marked by similar form and structure resulting from common ancestry.

**homogentisic acid** (2,5-Dihydroxyphenyl)acetic acid. An intermediate in the catabolism of tyrosine, it appears in the urine in alkaptonuria, in which its oxidation to maleylacetoacetate is deficient. Also *alkapton* (obs.), *alcapton* (obs.), *glycosuric acid*.

**homogentisuria** \-jen′tisoo′rē·ə\ The presence of homogentisic acid in the urine.

**homoglandular** \-glan′dyələr\ Of or relating to the same gland. Estrogen and progesterone, for example, have a *homoglandular* source (the ovary) in the female mammal.

**homogonic** \-gän′ik\ [HOMO- + GON-[2] + -IC ] Characterizing an alternative cycle in which larvae develop directly into infective parasitic forms instead of developing into free-living adults. Alternative homogonic and heterogonic cycles are seen in rhabditoid nematode worms. See also *STRONGYLOIDES*.

**homograft** \hō′mōgraft\ [HOMO- + GRAFT] ALLOGRAFT. **isogeneic h.** ISOGRAFT.

**homoio-** \hō′moi·ə-\ HOMEO-.

**homoioplasia** \hō′moi·əplā′zhə\ HOMEOPLASIA.

**homoiopodal** \hō′moi·äp′ədəl\ Describing or relating to neurons which have branches of one type only.

**homoiosmotic** \hō′moi·äzmät′ik\ Describing an aquatic animal that maintains an internal concentration of body fluids unlike that of the environment.

**homoiostasis** \hō′moi·əstā′sis\ HOMEOSTASIS.

**homoiothermal** \hō′moi·əthur′məl\ HOMEOTHERMIC.

**homoiothermic** \hō′moi·əthur′mik\ HOMEOTHERMIC.

**homoiotoxin** \hō′moi·ətäk′sin\ HOMEOTOXIN.

**homokaryon** \-kar′ē·än\ A cell that contains two or more genetically identical nuclei in a common cytoplasm. Compare HETEROKARYON.

**homokeratoplasty** \-ker′ətōplas′tē\ [HOMO- + KERATOPLASTY] Surgical exchange of a cornea from one individual to another of the same species.

**homolactic** \-lak′tik\ HOMOFERMENTATIVE.

**homolateral** \-lat′ərəl\ IPSILATERAL.

**homologous** \hōmäl′əgəs\ [Gk *homologos* (from *homologein* to agree, from *homo-* same + *legein* to say) in agreement, corresponding] **1** Resembling in structure and origin. In biology, of organs or structures having the same evolutionary history but divergent adaptation, such as the skeleton in the forelimb of a land vertebrate and that in the wing of a bat. Compare ANALOGOUS. **2** Obtained from an animal of the same species but not from the same individual as that providing the other constituents of the experiment or study: said especially of serum, tissue, cells, etc., under immunologic study. Also *isologous*. Compare AUTOLOGOUS, HETEROLOGOUS.

**homologue** \häm′əläg\ **1** Any organ or structure similar in structure and origin to that in another organism or series of organisms. Compare ANALOGUE. **2** HOMOLOGOUS CHROMOSOME.

**homology** \hōmäl′əjē\ [Gk *homologia* (from *homologos* in agreement; see HOMOLOGOUS) agreement, conformity] Similarity in structure and evolutionary development of organs or structures either in one individual or in two or a series of organisms; the state of being homologous. Compare ANALOGY. **metameric h.** HOMODYNAMY. **serial h.** HOMODYNAMY.

**homolysis** \hōmäl′isis\ ISOHEMOLYSIS.

**homomorphic** \-môr′fik\ In cytogenetics, of or relating to the synapsis of two chromosomes that are similar in shape and size, and are usually homologues, during meiosis. Also *homomorphous*.

**homonomous** \hōmän′əməs\ [Gk *homonomos* (from HOMO- + *nomos* custom, law) under the same law] Belonging to a set of similar structures: used especially of those structures that occur in series, such as ribs and fingers.

**homonymous** \hōmän′əməs\ [Gk *homōnymos* (from HOMO- + *onyma* name) having the same name] **1** Corresponding to the same side, as an image on the left projected by the left eye; uncrossed. **2** Designating or of the nature of an interrelated sequence of a muscle's nerve and motor response, as a muscle's reflex response elicited upon stimulating the nerve to that muscle. Compare HETERONYMOUS.

**homophene** \häm′əfēn\ [HOMO- + *-phene* (from Gk *phaine(sthai)* to appear); formed on the analogy of *homophone* (a word that sounds the same as a different word)] One of two or more spoken words that are indistinguishable to the deaf lip-reader but that may sound different to a hearer and have different meanings.

**homopolymer** \-päl′imər\ A polymer which is composed of only one type of monomer.

**homorganic** \hō′môrgan′ik\ [*hom(o)-* + ORGANIC] **1** Arising from the same organ. **2** Stemming from homologous organs.

**homoserine** $HOCH_2—CH_2—CH(NH_3^+)—COO^-$. 2-Amino-4-hydroxybutyric acid. An intermediate in the biosynthesis of threonine from aspartate in those organisms (not including man) that can make threonine. Symbol: Hse

**homoserine lactone** The cyclic compound formed from homoserine by ester formation between its carboxyl and hydroxyl groups. This formation occurs spontaneously in acid. A residue of homoserine lactone is found at the C terminus of a peptide formed by scission of polypeptide chains at methionine by the action of cyanogen bromide.

**homosexual** \-sek′shoo·əl\ [HOMO- + SEXUAL] **1** Characterized by homosexuality. **2** A homosexual individual.

**homosexuality** \-sek′shoo·al′itē\ [HOMO- + SEXUALITY] Preferential sexual attraction to members of one's own sex. Also *sexual inversion* (obs.). **ego-dystonic h.** Homosexuality in which the sexual attraction is unwanted and a source of distress. In addition, the subject seeks to acquire or increase heterosexual responsivity so that heterosexual relations can be initiated or maintained and homosexual inclinations forsaken. **latent h.** Homosexuality that is not expressed in overt sexual activity or even, in some cases, fully recognized as such by the subject. **unconscious h.** An extreme form of latent homosexuality in which the subject is attracted to members of his own sex but is not aware of it.

**homostimulation** \-stim′yəlā′shən\ The stimulation of an organ by a material from the same organ or from a homologous organ.

**homothermal** \-thur′məl\ HOMEOTHERMIC.

**homothermic** \-thur′mik\ HOMEOTHERMIC.

**homotonic** \-tän′ik\ ISOTONIC.

**homotopic** \-täp′ik\ In or involving the same or corresponding sites or parts of the body.

**homotransplant** \-trans′plant\ ALLOGRAFT.

**homotransplantation** \-trans′plantā′shən\ ALLOTRANSPLANTATION.

**homotropism** \hōmät′rəpizm\ [HOMO- + TROPISM] The property of a cell which causes similar cells to move toward or away from it.

**homotype** \häm′ətīp\ **1** Any part or organ with the same structure and function as another, especially in reversed symmetry, such as the hand. **2** A representative of a population whose characters most nearly approach the mean for that population. Compare HETEROTYPE.

**homotypic** \-tip′ik\ Pertaining to or exhibiting the characteristics of a homotype. Also *homotypical.*

**homovanillic acid** 3-Methoxy-4-hydroxymandelic acid. A metabolite of dopa, dopamine, and norepinephrine, found in urine.

**homozygosis** \-zīgō′sis\ The generation of an offspring that is homozygous at one or more specific loci by union of gametes having identical alleles at those loci.

**homozygosity** \-zīgäs′əitē\ In genetics, a condition in which one or more specific loci are homozygous.

**homozygote** \-zī′gōt\ A nonhaploid cell or organism that has identical alleles at a given locus.

**homozygous** \-zī′gəs\ [Gk *homozyg(os)* (from HOMO- + *zygon* a yoke) yoked together, paired, corresponding + -OUS] Characterized by identical alleles at a given locus or loci: said of nonhaploid cells or organisms. Compare HETEROZYGOUS.

**honeycomb** RETICULUM.

**hood** **1** A covering used in laboratories to provide a protected space. **2** In soft or argasid ticks, the anterior extension of the dorsal, leathery or wrinkled integument that covers the ventrally positioned mouthparts. A ventral groove or camerostome in the hood encloses the mouthparts. **tooth h.** DENTAL OPERCULUM.

**hook** **1** A long, thin surgical instrument with a curved, sharpened end. It is often used for retraction or fixation of tissues. **2** A double curved terminal device for an upper-limb prosthesis. One part is opened by the amputee using a steel cable, allowing grasping when it is closed. **dural h.** A small, sharp, hooked instrument for picking up the dura mater. **fixation h.** A surgical instrument used to retract or immobilize tissues during an operation. **h. of hamate bone** HAMULUS OSSIS HAMATI. **muscle h.** A surgical instrument with a right angled tip that may be positioned beneath an extraocular muscle to isolate and identify its insertion, for use in strabismus surgery. Also *squint hook.* **posterior palate h.** PALATE RETRACTOR. **tracheostomy h.** An instrument used in tracheostomy to hook forward and steady the trachea prior to incising it. It has a straight handle approximately 14 cm long, terminating in a fine sharp hook. **Tyrrell's h.** A very small angulated metal rod for use in eye surgery.

**hooklet** \hʊk′lit\ A small, clawlike rostellar structure of tapeworms, especially of the larval forms. The hooklets are arranged in various patterns that characterize families and genera. The hexacanth cestode embryo uses its six hooklets to claw out of its membrane sheath and to penetrate the gut wall of the host. • The larger, more robust holdfast structures of adult *Taenia* tapeworms are usually termed hooks rather than hooklets.

**hook-up** **1** The circuit arrangement of electrical equipment, cables, and electrodes for diagnosis or therapy. **2** A connection to a source of electricity, water, oxygen, suction, etc.

**hookworm** Any of various bloodsucking worms of the family Ancylostomatidae, which are parasitic in the intestine of humans and other vertebrates. Medically and veterinarily important genera include *Ancylostoma, Necator*, and *Uncinaria.* **American h.** NEW WORLD HOOKWORM. **European h.** OLD WORLD HOOKWORM. **New World h.** A hookworm of the species *Necator Americanus..* Also *American hookworm.* **Old World h.** A hookworm of the species *Ancylostoma duodenale.* Also *European hookworm.*

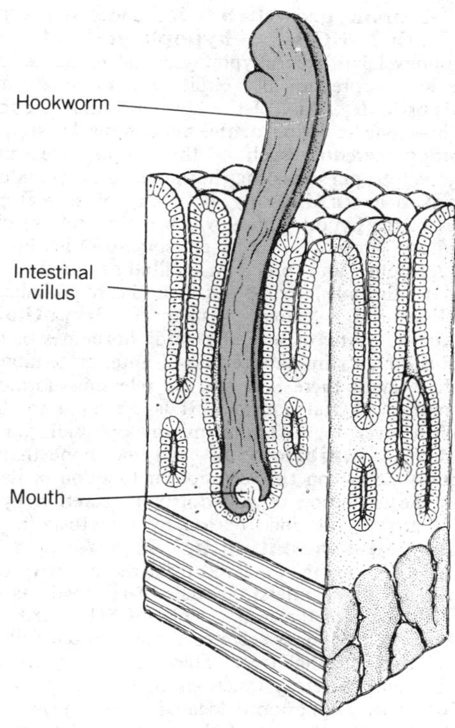


**Hookworm**

**Hoover** [Charles Franklin *Hoover,* U.S. physician, 1865–1927] **1** See under SIGN. **2** Grasset-Gaussel-Hoover sign. See under SIGN.

**Hoppe** [Hermann Henry *Hoppe,* U.S. neurologist, 1867–1929] Hoppe-Goldflam syndrome. See under MYASTHENIA GRAVIS.

**hora somni** At bedtime, used in prescription writing.

**hor. decub.** *hora decubitus* (L, at bedtime).

**hordenine** $C_{10}H_{15}NO$. 4-[2-(Dimethylamino)ethyl]phenol. A natural substance, present in malted barley, that is very similar to adrenaline in its pharmacologic activity. It is a sympathomimetic agent and it is used as a stimulant for the heart, a vasoconstrictor, and a bronchodilator.

**hordeolum** \hôrdē′ələm\ [New L, variant of Late L *hordeolus,* dim. of L *hordeum* barley, barleycorn] STYE.

**Horgan** [Edmund J. *Horgan,* U.S. surgeon, born 1884] Horgan's operation. See under TRANSANTRAL ETHMOIDECTOMY.

**hor. interm.** *horis intermediis* (L, in the intermediate hours).

**horizontalis** \hôr′īzäntā′lis\ Denoting a flat plane at right angles to a vertical plane, either the median or the coronal, with respect to the anatomical position of the body; horizontal.

**hormesis** \hôrmē′sis\ [Gk *hormēsis* (from *horm(an)* to set in motion + *-ēsis* -ESIS) rapid motion] The stimulating effect of small doses of any substance which in larger doses is inhibitory.

**hormonal** \hôr′mōnəl\ Of or relating to a hormone or hormones. Also *hormonic.*

# hormone

**hormone** \hôr′mōn\ [Gk *hormōn,* pres. part. of *horman* to set in motion, rouse, urge on] Any substance secreted by specialized cells in the endocrine glands or in clusters or diffusely spread through the brain, lungs, and gastrointestinal tract. These substances act upon specific target tissues more or less remote from the site of secretion or upon the regulation of metabolic processes throughout the organism. Also *internal secretion, incretion* (obs.). **adenohypophysial h.** A hormone secreted by the adenohypophysis (anterior pituitary), as growth hormone, prolactin, the gonadotropins, thyrotropin, adrenocorticotropin, or lipotropin. Also *anterior pituitary hormone.* **adipokinetic h.** *Older term* LIPOTROPIN. **adrenocortical h.** Any of several steroid hormones synthesized in and secreted by the adrenal cortex, suggested as comprising four classes. They are $C_{19}$ androgens, $C_{21}$ progestogens, $C_{21}$ corticosteroids, and perhaps $C_{18}$ estrogens. Also *cortical hormone.* **adrenocorticotropic h.** The adenohypophysial polypeptide hormone that regulates the structure and function of the adrenal cortex. A single chain of 39 amino acids, of 4567 daltons, it is controlled by the hypophysiotropic hormone, corticotropin-releasing hormone, and by the level of plasma cortisol, is secreted in a free-running circadian cycle, and is highly labile to external stimuli, increasing during stress. The hormone primarily stimulates the secretion of corticosteroids and androgens, having a lesser influence upon aldosterone. Adrenocorticotropic hormone is subnormally secreted in hypopituitarism and when corticosteroids are given medicinally, and excessively secreted in pituitary-dependent Cushing syndrome. As a pharmaceutical, most of its uses in inflammatory and allergic disease have been superseded by the introduction of the semisynthetic corticosteroids. Also *adrenocorticotropin, corticoptropin, corticotrophin, adrenocorticotrophin, adrenotropin, adrenotrophin, adrenotropic hormone* (seldom used), *acortan* (seldom used in the U.S.), *adrenotropic hormone, adrenocorticotropic peptide* (outmoded). Abbr. ACTH **androgenic h.** ANDROGEN. **anterior pituitary h.** ADENOHYPOPHYSIAL HORMONE. **antidiabetic h.** *Obs.* INSULIN. **antidiuretic h.** VASOPRESSIN. **Aschheim-Zondek h.** *Outmoded* LUTEINIZING HORMONE. **chondrotropic h.** *Outmoded* GROWTH HORMONE. **chorionic growth h.-prolactin** HUMAN PLACENTAL LACTOGEN. **chromaffin h.** *Older term* EPINEPHRINE. **chromatophorotropic h.** MELANOCYTE STIMULATING HORMONE. **circulatory h.** A hormonal substance that exerts its effects at a distant site via the bloodstream. This is in contrast to the products of enterochromaffin cells, which can only exert direct local effects on adjacent structures because they do not enter the circulatory system. **conjugated estrogen h.'s** CONJUGATED ESTROGENS. **corpus luteum h.** PROGESTERONE. **cortical h.** ADRENOCORTICAL HORMONE. **corticotropin releasing h.** A presumably peptide hormone of the hypothalamus that stimulates the release of adrenocorticotropin (ACTH) by adenohypophysial cells, whose own secretory rate is regulated by diurnal fluctuations in plasma cortisol values, plasma ACTH concentration, and stress. Also *corticoliberin.* Abbr. CRH **diabetogenic h.** A heterogenous substance identified in crude extracts of anterior pituitary tissue and found to induce hyperglycemia and act as an insulin antagonist. Most of the diabetogenic activity is probably due to growth hormone, some to adrenocorticotropin. **estrogenic h.** ESTROGEN. **fat-mobilizing h.** LIPOLYTIC HORMONE. **female h.** Estrogen or progesterone. *Popular.* **follicle stimulating h.** An anterior pituitary polypeptide hormone of 24 000–35 000 daltons, a sialic acid-containing gonadotropin which regulates the growth and maturation of the ovarian or graafian follicle and stimulates testicular spermatogenesis. For maximal effect on the male or female gonad this hormone requires also the presence of luteinizing hormone, the two hormones having a subunit in common. Pharmaceutical preparations from human pituitary extracts and postmenopausal urine are used in treatment of infertility in women. Also *gametogenic hormone* (seldom used), *gametokinetic hormone* (seldom used), *follicle-ripening hormone* (older term), *follicle stimulating principle* (older term), *thylakentrin* (older term). Abbr. FSH **follicle stimulating hormone releasing h.** A hypothalamic hormone specifically regulating the adenohypophysial release of follicle stimulating hormone (FSH). It is probably identical to gonadotropin releasing hormone which controls the release of both FSH and luteinizing hormone. Abbr. FSHRH **follicular h.** A hormone secreted by the ovarian or graafian follicle; estrogen. **galactopoietic h.** *Outmoded* PROLACTIN. **gametogenic h.** *Seldom used* FOLLICLE STIMULATING HORMONE. **gametokinetic h.** *Seldom used* FOLLICLE STIMULATING HORMONE. **gastrointestinal h.** Any of the hormones arising from specialized cells in the mucosa of the stomach and intestine and acting to control the motility and secretory activity of the gastrointestinal tract. The hormones include cholecystokinin, gastrin, secretin, vasoactive intestinal polypeptide, gastric inhibitory polypeptide, motilin, and bombesin. Also *gut hormone* (popular). **glycoprotein h.** Any polypeptide hormone containing sialic acid, as the anterior pituitary gonadotropins, thyrotopin, and chorionic gonadotropin. **gonadotropic h.** GONADOTROPIN. Abbr. GTH **gonadotropin releasing h.** A decapeptide, hypophysiotropic hormone which stimulates the release of follicle stimulating hormone (FSH) and luteinizing hormone from the anterior pituitary. It may also act on both gonadotropins, there being no separate releasing hormone for FSH. Also *luteinizing hormone releasing factor, luteinizing hormone releasing hormone, luliberin.* Abbr. GnRH **growth h.** **1** An adenohypophysial hormone that promotes and regulates somatic and skeletal growth and influences carbohydrate, fat, and protein metabolism. Human growth hormone is a polypeptide of about 21 500 daltons and containing 191 amino acids. It is secreted by specialized acidophil cells under the control of the hypothalamus, undergoing a periodic sleep-wake secretory cycle and responding briskly to many stimuli, being increased by stress and exercise, inhibited by obesity and glucocorticoids. Deprivation leads to dwarfism, excess to gigantism, acromegaly, and glucose intolerance. The pharmaceutical preparation from human or monkey but not other animal pituitary glands is used to treat human hypopituitary dwarfism. Also *somatotropin, somatotrophin, somatropin, chondrotropic hormone* (outmoded), *somatotropic hormone.* Abbr. GH **2** Any hormone that promotes growth. **growth hormone inhibiting h.** SOMATOSTATIN. Abbr. GHIH **growth hormone release inhibiting h.** SOMATOSTATIN. Abbr. GHRIH **growth hormone releasing h.** A hypothalamic releasing hormone which stimulates the secretion of growth hormone into the circulation by the adenohypophysis. Its chemical structure is not yet known. Also *somatotropin releasing hormone, somatotropin releasing factor.* Abbr. GHRH **gut h.** *Popular* GASTROINTESTINAL HORMONE. **human growth h.** See under GROWTH HORMONE. Abbr. HGH **hypophysial h.** Any adenohypophysial or neurohypophysial hormone, as growth hormone or vasopressin; any pituitary hormone. **hypophysiotropic h.** Any of the hormones that act to regulate the hormone secretion of the hypophysis by stimulating or inhibiting secretion, such as thyrotropin releasing hormone, gonadotropin releasing hormone, and somatostatin. **hypothalamic inhibitory h.** Any of several peptide hormones of the hypothalamus which inhibit release of anterior pituitary hormones, such as somatostatin (inhibiting growth hormone) and prolactin inhibitory hormone. It is conveyed to the adenohypophysis via the hypothalamic-hypophysial portal venous system. **hypothalamic releasing h.** Any of several peptide hormones of the hypothalamus which stimulate release of anterior pituitary hormones. In general there is a specific releasing hormone for each adenohypophysial hormone. It is conveyed to the adenohypophysis via the hypothalamic-hypophysial portal venous system. **inhibitory h.** Any hormone that exerts an inhibitory action on the secretion or function of its target tissue, as the inhibition of gonadotropin secretion by estrogen or of growth hormone release by somatostatin. **interstitial cell-stimulating h.** *Outmoded* LUTEINIZING HORMONE. • The name is derived from the property of stimulating the Leydig or interstitial cells of the testis as well as the corpus luteum of the ovary. Abbr. ICSH **intestinal h.** Any of the hormones secreted by specialized cells in the mucosa of the intestinal tract. They act mainly to regulate the motility and secretory functions of the gut itself. **intracellular h.** A hormone located or acting inside a cell. **juvenile h.** A secretion of the corpora allata and other tissues of insects, also found in certain plants. Acting in conjunction with ecdysone, juvenile hormones in insects ensure the normal preadult development. During the final nymphal or larval stage, the corpora allata are inactivated and ecdysone becomes dominant, leading to metamorphosis into the adult stage. Juvenile hormones are terpenoids, related esters of tridecadienoic acid. Also *neotenin.* **ketogenic h.** LIPOLYTIC HORMONE. **lactation h.** *Seldom used* PROLACTIN. **lactogenic h.** PROLACTIN. **lipolytic h.** Any hormone that stimulates the release of free fatty acids and glycerol from adipose tissue triglyceride by augmenting the formation of cyclic AMP which stimulates a protein kinase activating a hormone-sensitive lipase. These hormones include epinephrine, norepinephrine, adrenocorticotropin, glucagon, $\beta$-lipotropin, and arginine vasopressin. Growth hormone and cortisol stimulate delayed lipopysis. Also *ketogenic hormone, fat-mobilizing hormone.* **lipotropic h.** LIPOTROPIN. **luteal h.** PROGESTERONE. **luteinizing h.** An adenohypophysial gonadotropic hormone that stimulates ovulation, maintains progesterone secretion by the corpus luteum, and regulates secretion of testicular Leydig cells. It is a glycoprotein of 28 000 daltons, has an $\alpha$ unit in common with other glycopeptides, and a specific $\beta$ subunit. Under the control of hypothalamic gonadotropin releasing hormone, it undergoes the cyclic secretory variations of the menstrual cycle and more rapid diurnal oscillations. Also *interstitial cell-stimulating hormone* (outmoded), *Aschheim-Zondek hormone* (outmoded), *metakentrin* (older term), *luteinizing principle* (older term). Abbr. LH **luteinizing hormone releasing h.** GONADOTROPIN RELEASING HORMONE. Abbr. LHRH **luteotropic h.** PROLACTIN. **mammary stimulating h.** PROLACTIN. **mammogenic h.** PROLACTIN. **mammotropic h.** *Outmoded* PROLACTIN. **melanocyte stimulating h.** A specific pigmentary hormone secreted by the hypophysial intermediate lobe of lower forms, as amphibians, and stimulating the rearrangement of dermal melanin granules so as to produce darkening of the skin. In man, lacking a separate intermediate lobe, the adenohypophysis contains the $\beta$ form, a peptide of 2734 daltons and 22 amino acids which can also be radioimmunologically detected in plasma. $\beta$-melanocyte stimulating hormone in man is thought to be an extraction artifact of anterior pituitary $\beta$-lipotropin, not a distinct hormone. Also *melanophore stimulating hormone, chromatophorotropic hormone, intermedin, melanophore dilating principle.* Abbr. MSH **melanocyte stimulating hormone inhibitory h.** A hypothalamic hypophysiotropic hormone that inhibits the release of melanocyte stimulating hormone from the anterior pituitary. Such hormonal activity has been demonstrated but the hormone has not been identified chemically. Also *melanocyte stimulating hormone release inhibiting factor, intermediate lobe inhibiting factor.* **melanocyte stimulating hormone releasing h.** A hypothalamic releasing hormone which causes the release of melanocyte stimulating hormone from the anterior pituitary. Such hormonal activity has been demonstrated but the hormone has not been identified chemically. Also *melanocyte stimulating hormone regulatory hormone.* Abbr. MSHRH **melanophore stimulating h.** MELANOCYTE STIMULATING HORMONE. **morphogenetic h.** EVOCATOR. **morphogenic h.** A substance capable of bringing about changes in shape, form and structure of parts or the whole of a developing organism. Steroids exert a morphogenetic effect when they modify the course of development of the genital ducts and genitalia. **N. h.** Androgen, specifically adrenocortical androgen which stimulates nitrogen or nitrogen retention, as distinct from S. (sugar) hormone or glucocorticoid. An outmoded and seldom used term. Also *nitrogen hormone.* **orchidic h.** *Rare* TESTOSTERONE. **ovarian h.** A hormone secreted by the ovary; any estrogen or progestogen. **oxytocic h.** OXYTOCIN. **pancreatic hyperglycemic h.** *Obs.* GLUCAGON. **parathyroid h.** PARATHYRIN. **placental h.** Any hormone secreted or released by the placenta in pregnancy, including many estrogens, chorionic gonadotropin, and human placental lactogen. **placental growth h.** HUMAN PLACENTAL LACTOGEN. **posterior pituitary h.** Either of the hormones oxytocin and vasopressin, which come from the neurohypophysis (posterior part of the pituitary gland). **preproparathyroid h.** The initial hormonal substance synthesized in the cells of the parathyroid gland, the precursor of proparathyroid hormone and of parathyroid hormone. It contains 115 amino acids. **progestational h.** PROGESTERONE. **prolactin inhibitory h.** A hypothalamic hypophysiotropic hormone that inhibits the release of prolactin from the adenohypophysis. The principal component is dopamine. Abbr. PIH **prolactin releasing h.** A hypothalamic hypophysiotropic hormone that stimulates the release of prolactin from the anterior pituitary. It is a peptide but has not been identified chemically. Abbr. PRH **proparathyroid h.** An intermediate product in the biosynthesis of parathyroid hormone in the parathyroid gland. It contains 90 amino acids. **releasing h.** Any of the hormones that stimulate release of the pituitary hormones and thus regulate secretion; a hypophysiotropic hormone. Abbr. RH. **S. h.** *Older term* GLUCOCORTICOID. **sex h.** Any hormone affecting structure or function of a sexual organ or sexual behavior, especially testosterone and estrogen. **somatotropic h.** GROWTH HORMONE. **somatotropin releasing h.** GROWTH HORMONE RELEASING HORMONE. **steroid h.** A group of biologically and pharmaceutically important hormones secreted by the testis, ovary, adrenal cortex, and placenta, as the androgens, estrogens, glucocorticoids, and mineralocorticoid. **sympathetic h.** SYMPATHIN. **testicular h.** Any hormone secreted by the testis, specifically testosterone. Also *testis hormone.* **thyroid h.** Any of the active hormonal principles secreted by the thyroid gland, comprising thyroxine, triiodothyronine, and thyrocalcitonin. • In ordinary use the term refers to thyroxine or to thyroxine and triiodothyronine **thyroid stimulating h.** THYROTROPIC HORMONE. Abbr. TSH **thyrotropic h.** The adenohypophysial glycopeptide that regulates the growth, development, and secretory activity of the thyroid gland. It is a polypeptide having a molecular mass of about 28 000 daltons. It contains an $\alpha$ subunit structurally almost identical with those of follicle stimulating hormone, luteinizing hormone, and chorionic gonadotropin, and a specific $\beta$ subunit. The hormone stimulates many metabolic processes in the thyroid, including release of thyroxine and triiodothyronine from the thyroid follicles. Excessive thyrotropic hormone produces thyroid hyperplasia. The hormone is chiefly regulated by hypothalamic thyrotropin releasing hormone. Also *thyrotropin, thyrotrophin, thyroid stimulating hormone.* • *TSH* (from *thyroid stimulating hormone*) is often used as the abbreviation for *thyrotropic hormone,* since *TH* could be taken to refer to thyroid hormone. **thyrotropin releasing h.** The hypothalamic hypophysiotropic hormone that regulates the secretion of thyrotropic hormone. Its chemical structure is that of a tripeptide amide, 5-oxoprolylhistidyl prolineamide. Also *thyroid stimulating hormone releasing factor.* Abbr. TRH **tropic h.'s** Hormones that stimulate or regulate the function of other endocrine glands. Examples include the gonadotropic, thyrotropic, and adrenocorticotrophic hormones of the anterior pituitary. Also *trophic hormones* (older term).

**hormonic** \hôrmän′ik\ HORMONAL.

**hormonogenesis** \hôr′mənōjen′əsis\ [*hormon(e)* + *o* + GENESIS] The synthesis, production, or elaboration of a hormone or hormones. Also *hormonopoiesis.*

**hormonotherapy** \hôr′mənōther′əpē\ Treatment by the administration of hormones. Also *endocrinotherapy, incretotherapy* (outmoded).

**horn** [Middle English, from Old English, akin to L *cornu* horn] CORNU. **h. of Ammon** HIPPOCAMPUS. **anterior h. of lateral ventricle** CORNU ANTERIUS VENTRICULI LATERALIS. **anterior h. of spinal cord** CORNU ANTERIUS MEDULLAE SPINALIS. **coccygeal h.** CORNU COCCYGEUM. **cutaneous h.** A benign warty excrescence of the skin that may develop on a solar keratosis or other epidermal lesion. Also *warty horn, cornu cutaneum.* **dorsal h. of spinal cord** CORNU DORSALE MEDULLAE SPINALIS. **frontal h. of lateral ventricle** CORNU ANTERIUS VENTRICULI LATERALIS. **greater h. of hyoid bone** CORNU MAJUS OSSIS HYOIDEI. **iliac h.** A pointed bony projection arising from the back of the leaf of the iliac bones that is seen in the nail-patella syndrome. **inferior h. of cerebrum** CORNU INFERIUS VENTRICULI LATERALIS. **inferior h. of falciform margin** CORNU INFERIUS MARGINIS FALCIFORMIS. **inferior h. of lateral ventricle** CORNU INFERIUS VENTRICULI LATERALIS. **inferior h. of saphenous opening** CORNU INFERIUS MARGINIS FALCIFORMIS. **inferior h. of thyroid cartilage** CORNU INFERIUS CARTILAGINIS THYROIDEAE. **lateral h. of coccyx** Either of two transverse projections from the base of the coccyx. They represent rudimentary transverse processes of the first coccygeal vertebra and may articulate or fuse with the inferior lateral angle of the sacrum. **lateral gray h. of spinal cord** CORNU LATERALE MEDULLAE SPINALIS. **lateral h. of**

**spinal cord** CORNU LATERALE MEDULLAE SPINALIS. **lateral h. of uterus** 1 CORNU UTERI (DEXTRUM/SINISTRUM). 2 Either horn of a uterus bicornis. **lesser h. of hyoid bone** CORNU MINUS OSSIS HYOIDEI. **motor h.** CORNU ANTERIUS MEDULLAE SPINALIS. **posterior h. of lateral ventricle** CORNU POSTERIUS VENTRICULI LATERALIS. **posterior h. of spinal cord** CORNU DORSALE MEDULLAE SPINALIS. **pulp h.** A diverticulum of the pulp chamber beneath a cusp or mamelon of a tooth. **sacral h.** CORNU SACRALE. **sebaceous h.** A horny outgrowth from a sebaceous cyst. **superior h. of falciform margin** CORNU SUPERIUS MARGINIS FALCIFORMIS. **superior h. of hyoid bone** *Outmoded* CORNU MINUS OSSIS HYOIDEI. **superior h. of saphenous opening** CORNU SUPERIUS MARGINIS FALCIFORMIS. **superior h. of thymus** The conical proximal extremity of each of the two lobes of the thymus. **superior h. of thyroid cartilage** CORNU SUPERIUS CARTILAGINIS THYROIDEAE. **temporal h. of lateral ventricle** CORNU INFERIUS VENTRICULI LATERALIS. **uterine h.** CORNU UTERI (DEXTRUM/SINISTRUM). **ventral h. of spinal cord** CORNU ANTERIUS MEDULLAE SPINALIS. **warty h.** CUTANEOUS HORN.

**Horner** [Johann Friedrich *Horner*, Swiss ophthalmologist, 1831–1886] 1 See under PUPIL. 2 Claude Bernard-Horner syndrome, Bernard-Horner syndrome, Horner-Bernard syndrome. See under HORNER SYNDROME.

**Horner** [William Edmonds *Horner*, U.S. anatomist, 1793–1853] Horner's muscle. See under PARS LACRIMALIS MUSCULI ORBICULARIS OCULI.

**hornification** \hôr′nifikā′shən\ KERATINIZATION.

**hornskin** \hôrn′skin\ Thickening of the skin keratin in response to abnormal pressures or stresses.

**horny** \hôr′nē\ Resembling horn, especially in having a hard, rigid consistency. Also *keratic, corneous.*

**horopter** \hôräp′tər\ [Gk *hor(os)* a boundary + *optēr* one who looks or spies] The projection of corresponding retinal points into visual space; a concept of importance in explaining the perception of distance. Adj. horopteric. **Vieth-Müller h.** A conceptual spherical surface in space defined as the locus of spatial projection from the corresponding retinal points of the two eyes.

**horripilation** \hôr′ipilā′shən\ PILOERECTION.

**horror** [L, shuddering, dread, horror] 1 Intense fear and revulsion. 2 Intolerance (of), resistance (to): used primarily in Latin phrases. **h. autotoxicus** SELF-TOLERANCE. **h. fusionis** A pathologic change in binocular vision in which simultaneous macular alignment by the two eyes is impossible.

**horsefly** A large-bodied avidly bloodsucking fly of the genus *Tabanus* or other genus of the family Tabanidae. Also *horse fly.*

**horseshoe** An orthopedic surgical device that acts as a suspending support following the placement of Steinmann's pins or threaded wires.

**Horsfall** [Frank L. *Horsfall,* Jr., U.S. physician, 1906–1971] Tamm-Horsfall mucoprotein. See under MUCOPROTEIN.

**Horsley** [Sir Victor Alexander Haden *Horsley,* English surgeon and physiologist, 1857–1916] Horsley's bone wax. See under PUTTY.

**Hortega** [Pío del Río *Hortega,* Spanish-born anatomist active in Argentina, 1882–1945] 1 See under TUMOR, METHOD. 2 Hortega cells. See under MICROGLIA.

**hortobezoar** \hôr′təbēzôr′\ [L *hort(us)* vegetable garden + BEZOAR] PHYTOBEZOAR.

**Horton** [Bayard Taylor *Horton,* U.S. physician, born 1895] 1 Horton's vascular headache. See under MIGRAINOUS NEURALGIA. 2 Horton's arteritis. See under TEMPORAL ARTERITIS.

**hortungskörper** \hôr′tʊngskœr′pər\ [German *Hortung* accumulation + *Körper* body] Senile amyloid or other material found upon pathologic examinations of body organs in aged individuals.

**hor. un. spatio** *horae unius spatio* (L, at the end of one hour).

**hospice** \häs′pis\ [L *hospitium* a chamber for guests, lodging, hospitality. Compare HOSPITAL.] 1 A program or facility which provides palliative and supportive care for terminally ill patients and their families. 2 Originally, a shelter or short-term care facility for homeless or destitute people.

**hospital** [Old French (from L *hospitalis* pertaining to the accommodation of guests, from *hospes,* gen. *hospitis* a guest) a hostel, hospice] An institution equipped with inpatient facilities for the 24-hour care, diagnosis, and treatment of the sick and injured, usually for both medical and surgical conditions, and staffed with professionally trained medical practitioners. **closed h.** A hospital whose medical staff membership is not open to all physicians in the community. **field h.** A military hospital located in an area of troop activity such as a battle zone. **for-profit h.** See under PROPRIETARY HOSPITAL. **geriatric day h.** A facility attended by old people which provides some of the functions of a hospital but which does not provide overnight or weekend accommodation. • A term used in the United Kingdom, Australia, and New Zealand. Similar services exist in the United States, but are usually called simply "day care for the elderly." **government h.** A hospital that is owned, operated, and funded by a governmental authority. **maternity h.** A hospital that primarily provides obstetrical services. Also *lying-in hospital.* **mental h.** An inpatient facility for the care of patients with psychiatric disorders or developmental disabilities, or both. • Before the development of somatic treatments such as insulin coma and electroconvulsive treatment in the 1930s and neuroleptics, lithium, antidepressants, and other psychopharmacologic agents in the 1950s, mental hospitals were generally institutions for long-term care and protection. At the present time, most are oriented toward short-term, intensive treatment of acute episodes, in addition to longer-term custodial care for refractory patients who continue to be dangerous to themselves or others. **mobile army surgical h.** An easily transportable, usually temporary, hospital designed for use in military battlefield situations to treat injured soldiers. Abbr. MASH **open h.** A hospital whose medical staff membership is open to any physician in the community subject to meeting specified training and experience criteria. **private h.** A hospital that serves only private patients, thus excluding patients who do not have their own private physician and source of funding. **proprietary h.** A hospital owned by individuals or a corporation and operated for profit. A term used chiefly in the United States. • In the United Kingdom, India, and New Zealand, such a hospital is called a private hospital operated for profit. In the U.S., *for-profit hospital* is sometimes used as a variant of *proprietary hospital.* **psychogeriatric h.** A hospital designed to treat and care for people suffering from mental illnesses associated with old age. A term not used in the U.S. **public h.** An inpatient facility for medical and surgical care, in the United States usually short-term care, owned or operated by a governmental authority. **teaching h.** Any hospital that operates one or more teaching programs for medical, dental, or osteopathic students, interns, or residents. **voluntary h.** A nongovernmental, nonprofit hospital.

**hospitalism** \häs′pitəlizm′\ Anaclitic depression in infants associated with prolonged institutionalization, as in a hospital.

**hospitalization** \häs′pitəlīzā′shən\ The admission or stay of a patient in a hospital.

**host** [Old French *(h)oste,* from L *hospes,* gen. *hospitis* a host or guest; biological sense originated in German as *Wirt(h),* lit., a host, innkeeper] 1 An organism that harbors or provides nourishment, a habitat, or transport to another organism, whether symbiont, commensal, or parasite. 2 The recipient of any transplant from another organism. **accidental h.** A host not normally associated with a particular parasite. Also *incidental host.* **alternate h.** A facultative intermediate host. **biological intermediate h.** An intermediate host in which biologic or cyclic development takes place. Also *cyclic intermediate host.* Compare MECHANICAL INTERMEDIATE HOST. **dead-end h.** A human host infected by a parasite that is unable to complete its life cycle unless the human is consumed by another host in the transmission chain. Examples would be a human infected with *Trichinella, Echinococcus,* or tissue cysts of *Sarcocystis.* **definitive h.** The host in which a parasite or symbiont reaches adulthood, completes its development, or becomes sexually mature. Also *final host, primary host* (incorrect). **final h.** DEFINITIVE HOST. **incidental h.** ACCIDENTAL HOST. **intermediate h.** A host in which the symbiont or parasite undergoes larval or developmental stages or asexual multiplication. Also *intermediary host.* **maintenance h.** RESERVOIR HOST. **mechanical intermediate h.** An intermediate host in which the parasite or symbiont does not undergo development or reproduction, and transmission is by mechanical means. Tabanid flies, for example, can transmit many species of trypanosomes by direct inoculation from one host to another, with no intervening development. Compare BIOLOGICAL INTERMEDIATE HOST. **overwintering h.** An intermediate host or vector or a final host in which a parasite survives over the winter and can be transmitted to a new host the following spring. **paratenic h.** TRANSPORT HOST. **h. of predilection** The preferred or normal host of a parasite. **primary h.** 1 The first intermediate host, such as the snail host of digentic trematodes. 2 *Incorrect* DEFINITIVE HOST. **reservoir h.** A facultative host that serves as a reservoir of infection. See under RESERVOIR. Also *maintenance host, secondary host* (ambiguous), *reservoir.* **secondary h.** 1 A second intermediate host. 2 A host of secondary importance. 3 *Ambiguous* RESERVOIR HOST. **transfer h.** TRANSPORT HOST. **transport h.** An intermediate host in which maturation or cyclic development does not occur, but which carries the parasite to another host in which it does occur. It may be one of a succession of transport hosts, as exemplified in the second intermediate hosts of pseudophyllidean cestodes such as *Diphyllobothrium latum..* Also *paratenic host, transfer host.* See also PHORESIS.

**HOT** human old tuberculin.

**hot-box** An appliance usually of metal or wood designed to enclose a limb or the entire body excluding the head and equipped with an electrical system to produce dry heat. Temperatures for local treatment are 60–70°C. and for general heat treatment, 50–70°C. Also *hot air box, heat cabinet.*

**hot line** A telephone counseling service for people in crisis situations. A service will specialize in a particular condition, as in suicide or child abuse.

**house** / **halfway h.** Any facility that provides care designed to facilitate the transition between inpatient institutional care, such as for mental health, and outpatient community-based care. Also *interim accommodation center.* ● The term is used chiefly in the U.S., Canada, and New Zealand. It is known but less commonly used in the United Kingdom and Australia.

**housefly** A fly of the species *Musca domestica* (common housefly), or *Fannia canicularis* (lesser housefly). Also *house fly.*

**Houssay** [Bernardo Alberto *Houssay,* Argentinian physiologist, 1887–1971] 1 See under PHENOMENON. 2 Houssay-Biasotti syndrome. See under SYNDROME.

**Houston** [John *Houston,* Irish physician, 1802–1845] 1 Houston's valves. See under PLICAE TRANSVERSALES RECTI. 2 See under MUSCLE.

**Hovius** [Jacob *Hovius,* Dutch anatomist, 1710–1786] 1 See under PLEXUS. 2 Hovius membrane. See under COMPLEXUS BASALIS CHOROIDEAE. 3 Circulus venosus hovii. See under CIRCLE OF HOVIUS.

**Howard** [Benjamin Douglas *Howard,* U.S. physician, 1840–1900] See under METHOD.

**Howard** [John Eager *Howard,* U.S. physician, born 1902] Ellsworth-Howard test. See under HOWARD TEST.

**Howe** [Percy *Howe,* U.S. dentist, 1864–1950] Howe's silver nitrate. See under AMMONIACAL SILVER NITRATE SOLUTION.

**Howell** [William Henry *Howell,* U.S. physiologist, 1860–1945] Howell's bodies. See under HOWELL-JOLLY BODIES.

**Howship** [John *Howship,* English anatomist, 1781–1841] 1 Romberg-Howship symptom. See under SYMPTOM. 2 See under LACUNA.

**Hoyer** [Heinrich F. *Hoyer,* Polish anatomist and histologist, 1834–1907] Sucquet-Hoyer anastomosis. See under SUCQUET-HOYER CANAL.

**HP** House Physician.

**Hp** haptoglobin.

**HPFH** hereditary persistence of high fetal hemoglobin.

**HPI** history of present illness.

**HPL** human placental lactogen.

**HPLC** high-pressure liquid chromatography.

**HRA** 1 health risk appraisal. 2 Human Resources Administration.

**h.s.** *hora somni* (L, at bedtime).

**HSA** human serum albumin.

**5-HT** 5-hydroxytryptamine (serotonin).

**Ht** total hyperopia.

**HTLV** human T cell leukemia/lymphoma virus; human T cell lymphotrophic virus; human T cell leukemia virus; human lymphotrophic retrovirus

**Hubbard** [Leroy Watkins *Hubbard,* U.S. orthopedic surgeon, 1857–1938] See under TANK.

**Huber** [Johann Jacob *Huber,* Swiss anatomist, 1707–1778] See under GANGLION.

**hucklebone** \huk′əlbōn\ TALUS.

**Hudson** [Arthur Cyril *Hudson,* English ophthalmologist,1875–1962] Hudson's line. See under HUDSON-STÄHLI LINE.

**Hueck** [Alexander Friedrich *Hueck,* German anatomist, 1802–1842] Hueck's ligament. See under LIGAMENTUM PECTINATUM ANGULI IRIDOCORNEALIS.

**Huët** [G. J. *Huët,* Dutch physician, born 1879] Pelger-Huët nuclear anomaly. See under PELGER-HUËT ANOMALY.

**Hueter** [Karl *Hueter,* German surgeon, 1838–1882] See under SIGN, LINE.

**Hughes** [Charles Hamilton *Hughes,* U.S. neurologist, 1839–1916] See under REFLEX.

**Huguier** [Pierre Charles *Huguier,* French surgeon, 1804–1874] 1 Huguier's canal. See under ITER CHORDAE ANTERIUS. 2 See under CIRCLE, SINUS.

**Huhner** [Max *Huhner,* U.S. urologist, 1873–1947] See under TEST.

**hum** A dull, continuous sound, usually of unvarying tone. **venous h.** A continuous murmur heard to the right of the sternum and over the right jugular vein, especially in children. It may also be heard sometimes in adults, especially those who are anemic or pregnant. It is abolished by compression on the jugular vein or on assuming a recumbent posture. Also *humming-top murmur.*

**Human Tissue Act** See under UNIFORM ANATOMICAL GIFT ACT.

**humectant** **1** An agent that brings about a moistening effect. **2** Moist or damp.

**humectation** The process or act of moistening.

**humeral** \hyoo′mərəl\ Pertaining to the humerus.

**humeri** \hyoo′mərī\ Plural of HUMERUS.

**humerus** \hyoo′mərəs\ [L (akin to Gk *ōmos* the shoulder with upper arm), the shoulder of man and animal] [NA] The long bone of the arm, presenting an upper extremity carrying a rounded head for articulation with the scapula, a shaft, and a lower extremity with a condyle adapted to articulate with the radius and the ulna. **h. varus** An abnormally angulated humerus that curves toward the midline.

**humidifier** \hyoomid′ifī′ər\ A device that increases the moisture content of the air. Its use may be to increase the general ambient humidity or localized to a small area for purposes of breathing supersaturated air.

**humor** \hyoo′mər\ [Med L (from L, orig. *umor* dampness, moisture, a liquid), humor of the body] **1** Any of the four elemental body fluids believed by the ancients to be the physiologic and pathologic basis of health and disease. The humors are blood, phlegm, yellow bile, and black bile. **2** Any of various body fluids, especially the aqueous and vitreous humors of the eye. **aqueous h.** HUMOR AQUOSUS. **h. aquosus** [NA] A nutritive watery fluid that is formed by the ciliary processes and diffuses through the posterior and anterior chambers of the eye. It is reabsorbed into the venous system by filtering through the spaces of the iridocorneal angle into the sinus venosus sclerae, which communicates with the anterior ciliary veins. Besides serving as a refractive medium, it maintains the intraocular pressure and provides glucose, amino acids, and ascorbic acid to the avascular lens and cornea. Also *aqueous humor, aqueous, hydatoid, aqua oculi, intraocular fluid.* **crystalline h.** *Outmoded* LENS. **ocular h.** Either humor aquosus or humor vitreus. **vitreous h.** HUMOR VITREUS. **h. vitreus** [NA] The structureless gel within the loose network of collagen fibrils of the vitreous body of the eyeball. It is often equated with corpus vitreum. Also *vitreous humor, vitreous.*

**humoral** \hyoo′mərəl\ Pertaining to the humors, or certain fluids, of the body.

**humoralism** \hyoo′mərəlizm′\ The ancient doctrine that elemental body fluids (humors: blood, phlegm, yellow bile, and black bile) are the physiologic and pathologic basis of health and disease. Also *humorism, fluidism, humoral theory.*

**hump** / **buffalo h.** A nuchal and upper dorsal prominence seen in subjects with severe spontaneous or iatrogenic Cushing syndrome, caused by deposition of fat and upper dorsal kyphosis. Also *buffalo neck.*

**humpback** KYPHOSIS.

**Humphry** [George Murray *Humphry,* English surgeon, 1820–1896] Humphry's ligament. See under LIGAMENTUM MENISCOFEMORALE ANTERIUS.

**hunchback** KYPHOSIS.

**hunchbacked** KYPHOTIC.

**Hünermann** [Carl *Hünermann,* German physician, flourished mid-20th century] Hünermann's disease, Conradi-Hünermann syndrome. See under CHONDRODYSPLASIA PUNCTATA.

**Hung** [See-Lu *Hung,* U.S. scientist, flourished 20th century] Hung's method. See under FÜLLEBORN'S METHOD.

**hunger** [Old English *hungor*] A craving, usually for food. **affect h.** Insatiable demand for attention and affection, which may take the form of provocative antisocial behavior. It occurs in children who have suffered emotional deprivation. **air h.** KUSSMAUL RESPIRATION.

**Hunner** [Guy Leroy *Hunner,* U.S. surgeon, 1868–1957] Fenwick-Hunner ulcer. See under HUNNER'S ULCER.

**Hunt** [James Ramsay *Hunt,* U.S. neurologist, 1872–1937] **1** Hunt syndrome. See under RAMSAY HUNT SYNDROME. **2** Hunt striatal syndrome, Hunt's disease, Ramsey Hunt paralysis. See under JUVENILE PARALYSIS AGITANS. **3** Hunt's disease. See under DYSSYNERGIA CEREBELLARIS MYOCLONICA. **4** Hunt's paradoxical phenomenon. See under PHENOMENON.

**Hunt** [Reed *Hunt,* U.S. pharmacologist, 1870–1948] See under METHOD.

**Hunt** [William Edward *Hunt,* U.S. neurosurgeon, born 1921] Tolosa-Hunt syndrome. See under SYNDROME.

**Hunter** [Charles *Hunter,* Canadian physician, flourished 20th century] Hunter syndrome. See under MUCOPOLYSACCHARIDOSIS II.

**Hunter** [John *Hunter,* Scottish surgeon, 1728–1793] Hunter's canal. See under CANALIS ADDUCTORIUS.

**Hunter** [William *Hunter,* English botanist active in India, 1755–1812] See under GLOSSITIS.

**Hunter** [William *Hunter,* English anatomist, 1718–1783] **1** Bands of Hunter-Schreger. See under SCHREGER'S LINES. **2** Hunter's line. See under LINEA ALBA. **3** Hunter's ligament. See under LIGAMENTUM TERES UTERI.

**Huntington** [George *Huntington,* U.S. physician, 1850–1916] **1** See under SIGN. **2** Huntington's chorea. See under DISEASE.

**Hurler** [Gertrud *Hurler,* Austrian pediatrician, flourished early 20th century] **1** Hurler syndrome. See under MUCOPOLYSACCHARIDOSIS IH. **2** Hurler-Scheie syndrome. See under MUCOPOLYSACCHARIDOSIS IH/S. **3** Pseudo-Hurler's disease, pseudo-Hurler polydystrophy. See under MUCOLIPIDOSIS III. **4** Hurler-Scheie compound. See under COMPOUND.

**Hurst** [Edward Weston *Hurst,* English physician active in Australia, flourished 20th century] Hurst's disease. See under ACUTE HEMORRHAGIC LEUKOENCEPHALITIS.

**Hürthle** [Karl *Hürthle,* German histologist, 1860–1945] **1** See under CARCINOMA, TUMOR. **2** Hürthle cell adenoma. See under ONCOCYTIC ADENOMA.

**Huschke** [Emil *Huschke,* German anatomist, 1797–1858] **1** Auditory teeth of Huschke. See under DENTES ACUSTICI. **2** Vomerian cartilage of Huschke. See under CARTILAGO VOMERONASALIS. **3** See under CANAL. **4** Gastropancreatic folds of Huschke. See under FOLD. **5** Huschke's valve. See under PLICA LACRIMALIS. **6** Stria vascularis of Huschke. See under STRIA VASCULARIS DUCTUS COCHLEARIS.

**Hutchinson** [Sir Jonathan *Hutchinson,* English surgeon, 1828–1913] **1** Hutchinson's patch. See under SALMON PATCH. **2** Hutchinson's malignant lentigo. See under FRECKLE. **3** Hutchinson's mask. See under TABETIC MASK. **4** See under FACIES, NOTCH, PRURIGO, SIGN. **5** Hutchinson's tooth, hutchinsonian tooth, Hutchinson's incisors. See under SYPHILITIC TOOTH. **6** Hutchinson-Gilford syndrome. See under PROGERIA. **7** Hutchinson's disease. See under HUTCHINSON SUMMER PRURIGO. **8** Hutchinson syndrome. See under TRIAD. **9** Hutchinson-Boeck syndrome, Hutchinson-Boeck disease. See under SARCOIDOSIS.

**Huxley** [Thomas Henry *Huxley,* English biologist, 1825–1895] Huxley's membrane, Huxley sheath. See under LAYER.

**Huygens** [Christiaan *Huygens,* Dutch physicist, 1629–1695] **1** See under PRINCIPLE. **2** Huygen's ocular. See under HUYGENIAN EYEPIECE.

**HV** **1** hyperventilation. **2** herpes virus.

**HVL** half-value layer.

**hyal** \hī′əl\ HYOID.

**hyal-** \hī′əl-\ HYALO-.

**hyalin** \hī′əlin\ [Gk *hyal(os)* or *hyel(os),* a clear, transparent stone, oriental alabaster, crystal, glass + -IN] A clear homogeneous tissue formed as an eosinophilic product of amyloid degeneration. **hematogenous h.** The glassy, translucent material formed following platelet aggregation. *Older term.*

**hyaline** \hī′əlīn\ [Gk *hyalinos* made of crystal or glass] Nearly transparent, glasslike in appearance. Also *hyaloid.*

**hyalinization** \hī′əlin′īzā′shən\ The process by which a tissue or structure becomes dense, homogeneous, and glassy. It is usually associated with atrophy of cellular elements. Also *hyalinosis.* **tympanic h.** TYMPANOSCLEROSIS.

**hyalinosis** \hī′əlinō′sis\ [HYALIN + -OSIS] HYALINIZATION. **h. cutis** LIPOID PROTEINOSIS. **tympanic h.** TYMPANOSCLEROSIS.

**hyalitis** \hī′əlī′tis\ [HYAL- + -ITIS] Inflammation within the vitreous humor. Also *hyaloiditis.* **asteroid h.** ASTEROID HYALOSIS. **h. punctata** PUNCTATE HYALOSIS. **h. suppurativa** Purulent inflammation of the vitreous humor.

**hyalo-** \hī′əlō-\ [Gk *hyalos* glass] A combining form meaning (1) glassy, hyaline; (2)hyalin; (3) vitreous body or humor. Also *hyal-.*

**hyaloid** \hī′əloid\ [Gk *hyaloeidēs* glasslike, from *hyalo(s)* crystal, glass + *-eidēs* -like, -OID] **1** HYALINE. **2** Pertaining to the vitreous body or humor.

**hyaloiditis** \hī′əloidī′tis\ HYALITIS.

**hyaloidopathy** \hī′əloidäp′əthē\ [HYALOID + *o* + -PATHY] Any disease or deterioration of the vitreous humor. **asteroid h.** ASTEROID HYALOSIS.

**hyalomere** \hī′əlōmir′\ The granule-free, pale, clear peripheral zone of platelet cytoplasm. Compare GRANULOMERE.

***Hyalomma*** \hī′əläm′ə\ A genus of large, extremely hardy ixodid ticks of Asia and Africa, characterized by submarginal eyes, lack of body ornamentation, a long rostrum, and coalesced festoons. Life cycles are variable, with one, two, or three hosts, sometimes even variable within the same species. Members of this genus transmit many microorganisms pathogenic in humans and other animals, and they can also cause significant mechanical damage to hosts. Boutonneuse and Crimean hemorrhagic fever are among the diseases transmitted to humans by these ticks.

**hyalomucoid** HYALURONIC ACID.

**hyalonyxis** \hī′əlōnik′sis\ [HYALO- + Gk *nyxis* a pricking, piercing, stabbing] Incision of the vitreous body.

**hyaloplasm** \hī′əlōplazm′\ [HYALO- + -PLASM] The clear fluid portion of the protoplasm generally supported by the cytoreticulum. Also *cytohyaloplasm, cytolymph, cytosol, enchylema, endochylema, cell sap, interfilar substance.* **nuclear h.** KARYOLYMPH.

**hyaloserositis** \hī′əlōsir′ōsī′tis\ [HYALO- + SEROSITIS] **1** Inflammation of a serous membrane resulting in hyalinization. **2** Hyalinization and fibrosis of the capsule of an organ such as the spleen or liver. An obsolete usage. **progressive multiple h.** Progressive inflammation of the serous membranes, including the pericardium, pleura, and peritoneum, in which a fibrinous exudate gradually hyalinizes so that the inflamed areas acquire a thick, opaque, shiny, white or off-white coating.

**hyalosis** \hī′əlō′sis\ [HYAL- + -OSIS] Degenerative change of the vitreous body. **asteroid h.** The presence of numerous tiny white spheres composed of calcium soaps deposited upon the collagen framework of the vitreous humor as a result of a benign degenerative change. It is unassociated with systemic disease. Also *asteroid hyalitis, asteroid hyaloidopathy, Benson's disease.* **punctate h.** A condition of the vitreous humor in which multiple localized opacities exist. Also *hyalitis punctata.*

**hyaluronate lyase** The enzyme (EC 4.2.2.1) that catalyzes the breakdown of hyaluronic acid by an elimination reaction in which the *N*-acetylglucosamine residue is liberated as a new reducing end by cleavage of the oxygen it glycosylates from a glucuronate residue with the introduction of a double bond between C-4 and C-5 of the latter.

**hyaluronic acid** A major polysaccharide of connective tissue, consisting of alternate residues of D-glucuronic acid (glycosylated on O-4) and of *N*-acetylglucosamine (glycosylated on O-3). Also *hyalomucoid.*

**hyaluronidase** \hī′əlooran′idās\ An enzyme, produced by some strains of streptococci, that hydrolyzes hyaluronic acid. This reaction, in the ground substance of connective tissue, may promote spread of the microorganisms. Its presence in pathologic amounts in the joint fluid results in a reduced viscosity of the joint fluid. Also *spreading factor, Duran-Reynals factor, Reynals factor.* **h. for injection** A sterile enzyme powder derived from mammalian testes that is used to promote enzymatic hydrolysis of mucopolysaccharides and thus facilitate the rate of absorption of medical agents that are administered parenterally. It is suitable for either subcutaneous or intramuscular injection.

**hybaroxia** \hī′bəräk′sē·ə\ HYPERBARIC OXYGEN THERAPY.

**hybrid** \hī′brid\ [L *hybrida* or *hibrida* a cross-bred animal or person] **1** Any offspring of two parents with different genotypes. In this sense, all humans are hybrids. **2** An organism produced by the union of two parents of different species. Also *crossbreed.* **3** In experimental genetics, a cell formed by the fusion of two genetically distinct cells. **4** In molecular biology, a duplex nucleic acid formed *in vitro* between complementary DNA and RNA chains or DNA chains. **5** In population genetics, a group of organisms that results from the mating of genetically distinct populations. **$F_1$ h.** The offspring of a parental cross; a member of the first filial generation. **somatic h.** A cell formed by fusion of two cells from different organisms in tissue culture; heterokaryon. The inactivated Sendai virus increases the incidence of fusion in culture.

**hybridization** \hī′bridīzā′shən\ **1** The production of a hybrid cell, organism, or population through any of the numerous processes of fusing or mating genetically distinct parents or precursors. Also *crossbreeding.* **2** In molecular biology, the process of forming a double helix between DNA chains or DNA and RNA chains that are at least partially complementary. **cell h.** The process of the fusion of two somatic cells of different genotypes to produce a hybrid cell. **cross h.** In molecular biology, the hybridization of polynucleotide chains that are not perfectly complementary, as between species or strains. ***in situ* h.** A technique by which a known nucleic acid is applied to a cytologic preparation in which the DNA has been partially denatured. The conditions are then altered to promote annealing of the test nucleic acid to complementary sequences in the cell. The location of hybridization is usually detected by autoradiography. **molecular h.** A procedure used to compare the similarities of base sequences between two polynucleotide chains from different sources. The polynucleotide chains are heated to separate the single strands (melting). Recombination or annealing occurs upon slow cooling.

**hybridoma** \hī′bridō′mə\ [HYBRID + -OMA] A cell type formed by fusion of two or more different types of cells.

**hycanthone** $C_{20}H_{24}N_2O_2S$. 1-[[2-(Dimethylamino)ethyl]-amino]-4-(hydroxymethyl)-9*H*-thioxanthen-9-one. An antischistosomal drug that is given by parenteral injection, usually as the mesylate salt.

**hydatid** \hī′dətid\ [Gk *hydatis,* gen. *hydatidos* (from *hydōr* water) a drop of water, watery vesicle] **1** HYDATID CYST. **2** Any vesicle or cystlike structure that contains clear watery fluid. It may be a remnant of an embryonic structure or produced by larval parasites. **h. of Morgagni** **1** APPENDIX MORGAGNII. **2** APPENDIX TESTIS. **nonpedunculated h.** APPENDIX TESTIS. **pedunculated h.** APPENDIX OF THE EPIDIDYMIS. **pedunculated h. of Morgagni** **1** Any of the appendices vesiculosae epoöphori. **2** APPENDIX OF THE EPIDIDYMIS. **sessile h.** APPENDIX TESTIS. **sessile h. of Morgagni** APPENDIX TESTIS. **Virchow's h.** ALVEOLAR HYDATID CYST.

**hydatidiform** \hī′dətid′ifôrm\ Having the appearance of watery drops or a watery cyst.

**hydatidosis** \hī′dətidō′sis\ [HYDATID + -OSIS] ECHINOCOCCOSIS.

**hydatidostomy** \hī′dətidäs′təmē\ [HYDATID + *o* + -STOMY] A surgical procedure in which an opening is created in a hydatid cyst for the purpose of drainage. Such an opening may occur spontaneously, but it is rare.

***Hydatigena*** \hī′dətij′ənə\ *TAENIA.*

**hydatism** \hī′dətizm\ [Gk *hydat(is)* a drop of water, watery vesicle + -ISM] The sound caused by fluid movement in a body cavity.

**hydatoid** \hī′dətoid\ [Gk *hydatoeidēs* (from *hydōr,* gen. *hydato(s)* water + *-eidēs* -like, -OID) watery, aqueous] **1** *Outmoded* HUMOR AQUOSUS. **2** Pertaining to the aqueous humor. *Outmoded.*

**hydatorrhea** \hī′dətôrē′ə\ HYDRORRHEA.

**hydr-** \hīdr-\ HYDRO-.

**hydracetin** ACETYLPHENYLHYDRAZINE.

**hydradenitis** \hī′dradənī′tis\ HIDRADENITIS.

**hydradenoma** \hī′dradənō′mə\ HIDRADENOMA.

**hydraemia** *Brit.* HYDREMIA.

**hydragogue** [Gk *hydragōgos* (from *hydr-* water + *agōgos* inducing) bringing or producing water or a watery discharge] **1** Promoting or causing the expulsion of water, as from the gastrointestinal tract. **2** A cathartic that brings about a watery purgation.

**hydralazine** $C_8H_8N_4$. An antihypertensive agent that is administered orally or parenterally.

**hydramnios** \hīdram′nē·äs\ [HYDR- + New L *amnios,* irreg. from Gk *amnion* the membrane around a fetus] The presence of an abnormally large amount of amniotic fluid for a particular stage of pregnancy. It is commonly associated with fetal abnormality, maternal illnesses, such as diabetes mellitus, or with interference in normal fetal physiology by toxic or other substances. Also *hydramnion, polyhydramnios.*

**hydranencephaly** \hī′dranənsef′əlē\ [HYDR- + ANENCEPHALY] An extreme degree of hydrocephaly in which the lateral and third ventricles form essentially a single cerebral cavity enclosed within the three layers of meninges, the skull, and the skin. Cerebral hemispheres are largely reduced to basal ganglia and remnants of the choroid plexus, other nervous tissue presumably having succumbed to pressure atrophy from long-continued internal hydrocephalus. Other parts of the brain may appear to be developmentally normal but signs of pressure may be evident.

**hydrangiology** \hīdran′jē·äl′əjē\ LYMPHANGIOLOGY.

**hydrargyria** \hī′drärjir′ē·ə\ [*hydrargyr(um)* + -IA] MERCURY POISONING.

**hydrargyrism** \hīdrär′jirizm\ [*hydrargyr(um)* + -ISM] MERCURY POISONING.

**hydrargyromania** \hīdrär′jirōmā′nē·ə\ ERETHISM.

**hydrargyrosis** \hīdrär′jirō′sis\ [*hydrargyr(um)* + -OSIS] MERCURY POISONING.

**hydrargyrum** [New L, from Gk *hydrargyros* (from *hydr-* of or like water + *argyros* silver) quicksilver] MERCURY. **h. ammoniatum** AMMONIATED MERCURY. **hydrargyri subchloridum** CALOMEL.

**hydrarthrodial** \hī′drärthrō′dē·əl\ Of or relating to hydrarthrosis.

**hydrarthrosis** \hī′drärthrō′sis\ [HYDR- + ARTHROSIS] The presence of excessive synovial fluid within a joint. Also *hydrops articuli, articular dropsy.* **intermittent h.** A periodic swelling of a joint due to excessive synovial fluid.

**hydratase** Any enzyme catalyzing the reaction of a carbon-carbon double bond with water to add —OH to one carbon atom and —H to another, such as fumarate hydratase.

**hydrate** \hī′drāt\ A compound with water combined, usually reversibly.

**hydrated** \hī′drātid\ Having water added, usually by reversible chemical reaction.

**hydration** \hīdrā′shən\ **1** The addition of water, as by intravenous fluids to replace water lost from the body as a result of dehydration. **2** The binding of water molecules to ions or molecules in solution.

**hydraulics** \hīdrô′liks\ The branch of science and technology dealing with the mechanics of fluids, especially liquids, comprised of hydrostatics and hydrodynamics.

**hydremia** \hīdrē′mē·ə\ [HYDR- + -EMIA] An increase in the plasma volume of blood without a corresponding increase in the number of erythrocytes or hemoglobin concentration.

**hydrencephalocele** \hī′drensef′əlōsēl′\ HYDROENCEPHALOCELE.

**hydrencephalomeningocele** \hī′drensef′əlōməning′-gōsēl\ [HYDR- + ENCEPHALO- + MENINGOCELE] A hydrencephalocele specifically demonstrated to contain meninges. Also *hydroencephalomeningocele.*

**hydrencephalus** \hī′drensef′ələs\ HYDROCEPHALUS.

**hydrencephaly** \hī′drensef′əlē\ HYDROCEPHALUS.

**hydride** **1** Any compound of hydrogen with an element, particularly if the hydrogen is the more electronegative element. **2** The ion $H^-$.

**hydro-** \hī′drō-\ [Gk, combining stem of *hydōr* water] A combining form denoting (1) water or watery fluid; (2) water of hydration; (3) hydrogen. Also *hydr-.*

**hydroa** \hidrō′ə, hīdrō′ə\ [HYDR- + Gk *ōa,* pl. of *ōon* egg] Any condition characterized by vesicle formation. *Older term.* Also *hidroa.* **h. aestivale** *Older term* HUTCHINSON SUMMER PRURIGO. **h. vacciniforme** A rare photodermatosis of early childhood in which deep-seated umbilicated vesicles appear on exposed sites. After healing they leave large varioliform scars. In most subjects it persists into adult life.

**hydroblepharon** \-blef′ərän\ [HYDRO- + Gk *blepharon* an eyelid] A watery swelling of the eyelid.

**hydrocalicosis** [HYDRO- + New L *calic(is),* gen. of CALIX + -OSIS] A dilatation of a single renal calix, usually due to a congenital stricture or to an abnormal narrowing of the caliceal cup stalk.

**hydrocalix** \-kā′liks\ [HYDRO- + CALIX] Dilatation of a renal calix.

**hydrocarbon** \-kär′bən\ [HYDRO- + CARBON] A compound consisting only of the elements carbon and hydrogen. Squalene is the only important hydrocarbon metabolite in mammals. **chlorinated h.** A hydrocarbon containing a chlorine grouping in its molecular structure. Such compounds have many uses, particularly in pesticides or insecticides. Many are environmentally harmful because of their stability and undesirable ecological effects. **fluorinated h.** FLUOROCARBON. **halogenated h.** Any hydrocarbon molecule with one or more halogen atoms attached. Some such compounds are toxic and are used for the control of certain pest species. They are fat soluble and may accumulate in the food chain.

**hydrocardia** \-kär′dē·ə\ HYDROPERICARDIUM.

**hydrocele** \hī′drōsēl′\ [Gk *hydrokēlē* (from *hydro-* water + *kēlē* hernia or swelling) a scrotal hydrocele] An accumulation of serous fluid in a body cavity, especially between the visceral and parietal layers of the tunica vaginalis in the scrotum. It may be congenital. **bilocular h.** A collection of serous fluid in the tunica vaginalis testis or persistent processus vaginalis testis in the scrotum and/or inguinal regions of both sides. **cervical h.** BRANCHIAL CYST. **chylous h.** A type of hydrocele in which the liquid contents are milky white. **communicating h.** A hydrocele that communicates with the peritoneal cavity. **diffused h.** A collection of fluid diffused in spermatic cord tissue. **Dupuytren's h.** A bilocular hydrocele in which all or major parts of the processus vaginalis testis of both sides persist. **encysted h.** A small, localized hydrocele of the testis or epididymis situated at the point of reflection of the tunica vaginalis testis. **filarial h.** A hydrocele due to the presence, in the tunica vaginalis of the testicle, of microfilariae, usually of *Wuchereria bancrofti.* **funicular h.** A persistence of the embryonic saccus vaginalis testis in its upper extent but not continuously with the tunica vaginalis testis. It may be either a blind cyst beside the spermatic cord or an elongated sac continuous with the peritoneal cavity. **inguinal h.** A hydrocele accompanying an undescended testicle. It may be found in the inguinal canal or the pubic area. **scrotal h.** A hydrocele in the tunica vaginalis testis in the scrotum. **spermatic h.** The collection of spermatic fluid along the spermatic cord. **h. of the spermatic cord** An encysted hydrocele in that portion of the peritoneum surrounding the spermatic cord. It usually lies in the upper part of the scrotum or the inguinal canal. **h. spinalis** SPINA BIFIDA. **h. of the testis** A hydrocele of the testicular part of the tunica vaginalis. It is the commonest type of hydrocele. Also *hydrorchis.*

**hydrocelectomy** \-sēlek′təmē\ The surgical process of removing a hydrocele.

**hydrocenosis** \-sēnō′sis\ [HYDRO- + Gk *kenōsis* (from *kenos* empty) an emptying] A procedure by which an abnormal serous fluid accumulation is drained from the body.

**hydrocephalic** \-səfal′ik\ Describing, pertaining to, or affected by hydrocephalus.

**hydrocephalocele** \-sef′əlōsēl′\ HYDROENCEPHALOCELE.

**hydrocephaloid** \-sef′əloid\ Resembling hydrocephalus in having an apparently enlarged cranium, as is seen in some cases of starvation, but without any abnormal accumulation of cerebrospinal fluid.

**hydrocephalus** \-sef′ələs\ [New L, from Gk *hydrokephalon* (from *hydro-* water + *kephalē* head) hydrocephalus] Any condition in which there is an abnormally large volume of cerebrospinal fluid within the skull. Also *hydrencephalus,*

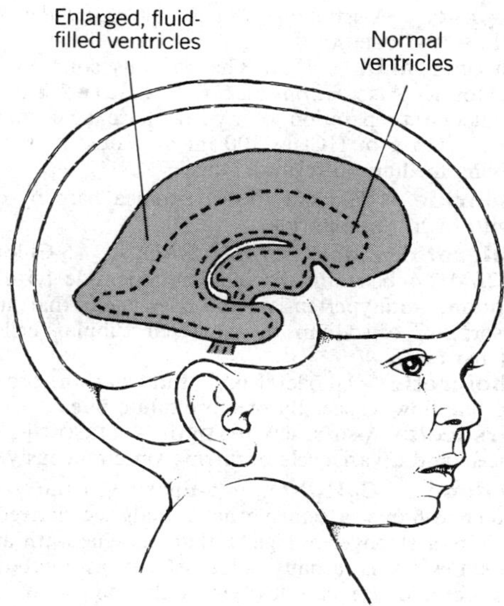


Hydrocephalus

*hydrencephaly, hydrocephaly, hydrocrania.* **communicating h.** Hydrocephalus in which there is obstruction to the flow of cerebrospinal fluid within the subarachnoid space. Also *external hydrocephalus, serous internal pachymeningitis.* **compensating h.** HYDROCEPHALUS EX VACUO. **congenital h.** Hydrocephalus due to developmental obstruction or stenosis of any of the passages through which cerebrospinal fluid normally passes. Also *primary hydrocephalus.* **external h.** COMMUNICATING HYDROCEPHALUS. **h. ex vacuo** The replacement of lost or atrophic brain tissue by cerebrospinal fluid, occurring as a compensatory mechanism to restore intracranial volume. Also *compensating hydrocephalus.* **hypertonic h.** Hydrocephalus with increased intracranial pressure. **internal h.** OBSTRUCTIVE HYDROCEPHALUS. **low-pressure h.** A form of communicating hydrocephalus identified as a cause of dementia, intermittent confusion, and gait disturbance, in which the cerebrospinal fluid pressure as measured by lumbar puncture is often low or normal. Also *normal-pressure hydrocephalus.* **noncommunicating h.** OBSTRUCTIVE HYDROCEPHALUS. **normal-pressure h.** LOW-PRESSURE HYDROCEPHALUS. **obstructive h.** Hydrocephalus due to a disease process or to a developmental or acquired lesion which causes obstruction to the normal flow of cerebrospinal fluid through the cerebral ventricular system. Also *internal hydrocephalus, noncommunicating hydrocephalus.* **occult h.** Hydrocephalus which is asymptomatic and produces no abnormal physical signs. **otitic h.** Benign intercranial hypertension occurring in association with otitis media and with thrombosis of one or more intercranial venous sinuses. **postmeningitic h.** Communicating hydrocephalus following meningitis. **post-traumatic h.** Hydrocephalus, usually of the communicating variety, developing as a sequel to head injury. **primary h.** CONGENITAL HYDROCEPHALUS. **thrombotic h.** Hydrocephalus resulting from intracranial venous sinus thrombosis. **toxic h.** Benign intracranial hypertension due to an exogenous or endogenous toxin.

**hydrocephaly** \-sef′əlē\ [French *hydrocéphalie* hydrocephalus] HYDROCEPHALUS.

**hydrochloric acid** HCl. The aqueous solution of hydrogen chloride. Also *muriatic acid.* **diluted h.** A diluted medicinal preparation of hydrochloric acid that contains 9.5 to 10.5 g of HCl in 100 ml of water. It is used as an acidifying medium in formulations.

**hydrochloride** The salt formed from a base by combination with hydrogen chloride.

**hydrochlorothiazide** $C_7H_8ClN_3O_4S_2$. 6-Chloro-3,4-dihydro-2*H*-1,2,4-benzothiadiazine-7-sulfonamide 1,1-dioxide, an important antihypertensive, diuretic agent that inhibits the reabsorption of sodium by the renal tubular cells. It is administered orally.

**hydrocholeretic** \-kō′ləret′ik\ Inducing or provoking increased bile flow, especially of more dilute bile.

**hydrocirsocele** \-sir′sōsēl\ [HYDRO- + CIRSO- + -CELE[1]] A hydrocele and a varicocele occurring simultaneously.

**hydrocodone** $C_{18}H_{21}NO_3$. 4,5-Epoxy-3-methoxy-17-methylmorphinan-6-one, a semisynthetic analgesic derived from codeine. It is a stronger analgesic than codeine with antitussive properties. It is usually administered as its bitartrate salt, and chronic use can lead to addiction. **h. resin complex** A combination of hydrocodone and a cationic resin for oral administration with slow release and absorption of the drug. The antitussive agent should act for about 12 hours after one dose in this formulation.

**hydrocolloid** \-käl′oid\ [HYDRO- + COLLOID] An elastic water-based impression material. **irreversible h.** A hydrocolloid, prepared by adding a powder to water, which can be used only once. **reversible h.** A thermoplastic hydrocolloid.

**hydrocolpocele** \-käl′pəsēl\ [HYDRO- + COLPO- + -CELE[2]] An accumulation of fluid other than blood or pus in the vagina. Such accumulation is usually dependent upon an imperforate hymen or atresia of the lower vaginal canal and is usually seen in the neonatal period. Also *hydrocolpos.*

**hydrocortamate** $C_{27}H_{41}NO_6$. An ester derivative of hydrocortisone that is used as a 0.5 percent ointment in the treatment of dermatologic conditions that respond to corticosteroids.

**hydrocortisone** \-kôr′tisōn\ CORTISOL.

**hydrocortisone acetate** The acetate ester of hydrocortisone (cortisol) at the C-21 position. It has the same uses as cortisol, the parent compound, and is given intra-articularly by soft-tissue injection and applied topically to the skin or conjunctiva.

**hydrocortisone sodium phosphate** The phosphate ester of hydrocortisone (cortisol). It has the same uses as the parent compound but has greater solubility in water. It is given intravenously and by intramuscular injection.

**hydrocortisone sodium succinate** The hemisuccinate ester sodium salt derivative of hydrocortisone. It has greater water solubility but is used for the same purposes as hydrocortisone. It is administered intravenously or intramuscularly.

**hydrocortisone tertiary-butylacetate** The tertiary butylacetate ester of hydrocortisone. It has the same uses as hydrocortisone. Also *hydrocortisone tebutate.*

**hydrocrania** \-krā′nē·ə\ [HYDRO- + *cran(i)-* + -IA] HYDROCEPHALUS.

**hydrocyanism** \-sī′ənizm\ [*hydro(gen)* + *cyan(ide)* + -ISM] Poisoning due to hydrogen cyanide. Toxic symptoms depend upon the dose, the form in which it is administered, and the route. With high concentrations, respiration ceases immediately. At lower concentrations, symptoms of muscular incoordination and decreased respiration develop more slowly, and may be fatal if left untreated.

**hydrocystadenoma** \-sis′tadənō′mə\ HIDROCYSTOMA.

**hydrocystoma** \-sistō′mə\ HIDROCYSTOMA.

**hydrodiascope** \-dī′əskōp\ A refracting device linked to the cornea with fluid, with the intent of subtracting the optical characteristics of the cornea from the refractive findings.

**hydrodiffusion** **1** The diffusion of a substance through water. **2** The diffusion of one liquid through another liquid.

**hydrodynamics** \-dīnam′iks\ The science and technology dealing with the motion of fluids and the forces they exert on solids within them.

**hydroencephalocele** \-ensef′əlōsēl′\ [HYDRO- + ENCEPHALOCELE] An encephalocele in which cerebrospinal fluid has accumulated either in meningeal spaces or in the ventricles of herniated brain, causing dilatation of the herniated mass. Also *encephalocystocele, encephalocystomeningocele, hydrencephalocele, hydrocephalocele.*

**hydroencephalomeningocele** \-ensef′əlōməning′gōsēl\ HYDRENCEPHALOMENINGOCELE.

**hydrofluoric acid** HF. Hydrogen fluoride and its solutions. It is strongly corrosive and a moderately strong acid.

**hydrogen** \hī′drəjən\ Element number 1, having atomic weight 1.0019. Hydrogen is the most abundant element in the universe but constitutes less than 0.22% of the total atoms on earth. It is a fuel sustaining the thermonuclear reactions in the sun and stars. It is the lightest of all gases, and only traces (less than 1 ppm) occur free in the atmosphere. It occurs chiefly in combination with oxygen in water. There are three isotopes. Hydrogen 1 (protium) has a natural abundance of 99.985%. The remaining 0.015% consists mostly of hydrogen 2 (deuterium). The one unstable isotope, hydrogen 3 (tritium) occurs naturally in minute traces. Hydrogen combines with other elements, often explosively. The valence is 1. As a constitutent of water and of most organic compounds, hydrogen is essential to life. See also DEUTERIUM, TRITIUM. Symbol: H **arseniuretted h.** ARSINE. **heavy h.** DEUTERIUM. **h. ion** The positively charged nucleus of the hydrogen atom; a proton. Acids have the ability to liberate hydrogen ions. Symbol: $H^+$ **radioactive h.** TRITIUM. **sulfuretted h.** *Obs.* HYDROGEN SULFIDE.

**hydrogen 2** DEUTERIUM.

**hydrogen 3** TRITIUM.

**hydrogen arsenide** ARSINE.

**hydrogenase** **1** The enzyme (EC 1.18.3.1) that catalyzes the reduction of ferredoxin by hydrogen gas. It is an iron-sulfur protein. **2** Any of various other enzymes that catalyze reductions by hydrogen gas. An outmoded usage.

**hydrogenate** \hī′drəjənāt′\ To add hydrogen to a molecule, usually by reaction with the atoms at either end of a double bond. It may be performed catalytically with hydrogen gas, or with numerous other reagents.

**hydrogenation** \-jənā′shən\ The process of adding hydrogen atoms to a compound, often using hydrogen gas. In nonbiological systems, it is frequently catalyzed by a noble metal or by one of its salts.

**hydrogen bromide** A colorless gas that browns on prolonged exposure to light, is dangerous to breathe, and is obtained by hydrolysis of phosphorus tribromide. Its saturated aqueous solution contains 66% HBr at 25°C. It is a strong acid and reducing agent, used for preparing bromides.

**hydrogen chloride** HCl. A gas, soluble in water and organic solvents. Its aqueous solution is hydrochloric acid. The commercial product is a concentrated solution about 12

M or 38% HCl, of density 1.19. It is a colorless liquid, which fumes in air and is highly corrosive with an irritant smell. When heated it loses hydrogen chloride until "constant boiling" hydrochloric acid is formed, of concentration about 6 M. Dilute solutions are used for preparing certain medicaments, especially hydrochlorides of alkaloids and other bases.

**hydrogenolysis** \-jənäl′isis\ A reaction in which the molecules of one reactant are broken into two parts, each containing one atom of hydrogen derived from the the other reactant, hydrogen gas.

**hydrogen peroxide** $H_2O_2$. A compound available in aqueous solution, but unstable when the solution is concentrated. It is both an oxidizing agent (being reduced to water) and a reducing agent (being oxidized to oxygen). It is produced when oxygen oxidizes the reduced form of many enzymes, particularly flavoproteins. The enzyme catalase converts it into water and oxygen, and peroxidases catalyze oxidations in which it is reduced to water. Also *peroxide.*

**hydrogen sulfate** ACID SULFATE.

**hydrogen sulfide** $H_2S$. A colorless, flammable, highly poisonous gas (boiling point −60°C) with a sweetish taste and an odor of rotten eggs. It owes its toxicity to its high affinity for iron compounds, such as cytochrome oxidase. It is used in the identification of metal ions, since many form insoluble sulfides. It is a reducing agent, being easily oxidized to sulfur, sulfur dioxide, and sulfuric acid. Colorless and photosynthetic sulfur bacteria use biologic and light energy respectively to decompose it to sulfur and to form a reducing agent of its hydrogen. Other bacteria, particularly those living in marine muds, form it from decomposing organic matter and sulfate. It can also be formed bacterially from cysteine derived from proteins. In low concentrations it causes irritation of mucous membranes, particularly of the eyes, leading to keratitis. In high concentrations it causes death from paralysis of the respiratory center. Also *sulfuretted hydrogen* (obs.), *hydrosulfuric acid, sulfur hydride, sulfhydric acid.*

**hydrohemarthrosis** \-hem′ärthrō′sis\ [HYDRO- + HEM- + ARTHROSIS] Hemorrhagic effusion of the joint.

**hydrohematosalpinx** \-hem′ətōsal′pingks\ [HYDRO- + HEMATO- + Gk *salpinx* tube] A collection of fluid and blood in an oviduct, usually due to damage by chronic salpingitis.

**hydrohystera** \-his′tərə\ [HYDRO- + Gk *hystera* the uterus] HYDROMETRA.

**hydrokinetic** \-kinet′ik\ Pertaining to the use of moving water or other fluid for therapeutic purposes, as in hydromassage.

**hydrokollag** \-käl′ag\ A graphite suspension that is used to study ciliary and lymphatic activity.

**hydrolase** Any enzyme that catalyzes the hydrolysis of its substrate.

**hydrolyase** Any enzyme that catalyzes the elimination of water from a molecule, usually with formation of a double bond, such as enolase.

**hydrolysate** The product or products of hydrolysis of a substance.

**hydrolysis** \hīdräl′isis\ [HYDRO- + LYSIS] A reaction in which bonds in the reactant are broken by reaction with water, with addition of a hydroxyl group and a hydrogen atom to the two atoms previously joined. Adj. hydrolytic. **papain h.** The hydrolysis of proteins using the protease obtained from the papaya plant. This enzyme is commonly used in immunologic research to split the IgG molecule into three parts (two Fab fragments and one Fc fragment).

**hydrolyze** \hī′drəlīz\ To split a substance into component parts with addition of the elements of water: to bring about the process of hydrolysis.

**hydroma** \hīdrō′mə\ HYGROMA.

**hydromassage** \-məsäzh′\ Therapeutic manipulation of soft tissues by means of agitated water, as in a whirlpool bath.

**hydromeningitis** \-men′injī′tis\ [HYDRO- + MENINGITIS] *Obs.* BENIGN INTRACRANIAL HYPERTENSION.

**hydromeningocele** \-məning′gōsēl\ A herniation of a fluid-filled sac of spinal or cranial meninges through a defect in the bony structures that normally prevent such protrusion.

**hydrometer** \hīdräm′ətər\ [HYDRO- + -METER] A meter used to determine a fluid's specific gravity.

**hydrometra** \-mē′trə\ [HYDRO- + Gk *mētra* the uterus] A collection of watery fluid or mucus in the uterus. Also *hydrohystera.*

**hydrometrocolpos** \-mē′trəkäl′pəs\ [HYDRO- + METRO- + Gk *kolpos* bosom, womb, fold] An accumulation of fluid other than blood or pus in the uterus and vagina. Such accumulation is usually contingent on an imperforate hymen or atresia of the lower vaginal canal.

**hydrometry** \hīdräm′ətrē\ [HYDRO- + -METRY] The determination of a fluid's specific gravity by using a hydrometer.

**hydromicrocephaly** \-mī′krəsef′əlē\ Microcephaly associated with a disproportionately large volume of cerebrospinal fluid.

**hydromorphone hydrochloride** $C_{17}H_{20}ClNO_3$. 4,5α-Epoxy-3-hydroxy-17-methylmorphinan-6-one hydrochloride, a chemically produced derivative of morphine with about 10 times the analgesic potency of morphine. It is given orally or by subcutaneous injection. Chronic use may lead to addiction.

**hydromphalus** \hīdräm′fələs\ [HYDR- + OMPHALUS] A cystic mass containing watery fluid associated with the umbilicus. The cyst is most likely a remnant of the embryonic vitelline duct or sac, or of the embryonic allantoic stalk.

**hydromyelia** \-mī·ē′lyə\ [HYDRO- + MYEL- + -IA] **1** A dilatation of the central canal of the spinal cord containing cerebrospinal fluid. **2** Any fluid-containing cavity within the spinal cord except those of syringomyelia. Also *hydrorachis.*

**hydromyelocele** \-mī·el′ōsēl\ [HYDRO- + MYELOCELE] The protrusion through a spina bifida of a fluid-filled sac enclosed by attenuated spinal cord tissue and associated meninges. The presence of cord tissue in the sac may be difficult to demonstrate, but its former presence may be inferred from the intact meninges.

**hydromyelomeningocele** \-mī′əlōməning′gōsēl\ A hydromyelocele with demonstrable spinal cord tissue in the wall of the fluid-filled sac protruding from a spina bifida.

**hydronephrosis** \-nefrō′sis\ [HYDRO- + NEPHROSIS] Dilatation of the renal pelvis and calices, and sometimes collecting ducts, secondary to obstruction of urine flow by calculi, tumors, neurologic disorders, or any of various congenital anomalies. Adj. hydronephrotic. **closed h.** Permanent hydronephrosis due to total obstruction of the ureter. **congenital h.** Hydronephrosis present at birth, sometimes due to atresia of ureters or the urethra or to hypertonicity of sphincters within the tract. **external h.** URINOMA. **infected h.** Hydronephrosis and an associated infection, usually caused by *E. coli,* with symptoms resembling those of severe pyelonephritis. Also *pyonephrosis.* **intermittent h.** Dilatation of the pelvis and calices due to intermittent, incomplete obstruction of ureters by an aberrant renal artery, movable kidney, calculi, etc. **perirenal**

**h.** URINOMA. **subcapsular h.** URINOMA.
**hydronium** *Outmoded* OXONIUM.
**hydroparasalpinx** \-par′əsal′pingks\ [HYDRO- + PARA- + SALPINX] The accumulation of serous fluid in any of the embryonic mesonephric duct or tube remnants associated with the oviduct.
**hydropedesis** \-pədē′sis\ HYPERHIDROSIS.
**hydropenia** \-pē′nē·ə\ [HYDRO- + -PENIA] A condition marked by an inadequate amount of water.
**hydropericarditic** \-per′ikärdit′ik\ Pertaining to or characterized by hydropericarditis.
**hydropericarditis** \-per′ikärdī′tis\ Pericarditis with liquid effusion into the pericardial sac.
**hydropericardium** \-per′ikär′dēəm\ The presence of an abnormally large volume of fluid in the pericardial sac. Also *hydrocardia, hydrops pericardii.*
**hydroperinephrosis** \-per′inefrō′sis\ [HYDRO- + PERI- + NEPHR- + -OSIS] The accumulation of fluid in the retroperitoneal connective tissue communicating with the renal pelvis.
**hydroperion** \-per′ē·än\ [HYDRO- + PERI- + Gk *(ō)on* egg] Fluid lying between the capsular and parietal portions of the decidua.
**hydroperitoneum** \-per′itənē′əm\ ASCITES.
**hydroperitonia** \-per′itō′nē·ə\ ASCITES.
**hydropexic** \-pek′sik\ [HYDRO- + *-pex(y)* + -IC] Of or relating to the incorporation of water into tissues.
**hydrophilic** \-fil′ik\ [HYDRO- + -PHILIC] Having an affinity for water: used of substances that are soluble in water or of chemical groups that raise the solubility in water of substances that contain them. Also *hydrophilous.*
**hydrophobia** \-fō′bē·ə\ [Gk (from *hydro-* water + *phobos* panic, terror) aversion to water, hydrophobia] **1** A clinical manifestation, usually of rabies, involving glottal spasm and paralysis of the muscles of deglutition and provoked by attempts to drink fluids or by the sight of fluids. **2** *Popular* RABIES. **paralytic h.** PARALYTIC RABIES.
**hydrophobic** \-fō′bik\ **1** Having low affinity for water. Hydrophobic groups have affinity for each other when they are in an aqueous environment, because of the tendency of their interface with water to diminish. Hydrocarbons are typically hydrophobic. **2** Relating to or characterized by hydrophobia.
**hydrophorograph** \fôr′əgraf\ [HYDRO- + PHORO- + -GRAPH] An apparatus for measuring the pressure or flow of a fluid.
**hydrophthalmia** \hī′dräfthal′mē·ə\ [HYDR- + OPHTHALMIA] BUPHTHALMOS.
**hydrophthalmos** \hī′dräfthal′məs\ [HYDR- + Gk *ophthalmos* the eye] BUPHTHALMOS.
**hydrophthalmus** \hī′dräfthal′məs\ [See HYDROPHTHALMOS.] BUPHTHALMOS.
**hydrophysometra** \-fī′sōmē′trə\ [HYDRO- + PHYSO- + Gk *mētra* the uterus] PNEUMOHYDROMETRA.
**hydropic** \hīdräp′ik\ [Gk *hydrōpikos* dropsical] Pertaining to or affected by hydrops or edema.
**hydropigenous** \-pij′ənəs\ [*hydrop(s)* + *i* + -GENOUS] Causing hydrops.
**hydroplasmia** \-plaz′mē·ə\ [HYDRO- + *plasm(a)* + -IA] A reduction in the osmolarity of blood plasma, due either to an increase in the water content or a decrease in the concentration of electrolytes and colloids. Also *hydroplasmy.*
**hydropleura** \-plUr′ə\ HYDROTHORAX.
**hydropneumatosis** \-n$^y$oo′mətō′sis\ [HYDRO- + PNEUMAT- + -OSIS] A condition characterized by the presence of fluid and gas within a tissue.
**hydropneumogony** \-n$^y$oomäg′ənē\ *Obs.* ARTHROGRAPHY.
**hydropneumopericardium** \-n$^y$oo′məper′ikär′dē·əm\ The presence of fluid and gas within the pericardial sac.
**hydropneumoperitoneum** \-n$^y$oo′məper′itənē′əm\ [HYDRO- + PNEUMO- + PERITONEUM] An intraperitoneal accumulation of air and fluid.
**hydropneumothorax** \-n$^y$oo′məthôr′aks\ The presence of air and watery fluid in the pleural cavity. Also *pneumohydrothorax, seropneumothorax.*
**hydrops** \hī′dräps\ [L (from Gk *hydrōps* dropsy, a dropsical person, from *hydōr* water), dropsy] An excessive accumulation of serous fluid in interstitial tissues or body cavities. **h. articuli** HYDRARTHROSIS. **Bart's hemoglobin h. fetalis** A form of α-thalassemia due to homozygosity for α-thalassemia-1 that is lethal during fetal life. Only hemoglobin Bart's is present in the blood of such a fetus. **h. of the cornea** Gross entry of aqueous humor into the cornea as a result of a rupture of the endothelium and Descemet's membrane, as may occur in keratoconus. **endolymphatic h.** **1** MENIÈRE'S DISEASE. **2** A distended state of the membranous labyrinth found in Menière's disease. **fetal h.** The abnormal accumulation of fluid in the tissues of a fetus or newborn infant, as in erythroblastosis fetalis. **hypertensive meningeal h.** BENIGN INTRACRANIAL HYPERTENSION. **labyrinthine h.** *Incorrect* MENIÈRE'S DISEASE. • The term is misleading as it implies involvement of the entire labyrinth when in fact only the endolymphatic compartment is involved. **h. pericardii** HYDROPERICARDIUM. **h. tubae** HYDROSALPINX. **h. tubae profluens** Vaginal secretion of profuse amounts of serous fluid originating in the fallopian tube. It may be a sign of a tubal carcinoma. **tympanic h.** SECRETORY OTITIS MEDIA.
**hydrorachis** \-rā′kis\ [HYDRO- + Gk *rhachis* the back, spine, backbone] HYDROMYELIA.
**hydrorchis** \hīdrôr′kis\ [HYDR- + Gk *orchis* testicle] HYDROCELE OF THE TESTIS.
**hydrorrhea** \hī′drôrē′ə\ [HYDRO- + -RRHEA] An excessive or copious discharge of water or other fluid. Also *hydatorrhea.* **h. gravidarum** Intermittent vaginal drainage of fluid during pregnancy. The fluid may come from the extra-amniotic space or may be amniotic fluid.
**hydrosalpinx** \-sal′pinks\ [HYDRO- + SALPINX] Distension of the fallopian tube by clear fluid, usually occurring as a result of closure of the fimbricated end of the tube by inflammation. Also *tubal dropsy, salpingian dropsy, hydrops tubae, sactosalpinx.*
**hydrosarcocele** \-sär′kəsēl\ Hydrocele and sarcocele combined.
**hydroscheocele** \hīdräs′kē·əsēl′\ [HYDR- + OSCHEOCELE] A scrotal hernia in which the hernial sac contains serous fluid.
**hydrospermatocele** \-spur′mətōsēl′\ SPERMATOCELE.
**hydrostomia** \-stō′mē·ə\ *Rare* PTYALISM.
**hydrosulfuric acid** HYDROGEN SULFIDE.
**hydrosyringomyelia** \-siring′gōmī·ē′lyə\ SYRINGOMYELIA.
**hydrotherapeutic** \-ther′əpyoo′tik\ Relating to hydrotherapy or hydrotherapeutics.
**hydrotherapeutics** \-ther′əpyoo′tiks\ The study of the therapeutic properties of water in all of its applications, including both internal and external.
**hydrotherapy** \-ther′əpē\ **1** Utilization of water by external application or by immersion as a primary therapeutic measure or adjunctive technique. **2** Therapeutic use of water by ingestion as in spa therapy. Also *water cure.*
**hydrothionemia** \-thī′ənē′mē·ə\ [HYDRO- + THION- +

-EMIA] The presence of hydrogen sulfide in blood, as in a person who has inhaled hydrogen sulfide gas.

**hydrothorax** \-thôr′aks\ [HYDRO- + THORAX] Watery fluid in the pleural cavity, usually due to heart failure or a state of generalized edema. Also *dropsy of chest, hydropleura.*

**chylous h.** CHYLOTHORAX.

**hydrotomy** \hīdrät′əmē\ [HYDRO- + -TOMY] A procedure in which tissues are separated or dissected free by injecting water or other fluid under high pressure.

**hydrotoxicity** \-täksis′itē\ WATER INTOXICATION.

**hydrotympanum** \-tim′pənəm\ SECRETORY OTITIS MEDIA.

**hydroureter** \hī′drōyUr′ətər\ [HYDRO- + URETER] Acquired dilatation of the ureter by fluid, usually due to obstruction of the urinary outflow tract or to vesicoureteral reflux. Also *hydroureterosis.*

**hydroureteronephrosis** \hī′drōyoorē′tərōnefrō′sis\ [HYDRO- + URETERO- + NEPHROSIS] Dilatation of kidney and ureter by fluid, usually due to obstruction of urinary outflow or to vesicoureteral reflux.

**hydroureterosis** \hī′drōyoorē′tərō′sis\ HYDROURETER.

**hydrovarium** \hī′drōver′ē·əm\ [HYDR- + New L *ovarium* (from L *ov(um)* egg + New L suffix *-arium*) ovary] Edema or cyst of the ovary.

**hydrox-** \hīdräks-\ HYDROXY-.

**hydroxamic acids** Derivatives of carboxylic acids, such as fatty acids or amino acids, in which a hydroxylamine bonds to the carbon of the carboxyl group, to give the structure R—CO—NH—OH. They are easily detected, and their spontaneous formation from thioesters allows these to be detected as metabolic intermediates.

**hydroxide** The ion $HO^-$ or a compound containing it.

**hydroxo-** [*hydrox(yl)* + *o*] A combining form used in inorganic chemistry to show that a hydroxide ion, $OH^-$, is a ligand in a complex.

**hydroxocobalamin** The cobalamin in which the sixth ligand of the cobalt is a hydroxide ion. It is an important form of vitamin $B_{12}$.

**hydroxy-** \hīdräk′sē-\ [HYDR- + OXY-[1]] A combining form designating the presence of a hydroxyl group, —OH, as a substituent in a molecule. Also *hydrox-*.

**3-hydroxyacyl-CoA dehydrogenase** The enzyme (EC 1.1.1.35) of fatty-acid catabolism responsible for the oxidation of a 3-hydroxyacyl-CoA to a 3-oxoacyl-CoA with transfer of hydrogen to $NAD^+$.

**hydroxyamphetamine** $C_9H_{13}NO$. *p*-(2-Aminopropyl)-phenol, an adrenergic agent that is applied topically to the conjunctiva as a mydriatic. The hydrochloride and hydrobromide salts are commonly used.

**hydroxyamphetamine hydrobromide** $C_9H_{13}NO{\cdot}HBr$. 4-(2-Aminopropyl)phenol hydrobromide, an adrenergic agent that is used as a mydriatic medication to the conjunctiva. It also acts as a nasal decongestant and, when given orally, is an effective pressor agent for the treatment of the carotid sinus syndrome, postural hypotension, and some types of heart block.

**11β-hydroxyandrostenedione** 11β-hydroxy-4-androstene-3,17-dione. A $C_{19}$ adrenal steroid, a weak androgen, and a major source with cortisol of the 11-oxygenated 17-ketosteroids in the urine.

**hydroxyapatite** $[Ca_3(PO_4)_2]_3{\cdot}Ca(OH)_2$. A compound whose crystals form a lattice that is embedded in the protein matrix of bones and teeth and contribute the major portion of rigid mineral structure to these structures. Also *bone-salt.*

**hydroxybenzene** PHENOL.

**3-hydroxybutyrate dehydrogenase** The enzyme (EC 1.1.1.30) that interconverts 3-hydroxybutyrate and acetoacetate, which uses $NAD^+$as hydrogen acceptor.

**3-hydroxybutyric acid** $CH_3$—CHOH—$CH_2$—CO-OH. An acid found in blood during ketosis, along with acetoacetic acid, from which it is formed by hydrogenation, and with acetone. Also *β-hydroxybutyric acid.* See also KETONE BODY.

**hydroxychloroquine sulfate** $C_{18}H_{26}ClN_3O{\cdot}H_2SO_4$. 7-Chloro-4-{4-[ethyl(2-hydroxyethyl)amino]- 1-methylbutyl-amino}-quinoline sulfate, the sulfate salt of a quinoline analog that is used as an antimalarial agent and as a suppressant drug for lupus erythematosus. It is also used in the treatment of rheumatoid arthritis and giardiasis. It is given orally.

**25-hydroxycholecalciferol** A precursor of 1,25-dihydroxycholecalciferol, which can act directly on intestine and kidney to enhance calcium absorption and retention. It is formed in the liver by hydroxylation of cholecalciferol (the main form of vitamin D).

**11-hydroxycorticosteroid** A steroid of the adrenal cortex containing an 11-hydroxyl group. Most corticosteroids contain such a group. This group is very unreactive, being axial and having access to it hindered by the neighboring methyl groups (C-18 and C-19).

**17-hydroxycorticosteroid** A steroid of the adrenal cortex containing a 17-hydroxyl group. The addition of this group converts corticosterone, the main adrenocortical hormone in the rat, into cortisol, the main such hormone in man.

**17-hydroxycorticosterone** CORTISOL.

**25-hydroxydihydrotachysterol** One of the most potent compounds synthesized from vitamin $D_2$ (ergocalciferol). It is used in the treatment of hypoparathyroidism and is often found to be more effective for this purpose than is vitamin $D_2$, as it causes a greater mobilization of bone.

**hydroxydione sodium** A compound related to adrenal steroids and once injected intravenously for the induction of general or basal anesthesia.

**25-hydroxyergocalciferol** A compound formed by hydroxylation of ergocalciferol, a minor form of vitamin D, in the same way as 25-hydroxycholecalciferol is formed from cholecalciferol.

**hydroxyestradiols** A large class of estradiol metabolites, comprising compounds with a hydroxyl group at the 2,6,15 and 2,6,16 positions. Some of these are further metabolized in the periphery to methoxyestrones.

**hydroxyestrin benzoate** ESTRADIOL BENZOATE.

**5-hydroxyindoleacetic acid** A metabolite of tryptophan found in urine.

**11-hydroxy-17-ketosteroid** A steroid likely to be androgenic, because of the carbonyl group at C-17 and the removal of the two-carbon side chain of adrenocortical hormones. It is also likely to be of adrenal origin, since the 11-hydroxyl group is present.

**hydroxyl** \hīdräk′sil\ [HYDR- + *ox(y)-*[1] + Gk *(h)yl(ē)* wood, material, stuff] The group formed from one hydrogen atom and one oxygen atom.

**hydroxylamine** 1 Any compound of general formula R—NH—OH where R is an alkyl radical. 2 $NH_2$—OH. An unstable compound forming colorless crystals, soluble in water and various organic solvents. It is a weak base (p*K* 7.97). Because of its instability its salts (hydrochloride, sulfate) are used as reducing agents or as reagents in organic chemistry. It is a nucleophile, and liberates thiols and alcohols from their esters. Sensitive tests exist for the hydroxamic acids formed, and this is used for assaying thioesters.

**hydroxylase** Any enzyme that replaces a hydrogen atom with a hydroxyl group, usually using molecular oxygen as oxidant. Such enzymes are monooxygenases if the second atom of oxygen is reduced to water, and they are dioxygenases if it is incorporated into the same substrate or into a second substrate. *Outmoded.*

**hydroxylation** \-lā′shən\ The process of replacing a hydrogen atom with a hydroxyl group.

**5-hydroxylysine** An amino acid present in collagen and some other proteins. It is produced by hydroxylation of lysine residues already incorporated into the protein. In some proteins the hydroxyl group is glycosylated.

**hydroxymethyglutaryl-CoA synthase** The enzyme (EC 4.1.3.5) that forms 3-hydroxy-3-methylglutaryl-CoA and coenzyme A from acetyl-CoA, acetoacetyl-CoA, and water. This reaction is a step both in the formation of isoprenoid compounds, including steroids and terpenses, and in the liberation of free acetoacetate.

**5-hydroxymethyl cytosine** Cytosine with a hydroxymethyl substituent on C-5. It occurs in certain forms of DNA, especially those of bacteriophages. It is made as part of the 2′-deoxycytidine 5′-phosphate molecule by transfer of the hydroxymethyl group from methylene-tetrahydrofolate.

**hydroxymethylglutaryl-CoA lyase** The enzyme (EC 4.1.3.4) that cleaves 3-hydroxy-3-methylglutaryl-CoA into acetoacetate and acetyl-CoA. This is the main reaction that forms free acetoacetate during ketosis.

**hydroxymethylglutaryl-CoA reductase** One of the enzymes responsible for the conversion of 3-hydroxy-3-methylglutaryl-CoA into mevalonate and coenzyme A. Two molecules of NADH are required by one such enzyme (EC 1.1.1.88), and two of NADPH by another (EC 1.1.1.34). The reaction is involved in the synthesis of isoprenoid compounds such as steroids.

**β-hydroxy-β-methylglutaryl-coenzyme A** HO-OC—$CH_2$—C(OH)($CH_3$)—$CH_2$—CO—coenzyme-A. A thioester formed by the action of hydroxymethylglutaryl-CoA synthase in the pathway of conversion of acetyl-CoA derived from fats into steroids and other isoprenoid compounds.

**hydroxymethyltransferase** Any enzyme that catalyzes the transfer of a hydroxymethyl group, HO—$CH_2$—, in exchange for a hydrogen atom. Such enzymes often use 5,10-methylenetetrahydrofolate as the donor of the hydroxymethyl group. The reaction is equivalent to the addition of formaldehyde.

**hydroxyphenamate** 2-Hydroxy-2-phenylbutyl carbamate. A carbamate with properties like those of meprobamate. It has been used as a minor tranquilizer for anxiety and tension states.

***p*-hydroxyphenylpyruvic acid** The 2-oxoacid formed from tyrosine by transamination. It is an intermediate in the pathway of tyrosine catabolism, in which it is degraded to homogentisic acid and carbon dioxide by reaction with oxygen catalyzed by 4-hydroxyphenylpyruvate dioxygenase.

**hydroxyphenyluria** \-fen′iloo′rē·ə\ Urinary excretion of phenylalanine and tyrosine. It occurs in premature infants deficient in ascorbic acid.

**17α-hydroxyprogesterone** 17α-Hydroxy-pregn-4-ene-3,20-dione, a$C_{21}$ steroid hormone, of great importance as an intermediate step between pregnenolone and cortisol in adrenocortical hormone biosynthesis. Also *α-progesterone.*

**hydroxyprogesterone caproate** 3,20-Dioxopregn-4-en-17α-yl hexanoate. It is used to treat functional uterine bleeding, dysmenorrhea, endometriosis, and threatened abortion. It is given intramuscularly and has a slow onset and prolonged effect for 7 to 17 days. Also *hypoprogesterone hexanoate.*

**hydroxyproline** An amino acid found in collagen, formed by hydroxylation of proline residues after they have been incorporated into the protein. Most of the hydroxyproline present is 4-hydroxyproline, but some is 3-hydroxyproline.

**hydroxyprolinemia** \-prō′linē′mē·ə\ An excess quantity of hydroxyproline in the blood, as in conditions of collagen degradation.

**hydroxyprolinuria** \-prō′linoo′rē·ə\ An excess quantity of hydroxyproline in the urine, as in conditions of collagen degradation.

**15-α-hydroxy prostaglandin dehydrogenase** An enzyme that inactivates prostaglandins by converting the 15-α-hydroxy groups to a ketone.

**8-hydroxyquinoline sulfate** A yellow powder, soluble in water, that is used in very low concentrations as a preservative in syrups, and in skin medications as an antibacterial and antifungal agent. Also *oxyquinoline sulfate.*

**hydroxystearin sulfate** A hydrophilic ointment base prepared by sulfating hydrogenated castor oil.

**11-hydroxysteroid** A steroid hydroxylated at C-11, usually a product of the adrenal cortex.

**hydroxystilbamidine isethionate** $C_{16}H_{16}N_4O{\cdot}2C_2H_6O_4S$. 2-Hydroxy-4,4′-diquanylstilbene diisethionate. A yellow powder used in the treatment of fungal and protozoan diseases. It is effective against leishmanial infections and North American blastomycosis.

**hydroxytetracycline** OXYTETRACYCLINE.

**5-hydroxytryptamine** See under SEROTONIN.

**5-hydroxytryptophan** The product of hydroxylation of tryptophan at C-5. It is an intermediate in the formation of serotonin (5-hydroxytryptamine), which is formed by its decarboxylation.

**hydroxyurea** $CH_4N_2O_2$. A white powder used to treat chronic granulocytic leukemia, melanoma, and inoperable tumors of the ovary. It inhibits DNA synthesis.

**hydroxyzine** $C_{21}H_{27}ClN_2O_2$. *N*-(4-Chlorobenzhydryl)-*N*′-(hydroxyethyloxyethyl)-piperazine. An antihistaminic drug with sedative properties. It is used as an antiemetic agent, for pre- and postoperative sedation, and for the treatment of anxiety and tension.

**hygiene** \hī′jēn, hī′ji·ēn\ [noun use of Gk *hygieinē*, fem. of *hygieinos* pertaining to or characterized by good health, from *hygieia* health, soundness, from *hygiēs* healthy, sound] The principles governing healthy development and the maintenance of health, and the practice of those principles. Also *hygienics.* **industrial h.** OCCUPATIONAL HYGIENE. • See note at OCCUPATIONAL HYGIENE. **mental h.** The totality of measures undertaken to deal with mental disorders through prevention, early detection, and treatment, and to improve the adaptation of patients to their social and occupational milieu. **occupational h.** A branch of occupational health which deals with the measurement, evaluation, and control of these environmental factors in the workplace to which exposure may be hazardous to health. Also *industrial hygiene.* • The term is used chiefly in the United Kingdom, Australia, and India. In New Zealand and Japan, *industrial hygiene* is the preferred term, and is also used in Britain. Neither term is used in the U.S. or South Africa.

**hygienic** \hī′jē·en′ik, hījē′nik\ **1** Of or relating to hygiene. **2** Conducive to health; sanitary.

**hygienics** \hī′jē·en′iks, hījē′niks\ HYGIENE.

**hygienist** \hījē′nist, hī′jənist\ One who specializes in hygiene, or in a specific branch of hygiene, as a dental hygienist. **dental h.** A skilled and sometimes licensed ancillary worker who assists a dentist and performs certain therapeutic and preventive services under the dentist's supervision.

**hygr-** \hīgr-\ HYGRO-.

**hygric** \hī′grik\ [HYGR- + -IC] **1** Concerning moisture. **2** Moist.

**hygro-** \hī′grō-\ [Gk *hygros* moist, wet, liquid] A combining form meaning moist, moisture. Also *hygr-*.

**hygroma** \hīgrō′mə\ [HYGR- + -OMA] **1** A cystic lymphangioma. **2** A fluid-filled tumor. Also *hydroma*. **acute traumatic subdural h.** A subdural hygroma forming over one or both cerebral hemispheres following head injury. **cystic h.** A congenital cystic lymphangioma of the neck. Also *hygroma cysticum, hygroma cysticum colli.* **subdural h.** A collection of cerebrospinal fluid in the subdural space.

**hygromatous** \hīgrō′mətəs\ Pertaining to a hygroma.

**hygrometer** \hīgräm′ətər\ [HYGRO- + -METER] An instrument used to measure the moisture of the atmosphere. Also *psychrometer.* **dew point h.** DEW POINT INDICATOR.

**hygroscopic** [*hygroscop(e)* (from HYGRO- + -SCOPE) an instrument that indicates changes in relative humidity by absorption of moisture + -IC] Capable of absorbing water from moist air.

**Hyl** Symbol for hydroxylysine.

**hyl-** \hīl-\ HYLO-.

**hyla** \hī′lə\ [Gk *hyl(ē)* wood, material, stuff, forest] A lateral evagination of the cerebral aqueduct (of Sylvius). Also *paraqueduct.*

**hyle-** \hī′lə-\ HYLO-.

**hylo-** \hī′lō-\ [Gk *hylē* wood, material, stuff] A combining form denoting matter, substance. Also *hyl-, hyle-*.

**hymen** \hī′mən\ [Gk *hymēn* a membrane] A thin crescentic or annular fold of mucous membrane that partially or completely occludes the vaginal orifice. It varies considerably in shape and extent and may be absent. Also *hymenal membrane.* **imperforate h.** A hymen without an opening. **septate h.** A hymen with two openings separated by a narrow band of tissue. Also *hymen septus.*

**hymenal** \hī′mənəl\ Pertaining to the hymen.

**hymenectomy** \hī′mənek′təmē\ [HYMEN + -ECTOMY] Excision of the hymen.

**hymenitis** \hī′mənī′tis\ [HYMEN + -ITIS] Inflammation of the hymen.

**hymenography** \hī′mənäg′rəfē\ HYMENOLOGY.

**hymenolepiasis** \hī′mənōlepī′əsis\ An infection or disease due to worms of the cestode genus *Hymenolepis.*

***Hymenolepis*** \hī′mənäl′əpis\ The largest genus of tapeworms in the order Cyclophyllidea and the type genus of the family Hymenolepididae, containing over 300 species, parasitic chiefly in aquatic birds and rodents. The genus has been subdivided by various taxonomists into a number of genera, placing the human parasite *H. nana* for example, in the genus *Vampirolepis,* while retaining unarmed species, including *H. diminuta,* in the type genus. ***H. diminuta*** The rat tapeworm, a common species found in rats and mice, and rarely in humans. The cysticercoid larvae occur in fleas, beetles, caterpillars, and other insects. Also *Taenia diminuta.* ***H. nana*** A species common in humans as well as in mice and rats; the dwarf mouse tapeworm. It is 7–80 mm long and is sometimes found in large numbers in the intestines, especially in children. The cysticercoid larvae can develop through all stages in a single host, or they may pass through a two-host cycle, with flour beetles or other insects as intermediate hosts. Human infections are usually asymptomatic, but in very heavy infections abdominal pain, diarrhea, insomnia, and other symptoms may occur. Rodent and human strains of the parasite appear to have developed. The rodent strain has been called *H. nana* var. *fraterna* or given the species designation *H. fraterna..* Also *Taenia minima, Taenia nana.*

**hymenology** \hī′mənäl′əjē\ [Gk *hymēn,* gen. *hymeno(s)* membrane + -LOGY] The study of the structural organization and functions of the membranes of the body. Also *hymenography.*

**Hymenoptera** \hī′mənäp′tərə\ [Gk *hymēn,* gen. *hymeno(s)* membrane + *ptera* wings] An order of holometabolous insects having locked pairs of membranous wings. It includes wasps, hornets, bees, and ants.

**hymenopteran** \hī′mənäp′tərən\ **1** Of or belonging to the insect order Hymenoptera. **2** A member of the order Hymenoptera.

**hymenotomy** \hī′mənät′əmē\ [HYMEN + *o* + -TOMY] Surgical incision in the hymen.

**hyo-** \hī′ō-\ [See HYOID.] A combining form meaning hyoid, or relating to the hyoid bone or hyoid arch.

**hyodeoxycholic acid** 3,6-Dihydroxycholanic acid. A bile acid whose conjugates are found in pig bile.

**hyoepiglottic** \hī′ō·ep′iglät′ik\ Pertaining to the hyoid bone and the epiglottis, specifically their connecting ligament. Also *hyoepiglottidean.*

**hyoglossal** \-gläs′əl\ [HYO- + GLOSSAL] Pertaining to the hyoid bone and the tongue. Also *glossohyal, glossohyoidal.*

**hyoid** \hī′oid\ [Gk *hyoeidēs* (from *(h)y,* orig. name of the letter upsilon ϒ υ + *-eidēs* -like, -OID) upsilon-shaped] **1** Shaped like the Greek letter upsilon or the Roman letter U, as the hyoid bone. **2** Pertaining to either the hyoid bone or, in comparative anatomy, the series of bones at the base of the tongue developed from the embryonic hyoid arch. Also *hyal.* **3** OS HYOIDEUM.

**hyolaryngeal** \-lərin′jē·əl\ Pertaining to the hyoid bone and the larynx.

**hyomandibular** \-mandib′yələr\ Pertaining to the first and second branchial arches and the groove or pouches lying between them.

**hyomental** \-men′təl\ Pertaining to the hyoid bone and the chin.

**hyoscine** SCOPOLAMINE.

**hyoscyamine** $C_{17}H_{23}NO_3$. 3α-Tropanyl *S*-(-)-tropate. An alkaloid obtained from *Hyoscyamus niger, Atropa belladonna,* and other sources. It is the levorotatory isomer of atropine, which is a racemic mixture. Its actions are like those of atropine, but its central and peripheral effects are more pronounced. It is an anticholinergic drug, can be given orally or parenterally, and is used in the treatment of asthma, bronchitis, and mental illness.

**hyoscyamine hydrobromide** The hydrobromide salt of hyoscyamine. It has the same properties and uses as atropine.

**hyoscyamine sulfate** The sulfate salt of hyoscyamine. It has the same properties and uses as atropine.

**hyosternal** \-stur′nəl\ Pertaining to the hyoid bone and the sternum.

**hyothyroid** \-thī′roid\ THYROHYOID.

**hyp-** \hīp-, hip-\ HYPO-.

**hypadrenia** \hī′padrē′nē·ə\ *Outmoded* HYPOADRENALISM.

**hypalbuminemia** \hī′palbyoo′minē′mē·ə \ HYPOALBUMINEMIA.

**hypalbuminosis** \hī′palbyoominō′sis\ HYPOALBUMINEMIA.

**hypalgesia** \hī′paljē′zē·ə\ [HYP- + ALGESIA] Reduction in sensitivity to pain. Also *hypalgia, hypoalgesia.* Adj. hypalgesic, hypalgetic.

**hypanakinesia** \hīpan′əkīnē′zhə\ HYPOKINESIA.

**hypanakinesis** \hīpan′əkīnē′sis\ HYPOKINESIA.

**hypaphrodisia** \hīpaf′rədē′zhə\ [HYP- + Gk *aphrodisia* sexual pleasures] SEXUAL ANESTHESIA.

**hyparterial** \hī′pärtir′ē·əl\ Situated below an artery. Also *hypoarterial.* Compare EPARTERIAL. • The term was first suggested and used with reference to the branches of the bronchi as related to the pulmonary artery.

**hypasthenia** \hī′pasthē′nē·ə\ [HYP- + ASTHENIA] A state of reduced strength. Compare HYPERSTHENIA.

**hypatonia** \hī′pətō′nē·ə\ HYPOTONIA.

**hypaxial** \hīpak′sē·əl\ **1** Below the axis of the vertebral column, usually with reference to quadrupedal forms, fish, etc.; ventral. **2** Below any axis.

**hypencephalon** \hī′pensef′əlän\ [HYP- + ENCEPHALON] The midbrain, pons, and medulla oblongata. *Obs.*

**hyper-** \hī′pər-\ [Gk (akin to English *over* and L *super*) over, above] A prefix meaning (1) over, above; (2) increased, excessive, too much or too many, above the normal. Compare HYPO-.

**hyperacidity** \-asid′itē\ [HYPER- + ACIDITY] Any condition characterized by a higher than normal concentration or quantity of acid. Also *peracidity.* **gastric h.** The secretion of increased amounts of acid by the stomach.

**hyperactivity** \-aktiv′itē\ Excessive activity especially as a part of minimal brain dysfunction. Also *hyperdynamia, hyperenergia, hyperergasia, hyperfunction.*

**hyperacuity** \-əkyoo′itē\ [HYPER- + ACUITY] Increased sharpness of sense perception.

**hyperacusis** \-əkoo′sis\ [HYPER- + -ACUSIS] A condition in which sounds are perceived as unduly loud. Also *hyperacusia.*

**hyperacute** \-əkyoot′\ Exceptionally acute or of explosive onset.

**hyperadiposis** \-ad′ipō′sis\ OBESITY.

**hyperadiposity** \-ad′ipäs′itē\ OBESITY.

**hyperadrenal** \-adrē′nəl\ [HYPER- + ADRENAL] Marked by excessive function or secretion of the adrenal, especially of the adrenal cortex; hyperadrenocortical.

**hyperadrenalemia** \-adrē′nəlē′mē·ə\ HYPEREPINEPHRINEMIA.

**hyperadrenalism** \-adrē′nəlizm\ [HYPERADRENAL + -ISM] Any excessive function of the adrenal gland, especially hyperadrenocorticism. *Imprecise.* Also *hyperadrenia* (outmoded).

**hyperadrenocortical** \-adrē′nōkôr′tikəl\ Of, caused by, or relating to hyperadrenocorticism.

**hyperadrenocorticism** \-adrē′nōkôr′tisizm\ The clinical condition induced by excessive amounts of glucocorticoids, either due to oversecretion of cortisol by the adrenal cortex in Cushing syndrome (hypercortisolism) or to long-term administration of any corticosteroid during treatment, as for an allergic or inflammatory disease. Also *hyperadrenocorticalism, hypercorticalism, hypercorticism.*

**hyperaemia** *Brit.* HYPEREMIA.

**hyperaeration** \-erā′shən\ [HYPER- + AERATION] HYPERVENTILATION.

**hyperaesthesia** *Brit.* HYPERESTHESIA.

**hyperalbuminemia** \-albyoo′minē′mē·ə\ A greater than normal concentration of albumin in plasma. Also *hyperalbuminosis, polyemia hyperalbuminosa.*

**hyperalcoholemia** \-al′kəhōlē′mē·ə\ ALCOHOLEMIA.

**hyperaldosteronemia** \-aldäs′tərōnē′mē·ə\ [HYPER- + *aldosteron(e)* + -EMIA] A greater than normal concentration of aldosterone in plasma.

**hyperaldosteronism** \-aldäs′tərōnizm\ ALDOSTERONISM.

**hyperaldosteronuria** \-aldäs′tərōnoo′rē·ə\ Excess excretion of aldosterone in the urine, associated with any condition that increases aldosterone secretion by the adrenal cortex.

**hyperalgesia** \-aljē′zē·ə\ [Gk *hyperalgēs* (from HYPER- + *algēs(is)* sense of pain, from *algein* to feel pain) suffering excessively + -IA] Excessive sensitivity to painful stimuli. Also *hyperalgia.* Adj. hyperalgesic, hyperalgetic. **auditory h.** A condition of the ear in which pain is experienced in response to auditory stimuli insufficiently intense to cause pain in the normal subject.

**hyperalgia** \-al′jə\ [HYPER- + -ALGIA] HYPERALGESIA.

**hyperalimentation** \-al′iməntā′shən\ Administration of nutritive substances in quantities exceeding the normal requirements of the individual; superalimentation. • *Hyperalimentation* is usually used to refer specifically to parenteral hyperalimentation or total parenteral nutrition. **parenteral h.** The intravenous administration of greater than the normally optimal amounts of essential nutrients. See also TOTAL PARENTERAL NUTRITION.

**hyperalimented** \-al′imen′tid\ Having received total parenteral nutrition.

**hyperaminoacidemia** \-am′inō·as′idē′mē·ə\ The presence of amino acids in the blood in greater than normal concentration.

**hyperaminoaciduria** \-am′inō·as′idoo′rē·ə\ Excess urinary excretion of amino acids, either specific or general. It is usually related to chronic nephritis or to specific defects in tubular reabsorption, as in the Fanconi syndrome.

**hyperammonemia** \-am′ənē′mē·ə\ [HYPER- + *ammon(ium)* + -EMIA] A greater than normal concentration of ammonium in plasma, commonly observed in patients with decompensation of liver function. Also *ammonemia.*

**hyperammonuria** \-am′ənoo′rē·ə\ Excess urinary excretion of ammonia, usually as a compensatory response to systemic acidosis.

**hyperamylasemia** \-am′ilāsē′mē·ə\ A greater than normal activity of amylase in plasma, as is commonly observed in acute pancreatitis. Also *diastemia.*

**hyperaphia** \-ā′fē·ə\ [HYPER- + Gk *(h)aph(ē)* a touching, touch + -IA] Increased sensitivity to touch. Also *hyperaphy, tactile hyperesthesia, hyperpselaphesia, oxyaphia.* Adj. hyperaphic.

**hyperazotemia** \-az′ōtē′mē·ə\ AZOTEMIA.

**hyperbaric** \-bar′ik\ [Gk *hyperbar(ys)* (from HYPER- + *barys* heavy) exceedingly heavy + -IC] At greater than atmospheric pressure.

**hyperbarism** \-bar′izm\ [*hyperbar(ic)* + -ISM] Any condition caused by exposure of the body to excessive ambient pressures, including adverse effects on body fluids, tissues, and cavities. An example is oxygen toxicity.

**hyperbetaalaninemia** \-bā′tə·al′əninē′mē·ə\ A rare, severe, inborn error of alanine metabolism presumably due to a deficiency of $\beta$-alanine-$\alpha$-ketoglutarate aminotransferase. The condition's profound mental retardation and seizures are accompanied by an abnormal accumulation of alanine and $\gamma$-aminobutyric acid in the plasma and the urine.

**hyperbetalipoproteinemia** \-bā′təlip′ōprō′tēnē′mē·ə\ Elevated concentration of $\beta$-lipoproteins in the blood. **familial h.** FAMILIAL HYPERCHOLESTEROLEMIA.

**hyperbicarbonatemia** \-bīkär′bōnətē′mē·ə\ An elevated concentration of bicarbonate in the blood or blood serum. Also *bicarbonatemia.*

**hyperbilirubinemia** \-bil′iroo′binē′mē·ə\ [HYPER- + BILIRUBIN + -EMIA] An increased concentration of bilirubin in the blood or blood serum, causing jaundice when sufficiently increased. **h. I** GILBERT SYNDROME. **con-**

**genital h.** CRIGLER-NAJJAR SYNDROME. **constitutional h.** GILBERT SYNDROME. **hereditary nonhemolytic h.** GILBERT SYNDROME.

**hyperblastosis** \-blastō′sis\ HYPERPLASIA.

**hyperbrachycephaly** \-brak′ēsef′əlē\ An abnormally great degree of brachycephaly, with a cephalic index exceeding 85.

**hypercalcemia** \-kalsē′mē·ə\ [HYPER- + CALC- + -EMIA] An elevated concentration of calcium in the blood or blood serum. Also *hypercalcinemia.* **idiopathic h.** A rare disease of infants, with symptoms of failure to thrive, constipation, thirst, and dehydration. A characteristic elfin facies is described. Serum calcium is raised and blood urea is high. Cardiac lesions such as aortic and pulmonary stenosis are often present. The disorder is thought to be due to an abnormal sensitivity to vitamin D. Few cases have been seen since about 1960.

**hypercalcinemia** \-kal′sinē′mē·ə\ HYPERCALCEMIA.

**hypercalcinuria** \-kal′sinoo′rē·ə\ HYPERCALCIURIA.

**hypercalcitoninemia** \-kal′sitō′ninē′mē·ə\ The presence of excessive calcitonin in the blood, as in the Sipple syndrome or multiple endocrine neoplasia type II. Detection of this abnormality is used as early evidence of dysfunction of the thyroidal parafollicular cells before a definite medullary carcinoma develops. Blood calcitonin concentrations are also raised, that is, above 100–200 pg/ml, in hypercalcemic states, oat cell carcinoma of the lung, carcinoma of the breast, and chronic renal disease.

**hypercalciuria** \-kal′siyoo′rē·ə\ [HYPER- + CALCIURIA] Excretion in the urine of more than 200 mg calcium per day on a diet containing 400 mg calcium per day. Nephrolithiasis is a common complication while nephrocalcinosis also may occur. Hypercalciuria may occur whenever hypercalcemia due to any cause is present. It may occur without hypercalcemia in renal tubular acidosis, normocalcemic hyperparathyroidism, or in an idiopathic form. Mechanisms for hypercalciuria include resorptive, absorptive, and renal hypercalciurias. Also *hypercalcinuria.* **absorptive h.** Hypercalciuria in which the primary mechanism is excessive absorption of calcium from the intestines, most commonly in primary or idiopathic hyperabsorption of calcium, but also in sarcoidosis and hypervitaminosis D. **idiopathic h.** Hypercalciuria either from idiopathic hyperabsorption of calcium for the intestines or idiopathic decreased renal tubular absorption of calcium. **renal h.** Hypercalciuria in which the primary mechanism is reduction of renal tubular reabsorption of calcium. The idiopathic form is the most common. Renal hypercalciuria also occurs in untreated renal tubular acidosis and in treated hyperparathyroidism. **resorptive h.** Hypercalciuria in which the primary mechanism is excess mobilization of skeletal calcium, as in primary hyperparathyroidism, malignancy of the bone, or in the active phases of degenerative bone diseases. **secondary h.** Hypercalciuria due to known causes such as primary hyperparathyroidism, renal tubular acidosis, bone malignancy, sarcoidosis, or hypervitaminosis D.

**hypercapnia** \-kap′nē·ə\ [HYPER- + CAPN- + -IA] An elevated concentration of carbon dioxide in the blood. Also *hypercarbia.*

**hypercapnic** \-kap′nik\ Relating to or characterized by hypercapnia.

**hypercarbia** \-kär′bē·ə\ HYPERCAPNIA.

**hypercarotenemia** \-kar′ətinē′mē·ə\ An elevated concentration of carotene in the blood or blood serum. The condition arises when one regularly eats very large amounts of foods rich in carotenoids, such as carrots. The plasma becomes orange-yellow and the skin can become tinged with the same color. It can be distinguished from jaundice as the eyes do not become yellow. The condition is benign, since vitamin A is not formed in toxic amounts in the body, and the skin reverts to its normal color on reducing the in take of carotenoids. Also *hypercarotenosis, aurantiasis, carotenemia* (imprecise), *carotinemia* (imprecise), *carotenosis, carotinosis, xanthemia.*

**hypercatabolism** \-kətab′əlizm\ A state of abnormally excessive breakdown of complex compounds into simpler substances.

**hypercellularity** \-sel′yəler′itē\ An increase in the number of cells within a structure such as the bone marrow or the renal glomeruli. Adj. hypercellular. **glomerular h.** An increase in the number of cells of the renal glomerulus caused by proliferation of intrinsic cells as well as infiltration by inflammatory cells. It is characteristic of certain forms of glomerulonephritis.

**hypercementosis** \-sē′mentō′sis\ [HYPER- + CEMENTOSIS] CEMENTOSIS.

**hyperchloremia** \-klôrē′mē·ə\ An elevated concentration of chloride in the blood or blood serum. Also *chloridemia.*

**hyperchloremic** \-klôrē′mik\ Relating to or characterized by hyperchloremia.

**hyperchlorhydria** \-klôrhid′rē·ə\ [HYPER- + CHLORHYDRIA] Excessive gastric secretion of hydrochloric acid, seen particularly in duodenal ulcer disease and the Zollinger-Ellison syndrome. Also *Rossbach's disease, hyperhydrochloria.*

**hyperchloridation** \-klôr′īdā′shən\ The creation of a state of excessive blood chloride content by the administration of sodium chloride.

**hyperchloruria** \-klôroo′rē·ə\ [HYPER- + *chlor(ide)* + -URIA] Excretion of greater than normal amounts of chloride in the urine. In general, chloride excretion approximates its intake, and parallels that of sodium. Hyperchloruria may be associated with excess chloride intake, diuretics, or spontaneous diuresis.

**hypercholesteremia** \-kōles′tərē′mē·ə\ HYPERCHOLESTEROLEMIA.

**hypercholesteremic** \-kōles′tərē′mik\ HYPERCHOLESTEROLEMIC.

**hypercholesterolemia** \-kōles′tərōlē′mē·ə\ [HYPER- + CHOLESTEROLEMIA] An elevated concentration of cholesterol in the blood or blood serum. Also *hypercholesterinemia, hypercholesteremia, cholesteremia, cholesterinemia.* **essential h.** FAMILIAL HYPERLIPOPROTEINEMIA TYPE III. **familial h.** A hereditary disorder of lipid metabolism of autosomal dominant transmittance, characterized by cutaneous and tendon xanthomas, premature arcus corneae, recurrent polyarthritis, accelerated atherosclerosis, and myocardial infarction in the fourth or fifth decade of life. Heterozygotes are relatively common, with a frequency of 1 in 500. The rare homozygotes have a qualitatively similar, but much more severe, condition, and often die in their teens. There is a marked increase in cholesterol of the low density lipoprotein (LDL) fraction. Serum concentration of high density lipoprotein is reduced. The disorder is due to a mutation in the LDL receptor of cell membranes, resulting in a functional deficiency of LDL receptors. Also *familial hyperlipoproteinemia type IIa, familial hyperbetalipoproteinemia, LDL-receptor disorder.*

**hypercholesterolemic** \-kōles′tərōlē′mik\ **1** Having a greater than normal cholesterol concentration: said of a blood specimen. **2** Denoting a person who has hypercholesterolemic blood. For defs. 1 and 2 also *hypercholesteremic.*

**hypercholesterolia** \-kōles′tərō′lyə\ Excessive cholesterol in bile.

**hypercholia** \-kō′lyə\ [Gk *hyperchol(os)* (from HYPER- + *cholē* bile) overcharged with bile + -IA] Excessive bile secretion.
**hyperchondroplasia** \-kän′drəplā′zhə\ [HYPER- + CHONDROPLASIA] The excessive formation of cartilage.
**hyperchromaffinism** \-krōmaf′inizm\ A disorder characterized by excessive secretion of chromaffin substances (sympathicomimetic agents) and associated with paroxysmal hypertension.
**hyperchromasia** \-krōmā′zhə\ HYPERCHROMATISM.
**hyperchromatic** \-krōmat′ik\ Characterized by intense coloration, either from natural pigments or from strong affinity for colored dyes. Also *hyperchromic.*
**hyperchromatin** \-krō′mətin\ Chromatin which stains with a blue aniline dye.
**hyperchromatism** \-krō′mətizm\ [HYPER- + CHROMAT- + -ISM] The increased or excessive staining capacity of a structure such as the nuclei of cancer cells, which stain excessively with hematoxylin owing to their increased nucleic acid (chromosomal) content. Also *hyperchromasia, hyperchromia.*
**hyperchromatopsia** \-krō′mətäp′sē·ə\ [HYPER- + CHROMAT- + -OPSIA] A disorder of visual perception in which everything the individual sees is colored or abnormally colored.
**hyperchromatosis** \-krō′mətō′sis\ Increased avidity for a stain. *Seldom used.*
**hyperchromia** \-krō′mē·ə\ **1** HYPERCHROMATISM. **2** The more intense staining, in blood films, of macrocytes when compared with normal erythrocytes. Also *macrocytic hyperchromia.* • The term in this latter sense has been used on analogy with *hypochromia,* but seldom. **macrocytic h.** HYPERCHROMIA.
**hyperchromic** \-krō′mik\ HYPERCHROMATIC.
**hyperchromicity** \-krōmis′itē\ An increase in the absorption of ultraviolet light by solutions of polynucleotides due to a loss of the secondary structure. The secondary structure can be lost as the nucleotide "melts" due to heating.
**hyperchylia** \-kī′lyə\ [HYPER- + CHYL- + -IA] GASTRIC HYPERSECRETION.
**hyperchylomicronemia** \-kī′lōmī′krənē′mē·ə\ CHYLOMICRONEMIA. **familial h.** FAMILIAL HYPERLIPOPROTEINEMIA TYPE I.
**hypercitruria** \-sitroo′rē·ə\ [HYPER- + *citr(ate)* + -URIA] Increased urinary excretion of citrate in alkalosis. The increased citrate enhances calcium solubility and thus may decrease or prevent calcium precipitation in urine and renal parenchyma.
**hypercoria** \-kôr′ē·ə\ HYPERKORIA.
**hypercorticalism** \-kôr′tikəlizm\ HYPERADRENOCORTICISM.
**hypercorticism** \-kôr′tisizm\ HYPERADRENOCORTICISM.
**hypercortisolism** \-kôr′tisəlizm\ The condition resulting from excessive endogenous production of cortisol or administration of exogenous cortisol or its congeners; hyperadrenocorticism.
**hypercryesthesia** \-krī′esthē′zhə\ [HYPER- + CRY- + -ESTHESIA] Extreme sensitivity to cold. Also *hypercryalgesia.*
**hypercupremia** \-kʸooprē′mē·ə\ [HYPER- + CUPR- + -EMIA] A greater than normal concentration of copper in blood.
**hypercupriuria** \-kʸoo′prēyoo′rē·ə\ Excretion of greater than usual amounts of copper in the urine. Hypercupriuria is a characteristic of hepatolenticular disease, and reflects the excess accumulation of copper in the body in this disease.
**hypercyanotic** \-sī·ənät′ik\ Characterized by extreme cyanosis.
**hypercyesis** \-sī·ē′sis\ SUPERFETATION.
**hypercythemia** \-sīthē′mē·ə\ ERYTHROCYTOSIS.
**hyperdactyly** \-dak′tilē\ POLYDACTYLY.
**hyperdiastole** \-dī·as′təlē\ Extreme dilatation of the heart during diastole. Also *hyperdiastoly.*
**hyperdicrotism** \-dik′rətizm\ A state of exaggerated dicrotism.
**hyperdiploid** \-dip′loid\ Having a chromosome complement slightly in excess of that found in the usual diploid state of a cell or an organism.
**hyperdipsia** \-dip′sē·ə\ Increased thirst and consequently an increased consumption of fluids.
**hyperdontia** \-dän′shə\ [HYPER- + *-(o)dontia*] POLYDONTIA.
**hyperdynamia** \-dīnam′ē·ə\ HYPERACTIVITY.
**hypereccrisia** \-əkris′ē·ə\ A state marked by excessive excretion. Also *hypereccrisis.*
**hyperechoic** \-ekō′ik\ [HYPER- + ECHOIC] Producing echoes of higher amplitude or density than the surrounding medium.
**hyperelastic** \-ilas′tik\ Characterized by an unusually increased state of elasticity.
**hyperemesis** \-em′əsis\ [HYPER- + EMESIS] Excessive or severe, protracted vomiting. **h. gravidarum** Excessive and persistent vomiting associated with pregnancy, usually experienced during the first trimester.
**hyperemetic** \-emet′ik\ Relating to or characterized by hyperemesis.
**hyperemia** \-ē′mē·ə\ [Gk *hyperaim(ein)* (from HYPER- + *(h)aima* blood) to be over-full of blood + -IA] An increase in the volume of blood in an affected part or tissue due to arterial or arteriolar dilatation. **active h.** Increase of blood flow to a segment of the body through vascular dilatation. **arterial h.** Increase in blood flow due to arterial dilatation. **Bier's passive h.** BIER'S TREATMENT. **collateral h.** A compensatory increase in arterial blood flow through preexisting collateral vessels as a consequence of the interruption of blood flow through the main artery supplying a part. **constriction h.** Passive hyperemia induced by a constriction, as by application of a tourniquet. Also *stauungs hyperemia.* See also BIER'S TREATMENT. **passive h.** An increase of blood in an area or part resulting from an obstruction to the blood's outflow path. **reactive h.** An increase of blood in a region following the restoration of the blood supply after a period of temporary arrest. **stauungs h.** CONSTRICTION HYPEREMIA.
**hyperendemic** \-endem′ik\ Endemic to a high degree; so prevalent and persistent in an area that the inhabitants are in effect exposed from birth, as can occur, for example, with malaria in certain regions or with yellow fever in some of the foci of that disease. Also *holoendemic.*
**hyperendocrinism** \-endäk′rinizm\ Excessive secretion of a hormone by an endocrine gland, or the condition resulting from it. Also *hyperhormonism.*
**hyperenergia** \-enur′jə\ HYPERACTIVITY.
**hypereosinophilia** \-ē′ōsinəfil′yə\ A marked increase in the number of eosinophils in the blood, often to $1 \times 10^9$ per liter or more.
**hyperepinephrinemia** \-ep′inef′rinē′mē·ə\ A greater than normal concentration of epinephrine in blood. Also *hyperadrenalemia.*
**hypererethism** \-er′əthism\ HYPERSENSITIVITY.
**hyperergasia** \-ərgā′zhə\ HYPERACTIVITY.
**hypererythrocythemia** \-irith′rəsīthē′mē·ə\ [HYPER- + *erythrocyt(e)* + -HEMIA] ERYTHROCYTOSIS.
**hyperesophoria** \-es′ōfôr′ē·ə\ [HYPER- + ESO- + PHO-

RIA] A combination of vertical and inward latent deviations of the eyes with respect to each other.

**hyperesthesia** \-esthē′zhə\ [HYPER- + ESTHESIA] Exaggerated sensibility. According to the organ or sensory pathway affected, hyperesthesia may be acoustic (auditory), gustatory, olfactory, optic, sexual, or tactile. Also *oxyesthesia.* Adj. hyperesthesic. **acoustic h.** DYSACUSIS. **auditory h.** DYSACUSIS. **gustatory h.** HYPERGEUSIA. **olfactory h.** HYPEROSMIA. **optic h.** A heightened sensitivity of the eye to brightness.

**hyperestrinemia** \-es′trinē′mē·ə\ HYPERESTROGENEMIA.

**hyperestrinism** \-es′trinizm\ HYPERESTROGENISM.

**hyperestrogenemia** \-es′trōjənē′mēə\ An increased concentration of estrogens in the blood or blood serum. Also *hyperestrinemia.*

**hyperestrogenism** \-es′trəjənizm\ A condition resulting from excessive estrogen secretion or exogenous administration of estrogens. Also *hyperestrinism, hyperfolliculinism.*

**hyperexophoria** \-ek′səfôr′ē·ə\ [HYPER- + EXOPHORIA] A combination of vertical and outward latent deviations of the eyes with respect to each other.

**hyperexplexia** \-eksplek′sē·ə\ Excessive jerking or jumping of the limbs and trunk on being startled.

**hyperextension** \-iksten′shən\ The excessive extension of a limb or a joint. Also *superextension.*

**hyperferremia** \-ferē′mē·ə\ [HYPER- + L *ferr(um)* iron + -EMIA] An increased concentration of iron in the blood or blood serum. Also *hyperferricemia.*

**hyperfibrinogenemia** \-fī′brinōjənē′mē·ə\ Increase in the concentration of plasma fibrinogen above normal.

**hyperfibrinolysis** \-fī′brinäl′isis\ Excessive fibrinolysis. **systemic h.** A coagulation disorder characterized by poor clot formation, rapid clot dissolution, and low plasma fibrinogen. It is the result of enhanced activity of plasma fibrinolysins and is considered part of the disorder of disseminated intravascular coagulation.

**hyperflexion** \-flek′shən\ An excessive flexion of a limb or a joint. Also *superflexion, overflexion.*

**hyperfolliculinism** \-fōlik′yələnizm\ [HYPER- + *folliculin* + -ISM] HYPERESTROGENISM.

**hyperfunction** HYPERACTIVITY.

**hypergalactia** \-gəlak′shə\ [HYPER- + GALACT- + -IA] Excessive secretion of breast milk. Also *hypergalactosis.* Adj. hypergalactous.

**hypergammaglobulinemia** \-gam′əgläb′yəlinē′mē·ə\ [HYPER- + *gamma globulin* + -EMIA] A greater than normal concentration of IgG immunoglobulin in blood, plasma, or serum. **M-component h.** Hypergammaglobulinemia due to an excess of monoclonal immunoglobulin.

**hypergenitalism** \-jen′ətəlizm\ Excessive growth or activity of the sexual organs: used especially in reference to precocious puberty.

**hypergeusia** \-joo′sē·ə\ [HYPER- + Gk *geus(is)* taste + -IA] Heightened taste perception. Also *gustatory hyperesthesia, hypergeusesthesia.*

**hypergigantosoma** \-jīgan′təsō′mə\ [HYPER- + GIGANTO- + Gk *sōma* body] *Older term* GIGANTISM.

**hyperglandular** \-glan′dyələr\ Of or characterized by excessive glandular secretion or size.

**hyperglobulia** \-glōbyoo′lē·ə\ [HYPER- + *globul(e)* + -IA] POLYCYTHEMIA VERA.

**hyperglobulinemia** \-gläb′yəlinē′mē·ə\ An elevated concentration of globulin in the blood or blood serum.

**hyperglobulism** \-gläb′yəlizm\ POLYCYTHEMIA VERA.

**hypergluconeogenesis** \-gloo′kōnē·ōjen′əsis\ [HYPER- + GLUCO- + NEOGENESIS] Excessive formation of carbohydrate from amino acids or fatty acids, a characteristic of hyperadrenocorticism. *Seldom used.* Also *hyperglyconeogenesis.*

**hyperglycaemia** *Brit.* HYPERGLYCEMIA.

**hyperglycemia** \-glīsē′mē·ə\ [HYPER- + GLYCEMIA] A greater than normal concentration of glucose in blood. Also *hyperglycosemia, hyperglycoplasmia.*

**hyperglycemic** \-glīsē′mik\ 1 Pertaining to, characterized by, or resulting from hyperglycemia. 2 Capable of increasing blood glucose concentration.

**hyperglyceridemia** \-glis′əridē′mē·ə\ [HYPER- + *glycerid(e)* + -EMIA] An increased concentration of glycerides, especially triglycerides, in the blood or serum.

**hyperglyceridemic** \-glis′əridē′mik\ 1 Pertaining to, characterized by, or resulting from hyperglyceridemia. 2 Capable of increasing blood glyceride concentration.

**hyperglycinemia** \-glī′sinē′mē·ə\ A congenital metabolic disorder marked by high blood levels of glycine and occurring in two forms, the ketotic form and the nonketotic form. The ketotic form is secondary to a number of organic acidemias, such as methylmalonic acidemia. The nonketotic form is due to a specific enzyme deficit. Patients show mental retardation, failure to thrive, and seizures but do not have episodic ketosis with neutropenia and thrombocytopenia, as in the ketotic form. Also *glycinemia.* **ketotic h.** The association of an elevated concentration of glycine in the plasma and urine with a presence of organic acids in the plasma. It occurs in several inborn errors of organic acid metabolism, especially the proprionic acidemias. **nonketotic h.** An autosomal recessive inborn error of glycine metabolism characterized by mental retardation, seizures, hypotonia, and lethargy, with onset and often death in infancy. The presumed basic defect is in glycine decarboxylation, perhaps in the enzyme glycine formiminotransferase.

**hyperglycinuria** [HYPER- + GLYCINURIA] GLYCINURIA.

**hyperglyconeogenesis** \-glī′kōnē′ōjen′əsis\ HYPERGLUCONEOGENESIS.

**hyperglycoplasmia** \-glī′kōplaz′mē·ə\ HYPERGLYCEMIA.

**hyperglycorrhachia** \-glī′kôrā′kē·ə\ [HYPER- + GLYCO- + -RRHACHIA] An abnormally high glucose content of the cerebrospinal fluid.

**hyperglycosemia** \-glī′kōsē′mē·ə\ HYPERGLYCEMIA.

**hyperglyoxylemia** \-glī·äk′silē′mē·ə \ Greater than normal concentration of glyoxylate in plasma, as may occur in thiamine deficiency.

**hypergonadism** \-gō′nədizm\ [HYPER- + GONAD + -ISM ] A condition resulting from untimely or excessive secretion of sex hormones by the gonads, and characterized by abnormally great somatic growth and precocious puberty.

**hypergonadotropic** \-gō′nədōträp′ik\ Having or characterized by excessive secretion of gonadotropic hormone or hormones, as in the hypergonadotropic eunuchoidism of the Klinefelter syndrome. Also *hypergonadotrophic.*

**hypergonia** \-gō′nē·ə\ The increased gonial angle of the mandible.

**hypergranulation** \-gran′yəlā′shən\ **juxtaglomerular cell h.** Abnormal increase in granules in juxtaglomerular cells reflecting renin hypersecretion and storage, often associated with hyperplasia and hypertrophy of the cells, and with large distorted nuclei.

**hyperguanidinemia** \-gwan′idinē′mē·ə\ Greater than normal concentration of guanidine in plasma.

**hyperhemoglobinemia** \-hē′mōglō′binē′mē·ə\ HEMOGLOBINEMIA.

**hyperhemolytic** \-hē′məlit′ik\ HEMOLYTIC.

**hyperheparinemia** \-hep′ərinē′mē·ə\ Greater than normal concentration of heparin in plasma, as occurs during therapeutic administration of heparin to prevent or retard formation of clots in blood vessels.

**hyperhidrosis** \-hidrō′sis\ [HYPER- + HIDROSIS] A state of increased sweating. Also *hidrorrhea, hyperidrosis, hydropedesis, polyhidrosis.* Adj. hyperhidrotic. **gustatory h.** AURICULOTEMPORAL SYNDROME. **h. unilateralis** HEMIHYPERHIDROSIS.

**hyperhistaminemia** \-his′təminē′mē·ə\ Very high concentration of histamine in blood or serum.

**hyperhormonism** \-hôr′mōnizm\ HYPERENDOCRINISM.

**hyperhydration** \-hidrā′shən\ [HYPER- + HYDRATION] A greater than normal amount of water in the body or any tissue.

**hyperhydrochloria** \-hī′drəklôr′ē·ə\ HYPERCHLORHYDRIA.

**hyperhypnosis** \-hipnō′sis\ [HYPER- + HYPNOSIS] HYPERSOMNIA.

**hyperhypophysism** \-hīpäf′isizm\ [HYPER- + *hypophys(is)* + -ISM] *Rare* HYPERPITUITARISM.

**hyperidrosis** \-īdrō′sis\ HYPERHIDROSIS.

**hyperimmune** \-imyoon′\ Having a high degree of immunity: usually said of an animal that has been repeatedly immunized.

**hyperimmunization** \-im′yənīzā′shən\ The induction of a high level of antibodies in the serum, especially by the administration of successive booster doses of antigen for the production of therapeutic antisera, as in horses and other animals. Also *hypervaccination.* **maternal h.** Hyperimmunization in a pregnant or postpartum mammalian female marked by increasing levels of circulating antibody and having the effect of ensuring that sufficient protection is passed from mother to offspring *in utero* via the placenta or to her nursing young via colostrum.

**hyperimmunoglobulinemia** \-im′yənōgläb′yəlinē′mē·ə\ An increase in immunoglobulin concentration of serum.

**hyperindicanemia** \-in′dik′ənē′mē·ə\ A very high concentration of indican in the blood.

**hyperinflation** \-inflā′shən\ An abnormal degree of distension of the lungs with air.

**hyperinnervation** \-in′ərvā′shən\ Abnormal, functionally effective connection of more than one axon with a given extrafusal muscle fiber, i.e., inclusion of the fiber in two or more motor units.

**hyperinsulinemia** \-in′sʸəlinē′mē·ə\ A very high concentration of insulin in the blood.

**hyperinsulinism** \-in′sʸəlinizm\ [HYPER- + INSULIN + -ISM] Abnormally increased secretion of insulin by the pancreatic islets, leading to hypoglycemia. **alimentary h.** Excess release of insulin following food ingestion, a postulated cause of reactive or functional hypoglycemia. **functional h.** Hyperinsulinism characterized by hypoglycemic attacks provoked by carbohydrate ingestion, not by the fasting state. Pancreatic islet cell adenoma is absent. **iatrogenic h.** Insulin overdosage resulting in hypoglycemia. The relative overdose may be due to error in insulin administration, failure to ingest a meal at the proper time, faulty timing of insulin dosage, brittle diabetes, or from unknown cause. The deliberate induction of hypoglycemic coma for treatment of schizophrenia is now obsolete.

**hyperinvolution** \-in′vəloo′shən\ [HYPER- + INVOLUTION] Excessive postpartum involution of the uterus of a nursing mother, resulting in a very small uterus. Also *superinvolution.*

**hyperiodemia** \-ī′ōdē′mē·ə\ [HYPER- + IOD- + -EMIA] A high concentration of iodide in blood or plasma or serum, for example a serum protein-bound iodine concentration in excess of 8 mg/100 ml.

**hyperirritability** \-ir′itəbil′itē\ A state of excessive reactivity or responsiveness to stimuli either from the internal or the external environments.

**hyperisotonic** \-ī′sōtän′ik\ [HYPER- + ISOTONIC] HYPERTONIC.

**hyperisotonicity** \-ī′sōtənis′itē\ HYPERTONICITY.

**hyperkalemia** \-kəlē′mē·ə\ [HYPER- + New L *kal(ium)* potassium + -EMIA] A high concentration of potassium in plasma, such as a concentration greater than 5 mEq/l. Also *hyperpotassemia, potassemia.* Also *hyperkaliemia.*

**hyperkaliemia** \-kal′i·ē′mē·ə\ HYPERKALEMIA.

**hyperkaluria** \-kəloo′rēə\ [HYPER- + New L *kal(ium)* potassium + -URIA] KALURESIS.

**hyperkeratinization** \-ker′ətin′īzā′shən\ HYPERKERATOSIS.

**hyperkeratosis** \-ker′ətō′sis\ [HYPER- + KERATOSIS] An excessive thickening of the horny layer of the epidermis. Also *hyperkeratinization.* Adj. hyperkeratotic. **bullous ichthyosiform h.** BULLOUS ICHTHYOSIFORM ERYTHRODERMA. **h. congenitalis palmaris et plantaris** PALMOPLANTAR KERATODERMA. **diffuse congenital h.** ICHTHYOSIS CONGENITA. **epidermolytic h.** Any of several forms of bullous ichthyotic skin disorders sharing onset prenatally or in early infancy and autosomal dominant inheritance. They include a generalized form (bullous ichthyosiform erythroderma) and a localized form (ichthyosis hystrix). **follicular h.** KERATOSIS PILARIS. **h. lacunaris pharyngis** KERATOSIS PHARYNGIS. **h. subungualis** Epithelial hyperplasia of the tissues beneath the nail plate. It is commonly seen in psoriasis and local chronic inflammatory conditions.

**hyperketonemia** \-kē′tōnē′mē·ə\ Very high concentration of ketones in plasma or serum, as in uncontrolled severe diabetes mellitus.

**hyperketonuria** \-kē′tōnoo′rē·ə\ KETONURIA.

**hyperkinemia** \-kīnē′mē·ə\ [HYPER- + KIN- + -EMIA ] A condition in which there is abnormally high blood flow.

**hyperkinemic** \-kīnē′mik\ **1** Characterized by or causing an abnormally high volume of blood flow. **2** An agent that increases the volume of blood flow.

**hyperkinesia** \-kīnē′zhə\ [HYPER- + KINESIA] **1** Abnormally intense motor activity, often associated with agitation. **2** Certain recurring or continuous involuntary movements seen in disease of the central nervous system, such as chorea and athetosis. For defs. 1 and 2 also *hyperkinesis, hyperpraxia.*

**hyperkinetic** \-kinet′ik\ **1** Characterized by abnormally intense motor activity, often associated with agitation; overactive. **2** Able to stimulate movements.

**hyperkoria** \-kôr′ē·ə\ [Gk *hyperkor(ēs)* (from *koros* satiety) overfull, satiated + -IA ] A feeling of satiety occurring before sufficient food has been consumed to meet the immediate needs of the body. *Seldom used.* Also *hypercoria.*

**hyperlactation** \-laktā′shən\ [HYPER- + LACTATION] Puerperal lactation that persists for a longer than usual time and is thought to be excessive in quantity. Also *superlactation.*

**hyperlacticacidemia** \-lak′tikas′idē′mē·ə\ Very high concentration of lactic acid in plasma.

**hyperlecithinemia** \-les′əithinē′mē·ə\ A greater than normal concentration of lecithin in blood.

**hyperlethal** Exceeding the minimum required for a lethal effect: said of a dosage of a drug or other agent.

**hyperleydigism** \-lī′digizm\ [HYPER- + *Leydig (cells)* + -ISM] Excessive increase in the activity of the Leydig cells of the testes; excessive secretion of testosterone.

**hyperlipaemia** *Brit.* HYPERLIPEMIA.

**hyperlipemia** \-līpē′mē·ə\ HYPERLIPIDEMIA. **essential familial h.** FAMILIAL HYPERLIPOPROTEINEMIA. **retention h.** *Obs.* FAMILIAL HYPERLIPOPROTEINEMIA TYPE I.

**hyperlipidemia** \-lip′idē′mē·ə\ [HYPER- + LIPID + -EMIA] A greater than normal concentration of lipids in blood plasma. Also *hyperlipemia, hyperlipoidemia, hyperliposis, lipemia* (imprecise). **carbohydrate-induced h.** A greater than normal concentration of lipids in the blood, especially of triglycerides, following ingestion of carbohydrates. The phenomenon is characteristic of familial hyperlipoproteinemia types IV and V. Also *carbohydrate-induced hyperlipemia, carbohydrate-induced hypertriglyceridemia.* **combined fat- and carbohydrate-induced h.** A form of hyperlipoproteinemia in which ingestion of fat or carbohydrates results in greater than normal plasma concentration of very low density lipoproteins and persistent chylomicronemia during fasting. **fat-induced h.** Greater than normal concentration of plasma lipids following ingestion of food containing fat. See also FAMILIAL HYPERLIPOPROTEINEMIA TYPE I. **mixed h.** A subtype of familial hyperlipoproteinemia type II, characterized by increased concentrations of serum low density lipoproteins and very low density lipoproteins during fasting. Also *familial hyperlipoproteinemia type IIb.*

**hyperlipoidemia** \-lip′oidē′mē·ə\ HYPERLIPIDEMIA.

**hyperlipoproteinemia** \-lip′ōprō′tēnē′mē·ə\ [HYPER- + LIPOPROTEIN + -EMIA] Greater than normal concentration of lipoprotein in blood, plasma, or serum. **acquired h.** Persistently greater than normal plasma concentration of lipoproteins that is nonhereditary in cause, secondary to some other disorder such as myxedema. **familial h.** Any of several genetic disorders of lipid metabolism characterized by increase in concentration of one or more types of serum lipoprotein. These disorders are classified as hyperlipoproteinemia types I, II, III, IV, and V. Also *essential familial hyperlipemia.* **familial mixed h.** A disorder of lipid metabolism that is of autosomal dominant transmittance in which affected members of a kindred may exhibit different serum lipid abnormalities like those of hyperlipoproteinemia types IIa, IIb, or V. **familial h. type I** A rare hereditary disorder of lipid metabolism, characterized by onset in childhood of xanthomas of skin, abdominal pain and pancreatitis, enlargement of liver and spleen, lipemic retinopathy, accelerated atherosclerosis, lipemic plasma, and marked increase in serum chylomicrons, extreme increase in serum triglycerides, and low concentration of serum cholesterol. Inheritance is autosomal recessive. Two different metabolic defects are responsible: in some families there is a deficiency of the enzyme lipoprotein lipase; in others there is a deficiency of apolipoprotein C-II, a cofactor of lipoprotein lipase, causing a functional deficiency of lipoprotein lipase. Also *familial hyperchylomicronemia, familial hypertriglyceridemia, endogenous hypertriglyceridemia, familial fat-induced hypertriglyceridemia, Bürger-Grütz syndrome, retention hyperlipemia* (obs.). **familial h. type II** Any of a number of disorders of lipid metabolism characterized by elevated serum cholesterol and low density lipoprotein, including familial hypercholesterolemia (type IIa) and mixed hyperlipidemia (type IIb). **familial h. type IIa** FAMILIAL HYPERCHOLESTEROLEMIA. **familial h. type IIb** MIXED HYPERLIPIDEMIA. **familial h. type III** A hereditary disorder of lipid metabolism of autosomal recessive transmittance, characterized by adult onset of cutaneous xanthomas, accelerated atherosclerosis, increase in serum very low density lipoprotein, marked increase in serum cholesterol and triglyceride. The metabolic defect is a deficiency of apoprotein E-3. Also *essential hypercholesterolemia* (outmoded), *xanthoma tuberosum* (outmoded), *xanthoma tuberosum multiplex, dysbetalipoproteinemia, broad-beta disease, floating beta disease.* **familial h. type IV** A disorder of lipid metabolism characterized by elevation of both plasma cholesterol and triglyceride levels secondary to an increase in the very-low density lipoprotein fraction. It occurs in response to a high carbohydrate diet in persons who are sensitive to this form of dietary induction. The genetics and metabolic defect are unknown. Also *familial hyperprebetalipoproteinemia, endogenous hypertriglyceridemia, familial hypertriglyceridemia.* See also CARBOHYDRATE-INDUCED HYPERLIPIDEMIA. **familial h. type V** A disorder of lipid metabolism characterized by adult onset of cutaneous xanthomas, sometimes by pancreatitis, peripheral neuropathy, hyperglycemia or abnormal glucose tolerance, increase in serum chylomicrons and triglycerides and very low density lipoproteins, but decrease in low density and high density lipoproteins. The disorder appears to have autosomal dominant transmittance, but penetrance is often incomplete. The metabolic defect is unknown. Affected relatives in a family may exhibit either type IV or type V hyperlipoproteinemia. A similar acquired lipoprotein abnormality may be seen in diabetes mellitus, alcoholism, nephrotic syndrome, or hypothyroidism.

**hyperliposis** \-lipō′sis\ HYPERLIPIDEMIA.

**hyperlithuria** \-lithoo′rē·ə\ HYPERURICURIA.

**hyperlordosis** \-lôrdō′sis\ An increase in the natural degree of lordosis.

**hyperluteinization** \-loo′tē·inīzā′shən\ **1** A condition in which an excessive number of graafian follicles of the ovary are luteinized, that is, are corpora lutea. **2** Abnormally long persistence of the luteal phase of the ovarian cycle.

**hyperlutemia** \-lootē′mē·ə\ [HYPER- + *lut(eo)-* + -EMIA] HYPERPROGESTERONEMIA.

**hyperlysinuria** \-lī′sinoo′rē·ə\ [HYPER- + *lysin(e)* + -URIA] Increased urinary excretion of lysine, a feature of persistent hyperlysinemia.

**hypermagnesemia** \-mag′nəsē′mē·ə\ An elevated concentration of magnesium in the blood or blood serum. Also *magnesemia.*

**hypermania** \-mā′nē·ə\ DELIRIOUS MANIA.

**hypermature** \-mətyoor′\ **1** Beyond the mature state. **2** Overripe.

**hypermedication** Excessive administration or use of therapeutic agents, either in the number of drugs taken, or in the amounts given.

**hypermegasoma** \-me′gəsō′mə\ [HYPER- + MEGA- + Gk *sōma* body] *Outmoded* GIGANTISM.

**hypermelanosis** \-mel′ənō′sis\ An excess of melanin pigmentation.

**hypermenorrhea** \-men′ôrē′ə\ [HYPER- + MENORRHEA] Frequent menstrual periods or an abnormal increase in the duration and/or amount of menstrual flow. Also *epimenorrhagia, epimenorrhea.*

**hypermetabolism** \-mətab′əlizm\ A state of excessive metabolic activity; an excessively high metabolic rate. **extrathyroidal h.** A state of excessive metabolic activity not attributable to hyperthyroidism.

**hypermetria** \-mē′trē·ə\ [Gk (from HYPER- + *metrein* to measure, reach) a going beyond measure] Motor incoordination such that movements overreach their target, as seen in cerebellar dysfunction. This can be noted in spontaneous movements but is often more obvious in actions rapidly executed on command, as in the finger-nose test or the heel-knee test.

**hypermetrope** \-met′rōp\ HYPEROPE.

**hypermetropia** \-mətrō′pē·ə\ [HYPER- + Gk *metron* a measure, rule, standard + -OPIA] HYPEROPIA.

**hypermetropic** \-məträp′ik\ HYPEROPIC.

**hypermicrosoma** \-mī′krəsō′mə\ Extreme generalized dwarfism.

**hypermimia** \-mim′ē·ə\ ECHOPRAXIA.

**hypermineralization** \-min′ərəlīzā′shən\ Excessive deposit of minerals in the body.

**hypermnesia** \-mnē′zhə\ [HYPER- + Gk *mnēs(is)* remembrance + -IA] Ability to recall material to a greater degree than is usual.

**hypermotility** \-mōtil′itē\ The capability of moving excessively.

**hypermyotonia** \-mī′ətō′nē·ə\ *Seldom used* HYPERTONIA.

**hypermyotrophy** \-mī·ät′rəfē\ A state of excessive muscular development.

**hypernasality** \-nāzal′itē\ The nasal quality imparted to speech when an undue proportion of the airflow passes through the nasal cavity, as may happen in cleft palate, following palatal paralysis, or as a result of surgery. Also *rhinolalia aperta*.

**hypernatremia** \nətrē′mē·ə\ [HYPER- + New L *natr(ium)* sodium + -EMIA] An elevated concentration of sodium in the blood or blood serum. Also *hypernatronemia*.

**hyperneocytosis** \-nē′əsītō′sis\ RETICULOCYTOSIS.

**hypernephroma** \-nefrō′mə\ [HYPER- + NEPHROMA] RENAL CELL CARCINOMA.

**hypernidation** \-nīdā′shən\ [HYPER- + NIDATION] More than one implantation, as in a multiple pregnancy.

**hypernitremia** \-nītrē′mē·ə\ An elevated concentration of nitrogen in the blood or blood serum.

**hypernutrition** \-nyootrish′ən\ [HYPER- + NUTRITION] Overeating or consuming more food than is required to meet the metabolic needs of the body, as a form of therapy. Hypernutrition is sometimes used in treating anorexic conditions by having the subject consume high-protein milk. Also *supernutrition*.

**hyperocclusion** \-äkloo′zhən\ [HYPER- + OCCLUSION] A tooth extrusion which causes premature contact.

**hyperoncotic** \-ängkät′ik\ **1** Marked by oncotic pressure that is greater than normal. **2** Of or relating to excessive swelling.

**hyperonychia** \-ənik′ē·ə\ [HYPER- + ONYCH- + -IA ] The presence of thickened or hypertrophic nails. Also *hyperonychosis*.

**hyperope** \hī′pərōp\ [HYPER- + -OPE] A person with hyperopia; a farsighted person. Also *hypermetrope*.

**hyperopia** \-ō′pē·ə\ [HYPER- + -OPIA] The refractive error in which additional dioptric power obtained by accommodation or by wearing a convex spectacle lens is needed in order to see clearly in the distance. Also *hypermetropia, farsightedness, far sight, long sight, longsightedness*. Adj. hyperopic. **absolute h.** That portion of hyperopia in excess of the amount of available accommodation and therefore uncorrectible by accommodative effort. **axial h.** Hyperopia caused by a relative shortness of the anteroposterior length of the eye. **curvature h.** Hyperopia caused by an increased convexity of the surfaces of the cornea or lens. Also *hyperopia of curvature*. **facultative h.** That portion of hyperopia that can be corrected by accommodative effort. **index h.** Hyperopia due to an increased refractive strength of the lens substance. **latent h.** The portion of hyperopia that cannot be measured without use of a cycloplegic drug for refraction. **manifest h.** The portion of hyperopia that may be readily measured by a noncycloplegic refraction. **relative h.** Hyperopia that induces excessive convergence, resulting in muscle imbalance.

**hyperopic** \-ō′pik\ Of or characterized by hyperopia. Also *hypermetropic, farsighted*.

**hyperorchidism** \-ôr′kidizm\ [HYPER- + *orchid(o)-* + -ISM] An abnormal increase in testicular function.

**hyperorexia** \-órek′sē·ə\ [HYPER- + Gk *orex(is)* a longing for + -IA] BULIMIA.

**hyperornithemia** \-ôr′nithē′mē·ə\ [HYPER- + *ornith(ine)* + -EMIA] A metabolic fault in which an excess of ornithine accumulates within the body. This results in gyrate atrophy of the choroid.

**hyperosmia** \-äz′mē·ə\ [HYPER- + *osm(o)-*[2] + -IA] Abnormally heightened olfactory perception. Also *hyperosphresis, olfactory hyperesthesia*.

**hyperosmolality** \-äz′mōlal′itē\ Having an osmolality greater than normal for body fluids.

**hyperosmolarity** \-äz′mōler′itē\ A state of high molecular density within a solution such that it will absorb water across a semipermeable membrane from a less dense solution.

**hyperosmotic** \-äzmō′tik\ Having a higher concentration of osmotically active solutes than a comparative solution.

**hyperosphresia** \-äsfrē′zhə\ HYPEROSMIA.

**hyperosteogenesis** \-äs′tē·əjen′əsis\ HYPEROSTOSIS.

**hyperostosis** \-ästō′sis\ [HYPER- + OSTOSIS] A hypertrophy of bone, either in the form of a local increase in size, such as an exostosis, or a generalized increase that involves a whole bone. Also *hyperosteogenesis*. **calvarial h.** A generalized irregular thickening of the cortex of the skull. It can take the form of the van Buchem syndrome or hyperostosis frontalis interna. **h. corticalis generalisata** VAN BUCHEM SYNDROME. **flowing h.** MELORHEOSTOSIS. **h. frontalis interna** Calvarial hyperostosis that affects only the inner wall of the frontal bone. It may be associated with obesity and hypertrichosis in middle-aged women. Also *Stewart-Morel syndrome, endocraniosis, Morel syndrome, Morgagni's hyperostosis, Morgagni-Stewart-Morel syndrome, Morgagni's disease, Morgagni syndrome*. **infantile h.** An intermittent inflammatory process characterized by multiple subperiosteal new bone formation points in the long bones, the mandible, and the clavicles, and resulting in swelling of the soft tissues. It is seen in young infants with pyrexia. Also *infantile cortical hyperostosis syndrome, Caffey's disease, Caffey syndrome, Caffey-Silverman syndrome, infantile cortical hyperostosis*. **Morgagni's h.** HYPEROSTOSIS FRONTALIS INTERNA. **senile ankylosing h. of spine** The generalized formation of new bone, with osteophytes most often bridging and forming within the interligamentous structures of the thoracic and upper lumbar vertebrae to produce a marked loss of movement and kyphosis. It is seen primarily in the elderly. Also *senile vertebral ankylosing hyperostosis*.

**hyperovarianism** \-ōver′ē·ənizm\ Excessive ovarian secretion of estrogen at any age. *Rare*.

**hyperoxaluria** \-äk′səloo′re·ə\ [HYPER- + OXALURIA] Increased excretion of oxalate in the urine, often a cause of calcium oxalate nephrolithiasis or nephrocalcinosis, or of chronic interstitial nephritis leading to renal failure. Hyperoxaluria may be genetic (primary), or secondary to ingestion or administration of excess amounts of oxalate precursors, or to intestinal diseases. **primary h.** The progressive deposition of calcium oxalate in the kidneys and other tissues (oxalosis) due to either of two inborn errors of oxalic acid metabolism, oxalosis I or oxalosis II. **primary h. type I** OXALOSIS I. **primary h. type II** OXALOSIS II.

**secondary h.** Increased oxalate in the urine, associated with intestinal disorders such as Crohn's disease or following ileal bypass surgery for obesity.

**hyperoxemia** \-äksē′mē·ə\ [HYPER- + *ox(y)-*$^2$ + -EMIA] Increased or excessive acidity of the blood or blood serum; acidosis.

**hyperoxia** \-äk′sē·ə\ [HYPER- + *ox(ygen)* + -IA] **1** Increased or excessive oxygen concentration. **2** Elevated oxygen tension in blood.

**hyperoxic** \-äk′sik\ Characteristic of, resulting from, or causing hyperoxia.

**hyperparasite** \-par′əsīt\ A parasite whose host is itself a parasite. **second degree h.** A parasite that exists within or preys on a hyperparasite. Complex interactions such as this sometimes occur in connection with biological control efforts involving hyperparasitic or parasitoid wasps, some of which parasitize one another while they are in a primary host, such as a scale insect.

**hyperparasitic** \-par′əsit′ik\ Parasitic upon a parasite. Also *biparasitic, paraneoxenous.*

**hyperparasitism** \-par′əsitizm\ Parasitism in which the host is itself parasitic upon yet another organism. Also *biparasitism, superparasitism.*

**hyperparasitoidism** \-par′əsitoi′dizm\ The phenomenon of a parasitoid preying upon another species of parasitoid.

**hyperparathyroidism** \-per′əthī′roidizm\ [HYPER- + PARATHYROID + -ISM] A condition resulting from excessive secretion of parathyroid hormone by the parathyroid glands, accompanied by hypercalcemia, hypophosphatemia, loss of calcium from bones, renal calculi, and gastrointestinal and mental disturbances. It is caused by hyperplasia, adenoma, and occasionally by a hormone-secreting cancer, as squamous cell carcinoma of the lung. Rarely, it is caused by carcinoma of the parathyroids. **acute h.** Sudden exacerbation of systemic symptoms of hypercalcemia occurring in the course of hyperparathyroidism, as constipation becoming ileus and lethargy coma. **primary h.** Hyperparathyroidism resulting from intrinsic disease of the parathyroid glands. **secondary h.** Excessive secretion of parathyroid hormone by the parathyroid glands in chronic renal insufficiency characterized by high serum phosphate concentration and low, normal, or subnormal calcium value. The cause is assumed to be failure of the diseased kidney to synthesize 1-$\alpha$-25-dihydroxycholecalciferol, the most active form of vitamin D, absence or deficiency of which leads to subnormal absorption of calcium from the gut and relative hypocalcemia, which stimulates parathyroid hormone oversecretion. **tertiary h.** A condition developing in the course of secondary hyperparathyroidism in which, after protracted oversecretion of parathyroid hormone in response to renal failure, the parathyroids become autonomous, and a state virtually identical to primary hyperparathyroidism develops, accompanied by high normal or excessive concentration of serum calcium. Treatment by parathyroidectomy is required.

**hyperpathia** \-path′ē·ə\ [HYPER- + PATH- + -IA] Abnormally enhanced sensitivity to pain, seen particularly in the thalamic syndrome and sometimes in lesions of peripheral nerves or of the spinothalamic tract. The sensation evoked by the painful stimulus is excessive and may persist after removal of the stimulus. Also *oxypathia, oxypathy.* Adj. hyperpathic. **thalamic h.** THALAMIC PAIN.

**hyperpepsia** \-pep′sē·ə\ GASTRIC HYPERSECRETION.

**hyperpepsinemia** \-pep′sinē′mē·ə\ An elevated concentration of pepsin in the blood.

**hyperpepsinia** \-pepsin′ē·ə\ Excessive production of pepsin by the stomach. See also GASTRIC HYPERSECRETION.

**hyperperistalsis** \-per′istal′sis\ Excessively active intestinal peristalsis.

**hyperphagia** \-fā′jə\ [HYPER- + -PHAGIA] BULIMIA.

**hyperphagic** \-fā′jik\ Characterized by eating to excess: said of animals whose satiety centers in the ventromedial nucleus of the hypothalamus have been damaged for experimental purposes.

**hyperphalangia** \-fəlan′jē·ə\ POLYPHALANGIA.

**hyperphalangism** \-fəlan′jizm\ POLYPHALANGIA.

**hyperphenylalaninemia** \-fen′ilal′əninē′mē·ə\ An elevated concentration of phenylalanine in the blood.

**hyperphoria** \-fôr′ē·ə\ [HYPER- + -PHORIA] A latent misalignment of the eyes in which the visual axis of an eye is higher than its fellow eye. This may be observed only when fusion is interrupted, as by covering one eye.

**hyperphosphatasemia** \-fäs′fatəsē′mē·ə\ Greater than normal concentration of phosphatase in blood.

**hyperphosphatasia** \-fäs′fətā′zhə\ A hereditary, autosomal recessive, chronic osteopathy characterized by an increased serum phosphatase concentration in the presence of normal serum calcium and phosphate concentrations. Also *juvenile Paget's disease.*

**hyperphosphatemia** \-fäs′fətē′mē·ə\ An elevated concentration of phosphate or phosphorus in the blood or blood serum.

**hyperphosphaturia** \-fäs′fətoo′rē·ə\ Increased excretion of inorganic phosphates in the urine, secondary to excess phosphate intake, to excess amounts of parathyroid or thyroid hormone, or to proximal tubular defects. It is sometimes associated with osteomalacia, defective growth in children, and a variety of other conditions.

**hyperphosphoremia** \-fäs′fôrē′mē·ə\ An elevated concentration of phosphorus compounds in the blood or blood serum.

**hyperpiesia** \-pī·ē′zhə\ [HYPER- + Gk *pies(is)* pressure, a squeezing + -IA] HYPERTENSION.

**hyperpiesis** \-pī·ē′sis\ HYPERTENSION.

**hyperpietic** \-pī·et′ik\ HYPERTENSIVE.

**hyperpituitarism** \-pit$^y$oo′itərizm\ [HYPER- + PITUITAR-ISM] Any condition characterized by excessive secretion of pituitary hormones, particularly those of the anterior pituitary, as acromegaly, Cushing's disease, or nonpuerperal galactorrhea associated with a prolactin-secreting microadenoma. Also *hyperhypophysism* (rare). **basophilic h.** Cushing's disease associated with basophil adenoma of the adenohypophysis, or more specifically, of the anterior pituitary corticotrophs. **eosinophilic h.** Pathologic overactivity of the eosinophil cells of the anterior pituitary (adenoma or hyperplasia), causing acromegaly or gigantism due to excessive secretion of growth hormone. *Seldom used.*

**hyperplasia** \-plā′zhə\ [HYPER- + -PLASIA] Increase in the number of cells in a tissue or organ with a concomitant increase in the size of the structure involved. It is a controlled, finite change, caused by known stimuli, and one that ceases when the causative stimulus stops. Also *hyperblastosis.* **angiofollicular mediastinal lymph node h.** BENIGN MEDIASTINAL LYMPH NODE HYPERPLASIA. **basal cell h.** An increase in the proportion of basal-type cells in a stratified, usually squamous epithelium. It is characteristic of the early stages of epithelial dysplasia. **benign mediastinal lymph node h.** A condition characterized by benign, solid, lymphoid masses occurring in the mediastinum of young adults. Histologically they are characterized by concentric perivascular aggregations of lymphocytes. Although usually asymptomatic, they may cause mechanical compression of vital structures. Surgical removal is the treatment of choice to prevent obstructive sequelae or neoplastic transformation. Also *angiofollicular mediastinal lymph node hyperplasia.* **congenital adrenocortical h.** An inherited metabolic disorder due to partial or complete lack of an enzyme, most commonly steroid 21-hydroxylase, in the synthesis of cortisol by the adrenal cotex. A reduced concentration of cortisol in plasma allows overproduction of adrenocorticotropic hormone by the anterior pituitary, leading to hypertrophy and hyperplasia of the adrenal cortex, and to excessive secretion of androgenic steroids. The affected male is born with enlarged penis, the female with enlarged clitoris and varying degrees of masculinization of the genitalia. Salt loss is an additional feature in some cases. Treatment is with cortisol or its analogs, together with salt replacement. Inheritance is autosomal recessive. Also *adrenogenital syndrome, androgenital syndrome* (seldom used), *congenital adrenal hyperplasia.* **congenital sebaceous gland h.** SEBACEOUS NEVUS. **cystic h.** Hyperplasia of glandular epithelium accompanied by cysts, resulting from a combination of retention of secretions and obstruction by the proliferated epithelium. It is most commonly seen in endometrium, breast, and prostate. Also *Swiss-cheese hyperplasia.* **cystic h. of the breasts** CYSTIC MASTOPATHY. **cystic-glandular h. of the endometrium** A form of endometrial hyperplasia characterized by proliferation of endometrial and stromal cells and cyst formation. It is most frequently seen at the time of the menopause or later and results from unremitting estrogenic stimulation. Also *Swiss-cheese endometrium.* **denture h.** Hyperplasia of the oral mucous membrane caused by repeated irritation from an ill-fitting denture. Also *inflammatory fibrous hyperplasia, denture hypertrophy.* **Dilantin gingival h.** A term used chiefly in the U.S. for DIPHENYLHYDANTOIN GINGIVITIS. **endometrial h.** An abnormal growth response in the endometrium due to excessive, unremitting or noncyclic, unopposed estrogenic stimulus. Also *hyperplasia endometrii.* **epiphyseal h.** DYSPLASIA EPIPHYSIALIS HEMIMELICA. **fibromuscular h.** See under FIBROMUSCULAR DISEASE. **focal adenomyomatous h. of the gallbladder** A focal lesion in the fundus of the gallbladder in which diverticuli are surrounded by fibrous and muscular tissue to form a tumorlike nodule. Also *adenomyoma* (incorrect). **focal nodular h. of the liver** A reactive or hamartomatous lesion of the liver characterized by the presence of one or several nodular, well circumscribed but not encapsulated hepatic nodules ranging in size from 1–15 cm. The lesion usually occurs in women of childbearing age and is generally asymptomatic and has a benign prognosis. **follicular h.** Increased numbers of secondary follicles with active germinal centers, detectable on microscopic examination of a lymph node. There may or may not be accompanying enlargement of the lymph node. **giant follicular h.** A peculiar form of lymph node hyperplasia characteristically involving the mediastinum but also found in the neck, axilla, and other sites. Large follicles are present within a mass of lymphoid tissue that may show prominent vascular proliferation and hyalinization, and sometimes plasma cells. **gingival h.** Enlargement of the gingiva produced by an increase in the number of its elements. Usually gingival hyperplasia is a plaque-associated gingivitis, more common in the young. A severe form may be found in patients on long-term diphenylhydantoin sodium therapy. **inflammatory fibrous h.** DENTURE HYPERPLASIA. **islet cell h.** A ribbonlike overgrowth, associated with excessive insulin secretion, of the $\beta$-cells of the pancreatic islets of Langerhans, and sometimes occurring as a part of multiple endocrine neoplasia Type I. **juxtaglomerular cell h.** Hyperplasia and hypertrophy of the juxtaglomerular cells of the kidney with consequent excessive secretion of renin, hyperangiotensinemia, aldosteronism, hypokalemia, alkalosis, insensitivity to the hypertensive action of angiotensin, and absence of hypertension. **juxtaglomerular h. with hyperaldosteronism** See under BARTTER SYNDROME. **ovarian stromal h.** THECOMATOSIS. **polar h.** Overdevelopment of the cranial or caudal end of an embryo, resulting in an abnormal fetus with two heads or three or four hind limbs. **polypoid h.** Focal hyperplasia of a tissue in which the affected area has the shape of a polyp. **pseudoepitheliomatous h.** Abundant proliferation of squamous epithelium simulating carcinoma. The lesion occurs over areas of chronic inflammation. Also *pseudocarcinomatous hyperplasia.* **Schwann h.** HEREDITARY HYPERTROPHIC INTERSTITIAL NEUROPATHY. **Swiss-cheese h.** CYSTIC HYPERPLASIA. **thymic medullary h.** A condition in which hyperplastic germinal centers are present in the medulla of the thymus. It is particularly common in myasthenia gravis.

**hyperplasmia** \plaz′mē·ə\ Increase in volume of blood plasma.

**hyperplasminemia** \-plaz′minē′mē·ə\ The abnormal emergence of the fibrinolytic enzyme plasmin in the blood, characteristic of disseminated intravascular coagulation.

**hyperplastic** \-plas′tik\ Pertaining to or characterized by hyperplasia.

**hyperploid** \hī′pərploid\ [HYPER- + -PLOID] Having a chromosome complement slightly in excess of that found in a complement having any integral multiple of the haploid set.

**hyperpnea** \hī′pərp·nē′ə\ [HYPER- + -PNEA] Excessively rapid or deep breathing. Adj. hyperpneic.

**hyperpnoea** *Brit.* HYPERPNEA.

**hyperpolarization** \-pō′ləriză′shən\ An increase in the transmembrane potential across nerve or muscle cells that occurs with an increased net difference in charge between the interior and exterior surfaces. **early h.** POSITIVE AFTER-POTENTIAL.

**hyperpolypeptidemia** \-päl′ipep′tidē′mē·ə\ An elevated concentration of polypeptides in the blood.

**hyperpotassemia** \-pät′asē′mē·ə\ HYPERKALEMIA.

**hyperpraxia** \-prak′sē·ə\ HYPERKINESIA.

**hyperprebetalipoproteinemia** \-prēbā′təlip′ōprō′tēnē′mē·ə\ An elevated concentration of prebetalipoproteins (very low density lipoproteins) in the blood or blood serum. Also *prebetalipoproteinemia.* **familial h.** FAMILIAL HYPERLIPOPROTEINEMIA TYPE IV.

**hyperprogesteronemia** \-prōjes′tərōnē′mē·ə\ An abnormally high concentration of progesterone in the blood. Also *hyperlutemia.*

**hyperprolactinemia** \-prōlak′tinē′mē·ə\ Raised concentration of prolactin in the blood, normal in pregnancy, lactation and response to stress, pathologic in pituitary adenomas, nonpuerperal galactorrhea, amenorrhea, and renal failure.

**hyperprolactinism** \-prölak′tinizm\ The presence of excessive levels of circulating prolactin, usually due either to an adenoma of the anterior pituitary gland or to stimulation with any of a number of drugs or conditions of physiologic stress. Normal levels are below 25 ng/ml.

**hyperprolinemia** \-prō′linē′mē·ə\ **1** An elevated concentration of proline in the blood. **2** A genetically determined metabolic disorder characterized by elevated plasma proline and increased urinary excretion of proline, hydroxyproline, and glycine, due to impairment of oxidation of proline. Clinical manifestations include mental retardation and renal dysfunction. For defs. 1 and 2 also *prolinemia.*

**familial h.** ENCEPHALOPATHY WITH PROLINEMIA.

**hyperprosessis** \-prōses′is\ [HYPER- + Gk *prosessis* for *prosexis* (from *prosechein* to turn one's attention to) attention] Exaggerated attentiveness. Also *hyperprosexia*.

**hyperproteinemia** \-prō′tēnē′mē·ə\ An elevated concentration of protein in the blood or blood serum.

**hyperpselaphesia** \hī′pərp·sel′əfē′zhə \ [HYPER- + Gk *psēlaphēs(is)* a touching, groping + -IA] HYPERAPHIA.

**hyperpyrexia** \-pīrek′sē·ə\ [HYPER- + PYREXIA] An excessively high body temperature, usually over 40.5°C (105°F). **fulminant h.** MALIGNANT HYPERPYREXIA. **heat h.** HEATSTROKE. **malignant h.** A familial disorder in which severe muscular pain and rigidity with hyperpyrexia, leading sometimes to a fatal termination, may be induced in susceptible individuals by various inhalational anesthetic agents, especially halothane, or by a muscular relaxant such as succinylcholine. Also *fulminant hyperpyrexia*.

**hyperreactive** \-rē·ak′tiv\ Exhibiting or pertaining to an excessive reaction to a stimulus.

**hyperreflexia** \-riflek′sē·ə\ [HYPER- + REFLEX + -IA] Exaggeration of reflexes. **autonomic h.** A condition in which there is an excessive autonomic response to visceral or somatic afferent stimuli.

**hyperresonance** \-rez′ənəns\ A greater than normal resonance.

**hypersaline** Characterized by increased or excessive salinity: used of treatment involving the administration of large doses of sodium chloride.

**hypersalivation** \-sal′ivā′shən\ PTYALISM.

**hypersecretion** \-sikrē′shən\ Excessive secretion, as of a gland. Also *supersecretion*. **gastric h.** Excessive production of mucus, acid, and/or pepsin by the gastric secretory cells. It occurs in the Zollinger-Ellison syndrome. Also *hyperchylia, hyperpepsia*.

**hypersegmentation** \-seg′məntā′shən\ The state of having many segments or lobes. **hereditary h. of neutrophils** UNDRITZ ANOMALY.

**hypersensibility** \-sen′səbil′itē\ Abnormally sharp sensory perception.

**hypersensitive** \-sen′sətiv\ Exhibiting hypersensitivity. Also *supersensitive*.

**hypersensitivity** \-sen′sitiv′itē\ [HYPER- + SENSITIVITY] **1** A state of reactivity where a subsequent exposure to an antigen produces a greater effect than that produced on the initial exposure. **2** Excessive reactivity to any stimulus. Also *hypererethism*. **atopic h.** ATOPY. **carotid sinus h.** Abnormal sensitivity of the carotid sinus, causing bradycardia or transient asystole and/or hypotension, which may result in syncope. **contact h.** Delayed (type 4) hypersensitivity reaction occurring in the skin at sites which have been in contact with agents that can bind to the skin to give rise to antigenic stimulation. Examples of substances that can induce contact hypersensitivity reactions are poison ivy (to which almost all exposed subjects react), and various drugs and cosmetics (to which comparatiely few react). Induction of contact hypersensitivy to dinitrochlorobenzene is used as a test of immune competence. **delayed h.** An increased sensitivity to a foreign agent which is cell-mediated. The lesions in which lymphocytes and macrophages are prominent do not appear before 24 hours after contact or injection of the foreign substance. This reactivity can be transferred by lymphocytes from the sensitized individual to an unsensitized individual. Also *type 4 hypersensitivity*. See also IMMUNOLOGICAL MECHANISMS OF TISSUE DAMAGE. **immediate h.** An increased sensitivity to a foreign agent, clinically manifest within minutes, characterized by the release of histamine and other pharmacologic mediators following the reaction of antigen with IgE antibody bound to mast cells. Serum of an affected individual that is introduced in another individual will allow immediate hypersensitivity to be produced in the second individual when challenged with the appropriate antigen. Also *immediate allergy, type 1 hypersensitivity*. See also IMMUNOLOGICAL MECHANISMS OF TISSUE DAMAGE. **type 1 h.** IMMEDIATE HYPERSENSITIVITY. **type 2 h.** Type 2 hypersensitivity reaction. See under IMMUNOLOGICAL MECHANISMS OF TISSUE DAMAGE. **type 3 h.** Type 3 hypersensitivity reaction. See under IMMUNOLOGICAL MECHANISMS OF TISSUE DAMAGE. **type 4 h.** DELAYED HYPERSENSITIVITY.

**hyperserotonemia** \-ser′ətōnē′mē·ə\ An elevated concentration of serotonin in the blood or blood serum.

**hypersomatotropism** \-sō′mətōtrō′pizm\ [HYPER- + *somatotrop(in)* + -ISM] **1** Excessive secretion of the anterior pituitary growth hormone. **2** ACROMEGALY.

**hypersomia** \-sō′mē·ə\ [HYPER- + Gk *sōma* body + -IA] GIGANTISM.

**hypersomnia** \-säm′nē·ə\ [HYPER- + *somn(i)-* + -IA] A pathologic state of prolonged sleep, from which the patient can be roused only partly and very briefly. Hypersomnia differs from narcolepsy in that the cause may be an identifiable organic disorder of cerebral structure and function. Also *hyperhypnosis, lethargy*. **continuous h.** A pathologic state of prolonged and uninterrupted sleep. This may be the principal symptom of such diseases as epidemic encephalitis or sleeping sickness, and can occur in patients with cerebral tumors, especially those situated in the third ventricular region or hypothalamus. **paroxysmal h.** Hypersomnia occurring in bouts which may last for several minutes or for several hours. Also *episodic hypersomnia*. **periodic h.** KLEINE-LEVIN SYNDROME.

**hypersplenism** \splē′nizm\ A pathologic increase in the normal splenic functions of sequestration and destruction of aged or damaged formed blood elements, often associated with enlargement of the organ. It is manifested as varying combinations of anemia, leukopenia, thrombocytopenia, and hyperplasia of corresponding precursors in the bone marrow. Also *hypersplenia*.

**hyperspongiosis** \-spän′jē·ō′sis\ An increase in the amount of substantia spongiosa ossium.

**hypersteatosis** \-stē′ətō′sis\ SEBORRHEA.

**hypersthenia** \-sthē′nē·ə\ [HYPER- + STHEN- + -IA ] A state of excessive strength. Compare HYPASTHENIA.

**hypersthenuria** \-sthenoo′rē·ə\ [HYPER- + STHEN- + -URIA] A condition characterized by a highly concentrated urine.

**hypersusceptibility** \-susep′tibil′itē\ Higher than normal susceptibility to a toxin or infectious agent.

**hypertelorism** \-tel′ərizm\ [HYPER- + Gk *tēlour(os)* (from *tēlou* far + *(ho)ros* boundary, limit) distantly bounded, broad + -ISM] **1** Abnormally increased distance between paired organs or parts. **2** ORBITAL HYPERTELORISM. **canthal h.** TELECANTHUS. **ocular h.** ORBITAL HYPERTELORISM. **orbital h.** The abnormally great interorbital distance associated with an enlarged sphenoid bone and sometimes with mental retardation and other developmental disorders such as craniofacial and cleidocranial dysostosis. Also *Greig syndrome, ocular hypertelorism, hypertelorism*.

**hypertensinase** ANGIOTENSINASE.

**hypertensinogen** \-tensin′əjən\ ANGIOTENSINOGEN.

**hypertension** Abnormally high tension or pressure: applied especially to systemic arterial or pulmonary arterial blood pressure. Also *hyperpiesis, hyperpiesia*. **accelerated h.** A form of hypertension characterized by extremely high arterial pressures and usually by papilledema, fundic hemorrhages and exudates, and rapidly progressing renal failure. It is associated with a very poor prognosis if no treatment is given. Also *malignant hypertension.* **adrenal h.** Hypertension as a consequence of adrenal disease. Also *suprarenal hypertension.* **arterial h.** Hypertension in the systemic arterial circuit. **benign h.** Hypertension in which the blood pressure is only modestly elevated in the absence of any secondary effects of the high blood pressure. • The term *benign* here is a misnomer, in that such cases often progress later to develop the serious complications of hypertension. **benign intracranial h.** A syndrome of high intracranial pressure associated with cerebral edema, sometimes resulting from intracranial venous sinus thrombosis but more often of undetermined cause. The cerebral ventricles are normal or smaller than normal in size and the course is benign unless papilledema damages vision. Also *pseudotumor cerebri, hypertensive meningeal hydrops, hydromeningitis* (obs.), *pseudoabscess.* **diastolic h.** Increased diastolic pressure in the systemic arteries, usually considered to be present in adults if 90 mmHg or greater when determined by the fifth phase of the Korotkoff sounds. **episodic h.** PAROXYSMAL HYPERTENSION. **essential h.** Hypertension for which no causative factor can be determined. Also *idiopathic hypertension, primary hypertension.* **gestational h.** Elevated blood pressure associated with pregnancy. **Goldblatt h.** 1 An experimental hypertension in animals caused by constriction of one or both renal arteries. 2 Hypertension in man secondary to renal artery stenosis. For defs. 1 and 2 also *Goldblatt phenomenon.* **idiopathic h.** ESSENTIAL HYPERTENSION. **intracranial h.** Increased intracranial pressure caused by a space-occupying lesion, cerebral edema, by obstructive or communicating hydrocephalus or by any process which increases the brain volume or pressure of the cerebrospinal fluid. The principal symptoms and signs are headache, vomiting, and papilledema. **malignant h.** ACCELERATED HYPERTENSION. **ocular h.** The presence of an intraocular pressure level higher than usually considered normal, but which has not yet resulted in any demonstrable visual field defects. Ocular hypertension is not necessarily benign, inasmuch as some cases progress to overt glaucomatous damage. The distribution of intraocular pressure levels in the normal population extends through a considerable range and overlaps with the range of pressures found in glaucoma. Classification of a given pressure (for example, greater than 22 mmHg) as representing glaucoma on the one hand or a normal value on the other is not possible without careful medical evaluation of both ocular function and structure. Also *hypertonia oculi.* **paroxysmal h.** A form of hypertension in which the blood pressure rises in paroxysms, characteristically associated with pheochromocytoma. Also *episodic hypertension.* **pituitary h.** Associated with disorders of the adenohypophysis, such as Cushing's disease and acromegaly. *Older term.* **portal h.** Elevation of portal vein pressure due to intrahepatic or extrahepatic cause, resulting in collateral circulation giving rise to esophageal and gastric varices or hemorrhoids, and in ascites, splenomegaly, and other manifestations. **primary h.** ESSENTIAL HYPERTENSION. **pulmonary h.** Increase in the pressure in the pulmonary circulation. Also *pulmonary artery hypertension.* **renal h.** Hypertension secondary to renal disease, renal artery stenosis, or obstruction of the urinary tract. Renin often is increased in renal veins of affected kidneys. **renin-dependent h.** Hypertension due to increased renin production in renal artery stenosis, renal parencyhmal disease, or in urinary tract obstruction. **renoprival h.** Hypertension in an anephric patient or in a patient whose kidneys do not function. Renoprival hypertension may result from fluid overload, absence of vasodepressor factors produced by the kidneys, or both. **renovascular h.** Hypertension secondary to stenosis of the main renal artery or its primary branches, or of an aberrant artery, usually due to atherosclerosis or fibromuscular hyperplasia. The renal artery rarely may be narrowed by extrinsic pressure, aneurysm, thrombosis, embolism, or arteritis. Renin is increased in renal venous blood from affected kidneys. The hypertension may be cured by surgical reconstruction of the affected artery, or by nephrectomy if the condition is unilateral. **secondary h.** Hypertension which is secondary to another disorder, such as renal disease, adrenal tumors, or coarctation of the aorta. Also *symptomatic hypertension.* **suprarenal h.** ADRENAL HYPERTENSION. **symptomatic h.** SECONDARY HYPERTENSION. **systolic h.** Increased systolic pressure in the systemic arteries, usually considered to be present if the systolic pressure is greater than 140 mmHg in adults. It is commonly accompanied by diastolic hypertension, but may be isolated in hyperthyroidism and in the elderly with rigid arteries due to arteriosclerosis. **transient h.** Hypertension that is evident only intermittently. **vascular h.** Abnormally high pressure in the blood vessels; hypertension. **venous h.** Increased venous pressure.

**hypertensive** \-ten′siv\ Affected by or pertaining to hypertension. Also *hyperpietic.*

**hypertestosteronism** \-testäs′tərōnizm\ Excessive secretion of testosterone from any source, as in Leydig cell tumor of the testis in prepubertal boys.

**hyperthecosis** \-thēkō′sis\ [HYPER- + *thec(a)* + -OSIS] The development of stromal hyperplasia and foci of luteinization in the ovary. Most patients are of age 20–30. **testoid h.** Diffuse hyperplasia and often focal luteinization of ovarian stromal cells associated with testosterone secretion, virilization, obesity, and sometimes diabetes.

**hyperthelia** \-thē′lē·ə\ [HYPER- + THEL- + -IA] POLYTHELIA.

**hyperthermalgesia** \-thur′maljē′sē·ə\ [HYPER- + THERMALGESIA] Excessive sensitivity to heat. Also *hyperthermesthesia, hyperthermoesthesia.*

**hyperthermia** \-thur′mē·ə\ [HYPER- + Gk *thermē* heat, feverish heat + -IA] Fever, especially therapeutic fever. Also *hyperthermy.* **malignant h.** See under MALIGNANT HYPERTHERMIA SYNDROME. **whole-body h.** The deliberate raising of body temperature for the treatment of disease. It may be used to enhance the effect of other therapeutic agents.

**hyperthermoesthesia** \-thur′mō·esthē′zhə\ HYPERTHERMALGESIA.

**hyperthermy** \-thur′mē\ HYPERTHERMIA.

**hyperthrombinemia** \-thräm′binē′mē·ə\ An elevated concentration or activity of thrombin in the blood.

**hyperthymism** \-thī′mizm\ An abnormal increase in activity of the thymus.

**hyperthyroid** \-thī′roid\ [HYPER- + THYROID] Of, characterized by, or resulting from hyperthyroidism.

**hyperthyroidism** \-thī′roidizm\ [HYPER- + THYROID + -ISM] 1 Excessive secretion by the thyroid gland of thyroxine or triiodothyronine or both, accompanied by increased rate of oxygen consumption, accelerated basal metabolic rate, thyroid enlargement, and systemic disturbances, the most prominent symptoms being weakness, weight loss, and nervousness. Also *thyroidism.* 2 *Ambiguous* GRAVES DISEASE. **apathetic h.** MASKED HYPERTHYROIDISM. **factitious h.** Hyperthyroidism produced by self-medication with thyroid hormone. **iatrogenic h.** Hyperthyroidism resulting from the administration of too much thyroid hormone in the course of medical treatment. **iodine-induced h.** Unexplained induction of true hyperthyroidism by ingestion of excessive iodine. Also *Jod-Basedow phenomenon, iod-Basedow.* **masked h.** Excessive secretion of thyroid hormone by the thyroid gland, usually in middle-aged or elderly persons, but without the typical signs and symptoms of hyperthyroidism. It is characterized by weakness, lethargy, and often by cardiac arrhythmia or congestive heart failure. Also *apathetic hyperthyroidism.* **primary h.** Hyperthyroidism due to intrinsic disease of the thyroid gland. **secondary h.** Hyperthyroidism due to stimulation of the thyroid gland by adenohypophysial oversecretion of thyrotropic hormone. The condition is very rare. Also *hyperthyrotropinism.*

**hyperthyroxinemia** \-thīräk′sinē′mē·ə\ An elevated concentration of thyroxine in the blood or blood serum.

**hypertonia** \-tō′nē·ə\ [*hyperton(ic)* + -IA] **1** Increased muscle tone. Also *hypertonus, hypermyotonia* (seldom used). Adj. hypertonic. **2** *Seldom used* HYPERTENSION. **h. oculi** OCULAR HYPERTENSION.

**hypertonic** \-tän′ik\ [Gk *hyperton(os)* (from HYPER- + *tonos* stretching, tension) strained to the utmost + -IC] **1** More than normally tonic, as the state of a muscle. **2** Having a greater tonicity than the solution with which it is compared. **3** Having an osmotic pressure higher than that of an isotonic solution or more concentrated than isotonic. Sodium chloride solutions are said to be hypertonic at concentrations of more than 0.45%, the point at which red blood cells undergo crenation. Also *hyperisotonic.*

**hypertonicity** \-tōnis′itē\ The property of being hypertonic. Also *hyperisotonicity.*

**hypertonus** \-tō′nəs\ HYPERTONIA.

**hypertrichosis** \-trikō′sis\ [HYPER- + TRICHOSIS] The growth of hair in any pattern which is excessive for the age, sex, and race of the subject. Also *hypertrichiasis.* Compare HIRSUTISM.

**hypertriglyceridemia** \-trīglis′əridē′mē·ə\ [HYPER- + TRIGLYCERIDE + -EMIA] An elevated concentration of triglycerides in the blood or blood serum. See also HYPERLIPOPROTEINEMIA. **alimentary h.** EXOGENOUS HYPERTRIGLYCERIDEMIA. **carbohydrate-induced h.** CARBOHYDRATE-INDUCED HYPERLIPIDEMIA. **endogenous h.** **1** FAMILIAL HYPERLIPOPROTEINEMIA TYPE I. **2** FAMILIAL HYPERLIPOPROTEINEMIA TYPE IV. **exogenous h.** A greater than normal concentration of triglycerides in plasma as a consequence of high triglyceride content of the diet or parenteral administration of large amounts of triglycerides. Also *alimentary hypertriglyceridemia.* **familial h.** **1** FAMILIAL HYPERLIPOPROTEINEMIA TYPE I. **2** FAMILIAL HYPERLIPOPROTEINEMIA TYPE IV. **familial fat-induced h.** FAMILIAL HYPERLIPOPROTEINEMIA TYPE I.

**hypertrophia** \-trō′fē·ə\ *Seldom used* HYPERTROPHY. **h. musculorum vera** A syndrome of generalized hypertrophy of the skeletal muscles. It is of multiple etiology, the causes including myotonia congenita and hypothyroidism.

**hypertrophic** Pertaining to or characterized by hypertrophy.

**hypertrophy** \hīpur′trəfē\ [HYPER- + Gk *trophē* nourishment, food] Increase in size of an organ or part due to an increase in the size of its individual cells. A common example is hypertrophy of the left ventricular myocardium as a result of systemic arterial hypertension. Also *hypertrophia* (seldom used), *simple hypertrophy.* **adaptive h.** Hypertrophy of the walls of a hollow organ as a result of increased resistance to the emptying function, as occurs in the left ventricle of the heart in aortic valve stenosis and in the urinary bladder in outflow obstruction due to prostatic gland enlargement. **adult h. of the pylorus** Acquired hypertrophy of the pylorus which presents in adults as partial or complete gastric outlet obstruction. It may be related in some cases to underlying peptic ulcer disease. Also *Billroth hypertrophy.* See also ADULT PYLORIC STENOSIS. **benign h. of the pons** Enlargement of the pons resulting from the presence of a slowly growing pontine glioma. **bilateral h. of masseters** A benign syndrome of unknown cause in which there is marked enlargement of both masseter muscles. **Billroth h.** ADULT HYPERTROPHY OF THE PYLORUS. **biventricular h.** Hypertrophy affecting both cardiac ventricles. **breast h. of the newborn** The enlargement of breast tissue common in infants of both sexes during the first week of life. It is sometimes associated with the secretion of a few drops of milk that may be released during this period. **cardiac concentric h.** Uniform hypertrophy of the ventricles. **cicatricial h.** The overproduction of fibrous connective tissue in a scar. **compensatory h.** Hypertrophy of a tissue or organ following damage or loss of a portion of such tissue. It is seen, for example, in the viable myocardium adjacent to an infarct, and in the remaining kidney following unilateral nephrectomy. Also *complementary hypertrophy, vicarious hypertrophy.* **compensatory h. of the heart** Hypertrophy of the heart as a response to increased work load as imposed by valvular heart disease or hypertension. **complementary h.** COMPENSATORY HYPERTROPHY. **concentric h.** Hypertrophy, especially of a cardiac chamber, characterized by increased thickness of the walls but without dilatation. **congenital h. of the bladder neck** MARION'S DISEASE. **denture h.** DENTURE HYPERPLASIA. **eccentric h.** Hypertrophy, especially of a cardiac chamber, characterized by normal or increased thickness of the walls and dilatation of the lumen. **false h.** PSEUDOHYPERTROPHY. **fibromuscular h.** FIBROMUSCULAR DISEASE. **functional h.** An increase in the size of an organ due to an increase in functional load or activity. Also *physiologic hypertrophy.* **hemangiectatic h.** KLIPPEL-TRENAUNAY-WEBER SYNDROME. **juxtaglomerular cell h.** Enlargement of the renal juxtaglomerular cells secondary to decreased blood flow. Associated degranulation reflects greater secretion than storage of renin. **mammary h.** Hypertrophy of one or both breasts, so excessive as to constitute a cosmetic or mechanical burden and require surgical correction. Also *barymazia.* **Marie's h.** Swelling of an extremity due to periostitis. **mulberry h.** See under HYPERTROPHIC RHINITIS. **physiologic h.** FUNCTIONAL HYPERTROPHY. **pseudomuscular h.** MUSCULAR PSEUDOHYPERTROPHY. **renal h.** Compensatory increase in mass and function of one kidney in response to absence or marked impairment of function of the contralateral kidney. This may be congenital or acquired, and occurs in transplanted kidneys. **simple h.** HYPERTROPHY. **true h.** Hypertrophy due to an increase in the size of all structural elements of an organ or part. **unilateral h.** Hypertrophy involving only one side of the body or of a portion of it, or one of a paired organ such as the kidney. **ventricular h.** Myocardial hypertrophy of a cardiac ventricle. **vicarious h.** COMPENSATORY HYPERTROPHY.

**hypertropia** \-trō′pē·ə\ [HYPER- + TROPIA] A constant deviation of alignment of the eyes in which the visual axis of one eye points in a direction higher than the other. The designation is applied to the higher of the two eyes, irrespective of which eye is used in fixation. Thus, in right hypertropia, the right eye is higher; in left hypertropia, the left.

**hypertyrosinemia** \-tī′rōsinē′mē·ə\ A greater than normal concentration of tyrosine in blood.

**hyperuresis** \-yoorē′sis\ [HYPER- + -URESIS] POLYURIA.

**hyperuricaciduria** \-yoo′rikas′idoo′rē·ə\ HYPERURICURIA.

**hyperuricemia** \-yoo′risē′mē·ə\ A greater than normal concentration of uric acid or urates in blood. Also *hyperuricacidemia, agremia* (older term)*, uricemia, uratemia, uricacidemia, lithemia.* Adj. hyperuricemic. **X-linked h.** HYPOXANTHINE PHOSPHORIBOSYLTRANSFERASE DEFICIENCY.

**hyperuricuria** \-yoo′rikyoo′rē·ə\ [HYPER- + URIC- + -URIA] Urinary excretion of more than 600 mg uric acid per day while on a low purine diet. It is associated with uric acid overproduction and hyperuricemia in some gouty patients, the Lesch-Nyhan syndrome, myeloproliferative disorders, polycythemia, hemolytic and certain other anemias, and some carcinomas, and may occur during treatment of gout with a uricosuric agent. Chronic hyperuricuria may result in uric acid calculi and gouty nephropathy, while acute hyperuricuria secondary to rapidly effective treatment of myeloproliferative disorders or large tumors may lead to precipitation of uric acid in the urinary tract with resultant acute renal failure. Also *hyperuricosuria, hyperlithuria, hyperuricaciduria.*

**hypervaccination** \-vak′sinā′shən\ HYPERIMMUNIZATION.

**hypervalinemia** \-val′inē′mē·ə\ A metabolic disorder, of which a single case has been described, characterized by retardation and vomiting, and by increased valine in both plasma and urine.

**hypervascular** \-vas′kyələr\ Having increased vascularity; very highly vascular.

**hyperventilation** \-ven′tilā′shən\ [HYPER- + VENTILATION] Pulmonary ventilation beyond that necessary for metabolism, causing excessive alveolar ventilation. Hyperventilation, often a reaction to anxiety or fear, results in progressive hypocapnia, producing symptoms of palpitations, dizziness or faintness, paresthesiae, and tetany. Also *overventilation, hyperaeration, overbreathing* (popular). **central neurogenic h.** Hyperventilation resulting from a lesion in the central nervous system. **hysterical h.** A syndrome of voluntary hyperventilation resulting from hysteria and usually occurring in young women, in which tetany and even syncope may occur.

**hypervitaminosis** \-vī′təminō′sis\ [HYPER- + VITAMIN + -OSIS] Adverse effects resulting from the consumption of excessive quantities of one or more vitamins. Also *supervitaminosis.* **h. A** A condition resulting from the ingestion of excessive amounts of vitamin A. It is characterized by loss of weight, soreness of the eyes, loss of hair, demineralization of the skeleton, and hemorrhages. The doses necessary to produce these effects are approximately 10 000 times the daily requirement and are therefore rarely encountered. **h. D** A condition resulting from the daily ingestion of excessive amounts of vitamin D. It increases excretion of blood phosphorus by the kidney, extracts calcium and phosphorus from bone, produces osteoporosis and causes deposition of calcium salts in the soft tissues.

**hypervitaminotic** \-vī′təminät′ik\ Relating to the excessive consumption of one or more vitamins.

**hypervolaemia** \-vōlē′mē·ə\ *Brit.* HYPERVOLEMIA.

**hypervolemia** \-vōlē′me·ə\ Greater than normal blood volume.

**hypervolemic** \-vōlē′mik\ Having or pertaining to greater than normal blood volume.

**hypesthesia** \hī′pesthē′zhə\ HYPOESTHESIA.

**hypha** \hī′fə\ [Gk *hyphē* (akin to English *web*) a web] (*pl.* hyphae) The unit of structure of most fungi, consisting of a tubular filament, combined into a complex network that makes up the thallus or body of a fungus. **apical h.** The growing tip of a fungal hypha and the region immediately behind it upon which it depends metabolically. **racquet h.** A specialized form of hypha consisting of a series of small paddleshaped units with the narrow end of each attached to the larger end of the preceding segment.

**hyphaema** *Brit.* HYPHEMA.

**hyphedonia** \hip′hēdō′nē·ə\ [*hyp(o)-* + *hēdon(ē)* pleasure + -IA] A state in which there is an inability to experience pleasure to a normal degree.

**hyphema** \hīfē′mə\ [New L *hyphaema* (from Gk *hyphaim(os)* suffused with blood, bloodshot, from *hyp-* under, up from under + *haima* blood) a sanguineous suffusion] The presence of free blood in the inferior portion of the anterior chamber of the eye. Being heavier than the aqueous humor, blood cells settle to the bottom, becoming oriented with a characteristic horizontal flat top as determined by gravity. This readily observable sign signifies the presence of serious intraocular pathology requiring prompt ophthalmological evaluation. Also *hyphemia.*

**hyphemia** \hīfē′mē·ə\ [HYP- + HEM- + -IA] *Obs.* ANEMIA.

**hyphylline** DYPHYLLINE.

**hypinosis** \hī′pinō′sis\ *Obs.* HYPOFIBRINOGENEMIA.

**hypn-** \hipn-\ HYPNO-.

**hypnagogic** **1** Sleep-producing; hypnotic. **2** Preceding sleep: used of images or dreams perceived during the transition between the waking state and sleep.

**hypnagogue** [HYPN- + -AGOGUE] **1** A hypnotic agent. **2** An agent causing sleepiness or drowsiness.

**hypnic** \hip′nik\ Describing, pertaining to, or inducing sleep.

**hypno-** \hip′nə-\ [Gk *hypnos* sleep] A combining form meaning sleep. Also *hypn-.*

**hypnoanesthesia** \hip′nə·an′esthē′zhə\ A trancelike state produced by hypnosis and sometimes suitable for performance of minor surgery.

**hypnocinematograph** \-sin′əmat′əgraf\ An instrument for recording movements made during sleep.

**hypnosis** \hipnō′sis\ [HYPN- + -OSIS] **1** A state of decreased general awareness but increased attention to a constricted area of rhythmic or repetitive stimulation, usually induced by another person, and distinguishable from sleep by the presence of catatonia and increased suggestibility. Also *hypnotic sleep, teleotherapeutics.* **2** The induction of a hypnotic state. Adj. hypnotic.

**hypnotherapy** \-ther′əpē\ The use of hypnosis as the major or sole modality of treatment. Also *hypnotic psychotherapy, Bernheim's therapy* (older term).

**hypnotic** \hipnät′ik\ [Gk *hypnōtikos* (from *hypnos* sleep) inclined to sleep, conducive to sleep, a hypnotic agent] **1** Inducing sleep or having an anodyne effect. **2** A sleep-producing or sedative agent. For defs. 1 and 2 also *dormifacient, soporific.* **3** Of, relating to, or resulting from hypnosis.

**hypo-** \hī′pō-\ [Gk *hypo* (akin to L *sub* under) under, below] **1** A prefix meaning (1) under, beneath; (2) diminished, deficient, too little or too few, below the normal. **2** In chemistry, a prefix designating an oxyacid or its salt with less oxygen than in the unprefixed compound. Compare HYPER-.

**hypoactive** \-ak′tiv\ Less than normally active.

**hypoacusis** \-əkyoo′sis\ [HYPO- + ACUSIS] Partial hearing loss.

**hypoadenia** \-ədē′nē·ə\ Subnormal function of a gland or glands. *Rare.*

**hypoadrenalemia** \-ad′rənalē′mē·ə\ Less than normal concentration of adrenal hormones and epinephrine in blood.

**hypoadrenalism** \-adrē′nəlizm\ [HYPO- + ADRENAL + -ISM] Any deficient function of the adrenal gland, especially hypoadrenocorticism. *Imprecise.* Also *hypadrenia* (outmoded), *hypoadrenia* (rare), *hyposuprarenalism* (seldom used).

**hypoadrenocortical** Of, caused by, or relating to hypoadrenocorticism.

**hypoadrenocorticism** \-adrē′nōkôr′tisizm\ The clinical condition induced by deficient secretion of hormones by the adrenal cortex, as in Addison's disease or panhypopituitarism. Also *hypoadrenocorticalism, hypocorticalism, hypocorticism.* **pituitary h.** SECONDARY HYPOADRENOCORTICISM. **secondary h.** Deficient secretion of adrenocortical hormones, particularly cortisol, due either to pituitary failure and subnormal secretion of adrenocorticotropin, suppression of the pituitary adrenocortical axis by exogenous corticosteroids, or, rarely, systemic disease, as Laennec cirrhosis of the liver. Also *pituitary hypoadrenocorticism.*

**hypoaesthesia** \-esthē′zhə\ *Brit.* HYPOESTHESIA.

**hypoagnathus** \-ag′nəthəs\ An individual with a much reduced or with no lower jaw.

**hypoalbuminemia** \-albyoo′minē′mē·ə\ Less than normal concentration of albumen in blood, plasma, or serum. Also *hypoalbuminosis, hypalbuminemia, hypalbuminosis.*

**hypoaldosteronemia** \-aldäs′tərōnē′mē·ə\ Less than normal concentration of aldosterone in blood, plasma, or serum.

**hypoaldosteronism** \-aldäs′tərōnizm\ [HYPO- + *aldosteron(e)* + -ISM] Deficient adrenocortical secretion of aldosterone, usually accompanying primary adrenocortical insufficiency or Addison's disease, and causing excessive renal salt wasting with depletion of blood volume, hyponatremia and hypotension. Also *aldosteronopenia.* **hyporeninemic h.** A disorder seen in elderly subjects and characterized by selective aldosterone deficiency and low plasma renin levels, hyperkalemia, and frequently hypertension. Possible causes are chronic renal disease, diabetes mellitus with autonomic neuropathy, and chronic overexpansion of blood volume. **isolated h.** A very rare form of primary adrenocortical insufficiency in which aldosterone secretion is subnormal or absent with normal secretion of other adrenocortical steroids, as cortisol.

**hypoalgesia** \-aljē′zē·ə\ HYPALGESIA.

**hypoalimentation** \-al′iməntā′shən\ [HYPO- + ALIMENTATION] Insufficient ingestion or administration of the essential nutrients needed to satisfy the metabolic needs of the body.

**hypoallergenic** \-al′ərjen′ik\ Not likely to induce an allergic reaction.

**hypoalphalipoproteinemia** \-al′fəlip′ōprō′tēnē′mē·ə\ ANALPHALIPOPROTEINEMIA.

**hypoaminoacidemia** \-am′inō·as′idē′mē·ə\ Less than normal concentration of amino acids in blood, plasma, or serum.

**hypoandrogenism** \-andräj′ənizm\ [HYPO- + ANDROGEN + -ISM] A deficiency of androgenic hormone or hormones, or the condition resulting from it.

**hypoarterial** \-ärtir′ē·əl\ HYPARTERIAL.

**hypobaric** \-bar′ik\ [HYPO- + BAR-[2] + -IC ] At less than normal atmospheric pressure.

**hypobarism** \-bar′izm\ [HYPO- + BAR-[2] + -ISM] Any condition which results from a decrease in ambient pressure to a level below that in body fluids, tissues, and cavities. Also *hypobaropathy.*

**hypobetalipoproteinemia** \-bā′təlip′ōprō′tēnē′mē·ə\ **1** Any reduction in $\beta$-lipoproteins in plasma. **2** A syndrome heritable as an autosomal dominant trait and characterized by reduced serum cholesterol and $\beta$-lipoprotein. Atherosclerosis is not a feature and longevity is either unaffected or increased. Other clinical features, including acanthocytosis, are inconsistent. Heterozygosity for the defect that causes abetalipoproteinemia has not been substantiated as the cause for hypobetalipoproteinemia. Also *familial hypobetalipoproteinemia.*

**hypobilirubinemia** \-bil′iroo′binē′mē·ə\ Less than normal concentration of bilirubin in blood, plasma, or serum.

**hypoblast** \hī′pōblast\ [HYPO- + -BLAST] A deeply placed germ layer, either in the general sense of endoderm or more often in primitive Amniota in the sense of entophyll. At the start of gastrulation the chick blastoderm consists of two layers, the epiblast above, the hypoblast beneath. The hypoblast arises at the posterior end of the area pellucida. It extends anteriorly until it lies beneath the whole of the area pellucida. Later the definitive endoblast invaginates through the anterior end of the primitive streak and becomes inserted into the sheet of hypoblast. Adj. hypoblastic.

**hypobranchial** \-brang′kē·əl\ Situated beneath the branchial arches.

**hypobromite** The ion $BrO^-$ and any salt containing it.

**hypobromous acid** HBrO. An acid that has not been isolated but is known in solution. Its salts are formed, together with bromides, when bromine is dissolved in alkali. It is a powerful oxidizing agent.

**hypocalcemia** \-kalsē′mē·ə\ Less than normal concentration of calcium in blood or serum. Adj. hypocalcemic. **neonatal h.** The decrease in serum calcium level which occurs during the first week of life. It is associated with an increase in the serum phosphorous level. Signs of tetany may become apparent in some infants where the calcium level falls below 2 mmol/l. This may occur with or without brief convulsive episodes. The hypocalcemia is considered to be secondary to a renal failure to clear phosphate. Since cow's milk contains more phosphorous than does human milk clinical symptoms are largely confined to artificially fed infants.

**hypocalcia** \-kal′sē·ə\ A state of reduced calcium content.

**hypocalcification** \-kal′sifikā′shən\ A decrease in the calcification process. **enamel h.** An abnormality in which the enamel is of normal thickness but is chalky and weak. It may be caused by fluorosis, or it may be hereditary.

**hypocalcipexy** \-kal′sipek′sē\ A state of reduced fixation of calcium.

**hypocalcitoninemia** \-kal′sitənē′mē·ə\ A concentration of calcitonin in the blood below the normal value of 5–100 pg/ml. Also *hypocalcitonemia.*

**hypocalciuria** \-kal′sēyoo′rē·ə\ Decreased urinary excretion of calcium. It is an inconstant sign of low dietary calcium intake, but is common during growth, pregnancy, and lactation, and in the intestinal malabsorption syndrome. The condition may be a sign of deficiency of parathyroid or thyroid hormones, or vitamin D. It also may occur during salt depletion or diuretic therapy.

**hypocapnia** \-kap′nē·ə\ [HYPO- + CAPN- + -IA] An abnormally low concentration of carbon dioxide in the blood. Also *hypocarbia.*

**hypocatalasemia** \-kat′əlāsē′mē·ə\ Less than normal activity of catalase in blood cells, especially in erythrocytes.

**hypocellularity** \-sel′yəler′itē\ A state characterized by an abnormally low number of cells, as seen in the bone marrow in aplastic anemia or following cancer chemotherapy. Adj. hypocellular.

**hypocenter** \hī′pōsen′tər\ That point on the surface of the earth that is directly at the center of a nuclear bomb explosion.

**hypoceruloplasminemia** \-seroo′lōplaz′minē′mē·ə\ A reduced concentration of plasma ceruloplasmin, as is usually found in Wilson's disease and Menkes disease and normally in the newborn.

**hypochloremia** \-klôrē′mē·ə\ Less than normal concentration of chloride in blood, plasma, or serum. Also *hypochloridemia, chloropenia.* Adj. hypochloremic.

**hypochlorhydria** \-klôrhī′drē·ə\ Diminished gastric secretion of hydrochloric acid. Also *hypohydrochloria.* Adj. hypochlorhydric.

**hypochloridation** \-klôr′idā′shən\ A level of chloride insufficient to accomplish the purpose for which it is intended.

**hypochloridemia** \-klôr′idē′mē·ə\ HYPOCHLOREMIA.

**hypochlorite** The ion $ClO^-$ and salts containing it.

**hypochloruria** \-klôroo′rē·ə\ Decreased urinary excretion of chloride, as in dietary salt restriction or accumulating edema. It may be secondary to excess chloride loss in gastric secretions or to secretion or administration of salt-retaining mineralocorticoid hormones.

**hypocholesterolemia** \-kōles′tərōlē′mē·ə\ A less than normal concentration of cholesterol in blood, plasma, or serum. Also *hypocholesteremia, hypocholesterinemia.* Adj. hypocholesterolemic, hypocholesteremic.

**hypocholia** \-kō′lyə\ [HYPO- + CHOL- + -IA] Diminished secretion of bile.

**hypochondria** \-kän′drē·ə\ HYPOCHONDRIASIS.

**hypochondriac** [Gk *hypochondriakos* relating to the hypochondrium or to diseases focused in that region.] **1** Pertaining to the regio hypochondriaca. **2** Pertaining to or characterized by hypochondriasis. **3** A person affected with hypochondriasis.

**hypochondriasis** \-kändrī′əsis\ [*hypochondr(iac)* + -IASIS] A somatoform disorder characterized by a misinterpretation of physical signs that leads to the belief of having a serious disease even though repeated evaluations can elicit no indications of physical disorder. Also *hypochondria, nosomania* (obs.), *nosophilia* (obs.), *somatophrenia, vapors* (obs.). Adj. hypochondriacal.

**hypochondrium** \-kän′drē·əm\ [New L, from Gk *hypochondrion* the region between the breastbone and the navel, from *hypo-* below + *chondros* (xiphoid) cartilage] REGIO HYPOCHONDRIACA (DEXTRA ET SINISTRA).

**hypochondroplasia** \-kän′drəplā′zhə\ A less severe form or variant of achondroplasia, with dwarfism that is not apparent until mid-childhood. It may be inherited as an autosomal dominant trait. Also *chondrohypoplasia* (obs.).

**hypochordal** \-kôr′dəl\ [HYPO- + Gk *chord(ē)* a cord, string of gut + -AL] Lying below or ventral to the notochord.

**hypochromasia** \-krōmā′zhə\ HYPOCHROMIA.

**hypochromatism** \-krō′mətizm\ **1** A less than usual intensity of color in any structure. **2** A fading of the chromatin of the cell nucleus.

**hypochromatosis** \-krō′mətō′sis\ **1** The condition of having less than the usual amount of color intensity. **2** A less than normal amount of chromatin in the cell nucleus.

**hypochromia** \-krō′mē·ə\ [HYPO- + CHROM- + -IA] A paler than normal appearance of erythrocytes when stained by a Romanowsky type stain and examined microscopically. The reduction in color intensity of such erythrocytes is due to diminution in their hemoglobin content. Also *hypochromemia, hypochromasia, oligochromasia.*

**hypochromic** \-krō′mik\ Exhibiting hypochromia. Hypochromic erythrocytes are characteristic of thalassemias, severe iron deficiency anemia, anemia of chronic disease, and sideroblastic anemias.

**hypochromicity** \-krōmis′itē\ A decrease in the absorption of ultraviolet light by a solution of polypeptide polynucleotide chains as the secondary structure is established.

**hypochromotrichia** \-krō′mətrik′ē·ə\ [HYPO- + CHROMO- + TRICH- + -IA] A reduced pigmentation of the hair, as is seen in protein malnutrition.

**hypochylia** \-kī′lyə\ [HYPO- + CHYL- + -IA] Diminished gastric secretion; insufficiency of chyle.

**hypocinesia** \-sīnē′zhə\ HYPOKINESIA.

**hypocinesis** \-sīnē′sis\ HYPOKINESIA.

**hypocitremia** \-sītrē′mē·ə\ Less than normal concentration of citrate in blood.

**hypocituria** \-sītroo′rē·ə\ [HYPO- + *citr(ate)* + -URIA] Decreased urinary excretion of citrate and increased potassium excretion during acidosis.

**hypocoagulability** \-kō·ag′ʸələbil′itē\ Retardation of the clotting process because of either a deficiency of one or more clotting factors or platelets, or the presence of coagulation inhibitors.

**hypocoagulable** \-kō·ag′ʸələbl\ Less able than normal to clot.

**hypocomplementemia** \-käm′pləməntē′mē·ə \ A condition in which there is less than normal activity of complement or any of the complement components of blood. The condition may be hereditary or acquired. Various immune complex diseases result in acquired deficiency of complement components. Also *acomplementemia.* Adj. hypocomplementemic.

**hypocorticalism** \-kôr′tikəlizm\ *Seldom used* HYPOADRENOCORTICISM.

**hypocorticism** \-kôr′tisizm\ *Seldom used* HYPOADRENOCORTICISM.

**hypocupremia** \-kʸoo prē′mē·ə\ [HYPO- + CUPR- + -EMIA] An abnormally low concentration of copper in the blood or blood serum.

**hypocyclosis** \-sīklō′sis\ [HYPO- + CYCL- + -OSIS] A deficient functioning of the ciliary muscle, resulting in an inadequacy of the accommodation of the eye. ● *Hypocyclosis* connotes a departure from normal and is not synonymous with *presbyopia,* which refers to the normal loss of accommodation that accompanies aging.

**hypodactyly** \-dak′tilē\ ECTRODACTYLY.

**hypoderm** \hī′pōdurm\ TELA SUBCUTANEA.

***Hypoderma*** \-dur′mə\ [HYPO- + DERMA] A genus of heel flies, or ox warble flies, (family Oestridae, sometimes placed in a separate family Hypodermatidae). The larvae (cattle grubs) migrate through the body of the host for about four months, reach the spinal cord, and eventually burrow to the skin. Parasitization of humansby various species has been reported, involving extensive visceral and dermal migration with severe painor discomfort, and sometimes temporary paralysis.

**hypodermatic** \-dərmat′ik\ SUBCUTANEOUS.

**hypodermic** \-dur′mik\ [HYPO- + -DERM + -IC] **1** SUBCUTANEOUS. **2** Applied or used beneath the skin: said especially of an injection or an instrument.

**hypodermis** \-dur′mis\ [HYPO- + DERMIS] TELA SUBCUTANEA.

**hypodermoclysis** \-dərmäk′lisis\ [HYPO- + DERMO- + Gk *klysis* a washing out, esp. by a clyster] Subcutaneous administration of fluids, most frequently used as an alternative to intravenous administration of replacement for body fluid loss or dehydration.

**hypodermomycosis** \-dur′məmīkō′sis\ [HYPO- + DERMO- + MYCOSIS] A subcutaneous fungal infection.

**hypodiploid** \-dip′loid\ Deficient in one or more chromosomes or chromosome segments compared to the diploid state: said of a cell or an individual.

**hypodipsia** \-dip′sē·ə\ [HYPO- + -DIPSIA] Diminished thirst with consequential reduction of fluid intake. Also *oligodipsia*.

**hypodontia** \hī′pōdän′shə\ [HYP- + -ODONTIA] The congenital condition of having fewer teeth than normal.

**hypodynamic** \-dīnam′ik\ Reduced in power or force; pertaining especially to reduced contractility of the heart.

**hypoeccrisia** \-ekris′ē·ə\ The state of decreased secretion. Also *hypoeccrisis*. Adj. hypoeccritic.

**hypoechoic** \-ekō′ik\ [HYPO- + ECHOIC] Producing echoes of lower amplitude or density than the surrounding medium.

**hypoeosinophilia** \hī′pō·ē′ōsin′əfil′yə\ [HYPO- + EOSINOPHIL + -IA] EOSINOPENIA.

**hypoepinephrinemia** \-ep′inef′rinē′mē·ə\ An abnormally low concentration of epinephrine in the blood.

**hypoergia** \hī′pō·ur′jə\ [HYPO- + *(all)erg(en)* + -IA] Reduced sensitivity to allergens; hyposensitivity. Also *hypoergy*. Adj. hypoergic.

**hypoesophoria** \-es′ōfôr′ē·ə\ [HYPO- + ESO- + PHORIA] A latent deviation of ocular alignment characterized by the lower eye turning inward, toward the nose.

**hypoesthesia** \-esthē′zhə\ [HYPO- + ESTHESIA] Reduction in sensitivity. Also *hypesthesia*. Adj. hypoesthetic, hypesthetic. **olfactory h.** HYPOSMIA. **tactile h.** A reduced perception of touch. Also *amblyaphia*.

**hypoestrogenemia** \-es′trəjənē′mē·ə\ Abnormally low concentrations of estrogens, as estrone or estradiol or both, in the blood. Also *hypoestrinemia* (older term).

**hypoestrogenism** \-es′trəjənizm\ [HYPO- + ESTROGEN + -ISM] Subnormal or deficient ovarian secretion of estrogens, or the condition resulting from it. Also *hypoestrinism* (older term).

**hypoexcitability** \-iksī′təbil′itē\ A state of reduced excitability, either of the whole person, or of neurons or other nervous structures and pathways.

**hypoexcitable** \-iksī′təbl\ Inadequately or subnormally reactive to normally exciting stimuli.

**hypoexophoria** \-ek′səfôr′ē·ə\ [HYPO- + EXO- + PHORIA] A latent deviation of ocular alignment characterized by the lower eye turning outward, toward the ear.

**hypoferremia** \-ferē′mē·ə\ [HYPO- + L *ferr(um)* iron + -EMIA] An abnormally low concentration of iron in the blood or blood serum. Also *oligosideremia*.

**hypoferrism** \-fer′izm\ IRON DEFICIENCY.

**hypofibrinogenemia** \-fī′bröjənē′mē·ə\ Reduced concentration of plasma fibrinogen. Also *fibrinogenopenia, hypinosis* (obs.).

**hypofunction** Reduced function of an organ, tissue, or system, often signifying function at a subnormal level, as of an endocrine gland. **convergence h.** Deficient amplitude of ocular convergence. Also *insufficiency of the interni*. **divergence h.** Deficient amplitude of ocular divergence. Also *insufficiency of the externi*.

**hypogalactia** \-gəlak′shə\ [HYPO- + GALACT- + -IA] Reduced milk formation.

**hypogalactous** \-gəlak′təs\ In a state of reduced milk formation.

**hypogammaglobulinemia** \-gam′əglō′byəlinē′mē·ə\ [HYPO- + *gamma globulin* + -EMIA] A condition of immunologic deficiency marked by abnormally low levels or the virtual absence of immunoglobulins in the blood, causing increased vulnerability to infectious diseases. Also *agammaglobulinemia*. Adj. hypogammaglobulinemic. **acquired h.** Hypogammaglobulinemia which is due to causes other than genetic defects in antibody formation and which becomes manifest after early childhood. **congenital h.** INFANTILE SEX-LINKED HYPOGAMMAGLOBULINEMIA. **infantile sex-linked h.** A congenital disorder affecting male infants, in which all classes of immunoglobulins may be deficient, with subnormal plasma concentrations. The affected infant is prone to infections, particularly respiratory, due to bacterial pathogens and especially *Pneumocystis carinii*. Replacement therapy with regular injections of plasma protein derivatives rich in immunoglobulin G is partially effective. Also *Bruton's disease, congenital hypogammaglobulinemia, X-linked hypogammaglobulinemia, Bruton type agammaglobulinemia*. **lymphopenic h.** SEVERE COMBINED IMMUNODEFICIENCY. **physiologic h.** The normal fall in plasma concentration of immunoglobulin which occurs during the first three to six months after birth. It is due to a delay before the start of synthesizing immunoglobulin G (IgG). **primary h.** Hypogammaglobulinemia resulting from defects in or diseases of the normal antibody-forming mechanism. **secondary h.** Hypogammaglobulinemia resulting from nonimmunologic disease, as from conditions causing protein loss into the gut or urine, certain drugs, infections, or malnutrition. **Swiss type h.** SEVERE COMBINED IMMUNODEFICIENCY. **transient h. of infancy** The low plasma level of immunoglobulin, particularly IgG, that normally occurs at about three months of life because in early infancy the amount of immunoglobulin received through the placenta before birth is catabolized more rapidly than new immunoglobulin is formed. **X-linked h.** INFANTILE SEX-LINKED HYPOGAMMAGLOBULINEMIA.

**hypogastric** \-gas′trik\ [HYPO- + GASTRIC] **1** Pertaining to the hypogastrium. **2** Below the stomach.

**hypogastrium** \-gas′trē·əm\ [New L, from Gk *hypogastrion* (from HYPO- + *gastēr* belly) the lower part of the belly] REGIO PUBICA.

**hypogastropagus** \-gasträp′əgəs\ [*hypogastr(ium)* + -PAGUS] Equal conjoined twins joined in the hypogastric regions.

**hypogastroschisis** \-gasträs′kisis\ [*hypogastr(ium)* + -SCHISIS] The developmental failure of the abdominal wall to close in the region below the umbilicus and above the pubis.

**hypogenesis** \-jen′əsis\ [HYPO- + GENESIS] Failure of development or growth of an embryo, fetus, or a part of it. Adj. hypogenetic. **polar h.** Specific underdevelopment at the cephalic or caudal ends of the body, or both.

**hypogenitalism** \-jen′ətəlizm\ [HYPO- + GENITAL + -ISM] Underdevelopment of the genitalia owing to hypogonadism.

**hypogeusia** \-joo′sē·ə\ [HYPO- + Gk *geus(is)* taste + -IA] Diminished acuity of taste perception. Because of the close association of the senses of taste and smell, patients with anosmia will usually complain of hypogeusia although the sense of taste may be shown to be unaffected.

**hypoglandular** \-glan′dyələr\ Characterized by subnormal or deficient glandular secretion.

**hypoglobulia** \-glōbyoo′lē·ə\ [HYPO- + *globul(e)* + -IA] An abnormally low concentration of erythrocytes in the blood, or of erythrocyte precursors in the bone marrow.

**hypoglossal** \-gläs′əl\ [Gk *hypoglōss(os)* (from HYPO- + *glōssa* tongue) under the tongue + -AL] Below the tongue.

**hypoglossis** \-gläs′is\ HYPOGLOTTIS.

**hypoglossus** \-gläs′əs\ NERVUS HYPOGLOSSUS.

**hypoglottis** \-glät′is\ [Gk *hypoglōttis* or *hypoglōssis* (from HYPO- + *glōtta* or *glōssa* tongue) the underside of the tongue] The inferior surface of the tongue. Also *hypoglossis.*

**hypoglycaemia** *Brit.* HYPOGLYCEMIA.

**hypoglycemia** \-glīsē′mē·ə\ [HYPO- + GLYCEMIA] Subnormal concentration of glucose in the blood. It may be caused by pancreatic islet cell overactivity, overdosage of insulin, intestinal malabsorption, or hepatic or endocrine disease. It produces symptoms of headache, tremor, sweating, blanching, mental and emotional disturbances (faintness, impaired concentration and memory), convulsions, and coma. Adj. hypoglycemic. **fasting h.** Pathologically low blood glucose concentration in the fasting state, that is, after a 48 to 72 hour fast. It is characteristic of the hypoglycemia of organic as opposed to functional disease, and is found in insulinoma, very severe hepatic disease, sprue, advanced malnutrition, Addison's disease, and panhypopituitarism. **functional h.** REACTIVE HYPOGLYCEMIA. **leucine-induced h.** Hypoglycemia of infants, induced by most proteins, which contain leucine. A familial disease, it is transmitted as an autosomal recessive. **mixed h.** Hypoglycemia with the characteristics of both fasting and reactive hypoglycemia, marked by low blood sugar when fasting and after a carbohydrate feeding. It is found in some patients with infantile hypoglycemia, Addison's disease, panhypopituitarism, and insulinoma. **reactive h.** Hypoglycemia occurring in response to a carbohydrate feeding, due to abnormally increased insulin secretion. It is found in functional hypoglycemia, sometimes in the postgastrectomy syndrome, and after the excessively rapid absorption of carbohydrate in thyrotoxicosis. Also *functional hypoglycemia.*

**hypoglycemic** \-glīsē′mik\ **1** Of, relating to, or characterized by hypoglycemia. **2** Acting to lower the level of glucose in the blood, as *hypoglycemic agent.*

**hypoglycorrhachia** \-glī′kôrā′kē·ə\ [HYPO- + GLYCO- + -RRHACHIA] An abnormally small glucose content of the cerebrospinal fluid.

**hypogonadal** \-gän′ədəl\ Having or pertaining to hypogonadism.

**hypogonadism** \-gō′nədizm\ [HYPO- + GONAD + -ISM] The condition resulting from subnormal secretion of sex hormones by the gonads, with consequent retardation of growth, eunuchoidism, and failure of the secondary sex characters to develop. Also *hypogonadia* (older term). **h. with anosmia** KALLMANN SYNDROME. **familial hypogonadotropic h.** Failure of secondary sexual characters to develop owing to isolated deficiency of anterior pituitary secretion of gonadotropin. It appears to be inherited as an autosomal recessive trait. **hypogonadotropic h.** Hypogonadism owing to deficient anterior pituitary secretion of gonadotropic hormones. Also *secondary hypogonadism.* **pituitary h.** Hypogonadism resulting from disease of the anterior pituitary with deficient secretion of gonadotropic hormones. **primary h.** Insufficient development, hormone secretion, and gamete production by the gonads due to intrinsic gonadal disease, as contrasted to hypergonadotropic hypogonadism (secondary hypogonadism). **secondary h.** HYPOGONADOTROPIC HYPOGONADISM.

**hypogonadotrophic** \-gän′ədōträf′ik\ HYPOGONADOTROPIC.

**hypogonadotrophism** \-gän′ədōträf′izm\ HYPOGONADOTROPISM.

**hypogonadotropic** \-gän′ədōträp′ik\ Of or characterized by hypogonadotropism. Also *hypogonadotrophic.*

**hypogonadotropism** \-gän′ədōträp′izm\ [HYPO- + *gonadotrop(in)* + -ISM] Subnormal or deficient secretion of the gonadotropic hormones of the anterior pituitary, or the condition resulting from it. Also *hypogonadotrophism.*

**hypogranulocytosis** \-gran″yəlōsītō′sis\ GRANULOCYTOPENIA.

**hypohidrosis** \-hidrō′sis\ [HYPO- + HIDROSIS] Diminished sweating. Also *hidroschesis, oligohidrosis, hypoidrosis.*

**hypohidrotic** \-hidrät′ik\ A substance that inhibits sweating.

**hypohormonal** \-hôr′mōnəl\ [HYPO- + HORMONAL] Marked by insufficient secretion of a hormone or hormones.

**hypohyal** \-hī′əl\ The hyoid element that lies between the ceratohyal and basihyal of the hyoid apparatus. It is derived from the anterior end of the distal part of the cartilage of the second branchial arch, and it forms the lesser horn of the hyoid bone in the human adult.

**hypohydration** \-hīdrā′shən\ [HYPO- + HYDR- + -ATION] A state of decreased water content.

**hypohydrochloria** \-hī′drəklôr′ē·ə\ HYPOCHLORHYDRIA.

**hypohypnotic** \-hipnät′ik\ Relating to light sleep.

**hypohypophysism** \-hīpäf′isizm\ [HYPO- + *hypophys(is)* + -ISM] *Rare* HYPOPITUITARISM.

**hypoidrosis** \-hī′pō·idrō′sis\ HYPOHIDROSIS.

**hypoinsulinemia** \-in′syəlinē′mē·ə\ [HYPO- + INSULIN + -EMIA] The condition of having a subnormal concentration of insulin in the blood relative to the blood glucose concentration. A degree of hypoinsulinemia is present in all patients with diabetes mellitus.

**hypoinsulinism** \-in′syəlinizm\ [HYPO- + INSULIN + -ISM] The incapacity to secrete normal amounts of insulin, as in diabetes mellitus.

**hypoisotonic** \-ī′sōtän′ik\ HYPOTONIC.

**hypokalemia** \-kəlē′mē·ə\ [HYPO- + New L *kal(ium)* potassium + -EMIA] An abnormally low concentration of potassium in the blood or blood serum. It may be congenital, as in familial periodic paralysis, or acquired through intestinal or renal loss. Manifestations may include muscle weakness or paralysis, electrocardiographic abnormalities, and impairment of renal tubular function. Also *hypopotassemia, hypokaliemia.*

**hypokalemic** \-kəlē′mik\ **1** Pertaining to or resulting from hypokalemia. Also *hypopotassemic.* **2** Any substance which lowers potassium content of blood or tissue.

**hypokaliemia** \-kal′i·ē′mē·ə\ HYPOKALEMIA.

**hypokinemia** \-kīnē′mē·ə\ [HYPO- + KIN- + -EMIA] Reduced cardiac output.

**hypokinesia** \-kīnē′zhə\ A reduction in motor activity or in the range of movement of the body or limbs. Also *hypanakinesia, hypanakinesis, hypokinesis, hypocinesis, hypocinesia.* Adj. hypokinetic.

**hypolarynx** \-ler′ingks\ The lower part of the laryngeal cavity, extending from the vocal folds to the level of the lower border of the cricoid cartilage.

**hypolemmal** \-lem′əl\ Pertaining to hypolemma.

**hypolethal** \-lē′thəl\ Describing a mutant allele that may reduce fitness of the organism without totally eliminating the possibility of reproduction.

**hypoleukocytic** \-loo′kəsit′ik\ LEUKOPENIC.

**hypoleydigism** \-lī′digizm\ [HYPO- + *Leydig (cells)* + -ISM] Deficient secretion of androgen (testosterone) by the testicular interstitial cells of Leydig.

**hypolipemia** \-līpē′mē·ə\ [HYPO- + LIP- + -EMIA] An abnormally low concentration of fat in the blood or blood serum.

**hypolipoproteinemia** \-lip′ōprō′tēnē′mē·ə\ An abnormally low concentration of lipoprotein in the blood or blood serum. See also HYPOBETALIPOPROTEINEMIA, ABETALIPROTEINEMIA, ANALPHALIPOPROTEINEMIA.

**hypoliposis** \-lipō′sis\ An abnormally low concentration of lipids in the blood or tissues.

**hypolutemia** \-l^yootē′mē·ə\ [HYPO- + *lut(eo)-* + -EMIA] An abnormally low concentration of progesterone in the blood or blood serum.

**hypolymphemia** \-limfē′mē·ə\ LYMPHOCYTOPENIA.

**hypomagnesemia** \-mag′nəsē′mē·ə\ An abnormally low concentration of magnesium in the blood or blood serum, manifested chiefly by muscular hyperirritability.

**hypomania** \-mā′nē·ə\ [HYPO- + -MANIA] A relatively mild form of mania characterized by elated mood, restlessness and irritability, overproductivity, distractibility and an increase in ideas and the rate of speech. Also *submania*.

**hypomastia** \-mas′tē·ə\ [HYPO- + MAST- + -IA] Congenital underdevelopment of the female breast. Also *hypomazia*.

**hypomelanism** \-mel′ənizm\ A state of reduced skin pigmentation. **dominant oculocutaneous h.** An autosomal dominant hereditary disorder, similar to albinism, in which the iris is translucent when light is passed through it and the skin is hypersensitive to ultraviolet radiation.

**hypomelanosis** \-mel′ənō′sis\ [HYPO- + MELANOSIS] A reduced melanin pigmentation of the skin. **hereditary h.** A reduced melanin pigmentation that is of hereditary origin. **idiopathic guttate h.** The development of small macules of hypomelanosis. It is a common but inconspicuous condition that begins in late childhood.

**hypomenorrhea** \-men′ôrē′ə\ [HYPO- + MENORRHEA] Diminution in the amount of flow or a shortening of the duration of menstruation.

**hypomere** \hī′pōmir\ [HYPO- + -MERE] The part of the mesoderm in an embryo that gives rise to the mesothelial lining of the serous cavities. It is derived from lateral plate mesoderm.

**hypomery** \hīpäm′ərē\ [HYPO- + *-mer(e)* + -Y] Diminution in the number of the primitive embryonic segments.

**hypomesosoma** \-mes′əsō′mə\ A stature that is shorter than the median percentile.

**hypometabolism** \-mətab′əlizm\ A state of reduced metabolic activity; a reduced rate of metabolism. **euthyroid h.** A state of reduced metabolic activity in the presence of normal thyroid function.

**hypometria** \-mē′trē·ə\ [HYPO- + Gk *metr(on)* a measure + -IA] A form of dysmetria in which movement of a limb falls short of the intended target.

**hypometropia** \-mētrō′pē·ə\ [HYPO- + Gk *metr(on)* measure + -OPIA] *Seldom used* MYOPIA.

**hypomicrosoma** \-mī′krəsō′mə\ The smallest stature within the normal percentiles.

**hypomineralization** \-min′əral′īzā′shən\ A state marked by a deficiency of minerals in the body.

**hypomorph** \hi′pōmôrf\ [HYPO- + -MORPH] **1** An individual who is short in standing height in proportion to sitting height. This results from a lower limb length that is proportionally shorter than trunk length. Adj. hypomorphic. **2** An allele of reduced effect compared to the wild-type allele. The protein product, for example, would have reduced, but not absent, enzymatic activity. Also *leaky gene, leaky allele*.

**hypomotility** \-mōtil′itē\ A condition marked by levels of movement that are less than normal.

**hyponanosoma** \-nan′ōsō′mə\ An extreme degree of dwarfism.

**hyponasality** \-nāzal′itē\ The nasal quality of speech when there is an obstruction to normal airflow through the nose, particularly for the nasal consonants such as *m* or *n*. Also *rhinolalia clausa, denasality*.

**hyponatremia** \-nətrē′mē·ə\ [HYPO- + New L *natr(ium)* sodium + -EMIA] An abnormally low concentration of sodium in the blood serum. Adj. hyponatremic.

**hyponatruria** \-nətroo′rē·ə\ Decreased urinary excretion of sodium, as in dietary salt restriction or accumulating edema, or secondary to increased secretion or to administration of salt-retaining mineralocorticoid hormones.

**hyponoderma** \-nədur′mə\ *Obs.* CUTANEOUS LARVA MIGRANS.

**hyponomoderma** \-näm′ədur′mə\ *Obs.* CUTANEOUS LARVA MIGRANS.

**hyponychium** \-nik′e·əm\ [New L, from HYP- + ONYCH- + *-ium*, noun suffix] [NA] The part of the fingertip that extends from the distal end of the nail bed to the distal crease on the palmar aspect of the finger. It corresponds to the pulp of the finger.

**hyponychon** \hīpän′ikän\ [irreg. from HYP- + Gk *onyx*, gen. *onychos*, talon, claw, nail] An ecchymosis that lies beneath a fingernail or toenail.

**hypo-oncotic** \-ängkät′ik\ Marked by oncotic pressure that is less than the normal.

**hypo-osmosis** \-äzmō′sis\ The reduced movement of a solvent as a result of a diminished difference in osmotic activity between two solutions.

**hypo-osmotic** \-äzmät′ik\ Having a lower concentration of osmotically active solutes than a comparative solution.

**hypo-ovarianism** \-ōver′ē·ənizm\ HYPOVARIANISM.

**hypopallesthesia** \-pal′esthē′zhə\ [HYPO- + PALLESTHESIA] Abnormal reduction in sensitivity to applied vibration.

**hypopancreatism** \-pan′krē·ətizm\ Pancreatic hyposecretion or insufficiency.

**hypoparathyroid** \-par′əthī′roid\ Of, relating to, or characteristic of hypoparathyroidism.

**hypoparathyroidism** \-par′əthī′roidizm\ [HYPO- + PARATHYROID + -ISM] The condition resulting from subnormal or absent secretion of parathyroid hormone by the parathyroid glands, most often due to inadvertent parathyroidectomy or injury to the glands during thyroid surgery. The idiopathic form is rare and may have an autoimmune basis. It is sometimes associated with pernicious anemia, Addison's disease, or ovarian failure. Hypoparathyroidism is characterized by hypocalcemia, high serum phosphorous, low levels of plasma, immunoreactive parathyroid hormone, increased bone density, cataracts, tetany, convulsions, ectopic calcifications, and mental disturbances. There may be associated abnormalities of skin, nails, hair, and teeth. Also *parathyroid insufficiency*. **familial h.** Any of three forms of hereditary hypoparathyroidism, comprising neonatal hypoparathyroidism, an X-linked recessive disorder occurring only in males; the familial disorder without Addison's disease and moniliasis, an autosomal recessive disorder often associated with consanguinity; and the familial disorder with Addison's disease and mucocutaneous moniliasis, an autosomal recessive disorder sometimes associated with other autoimmune disorders, as pernicious anemia, thyroiditis or ovarian failure. Familial hypoparathyroidism constitutes about 25 percent of cases of hypoparathyroidism.

**hypopepsia** \-pep′sē·ə\ Diminished gastric secretion. Adj. hypopeptic.

**hypoperistalsis** \-per′istal′sis\ Diminished or inadequate peristalsis.

**hypoperistaltic** \-per′istal′tik\ Relating to or characterized by hypoperistalsis.

**hypopexia** \-pek′sē·ə\ [HYPO- + *-pex(y)* + -IA] The reduced fixation of a substance into tissues. Also *hypopexy*.

**hypophalangism** \-fəlan′jizm\ [HYPO- + *phalang(es)*, pl. of PHALANX + -ISM] A condition of having fewer than the normal number of phalanges.

**α-hypophamine** *Seldom used* OXYTOCIN.
**β-hypophamine** *Seldom used* VASOPRESSIN.
**hypopharyngoscope** \-fəring′gəskōp\ ESOPHAGEAL SPECULUM.
**hypopharyngoscopy** \-far′ing·gäs′kəpē\ The examination of the interior of the hypopharynx, often combined with the examination of the cricopharyngeal region and the upper esophagus.
**hypopharynx** \-far′ingks\ PARS LARYNGEA PHARYNGIS.
**hypophonia** \-fō′nē·ə\ [HYPO- + PHON- + -IA] The weak or thin voice, or whisper, resulting from impaired respiratory or vocal fold activity.
**hypophoria** \-fôr′ē·ə\ [HYPO- + -PHORIA] A latent, downward deviation of one eye, spontaneously corrected by the fusion mechanisms. The specified eye is the deviating lower eye. Thus, in right hypophoria, the right eye tends to deviate downward and the left to fix; in left hypophoria, the left eye tends to deviate downward and the right eye to fix.
**hypophosphatasia** \-fäs′fətā′zhə\ An inherited deficiency of alkaline phosphatase. Severe forms occur in infancy and childhood and are inherited as autosomal recessive traits. Features include severe undermineralization of the skeleton and stillbirth in the most severe cases, irritability, seizures, rachitic skeletal changes, premature loss of teeth, and susceptibility to bleeding and infection. The adult-onset form is inherited as an autosomal dominant trait and features bone fragility, osteoporosis, and premature loss of teeth.
**hypophosphatemia** \-fäs′fətē′mē·ə\ [HYPO- + PHOSPHATEMIA] Less than normal concentration of phosphate in blood, plasma, or serum. Also *hypophosphoremia.* **familial h.** FAMILIAL HYPOPHOSPHATEMIC RICKETS. **hereditary h.** X-LINKED HYPOPHOSPHATEMIA. **renal h.** FAMILIAL HYPOPHOSPHATEMIC RICKETS. **X-linked h.** The most common form of familial hypophosphatemic rickets, inherited as an X-linked dominant trait, and characterized by radiologic rickets and osteomalacia, slow growth, bowed legs, hypophosphatemia, decreased renal tubular phosphate reabsorption, and normal plasma calcium and parathyroid hormone. The biochemical defect is unclear. Also *familial vitamin D resistant rickets, hereditary hypophosphatemia, phosphate diabetes* (obs.).
**hypophosphaturia** \-fäs′fətoo′rē·ə\ Decreased urinary excretion of inorganic phosphates when dietary phosphate intake is low, but more commonly when phosphates are bound in the gastrointestinal tract by nonabsorbable antacids. It is also caused by normal somatic growth, pregnancy, lactation, hypoparathyroidism, Addison's disease, and sodium depletion.
**hypophosphoremia** \-fäs′fôrē′mē·ə\ HYPOPHOSPHATEMIA.
**hypophrenia** \-frē′nē·ə\ [HYPO- + -PHRENIA] MENTAL RETARDATION.
**hypophrenium** \-frē′nē·əm\ The part of the peritoneal cavity between the diaphragm above and the transverse colon and mesocolon below. It comprises all the subphrenic and subhepatic recesses and the omental bursa. *Outmoded.* Also *supracolic space, supraomental region, subphrenic region.*
**hypophyseal** \-fizē′əl, -fiz′e·əl\ HYPOPHYSIAL.
**hypophysectomize** \-fizek′təmīz\ [*hypophys(is)* + -ECTOMIZE ] To excise or destroy the hypophysis.
**hypophysectomy** \-fizek′təmē\ [*hypophys(is cerebri)* + -ECTOMY] The excision or destruction of the hypophysis cerebri. Among the indications are certain pituitary tumors, particularly chromaphobe adenomas, and certain endocrine disorders, particularly acromegaly and Cushing's disease. The operation as a means of relieving advanced breast cancer and carcinoma of the prostate has been largely superseded by chemotherapy and hormone therapy. The surgical approach may be transcranial or extracranial (as in transeptal and transethmoidal hypophysectomy). Also *hypophysiectomy.* **trans-sphenoidal h.** An operation for removal of the pituitary by traversing the sphenoid sinus and removing the floor of the sella turcica. It is now performed with the aid of a surgical microscope. To prevent cerebrospinal-fluid leakage the operation attempts to preserve the diaphragma sellae, uses material to pack the cavity of the sella turcica, and employs a substituting material for replacing the defect in the floor of the sella.
**hypophysial** \-fiz′ē·əl\ Of or relating to the pituitary gland (hypophysis). Also *hypophyseal.*
**hypophysiectomy** \-fiz′ē·ek′təmē\ HYPOPHYSECTOMY.
**hypophysin** **1** The hormone of the posterior pituitary gland. Rarely used in this sense. **2** An extract of bovine pituitary gland containing oxytocin and vasopressin.
**hypophysiotropic** \-fiz′ē·əträp′ik\ Acting upon the pituitary gland (hypophysis cerebri), as the hypothalamic hypophysiotropic hormones. Also *hypophysiotrophic.*
**hypophysis** \hīpäf′isis\ [Gk (from *hypophyesthai* to grow or be attached below, from HYPO- + *phyein* to grow) a growth or attachment underneath] [NA] An unpaired, ovoid body that lies below the hypothalamus in the pituitary fossa of the sella turcica; the pituitary gland. Also *hypophysis cerebri.* **accessory h.** One or more rests of adenohypophyseal tissue up to 5 mm in diameter found near the junction of the sphenoid and the vomer in relation to the site of the embryologic craniopharyngeal canal. In man they often merge with the mucous glands in the nasopharynx. They may hypertrophy and become functional if the hypophysis is destroyed. Also *pharyngeal hypophysis.* **h. cerebri** HYPOPHYSIS. **pharyngeal h.** ACCESSORY HYPOPHYSIS.
**hypophysitis** \hīpäf′isī′tis\ [*hypophys(is cerebri)* + -ITIS] Inflammation of the pituitary gland.
**hypopiesia** \-pī·ē′zhə\ HYPOTENSION.
**hypopiesis** \-pī·ē′sis\ HYPOTENSION.
**hypopietic** \-pī·et′ik\ HYPOTENSIVE.
**hypopituitarism** \-pit^y^oo′itərizm\ [HYPO- + PITUITARISM] Deficient secretion of anterior pituitary hormones. Hypopituitarism may result from postpartum necrosis of the pituitary gland as in the Sheehan syndrome, to tumors, to surgical hypophysectomy, or to sudden infarction of the gland (pituitary apoplexy). It is associated with varying degrees of stunted growth and with gonadal, thyroidal, and adrenocortical deficiency. Also *anterior pituitary insufficiency, hypophysial dystrophy, hypohypophysism* (rare), *pituitary insufficiency, subpituitarism.* **postpartum hemorrhagic h.** SHEEHAN SYNDROME.
**hypopituitary** \-pit^y^oo′iter′ē\ Of or characteristic of hypopituitarism.
**hypoplasia** \-plā′zhə\ [HYPO- + -PLASIA] An underdevelopment of a tissue, organ, or region of the body. It implies fewer than the usual number of cells. Also *microgenesis.* Compare AGENESIS, APLASIA, DYSPLASIA. **h. of the aortic tract complexes** See under HYPOPLASTIC LEFT HEART SYNDROME. **cartilage-hair h.** METAPHYSEAL CHONDRODYSPLASIA, McKUSICK TYPE. **congenital generalized muscular h.** A syndrome marked by generalized muscle hypoplasia, with onset at birth with generalized muscular weakness, hypotonia, and delay in walking and in reaching other physical milestones. There are no other constitutional abnormalities, and the deep tendon reflexes are usually normal. It is now known that this is a syndrome of multiple etiology and not a specific disease. The condition

often tends to improve spontaneously. Also *Krabbe syndrome, Krabbe's disease, congenital universal muscular hypoplasia.* **craniofacial h.** Congenital underdevelopment of the cranial and facial bones frequently associated with other malformations. **h. cutis congenita** 1 Developmental ectodermal dysplasia involving absence or deficiency of hair, nails, and glands of the skin. 2 Any developmental dysplasia or hypoplasia of the skin. **enamel h.** A hereditary abnormality in which the enamel is defective in thickness or structure. What enamel is present may be of normal structure and calcification. The condition is most often seen as pits on what are normally smooth surfaces. The pits may become carious. Also *hereditary enamel hypoplasia.* **focal dermal h.** An X-linked, dominant, congenital syndrome of asymmetric scarlike regions and hyperpigmented streaks on the skin, isolated herniations of subcutaneous fat, papillomas of the lips, mouth, and anogenital area; sparse hair, dysplastic nails, digital anomalies, ear malformations with conductive deafness, and osteopathia striata. Mental retardation and dental, palatal, and cardiac anomalies also occur. The syndrome is usually lethal *in utero* in males, producing an increased miscarriage rate in affected women. Also *Goltz syndrome.* **granulocytic h.** Reduction in the rate of formation of granulocytes by bone marrow. **hereditary brown h. of enamel** AMELOGENESIS IMPERFECTA. **hereditary enamel h.** ENAMEL HYPOPLASIA. **lobular h.** LOBULAR APLASIA. **nasomaxillary h.** The underdevelopment of the structures forming the nose and the upper jaw. **oligonephronic h.** Renal underdevelopment characterized by reduced numbers of nephrons. **pluricystic h.** Renal underdevelopment associated with numerous cysts, as is seen in polycystic kidney. **h. of the right ventricle** A congenital abnormality of the right ventricular wall, which may be so underdeveloped that it has no muscular tissue and is paper thin. Also *parchment heart.* See also UHL'S ANOMALY. **h. of tooth** Defective formation of a tooth, most often of the enamel, but occasionally of the dentin.

**hypoploid** \hī′pōploid\ [HYPO- + -PLOID] Having a chromosome complement which is aneuploid through loss of chromosomes from the usual integral number of sets: usually said of a complement slightly less than an integral multiple, as in hypodiploid.

**hypopnea** \hī′päp·nē′ə\ [HYPO- + -PNEA] Slow and shallow breathing. Also *oligopnea.*

**hypopnoea** *Brit.* HYPOPNEA.

**hypopotassemia** \-pät′asē′mē·ə\ HYPOKALEMIA.

**hypopotassemic** \-pät′asē′mik\ HYPOKALEMIC.

**hypopotentia** \-pōten′shə\ 1 Reduced electrical activity of the cerebral cortex. 2 Weakness. *Outmoded.*

**hypoproaccelerinemia** \-prō′aksel′ərinē′mē·ə\ [HYPO- + PROACCELERIN + -EMIA] Factor V deficiency in plasma.

**hypoproconvertinemia** \-prō′kənvur′tinē′mē·ə\ [HYPO- + PROCONVERTIN + -EMIA] A condition marked by low plasma factor VII activity, which may result from administration of coumarin anticoagulants, from severe liver disease, or from a genetic disorder. **hereditary h.** FACTOR VII DEFICIENCY.

**hypoprogesterone hexanoate** HYDROXYPROGESTERONE CAPROATE.

**hypoproteinemia** \-prō′tēnē′mē·ə\ [HYPO- + PROTEINEMIA] Less than normal concentration of protein in blood, plasma, or serum. **chronic idiopathic h. in the child** Unexplained hypoproteinemia in a young child, often presenting as edema. Investigation usually reveals a chronic gastrointestinal disorder, such as celiac disease, lymphangiectasis, or ulcerative colitis.

**hypoproteinemic** \-prō′tēnē′mik\ Marked by a less-than-normal protein concentration in the plasma.

**hypoproteinia** \-prō′tē·in′ē·ə\ An abnormally low level of protein in the blood plasma due to a very low intake from the diet or arising from a disease state such as nephrosis, or liver disease.

**hypoprothrombinemia** \-prōthräm′binē′mē·ə \ A less than normal activity or concentration of prothrombin in blood. Also *prothrombinopenia.*

**hypopus** \hīpō′pəs\ [Gk *hypopous* furnished with feet] (*pl.* hypopi) An unusual transport stage in the life cycle of certain grain mites (order Acariformes, suborder Astigmata), in which a distinctive body form develops between the first and second nymphal stages. In some species phoretic or active hypopi occur, adapted for clinging to arthropods or mammals. Another type is a passive form, the dauernymph, which is able to use air currents for dispersal or which is simply a waiting stage.

**hypopyon** \hīpō′pē·än\ [Gk (from *hypopy(os)* suppurative, from *hyp-* under, up from under + *pyon* pus) a suppurating ulcer] The sedimentation of white blood cells into the inferior portion of the anterior chamber of the eye, where a flat-topped gravity line is formed. This inferior white deposit is an easily observed sign of serious intraocular inflammation.

**hyporeactive** \-rē·ak′tiv\ Exhibiting a reduced responsiveness to stimulation.

**hyporeflexia** \-riflek′sē·ə\ Reduction or weakening of reflexes. Also *hyporeflectivity.*

**hyporiboflavinosis** \-rī′bōflā′vinō′sis\ RIBOFLAVIN DEFICIENCY.

**hyposarca** \-sär′kə\ ANASARCA.

**hyposcheotomy** \hīpäs′kē·ät′əmē\ [HYP- + OSCHEO- + -TOMY] Incision of a hydrocele at the inferior portion of the tunica vaginalis testis.

**hyposcleral** \-sklir′əl\ [HYPO- + SCLERAL] Situated between the sclera and the choroid.

**hyposecretion** \-sikrē′shən\ [HYPO- + SECRETION] Subnormal secretion, as of a substance or hormone by a gland.

**hyposensitivity** \-sen′sətiv′itē\ [HYPO- + SENSITIVITY] A state in which an immune individual reacts with diminished response on subsequent exposure to a specific antigen to which he has been previously sensitized.

**hyposensitization** \-sen′sətīzā′shən\ The induction of a state of hyposensitivity.

**hyposensitize** \sen′sətīz\ To subject to repeated and gradually increasing doses of a sensitizing allergen to induce a state hyposensitivity for that specific allergen.

**hyposmia** \hīpäz′mē·ə\ [HYP- + *osm(o)-*$^2$ + -IA] Subnormal olfactory perception. Also *hyposphresia, olfactory hypoesthesia.*

**hyposomatotropism** \-sō′mətōtrō′pizm\ [HYPO- + SOMATO- + TROPISM] 1 Deficient or absent adenohypophysial secretion of growth hormone, or the condition resulting from it. 2 Hypopituitary dwarfism of children. See under HYPOPHYSIAL DWARF.

**hyposomia** \-sō′mē·ə\ [HYPO- + *som(a)* + -IA] A condition marked by an underdeveloped body.

**hyposomnia** \-säm′nē·ə\ INSOMNIA.

**hypospadias** \-spā′dē·as\ [Gk (from *hypospan* to pull out from under, from HYPO- + *span* to pull away, draw off) an individual with hypospadias] A developmental defect of the urethra in which the urethral folds have failed to unite to complete the ventral wall of the urethra. The defect may involve only localized segments of a major portion of the urethra. Urine is discharged at the most proximal point of the defect. **balanic h.** Hypospadias on or near the glans penis. Also *coronal hypospadias, glandular hypospadias.*

**female h.** Hypospadias in the female, allowing leakage or discharge of urine into the lower vagina. **glandular h.** BALANIC HYPOSPADIAS. **penile h.** Hypospadias in the male at any point in or throughout the length of the penile urethra. **penoscrotal h.** Hypospadias occurring either separately or continuously on both the ventral aspect of the penis and at the midline of the scrotum. **perineal h.** Hypospadias in which the entire scrotum is cleft by an extensive defect in the base of the penile urethra and in more or less of the urethra on the shaft of the penis. The testes often do not descend and the penis may be rudimentary, with a chordee.

**hyposphresia** \hī′päsfrē′zhə\ HYPOSMIA.

**hypostasis** \hīpäs′təsis\ [Gk *hypostasis* (from *hypo-* under + *stasis* a standing) deposited matter, sediment] **1** The settling or pooling of a fluid or suspended solid due to gravity; especially, stasis of the circulation in a dependent part or organ. **2** The failure of the usual phenotypic expression of a gene when in the presence of another gene that is epistatic toward it.

**hypostatic** \-stat′ik\ **1** Of or characterized by hypostasis. **2** Failing to be expressed phenotypically when in the presence of an epistatic gene: said of a gene.

**hyposteatosis** \-stē·ətō′sis\ OLIGOSTEATOSIS.

**hyposthenia** \hī′pästhē′nē·ə\ A state of reduced strength; weakness.

**hypostheniant** \hī′pästhē′nē·ənt\ Any substance that brings about hyposthenia.

**hyposthenuria** \hī′pästhēnoo′rē·ə\ [HYPO- + STHEN- + -URIA] Impaired ability of the kidneys to concentrate urine appropriately in response to fluid deprivation or administration of antidiuretic hormone. It may be measured by the relative density of urine under conditions of known fluid deficit or by the urine-to-plasma osmolality ratio.

**hypostome** \hī′pōstōm\ [HYPO- + Gk *stom(a)* mouth] An organ of attachment in the tick capitulum. Centrally located and covered with spines, it allows the tick to anchor itself while feeding.

**hypostomia** \-stō′mē·ə\ [HYPO- + STOM- + -IA] Microstomia in which the oral orifice tends to be a small sagittal slit rather than a transverse one.

**hypostosis** \hī′pästō′sis\ [HYP- + OSTOSIS] A decreased development of bone.

**hyposulfite** *Outmoded* DITHIONITE.

**hyposuprarenalism** \-soo′prərē′nəlizm\ [HYPO- + SUPRARENAL + -ISM] *Seldom used* HYPOADRENALISM.

**hypotelorism** \-tel′ərizm\ [HYPO- + *-telorism* as in HYPERTELORISM] Abnormal closeness of paired organs or parts.

**hypotension** \-ten′shən\ [HYPO- + TENSION] Abnormally low tension or pressure, especially blood pressure. Also *hypopiesis, hypopiesia.* **arterial h.** Abnormally low systemic arterial pressure. **chronic orthostatic h.** SHY-DRAGER SYNDROME. **controlled h.** INDUCED HYPOTENSION. **familial orthostatic h.** The Shy-Drager syndrome involving more than one member of a family. **induced h.** Hypotension intentionally produced, either by mechanical or by pharmacological means, usually for the purpose of reducing blood loss in surgery. Also *controlled hypotension.* **intracranial h.** Reduced intracranial pressure. **orthostatic h.** Hypotension on assuming the upright posture, commonly manifested by faintness or syncope. It is a feature of certain disorders of the autonomic nervous system and also of treatment with certain antihypertensive agents. Also *postural hypotension.* **spinal h.** Hypotension resulting from the block of sympathetic nerve fibers during spinal anesthesia or spinal cord trauma. **vascular h.** Hypotension as a consequence of vascular dilatation. **ventricular h.** Reduction in the pressure of the cerebrospinal fluid in the cerebral ventricles following cranial surgery or head injury or occurring in states of dehydration, but most often following lumbar puncture or occurring in conditions causing extracranial leakage of cerebrospinal fluid. The principal symptoms are headache, which is worse when the patient stands or sits up, vomiting, and stiffness of the neck.

**hypotensive** \-ten′siv\ Characterized by or causing abnormally low tension or pressure, especially blood pressure. Also *hypopietic.*

**hypothalamic** \-thalam′ik\ Describing, pertaining to, or affecting the hypothalamus.

**hypothalamotomy** \-thal′əmät′əmē\ [*hypothalam(us)* + *o* + -TOMY] Incision into the hypothalamus or into the floor of the third ventricle.

**hypothalamus** \-thal′əməs\ [HYPO- + THALAMUS] [NA] A subdivision of the diencephalon that extends from the lamina terminalis to the mamillary bodies and comprises the ventrolateral wall and floor of the third ventricle below the hypothalamic sulcus. It can be divided into three zones (supraoptic, infundibulotuberal, and mamillary) and contains various groups of nuclei which exert control over autonomic functions, water balance, regulation of body temperature, appetite and food intake, sleep, and certain endocrine functions, including the neurosecretory control of the adenohypophysis and neurohypophsysis.

**hypothenar** \hīpäth′ənär, hī′pōthē′när\ [Gk (from HYPO- + THENAR) any of the marginal eminences of the palm] [NA] The elongated eminence along the ulnar border of the palm of the hand, produced mainly by the three intrinsic muscles that abduct, flex and oppose the fifth digit. Also *hypothenar eminence, antithenar.*

**hypothermal** \-thur′məl\ Descriptive of a body temperature below the normal.

**hypothermia** \-thur′mē·ə\ [HYPO- + Gk *therm(ē)* heat, feverish heat + -IA] A body temperature below the normal value of 98.6°F or 37°C. Clinically, hypothermia is not important unless the body temperature declines to 91–92°F or about 33°C. Also *hypothermy.* **accidental h.** Hypothermia caused by exposure to a cold environment and characterized by a dangerous fall in body temperature. It occurs most often in infants and in the elderly. **endogenous h.** Hypothermia caused by bodily disease or dysfunction rather than exogenous causes. **induced h.** Reduction in body temperature intentionally produced, for therapeutic purposes or as an adjunct to surgical techniques in which a reduction in body metabolism is helpful. **moderate h.** Hypothermia in which the body temperature is reduced to a range of 23–32°C. **profound h.** Body temperature of 12–20°C. **regional h.** Local cooling of an ischemic organ by refrigeration or perfusion with cold blood to reduce its metabolic requirements.

**hypothermy** \-thur′mē\ HYPOTHERMIA.

**hypothesis** \hīpäth′əsis\ [Gk *hypothesis* (from *hypotithenai* to place under, lay down, presuppose) a groundwork, assumption, principle] An assumption advanced to explain phenomena subject to tests that confirm, modify, or disprove it, or to serve as a basis for further experimentation or argument. **anniversary h.** A hypothesis stating that if a person who loses a parent during childhood, who later marries and has children, who still later is hospitalized for a first episode of mental illness, is likely to have that first episode at the time that his eldest child is within a year of his own age when he lost his parent. **biogenic amine h.** The theory that the biogenic amines are significant and perhaps even etiologic factors in the development of the major affective disorders and schizophrenia. The catecholamine hypothesis of affect disorders states that depressions are associated with a relative or absolute deficiency of catecholamines in functionally important sites in the brain. The permissive hypothesis of affect disorders states that a defect in central indolaminergic transmission permits affect disorder but is not enough to cause it. When superimposed on the indolamine defect, excess catecholamine produces mania while deficiency produces depression. The dopamine hypothesis of schizophrenia states that excess dopaminergic activity in the brain causes, precipitates, provokes, or exaggerates schizophrenic symptoms. **Buergi's h.** A theory that if two drugs have identical pharmacologic effects, their combined activity will be more than additive, when given simultaneously, if they have different mechanisms of pharmacologic action. Also *Buergi's theory.* **cardionector h.** The hypothesis that two pacemaker regions in the heart, the sinoatrial node (atrionector) and the atrioventricular node (ventriculonector), control the heart rhythm. *Obs.* **cascade h. of coagulation** An explanation of the sequence of events in coagulation in which the product of each step is a protease that activates the ensuing step by converting an inactive plasma protein to an active protease that in turn activates the next step. See diagram at COAGULATION. **catecholamine h.** See under BIOGENIC AMINE HYPOTHESIS. **chemiosmotic h.** The hypothesis that the action of the respiratory chain leads to the formation of a gradient in chemical potential of hydrogen ions across the membrane containing that respiratory chain, e.g. the mitochondrial membrane of eukaryotes, and that the passage of hydrogen ions down this gradient is used to drive chemical reactions, such as the condensation of ADP and orthophosphate to form ATP. The difference in chemical potential of the hydrogen ions consists of two parts, the pH difference and the difference in electrical potential across the membrane. The hypothesis was formulated to explain the coupling of oxidation to ATP formation by mitochondria, but it has also been extended to ATP formation in photosynthesis and to membrane transport by bacteria. **dopamine h.** See under BIOGENIC AMINE HYPOTHESIS. **Harrower's h.** The proposal that certain organ abnormalities may be ascribed to the defective supply of hormones on which the proper functioning of the organ depends. **inactive X h.** LYON PHENOMENON. **intact nephron h.** The hypothesis that chronic renal failure is characterized by a progressive decrease in the number of functioning nephrons rather than from separate impairment of the function of glomeruli and tubules. As nephrons decrease in number those remaining are thought to undergo structural and functional hypertrophy. **Lyon h.** LYON PHENOMENON. **Lyon-Russell h.** LYON PHENOMENON. **Makeham's h.** The proposal that death is due to both chance, which is constant, and the inability to prevent destruction, a factor that increases geometrically with age. **master-slave h.** The concept, now largely disproven, that structural genes are present in multiple, tandemly repeated copies in the genome. One copy is the master and serves as a corrective template for the other copies (the slaves) during each replication of the chromosome, a process termed rectification. The hypothesis was advanced by H.G. Callan in the 1960s and sought to account for the immense variation in nuclear DNA content among closely related organisms. **multiple factor h.** QUANTITATIVE INHERITANCE. **null h.** In statistics, the assumption that a measured difference between two samples of the same population is purely accidental, rather than being the result of some systematic variation. **one gene-one enzyme h.** The concept that each gene specifies a single enzyme. Although of historical importance, this hypothesis has been superseded by the one gene-one polypeptide hypothesis. **one gene-one polypeptide h.** The concept that each gene specifies a sequence in mRNA that directs the translation of one functional polypeptide. **Orgel's h.** ERROR CATASTROPHE. **permissive h. of affective disorders** See under BIOGENIC AMINE HYPOTHESIS. **polarization h.** The hypothesis that blastomeres at the 8-cell stage "recognize" an asymmetry of cell contacts by developing a polarized phenotype with an axis normal to the points of contact. The polarity is stable throughout division to the 16-cell stage yielding distinguishable superficial and deep subpopulations of cells. Continuing interactions between these cell subpopulations cause increasingly divergent differentiation to generate trophectoderm and inner cell mass tissues at the 32-cell stage. **polyneme h.** The hypothesis that a chromatid consists of more than one molecule of DNA. This concept has now been generally supplanted by the unineme hypothesis. **self-marker h.** A hypothesis to explain self/nonself discrimination by proposing that the body's own antigens carry markers which are recognized as self by immunologically competent cells. The latter cells are then inhibited from responding against those antigens which carry the self-marker. No molecular basis for the theory was proposed. **sliding-filament h.** The hypothesis that the basic mechanism responsible for the contractile force and shortening of muscle tissue depends upon longitudinally arranged and interdigitating actin and myosin filaments which, through activation of cross-bridges, increase the overlap along their lengths and so shorten the sarcomere. **structural h.** The hypothesis that the psyche has three divisions, id, ego, and superego. Also *structural theory.* **topographic h.** The hypothesis that the psyche has three divisions, conscious, preconscious, and unconscious. **trade-off h.** The hypothesis that as renal function declines various compensatory changes tend to maintain the concentration of solutes in body fluids at near normal levels, at the expense of some other organs or organ systems. This is based on the retention of phosphate as glomerular filtration rate decreases, which in turn causes an increase in the secretion of parathyroid hormone. The increased parathyroid hormone inhibits proximal reabsorption of phosphate, thus returning the plasma phosphate level to normal. However, the persistent increase in parathyroid hormone mobilizes calcium from the bones and thus leads to the osteodystrophy of chronic renal failure. In this manner, maintainence of a normal plasma phosphate level is "traded-off" for secondary hyperparathyroidism and renal osteodystrophy. **triplet h.** The hypothesis that a sequence of three nucleotides in the deoxyribonucleic acid molecule (a codon), carries the genetic information needed to place a specific amino acid in a polypeptide chain. **unineme h.** The concept, generally accepted for all eukaryotes, that one double helix of DNA extends from one end of a chromatid to the other. **unitarian h.** The theory, now obsolete, that antibody is a single species of immunoglobulin regardless of the types of reaction seen with various antigens. Also *unitarian theory of antibodies.* **wobble h.** The hypothesis which states that the terminal nucleotide (3′) in a codon may be either of the two purines without altering the amino acid incorporated into the polypeptide chain, or in other codons either of two pyrimidines without altering specificity. The specificity of the codon is dependent on the first two nucleotides, with some freedom in the third nucleotide. The wobble is dependent on the geometry of the ribosome.

**hypothromboplastinemia** \-thräm′bəplas′tinē′mē·ə\

[HYPO- + THROMBOPLASTIN + -EMIA] A deficiency of one of the hemophilic factors, VIII, IX, or XI.

**hypothyroid** \-thī′roid\ [HYPO- + THYROID] Of, relating to, or characteristic of hypothyroidism. Also *athyreotic* (seldom used).

**hypothyroidism** \-thī′roidizm\ [HYPOTHYROID + -ISM] Deficient hormone secretion by the thyroid gland, or the condition resulting from it. In infants, hypothyroidism leads to cretinism. In adults, it is characterized by lowered oxygen consumption, a slowed basal metabolic rate, sluggishness, lethargy, pallor, menstrual disorders, and disturbances in mentation. In advanced stages, myxedema ensues and coma may follow. The commonest form of thyroid gland failure may have an autoimmune basis. Also *thyroid insufficiency, subthyroidism, thyroprivia, athyreosis* (seldom used), *athyroidism* (seldom used). **familial goitrous h.** FAMILIAL GOITER. **hypothalamic h.** Hypothyroidism due to failure of hypothalamic thyrotropin releasing hormone secretion, which leads to hyposecretion of adenohypophysial thyrotropin, causing atrophy and diminished elaboration of thyroid hormones by the thyroid gland. Also *tertiary hypothyroidism, hypothalamic myxedema, tertiary myxedema.* **infantile h.** CRETINISM. **postoperative h.** Hypothyroidism following surgical removal of all or part of the thyroid gland. Also *postablative hypothyroidism.* **primary h.** Hypothyroidism due to disease of the thyroid gland itself, as in idiopathic atrophy of the gland (Gull's disease). **tertiary h.** HYPOTHALAMIC HYPOTHYROIDISM. **thyroprivic h.** Hypothyroidism due to loss or atrophy of thyroid gland tissue with hyposecretion of thyroid hormone; primary hypothyroidism.

**hypotonia** \-tō′nē·ə\ [HYPO- + Gk *ton(os)* (from *teinein* to stretch, strain, draw tight) a tightening, rope, sinew, force + -IA] Reduction in muscle tone. Also *hypotony, hypatonia.* **benign congenital h.** Diffuse hypotonia of the skeletal musculature present from birth accompanied by delayed physical development and showing a tendency to spontaneous improvement and sometimes complete recovery. This is now known to be a syndrome of multiple etiology and not a single disease entity. Also *benign infantile hypotonia.* **infantile h.** FLOPPY INFANT SYNDROME. **h. oculi** OCULAR HYPOTONY.

**hypotonic** \-tän′ik\ **1** Less than normally tonic, as the state of a muscle. **2** Having an osmotic pressure less than that of an isotonic solution or less concentrated than isotonic. Also *hypoisotonic.*

**hypotonicity** \-tōnis′itē\ A condition in which the effective osmotic pressure of a body fluid is lower than that in surrounding tissues.

**hypotonus** \-tō′nəs\ [HYPO- + TONUS] A reduced force or tension exerted by a muscle while the muscle is in the relaxed state.

**hypotony** \hīpät′ənē\ HYPOTONIA. **ocular h.** Abnormally soft intraocular pressure, as may occur in the presence of a perforating wound or a diminished rate of formation of the aqueous humor. Also *hypotonia oculi.*

**hypotoxicity** \-täksis′itē\ [HYPO- + TOXICITY] Low or moderate toxicity.

**hypotransferrinemia** \-trans′ferinē′mē·ə\ Less than normal concentration of transferrin in plasma or serum, as occurs in many chronic disorders, malignancies, infectious diseases, rheumatoid arthritis, and chronic renal disease.

**hypotrichiasis** \-trikī′əsis\ HYPOTRICHOSIS.

**hypotrichosis** \-trikō′sis\ [HYPO- + TRICHOSIS] Any condition marked by a partial lack of hair. Also *hypotrichiasis, oligotrichy.*

**hypotrophy** \hīpät′rəfē\ [HYPO- + TROPH- + -Y] Wasting or reduction in size.

**hypotropia** \-trō′pē·ə\ [HYPO- + TROPIA] A vertical misalignment of the eyes. The specified eye is the deviating lower eye. Thus, in right hypotropia, the right eye is the nonfixing, downward-directed eye; in left hypotropia, the left.

**hypotympanum** \-tim′pənəm\ The part of the tympanic cavity below the level of the tympanic membrane, bounded inferiorly by the paries jugularis. *Outmoded.*

**hypouricuria** \hī′pōyoo′rikyoo′rē·ə \ [HYPO- + -URIC + -URIA ] Decreased urinary excretion of uric acid. The hyperuricemia of most patients with gout results from increased reabsorption of uric acid from the glomerular filtrate by the renal tubule cells, often due to inherited enzyme defects. Secondary causes of hypouricuria include increased plasma organic acids which inhibit tubular reabsorption of uric acid, as in starvation, ketosis, of lactic acid acidosis. Volume depletion due to any cause, including diuretics, and renal failure also are common causes of hypouricuria. Also *hypouricosuria.*

**hypovarianism** \-ver′ē·ənizm\ Deficient hormone secretion by the ovary. Also *hypo-ovarianism.*

**hypovasopressinemia** \-vā′sōpres′inē′mē·ə\ Less than normal concentration of vasopressin in blood, as in pituitary insufficiency or diabetes insipidus.

**hypoventilation** \-ven′tilā′shən\ [HYPO- + VENTILATION] Insufficient ventilation of the alveoli of the lungs to maintain normal levels of oxygen and/or carbon dioxide in arterial blood. **central h.** Hypoventilation due to disease or dysfunction of the brainstem. **chronic alveolar h.** Hypoventilation often resulting from chronic neuromuscular disease giving rise to weakness of the respiratory muscles and carbon dioxide retention, with consequential headache, drowsiness, and confusion. **primary alveolar h.** Hypoventilation occurring in a patient with normal ventilatory function, due to a deficiency in the brainstem regulation of breathing.

**hypovigility** \-vijil′itē\ Diminished responsivity to or awareness of external stimuli.

**hypovitaminosis** \-vī′təminō′sis\ [HYPO- + VITAMIN + -OSIS] A disorder due to a deficiency of one or more vitamins. Also *avitaminosis* (imprecise).

**hypovolaemia** *Brit.* HYPOVOLEMIA.

**hypovolemia** \-vōlē′mē·ə\ [HYPO- + *vol(ume)* + -EMIA] Abnormal reduction in the circulating blood volume.

**hypovolemic** \-vōlē′mik\ Related to or characterized by hypovolemia.

**hypovolia** \-vō′lyə\ A reduced volume or diminished water content.

**hypoxaemia** *Brit.* HYPOXEMIA.

**hypoxanthine** 4-Hydroxypurine and its keto tautomer. It is produced by the hydrolysis of adenine when this is catabolized. Xanthine oxidase converts it, via xanthine, into uric acid, which is excreted in man, although most other mammals break it down further. Also *adenine hypoxanthine.*

**hypoxanthine-guanine-phosphoribosyl-transferase** The enzyme responsible for purine salvage, whereby guanine and hypoxanthine are converted to guanilic acid and inosinic acid. The absence of this enzyme results in an accumulation of uncombined phosphoribosyl-l-pyrophosphate, which causes an acceleration in purine production and an excess in uric acid production.

**hypoxemia** \hī′päksē′mē·ə\ [HYP- + *ox(ygen)* + -EMIA] Reduced oxygen concentration in arterial blood.

**hypoxia** \hīpäk′sē·ə\ [HYP- + *ox(ygen)* + -IA] Inadequate oxygen concentration in body tissues. Also *suboxidation* (rare). **anemic h.** Less than normal oxygen content of blood due to decreased hemoglobin concentration of blood. **circulatory h.** Impaired oxygen delivery to tissues due to decreased blood flow. **diffusion h.** Hypoxia that may result at termination of nitrous oxide-oxygen anesthesia, believed to be the result of outward diffusion of nitrous oxide reducing the concentration of oxygen in alveoli. **histotoxic h.** A condition marked by a reduced ability of a tissue to utilize oxygen. **hypoxic h.** A reduced supply of oxygen to tissues due to a reduced partial pressure of oxygen in the blood.

**hypoxic** \hīpäk′sik\ [HYP- + *ox(ygen)*] Marked by a reduced oxygen supply.

**hypoxidosis** \hīpäk′sidō′sis\ [HYP- + OXIDOSIS] A reduction of cell function or activity due to an inadequate oxygen supply.

**hypsarrhythmia** \hip′səriTH′mē·ə\ [*hyps(o)-* + ARRHYTHMIA] In electroencephalography, a pattern of continuous generalized irregular wave and spike activity occurring in children. This pattern is not specific. It may be seen in various forms of cerebral lipidosis, in some other neuronal storage diseases and in tuberous sclerosis, but most often occurs in infants suffering from infantile massive spasm. These attacks are often very frequent. They may be partially responsive to ACTH treatment, but most affected infants become severely mentally retarded. Similar appearances in the EEG may occur in adults with Creutzfeldt-Jakob disease. Also *hypsarhythmia.*

**hypsi-** \hip′sē-\ HYPSO-.

**hypso-** \hip′sō-\ [Gk *hypsos* height; Gk *hypsi* on high, aloft] A combining form meaning height, high. Also *hypsi-*.

**Hyrtl** [Joseph *Hyrtl*, Austrian anatomist, 1811–1894] **1** Hyrtl's foramen. See under PORUS CROTAPHITICOBUCCINATORIUS. **2** Hyrtl's anastomosis. See under LOOP. **3** Hyrtl's recess. See under RECESSUS EPITYMPANICUS.

**hyster-** \hister-\ HYSTERO-.

**hystera** \his′tərə\ [Gk, the uterus] UTERUS.

**hysteratresia** \his′tərətrē′zhə\ Atresia of the uterine lumen. It is usually a result of inflammation. Developmental atresia occurs when a paramesonephric duct fails to join with the urogenital sinus, thereby leaving an oviduct and part of the uterus isolated from the rest of the female genital tract.

**hysterectomy** \his′tərek′təmē\ [HYSTER- + -ECTOMY] Surgical removal of the uterus. Also *metrectomy.* **abdominal h.** Removal of the uterus through an incision in the abdominal wall. Also *supravaginal hysterectomy, celiohysterectomy.* **abdominovaginal h.** Surgical removal of the uterus from a combined abdominal and vaginal approach. **cesarean h.** Removal of the uterus at the time of cesarean section. Also *radical caesarian section, Porro hysterectomy.* **complete h.** Removal of the uterine fundus and cervix. Also *panhysterectomy, total hysterectomy.* **partial h.** SUBTOTAL HYSTERECTOMY. **Porro h.** CESAREAN HYSTERECTOMY. **radical h.** Removal of the uterus, upper vagina, and parametrium for cancer. **subtotal h.** Removal of the uterus at or above the level of the internal os. Also *partial hysterectomy, supracervical hysterectomy.* **supracervical h.** SUBTOTAL HYSTERECTOMY. **supravaginal h.** ABDOMINAL HYSTERECTOMY. **total h.** COMPLETE HYSTERECTOMY. **vaginal h.** Surgical removal of the uterus through the vagina. Also *colpohysterectomy.*

**hysteremphysema** \his′tərem′fəsē′mə\ [HYSTER- + EMPHYSEMA] Gas in the uterus.

**hysteresis** \his′tərē′sis\ [Gk *hysterēsis* (from *hysterein* to be behind, come later, from *hysteros* coming after) a coming short, want, need] The dependence of a system output on the history and direction of the input. The mechanical hysteresis of the lung causes different transpulmonary pressures after inspiration and expiration. The thermal hysteresis of a reversible colloid causes differing temperatures of gelation and liquefaction. The magnetization of a magnetic material differs for increasing and decreasing magnetic forces. **protoplasmic h.** A condition in which the protoplasm becomes less dispersed due to a loss of water and a reduction of electrical charge, postulated as a cause of cell senescence.

**hystereurynter** \his′təryoorin′tər\ [HYSTER- + Gk *euryn(ein)* to widen, dilate (from *eurys* wide) + *-tēr*, agentive suffix] METREURYNTER.

**hystereurysis** \his′təryoo′riris\ [HYSTER- + Gk *eury(nein)* to widen, dilate (from *eurys* wide) + *-sis*, derivative noun suffix] Dilatation of the cervix.

**hysteria** \histir′ē·ə\ [Gk *hyster(a)* the uterus + -IA. See HYSTERIC.] **1** See under CONVERSION HYSTERIA. **2** See under ANXIETY HYSTERIA. **3** Any of various disorders characterized by conversion symptoms, such as paralysis, tremor, anesthesia, vomiting, amnesia, somnambulism, fugue, or other dissociation manifestations. *Outmoded.* Also *hysterical neurosis.* • *Hysteria* is no longer recognized as a separate clinical entity without qualification. **anxiety h.** A phobic disorder, consisting of a specific, persistent, and irrational fear that leads to avoidance of all situations in which the feared object may be encountered and significant constriction of usual activities. The fear comes to dominate the patient's entire life. In time, it often spreads to include more than the original object as well as anticipatory fear that the anxiety or panic associated with exposure to the object may recur spontaneously. Also *phobic neurosis, phobism* (outmoded), *phobic reaction.* **conversion h.** A disorder, without detectable organic basis, characterized by a motor, sensory, or visceral physical manifestation, such as paralysis, tic, paresthesia, or vomiting, or a mental manifestation such as amnesia, fugue, depersonalization, or multiple personality. The subject displays a surprisingly calm mental attitude concerning his symptoms. Also *somatic conversion, hysteroneurosis, conversion neurosis.*

**hysteric** \hister′ik\ [Gk *hysterikos* (from *hystera* uterus) uterine, suffering from a uterine disorder, hysterical (supposedly manifesting a uterine disorder)] **1** A person suffering from hysteria. **2** HYSTERICAL.

**hysterical** \hister′ikəl\ Characterized by hysteria. Also *hysteric.*

**hystero-** \his′tərō-\ [Gk *hystera* uterus] A combining form meaning (1) the uterus; (2) hysteria. Also *hyster-*.

**hysterocolpectomy** \-kälpek′təmē\ [HYSTERO- + COLP- + -ECTOMY] Removal of the uterus and vagina. Also *panhysterocolpectomy.*

**hysterocolposcope** \-käl′pəskōp\ [HYSTERO- + COLPO- + -SCOPE] An instrument for viewing the vagina, cervix, and uterine cavity.

**hysterocystocleisis** \-sis′təklī′sis\ [HYSTERO- + CYSTO- + -CLEISIS] An operation in which the uterus is used to aid the closure of a vesicovaginal fistula. Also *Bozeman's operation.*

**hysteroedema** \his′tərō·ēdē′mə\ Swelling of the uterus from edema.

**hysterograph** \his′tərōgraf′\ [HYSTERO- + -GRAPH] A device which measures the strength of uterine contractions.

**hysterolith** \his′tərōlith′\ [HYSTERO- + -LITH] A stone or calcification in the uterus.

**hysterometer** \his′təräm′ətər\ [HYSTERO- + -METER] UTERINE SOUND.

**hysterometry** \his′təräm′ətrē\ [HYSTERO- + -METRY]

The process of measuring uterine size. Also *uterometry*.

**hysteroneurosis** \-nʸUrō′sis\ CONVERSION HYSTERIA.

**hysteropathy** \his′tərăp′əthē\ [HYSTERO- + -PATHY] METROPATHY.

**hysteropexy** \his′tərōpek′sē\ [HYSTERO- + -PEXY] The operative fixation of an abnormally positioned uterus. Also *uterofixation, uteropexy, metropexy*.

**hysteropia** \-ō′pē·ə\ [HYSTER- + -OPIA] The presence of visual symptoms caused by hysteria. Characteristically, these are variable even within a very short time of examination and are readily influenced by suggestion. Bizarre, nonphysiologic visual field constrictions of tunnel configuration are common. Inability to see during stressful situations is the typical complaint. The affected person shows little concern over this visual loss, in contrast to the apprehension that most patients show when suffering from an organic loss of sight.

**hysteroplasty** \his′tərōplas′tē\ [HYSTERO- + -PLASTY] UTEROPLASTY.

**hysteropsychosis** \-sīkō′sis\ HYSTERICAL PSYCHOSIS.

**hysteroptosia** \his′tərăptō′zhə\ [HYSTERO- + Gk *ptōs(is)* a fall, falling + -IA] PROLAPSE OF UTERUS.

**hysteroptosis** \his′tərăptō′sis\ [HYSTERO- + -PTOSIS] PROLAPSE OF UTERUS.

**hysterosalpingectomy** \-sal′pinjek′təmē\ Removal of the uterus and an oviduct. Also *panhysterosalpingectomy*.

**hysterosalpingography** \-sal′ping·găg′rəfē\ [HYSTERO- + SALPINGO- + -GRAPHY] Radiographic examination of the uterus and fallopian tubes following the instillation of opaque contrast medium via the cervical os. Also *hysterotubography, uterosalpingography, uterotubography*.

**hysterosalpingo-oophorectomy** \-salping′gō-ō′əfôrek′təmē\ [HYSTERO- + SALPINGO- + OOPHORECTOMY] Surgical removal of the uterus, fallopian tubes, and ovaries. Also *hysterosalpingo-oothectomy, panhysterosalpingo-oophorectomy*.

**hysterosalpingostomy** \-sal′ping·găs′təmē\ [HYSTERO- + SALPINGO- + -STOMY] A reimplantation of a partially occluded oviduct for the purpose of establishing fertility.

**hysterosalpinx** \-sal′pingks\ TUBA UTERINA.

**hysteroscope** \his′tərōskōp′\ [HYSTERO- + -SCOPE] A transcervical instrument for examining the uterine cavity. Also *metroscope, uteroscope*.

**hysteroscopy** \his′tərăs′kəpē\ [HYSTERO- + -SCOPY] Inspection of the uterine cavity.

**hysterostat** \his′tərōstat′\ [HYSTERO- + -STAT] A device in which are placed sealed sources of radioactive substances, such as radium, for intrauterine insertion. It is used in radiation therapy for cancer of the uterus.

**hysterostomatomy** \-stōmat′əmē\ [HYSTERO- + *stoma(t)-* + -TOMY] Surgical enlargement of the os uteri by an incision.

**hysterothermometry** \-thərmăm′ətrē\ UTEROTHERMOMETRY.

**hysterotomy** \his′tərăt′əmē\ [HYSTERO- + -TOMY] Incision into the uterus extending into the uterine cavity. It may be performed vaginally or transabdominally. Also *uterotomy, metrotomy, metratomy*.

**hysterotracheloplasty** \-trā′kəlōplas′tē\ TRACHELOPLASTY.

**hysterotubography** \-tʸoobăg′rəfē\ HYSTEROSALPINGOGRAPHY.

**hysterythrine** \hister′ithrin\ *Outmoded* ESTROGEN.

**Hz** Symbol for the unit, hertz.

# I

**I** 1 Symbol for the element, iodine. 2 Symbol for isoleucine. 3 Symbol for inosine.

***i-*** iso-.

**-ia** \-ē·ə\ [L and Gk suffix commonly used for derivative abstract nouns] 1 A suffix meaning state or condition: used especially in the names of diseases or pathologic conditions. 2 A suffix used in taxonomic names.

**iamatology** \ī·am′ətăl′əjē\ [Gk *iama*, gen. *iamato(s)*, a means of healing + -LOGY] The science of medical cures and remedies.

**IANC** International Anatomical Nomenclature Committee. (The Committee which prepares the *Nomina Anatomica*).

**-iasis** \-ī′əsis\ [Gk, verb-stem ending *-ia-* + noun-forming suffix *-sis*] A suffix usually denoting a disease or infection from a (specified) cause, as in *amebiasis* (amebas), *schistosomiasis* (schistosomes), *cholelithiasis* (gallstones). ● In modern coinages *-iasis* tends to be used especially for infection by protozoan or metazoan parasites, but there are exceptions such as *candidiasis* and *hypochondriasis*. Words inherited from ancient Greek include some prototypes of the modern use of the suffix, e.g., *drakontiasis* (guinea worm disease), while in others the suffix has a simulative force, e.g., *elephantiasis*.

**iatr-** \ī·atr-\ IATRO-.

**iatraliptic** \ī′atrəlip′tik\ [Gk *iatraleiptik(ē)* (from *iatr(os)* surgeon + *aleiptik(os)* pertaining to an anointer, from *aleiphein* to anoint with oil) the practice of surgery by anointing, friction, or exercise] Relating to the administration of medicinal substances by surface application to the skin.

**iatreusiology** \ī′atroo′sē·ăləjē\ [Gk *iatreusi(s)* a means of healing + *o* + -LOGY] The science of therapeutics.

**iatreusis** \ī′atroo′sis\ [Gk, a means of healing] Medical treatment.

**iatric** \ī·at′rik\ [Gk *iatrikos* (from *iatros* a physician, healer) pertaining to or skilled in healing or medicine] Of or pertaining to a physician or to medicine.

**-iatrics** \-ī·at′riks\ [See IATRIC.] A combining form meaning medical care or treatment.

**iatro-** \ī·at′rō-, ī′atrō-\ [Gk *iatros* physician; *iatreia* medical treatment] A combining form meaning physician or medicine. Also *iatr-*.

***Iatrobdella*** \ī′atrōdel′ə\ *HIRUDO*

**iatrochemistry** \ī′atrōkem′istrē\ The study of the relation between chemistry and medicine, especially in connection with the 17th-century doctrine that attributed to chemical substances a key role in physiologic processes and disease. Also *chemiatry*.

**iatrogenic** \ī′atrəjen′ik\ [IATRO- + -GENIC] 1 Pertaining to or describing a complication, injury, unfavorable result, or other problem which can be directly attributed to medical care. 2 Pertaining to or describing any effect upon a patient resulting from the action of a physician.

**iatrology** \ī′atrăl′əjē\ [IATRO- + -LOGY] Medical science.

**iatrotechnical** \ī'atrətek'nikəl\ Pertaining to the techniques of medical practice.
**-iatry** \-ī'ətrē\ [Gk *iatreia* the practice of healing] A combining form meaning medical treatment.
**IB** 1 immune body (antibody). 2 inclusion body.
**IBC** iron-binding capacity.
**-ible** \-ibl\ -ABLE.
**ibogaine** $C_{20}H_{26}N_2O$. An alkaloid obtained from the root of the African plant *Tabernanthe iboga* and species of *Peschiera* and *Voacanga*. It is said to prevent fatigue and has been used as a possible antidepressant drug, but it may produce serious psychological disturbances.
**ibufenac** $C_{12}H_{16}O_2$. 4-(2-Methylpropyl)benzeneacetic acid. An analgesic drug formerly used in the treatment of rheumatoid arthritis. It was found to cause jaundice.
**ibuprofen** $C_{13}H_{18}O_2$. α-Methyl-4-(2-methylpropyl)-beneneacetic acid. A nonsteroidal anti-inflammatory agent with antipyretic and analgesic properties. It is employed in the treatment of rheumatoid and osteoarthritis by oral administration.
**IC** 1 internal conversion. 2 intermittent claudication.
**-ic** \-ik\ [Gk *-ik(os)*, adj. suffix] 1 A suffix meaning pertaining to or characterized by. 2 In chemistry, a suffix applied to names of elements to indicate that they are in their higher oxidation state. It is also used in forming names of acids. Compare -OUS.
**ICC** intensive coronary care.
**ICD** 1 International Classification of Diseases (of the World Health Organization). 2 ischemic coronary disease. 3 intrauterine contraceptive disease.
**ICDA** International Classification of Diseases Adapted (for use in the United States).
**ice** The solid state of water. **dry i.** SOLID CARBON DIOXIDE.
**ichnogram** \ik'nəgram\ [Gk *ichno(s)* footstep, track + -GRAM] FOOTPRINT.
**ichor** \ī'kôr\ [Gk *ichōr* the watery part of blood or of milk, serum, lymph, impure discharge] A thin, serous discharge from a wound or an ulcer. *Obs.* Adj. ichorous.
**ichoremia** \ī'kôrē'mē·ə\ SEPTICEMIA.
**ichorrhemia** \ī'kôrē'mē·ə\ SEPTICEMIA.
**ichthammol** \ik'thamôl\ A darkly colored, viscous fluid obtained from the distillation of particular bituminous schists, sulfonation of the distillate, and subsequent neutralization of the product with ammonia. It is used as a topical anti-infective medication for skin diseases. Also *ammonium ichthyosulfonate.*
**ichthyo-** \ik'thē·ō-\ [Gk *ichthys* fish] A combining form meaning fish.
**ichthyoid** \ik'thē·oid\ Fishlike; fish-shaped.
**ichthyolsulfonate** An ichthammol derivative, a salt form of ichthyolsulfonic acid. It was formerly used as a dermatologic medication due to its demulcent and emmolient properties.
**ichthyosarcotoxin** \-sär'kətäk'sin\ [ICHTHYO- + SARCO- + TOXIN] A substance that occurs in the flesh of certain fishes, which causes it to be poisonous upon ingestion.
**ichthyosarcotoxism** \-sär'kətäk'sizm\ A pathological condition caused by ingestion of the flesh of fishes that contains ichthyosarcotoxin. Clinical signs of poisoning are numbness of the lips, tongue, and throat, followed shortly by nausea, vomiting, abdominal pain, and diarrhea. Later symptoms are nervousness, muscle pain, sore teeth, visual disturbances, and convulsions. Some deaths have been reported due to respiratory paralysis.
**ichthyosis** \ik'thē·ō'sis\ [*ichthy(o)-* + -OSIS] Any of a group of disorders of keratinization that are characterized by dryness and fine scaling. Also *fish-skin disease.* **acquired i.** Nonhereditary ichthyosis, often occurring as a manifestation of systemic disease, particularly neoplastic disease. **i. congenita** A rare, severe form of ichthyosis in which grossly hyperkeratotic lesions are present at birth. Also *diffuse congenital hyperkeratosis, keratosis universalis congenita.* **i. cornea** ICHTHYOSIS HYSTRIX. **i. fetalis** 1 Gross ichthyosis present at birth. 2 Any ichthyosis present in the fetus. **i. hystrix** Autosomal dominant dermatoses that share congenital or perinatal onset of hyperkeratotic quill-like projections. In the Lambert type, only rudimentary tonofilaments occur. In the Curth-Macklin type, concentric unbroken shells of abnormal tonofilaments cluster around the nucleus. Also *ichthyosis cornea, ichthyosis spinosa.* **lamellar i.** A hereditary disorder of keratinization characterized by diffuse erythema and large lamellar scales. **i. linearis circumflexa** A rare form of hereditary icthyosis, presenting at or soon after birth, and characterized by a generalized erythema and scaling, with some lesions having a thickened horny serpiginous border. **i. palmaris** PALMAR KERATODERMA. **senile i.** The dryness and scaling of the skin associated with old age. **sex-linked recessive i.** An inherited ichthyosis determined by a sex-linked recessive gene. Unlike ichthyosis vulgaris, it does not spare the flexures. Also *X-linked ichthyosis.* **i. simplex** ICHTHYOSIS VULGARIS. **i. spinosa** ICHTHYOSIS HYSTRIX. **i. vulgaris** The common form of ichthyosis. It is of autosomal dominant inheritance. Also *ichthyosis simplex.* **X-linked i.** SEX-LINKED RECESSIVE ICHTHYOSIS.
**ichthyotoxicology** \-täk'sikäl'əjē\ [ICHTHYO- + TOXICOLOGY] The study of the natural toxins present in fish.
**icosa-** \īkō'sə-\ [Gk *eikos(i)* (*eikosin* before a vowel) twenty + *a-*] A combining form meaning twenty. Also *eicosa-.*
**icosanoid** \īkō'sənoid\ Any of a large number of fatty acids that are 20 carbons in length, including arachidonic acid, prostaglandins, thromboxanes, and related compounds.
**icosapentaenoic acid** An unsaturated fatty acid, twenty carbons in length, that contains five double bonds. It is a precursor of some prostaglandins, such as $PGI_2$.
**icosatrienoic acid** An unsaturated fatty acid twenty carbons in length that contains three double bonds. It is a precursor of some prostaglandins.
**-ics** \-iks\ [L suffix *-icus* and Gk suffix *-ikos*] A suffix (forming nouns from words originally adjectives) meaning (1) a study or discipline, as a science or branch of science; (2) practice, method, manner.
**ICSH** interstitial cell-stimulating hormone (luteinizing hormone).
**ICT** 1 insulin coma therapy. 2 inflammation of connective tissue.
**ictal** \ik'təl\ Describing or pertaining to an ictus.
**icteric** \ikter'ik\ [Gk *ikterikos* jaundiced] Relating to or characterized by the presence of icterus, or jaundice.
**ictero-** \ik'tərō-\ [Gk *ikteros* jaundice] A combining form denoting jaundice.
**icteroanemia** \ik'tərō·anē'mē·ə\ Anemia associated with jaundice.
**icterogenic** \-jen'ik\ [ICTERO- + -GENIC] Causing or contributing to the development of jaundice.
**icteroid** \ik'təroid\ [*icter(us)* + -OID] Jaundicelike; characterized by a yellow color.
**icterus** \ik'tərəs\ [New L, from Gk *ikteros* jaundice] JAUNDICE. **benign familial i.** GILBERT SYNDROME. **i. castrensis gravis** Icteric leptospirosis occurring among troops in camp. **chronic familial i.** HEREDI-

I J K

TARY SPHEROCYTOSIS. **congenital familial i.** HEREDITARY SPHEROCYTOSIS. **congenital hemolytic i.** HEREDITARY SPHEROCYTOSIS. **familial hemolytic i.** HEREDITARY SPHEROCYTOSIS. **i. gravis** An acute destructive disease of the liver; massive liver necrosis. **i. gravis neonatorum** ERYTHROBLASTOSIS FETALIS. **i. infectiosus** ICTERIC LEPTOSPIROSIS. **i. neonatorum** **1** PHYSIOLOGIC JAUNDICE. **2** A rare, congenitally induced jaundice due to occlusion of the common bile duct or to congenital malformation of the liver. Also *jaundice of the newborn.* **nuclear i.** KERNICTERUS. **i. praecox** Mild jaundice that occurs during a newborn's first 24 hours, due to ABO blood group incompatibility of mother and fetus. **spirochetal i.** ICTERIC LEPTOSPIROSIS.

**Ictotest** A tablet containing sulfosalicylic acid and *p*-nitrobenzene diazonium *p*-toluene sulfonate that is used to detect bilirubin in urine. A purple discoloration constitutes a positive result. A proprietary name.

**ictus** \ik′təs\ [L (from *ictus,* past part. of *icere* to beat, stab, strike), a stroke, blow, stab, hit] An event of sudden onset, such as a stroke or cerebrovascular accident. Adj. ictal. **i. cordis** HEARTBEAT. **i. paralyticus** A stroke causing paralysis. **i. sanguinis** CEREBRAL HEMORRHAGE.

**ICU** intensive care unit.

**ID** **1** infective dose. **2** intradermal. **3** infectious disease(s). **4** inside diameter.

**$ID_{50}$** **1** minimal infecting dose. **2** median infective dose.

**id** \id\ [L (neut. sing. of *is* he), it] That portion of the psychic apparatus which precedes the ego and superego and contains the psychic representatives of the drives and all the phylogenetic acquisitions. The processes of the id are completely unconscious and its operation is governed by the pleasure principle and the primary process.

**id.** *idem* (L, the same).

**-id¹** \-id\ [Gk adj. and noun suffix *-is,* gen. *-id(os)* belonging to or descendant of] A suffix meaning belonging to or a member of a broader category that includes the category designated by the stem, as *hominid* (including *Homo, hominhumans*), *lipid* (including *lip(o)-* fats).

**-id²** \-id\ [from -ID¹] **1** A suffix designating a superficial manifestation, usually cutaneous, of a (specified) underlying disease, as *tuberculid,* (from *tuberculosis*). Also *-ide.* **2** A suffix designating (1) a structural element or component, as *chromatid;* (2) a mandibular tooth element corresponding to a (specified) maxillary element, as *trigonid* (from *trigone*).

**-idae** \-idē\ [-ID¹ + *-ae,* fem. pl. suffix] A suffix designating a family in zoological taxonomy, or a subclass in botanical taxonomy.

**IDDM** insulin-dependent diabetes mellitus.

**-ide¹** \-īd\ [French (from L *-idus,* adj. suffix); first used chemically in *oxide* (now *oxyde*), by analogy from *acide* acid] **1** A combining form used in chemistry for a binary compound to signify the more electronegative of the two elements. It replaces the ending of the name of one of them, e.g. sodium and chlorine give sodium chloride. **2** A combining form used in chemistry to signify negative ions formed from an atom by the gain of one or more electrons, e.g. chloride for $Cl^-$. By extension it signifies other anions formed by loss of hydrogen ions, e.g. amide for $NH_2^-$, acetylide for $HC{\equiv}C^-$, methanide for $CH_3^-$. Amines are also considered to become amides when acylated. • When *-ide* replaces *-e* at the end of the name of a sugar ending in *-ose,* it signifies glycoside formation. Several other words contain the ending, e.g. *nucleoside, lactide,* and here the relationship to the original meaning is more distant.

**-ide²** \-īd, -id\ -ID².

**idea** [L (from Gk *idea,* from *idein* to see), a form or image present to the mind, idea, form] Any mental image or thought. **fixed i.** IDÉE FIXE. **imperative i.** OBSESSION. **i. of reference** A delusion in which the subject believes that anything that happens in the world has a specific meaning for him or has been done only because of him. Most commonly, an idea of reference accompanies a delusion of persecution. Also *delusion of reference, self-referential delusion, referential idea.* **ruminative i.** OBSESSION.

**idée fixe** \ēdā′fēks′\ A delusion that tends to have a dominating impact on behavior. Also *fixed idea.*

**identification** **1** The act of identifying or the means by which an identity is established. **2** In psychoanalytic psychology, an unconscious, intrapsychic process in which a part of the self is transformed into a facsimile of one or more external objects, and the subject then begins to think, feel, or act as he imagines the external object would do. Identification is a primitive method of recognizing reality that provides a means of rendering the frightening unknown into the tolerable familiar. **3** In developmental psychology, the assimilation of parental values in the child, assisting the gradual formation of a sense of self. **firearms i.** FORENSIC BALLISTICS. **projective i.** A dual process of attributing one's own impulses to another and then fearing that the other will turn that impulse, often aggression, against oneself.

**identity** [French *identité* (from L *idem* the same one, the same, from *is* he) identity] The image, concept, or inner conviction that one has of oneself, whether as a whole or in relation to particular functions or roles, as in *body indentity, gender identity, mental* or *psychological identity, social identity,* etc. **body i.** BODY IMAGE. **core gender i.** The inner conviction that one is male, female, ambivalent, or neutral. It is established in accordance with the sex of assignment and of rearing and becomes evident by 18 months of age. By the age of 30 months, it is generally irreversible. Also *gender identity.* **ego i.** Delineation of the physical and mental self as distinct from the external world; the existence of a persistent and coordinate system that distinguishes between the self and the environment and situates the self in relation to the environment. **gender i.** CORE GENDER IDENTITY. **sexual i.** The biologically determined sex of a person, no matter what form that same person's core gender identity and gender role may take.

**ideo-** \ī′dē-ō-\ [Gk *idea* idea, form] A combining form meaning idea, mental.

**ideokinetic** \-kinet′ik\ IDEOMOTOR.

**ideomotion** \-mō′shən\ Muscular activity aroused by an idea or thought; involuntary movement associated with mental activity, as moving the lips while reading. Also *ideomotor phenomenon.*

**ideomotor** \-mō′tər\ Initiated directly by an idea: said of a motor response or action, usually those involuntary, tentative, and diminished body movements that are evoked by thought processes rather than by sensory stimulation. Also *ideomuscular, ideokinetic.*

**ideovascular** \-vas′kyələr\ Denoting vascular changes stemming from mental activity.

**idio-** \id′ē-ō-\ [Gk *idios* one's own, personal] A combining form meaning applying to or originating within oneself, personal, individual.

**idiochromosome** \-krō′məsōm\ SEX CHROMOSOME.

**idiocrasy** \id′ē-äk′rəsē\ IDIOSYNCRASY.

**idiocratic** \-krat′ik\ IDIOSYNCRATIC.

**idiocy** \id′ē-əsē\ [*idio(t)* (from Med French, ignorant, silly, from L *idiota* an ignoramus, layman, from Gk *idiōtēs* an ignoramus, layman, private individual, from *idios* private, one's own) + English *-cy*, abstract noun suffix] Profound mental retardation, with an IQ below 25. *Outmoded.* **amaurotic familial i.** Any of various neurodegenerative disorders. An ambiguous, obsolete, and regrettable term. See under TAY-SACHS DISEASE, CEROID-LIPOFUSCINOSIS. **infantile amaurotic familial i.** *Obs.* TAY-SACHS DISEASE. **spastic amaurotic axonal i.** *Obs.* INFANTILE NEUROAXONAL DYSTROPHY. **xerodermic i.** *Outmoded* DE SANCTIS-CACCHIONE SYNDROME.

**idioglossia** \-gläs′ē·ə\ [Gk *idioglōss(os)* (from IDIO- + *glōssa* tongue, language) peculiar in speech + -IA] **1** The speech of a deaf child which may be intelligible to its parents but not to others. **2** A form of developmental dysarthria characterized by frequent consonant substitutions and showing a tendency to spontaneous improvement. Adj. idioglottic.

**idioglottic** \-glät′ik\ Of, pertaining to, or suffering from idioglossia.

**idiogram** \id′ē·əgram′\ A diagram, drawn to scale, that represents a single chromosome or the entire karyotype. Ordinarily, chromosome bands (according to standard conventions and stage of mitosis or meiosis), the centromere, and any secondary constrictions and satellites are included.

**idiographic** \-graf′ik\ [IDIO- + GRAPH- + -IC] Referring to the value of a variable, such as pulse rate or blood pressure, for an individual at a given time as compared with the personal norm or baseline value of that variable for that individual.

**idiometritis** \mētrī′tis\ [IDIO- + METRITIS] MYOMETRITIS.

**idiomiasma** \-mē·az′mə\ A self-produced offensive odor.

**idionodal** \-nō′dəl\ Arising in the atrioventricular node itself; junctional: applied particularly to cardiac rhythms.

**idiopathic** \-path′ik\ [IDIO- + PATH- + -IC] Having no known cause: said of a disease or other pathologic condition. ⟨"Originally, when it first came into the language of medicine, the term had a different, highly theoretical meaning. It was assumed that most human diseases were intrinsic, due to inbuilt failures of one sort or another, things gone wrong with various internal humors. The word 'idiopathic' was intended to mean, literally, a disease having its own origin, a primary disease without any external cause." —Lewis Thomas, *The Medusa and the Snail*, 1979⟩ Also *idiopathetic, autopathic* (seldom used).

**idiopathy** \id′ē·äp′əthē\ [IDIO- + -PATHY] A disease of spontaneous origin or without apparent external cause.

**idioreflex** \-rē′fleks\ A self-induced reflex.

**idiosyncrasy** \-sin′krəsē\ [Gk *idiosynkrasia* (from IDIO- + *synkrasis* constitution, temperament, from *syn-* together + *krasis* blending, mixture, from *kera(nnynai)* to mix, temper) a peculiar physical or mental set] **1** A property or characteristic peculiar to an individual's physical or mental constitution. Also *idiocrasy.* **2** An unusual or exaggerated reaction to a drug or food that is due to some inherent characteristic of the responder's metabolism and not to allergy (or immunologic response to the drug or food). Idiosyncratic reactions occur on first exposure to the drug or food in contrast to the requirement of immunologic reactions for presensitization.

**idiosyncratic** \-sinkrat′ik\ Of the nature of an idiosyncrasy; peculiar to an individual's physical or mental constitution. Also *idiocratic.*

**idiot savant** \ēdē·ō′ sävän′\ [French, lit., a wise idiot] A mentally retarded person of any grade who has a special but limited talent of some sort, most often a memory for the details of music or an ability to make rapid arithmetic calculations.

**idiotope** \id′ē·ətōp′\ [IDIO- + Gk *top(os)* a place] An epitope on the variable region of an antibody molecule that can be recognized by the combining site of other antibodies in the same animal species.

**idiotopy** \id′ē·ətäp′ē\ The interrelationships of the positions of parts of an organ.

**idiotype** \id′ē·ətīp′\ The antigenic determinants, associated with the hypervariable regions in the variable domains of antibody molecules, which characterize individual antibodies; the set of idiotopes of the antibody produced by a given clone of cells. Similar antigenic determinants have been described on T cells and presumably occur in the T cell receptor. It is a central tenet of the network theory of immune regulation that all antibodies are anti-idiotypes in addition to reacting with other antigens.

**idioventricular** \-ventrik′yələr\ Arising in the ventricles themselves, or pertaining to or affecting the cardiac ventricles alone. See also IDIOVENTRICULAR RHYTHM.

**-idium** \-id′ē·əm\ [New L (from Gk *-idion* diminishing suffix), suffix denoting smaller or lesser] A suffix meaning a smaller or lesser one.

**idolomania** \ī′dōləmā′nē·ə\ [*idol* + *o* + -MANIA] FETISHISM.

**idose** The aldohexose with the opposite configuration to glucose at C-2, C-3, and C-4. Thus the inversion of configuration at these three carbon atoms of D-glucose would yield D-idose, whereas inversion at C-5 of D-glucose yields L-idose. Residues of L-iduronic acid are produced in heparin by this latter route from glucuronic residues.

**idoxuridine** $C_9H_{11}IN_2O_5$. A pyrimidine analogue of the structure 2-deoxy-5-iodo-uridine. It is a white powder used as an antiviral agent in the treatment of herpes simplex keratitis. It inhibits viral DNA synthesis, and is applied topically to the conjunctiva. Also *5-iododeoxyuridine.* Abbr. IDU

**IDS** inhibitor of DNA synthesis.

**IDU** idoxuridine.

**iduronate** The anion, salt, or ester of iduronic acid, formed by the oxidation of C-6 of idose to —COOH.

**iduronic acid** The substance produced by oxidation of C-6 of idose to form a carboxyl group. Residues of L-iduronic acid occur in heparin, where they are produced from D-glucuronic residues by inversion at C-5.

**IEM** **1** immune electron microscopy. **2** inborn error of metabolism.

**IEP** **1** isoelectric point. **2** isoelectric precipitation.

**IF** **1** intrinsic factor. **2** interferon. **3** interstitial fluid. **4** initiation factor (in protein synthesis).

**Ig** immunoglobulin.

**IgA** immunoglobulin A.

**IgD** immunoglobulin D.

**IgE** immunoglobulin E.

**IgG** immunoglobulin G.

**IgM** immunoglobulin M.

**ignatia** \ignā′shē·ə\ The dried and ripened seeds of *Strychnos ignatii*, containing alkaloids such as strychnine and brucine, as well as igasuric acid and loganin. It is used in the preparation of certain bitter tonics.

**igniextirpation** \ig′nē·eks′tərpā′shən\ [L *igni(s)* fire + EXTIRPATION] A surgical procedure in which one or more organs are removed by use of a cautery.

**ignioperation** \ig′nē·äp′ərā′shən\ Any surgical procedure in which a hot cautery is used to perform all or part of the operation.

**ignipedites** \ig′nipedī′tis\ [New L, from L *ignipes*, gen. *ignipedis* (from *igni(s)* fire + *pes* foot) fire-footed] BURNING FEET.

**ignisation** \ig′nisā′shən\ [L *ignis* fire, heat + -ATION ] HEAT EXHAUSTION.

**IH** infectious hepatitis.

**IK** Immune Körper (German, immune bodies).

**IL** interleukin.

**Il** Symbol for the element, illinium, now called promethium.

**il-** \il-\ **1** IN-[1]. **2** IN-[2].

**ILA** insulinlike activity.

**Ile** Symbol for isoleucine.

**-ile** \-il, -īl\ [L *-ilis,* suffix denoting relating to, proper to, of] A suffix meaning of, like, relating to, or capable of.

**ileac** \il′ē·ak\ **1** Relating to or characterized by ileus. **2** ILEAL.

**ileal** \il′ē·əl\ Pertaining to the ileum. Also *ileac.*

**ileectomy** \il′ē·ek′təmē\ [*ile(o)-* + -ECTOMY] A surgical procedure in which all or a part of the distal small bowel is removed.

**ileitis** \il′ē·ī′tis\ [*ile(o)-* + -ITIS] Inflammation of the ileum. **backwash i.** Mucosal changes in the ileum consisting of colonic metaplasia and also inflammatory changes typical of ulcerative colitis. This condition is found in patients with ulcerative colitis. **distal i.** TERMINAL ILEITIS. **regional i.** Crohn's disease involving the ileum. **terminal i.** Crohn's disease involving the terminal ileum. Also *distal ileitis.*

**ileo-** \il′ē·ō-\ [Med L *ileum.* See ILEUM.] A combining form denoting the ileum.

**ileocecostomy** \-sēkäs′təmē\ [ILEO- + CECO- + -STOMY] A surgical procedure creating an opening between the distal small bowel and the cecum. Such an opening may rarely result spontaneously from inflammatory, neoplastic, or traumatic causes.

**ileocecum** \-sē′kəm\ The ileum and the cecum considered as a single entity.

**ileocolic** \-kō′lik\ Pertaining to the ileum and the colon, usually the ascending colon. Also *ileocolonic, coloileal.*

**ileocolitis** \-kōlī′tis\ [ILEO- + COLITIS] **1** Mucous membrane inflammation of the ileum and colon. **2** Crohn's disease involving both the ileum and the colon.

**ileocolonic** \-kōlän′ik\ ILEOCOLIC.

**ileocolostomy** \-kōläs′təmē\ [ILEO- + COLO- + -STOMY] A surgical procedure creating an opening between the distal small bowel and the large bowel, following resection or bypass. Such an opening may rarely occur spontaneously following neoplastic, inflammatory, or traumatic disease.

**ileocolotomy** \-kōlät′əmē\ [ILEO- + COLO- + -TOMY ] A surgical procedure in which an incision is made into the distal small bowel and large bowel. A similar result may rarely be produced by trauma.

**ileocystoplasty** \-sis′təplas′tē\ A surgical procedure in which a defect in the urinary bladder wall is repaired with a small defunctionalized loop of distal small bowel.

**ileocystostomy** \-sistäs′təmē\ A surgical procedure creating an opening between the distal small bowel and the urinary bladder.

**ileoileostomy** \il′ē·ō·ilē·äs′təmē\ [ILEO- + ILEO- + -STOMY] A surgical procedure creating an opening between two sections of distal small bowel following resection or bypass. Such an opening may rarely result from neoplastic, inflammatory, or traumatic causes.

**ileojejunitis** \-jē′joonī′tis\ The involvement of the ileum, in part or totally, and the jejunum with a chronic inflammatory condition.

**ileopexy** \il′ē·ōpek′sē\ [ILEO- + -PEXY] A surgical procedure in which the distal small bowel is suspended and fixed to prevent ptosis or torsion.

**ileoproctostomy** \-präktäs′təmē\ [ILEO- + PROCTOSTOMY] A surgical procedure creating an opening between the distal small bowel and the rectum following a colonic resection or bypass. Such an opening may rarely result spontaneously from neoplastic, inflammatory, or traumatic causes. Also *ileorectostomy.*

**ileorrhaphy** \il′ē·ôr′əfē\ [ILEO- + -RRHAPHY] A surgical procedure in which sutures are placed into the distal small bowel for purposes of plication or repair.

**ileosigmoidostomy** \-sig′moidäs′təmē\ [ILEO- + SIGMOIDOSTOMY] A surgical procedure creating an opening between the distal small bowel and the sigmoid colon following bypass or resection of the colon. Such an opening may rarely result from neoplastic, traumatic, or inflammatory causes.

**ileostomy** \il′ē·äs′təmē\ [ILEO- + -STOMY] A surgical procedure in which a loop or end of the distal small bowel is brought out through an opening in the abdominal wall following colonic bypass or resection. Such a protrusion may rarely result spontaneously from an inflammatory, neoplastic, or traumatic process. **end i.** An exteriorization on the abdominal wall of the divided proximal ileum.

**ileotomy** \il′ē·ät′əmē\ [ILEO- + -TOMY] A surgical procedure in which an incision is made into the distal small bowel.

**ileotransversostomy** \-trans′vərsäs′təmē\ ILEOTRANSVERSE COLOSTOMY.

**ileotyphlitis** \-tiflī′tis\ [ILEO- + TYPHL-[1] + -ITIS] Inflammation of the ileum and the cecum.

**ileum** \il′ē·əm\ [Med L (prob. from L *ile,* a sing. of *ilia* the inguinal regions and groin) the iliac (or pelvic) intestine; or (influenced by Gk *eilein* to bind, wind, roll up) the convoluted intestine] [NA] The distal three-fifths of the small intestine, continuous with the jejunum proximally and ending at the junction of the cecum and the ascending colon. It is attached to the posterior abdominal wall by the mesentery and most of it is situated in the hypogastric and pelvic regions. Its wall is thinner than that of the jejunum, and it contains characteristic aggregated lymph follicles.

**ileus** \il′ē·əs\ [L, from Gk *ileos* or *eileos* (from *eilein* to stop, hinder, bind, wind, roll up) intestinal stasis or obstruction] **1** Slowing or stoppage of the transit of intestinal contents due to diminished or absent bowel motility. **2** Any intestinal obstruction. **adynamic i.** Intestinal obstruction due to a lack of intestinal motility. **angiomesenteric i.** SUPERIOR MESENTERIC ARTERY SYNDROME. **dynamic i.** Intestinal obstruction due to spasm of some part of the intestinal musculature. Also *hyperdynamic ileus, spastic ileus.* **hyperdynamic i.** DYNAMIC ILEUS. **mechanical i.** Intestinal obstruction from a mechanical cause such as a gallstone, hernia, adhesion, volvulus, or foreign body. Also *occlusive ileus.* **meconium i.** Intestinal obstruction in neonates as the result of a mass of thickened meconium. It is commonly due to cystic fibrosis. **occlusive i.** MECHANICAL ILEUS. **paralytic i.** Ileus as the result of inhibition of bowel motility. Also *ileus paralyticus.* **spastic i.** DYNAMIC ILEUS. **i. subparta** Intestinal obstruction due to the pressure of a pregnant uterus on the colon. **terminal i.** Obstruction of the terminal part of the small intestine.

**ilia** \il′ē·ə\ Plural of ILIUM.

**iliac** \il′ē·ak\ Pertaining to the ilium.

**ilicin** \ī′ləsin\ A bitter principle isolated from the leaves of *Ilex aquifolium,* the European holly.

**ilio-** \il′ē·ō-\ [New L *ilium.* See ILIUM.] A combining form denoting the ilium.

**iliococcygeal** \-käksij′ē·əl\ Pertaining to the ilium and the coccyx.
**iliococcygeus** \-käksij′ē·əs\ MUSCULUS ILIOCOCCYGEUS.
**iliocolotomy** \-kōlät′əmē\ [ILIO- + COLOTOMY] An incision into the colon in the iliac region.
**iliocostal** \-käs′təl\ Pertaining to the ilium and the ribs, specifically the muscles between them.
**iliocostocervicalis** \-käs′tōsur′vikā′lis\ Denoting the iliocostalis cervicis and iliocostalis thoracis muscles. *Outmoded.*
**iliodorsal** \-dôr′səl\ Of or pertaining to the posterior, or gluteal, surface of the ilium.
**iliofemoral** \-fem′ərəl\ Pertaining to the ilium and the femur, or to the iliac region and the thigh.
**iliofemoroplasty** \-fem′əroplas′tē\ A surgical procedure in which a reconstruction of the iliac and femoral arteries is performed.
**iliohypogastric** \-hī′pōgas′trik\ Pertaining to the iliac and hypogastric regions.
**ilioinguinal** \-ing′gwənəl\ Pertaining to the iliac and inguinal regions.
**iliolumbar** \-lum′bər\ **1** Pertaining to the iliac and the lumbar regions. **2** Pertaining to the flank and the loin.
**iliopagus** \il′ē·äp′əgəs\ [ILIO- + -PAGUS] Equal conjoined twins with union restricted to the iliac region.
**ilioparasitus** \-par′əsī′təs\ Unequal conjoined twins with the parasitic member attached at the iliac region of the host. Also *iliopagus parasiticus.*
**iliopectineal** \-pektin′ē·əl\ Pertaining to the ilium and the pecten of the pubic bone.
**iliopelvic** \-pel′vik\ Pertaining to the iliac region and the pelvis, or to the iliacus muscle and the pelvic cavity.
**ilioperoneal** \-per′ənē′əl\ Pertaining to the ilium and the fibula, or to the inguinal region and the lateral compartment of the leg.
**iliopsoas** \il′ē·ōsō′as\ MUSCULUS ILIOPSOAS.
**iliopubic** \-pyoo′bik\ Pertaining to the ilium and the pubis or pubes; iliopectineal.
**iliosacral** \-sā′krəl\ Pertaining to the ilium and the sacrum.
**iliosciatic** \-sī·at′ik\ Pertaining to the ilium and the ischium.
**ilioscrotal** \-skrō′təl\ Of or pertaining to the ilium and the scrotum.
**iliospinal** \-spī′nəl\ Pertaining to the ilium and the vertebral column.
**iliothoracopagus** \-thôr′əkäp′əgəs\ [ILIO- + THORACO- + -PAGUS] Equal conjoined twins with union extending from the thoracic to the iliac regions.
**iliotibial** \-tib′ē·əl\ Pertaining to or connecting the ilium and the tibia.
**iliotrochanteric** \-trō′kanter′ik\ Pertaining to the ilium and a trochanter, usually the greater trochanter of femur.
**ilioxiphopagus** \-zifäp′əgəs\ [ILIO- + *xipho(id)* + -PAGUS] Equal conjoined twins with union extending from the xiphoid to the iliac regions.
**-ility** \-il′itē\ [L *-ilitas* a noun-forming suffix denoting quality or condition] A suffix denoting a quality or condition.
**ilium** \il′ē·əm\ [New L, short for *os ilium* (from L *os* bone + *ilium*, gen. pl. of *ilia* the iliac regions and groin) the iliac bone] [NA] OS ILII. ● Both *os ilium* and *os ilii* are grammatically allowable. *Ilium* in *os ilium* is genitive plural because in classical Latin the singular of this term was almost never used. The rare singular (nominative *ilium* or *ile*, genitive *ilii*) is considered logically preferable in this phrase, however, since *os* is singular, referring to each of the bilaterally paired bones separately, while the plural *ilia* (gen. *ilium*) designates the iliac regions on both sides together.
**ill** [Middle English, from Old Norse *illr* ill] **1** Not well; sick. **2** A disorder or disease: used especially in veterinary medicine.
**illinition** \il′inish′ən\ [L *illin(ere)* (from *in-* in, on + *linere* to rub, smear) to rub in, smear on + -ITION] Friction of the skin to facilitate absorption of a medicinal substance; inunction.
**illness** **1** The state of being ill. **2** A disorder producing such a state; a disease. **functional i.** Disturbance or variation in the way in which an organ or body system functions, with no evidence of alteration of that organ's structure. Psychogenic illnesses are functional, but not all functional illnesses are psychogenic. **psychosomatic i.** PSYCHOSOMATIC DISORDER. **radiation i.** RADIATION SICKNESS. **terminal i.** An illness from which the patient is not expected to recover and which is expected to be the proximate cause of death.
**illumination** [Late L *illuminatio* (from L *illuminare* to throw light on, from *in-* in, on + *luminare* to light up, make bright, from *lumen* a light, brightness) lighting, illumination] The act or process of casting light on an object, as that seen under a microscope, or in an enclosed space, as within a body cavity, to render it visible for examination. **axial i.** The transmission or reflection of light along the optical axis of the objective and eyepiece of a microscope. Also *central illumination.* **central i.** AXIAL ILLUMINATION. **contact i.** A method of inspecting the interior of the eye by means of light transmitted from a source touching the eye. This is most useful as a method of producing retroillumination, or backlighting, of the area under observation. **critical i.** In microscopy, the focusing of light from the source precisely upon the object to be observed. The image of the light source falls at the plane and location of the object observed. **dark-field i.** The illumination of an object by light rays striking it only from the periphery. The central or vertically oriented light is obstructed, causing the field to appear dark and the object to appear bright as it scatters or reflects the peripherally incident light. Also *dark-ground illumination.* **direct i.** In microscopy, illumination by a light source situated above the object being observed, with the light reflected upward through the optical system. Also *surface illumination.* **lateral i.** Illumination by light from a source whose axis is diagonal to the optical axis of the microscope. Also *oblique illumination.* **oblique i.** LATERAL ILLUMINATION. **orthogonal i.** Illumination for microscopic examination using light rays that are perpendicular to the axis of observation. **surface i.** DIRECT ILLUMINATION.
**illusion** [L *illusio* (from *illudere* to fool, trick, from *ludere* to play) trickery, ridicule] **1** A false perception of the actual appearance or character of an object. **2** Any perception based on erroneous interpretation of sensory stimuli. **autokinetic i.** The apparent movement of a pinpoint of light when regarded continuously in a darkened room. **i.'s of doubles** CAPGRAS SYNDROME. **epileptic i.** A perceptual disorder which is the basic, often the initial, and sometimes the only, symptom of an attack of focal epilepsy, and which is caused by epileptic discharge arising in part of the temporal cortex. According to the exact area involved, one can distinguish between perceptual illusions, in which the object in question is perceived in a distorted manner, and agnosic illusions, in which the object in question is perceived correctly but not recognized, thus giving rise either to déjà vu or jamais vu. Perceptual illusions can be classified, according to the sense involved, into somatosensory, vi-

sual, auditory, vertiginous, olfactory, and gustatory epileptic illusions. The dreamlike epileptic state is a prolonged epileptic illusional condition. Also *illusional aura.* **Fregoli's i.** The belief that a persecutor has assumed the guise of various people whom the subject encounters routinely. Also *Fregoli's phenomenon, illusion of negative double.* **optical i.** A false visual interpretation. The cerebral perception of patterns and designs is subject to variable interpretations, depending upon associated forms and perspectives. Thus, a given line may seem spontaneously to change from the background to the foreground of a drawing, causing the shape to turn inside out. In other examples, perceptions of distance and shape may be changed. Alternatively, optical devices may be used to produce distortions of space, as with anisokonic lenses.

**IM** 1 intramuscularly (injection site). 2 internal medicine. 3 infectious mononucleosis.

**im** intramuscularly (injection site).

**im-** \im-\ 1 IN-[1]. 2 IN-[2].

**image** [French, from L *imago,* gen. *imaginis* (akin to *imitare* to imitate, copy) a likeness, reflection, image, copy] The physical reproduction or mental picture of an object. **accidental i.** AFTERIMAGE. **acoustic i.** AUDITORY IMAGE. **auditory i.** A conception of something previously heard. Also *acoustic image.* **body i.** The image or concept that one holds of one's self and one's body as an object in space. Also *body identity.* **direct i.** VIRTUAL IMAGE. **double i.** See under DIPLOPIA. **eidetic i.** See under EIDETIC. **erect i.** VIRTUAL IMAGE. **false i.** The incorrectly localized double image originating from the nonfixing eye in strabismus. There is no real object in space corresponding to the apparent location of the false image. **gamma i.** SCINTISCAN. **incidental i.** AFTERIMAGE. **inverted i.** REAL IMAGE. **mirror i.** The reflection of an object in a mirror, with particular reference to its side to side reversal from the original object. Also *lateral inversion.* **motor i.** Self-awareness of the entire body with regard to motor function. **negative i.** See under NEGATIVE AFTERIMAGE. **optical i.** An image formed by the projection of light rays through a lens system which reassembles them at a point of focus where they may be perceived as a visual replica of an object. **pulse echo i.** A two-dimensional image achieved by sending pulses of ultrasound into the body and processing and displaying reflected echoes from tissue interfaces and parenchyma as an anatomic image. **Purkinje i.'s** The four images resulting from reflection of light by the front and back surfaces of the cornea and the lens of the eye. Also *Purkinje-Sanson mirror images, Sanson's images.* **real i.** An image formed at the intersection of convergent light rays and which may be visibly displayed on a surface. Also *inverted image.* **retinal i.** The real image projected upon the retina. The quality of this image is dependent upon such components of the object-image relationship as the refractive status of the eye, accommodation, corrective lenses, and clarity of the ocular media. **Sanson's i.'s** PURKINJE IMAGES. **specular i.** 1 An image caused by a reflecting surface. 2 The fine detail of a surface that may be perceived by observation of light reflected from the surface. The endothelial cells of the living cornea, for example, may be studied in microscopic detail by the technique of specular reflection. **tactile i.** The three dimensional concept elicited by palpation of an object. **true i.** The correctly localized image of the double images in strabismus. It originates from the fixing eye. The real object in space corresponds to the apparent location of the true image. **virtual i.** An image situated at the theoretical point of intersection of light rays but which cannot be displayed on a surface, as that seen in a plane mirror. Also *direct image, erect image.*

**imagery** \im′ijrē\ An inner evocation of some prior perceptual experience that retains many of the sensory qualities of the external stimuli giving rise to the original experience.

**imaging** \im′ijing\ The process of obtaining or producing an image. **dynamic i.** Imaging in which a rapid sequence of static images is used for real-time display of moving structures. **magnetic resonance i.** An imaging technique, based on the application of the principle of nuclear magnetic resonance, in which a patient is placed in a strong magnetic field. Radio-frequency signals are then used to distinguish between nuclei of the same element, usually hydrogen, in different types of tissue. Variations in magnetic field strength determine the location of the signals, and a computer reconstructs an image of the tissues. Abbr. MRI **pulse echo i.** Imaging of normally nonvisible tissues and tissue interfaces by ultrasonic pulse echo technique. See also PULSE ECHO IMAGE. **static i.** Imaging in which a single still image is produced. **stop-action i.** Imaging of cyclical motion in such a way as to produce a stationary representation. This is accomplished by repetitively imaging at the same point in time of the repetitive cycle, for example with a stroboscope. **through-transmission i.** Imaging by transmission of an interrogating beam through the specimen and receiving on a far surface.

**imago** \imā′gō\ [L, an image. See IMAGE.] The adult, sexually mature stage in the life cycle of an insect.

**imagocide** \imā′gōsīd′\ A chemical agent that destroys the adult stage of the insect, most often adult malarial parasites.

**imbalance** [IM- + BALANCE] Lack of balance, whether in motor activities or in the activities of various organs, glands, viscera, or systems. **autonomic i.** Any disorder of the autonomic nervous system in which there is unequal activity of the sympathetic and parasympathetic systems. Also *vasomotor imbalance.* **gene i.** Any situation in which the number of alleles being expressed at one or more loci has deleterious consequences on phenotype, and in aneuploidy. It is a potential complication of abnormal gene dosage. **sex chromosome i.** Any karyotype in which an abnormal number of entire or partial sex chromosomes is present. The most common examples in humans are 47,XXX; 47,XXY; and 47,XYY. **vasomotor i.** AUTONOMIC IMBALANCE.

**imbed** \imbed′\ EMBED.

**imbibition** \im′bibish′ən\ [L *imbibitus,* past part. of *imbibere* (from *im-* -IN + *bibere* to drink) to drink in] The absorption of a liquid by a gel, solid, or organized body.

**imbricate** \im′brikāt\ [Late L *imbricat(us),* past part. of *imbricare* (from L *imbrex,* gen. *imbricis* a gutter tile) to furnish with gutter tiles] To cause to overlap, as tissue: used in surgery to denote the intentional overlapping of adjacent tissues in order to improve contour or tensile strength.

**imbrication** \im′brikā′shən\ The overcrowding of incisor teeth in the same arch.

**Imerslund** [Olga *Imerslund,* Scandinavian physician, flourished 20th century] Imerslund-Najman-Gräsbeck syndrome. See under IMERSLUND SYNDROME.

**imidamine** ANTAZOLINE.

**imidazole** $C_3H_4N_2$. The heterocyclic aromatic base whose molecules contain a five-membered ring consisting of two nitrogen atoms at positions 1 and 3, one of them carrying a hydrogen atom, and three CH groups. It is a weak base (p*K* 7.2) and a very weak acid (p*K* 14.2). It is used as a buffer and as a basic catalyst, and it is the functional component of histidine residues in proteins. Also *glyoxalin* (outmoded), *iminazole* (outmoded).

**imide** \im′īd, im′id\ A compound containing the NH group joined to two CO groups. Such a compound is stable only if the grouping is part of a ring.

**imine** \im′īn\ Any compound formed by condensation of a primary amine (or ammonia), R—$NH_2$, with a carbonyl compound, R′—CO—R″, to give the structure R—N=CR′R″. Several enzymes, such as aldolase, combine with their substrates by reversible imine formation. Also *Schiff base, azomethine.*

**imino-** \imē′nō-, im′inō-\ [variant of AMINO-] A prefix indicating the bivalent =NH group, as in iminodiacetic acid, HN(—$CH_2$—COOH)$_2$.

**iminoglycinuria** \im′inōglī′sinoo′rē·ə \ The urinary excretion of the imino acids, proline and hydroxyproline, and the amino acid glycine. It occurs normally in newborns until renal transport mechanisms mature, and abnormally in the Fanconi syndrome, in hyperprolinemia, in hyperhydroxyprolinemia, and in benign familial iminoglycinuria. Also *proline-hydroxyproline-glycinuria.* **familial i.** A benign, autosomal, recessive phenotype characterized by iminoglycinuria. **familial renal i.** A familial defect in renal tubular transport that leads to increased excretion of L-proline, glycine, and the imino acids. Transmitted as an autosomal recessive trait, the condition usually is benign, but may be associated with decreased intestinal absorption of the same imino acids, seizures, and mental retardation.

**imipramine hydrochloride** $C_{19}H_{24}N_2·HCl$. 10,11-Dihydro-*N,N*-dimethyl-5*H* dibenz[*b,f*]azepine-5-propanamine monohydrochloride. A member of the class of tricyclic antidepressant drugs. It is used in the treatment of depression and in enuresis, and is given orally.

**Imlach** [Francis *Imlach*, Scottish anatomist and surgeon, 1819–1891] Imlach's fat plug. See under PLUG.

**immedicable** \imed′ikəbl\ Not subject to being cured by medical practice.

**immersion** \imur′shən\ [L *immersio* (from *immersus*, past part. of *immergere* to plunge into, immerse, sink, from *im-* in, into + *mergere* to put under water, dip) a plunging into] **1** The placing of a body or part entirely in water or another liquid. **2** In microscopy, the interposition of a liquid between the objective lens and the object under examination so that the liquid bathes both surfaces. **cold i.** A syndrome consisting of hypothermia and sometimes frostbite resulting from prolonged contact of a part or the whole of the body with a cold liquid. **oil i.** The use of oil as the immersion fluid in microscopy between the objective lens and the object examined. **water i.** The use of water as the immersion fluid in microscopy between the objective lens and the object examined.

**immigration** In population genetics, the introduction of genes through reproduction by individuals foreign to a breeding population.

**immiscible** \imis′əbl\ Possessing qualities that prevent mixing; unmixable.

**immobilize** \imō′bilīz\ To make immovable, as a fractured limb with a splint; fix in place.

**immune** \imyoon′\ [L *immunis* (from *im-*, *in-* not, un-, without + *munus* duty, task, service) exempt] **1** Characterized by a high degree of resistance to a specific pathogen or other foreign substance, either antibody-mediated resistance or resistance manifested as delayed hypersensitivity (T cell-mediated). **2** Pertaining to or producing immunity or antibody activity, as *immune response, immune serum, immune complex.*

**immunifaction** \im′yənifak′shən\ IMMUNIZATION.

**immunity** \imyoo′nitē\ [L *immunitas* (from *immunis* exempt; see IMMUNE) exemption] A state of increased resistance against the harmful effects of a noxious agent, as an infectious agent or toxin. Immunity can be innate or acquired. Acquired immunity may be humoral or cellular in origin and may be achieved as a result of a host's response to a prior disease or infection, or it may be produced in a host by means of immunization. **acquired i.** Immunity to infectious disease gained during one's lifetime, not inherited. It may be active or passive, with active immunity the result when antibody (or specifically reactive lymphocytes) is produced by the individual's immune system in response to a naturally acquired infection or to vaccination, and passive immunity the result when antibody is transferred to the individuals from another, immune human or animal host. Passive immunity can also be transferred with lymphocytes from an immune syngeneic animal. **active i.** Acquired immunity in which specific antibody (or specifically reactive lymphocytes) is produced by the individual's own immune system in response to a naturally acquired infection or to vaccination. **adoptive i.** Passive immunity of the cell-mediated type following the administration of sensitized lymphocytes from an immune donor. **artificial i.** Active or passive immunity, produced artificially, as distinguished from naturally acquired immunity. The administration of an antitoxin is an example of artificial immunity. **cell-mediated i.** Those manifestations of the immune response that are brought about by cells, in particular by T lymphocytes and macrophages. Also *cellular immunity.* Abbr. CMI **community i.** HERD IMMUNITY. **congenital i.** The immunity an individual has at birth. **cross i.** Immunity to a disease occurring subsequent to either natural infection or immunization with a different, but usually closely related, organism or toxin. **familial i.** NATURAL IMMUNITY. **functional i.** PROTECTIVE IMMUNITY. **genetic i.** NATURAL IMMUNITY. **herd i.** The epidemiologic concept that a population can be more resistant to the spread of a disease than would be suggested by the immunities of its members. Also *community immunity.* **humoral i.** Those manifestations of the immune response that are brought about by components of plasma, in particular antibodies and complement, and do not require the presence of cells. Humoral immunity does, however, recruit cells secondarily in a number of situations. **induced i.** Immunity acquired as a result of either active or passive immunization. **inherent i.** NATURAL IMMUNITY. **inherited i.** NATURAL IMMUNITY. **innate i.** NATURAL IMMUNITY. **intrauterine i.** Fetal immunity acquired by the passage of maternal immunoglobulins across the placenta and into the fetal circulation. Also *placental immunity.* **local i.** Immunity confined chiefly to a particular organ, part, or kind of tissue. **maternal i.** Passive immunity transferred humorally from mother to offspring before or after birth. In man and other primates, maternal immunoglobulins pass into the fetal circulation by crossing the placenta. Also *natural immunity.* **natural i.** **1** Immunity to a microorganism that does not require prior experience of the organism and does not depend on the generation of specific lymphocytes or the formation of specific antibody. Also *innate immunity, native immunity, inherited immunity, inherent immunity, natural resistance, genetic immunity, familial immunity, autarcesis, occult immunization* (rare). **2** MATERNAL IMMUNITY. **naturally acquired i.** Immunity acquired by fortuitous exposure to an antigen and not by deliberate immunization. **nonspecific i.** Resistance to infection resulting from any mechanism other

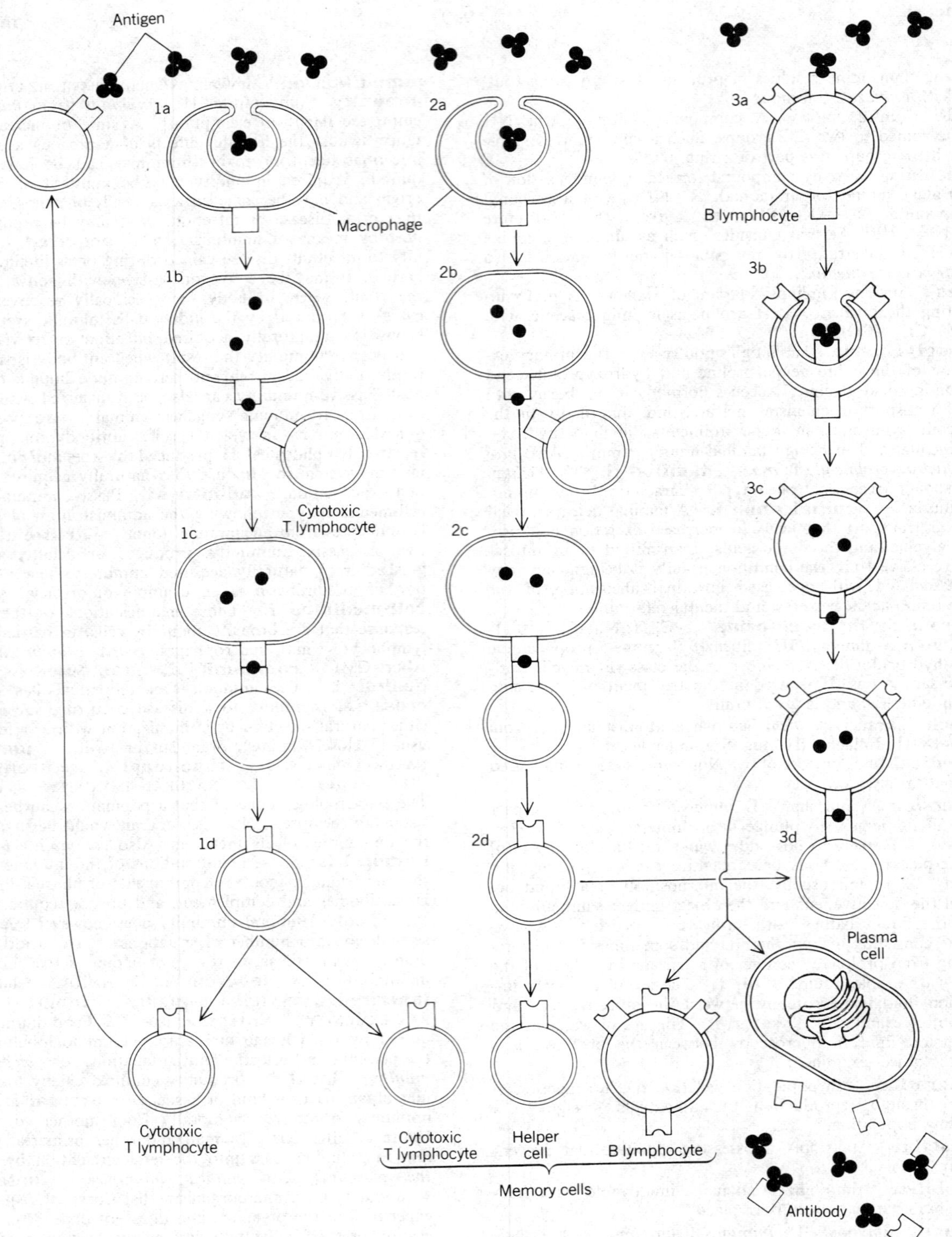


**Immunity** *Cell-mediated:* (1a) Macrophage endocytizes antigen. (1b) Antigen is broken down and pieces are displayed on cell membrane. Cytotoxic T lymphocyte is attracted. (1c) Cytotoxic T lymphocyte is sensitized to this specific antigen. (1d) T lymphocyte proliferates, producing daughter cells that are exact clones and thereby ready to attack antigen or to be memory cytotoxic T lymphocytes. (2a) Macrophage endocytizes antigen. (2b) Antigen is broken down and pieces are displayed on cell membrane. Helper cell (helper T lymphocyte) is attracted. (2c) Helper cell is sensitized to this specific antigen. (2d) Helper cell proliferates into memory helper cells or interacts with B lymphocytes. *Humoral:* (3a) Receptor on B lymphocyte captures antigen. Receptor and antigen enter B lymphocyte by endocytosis. (3c) Antigen is broken down and pieces are displayed on B lymphocyte membrane. (3d) Interaction between B lymphocyte and helper cell causes B lymphocyte to proliferate, producing either memory B lymphocytes or plasma cells that produce antigen-specific antibodies.

than the formation of antibodies and the generation of antigen-reactive lymphocytes. **passive i.** Acquired immunity in which specific antibody is transferred to the individual from another, already immune human or animal host (as from mother to fetus) or by injection with serum. In inbred strains of animals or in identical twins, passive immunity can also be conferred by transfer of lymphocytes from an immune donor. Also *passive protection.* **phagocytic i.** An inherent defense system that is based on the ability of macrophages and neutrophil polymorphs to ingest and destroy infective agents. **placental i.** INTRAUTERINE IMMUNITY. **preemptive i.** Immunity conferred by the interference phenomenon: cells infected with one virus may be insusceptible to superinfection with another. **protective i.** Immunity following administration of an antigen which stimulates antibodies or cellular immunity protective against a disease or an allergic state. Also *functional immunity.* **residual i.** Immunity of indeterminate duration following the disappearance of an infection. **specific i.** Immunity resulting from the formation of antibodies or the generation of specifically reactive lymphocytes against a particular antigen. It may occur following natural infection or as a result of immunization. **superinfection i.** In bacteriophage-infected cells, an alteration in the cell surface that prevents superinfection with another bacteriophage strain. **toxin-antitoxin i.** Acquired immunity brought about by subcutaneous inoculation with a toxin combined with its specific antitoxin. This method was developed as a form of diphtheria prophylaxis in the late nineteenth century. **transplantation i.** The development of an immune response on the part of the host to transplanted allogenic tissue.

**immunization** \im'yoonīzā'shən\ [*immun(o)-* + *-iz(e)* + -ATION] The act or process of making a subject immune, as to decrease susceptibility to infection. Also *immunifaction.* **active i.** The induction of active immunity by the administration of antigen. Also *active sensitization, isopathic immunization.* **occult i.** *Rare* NATURAL IMMUNITY. **passive i.** The conferring of passive immunity by the administration of antibody or, less frequently, of syngeneic, specifically reactive lymphocytes. Also *passive sensitization.* **prophylactic i.** Immunization that prevents disease.

**immunize** \im'yənīz\ [*immun(e)* + -IZE] To make immune.

**immuno-** \im'yənō-\ [L *immunis* exempt. See IMMUNE.] A combining form meaning immune, immunity.

**immunoadsorbent** \-adsôr'bənt\ IMMUNOSORBENT.

**immunoadsorption** \-adsôrp'shən\ A technique for the separation or quantification of an antibody from a serum or mixture, or of an antigen from a solution. The material sought is brought into contact with a solid phase that has the specific antigen or antibody on its surface. The specific antigen-antibody reaction attaches the material to the solid phase, resulting in physical separation from the original fluid medium. The adsorbed material can then be measured, eluted, purified, or otherwise manipulated in relatively pure form.

**immunoagglutination** \-əgloo'tinā'shən\ Clumping of blood cells or other antigen-bearing particulate matter induced by their reactivity with a corresponding antibody.

**immunoassay** \-as'ā\ [IMMUNO- + ASSAY] The measurement of a material by means of an antigen-antibody reaction that can be precisely quantified. Radioimmunoassay, enzyme-multiplied procedures, and rocket immunoelectrophoresis are frequently used techniques. Also *immune assay.* **enzyme-multiplied i.** A competitive binding technique employing an antibody specific for the substance being measured and a readily detectible enzyme that is coupled to a known quantity of the analyte in reagent form. The reaction of the antibody with the analyte inactivates the attached enzyme. The quantity of analyte in the unknown is calculated from the proportion of inactivated enzyme in the aliquot of indicator material.

**immunobiology** \-bī·äl'əjē\ The study of the immunologic factors that affect the growth, development, and health of biological organisms.

**immunoblast** \im'yənōblast'\ A transformed B lymphocyte or T lymphocyte with pyroninophilic cytoplasm and a centrally placed nucleolus. Such cells are capable of differentiating further to form either plasma cells or committed T lymphocytes. Also *pyroninophilic blast cell.*

**immunochemical** \-kem'ikəl\ Of or relating to immunochemistry; involving the chemical aspects of immunologic phenomena.

**immunochemistry** \-kem'istrē\ The study of the chemical basis of the antigen-antibody reaction and other immunologic responses. Also *chemoimmunology.*

**immunocompetence** \-käm'pətəns\ The property of being immunocompetent; the capacity to respond immunologically to an antigen. Also *immunologic competence.*

**immunocompetent** \-käm'pətənt\ Capable of responding immunologically to an antigen, as by producing antibodies or by developing cell-mediated immunity.

**immunocompromised** \-käm'prəmīzd\ In a state of diminished or impaired immunity, such as may be brought on by cytotoxic chemotherapy or irradiation or by certain disease processes.

**immunoconglutinin** \-kəngloo'tinin\ An anticomplement antibody produced in the body which binds the individual's own complement components, usually when bound at a complement fixation site. These antibodies react with bound C3 and bound C4. Also *autoanticomplement.*

**immunocyte** \im'yənōsīt'\ A lymphoid cell capable of reacting with antigen to induce antibody synthesis or cell-mediated immunity. Also *immunologically competent cell, immunocompetent cell, I cell.*

**immunocytoadherence** \-sī'tō·ədhir'əns\ A means of determining cell surface properties, in which receptors or immunoglobulins on the surface of one cell population cause cells with corresponding molecular configurations on their surface to adhere in rosettes around the indicator cells.

**immunocytochemistry** \-sī'təkem'istrē\ A histologic and cytologic process in which antigens can be identified using specific antibodies labeled with fluorescein or enzymes that can give a colored reaction product. Also *immunohistochemistry.*

**immunocytology** \-sītäl'əjē\ The branch of histology that employs immunologic probes in studying cells and their origins, structure, function, and pathology.

**immunodeficiency** \-difish'ənsē\ [IMMUNO- + DEFICIENCY] Any deficiency in the capacity to respond immunologically, as by defective production of humoral or cell-mediated immunity. Also *immunologic deficiency.* **acquired primary i.** Abnormal lack of resistance to infection due to disorder of the immunological apparatus and first appearing after early childhood. **combined i.** Immunodeficiency involving both humoral and cell-mediated immunity. See also SEVERE COMBINED IMMUNODEFICIENCY. **common variable i.** The most frequent form of primary immunodeficiency which includes sporadic cases of congenital immunodeficiency not falling into a recognized category and most cases of acquired primary immunodeficiency. Antibody deficiency disease is the most common manifestation, but abnormalities of T cells as well as of B cells can be found. It is likely to represent a mixture of different diseases which have not so far been clearly delineated. **severe combined i.** A group of disorders in which both antibody formation and cellular immunity are highly deficient, usually occurring in infants. The disease is associated with a propensity to overwhelming infections in early life, often due to *Pneumocystis carinii* or other organisms of low pathogenicity, and unless corrected by bone marrow grafting is fatal. The primary defect in most cases is unknown, but a proportion is due to homozygous deficiency of adenine deaminase. Also *severe combined immunodeficiency disease, combined immunodeficiency disease, combined immunodeficiency syndrome, Swiss type agammaglobulinemia, Swiss type hypogammaglobulinemia, Swiss type immunodeficiency, lymphopenic agammaglobulinemia, lymphopenic hypogammaglobulinemia.* Abbr. SCID **Swiss type i.** SEVERE COMBINED IMMUNODEFICIENCY. **i. with thymoma** A primary immunodeficiency which develops in older adults in association with benign tumors of the thymus and is characterized by agammaglobulinemia and defective antibody formation. Persons with this disorder have little or no resistance to bacterial, viral, and fungal infections and are subject to frequent, recurrent infections. Also *Good syndrome* (outmoded). **thymus-dependent i.** Those immunity deficiency states that arise from a failure of thymus function. Congenital absence of the thymus, as occurs in nude mice or in DiGeorge syndrome in man, is associated with absence or serious deficiency of peripheral T cells and a consequent failure of cell-mediated immunity. Homozygous deficiency of purine nucleotide phosphorylase also produces selective T cell defects in man. Clinically, thymus-dependent immunodeficiency is associated particularly with unusually severe or persistent viral exanthematous disease and infection with *Candida*. Removal or destruction of the thymus after infancy produces no obvious immunodeficiency. Also *thymus-dependent deficiency.* **X-linked i. with undue susceptibility to Epstein-Barr virus** A rare disease of apparently immunologically normal males who, upon first infection with the Epstein-Barr virus, develop fulminating infectious mononucleosis, agammaglobulinemia, or B-cell lymphoma, or bone-marrow aplasia. It shows the inheritance characteristic of X chromosome genetic defects. Also *X-linked lymphoproliferative syndrome, X-linked progressive combined variable immunodeficiency.* **X-linked progressive combined variable i.** X-LINKED IMMUNODEFICIENCY WITH UNDUE SUSCEPTIBILITY TO EPSTEIN-BARR VIRUS.

**immunodeficient** \-defish′ənt\ Deficient in the capacity to respond immunologically; characterized by an immunodeficiency.

**immunodepression** \-dipresh′ən\ IMMUNOSUPPRESSION.

**immunodiffusion** \-difyoo′zhən\ [IMMUNO- + DIFFUSION] A precipitin technique in which an antigen and an antibody diffuse through a gel medium, producing precipitin lines at those sites where the antigen and antibody concentrations are optimal for precipitation of insoluble complexes. This basic principle is used, either alone or in combination with electrophoretic principles, in a variety of qualitative, semiquantitative, and quantitative techniques such as radial diffusion and immunoelectrophoresis. Also *diffusion test, immunodiffusion test.* **radial i.** A technique for quantifying antigen in a solution. A measured quantity of the antigen is placed in a well in an agar plate containing a uniformly distributed antibody. As the antigen diffuses outward, a precipitin ring forms where antigen and antibody concentrations are optimal. The radius of the ring is proportional to the antigen concentration. Absolute figures can be derived by comparison with ring sizes observed when using standards of known concentration. Abbr. RID

**immunodominant** \-däm′ənənt\ **1** Describing those antigenic determinants in a molecule, or those components in an antigenic mixture, to which an immune response is produced preferentially. **2** Contributing a disproportionately large amount of binding energy in an antigen-antibody reaction. For example, the monosaccharide unit determining the antigenic specificity of a polysaccharide is immunodominant, as is the action of haptens.

**immunoelectrophoresis** \-ilek′trōfôrē′sis\ [IMMUNO- + ELECTROPHORESIS] A semiquantitative analytic technique in which electrically charged molecules, usually proteins, are separated by electrophoresis in an agar gel and then further characterized by the precipitin lines developing after suitable antibodies are introduced into the gel. Also *immunophoresis.* Abbr. IE **counter i.** See under COUNTERIMMUNOELECTROPHORESIS. **crossed i.** TWO-DIMENSIONAL IMMUNOELECTROPHORESIS. **rocket i.** A technique for quantifying proteins that employs both the immunodiffusion of an antigen into an antibody-containing gel and the electrophoretic stimulation of protein migration. Test samples and standards of known concentration are placed in wells and then current is applied to speed and direct the migration into agarose that contains a uniformly distributed antibody to the protein being measured. Convex precipitin arcs, which resemble the shape of a rocket, form at a distance from the origin that is determined by the concentration of protein present. Also *Laurell rocket test, Laurell crossed immunoelectrophoresis.* **two-dimensional i.** Crossed electrophoresis in which the antiserum to the migrating proteins is introduced with the second application of current, producing precipitin arcs that move perpendicularly to the initial direction of protein migration. Also *crossed immunoelectrophoresis.*

**immunofiltration** \-filtrā′shən\ [IMMUNO- + FILTRATION] Immunoadsorption in which the fluid material is filtered through a column containing the immunosorbent. Also *electrosyneresis.* **analytical i.** ANTIBODY AFFINITY CHROMATOGRAPHY.

**immunofluorescence** \-floo′əres′əns\ [IMMUNO- + FLUORESCENCE] A technique in which antigen or antibody is coupled with a fluorochrome dye (i.e., fluorescein isothiocyanate or rhodamine) and used to localize the site of an immune reaction. It is used in tissue sections, cell or bacterial smears, and flow cytometry. **direct i.** Immunofluorescence in which antigens in tissue sections or cell surfaces are localized with a fluorochrome-conjugated antibody specific for that tissue constituent. Also *single-layer immunofluorescence technique.* **indirect i.** A two-step technique for detecting antibodies reactive against cellular antigens. The unmodified serum is incubated with fixed cells containing the antigen. The specific antibody, if present, attaches to antigen sites. The presence of attached antibody is detected by adding fluorochrome-labeled antiglobulin serum, which attaches to the previously fixed antibody and produces a marker visible by fluorescent microscopic examination. Also *double layer fluorescent antibody technique.*

**immunogen** \imyoo′nəjən\ [IMMUNO- + -GEN] ANTIGEN.

**immunogenetic** \-jənet′ik\ Pertaining to or characterized by the interplay between immunology and genetics.

**immunogenetics** \-jənet′iks\ **1** The study of genetic mechanisms of immunologic control, expression, and disease. **2** The application of immunologic methods, such as monoclonal antibodies, to genetic investigations.

**immunogenic** \-jen′ik\ [IMMUNO- + -GENIC] Capable of inducing an immune response: often said of antigens.

**immunogenicity** \-jənis′itē\ The capacity of an antigen

to induce an immune response. Also *antigenicity.*

**immunoglobulin** \-gläb′yəlin\ A family of proteins having antibody activity. Immunoglobulins are composed of a basic structural unit comprising two identical heavy and two identical light chains linked together by disulfide bonds. There are five distinct kinds of heavy chains which form the basis for the five classes of immunoglobulins (IgA, IgD, IgE, IgG, IgM). Subclasses of IgG, IgA, and IgM with related but different heavy chains also occur. In addition, there are two different light chains designated κ and λ which are found in all classes. Also *immune globulin, immunoprotein, gamma globulin.* **i. A** The class of immunoglobulin which is secreted in saliva, mucus, and other external secretions and reacts with viruses, bacteria, and other antigens to protect epithelial cells. IgA monomer has a molecular weight of 170 000. Molecules of IgA are commonly linked by an additional J chain to form IgA dimers. Prior to secretion, a secretory piece, formed in epithelial cells, is attached to each IgA monomer, and the secretory immunoglobulin so formed then has a molecular weight of about 400 000. In serum, IgA is a monomer with a normal concentration of 150–400 mg/dl. IgA does not pass the placenta into the fetal circulation. It usually does not fix complement. In humans there are at least two subclasses of IgA. Also *gamma-A globulin* (obs.)*, secretory immunoglobulin, exocrine immunoglobulin, beta-2a globulin* (obs.). Abbr. IgA **Bence-Jones monoclonal i.** BENCE JONES PROTEIN. **i. D** The class of immunoglobulin which is found on the surface of B lymphocytes. It occurs in human plasma at low concentrations (0.3–40 mg/100 ml), primarily in the intravascular space. It has a molecular weight of 150 000. Also *gamma-D globulin* (obs.). Abbr. IgD **i. E** The class of immunoglobulin which has reaginic or homocytotropic antibody activity. It occurs in normal human plasma at very low concentrations (300 ng/ml). The concentration is greater in the presence of atopic allergy. It has a molecular weight of 196 000 and a high carbohydrate content. Also *gamma-E globulin* (obs.). Abbr. IgE **exocrine i.** IMMUNOGLOBULIN A. **i. G** The class of immunoglobulin present in largest amount in plasma and which fixes complement and crosses the placenta. It occurs in normal human plasma at concentrations of 800–1600 mg/100 ml. It has a molecular weight of 150 000. Four subclasses, called IgG1, IgG2, IgG3, and IgG4, have been identified. Also *gamma-G globulin* (obs.)*, human gamma globulin.* Abbr. IgG **i. M** The class of immunoglobulin which is active against bacteria or erythrocytes and in certain pathologic states may be active against autologous antibody. It occurs in normal human plasma at concentrations of 50–200 mg/ml. It is composed of a cyclic pentameter of five basic units of heavy and light chains linked by disulfide bonds. Its heavy chain is larger than that of other immunoglobulins. Because of its size, it does not cross the placental barrier in man. It has a molecular weight of 900 000. Also *gamma-M globulin* (obs.)*, beta-2M globulin* (obs.)*, γ macroglobulin* (obs.). Abbr. IgM **monoclonal i.** Immunoglobulin derived from a single cell or clone. It may be present in the serum of patients with multiple myeloma, in which case antibody specificity is rarely identifiable, or it may be an antibody deliberately produced and harvested by hybridoma techniques. **secretory i.** IMMUNOGLOBULIN A. **surface i.** Immunoglobulin present on the cell membrane, an important characteristic of a β-lymphocyte.

**immunoglobulinopathy** \-gläb′yəlinäp′əthē\ GAMMOPATHY.

**immunohematology** \-hē′mətäl′əjē\ The study of the humoral and cellular immune mechanisms as these relate to the pathogenesis, diagnosis, or treatment of diseases of blood and hematopoietic tissues. Blood banking is part of the field of immunohematology.

**immunohistochemistry** \-his′təkem′istrē\ IMMUNOCYTOCHEMISTRY.

**immunologic** \-läj′ik\ Of or relating to immunology. Also *immunological.*

**immunologist** \im′yənäl′əjist\ A specialist in immunology.

**immunology** \im′yənäl′əjē\ [IMMUNO- + -LOGY] The science concerned with the phenomena that allow an animal to respond to a subsequent exposure to a foreign substance in a way that is distinct from the way it responds to the initial exposure to that same substance. The modified response is specific for the particular foreign substance and can be elicited after long intervals (months or years) from the initial exposure. Immunology may be considered the study of the phenomena that enable organisms to distinguish self from nonself macromolecules and to respond specifically to foreign macromolecules. The formation of antibodies and the generation of antigen-reactive lymphocytes are the two principal phenomena studied. All aspects of these two phenomena and the effector mechanisms that they can recruit are included in the science of immunology.

**immunopathologic** \-path′əläj′ik\ Of or relating to immunopathology.

**immunopathology** \-pəthäl′əjē\ That part of the science of immunology that is concerned with the role of immune reactions in the pathogenesis, diagnosis, and treatment of disease.

**immunoperoxidase** See under STAIN.

**immunophoresis** \-fôrē′sis\ IMMUNOELECTROPHORESIS.

**immunoprecipitation** \-prisip′itā′shən\ Precipitation produced by the introduction of a specific antibody to a soluble antigen. Also *precipitation.*

**immunoprecipitin** \-prisip′itin\ *Older term* PRECIPITIN.

**immunoproliferative** \-prōlif′ərā′tiv\ Marked by an increase in the number of cells that play a role in antibody formation, i.e. lymphocytes and plasma cells. Immunoproliferative disorders include malignant lymphomas, lymphocytic leukemias, and multiple myeloma.

**immunoprophylaxis** \-prō′filak′sis\ Disease prevention by immunologic means. Active immunoprophylaxis involves the administration of antigens to stimulate the host's own immune system. Passive immunoprophylaxis involves the administration of antibody (or, in inbred species or identical twins, of lymphocytes) from an immune donor.

**immunoprotein** \-prō′tē·in\ IMMUNOGLOBULIN.

**immunoreaction** \-rē·ak′shən\ IMMUNE RESPONSE.

**immunoreactive** \-rē·ak′tiv\ Having the capacity to participate in an antigen-antibody reaction: often applied to hormones where assays of the immunoreactive material may not always parallel assay of the functional hormone.

**immunoreactivity** \-rē′aktiv′itē\ The capability for or degree of interaction between antigen and antibody or antigen and lymphocyte or plasma cell. **gastrointestinal glucagonlike i.** Extrapancreatic material detected by immunoassays for glucagon. It is of incompletely known structure and function, produced by mucosal cells of the postduodenal bowel, as in the dog. It is distinct from gastric glucagon. Abbr. GLI

**immunoselection** \-silek′shən\ The survival of certain cell lines based on their ability to escape the cytotoxic actions of antibody or immune lymphoid cells.

**immunosenescence** \-senes′əns\ The decline in immune function that occurs with advancing age. This decline has been held as the cause of many manifestations of aging, but on the basis of little substantive evidence.

**immunosmoelectrophoresis** \im'yənäz'mō·ilek'trəfôr-ē'sis\ COUNTERIMMUNOELECTROPHORESIS.

**immunosorbent** \-sôr'bənt\ The insoluble or solid form of an antigen or antibody that is used in immunoadsorption. Also *immunoadsorbent.*

**immunosuppressant** \-səpres'ənt\ Any substance capable of inhibiting or depressing the immune response to an antigen, an immunosuppressive substance.

**immunosuppression** \-səpresh'ən\ The inhibition or suppression of the immune response, as by antimetabolites or irradiation, or by the administration of antilymphocytic sera or cyclosporine to prevent the rejection of grafts or organ transplants; or by infection, as in acquired immune deficiency syndrome (AIDS). Also *immunodepression.*

**immunosurveillance** \-sərvā'ləns\ IMMUNOLOGIC SURVEILLANCE.

**immunotherapy** \-ther'əpē\ [IMMUNO- + THERAPY] **1** The treatment of disease by the administration to the patient of antibody raised in another individual or another species (passive immunotherapy) or by immunizing the patient with antigens appropriate to the disease (active immunotherapy). **2** Therapy, used especially in the treatment of cancer, intended to stimulate the effector mechanisms of the immune response nonspecifically. **adoptive i.** Treatment of disease by the administration of specific antibody raised in either another species or another individual of the same species, or by the administration of lymphocytes reactive to a particular antigen obtained from a (preferably syngeneic) member of the same species.

**immunotolerance** \-täl'ərəns\ IMMUNOLOGIC TOLERANCE.

**immunotolerant** \-täl'ərənt\ Characterized by immunologic tolerance.

**immunotoxicology** \-täk'sikäl'əjē\ **1** The study of immunologic methods for directing toxic molecules to specific target sites, as by using antibody-toxin conjugates. **2** The study and assay of toxic molecules by immunologic techniques.

**immunotransfusion** \-transfyoo'zhən\ The use of blood or blood components from a donor who has developed an appropriate immune response to a particular pathogen. This is a form of adoptive immunotherapy. Also *phylactotransfusion.*

**IMP** inosine monophosphate (inosinic acid).

**impact** \(1,2) impakt'; (3) im'pakt\ [L *impact(us),* past part. of *impingere* to hit, throw against, fasten] **1** To press firmly into a space, as food between the teeth. **2** To jam forcibly together as a result of trauma, as the ends of bones. **3** The force that a moving body imparts to another upon colliding with it.

**impacted** \impak'tid\ **1** Pressed firmly into a space, as food between two teeth. **2** Prevented from erupting by some obstacle: said of a tooth. **3** Forcibly jammed together as a result of trauma, as the fractured ends of bones: said of a fracture.

**impaction** \impak'shən\ [L *impactio,* from *impactus,* past part. of *impingere* to thrust, drive against] The condition of being impacted. **ceruminal i.** IMPACTED CERUMEN. **dental i.** A condition in which a tooth is prevented from erupting by an obstacle such as another tooth. **fecal i.** A mass of compressed, often inspissated and hard feces found in the sigmoid colon or rectum. **mucoid i.** Obstruction of a bronchus by mucuslike material.

**impaired** \imperd'\ Acting under a handicap, as that arising from drug or alcohol abuse, that is likely to diminish significantly the effectiveness or competence of performance with respect to the medical service rendered, as *impaired physician.* • The term is used in this sense in India and New Zealand as well as the United States. In the United Kingdom, *sick,* as in *sick doctor,* is sometimes used with this sense, but *impaired* is not used.

**impairment** \imper'mənt\ [Old French *empeirier* (from Vulgar L *impejorare,* from L *im-* intensive + *pejorare* to make worse, from *pejor* worse) to diminish, lessen + -MENT] **1** A partial disability or loss of function; a functional deficit. **2** Diminution or reduction below normal, as applied, for example, to resonance on percussion or to loudness of breath or voice sounds on auscultation of the chest. **conductive hearing i.** CONDUCTIVE HEARING LOSS. **hearing i.** HEARING LOSS.

**impalpable** \impal'pəbl\ Impossible to perceive by touch.

**impar** \im'pär\ [L (from *im-* IM-[2] + *par* equal, a pair), unequal] Unpaired; azygous.

**impatency** \impā'tənsē\ The state of being closed or blocked.

**impatent** \impā'tənt\ Closed or blocked; not patent.

**impedance** \impē'dəns\ [L *imped(ire)* (from *im-* in, into + *pes,* gen. *pedis,* foot) to entangle, hinder, impede + -ANCE] **1** The opposition to flow from an alternating source at a given frequency. **2** In electricity, the sum, in quadrature, of the resistance and the reactance, which is composed of capacitance and inductance. **3** In fluid flow, the sum, in quadrature, of the viscous resistance and the reactance, which is composed of compliance and inertance. **4** In acoustics, the product of the velocity of sound and the density. **acoustic i.** The opposition to the flow of sound energy in a mechanical system such as the tympanic membrane and ossicular chain, its measurement being related to the wavelength of the sound and the inertia, stiffness, and mass of the system. Also *ear impedance.* **characteristic acoustic i.** Density multiplied by the sound speed of a medium. **ear i.** ACOUSTIC IMPEDANCE. **specific acoustic i.** The ratio of sound pressure to particle velocity.

**imperception** \impərsep'shən\ Impaired perception in any sensory modality.

**imperforate** \impur'fərət\ [IM-[2] + L *perforat(us),* past part. of *perforare* to pierce, form by boring] Lacking a normal orifice.

**imperforation** \impur'fərā'shən\ [IM- + PERFORATION] A failure of a normal opening to occur in an organ during embryonic development.

**impermeable** \impur'mē·əbl\ Not permeable; incapable of being penetrated by a fluid, as a gas.

**impersistence** \im'pərsis'təns\ **motor i.** Inability to sustain any motor act or movement.

**impervious** \impur'vē·əs\ Not permitting passage, as of fluids or light; blocking penetration.

**impetigo** \im'pətī'gō\ [L (from *impetere* to attack, assault), a skin infection] A contagious bullous, crusted, or pustular eruption of the skin that is caused by streptococci and/or staphylococci. Also *impetigo vulgaris, impetigo contagiosa.* **Bockhart's i.** A staphylococcal infection of the skin characterized by superficial follicular pustules. Also *superficial pustular perifolliculitis.* **bullous i.** Impetigo of the newborn characterized by predominantly bullous lesions. Also *impetigo bullosa, impetigo neonatorum.* **chronic symmetric i.** Extensive impetigo that affects the trunk. **circinate i.** Impetigo in which the lesions are grouped in a coiled configuration. **i. contagiosa** IMPETIGO. **i. herpetiformis** *Outmoded* PUSTULAR PSORIASIS. **miliary i.** PUSTULAR MILIARIA. **i. neonatorum** BUL-

LOUS IMPETIGO. **i. pityroides** PITYRIASIS ALBA. **i. vulgaris** IMPETIGO.

**implant** \im′plant, implant′\ [L *im-* in + PLANT] **1** To insert into the body, usually at operation, as to preserve or restore function or to maintain configuration or for other therapeutic purposes. **2** An object so inserted. **carcinomatous i.'s** The growth of carcinoma from cells transferred from another site, as on peritoneal surfaces from an ovarian primary tumor. **cartilaginous i.** Cartilage, usually autogenous tragal cartilage, implanted into the middle ear for a variety of tympanoplastic and other therapeutic procedures. **cochlear i.** An electrode, usually a multichannel electrode, implanted into the inner ear, less often into the middle ear, in an attempt to restore a modicum of hearing to someone deafened as the result of the total loss of cochlear function. **dental i.** ORAL IMPLANT. **deoxycortone acetate i.** A formulation as a cylinder or tablet of deoxycortone acetate suitable for subcutaneous administration to provide slow, sustained release of the drug. **diodontic i.** ENDODONTIC IMPLANT. **dynamic i.** A significant idea that is introduced into the subject's consciousness with the expectation that he will assimilate the idea and reorganize his thinking and behavior accordingly. **endodontic i.** An endosteal implant inserted through the root canal of a tooth for the purpose of splinting the tooth.

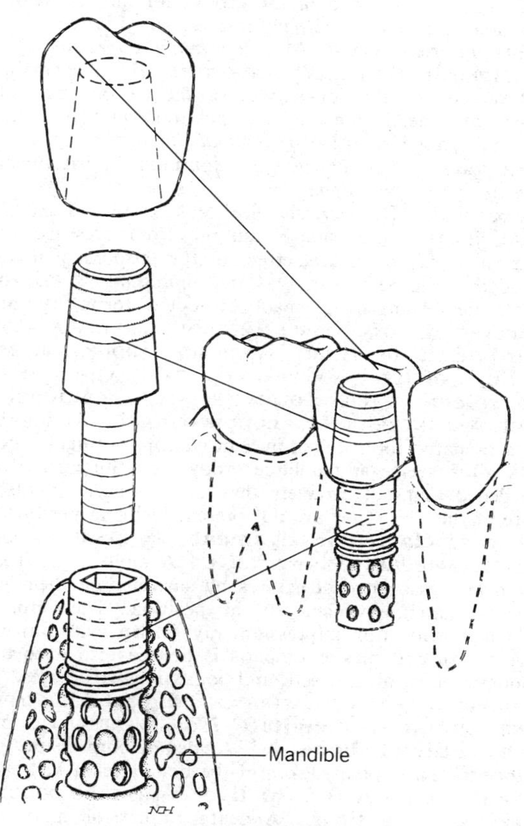


**Endosteal implant**

Also *diodontic implant.* **endometrial i.'s** ENDOMETRIOSIS. **endosteal i.** An oral implant entering, and surrounded by, bone. The infrastructure may consist of wedge-shaped blades which fit into longitudinal grooves cut into the bone. In the case of single tooth implants, it may be a simple spiral or perforated structure which fits into a tooth socket or prepared substitute. Also *endosseous implant.* **hormone i.** A fused or compressed hormone formulation in the shape of a cylinder or tablet suitable for subcutaneous or intramuscular placement. Slow release of the hormone is provided by this route of administration. **intraosseous i.** A metal implant for intraosseous fixation of fractures. **magnetic i.** An oral implant completely buried in the bone. Its function is to improve the retention of a denture by the mutual attraction between it and another magnet attached to the denture. **needle endosteal i.** PIN ENDOSTEAL IMPLANT. **oral i.** An insert of biologic or alloplastic material in the hard or soft oral tissues for cosmetic purposes or to support or retain a denture, bridge, or crown. Also *dental implant, ventplant.* **pin endosteal i.** An oral implant of which the infrastructure is a number of pins driven into the bone at various angles. Also *needle endosteal implant, pin implant.* **subperiosteal i.** An oral implant made to fit the surface of the bone and covered, apart from the necks of the abutments, with mucoperiosteum.

**implantation** \implantā′shən\ [IMPLANT + -ATION] **1** The attachment of the fertilized ovum to, or penetration into, an organ where it develops during gestation. Implantation almost always takes place in the uterus on the receptive mucous lining or endometrium. Penetration is accompanied by destruction of endometrial tissue. Exceptionally (about 0.1%), it occurs outside the uterus (ectopic pregnancy) in the lining of the uterine tube or even in some other intra-abdominal organ, such as the ovary. Implantation generally occurs when the fertilized ovum has reached the blastocyst stage, or at the start of gastrulation after the appearance of secondary mesoderm. Also *nidation.* **2** The surgical fixation or insertion of a tissue such as muscle, tendon, nerve, or bone to establish a new union. **3** The act or process of placing a surgical implant. **central i.** SUPERFICIAL IMPLANTATION. **circumferential i.** SUPERFICIAL IMPLANTATION. **delayed i.** A pause in development of the blastocyst, which in many mammalian species remains unimplanted inside the uterine horn for varying periods. **eccentric i.** Implantation of the ovum in which the chorionic sac lies for a time in a fold or pocket of the uterine mucosa where it eventually implants by destruction of some tissue and becomes closed off from the main uterine cavity, as in the mouse and rat. **endometrial i.** The process whereby the blastocyst penetrates and becomes fixed in the endometrium. **interstitial i.** Implantation of the ovum in which the ovum penetrates into the substance of the uterine mucosa, as in the hedgehog, guinea pig, and some primates, including man. **intrafollicular i.** Ectopic implantation of an embryo within an ovarian (graafian) follicle which occurs following spontaneous (parthenogenetic) activation and intrafollicular development of an ovarian oocyte. This phenomenon has been reported in various mammalian species, but most commonly in the LT/SV strain of mice, and is the likely origin of most ovarian teratocarcinomas where development becomes disorganized shortly after the blastocyst stage. **juxtafollicular i.** The ectopic embedding of the blastocyst near to or adjoining an ovarian (graafian) follicle. **nerve i.** Grafting by insertion of a nerve into muscle. **periosteal i.** A surgical procedure in which the tendon from one or more functional muscles is inserted into the periosteum to take the place of a nonfunctional muscle. **superficial i.** Implantation of the ovum in which the chorionic sac (the outer surface of the expanding blastocyst) makes a simple contact with the uterine mucosa, as in the pig, sheep, cow, horse, dog, cat, and some primates. Also *central implantation, circumferential implantation.* **tooth i.** The surgical insertion of a structure or material into or on the bone of the jaw to support a dental restoration, for cosmetic correction, or for the immobilization of a fracture.

**implantology** \im'plantäl'əjē\ **oral i.** The study of the implantation of teeth or implants.

**implosion** \implō'zhən\ [IM-[1] + *plos(us)* for *plausus,* past part. of *plaudere* to clap, beat + -ION] A therapeutic technique in which the phobic patient imagines the object or situation he fears.

**impotence** \im'pətəns\ [L *impotentia* (from *impotens,* gen. *impotentis* powerless, from *in-* not + *potens* potent, capable, pres. part. of *posse* to be able) weakness, helplessness] A dysfunction in which the male is unable to perform the sexual act. It may be of psychosexual or organic origin. Also *impotency, improcreance, invirility* (obs.). **functional i.** PSYCHIC IMPOTENCE. **organic i.** Impotence resulting from any organic disorder of the sexual apparatus, its innervation, or its blood supply. Also *secondary impotence.* **orgastic i.** Failure of either the male or female to achieve orgasm, despite adequacy of response in earlier phases of the sexual act. Also *anorgasmy.* **paretic i.** Impotence due to a lesion of the spinal cord or any other part of the central nervous system. **psychic i.** A psychosexual dysfunction consisting of inability of the male to perform sexual intercourse despite sexual desire and despite the lack of any organic condition that affects genital structure or function. Also *functional impotence, primary impotence, psychogenic impotence.* **secondary i.** ORGANIC IMPOTENCE. **symptomatic i.** Impotence due to a lesion of the afferent (perineal nerve) components of the reflex arcs concerned with erection and ejaculation.

**impotency** \im'pəten'sē\ IMPOTENCE.

**impregnate** \impreg'nāt\ **1** To make pregnant; fertilize. **2** To permeate; saturate.

**impregnation** \im'pregnā'shən\ **1** The act of impregnating or making pregnant; fertilization. Also *ingravidation.* **2** The process of saturating a substance or the condition resulting from it. **artificial i.** ARTIFICIAL INSEMINATION.

**impressio** \impres'ē·ō\ [L (from *impressus,* past part. of *imprimere* to press into, stamp into, from *im-* into + *premere* to press), a pressing in or into, stamping into] (*pl.* impressiones) A concave depression or indentation in the surface of an organ or structure produced by the contact of another, as of the surface of the liver in contact with the stomach. Also *impression.* **i. cardiaca hepatis** [NA] A shallow depression on the superior portion of the diaphragmatic surface of the liver, related to the heart through the diaphragm. Also *cardiac impression of liver.* **i. cardiaca pulmonis** [NA] A deep concavity on the mediastinal part of the medial surface of each lung, more pronounced on the left, for accommodation of the heart and pericardium. Also *cardiac impression of lung.* **i. colica hepatis** [NA] A variable hollow on the visceral surface of the right lobe of the liver, adjacent to the inferior border and to the right of the gallbladder, and related to the right flexure of the colon. Also *colic impression of liver.* **impressiones digitatae** [NA] Faint hollow markings on the inner surface of the cranium produced by the cerebral gyri. Also *digitate impressions, digital impressions.* **i. duodenalis hepatis** [NA] A small, shallow depression on the visceral surface of the right lobe of the liver, wedged between the colic and the renal impressions to the right of the neck and adjacent part of the gallbladder and produced by the junction of the superior and descending parts of the duodenum. Also *duodenal impression of liver.* **i. esophagealis hepatis** [NA] A small, shallow depression on the posterior aspect of the left lobe of the liver to the left of the upper end of the fissure for ligamentum venosum and related to the abdominal part of the esophagus. Also *esophageal impression of the liver.* **i. gastrica hepatis** [NA] A large concavity, occupying most of the visceral surface of the left lobe and continuing on to the anterior part of the quadrate lobe of the liver, related to the anterior surface and pyloric part of the stomach respectively. Also *gastric impression of liver.* **i. ligamenti costoclavicularis** [NA] A rough raised area on the inferior surface of the medial, or sternal, end of the clavicle for the attachment of the costoclavicular ligament. Also *impression of costoclavicular ligament, rhomboid impression of clavicle.* **i. petrosa pallii** A shallow indentation on the inferior surface of the temporal lobe made by the superior ridge of the petrous portion of the temporal bone. Also *impressio petrosa cerebri, petrous impression.* **i. renalis hepatis** [NA] A large hollow on the posterior part of the visceral surface of the right lobe of the liver, bounded posteriorly by the inferior layer of the coronary ligament, medially by the duodenal impression, and anteriorly by the colic impression, and related to most of the anterior surface of the right kidney below the suprarenal gland. Also *renal impression of liver.* **i. suprarenalis hepatis** [NA] A small depression on the "bare area" of the posterior surface of the right lobe of the liver, to the right of the lower end of the groove for inferior vena cava and superomedial to the renal impression. It is related to the right suprarenal gland. Also *suprarenal impression of liver.* **i. trigeminalis ossis temporalis** [NA] A small, oval hollow on the anterior surface of the petrous part of the temporal bone, just behind its apex, on which rests the trigeminal ganglion. Also *trigeminal impression of temporal bone, fossa of gasserian ganglion* (outmoded), *trigeminal impression for gasserian ganglion.*

**impression** [L *impressio.* See IMPRESSIO.] **1** IMPRESSIO. **2** An imprint of a shape resulting from pressure applied against a plastic surface, often for the purpose of making a mold that can be cast, as a *dental impression.* **anatomic i.** A dental impression made without distorting the tissues. **cardiac i. of liver** IMPRESSIO CARDIACA HEPATIS. **cardiac i. of lung** IMPRESSIO CARDIACA PULMONIS. **colic i. of liver** IMPRESSIO COLICA HEPATIS. **colic i. of spleen** FACIES COLICA SPLENIS. **composite i.** SECTIONAL IMPRESSION. **copper-ring i.** An impression of a prepared tooth taken in a fitted copper ring. **costal i.'s** Transverse and oblique grooves on the surface of the hardened lungs of cadavers that are produced by the pressure of the ribs. They are not present in living persons. **i. of costoclavicular ligament** IMPRESSIO LIGAMENTI COSTOCLAVICULARIS. **dental i.** A mold made from the teeth and associated structures by surrounding them with a plastic material which sets in position. The impression, which is held in an impression tray, is then withdrawn from the mouth and plaster of paris is poured into it to form a model or cast of the teeth and contiguous structures. **digastric i.** FOSSA DIGASTRICA. **digital i.'s** IMPRESSIONES DIGITATAE. **digitate i.'s** IMPRESSIONES DIGITATAE. **direct bone i.** A dental impression, for a subperiosteal implant, taken of the bone after it has been exposed. **duodenal i. of liver** IMPRESSIO DUODENALIS HEPATIS. **elastic i.** A dental impression made with a material which when set yields enough to permit its removal from undercuts and which then returns to its original set shape. **esophageal i. of liver** IMPRESSIO ESOPHAGEALIS HEPATIS. **fluid wax i.** A dental impression which has been corrected by the addition of wax in a fluid state and then returned to the mouth. **functional i.** A dental impression taken with the supporting tissues compressed and the orofacial muscles active. Also *registration of functional form, mucodisplacement impression.* **gastric i. of liver** IMPRESSIO GASTRICA HEPATIS. **gastric i. of spleen** FACIES GASTRICA SPLENIS. **meningeal i.** FOVEOLAE GRANULARES. **mucodisplacement i.** FUNCTIONAL IMPRESSION. **mucostatic i.** A dental impression causing minimal mucosal displacement. **petrous i.** IMPRESSIO PETROSA PALLII. **renal i. of liver** IMPRESSIO RENALIS HEPATIS. **rhomboid i. of clavicle** IMPRESSIO LIGAMENTI COSTOCLAVICULARIS. **sectional i.** A dental impression, usually for a partial denture, made in sections so that a material which is rigid when set can be withdrawn from undercuts and reassembled in the impression tray for casting. Also *composite impression.* **suprarenal i. of liver** IMPRESSIO SUPRARENALIS HEPATIS. **trigeminal i. for gasserian ganglion** IMPRESSIO TRIGEMINALIS OSSIS TEMPORALIS. **trigeminal i. of temporal bone** IMPRESSIO TRIGEMINALIS OSSIS TEMPORALIS.

**impressiones** \impres'ē·ō'nēz\ Plural of IMPRESSIO.

**impressorium** \im'presôr'ē·əm\ SENSORIUM.

**imprinting** A mode of rapid learning by some animals depending on very brief and very early exposure to adults, usually parents, such as the following behavior of birds soon after hatching.

**improcreance** \imprō'krē·əns\ IMPOTENCE.

**impulse** \im'puls\ [L *impulsus* (from *impellere* to push, drive, impel, from *im-* into, toward + *pellere* to set in motion) a setting in motion, moving, impulse] **1** A sudden urge to act in response to subjective or external stimuli: used especially of behavior viewed as powerfully motivated, compulsive, or irrational. **2** Any driving force. **3** A nerve impulse. **apex i.** APEX BEAT. **apical i.** APEX BEAT. **cardiac i.** The visible or palpable thrust of the heart against the chest wall; apex beat. Also *pulsus cordis.* **ectopic i.** An electrical impulse arising in any part of the heart other than the sinuatrial node. **enteroceptive i.'s** Nerve impulses derived from the viscera. **exteroceptive i.'s** Nerve impulses derived from sense organs of the skin and distance receptors. **involuntary i.** REFLEX ACT. **nerve i.** A rapid, electrochemical, conducted event propagated in nerve fibers. Also *neural impulse.* **proprioceptive i.'s** Nerve impulses derived from receptors in muscles, tendons, and joints.

**imu** \ē'moo\ [Ainu] A culture-specific syndrome of the Ainu of Japan consisting of hyperkinesia, catalepsy, echolalia, echopraxia, and command automatism. It appears almost exclusively in adult females.

**imus** \ī'məs\ [L, irreg. superl. of *inferus* lower] Lowest.

**IMViC** A set of tests used to distinguish various Enterobacteriaceae, and especially to distinguish coliforms of fecal origin from *Enterobacter* species. The tests are for indole production, methyl red color change with pH, Voges-Proskauer reaction for acetoin, and citrate utilization.

**In** Symbol for the element, indium.

**in-[1]** \in-\ [L preposition *in* (in all combinations with L words *in-* becomes *im-* before *b, m, p; il-* before *l, ir-* before *r*; with English words *in-* may remain unchanged regardless of following letter) in, on, into] **1** A prefix meaning (1) in, into, toward; (2) becoming or causing to become. **2** A prefix denoting intensity or emphasis. Also *il-, im-, ir-.*

**in-[2]** \in-\ [L prefix *in-* (regularly *im-* before *b, m, p; il-* before *l; ir-* before *r*) not] A prefix meaning not, non-, un-, or lacking. Also *il-, im-, ir-.*

**-in** \-in, -ən\ [modification of -INE] A suffix used in the names of many kinds of biologic substances, such as enzymes (*pepsin, kallikrein*), plasma proteins (*albumin, globulin*), hormones (*bradykinin, gonadotropin*), tissue or cell components (*myosin, chromatin*), antibodies (*hemolysin, agglutinin*), and pharmaceutical principles and antibiotics (*tuberculin, streptomycin*).

**-ina** \-ē'nə, -ī'nə\ [fem. sing. or neut. pl. of L *-inus* combining form denoting belonging to] A suffix used in some biological taxonomic names.

**inaction** **1** Lack of action. **2** Sluggish response to a stimulus.

**inactivate** \inak'tivāt\ To make biologically inactive, as viruses or bacteria, toxins, or serum complement, by any of various means, such as by physical means (exposure to x rays, ultraviolet irradiation, or heating), or by exposure to chemical agents or to immunologic antagonists.

**inactivation** \inak'tivā'shən\ The process by which a substance or agent, as a virus, a toxin, or enzyme, is rendered biologically inactive, or the condition thus effected by such a process. **paternal-X i.** The nonrandom inactivation of the X chromosome that is derived from the father in the somatic cells of females of some species, including marsupials. **random-X i.** The inactivation of most of one of the two X chromosomes present in the homogametic sex, such as human females, as a mechanism of dosage compensation. The selection of which X chromosome becomes inactive occurs randomly in normal cells.

**inactivator** \inak'tivā'tər\ **C3b i.** *Outmoded* FACTOR I. • The reference is to factor I (the letter, not the roman numeral).

**inagglutinable** \in'əgloo'tinəbl\ Not capable of being agglutinated.

**inanimate** \inan'imət\ Lacking life; not animate.

**inanition** \in'ənish'ən\ [Late L *inanitio,* from L *inanire* to empty, from *inanis* empty] Any disorder of the body due to the insufficient intake of one or more essential nutrients including water, as vitamin deficiency diseases, starvation, kwashiorkor, marasmus, goiter, and anemia.

**inarticulate** \in'ärtik'yəlit\ **1** Incapable of producing the sounds of intelligible speech. **2** Unable to speak easily or well; uncommunicative.

**in articulo mortis** \in ärtik'yəlō môr'tis\ [L *in* in + *articulo,* ablative of *articulus* juncture, fit moment + *mortis,* gen. of *mors* death] At the exact moment of death.

**inassimilable** \in'əsim'iləbl\ Not capable of being assimilated, as ingested nutrients.

**inattention** \in'əten'shən\ Lack of attention. **sensory i.** INATTENTION PHENOMENON.

**inborn** **1** HEREDITARY. **2** CONGENITAL.

**inbred** Characterized by inbreeding; describing a population in which the occurrence of consanguineous matings has been relatively high.

**inbreeding** **1** The selective crossing of related plants or animals. Compare OUTBREEDING. **2** A mating system, whether directed or occurring in nature, in which mates are on average more closely related than expected on the basis of random selection. Also *intermarriage* (popular), *linebreeding.*

**incanous** \inkā'nəs\ [L *incanus* gray-white] Having a grayish white hue.

**incaparina** \inkap'ərē'nə\ [*I(nstitute of) N(utrition of) C(entral) A(merica and) P(anama)* + L *(f)arina* flour] A dietary supplement containing 27.5% protein used in the prevention and treatment of protein-calorie malnutrition, including kwashiorkor. Different formulas exist but all have the same protein content.

**incarceration** \inkär′sərā′shən\ [Late L *incarceratio* imprisonment, from L *in* IN + *carcer* prison + *-atio* -ATION] Abnormal enclosure or confinement of a part.

**incarnatio** \in′kärnā′shō\ [Late L, from *incarnatus,* past part. of *incarnare* to clothe with flesh, from L *-in* -IN[1] + *caro,* gen. *carnis,* flesh] INGROWING NAIL.

**incarnative** \inkär′nətiv\ **1** Promoting formation of granulation tissue. **2** Any agent that increases the formation of granulation tissue.

**incendiarism** \insen′dē·ərizm\ [L *incendiar(ius)* (from *incendium* fire, heat) an incendiary + -ISM] PYROMANIA.

**inceptus** \insep′təs\ [L, from *inceptus,* past part. of *incipere* to begin, undertake] ANLAGE.

**incertae sedis** \insur′tē sē′dis\ Of uncertain affiliation: used in taxonomy.

**incest** \in′sest\ [L *incest(um)* (from neut. of *incestus* unchaste, polluted, from *in-* not + *castus* chaste, pure) impurity, incest] Sexual intercourse between two persons who are close blood relatives.

**inch** [Old English *ince,* from L *uncia* the twelfth part of any whole] A unit of length equal to $^1/_{36}$ yard; $^1/_{12}$ foot; 2.54 centimeters exactly. Symbol: in

**inchação** \ēɴ′shasouɴ′\ [Portuguese, a swelling (referring to the edema of wet beriberi)] A Brazilian term for BERIBERI.

**incidence** \in′sidəns\ [Late L *incidentia* (from *incidere* to happen, befall, drop into, from *in-* in, on, into + *cadere* to fall) a happening, occurrence] The number of cases of a disease, abnormality, accident, etc., arising in a defined population during a stated period, expressed as a proportion, such as *x* cases per 1000 population per year. Also *incidence rate, attack rate.*

**incident** \in′sidənt\ Falling upon, or impinging on, as *incident light.*

**incipient** \insip′ē·ənt\ [L *incipiens,* gen. *incipientis,* pres. part. of *incipere* to begin] About to appear or come into existence; initial, as a stage of illness.

**incisal** \insī′zəl\ **1** Relating to an incisor tooth. **2** Relating to the cutting edge of an incisor tooth.

**incise** \insīz′\ [L *incis(us),* past part. of *incidere* to cut into, from *in-* into + *caedere* to cut] To cut into or divide with a knife, scissors, or other sharp instrument during a surgical procedure.

**incision** \insizh′ən\ [*incis(e)* + -ION] A surgical cut with a sharp instrument into the body that results in a division of tissue and creation of a wound. **Battle's i.** A vertical incision through the paramedian part of the anterior abdominal wall in which the anterior and posterior parts of the rectus sheaths are longitudinally divided and the muscles are retracted. Also *Battle-Jalaguier-Kammerer incision, lateral rectus incision.* **collar i.** A surgical incision of one of the natural transverse creases of the skin of the front of the neck, particularly such an incision based on the midline low in the neck. The object of such an incision is to ensure that the scar, by coinciding with a natural crease, will be inconspicuous. **confirmatory i.** An incision into an organ, tissue, or mass for diagnostic purposes. **cruciate i.** A surgical incision in the shape of a cross, frequently employed for drainage procedures. **decompression i.** An incision to relieve pressure within a tight body compartment. In the case of burns this may be made through the skin, and in other forms of trauma or vascular compromise it may be made through the investing muscle fascia. **double-Y i.** HAYES MARTIN INCISION. **Dührssen's i.'s** Longitudinal incisions in the uterine cervix utilized to facilitate vaginal delivery of a fetus. **endaural i.** **1** A surgical incision, used in middle-ear surgery, made within the confines of the external ear in contrast to the classic postauricular incision. **2** An extracartilaginous incision which consists of a curved incision down to bone at the entrance to the external auditory meatus posteriorly, in front of the anterior edge of the conchal cartilage. The incision continues with an extension upwards and forwards between the tragus and the ascending portion of the helix, this part remaining superficial to the temporalis fascia. **Fergusson's i.** WEBER-FERGUSSON INCISION. **Gluck i.** A skin incision in the front of the neck performed for total laryngectomy. It consists of three parts: a gently curved transverse incision convex downward at the level of the hyoid bone, a second shorter curved transverse incision convex upward at the level of the second tracheal ring, and a vertical incision in or to one side of the midline joining the transverse incisions. Though still employed, the incision has been modified. **Hayes Martin i.** A composite skin incision on one side of the neck, utilized for total laryngectomy combined with radical neck dissection. It consists of three parts: a shallow V-shaped incision convex downward extending from the tip of the mastoid process to a point beneath the tip of the chin, a second incision in the form of an inverted V based on the clavicle and, the third, a vertical incision joining the nearest points of the other two. Also *double-Y incision.* **hockey stick i.** An incision consisting of two joined straight incisions that form an obtuse angle. It is usually made to extend an otherwise inadequate incision. **Howarth's i.** A curved incision approximately 3.5 cm in length carried down to bone, approximately 1 cm medial to the inner canthus of the eye, and extending downward from a point just below the inner end of the eyebrow. It originated as the first step in frontoethmoidectomy but has since been used in a number of other surgical procedures including transsphenoidal hypophysec-

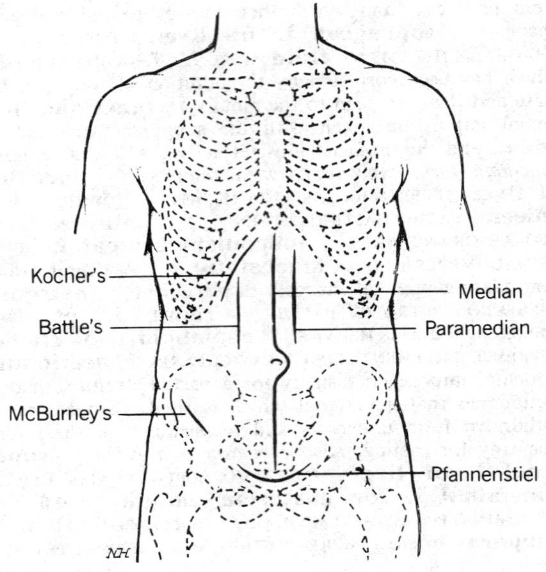

Surgical incisions

tomy. Also *Lynch incision.* **Kehr's i.** A long midline incision through the abdominal wall, beginning at the xiphoid cartilage, passing around the umbilicus, and continuing to the pubis. **Kocher's i.** A right subcostal incision in the abdominal wall two finger breadths below and parallel to the costal margin. **lateral rectus i.** BATTLE'S INCISION. **Lynch i.** HOWARTH'S INCISION. **MacFee i.'s** Two parallel transverse incisions, one at the base of the neck and the other just below the jaw line, utilized during radical neck dissection. **mastoid i.** POSTAURICULAR INCISION. **McBurney's i.** A surgical incision for appendectomy in the right lower quadrant of the anterior abdominal wall parallel to the fibers of the external oblique muscle through a point one third the distance between the umbilicus and the anterior superior iliac spine. All of the underlying muscles are split rather than incised. This was originally developed as a drainage incision for acute appendicitis. **median i.** An incision along all or part of the midline of the anterior abdominal wall. **paramedian i.** A surgical incision in the anterior abdominal wall parallel to the rectus muscle and away from the midline. **paravaginal i.** A surgical incision made into the vagina and perineum designed to increase the diameter of the vaginal outlet. **Pfannenstiel's i.** A lower abdominal curvilinear transverse incision through the skin, followed by a midline fascial and peritoneal incision. **postauricular i.** An incision made behind the ear to provide surgical access to the interior of the mastoid process and, frequently, thereby to the tympanic cavity and its contents. At one time, the skin incision was carried through the periosteum down to bone, but increasingly surgeons have incised the periosteum separately backward of the skin incision to create a separate periosteal flap. Also *postaural incision, mastoid incision.* **rectus i.** Any surgical incision into the abdominal wall that passes through the rectus muscle on one or both sides of the midline. **relief i.** An incision, usually made into fascia, that releases tension on a suture line or within a tissue. Also *relieving incision.* **Robertson i.** A surgical procedure for treating hypertrophic pyloric stenosis, in which a transverse incision is made opposite the eighth costal cartilage. The underlying muscles are split according to fiber direction, and a transverse peritoneal incision is made. **Ruddy's i.** A curved surgical incision, through the mucoperiosteum of the hard palate, used as an approach for the correction of congenital choanal atresia. **Schuchardt's i.** A large paravaginal incision used in preparation for a radical vaginal hysterectomy. **Sorensen i.** A skin incision in the front of the neck frequently used for laryngectomy. It is a symmetrical U-shaped incision centered on the midline, following the anterior border of the sternomastoid muscle on either side from the level of the hyoid bone above to the level of the third ring of the trachea below where the lateral limbs of the incision are united by a short transverse incision convex downwards. **Weber-Fergusson i.** An incision that courses through the upper lip, along the side of the nose, and then along the inferior orbital rim. The cheek and lip can then be reflected to the side permitting wide exposure of the maxilla, as is needed during total maxillectomy. Also *Fergusson's incision.* **Wilde's i.** An obsolete procedure involving an incision into the swelling behind the ear carried down to the mastoid bone, for the relief of mastoiditis. It has been replaced by mastoidectomy.

**incisive** \insī′siv\ **1** Cutting; penetrating. **2** Relating to the incisor teeth or to the os incisivum.

**incisor** \insī′zər\ [*incis(e)* + -OR] A tooth situated in front of the canines. In human dentition, one of the four most anterior teeth in either jaw. Also *cutting tooth, incisor tooth.* **central i.** The incisor nearest to the midsagittal plane in each quadrant. Also *first incisor, medial incisor.* **first i.** CENTRAL INCISOR. **Hutchinson's i.'s** See under SYPHILITIC TOOTH. **lateral i.** The incisor situated distal to the first incisor and mesial to the canine. Also *second incisor.* **medial i.** CENTRAL INCISOR. **second i.** LATERAL INCISOR.

**incisura** \in′sīsyoo′rə\ [L (from *incidere* to cut into, from *in-* into + *caedere* to cut, fell) a cut, groove] (*pl.* incisurae) A notch, depression, or indentation, often on the edge of a structure. Also *incisure, notch.* **i. acetabuli** [NA] A gap between the inferior ends of the lunate surface of the acetabulum of the hip bone which is bridged by the transverse ligament to form the cotyloid foramen. Also *incisure of acetabulum, acetabular notch, cotyloid notch, cotyloid incisure.* **anacrotic i.** ANACROTIC NOTCH. **i. angularis gastrica** [NA] A depression at the most dependent point of the lesser curvature of the stomach, usually at the junction of its upper two thirds and lower one third. It separates the body of the stomach on the left from the pyloric antrum on the right. Its position varies with the degree of distension of the stomach and with the inherent shape of the stomach. Also *incisura angularis ventriculi, gastric notch, angulus of stomach, angular notch, angular sulcus, angular incisure.* **i. angularis ventriculi** INCISURA ANGULARIS GASTRICA. **i. anterior auris** [NA] A marked notch separating the crus of the helix from the tragus of the external ear, occasionally surmounted by the supertragic tubercle. Also *anterior incisure of ear, anterior auricular groove, anterior notch of ear.* **i. apicis cordis** [NA] A small notch on the right margin of the heart just to the right of the apex where the anterior interventricular sulcus on the sternocostal surface becomes continuous with posterior interventricular sulcus on the diaphragmatic surface. Also *incisure of apex of heart, notch of apex of heart.* **i. cardiaca pulmonis sinistri** [NA] A wide notch in the anterior margin of the superior lobe of the left lung, just above the lingula and anterior to the cardiac fossa occupied by the heart and pericardium. Also *cardiac incisure of left lung, cardiac notch of left lung, fovea cardiaca.* **i. cardiaca gastrica** [NA] The acute-angled notch at the junction of the left margin of the esophagus and the greater curvature of the stomach, above the level of which the fundus is located. Also *cardiac incisure of stomach, cardiac notch of stomach.* **incisurae cartilaginis meatus acustici** [NA] Two or three fissures in the anterior wall of the cartilaginous part of the external acoustic meatus providing mobility of the ear. Also *Santorini's clefts, Santorini's fissures, Duverney's fissures, incisures of Duverney.* **i. cerebelli anterior** The broad indentation on the anterior surface of the cerebellum, overlying the inferior colliculus and the superior cerebellar peduncle. Also *anterior cerebellar notch.* **i. cerebelli posterior** The narrow indentation behind the cerebellar hemispheres containing the falx cerebelli. Also *posterior cerebellar notch, marsupial notch* (obs.). **i. clavicularis sterni** [NA] The oval, concave articular surface on either side of the jugular notch on the superior margin of the manubrium sterni for receiving the medial end of the clavicle and the intervening articular disk. Also *clavicular incisure of sternum, clavicular notch of sternum, clavicular facet.* **incisurae costales sterni** [NA] Notches on the lateral borders of the sternum, seven on each side, for articulation with the first seven costal cartilages. Also *costal incisures of sternum, costal foveae of sternum, costal notches of sternum, articular foveae for rib cartilages, lateral facets of sternum, costal facets of sternum, articular facets for rib cartilages.* **i. ethmoidalis ossis frontalis** [NA] A wide, quadrangular space between the orbital parts of the frontal bone occupied by the cribriform plate of the ethmoid bone articulating in the frontoethmoidal suture. Also *ethmoidal incisure of frontal bone, ethmoidal notch of frontal bone, notch of ethmoid.* **i. fastigii** A transverse notch seen on the ventricular surface during fetal development of the cerebellar lamina. **i. fibularis tibiae** [NA] A triangular notch on the lateral surface of the distal end of the tibia, the rough upper part of which receives the attachment of the lower end of the interosseous membrane while the lower part may be covered with articular cartilage for articulation with the lower end of the fibula. Also *fibular incisure of tibia, fibular notch of tibia.* **i. frontalis** [NA] A minute notch occasionally present medial to the supraorbital notch or foramen and transmitting a diploic branch of the supraorbital artery and a frontal branch of supraorbital nerve to the frontal sinus. The notch may be bridged over by bone, converting it into foramen frontale. Also *frontal incisure, frontal notch, supraorbital notch, notch of frontal bone.* **i. interarytenoidea laryngis** [NA] A small notchlike prolongation of the aditus laryngis posteriorly between the corniculate cartilages and the apices of the arytenoid cartilages on each side as far back as the interarytenoid fold of mucosa. Also *interarytenoid incisure of larynx, interarytenoid notch.* **i. interlobaris pulmonis** Either fissura obliqua pulmonis or fissura horizontalis pulmonis dextri. **i. intertragica** [NA] A deep notch between the tragus and the antitragus just above the lobe of the ear pinna. Also *intertragic incisure, intertragic notch, incisura tragica, intertragic incisure of ear.* **i. ischiadica major** [NA] A wide, deep notch in the posterior border of the ilium, above, and the ischium, below, extending from the posterior inferior iliac spine to the sciatic, or ischial, spine, and converted into a foramen by the sacrotuberous and sacrospinous ligaments. Also *greater ischiadic incisure, greater ischiatic notch, greater sciatic notch.* **i. ischiadica minor** [NA] A shallow notch on the posterior margin of the ischium, limited by the sciatic, or ischial, spine above and the upper end of the ischial tuberosity below, and converted into a foramen by the sacrotuberous and sacrospinous ligaments. Also *lesser ischiadic incisure, lesser ischiadic notch, lesser sciatic notch.* **i. jugularis ossis occipitalis** [NA] An indentation on the front of the jugular process of the occipital bone, forming the posterior part of the jugular foramen. The notch is subdivided by the intrajugular process. Also *jugular incisure of occipital bone, jugular notch of occipital bone.* **i. jugularis ossis temporalis** [NA] A large, ellipsoid notch on the inferior surface of the petrous part of the temporal bone, posterior to the external carotid foramen, forming the anterior and lateral parts of the jugular foramen and containing the superior bulb of the internal jugular vein. Also *jugular incisure of temporal bone, jugular notch of temporal bone.* **i. jugularis sterni** [NA] A concavity in the center of the superior border of the manubrium sterni, bounded by the clavicular notch on each side. Also *jugular incisure of sternum, jugular notch of sternum, suprasternal notch, sternal notch, sternal incisure, interclavicular incisure, interclavicular notch, presternal notch.* **i. lacrimalis maxillae** [NA] A narrow, vertical depression located anteriorly on the medial border of the orbital surface of the maxilla where the lacrimomaxillary suture is in the fossa for the lacrimal sac adjacent to the orbital orifice of the nasolacrimal duct. Also *lacrimal incisure of maxilla, lacrimal notch of maxilla, lacrimal notch.* **i. ligamenti teretis** [NA] A notch of varying size and depth in the inferior border of the liver slightly to the right of the median plane, continuous posteriorly with the fissure for ligamentum teres and containing the ligamentum teres. Also *umbilical incisure, umbilical notch, notch of ligamentum teres, interlobar notch.* **i. mandibulae** [NA] A deep concavity in the superior border of the ramus of the mandible, between the coronoid and condylar processes, through which the masseteric nerve and vessels pass. Also *incisure of mandible, mandibular notch, sigmoid incisure of mandible.* **i. mastoidea ossis temporalis** [NA] A deep longitudinal furrow, medial to the base of the mastoid process of the temporal bone and lateral to the groove for occipital artery, to which the posterior belly of the digastric muscle is attached. Also *mastoid incisure of temporal bone, mastoid notch, mastoid groove, digastric groove, digastric notch, digastric incisure of temporal bone, digastric fossa, incisura mastoidea.* **i. nasalis maxillae** [NA] A large concavity on the medial border of the anterior surface of the body of the maxilla, forming the lateral and inferior margin of the piriform aperture, the lower end of which continues anteriorly to meet the opposite side at the anterior nasal spine. Also *nasal incisure of maxilla, nasal notch of maxilla.* **i. pancreatis** [NA] A groove between the head and the neck of the pancreas inferiorly where the uncinate process hooks posterior to the superior mesenteric vessels. Also *pancreatic notch, inferior notch of neck of pancreas.* **i. parietalis ossis temporalis** [NA] The angle, or notch, formed by the posterior part of the superior border of the squamous part of the temporal bone meeting the mastoid part. It is located at the posterior end of the petrosquamous suture internally and the squamomastoid suture externally. Also *parietal incisure of temporal bone, parietal notch of temporal bone, parietosphenoid fissure.* **i. preoccipitalis** [NA] The ventrolateral notch demarcating the caudal limit of the temporal lobe and the rostral boundary of the occipital lobe. Also *preoccipital notch, preoccipital incisure.* **i. pterygoidea** [NA] The angular fissure separating the lower parts of the medial and lateral plates of the pterygoid process of the sphenoid bone, the margins of which articulate with the pyramidal process of the palatine bone. Also *pterygoid fissure, pterygoid notch, fissura pterygoidea, palatine incisure, pterygoid incisure.* **i. radialis ulnae** [NA] A shallow concavity on the lateral surface of the coronoid process of the ulna for articulation with the circumference of the head of radius, while the anterior and posterior edges of the notch provide attachment for the annular ligament. Also *radial incisure of ulna, radial notch of ulna, lesser sigmoid cavity of ulna.* **i. scapulae** [NA] A deep notch on the superior margin of the scapula at its junction with the coracoid process. The notch is bridged over by the superior transverse scapular ligament, over which the suprascapular vessels pass and deep to which the suprascapular nerve runs. Also *incisure of scapula, scapular notch, suprascapular notch, suprascapular incisure.* **i. sphenopalatina ossis palatini** [NA] A narrow gap between the orbital and the sphenoidal processes at the top of the perpendicular plate of the palatine bone which is converted into a foramen by the body of the sphenoid bone coming into contact with the processes superiorly. The gap lies between the pterygopalatine fossa laterally and the posterior part of the nasal cavity near its roof medially. Also *sphenopalatine incisure of palatine bone, sphenopalatine notch of palatine bone, palatine incisure of Henle, palatine notch of palatine bone, incisura sphenopalatina.* **i. supraorbitalis** [NA] A small notch, often converted to a bony foramen, at the junction of the rounded medial one third and the sharp lateral two thirds of the supraorbital margin of the frontal bone for the transmission of the supraorbital nerve and vessels. Also *supraorbital incisure, supraorbital notch.* **i. temporalis** The notch between the uncus and the tip of the temporal lobe. Also *temporal in-*

*cisure.* **i. tentorii** [NA] The large, oval opening that contains the midbrain and the anterior part of the superior surface of the vermis of the cerebellum. It is bounded anteriorly by the dorsum sellae of the sphenoid bone and laterally and posteriorly by the concave, free margin of the tentorium cerebelli. Also *tentorial notch, incisure of tentorium of cerebellum, incisure of cerebellum, tentorial hiatus, foramen ovale of Pacchioni.* **i. terminalis auris** [NA] A deep notch almost completely separating the cartilage of the auricle from that of the external acoustic meatus. Also *terminal incisure of ear, terminal notch of auricle.* **i. thyroidea inferior** [NA] A shallow notch in the inferior margin of the thyroid cartilage at the junction of the laminae in the midline, where the median cricothyroid ligament is attached. Also *inferior thyroid incisure, inferior thyroid notch.* **i. thyroidea superior** [NA] A deep V-shaped notch situated anteriorly in the midline between the superior margins of the laminae of the thyroid cartilage and just above the laryngeal prominence. Also *superior thyroid incisure, superior thyroid notch.* **i. tragica** INCISURA INTERTRAGICA. **i. trochlearis ulnae** [NA] A deep concave notch at the upper end of the ulna formed by the superior surface of the coronoid process and the anterior surface of olecranon for articulation with the trochlea of the humerus. It is unevenly divided by a longitudinal ridge fitting the groove on the trochlea. Also *trochlear notch of ulna, trochlear incisure of ulna, semilunar fossa of ulna, sigmoid fossa of ulna, greater sigmoid cavity of ulna.* **i. tympanica** [NA] A gap in the superior part of the tympanic sulcus of the temporal bone occupied by the pars flaccida of the tympanic membrane above the malleolar folds. Also *tympanic notch, Rivinus incisure, notch of Rivinus, rivinian notch, tympanic incisure, rivinian segment, segment of Rivinus.* **i. ulnaris radii** [NA] A concavity on the medial surface of the lower end of radius for articulation with the circumference of the head of ulna in the inferior radioulnar joint. Also *ulnar incisure of radius, ulnar notch of radius, sigmoid cavity of radius.* **i. vertebralis inferior** [NA] A notch on the inferior border of the pedicle of a vertebra, forming the upper part of an intervertebral foramen. Also *inferior vertebral incisure, inferior vertebral notch, greater vertebral incisure.* **i. vertebralis superior** [NA] A notch on the superior border of the pedicle of a vertebra, forming the lower part of an intervertebral foramen. Also *superior vertebral incisure, superior vertebral notch, lesser vertebral incisure.*

**incisurae** \in′sīsyoo′rē\ Plural of INCISURA.

**incisural** \insī′zhərəl\ Pertaining to an incisura.

**incisure** \insī′zhər\ [L *incisura.* See INCISURA.] INCISURA. **i. of acetabulum** INCISURA ACETABULI. **angular i.** INCISURA ANGULARIS GASTRICA. **anterior i. of ear** INCISURA ANTERIOR AURIS. **i. of apex of heart** INCISURA APICIS CORDIS. **cardiac i. of left lung** INCISURA CARDIACA PULMONIS SINISTRI. **cardiac i. of stomach** INCISURA CARDIACA GASTRICA. **i. of cerebellum** INCISURA TENTORII. **clavicular i. of sternum** INCISURA CLAVICULARIS STERNI. **costal i.'s of sternum** INCISURAE COSTALES STERNI. **cotyloid i.** INCISURA ACETABULI. **digastric i. of temporal bone** INCISURA MASTOIDEA OSSIS TEMPORALIS. **i.'s of Duverney** INCISURAE CARTILAGINIS MEATUS ACUSTICI. **ethmoidal i. of frontal bone** INCISURA ETHMOIDALIS OSSIS FRONTALIS. **fibular i. of tibia** INCISURA FIBULARIS TIBIAE. **frontal i.** INCISURA FRONTALIS. **greater ischiadic i.** INCISURA ISCHIADICA MAJOR. **greater vertebral i.** INCISURA VERTEBRALIS INFERIOR. **inferior thyroid i.** INCISURA THYROIDEA INFERIOR. **inferior vertebral i.** INCISURA VERTEBRALIS INFERIOR. **interarytenoid i. of larynx** INCISURA INTERARYTENOIDEA LARYNGIS. **interclavicular i.** INCISURA JUGULARIS STERNI. **intertragic i.** INCISURA INTERTRAGICA. **intertragic i. of ear** INCISURA INTERTRAGICA. **jugular i. of occipital bone** INCISURA JUGULARIS OSSIS OCCIPITALIS. **jugular i. of sternum** INCISURA JUGULARIS STERNI. **jugular i. of temporal bone** INCISURA JUGULARIS OSSIS TEMPORALIS. **lacrimal i. of maxilla** INCISURA LACRIMALIS MAXILLAE. **i.'s of Lanterman-Schmidt** SCHMIDT-LANTERMAN INCISURES. **lesser ischiadic i.** INCISURA ISCHIADICA MINOR. **lesser vertebral i.** INCISURA VERTEBRALIS SUPERIOR. **i. of mandible** INCISURA MANDIBULAE. **mastoid i. of temporal bone** INCISURA MASTOIDEA OSSIS TEMPORALIS. **nasal i. of frontal bone** MARGO NASALIS OSSIS FRONTALIS. **nasal i. of maxilla** INCISURA NASALIS MAXILLAE. **palatine i.** INCISURA PTERYGOIDEA. **palatine i. of Henle** INCISURA SPHENOPALATINA OSSIS PALATINI. **parietal i. of temporal bone** INCISURA PARIETALIS OSSIS TEMPORALIS. **preoccipital i.** INCISURA PREOCCIPITALIS. **pterygoid i.** INCISURA PTERYGOIDEA. **radial i. of ulna** INCISURA RADIALIS ULNAE. **Rivinus i.** INCISURA TYMPANICA. **i. of scapula** INCISURA SCAPULAE. **Schmidt-Lanterman i.'s** Oblique channels of Schwann cell cytoplasm extending across the myelin sheaths of peripheral nerves. Also *incisures of Lanterman-Schmidt, Schmidt-Lanterman clefts, Lanterman's clefts.* **sigmoid i. of mandible** INCISURA MANDIBULAE. **sphenopalatine i. of palatine bone** INCISURA SPHENOPALATINA OSSIS PALATINI. **sternal i.** INCISURA JUGULARIS STERNI. **superior thyroid i.** INCISURA THYROIDEA SUPERIOR. **superior vertebral i.** INCISURA VERTEBRALIS SUPERIOR. **supraorbital i.** INCISURA SUPRAORBITALIS. **suprascapular i.** INCISURA SCAPULAE. **i. of talus** SULCUS TENDINIS MUSCULI FLEXORIS HALLUCIS LONGI TALI. **temporal i.** INCISURA TEMPORALIS. **i. of tentorium of cerebellum** INCISURA TENTORII. **terminal i. of ear** INCISURA TERMINALIS AURIS. **trochlear i. of ulna** INCISURA TROCHLEARIS ULNAE. **tympanic i.** INCISURA TYMPANICA. **ulnar i. of radius** INCISURA ULNARIS RADII.

**incitant** \insī′tənt\ The causative agent of a disorder or condition, such as the agent that triggers an allergic response.

**inclinatio** \in′klinā′shō\ [L (from *inclinatus,* past part. of *inclinare* to incline, bend), an inclining, leaning, bending] A leaning, bending, or sloping with respect to a particular plane. Also *inclination, incline.* **i. pelvis** [NA] The angle between the plane of the superior aperture of the pelvis and the horizontal plane, which, in the standing anatomical position, varies in individuals from 50° to 60°. Also *inclination of pelvis, pelvic inclination, pelvic incline, incline of pelvis, angle of inclination, angle of pelvis, pelvivertebral angle.*

**inclination** \in′klinā′shən\ [INCLINE + -ATION] INCLINATIO. **axial i.** The inclination of a tooth relative to the vertical. The inclination is usually described as mesial, distal, lingual, labial or buccal. Also *inclination of tooth.* **lateral condylar i.** The direction of movement of the head of the condyle on the balancing side when the mandible is swung laterally. **pelvic i.** INCLINATIO PELVIS. **i. of pelvis** INCLINATIO PELVIS. **i. of tooth** AXIAL INCLINATION.

**inclinationes** \in′klināshō′nēz\ Plural of INCLINATIO.

**incline** \inklīn′\ [L *inclinare* (*in-* in + obsolete *clinare* to bend, lean, from Gk *klinein* to make a thing slope or slant, to make recline) to incline, bend, curve] INCLINATIO. **pelvic i.** INCLINATIO PELVIS. **i. of pelvis** INCLINATIO PELVIS.

**inclinometer** \inklinäm′ətər\ A device to measure the axis of astigmatism.

**inclusion** \inkloo′zhən\ [L *inclusio* (from *includere* to shut up, confine, from *in-* in + *claudere* to close, shut) a shutting up, confinement] **1** The state of being included or enclosed. **2** Something included or enclosed, as within a cell. **cell i.** **1** A foreign body contained within a cell. **2** A storage substance, a pigment, or a metabolic product found as a granule or vesicle in a cell. **fetal i.** A parasitic and usually incomplete member of a pair of unequal conjoined twins enclosed within the body of the host twin. **Guarnieri's i.'s** GUARNIERI BODIES. **intranuclear i.'s** Foreign matter found within a cell nucleus, usually representing viral material. **leukocyte i.'s** Small, round or oval, gray-blue bodies found in the cytoplasm of neutrophils in severe infections, burns, septicemia, and toxic conditions. They are common in scarlet fever, but contrary to earlier beliefs are not specific for this disease. They are comprised of RNA fibrils in an area free of specific granules. They are also seen occasionally in thrombocytopenic purpura, myeloproliferative syndromes, chronic myelogenous leukemia, pernicious anemia, and hemolytic anemia. They are a permanent morphologic feature of the May-Hegglin anomaly of platelets. **Walthard's i.'s** WALTHARD'S CELL NESTS.

**incoagulability** \in′kō·ag′yələbil′itē\ A state characterized by the inability of blood or plasma to clot. Absolute incoagulability is rare.

**incoagulable** \in′kō·ag′yələbl\ Exhibiting incoagulability.

**incomitance** \inkō′mitəns\ [IN-[2] + COMITANCE] The characteristic of strabismus whereby the amount of ocular misalignment changes with different positions of gaze. Adj. incomitant.

**incompatibility** \in′kəmpat′ibil′itē\ The quality of being incompatible, as drugs whose interaction renders them ineffective or harmful, or blood types which in combination induce an undesirable immunologic reaction in the host. **ABO i.** Lack of compatibility of cells bearing the ABO blood group when mixed with serum containing the corresponding, naturally occurring isoantibodies. The lack of compatibility is manifested *in vivo* by hemolysis. **chemical i.** Chemical unmixability, e.g., of oil and water. **physiologic i.** Unsuitability for being administered together because of antagonistic pharmacologic actions. **therapeutic i.** Unsuitability for combination, as of drugs administered at the same time.

**incompatible** \in′kəmpat′ibəl\ Having an adverse or unwanted effect if combined or used together, as drugs, blood types, or other substances.

**incompetence** \inkäm′pətəns\ [L *in-* not + COMPETENCE] Failure of an organ, part, or system to meet an accepted standard for quality of function, often of a specific physiologic function; substandard function; insufficiency. **aortic i.** AORTIC REGURGITATION. **ileocecal i.** The lack of function of the ileocecal valve allowing for cephalad flow of fecal material into the small bowel. Also *ileocolic incompetence, ileocecal insufficiency.* **ileocolic i.** ILEOCECAL INCOMPETENCE. **valvular i.** Incompetence of a cardiac valve due to inadequate closure, resulting in valvular regurgitation. **velopharyngeal i.** VELOPHARYNGEAL INSUFFICIENCY.

**incompetent** \inkäm′pətənt\ **1** Characterized by incompetence; substandard in function; insufficient. **2** Held to be unable to enter into certain contractual relationships or to make certain kinds of decisions independently. A legal term.

**incongruence** \inkäng′groo·əns\ [L *in-* not + *congruentia* (from *congruens,* gen. *congruentis,* agreeing + *-ia* -IA) conformity, symmetry] A characteristic of binocular visual field defects in which the defects are disimilar in the two eyes. Adj. incongruent.

**incontinence** \inkän′tinəns\ [L *incontinentia.* See INCONTINENTIA.] **1** Absence of voluntary control of an excretory function, especially defecation or urination. Also *incontinentia.* **2** Willing or unwilling lack of restraint of one's appetites or impulses. **fecal i.** The inability to voluntarily control the anal sphincters, resulting in involuntary release of flatus and stool. Also *rectal incontinence, incontinentia alvi.* **intermittent i.** Urinary incontinence which is not continuous but is characterized by lack of voluntary inhibitory response to stress on the bladder or to sudden movement. It is one manifestation of the neurogenic bladder. **overflow i.** Dribbling of urine due to pressure in a full, overdistended bladder. Also *paradoxical incontinence.* **paradoxical i.** OVERFLOW INCONTINENCE. **paralytic i.** Incontinence due to an inoperative or paralyzed sphincter, resulting from disease or dysfunction of the central nervous system. Also *sphincteric incontinence.* **passive i.** Urinary incontinence in which, because emptying cannot occur normally or voluntarily, urine dribbles out under the pressure of a full bladder. **rectal i.** FECAL INCONTINENCE. **sphincteric i.** PARALYTIC INCONTINENCE. **stress i.** Discharge of urine or feces due to increased intra-abdominal pressure, as in coughing, straining, or sudden movement. **urinary i.** Inability to control urination, with resultant repeated or continuous involuntary passage of urine.

**incontinent** \inkän′tinənt\ Exhibiting or characterized by incontinence.

**incontinentia** \in′käntinen′shə\ [L (from *incontinens,* gen. *incontinentis,* intemperate, immoderate, incontinent, from *in-* not + *continens,* pres. part. of *continere* to hold or keep together, hold), inability to restrain one's desires, incontinence] INCONTINENCE. **i. alvi** FECAL INCONTINENCE. **i. pigmenti** An X-linked dominant syndrome of neonatal onset characterized by progressive skin lesions leading to swirling patterns of hyperpigmentation, alopecia of the crown of the head, ocular changes including optic atrophy, absent or malformed teeth, mental retardation, and seizures. A paucity of affected males and an increased miscarriage rate among affected women are consistent with this disorder's being lethal *in utero* in hemizygous males. Also *Bloch-Sulzberger syndrome.*

**incoordination** \in′kō·ôr′dinā′shən\ Lack of coordination, whether in motor activities (ataxia) or in the activities of various organs, glands, or viscera. **first-degree uterine i.** PRIMARY UTERINE INERTIA. **second-degree uterine i.** SECONDARY UTERINE INERTIA.

**incorporation** \inkôr′pərā′shən\ [Late L *incorporatio,* from *incorporare* to incorporate, from L *in-* IN[1] + *corpus,* gen. *corporis* body] In psychoanalytic psychology, assimilation of external objects into the self, usually applied to the earliest phase of object recognition when everything pleasurable is something to swallow. Less commonly, incorporation is equated with identification or introjection, or both.

**incostapedial** \ing′kōstəpē′dē·əl\ INCUDOSTAPEDIAL.

**incretin** \inkrē′tin\ *Seldom used* SECRETIN.

**incretion** \inkrē′shən\ *Obs.* HORMONE.

**incretotherapy** \inkrē′təther′əpē\ *Outmoded* HORMONOTHERAPY.

**incross** \in′kräs\ In experimental genetics, the mating of two organisms that are both homozygous at a given locus for the same allele.

**incrustation** \in′krustā′shən\ CRUST.
**incubate** \in′kyəbāt\ [See INCUBATION.] To maintain a microbiologic culture or a preparation of biological or chemical materials at a fixed temperature.
**incubation** \in′kyəbā′shən\ [L *incubatio* (from *incubare* to lie or sit on, brood, from *in-* in, on + *cubare* to lie, recline) brooding, incubation] **1** The maintenance of microbiologic cultures or of preparations of biologic or chemical material at a fixed temperature for a prescribed period of time. **2** The development of an infectious disease in a host from the time the infecting agent is introduced into the body until the first clinical features manifest themselves. **3** The maintenance of a newborn infant in an environment controlled for temperature and atmospheric conditions, used especially for premature or sick newborns.
**incubator** \in′kyəbā′tər\ A device in which fixed temperature and atmospheric conditions can be maintained, used for incubation of biologic or chemical materials and in pediatrics to provide a controlled environment for the care of premature or sick newborns.
**incubus** \in′kyəbəs\ [Late L (from *incubare* to lie upon, from *cubare* to lie) a demon that lies upon persons in their sleep] A nightmare, especially one in which a woman dreams that a man or devil has entered her bed to have intercourse with her.
**incudal** \ing′koodəl\ Pertaining to the incus.
**incudius** \ingkyoo′dē·əs\ LIGAMENTUM MALLEI ANTERIUS.
**incudomalleal** \ing′kyədōmal′ē·əl\ MALLEOINCUDAL.
**incudostapedial** \ing′kyədōstāpē′dē·əl\ Pertaining to the incus and the stapes. Also *incostapedial.*
**incuneation** \ingkyoo′nē·ā′shən\ GOMPHOSIS.
**incurable** \inkyoo′rəbl\ Admitting of no cure; not curable.
**incus** \ing′kəs\ [L (from *incudere* to stamp, strike), anvil] (*pl.* incudes) [NA] The middle of the three auditory ossicles of the middle ear. It has a cuboid body that articulates anteriorly with the head of the malleus, a long crus that terminates in the lentiform process for articulation with the head of the stapes, and a short crus which is attached to the fossa incudis. Also *anvil, stithe* (outmoded).
**incyclodeviation** \insī′klədē′vē·ā′shən\ [IN-[1] + CYCLODEVIATION] Torsional displacement of an eye on its anteroposterior axis so that its upper (12 o'clock) part is rotated inward in the direction of the nose. Also *positive torsion.*
**incyclophoria** \insī′kləfôr′ē·ə\ [IN-[1] + CYCLOPHORIA] A latent tendency to torsion of the eye, the superior portion turning nasalward.
**incyclotropia** \insī′klətrō′pē·ə\ [IN-[1] + CYCLOTROPIA] A manifest tendency to torsion of the eye, the superior portion turning nasalward.
**incyclovergence** \insī′kləvur′jəns\ [IN-[1] + CYCLO- + VERGENCE] Inward torsion of the top of both eyes.
**in d.** *in dies* (L, meaning daily), used in prescription writing.
**indemnity** \indem′nitē\ [L *indemnitas* (from *indemn(is)* suffering no financial loss, from *-in* not + *damnum* damage, harm, + *-itas* -ITY) security from loss] The agreement of an insurer to provide health insurance benefits in the form of cash payments to, or on behalf of, a beneficiary for services provided, rather than the provision of the services themselves.
**indentation** \in′dentā′shən\ [L *in-* into + *dens,* gen. *dentis,* tooth + -ATION] **1** The formation of notches in an edge or pits in a surface. **2** A notch or pit. **aortic i. of esophagus** AORTIC NARROWING OF ESOPHAGUS. **i. of Hahn** An anterior defect of the vertebral body seen on the lateral radiograph of the vertebral column of the young child, giving to the vertebra a "turtle head" appearance. It may persist in the adult as a fine medial vertebral canal in one or more vertebrae. **i. of the tongue** The impression made on the surface of the tongue by the occlusal surfaces of the teeth. It is caused by the development of rigor mortis in the muscles of mastication.
**independence** / **statistical i.** A lack of statistical bearing of the outcome of one eventuality on that of the outcome of another. Two events are statistically independent if the probability of both occurring is equal to the product of the separate probabilities of the occurrence of each.

# index

**index** \in′deks\ [L (from *indicare* to disclose, reveal, from IN-[1] + *dicare* to show, dedicate) an informer, indicator] (*pl.* indices, indexes) **1** The second finger of the hand. Also *indicator, index finger, digitus secundus, digitus demonstrativus, forefinger, digitus II.* **2** Anything used to indicate or point out. **3** Any numerical characteristic developed for use in the analysis of quantitative information; specifically, a number expressing the magnitude of a given quantity as a ratio of that of another quantity of similar kind, or of itself at some other period, these latter in each case being given by convention the value 100 (or other power of ten) in the scale of relative values. **absolute refractive i.** The ratio between the velocity of light in a vacuum and the velocity of light in the designated medium. **alpha i.** The proportion of time during which alpha rhythms are recorded by an electroencephalograph during any single recording. **alveolar i.** A measure of the degree of prognathism of a skull: (basion-nasion length × 100)/basion–alveolar point length. **Ayala's i.** AYALA'S QUOTIENT. **basilar i.** A measure of the relationship between the basion and the auricular point to the maximum length of the skull: (basion–alveolar point × 100)/maximum length. **Becker-Lennhoff i.** LENNHOFF'S INDEX. **Boedecker's i.** The ratio of the number of carious tooth surfaces in a mouth to the number of tooth surfaces at risk. **breadth-height i.** A measure of the relationship between the maximum breadth and the maximum height of the head: (breadth × 100)/height. **Broders i.** BRODERS CLASSIFICATION. **Brugsch i.** The chest circumference × 100 divided by the length of the body. **cardiac i.** The cardiac output of blood per unit of time divided by the body surface area. **cardiothoracic i.** The ratio between the greatest transverse diameter of the heart and the greatest transverse diameter of the chest as measured on a PA chest x ray. This is normally less than 1:2 in the adult and children over four years. **centromeric i.** In cytogenetics, a measure of relative centromere position, *C.* If *p* is the length of the short chromosome arm and *q* the length of the long arm, *C* equals *p* divided by the sum of *p* and *q,* multiplied by 100. **cephalic i.** A measure of the relationship between the maximum breadth of the head and and the maximum length of the head: (maximum head breadth × 100)/maximum head length. **cephalic height i.** A measure of the relationship between the height of the head and its length: (vertex–auricular point × 100)/glabella-opisthocranion. **cerebral i.** A measure of the relationship between the maximum transverse diameter to the maximum anteroposterior length of the cranial cavity: (maximum internal breadth × 100)/maximum anteroposterior internal length. **chemotherapeutic i.** THERAPEUTIC INDEX. **coliform i.** COLIFORM TEST. **color i.** An index of the hemoglobin concentration of erythrocytes that was once widely used, but is now obsolete. The color index was obtained by dividing hemoglobin concentration by the erythrocyte count and multiplying the quotient by 0.345. The factor was used to make the color index of normal blood approximately 1.0. The color index has been supplanted by measurement of mean corpuscular hemoglobin. Also *cell color ratio.* **Colour Index** A joint publication of the English Society of Dyers and Colourists and the American Association of Textile Chemists and Colorists that lists and characterizes dyes and stains and assigns to each a number (CI number). The index permits appropriate classification and allows accurate identification. Abbr. CI **combined thyroid hormone i.** A calculated value that reflects overall biologic effects of thyroid gland secretion, achieved by combining the values of free thyroxine index, free triiodothyronine index, and thyroid-binding globulin activity expressed by percentage of resin uptake. Because it corrects for hormonal or drug-induced alterations of thyroid-binding globulin activity, it appears to give more precise distinction among hypothyroid, euthyroid, and hyperthyroid states than the free hormone index for either thyroxine or triidothyronine. **community periodontal i. of treatment needs** A method of assessing the requirement for periodontal treatment based on bleeding, calculus formation, and depth of pockets, utilizing the WHO periodontal probe. The mouth is divided into sextants and the worst condition in each is coded as follows: a pocket of 6 mm or more is code 4; a pocket of 4–5 mm is code 3; supragingival or subgingival calculus is code 2, bleeding after probing is code 1; and no symptoms is code 0. **cranial i.** A measure of the relationship between the maximum breadth to the maximum length of the skull: (maximum breadth × 100)/maximum length. Also *length-breadth index.* **def i.** An index of the effects of caries on the deciduous dentition. A tooth has a positive score if it is decayed (d), extraction is indicated (e), or it contains a filling (f). Missing teeth, not known to have been extracted, are ignored because of normal exfoliation. Also *def rate, def.* **dental i.** A measure of the relationship between the length of the tooth row and the basion-nasion length: (length of tooth row × 100)/basion-nasion length. Also *Flower's index.* **DMF i.** An index of the effects of caries on the permanent dentition. Decayed, missing and filled teeth are counted as equals. A tooth is given a positive score if is decayed, has been extracted because of caries, or is filled. Also *DMF rate, DMF.* • This index is also called DMFT to distinguish it from a related, more refined index, DMFS, in which the surfaces involved are counted. **effective temperature i.** An index of apparent warmth relating the temperature, movement, and humidity of air. **erythrocyte indices** A set of calculated figures for cell size, hemoglobin content, and hemoglobin concentration of individual red blood cells. They include mean cell volume, mean cell hemoglobin, and mean cell hemoglobin concentration. **facial i.** Either of two measures of the relationship between the length of the face to its width: (nasion–alveolar point × 100)/maximum bizygomatic width = superior facial index, or (nasion–mental tubercle × 100)/maximum bizygomatic width = total facial index. **fatigue i.** The ratio between the muscle tension remaining after a test period of tetanic stimulation to the value present initially. Generally the stimulus consists of repeated brief trains of pulses. **Flower's i.** DENTAL INDEX. **free thyroxine i.** The product of the serum total thyroxine concentration and the triiodothyronine resin uptake. Since this product is proportional to the serum free thyroxine concentration over a wide range of values, the derived figure provides a valid index of free thyroxine concentration. Abbr. FTI **free triiodothyronine i.** An indicator of the serum concentration of free triiodothyronine based on calculations similar to those used for determining the free thyroxine index. The tests in common use correct for abnormalities in thyroxine-binding globulin. **gnathic i.** The ratio between the distance from the basion to the prosthion multiplied by 100 and the distance between the basion and the nasion, an index of prominence of the maxilla. **hair i.** A mathematical expression of the shape of the hair, obtained by dividing the least diameter of a hair by the greatest diameter and multiplying by 100. **hemophagocytic i.** PHAGOCYTIC INDEX. **juxtaglomerular i.** A morphologic estimation of the degree of cytoplasmic granularity of the juxtaglomerular cells, and therefore an indirect assessment of renin content. **Kaup i.** An expression of the relationship between body weight and stature: body weight divided by the square of the body length. **Langelier's i.** The hydrogen ion concentration of a water when in equilibrium with its calcium carbonate content. **length-breadth i.** CRANIAL INDEX. **Lennhoff's i.** Sternal notch to pubic symphysis length × 100, divided by the maximum circumference of abdomen. Also *Becker-Lennhoff index.* **Macdonald i.** The proportion of a population of children with enlarged spleen in which malarial parasites are also found on microscopic examination of blood. **maturation i.** A cytologic evaluation of vaginal cells in which there is a calculated ratio of parabasal, intermediate, and superficial cells. **i. of mental deterioration** A measure of the degree of psychologic or intellectual deficit produced by the condition under study, often expressed as a deterioration quotient or ratio obtained by comparing relatively stable functions such as vocabulary retention with relatively unstable functions, such as digit symbol or arithmetic abilities. **mitotic i.** The proportion of a population of cells that are in mitosis at a given point in time. **nucleoplasmic i.** The ratio obtained by dividing the volume of the nucleus of a cell by the cytoplasmic volume. **obesity i.** A method of estimating the degree of overweight in which body weight is divided by body volume. **opsonic i.** A measure of the opsonizing antibodies to a given microorganism, obtained by comparing the number of bacteria phagocytized by leukocytes in the presence of the test serum or of serum from a normal individual. Also *opsonocytophagic index.* **optical i.** An index of microscope objectives. It reflects both the magnification and the numerical aperture of the lenses involved. **parasite i.** The proportion of individuals in a population in which malarial parasites are found on examination of blood smears. **pelvic i.** A value based on comparative measurements of the conjugate and transverse diameters of the maternal pelvis as a means of estimating whether or not cephalopelvic disproportion is likely. Also *pelvic inlet index.* **periodontal i.** A weighted index of periodontal disease used extensively for epidemiological surveys. Scores are recorded for gingivitis, the presence of pockets, and mobility with loss of function. Also *Russell index.* Abbr. PI **periodontal disease i.** An index based on a clinical examination around six teeth: the upper right first molar, upper left central incisor and first bicuspid, lower left first molar, lower right central incisor and first bicuspid. Also *Ramfjord index.* Abbr. PDI **phagocytic i.** The mean number of bacteria in leukocyte cytoplasm after incubation of washed leukocytes and serum with the bacteria to be tested. The index reflects the presence of antibodies to the bacteria in the serum and the ability of leukocytes to ingest the bacteria. Also *hemophagocytic index.* **physiognomonic upper face i.** The relationship between the height and breadth of the upper face: (nasion-stomion × 100)/maximum bizygomatic breadth. **Pirquet's i.** An estimate of nutritional status in infants and children based on measurement of weight and sitting height. A value below 94 pelidisi indicates the child is undernourished, between 95 and 100, the nutritional status is good, and over 101, overnutrition is apparent. **PMA i.** An index of gingivitis: scores are recorded for inflammation of the papilla (P), the labial gingival margin (M) and the attached gingiva (A). **Pont's i.** An index relating the inclusive width of the four incisors, the distance between the left and right first premolars, and the distance between the left and right first molars. **profunda-popliteal collateral i.** A determination of the adequacy of profunda collaterals when the superficial femoral artery is occluded. It is suggested as a means for determining whether lower extremity revascularization can be accomplished with an inflow procedure alone, or whether outflow must be augmented as well. **pulsatile i.** An objective measure of the effect of a proximal stenosis upon an arterial waveform. It is the quotient peak-to-peak waveform excursion divided by mean velocity. **Ramfjord i.** PERIODONTAL DISEASE INDEX. **recession i.** An assessment of chronic periodontal disease obtained by counting the number of teeth where gingival recession has exposed the cementoenamel junction. It is expressed as a percentage of the total teeth in the mouth. Abbr. RI **refractive i.** The ratio between the velocity of light in air and the velocity of light in a designated medium. **Russell i.** PERIODONTAL INDEX. **saturation i.** An obsolete expression of hemoglobin concentration within erythrocytes, obtained by dividing the percentage of standard of hemoglobin by the percentage of standard of hematocrit. The normal value was 0.97–1.02. **spleen i.** The proportion of individuals in a population that have enlarged spleens, as used in malaria surveys. This index is generally based on the examination of children, which has been found to be a useful indicator of malaria in the entire population. **superior facial i.** See under FACIAL INDEX. **tension-time i.** The product of heart rate and the time interval of ventricular systolic pressure. **therapeutic i.** A measure of drug safety, given by the ratio of the median lethal dose ($LD_{50}$) divided by the median effective dose ($ED_{50}$). The larger the ratio, the safer the drug. This ratio, however, does not include allowance for the differences in distribution of the population about these median values, and may not show the differences between the doses required for effectiveness in most of the population and the dose required for toxicity in a few individuals. Also *chemotherapeutic index, therapeutic ratio, curative ratio.* **trunk i.** The relationship between the length and breadth of the trunk: (biacromial breadth × 100)/maximum sitting height at suprasternale. **urea i.** AMBARD'S FORMULA. **Youden's i.** An index for rating the accuracy of diagnostic tests. The index is the figure obtained by subtracting one from the sum of the specificity and the sensitivity.

**indican** \in′dikan′\ [L *indic(um)* indigo + -AN] The plant glucoside whose aglycon, indoxyl, is oxidized by air to yield the dye indigo.

**indicanemia** \in′dikənē′mē·ə\ The presence of indican of animal origin in the blood.

**indicant** \in′dikənt\ 1 Providing an indication. 2 Something that serves as an indication, as a symptom that indicates a diagnosis.

**indicanuria** \in′dikənoo′rē·ə\ [INDICAN + -URIA] The presence of excessive amounts of indican in the urine.

**indication** \in′dikā′shən\ 1 A symptom, sign, or circumstance that points to a specific treatment for an illness. Also *indicatio.* 2 A mode of treatment indicated as appropriate or necessary based on an evaluation of the condition and history of the patient and the nature of his illness.

**indicator** \in′dikā′tər\ [L (from *indicatus,* past part. of *indicare* to show, reveal, + *-or* -OR), that which or one who indicates or values. See INDEX.] 1 INDEX. 2 MUSCULUS EXTENSOR INDICIS. 3 A substance used to produce color in response to a specific metabolic activity such as fermentation or acid production. 4 A strain of microorganisms used to test for the presence of a substance, as in bioautography. 5 A phage-sensitive strain used to test for release of a phage by a lysogenic strain. **anaerobic i.** A solution whose appearance reflects the oxygen status of its environment. **dew point i.** A device that measures the moisture content of a gas by recording the temperature at which condensation occurs as the vapor is cooled. Also *dew point hygrometer.* **fluorescent i.** An indicator that is labeled with fluorescein or some other fluorescent substance. It is used to localize materials in fluorescence microscopy or to permit titrimetric examination, under ultraviolet light, of materials that are turbid or highly pigmented in ordinary light. **oxidation-reduction i.** A substance whose color changes with differences in oxidation potential. Also *redox indicator.* **pH i.** A substance that undergoes a color change with a change in pH. It is used in titration and as a means for visual estimation of the pH of solutions or substances. **proportional mortality i.** The percentage of all deaths in a population during a given period that occur at age 50 years or over, proposed by WHO in 1957 as a simple but effective index to distinguish countries of differing levels of health. **radioactive i.** RADIOACTIVE TRACER. **redox i.** OXIDATION-REDUCTION INDICATOR. **universal i.** A mixture of indicator substances compounded so that distinct colors will develop at different points along a range of pH values.

**indices** \in′disēz\ Plural of INDEX.

**indicophose** \in′dikōfōs′\ [L *Indic(um)* a blue pigment from India, indigo + *o* + Gk *phōs* light, daylight] A blue subjective light sensation.

**indifférence** \eNdifäräNs′\ [French, indifference] **la belle i.** A situation seen in patients with conversion hysteria, where the patient exhibits an apparent lack of concern about the accompanying disabling symptoms. Also *belle indifférence.*

**indigent** \in′dijənt\ **medically i.** Having inadequate financial resources to pay for or otherwise obtain medical care without depriving oneself or one's family of the other basic necessities of life.

**indigestion** \in′dijes′chən\ 1 Inadequate or disordered digestion of food in the alimentary canal. 2 Gastric or abdominal discomfort experienced after eating. *Popular.*

**indigitation** \indij′itā′shən\ [*indigitat(e)* (from L *digitus* finger) to interlock the fingers of the two hands + -ION] An invagination, intussusception, or interlocking structure.

**indigo** \in′digo\ [Portuguese, from L *indicum* (from *indicus* of India) a blue pigment imported from India] A blue dye that was originally derived from plants of the genera *Isatis* and *Indigofera* by fermentation of the plant glucoside indican. It is now commercially obtained and is used in both histological and cytologic techniques as a counterstain. Also *indigo blue.*

**indigopurpurine** A purple coloration present in the

urine due to the presence of indoxyl sulfate, the conjugate of indoxyl derived from tryptophane.

**indirubin** \in'diroo'bin\ A red pigment sometimes seen in urine as a result of oxidation of indoxyl to isatin which then combines with unaltered indoxyl.

**indirubinuria** \in'diroo'binoo'rē·ə\ The presence of indirubin in the urine, producing red urine.

**indisposition** \in'dispəzish'ən\ A slight illness or feeling of being unwell. *Popular.*

**indium** \in'dē·əm\ [L *indicum* indigo] A soft metallic element having atomic number 49 and atomic weight 114.82. It is found in ores of zinc and other metals. There are two naturally occurring stable isotopes. Some 20 radioactive isotopes are known. Indium has various technologic applications. Symbol: In

**indium 111** The radioactive isotope of indium of atomic mass 111, having a half-life of 2.83 days and gamma ray energies of 171 and 245 keV. Symbol: $^{111}In$

**indium 113m** A radioactive form of indium, with a half-life of 1.7 hours, which decays by isomeric transition, emitting gamma rays of 391.7 keV. Indium 113m is generator-produced from the parent tin 113. When labeled to appropriate substances, it can be used for blood-pool, liver-spleen, lung, and brain scanning.

**individualization** \in'divid'yoo·əlīzā'shən\ The process of becoming an independent organism separated from the support of mother or surrogate or from a similar organism, as in the separation of conjoined twins.

**individuation** \-in'divid'yoo·ā'shən\ **1** In embryology, an inductive process which results in the formation of complete or entire organic structures. **2** The behavioral principle that wholes emerge prior to partial patterns distinguishable as subunits of the total pattern; in popular usage, the gradual definition of an individual, as growth and experience combine to produce a unique person. **3** Jung's treatment procedure which moves through successive layers of psychologic conflict to reach the inner core, the self.

**indocyanine green** A nontoxic, nonirritating dye used to measure hepatic excretory function. When injected intravenously, it is bound to plasma proteins. It is removed and excreted solely by hepatocellular action, with no enterohepatic recirculation. Plasma levels are measured spectrophotometrically at an absorbance peak of 805 nm. The normal plasma decay curve has a half-life of 3.8 minutes.

**indole** The heterocyclic compound whose molecules contain a benzene ring fused to C-2 and C-3 of a pyrrole ring. It is not very basic, and when protonated by strong acids it loses its aromatic character and is then easily oxidized. Tryptophan and many alkaloids are substituted indoles.

**indole-3-acetic acid** A plant hormone, or auxin, which evokes the faster lengthening of growing tips on the side away from light, and hence the phototropic response. It is derived from tryptophan. Also *heteroauxin* (obs.).

**indolent** \in'dələnt\ [Late L *indolens*, gen. *indolentis* (from *in-* not + *dolere* to feel or cause pain) free from pain, causing no pain] **1** Characterized by slow progression, as of a disease process or a tumor of low malignancy. **2** Causing little or no pain.

**indolylacryloylglycine** A conjugate of indolyacrylic acid and glycine formed as a product of the colonic fermentation of tryptophan. It is found in abnormal quantities in the urine of patients with Hartnup disease following the ingestion of large doses of tryptophan.

**indomethacin** $C_{19}H_{16}ClNO_4$. 1-(4-Chlorobenzoyl)-5-methoxy-2-methyl-1*H*-indole-3-acetic acid. An agent with anti-inflammatory, antipyretic, and analgesic properties. It is used in the treatment of several types of arthritis, including rheumatoid arthritis, osteoarthritis of the hip, and gouty arthritis. It is given orally.

**indophenol** \in'dōfē'nôl\ **1** Any of a series of colored compounds of the quinone-imine group that do not readily form salts with mineral acids and whose halogenated substitution products are used as pH indicators, losing color in the reduced state. **2** The specific compound consisting of the imine formed between *p*-benzoquinone and *p*-hydroxyaniline, the simplest of the indophenol series.

**indoxyl** 2-Hydroxyindole. It is released from the plant glucoside indican by hydrolysis. It is oxidized by the air to the dye indigo. Some indoxyl is formed from tryptophan by intestinal bacteria and is excreted in the urine as its sulfate.

**indoxylemia** \indäk'silē'mē·ə\ The presence of indole oxidation products in the blood.

**induced** \ind'ʸoost'\ Brought about, especially by intervention, as *induced labor.*

**inducer** \ind'ʸoo'sər\ A small molecule that accelerates the transcription of particular genes by binding to a regulatory protein.

**inductance** \induk'təns\ [See INDUCTION.] The property of an electric circuit by which a changing current induces in the same or a neighboring circuit an electromotive force proportional to the rate of change of the current, expressed in henrys.

**induction** \induk'shən\ [L *inductio* (from *inductus*, past part. of *inducere* to lead in, introduce, induce) a bringing or leading in or into, intention, induction] **1** In embryology, the production of a specific morphogenetic effect, or the determination of the developmental fate of a cell or tissue, in the developing embryo through the influence of chemical substances (evocators) produced within and released by another cell or tissue. **2** In microbiology, the process by which a foodstuff or metabolite stimulates the formation of a protein related to its metabolism. This is a major mechanism in enzyme adaptation. **3** Any change in the composition or behavior of a cell in response to an environmental stimulus, such as lysis by ultraviolet activation of a potentially lytic prophage. **4** That phase of inhalation anesthesia from the start to attainment of a surgical plane of anesthesia. **autonomous i.** Induction in which the cells which produce the inducing substance do not themselves become incorporated into the resultant tissue or organ so formed. Compare COMPLEMENTARY INDUCTION. **complementary i.** A particular type of induction in which the cells which produce the inducing substance become incorporated into the resultant tissue or organ so formed. Compare AUTONOMOUS INDUCTION. **enzyme i.** The increase in the rate of biosynthesis of an enzyme in response to a stimulus. It differs from, but is physiologically complementary to, the increase of activity of preexisting enzyme as a control mechanism. **medical i. of labor** Induction of labor through the use of oxytocic drugs. **Spemann's i.** The original demonstration of the controlling influence of localized parts of the early embryo on the morphogenetic development of neighboring tissues or parts. This effect was later shown to be due to the production and diffusion of chemical substances (inductors) from these parts. **spinal i.** The process in the spinal cord by which activity in one nerve cell or group of cells lowers the threshold of activity in other nerve cells. **surgical i. of labor** Induction of labor by artificial rupture of the fetal membranes.

**inductor** \induk'tər\ **1** A tissue which elaborates a chemical substance during embryonic development that determines the developmental fate of a nother cell or tissue. The ability of a cell or tissue to respond in this way is a demonstration of its competence. Also *evocator, organizer.*

2 ORGANIZER. 3 A coil of wire, with or without a magnetic core, for introducing inductance into an electrical circuit. **gene i.** A substance, such as a nutrient, in the cell's environment which allows an operon to be transcribed. The inductor may function by the inactivation of a repressor protein.

**indulin black** A synthetic dye with a black guinone-imine chromatophore used as a background stain in the study of bacteria and in the staining of tissue of the central nervous system. Also *indulin.*

**indurated** \in′d$^y$ərā′tid\ Hardened, or characterized by an increase in consistency.

**induration** \in′dyoorā′shən\ [Late L *induratio* (from L *indurare* to make hard, from *durus* hard) a hardening] The hardening of normally soft tissues or organs due to inflammation or infiltration. **black i.** Dark pigmentation and fibrosis of the lung due to anthracosis. **brawny i.** Hardening of soft tissues caused by chronic inflammation. **fibroid i.** CIRRHOSIS. **granular i.** Cirrhosis. **phlebitic i.** Induration of the skin of the leg as a consequence of chronic phlebitis, occurring initially around phlebitic veins of the lower leg, but sometimes extending to form large plaques on legs with chronic venous insufficiency. **plastic i. of penis** PEYRONIE'S DISEASE. **rigid i. of the bladder neck** MARION'S DISEASE.

**indurative** \in′d$^y$ərā′tiv\ Characterized by or pertaining to induration.

**indusium** \ind$^y$oo′zē·əm\ [L, an outer tunic] INDUSIUM GRISEUM. **i. griseum** [NA] The dorsal continuation of the hippocampus, lying above the corpus callosum and continuous with the lower margin of the cingulate gyrus. Also *hippocampal rudiment, gyrus epicallosus, indusium.*

**indwelling** \in′dweling\ Remaining in place in the body, as to provide drainage or to allow administration of nutrients or drugs: said especially of a catheter or similar tubular implement.

**-ine** [L adj. suffix *-inus* and Gk *-inos*] 1 A suffix meaning (1) composed of or pertaining to, as in *crystalline, uterine*; (2) belonging to a zoological subfamily with a corresponding name ending in *-inae,* as *culicine* (of the subfamily Culicinae). 2 An ending of the names of many chemical substances, including amino acids and amines, but with no precise definition. It may also be part of some more complex suffixes, e.g. -olidine, which signifies a 5-membered saturated ring containing nitrogen.

**inebriant** \inē′brē·ənt\ Producing inebriation; intoxicating.

**inebriation** \inē′brē·ā′shən\ [L *inebriatio* (from L *inebriare* to make drunk, from *ebrius* drunk) intoxication, drunkenness] A stuporous state induced by ingesting an intoxicating substance, especially alcohol, characterized by motor incoordination and slurred speech; drunkenness.

**inert** \inurt′\ Having little or no tendency to react chemically.

**inertia** \inur′shə\ [L (from *iners,* gen. *inertis* lacking skill, idle, inactive (from *in-* not, lacking + *ars,* gen. *artis* skill, art) disinclination for activity, indolence] 1 The property of matter that causes it to continue in a state of rest or uniform motion in a straight line unless acted upon by an external force. 2 A state of little or no action or movement. **primary uterine i.** Abnormal uterine contractions probably synonymous with the latent phase of labor or false labor but characterized by failure to progress in labor. Inherent musculature weakness or faulty innervation is felt to be etiologic if such contractions persist for prolonged periods of time. Also *first-degree uterine incoordination.* **psychic i.** FIXATION. **secondary uterine i.** Abnormal uterine contractions characterized by poor intensity attributed to exhaustion of the uterine musculature due to protracted uterine activity. Also *second-degree uterine incoordination.* **uterine i.** Abnormal contraction of the uterus during or just preceding labor.

**inexcitable** \in′iksī′təbl\ Incapable of responding to stimulation. Also *unirritable.*

**in extremis** \in ikstrē′mis\ [L *in* in + *extremis,* ablative pl. of *extremum* the last stage] At the point of death.

**inf.** *infunde* (L, pour in).

**infancy** [L *infantia* inability to speak, infancy. See INFANT.] The period from birth to about one year of age.

**infant** [L *infans,* gen. *infantis* (pres. part. of assumed *infari,* from *in-* not + *fari* to say, speak), speechless, young, little, childish; as substantive, a little child, infant] A child from birth to about one year of age. **floppy i.** See under FLOPPY INFANT SYNDROME. **i. Hercules** A young male child exhibiting marked hypertrophy or pseudohypertrophy of skeletal muscles and therefore having the superficial and deceptive appearance of extraordinary muscular development. It is most often seen in Duchenne type muscular dystrophy, less often in myotonia congenita. **immature i.** A premature infant born before 27 weeks of gestational age measured from the first day of the last menstrual period. **liveborn i.** A fetus that is born alive. **mature i.** TERM INFANT. **newborn i.** See under NEONATE. **postmature i.** An infant born after 42 weeks of gestation measured from the first day of the last menstrual period. The fetus may show a normal growth rate or may be of a reduced birth weight with loss of soft tissue mass. Also *post-term infant.* **premature i.** An infant having a birth weight less than 2500 grams and born after a gestation period of less than 38 weeks from the first day of the last menstrual period. The low birth weight is a result of normal fetal growth for an abnormally short period of time. Also *preterm infant.* **stillborn i.** An infant born without evidence of life. **term i.** An infant born between 38 and 42 weeks of gestational age measured from the first day of the last menstrual period and having a weight greater than 2500 grams. Also *mature infant.*

**infanticide** \infan′tisīd\ [INFANT + *i* + -CIDE] 1 The killing of an infant. The period of infancy as defined in such cases is usually designated as the time from birth through the first year of life, but varies slightly from jurisdiction to jurisdiction. 2 One who commits infanticide.

**infantile** 1 Of or characteristic of infants or infancy. 2 Relating to behavioral or developmental characteristics like those of infancy.

**infantilism** \infan′tilizm\ [*infantil(e)* + -ISM] The persistence of physical and/or mental characteristics of childhood into adult life. • In endocrinologic contexts, the term *infantilism* is outmoded. **celiac i.** INFANTILE CELIAC DISEASE. **Herter's i.** INFANTILE CELIAC DISEASE. **hypophysial i.** *Older term* HYPOPHYSIAL DWARFISM. **idiopathic i.** *Older term* HYPOPHYSIAL DWARFISM. **intestinal i.** INFANTILE CELIAC DISEASE. **Lévi-Lorain i.** *Outmoded* HYPOPHYSIAL DWARFISM. **Lorain's i.** *Outmoded* HYPOPHYSIAL DWARFISM. **myxedematous i.** *Older term* CRETINISM. **pituitary i.** *Older term* HYPOPHYSIAL DWARFISM. **proportionate i.** *Older term* HYPOPHYSIAL DWARFISM. **renal i.** Stunted growth due to renal osteodystrophy in the early years of life. **sexual i.** Failure of the secondary sex characters to develop, as in hypophysial dwarfism. **thyroid i.** *Seldom used* CRETINISM.

**infarct** \in′färkt\ [L *infarctus* (past part. of *infarcire* to stuff or cram into, from *in-* into + *farcire* to fill up, stuff) stuffed in, crammed in] A discrete, usually wedge-shaped area of ischemic coagulative necrosis caused by interruption of blood flow. The apex of the wedge usually points toward the point of vascular occlusion. **anemic i.** An infarct caused by arterial occlusion. They are distinctly pale in gross appearance because they result from ischemic coagulative necrosis affecting an organ with a single arterial blood supply. Also *pale infarct, white infarct.* **aseptic i.** BLAND INFARCT. **bilirubin i.** An infarct containing bilirubin crystals found in the renal pyramids, usually in the newborn. **bland i.** An infarct that is not contaminated by infectious microorganisms. Also *aseptic infarct.* **Brewer's i.'s** Conical dark red areas seen on section of the kidney in pyelonephritis. They are not considered true infarcts. **cerebral i.** An infarct of cerebral tissues. It may be either anemic or hemorrhagic. The cause is usually atherosclerotic occlusion with or without thrombosis or thromboembolism from a remote source. In their evolution, cerebral infarcts undergo liquefaction and cystic transformation with permanent loss of brain parenchyma. **cystic i.** An infarct that has undergone liquefaction and cystic transformation as, for example, in old cerebral infarcts. **embolic i.** An infarct caused by embolic occlusion of an artery. **hemorrhagic i.** An infarct that appears red due to interstitial hemorrhage throughout the necrotic area. This is usually the result of venous occlusion or arterial occlusion in organs that have a double blood supply. It may also follow the reestablishment of blood flow after the ischemic tissue has undergone necrosis. Also *red infarct, red softening.* **infected i.** SEPTIC INFARCT. **kidney i.** RENAL INFARCT. **mesenteric i.** Necrosis of the intestine and mesentery resulting from the impairment of the intestinal blood supply within the mesentery. **pale i.** ANEMIC INFARCT. **placental i.** An area of ischemic necrosis located in the substance of a placenta. **pulmonary i.** Dead lung tissue resulting from obstruction of its blood supply. **red i.** HEMORRHAGIC INFARCT. **renal i.** Necrosis secondary to ischemia due to interruption of arterial or venous circulation of the kidneys. Arterial obstruction usually is secondary to arteriosclerotic narrowing of a renal artery or to emboli. Obstruction of arcuate or larger arteries may cause infarction. Vasculitis, aneurysm, compression by tumors, or trauma also may precipitate renal infarcts. Venous thrombosis secondary to hypercoagulable states, dehydration, or some kidney diseases such as membranous glomerulonephritis also, on rare occasions, may contribute to renal infarction. Clinically, renal infarction is characterized by lumbar pain, transient proteinuria and hematuria, and renal function impairment. Renal infarction leads to scarring and contracted depressions. Also *kidney infarct, infarcted kidney.* **septic i.** An infarct that is contaminated by infectious microorganisms. Such infarcts may result from necrosis of a previously infected area, or by the seeding of a developing infarct with microorganisms contained in emboli of vegetations from infected heart valves. These infarcts commonly progress to abscess formation. Also *infected infarct, inflammatory infarct* (incorrect and seldom used). **thrombotic i.** An infarct that is due to vascular occlusion by a thrombus. **uric acid i.** The presence of yellow streaks in the tips of the renal papillae of newborn infants. The streaks are caused by uric acid crystals in the terminal collecting ducts, but infarction is not present. This appears to be a normal physiologic condition of unknown explanation. • This term is inappropriate but nevertheless accepted. **white i.** ANEMIC INFARCT.

**infarction** \infärk'shən\ The process of infarct formation. **acute myocardial i.** The acute phase of a myocardial infarction. **anterior myocardial i.** Myocardial infarction involving the anterior wall of the heart, revealed in the electrocardiogram by involving most of the leads from $V_1$ to $V_6$. **anterolateral myocardial i.** Infarction affecting the lateral wall of the heart, revealed on the electrocardiogram by changes in $V_5$ and $V_6$ and in leads I and aVL. **anteroseptal myocardial i.** Infarction involving the anterior wall and septum of the heart and revealed in the electrocardiogram by changes in $V_1$ to $V_4$. **apical myocardial i.** Infarction involving the apex of the heart. **atrial myocardial i.** Myocardial infarction involving one or both of the atria. **cardiac i.** MYOCARDIAL INFARCTION. **diaphragmatic myocardial i.** INFERIOR MYOCARDIAL INFARCTION. **high lateral myocardial i.** Myocardial infarction involving the high lateral wall of the ventricle and sometimes only revealed in the electrocardiogram in leads such as aVL and the high lateral leads. Also *lateral myocardial infarction.* **inferior myocardial i.** Infarction involving the inferior surface of the myocardium and usually revealed on the electrocardiogram best in leads II, III, and aVF. It is usually due to occlusion of the right coronary artery, but may result from circumflex artery occlusion. Also *diaphragmatic myocardial infarction, posterior myocardial infarction* (incorrect and outmoded). **inferolateral myocardial i.** Infarction affecting both the inferior and lateral surfaces of the heart and revealed on the electrocardiogram by changes in leads II, III, aVF, $V_5$ and $V_6$. **lateral myocardial i.** HIGH LATERAL MYOCARDIAL INFARCTION. **myocardial i.** An acute necrotic process of the myocardium resulting from of sudden loss of blood supply to the affected tissue. It is usually associated with thrombosis, but embolism, rupture of a plaque, and coronary arterial spasm may all be factors in its genesis. Also *cardiac infarction.* **pituitary i.** An acute vascular accident accompanying thrombus, embolus, or vasospasm of the blood vessels of the hypothalamic-adenohypophysial portal venous system, leading to ischemic necrosis with or without hemorrhage into the adenohypophysis, and sometimes also involving the neurohypophysis. The lesion characterizes the Sheehan syndrome. It may occur in five to ten percent of cases of pituitary tumor and in a small number of cases of diabetes mellitus. Other precipitating causes are anticoagulation therapy, radiotherapy of the pituitary fossa, and basilar fractures of the skull. Impairment of pituitary function is variable. The lesion may figure in the pathogenesis of empty-sella syndrome. The clinical syndrome associated with pituitary infarction is sometimes called pituitary apoplexy. **posterior myocardial i.** **1** Infarction involving the posterior wall of the left ventricle. It is not readily visualized on the electrocardiogram but is often associated with lateral and inferior changes and also with the development of a dominant R wave in $V_1$. **2** An incorrect and outmoded term for INFERIOR MYOCARDIAL INFARCTION. **posterolateral myocardial i.** Infarction affecting posterior and lateral walls of the heart. **pulmonary i.** Infarction in a lung, commonly resulting from obstruction of the blood supply by an embolus. **renal i.** RENAL INFARCT. **right ventricular i.** Infarction involving the wall of the right ventricle. It is virtually always associated with an inferior myocardial infarction. Transient ST segment elevation may be seen in the right precordial leads. **septal myocardial i.** Infarction involving the interventricular septum. It usually produces changes in leads $V_1$ to $V_4$. **silent myocardial i.** Myocardial infarction occurring in the absence of the characteristic symptoms. **subendocardial i.** Infarction involving only that part of the myocardium which is adjacent to the endocardium.

**through-and-through myocardial i.** TRANSMURAL MYOCARDIAL INFARCTION. **transmural myocardial i.** Infarction involving the full thickness of the myocardium. Also *through-and-through myocardial infarction.* • The term *transmural* is sometimes used inaccurately to describe any infarction associated with pathological Q waves, which were at one time thought to indicate infarction through the full thickness, though it is now known that this is not necessarily the case.

**infect** [L *infect(us),* past part. of *inficere* to infect. See INFECTION.] **1** To invade and become established in or on (the body of a host): said of pathogenic microorganisms and internal parasites, such as bacteria, viruses, fungi, protozoa, helminths, and sometimes arthropods. **2** To transmit an infection to; contaminate with an infectious agent.

**infection** [Late L *infectio* (from *inficere* to dip in, dye, stain, discolor, taint, infect, from *in-* into + *facere* to make, treat, prepare) contamination, corruption] **1** The process whereby pathogenic organisms become established and multiply in or on the body of a host. **2** The state resulting from this process, which often includes local or systemic disease with cellular or systemic injury. **air-borne i.** Infection caused by microorganisms carried on droplets of moisture or particles suspended in the air and which usually gain access to the host through inhalation. Also *aerial infection.* **autochthonous i.** Infection by organisms indigenous or native to the environment. **concurrent i.** Simultaneous infections by two or more causative agents. Also *complex infection.* **contact i.** An infection resulting from direct contact with an infected person or animal. Also *direct infection.* Compare INDIRECT INFECTION. **covert i.** Any clinically inapparent infection, which may be either dormant or latent. Also *inapparent infection, silent infection, subclinical infection.* **cross i.** An infection spread from one person or animal to another person or animal. • The term is sometimes reserved for infections contracted in hospital. **cryptogenic i.** An infection in which the origin or entry point of the causative agent is unknown. **diaplacental i.** Infection transmitted to the embryo or fetus through the placenta. **direct i.** CONTACT INFECTION. **dormant i.** An infection in which a pathogenic microorganism can be recovered from the host but is not at that time causing symptomatic disease in that individual. If the organism is shed the individual is called a carrier. **droplet i.** An infection caused by the inhalation of liquid particles containing infective organisms. **dust-borne i.** An infection caused by the inhalation of dust particles carrying pathogenic microorganisms. **ectogenous i.** EXOGENOUS INFECTION. **endogenous i.** Infection by organisms already present in or on the host as components of its normal flora and fauna or as pathogens in a dormant state. Compare EXOGENOUS INFECTION. **exogenous i.** An infection due to a pathogen which originated outside the body of the host. Also *ectogenous infection.* Compare ENDOGENOUS INFECTION. **focal i.** An infection which is confined to a single site, such as the prostatic bed or sinuses. • In the past certain systemic diseases were often erroneously attributed to focal infections. **germinal i.** Infection transmitted to offspring as a result of infection of the sperm or ovum of a parent. **inapparent i.** COVERT INFECTION. **indirect i.** An infection transmitted by an intermediary such as food, water, air or fomes rather than transmitted directly from host to host. Compare CONTACT INFECTION. **intercurrent i.** An infection occurring during the course of another infection. **invasive burn i.** A bacterial or fungal infection of a burn wound that has invaded the living tissue under the area of necrotic skin. It is a harbinger of systemic sepsis. **latent i.** **1** An infection in which the causative agent (the tubercle bacillus, for example) cannot be recovered from a patient although its continued presence can be inferred from continuing immunologic reactivity or, retrospectively, from the later emergence of overt illness. **2** An infection with certain viruses where the viral genome becomes integrated into the cellular DNA of host cells and is replicated at cell division but where no virions are formed. Such latent infections (for example, with herpes simplex virus) may become reactivated to give a productive infection. **local i.** An infection confined to a definite area or tissue. **metastatic i.** An infection which is transferred from an original focus to another part or parts of the body by conveyance of the pathogen in the blood or lymph. **nonspecific i.** An infection in which a specific causative organism has not been identified. **nosocomial i.** An infection acquired in a hospital or other health-care facility. **opportunistic i.** An infection in a patient with diminished resistance by an organism that is ordinarily a harmless commensal. **phycomycotic i.** MUCORMYCOSIS. **puerperal i.** An infection of the birth canal occurring during the postpartum period. **pyogenic i.** An infection due to pus-producing organisms, especially *Staphylococcus aureus* and *Streptococcus pyogenes.* **retrograde i.** An infection that spreads up a tube or duct in a direction contrary to the flow of secretions or excretions. **secondary i.** **1** An infection complicating a prior infection. **2** An infection complicating another underlying disease, as, for example, bacterial pneumonia occurring in a patient with bronchial carcinoma. **silent i.** COVERT INFECTION. **slow i.** An infection in which there is a lengthy period of incubation and/or latency (months or years) followed by the appearance of illness which may be severe and associated with life-threatening signs and symptoms. Such infections are usually of viral origin and include kuru, subacute sclerosing panencephalitis, progressive multifocal leukoencephalopathy, and scrapie in sheep. **subclinical i.** COVERT INFECTION. **water-borne i.** An infection in which the pathogenic organisms are transmitted by water used for drinking, bathing, or other purposes. **zoogenic i.** **1** An infection of humans for which there is an animal reservoir. **2** Infection by an animal organism, as, for example, by a parasite helminth.

**infectious** **1** Caused by infection with pathogenic organisms: said of diseases. **2** Capable of causing an infection; infective. **3** Capable of being spread from one host to another, with or without direct contact.

**infectiousness** \infek′shəsnis\ The state or quality of being able to cause or to communicate infection. Also *infectivity.*

**infective** \infek′tiv\ Capable of causing infection.

**infectivity** \in′fektiv′itē\ INFECTIOUSNESS.

**infecundity** \in′fēkun′ditē\ [IN-[2] + FECUNDITY] Inability to become pregnant.

**inferent** \in′fərənt\ AFFERENT.

**inferior** Lower; near or toward the bottom: used in human anatomy with reference to the upright posture and designating structures or parts relatively near the caudal end of the body as compared with others nearer the cranial (cephalic) end.

**infero-** \in′fərō-\ [L *inferus* below, low] A combining form meaning inferior.

**inferocostal** \-käs′təl\ INFRACOSTAL.

**inferofrontal** \-frän′təl\ Denoting the inferior portion of the frontal lobe.

**inferolateral** \-lat′ərəl\ Situated below and at or toward the side.

**inferomedial** \-mē′dē·əl\ Situated below and at or toward the median plane.

**inferomedian** \-mē′dē·ən\ Situated below and in the middle.

**inferoparietal** \-pəri′ətəl\ Denoting the inferior parietal lobule of the cerebrum, including the angular and supramarginal gyri.

**inferoposterior** \-pästir′ē·ər\ Situated below and behind.

**infertility** \in′fərtil′itē\ [L *in-* not + FERTILITY] **1** Inability to conceive; inability to become pregnant. **2** Inability to impregnate. **primary i.** Infertility of a couple in which the woman has never conceived. **secondary i.** Current infertility of a couple although the woman has previously had at least one pregnancy.

**infest** \infest′\ [L *infest(are)* to attack, damage, infest] **1** To dwell in or invade (a habitat or locality): said of populations of disease vectors or other pestiferous organisms. **2** To dwell on or in (a host): said of populations of metazoan parasites, especially ectoparasites.

**infestation** \in′festā′shən\ [Late L *infestatio* (from L *infestatus,* past part. of *infestare* to molest) a molesting, infestation] The invasion or inhabitation of a place, or of a host organism, by a population of pests or parasites. • The term *infection,* rather than *infestation,* is normally used for the invasion or inhabitation of a host by noxious microorganisms, and many consider *infection* the only correct term to use in reference to larger internal parasites as well, limiting *infestation* of a host to surface-dwelling parasites such as lice, fleas, or ticks.

**infestive** \infes′tiv\ Likely or apt to cause an infestation.

**infibulation** \infib′yəlā′shən\ The practice of fastening by stitches or clasps the labia majora in girls or the prepuce in boys in order to prevent copulation.

**infiltrate** \infil′trāt, in′filtrāt\ [L *in-* into + FILTRATE] The extracellular accumulation of fluids, cells, or other materials as a result of a pathologic process. **Assmann's tuberculous i.** ASSMANN FOCUS. **leukemic i.** The accumulation of leukemic cells within any organ other than the bone marrow. Common sites include the liver, spleen, lymph nodes, and meninges.

**infiltration** \in′filtrā′shən\ [L *in-* into + FILTRATION] The extracellular accumulation within a tissue or organ of any material or cell type that is not a normal component of that tissue. **calcareous i.** CALCIFICATION. **calcium i.** CALCIFICATION. **cellular i.** The permeation or accumulation of cells within tissues that are distant from their point of origin. **epituberculous i.** Infiltration of lung tissue related to large tuberculous lymph nodes, seen in children with tuberculosis. **glycogen i.** The vacuolated or empty appearance of the nucleus and/or cytoplasm of cells due to excessive accumulation of glycogen, as may occur in diabetes mellitus, glycogen-storage disease, or in patients receiving glucose-rich intravenous infusions. **inflammatory i.** An accumulation of the effector cells of inflammation, mostly granulocytes, macrophages, and lymphocytes. **lymphocytic i. of skin** A benign disorder of unknown origin that is characterized by the development of reddish brown plaques. Histologically it appears as an intense lymphocytic infiltration of the dermis. The condition affects men primarily. Also *Jessner-Kanof disease.* **pulmonary i. with eosinophilia** LÖFFLER SYNDROME. **round-cell i.** The accumulation of mononuclear cells such as monocytes and lymphocytes, usually associated with viral infections and chronic inflammation. **urinous i.** An infiltration of urine resulting from a break in the continuity of the wall of the ureter or bladder. It may be caused by cancer, trauma, or inflammation.

**infirm** \infurm′\ [L *infirm(us)* weak, feeble] Weak or enfeebled, as by a chronic condition: used especially of the old.

**infirmary** \infur′mərē\ [Med L *infirmarium* (from L *infirm(us)* not strong, infirm + *-arium* -ARY) infirmary] A primary or short-term medical care facility, usually serving a larger institution. • The term was originally applied to that part of a monastery or other institution where the sick or infirm were cared for, and is still used in this sense, as in *school infirmary,* but is now also used more broadly of much larger health-care facilities, even of large hospitals.

**infirmity** \infur′mitē\ [L *infirmitas* weakness, feebleness] **1** A condition that produces prolonged weakness or enfeeblement, especially in the aged. **2** Weakness; feebleness.

**inflammation** [L *inflammatio* (from *inflammatus,* past part. of *inflammare* to set on fire, excite, rouse, from *in-* in + *flamma* flame, fire, ardor) an inflaming, kindling, inflammation] The localized response of vascularized tissues to injury caused by chemical, physical, or biological agents. Clinically, the cardinal signs of inflammation include redness, swelling, heat, pain, loss of function, and fever. Events that follow injury include vasodilation, stasis, leukocytic margination and emigration, and exudation of leukocytes and plasma. The purpose of inflammation is to dilute, contain and destroy the injurious agent. The exact nature of this response, and the healing that follows it, depend on several factors, including the nature and extent of the injury, the tissue injured, and the responsiveness of the organism. **acute i.** Inflammation of sudden onset, usually characterized by the cardinal signs (swelling, heat, redness, pain, and fever) clinically, and by predominately vascular and exudative responses pathologically. **adhesive i.** Inflammation in which the amount of fibrin in the exudate is sufficient to stimulate, in the healing stage, the formation of fibrous adhesions between adjacent structures such as the pleural or pericardial surfaces. **allergic i.** Inflammation resulting from a hypersensitivity reaction. **atrophic i.** A form of chronic inflammation that results in excessive fibrous tissue formation that retracts and atrophies and compresses the intervening parenchymal tissue. Also *sclerosing inflammation.* **bacterial i.** Inflammation caused by bacterial infection. **chemical i.** Inflammation due to a chemical injury to tissues. **chronic i.** Inflammation that is persistent over time, due to the continuation of an acute stimulus, repeated bouts of acute inflammation, or the continuation over time of a low-grade, subclinical focus. It is characterized by mononuclear cell infiltration and the proliferation of fibroblasts, and frequently leads to scarring. **diffuse i.** Inflammation that involves most of an organ or tissue in a homogeneous manner. **disseminated i.** Inflammation affecting several distinct foci throughout the body. **fibrinopurulent i.** A form of acute inflammation whose exudate is mainly composed of fibrin and pus. **focal i.** Inflammation that is localized in a discrete area. **granulomatous i.** Chronic inflammation characterized by granuloma formation and the presence of giant cells, as in tuberculosis. **hyperplastic i.** A form of chronic inflammation associated with an exaggerated repair process that often results in abundant fibrovascular scar tissue. Also *productive inflammation.* **hypertrophic i.** Inflammation characterized by an increase in size of the cellular elements of the affected tissue. **interstitial i.** Inflammation of the stroma, or interstitium, of an organ with relative sparing of the parenchymatous elements. **obliterative i.** Inflammation that results in the obliteration or replacement of a structure with scar tissue. **parenchymatous**

**i.** Inflammation of the parenchymal cells of an organ, with relative sparing of its stromal connective tissue framework. **productive i.** HYPERPLASTIC INFLAMMATION. **pseudomembranous i.** Acute inflammation of a mucosal surface that is characterized by the formation of a friable membrane on the affected mucosa. The membrane is composed of precipitated fibrin, polymorphonuclear leukocytes, and necrotic epithelial cells. This response is the result of powerful necrotizing toxins, such as diphtheria toxin. **purulent i.** SUPPURATIVE INFLAMMATION. **sclerosing i.** ATROPHIC INFLAMMATION. **serofibrinous i.** Inflammation characterized by a serous exudate containing a relatively large amount of fibrin. **serous i.** Inflammation characterized by an exudate comprised mostly of serum and lacking significant cellular infiltration. **simple i.** Inflammation devoid of distinguishing features such as pus formation. **specific i.** Inflammation that is caused by a single, identified agent, usually a microorganism. **subacute i.** Inflammation that is intermediate between acute and chronic in the duration and characteristics of the response. **suppurative i.** Inflammation that is characterized by pus formation, such as that caused by pyogenic bacteria. Also *purulent inflammation.* **toxic i.** Inflammation caused by a poison, which may be bacterial products, such as exotoxins, or chemical compounds, such as chlorinated hydrocarbons. **ulcerative i.** Inflammation accompanied by sloughing of the inflamed necrotic tissue, resulting in a local defect, or ulceration, in the surface of the affected area.

**inflammatory** \inflam′ətôr′ē\ Characterized by or resulting from inflammation.

**inflation** [L *inflatio* (from *inflatus,* past part. of *inflare* to inflate, cause to swell) an inflating] **1** The condition of being distended, as with a gas or fluid. **2** The process of becoming distended.

**inflected** \inflek′tid\ INFLEXED.

**inflection** \inflek′shən\ The act of bending inward or the state of being bent inward. Also *inflexion.*

**inflexed** \inflekst′\ Bent or curved inward. Also *inflected.*

**inflexion** \inflek′shən\ INFLECTION.

**inflow** The adequacy of arterial perfusion into an arterial segment.

**influenza** \in′floo·en′zə\ [Italian (from Med L *influentia* influx, influence, astral influence) influence, contagion, epidemic; first used in English in reference to the European influenza epidemic of 1743] An acute respiratory disease of viral origin which is distributed worldwide and often occurs in widespread epidemics. It is characterized by fever, headache, myalgia, and prostration and occurs with rapid onset. Complications such as bronchitis and bacterial pneumonia are common. Two serologically distinct viruses cause the disease, influenza virus A and influenza virus B. These viruses, particularly A, periodically undergo changes in antigenic composition and as a result, world populations become newly susceptible to the disease. New serologic types and the illnesses they cause are designated according to where they are first identified, for example, Hong Kong influenza, Asian influenza and Russian influenza. Also *flu* (popular), *grippe* (older term), *grip* (older term). **i. A** Influenza caused by a serotype of the type A influenza virus. It is the most widespread and frequently occurring influenza type. **i. B** Influenza caused by the type B influenza virus. Although less frequently a cause of epidemics than influenza A, it produces illness indistinguishable from that produced by influenza A and it contributes to excess mortality. It is also associated as an antecedent infection with the Reye syndrome. **i. C** A mild respiratory infection caused by the type C influenza virus and resembling the common cold. This illness is not influenza in the clinical or epidemiological sense of the term. **clinical i.** An infection which clinically resembles influenza but for which the specific pathogen has not been identified. It is characterized by the abrupt onset of fever, headache, muscle ache, and cough in winter months. **swine i.** An acute influenzal illness caused by influenza A virus, subtype Hsw1N1. It affects swine, is transmissible to man, and is often highly contagious among members of these two populations. This particular type of influenza was responsible for the great pandemic of 1918–1919, which killed 21 000 000 persons worldwide in three waves of disease. Reports of isolated cases of human infection and a small outbreak among recruits at a U.S. military base in 1975–1976 prompted development of a vaccine and a national immunization program. However, the infection did not spread and no epidemics occurred. Also *Spanish influenza.*

**influenzal** \in′floo·en′zəl\ Pertaining to influenza.

**infold** [IN-[1] + *fold*] To fold inward so as to be self-enclosing, either surgically (as for a lesion) or developmentally (as an embryonic structure).

**information** / **genetic i.** GENETIC CODE. **sensory i.** Afferent input to the central nervous system, essential for sensory experience.

**infra-** \in′frə-\ [L *infra* (for *infera*) below, beneath, under] A prefix meaning below, beneath.

**infra-alveolar** \-alvē′ələr\ **1** Below an alveolus. **2** Below the alveolar part of the mandible.

**infra-auricular** \-ôrik′yələr\ Below the ear pinna.

**infracardiac** \-kär′dē·ak\ Below the heart or the level of the heart.

**infracerebral** \-ser′əbrəl\ Beneath the cerebrum.

**infraclavicular** \-klavik′yələr\ Below the clavicle. Also *subclavicular.*

**infraclinoid** \-klī′noid\ Below any clinoid process of the sphenoid bone.

**infraclusion** \-kloo′zhən\ [INFRA- + *(oc)clusion*] The failure of a tooth to erupt fully to the height of its neighbors.

**infracortical** \-kôr′tikəl\ Beneath the cortex of an organ; subcortical.

**infracostal** \-käs′təl\ Below a rib or the ribs. Also *inferocostal.*

**infracotyloid** \-kät′iloid\ Below the acetabulum.

**infraction** \infrak′shən\ [L *infractio* (from *infractus,* past part. of *infringere* to break, break into pieces, dishearten, interrupt) a breaking into pieces, weakening, dejection] INCOMPLETE FRACTURE. **Freiberg's i.** KÖHLER SECOND DISEASE.

**infracture** \infrak′chər\ INCOMPLETE FRACTURE.

**infraduction** \-duk′shən\ [INFRA- + DUCTION] The rotation of one eye downward. Also *deorsumduction.*

**infrageniculate** \-jənik′yəlāt\ **1** Below the knee. **2** Below the geniculum of the facial nerve.

**infragenual** \-jen′oo·əl\ INFRAPATELLAR.

**infraglenoid** \-glē′noid\ Below the glenoid cavity of the scapula. Also *subglenoid.*

**infraglottic** \-glät′ik\ Below the glottis. Also *subglottic.*

**infrahyoid** \-hī′oid\ Below the hyoid bone. Also *subhyoid, subhyoidean.*

**inframammary** \-mam′ərē\ Below the mammary gland or the breast, submammary.

**inframandibular** \-mandib′yələr\ Below the mandible; submandibular.

**inframarginal** \-mär′jənəl\ Below any margin or border.

**inframaxillary** \-mak′siler′ē\ Below the maxilla; submaxillary. • The term was formerly used to refer to either the mandibular or the inframandibular area.

**infranatant** \-nā′tənt\ [INFRA- + L *natans*, gen. *natantis*, pres. part. of *natare* to swim, float] **1** Denoting a fluid that, because of its greater density, settles below a layer of solids or other fluid after the mixture is subjected to centrifugation or sedimentation by gravity. **2** An infranatant fluid. For defs. 1 and 2 also *subnatant*. Compare SUPERNATANT.

**infranuclear** \-n$^{y}$oo′klē·ər\ Denoting an axonal process originating in a nuclear neuronal aggregate, especially with respect to the functional changes resulting from interruption of motor nerves, in contrast to damage to the cell bodies and the descending axons impinging upon them.

**infraorbital** \-ôr′bitəl\ Located below the orbit. Also *suborbital*.

**infrapatellar** \-pətel′ər\ Below the patella, referring particularly to the infrapatellar synovial fold and its contained pad of fat. Also *infragenual, subpatellar*.

**infrared** \-red′\ [INFRA- + RED] That portion of the electromagnetic spectrum having wavelengths longer than the red part of the visible spectrum and shorter than microwaves, from 0.77 to 300 micrometers.

**infrascapular** \-skap′yələr\ Below the scapula.

**infrasound** \in′frəsound′\ Wave motion with a frequency too low (below about 20 hertz) to be perceived as sound. Adj. infrasonic.

**infraspecific** \-spəsif′ik\ [INFRA- + SPECIFIC] Pertaining to a category of organisms within a species, as a variety or subspecies.

**infraspinous** \-spī′nəs\ Below any spinous process or spine, such as of the scapula or of a vertebra. Also *subspinous*.

**infrastructure** \in′frəstruk′chər\ **implant i.** The part of an oral implant which is embedded in the bone or covered with mucoperiosteum. Also *implant substructure*.

**infratemporal** \-tem′pərəl\ Below the temporal fossa of the skull.

**infratentorial** \-tentôr′ē·əl\ Situated below the tentorium cerebelli in the posterior cranial fossa.

**infrathoracic** \-thôras′ik\ Below the thorax.

**infratonsillar** \-tän′silər\ Below the palatine tonsil.

**infratracheal** \-trā′kē·əl\ Below the trachea.

**infratrochlear** \-träk′lē·ər\ Below a trochlea, particularly that of the superior oblique muscle of the eye.

**infraturbinal** \-tur′binəl\ CONCHA NASALIS INFERIOR.

**infraversion** \-vur′zhən\ [INFRA- + VERSION] **1** The downward turning of both eyes simultaneously. Also *deorsumversion, downgaze*. **2** INFRACLUSION.

**infravesical** \-ves′ikəl\ Below the urinary bladder.

**infrazygomatic** \-zī′gəmat′ik\ Below the zygomatic, or cheek, bone.

**infundibula** \in′fundib′yələ\ Plural of INFUNDIBULUM.

**infundibular** \in′fundib′yələr\ **1** Pertaining to, resembling, or having the characteristics of an infundibulum. **2** Denoting the infundibulum hypothalami.

**infundibulectomy** \in′fundib′yəlek′təmē\ [*infundibul(um)* + -ECTOMY] Excision of the infundibular region of the right ventricle in subvalvar pulmonary stenosis, especially in the tetralogy of Fallot. **Brock's i.** TRANSVENTRICULAR CLOSED VALVOTOMY.

**infundibuloma** \in′fundib′yəlō′mə\ [*infundibul(um)* + -OMA] A tumor of the infundibulum of the pituitary.

**infundibulo-ovarian** \in′fundib′yəlō-ōver′ē·ən\ Pertaining to the infundibulum of the uterine tube and the ovary.

**infundibulum** \in′fundib′yələm\ [L (from *infundere* to pour in, from *fundere* to pour) a funnel] (*pl.* infundibula) **1** Any funnel-shaped structure or passage. **2** INFUNDIBULUM HYPOTHALAMI. **3** CONUS ARTERIOSUS. **cardiac i.** CONUS ARTERIOSUS. **i. ethmoidale** [NA] A deep, crescentic groove in the lateral wall of the middle nasal meatus, formed by the medial surface of the ethmoidal labyrinth. The groove lies anterior to hiatus semilunaris, below bulla ethmoidalis, and above the uncinate process.At its middle it receives the ostium of the maxillary sinus, while anteriorly are the openings of the anterior ethmoidal cells and the opening of either the frontal sinus or the frontonasal duct. It may end blindly in the anterior ethmoidal cells. Also *ethmoidal infundibulum*. **i. of frontal sinus** FRONTONASAL DUCT. **i. of heart** CONUS ARTERIOSUS. **i. of hypophysis** INFUNDIBULUM HYPOTHALAMI. **i. hypothalami** [NA] The funnel-shaped, hollow stalk of the posterior lobe of the pituitary gland, extending forward from the rostral tuber cinereum of the hypothalamus. Also *hypophysial stalk, neural stalk, infundibulum of hypophysis, infundibulum of hypothalamus, infundibulum, peduncle of hypophysis* (obs.), *pituitary stalk, infundibular nucleus, infundibular process*. **i. pulmonis** Any of the ductuli alveolares in the substance of the lung. Also *infundibulum of lung*. **i. tubae uterinae** [NA] The funnel-shaped dilatation at the lateral, or abdominal, end of the uterine tube, from the margins of which the fimbriae diverge. Also *infundibulum of uterine tube*. **i. of urinary bladder** FUNDUS VESICAE URINARIAE. **i. of uterine tube** INFUNDIBULUM TUBAE UTERINAE.

**infused** Placed in an aqueous or other suitable solution, as a substance, to extract the soluble portion.

**infusible** **1** Incapable of being melted or fused. **2** Capable of being infused.

**infusion** [L *infusio* (from *infusus*, past part. of *infundere* to pour in or into, impart, instill) a pouring in or into, imparting] **1** The addition of water or other suitable liquid to a substance to obtain an extract of its soluble components. **2** The steeping of a therapeutic agent in order to extract its medicinally active ingredients. **3** The administration of a fluid other than blood into a vein for therapeutic purposes, e.g., the intravenous administration of saline. **4** A solution containing the water-soluble principles of a vegetable drug. Also *infusum*. **5** A solution to be administered intravenously by infusion for therapeutic purposes. **amniotic fluid i.** AMNIOTIC FLUID EMBOLISM. **cold i.** The extraction of a drug or drug source with cold water to obtain the active material. **drop i.** Administration of a medication, such as an intravenous fluid, by slow, drop-by-drop injection. **saline i.** The procedure of introducing saline solution into the body parenterally.

**infusodecoction** \infyoo′zōdikäk′shən\ A preparation containing both a decoction and an infusion of a source of a medicinal material.

**Infusoria** \in′fyəsôr′ē·ə\ [New L (from *infusoria*, neut. pl. of *infusorius*, pertaining to infusions, from L *infus(us)*, past part. of *infundere* to pour into, + *-orius* -ORY)] *Outmoded* CILIATA

**infusum** INFUSION.

**-ing** \-ing\ [Old English *-ing, -ung*, suffix forming gerunds and nouns from verbs] A suffix used to indicate the present participle in verbs and to form nouns and gerunds from verbs with the meaning of an act or result of doing (the action expressed in the verb).

**ingesta** \injes′tə\ [L, neut. pl. of *ingestus*, past part. of *ingerere* to take in] Material that has been swallowed or is intended for swallowing. Also *ingestant*.

**ingestion** \injes′chən\ [Late L *ingestio* (from L *ingerere* to pour in, take in, from *in-* in + *gerere* to carry, perform, do) a taking in] The process of taking materials into the gastrointestinal tract through the mouth.

**Ingrassia** [Giovanni Filippo *Ingrassia*, Italian anatomist, 1510–1580] **1** Apophysis of Ingrassia. See under ALA MINOR OSSIS SPHENOIDALIS. **2** Wings of Ingrassia. See under WINGS OF SPHENOID BONE.

**ingravescent** \ingrəves′ənt\ Becoming more severe.

**ingravidation** \in′grəvidā′shən\ IMPREGNATION.

**ingrowth** A process progressing inward from the surface.

**inguen** \ing′gwen\ [L (akin to Gk *adēn* a gland) the groin, a swelling in the groin] GROIN.

**inguinal** \ing′gwinəl\ Pertaining to the groin, or inguen.

**inguino-** \ing′gwənō-\ [L *inguen*, gen. *inguinis* groin] A combining form denoting the groin.

**inguinoabdominal** \-abdäm′inəl\ Pertaining to or located in the groin and the abdomen.

**inguinocele** \ing′gwinōsel′\ A pathologic swelling found in the groin or inguinal region.

**inguinocrural** \-kroo′rəl\ Pertaining to or located in the groin and the thigh.

**inguinolabial** \-lā′bē·əl\ Pertaining to or located in the groin and the labium majus.

**inguinoscrotal** \-skrō′təl\ Pertaining to or located in the groin and the scrotum.

**INH** A proprietary name for isoniazid.

**inhalant** \inhā′lənt\ An agent or medicinal substance that is administered in a vaporous form into the upper respiratory passages. Also *inhalent.* **antifoaming i.** A medicinal agent administered in the form of a vapor for the purpose of preventing the accumulation of foam in the respiratory passages of patients suffering from pulmonary edema.

**inhalation** \in′həlā′shən\ **1** The process of drawing materials into the lungs through the respiratory passages. **2** An agent suitable for administration through the respiratory passages into the lungs; inhalant. **naphtha i.** Intoxication from inhaling any of various organic solvents. The acute response consists of a brief euphoria, excitement and giddiness, followed by central nervous system depression. **smoke i.** A syndrome that occurs following inhalation of the by-products of combustion. These by-products, besides carbon monoxide are tissue-toxic, and can produce severe respiratory distress and pulmonary damage. Diagnosis can be made from history of closed space fire and elevated carbon monoxide levels. The syndrome is particularly lethal in combination with cutaneous burns, approximately doubling the mortality for burns of any size.

**inhale** [L *in-* in + *halare* to breath, exhale] To draw materials into the lungs through the mouth or nasal passages. Also *inspire.*

**inhalent** INHALANT.

**inhaler** **1** A device to administer medicinal agents in a vapor phase into the respiratory system by inhalation. **2** A mask or face covering that prevents smoke or other particulate matter from entering the respiratory tract by inhalation. It may also be used to protect against breathing cold or damp air.

**inheritance** \inher′itəns\ [Anglo-French *enheritance* (from Old French *enheriter* to designate as heir, from *en-* IN-[1] + *heriter,* from Late L *hereditare* to inherit, from L *heres,* gen. *heredis* an heir) heirship, becoming an heir] **1** The acquisition by offspring of characters transmitted through the parents' genes. Also *transmission.* **2** Those characters which are transmitted from parent to offspring through the genes. **autosomal i.** The transmission of a phenotype determined by a gene located on an autosome. Also *autosomal heredity.* **biparental i.** Transmission to offspring of phenotypes present in both parents. *Seldom used.* **blending i.** The appearance in offspring of phenotypes that appear intermediate in qualitative or quantitative characteristics to those of the parents. Compare MENDELIAN INHERITANCE. **cytoplasmic i.** The transmission of phenotypes, usually found in the mother, that are controlled or determined by genes not part of the nuclear chromosome set. Such phenotypes are characterized by nonsegregation and constancy of the phenotype in backcrosses to the parents. It is due to mitochondrial DNA (in most animals), non-nuclear DNA-containing plasmids, or chloroplast DNA. Also *mitochondrial inheritance, maternal inheritance, extranuclear inheritance, extrachromosomal inheritance, matrilinear inheritance.* **dominant i.** The appearance of a phenotype in relatives who are heterozygous for a mutant allele. Characteristics of this form of transmission of traits are a vertical pattern in a pedigree, with multiple affected generations; an equality of frequency and severity of effect between males and females; a 50 percent chance of transmitting the phenotype from an affected parent to each offspring; and a possibility of cases arising from a sporadic germinal mutation in a parent. A paternal age effect is often demonstrated in sporadic cases. Also *dominant heredity.* **extrachromosomal i.** CYTOPLASMIC INHERITANCE. **extranuclear i.** CYTOPLASMIC INHERITANCE. **galtonian i.** QUANTITATIVE INHERITANCE. **holandric i.** The appearance of a trait, determined at least in part by a gene or genes, that arises only in males. In humans, it is usually due to a locus on the Y chromosome. **hologynic i.** The appearance of a trait, determined at least in part by a gene or genes, that arises only in females. In humans, examples are X-linked dominant traits that are lethal *in utero* in males,

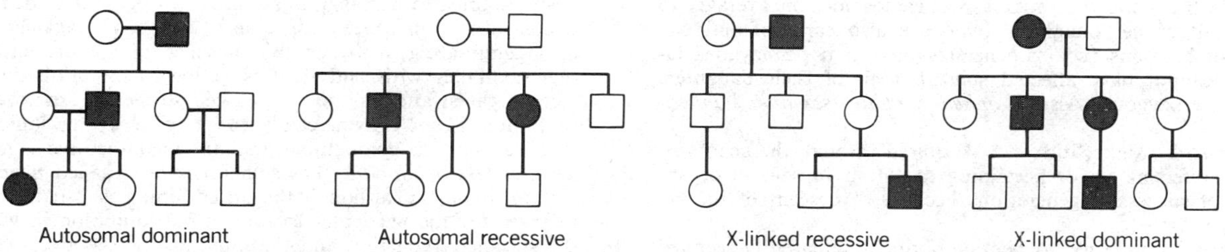


**Major modes of mendelian inheritance** □ Male; ○ female; ■ male exhibiting trait; ● female exhibiting trait.

traits such as hydrometrocolpos which are sex-limited, and structural abnormalities of the X chromosome that result in defective segregation. **maternal i.** CYTOPLASMIC INHERITANCE. **matrilinear i.** CYTOPLASMIC INHERITANCE. **mendelian i.** The transmission of phenotypes from parent to offspring in accordance with mendelian theory. Also *monogenic inheritance, unit inheritance, monofactorial inheritance, particulate inheritance.* Compare BLENDING INHERITANCE. **mitochondrial i.** CYTOPLASMIC INHERITANCE. **monofactorial i.** MENDELIAN INHERITANCE. **monogenic i.** MENDELIAN INHERITANCE. **mosaic i.** In an individual, with respect to a given trait, the transmission of some proportion of the cells with a phenotype determined by a paternal allele and the rest of the cells with a phenotype determined by a maternal allele. This is seen with X-linked traits in mammalian females. **multifactorial i.** **1** The transmission of a phenotype, the presence and nature of which are determined by multiple genes and environmental factors. **2** The transmission of a phenotype that is determined by multiple genes and environmental factors, but that holds to the following empiric rules: the appearance or severity often differs between the sexes; the occurrence is greater in first-degree relatives than in second-degree relatives, which, in turn, is greater than in third-degree relatives; the risk of recurrence in offspring is greater if the affected parent is of the less commonly affected sex; and the average risk of recurrence in offspring approximates the square root of the population prevalence. **particulate i.** MENDELIAN INHERITANCE. **polygenic i.** The transmission of a phenotype that is determined by several, often many, genes. It is an essential component of multifactorial inheritance. **quantitative i.** The transmission of a metrical phenotype, usually one that exhibits continuous variation in the population, such as height. The phenotype is determined by the cumulative and inseparable action of many genes. Also *galtonian inheritance, multiple factor hypothesis.* **quasidominant i.** The transmission of a phenotype through multiple generations of a family in a pattern that is consistent with autosomal dominant inheritance but is in fact due to mating of a homozygous affected individual with a heterozygous carrier of a recessive trait. Such inheritance is rare except when the mutant allele frequency is high or consanguinity is common. **recessive i.** The transmission of a phenotype, determined by a single genetic locus in diploid organisms, that is present only when that locus is homozygous for the responsible allele. **sex-linked i.** **1** The transmission of a phenotype that is determined by one or more loci on one of the sex chromosomes. **2** *Imprecise* X-LINKED INHERITANCE. **unit i.** **1** The transmission of a phenotype that is apparently unaltered through successive generations. **2** MENDELIAN INHERITANCE. **X-linked i.** The transmission of a phenotype that is determined by a gene located on the X chromosome. Characteristics of this form of inheritance are: males are more severely or obviously affected than females; a heterozygous (carrier) female transmits the mutant X-chromosome, on average, to one half of her daughters (who are also carriers) and one half of her sons (who are hemizygous); and hemizygous fathers cannot have affected sons, but all of their daughters are heterozygous. Also *X-linked heredity, sex-linked inheritance.*

**inherited** \inher′itid\ **1** Acquired through the genotype. **2** Of, referring to, or pertaining to a trait present in organisms of successive generations because of descent of the genotype.

**inhibin** \inhib′in\ A peptide hormone apparently secreted by the Sertoli cells of the seminiferous tubules of the testis and acting to suppress or inhibit the release of anterior pituitary follicle-stimulating hormone (FSH). Loss of inhibin secretion presumably accounts for the raised FSH secretion observed in disorders of the testis associated with tubular destruction, such as the Klinefelter syndrome and myotonic muscular dystrophy.

**inhibit** \inhib′it\ To restrain or suppress.

**inhibiter** \inhib′itər\ INHIBITOR.

**inhibition** \in′hibish′ən\ [L *inhibitio* (from *inhibitus,* past part. of *inhibere* to hold in, hold back, restrain, from *in-* in + *habere* to have, hold) a restraining] **1** The diminishing or total suppression of a function or activity of the nervous system. **2** In chemistry, the phenomenon whereby certain substances can slow or stop a reaction. **3** Unconscious restriction of an impulse or its manifestations. **4** A restriction or suppression of thought or behavior not dependent on any known neural mechanism. **allogeneic i.** A phenomenon in which the interaction of lymphocytes differing at the major histocompatibility locus depresses the reactivity of the lymphocytes to other antigens. **allosteric i.** Inhibition of an enzyme by an allosteric effector. The flux through many reaction pathways is controlled by allosteric inhibition of an enzyme early in the pathway by the final product of the pathway. **antidromic i.** RECURRENT INHIBITION. **autogenous i.** A reflex inhibition taking place at the point of stimulation. **central i.** The suppression of excitation of the neurons within the central nervous system. **competitive i.** Enzyme inhibition in which the inhibitor raises the Michaelis constant ($K^m$) without affecting the limiting rate ($V$) of the catalyzed reaction that is approached at high substrate concentration. The inhibition is said to have a competitive component if the inhibitor diminishes $V/K^m$. The simplest mechanism proposed for competitive inhibition is that the inhibitor and substrate compete for the same site on the enzyme, which cannot bind both at once. **contact i.** **1** A cessation of the increase in cell numbers when the population density allows physical contact between cells. Also *density-dependent inhibition.* **2** A cessation of movement of cells and inhibition of the undulatory behavior of the lamellipodia when two cells in a culture come into contact. **end-product i.** Inhibition of a process by the final product that it forms. In metabolic sequences, end-product inhibition is usually exerted on the first step of the sequence. **enzyme i.** The suppression of enzyme activity by the reversible, and usually noncovalent, binding of a substance to the enzyme. **feedback i.** Inhibition of a step in a pathway by a product of that pathway. This provides a mechanism for controling the rate of a metabolic pathway. **fertility i.** Decreased formation of sex pili by cells carrying the F factor, when superinfected with an R factor forming a repressor with the same specificity. R factors are thus classified into $fi^+$ and $fi^-$. **hemagglutination i.** An immunologic procedure capable of demonstrating the presence of either an antigen or antibody, employing as its end point the inhibition of previously established hemagglutination. It can be used to demonstrate the presence of an antibody against a hemagglutinating virus, or the presence of soluble antigen that combines with and inhibits action of an antibody directed against antigens on the red cell surface. **mixed i.** Inhibition of an enzyme-catalyzed reaction by an inhibitor that has both a competitive and an uncompetitive component. • *Mixed inhibition* has sometimes been called *noncompetitive inhibition,* although the latter term has usually been reserved for the particular case of mixed inhibition in which the specificity constant and the limiting velocity are lowered by the same factor. **motor i.** A suppression of motor activity; a state of persistent reduction in motor activity resulting in immobility, weakness, or diminished speed of execution of movements and actions. This must be differentiated from fading, in which there is progressive diminution followed by total cessation of the movement, and from bradykinesia, which is simply an abnormal slowness of movement. **noncompetitive i.** 1 See under MIXED INHIBITION. 2 Inhibition of an enzyme-catalyzed reaction in which the inhibitor diminishes the limiting rate ($V$) that the reaction approaches at high substrate concentration without affecting the Michaelis constant ($K_m$). This type of inhibition is rare. **potassium i.** Cardiac arrest as a result of potassium infusion. **proactive i.** The inhibiting effect of prior learning on material to be learned later. This effect is found especially in studies of verbal learning. The rate of learning is faster for elements appearing early in a sequence to be mastered than for those coming later. **reciprocal i.** Suppression of excitability of the motor neurons or reflex responses of one muscle or synergist group when an antagonist muscle is reflexly facilitated. The classic example is the inhibition of activity in a flexor when a stretch reflex is elicited in an antagonist extensor muscle. **recurrent i.** The reduction of neuron discharge via a feedback circuit involving axon collaterals that excite interneurons, e.g., Renshaw cells, which provide inhibitory control. Also *Renshaw inhibition, antidromic inhibition.* **reflex i.** A consistent negative response to a stimulus involving two or more neurons, especially muscle relaxation or a reduction of impulse discharge. **Renshaw i.** RECURRENT INHIBITION. **retroactive i.** The inhibition of recall of something once learned by the action of something learned later, especially if there is a degree of similarity between the learned elements. **substrate i.** The phenomenon of decrease in the rate of an enzyme-catalyzed reaction with increasing concentration of substrate. Such a decrease may occur at high substrate concentrations after the usual increase of rate with concentration at lower values of the concentration. **uncompetitive i.** Enzyme inhibition in which the inhibitor diminishes to the same degree both the limiting rate ($V$) of the catalyzed reaction that is approached at high substrate concentration and the Michaelis constant ($K^m$) for the substrate. Inhibition is said to have an uncompetitive component when the inhibitor diminishes $V$. **Wedensky i.** A nerve conduction block resulting from previous high frequency electrical stimulation.

**inhibitor** \inhib′itər\ 1 Anything that causes inhibition. 2 Denoting a neuron which inhibits the activity of the organ or structure which it innervates. 3 In biochemistry, any substance that diminishes the rate of an enzymatic reaction, such as competitive inhibitors, noncompetitive inhibitors, or allosteric inhibitors. Also *inhibiter.* **ACE i.** ANGIOTENSIN CONVERTING ENZYME INHIBITOR. **active-site-directed irreversible i.** An inhibitor of an enzyme-catalyzed reaction that binds to the active site of the enzyme, usually because it is similar in properties to the natural substrate, and there reacts with the enzyme irreversibly. **aldosterone i.** A drug or medicinal agent capable of inhibiting or antagonizing the effects of aldosterone on the renal tubules of the nephron. **angiotensin converting enzyme i.** Any of a class of drugs that inhibit the enzyme kininase II (dipeptidyl carboxypeptidase). Inhibition of kininase II results in decreased formation of angiotensin II and also results in decreased breakdown of bradykinin. Drugs in this class are used in the treatment of hypertension and congestive heart failure. Also *ACE inhibitor.* **C1-i.** A stoichiometric inhibitor of C1 and of a number of other serine proteases, including plasmin, kallikrein, and factors XIIa and XIa of the clotting system. It is the only inhibitor of C1 in plasma. Heterozygous deficiency of C1-inhibitor is associated with hereditary angioedema. **cholesterol i.** A drug or agent capable of inhibiting the synthesis of cholesterol and reducing its concentration in the blood. **competitive i.** A substance that inhibits an enzyme reversibly by binding to it in competition with the substrate, since the enzyme cannot bind both substrate and inhibitor simultaneously. The degree of inhibition is therefore diminished as the substrate concentration is increased. Such inhibitors are usually substrate analogues that bind to the enzyme at the substrate-binding site. **irreversible i.** An inhibitor of an enzyme-catalyzed reaction whose effect is not reversed by removing unreacted inhibitor from the enzyme. Although this may sometimes be due to very tight binding, so that no dissociation can normally be observed, it is more often due to an irreversible reaction that leads to a covalent compound between enzyme and inhibitor. **noncompetitive i.** A substance that inhibits an enzyme reversible in such a way that the degree of inhibition is independent of the concentration of substrate. **reversible i.** An inhibitor of an enzyme-catalyzed reaction whose action is reversed by removing the inhibitor. It acts by binding to the enzyme, but the binding is reversible, so that lowering the concentration of free inhibitor allows dissociation to regenerate unligated, active enzyme.

**inhomogeneity** \in′hō′məjənē′itē\ 1 The property of being inhomogeneous. 2 The difference between one part of inhomogeneous material and others. 3 A part that so differs.

**inhomogeneous** \in′hō′məjē′nē·əs\ Possessing differences between its different parts. In an inhomogeneous substance, the molecules differ, so that the substance is not a pure compound.

**iniad** \in′ē·ad\ Toward the inion.

**inial** \in′ē·əl\ Pertaining to the inion.

**iniencephaly** \in′ē·ensef′əlē\ [Gk *ini(on)* back of the head, nape of the neck + ENCEPHAL- + -Y] A developmental defect in which the occipital part of the cranium and upper spinal regions fail to close about the neural tube, thus permitting exposure of brain and cord tissue. The condition often involves extreme retroflection of the head combined with variable degrees of cervical rachischisis.

**inion** \in′ē·än\ [Gk *inion* (dim. of *is,* gen. *inos,* strength, a nerve, sinew, muscle) the sinews between occiput and back, the back of the head, nape of the neck] [NA] The most prominent point of the external occipital protuberance in the midline, used in craniometry.

**iniopagus** \in′ē·äp′əgəs\ [Gk *inio(n)* the back of the head + -PAGUS] A pair of equal conjoined twins with union at the occipital region.

**initiation** \inish′ē·ā′shən\ The initial carcinogenic event in a tissue or cell caused by a tumor-producing substance.

**inject** To instill or infuse (a fluid) into an artery, vein, organ, body cavity, or tissue region.

**injectable** 1 Suitable for injection. 2 A preparation of a drug or agent designed to be given by injection.

**injection** [L *injectio* (from *in(j)icere* to throw in, lay on, introduce, infuse, inject, from *in-* in + *jacere* to throw) the act of throwing in, infusing, injecting] 1 The administration of a medicinal or nutritional substance into the subcutaneous tissue, muscular tissue, the veins, or one of the body canals or orifices, such as the vagina, rectum, or urethra. Also *injectio.* 2 A condition of visible hyperemia, as *conjunctival injection.* **adrenal cortex i.** An aqueous solution containing the active principles of the adrenal cortex steroids. It was formerly used for the treatment of Addison's disease, but it has been superseded by hydrocortisone and other preparations of adrenal steroids. **anatomical i.**

The injection of one of several formulae of special fluids, and occasionally dyes, into vessels, cavities, or organs of a cadaver so as to preserve the body for dissection or to facilitate demonstration. **coarse i.** An anatomic injection that involves only the large vessels. **depot i.** An injection of a medical agent in a vehicle that causes slow release of the substance from the injection site over a prolonged interval. **dextrose i.** A sterile solution of dextrose in water suitable for parenteral administration of dextrose as a nutrient or as fluid replacement. **endermic i.** INTRADERMAL INJECTION. **epifascial i.** A procedure in which liquid is forced through a needle into a fascial plane. **fine i.** An anatomic injection that reaches the smallest vessels. **fructose i.** A sterile solution of fructose in water given parenterally for nutritional needs or fluid replacement. **gelatin i.** An anatomic injection in which gelatin forms the basic ingredient in order to prevent the tissues from becoming too hard. **hypodermic i.** SUBCUTANEOUS INJECTION. **insulin i.** A sterile, neutralized solution of the active principle of the pancreatic islet cells that affects the metabolism of glucose. It acts promptly as a hypoglycemic agent in the treatment of diabetes mellitus. Also *neutral insulin, regular insulin.* **intradermal i.** An injection into the corium, or substance of the skin. Also *endermic injection, intracutaneous injection, intradermic injection.* **intramuscular i.** An injection made into the body of a muscle. **intrathecal i.** An injection into the subarachnoid space, as of gas, contrast material, anesthetic agent, or medication. **intravascular i.** An injection made directly into a blood vessel. **iron-dextran i.** A sterile, colloidal solution of ferric hydroxide and low molecular weight dextrans suitable for parenteral administration of iron. Also *iron dextran complex.* **iron sorbitex i.** A sterile, brown, colloidal solution composed of a complex of ferric iron, sorbitol, and citric acid. It is stabilized with dextran and sorbitol. It is used as a parenteral form of iron for the treatment of iron deficiency anemia where oral treatment is not possible or is ineffective. **jet i.** The injection of a drug through the skin by a very fine jet of solution under high pressure. **lactated Ringer's i.** A sterile solution containing calcium chloride, potassium chloride, sodium chloride, and sodium lactate in water for parenteral infusion to replenish fluid and electrolyte loss. Also *Ringer's lactate.* **oxytocin i.** A clear, sterile, aqueous solution containing the active principle of the posterior pituitary, which may be prepared from domestic animals or by synthesis. It is used to stimulate uterine contractions and for the control of postpartum hemorrhage. **parathyroid i.** A sterile aqueous solution containing the water-soluble principles obtained from bovine parathyroid glands. It is administered parenterally to maintain normal levels of calcium in the blood. Also *parathyroid extract, parathyroid solution.* **parenchymatous i.** An injection made into the substance of an organ. **posterior pituitary i.** A sterile aqueous solution containing the water-soluble principles of the posterior lobe of the pituitary gland from domestic animals. It is administered parenterally for its oxytocic properties and the treatment of diabetes insipidus. Also *pituitary solution, posterior pituitary solution, liquor pituitarii posterii.* **preservative i.** An anatomic injection that preserves the cadaver or any specimen and prevents decomposition. **protamine sulfate i.** A sterile solution of protamine sulfate in sodium chloride injection. It is used to neutralize the anticoagulant effect of heparin and prevent hemorrhage from heparin overdosage. **protein hydrolysate i.** A sterile solution of amino acids and small peptides derived by hydrolysis of casein, lactalbumin, or other suitable protein sources. It is used as a parenteral nutrient replacement for oral protein intake. **repository i.** The injection of a medication in a formulation that permits slow absorption and a prolonged drug effect. **Ringer's i.** A sterile solution containing sodium chloride, potassium chloride, and calcium chloride in water. It is used parenterally to replace fluid and electrolyte loss. **sclerosing i.** The injection into a blood vessel, usually a varicose vein, of a substance which causes obliteration of the vessel. See also INJECTION SCLEROTHERAPY. **sodium chloride i.** A sterile, isotonic aqueous solution of sodium chloride. It is used as a parenteral injection to replace the loss of fluid and electrolytes, and as a vehicle for the administration of other therapeutic agents. **subcutaneous i.** An injection into the loose connective tissue beneath the skin using a needle or syringe. Also *hypodermic injection.* **Teflon i. of vocal cord** The injection of a measured amount of Teflon paste lateral to the conus elasticus in cases of unilateral abduction of the vocal cord and imperfect glottic closure, the object being to compel the affected cord towards the midline. **trigger point i.** Infiltration of trigger points with local anesthetics and/or cortisone to relieve muscle spasm. **vasopressin i.** A sterile, aqueous solution containing the pressor principle of the posterior pituitary. It is prepared from the glands of domestic animals or from synthetic material. It is used as a diuretic medication.

**injector** An instrument, such as a syringe, used to inject solutions into body organs or tissues. **jet i.** A high-pressure syringelike apparatus used to instill doses of drugs hypodermically without using a needle to puncture the skin.

**injure** [back-formation from *injury.* See INJURY.] To harm or hurt; disrupt the integrity or function of a tissue or organ by external, usually mechanical, means.

**injury** [L *injuria* (from *in-* not + *jus,* gen. *juris,* justice, right, law) a thing done unjustly, injury] A disruption of the integrity or function of a tissue or organ by external means, which are usually mechanical but can also be chemical, electrical, thermal, or radiant. **air-blast i.** An injury caused by the rapid expansion of air. Common examples include explosions and direct injection of compressed air into the body in industrial accidents. **atmospheric blast i.** An injury resulting from rapid changes in pressure of the ambient air, as in an explosion. It may also result from sudden decompression, as in high altitude aircraft accidents. **birth i.** Bodily damage suffered by an infant as a result of the birth process. **blunt i.** A mechanical injury produced by the impact of a blunt instrument that tears, shears, or crushes tissue in contrast to an incision injury. The three basic forms are lacerations, contusions, and abrasions. **bucket-handle i.** BUCKET-HANDLE TEAR. **bumper i.** BUMPER FRACTURE. **closed head i.** An injury to the brain without an associated skull fracture. **cold i.** An injury resulting when the circulation of a part is insufficient to protect the cells from damage by a cold environment. The severity of the injury is proportional to the adequacy of the circulation in relation to the temperature of the environment. If the environment is wet, trench foot results, or if dry, frostbite results. **compression i.** CRUSH INJURY. **contrecoup i.** An injury caused by a blow to the brain but found on the side opposite the blow. The blow starts the brain in motion and momentum is stopped by the opposite side of the skull, creating damage to the brain at that opposite point. Although such lesions can occur in a fluid-filled organ, a contrecoup other than to the brain is quite rare. Also *counterstroke, contrecoup contusion.* **coup i. of brain** Contusion or laceration of the brain substance underlying the point of impact upon the skull.

**coup-contrecoup i.** Contusion or laceration of the brain substance both on the side of the impact and on the opposite side. **crush i.** A tissue or organ injury caused by severe squeezing or pressure. The squeezing may be purely mechanical or it may be due to sudden expansion of liquid or gas, as in an explosion or the passage of a high-velocity missile. The damage is not usually evident immediately or at the time of initial examination. Intense swelling occurs in the crushed part, and unless compartments are decompressed, further tissue damage may occur from vascular compromise. Also *compression injury.* **deceleration i.** An injury that occurs when there is a sudden deceleration and stopping of a moving vehicle, as in an automobile or aircraft crash. The magnitude of the injury is related to the deceleration force to which the individual is subjected. The force is directly proportional to the square of the vehicle speed and inversely proportional to the stopping distance. The most serious of these is traumatic rupture of the thoracic aorta at the point where the arch meets the descending aorta. **high-explosive i.** An injury caused by the sudden change in atmospheric pressure resulting from the instantaneous reaction of unstable compounds. The injuries result both from the blast and from flying debris. Also *shell injury.* **hyperextension-hyperflexion i.** An injury to a joint caused by forcibly moving the joint beyond its normal range. See also WHIPLASH INJURY. **immersion blast i.** A blast injury caused by an underwater explosion from a mine or depth charge to anyone in the water near the explosion. Because water is not compressible the shock wave is transmitted over long distances with almost undiminished force. Such injuries may be more severe than those caused by comparable explosions transmitted through the atmosphere. **internal i.** Injury to organs or tissues within body cavities. **neonatal cold i.** The effect of hypothermia in the newborn infant. There is gradually increasing lethargy and failure to feed. The body temperature falls below 32°C (89.6°F), leading to hardening of the subcutaneous tissue of the buttocks and thighs (sclerema), although the face remains misleadingly rosy. The blood sugar is low. Treatment requires slow rewarming, but the mortality is high. **occupational i.** An injury which arises out of and in the course of work. In some countries, injuries received traveling to and from work or occurring at the place of work outside working hours are also classified as occupational for purposes of claiming compensation. **open head i.** An injury to the brain associated with a fracture of the skull, especially with compound or depressed fractures or with indriven fragments of bone, hair, or foreign material. **patterned i.** A wound, most commonly resulting from blunt force, in which an impression of the wound-producing instrument's surface remains on the skin. **shell i.** HIGH-EXPLOSIVE INJURY. **soft tissue i.** Any injury to muscle, fascia, tendon, ligament, skin, fat, or other nonosseous, noncartilaginous tissue of the body. **steering wheel i.** An injury to the anterior chest wall and/or the mediastinal contents resulting from forcible contact with the steering wheel of a motor vehicle during sudden deceleration. **straddle i.** An injury to the perineum and/or the pelvis caused by a fall directly onto the perineum. Injury results because the force of the fall is not dispersed through the lower extremities. **vital i.** In forensic medicine, an antemortem injury occurring at a sufficient interval prior to death to initiate tissue and organ reactions such as hemorrhage, coagulation, inflammation, swelling, and initial or partial healing of the injured tissue. **whiplash i.** Injury to the soft tissues (muscles and ligaments) supporting the cervical spine, usually in the area of the third and fourth cervical vertebrae (C-3 and C-4). It is usually caused by sudden hyperextension of the neck in a rear-end motor vehicle collision as the supported body is accelerated and the unsupported head initially remains stationary. The head reaches the end of its travel and then snaps forward, doing further damage. Objective assessment of injury is difficult, and such injuries are a frequent cause of legitimate as well as spurious claims for damages following such accidents. **wringer i.** An injury, usually to an extremity, in which there is an avulsion of the skin from its blood supply as might be caused by the extremity being drawn through a wringer.

**inlay** [IN-[1] + *lay*] A restoration, made out of the mouth to fit in a prepared tooth cavity and fixed in place by a thin layer of dental cement. An inlay is usually made of cast gold alloy, but fused porcelain has also been used. **bone i.** The grafting of bone into a slot or gutter. **epithelial i.** INLAY GRAFT. **skin graft i.** INLAY GRAFT.

**inlet** A space or passage leading into a cavity. **pelvic i.** APERTURA PELVIS SUPERIOR. **thoracic i.** **1** The superior mediastinum and the base of the neck, through which pass the great brachiocephalic vessels. **2** APERTURA THORACIS SUPERIOR.

**INN** International Nonproprietary Names.

**innate** \inātʹ\ [L *innat(us)* (past part. of *innasci* to be born or spring up in a place) inborn, innate] Inborn; hereditary.

**innervate** \inʹərvāt\ To supply with nerve fibers or a nerve stimulus, as to a neuron, muscle, or gland.

**innervation** \inʹərvāʹshən\ [L *in-* in + NERVE + -ATION] The distribution of nerve fibers or a neural stimulus to a neuron, muscle, or gland. **double i.** Nerve fiber distribution from two distinct sources, such as autonomic innervation by sympathetic and parasympathetic axons or a muscle by two nerves of differing origin. **multiple i.** The presence of more than one motor endplate on a given muscle fiber. **plurisegmental i.** Innervation of a single structure, such as a muscle, by two or more consecutive segments of the spinal cord. **polyneuronal i.** Innervation by more than one neuron, as is characteristic of ordinary muscle fibers at one stage in the development of a mammal, and of intrafusal muscle fibers in the adult. **reciprocal i.** Innervation of muscle antagonist pairs whereby the agonist is excited and its antagonist inhibited to achieve synchronized contraction and relaxation. Also *Sherrington's law.*

**innidiation** \inidʹē·āʹshən\ [IN-[1] + L *nid(us)* nest + *i* + -ATION] The growth and proliferation of cells in a region of the body to which they have been transported in a metastatic process.

**innocent** Not inherently harmful; benign.

**innominate** \inämʹināt\ [Late L *innominat(us)* (from L *in-* IN-[2] + *nominatus,* past part. of *nominare* to name, from *nomen* a name) unnamed, nameless] Nameless or unnamed: applied to certain anatomic structures.

**innominatum** \inämʹināʹtəm\ (*pl.* innominata) OS COXAE.

**innoxious** \inäkʹshəs\ Safe; harmless.

**Ino** Symbol for the nucleoside inosine.

**ino-** \inʹō-\ [Gk *is,* gen. *ino(s)* sinew, tendon, fiber] A combining form denoting (1) fiber, fibrous tissue; (2) muscle fibers, muscle; (3) fibrin, fibrinous coagulation. • In oncology *ino-* has been combined with a variety of terms to indicate combinations of fibrous tissue with the other tumor elements, as in *inomycoma, inomyxoma, inoneuroma, inoleiomyoma, inoglioma,* and *inochondroma.* All are obsolete.

**inocula** \inäkʹyələ\ Plural of INOCULUM.

**inoculate** \inäkʹyəlāt\ [See INOCULATION.] **1** To introduce microorganisms into (culture media, tissue culture, on animal, soil, etc.) for the purposes of growth and identification of the organism. **2** To introduce infectious material or noninfectious antigenic material parenterally into (the body) in order to stimulate a protective immune response.

**inoculation** \inäk′yəlā′shən\ [L *inoculatio* (from *inoculare* to implant a bud into, from *oculus* an eye, a bud used in grafting plants) bud implantation] Introduction of a microorganism or other antigenic material into an organism or a culture medium, usually in order to stimulate a protective immune response or to study the cultured substance.

**inoculative** \inäk′yəlā′tiv\ Pertaining to or done by inoculation: said especially of the mode of transmission of an infective agent or a venom, as by the sting or bite of an animal.

**inoculum** \inäk′yələm\ [New L, from *inocul(are)* to inoculate + *-um,* noun suffix] **1** The substance inoculated into culture or into an experimental animal. **2** A substance injected into an organism by natural means, as by a mosquito bite or a bee sting.

**inocyte** \in′ōsīt\ [INO- + -CYTE] FIBROBLAST.

**inogenesis** \-jen′əsis\ Fibrous tissue formation.

**inogenous** \inäj′ənəs\ Derived from or producing fibrous tissue.

**inoperable** \inäp′ərəbl\ [IN-[2] + OPERABLE] Describing a disease or condition, or a stage thereof, that would not be improved by surgical intervention.

**inopexia** \-pek′sē·ə\ A tendency to accelerated coagulation; a hypercoagulable state. *Seldom used.* Adj. inopectic.

**inorganic** \in′ôrgan′ik\ **1** Denoting compounds that do not contain carbon-carbon and carbon-hydrogen bonds. **2** Denoting the chemistry of inorganic compounds.

**inosculate** \inäs′kyəlāt\ [IN-[1] + *oscul(um)* + -ATE] To link by small openings; anastomose.

**inosculation** \inäs′kyəlā′shən\ [*inosculat(e)* + -ION] ANASTOMOSIS.

**inose** INOSITOL.

**inosemia** \-sē′mē·ə\ The presence of inositol in blood.

**inosine** \in′ōsin\ A nucleoside resulting from the deamination of adenosine.

**inosinic acid** Inosine 5′-phosphate. It can be formed from adenylic acid by biologic deamination with release of ammonia, or by deamination *in vitro* with nitrous acid.

**inosite** INOSITOL.

**inositide** Any of various compounds of inositol, usually a lipid such as phosphatidylinositol.

**inositol** $C_6H_{12}O_6$. The compound formed by a ring of six —CHOH— groups. It is found combined in phospholipids, e.g. as phosphatidylinositol. The main isomer found naturally is *myo*-inositol, which has the two hydroxyl groups on C-4 and C-6 on the opposite side of the plane of the ring from the other four. Its biosynthesis is as its 1-phosphate, which is formed by cyclization of glucose 6-phosphate with inversion at C-5 of the glucose residue (C-2 of the inositol residue). Its hexaphosphate is phytic acid. Also *inose, inosite, antialopecia factor, mouse antialopecia factor.*

**inositol niacinate** $C_{42}H_{30}N_6O_{12}$. *myo*-Inositol hexa-3-pyrimidinecarboxylate. A polyester of inositol and nicotinic acid. It has been used therapeutically as a peripheral vasodilator in the treatment of peripheral vascular disease. It is given orally.

**inosituria** \-sit$^y$oo′rē·ə\ [*inosit(ol)* + -URIA] The appearance of inosinic acid in the urine of a subject in shock. Also *inosuria.*

**inostosis** \in′ästō′sis\ [IN-[1] + OST- + -OSIS ] The re-formation of bone in an area of damage.

**inosuria** \-soo′rē·ə\ INOSITURIA.

**inotropic** \-träp′ik\ [INO- + -TROPIC[1]] Affecting the force or speed of muscular contraction either by enhancing or inhibiting it.

**inpatient** \in′pāshənt\ [*in* + PATIENT] **1** An individual admitted to a health care institution, usually for a period including at least one overnight stay. **2** Pertaining to or serving inpatients. Compare OUTPATIENT.

**input** Anything that is put into a system, such as data into a computer, a signal into an amplifier, or a stimulus into an animal.

**inquest** \in′kwest\ [Late L *inquesta* (from *inquesta,* past part. of *inquirere* to search into, from L *in* into + *quaerere* to search) a searching into] CORONER'S INQUEST. **coroner's i.** A judicial inquiry, convened by a coroner and usually conducted before a jury, into the manner of death of an individual whose death occurred suddenly under suspicious, unusual, or violent circumstances. The performance of forensic autopsies has greatly reduced the need for inquests. In many jurisdictions, however, it remains a legal requirement that all deaths in penal institutions, foster homes, mental institutions, etc. be subjected to an inquest. Also *inquest.*

**inquisition** \in′kwizish′ən\ [L *inquisitio* (from *inquisitus,* past part. of *inquirere* to seek for, examine) an inquiry] Any judicial inquiry, particularly one made to determine mental competence.

**insaccation** \in′sakā′shən\ The condition of being surrounded by a sac.

**insane** \insān′\ [L *insan(us)* (from *in-* not + *sanus* sound, sane) not well, diseased in mind, insane] Of or pertaining to unsoundness of mind or insanity. • The term is no longer used in psychiatry except in legal contexts. **i. on arraignment** Designating an individual found incompetent to stand trial by reason of mental disorder or legal insanity. A term used only in the U.S. Also *unfit to plead* (British and New Zealand usage). **criminally i.** Describing a person who has committed a crime and who suffers or did at the time suffer mental illness of enough severity to reduce or abolish responsibility for his action: a legal or judicial finding.

**insanity** \insan′itē\ [L *insanitas* (from *insan(us)* insane + *-itas* -ITY) insanity] As determined by a court of law, a mental disorder of such a nature or degree as to interfere with the subject's capacity to discharge his legal responsibilities. **affective i.** *Obs.* AFFECTIVE PSYCHOSIS. **alcoholic i.** *Outmoded* ALCOHOLIC PSYCHOSIS. **collective i.** SHARED DELUSION. **communicated i.** SHARED DELUSION. **criminal i.** The state of mind resulting from a mental defect or disorder and which was present when an individual committed a crime and rendered him unable to understand the wrongfulness of his conduct or to conform his conduct to the requirements of the law. **degenerative i.** *Obs.* SENILE DEMENTIA. **double i.** FOLIE À DEUX. **doubting i.** FOLIE DU DOUTE. **imposed i.** SHARED DELUSION. **induced i.** SHARED DELUSION. **intermittent i.** *Obs.* MANIC-DEPRESSIVE PSYCHOSIS. **manic-depressive i.** *Obs.* MANIC-DEPRESSIVE PSYCHOSIS. **partial i.** In the legal system, a mental disorder that limits the subject's responsibility for his actions but which is not severe enough to render him totally free of responsibility. **periodic i.** *Obs.* MANIC-DEPRESSIVE PSYCHOSIS. **puerperal i.** POSTPARTUM PSYCHOSIS. **recurrent i.** *Obs.* MANIC-DEPRESSIVE PSYCHOSIS. **senile i.** SENILE DEMENTIA. **simultaneous i.** FOLIE À DEUX. **toxic i.** A state of mental confusion due to the ingestion of an animal poison or plant poison, alcohol, opium, heroin, cocaine, or other hallucinogenic agent. It may also be precipitated by drug withdrawal or certain metabolic disorders.

**inscriptio** \inskrip′shē·ō\ [L (from *inscribere* to inscribe, from *in-* into, on + *scribere* to mark, trace, write) an inscription, marking] (*pl.* inscriptiones) INSCRIPTION. **i. tendinea** INTERSECTIO TENDINEA. **inscriptiones tendineae musculi recti abdominis** INTERSECTIONES TENDINEAE MUSCULI RECTI ABDOMINIS.

**inscription** [L *inscriptio*. See INSCRIPTIO.] **1** The main section of a prescription, in which are listed the drug ingredients and the amounts of each to be compounded. **2** A mark or line. Also *inscriptio*. **tendinous i.** INTERSECTIO TENDINEA. **tendinous i.'s of rectus abdominis muscle** INTERSECTIONES TENDINEAE MUSCULI RECTI ABDOMINIS.

**insect** [L *insectum* (from *insectus* indented, incised, from *insecare* to incise, from *in-* into + *secare* to cut, divide) an insect or similar arthropod; translation of Gk *entomon*. See ENTOMO-.] A member of the class Insecta.

**Insecta** \insek′tə\ [pl. of L *insectum*. See INSECT.] A class of arthropods, the largest group of animals known, whose members have three pairs of jointed legs and are characteristically divided into three anatomical portions: head, thorax, and abdomen. Many members are parasitic and others serve as intermediate hosts for human and animal pathogens.

**insecticide** \insek′tisīd\ [INSECT + *i* + -CIDE] Any substance that kills insects. Insecticides are widely used in agriculture to increase crop production and in disease control. Many are highly toxic and can give rise to hazardous exposures in both occupational and nonoccupational situations. The toxic dose and clinical picture vary with the compound. • By U.S. statute, an *insecticide* is "any substance or mixture of substances intended for preventing, destroying, repelling, or mitigating any insects which may be present in the environment whatsoever." It thus embraces a broader range of effect than that employed in ordinary usage.

**insectifuge** \insek′tifyooj\ An insect repellent.

**insectivore** \insek′tivôr\ [INSECT + *i* + English *-vore*, combining form from L *vorare* to swallow, devour] **1** Any organism that feeds on insects. **2** Any member of the order Insectivora such as shrews, moles, and hedgehogs.

**insectivorous** \in′sektiv′ərəs\ [*insectivor(e)* + -OUS] Characterized by a diet of insects.

**insectology** \in′sektäl′əjē\ [INSECT + *o* + -LOGY] ENTOMOLOGY.

**insemination** \insem′inā′shən\ [L *insemin(are)* (from *in-* in + *seminare* to sow, plant, beget, from *semen* seed, sperm) to implant, impregnate + -ATION] The deposit of semen in the female genital tract. Also *semination*. **artificial i.** Introduction of semen into the female genital tract by means of a suitably designed instrument. Also *artificial fecundation, artificial impregnation*. **donor i.** Artificial insemination utilizing semen from a male other than the female's husband. Also *heterologous insemination*. Abbr. A.I.D.

**insenescence** \in′senes′əns\ The condition of growing old without the usual signs of aging. Adj. insenescent.

**insensible** \insen′sibəl\ **1** UNCONSCIOUS. **2** Without the awareness of the senses.

**insert** \(1,3) insurt′; (2) in′surt\ [L *insertus* (past part. of *inserere* to put, bring, or introduce into, insert, mix, connect) put, brought, or introduced into] **1** To put in or implant. **2** Something that is put in or implanted. **3** To attach, as a tendon to a bone. **package i.** The labeling included with a prescription drug shipped to the pharmacist by the manufacturer and which may be required by law in certain jurisdictions to contain specific types of information.

**insertio** \insur′shō\ [L, from *insertus*. See INSERT.] INSERTION.

**insertion** [L *insertio*. See INSERTIO.] The more movable attachment of a muscle during the principal action of that muscle, usually the distal end of a muscle's attachment to a bone and the point on which the force of a muscle is applied. Also *insertio*. **parasol i.** Separation of the umbilical vessel some distance from the center of the placenta so that they spread out like the ribs of an umbrella or parasol. **velamentous i.** The attachment of the umbilical cord to the placenta so that the umbilical vessels ramify some distance from the placental margin and diverge on the chorion before reaching the substance of the placenta.

**insidious** \insid′ē·əs\ Denoting the progression of a disease process that gives little or no symptomatic indication of its severity.

**insight** In psychiatry, awareness and acknowledgment that one's symptoms or complaints represent some disorder or abnormality, and some degree of understanding of the relationship between probable causes or predisposing factors and the ensuing dysfunction.

***in situ*** \in sī′too, sit′oo\ [L, from *in* in + *situ*, ablative of *situs* place. See SITUS.] **1** In its original or normal position. **2** Not invasive: applied especially to carcinomas which have not invaded beyond their original epithelial confines.

**insolation** \in′sōlā′shən\ [L *insolatio* (from *insolatus*, past part. of *insolare* to place in the sun, from *in-* IN-[1] + *sol* the sun) a placing in the sun] SUNSTROKE. **hyperpyrexial i.** *Obs.* SUNSTROKE.

**insoluble** \insäl′yəbl\ Not capable of being dissolved in the solvent medium under consideration.

**insomnia** \insäm′nē·ə\ [L (from *insomnis* sleepless, from *in-* not + *somnus* sleep) sleeplessness] A sleep disorder in which the individual is unable to initiate or to maintain sleep. Also *hyposomnia, sleeplessness, agrypnia* (seldom used), *anhypnia* (obs.), *asomnia* (obs.).

**inspection** Careful visual examination, as of the body or a part.

**inspersion** \inspur′zhən\ The sprinkling around of a liquid or the scattering about of a powder.

**inspiration** The act or process of breathing in; in humans, the taking in of air into the lungs as part of the process of respiration. **crowing i.** INSPIRATORY STRIDOR.

**inspirator** A respirator or inhaler.

**inspire** INHALE.

**inspissant** \inspis′ənt\ Any agent that decreases the liquidity of a body fluid by extracting water.

**inspissate** \inspis′āt\ [Late L *inspissare* (from L *in-*, intensive prefix, + *spissare* to thicken, from *spissus* dense, thick) to thicken] To bring about a decreased liquidity in (a body fluid) by the extraction of water.

**instep** The highest part of the medial longitudinal arch on the dorsum of the foot.

**instillation** \in′stilā′shən\ The delivery of a liquid, drop-by-drop, into some body cavity or part.

**instillator** \in′stilā′tər\ A medicine dropper.

**instinct** \in′stingkt\ [L *instinctus* (akin to *(in)stigare* to incite, arouse) instigation, prompting, inspiration, excitement] A complex unlearned response that is usually genetically determined and species-specific. **death i.** In psychoanalytic psychology, a biologic tendency, under the control of the repetition-compulsion principle, toward self-destruction and the destruction of anything, whether arising from outside or inside the organism, that threatens to disturb the status quo. Also *ego instinct, aggressive instinct, Thanatos.* **sexual i.** In psychoanalytic psychology, an instinct hypothesized to be under the control of the pleasure principle and its primary function being the preservation of life. Also *eros, life instinct.*

**institutionalization** \in′stit$^y$oo′shənəlīzā′shən\ Commitment of an individual to a custodial or health care facility.

**instruction** A code that tells a computer to perform arithmetic and logic functions, control peripheral devices, or indicate succeeding instructions.

**instrument** [L *instrumentum* (from *instruere* to put together, set in order, erect, build in or into + *-mentum* -MENT) a tool, implement, furniture, utensils] An implement or tool. **hand i.** An instrument held in and worked by the hand as opposed to a rotary instrument which is held in a handpiece and is driven by an external power source. **plugging i.** A dental instrument used for condensing. It may be worked by hand or by engine. Also *nib instrument.* **stereotaxic i.** STEREOTAXIC APPARATUS.

**instrumentarium** \in′strəmenter′ē·əm\ [Med L (from L *instrument(um)* tool, instrument + *-arium* -ARY), a case for carrying or storing papers] The instruments or other equipment required for a given surgical or medical procedure.

**instrumentation** \in′strəmentā′shən\ [INSTRUMENT + -ATION] 1 The set of instruments that measure, monitor, record, control, and treat subject variables. 2 The use of instruments.

**insuccation** \in′sukā′shən\ The process of soaking, as in the treatment of a crude drug source to obtain an extract for further purification of the active principle.

**insufficiency** \in′səfish′ənsē\ [L *insufficientia* (from *in-* not + *sufficientia* sufficiency, from *sufficiens,* gen. *sufficientis,* pres. part. of *sufficere,* to afford, supply, be sufficient, from SUB- + L *facere* to do, make) insufficiency] A failure of an organ, part, or system to perform at a normal or adequate level of function; relative ineffectuality of function. Also *insufficientia.* **active i.** A limitation of the contraction of a muscle stemming from the approximation of its origin and insertion. **acute adrenocortical i.** ADDISONIAN CRISIS. **acute coronary insuffiencey** UNSTABLE ANGINA. **adrenocortical i.** 1 Failure of adrenocortical secretion of steroid hormones due to any cause, such as bilateral total adrenalectomy, primary disease of the adrenal cortex (as autoimmune or tuberculous infiltration of the gland), or hypopituitarism. Also *capsular insufficiency* (older term). 2 ADDISON'S DISEASE. **anterior pituitary i.** HYPOPITUITARISM. **aortic i.** AORTIC REGURGITATION. **basilar i.** VERTEBROBASILAR SYNDROME. **capsular i.** *Older term* ADRENOCORTICAL INSUFFICIENCY. **cardiac i.** HEART FAILURE. **chronic adrenocortical i.** ADDISON'S DISEASE. **chronic renal i.** A disorder characterized by progressive decrease in renal function, including the glomerular filtration rate, over months or years. Urea and other nonprotein nitrogenous substances increase in the blood. A large number of other biochemical abnormalities gradually develop along with anemia, osteodystrophy, hypertension, anorexia, and many other signs and symptoms of the uremic syndrome. **i. of the externi** DIVERGENCE HYPOFUNCTION. **gastric i.** Deficient ability of the stomach to empty itself, resulting in dilatation. Also *gastromotor insufficiency.* **ileocecal i.** ILEOCECAL INCOMPETENCE. **i. of the interni** CONVERGENCE HYPOFUNCTION. **mitral i.** See under MITRAL REGURGITATION. **pancreatic i.** Inadequate production or release of pancreatic enzymes, resulting in inadequate digestion of nutrients and in abdominal symptoms. **parathyroid i.** HYPOPARATHYROIDISM. **pituitary i.** HYPOPITUITARISM. **placental i.** Abnormal growth or function of the placenta due to inadequate oxygenation or nutrition, so that it is often unable to sustain adequately the developing fetus. **post-traumatic pulmonary i.** ADULT RESPIRATORY DISTRESS SYNDROME. **primary adrenocortical i.** ADDISON'S DISEASE. **pulmonary i.** 1 Failure of the lungs to maintain normal levels of oxygen and/or carbon dioxide in arterial blood. 2 Regurgitation of the pulmonic valve. **pyloric i.** A condition characterized by inadequate closure of the pyloric valve, resulting in too rapid emptying of the stomach or in duodenogastric reflux. **secondary adrenocortical i.** Adrenocortical insufficiency resulting from hypopituitarism. Also *secondary adrenocortical failure.* **thyroid i.** HYPOTHYROIDISM. **tricuspid i.** See under TRICUSPID REGURGITATION. **uterine i.** Abnormal or inadequate uterine contractions during labor which do not effectively dilate the cervix. **valvular i.** See under VALVULAR REGURGITATION. **velopharyngeal i.** Imperfect closure of the palatopharyngeal sphincter on swallowing or while speaking. Important causes include a variety of neurologic diseases producing paralysis of the palate or of the palate and pharynx, and cleft palate. Also *velopharyngeal incompetence.* **venous i.** Impairment of venous return as a result of incompetence of the venous valves. **vertebral i.** VERTEBROBASILAR SYNDROME. **vertebrobasilar i.** VERTEBROBASILAR SYNDROME.

**insufficientia** \in′səfish′ē·en′shə\ INSUFFICIENCY.

**insufflate** \in′səflāt, insuf′lāt\ [See INSUFFLATION.] To blow, or deliver under pressure (air, gas, vapor, or particulate matter) into (a chamber or body cavity).

**insufflation** \in′səflā′shən\ [L *insufflatio* (from *insufflatus,* past part. of *insufflare* to blow on or into, from *in-* in + *sufflare* to blow at or against, inflate, from SUB- + L *flare* to blow, breathe) a blowing into] 1 The delivery under pressure of air, gas, vapor, or particulate matter into a chamber or cavity of the body, as, for example, the delivery of air to the lungs in artificial respiration. 2 An inhalant or other substance to be insufflated. **presacral i.** An outmoded radiographic technique characterized by injection of gas, usually carbon dioxide, through a needle placed into retrorectal space for radiologic visualization of the kidneys, adrenal glands, and other retroperitoneal structures. **tubal i.** The transcervical instillation of carbon dioxide gas in order to allow distension and subsequent passage of the gas from the fimbriae of the fallopian tubes into the peritoneal cavity. The procedure is most commonly utilized to determine patency of the fallopian tubes.

**insula** \in′s$^y$ələ\ [L, an island] (*pl.* insulae) 1 [NA] The expanded area of cerebral cortex at the depth of the lateral sulcus, delimited below by the underlying claustrum. Also *lobus insularis, insula of Reil, island of Reil, caudate lobe of cerebrum* (obs.). 2 A body of tissue or cluster of cells embedded in another kind of tissue. **insulae pancreaticae** ISLETS OF LANGERHANS.

**insulae** \in′s$^y$əlē\ Plural of INSULA.

**insular** \in′s$^y$ələr\ 1 Of or relating to the insula. 2 Of or relating to the islets of Langerhans.

**insulate** \in′s$^y$əlāt\ To separate conductors by a material of poor conductivity to minimize the passage of electricity, heat, or sound.

**insulin** \in′s$^y$əlin\ [*insul(a)* + -IN] A peptide hormone synthesized and secreted by the beta cells of the pancreatic islets of Langerhans, the principal fuel-metabolizing hormone of mammals. It is a polypeptide having two chains (the A chain of 21 amino acids and the B chain of 30 amino acids) linked by two disulfide bonds, and having a molecular weight of 5734. The hormone accelerates the transport of glucose, amino acids, and potassium across cell membranes, and elicits the release of one or more intracellular second messengers, with consequent changes in the levels of enzyme action and other activities, thereby regulating carbohydrate, lipid, and amino acid metabolism. Diabetes mellitus is the result of insulin deficiency. Preparations of the crystalline or chemically modified or bound hormone derived from hog or beef pancreas are used in treating the human disease. Also *insuline* (obs.), *antidiabetic hormone* (obs.). **dealinated i.** A derivative of porcine insulin prepared by the removal of the alanine residue at the C-terminal end of the B chain. Replacement by phenylalanine yields human insulin. Porcine insulin so treated is biologically active and useful in instances where antibodies to porcine or bovine insulin have reduced the effectiveness of those preparations. **depot i.** A preparation of insulin that is slowly absorbed from the site of injection. **globin zinc i.** A combination of insulin, globin, and zinc, with an intermediate time of onset of action and a duration of activity between regular insulin and protamine zinc insulin. Also *globin insulin.* **hexamine i.** A combination of hexamethylenetetramine and insulin that is no longer used. **immunoreactive i.** The insulin measured by immunoassay rather than by its hormonal activity. Immunoassays detect both insulin and proinsulin, but not the various nonsuppressible insulinlike activities of human plasma. **i. lente** INSULIN ZINC SUSPENSION. **neutral i.** INSULIN INJECTION. • The terms are now equivalent, but previously insulin injection was not neutralized, and this distinction was of importance because of the greater stability of the neutralized preparation. **pectin i.** A combination of insulin and pectin that is no longer used. **plant i.** Any substance obtained from plant material that produces a hypoglycemic effect in experimental animals. Also *vegetable insulin.* **protamine i.** A combination of insulin with protamine but without zinc, no longer used clinically. Also *insulin protaminate.* Abbr. PI **protamine zinc i.** A sterile suspension of insulin in buffered water to which zinc chloride and protamine sulfate have been added. It is administered by injection. Also *zinc protamine insulin, protamine zinc insulin suspension.* **regular i.** INSULIN INJECTION. **synalbumin i.** A postulated antagonist of insulin that is present in the blood of some diabetics and is believed to be a polypeptide related to the B chain of insulin associated with serum albumin. **three-to-one i.** A combination of regular insulin and protamine zinc insulin in a ratio of these two activities of 3:1. Such combinations have been largely replaced by combinations of amorphous and crystalline insulins and limited concentrations of zinc, to obtain both rapid onset and prolonged duration of insulin activity. **vegetable i.** PLANT INSULIN. **zinc protamine i.** PROTAMINE ZINC INSULIN.

**insuline** \in′sʸəlin\ *Obs.* INSULIN.

**insulinlipodystrophy** \in′sʸəlinlip′ōdis′trəfē\ Atrophy of fat at the sites of insulin injection.

**insulinoid** \in′sʸəlinoid′\ Having hypoglycemic properties like insulin.

**insulinoma** \in′sʸəlinō′mə\ [INSULIN + -OMA] A tumor of the beta cells of the pancreatic islets. Such tumors are usually benign and are characterized by excessive secretion of insulin with consequent severe hypoglycemia. Also *insuloma.*

**insulinopenia** \-in′sʸəlin′ōpē′nē·ə\ [INSULIN + *o* + -PENIA] Relative or absolute lack of insulin, as in diabetes mellitus or following pancreatectomy. Adj. insulinopenic.

**insulinoprivic** \in′sʸəlin′ōpriv′ik\ [insulin + *o* + L *priv(us)* deprived of + -IC] Lacking insulin; marked by insulinopenia.

**insulin protaminate** PROTAMINE INSULIN.

**insuloma** \in′sʸəlō′mə\ INSULINOMA.

**insult** [French *insult(er)* (from L *insultare* to leap upon or against, scoff at, insult, from *in-* in, on +*saltare* to leap) to offend by hurtful words] A stressful stimulus which is not necessarily injurious in favorable circumstances but which, with repetition or in combination with other factors, may result in injury.

**insurance** A contractual relationship between an insurer and another party under which the insurer agrees to reimburse or otherwise provide compensation for a loss, should one occur, in exchange for the payment of a fee. **catastrophic health i.** Health insurance which provides protection against the high cost of treating severe or lengthy illness or disability; major medical. **disability income i.** A form of health insurance that provides periodic payments to replace income when the insured is unable to work as the result of injury or illness. **health i.** Insurance against loss by disease, bodily injury, or illness, and related health care needs. **professional liability i.** Insurance purchased by a health care provider to protect against the risk of or actual financial loss on the part of the provider due to damages awarded as a result of the provider's negligent acts. Also *malpractice insurance.* **supplemental health i.** Health insurance which covers medical expenses not covered by separate health insurance already held by the insured.

**intake** The entry into the body of a solid, liquid, or gaseous substance. **acceptable daily i.** **1** The amounts of the various nutrients that need to be consumed to satisfy a person's metabolic needs. **2** The maximum amount of a substance added to food that can be consumed without causing a health hazard. Abbr. ADI **caloric i.** The caloric value of substances taken into the body. **conditional daily i.** The amount of a given food absorbed per day by the body. **daily i.** The amount of any given food substance consumed per day. Also *unconditional daily intake.* **provisional total weekly i.** The amount of food expected to be consumed by a person given an itemized dietary regimen. **total daily i.** The absolute amount of all nutrients consumed per day. **unconditional daily i.** DAILY INTAKE.

**Intal** A proprietary name for disodium chromoglycate.

**integration** \in′təgrā′shən\ [L *integratio* (from *integrare* to make whole, renew, heal, from *integer* whole, complete, intact, from IN-[2] + *tangere* to touch, affect) a renewing, restoration] **1** The amalgamation of different parts into a coordinated whole. **2** In microbiology or cell biology, the incorporation of a piece of DNA, often a viral genome or a plasmid, into a chromosome. **3** In psychology, the process of making integral the several contributing elements or characteristics of a subject. **nervous i.** The process by which a neuron or set of neurons provides an output or behavior in response to the synaptic interactions of inputs. **structural i.** ROLFING.

**integument** \integ′yəmənt\ INTEGUMENTUM. **common i.** INTEGUMENTUM COMMUNE. **spore i.** The envelope of a bacterial spore, consisting of the core membrane, cortex, coat, and exosporium.

**integumentary** \integ′yəmen′tərē\ **1** Pertaining to the integumentum commune. **2** Providing a covering.

**integumentum** \integ′yəmen′təm\ [L (from *in-* IN-[1] + *tegumentum*, also *tegmentum* a covering, protection, from *teg(ere)* to cover + *-mentum* -MENT), a covering, integument] A covering or investing layer of a part or the body. Also *integument.* • The term is often used instead of *integumentum commune.* **i. commune** [NA] The layer enveloping the whole body, i.e., the skin, comprising epidermis and dermis, and all appendages such as hairs, nails, sweat and sebaceous glands, and mammary glands. Also *common* *integument, cutaneous system, integumentary system, dermoid system* (seldom used), *dermal system* (seldom used).

***in tela*** \in tē′lə\ [L *in* in + *telā,* ablative of TELA] Within membranous connective tissue: said especially of preparations for the light microscope.

**intellectualization** \in′telek′choo·əlīzā′shən\ An attempt to analyze a personal problem in purely intellectual terms, to the neglect or exclusion of affective considerations that would be normal under the circumstances. It is often a defensive measure by which the individual can achieve some degree of insulation against the feelings of emotional hurt that would otherwise be experienced.

**intelligence** [L *intelligentia* or *intellegentia* (from *intelligens, intellegens,* gen. *intelligentis, intellegentis,* pres. part. of *intelligere, intellegere* to understand, perceive, know, from INTER- + L *legere* to collect, pick up, read) perception, understanding, intellect] **1** A quality of behavior demonstrating the degree to which an organism is able to learn quickly and to adopt responses rapidly and effectively when faced with novel situations. **2** The ability to manipulate symbols and to grasp abstract relationships in problem-solving and to respond flexibly to changing demands within a given context. Human intelligence would encompass the collective repertory of cognitive powers possessed by an individual which can be brought to bear on the solution of difficult and complex problems, such as reason, insight, foresight, judgment, or imagination. **artificial i.** The programming of a computer to perform functions that are normally associated with human intelligence, such as learning, reasoning, and decision-making.

**intensification** \inten′sifikā′shən\ An increase in intensity. **image i.** In radiology, the method of increasing the brightness of fluoroscopic image by means of an image intensifier tube.

**intensity** \inten′sitē\ [*intens(e)* + -ITY] The magnitude or strength of a variable, such as brightness, ionizing radiation, sound, electric field, or magnetic field. **intrauterine i.** The strength of intrauterine pressure that occurs with a uterine contraction during labor. **luminous i.** The luminous flux incident on a small surface which lies in a specified direction from a light source and is normal to this direction, divided by the solid angle (in steradians) which the surface subtends at the source of light. Also *light intensity.* **pulse average i.** Intensity averaged over the pulse duration. **spatial average i.** Intensity averaged over the transducer area or the ultrasound beam cross-sectional area. **spatial average temporal average i.** Intensity averaged over the cross-sectional area of an ultrasound transducer beam and over the pulse repetition period. **spatial peak i.** Intensity at the point in an ultrasound beam where it is maximum. **spatial peak temporal average i.** Intensity averaged over the ultrasound pulse repetition period at the point in the beam where it is maximum. **temporal average i.** Intensity averaged over an ultrasound pulse repetition period. **temporal peak i.** The maximum intensity reached in an ultrasound pulse repetition period. **threshold i.** The stimulus magnitude necessary for tissue excitation or sensory detection.

**intensive** \inten′siv\ Marked by intensity; specifically, requiring special attention or strong measures, as *intensive care.*

**intent** \intent′\ **criminal i.** The intent to do harm, as evidenced by the commission of a criminal act, or the mental ability to form such an intention, or both, frequently an important consideration in establishing responsibility of a person accused of having committed such an act. Also *mens rea.*

**intention** A manner of healing of wounds and incisions, such as healing by first intention.

**inter-** \in′tər-\ [L *inter* between, among] A prefix meaning (1) between or among; (2) mutual, shared, combined.

**interacinar** \-as′inər\ Between acini. Also *interacinous.*

**interaction** [INTER- + ACTION] In statistics, the relationship obtaining between two independent variables when their joint effect on the dependent variable is greater than that of the sum of the effects of both acting separately. **complementary i.** Nonallelic gene interaction in which the phenotype produced is distinct from that of either gene separately. **heme-heme i.** Interaction between two heme groups. Such interactions occur in hemoglobin, where oxygenation (or deoxygenation) of one heme facilitates the oxygenation (or deoxygenation) of others. The interactions are indirect, since they are effected by alterations in the structural configuration of the globin chains rather than of their heme components. **ion-dipole i.** An interaction or attraction between a neutral molecule and an ion. The ion-dipole interactions are weak and the forces decrease rapidly as the interacting groups are moved apart. **primary i.** The binding of antibody to antigen, regardless of whether it can be detected serologically.

**interalveolar** \-alvē′ələr\ Between alveoli, particularly those of the lung.

**interamnios** \-am′nē·äs\ [INTER- + New L *amnios,* variant of AMNION] A cavity between the amnion and the embryophore in the eggs of mammals showing inversion of germ layers.

**interannular** \-an′yələr\ Between two ringlike structures or constrictions.

**interapophyseal** \-ap′ōfiz′ē·əl\ Between two bony processes or projections.

**interarticular** \-ärtik′yələr\ Between the articular surfaces of a joint or between two joints.

**interarytenoid** \-ar′ətē′noid\ Between the two arytenoid cartilages of the larynx. Also *interarytenoidal.*

**interatrial** \-ā′trē·əl\ Between the atria of the heart. Also *interauricular.*

**interauricular** \-ôrik′yələr\ **1** Between the auricles of the external ears. **2** Between the auricles of the atria.

**interaxonal** \-ak′sənəl\ Between axons, with reference to the Schwann cell processes and endoneurial collagen in peripheral nerves.

**interbands** The regions of a polytene chromosome between the cytologic bands.

**interbrain** [INTER- + BRAIN] DIENCEPHALON.

**intercalary** \intur′kəler′ē\ Inserted between; additional, interposed, as intercalary ducts of compound exocrine glands and intercalated disks of cardiac muscle. Also *intercalated, intercalate.*

**intercarotid** \-kərät′id\ Between the external and internal carotid arteries. Also *intercarotic.*

**intercarpal** Between carpal bones.

**intercartilaginous** \-kär′tilaj′inəs\ Located between, or connecting, cartilages. Also *interchondral.*

**intercavernous** \-kav′ərnəs\ **1** Between two cavities. **2** Between or connecting the two cavernous sinuses.

**intercellular** \-sel′yələr\ Between and among cells.

**interchange** In cytogenetics, any redistribution of chromatin, which is detectable microscopically, between or among chromosomes or between chromatids, such as translocations and sister chromatid exchanges.

**interchondral** \-kän′drəl\ INTERCARTILAGINOUS.

**intercilium** \-sil′ē·əm\ **1** GLABELLA. **2** The gap between the eyebrows.

**interclinoid** \-klī′noid\ Between the clinoid processes of the sphenoid bone, either between anterior and posterior or across the midline. Also *interclinoidal.*

**intercondylar** \-kän′dilər\ Between any two condyles. Also *intercondylous, intercondyloid.*

**intercornual** \-kôr′n$^y$oo·əl\ Lying between cornua.

**intercoronoideal** \-kôr′ənoi′dē·əl\ Between the right and the left coronoid processes of the mandible.

**intercostal** \-käs′təl\ Between the ribs.

**intercourse** Exchange or communication between people. **sexual i.** COITUS.

**intercoxal** \-käk′səl\ Between the hips or the hip bones.

**intercricothyrotomy** \-krī′kōthīrät′əmē\ CRICOTHYROTOMY.

**intercristal** \-kris′təl\ Between two crests, particularly those of the ilia of the hip bones: applied to measurement of the distance between them or to the level of the plane between their highest points.

**intercross** The mating of diploid individuals who are both heterozygous for one or more of the same alleles at given loci.

**intercrural** \-kroo′rəl\ **1** Between any two crura. **2** Between the legs.

**intercurrent** \-kur′ənt\ Denoting a disease process affecting a patient already suffering from a preexisting illness.

**intercuspal** \-kus′pəl\ Pertaining to the relationship, or fit, of the cusps of the teeth of the upper or lower jaw against those on the teeth of the opposite jaw.

**intercuspation** \-kuspā′shən\ [INTER- + CUSP + -ATION] The fitting of the cusps of the teeth of one arch into the fossae and occlusal embrasures of the opposing arch.

**interdeferential** \-def′əren′shəl\ Between the two ductus deferentes.

**interdental** \-den′təl\ Describing the space or position between adjacent teeth in the same jaw. Also *interproximal.*

**interdigit** \-dij′it\ The part of the hand or foot between any two adjacent digits.

**interdigital** \-dij′itəl\ Between any two adjacent fingers or toes.

**interdigitation** \-dij′itā′shən\ The state of being interlocked or interwoven in elongated or fingerlike processes.

**interface** \in′tərfās\ [INTER- + FACE] **1** In a biological system, the junctional layer between two different materials. **2** The point in a process where independent systems interact. **dermoepidermal i.** DERMOEPIDERMAL JUNCTION. **gamma camera i.** The electronic equipment that functionally connects a gamma camera to a computer and serves to convert the analog signals generated by the camera to digital signals compatible with the computer format.

**interfemoral** \-fem′ərəl\ Between the thighs.

**interference** \-fir′əns\ [*interfer(e)* + -ENCE] **1** The combination of two or more wave disturbances, differing in frequency or in direction of propagation, acting at the same point, to produce a net disturbance. **2** In the presence of atrioventricular dissociation, the interruption of the regular rhythm of one pair of chambers by activation deriving from the other, most often of the ventricles (ventricular capture) by an impulse deriving from the atria. **3** In genetics, any statistically significant alteration in cross-over frequency from randomness. Chromosome interference may be either positive or negative, depending on whether a given cross-over decreases or increases, respectively, the frequency of another cross-over. Also *chiasma interference.* **4** See under OCCLUSAL INTERFERENCE. **chiasma i.** INTERFERENCE. **cuspal i.** The presence of tooth contacts which prevent a normal path of closure or cause instability of a denture. **initial i.** PREMATURE INTERFERENCE. **interceptive occlusal i.** PREMATURE INTERFERENCE. **interchromosomal i.** Balancing of negative interference in one pair of homologues by positive interference in another such that the overall cross-over frequency is less altered than in either situation alone. **occlusal i.** A contact between antagonistic teeth which prevents proper closure or function. **premature i.** Occlusal interference during closure in centric position. Also *initial interference, interceptive occlusal interference.*

**interferon** \-fir′än\ A protein produced in organisms infected by viruses, and effective at protecting those organisms from other virus infections. In the presence of a double-stranded RNA, such as viral RNA, it stimulates the synthesis of 2′,5′-linked oligonucleotides of adenylate, carrying a 5′-triphosphate group, and these stimulate a ribonuclease that degrades messenger RNA. Also, in the presence of double-stranded RNA, it stimulates a kinase that phosphorylates an initiation factor and thereby inactivates it. Interferon therefore suppresses protein biosynthesis by two mechanisms. **$\alpha$ i.** Any of a number of closely related antiviral proteins synthesized by many types of cell in response to viral infections or to a variety of inducers (e.g. double-stranded DNA). Lymphoblastoid cells are a good source of $\alpha$ interferon, which has been purified from them. All $\alpha$ interferons show a characteristic resistance to acid pH. Also *lymphoblastoid cell interferon.* **$\beta$ i.** A particular molecular species of interferon that shares most of its properties, including acid stability, with $\alpha$ interferons. It is synthesized by many types of cell in response to virus infection, but was first isolated from fibroblast cells. Also *fibroblast interferon.* **$\gamma$ i.** The variety of interferon that is produced by sensitized T lymphocytes on stimulation by specific antigens. Besides its action in preventing viral replication, it is a macrophage-activating factor. It is structurally quite distinct from the classical interferons ($\alpha$ interferon and $\beta$ interferon). Also *immune interferon.* **antigenic i.** Interferon measured by reaction with specific antibody rather than by its biologic activity. Also *immunoreactive interferon.* **fibroblast i.** $\beta$ INTERFERON. **immune i.** $\gamma$ INTERFERON. **immunoreactive i.** ANTIGENIC INTERFERON. **lymphoblastoid cell i.** $\alpha$ INTERFERON.

**interfibrillar** \-fī′brilər\ Between and among fine fibers. Also *interfibrillary.*

**interfrontal** \-frun′təl\ Between the two unfused frontal bones, with reference to the frontal, or metopic, suture.

**interganglionic** \-gang′glē·än′ik\ Denoting connections, which have been shown to be nonexistent, between sensory ganglion cells. *Outmoded.*

**intergemmal** \-jem′əl\ Between two or more gemmae, or bulblike structures, such as taste buds.

**intergenic** \-jē′nik\ **1** Pertaining to a region of DNA or chromosome that is located between two genetic loci, but not necessarily involving either. **2** Of or relating to a mutation that is located between two genetic loci, but not necessarily involving either. **3** Designating a mutation which affects the expression of two juxtaposed loci.

**intergluteal** \-gloo′tē·əl\ Between the buttocks; internatal.

**intergonial** \-gō′nē·əl\ Between the gonia, or angles of the mandible.

**intergrade** \in′tərgrād\ A stage of transition between two other stages.

**intergranular** \-gran′yələr\ Situated within the granule cell layers of the cerebrum or cerebellum.

**intergyral** \-jī′rəl\ Connecting or situated between cerebral gyri.

**interhemispheric** \-hem′isfer′ik\ Situated or occurring

between, or connecting, the cerebral hemispheres.

**interictal** \-ik′təl\ [INTER- + ICTAL] Present or occurring between attacks. Also *interparoxysmal.*

**interior** Located on or toward the inside.

**interischiadic** \-is′kē·ad′ik\ Between the two ischia, particularly their tuberosities. Also *intersciatic.*

**interjugal** \-joo′gəl\ **1** Between the zygomatic processes. **2** Between right and left jugale, a measurement used in craniometry.

**interkinesis** \-kīnē′sis\ [INTER- + KINESIS] The interval between cell divisions, especially the first and second meiotic divisions.

**interlabial** \-lā′bē·əl\ **1** Between the lips. **2** Between the labia.

**interleukin-1** \-loo′kin\ A mediator produced by macrophages which acts upon lymphocytes enhancing their capacity to respond to antigens. Interleukin-1 is also believed to be the same as endogenous pyrogen and as catabolin and to be responsible for inducing the increased synthesis of many acute phase proteins during an inflammatory response *in vivo.* Also *lymphocyte-activating factor.* Abbr. IL-1

**interleukin-2** A lymphokine that supports growth and differentiation of thymus-derived cells and plaque-forming cells. Also *T-cell growth factor.* Abbr. IL-2

**interlobar** \-lō′bər\ Between the lobes of any structure or organ.

**interlobular** \-läb′yələr\ Between the lobules of a structure or organ.

**interlocking** The locking together of twins by the chins where the first twin presents as a breech and the second one presents as a vertex. Also *compaction, head locking.*

**intermalar** \-mal′ər\ Between the zygomatic bones.

**intermalleolar** \-məlē′ələr\ Between the medial and the lateral malleolus.

**intermamillary** \-mam′iler′ē\ **1** Between the nipples of the breasts, with reference to an imaginary line between them. **2** INTERMAMMARY.

**intermammary** \-mam′ərē\ Between the breasts. Also *intermamillary.*

**intermarginal** Between two margins or borders.

**intermarriage** **1** *Popular* INBREEDING. **2** The marriage of individuals of different races, cultures, religions, or other groups.

**intermaxilla** \-maksil′ə\ OS INCISIVUM.

**intermaxillary** \-mak′siler′ē\ Between the two maxillae.

**intermediate** **1** Occurring at or representing a middle position between others more extreme; halfway. **2** INTERMEDIUS. **3** A substance formed from the reactant in a chemical reaction and then transformed into the product.

**intermedin** \-mē′din\ [after *pars intermedia,* the intermediate lobe of the pituitary gland, the site of the hormone in amphibia, reptiles, and other forms] MELANOCYTE STIMULATING HORMONE.

**intermediolateral** \-mē′dē·ōlat′ərəl\ Intermediate and on the lateral side.

**intermediomedial** \-mē′dē·ōmē′dē·əl\ Intermediate and on the medial side.

**intermedius** \-mē′dē·əs\ Denoting the middle of three structures, the other two being on either side of it, the one being nearest and the other furthest from the median plane; intervening; between two extremes. Also *intermediate.*

**intermenstrual** \-men′stroo·əl\ Between the menses or menstrual periods.

**intermetacarpal** \-met′əkär′pəl\ Between metacarpal bones.

**intermetatarsal** \-met′ətär′səl\ Between metatarsal bones.

**intermitotic** \-mītät′tik\ Pertaining to the period and the events occurring between mitotic divisions.

**intermittence** \-mit′əns\ Occurrence at intervals rather than continuously; interruptedness: commonly used with reference to the occasional dropping of heart beats or pulses. Also *intermittency.*

**intermittent** \-mit′ənt\ Occurring at intervals rather than continuously.

**intermural** Between the walls of an organ or organs of the body. Also *interparietal.*

**intermuscular** Between muscles, as of a septum.

**intern** \in′turn\ [French *interne* (from L *internus* internal) a resident student] An individual in professional training in a health care field, usually immediately after the awarding of the degree but before independent practice. Also *interne.*

**internal** [L *intern(us)* inner + -AL] Situated or occurring on the inside of a part, organ, or body; interior. • Occasionally used, incorrectly, to describe a medial position.

**internalization** \intur′nəlīzā′shən\ The process hypothesized to account for an individual's incorporation of the mores and standards of conduct of his society. Moral values, attitudes, and opinions are learned from others, primarily from parents, and these internalized principles then substitute for outer controls in the guidance of behavior.

**internarial** \-ner′ē·əl\ Between the nostrils. Also *internasal.*

**internasal** \-nā′zəl\ **1** Between the nasal bones or cartilages. **2** INTERNARIAL.

**internatal** \-nā′təl\ Between the buttocks, or nates; intergluteal.

**internation** \in′turnā′shən\ [*intern* (v.) + -ATION] The confinement of an individual, ordered by law, in a specified institution such as a prison or psychiatric hospital.

**International Classification of Diseases** A list of diseases, injuries, and causes of death, arranged under numbered categories according to etiology and anatomic localization and intended to ensure by international agreement comparability of mortality and morbidity statistics. Although every morbid condition can be assigned to a category, each does not necessarily have a category of itself. Contrary, therefore, to what is often assumed, the list does not constitute a nomenclature of diseases and injuries but a classification intended primarily for statistical use. Originally produced at the International Statistical Congress of Paris, in 1855, with various subsequent modifications, the Classification now undergoes a decennial revision under the auspices of the World Health Organization. The most recent edition, ICD-9, became effective in January 1979. Abbr. ICD

**International Health Regulations** A set of regulations introduced by the World Health Organization in 1969, with subsequent amendments, to replace the International Sanitary Regulations. They are binding on member states of WHO, unless specific reservations have been formally entered, and lay down the maximum measures that may be imposed on international traffic when there is a risk of transmission of a disease subject to be dealt with under the regulations. The regulations also deal with preventive arrangements at ports and airports and provide for the international surveillance of other diseases such as influenza and salmonellosis.

**International Nonproprietary Names** The nonproprietary names recommended by the World Health Organization for any drug. Lists of such names are published regularly. Abbr. INN

**International Pharmacopeia** A collection of specifications prepared by the World Health Organization for the quality control of pharmaceutical products which would enable all countries to establish standards in common. It differs from national pharmacopeias in that it lacks legal force. Each member state of the World Health Organization is, however, authorized to incorporate any part of the International Pharmacopeia in its own national pharmacopeia or to adopt it *in toto* as its national pharmacopeia.

**International System of Units** See under SYSTÈME INTERNATIONAL D'UNITÉS.

**interne** \inturn′\ INTERN.

**interneural** \-n$^y$Ur′əl\ Between the vertebral, or neural, arches.

**interneuron** \-n$^y$Ur′än\ [INTER- + NEURON] Any neuron in a neural chain other than a primary afferent ganglion cell or a motor fiber innervating muscle. Also *internuncial cell, connector neuron, intercalary neuron, internuncial neuron.* **inhibitory i.** A short-axon neuron whose excitation produces an inhibitory postsynaptic potential on a nearby neuron, such as the Renshaw cells of the spinal cord.

**interneuronal** \-n$^y$Urō′nəl\ Pertaining to interneurons and their action.

**internist** \in′turnist, intur′nist\ A physician specializing in internal medicine.

**internodal** \-nō′dəl\ Situated between nodes. Also *internodular.*

**internode** \in′tərnōd\ INTERNODAL SEGMENT. **i. of Ranvier** INTERNODAL SEGMENT.

**internodular** \-näd′yələr\ **1** Between two nodules. **2** INTERNODAL.

**internship** \in′tərnship\ [INTERN + *-ship*] A period of training in a health care field such as medicine, usually following the awarding of a professional degree but preceding residency or independent practice.

**internuclear** \-n$^y$oo′klē·ər\ Situated between nuclei: used especially of nuclear groups in the central nervous system.

**internuncial** \-nun′sē·əl\ [L *internunti(us)* (from INTER- + *nuntium* message) a messenger, go-between + -AL] Denoting an intermediary neural effect mediated between nerve cells or centers through the action of interneurons.

**internus** \intur′nəs\ Internal.

**interoception** \in′tərōsep′shən\ [*inter-* as in *interior* + *o* + *(re)ception*] VISCERAL SENSE.

**interoceptive** \in′tərōsep′tiv\ Denoting the internal receptive apparatus associated with viscera and mediating internal sensation.

**interoceptor** \in′tərōsep′tər\ A sense organ located in the viscera.

**interoinferiorly** Inward and below or downward.

**interolivary** \-äl′iver′ē\ Situated between the paired inferior olivary bodies of the medulla oblongata.

**interorbital** \-ôr′bətəl\ Between the orbits.

**interosseal** \-äs′ē·əl\ **1** Denoting the interosseous muscles. **2** INTEROSSEOUS.

**interosseous** \-äs′ē·əs\ Connecting or located between bones, particularly with reference to muscles, nerves, and vessels. Also *interosseal.*

**interpalatine** \-pal′ətīn\ Between the palatine bones.

**interpalpebral** \-pal′pəbrəl\ Situated between the upper and lower eyelid. The interpalpebral aperture is the opening for the eye.

**interparietal** \-pərī′ətəl\ **1** Between the parietal bones. **2** INTERMURAL. **3** Between certain gyri of the parietal lobe of the cerebrum.

**interparoxysmal** \-par′äksiz′məl\ [INTER- + PAROXYSMAL] INTERICTAL.

**interpediculate** \-pədik′yəlāt\ Between pedicles of a vertebra or vertebrae.

**interpeduncular** \-pədungk′yələr\ Situated between paired peduncles, like the fossa separating the cerebral peduncles from the nucleus interpeduncularis.

**interphalangeal** \-fəlan′jē·əl\ Between contiguous phalanges of a finger or toe.

**interphase** \in′tərfāz\ The phase of the cell cycle between cell divisions, during which much of the synthesis of cellular constituents occurs. Interphase is divided into the following stages: $G_1$, a period immediately after mitosis or meiosis, during which no DNA synthesis is occurring; S, during which DNA synthesis occurs; and $G_2$, after DNA synthesis and before the onset of division.

**interplant** \in′tərplant\ The insertion of a part or piece of one embryo into a reasonably indifferent environment of another, such as the coelom or the chorioallantoic membrane.

**interpleural** \-plUr′əl\ Between the pleurae, or between two layers of a pleural sac.

**interpleuricostal** \-plUr′ikäs′təl\ Between a pleural sac and the surrounding ribs.

**interpolated** \intur′pəlā′tid\ **1** Obtained or implanted by interpolation. **2** Inserted; intercalated.

**interpolation** \intur′pəlā′shən\ [L *interpolatio* (from *interpolare* to process, work over, touch up, from INTER- + *pol-* as in *polire* to polish) refurbishment, touching up] **1** Estimation of the value taken by a function at points intermediate between two known values. In the simplest form of interpolation it is assumed that the dependent variable is directly proportional to the independent variable, and in this case the interpolation is said to be linear. **2** In surgery, the insertion of a flap between two or more structures.

**interposition** A putting between; the condition of being interposed.

**interpretation** \-prətā′shən\ [L *interpretatio* (from *interpretari* to interpret, explain, from *interpres,* gen. *interpretis,* an agent, mediator, negotiator, from INTER- + root of *pretium* worth, value) interpretation] The therapist's description or formulation of the significance of a patient's productions during psychoanalytic treatment, often presented as a hypothesis to explain contradictions or inconsistencies in the patient's behavior or feelings.

**interpreter** \intur′prətər\ A specialized computer program that translates each line of a high-level language such as BASIC into machine language and executes the specified instruction before going on to the next instruction.

**interproximal** \-präk′siməl\ INTERDENTAL.

**interpterygoid** \in′tərter′igoid\ Between the pterygoid processes of the sphenoid bone.

**interpubic** \-pyoo′bik\ Between the pubic bones.

**interpyramidal** \-piram′idəl\ **1** Situated within the pyramidal tract. **2** Situated between the paired pyramids of the medulla oblongata.

**interrenal** \-rē′nəl\ Between the kidneys.

**interrupted** Broken in continuity; characterized by intervals of discontinuity; irregular.

**interrupter** / **ground fault circuit i.** A special circuit breaker that disconnects the source of electric power when a ground fault (leakage path) greater than about six milliamperes occurs. Safety codes require their use in wet areas such as bathrooms, swimming pools, and hydrotherapy areas to prevent electrocution.

**interscapilium** \-skəpil′ē·əm\ INTERSCAPULUM.

**interscapulum** \-skap′yələm\ The area between the scapulae. Also *interscapilium.*

**intersciatic** \-sī·at′ik\ INTERISCHIADIC.

**intersectio** \-sek′shō\ [L, from *intersecare* to cut through, from INTER- + *secare* to cut, divide] (*pl.* intersectiones) A site of meeting or crossing of two structures; a division or separation. Also *intersection.* **i. tendinea** [NA] A fibrous band that extends transversely or obliquely across a muscle belly, dividing it, wholly or partly, into segments. Also *inscriptio tendinea, tendinous intersection, tendinous inscription, aponeurotic intersection.* **intersectiones tendineae musculi recti abdominis** [NA] Fibrous bands, usually three in number, that pass transversely or obliquely across the rectus abdominis muscle, one being at the level of the umbilicus, a second opposite the tip of the xiphoid process, and a third being midway between the former two. They extend partly or totally through the substance of the muscle and are fixed to the anterior lamina of the rectus sheath. Also *tendinous intersections of rectus abdominis muscle, inscriptiones tendineae musculi recti abdominis, tendinous inscriptions of rectus abdominis muscle.*

**intersection** [L *intersectio.* See INTERSECTIO.] INTERSECTIO. **aponeurotic i.** INTERSECTIO TENDINEA. **tendinous i.** INTERSECTIO TENDINEA. **tendinous i.'s of rectus abdominis muscle** INTERSECTIONES TENDINEAE MUSCULI RECTI ABDOMINIS.

**intersectiones** \-sekshō′nēz\ Plural of INTERSECTIO.

**intersegmental** \-segmen′təl\ **1** Placed between two segments. **2** In embryology, lying between two metameres.

**interseptal** \-sep′təl\ Between septa, or partitions.

**interseptum** \-sep′təm\ DIAPHRAGMA.

**intersex** An individual exhibiting ambiguous sexual characteristics, largely with respect to anatomical or behavioral traits. • The term is used in a more general sense than hermaphrodite or gynandromorph. **female i.** FEMALE PSEUDOHERMAPHRODITE. **male i.** MALE PSEUDOHERMAPHRODITE. **true i.** TRUE HERMAPHRODITE.

**intersexual** \-sek′shoo·əl\ Pertaining to or having the characteristics of intersexuality.

**intersexuality** \-sek′shoo·al′itē\ Any combination of male and female genetic, chromosomal, morphologic, hormonal, gonadal, and behavorial characteristics within the same individual; sexual ambiguity due to any cause. **female genital i.** Ambiguity of internal or external genitalia due to any cause in a genotypic female. **gonadal i.** TRUE HERMAPHRODITISM. **male genital i.** Ambiguity of internal or external genitalia due to any cause in a genotypic male.

**intersigmoid** \-sig′moid\ Between two parts of the sigmoid colon.

**interspace** \in′tərspās\ A gap or area between two similar structures, such as the space between two ribs, or between two lobules of an organ. **dineric i.** The region of contact between two liquids.

**interspinal** \-spī′nəl\ Between two spines or spinous processes. Also *interspinous.*

**interstice** \intur′stis\ [L *interstitio* (from *intersistere* to pause, from INTER- + *sistere* to cause to stand or stop, from *stare* to stand) an interval, intermission] **1** Any small gap or space in the structure of a tissue or organ. **2** A crevice or interval between parts of the body. Also *interstitium.*

**interstitial** \-stish′əl\ Pertaining or belonging to interstices or interspaces of a tissue or organ.

**interstitium** \-stish′ē·əm\ **1** INTERSTICE. **2** INTERSTITIAL TISSUE.

**intertarsal** \tär′səl\ Between tarsal bones.

**intertendinous** \-ten′dinəs\ Between tendons.

**intertragic** \-trā′jik\ Between the tragus and the antitragus of the pinna.

**intertransversalis** \-trans′vərsā′lis\ Any one of the musculi intertransversarii. Also *intertransversarius.*

**intertransverse** \-transvurs′\ Between transverse processes of the vertebrae.

**intertriginous** \-trij′inəs\ Pertaining to intertrigo, or to sites anatomically susceptible to intertrigo.

**intertrigo** \-trē′gō, -trī′gō\ [L (from *inter-* between + *tri(tus),* past part. of *terere* to rub + *-(i)go,* suffix forming nouns from verbs, often indicating diseased condition), a sore place caused by chafing] Erythema or eczema that affects apposed skin surfaces, as in flexurae or beneath a pendulous breast. Adj. intertriginous.

**intertrochanteric** \-trō′kanter′ik\ Between the greater and lesser trochanters of the femur.

**intertubercular** \-t$^y$ubur′kyələr\ Between tubercles.

**interureteric** \-yoo′rəter′ik\ Between the ureters. Also *interureteral.*

**interuteroplacental** \-yoo′tərōpləsen′təl\ [INTER- + UTERO- + PLACENTAL] Located or occurring between the uterus and placenta.

**intervaginal** \-vaj′ənəl\ Between sheaths.

**interval** \in′tərvəl\ [L *intervallum* (from INTER- + L *vallum* a palisade made from stakes and set up on a rampart) a space between two palisades, an intervening space, interval] A gap between two parts or structures; a period between two points in time. **a-c i.** The interval between the onset of the a wave and that of the c wave of the jugular pulse. **A-H i.** The time between the onset of the atrial deflection and the His bundle deflection. This is normally between 50 and 150 milliseconds. **atrioventricular i.** The interval between the onset of atrial systole and that of ventricular systole. Also *A-V interval, auriculoventricular interval.* **auriculoventricular i.** ATRIOVENTRICULAR INTERVAL. **A-V i.** ATRIOVENTRICULAR INTERVAL. **BH i.** The duration of His bundle deflection. **cardio-arterial i.** The interval between the onset of the apex beat and that of the radial pulse. **confidence i.** In statistics, the interval, as calculated from observations on a random sample, within which will lie, with a degree of probability specified in advance, the true value of a given population parameter. The complement of the probability is an index of the risk of being in error when regarding the interval so defined as containing the true value. A commonly observed convention is to accept a risk of error of 5% or 1%. The boundary values of the interval are termed confidence limits. **coupling i.** The interval between the onset of a QRS complex in sinus rhythm and that of a succeeding premature beat, usually expressed in hundredths of a second or milliseconds. **H-V i.** The time from the onset of the earliest His bundle deflection to the earliest component of ventricular depolarization. **induction-delivery i.** The period of time between starting an induction of labor and the delivery of the infant. **interectopic i.** The interval between two successive ectopic beats. **interstimulus i.** In classical conditioning, the time elapsing between the onset of a conditioned stimulus and the onset of the paired unconditioned stimulus. **intertrial i.** The interval between successive presentations of any kind of stimuli, such as words in a list of nonsense syllables. **isovolumetric i.** The period during which the cardiac ventricle is contracting but its volume remains the same; the period between the onset of mechanical systole and the opening of the semilunar valves. Also *isometric interval, presphygmic interval.* **lucid i.** **1** A period of relative freedom from confusion, hallucinations, delusions, and other grossly psychotic symptoms, as may occur during organic deliria as well as acute schizophrenic episodes. **2** In forensic medicine, a sufficient restoration of reason so that the subject is able to comprehend and perform an action with such memory, perception, and judgment as to be held legally responsible for the action. **P-A i.** The time between the earliest deflection of the P wave and the deflection caused by depolarization of the lower atrial septum in intracardiac electrography. **P-J i.** The interval between the onset of the P wave of the electrocardiogram and the junction (J) between the terminal part of the S wave and the ST segment. **postmortem i.** In forensic medicine, the amount of time between a person's death and the discovery of the body. The determination of this period is never exact except under circumstances in which death is witnessed. In unwitnessed deaths, the estimate is made by an assessment of the development of algor, rigor, and livor mortis and by vitreous humor analysis and other tests and examinations. **P-P i.** The interval between two successive P waves. **P-R i.** The interval between the onset of the P wave and the beginning of the QRS complex, whether this be a Q wave or an R wave. It is usually between 0.12 and 0.20 second. **presphygmic i.** ISOVOLUMETRIC INTERVAL. **Q-R i.** The interval between the onset of the QRS complex and the peak of the R wave. **QRS i.** The interval between the onset of the Q wave and the termination of the S wave. **Q-T i.** The interval between the onset of the Q wave and the termination of the T wave, representing the duration of ventricular depolarization and repolarization. Also *QRST interval.* **$S_2$-OS i.** The interval between the second heart sound and the opening snap in mitral stenosis. The shorter the interval, the more severe the stenosis is apt to be.

**intervention** \-ven′shən\ [Late L *interventio* (from *interventus,* past part. of *intervenire* to come between) an intervening] Any procedure implemented to assist or educate a patient in preserving or improving his health or well-being.

**interventricular** \-ventrik′yələr\ Between ventricles.

**interview** / **stress i.** A psychiatric evaluation session in which the interviewer deliberately avoids the usual ways of reducing the subject's anxiety in order to heighten pressure and have it released within the controlled environment of the interview.

**intervillous** \-vil′əs\ Among or between villi.

**interzonal** \-zō′nəl\ Between zones, as the fibers connecting chromatids during anaphase of mitosis.

**intestinal** \intes′tinəl\ Concerning the intestine.

**intestine** \intes′tin\ [L *intestinum.* See INTESTINUM.] The tubular portion of the digestive apparatus which extends from the pylorus of the stomach to the anus. It is divided into the small intestine and the large intestine. Also *bowel, gut, intestinum.* **blind i.** CAECUM. **large i.** INTESTINUM CRASSUM. **mesenterial i.** INTESTINUM TENUE MESENTERIALE. **preoral i.** The part of the embryonic intestine in front of the buccopharyngeal membrane and forming the deep part of the stomodeum. **small i.** INTESTINUM TENUE.

**intestinum** \in′testī′nəm\ [L (substantive from *intestinus* internal, from *intus* inside, inward) bowel, gut] INTESTINE. **i. crassum** [NA] The distal portion of the intestine which extends from the termination of the ileum to the anus. It is divided into the cecum with the vermiform appendix, the colon, the rectum, and the anal canal. It is arranged to surround the small intestine and functions mainly in the absorption of fluid and solutes. It differs from the small intestine in several ways including its wider caliber and the presence of taeniae coli, haustrations, plicae semilunares coli, and appendices epiploicae. Also *large intestine.* **i. tenue** [NA] The convoluted proximal portion of the intestine which extends from the pyloric orifice to the ileocecal valve. It is divided into duodenum, jejunum, and ileum, of which the latter two are suspended from the posterior abdominal wall by the mesentery. It is situated in the central and lower portions of the abdominal cavity and is surrounded by the large intestine. Its major functions include the continued digestion of food by intestinal juices and the absorption of nutrients into the blood and lymph vessels, for which the mucosal surface is considerably increased by the formation of the plicae circulares and the villi. Also *small intestine, enteron.* **i. tenue mesenteriale** The portion of the small intestine that is suspended from the posterior abdominal wall by the mesentery, namely, jejunum and ileum. Also *mesenterial intestine.*

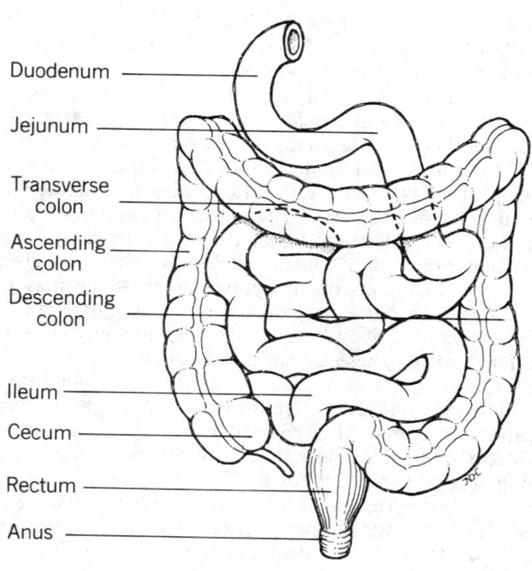


**Intestines**

**intima** \in′timə\ [L, fem. sing. of *intimus* innermost, superl. of assumed *interus* inward (the comparative is *interior* inner, interior)] **1** Denoting an innermost layer. **2** TUNICA INTERNA VASORUM.

**intimal** \in′timəl\ Pertaining to the tunica intima of a blood vessel.

**intimectomy** \in′timek′təmē\ [*intim(a)* + -ECTOMY] Removal of a portion of the intima of an artery.

**intimitis** \in′timī′tis\ [*intim(a)* + -ITIS] Inflammation of the intima of an artery or vein; endangiitis.

**intoe** \in′tō\ A deformity of the foot in which, when walking or standing, the foot turns inward. It can arise from metatarsus varus, tibial torsion, or persistence of the fetal alignment.

**intolerance** \intäl′ərəns\ [L *intolerantia* (from *in-* not + *tolerantia* patience, endurance) lack of patience. See TOLERANCE] **1** Inability or unwillingness to accept or withstand. **2** A tendency to react hypersensitively, as to a drug. **congenital lactose i.** A condition of diarrhea and a failure to thrive due to the malabsorption of lactose. In some it is due to congenital deficiency of lactase, which is inherited as an autosomal recessive trait. In others it is due to an autosomal dominant, more severe disorder associated with lactosuria. **disaccharide i.** An inability to digest one or more disaccharides, leading to symptoms of bloating, abdominal discomfort, nausea, vomiting, and explosive, acidic diarrhea when the offending sugar is ingested. This arises as a result of a deficiency in the disaccharidases present in the brush border membrane of the intestinal villi. Human jejunal mucosa contains five maltases, two sucrases, two lactases and an α-dextrinase. Such a deficiency can arise as a primary, inherited enzyme defect or an acquired defect secondary to another disease such as kwashiorkor, celiac disease, giardiasis, sprue, acute enteric infections, and cystic fibrosis. **hereditary fructose i.** A rare, inherited, metabolic disorder due to an absence of the enzyme 1-phosphate aldolase from the liver. This leads to interference with several aspects of carbohydrate metabolism, including that of glycogen breakdown, with consequent hypoglycemia which may be severe. Symptoms consisting of vomiting, sweating, and convulsions occur after sucrose or fructose are introduced into an infant's diet. These disappear if glucose is given. Older children and adults may have epigastric pain, bloating, diarrhea, and hepatomegaly. Symptoms are brought on acutely by eating fruit or food sweetened with cane sugar (sucrose). Symptoms are reversible and competely preventable by excluding fructose from the diet. The inheritance is autosomal recessive. Also *fructose intolerance, fructokinase deficiency.* Abbr. HFI. **hereditary galactose i.** GALACTOSEMIA. **lactose i.** Inadequate capacity of the intestine to hydrolyze lactose, resulting in a syndrome of abdominal discomfort, cramps, and watery diarrhea, mostly occurring within thirty minutes to a few hours after ingesting milk or milk products. It may be genetic or occur in association with other gastrointestinal disorders. Also *milk intolerance.* **leucine i.** Intolerance of the branched-chain amino acid leucine, one of the causes of hypoglycemia in early infancy. Ingestion of leucine causes a rapid fall in blood sugar. It also occurs in maple sugar urine disease, the dietetic control of which requires regulating the amounts of the three branched-chain amino acids, leucine, valine, and isoleucine. **lysine i.** An autosomal recessive disorder that is caused by a deficiency of L-lysine:NAD-oxido-reductase. It is evident in infancy, and it is characterized by vomiting, coma, and hyperammonemia. A low-protein diet to restrict lysine constitutes treatment. **milk i.** LACTOSE INTOLERANCE.

**intonation** \in'tōnā'shən\ [Med L *intonatio* (from *intonare* to utter in a singing tone, to intone, from L *in-* IN-[1] + *tonus* a sound) an intoning] **1** The patterned pitch variations that characterize utterances in a particular language or of a particular speaker. **2** The quality of musical tone production with respect to accuracy of pitch. **3** The quality of voice production with respect to its tonal characteristics. **nasal i.** NASAL RESONANCE.

**intorsion** \intôr'shən\ Rotation of the eye upon its anteroposterior axis so that the upper part of the eye approaches the midline of the body. Also *conclination.*

**intorter** \intôr'tər\ [L *intort(us),* past part. of *intorquere* to turn around, twist + -ER] An extraocular muscle that turns the eye on its anteroposterior axis so that the upper part of the eye moves nasalward.

**intoxation** \in'täksā'shən\ *Seldom used* INTOXICATION.

**intoxicant** \intäk'sikənt\ A substance that produces intoxication or drunkenness.

**intoxication** \intäk'sikā'shən\ [Med L *intoxicatio* (from *intoxicare* to poison, from IN-[1] + L *toxicum* a poison) poisoning. See TOXIC.] **1** The action of an absorbed and diffused toxic substance upon an organism, or the resultant pathological state of the organism; poisoning. Also *toxication, intoxation* (seldom used). **2** Drunkenness; acute alcoholism or a clinically similar condition. **anaphylactic i.** ANAPHYLACTIC SHOCK. **citrate i.** A condition that may develop from blood transfusions in which citrate has been used as an anticoagulant. Tetany may result from the citrate combining with the blood calcium, thereby reducing the concentration of ionized calcium. **digitalis i.** Poisoning with one of the digitalis alkaloids. Overdosage causes increased cardiac irritability and irregularities, gastrointestinal and visual disturbances, and occasionally, bizarre neurologic symptoms and psychoses in later stages of intoxication. **intestinal i.** Intoxication from the production and accumulation of toxins formed in the intestine. Also *autointoxication, intestinal autointoxication.* **manganese i.** A syndrome resembling parkinsonism which results from chronic exposure to the dust of manganese ores and which is seen almost exclusively in miners of the metal and those handling the ores in factories. **pathologic i.** Idiosyncratic hypersensitivity to alcohol, a small amount of which precipitates extreme excitement with persecutory ideas and aggressive, destructive, and sometimes homicidal outbursts. The reaction lasts several hours and ends with the subject falling into a deep sleep from which he wakes with total amnesia for the episode. Also *alcoholic fury, mania a potu, alcoholic mania.* **roentgen i.** RADIATION SICKNESS. **serum i.** SERUM SICKNESS. **water i.** An excessive water content in the body. Also *hydrotoxicity.*

**intra-** \in'trə-\ [L *intra* (for *intera*) within, inside] A prefix meaning within, inside.

**intra-abdominal** \-abdäm'ənəl\ Situated or occurring within the abdomen.

**intra-arachnoid** \-ərak'noid\ Situated within the trabeculae of the arachnoid in the subarachnoid space.

**intra-arterial** \-ärtir'ē·əl\ Within an artery or arteries.

**intra-articular** \-ärtik'yələr\ Within a joint cavity.

**intra-atrial** \-ā'trē·əl\ Within an atrium or the atria of the heart.

**intra-aural** \-ôr'əl\ Within the ear.

**intra-auricular** \-ôrik'yələr\ Within an auricle of the ear or the atrium of the heart.

**intrabuccal** \-buk'əl\ **1** Within the mouth. **2** Within the mass of the cheek.

**intracaliceal** \-kal'isē'əl\ Within a renal calix.

**intracapsular** \-kap's$^y$ələr\ Within a capsule, particularly of a joint.

**intracardiac** Within the heart. Also *intracordal.*

**intracarpal** Within the wrist or among wrist bones.

**intracartilaginous** \-kär'tilaj'ənəs\ Located or formed within cartilage or cartilaginous tissue. Also *endochondral, enchondral, intrachondral, intrachondrial.*

**intracatheter** \-kath'ətər\ [INTRA- + CATHETER] A plastic tube introduced through a metal needle into a vein or artery and used for fluid infusion, drug injection, sampling blood, or keeping track of pressures.

**intracavernous** Within a cavernous sinus of the skull.

**intracavitary** \-kav'iter'ē\ Within the cavity of an organ or part.

**intracelial** \-sē'lē·əl\ Within any of the body cavities; endoceliac.

**intracellular** \-sel'yələr\ Within a cell. Also *endocellular.*

**intracerebral** \-ser'əbrəl\ Within the cerebrum.

**intracervical** \-sur'vikəl\ Within any cervical canal, particularly that of the cervix uteri.

**intrachange** \in'trəchānj\ HOMOSOMAL ABERRATION.

**intrachondral** \-kän'drəl\ INTRACARTILAGINOUS.

**intrachondrial** \-kän'drē·əl\ INTRACARTILAGINOUS.

**intrachordal** \-kôr'dəl\ [INTRA- + CHORDAL] Situated or occurring inside the notochord.

**intrachorionic** \-kôr'ē·än'ik\ Situated or occurring within the chorion.

**intracolic** \-kō'lik\ Situated or occurring within the colon.

**intracordal** \-kôr′dəl\ INTRACARDIAC.

**intracoronal** \-kôr′ənəl\ Situated within the crown of a tooth: used especially of an attachment placed in a prepared cavity.

**intracorporeal** \-kôrpôr′ē·əl\ Located or occurring within a body. Also *intracorporal*.

**intracorpuscular** \-kôrpus′kyələr\ Located inside a corpuscle, especially inside an erythrocyte. Hemolytic disorders may be divided into those of intracorpuscular and those of extracorpuscular cause. Also *endocorpuscular*.

**intracostal** \-käs′təl\ On the internal surface of a rib or ribs.

**intracranial** \-krā′nē·əl\ Within the skull or cranium.

**intractable** \intrak′təbl\ [L *intractabilis* (from *in-* not + *tractabilis* manageable, from *tractare* to handle, deal with, from *trahere* to pull, attract) unmanageable] Resistant to therapy.

**intracystic** \-sis′tik\ Occurring within a cyst or within the urinary bladder.

**intracytoplasmic** \-sī′təplaz′mik\ Located in the cytoplasm of a cell.

**intradermal** \-dur′məl\ Situated within the dermis. Also *intradermic*.

**intradermoreaction** \-dur′mōrē·ak′shən\ INTRACUTANEOUS REACTION.

**intraduct** \in′trədukt\ Within a duct or ducts. Also *intraductal*.

**intradural** \-d^yoo′rəl\ Situated within or below the dura mater of the brain or spinal cord.

**intraembryonic** \in′trə·em′brē·än′ik\ [INTRA- + EMBRYONIC] Situated or occurring within the embryo.

**intraepidermal** \in′trə·ep′idur′məl\ Situated within the epidermis. Also *intraepidermic*.

**intraerythrocytic** \in′trə·irith′rəsit′ik\ Located within the cytoplasm of erythrocytes.

**intrafebrile** \-feb′ril\ Occurring during the febrile phase of a disease. Also *intrapyretic*.

**intrafissural** \-fish′ərəl\ Within a fissure of the cerebral cortex.

**intrafusal** \-fyoo′zəl\ Denoting the striated muscle fibers situated within the fusiform capsule of a muscle spindle.

**intragastric** \-gas′trik\ Found or occurring within the stomach.

**intragemmal** \-jem′əl\ Within any gemma or bulblike structure, such as a taste bud.

**intragenic** \-jē′nik\ **1** Pertaining to a region of DNA or chromosome entirely within a genetic locus. **2** Referring to a mutation, particularly a deletion or an insertion, that is located entirely within a given locus.

**intraglandular** Within a gland or glandular tissue.

**intragluteal** \-gloo′tē·əl\ Within the buttock or the gluteal region.

**intragyral** \-jī′rəl\ Within a gyrus of the cerebral cortex.

**intrahepatic** \-hepat′ik\ Within the liver.

**intrahyoid** \-hī′oid\ Occurring within the hyoid bone, as accessory thyroid glands.

**intraictal** \in′trə·ik′təl\ [INTRA- + ICTAL] Present or occurring during an attack.

**intrajugular** \-jug′yələr\ Within the jugular fossa, notch, process, foramen, or vein.

**intralaryngeal** \-larin′jē·əl\ Within the larynx.

**intralesional** \-lē′zhənəl\ Present within a lesion.

**intraleukocytic** \-loo′kōsit′ik\ Located within the cytoplasm of leukocytes.

**intralingual** \-ling′gwəl\ Within the tongue.

**intraluminal** \-loo′minəl\ Within the lumen of any tubular structure, such as an artery or the intestine.

**intramammary** \-mam′ərē\ Within the mammary gland or breast.

**intramarginal** \-mär′jənəl\ Within the margin or edge of any structure or organ.

**intramatrical** \-mat′rikəl\ Situated within a matrix.

**intramedullary** \-med′yəler′ē\ Within or into any medulla, marrow, or myelin sheath.

**intramembranous** \-mem′brənəs\ Within the layers of a membrane.

**intrameningeal** \-mənin′jē·əl\ Situated within the meninges surrounding the brain and spinal cord.

**intramenstrual** \-men′stroo·əl\ Occurring within the menstrual period.

**intramucosal** \-myookō′səl\ Within the layers of a mucous membrane.

**intramural** \myoo′rəl\ Within the substance or the boundary of the wall of any organ or cavity. Also *intraparietal*.

**intramuscular** \-mus′kyələr\ Within or into a muscle. Abbr. IM

**intranasal** \-nā′zəl\ Within the nose.

**intraneural** \-n^yUr′əl\ **1** Within or extending into a nerve. **2** Within or extending into the central nervous system. **3** Within or extending into the cytoplasm of a neuron or one of its processes. Also *intraneuronal*.

**intranuclear** \-n^yoo′klē·ər\ Situated or occurring within the nucleus.

**intraocular** \-äk′yələr\ [INTRA- + OCULAR] Located or occurring within the eyeball.

**intraoperative** \-äp′ərətiv\ [INTRA- + OPERATIVE] Pertaining to the period of time between the beginning and the completion of a surgical procedure.

**intraoral** \in′trə·ôr′əl\ Within the mouth.

**intraosseous** \in′trə·äs′ē·əs\ Within a bone or bony tissue. Also *intraosteal*.

**intraparenchymatous** \-par′ənkim′ətəs\ Within the parenchyma of a gland or an organ.

**intraparietal** \-pərī′ətəl\ **1** INTRAMURAL. **2** Within the parietal lobe of the cerebrum; specifically, denoting the intraparietal sulcus.

**intrapartum** \-pär′təm\ [INTRA- + *partum*, accusative of *partus* a birth, begetting] Occurring during labor or delivery.

**intrapericardial** \-per′ikär′dē·əl\ Within the pericardium or the pericardial cavity.

**intraperineal** \-per′ənē′əl\ Within the structures of the perineum.

**intraperitoneal** \-per′itənē·′əl\ Within the cavity of the peritoneum.

**intrapial** \-pē′əl\ Lying within or covered by the pia mater.

**intrapleural** \-plUr′əl\ Within the pleura or pleural cavity.

**intrapulmonary** \-pul′məner′ē\ Within the lung or lungs.

**intrapyretic** \-pīret′ik\ INTRAFEBRILE.

**intrarenal** \-rē′nəl\ Within the kidney.

**intraretinal** \-ret′ənəl\ Located within the retina.

**intrasegmental** Within a segment, such as of the spinal cord.

**intrasellar** \-sel′ər\ Within the sella turcica of the sphenoid bone.

**intraspinal** \-spī′nəl\ Within the vertebral column, the vertebral canal, or the spinal cord.

**intraspinous** \-spī′nəs\ Within a spinous process, as of a vertebra.

**intrastitial** \-stish′əl\ Situated within the fibers or cells of a tissue.
**intrastromal** \-strō′məl\ Within the stroma, or framework, of an organ.
**intrasynovial** \-sinō′vē·əl\ Within the synovial membrane of a joint cavity or the synovial sheath of a tendon.
**intrathecal** \-thē′kəl\ **1** Within a sheath. **2** Within the subarachnoid space; intradural.
**intrathenar** \-thē′när\ Pertaining to the shallow sulcus between the thenar and the hypothenar eminences in the palm of the hand.
**intrathoracic** ENDOTHORACIC.
**intratubal** \-t$^y$oo′bəl\ Within a tube or tubular structure, particularly the uterine tube.
**intratubular** \-t$^y$oo′byələr\ Within a tubule or tubules of an organ.
**intratympanic** \-timpan′ik\ Within the tympanic cavity.
**intraurethral** \-yoorē′thrəl\ Within the urethra. Also *endourethral.*
**intrauterine** \-yoo′tərin\ Within the uterus.
**intravasation** \intrav′əsā′shən\ [INTRA- + VAS + -ATION ] The entry or introduction of foreign matter into a vein or artery.
**intravascular** \-vas′kyələr\ Within a vessel or vessels, particularly blood and lymphatic vessels.
**intravenous** \-vē′nəs\ **1** Within a vein or veins. **2** Into a vein. Abbr. IV
**intravertebral** \-vur′təbrəl\ Within the vertebral column or canal.
**intravesical** \-ves′ikəl\ Within the bladder, particularly the urinary bladder.
**intravital** \-vī′təl\ **1** Found or occurring during life. **2** Used, or capable of being used, on the cells or tissues of living organisms: said of a stain. For defs. 1 and 2. also *intravitam.* Compare SUPRAVITAL.
**intravitam** INTRAVITAL.
***intra vitam*** \in′trə vī′təm\ [L *intra* within, inside + *vitam,* accus. sing. of *vita* life] During life.
**intravitelline** \-vītel′īn\ Situated inside the vitellus.
**intravitreous** \-vit′rē·əs\ Located or occurring within the vitreous cavity. Also *intravitreal.*
**intrinsic** \intrin′sik, intrin′zik\ [L *intrinsecus* (from *int(e)r* within + *-im,* adv. suffix, + *secus* beside; ending *-ec(us)* assimilated in English to -IC) from inside, internally] **1** Originating within the organism; endogenous. **2** Situated within and forming an integral part of the organ served: said of anatomic structures. Compare EXTRINSIC.
**intro-** \in′trə-\ [L *intro* (for *intero*) inward, within] A prefix meaning into, inward, being directed within.
**introducer** \-d$^y$oo′sər\ Any instrument designed to facilitate the introduction of some other instrument or appliance. For example, the introducer of a tracheostomy tube converts the blunt open end of the tube into a smooth, rounded tip and provides a handle.
**introflexion** \-flek′shən\ A bending or flexing inward.
**introgastric** \-gas′trik\ Moved or transported into the stomach.
**introitus** \intrō′itəs\ [L (from INTRO- + L *itus* past part. of *ire* to go) a going in, entrance] The opening into a cavity, canal, or hollow organ.
**introjection** \-jek′shən\ [INTRO- + *(pro)jection*] An unconscious defense mechanism of the ego consisting of incorporation or assimilation of an external object into one's ego, a part of which is thereby transformed into the representation of that object so that what originally occurred between the real object and self now occurs between the introjected object and self.
**intromission** \-mish′ən\ [L *intromissus,* past part. of *intromittere* (from *intro-* inward, within + *mittere* to send, cause to go) to send into or to] **1** The act of inserting the penis into the vagina in coitus. **2** Introduction or insertion of an object or part within something else.
**intron** \in′trän\ [*intr(a)-* + -ON] A region of a gene that lies between exons and is transcribed into RNA, but later is spliced out and does not code for translated gene product. Also *intervening sequence.* Compare EXON.
**intropunitive** \-pyoo′nitiv\ [INTRO- + PUNITIVE] Denoting a self-punishing reaction to frustration characterized by self-blame and feelings of shame, guilt, or humiliation.
**introrsus** \intrôr′səs\ [L (from INTRO- + *(v)orsus,* variant of *versus* turned) inward, inwardly] Turned inward or toward the center.
**introsusception** \-susep′shən\ INTUSSUSCEPTION.
**introversion** \-vur′zhən\ [New L *introversio* (from INTRO- + L *ver(tere)* to turn) a turning inward] The dynamic process in personality development by which the psychic energy of the individual is directed inwardly toward the self.
**introversion-extroversion** A hypothetical bipolar dimension of the personality which attempts to classify individuals along a continuum varying from complete absorption in the self, to a complete outer-directedness towards external objects and other people.
**introvert** \in′trəvurt\ [INTRO- + L *vert(ere)* to turn] One whose personality is turned primarily inward, whose interests are vested more in personal thoughts, feelings, and experiences than in the world of external objects, other people, or social concerns.
**intrude** [L *intrudere* (from *in-* in + *trudere* to thrust) to push or thrust in] To move a tooth into the bone in the direction of its root.
**intrusion** Inward protrusion, thrusting, or penetration.
**intubate** \in′t$^y$oobāt\ [IN-[1] + *tub(e)* + -ATE] To introduce a tube into.
**intubation** \in′t$^y$oobā′shən\ [L *in-* in + TUBE + -ATION] The introduction of a tube, as into a vessel or orifice. **aqueductal i.** The introduction of a catheter through the aqueduct of Sylvius. **blind nasal i.** Nasal intubation in which the physician uses tactile and visual senses and the breathing sounds made by the patient as a guide, thus obviating the use of a laryngoscope. A topical or general anesthetic is applied prior to this procedure. **blind nasotracheal i.** Nasotracheal intubation in which the physician does not have direct vision of the trachea. **nasal i.** The passage of a tube, via the nose, into the trachea or stomach. **nasotracheal i.** The passage of a tube into the trachea via the nose, either blindly or under direct vision. **oral i.** The passage of a tube into the stomach or trachea via the mouth, done under direct vision. **orotracheal i.** The passage of a tube, via the mouth, into the trachea done under direct vision.
**intubator** \in′t$^y$oobā′tər\ One who performs intubation.
**intuition** \in′t$^y$oo·ish′ən\ [Late L *intuitio* (from L *intuitus,* past part. of *intueri* to look at or upon) a beholding, contemplation] Judgment, perception, or knowledge that arrives in consciousness without prior, conscious, systematic thinking or reflection. The meaning of the data that are directly apprehended often contains an emotional component and is notable for its immediacy and the absence of any need for cogitation.
**intumesce** \in′t$^y$oomes′\ TUMEFY.
**intumescence** \in′t$^y$oomes′əns\ **1** INTUMESCENTIA. **2** The process of swelling.
**intumescentia** \int$^y$oo′məsen′shə\ [L *intumenscens,* gen.

*intumescent(is)*, pres. part. of *intumescere* to swell up, rise, project (from *tumere* to be swollen) + *-ia*, noun suffix] A swelling or enlargement. **i. cervicalis** [NA] The cervical enlargement of the spinal cord, reaching its maximum thickness at the level of the fifth and sixth cervical vertebrae. It contains the motoneurons, interneurons, and fiber connections for $C_5$–$T_1$ spinal roots. Also *cervical enlargement.* **i. ganglioformis** A swelling in the shape of a ganglion. **i. lumbalis** [NA] The lumbar enlargement of the spinal cord beginning at the level of the tenth thoracic vertebra, reaching its maximum thickness at the level of the first lumbar vertebra and tapering caudally. It includes central neurons and connects for $L_4$–$S_3$ spinal roots. Also *lumbar enlargement.* **i. tympanica** A swelling of the tympanic branch of the glossopharyngeal nerve lacking ganglion cells. Also *Valentin pseudoganglion.*

**intussusception** \in'tususep'shən\ [L *intus* within, inside + *susceptio* (from *suscipere* to receive, take up, from *capere* to take) reception, taking on] The invagination or telescoping of one segment of the intestine within a neighboring segment, most commonly the ileum into the colon. Also *intro-susception.* **agonic i.** POSTMORTEM INTUSSUSCEPTION. **appendicular i.** The intussusception of the vermiform appendix upon itself. This mostly occurs in infancy and early childhood. **double i.** The occurrence of a second intussusception proximal to the first so that the mass formed by the first intussusception is enveloped by the second. **enterocolic i.** An intussusception of both the terminal ileum and the right colon such that the terminal ileum passes distally through the ileocecal valve into the cecum or colon. **ileal i.** An intussusception involving two segments of the ileum. **ileocecal i.** An enterocolic intussusception with the passage of the ileum into the cecum. **jejunogastric i.** A post-gastrojejunostomy complication involving the intussusception of either an efferent or afferent loop of bowel into the stomach. **postmortem i.** The development of an intestinal intussusception during the early postmortem interval. Also *agonic intussusception.* **retrograde i.** Intussusception of distal bowel into a proximal segment.

**intussusceptum** \in'tususep'təm\ A segment of intestine which has prolapsed into an immediately adjacent portion of intestine.

**intussuscipiens** \in'tususip'ē·əns\ A segment of intestine into which an immediately adjacent portion of intestine has prolapsed.

**inulin** \in'yəlin\ A vegetable polysaccharide composed of fructofuranose units in a polymer form. It is used as a test substance to evaluate renal excretory function.

**inunction** \inungk'shən\ [L *inunctio* (from *inunguere* to rub in, from *unguere* to anoint) an anointing or rubbing in] **1** Surface application of an ointment with friction to facilitate penetration into the skin. Also *perfrication.* **2** An ointment or other medication to be applied with friction. Also *inunctum.*

**inunctum** \inungk'təm\ INUNCTION.

***in utero*** \in yoo'tərō\ [L *in* in + *utero*, ablative of UTERUS] Situated within the uterine cavity.

***in vacuo*** \in vak'yoo·ō\ [L *in* in + *vacuo*, ablative of *vacuum* (substantive from neut. sing. of *vacuus* empty, void) a vacuum] **1** Taking place in a vacuum. **2** Designating events or actions that occur seemingly without causal relationship to any other event.

**invade** To penetrate or spread into injuriously, as infectious organisms or diseased tissue.

**invaginate** \invaj'ināt\ [See INVAGINATION.] To infold (one portion of a structure) so that it becomes ensheathed within the structure.

**invagination** \invaj'inā'shən\ [L *in-* in + L *vagin(a)* sheath + -ATION] **1** A type of gastrulation in which part of the blastoderm of an early embryo folds inward so that the hollow sphere becomes a double-walled cup. **2** The portion of the structure so ensheathed. **basilar i.** PLATYBASIA. **i. of enamel** DENS INVAGINATUS. **mammary i.** The primitive epithelial invagination, which during the eighth week in human development develops internally from the surface of the skin to form the galactiferous ducts.

**invaginator** \invaj'inā'tər\ [See INVAGINATION.] A surgical instrument that is used to fold in one portion of a structure onto another portion of the same structure.

**invalid** \in'vəlid\ [L *invalidus* (from *in-* IN-[2] + *validus* strong, from *valere* to be strong, have force) weak, powerless] **1** Suffering from a disabling condition. **2** A person whose condition is disabling, as from chronic illness, infirmity, or injury.

**invalidism** \in'vəlidizm'\ [INVALID + -ISM] The condition of being an invalid, especially when of long duration.

**invasion** The infiltration of adjacent tissues by a disease process, usually cancer.

**invasive** \invā'siv\ [Med L *invasivus* (from L *invadere* to come on, attack, invade, from *vadere* to advance, proceed) tending to invade] **1** Marked by invasiveness; tending to spread to other tissues. **2** Involving the penetration of a body cavity or the skin; used especially of a therapeutic or diagnostic procedure.

**invasiveness** \invā'sivnis\ **1** The aspect of pathogenicity involving penetration into a tissue or stable attachment to an epithelial surface, thus promoting spread in the body. **2** The quality of being invasive, as a therapeutic or diagnostic procedure.

**inventory** \in'vəntôr'ē\ [Med L *inventor(ium)* (irreg. from Late L *inventarium* a finding out, from *invent(us)*, past part. of *invenire* to find, obtain information on + *-arium* -ARY) a finding information on + -Y] A list of questions to be answered to determine the presence or absence of certain interests, behaviors, or attitudes. **Maudsley personality i.** A questionnaire consisting of a variety of items about characteristic personal behaviors and interpersonal reactions. It is designed to measure two dimensions of personality held to be basic: neuroticism and introversion-extroversion. **Minnesota multiphasic personality i.** A widely used paper-and-pencil personality test in which the subject marks 550 items, concerning behavior, feelings, abnormal symptoms, social attitudes, or reactions, as "agree," "disagree," or "cannot say." Also *Minnesota multiphasic personality test.*

**invermination** \invur'minā'shən\ [IN-[1] + VERMIN + -ATION] Infestation by vermin.

**Inversine** A proprietary name for mecamylamine hydrochloride.

**inversion** \invur'zhən\ [L *inversio* (from *inversus*, past part. of *invertere* to turn over, transpose, alter, from *in-* in + *vertere* to turn) a transposition, reversal] **1** The condition of being inside out, upside down, or out of place or usual position. **2** Any developmental reversal of the usual position, sidedness, or relationship of organs or parts. It occurs most commonly in the viscera, as in situs inversus viscerum. **3** The conversion of a chiral center in a molecule into its enantiomeric configuration. **4** An alteration in a section of DNA that reverses the direction of transcription. Inversion plays a key role in the regulation of a number of bacterial genes, such as those involved in phase variation in *Salmonella.* **i. of the bladder** A partial or complete inversion of the urinary bladder through the urethral meatus due to relaxation of the vesical outlet. It is in many cases a result of straining during urination. **chromosome i.** A chromosome aberration in which one portion of the chromatid is rotated 180° about its longitudinal midpoint. The phenotype may or may not be affected. **forced i.** Iatrogenic inversion of the uterus caused by undue traction on the umbilical cord or excessive fundal pressure in an effort to deliver a placenta following delivery of an infant. **i. of gradient** Abnormal uterine contractions during labor which start in the lower uterine segment and spread toward the fundus. Normally contractions start in the fundus and spread toward the lower uterine segment. **lateral i.** MIRROR IMAGE. **paracentric i.** A chromosome aberration in which a portion of one chromosome arm, not including the centromere, is inverted. **pericentric i.** A chromosome aberration in which a portion of both chromosome arms and the centromere is inverted. **sexual i.** *Obs.* HOMOSEXUALITY. **sound i.** SONOINVERSION. **spontaneous i.** The turning inside out of the uterus as a natural occurrence during or following placental delivery as opposed to its occurrence as a complication of too vigorous traction on the umbilical cord to speed placental delivery (forced inversion). **thermic i.** A reversal of the normal circadian rhythm of body temperature that results in the temperature being at its highest in the morning. **i. of uterus** Abnormal turning of the uterus inside out so that the internal surface of the corpus uteri lies in or outside of the vagina. Also *metranastrophe.* **visceral i.** SITUS INVERSUS VISCERUM.

**inversus** \invur′səs\ [L, past part. of *invertere* to turn about, change, invert] Denoting a reversal of the normal position or relations of a structure or an organ, from right side to left side, or vice versa, or upside down; transposition of viscera.

**invert** \in′vurt\ *Older term* HOMOSEXUAL.

**invertase** β-D-Fructofuranosidase, an enzyme especially important for its hydrolysis of sucrose to glucose and fructose. The mixture produced was once known as invert sugar, owing to its possessing an optical rotation of opposite sign to that of the sucrose substrate. *Outmoded.* Also *invertin.*

**invertebrate** \invur′təbrət\ **1** Any animal that lacks a nerve cord, or in which the nerve cord is not enclosed in a skeletal backbone. **2** Any animal that is not classified as a member of the chordate subphylum Vertebrata.

**invertin** INVERTASE.

**invertor** \invur′tər\ A muscle responsible for turning a part, such as the foot, inward.

**invest** To surround, envelop, or ensheath with a particular material.

**investing** The act of surrounding a wax pattern or any solid form with a setting material so as to make a mold. **vacuum i.** The subjecting of a dental investment mixture to a vacuum in order to remove air bubbles.

**investment** [L *invest(ire)* (from *in-* in + *vestire* to cover, clothe, from *vestis* a garment, clothing, akin to Gk *esthēs* a garment) to clothe + -MENT] **1** An outer covering, enveloping material, or sheath. **2** The setting material used to surround a wax pattern in the making of a mold, especially refractory material used in casting. For defs. 1 and 2 also *investiture.* **emotional i.** CATHEXIS. **fibrous i.** A fibrous connective tissue layer surrounding a structure but separate from its capsule. **hygroscopic i.** An investment using the property of hygroscopic expansion to compensate for the contraction of the cast on cooling. **myelin i.** MYELIN SHEATH.

**inveterate** \invet′ərit\ [L *inveterat(us),* past part. of *inveterare* (from *in-* IN-[1] + *vetus,* gen. *veteris,* old, of long standing) to become old, last a long time] Long-standing, chronic, and resistant to cure or correction.

**invirility** \in′viril′itē\ *Obs.* IMPOTENCE.

***in vitro*** \in vē′trō\ [L *in* in + *vitro,* ablative of *vitrum* glass] Describing a biological event that occurs in a laboratory in an artificial environment. Compare *IN VIVO.*

***in vivo*** \in vē′vō\ [L *in* in + *vivo,* ablative of *vivum* that which is living, from neut. sing. of *vivus* living] Describing a biological event that occurs in an intact animal or in the natural environment. Compare *IN VITRO.*

**involucrum** \in′vōloo′krəm\ [L (from *involvere* to wrap up, envelop, cover), a wrapper, covering] **1** A surrounding sheath or membrane. Also *involucre.* **2** The growth of new bone that forms around necrosed bone (sequestrum).

**involuntary** \inväl′ənter′ē\ **1** Not voluntary. **2** In psychiatry, not consciously desired.

**involute** \in′vōloot\ To infold within another structure.

**involution** \in′vōloo′shən\ [L *involutio* (from *involutus,* past part. of *involvere* to roll in, envelop, from *in-* in + *volvere* to roll, turn) an enveloping] **1** An infolding. **2** A return to a former state. **3** Retrogression or decay. **4** CATABOLISM. **buccal i.** The turning inward of ectoderm as the primitive oral cavity is formed in the embryo. **pituitary i.** The first sign of Rathke's pouch as an upgrowth from the roof of the buccal cavity which will form the anterior lobe of the pituitary gland. **i. of the uterus** The gradual restoration to normal size of the uterus following a pregnancy.

**involvement** \invälv′mənt\ [L *involvere* to to roll in, envelop, cover, from *in-* in + *volvere* to roll, turn + -MENT] The inclusion in a disease process of a part not previously affected. **bifurcation i.** The extension of a periodontal pocket between the roots of a two-rooted tooth. **trifurcation i.** The extension of a periodontal pocket between the roots of a three-rooted tooth.

**iod-** IODO-.

**iodalbumin** Albumin containing covalently linked iodine in tyrosyl residues. It is a source of iodine and has properties like those of thyroglobulin, although it is much less active.

***Iodamoeba beutschlii*** \ī·ō′dəmē′bə bʏch′lē·ī\ A species of ameba parasitic in the large intestine of humans. The trophozoites range from 5 to 20 μm in diameter and are infrequently found in feces. Cysts, ranging from 5 to 14 μm in diameter, are of irregular shape, uninucleate, and thick-walled, with a compact mass of glycogen that stains deeply with iodine solution. Cysts are the infective forms passed in feces. The organism is normally not pathogenic in man.

**iod-Basedow** \ī′ōd-bas′ədō\ [*iod(ine-induced)* + *Basedow('s disease)*] IODINE-INDUCED HYPERTHYROIDISM.

**iodemia** \ī′ōdē′mē·ə\ The presence of iodine or iodide in blood, plasma, or serum.

**iodide** **1** The ion $I^-$ or a salt that contains it. **2** Iodine in covalent combination, e.g. iodomethane, $CH_3$—I, may be called methyl iodide.

**iodinate** To add iodine to a compound, usually in substitution for hydrogen, but sometimes by simple addition.

**iodine** \ī′ədīn\ A nonmetallic element of the halogen group, having atomic number 53 and atomic weight 126.9045. It consists of lustrous blackish crystalline flakes that volatilize at room temperature, forming a violet vapor with a strong odor. Iodine occurs in salt deposits and in sea water, where it is concentrated in the fronds of seaweeds. Inland areas are often deficient in iodine. The only isotope found in nature is the stable iodine 127. Valences are 1, 3, 5, and 7. Iodine is insoluble in water but soluble in an aqueous solution of potassium or sodium iodide. Its characteristic reaction with starch, the formation of a dark blue compound, provides a simple test for either starch or iodine. Iodine is an essential constituent of thyroid hormones and small amounts of iodine are essential in the diet. Symbol: I **butanol-extractable i.** Iodine, largely deriving from thyroid hormones, that is separated from serum by extraction with butanol, a step that eliminates some but not all of the interfering compounds that render the protein-bound iodine level inaccurate as a measurement of circulating thyroxine. This test is now supplanted by direct measurement of thyroxine. Abbr. BEI **protein-bound i.** Iodine present in serum and precipitated with serum proteins. Although largely derived from thyroid hormones, protein-bound iodine values also include inorganic iodides, abnormal iodinated proteins, and exogenous iodine-containing materials. It was formerly measured to indicate circulating thyroxine levels, but is now supplanted by direct measurement of thyroxine. Abbr. PBI **radioactive i.** Any iodine isotype other than iodine 127, which is stable. Three of these have been useful as diagnostic and therapeutic tools in diseases of the thyroid gland. The one in longest use is eight-day iodine 131, but it has been replaced to some extent by three-hour iodine 123 and iodine 125. Also *radioiodine.*

**iodine 131** A radioactive isotope of iodine emitting beta and gamma radiation. As the radioactive element itself, it is used for thyroid imaging and function tests. It can also be used as a marker for renal imaging (sodium iodohippurate I-131), hepatobiliary imaging (rose bengal I-131), and for many other labeled agents. In therapeutic doses, it is used in the treatment of hyperthyroidism and thyroid carcinoma. Physical half-life is 8.04 days. Symbol: $^{131}I$

**iodine-fast** Describing hyperthyroidism unresponsive to treatment with iodine.

**iodine green** A chromatin stain containing triphenylmethane. Also *Hoffman green.*

**iodinin** $C_{12}H_8N_2O_4$. 1,6-phenazinediol 5,10-dioxide, a purple chemical isolated from *Chromobacterium iodinum.* It has antibiotic activity against staphylococci, streptococci, and some Gram-negative bacteria.

**iodinophil** \ī′ōdin′əfil\ **1** Readily combining with or staining with iodine. Also *iodinophilous.* **2** An iodinophil cell or other tissue constituent. Also *iodophil.*

**iodipamide** $C_{20}H_{14}I_6N_2O_6$. 3,3′-[(1,6-Dioxo-1,6-hexanediyl)diimino]bis[2,4,6-triiodobenzoic acid]. A contrast substance for radiographic visualization of the biliary system.

**iodism** \ī′ədizm\ Poisoning from the chronic ingestion of iodine or its compounds, or from intensive, repeated therapy. Symptoms are coryza, ptyalism, headache, and skin eruptions.

**iodize** To treat with iodine and incorporate or attach (iodine) to a product; iodinate.

**iodo-** [Gk *iōdēs* (from *ion* violet) violet-colored] **1** A combining form meaning violet. **2** A combining form meaning (1) iodine; (2) substitution of iodine for hydrogen in a chemical compound. Also *iod-.*

**iodoacetamide** I—CH$_2$—CO—NH$_2$. A reagent often used for alkylating thiol groups in proteins. Their ionized form, R—S$^-$, attacks its methylene group, expelling I$^-$ to form R—S—CH$_2$—CO—NH$_2$.

**iodoacetic acid** I—CH$_2$—COOH. An acid forming colorless crystals, soluble in alcohol and ether, which darken on keeping, especially in the light, with release of iodine, so that pure samples need to be freshly recrystallized. It is a moderately strong acid (p*K* 3.1). It carboxymethylates nucleophiles, especially the thiol group, and inhibits thiol enzymes by the reaction: R—SH + I—CH$_2$—COO$^-$ → R—S—CH$_2$—COO$^-$ + H$^+$ + I$^-$.

**iodoantipyrine** A freely diffusible radioisotope-labeled tracer used to measure the blood flow in skin and other tissues.

**iodobrassid** $C_{24}H_{44}I_2O_2$. 13,14-Diiodo-13-docosenic acid ethyl ester. A source of iodine for iodide therapy and a radiopaque contrast medium.

**iodocasein** An iodinated casein preparation containing 5.7% iodine, attached to the tyrosine residues. It has thyroxinelike activity.

**iodochlorhydroxyquin** $C_9H_5ClINO$. 5-Chloro-7-iodo-8-quinolinol. A brownish yellow powder, prepared as a powder, cream, or ointment, in suppositories, or as enteric-coated tablets. It has a direct amebicidal action and is used to treat acute and chronic intestinal amebiasis. It has also been used to treat *Trichomonas, Candida,* and various dermatitis infections by local or tropical application. It has also been used in dusting powders on wounds, ulcers, and burns of the skin. Also *clioquinol.*

**iodocholesterol** Cholesterol that has been labeled with one or more iodine atoms. The iodine may be radioactive (radioiodinated cholesterol).

**5-iododeoxyuridine** IDOXURIDINE.

**iodoform** \ī·ō′dəfôrm\ $CHI_3$. A compound containing approximately 96% iodine. It is a yellow, crystalline powder and has been used topically as an anti-infective agent. It is known to be toxic in some cases. Also *triiodomethane.*

**iodogorgonine** An iodinated protein from corals which produces diiodotyrosine upon hydrolysis.

**iodohippurate sodium** A compound used for studying renal function when labeled with an appropriate radionuclide. It has also been used as a radiopaque compound for urography.

**iodophendylate** IOPHENDYLATE.

**iodophil** \ī′ōdōfil′\ IODINOPHIL.

**iodophilia** \ī′ōdōfil′yə\ An affinity for iodine or iodide, characteristic of starch and amyloid. Although iodophilia is said to be characteristic of neutrophil leukocytes in certain pathologic states, such as toxemia, it is not currently considered of diagnostic value. *Rare.*

**iodophor** A high molecular weight carrier, such as polyvinylpyrrolidone, which holds iodine and is used pre-operatively as a disinfectant on the skin.

**iodoprotein** \ī′ōdōprō′tē·in\ An endogenous protein of the serum in which iodine is covalently bound within the peptide sequence. It is measured by the difference between protein-bound iodine and serum thyroxine. Its concentration is often raised in Hashimoto's disease and subacute thyroiditis, and sometimes in thyroid cancers and nontoxic goiter.

**iodopsin** \ī′ōdäp′sin\ [IOD- + *opsin* as in *rhodopsin*] The retinal visual pigment of the cone photoreceptors, responsible for day vision. Also *visual violet.* Compare RHODOPSIN.

**iodopyracet** $C_{11}H_{16}I_2N_2O_5$. Diethanolammonium-3,5-diiodo-4-pyridone-*N*-acetate. A compound which is radiopaque due to its iodine content. It is used in urographic procedures.

**iodoquinol** DIIODOHYDROXYQUIN.

**iodostick** An applicator composed of iodine and potassium iodide. it is used topically as an antiseptic.

**iodosulfate** A combination of iodine and sulfuric acid with a basic compound to yield a complex salt of these two acidic components.

**iodotherapy** \ī′ōdōther′əpē\ [IODO- + THERAPY] Treatment with iodine or iodides. *Older term.*

**iodothiouracil** 5-Iodo-2-thiouracil. An iodine-containing derivative of thiouracil which has an advantage over the latter because preoperative iodine administration is no longer necessary. It is given orally as the sodium salt.

**iodothyroglobulin** *Seldom used* THYROGLOBULIN.
**iodothyronine** \ī′ōdōthī′rē·in\ A compound formed by the oxidative coupling of two iodotyrosines through an ether linkage in the *para* configuration. Compounds of this class comprise the thyroid hormones, thyroxine, triiodothyronine, and their metabolites.
**iodotyrosine** Tyrosine iodinated *ortho* to its hydroxyl group. The term is sometimes used to include the tyrosine doubly iodinated. These two compounds are precursors of thyroxine and triiodithyronine, the thryoid hormones.
**iodoxyquinolinesulfonic acid** An amebicidal agent given in a mixture with sodium bicarbonate as chiniofon, or as chiniofon sodium.
**ion** \ī′än\ [Gk *iōn,* pres. part. neut. of *ienai* to go] An atom or radical that is electrically charged as a result of having lost or gained one or more electrons.
**-ion** [L *-io,* gen. *-ionis,* suffix denoting an act or process, the result thereof, a condition or state, or thing acted upon] A noun suffix denoting action, process, or result.
**ionization** \ī′ənīzā′shən\ [ION + *-iz(e)* + -ATION] **1** Dissociation into charged atoms or groups of atoms by electrolytes in aqueous solution. **2** Production of charged atoms or molecules in a gas by electric discharge or by irradiation. **avalanche i.** A process occurring among gaseous ions in an ionization chamber radiation detector. Given an adequate mean free path, a primary ion caused by the incident radiation can be accelerated by the applied voltage to the point where its collisions produce several other ions, whereupon each secondary ion does the same thing, and so on, causing an "avalanche." The multiplication of ions can be millionfold or more. Also *Townsend avalanche, avalanche, Townsend ionization.*
**ionize** \ī′ənīz\ To undergo or cause to undergo ionization.
**ionometer** \ī′ōnäm′ətər\ [ION + *o* + -METER] Any apparatus which measures the intensity or quantity of radiation by measuring the ionization it produces. Also *iontoquantimeter, iontoradeometer.*
**ionometry** \ī′ōnäm′ətrē\ [ION + *o* + -METRY] Measurement of ionizing radiation.
**ionopherogram** \ī′ənōfer′əgram\ ELECTROPHORETOGRAM.
**ionophore** \ī·än′əfôr\ [ION + *o* + -PHORE] An antibiotic that carries specific ions across a membrane, such as the plasma membrane of bacterial or animal cells or the mitochondrial membrane. Examples of ionophores are valinomycin and alamethicin.
**ionophoresis** \ī′ənōfôrē′sis\ The electrophoresis of small molecules.
**ionophose** \ī′ənōfōs′\ [Gk *ion* the violet + *o* + *phōs,* contraction of *phaos* light] A violet-colored subjective light sensation.
**iontherapy** \ī′änther′əpē\ *Seldom used* IONTOPHORESIS.
**iontophoresis** \ī·än′tōfôrē′sis\ [Gk *ionto(s),* gen. of *iōn,* pres. part. of *ienai* to go + -PHORESIS] The tranference of ions into the body by an electromotive force for purposes of local or systemic medicinal effect. Also *galvanoionization, iontotherapy.*
**iontophoretic** \ī·än′tōfôret′ik\ Relating to iontophoresis.
**iontoquantimeter** \ī·än′tōkwôntim′ətər\ IONOMETER.
**iontoradeometer** \ī·än′tôrā′dē·äm′ətər\ IONOMETER.
**iontotherapy** \ī·än′tōther′əpē\ IONTOPHORESIS.
**IOP** intraocular pressure.
**iophendylate** $C_{19}H_{29}IO_2$. An iodine-containing, oily radiopaque medium that has been used diagnostically for both the examination of the biliary tract and for myelography. Also *ethyl iodophenylundecylate, iodophendylate.*
**iopydol** $C_8H_9I_2NO_3$. 1-(2,3-Dihydroxypropyl)-3,5-diiodo-4(1*H*)-pyridinone. A radiopaque material used diagnostically in bronchoscopy to visualize the bronchial structures.
**iopydone** $C_5H_3I_2NO$. 3,5-Diiodo-4(1*H*)-pyridinone. A radiopaque agent used diagnostically in bronchography.
**iothalamate** A salt of iothalamic acid. The meglumine and sodium salts are the main forms used diagnostically as radiopaque agents.
**iothalamic acid** $C_{11}H_9I_3N_2O_4$. 5-Acetamido-2,4,6-triiodo-*N*-methylisophthalamic acid, the meglumine and sodium salts of which are used in radiology as water-soluble contrast media, such as in intravenous urography.
**iothiouracil** $C_4H_3IN_2OS$. 5-Iodo-2-thiouracil. An agent used in the treatment of hyperthyroidism. It acts as a thyroid inhibitor, and it is used when a surgical thyroidectomy is contraindicated.
**IP** intraperitoneally (injection site).
**ipecac** \ip′əkak\ [short for Brazilian Portuguese *ipecacuanha,* from Tupi *ïpekakwaña* (from *ïpeka* duck + *akwaña* penis) lit., duck's penis] The dried roots and rhizome of *Cephaelis ipecacuanha* or *C. acuminata,* which is used as an emetic and amebicidal drug. Also *ipecacuanha.*
**ipodate sodium** An iodinated compound used for radiologic cholangiography and cholecystography. It is thought to increase $T_3$ uptake. Also *sodium ipodate.*
**ipomea** A cathartic medication obtained from the dried root of *Ipomoea orizabensis.* Also *orizaba jalap root.*
**IPPB** intermittent positive pressure breathing.
**ipratropium bromide** $C_{20}H_{30}BrNO_3$. 3-(3-Hydroxy-1-oxo-2-phenylpropoxy)-8-methyl-8-(1-methylethyl)-8-azoniabicyclo[3.2.1]octane bromide. An anticholinergic agent used in the treatment of asthma. Since it is a charged molecule, it does not appear to cross the blood-brain barrier and therefore may have fewer side effects on the central nervous system than atropine. It is administered by inhalation and may occasionally cause dryness of the oropharynx.
**iprindole** $C_{19}H_{28}N_2$. 6,7,8,9,10,11-Hexahydro-*N,N*-dimethyl-5*H*-cyclooct[*b*]indole-5-propanamine. An agent with pharmacologic actions like those of imipramine. It is used as an antidepressant drug in the form of the hydrochloride.
**iproniazid** $C_9H_{13}N_3O$. 4-Pyridinecarboxylic acid 2-(1-methylethyl)hydrazide. An antidepressant agent chemically related to isoniazid. It is an inhibitor of monoamine oxidase and it has antituberculosis activity. It is not regularly used to treat tuberculosis, however, because its toxicity is greater than that of other agents now available.
**ipsefact** \ip′səfakt\ [L *ipse* self + *fact(um)* a thing made, from neut. sing. of *factus,* past part. of *facere* to make] Any portion or aspect of an animal's habitat or environment created by its own behavior, such as nests, beehives, and prairie dog villages.
**ipsilateral** \ip′silat′ərəl\ Located on or affecting the same side. Also *ipselateral* (outmoded spelling), *homolateral, isolateral.* Compare CONTRALATERAL.
**IPSP** inhibitory postsynaptic potential.
**IPTG** isopropyl thiogalactoside.
**IQ** intelligence quotient.
**Ir** Symbol for the element, iridium.
**ir-** \ir-\ **1** IN-[1]. **2** IN-[2].
**IRC** inspiratory reserve capacity (inspiratory reserve volume).
**IRI** immunoreactive insulin.
**irid-** \ī′rid-, ir′id-\ IRIDO-.
**iridal** \ī′ridəl, ir′idəl\ IRIDIC.
**iridauxesis** \ī′ridôksē′sis\ [IRID- + AUXESIS] Thickening of the iris.

**iridavulsion** \ī′ridəvul′shən\ [IRID- + AVULSION] IRIDODIALYSIS.
**iridectasis** \ī′ridek′təsis\ [IRID- + ECTASIS] Prolapse of the iris through a wound or incision.
**iridectome** \ī′ridek′tōm\ [IRID- + -ECTOME] A surgical instrument for cutting the iris.
**iridectomesodialysis** \ī′ridek′tōmē′sōdī·al′isis\ [IRID- + ECTO- + MESO- + DIALYSIS] A combination of excision of a portion of the iris and freeing of pupillary adhesions.
**iridectomy** \ī′ridek′təmē\ [IRID- + -ECTOMY] The surgical removal of a portion of the iris. **buttonhole i.** PERIPHERAL IRIDECTOMY. **optical i.** Excision of a central portion of the iris with the intent of enhancing the entry of light into the eye. **peripheral i.** Excision of a very small portion of the peripheral iris, with preservation of the pupil. Also *coretomedialysis, buttonhole iridectomy, stenopeic iridectomy.*
**iridencleisis** \ir′idenklī′sis\ [IRID- + EN- + -CLEISIS] Incarceration of a tongue of iris in a limbal wound with the intention of creating an artificial channel for drainage of aqueous from the eye, in management of glaucoma.
**irideremia** \ir′idərē′mē·ə\ [IRID- + Gk *erēmia* want of, absence] ANIRIDIA.
**irides** \ir′idēz\ Plural of IRIS.
**iridesis** \īrid′əsis\ [*iri(d)-* + -DESIS] Iris inclusion surgery for glaucoma, in which the iris is interposed in a corneoscleral incision to block its closure. Also *iridodesis.*
**iridic** \īrid′ik\ [IRID- + -IC] Of or relating to the iris. Also *iritic, iridal, iridial, iridian.*
**iridium** \īrid′ē·əm\ A metallic element having atomic number 77 and atomic weight 192.22. It occurs uncombined in nature along with platinum and other metals. It is heavier than any other known element except osmium, and is the most corrosion-resistant metal. Symbol: Ir
**irido-** \ī′ridō-, ir′idō-\ [Gk *iris* (genitive *iridos*) rainbow, iris] A combining form denoting the iris. Also *irid-*.
**iridoavulsion** \ir′idō·əvul′shən\ [IRIDO- + AVULSION] IRIDODIALYSIS.
**iridocapsulitis** \-kap′s^yəlī′tis\ [IRIDO- + CAPSULITIS] Inflammation of the iris and lens capsule.
**iridocapsulotomy** \-kap′s^yəlät′əmē\ [IRIDO- + CAPSULOTOMY] Surgical excision of a portion of the iris and adherent lens capsule.
**iridocele** \īrid′əsēl\ [IRIDO- + -CELE[1]] Prolapse of the iris through a wound in cornea or limbus. Also *myiocephalon* (outmoded), *myiocephalum* (outmoded).
**iridochoroiditis** \-kôr′oidī′tis\ [IRIDO- + CHOROIDITIS] UVEITIS.
**iridoconstrictor** \-kənstrik′tər\ [IRIDO- + CONSTRICTOR] The sphincter muscle of the iris or any autonomic stimulus that activates it.
**iridocorneosclerectomy** \-kôr′nē·ōsklirek′təmē\ [IRIDO- + *corne(a)* + *o* + SCLER- + -ECTOMY] A glaucoma operation consisting of excision of a portion of the limbus and underlying iris.
**iridocyclectomy** \-sīklek′təmē\ [IRIDO- + CYCL- + -ECTOMY] Excision of a portion of iris and ciliary body, as for a neoplasm.
**iridocyclitis** \-sīklī′tis\ [IRIDO- + CYCLITIS] Inflammation of the iris and ciliary body. Also *anterior uveitis.* **heterochromic i.** A mild, persistent anterior uveitis associated with a developmental melanin deficiency of the affected eye.
**iridocyclochoroiditis** \-sī′kləkôr′oidī′tis\ [IRIDO- + CYCLO- + CHOROIDITIS] UVEITIS.
**iridodesis** \ir′idäd′əsis\ [IRIDO- + -DESIS] IRIDESIS.
**iridodialysis** \-dī·al′isis\ [IRIDO- + DIALYSIS] A tearing of the iris from its base upon the ciliary body. Also *iridoavulsion, iridavulsion.*
**iridodiastasis** \-dī·as′təsis\ [IRIDO- + DIASTASIS] Absence of a portion of the iris at its peripheral base.
**iridodilator** \-dī′lātər\ **1** MUSCULUS DILATOR PUPILLAE. **2** A neurochemical acting to innervate this muscle.
**iridodonesis** \-dōnē′sis\ [IRIDO- + Gk *don(ein)* to shake + -ESIS] Tremulousness of the iris, which results when the physical support of the lens is lost, as following dislocation of the lens or cataract extraction.
**iridokeratitis** \-ker′ətī′tis\ [IRIDO- + KERATITIS] Inflammation of the iris and cornea.
**iridokinetic** \-kinet′ik\ Pertaining to movement of the iris.
**iridolysis** \ir′idäl′isis\ [IRIDO- + LYSIS] A freeing of the iris from synechiae.
**iridomesodialysis** \-mē′sōdī·al′isis\ [IRIDO- + MESO- + DIALYSIS] A freeing of the iris from adhesions affecting the pupil margin.
**iridomotor** \-mō′tər\ Pertaining to or causing movement of the iris.
**iridoncus** \ir′idäng′kəs\ [IRID- + -ONCUS] A tumor of the iris.
**iridoplegia** \-plē′jə\ [IRIDO- + -PLEGIA] Loss of motor function of the iris. Also *iridoparalysis, pupilloplegia.* **accommodation i.** Loss of the pupillary reaction component of the accommodation-convergence reflex.
**iridorhexis** \ir′idôrek′sis\ [IRIDO- + -RHEXIS] Tearing or rupture of the iris.
**iridoschisis** \ir′idäs′kisis\ [IRIDO- + -SCHISIS] A splitting of the frontal plane of mesodermal layers of the iris, usually as a spontaneous degenerative change.
**iridosclerotomy** \-sklirät′əmē\ [IRIDO- + SCLEROTOMY] An incision through sclera and iris, as for acute angle-closure glaucoma.
**iridosis** \ir′idō′sis\ IRIDOTASIS.
**iridosteresis** \-stirē′sis\ [IRIDO- + Gk *sterēsis* loss] Absence of all or most of the iris owing to trauma, disease, or developmental cause.
**iridotasis** \ir′idät′əsis\ [IRIDO- + Gk *tasis* a stretching, straining] Incarceration of iris in a corneoscleral incision. Also *iridosis.*
**iridotome** \ir′idōtōm′\ [IRIDO- + -TOME] A surgical instrument designed for incising the iris.
**iridotomy** \ir′idät′əmē\ [IRIDO- + -TOMY] A cut into the iris without removal of tissue. This is performed during cataract extraction as a prophylactic measure against possible pupillary blockage by the vitreous humor. Also *iritomy, irotomy.*
**iris** \ī′ris\ [Gk, rainbow, halo, iris] (*pl.* irides) [NA] The visible, colored portion of the vascular tunic of the eye, in front of the lens, functioning as a diaphragm and encompassing a central orifice (pupil) whose size is regulated by sphincter and dilator muscles to control the passage of light. It is lined posteriorly by a double layer of pigmented epithelial cells and is attached at the margins to the ciliary body. Adj. iridic, iridal, iridial, iridian. **i. bombé** Forward displacement of the midportion of the iris due to a pupillary block that occludes aqueous flow into the anterior chamber. Also *umbrella iris.* **tremulous i.** See under IRIDODONESIS. **umbrella i.** IRIS BOMBÉ.
**iritic** \īrit′ik\ Pertaining to or characterized by iritis.
**iritis** \īrī′tis\ [*ir(is)* + -ITIS] Inflammation of the iris. **plastic i.** Iritis that results in fibrinous outpouring into the aqueous. **serous i.** Iritis associated with leakage of plasma proteins into the aqueous. **spongy i.** Iritis associated with fibrin clots in the anterior chamber.

**iritoectomy** \īr′itō·ek′təmē\ [*irito-* (irreg. for IRIDO-) + -ECTOMY] Excision of secondary cataract and adherent iris.
**iritomy** \īrit′əmē\ IRIDOTOMY.
**irium** A hard, white, metallic element having atomic number 77, and atomic weight 192.2. Symbol: Ir
**iron** Element number 26, having atomic weight 55.847. By weight, iron is the fourth most abundant element in the lithosphere, where it is found combined with oxygen. The core of the earth is believed to be largely molten iron. Ordinary iron is a mixture of four stable isotopes. Valences are 2, 3, 4, and 6. The metal has been central to technology from prehistoric times. Its compounds figure in such plant and animal life processes as photosynthesis, oxygen transport, and the action of many enzymes. Symbol: Fe Adj. ferric, ferrous. **i. and ammonium citrate** A combination of ferric citrate and ammonium citrate, soluble in water and often used to treat iron deficiency anemia. Also *ferric ammonium citrate.* **i. and ammonium sulfate** A combination of ferric iron and ammonium sulfate as a complex salt, $FeNH_4(SO_4)_2 \cdot 12H_2O$. It is used as an astringent and styptic medication. Also *ferric ammonium sulfate.* **i. and ammonium tartrate** Reddish-brown scales composed of ferric ammonium tartrate. It is used as a convenient source of iron for the treatment of iron deficiency anemia. **available i.** The component of dietary iron which can be absorbed from the gastrointestinal tract. **nonheme i.** Iron that is not part of the heme group: describing particularly the iron-sulfur proteins. These contain iron bound, often in a complex with $S^{2-}$ions, to cysteine residues of the protein in their deprotonated form. **Quevenne's i.** REDUCED IRON. **i. and quinine citrate** A complex ammonium quinine ferric citrate containing 14.5–15.5% anhydrous quinine and 12–14% iron. It has been used as a tonic. **reduced i.** A fine, black powder of metallic iron prepared from iron salts by reduction with hydrogen under standard conditions. It is insoluble in water, but dissolves in dilute mineral acids. It has the same uses as iron salts, but its bioavailability is limited and variable. Also *Quevenne's iron.*
**iron 55** A radioisotope of iron. It decays by electron capture, emitting characteristic x rays of 5.9 keV. Physical half-life is 2.7 years. Symbol: $^{55}Fe$
**iron 59** A radioisotope of iron, emitting beta and gamma rays. Physical half-life is 45 days. Symbol: $^{59}Fe$
**iron acetate** $Fe(O_2CCH_3)_3$. An iron salt of limited value as an astringent agent.
**iron adenylate** A form of iron used for parenteral (intramuscular) administration.
**iron ascorbate** A soluble complex of reduced iron and ascorbic acid that is used for the treatment of iron deficiency anemia. Also *iron cevitaminate.*
**iron choline citrate** FERROCHOLINATE.
**iron citrate** FERRIC CITRATE.
**iron dextrin** A sterile, clear, dark brown solution containing a complex of ferric hydroxide and partially hydrolyzed dextrin in water suitable for intravenous administration.
**iron gluconate** FERROUS GLUCONATE.
**iron glycerophosphate** FERRIC GLYCEROPHOSPHATE.
**iron hematoxylin** A hematoxylin solution containing an iron salt that acts as both an oxidizing agent and a mordant.
**iron hypophosphite** FERRIC HYPOPHOSPHITE.
**iron iodide** FERROUS IODIDE.
**iron lactate** FERROUS LACTATE.
**iron magnesium sulfate** A mixture of ferrous sulfate and magnesium sulfate used in the treatment of iron-deficiency anemia.
**iron malate** A preparation of iron in apple juice used as an oral form of iron treatment for anemia.
**iron oleate** An iron salt of oleic acid that is a waxy, solid preparation. It is used as an astringent.
**iron phosphate** A mixture of ferric and ferrous phosphates that has been used to treat iron-deficiency anemias. **soluble i.** Ferric phosphate made soluble by the addition of sodium citrate. It has been used in the treatment of iron-deficiency anemia.
**iron protosulfate** FERROUS SULFATE.
**iron pyrophosphate** $Fe_4(P_2O_7)_3 \cdot 9H_2O$. A salt of iron, insoluble in water, that has been used as a nutrient source of iron to prevent anemia.
**iron sorbitex** A sterile, brown, colloidal solution containing ferric iron, sorbitol, and citric acid, stabilized with dextrin and sorbitol. It can be used intramuscularly in the treatment of iron-deficiency anemia, but should not be given intravenously.
**iron subcarbonate** An amorphous powder consisting mostly of iron hydroxide.
**iron sulfate** FERROUS SULFATE.
**iron valerianate** $FeC_5H_9O_2(OH)_2$. A ferric salt of valeric acid, insoluble in water, that has been used in the treatment of iron deficiency anemia.
**irotomy** \īrät′əmē\ IRIDOTOMY.
**irradiate** \irā′dē·āt\ [L *irradiare* (from *ir-* in, on + *radiare* to shine, emit rays of light, from *radius* ray) to shine upon, illumine] To expose to ionizing radiation, as for diagnosis, treatment, or sterilization, or by accident.
**irradiation** \irā′dē·ā′shən\ [*irradiat(e)* + -ION] **1** In radiology, treatment by ionizing radiations. **2** LUMINESCENCE. **interstitial i.** Therapeutic irradiation by the insertion, in the tissue, of an encapsulated radioactive nuclide such as radium, cobalt 60, etc. **intracavitary i.** INTRACAVITARY RADIOTHERAPY. **painful i.** The propagation or extension of pain into a region which may be near to, or less often far from, its origin, as in propagation of the chest pain of angina pectoris, which is usually retrosternal, into the left or both shoulders and arms or into the neck and jaw. **ultraviolet blood i.** A method of irradiation consisting of the extracorporeal exposure of blood to ultraviolet light.
**irreducible** \ir′əd^y oo′sibl\ **1** Impossible to be lowered by the application of current knowledge or techniques, as an irreducible infection rate. **2** Not able to be corrected further.
**irregular** **1** Not regular, orderly, or proper. **2** Occurring at uneven intervals, as *irregular heartbeat.*
**irremediable** \ir′əmē′dē·əbl\ Not capable of being remedied; lacking a remedy.
**irrespirable** \ir′əspī′rəbl\ Unsuitable for breathing: said of air or gas that will not support the respiratory processes, or is toxic, or of aerosols in which the particle size is too large.
**irresponsibility** / **criminal i.** Exemption from responsibility for criminal conduct due to mental illness or defect which can be demonstrated to have been present in an individual at the time a criminal act was committed. Compare CRIMINAL RESPONSIBILITY.
**irresuscitable** \ir′əsus′itəbl\ [IR- + L *resuscit(are)* to revive + -ABLE] Denoting a shock state or injury so severe that currently known treatment cannot restore enough vital function to prevent death.
**irreversibility** \ir′əvur′sibil′itē\ The quality of being unable to return to its original form or state. **i. of conduction** The theory that conduction can occur in one di-

rection only in a reflex arc. This principle is physiologically unsound with respect to nerve fibers which are capable of antidromic conduction, but holds for transmission through the synapse which occurs in one direction only.

**irrigant** A fluid used to flush out or irrigate a cavity or surface.

**irrigate** \ir′igāt\ [L *irrigare* (from *ir-*, *in-*, intensive prefix + *rigare* to water, soak, bathe) to flood, drench, irrigate] To flush thoroughly, especially a cavity or wound, with a fluid to rid of unwanted substances.

**irrigation** \ir′igā′shən\ [L *irrigatio* (from *irrigare*; see IRRIGATE) flooding, irrigation] The process of flushing a cavity or wound thoroughly with water, salt solution, or medicated fluid, as to wash out debris, foreign material, or dead tissues. **continuous i.** Irrigation performed with an uninterrupted stream of fluid.

**irrigator** \ir′igā′tər\ Any of a number of devices used for irrigation. Examples are syringes, tubing connected to a bottle elevated for gravity flow, and pumps that provide continuous or pulsatile flow.

**irrigoradioscopy** \ir′igôrā′dē·äs′kəpē\ [L *irrig(are)* to water, conduct water to + *o* + RADIOSCOPY] Fluoroscopy of the large bowel during the administration of a contrast enema. Also *irrigoscopy*.

**irrigoscopy** \ir′igäs′kəpē\ IRRIGORADIOSCOPY.

**irritability** \ir′itəbil′itē\ EXCITABILITY. **electric i.** Responsiveness to electric current. **myotatic i.** Responsiveness of muscle to transient muscle stretch. **specific i.** LAW OF SPECIFIC IRRITABILITY. **uterine i.** An increased propensity for uterine contractions following any type of stimulus.

**irritable** \ir′itəbl\ **1** Capable of reacting to a stimulus. **2** Hypersensitive to stimulation.

**irritant** \ir′itənt\ An agent that causes irritation or inflammation. **primary i.** An agent or substance capable of producing inflammation on first contact with a tissue, especially the skin.

**irritation** [L *irritatio* (from *irritatus*, past part. of *irritare* to stir up, incite, excite) a stirring up, provoking, incitement] **1** The response of excitable tissue to a stimulus. **2** The incipient inflammatory response of tissue to a noxious stimulus. **3** The application of a stimulus or excitation. **cerebral i.** **1** The state produced by any lesion or disease which irritates brain cells. **2** The clinical state of irritability or intolerance of interference which may result from brain injury or disease. **meningeal i.** Irritation of the meninges due to meningitis or hemorrhage and giving rise to headache and neck stiffness. **spinal i.** Spinal rigidity and pain due to a lesion or disease in the spinal column or canal. **sympathetic i.** Inflammation of an organ as a consequence of inflammation of a related organ, typically seen in one eye following trauma or surgery to the other.

**irritative** \ir′itā′tiv\ *Obs.* EXCITATORY.

**Irvine** [A. Ray *Irvine*, Jr., U.S. ophthalmologist, born 1917] See under SYNDROME.

**Irving** [Frederick Carpenter *Irving*, U.S. obstetrician, born 1883] See under OPERATION.

**IS** **1** intercostal space. **2** intraspinal. **3** immune serum.

**Isaacs** [Charles Edward *Isaacs*, U.S. physiologist, 1811–1860] Isaacs-Ludwig arteriole. See under ARTERIOLE.

**isauxesis** \ī′sôksē′sis\ [*is(o)-* + AUXESIS] A proportionate equality of growth between parts and the whole.

**ischaemia** *Brit.* ISCHEMIA.

**ischemia** \iskē′mē·ə\ [Gk *ischaim(os)* (from *isch(ein)* to restrain, check + *(h)aima* blood) staunching blood, styptic + -IA] Inadequate blood flow to a part or organ. **mesenteric i.** The impairment of blood supply to a part of the small or large bowel leading to impairment of cellular function but not to cell death. **postural i.** Reduction of the blood flow in a limb or part thereof during a surgical procedure, by elevating it above the level of the heart. **renal i.** Decreased blood perfusion of the kidney, either from organic causes, such as stenosis of the main renal artery or its primary branches due to atherosclerosis or fibromuscular disease, to arteriolar nephrosclerosis, or to functional prerenal situations such as heart failure, hypovolemia, or shock. **i. retinae** Inadequate retinal circulation due to shock following profuse blood loss. **subendocardial i.** Inadequate blood flow to a part of the myocardium adjacent to the endocardium. **subepicardial i.** Inadequate blood flow to the myocardium subjacent to the pericardium. **transient cerebral i.** TRANSIENT ISCHEMIC ATTACK. Abbr. TCI **vasospasm cerebral i.** A temporary reduction of cerebral blood supply as a result of spasm of nutrient arteries.

**ischemic** \iskē′mik\ Characterized by or affected with ischemia.

**ischi-** \is′kē-\ ISCHIO-.

**ischia** \is′kē·ə\ Plural of ISCHIUM.

**ischial** \is′kē·əl\ Of or relating to the ischium or the hip joint; sciatic. Also *ischiadic, ischiatic, ischiac*.

**ischiatitis** \is′kē·ətī′tis\ *Obs.* SCIATICA.

**ischidrosis** \is′kidrō′sis\ ANHIDROSIS.

**ischiectomy** \is′kē·ek′təmē\ [ISCHI- + -ECTOMY] The surgical removal of all or part of one or both hips.

**ischio-** \is′kē·ō-\ [Gk *ischion* hip joint, hip] A combining form denoting the ischium. Also *ischi-*.

**ischiobulbar** \-bul′bər\ Pertaining to the ischium and the bulb of the penis.

**ischiocapsular** \-kap′s$^y$ələr\ Pertaining to the ischium and the capsule of the hip joint.

**ischiocavernous** \-kav′ərnəs\ Pertaining to the ischium and the corpus cavernosum penis or clitoridis.

**ischiocele** \is′kē·əsēl′\ SCIATIC HERNIA.

**ischiococcygeus** \-käksij′ē·əs\ MUSCULUS COCCYGEUS.

**ischiomelus** \is′kē·äm′ələs\ [ISCHIO- + Gk *melos* a limb] Unequal conjoined twins in which the parasitic member is represented mainly by an extra arm or leg attached to the host in the pelvic region.

**ischiopagus** \iskē·äp′əgəs\ [ISCHIO- + -PAGUS] Equal conjoined twins united in the ischial region. **i. parasiticus** Unequal conjoined twins with the parasitic member attached at the ischial region of the host. **i. tetrapus** An ischiopagus parasiticus with four feet, the parasitic member being represented largely by an extra pair of lower extremities. **i. tripus** An ischiopagus parasiticus with three feet, the parasitic member being represented by a single lower extremity with or without variable other parts.

**ischiopubis** \-pyoo′bis\ **1** The ischium and the pubis considered as a single unit. **2** The junction of the ischium and the pubis.

**ischiothoracopagus** \-thôr′əkäp′əgəs\ [ISCHIO- + THORACO- + -PAGUS] Equal conjoined twins united from the thorax to the pelvis. The pelvic union more often involves the ilium than the ischium.

**ischium** \is′kē·əm\ [L, from Gk *ischion* hip joint, hip, ischium] OS ISCHII.

**ischogyria** \is′kōjī′rē·ə\ [Gk *isch(ein)* to check, hold back, stop + *o* + *gyr(us)* + -IA] A jagged or nodular appearance of cerebral gyri as seen sometimes in tuberous sclerosis.

**ischospermia** \is′kōspur′mē·ə\ [Gk *isch(ein)* to hold, check + *o* + SPERM- + -IA] The retention of semen, or the suppression of semen excretion.

**ischuria** \iskyoo′rē·ə\ [Gk *ischouria* (from *isch(ein)* to hold, retain + *ouron* urine) retention of urine] URINARY RETENTION. **i. paradoxa** Excessive dilatation of the bladder from urine, although the passing of urine continues. **i. spastica** Retention of urine due to spasm of the bladder sphincter.

**-ise** \-īz\ *Brit.* -IZE.

**iseiconia** \ī′sīkō′nē·ə\ ISEIKONIA.

**iseiconic** \ī′sīkän′ik\ ISEIKONIC.

**iseikonia** \ī′sīkō′nē·ə\ [*is(o)-* + Gk *eikōn* image, likeness + -IA] Equality of image size perceived by the two eyes. Also *iso-iconia.* Also *iseiconia.*

**iseikonic** \ī′sīkän′ik\ Characterized by or pertaining to iseikonia; relating to equal size of the images perceived by the two eyes. Also *iso-iconic, iseiconic.*

**Ishihara** [Shinobu *Ishihara,* Japanese ophthalmologist, 1879–1963] See under TEST.

**island** [Old English *īgland*] ISLET. **blood i.** An aggregate of mesenchymal cells in the embryo that give rise to primitive blood vessels and the first blood cells. Collectively, blood islands are known as angioblastema. Also *Wolff's island, Pander's island.* **bone i.** Isolated piece of bone found with either normal cortical or cancellous bone. **i.'s of Calleja** Dense clusters of granular and polymorphic neurons in the cortex of the anterior perforated space within the tuberculum olfactorium. Also *Calleja's islets, olfactory islands.* **cartilage i.** A residual area of cartilaginous tissue that remains within bony tissue following endochondral ossification. **i.'s of Langerhans** ISLETS OF LANGERHANS. **olfactory i.'s** ISLANDS OF CALLEJA. **Pander's i.** BLOOD ISLAND. **i. of Reil** INSULA. **skin i.** EPITHELIAL BUD. **Wolff's i.** BLOOD ISLAND.

**islet** \ī′lət\ [Middle French *islette* (from *isle* island, from L *insula* island, + *-ette* French diminishing suffix) a small island] A small cluster of cells with a similar or related function. Also *island.* **Calleja's i.'s** ISLANDS OF CALLEJA. **i.'s of Langerhans** Localized clusters of endocrine cells scattered through the acinar substance of the pancreas. They contain alpha, beta, and delta cells that secrete, respectively, glucagon, insulin, and gastrin. Also *islands of Langerhans, pancreatic islets, insulae pancreaticae.* **pancreatic i.'s** ISLETS OF LANGERHANS. **Walthard's i.'s** Small, glistening nodules found on the surface of the fallopian tubes. They are composed of serosal cells that have become hyperplastic or metaplastic. They are benign, and must be distinguished from tumor implants.

**-ism** \-izm\ [Gk *-ismos,* suffix for nouns derived from verbs ending in *-izein* -IZE] A suffix meaning (1) act or process; (2) state or condition; (3) abnormal condition, anomaly; (4) doctrine of belief or system of practice.

**iso-** \ī′sō-\ [Gk *isos* equal] **1** A combining form meaning equal, equivalent. **2** A prefix used in chemical nomenclature to indicate a slight difference, most commonly to indicate chain branching. Thus, whereas the propyl group is $CH_3$—$CH_2$—$CH_2$—, the isopropyl group is $(CH_3—)_2CH$—. Abbr. *i-*

**isoallele** \ī′sō·əlēl′\ An allele that is distinguishable from another, which is usually the wild type, only by its effect on the phenotype when it is present with certain mutant alleles in heterozygotes or by its DNA sequence.

**isoalloxazine** The compound whose molecule provides the basic ring system of flavins. It consists of three rings. The central one is pyrazine, with a benzene ring fused to one of its C-C bonds, and a uracil ring to the other. In flavins, the benzene ring carries two methyl substituents, and one nitrogen atom of the central ring is substituted with ribitol.

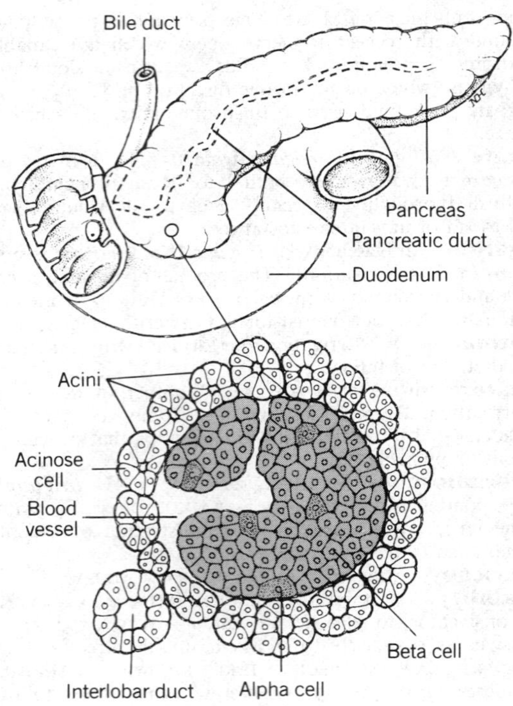


**Islet of Langerhans**

This ring system can undergo reversible hydrogenation.

**isoalloxazine mononucleotide** FLAVIN MONONUCLEOTIDE.

**isoamylethylbarbituric acid** AMOBARBITAL.

**isoamyl nitrite** AMYL NITRITE.

**isoandrosterone** \-andräs′tərōn\ EPIANDROSTERONE.

**isoantibody** \-an′tibäd′ē\ *Outmoded* ALLOANTIBODY.

**isoantigen** \-an′təjən\ *Outmoded* ALLOANTIGEN. **H i.** One of the antigens of the ABH blood groups, expressed predominantly in type O individuals and to a lesser degree in type B, A, and AB individuals.

**isobar** \ī′səbär\ Any of two or more nuclides having the same mass number but different atomic numbers, such as uranium 235 and neptunium 235.

**isobody** \ī′sōbäd′ē\ *Outmoded* ALLOANTIBODY.

**isobucaine hydrochloride** $C_{15}H_{23}NO_2 \cdot HCl$. 2-Isobutylamino-2-methylpropylbenzoate hydrochloride. A white, crystalline powder which is used as a local anesthetic for dental anesthesia.

**isobutylallylbarbituric acid** BUTALBITAL.

**isocaloric** \-kəlôr′ik\ EQUICALORIC.

**isocarboxazid** $C_{12}H_{13}N_3O_2$. 5-Methyl-3-isoxazolecarboxylic acid 2-benzylhydrazide. It is a monoamine oxidase inhibitor and used in the treatment of depressed patients who are refractory to tricyclic antidepressant drugs, or in patients in which the tricyclic antidepressants are contraindicated.

**isocholesterol** LANOSTEROL.

**isochromosome** \-krō′məsōm\ A mediocentric chromosome with homologous arms, probably resulting from an abnormal transverse division of the centromere during meiosis.

**isochronia** \-krō′nē·ə\ [ISO- + CHRON- + -IA] **1** ISOCHRONISM. **2** A correspondence in time, rate, or frequency, as between biological processes.

**isochronism** \īsäk′rənizm\ The condition of nerve and muscle possessing the same chronaxy (i.e. excitability). Also *isochronia, law of isochronism, Lapicque's law.*

**isocitrate dehydrogenase** The enzyme (EC 1.1.1.41), of the citric acid cycle, that converts the CHOH group of isocitrate into a carbonyl group with concomitant reduction of $NAD^+$. The initial product undergoes decarboxylation to form 2-oxoglutarate before it dissociates from the enzyme. There is also an NADP-linked enzyme (EC 1.1.1.42), which is cytosolic.

**isocitrate lyase** The enzyme (EC 4.1.3.1) that converts isocitrate into succinate and glyoxylate. It is found in microorganisms, some worms, and plants, but not in mammals, and is part of the glyoxylate cycle, which effects the net conversion of fat into carbohydrate. Also *isocitratase* (outmoded).

**isocitric acid** HOOC—$CH_2$—CH(COOH)—CHOH—COOH. 1-Hydroxypropane-1,2,3-tricarboxylic acid. The natural compound is the 1*R*,2*S* isomer. It is an intermediate in the citric acid cycle, being produced from citrate by the enzyme aconitase, and being converted into 2-oxoglutarate by the enzyme isocitrate dehydrogenase. It is also an intermediate in the glyoxylate cycle in plants, where it is split by isocitrate lyase to form glyoxylate and succinate.

**isocomplement** \-käm′plimənt\ Complement derived from serum of a member of the same species or the same individual that also was a source of antibody.

**isocoria** \-kôr′ē·ə\ [ISO- + *cor(e)-* + -IA] Equality of pupil size.

**isocortex** \-kôr′teks\ The portion of the cerebral cortex that is most complex in structure and considered phylogenetically most recent. It is characteristically six-layered, and covers the lateral cerebral hemispheres. All other cortical areas contain fewer layers and are located medially. Also *neopallium, neocortex, homogenetic cortex, homotypic cortex, eulaminate cortex* (older term), *nonolfactory cortex* (outmoded).

**isocyanate** The group —N═C═O or a compound that contains it. Such compounds are hydrolyzed slowly by water, and they react with amines to form urea derivatives.

**isocytosis** \-sītō′sis\ Uniformity of cell size, especially of erythrocytes. Compare ANISOCYTOSIS.

**isodiagnosis** \-dī′əgnō′sis\ The diagnosis of a subclinical or inapparent infection by inoculation of a susceptible laboratory animal with blood from the patient suspected of having the condition.

**isodose** \ī′sədōs\ [ISO- + DOSE] In radiotherapy, designating a curve or surface in which all the points receive the same dose of radiation.

**isodynamic** \-dīnam′ik\ [ISO- + DYNAMIC] Possessing the same force or power. Also *isoenergetic, isodynamogenic.*

**isoelectric** \ī′sō·ilek′trik\ Possessing the same electric potential, as ions having the same electric charge; isopotential.

**isoelectronic** \-il′ekträn′ik\ Having the same number and arrangement of electrons. The ammonium ion is, for example, isoelectronic with the methane molecule.

**isoenergetic** \-en′ərjet′ik\ [ISO- + ENERGETIC] ISODYNAMIC.

**isoenzyme** \-en′zīm\ One of different forms of an enzyme, all judged to be the same enzyme by the fact that they catalyze the same reaction. The term was originally used for enzymes that differed in any way, usually because they were separable by electrophoresis or isoelectric focusing, but it has since become restricted to forms that differ by genetically determined differences in amino-acid sequence, rather than those that differ by modification of the same sequence, as by loss of amide nitrogen. Also *isozyme.*

**isoephedrine** PSEUDOEPHEDRINE.

**isoerythrolysis** \ī′sō·irithräl′isis\ The destruction of red cells by alloantibodies. **neonatal i.** Destruction of neonate red cells by alloantibodies, generally of maternal origin, as in hemolytic disease of the newborn.

**isoetharine** $C_{13}H_{21}NO_3$. 3,4-Dihydroxy-α-[1-(isopropylamino)propyl]benzyl alcohol. An adrenergic drug used for the treatment of bronchial asthma and as a bronchiolar dilator.

**isoflurophate** DIISOPROPYL FLUOROPHOSPHATE.

**isogame** \īsäg′əmē\ ISOGAMY.

**isogamete** \-gam′ēt\ [ISO- + GAMETE] A gamete similar in size and form to the cell with which it unites.

**isogametic** \-gəmet′ik\ Producing similar gametes that fuse in syngamy. Some protozoa and algae are isogametic.

**isogamety** \-gam′ətē\ The production of gametes by a homogametic individual, with all gametes having the same sex chromosome. It is the situation found in the normal human female.

**isogamous** \īsäg′əməs\ Reproducing by fusion of gametes which are similar in size and form.

**isogamy** \īsäg′əmē\ [ISO- + GAM- + -Y] Reproduction in which the two uniting gametes are similar in size, shape, and motility. Also *microgamy.* Also *isogame.*

**isogeneic** \-jənē′ik\ Of or relating to transplantation of tissues in which the donor and the host are genetically identical, as in grafts between monozygous twins. Also *isologous, isoplastic.*

**isogenic** \-jen′ik\ **1** Of or relating to two or more cells, clones, tissues, or individuals that have the same genotypes. Also *syngeneic.* **2** Pertaining to two or more cells, clones, tissues, or individuals that have the same genotype at specific loci. For defs. 1 and 2 also *isologous.*

**isogenous** \īsäj′ənəs\ Originating from one cell.

**isograft** \ī′səgraft\ A graft transferred from one individual to another individual who is genetically identical, as in identical twins or animals so highly inbred that they have complete compatibility of genes. Also *isogeneic homograft, syngraft, isogeneic graft, isologous graft, isoplastic graft, syngeneic graft, isotransplant.*

**isohemolysin** \-hēmäl′isin\ Antibody directed against an antigen found in the same species and capable of inducing red cell destruction.

**isohemolysis** \-hēmäl′isis\ Hemolysis caused by antierythrocyte antibodies formed in response to stimulation by antigens of another member of the same species. Also *homolysis.* Adj. isohemolytic.

**isohydruria** \-hīdroo′rē·ə\ The excretion of urine at a fixed pH.

**iso-iconia** \-īkō′nē·ə\ ISEIKONIA.

**iso-iconic** \-īkän′ik\ ISEIKONIC.

**isoimmunization** \-im′yənīzā′shən\ Immunization following exposure to antigens originating in a genetically different member of the same species. **Rh i.** Isoimmunization resulting from exposure to an Rh antigen, formerly the most common cause of hemolytic disease of the newborn. See also RH ANTIGEN.

**isoindicial** \ī′sō·indish′əl\ Within a medium of progressively changing refractive index, such as the crystalline lens, referring to a zone or region within which the index of refraction is the same.

**isolabeling** \-lā′bəling\ The appearance of radioactive

precursors of DNA synthesis (usually tritiated thymidine) in both daughter chromatids at the second metaphase after the labelled precursor is administered. It is the consequence of sister chromatid exchange.

**isolate** [French *isolé* (from Italian *isolato* like an island, from *isola* an island, from L *insula* island) separated, little frequented, insulated + -ATE] **1** To separate from other chemicals, materials, objects, persons or other living organisms a population or group of one kind. **2** Any isolated substance, organism, population, etc.

**isolateral** \-lat′ərəl\ **1** Having sides that are equal or identical. **2** IPSILATERAL.

**isolation** [*isolat(e)* + -ION] The condition of being set apart from others, as to minimize the risk of being infected or of spreading infection. **ethologic i.** **1** The inability of members of a population to reproduce because of profound differences in mating behavior. **2** The inability of related species to produce hybrids due to different mating behavior. **sensory i.** SENSORY DEPRIVATION.

**isolator** **1** A surgical instrument that functions to separate one region of tissue from another. **2** A person whose function is to preserve separation of one region of tissue from another during operative procedures. **surgical i.** A large plastic bag in which the patient and operative team are placed during a surgical procedure in order to prevent infective contamination of the patient.

**isolecithal** \-les′ithəl\ [ISO- + LECITHAL] MIOLECITHAL.

**isoleucine** \-loo′sēn\ $CH_3$—$CH_2$—$CH(CH_3)$—CH $(NH_3{}^+)$—$COO^-$. One of the 20 amino acids that are incorporated in proteins. It is essential in the human diet. The name is restricted to the 2*S*,3*S* compound (L-isoleucine) and its enantiomer, the 2*R*,3*R* compound, the other two diastereoisomers being known as alloisoleucine. Symbol: Ile

**isologous** \īsäl′əgəs\ **1** ISOGENIC. **2** ISOGENEIC. **3** HOMOLOGOUS.

**isomer** \ī′səmər\ [Gk *isomerēs* (from *iso(s)* equal + *meros* part) having equal parts] **1** One of two or more substances whose molecules possess equal numbers of each type of atom they contain, such as $CH_3$—$CH_2$—OH and $CH_3$—O—$CH_3$, both $C_2H_6O$ but having very different properties. The term is applied especially to closely related substances, such as citric acid and isocitric acid, that differ in the locations of —OH and an —H in their molecules. **2** Any of two or more atomic nuclei which have the same number of protons and neutrons but different energy states, such as technetium 99 and technetium 99m. ***cis-trans* i.** Either of two stereoisomers that differ only in having certain atoms located on different sides of a specified plane. The plane is usually that of a double bond or a ring. Also *geometric isomer.* **conformational i.** Any of two or more isomers that can be interconverted without bond breakage, but which nevertheless are in conformations to which their atoms return spontaneously after small displacements. Conformational isomers often interconvert fairly rapidly. Also *conformer.* **geometric i.** *CIS-TRANS* ISOMER. **optical i.** ENANTIOMER.

**isomerase** \īsäm′ərās\ Any enzyme which converts a substrate to its isomer.

**isomeric** \-mer′ik\ Being in the relation of isomers: said of substances. also *isomerous.*

**isomerism** \īsäm′ərizm\ The phenomenon that molecules can differ when they contain the same numbers of the same atoms. **optical i.** The phenomenon of molecules differing by being the mirror images of each other (enantiomers). Such isomers rotate the plane of polarized light in opposite directions.

**isomerization** \īsäm′ərīzā′shən\ The conversion of one isomer into another.

**isomerous** \īsäm′ərəs\ ISOMERIC.

**isomethadone** $C_{21}H_{27}NO$. 6-(Dimethylamino)-5-methyl-4,4-diphenyl-3-hexanone. A compound similar to methadone in structure and in pharmacologic properties. It is an analgesic with addicting properties if taken chronically.

**isometheptene** $C_9H_{19}N$. *N*,1,5-Trimethyl-4-hexenylamine. An adrenergic drug used as an antispasmodic for intestinal, biliary, or ureteral spasm or colic.

**isometheptene mucate** $C_{24}H_{48}N_2O_8$. The mucate derivative of isometheptene. It has the same adrenergic properties and uses as the parent drug.

**isometric** \-met′rik\ [ISO- + METRIC] Possessing the same length or dimensions, as a muscle contraction in which the force is increased without a change in length.

**isometrics** \-met′riks\ Movements or exercises in which the muscles are tensed without motion at the joints they bridge.

**isometropia** \-metrō′pē·ə\ [ISO- + Gk *metr(on)* measure + -OPIA] A similar refraction state in each eye.

**isomicrogamete** \-mī′krəgam′ēt\ [ISO- + MICRO- + GAMETE] A small gamete that is equal in size to the cell with which it conjugates. Such gametes are produced by some protozoa.

**isomorph** \ī′səmôrf\ *Outmoded* ALLELE.

**isomorphic** \-môr′fik\ ISOMORPHOUS.

**isomorphism** \-môr′fizm\ The property of being morphologically similar.

**isomorphous** \-môr′fəs\ [ISO- + MORPH- + -OUS] Occurring in the same form. Also *isomorphic.*

**isoniazid** \-nī′əzid\ $C_6H_7N_3O$. 4-Pyridinecarboxylic acid hydrazide. A crystalline solid, soluble in water and alcohol, practically insoluble in ether and benzene, used in the treatment of tuberculosis. Also *isonicotinic acid hydrazide, isonicotinoylhydrazine.*

**isonicotinic acid** Pyridine-4-carboxylic acid, an isomer of nicotinic acid. Its hydrazide inhibits pyridoxal-containing enzymes, particularly in some bacteria. Its consequent toxicity to them is the basis of the use of the hydrazide in treating tuberculosis.

**isonicotinic acid hydrazide** ISONIAZID.

**isonicotinoylhydrazine** ISONIAZID.

**isonipecaine** MEPERIDINE HYDROCHLORIDE.

**isonormocytosis** \-nôr′məsītō′sis\ Having a normal total leukocyte count and normal proportions of different classes of leukocytes.

**iso-oncotic** \-ängkät′ik\ Possessing the same oncotic pressure.

**iso-osmotic** \-äzmät′ik\ ISOSMOTIC.

**isopentenyl diphosphate** $CH_2$═$C(CH_3)$—$CH_2$—$CH_2$ —O—PO(OH)—O—$PO(OH)_2$. 3-Methylbut-3-enyl diphosphate. This substance is formed from diphosphomevalonic acid by a decarboxylation and elimination linked with the hydrolysis of ATP, in an early step of the pathway by which steroids and other terpenses are made. Also *isopentenyl pyrophosphate.*

**isopentenyldiphosphate isomerase** The enzyme (EC 5.3.3.2) that catalyzes the interconversion of isopentenyl diphosphate (3-methylbut-3-enyl diphosphate) and dimethylallyl diphosphate (3-methylbut-2-enyl phosphate). In a further reaction of the pathway of terpene and steroid biosynthesis, isopentenyl and dimethylallyl diphosphates condense with the formation of the $C_{10}$-compound, geranyl diphosphate, and the release of inorganic diphosphate.

**isopentenyl pyrophosphate** ISOPENTENYL DIPHOSPHATE.

**isophan** \ī′səfan\ [Gk *isophanēs* (from *iso(s)* equal, same + *-phanēs* -appearing, from *phainesthai* to appear) appearing alike] PHENOCOPY.

**isophene** \ī′səfēn\ [ISO- + PHENE] GENOCOPY.

**isophoria** \-fôr′ē·ə\ [ISO- + -PHORIA] **1** A constant balance of ocular muscles regardless of the position of the eyes. **2** Alignment of the visual axes of the two eyes on the same horizontal plane so that there is no hyperphoria or hypophoria.

**isophotometer** \-fōtäm′ətər\ [ISO- + PHOTOMETER] A device for locating points of equal density on a radiograph or another type of film.

**isoplastic** \-plas′tik\ ISOGENEIC.

**isopotential** \-pəten′shəl\ Possessing the same potential force or energy; having the same ability to do work.

**isopregnenone** DYDROGESTERONE.

**isoprenaline** ISOPROTERENOL.

**isoprene** $CH_2{=}CH{-}C(CH_3){=}CH_2$. 2-Methylbuta-1,3-diene. A hydrocarbon that is the fundamental unit from which many natural products, including steroids, are built.

**isoprenoid** Any substance biosynthesized from $C_5$-units with the isoprene skeleton. Such compounds include squalene, the precursor of steroids, and terpenes. Isopentenyl diphosphate and dimethylallyl diphosphate are the two precursors of the $C_5$-units present in more complex molecules.

**Isoprinosine** $C_{52}H_{78}N_{10}O_{17}$. A drug which stimulates T cells and lymphocytes *in vitro* and *in vivo*, and has been reported to have some antiviral activity *in vitro*. A proprietary name.

**isopropamide iodide** $C_{23}H_{33}IN_2O$. γ-(Aminocarboxyl)-*N*-methyl-*N*-*N*-bis(1-methylethyl)-γ-phenylbenzene propanaminium iodide. An anticholinergic agent used to treat peptic ulcer. It is given orally.

**isopropyl** $(CH_3{-})_2CH{-}$. The group formed by removing a hydrogen atom from C-2 of propane. Also *propyl*.

**isopropylarterenol** ISOPROTERENOL.

**isopropylepinephrine** ISOPROTERENOL.

**isopropyl meprobamate** CARISOPRODOL.

**isopropyl myristate** $C_{17}H_{34}O_2$. An ester used in topical medicinal preparations because of its ability to promote absorption of externally applied drugs through the skin.

**isopropyl thiogalactoside** A synthetic galactoside derivative containing sulfur instead of oxygen as the glycosylated atom. It is used as an inducer of the formation of bacterial enzymes of galactoside metabolism, specifically those controlled by the *lac* operon.

**isoproterenol** $C_{11}H_{17}NO_3$. 3,4-Dihydroxy-α-[(isopropylamino)methyl]benzyl alcohol. A synthetic adrenergic agent similar to epinephrine, with a propyl group replacing the methyl group. It is a potent cardiac stimulant and bronchodilator. As the hydrochloride, it is given by inhalation, sublingually, or parenterally for treatment of bronchial asthma. It is used also for some cardiac conditions responding to these drugs. Also *isoprenaline, isopropylarterenol, isopropylepinephrine*.

**isopter** \īsäp′tər\ [*is(o)-* + *-opter* as in *diopter*] A line on a visual field chart passing through points of equal visual acuity.

**isopyknosis** \-piknō′sis\ [ISO- + PYKN- + -OSIS] A state of equivalent condensation of chromatin, as applied particularly to comparisons between and within chromosomes.

**isorhythmic** \-riTH′mik\ Having a constant, invariable rhythm.

**isoriboflavin** $C_{17}H_{20}N_4O_6$. 8-Demethyl-6-methylriboflavin. An antimetabolite of riboflavin which has methyl groups on the 6 and 5 positions, rather than 6 and 7 positions of the isoalloxazine nucleus. It has been used to produce a riboflavin deficiency in experimental animals.

**isorrhea** \ī′sôrē′ə\ [ISO- + -RRHEA] A homeostasis of body fluid volume and composition.

**isosensitize** \-sen′sətīz\ AUTOSENSITIZE.

**isoserotherapy** \-sir′ōther′əpē\ Therapy involving injections of isoserum.

**isoserum** \-sir′əm\ Serum taken from a person who is convalescing from the same disease as that of the patient to be treated with such serum.

**isosmotic** \ī′säzmät′ik\ Having equal osmotic pressure: used of two fluids. Also *iso-osmotic*.

**isosorbide** $C_6H_{10}O_4$. 1,4:3,6-Dianhydro-D-glucitol. A derivative of sorbitol used as an osmotic diuretic agent. It also reduces the intraocular pressure and is used to lower the tension quickly in glaucoma.

**isosorbide dinitrate** $C_6H_8N_2O_8$. 1,4:3,6-Dianhydro-D-glucitol dinitrate. A form of nitrate used to dilate the coronary vessels of the heart. It is given in tablets for sublingual absorption and in sustained-release oral tablets, the latter being considerably less effective.

***Isospora*** \īsäs′pôrə\ A genus of monoxenous coccidian parasites in the suborder Eimeriina, found chiefly in mammals, but also in birds, amphibians, and reptiles. The mature oocysts, found in feces, contain two sporocysts, each with four sporozoites. ***I. belli*** A species found in the small intestine of humans in the tropics, and probably throughout the world. The infection, known as coccidiosis, is usually asymptomatic and self-limiting, but has been associated with mucous diarrhea or steatorrhea, anorexia, nausea, and, in some cases, colicky abdominal pain and malabsorption. ***I. hominis*** *SARCOCYSTIS HOMINIS*.

**isosporiasis** \-spôrī′əsis\ [*Isospor(a)* + -IASIS] Infection by sporozoans of the genus *Isospora*, which are found in the intestines of a wide variety of animals and which occasionally infect man. Also *isosporosis*. See also COCCIDIOSIS.

**isosporosis** \-spôrō′sis\ ISOSPORIASIS.

**isostere** A compound similar to another compound in the shape of its molecule but differing from it in chemical structure. Isosteres of natural compounds are often useful as research tools, since they may bind to enzymes and other receptors for the natural compounds.

**isosthenuria** \īsäs′thēnoo′rē·ə\ [ISO- + STHEN- + -URIA] Excretion of urine with a fixed relative density ($\pm 1.010$) under all circumstances. It is a sign of advanced renal failure.

**isotel** \ī′sətel\ [ISO- + Gk *tel(os)* end, completeness, fulfillment] A dietary factor which can effectively replace another essential nutrient.

**isothermagnosia** \-thur′magnō′zhə\ [ISO- + THERM- + AGNOSIA] **1** Inability to distinguish between heat and cold. **2** An abnormality of sensation in which the patient perceives pain, heat, and cold as a feeling of heat.

**isothermal** \-thur′məl\ ISOTHERMIC.

**isothermic** \-thur′mik\ [ISO- + THERM- + -IC] Possessing the same temperature. Also *isothermal, synthermal*.

**isothiazine hydrochloride** ETHOPROPAZINE HYDROCHLORIDE.

**isothipendyl** $C_{16}H_{19}N_3S$. 10-(2-Dimethylamino-2-methylethyl)-10*H*-pyrido[3,2-*b*][1,4]benzothiazine. An antihistamic agent often given in the hydrochloride salt form. It is a potent, but short acting antihistaminic medication, given by oral or parenteral routes for severe allergies.

**isotone** \ī′sətōn\ Any of two or more atomic nuclei which have the same number of neutrons but different atomic numbers and different mass numbers such as $^{30}_{14}Si$, $^{31}_{15}P$, and $^{32}_{16}S$.

**isotonic** \-tän′ik\ **1** Denoting a fluid exerting the same osmotic pressure as another fluid with which it is being compared and in which cells can be immersed without changing their size and shape. **2** Maintaining a uniform muscle tone. For defs. 1 and 2 also *homotonic.*

**isotonicity** \-tōnis′itē\ The quality of being isotonic.

**isotope** \ī′sətōp\ [Gk *iso(s)* same + *topos* place: occupying the same place in the periodic table] Any of several atoms which have the same number of protons, and thus are members of the same element, but have different numbers of neutrons. Thus $^{129}I$ and $^{131}I$ are isotopes of iodine. • At one time *isotope* was widely but incorrectly used to refer to any radioactive atom, for which the preferred term is now *radioactive nuclide* or *radionuclide,* unless reference is made specifically to two nuclides of the same element. Adj. isotopic. **heavy i.** An isotope of greater nuclear mass than that of the naturally most abundant isotope of the element concerned, or the more massive of two naturally occurring isotopes. Although many radioactive isotopes are heavier than their naturally most abundant forms, e.g. $^{3}H$ or $^{14}C$ compared with $^{1}H$ or $^{12}C$, the term is often used specifically for isotopes that do not emit radiation, e.g. $^{2}H$, $^{13}C$, $^{15}N$, or $^{18}O$. **radioactive i.** *Incorrect* RADIONUCLIDE. **stable i.** An isotope that does not transmute into another element; a nonradioactive isotope.

**isotoxic** \-täk′sik\ HOMEOTOXIC.

**isotoxin** \-täk′sin\ [ISO- + TOXIN] HOMEOTOXIN.

**isotransplant** \-trans′plant\ ISOGRAFT.

**isotretinoin** The 13-cis isomer of tretinoin (retinoic acid), an agent used orally in the treatment of nodular cystic acne. It may work through inhibition of sebaceous gland function. Its side effects include dry skin, hyperostosis, and elevation of triglycerides. It is contraindicated during pregnancy, as it is a teratogen.

**isotropic** \-träp′ik\ [ISO- + -TROPIC[1]] Having physical properties that are independent of direction in the material.

**isotypical** \-tip′ikəl\ Of the same type.

**isovaleric acid** $(CH_3)_2CH—CH_2—COOH$. 3-Methylbutyric acid. It contains the carbon chain of the amino acid valine.

**isovalericacidemia** \-valer′ikas′idē′mē·ə\ An inborn error of metabolism of the branched-chain amino acid leucine. The basic defect is thought to be a deficiency of the enzyme isovaleryl-CoA dehydrogenase. Serum isovaleric acid levels are markedly elevated, with clinical consequences appearing as psychomotor retardation, an objectionable body odor that resembles sweaty feet, and a tendency for developing dehydration, acidosis, and coma. The condition is inherited as an autosomal recessive trait. Also *Sidbury syndrome, odor-of-sweaty-feet syndrome, sweaty feet syndrome.*

**isoxazolyl penicillin** A group of semisynthetic penicillins that are resistant to penicillinase and to acid hydrolysis. They include cloxacillin, dicloxacillin, flucloxacillin, and oxacillin.

**isoxsuprine hydrochloride** $C_{18}H_{23}NO_3·HCl$. *p*-Hydroxy-α-[1-[(1-methyl-2-phenoxyethylamino]ethyl]benzyl alcohol hydrochloride. A white, crystalline powder, sparingly soluble in water, used as a vasodilator in the treatment of peripheral vascular disease associated with arteriosclerosis.

**isozyme** \ī′sōzīm\ ISOENZYME.

**-ist** \-ist\ [Gk suffix *-istēs* from verb termination *-izein* denoting to perform an act + *-tēs* forming agent nouns] A suffix denoting a person engaged in a profession or activity.

**isthmectomy** \ismek′təmē\ [*isthm(us)* + -ECTOMY] A surgical procedure in which a narrow bridge of tissue connecting two larger tissue masses is excised, as removal of the thyroid isthmus. Also *median strumectomy.*

**isthmi** \is′mī\ Plural of ISTHMUS.

**isthmian** \is′mē·ən\ Pertaining to any anatomical isthmus. Also *isthmic.*

**isthmoid** \is′moid\ Resembling an anatomical isthmus.

**isthmus** \is′məs\ [Gk *isthmos* a neck, narrow passage, isthmus] **1** A narrow strip of tissue connecting the larger structures or parts of an organ. **2** A short narrow passage or constriction connecting two cavities or canals. **i. aortae** [NA] A narrowing of the lumen of the aorta, especially marked in the fetus, between the final site of origin of the left subclavian artery and the attachment of the ductus arteriosus, which becomes the ligamentum arteriosum after birth. The constriction occasionally persists in the adult. Also *isthmus of aorta, aortic isthmus.* **i. of auditory tube** ISTHMUS TUBAE AUDITIVAE. **i. of auricle** ISTHMUS CARTILAGINIS AURIS. **i. cartilaginis auris** [NA] A narrow strip of cartilage joining the cartilage of the auricle of the external ear to that of the external acoustic meatus. Also *isthmus of cartilage of auricle, isthmus of auricle, isthmus of cartilaginous part of ear.* **i. of cingulate gyrus** ISTHMUS GYRI CINGULI. **i. of external auditory meatus** A very narrow segment of the osseous part of the external acoustic meatus that is situated at the junction of the outer three fourths and the inner one fourth of the meatus. **i. faucium** [NA] The slightly narrowed opening between the oral cavity and the oral pharynx, bounded superiorly by the free border of the palatal velum and the uvula, laterally by the palatoglossal arches, and inferiorly by the dorsum of the tongue. Also *isthmus of fauces.* **i. glandulae thyroideae** [NA] A horizontal strip of thyroid tissue, of varying size, anterior to the upper part of the trachea, connecting the lower parts of the lateral lobes of the thyroid gland. Occasionally the pyramidal lobe is attached to it. Also *isthmus of thyroid gland.* **gyral i.** A narrow bridge interposed between two gyri of the cerebral cortex. **i. gyri cinguli** [NA] The constriction of the cingulate gyrusbehind and below the splenium of the corpus callosum at its transition to the parahippocampal gyrus. Also *isthmus gyri fornicati, isthmus of limbic lobe, isthmus of cingulate gyrus.* **i. gyri fornicati** ISTHMUS GYRI CINGULI. **i. hippocampi** The narrow retrosplenial cortex bridging the cingulate gyrus and the parahippocampal gyrus. **i. of His** ISTHMUS RHOMBENCEPHALI. **i. of limbic lobe** ISTHMUS GYRI CINGULI. **i. prostatae** [NA] A band of fibromuscular tissue that joins the right to the left lobe of the prostate in front of the urethra. Also *isthmus of prostate.* **i. rhombencephali** The constriction formed in fetal development by a bend in the neural tube at the juncture of the rhombencephalon and mesencephalon. Also *isthmus of His.* **i. of thyroid gland** ISTHMUS GLANDULAE THYROIDEAE. **i. tubae auditivae** [NA] The narrowest part of the auditory tube, occurring at the junction of the osseous and cartilaginous portions. Also *isthmus of auditory tube.* **i. tubae uterinae** [NA] The narrow, cordlike medial one third of the uterine tube, lying between its ampulla and the wall of the uterus. Also *isthmus of uterine tube.* **i. uteri** [NA] The transverse constriction between the cervix and the body of the uterus. Also *isthmus of uterus.* **i. of uterine tube** ISTHMUS TUBAE UTERINAE. **i. of uterus** ISTHMUS UTERI. **i. of Vieussens** LIMBUS FOSSAE OVALIS.

**isuria** \īsʸoo′rē·ə\ [*is(o)-* + UR- + -IA] The excretion of urine at a rate that remains constant over time.

**itch** [(substantive) Middle English *icche,* from Old English *gicce;* (verb) Middle English *icchen,* from Old English *giccan*] **1** A sensation that elicits the desire to scratch; pruritus. **2** A skin disorder characterized by an itch. **3** *Popular* SCABIES. **barbers' i.** Infections and other disorders of the skin of the beard area in men, including ringworm, bacterial folliculitis, and pseudofolliculitis. *Imprecise.* **bath i.** Pruritus caused by soap. **clam diggers' i.** SCHISTOSOME DERMATITIS. **filarial i.** ONCHOCERCAL DERMATITIS. **ground i.** An irritable eruption of the skin of the feet that is caused by penetration by hookworm or *Strongyloides* larvae. Also *water itch, swamp itch, uncinarial dermatitis.* **gym i.** TINEA CRURIS. **jock i.** *Popular* TINEA CRURIS. **kabure i.** SCHISTOSOMIASIS. **Norway i.** NORWEGIAN SCABIES. **poultryman's i.** A dermatitis caused by the chicken mite, *Dermanyssus gallinae.* **sarcoptic i.** SARCOPTIC SCABIES. **Sawah i.** An East Indian term for SCHISTOSOMIASIS. **seven-year i.** SCABIES. **summer i.** HUTCHINSON SUMMER PRURIGO. **swamp i.** GROUND ITCH. **swimmers' i.** SCHISTOSOME DERMATITIS. **warehouseman's i.** Dermatitis caused by exposure to mites that infest food. Warehouse workers are most at risk, but other wholesale and retail food handlers may also be affected. **water i.** GROUND ITCH. **winter i.** WINTER PRURIGO.

**itching** [ITCH + -ING] PRURITUS.

**-ite** \\-īt\\ [Gk-*itēs* (feminine *-itis*) suffix denoting resembling, of the nature of; also L *-itus* general past participle ending; also arbitrary variant of *-ate* from L *-atus* past participle ending] **1** A suffix meaning (1) substance of or derived from (something specified); (2) constituent or division, especially an early developmental stage of an anatomic part. **2** A suffix designating an anion, salt, or ester containing less oxygen than that contained in another anion, salt, or ester based on the same element, as nitrite, $NO_2^-$ in contrast with nitrate, $NO_3^-$.

**iter** \\ī′tər\\ [L (gen. *itineris;* from *itus,* past part. of *ire* to go), a going along, walk, road, way, path] A tubular passage or channel between two structures or parts. **i. ad infundibulum** The median tubular passage of the infundibular stalk connecting the hypothalamic third ventricle with the pituitary. **i. a tertio ad quartum ventriculum** AQUEDUCTUS CEREBRI. **i. chordae anterius** A foramen situated at the inner end of the petrotympanic fissure that transmits the chorda tympani from the cavity of the middle ear to the deep face. Also *Huguier's canal, Civinini's canal.* **i. chordae posterius** CANALICULUS CHORDAE TYMPANI. **i. of Sylvius** AQUAEDUCTUS CEREBRI.

**iteral** \\ī′tərəl\\ Pertaining to an iter.

**iterative** \\it′ərā′tiv\\ [Late L *iterativus* (from L *iterat(us),* past part. of *iterare* to repeat + *-ivus* -IVE) repetitive] Repeatedly executing a series of operations or instructions until some condition is satisfied: said of a procedure or computer program.

**ithyokyphosis** \\ith′ē·ōkīfō′sis\\ [Gk *ithy(s)* straight ahead + *o* + KYPHOSIS] A backward projection of the spine with no accompanying lateral deviation.

**-itides** \\-it′idēz\\ Plural of -ITIS.

**-ition** \\-ish′ən\\ [L verb-stem ending *-i-* + noun-forming suffix *-tio,* gen. *-tionis*] A noun suffix denoting an action, process, or result.

**-itis** \\-ī′tis\\ [Gk, fem. of adj. suffix *-itēs*] (*pl.* -itides) A suffix meaning inflammation, or a disease characterized by inflammation, of a (specified) organ or part. • Words with this suffix in Greek were originally adjectives, for example, *arthritēs,* fem. *arthritis,* pertaining to joints, articular: *arthritis nosos* joint disease. With omission of *nosos* (disease) as "understood," such words became nouns. The suffix was not specialized in the sense of "inflammation" until its proliferation in modern times; Greek *nephritis,* for example, usually implied kidney stones. Most of the prototype *-itis* words, however, did happen to designate inflammatory diseases, and this fact set the pattern for the modern usage. See also note at -OSIS.

**Ito** [Hayazo *Ito,* Japanese pathologist, born 1865] Ito-Reenstierna reaction. See under ITO-REENSTIERNA TEST.

**Ito** [Minoru *Ito,* Japanese dermatologist, flourished 20th century] See under NEVUS.

**ITP** idiopathic thrombocytopenic purpura.

**Itsenko** [N. N. *Itsenko,* Russian physician, flourished mid-20th century] Itsenko's disease. See under CUSHING SYNDROME.

**-ity** \\-itē\\ [L *-itas,* suffix forming nouns from adjectives and denoting state or condition] A suffix denoting state or condition.

**IU** **1** international unit. **2** immunizing unit. **3** intrauterine.

**IUCD** intrauterine contraceptive device.

**IUD** intrauterine device.

**IV** **1** intravenous(ly). **2** intravertebral.

**Ivalon** A proprietary name for polyvinyl alcohol

**IVC** inferior vena cava.

**-ive** \\-iv\\ [L *-ivus,* adjectival suffix] A suffix meaning (1) doing or tending to do (something specified), as *invasive, curative;* (2) an agent that does or tends to do (something specified), as *fixative, sedative.*

**ivermectin** \\ī′vurmek′tin\\ One of a class of potent antiparasitic drugs, the avermectins, used against a wide variety of nematodes and arthropods. It is the 22,23-dihydro derivative of avermectin B1, which is a macrocyclic lactone produced by *Actinomyces avermitilis.* The antiparasitic activity apparently is associated with blocking neuromuscular transmission mediated by $\gamma$-aminobutyric acid. It is used currently to control parasites of domestic animals, but its use may be extended to man.

**IVP** **1** intravenous pyelogram. **2** intraventricular pressure.

**IVT** intravenous transfusion.

**Ivy** [Andrew Conway *Ivy,* U.S. physiologist, 1893–1978] Ivy's method. See under IVY BLEEDING TIME TEST.

**Ivy** [Robert H. *Ivy,* U.S. oral and plastic surgeon, 1881–1974] Ivy loop wiring. See under EYELET WIRING.

**ivy** **1** Any of various members of the genus *Hedera,* which is composed primarily of climbing plants. **2** See under POISON IVY. **poison i.** **1** Any of several plants of the genus *Toxicodendron* (especially *T. radicans*) widely distributed in North America and occurring also in South Africa, producing contact dermatitis with itching and in severe cases blistering. Smoke from the burning plant is also toxic. **2** Dermatitis resulting from contact or exposure to the toxin of the poison ivy plant.

**Iwanoff** [Wladimir *Iwanoff,* Russian ophthalmologist, born 1861] Iwanoff cysts. See under CYST.

***Ixodes*** \\iksō′dēz\\ [Gk *ixōdēs* (from *ixos* mistletoe, birdlime, sticky substance, akin to L *viscus* or *viscum,* same meanings) like birdlime, sticky] The largest genus of ixodid or hard ticks, consisting of about 250 species, 40 from North America. They are all three-host ticks. Many are ectoparasites of man and domestic and wild mammals, causing severe reactions by their bites, and transmitting a number of disease agents. ***I. dammini*** The principal vector in the northeastern United States of *Borrelia burgdorferi,* the spirochete that causes Lyme disease; the deer tick. The larval and nymphal stages feed on many kinds of mammals but especially rodents, while the adults prefer large mammals such as deer. All stages are known to attack humans. ***I. hexagonus*** A species found on domestic and wild carnivores in Africa and Europe, and implicated in transmission of tick-borne encephalitis virus and several human cases of tick paralysis in Europe. ***I. holocyclus*** An Australian species, the scrub tick, commonly found on wild rodents, but which often infests dogs, cats, other domestic animals, birds, and humans. It secretes a toxin that causes ascending flaccid paralysis and death from respiratory failure. One tick can cause death of a dog. Larger animals are unlikely to be affected. It is also the probable vector of Queensland tick typhus. ***I. pacificus*** The California black-legged tick, a species common on cattle and deer in California. It readily attacks man. It is considered a possible vector of tularemia in humans, and is a cause of tick paralysis. ***I. persulcatus*** A low-temperature-tolerant Eurasian species, the taiga tick, which is a vector of Russian spring-summer encephalitis, Omsk hemorrhagic fever virus, Absettarov virus, and Kemerovo virus in western Siberia. It plays an important role in the transmission of viruses to man and of bovine babesiosis in cattle. It is associated with a wide variety of small forest mammals and birds in its larval stages, and with larger domestic and wild animals as an adult tick. ***I. ricinus*** The European castor bean tick, one of the most important viral and babesiosis vectors in this large genus. It is parasitic on sheep, cattle, and many wild animals. Larvae are found on a great range of small mammals and birds. It transmits a variety of disease agents including the virus of louping ill, Omsk hemorrhagic fever virus (the Bukovinian agent), Absettarov virus, Tribec virus, central European tick-borne encephalitis virus, and the Uukuniemi group viruses. It is also the vector of *Babesia bovis,* possibly of the Japanese B encephalitis virus, and is the etiologic agent of tularemia. ***I. scapularis*** An American species, the black-legged or shoulder tick closely related to *I. ricinus* and *I. persulcatus* of Europe. This species is found in the eastern United States and frequently attacks man, inflicting a painful bite. It is closely related to the recently described vector of human babesiosis caused by *Babesia microti* and occurring in Massachusetts.

**ixodiasis** \isk'ōdī'əsis\ [*Ixod(es)* + -IASIS] **1** Any disease caused by tick bites. **2** Infestation with ticks. Also *ixodism.*

**ixodid** \iksäd'id\ **1** Pertaining or belonging to the family Ixodidae. **2** A tick of the family Ixodidae.

**Ixodidae** \iksäd'idē\ [*Ixod(es)* + -IDAE] A family of ticks (order Acarina, suborder Ixodides) comprising some 660 species in 14 genera; the hard ticks. They are characterized by a rigid body form and the presence of a scutum. Many have a three-host life cycle with larvae on rodents or small birds, nymphs on intermediate-sized mammals, and adults on larger mammals, especially ruminants. It includes the genera *Amblyomma, Anocentor, Aponomma, Boophilus, Demacentor, Haemaphysalis, Hyalomma, Ixodes, Margaropus, Nosomma,* and *Rhipicephalus.* See illustration at TICK.

**ixodism** \iks'ōdizm\ IXODIASIS.

**-ize** \-īz\ [Gk *-izein* infinitive verb termination meaning to perform an act] A suffix meaning to subject to. Also *-ise* (British spelling).

# J

**J** **1** Symbol for the unit, joule. **2** Symbol for Joule's equivalent.

**Jaboulay** [Mathieu *Jaboulay,* French surgeon, 1860–1913] **1** Jaboulay's amputation. See under INTERPELVIABDOMINAL AMPUTATION. **2** Jaboulay's operation. See under INTERPELVIABDOMINAL AMPUTATION.

**Jaccoud** [François-Sigismond *Jaccoud,* French physician, 1830–1913] See under FEVER.

**jacket** [French *jaquette,* dim. of *jaque* a medieval short cloak, after *Jaques* an appellation for a peasant] A device that surrounds the torso and provides support and/or immobilizes the body. **Minerva j.** A closely molded plaster-of-Paris jacket that extends from the iliac crest to the external occiput. • The term is named after *Minerva,* the Roman goddess of wisdom. **plaster-of-Paris j.** A Minerva jacket that does not encompass the neck and occiput. It is used for spinal fractures and for correcting deformities.

**Jackson** [Chevalier Q. *Jackson,* U.S. otolaryngologist, 1865–1958] Jackson's safety triangle. See under TRIANGLE.

**Jackson** [John Hughlings *Jackson,* English neurologist, 1835–1911] **1** Bravais-Jacksonian epilepsy. See under JACKSONIAN EPILEPSY. **2** See under THEORY, SIGN. **3** Jackson's rule. See under LAW. **4** Jackson syndrome, Jackson-Mackenzie syndrome. See under JACKSON'S PARALYSIS.

**jacksonism** \jak'sənizm\ [after John Hughlings *Jackson,* English neurologist, 1835–1911 + -ISM] *Seldom used* JACKSONIAN MARCH.

**Jacob** [Arthur *Jacob,* Irish ophthalmologist, 1790–1874] Jacob's membrane. See under STRATUM NEUROEPITHELIALE RETINAE.

**Jacobaeus** [Hans Christian *Jacobaeus,* Swedish physician, 1879–1937] See under OPERATION.

**Jacobson** [Julius *Jacobson,* German ophthalmologist, 1828–1889] Jacobson's retinitis. See under RETINITIS SYPHILITICA.

**Jacobson** [Ludvig Levin *Jacobson,* Danish anatomist, 1783–1843] **1** Jacobson's plexus. See under PLEXUS TYMPANICUS. **2** Jacobson's nerve, tympanic nerve of Jacobson. See under NERVUS TYMPANICUS. **3** Ramus tubae plexus tympanici jacobsoni. See under RAMUS TUBARIUS PLEXUS TYMPANICI. **4** Organ of Jacobson. See under VOMERONASAL ORGAN. **5** Jacobson's canal, canal for Jacobson's nerve. See under CANALICULUS TYMPANICUS. **6** Jacobson's cartilage. See under CARTILAGO VOMERONASALIS. **7** Nucleus supraspinalis of Jacobson. See under SUPRASPINAL NUCLEUS.

**Jacod** [Maurice *Jacod,* French physician, born 1880] Jacod syndrome, Jacod-Negri syndrome. See under PETROSPHENOID SYNDROME.

**Jacquemier** [Jean Marie *Jacquemier,* French obstetrician, 1806–1879] See under SIGN.

**Jacques** [Paul *Jacques,* French physician, flourished late 19th century] See under PLEXUS.

**Jacquet** [Leonard Marie Lucien *Jacquet,* French dermatologist, 1860–1914] See under ERYTHEMA.

**jactitation** \jak′titā′shən\ [Late L *jactitatio* (from L *jactitatus*, past part. of *jactitare* to throw out, display) a making a show, displaying] **1** The tossing, restless, to-and-fro movements of a delirious subject. **2** Any irregular jerking, twitching, and repetitive movements of the trunk and limbs, such as the movements of focal motor epilepsy. Also *jactatio, jactation*. **periodic j.** CHOREA.

**Jadassohn** [Josef *Jadassohn*, German dermatologist, 1863–1936] **1** Jadassohn-Lewandowsky syndrome. See under PACHYONYCHIA CONGENITA. **2** Jadassohn-Lewandowsky syndrome. See under PALMOPLANTAR KERATODERMA. **3** Jadassohn's macular atrophy. See under ATROPHY. **4** Jadassohn's test. See under IRRIGATION TEST.

**Jaffe** [Henry Lewis *Jaffe*, U.S. pathologist, born 1907] Jaffe's disease, Jaffe-Lichtenstein disease, Jaffe-Lichtenstein syndrome. See under FIBROUS DYSPLASIA.

**Jaffé** [Max *Jaffé*, Russian physician, 1841–1911] Jaffé reaction. See under TEST.

**Jakob** [Alfons *Jakob*, German physician, 1884–1931] Jakob-Creutzfeldt disease, Jakob's disease, Jakob spastic pseudosclerosis, Creutzfeldt-Jakob presenile encephalopathy, Creutzfeldt-Jakob syndrome. See under CREUTZFELDT-JAKOB DISEASE.

**Jalaguier** [Adolphe *Jalaguier*, French surgeon, 1853–1924] Battle-Jalaguier-Kammerer incision. See under BATTLE'S INCISION.

**jalap** \jal′əp\ [Spanish *jalapa*, named after the city of Jalapa in the state of Veracruz, Mexico] The resinous material present in the dried roots of *Exogonium purga* and various *Ipomocu* species. The powdered material or a tincture derived from the resin have been used as a cathartic. Also *jalap resin*.

**jamais vu** \zhämā′ vʏ′, vyoo′, voo′\ [French *jamais* never + *vu*, past part. of *voir* to see] A form of paramnesia consisting of a powerful sense of unreality or depersonalization and a feeling that one has never before seen what is being perceived, even though the visual experience, as of a domestic scene, is one that ought to be familiar to the subject. It often occurs as a manifestation of temporal lobe epilepsy, but sometimes in states of emotional disturbance or anxiety (the phobic anxiety-depersonalization syndrome) in which the patient feels curiously detached from his environment as if in a dream or unreal world. Hence this is sometimes an epileptic illusion which, if prolonged, gives a so-called epileptic dreamy state.

**James** [G. C. W. *James*, U.S. physician, flourished 20th century] Swyer-James-Macleod syndrome, Swyer-James syndrome. See under MACLEOD SYNDROME.

**James** [William *James*, U.S. psychologist and philosopher, 1842–1910] James-Lange-Sutherland theory. See under JAMES-LANGE THEORY.

**Jampel** [Robert Steven *Jampel*, U.S. ophthalmologist, born 1926] Schwartz-Jampel syndrome. See under CHONDRODYSTROPHIC MYOTONIA.

**Janet** [Pierre Marie Felix *Janet*, French psychologist and neurologist, 1859–1947] **1** Janet's disease. See under PSYCHASTHENIA. **2** See under PSYCHOLOGY.

**janiceps** \jan′iseps\ [after *Jan(us)* a two-faced Roman god + *i* + L *-ceps*, combining form from *caput* head] Equal conjoined twins united at the head, with two faces oriented in different directions. Also *janus*. **j. asymmetrus** Janiceps with one of the two faces imperfectly formed. Also *syncephalus asymmetros*. **j. parasiticus** Unequal conjoined twins in which the parasitic member consists primarily of a head with recognizable facial features.

**Janin** [Joseph *Janin*, French physician, born 1864] Janin's tetanus. See under CEPHALIC TETANUS.

**Jansen** [Albert *Jansen*, German otologist, 1859–1933] See under FORCEPS.

**Jansen** [Murk *Jansen*, Dutch orthopedic surgeon, 1867–1935] See under DISEASE.

**Jansky**

**janus** \jā′nəs\ [See JANICEPS.] JANICEPS.

**jar**[1] A vessel with a wide mouth, usually of glass or earthenware. **anaerobic j.** A closed container with a device for eliminating molecular oxygen. It is used for incubating plates inoculated with anaerobic bacteria. **bell j.** A bell-shaped enclosure that is usually made of glass and is placed over or around a substance or device. It is used most often in procedures that involve gases or vacuums. **candle j.** A convenient means of providing an atmosphere of elevated carbon dioxide content when required for the growth of certain bacteria: a candle is lit in a jar containing the inoculated plates, the jar is sealed, and the candle extinguishes itself when part of the oxygen present is converted to carbon dioxide. **Coplin j.** A wide-mouthed glass container with a rectangular internal cross-section and vertically oriented grooves on two sides. It is used to immerse microscope slides in staining solutions.

**jar**[2] [onomatopoeic] A jolt or wrenching movement.

**jargon** \jär′gən\ [Middle English *jargoun*, from Middle French *jargon* (of imitative origin) a chattering, as of birds] In aphasia, the combination of syllables or segments of speech into fluent but meaningless gibberish.

**jargonagraphia** \jär′gənəgraf′ē·ə\ JARGON AGRAPHIA.

**jargonaphasia** \jär′gənəfā′zhə\ JARGON APHASIA.

**jargonorrhea** \jär′gənôrē′ə\ JARGON APHASIA.

**Jarisch** [Adolf *Jarisch*, Austrian dermatologist, 1850–1902] **1** Jarisch-Herxheimer reaction. See under HERXHEIMER REACTION. **2** Bezold-Jarisch effect, Bezold-Jarisch reflex. See under BEZOLD REFLEX.

**Jarjavay** [Jean François *Jarjavay*, French physician, 1815–1868] Jarjavay's ligaments. See under LIGAMENT.

**Jarvik** [Robert Koffler *Jarvik*, U.S. biomedical engineer and physician, born 1946] Jarvik heart. See under ARTIFICIAL HEART.

**jaundice** \jôn′dis, jän′-\ [Middle English *jaundis*, from Old French *jaunisse* jaundice, from *jaune* yellow, from L *galbinus* greenish yellow] Yellow discoloration of the skin and mucous membranes resulting from hyperbilirubinemia and subsequent deposition of bile pigment in the involved structure. Also *icterus*. **acholuric j.** HEMOLYTIC JAUNDICE. **breast-milk j.** Severe hyperbilirubinemia due to raised concentration of unconjugated bilirubin in nursing infants two to four weeks postpartum. The cause appears to be a steroidal agent in breast milk that interferes with the action of hepatic glucuronyl transferase in the infant. **cholestatic j.** Jaundice due to a reduction in bile flow, either because of hepatocyte necrosis with reduction of all liver cell functions, or because of interference with the excretory function of the liver cell only, with preservation of other functions. **congenital hemolytic j.** HEREDITARY SPHEROCYTOSIS. **congenital nonhemolytic j.** **1** Any condition in which neonatal jaundice occurs in the absence of hemolysis. **2** CRIGLER-NAJJAR SYNDROME. **congenital obliterative j.** Obstructive jaundice of the newborn associated with the absence or nonpatency of the hepatic bile duct system. It is uncertain whether the condition is genetic or caused by intrauterine infection. **constitutional j.** GILBERT SYNDROME. **Crigler-Najjar j.** CRIGLER-NAJJAR SYNDROME. **epidemic catarrhal j.** *Outmoded* HEPATITIS A. **hemolytic j.** Jaundice due to increased destruction of erythrocytes and characterized by the absence of bilirubin in the urine and increase in the indirect-reacting bilirubin concentration in blood. Also *acholuric jaundice.* **hemorrhagic j.** ICTERIC LEPTOSPIROSIS. **hepatocanalicular j.** HEPATOCELLULAR JAUNDICE. **hepatocellular j.** Jaundice resulting from intrinsic disease of the liver cells rather than hemolysis or obstruction of the biliary drainage system. Also *parenchymatous jaundice, hepatocanalicular jaundice.* **homologous serum j.** HEPATITIS B. **human serum j.** HEPATITIS B. **infectious j.** Viral or leptospiral hepatitis. An ambiguous term. Also *infective jaundice.* **latent j.** Hyperbilirubinemia without visible yellow staining of skin or mucous membranes. Also *occult jaundice.* **leptospiral j.** ICTERIC LEPTOSPIROSIS. **mechanical j.** OBSTRUCTIVE JAUNDICE. **j. of the newborn** ICTERUS NEONATORUM. **nonhemolytic j.** Jaundice due to liver disease rather than hemolysis. **nonobstructive j.** Jaundice that is due to any cause other than stoppage of the flow of bile from the liver to the small intestine. **nuclear j.** KERNICTERUS. **obstructive j.** Jaundice due to anatomic obstruction of the biliary drainage system at any level. Also *mechanical jaundice.* **occult j.** LATENT JAUNDICE. **parenchymatous j.** HEPATOCELLULAR JAUNDICE. **physiologic j.** The mild jaundice common in newborn infants from the second or third day and which usually disappears within a week. The main cause is the low activity of the liver enzyme glucuronyl transferase at birth. Thus, bilirubin released by red cell breakdown is only slowly changed to a conjugated form which enables it to be excreted. Also *icterus neonatorum, Ritter's disease.* **relapsing epidemic j.** *Outmoded* CHRONIC ACTIVE HEPATITIS. **retention j.** Jaundice resulting from production of bilirubin in excess of the liver's ability to excrete it, as from hemolysis. **spirochetal j.** ICTERIC LEPTOSPIROSIS. **syringe j.** SERUM HEPATITIS. **toxic j.** Jaundice due to acute or chronic exposure to toxic chemical agents. Also *toxemic jaundice.* **transfusion j.** SERUM HEPATITIS.

**jaw** [Middle English *jowe, jawe*; of unknown origin, perh. akin to *chew, chaw* or from Middle French *joue* cheek] Either of two bony or cartilaginous structures of the face supporting the teeth and forming the framework of the mouth in most vertebrates. In humans, they are entirely bony in adults and used in opening and closing the mouth, chewing, and adjusting the size and shape of the oral cavity for speech. The upper jaw comprises the two maxillae, and the lower jaw, the mandible. • The term is commonly used for the mouth region. **bird-beak j.** A facial deformity produced by forward protrusion of the upper jaw and teeth. **cleft j.** A midline cleft or hypoplastic groove involving the chin or the entire lower jaw. The mandible is variably affected, from minimal notching to complete separation at the midline. **crackling j.** Crepitus arising from a diseased meniscus of the temporomandibular joint when the jaw is opened or closed. Also *snapping jaw.* **Hapsburg j.** 1 MANDIBULAR PROGNATHISM. 2 A prominence of the jaw that is transmitted as an autosomal dominant trait, as seen in the Hapsburg royal house of Europe. **inferior j.** MANDIBULA. **lock j.** See under LOCKJAW. **locked j.** TRISMUS. **lower j.** MANDIBULA. **lumpy j.** See under ACTINOMYCOSIS. **parrot j.** A facial deformity produced by the forward projection of the incisor teeth. **phossy j.** A condition caused by chronic yellow phosphorous poisoning and characterized by periostitis with suppuration, ulceration, necrosis, and severe deformity of the mandible. It is a most distressing disease because it is painful and accompanied by a foul, fetid discharge which makes its victim unendurable to others. It occurred among workers making matches before the use of yellow phosphorous was prohibited, and the condition is now mainly of historical interest. Also *phosphonecrosis, phosphorus necrosis, mandibular necrosis.* **snapping j.** CRACKLING JAW. **upper j.** MAXILLA.

**jawbone** 1 MANDIBULA. 2 A bone of the upper or lower jaw, usually the mandible. Also *jaw bone.*

**jaw-limb** In tonic torsion of the head to one side, the arm or forelimb toward which the jaw is rotated.

**jaw winking** MARCUS GUNN SYNDROME.

**Jefferson** [Sir Geoffrey *Jefferson*, English neurosurgeon, born 1886] Jefferson syndrome. See under INFRACLINOID SYNDROME.

**Jeghers** [Harold *Jeghers*, U.S. physician, born 1904] Peutz-Jeghers syndrome. See under SYNDROME.

**jejunal** \jəjoo′nəl\ Pertaining to the jejunum.

**jejunectomy** \jē′joonek′təmē\ [*jejun(o)-* + -ECTOMY] A surgical procedure in which the proximal part of the small intestine is resected, usually in association with a reanastomosis.

**jejunitis** \jē′joonī′tis\ [*jejun(o)-* + -ITIS] An inflammatory process involving the jejunum.

**jejuno-** \jəjoo′nō-\ [L *jejunus* empty, hungry] A combining form denoting the jejunum.

**jejunocecostomy** \-sēkäs′təmē\ A surgical procedure creating an opening between the proximal part of the small bowel and the cecum after a bypass or resection of the intervening bowel. Such an opening may rarely occur spontaneously following trauma or inflammatory or neoplastic disease.

**jejunocolostomy** \-kōläs′təmē\ A surgical procedure creating an opening between the proximal small intestine and the large intestine following a resection or bypass. Such an opening may rarely result from trauma or inflammatory or neoplastic disease.

**jejunogastric** \-gas′trik\ Relating to the jejunum and the stomach; gastrojenunal.

**jejunoileitis** \jəjoo′nō·il′ē·ī′tis\ An inflammatory process involving both the jejunum and the ileum.

**jejunoileostomy** \jəjoo′nō·il′ē·äs′təmē\ A surgical procedure that creates an opening between the proximal and distal parts of the small bowel following a resection or bypass of the intervening bowel. Such an opening may rarely result spontaneously from traumatic, neoplastic, or inflammatory causes.

**jejunoileum** \jəjoo′nō·il′ē·əm\ The jejunum and ileum considered as a unit.

**jejunojejunostomy** \-jē′joonäs′təmē\ A surgical procedure to create an opening between two loops of the proximal small bowel following resection or bypass. Such an opening may rarely result spontaneously from traumatic, neoplastic, or inflammatory causes.

**jejunoplasty** \jəjoo′nəplas′tē\ [JEJUNO- + -PLASTY] A surgical procedure in which the proximal part of the small bowel is repaired or plicated.

**jejunorrhaphy** \jē′joonôr′əfē\ [JEJUNO- + -RRHAPHY] A surgical procedure in which the proximal part of the small bowel is sutured.

**jejunostomy** \jē′joonäs′təmē\ [JEJUNO- + -STOMY] A surgical procedure creating an opening in the proximal part of the small bowel that communicates with the skin. Such an opening may rarely result from traumatic, neoplastic, or inflammatory causes. Also *nesteostomy, nestiostomy.*

**jejunotomy** \jē′joonät′əmē\ [JEJUNO- + -TOMY] A surgical procedure in which an incision is made into the proximal part of the small bowel.

**jejunum** \jəjoo′nəm\ [L *(intestinum) jejunum* empty intestine, a translation of Gk *nēstis* fasting, empty, from the belief that this portion of the intestine was always found empty after death] [NA] The proximal two-fifths of the small intestine, extending from the duodenojejunal flexure to its junction with the ileum, and arranged in coils or loops suspended from the posterior abdominal wall by the mesentery. Typically, it has larger villi and is thicker and more vascular than the ileum.

**Jellinek** [Stefan *Jellinek*, Austrian physician, born 1871] Jellinek symptom. See under SIGN.

**jelly** [French *gelée* (past part. of *geler* to freeze into ice, from L *gelare* to freeze) jelly, frost] A semisolid, colloidal gelatinous substance that is often clear or nearly translucent. **cardiac j.** A gelatinous material, probably of mucopolysaccharide nature, occupying the space between endocardium and myocardium in the early embryonic heart tube. It is thought to be responsible for preventing regurgitation of blood before identifiable valves are present. Subsequently, it accumulates as subendocardial cushions in restricted parts of the heart such as the atrioventricular canal and the truncus arteriosus and eventually is invaded by fibrous connective tissue to contribute to definitive cardiac valves and septa. Elsewhere it disappears in step with the differentiation of the muscle fibers. **contraceptive j.** A spermicidal medication of jellylike consistency used alone or in conjunction with a mechanical barrier as a means of preventing sperm from reaching an ovum. Similar preparations are formulated as medicated creams and foams. **electrode j.** Jelly used in electrocardiography, electroencephalography, and surface electromyography to improve contact between the electrode and the skin. **enamel j.** STELLATE RETICULUM. **mineral j.** PETROLATUM. **petroleum j.** PETROLATUM. **Wharton's j.** Mucous tissue peculiar to the umbilical cord. It has few fibers but is rich in mucoid (mucopolysaccharide) jelly and differentiates from the primitive extraembryonic mesenchyme included in the cord at the time of its formation. It is the only part that remains of the primitive extraembryonic mesenchyme itself representing the magma rectulare of the blastocoel.

**Jena Nomina Anatomica** A revision of the 1933 Birmingham Revision (BR) of the Basle Nomina Anatomica (1895), prepared and adopted by German anatomists at Jena in 1936 and now superseded by several revisions of Nomina Anatomica.

**Jendrassik** [Ernö *Jendrassik*, Hungarian physician, 1858–1936] See under MANEUVER.

**Jenner** [Edward *Jenner*, English physician, 1749–1823] **1** Jennerian vaccination. See under VACCINATION. **2** Jennerian vaccine. See under SMALLPOX VACCINE.

**Jensen** [Edmund *Jensen*, Danish ophthalmologist, 1861–1950] See under CHOROIDITIS, DISEASE.

**Jensen** [Sigurd Orla *Jensen*, Danish bacteriologist, born 1870] Löwenstein-Jensen agar, Löwenstein-Jensen medium. See under AGAR.

**jerk** A momentary, involuntary movement, usually of an extremity or the head. **Achilles j.** ACHILLES TENDON REFLEX. **ankle j.** ACHILLES TENDON REFLEX. **biceps j.** BICEPS REFLEX. **crossed adductor knee j.** Adduction of the thigh in response to elicitation of the patellar reflex in the contralateral limb. **crossed knee j.** Contraction of the quadriceps in response to tapping the patellar tendon on the contralateral leg. **elbow j.** TRICEPS REFLEX. **epileptic j.** INFANTILE MASSIVE SPASM. **finger j.** HOFFMAN'S REFLEX. **jaw j.** Brisk contraction of the muscles of mastication when the chin of the partially opened and lax jaw is tapped. It is mediated by the trigeminal nerve. Also *jaw reflex, mandibular reflex, jaw jerk reflex, chin reflex, chin-jerk reflex*. **knee j.** PATELLAR REFLEX. **massive myoclonic j.** INFANTILE MASSIVE SPASM. **myoclonic j.** MYOCLONUS. **nystagmoid j.'s** Transient, lateral, jerking movements of the eyes, which are not sustained and may be seen on extreme lateral gaze. They are neither as regular nor as repetitive as true nystagmus and are of no pathologic significance. Also *deviational nystagmus, end-point nystagmus, end-position nystagmus*. **pendular knee j.** The type of knee jerk seen in patients with chorea in which there is hypotonia and impaired inhibition in that the leg swings backwards and forwards several times like a pendulum after a single blow on the patellar tendon. Also *pendulousness of the legs test*. **quadriceps j.** PATELLAR REFLEX. **supinator j.** BRACHIORADIALIS REFLEX. **tendon j.** TENDON REFLEX. **triceps surae j.** ACHILLES TENDON REFLEX.

**Jervell** [Anton *Jervell*, Norwegian cardiologist, born 1901] Jervell and Lange-Nielsen syndrome. See under SYNDROME.

**Jeune** [Mathis *Jeune*, French pediatrician, born 1910] Jeune syndrome. See under ASPHYXIATING THORACIC DYSTROPHY.

**Jewett** [Eugene Lyon *Jewett*, U.S. surgeon, born 1900] See under OPERATION, NAIL.

**jigger** CHIGOE.

**jitter** Small, rapid irregularities in echo location on an ultrasound display due to electronic noise, mechanical disturbances, and other variables.

**JNA** Jena Nomina Anatomica.

**Jobert de Lamballe** [Antoine Joseph *Jobert de Lamballe*, French surgeon, 1799–1867] Jobert's fossa. See under FOSSA.

**Jobling** [James Wesley *Jobling*, U.S. pathologist, 1876–1961] Flexner-Jobling carcinosarcoma. See under CARCINOSARCOMA.

**Johansson** [Sven Christian *Johansson*, Swedish surgeon, born 1880] Sinding-Larsen-Johansson disease. See under LARSEN-JOHANSSON DISEASE.

**Johne** [Heinrich Albert *Johne*, German veterinarian, 1839–1910] Johne's bacillus. See under *MYCOBACTERIUM PARATUBERCULOSIS*.

**Johnson** [Frank B. *Johnson*, U.S. pathologist, born 1919] Dubin-Johnson syndrome. See under SYNDROME.

**Johnson** [Frank Chambliss *Johnson*, U.S. pediatrician, 1894–1934] Stevens-Johnson disease. See under STEVENS-JOHNSON SYNDROME.

**Johnson** [Treat Baldwin *Johnson*, U.S. chemist, 1875–1947] Wheeler and Johnson test. See under TEST.

# joint

**joint** [Old French *joint* (from L *junct(us)*, past part. of *jungere* to join, unite) a joining of two things] ARTICULATIO. **acromioclavicular j.** ARTICULATIO ACROMIOCLAVICULARIS. **amphidiarthrodial j.** AMPHIDIARTHROSIS. **ankle j.** ARTICULATIO TALOCRURALIS. **anterior talocalcanean j.** ARTICULATIO TALOCALCANEONAVICULARIS. **arthrodial j.** ARTICULATIO PLANA. **arycorniculate j.** The cartilaginous, sometimes synovial, joint between the apex of each arytenoid cartilage and the corresponding corniculate cartilage. **atlantoaxial j.** Either articulatio atlantoaxialis lateralis or articulatio atlantoaxialis mediana. **atlanto-occipital j.** ARTICULATIO ATLANTO-OCCIPITALIS. **ball-and-socket**

**j.** ARTICULATIO SPHEROIDEA. **biaxial j.** A variety of joint that permits totally independent movements around two axes at right angles to each other and possesses two degrees of freedom, such as condyloid and saddle-shaped joints. **bilocular j.** A variety of synovial joint in which the intra-articular disk divides the joint into two distinct cavities, such as the temporomandibular joint. **Budin's j.** SYNCHONDROSIS INTRAOCCIPITALIS POSTERIOR. **calcaneocuboid j.** ARTICULATIO CALCANEOCUBOIDEA. **capitular j.** ARTICULATIO CAPITIS COSTAE. **carpometacarpal j.'s** ARTICULATIONES CARPOMETACARPALES. **cartilaginous j.** ARTICULATIO CARTILAGINEA. **Charcot's j.** NEUROGENIC ARTHROPATHY. **Chopart's j.** ARTICULATIO TARSI TRANSVERSA. **Clutton's j.** Painless joint effusions seen in congenital syphilis. **coccygeal j.** ARTICULATIO SACROCOCCYGEA. **cochlear j.** A hinge joint that also allows some rotation or lateral deviation because the cylindrical axis of the condyle tends to be spiral in section rather than a simple arc of a circle. Also *cochlear articulation.* **composite j.** ARTICULATIO COMPOSITA. **compound j.** ARTICULATIO COMPOSITA. **condylar j.** ARTICULATIO BICONDYLARIS. **condyloid j.** *Imprecise* ARTICULATIO BICONDYLARIS. **costochondral j.'s** ARTICULATIONES COSTOCHONDRALES. **costotransverse j.** ARTICULATIO COSTOTRANSVERSARIA. **costovertebral j.'s** ARTICULATIONES COSTOVERTEBRALES. **cotyloid j.** Either articulatio spheroidea or articulatio coxae. The latter use is outmoded. **cricoarytenoid j.** ARTICULATIO CRICOARYTENOIDEA. **cricothyroid j.** ARTICULATIO CRICOTHYROIDEA. **Cruveilhier's j.** 1 ARTICULATIO ATLANTOAXIALIS MEDIANA. 2 ARTICULATIO ATLANTO-OCCIPITALIS. **cubital j.** ARTICULATIO CUBITI. **cuboideonavicular j.** A fibrous joint connecting the navicular and cuboid bones by dorsal, plantar, and interosseous ligaments, the movements being limited to gliding. **cuneocuboid j.** ARTICULATIO CUNEOCUBOIDEA. **cuneometatarsal j.'s** ARTICULATIONES TARSOMETATARSALES. **cuneonavicular j.** ARTICULATIO CUNEONAVICULARIS. **diarthrodial j.** ARTICULATIO SYNOVIALIS. **dry j.** 1 A joint lacking normal synovial fluid. 2 In chronic arthritis, a joint characterized predominantly by fibrosis rather than proliferative synovitis with joint effusion. **elbow j.** ARTICULATIO CUBITI. **ellipsoidal j.** ARTICULATIO ELLIPSOIDEA. **enarthrodial j.** ARTICULATIO SPHEROIDEA. **false j.** PSEUDARTHROSIS. **femoropatellar j.** That portion of the knee joint in which the articular facets on the posterior surface of the patella articulate with the patellar surface of the femur, sharing the same articular cavity with the tibiofemoral portion. Also *patellofemoral articulation.* **femorotibial j.** That portion of the knee joint in which the two condyles of the femur articulate with the superior articular surface of the tibia, sharing the same articular cavity with the femoropatellar portion. **fibrocartilaginous j.** SYMPHYSIS. **flail j.** A joint in which there is pathological mobility and instability that is caused by a loss of motor power in the surrounding muscles. **freely movable j.** ARTICULATIO SYNOVIALIS. **ginglymoid j.** GINGLYMUS. **gliding j.** ARTICULATIO PLANA. **hemophilic j.** Painful hemarthrosis progressing to degenerative changes and limited motion, characteristic of inadequately treated hemophilias. **hinge j.** GINGLYMUS. **hip j.** ARTICULATIO COXAE. **humeroradial j.** ARTICULATIO HUMERORADIALIS. **humeroulnar j.** ARTICULATIO HUMEROULNARIS. **immovable j.** ARTICULATIO FIBROSA. **incudomalleolar j.** ARTICULATIO INCUDOMALLEARIS. **incudostapedial j.** ARTICULATIO INCUDOSTAPEDIA. **inferior radioulnar j.** ARTICULATIO RADIOULNARIS DISTALIS. **inferior sternal j.** SYNCHONDROSIS XIPHOSTERNALIS. **inferior tibiofibular j.** SYNDESMOSIS TIBIOFIBULARIS. **interarticular j.'s** ARTICULATIONES ZYGAPOPHYSIALES. **intercarpal j.'s** ARTICULATIONES INTERCARPALES. **interchondral j.'s** ARTICULATIONES INTERCHONDRALES. **intercuneiform j.'s** ARTICULATIONES INTERCUNEIFORMES. **intermetacarpal j.'s** ARTICULATIONES INTERMETACARPALES. **interphalangeal j.'s** Either articulationes interphalangeales manus or articulationes interphalangeales pedis. **jaw j.** ARTICULATIO TEMPOROMANDIBULARIS. **knee j.** ARTICULATIO GENUS. **ligamentous j.** SYNDESMOSIS. **Lisfranc's j.'s** ARTICULATIONES TARSOMETATARSALES. **lumbosacral j.** ARTICULATIO LUMBOSACRALIS. **j.'s of Luschka** A series of small synovial joints between the raised bony lips on the lateral sides of the bodies of contiguous cervical vertebrae, i.e., between the lips on the lower surface of one vertebra and those on the upper surface of the subjacent vertebra. They develop in childhood at the age of about ten years. Medial to each is the intervertebral disk and laterally is a capsular ligament. Some authorities believe that they are not synovial joints but merely clefts in the intervertebral disks. **mandibular j.** ARTICULATIO TEMPOROMANDIBULARIS. **manubriosternal j.** SYNCHONDROSIS MANUBRIOSTERNALIS. **mediocarpal j.** ARTICULATIO MEDIOCARPALIS. **metacarpophalangeal j.'s** ARTICULATIONES METACARPOPHALANGEALES. **metatarsophalangeal j.'s** ARTICULATIONES METATARSOPHALANGEALES. **midcarpal j.** ARTICULATIO MEDIOCARPALIS. **midtarsal j.** ARTICULATIO TARSI TRANSVERSA. **mixed j.** A type of joint in which characteristics of different varieties of joints are found. **mortise j.** ARTICULATIO TALOCRURALIS. **movable j.** Articulatio synovialis, or, to a lesser extent, articulatio cartilaginea. **multiaxial j.** ARTICULATIO SPHEROIDEA. **peg-and-socket j.** GOMPHOSIS. **pisotriquetral j.** ARTICULATIO OSSIS PISIFORMIS. **pivot j.** ARTICULATIO TROCHOIDEA. **plane j.** ARTICULATIO PLANA. **polyaxial j.** ARTICULATIO SPHEROIDEA. **posterior talocalcanean j.** ARTICULATIO SUBTALARIS. **radiocarpal j.** ARTICULATIO RADIOCARPALIS. **rotary j.** ARTICULATIO TROCHOIDEA. **sacrococcygeal j.** ARTICULATIO SACROCOCCYGEA. **sacroiliac j.** ARTICULATIO SACROILIACA. **saddle j.** ARTICULATIO SELLARIS. **saddle-shaped j.** ARTICULATIO SELLARIS. **sellar j.** ARTICULATIO SELLARIS. **shoulder j.** ARTICULATIO HUMERI. **simple j.** ARTICULATIO SIMPLEX. **skin j.** FLEXURE LINE. **slightly movable j.** ARTICULATIO CARTILAGINEA. **slip j.** A connector fitted into the proximal end of an endotracheal tube for attachment to a breathing circuit. **socket j. of tooth** GOMPHOSIS. **spheno-occipital j.** SYNCHONDROSIS SPHENO-OCCIPITALIS. **spheroidal j.** ARTICULATIO SPHEROIDEA. **sternoclavicular j.** ARTICULATIO STERNOCLAVICULARIS. **sternocostal j.'s** ARTICULATIONES STERNOCOSTALES. **subtalar j.** ARTICULATIO SUBTALARIS. **superior radioulnar j.** ARTICULATIO RADIOULNARIS PROXIMALIS. **superior sternal j.** SYNCHONDROSIS MANUBRIOSTERNALIS. **superior tibiofibular j.** ARTICULATIO TIBIOFIBULARIS. **suture j.** SUTURA. **synovial j.** ARTICULATIO SYNOVIALIS. **talocalcaneal j.** Either the posteroinferior part of the articulatio talocalcaneonavicularis or the articulatio subtalaris. **talocalcaneonavicular j.** ARTICULATIO TALOCALCANEONAVICULARIS. **talocrural j.** ARTICULATIO TALOCRURALIS. **talonavicular j.** The portion of the talocalcaneonavicular joint that combines with the calcaneocuboid articulation to form the transverse

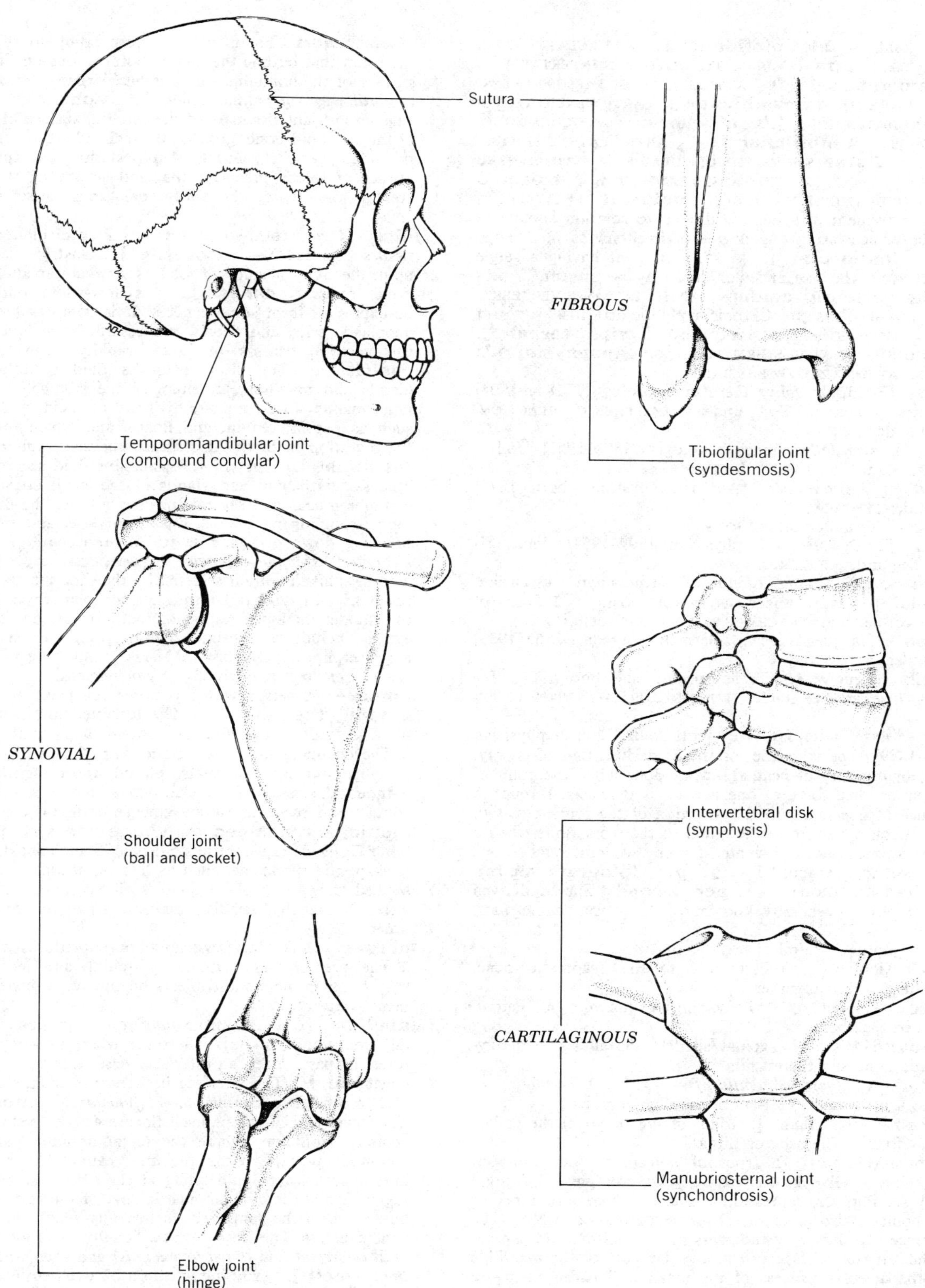
Sutura
FIBROUS
Temporomandibular joint
(compound condylar)
Tibiofibular joint
(syndesmosis)
SYNOVIAL
Intervertebral disk
(symphysis)
Shoulder joint
(ball and socket)
CARTILAGINOUS
Manubriosternal joint
(synchondrosis)
Elbow joint
(hinge)

**Joints**

tarsal joint. **talotibiofibular j.** ARTICULATIO TALOCRURALIS. **tarsal j.'s** ARTICULATIONES INTERTARSEAE. **tarsometatarsal j.'s** ARTICULATIONES TARSOMETATARSALES. **temporomandibular j.** ARTICULATIO TEMPOROMANDIBULARIS. **j.'s of thorax** ARTICULATIONES THORACIS. **tibiofibular j.** 1 ARTICULATIO TIBIOFIBULARIS. 2 SYNDESMOSIS TIBIOFIBULARIS. **transverse tarsal j.** ARTICULATIO TARSI TRANSVERSA. **trochoid j.** ARTICULATIO TROCHOIDEA. **uniaxial j.** A joint in which movement of a bone is limited to rotation about one axis only, possessing one degree of freedom, as in a hinge joint. **unilocular j.** A synovial joint having a single cavity, even when an articular disk may be present. **j.'s of the vertebral column** ARTICULATIONES VERTEBRALES. **von Gies j.** Chronic syphilitic arthritis. **wrist j.** ARTICULATIO RADIOCARPALIS. **xiphisternal j.** SYNCHONDROSIS XIPHOSTERNALIS. **zygapophysial j.'s** ARTICULATIONES ZYGAPOPHYSIALES.

**Jolly** [Friedrich *Jolly,* German neurologist, 1844–1904] 1 Jolly's reaction. See under MYASTHENIC REACTION. 2 See under SIGN.

**Jolly** [Justin *Jolly,* French histologist, 1870–1953] Jolly's bodies. See under HOWELL-JOLLY BODIES.

**Jonas** [Siegfried *Jonas,* Austrian physician, born 1874] See under SYMPTOM.

**Jones** See under BENCE JONES.

**Jones** [T. D. *Jones,* U.S. physician, 1899–1954] Jones criteria. See under CRITERION.

**Jonnesco** [Thoma *Jonnesco,* Rumanian physician, 1860–1926] 1 See under OPERATION, FOSSA. 2 Fossa of Jonnesco. See under RECESSUS DUODENALIS SUPERIOR.

**Joseph** [Jacques *Joseph,* German surgeon, 1865–1934] See under OPERATION.

**Joseph** [Rene *Joseph,* French pediatrician, born 1907] Joseph's disease. See under ENCEPHALOPATHY WITH PROLINEMIA.

**joule** \jool\ [after James Prescott *Joule,* English physicist, 1818–1889] Special name for the SI derived unit of energy, work, or quantity of heat; the work done when the point of application of a force of one newton is displaced through a distance of one meter in the direction of the force; equal to one newton meter. It is also equal to the work done when a power of one watt is dissipated for one second; equal to one watt second. Symbol: J **j. per kilogram-second** WATT PER KILOGRAM. **j. per second** The SI derived unit of power, generally known by the special name watt. Symbol: J/s, $J{\cdot}s^{-1}$

**juga** \joo′gə\ Plural of JUGUM.

**jugal** \joo′gəl\ 1 Pertaining to the zygomatic bone. 2 Uniting; yoked together.

**jugate** \joo′gāt\ 1 Possessing a jugum. 2 Paired. 3 Joined together.

**jugomaxillary** \joo′gōmak′siler′ē\ Pertaining to the zygomatic bone and the maxilla.

**jugular** \jug′yələr\ [*jugul(um)* + -AR] 1 Pertaining to the neck or throat. 2 Any of the jugular veins.

**jugulum** \joo′gələm\ [L (dim. of *jugum* yoke) the collarbone, throat] The neck or throat.

**jugum** \joo′gəm\ [L (root of *jungere* to join, connect, yoke, akin to Gk *zygon* a yoke) a yoke, crosspiece] (*pl.* juga) [NA] A ridge or depression connecting two structures or two points. Also *yoke.* **juga alveolaria** [NA] The eminences produced by the roots of the incisors and canines on the anterior surface of the alveolar part of the mandible and the alveolar process of the maxilla. Between them are depressions corresponding to the interalveolar septa. Also *alveolar eminences, alveolar yokes.* **juga cerebralia ossium cranii** Faint ridges corresponding to the sulci of the brain that outline the digitate impressions on the internal surface of the cranium. Also *cerebral ridges of cranial bones, cerebral crests of cranial bones.* **j. sphenoidale** [NA] The smooth anterior part of the cerebral surface of the body of the sphenoid bone, grooved on each side of the midline by the olfactory tracts and limited posteriorly by the anterior border of sulcus prechiasmatis, and separating the anterior cranial fossa from the sphenoidal sinus. Also *sphenoidal yoke.*

**juice** [L *jus* broth, soup] 1 Any fluid of plant or animal tissues. 2 SUCCUS. **appetite j.** Gastric juice secreted upon the sight or smell of food as a vagally mediated conditioned reflex. **cancer j.** A yellow-white fluid that can be expressed from some cancers. It is comprised of plasma, neoplastic cells, and debris, and results from liquefaction of the necrotic centers of large, rapidly growing tumors. **gastric j.** The clear, colorless fluid secretion of the glands and mucosal epithelium of the stomach which contains mainly water, mucus, hydrochloric acid, and enzymes, such as pepsin, rennin, and lipase, and which functions in the digestion of food. Also *succus gastricus, liquor gastricus.* **intestinal j.** The colorless, alkaline fluid secretion of the mucosal epithelium and glands of the small intestine which contains mucus and several enzymes used in the digestion of food, including peptidases, lipase, amylase, and enzymes for breaking down disaccharides to monosaccharides. Also *succus entericus, liquor entericus.* **pancreatic j.** The clear, colorless, alkaline fluid secreted by the exocrine glands of the pancreas and discharged through the pancreatic ducts into the duodenum for digestion of food. It contains several enzymes including trypsin, chymotrypsin, carboxypeptidase, amylase, lipase, DNAase, RNAase, and phospholipase A. Also *succus pancreaticus, liquor pancreaticus.*

**jumper** A person with myoclonic epilepsy.

**jumping the bite** 1 The forcible movement forward of a retruded mandible to obtain a normal occlusion. 2 The changing of cuspal relationships in centric occlusion, as when moving a lingually placed upper incisor buccally without disoccluding it, causing a temporary premature contact and occlusion of convenience until it is in place.

**jumping Frenchmen of Maine** A syndrome resembling Gilles de la Tourette syndrome. Some consider it a culture-specific syndrome, such as lata, as it was originally described in a group of inhabitants of the state of Maine who were of French Canadian descent. Also *jumper disease of Maine.*

**jumps** 1 Jerking, twitching, or choreiform movements. 2 The premonitory muscular twitching and jerking which may occur in alcoholic subjects on the verge of delirium tremens. *Imprecise.*

**junction** [L *junctio* (from *jungere* to join, connect) a joining, connection, union] The place where two organs, structures, or parts meet; an interface. Also *junctura.* **amelodentinal j.** The interface between the enamel and dentin of a tooth. Also *dentinoenamel junction.* **anorectal j.** The lower end of the perineal flexure at the level of the urogenital diaphragm, where the rectal ampulla narrows and continues posteriorly as the anal canal. The puborectalis muscle forms a palpable sling at the sides and back of this region, while the circular muscle coat of the rectum thickens here to form the sphincter ani internus which surrounds the anal canal. • This term is occasionally used synonymously with *anorectal line (linea anorectalis)* and even with *pectinate line.* **cell j.** Any modification of a cell surface that provides cohesion between adjacent cells. **cementodentinal j.** The interface between the cementum and dentin of a tooth. Also *dentinocemental junction.* **cemento-enamel j.** The boundary between the cementum and enamel of a tooth. In animals which do not have coronal cementum, it forms the cervical line demarcating the anatomical crown from the root. **cervicomedullary j.** That part of the neuraxis where the cervical spinal cord becomes medulla oblongata; the zone of transition between the rostral part of the spinal cord and the caudal part of the brainstem. **choledochoduodenal j.** The site, just below the middle of the descending part of the duodenum, where the bile and the main pancreatic ducts join to form the hepatopancreatic ampulla before it narrows to open on the major duodenal papilla. However, the ducts may open separately on the papilla. **dentinocemental j.** CEMENTODENTINAL JUNCTION. **dentinoenamel j.** AMELODENTINAL JUNCTION. **dermoepidermal j.** The interdigitating interface between the epidermis and the papillary layer of the corium, or dermis, where the perpendicular papillae fit into corresponding pits on the deep surface of the epidermis. Also *dermoepidermal interface.* **esophagogastric j.** The interface, about 2.5 cm below the diaphragm, where the abdominal part of the esophagus becomes confluent with the stomach, marked internally by an abrupt transition from the stratified squamous epithelium of the esophagus to the simple columnar epithelium of the stomach, and externally, on the left, by the cardiac notch. Internally the junction is visible as a notched line, the esophagus being smooth and pinkish-gray in comparison with the pitted, honeycomblike, red gastric mucosa. **fibromuscular j.** The site of the blending of the thick smooth muscle layer of the wall of the body of the uterus with the dense fibrous tissue of the cervix uteri. **gap j.** A type of intercellular junction which allows communication between cells by affording passage to small molecules and ions. At gap junctions the space between plasma membranes of adjacent cells is about 30 Å, and cylinders with an inside diameter of 20 Å run as a pipeline between the cytoplasm of the two cells. The cylinders are each composed of 12 protein subunits, six associated with each plasma membrane. Also *nexus.* **intermediate j.** ZONULA ADHERENS. **intermembrane j.** ZONE OF ADHESION. **iridociliary j.** MARGO CILIARIS IRIDIS. **j. of the lips** 1 COMMISSURA LABIORUM ORIS. 2 ANGULUS ORIS. **mucocutaneous j.** The site where the skin becomes confluent with a mucous membrane, such as the lips of the mouth and the anus. **mucogingival j.** A scalloped linear boundary between the attached gingiva and the nonkeratinized lining mucosa of the sulcus. **myoneural j.** MOTOR ENDPLATE. **myotendinal j.** MUSCLE-TENDON ATTACHMENT. **neuromuscular j.** MOTOR ENDPLATE. **osseous j.** ARTICULATIO. **pentilaminar j.** TIGHT JUNCTION. **rectosigmoid j.** The site of union of the lower end of the sigmoid colon with the rectum which is situated in the median plane at the level of the third sacral vertebra. **root-cord j.** The site of junction of the spinal roots with the substance of the spinal cord. Also *cornuradicular zone.* **sclerocorneal j.** LIMBUS CORNEAE. **ST j.** J POINT. **tendinous j.'s** CONNEXUS INTERTENDINEUS. **tight j.** A region where the plasma membranes of two adjacent cells are closely apposed, preventing the movement of materials between the cells. When observed by electron microscopy, the outer dark layer of the plasma membranes of the adjacent cells form a common layer. The junction may be a zone around the cell (zonula occludens) or only a point (macula occludens). Also *pentilaminar junction.* **tympanostapedial j.** SYNDESMOSIS TYMPANOSTAPEDIA. **ureteropelvic j.** The site at which the renal pelvis becomes continuous with the ureter, often marked by a slight constriction outside the hilum. **ureterovesical j.** The site of the oblique passage of the ureter through the wall of the urinary bladder, into which it opens by a slitlike ostium. Also *ureterotrigonal complex.*

**junctura** \jungktyoo′rə\ [L (from *jungere* to join, connect + *-ura* -URE) a joining, uniting, joint, seam] (*pl.* juncturae) 1 [NA] JUNCTION. 2 *Outmoded* ARTICULATIO. **j. cartilaginea** ARTICULATIO CARTILAGINEA. **juncturae cinguli membri inferioris** ARTICULATIONES CINGULI MEMBRI INFERIORIS. **juncturae cinguli membri superioris** ARTICULATIONES CINGULI MEMBRI SUPERIORIS. **j. fibrosa** ARTICULATIO FIBROSA. **j. lumbosacralis** ARTICULATIO LUMBOSACRALIS. **j. ossium** ARTICULATIO. **juncturae ossium** Articulations; joints. **j. sacrococcygea** ARTICULATIO SACROCOCCYGEA. **j. synovialis** ARTICULATIO SYNOVIALIS. **juncturae tendinum** CONNEXUS INTERTENDINEUS. **juncturae zygapophyseales** ARTICULATIONES ZYGAPOPHYSIALES.

**juncturae** \jungktyoo′rē\ Plural of JUNCTURA.

**Jung** [Karl Gustav *Jung*, Swiss anatomist, 1793–1864] Jung's muscle. See under MUSCULUS PYRAMIDALIS AURICULAE.

**jungian** \yUng′ē·ən\ [Carl Gustav *Jung*, Swiss psychologist and psychiatrist, 1875–1961] Pertaining to the theories proposed by or associated with Carl Jung.

**juniper** \joo′nipər\ The dried, ripe fruit of the evergreen shrub *Juniperus communis* of the Coniferae family. An infusion of the berries is diuretic. Its volatile oil is used as a diuretic, urinary antiseptic, and carminative.

**Junius** [Paul *Junius*, German ophthalmologist, born 1871] Kuhnt-Junius disease, Kuhnt-Junius degeneration. See under DISCIFORM MACULAR DEGENERATION.

**jurisprudence** \joo′risproo′dəns\ The science of law, or a particular system or division of law. **dental j.** FORENSIC DENTISTRY. **medical j.** 1 The philosophy, principles, doctrines, and statutes of law and justice as they apply to and govern various aspects of medical practice, particularly the relationships between patients and medical practitioners as well as the relationship of medical practitioners to each other. 2 FORENSIC MEDICINE.

**jury** / **coroner's j.** A jury that inquires into the cause and manner of sudden, unusual, unattended, or violent deaths to determine whether unlawful activity was involved in the death and, if so, to issue appropriate indictments. It is assembled at the request of a coroner. Also *inquest jury.*

**Juster** [Emile *Juster*, French neurologist, flourished 20th century] See under REFLEX.

**justo major** \jus′tō mā′jər\ [L (from *justo,* ablative of *justum* what is right + *major* larger), larger than right] GIANT PELVIS.

**justo minor** \jus′tō mī′nər\ [L (from *justo,* ablative of *justum* what is right + *minor* less, smaller), smaller than is right] PELVIS JUSTO MINOR.

**juvenile** [L *juvenil(is)* (from *junven(is)* young, young man, young people + *ilis* -ILE) youthful, juvenile] 1 Of or relating to youth or to an early period of development. 2 A juvenile specimen or individual.

**juxta-articular** \juks′tə-ärtik′yələr\ Near or adjacent to a joint.

**juxtacortical** \juks′təkôr′dikəl\ Near or adjacent to the cortex of an organ or a structure.

**juxtaglomerular** \juks′təglōmer′ʸələr\ Near or adjacent to a renal glomerulus.

**juxtallocortex** \juks′talōkôr′teks\ [L *juxt(a)* next to + ALLOCORTEX] The cerebral cortex transitional between typical allocortex and isocortex.

**juxtapapillary** \juks′təpap′iler′ē\ [L *juxta* + *papill(a)* + -ARY] Adjacent to the optic disk.
**juxtaposition** \juks′təpəzish′ən\ A side by side position; apposition.
**juxtapyloric** \juks′təpīlôr′ik\ Near or adjacent to the pylorus or the pyloric portion of the stomach.
**juxtaspinal** \juks′təspī′nəl\ Near or adjacent to the vertebral column.

# K

**K** 1 Symbol for the element, potassium. 2 Symbol for the unit, kelvin. 3 Symbol for lysine.
**K.** cathode.
**k** Symbol for kilo-: used with SI units.
$K_m$ Symbol for the quantity, Michaelis constant.
$\kappa$ Symbol for the quantity, magnetic susceptibility.
**Kaes** [Theodor *Kaes*, German neurologist, 1852–1913] Band of Kaes-Bekhterev, Kaes feltwork, line of Kaes, layer of Kaes-Bekhterev, stripe of Kaes-Bekhterev. See under BEKHTEREV'S LAYER.
**kafindo** \käfin′dō\ ONYALAI.
**Kahlbaum** [Karl Ludwig *Kahlbaum*, German physician, 1828–1899] 1 Kahlbaum syndrome, Kahlbaum's disease. See under CATATONIC STUPOR. 2 Kahlbaum-Wernicke syndrome. See under PRESBYOPHRENIA.
**Kahler** [Otto *Kahler*, German physician, 1849–1893] See under LAW.
**kaino-**[1] \kī′nō-\ CENO-[1].
**kaino-**[2] \kī′nō-\ CENO-[2].
**kak-** \kak-\ CACO-.
**kakesthesia** \kak′esthē′zhə\ CACESTHESIA.
**kakidrosis** \kak′idrō′sis\ BROMHIDROSIS.
**kako-** \kak′ə-\ CACO-.
**kakosmia** \kakäz′mē·ə\ CACOSMIA.
**kala-azar** \kä′lə-äzär′\ [Hindi *kālā* black + *āzār* disease] An acute, infectious, systemic disease characterized by irregular fever of long duration, splenomegaly, hepatomegaly, hyperglobulinemia, and progressive emaciation. Leukopenia and anemia result from bone-marrow infiltration, and lymphadenopathy, malaise, and secondary infections are frequent accompaniments. If untreated, death may occur. The disease is caused by the protozoan parasite *Leishmania donovani* and transmitted by sandfly bites (*Phlebotomus* species and related genera). The organism lives and multiplies throughout the reticuloendothelial system. Kala-azar is widespread and occurs with local differences in India, Kenya, the Sudan, China, Brazil, and the USSR. Also *visceral leishmaniasis, Assam fever, Dumdum fever, febrile tropical splenomegaly, old world leishmaniasis, black sickness.* **Mediterranean k.** A variant of kala-azar which occurs on the Mediterranean littoral, especially in Greece and Portugal, and usually affects infants and children. It is caused by *Leishmania infantum* which is antigenically identical to *L. donovani*.. Also *infantile leishmaniasis.*
**kalafungin** An antibiotic from *Streptomyces tanashiensis* var. *kala*. It has antifungal properties.
**kaliopenic** \kal′ē·ōpē′nik\ [New L *kali(um)* potassium + *o* + *-pen(ia)* + -IC] Deficient in potassium.
**Kalischer** [Siegfried *Kalischer*, German physician, born 1862] Kalischer's disease, Sturge-Kalischer-Weber syndrome. See under STURGE-WEBER SYNDROME.
**kallidin** Either of two peptides, bradykinin and lysylbradykinin, released by the action of the enzyme kallikrein from a plasma protein. The 9-residue peptide bradykinin is sometimes known as kallidin-9 or kallidin I, whereas the 10-residue peptide lysyl-bradykinin is sometimes known as kallidin-10 or kallidin II.
**kallikrein** \kal′ikrē′in\ [Gk *kallikre(as)* pancreas, sweetbread (from *kall(os)* beautiful + *kreas* meat) + -IN] The enzyme (EC 3.4.21.8) that releases bradykinin or lysyl-bradykinin from the plasma protein kininogen. At least three types, characteristic of plasma, pancreas, and kidney, are physiologically important. They are proteinases with a preference for splitting on the C-terminal side of arginine and lysine residues. Also *kininogenase, callicrein.*
**kallikreinogen** \kal′əkrē′inəjən\ PREKALLIKREIN.
**Kallmann** [Franz Josef *Kallmann*, German-born U.S. geneticist and psychiatrist, 1897–1965] See under SYNDROME.
**kaluresis** \kal′ʸooré′sis\ [New L *kal(ium)* potassium + -URESIS] Increased urinary excretion of potassium secondary to hyperkalemia, adrenocortical hyperfunction, or administration of adrenocortical hormones or any of many diuretic agents. Also *hyperkaluria, kaluria.*
**kaluretic** \kal′ʸooret′ik\ 1 Pertaining to or causing kaluresis. 2 Any agent or condition that increases renal excretion of potassium.
**kaluria** \kal′ʸoo′rē·ə\ KALURESIS.
**Kammerer** [Frederic *Kammerer*, U.S. surgeon, 1856–1928] Battle-Jalaguier-Kammerer incision. See under BATTLE'S INCISION.
**kanamycin** \kan′əmī′sin\ $C_{18}H_{36}N_4O_{11}$. An antibiotic produced by *Streptomyces kanamyceticus* which is active against many Gram-positive and Gram-negative bacteria. Excessive or prolonged use may cause irreversible damage to the eighth cranial nerve. The sulfate salt has been most commonly used, but resistant organisms, hypersensitivity, and ototoxicity have limited its usefulness.
**Kanavel** [Allen Buckner *Kanavel*, U.S. surgeon, 1874–1938] 1 See under SIGN, TRIANGLE. 2 Lumbrical canals of Kanavel. See under CANAL. 3 Kanavel's cockup splint. See under SPLINT.
**Kandinsky** [Victor Chrisanfovic *Kandinsky*, Russian psychiatrist, 1825–1890] Clérambault-Kandinsky syndrome. See under CLÉRAMBAULT-KANDINSKY COMPLEX.
**Kandori** [Fumio *Kandori*, Japanese ophthalmologist, born 1904] Kandori's flock retina. See under RETINA.
**kaninloma** \kā′ninlō′mə\ GANGOSA.
**Kanner** [Leo *Kanner*, Austrian-born U.S. child psychiatrist, born 1894] Kanner syndrome. See under EARLY INFANTILE AUTISM.
**Kanter** [Aaron Elias *Kanter*, U.S. gynecologist, born 1893] See under SIGN.
**Kantor** [John Leonard *Kantor*, U.S. physician, 1890–1947] Kantor sign. See under STRING SIGN.
**kanyemba** \känyem′bə\ [native language of southern Africa] A severe necrotic inflammatory disorder of the colon and rectum seen in mountain regions of Malawi, Zambia, and South America.
**kaodzera** \kä′ōdzir′ə\ [Bantu] RHODESIAN TRYPANOSOMIASIS.
**kaolin** \kā′əlin\ [Chinese *gāolíngtǔ* Kao-ling earth, first

obtained from a hill called Gāolǐng (Kao-ling) (from *gāo* high + *lǐng* ridge) in Jiangxi (Kiangsi) province, China] $Al_2O_3 \cdot 2SiO_2 \cdot 2H_2O$. Hydrated aluminum silicate, found in natural deposits. It is used as an absorbent, in filters to clarify liquids, and as a constituent of dusting powders. Also *bolus alba, terra alba*.

**kaolinosis** \kā′ōlinō′sis\ Pneumoconiosis resulting from inhalation of kaolin dust.

**Kaposi** [Moritz *Kaposi*, Hungarian-born Austrian dermatologist, 1837–1902] **1** Kaposi's disease, multiple hemorrhagic hemangioma of Kaposi. See under KAPOSI SARCOMA. **2** Xeroderma of Kaposi. See under XERODERMA PIGMENTOSUM. **3** Kaposi's varicelliform eruption. See under ERUPTION.

**kaps-** \kaps-\ CAPS-.

**karakurt** \kä′rəkoort′\ [Turki, from *kara* black + *kurt* wolf] A spider of the species *Latrodectus lugubris*, a central Asian variant of the venomous black widow.

**karaya** \kär′äyä\ STERCULIA GUM.

**Karr** [Walter Gerald *Karr*, U.S. biochemist, born 1892] See under METHOD.

**Kartagener** [Manes *Kartagener*, Swiss physician, born 1897] Kartagener's triad. See under SYNDROME.

***Karyamoebina falcata*** \kär′ē·am′ēbī′nə falkā′tə\ *ENTAMOEBA HISTOLYTICA*.

**karyapsis** \kär′ē·ap′sis\ [*kary(o)-* + Ionic Gk *apsis* a juncture, knot, arch] The fusion of nuclei following cell conjugation.

**karyo-** \kar′ē·ō-\ [Gk *karyon* nut, kernel] A combining form meaning nucleus. Also *caryo-*.

**karyoclasis** \kar′e·äk′ləsis\ [KARYO- + -CLASIS] NUCLEORRHEXIS. Adj. karyoclastic.

**karyogamy** \kar′ē·äg′əmē\ [KARYO- + GAM- + -Y] The fusion of nuclei, the ultimate event of fertilization. The result of karyogamy is the reestablishment of the diploid number of chromosomes in the zygote. Adj. karyogamic.

**karyogonad** \-gō′nad\ [KARYO- + GONAD] MICRONUCLEUS.

**karyokinesis** \-kinē′sis\ [KARYO- + Gk *kinēsis* movement] Division of the cell nucleus by mitosis. Adj. karyokinetic. **asymmetric k.** A mitotic division in which the chromosome complement is unequally distributed to the two daughter cells. **hyperchromatic k.** A nuclear division in which the number of chromosomes involved is greater than the normal number. **hypochromatic k.** A nuclear division in which the number of chromosomes involved is lower than the normal number.

**karyolobic** \-lō′bik\ Having a lobate nucleus: said of a cell.

**karyolobism** \-lō′bizm\ The condition in which the cell nucleus has a number of lobes, as the nucleus of a neutrophil leukocyte.

**karyology** \kar′ē·äl′əjē\ The study of the cell nucleus, its organelles, structures, and functions. Also *nuclear cytology*.

**karyolymph** \kar′ē·əlimf′\ [KARYO- + LYMPH] The fluid content of the cell nucleus. Also *nuclear hyaloplasm, nuclear sap, nucleolymph*.

**karyolysis** \kar′ē·äl′isis\ [KARYO- + LYSIS] **1** Dissolution of the nucleus so that it no longer takes a basic stain. **2** The disappearance of the interphase nucleus during the early prophase of mitosis. Adj. karyolytic.

**karyomegaly** \-meg′əlē\ [KARYO- + -MEGALY] A slight, uniform increase in nuclear size in the cells of a tissue.

**karyomere** \kar′ē·əmir′\ [KARYO- + Gk *meros* a portion, part] Any of a series of small nuclei resulting when chromosomes which are widely spaced on the spindle diverge at anaphase. This condition occurs commonly during cleavage in some animal cells and can be induced chemically in others.

**karyometry** \kar′ē·äm′ətrē\ [KARYO- + -METRY] The measurement of the nuclei of cells.

**karyomitosis** \-mītō′sis\ MITOSIS.

**karyomitotic** \-mitāt′ik\ MITOTIC.

**karyon** \kar′ē·än\ [Gk, a kernel] The nucleus of a cell. Also *karyoplast*.

**karyonide** \kar′ē·ənīd′\ Any of the nuclei in a clone, all nuclei being derived from a single nucleus.

**karyophage** \kar′ē·əfāj′\ [KARYO- + -PHAGE] An intracellular protozoan parasite that feeds on the nucleus of the host cell.

**karyoplasm** \kar′ē·əplazm′\ NUCLEOPLASM.

**karyoplasmic** \-plaz′mik\ Pertaining to karyoplasm.

**karyoplast** \kar′ē·əplast′\ [KARYO- + -PLAST] KARYON.

**karyopyknosis** \-piknō′sis\ Shrinkage of nuclei and condensation of the chromatin into structureless masses, as in squamous epithelium when it forms cornified epithelium. Adj. karyopyknotic.

**karyorrhexis** \kar′ē·ôrek′sis\ [KARYO- + -RRHEXIS] NUCLEORRHEXIS. Adj. karyorrhectic.

**karyosome** \kar′ē·əsōm′\ [KARYO- + Gk *sōm(a)* body] A mass of aggregated chromatin material in an interphase nucleus. It is often confused with the nucleolus. Also *net knot, chromatin nucleolus, false nucleolus, pseudonucleolus, chromatin reservoir, chromocenter*.

**karyostasis** \kar′ē·äs′təsis\ [KARYO- + STASIS] The nondividing condition of the cell nucleus during interphase.

**karyotype** \kar′ē·ətīp′\ The particular chromosome complement of an individual as defined by the number, size, and centromere position of the chromosomes, usually in mitotic metaphase. See also IDIOGRAM. Adj. karyotypic.

**Kasabach** [Haig Haigouni *Kasabach*, U.S. physician, 1898–1943] Kasabach-Merritt syndrome. See under SYNDROME.

**Kasanin** [Jacob Sergi *Kasanin*, U.S. psychologist, 1897–1946] Hanfmann-Kasanin test. See under TEST.

**Kast** [Alfred *Kast*, German internist, 1856–1903] Kast syndrome. See under MAFFUCCI SYNDROME.

**Kastert** [Josef *Kastert*, German orthopedic surgeon, born 1910] Hoffa-Kastert disease. See under HOFFA'S DISEASE.

**kat-** \kat-\ CATA-.

**kata-** \kat′ə-\ CATA-.

**katabolism** \kətab′əlizm\ CATABOLISM.

**katal** The special name for the unit of catalytic activity equal to one mole per second. With reference to the concentration of enzymatic activity, a katal is the amount of enzyme that catalyzes the transformation of substrate at a rate of one mole per second. Symbol: kat **k. per liter** The unit of catalytic concentration or concentration of enzymatic activity. Symbol: kat/l, $kat \cdot l^{-1}$

**kataphylaxis** \-fīlak′sis\ CATAPHYLAXIS.

**Katayama** [Kunika *Katayama*, Japanese physician, 1856–1931] Katayama disease. See under KATAYAMA SYNDROME.

***Katayama*** \kä′təyä′mə\ *ONCOMELANIA*.

**kath-** \kath-\ CATA-.

**katine** $C_9H_{13}NO$. *d*-Norpseudoephedrine. An alkaloid isolated from *Catha edulis*. It has an effect on the central nervous system like that of cocaine, but no local anesthetic properties, and it has been used as an anorectic agent. The leaves (catha) are used for tea and chewed in several regions of Africa.

**kation** \kat′ī·ən\ CATION.

**Kato** [Kan *Kato*, Japanese scientist, born 1879] See under TEST.

**katolysis** \kətäl′isis\ [Gk *katō* below + LYSIS] A partial digestion or breakdown.

**kava** \kä′və\ **1** An intoxicating, addictive beverage prepared from the roots of *Piper methysticum.* **2** The dried roots and rhizome of *P. methysticum,* which contain kawain. Also *kava-kava, ava-kava, ava.*

**kavaism** \kä′və·izm\ A condition resulting from the abuse of kava, or ava, a beverage prepared from the dried rhizome and roots of *Piper methysticum* in Polynesia. Symptoms are muscular weakness and mental confusion, progressing to convulsions or paralysis.

**Kawasaki** [T. *Kawasaki,* Japanese pediatrician, flourished 20th century] Kawasaki disease. See under SYNDROME.

**Kayser** [Bernhard *Kayser,* German ophthalmologist, 1869–1954] **1** Kayser-Fleischer ring. See under RING. **2** Kayser's disease. See under WILSON'S DISEASE.

**Kazanjian** [Varaztad Hovhannes *Kazanjian,* Armenian-born U.S. otorhinolaryngologist, born 1879] Kazanjian procedure. See under RIDGE EXTENSION.

**KCT** kathodal (cathodal) closure tetanus.

**kDa** Symbol for kilodalton.

**KDO** ketodeoxyoctonate.

**Keating-Hart** [Walter-Valentin *Keating-Hart,* French physician, 1870–1922] See under TREATMENT.

**kedani** \kedä′nē\ [Japanese (from *ke* hair + *dani* tick, mite) hairy mite] A Japanese term for CHIGGER.

**Keeler** [Leonard *Keeler,* U.S. criminologist, 1903–1949] Keeler's lie polygraph. See under POLYGRAPH.

**Kehr** [Hans *Kehr,* German surgeon, 1862–1916]

**Kehrer** [Ferdinand Adalbert *Kehrer,* German physician, born 1883] **1** Kehrer-Adie syndrome. See under ADIE SYNDROME. **2** Kehrer's reflex. See under EXTERNAL AUDITORY MEATUS REFLEX.

**keel** / **McNaught k.** A small, flanged, metal plate inserted between the anterior parts of the vocal cords at the conclusion of certain laryngeal operations and removed only when it is judged that there is no longer a risk of cicatricial stenosis.

**Keeler** [Leonard *Keeler,* U.S. criminologist, 1903–1949] Keeler's lie polygraph. See under POLYGRAPH.

**Kehr** [Hans *Kehr,* German surgeon, 1862–1916] See under INCISION.

**Kehrer** [Ferdinand Adalbert *Kehrer,* German physician, born 1883] **1** Kehrer-Adie syndrome. See under ADIE SYNDROME. **2** Kehrer's reflex. See under EXTERNAL AUDITORY MEATUS REFLEX.

**Keith** [Sir Arthur *Keith,* Scottish anatomist, 1866–1955] Keith's node, sinuatrial node of Keith and Flack, Keith-Flack node, Keith's bundle. See under NODUS SINUATRIALIS.

**kelis** \kē′lis\ *Obs.* MORPHEA.

**Kellie** [George *Kellie,* Scottish anatomist, flourished late 18th century] Monro-Kellie doctrine. See under DOCTRINE.

**Kelly** See under BROWN KELLY.

**Kelly** [Howard Atwood *Kelly,* U.S. gynecologist, 1858–1943] See under OPERATION, SPECULUM.

**keloid** \kē′loid\ [French *kéloïde* (later *chéloïde*), from Gk *kēl(ē)* tumor, swelling or *chēl(ē)* claw, hoof + French *-oïde* -OID] A firm, scarlike nodule of the skin, composed of fibrous tissue with broad bands of homogeneous acidophilic collagen. It develops as a response to trauma that may be trivial and far exceeds the physiologic needs appropriate to the site and the degree of injury. It is usually found in heavily pigmented people, and, unlike a hyperplastic scar, it tends to recur. Also *cheloid.* **acne k.** A keloid that forms at the nape of the neck as a result of keloid acne. **Addison's k.** MORPHEA. **Alibert's k.** A keloid formed by the hypertrophy of a scar rather than as a response to trauma. Also *cicatricial keloid, false keloid.*

**kelotomy** \kēlät′əmē\ [Gk *kēl(ē)* a rupture, hernia + *o* + -TOMY] HERNIOTOMY.

**Kelvin** [William Thomson (Lord *Kelvin*), English physicist, 1824–1907] See under SCALE, THERMOMETER.

**kelvin** \kel′vən\ [after William Thomson, Lord *Kelvin,* British physicist, 1824–1907] **1** The SI base unit of thermodynamic temperature, defined as the fraction $^{1}/_{273.16}$ of the thermodynamic temperature of the triple point of water. Also *degree absolute, degree kelvin* (outmoded). Symbol: K **2** A unit of electrical energy equal to the kilowatt-hour. An obsolete unit.

**Kemadrin** A proprietary name for procyclidine hydrochloride.

**Kennedy** [Edward *Kennedy,* U.S. dentist, born 1883] **1** Kennedy bar. See under CONTINUOUS BAR RETAINER. **2** See under CLASSIFICATION.

**Kennedy** [Robert Foster *Kennedy,* U.S. neurologist, 1884–1952] Kennedy syndrome. See under FOSTER KENNEDY SYNDROME.

**Kenny** [Elizabeth *Kenny,* Australian nurse, 1886–1952] Kenny's treatment. See under METHOD.

**keno-** \kē′nō-\ CENO-[3].

**Kent** [Albert Frank Stanley *Kent,* English physiologist, 1863–1958] Kent's bundle, Kent-His bundle, bundle of Stanley Kent. See under FASCICULUS ATRIOVENTRICULARIS.

**Kepone** A proprietary name for chloredecone

**Keq** Symbol for equilibrium constant.

**Kerandel** [Jean François *Kerandel,* French physician, 1873–1934] Kerandel sign. See under SYMPTOM.

**kerat-** \kerət-\ KERATO-.

**keratectasia** \ker′ətektā′zhə\ [KERAT- + ECTASIA] A localized thinning and protrusion of the cornea; a forward bulging of part of the corneal curvature. Also *corneal ectasia.*

**keratectomy** \ker′ətek′təmē\ [KERAT- + -ECTOMY] Excision of a portion of the cornea. Also *ceratectomy.*

**keratic** \kerat′ik\ HORNY.

**keratin** \ker′ətin\ [KERAT- + -IN] A scleroprotein or albuminoid found in horny tissues such as hair, nails, feathers, and scales. Keratins are insoluble in water, in dilute acids, and in dilute alkalis, and are generally not digested by proteolytic enzymes. Keratins have a high sulfur content. The amino acids cystine and arginine generally predominate. Also *ceratin.* **false k.** PSEUDOKERATIN.

**keratinase** \ker′ətinās\ A keratin-hydrolyzing enzyme that catalyzes the breakdown of keratin.

**keratinization** \ker′ətin′īzā′shən\ The formation of keratin, as in the development of a horny layer of tissue. Also *cornification, hornification.*

**keratinocyte** \kerat′inōsīt′\ A cell of the epidermis that produces keratin.

**keratinoid** **1** Resembling keratin. **2** A pill or tablet having keratin as an enteric coating.

**keratitic** \ker′ətit′ik\ Pertaining to the cornea; corneal.

**keratitis** \ker′ətī′tis\ [KERAT- + -ITIS] Inflammation of the cornea. Also *ceratitis.* **actinic k.** Corneal epithelial damage from the ultraviolet rays of the sun. **k. arborescens** DENDRITIC KERATITIS. **band k.** BAND KERATOPATHY. **k. bandelette** BAND KERATOPATHY. **k. bullosa** A condition characterized by the formation of blebs and vesicles on the corneal epithelium. **deep k.** Inflammation of the posterior stromal and Descemet's layers of the cornea. Also *keratitis profunda.* **dendritic k.** Linear and branching corneal ulceration due to herpes simplex or herpes zoster. Also *dendriform keratitis, keratitis arborescens.* **Dimmer's k.** KERATITIS NUMMULARIS.

**disciform k.** Stromal scarring and infiltration from herpes. Also *keratitis disciformis.* **exfoliative k.** Loss of the corneal epithelium due to inflammation of the cornea. **exposure k.** EXPOSURE KERATOPATHY. **fascicular k.** Progressive, ulcerative corneal damage associated with localized vascularization. **k. filamentosa** Corneal irritation, usually from inadequate lubrication, that causes strands of epithelial cells to hang from the corneal surface. **herpetic k.** Corneal infection with herpes simplex or herpes zoster. **interstitial k.** Inflammation of the deep corneal stroma, often due to congenital syphilis. **lagophthalmic k.** EXPOSURE KERATOPATHY. **mycotic k.** Corneal infection with a fungus, commonly *Aspergillus, Fusarium,* or *Candida..* **necrogranulomatous k.** A severe corneal disorder in which focal infiltrates of inflammatory cells break down and ulcerate. **neuroparalytic k.** Corneal damage resulting from loss of sensitivity due to trigeminal nerve damage. Infrared lacrimation may be a contributing factor. Also *neurotrophic keratitis, neuropathic keratitis, neuroparalytic ophthalmia.* **k. nummularis** A mild inflammation of the cornea in which small superficial disk-shaped opacities exist. Also *Dimmer's keratitis.* **k. petrificans** Calcification of the corneal surface. **k. profunda** DEEP KERATITIS. **punctate k.** The presence of multiple small erosions of the corneal epithelium. Also *keratitis punctata, superficial punctate keratitis.* **k. ramificata superficialis** The loss of the superficial corneal epithelium resulting from exposure to tropical conditions. *Rare.* **sclerosing k.** Opacification of the cornea continuous with the white sclera, due to inflammation. **senile guttate k.** Endothelial dystrophy, with Hassall-Henle bodies on Descemet's membrane. **serpiginous k.** A chronic, ulcerative corneal inflammation occurring in older persons. **k. sicca** Corneal damage secondary to deficient lacrimal secretion. **superficial punctate k.** PUNCTATE KERATITIS. **vascular k.** Keratitis characterized by the invasion of blood vessels in the cornea. **vesicular k.** Keratitis characterized by the presence of multiple, localized, fluid spaces between the corneal epithelium and Bowman's membrane. **xerotic k.** Corneal damage due to pathologic dryness, as in vitamin A deficiency. **zonular k.** BAND KERATOPATHY.

**kerato-** \ker′ətō-\ [Gk *keras,* combining stem *kerat(o)-* horn; *kerato(eides chitōn)* horny coat of the eye, cornea] A combining form denoting (1) the cornea; (2) horny tissue; (3) a horn or hornlike structure. Also *kerat-, cerat-, cerato-.*

**keratoacanthoma** \-ak′anthō′mə\ [KERATO- + ACANTHOMA] A rapidly growing benign squamous cell, tumorlike lesion occurring predominantly in exposed skin and forming a nodule with a central crater filled with keratin. It occurs especially in individuals exposed to sunlight, tar, and other environmental carcinogens. The crateriform nodule enlarges for 3–4 weeks after which it decreases in size and is eventually shed, to be followed by a distinctive scar. This spontaneous recovery takes place in the vast majority of keratoacanthomas, but occasional transformation to squamous cell carcinoma occurs, notably with lesions of the pinna and lower lip and more particularly in the very elderly. Also *Ackerman's tumor.*

**keratoangioma** \-an′jē·ō′mə\ ANGIOKERATOMA.

**keratocele** \ker′ətōsēl′\ [KERATO- + -CELE[1]] DESCEMETOCELE.

**keratocentesis** \-sentē′sis\ [KERATO- + CENTESIS] Surgical puncture of the cornea for diagnostic aspiration of aqueous from the anterior chamber.

**keratoconjunctivitis** \-kənjunk′tivī′tis\ [KERATO- + CONJUNCTIVITIS] Inflammation of both the cornea and conjunctiva. **epidemic k.** An acute infectious conjunctivitis usually caused by adenovirus types 8 and 19 and characterized by scanty exudate and development of corneal subepithelial infiltrations 7–10 days after the onset of inflammation. Epidemic outbreaks have occurred, with one of the first large-scale epidemics involving shipyard workers. Also *shipyard keratoconjunctivitis, shipyard eye, shipyard conjunctivitis, Sander's disease.* **flash k.** Irritation of the cornea and conjunctiva by ultraviolet radiation from welding, particularly electric-arc welding. **phlyctenular k.** Superficial sector allergic response of the cornea and conjunctiva. Also *phlyctenular ophthalmia.* **shipyard k.** EPIDEMIC KERATOCONJUNCTIVITIS. **k. sicca** XEROPHTHALMIA. **superior limbic k.** Inflammation of the superior cornea and adjacent conjunctiva of unknown etiology. **vernal k.** An allergic response of the conjunctiva and cornea occurring primarily in children, with a tendency to be more severe in the spring. It is characterized by giant papillary formation on the palpebral conjunctiva. Also *spring ophthalmia.* **viral k.** Any keratoconjunctivitis caused by adenoviruses or other viruses. The epidemic form is usually caused by adenoviruses types 1–3, 7–9, and 19.

**keratoconus** \-kō′nəs\ [KERATO- + L *conus* a cone] A dystrophy in which the central cornea becomes thin and ectatic, to form a symmetrical, conical protrusion. Also *conical cornea, sugar-loaf cornea.* **congenital k.** A developmental anomaly of corneal curvature in which the central cornea is thinned and conical in shape.

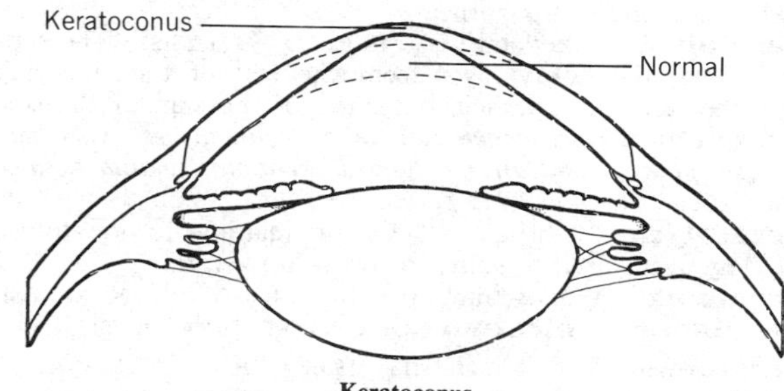


**Keratoconus**

**keratocricoid** \-krī′koid\ CERATOCRICOID.

**keratocyst** \ker′ətōsist′\ [KERATO- + CYST] A dental cyst lined by keratinizing epithelium. The probable origin is from the dental lamina and there is a risk of recurrence unless enucleation is thorough.

**keratocyte** \ker′ətōsīt′\ **1** An abnormally shaped erythrocyte that has two hornlike projections on the same side. Keratocytes may be found in blood films from persons who have been exposed to drugs or toxins that cause oxidative injury to erythrocytes, such as dapsone. Also *bite cell.* **2** A stromal cell of the cornea.

**keratoderma** \-dur′mə\ [KERATO- + -DERMA] The thickening of the horny layer of the epidermis. Also *keratodermia.* **k. blennorrhagicum** The distinctive warty lesions of the skin that are symptomatic of the Reiter syndrome, occurring typically on the soles of the feet and the nail beds and palms of the hand, and often elsewhere. Also *keratosis blennhorrhagica.* **k. climactericum** A circumscribed palmoplantar keratoderma that occurs among women of middle age. It has been ascribed without evidence to menopausal hormonal changes. **palmar k.** An in-TEST.

creased thickness in the palmar skin. It may be diffuse, striated, or papular, or it may be confined to areas of pressure. Also *ichthyosis palmaris.* **palmoplantar k.** A thickening of the horny layer of the palms and soles. Also *symmetric keratoderma, Jadassohn-Lewandowsky syndrome.* **plantar k.** Increased thickness of the plantar skin. The increase may be diffuse, striate, or papular, or confined to areas of pressure. Also *ichthyosis plantaris.* **punctate k.** A form of hereditary palmoplantar keratoderma in which the lesions are circumscribed keratoses. Also *keratosis punctata.* **symmetric k.** PALMOPLANTAR KERATODERMA.

**keratodermatocele** \-dərmat′əsēl\ [KERATO- + DERMATOCELE] DESCEMETOCELE.

**keratodermia** \-dur′mē·ə\ KERATODERMA. **k. plantaris sulcata** PITTED KERATOLYSIS.

**keratoectasia** \-ektā′zhə\ [KERATO- + ECTASIA] A forward bulging of thinned cornea without the iris being adherent posteriorly.

**keratogenesis** \-jen′əsis\ The formation of keratin.

**keratoglobus** \-glō′bəs\ [KERATO- + GLOBUS] MEGALOCORNEA.

**keratohyal** \-hī′əl\ CERATOHYAL.

**keratohyalin** \-hī′əlin\ The hyaline material found in the granular layer of the epidermis.

**keratoid** \ker′ətoid\ [Gk *keratoeidēs* (from *kera(s)* horn; see KERATO-) horny, hornlike] **1** Horny or scaly. **2** Resembling or pertaining to the cornea.

**keratoiridoscope** \-īrid′əskōp\ BIOMICROSCOPE.

**keratoleukoma** \-lookō′mə\ [KERATO- + LEUKOMA] A white scarring of the cornea.

**keratolysis** \ker′ətäl′isis\ [KERATO- + LYSIS] The separation of the horny layer from the rest of the epidermis. **pitted k.** A superficial infection of the skin of the soles by species of *Corynebacterium* or of *Actinomyces.* Also *keratolysis plantare sulcatum, chaluni, keratoma plantare sulcatum* (obs.), *keratodermia plantaris sulcata.*

**keratolytic** \-lit′ik\ **1** Of or relating to keratolysis. **2** Any agent used to soften or break up keratin.

**keratoma** \ker′ətō′mə\ [KERAT- + -OMA] KERATOSIS. **k. plantare sulcatum** *Obs.* PITTED KERATOLYSIS.

**keratomalacia** \-məlā′shə\ [KERATO- + MALACIA] A wasting and opacification of the cornea classically associated with vitamin A deficiency, but also occurring with other nutritional or metabolic defects.

**keratomata** \ker′ətō′mətə\ Plural of KERATOMA.

**keratome** \ker′ətōm\ KERATOTOME.

**keratometer** \ker′ətäm′ətər\ A device for measuring the anterior curvatures of the cornea, of particular use in evaluating astigmatism and in fitting contact lenses. Also *ophthalmometer.*

**keratometry** \ker′ətäm′ətrē\ [KERATO- + -METRY] The measurement of corneal curvature. Also *ophthalmometry.* Adj. keratometric.

**keratomileusis** \-mīloo′sis\ [KERATO- + Gk *(s)mileusis* the act of carving] A surgical modification of the corneal curvature in order to change refractive error; refractive keratoplasty.

**keratomycosis** \-mīkō′sis\ [KERATO- + MYCOSIS] A fungous infection of the cornea.

**keratonyxis** \-nik′sis\ [KERATO- + Gk *nyxis* a pricking] Surgical perforation of the cornea.

**keratopathy** \ker′ətäp′əthē\ [KERATO- + -PATHY] A noninflammatory corneal disease. **band k.** A superficial, interpalpebral, corneal calcification usually associated with severe general degeneration of an eye. Also *band keratitis, keratitis bandelette, zonular keratitis.* **exposure k.** Keratopathy due to faulty lid closure. Also *exposure keratitis, lagophthalmic keratitis.*

**keratoplasty** \ker′ətōplas′tē\ [KERATO- + -PLASTY] **1** The replacement of a faulty cornea by a portion of a normal cornea obtained from another eye. Also *corneal transplantation.* **2** Any plastic operation on the cornea. **lamellar k.** Transplantation of only partial thickness of the cornea. **optic k.** Corneal transplantation to improve eyesight. **tectonic k.** Corneal transplantation for structural reasons, as in infections or traumatic loss of tissue.

**keratoscleritis** \-sklirī′tis\ [KERATO- + SCLERITIS] Inflammation of the cornea and sclera.

**keratoscope** \ker′ətōskōp′\ A device to observe or measure corneal curvature.

**keratoscopy** \ker′ətäs′kəpē\ [KERATO- + -SCOPY] Observation or measurement of corneal curvature.

**keratosis** \ker′ətō′sis\ [KERAT- + -OSIS] A benign horny lesion. It is usually actinic or seborrheic in origin. Also *keratoma.* **actinic k.** An erythematous scaly lesion of the skin that is provoked by prolonged exposure to sunlight. Also *solar keratosis, senile keratosis.* **aural k.** CHOLESTEATOMA. **k. blennorrhagica** KERATODERMA BLENNORRHAGICUM. **k. follicularis** A hereditary disorder of keratinization characterized by the widespread development of dyskeratotic follicular papules. Also *Darier's disease, keratosis vegetans* (obs.), *psorospermosis.* **k. follicularis decalvans** Keratosis follicularis that results in the destruction of the follicles and subsequent alopecia. **inverted follicular k.** A hyperkeratotic papule arising as a result of an abnormality in growth of hair follicle epithelium. It is a benign lesion. **k. labialis** Actinic keratosis occurring on the mucous membrane of the lip. **k. nigricans** ACANTHOSIS NIGRICANS. **k. obliterans** KERATOSIS OBTURANS. **k. obturans** A disease of the external ear in which the canal becomes obstructed and sometimes expanded by a firm mass of keratin, epidermic scales, and cerumen. Also *keratosis obliterans, wax keratosis.* **k. pharyngis** A disease of unknown pathogenesis, affecting the epithelial covering of the lymphoid tissue of the fauces and pharynx. It is characterized by grayish white horny spicules scattered over the palatine or lingual tonsils or the adenoids or pharyngeal lymphoid nodules, but most often over the palatine tonsils. The disease causes few if any symptoms and eventually resolves spontaneously. Also *hyperkeratosis lacunaris pharyngis, pharyngitis keratosa.* **k. pilaris** Hyperkeratosis of the hair follicles which gives rise to small horny papules, visible most often on the extensor aspect of the limbs. Also *follicular hyperkeratosis, keratosis pilaris rubra.* **k. pilaris atrophicans** Follicular keratosis in which the horny plugs are succeeded by atrophic scars. **k. pilaris rubra** KERATOSIS PILARIS. **k. punctata** PUNCTATE KERATODERMA. **seborrheic k.** A benign tumor, common among the elderly, that is formed of immature epidermal cells. Also *acanthosis seborrheica, verruca seborrheica.* **senile k.** ACTINIC KERATOSIS. **solar k.** ACTINIC KERATOSIS. **k. universalis congenita** ICHTHYOSIS CONGENITA. **k. vegetans** *Obs.* KERATOSIS FOLLICULARIS. **wax k.** KERATOSIS OBTURANS.

**keratosulfate** A polysaccharide of connective tissue. It consists of alternate residues of $\beta$-D-galactose, glycosylated on O-3, and $\beta$-D-*N*-acetylglucosamine 6-sulfate, glycosylated on O-4.

**keratosulfaturia** \-sul′fətoo′rē·ə\ The excretion of excessive keratosulfates in the urine. It is symptomatic of mucopolysaccharidosis IV.

**keratotome** \ker′ətōtōm′\ [KERATO- + -TOME] A triangular surgical knife designed to cut through the cornea to enter the anterior chamber. Also *keratome.*

**keratotomy** \ker′ətät′əmē\ [KERATO- + -TOMY] An incision in the cornea. **delimiting k.** Incision of the cornea with the hope of preventing progression of an ulcer. **radial k.** A technique of refractive keratoplasty in which a series of radial incisions are made in the peripheral cornea in order to flatten the corneal curvature, thereby reducing myopia. The procedure gives inconstant and variable results and leaves permanent corneal scars, and is therefore considered controversial.

**Kerckring** [Thomas Theodor *Kerckring*, Dutch anatomist, 1640–1693] **1** See under CENTER, OSSICLE. **2** Kerckring's folds of small intestine, Kerckring's valves. See under PLICAE CIRCULARES. **3** Nodules of Kerckring. See under NODULI VALVULARUM SEMILUNARIUM VALVAE AORTAE.

**kerectomy** \kerek′təmē\ KERATECTOMY.

**kerion** \kir′ē·än\ [Gk *kērion* (from *kēros* beeswax) a honeycomb, a honeycomblike cutaneous lesion] A highly inflammatory, purulent ringworm infection usually occurring on the scalp, beard area, or limb where there are coarse follicles. It is typically caused by a dermatophyte contracted from an animal or from the soil. Also *tinea kerion*.

**Kerley** [Peter James *Kerley*, English radiologist, born 1900] Kerley's lines. See under LINE.

**kernicterus** \kurnik′tərəs\ [German *Kernikterus* (from *Kern* a kernel, nucleus, core + *Ikterus* jaundice) nuclear jaundice] Damage to the globus pallidus, putamen, and caudate nucleus and to the cerebral cortical gray matter and cerebellar and brainstem nuclei, with deep yellow staining of the affected areas resulting from high levels of serum bilirubin. Clinical manifestations include deafness, mental retardation, and athetosis. The condition has usually but not invariably been the result of hemolytic jaundice due to Rh incompatibility. Also *bilirubin encephalopathy, nuclear icterus, nuclear jaundice*.

**Kernig** [Vladimir Michailovich *Kernig*, Russian physician, 1840–1917] See under SIGN.

**Kerr** See under MUNRO KERR.

**Kerr** [Harry Hyland *Kerr*, U.S. surgeon, born 1881] Parker-Kerr suture. See under SUTURE.

**ketamine hydrochloride** $C_{13}H_{16}ClNO$. A fast-acting general anesthetic administered intravenously or intramuscularly. It is related to the hallucinogen phencycladine. It produces dissociation in the central nervous system with a lack of awareness. It is a competent analgesic but reflexes and strong sympathetic response are retained.

**ketimine** An imine formed between a ketone and an amine, as between enzyme-bound pyridoxamine phosphate and a 2-oxoacid in an aminotransferase. Compare ALDIMINE.

**keto-** \kē′tō-\ [from *ketone*. See KETONE.] A combining form indicating the presence of a carbonyl group. • Although *keto-* was once used in systematic nomenclature, the form *oxo-* is now used in its place to signify replacement of $CH_2$ by CO, but the word *keto* is still used to designate a class of substance. Thus, 2-oxoglutaric acid is a keto acid. It is sometimes used in carbohydrate nomenclature to signify replacement of CHOH by CO.

**keto acid** A substance containing both a carbonyl group and an acidic group. 2-Oxoacids, formed by oxidation of carbohydrates and of branched-chain amino acids, as well as by transamination of amino acids, are the most biologically important keto acids.

**ketoacidosis** \-as′idō′sis\ A metabolic acidosis associated with an accumulation of ketone bodies that are characteristic of uncontrolled diabetes mellitus. **diabetic k.** Ketoacidosis resulting from uncontrolled diabetes mellitus. The precipitating cause may be failure to take insulin, infection, or acute stressful illness. The clinical picture is one of severe dehydration, prostration, fever, hypotension, hyperpnea, and, if untreated, shock and death. Also *diabetic acidosis*.

**ketoaciduria** \-a′sidoo′rē·ə\ KETONURIA. **branched chain k.** MAPLE SYRUP URINE DISEASE.

**$\beta$-ketoacyl-ACP reductase** 3-OXOACYL-ACP REDUCTASE.

**3-ketoacyl-CoA thiolase** *Outmoded* ACETYL-COA ACETYLTRANSFERASE.

**ketoaminoacidemia** \-am′inō·as′idē′mē·ə\ MAPLE SYRUP URINE DISEASE.

**ketodeoxyoctonate** Usually 2-keto-3-deoxyoctonate. It is an octose sugar, oxidized to the carboxylic acid at C-1, and to the ketone at C-2, and reduced to $CH_2$ at C-3. It is alternatively described as a 3-deoxyoctulosonic acid, or more strictly as a 2-dehydro-3-deoxyoctonic acid. It occurs in the pyranose form, with O-6 bound to C-2. The compound with the mannose configuration at C-4 to C-7 is important in the linking of the antigenic branched polysaccharides of bacterial cell walls to the core lipopolysaccharide structure. Abbr. KDO

**ketogenesis** \-jen′əsis\ The formation of the ketones acetoacetate, acetone, and $\beta$-hydroxybutyrate.

**2-ketogluconate** The compound formed when the hydroxyl group on the number 2 carbon of gluconic acid is oxidized to a ketone group.

**$\alpha$-ketoglutarate dehydrogenase** *Outmoded* OXOGLUTARATE DEHYDROGENASE.

**$\alpha$-ketoglutaric acid** *Outmoded* 2-OXOGLUTARIC ACID.

**ketolytic** \-lit′ik\ Capable of destroying ketones, particularly of lowering the blood concentration of ketone bodies.

**ketonaemia** *Brit.* KETONEMIA.

**ketone** \kē′tōn\ [German *Keton*, irreg. coinage from *Azeton* acetone] A compound containing a carbonyl group, CO, bonded to two other carbon atoms. Ketones are typically less reactive than aldehydes, because the two alkyl groups are usually electron-donating and diminish the electrophilic reactivity of the carbonyl group.

**ketonemia** \-nē′mē·ə\ ACETONEMIA.

**ketonic** \kētō′nik\ Related to a ketone. A ketonic substance contains the carbonyl group, but often contains other functional groups.

**ketonuria** \kē′tōnʸoo′rē·ə\ The excretion of ketone bodies in the urine, as seen in starvation, fever, and diabetes mellitus. Also *ketoaciduria, ketosuria, hyperketonuria, acetonuria* (seldom used), *oxonuria* (seldom used).

**ketoplasia** \-plā′zhə\ [KETO- + -PLASIA] The formation of ketone bodies.

**ketose** A sugar that is a ketone, in distinction from an aldose, which is a sugar that is an aldehyde. All monosaccharide molecules consist of a chain of carbon atoms. One of these carbon atoms is in a carbonyl group, and each of the others carries a hydroxyl group. Hence the carbonyl group of a ketose is not at the end of the chain. All natural ketoses known are uloses, i.e. the second atom in the chain is in the carbonyl group.

**ketosis** \kētō′sis\ [*ket(o)-* + -OSIS] A disordered metabolic state occurring in starvation, acute alcoholism, and uncontrolled diabetes mellitus, characterized by the accumulation of ketone bodies in cells, extracellular fluid, and plasma. The biochemical basis is incomplete combustion of long-chain fatty acids to carbon dioxide and water. Adj. ketotic.

**ketosteroid** A steroid that is a ketone.

**17-ketosteroid** A steroid with a carbonyl group at C-17. Measurements of neutral 17-ketosteroids are taken to indicate metabolites of androgens, because C-21 steroids derived from progesterone and corticosteroids cannot possess the 17-carbonyl group, and estrogens are phenolic and so are not neutral, i.e. they are extracted from an organic solvent by alkali before the test is made.

**ketosuria** \\-soo′rē·ə\\ KETONURIA.

**β-ketothiolase** *Outmoded* ACETYL-COA ACYLTRANSFERASE.

**ketotic** \\kētät′ik\\ Of, relating to, or characteristic of ketosis.

**Key** [Ernst Axel Henrik *Key,* Swedish anatomist, 1832–1901] Key-Retzius sheath. See under ENDONEURIUM.

**key** / **determinative k.** A diagram of the properties of various bacteria which enables one to identify a species by tracing its properties through successive forks in a branching tree.

**keyway** **1** The dovetailed part of a prepared cavity in a tooth, designed to improve retention of the restoration. **2** The dovetailed groove in the female part of a precision attachment.

**kg** Symbol for the unit, kilogram.

**khat** \\kat\\ CATHA.

**KHN** Knoop hardness number.

**kHz** Symbol for the unit, kilohertz.

**kibisitome** \\kībis′ətōm\\ [Gk *kibisi(s)* a pocket, pouch + -TOME] A surgical device for cutting the capsule of the crystalline lens.

**kick** / **atrial k.** Forceful contraction of the atrium which leads to distension and rise in pressure in the ventricle, especially in the presence of ventricular hypertrophy as in aortic stenosis or hypertension. It is associated with a marked a wave in the apexcardiogram and a fourth heart sound.

**kidney** [Middle English *kidenei,* of unknown origin] Either of a pair of organs in the dorsal area of the abdominal cavity of vertebrates which function to excrete waste products and to maintain fluid, electrolyte, and acid-base homeostasis; ren. **amyloid k.** RENAL AMYLOIDOSIS. **artificial k.** *Popular* HEMODIALYZER. **atrophic k.** RENAL ATROPHY. **cake k.** A form of fused kidney characterized by a lobular anterior renal surface, from which the ureters arise, and a smooth concave posterior surface. It is usually situated in the pelvis. **coarsely granular k.** A kidney with large, depressed, irregular scars on its surface, with irregular elevations between the scars, usually associated with arterionephrosclerosis. **congenital double k.** Reduplication of the ureter, renal pelvis and kidney occurring to a varying degree (usually incomplete), resulting from a reduplication of the embryologic ureteric bud. It may be associated with other urogenital anomalies. Although usually asymptomatic, the congenital duplication of these structures may make them prone to infection, obstruction, and calculus formation. **congested k.** Excess blood in the kidney, usually secondary to congestive heart failure or obstruction of the vena cava or renal veins. Renal function may be moderately decreased, but it returns to normal when the heart failure or obstruction responds to treatment. Also *cyanotic kidney* (seldom used). **contracted k.** A small, shrunken kidney with a finely and coarsely granular surface and a thick adherent capsule. Scattered elevations 0.5 to 2 cm long separated by deep, wedge-shaped scars may be present, while small cysts are common. Many chronic glomerular, vascular, or interstitial diseases may lead to contracted kidneys and uremia. **crush k.** Acute tubular necrosis secondary to shock resulting from severe crushing injuries. **cyanotic k.** *Seldom used* CONGESTED KIDNEY. **cystic k.** A kidney marked by the presence of one or more cysts. **definitive k.** METANEPHROS. **disk k.** A disk-shaped excretory organ formed by fusion of both poles of the renal anlagen. Also *doughnut kidney.* See also RENAL FUSION. **dystopic k.** A congenital anomaly in which one or both kidneys are in an abnormal position, held in place by anomalous blood vessels which persisted from early fetal life. The abnormally placed kidney usually is deformed and small. It may be located in the pelvis, sacroiliac area, thorax or elsewhere. It is more common in males, and may be associated with other congenital anomalies. Also *renal ectopia, ectopic kidney.* **fatty k.** A large, white kidney with increased lipid content, usually associated with the nephrotic syndrome. The medulla is darker than the cortex. Also *large white kidney.* **finely granular k.** A kidney sometimes seen when the capsule is stripped off at autopsy. Small, pale, surface elevations of approximately 0.2 cm or less are separated by darker, shallow depressions. The elevations represent dilated tubules, the depressions atrophy and scarring. **flea-bitten k.** A kidney with pinhead-sized red spots scattered irregularly over the surface, sometimes seen in the focal glomerulonephritis of subacute bacterial endocarditis. **floating k.** *Popular* NEPHROPTOSIS. **fused k.** A congenital anomaly characterized by fusion of both kidneys at the upper or lower pole (horseshoe kidney), at both poles (disk or doughnut kidney), along the entire length (cake kidney), or at the contralateral upper and lower poles (sigmoid kidney), or location of both kidneys on one side, with fusion between the lower and upper poles (tandem kidney). Fused kidneys are usually in the pelvis or at level of the fifth lumbar vertebra. The vascular supply and course of the ureters also usually are anomolous. It is caused by adherence during embryogenesis of the metanephric organs after they have passed through the crotch between the embryonic umbilical arteries in ascending from their pelvic site of origin. Fused kidneys are susceptible to calculi, hydronephrosis, and infection. Also *renal fusion.* **Goldblatt k.** A kidney in which, in experimental animals, the renal artery has been constricted, producing hypertension. **gouty k.** URATE NEPHROPATHY. **granular k.** A kidney characterized by elevations separated by depressed scars and distributed over the renal surface, which may be fine or coarse. **horseshoe k.** A form of fused kidney in which the kidneys are fused at either the upper or, more commonly, the lower poles. There may also be some caudal ectopia and hyporotation. This condition is associated with an increased risk of calculi, hydronephrosis, and infection. **infarcted k.** RENAL INFARCT. **lardaceous k.** RENAL AMYLOIDOSIS. **large white k.** FATTY KIDNEY. **medullary sponge k.** A congenital anomaly affecting one or, much more commonly, both kidneys, in which a large number of small cysts arise from the calices or collection ducts in the pyramids. The condition usually is asymptomatic, the diagnosis being made on characteristic changes in the intravenous pyelogram. In a few patients calculi, recurrent infections, or recurrent hematuria may complicate the condition. However, prognosis is good and life expectancy is normal. Also *sponge kidney.* **monopyramidal k.** UNILOBAR KIDNEY. **movable k.** NEPHROPTOSIS. **multilobar k.** A kidney consisting of more than one lobe, up to 18 having been reported in humans. **mural k.** An uncommon anomalous condition in which the kidney is situated in a peritoneal pouch in the abdominal wall. **myeloma k.** A complication of multiple myeloma characterized by diffuse atrophy of tubules associated with dense casts and multinucleated giant cells, and by an interstitial nephritis often leading to uremia. Myeloma kidney is almost always associated with Bence Jones proteinuria. Bence Jones protein has been demonstrated to have a toxic effect on renal tubule cells. Excretion of other proteins is usual, and may be great enough to lead to the nephrotic syndrome. **palpable k.** A kidney that can be palpated in a flank. In adults a palpable kidney usually indicates an enlarged kidney. **pelvic k.** A kidney abnormally located in the pelvic cavity, often a fused kidney. **primitive k.** PRONEPHROS. **sclerotic k.** NEPHROSCLEROSIS. **sigmoid k.** A type of fused kidney in which the two kidneys are fused at their upper and lower contralateral poles. Also *lump kidney, tandem kidney.* **single k.** Fused kidneys in which there is little external indication of their original duality and in which a single irregular mass at any of several locations serves the functional role of the two normal organs. Two ureters usually emerge from separate sites on the surface. **solitary k.** A single kidney, either congenital or due to surgical removal. **sponge k.** MEDULLARY SPONGE KIDNEY. **sulfa k.** SULFONAMIDE TOXICITY. **unilateral k.** The one existing kidney in unilateral renal agenesis, usually located at the approximate normal level of the kidney of that side. **unilateral fused k.** A fused kidney lying on one or the other side of the vertebral column, usually at or near the vertebral level of the normal kidney of that side. **unilobar k.** A kidney containing a single lobe; a rare, abnormal condition in a human kidney, which normally contains 5 to 11 lobes each comprising a pyramid, protruding into the calix region, and associated cortex. In some species, such as the beaver and the pig, a single lobe is the typical appearance. Also *monopyramidal kidney.* **waxy k.** *Rare* RENAL AMYLOIDOSIS.

**Kielland** [Christian *Kielland,* Norwegian gynecologist, 1871–1941] See under FORCEPS.

**Kien** [Alphonse-Marie-Joseph *Kien,* German physician, flourished 19th century] Kussmaul-Kien respiration. See under KUSSMAUL RESPIRATION.

**Kienböck** [Robert *Kienböck,* Austrian physician, 1871–1953] See under DISEASE, DISLOCATION.

**Kiernan** [Francis *Kiernan,* Irish-born British physician, 1800–1874] Kiernan spaces. See under PORTAL CANAL.

**kieselguhr** \kē′zəlgoor′\ [German *Kiesel* quartz, hard stone, flint + *Guhr* loose earth deposited in cavities by water] DIATOMACEOUS EARTH.

**Kieser** [Willibald *Kieser,* German physician, flourished mid-20th century] Turner-Kieser syndrome. See under NAIL-PATELLA SYNDROME.

**Kiesselbach** [Wilhelm *Kiesselbach,* German laryngologist, 1839–1902] Kiesselbach space. See under AREA.

**Kilian** [Hermann Friedrich *Kilian,* German gynecologist, 1800–1863] See under LINE.

**Killian** [Gustav *Killian,* German laryngologist, 1860–1921] **1** Killian's tubes. See under TUBE. **2** Killian's operation. See under KILLIAN FRONTAL SINUS OPERATION. **3** See under DEHISCENCE. **4** Killian nasal speculum. See under SPECULUM.

**killing / mercy k.** See under EUTHANASIA.

**kilo-** \kil′ə-, kil′ō-\ [Gk *chilioi* one thousand] A combining form denoting $10^3$, one thousand: used with SI units. Symbol: k

**kilobecquerel** \-bek′ərəl\ [KILO- + BECQUEREL] A unit of activity of a radionuclide equal to $10^3$ becquerel. Symbol: kBq

**kilocalorie** \-kal′ərē\ [KILO- + CALORIE] A unit of quantity of heat equal to $10^3$ calories; 4.2 kilojoules approximately. Symbol: kcal

**kilocurie** \-kyoo′rē\ [KILO- + CURIE] A unit of activity of a radionuclide or of a radioactive source equal to $10^3$ curies; $3.7 \times 10^{13}$ becquerels, exactly. Symbol: kCi

**kilocycle** \-sī′kl\ [KILO- + CYCLE] See under KILOCYCLE PER SECOND. **k. per second** A unit of frequency equal to $10^3$ cycles per second; $10^3$ hertz. Symbol: kc/s • The term *kilohertz,* a unit with the same meaning, is more commonly used than *kilocycle per second. Kilocycle* is often but incorrectly used for *kilocycle per second.*

**kilodalton** \-dôl′tən\ A unit of mass equal to 1000 daltons. It is used to describe a molecule with a molar mass of 1 kg/mol, and a relative molecular mass of 1000. This unit is widely used in biochemistry. Symbol: kDa

**kiloelectronvolt** \kil′ō·ilek′trənvōlt′\ A unit of energy equal to $10^3$ electronvolts. Symbol: keV

**kilogram** \-gram\ [KILO- + GRAM] The SI base unit of mass, equal to $10^3$ grams; 2.2046 pounds. It is equal to the mass of the international prototype of the kilogram, a solid cylinder of platinum-iridium in the custody of the Bureau International des Poids et Mesures, Sèvres, France. The kilogram is also the unit of weight used in commercial trading. Symbol: kg

**kilogram-calorie** CALORIE.

**kilogram-force** The technical unit of force in the metric gravitational system of units, being that force which, acting on a mass of one kilogram, gives to it an acceleration equal to the internationally agreed acceleration of free fall, 9.806 65 meters per second squared; 9.806 65 newtons. Also *kilopond* (German usage). Symbol: kgf

**Kiloh** [Leslie Gordon *Kiloh,* Australian physician, flourished 20th century] Kiloh-Nevin syndrome. See under OCULAR MYOPATHY.

**kilohertz** \-hurts\ A unit of frequency equal to $10^3$ hertz. Symbol: kHz

**kilohm** \kil′ōm′\ A unit of electrical resistance equal to $10^3$ ohms. Also *kiloohm.* Symbol: kΩ

**kiloohm** \kil′ə·ōm\ KILOHM.

**kilopond** \-pänd\ [KILO- + POND] The German term for KILOGRAM-FORCE. Symbol: kp

**Kimmelstiel** [Paul *Kimmelstiel,* German-born physician, 1900–1970] **1** Kimmelstiel-Wilson syndrome. See under DIABETIC GLOMERULOSCLEROSIS. **2** Kimmelstiel-Wilson lesion. See under LESION.

**kin-** \kin-, kīn-\ KINE-.

**kinaesthesia** *Brit.* KINESTHESIA.

**kinaesthesiometer** *Brit.* KINESTHESIOMETER.

**kinanaesthesia** *Brit.* KINANESTHESIA.

**kinanesthesia** \kin′anesthē′zhə\ [KIN- + ANESTHESIA] Loss of position and joint sense and of deep pressure sensation, resulting in the inability to perceive movement at joints, especially in the limbs. Also *cinanesthesia.*

**kinase** \kī′nās, kin′ās\ Any enzyme that transfers a phospho group from ATP or from another nucleoside triphosphate onto a hydroxyl group to form a phosphate or onto an amino group to form a phosphoramidate.

**kindling** A neurological phenomenon characterized by the relatively enduring reduction in threshold of a function or of neuronal activity by a brain structure following a period of sustained activation of a distant locus with which the structure has neuronal connections. Often the distant locus is the contralateral homologue of the affected structure. Activation of the distant site may occur through pathologic change or may be induced experimentally by electrical or chemical stimuli.

**kine-** \kin′ə-, kī′nə-\ [Gk *kinein* to move] A combining form meaning movement, motion. Also *cine-, kin-, cin-.*

**kinematics** \kin′əmat′iks\ [French *cinématique* (from Gk *kinēma,* gen. *kinēmatos,* motion + French *-ique* -ICS) the part of mechanics that studies motion] The science of motion without reference to force or mass. Also *cinematics.*

**kineplasty** \kin′əplas′tē\ [KINE- + -PLASTY] A method of amputation, usually of the upper extremity of man, in which the muscles and tendons in the stump are arranged so that they can transmit movements through a mechanical prosthesis. Skin grafts or flaps are often used to isolate the tendons or muscles. Also *kineplastics*.

**kinesalgia** \kin′əsal′jə\ Pain evoked by movement. Also *kinesialgia, cinesalgia*.

**kinescope** \kin′əskōp\ [KINE- + -SCOPE] A device for refraction based upon the principle of subjective movement of an object positioned in front of the pupil.

**kinesi-** \kīnē′sē-\ KINESIO-.

**kinesia** \kīnē′zhə\ [*kines(i)-* + -IA] **1** MOTION SICKNESS. **2** A condition characterized by movement or increased activity. **paradoxical k.** Transient disappearance of akinesia, chiefly in parkinsonism, with the concomitant appearance of rapid movements, such as running, boxing, etc. Also *kinesia paradoxa*.

**kinesialgia** \kīnē′sē·al′jə\ KINESALGIA.

**kinesiatrics** \kīnē′sē·at′riks\ KINESITHERAPY.

**kinesic** \kīnē′sik\ KINETIC.

**kinesigenic** \-jen′ik\ Produced by movement. Also *kinesogenic*.

**kinesimeter** \kī′nēsim′ətər\ An instrument used for measuring bodily movements. Also *cinometer*.

**kinesio-** \kīnē′sē·ō-\ [Gk *kinēsis* movement] A combining form meaning movement, motion. Also *cinesio-, kinesi-, cinesi-, kineso-, cineso-*.

**kinesiodic** \kinē′sē·äd′ik\ KINESODIC.

**kinesiology** \kinē′sē·äl′əjē\ The study of muscular movements of the body and of its parts, especially with reference to therapy. Also *kinology, cinology*.

**kinesiotherapy** \-ther′əpē\ KINESITHERAPY.

**kinesis** \kīnē′sis\ [Gk *kinēsis* movement] (*pl.* kineses) **1** Generalized movements of an organism or population of organisms, especially in response to an environmental stimulus, such as light. **2** MOTION SICKNESS.

**kinesitherapy** \kīnē′sēther′əpē\ [KINESI- + THERAPY] The therapeutic use of muscle or body movements administered as a course of exercises. Also *kinesiotherapy, kinetotherapy, kinesotherapy, kinesiatrics*.

**kineso-** \kīnē′sō-\ KINESIO-.

**kinesodic** \kin′ēsäd′ik\ Concerning the conduction of impulses in motor nerves. Also *kinesiodic*.

**kinesogenic** \-jen′ik\ **1** KINETOGENIC. **2** KINESIGENIC.

**kinesotherapy** \-ther′əpē\ KINESITHERAPY.

**kinesthesia** \kin′esthē′zhə\ [KIN- + ESTHESIA] The sensation or perception of movement of the body or its parts. Also *kinesthesis, kinesthetic sense, kinesthetic sensation, kinesthetic sensibility*. Compare PROPRIOCEPTION. • The term is often imprecisely used to include sensations of static position, loading, or resistance to movement.

**kinesthesiometer** \kin′esthē′zē·äm′ətər\ An instrument for testing joint sense.

**kinesthesis** \kin′esthē′sis\ KINESTHESIA.

**kinetic** \kinet′ik\ [Gk *kinētikos* putting in motion, stirring up, from *kinēsis* a moving, motion, from *kinein* to move, set in motion] **1** Relating to or characterized by motion. Also *kinesic*. **2** Of or relating to kinetics.

**kinetics** \kinet′iks\ [See KINETIC.] **1** The branch of science dealing with the production of movement and the rate of change, acceleration, and deceleration of bodies in motion in relation to the forces acting on them. **2** The study or description of chemical reactions with respect to the rates at which they proceed and the factors that affect these rates. **3** The study or description of routes taken and changes undergone by substances in biologic systems as they are absorbed, distributed, metabolized, and excreted. **first-order k.** The kinetics characteristic of first-order reactions. In these reactions the rate is proportional to the concentration of reactant, and the logarithm of this concentration falls linearly with time. In a given interval a constant fraction of reactant disappears. **Michaelis k.** The relationship between the rate of an enzyme-catalyzed reaction and the concentration of free substrate that is expressed by the Michaelis-Menten equation. Also *Michaelis-Menten kinetics*. **pre-steady-state k.** The study of the rates of enzyme-catalyzed reactions under conditions when it cannot be assumed that the concentration of enzyme-substrate complex is constant. For much of the course of the reaction this constancy may be assumed, but at early stages after mixing enzyme and substrate the concentration of this complex must rise, and the study of the rate it does so can reveal some rate constants that cannot be determined from measurements made once the steady state has been reached. Also *transient kinetics*.

**kinetin** 6-Furfurylaminopurine, a purine that acts as a growth factor in plants which at low concentrations increases the mitotic rate in meristems, generally by reducing the duration of the interphase. It may not occur in nature.

**kinetism** \kin′ətizm\ The ability to produce muscular activity.

**kineto-** \kīnet′ō-\ [Gk *kinētikos* (from *kinein* to move) putting in motion] A combining form meaning movement, motion. Also *cineto-*.

**kinetocardiogram** \-kär′dē·əgram′\ A record of the low-frequency vibrations of the anterior chest wall over the cardiac region. Also *precordial cardiogram*.

**kinetochore** \kīnet′əkôr\ CENTROMERE.

**kinetogenic** \-jen′ik\ Causing movement. Also *kinesogenic*.

**kinetography** \kī′nətäg′rəfē\ The process of recording movement. Also *kinetoscopy*.

**kinetoplasm** \kīnet′əplazm\ **1** The highly contractile portion of the cell cytoplasm. **2** A region of the cytoplasm of a neuron which contains chromophilic material.

**kinetoplast** \kīnet′əplast\ [KINETO- + -PLAST] A DNA-rich organelle forming part of the cytoplasmic kinetic complex of certain protozoans, such as the flagellates (order Kinetoplastida, subphylum Mastigophora). The kinetoplast is included within a single large mitochondrion extending the length of the body. It is associated with the basal granule (kinetosome) from which the flagellum arises. It is also closely associated with the parabasal body, which appears to be related to nuclear division. The exact function of each of these entities is uncertain, and some authorities consider the entire complex to form a single kinetoplast. Also *motion nucleus*.

**Kinetoplastida** \-plas′tidə\ [KINETOPLAST + *-ida*, suffix denoting a taxonomic order] An order of flagellate protozoa in the class Zoomastigophorea, subphylum Mastigophora, characterized by one or two anterior flagella and a single mitochondrion extending the length of the body, with a conspicuous DNA-containing kinetoplast near the flagellar kinetosomes. The order contains the suborders Bodonina (typical genera: *Bodo, Cryptobia, Rhynchomonas)* and Trypanosomatina (genera *Leishmania, Trypanosoma)*. Most species are parasitic. Also *Protomastigida* (former name).

**kinetoscope** \kīnet′əskōp\ An instrument for making serial photographs of movements.

**kinetoscopy** \kī′nətäs′kəpē\ KINETOGRAPHY.

**kinetosome** \kīnet′əsōm\ [KINETO- + -SOME] BASAL BODY.

**kinetotherapy** \-ther′əpē\ KINESITHERAPY.

**King** [Brien Thaxton *King*, U.S. surgeon, born 1886] See under OPERATION.

**kingdom** A taxonomic group that is the primary category in the classification of organisms.

**kinin** \kī′nin\ [KIN- + -IN] A basic peptide released from a plasma protein by proteolysis in the allergic response, and capable of causing vasodilatation and contraction of smooth muscle. **venom k.** A peptide in the venom of certain insects that acts on blood vessels, smooth muscles, and certain nerve endings. **wasp k.** A peptide in wasp venom which induces rapid and intense pain.

**kininogen** \kinin′əjən\ A protein that, upon cleavage by a kininogenase such as kallikrein, forms kinins. Two kininogens are recognized: high molecular weight kininogen, which yields bradykinin following kallikrein cleavage, and low molecular weight kininogen, which yields kallidin following cleavage. **high molecular weight k.** A plasma protein of 110 000 MW that normally exists in plasma in a 1:1 complex with prekallikrein. The complex is a cofactor in the activation of coagulation factor XII. The product of this reaction, factor XIIa, in turn activates prekallikrein to kallikrein, which cleaves high molecular weight kininogen to form bradykinin, a vasodilator, and two other fragments that accelerate coagulation. **low molecular weight k.** A protein of 50 000 MW that occurs in various normal tissues and which, upon cleavage by kallikrein or other kininogenase, forms kallidin. Kallidin, in turn, is converted to bradykinin.

**kininogenase** \kī′ninäj′ənās\ KALLIKREIN.

**kink** A sharp twist or bend. **ileal k.** Obstruction of the terminal ileum due to kinking of Lane's band, an anomalous membrane connecting the ileum and mesentery to the cecum. Also *Lane's kink*.

**Kinnier Wilson** See under WILSON.

**kino-** \kī′nō-\ [Gk *kinein* to move] A combining form meaning movement, motion. Also *cino-*.

**kinocilium** \-sil′ē·əm\ [KINO- + CILIUM] (*pl.* kinocilia) A cytoplasmic filament that is motile and extends out from the plasma membrane or free surface of a cell.

**kinology** \kīnäl′əjē\ KINESIOLOGY.

**kinomere** \kī′nəmir\ CENTROMERE.

**kinomometer** \kī′nōmäm′ətər\ An instrument that measures the range of motion.

**kinosphere** \kī′nōsfir\ [KINO- + SPHERE] ASTER.

**kinship** **1** Relatedness among individuals or groups based on consanguinity or on connection through marriage. **2** A group of individuals whose relatedness is based on consanguinity.

**kiono-** \kī′ənō-\ CIONO-.

**Kirk** [Norman Thomas *Kirk*, U.S. surgeon, 1888–1960] See under AMPUTATION.

**kirromycin** \kir′ōmī′sin\ An antibiotic that blocks release of EFTu·GDP from the ribosome, thus preventing completion of the initiation step in protein synthesis in bacteria.

**Kirschner** [Martin *Kirschner*, German surgeon, 1879–1942] **1** See under WIRE, APPARATUS. **2** Kirschner wire splint. See under SPLINT.

**Kisch** [Bruno *Kisch*, German physiologist, 1890–1966] Kisch reflex. See under EXTERNAL AUDITORY MEATUS REFLEX.

**kitasamycin** An antibiotic compound from *Streptomyces kitasatoensis*, with properties much like those of erythromycin.

**kiting** \kī′ting\ Falsification of a prescription by increasing the quantity of the drug prescribed.

**Kjeldahl** [Johan Gustav Christoffer *Kjeldahl*, Danish chemist, 1849–1900] Kjeldahl's method, macro-Kjeldahl method. See under TEST.

**kkat** Symbol for the unit, kilokatal.

**Klauder** [Joseph Victor *Klauder*, U.S. dermatologist, 1888–1962] See under SYNDROME.

**Klebs** [Theodor Albrecht Edwin *Klebs*, German pathologist and bacteriologist, 1834–1913] Klebs-Löffler bacillus. See under *CORYNEBACTERIUM DIPHTHERIAE*.

***Klebsiella*** \kleb′zē·el′ə\ [after T. A. E. *Klebs*, German pathologist and bacteriologist, 1834–1913] A genus of Enterobacteriaceae closely related metabolically to *Enterobacter*, but differing in its range of surface antigens and in often being a primary pathogen. ***K. ozaenae*** A species that causes a progressive fetid atrophy of the nasal mucosa. ***K. pneumoniae*** The most important human pathogen of the *Klebsiella* group. It forms an unusually large capsule of various serologic types. It is an occasional component of the normal throat flora, a secondary invader in chronic pulmonary infection, and a primary cause of severe pneumonia and of urinary-tract infection. Also *Friedlaender's bacillus* (older term). ***K. rhinoscleromatis*** A species that causes a destructive granuloma of the nose and pharynx.

**Kleine** [Willi *Kleine*, German psychiatrist, flourished 20th century] Kleine-Levin syndrome. See under SYNDROME.

**-kleisis** \-klē′sis, -kləsis\ -CLEISIS.

**Kleist** [Karl *Kleist*, German neurologist and physician, born 1879] **1** See under CLASSIFICATION, SIGN. **2** Kleist's opposition motor phenomenon. See under MAYER-REISCH PHENOMENON.

**Klemm** [Paul *Klemm*, Russian physician, 1861–1921] Klemm's tetanus. See under CEPHALIC TETANUS.

**Klemperer** [Felix *Klemperer*, German physician, 1866–1931] See under TUBERCULIN.

**Klemperer** [Georg *Klemperer*, German physician, 1865–1946] **1** Klemperer's disease. See under BANTI'S DISEASE. **2** See under TUBERCULIN.

**kleptomania** \klep′təmā′nē·ə\ [Gk *klept(ein)* to steal + *o* + -MANIA] A disorder of impulse control consisting of stealing. It is senseless in that the objects are not taken for use or for their value. Also *cleptomania*.

**Kleyn** [Adrianus Paulus Huibertus Antoine de *Kleyn*, Dutch otorhinolaryngologist, flourished mid-20th century] Van der Hoeve-Kleyn syndrome. See under SYNDROME.

**KLHC** keyhole-limpet hemocyanin.

**Kligler** [Israel J. *Kligler*, U.S. bacteriologist, 1889–1943] See under AGAR.

**Klinefelter** [Harry Fitch *Klinefelter*, Jr., U.S. physician, born 1912] See under SYNDROME.

**Klippel** [Maurice *Klippel*, French neurologist, 1858–1942] **1** Klippel-Feil sign. See under SIGN. **2** Klippel-Feil syndrome. See under SYNDROME. **3** Klippel-Feil malformation. See under MALFORMATION. **4** Klippel-Trenaunay syndrome. See under KLIPPEL-TRENAUNAY-WEBER SYNDROME.

**kliseometer** \klis′ē·äm′ətər\ CLISEOMETER.

**Kluge** [Karl Alexander Ferdinand *Kluge*, German obstetrician, 1782–1844] Kluge sign. See under CHADWICK SIGN.

**Klumpke** [Augusta Dejerine-*Klumpke*, French neurologist, 1859–1927] Dejerine-Klumpke paralysis, Klumpke's paralysis, Klumpke-Dejerine syndrome, Klumpke-Dejerine paralysis. See under DEJERINE-KLUMPKE SYNDROME.

**Klüver** [Heinrich *Klüver*, German-born U.S. neurologist, born 1897] Klüver-Bucy syndrome. See under SYNDROME.

**Knapp** [Herman Jakob *Knapp*, U.S. ophthalmologist, 1832–1911] Knapp streak, Knapp stria. See under ANGIOID STREAK.

**Knaus** [Hermann Hubert *Knaus*, Austrian physiologist, born 1892] **1** See under RULE. **2** Ogino-Knaus method. See under METHOD.

**kneading** \nē′ding\ A massage technique in which the muscles are grasped and pressed in a manner similar to kneading dough. Also *pétrissage.*

**knee** [Old English *cnēow;* akin to L *genu* knee and Gk *gony* knee] The articulation of the lower limb that joins the femur, patella, and tibia, along with the region surrounding this articulation; genus; articulatio genus. **back k.** GENU RECURVATUM. **beat k.** Bursitis and/or cellulitis due to prolonged pressure and friction on the knee. It occurs in miners who are obliged to work in a kneeling position. A similar condition may affect the elbow. **Brodie's k.** BRODIE'S DISEASE. **conventional single axis k.** A simple low-cost prosthetic knee mechanism that provides for a constant friction or braking action during the swing phase of locomotion. **housemaids' k.** A prepatellar bursitis caused by excessive kneeling on a hard surface, as found among household workers who regularly scrub floors. A similar condition may affect clergymen and nuns. **hydraulic k.** A complex prosthetic knee that allows for variations in swing more closely duplicating the normal movement of the lower extremity than does the conventional single axis knee. **k. of internal capsule** GENU CAPSULAE INTERNAE. **little k. of facial canal** GENICULUM CANALIS FACIALIS. **locked k.** The inability to extend fully the knee because of the presence of a loose body in the joint, a tear of a meniscus, or patellofemoral derangement. **rugby k.** OSGOOD-SCHLATTER DISEASE.

**kneecap** PATELLA.

**knife** [Old English *cnīf*] Any surgical instrument with one or more sharp blades, designed in many shapes and configurations and used to incise tissues. **Ballenger swivel k.** An instrument for removing large portions of the quadrilateral cartilage in submucous resection of the nasal septum. The small knife blade, set at right angles at the end of the divided shaft, swivels so as to remain in line with the direction of thrust. **Blair k.** A long, straight-edged knife used for the free-hand harvesting of split-thickness skin grafts. **button k.** A small-bladed knife used for cutting cartilage. **cautery k.** A modified scalpel that utilizes current from an electric cautery. Also *electric knife, electrosurgical knife, endotherm knife.* **gold k.** **1** A dental hand instrument used for trimming gold foil restorations. **2** A large knife used to cut gold foil into small pieces for insertion into a tooth cavity. **Humby k.** A knife for harvesting split-thickness skin grafts or excising burned tissue, having a roller guide for adjusting the thickness of the graft. **lenticular k.** A knife designed for surgical procedures on or about the lens of the eye. **meniscectomy k.** A knife with a short, sharp cutting edge that is used to excise the peripheral attachment of a torn meniscus. **Thiersch k.** A specially designed knife for cutting partial-thickness skin grafts.

**Knight** [James *Knight,* U.S. physician, born 1810] **1** See under BRACE. **2** Knight-Taylor brace. See under BRACE.

**knismogenic** \nis′məjen′ik\ [Gk *knismo(s)* a tickling, itching + -GENIC] Giving rise to a sensation of tickling.

**knob** A rounded protuberance or mass. **aortic k.** The prominence caused by the aortic arch in a chest radiograph. **basal k.** A node or swelling at the cell surface from which the cilium projects. **double aortic k.** Persistence of two aortic arches, resulting from a variation in development of the primitive vascular arches. **embryonic k.** The part of the inner cell mass consisting of the primary ectoderm and endoderm after the migration of the parietal endodermal cells, which are involved in the formation of the yolk sac, has occurred. In some mammals, notably the rodents, this represents the earliest stage of egg cylinder formation. **synaptic k.** END FOOT.

**knock / pericardial k.** A clicking sound occasionally heard on auscultation of the heart after penetrating trauma to the pericardium.

**knock-knee** GENU VALGUM.

**knokkelkoorts** [Dutch *knokkel* knuckle + *koorts* fever] A Dutch term for DENGUE, used in Indonesia.

**knot** [Old English *cnotta*] **1** An interlacing or looping of a string, thread, rope, or strip of material such as may be used in attaching or securing it to another structure. **2** A knoblike mass, such as a node; a clump of cells, vessels, or nerves suggestive of a knot. **clove-hitch k.** A knot in which two continguous loops are applied around the end of a limb to permit traction on the part for reduction of a dislocation or for immobilizing fractures. **double k.** FRICTION KNOT. **false k.** A varicosity of umbilical cord vessels, giving the appearance of a knot. **friction k.** A knot used in surgical procedures that is made by twisting the ends of the suture twice rather than once before the knot is tied. Also *double knot, surgical knot.* **granny k.** A surgical knot consisting of two separate knots placed in such a way that the two knots may slide on the suture when pressure is applied. **Hensen's k.** A primitive node at the cephalic end of the primitive streak. Also *protochordal knot.* **net k.** KARYOSOME. **primitive k.** HENSEN'S NODE. **protochordal k.** HENSEN'S KNOT. **square k.** A surgical double knot in which the two throws of the knot lie in the same plane, thus preventing slippage. Also *sailor's knot, reef knot.* **stay k.** A surgical knot made with two or more square-knotted sutures. **surgical k.** FRICTION KNOT. **syncytial k.** A multinucleated mass on the outer aspect of the chorionic trophoblast in the established placenta. **true k.** An actual knot in the umbilical cord that occurs as a result of intrauterine movement of the fetus. Also *knot of umbilical cord.*

**knuckle** [Middle English *knokel* (prob. from Middle Low German *knökel,* dim. of *knoke* a bone) protuberance at a joint] **1** A prominence produced by the posterior aspect of any interphalangeal or metacarpophalangeal joint when the finger is flexed or the hand is clenched. **2** Any of various anatomical structures resembling such a flexed, knoblike prominence. **aortic k.** The terminal part of the arch of the aorta seen above the heart as a rounded shadow, usually to the left of the vertebral column, in anteroposterior radiographs. **cervical aortic k.** An anomaly of the aortic arch when it extends into the neck, forming an anteroposterior arch, for varying distances as high as the hyoid bone.

**Kobelt** [George Ludwig *Kobelt,* German physician, 1804–1857] **1** Kobelt's tubes. See under TUBE. **2** Kobelt's tubules. See under TUBULE.

**Köbner** [Heinrich *Köbner,* German dermatologist, 1838–1904] Köbner's phenomenon. See under ISOMORPHIC EFFECT.

**KOC** kathodal (cathodal) opening contraction.

**Koch** [Heinrich Herman Robert *Koch,* German bacteriologist, 1843–1910] **1** Koch's postulates. See under LAW. **2** Koch-Weeks conjunctivitis. See under ACUTE CONTAGIOUS CONJUNCTIVITIS. **3** Koch-Weeks bacillus. See under *HAEMOPHILUS AEGYPTIUS.* **4** Koch's lymph. See under OLD TUBERCULIN.

**Koch** [Walter *Koch,* German surgeon, born 1880] Koch's node. See under NODUS ATRIOVENTRICULARIS.

**Kocher** [Emil Theodor *Kocher,* Swiss surgeon, 1841–1917] **1** See under INCISION, FORCEPS, MANEUVER. **2** Kocher's reflex. See under TESTICULAR COMPRESSION REFLEX. **3** Kocher-Debré-Semelaigne syndrome. See under DEBRÉ-SEMELAIGNE SYNDROME.

**kocherization** \kō′kərīzā′shən\ [after Emil Theodor *Kocher,* Swiss surgeon, 1841–1917 + *-iz(e)* + -ATION] The surgical technique of reflecting the second portion of the duodenum and head of the pancreas, commonly used to facilitate the transduodenal exposure of the ampulla of Vater.

**Kocks** [Joseph *Kocks,* German surgeon, 1846–1916] See under OPERATION.

**Koerber** [Hermann *Koerber,* German ophthalmologist, born 1878] Koerber-Salus-Elschnig syndrome. See under AQUEDUCT OF SYLVIUS SYNDROME.

**Koester** [Karl *Koester,* German pathologist, 1843–1904] See under NODULE.

**Kogoj** [Franjo *Kogoj,* Yugoslavian dermatologist, born 1894] Spongiform pustule of Kogoj. See under PUSTULE.

**Köhler** [Alban *Köhler,* German roentgenologist, 1874–1947] **1** See under DISEASE. **2** Köhler's second disease. See under DISEASE. **3** Köhler-Pellegrini-Stieda disease. See under PELLEGRINI-STIEDA DISEASE.

**Kohlrausch** [Otto Ludwig Bernhard *Kohlrausch,* German physician, 1811–1854] **1** Kohlrausch folds, Kohlrausch valves. See under PLICAE TRANSVERSALES RECTI. **2** Kohlrausch veins. See under VEIN.

**Kohn** [Hans N. *Kohn,* German pathologist, born 1866] See under PORE.

**koilo-** \koi′lō-\ [Gk *koilos* (adjective) hollow] A combining form meaning hollow in shape, concave.

**koilocytosis** \-sītō′sis\ [KOILO- + CYT- + -OSIS ] A cell conformation that is characterized by concavity of the cell membrane, as seen in the normal mature red blood cell.

**koilonychia** \koi′lōnik′ē·ə\ [*koil(o)-* + ONYCH- + -IA] The presence of spoon-shaped nails, with a concave surface.

**koilorrhachic** \koi′lôrak′ik\ [KOILO- + *rrach(i)-* + -IC] Exhibiting a reversal of normal lumbar lordosis such that the spine appears concave in the lumbar region when viewed anteriorly.

**koino-** \koi′nō-\ CENO-[2].

**koktigen** A vaccine prepared by boiling a suspension of bacteria in isotonic saline for 30 minutes.

**Kölliker** [Rudolf Albert von *Kölliker,* Swiss anatomist and physiologist, 1817–1905] **1** Kölliker's nucleus. See under SUBSTANTIA INTERMEDIA CENTRALIS MEDULLAE SPINALIS. **2** Kölliker's layer. See under STROMA IRIDIS. **3** Kölliker's gland. See under GLANDULA OLFACTORIA. **4** Kölliker's membrane. See under MEMBRANA RETICULARIS DUCTUS COCHLEARIS.

**Kollmann** [Arthur *Kollmann,* German urologist, born 1858] See under DILATOR.

**kolp-** \kälp-\ COLPO-.

**kolpo-** \käl′pō-\ COLPO-.

**Kondoleon** [Emmanuel *Kondoleon,* Greek surgeon, 1879–1939] See under OPERATION.

**König** [Franz *König,* German surgeon, 1832–1910] **1** König's disease. See under OSTEOCHONDRITIS DISSECANS. **2** See under OPERATION.

**koniocortex** \kō′nē·ōkôr′teks\ [Gk *koni(a)* dust + *o* + CORTEX] The areas of the cerebral cortex, especially the sensory areas, containing a thick granular layer. Also *coniocortex.*

**Koplik** [Henry *Koplik,* U.S. pediatrician, 1858–1927] **1** Koplik sign, Koplik's spots. See under SPOT. **2** Koplik stigma of degeneration. See under STIGMA.

**kopr-** \käpr-\ COPRO-.

**kopro-** \käp′rə-\ COPRO-.

**Korff** [Karl von *Korff,* German anatomist and histologist, flourished 20th century] Korff's fibers. See under FIBER.

**Kornzweig** [Abraham Leon *Kornzweig,* U.S. physician, born 1900] Bassen-Kornzweig disease, Bassen-Kornzweig syndrome. See under ABETALIPOPROTEINEMIA.

**Korotkoff** [Nikolai Sergeivich *Korotkoff,* Russian physician, 1874–1920] **1** See under METHOD. **2** Korotkoff sounds. See under SOUND.

**Korsakoff** [Sergei Sergeivich *Korsakoff,* Russian psychiatrist, 1854–1900] **1** Korsakoff's disease, Korsakoff syndrome. See under PSYCHOSIS. **2** Wernicke-Korsakoff syndrome. See under WERNICKE-KORSAKOFF PSYCHOSIS.

**Kostmann** [Rolf *Kostmann,* Swedish physician, born 1909] **1** Kostmann's disease. See under FANCONI'S ANEMIA. **2** Kostmann's disease. See under CONGENITAL NEUTROPENIA.

**koumiss** \koo′mis\ [Tatar *kumyz*] **1** Originally, a fermented alcoholic drink made from mare's milk by Tatars. **2** A powder preparation containing yeast and lactic-acid producing organisms, used to make fermented milk drinks for dietary purposes from cow's milk, or a beverage so made. Also *lac fermentum.*

**Koyanagi** [Yoshizo *Koyanagi,* Japanese ophthalmologist, 1880–1954] Vogt-Koyanagi syndrome. See under SYNDROME.

**Kozhevnikov** [Aleksei Yakovlevich *Kozhevnikov,* Russian neurologist, 1836–1902] Kozhevnikov's disease, Kozhevnikov's epilepsy, Kozhevnikov syndrome. See under CONTINUOUS PARTIAL EPILEPSY.

**KP** **1** keratitic precipitates. **2** keratitis punctata.

**kPa·s/l** Symbol for the unit, kilopascal second per liter.

**kPa·s·l**$^{-1}$ Symbol for the unit, kilopascal second per liter.

**Kr** Symbol for the element, krypton.

**Krabbe** [Knud H. *Krabbe,* Danish neurologist, 1885–1961] **1** Krabbe syndrome. See under CONGENITAL GENERALIZED MUSCULAR HYPOPLASIA. **2** Krabbe's leukodystrophy, Krabbe type diffuse sclerosis. See under DISEASE. **3** Christensen-Krabbe disease, Christensen-Krabbe progressive infantile cerebral poliodystrophy. See under KRABBE'S DISEASE.

**Kraepelin** [Emil *Kraepelin,* German psychiatrist, 1856–1926] See under CLASSIFICATION.

**krait** \krāt\ [Hindi *karait*] Any venomous snake of the elapid genus *Bungarus.*

**Kraske** [Paul *Kraske,* German surgeon, 1851–1930] See under OPERATION.

**kraurosis** \krôrō′sis\ **k. penis** BALANITIS XEROTICA OBLITERANS. **k. vulvae** Primary atrophy of the vulva.

**Krause** [Fedor *Krause,* German surgeon, 1857–1937] **1** Krause-Wolfe graft, Wolfe-Krause graft. See under FULL-THICKNESS GRAFT. **2** Hartley-Krause operation. See under OPERATION.

**Krause** [Karl Friedrich Theodor *Krause,* German anatomist, 1797–1868] **1** Krause glands. See under GLAND. **2** Krause glands. See under GLANDULAE LACRIMALES ACCESSORIAE. **3** Krause glands. See under GLANDULAE CONJUNCTIVALES. **4** Krause ligament. See under LIGAMENTUM TRANSVERSUM PERINEI. **5** Krause valve. See under BÉRAUD'S VALVE.

**Krause** [Wilhelm *Krause,* German anatomist, 1833–1910] **1** Krause line. See under Z BAND. **2** Krause bone. See under OS ACETABULI. **3** Ulnar collateral nerve of Krause. See under NERVE. **4** Bulbs of Krause. See under CORPUSCULA BULBOIDEA.

**krebiozen** A substance, isolated from the blood of horses previously injected with *Actinomyces bovis,* that was claimed to cure cancer. The major component in the preparations was identified as creatine. Its use has been prohibited in the United States by the Food and Drug Administration.

**Krebs** [Sir Hans Adolf *Krebs,* German-born English biochemist, born 1900] **1** Krebs cycle. See under TRICARBOX-

YLIC ACID CYCLE. **2** Krebs-Henseleit cycle. See under UREA CYCLE. **3** Krebs-Ringer solution. See under SOLUTION.

**kreotoxin** \krē′ōtäk′sin\ [Gk *kre(as)* meat + *o* + TOXIN] A toxin in meat produced by microorganisms. Also *creatoxin, creotoxin.*

**Kretschmann** [Friederick *Kretschmann,* German otologist, 1858–1934] See under SPACE.

**Kristeller** [Samuel *Kristeller,* German gynecologist, 1820–1900] Kristeller technique. See under KRISTELLER'S MANEUVER.

**Krogh** [Schack August Steenberg *Krogh,* Danish physiologist, 1874–1949] See under APPARATUS.

**Kromayer** [Ernst L. F. *Kromayer,* German dermatologist, 1862–1933] See under LAMP.

**Krompecher** [Edmund *Krompecher,* Hungarian pathologist, 1870–1926] Krompecher's tumor, Krompecher's carcinoma. See under BASAL CELL CARCINOMA.

**Kronecker** [Karl Hugo *Kronecker,* Swiss pathologist, 1839–1914] **1** See under PUNCTURE. **2** Kronecker center. See under CARDIOINHIBITORY CENTER.

**Krönlein** [Rudolf U. *Krönlein,* Swiss surgeon, 1847–1910] See under OPERATION.

**Krukenberg** [Adolph *Krukenberg,* German anatomist, 1816–1877] Krukenberg's veins. See under VENAE CENTRALES HEPATIS.

**Krukenberg** [Friedrich Ernst *Krukenberg,* German pathologist, 1871–1946] **1** See under TUMOR. **2** Axenfeld-Krukenberg spindle. See under KRUKENBERG SPINDLE.

**Krukenberg** [Herman *Krukenberg,* German surgeon, born 1863] Krukenberg's hand. See under ARM.

**Krumwiede** [Charles *Krumwiede,* U.S. physician, 1879–1930] Krumwiede triple sugar agar. See under AGAR.

**krypto-** \krip′tə-\ CRYPTO-.

**krypton** \krip′tän\ A rare gas having atomic number 36, atomic weight 83.80. It is present in the atmosphere in a concentration of about one part per million. Six stable isotopes occur in nature and 15 unstable isotopes have been reported. Long believed to be inert chemically, krypton forms a few compounds with fluorine. The most notable of the few uses of krypton is based on the wavelength of the orange-red line in the spectrum of krypton 86, which has been adopted as the basic standard of length in defining the meter. Symbol: Kr

**krypton 85** A radioactive isotope of krypton, emitting beta and gamma radiation. It has been used in the study of respiratory exchange, cardiac output, and peripheral blood flow. Physical half-life is 10.6 years. Symbol: $^{85}$Kr

**17-KS** 17-ketosteroid.

**KSC** kathodal (cathodal) closing contraction.

**KST** kathodal (cathodal) closing tetanus.

**KUB** A roentgenogram of the abdomen designed to reveal abnormalities of the kidneys, ureters, or bladder; a scout film of the abdomen.

**Kufs** [H. *Kufs,* German psychiatrist, 1871–1955] Kufs disease. See under ADULT CEROID-LIPOFUSCINOSIS.

**Kugelberg** [Eric Klas Henrik *Kugelberg,* Swedish neurologist, born 1913] Kugelberg-Welander disease, Kugelberg-Welander syndrome. See under JUVENILE FAMILIAL MUSCULAR ATROPHY.

**Kühne** [Wilhelm Friedrich *Kühne,* German physiologist and histologist, 1837–1900] **1** Kühne's terminal plates. See under PLATE. **2** Kühne's muscular phenomenon. See under PHENOMENON. **3** Kühne's fiber. See under MUSCLE SPINDLE.

**Kuhnt** [Hermann *Kuhnt,* German ophthalmologist, 1850–1925] **1** Kuhnt-Szymanowski procedure. See under KUHNT-SZYMANOWSKI OPERATION. **2** See under MENISCUS, TISSUE. **3** Kuhnt-Junius disease, Kuhnt-Junius degeneration. See under DISCIFORM MACULAR DEGENERATION. **4** Kuhnt spaces. See under SPACE. **5** Kuhnt's postcentral vein. See under VEIN.

**Kulchitsky** [Nicholas *Kulchitsky,* Russian histologist, 1856–1925] **1** Kulchitsky cell carcinoma. See under CARCINOID. **2** Kulchitsky cell. See under ARGENTAFFIN CELL.

**Kümmell** [Hermann *Kümmell,* German surgeon, 1852–1937] Kümmell-Verneuil disease, Kümmell spondylitis. See under KÜMMELL'S DISEASE.

**Kunkel** [Henry George *Kunkel,* U.S. physician, born 1916] See under SYNDROME.

**Küntscher** [Gerhard *Küntscher,* German surgeon, 1902–1972] See under NAIL.

**Kupffer** [Karl Wilhelm von *Kupffer,* German anatomist, 1829–1902] **1** Kupffer cell sarcoma. See under SARCOMA. **2** Von Kupffer cell. See under KUPFFER CELL.

**Kurie** [Franz Newell Devereux *Kurie,* U.S. physicist, born 1907] See under PLOT.

**Kurloff** [Mikhail Georgievich *Kurloff,* Russian physician, 1859–1932] See under CELL.

**kuru** \koo′roo\ [Papuan] A transmissible spongiform encephalopathy due to a slow infection believed to be caused by a prion, found only among the Fore people in the eastern highlands of Papua New Guinea. After a very long incubation period (10–20 years), the disease presents as progressive cerebellar ataxia with tremor of the head, trunk, and limbs, dysarthria, and dementia. Death usually ensues in 3–9 months. At autopsy, the vermis cerebelli and its afferent and efferent connections show marked degenerative changes. Kuru was seen principally in Fore women and children, the traditional participants in a cannibalistic mourning rite involving consumption of a dead kinsman, with infection resulting from autoinoculation from ingestion of infected brain tissue. As cannibalism among the Fore has ceased, the disease is now rare. Little is known about the agent, which is extremely small, highly resistant to activation, and similar to the agents of other slow infections such as scrapie and Creutzfeldt-Jakob disease. The agent is transmissible by peripheral or intracerebral inoculation to chimpanzees, some monkeys, ferrets, and mink.

**Küss** [Emil *Küss,* German physiologist, 1815–1871] See under EXPERIMENT.

**Kussmaul** [Adolf *Kussmaul,* German physician, 1822–1902] **1** Kussmaul breathing, Kussmaul symptom, Kussmaul-Kien respiration. See under KUSSMAUL RESPIRATION. **2** Kussmaul-Maier disease, Kussmaul disease. See under POLYARTERITIS NODOSA. **3** Kussmaul's pulse. See under SIGN. **4** Kussmaul paralysis, Kussmaul-Landry paralysis. See under LANDRY'S PARALYSIS.

**Küstner** [Heinz *Küstner,* German gynecologist, born 1897] Prausnitz-Küstner test. See under PRAUSNITZ-KÜSTNER REACTION.

**Küstner** [Otto Ernst *Küstner,* German gynecologist, 1849–1931] See under SIGN.

**kuttarosome** \kutär′əsōm\ [Gk *kyttaro(s)* a hollow, cell of a honeycomb, pinecone + *sōm(a)* body] A multilayered structure, at the outer segments of the retinal rods and cones, that acts as a receptor of light energy. Also *photoreceptor lamella.*

**Kveim** [Morton Ansgar *Kveim,* Norwegian physician, born 1892] Kveim antigen. See under KVEIM-SILTZBACH TEST.

**kvp** kilovolt peak.

**kwashiorkor** \kwä′shē·ôr′kôr, -ôrkôr′\ [Ga (language of Accra and vicinity, Ghana) *kwashiɔkɔ́* (from *Kwashi,* a boy's name, + Akan *(k)ɔkɔ́* red, light-complexioned) "Red Kwashi," a nickname; prob. orig. a euphemistic reference to the depigmented hair] A severe form of malnutrition characterized by edema, anemia, impaired growth, diarrhea, a crazy-paving dermatosis, and brittle, red hair. The pancreas and the liver are particularly involved, the liver is infiltrated to an excessive degree with fat, and serum albumin is severely depressed. Secondary infections are common and can cause the patient to go into negative nitrogen balance if the protein intake is borderline. Untreated, there is a very high death rate. Kwashiorkor is found especially in children (peak age one to four years) in tropical countries where children are weaned onto food with a very low protein content. It is particularly common where maize, rice, yams, cassava, and plantain are staple foods. Secondary forms of the disease exist in both children and adults and are usually superimposed on a disease associated with gross catabolism, such as tuberculosis. Also *malignant malnutrition, pluridefіciency syndrome, fatty liver of Brahmin children* (used in India), *protein malnutrition, deposed child syndrome.* **marasmic k.** A clinical condition midway between the two extreme forms of protein-calorie malnutrition, kwashiorkor and marasmus. It frequently develops in a child who is subject to a severe caloric restriction and marginal protein intake, and who develops a systemic or intestinal infection. Acute protein deficiency results. The child characteristically shows loss of subcutaneous fat, muscle wasting, and severe dehydration. Following treatment, the characteristics of kwashiorkor disappear but the child is still grossly emaciated.

**kyan-** \kī′ən-\ CYANO-.

**kyano-** \kī′ənō-\ CYANO-.

**kyllosis** \kilō′sis\ [Gk *kyllo(s)* crippled, halt + -SIS] Any deformity of the foot, but particularly talipes.

**kymatism** \kī′mətizm\ [Gk *kyma*, gen. *kymatos*, anything swollen + -ISM] MYOKYMIA.

**kymograph** \kī′məgraf\ [Gk *kym(a)* (from *kyein* to hold, contain, carry in the womb) anything swollen, the swell of the sea, a wave, billow + *o* + -GRAPH] An instrument that records oscillating motion or pressure. Also *cymograph, kymocyclograph.* **x-ray k.** A device for recording the movement of the heart or other types of motion on a single x-ray film. It contains a lead sheet with multiple parallel slits 1 mm wide and 1 cm apart. The lead sheet, placed on an x-ray cassette, moves 1 cm in its logitudinal direction during x-ray exposure to the heart in order to record on x-ray film pulsation amplitude and direction from many points of the cardiac border. Also *multiple slit kymograph.*

**kymography** \kīmäg′rəfē\ The use of a kymograph to record oscillating motion. **roentgen k.** A roentgenographic technique for recording on a single x-ray film the extent and rate of movements of the borders of an organ or structure. Abbr. RKY

**kynurenic acid** 4-Hydroxyquinoline-2-carboxylic acid. It is an intermediate in one pathway of tryptophan catabolism. Transamination of kynurenine gives a 2-oxoacid that cyclizes spontaneously to form kynurenic acid. This loses its hydroxyl group to form quinoline-2-carboxylic acid (quinaldic acid), which is found in urine. Kynurenic acid may be present in the urine in increased quantities in certain hereditary disorders of metabolism.

**kynureninase** The enzyme (EC 3.7.1.3) that hydrolyzes kynurenine to form anthranilate, i.e. *o*-aminobenzoate, and alanine. It contains pyridoxal phosphate, and is on one of the pathways of tryptophan catabolism.

**kynurenine** 2-Amino-4-(2-aminophenyl)-4-oxobutyric acid. It is an intermediate in the catabolism of tryptophan. It is broken down in various ways, partly by hydroxylation at C-3 of its phenyl group followed by hydrolysis to alanine and 2-amino-3-hydroxybenzoate.

**kyphorachitis** \kī′fôrəkī′tis\ A curvature of the vertebral column and thorax to create an exaggerated anterior concavity or posterior hump as a result of rickets. The pelvis may also be involved in the abnormal anterior curvature.

**kyphos** \kī′fäs\ [Gk *kyphos* crookedness, esp. a hump] **1** An abnormal spinal curvature with anterior concavity. **2** A hump.

**kyphoscoliosis** \kī′fōskō′lē·ō′sis\ The combined deformity of kyphosis and scoliosis in the thoracic spine. Adj. kyphoscoliotic.

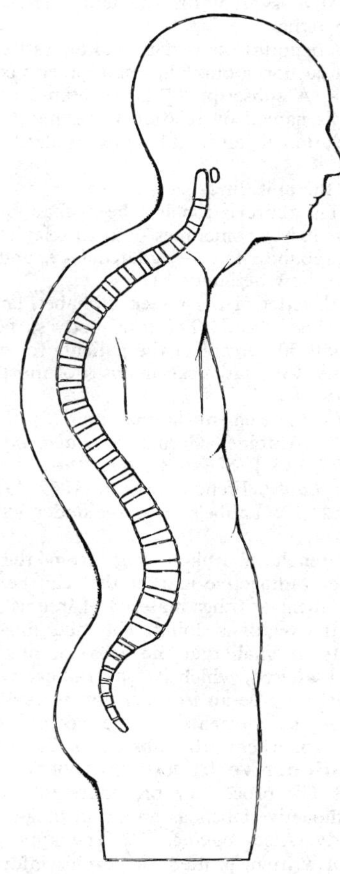

Kyphosis

**kyphosis** \kīfō′sis\ [Gk *kyphōsis* (from *kyphos* bent or bowed forward, stooping, from *kyptein* to bend forward, stoop) a humpbacked condition] An excessive flexion of the thoracic spine that results in marked convexity when viewed from the side. Also *cyrtosis, round back deformity, rachiocyphosis, rachiokyphosis, hunchback, humpback, anterior curvature.* **angular k.** A sharp, anterior flexion of several segments of the thoracic spine that have been diseased by tumor or infection or deformed by trauma. **k. dorsalis juvenilis** SCHEUERMANN'S KYPHOSIS. **juvenile k.** SCHEUERMANN'S KYPHOSIS. **post-traumatic k.** An angular flexion deformity of the spine that follows a crush injury of one or more vertebral bodies. **Scheuermann's k.** Osteochondritis of the epiphyses of the vertebral bodies. Also *juvenile kyphosis, kyphosis dorsalis juvenilis, Scheuermann's disease, vertebral epiphysitis, osteochondritis deformans juvenilis dorsi.*

**kyphotic** \kīfät′ik\ 1 Of or relating to kyphosis. 2 Exhibiting kyphosis. Also *hunchbacked.*

**kyrtorrhachic** \kir′tôrak′ik\ [Gk *kyrto(s)* curved, bent, humped + *rrhach(i)-* + -IC] Exhibiting lumbar lordosis such that the spine appears convex in the lumbar region when viewed from the side.

**kystho-** \kisthə-\ [Gk *kysthos* a hollow] A combining form designating the vagina. An obsolete form. Also *kysth-.*

**kyto-** \kī′tə-\ CYTO-.

# L

**L** 1 Alternative symbol for the unit, liter. 2 Symbol for leucine. 3 lethal.

L- A prefix denoting a certain configuration of atoms around a chiral carbon atom. The enantiomeric configuration is designated D-. A subscript "s" is sometimes used to show that the center is named by relation to serine, or a subscript "g" to show relation to glyceraldehyde, to clarify the configuration.

**l** Symbol for the unit, liter.

***l*-** levo-. • This abbreviation has been abandoned because of ambiguity, as it was sometimes used to refer to optical rotation of a compound, now designated (−), and sometimes to configuration, now designated L.

**λ** The eleventh letter of the Greek alphabet, lambda.

**LA50** [from *lethal area.*] The total body surface size of a burn that will kill 50 percent of the patients (or experimental animals). It is used in statistical analyses of mortality figures for burn patients.

**La** Symbol for the element, lanthanum.

**Labarraque** [Antoine Germaine *Labarraque,* French apothecary, 1777–1850] See under SOLUTION.

**Labbé** [Leon *Labbé,* French surgeon, 1832–1916] 1 See under TRIANGLE. 2 Labbé's vein. See under VENA ANASTOMOTICA INFERIOR.

**label** [Old French, a ribbon, rag, from the Germanic] 1 A chemical or radioactive marker that can be attached to some pharmaceutical or other material of interest, the vector, to show what the vector is doing. The label must be detectable in amounts so small that the behavior of the vector is not significantly altered, which is why radioactive labels are useful. The label may be an isotope, not necessarily radioactive, of one of the elements in the vector. Also *tracer.* 2 To add such a marker to (a substance). For defs. 1 and 2 also *tag.* **radioactive l.** RADIOACTIVE TRACER.

**labeling** 1 The process or procedure followed in using chemical or radioactive labels as an aid in diagnosis or in experimental study. Also *tagging.* 2 The appending or accompaniment of written, printed, or graphic information to a food, drug, medical device, equipment or cosmetic, the content of which may be specified by law. **affinity l.** A method of identifying functional groups, such as enzymes, in macromolecules by allowing them to react with synthetic compounds that resemble the substance with which they bind biologically, such as substrate or allosteric effector, but which also contains a reactive grouping capable of rapidly forming a covalent bond with a group at or near the binding site of the macromolecule. **ferritin l.** The technique of identifying substances in electron micrographs by treating the specimen with antibodies specific to the substances to be identified after attaching these antibodies to ferritin. The ferritin may be identified by its high electron density, which is due to its high content of iron. **isotope l.** The technique of using a labeled compound in an experiment so that the products made from it may be identified. The labeled compound is a mixture of the ordinary compound with the substance in which an unusual isotope replaces one or more of its atoms. For example, ethanol might be mixed with ($^{18}$O)ethanol (the parentheses indicating isotope substitution) to give [$^{18}$O]ethanol (the square brackets indicating isotope labeling). Appearance of $^{18}$O in another compound would then indicate that it originated from the ethanol added. **peroxidase l.** A technique for iodinating tyrosine residues in proteins with $^{131}$I-labeled iodine. Since it is inconvenient and dangerous to handle the radioactive isotope in the form of volatile di-iodine, in this technique it is added as the iodide ion, which is not volatile. A low concentration of the $I_2$ species is then produced in solution by oxidizing the iodide with hydrogen peroxide in the presence of the enzyme iodide peroxidase, which is found in milk. The di-iodine then reacts with tyrosine residues. **pulse l.** An experimental technique in which cells are exposed for a short time to a compound labeled with a radioactive nuclide, followed by a "chaser" (a large quantity of the same compound without the label). The emitted radiation can then be followed as the compound is metabolized. **spin l.** The insertion into a molecule of a stable radical. The radical possesses an unpaired electron, and hence net spin. This can be observed by electron paramagnetic resonance, so that the radical acts as a reporter group, because the environment of the molecule interacts with the spin of the radical.

**Labhart** [A. *Labhart,* Swiss physician, flourished mid-20th century] Prader-Labhart-Willi syndrome. See under PRADER-WILLI SYNDROME.

**labia** \lā′bē·ə\ Plural of LABIUM.

**labial** \lā′bē·əl\ 1 Pertaining to the lip or lips or any labium. 2 Toward or facing the lips.

**labialism** \lā′bē·əlizm\ [LABIAL + -ISM] Undue use of bilabial consonants, that is /b/, /p/, sometimes /w/, and the /β/ and /ϕ/ sounds which are not used in English, usually as substitutions for sounds involving the tongue, such as /d/, /z/ or /g/, which the speaker cannot produce.

**labile** \la′bīl, -bil\ [L *labilis* (from *labi* to glide, slip, fall) gliding, smooth] 1 Easily or spontaneously changed; responding readily to conditions inducing change; unstable. 2 In psychiatry, referring to emotions that are inordinately changeable.

**lability** \ləbil′itē\ [*labil(e)* + -ITY] The property of being easily changed or destroyed, often by some specified agent, such as heat.

**labio-** \lā′bē·ō-\ [L *labium* lip] A combining form meaning labial, labium, or lip.

**labioalveolar** \-alvē′ələr\ 1 Pertaining to the lip and the dental alveoli. 2 Relating to the labial aspect of a dental alveolus.

**labiocervical** \-sur′vikəl\ Pertaining to the labial aspect of the neck of a tooth.

**labioplasty** \lā′bē·əplas′tē\ [LABIO- + -PLASTY] **1** Any plastic operation on the labium majus or the labium minus. **2** CHEILOPLASTY.

**labiotenaculum** \-tənak′yələm\ [LABIO- + TENACULUM] An instrument used for holding a lip or lips, as the labia majora.

**labium** \lā′bē·əm\ [L, a lip] (*pl.* labia) **1** [NA] A lip or lip-shaped structure; a fleshy margin or fold. **2** A posterior mouthpart of certain insects, analogous to a lower lip. Compare LABRUM. **l. anterius ostii uteri** [NA] The anterior lip of the external os of the uterus, thicker and shorter than the posterior lip, both being more obvious in multiparous women in whom the os has become a transverse slit and is no longer rounded as in nulliparous women. It is closely related to the posterior wall of the vagina. Also *anterior lip of ostium of uterus, anterior lip of cervix of uterus.* **l. externum cristae iliacae** [NA] The outer margin or lip of the iliac crest that provides attachment along its whole length for fascia lata as well as for the tensor fasciae latae muscle from the anterior third, the lower fibers of the external oblique muscle of abdomen along the anterior two thirds, and the lowest fibers of the latissimus dorsi muscle from the posterior one-third. At the junction of the anterior and middle thirds the prominent tubercle of the crest is located. Also *external lip of iliac crest.* **l. inferius oris** [NA] The fleshy lower margin or fold of the oral fissure, formed internally of mucous membrane and externally of skin, which surround the orbicularis oris muscle, vessels, nerves, areolar tissue, and small salivary glands. Externally it extends to the mentolabial sulcus which separates it from the chin. Also *lower lip, inferior lip.* **l. internum cristae iliacae** [NA] The inner margin, or lip, of the iliac crest that provides attachment for the fascia iliaca and lower fibers of the transversus abdominis muscle along its anterior two thirds, for the lumbodorsal fascia and quadratus lumborum muscle just posterior to them, and for part of the erector spinae muscle posteriorly. Also *internal lip of iliac crest.* **l. laterale lineae asperae femoris** [NA] The outer lip of linea aspera of femur, continuous with the gluteal tuberosity superiorly and with the lateral supracondylar line bounding the popliteal surface inferiorly, and providing attachment, from medial to lateral side, to the short head of the biceps femoris muscle, the lateral intermuscular septum, and the fused vastus lateralis and vastus intermedius muscles. Also *lateral lip of linea aspera of femur, external lip of linea aspera of femur.* **l. limbi tympanicum laminae spiralis** [NA] The extended and tapering lower part of the C-shaped, periosteal-formed sulcus spiralis internus, within the duct of the cochlea, which is perforated by foramina for branches of the cochlear nerve and by means of which the basilar membrane is attached to the tympanic lip of the osseous spiral lamina. Also *tympanic lip of limb of spiral lamina.* **l. limbi vestibulare laminae spiralis** [NA] The upper part of the C-shaped, periosteal-formed sulcus spiralis internus, within the duct of the cochlea, produced by the projecting edge of the limbus laminae spiralis to which the inner, thin part of the membrana tectoria is attached. The upper surface of the lip has furrows separated by projections, forming the auditory teeth. Also *vestibular lip of limb of spiral lamina, crista spiralis, spiral crest, lamina dentata.* **labia majora** The greater lips of the pudendum. See under LABIUM MAJUS PUDENDI. **l. majus pudendi** [NA] One of two prominent, elongated and rounded cutaneous folds, one on either side of the rima pudendi of the vulva, extending from the mons pubis anteriorly, where they meet to form the anterior commissure, to a short distance in front of the anus posteriorly where they form the posterior commissure. Each is separated from the medial surface of the thigh by a deep cleft, and the external surface of each is covered with hairs while the internal surface is smooth, bearing numerous openings of sebaceous glands. Between the two surfaces is a varying amount of fat, areolar tissue and dartos muscle fibers. Also *greater lip of pudendum.* **l. mediale lineae asperae femoris** [NA] The inner lip of the linea aspera of femur, continuous superiorly with the spiral line and then the intertrochanteric line, and inferiorly with the medial supracondylar line, and having the medial intermuscular septum attached to it. Lateral to the septum the adductor longus muscle and medially the the vastus medialis muscle are attached. Also *medial lip of linea aspera of femur.* **labia minora** The lesser lips of the pudendum. See under LABIUM MINUS PUDENDI. **l. minus pudendi** [NA] One of two thin cutaneous folds located on either side of the external openings of the vagina and urethra and between the labia majora. Anteriorly each one splits into two folds to meet those of the opposite side anterior and posterior to the free end of the clitoris. Posteriorly each either blends with the corresponding labium majus or, in the virginal state, becomes joined to the other by a fold of skin, frenulum labiorum pudendi. The labium is smooth and pigmented, devoid of hair and fat, and contains areolar tissue, blood vessels, and small sebaceous and sweat glands. Also *lesser lip of pudendum, nympha.* **labia oris** [NA] The fleshy upper and lower borders of the rima oris that form the front wall of the oral cavity and are continuous laterally with the cheeks; the lips. Internally they are separated from the teeth and gums by the vestibule. **l. posterius ostii uteri** [NA] The posterior lip of the external os of the uterus, thinner and longer than the anterior lip, both being more obvious in multiparous women in whom the os has become a transverse slit and is no longer rounded as in nulliparous women. It is closely related to the posterior wall of the vagina. Also *posterior lip of ostium of uterus, posterior lip of cervix of uterus.* **l. superius oris** [NA] The fleshy upper border of the oral fissure, formed internally of mucous membrane and externally of skin which surround orbicularis oris muscle, vessels, nerves, areolar tissue and small salivary glands. Superiorly it extends as far as the nose, and laterally it is separated from the cheek by the nasiolabial sulcus. Internally it is separated from the teeth and gums by the vestibule. Also *upper lip, superior lip.* **l. urethrae** One of the two lateral margins of the slightly elevated and irregular external ostium of the urethra.

**labor** [L, work, toil, travail] The process which, by the utilization of uterine musculature contractions as a force, results in the delivery of the products of conception of a pregnancy from the uterus and through the vaginal outlet. Customarily, labor is divided into three stages: the first, from onset of purposeful uterine contractions until full dilatation of the cervix; the second, from full cervical dilatation until vaginal delivery of the fetus; and the third, from delivery of the fetus through delivery of the placenta. **active l.** ACTIVE PHASE. **arrested l.** Labor that has failed to progress at an expected rate given the particular characteristics of fetus and mother. **artificial l.** INDUCED LABOR. **atonic l.** Labor that is prolonged due to hypotonic uterine dysfunction. **complicated l.** Abnormal labor resulting from cephalopelvic disproportion, fetal distress, third trimester hemorrhage, or some other untoward complication. **delayed l.** POSTMATURE LABOR. **dry l.** Labor that occurs following premature rupture of the fetal membranes with subsequent escape of amniotic fluid from the uterine cavity. Also *xerotocia*. **false l.** Uterine contractions that mimic those of labor but do not result in any measurable progress. Also *mimetic labor, spurious labor*. **habitual premature l.** Premature labor occurring in at least three successive pregnancies. **immature l.** Labor occurring in a pregnancy between 20 and 27 weeks after the first day of the last menstrual period. **induced l.** Labor that is initiated by artificial means, as by the artificial rupture of the fetal membranes or through the administration of oxytocic drugs. Also *artificial labor*. **inert l.** Ineffective labor due to uncoordinated uterine contractions. **mimetic l.** FALSE LABOR. **missed l.** Uterine contractions occurring at or near term, followed by fetal death and cessation of all uterine contractions. The fetus may be retained *in utero* for months in some instances. **normal l.** Labor that results in cervical effacement, cervical dilatation, and descent of the fetus such that vaginal delivery occurs. For primiparas the duration is about 14 hours, while for multiparas the duration is about 8 hours. **obstructed l.** Labor that fails to progress due to cephalopelvic disproportion. **postmature l.** Labor occurring after a gestation of more than 42 weeks measured from the first day of the last menstrual period. Also *delayed labor, postponed labor*. **precipitate l.** Labor that proceeds so rapidly that there is some danger of maternal or fetal harm due to inability to control delivery. **premature l.** Labor occurring less than 38 weeks after the first day of the last menstrual period. **prolonged l.** Labor of duration longer than expected. Labor is said to be prolonged if the latent phase continues more than 20 hours in a nullipara or 14 hours in a multipara. In the active phase, labor is said to be prolonged if cervical dilatation occurs at a rate of less than 1.2 cm per hour in a nullipara or 1.5 cm per hour in a multipara. Also *protracted labor*. **spontaneous l.** Labor that occurs naturally without the use of instruments or oxytocic drugs. **spurious l.** FALSE LABOR. **stages of l.** See under STAGE. **stimulation of l.** See under STIMULATION. **trial of l.** See under TRIAL.

**laboratorian** \lab′ərətôr′ē·ən\ An individual whose professional concerns lie in the laboratory rather than in clinical areas. The title applies to professional workers across a spectrum of educational levels.

**laboratory** [Med L *laborat(orium)* (from L *laborat(us)*, past part. of *laborare* to labor + *-orium* -ORY) a room for scientific research or experiment] **1** The space and the equipment used to perform experimental and analytical tests. **2** A group of persons engaged in testing, especially those associated with a discrete organizational entity.

**labour** *Brit.* LABOR.

**labra** \lā′brə\ Plural of LABRUM.

**labrocyte** \lā′brəsīt\ MAST CELL.

**labrum** \lā′brəm\ [L (akin to *lambere* to lick) a lip, edge, rim] (*pl.* labra) **1** A brim or liplike structure. **2** An anterior mouthpart of certain insects, analogous to an upper lip. Compare LABIUM. **l. acetabulare** [NA] A triangular rim of fibrocartilage, the base of which is fixed to the margin of the acetabulum, deepening its cavity. Inferiorly it stretches across the acetabular notch as the transverse ligament. The free edge of the labrum grips the head of the femur. Also *acetabular lip, circumferential cartilage, border of acetabulum, cotyloid fibrocartilage, cotyloid ligament, fibrocartilaginous lip of acetabulum, acetabular labrum*. **l. glenoidale** [NA] A triangular rim of fibrocartilage, the base of which is fixed to the circumference of the glenoid cavity of the scapula, deepening it. Superiorly it is continuous with the tendon of the long head of the biceps brachii muscle. Also *glenoid lip, circumferential cartilage, glenoid labrum*.

**laburinine** CYTISINE.

**labyrinth** \lab′ərinth\ [L *labyrinthus*. See LABYRINTHUS.] A complex of interconnecting cavities or canals; labyrinthus. **acoustic l.** COCHLEA. **bony l.** LABYRINTHUS OSSEUS. **cortical l.** PARS CONVOLUTA LOBULI CORTICALIS RENALIS. **l. of ethmoid** LABYRINTHUS ETHMOIDALIS. **ethmoidal l.** LABYRINTHUS ETHMOIDALIS. **Ludwig's l.'s** Spaces between the renal columns and the cortical arches. **membranous l.** LABYRINTHUS MEMBRANACEUS. **osseous l.** LABYRINTHUS OSSEUS. **renal l.** PARS CONVOLUTA LOBULI CORTICALIS RENALIS. **Santorini's l.** PLEXUS VENOSUS PROSTATICUS. **l. of vestibule** LABYRINTHUS VESTIBULARIS.

**labyrinthectomy** \lab′ərinthek′təmē\ Surgical destruction, either partial or complete, of the sensory elements of the labyrinth, chiefly for the relief of Menière's disease. Techniques used include the injection of absolute alcohol into the labyrinth, membranous labyrinthectomy, and the use of diathermy, ultrasound, and cryosurgery. Also *vestibulectomy*. **membranous l.** Labyrinthectomy effected by avulsing the membranous lateral semicircular canal. The osseous lateral semicircular canal is exposed by mastoidectomy and opened to reveal the contained membranous canal which is avulsed together with the ampulla. **transtympanic l.** Labyrinthectomy effected by transtympanic avulsion of the utricle. The stapes is exposed by tympanotomy and either removed or turned aside. The utricle, drawn into view with a small hook, is then avulsed using fine forceps. **ultrasonic l.** Selective destruction of the vestibular labyrinth by means of ultrasound, used for relief of Menière's disease. The object is to conserve hearing while destroying the source of the vertigo.

**labyrinthi** \lab′ərin′thī\ Plural of LABYRINTHUS.

**labyrinthine** \lab′ərin′thīn\ Relating to a labyrinth, especially to that of the inner ear.

**labyrinthitis** \lab′ərinthī′tis\ [LABYRINTH + -ITIS] Inflammation of the inner ear. Also *otitis interna* (rare). **circumscribed l.** A disorder in which transient vertigo is associated with a fistula between the middle and inner ears. The fistula may be caused by cholesteatoma or may occur accidentally during mastoid surgery or deliberately as in stapedectomy or fenestration. The true cause of vertigo will often be perilymph leakage rather than inflammation of the labyrinth. Also *perilabyrinthitis* (imprecise). **serous l.** Nonsuppurative labyrinthitis, occurring especially in the presence of a fistula between the middle-ear cleft and the periotic labyrinth, characteristically at the site of the lateral semicircular canal. **suppurative l.** An infection of the inner ear caused by pus-forming organisms and usually resulting in a dead ear. In most cases the labyrinthitis is a complication of chronic suppurative otitis media, the infection reaching the inner ear by one of a number of routes. **traumatic l.** Labyrinthitis complicating head injury, where a fracture line passes through the inner ear, or complicating aural surgery. Most cases result in a dead ear.

**labyrinthotomy** \lab′ərinthät′əmē\ [LABYRINTH + *o* + -TOMY ] A double vestibulotomy once used in the treatment of suppurative labyrinthitis. Access to the inner ear was gained both through the foramen vestibuli and by an opening in the osseous lateral semicircular canal.

**labyrinthus** \lab′ərin′thəs\ [L (from Gk *labyrinthos* labyrinth, maze, anything of spiral or twisted shape), a labyrinth, esp. the one in Crete built by Daedalus] (*pl.* labyrinthi) [NA] A complex of interconnecting cavities or canals; a labyrinth. **l. ethmoidalis** [NA] A roughly oblong mass of thin-walled air cells between two parallel vertical plates of bone, suspended from the lateral part of the cribriform plate and situated on each side of the perpendicular plate of the ethmoid bone. The lateral or orbital plate forms part of the medial wall of the orbit while the vertical medial plate is part of the lateral wall of the nasal cavity and has the superior and middle nasal conchae projecting medially into the cavity. Also *ethmoidal labyrinth, labyrinth of ethmoid, lateral mass of ethmoid bone.* **l. membranaceus** [NA] A closed system of communicating membranous sacs and ducts situated within the bony labyrinth of the internal ear, containing endolymph, surrounded by perilymph, and having the branches of the vestibulocochlear nerve distributed in its walls. It comprises the labyrinthus vestibularis formed by the utricle, saccule, and three semicircular ducts, and the labyrinthus cochlearis, formed by the duct of the cochlea. Also *membranous labyrinth.* **l. osseus** [NA] The system of bony cavities of the internal ear lodged in the petrous part of the temporal bone and connected to the middle ear by the fenestra vestibuli and fenestra cochleae in the intervening wall. It is divided into the vestibulum, the canales semicirculares ossei, and the cochlea and it communicates with the cranial cavity by the meatus acusticus internus, which transmits the vestibulocochlear nerve to it. It is lined by periosteum and houses the membranous labyrinth, from which it is separated by the perilymph in the perilymphatic space. Also *bony labyrinth, osseous labyrinth, bony canals of ear.* **l. vestibularis** [NA] The portion of the membranous labyrinth of the internal ear comprising the sacculus and utriculus and their connections and the three semicircular canals. It is the component of the inner ear concerned with the direction of linear and rotational acceleration. Also *labyrinth of vestibule, vestibular system, labyrinthine system, vestibular organ, endovestibular system.*

**lac[1]** [L (gen. *lactis*; akin to Gk *gala*, gen. *galaktos*, milk), milk, the juice of herbs, a milky color] Natural milk or any medication resembling milk. **l. coactum** Curdled milk. **l. defloratum** Skimmed milk. **l. femininum** Human milk. **l. fermentum** KOUMISS. **l. sulfuris** PRECIPITATED SULFUR. **l. vaccinum** Cow's milk.

**lac[2]** [Persian *lak* and Hindi *lākh* lac, from Sanskrit *lākṣā*, variant of *rākṣā* a resin from which a crimson dye is obtained.] The reddish, resinous secretion of the scale insect *Laccifer (Tachardia) lacca,* produced after the insects suck the sap of various resiniferous trees, chiefly in India. Varying in color and occasionally bleached or dewaxed, it is the basis of lacquer, has a great many industrial uses, and is used for the enteric coating of pills and tablets. A variety produced by *Coccus lactis* in India is used in dentistry and surgery. Also *shellac, lacca.*

**Lacassagne** [Antoine Marcelin *Lacassagne,* French physician, born 1884] Regaud and Lacassagne technique. See under PARIS TECHNIQUE.

**lacca** [Italian and New Latin, from Persian *lak,* lac[2].] LAC[2].

**lacerate** \las′ərāt\ [See LACERATION.] To tear by blunt force and produce a torn, irregular, ragged wound.

**laceration** \las′ərā′shən\ [L *laceratio* (from *lacerare* to hew, tear to pieces, mangle, from *lacer* hewn, mangled, torn in pieces) a hewing, tearing, mangling] **1** An injury produced by a blunt instrument in which the skin and/or soft tissues are torn by the crushing and shearing forces produced at impact. Lacerations are characterized by ragged, irregular margins, surrounding contusion, marginal abrasion, tissue bridging in the wound depths, and undermining of the sound in the direction of the blunt force. **2** The act of producing a laceration. **brain l.** Laceration of any part of the brain due to head injury. **dicing l.'s** DICING ABRASIONS. **first-degree obstetric l.** An obstetric laceration of the perineum involving the fourchette, the vaginal mucosa, and adjacent skin but not the underlying fascia and muscle. **fourth-degree obstetric l.** An obstetric laceration of the perineum which extends from the vaginal canal to and through the rectal canal and involves underlying fascia and musculature. **obstetric l.** LACERATION OF THE PERINEUM. **l. of the perineum** A laceration that occurs during vaginal delivery and involves the perineum of the mother. Also *obstetric laceration.* **second-degree obstetric l.** An obstetric laceration of the perineum which involves the skin, vaginal mucosa, and underlying fascia and musculature but does not involve the anal sphincter or extend into the rectal canal. **third-degree obstetric l.** An obstetric laceration of the perineum which involves the skin, vaginal mucosa, underlying fascia and musculature, including the anal sphincter, but does not extend into the anal canal.

**lacertus** \ləsur′təs\ [L, the upper part of the arm] (*pl.* lacerti) A fibrous band or bundle. **l. cordis** Any one of the trabeculae carneae cordis. **l. fibrosus musculi bicipitis brachii** APONEUROSIS MUSCULI BICIPITIS BRACHII. **l. musculi recti lateralis bulbi** [NA] A fascial band extending from the sheath of the lateral rectus muscle of the orbit to a small tubercle on the orbital surface of the zygomatic bone, and considered to check excessive movement of the muscle. Also *lateral check ligament of eyeball.*

***Lachesis*** \lak′əsis\ A genus of venomous snakes of the family Crotalidae, distributed in South America. It includes *L. mutus,* the bushmaster.

**lacinia** \ləsin′ē·ə\ *Outmoded* FIMBRIA.

**lacmus** \lak′məs\ LITMUS.

**lacrima** \lak′rimə\ [L, also *lachryma, lacruma,* prob. alter. of earlier *dacruma,* from Gk *dakryma* something wept for, tears, from *dakry* a tear (akin to common Germanic *tahr-,* English *tear*) a tear, weeping] The fluid of tears, which is an isotonic sodium chloride solution of low protein content with a pH of about 7.4. It contains lysozyme, a bactericidal enzyme.

**lacrimae** \lak′rimē\ Plural of LACRIMA.

**lacrimal** \lak′riməl\ [*lacrim(a)* + -AL] Relating to the tears or to their secretory and drainage apparatus.

**lacrimation** \lak′rimā′shən\ [L *lacrimatio* (from *lacrimare* to shed tears, from *lacrima* a tear) weeping] The production of tears.

**lacrimator** \lak′rimā′tər\ [L *lacrim(a)* a tear + -ATOR] TEAR GAS.

**lacrimatory** \lak′rimətôr′ē\ Producing tears or associated with lacrimation.

**lacrimonasal** \lak′rimōnā′zəl\ Pertaining to the lacrimal apparatus and the nose; nasolacrimal.

**lacrimotome** \lak′rimətōm\ [L *lacrim(a)* a tear + *o* + -TOME] A surgical device for cutting the lacrimal ducts or sacs.

**lacrimotomy** \lak′rimät′əmē\ [L *lacrim(a)* a tear + *o* + -TOMY] Incision into the lacrimal duct or sac.

**lact-** \lakt-\ LACTO-.

**lactacidemia** \laktas′idē′mē·ə\ LACTICACIDEMIA.

**lactaciduria** \laktas′idoo′rē·ə\ The presence of lactic acid in the urine.

**lactagogue** \lak′təgäg\ [LACT- + -AGOGUE] GALACTAGOGUE.

**lactalbumin** Any of a group of proteins found in milk that are not precipitated by half-saturation with ammonium sulfate. One such is α-lactalbumin, which is a component of the enzyme lactose synthase. In its absence the other component of the enzyme catalyzes transfer of a β-galactosyl group from UDPgalactose onto O-4 of *N*-acetylglucosamine. In its presence, the recipient is glucose and the product is lactose.

**lactam** 1 A cyclic amide. 2 The tautomer containing the group —NH—CO—, which may be written $—NH^{+}═C(—O^{-})—$, as opposed to the tautomer containing the group —N═C(—OH)—, in heterocyclic bases such as uracil and cytosine.

**β-lactam** See under β-LACTAM ANTIBIOTIC.

**β-lactamase** Any bacterial enzyme that hydrolyzes the β-lactam bond in β-lactam antibiotics, resulting in the loss of antimicrobial activity. Specificities for various penicillins and cephalosporins vary. The enzyme may be membrane-bound, excreted, or periplasmic, and it may be coded for by a chromosomal gene or by a plasmid.

**lactase** β-D-Galactosidase. Lactose is one of its most important natural substrates. *Outmoded.*

**lactate** \lak′tāt\ 1 To produce breast milk. 2 The anion, or a salt, or an ester, of lactic acid. **Ringer's l.** LACTATED RINGER'S INJECTION.

**lactate dehydrogenase** An enzyme (EC 1.1.1.27) that catalyzes the reaction: lactate + $NAD^{+}$ ⇌ pyruvate + NADH + $H^{+}$. The equilibrium of the reaction greatly favors lactate and $NAD^{+}$ at neutral pH. In this direction the reaction allows muscle glycolysis to occur under anaerobic conditions, the lactate passing into the blood as it is formed. The enzyme is a tetramer consisting of two types of chain. The first (type 1, or α, or H) is predominant in the enzyme from heart muscle, and the other (type 2, or β, or M) is predominant in the enzyme from skeletal muscle. The five tetrameric forms, $H_4$, $H_3M$, $H_2M_2$, $HM_3$, and $M_4$, may be separated by electrophoresis. The different forms have different kinetic characteristics. Thus forms with M chains predominating are less inhibited by high pyruvate concentrations, which may occur in anaerobic skeletal muscle but are unlikely to be present in heart muscle. The enzyme acts on (*S*)-lactate. Dehydrogenases acting on (*R*)-lactate also exist.

**lactate racemase** An enzyme (EC 5.1.2.1) that interconverts (*S*)-lactate and (*R*)-lactate. It enables animals to metabolize (*R*)-lactate, which is mainly of bacterial origin.

**lactation** \laktā′shən\ [LACT- + -ATION] 1 The secretion of milk. Also *galactosis.* 2 The period during which secretion of milk occurs. Adj. lactational.

**lacteal** \lak′tē·əl\ [L *lacte(us)* (from *lac*, gen. *lactis*, milk) milky, pertaining to milk + English -AL] 1 Of or relating to milk. 2 A lacteal vessel; one of the chyliferous lymphatic capillaries of the small intestine. **central l.** The central lymphatic capillary of an intestinal villus, important in the absorption of chyle.

**lactein** \lak′tē·in\ [*lacte(us)* made of milk, milky + -IN] CONDENSED MILK.

**lactescent** \laktes′ənt\ Describing blood serum that displays a milky or opalescent character.

**lacti-** \lak′tē-\ LACTO-.

**lactic** [LACT- + -IC] 1 Pertaining to milk. 2 Producing lactic acid, as in fermentations.

**lactic acid** $CH_3$—CHOH—COOH. The product of anaerobic glycolysis by milk-souring bacteria and in animal tissues. It is formed when muscles are strenuously exercised. It is formed by the action of lactate dehydrogenase on pyruvate, and this reaction reoxidizes NADH to supply the $NAD^{+}$ needed in glycolysis. The same reaction occurs in the reverse direction, particularly in liver, reconverting lactate into pyruvate at the start of its reconversion into carbohydrate. (*S*)-Lactate is the isomer involved in animal tissues. (*R*)-Lactate is formed by many species of bacteria. Also *sarcolactic acid.*

**D-lactic acid** The form of lactic acid produced from methylglyoxal and NADPH by some microorganisms.

**L-lactic acid** The form of lactic acid produced from pyruvate by the action of lactate dehydrogenase and NADH. It has the *S* configuration at C-2.

**lacticacidemia** \lak′tikas·idē′mē·ə\ Greater than normal concentration of lactic acid in blood, plasma, or serum. Also *lactacidemia, lacticemia.*

**lactiferous** \laktif′ərəs\ Capable of producing, transporting, or secreting milk. Also *galactophorous.*

**lacto-** \lak′tō-\ [L *lac* (genitive *lactis*) milk] A combining form denoting (1) milk; (2) lactic acid. Also *lact-, lacti-.*

**lactobacilli** \-bəsil′ī\ Plural of LACTOBACILLUS.

***Lactobacillus*** \-bəsil′əs\ [LACTO- + BACILLUS] A genus of Gram-positive, nonsporulating, anaerobic or facultative rods of the family Lactobacillaceae. Growth requirements are complex. Various species are homofermentative or heterofermentative, producing D- or L- or DL-lactic acid. Major species include *L. delbrueckii, L. leichmannii, L. lactis, L. bulgaricus, L. helveticus, L. casei,* and *L. plantarum.* Some species are found in the human mouth, intestine, and vagina. In metabolism and distribution, lactobacilli are very much like the Gram-positive cocci of the family Streptococcaceae. ***L. acidophilus*** A homofermentative lactobacillus that is prominent in infants' feces and has also been isolated from the human mouth and vagina. ***L. bifidus*** *Obs.* *BIFIDOBACTERIUM.* ***L. salivarius*** An organism isolated from the mouth of humans and of some lower animals.

**lactobacillus** \-bəsil′əs\ (*pl.* lactobacilli) A microorganism of the genus *Lactobacillus.*

**lactocele** \lak′təsēl\ GALACTOCELE.

**lactoferrin** \-fer′in\ An iron-binding protein of milk, other tissue fluids, and neutrophils that chelates iron, thereby retarding bacterial proliferation.

**lactoflavin** The original name for RIBOFLAVIN.

**lactogen** \lak′təjən\ [LACTO- + -GEN] Any agent that stimulates lactation, such as prolactin. **human placental l.** A polypeptide hormone, structurally related to human growth hormone and prolactin, secreted by the placenta and disappearing from maternal circulation within 48 hours after parturition. The hormone has several effects, growth-stimulating, lactogenic, and luteotropic, and it may be important in the maintenance and growth of the fetus. The concentration in plasma is raised in molar pregnancy and choriocarcinoma. Also *human chorionic somatomammotropin, placental growth hormone, chorionic growth hormone-prolactin, galactagogin, somatomammotropin, human chorionic somatomammotropin.* Abbr. HPL.

**lactogenesis** \-jen′əsis\ The production of milk by the mammary glands. Also *galactopoiesis.*

**lactogenic** \-jen′ik\ Stimulating lactation; enhancing the production of milk. Also *galactopoietic.*

**lactoglobulin** A protein present in milk. It has a subunit molecular mass of 18 kDa, and in most species forms dimers, which may associate further. In cow's milk it has a concentration of about 3 g/l, second only to casein among the milk proteins. Also *β-lactoglobulin.*

**lactolin** \lak′təlin\ [LACTO- + *l* + -IN] CONDENSED MILK.

**lactone** An internal cyclic ester within an organic molecule, formed by the elimination of water from a carboxyl group and combination with an alcoholic hydroxyl nearby.

**γ-lactone** A compound that contains a five-membered ring of atoms including the —CO—O— group. It is the lactone formed between a carboxyl group and the γ-hydroxyl group of an acid.

**lactoperoxidase** The iodide peroxidase found in milk. It is a hemoprotein.

**lactophosphate** A salt of both lactic acid and phosphonic acid, using the same base component.

**lactoprecipitin** A precipitin that precipitates the casein of milk. It is produced in the serum of an animal by injecting milk of another species.

**lactorrhea** \lak'tôrē'ə\ [LACTO- + -RRHEA] GALACTORRHEA.

**lactose** [*lact(o)-* + -OSE[2]] 4-*O*-$\beta$-D-Galactosyl-D-glucose. It is the main sugar of milk. It is hydrolyzed by $\beta$-galactosidase to galactose and glucose. A genetic inability to continue production of this enzyme into adult life is common in many parts of the world, especially in hot countries where milk has not normally been in the adult diet. People with this inability suffer discomfort after drinking milk, as the lactose is not hydrolyzed and absorbed but instead provides nutrient for gas-forming intestinal flora. Also *saccharum lactis, milk sugar* (outmoded).

**lactoserum** The serum of an animal previously injected with milk from another species. The serum contains lactoprecipitin, which precipitates milk casein.

**lactose synthase** The enzyme (EC 2.4.1.22) that catalyzes the synthesis of lactose by galactosylating glucose using UDPgalactose as donor. It is found in milk and in mammary glands. It consists of two proteins, one of which is by itself capable of galactosylating *N*-acetylglucosamine to form *N*-acetyllactosamine, but not glucose, and the other, from which it dissociates fairly easily, modifies its specificity so that it galactosylates glucose. The modifying protein has proved identical with that previously described as $\alpha$-lactalbumin.

**lactosuria** \-soo'rē·ə\ The presence of lactose in the urine.

**lactotoxin** \-täk'sin\ [LACTO- + TOXIN] Any toxic substance formed in milk.

**lactovegetarian** \-vej'əter'ē·ən\ [LACTO- + *vegetarian*] One whose diet consists of vegetables, fruit, and milk.

**lactulum unguis** \lak't[y]ələm ung'gwis\ MATRIX UNGUIS.

**lacuna** \lək[y]oo'nə\ [L (from *lacus* a lake, cistern, basin) a ditch, pool, cleft, gap] (*pl.* lacunae) **1** A space or cavity between cells or structures or within a structure; a small depression or pit in a surface. **2** An abnormal gap or discontinuity. For defs. 1 and 2 also *lacune.* **absorption l.** HOWSHIP'S LACUNA. **air l.** A small air-filled space, such as the cortical fusi of the hair shaft. **Blessig's lacunae** Blessig cysts. **cartilage l.** One of the spaces within cartilaginous tissue which house the formative cells or chondrocytes. Also *cartilage space.* **cerebral lacunae** Tiny cavities, often measuring no more than a millimeter or two in diameter, found within the gray or white matter of the cerebrum and almost invariably resulting from minute areas of infarction due to occlusion of one or more small cerebral arteries. Hypertension is the most common cause, and several specific syndromes of so-called lacunar strokes have been defined. **Howship's l.** A rounded pit or defect on the surface of bony tissue that is usually occupied by one or more osteoclasts. It is believed to be a site of bone resorption. Also *absorption lacuna.* **intervillous l.** INTERVILLOUS SPACE. **lacunae laterales** [NA] The venous network within the dura mater through which arachnoid villi project into the superior sagittal sinus. Also *parasinoidal lacunae, parasinoidal sinus.* **l. magna** A pitlike recess in the roof of the fossa navicularis urethrae from which it is separated by the valvula fossae navicularis. Also *Guérin sinus.* **lacunae of Morgagni** Lacunae urethrales in the male urethra. Also *mucous sinuses of male urethra.* **l. musculorum** [NA] The space between the inguinal ligament and the hip bone, lateral to the iliopectineal arch and transmitting the iliopsoas muscle and femoral nerve into the thigh. Also *lacuna of muscles, muscular compartment, iliac canal.* **osseous lacunae** Small spaces within bony tissue that contain the osteocytes and are connected to each other by fine radiating channels or canaliculae. **parasinoidal lacunae** LACUNAE LATERALES. **trophoblastic lacunae** Small spaces that develop in the syncytial trophoblast of the developing human placenta and fuse to form the intervillous space. **lacunae urethrales** [NA] Pitlike recesses of varying size in the mucous membrane of the spongy part of the urethra in the male and the entire urethra in the female. It is considered that some are the wide ostia of the urethral glands. Also *urethral lacunae, lacunae of urethra.* **l. vasorum** [NA] The space between the inguinal ligament and the hip bone, medial to the iliopectineal arch and lateral to the lacunar ligament, transmitting the femoral sheath and its contents. Also *lacuna of vessels, venous lacuna.*

**lacunae** \lək[y]oo'nē\ Plural of LACUNA.

**lacunar** \lək[y]oo'nər\ Relating to a lacuna or characterized by lacunae.

**lacune** \lək[y]oon'\ LACUNA.

**lacunula** \lək[y]oon'yələ\ A very small lacuna. Also *lacunule.*

**lacus** \lā'kəs\ [L, a lake, cistern, basin] (*pl.* lacus) A space in which fluid collects; lake. **l. lacrimalis** LACRIMAL LAKE.

**Ladd** [William Edwards *Ladd,* U.S. pediatric surgeon, 1880–1967] **1** Ladd's bands. See under BAND. **2** See under PROCEDURE.

**Ladd-Franklin** [Christine *Ladd-Franklin,* U.S. psychologist and logician, 1847–1930] Ladd-Franklin theory. See under THEORY.

**Ladin** [Louis Julius *Ladin,* U.S. obstetrician, born 1862] Ladin sign. See under HEGAR SIGN.

***Laelaps*** \lē'laps\ ECHINOLAELAPS.

**Laennec** [René Theophile Hyacinthe *Laennec,* French physician, 1781–1826] Laennec's disease. See under CIRRHOSIS.

**laetrile** \lā'ətril\ [*lae(vorotaryni)trile,* from LAEVO- + *rotary* + *nitrile*] A preparation of amygdalin, a cyanide-containing substance obtained from the pits of apricots, peaches, and bitter almonds. Though sometimes promoted as a cancer treatment, no responsible scientist has been able to find any valid basis to the theory that it has an antineoplastic effect. Also *vitamin* $B_{17}$.

**laevo-** \lē'vō-\ *Brit.* LEVO-.

**laevocardia** *Brit.* LEVOCARDIA.

**LAF** lymphocyte-activating factor.

**Lafora** [Gonzalo Rodriguez *Lafora,* Spanish neurologist, 1887–1971] **1** Lafora's bodies. See under BODY. **2** Myoclonic epilepsy with Lafora bodies, Lafora's disease, Lafora body disease. See under PROGRESSIVE MYOCLONIC EPILEPSY.

**lag** **1** A slowness to act or react. **2** The interval between an expected action or reaction and its occurrence. **anaphase l.** A retarded movement of chromosomes during mitosis. If homologous chromosomes do not separate far enough or fast enough, the daughter cells will be aneuploid for the involved chromosomes. Also *lagging.* **eyelid l.** Failure of the upper eyelid to descend promptly and steadily when the gaze is directed downward. Instead the eyelid moves belatedly and jerkily, a sign of Graves disease. Also *lid lag, Graefe sign, von Graefe sign, Boston sign.* **globe l.** An ocular sign of Graves disease. In the act of looking upward, the patient's upper eyelid pulls back faster than the eyeball is raised, thus exposing the sclera above the iris. Also

*Kocher sign, Kocher symptom.* **jet l.** An alteration in biologic rhythm due to rapid transport, as by jet aircraft, from one time zone to another. Patterns of sleep and wakefulness and of hunger and satiety are often temporarily disrupted, producing disorientation and fatigue. Also *flying fatigue.* **lid l.** EYELID LAG. **phenomic l.** A period of multiplication in a mutated cell in which the premutational phenome is diluted and is replaced by a phenome corresponding to the mutated genome. Several generations are required before an auxotrophic mutation is phenotypically expressed. **phenotypic l.** An interval between the occurrence of a mutation and its phenotypic expression in bacteria. Its components are stabilization of the mutation by its replication on a complementary strand, nuclear segregation, and phenomic lag.

**lagena** \ləjē′nə\ [L, a flagon, flask, bottle] (*pl.* lagenae) CAECUM CUPULARE DUCTUS COCHLEARIS.

**lagging** ANAPHASE LAG.

**lagnosis** \lagnō′sis\ [Gk *lagn(os)* lustful + -OSIS] SATYRIASIS.

***Lagochilascaris minor*** \lag′ōkīlas′kəris\ A small nematode (male 9 mm; female 15 mm) of the family Ascarididae, found in subcutaneous, tonsillar, and mastoid abscesses of humans in Trinidad and Suriname. It probably occurs normally in the intestines of South American felids. Treatment is with diethylcarbamazine.

**lagophthalmos** \lag′äfthal′məs\ [Gk *lag(ōs)* a hare + *ophthalmos* the eye] Inability to close the eyelids completely, as in facial nerve paralysis. Also *oculus leporinus, hare's eye.* Also *lagophthalmus.*

**lake**[1] [L *lacus.* See LACUS.] A small collection of fluid or the space in which it collects; lacus. **capillary l.** The total volume of blood contained in the capillary beds. **lacrimal l.** The pool of tears normally existing in the medial portion of the lower cul-de-sac. Also *lacus lacrimalis.* **marginal l.'s** Dilated regions of the peripheral part of the intervillous space of the human placenta which merge medially with the subchorial space.

**lake**[2] [Persian *lak* lac. See LAC[2].] **1** Any of a class of pigments, originally red or purplish red but now including various colors, produced by precipitation of a soluble natural or synthetic dye with a metallic compound. Some lakes are used as coloring agents in foods and in medicinal tablets and capsules. **2** *Seldom used* HEMOLYZE.

**Laki** [Koloman *Laki,* Hungarian-born U.S. physiologist, born 1909] Laki-Lorand factor. See under FACTOR XIII.

**-lalia** \-lā′lyə\ [Gk *lalia* (from *lalein* to prate, chatter, speak) talking, chattering] A combining form designating a disorder involving speech.

**Lallemand** [Claude François *Lallemand,* French surgeon, 1790–1854] Lallemand-Trousseau bodies, Trousseau-Lallemand bodies. See under BENCE JONES CYLINDERS.

**lalo-** \lal′ō-\ [Gk *lalein* to prate, chatter, speak] A combining form denoting speech.

**lalorrhea** \lal′ôrē′ə\ [LALO- + -RRHEA] LOGOMANIA.

**Lamarck** [Jean Baptiste Pierre Antoine de Monet *Lamarck,* French naturalist, 1744–1829] See under THEORY.

**lamarckism** \ləmär′kizm\ [after Jean Baptiste Pierre Antoine de Monet *Lamarck,* French naturalist, 1744–1829 + -ISM] LAMARCK'S THEORY.

**Lamaze** [Fernand *Lamaze,* French obstetrician, 1890–1957] See under METHOD.

**lambda** \lam′də\ **1** The name of the eleventh letter of the Greek alphabet. Symbol: λ **2** A craniometric point marking the position of the occipital fontanel situated at the junction of the sagittal and lambdoid sutures.

**lambdoid** \lam′doid\ Shaped like or relating to the Greek letter lambda (λ). Also *lambdoidal.*

**Lambert** [Edward Howard *Lambert,* U.S. physiologist, born 1915] Eaton-Lambert syndrome. See under LAMBERT-EATON SYNDROME.

**Lambert** [Johann Heinrich *Lambert,* German mathematician, 1728–1777] **1** Lambert law, Lambert-Holzknecht law. See under LAW. **2** Beer-Lambert law. See under BEER'S LAW.

**lambert** \lam′bərt\ [after Johann Heinrich *Lambert,* German mathematician and physicist, 1728–1777] The CGS unit of illuminance equal to one lumen per square centimeter; $10^4$ lumen per square meter; $10^4$ lux. Symbol: La

***Lamblia*** \lam′blē·ə\ GIARDIA. ***L. intestinalis*** *GIARDIA LAMBLIA.*

**lambliasis** \lamblī′əsis\ Infection caused by *Giardia lamblia.* Also *lambliosis.* See also GIARDIASIS.

**Lambotte** [Albin *Lambotte,* Belgian surgeon, 1866–1912] See under TREATMENT.

**lamella** \ləmel′ə\ [L (dim. of *lamina*) a small metal plate, disk, wafer] (*pl.* lamellae) **1** A thin plate, layer, or sheet, as of compact bone. **2** A medicated disk to be inserted under the eyelid, consisting of an alkaloid drug, contained in a mixture of gelatin, glycerine, and distilled water. Also *lamel.* **annulate lamellae** Flattened lamellar stacks, having fenestrae (windows) similar to nuclear pores located in the cytoplasm of some cells. The annulate lamellae are believed to arise as blebs from the nuclear envelope. **articular l.** A layer of smooth compact bone to which articular cartilage is firmly attached. **circumferential l.** One of a varying number of layers of bone encircling either the external surface of compact bone (lamella circumferentialis externa) or the internal surface lining the wall of the marrow cavity (lamella circumferentialis interna). **l. circumferentialis externa** See under CIRCUMFERENTIAL LAMELLA. **l. circumferentialis interna** See under CIRCUMFERENTIAL LAMELLA. **concentric l.** One of a number of concentric layers (4 to 20) of bony tissue surrounding a central Haversian canal, or canalis centralis osteoni, and its contained neurovascular bundle. **cornoid l.** A parakeratotic horny structure histologically characteristic of porokeratosis of Mibelli. **elastic l.** One of the layers of elastic tissue that form part of the tunica media of an artery. The elastic lamellae are particularly prominent in the larger arteries. Also *elastic lamina, elastic membrane.* **enamel l.** One of the microscopic layers of organic material that run through tooth enamel to reach the dentine layer. **endosteal l.** One of the circumferential lamellae under the endosteum lining the wall of the marrow cavity. **interstitial l.** One of the curved bony layers occupying the irregular intervals between the haversian systems or osteons. These bony layers are the remains of older osteons partly resorbed during bone remodeling. Also *lamella interstitialis.* **osseous l.** One of a series of contiguous thin layers of bone matrix that comprises the basic structural unit of bone, such as a concentric or circumferential lamella. Also *lamella ossea.* **periosteal l.** A bony layer at the external surface of a bone adjacent to the periosteum. **photoreceptor l.** KUTTAROSOME. **posterior border l. of Fuchs** COMPLEXUS BASALIS CHOROIDEAE. **triangular l.** TELA CHOROIDEA VENTRICULI TERTII. **vitreous l.** COMPLEXUS BASALIS CHOROIDEAE.

**lamellae** \ləmel′ē\ Plural of LAMELLA.

**lamellar** \ləmel′ər\ Pertaining to, composed of, or characterized by lamellae.

**lamellipodia** \ləmel′ēpō′dē·ə\ (*sing.* lamellipodium) Broad flattened projections from the leading edge of a cell, such as fibroblast, when growing in tissue culture. The lamellipodia are ruffled in appearance and have an undulating motion. Microfilaments are abundant, especially at points of adhesion to the substrate.

# lamina

**lamina** \lam′inə\ [L, a plate or thin sheet of metal, wood, or other material] (*pl.* laminae) A thin, flat layer or plate; a scale. **l. affixa** [NA] The tela choroidea of the medial wall of the lateral ventricle that fuses during development in the midline, attaches to the dorsal surface of the thalamus overlying the stria terminalis, and covers the thalamostriate and choroid veins. **alar l.** That part of the lateral wall of the neural tube of the embryo lying between the sulcus limitans and the roof plate of the tube. Formed by proliferation of the germinal cells of the ependymal zone, the neuroblasts of each alar lamina become the receptor cells of the posterior horns of the spinal cord and sensory cells in the medulla. Also *lamina alaris, flügelplatte, dorsolateral plate, wing plate, encephalic region, epencephalic region, dorsal zone of His.* **laminae albae cerebelli** [NA] The myelinated fiber bundles underlying the cerebellar cortex. Also *laminae medullares cerebelli, white laminae of cerebellum.* **anterior limiting l.** LAMINA LIMITANS ANTERIOR CORNEAE. **l. anterior vaginae musculi recti abdominis** [NA] The anterior layer of the sheath of the rectus abdominis muscle, extending from the costal margin to the symphysis pubis and formed in its entirety by the aponeurosis of the external oblique muscle which is strengthened by the anterior lamina of the internal oblique muscle in its upper two thirds and by the aponeuroses of the internal oblique and transversus abdominis muscles in its lower one third. Also *anterior layer of the rectus abdominis sheath.* **l. arcus vertebrae** [NA] One of two broad symmetrical plates of bone that fuse at their junction with the spinous process to form the posterior wall of the vertebral arch, each extending laterally to the base of the transverse process where each fuses with the corresponding pedicle. Also *lamina of vertebral arch.* **basal l.** That part of the lateral wall of the neural tube of the embryo lying between the sulcus limitans and the floor plate of the tube. Formed by proliferation of the germinal cells of the ependymal zone, the neuroblasts of each basal lamina become the motor cells of the anterior horns of gray matter of the spinal cord and the motor cells in the medulla. Also *ventrolateral plate, hypencephalic region, ventral zone of His, lamina basalis, grundplatte.* **basal l. of choroid** COMPLEXUS BASALIS CHOROIDEAE. **l. basalis** BASAL LAMINA. **l. basalis choroideae** COMPLEXUS BASALIS CHOROIDEAE. **basement l.** BASEMENT MEMBRANE. **l. basilaris ductus cochlearis** [NA] The fibrous membrane of the floor of the cochlear duct extending from the tympanic lip of the osseous spiral lamina to the crista basilaris of the spiral ligament of the lateral wall, supporting the spiral organ of Corti within the duct and completing the roof of the scala tympani. Also *basilar membrane of cochlear duct, basilar membrane envelope.* **bony spiral l.** LAMINA SPIRALIS OSSEA. **Bowman's l.** LAMINA LIMITANS ANTERIOR CORNEAE. **buccal l.** LATERAL ENAMEL STRAND. **buccogingival l.** VESTIBULAR LAMINA. **l. cartilaginis cricoideae** [NA] The flat, quadrate posterior expansion of the signet-ring-shaped cricoid cartilage, its anterior surface forming much of the posterior wall of the larynx, and its posterior surface providing attachment to the posterior cricoarytenoid muscles and ligaments. The arytenoid cartilages articulate with the superior border of the lamina. Also *lamina of cricoid cartilage.* **l. cartilaginis lateralis tubae auditivae** [NA] The narrow lateral plate of the troughlike, bent superior part of the cartilaginous portion of the auditory tube. Also *lateral cartilaginous layer, lateral lamina of cartilage of auditory tube.* **l. cartilaginis medialis tubae auditivae** [NA] The broad medial plate of the troughlike, bent superior part of the cartilaginous portion of the auditory tube. Also *medial cartilaginous layer, medial lamina of cartilage of auditory tube.* **l. cartilaginis thyroideae dextra/-sinistra** [NA] One of a pair (right and left) of quadrate-shaped plates of the thyroid cartilage, widely separated posteriorly and fused in the midline anteriorly to form the laryngeal prominence surmounted by the thyroid notch. The posterior border has two slender projections, the superior and inferior cornua. The smooth internal surface, lined by mucous membrane, encloses the specialized vocal apparatus while the external surface provides attachment for muscles. Also *lamina of thyroid cartilage.* **l. choriocapillaris** *Outmoded* LAMINA CHOROIDOCAPILLARIS. **l. choroidea epithelialis thalami** The lamina epithelialis of the superior and medial surface of the thalamus. **l. choroidea epithelialis ventriculi lateralis** The ependymal cell layer of the choroid plexus lining the lateral cerebral ventricles. **l. choroidea epithelialis ventriculi quarti** The ependymal cell lining of the roof of the fourth ventricle overlying the rostral medulla oblongata. **l. choroidocapillaris** [NA] A layer of capillaries forming a network in the choroid in which the choroidal arteries end and which is separated from the retina by Bruch's membrane. The spaces in the network are very small posteriorly but become larger anteriorly and contain elastic and collagenous fibers. Near the ciliary body the capillaries join those of the ciliary processes. Also *choriocapillaris, lamina choriocapillaris* (outmoded), *membrana choriocapillaris, Ruysch membrane, Ruysch tunic, ruyschian membrane, choriocapillary layer.* **cribriform l.** *Outmoded* FASCIA CRIBROSA. **l. cribrosa** Either lamina cribrosa ossis ethmoidalis or lamina cribrosa sclerae. **l. cribrosa ossis ethmoidalis** [NA] The perforated horizontal plate of the ethmoid bone, forming part of the roof of the nasal cavity and occupying the ethmoidal notch of the frontal bone. Attached inferiorly are the labyrinth on each side and the perpendicular plate in the center, above which the crista galli projects superiorly. The plate is perforated by numerous branches of the olfactory nerves, which are connected to the olfactory bulbs superior to it. The gyrus rectus is also above the plate. Also *cribriform plate of ethmoid bone, cribrum, sieve bone.* **l. cribrosa sclerae** [NA] The posterior circular, sievelike area of the sclera which is pierced by the nerve bundles of the optic nerve. At its periphery the sclera is continuous with the fibrous sheath of the nerve. At the center of the area there is a large opening for the central artery and vein of the retina. This is the weakest part of the sclera which may bulge outward if the intraocular pressure becomes raised. Also *perforated layer of sclera.* **l. of cricoid cartilage** LAMINA CARTILAGINIS CRICOIDEAE. **l. densa** *Outmoded* GLOMERULAR BASEMENT MEMBRANE. **dental l.** A flat band of epithelial cells that develops in embryos as a medially placed strip from the primary dental band of the mandibular arch and opposed surface of the maxillary process. The dental organs (tooth germs) develop at intervals along the dental lamina to give rise to the primary and secondary dentition. Also *primitive dental groove,* *lamina dentalis.* **l. dentata** LABIUM LIMBI VESTIBULARE LAMINAE SPIRALIS. **l. dura** A dense linear radiographic image of the bone which lines the socket of a tooth. **elastic l.** ELASTIC LAMELLA. **l. elastica anterior bowmani** *Outmoded* LAMINA LIMITANS ANTERIOR CORNEAE. **l. episcleralis** [NA] The loose fibroelastic tissue which forms the outermost layer of the sclera and is continuous externally with the dense connective tissue of the vagina bulbi, while its inner surface blends with the substantia propria sclerae. Also *episcleral lamina.* **l. epithelialis** The modified layer of ependymal cells forming the ventricular surface of the tela choroidea. **l. externa cranii** [NA] The dense outer layer of compact bone of the flat cranial bones. It encloses the diploë and certain paranasal sinuses between it and the inner layer. Also *outer plate of cranial bones, outer table of bones of skull, lamina externa.* **external elastic l.** A fenestrated layer of elastic tissue that represents the boundary between the tunica media and the tunica adventitia of an artery. Also *external elastic membrane, Henle's elastic membrane.* **external medullary l. of thalamus** See under LAMINAE MEDULLARES THALAMI. **external plexiform l.** STRATUM PLEXIFORME EXTERNUM. **fibrocartilaginous interpubic l.** DISCUS INTERPUBICUS. **foliate l.** A laminated connective tissue sheath present in some melanocytic nevi. **l. fusca sclerae** [NA] The thin, pigmented innermost layer of the sclera, composed of small bundles of collagen fibers and many elastic fibers between which are branching chromatophores containing melanin. Its inner surface has grooves for the ciliary vessels and nerves. Also *membrana fusca.* **hepatic l.** A sheet or layer of liver cells that lies between adjacent sinusoids. **l. horizontalis ossis palatini** [NA] The quadrilateral horizontal plate of the palatine bone which articulates anteriorly with the palatine process of the maxilla so that its palatal surface forms the posterior part of the hard palate and its nasal surface forms the back of the floor of the nasal cavity on each side. Also *horizontal plate of palatine bone,.* **l. interna cranii** [NA] The dense internal layer of compact bone of the flat cranial bones. It lies on the inner aspect of the diploë and, in certain parts, of the paranasal sinuses. Also *inner plate of cranial bones, inner table of bones of skull, lamina interna, inner table.* **internal elastic l.** The innermost layer of elastic tissue in the wall of an artery. It forms the boundary between the tunica interna and the tunica media. Also *internal elastic coat of artery.* **internal medullary l. of thalamus** See under LAMINAE MEDULLARES THALAMI. **internal plexiform l.** STRATUM PLEXIFORME INTERNUM. **labial l.** The ectodermal precursor demarcating the lips from the gums, at first in the form of a semicircular band along the upper and lower jaws of a developing embryo. The lateral portion of the labial lamina, sometimes called the vestibular lamina, becomes grooved (vestibular groove), and the grooves deepen to give rise to the vestibule of the mouth. Also *primary labial groove, labiogingival lamina, lip furrow band.* **labiodental l.** One of the ectodermal ingrowths that give rise to the dental and labiogingival laminae. **labiogingival l.** LABIAL LAMINA. **lateral l. of cartilage of auditory tube** LAMINA CARTILAGINIS LATERALIS TUBAE AUDITIVAE. **l. lateralis processus pterygoidei** [NA] The broad, short and everted lateral plate of each of the two pterygoid processes projecting down from the junctions of the body and greater wings of the sphenoid bone. The outer surface is part of the medial wall of the infratemporal fossa and gives attachment to the lateral pterygoid muscle, while the inner surface is separated from the medial plate by the pterygoid fossa and gives attachment to the medial pterygoid muscle. The upper portion of the anterior border forms the posterior margin of the pterygomaxillary fissure. Also *lateral plate of pterygoid process, lateral pterygoid plate, lateral pterygoid lamina, external pterygoid plate* (outmoded). **lateral medullary l.** LAMINA MEDULLARIS LATERALIS CORPORIS STRIATI. **lateral medullary l. of lentiform nucleus** LAMINA MEDULLARIS LATERALIS NUCLEI LENTIFORMIS. **lateral pterygoid l.** LAMINA LATERALIS PROCESSUS PTERYGOIDEI. **l. limitans anterior corneae** [NA] The layer of tightly interwoven fibrils which is situated directly underneath the corneal epithelium and is considered to be a modified layer of the underlying substantia propria but without fibroblasts. Also *anterior limiting lamina, lamina elastica anterior bowmani* (outmoded), *Bowman's membrane, Bowman's layer, anterior elastic layer, Reichert's membrane, ectocornea.* **l. limitans posterior corneae** [NA] The thin, homogeneous, transparent membrane separating the substantia propria from the epithelium posterius of the cornea, of the latter of which it is considered to be the basement membrane. At the circumference of the cornea it breaks up into the trabecular meshwork on the inner wall of sinus venosus sclerae. Also *Descemet's membrane, Demours membrane, posterior elastic layer, Duddell's membrane, vitreous membrane.* **l. limitans tubuli seminiferi convoluti** The limiting membrane that surrounds the cellular wall of a convoluted seminiferous tubule. It comprises a basement membrane surrounded by an envelope of loose connective tissue containing a single continuous layer of myoid cells, the stratum myoideum. **medial l. of cartilage of auditory tube** LAMINA CARTILAGINIS MEDIALIS TUBAE AUDITIVAE. **l. medialis processus pterygoidei** [NA] The long, narrow inner plate of each of the two pterygoid processes projecting down from the junctions of the body and greater wings of the sphenoid bone. It fuses anteriorly with the lateral plate to form the pterygoid fossa between them. Its medial surface helps to form the corresponding posterior aperture of the nose. Extending inferiorly from the plate is a hooklike process, or hamulus, around which the tendon of the tensor veli palatini muscle passes, while superiorly the plate is prolonged along the inferior surface of the body of the sphenoid as the vaginal process. The posterior border provides attachment for part of the superior constrictor muscle of the pharynx. Also *medial plate of pterygoid process, medial pterygoid plate, internal pterygoid plate* (outmoded). **medial medullary l.** LAMINA MEDULLARIS MEDIALIS CORPORIS STRIATI. **laminae mediastinales** The reflections of the mediastinal pleura at the right and left sides of the mediastinum. They extend over the pericardium, to which they adhere, and over the other structures of the mediastinum. **laminae medullares cerebelli** LAMINAE ALBAE CEREBELLI. **laminae medullares thalami** Two bands of myelinated fibers associated with the thalamus. The outer or external medullary lamina surrounds the lateral and ventral surfaces, and the inner or internal medullary lamina separates the medial from the ventrolateral tier of nuclei. Also *medullary laminae of thalamus.* **l. medullaris lateralis corporis striati** [NA] The band of myelinated fibers coursing between the medial and lateral segments of the globus pallidus. Also *lateral medullary lamina.* **l. medullaris lateralis nuclei lentiformis** [NA] The nerve bundle lateral to the nucleuslentiformis. Also *lateral medullary lamina of lentiform nucleus.* **l. medullaris medialis corporis striati** [NA] The layer of myelinated fibers coursing between the globus pallidus and the putamen. Also *medial medullary lamina.* **l. medullaris transversa corporis quadrigemini**

STRATUM ALBUM PROFUNDUM CORPORIS QUADRIGEMINI. **medullary laminae of lentiform nucleus** Lamina medullaris lateralis nuclei lentiformis and lamina medullaris medialis nuclei lentiformis. **medullary laminae of thalamus** LAMINAE MEDULLARES THALAMI. **l. membranacea tubae auditivae** [NA] A membranous connective tissue layer extending between the free edges of the medial and lateral plates of the troughlike cartilaginous portion of the auditory tube, completing it inferiorly and laterally. Also *membranous layer of auditory tube.* **l. mesenterii propria** *Outmoded* COMMON DORSAL MESENTERY. **l. modioli** [NA] The upper part of lamina spiralis ossea. **l. muscularis mucosae** A thin layer of smooth muscle in the wall of most parts of the digestive tube, located between the lamina propria mucosae and the loose connective tissue of the tela submucosa. **l. muscularis mucosae coli** Lamina muscularis mucosae intestini crassi as observed in the colon. **l. muscularis mucosae esophagi** [NA] The thin layer of longitudinal muscle fibers and some elastic fibers located external to the lamina propria mucosae of the esophagus. This muscular lamina and the tela submucosa form longitudinal folds in the lumen which flatten out during the swallowing of food. **l. muscularis mucosae gastricae** [NA] The thin layer of smooth muscle, consisting of an inner circular and an outer longitudinal layer and, in some areas, of an additional outer circular layer, located in the wall of the stomach between the lamina propria mucosae and the tela submucosa. The inner circular layer may send fibers between the glands to the mucosal surface, the contraction of which flattens the longitudinal folds of the mucosa in the presence of food. **l. muscularis mucosae intestini crassi** [NA] A well-developed layer of smooth muscle in the mucous membrane of the large intestine, composed of outer longitudinal and inner circular fibers. It is situated between the lamina propria muscosae and the tela submucosa. It may be irregular or lacking at the sites of lymphatic nodules. Occasionally thin bundles of muscle cells extend toward the surface epithelium. **l. muscularis mucosae intestini tenuis** [NA] The regular and well-developed layer of smooth muscle of the wall of the small intestine located between the lamina propria mucosae and the tela submucosa. **l. muscularis mucosae recti** [NA] The well-developed layer of smooth muscle deep in the tunica mucosa of the rectum, which has the same characteristics as the lamina muscularis mucosae coli, except that the rectal mucosa presents folds in the lumen. **nuclear fibrous l.** A fibrillar layer that is applied to the internal aspect of the inner nuclear membrane. **l. orbitalis ossis ethmoidalis** [NA] A vertical, oblong bony plate which forms the lateral surface of the ethmoidal labyrinth and a large part of the medial wall of the orbit. It articulates with the lacrimal bone anteriorly, the sphenoid bone posteriorly, the orbital part of the frontal bone superiorly and the maxilla and palatine bone inferiorly. Also *orbital lamina, orbital plate of ethmoid bone, os planum.* **palatine l. of maxilla** PROCESSUS PALATINUS MAXILLAE. **l. parietalis pericardii** [NA] The outer layer of serous pericardium that is reflected off the great vessels and heart to line the fibrous pericardium of the cavity in which the heart lies. Also *parietal layer of serous pericardium, parietal pericardium, parietal layer of pericardium.* **l. parietalis tunicae vaginalis testis** [NA] The outer layer of tunica vaginalis testis. It is reflected from the testis and from a short way up the front and medial side of the spermatic cord on to the internal surface of the scrotum, where it adheres to the internal spermatic fascia. Also *parietal layer of tunica vaginalis of testis.* **periclaustral l.** CAPSULA EXTERNA. **l. perpendicularis ossis ethmoidalis** [NA] The thin quadrilateral plate of the ethmoid bone, descending vertically from the crista galli at its junction with the cribriform plate to form the upper part of the nasal septum and join the septal cartilage below. The posterior margin articulates with the vomer inferiorly and with the sphenoidal crest superiorly. Also *perpendicular lamina of ethmoid bone, perpendicular plate of ethmoid bone.* **l. perpendicularis ossis palatini** [NA] The thin quadrangular vertical part of the palatine bone, the anterior border of which articulates with the maxilla and the inferior nasal concha so that its nasal surface forms part of the lateral wall of the nasal cavity, while its lateral, or maxillary, surface forms part of the posterior wall of maxillary sinus and the medial wall of the pterygopalatine fossa and has a deep vertical groove, the greater palatine groove, posteriorly. The superior border has the orbital process in front, the sphenoidal process posteriorly and the sphenopalatine notch between them. Also *perpendicular plate of palatine bone, vertical plate of palatine bone.* **posterior membranous l. of trachea** PARIES MEMBRANACEUS TRACHEAE. **l. posterior vaginae musculi recti abdominis** [NA] The posterior layer of the sheath of the rectus abdominis muscle. It is formed by the posterior lamina of the aponeurosis of the internal oblique muscle blending with the aponeurosis of the transversus abdominis muscle, extending from the costal margin to the arcuate line about halfway between the umbilicus and symphysis pubis. Also *posterior layer of rectus sheath.* **l. pretrachealis fasciae cervicalis** [NA] A layer of deep cervical fascia continuous with the investing layer behind the sternocleidomastoid muscle. It passes in front of the trachea and larynx, ensheathing the infrahyoid muscles and forming a sheath around the thyroid gland. Superiorly it is attached to the hyoid bone and laterally it forms the carotid sheath and blends with the buccopharyngeal fascia. Inferiorly it extends to the back of the manubrium sterni becoming continuous with the fibrous covering of the aorta and of the pericardium. Also *middle layer of cervical fascia, pretracheal fascia, pretracheal layer, cervical visceral fascia.* **l. prevertebralis fasciae cervicalis** [NA] The circular layer of deep cervical fascia that covers the prevertebral and scalene muscles, forming a fascial floor for the posterior triangle of the neck. Posteriorly it is continuous with the ligamentum nuchae, attaching to the external occipital protuberance and the spine of the seventh cervical vertebra. Anteriorly it lies behind the pharynx, the esophagus, and the carotid sheath, to which it is attached by fibroareolar tissue. Inferiorly it extends into the superior mediastinum to blend with the anterior longitudinal ligament. Also *prevertebral fascia, fascia prevertebralis.* **l. profunda fasciae temporalis** [NA] The inner, or deep, layer of the aponeurotic fascia over the temporalis muscle that is attached to the medial surface of the zygomatic arch, just above which it is connected to the superficial layer by dense, fibrous tissue and separated by fat and vessels. It provides origin to fibers of the temporalis muscle. **l. profunda musculi levatoris palpebrae superioris** MUSCULUS TARSALIS SUPERIOR. **proper l. of mesentery** *Outmoded* COMMON DORSAL MESENTERY. **l. propria** LAMINA PROPRIA MUCOSAE. **l. propria mucosae** [NA] A layer of connective tissue between the superficial epithelium and the underlying lamina muscularis mucosae of the alimentary tract. Also *lamina propria, proper mucous membrane, mucoderm.* **reticular l. of the cochlea** MEMBRANA RETICULARIS DUCTUS COCHLEARIS. **l. reticularis** MEMBRANA RETICULARIS DUCTUS COCHLEARIS. **reticular l. of the spiral organ** MEMBRANA RETICU-

LARIS DUCTUS COCHLEARIS. **laminae of Rexed** A group of cytoarchitectural layers and zones of the spinal gray matter which have provided an anatomically consistent and physiologically meaningful way of grouping spinal neurons. These consist of laminae I–IX arranged in the dorsoventral direction and a centrally situated lamina X. Also *Rexed's layers.* **l. rostralis** The thin median bridge extending from the rostrum of the corpus callosum down to the lamina terminalis. It comprises the median reflection of pia mater, and contrary to some earlier beliefs does not contain commissural fibers. Also *rostral lamina, taeniola corporis callosi of Reil.* **l. septi pellucidi** [NA] The vertical neural laminae separated by a space, the cavum septi pellucidi. The lamina contains the medial and lateral nuclei of the septum pellucidum and fibers of the fornix. Also *lamina of septum pellucidum.* **l. spiralis ossea** [NA] The ledge of bone projecting from the modiolus of the cochlea and winding screwlike around it, partially dividing the cochlear canal into an upper passage, or scala vestibuli, and a lower one, or scala tympani. It ends at the apex in the hooklike hamulus. It comprises an upper and a lower lamella between which minute canals transmit fibers of the cochlear nerve to its edge and the organ of Corti. Also *bony spiral lamina, spiral plate.* **l. spiralis secundaria** [NA] A bony ridge projecting inwards from the outer wall of the lower part of the first turn of the cochlea, opposite the osseous spiral lamina but not reaching it. Also *secondary spiral plate.* **submucous l. of stomach** A layer of loose connective tissue that contains vessels and autonomic nerves. It is situated between the main muscle layer externally and the mucosal layer internally. Also *vascular lamina of stomach.* **l. superficialis fasciae cervicalis** [NA] The superficial, or investing, layer of deep fascia of the neck, fused posteriorly with the ligamentum nuchae, surrounding the trapezius muscle and covering the posterior triangle of the neck, then investing the sternocleidomastoid muscle, anterior to which it covers the anterior triangle of the neck and becomes continuous with the corresponding layer of the opposite side at the midline. Inferiorly it is attached to the clavicle and manubrium sterni while superiorly it attaches to the superior nuchal line and the body of the mandible and extends over the parotid gland to the masseteric fascia, as well as attaching to the symphysis menti and the hyoid bone. Also *external cervical fascia, superficial lamina of cervical fascia, investing layer of cervical fascia.* **l. superficialis fasciae temporalis** [NA] The superficial layer of the aponeurotic fascia covering the temporalis muscle that is attached to the outer surface of the zygomatic arch, above which it is connected to the deep layer by dense, fibrous tissue. The superficial temporal vessels and the auriculotemporal nerve cross it superficially while deep to it the middle temporal artery and fatty and areolar tissue may be found. **l. superficialis musculi levatoris palpebrae superioris** [NA] The fibrous, aponeurotic superior layer of the levator palpebrae superioris muscle of the orbit that is inserted partly into the anterior surface of the superior tarsus, and partly into the skin of the upper eyelid after passing through fibers of the orbicularis oculi muscle. **l. suprachoroidea** [NA] A thin layer of pigmented, nonvascular, obliquely directed lamellae which is situated on the external surface of the choroid and connected to the lamina fusca sclerae. Each lamella consists of a meshwork of delicate collagen and elastic fibers within which are branching melanocytes, ganglionic neurons and nerve fibers. Also *suprachoroid lamina, suprachoroidea.* **l. tecti mesencephali** The roof of the mesencephalon, consisting of laminae of fibers and nerve cells. In submammalian forms, it forms the roof of the optocoele. In mammals it refers to the superior and inferior colliculi (corpora quadrigemina). Also *quadrigeminal plate, tectal lamina of mesencephalon.* **l. terminalis** [NA] A membrane formed in the developing embryo by the closure of the anterior neuropore at the cephalic end of the early neural tube. In the adult brain the lamina terminalis remains as a thin layer of gray matter, derived from the telencephalon, that extends from the superior surface of the optic chiasma to the rostrum of the corpus callosum. It forms part of the anterior wall of the third ventricle. Also *terminal lamina of hypothalamus, terminal plate.* **l. of thyroid cartilage** LAMINA CARTILAGINIS THYROIDEAE DEXTRA/SINISTRA. **l. tragi** [NA] The arched longitudinal lamina of cartilage of the tragus of the auricle, quite separate from the cartilage of the auricle and attached to the outer margin of the cartilage of the external auditory meatus. Also *lamina tragica.* **ungual laminae** CRISTAE MATRICIS UNGUIS. **vascular l. of stomach** SUBMUCOUS LAMINA OF STOMACH. **l. vasculosa choroideae** [NA] The outermost layer of the choroid proper which consists of the branches of the short posterior ciliary arteries extending anteriorly, a venous plexus which converges in whorls on the vorticose veins, and a loose connective tissue containing melanocytes. It is situated between the lamina suprachoroideae externally and the lamina choroidocapillaris deep to it. The vessels tend to diminish in size from the outer to the inner aspects of this layer. Also *vascular layer of choroid, Haller's layer, Haller's membrane.* **l. of vertebral arch** LAMINA ARCUS VERTEBRAE. **vestibular l.** That part of the labial lamina, extending backwards between the developing cheek and gums, that will split to form the vestibule of the mouth. Also *buccogingival lamina.* **l. visceralis pericardii** [NA] The layer of the serous pericardium that closely invests the heart and the beginning of the aorta and pulmonary trunk. Also *epicardium, visceral layer of pericardium, visceral pericardium.* **l. visceralis tunicae vaginalis testis** [NA] The layer of the tunica vaginalis testis that closely invests the testis on its medial and lateral surfaces and anterior border and also covers the lateral and medial aspects of the epididymis as well as the upper surface of its head. Also *visceral layer of tunica vaginalis of testis.* **white laminae of cerebellum** LAMINAE ALBAE CEREBELLI. **zonal l.** STRATUM MOLECULARE. **l. zonalis of cerebellum** STRATUM MOLECULARE CEREBELLI.

**laminae** \lam′inē\ Plural of LAMINA.

**laminagraph** \lam′inəgraf′\ [LAMINA + -GRAPH] X-ray equipment for doing body section roentgenography. Also *laminograph.*

**laminagraphy** \lam′inäg′rəfē\ [LAMINA + -GRAPHY] BODY SECTION ROENTGENOGRAPHY.

**laminar** \lam′inər\ Consisting of, arranged in, or pertaining to laminae; laminated.

**laminarin sulfate** The sulfated form of a polysaccharide from a seaweed, *Laminaria,* having anticoagulant properties, like heparin. Also *laminaran.*

**laminated** \lam′inā′tid\ Consisting of or arranged in layers or laminae. Also *laminate.*

**lamination** \lam′inā′shən\ A layered arrangement or formation.

**laminectomy** \lam′inek′təmē\ [*lamin(a)* + -ECTOMY] Excision of the posterior arches and spinous processes of a vertebra. Also *rachiotomy, spondylotomy, rachitomy.*

**laminograph** \lam′inəgraf′\ LAMINAGRAPH.

**laminography** \lam′inäg′rəfē\ [*lamin(a)* + *o* + -GRAPHY] BODY SECTION ROENTGENOGRAPHY.

**laminotomy** \lam′inät′əmē\ [*lamin(a)* + *o* + -TOMY]

The division or partial removal of vertebral laminae.

**lamp** A device for producing light artificially for illumination. **carbon arc l.** A lamp that produces intense white light by electric discharge between carbon rod electrodes. **Eldridge-Green l.** A color-vision testing device using spectral filters. **Finsen l.** A carbon arc lamp producing concentrated ultraviolet radiation at 50 volts and 50 amperes and utilized for dermatological treatment, particularly lupus vulgaris. **Kromayer l.** A hand-held, water- or air-cooled mercury quartz ultraviolet lamp for localized application of intense bactericidal wave length, utilized in the treatment of skin ulcers. **mercury vapor l.** A carbon arc lamp in which the electric arc is enclosed in a quartz burner containing mercury vapor, producing ultraviolet radiation that may be used therapeutically for general irradiation of large body areas, artificially duplicating the effect of sunlight, or adapted for focal application as a Kromayer lamp. **mignon l.** A tiny surgical instrument with a light at the end, used during endoscopic procedures. **quartz l.** A mercury vapor lamp emitting ultraviolet light. Two types exist, cold quartz, operating at low vapor pressure and low intensity, producing shorter wave lengths (Kromayer lamp), and hot quartz, operating under high vapor pressure and high intensity at a relatively high temperature, producing longer wave lengths (sun lamp). **Simpson l.** An electric arc lamp emitting heat rays and visible and ultraviolet light. One electrode is made from tungstenate of iron and the other from manganese. Also *Simpson light.* **slit l.** A combination of a microscope and a narrow beam of collimated light, used to observe the eye. Also *corneal microscope, slit lamp microscope.* **sun l.** Any lamp used for irradiation or sunbathing purposes that emits radiation which simulates that of the sun in some respect, especially in the ultraviolet range. **Wood's l.** A device for producing ultraviolet rays (Wood's light) filtered through nickel glass and peaking at 365 nm, which gives a characteristic fluorescence in the presence of some microbial agents. It is commonly used to demonstrate *Microsporum* species in the hair of children. Infected hair has a bright green fluorescence. A pink fluorescence appears in skin lesions of erythrasma, a gold fluorescence in areas of pityriasis versicolor, and a bright green in wounds, lesions, and toe webs of *Pseudomonas.* Wood's light is invaluable in controlling outbreaks of *Microsporum* infection. However, some fungi causing tinea capitis (ringworm of the scalp), such as *Trichophyton tonsurans,* produce no fluorescence when subjected to ultraviolet light.

**Lamy** [Maurice Emile Joseph *Lamy,* French physician, born 1895] **1** Maroteaux-Lamy disease. See under DISEASE. **2** Maroteaux-Lamy syndrome. See under MUCOPOLYSACCHARIDOSIS VI.

**lance** **1** To incise tissue with a lancet for purposes of drainage. **2** LANCET.

**Lancefield** [Rebecca Craighill *Lancefield,* U.S. bacteriologist, born 1895] See under CLASSIFICATION.

**Lancereaux** [Étienne *Lancereaux,* French physician, 1829–1910] Lancereaux-Mathieu disease. See under ICTERIC LEPTOSPIROSIS.

**lancet** \lan′sət\ [Middle French *lancette* (dim. of Old French *lance,* from L *lancea* a lance, spear, perh. of Celtic origin) a small lance, lancet] A small surgical blade, usually with two honed edges, used for making small drainage incisions. Also *lance.* **abscess l.** A surgical knife with one convex and one concave cutting edge that is used for drainage of an abscess. **spring l.** A surgical blade, usually concealed in a case, that is released and activated by a spring. **thumb l.** A short surgical knife that has a blade which folds back into a metallic sheath.

**lancinating** \lan′sinā′ting\ [L *lancinat(us),* past part. of *lancinare* (akin to *lacer* hewn, mangled) to tear in pieces, lacerate + -ING] Describing a sudden sharp and transient pain.

**Lancisi** [Giovanni Maria *Lancisi,* Italian physician, 1654–1720] Longitudinal nerves of Lancisi. See under NERVES OF LANCISI.

**Landau** [Leopold *Landau,* German gynecologist and obstetrician, 1848–1920] See under REFLEX.

**landmark** A specified and recognized anatomical marking or structure that is used in locating other structures or as a reference point in making measurements.

**Landolt** [Edmund *Landolt,* French ophthalmologist, 1846–1926] **1** See under OPERATION, RING. **2** Landolt ring chart. See under CHART.

**Landor** [J. V. *Landor,* English physician, flourished 20th century] Hawes-Pallister-Landor syndrome. See under STRACHAN-SCOTT SYNDROME.

**Landouzy** [Louis Theophil Joseph *Landouzy,* French physician, 1845–1917] **1** Landouzy-Grasset law. See under LAW. **2** Landouzy-Dejerine atrophy, Landouzy-Dejerine myopathy, Duchenne-Landouzy dystrophy, Dejerine-Landouzy dystrophy, Landouzy's dystrophy, Landouzy-Dejerine dystrophy. See under FACIOSCAPULOHUMERAL MUSCULAR DYSTROPHY. **3** Landouzy's disease. See under ICTERIC LEPTOSPIROSIS.

**Landry** [Jean Baptiste Octave *Landry,* French physician, 1826–1865] **1** Landry-Guillain-Barré syndrome. See under GUILLAIN-BARRÉ SYNDROME. **2** Kussmaul-Landry paralysis, Landry syndrome. See under LANDRY'S PARALYSIS.

**Landsberg** [J. W. *Landsberg,* U.S. hematologist, born 1907] Wintrobe and Landsberg method. See under METHOD.

**Landsteiner** [Karl *Landsteiner,* Austrian-born U.S. pathologist, 1868–1943] **1** Donath-Landsteiner cold autoantibody. See under DONATH-LANDSTEINER ANTIBODY. **2** Donath-Landsteiner syndrome. See under PAROXYSMAL COLD HEMOGLOBINURIA. **3** Donath-Landsteiner test. See under TEST. **4** See under CLASSIFICATION.

**Landström** [John *Landström,* Swedish surgeon, 1869–1910] See under MUSCLE.

**Landzert** [Theodor *Landzert,* German anatomist, died 1889] **1** Landzert's fossa, Gruber-Landzert fossa. See under RECESSUS PARADUODENALIS. **2** Gruber-Landzert fossa. See under FOSSA.

**Lane** [Clayton Arbuthnot *Lane,* British parasitologist active in India, born 1868] Lane method. See under DIRECT CENTRIFUGAL FLOTATION METHOD.

**Lane** [John Edward *Lane,* U.S. dermatologist, 1872–1933] Lane's disease. See under ERYTHEMA PALMARE HEREDITARIUM.

**Lane** [Sir William Arbuthnot *Lane,* English surgeon, 1856–1943] **1** Lane's kink. See under ILEAL KINK. **2** Lane's band. See under GENITOMESENTERIC BAND. **3** Lane plates. See under PLATE.

**Lange** [Carl *Lange,* German physician, born 1883] Lange's reaction, Lange's test. See under COLLOIDAL GOLD TEST.

**Lange** [Carl Georg *Lange,* Danish psychologist, 1834–1900] James-Lange-Sutherland theory. See under JAMES-LANGE THEORY.

**Langenbeck** [Bernhard Rudolph Konrad von *Langenbeck,* German surgeon, 1810–1887] **1** See under TRIANGLE. **2** Langenbeck flap. See under VON LANGENBECK'S BIPEDICLED MUCOPERIOSTEAL FLAP.

**Langendorff** [Oscar *Langendorff,* German physiologist, 1853–1908] Langendorff's method. See under PREPARATION.

**Lange-Nielsen** [Fredrik *Lange-Nielsen*, Norwegian cardiologist, flourished mid-20th century] Jervell and Lange-Nielsen syndrome. See under SYNDROME.

**Langer** [Karl Ritter von *Langer*, Austrian anatomist, 1819–1887] **1** Langer's axillary arch. See under PECTORODORSALIS MUSCLE. **2** Langer's lines. See under CLEAVAGE LINES.

**Langerhans** [Paul *Langerhans*, German pathological anatomist, 1847–1888] **1** Islands of Langerhans. See under ISLETS OF LANGERHANS. **2** Langerhans cell granule. See under GRANULE.

**Langhans** [Theodor *Langhans*, German anatomist, 1839–1915] **1** Langhans layer. See under CYTOTROPHOBLAST. **2** See under STRIA, CELL. **3** Langhans cell. See under LANGHANS GIANT CELL.

**Langley** [John Newport *Langley*, English physiologist, 1852–1925] **1** Langley's nerves. See under PILOMOTOR NERVES. **2** See under GANGLION.

**Langmuir** [Irving *Langmuir*, U.S. chemist, 1881–1957] See under TROUGH.

**language** Any system making use of word symbols to convey meaning to other individuals and, possibly, to influence their behavior. The signals of any language system, whether they are spoken, written, or conveyed by gesture, are learned, and they permit an exchange of information with any other individual who has also learned the rules of that system.

**Lannelongue** [Odilon Marc *Lannelongue*, French surgeon, 1840–1911] **1** Foramina of Lannelongue. See under FORAMEN. **2** Foraminula of Lannelongue. See under FORAMINA VENARUM MINIMARUM CORDIS.

**Lannois** [Maurice *Lannois*, French otorhinolaryngologist, born 1856] Gradenigo-Lannois syndrome. See under GRADENIGO SYNDROME.

**lanolin** A waxy, fatty secretion of the sebaceous glands of the sheep, which is deposited on the wool fibers. It contains about 25–30% water and is used as an ointment base. Also *wool fat*. **anhydrous l.** A yellowish, semisolid fat, obtained from sheep's wool, that is practically insoluble in water but can be mixed with water to form a stable emulsion. It is used as an ointment base. Also *adeps lanae*.

**lanosterol** A sterol originally found in wool fat. It differs from cholesterol by possessing two methyl groups on C-4 and one on C-14, by the absence of a double bond at C-5, and by the presence of two at C-8 and C-24. It is the first steroid made in the pathway by which squalene is converted into sterols in animals. Cycloartenol plays a similar role in plants. It is made by the action of lanosterol synthase on squalene 2,3-epoxide. Also *isocholesterol*.

**lanosterol synthase** The enzyme (EC 5.4.99.7) responsible for the biosynthesis of the steroid ring in animals. It isomerizes squalene 2,3-epoxide with formation of four rings.

**Lanterman** [A. J. *Lanterman*, U.S. anatomist active in France, flourished late 19th century] **1** Schmidt-Lanterman segment. See under MEDULLARY SEGMENT. **2** Lanterman's clefts, Schmidt-Lanterman clefts, incisures of Lanterman-Schmidt. See under SCHMIDT-LANTERMAN INCISURES.

**lanthanum** \lan′thənəm\ Element number 57, having atomic weight 138.9055. It is a soft, silvery white metal, the first member of the lanthanide series of elements. The valence is 3. Lanthanum and its compounds are somewhat toxic. Symbol: La

**lanthopine** A minor alkaloid of opium.

**lanugo** \lanoo′gō\ [L, soft, tender hair or down] The fine downy hairs, devoid of a medulla, that cover the skin of a human fetus, except for the palms and soles, at about midterm. They are mostly shed before birth and are replaced on the trunk and limbs by the fine secondary hairs of the vellus during the first few months after birth, and by longer and coarser terminal hair on the scalp. Also *down*. Adj. lanuginous. • The term *lanugo* is often misused for the vellus hair.

**Lanz** [Otto *Lanz*, Swiss-born surgeon active in the Netherlands, 1865–1935] **1** See under POINT. **2** Lanz line. See under INTERSPINAL LINE.

**LAP** leukocyte alkaline phosphatase.

**lapactic** PURGATIVE.

**lapar-** \lap′ər-\ LAPARO-.

**laparectomy** \lap′ərek′təmē\ [LAPAR- + -ECTOMY] A surgical procedure in which part or all of the abdominal wall is excised and then reconstructed. It is usually performed to correct laxity but may be done because of a neoplasm, inflammation, or trauma.

**laparo-** \lap′ərō-\ [Gk *lapara* the soft part of the body between ribs and hip, flank, loin] A combining form denoting (1) the flank or loin; (2) the abdominal wall. Also *lapar-*.

**laparocele** \lap′ərōsēl′\ VENTRAL HERNIA.

**laparocholecystotomy** \-kō′ləsistät′əmē\ [LAPARO- + CHOLECYSTOTOMY] CHOLECYSTOTOMY.

**laparocolectomy** \-kōlek′təmē\ COLECTOMY.

**laparocolostomy** \-kōläs′təmē\ A colostomy with the opening on the lateral or anterolateral wall of the abdomen.

**laparocolotomy** \-kōlät′əmē\ COLOTOMY.

**laparocystectomy** \-sistek′təmē\ A surgical procedure in which an intra-abdominal cyst is removed by way of an abdominal wall incision.

**laparocystidotomy** \-sis′tidät′əmē\ An incision into the urinary bladder made by a suprapubic approach.

**laparocystotomy** \-sistät′əmē\ [LAPARO- + CYSTOTOMY] SUPRAPUBIC CYSTOTOMY.

**laparoenterostomy** \-en′təräs′təmē\ An enterostomy through the abdominal wall.

**laparoenterotomy** \-en′tərät′əmē\ A surgical incision through the abdominal wall and into the small bowel. Also *celioenterotomy*.

**laparogastroscopy** \-gasträs′kəpē\ An exploratory operation in which the interior of the stomach is inspected after laparogastrotomy.

**laparogastrotomy** \-gasträt′əmē\ A surgical incision through the abdominal wall and into the stomach. Also *celiogastrotomy*.

**laparohepatotomy** \-hep′ətät′əmē\ Incision of the liver through a laparotomy.

**laparoileotomy** \lap′ərō·il′ē·ät′əmē\ Incision of the ileum through a laparotomy.

**laparomyomectomy** \-mī′əmek′təmē\ ABDOMINAL MYOMECTOMY.

**laparomyomotomy** \-mī′əmät′əmē\ [LAPARO- + MYOMOTOMY] CELIOMYOMOTOMY.

**laparonephrectomy** \-nefrek′təmē\ A nephrectomy done via either an abdominal or a lumbar incision.

**laparorrhaphy** \lap′ərôr′əfē\ The repair or strengthening of the abdominal wall by means of sutures. Also *celiorrhaphy, laparorrhaphia*.

**laparoscope** \lap′ərəskōp′\ [LAPARO- + -SCOPE] An endoscope designed for examination of the peritoneal cavity, especially the surface of the liver. Also *peritoneoscope*.

**laparoscopy** \lap′əräs′kəpē\ [LAPARO- + -SCOPY] Endoscopic examination of the peritoneal cavity and surface of accessible abdominal organs by means of a laparoscope. Also *peritoneoscopy*.

**laparosplenotomy** \-splēnät′əmē\ A surgical procedure resecting all or part of the spleen through an abdominal incision. Also *splenolaparotomy*.

**laparotomy** \lap′ərät′əmē\ [LAPARO- + -TOMY] **1** A

surgical incision through the abdominal flank. 2 *Imprecise* CELIOTOMY.

**laparotyphlotomy** \-tiflät′əmē\ Incision of the cecum through a laparotomy.

**lapathin** CHRYSOPHANIC ACID.

**Lapham** [Maxwell Edward *Lapham*, U.S. obstetrician, born 1899] Friedman-Lapham test. See under FRIEDMAN TEST.

**Lapicque** [Louis *Lapicque*, French physiologist, 1866–1952] Lapicque's law. See under ISOCHRONISM.

**lapis** [L, a stone] A stone: used in alchemy for any non-volatile material. **l. albus** Native calcium silicofluoride, or the precipitated compound. **l. calaminaris** CALAMINE. **l. imperialis** SILVER NITRATE. **l. infernalis** SILVER NITRATE. **l. lunaris** SILVER NITRATE.

**Laplace** [Pierre-Simon *Laplace*, French mathematician, astronomer, and physicist, 1749–1827] 1 See under LAW. 2 Laplace-Gauss distribution. See under NORMAL DISTRIBUTION.

**lapsus** \lap′səs\ [L, a fall, slip] A lapse or slip, as of memory. **l. linguae** Slip of the tongue.

**lard** [L *lardum*, also *laridum* the fat of bacon, fat] Purified fat from the omentum of the hog. It has been used in the compounding of ointments, but has been superseded by more stable vehicles. Also *adeps, adeps praeparatus.* **benzoinated l.** ADEPS BENZOINATUS. **leaf l.** Lard prepared from the perirenal fat. **l. oil** An oil obtained from lard that is used for some pharmaceutical purposes.

**lariat** \lar′ē·ət\ A structure that forms during processing of mRNA in which one end of the molecule forms a covalent bond with a nucleotide at a consensus sequence within a transcribed intron, forming a loop with a tail, to resemble a rope lariat. The structure is important in proper splicing of mRNA to the mature molecule that directs translation.

**Larmor** [Sir Joseph *Larmor*, Irish mathematician and physicist, 1857–1942] See under FREQUENCY, EQUATION.

**Laron** [Zvi *Laron*, Israeli pediatric endocrinologist, born 1927] See under DWARF.

**Larrey** [Baron Dominique Jean *Larrey*, French surgeon, 1766–1842] 1 Larrey space, Larrey's cleft. See under MORGAGNI'S FORAMEN. 2 Larrey-Weil disease. See under ICTERIC LEPTOSPIROSIS.

**Larsen** [Christian Magnus Falsen Sinding-*Larsen*, Norwegian physician, 1866–1930] Larsen's disease, Sinding-Larsen-Johansson disease. See under LARSEN-JOHANSSON DISEASE.

**Larsen** [Loren Joseph *Larsen*, U.S. orthopedic surgeon, born 1914] See under SYNDROME.

**Larsson** [Tage Konrad Leopold *Larsson*, Swedish scientist, born 1905] Sjögren-Larsson syndrome. See under SYNDROME.

**larva** \lär′və\ [L (akin to *lar* a tutelary god), a ghost, specter, mask] (*pl.* larvae) 1 A usually motile feeding and developing stage in the life cycle of holometabolous insects which follows the egg stage and precedes the pupa. Larvae of some kinds of insects are known as caterpillars, maggots, grubs, and worms. 2 An early nymphal stage of various hemimetabolous insects and other arthropods, or a morphologically distinct early stage of certain other invertebrates such as helminths, or of vertebrates such as some amphibians and fishes, which in an immature stage of development do not resemble the adult form but which will undergo a metamorphic transformation to assume it. **filariform l.** The infective or third-stage larva of certain parasitic nematodes such as *Strongyloides, Ascaris,* hookworms, and others that have larvae that penetrate or migrate through the body of the host to reach the intestine where the final molt, maturation, and completion of the life cycle occur. **rat-tailed l.** RAT-TAIL MAGGOT.

**larvaceous** \lärvā′shəs\ LARVATE.

**larva currens** \lär′və kur′əns\ A rapidly spreading skin infestation by the larva of *Strongyloides stercoralis,* which produces a rapidly progressing linear urticarial trail in the skin, usually starting at or near the anus. It may be caused by zoonotic species of *Stronglyloides,* such as *S. fuelleborni* in Southeast Asia (from primates) or *S. procyonis* in the United States (from raccoons).

**larvae** \lär′vē\ Plural of LARVA.

**larval** \lär′vəl\ [*larv(a)* + -AL] Pertaining to or resembling larvae.

**larva migrans** \lär′və mī′granz\ A migratory phase of the life cycle of helminths, warble flies, and other parasites. It usually applies to parasites in an abnormal host or site where the wandering is random. Examples are seen in human cutaneous larva migrans by dog or cat hookworm larvae and human visceral larva migrans by dog or cat ascarid larvae. **cutaneous l.** Larva migrans in the skin, as for example the linear eruption caused by hookworm larvae. Also *creeping eruption, dermatitis linearis migrans.* **visceral l.** A disorder caused by visceral migration of the larva of *Toxocara, Toxascaris,* and other nematodes not adapted to man, so the normal migratory pathway from the intestine to liver, heart, lungs, trachea, mouth and back to the intestine is not completed. The worms leave the bloodstream and wander to the viscera until they are encapsulated usually within a few weeks to several months. Dog and cat ascarids are frequently responsible, such as *Toxacara canis, T. cati, Toxascaris leonina.* Clincal features are hypereosinophilia, hepatomegaly, and pneumonitis. Also *nonpatent nematodiasis.*

**larvate** \lär′vāt\ Masked, concealed or hidden. Also *larvaceous.* • Used in describing a symptom, disease, or condition with atypical features

**larvicide** A medication effective against the larval forms of insects. **Panama l.** A larvicidal mixture against mosquito larvae, containing carbolic acid, rosin, and caustic soda.

**larviparous** \lärvip′ərəs\ [*larv(a)* + *i* + L *par(ere)* to bear or beget young + -OUS] Depositing hatched larvae rather than eggs: a characteristic of insects such as certain myiasis flies. See also PUPIPAROUS.

**larviposition** \lär′vēpəzish′ən\ [*larv(a)* + *i* + *(de)position*] The deposition of larvae, particularly in the tissues of a host.

**laryng-** \ləring-\ LARYNGO-.

**laryngeal** \larin′jē·əl\ Pertaining to the larynx.

**laryngectomy** \lar′ənjek′təmē\ [LARYNG- + -ECTOMY] Excision of part or all of the larynx. • When not qualified, the term is widely used to mean total laryngectomy. **frontolateral partial l.** An operation similar to lateral partial laryngectomy employed when the tumor to be excised spreads across the anterior laryngeal commissure to involve the front end of the contralateral vocal cord. **lateral partial l.** Partial laryngectomy for small tumors localized to the membranous part of one vocal cord. The larynx is opened by the laryngofissure approach and the tumor removed with a surrounding margin of healthy tissue. The procedure may also involve the excision of part of the cartilaginous thyroid ala adjacent to the tumor. Also *laryngofissure.* **partial l.** One of a number of varieties of laryngectomy in which a large part of the larynx is spared and the laryngeal airway and, thus, laryngeal voice preserved. **supraglottic l.** HORIZONTAL HEMILARYNGECTOMY. **total l.** Laryngectomy of the most radical kind, necessitating removal of the whole larynx along with a variable amount of the upper trachea and, usually, the hyoid bone and preepiglottic tissues. The establishment of a permanent end tracheostome is an inevitable consequence. The indication in all but the exceptional case is malignant disease of the larynx or laryngopharynx too extensive for more limited procedures. Technical variations, for instance the excision of the homolateral thyroid lobe, may be required by the extent of the disease, which may also determine the need for removal of part of the pharynx (pharyngolaryngectomy) or radical neck dissection for lymph node metastasis.

**laryngismus** \lar′injiz′məs\ [New L, from LARYNG- + L *-ismus* -ISM] LARYNGOSPASM. **l. stridulus** Brief, nocturnal attacks of laryngospasm, usually in children, often waking the patient from sleep. There is neither evidence of other laryngeal abnormality nor, characteristically, of intercurrent disease. Also *false croup, pseudocroup.*

**laryngitis** \lar′ənjitis\ [LARYNG- + -ITIS] Inflammation of the lining of the larynx. The principal symptom is hoarseness. Adj. laryngitic. **acute catarrhal l.** SIMPLE LARYNGITIS. **acute spasmodic l.** LARYNGITIS STRIDULOSA. **atrophic l.** Laryngitis in which the lining of the larynx is dry and crusted and sometimes atrophic. It is a rare disease today, although once common, usually occurring as a complication of atrophic rhinitis or, occasionally, chronic suppurative sinusitis. Also *laryngitis sicca.* **catarrhal l.** Laryngitis characterized by a catarrhal reaction of the mucosa in the absence of other specific features. **chronic hyperplastic l.** A variety of chronic nonspecific laryngitis in which the nonkeratinized squamous epithelium of the vocal cords and often the respiratory epithelium of the vestibular folds have undergone hyperplastic changes often with metaplasia and keratinization. The well-established condition is regarded as precancerous. **chronic nonspecific l.** Laryngitis of a chronic nature which cannot be easily ascribed to a specific cause, such as tuberculosis or syphilis, nor can the manifestations be easily circumscribed, as in the case of polyps or contact pachydermia. Metaplasia and hyperplasia of the laryngeal lining are characteristic and may possibly be caused by vocal abuse or abuse of alcohol and tobacco. Chronic infection elsewhere in the respiratory tract is present in more than half the cases. **diphtheritic l.** LARYNGEAL DIPHTHERIA. **edematous l.** Edema of the larynx which presents as a feature of various types of laryngitis, both infective and noninfective, as well as a complication of major surgery of the floor of the mouth, radiotherapy to the larynx and pharynx, and adjacent severe infection such as Ludwig's angina and peritonsillar abscess. It was once regarded as a separate disease entity. **membranous l.** Laryngitis, usually acute, characterized by pseudomembrane formation and presenting with hoarseness, stridor, and obstruction to the laryngeal airway. The most common cause is laryngeal diphtheria but infection with $\beta$-hemolytic streptococcus or *Pseudomonas aeruginosa* may be responsible. Noninfective causes include inhalation of hot gases by the victims of fires, and of certain poisonous gases. **l. sicca** ATROPHIC LARYNGITIS. **simple l.** Acute infective laryngitis complicating the common upper respiratory tract infections, in particular the common cold. Also *acute catarrhal laryngitis.* **l. stridulosa** Acute laryngitis occurring in children, characterized by brief attacks of laryngospasm that are usually nocturnal. The attacks resolve spontaneously over a short period of time. Also *acute spasmodic laryngitis, spasmodic croup, false croup, pseudocroup.* See also LARYNGISMUS STRIDULUS. **subglottic l.** Laryngitis affecting especially the subglottic larynx, seen particularly in children. Subglottic edema occurs frequently and is responsible for the characteristic respiratory obstruction. **supraglottic l.** Inflammation of the supraglottic larynx, particularly that due to *Haemophilus influenzae* type B. It can occur at any age, complicating *H. influenzae* bacteremia, but it usually and characteristically occurs in childhood. The epiglottis, aryepiglottic folds, and other parts above the vocal cords become greatly swollen and quickly threaten the patient with asphyxia. It responds well to correct antibiotic therapy but intubation or tracheostomy may be urgently required. Also *epiglottitis.* **syphilitic l.** Laryngitis occurring sometimes during the secondary stage of syphilis and, rarely, during the tertiary stage. In secondary syphilis the typical mucous patches may be observed on the vocal cords, epiglottis, or ventricular bands. **tuberculous l.** Laryngitis caused by infection with *Mycobacterium tuberculosis,* still seen as a complication of pulmonary tuberculosis in the many parts of the world where the latter disease remains a major problem. The protean clinical features may cause confusion with other laryngeal granulomata and even carcinoma of the larynx. Also *laryngeal tuberculosis.*

**laryngo-** \ləring′gō-\ [Gk *larynx* (genitive *laryngos*) larynx] A combining form denoting the larynx. Also *laryng-.*

**laryngocele** \ləring′gōsēl′\ [LARYNGO- + -CELE[1]] An air-containing pouch, usually bilateral, formed by the ballooning of a sacklike expansion of the ventricular saccule of the larynx. It is normally present in certain higher primates which are able to distend them at will by an expiratory effort. In man, it occurs rarely and as an occupational hazard, particularly in glassblowers and wind-instrument players. **external l.** The commoner variety of laryngocele that presents intermittently as a swelling in the subhyoid region of the neck as the result of the herniation of the distended ventricular saccule through the thyrohyoid membrane. **internal l.** A rare variety of laryngocele presenting as a cystlike swelling at the entrance to the larynx above the vocal cord, diagnosed by demonstrating on x ray an air-containing sac distensible by the Valsalva maneuver. Also *ventricular laryngocele.*

**laryngofissure** \-fish′ər\ **1** LATERAL PARTIAL LARYNGECTOMY. **2** A surgical approach to the interior of the larynx by a midline incision carried through the cricothyroid membrane and the angle of the thyroid cartilage. Also *laryngofission, median laryngotomy, thyrochondrotomy, thyrofissure.*

**laryngogram** \ləring′gōgram\ **1** Any x-ray film showing details of the larynx, particularly films using contrast techniques. See also LARYNGOGRAPHY. **2** ELECTROLARYNGOGRAM.

**laryngography** \lar′ing·gäg′rəfē\ **1** Radiography, usually contrast radiography, of the larynx. The structures are outlined not only by the air in the larynx and pharynx but also by a radiopaque medium such as Dionosil aqueous injected over the back of the tongue. The larynx may be screened or various films taken at rest or during the Valsalva maneuver. It is of particular value in demonstrating the presence of laryngeal tumors, paralysis, and stenosis. **2** ELECTROLARYNGOGRAPHY.

**laryngohypopharynx** \-hī′pōfar′ingks\ The walls of the pars laryngea pharyngis and the aditus laryngis considered together. *Outmoded.*

**laryngologist** \ler′ing·gäl′əjist\ An otorhinolaryngologist especially interested and experienced in laryngology and, therefore, everything concerned with the voice.

**laryngology** \ler′ing·gäl′əjē\ [LARYNGO- + -LOGY] The branch of otorhinolaryngology concerned particularly with the larynx.

**laryngomalacia** \-məlā′shə\ [LARYNGO- + MALACIA]

A flaccid condition of the supraglottic larynx found in a small proportion of newborn infants and responsible for inspiratory stridor. It tends to improve spontaneously as the child grows. Also *chondromalacia of the larynx*.

**laryngopathy** \lar′ing·gäp′əthē\ [LARYNGO- + -PATHY] Any disease of the larynx.

**laryngopharyngeal** \-fərin′jē·əl\ Pertaining to the laryngopharynx or laryngeal part of the pharynx.

**laryngopharyngectomy** \-far′injek′təmē\ PHARYNGOLARYNGECTOMY.

**laryngopharyngitis** \-far′injī′tis\ Inflammation involving both the larynx and pharynx. The laryngitis occurs as a complication of the pharyngitis. Also *pharyngolaryngitis*.

**laryngopharynx** \-far′ingks\ PARS LARYNGEA PHARYNGIS.

**laryngoplasty** \ləring′gōplas′tē\ [LARYNGO- + -PLASTY] Any operation designed to reconstruct the larynx. It is usually done to improve the airway, as in cases of bilateral laryngeal abductor paralysis.

**laryngorhinology** \-rīnäl′əjē\ RHINOLARYNGOLOGY.

**laryngoscleroma** \-sklirō′mə\ Scleroma of the larynx. It occurs rarely secondary to rhinoscleroma with pharyngeal involvement. Induration rather than ulceration occurs and obstruction to the airway has been reported. Healing with marked scarring and distortions is characteristic as is the case in other granulomatous diseases.

**laryngoscope** \ləring′gəskōp\ [LARYNGO- + -SCOPE] An instrument for inspecting the interior of the larynx. **Macintosh l.** A laryngoscope for tracheal intubation. The curved tongue blade is designed so that the tip comes to rest between the base of the tongue and the epiglottis and is cut away on one side to afford the optimum view of the vocal cords. A lightbulb powered by a battery is located just beyond the midpoint of the blade.

**laryngoscopy** \lar′ing·gäs′kəpē\ [LARYNGO- + -SCOPY] The inspection of the interior of the larynx. Adj. laryngoscopic. **direct l.** Laryngoscopy using a rigid instrument that permits a direct view of the interior of the larynx. **fiberoptic l.** Laryngoscopy using a flexible fiberoptic nasopharyngoscope. This technique is particularly suitable for use on outpatients as an adjunct to indirect laryngoscopy or when the indirect method has proven unsuccessful. **indirect l.** Laryngoscopy using a special mirror held at the back of the mouth so as to reflect light into the interior of the larynx and reflect the image back to the examiner. Also *mirror laryngoscopy*. **suspension l.** A kind of direct laryngoscopy, usually carried out on the anesthetized patient, in which the laryngoscope is held in place mechanically so as to free both hands of the surgeon for any required operative procedure on the interior of the larynx thus exposed.

**laryngospasm** \ləring′gəspazm\ Reflex spasm of the laryngeal sphincter, particularly the glottic sphincter, initiated typically by the threat of inhalation of foreign material into the lower air passages. Thus, secretions, blood, or a foreign body reaching the laryngeal inlet or, especially, the vocal cords will precipitate such spasm. The reflex is particularly brisk in children. It also occurs as a symptom of a number of other diseases, such as tabes dorsalis and tetanus. While the spasm persists the inspiration of air is impossible or very difficult and then accompanied by marked stridor. Also *glottic spasm, laryngismus*.

**laryngostenosis** \-stenō′sis\ LARYNGEAL STENOSIS.

**laryngostomy** \lar′ing·gäs′təmē\ [LARYNGO- + -STOMY] The surgical establishment of an opening into the subglottic larynx maintained by the presence of an oval-section laryngotomy tube for the relief of upper airway obstruction. Although indicated occasionally in an emergency, for the most part laryngostomy has been superseded by tracheostomy or endotracheal intubation.

**laryngostroboscope** \-sträb′əskōp\ A stroboscope adapted for use in laryngoscopy. In particular, it enables the movements of the vocal cords to be studied in detail by showing them in slow motion or arrested in the desired phase.

**laryngostroboscopy** \-strəbäs′kəpē\ Study of the vocal cord in action by indirect laryngoscopy using the laryngostroboscope.

**laryngotome** \ləring′gətōm\ [LARYNGO- + -TOME] An instrument for performing laryngotomy, usually comprising a curved trocar and a cannula of oval cross section.

**laryngotomy** \lar′ing·gät′əmē\ [LARYNGO- + -TOMY] 1 Surgical incision of the larynx. 2 CRICOTHYROTOMY. **inferior l.** CRICOTHYROTOMY. **median l.** LARYNGOFISSURE. **superior l.** Opening of the larynx through the thyrohyoid membrane. This procedure should be properly regarded as a pharyngotomy. Also *subhyoid laryngotomy, thyrohyoid laryngotomy*.

**laryngotracheal** \-trā′kē·əl\ Pertaining to both the larynx and trachea.

**laryngotracheitis** \-trā′kē·ī′tis\ 1 LARYNGOTRACHEOBRONCHITIS. 2 Inflammation of the larynx and trachea.

**laryngotracheobronchitis** \-trā′kē·ōbrängkī′tis\ Inflammation of the larynx, trachea, and bronchial tree but particularly such inflammation occurring in the very young as an acute illness due to one of a number of viruses, especially the parainfluenza virus type 1 and the measles virus. The characteristic slowly progressive respiratory obstruction is due chiefly to subglottic swelling and the tenacious secretions occupying the airways. Also *laryngotracheitis*.

**laryngotracheobronchoscopy** \-trā′kē·ōbräng-käs′kəpē\ The endoscopic examination of the interior of the larynx and of the tracheobronchial tree.

**laryngotracheoscopy** \-trā′kē·äs′kəpē\ The examination of the interior of the larynx and trachea, usually by endoscopic means.

**laryngotracheotomy** \-trā′kē·ät′əmē\ CRICOTRACHEOTOMY.

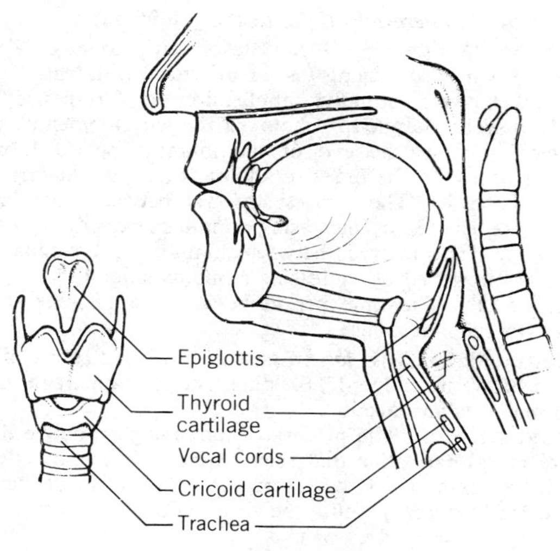


**Larynx**

**larynx** \lar′ingks\ [Gk *larynx,* gen. *laryngos,* the larynx or upper part of the windpipe] [NA] A tubular organ which extends vertically from the root of the tongue opposite the hyoid bone to the trachea and is composed of a framework of cartilages held together by ligaments and membranes which are acted on by both extrinsic and intrinsic muscles. It is covered by skin and fasciae and is situated posteromedial to the infrahyoid muscles and is lined internally by mucous membrane which forms the true and false vocal folds. It lies anterior to the pharynx with which it is continuous through its inlet or aditus. It forms the organ of phonation and serves as an air passage to the lungs and a sphincteric mechanism to guard the trachea. Also *voice box.* **artificial l.** One of a number of mechanical or electronic devices designed to assist with the production of voice after total laryngectomy.

**Lasègue** [Ernest C. *Lasègue,* French physician, 1816–1883] **1** Lasègue's test. See under LASÈGUE SIGN. **2** Lasègue's maneuver. See under NERI SIGN.

**laser** \lā′zər\ [*l(ight) a(mplification by) s(timulated) e(mission of) r(adiation)*] A device that produces an intense, small, nondiverging beam of coherent electromagnetic radiation in the ultraviolet, visible, or infrared regions of the spectrum. It is used in retinal welding, microsurgery, cauterization, tumor therapy, and diagnosis of deep pathologic lesions. Exposure of any part of the body surface to a laser beam can cause injury. The eye is especially vulnerable to its thermal and photochemical effects. **carbon dioxide l.** A laser used to remove lesions of the skin or other superficial organs by burning them away. It operates at a wavelength of 10.6 $\mu$m and provides a very high output of 50–500 watts. **argon l.** A laser using the coherent emission spectrum of light emitted by argon. This light is blue-green and is readily absorbed by red hemoglobin, thus allowing the use of the argon laser in coagulation of bleeding sites in surgery.

**lata** \lä′tə\ [Malay] An acute catatonoid reaction first described in Malaya, consisting of echopraxia, automatic obedience, and coprolalia. It is most frequent in women below the age of 20 years. Also *latah.*

**Latarjet** [André *Latarjet,* French anatomist, born 1877] **1** Hypogastric nerve of Latarjet. See under NERVUS HYPOGASTRICUS DEXTER ET SINISTER. **2** Latarjet's vein. See under VENA PREPYLORICA.

**lat. dol.** *lateri dolenti* (L, to the painful side).

**latency** \lā′tənsē\ **1** A state of being latent or a period during which something (as an infection) is latent. **2** The period between stimulus application and response onset. **3** In psychoanalytic psychology, the developmental period extending from the end of the infantile period (normally about age 5) to the onset of adolescence. Also *latency phase.* **absolute l.** The shortest interval between stimulus and response, elicited by increasing stimulus strength. **reducible l.** The interval between stimulus and response that can be shortened by increasing stimulus magnitude. **total reflex l.** The time period between an afferent stimulus and the reflex response.

**latent** \lā′tənt\ [L *latens,* gen. *latentis,* pres. part. of *latere* to be low, lie hidden] Existing but not apparent; hidden; dormant, as an infection.

**latentiation** The process of modifying an active drug to a chemical derivative that then requires absorption, distribution, or metabolism to restore the active form of the drug. The modification permits the slow release or gradual formation of the active drug *in vivo.*

**laterad** \lat′ərəd\ Toward a side; sidewards; laterally.

**lateral** \lat′ərəl\ [L *lateralis* (from *latus,* gen. *lateris* the side, flank) of or on the side of the body] **1** Of, at, or toward the side. **2** Farther toward the right or left, as compared with other structures or parts that are nearer the midline or median plane of the body. Compare MEDIAL. **left l.** In roentgenography, describing a lateral projection with the patient's left side closest to the film. **right l.** In roentgenography, describing a lateral projection with the patient's right side closest to the film.

**lateralis** \lat′ərā′lis\ Lateral. Also *externus* (outmoded and incorrect).

**laterality** \lat′əral′itē\ [LATERAL + -ITY] A relationship or tendency towards one side. **crossed l.** **1** The predominant control of motor acts by the contralateral cerebral hemisphere. **2** Paired interactions between right and left sides, as associated mirror movements. **dominant l.** Preferential use of right or left for any structure. **mixed l.** Preferential use of opposite sides in various paired structures in a given individual.

**lateralization** \lat′ərəl′īzā′shən\ **1** The tendency to perform an act predominantly on the left or right side of the body. **2** Laterally asymmetrical functional localization in the central nervous system. **sound l.** The ability of the listener to determine the side on which a sound stimulus has occurred. The neurophysiology is complex and different processes are involved for low and high frequency tones, partly as a result of the relation of the wavelength of the sound to the diameter of the head.

**latericumbent** \lat′ərikum′bənt\ In a lateral recumbent position; lying on one's side.

**latero-** \lat′ərō-\ [L *latus* (genitive *lateris*) side, flank] A combining form meaning lateral.

**laterodetrusion** \-ditroo′zhən\ [LATERO- + *detrusion,* from L *detrusus,* past part. of *detrudere* to push downward or outward] The lateral and opening movement of the mandible at the beginning of the masticatory cycle.

**laterodorsal** \-dôr′səl\ DORSOLATERAL.

**lateroduction** \-duk′shən\ Lateral movement, especially of an eye.

**lateroflexion** \-flek′shən\ [LATERO- + FLEXION] A bending to one side of the body.

**laterognathism** \lat′ərōnath′izm\ The deviation of the chin to one side or the other due to underdevelopment or overdevelopment of one side of the mandible.

**lateromarginal** \-mar′jənəl\ Situated on the outer edge or border.

**lateropulsion** \-pul′shən\ Involuntary deviation to one side when walking.

**lateroretrusive** \-ritroo′siv\ Describing movement of the mandible involving lateral and backward components.

**laterosellar** \-sel′ər\ At or to the side of the sella turcica.

**laterotorsion** \-tôr′shən\ A twisting to one side, especially rotation of an eye in a lateral direction from the twelve o'clock meridian.

**laterotrusion** \-troo′zhən\ [LATERO- + TRUSION] Outward transtrusion. Also *side-shift.*

**lateroversion** \-vur′zhən\ A turning or deflection to one side, as of the uterus.

**lathyrism** \lath′irizm\ [*Lathyr(us)* + -ISM] Spastic paraparesis with sensory impairment in the lower limbs, resulting from the ingestion of peas of the genus *Lathyrus.* The condition is seen especially in parts of India. Turkeys fed a diet containing seeds of *L. odoratus* died of hemorrhage because of rupture of the aorta. The active principle is $\beta$-aminoproprionitrile. Adj. lathyritic.

**lathyrogenic** Capable of producing lathyrism.

**latissimocondylaris** \lətis′imōkän′diler′is\ An uncommon variation of the latissimus dorsi muscle, of which a tendinous slip may be inserted into the brachial fascia, triceps muscle, lateral epicondyle of humerus, or other neighboring structures. Often present in some lower animals, the tendinous slip in humans is usually inserted into the brachial fascia or long head of triceps muscle. Also *latissimocondyloideus, dorsoepitrochlearis.*

**latissimus** \lətis′iməs\ Widest; usually used in reference to wide, flat muscles.

**latrodectism** \lat′rōdek′tizm\ [*Latrodect(us)* + -ISM] Poisoning by the venom of spiders of the genus *Latrodectus.* The most dangerous is the black widow. The bite produces localized pain, muscle spasms, and paresthesia. Severe poisoning may result in coma, respiratory paralysis, and cardiovascular collapse.

***Latrodectus*** \lat′rōdek′təs\ A genus of poisonous spiders of the family Theridiidae, the comb-footed spiders, of cosmopolitan distribution. ***L. mactans*** The black widow spider, a highly venomous species found in the southern U.S., and in warmer parts of the Americas and in similar climatic zones of other continents. The fully-grown female has a bright red hourglass-shaped mark on the ventral side of the abdomen. The male lacks this mark and is not venomous. The toxic fraction of the venom of the female is a neurotoxic labile protein which causes ascending motor paralysis and destruction of peripheral nerve endings.

**LATS** long-acting thyroid stimulator.

**lattice** / **space l.** A three-dimensional grid or other orderly structure, as that which characterizes the arrangement of atoms in a crystal.

**latus** \lā′təs\ [L, the flank] (*pl.* latera.) The side of the trunk between the lowest rib and the iliac crest; the flank.

**Latzko** [Wilhelm *Latzko,* Austrian gynecologist and obstetrician, 1863–1945] See under OPERATION, SECTION.

**Lauber** [Hans *Lauber,* Swiss-born ophthalmologist active in Austria, born 1876] Lauber's disease. See under FUNDUS ALBIPUNCTATUS.

**laudanidine** The *l*-isomer of laudanine, an alkaloid from opium.

**laudanine** $C_{20}H_{25}NO_4$. The *dl*-forms of a minor alkaloid from opium that remain in solution in the usual process for extracting morphine from opium.

**laudanum** \lô′dənəm\ [New L (alter. of L *ladanum,* from Gk *ladanon,* a kind of gum resin), a name given by Paracelsus to a remedy of secret ingredients, prob. including opium] OPIUM TINCTURE.

**laugh** 1 To produce laughter. 2 LAUGHTER. **canine l.** RISUS SARDONICUS. **sardonic l.** RISUS SARDONICUS.

**laughter** The sound and accompanying facial and other movements that express amusement, exultation, or scorn. It is prompted by amusement, exultation, scorn, or nervous stimulation such as occurs in tickling. Also *laugh, risus.*

**Laugier** [Stanislas *Laugier,* French surgeon, 1799–1872] See under SIGN.

**Laumonier** [Jean-Baptiste-Philippe-Nicolas-René *Laumonier,* French surgeon, 1749–1818] Laumonier's ganglion. See under INFERIOR CAROTID GANGLION.

**Launois** [Pierre Emile *Launois,* French physician, 1856–1914] 1 Launois syndrome. See under PITUITARY GIGANTISM. 2 Launois-Cléret syndrome. See under FRÖHLICH SYNDROME.

**Laurence** [John Zacharias *Laurence,* English physician, 1830–1874] Laurence-Moon syndrome. See under SYNDROME.

**Laurens** [Georges *Laurens,* French surgeon, flourished 20th century] See under OPERATION.

**laureth 9** A mixture of polyethylene glycol monododecyl ethers with an average value of nine ethylene oxide groups per molecule. The compound is used as a pharmaceutical aid and as a spermicide.

**lauric acid** $CH_3—[CH_2]_{10}—COOH$. Dodecanoic acid. It is one of the fatty acids commonly found in natural fats such as butter.

**Lauth** [Ernest Alexandre *Lauth,* French anatomist and physiologist, 1803–1837] Lauth's canal. See under SINUS VENOSUS SCLERAE.

**Lauth** [Thomas *Lauth,* German anatomist and surgeon, 1758–1826] 1 See under LIGAMENT. 2 Lauth's ligament. See under LIGAMENTUM ARCUATUM PUBIS.

**LAV** lymphadenopathy-associated virus.

**lavage** \ləväzh′\ [French (from *laver* to wash, from L *lavare* to wash) a washing, cleaning by irrigation] 1 The washing out, especially by irrigation, of a hollow organ, or cavity, such as the stomach, bowel, or bladder. Also *lavation, lavement* (obs.). 2 The purification of a solid, liquid, or gas by means of a substance or solution that is not itself contaminated and will not dissolve or decompose the substance to be purified. **bronchoalveolar l.** A technique for obtaining cells from bronchioles and alveoli of the lungs by instillation of sterile fluid through a fiberoptic bronchoscope into a lobe and subsequent removal by suction. The technique may be of diagnostic value or be used to evaluate the effectiveness of treatment. **gastric l.** A procedure used to remove the contents of the stomach, as for example after ingestion of a toxic substance. **intestinal l.** A form of dialysis in which fluids are instilled and withdrawn in the small intestine in order to remove waste products from the blood across the intestinal mucosa. **peritoneal l.** The instillation and retrieval of a physiologic solution in the peritoneal cavity in order to examine the effluent for abnormal cells, bacteria, or evidence of internal bleeding following trauma.

**lavation** \lavā′shən\ 1 An act of washing or cleansing. 2 LAVAGE.

**lavender** *Lavandula officinalis,* a perennial shrub of the Labiatae family. The flowers are the source of lavender oil, a volatile oil that contains linalyl acetate, geraniol, linalool, limonene, pinene, and cineol. It is used in perfumes, as a flavoring, as a carminative and aromatic, and as an insect repellent.

**Laveran** [Charles Louis Alphonse *Laveran,* French army surgeon, 1845–1922] Laveran bodies. See under BODY.

***Laverania*** \lav′ərā′nē·ə\ A former genus, now considered a subgenus, that includes *Plasmodium falciparum* as opposed to the other human plasmodia. ***L. falcipara*** *PLASMODIUM FALCIPARUM.*

# law

**law** [Old English *lagu*] A description of phenomena so thoroughly tested and accepted that it can be relied on as a principle governing like phenomena. See also entries under PRINCIPLE and RULE. **Adrian-Bronk l.** ALL-OR-NONE LAW. **all-or-none l.** The response of muscle and nerve cells to stimuli at or above threshold is maximal, but to stimuli below threshold is nil, i.e., no response of intermediate level is obtainable by subthreshold stimuli. The law is applicable to individual neurons or muscle cells, but not to the aggregate comprising a nerve or muscle. Also *all-or-nothing law of excitation, Adrian-Bronk law, Bowditch's law.* **antisubstitution l.'s** Regulations concerning the substitution of generic, alternative drugs for proprietary or brand name drugs by the pharmacist. If the physician specifies a proprietary drug and adds "DAW" (Dispense as Written) in writing on the prescription, the pharmacist is forbidden in most jurisdictions to substitute a generic drug. **Arndt's l.** The doctrine that physiological activity is excited by weak stimuli, optimal with moderate stimuli, and curtailed by strong stimuli. Also *Arndt-Schultz law.* **l.'s of articulation** Rules for setting up teeth in dentures to ensure occlusal balance. **Avogadro's l.** Equal volumes of different gases, observed at the same temperature and pressure, contain the same number of molecules. **Babinski's l.** A law defining the response to the galvanic test of normal subjects compared with those with labyrinthine disease. The normal subject inclines to the side of the positive pole, whereas someone with labyrinthine disease, tending to fall to one side, will incline that way on galvanic stimulation. Where the disease has destroyed the labyrinth, there will be no response. *Outmoded.* **Baer's l.** LAW OF VON BAER. **Baumès l.** COLLES LAW. **Beer's l.** The law relating the intensity, *I*, of light or other electromagnetic radiation to the length *l* of absorbing solution through which the radiation has passed and the concentration, *c*, of absorbing solute. It states that $\log(I/I_0) = \epsilon{\cdot}l{\cdot}c$, where $I_0$ is the incident intensity, and $\epsilon$ is an empirical constant, the molar absorption coefficient. The law only holds for monochromatic radiation. Also *Beer-Lambert law.* **Behring's l.** Immunity may be passively transferred to a nonimmune person by injection of transfusion of serum or blood from an immunized person. **Bell-Magendie l.** The concept that the dorsal spinal roots conduct sensory activity toward the spinal cord and the ventral roots conduct to muscle. Also *Bell's law, Magendie's law.* **Bergonié-Tribondeau l.** A law expressing the mode of variation of tissue sensitivity to x rays: the sensitivity of a cell to x rays is directly proportional to its ability to reproduce and inversely proportional to its degree of differentiation. **biogenetic l.** RECAPITULATION THEORY. **Bowditch's l.** ALL-OR-NONE LAW. **Boyle's l.** The volume of a fixed mass of gas is inversely proportional to the pressure on it, provided that the temperature remains constant. Also *Mariotte's law.* **Briggs l.** A Massachusetts state law establishing compulsory and impartial psychiatric examination of all those defendants either accused of capital crimes, previously convicted of more than one other offense, or previously convicted of a felony. The examination is conducted by a panel of experts who make determinations regarding mental status and the presence or absence of mental disorders which could exempt defendants from criminal responsibility. **Broadbent's l.** Lesions of the corticospinal tract in the cerebral hemisphere produce less marked paralysis of contralateral muscles (such as those of the face) which are usually involved in simultaneous bilateral movements than of muscles which are more often unilateral (those of the limbs). **Buhl-Dittrich l.** The assumption that in every instance of acute miliary tuberculosis there is a preexisting caseous focus. **Bunge's l.** The secretory cells of the mammary gland take minerals from the plasma in the exact proportion necessary for the optimum development of the offspring. **Cannon's l. of denervation** When an efferent neuron is destroyed, hypersensitivity to the neurotransmitter substance which it normally releases develops in the denervated target organ; the hypersensitivity of denervation. **Charles l.** The volume of a fixed weight of a gas at constant pressure is directly proportional to its absolute temperature. **Colles l.** A child with congenital syphilis does not infect its mother. It became clear later that the reason for the apparent paradox is that the mother was already infected and passed the disease to the child. Also *Baumès law, Colles-Baumès law.* **Collin's l.** After removal of a tumor in infancy or childhood, if metastasis or recurrence does not develop within a period equal to the age of the patient plus nine months, the risk of such a development is small. **l. of contrary innervation** Living functions are maintained by the constant opposing forces of activation and inhibition; the concept of dualistic innervation. Also *Meltzer's law.* **Courvoisier's l.** A principle differentiating physical findings in benign and malignant causes of obstructive jaundice: obstruction of the common bile duct by a gallstone rarely results in dilatation of the gallbladder, whereas obstruction due to cancer or other causes commonly results in gallbladder dilatation. See also COURVOISIER SIGN. **Dale-Feldberg l.** Each neuron releases only a single neurotransmitter from all its terminals. This law has been challenged in the light of recent data. **Dalton's l.** In a mixture of gases, the total pressure is equal to the sum of the partial pressures of the constituents. **Deiter's l.** The doctrine, first enunciated in 1865, that all nerve fibers are long processes of nerve cells. **l. of denervation** See under CANNON'S LAW OF DENERVATION. **l. of diffusion** **1** The principle that the diffusion rate of a substance is a function of the difference in concentration between two given points. **2** The principle that a central neural process can be broadly distributed in its effects. **l. of dissolution** JACKSON'S LAW. **Donders l.** The amount of cyclotorsion of the eye at any given line of fixation of the eyes with respect to the head is always the same regardless of the manner of adoption of that line of fixation. **DuBois-Reymond's l.** The principle that the rate of change rather than the absolute magnitude of an electrical stimulus determines the excitability threshold of a muscle or nerve. Also *law of excitation.* **Edinger's l.** Neuronal functioning enhances growth, but if not sustained or excessive can lead to atrophy and degeneration. **l. of effect** The empirical generalization that a behavioral response which leads to a successful outcome is associated more rapidly to the stimuli which accompany or immediately precede it, and that learning is slow or does not occur at all if the response to such stimuli is followed by an annoying or unsuccessful outcome. **Einthoven's l.** The potential in lead II of the electrocardiogram is equal to the arithmetic sum of the potentials from leads I and III. Lead I is measured between the left arm and the right arm, lead II between the left leg and the right arm, and lead III between the left leg and the left arm. See also STANDARD LEAD. **Ewald's l.'s** Two laws defining the effect of endolymph flow in the semicircular canals of the inner ear on reflex movements of the head and eyes. The first is that the movement of the endolymph in the horizontal semicircular canal causes a slow movement of the eyes or head in the direction of the endolymph current, and the second is that in the horizontal canal the current towards the ampulla is a stronger stimulus than the current away from the ampulla. **l. of excitation** DUBOIS-REYMOND'S LAW. **l. of exponential decay** A law expressing the relationship of radioactive decay to time: for any radioactive nuclide, the change in activity can be expressed by the relation $A_t = A_o e^{-\lambda t}$ where $A_t$ is the activity remaining from an initial activity $A_o$ after a time t, and $\lambda$ is the fractional decay per unit time, known as the decay constant. **l. of facilitation** Impulse activity over a synaptic pathway by repetition. **Faget's l.** Lack of correlation between body temperature and heart rate in yellow fever. There is either a bradycardia associated with a constant temperature, or a normal heart rate with a rising temperature. A similar dissociation may occur in *Salmonella typhi* infections. Also *Faget sign*. **Farr's l.** The statement that "subsidence is a property of all zymotic diseases," meaning that a curve representing the incidence of an epidemic disease rises steeply at first, levels off somewhat as it nears its peak, and falls more steeply than it rose. **Fechner's l.** The principle that the magnitude of sensation increases logarithmically with stimulus intensity. Also *range of sensibility*. **Ferry-Porter l.** The critical frequency of a flickering light, above which the flickering is no longer perceptible, is directly proportional to the logarithm of the light intensity. **Fildes l.** A syphilitic reagin in the blood of a newborn infant is diagnostic of syphilis in the mother. **l. of filial regression** GALTON'S LAW OF REGRESSION. **Fitz l.** A clinical principle for diagnosis of acute pancreatitis: acute pancreatitis should be strongly suspected when a previously healthy person experiences sudden onset of severe epigastric pain, vomiting, and prostration which is followed within a day by abdominal distension, tympany, and guarding, in the presence of a slight fever. **Flatau's l.** The principle that the longer ascending and descending tracts of the spinal cord tend to be displaced peripherally by shorter axons arriving or terminating at other levels. **Flechsig's myelogenetic l.** MYELOGENETIC LAW. **Fuerbringer's l.** The developmental origin of a muscle can be determined from its nerve supply based on the fundamental pattern of innervation of muscles established in the embryo. **Galton's l. of regression** A principle of quantitative genetics that holds the average value of a given multifactorial trait in offspring approaches the mean of the trait in the parents. Also *Galton's law, law of filial regression, law of regression*. **Gay-Lussac's l.** At constant pressure the volume of a fixed mass of gas increases by the same fraction for each degree rise in temperature. **Geiger-Nuttall l.** A rule referring to radioactive disintegration by alpha emission: in any radioactive series, the logs of the ranges of the alpha particles are linearly related to the logs of the decay constants. **Giraud-Teulon l.** The perceived location of a binocularly seen image is at the intersection of the projection of the visual axes from the corresponding retinal points that are stimulated. **Gompertz l.** The principle that there is a positive correlation that can be quantified between the probability of death from a disease and increasing age. **Goodell's l.** GOODELL SIGN. **Good Samaritan l.** Any law designed to shield from subsequent legal action those who voluntarily try to help a victim of an accident or illness in an emergency. The legislation is intended to encourage citizens to help strangers in distress. Most states of the United States have enacted such legislation. A term used chiefly in the U.S. **Graham's l.** The rate of diffusion of a gas is inversely proportional to the square root of its density. **Grasset's l.** LANDOUZY-GRASSET LAW. **l. of gravitation** See under NEWTON'S LAW OF GRAVITATION. **Gudden's l.** Upon division of an axon, some degeneration of the nerve fiber spreads centripetally towards the neuronal cell body. **Gull-Toynbee l.** In mastoiditis, intracranial spread of infection usually involves the cerebellum, whereas in otitis media, which particularly involves the tympanic antrum, upward spread into the temporal lobe is more common. Also *Toynbee's law*. **Gunn's l.** To reduce a dislocation, the joint must be placed as at the time of the injury. A force can then be applied in the direction opposite to that of the dislocating force. **Haeckel's l.** RECAPITULATION THEORY. **Haldane's l.** A principle of genetics that pertains to hybrid offspring of two species. If one sex of the hybrids is sterile or absent, then that sex is heterogametic. **Hardy-Weinberg l.** A mathematical formulation of the relationship between allele frequency and genotype frequency at genetic equilibrium in a large, randomly breeding population not subject to such influences as mutation, drift, and migration that disturb equilibrium. If the frequencies of alleles A and a are $p$ and $q$, respectively, and if $p + q = 1$ at equilibrium, the frequencies of genotypes AA, Aa, and aa are $p^2$, $2pq$, and $q^2$, respectively. **l. of the heart** STARLING'S LAW. **Hecker's l.** With each successive delivery of a multipara, the infant's weight tends to exceed that of its immediate predecessor by about 200 grams. **Hellin's l.** A statement of the statistical probability of multiple pregnancies: about one in 89 pregnancies results in twins. For triplets, the ratio is one in $89^2$, and for each higher order the probability decreases by a factor of 89. Also *Hellin-Zeleny law*. **Henry's l.** The weight of a gas dissolved in a liquid is directly proportional to the pressure of that gas. **Heymans l.** A simultaneous stimulus of vision will proportionately increase the threshold of a visual stimulus. **Hilton's l.** The principle that a nerve trunk supplying a joint also contains axons innervating the muscles acting upon that joint and the skin overlying the articular insertions of those muscles. **l. of independent assortment** See under MENDEL'S LAWS. **l. of the intestines** The physiologic principle that explains the coordinated caudad progression of intestinal contents: the presence of a bolus in the intestine induces contraction cephalad and relaxation caudad to it. **l. of inverse square** A rule expressing the effect of distance on x-ray or gamma ray intensity: the intensity of radiation emitted from a point source varies inversely as the square of the distance from that source. **l. of isochronism** ISOCHRONISM. **Jackson's l.** Those cerebral functions which are the last to be acquired in the course of evolution are the first to be lost when the cerebral cortex is damaged, and they are last to reappear during recovery. Also *law of dissolution, Jackson's rule*. **Kahler's l.** The successive addition of dorsal root fibers in the dorsal column results in a somatotopic pattern wherein each successive rostral spinal input forms a mediolateral sequence by adding to the lateral surface of the tract. **Koch's l.** The rule that four conditions must be satisfied to establish the causative organism of a specific disease: the organism must be present in every case of the disease; the organism must be isolated and grown in pure culture; the pure culture must produce the disease when it is inoculated into a susceptible animal; and the organism must be recovered from the infected animal and grown again in pure culture. Also *Koch's postulates, law of specificity of bacteria*. **Lambert's cosine l.** A law expressing the mode of variation of radiation intensity for parallel rays on an absorbing surface: the intensity varies as the cosine of the angle of incidence. **Lambert-Holzknecht l.** The basic principle of superficial radiotherapy: in order to obtain a homogeneous dose on the surface of an entire area of irradiated field, the source-skin distance must be at least equal to if not greater than twice the greatest diameter of the field. **Landouzy-Grasset l.** Where there is a unilateral cerebral lesion, the head turns towards the side of the lesion in a case of flaccid hemiplegia, and towards the side of the affected limbs in a case of spastic hemiplegia. *Seldom used*. Also *Grasset's law*. **Lapicque's l.** ISOCHRONISM. **Laplace's l.** The transmural pressure in a free sphere or cylinder is directly proportional to the circumferential tension in the wall and inversely proportional to the radius, the factor of proportionality for tension being 2 for a sphere and unity for a cylinder. **Leopold's l.** A law expressing a relation between the configuration of the oviducts and implantation: with posterior uterine wall implantation of the placenta, the oviducts curve anteriorly, while with anterior wall implantation the oviducts turn backwards and are parallel to the body axis when the mother is recumbent. **Levret's l.** In cases of placenta previa, the umbilical cord is usually inserted marginally. **Listing's l.** When the fixation of the eye changes, the angle of rotation in the new position is the same as if the eye had arrived at this position by turning on a fixed axis perpendicular to the original and new positions of the line of fixation. **Louis's l.** The propositions that pulmonary tuberculosis usually originates in the left lung, and that tuberculosis in any part of the body is accompanied by localization in the lung. **Magendie's l.** BELL-MAGENDIE LAW. **Mariotte's l.** BOYLE'S LAW. **Meltzer's l.** LAW OF CONTRARY INNERVATION. **Mendel's l.'s** A set of three principles of genetics. The first law, known as the principle of uniformity in $F_1$, holds that, in a mating between one parent having a dominant phenotype due to homozygosity for an allele and the other parent having a recessive phenotype controlled by a different allele at the same locus, all offspring will be heterozygotes and express the dominant phenotype. This uniformity is independent of which parent was dominant and which recessive. The second law, the principle of segregation, holds that alleles separate, or segregate, at meiosis and are carried in different gametes. The third law, the principle (or law) of independent assortment, holds that the allele pairs of unlinked loci are transmitted to gametes, or assorted, independently. Also *mendelian law.* **Meyer's l.** The internal structure of a mature bone provides the greatest resistance with the least possible amount of material. **Müller's l.** LAW OF SPECIFIC IRRITABILITY. **Müller-Haeckel l.** RECAPITULATION THEORY. **myelogenetic l.** The order in which nerve fibers become myelinated is determined by the order in which they appear phylogenetically and become functional. The earliest to myelinate are ventral nerve root fibers, then dorsal root fibers, and central nervous system tract fibers later on. Pyramidal tract fibers myelinate late, about the first or second year after birth in man. Also *Flechsig's myelogenetic law.* **Naegeli's l.** The proposition that a disease with eosinophilic leukocytes present in half-normal, normal, or increased numbers cannot be typhoid fever. The presence of even a small number of eosinophils makes a diagnosis of typhoid questionable. **Nernst's l.** The threshold for electrical excitation of muscle varies in proportion to the square root of stimulus frequency. **Newton's l. of gravitation** The principle that two bodies of matter attract each other with a force proportional to the product of their masses and inversely proportional to the square of the distance between them. **Nysten's l.** Rigor mortis develops first in the masticatory muscles and then sequentially in the musculature of the neck, upper extremities, trunk, and finally the lower extremities. **Ohm's l.** The voltage across a resistor is equal to the product of the magnitude of the current flowing through it and a property of the resistor called resistance. **Pajot's l.** A law explaining the manner of presentation of the fetus during labor: the shape of a cavity governs to some extent the position of an object within it, especially if the contained object is of a sizable mass. The law explains why a vertex presentation of a fetus is the usual one. **l. of parsimony** OCCAM'S RAZOR. **Poiseuille's l.** The rate of flow of liquid in a tube is directly proportional to the pressure drop along the tube and to the fourth power of the radius of the tube, and is inversely proportional to the length of the tube and to the viscosity of the fluid. Also *Poiseuille's equation.* **Profeta's l.** A clinically syphilis-free baby born of a syphilitic mother is immune to the disease. This was later refuted when it was found that the child had been infected from birth but the infection was in a latent or unrecognized form. **psychophysical l.** 1 WEBER-FECHNER LAW. 2 The subjective magnitude of each sensation is a specific power (i.e., an exponential) function of stimulus magnitude. **l. of referred pain** The doctrine that referred pain can only arise from excitation of nociceptor axons. **l. of regression** GALTON'S LAW OF REGRESSION. **l. of relativity** The relationship of altering subjective sensation magnitude by comparing simultaneous versus successive stimuli of the same magnitude. **Rosenbach's l.** Extensor muscles of the limbs are involved before the flexor muscles in disorders of spinal anterior horn cells or peripheral nerves. **Schroeder van der Kolk's l.** In a mixed peripheral nerve, sensory fibers are distributed to regions moved by motor fibers of the same nerve. Also *van der Kolk's law.* **l. of segregation** See under MENDEL'S LAWS. **Semon's l.** A law purporting to explain the inconstant position assumed by the vocal cords when their motor nerve supply is affected by disease or injury: in progressive organic lesions of the motor nerve supply of the intrinsic laryngeal muscles, the function of abduction is lost before that of adduction. **Sherrington's l.** RECIPROCAL INNERVATION. **l. of specific energies** LAW OF SPECIFIC IRRITABILITY. **l. of specific irritability** The doctrine proposed by Johannes Müller that each nerve is excited via sense organs responsive to a specific form of energy, and that its excitation, because of its connections, can only give rise to one modality of sensation regardless of whether the nerve is electrically or mechanically excited, e.g., excitation of the optic nerve by any means can only lead to visual sensory impressions. Also *doctrine of specific nerve energies, Müller's law, specific irritability, specific nerve energy, law of specific energies.* **l. of specificity of bacteria** KOCH'S LAW. **Starling's l.** As a general rule, the energy of contraction of cardiac muscle fibers is proportional to their length at the start of contraction. Also *law of the heart.* **Teevan's l.** Fractures of bones occur in lines of extension and in the line of compression. **Toynbee's l.** GULL-TOYNBEE LAW. **van der Kolk's l.** SCHROEDER VAN DER KOLK'S LAW. **Virchow's l.** Tumor cells are derived from preexisting normal cells. **l. of von Baer** The concept of embryogenic recapitulation according to which the forms of higher animals pass during their development through stages recalling those of lower forms. Also *Baer's law.* • K. E. von Baer (1792-1876) was the father of modern embryology. He discovered the mammalian ovum in 1827 and described many embryologic structures, including the germ layers. **Vulpian's l.** When a part of the brain is destroyed, its functions may be adopted by the surviving parts. **Waller's l.** If sensory fibers are divided in a spinal root proximal to the ganglion, the fibers between the lesion and the ganglion remain intact while those between the lesion and the spinal cord degenerate. Also *wallerian law.* **Weber's l.** The smallest discriminable intensity increment is a fixed fraction of the comparison stimulus magnitude for all sensory systems, i.e., $\Delta I/I$-constant. **Weber-Fechner l.** For any sensory system the incremental threshold changes in relation to the background intensity in such a way that the ratio of increment ($\Delta I$) to the background intensity (I) is always constant. Also *psychophysical law.* **Wien's displacement l.** A law expressing the relationship of the wavelength of maximal intensity to the temperature of an object capable of absorbing and emitting radiations of all wavelengths: the wavelength of maximal intensity becomes shorter as the temperature increases. Wavelength times temperature equals a constant: 0.2898 cm-deg. **Wolff's l.** The internal structure and external shape of a bone develop in response to the change in function and to the forces acting upon it.

**Lawrence** [Robert Daniel *Lawrence, English physician, flourished 20th century*] **1** Lawrence-Seip syndrome, Seip-Lawrence syndrome. See under SEIP SYNDROME. **2** Lawrence syndrome. See under ACQUIRED GENERALIZED LIPODYSTROPHY.

**lawrencium** \lôren′sē·əm\ A synthetic element of the actinide series, having atomic number 103 and mass number 257. Several isotopes have been reported, the maximum half-life being 35 seconds. Symbol: Lr

**lawsone** \lô′sōn\ $C_{10}H_6O_3$. 2-hydroxy-1,4-naphthoquinone. An agent isolated from the leaves of *Lawsonia inermis* that has the ability to act as a sunscreen.

**laxation** \laksā′shən\ [L *laxatio* (from *laxatus,* past part. of *laxare* to loosen, disengage, deliver) a loosening, relaxing] DEFECATION.

**laxative** \lak′sətiv\ [Med L *laxativus* (from L *laxatus,* past part. of *laxare* to loosen + *-ivus* -IVE) loosening, lessening. See also LAXATOR.] **1** Tending to promote the onset of defecation; stimulating a bowel movement. **2** A laxative agent; a mild cathartic.

**laxator** \laksā′tər\ [L *laxat(us)* (past part. of *laxare* to enlarge, widen, loosen, slacken, relax; Gk *lagaroun* to become slack, loose) enlarged, widened, loosened, freed + -OR] Something that loosens or relaxes. An outmoded term in anatomy.

**laxity** \lak′sitē\ [L *laxit(as)* (from *lax(us)* slack, loose, spacious + *-itas* -ITY) spaciousness, wideness, looseness + -Y] The capability of either normal free motion or greater than normal motion, as of a joint; looseness. **congenital l. of ligaments** A familial disorder, often observed in families of contortionists in whom a remarkable range of movement at many joints is possible, which is believed to be due to ligamentous laxity present from birth.

# layer

**layer** [Middle English *leyer,* from *leyen* to lay] A sheet of tissue of more or less uniform thickness, commonly one of several superimposed sheets; a lamina or a stratum. **l. I** STRATUM MOLECULARE. **l. II** EXTERNAL GRANULAR LAYER OF CEREBRUM. **l. III** LAYER OF SMALL PYRAMIDAL CELLS. **l. IV** INTERNAL GRANULAR LAYER. **l. V** INTERNAL PYRAMIDAL LAYER. **l. VI** MULTIFORM LAYER. **adamantine l.** ENAMEL. **ameloblastic l.** A layer of cells which are derived from the inner enamel epithelium and which produce the enamel of a tooth. Also *enamel layer.* **anterior elastic l.** LAMINA LIMITANS ANTERIOR CORNEAE. **anterior limiting l. of iris** FACIES ANTERIOR IRIDIS. **anterior l. of the rectus abdominis sheath** LAMINA ANTERIOR VAGINAE MUSCULI RECTI ABDOMINIS. **Baillarger's l.** A horizontal band of myelinated fibers in the internal granular layer of the cerebral neocortex, often called the inner line of Baillarger. See also BAILLARGER'S LINES. **basal l.** **1** COMPLEXUS BASALIS CHOROIDEAE. **2** STRATUM BASALE ENDOMETRII. **basal l. of epidermis** A single layer of columnar cells that form the deepest layer of the germinative part of the epidermis. The cells are perpendicular to a basement membrane and contain mitoses and occasional pigment cells or chromatocytes. **basement l.** BASEMENT MEMBRANE. **Bekhterev's l.** A narrow band or plexus of horizontal myelinated fibers at the margin of the external granular and external pyramidal layers (layers II and III) of the cerebral cortex. Also *line of Kaes* (outmoded), *Bekhterev's band* (outmoded), *band of Kaes-Bekhterev* (outmoded), *Kaes feltwork, layer of Kaes-Bekhterev, supraradial plexus, stria kaesbekhterevi, stripe of Kaes-Bekhterev.* **blastodermic l.** GERM LAYER. **Bowman's l.** LAMINA LIMITANS ANTERIOR CORNEAE. **Bruch's l.** COMPLEXUS BASALIS CHOROIDEAE. **buffy l.** BUFFY COAT. **cambium l.** **1** A condensation of loose connective tissue at its interface with a different layer or structure. **2** STRATUM OSTEOGENETICUM. **l.'s of cerebellar cortex** The laminar pattern found in the superficial part of the cerebellum, comprising an outer molecular layer, a Purkinje cell layer, and a broad granule cell layer containing a variety of cell types. These layers overlie the white matter, which is devoid of neuron cell bodies. **choriocapillary l.** LAMINA CHOROIDOCAPILLARIS. **circular l. of eardrum** STRATUM CIRCULARE MEMBRANAE TYMPANI. **circular l. of muscular tunic of colon** STRATUM CIRCULARE TUNICAE MUSCULARIS COLI. **circular l. of muscular tunic of rectum** STRATUM CIRCULARE TUNICAE MUSCULARIS RECTI. **circular l. of muscular tunic of small intestine** STRATUM CIRCULARE TUNICAE MUSCULARIS INTESTINI TENUIS. **circular l. of muscular tunic of stomach** STRATUM CIRCULARE TUNICAE MUSCULARIS GASTRICAE. **circular l. of tympanic membrane** STRATUM CIRCULARE MEMBRANAE TYMPANI. **claustral l.** *Outmoded* CLAUSTRUM. • It is so named because the claustrum was once believed to constitute a separate layer of cortex. **clear l. of skin** STRATUM LUCIDUM EPIDERMIDIS. **columnar l.** **1** STRATUM NEUROEPITHELIALE RETINAE. **2** MANTLE LAYER. **compact l.** STRATUM COMPACTUM ENDOMETRII. **cortical l.** CORTEX. **cremasteric l.** CREMASTERIC COAT OF TESTIS. **cutaneous l. of tympanic membrane** STRATUM CUTANEUM MEMBRANAE TYMPANI. **cuticular l.** In the skin, a single layer of scaly cells with atrophic nuclei that is closely applied to the outside of the hair root. Also *epidermicula.* **deep l. of triangular ligament** FASCIA DIAPHRAGMATIS UROGENITALIS SUPERIOR. **deep l. of urogenital diaphragm** FASCIA DIAPHRAGMATIS UROGENITALIS SUPERIOR. **dense l.** GLOMERULAR BASEMENT MEMBRANE. **dermic l.** STRATUM CUTANEUM MEMBRANAE TYMPANI. **enamel l.** AMELOBLASTIC LAYER. **ependymal l.** An internal layer of cells of the primitive neural tube bounding the central canal. The ependymal cells abut against an internal limiting membrane next to the canal while their processes extend peripherally. The thick pseudostratified epithelium present in the recently closed neural tube is known as the neuroepithelial layer. Later on the mantle and marginal layers or zones will appear, to give rise to the grey and white matter. Also *ependymal zone.* **epitrichial l.** The outermost layer of the embryonic epidermis which, after the sixth month of intrauterine life, is loosened by the growth of lanugo and contributes to the vernix caseosa as the epitrichium. **external granular l. of cerebrum** The most superficial neuronal layer of cerebral neocortex, containing numerous densely packed small neurons (granule cells) and few myelinated fibers. Also *layer II.* **external pyramidal l.** LAYER OF SMALL PYRAMIDAL CELLS. **fatty l. of perineum** SUPERFICIAL LAYER OF FASCIA OF PERINEUM. **fibrous l. of articular capsule** MEM-

BRANA FIBROSA CAPSULAE ARTICULARIS. **functional l. of endometrium** STRATUM FUNCTIONALE ENDOMETRII. **fusiform l.** MULTIFORM LAYER. **ganglionic l. of cerebellum** STRATUM GANGLIOSUM CEREBELLI. **ganglionic l. of optic nerve** STRATUM GANGLIONARE RETINAE. **ganglionic l. of retina** STRATUM GANGLIONARE RETINAE. **Gennari's l.** GENNARI'S BAND. **germ l.** One of the three basic layers or laminae of cells of the early embryo: ectoderm (outer skin), mesoderm (middle skin), and endoderm (inner skin). The tissues of the body are derived from the germ layers and the fate of each layer is

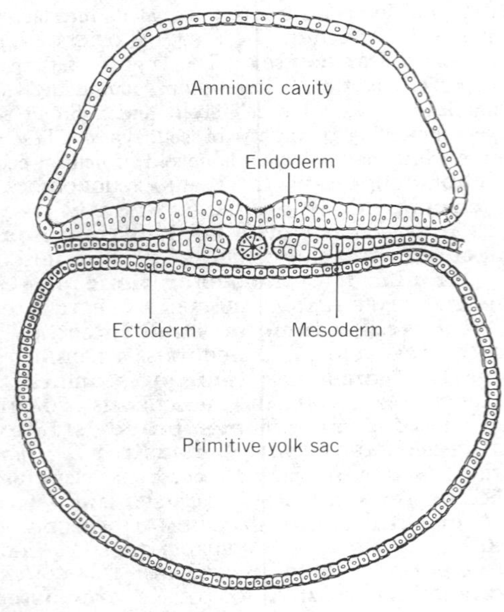


**Germ layers**

fairly well defined, though not as specifically as formerly believed. The layers may be considered as assembly areas from where the parts of the embryo will emerge at the right position and in the right order. Also *blastodermic layer.* **germinative l.** A layer of cells within which new cells are formed. **germinative l. of epidermis** The zone of the epidermis in which the generation of new epidermal cells occurs. It is the stratum basale epidermidis and stratum spinosum epidermidis combined. **germinative l. of nail** STRATUM GERMINATIVUM UNGUIS. **granular l.** INTERNAL GRANULAR LAYER. **granular-cell l.** GRANULE LAYER. **granular l. of cerebellum** STRATUM GRANULOSUM CEREBELLI. **granular l. of epidermis** The deeper of the keratinizing layers of the epidermis, lying between the stratum spinosum of the germinative layers and the more superficial stratum lucidum. The cells derive from the stratum spinosum, become flattened, contain pyknotic nuclei, and synthesize keratohyalin granules. Also *keratohyaline layer.* **granular l. of follicle of ovary** STRATUM GRANULOSUM FOLLICULI OVARICI SECUNDARII. **granular l. of Tomes** A narrow zone in the peripheral region of the dentin of a root which has a granular appearance in ground sections of teeth. **granule l.** The layer of densely packed small neurons (granule cells) of the cerebral and cerebellar cortex. They constitute the principal zone of termination of afferent fibers. Also *granular-cell layer.* **gray l. of superior colliculus** STRATUM GRISEUM COLLICULI SUPERIORIS. **half-value l.** An index of photon beam radiation quality. It is the thickness of appropriate attenuating material which, when inserted in a narrow beam, reduces its intensity in half. Also *half-value thickness, half-thickness, half-layer, half-thickness layer.* Abbr. Hvl **Haller's l.** LAMINA VASCULOSA CHOROIDEAE. **Henle's l.** A darkly staining layer that forms the outer portion of the inner root sheath of a hair. **Henle's fiber l.** An outer sublayer of the external plexiform lamina around the fovea centralis. It is formed by horizontally stretched inner rod and cone fibers and corresponding parts of Müller's fibers. **Henle's nervous l.** ENTORETINA. **horny l. of epidermis** STRATUM CORNEUM EPIDERMIDIS. **horny l. of nail** STRATUM CORNEUM UNGUIS. **Huxley's l.** The two layers of cells that are immediately external to the inner root sheath cuticle of a hair. Also *Huxley sheath, Huxley's membrane.* **inferior l. of pelvic diaphragm** FASCIA DIAPHRAGMATIS PELVIS INFERIOR. **inferior l. of urogenital diaphragm** MEMBRANA PERINEI. **infragranular l.** A cell layer of the human fetal cerebral cortex that appears about the sixth month deep to the inner granular layer and gives rise to the ganglionic layer. **inner muscular l. of stomach** STRATUM CIRCULARE TUNICAE MUSCULARIS GASTRICAE. **inner neuroblastic l.** The layer of the embryonic retina giving rise to ganglion cells, amacrine, and sustentacular cells. **inner nuclear l.** STRATUM NUCLEARE INTERNUM. **inner plexiform l. of the retina** STRATUM PLEXIFORME INTERNUM. **internal granular l.** The layer of cerebral neocortex consisting of densely packed, small stellate neurons (granule cells). It is the main recipient zone of specific thalamocortical afferent terminals, and is consequently best developed in the sensory areas. Also *granular layer, layer IV.* **internal medullary l.'s of optic thalamus** The two bands (fused in part) of myelinated axons separating the medial from the lateral and ventral thalamic nuclear groups and containing the intralaminar nuclei. **internal pyramidal l.** The lamina of cerebral neocortex containing the largest pyramidal neurons, which are especially large and conspicuous in the motor areas. Also *layer V, Meynert's layer.* **investing l. of cervical fascia** LAMINA SUPERFICIALIS FASCIAE CERVICALIS. **l. of Kaes-Bekhterev** BEKHTEREV'S LAYER. **keratohyaline l.** GRANULAR LAYER OF EPIDERMIS. **Kölliker's l.** STROMA IRIDIS. **Langhans l.** CYTOTROPHOBLAST. **lateral cartilaginous l.** LAMINA CARTILAGINIS LATERALIS TUBAE AUDITIVAE. **longitudinal l. of muscular tunic of colon** STRATUM LONGITUDINALE TUNICAE MUSCULARIS COLI. **longitudinal l. of muscular tunic of rectum** STRATUM LONGITUDINALE TUNICAE MUSCULARIS RECTI. **longitudinal l. of muscular tunic of small intestine** STRATUM LONGITUDINALE TUNICAE MUSCULARIS INTESTINI TENUIS. **longitudinal l. of muscular tunic of stomach** STRATUM LONGITUDINALE TUNICAE MUSCULARIS GASTRICAE. **malpighian l.** The main portion of the epidermis, which is composed of squamous cells that are connected by numerous intercellular bridges, or desmosomes. Also *Renaut's layer.* **mantle l.** The middle layer of the neural tube, lying between the germinal layer inside it and the marginal layer outside. As the neural tube differentiates, the cell derivatives of the original neuroepithelial layer settle in different zones of the wall. All the neuroblasts, supported by numerous but not all glial precursors, occupy the mantle layer. Also *mantle zone, columnar layer.* **marginal l.** The outermost layer of the neural tube at the start of its development, which includes few cell bodies, but mostly nerve fibers and prolongations of the interlacing neuroglia. Separated by an external limiting membrane from a dense mesenchymatous layer (future leptomeninges), it surrounds the mantle layer (future gray matter) and itself will develop into the white matter of the spinal cord. Also *marginal zone.* **matching l.** Material placed in front of the face of an ultrasound transducer element to reduce the reflection of sound at the transducer surface. **medial cartilaginous l.** LAMINA CARTILAGINIS MEDIALIS TUBAE AUDITIVAE. **membranous l. of the perineum** The thin, but strong, aponeurotic deep layer of the superficial fascia of the perineum, continuous with the membranous, or Scarpa's, layer of superficial fascia of the lower abdominal wall, the tunica dartos and the fascia of the penis. It is attached to the ischiopubic rami laterally, and to the posterior, or inferior, border of the perineal membrane and the perineal body posteriorly. Deep to it is the superficial perineal pouch. **Meynert's l.** INTERNAL PYRAMIDAL LAYER. **middle l. of cervical fascia** LAMINA PRETRACHEALIS FASCIAE CERVICALIS. **molecular l.** STRATUM MOLECULARE. **molecular l. of cerebellar cortex** STRATUM MOLECULARE CEREBELLI. **molecular l. of cerebellum** STRATUM MOLECULARE CEREBELLI. **molecular l. of olfactory bulb** The ill-defined external plexiform layer of the olfactory bulb. It lies between the layer of synaptic glomeruli and interglomerular spaces externally and the mitral cell layer centrally, and contains tufted cells which diminish in size throughout the layer towards the glomeruli. Some authorities include the mitral cells, which are analogous to but larger than the tufted cells, in this layer. **monomolecular l.** MONOLAYER. **mucous l. of tympanic membrane** STRATUM MUCOSUM MEMBRANAE TYMPANI. **multiform l.** The deepest neuronal layer of the cerebral neocortex, containing predominantly spindle-shaped (fusiform) cells. It is bordered below by the white matter and above by the internal pyramidal layer. It is distinctively pierced by bundles of radial axons, and gives rise to many short association fibers. In some earlier schemes it was subdivided into layers VI and VII (Vogt) to distinguish the cells scattered at the border of the white matter. Also *fusiform layer, spindle-celled layer, layer VI.* **muscular l. of fallopian tube** TUNICA MUSCULARIS TUBAE UTERINAE. **nervous l.** STRATUM NERVOSUM RETINAE. **neuroepithelial l.** The single layer of cells that comprises the neural plate and its derivative, the early neural tube. Subsequently, as the neural tube thickens, the cells of the neuroepithelial layer proliferate and give rise to precursors of neurons, ependyma, and glial cells. **neuroepithelial l. of retina** STRATUM NEUROEPITHELIALE RETINAE. **l. of Nitabuch** MEMBRANE OF NITABUCH. **odontoblastic l.** The pseudostratified layer of large, elongated and radially arranged cells that line a tooth's pulp cavity adjacent to the dentin and send protoplasmic processes, or fibers of Tomes, into the dentinal tubules. The cells contain mitochondria and a Golgi net. **Oehl's l.** STRATUM LUCIDUM EPIDERMIDIS. **Ollier's l.** STRATUM OSTEOGENETICUM. **osteoblastic l.** STRATUM OSTEOGENETICUM. **osteogenetic l.** STRATUM OSTEOGENETICUM. **outer neuroblastic l.** The layer of the embryonic retina giving origin to the photoreceptive elements, the rods and cones, and the bipolar neurons. **outer nuclear l.** STRATUM NUCLEARE EXTERNUM. **outer plexiform l. of the retina** STRATUM PLEXIFORME EXTERNUM. **papillary l. of corium** STRATUM PAPILLARE CORII. **parietal l. of pelvic fascia** FASCIA PELVIS PARIETALIS. **parietal l. of serous pericardium** LAMINA PARIETALIS PERICARDII. **parietal l. of tunica vaginalis of testis** LAMINA PARIETALIS TUNICAE VAGINALIS TESTIS. **perforated l. of sclera** LAMINA CRIBROSA SCLERAE. **pericyte l.** PERITHELIUM. **peripheral l.** STRATUM MOLECULARE. **pigmented l. of ciliary body** EPITHELIUM PIGMENTOSUM PARTIS CILIARIS RETINAE. **pigmented l. of ciliary part of retina** EPITHELIUM PIGMENTOSUM PARTIS CILIARIS RETINAE. **pigmented l. of iris** EPITHELIUM POSTERIUS PIGMENTOSUM PARTIS IRIDICAE RETINAE. **pigmented l. of optic part of retina** STRATUM PIGMENTOSUM PARTIS OPTICAE RETINAE. **pigmented l. of retina** STRATUM PIGMENTOSUM PARTIS OPTICAE RETINAE. **plexiform l.** 1 Either stratum plexiforme externum or stratum plexiforme internum. 2 STRATUM MOLECULARE. **Polyak l.** The horizontal cell layer of the retina. **posterior l. of rectus sheath** LAMINA POSTERIOR VAGINAE MUSCULI RECTI ABDOMINIS. **pretracheal l.** LAMINA PRETRACHEALIS FASCIAE CERVICALIS. **prickle-cell l.** STRATUM SPINOSUM EPIDERMIDIS. **primitive l.** The internal layer of the neuroepithelium of the optic cup, which gives rise to the outer and inner neuroblastic layers. **Purkinje l.** STRATUM GANGLIOSUM CEREBELLI. **l. of pyramidal cells** A lamina of large, pyramidal neurons in the cerebral cortex, especially the internal pyramidal layer (layer V) of neocortex or the main neuronal lamina of the hippocampal and dentate gyri. **radiate l. of tympanic membrane** STRATUM RADIATUM MEMBRANAE TYMPANI. **Rauber's l.** PRIMITIVE ECTODERM. **Renaut's l.** MALPIGHIAN LAYER. **reticular l. of corium** STRATUM RETICULARE CORII. **Rexed's l.'s** LAMINAE OF REXED. **l. of rods and cones** STRATUM NEUROEPITHELIALE RETINAE. **Rohr's l.** Fibrinoid stria in the juxtaintervillous portion of the basal plate of a human placenta, often closely related to Nitabuch's membrane. **Sattler's l.** The part of the lamina vasculosa choroideae which is close to the lamina choroidocapillaris and contains the smaller caliber blood vessels. **sclerotogenous l.** SKELETOGENOUS LAYER. **second half-value l.** That thickness of absorbing medium required to reduce the intensity of penetrating radiation by one half, subsequent to a reduction by one half of the original radiation intensity by the primary absorbing medium. **skeletogenous l.** The mesoderm around the notochord that gives rise to the axial skeleton. Also *sclerotogenous layer.* **slime l.** 1 A loosely adherent bacterial capsule. 2 A layer of dextran or levan which promotes adherence of some bacteria. **sluggish l.** STILL LAYER. **l. of small pyramidal cells** The lamina of supragranular pyramidal cells in the cerebral neocortex containing numerous granule and Martinotti neurons intermingled in a gradient of pyramidal neurons decreasing in size towards the surface. In myelin-stained preparations this layer displays the horizontal band of Kaes-Bechterev. Also *external pyramidal layer, layer III.* **somatic l.** SOMATOPLEURE. **spindle-celled l.** MULTIFORM LAYER. **spinous l. of epidermis** STRATUM SPINOSUM EPIDERMIDIS. **splanchnic l.** SPLANCHNOPLEURE. **spongy l.** STRATUM SPONGIOSUM ENDOMETRII. **still l.** The relatively slow moving layer of blood adjacent to the wall of a capillary. Also *sluggish layer.* **subcallosal l.** A layer of myelinated axons on the inferior surface of the corpus callosum. **subcutaneous l.** TELA SUBCUTANEA. **subendocardial l.** A layer of loose connective tissue that binds the endocardium to the myocardium, is continuous with the myocardial interstitial tissue, and contains blood vessels, nerves, and conducting fibers of the heart. It lies deep to the subendothelial layer. **subendothelial l.** A thin collagenous layer deep to the lining endothelium of the endocardium and of the large and medium caliber vessels, containing a few fibroblasts and elastic fibers. **subepicardial l.** A thin collagenous layer with elastic fibers, blood vessels, and nervous elements between the mesothelial layer of the epicardium and the underlying myocardium. **submantle l.** A fine layer of dentin with interglobular spaces just deep to the peripheral layer of cover dentin at its junction with the circumpulpar dentin. It is analagous to the granular layer of Tomes in the root of the tooth. **submucous l.** TELA SUBMUCOSA. **subodontoblastic l.** A layer of the peripheral pulp of the tooth, deep to the odontoblasts and best seen in older teeth. It is characterized by absence of cells, the fibrous tissue and cell processes forming a clear cell-free zone. In a young tooth, a capillary plexus is found in this zone, as well as branches from longitudinal myelinated fibers in the pulp forming a plexus (of Raschkow) here. Also *Weil's basal layer.* **subpapillary l.** A vascular layer deep to the papillary layer at its junction with the reticular layer of the dermis where the rete subpapillare is found. **subserous l.** TELA SUBSEROSA. **subserous l. of peritoneum** TELA SUBSEROSA PERITONEI. **superficial l. of fascia of perineum** The fatty, or superficial, layer of the superficial fascia of the perineum, continuous anteriorly either with the fat-free tunica dartos and fascia of the penis or with the labia majora where it contains a lot of fat, laterally with superficial fascia on the medial side of the thighs, and posteriorly with the perianal superficial fascia. Also *fatty layer of perineum.* **superficial gray l.** STRATUM GRISEUM COLLICULI SUPERIORIS. **superficial l. of triangular ligament** MEMBRANA PERINEI. **superficial l. of urogenital diaphragm** MEMBRANA PERINEI. **superior l. of pelvic diaphragm** FASCIA DIAPHRAGMATIS PELVIS SUPERIOR. **superior l. of urogenital diaphragm** See under SPATIUM PERINEI PROFUNDUM. **supragranular l.** The neuronal lamina above the internal granular layer of the cerebral neocortex. It is the zone above the principal zone of specific afferent fiber termination, and generally recognized as comprising layers II and III, which are difficult to separate in some cortical areas (e.g., the limbic cortex). **synovial l. of articular capsule** MEMBRANA SYNOVIALIS CAPSULAE ARTICULARIS. **vascular l. of choroid** LAMINA VASCULOSA CHOROIDEAE. **vascular l. of testis** TUNICA VASCULOSA TESTIS. **vessel l. of the iris** STRATUM VASCULOSUM IRIDIS. **visceral l. of pelvic fascia** FASCIA PELVIS VISCERALIS. **visceral l. of pericardium** LAMINA VISCERALIS PERICARDII. **visceral l. of tunica vaginalis of testis** LAMINA VISCERALIS TUNICAE VAGINALIS TESTIS. **Waldeyer's l.** 1 GERMINAL EPITHELIUM. 2 EPITHELIUM SUPERFICIALE OVARII. **Weil's basal l.** SUBODONTOBLASTIC LAYER. **yellow l.** BUFFY COAT. **zonal l. of cerebellum** STRATUM MOLECULARE CEREBELLI. **zonal l. of quadrigeminal body** STRATUM ZONALE CORPORIS QUADRIGEMINI. **zonal l. of thalamus** STRATUM ZONALE THALAMI.

**lazaretto** \lazəret′ō\ [alteration (because of *Lazarus,* the New Testament person afflicted with sores) of Italian *Nazareto* Nazareth, from Santa Maria di *Nazaret,* an important hospital in Venice] 1 A hospital for isolating cases of infectious disease. 2 A building used for housing persons being kept in quarantine.

**lb** Symbol for the unit, pound.

**LBF** *Lactobacillus bulgaricus* factor (folic acid).

**lb tr** Symbol for the unit, pound troy.

**LCM** lymphocytic choriomeningitis.

**LD** 1 lethal dose. 2 light difference (eye examination).

**$LD_{50}$** median lethal dose.

**$LD_{100}$** The dose of biologically active material, usually a drug, a toxin, or a microorganism, that causes death in all exposed subjects. Also *invariably lethal dose.*

**LDH** lactate dehydrogenase.

**LDL** 1 low-density lipoprotein. 2 loudness discomfort level.

**LDV** laser Doppler velocimetry.

**LE** lupus erythematosus.

**leach** \lēch\ [prob. Old English *leccan* to wet, irrigate] 1 To separate constituents of (a mixture) by contact with a solvent in which only some of the constituents are soluble, often used to harvest the soluble material. 2 To remove (the soluble portion) of a mixture.

**lead[1]** \led\ [Old English *lēad*] Element number 82, having atomic weight 207.2. Lead is a soft, bluish white metal with specific gravity 11.35, easily separated from its ores and sometimes found in elemental form. Four stable isotopes are found in nature, the end products of the uranium, thorium, and actinium disintegration series. Seventeen unstable isotopes are known. Lead is corrosion resistant and it is an effective absorber of sound and a wide range of electromagnetic radiation. It is universally used as a shield against x rays and other hazardous radiation. Its compounds have many applications in technology, in storage batteries, gasoline, paints, etc. It is a cumulative poison, and lead pollution becomes an endemic health hazard in some environments. Symbol: Pb **radioactive l.** Any of the radioactive isotopes of lead that either occur in nature as intermediates in the uranium, neptunium, thorium, or actinium series or are artificially produced. Also *radiolead.*

**lead[2]** \lēd\ [Middle English *lede* a leading, from *leden* to lead, from Old English *lǣden* to cause to go] 1 Any of the electrical connections used for recording a biopotential, such as an electrocardiogram. 2 Any of the records made from specific sites or pair of connections. **bipolar l.** A lead in which each of two sites of location of the electrodes contributes significantly to the record, as in the standard leads I, II, and III. **CF l.** A chest lead with the indifferent electrode attached to the left leg. **chest l.** An electrocardiographic lead in which the exploring electrode is placed on the chest. See also V LEAD. Also *precordial lead, Wilson's lead.* **CL l.** A chest lead with the indifferent electrode attached to the left arm. **CM l.** A chest lead with the indifferent electrode placed on the manubrium sterni. **CR l.** A chest lead with the indifferent electrode attached to the right arm. **electroencephalographic l.** An electrical connection of two wires to two electrodes on the scalp that measures the cerebral activity between them. Normally many leads simultaneously record from many pairs of electrodes. **esophageal l.** An electrocardiographic lead in which the electrode is placed in the esophagus. **limb l.** Any of the electrocardiographic leads in which the exploring electrode or both electrodes are placed on the limbs: leads I, II, or III, or aVR, aVL, or aVF. **precordial l.** CHEST LEAD. **standard l.** One of the three bipolar leads that were regarded as standard in the early days of electrocardiography: lead I (right arm–left arm), lead II (left leg–right arm), and lead III (left leg–left arm). Also *standard limb lead, standard extremity lead.* **unipolar l.** A lead in which one electrode is an exploring electrode and the other is an indifferent electrode with effective zero input, such as the Wilson central terminal. **unipolar limb l.** A unipolar lead in which the exploring electrode is attached to one of the limbs, as aVR (right arm), aVL (left arm), or aVF (left leg). **V l.** A unipolar electrocardiographic lead in which the exploring electrode is on the chest. The locations of the most commonly used V leads are as follows: $V_1$ and $V_2$ are in the fourth intercostal space, to the right and left of the sternum, respectively. $V_3$ is midway between $V_2$ and $V_4$, the latter being in the fifth intercostal space on the midclavicular line. $V_5$, on the left anterior axillary line, and $V_6$, on the midaxillary line, are both on the same horizontal level as $V_4$. **Wilson's l.** CHEST LEAD.

**Leadbetter** [Guy Whitman *Leadbetter*, U.S. orthopedic surgeon, 1893–1945] See under MANEUVER.

**lead zirconate titanate** A piezoelectric ceramic material used in ultrasonic transducers. Symbol: PZT

**leaf** [Old English *lēaf*, akin to L *liber* inner bark of a tree] A plant stem appendage that functions in transpiration and photosynthesis. **anterior mesodermal l.** The more anterior half of the portion of the iris of mesodermal origin. This portion of the iris does not extend to the pupil, but stops at an irregular border midway between the pupil edge and the iris base. **digitalis l.** The dried leaf of *Digitalis purpurea*, the purple foxglove. This the common form of digitalis, which was prescribed for many years as powdered digitalis leaf. It has been standarized as a reference of activity for other crude digitalis preparations. The availability of the purified digitalis glycosides has gradually replaced the use of the crude leaf preparations in most countries. ***Digitalis lantana* l.** The dried leaf of *Digitalis lantana*, which contains cardioactive glycosides and is more potent than digitalis leaf. Also *woolly foxglove, Austrian foxglove.*

**leaflet** A small structure resembling a leaf, such as a cusp of a valvule of a heart valve.

**Leão** [A. A. P. *Leão*, Brazilian physiologist, born 1914] Leão spreading depression. See under DEPRESSION.

**learning** [Old English *leornung*, from *leornian* to learn + *-ung* -ING] The acquired responses of an organism that are the result of experience, especially of repeated experience or practice, and of such deliberate modification procedures as classical or operant conditioning. Temporary behavioral changes that are the consequence of physiologic fluctuations, such as sensory adaptation, disease, fatigue, or drug effects are not regarded as instances of learning, nor are those maturational changes rooted directly in genetic influences. **avoidance l.** That type of training in which an experimental animal learns to make a particular instrumental response to prevent the occurrence of a noxious stimulus. The response is usually to some warning signal that just precedes the delivery of a painful or punishing stimulus. **conditioning l.** CONDITIONING. **discriminative l.** The learning of responses to selected stimuli through the application of differential reinforcement. **escape l.** Learning which is reinforced by subjecting the experimental animal to noxious or painful stimuli which the animal can escape by making a particular response. **immunologic l.** The progressive changes in the nature of the antibodies formed (including increased avidity) following antigenic stimulation. **incidental l.** Learning or remembering that takes place without any obvious intent or particular purpose, and without any formal instruction to learn or remember, or any evident motive to learn. **motor l.** Learning of tasks that involve the processes of skeletomuscular action rather than ideation. Motor and ideational learning are not, however, mutually exclusive processes. **perceptual l.** Learning in which the principal task or feature is a modification in the way things are perceived. **programed l.** Self-instruction using a set of materials specially selected to allow the learner to determine the pace. **state-dependent l.** Learning which takes place while the person is in a particular physiologic state and can most readily be recalled when the person is once again in the same state, such as a state induced by a dissociative drug or alcohol.

**leash** A cordlike group of nerves, blood vessels, fibers, or similar structures.

**Leber** [Theodor von *Leber*, German ophthalmologist, 1840–1917] **1** Leber's optic atrophy, von Leber's atrophy. See under ATROPHY. **2** See under DISEASE. **3** Leber's corpuscle. See under HASSALL'S CORPUSCLE. **4** Amaurosis congenita of Leber. See under AMAUROSIS. **5** Leber's plexus. See under HOVIUS PLEXUS.

**lecanosomatopagus** \lek′ənōsō′mətäp′əgəs\ [Gk *lecan(ē)* a dish + *o* + SOMATO- + -PAGUS] Equal conjoined twins united throughout all or most of the trunk, including the pelvis. This condition is a form of dicephaly, the head being duplicated fully and the trunk only partially.

**Lecat** [Claude Nicolas *Lecat*, French surgeon, 1700–1768] See under GULF.

**lecith-** \les′ith-\ [Gk *lekithos* pulse porridge, yolk of an egg] A combining form denoting the yolk of an egg.

**lecithal** \les′ithəl\ [LECITH- + -AL] Possessing yolk. Eggs are classified according to the amount of yolk present, and range from microlecithal (having little yolk) to megalethical (having much yolk).

**lecithin** \les′ithin\ PHOSPHATIDYLCHOLINE.

**lecithinase** *Obs.* PHOSPHOLIPASE.

**lecithin:cholesterol acyl transferase** A normally occurring plasma enzyme that esterifies cholesterol in the reaction: lecithin + cholesterol $\xrightarrow{\text{LCAT}}$ lysolecithin + cholesteryl ester. Abbr. LCAT

**lecithinemia** \les′ithinē′mē·ə\ The presence of lecithin in blood.

**lecitho-** \les′ithō-\ LECITH-.

**Leclanché** [Georges *Leclanché*, French chemist, 1839–1882] See under CELL.

**lectin** \lek′tin\ [L *lect(us)*, past part. of *legere* to pick, select + -IN; so called because of specificity (selectivity) for particular binding sites] **1** A hemagglutinating protein substance present in the saline extracts of the seeds of certain plants. Lectins bind specifically to certain sugars and oligopolysaccharides, including certain glycoproteins present on the surface of many mammalian cells. Some lectins have specific binding properties for certain lymphocyte subsets and are thus extensively used as mitogens in immunologic experiments. Their reaction usually requires divalent cations. **2** Any protein other than an antibody that binds to a specific carbohydrate group. Lectins in this sense of the term may be of animal, plant, or microbial origin. They are important determinants of microbial adherence in infection. Adj. lectinic.

**ledbänder** \led′bandər\ BÜNGNER'S BANDS.

**Lederer** [Max *Lederer*, U.S. pathologist, 1885–1952] Lederer-Brill anemia. See under LEDERER'S ANEMIA.

**Lee** [Robert *Lee*, English gynecologist and obstetrician, 1793–1877] Lee's ganglion. See under CERVICAL GANGLION OF UTERUS.

**leech** [Old English *lǣce* a healer, physician] **1** An annelid worm of the class Hirudinea, especially an aquatic, blood-sucking member of such genera as *Hirudo, Limnatis, Dinobdella*, or *Haemopis*. Most leeches are aquatic scavengers or predators of snails, insects, annelids, or other soft-bodied aquatic animals. Land leeches, *Haemadipsa* species, are notorious pests in southeast Asian rainforests. Also *sanguisuga*. **2** To apply leeches to (the body of a patient) for

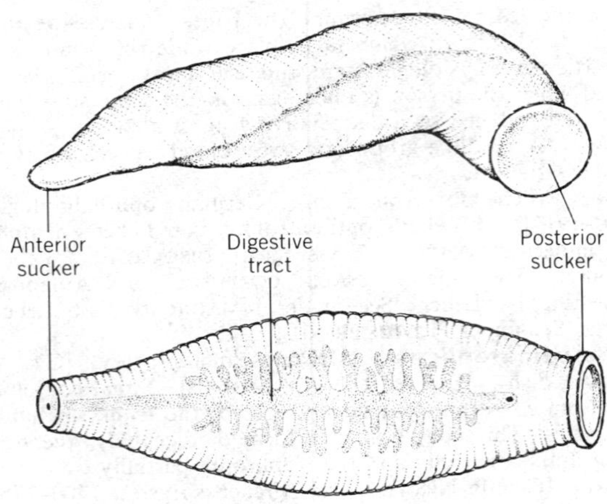


**Leech** *(Hirudo medicinalis)*

bloodletting, reduction of hematomas or varicosities, or other therapeutic purposes. **3** A practitioner of leeching; formerly, a physician. **American l.** A leech of the species *Macrobdella decora.* **medicinal l.** A leech of the species *Hirudo medicinalis.*

**Leede** [Carl Stockbridge *Leede*, U.S. physician, born 1882] Rumpel-Leede sign, Rumpel-Leede test, Leede-Rumpel phenomenon. See under RUMPEL-LEEDE PHENOMENON.

**Leeuwenhoek** [Antony van *Leeuwenhoek*, Dutch microscopist, 1632–1723] Leeuwenhoek's canal. See under HAVERSIAN CANAL.

**Lefèvre** [Paul *Lefèvre*, French dermatologist, flourished 20th century] Papillon-Lefèvre syndrome. See under SYNDROME.

**Le Fort** [Leon Clement *Le Fort*, French surgeon, 1829–1893] **1** See under OPERATION, FRACTURE. **2** Le Fort I osteotomy, Le Fort II osteotomy, Le Fort III osteotomy. See under OSTEOTOMY.

**leg** [Middle English, from Old Norse *leggr* leg, hollow bone of arm or leg] **1** In human anatomy, the portion of the lower limb between the knee and the ankle joint; crus. **2** In common usage, the whole lower limb including or excluding the foot. **bandy l.** GENU VARUM. **bayonet l.** Genu recurvatum combined with ankylosis. **cross l.** SCISSOR LEG. **jimmy l.'s** RESTLESS LEGS SYNDROME. **jitter l.'s** RESTLESS LEGS SYNDROME. **milk l.** PHLEGMASIA ALBA DOLENS. **scissor l.** A pattern of weight bearing and walking in which the legs cross over each other. It is seen in spasticity, particularly of the adductor muscles, and in cerebral palsy. Also *cross leg.* **white l.** PHLEGMASIA ALBA DOLENS.

**Legal** [Emmo *Legal*, German physician, 1859–1922] Legal's disease. See under GLOSSOPHARYNGEAL NEURALGIA.

**Legendre** [Gaston-Lucien-Joseph *Legendre*, French physician, born 1887. The spelling *Le Gendre* is erroneous.] Le Gendre sign. See under SIGN.

**Legg** [Arthur Thornton *Legg*, U.S. surgeon, 1874–1939] Legg's disease, Legg-Calvé-Perthes disease. See under PERTHES DISEASE.

***Legionella*** \lē′jənel′ə\ A genus of bacteria that includes *L. pneumophila,* the agent of legionnaire's disease, and, tentatively, various other species related to it such as the Pittsburgh pneumonia agent, *L. pittsburghensis* (alternatively classified as *Tatlockia micdadei*). ***L. pneumophila*** A thin, nonmotile, nonspore-forming, Gram-negative rod that causes epidemics and sporadic cases of severe pneumonia (legionnaire's disease). Its growth *in vitro* requires a medium rich in cysteine and iron. In some epidemics the organism has been spread from soil or from the cooling water in air-conditioning systems.

**legionellosis** \lē′jənelō′sis\ Any disease caused by bacteria of the genus *Legionella.*

**Leichtenstern** [Otto Michael Ludwig *Leichtenstern*, German physician, 1845–1900] **1** Leichtenstern's encephalitis, Strümpell-Leichtenstern encephalitis. See under ACUTE HEMORRHAGIC LEUKOENCEPHALITIS. **2** Strümpell-Leichtenstern disease. See under ACUTE INFANTILE HEMIPLEGIA.

**Leifson** [Einar *Leifson*, U.S. bacteriologist, born 1902] Leifson's flagella stain. See under STAIN.

**Leigh** [Archibald Denis *Leigh*, English neuropathologist, born 1915] Leigh's necrotizing encephalomyelopathy, Leigh's disease, Leigh's encephalopathy. See under SUBACUTE NECROTIZING ENCEPHALOPATHY.

**Leiner** [Karl *Leiner*, Austrian pediatrician, 1871–1930] See under DISEASE.

**leio-** \lī′ō-\ [Gk *leios* smooth] A combining form meaning smooth. Also *lio-.*

***Leiognathus bacoti*** \lī′ōnath′əs bəkō′tē\ *ORNITHONYSSUS BACOTI.*

**leiomyoblastoma** \-mī′əblastō′mə\ A smooth muscle tumor with polygonal cells having pale or clear cytoplasm. It is usually benign. It is most frequently found in the stomach and intestines. Also *epithelioid leiomyoma.*

**leiomyoma** \-mī-ō′mə\ [LEIO- + MYOMA] A benign tumor of smooth-muscle cells typically showing little variation in their appearance. Mitotic activity is very low. Collagen formation may be excessive, obscuring the muscular nature of the tumor. It can be found in a variety of sites but is most frequent in the uterus. Also *fibroid, fibromyoma, myofibroma.* **bizarre l.** A leiomyoma with large, bizarrely shaped cells. Mitoses are rare. **l. cutis** A cutaneous nodule containing smooth muscle tissue. Also *dermatomyoma.* **epithelioid l.** LEIOMYOBLASTOMA. **multiple cutaneous l.** Multiple cutaneous nodules containing smooth muscle tissue. **parasitic l.** A leiomyoma, usually uterine, which detaches from the uterine serosa and grows on the peritoneum at another site. **l. of the seminal vesicles** A rare, benign, smooth-muscle tumor of the seminal vesicle. It may clinically resemble a vesicular cyst. **l. uteri** Leiomyoma of the uterus, the most frequent site of this tumor. Also *fibromyoma uteri.* **vascular l.** ANGIOMYOMA. **Zenker's l.** LEIOMYOSARCOMA.

**leiomyomatosis** \-mī′ōmətō′sis\ [*leiomyomat(a),* pl. of LEIOMYOMA, + -OSIS] Multiple widespread leiomyomas.

**leiomyosarcoma** \-mī′əsärkō′mə\ [LEIO- + MYO- + SARCOMA] A malignant tumor of smooth-muscle cells, which, in its well-differentiated forms, closely simulates leiomyoma. The most important distinguishing feature is the presence of mitotic figures. It may occur at a number of body sites such as the uterus and the stomach. Also *Zenker's leiomyoma.*

**leipo-** \lī′pō-\ [Gk *leip(ein)* to leave, lack] A combining form meaning lack, loss.

**Leishman** [Sir William Boog *Leishman*, British surgeon, 1865–1926] **1** Leishman's nodules. See under NODULE. **2** Leishman-Donovan body. See under AMASTIGOTE. **3** Leishman's chrome cells. See under CELL. **4** See under STAIN, ANEMIA.

***Leishmania*** \lēshman′ē·ə\ [after Sir William B. *Leishman,* British surgeon, 1865–1926 + -IA] A genus of flagellate protozoa (family Trypanosomatidae, order Kinetoplastida) found in the macrophages of vertebrate hosts in the amastigote form, and in invertebrate hosts (or cultures) in the promastigote form. Most species are morphologically indistinguishable. They may be differentiated on the basis of developmental pattern in the sandflies that are their intermediate hosts, clinical manifestations, geographic distribution, and biochemical or physicochemical characteristics, such as enzyme electrophoretic patterns, kinetoplast DNA analysis, and DNA buoyant density measurements. ***L. aethiopica*** A species responsible for cutaneous leishmaniasis in the Ethiopian highlands and on the slopes of Mt. Elgon in Kenya. It is frequently seen as blind swellings of the nose and upper lip without ulceration and with few parasites. A diffuse form is occasionally seen among anergic patients. Reservoir hosts are rock hyraxes (*Procavia* spp.) and the vector sandflies are *Phlebotomus longipes* and *P. pedifer.* ***L. brasiliensis*** A species or complex of species that includes the causative agents of mucocutaneous leishmaniasis. Also *Leishmania braziliensis.* ***L. brasiliensis pifanoi*** See under *LEISHMANIA PIFANOI.* ***L. braziliensis*** *LEISHMANIA BRASILIENSIS.* ***L. chagasi*** The South American agent of kala-azar, formerly thought to be a variant of the Asian *L. donovani,* but now considered likely to be an endemic form originally from the Amazon basin and subsequently spread through much of South America. Reservoirs are wild and domestic canids, and vectors are various species of the sandflies *Lutzomyia* and *Psychodopygus.* ***L. donovani*** The agent of the Old World visceral leishmaniasis, or kala azar, found in the Mediterranean region the south-central Soviet Union, India, northern China, and central and eastern Africa. In each region the disease has its own clinical characteristics, sandfly vectors, and animal reservoirs, if any. It has been proposed that the agents in each area be recognized as distinct subspecies. ***L. enrietti*** A species infecting guinea pigs in Brazil and now widely used in research into immunity in leishmaniasis. This is the only species of *Leishmania* that is readily distinguishable from those species infecting man. ***L. guyanensis*** A species of the *L. brasiliensis* complex (sometimes treated as a subspecies, *L. brasiliensis guyanensis*) that causes a form of New World cutaneous leishmaniasis called pian bois, forest yaws, bay sore, or buba, found in forest regions of Guyana, and in northern Pará and Amazonas states and Roraima territory in Brazil. Moderate ulceration is produced, sometimes with metastatic spread over the body via the lymphatics. Espundia is rare. Reservoir hosts are arboreal rodents, and the vector is *Lutzomyia umbratilis.* ***L. infantum*** A species, sometimes treated as a subspecies of *L. donovani,* that causes visceral leishmaniasis primarily in infants in regions of the Mediterranean. Sandflies of the *Phlebotomus major* group are the vectors and the reservoir host is the dog and, in some areas, other canids. Infection is usually limited to children under two years old. ***L. major*** See under *LEISHMANIA TROPICA.* ***L. mexicana*** A species, or species group, that includes the causative agent of chiclero ulcer, a form of New World cutaneous leishmaniasis found among workers in chicle gum and mahogany forests in southeastern Mexico and Guatemala. The vector is the sandfly *Lutzomyia flaviscutellata,* and reservoir hosts include various marsupials, primates, and rodents, especially the arboreal spiny rat *Proechimys guyanensis.* ***L. peruviana*** A species, sometimes regarded as a subspecies of *L. brasiliensis,* that causes uta, the only form of New World cutaneous leishmaniasis that is not characteristically restricted to forest regions. It occurs in the high arid valleys of the Andes in Peru, Bolivia, and Argentina. The sandfly vectors are probably *Lutzomyia verrucarum* and/or *L. peruensis,* and dogs are reservoir hosts. ***L. pifanoi*** A species that causes diffuse cutaneous leishmaniasis, first described in Venezuela and also known in the Amazon basin and in Mato Grosso in Brazil. The vector is the sandfly *Lutzomyia flaviscutellata* and the reservoir hosts are arboreal rodents. Now considered a distinct species by many workers, it is also commonly classified as a subspecies of *Leishmania mexicana (L. m. pifanoi),* and formerly as a subspecies of *L. brasiliensis (L. b. pifanoi).* ***L. tropica*** The causative agent of Old World cutaneous leishmaniasis, or oriental sore. It is found in the Mediterranean littoral, the Middle East, India, Pakistan, and the southern USSR. It has also been reported in western Africa. Two forms of *L. tropica* have been described. *L. major* (formerly *L. t. major*) is the agent of moist, or rural, oriental sore, a zoonosis. *L. tropica* (formerly *L. t. minor*) is the agent of dry, urban, or classical oriental sore (variously known as Aleppo, Baghdad, or Delhi boil, bouton d'orient, bouton de Biskra, and by many other names), an anthroponotic disease. Various sandflies of the genus *Phlebotomus* serve as vectors, chiefly *P. papatasi* and *P. sergenti.* Various rodents serve as reservoirs of *L. major,* whereas *L. tropica* is largely dependent on human-sandfly-human or dog-sandfly-human transmission.

**leishmania** (*pl.* leishmaniae) **1** *Older term* AMASTIGOTE. **2** A member of the genus *Leishmania.* .

**leishmanial** \lēshman′ē·əl\ **1** Pertaining to or caused by organisms of the genus *Leishmania.* **2** Pertaining to the amastigote or "leishmania" stage of certain other flagellate protozoans such as *Trypanosoma cruzi.*

**leishmaniasis** \lēsh′mənī′əsis\ [*Leishman(ia)* + -IASIS] Any of a group of infectious diseases caused by flagellate protozoan parasites of the genus *Leishmania* and transmitted to man by sandflies of the genera *Phlebotomus* and *Lutzomyia.* This group includes a visceral form of the disease (kala-azar), several cutaneous forms, and a mucocutaneous form. Also *leishmaniosis.* **American l.** MUCOCUTANEOUS LEISHMANIASIS.

**leishmanicidal** **1** Effective against *Leishmania.* **2** A leishmanicidal drug.

**leishmaniosis** \lēsh′manē·ō′sis\ LEISHMANIASIS.

**leishmanoid** \lish′mənoid\ [*leishman(ia)* + -OID] POST-KALA-AZAR DERMAL LEISHMANOID. **dermal l.** POST-KALA-AZAR DERMAL LEISHMANOID. **post-kala-azar dermal l.** A cutaneous lesion, usually on the face, in which leishmaniae are present. It is evidence of post-kala-azar dermal leishmaniasis, and has been reported in India, Kenya, and the Sudan. It is usually cured by antimony therapy. Also *leishmanoid, dermal leishmanoid.*

**Leitner** [Stefan J. *Leitner,* Swiss physician, born 1903] See under SYNDROME.

***Lelaps*** \lē′laps\ *ECHINOLAELAPS.*

**lema** \lē′mə\ [Gk *lēmē* a humor in the corners of the eye, gum, rheum] Secretions of the tarsal glands. Also *sebum palpebrale.*

**Lembert** [Antoine *Lembert,* French surgeon, 1802–1851] Czerny-Lembert suture. See under SUTURE.

**lememia** \lēmē′mē·ə\ [Gk *loim(os)* plague, deadly infection + -EMIA] The presence of plague bacilli *(Yersinia pestis)* in the blood.

**Lemli** [Luc *Lemli,* U.S. pediatrician, flourished 20th century] Smith-Lemli-Opitz syndrome. See under SYNDROME.

**lemma** \lem′ə\ [Gk (from *le(pein)* to peel + *-ma,* derivative noun suffix) a peel, husk] A layer or covering: used especially to describe cell membranes, as a sarcolemma.

**lemmoblast** \lem′əblast\ A cell derived from the embryonic neural crest cells which gives rise to a neurilemma cell. Also *lemnoblast.*
**lemmocyte** \lem′əsīt\ A cellular derivative of the neural crest and precursor of a neurilemma cell. Also *lemnocyte.*
**lemmocytoma** \lem′əsītō′mə\ [*lemmocyt(e)* + -OMA] NEURILEMMOMA.
**lemnisci** \lemnis′ī\ Plural of LEMNISCUS.
**lemniscus** \lemnis′kəs\ [L (from Gk *lēmniskos* a ribbon, fillet), a ribbon hanging from a victor's wreath, crown, or garland] (*pl.* lemnisci) A ribbon, band, fillet, or bundle of axons. Also *fillet.* **l. lateralis** [NA] A longitudinal tract of auditory system axons, originating in the cochlear nuclei and trapezoid body, that crosses and ascends in the lateral pontine tegmentum and terminates in the inferior colliculus and the thalamic medial geniculate body. Also *lateral lemniscus, acoustic lemniscus.* **l. medialis** [NA] A large, myelinated tract emerging from the nuclei gracilis and cuneatus, descending in an arc as the internal arcuate fibers, and crossing above the pyramidal tracts in the medulla oblongata. It ascends as a compact bundle terminating principally in the opposite ventrobasal thalamic nucleus. Each axon conveys impulses activated by a specific type of mechanoreceptor and from a restricted contralateral receptive field, chiefly cutaneous. It is the largest somatosensory tract in the brain and subserves tactile sensibility and position sense. Also *sensory lemniscus, medial lemniscus, lemniscus.* **optic l.** *Obs.* TRACTUS OPTICUS. **sensory l.** LEMNISCUS MEDIALIS. **spinal l.** *Seldom used* SPINOTHALAMIC TRACT. **l. spinalis** *Seldom used* SPINOTHALAMIC TRACT. **l. trigeminalis** [NA] A large band of myelinated axons originating mainly from the principal trigeminal sensory nucleus and with contributions from all sectors of the spinal trigeminal nucleus. Its fibers cross in the pons and join the lemniscus medialis, terminating in the medial sector of the thalamic ventrobasal nucleus. This large tract conveys tactile sensory information from facial skin and the oral cavity, and is considered the trigeminal homologue of the lemniscus medialis. A separate, uncrossed component conveying tactile activity from the oral and perioral regions to the ipsilateral ventral thalamus via a dorsal course is called the dorsal trigeminal lemniscus or tract, the homolateral trigeminal tract, and Wallenberg's bundle or tract. Also *trigeminal lemniscus, trigeminothalamic tract, central tract of cranial nerves, central tract of trigeminal nerve.*
**lemnoblast** \lem′nəblast\ LEMMOBLAST.
**lemnocyte** \lem′nəsīt\ LEMMOCYTE.
**lemoparalysis** \lē′mōpəral′isis\ [Gk *laimo(s)* the throat, gullet + PARALYSIS] ESOPHAGEAL PARALYSIS.
**Lendrum** [A. C. *Lendrum,* Scottish pathologist, flourished 20th century] Lendrum's inclusion body stain. See under STAIN.
**length** Linear extent from one point to another. **arch l.** The distance between the most posterior teeth in either the upper or lower jaw, measured around the periphery of the dental arch. **cranial l.** The length of the skull between the glabella and the inion. **crown-heel l.** The length of an embryo, fetus, or infant, stretched out and measured from the top of the head to the heel of the foot. **crown-rump l.** The distance from the top of the head to the buttocks, used in describing an embryo, fetus, or infant. **dental l.** The overall length of a dental quadrant. **focal l.** The distance at which a lens converges or appears to diverge parallel light. **foot l.** The heel-to-toe measurement taken of a fetus to estimate its age. This measurement at times has an advantage in that distortion of the fetus can cause inaccuracy in other measurements. **l. of generation** The average age in a cohort of mothers at which one first bears a daughter. **l. of gestation** The duration of a pregnancy as measured, usually in weeks, from the first day of the last normal menstrual cycle. **mean l. of life** The average length of life given certain defined rates of mortality. Also *expectation of life at birth.* **pulse l.** PULSE DURATION. **sitting l.** The distance between the vertex of the head and the coccyx. It is approximately equivalent to the crown-rump length used in measurement of embryos, fetuses, and infants. **stem l.** The distance between the vertex of the head and the midpoint of a line joining the ischial tuberosities. **wave l.** See under WAVELENGTH.
**Lenhossek** [Joseph von *Lenhossek,* Hungarian anatomist, 1818–1888] Lenhossek's fibers. See under STILLING'S FIBERS.
**lenitive** **1** Soothing. **2** A lenitive agent.
**Lennhoff** [Rudolf *Lennhoff,* German physician, 1866–1933] **1** See under SIGN. **2** Becker-Lennhoff index. See under LENNHOFF'S INDEX.
**Lennox** [William Gordon *Lennox,* U.S. physician, 1884–1960] Lennox syndrome. See under LENNOX-GASTAUT SYNDROME.
**Lenoir** [Camille-Alexandre-Henri *Lenoir,* French anatomist, born 1867] See under FACET.
**lens** [L, gen. *lentis,* a lentil] **1** A medium bound by two surfaces that refracts light rays. **2** [NA] A transparent, biconvex disk situated between the iris anteriorly and the vitreous body behind. It is encased in a capsule and held in position at its equator by the ciliary zonule. Almost spherical at birth, it becomes fairly convex in the adult, the anterior surface being less convex than the posterior surface, and it flattens in old age. The shape also changes during near and far accommodation. As a refractive medium, it focuses rays of light on the retina. Its substance comprises a soft cortex and a firm, central nucleus. Also *crystalline lens, lens crystallina, crystalline humor* (outmoded), *phacoid.* Adj. lenticular. **achromatic l.** A lens corrected for chromatic aberration. Also *achromat.* **acoustic l.** A device that focuses sound, analogous to an optical lens that focuses light. **aniseikonic l.** A lens that changes the size of an image without altering the focal distance. **aplanatic l.** A lens corrected for spherical aberration. **concavoconvex l.** A lens with negative dioptric power on a concave surface, and plus dioptric power on the other, convex surface. **contact l.** A lens that fits directly upon the cornea. **converging l.** PLUS LENS. **convexoconcave l.** A lens with plus dioptric power on a convex surface, and minus dioptric power on the other, concave surface. **l. crystallina** LENS. **crystalline l.** LENS. **cylindrical l.** An optical lens having its greatest strength along one meridian, designed to correct astigmatism. Also *cylinder.* **decentered l.** A lens positioned with its optical center off the axis of the optical system to cause a prismatic effect and correct for muscle imbalance. **diverging l.** MINUS LENS. **electron l.** An electromagnetic device that is used to focus a beam of electrons within an electron microscope. **flat l.** A lens with one plane surface or with opposite surfaces both equally concave or convex. **Hruby l.** A minus 55 diopter lens designed to permit biomicroscopic viewing of the ocular fundus. **immersion l.** An objective lens intended for direct contact with an immersion fluid. **iseikonic l.** A lens that changes the size of an object to correct for aniseikonia. **meniscus l.** A deeply curved concavoconvex lens. **meter l.** A lens with a power of one diopter plus. **minus l.** A lens that diverges rays of light; a lens having minus dioptric power. Also *negative lens, diverging lens.*

**omnifocal l.** A bifocal lens in which the curvature of the lens is such that dioptric power increases gradually toward the lens periphery, thereby providing a continuous range of focal distances from which the user can select the one best suited for a chosen working distance at any given time. Also *progressive lens.* **orthoscopic l.** A lens corrected for spherical aberrations. **photochromic l.** A lens that darkens upon exposure to ultraviolet and is used in sunglasses. **plus l.** A lens that converges rays of light; a lens having plus dioptric power. Also *positive lens, converging lens.* **progressive l.** OMNIFOCAL LENS. **spherical l.** A lens with plus or minus dioptric power, but no cylindrical power. **spherocylindrical l.** TORIC LENS. **toric l.** A concavoconvex or convexoconcave lens with a cylinder ground on its outer surface for the correction of astigmatism. Also *spherocylindrical lens, spherocylinder.*

**lensectomy** \lenzek′təmē\ LENTECTOMY.

**lensometer** \lenzäm′ətər\ A device for measurement of lens strength.

**lentectomy** \lentek′təmē\ [L *lens,* gen. *lent(is)* lentil, lens + -ECTOMY] Surgical removal of the crystalline lens. Also *lensectomy.*

**lenticel** \len′tisēl\ A lens-shaped or lentil-shaped gland, particularly one found at the root of the tongue.

**lenticonus** \len′tikō′nəs\ [LENS + L *conus* a cone] LENTIGLOBUS.

**lenticula** \lentik′yələ\ [L, dim. of *lens,* gen. *lentis,* a lentil, freckle] NUCLEUS LENTIFORMIS.

**lenticular** \lentik′yələr\ [L *lenticularis* (from *lenticula* a lentil) of or like a lentil] **1** Lens-shaped or lentil-shaped; lentiform. **2** Pertaining to a lens. **3** Pertaining to the nucleus lentiformis.

**lenticuli** \lentik′yəlī\ Plural of LENTICULUS.

**lenticulostriate** \lentik′yəlōstrī′āt\ **1** Pertaining to the lenticular nucleus and the corpus striatum. **2** Denoting the largest of the striate branches of the middle cerebral artery, one of the most frequent sites of cerebral arterial occlusion.

**lenticulothalamic** \lentik′yəlōthalam′ik\ Pertaining to the lenticular nucleus and the thalamus.

**lenticulus** \lentik′yələs\ [L (dim. of *lens,* gen. *lentis,* a lentil), a little lentil] A small lens.

**lentiform** \len′tifôrm\ **1** Shaped like a lentil or the lens of an eye. **2** NUCLEUS LENTIFORMIS.

**lentigines** \lentij′inēz\ Plural of LENTIGO.

**lentiginosis** \lentij′inō′sis\ [L *lentigo,* gen. *lentigin(is)* (see LENTIGO) + -OSIS] The presence of lentigines in exceptionally large numbers or in a distinctive distribution. **cardiomyopathic l.** MULTIPLE LENTIGINES SYNDROME.

**lentiglobus** \len′tiglō′bəs\ [L *lens,* gen. *lentis,* a lentil + GLOBUS] An anomalous conical or spheroidal elevation on the surface of the crystalline lens. Also *lenticonus.*

**lentigo** \lentī′gō\ [L (gen. *lentiginis;* from LENS), a lentil-shaped spot] (*pl.* lentigines.) A small brown macule that results from an increased number of melanocytes at the dermoepidermal junction. **l. aestiva** FRECKLE. **Hutchinson's malignant l.** HUTCHINSON'S MELANOTIC FRECKLE. **l. maligna** HUTCHINSON'S MELANOTIC FRECKLE. **malignant l.** HUTCHINSON'S MELANOTIC FRECKLE.

**lentigomelanoma** \lentī′gōmel′ənō′mə\ [LENTIGO + MELANOMA] A malignant melanoma arising in a lentigo.

**lentigomelanosis** \lentī′gōmel′ənō′sis\ [LENTIGO + MELANOSIS] A localized, irregular, brownish black pigmentation produced by a senile lentigo.

**lentitis** \lentī′tis\ [L *lens,* gen. *lentis,* a lentil + -ITIS] PHAKITIS.

**lentivirus** \len′tivī′rəs\ A slow virus belonging to the *Lentivirus* genus and Lentivirinae subfamily of the Retroviridae. Maedi and visna viruses are members of this genus.

**Leonardo** [*Leonardo* da Vinci, Italian scientist, artist, engineer, and inventor 1452–1519] Leonardo's band. See under TRABECULA SEPTOMARGINALIS.

**leontiasis** \lē′əntī′əsis\ [Gk *leōn,* gen. *leontos,* a lion + -IASIS] *Obs.* LEONINE FACIES. **l. ossea** LEONTIASIS OSSIUM. **l. ossea generalisata** VAN BUCHEM SYNDROME. **l. ossium** A bilateral, symmetric hypertrophy of the bones of the face and cranium of unknown etiology. It results in a lion-like facial expression which must be differentiated from the leonine face of lepromatous leprosy. Also *leontiasis ossea.*

**Leopold** [Christian Gerhard *Leopold,* German physician, 1846–1911] **1** See under LAW. **2** Leopold's maneuvers. See under MANEUVER.

**leper** \lep′ər\ [French *lèpre* (from Gk *lepra* leprosy, from *lepra,* fem. of *lepros* scaly) leprosy. English *leper* formerly meant the disease itself, afflicting a leprous person] A person suffering from leprosy. Also *lazar.* • The term is rarely used by the medical profession because of its alternative definition as a tainted or objectionable person.

**lepido-** \lep′idō-\ [Gk *lepis* (genitive *lepidos*) scale, husk, shell] A combining form meaning scale, flake.

**Lepidoptera** \lep′idäp′tərə\ [LEPIDO- + Gk *ptera* (pl. of *pteron* a feather) feathers, wings] An order of holometabolous insects characterized by wings covered with scales; the moths and butterflies.

**Lépine** [Jean *Lépine,* French physician, born 1876] Lépine-Froin syndrome. See under FROIN SYNDROME.

**leporipoxvirus** \lep′ôrēpäks′vī′rəs\ [L *lepus,* gen. *leporis,* a hare + POX + VIRUS] Any virus of the genus *Leporipoxvirus* in the family Poxviridae. They cause myxomas and fibromas in leporids and squirrels. The virions are enveloped, brick-shaped, 218–270 nm, contain double-stranded DNA, and are inactivated by ether. Serological cross-reactivity among species is common. Mechanical transmission by mosquitoes frequently occurs. Myxoma virus is the type species.

**lepothrix** \lep′əthriks\ [Gk *lepo(s)* husk, rind, scale + *thrix* hair] A superficial *Corynebacterium* infection of the axillary or pubic hair in which red, yellow, or black nodules or sheaths form on the hair shafts. Also *trichomycosis chromatica, trichomycosis nodosa.* • This condition was originally thought to be a fungal infection, giving rise to the *trichomycosis* misnomers.

**lepra** \lep′rə\ [L, from Gk (from *lepros* scaly, scabby, from *lepis* scales, flakes) any of various skin diseases, prob. usually psoriasis] **1** LEPROSY. **2** *Obs.* PSORIASIS. **l. alba** Macular leprosy that is characterized by hypopigmented lesions. **l. alphos** PSORIASIS. **l. graecorum** LEPROSY. **l. manchada** LUCIO PHENOMENON. **l. minor** Tuberculoid leprosy manifested by small, discrete lesions. **Willan's l.** PSORIASIS CIRCINATA.

**leprolin** \lep′rəlin\ A preparation of tissue containing *Mycobacterium leprae* used in the early twentieth century in attempts to induce immunity to leprosy.

**leprologist** \lepräl′əjist\ A specialist in the diagnosis and treatment of leprosy.

**leprology** \lepräl′əjē\ [*lepro(sy)* + -LOGY] The study of leprosy.

**leproma** \leprō′mə\ [*lepr(a)* + -OMA] A histiocytic cellular reaction characteristic of lepromatous leprosy. A diagnostic feature is the demonstration of leprosy bacilli following suitable staining.

**lepromatosis** \lep′rōmətō′sis\ [LEPROMA + *t* + -OSIS] See under LUCIO PHENOMENON.

**lepromatous** \leprō′mətəs\ 1 Pertaining to or characterized by lepromas. 2 Affected with lepromatous leprosy.

**lepromin** \lep′rəmin\ [*leprom(a)* + -IN] The material used in the lepromin test, of which there are two preparations in common use: leprominum integrale (Mitsuda-type) and Dharmendra lepromin. Also *Mitsuda antigen*.

**leprostatic** Inhibitory to the growth of *Mycobacterium leprae*, the organism that causes leprosy.

**leprosy** \lep′rəsē\ [assumed Med L *leprosia* (from *lepros(us)* leprous, from *lepra;* see LEPRA) leprosy or any of several similar diseases] A chronic mycobacterial disease that is sometimes infectious. It primarily affects the peripheral nervous system and secondarily involves the skin and certain other tissues. Also *Hansen's disease, hanseniasis* (rare), *lepra graecorum, lepra*. **borderline l.** Leprosy affecting persons possessing a moderate degree of cell-mediated immunity to *Mycobacterium leprae*. Because immunity is unstable the leprosy is able to upgrade to the tuberculoid pole or downgrade to the lepromatous pole. **cutaneous l.** Leprosy manifested by one or more skin lesions in the absence of clinical evidence of involvement of other tissues. *Rare*. • The term is a misnomer because nerve involvement occurs in all cases of leprosy even though clinical evidence of nerve damage is lacking. **histoid l.** Leprosy characterized by skin nodules that are firm, shiny, glistening, and sometimes erythematous, as in hyperactive lepromatous leprosy. These skin nodules may be seen in new patients or in relapsed cases, and the classical histological finding is of spindle-shaped histiocytes containing large numbers of leprosy bacilli. **lepromatous l.** Leprosy affecting persons with depressed cell-mediated immunity to *Mycobacterium leprae*. As a result leprosy bacilli are widely disseminated in the tissues. Also *virchowian leprosy*. Abbr. LL **Lucio l.** A diffuse, non-nodular variant of lepromatous leprosy rarely encountered outside Mexico and Central America. **macular l.** Leprosy characterized by skin lesions that are entirely composed of macules. These flat lesions cannot be felt by the examiner's finger. **polar lepromatous l.** Lepromatous leprosy which is immunologically stable. There is no evolution to a different type, hence the leprosy is termed polar. Abbr. LLp **pure neural l.** Leprosy characterized by one or more palpably thickened nerves, with or without signs of nerve dysfunction, that occur in the absence of skin lesions. **reactional l.** LEPRA REACTION. **spotted l.** LUCIO PHENOMENON. **subclinical l.** Infection with *Mycobacterium leprae* that is apparent only by immunologic testing and is acquired by contact with infectious leprosy. There are no clinical manifestations and only a very small proportion of infected persons develop clinical disease, confirming that the rate of transmission of *Mycobacterium leprae* is very significantly higher than the disease attack rate. **subpolar lepromatous l.** Lepromatous leprosy that has previously undergone a borderline phase. It is immunologically unstable and may upgrade to the borderline type. Abbr. LLs **tuberculoid l.** Leprosy that affects persons possessing good cell-mediated immunity to *Mycobacterium leprae*. Clinical manifestations are few and leprosy bacilli are scanty or absent in the tissues. **virchowian l.** LEPROMATOUS LEPROSY. • In the new leprosy terminology officially approved in Brazil, the term *virchowian* has replaced *lepromatous*, but the change has received little general acceptance in the English-speaking world.

**leprotic** \leprät′ik\ Of or relating to leprosy. Also *leprous*.

**leprous** \lep′rəs\ [*lepr(a)* + -OUS] LEPROTIC.

**-lepsia** \-lep′sē·ə\ -LEPSIS.

**-lepsis** \-lep′sis\ [Gk *lēpsis* (akin to *lambanein* to take hold of, seize) a taking, seizing] A combining form meaning a seizure.

**-lepsy** \-lepsē\ -LEPSIS.

**lept-** \lept-\ LEPTO-.

**leptazol** PENTYLENETETRAZOLE.

**lepto-** \lep′tō-\ [Gk *leptos* thin, fine, slender, delicate] A combining form meaning fine, slender, delicate, weak. Also *lept-*.

**leptocyte** \lep′təsīt\ An erythrocyte that is thinner than normal and hence appears hypochromic. It is commonly observed in iron deficiency anemia, thalassemias, chronic inflammatory disorders, and other conditions.

**leptocytic** \-sit′ik\ Pertaining to leptocytes.

**leptocytosis** \-sītō′sis\ The presence of numerous leptocytes in blood.

**leptodactyly** \-dak′tilē\ [LEPTO- + DACTYL- + -Y ] An unusual slenderness or elongation of the fingers and toes.

**leptomeninges** \-mənin′jēz\ [New L (from LEPTO- + *meninges*) the thin or delicate meninges] (*sing.* leptomeninx) The arachnoidea and pia mater together. Also *arachnopia* (obs.), *pia-arachnoid, piarachnoid*.

**leptomeningioma** \-mənin′jē·ō′mə\ [*leptomening(es)* + *i* + -OMA] A tumor of the leptomeninges.

**leptomeningitis** \-men′inji′tis\ Inflammation of the leptomeninges. Also *meninginitis, subarachnoiditis, pia-arachnitis, piarachnitis*. See also MENINGITIS. **sarcomatous l.** Diffuse sarcomatous infiltration in the meninges and subarachnoid space.

**leptomeningopathy** \-men′ing·gäp′əthē\ [LEPTO- + MENINGO- + -PATHY] Any disease of the leptomeninges.

**leptomeninx** \-mē′ningks\ Singular of LEPTOMENINGES.

**leptonema** \-nē′mə\ A very thin, threadlike form, as taken by the chromosomes during the leptotene stage of meiosis.

**leptopellic** \-pel′ik\ Having an unusually narrow pelvis.

**leptophonia** \-fō′nē·ə\ [LEPTO- + PHON- + -IA] A weak, thin quality to the voice, resulting from general debility or certain myopathic or neurologic conditions. Also *microphonia*.

**leptoprosopia** \-prōsō′pē·ə\ [LEPTO- + PROSOP- + -IA] An extreme narrowness of the face.

***Leptopsylla segnis*** \-sil′ə seg′nis\ The cosmopolitan European mouse flea, also commonly found on rats. It is able to transmit plague, but is a poor vector as it bites humans rarely. Also *Ctenopsyllus segnis*.

**leptoscope** \lep′təskōp\ An optical instrument used to measure the thickness of a thin film, such as the plasma membrane.

***Leptospira*** \lep′təspī′rə\ [LEPTO- + Gk *speira* anything wound or wrapped around a thing] A genus of coiled, aerobic spirochetes. See under *LEPTOSPIRA INTERROGANS*. ***L. biflexa*** A saprobic leptospire found in streams. It carries a genus-specific antigen used in the diagnosis of leptospiral infection. ***L. interrogans*** A species of spirochete with a very tight coil, the body often being bent at the ends in the form of a hook. It can be grown aerobically in complex media containing fatty acids. Wild rodents and domestic animals are the reservoir, often shedding the organisms in the urine during a mild, chronic illness. The human illness varies from subclinical to a severe disease with jaundice, albuminuria, and hemorrhages (Weil's disease). Many strains may be differentiated, whether antigenically, by G + C content of the DNA, or by origin. All the pathogens are classified in the one species, with serotypes such as *icterohaemorrhagiae* from rats, *canicola* from dogs, etc. • The epithet *interrogans* derives from the resemblance of the organism to a question mark. ***L. interrogans* serotype *autumnalis*** A leptospire originally isolated in Japan and shown serologically to have been the cause of an epidemic of pretibial fever at Fort Bragg.

**leptospire** \lep′təspī′r\ An organism of the genus *Leptospira.* Adj. leptospiral.

**leptospirosis** \lep′təspīrō′sis\ [*Leptospir(a)* + -OSIS] Infection by spirochetes of the genus *Leptospira,* of which there are more than 170 serotypes. The major diseases in man are caused by *L. icterohaemorrhagiae* and *L. canicola.* Many kinds of mammals serve as reservoirs of infection, especially rats and dogs. The bacteria are excreted in the animals' urine, and infection is acquired through cuts and abrasions in the skin. The disease has multiple clinical presentations. **anicteric l.** A common, relatively mild form of leptospirosis characterized by fever, headache, myalgia, nausea, malaise, and, rarely, circulatory collapse. Jaundice is absent and hepatomegaly is rare. The disease may be biphasic, with the first stage lasting three to seven days and the second, or immune, stage lasting one to three days. Fever may not be present in the second stage. Also *benign leptospirosis.* **l. hebdomadis** NANUKAYAMI. **icteric l.** The severe form of leptospirosis, characterized by biphasic fever, muscle pain, bleeding tendencies, gastrointestinal symptoms, and commonly also jaundice, azotemia, anemia, and disturbances of consciousness resulting from liver and kidney impairment. It may be caused by almost any serotype of *Leptospira interrogans.* Once common among sewer and abattoir workers and laborers in rice paddies, it now occurs primarily in young people exposed to contaminated water during outdoor recreation. Also *Weil's disease, leptospirosis icterohemorrhagica, leptospiral jaundice, icterohemorrhagic fever, spirochetal jaundice, spirochetal icterus, icterus infectiosus, hemorrhagic jaundice, icterogenic spirochetosis* (obs.), *spirochetosis icterohemorrhagica, Fiedler's disease, Larrey-Weil disease, Landouzy's disease, Lancereaux-Mathieu disease, Mathieu's disease, Wassilieff's disease, bilious typhoid* (outmoded), *Mediterranean yellow fever* (outmoded).

**leptotene** \lep′tətēn\ The first stage in the first prophase of meiosis, in which chromosomes first become visible as thin threads.

***Leptotrombidium*** \-trämbid′ē·əm\ A genus of chigger mites in the family Trombiculidae, formerly considered a subgenus of *Trombicula.* It probably includes all known vectors of *Rickettsia tsutsugamushi,* the causative agent of scrub typhus. The principal species that transmit this disease include *L. akamushi (Trombicula akamushi, Microtrombidium akamushi),* which is the vector of classical Japanese scrub typhus.

***Leptus*** \lep′təs\ A pseudogenus of chiggers, or larval trombiculid mites. *L. autumnalis,* for example, is the larva of *Trombicula autumnalis* and *L. akamushi* is the larva of *Leptotrombidium akamushi.* It also includes some larval forms of which the adult stage has not been identified and which are therefore not yet assigned to a true genus and species.

**Leq** loudness equivalent: the equivalent continuous sound level of noise, measured on the dB(A) scale, used in the investigation of noise levels as these affect the community and place of work, and in the experimental investigation of noise-induced hearing loss.

**Léri** [Andre *Léri,* French physician, 1875–1930] **1** See under SIGN. **2** Léri's disease. See under MELORHEOSTOSIS. **3** Léri's pleonosteosis, Léri-Weill syndrome. See under DYSCHONDROSTEOSIS.

**Leriche** [René *Leriche,* French surgeon, 1879–1955] **1** Leriche costoclavicular outlet syndrome. See under SCALENUS ANTERIOR SYNDROME. **2** See under TREATMENT. **3** Leriche's disease. See under POST-TRAUMATIC OSTEOPOROSIS.

**Lermoyez** [Marcel *Lermoyez,* French otolaryngologist, 1858–1929] See under SYNDROME.

**Leroy** [Emile *Leroy,* French physician, born 1873] Fiessinger-Leroy-Reiter syndrome. See under REITER SYNDROME.

**les** **1** local excitatory state. **2** lower esophageal sphincter (cardiac sphincter).

**lesbian** \lez′bē·ən\ [Gk *Lesbi(os)* pertaining to the Gk island of Lesbos and to its people + English *-an,* adjectival suffix] **1** A female homosexual. **2** Characterized by female homosexuality.

**Leser** [Edmund *Leser,* German surgeon, 1853–1916] Leser-Trélat sign. See under SIGN.

**lesion** \lē′zhən\ [L *laesio* (from *laesus,* past part. of *laedere* to strike, injure) a hurting, harming] A pathologic alteration in the structure or function of a tissue or organ. **Armanni-Ebstein l.** A morphologic change occasionally seen in the kidney of diabetes mellitus patients. The tubule cells appear markedly vacuolated due to the accumulation of glycogen. Also *Ebstein's lesion.* **Bracht-Wächter l.'s** Microscopic foci of myocardial necrosis, seen in bacterial endocarditis and resulting from either coronary embolization or endarteritis. **capsular drop l.** HYALINE LESION. **caviar l.** Venous ectasia of the undersurface of the tongue. **central l.** Any lesion of the central nervous system. **coin l.** A lesion in the lung which appears radiographically as a discrete disk of opacity. **complement l.** The consequence of the insertion of the membrane complex of complement into a membrane. It is characterized functionally by the formation of a transmembrane channel and morphologically by a characteristic ring-shaped appearance on electron microscopy. **compressive l. of the lumbosacral region** A mass lesion within the lumbar or sacral spinal canal, as that found in herniated nucleus pulposus or in tumor. It is usually identified by symptoms of pain or weakness attributable to injury to the lumbar or sacral nerve roots. **Councilman l.** COUNCILMAN BODIES. **destructive l.** A lesion which results in the death of the affected tissue or organ. **diffuse l.** A poorly localized lesion. **discharging l.** Any brain lesion which gives rise to focal electrical discharge in the electroencephalogram or to focal epilepsy. **Ebstein's l.** ARMANNI-EBSTEIN LESION. **focal l.** A circumscribed, well-localized lesion. **functional l.** A lesion characterized by an alteration of function of the affected part. **Ghon's primary l.** GHON TUBERCLE. **gross l.** A lesion visible to the naked eye. Also *macroscopic lesion.* **hepatic veno-occlusive l.** Occlusion of the hepatic veins, a rare condition usually caused by tumor or thrombus arising locally or by extension from the inferior vena cava. Other reported causes are thrombophlebitis migrans and clotting diseases such as polycythemia rubra vera. Membranous obliteration of the hepatic segment of the vena cava has also been described. **herpetiform l. of Cole** The initial cutaneous or mucosal vesicular lesion of lymphogranuloma venereum. **histologic l.** A lesion too small to be seen with the naked eye. **hyaline l.** Hyaline accumulations in the lumina of one or more capillary peripheral loops in the glomerular capsule, or in the glomerular space, often found in but not specific for diabetic glomerulopathy. Also *fibrin cap, fibrinoid cap, capsular drop lesion.* See also GLOMERULAR DEPOSITS, DIABETIC GLOMERULOSCLEROSIS. **indiscriminate l.** A lesion affecting multiple organs, regions, or tissues. **initial syphilitic l.** HARD CHANCRE. **irritative l.** A lesion that results in stimulation of the affected part. **jet l.** A focus of endocardial fibrosis caused by the trauma of repeated jet-like streams of blood directed at the focus, due to incompetence or stenosis of a cardiac valve. **Kimmelstiel-Wilson l.** Round hyaline deposits in glomerular mesangial areas, characteristic of but not specific for diabetic glomerulosclerosis. **local l.** Any lesion of the central nervous system restricted to a particular area and giving rise to focal neurologic signs. **local glomerular l.** SEGMENTAL GLOMERULAR LESION. **lower motor neuron l.** Any lesion involving lower as distinct from upper motor neurons. **macroscopic l.** GROSS LESION. **mass l.** Any large space-occupying lesion, particularly in the central nervous system, such as a tumor, hematoma, or abscess. **molecular l.** A lesion demonstrable at the molecular level. The lesion itself is thus not visible, although its effects on the tissue may be apparent. **onion scale l.'s** Replication of the arterial laminae, specifically of the splenic arterioles, giving the histologic appearance in cross-section of concentric circles resembling a sliced onion. These lesions are characteristic of systemic lupus erythematosus, but may be seen in vasculitis and hypertension. **organic l.** A lesion that produces an alteration in the structure of the affected organ or tissue. Also *structural lesion*. **partial l.** A lesion that is present in only a part of the affected tissue or organ. • Frequently used to describe lesions that affect only part of a conducting tract in neurological disorders. **precancerous l.** A morphologically altered tissue that has a greater risk of becoming a cancer than its normal counterpart, as in epithelial dysplasia, Barrett's esophagus, or adenoma of the colon. **retrocochlear l.** A lesion behind the cochlea, that is, central to the cochlea on the vestibular pathway. In patients with vertigo and/or sensorineural deafness it is critically important to differentiate between cochlear and retrocochlear lesions if, for instance, cases of Menière's disease, a cochlear lesion, are to be separated from cases of acoustic neuroma, a retrocochlear lesion. **ring-wall l.** A small area of organized perivascular hemorrhage in the brain, surrounded by glial proliferation. **Scheibe l.** A lesion of the cochlea and saccule suspected of being the most common cause of congenital genetic deafness. The sensory epithelium of the organ of Corti and the saccular macula is represented simply by a mass of entirely undifferentiated cells. **segmental glomerular l.** Any lesion involving part of a glomerulus. Also *local glomerular lesion*. **structural l.** ORGANIC LESION. **swan-neck tubular l.** A distortion of the proximal convoluted tubule caused by thinning and shortening of the first portion of the proximal tubule, often present in congenital nephrosis. It may be suspected by histologic study but can be definitively demonstrated by microdissection. **systemic l.** A lesion that may involve multiple organ systems, such as fibrin thrombi occluding multiple capillary beds in disseminated intravascular coagulation. **trophic l.** A lesion that results from altered nutrition of the affected part. **tumorlike l.** A non-neoplastic lesion resembling a neoplasm. Also *pseudotumor, false tumor*. **wire-loop l.** Thickened glomerular capillary walls that look like stiff wire loops in histologic sections, frequently seen in but not specific for lupus nephropathy.

**Lesshaft** [Pyotr Frantsovich *Lesshaft*, Russian anatomist, 1836–1909] Lesshaft space. See under SUPERIOR LUMBAR TRIANGLE.

**LET** linear energy transfer.

**let-down** The movement of newly formed milk from the alveoli to the ducts of the mammary gland.

**lethal** \lē'thəl\ [L *letalis* or *lethalis* (from *let(um)* death, ruin, akin to *delere* to destroy, blot out + *-alis* -AL) deadly, mortal] Causing or capable of causing death; deadly.

**lethality** \lēthal'itē\ [*lethal* + -ITY] FATALITY RATE.

**lethargogenic** 1 Producing lethargy. 2 A drug or agent that produces lethargy.

**lethargus** \lēthär'gəs\ [L, lethargy, morbid drowsiness] 1 GAMBIAN TRYPANOSOMIASIS. 2 RHODESIAN TRYPANOSOMIASIS.

**lethargy** \leth'ərjē\ [Late L *lethargia* (from L *lethargus* drowsiness, morbid sleepiness, from Gk *lēthargos* forgetful, lethargic, from *lēthē* forgetfulness) lethargy, forgetfulness] 1 A state of excessive fatigue or retardation, with diminished physical or mental activity. This can be due to organic disease or dysfunction of the nervous system or to mental illness, such as depression. 2 HYPERSOMNIA. **African l.** 1 GAMBIAN TRYPANOSOMIASIS. 2 RHODESIAN TRYPANOSOMIASIS. **hypnotic l.** A state of apparent sleep or stupor induced by hypnosis. Also *hypnotic trance, hysteric lethargy, induced lethargy, induced trance*. **hysteric l.** HYPNOTIC LETHARGY. **induced l.** HYPNOTIC LETHARGY. **lucid l.** Retention of consciousness and of the power of speech with inability to move as in sleep paralysis or, less commonly, in hysteric dissociation states.

**letheral** \lē'thərəl\ [Gk *lēthē* forgetfulness + *r* + -AL] AMNESIC.

**lethologica** \leth'əläj'ikə\ [Gk *lēth(ē)* forgetfulness + *o* + *logika*, neut. pl. of *logikos* pertaining to speech or reason] NOMINAL APHASIA.

**Letterer** [Erich *Letterer*, German pathologist, born 1895] Letterer-Siwe disease. See under DISEASE.

**Leu** Symbol for leucine.

**leuc-** \loos-, look-\ LEUKO-.

**leucemia** \loosē'mē·ə\ LEUKEMIA.

**leucine** \loo'sēn\ [LEUC- + -INE; so called from its white crystalline form] $(CH_3)_2CH—CH_2—CH(NH_2)COOH$. One of the nutritionally essential amino acids for man and other higher animals. Also *aminoisocaproic acid* (obs.).

**leucine aminopeptidase** The cytosolic aminopeptidase found in mammals. It is a zinc-containing enzyme that hydrolyzes peptides, removing the N-terminal residue, provided that this is not arginine or lysine. It is often used for determining the sequences of peptides.

**[4-leucine] oxytocin** A synthetic neurohypophysial peptide, an analogue of oxytocin. It induces renal excretion of sodium, potassium and chloride, and also opposes the antidiuretic action of arginine vasopressin.

**leucitis** \loosī'tis\ [LEUC- + -ITIS] SCLERITIS.

**leuco-** \loo'kō-\ LEUKO-.

**leucocidin** *Brit.* LEUKOCIDIN.

**leucocyte** *Brit.* LEUKOCYTE.

**leucocytosis** *Brit.* LEUKOCYTOSIS.

**leucoderma** *Brit.* LEUKODERMA.

**leucofluorescein** The product of fluorescein after reduction with zinc powder in acidic solution. It is used in solution as a diagnostic aid to detect corneal damage or injury. Also *fluorecin*.

**leucoma** *Brit.* LEUKOMA.

**leuconychia** \-nik'ē·ə\ *Brit.* LEUKONYCHIA.

**leucopenia** \-pē'nē·ə\ *Brit.* LEUKOPENIA.

**leucoplakia** *Brit.* LEUKOPLAKIA.

**leucopoiesis** \-poi·ē'sis\ *Brit.* LEUKOPOIESIS.

**leucorrhoea** \loo'kôrē'ə\ *Brit.* LEUKORRHEA.

**leucotomy** \lookät'əmē\ *Brit.* LEUKOTOMY.

**leucovorin** \-vôr'in\ FOLINIC ACID.

**leucovorin calcium** The calcium salt of folinic acid (leucovorin). It is used to counteract the toxic effects of folic acid antagonists. It is also used in the treatment of megaloblastic anemias and as an adjunct to cyanocobalamin in the treatment of pernicious anemia.

**leuk-** \look-\ LEUKO-.

**leukaemia** *Brit.* LEUKEMIA.
**leukagglutinin** \loo′kəgloo′tinin\ LEUKOAGGLUTININ.
**leukapheresis** \loo′kəferē′sis\ Selective removal of leukocytes by hemapheresis. It may be performed to obtain leukocyte donation or as a therapeutic measure in patients with elevated peripheral blood white cells where the cells are likely to cause cerebral white cell infarcts as in the acute "blast crisis" phase of chronic granulocytic leukemia.
**leukemia** \lookē′mē·ə\ [LEUK- + -EMIA] A malignant proliferation of blood leukocytes, usually characterized by leukocytosis and infiltration of other organs by the leukemic cells, ultimately causing death. Several distinct types of leukemia are recognized, including acute lymphocytic, acute myelogenous, acute monocytic, acute myelomonocytic, acute promyelocytic, erythroleukemia, chronic myelogenous, and chronic lymphocytic. Also *Bennett's disease, hemosarcoma* (obs.), *medullosis* (obs.), *hemocytoblastoma, leukocytic sarcoma.* Also *leucemia.* **acute l.** Any of several acute forms of leukemia, such as acute lymphocytic leukemia, acute granulocytic leukemia, acute monocytic leukemia, acute myelomonocytic leukemia, acute erythroleukemia, or acute promyelocytic leukemia. Also *blast cell leukemia, Bennet syndrome.* See also FRENCH-AMERICAN-BRITISH CLASSIFICATION. **acute basophilic l.** A very rare form of acute granulocytic leukemia in which the myeloblasts or other granulocyte precursors show signs of differentiation into basophils, such as the presence of a few very large basophilic granules in the cytoplasm of cells beyond the progranulocyte stage. **acute eosinophilic l.** A rare form of acute granulocytic leukemia in which the myeloblasts or other granulocyte precursors exhibit signs of differentiation into eosinophils, such as the presence of a few large eosinophilic granules in the cytoplasm. **acute granulocytic l.** An acute leukemia characterized by a predominance of myeloblasts in the peripheral blood and bone marrow. Also *myeloblastic leukemia, acute myeloid leukemia, myeloblastic leukosis* (rare), *acute myelocytic leukemia.* **acute lymphocytic l.** An acute leukemia that is distinguished by the presence of large numbers of lymphoblasts in the blood and bone marrow. Also *acute lymphoid leukemia, acute lymphoblastic leukemia, acute lymphogenous leukemia, lymphoblastic leukemia.* See also FRENCH-AMERICAN-BRITISH CLASSIFICATION. **acute myelocytic l.** ACUTE GRANULOCYTIC LEUKEMIA. **acute myeloid l.** ACUTE GRANULOCYTIC LEUKEMIA. **acute nonlymphocytic l.** Any acute leukemia that is distinguished by the presence of large numbers of immature cells (usually blasts) other than lymphoblasts in the blood. Included are acute granulocytic leukemia, progranulocytic leukemia, myelomonocytic leukemia, acute monocytic leukemia, and acute erythroleukemia. See also FRENCH-AMERICAN-BRITISH CLASSIFICATION. **acute promyelocytic l.** An uncommon type of acute granulocytic leukemia in which atypical promyelocytes are the predominant leukocytes. The atypical promyelocytes have fewer of the prominent dense primary cytoplasmic granules that characterize promyelocytes, and they often have large numbers (5–20) of Auer rods that may be arranged in sheaves or "faggots." This leukemia is typically associated with deficiencies of clotting factors due to intravascular coagulation and with a cytogenetic abnormality in the leukemic cells that is a 15;17 translocation, i.e. t(15;17)(q26;q22). **aleukemic l.** Acute leukemia in which leukemic cells ("blasts") are not present in blood, nor is there leukocytosis. Often there is pancytopenia. Diagnosis is made by examination of bone marrow. *Rare.* Also *aleukocythemic leukemia, leukopenic leukemia, cryptoleukemia.* **basophilic l.** A rare form of leukemia in which there is a very marked increase in basophils in blood and bone marrow. It is considered a variant of chronic granulocytic leukemia. **blast cell l.** ACUTE LEUKEMIA. **chronic granulocytic l.** A neoplastic disorder of the blood granulocytes that usually occurs in persons of age 30–50 years, and is characterized by splenomegaly, increase in the number of granulocytes in blood and bone marrow to values as high as $500 \times 10^9$/l, thrombocytosis that may be very marked, absent or nearly absent leukocyte alkaline phosphatase, and a distinctive cytogenetic abnormality of granulocytes, the Philadelphia ($Ph^1$) chromosome: t(9;22)(p34;q11). Approximately 10% of cases that have the other features of chronic granulocytic leukemia lack the chromosomal anomaly; the taxonomic status of "Philadelphia chromosome negative chronic granulocytic leukemia" is unresolved. Also *chronic myeloid leukemia, chronic myelocytic leukemia, splenomyelogenous leukemia, mature cell leukemia, medullary leukemia,.* **chronic lymphocytic l.** A neoplastic disorder of adults characterized by marked increase in mature lymphocytes in blood, often by enlargement of lymph nodes and spleen, and by duration of months to years. Also *lymphocytic leukemia, chronic lymphatic leukemia.* **chronic myelocytic l.** CHRONIC GRANULOCYTIC LEUKEMIA. **chronic myeloid l.** CHRONIC GRANULOCYTIC LEUKEMIA. **l. cutis** Involvement of the skin, particularly the dermis, by leukemia. This condition is seen particularly in the Sézary syndrome, but also in chronic lymphocytic and acute leukemias. Also *lymphodermia perniciosa* (obs.). **embryonal l.** STEM CELL LEUKEMIA. **eosinophilic l.** A very rare form of leukemia in which eosinophilia of peripheral blood and bone marrow is associated with an excessive number of myeloblasts (e.g. 10% or more of the granulocytic cells) in bone marrow or blood or both. **feline l.** An acute lymphocytic leukemia that occurs in cats infected with the feline leukemia virus. In addition to leukemia, this virus infection of cats may cause thymoma, lymphosarcoma, fibrosarcoma, hypoplastic anemia, or an immunodeficiency syndrome that mimics in many of its features the human acquired immunodeficiency sydrome (AIDS), including the propensity to fatal infections with opportunistic microorganisms. **granulocytic l.** A leukemia in which the predominant cells are of the granulocytic cell line, i.e. polymorphonuclear leukocytes and their precursors. The term includes chronic granulocytic leukemia, in which granulocytes of all stages of maturation are present in blood, and acute granulocytic leukemia, in which myeloblasts are markedly increased in blood and bone marrow. Also *myelogenous leukemia, myeloid leukemia, myeloleukemia, myeloid granulocytic leukemia, myelocytic leukemia, neutrophilic leukemia, polymorphocytic leukemia.* **Gross l.** A murine leukemia of experimental importance, for which the causative virus can be transmitted by inoculation from one species to another. **hairy cell l.** LEUKEMIC RETICULOENDOTHELIOSIS. **hemoblastic l.** STEM CELL LEUKEMIA. **hemocytoblastic l.** STEM CELL LEUKEMIA. **histiocytic l.** **1** The leukemic phase of histiocytic medullary reticulosis. **2** SCHILLING'S LEUKEMIA. See under MONOCYTIC LEUKEMIA. **leukopenic l.** ALEUKEMIC LEUKEMIA. **lymphoblastic l.** ACUTE LYMPHOCYTIC LEUKEMIA. **lymphocytic l.** CHRONIC LYMPHOCYTIC LEUKEMIA. **lymphoid l.** Any neoplastic proliferation of lymphoid cells in the blood and marrow, including acute lymphocytic leukemia and chronic lymphocytic leukemia. Also *lymphogenous leukemia.* **lymphosarcoma cell l.** A type of lymphatic leukemia characterized by numerous large lymphocytes with prominent, usually single, nucleoli. It is often considered a variant of chronic lymphocytic leukemia. Also *lymphosarcoleukemia.* **mast**

**cell l.** A malignant proliferation of mast cells; a leukemic phase of systemic mastocytosis. Also *malignant mastocytosis.* **mature cell l.** CHRONIC GRANULOCYTIC LEUKEMIA. **medullary l.** CHRONIC GRANULOCYTIC LEUKEMIA. **megakaryocytic l.** 1 A variant of chronic granulocytic leukemia in which megakaryocytic proliferation and thrombocytosis predominate. 2 ESSENTIAL THROMBOCYTHEMIA. **micromyeloblastic l.** A variety of acute granulocytic leukemia in which the predominant cell is a small myeloblast, resembling a lymphocyte and best distinguished by histochemistry. **monocytic l.** Neoplastic proliferation of monocytes, a broad category which combines two varieties: Naegeli type acute myelomonocytic leukemia, in which cells are relatively smaller and exhibit some myeloblastic characteristics, and Schilling's leukemia, in which cells are larger and more typically monocytoid or even histiocytic. Also *monocytoma, monoblastoma.* **myeloblastic l.** ACUTE GRANULOCYTIC LEUKEMIA. **myelocytic l.** GRANULOCYTIC LEUKEMIA. **myelogenous l.** GRANULOCYTIC LEUKEMIA. **myeloid l.** GRANULOCYTIC LEUKEMIA. **myeloid granulocytic l.** GRANULOCYTIC LEUKEMIA. **myelomonocytic l.** A leukemia that is commonly subacute, but may be acute, and which is characterized by the presence in blood and bone marrow of numerous cells that have features both of myeloblasts and monocytes. These cells give positive reactions with nonspecific esterase stain (a monocyte stain) and with chloroacetate esterase stain (a granulocyte stain), and they may be peroxidase positive. In the French-American-British classification this condition is acute nonlymphocytic leukemia M4. **Naegeli type acute myelomonocytic l.** An acute monocytic leukemia in which many of the leukemic cells resemble myeloblasts. It is type M-4 in the French-American-British classification. **neutrophilic l.** GRANULOCYTIC LEUKEMIA. **plasma cell l.** A malignant disorder of plasma cells characterized by large numbers of plasma cells in blood as well as in bone marrow. Plasma cells exceed $1 \times 10^9/l$ in blood of persons with this disorder. **polymorphocytic l.** GRANULOCYTIC LEUKEMIA. **progranulocytic l.** PROMYELOCYTIC LEUKEMIA. **promyelocytic l.** A variety of myeloblastic leukemia in which promyelocytes predominate. It is often complicated by coagulation abnormalities. It is type M-3 in the French-American-British classification. Also *progranulocytic leukemia.* **Rieder cell l.** A variety of acute granulocytic leukemia in which the myeloblasts have indented nuclei (Rieder cells). **Schilling's l.** The acute form of monocytic leukemia. It is type M-5 in the French-American-British classification. Also *histiocytic leukemia.* **splenic l.** Any instance of leukemia accompanied by significant splenomegaly. *Imprecise.* **splenomyelogenous l.** *Obs.* CHRONIC GRANULOCYTIC LEUKEMIA. **stem cell l.** An acute leukemia in which the primitive blast cells cannot be classified as lymphoblasts, myeloblasts, or monoblasts, but may be presumed to represent the common precursor of all three cell lines. Also *embryonal leukemia, undifferentiated cell leukemia, hemoblastic leukemia, hemocytoblastic leukemia.*

**leukemic** \lookē′mik\ Having or pertaining to leukemia.

**leukemid** \lookē′mid\ [*leukem(ia)* + -ID[2]] A nonspecific cutaneous lesion containing infiltrates of leukemia cells, seen in patients with leukemia.

**leukemogen** \lookē′məjən\ Any substance or condition that promotes the development of leukemia, including chemicals such as benzene, all forms of ionizing radiation, and some viruses.

**leukemogenesis** \lookē′mōjen′əsis\ The process or mechanism of the development of leukemia.

**leukemogenic** \lookē′mōjen′ik\ Having the property of promoting the occurrence of leukemia.

**leukemoid** \lookē′moid\ Having features resembling those of leukemia, such as marked leukocytosis or the appearance of immature leukocytes in blood or bone marrow. Leukemoid reactions may occur in the course of some infections, as in miliary tuberculosis.

**leukencephalitis** \loo′kensef′əlī′tis\ LEUKOENCEPHALITIS.

**leukin** \loo′kin\ LEUKOCYTIC ENDOLYSIN.

**leuko-** \loo′kō-\ [Gk *leukos* light, bright, white] A combining form meaning (1) white or colorless; (2) leukocyte. Also *leuco-, leuk-, leuc-.*

**leukoagglutinin** \-əgloo′tinin\ Any antibody that causes clumping of leukocytes. Also *leukagglutinin.*

**leukoblastosis** \-blastō′sis\ Any malignant proliferative disorder of white blood cells, including leukemias and lymphomas.

**leukocidin** \-sī′din\ [LEUKO- + *-cid(e)* + -IN] A complement-fixing antileukocyte antibody that, in the presence of complement, will cause the leukocytes to be killed.

**leukocoria** \-kôr′ē·ə\ LEUKOKORIA.

**leukocytal** \-sī′təl\ *Seldom used* LEUKOCYTIC.

**leukocyte** \loo′kōsīt\ [LEUKO- + -CYTE] Any of several nucleated cells that occur in blood or tissue fluid, exclusive of erythrocytes and erythrocyte precursors. Major classes of leukocytes are lymphocytes, monocytes, neutrophils, eosinophils, and basophils. Also *white cell, white blood cell, white*

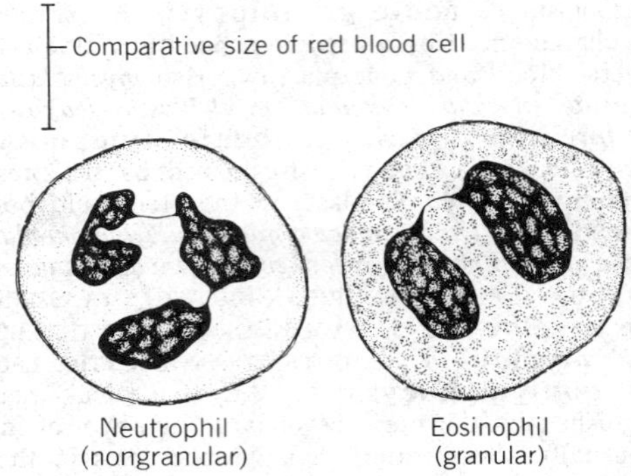


**Leukocytes**

*corpuscle, white blood corpuscle, amebocyte* (rare), *amoebocyte* (rare). **acidophilic l.** See under EOSINOPHIL. **agranular l.'s** Leukocytes that do not have cytoplasmic granules. Included are, principally, lymphocytes and monocytes, but also plasma cells, lymphoblasts, myeloblasts, and monoblasts. Also *nongranular leukocytes.* **cystinotic l.** A monocyte or neutrophil that contains cystine in prominent lysosomes as a manifestation of the hereditary metabolic disorder cystinosis. **endothelial l.** MACROPHAGE. **eosinophilic l.** See under EOSINOPHIL. **globular l.** A small lymphocyte observed in the subepithelial layers of the crypts of the intestinal mucosa. It has cytoplasmic globules which are eosinophilic. Also *globule leukocyte.* **granular l.** GRANULOCYTE. **heterophil l.** NEUTROPHIL. **hyaline l.** *Obs.* MONOCYTE. **lymphoid l.** LYMPHOCYTE. **motile l.** Any leukocyte that shows pseudopodia and ameboid movement in supravital, or wet, nonfixed preparations. All viable leukocytes are motile or potentially motile. **neutrophil l.** NEUTROPHIL. **nonfilament polymorphonuclear l.** Any leukocyte of the polymorphonuclear class that does not have two or more nuclear lobes connected by fine strands of chromatin. Included are band neutrophils, metamyelocytes, myelocytes, promyelocytes, and myeloblasts. **nongranular l.'s** AGRANULAR LEUKOCYTES. **nonmotile l.** A leukocyte lacking ameboid movement capability. **polymorphonuclear l.** A blood leukocyte that has a distinctly segmented or lobulated nucleus, the lobules being separated by a thin strand of chromatin. Included are segmented neutrophils, eosinophils, and basophils. Also *lobocyte, polymorphocyte, segmented leukocyte.* **Türk's irritation l.** TÜRK CELL.

**leukocythemia** \-sīthē'mē·ə\ LEUKOCYTOSIS.

**leukocytic** \-sit'ik\ Pertaining to or characteristic of leukocytes. Also *leukocytal* (seldom used).

**leukocytoblast** \-sī'təblast\ The earliest recognizable leukocyte precursor. It may be a lymphoblast, monoblast, or myeloblast.

**leukocytogenesis** \-sī'təjen'əsis\ LEUKOPOIESIS.

**leukocytoid** \-sī'toid\ Resembling, or characteristic of, leukocytes.

**leukocytolysis** \-sītäl'isis\ LEUKOLYSIS.

**leukocytolytic** \sī'təlit'ik\ LEUKOLYTIC.

**leukocytoma** \-sītō'mə\ Any of various tumorous accumulations of leukocytes, including chloroma, granulocytic sarcoma, and lymphoma.

**leukocytometer** \-sītäm'ətər\ A finely calibrated glass chamber which, used with a microscope, permits enumeration of leukocytes in accurately diluted samples of blood or other body fluids.

**leukocytopenia** \-sī'təpē'nē·ə\ LEUKOPENIA.

**leukocytophagy** \-sītäf'əjē\ The phagocytosis of leukocytes by cells of the monocyte-macrophage system.

**leukocytoplania** \-sī'təplā'nē·ə\ LEUKOPEDESIS.

**leukocytopoiesis** \-sī'təpoi·ē'sis\ LEUKOPOIESIS.

**leukocytosis** \-sītō'sis\ [*leukocyt(e)* + -OSIS] Any condition marked by increased concentration of leukocytes in the blood, including absolute lymphocytosis and absolute neutrophilia. Also *absolute leukocytosis, leukocythemia.* **agonal l.** TERMINAL LEUKOCYTOSIS. **basophilic l.** Leukocytosis due to increased basophilic granulocytes. Also *basocytosis.* **digestive l.** A mild, transient leukocytosis which normally follows ingestion of food. **eosinophilic l.** An increase in eosinophilic leukocytes in the peripheral blood. **lymphocytic l.** Leukocytosis due to an increase of lymphocytes in the peripheral blood. **mononuclear l.** Leukocytosis due to an increase of monocytes in the peripheral blood. **neutrophilic l.** Leukocytosis due to an increase of neutrophils in the peripheral blood. Also *pure leukocytosis.* **l. of the newborn** The normal leukocytosis observed during the first four days of life, reflecting transient increases in neutrophil numbers up to 30 000 per $mm^3$. **pathologic l.** Leukocytosis due to infection, inflammation, or other disease. **physiologic l.** Leukocytosis due to normal physiologic stimuli, including exercise or other nonpathologic factors. **pure l.** NEUTROPHILIC LEUKOCYTOSIS. **terminal l.** An elevation in the number of leukocytes in blood that occurs as a person dies. Also *agonal leukocytosis.* **toxic l.** An increase in the number of leukocytes in blood in response to severe infection.

**leukocytotactic** \-sī'tətak'tik\ Having the property of attracting the migration of leukocytes.

**leukocytotaxis** \-sī'tətak'sis\ The migration of leukocytes to a site of inflammation or injury. Also *leukocytotaxia.*

**leukocytotherapy** \-sī'təther'əpē\ Treatment by injection of leukocytes, for example, transfusion of granulocytes.

**leukocytotoxin** \-sī'tətäk'sin\ Any substance that selectively damages leukocytes. Also *leukotoxin.*

**leukocytotropic** \-sī'tətrāp'ik\ Having an affinity for leukocytes.

**leukocyturia** \-sītoo'rē·ə\ The presence of a greater than normal number of leukocytes in the urine, as in pyelonephritis.

**leukoderma** \-dur'mə\ [LEUKO- + DERMA] Lack of normal pigmentation of the skin. Also *leukopathia, leukopathy, leukodermia.* **l. colli** VENEREAL COLLAR. **congenital l.** The presence of patchy areas of skin depigmentation that are noticeable at or shortly after birth, as is seen in the Waardenburg syndrome. The condition is phenotypically similar to vitiligo, an acquired phenomenon.

**leukodermia** \-dur'mē·ə\ LEUKODERMA.

**leukodystrophia cerebri progressiva** \-distrō'fē·ə ser'əbrī\ PROGRESSIVE CEREBRAL LEUKODYSTROPHY.

**leukodystrophy** \-dis'trəfē\ [LEUKO- + DYSTROPHY] A group of diseases of the central nervous system, marked anatomically by lesions of the white matter of the cerebral hemispheres and sometimes involving myelin within the cerebellum and peripheral nerves. These diseases result in progressive demyelination, and most are due to inborn errors of lipid metabolism. Among the leukodystrophies are metachromatic leukodystrophy, Krabbe's disease, and Pelizaeus-Merzbacher disease. **cerebral l.** ADRENOLEUKODYSTROPHY. **dysmyelinogenic l.** ALEXANDER'S DISEASE. **globoid l.** KRABBE'S DISEASE. **globoid cell l.** KRABBE'S DISEASE. **Krabbe's l.** KRABBE'S DISEASE. **melanodermic l.** ADRENOLEUKODYSTROPHY. **metachromatic l.** A form of progressive cerebral leukodystrophy, of autosomal recessive inheritance, usually beginning in childhood and marked clinically by progressive dementia and progressive spastic tetraplegia with contractures. Morphologically, there is diffuse degeneration of the white matter of the brain, with degeneration of the oligodendroglia and accumulation of degenerate myelin products which stain metachromatically with toluidine blue. The condition is now known to be due to sulfatide accumulation due to an inherited deficiency of aryl sulfatase which can be demonstrated in the leukocytes. The peripheral nerves are generally affected, showing signs of a polyneuropathy. A form of late onset producing a fatuous euphoric dementia and polyneuropathy has been described in adults. Also *Scholz-Bielschowsky-Henneberg diffuse cerebral sclerosis, Scholz disease, Scholz cerebral sclerosis, Scholz-Greenfield disease, Scholz metachromatic leukoencephalitis, Greenfield syndrome, van Bogaert-Nyssen-Pfeiffer disease, metachromatic leukoencephalopathy, sulfatide lipidosis, cerebroside sulfatase deficiency.* **progressive cerebral l.** Any of the progressive demyelinating or dysmyelinating leukodystrophies involving the cerebral hemispheres. Also *leukodystrophia cerebri progressiva.* **spongiform l.** CANAVAN'S DISEASE. **sudanophilic l.** Any of a group of demyelinating leukodystrophies, including Schilder's disease, in which the degenerating lipid is sudanophilic.

**leukoencephalitis** \-ensef'əlī'tis\ Any form of encephalitis involving predominantly the cerebral white matter rather than the gray. Also *leukencephalitis.* • The term, though outmoded, is still sometimes used to embrace the various forms of postinfective encephalomyelitis. **acute hemorrhagic l.** An exceptionally acute form of acute disseminated encephalomyelitis characterized clinically by rapidly advancing coma, occasionally convulsions, and sometimes focal neurologic signs, including hemiplegia. Pathologically, there is widespread perivascular demyelination with areas of hemorrhage and cellular infiltration around blood vessels largely in the cerebral white matter. Sometimes the lesions are more severe in one cerebral hemisphere than the other, thus accounting for unilateral neurologic signs. Many cases are fatal, and in those who recover there may be significant neurologic residua. Also *acute hemorrhagic leukoencephalopathy, acute necrotizing hemorrhagic leukoencephalopathy, Leichtenstern's encephalitis, Strümpell-Leichtenstern encephalitis, Hurst's disease.* See also BRAIN PURPURA. **concentric periaxial l.** BALÓ'S DISEASE. **Scholz metachromatic l.** METACHROMATIC LEUKODYSTROPHY. **subacute sclerosing l.** SUBACUTE SCLEROSING PANENCEPHALITIS. **van Bogaert sclerosing l.** SUBACUTE SCLEROSING PANENCEPHALITIS.

**leukoencephalopathy** \-ensef′əläp′əthē\ [LEUKO- + ENCEPHALOPATHY] Any disease of the white matter of the brain. Also *leukoencephaly.* **acute hemorrhagic l.** ACUTE HEMORRHAGIC LEUKOENCEPHALITIS. **acute necrotizing hemorrhagic l.** ACUTE HEMORRHAGIC LEUKOENCEPHALITIS. **metachromatic l.** METACHROMATIC LEUKODYSTROPHY. **progressive multifocal l.** Progressive multifocal demyelination in cerebral white matter giving rise to dementia, spastic paralysis, and sometimes blindness and resulting from opportunistic infection with papova viruses (e.g., polyoma viruses) in patients suffering from immune deficiency states associated with systemic diseases, particularly malignant lymphomas. Also *multifocal leukoencephalopathy, progressive multifocal encephalopathy.* Abbr. PML **subacute sclerosing l.** SUBACUTE SCLEROSING PANENCEPHALITIS.

**leukoencephaly** \-ensef′əlē\ LEUKOENCEPHALOPATHY.

**leukoerythroblastosis** \-irith′rəblastō′sis\ The presence in blood of numerous normoblasts together with immature cells of the granulocytic series. See also MYELOPHTHISIC ANEMIA.

**leukokeratosis** \-ker′ətō′sis\ LEUKOPLAKIA. **congenital oral l.** ORAL FAMILIAL WHITE FOLDED DYSPLASIA.

**leukokinetics** \-kinet′iks\ The study of the formation, circulation, and fate of leukocytes, usually by use of a radioactive tracer.

**leukokoria** \-kôr′ē·ə\ [LEUKO- + Gk *kor(ē)* the pupil of the eye + -IA] A disorder causing a white reflex of the pupil, as in retinopathy of prematurity. Leukokoria does not include cataract, but only conditions posterior to the crystalline lens. Also *leukocoria.*

**leukolysis** \lookäl′isis\ The destruction of leukocytes. Also *leukocytolysis.*

**leukolytic** \-lit′ik\ Relating to, characteristic of, or resulting from leukolysis. Also *leukocytolytic.*

**leukoma** \lookō′mə\ [Gk *leukōma* (from *leukos* white) a white spot in the eye] A dense white scar of the cornea. **l. adhaerens** A dense white corneal scar associated with an anterior synechia.

**leukomatous** \lookō′mətəs\ Having or pertaining to leukoma.

**leukomelanoderma** \-mel′ənōdur′mə\ MELANOLEUKODERMA.

**leukonychia** \-nik′ē·ə\ [LEUK- + ONYCHIA] White nails that are attributable to a whitening of the nail plate. Also *onychopacity, gift spots.* **l. striata** Transverse white lines of the nail plate.

**leukopathia** \-path′ē·ə\ [*leukopathy.* See LEUKOPATHY.] LEUKODERMA. **acquired l.** VITILIGO. **congenital l.** ALBINISM.

**leukopathy** \lookäp′əthē\ [LEUKO- + -PATHY] LEUKODERMA. **symmetric progressive l.** Punctate leukoderma that develops in young adults on the shins and the extensor aspects of the arms.

**leukopedesis** \-pēdē′sis\ [LEUKO- + Gk *pēdēsis* a leaping] The migration of leukocytes through the walls of blood vessels or through other tissues. It is a form of diapedesis. Also *leukocytoplania.*

**leukopenia** \-pē′nē·ə\ [LEUKO- + -PENIA] An abnormal decrease in the number of leukocytes in the blood. Also *leukocytopenia, oligoleukocythemia, oligoleukocytosis.* **basophilic l.** An abnormal decrease in the number of basophils in the circulating blood. **congenital l.** CONGENITAL NEUTROPENIA. **eosinophilic l.** An abnormal decrease in the number of eosinophiles in the circulating blood. **lymphocytic l.** LYMPHOCYTOPENIA. **malignant pernicious l.** AGRANULOCYTOSIS. **monocytic l.** MONOCYTOPENIA. **neutrophilic l.** NEUTROPENIA.

**leukopenic** \-pē′nik\ Pertaining to, characterized by, or resulting from leukopenia. Also *hypoleukocytic.*

**leukophagocytosis** \-fag′əsītō′sis\ The ingestion of leukocytes by phagocytes.

**leukoplakia** \-plā′kē·ə\ [LEUKO- + Gk *plax,* gen. *plakos,* anything flat and broad, a flat stone, plate + -IA] A lesion of the mucous membrane characterized by white patches due to epithelial hyperplasia with keratosis. It chiefly affects the tongue, cheeks, and gums but also the mucosa of the upper respiratory tract, particularly the larynx, the urinary bladder, and the female genitalia. It is a macroscopic and clinical diagnosis. Many sources of chronic irritation, including smoking, alcohol, and syphilis, have been blamed. Many such lesions are premalignant while others are examples of carcinoma *in situ.* Some are completely innocuous. This assessment must be made microscopically. Also *leukoplasia, leukokeratosis, smokers' patch.* **l. of the larynx** Leukoplakia involving the lining of the larynx. It is frequently a feature of chronic hyperplastic laryngitis. The vocal cords are most often the site but areas normally lined by respiratory epithelium, such as the vestibular folds, may be affected when epithelial metaplasia into squamous epithelium precedes keratinization.

**leukoplakic** \-plā′kik\ Affected by, resembling, or due to leukoplakia.

**leukoplasia** \-plā′zhə\ LEUKOPLAKIA.

**leukopoiesis** \-poi·ē′sis\ [LEUKO- + -POIESIS] The formation, growth, and maturation of leukocytes. Also *leukocytogenesis, leukocytopoiesis.*

**leukopoietic** \-poi·et′ik\ **1** Concerning or characterized by leukopoiesis. **2** An agent capable of stimulating leukopoiesis.

**leukoprophylaxis** \-prō′filak′sis\ Augmenting of the number of leukocytes in the blood by granulocyte transfusion before surgery to reduce the risk of infection. *Seldom used.*

**leukopsin** \lookäp′sin\ The colorless product of bleaching of rhodopsin.

**leukorrhea** \loo′kôrē′ə\ [LEUKO- + -RRHEA] A gynecologic disorder characterized by an abnormal, whitish, nonbloody discharge from the genital tract. Also *fluor albus.*

**leukorrheal** \loo′kôrē′əl\ Pertaining to or associated with leukorrhea.

**leukosarcomatosis** \-sär′kōmətō′sis\ The presence of multiple tumor masses consisting of leukemic cells. *Seldom used.*

**leukoscope** \loo′kəskōp\ [LEUKO- + -SCOPE] A color-vision testing instrument that mixes spectral colors to form white.

**leukosis** \lookō′sis\ [LEUK- + -OSIS] Excess proliferation, usually malignant, of one or more leukocyte varieties. It includes lymphoproliferation and myeloproliferation. **avian l. complex** See under COMPLEX. **myeloblastic l.** *Rare* ACUTE GRANULOCYTIC LEUKEMIA.

**leukotactic** \-tak′tik\ Capable of attracting leukocytes, usually to an inflammatory focus.

**leukotaxine** \-tak′sin\ A cell-free nitrogenous material prepared from inflammatory exudates and inflamed tissues that increases capillary permeability and attracts leukocytes. Also *leukotaxin.* • Greater definition of chemoattractants in recent years has made this term obsolete.

**leukotaxis** \-tak′sis\ The active, ameboid, unidirectional migration of leukocytes toward an attractant, as in an inflammatory focus.

**leukotherapy** \-ther′əpē\ The administration by transfusion of leukocytes obtained from donor blood. Also *granulocyte transfusion.* **preventive l.** Transfusion of leukocytes obtained from donor blood to prevent bacterial infection, as when the recipient's blood neutrophil count is less than $0.5 \times 10^9$/l.

**leukotic** \lookät′ik\ Pertaining to or affected by leukosis.

**leukotome** \loo′kətōm\ [LEUKO- + -TOME] An instrument for dividing the white fibers of the cerebrum in performing a lobotomy.

**leukotomy** \lookät′əmē\ [LEUKO- + -TOMY] A chiefly British term for FRONTAL LOBOTOMY. **transorbital l.** A chiefly British term for TRANSORBITAL LOBOTOMY.

**leukotoxin** \-täk′sin\ LEUKOCYTOTOXIN.

**leukotrienes** \-trī′ēnz\ A group of icosanoid compounds derived from 5-hydroperoxy-6,8,11,14-icosatetraenoic acid, and thus ultimately from arachidonic acid, that are mediators of the inflammatory reaction. Leukotriene $A_4$ is an unstable intermediate that is converted to leukotriene $B_4$, which is a chemoattractant for and an aggregator of neutrophils. Leukotrienes $C_4$, $D_4$, and $E_4$ play roles in anaphylaxis (and were formerly called the slow reacting substance of anaphylaxis).

**Levaditi** [Constantin *Levaditi,* Rumanian bacteriologist, 1874–1928] See under METHOD.

**levallorphan tartrate** $C_{19}H_{25}NO{\cdot}C_4H_6O_6$. 9a-Allylmorphinan-3-ol-hydrogen tartrate, the tartrate salt form of levallorphan, a white crystalline powder. It is used as a narcotic antagonist, particularly to treat respiratory depression caused by narcotic administration. It is given parenterally.

**levamfetamine** $C_9H_{13}N$. *l*-α-methylbenzeneethanamine. This form has actions similar to racemic amphetamine, but is less potent than either the racemic or dextrorototory forms of amphetamine. Also *levamphetamine.*

**levamfetamine succinate** $C_9H_{13}N{\cdot}C_4H_6O_4$. The succinate salt of levamfetamine (or amphetamine). It is employed therapeutically in the treatment of narcolepsy and hyperkinesis. It is also used as an anorexic agent in the treatment of obesity. It is given orally.

**levamisole hydrochloride** $C_{11}H_{12}N_2S{\cdot}HCl$. (*S*)-2,3,5,6-Tetrahydro-6-phenylimidazo[2,1-*b*]thiazole monohydrochloride. The *l*- form of tetramisole, with anthelmintic properties. It is used orally to treat roundworm, hookworm, and *Strongyloides* infections, and is also employed as an investigational drug in the treatment of cancer as an immunopotentiator agent.

**levamphetamine** LEVAMFETAMINE.

**levarterenol** \lev′ärter′ənôl\ NOREPINEPHRINE.

**levator** \levā′tər\ [L *levat(us)* (past part. of *levare* to lift, raise, elevate, from *levis* light in weight) + *-or* -OR] (*pl.* levatores) **1** A muscle that raises or lifts up the part into which it is inserted. **2** A surgical instrument used to elevate fragments of bone, especially of the skull. **l. claviculae** An occasional detached slip of musculus levator scapulae that arises from the transverse processes of the upper two or the lower cervical vertebrae and is inserted on the lateral end of the clavicle. It is commonly found in many nonhuman vertebrates. Also *omocervicalis.*

**levatores** \lev′ətôr′ēz\ Plural of LEVATOR.

**LeVeen** [Harry H. *LeVeen,* U.S. surgeon, born 1914] See under VALVE.

**level** [L *libella* (dim. of *libra* a level, pair of scales, balance) a level, plumb line] **1** A position or value relative to others in a scale; extent or degree. **2** In neuroanatomy, a plane or stage of complexity in the cerebrospinal axis, usually referring to geographic position as well as operational complexity. **l. of anesthesia** **1** The relative depth of narcosis in general anesthesia. **2** The segmental height of spinal or epidural anesthesia. **bone conduction hearing l.** The auditory threshold of a subject as measured by bone conduction. Also *sensorineural acuity level.* **l.'s of brightness** A range of illuminance levels recommended for various tasks or work areas. The levels recommended by the Illuminating Engineering Society of Great Britain range from 3000 lux for minute work to 150 lux for an area with no continuous work. For routine work which is not fine the value is 500 lux. Individual needs have to be considered when choosing levels for particular tasks. **complement l.** The serum quantity of either a specified complement component, such as C3, or of the total functional sequence of complement proteins, specified by the function tested, as whole hemolytic complement. **continuous noise l.** The average or the minimum level of noise measured by a sound level meter during a specified period, such as during working hours. It is important for hearing conservation programs in those locations where there are high levels of ambient noise. **developmental l.** The division of the lifespan according to chronologic age, corresponding with major advancements in biopsychosocial organization. One system, for example, recognizes the neonatal period, from birth to one month; infancy, from one month to one year; childhood, from one year to puberty; adolescence, from puberty to 18 or 21 years; adulthood, from 21 to 65 years; senium, after 65 years of age. **isoelectric l.** BASELINE. **loudness discomfort l.** The level of loudness at which the subject complains of discomfort as the intensity of the sound is increasing. It is usually estimated on the pure tone audiometer and expressed in dB HL. Also *threshold of discomfort.* **masking zero reference l.** The reference intensity for a noise, wide or narrow band, used for masking in audiometric investigations. **no adverse effect l.** The dose level at and below which a substance or mixture of substances produces no harmful effect in a biologic system. **no detectable effect l.** NO OBSERVABLE EFFECT LEVEL. **no effect l.** NO OBSERVABLE EFFECT LEVEL. **noise l.** The intensity of ambient noise or of a particular noise. The conditions under which the noise is being measured need to be specified. Important features of noise measurement are its minimum continuous level, the duration and temporal pattern of the maxima, and the spectral distribution of acoustic energy. **noise emission l.** The level of noise measured at a specified distance from a noise-producing source such as an engine or machine. **no observable effect l.** The subthreshold dose level at and below which no adverse effects from the given substance can be observed. Also *no detectable effect level, no effect level.* **sensation l.** The magnitude of acoustic energy required for sensory detection. **sensorineural acuity l.** BONE CONDUCTION

HEARING LEVEL. **serum transaminase l.** The serum quantity of either glutamic oxalacetic transaminase or glutamic pyruvate transaminase, used as a measure of tissue damage. **sound pressure l.** The acoustic force applied to the unit area of a sound-sensitive instrument such as a microphone. Its measure is a ratio of this force to the reference sound pressure of 20 $\mu$Pa and recorded in dB SPL. Abbr. SPL **threshold l.** The lowest dose level of a test substance required to elicit a response. **tonal l.** The auditory threshold for pitch discrimination.

**leveling** \lev′əling\ The tendency, in recall, to simplify the events and to leave out details, remembering the content of experience as being more balanced and regular than actually was the case.

**Leventhal** [Michael Leo *Leventhal,* U.S. obstetrician and gynecologist, 1901–1971] Stein-Leventhal syndrome. See under SYNDROME.

**Lévi** [Leopold *Lévi,* French endocrinologist, 1868–1933] **1** Lévi-Lorain infantilism, Lorain-Lévi syndrome, Lévi-Lorain type. See under HYPOPHYSIAL DWARFISM. **2** Lévi-Lorain dwarf, Lorain-Lévi dwarf. See under HYPOPHYSIAL DWARF.

**Levin** [Max *Levin,* Russian-born U.S. neurologist, born 1901] Kleine-Levin syndrome. See under SYNDROME.

**Levine** [Max *Levine,* Polish-born U.S. bacteriologist, born 1889] Levine's EMB agar, Levine's eosin-methylene blue agar. See under EOSIN-METHYLENE BLUE AGAR.

**Levine** [Samuel A. *Levine,* U.S. physician and cardiologist, 1891–1966] **1** Levine's clenched-fist sign. See under CLENCHED FIST SIGN. **2** Lown-Ganong-Levine syndrome. See under SHORT PR SYNDROME.

**levo-** \lē′vō-\ [L *laevus* (akin to Gk *laios* left) left, to the left] **1** A combining form meaning left, to or on the left. **2** In stereochemistry, a combining form designating the levorotatory enantiomer of a substance. Also *laevo-* (British spelling). Compare DEXTRO-. Symbol: (−)

**levoangiocardiography** \-an′jē·ōkär′dē·äg′rəfē\ Angiographic examination of the chambers of the left side of the heart.

**levocardia** \-kär′dē·ə\ [LEVO- + -CARDIA] The presence of a normally positioned heart on the left side in an individual with situs inversus of other asymmetrical viscera. Associated malformations are often found in the heart and aortic arch. **mixed l.** A congenital malformation in which the heart, located in the left chest, has discordant atrial and ventricular chambers, that is, either normally arranged atria and mirror-image ventricles, or mirror-image atria and normally arranged ventricles. Most frequently it is found also with ventriculoarterial discordance and is then known as "congenitally corrected transposition."

**levoclination** \-klīnā′shən\ [LEVO- + *(in)clination*] LEVOCYCLODUCTION.

**levocondylism** \-kän′dilizm\ [LEVO- + *condyl(e)* + -ISM] Leftward deviation of the mandibular condyles.

**levocycloduction** \-sī′kləduk′shən\ [LEVO- + CYCLODUCTION] Cyclotorsion of the eye to the left (with respect to 12 o'clock). Also *levoclination.*

**levocycloversion** \-sī′kləvur′zhən\ [LEVO- + CYCLOVERSION] Simultaneous cyclotorsion of both eyes to the left (with respect to twelve o'clock).

**levodopa** $C_9H_{11}NO_4$. 3-Hydroxyl-L-tyrosine. The levorotatory isomeric form of dopa. It is administered orally in the treatment of Parkinson's disease. Also *L-dopa.*

**levoduction** \-duk′shən\ [LEVO- + DUCTION] The turning of an eye to the left side.

**levonordefrin** *L*-3,4-Dihydroxynorephedrine. A white, odorless, crystalline powder, practically insoluble in water, usually used as the hydrochloride salt. It is used as a vasoconstrictor in dentistry in a concentration of 1:20 000 in solutions of local anesthetic agents.

**levorotatory** \-rō′tətôr′ē\ Capable of rotating the plane of polarized light counterclockwise, when viewed towards the light source. Compare DEXTROROTATORY. Symbol: *l*-, (−)

**levorphanol** L-3-Hydroxy-*N*-methylmorphinan. It is used as a narcotic analgesic similarly to morphine, and is usually given as the tartrate salt.

**levorphanol tartrate** $C_{17}H_{23}NO{\cdot}C_4H_6O_6{\cdot}2H_2O$. 9a-Methylmorphinan-3-ol hydrogen tartrate dihydrate, a synthetic narcotic possessing analgesic properties. It is a white crystalline powder and is administered subcutaneously or orally.

**levothyroxine sodium** $C_{15}H_{10}I_4NNa_4{\cdot}H_2O$. The sodium salt of L-thyroxine hydrate. It is used as replacement therapy in patients with reduced or nonexistent thyroid function. It is a yellow, hygroscopic powder which is given orally.

**levotorsion** \-tôr′shən\ [LEVO- + TORSION] Cyclorotation of the eye to the left (with respect to twelve o'clock).

**levoversion** \-vur′zhən\ [LEVO- + VERSION] Conjugate rotation of both eyes to the left.

**levoxadrol hydrochloride** $C_{20}H_{24}ClNO_2$. 2,2-Diphenyl-4-(2-piperidyl)-1,3-dioxolane. It is the L-isomer of dioxadiol hydrochloride. It is used as a local anesthetic and smooth muscle relaxant drug.

**Levret** [André *Levret,* French obstetrician, 1703–1780] See under MANEUVER, LAW.

**levulinate** A salt or ester derivative of levulinic acid.

**levulinic acid** $CH_3$—CO—$CH_2$—$CH_2$—COOH. 4-Oxopentanoic acid. It is formed by heating hexoses in concentrated hydrochloric acid. Its identification as a product of the ozonolysis of rubber provided a vital clue to the head-to-tail nature of the isoprene units in that polymer. It is best known as its derivative aminolevulinic acid, an intermediate in the biosynthesis of porphyrins.

**levulose** \lev′yəlōs\ *Outmoded* FRUCTOSE. • This name was originally given because, in contrast to glucose, it is levorotatory.

**levulosemia** \lev′yəlōsē′mē·ə\ FRUCTOSEMIA.

**Levy** [Robert Louis *Levy,* U.S. physician, 1888–1974] Levy, Rowntree, and Marriott method. See under METHOD.

**Lévy** [Gabrielle *Lévy,* French neurologist, 1886–1935] Lévy-Roussy syndrome. See under ROUSSY-LÉVY SYNDROME.

**Lewandowsky** [Felix *Lewandowsky,* German dermatologist, 1879–1921] **1** Nevus elasticus of Lewandowsky. See under NEVUS. **2** Jadassohn-Lewandowsky syndrome. See under PACHYONYCHIA CONGENITA. **3** Jadassohn-Lewandowsky syndrome. See under PALMOPLANTAR KERATODERMA. **4** Lewandowsky-Lutz disease. See under EPIDERMODYSPLASIA VERRUCIFORMIS.

**Lewis** [Gilbert Newton *Lewis,* U.S. chemist, 1875–1946] See under BASE, ACID.

**Lewis** [Sir Thomas *Lewis,* English cardiologist 1881–1945] **1** Lewis and Pickering test. See under TEST. **2** H factor of Lewis. See under FACTOR. **3** Lewis reaction, triple response of Lewis. See under WHEAL-FLARE REACTION.

**Lewisohn** [Richard *Lewisohn,* U.S. surgeon, 1875–1961] See under METHOD.

**Lewy** [Frederic H. *Lewy,* German-born neurologist active in the U.S., 1885–1950] Lewy bodies. See under BODY.

**Leyden** [Ernst Victor von *Leyden,* German physician, 1832–1910] **1** Leyden's ataxia. See under DIABETIC PSEUDOTABES. **2** See under DISEASE. **3** Leyden-Möbius dystrophy. See under LIMB-GIRDLE MUSCULAR DYSTROPHY.

**Leydig** [Franz von *Leydig,* German anatomist, 1821–1908] **1** Sertoli-Leydig cell tumor. See under TUMOR. **2** Interstitial cells of Leydig. See under LEYDIG CELLS.

**leydigarche** \lī'digär'kē\ [*Leydig (cells)* + Gk *archē* a beginning] The onset of gonadal function in the male. *Seldom used.*

**Lf** [abbreviated from Latin *limes* limit, and *flocculation*] See under LF DOSE.

**LFA** left frontoanterior position (of a fetus). See under BROW ANTERIOR POSITION.

**LFD** least fatal dose.

**L-forms** Slowly growing, spherical cells of certain bacterial species that have lost the rigid murein layer. They are formed either spontaneously or after exposure to an agent that impairs wall synthesis. Some are due to mutations and revert slowly if at all. Others are due to undefined phenotypic changes, and their reversion is promoted by $Mg^{2+}$ and by a high concentration of agar. Their relation to disease is uncertain. Also *L-phase variants.* • *L* is derived from Lister Institute.

**LFP** left frontoposterior position (of a fetus). See under BROW POSTERIOR POSITION.

**LFT** left frontotransverse position (of a fetus). See under BROW TRANSVERSE POSITION.

**LH** luteinizing hormone.

**Lhermitte** [Jean *Lhermitte,* French physician, 1877–1959] 1 Claude and Lhermitte syndrome. See under HYPOTHALAMIC SYNDROME. 2 See under SIGN.

**LHRF** luteinizing hormone releasing factor (gonadotropin releasing hormone).

**LHRH** luteinizing hormone releasing hormone.

**Li** Symbol for the element, lithium.

**liability** \lī'əbil'itē\ **professional l.** 1 The obligation of professional practitioners such as physicians to assume responsibility for payment of damages resulting from their negligent acts in the care of patients. 2 The obligation of professional practitioners such as physicians to provide health care that adequately meets recognized standards of quality.

**libido** \libē'dō, libī'dō\ [L (from *libere* to please, be wanted, akin to English *love*) desire, passion, sexual appetite] The energy of the sexual drive in Freud's psychoanalytic psychology. It is often used to include the energy of the aggressive drive as well. **ego l.** Libidinal energy that cathects the ego itself, as in narcissism. **object l.** Libidinal energy that cathects objects other than the self.

**Libman** [Emanuel *Libman,* U.S. physician, 1872–1946] Libman-Sacks disease, Libman-Sacks syndrome. See under LIBMAN-SACKS ENDOCARDITIS.

**library / gene l.** A number of independently cloned DNA fragments which theoretically contain at least one copy of each gene of the organism from which the DNA was obtained.

**Librium** A proprietary name for chlordiazepoxide hydrochloride.

**lice** Plural of LOUSE.

**lichen** \lī'kən\ [Gk *leichēn,* also *lichēn* a tree moss, lichen, lichenlike eruption on the skin, scurvy, blight, canker] 1 LICHEN PLANUS. 2 Any skin lesion that resembles lichen planus. **l. albus** LICHEN SCLEROSUS ET ATROPHICUS. **l. amyloidosus** The most common form of cutaneous amyloidosis, consisting of discrete, firm, hemispherical papules. The papules are brown or yellow in color, smooth, and shining. In some cases, scaling may exist. The condition most often involves the lower legs. Also *lichenoid amyloidosis.* **l. axillaris** FOX-FORDYCE DISEASE. **l. corneus hypertrophicus** Hyperkeratotic lichen planus. **follicular l. planus** LICHEN PLANOPILARIS. **hypertrophic l. planus** Chronic hyperkeratotic lesions of lichen planus that are most frequently seen on the lower leg. Also *lichen planus hypertrophicus, lichen ruber verrucosus, lichen planus verrucosus.* **l. planopilaris** Lichen planus in which the typical lesions are associated with follicular lesions that cause follicular destruction and cicatricial alopecia. Also *lichen pilaris, follicular lichen planus.* **l. planus** A common skin disease of unknown cause, characterized by an eruption of violaceous papules, which are of variable morphology and extent. Also *lichen ruber planus, Wilson's lichen, lichen.* **l. planus hypertrophicus** HYPERTROPHIC LICHEN PLANUS. **l. planus morpheicus** LICHEN SCLEROSUS ET ATROPHICUS. **l. planus verrucosus** HYPERTROPHIC LICHEN PLANUS. **l. ruber planus** LICHEN PLANUS. **l. ruber verrucosus** HYPERTROPHIC LICHEN PLANUS. **l. sclerosus et atrophicus** A superficial form of scleroderma which may be widely distributed, but affects most frequently the penis or the vulva. Also *lichen albus, lichen planus morpheicus.* **l. scrofulosorum** A tuberculid consisting of grouped lichenoid follicular papules. Also *papular scrofuloderma, tuberculosis lichenoides.* **l. simplex** A response in some predisposed skins to rubbing. It is seen as isolated lesions, mainly on the nape of the neck and the lateral aspects of the lower leg in men. It often complicates eczema of any origin. In many cases no history of any preceeding disease is known, but some cause must have brought on the irritation that led to the scratching or rubbing. Also *circumscribed neurodermatitis, Vidal's disease.* **l. striatus** A linear inflammatory dermatosis of unknown origin, occurring principally on a limb and in childhood. It resolves spontaneously after weeks or months. Also *linear dermatitis.* **l. tropicus** MILIARIA RUBRA. **Wilson's l.** LICHEN PLANUS.

**lichenification** \lī'kənifikā'shən\ [LICHEN + *i* + -FICATION] Thickening of the epidermis with increased prominence of the surface markings of the skin that is produced by repeated rubbing. Also *eczema hypertrophicum.*

**licheniformin** Any of a group of antibiotics isolated from *Bacillus subtilis.* Their properties resemble those of subtilin.

**lichenoid** \lī'kənoid\ Resembling lichen planus. Also *lichenous.*

**Lichtheim** [Ludwig *Lichtheim,* German physician, 1845–1928] 1 See under APHASIA, TEST. 2 Proust-Lichtheim maneuver. See under MANEUVER. 3 Lichtheim plaques. See under PLAQUE. 4 Dejerine-Lichtheim phenomenon, Lichtheim's phenomenon. See under LICHTHEIM SIGN.

**licorice** GLYCYRRHIZA.

**lid** [Old English *hlid* lid, gate] EYELID. **granular l.'s** MARGINAL BLEPHARITIS.

**Liddell** [Edward George Tandy *Liddell,* English physiologist, born 1895] Liddell-Sherrington reflex. See under REFLEX.

**lidocaine** $C_{14}H_{22}N_2O$. 2-(Diethylamino)-*N*-(2,6-dimethylphenyl)acetamide. A white, crystalline powder, practically insoluble in water, very soluble in alcohol and chloroform, very soluble in ether and in oils. It is a local anesthetic applied in sprays and creams to skin and mucous membranes. Also *lignocaine.*

**lidocaine hydrochloride** $C_{14}H_{22}N_2O{\cdot}HCl{\cdot}H_2O$. A monohydrate, white, crystalline powder, soluble in water and alcohol and insoluble in ether. Injectable as a water-soluble local anesthetic, it is more potent than procaine, and has antiarrhythmic and anticonvulsant properties as well.

**lidoflazine** 4-[4,4-Bis(*p*-fluorophenyl)butyl]-1-piperazine aceto-2′,6′-xylidide. An agent with coronary vasodilator and cardiac stimulant properties.

**lie** [Old English *licgan* to lie, akin to L *lectus* a bed, Gk *lechos* a bed] The relationship of the long axis of the fetus to that of the mother. **longitudinal l.** A lie in which the long axis of both mother and fetus are in the same plane during labor. **oblique l.** A lie in which the long axes of mother and fetus cross each other at an angle of 45° during labor. **transverse l.** A lie in which the long axes or mother and fetus cross at an angle of 90° during labor. Except in very special circumstances, the fetus cannot be delivered vaginally in this situation. Also *cross birth, torso presentation, transverse presentation, trunk presentation.*

**Lieberkühn** [Johannes Nathanael *Lieberkühn*, German anatomist, 1711–1756] Lieberkühn's follicles, glands of Lieberkühn, crypts of Lieberkühn. See under GLANDULAE INTESTINALES.

**Liebermann** [Carl Theodore *Liebermann*, German chemist, 1842–1914] Burchard-Liebermann test, Burchard-Liebermann reaction, Liebermann-Burchard reaction. See under LIEBERMANN-BURCHARD TEST.

**lien** \lī′ən\ [L (akin to Gk *splēn* the spleen), the spleen] SPLEN. **l. accessorius** SPLEN ACCESSORIUS. **l. mobilis** FLOATING SPLEEN. **l. succenturiatus** SPLEN ACCESSORIUS.

**lien-** \lī′ən-, lī-ēn′-\ LIENO-.

**lienal** \lī′ənəl\ [LIEN + -AL] Pertaining to the spleen; splenic.

**lienculus** \lī·en′kyələs\ SPLEN ACCESSORIUS.

**lienectomy** \lī′ənek′təmē\ [LIEN- + -ECTOMY] SPLENECTOMY.

**lienitis** \lī′ənī′tis\ SPLENITIS.

**lieno-** \lī-ē′nō-\ [L *lien* and *lienis* (prob. akin to Gk *splēn*) spleen] A combining form denoting the spleen. Also *lien-*.

**lienography** \lī′ənäg′rəfē\ [LIENO- + -GRAPHY] SPLENOGRAPHY.

**lienomalacia** \-məlā′shə\ SPLENOMALACIA.

**lienomedullary** \-med′yəler′ē\ SPLENOMEDULLARY.

**lienomyelogenous** \-mī′əläj′ənəs\ SPLENOMEDULLARY.

**lienomyelomalacia** \-mī′əlōməlā′shə\ SPLENOMYELOMALACIA.

**lienorenal** \-rē′nəl\ Pertaining to the spleen and the kidney; splenonephric; splenorenal.

**lientery** \lī′enter′ē\ [Gk *leienteria* (from *lei(os)* smooth, soft + *enter(on)* intestine) a passing of one's food undigested] Diarrhea in which the feces contain undigested food. Adj. lienteric.

**lienunculus** \lī′ənung′kyələs\ SPLEN ACCESSORIUS.

**Lieutaud** [Joseph *Lieutaud*, French physician, 1703–1780] 1 Lieutaud's triangle, Lieutaud's trigone. See under TRIGONUM VESICAE. 2 Lieutaud's uvula, Lieutaud's luette. See under UVULA VESICAE.

**LIF** 1 leukocyte migration inhibition factor. 2 left iliac fossa.

**life** [Old English *līf*] The condition that distinguishes organisms from inorganic substances, characterized especially by metabolism and the capacity to grow and reproduce. **antenatal l.** Existence before birth, especially of the conceptus in viviparous animals in the intrauterine period. **average l.** MEAN EFFECTIVE LIFE. **embryonic l.** The functional activity or the period of functional activity at the embryo stage of development. In humans it is usually restricted to the first eight weeks of intrauterine life. **fetal l.** The functional activity or the period of functional activity at the fetal stage of development. In humans it is usually restricted to the period of intrauterine life that follows the first eight weeks. **intrauterine l.** The functional activity or the period of functional activity associated with development of an animal *in utero.*. Also *uterine life.* **mean effective l.** The mean duration of existence of molecules, particles, or constituents of specified decaying nuclides, chemical substances, or biologic systems, the rate of decay often decreasing as an exponential curve. Also *mean life, average life, mean time.* **potential years of l. lost** A measure of the estimated effect that early deaths from a specified cause have on a given population compared to that population's normal life expectancy. Abbr. PYLL **uterine l.** INTRAUTERINE LIFE. **vegetative l.** 1 The level of functional activity attributable to plants. 2 The automatic functional activity associated with mechanisms, such as metabolism and reproduction, that are essential for continued existence.

**lig.** ligament; ligamentum.

# ligament

**ligament** \lig′əmənt\ [L *ligamentum*. See LIGAMENTUM.] LIGAMENTUM. **accessory l.** A fibrous band that strengthens the capsule of a joint, either external or internal to it. **accessory atlantoaxial l.** A fibrous band extending between the lateral mass of the atlas near the lower attachment of the transverse ligament and the body of the axis adjacent to the base of the dens, thereby strengthening each of the lateral atlantoaxial joints posteromedially. **accessory patellar l.'s** Ligamentum meniscofemorale anterius and ligamentum meniscofemorale posterius. **acromioclavicular l.** LIGAMENTUM ACROMIOCLAVICULARE. **alar l.'s** LIGAMENTA ALARIA. **alveolodental l.** PERIODONTIUM. **annular l. of base of stapes** LIGAMENTUM ANNULARE STAPEDIS. **annular l.'s of digits of foot** PARS ANNULARIS VAGINAE FIBROSAE DIGITORUM PEDIS. **annular l.'s of digits of hand** PARS ANNULARIS VAGINAE FIBROSAE DIGITORUM MANUS. **annular l. of femur** ZONA ORBICULARIS ARTICULATIONIS COXAE. **annular l.'s of fingers** PARS ANNULARIS VAGINAE FIBROSAE DIGITORUM MANUS. **annular l. of radius** LIGAMENTUM ANNULARE RADII. **annular l. of stapes** LIGAMENTUM ANNULARE STAPEDIS. **annular l.'s of tendon sheaths of fingers** PARS ANNULARIS VAGINAE FIBROSAE DIGITORUM MANUS. **anococcygeal l.** LIGAMENTUM ANOCOCCYGEUM. **anterior l. of the ankle joint** The thin anterior part of the capsule of the talocrural joint attached to the articular margins of the tibia and malleoli superiorly and to the talus inferiorly. **anterior annular l. of tarsus** *Outmoded* RETINACULUM MUSCULORUM EXTENSORUM PEDIS INFERIUS. **anterior atlanto-occipital l.** MEMBRANA ATLANTO-OCCIPITALIS ANTERIOR. **anterior auricular l.** LIGAMENTUM AURICULARE ANTERIUS. **anterior carpometacarpal l.'s** LIGAMENTA CARPOMETACARPALIA PALMARIA. **anterior costocentral l.** LIGAMENTUM CAPITIS COSTAE RADIATUM. **anterior cruciate l.** LIGAMENTUM CRUCIATUM ANTERIUS GENUS. **anterior cruciate l. of knee** LIGAMENTUM CRUCIATUM ANTERIUS GENUS. **anterior l. of head of fibula** LIGAMENTUM CAPITIS FIBULAE ANTERIUS. **anterior l. of head of rib** LIGAMENTUM CAPITIS COSTAE RADIATUM. **anterior longitudinal l.** LIGAMENTUM LONGITUDINALE ANTERIUS. **anterior l. of malleus** LIGAMENTUM MALLEI ANTERIUS. **anterior meniscofemoral l.** LIGAMENTUM MENISCOFEMORALE ANTERIUS. **anterior petrosphenoid l.** SYNCHON-

DROSIS SPHENOPETROSA. **anterior radiocarpal l.** LIGAMENTUM RADIOCARPALE PALMARE. **anterior l. of radiocarpal joint** LIGAMENTUM RADIOCARPALE PALMARE. **anterior sacrococcygeal l.** LIGAMENTUM SACROCOCCYGEUM ANTERIUS. **anterior sacroiliac l.'s** LIGAMENTA SACROILIACA ANTERIORA. **anterior sacrosciatic l.** LIGAMENTUM SACROSPINALE. **anterior sternoclavicular l.** LIGAMENTUM STERNOCLAVICULARE ANTERIUS. **anterior talocalcaneal l.** LIGAMENTUM TALOCALCANEUM ANTERIUS. **anterior talofibular l.** LIGAMENTUM TALOFIBULARE ANTERIUS. **anterior talotibial l.** PARS TIBIOTALARIS ANTERIOR LIGAMENTI MEDIALIS. **anterior tibiofibular l.** LIGAMENTUM TIBIOFIBULARE ANTERIUS. **anterior true l. of bladder** 1 LIGAMENTUM PUBOPROSTATICUM. 2 LIGAMENTUM PUBOVESICALE. **apical l. of dens** LIGAMENTUM APICIS DENTIS AXIS. **apical dental l.** LIGAMENTUM APICIS DENTIS AXIS. **apical odontoid l.** LIGAMENTUM APICIS DENTIS AXIS. **Arantius l.** LIGAMENTUM VENOSUM. **arcuate l. of knee** LIGAMENTUM POPLITEUM ARCUATUM. **arcuate popliteal l.** LIGAMENTUM POPLITEUM ARCUATUM. **arcuate pubic l.** LIGAMENTUM ARCUATUM PUBIS. **Arnold's l.** LIGAMENTUM INCUDIS SUPERIUS. **arytenoepiglottic l.** PLICA ARYEPIGLOTTICA. **l.'s of auditory ossicles** LIGAMENTA OSSICULORUM AUDITUS. **l.'s of auricle** LIGAMENTA AURICULARIA. **Barkow's l.** 1 Vertical fibers of the part of the capsule of the elbow joint that pass through the pad of fat in the olecranon fossa of the humerus. 2 The anterior and posterior portions of the fibrous capsule of the elbow joint. **Bellini's l.** The fibrous bandlike extension of the ischiofemoral ligament to the greater trochanter of the femur. **Béraud's l.** A fibrous band connecting the upper part of the pericardium to the front of the third thoracic vertebra and the disk below it and occasionally to the prevertebral cervical fascia. Also *pericardiovertebral ligament*. **Berry's l.** LIGAMENTUM THYROHYOIDEUM LATERALE. **Bertin's l.** LIGAMENTUM ILIOFEMORALE. **bifurcate l.** LIGAMENTUM BIFURCATUM. **bifurcated l.** LIGAMENTUM BIFURCATUM. **Bigelow's l.** LIGAMENTUM ILIOFEMORALE. **bigeminate l.'s of Arnold** LIGAMENTA TARSOMETATARSALIA DORSALIA. **l. of Botallo** LIGAMENTUM ARTERIOSUM. **Bourgery's l.** LIGAMENTUM POPLITEUM OBLIQUUM. **broad l. of liver** LIGAMENTUM FALCIFORME HEPATIS. **broad l. of uterus** LIGAMENTUM LATUM UTERI. **Brodie's l.** TRANSVERSE HUMERAL LIGAMENT. **Burns l.** MARGO FALCIFORMIS HIATUS SAPHENUS. **calcaneocuboid l.** LIGAMENTUM CALCANEOCUBOIDEUM. **calcaneofibular l.** LIGAMENTUM CALCANEOFIBULARE. **calcaneonavicular l.** LIGAMENTUM CALCANEONAVICULARE. **calcaneotibial l.** PARS TIBIOCALCANEUS LIGAMENTI MEDIALIS. **Caldani's l.** LIGAMENTUM CORACOCLAVICULARE. **Campbell's l.** SUSPENSORY LIGAMENT OF AXILLA. **Camper's l.** DIAPHRAGMA UROGENITALE. **capsular l.'s** 1 LIGAMENTA CAPSULARIA. 2 Articular capsules. See under CAPSULA ARTICULARIS. **capsular l. of hip joint** CAPSULA ARTICULARIS COXAE. **Carcassonne's l.** MEMBRANA PERINEI. **caroticoclinoid l.** An interclinoid ligament between the anterior and the middle clinoid processes on either side of the body of the sphenoid bone, often ossified and converted into a foramen transmitting the internal carotid artery. **carpal dorsal l.'s** LIGAMENTA INTERCARPALIA DORSALIA. **Casser's l.** LIGAMENTUM MALLEI LATERALE. **casserian l.** LIGAMENTUM MALLEI LATERALE. **caudal l. of common integument** RETINACULUM CAUDALE. **cemental l.** PERIODONTIUM. **ceratocricoid l.** LIGAMENTUM CERATOCRICOIDEUM. **check l.** A ligament that checks or limits the movement of a muscle or joint; specifically, one of the check ligaments of the axis (ligamenta alaria), or of the eyeball, medial and lateral (lacertus musculi recti lateralis bulbi). **check l.'s of axis** LIGAMENTA ALARIA. **chondroxiphoid l.'s** LIGAMENTA COSTOXIPHOIDEA. **l. of Chopart** LIGAMENTUM BIFURCATUM. **circular l.** PERIODONTIUM. **l. of Civinini** LIGAMENTUM PTERYGOSPINALE. **Cloquet's l.** RUDIMENT OF VAGINAL PROCESS. **collateral l.'s** LIGAMENTA COLLATERALIA. **collateral l.'s of interphalangeal articulations of foot** LIGAMENTA COLLATERALIA ARTICULATIONUM INTERPHALANGEARUM PEDIS. **collateral l.'s of interphalangeal articulations of hand** LIGAMENTA COLLATERALIA ARTICULATIONUM INTERPHALANGEARUM MANUS. **collateral l.'s of interphalangeal joints of foot** LIGAMENTA COLLATERALIA ARTICULATIONUM INTERPHALANGEARUM PEDIS. **collateral l.'s of interphalangeal joints of hand** LIGAMENTA COLLATERALIA ARTICULATIONUM INTERPHALANGEARUM MANUS. **collateral l.'s of joints of fingers** LIGAMENTA COLLATERALIA ARTICULATIONUM INTERPHALANGEARUM MANUS. **collateral l.'s of joints of toes** LIGAMENTA COLLATERALIA ARTICULATIONUM INTERPHALANGEARUM PEDIS. **collateral l.'s of metacarpophalangeal articulations** LIGAMENTA COLLATERALIA ARTICULATIONUM METACARPOPHALANGEARUM. **collateral l.'s of metatarsophalangeal articulations** LIGAMENTA COLLATERALIA ARTICULATIONUM METATARSOPHALANGEARUM. **collateral l.'s of midcarpal joint** Short ligaments on the radial and ulnar sides of the midcarpal joint. The radial ligament is the stronger and more distinct of the two and runs between the scaphoid and trapezium while the ulnar ligament connects the triquetrum and the hamate. They are continuous with the corresponding collateral ligaments of the wrist joint. **Colles l.** LIGAMENTUM REFLEXUM. **common l. of knee of Weber** LIGAMENTUM TRANSVERSUM GENUS. **conoid l.** LIGAMENTUM CONOIDEUM. **Cooper's l.** 1 LIGAMENTUM PECTINEALE. 2 CHORDA OBLIQUA. 3 One of the ligamenta suspensoria mammaria. **Cooper suspensory l.'s** LIGAMENTA SUSPENSORIA MAMMARIA. **coracoacromial l.** LIGAMENTUM CORACOACROMIALE. **coracoclavicular l.** LIGAMENTUM CORACOCLAVICULARE. **coracohumeral l.** LIGAMENTUM CORACOHUMERALE. **corniculopharyngeal l.** A fibroelastic band extending from the corniculate cartilage inferiorly toward the midline, where it joins the pharyngeal mucosa and the corresponding opposite ligament behind the transverse and oblique arytenoid muscles to form the cricopharyngeal ligament which descends centrally. Also *cricosantorinian ligament*. **coronary l. of the knee** Fibers of the deep surface of the fibrous capsule of the knee joint that are attached to the peripheral margins of the medial and lateral menisci and to the corresponding margins of the condyles of the tibia, to which each meniscus is firmly held by each ligament. **coronary l. of liver** LIGAMENTUM CORONARIUM. **costoclavicular l.** LIGAMENTUM COSTOCLAVICULARE. **costocolic l.** LIGAMENTUM PHRENICOCOLICUM. **costopericardiac l.** An extension of one of the bands of the sternopericardiac ligaments to the posterior aspect of the first sternocostal joint. Also *Lannelongue's ligament*. **costotransverse l.** LIGAMENTUM COSTOTRANSVERSARIUM. **costovertebral l.** LIGAMENTUM CAPITIS COSTAE RADIATUM. **costoxiphoid l.'s** LIGAMENTA COSTOXIPHOIDEA. **cotyloid l.** LABRUM ACETABULARE. **Cowper's l.** FASCIA PECTINEA.

**cricopharyngeal l.** LIGAMENTUM CRICOPHARYNGEUM. **cricopharyngeal l. of Luschka** LIGAMENTUM CRICOPHARYNGEUM. **cricosantorinian l.** 1 LIGAMENTUM CRICOPHARYNGEUM. 2 CORNICULOPHARYNGEAL LIGAMENT. **cricothyroid l.** LIGAMENTUM CRICOTHYROIDEUM MEDIANUM. **cricotracheal l.** LIGAMENTUM CRICOTRACHEALE. **cricotracheal l. of Luschka** A median thickening of the ligamentum cricotracheale. *Outmoded.* **crucial l.'s of fingers** PARS CRUCIFORMIS VAGINAE FIBROSAE DIGITORUM MANUS. **cruciate l.'s** LIGAMENTA CRUCIATA GENUS. **cruciate l. of atlas** LIGAMENTUM CRUCIFORME ATLANTIS. **cruciate l.'s of fingers** PARS CRUCIFORMIS VAGINAE FIBROSAE DIGITORUM MANUS. **cruciate l.'s of knee** LIGAMENTA CRUCIATA GENUS. **cruciate l.'s of toes** PARS CRUCIFORMIS VAGINAE FIBROSAE DIGITORUM PEDIS. **cruciform l. of atlas** LIGAMENTUM CRUCIFORME ATLANTIS. **crural l.** LIGAMENTUM INGUINALE. **Cruveilhier's l.'s** LIGAMENTA PLANTARIA ARTICULATIONUM METATARSOPHALANGEALIUM. **cysticoduodenal l.** An occasionally persisting remnant of the embryonic ventral mesentery extending between the gallbladder and the first or second portion of the duodenum or the pylorus. Also *cystoduodenal ligament, cholecystoduodenal band, cholecystoduodenocolic fold.* **deep dorsal sacrococcygeal l.** LIGAMENTUM SACROCOCCYGEUM POSTERIUS PROFUNDUM. **deep transverse metacarpal l.** LIGAMENTUM METACARPEUM TRANSVERSUM PROFUNDUM. **deep transverse metatarsal l.** LIGAMENTUM METATARSALE TRANSVERSUM PROFUNDUM. **deep transverse palmar l.** LIGAMENTUM METACARPEUM TRANSVERSUM PROFUNDUM. **deltoid l. of ankle** LIGAMENTUM MEDIALE ARTICULATIONIS TALOCRURALIS. **deltoid l. of elbow** LIGAMENTUM COLLATERALE ULNARE. **deltoid l. of talocrural joint** LIGAMENTUM MEDIALE ARTICULATIONIS TALOCRURALIS. **Denonvilliers l.** SEPTUM RECTOVESICALE. **dental l.** The horizontal group of fibers of the periodontium attached to the neck of a tooth. **dentate l. of spinal cord** LIGAMENTUM DENTICULATUM. **denticulate l.** LIGAMENTUM DENTICULATUM. **Denucé's l.** LIGAMENTUM QUADRATUM. **diaphragmatic l.** An involuted remnant of the cranial genital fold in the embryo. In the female it becomes the suspensory ligament of the ovary. **digital vaginal l.'s** Vaginae fibrosae digitorum manus and vaginae fibrosae digitorum pedis. **distal intermetacarpal l.** LIGAMENTUM METACARPEUM TRANSVERSUM PROFUNDUM. **distal plantar intermetatarsal l.** LIGAMENTUM METATARSALE TRANSVERSUM PROFUNDUM. **dorsal l.'s of bases of metacarpal bones** LIGAMENTA METACARPALIA DORSALIA. **dorsal l.'s of bases of metatarsal bones** LIGAMENTA METATARSALIA DORSALIA. **dorsal calcaneonavicular l.** LIGAMENTUM CALCANEONAVICULARE DORSALE. **dorsal carpal l.** RETINACULUM EXTENSORUM MANUS. **dorsal carpometacarpal l.'s** LIGAMENTA CARPOMETACARPALIA DORSALIA. **dorsal cuboideonavicular l.** LIGAMENTUM CUBOIDEONAVICULARE DORSALE. **dorsal cuneocuboid l.** LIGAMENTUM CUNEOCUBOIDEUM DORSALE. **dorsal cuneonavicular l.'s** LIGAMENTA CUNEONAVICULARIA DORSALIA. **dorsal intercarpal l.'s** LIGAMENTA INTERCARPALIA DORSALIA. **dorsal intercuneiform l.'s** LIGAMENTA INTERCUNEIFORMIA DORSALIA. **dorsal intermetacarpal l.'s** LIGAMENTA METACARPALIA DORSALIA. **dorsal intermetatarsal l.'s** LIGAMENTA METATARSALIA DORSALIA. **dorsal intertarsal l.'s** LIGAMENTA TARSI DORSALIA. **dorsal metacarpal l.'s** LIGAMENTA METACARPALIA DORSALIA. **dorsal metatarsal l.'s** LIGAMENTA METATARSALIA DORSALIA. **dorsal radiocarpal l.** LIGAMENTUM RADIOCARPALE DORSALE. **dorsal l. of radiocarpal joint** LIGAMENTUM RADIOCARPALE DORSALE. **dorsal sacroiliac l.'s** LIGAMENTA SACROILIACA DORSALIA. **dorsal talonavicular l.** LIGAMENTUM TALONAVICULARE. **dorsal tarsometatarsal l.'s** LIGAMENTA TARSOMETATARSALIA DORSALIA. **dorsal l.'s of tarsus** LIGAMENTA TARSI DORSALIA. **dorsal l. of wrist** RETINACULUM EXTENSORUM MANUS. **Douglas l.** PLICA RECTOUTERINA. **l. of ductus venosus** LIGAMENTUM VENOSUM. **duodenohepatic l.** LIGAMENTUM HEPATODUODENALE. **epihyal l.** LIGAMENTUM STYLOHYOIDEUM. **external arcuate l. of diaphragm** *Outmoded* LIGAMENTUM ARCUATUM LATERALE. **external intercostal l.** MEMBRANA INTERCOSTALIS EXTERNA. **external lateral l. of knee** LIGAMENTUM COLLATERALE FIBULARE. **external lateral l. of temporomandibular joint** LIGAMENTUM LATERALE ARTICULATIONIS TEMPOROMANDIBULARIS. **external lateral l. of wrist joint** LIGAMENTUM COLLATERALE CARPI RADIALE. **extracapsular accessory l.'s** Any supplementary supportive ligaments distinct from and external to an articular capsule which are additional to its usual extracapsular ligaments. **falciform l.** PROCESSUS FALCIFORMIS LIGAMENTI SACROTUBERALIS. **falciform l. of liver** LIGAMENTUM FALCIFORME HEPATIS. **false l.** 1 The peritoneum reflected from the superior surface and apex of the urinary bladder to either the anterior abdominal wall or the walls of the pelvis. Occasionally this is divided into superior, lateral, and posterior false ligaments. 2 Any ligament that is actually a peritoneal fold and not truly ligamentous in structure. **Ferrein's l.** LIGAMENTUM LATERALE ARTICULATIONIS TEMPOROMANDIBULARIS. **fibrous l.'s of breast** LIGAMENTA SUSPENSORIA MAMMARIA. **fibular collateral l.** LIGAMENTUM COLLATERALE FIBULARE. **flaval l.'s** LIGAMENTA FLAVA. **Flood's l.** The superior glenohumeral ligament of the shoulder joint. See also LIGAMENTA GLENOHUMERALIA. **fundiform l. of penis** LIGAMENTUM FUNDIFORME PENIS. **gastrocolic l.** 1 LIGAMENTUM GASTROCOLICUM. 2 A segment of the dorsal mesogastrium in the embryo which is attached along the inferior border (greater curvature) of the stomach and forms the anterior peritoneal sheet, doubled, of the omental bursa, and is finally included within the greater omentum. **gastrohepatic l.** LIGAMENTUM HEPATOGASTRICUM. **gastrolienal l.** LIGAMENTUM GASTROSPLENICUM. **gastrophrenic l.** LIGAMENTUM GASTROPHRENICUM. **gastrosplenic l.** LIGAMENTUM GASTROSPLENICUM. **genitoinguinal l.** The ridge extending from the caudal pole of the gonad to the inguinal region of the embryo, through which it passes to the ipsilateral labioscrotal fold. The gubernaculum differentiates within the ridge and constitutes a potential pathway for the descent of the gonad. Also *ligamentum genitoinguinale, inguinal fold, caudal genital fold.* **Gerdy's l.** SUSPENSORY LIGAMENT OF AXILLA. **Gillette suspensory l.** TENDO CRICOESOPHAGEUS. **Gimbernat's l.** LIGAMENTUM LACUNARE. **gingivodental l.** The dentogingival fibers of the periodontal membrane. **glenohumeral l.'s** LIGAMENTA GLENOHUMERALIA. **glenoid l.'s of Cruveilhier** LIGAMENTA PLANTARIA ARTICULATIONUM METATARSOPHALANGEALIUM. **Günz l.** A layer of the obturator membrane. **hammock l.** A slinglike arrangement of collagen fibers that separate the apex of the developing root of a tooth from the fundus of its socket. Although original descriptions suggested otherwise, it is not attached to bone. **l. of head**

**of femur** LIGAMENTUM CAPITIS FEMORIS. **Helmholtz l.** 1 A band of fibers of the anterior ligament of the malleus attached to the greater tympanic spine of the tympanic notch. 2 The posterior part of the lateral ligament of the malleus. **l.'s of Helvetius** LIGAMENTA PYLORI. **Henle's l.** A fascial expansion of the lowermost part of the rectus abdominis muscle tendon or sheath, or of part of the aponeurosis of the transversus abdominis muscle that reinforces the deep surface of the conjoined tendon, or falx inguinalis. See also HENLE'S BAND. **Hensing's l.** LIGAMENTUM PHRENICOCOLICUM. **hepatic l.'s** Peritoneal folds between the liver and surrounding structures. **hepatocolic l.** LIGAMENTUM HEPATOCOLICUM. **hepatocystocolic l.** An occasional extension of the hepatocolic ligament to the gallbladder. **hepatoduodenal l.** LIGAMENTUM HEPATODUODENALE. **hepatoesophageal l.** LIGAMENTUM HEPATOESOPHAGEUM. **hepatogastric l.** LIGAMENTUM HEPATOGASTRICUM. **hepatogastroduodenal l.** OMENTUM MINUS. **hepatorenal l.** LIGAMENTUM HEPATORENALE. **Hesselbach's l.** LIGAMENTUM INTERFOVEOLARE. **Hey's l.** MARGO FALCIFORMIS HIATUS SAPHENUS. **Holl's l.** A ligamentous band joining the two corpora cavernosa clitoridis anterior to the external urethral ostium. **Hueck's l.** RETICULUM TRABECULARE SCLERAE. **Humphry's l.** LIGAMENTUM MENISCOFEMORALE ANTERIUS. **Hunter's l.** LIGAMENTUM TERES UTERI. **hyaloideocapsular l.** Circular fibers adhering the posterior surface of the capsule of the lens of the eye to the vitreous body. **hyoepiglottic l.** LIGAMENTUM HYOEPIGLOTTICUM. **hypsiloid l.** LIGAMENTUM ILIOFEMORALE. **iliofemoral l.** LIGAMENTUM ILIOFEMORALE. **iliolumbar l.** LIGAMENTUM ILIOLUMBALE. **iliopectineal l.** ARCUS ILIOPECTINEUS. **iliotibial l. of Maissiat** TRACTUS ILIOTIBIALIS. **iliotrochanteric l.** The lateral band of the iliofemoral ligament, extending between the anterior superior iliac spine and the greater trochanter and adjacent upper end of the intertrochanteric line of the femur. **inferior arcuate l. of pubis** LIGAMENTUM ARCUATUM PUBIS. **inferior calcaneonavicular l.** LIGAMENTUM CALCANEONAVICULARE PLANTARE. **inferior l. of epididymis** LIGAMENTUM EPIDIDYMIDIS INFERIUS. **inferior glenohumeral l.** See under LIGAMENTA GLENOHUMERALIA. **inferior metatarsophalangeal l.'s** LIGAMENTA PLANTARIA ARTICULATIONUM METATARSOPHALANGEALIUM. **inferior l. of neck of rib of Henle** LIGAMENTUM COSTOTRANSVERSARIUM. **inferior pubic l.** LIGAMENTUM ARCUATUM PUBIS. **inferior sternopericardial l.** See under LIGAMENTA STERNOPERICARDIACA. **inferior transverse l. of scapula** LIGAMENTUM TRANSVERSUM SCAPULAE INFERIUS. **inferior l. of tubercle of rib** LIGAMENTUM COSTOTRANSVERSARIUM LATERALE. **infundibulo-ovarian l.** FIMBRIA OVARICA. **infundibulopelvic l.** LIGAMENTUM SUSPENSORIUM OVARII. **inguinal l.** LIGAMENTUM INGUINALE. **inguinal l. of Cooper** LIGAMENTUM PECTINEALE. **interchondral l.** Either the medial or the lateral ligament which strengthens the thin fibrous capsule of each interchondral joint. **interclavicular l.** LIGAMENTUM INTERCLAVICULARE. **interclinoid l.** A band of dura mater extending between any two clinoid processes on either side of the body of the sphenoid bone. The caroticoclinoid ligament is an example. **intercornual l.** LIGAMENTUM SACROCOCCYGEUM LATERALE. **interfoveolar l.** LIGAMENTUM INTERFOVEOLARE. **interlaminar l.'s** LIGAMENTA FLAVA. **internal arcuate l. of diaphragm** *Outmoded* LIGAMENTUM ARCUATUM MEDIALE. **internal intercostal l.** MEMBRANA INTERCOSTALIS INTERNA. **internal lateral l. of knee** LIGAMENTUM COLLATERALE TIBIALE. **internal lateral l. of wrist joint** *Outmoded* LIGAMENTUM COLLATERALE CARPI ULNARE. **interosseous l.'s of bases of metacarpal bones** LIGAMENTA METACARPALIA INTEROSSEA. **interosseous l.'s of bases of metatarsal bones** LIGAMENTA METATARSALIA INTEROSSEA. **interosseous l.'s of carpal bones** LIGAMENTA INTERCARPALIA INTEROSSEA. **interosseous cuboideonavicular l.** A ligament composed of strong transverse fibers which connects the nonarticular parts of the adjacent surfaces of the cuboid and navicular bones. **interosseous cuneometatarsal l.'s** LIGAMENTA CUNEOMETATARSALIA INTEROSSEA. **interosseous intercarpal l.'s** LIGAMENTA INTERCARPALIA INTEROSSEA. **interosseous intercuneiform l.'s** LIGAMENTA INTERCUNEIFORMIA INTEROSSEA. **interosseous intermetacarpal l.'s** LIGAMENTA METACARPALIA INTEROSSEA. **interosseous intermetatarsal l.'s** LIGAMENTA METATARSALIA INTEROSSEA. **interosseous intertarsal l.'s** LIGAMENTA TARSI INTEROSSEA. **interosseous metacarpal l.'s** LIGAMENTA METACARPALIA INTEROSSEA. **interosseous metatarsal l.'s** LIGAMENTA METATARSALIA INTEROSSEA. **interosseous sacroiliac l.'s** LIGAMENTA SACROILIACA INTEROSSEA. **interosseous talocalcaneal l.** LIGAMENTUM TALOCALCANEUM INTEROSSEUM. **interosseous l.'s of tarsus** LIGAMENTA TARSI INTEROSSEA. **interspinal l.'s** LIGAMENTA INTERSPINALIA. **interspinous l.'s** LIGAMENTA INTERSPINALIA. **intertransverse l.'s** LIGAMENTA INTERTRANSVERSARIA. **intertransverse l.'s of vertebral arch** LIGAMENTA INTERTRANSVERSARIA. **intra-articular l.'s** LIGAMENTA INTRACAPSULARIA. **intra-articular costovertebral l.** LIGAMENTUM CAPITIS COSTAE INTRA-ARTICULARE. **intra-articular l. of head of rib** LIGAMENTUM CAPITIS COSTAE INTRA-ARTICULARE. **intra-articular sternocostal l.** LIGAMENTUM STERNOCOSTALE INTRA-ARTICULARE. **intrinsic l.** A taut ligament between two points on the same bone or on another anatomical structure. **intrinsic l.'s of the auricle** A number of short fibrous bands connecting some projections of the cartilage of the auricle of the ear, the main ones being between the tragus and the helix, thereby completing the meatus anteriorly and bounding the concha, and between the tail of the helix and the anthelix. There are also a few less conspicuous bands on the cranial surface of the auricle. **ischiofemoral l.** LIGAMENTUM ISCHIOFEMORALE. **Jarjavay's l.'s** The uterosacral ligament and the rectovaginal fold. **Krause's l.** LIGAMENTUM TRANSVERSUM PERINEI. **laciniate l.** RETINACULUM MUSCULORUM FLEXORUM PEDIS. **lacunar l.** LIGAMENTUM LACUNARE. **lacunar l. of Gimbernat** LIGAMENTUM LACUNARE. **Lannelongue's l.** COSTOPERICARDIAC LIGAMENT. **lateral l. of the ankle joint** A strengthening capsular ligament on the lateral side of the talocrural joint comprising three fascicles attached to the lateral malleolus and described as separate ligaments, namely, ligamentum talofibulare anterius, ligamentum talofibulare posterius, and ligamentum calcaneofibulare between them. Also *lateral ligament of the ankle, lateral ligament of talocrural joint.* **lateral arcuate l.** LIGAMENTUM ARCUATUM LATERALE. **lateral atlanto-occipital l.** LIGAMENTUM ATLANTO-OCCIPITALE LATERALE. **lateral l.'s of the bladder** Thickenings of fibroareolar tissue connecting the sides of the urinary bladder to the tendinous arch of the pelvic fascia on each side. **lateral cervical l.** A bandlike condensation of pelvic fascia at the base of the broad ligament of the uterus, extending from the side of the cervix and the upper end and lateral fornix of the vagina to the fibroareolar tissue around the blood vessels on the lateral wall of the pelvis. It is one of the important supporting ligaments of the uterus. **lateral check l. of eyeball** LACERTUS MUSCULI RECTI LATERALIS BULBI. **lateral costotransverse l.** LIGAMENTUM COSTOTRANSVERSARIUM LATERALE. **lateral l. of elbow** LIGAMENTUM COLLATERALE RADIALE. **lateral l.'s of joints of fingers** LIGAMENTA COLLATERALIA ARTICULATIONUM INTERPHALANGEARUM MANUS. **lateral l.'s of joints of toes** LIGAMENTA COLLATERALIA ARTICULATIONUM INTERPHALANGEARUM PEDIS. **lateral l. of knee** LIGAMENTUM COLLATERALE FIBULARE. **lateral l. of malleus** LIGAMENTUM MALLEI LATERALE. **lateral metacarpophalangeal l.'s** LIGAMENTA COLLATERALIA ARTICULATIONUM METACARPOPHALANGEARUM. **lateral l.'s of metacarpophalangeal joints** LIGAMENTA COLLATERALIA ARTICULATIONUM METACARPOPHALANGEARUM. **lateral metatarsophalangeal l.'s** LIGAMENTA COLLATERALIA ARTICULATIONUM METATARSOPHALANGEARUM. **lateral l.'s of metatarsophalangeal joints** LIGAMENTA COLLATERALIA ARTICULATIONUM METATARSOPHALANGEARUM. **lateral occipitoaxial l.'s** LIGAMENTA ALARIA. **lateral palpebral l.** LIGAMENTUM PALPEBRALE LATERALE. **lateral puboprostatic l.** The lateral extension of ligamentum puboprostaticum. **lateral l. of rectum** The fascia around the middle rectal vessels which passes from the posterolateral wall of the true pelvis to each side of the rectum at the level of the third sacral vertebra. **lateral sacrococcygeal l.** LIGAMENTUM SACROCOCCYGEUM LATERALE. **lateral talocalcaneal l.** LIGAMENTUM TALOCALCANEARE LATERALE. **lateral l. of talocrural joint** LATERAL LIGAMENT OF THE ANKLE JOINT. **lateral l. of temporomandibular articulation** LIGAMENTUM LATERALE ARTICULATIONIS TEMPOROMANDIBULARIS. **lateral thyrohyoid l.** LIGAMENTUM THYROHYOIDEUM LATERALE. **lateral true l. of bladder** LIGAMENTUM PUBOPROSTATICUM. **Lauth's l.** 1 Some fibers of the alar ligaments of the axis that form a transverse band behind the dens and above the transverse ligament of the atlas, extending from one edge of the foramen magnum to the other. 2 LIGAMENTUM ARCUATUM PUBIS. **left phrenicocolic l.** LIGAMENTUM PHRENICOCOLICUM. **left triangular l. of liver** LIGAMENTUM TRIANGULARE SINISTRUM HEPATIS. **lienophrenic l.** LIGAMENTUM SPLENORENALE. **lienorenal l.** LIGAMENTUM SPLENORENALE. **Lisfranc's l.** One of the ligamenta cuneometatarsea interossea, namely, the strong band between the lateral surface of the medial cuneiform bone and the medial aspect of the base of the second metatarsal bone, which separates the medial from the intermediate tarsometatarsal articulation. **Lockwood suspensory l.** SUSPENSORY LIGAMENT OF EYEBALL. **long plantar l.** LIGAMENTUM PLANTARE LONGUM. **long posterior sacroiliac l.** See under LIGAMENTA SACROILIACA DORSALIA. **lumbocostal l.** LIGAMENTUM LUMBOCOSTALE. **lumbocostal l. of Henle** LIGAMENTUM LUMBOCOSTALE. **l.'s of Luschka** LIGAMENTA STERNOPERICARDIACA. **l. of Maissiat** TRACTUS ILIOTIBIALIS. **l.'s of malleus** The ligaments attaching the malleus to the walls of the middle ear, namely, ligamentum mallei anterius, ligamentum mallei laterale, and ligamentum malleus superius. **Mauchart's l.'s** LIGAMENTA ALARIA. **l. of Mayer** LIGAMENTUM CARPI RADIATUM. **Meckel's l.** MECKEL'S BAND. **medial arcuate l.** LIGAMENTUM ARCUATUM MEDIALE. **medial check l. of eyeball** A strong, triangular expansion extending medially from the junction of the bulbar sheath and the tubular sheath of the medial rectus muscle of the bulb to the lacrimal bone. It checks the action of the muscle. **medial l. of elbow joint** LIGAMENTUM COLLATERALE ULNARE. **medial palpebral l.** LIGAMENTUM PALPEBRALE MEDIALE. **medial puboprostatic l.** The medial extension of ligamentum puboprostaticum. **medial talocalcaneal l.** LIGAMENTUM TALOCALCANEARE MEDIALE. **medial l. of temporomandibular joint** LIGAMENTUM MEDIALE ARTICULATIONIS TEMPOROMANDIBULARIS. **medial umbilical l.** LIGAMENTUM UMBILICALE MEDIALE. **medial l. of wrist** LIGAMENTUM COLLATERALE CARPI ULNARE. **median arcuate l.** LIGAMENTUM ARCUATUM MEDIANUM. **median thyrohyoid l.** LIGAMENTUM THYROHYOIDEUM MEDIANUM. **median umbilical l.** LIGAMENTUM UMBILICALE MEDIANUM. **metacarpal interosseous l.'s** LIGAMENTA METACARPALIA INTEROSSEA. **middle cricothyroid l.** LIGAMENTUM CRICOTHYROIDEUM MEDIANUM. **middle glenohumeral l.** See under LIGAMENTA GLENOHUMERALIA. **middle thyrohyoid l.** LIGAMENTUM THYROHYOIDEUM MEDIANUM. **middle umbilical l.** LIGAMENTUM UMBILICALE MEDIANUM. **l. of neck of rib** LIGAMENTUM COSTOTRANSVERSARIUM. **nephrocolic l.** Fibrous strands of areolar tissue between the perirenal fascia anterior to the lower pole of each kidney and areolar tissue on the posterior aspect of the ascending and the descending colon related to corresponding kidneys. **nuchal l.** LIGAMENTUM NUCHAE. **oblique l.** CHORDA OBLIQUA. **oblique l. of Cooper** CHORDA OBLIQUA. **oblique l. of elbow joint** CHORDA OBLIQUA. **oblique l. of forearm** CHORDA OBLIQUA. **oblique popliteal l.** LIGAMENTUM POPLITEUM OBLIQUUM. **oblique l. of superior radioulnar joint** CHORDA OBLIQUA. **occipitoaxial l.** MEMBRANA TECTORIA. **occipito-odontoid l.'s** LIGAMENTA ALARIA. **odontoid l.'s of axis** LIGAMENTA ALARIA. **orbicular l. of radius** LIGAMENTUM ANNULARE RADII. **ovarian l.** LIGAMENTUM OVARII PROPRIUM. **l. of ovary** LIGAMENTUM OVARII PROPRIUM. **palmar l.'s** LIGAMENTA PALMARIA ARTICULATIONUM METACARPOPHALANGEALIUM. **palmar carpometacarpal l.'s** LIGAMENTA CARPOMETACARPALIA PALMARIA. **palmar intercarpal l.'s** LIGAMENTA INTERCARPALIA PALMARIA. **palmar intermetacarpal l.'s** LIGAMENTA METACARPALIA PALMARIA. **palmar metacarpal l.'s** LIGAMENTA METACARPALIA PALMARIA. **palmar metacarpophalangeal l.'s** LIGAMENTA PALMARIA ARTICULATIONUM METACARPOPHALANGEALIUM. **palmar radiocarpal l.** LIGAMENTUM RADIOCARPALE PALMARE. **palmar ulnocarpal l.** LIGAMENTUM ULNOCARPALE PALMARE. **patellar l.** LIGAMENTUM PATELLAE. **pectinate l. of iridocorneal angle** RETICULUM TRABECULARE SCLERAE. **pectineal l.** LIGAMENTUM PECTINEALE. **pectineal l. of Cooper** LIGAMENTUM PECTINEALE. **pericardiovertebral l.** BÉRAUD'S LIGAMENT. **perineal l. of Carcassonne** MEMBRANA PERINEI. **periodontal l.** PERIODONTIUM. **peritoneal l.** A fold or double layer of peritoneum which connects an organ either to another organ or to the abdominal or pelvic walls. It may contain extraperitoneal connective tissue, vessels, or nerves. **Petit's l.** UTEROSACRAL LIGAMENT. **Pétrequin's l.** A small tract of intercrural fibers that are attached to the inguinal ligament. **petrosphenoid l.** A fibrous band between the lateral edge of the dorsum sellae at the posterior clinoid process and the superior margin of the petrous part of the temporal bone near its medial end. Also *petroclinoid ligament.* **pharyngeal l.** RAPHE PHARYNGIS. **phrenicocolic l.** LIGAMENTUM PHRENICOCOLICUM. **phrenicolienal l.** LIGAMENTUM SPLENORENALE. **phrenicosplenic l.** LIGAMENTUM SPLENORENALE. **phrenocolic l.** LIGAMENTUM PHRENICOCOLICUM. **pisohamate l.** LIGAMENTUM PISOHAMATUM. **pisometacarpal l.** LIGAMENTUM PISOMETACARPEUM. **plantar l.'s** LIGAMENTA PLANTARIA ARTICULATIONUM METATARSOPHALANGEALIUM. **plantar l.'s of bases of metatarsal bones** LIGAMENTA METATARSALIA PLANTARIA. **plantar calcaneocuboid l.** LIGAMENTUM CALCANEOCUBOIDEUM PLANTARE. **plantar calcaneonavicular l.** LIGAMENTUM CALCANEONAVICULARE PLANTARE. **plantar cuboideonavicular l.** LIGAMENTUM CUBOIDEONAVICULARE PLANTARE. **plantar cuneocuboid l.** LIGAMENTUM CUNEOCUBOIDEUM PLANTARE. **plantar cuneonavicular l.'s** LIGAMENTA CUNEONAVICULARIA PLANTARIA. **plantar intercuneiform l.'s** LIGAMENTA INTERCUNEIFORMIA PLANTARIA. **plantar intermetatarsal l.'s** LIGAMENTA METATARSALIA PLANTARIA. **plantar intertarsal l.'s** LIGAMENTA TARSI PLANTARIA. **plantar metatarsal l.'s** LIGAMENTA METATARSALIA PLANTARIA. **plantar metatarsophalangeal l.'s** LIGAMENTA PLANTARIA ARTICULATIONUM METATARSOPHALANGEALIUM. **plantar tarsometatarsal l.'s** LIGAMENTA TARSOMETATARSALIA PLANTARIA. **plantar l.'s of tarsus** LIGAMENTA TARSI PLANTARIA. **popliteal arcuate l.** LIGAMENTUM POPLITEUM ARCUATUM. **posterior annular l. of carpus** RETINACULUM EXTENSORUM MANUS. **posterior atlanto-occipital l.** MEMBRANA ATLANTO-OCCIPITALIS POSTERIOR. **posterior auricular l.** LIGAMENTUM AURICULARE POSTERIUS. **posterior carpometacarpal l.'s** LIGAMENTA CARPOMETACARPALIA DORSALIA. **posterior cricoarytenoid l.** LIGAMENTUM CRICOARYTENOIDEUM POSTERIUS. **posterior cruciate l.** LIGAMENTUM CRUCIATUM POSTERIUS GENUS. **posterior cruciate l. of knee** LIGAMENTUM CRUCIATUM POSTERIUS GENUS. **posterior false l.'s of bladder** SACROGENITAL FOLD. **posterior l. of head of fibula** LIGAMENTUM CAPITIS FIBULAE POSTERIUS. **posterior l. of incus** LIGAMENTUM INCUDIS POSTERIUS. **posterior longitudinal l.** LIGAMENTUM LONGITUDINALE POSTERIUS. **posterior meniscofemoral l.** LIGAMENTUM MENISCOFEMORALE POSTERIUS. **posterior meniscofemoral l. of Wrisberg** LIGAMENTUM MENISCOFEMORALE POSTERIUS. **posterior oblique l. of knee** LIGAMENTUM POPLITEUM OBLIQUUM. **posterior l. of pinna** LIGAMENTUM AURICULARE POSTERIUS. **posterior l. of radiocarpal joint** LIGAMENTUM RADIOCARPALE DORSALE. **posterior sacrococcygeal l.** Either ligamentum sacrococcygeum posterius profundum or ligamentum sacrococcygeum posterius superficiale. **posterior sternoclavicular l.** LIGAMENTUM STERNOCLAVICULARE POSTERIUS. **posterior talocalcaneal l.** LIGAMENTUM TALOCALCANEUM POSTERIUS. **posterior talofibular l.** LIGAMENTUM TALOFIBULARE POSTERIUS. **posterior talotibial l.** PARS TIBIOTALARIS POSTERIOR LIGAMENTI MEDIALIS. **posterior tibiofibular l.** LIGAMENTUM TIBIOFIBULARE POSTERIUS. **posterior l. of uterus** RECTOVAGINAL FOLD. **Poupart's l.** LIGAMENTUM INGUINALE. **preurethral l. of Waldeyer** LIGAMENTUM TRANSVERSUM PERINEI. **proper l. of the ovary** LIGAMENTUM OVARII PROPRIUM. **proximal intermetacarpal l.'s** Any of three groups of ligaments: (1) ligamenta metacarpalia dorsalia; (2) ligamenta metacarpalia palmaria; (3) ligamenta metacarpalia interossea. **proximal posterior intermetatarsal l.'s** LIGAMENTA METATARSALIA DORSALIA. **pterygomandibular l.** RAPHE PTERYGOMANDIBULARIS. **pterygospinal l.** LIGAMENTUM PTERYGOSPINALE. **pterygospinous l.** LIGAMENTUM PTERYGOSPINALE. **pubic arcuate l.** LIGAMENTUM ARCUATUM PUBIS. **pubocapsular l.** LIGAMENTUM PUBOFEMORALE. **pubofemoral l.** LIGAMENTUM PUBOFEMORALE. **puboprostatic l.** LIGAMENTUM PUBOPROSTATICUM. **puborectal l.** 1 LIGAMENTUM PUBOPROSTATICUM. 2 LIGAMENTUM PUBOVESICALE. **pubovesical l.** LIGAMENTUM PUBOVESICALE. **pulmonary l.** LIGAMENTUM PULMONALE. **quadrate l.** LIGAMENTUM QUADRATUM. **quadrate l. of Denucé** LIGAMENTUM QUADRATUM. **radial carpal collateral l.** LIGAMENTUM COLLATERALE CARPI RADIALE. **radial collateral l.** LIGAMENTUM COLLATERALE RADIALE. **radial collateral l. of carpus** LIGAMENTUM COLLATERALE CARPI RADIALE. **radial collateral l. of elbow joint** LIGAMENTUM COLLATERALE RADIALE. **radial collateral l. of wrist** LIGAMENTUM COLLATERALE CARPI RADIALE. **radiate l.** LIGAMENTUM CAPITIS COSTAE RADIATUM. **radiate carpal l.** LIGAMENTUM CARPI RADIATUM. **radiate l. of head of rib** LIGAMENTUM CAPITIS COSTAE RADIATUM. **radiate l. of Mayer** LIGAMENTUM CARPI RADIATUM. **radiate sternocostal l.'s** LIGAMENTA STERNOCOSTALIA RADIATA. **radiate l. of wrist** LIGAMENTUM CARPI RADIATUM. **rectouterine l.** Musculus rectouterinus within the plica rectouterina. **reflected l.** LIGAMENTUM REFLEXUM. **reflex l. of Gimbernat** LIGAMENTUM REFLEXUM. **reflex inguinal l.** LIGAMENTUM REFLEXUM. **reinforcing l.** Any ligament that strengthens the capsule of a joint. **Retzius l.** The stem portion of the Y-shaped inferior extensor retinaculum. See also RETINACULUM MUSCULORUM EXTENSORUM PEDIS INFERIUS. **rhomboid l. of clavicle** LIGAMENTUM COSTOCLAVICULARE. **right triangular l. of liver** LIGAMENTUM TRIANGULARE DEXTRUM HEPATIS. **ring l. of hip joint** ZONA ORBICULARIS ARTICULATIONIS COXAE. **Robert's l.** LIGAMENTUM MENISCOFEMORALE POSTERIUS. **round l. of elbow joint** CHORDA OBLIQUA. **round l. of femur** LIGAMENTUM CAPITIS FEMORIS. **round l. of liver** LIGAMENTUM TERES HEPATIS. **round l. of uterus** LIGAMENTUM TERES UTERI. **sacrospinal l.** LIGAMENTUM SACROSPINALE. **sacrospinous l.** LIGAMENTUM SACROSPINALE. **sacrotuberal l.** LIGAMENTUM SACROTUBERALE. **sacrotuberous l.** LIGAMENTUM SACROTUBERALE. **Santorini's l.** LIGAMENTUM CRICOPHARYNGEUM. **Sappey's l.** A thickening of the posterior wall of the articular capsule of the temporomandibular joint, formed by a thick layer of loose and vascularized connective tissue fusing the articular disk to the capsule. Also *retrodiscal pad.* **l. of Scarpa** CORNU SUPERIUS MARGINIS FALCIFORMIS. **scrotal l. of testis** GUBERNACULUM TESTIS. **Sebileau suspensory l.'s** SUSPENSORY APPARATUS OF THE PLEURA. **serous l.** LIGAMENTUM SEROSUM. **short plantar l.** LIGAMENTUM CALCANEOCUBOIDEUM PLANTARE. **short posterior sacroiliac l.** See under LIGAMENTA SACROILIACA DORSALIA. **l.'s of the skull** Fibrous bands linking bones of the cranial base to each other or to bones below it, for example, the stylohyoid, stylomandibular, pterygospinous and sphenomandibular ligaments. **Soemmering's l.** Fibrous tissue connecting the convex border of the orbital part of the lacrimal gland to the orbital periosteum. **sphenomandibular l.** LIGAMENTUM SPHENOMANDIBULARE. **sphenomandibular l. proper** The portion of the sphenomandibular ligament that is attached to the spine of the sphenoid. **spinoglenoid l.** LIGAMENTUM TRANSVERSUM SCAPULAE INFERIUS. **spiral l. of cochlea** LIGAMENTUM SPIRALE COCHLEAE. **spring l.** LIGAMENTUM CALCANEONAVICULARE PLANTARE. **Stanley's cervical l.** RETINACULUM CAPSULAE ARTICULARIS COXAE. **stapedial l.** LIGAMENTUM ANNULARE STAPEDIS. **sternocostal l.'s** LIGAMENTA STERNOCOSTALIA RADIATA. **sternopericardiac l.'s** LIGAMENTA STERNOPERICARDIACA. **sternopericardial l.'s** LIGAMENTA STERNOPERICARDIACA. **stylohyoid l.** LIGAMENTUM STYLOHYOIDEUM. **stylomandibular l.** LIGAMENTUM STYLOMANDIBULARE. **subflaval l.'s** LIGAMENTA FLAVA. **subpubic l.** LIGAMENTUM ARCUATUM PUBIS. **superficial dorsal sacrococcygeal l.** LIGAMENTUM SACROCOCCYGEUM POSTERIUS SUPERFICIALE. **superficial transverse metacarpal l.** LIGAMENTUM METACARPALE TRANSVERSUM SUPERFICIALE. **superficial transverse metatarsal l.** LIGAMENTUM METATARSALE TRANSVERSUM SUPERFICIALE. **superior auricular l.** LIGAMENTUM AURICULARE SUPERIUS. **superior costotransverse l.** LIGAMENTUM COSTOTRANSVERSARIUM SUPERIUS. **superior l. of epididymis** LIGAMENTUM EPIDIDYMIDIS SUPERIUS. **superior glenohumeral l.** See under LIGAMENTA GLENOHUMERALIA. **superior l. of incus** LIGAMENTUM INCUDIS SUPERIUS. **superior l. of malleus** LIGAMENTUM MALLEI SUPERIUS. **superior l. of pinna** LIGAMENTUM AURICULARE SUPERIUS. **superior pubic l.** LIGAMENTUM PUBICUM SUPERIUS. **superior sternopericardial l.** See under LIGAMENTA STERNOPERICARDIACA. **superior transverse l. of scapula** LIGAMENTUM TRANSVERSUM SCAPULAE SUPERIUS. **suprascapular l.** LIGAMENTUM TRANSVERSUM SCAPULAE SUPERIUS. **supraspinal l.** LIGAMENTUM SUPRASPINALE. **supraspinous l.** LIGAMENTUM SUPRASPINALE. **suspensory l. of axilla** The fused laminae of the clavipectoral fascia extending between the lower border of the pectoralis minor muscle and the axillary fascia covering the floor of the axilla. Also *Campbell's ligament, Gerdy's ligament.* **suspensory l.'s of breast** LIGAMENTA SUSPENSORIA MAMMARIA. **suspensory l. of clitoris** LIGAMENTUM SUSPENSORIUM CLITORIDIS. **suspensory l. of duodenum** MUSCULUS SUSPENSORIUS DUODENI. **suspensory l. of eyeball** A thickening of the lower part of the bulbar sheath which is formed by the medial and lateral check ligaments of the eyeball fusing with the margins of the sheath of the inferior rectus muscle of the bulb, forming a broad sling below the eyeball and limiting certain of its movements. Also *Lockwood suspensory ligament.* **suspensory l. of lens** ZONULA CILIARIS. **suspensory l.'s of mammary gland** LIGAMENTA SUSPENSORIA MAMMARIA. **suspensory l. of ovary** LIGAMENTUM SUSPENSORIUM OVARII. **suspensory l. of penis** LIGAMENTUM SUSPENSORIUM PENIS. **sutural l.** A layer of connective tissue in the sutural gap between any two skull bones, continuous at the margins with periosteum both outside and inside the skull. Also *sutural membrane, intersutural membrane.* **synovial l.** A large fold of synovial membrane inside the capsule of a joint. **talonavicular l.** LIGAMENTUM TALONAVICULARE. **temporomandibular l.** LIGAMENTUM LATERALE ARTICULATIONIS TEMPOROMANDIBULARIS. **Teutleben's l.** LIGAMENTUM PULMONALE. **Thompson's l.** DEEP CRURAL ARCH. **thyroepiglottic l.** LIGAMENTUM THYROEPIGLOTTICUM. **thyrohyoid l.** LIGAMENTUM THYROHYOIDEUM LATERALE. **tibial collateral l.** LIGAMENTUM COLLATERALE TIBIALE. **tibiofibular l.** SYNDESMOSIS TIBIOFIBULARIS. **tibionavicular l.** PARS TIBIONAVICULARIS LIGAMENTI MEDIALIS. **Toynbee's l.** LIGAMENTUM MALLEI ANTERIUS. **tracheal annular l.'s** LIGAMENTA ANNULARIA TRACHEALIA. **transverse l. of acetabulum** LIGAMENTUM TRANSVERSUM ACETABULI. **transverse l. of atlas** LIGAMENTUM TRANSVERSUM ATLANTIS. **transverse humeral l.** A ligamentous thickening of the capsule of the shoulder joint extending between the greater and the lesser tubercles of the humerus, converting the intertubercular sulcus into a canal for the tendon of the long head of biceps brachii as it emerges from the capsule. Also *Brodie's ligament.* **transverse l. of knee** LIGAMENTUM TRANSVERSUM GENUS. **transverse l. of leg** RETINACULUM MUSCULORUM EXTENSORUM PEDIS SUPERIUS. **transverse pelvic l.** LIGAMENTUM TRANSVERSUM PERINEI. **transverse l. of pelvis** LIGAMENTUM TRANSVERSUM PERINEI. **transverse perineal l.** LIGAMENTUM TRANSVERSUM PERINEI. **transverse tibiofibular l.** The lower, deep part of the posterior tibiofibular ligament, extending from the lateral malleolar fossa to the posterior articular margin of the medial malleolus and articulating anteriorly with the talus. **trapezoid l.** LIGAMENTUM TRAPEZOIDEUM. **l. of Treitz** MUSCULUS SUSPENSORIUS DUODENI. **triangular l. of Colles** MEMBRANA PERINEI. **tubopharyngeal l. of Rauber** PLICA SALPINGOPHARYNGEA. **Tuffier's inferior l.** The distal part of the mesentery extending into the iliac fossa. **ulnar carpal l.** LIGAMENTUM COLLATERALE CARPI ULNARE. **ulnar carpal collateral l.** LIGAMENTUM COLLATERALE CARPI ULNARE. **ulnar collateral l. of carpus** LIGAMENTUM COLLATERALE CARPI ULNARE. **ulnar collateral l. of elbow joint** LIGAMENTUM COLLATERALE ULNARE. **ulnar collateral l. of wrist** LIGAMENTUM COLLATERALE CARPI ULNARE. **uteropelvic l.'s** Fibromuscular bands at the base of the broad ligament of the uterus extending from each side of the uterus and the vagina to the fascia on the obturator internus and levator ani muscles on the lateral pelvic wall. They include, for example, the lateral cervical ligament. **uterosacral l.** A band of fibrous tissue and smooth muscle fibers within the rectouterine fold, extending backward on each side from the cervix uteri to the front of the sacrum. Also *Petit's ligament.* **uterovesical l.** A peritoneal fold extending from the junction of the cervix and the body of the uterus anteriorly to the the upper surface of the urinary bladder. Also *vesicouterine ligament.* **vaginal l.'s of fingers** VINCULA TENDINUM DIGITORUM MANUS. **l.'s of Valsalva** LIGAMENTA AURICULARIA. **venous l. of liver** LIGAMENTUM VENOSUM. **ventral sacrococcygeal l.** LIGAMENTUM SACROCOCCYGEUM ANTERIUS. **ventral sacroiliac l.'s** LIGAMENTA SACROILIACA ANTERIORA. **ventricular l. of larynx** LIGAMENTUM VESTIBULARE. **vertebropelvic l.** Any of three ligaments: (1) ligamentum iliolumbale; (2) ligamentum sacrospinale; (3) ligamentum sacrotuberale. **vertebropericardial l.** Fibrous tissue intervening between the posterior surface of the fibrous pericardium and the vertebral column from the sixth cervical vertebra to the fourth thoracic vertebra. **l. of Vesalius** LIGAMENTUM INGUINALE. **vesicopubic l.** LIGAMENTUM PUBOVESICALE. **vesicoumbilical l.** LIGAMENTUM UMBILICALE MEDIANUM. **vesicouterine l.** UTEROVESICAL LIGAMENT. **vestibular l.** LIGAMENTUM VESTIBULARE. **vocal l.** LIGAMENTUM VOCALE. **volar l.'s of bases of metacarpal bones** LIGAMENTA METACARPALIA PALMARIA. **volar carpal l.** The superficial part of the flexor retinaculum which overlies the ulnar nerve and vessels. *Outmoded.* **volar carpometacarpal l.'s**

LIGAMENTA CARPOMETACARPALIA PALMARIA. **volar intercarpal l.'s** LIGAMENTA INTERCARPALIA PALMARIA. **volar radiocarpal l.** LIGAMENTUM RADIOCARPALE PALMARE. **Weitbrecht's l.** CHORDA OBLIQUA. **Winslow's l.** LIGAMENTUM POPLITEUM OBLIQUUM. **Wrisberg's l.** LIGAMENTUM MENISCOFEMORALE POSTERIUS. **xiphicostal l.'s of Macalister** LIGAMENTA COSTOXIPHOIDEA. **yellow l.'s** LIGAMENTA FLAVA. **l. of Zaglas** Part of the posterior sacroiliac ligament extending from the posterior superior iliac spine to the lateral crest of the second sacral vertebra. **Zinn's l.** ANNULUS TENDINEUS COMMUNIS. **zonular l.** ANNULUS TENDINEUS COMMUNIS.

**ligamenta** \lig′əmen′tə\ Plural of LIGAMENTUM.

**ligamentopexy** \lig′əmen′təpek′sē\ [LIGAMENT + *o* + -PEXY] A surgical procedure in which one or more ligaments are shortened, plicated, or strengthened. This operation, performed on the uterine round ligaments, is now rarely undertaken. Also *ligamentopexis.*

**ligamentous** \lig′əmen′təs\ Pertaining to, resembling, or having the characteristics of a ligament.

# ligamentum

**ligamentum** \lig′əmen′təm\ [L (from *liga(re)* to bind, tie + *-mentum* -MENT) a band, bandage] (*pl.* ligamenta) **1** [NA] A band, sheet, or local thickening of fibrous connective tissue in which the predominantly collagenous, as well as elastic, fibers are regularly oriented in thick bundles. It may occur inside a joint capsule, outside a capsule, or replacing a capsule, and is attached to two or more bones of a joint, strengthening, supporting, and limiting its movements. **2** [NA] A fibrous band, a fascial condensation, or a fold of peritoneum attached to an organ or organs, supporting it or them. **3** A fibrous remnant of an embryological or fetal tissue or organ. For defs. 1, 2, and 3 also *ligament.* **l. acromioclaviculare** [NA] A broad fibrous band covering the superior part of the capsule of the acromioclavicular joint, extending from the acromial end of the clavicle to the superior surface of the acromion and strengthened by the aponeuroses of the trapezius and deltoid muscles. Also *acromioclavicular ligament.* **ligamenta alaria** [NA] Two rounded cords extending from the sides of the dens of the axis to rough surfaces medial to the condyles of the occipital bone. They are relaxed when the head is extended, but tighten on flexion so as to limit the movement. Also *alar ligaments, check ligaments of axis, check ligaments of odontoid, Mauchart's ligaments, occipito-odontoid ligaments, lateral occipitoaxial ligaments.* **l. annulare bulbi** RETICULUM TRABECULARE SCLERAE. **l. annulare radii** [NA] A thick band encircling the head of the radius and forming three-fourths of an osseofibrous ring by its attachment to the anterior and posterior margins of the radial notch. Its inner surface is lined with cartilage for articulation with the circumference of the head of the radius. Its fibers blend with the capsule of the elbow joint and with some surrounding ligaments and muscles. Also *orbicular ligament of radius, annular ligament of radius.* **l. annulare stapedis** [NA] A ring of elastic fibers encircling the base of the stapes and holding it to the margin of the fenestra vestibuli as well as serving as a hinge on which the base moves during contraction of the stapedius muscle. Also *annular ligament of stapes, annular ligament of base of stapes, stapedial ligament.* **ligamenta annularia trachealia** [NA] Fibrous membranes, composed of collagen and intermingled elastin fibers, continuous with the perichondrium of adjacent tracheal rings, linking them and connecting the ends of the incomplete rings posteriorly. Also *tracheal annular ligaments.* **l. anococcygeum** [NA] A fibromuscular band, comprising fibers of the subcutaneous part of the external anal sphincter and of connective tissue, attached to the posterior aspect of the dermis of the anus and to the tip of the coccyx. Also *anococcygeal ligament, Symington's body.* **l. apicis dentis axis** [NA] A narrow fibrous band extending from the tip of the dens of the axis to the anterior border of the foramen magnum and located between the alar ligaments. It is tightened by extension of the head. Also *apical dental ligament, apical odontoid ligament, apical ligament of dens.* **l. arcuatum laterale** [NA] A thickened transverse band in the fascia of the quadratus lumborum muscle, or anterior lamella of thoracolumbar fascia, attached laterally to the lower border of the twelfth rib and medially to the front of the transverse process of the first lumbar vertebra, serving as an origin of the diaphragm. Also *lateral arcuate ligament, lateral lumbocostal arch, lateral lumbocostal arch of Haller, arcus lumbocostalis lateralis, external arcuate ligament of diaphragm* (outmoded). **l. arcuatum mediale** [NA] A horizontal ligamentous band in the psoas fascia attached laterally to the front of the transverse process of the first lumbar vertebra and medially to the body of the first or second lumbar vertebra where it is continuous with the outer side of the corresponding crus of the diaphragm, serving as an origin of the diaphragm. Also *medial arcuate ligament, medial lumbocostal arch, medial lumbocostal arch of Haller, arcus lumbocostalis medialis, internal arcuate ligament of diaphragm* (outmoded). **l. arcuatum medianum** [NA] The tendinous arch joining the crura of the diaphragm in the median plane in front of the aorta. Also *median arcuate ligament.* **l. arcuatum pubis** [NA] A thick fibrous arch across the inferior surface of the body of the pubis on each side, attached to the interpubic disk superiorly and to the inferior pubic rami laterally. It forms the apex of the pubic arch. Also *arcuate pubic ligament, inferior pubic ligament, subpubic ligament, inferior arcuate ligament of pubis, pubic arcuate ligament, Lauth's ligament.* **l. arteriosum** [NA] The thick cordlike remnant of the closed ductus arteriosus, extending from the left pulmonary artery, near its origin, to the concavity of the arch of the aorta. Also *ligament of Botallo.* **l. atlanto-occipitale laterale** [NA] A ligament lateral to and strengthening the capsule of the atlanto-occipital joint which extends craniomedially from the transverse process of the atlas, lateral to the foramen transversarium, to the inferior surface of the jugular process of the occipital bone. Also *lateral atlanto-occipital ligament.* **l. auriculare anterius** [NA] An extrinsic ligament of the ear attaching the helix and the tragus of the auricle to the root of the zygoma. Also *anterior auricular ligament.* **l. auriculare posterius** [NA] An extrinsic ligament of the ear extending between the posterior aspect of the concha of the auricle and the mastoid process of the temporal bone. Also *posterior auricular ligament, posterior ligament of pinna.* **l. auriculare superius** [NA] An extrinsic ligament of the ear extending between the spine of the helix and the upper margin of the bony external acoustic meatus. Also *superior auricular ligament, superior ligament of pinna.* **ligamenta auricularia** [NA] The three extrinsic ligaments, namely, anterior, posterior, and superior, that attach the auricle to the side of the head. Also *ligaments of auricle, ligaments of Valsalva.* **ligamenta basium** Ligaments connecting the bases of the metacarpal bones in the intermetacarpal articulations, and of the metatarsals in the intermetatarsal articulations: ligamenta metacarpalia (dorsalia, palmaria, and interossea) and ligamenta metatarsalia (dorsalia, plantaria, and interossea). **l. bifurcatum** [NA] A strong short band, the stem of which is attached posteriorly to the anterior part of the superior surface of the calcaneus while anteriorly it bifurcates into two, namely, the calcaneocuboid and calcaneonavicular ligaments. Also *bifurcate ligament, bifurcated ligament, ligament of Chopart.* **l. calcaneocuboideum** [NA] The anterolateral portion of the bifurcated ligament that is attached distally to the dorsal part of the medial aspect of the cuboid bone, helping to secure the first to the second row of tarsal bones. Also *calcaneocuboid ligament.* **l. calcaneocuboideum plantare** [NA] A short broad band extending from the anterior tubercle and adjacent anterior area of the calcaneus to the contiguous plantar surface of the cuboid bone. This powerful ligament tends to prevent flattening of the lateral longitudinal arch of the foot. Also *plantar calcaneocuboid ligament, short plantar ligament.* **l. calcaneofibulare** [NA] A long, cordlike band extending posteriorly from the hollow anterior to the apex of the lateral malleolus of the fibula down to the tubercle near the middle of the lateral surface of the calcaneus. With the anterior and posterior talofibular ligaments, it forms the lateral ligament of the talocrural joint. Also *calcaneofibular ligament.* **l. calcaneonaviculare** [NA] The anteromedial portion of the bifurcated ligament that is attached distally to the dorsolateral part of the navicular bone. Also *calcaneonavicular ligament, calcaneonavicular part of bifurcated ligament.* **l. calcaneonaviculare dorsale** The dorsal fibers of the ligamentum calcaneonaviculare, no longer considered separately from the main ligament. *Outmoded.* Also *dorsal calcaneonavicular ligament.* **l. calcaneonaviculare plantare** [NA] A broad, thick, and strong band extending between the anterior margin of the sustentaculum tali of the calcaneus and the plantar aspect of the navicular bone, supporting the head of talus on its dorsal surface. Also *plantar calcaneonavicular ligament, spring ligament, inferior calcaneonavicular ligament.* **l. capitis costae intra-articulare** [NA] A short, flat band stretching transversely from the crest separating the two articular facets on the head of a rib to the adjacent intervertebral disk, dividing the joint cavity into two compartments. It is absent in the joints of the first, tenth, eleventh, and twelfth ribs. Also *intra-articular ligament of head of rib, intra-articular costovertebral ligament.* **l. capitis costae radiatum** [NA] Fibers attached to the anterior surface of the head of a rib and radiating medially to the body of the vertebra above, to that of the vertebra below, and to the intervertebral disk in between. Also *radiate ligament of head of rib, anterior ligament of head of rib, anterior costocentral ligament, costovertebral ligament, radiate ligament.* **l. capitis femoris** [NA] A flat triangular intracapsular band attached by its apex to the anterosuperior part of the fovea on the head of the femur and by its base to each side of the acetabular notch and the inferior border of the transverse ligament in between. It is surrounded by synovial membrane and it tightens when the hip joint is semiflexed or adducted. Also *ligament of head of femur, round ligament of femur.* **l. capitis fibulae anterius** [NA] A broad band extending upwards and obliquely from the front of the head of the fibula to the lateral condyle of the tibia and fused on its deep surface with the capsule of the superior tibiofibular joint. Also *anterior ligament of head of fibula.* **l. capitis fibulae posterius** [NA] A thick band extending upwards and obliquely from the back of the head of the fibula to the lateral condyle of the tibia deep to the tendon of the popliteus muscle. Its deep surface is fused with the capsule of the superior tibiofibular joint. Also *posterior ligament of head of fibula.* **ligamenta capsularia** [NA] Ligamentous thickenings in the fibrous layer of articular capsules. Also *capsular ligaments.* See also MEMBRANA FIBROSA CAPSULAE ARTICULARIS. **l. carpi radiatum** [NA] A group of ligamentous fascicles on the palmar aspect of the carpus radiating from the head of the capitate bone to surrounding bones of the midcarpal joint. Also *radiate carpal ligament, radiate ligament of Mayer, radiate ligament of wrist, ligament of Mayer.* **ligamenta carpometacarpalia dorsalia** [NA] A group of fibrous bands strengthening the articular capsules between the distal row of carpal bones and the bases of the metacarpal bones on their posterior surfaces. Also *dorsal carpometacarpal ligaments, posterior carpometacarpal ligaments.* **ligamenta carpometacarpalia palmaria** [NA] A group of fibrous bands strengthening the articular capsules between the distal row of carpal bones and the bases of the metacarpal bones on their anterior, or palmar, surfaces. Also *palmar carpometacarpal ligaments, anterior carpometacarpal ligaments, volar carpometacarpal ligaments.* **l. ceratocricoideum** [NA] An external accessory ligament which strengthens the fibrous capsule of the cricothyroid joint. Also *ceratocricoid ligament.* **l. collaterale carpi radiale** [NA] A short, rather weak band lying deep to the radial artery and extending between the tip of the styloid process of the radius and the lateral side of the scaphoid and trapezium bones. Also *radial carpal collateral ligament, radial collateral ligament of carpus, radial collateral ligament of wrist, external lateral ligament of wrist joint.* **l. collaterale carpi ulnare** [NA] A strong short band attached proximally to the tip of the styloid process of the ulna and distally by two fasciculi, one to the pisiform bone and one to the medial aspect of triquetrum. Also *ulnar carpal collateral ligament, ulnar carpal ligament, ulnar collateral ligament of carpus, ligamentous funiculus, ulnar collateral ligament of wrist, medial ligament of wrist, internal lateral ligament of wrist joint* (outmoded). **l. collaterale fibulare** [NA] A strong fibrous band extending from the lateral epicondyle of the femur to the head of the fibula anterior to its apex. Also *fibular collateral ligament, lateral ligament of knee, external lateral ligament of knee.* **l. collaterale radiale** [NA] A strong triangular band attached proximally by its apex to the lower part of the lateral epicondyle of the humerus and distally by its base to the annular ligament of the radius and the supinator crest of the ulna. Also *radial collateral ligament, lateral ligament of elbow, radial collateral ligament of elbow joint.* **l. collaterale tibiale** [NA] A broad fibrous band, posteromedial to the knee joint, extending from the medial epicondyle of the femur, below the adductor tubercle, to the medial condyle and adjacent shaft of the tibia, and having its deep surface firmly attached to the medial meniscus and capsule of the knee joint. Also *tibial collateral ligament, internal lateral ligament of knee.* **l. collaterale ulnare** [NA] A strong triangular band on the medial side of the elbow joint, attached proximally at its apex to the anterior and inferior surfaces of the medial epicondyle and divisible distally into three parts: an anterior part attached to the upper end of the medial edge of the coronoid process of the ulna, a posterior part attached to the medial surface of the olecranon, and an intermediate part between these two parts attached to the oblique band between the coronoid and olecranon processes. Also *ulnar collateral ligament of elbow joint, medial ligament of elbow joint, deltoid ligament of elbow.* **ligamenta collateralia** [NA] Thick fibrous bands that are located on the sides of uniaxial hinge joints such as the interphalangeal, humeroulnar, and knee joints. They help strengthen the joint capsules and control movement. Also *collateral ligaments.* **ligamenta collateralia articulationum interphalangearum manus** [NA] Strong, thick cords placed obliquely on the sides of the interphalangeal joints of the fingers, extending from the posterolateral surface of the distal end of the proximal bone to the anterolateral aspect of the base of the distal bone. Posteriorly the fibers join the expansion of the extensor tendon of each finger. The ligaments are always tense, preventing lateral movements. Also *collateral ligaments of interphalangeal articulations of hand, collateral ligaments of joints of fingers, lateral ligaments of joints of fingers, collateral ligaments of interphalangeal joints of hand.* **ligamenta collateralia articulationum interphalangearum pedis** [NA] Strong fibrous cords placed obliquely on the sides of the interphalangeal joints of the toes, extending from a small depression on the side of the head of the more proximal bone to a rough edge on the side of the base of the distal bone. Also *collateral ligaments of interphalangeal articulations of foot, collateral ligaments of joints of toes, lateral ligaments of joints of toes, collateral ligaments of interphalangeal joints of foot.* **ligamenta collateralia articulationum metacarpophalangearum** [NA] Strong fibrous cords placed obliquely on the sides of the metacarpophalangeal joints, extending from a posterior tubercle and depression on each side of the head of the metacarpal bone to the corresponding anterolateral side of the base of the proximal phalanx. The fibers connect posteriorly with the extensor expansion and anteriorly with the palmar ligament of each finger. In the thumb, the ligaments also attach to the sesamoid bones. Also *collateral ligaments of metacarpophalangeal articulations, lateral ligaments of metacarpophalangeal joints, lateral metacarpophalangeal ligaments.* **ligamenta collateralia articulationum metatarsophalangearum** [NA] Strong fibrous cords placed obliquely on the sides of the metatarsophalangeal joints, extending from a tubercle on each side of the posterior aspect of the head of the metatarsal bone to the corresponding anterolateral side of the base of the proximal phalanx. Also *collateral ligaments of metatarsophalangeal articulations, lateral ligaments of metatarsophalangeal joints, lateral metatarsophalangeal ligaments.* **l. conoideum** [NA] The triangular, posteromedial part of the coracoclavicular ligament, attached superiorly by its base to the conoid tubercle and an adjoining line medial to it on the inferior surface of the clavicle and inferiorly by its apex to the posteromedial edge of the root of the coracoid process at the scapular notch. Also *conoid ligament.* **l. coracoacromiale** [NA] A strong triangular band attached at its apex near the tip of the acromion anterior to the articular surface for the clavicle and by its base to the lateral margin of the coracoid process, forming an arch over the shoulder joint and deep to the deltoid muscle. Also *coracoacromial ligament.* **l. coracoclaviculare** [NA] A strong band holding the lateral end of the clavicle to the underlying coracoid process of the scapula and consisting of two parts, the conoid and the trapezoid ligaments, separated from each other by fat or a bursa. Also *coracoclavicular ligament, Caldani's ligament.* **l. coracohumerale** [NA] A broad band, partly fused with the capsule of the shoulder joint, extending inferolaterally from the lateral side of the root of the coronoid process of the scapula to the anterior aspect of the greater tubercle of the humerus. Also *coracohumeral ligament.* **l. coronarium** [NA] The peritoneal reflection from the diaphragm to the superior and posterior surfaces of the liver, comprising an upper and a lower layer that are separated by part of the right lobe devoid of peritoneum, the bare area, and continuous with the right triangular ligament. To the left, the upper layer is continuous with the right layer of the falciform ligament while the lower layer becomes continuous with the posterior layer of the hepatogastric ligament. Also *coronary ligament of liver.* **l. costoclaviculare** [NA] A strong V-shaped band extending inferomedially from the inferior surface of the sternal end of the clavicle to the superior surface of the first rib and adjacent cartilage, and comprising two laminae, anterior and posterior, that fuse laterally and are continuous medially with the capsule of the sternoclavicular joint. Also *costoclavicular ligament, rhomboid ligament of clavicle.* **l. costotransversarium** [NA] A short, wide band of fibers that is attached anteriorly to the posterior aspect of the neck of a rib and posteriorly to the anterior surface of the adjacent transverse process. Also *costotransverse ligament, inferior ligament of neck of rib of Henle, ligament of neck of rib.* **l. costotransversarium laterale** [NA] A powerful, short fibrous band extending upward and laterally from the tip of the transverse process of a vertebra to the nonarticular part of the tubercle of the adjacent rib. It is absent on the eleventh and twelfth ribs. Also *lateral costotransverse ligament, inferior ligament of tubercle of rib.* **l. costotransversarium superius** [NA] A strong, broad fibrous band consisting of two layers. The anterior layer extends from the crest on the superior margin of the neck of a rib to the inferior margin of the transverse process above it, being continuous with the medial margin of the internal intercostal membrane. The posterior layer extends medially from the posterior surface of the neck of a rib to the transverse process above it. The ligament is absent on the first rib. Also *superior costotransverse ligament.* **ligamenta costoxiphoidea** [NA] Inconstant fibrous bands, varying in length and breadth, that connect the front and back of the xiphoid process to corresponding surfaces of the seventh, and occasionally the sixth, costal cartilages. Also *costoxiphoid ligaments, xiphicostal ligaments of Macalister, chondroxiphoid ligaments.* **l. cricoarytenoideum posterius** [NA] A strong, short band reinforcing the cricoarytenoid joint and extending from the upper border of the lamina of the cricoid cartilage to the medial surface of the base and muscular process of the arytenoid cartilage, fixing and limiting the forward movements of the latter. Also *posterior cricoarytenoid ligament.* **l. cricopharyngeum** [NA] A single band extending downward in the median plane from the junction of the right and left corniculopharyngeal ligaments and the pharyngeal mucosa to the cricoid lamina and the pharyngeal mucosa. Also *cricopharyngeal ligament, cricosantorinian ligament, Santorini's ligament, cricopharyngeal ligament of Luschka.* **l. cricothyroideum medianum** [NA] The midline band of yellow elastic tissue connecting the cricoid cartilage to the lower margin of the thyroid cartilage. Laterally it is continuous with the conus elasticus (cricovocal membrane), the upper edge of which is the ligamentum vocale. Also *cricothyroid ligament, middle cricothyroid ligament.* **l. cricotracheale** [NA] A fibrous ring linking the lower border of the cricoid cartilage to the first cartilaginous ring of the trachea and continuous inferiorly with the tracheal annular ligaments. Also *cricotracheal ligament, cricotracheal membrane.* **ligamenta cruciata genus** [NA] Strong intracapsular ligaments that cross each other in the intercondylar region of the knee joint posterior to its center, and called ligamentum cruciatum anterius genus and ligamentum cruciatum posterius genus. Also *cruciate ligaments of knee, cruciate ligaments.* **l. cruciatum anterius genus** [NA] A thick cordlike band within the knee joint extending from the anterior intercondylar area of the tibia to the posterior part of the medial aspect of the lateral condyle of the femur. Although taut in all positions, it prevents forward gliding of the tibia on the femur. Also *anterior cruciate ligament of knee, anterior cruciate ligament.* **l. cruciatum posterius genus** [NA] A strong band, shorter than the anterior cruciate ligament, extending from the posterior intercondylar area of the tibia to the front of the lateral aspect of the medial condyle of the femur. It is taut in all positions and prevents backward gliding of the tibia on the femur. Also *posterior cruciate ligament of knee, posterior cruciate ligament.* **l. cruciforme atlantis** [NA] A cross-shaped fibrous band in which the transverse ligament of atlas forms a horizontal bar posterior to the dens where it sends ascending and descending longitudinal bundles to be attached superiorly on the internal aspect of the anterior margin of the foramen magnum, between the apical ligament of dens and the membrana tectoria, and inferiorly to the posterior surface of the body of the axis, respectively. Also *cruciform ligament of atlas, cruciate ligament of atlas.* **l. cuboideonaviculare dorsale** [NA] A fibrous band strengthening the transverse articulation of the tarsus and extending laterally and distally from the dorsal surface of the navicular to the medial side of the cuboid bone. Also *dorsal cuboideonavicular ligament.* **l. cuboideonaviculare plantare** [NA] A strong band strengthening the transverse articulation of the tarsus and extending transversely from the medial side of the plantar surface of the cuboid to the plantar surface of the navicular bone. Also *plantar cuboideonavicular ligament.* **l. cuneocuboideum dorsale** [NA] A fibrous band between the dorsal surfaces of the lateral cuneiform and the cuboid bones. Proximally it may blend with the dorsal cuboideonavicular and cuneonavicular ligaments. Also *dorsal cuneocuboid ligament.* **l. cuneocuboideum interosseum** [NA] Strong fibers connecting the adjacent nonarticular surfaces of the lateral cuneiform and cuboid bones. Also *interosseous cuneocuboid ligament.* **l. cuneocuboideum plantare** [NA] A fibrous band connecting the plantar surfaces of the lateral cuneiform and cuboid bones, reinforced by slips from the tendon of the tibialis posterior muscle. Also *plantar cuneocuboid ligament.* **ligamenta cuneometatarsalia interossea** [NA] Fibrous bands, usually three in number, connecting the cuneiform bones to the bases of adjoining metatarsal bones. The strongest is the one between the lateral surface of medial cuneiform and the medial surface of the base of the second metatarsal bone. The second band joins the lateral cuneiform to the second metatarsal, and the third band connects the lateral cuneiform with the bases of the third and fourth metatarsal bones. Also *interosseous cuneometatarsal ligaments.* **ligamenta cuneonavicularia dorsalia** [NA] Strong bands, usually fusing into a continuous band, connecting each of the dorsal surfaces of the three cuneiform bones to the navicular bone. The band to the medial cuneiform sends fasciculi medially to join the plantar cuneonavicular ligaments. Also *dorsal cuneonavicular ligaments.* **ligamenta cuneonavicularia plantaria** [NA] Strong bands, usually fusing into a continuous band, connecting each of the plantar surfaces of the three cuneiform bones to the navicular bone, and reinforced by slips of the tendon of tibialis posterior muscle. Also *plantar cuneonavicular ligaments.* **l. denticulatum** [NA] One of a series of flattened triangular bands of epipial tissue attached medially to the lateral surface of the spinal cord midway between the dorsal and ventral roots and lateral to the dural sheath. 18 to 24 ligaments anchor the spinal cord to the dura and alternate with the dural evaginations marking the exit of the cervical, thoracic, and first lumbar spinal nerves. Also *denticulate ligament, dentate ligament of spinal cord.* **l. epididymidis inferius** [NA] A fold of the visceral layer of the tunica vaginalis at the lower end of the sinus epididymidis passing from the testis over the tail of the epididymis to become continuous with the parietal layer. Also *inferior ligament of epididymis.* **l. epididymidis superius** [NA] A fold of the visceral layer of the tunica vaginalis at the upper end of the sinus epididymidis passing from the testis over the head of the epididymis to become continuous with the parietal layer. Also *superior ligament of epididymis.* **ligamenta extracapsularia** [NA] Ligaments that are outside the capsule of a synovial joint and sometimes separated from it. **l. falciforme hepatis** [NA] A midline crescentic fold of peritoneum, the ventral part of the primitive ventral mesogastrium, connecting the liver to the diaphragm and the anterior abdominal wall above the umbilicus, and containing the ligamentum teres and paraumbilical veins in its free edge which is attached to the inferior border of the liver. On the superior surface of the liver the two layers separate and the right layer becomes continuous with the upper layer of the coronary ligament while the left layer is continuous with the anterior layer of the left triangular ligament of liver. Also *falciform ligament of liver, broad ligament of liver.* **ligamenta flava** [NA] A series of plates of yellow elastic tissue forming elastic syndesmoses between the laminae of adjacent vertebrae and extending from the posterior arch of the atlas to the first sacral vertebra. They are thinnest in the neck and thickest in the lumbar region. They facilitate flexion and steady the vertebrae during regaining the erect position from a flexed one. Also *flaval ligaments, yellow ligaments, interlaminar ligaments, subflaval ligaments.* **l. fundiforme penis** [NA] A thickened elastic band of the membranous layer of the superficial fascia adherent to the lower part of the linea alba and the top of the symphysis pubis that extends to the dorsum of the penis and splits around it, reuniting below it to attach to the septum of the scrotum. Also *fundiform ligament of penis.* **l. gastrocolicum** [NA] The portion of the greater omentum that extends from the greater curvature of the stomach to the transverse colon, fusing with its anterior surface. It is continuous superiorly with the gastrosplenic ligament and to the left with the phrenicocolic ligament. Also *gastrocolic ligament.* **l. gastrophrenicum** [NA] A short fold, formed by the merging of the splenorenal and gastrosplenic ligaments, which passes forward from the diaphragm to the posterior surface of the fundus of the stomach, the two layers separating around the esophagus. It is essentially an upper portion of the greater omentum. Also *gastrophrenic ligament.* **l. gastrosplenicum** [NA] The part of the greater omentum that extends from the greater curvature on the left side of the fundus and adjoining part of the body of the stomach to the hilum of the spleen. Also *gastrosplenic ligament, gastrolienal ligament.* **l. genitoinguinale** GENITOINGUINAL LIGAMENT. **ligamenta glenohumeralia** [NA] Three variable fibrous bands, superior, middle, and inferior, projecting on the inner aspect of the front of the capsule of the shoulder joint and extending from the edge of the glenoid cavity and labrum glenoidale to the lesser tubercle and adjoining inferior part of the neck of the humerus. Also *glenohumeral ligaments.* **l. hepatocolicum** [NA] An occasional prolongation inferiorly of the hepatoduodenal ligament to the transverse colon and right colic flexure. Also *hepatocolic ligament.* **l. hepatoduodenale** [NA] The right portion of the lesser omentum, extending from the porta hepatis to the first part of the duodenum, forming the anterior boundary of the epiploic foramen. Also *hepatoduodenal ligament, duodenohepatic liga-*

*ment.* **l. hepatoesophageum** The left margin of the lesser omentum extending between the liver and the abdominal part of the esophagus. Also *hepatoesophageal ligament.* **l. hepatogastricum** [NA] The upper, major part of the lesser omentum, extending between the lesser curvature of the stomach and the fissure for ligamentum venosum of the liver. Also *hepatogastric ligament, gastrohepatic ligament.* **l. hepatorenale** [NA] An occasional prolongation inferiorly of the lower layer of the coronary ligament of the liver on to the right kidney just to the right of the epiploic foramen. Also *hepatorenal ligament.* **l. hyoepiglotticum** [NA] A broad elastic sheet connecting the anterior surface of the upper part of the epiglottis to the superior margin of the body of the hyoid bone and to its greater horn. Also *hyoepiglottic ligament, hyoepiglottic membrane.* **l. iliofemorale** [NA] A strong inverted Y-shaped band attached proximally to the lower part of the anterior inferior iliac spine and distally to the anterior surface of the greater trochanter and the intertrochanteric line of the femur. The central portion is weak and the medial band is strong. The lateral band is often called the iliotrochanteric ligament. The ligament is fused with the capsule of the hip joint anteriorly, supporting the weight of the body in the erect posture, with minimal muscular action, and limiting hyperextension and lateral rotation. Also *iliofemoral ligament, hypsiloid ligament, Bigelow's ligament, Bertin's ligament.* **l. iliolumbale** [NA] A strong triangular band extending from a long attachment on the internal aspect of the iliac crest to the anteroinferior part of the transverse process of the fifth, and often the fourth, lumbar vertebra. Also *iliolumbar ligament.* **l. iliopectineale** ARCUS ILIOPECTINEUS. **l. incudis posterius** [NA] A short fibrous band connecting the tip of the short process of the incus to the fossa incudis on the posterior wall of the tympanic cavity. Also *posterior ligament of incus.* **l. incudis superius** [NA] A fold of mucous membrane extending upward from the body of the incus to the roof of the epitympanic recess of the middle ear. Also *superior ligament of incus, Arnold's ligament.* **l. inguinale** [NA] The free and upturned, hammocklike, lower edge of the aponeurosis of the external oblique muscle extending from the anterior superior iliac spine to the pubic tubercle and pecten pubis, curved convex downward and attached to the fascia lata. The lateral part is strengthened by iliac fascia while the medial part forms the inguinal canal. Also *inguinal ligament, arcus inguinalis, crural ligament, Poupart's ligament, crural arch, ligament of Vesalius.* **ligamenta intercarpalia dorsalia** [NA] Transverse bands connecting the dorsal surfaces of the carpal bones in the proximal row and of those in the distal row, as well as short, irregular bundles between the proximal and distal rows. Also *dorsal intercarpal ligaments, carpal dorsal ligaments.* **ligamenta intercarpalia interossea** [NA] Short, variable bands connecting the adjacent surfaces of the proximal and of the distal carpal bones. Also *interosseous intercarpal ligaments, interosseous ligaments of carpal bones.* **ligamenta intercarpalia palmaria** [NA] Transverse bands connecting the palmar surfaces of the proximal row and of the distal row of carpal bones, as well as short, irregular bundles between the bones of the proximal and those of the distal row. Also *palmar intercarpal ligaments, volar intercarpal ligaments.* **l. interclaviculare** [NA] A strong, flat, curved fibrous band connecting the posterosuperior parts of the sternal ends of the two clavicles. Also *interclavicular ligament.* **ligamenta intercuneiformia dorsalia** [NA] Transverse fibrous bands connecting the dorsal surfaces of the three cuneiform bones. Also *dorsal intercuneiform ligaments.* **ligamenta intercuneiformia interossea** [NA] Strong, deep fibrous ligaments which connect the intermediate cuneiform with the lateral and medial cuneiform bones, occupying the total vertical depth between the nonarticular surfaces of the adjoining bones and blending with the plantar and dorsal cuneonavicular ligaments. Also *interosseous intercuneiform ligaments.* **ligamenta intercuneiformia plantaria** [NA] Transverse fibrous bands connecting the plantar surfaces of the three cuneiform bones and reinforced by slips from the tendon of the tibialis posterior muscle. Also *plantar intercuneiform ligaments.* **l. interfoveolare** [NA] A thickened band of the transversalis fascia, occasionally containing muscle fibers, extending from the lower margin of the transversus abdominis muscle to the superior ramus of the pubis, or, occasionally to blend with the femoral sheath. The band passes medial to the deep inguinal ring. Also *interfoveolar ligament, Hesselbach's ligament, semilunar fold of transversalis fascia.* **ligamenta interspinalia** [NA] Fibrous membranes located between the spines of the vertebrae, extending obliquely from the root of one spine to the tip of the adjacent spine and continuous with the ligamenta flava anteriorly and the supraspinous ligaments posteriorly. They are best developed in the lumbar region and least in the neck. Also *interspinal ligaments, interspinous ligaments.* **ligamenta intertransversaria** [NA] Weak fibrous bands or bundles extending between the tips of adjacent transverse processes of vertebrae, best developed in the lumbar region and replaced by the intertransverse muscles in the neck. Also *intertransverse ligaments, intertransverse ligaments of vertebral arch.* **ligamenta intracapsularia** [NA] Ligaments situated inside the capsule of a joint but excluded from the joint cavity by folds of synovial membrane, such as the cruciate ligaments of the knee. Also *intra-articular ligaments.* **l. ischiofemorale** [NA] A strong triangular band posterior to the capsule of the hip joint, spiraling superolaterally behind the neck of the femur from its attachment on the body of the ischium, behind and below the acetabulum, to the greater trochanter and trochanteric fossa, while some of the lateral and deeper fibers are continuous with the zona orbicularis. It helps to prevent excessive medial rotation. Also *ischiofemoral ligament.* **l. lacunare** [NA] The triangular extension of the medial end of the inguinal ligament to the medial part of the pecten pubis along which it extends laterally to blend with the pectineal fascia. The apex is attached to the pubic tubercle and its laterally directed concave base forms the medial border of the femoral ring. Its superior, abdominal surface forms the floor of the inguinal canal medially. Also *lacunar ligament, Gimbernat's ligament, lacunar ligament of Gimbernat, pectineal part of inguinal ligament.* **l. laterale articulationis temporomandibularis** [NA] A strong, oblique fibrous band, closely related to the lateral surface of the capsule of the temporomandibular joint, extending downward and posteriorly from its attachment on the lateral surface and crest of the tubercle on the root of the zygoma to the lateral surface and back of the mandibular neck while the deeper, medial fibers attach to the articular disk and lateral aspect of the mandibular condyle. Also *lateral ligament of temporomandibular articulation, temporomandibular ligament, Ferrein's ligament, external lateral ligament of temporomandibular joint.* **l. latum uteri** [NA] A transverse fold of peritoneum extending from each lateral surface of the uterus and supravaginal cervix to the lateral walls of the pelvic cavity. The two layers are continuous at the superior, free border which contains the uterine tube, while they diverge near the superior surface of levator ani muscle. The ligament is divided into mesosalpinx, mesovarium and mesometrium.

Also *broad ligament of uterus.* **l. longitudinale anterius** [NA] A strong band, of variable width and composed of several layers of longitudinal fibers, extending down the front of the bodies of the vertebrae from the basilar part of the occipital bone to the front of the first sacral segment. It is fixed to the intervertebral disks and the upper and lower margins of the vertebral bodies, the superficial fibers extending over several vertebrae while the deep ones pass from one vertebra to the next. Also *anterior longitudinal ligament.* **l. longitudinale posterius** [NA] A strong band, of variable width and composed of several layers of longitudinal fibers, extending down the posterior surfaces of the bodies of the vertebrae inside the vertebral canal from the axis, where it is continuous superiorly with the membrana tectoria, to the first two segments of the sacrum. It is fixed to the intervertebral disks and the upper and lower margins of the vertebral bodies, narrowing over the center of the bodies from which it is separated by veins. Its superficial fibers span several vertebrae while the deep fibers attach to contiguous vertebrae. Also *posterior longitudinal ligament.* **l. lumbocostale** [NA] A strong band of fibers connecting the neck of the twelfth rib to the base of the transverse process of the first lumbar vertebra, in series with the superior costotransverse ligaments. Also *lumbocostal ligament, tendinous arch of lumbodorsal fascia, lumbocostal ligament of Henle.* **l. mallei anterius** [NA] A band extending from the neck of the malleus near the anterior, or long, process to the anterior tympanic wall, some fibers (Meckel's band) continuing through the adjacent petrotympanic fissure to the angular spine of the sphenoid bone. A few fibers may reach the sphenomandibular ligament. Also *anterior ligament of malleus, Toynbee's ligament, incudius, Casser's muscle, casserian muscle.* **l. mallei laterale** [NA] A short, triangular band extending from the head of the malleus to the posterior margin of the tympanic notch. Also *lateral ligament of malleus, Casser's ligament, casserian ligament.* **l. mallei superius** [NA] A fine, round band that ascends from the head of the malleus to the roof of the epitympanic recess of the middle ear. Also *superior ligament of malleus.* **l. mediale articulationis talocruralis** [NA] A strong triangular band on the medial side of the talocrural joint, attached proximally to the tip and anterior and posterior margins of the medial malleolus and passing inferiorly in four bands, namely, pars tibionavicularis, pars tibiocalcanea, pars tibiotalaris anterior, and pars tibiotalaris posterior, to the tarsal bones. Also *deltoid ligament of ankle, deltoid ligament of talocrural joint.* **l. mediale articulationis temporomandibularis** [NA] A horizontal fibrous band that strengthens the capsule on the medial side of the temporomandibular joint and prevents backward displacement of the mandibular condyle. Also *medial ligament of temporomandibular joint.* **l. meniscofemorale anterius** [NA] An oblique fasciculus extending from the posterior part of the lateral meniscus to the medial condyle of the femur and passing anterior to and blending with the posterior cruciate ligament. Also *anterior meniscofemoral ligament, Humphry's ligament.* **l. meniscofemorale posterius** [NA] A strong fasciculus extending from the posterior extremity of the lateral meniscus to the medial condyle of the femur and passing posterior to and blending with the posterior cruciate ligament. Also *posterior meniscofemoral ligament, Robert's ligament, Wrisberg's ligament, posterior meniscofemoral ligament of Wrisberg.* **l. metacarpale transversum superficiale** [NA] A transverse band of fibers in the superficial fascia across the webs of the fingers, attached to the skin of the webs as well as to the fifth metacarpal bone. Also *superficial transverse metacarpal ligament.* **ligamenta metacarpalia dorsalia** [NA] Short transverse bands connecting the dorsal surfaces of the bases of the second to fifth metacarpal bones to each other. Also *dorsal metacarpal ligaments, dorsal ligaments of bases of metacarpal bones, dorsal intermetacarpal ligaments.* **ligamenta metacarpalia interossea** [NA] Short fibrous bands connecting the apposed surfaces, distal to the articular facets, of the bases of the medial four metacarpal bones. Also *interosseous metacarpal ligaments, interosseous intermetacarpal ligaments, interosseous ligaments of bases of metacarpal bones, metacarpal interosseous ligaments.* **ligamenta metacarpalia palmaria** [NA] Short transverse bands connecting the palmar surfaces of the bases of the second to fifth metacarpal bones to each other. Also *palmar metacarpal ligaments, palmar intermetacarpal ligaments, volar ligaments of bases of metacarpal bones.* **l. metacarpeum transversum profundum** [NA] A series of short fibrous bands connecting the palmar ligaments of the second to fifth metacarpophalangeal joints, forming a continuous transverse band fused proximally to fascia of the interosseous muscles and to digital slips of the palmar aponeurosis and, on the sides of the joints, joining the transverse band of the dorsal digital expansion. Also *deep transverse metacarpal ligament, deep transverse palmar ligament, distal intermetacarpal ligament.* **l. metatarsale transversum profundum** [NA] A series of short fibrous bands connecting the plantar ligaments of the metatarsophalangeal joints, forming a continuous transverse band that fuses with the sheaths of the flexor tendons and receives slips from digital bands of the plantar aponeurosis. Also *deep transverse metatarsal ligament, distal plantar intermetatarsal ligament.* **l. metatarsale transversum superficiale** [NA] Transverse bands in the superficial fascia of the sole of the foot linking the webs of the toes and attached to the skin of the webs. Also *superficial transverse metatarsal ligament.* **ligamenta metatarsalia dorsalia** [NA] Transverse membranous bands connecting the dorsal surfaces of the bases of the four lateral metatarsal bones, strengthening the capsules of the intermetatarsal joints. Also *dorsal metatarsal ligaments, dorsal ligaments of bases of metatarsal bones, proximal posterior intermetatarsal ligaments, dorsal intermetatarsal ligaments.* **ligamenta metatarsalia interossea** [NA] Strong transverse bands connecting the nonarticular parts of the adjacent surfaces of the bases of the lateral four metatarsal bones. Also *interosseous metatarsal ligaments, interosseous ligaments of bases of metatarsal bones, interosseous intermetatarsal ligaments.* **ligamenta metatarsalia plantaria** [NA] Transverse membranous bands connecting the plantar surfaces of the bases of the four lateral metatarsal bones, strengthening the capsules of the intermetatarsal joints. Also *plantar metatarsal ligaments, plantar ligaments of bases of metatarsal bones, plantar intermetatarsal ligaments.* **l. nuchae** [NA] A midline fibroelastic band extending from the external occipital protuberance and crest to the spine of the seventh cervical vertebra, its deep surface being attached to the occipital bone, posterior tubercle of atlas, and the tips of the spines of the cervical vertebrae. It is homologous with the supraspinous and interspinous ligaments with which it is continuous inferiorly. Also *nuchal ligament.* **ligamenta ossiculorum auditus** [NA] Either bands of collagen fibers or vascularized folds of mucous membrane that connect the malleus, incus, and stapes to the walls of the tympanic cavity. Also *ligaments of auditory ossicles.* **l. ovarii proprium** [NA] A fibromuscular cord located between the layers of the broad ligament of the uterus and connecting the uterine, or inferior, extremity of the ovary to the lateral angle of the uterus below and posterior to the attachment of the uterine tube. Also *ovarian ligament, proper ligament of the ovary, ligament of ovary.* **ligamenta palmaria articulationum interphalangealium manus** [NA] Fibrocartilaginous bands anterior to the interphalangeal joints of the hand, similar to, but thinner than, those of the metacarpophalangeal joints. They are joined laterally to the collateral ligaments and are grooved by the flexor tendons. **ligamenta palmaria articulationum metacarpophalangealium** [NA] Thick fibrocartilaginous bands anterior to the metacarpophalangeal joints, firmly attached to the margins of the bases of the phalanges but only united by areolar tissue to the metacarpals, and joined laterally to the collateral ligaments and deep transverse metacarpal ligament. Anteriorly they are grooved by the flexor tendons which are held in the grooves by their fibrous sheaths. Also *palmar ligaments, palmar metacarpophalangeal ligaments.* **l. palpebrale laterale** [NA] A thick fibrous band lying deep to a muscular raphe and fixing the lateral ends of the tarsal plates of the eyelids to a tubercle on the zygomatic bone just within the orbital margin. Also *lateral palpebral ligament.* **l. palpebrale mediale** [NA] A strong fibrous band, formed by a slip from the medial end of each tarsus, that passes medially in front of the lacrimal sac to become attached to the frontal process of the maxilla and its anterior lacrimal crest. Some deep fibers attach to the posterior lacrimal crest of the lacrimal bone. Also *medial palpebral ligament.* **l. patellae** [NA] The flattened continuation of the common tendon of the quadriceps femoris muscle extending from the apex and inferior margins of the patella to the upper part of the tuberosity of the tibia. Its deep surface is fused to the capsule of the knee joint, being separated from the synovial membrane by the infrapatellar pad of fat. Also *patellar ligament.* **l. pectinatum anguli iridocornealis** RETICULUM TRABECULARE SCLERAE. **l. pectineale** [NA] A strong fibrous band extending laterally from the base of the lacunar ligament along the pecten pubis where it fuses with the pectineal fascia and periosteum, as well as with the lateral extensions of the conjoint tendon and adminiculum lineae albae. Also *pectineal ligament, Cooper's ligament, inguinal ligament of Cooper, pectineal ligament of Cooper.* **l. phrenicocolicum** A triangular fold of peritoneum extending from the left colic flexure to the diaphragm opposite the left tenth and eleventh ribs, against which the lower pole of the spleen may rest. Also *phrenicocolic ligament, phrenocolic ligament, costocolic ligament, Hensing's ligament, Hensing's fold, costocolic fold, left phrenicocolic ligament.* **l. pisohamatum** [NA] One of the prolongations of the tendon of insertion of the flexor carpi ulnaris muscle, extending from the pisiform bone to the hook of the hamate bone. Also *pisohamate ligament.* **l. pisometacarpeum** [NA] One of the prolongations of the tendon of insertion of the flexor carpi ulnaris muscle, extending from the pisiform bone to the base of the fifth metacarpal bone. Also *pisometacarpal ligament.* **l. plantare longum** [NA] A long, broad band attached proximally to the inferior surface of calcaneus anterior to the medial and lateral processes of the tuberosity, while distally the deep fibers attach to the plantar surface of the cuboid bone and the superficial fibers attach to the bases of the second through fifth metatarsal bones. Also *long plantar ligament.* **ligamenta plantaria articulationum interphalangealium pedis** [NA] Fibrocartilaginous bands anterior to the interphalangeal joints of the toes, similar to, but thinner than, those of the metatarsophalangeal joints. They are joined laterally to the collateral ligaments and are grooved by the flexor tendons. **ligamenta plantaria articulationum metatarsophalangealium** [NA] Thick fibrous, sometimes fibrocartilaginous, pads on the plantar surfaces of the metatarsophalangeal joints, firmly attached to the margins of the bases of the phalanges, deepening the articular surfaces, but only loosely joined to the metatarsals, and united laterally to the collateral ligaments and the deep transverse metatarsal ligaments. Their plantar aspects are grooved by the flexor tendons which are held in the grooves by their fibrous flexor sheaths. Also *plantar ligaments, Cruveilhier's ligaments, inferior metatarsophalangeal ligaments, glenoid ligaments of Cruveilhier, plantar metatarsophalangeal ligaments.* **l. popliteum arcuatum** [NA] A broad band of fibers attached to the apex of the head of the fibula from which it arches upwards superficial to the popliteus tendon and divides into two bands: one passes medially to blend with the oblique popliteal ligament and attach to the intercondylar area of the tibia, while the other band becomes the short lateral ligament. Also *arcuate popliteal ligament, popliteal arch, arcuate ligament of knee, popliteal arcuate ligament.* **l. popliteum obliquum** [NA] An oblique expansion of the tendon of the semimembranosus muscle near its insertion, extending upwards and laterally to blend with the joint capsule and to attach to the lateral epicondyle of the femur where it unites with the lateral head of the gastrocnemius muscle. Also *oblique popliteal ligament, posterior oblique ligament of knee, Bourgery's ligament, Winslow's ligament.* **l. pterygospinale** [NA] A fibrous band, occasionally replaced by muscle fibers, extending between the posterior margin of the lateral pterygoid lamina and the spine of the sphenoid. Occasionally it ossifies to form a bony foramen through which muscular branches of the mandibular nerve pass. Also *pterygospinal ligament, pterygospinous ligament, ligament of Civinini.* **l. pubicum superius** [NA] A transverse band of yellow fibers above the symphysis pubis extending along the pubic crest on either side as far as the pubic tubercle, and fusing in the midline with the interpubic disk. Also *superior pubic ligament.* **l. pubofemorale** [NA] A triangular band, the base of which is attached to the obturator crest, the iliopubic eminence, and the superior pubic ramus, while distally it unites with the capsule of the hip joint anteriorly and with the deep aspect of the medial band of the iliofemoral ligament. Also *pubofemoral ligament, pubocapsular ligament.* **l. puboprostaticum** [NA] A thickened sheet of endopelvic fascia in the male that extends from the base of the prostate and the neck of the bladder anteriorly to the parietal fascia on the back of the pubis (formerly called ligamentum puboprostaticum medium) and laterally to the arcus tendineus fasciae pelvis (formerly called ligamentum puboprostaticum laterale). It is equivalent to ligamentum pubovesicale in the female. Also *puboprostatic ligament, anterior true ligament of bladder, lateral true ligament of bladder, puborectal ligament.* **l. pubovesicale** [NA] A thickened sheet of endopelvic fascia in the female that extends from the neck of the bladder anteriorly to the parietal fascia on the back of the pubis (formerly called ligamentum pubovesicale medium) and laterally to the arcus tendineus fasciae pelvis (formerly called ligamentum pubovesicale laterale). It is equivalent to ligamentum puboprostaticum in the male. Also *pubovesical ligament, vesicopubic ligament, puborectal ligament, anterior true ligament of bladder.* **l. pulmonale** [NA] A reflected fold of mediastinal pleura extending from the anterior and posterior surfaces of the structures in the root of the lung down along the mediastinal surface of the lung behind the cardiac impression to the diaphragm where it ends in a free falciform border. It helps to hold the lung in position. Also *pulmonary ligament, Teutleben's ligament.* **liga-**

**menta pylori** Thickened longitudinal muscle bands along the anterior and posterior walls of the pyloric antrum, most of the muscle fibers passing deep to end in the pyloric sphincter. *Outmoded.* Also *ligaments of Helvetius, taeniae pylori.* **l. quadratum** [NA] A thin fibrous membrane extending from the distal margin of the radial notch of the ulna to the neck of the radius and closing the synovial membrane over the inferomedial aspect of the proximal radioulnar joint. Also *quadrate ligament, Denucé's ligament, quadrate ligament of Denucé.* **l. radiocarpale dorsale** [NA] A thin fibrous sheet extending over the back of the radiocarpal joint from the posterior margin of the distal end of the radius and the edge of the articular disk to the proximal row of carpal bones and blending with the dorsal intercarpal ligaments. Also *dorsal radiocarpal ligament, dorsal ligament of radiocarpal joint, posterior ligament of radiocarpal joint.* **l. radiocarpale palmare** [NA] A thick membranous band in front of the radiocarpal joint extending from the anterior margin of the styloid process and distal end of the radius to the anterior surfaces of the proximal row of carpal bones, blending with the anterior intercarpal ligaments. Also *palmar radiocarpal ligament, volar radiocarpal ligament, anterior ligament of radiocarpal joint, anterior radiocarpal ligament.* **l. reflexum** [NA] According to some authorities, a poorly developed expansion of the lateral crus of the inguinal ligament, passing medially and upward behind the medial end of the superficial inguinal ring in front of the conjoint tendon, feebly reinforcing the posterior wall of the inguinal canal, and interweaving with like fibers of the opposite side in the linea alba. Others describe it as a poorly developed triangular band of the external oblique aponeurosis of one side that crosses the midline, passing behind the superficial inguinal ring of the opposite side to be attached to the pectineal line. It is seldom independent, usually being fused with the external oblique aponeurosis or with the conjoint tendon. Also *reflex inguinal ligament, Colles ligament, reflex ligament of Gimbernat, reflected ligament, triangular fascia of abdomen, triangular fascia of Quain.* **l. sacrococcygeum anterius** [NA] A series of fibers, considered to be the termination of the anterior longitudinal ligament, extending anterior to the sacrococcygeal joint from the lowest segment of the sacrum to the coccyx. Also anterior sacrococcygeal ligament, ventral sacrococcygeal ligament. **l. sacrococcygeum laterale** [NA] A broad band, similar to an intertransverse ligament, that extends from the lateral inferior margin of the sacrum to the transverse process of the first coccygeal vertebra, forming a foramen for the ventral branch of the fifth sacral nerve. Also *lateral sacrococcygeal ligament, intercornual ligament.* **l. sacrococcygeum posterius profundum** [NA] A fibrous band extending from the dorsal surface of the fifth sacral vertebra to the back of the coccyx, representing the posterior longitudinal ligament with which it may be continuous superiorly. Also *deep dorsal sacrococcygeal ligament.* **l. sacrococcygeum posterius superficiale** [NA] A flat band continuous with the supraspinous ligament and extending downward from the margin of the sacral hiatus to the dorsal surface of the coccyx covering the lower part of the sacral canal. Also *superficial dorsal sacrococcygeal ligament.* **ligamenta sacroiliaca anteriora** [NA] Fibrous thickenings of the anterior and inferior parts of the capsule of the sacroiliac joint, especially strong opposite the arcuate line. Also *anterior sacroiliac ligaments, ventral sacroiliac ligaments.* **ligamenta sacroiliaca dorsalia** [NA] A series of thick fibrous bands posterior to the sacroiliac joint extending from the lateral sacral crest to the tuberosity of the ilium, the iliac crest, and the posterior iliac spines. The direction of different bands is irregular and the series is often divided into an upper, deep group (the short posterior sacroiliac ligament) and the lower, more superficial group (the long posterior sacroiliac ligament) which is continuous with the sacrotuberous ligament. Also *dorsal sacroiliac ligaments.* **ligamenta sacroiliaca interossea** [NA] Short, strong fibrous bands, deep to the posterior sacroiliac ligaments, extending from the iliac tuberosity to the sacral tuberosity just posterior to the auricular surface. Also *interosseous sacroiliac ligaments.* **l. sacrospinale** [NA] A thin triangular fibrous band attached by its apex to the margins and pelvic surface of the ischial spine and by its base to the lateral margin and pelvic surface of the lower part of the sacrum and the coccyx. Also *sacrospinal ligament, sacrospinous ligament, anterior sacrosciatic ligament.* **l. sacrotuberale** [NA] A long, strong, somewhat triangular-shaped fibrous band extending from the posterior superior and inferior iliac spines and the lateral margins and dorsal surfaces of the last three sacral and first two coccygeal vertebrae to the medial margin of the ischial tuberosity and of the ischial ramus. Also *sacrotuberal ligament, sacrotuberous ligament.* **l. serosum** Any fold of a serous membrane, particularly peritoneum, that supports or connects an organ or part and transmits blood vessels and nerves. *Outmoded.* Also *serous ligament.* **l. sphenomandibulare** [NA] A thin fibrous remnant of Meckel's cartilage lying medial to the capsule of the temporomandibular joint and extending from the spine of the sphenoid bone and the area adjacent to the petrotympanic fissure to the lingula and the back of the mylohyoid groove of the mandible. Also *sphenomandibular ligament.* **l. spirale cochleae** [NA] A ridge of thickened and altered periosteum supporting the lateral wall of the cochlear duct and having the basilar membrane attached to it. Also *spiral ligament of cochlea.* **l. splenorenale** [NA] A peritoneal fold, comprising a left layer (parietal layer of greater sac) passing from the abdominal wall to the front of the left kidney, where it meets the right layer (from the lesser sac) from the front of the pancreas, extending to the hilum of the spleen and merging into the gastrophrenic ligament. Also *lienorenal ligament, lienophrenic ligament, phrenicolienal ligament, phrenicosplenic ligament.* **l. sternoclaviculare anterius** [NA] A broad band blending with the anterior surface of the capsule of the sternoclavicular joint and extending from the anterior and superior margins of the medial end of the clavicle to the front of the upper border of the manubrium sterni and the adjacent costal cartilage. Also *anterior sternoclavicular ligament.* **l. sternoclaviculare posterius** [NA] A fibrous band blending with the posterior surface of the capsule of the sternoclavicular joint and extending from the posterior margin of the medial end of the clavicle to the posterior surface of the adjacent upper margin of the manubrium sterni. Also *posterior sternoclavicular ligament.* **l. sternocostale intra-articulare** [NA] An inconstant fibrocartilaginous band connecting the cartilage of the second rib to the fibrocartilage joining the manubrium to the body of the sternum, and dividing the joint into two compartments. Also *intra-articular sternocostal ligament.* **ligamenta sternocostalia radiata** [NA] Thin, triangular bands radiating from the anterior and the posterior surfaces of the medial ends of the costal cartilages of the true ribs to corresponding adjacent surfaces of the sternum. Also *radiate sternocostal ligaments, sternocostal ligaments, radiating fibers of anterior chondrosternal ligaments.* **ligamenta sternopericardiaca** [NA] Two variable bands of dense fibrous tissue fixing the fibrous pericardium to the upper and lower parts of the posterior surface of the sternum. Also *sternopericardiac ligaments, sternopericardial ligaments, ligaments of Luschka.* **l. stylohyoideum** [NA] A slender fibrous cord extending from the tip of the styloid process of the temporal bone to the lesser cornu of the hyoid bone and providing partial origin for the middle constrictor of the pharynx. Also *stylohyoid ligament, epihyal ligament.* **l. stylomandibulare** [NA] A thin process of the deep cervical fascia attached proximally to the tip of the styloid process of the temporal bone and distally to the angle and posterior margin of the ramus of the mandible between the masseter and medial pterygoid muscles. It separates the parotid gland from the submandibular gland. Also *stylomandibular ligament.* **l. supraspinale** A longitudinal band of variable thickness connecting the tips of the spines of the vertebrae and extending from the second cervical vertebra to the median sacral crest where it is continuous with the superficial dorsal sacrococcygeal ligament. Superiorly it is continuous with ligamentum nuchae. Also *supraspinal ligament, supraspinous ligament.* **ligamenta suspensoria mammaria** [NA] The coarse connective tissue strands connecting the glandular tissue of the upper part of the mammary gland to both the dermis of the overlying skin and the underlying pectoral fascia, resembling retinacula cutis. Also *suspensory ligaments of mammary gland, suspensory ligaments of breast, fibrous ligaments of breast, Cooper suspensory ligaments.* **l. suspensorium clitoridis** [NA] A fibrous band connecting the dorsum of the body of the clitoris to the arcuate pubic ligament and symphysis pubis. Also *suspensory ligament of clitoris.* **l. suspensorium ovarii** [NA] The part of the broad ligament of uterus that extends from the tubal end of the ovary and the infundibulum of the uterine tube to the lateral wall of the pelvis, transmitting the ovarian blood vessels, nerves, and lymph vessels. Also *suspensory ligament of ovary, infundibulopelvic ligament, Clado's band.* **l. suspensorium penis** [NA] A triangular fibroelastic band, deep to the fundiform ligament, attached above to the front of symphysis pubis and below to the fascia around the penis. Also *suspensory ligament of penis.* **l. talocalcaneare laterale** [NA] A short band extending downward and posteriorly, from the talus just anteroinferior to the lateral malleolar surface, to the lateral surface of the calcaneus anterior to the attachment of the calcaneofibular ligament. Also *lateral talocalcaneal ligament.* **l. talocalcaneare mediale** [NA] A narrow band extending obliquely downward from the medial tubercle of the talus to the calcaneus behind the sustentaculum tali and blending with the medial ligament of the talocrural joint. Also *medial talocalcaneal ligament.* **l. talocalcaneum anterius** A fibrous band extending from the anterolateral aspect of the neck of the talus to the superior surface of the calcaneus. Also *anterior talocalcaneal ligament.* **l. talocalcaneum interosseum** [NA] A broad band occupying the sinus tarsi and running obliquely and laterally from the roof of sulcus tali to sulcus calcanei. It strengthens the capsules of both the talocalcaneonavicular joint and the subtalar joint. Also *interosseous talocalcaneal ligament.* **l. talocalcaneum posterius** A short band radiating from the lateral tubercle of the talus to the proximal medial aspect of the calcaneus. Also *posterior talocalcaneal ligament.* **l. talofibulare anterius** [NA] A narrow band extending from the anterior margin of the lateral malleolus to the lateral aspect of the talus anterior to the malleolar surface. Also *anterior talofibular ligament.* **l. talofibulare posterius** [NA] A thick horizontal band extending from the posterior border and fossa of the lateral malleolus to the lateral tubercle of the posterior process of the talus. Also *posterior talofibular ligament.* **l. talonaviculare** [NA] A broad, thin band extending from the dorsolateral surface of the neck of the talus to the dorsal surface of the navicular bone. Also *talonavicular ligament, dorsal talonavicular ligament.* **ligamenta tarsi dorsalia** [NA] The ligaments that connect the tarsal bones on their dorsal surfaces, including the talonavicular, intercuneiform, cuneocuboid, cuboideonavicular, and bifurcate ligaments. Also *dorsal ligaments of tarsus, dorsal intertarsal ligaments.* **ligamenta tarsi interossea** [NA] The ligaments connecting the adjoining surfaces of the tarsal bones, including the interosseous cuneocuboid, talocalcaneal, and intercuneiform ligaments. Also *interosseous ligaments of tarsus, interosseous intertarsal ligaments.* **ligamenta tarsi plantaria** [NA] The ligaments that bind the tarsal bones on their plantar surfaces, including the long plantar, calcaneocuboid, calcaneonavicular, cuneonavicular, cuboideonavicular, cuneocuboid, and intercuneiform ligaments. Also *plantar ligaments of tarsus, plantar intertarsal ligaments.* **ligamenta tarsometatarsalia dorsalia** [NA] Short fibrous bundles extending distally from the cuboid and the three cuneiform bones to the bases of the metatarsal bones on their dorsal surfaces. Also *dorsal tarsometatarsal ligaments, bigeminate ligaments of Arnold.* **ligamenta tarsometatarsalia plantaria** [NA] Longitudinal and oblique bands binding the plantar surfaces of the cuboid and the three cuneiform bones to the bases of the metatarsal bones. Also *plantar tarsometatarsal ligaments.* **l. teres hepatis** [NA] A fibrous cord, the remnant of the obliterated umbilical vein, extending from the umbilicus to the anterior border of the liver in the free margin of the falciform ligament and ending in the left branch of the portal vein at the left side of the porta hepatis. Also *round ligament of liver.* **l. teres uteri** [NA] A narrow fibrous band attached proximally to the lateral angle of the uterus on each side, passing between the two layers of the broad ligament anteroinferior to the uterine tube to enter the deep inguinal ring and leave the inguinal canal through the superficial ring, ending in the labium majus by becoming continuous with the connective tissue. Near the uterus it also contains muscle fibers. It is homologous with part of the gubernaculum testis. Also *round ligament of uterus, Hunter's ligament.* **l. testis** A ligament in the embryo developing within the caudal genital ridge to form the cranial portion of the gubernaculum. **l. thyroepiglotticum** [NA] An elastic band firmly connecting the stalk, or petiole, of the lower end of the epiglottis to the back of the thyroid cartilage in the midline just below the superior notch. Also *thyroepiglottic ligament.* **l. thyrohyoideum laterale** [NA] The elastic, cordlike posterior edge of the thyrohyoid membrane extending from the superior cornu of the thyroid cartilage to the greater cornu of the hyoid bone. Also *lateral thyrohyoid ligament, Berry's ligament, thyrohyoid ligament.* **l. thyrohyoideum medianum** [NA] The median elastic thickening of the thyrohyoid membrane extending upward behind the body of the hyoid bone from the superior notch of the thyroid cartilage to the superior margin of the hyoid bone, a bursa interposing between the latter and the band. Also *median thyrohyoid ligament, middle thyrohyoid ligament.* **l. tibiofibulare anterius** [NA] A strong triangular band in front of the tibiofibular syndesmosis extending downward and laterally from the distal end of the tibia at the anterior margin of the fibular notch to the adjacent margin of the lateral malleolus. Also *anterior tibiofibular ligament.* **l. tibiofibulare posterius** [NA] A fibrous band situated diagonally behind the tibiofibular syndesmosis and extending from the posterior margin of the fibular notch at the distal end of the tibia to the adjacent posterior margin of the lateral malleolus. Also *posterior tibiofibular ligament.* **l. transversum acetabuli** [NA] A fibrous band of decussating fibers spanning the acetabular notch, converting it into a foramen, and attached to the margin of the acetabulum on each side of the notch and continuous with the acetabular labrum. It is also attached to the ligament of the head of femur and the capsule of the hip joint. Also *transverse ligament of acetabulum.* **l. transversum atlantis** [NA] A powerful, thick fibrous band, attached at each end to a tubercle on the medial surface of the lateral mass of the atlas, converting the ring of the atlas into a small anterior portion for the dens of the axis with which it articulates and a larger posterior portion for the spinal cord and its membranes. It forms the horizontal bar of the cruciform ligament of the atlas. Also *transverse ligament of atlas.* **l. transversum genus** [NA] A fibrous cord of variable thickness connecting the anterior convex margin of the lateral meniscus of the knee joint to the anterior extremity of the medial meniscus. It is occasionally absent. Also *transverse ligament of knee, common ligament of knee of Weber.* **l. transversum perinei** [NA] A thickening at the line of fusion of the anterior margin of the perineal membrane and the endopelvic fascia deep to it, extending transversely between the inferior pubic rami and lying below the dorsal vein and nerves of penis or clitoris. Also *transverse perineal ligament, transverse pelvic ligament, Krause's ligament, transverse ligament of plevis, preurethral ligament of Waldeyer.* **l. transversum scapulae inferius** [NA] A thin membranous band extending, when present, from the lateral margin of the spine of the scapula to the margin of the glenoid cavity. Also *inferior transverse ligament of scapula, spinoglenoid ligament.* **l. transversum scapulae superius** [NA] A fibrous band bridging the scapular notch, converting it into a foramen for the suprascapular nerve and extending from the lateral end of the superior margin to the base of the coracoid process. Also *superior transverse ligament of scapula, suprascapular ligament.* **l. trapezoideum** [NA] The broad anterolateral part of the coracoclavicular ligament, extending from a ridge on the medial margin of the coracoid process to an oblique ridge running anterolaterally from the conoid tubercle on the inferior surface of the lateral end of the clavicle. It is separated from the conoid ligament by fat or a bursa. It limits anterior movement of the scapula. Also *trapezoid ligament.* **l. triangulare dextrum hepatis** [NA] A triangular fold of peritoneum connecting the right lobe at the apex of the bare area of the liver to the diaphragm and formed by the fusion of the superior and the inferior layers of the coronary ligament. Also *right triangular ligament of liver.* **l. triangulare sinistrum hepatis** [NA] A long fold of peritoneum connecting the superior surface of the left lobe of the liver to the diaphragm, its anterior layer being continuous with the left layer of the falciform ligament while the posterior layer continues as the anterior layer of the lesser omentum. The two layers are in close contact and become continuous with each other at the left free border. Also *left triangular ligament of liver.* **l. ulnocarpale palmare** [NA] A rounded fibrous bundle extending from the styloid process of the ulna and the front of the articular disk to the palmar surfaces of the carpal bones, particularly the lunate and triquetrum. Also *palmar ulnocarpal ligament.* **l. umbilicale mediale** [NA] A fibrous cord, the remnant of the obliterated umbilical artery beyond the origin of the superior vesical artery from the internal iliac artery, lying within a fold of peritoneum, the medial umbilical fold, extending from the pelvis along the lateral wall of the bladder and the posterior surface of the anterior abdominal wall to the umbilicus. Also *medial umbilical ligament, obliterated hypogastric artery.* **l. umbilicale medianum** [NA] The fibrous remnant of the urachus between the apex of the bladder and the umbilicus that raises up a fold of peritoneum, the median umbilical fold, on the posterior surface of the anterior abdominal wall. Also *median umbilical ligament, middle umbilical ligament, vesicoumbilical ligament.* **l. vaginale** *Outmoded* RUDIMENT OF VAGINAL PROCESS. **l. venosum** [NA] The fibrous remnant of the obliterated ductus venosus connecting the left branch of the portal vein to the inferior vena cava or the left hepatic vein and occupying a fissure on the posterior aspect of the liver. Also *venous ligament of liver, Arantius ligament, ligament of ductus venosus.* **l. vestibulare** [NA] A narrow fibrous band within the vestibular fold and extending posteriorly from the angle of the thyroid cartilage to the anterolateral surface of the arytenoid cartilage just above the vocal process. Also *vestibular ligament, ventricular ligament of larynx.* **l. vocale** [NA] The thickened free upper edge of the lateral part of the cricothyroid ligament, extending from the thyroid angle to the tip of the vocal process of the arytenoid cartilage, and lying alongside the vocalis muscle within the vocal fold. It is composed of yellow elastic tissue. Also *vocal ligament.*

**ligand** \lig′ənd, lī′gənd\ [L *ligand(us)*, gerundive of *ligare* to bind] Any one of several molecules or ions, identical or different, that bind to the same central entity. For example, the nitrogen atoms and the oxygen molecule bind to the iron of hemoglobin. The hydrogen ions that bind to the same protein molecule are another example. **cell l.'s** Molecules associated with cell surfaces which interact and link the cells together. Ligands are found on surfaces of embryonic cells and are responsible for the adhesiveness of specific cells.

**ligase** \lī′gās\ SYNTHETASE.

**ligate** \lī′gāt\ [L *ligat(us)*, past part. of *ligare* to bind, tie] **1** To tie or compress with a suture, as a vessel or other tissue. **2** To bind together, as one molecule (the ligand), which is considered peripheral, to another (such as a metal ion or a protein) which is considered central.

**ligation** \līgā′shən\ [L *ligatio* (from *ligare* to bind, tie) a binding, tying] A surgical procedure in which a suture is placed around a tissue, usually a vessel, in order to tie off or obliterate the lumen. **immediate l.** A surgical procedure in which a ligature is tied directly on a vessel without incorporating any surrounding tissue. . *Outmoded.* **mediate l.** A surgical procedure in which a ligature is tied around a vessel along with a small amount of surrounding tissue. *Obs.* **proximal l.** A surgical procedure in which a suture is used to tie off or obliterate the proximal or near end of a vessel, duct, or other hollow organ; ligature of the upstream end of a vessel or duct. **quadruple l.** A method for controlling an arteriovenous fistula by which the two arterial and two venous components of the fistula are ligated. It is a less favored approach, because distal perfusion is dependent upon collateral flow around the operative site. **saphenous l.** A surgical procedure in which one or more sutures are passed around the saphenous vein, usually at the saphenofemoral junction, as a treatment for venous incompetence of the leg. **surgical l.** The fixing of a ligature around the neck of an unerupted tooth so that tractioncan be applied to it. **tooth l.** The tying together of two or more teeth with fine wire or thread either for splinting or for orthodontic movement. **tubal l.** A surgical procedure in which one or both fallopian tubes are tied and cut or crushed for the purpose of sterilization.

**ligator** \lī′gātər\ [*ligat(e)* + -OR] A surgical instrument used to facilitate the ligation of deep, small, and otherwise inaccessible structures.

**ligature** \lig′əchər\ [L *ligatura* (from *ligatus*, past part. of *ligare* to bind + *-ura* -URE) a band, tie] A suture that is tied around a tissue or vessel in order to obliterate the lumen. It may be made of any naturally occurring or synthetic material. **double l.** A pair of ligatures tied around the same structure, usually in close approximation, to ensure against leakage. **grass-line l.** A ligature, used in tooth ligation, which has the property of shrinking when wetted and so tightening. **l. in continuity** Placement and tying of ligatures on tissue prior to incising between the ligatures. **interlocking l.** A ligature in which the loops of successive stitches interlock. Also *interlacing ligature*. **occluding l.** A suture that is tied about a vessel to obliterate the blood flow distally. **Stannius l.** A thread tied around the heart of cold-blooded animals either at the sinoatrial junction (first Stannius ligature) or in the atrioventricular groove (second Stannius ligature). It is used in experiments demonstrating the different degrees of inherent rhythmicity in sinus, atrial, and ventricular tissues.

**light** [Old English *lēoht*, akin to L *lux* daylight, light, brightness and to Gk *leukos* bright, white] **1** Electromagnetic radiation to which the human eye is sensitive, comprising the wavelength range from 400 to 700 nm. Both limits are poorly defined. **2** Electromagnetic radiation with wavelengths outside the visible limits, but excited by similar means. The portion with wavelengths longer than the visible is called infrared light, that with shorter, ultraviolet. **actinic l.** Sunlight capable of producing chemical changes in the skin. **l. chaos** INTRINSIC LIGHT. **coherent l.** Light from a laser, which has a single frequency, whose waves are in phase in space and time, and which travels in intense parallel beams with very small divergence. **idioretinal l.** INTRINSIC LIGHT. **intrinsic l.** The variable phosphenes spontaneously seen in darkness. Also *idioretinal light, light chaos*. **Simpson l.** SIMPSON LAMP. **Wood's l.** Ultraviolet light produced by Wood's lamp, used to detect the presence of certain microbial agents in the hair, especially of children. See also WOOD'S LAMP.

**lightening** The descent of the fetus deeper into the pelvis, resulting in a decrease in the fundal height. Lightening occurs a few days or weeks before labor, due to physiologic changes of the uterus.

**Lightwood** [Reginald *Lightwood*, English pediatrician, flourished 20th century] See under SYNDROME.

**Lignac** [Georges Otto Emile *Lignac*, Dutch pediatrician, 1891–1954] Lignac's disease, Lignac-Fanconi syndrome. See under CYSTINOSIS.

**lignocaine** LIDOCAINE.

**ligula** \lig′yələ\ [L (variant of *lingula*, dim. of *lingua* tongue), a little tongue or strap] A narrow band of white matter in the brainstem connecting the nucleus gracilis to the inferior cerebellar peduncle and closely related to the most lateral part of the floor of the fourth ventricle. Also *ligule*.

***Limax*** \lī′maks\ [L, a slug, snail] A genus of common shell-less gastropods or land slugs in the family Limacidae which serve as the intermediate hosts for various helminth parasites, such as the nematode *Angiostrongylus*. Several species have become established in the United States, and are now widespread garden pests, for example, *L. maximus* and *L. flavus*.

**limb** [Old English *lim*] **1** An arm, leg, or appendage projecting from the trunk of a body; membrum. **2** Any of various internal anatomical structures resembling or suggestive of such an appendage; crus. **3** A segment, defined by its slope or orientation, of a linear structure or graph. **anacrotic l.** The ascending limb of the arterial pressure pulse wave. **aneurogenic l.** A limb bud of an early embryo into which no nerve has yet grown. When a limb bud appears, the nerves of the segments opposite to where it is formed grow out into its mesenchyme to innervate muscles and the skin segments forming the limb. **anterior l. of internal capsule** The most anterior part of the internal capsule, separating the head of the caudate nucleus from the lentiform nucleus. **anterior l. of stapes** CRUS ANTERIUS STAPEDIS. **l.'s of anthelix** CRURA ANTHELICIS. **ascending l.** See under LOOP OF HENLE. **catacrotic l.** The descending limb of the arterial pressure pulse wave. **descending l.** See under LOOP OF HENLE. **inferior l.** MEMBRUM INFERIUS. **long l. of incus** CRUS LONGUM INCUDIS. **lower l.** MEMBRUM INFERIUS. **pelvic l.** MEMBRUM INFERIUS. **phantom l.** The perception by an amputee of sensations, often interpreted as pain, that appear to issue from a limb when in fact the limb has been amputated. It is a neurologic phenomenon originating in the transected peripheral nerve endings. Also *stump hallucination, pseudomelia*. **posterior l. of internal capsule** The most posterior part of the internal capsule lying lateral to the thalamus and lentiform nucleus. **posterior l. of stapes** CRUS POSTERIUS STAPEDIS. **short l. of incus** CRUS BREVE INCUDIS. **superior l.** MEMBRUM SUPERIUS. **thick ascending l.** The ascending limb of a Henle's loop of a subcapsular nephron, which is much shorter and thicker than that of a juxtaglomerular nephron. It forms the U-turn and the descending limb may be thin and very short. Such a loop only extends into the outer part of the medulla and produces the zonation of the medulla. **thick descending l.** A descending limb of Henle's loop which develops thick squamous cells in a short loop from a subcapsular nephron. **thick l. of the loop of Henle** See under THICK ASCENDING LIMB. **thin l. of the loop of Henle** The descending limb of a loop of Henle. See under LOOP OF HENLE. **thoracic l.** MEMBRUM SUPERIUS. **upper l.** MEMBRUM SUPERIUS.

**limbal** \lim′bəl\ Pertaining to a limbus, especially the limbus corneae of the eye.

**limbi** \lim′bī\ Plural of LIMBUS.

**limbic** \lim′bik\ **1** Denoting a limbus. **2** In the brain, denoting anatomically the limbic lobe (of P. Broca) constituting the cerebral cortex forming the hilus of each hemisphere.

**limbous** \lim′bəs\ Overlapping.

**limbus** \lim′bəs\ [L, the hem, welt, border of a garment] (*pl.* limbi) An edge, border, or fringe. Adj. limbal, limbic. **l. chorioideus** The infolded part of the ependyma in the developing medial wall of the archipallium. Between the infolded lips of this double-layered ependymal fold vascular mesodermal tissue grows to form the choroid plexus of the lateral ventricle. *Outmoded.* **l. corneae** [NA] The line of junction between the cornea and the sclera which is marked on the surface of the eyeball by the sulcus sclerae. It also marks the junction of the cornea and the conjunctiva. Also *limbus of cornea, sclerocorneal junction.* **l. corticalis** A region of the medial wall of the developing telencephalon covered by a layer of cortical cells that eventually forms the subiculum, dentate gyrus, induseum griseum, and striae Lancisii. *Outmoded.* **l. fossae ovalis** [NA] The well-marked crescentic edge of the fossa ovalis on the interatrial septum in the right atrium of the heart, representing the margin of the septum secundum of the embryonic heart. Its anterior part is continuous with the valve of the inferior vena cava. Also *annulus ovalis, Vieussens annulus, border of oval fossa, limbus of Vieussens, isthmus of Vieussens, ring of Vieussens.* **l. laminae spiralis osseae** [NA] Thickened periosteum on the upper plate of the osseous spiral lamina, projecting into the duct of the cochlea and ending laterally as the sulcus spiralis internus. Also *zona cartilaginea*. **l. medullaris** That part of the developing medial wall of the telencephalon that is not covered by cortical cells and eventually develops into the fimbria hippocampi. *Outmoded.* **l. membranae tympani** The thickened margin of the tympanic membrane attached by the annulus fibrocartilagineus to the tympanic sulcus of the temporal bone. **limbi palpebrales anteriores** [NA] The rounded anterior edges of the free margin of the upper and lower eyelids. They bear the eyelashes, or cilia. **limbi palpebrales posteriores** [NA] The sharp posterior edges of the free margin of the upper and lower eyelids. They rest on the surface of the eyeball and mark the junction of the skin and palpebral conjunctiva. Along them are the single rows of minute openings of the tarsal glands. **l. of the sphenoid bone** The sharp anterior edge of the sulcus prechiasmaticus on the superior surface of the body of the sphenoid bone. Also *limbus sphenoidalis*. **l. of Vieussens** LIMBUS FOSSAE OVALIS.

**lime** [Old English *līm* cement, birdlime, akin to L *limus* mud, slime] Either calcium oxide or calcium hydroxide. **slaked l.** CALCIUM HYDROXIDE.

**limen** \lī′mən\ [L (akin to *limes* a limit, boundary), a threshold, lintel, entrance] A threshold or boundary. **difference l.** DIFFERENCE THRESHOLD. **l. insulae** [NA] The zone of junction, on the inferior surface of the cerebral hemisphere, between the cortex of the insula and that of the frontal lobe. Also *gyrus of Retzius*. **l. nasi** [NA] A curved ridge demarcating the junction of the skin of the vestibule and the mucous membrane of the nasal cavity proper. It corresponds to the superior margin of the lower nasal cartilage. Also *threshold of nose*.

**limes zero** The largest amount of toxin which, when mixed with one standard unit of the corresponding antitoxin and administered by subcutaneous injection to a 250-gram guinea pig, will produce no observable reaction. Also *limes nul dose*. Symbol: $L_0$

**limina** \lim′inə\ Plural of LIMEN.

**liminal** \lim′inəl\ [L *limen*, gen. *liminis*, threshold + -AL] Pertaining to the threshold of sensation.

**liminometer** \lim′inäm′ətər\ [L *limen*, gen. *liminis*, threshold + *o* + -METER] An instrument capable of measuring the intensity of a stimulus applied to a tendon in order to evoke a reflex as well as the threshold intensity which will just evoke a reflex.

**limit** [L *limes*, gen. *limitis* boundary path, boundary] A value or condition regarded as an end point or boundary. **Anstie's l.** The amount of absolute alcohol that may be taken without injury, as interpreted by the life insurance industry. This is equivalent to about 1.5 oz per day for adults, or approximately 3 oz per day of whiskey, brandy, rum, or gin. Also *Anstie's rule*. **elastic l.** The greatest degree to which a pliable material may be stretched without impairing its ability to return to its original dimensions. **emergency exposure l.** The maximum concentration of a highly dangerous toxic material to which a volunteer can be exposed following a disaster or accident, on the assumption that any health impairment incurred would be reversible and that the possibility of such impairment would be justifiable on the grounds of saving human life. **exposure l.** The airborne concentration of a dust, gas, or fume in the workplace to which an individual may be safely exposed for a specified period of time. Exposure limits vary in the degree of protection offered. **quantum l.** MINIMUM WAVELENGTH.

**limophthisis** Wasting due to a diminished food intake fasting.

**limosis** [Gk *limo(s)* hunger, famine + -SIS] An abnormally large appetite.

**limotherapy** [Gk *limo(s)* hunger, want of food + THERAPY] The treatment of disease by restricting food intake. It is used in obesity to force the body to metabolize some of its own adipose tissue. At one time it was used in cancer treatment as it was believed that deprivation of food led to starvation of the tumor. This belief has now dissappeared from modern medical practice.

**limp** [Middle English *lympen*, from Old English *limpan* to happen] An abnormality of gait such that full weight bearing is not applied to one of the lower extremities; commonly, a type of walking produced by pain or sensitivity in the leg or foot.

***Limulus*** \lim′yələs\ A genus of arthropods of the class Merostomata; the horseshoe crab. Amebocytes from the organism are used in a highly sensitive test for endotoxin.

**lincomycin** $C_{18}H_{34}N_2O_6S$. An antibiotic from a variant strain of *Streptomyces lincolnensis*. It acts primarily on Gram-positive bacteria.

**lincomycin hydrochloride** $C_{18}H_{34}N_2O_6S{\cdot}HCl{\cdot}H_2O$. The monohydrate, monohydrochloride salt of lincomycin. It is used as an antibiotic against susceptible strains of streptococci, pneumococci, and staphylococci. It can be administered intramuscularly and intravenously.

**lincture** ELECTUARY.

**linctus** ELECTUARY.

**lindane** \lin′dān\ $C_6H_6Cl_6$. The gamma isomer of hexachlorocyclohexane. A white, crystalline powder with a slightly musty odor, widely used as an insecticide. Serious poisoning and fatalities have occurred from its improper use. It acts as a systemic poison, causing lassitude, headache, limb pains, intestinal colic, and diarrhea. Convulsions and other disorders of the central nervous system may follow. Also *gammexane, gamma benzene hexachloride*.

**Lindbergh** [Charles Augustus *Lindbergh*, U.S. aviator, 1902–1974] **1** Carrel-Lindbergh pump. See under PUMP. **2** Lindbergh pump. See under PUMP.

**Lindemann** [August *Lindemann*, German surgeon, born 1880] See under METHOD.

**Lindner** [Karl David *Lindner*, Austrian ophthalmologist, 1883–1961] Lindner's initial bodies. See under MIYAGAWA BODIES.

**Lindqvist** [Johan Torsten *Lindqvist*, Swedish physician, born 1906] Fahraeus-Lindqvist effect. See under EFFECT.

# line

**line** [L *linea*. See LINEA.] **1** A connection between two points or a boundary between two areas. **2** A long thin mark, ridge, or crease on the surface of a structure; linea. **3** A strain of organisms, cells, or other living material descended from the same ancestor or precursor. **accretion l.'s** INCREMENTAL LINES. **ala-tragal l.** CAMPER'S LINE. **Amberg's l.** A line bisecting the angle between the anterior margin of the mastoid process and the temporal line. It indicates the location of the transverse sinus for certain surgical procedures. Also *lateral sinus line*. **anocutaneous l.** The line of junction of the perianal skin and the stratified squamous epithelium of the lower part of the anal canal, a level where the hair follicles cease. Also *linea anocutanea*. See also PECTINATE LINE. **anorectal l.**

LINEA ANORECTALIS. **anterior axillary l.** LINEA AXILLARIS ANTERIOR. **anterior gluteal l.** LINEA GLUTEA ANTERIOR. **anterior median l.** LINEA MEDIANA ANTERIOR. **arcuate l. of ilium** LINEA ARCUATA OSSIS ILII. **arcuate l. of innominate bone** LINEA ARCUATA OSSIS ILII. **arcuate l. of pelvis** LINEA TERMINALIS PELVIS. **arcuate l. of sheath of rectus abdominus muscle** LINEA ARCUATA VAGINAE MUSCULI RECTI ABDOMINIS. **Arlt's l.** A horizontal scar of the upper palpebral conjunctiva that is almost pathognomic of chronic trachoma. **auriculobregmatic l.** A line extending from the auricular point to the bregma. **axial l.'s** In the limbs, the dorsal and ventral lines that represent contact between nonconsecutive dermatome areas. **Baillarger's l.'s** Two myelinated, horizontal laminae visible in vertical sections through the cerebral cortex as pale bands running parallel to the pial surface and composed of an inner and an outer band. They lie in the fifth and fourth cortical layers, respectively, and apparently reflect the profusion of corticipetal arborizations in these areas. These laminar bands vary in conspicuousness in different cortical areas. In the area striata of visual cortex, the outer band (Gennari's band) is unusually prominent. In agranular cortex, both lines are usually absent. Also *Baillarger's bands, Baillarger stripes, Baillarger striations, striae of Baillarger, interradial plexus.* **base l.** A line connecting the orbitale and the superior border of the external auditory meatus and extending to the median line of the occipital bone. It is used as the basis of the Frankfort horizontal plane in craniometric studies, and approximates the base of the skull. Also *Reid's base line, Reid's baseline.* **base-apex l.** A line that is perpendicular to the base of a prism and bisects the prism's refracting angle. **basinasal l.** A line joining basion to nasion. Also *nasobasilar line.* **basiobregmatic l.** A line joining basion to bregma, used in craniometry to measure the height of the cranium. **Baudelocque's l.** EXTERNAL CONJUGATE. **Beau's l.'s** Superficial transverse depressions in the nail plates that appear several weeks after an acute illness. **biauricular l.** A line connecting the two external auditory meatuses across the vertex of the skull. **bi-iliac l.** A line joining the widest points between the two iliac crests. **bismuth l.** A black line at the gingival margin caused by the deposition of bismuth sulfide from the ingestion of bismuth salts and their reaction with sulfur-containing products of dental plaque. **blue l.** LEAD LINE. **Borsieri's l.** A white line that quickly turns red, produced by drawing the finger across the skin: supposedly an early sign of scarlet fever. Also *Borsieri sign.* **Brödel's l.** A longitudinal line just posterior to the outer convex border of the kidney, considered to be a bloodless zone between the areas of distribution of the anterior and the posterior branches of the renal artery. However, in fact, the areas supplied by the vessels overlap and the linear zone is only relatively avascular. **Brödel's white l.** A longitudinal pale zone located along the anterior aspect of the outer convex border of the kidney. **Bryant's l.** A horizontal line drawn, with the subject in the supine position, from the greater trochanter of the femur to a vertical line, which it meets at right angles, from the anterior superior iliac spine to the table underneath the person. It is the base of Bryant's triangle. **Burton's l.** BURTON SIGN. **calcification l.'s** INCREMENTAL LINES. **Camper's l.** A line drawn from the base of the anterior nasal spine, or subnasale, to the upper border of the tragus of the ear, or tragion. Also *ala-tragal line, Camper's plane.* **cell l.** A population of cells established as a primary culture and propagated in tissue culture. **cement l.** In bony tissue, a line of reversal of bone growth. It marks the junction between adjacent osteons. The increased basophilia of the line is due to a high inorganic matrix content. **Chamberlain's l.** A line drawn on a lateral radiograph of the skull joining the posterior end of the hard palate to the posterior margin of the foramen magnum. In the normal individual the odontoid process of the axis should not extend above this line. **chorionic plate l.** The dense ultrasound echo line between the placental echo pattern and the uterine cavity along the placental border. **cleavage l.'s** Fine linear clefts in the skin, produced by the parallel bundles of connective tissue in the reticular layer, along which the skin more easily splits especially when incised. The direction of the bundles varies in different parts of the body, generally paralleling lines of tension and compression due to ordinary movements. Also *Langer's lines, tension lines.* **Conradi's l.** A line drawn between the base of the xiphisternum and the apex of the heart, to indicate the normal upper margin of the left lobe of the liver. **contour l.'s** LINES OF OWEN. **costophrenic septal l.'s** Fine horizontal lines seen mainly in the costophrenic region on the chest radiograph in pulmonary edema and several other conditions. **Crampton's l.** A line of incision drawn from the tip of the twelfth costal cartilage to a point just above the iliac crest and then anteriorly to a point just inferomedial to the anterior superior iliac spine. It is used for an extraperitoneal approach to ligate the common iliac artery. **Czermak's l.'s** Lines visible in histologic sections of dentin produced by rows of interglobular spaces. **l. of demarcation** An ill-defined, irregular line that separates infarcted or gangrenous tissue from healthy tissue. The line becomes more distinct with time as granulation tissue develops. Also *surface demarcation.* **dentate l.** PECTINATE LINE. **developmental l.** DEVELOPMENTAL GROOVE. **l. of Douglas** LINEA ARCUATA VAGINAE MUSCULI RECTI ABDOMINIS. **Duhot's l.** A line connecting the anterior superior iliac spine to the apex of the sacrum. **ectental l.** The line of junction between ectoderm and entoderm. **Egger's l.** The circular attachment of the hyaloideocapsular ligament to the posterior periphery of the crystalline lens capsule. **epiphyseal l.** 1 LINEA EPIPHYSIALIS. 2 A radiolucent line seen on a radiograph at the growing end of the diaphysis of a long bone representing a zone of cartilage next to a layer of new bone of the metaphysis. **external oblique l.** A ridge on the lateral surface of the mandible which extends downwards and forwards from the anterior edge of the coronoid process and becomes indistinct in the region of the first permanent molar tooth. **Farre's white l.** A pale straight line along the mesovarian border of the ovary where the mesovarium meets the germinal epithelium of the ovary. **Feiss l.** A line drawn from the distal tip of the medial malleolus to the plantar aspect of the first metatarsophalangeal joint. **finish l.** The line made by the meeting of a bevel with the surface of the tooth. It indicates the margin of a restoration to the technician making a wax pattern. **fissural l.** A fine linear density seen on a chest x ray representing the pleura seen tangentially within the fissures separating pulmonary lobes. It is usually made up of two layers of pleura. **l. of fixation** An imaginary line from the fovea to the object of regard. **Fleischner l.** Linear density seen on a chest x ray representing atelectasis of a small area of lung. It is usually associated with decreased diaphragmatic motion, thoracic trauma, subphrenic disease, or pulmonary embolus, but can be seen also in normal people with high diaphragms. Also *platelike atelectasis, discoid atelectasis.* **flexure l.** Any one of several furrows in the skin produced by folds in the dermis resulting from compression by constant joint movements, and indicative of planes of anchorage to the underlying deep fascia. During joint movements the skin on each side of a line is folded passively, making the line more prominent. These lines are conspicuous anterior to the wrist joint, on the palms, the soles, and the digits. In the palm there are usually two curved horizontal and at least two longitudinal lines. Also *skin joint, flexion crease.* **Fränkel's l.** WHITE LINE OF FRÄNKEL. **fulcrum l.** One of the hypothetical lines about which a partial denture tends to rotate during mastication. The principle fulcrum lines are vertical, horizontal fore and aft, and horizontal cross-arch. **Gant's l.** A demarcation on the proximal femoral shaft just below the greater trochanter. It serves as a landmark during surgical exploration. **l. of Gennari** GENNARI'S BAND. **germ l.** 1 In an individual, all cells derived from the embryonic cells that have the potential for forming gametes. 2 In a species, the linkage of related individuals through germ cells. Also *germ track.* **Gottinger's l.** A line parallel to the superior margin of the zygomatic arch. **Granger l.** A curved line on a specially angled posteroanterior roentgenogram of the skull, representing the superior surface of the sphenoid bone. It is used to localize and demonstrate the optic groove. **growth arrest l.** A metaphyseal transverse line of increased radiodensity that is seen on radiography of a long bone. It represents a zone of increased calcification resulting usually from growth arrest due to malnutrition or disease. Also *Harris line.* **Haller's l.** *Obs.* FISSURA MEDIANA ANTERIOR MEDULLAE SPINALIS. **Harris l.** GROWTH ARREST LINE. **health l.** *Popular* MUCOGINGIVAL JUNCTION. **highest nuchal l.** LINEA NUCHAE SUPREMA. **Hilton's white l.** The mucocutaneous junction between the upper border of the stratified squamous epithelium of the anal canal and the stratified columnar or cuboidal epithelium, slightly below the pectinate line. Common clinical usage, however, equates this with the pectinate line, that is, the clinical anorectal junction. Some consider this line to lie at the level of an intermuscular septum between the internal sphincter and the subcutaneous part of the external sphincter of the anus. See also PECTINATE LINE. **Holden's l.** A flexure line in the inguinal region between the anterior superior iliac spine and the greater trochanter of the femur, crossing the position of the capsule of the hip joint. **Hudson-Stähli l.** A linear, subepithelial corneal deposit of hemosiderin, occurring as a normal aging process. Also *Hudson's line, pigmented line of the cornea, Stähli's pigment line.* **Hueter's l.** The line drawn between the medial epicondyle of the humerus and the top of the olecranon when the elbow is extended. **Hunter's l.** LINEA ALBA. **iliopectineal l.** 1 The posterior continuation of pecten pubis as far as the iliopubic eminence or beyond, being part of the terminal line. Also *linea iliopectinea* (outmoded). 2 LINEA ARCUATA OSSIS ILII. **imbrication l.'s** See under PICKERILL'S IMBRICATION LINES. **incremental l.'s** The lines visible in histologic sections of teeth and bone which reflect the rhythmic formation of mineralized tissues. Also *accretion lines, calcification lines, recessional lines.* **inferior gluteal l.** LINEA GLUTEA INFERIOR. **inferior nuchal l.** LINEA NUCHAE INFERIOR. **inferior temporal l. of parietal bone** LINEA TEMPORALIS INFERIOR OSSIS PARIETALIS. **inflating l.** A tube used to inflate a pilot balloon on a tracheal or tracheostomy tube. **infracostal l.** SUBCOSTAL LINE. **infrascapular l.** A line drawn horizontally through the tips of the inferior angles of the two scapulae. **intercondylar l.** LINEA INTERCONDYLARIS FEMORIS. **intercondyloid l.** LINEA INTERCONDYLARIS FEMORIS. **intermediate l. of iliac crest** LINEA INTERMEDIA CRISTAE ILIACAE. **interspinal l.** A line drawn across the abdomen between the two anterior superior iliac spines, to help demarcate the interspinal plane. Also *Lanz line.* **intertrochanteric l.** LINEA INTERTROCHANTERICA. **intertubercular l.** A line drawn across the surface of the abdomen between the tubercles of the iliac crests, helping to demarcate the transtubercular plane. **isoeffect l.'s** In radiotherapy, lines on a chart showing the location of doses producing equal effects on the tissues. **isoelectric l.** BASELINE. **l. of Kaes** *Outmoded* BEKHTEREV'S LAYER. **Kerley's l.'s** Thin linear soft-tissue densities, a few centimeters long, of the lungs, seen on roentgenograms of the chest and thought to represent thickened interlobular septa. Kerley's B lines are located peripherally, especially at the costophrenic sulci, often arranged horizontally in stepladder fashion. Kerley's A lines are located centrally and run obliquely. Kerley's C lines are tiny lacelike densities in the midzones of the lungs. Kerley's lines are seen with interstitial pulmonary edema and pulmonary fibrosis. **Kilian's l.** A transverse line through the promontory of the sacrum. **Krause l.** Z BAND. **Langer's l.'s** CLEAVAGE LINES. **Lanz l.** INTERSPINAL LINE. **lateral l.** LINEA MEDIOCLAVICULARIS. **lateral sinus l.** AMBERG'S LINE. **lateral sternal l.** LINEA STERNALIS. **lead l.** A blue or blue-black pigmentation within the marginal gingiva caused by lead intoxication. It is found around teeth with heavy deposits of dental plaque, and precipitation within the soft tissues of dark metallic salts (probably sulfides) from reaction with absorbed products of plaque metabolism as the likely mechanism. Also *blue line, halo saturninus.* See also BURTON SIGN. **mamillary l.** LINEA MAMILLARIS. **mammary l.** 1 MAMMARY RIDGE. 2 A horizontal line drawn between the nipples of the breasts. **McKee's l.** A line of incision drawn from the tip of the eleventh costal cartilage to a point one and a half inches medial to the anterior superior iliac spine and then across to a point just above the position of the superficial inguinal ring. It is used for an extraperitoneal approach for ligation of the common iliac artery. **median nuchal l.** CRISTA OCCIPITALIS EXTERNA. **mercurial l.** A dark line of variable color at the gingival margin caused by the ingestion of mercurial salts. It sometimes used to be seen in patients being treated for syphilis with mercury. **Meyer's l.** An axial line through the big toe that, when projected backwards, will pass through the center of the heel in a normal foot. **midaxillary l.** LINEA AXILLARIS MEDIA. **midclavicular l.** LINEA MEDIOCLAVICULARIS. **middle nuchal l.** CRISTA OCCIPITALIS EXTERNA. **middle l. of scrotum** RAPHE SCROTI. **midspinal l.** A vertical line drawn down the center of the vertebral column in the median plane. **midsternal l.** A vertical line drawn down the center of the sternum. **milk l.** MAMMARY RIDGE. **Monro-Richter l.** A line drawn between the umbilicus and the left anterior superior iliac spine. Also *Monro's line.* **Morgan's l.** A crease below the lower eyelids in atopic dermatitis. Also *Dennie sign.* **Moyer's l.** A line drawn between the midpoint of the body of the third sacral vertebra and a point midway between the two anterior superior iliac spines. **mylohyoidean l.** LINEA MYLOHYOIDEA MANDIBULAE. **mylohyoid l. of mandible** LINEA MYLOHYOIDEA MANDIBULAE. **nasobasilar l.** BASINASAL LINE. **nasolabial l.** A line drawn between the ala of the nose and the angle of the mouth on the same side. **nasosubnasal l.** A line drawn between the nasion and the subnasal point. **Nélaton's l.** A line drawn from the anterior superior iliac spine to the most prominent part of the ischial tuberosity, passing through the top of the greater trochanter of the femur normally when the thigh is partly flexed. Also *Roser's line.* **neonatal l.** A prominent incremental line found in enamel and in dentin. It is caused by a retardation in the formation of these tissues during the postpartum period. Also *neonatal ring.* **nipple l.** LINEA MAMILLARIS. **Obersteiner-Redlich l.** OBERSTEINER-REDLICH SPACE. **oblique l.** A line placed obliquely on a structure in the anatomical position. **oblique l. of mandible** LINEA OBLIQUA MANDIBULAE. **oblique l. of radius** The proximal part of the anterior margin of the radius extending from the anterolateral part of the radial tuberosity to the middle of the junction of the anterior and lateral surfaces just above the rough tuberosity for the insertion of the pronator teres muscle. **oblique l. of thyroid cartilage** LINEA OBLIQUA CARTILAGINIS THYROIDEAE. **obturator l.** A line normally crossing the obturator fascia internal to the acetabulum, as seen on an anteroposterior radiograph. **l. of occlusion** PLANE OF OCCLUSION. **Ogston's l.** A line drawn from the adductor tubercle to the intercondylar fossa of the femur. **omphalospinous l.** A line drawn between the umbilicus and the anterior superior iliac spine. Also *umbilicoiliac line.* **orthostatic l.'s** Flexure lines in the neck accommodating flexion and extension movements. **Ouchterlony l.** The precipitin line formed when antigen and antibody combine in optimal proportions in immunodiffusion in agar gel. **l.'s of Owen** The incremental lines in dentin caused by minor bends in the dentinal tubules. Also *contour lines.* **parasternal l.** LINEA PARASTERNALIS. **Pastia's l.'s** Transverse red lines which appear in skin creases at the inside of the elbow, wrists, and inguinal areas in the early stages of scarlet fever. They persist throughout the disease and may be of some late diagnostic value. Also *Pastia sign, Thomson sign.* **pectinate l.** An uneven horizontal line formed by the continuity between the anal valves and the bases of the rectal columns about 2 cm above the anal opening. Clinicians consider this to be the upper boundary of the anal canal at the clinical anorectal junction; however, anatomists view the line as being in the middle of the anal canal. The line has commonly been considered to lie at the junction of the endodermal part of the anal canal and the ectodermal proctodeum, but there is evidence that this union is situated lower down. Various authors have also considered the anocutaneous and anorectal lines to be the same as the pectinate line, producing confusion. Also *dentate line, dentate margin.* **pectineal l.** 1 PECTEN OSSIS PUBIS. 2 LINEA PECTINEA FEMORIS. **Pickerill's imbrication l.'s** Transverse grooves on the surface of enamel. They are especially numerous towards the neck of a tooth. **pigmented l. of the cornea** HUDSON-STÄHLI LINE. **pleuroesophageal l.** On an anteroposterior or posteroanterior chest roentgenogram, a vertical line of soft-tissue density to the left of the thoracic spine, representing the zone of contact of the left lung with the esophagus. **Poirier's l.** A line drawn from the nasion to the lambda, passing 5 mm above the external auditory meatus. **popliteal l. of femur** LINEA INTERCONDYLARIS FEMORIS. **popliteal l. of tibia** LINEA MUSCULI SOLEI. **posterior axillary l.** LINEA AXILLARIS POSTERIOR. **posterior gluteal l.** LINEA GLUTEA POSTERIOR. **posterior median l.** LINEA MEDIANA POSTERIOR. **Poupart's l.** A line drawn on the surface of the abdomen passing vertically through the midpoint of the inguinal ligament and parallel to the median plane. Used to help demarcate regions of the abdomen, it approximates the lower extension of the midclavicular, or lateral, line (linea medioclavicularis). **precentral l.** An oblique line drawn on the surface of the head extending anteroinferiorly from the median plane at an angle of about 70° from the midpoint between glabella and inion. It approximates the position of the precentral sulcus. **profile l.** CAMPER'S LINE. **protrusive l.** A central line on a pantographic tracing. **pure l.** A strain of organisms that is produced by self-fertilization of apomixic plants or by continual inbreeding of a sexual species. It is genetically pure, except for random, sporadic mutation. Each individual is homozygous at each locus and has the same genotype as every other individual of the strain. **radial longitudinal l.** LINEA VITALIS. **recessional l.'s** INCREMENTAL LINES. **Reid's base l.** BASE LINE. **Retzius l.'s** STRIAE OF RETZIUS. **Robson's l.** A line drawn from either nipple to the umbilicus. **Roser's l.** NÉLATON'S LINE. **Salter's l.'s** Incremental lines visible in histologic sections of cementum. **scan l.** A line produced on a cathode ray tube by moving an electron beam spot at constant speed. **scapular l.** LINEA SCAPULARIS. **Schoemaker's l.** A line drawn between the greater trochanter of the femur and the anterior superior iliac spine, the projection of which normally passes above the umbilicus. **Schreger's l.'s** Lines seen in longitudinal sections of human enamel when viewed by reflected light. Also *bands of Schreger, bands of Hunter-Schreger, Schreger striae.* **Schwalbe's l.** The peripheral edge of Descemet's membrane, as observed by gonioscopy. See also SCHWALBE'S RING. **semicircular l. of Douglas** LINEA ARCUATA VAGINAE MUSCULI RECTI ABDOMINIS. **semilunar l.** LINEA SEMILUNARIS. **semilunar l. of Spieghel** LINEA SEMILUNARIS. **septal l.'s** Lines on a chest roentgenogram representing thickened interlobular septa, such as Kerley B lines. **Shenton's l.** A smooth curve drawn on an anteroposterior roentgenogram of the normal hip, extending from the upper border of the obturator foramen to the medial cortex of the neck of the femur. Also *Shenton's arch, Skinner's line.* **l. of sight** An imaginary line from the fixation point to the center of the pupil. **simian l.** A major flexion crease that completely traverses the human palm. It is found as a normal variant as well as with increased frequency in some syndromes, especially the Down syndrome. Also *simian crease.* **Skinner's l.** SHENTON'S LINE. **soleal l. of tibia** LINEA MUSCULI SOLEI. **Spieghel's l.** LINEA SEMILUNARIS. **spigelian l.** LINEA SEMILUNARIS. **Spigelius l.** LINEA SEMILUNARIS. **spiral l. of femur** A curved line continuous above with the lower end of the intertrochanteric line and below with the medial lip of linea aspera femoris. It forms the medial boundary of the insertion of the iliacus muscle. Also *linea spiralis* (outmoded). **Stähli's pigment l.** HUDSON-STÄHLI LINE. **sternal l.** LINEA STERNALIS. **sternomastoid l.** A line along the anterior margin of the sternocleidomastoid muscle from the medial end of the clavicle to the mastoid process of the temporal bone. **subcostal l.** A line drawn across the lowest points on the tenth costal cartilages on the anterior surface of the trunk. It is the level of the subcostal plane. Also *infracostal line.* **superior nuchal l.** LINEA NUCHAE SUPERIOR. **superior temporal l. of parietal bone** LINEA TEMPORALIS SUPERIOR OSSIS PARIETALIS. **supracondylar l.'s** Two diverging lines, medial and lateral, on the posterior surface of the lower third of the shaft of the femur, bounding the popliteal surface and continuous above with the medial and lateral lips of the linea aspera while ending inferiorly at the adductor tubercle and lateral epicondyle, respectively. They serve as the partial attachments of muscles and intermuscular septa. **supreme**

**nuchal l.** LINEA NUCHAE SUPREMA. **survey l.** A line joining the points of height of contour on the teeth. Also *clasp guideline.* **suture l.** 1 The site of anastomosis of two luminal structures, as the juncture of two blood vessels. 2 Any site where two tissue edges have been brought together by sutures. **Sydney l.** The proximal transverse flexure line in the palm that reaches the ulnar border of the hand. Also *Sydney crease.* **temporal l. of frontal bone** LINEA TEMPORALIS OSSIS FRONTALIS. **tension l.'s** CLEAVAGE LINES. **terminal l. of pelvis** LINEA TERMINALIS PELVIS. **thyroid red l.** An erythematous streak caused by irritation of the skin on the anterior neck and upper thorax in hyperthyroid patients. **Topinard's l.** A line connecting the glabella and the gnathion. **tram l.'s** Thin parallel lines on a chest radiograph, representing peribronchial interstitial thickening best seen in the central aspects of the lower lung fields, due to chronic inflammation. **transverse l.'s of sacrum** LINEAE TRANSVERSAE OSSIS SACRI. **trapezoid l.** LINEA TRAPEZOIDEA. **triradiate l.'s** Linear sutures that develop in the embryonic lens because of the less than interpolar length of lens fibers. They give rise to complex lens stars with from three to as many as nine rays. **Trümmerfeld l.** The zone of rarefaction at the growing end of the shaft of a long bone, seen in infantile scurvy. It sometimes leads to fracture and displacement of the epiphysis. **type l.** Either of two diverging epidermal ridges seen in fingerprints. **Ullmann's l.** In the displacement of spondylolisthesis, a vertical line that, when drawn upward from the anterior edge of the first sacral segment, will pass through the body of the fifth lumbar vertebra. **umbilicoiliac l.** OMPHALOSPINOUS LINE. **l. of Venus** The main flexure line across the anterior aspect of the wrist. **Veslingius l.** RAPHE SCROTI. **vibrating l.** An imaginary line demarcating the hard palate from the movable tissues of the soft palate. **Virchow's l.** A line from nasion to lambda. **visual l.** VISUAL AXIS. **Wagner's l.** A curved, pale line at the junction of the epiphysis and the diaphysis of a long bone produced by provisional calcification in the cartilaginous plate. **Weiger's l.** The circular line of attachment of the vitreous body to the posterior surface of the lens, which is located towards the lens periphery. **white l.** LINEA ALBA. **white l. of Fränkel** A roentgenographic sign of scurvy, consisting of a line of increased radiodensity in the metaphysis at the provisional zone of calcification. Also *Fränkel's line.* **white l. of pelvic fascia** ARCUS TENDINEUS FASCIAE PELVIS. **white l. of pharynx** RAPHE PHARYNGIS. **Wimberger's l.** A zone of increased radiodensity at the periphery of the epiphysis, seen typically in scurvy. **working l.** A lateral line on a pantographic tracing. **Y l.** A horizontal line drawn through the Y cartilages of the hips on an anteroposterior radiograph of the pelvis to assess acetabular angles. **Z l.** Z BAND. **l.'s of Zahn** Striations on the surface of a blood clot due to the layering of platelet aggregates. Also *Zahn's ribs.* **Zöllner's l.'s** An optical illusion of converging and diverging lines.

**linea** \lin′ē·ə\ [L (from *lineus* made of flax, from *linum* flax, linen, thread) a thread, string, line] (*pl.* lineae) A long thin mark, ridge, or crease on the surface of a structure; a line. **l. alba** [NA] A midline tendinous band extending from the xiphoid process to the symphysis pubis and formed by the aponeuroses of the external oblique, internal oblique and transversus muscles of the abdomen fusing and decussating with each other and with corresponding aponeuroses of the opposite side. It is interrupted by the umbilicus. Also *white line, Hunter's line.* **l. anocutanea** ANOCUTANEOUS LINE. **l. anorectalis** [NA] A vague annular region of the lumen of the large intestine usually at or below the level of the anorectal junction. It is commonly considered to be about 4 cm above the anocutaneous line and about 1.5 cm above the pectinate line, approximating the upper end of the anal columns. In this region the intestinal glands shorten and disappear and the circular muscle coat of the rectum thickens to form the upper end on the sphincter ani internus. Also *anorectal line.* • Originally this term referred to the lower limit of the simple columnar epithelium of the rectal mucosa, which is usually lower than the level of the anorectal junction. Nevertheless, it is occasionally used synonymously with *anorectal junction.* **l. arcuata ossis ilii** [NA] The thick, rounded continuation anteriorly of the anteroinferior end of the medial border of the ilium, where the latter meets the anterior angulation of the auricular surface, extending to the iliopubic eminence as the iliac portion of the terminal line and separating the iliac fossa from the internal surface of the body of the ilium in the true pelvis. It forms part of the lateral wall of the inlet of the minor pelvis, and transmits compression forces from the trunk to the lower limb. Also *arcuate line of ilium, iliopectineal crest of iliac bone, iliopectineal line, arcuate line of innominate bone.* **l. arcuata vaginae musculi recti abdominis** [NA] The concave lower margin of the posterior wall of the rectus sheath, located about midway between the umbilicus and the pubic symphysis, below which all three aponeuroses of the abdominal muscles pass anterior to the rectus abdominis muscle. The inferior epigastric vessels pass anterior to the line. Also *arcuate line of sheath of rectus abdominis muscle, semicircular line of Douglas, line of Douglas, Douglas fold.* **l. aspera femoris** [NA] A rough, crestlike ridge buttressing the middle third of the posterior surface of the shaft of the femur, comprising medial and lateral lips and resisting compression forces produced by the anterior curvature of the femur. It provides attachment for muscles and intermuscular septa of the thigh. Also *femoral crest.* **lineae atrophicae** STRIAE ATROPHICAE. **l. axillaris anterior** [NA] A vertical line, parallel to the median plane, extending downward from the medial end of the anterior fold of the axilla along the side of the trunk. Also *anterior axillary line.* **l. axillaris media** [NA] A vertical line, parallel to the anterior and the posterior axillary lines and midway between them, usually passing through the apex of the axilla. Also *midaxillary line, linea medio-axillaris.* **l. axillaris posterior** [NA] A vertical line, parallel to the median plane, extending downward from the medial end of the posterior fold of the axilla along the side of the thorax. Also *posterior axillary line.* **l. epiphysialis** [NA] A line seen on the surface in a mature bone at the junction between the epiphysis and the metaphyseal end of the diaphysis. It corresponds to the level of the perichondrial ring around the epiphyseal plate in an immature bone. Also *epiphyseal line.* **l. fusca** A band of pigmentation along the frontal hair margin. It may be associated with cerebral inflammatory or neoplastic lesions. **l. glutea anterior** [NA] The middle of three curved ridges on the gluteal surface of the ala of the ilium extending from a point on the iliac crest 2–3 cm behind the anterior superior iliac spine to the middle of the superior margin of the greater sciatic notch. Between this line and the crest, the gluteus medius muscle arises. Also *anterior gluteal line.* **l. glutea inferior** [NA] The most anterior, and least distinct, of three curved ridges on the gluteal surface of the ala of the ilium, extending backwards from the notched margin below the anterior inferior iliac spine to the front angulation of the greater sciatic notch. Most of the area between the anterior

## Contents of Color Plate Section



Scientific support: P. Posel

* Mrs. Siri Mills (Munich) provided the drawings; partly based on work by E. Lepier, K. Endtresser, L. Schrott (from Pernkopf, *Atlas of Topographic and Applied Human Anatomy*; Munich 1963, 1979).

## Skeleton

**Head**
1 Os frontale (fronal bone)
2 Os nasale (nasal bone)
3 Vomer
4 Maxilla
5 Mandibula (mandible)
6 Angulus mandibulae (angle of mandible)
7 Os zygomaticum (zygomatic bone)
8 Fissura orbitalis superior (superior orbital fissure)
9 Foramen supraorbitale (supraorbital foramen)
10 Foramen infraorbitale (infraorbital foramen)
11 Foramen mentale (mental foramen)

**Vertebral column** (in part)
12 Discus intervertebralis (intervertebral disk)
13 Vertebra prominens (7th cervical vertebra)
14 Vertebra thoracica I (1st thoracic vertebra)

**Thoracic cage**
15 Costae verae, I–VII (true ribs)
16 Costae spuriae, VIII–XII (false ribs)
17 Costae fluitantes, XI–XII (floating ribs)
18 Arcus costalis (costal arch)
19 Apertura thoracis superior (upper thoracic opening)
20 Apertura thoracis inferior (lower thoracic opening); angulus infrasternalis (infrasternal angle)
21 Incisura jugularis sterni (jugular notch of sternum)
22 Manubrium sterni
23 Corpus sterni (body of sternum)
24 Processus xiphoideus (xiphoid process)

**Shoulder girdle**
25 Clavicula (clavicle)
*26–35 Scapula:*
26 Facies costalis (costal surface); fossa subscapularis (subscapular fossa)
27 Facies posterior (posterior surface)
28 Spina scapulae (spine of scapula)
29 Acromion
30 Processus coracoideus (coracoid process)
31 Ligamentum coracoacromiale (coracoacromial ligament)
32 Incisura scapulae (scapular notch)
33 Fossa supraspinata (supraspinous fossa)
34 Fossa infraspinata (infraspinous fossa)
35 Cavitas glenoidalis (glenoid cavity)
36 Ligamenta glenohumeralia (glenohumeral ligaments)

**Upper limb**
37 Humerus
38 Caput humeri (head of humerus)
39 Tuberculum majus (greater tubercle)
40 Tuberculum minus (lesser tubercle)
41 Sulcus intertubercularis (intertubercular sulcus)
42 Epicondylus medialis (medial epicondyle)
43 Epicondylus lateralis (lateral epicondyle)
44 Capitulum humeri (little head of humerus)
45 Trochlea humeri (trochlea of humerus)
46 Capsula articularis cubiti (elbow joint capsule); ligamenta collateralia ulnare et radiale (ulnar and radial collateral ligaments)
47 Ulna and radius in pronation
48 Ulna and radius in supination
49 Radius
50 Caput radii (head of radius)
51 Tuberositas radii (radial tuberosity)
52 Processus styloideus radii (styloid process of radius)
53 Ulna
54 Processus coronoideus ulnae (coronoid process of ulna)
55 Processus styloideus ulnae (styloid process of ulna)
56 Ligamentum collaterale carpi radiale (radial collateral ligament of wrist)
*57–63 Ossa carpi (carpal bones):*
57 Os scaphoideum (scaphoid bone)
58 Os lunatum (lunate bone)
59 Os triquetrum (triquetral bone); pisiform not shown
60 Os trapezium
61 Os trapezoideum (trapezoid bone)
62 Os capitatum (capitate bone)
63 Os hamatum (hamate bone)
64 Ossa metacarpi (metacarpal bones)
65 Ossa digitorum manus (phalanges)

**Vertebral column** (in part)
*66–72 Structure of a vertebra:*
66 Corpus vertebrae (body of vertebra)
67 Arcus vertebrae (vertebral arch)
68 Foramen vertebrale (vertebral foramen)
69 Processus spinosus (spinous process)
70 Processus transversus (transverse process)
71 Processus articularis superior (superior articular process)
72 Processus costalis (costal process)
73 Vertebra lumbalis I (1st lumbar vertebra)
74 Ligamentum longitudinale anterius (anterior longitudinal ligament)
75 Promontorium ossis sacri (promontory of sacrum)
76 Os sacrum; vertebrae sacrales I–V (sacrum; sacral vertebrae)
77 Ligamentum iliolumbale (iliolumbar ligament)
78 Os coccygis; vertebrae coccygeae I–IV (coccyx; coccygeal vertebrae)

**Pelvis; os coxae** (hip bone)
79 Os ilii (ilium)
80 Crista iliaca (iliac crest)
81 Spina iliaca anterior superior (anterior superior iliac spine)
82 Ligamentum inguinale (inguinal ligament)
83 Ligamentum sacrospinale (sacrospinal ligament)
84 Ligamentum sacrotuberale (sacrotuberal ligament)
85 Foramen obturatum (obturator foramen)
86 Articulatio sacroiliaca (sacroiliac joint)
87 Os ischii (ischium)
88 Os pubis (pubic bone)
89 Symphysis pubica (pubic symphysis)
90 Tuberculum pubicum (pubic tubercle)

**Lower limb**
*91–92 Capsula articularis coxae (hip joint capsule) and ligaments*
91 Ligamentum pubofemorale (pubofemoral ligament)
92 Ligamentum iliofemorale (iliofemoral ligament)
93 Os femoris (femur)
94 Caput ossis femoris (head of femur)
95 Collum ossis femoris (neck of femur)
96 Trochanter major (greater trochanter)
97 Trochanter minor (lesser trochanter)
98 Epicondylus medialis (medial epicondyle)
99 Condylus medialis femoris (medial condyle of femur)
100 Condylus lateralis femoris (lateral condyle of femur)
101 Patella
102 Capsula articularis genus (knee joint capsule)
103 Ligamentum patellae (patellar ligament)
104 Retinaculum patellae laterale (lateral patellar retinaculum)
105 Retinaculum patellae mediale (medial patellar retinaculum)
106 Ligamentum collaterale tibiale (tibial collateral ligament)
107 Ligamentum collaterale fibulare (fibular collateral ligament)
108 Tibia
109 Condylus medialis tibiae (medial condyle of tibia)
110 Tuberositas tibiae (tuberosity of tibia)
111 Malleolus medialis (medial malleolus)
112 Fibula
113 Caput fibulae (head of fibula)
114 Malleolus lateralis (lateral malleolus)
115 Membrana interossea cruris (interosseous membrane of leg)
116 Capsula articularis talocruralis (capsule of ankle joint); ligamentum mediale articulationis talocruralis (deltoid ligament of ankle)
*117–122 Ossa tarsi (tarsal bones) (calcaneus not shown)*
117 Talus (ankle bone)
118 Os cuboideum (cuboid bone)
119 Os naviculare (navicular bone)
120 Os cuneiforme mediale (medial cuneiform bone)
121 Os cuneiforme intermedium (intermediate cuneiform bone)
122 Os cuneiforme laterale (lateral cuneiform bone)
123 Ossa metatarsi (metatarsal bones)
124 Ossa digitorum pedis (phalanges)

## Skeleton

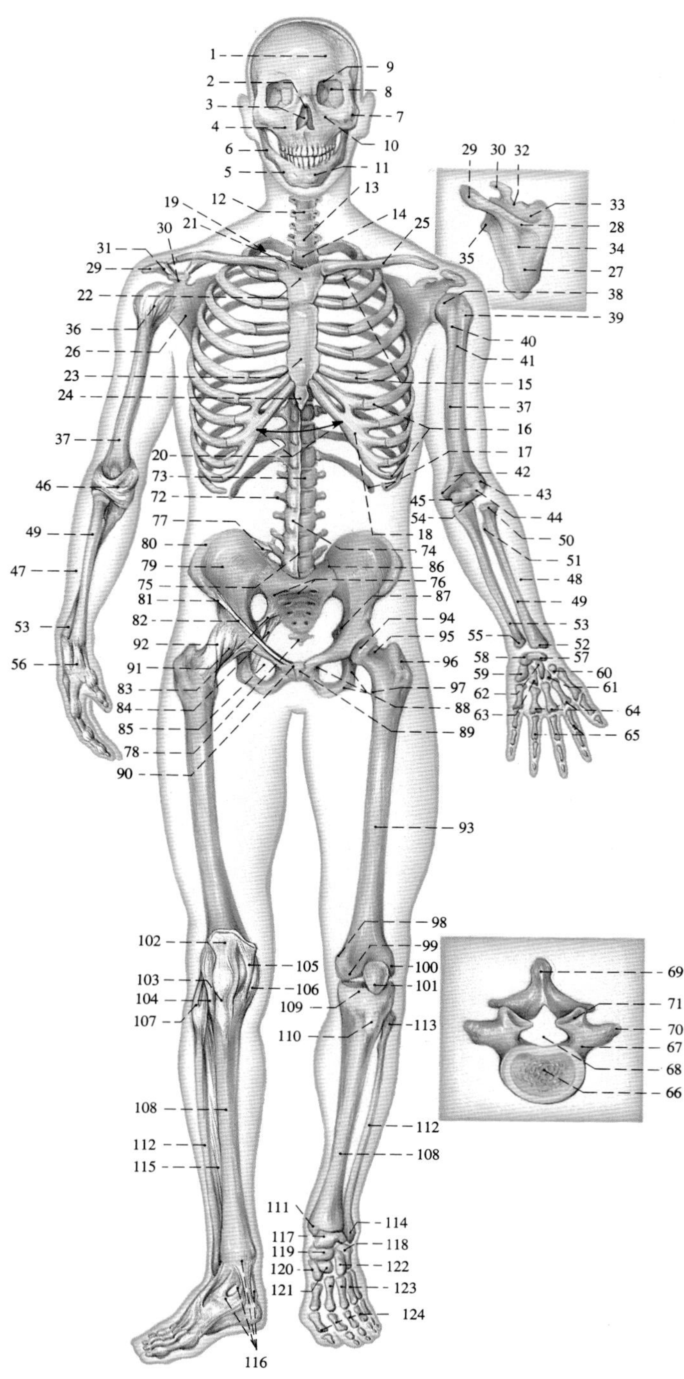

III

## Muscles of the back

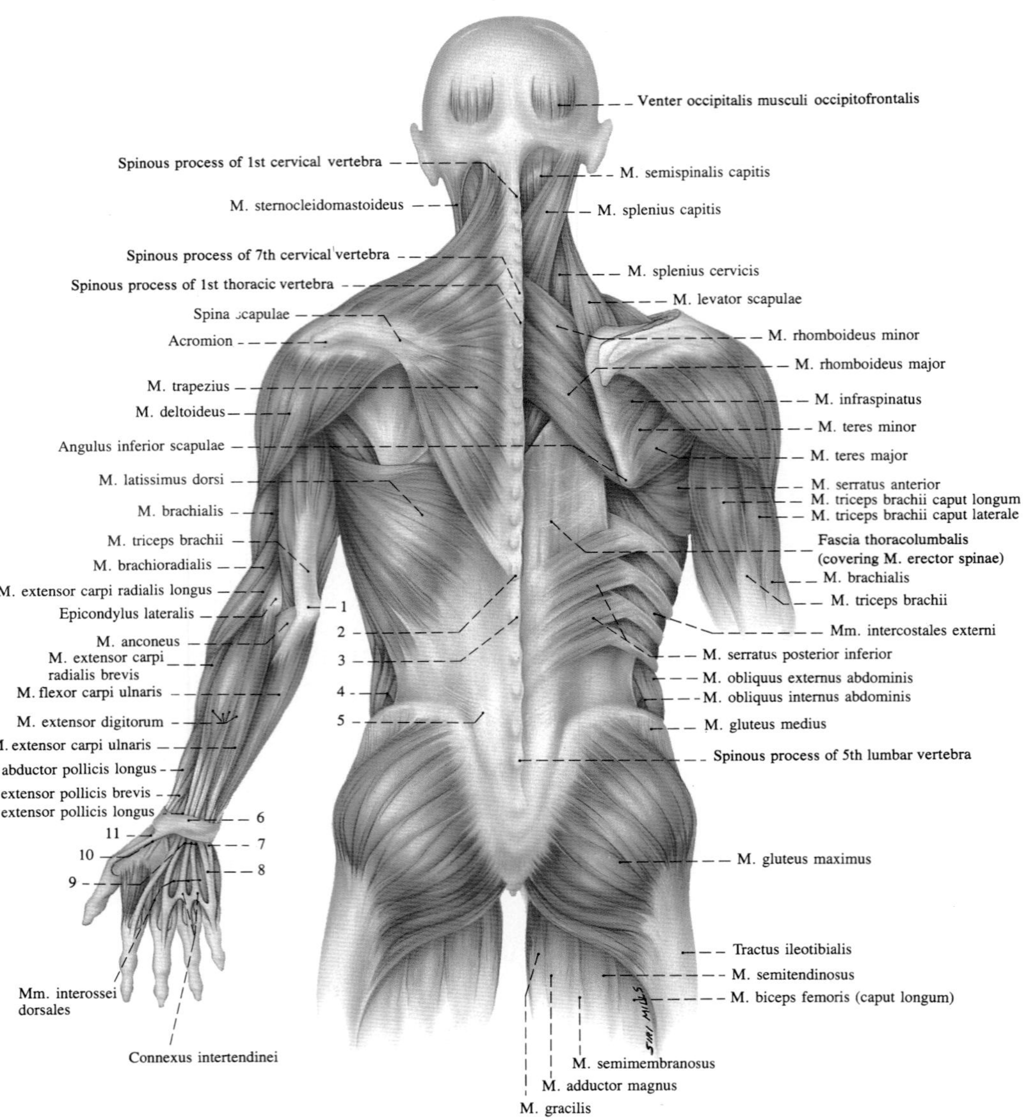


1 Olecranon
2 Spinous process of 12th thoracic vertebra
3 Spinous process of 1st lumbar vertebra
4 Trigonum lumbale
5 Fascia thoracolumbalis (covering M. erector spinae)
6 Retinaculum extensorum
7 Tendon of M. extensor carpi ulnaris
8 Tendon of M. extensor digiti minimi
9 Tendons of M. extensor indicis and M. extensorum digitorum
10 Tendon of M. extensor carpi radialis longus
11 Tendon of M. extensor policis longus

# Head

## Paramedian section through facial portion of the head and through the neck

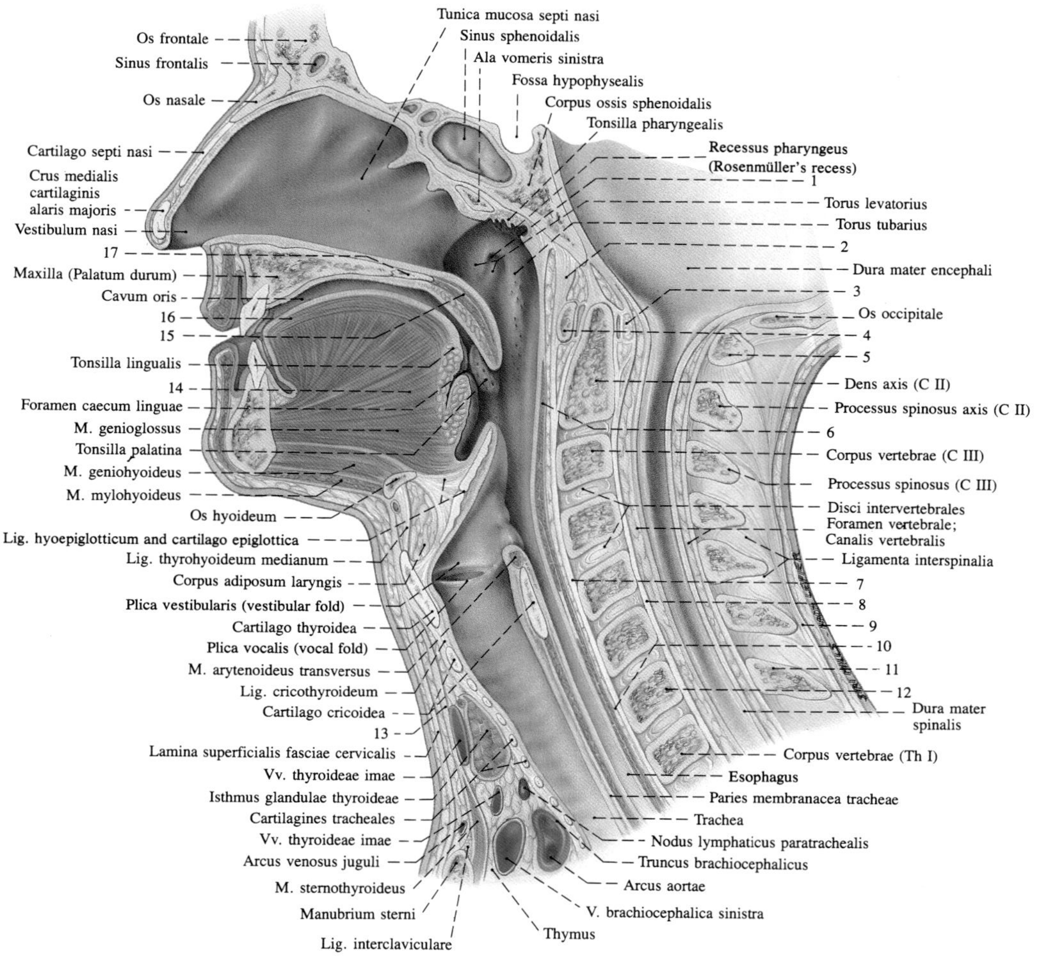


1 Ostium pharyngeum tubae auditivae
2 Membrana atlanto-occipitalis anterior
3 Lig. transversum atlantis (Lig. cruciforme atlantis)
4 Arcus anterior atlantis (C I)
5 Arcus posterior atlantis (C I)
6 M. constrictor pharyngis superior
7 Lig. longitudinale anterius
8 Lig. longitudinale posterius
9 Lig. supraspinale, Lig. nuchae
10 Spatium retroesophageum and lamina prevertebralis fasciae cervicalis
11 Processus spinalis (C VII)
12 Corpus vertebrae (C VII)
13 Lamina praetrachealis fasciae cervicalis
14 Corpus linguae with septum linguae
15 Velum palatinum (Palatum molle)
16 M. longitudinalis superior linguae
17 Os palatinum (Palatum durum)

## Brain: basal and lateral aspects
### Cranial nerves and branches of arteries supplying blood to the brain

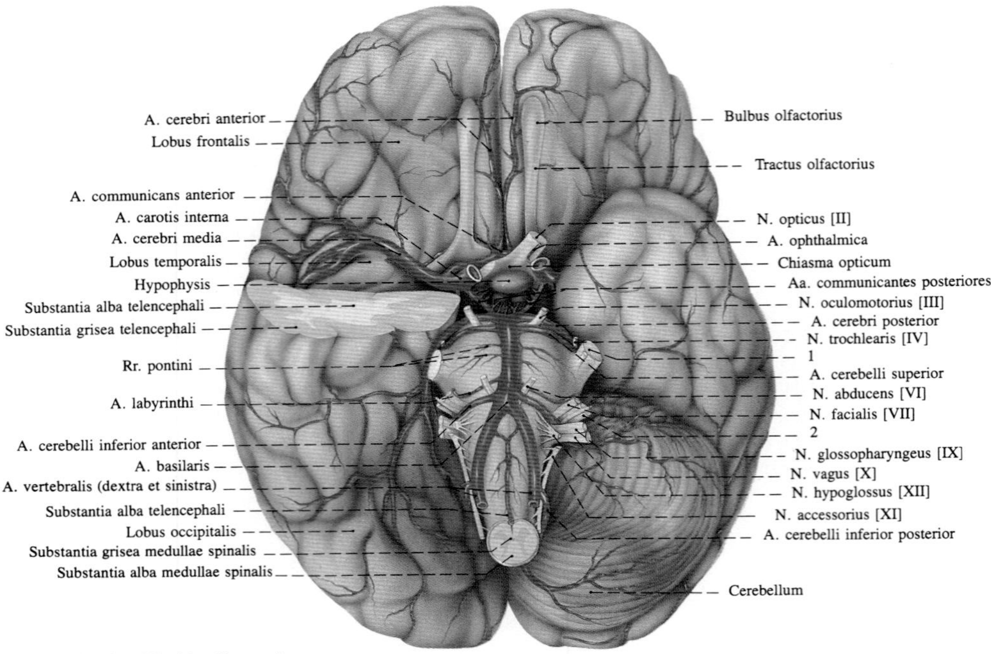


1 N. trigeminus [V] with radix motoria
2 N. vestibulocochlearis [VIII] and N. intermedius

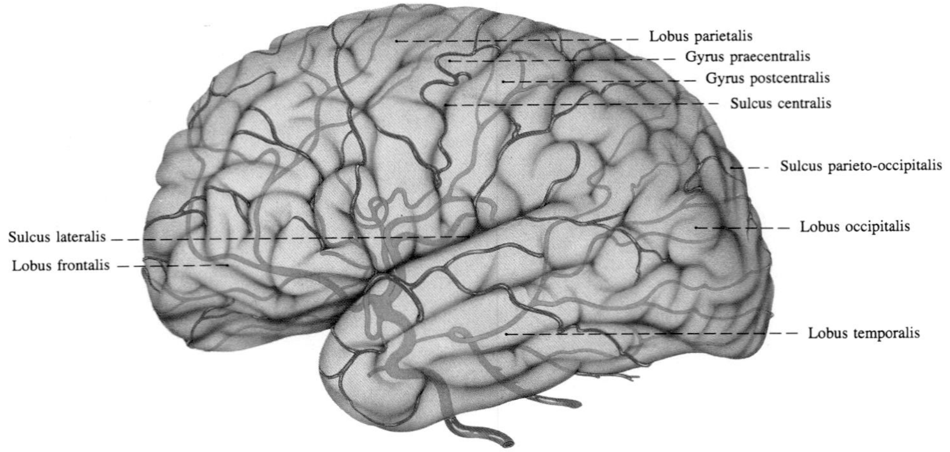

## Brain: telencephalon and frontal section

**Left hemisphere of the telencephalon showing sulci and gyri and ventricular system of the adult brain**

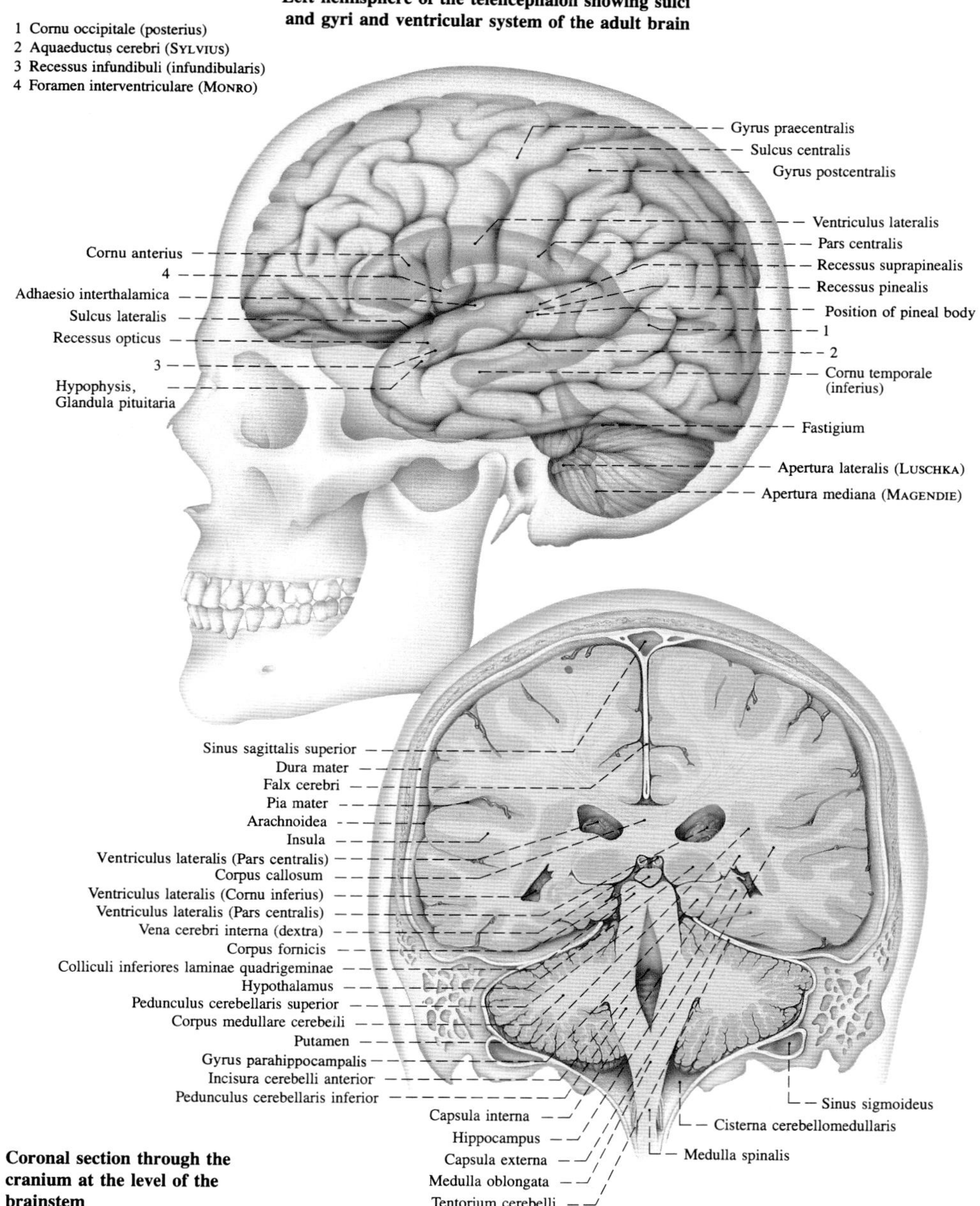


**Coronal section through the cranium at the level of the brainstem**

## Cranial nerve nuclei

**a) Motor** (red), **parasympathetic** (ocher), **and sensory** (blue) **nuclei in the tegmentum of the lower brainstem, with their peripheral connections.** The corresponding cranial nerves are designated by Roman numerals I–XII. (Schematic, lateral view; after M. Clara.)

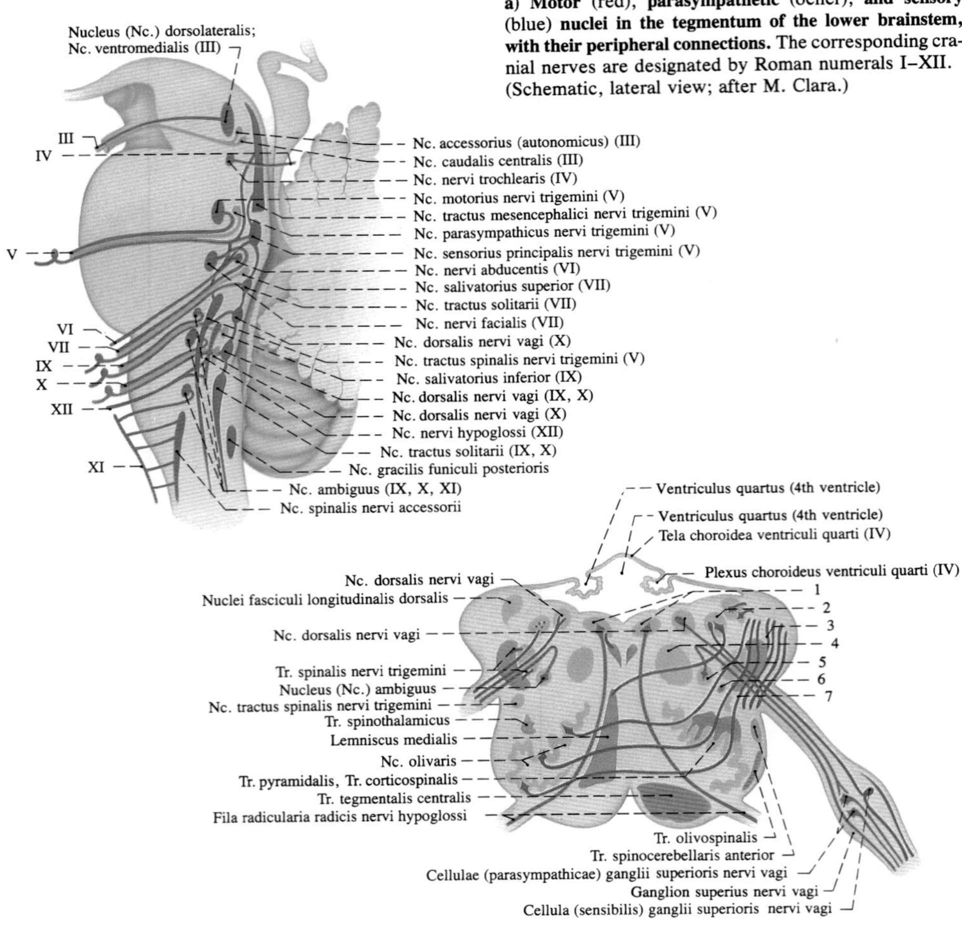


**b) Structure of the medulla oblongata in the region of the caudal portion of the rhomboid fossa.**
(Schematic transverse section; descending tracts in red, ascending in blue.)

1 Nc. nervi hypoglossi
2 Tractus (et nucleus tractus) solitarius
3 Tractus (Tr.) spinocerebellaris posterior
4 Formatio reticularis
5 Nucleus (Nc.) ambiguus
6 Tr. rubrospinalis
7 Fibrae olivocerebellares

**c) Structure of the medulla oblongata at the level of pyramidal decussation.**
(Schematic transverse section; descending tracts in red, ascending in blue.) ▼

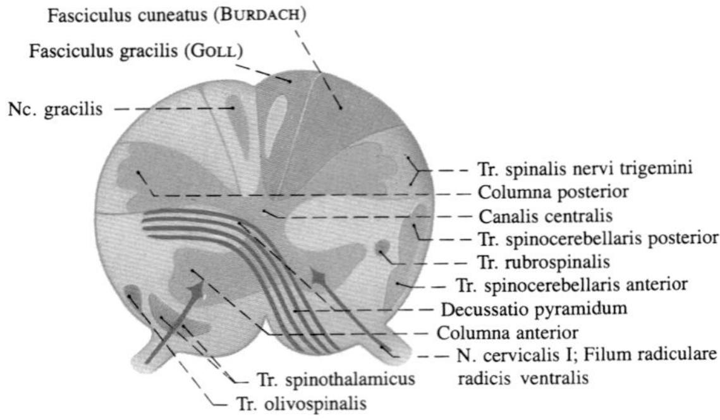

# Spinal cord

**Position of the spinal cord in the vertebral canal.**
(Different colors indicate spinal cord segments and nerve roots in relation to segments of the vertebral column.)

Cervical segments: ocher
Thoracic segments: red
Lumbar segments: green
Sacral segments: crimson
Coccygeal segment: white

**The sympathetic trunk and its relationship to the spinal nerves and their branches**

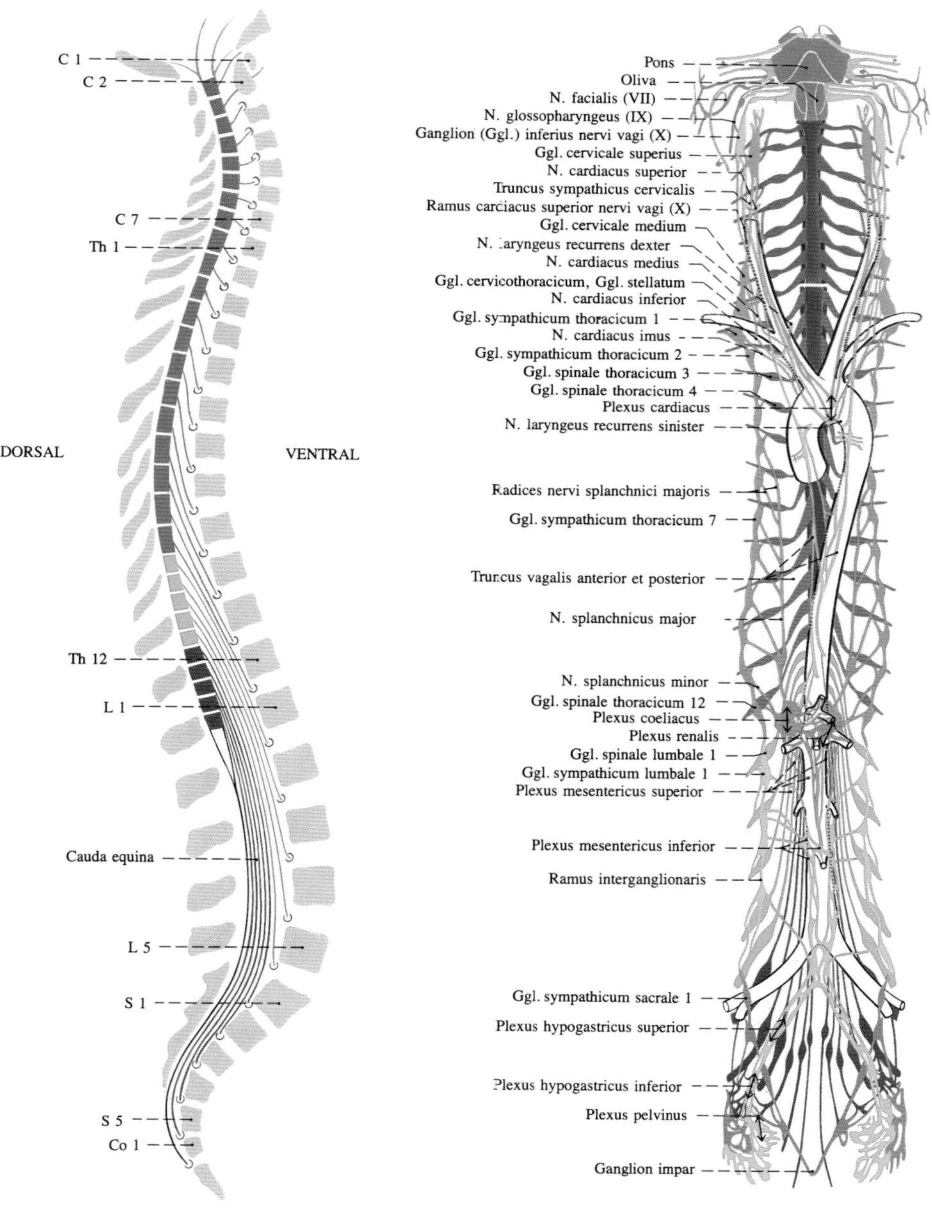

# Ear

## Lateral view of right external ear

## Auditory ossicles of the right middle ear in their natural position

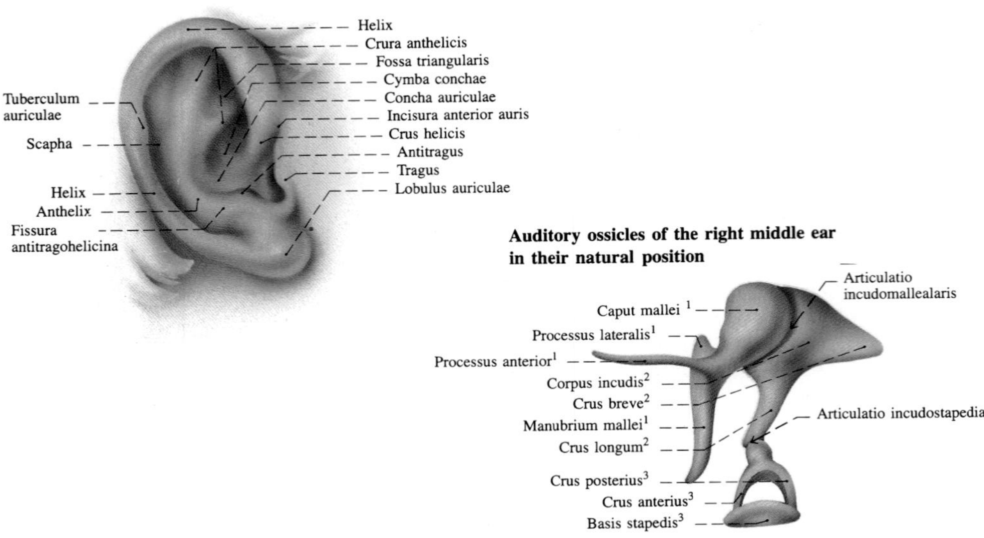


## Right tympanic membrane, external aspect

(Otoscopy of living subject)

## Topographic view of portions of the organ of hearing and equilibrium (organum vestibulocochleare) situated within the right temporal bone

Red: Meatus acusticus externus (external auditory canal)
Green: Auris media (middle ear)
Blue: Auris interna (inner ear)

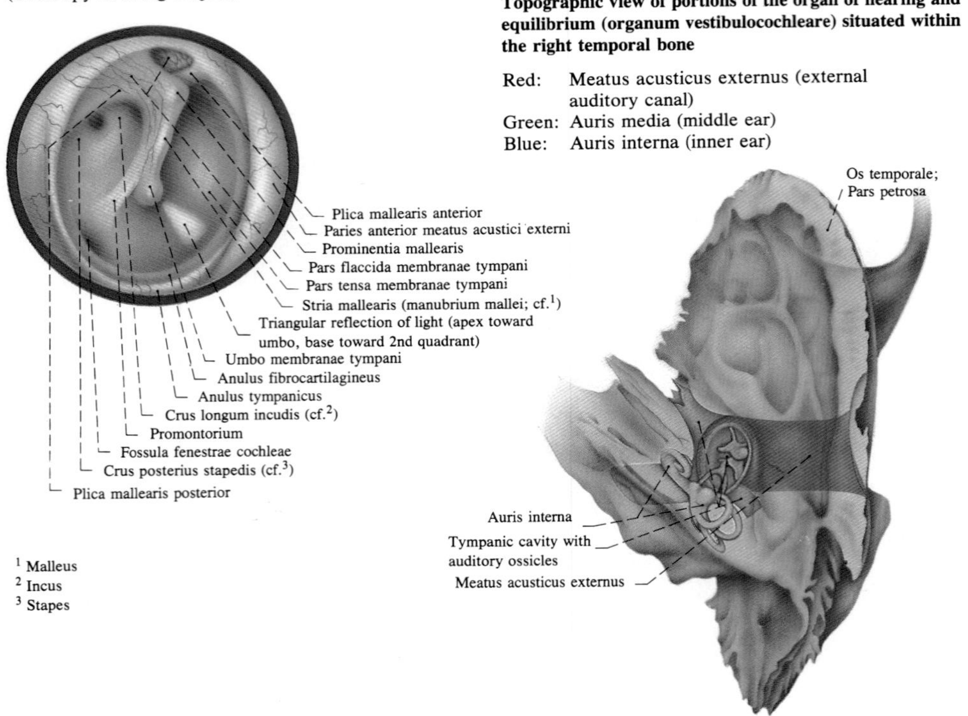


[1] Malleus
[2] Incus
[3] Stapes

X

## Ear

### Middle and inner ear of the right side of the head (general view)

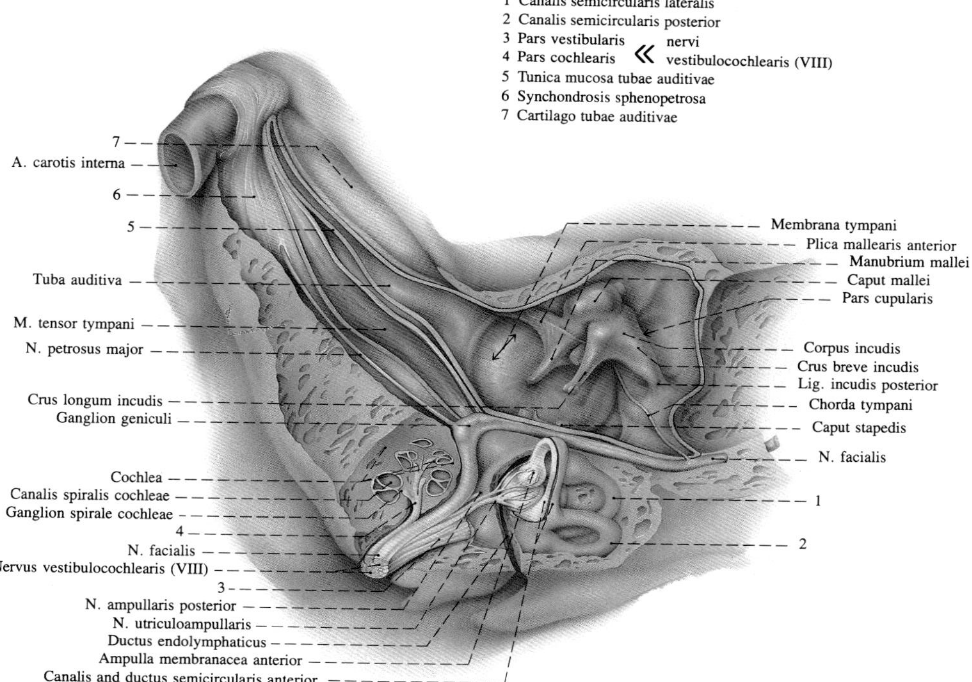


### Computed tomogram of the external auditory canal with sections of the inner ear*

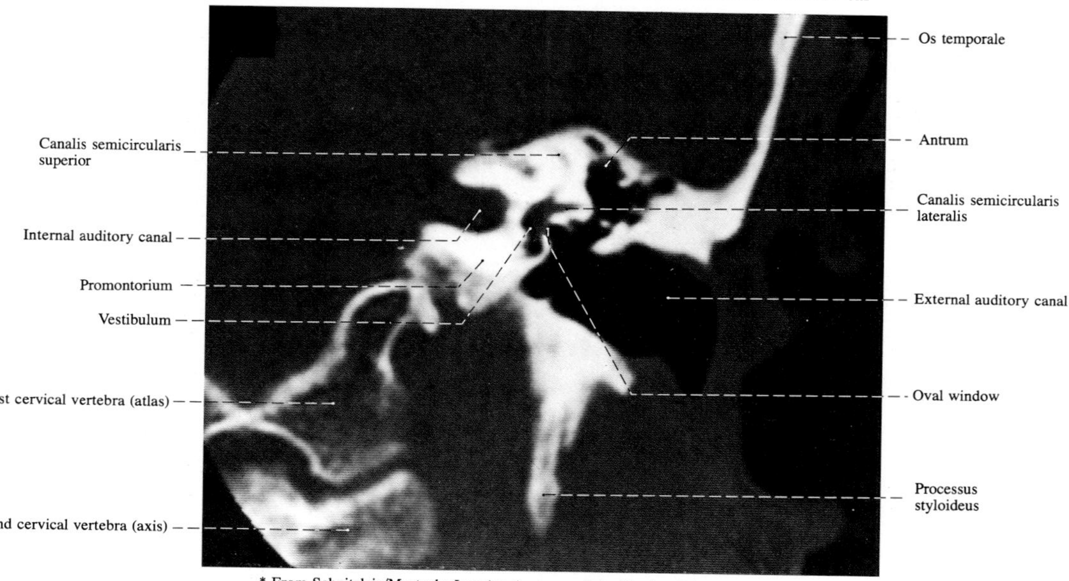


* From Schnitzlein/Murtagh: *Imaging Anatomy of the Head and Spine* (Munich, 1985)

## Eye

**Horizontal meridional section of the right human ocular bulb**

(Schematic. Tunica fibrosa: orange; tunica vasculosa: blue; tunica interna: yellow.)

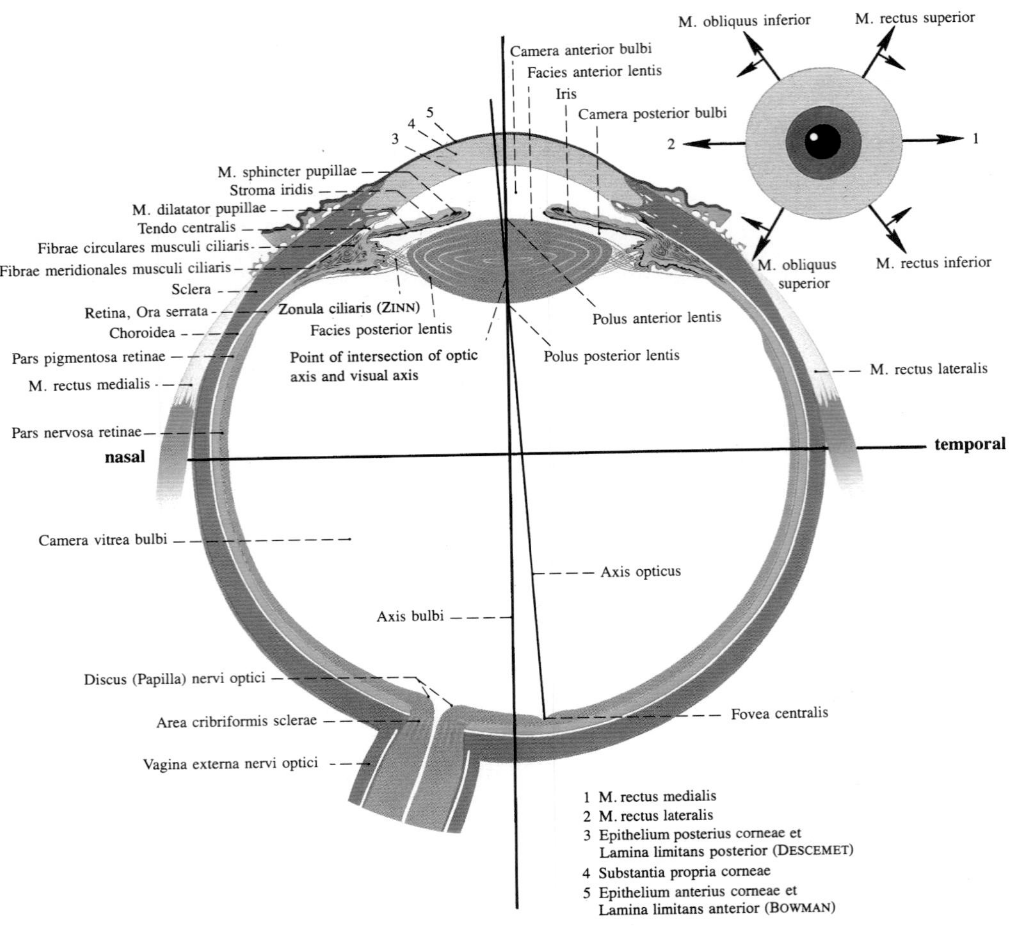


**Muscles of the right eye** (view from above)

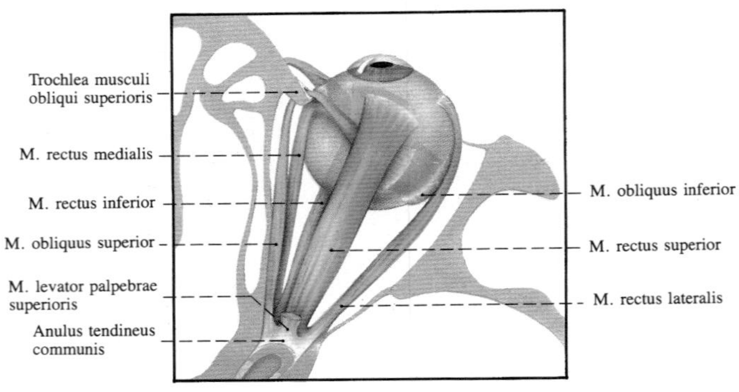

**Schematic illustration of the individual functional phases of the heart during a cardiac cycle**

1 Vv. pulmonales sinistrae
2 Left atrium
3 Ventricular level
4 Left ventricle
5 Right ventricle
6 V. cava inferior
7 Right atrium
8 V. cava superior
9 Aorta
10 Truncus pulmonalis

I Filling phase

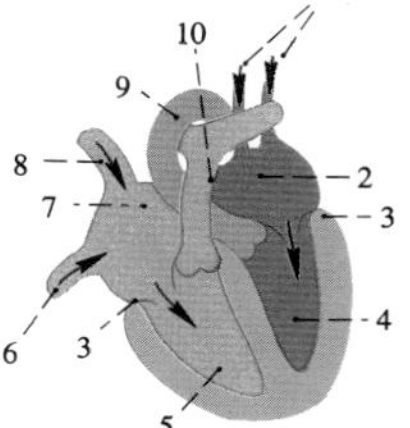


II Atrial contraction

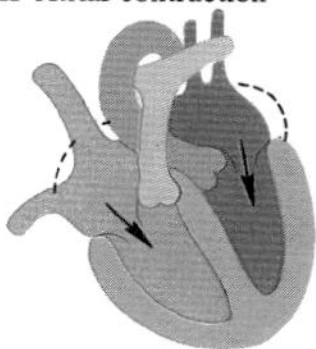

III Ventricular contraction

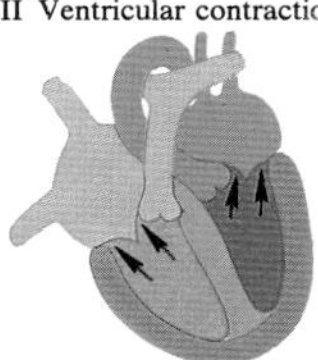

IV Ejection phase

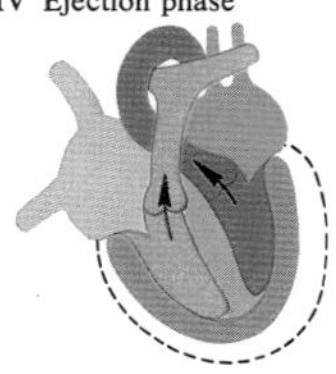

V Relaxation phase

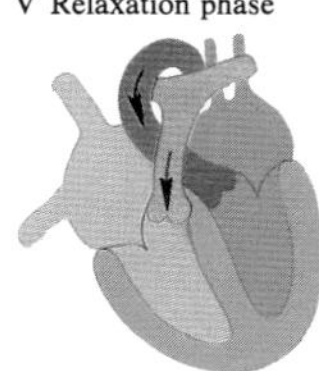

# Heart

## Cardiac vessels

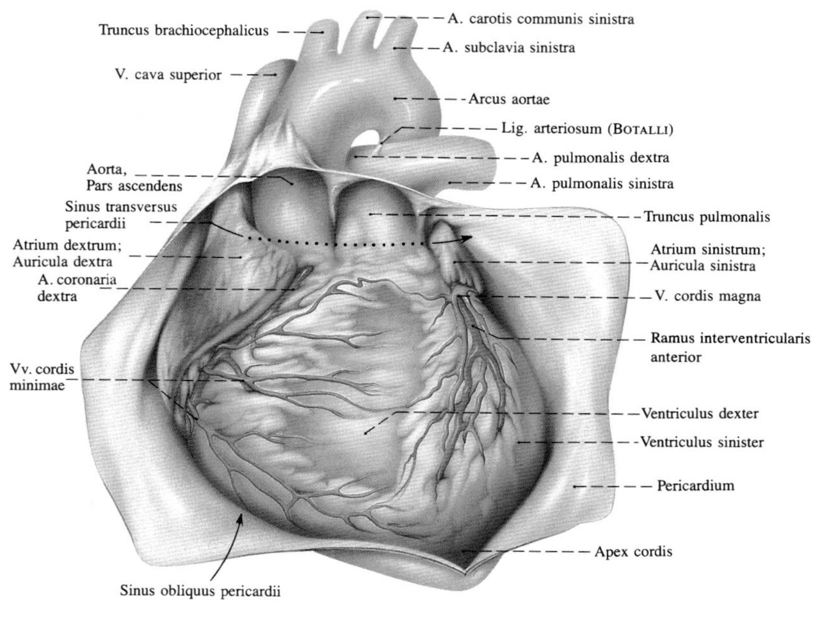


## Section above ventricular level with heart valves

[1] Pulmonary valve
[2] Aortic valve
[3] Tricuspid valve
[4] Mitral valve
[5] Coronary vessels

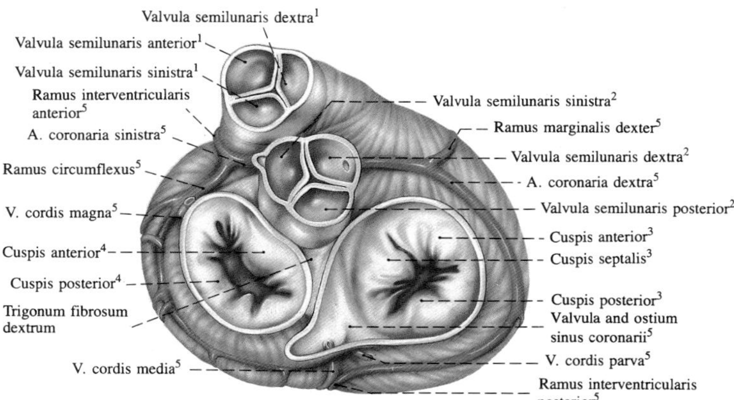

# Lung
## Bronchial system and fine structure

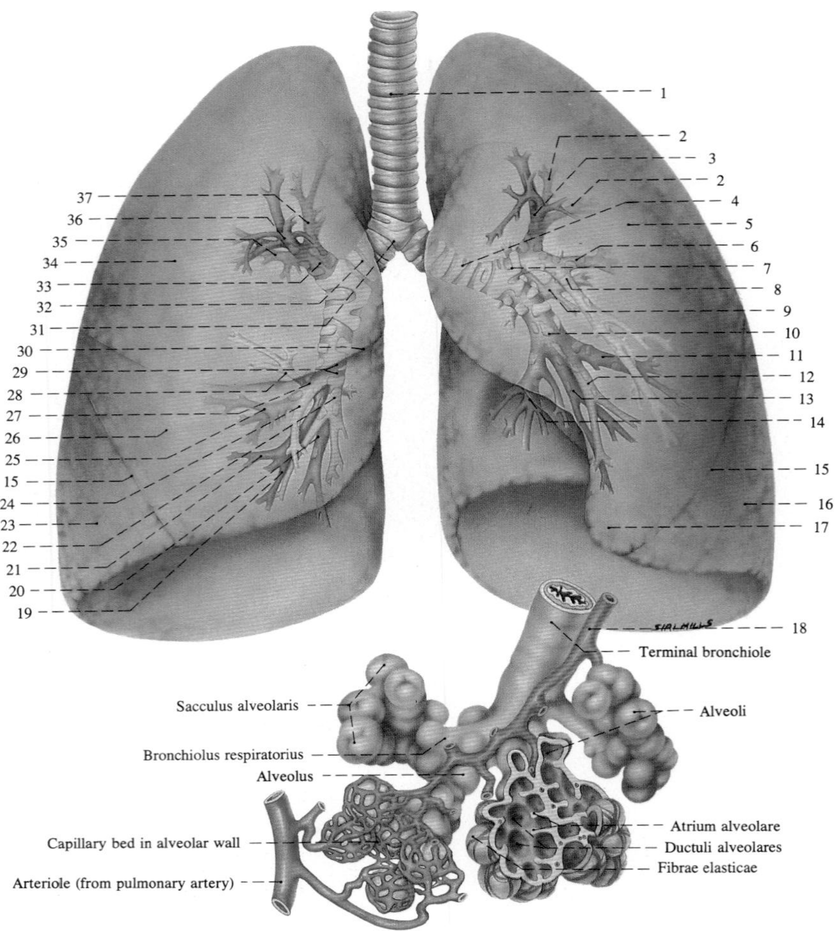


1 Trachea
4 Bronchus principalis sinister
5 Lobus superior
15 Fissura obliqua
16 Lobus inferior
17 Lingula
23 Lobus inferior
26 Lobus medius pulmonis dextri
30 Fissura horizontalis
31 Bifurcatio tracheae
32 Bronchus principalis dexter
33 Bronchus lobaris superior dexter
34 Lobus superior

*35, 36, 37 Segmental bronchi of right upper lobe*
27 Bronchus lobaris medius dexter
35 Bronchus segmentalis posterior
36 Bronchus segmentalis anterior
37 Bronchus segmentalis apicalis

*24, 25 Segmental bronchi of right middle lobe*
24 Bronchus segmentalis medialis
25 Bronchus segmentalis lateralis
29 Bronchus lobaris inferior dexter

*19–22, 28 Segmental bronchi of right lower lobe*
7 Bronchus lobaris superior sinister
19 Br. segmentalis basalis lateralis
20 Br. segmentalis basalis posterior
21 Br. segmentalis basalis anterior
22 Br. segmentalis basalis medialis
28 Br. segmentalis apicalis

*2, 3, 6, 8 Segmental bronchi of left upper lobe*
2 Bronchi segmentales apicoposteriores
3 Bronchus segmentalis anterior
6 Bronchus lingularis superior
8 Bronchus lingularis inferior
10 Bronchus lobaris inferior sinister

*9, 11–14 Segmental bronchi of left lower lobe*
9 Bronchus segmentalis apicalis
11 Bronchus segmentalis basalis anterior
12 Br. segmentalis basalis medialis (inconstant)
13 Br. segmentalis basalis lateralis
14 Br. segmentalis basalis posterior
18 Pulmonary venule

## Ventral view and viscera

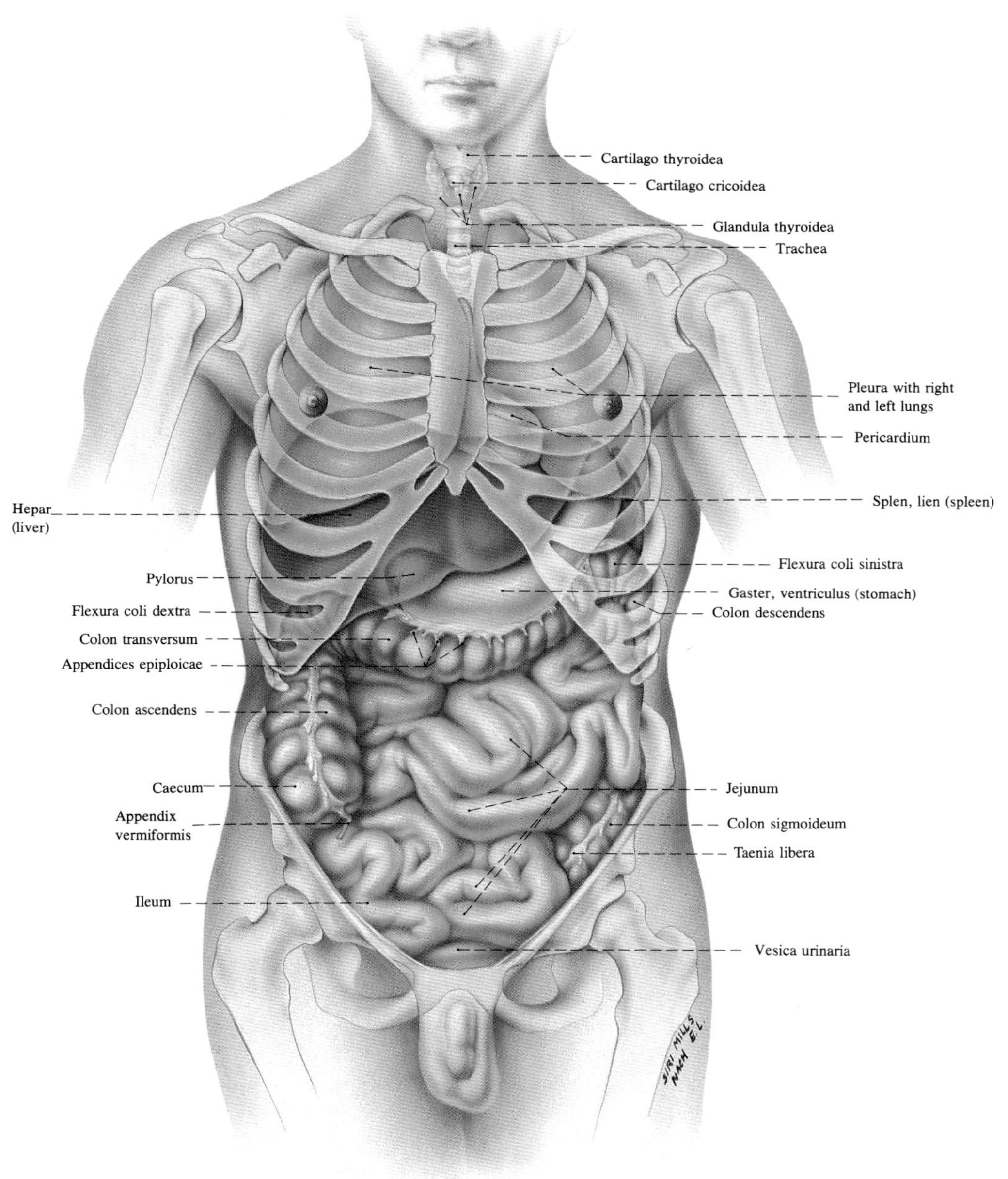


XV

## Urogenital tract

### Internal female genital tract (right adnexa displayed)

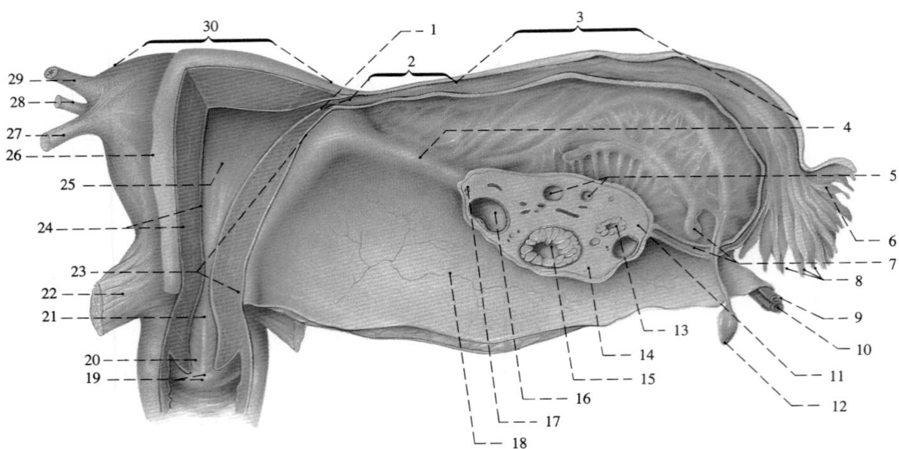


The right side of the uterus, the adjacent part of the vagina, and the right uterine tube are opened from the dorsal aspect. The right ovary is shown in frontal section.

*Tuba uterina (oviduct or fallopian tube)*
1 Pars uterina tubae
2 Isthmus tubae uterinae
3 Ampulla tubae uterinae
4 Lig. ovarii proprium
6 Infundibulum tubae uterinae (with ostium abdominale tubae uterinae)
7 Fimbria ovarica
8 Fimbriae tubae
9 Vena ovarica
10 Arteria ovarica
12 Appendix vesiculosa epoöphori
18 Ligamentum (Lig.) latum uteri

*Ovary*
5 Folliculi ovarii primarii
11 Extremitas tubaria
13 Corpus albicans
14 Stroma ovarii
15 Corpus luteum
16 Folliculus ovaricus vesiculosus (graafian follicle)
17 Extremitas uterina

*Uterus*
19 Ostium uteri (dimple-shaped in nullipara, slit-shaped in parous uterus)
20 Portio vaginalis uteri
21 Canalis cervicis uteri
22 Lig. sacrouterinum
23 Corpus uteri
24 Myometrium
25 Endometrium
26 Perimetrium
27 Lig. ovarii proprium
28 Lig. teres uteri
29 Tuba uterina
30 Fundus uteri

### Sagittal section through female pelvis (schematic)

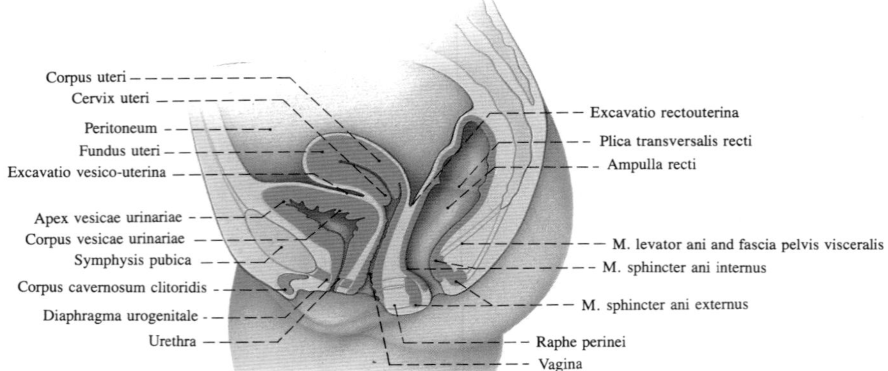

# Urogenital tract

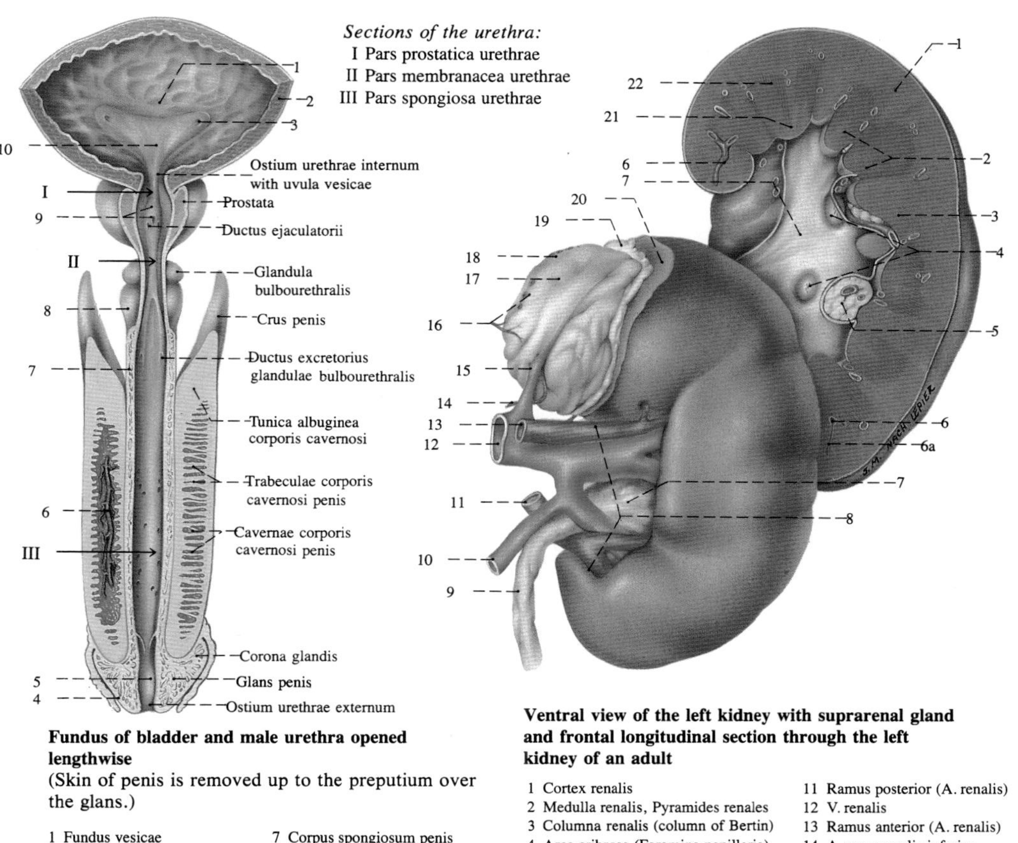


**Fundus of bladder and male urethra opened lengthwise**

(Skin of penis is removed up to the preputium over the glans.)

1 Fundus vesicae
2 M. detrusor vesicae
3 Ostium ureteris
4 Praeputium
5 Fossa navicularis urethrae
6 A. profunda penis
7 Corpus spongiosum penis
8 Bulbus penis
9 Colliculus seminalis with utriculus prostaticus
10 Trigonum seminalis

**Ventral view of the left kidney with suprarenal gland and frontal longitudinal section through the left kidney of an adult**

1 Cortex renalis
2 Medulla renalis, Pyramides renales
3 Columna renalis (column of Bertin)
4 Area cribrosa (Foramina papillaria)
5 Corpus adiposum sinus renalis
6 A. interlobaris
6a Aa. arcuatae
7 Pelvis renalis
8 Hilum renale
9 Ureter sinister
10 V. testicularis sinistra
11 Ramus posterior (A. renalis)
12 V. renalis
13 Ramus anterior (A. renalis)
14 A. suprarenalis inferior
15 V. suprarenalis
16 Aa. suprarenales mediae
17 Glandula suprarenalis
18 Aa. suprarenales superiores
19 Capsula adiposa renis
20 Capsula fibrosa renis
21 Basis pyramidis; Medulla renalis
22 Papilla renalis; Medulla renalis

**Sagittal section through the male pelvis (schematic)**

Peritoneum
Corpus vesicae urinariae
Apex vesicae urinariae
Prostata
Symphysis pubica
Ductus ejaculatorius
Corpus cavernosum penis
Corpus spongiosum
Scrotum
Glans penis
Praeputium
Excavatio rectovesicalis
Plica transversalis recti (Kohlrausch fold)
Ampulla recti
M. levetor ani and fascia pelvis visceralis
M. sphincter ani externus
M. sphincter ani internus
Diaphragma urogenitale

# Ocular fundus

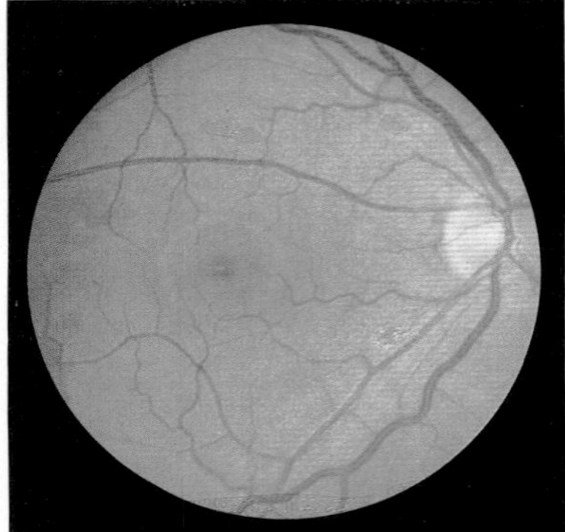

**Normal ocular fundus** (right eye)

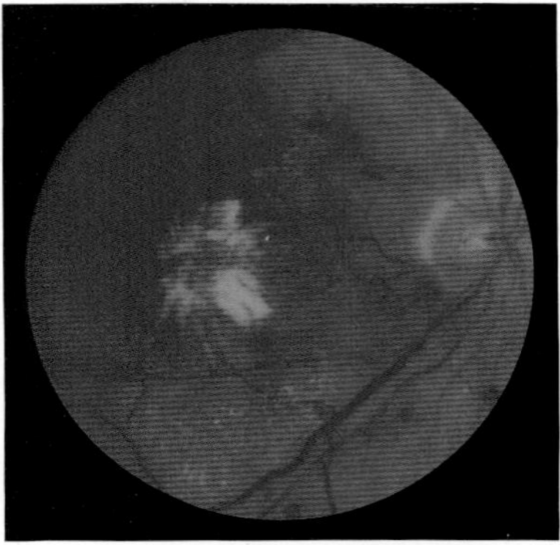

**Hypertonic fundus** with occlusion of several venous branches (right eye)

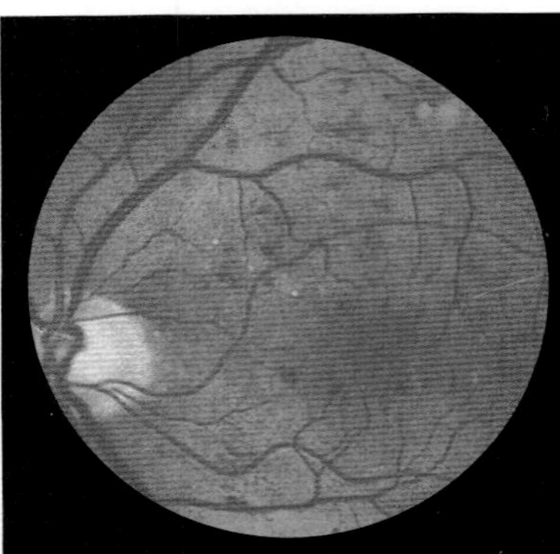

**Diabetic retinopathy** with multiple flea-bite type hemorrhages and microaneurysms (left eye)

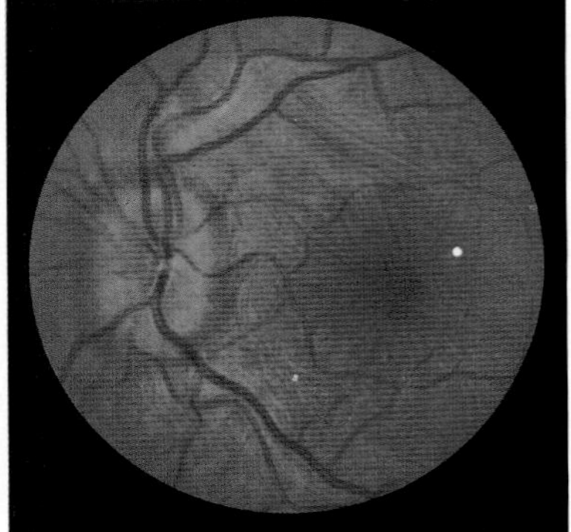

**Papilledema** with conspicuous retinal folding (left eye)

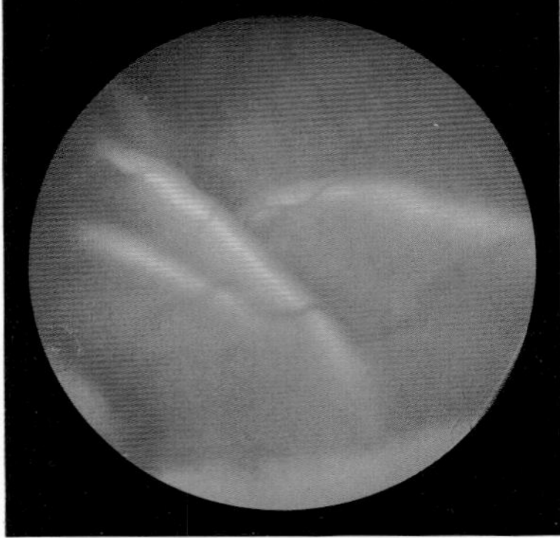

**Retinal detachment** with retinal folds and bayonetlike kinking of vessels (left eye)

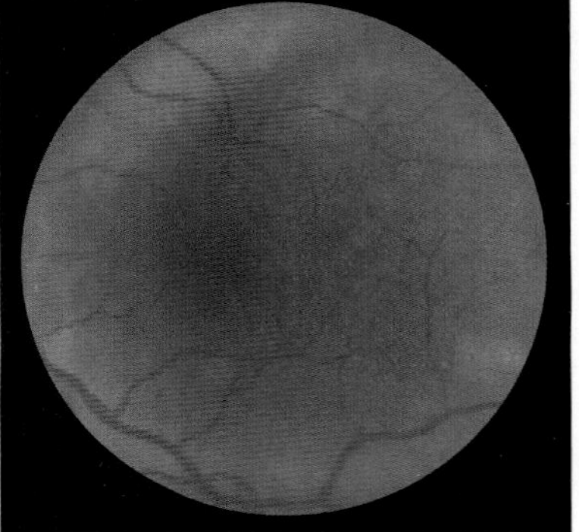

**Melanoma** of the choroid (left eye)

From Sauter/Straub/Truss/Kossmann: *Atlas of the Ocular Fundus*, 3rd edition; Munich, 1984

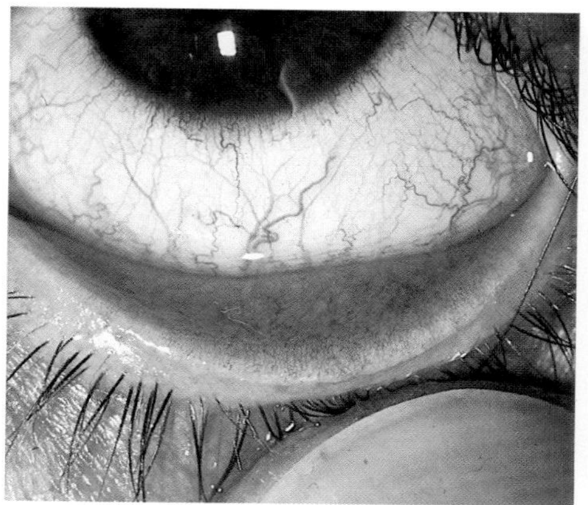

**Conjunctivitis** (herpes zoster)

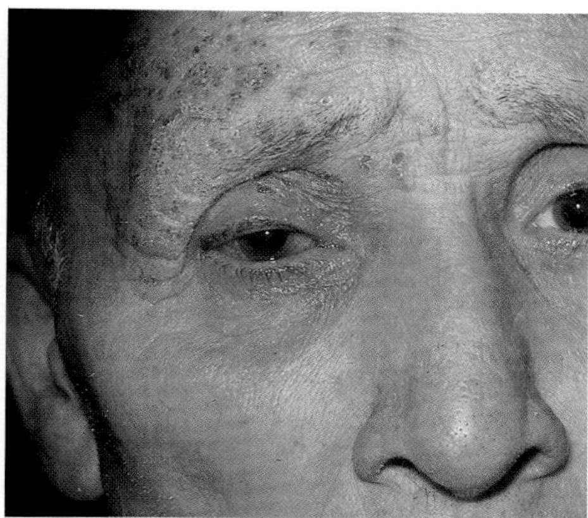

**Herpes zoster ophthalmicus**

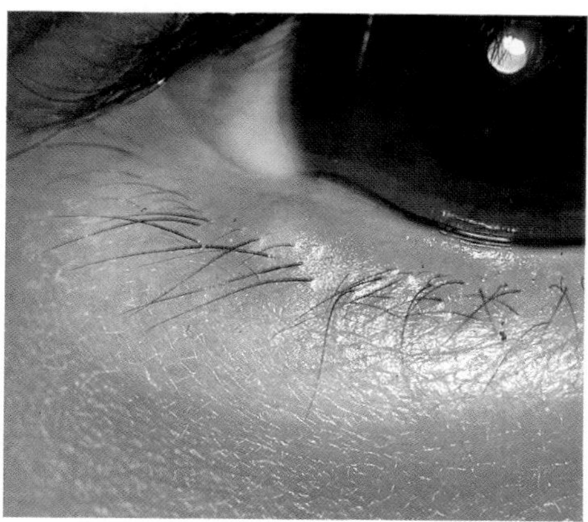

**Stye** (staphylococci)

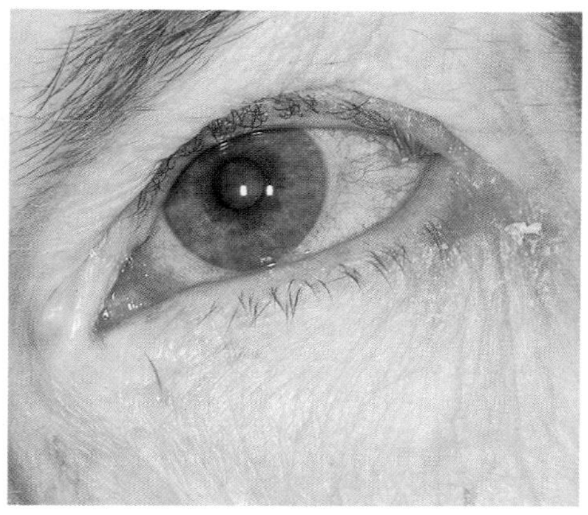

**Blepharitis angularis** *(Staphylococcus aureus)*

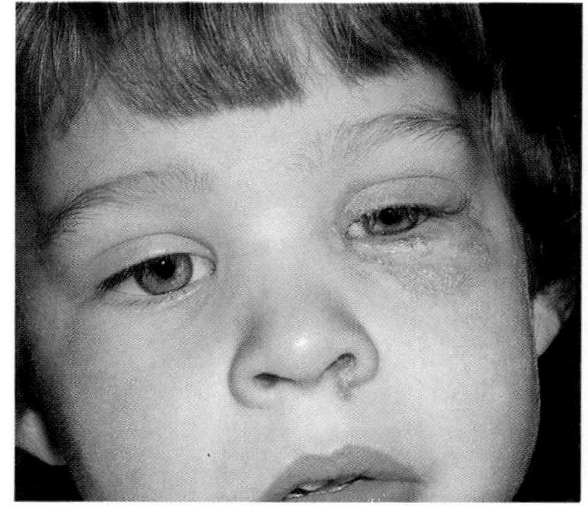

**Impetigo** (β-hemolytic streptococci)

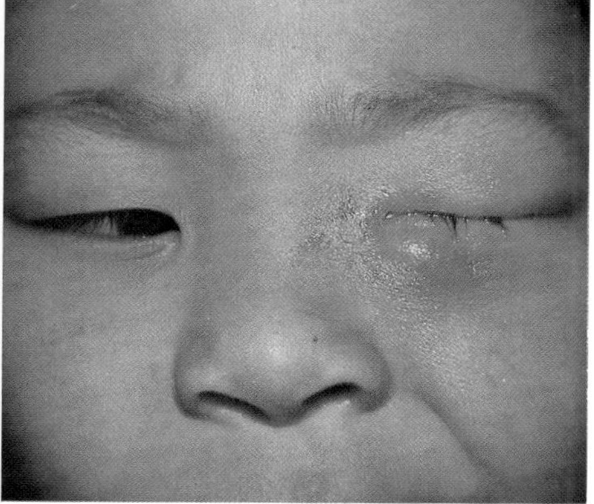

**Dacryocystitis** *(Haemophilus influenzae)*

From Ostler/Dawson/Okumoto: *Color Atlas of Infectious and Inflammatory Diseases of the External Eye:* Munich, 1987

Blood cells: developmental series (simplified scheme)

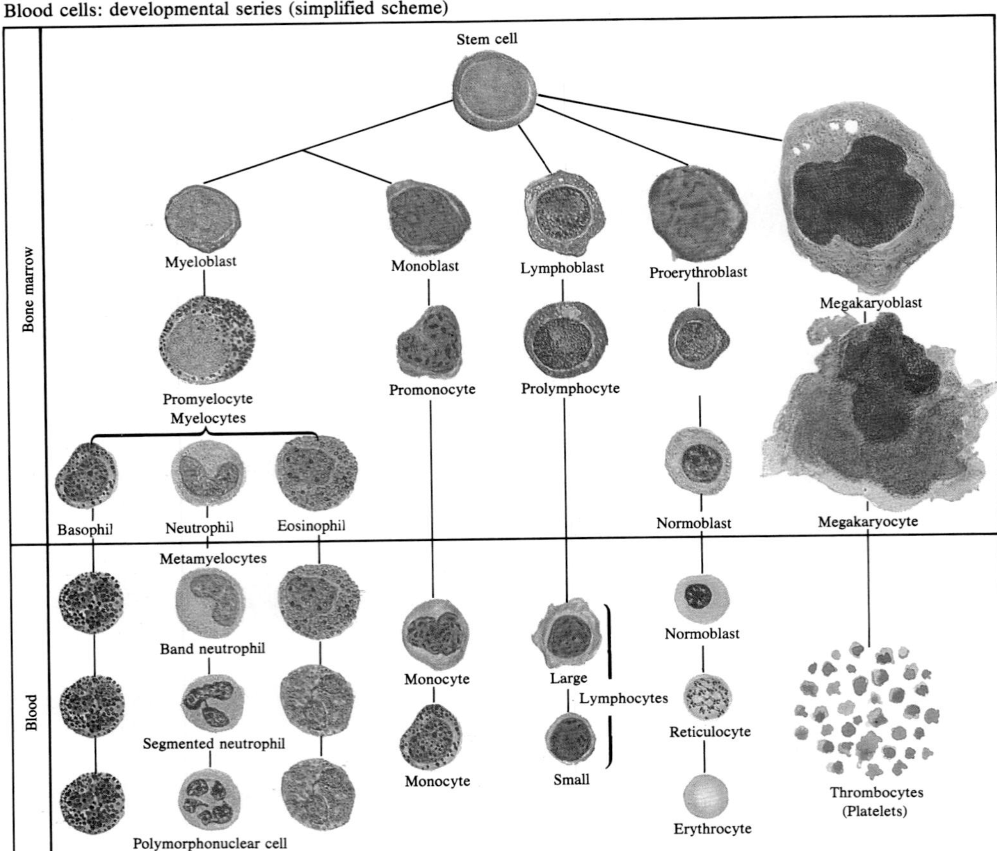


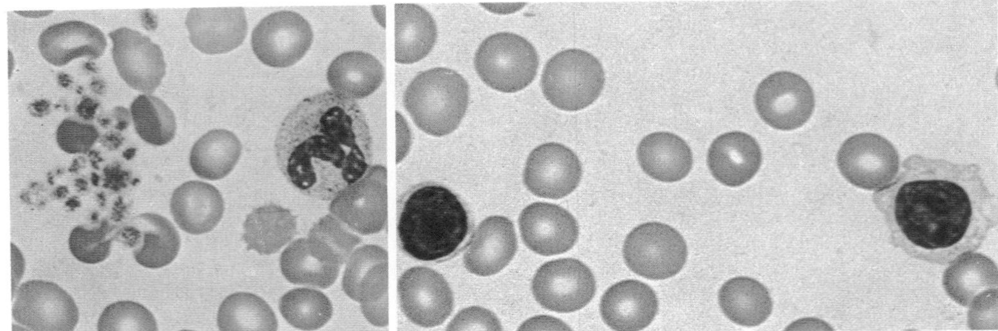

Normal hemogram with thrombocyte (left) and a granulocyte (right)

Normal hemogram with a small lymphocyte (left) and a large lymphocyte (right)

**Color scintigraphy**
Dr. H. Gremmel, Kiel

Scintigraphy of the interior cardiac space using 370 MBq $^{99m}$Tc and Zn(II) as agent. Dynamic study with the gamma camera. Sectional visualization is of the heart and the adjacent large vessels.

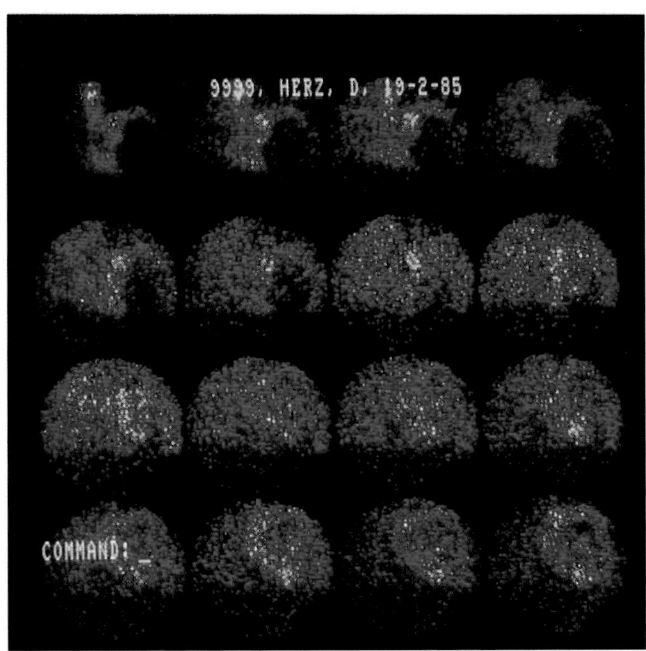


Scintigraphy of the interior cardiac space. Visualization is of the atria and ventricles of the left heart as well as the adjacent large vessels, using the gamma camera; no pathological findings

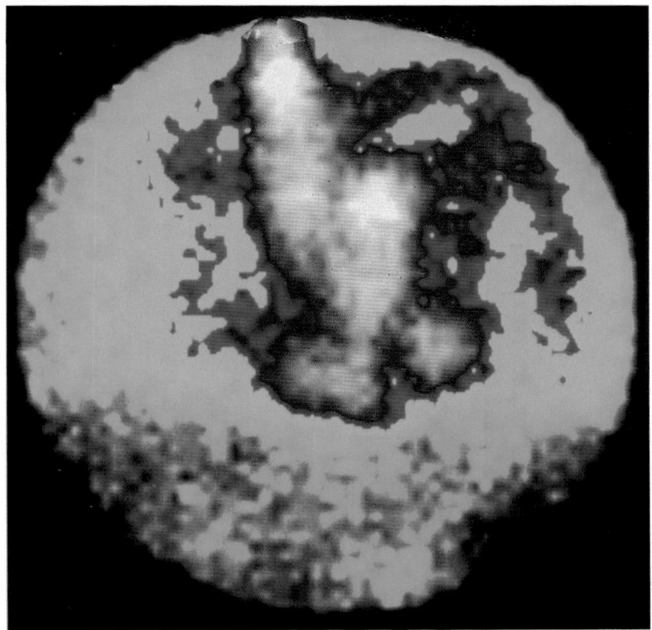

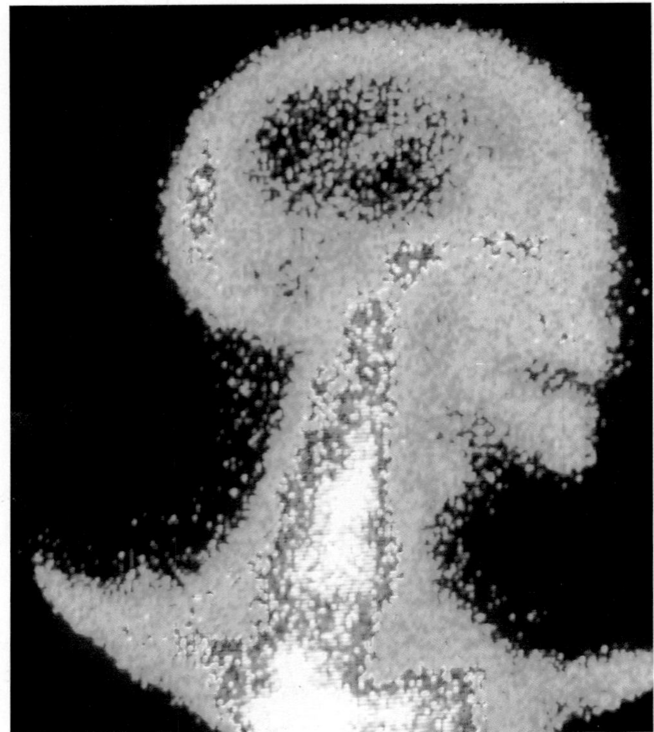

Bone scintigraphy of the skull and cervical spine using 555 MBq $^{98m}Tc$ with Teceos®
Scan is in left lateral projection with the gamma camera; no pathological findings.

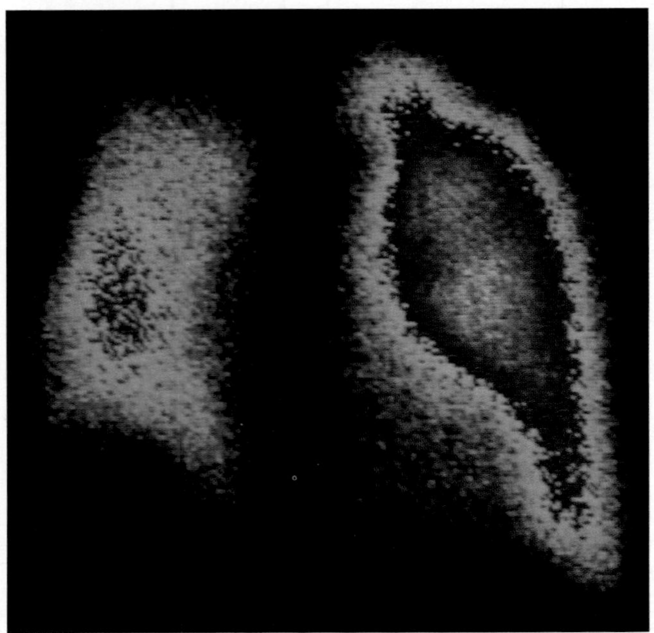

Pulmonary perfusion scintigraphy using 111 MBq $^{99m}Tc$ and microspheres. Collimation picture in ventral projection with the gamma camera shows hypoperfusion on the right side with pneumothorax.

Liver scintigraphy
111 MBq $^{99m}$Tc with sodium phytate.
Collimation picture in ventral projection with the gamma camera, no pathological findings.

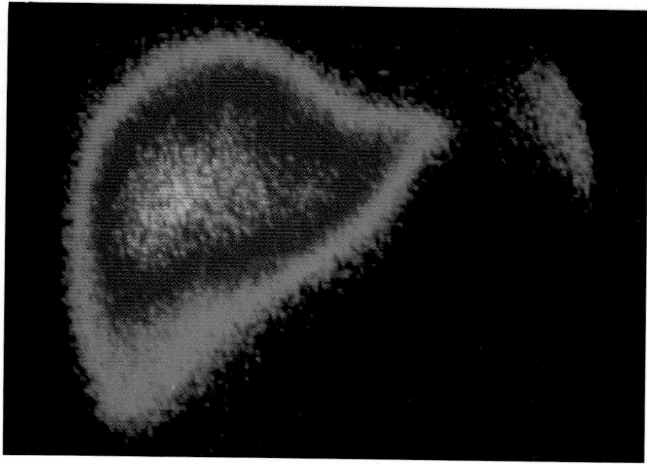

## Color Doppler echocardiography

Dr. D. A. REDEL, Bonn

The color Doppler echocardiography displays the blood flow in color pictures; these pictures are integrated in the conventional two-dimensional echocardiogram which provides a view of the heart structures (walls and valves). The flow velocities are displayed across a sectorial field from maximal 90° up to 32 000 dots, virtually in real time. **Blood flow direction** and **relative flow velocity** as well as **turbulences** are recorded. The flow direction toward the transducer is indicated in warm colors (red or yellow), the flow direction away from the transducer in cool colors (blue or green). An increase in the flow velocity is visualized by increased brightness of colors. If, as a result, penetration depth of the maximal velocity range (the Nyquist limit) is exceeded, a reversal occurs to complementary colors (alias effect), as in illustrations 2 and 4. The alias effect always indicates high velocities. The variance of the instant velocities is a measure of blood flow turbulences as seen in cardiac defects and is visualized by admixture of green to red (resulting in yellow) and green to blue (resulting in turquoise).

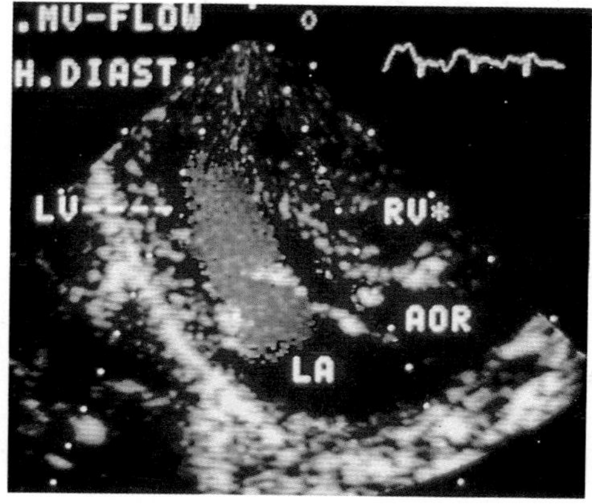


1. Normal diastolic inflow into left ventricle (LV) from left atrium (LA) across the mitral valve, flow direction is toward the transducer; uniform red color of the inflow tract indicates normal diastolic filling of the ventricle. The aortic valve (aortic root = AOR) is closed, the right ventricle is located in the right picture (RV). The sectional plane is parasternal long axis.

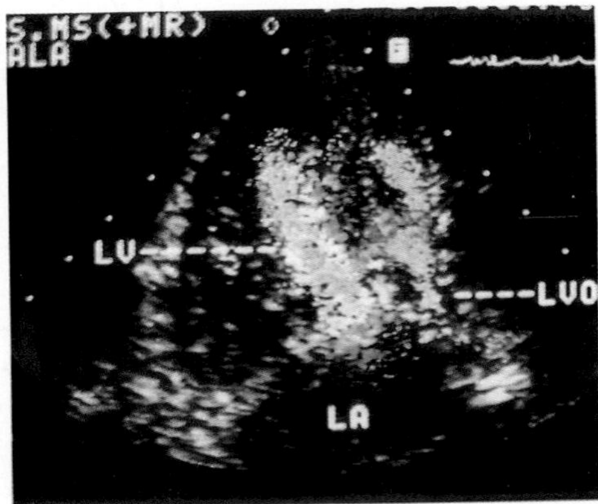


2. Diastolic inflow pattern with mitral stenosis. The so-called candle flame phenomenon is typical, composed of a center field reversed to the complementary color (blue-turquoise). The center field is surrounded by a red-yellow edging, which indicates the actual forward flow direction. Filling of the ventricular outflow tract (LVO) is indicated by the blue color.

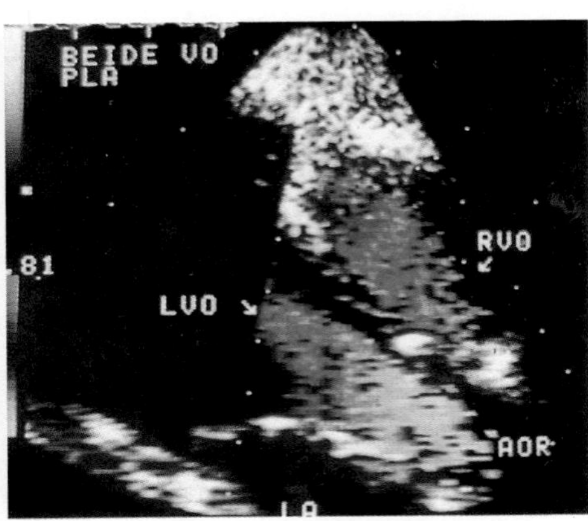


3. Normal systolic outflow from the left ventricle across the left ventricular outflow tract, across the opened aortic valve into the aortic root. Simultaneously the right ventricle empties across the outflow tract (VO) into the pulmonary artery, located above this plane and thus not projected. A distinct velocity increase in the aortic root is visible due to increased color brightness. Turbulences and swirls do not develop. The sectional plane is a parasternal long axis.

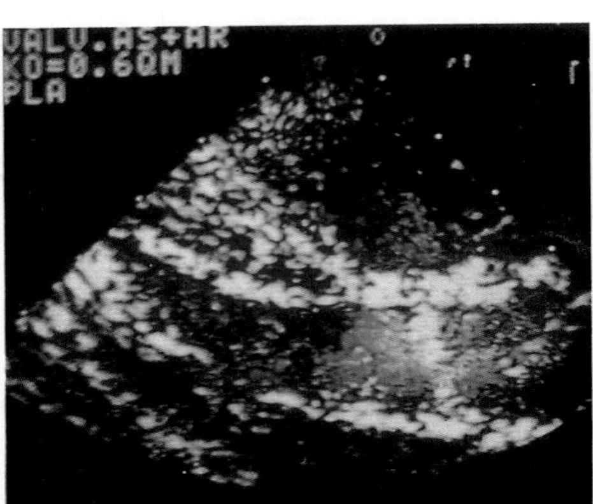


4. Severe aortic valve stenosis in the parasternal long axial section. The narrow base systolic outflow across the aortic valve (blue) into the aortic root is visible as yellow swirls bilateral to the blue jets.

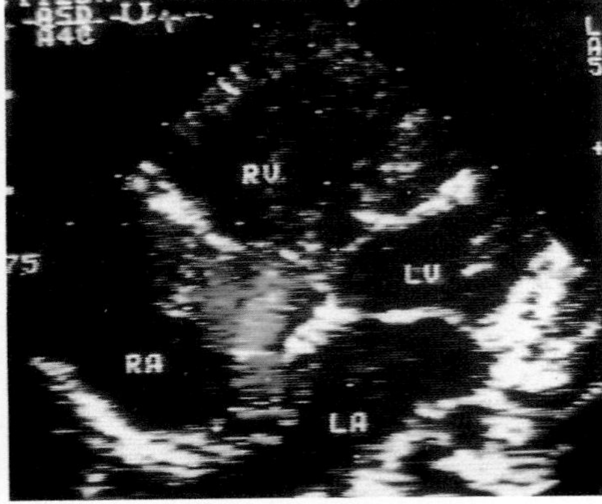


5. Left-right shunt across an atrial septal defect of the Botallo's foramen type, in apical four-chamber view in late systole. The yellow area shows blood passage from the left atrium (LA) to the right atrium (RA) caused by a defect in the interatrial septum. The valves between the atria and ventricles (RV, LV) are still closed.

and the inferior lines gives rise to the gluteus minimus muscle. Also *inferior gluteal line.* **l. glutea posterior** [NA] The posterior, and shortest, of three curved ridges on the gluteal surface of the ala of the ilium, extending downwards from a point on the iliac crest about 5 cm in front of the posterior superior iliac spine to the superior margin of the greater sciatic notch just in front of the posterior inferior iliac spine. A small portion of gluteus maximus muscle arises behind this line. Also *posterior gluteal line.* **l. iliopectinea** *Outmoded* ILIOPECTINEAL LINE. **l. intercondylaris femoris** [NA] A faint transverse ridge separating the posterior part of the intercondylar fossa of the femur from the popliteal surface and providing attachment for the capsule of the knee joint. Also *intercondylar line, intercondyloid line, popliteal line of femur.* **l. intermedia cristae iliacae** [NA] A narrow strip between the outer and the inner lips of the iliac crest, the anterior two-thirds of which provides partial origin for the internal oblique muscle of the abdomen. Also *intermediate line of iliac crest.* **l. intertrochanterica** [NA] A prominent oblique ridge separating the anterior surface of the neck of the femur from the shaft, extending inferomedially from a tubercle at the anterosuperior part of the greater trochanter to a point anterior to the lesser trochanter, where it becomes continuous with the spiral line. The iliofemoral ligament and the capsule of the hip joint are attached to it. Also *intertrochanteric line, anterior intertrochanteric crest.* **l. mamillaris** [NA] A vertical line, parallel to the median plane, passing through the nipple of either breast. Because of the variable position of the nipple, it is untenable to equate it with the linea medioclavicularis, with which it occasionally overlaps. Also *mamillary line, nipple line.* **l. mediana anterior** [NA] A vertical line on the anterior surface of the body along the median plane, dividing the body into equal right and left halves. Also *anterior median line.* **l. mediana posterior** [NA] A vertical line on the posterior surface of the body along the median plane, dividing the body into equal right and left halves. Also *posterior median line.* **l. medio-axillaris** LINEA AXILLARIS MEDIA. **l. medioclavicularis** [NA] A vertical line, parallel to the median plane, passing through the midpoint between the jugular notch and the tip of the acromion and extending down the trunk on each side to cross the inguinal ligament midway between the anterior superior iliac spine and the symphysis pubis. Occasionally it may coincide with the mamillary line but by definition it is not the same. Also *midclavicular line, lateral line.* See also POUPART'S LINE. **l. musculi solei** [NA] An oblique ridge on the posterior surface of the tibia extending downward and medially from the fibular facet to the medial border about one-third of the distance from the upper end. Attached to it are the soleus muscle and its fascia, the popliteal fascia and the fascia covering the deep muscles of the leg. Also *soleal line of tibia, popliteal line of tibia.* **l. mylohyoidea mandibulae** [NA] An oblique ridge on the medial surface of the body of the mandible extending from a point behind the third molar tooth just below the alveolar margin to the lower end of the symphysis menti below the mental spine. It provides attachment for the mylohyoid muscle, helping to form the floor of the mouth, and posteriorly for part of the superior constrictor muscle of the pharynx and for the pterygomandibular raphe. Also *mylohyoid line of mandible, mylohyoidean line, mylohyoid ridge.* **l. nigra** The linea alba of the abdomen during pregnancy, when it becomes pigmented. **l. nuchae inferior** [NA] A curved bony ridge on the external surface of the squamous part of the occipital bone extending laterally from the midpoint of the external occipital crest to the jugular process and providing attachment for the upper margins of the rectus capitis posterior major and minor muscles. Also *inferior nuchal line.* **l. nuchae superior** [NA] A curved bony ridge on the external surface of the squamous part of the occipital bone extending laterally from the external occipital protuberance towards the lateral angle and providing attachment for the trapezius muscle medially and the sternocleidomastoid muscle laterally. Also *superior nuchal line.* **l. nuchae suprema** [NA] A faint curved bony ridge on the external surface of the squamous part of the occipital bone extending laterally from the external occipital protuberance above the superior nuchal line and providing attachment for the galea aponeurotica. Also *highest nuchal line, supreme nuchal line.* **l. obliqua cartilaginis thyroideae** [NA] A curved line on the external surface of the lamina of the thyroid cartilage extending anteroinferiorly between the superior and the inferior tubercles and providing attachment to the sternothyroid and thyrohyoid muscles and the inferior constrictor muscle of the pharynx. Also *oblique line of thyroid cartilage, oblique crest of thyroid cartilage.* **l. obliqua mandibulae** [NA] An indefinite ridge on the outer surface of the body of the mandible extending backwards and upwards from the mental tubercle to the lower end of the anterior margin of the ramus, and providing attachment, anteriorly, for the depressor muscles of the mouth. Also *oblique line of mandible.* **l. parasternalis** [NA] A vertical line drawn on the anterior surface of the trunk midway between and parallel to the sternal and midclavicular lines. Also *parasternal line.* **l. pectinea femoris** [NA] A slight ridge on the posteromedial aspect of the upper part of the shaft of the femur, descending from the base of the lesser trochanter to the top of the linea aspera and lying between the spiral line medially and the gluteal tuberosity laterally. The pectineus muscle is attached to it. Also *pectineal line, pectineal crest of femur.* **l. scapularis** [NA] A vertical line drawn through the inferior angle of the scapula and parallel to the median plane. Also *scapular line.* **l. semilunaris** An irregularly curved groove on the abdominal surface outlining the lateral margin of each rectus abdominis muscle and extending from the tip of the ninth costal cartilage to the pubic tubercle. It is best seen in lean, muscular individuals. Also *semilunar line, Spieghel's line, Spigelius line, spigelian line, semilunar line of Spieghel.* **l. spiralis** *Outmoded* SPIRAL LINE OF FEMUR. **l. splendens** A reduplication of pia mater in the fissura mediana anterior medullae spinalis forming a sheath for the anterior spinal artery. *Seldom used.* **l. sternalis** [NA] A vertical line corresponding to the lateral sternal margin on the anterior surface of the thorax. Also *sternal line, lateral sternal line.* **l. temporalis inferior ossis parietalis** [NA] The lower of two curved transverse lines, convex upwards, crossing the middle of the external surface of the parietal bone, to which the temporalis muscle is attached. Also *inferior temporal line of parietal bone.* **l. temporalis ossis frontalis** [NA] A prominent line curving back from the zygomatic process of the frontal bone and soon dividing into superior and inferior lines that are continuous with the two lines traversing the parietal bone. Also *temporal line of frontal bone, temporal crest of frontal bone, external frontal crest, temporal ridge.* **l. temporalis superior ossis parietalis** [NA] The upper of two curved transverse lines, convex upwards, crossing the middle of the external surface of the parietal bone and providing attachment for the temporal fascia. Also *superior temporal line of parietal bone.* **l. terminalis pelvis** [NA] A ridge on the inner surface of the side walls of the bony pelvis, comprising the arcuate line posteriorly, the iliopectineal line and pecten pubis laterally, and crest of pubis anteriorly on each side, continuous with the promontory of the sacrum posteriorly and dividing the false, or major, pelvis above from the true, or minor, pelvis below. It forms most of the boundary of the superior aperture, or inlet, of the minor pelvis. Also *terminal line of pelvis, iliopectineal crest of pelvis, arcuate line of pelvis.* **lineae transversae ossis sacri** [NA] Four transverse ridges on the pelvic surface of the sacrum extending between the paired pelvic sacral foramina as lines of fusion between the bodies and representing the positions of the former intervertebral disks. Also *transverse lines of sacrum, transverse ridges of sacrum.* **l. trapezoidea** [NA] A narrow ridge running anterolaterally from the conoid tubercle on the posterior border of the inferior surface of the lateral third of the clavicle and providing attachment for the trapezoid ligament, a part of the coracoclavicular ligament. Also *trapezoid line.* **l. visus** VISUAL AXIS. **l. vitalis** A flexure line encircling the thenar eminence on the palm of the hand. Also *radial longitudinal line.*

**lineae** \lin′i·ē\ Plural of LINEA.

**lineage** \lin′ē·ij\ [French *lignage* (from *ligne* line, from LINEA) race, lineage] **1** The direct descendants of an individual. **2** The line of descent of a strain of cells cultured *in vitro.* **sympathetic cell l.** Categories of cells derived from the neural crest epithelium and including the following types: sympathogonia, unipolar sympathoblasts, multipolar sympathetic neurons, paraganglionic cells.

**lineal** \lin′ē·əl\ Of or relating to direct descent, as in a pedigree.

**linear** \lin′ē·ər\ Relating to or having the properties of a line. Also *lineal.*

**linebreeding** INBREEDING.

**liner** A protective or insulating layer applied to a surface, especially to the inside of a container or cavity. **cavity l.** A thin layer of varnish placed in a prepared dental cavity before placing the cement base. Also *cavity primer, cavity varnish.* **soft l.** A soft material for application to the fitting surfaces of dentures. It may be a synthetic elastomer or a plasticized acrylic polymer. Also *soft lining.*

**Lineweaver** [Hans *Lineweaver,* U.S chemist, born 1907] Lineweaver-Burk equation. See under LINEWEAVER-BURK PLOT.

**Ling** [Per Henrik *Ling,* Swedish hygienist, 1776–1839] Ling's method. See under SWEDISH GYMNASTICS.

**lingism** \ling′izm\ SWEDISH GYMNASTICS.

**lingua** \ling′gwə\ [L (alter. of earlier *dingua,* akin to English *tongue*) tongue, speech, language. (The dialect variant *l-* prob. replaced *d-* by assimilation to *lingere* to lick.)] [NA] A muscular organ covered with mucous membrane on its upper and lower surfaces, situated in the floor of the mouth and the anterior wall of the pharynx, and involved in mastication, swallowing, taste, and speech; the tongue. It is composed of three layers of intrinsic muscles which alter its shape, and it is connected to the mandible, hyoid bone, styloid process, and palate by four pairs of extrinsic muscles which can move it in all directions. The motor nerve is the hypoglossal nerve, while sensory and taste innervation come from the fifth, seventh, and ninth cranial nerves. Also *glossa.* **l. cerebelli** The most anteroventral portion of the cerebellar vermis, bounded inferiorly by the superior medullary velum and superiorly by the lobus centralis. **l. nigra** BLACK HAIRY TONGUE. **l. villosa nigra** BLACK HAIRY TONGUE.

**lingua-** \ling′gwə-\ LINGUO-.

**linguae** \ling′gwē\ Plural of LINGUA.

**lingual** \ling′gwəl\ **1** Relating to the tongue; lingualis. **2** Resembling or suggestive of a tongue; linguiform. **3** Next to or in the direction of the tongue.

**linguale** \ling·gwā′lē\ In craniometry, the highest point on the lingual surface of symphysis menti.

***Linguatula*** \ling·gwat′ʸələ\ [Late L *linguatus* tongued + -ULA *-ule*] A genus of bloodsucking parasites, the tongue worms, of the phylum Pentastomida (family Linguatulidae, order Porocephalida), which are endoparasitic as adults in the lungs, sinuses, and other air passages of various animals, including man. Larvae are found in the digestive organs and lungs of a wide variety of hosts. Also *Pentastoma.*

**linguatuliasis** \ling·gwat′yəlī′əsis\ [*Linguatul(a)* + -IASIS] Infection with pentastome parasites of the genus *Linguatula.* Also *linguatulosis.*

**linguatulid** \ling·gwat′yəlid\ [*Linguatul(ida)* + -ID[1]] **1** Pertaining or belonging to the family Linguatulidae. **2** A pentastome worm of the family Linguatulidae.

**Linguatulidae** \ling′gwatʸ oo′lidē\ A family of parasites in the order Porocephalida, class or phylum Pentostomida. Having a flattened body resembling acanthocephalan worms, they are parasitic in the nasal cavities of dogs, cats, and other carnivores in the adult form, and in the tissues of rodents, herbivores, and many other animals in the larval (or nymphal) form. Both forms have been reported from humans, the larval form from ingestion of eggs, the adult form from ingestion of raw or undercooked liver or other organs.

**linguatulosis** \ling·gwat′yəlō′sis\ LINGUATULIASIS.

**lingula** \ling′gyoolə\ [L, dim. of LINGUA] A small structure or process shaped like or suggestive of a tongue. • When used without modifiers the term commonly refers to lingula cerebelli. **l. cerebelli** [NA] The most anterior and ventral portion of the vermis of the cerebellum. It is the medial component of the anterior lobe, and receives the attachment of the superior medullary velum. Also *lingula of cerebellum.* **l. of left lung** LINGULA PULMONIS SINISTRI. **l. mandibulae** [NA] A small projection of bone anteromedial to the mandibular foramen on the medial surface of the ramus of the mandible, providing attachment to the sphenomandibular ligament. Also *lingula of mandible, spine of Spix.* **l. pulmonis sinistri** [NA] An occasional projection of the lower end of the anterior border of the superior lobe of the left lung, just below the cardiac notch and above the oblique fissure. Also *lingula of left lung.* **l. sphenoidalis** [NA] A narrow bony projection between the posterior part of the lateral surface of the body of the sphenoid bone and the greater wing of the sphenoid, forming the lateral margin of the back of the carotid sulcus and roofing the posterior opening of the pterygoid canal. Also *lingula of sphenoid, sphenoidal lingula.*

**lingulae** \ling′gyəlē\ Plural of LINGULA.

**lingular** \ling′gyələr\ Pertaining to a lingula or lingula-like process.

**lingulate** \ling′gyəlāt\ Like a tongue or a lingula; linguiform.

**lingulectomy** \ling′gyəlek′təmē\ [*lingul(a)* + -ECTOMY] Removal of the lingula of the left upper lobe of the lung.

**linguo-** \ling′gwō-\ [L *lingua* tongue, language] A combining form denoting the tongue or relationship to the tongue. Also *lingua-.*

**linguocervical** \-sur′vikəl\ Pertaining to the lingual aspect of the neck of a tooth. Also *cervicolingual.*

**linguoclination** \-klinā′shən\ [LINGUO- + *(in)clination*] The inclination of a tooth in the lingual direction.

**linguoclusion** \-kloo′zhən\ [LINGUO- + *(oc)clusion*] Linguoversion of a group of teeth.

**linguodental** \-den′təl\ [LINGUO- +DENTAL] Relating to both the tongue and the teeth.

**linguopapillitis** \-pap′ilī′tis\ Inflammation of the lingual papillae, particularly along the edges of the tongue. An unspecific and seldom used term.
**linguoplacement** \-plās′mənt\ LINGUOVERSION.
**linguoplate** \ling′gwōplāt\ [LINGUO- + PLATE] A major connector in a partial denture which covers the gingivae and the cingula of the anterior teeth.
**linguoversion** \-vur′zhən\ [LINGUO- + VERSION] The deviation of a tooth from the arch towards the tongue. Also *linguoplacement, lingual placement.*
**liniment** [L *linimentum.* See LINIMENTUM.] An oily liquid preparation, applied externally or to the gums. It may be a solution, suspension, or emulsion; and used as a counterirritant, anodyne, or cleansing agent. **ammoniated l. of camphor** A liniment containing 12% camphor, strong ammonia solution, and lavender oil in alcohol. **l. of belladonna** A liniment prepared by percolating belladonna root with 80% alcohol, followed by the addition of camphor. **camphor l.** A liniment containing 20% camphor in arachis oil. Also *camphorated oil.* **medicinal soft soap l.** GREEN SOAP TINCTURE.
**linimentum** [L (from *lin(ere)* to smear + *i* + *-mentum* -MENT), an ointment, anointing] Liniment. **l. saponis mollis** GREEN SOAP TINCTURE.
**linin** A substance that forms fine threadlike structures to which nuclear chromatin granules appear to be attached. An obsolete term.
**lining** 1 A cement base under a dental restoration. A British usage. 2 An extra layer on the fitting surface of a denture. **soft l.** SOFT LINER.
**linitis** \linī′tis\ [Gk *lin(on)* a thing made of flax, thread, fishing net, linen + -ITIS] Inflammation of the stomach. *Older term.* **l. plastica** A thickening and stiffening of the wall of the stomach due to diffuse mural infiltration by a poorly differentiated scirrhous carcinoma. Also *sclerotic stomach, gastric sclerosis.*
**link / salt l.** The attraction between two ions of opposite charge, i.e. the same type of bond as between the ions of a salt crystal. The term often applies to this attraction between two amino-acid side chains of a protein.
**linkage** The tendency for genes, during breeding, not to segregate entirely at random but in daughter cells to remain associated in their original combinations. In eukaryotic cells, linkage usually indicates that the linked genes are carried on the same chromosome. Linkage analysis is the experimental determination of the degree to which genetic markers tend to remain together during recombination. This is inversely proportional to the distance that separates these genes from each other. That is, the greater the degree of random segregation of two genes, the less the linkage, and the more recombination between them. When the chance of recombination between two genes is 50 percent, segregation is random, and the genes are unlinked, although they might still be syntenic. **record l.** The systematic linking of all relevant items of information relating to each individual in a population or group so as to provide a cumulative and up-to-date record of the significant health events, such as hospitalizations and immunization and vaccination procedures, affecting the individual. • Record linkage is practiced chiefly in the U.S., United Kingdom, and Canada, although it is known and sometimes made use of in New Zealand and India. **sex l.** 1 An inheritance in which a phenotype is determined by a genetic locus on a sex chromosome. In humans, nearly all such phenotypes are X-linked. 2 A genetic locus that occurs on a sex chromosome. It is designated by specifying the chromosome on which the linkage occurs. **Y l.** Linkage associated with loci on the Y chromosome.
**Linodil** A proprietary name for inositol niacinate.
**linoleic acid** $CH_3—[CH_2]_4—CH═CH—CH_2—CH═CH—[CH_2]_7—COOH$. An essential fatty acid. It is produced in plants as its coenzyme-A derivative by insertion of the 12-13 double bond in the *cis* configuration. It (or other polyunsaturated fatty acids with which it is interconvertible, such as linolenic acid and arachidonic acid) is required in the mammalian diet, especially as a precursor of prostaglandins.
**linolenic acid** $CH_3—[CH_2—CH═CH—]_3—[CH_2]_7—COOH$. An essential fatty acid, interconvertible with arachidonic acid and linoleic acid, required for prostaglandin synthesis.
**linseed** The dried ripe seed of *Linum usitatissium,* flax. It contains mucilage, protein, and a fixed oil (linseed oil) which constitutes 30 to 40 percent of the seed. If taken internally, the oil acts as a demulcent and laxative. Also *linum.*
**Linser** [Paul *Linser,* German dermatologist, born 1871] See under METHOD.
**Linstowiidae** A family of small to medium-sized tapeworms (order Cyclophyllidea, subclass Cestoda) that are parasitic in reptiles, birds, and mammals, including humans. Genera of medical importance as rarely reported parasites of man include *Oochoristica* and *Inermicapsifer.* They inhabit the intestine but their effects, if any, are unknown.
**lint** A surgical dressing material originally made of scrapings from linen cloth but now made of a specially finished fabric. Also *charpie.*
**Linton** [Robert Ritchie *Linton,* U.S. surgeon, born 1900] See under PROCEDURE.
**linum** \lin′əm\ LINSEED.
**Linzenmeier** [Georg *Linzenmeier,* German physician, born 1882] See under TEST.
**lio-** \lī′ō-\ LEIO-.
**lip** [Old English *lippa,* akin to L *labium* lip and *labrum* lip, edge, rim] 1 Either the upper or the lower fleshy fold forming the movable anterior wall of the mouth cavity and surrounding the oral fissure; labium oris. 2 Any projecting liplike margin or edge; labium; labrum. **acetabular l.** LABRUM ACETABULARE. **anterior l. of cervix of uterus** LABIUM ANTERIUS OSTII UTERI. **anterior l. of ostium of uterus** LABIUM ANTERIUS OSTII UTERI. **cleft l.** A developmental defect consisting of a notch, fur-

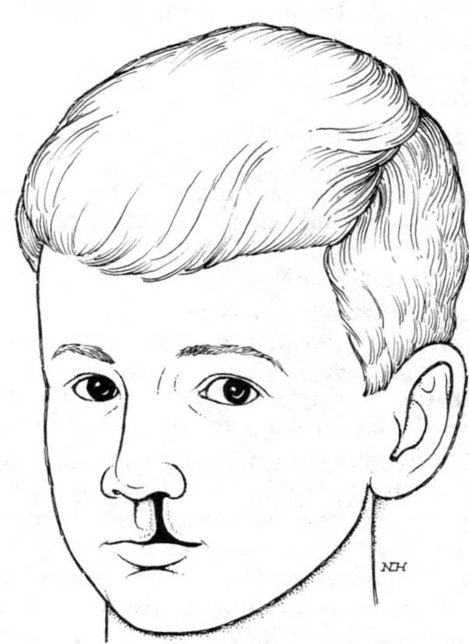

Cleft lip

row, or open fissure of the upper lip with or without associated cleft of the maxilla. The cleavage is usually on one side of the philtrum and premaxilla. It is sometimes bilateral, in which case a segment of lip and associated premaxilla are relatively set apart on the midline. Rarely, the midline segments are absent, and then the midline cleft bears some resemblance to that of a hare. It results from the failure of the embryonic medial nasal and maxillary processes to unite in normal embryogenesis. It is often associated with cleft palate, and infrequently with genal or oblique facial cleft. Also *harelip, cheiloschisis.* **dorsal l. of blastopore** In amphibians, the dorsal edge of the blastopore, formed by invagination. It appears precociously at the start of the invagination process at gastrulation and in essence marks the appearance of the notochord. The cells of the dorsal lip have been shown to possess organizing powers. **double l.** A fold of tissue on the inner side of the lip resembling a second lip. Habitual sucking between the teeth may be a factor in its development. **external l. of iliac crest** LABIUM EXTERNUM CRISTAE ILIACAE. **external l. of linea aspera of femur** LABIUM LATERALE LINEAE ASPERAE FEMORIS. **fibrocartilaginous l. of acetabulum** LABRUM ACETABULARE. **glenoid l.** LABRUM GLENOIDALE. **greater l. of pudendum** LABIUM MAJUS PUDENDI. **inferior l.** LABIUM INFERIUS ORIS. **internal l. of iliac crest** LABIUM INTERNUM CRISTAE ILIACAE. **lateral l.'s of blastopore** The two lateral edges of the blastopore which extend from the dorsal lip to the ventral lip. **lateral l. of linea aspera of femur** LABIUM LATERALE LINEAE ASPERAE FEMORIS. **lesser l. of pudendum** LABIUM MINUS PUDENDI. **lower l.** LABIUM INFERIUS ORIS. **medial l. of linea aspera of femur** LABIUM MEDIALE LINEAE ASPERAE FEMORIS. **posterior l. of cervix of uterus** LABIUM POSTERIUS OSTII UTERI. **posterior l. of ostium of uterus** LABIUM POSTERIUS OSTII UTERI. **rhombic l.** The lateral edge of the embryonic rhombencephalon. **superior l.** LABIUM SUPERIUS ORIS. **tapir l.'s** TAPIR MOUTH. **tympanic l. of limb of spiral lamina** LABIUM LIMBI TYMPANICUM LAMINAE SPIRALIS. **upper l.** LABIUM SUPERIUS ORIS. **ventral l. of blastopore** The ventral edge of the blastopore, appearing after the dorsal lip and to which it will be united by the lateral lips. **vestibular l. of limb of spiral lamina** LABIUM LIMBI VESTIBULARE LAMINAE SPIRALIS.

**lip-** \lip-\ LIPO-.

**lipa-** \lip′ə-\ LIPO-.

**lipacidemia** \-asidē′mē·ə\ The presence of fatty acid in blood.

**lipaciduria** [LIP- + ACIDURIA] Urinary excretion of fatty acids, which is increased in ketoacidosis. A rarely used term.

**lipaemia** *Brit.* LIPEMIA.

**liparocele** \lip′ərōsēl\ LIPOCELE.

**liparodyspnea** \lip′ərōdispnē′ə\ Difficulty in breathing secondary to obesity.

**liparomphalus** \lip′əräm′fələs\ [Gk *lipar(os)* oily, fat + *omphalos* the navel] A lipoma of the umbilicus.

**lipase** \lip′ās\ Any enzyme that catalyzes the hydrolysis of a fat. **pancreatic l.** The lipolytic digestive enzyme secreted by the exocrine pancreas. It is a triacylglycerol lipase (EC 3.1.1.3). Also *pancreatolipase.*

**lipectomy** \lipek′təmē\ [LIP- + -ECTOMY] The excision of a mass of subcutaneous adipose tissue. It is usually from the abdominal wall but it may be taken from any part of the body. Also *adipectomy.* **suction l.** A lipectomy performed by means of a vacuum device, usually utilized in the region of the hips and thighs. The device is applied through a metal cannula which is inserted into the subcutaneous tissue through a small incision. **submental l.** A cosmetic operation for the removal of excessive fat beneath the chin.

**lipemia** \lipē′mē·ə\ [LIP- + -EMIA] **1** *Imprecise* HYPERLIPIDEMIA. **2** Greater than normal turbidity of plasma due to the presence of lipids. **alimentary l.** Transient lipemia developing after consumption of lipid-rich food. It is due largely to increase in the number of chylomicrons. Also *postprandial lipemia.* **diabetic l.** Raised plasma values of triglycerides in uncontrolled diabetes mellitus. Many physiologic events combine to raise triglycerides, largely insulin lack, low levels of lipoprotein lipase, and low plasma postheparin lipolytic activity. Insulin repletion reverses these processes. **postprandial l.** ALIMENTARY LIPEMIA. **l. retinalis** A creamy or milky appearance of the retinal blood vessels due to marked hyperlipemia of any cause.

**lipemic** \lipē′mik\ **1** Having increased concentration of lipids in serum or plasma. **2** Having a cloudy or milky appearance: used of a plasma or serum specimen.

**lipfanogen** \lipfan′əjən\ Any substance which, when taken up by cells, results in formation of globules of fat in the cytoplasm of the cell.

**lipid** \lip′id\ [LIP- + -ID[1]] Any natural compound soluble in apolar but not in polar solvents. Lipids usually contain residues of fatty acids, one-chain alcohols, steroids, or sphingoids. Lipids therefore include fats and phospholipids. Also *lipoid* (outmoded). **Gaucher l.** CEREBROSIDE. **Niemann-Pick l.** SPHINGOMYELIN. **skin surface l.** The lipid found on the skin surface. In the human this is composed mainly of sebum from the sebaceous glands, with a small contribution from the keratinizing epidermis and traces derived from exogenous sources, such as soaps and cosmetics.

**lipid A** The endotoxic component of lipopolysaccharide, consisting of a $\beta$-1,6-D-glucosamine disaccharide with all of its OH groups substituted (with two phosphates, a ketodeoxyoctonate trisaccharide link to the O antigen, and three fatty acids) and its $NH_2$ groups substituted with hydroxymyristic acid.

**lipidolysis** \lip′idäl′isis\ LIPOLYSIS.

**lipidosis** \lip′idō′sis\ [LIPID + -OSIS] Any disorder of lipid metabolism in which abnormal amounts of lipid are stored within cells of the reticuloendothelial system. Also *lipid storage disease.* **cerebral l.** Any of a group of genetically determined disorders in which abnormal amounts of lipid are stored within brain neurons. Also *familial cerebral lipidosis.* **ganglioside l.** GANGLIOSIDOSIS. **neurovisceral l.** $GM_1$ GANGLIOSIDOSIS. **sphingomyelin l.** NIEMANN-PICK DISEASE. **sulfatide l.** METACHROMATIC LEUKODYSTROPHY.

**lipiduria** \lip′idoo′rē·ə\ The presence of fat in the urine, as neutral fat bodies floating in the urine, oval fat bodies which appear yellow or black under reduced light and which may be single or aggregated, casts with inclusion fat or fatty cells, renal tubular epithelial cells containing neutral fat which stain red with Sudan III or oil red, or degenerating fatty vacuoles. It is characteristic of but not specific for the nephrotic syndrome. Also *lipuria.*

**lipo-** \lip′ō-, lī′pō-\ [Gk *lipos* fat, lard, oil] A combining form meaning fat or lipid. Also *lip-, lipa-.*

**lipoadenoma** \-ad′ənō′mə\ [LIPO- + ADEN- + -OMA] A rare tumor, typically of the parathyroid, composed of an intimate admixture of glandular and fatty tissue. Also *adenolipoma.*

**lipoamide** The amide of lipoic acid, which is the cyclic disulfide formed by oxidation of 6,8-dimercaptooctanoic acid. Since lipoic acid occurs in enzymes in amide combination with the side chain of a lysine residue, enzymes that catalyze conversions of the lipoyl group often act also on free lipoamide.

**lipoamide reductase** DIHYDROLIPOAMIDE DEHYDROGENASE.

**lipoarthritis** \-ärthrī′tis\ Arthritis associated with any one of several types of lipid storage disorders or hyperlipidemia.

**lipoatrophy** \-at′rəfē\ **1** Atrophy of adipose tissue, as at subcutaneous sites of insulin injection. **2** LIPODYSTROPHY.

**lipoblast** \lip′əblast\ [LIPO- + -BLAST] A cell, originating in connective tissue, which becomes a fat cell. The cell usually has a polyhedral shape and contains numerous small lipid droplets.

**lipoblastoma** \-blastō′mə\ A localized lesion or form of lipoblastomatosis.

**lipoblastomatosis** \-blas′tōmətō′sis\ [LIPOBLAST + -OMA + *t* + -OSIS] A benign lobulated tumor of fetal fat cells seen primarily in infants. It may be localized or diffuse.

**lipocele** \lip′əsēl\ [LIPO- + -CELE[1]] A hernia containing fatty tissue. Also *adipocele, liparocele.*

**lipochromemia** \-krōmē′mē·ə\ A greater than normal concentration of carotenoid pigments in blood, as in hypercarotenemia.

**lipoclasis** LIPOLYSIS.

**lipoclastic** \-klas′tik\ LIPOLYTIC.

**lipocyte** \lip′əsīt\ [LIPO- + -CYTE] FAT CELL.

**lipodermatosclerosis** \-dur′mətōsklirō′sis\ A brawny, pigmented fibrosis of the skin and subcutaneous tissues of the lower leg that results from chronic venous stasis. Also *liposclerosis.*

**lipodystrophy** \-dis′trəfē\ [LIPO- + DYSTROPHY] A condition characterized by abnormal fat metabolism. Also *lipodystrophia.* **acquired generalized l.** A form of lipodystrophy that often develops after another illness or pregnancy. Characterized by loss of body fat (unlike the congenital form the face may be spared), accelerated linear growth, liver enlargement, nephrotic syndrome, hyperglycemia with insulin resistance, hypertriglyceridemia, and increased metabolic activity with normal thyroid function. Also *Lawrence syndrome.* **acquired partial l.** PROGRESSIVE LIPODYSTROPHY. **cephalothoracic l.** Lipodystrophy involving the head and thorax. **congenital l.** SEIP SYNDROME. **familial generalized l.** SEIP SYNDROME. **familial l. of limbs and trunk** A rare familial lipodystrophy of the limbs and lower trunk, sparing the face, neck, and upper trunk, inherited as a dominant trait. The condition chiefly affects women, with onset at puberty. Also *reverse partial lipodystrophy, Köbberling-Dunnigan syndrome.* **generalized l.** SEIP SYNDROME. **inferior l.** Lipodystrophy involving the lower limbs. **insulin l.** Atrophy of subcutaneous fat at sites of insulin injection. Also *insulin-induced lipodystrophy.* **intestinal l.** WHIPPLE'S DISEASE. **progressive l.** The commonest form of lipodystrophy, usually characterized by a progressive symmetric loss of fat from the face and upper body and abnormal deposition of fat about the buttocks and thighs. Females are more often affected than males. Insulin resistance and endogenous hyperlipemia are generally present. Also *acquired partial lipodystrophy, Barraquer-Simons syndrome.* **reverse partial l.** FAMILIAL LIPODYSTROPHY OF LIMBS AND TRUNK. **total l. and acromegaloid gigantism** SEIP SYNDROME. **trochanteric l.** RIDING BREECHES DEFORMITY.

**lipoferous** \lipäf′ərəs\ [LIPO- + -FEROUS] Capable of combining with fat for transport purposes.

**lipofibroma** \-fībrō′mə\ [LIPO- + FIBROMA] FIBROLIPOMA.

**lipofuscin** \-fyus′in\ A brown pigment partially soluble in a fat, occurring in granules in cells, such as nerve or muscle cells, as a result of the fusion of a lysosome with an endocytic vesicle, the undigested material remaining being primarily lipofuscin. An estimate of the age of an animal can often be made based on the number of lipofuscin granules. Also *age pigment.*

**lipogenic** \-jen′ik\ Of or relating to the production of fat. Also *adipogenic, adipogenous, lipogenous, lipoplastic, lipogenetic.*

**lipogranuloma** \-gran′yəlō′mə\ A granulomatous inflammation of the subcutaneous fat. Also *oleoma.*

**lipogranulomatosis** \-gran′yəlōmətō′sis\ A rare metabolic disorder in which ceramides and gangliosides accumulate, as a result of ceramidase deficiency, within neurons and glial cells of the central nervous system, resulting in mental and motor retardation and a fatal outcome usually by the age of two years. Subcutaneous nodules and skin lesions are also seen. Also *Farber's disease, disseminated lipogranulomatosis.*

**lipohemarthrosis** \-hem′ärthrō′sis\ A joint abnormality characterized by synovial fluid containing both fat droplets and blood, as occurs in a bone fracture involving the joint.

**lipohyalin** \-hī′əlin\ Lipoid material sometimes found in hyalinized beta cells of the pancreatic islets of Langerhans in diabetes mellitus.

**lipoic acid** The acid formed by oxidation of the thiol groups of 6,8-dimercaptoocatanoic acid to a disulfide, so that a five-membered ring is formed. It is a component of the 2-oxo acid dehydrogenase complexes, and becomes reductively acylated in the course of the reaction in which, for example, pyruvate or 2-oxoglutarate is converted into acetyl-CoA or succinyl-CoA, respectively, with elimination of carbon dioxide, consumption of coenzyme A, and reduction of NAD. Lipoic acid occurs in amide linkage with lysine residues of one of the enzymes of the complex. Also *thioctic acid.*

**lipoid** \lip′oid\ [LIP- + -OID] **1** Of or like fat. **2** *Outmoded* LIPID. **Forssman's l.** FORSSMAN ANTIGEN.

**lipoidosis** \lip′oidō′sis\ [LIPOID + -OSIS] Any disturbance of fat metabolism. See also LIPIDOSIS. **arterial l.** ATHEROSCLEROSIS.

**lipoidproteinosis** \lip′oidprō′tēnō′sis\ LIPOID PROTEINOSIS.

**lipoiduria** \lip′oidoo′rē·ə\ LIPIDURIA.

**lipolysis** \lipäl′isis\ [LIPO- + LYSIS] The hydrolysis of fat into free fatty acids and glycerol, often with release of free fatty acids into the plasma. Also *adipolysis, steatolysis, lipidolysis, lipoclasis.*

**lipolytic** \-lit′ik\ Of or relating to the breakdown of fat. Also *adipolytic, lipoclastic, steatolytic.*

**lipoma** \lipō′mə\ [LIP- + -OMA] A benign growth of mature adipose tissue cells showing no evidence of cellular atypia. It may occur at a variety of sites, such as skin and intestines. Also *pimeloma, adipose tumor, fatty tumor, adipoma* (obs.). **l. arborescens** A lipomatous transformation of the synovium, producing a villous form. **calcified l.** A lipoma containing deposits of calcium, usually the result of fat necrosis. **l. of corpus callosum** A rare tumor of the corpus callosum which gives rise to a typical radiologic appearance because of calcification within the tumor. **diffuse l.** An unencapsulated lipoma. **diffuse symmetrical l.'s of the neck** A condition characterized by diffuse and symmetrical, benign adipose tumors in the neck and occasionally on the trunk. It occurs mostly in adult males and usually does not affect the general health. Also *Madelung's disease.* **fetal fat cell l.** HIBERNOMA. **l. fibrosum** FIBROLIPOMA. **intramuscular l.** A benign proliferation of mature adipose tissue infiltrating striated muscle. Also *infiltrating lipoma.* **lumbosacral l.** A lipoma in the lumbosacral region, usually overlying a spina bifida. **l. myxomatodes** MYXOLIPOMA. **nevoid l.** ANGIOLIPOMA. **renal l.** A benign adipose tissue tumor of the renal cortex. **l. of the spermatic cord** A benign growth of adipose tissue of the spermatic cord which may show considerable swelling in the inguinal region and extend down to the scrotum, resembling an inguinal hernia. **spinal l.** An intradural lipoma within the spinal cord, usually seen in association with spinal dysraphism and spina bifida. **telangiectatic l.** ANGIOLIPOMA.

**lipomatoid** \lipō′mətoid\ [LIPOMA + *t* + -OID] Resembling a lipoma.

**lipomatosis** \-mətō′sis\ [LIPOMA + *t* + -OSIS] 1 The presence of multiple or diffuse lipomas. 2 Replacement of atrophic or destroyed parenchyma of an organ, as the kidney, by adipose tissue. Also *liposis.* **diffuse l.** A diffuse, infiltrating proliferation of mature adipose tissue showing no evidence of cellular atypia. Large examples of this lesion may involve sizable portions of an extremity or the trunk. It chiefly affects children and is exceedingly rare during adult life. **l. dolorosa** The presence of multiple painful lipomas. The pain often appears in one lipoma after another. Also *lipomatosis neurotica.* **medullary l.** Proliferation of renal hilar fat, a benign condition discovered incidentally on autopsy. **l. neurotica** LIPOMATOSIS DOLOROSA.

**lipomatous** \lipō′mətəs\ Pertaining to a lipoma.

**lipomeningocele** \-məning′gōsēl\ [LIPO- + MENINGOCELE] A lipoma within the cauda equina. It is often associated with spina bifida.

**lipometabolism** \-mətab′əlizm\ [LIPO- + METABOLISM] The metabolism of fat.

**lipomicron** \-mī′krän\ CHYLOMICRON.

**lipomphalus** \lipäm′fələs\ A fat hernia of the umbilicus.

**lipomucopolysaccharidosis** \-myoo′kōpäl′ēsak′əridō′sis\ MUCOLIPIDOSIS.

**lipomyohemangioma** \-mī′əhēman′jē·ō′mə\ [LIPO- + MYO- + HEMANGIOMA] ANGIOMYOLIPOMA.

**lipomyxoma** \-miksō′mə\ MYXOLIPOMA.

**lipomyxosarcoma** \-mik′sōsärkō′mə\ [LIPO- + MYXO- + SARCOMA] MYXOID LIPOSARCOMA.

***Liponyssoides*** \-nisoi′dēz\ A genus of bloodsucking mites, ectoparasites of mammals. The mouse mite, *L. sanguineus,* transmits *Rickettsia akari* accidentally to humans, causing rickettsialpox. Also *Allodermanyssus.*

***Liponyssus*** \-nis′əs\ [LIPO- + New L *-nyssus,* suffix formed from Gk *nyssein* or *nyttein* to prick, spur, pierce] ORNITHONYSSUS.

**lipopenia** \-pē′nē·ə\ [LIPO- + -PENIA] A deficiency of fat occurring in the body.

**lipopexia** \-pek′sē·ə\ The deposition of fat in the tissues.

**lipophage** \lip′əfāj\ A cell which takes in fat from its environment.

**lipophagy** \lipäf′əjē\ [LIPO- + *-phag(ia)* + -Y] The dissolution of adipose tissue and engulfment of the lipid by phagocytic cells. Also *lipophagia.*

**lipophilia** \-fil′yə\ An attraction for fat.

**lipophilic** \-fil′ik\ Fat-soluble: used especially to describe the affinity of certain dyes for lipid substances.

**lipophore** \lip′əfôr\ [LIPO- + -PHORE] A pigmented cell whose color is caused by lipochrome pigment.

**lipoplastic** \-plas′tik\ LIPOGENIC.

**lipopolysaccharide** \-päl′isak′ərīd\ Any substance of whose molecule is part a polysaccharide and part a lipid. Such substances are found as components of bacterial cell walls. They are frequently antigenic.

**lipoprotein** \-prō′tē·in\ [LIPO- + PROTEIN] Any complex or compound of lipids with proteins. The lipoproteins of blood plasma are generally classified on the basis of density (lipid content) as very low density, low density, and high density lipoproteins, and are important in lipid transport. Other lipoproteins are important components of membranes. **high-density l.** Any plasma lipoprotein of density in the range 1.061– 1.21 g/ml. Such lipopr oteins contain about 50% protein, 25% phospholipid, 20% cholesterol, and 5% fat. They are longer lived than lipoproteins of lower density, with half-lives of some days. They originate in both liver and intestine. High concentrations have inverse correlation with cardiovascular disease, and this may be related to their function of cholesterol transport. **low-density l.** A lipoprotein containing relatively large amounts of cholesterol, average quantities of protein and phospholipid, and little triglyceride. Abbr. LDL **plasma l.** Any of the various complexes of lipid and protein which occur in blood plasma. **very-low-density l.** Any lipoprotein of the blood plasma of density below 1.006 g/ml. The lipid is about 55% fat, 25% cholesterol and its esters, and 20% phospholipid. Such lipoproteins are formed in both liver and intestinal mucosa, and are responsible for the transport of fat from these tissues. This fat can be converted, for utilization, into fatty acids by lipoprotein lipase.

**lipoprotein lipase** The enzyme (EC 3.1.1.34) that catalyzes the hydrolysis of fat to fatty acid and glycerol. It owes its ability to hydrolyze lipoprotein, e.g. very-low-density lipoprotein of the blood, rather than fat in other environments, to its activation by one of the apoproteins of blood lipoprotein. It is bound by glycosaminoglycan to capillary walls, and its action enables cells to obtain fatty acid from blood lipoproteins. Also *clearing factor.*

**lipoproteinosis** \-prō′tēnō′sis\ LIPOID PROTEINOSIS.

**liposarcoma** \-särkō′mə\ [LIPO- + SARCOMA] A malignant tumor of adipose tissue. Atypical lipoblasts in varying stages of differentiation are characteristic. It may occur in a variety of sites but especially in soft tissue and retroperitoneum. Its behavior appears to vary with its degree of differentiation. It can be subtyped according to whether the predominant cell pattern is well-differentiated, myxoid (embryonal), round cell, pleomorphic (poorly differentiated), or mixed. **myxoid l.** A liposarcoma containing a predominant myxomatous component. Also *embryonal liposarcoma, lipomyxosarcoma, myxoliposarcoma, myxolipofibrosarcoma.*

**lipose** \lip′ōs\ Any lipase present in blood plasma. Also *liposin.*

**liposis** \lipō′sis\ LIPOMATOSIS. **general l.** Diffuse fatty infiltration of cells.

**liposome** \lip′əsōm\ A small vesicular structure which forms spontaneously when phospholipids are placed in water. The phospholipids form bimolecular layers, with the hydrophobic portion of the molecules facing toward the middle of the layer and the hydrophilic portions of the molecules facing outward. The bilipid layers form multiple-layered spheres, the phospholipid bilayers being separated by an aqueous phase.

**lipoteichoic acid** The type of teichoic acid found in bacterial membranes, as opposed to bacterial walls. It contains a lipid as a terminal part of the molecule. Also *membrane teichoic acid.*

**lipotrophic** \-träf′ik\ [LIPO- + -TROPHIC] Stimulating the formation of fat.

**lipotropin** \-trō′pin\ [LIPO- + *-trop(ic)*[1] + -IN] Any hormone that causes release of fatty acid from the fat of adipose tissue. Several pituitary hormones have this effect. Also *lipotropic hormone, adipokinetic hormone* (older term).

**β-lipotropin** A single-chain polypeptide hormone containing 91 amino acids, isolated from the anterior pituitary of several species, including man. It has weak lipolytic, melanophorotropic, and adrenocorticotropic properties, but its principal significance is its function as a prohormone for the endorphins, enkephalins, and melanocyte stimulating hormone.

**γ-lipotropin** A single-chain polypeptide hormone containing 58 amino acids, isolated from the anterior pituitary of several species, including sheep and cattle. It has weak lipolytic properties. The physiologic role of the hormone is not yet known.

**lipotuberculin** \-tʸUbur′kyəlin\ A tuberculin preparation containing in emulsion or solution the fatty component of the tubercle bacillus, *Mycobacterium tuberculosis.*.

**lipovaccine** \-vak′sin, -vaksēn′\ [LIPO- + VACCINE] A vaccine prepared by suspending the microorganisms in vegetable oil. Absorption of antigenic material is thereby delayed.

**lipoxenous** \lipäk′sənəs\ Relating to or characterized by lipoxeny.

**lipoxeny** \lipäk′sənē\ [Gk *lip(ein),* 2nd aorist inf. of *leipein* to desert in danger, forsake + *xen(os)* a host, guest + -Y] The process or phenomenon of desertion of the host by a parasite upon completion of the parasite's development.

**lipoxygenase** The enzyme (EC 1.13.11.12) that catalyzes the oxidation of linoleate, and of similar substances that contain the grouping —CH=CH—$CH_2$—CH=CH—, with uptake of molecular oxygen, to give the grouping —CH(—O—OH)—CH=CH—CH=CH—. Also *lipoxidase* (outmoded).

**lipoxysm** \lipäk′sizm\ [LIP- + OXY-[2] + *-(i)sm*] A condition resulting from the ingestion of excessive amounts of fatty acids, such as oleic acid.

**lippa** \lip′ə\ [New L, from L *lippus,* blear-eyed (akin to Gk *lipos* fat, grease)] BLEPHARITIS.

**Lippes** [Jacob *Lippes,* U.S. obstetrician, born 1924] See under LOOP.

**lipping** \lip′ing\ **1** A bony spur in the juxta-articular area secondary to degenerative arthritis. **2** *Seldom used* CODMAN'S TRIANGLE.

**lippitude** \lip′itʸood\ [L *lippitudo* (from *lippus* blear-eyed) a condition in which the eyes are watery and inflamed] BLEPHARITIS.

**lip-print** An impression of the pattern of the ridges, cracks, and wrinkles of the lip surfaces, made by applying ink or other staining material to the lips which are then blotted on a white card or paper. As a method of identification, it has limited application since the lip surfaces change with age and season.

**Lipschütz** [Benjamin *Lipschütz,* Austrian dermatologist, 1878–1931] Lipschütz ulcer. See under DISEASE.

**lipsis animi** SYNCOPE.

**lipuria** \lipoo′rē·ə\ LIPIDURIA.

**liq.** *liquor* (L, liquid).

**liq dr** Symbol for the unit, liquid dram.

**liq oz** Symbol for the unit, liquid ounce.

**liq pt** Symbol for the unit, liquid pint.

**liq qt** Symbol for the unit, liquid quart.

**Liquamar** A proprietary name for phenprocoumon.

**liquefaction** \lik′wəfak′shən\ [Late L *liquefactio* (from L *liquefacere* to make fluid, from *liquere* to be fluid + *facere* to make) a making fluid] The process of becoming or making liquid, often due to hydrolysis of structural macromolecules.

**liquid** [L *liquidus* (from *liquere* to be clear, liquid, molten) clear, liquid, molten] **1** Being in a state that is fluid but not dispersed; neither solid nor gaseous. **2** A liquid substance. **Altmann's l.** ALTMANN'S FLUID. **Flemming's l.** FLEMMING'S FIXING FLUID. **Thoma's l.** THOMA'S FLUID.

**liquor** \lik′ər, lik′wôr\ [L (from *liquere* to be liquid) liquidity, a liquid] **1** A liquid or fluid. **2** In anatomy, a fluid secretion that is produced by certain tissues, such as the antrum of an ovarian follicle and the choroid plexus of the brain. It is usually nutritive. **3** In pharmacy, an aqueous solution of any nonvolatile substance, or an aqueous solution of a gas. **l. amaranthi** AMARANTH SOLUTION. **l. ammoniae dilutus** DILUTED AMMONIA SOLUTION. **l. ammoniae fortis** STRONG AMMONIA SOLUTION. **l. amnii** AMNIOTIC FLUID. **l. cerebrospinalis** [NA] A clear, colorless fluid that circulates within the four ventricles of the brain and the subarachnoid spaces surrounding the brain and spinal cord. An ultrafiltrate of the blood secreted by the choroid plexus in the lateral third and fourth ventricles, it is largely resorbed into the venous system via the arachnoid villi. Also *cerebrospinal fluid, neurolymph* (seldom used). **l. chloridorum trium isotonicus** RINGER SOLUTION. **l. chorii** Fluid present in the early embryo within the confines of the chorion but outside the developing embryo and amniotic cavity. **l. entericus** INTESTINAL JUICE. **l. folliculi** FOLLICULAR FLUID. **l. formaldehydi** FORMALDEHYDE SOLUTION. **l. gastricus** GASTRIC JUICE. **l. hydrogenii peroxidi** HYDROGEN PEROXIDE SOLUTION. **l. iodi fortis** STRONG IODINE SOLUTION. **l. pancreaticus** PANCREATIC JUICE. **l. pericardii** PERICARDIAL FLUID. **l. pituitarii posterii** POSTERIOR PITUITARY INJECTION. **l. plumbi subacetatis fortis** Strong lead acetate solution. **l. prostaticus** SUCCUS PROSTATICUS. **l. sanguinis** PLASMA. **l. of Scarpa** ENDOLYMPHA. **l. seminis** The fluid component of semen.

**liquores** \likwôr′ēz\ Plural of LIQUOR.

**liquorice** GLYCYRRHIZA.

**Lisfranc** [Jacques *Lisfranc,* French surgeon, 1790–1847] **1** Lisfranc's joints. See under ARTICULATIONES TARSOMETATARSALES. **2** See under DISLOCATION, LIGAMENT, FRACTURE. **3** Lisfranc's operation. See under AMPUTATION. **4** Lisfranc's tubercle. See under TUBERCULUM MUSCULI SCALENI ANTERIORIS.

**lisp** [Middle English *lysp(en), wlisp(en)* to lisp, from Old English *-wlispian,* from *wlisp, wlips* a lisping] **1** Defective production of the sibilant sounds of speech such as *s* and *z,* which tend to be replaced by *th* sounds, with a tendency for the tongue tip to protrude past the upper central teeth. **2** To speak with a lisp.

**Lissauer** [Heinrich *Lissauer,* German neurologist, 1861–1891] Lissauer's marginal zone. See under TRACTUS DORSOLATERALIS.

**lissencephaly** \lis′ensef′əlē\ [Gk *liss(os)* smooth + ENCEPHAL- + -Y] AGYRIA.

**lissive** \lis′iv\ [Gk *liss(os)* smooth + -IVE ] Having the property of relieving muscle spasm.

**list** A lateral deviation of the trunk.

**listening / dichotic l.** An experimental procedure in which different stimuli or different messages are simultaneously presented to two ears as a means of examining selective attention.

**Lister** [Joseph *Lister,* English surgeon, 1827–1912] **1** Lister's method. See under LISTERISM. **2** Lister's tubercle. See under TUBERCULUM DORSALE RADII.

***Listeria monocytogenes*** \lister′ē·ə män′əsītäj′ənēz\ A small, Gram-positive, motile, aerobic to microaerophilic, asporogenous rod, tending to grow in chains, palisades, or filaments and easily mistaken for a diphtheroid. Several O and H antigenic types are recognized. It is a parasite in many vertebrates and invertebrates and is also found in soil and in rotting vegetation. In humans it most often causes a purulent meningitis (especially in debilitated patients), or intrauterine or perinatal infection.

**listerism** \lis′tərizm\ [after Baron Joseph *Lister,* English surgeon, 1827–1912 + -ISM] The practice and procedures of aseptic and antiseptic surgery, developed originally by Joseph Lister. Also *Lister's method.*

**Listing** [Johann Benedikt *Listing,* German physicist, 1808–1882] See under LAW.

**Liston** [Robert *Liston,* English surgeon, 1794–1847] Liston scissors. See under SHEARS.

**liter** \lē′tər\ [French *litre* (from *litron* former measure of capacity containing a sixteenth of a bushel, irreg. from Med L and Gk *litra* a pound of twelve ounces) a liter, liter measure] A unit of volume or capacity equal to $10^3$ cubic centimeters or $10^{-3}$ cubic meter: used in conjunction with SI units. A liter is equivalent to 1.0567 liquid quarts or 33.814 (US) fluid ounces. Also *litre.* Symbol: l, L ● In Great Britain and in international usage, the spelling *litre* is preferred, but in the United States *liter* is the usual spelling. The symbol l is preferred over L except in those instances where it might be confused with the numeral 1. **l. per centimeter of water** A unit of compliance and dynamic compliance equal to $1.019\ 72 \times 10^{-3}$ meter cubed per pascal: used especially in connection with respiratory ducts. Symbol: $l/cmH_2O$

**lith-** \lith-\ LITHO-.

**-lith** \-lith\ [Gk *lithos* stone] A combining form meaning (1) stone; (2) calculus.

**lithaemia** *Brit.* LITHEMIA.

**lithagogectasia** \lith′əgō′jektā′zhə\ LITHECTASY.

**lithagogue** \lith′əgäg\ [LITH- + -AGOGUE] Any remedy that enhances the removal of concretions or calculi.

**lithangiuria** \lith′anjēyoo′rē·ə\ [LITH- + ANGI- + -URIA] The presence of calculi in the urinary tract.

**lithectasy** \lithek′təsē\ [LITH- + *ectas(ia)* + -Y] A surgical procedure in which a renal stone is extracted with a specially designed instrument through a surgically dilated urethra. Also *lithagogectasia.*

**lithemia** \lithē′mē·ə\ [LITH- + -EMIA] HYPERURICEMIA.

**lithiasis** \lithī′əsis\ [Gk (from *lithos* a stone) kidney stone disease] The development of calculi, usually in the gallbladder or kidneys. Formation of such calculi usually results from increased concentration in the bile or urine of substances contained within the stone, as well as favorable local physicochemical conditions. Also *calculosis.* **l. conjunctivae** Calcifications of the conjunctival crypts. **renal l.** NEPHROLITHIASIS.

**lithic** \lith′ik\ Pertaining to calculi.

**lithicosis** \lith′ikō′sis\ PNEUMOCONIOSIS.

**lithium** \lith′ē·əm\ Element number 3, having atomic weight 6.941. It is the lightest of all metals, with specific gravity 0.534. The first member of the alkali series, it is never found free in nature. There are numerous industrial applications and some pharmaceutical uses for the element. It does not appear to be essential to any organism. Symbol: Li

**lithium antimoniothiomalate** ANTHIOLIMINE.

**lithium carbonate** $Li_2CO_3$. A white, granular powder used as a source of lithium ions in the treatment of mania and the prophylaxis of manic depression and depression. Lithium ions compete with sodium ions, but the mechanism of its beneficial effects in depression is not known.

**litho-** \lith′ə-\ [Gk *lithos* stone] A combining form meaning (1) stone; (2) calculus. Also *lith-.*

**lithocenosis** \-sēnō′sis\ LITHOLAPAXY.

**lithocholic acid** 3α-Hydroxy-5β-cholanic acid. It is found in small amounts in mammalian bile, conjugated with glycine and taurine.

**lithoclast** \lith′əklast\ LITHOTRITE.

**lithoclasty** \lith′əklas′tē\ LITHOLAPAXY.

**lithoconion** \-kō′nē·än\ LITHOTRITE.

**lithocystotomy** \-sistät′əmē\ [LITHO- + CYSTO- + -TOMY] A surgical procedure in which solitary or multiple stones are removed from the bladder through an incision and under direct vision.

**lithogenesis** \-jen′əsis\ The formation of a calculus.

**lithogenous** \lithäj′ənəs\ [LITHO- + -GENOUS] Causing or capable of causing calculus formation.

**lithokelyphopedion** \-kel′ifōpē′dē·än\ A lithopedion with calcified membranes surrounding it.

**lithokonion** \-kō′nē·än\ LITHOTRITE.

**litholabe** \lith′əlāb\ [LITHO- + Gk *labē* a grip, handle] A surgical instrument designed to hold a bladder calculus in order to aid in its removal or fragmentation.

**litholapaxy** \lithäl′əpak′sē\ [LITHO- + Gk *lapax(is)* (from *lapassein* to empty, evacuate) an emptying, evacuation + -Y] A surgical procedure consisting of crushing a stone or stones within the urinary system and immediately irrigating to remove the fragments. Also *lithoclasty, lithotripsy, lithotrity, Civiale's operation, lithocenosis.*

**lithology** \lithäl′əjē\ [LITHO- + -LOGY] The science of the formation, effects, and treatment of calculi.

**litholysis** \lithäl′isis\ [LITHO- + LYSIS] Fragmentation or dissolution of stones in the urinary bladder.

**litholyte** \lith′əlīt\ An instrument designed to administer stone-dissolving agents directly inside the bladder.

**litholytic** \-lit′ik\ Stone-dissolving; tending to dissolve calculi, especially in the bladder.

**lithomyl** \lith′əmil\ LITHOTRITE.

**lithonephrotomy** \-nefrät′əmē\ NEPHROLITHOTOMY.

**lithontriptic** \lith′äntrip′tik\ LITHOTRIPTIC.

**lithopaedion** *Brit.* LITHOPEDION.

**lithopedion** \-pē′dē·än\ [LITHO- + Gk *paidion* a young child, dim. of *pais* a child] A retained fetus, whether extrauterine or intrauterine, which has undergone calcification. Also *calcified fetus, mummified fetus, osteopedion.*

**lithoscope** \lith′əskōp\ [LITHO- + -SCOPE] An instrument used for visual examination of calculi in the urinary bladder.

**lithosis** \lithō′sis\ PNEUMOCONIOSIS.

**lithotome** \lith′ətōm\ [LITHO- + -TOME] A knife specifically designed to perform lithotomies.

**lithotomy** \lithät′əmē\ [Gk *lithotomia* (from *litho(s)* stone + *tom(ē)* a cut) cutting for urinary stones.] An incision into a duct or organ for the purpose of removing stones. **high l.** SUPRAPUBIC LITHOTOMY. **lateral l.** A lithotomy to remove urinary bladder stones employing an incision in the perineum immediately lateral to the raphe perinei. **marian l.** MEDIAN LITHOTOMY. **median l.** A surgical incision into the raphe perinei for the purpose of removing bladder stones. Also *marian lithotomy, prerectal lithot-*

*omy, Allarton's operation, sectio mediana.* **mediolateral l.** Any combination of incisions on or immediately lateral to the raphe perinei for the purpose of stone removal. **perineal l.** Any surgical incision into the perineum for the purpose of stone removal. Also *celsian operation.* **prerectal l.** MEDIAN LITHOTOMY. **suprapubic l.** The removal of a bladder calculus by an incision above the pubis. **vaginal l.** A surgical incision made through the vagina into the bladder for the purpose of stone removal. Also *vesicovaginal lithotomy.* **vesicovaginal l.** VAGINAL LITHOTOMY.

**lithotony** \lithät′ənē\ [LITHO- + *ton(o)-* + -Y] A surgical procedure in which a bladder fistula is created for the purpose of urinary stone removal.

**lithotresis** \-trē′sis\ [LITHO- + Gk *trēsis* a perforation] A surgical procedure in which holes are drilled into a calculus to facilitate its removal. **ultrasonic l.** A procedure in which ultrasonic waves are used to facilitate the removal of urinary stones.

**lithotripsy** \lith′ətrip′sē\ [LITHO- + -TRIPSY] LITHOLAPAXY. **electrohydraulic l.** The breaking up of kidney stones by using an electric discharge directly to the stone. **extracorporeal shock-wave l.** Lithotripsy utilizing shock waves in a water-filled tub to pulverize kidney stones in a patient partially submerged in the tub. Surgery is avoided if the fragments pass spontaneously. The device utilizing this technique is usually called an extracorporeal shock-wave lithotriptor.

**lithotriptic** \-trip′tik\ **1** Of or relating to lithotripsy. Also *lithontriptic.* **2** A device utilizing shock waves to break up kidney stones without surgical intervention.

**lithotriptor** \lith′ətrip′tər\ LITHOTRITE. **extracorporeal shock-wave l.** See under EXTRACORPOREAL SHOCK-WAVE LITHOTRIPSY.

**lithotriptoscope** \-trip′təskōp\ A surgical instrument which is used to pulverize a bladder calculus under direct vision. Also *cystoscopic lithotrite.*

**lithotriptoscopy** \-triptäs′kəpē\ A surgical procedure in which bladder stones are crushed and flushed out under direct vision.

**lithotrite** \lith′ətrīt\ [LITHO- + L *tritus,* past part. of *terere* to rub, wear away; Gk *teirein* to rub, rub away, wear away and *tribein* to rub, grind down] A surgical instrument designed to crush or to fragment stones and thereby facilitate spontaneous or operative removal. Also *lithoclast, lithokonion, lithoconion, lithomyl, lithotriptor.* **cystoscopic l.** LITHOTRIPTOSCOPE. **electrohydraulic l.** A flexible electrode placed next to a urinary calculus to fracture it into smaller pieces by applying a high-voltage spark.

**lithotrity** \lithät′ritē\ [LITHO- + L *trit(us),* past part. of *terere* to rub + -Y ] LITHOLAPAXY.

**lithuresis** \lith′yoorē′sis\ [LITH- + URESIS] **1** Excess urinary excretion of uric acid. **2** The passage, usually painless, of tiny calculi (gravel) during urination.

**lithureteria** \lith′yoorəter′ē·ə\ [LITH- + URETER- + -IA] Calculi formation in the ureter.

**litmus** \lit′məs\ [Old Norse *litmose* (from *litr* color + *mosi* moss) a lichen used in dyeing] A natural pigment, obtained from lichens whose major principle is azolitmin. It is used primarily in paper strips as a pH indicator, being red at an acid pH below 4.5 and blue at an alkaline pH above 8.3. Also *turnsol, lacmus.*

**litre** \lē′tər\ LITER.

**Litten** [Moritz *Litten,* German physician, 1845–1907] Litten's diaphragm phenomenon, Litten sign. See under DIAPHRAGM PHENOMENON.

**Little** [James Lawrence *Little,* U.S. physician, 1836–1885] Little's area. See under KIESSELBACH'S AREA.

**Little** [William John *Little,* English surgeon, 1810–1894] **1** See under DISEASE. **2** Little's paralysis. See under ACUTE ANTERIOR POLIOMYELITIS.

**Littre** [Alexis *Littre,* French anatomist, 1658–1726] **1** See under SPACE. **2** Littre's crypts, Littre's glands. See under GLANDULAE PREPUTIALES. **3** Littre's crypts, Littre's glands. See under GLANDULAE URETHRALES URETHRAE MASCULINAE.

**littritis** \litrī′tis\ [after Alexis *Littre,* French anatomist and physician, 1658–1726 + -ITIS] Inflammation of Littre's glands, manifesting itself as an abscess which can open under the skin or in the urethra and result, in men, in a fistula of the urethra.

**Litzmann** [Karl Konrad Theodor *Litzmann,* German gynecologist, 1815–1890] Litzmann's obliquity. See under POSTERIOR ASYNCLITISM.

**live-born** An infant that is born alive, in contradistinction to one that is stillborn.

**livedo** \livē′dō\ [L (from *livere* to be blue or bluish), lividness] A discoloration or erythema of the skin that follows the reticulate pattern of the cutaneous vascular network. Also *suggillation* (obs.). **l. annularis** LIVEDO RETICULARIS. **l. calorica** Livedo reticularis due to heat. **l. reticularis** A mottled bluish or livid discoloration of the skin in a network pattern, an accentuation of the normal vascular pattern of the skin, with dilatation of the capillaries and small venules. It is a benign condition that may be due to either arterial and arteriolar constriction of diverse causation, aggravated by cold, or to external heat which selectively damages the dark part of the network with its more precarious blood supply. Also *livedo annularis.* **l. telangiectatica** Livedo reticularis in which the small vessel dilatation is gross enough to cause visible telangiectases.

**livedoid** \liv′idoid\ [*lived(o)* + -OID] **1** Resembling livedo. **2** Of or relating to livedo.

**liver** [Old English *lifer*] A large gland located in the upper right quadrant of the abdomen immediately beneath the diaphragm; hepar. As an exocrine gland it secretes bile. Its other major functions are the synthesis of plasma proteins, heparin, fibrinogen, and prothrombin; the destruction of red cells; detoxification; the metabolism of proteins, carbohydrates, and fats; and the storage of glycogen and other important substances. For a further discussion of the anatomy of the liver, see *hepar.* **amyloid l.** A liver infiltrated with amyloid. The liver becomes enlarged and appears pale gray and waxy. Microscopically, the deposits appear as an amorphous, eosinophilic substance deposited primarily in the space of Disse, between the hepatocytes and the sinusoidal endothelial cells. The continued accumulation of amyloid results in progressive atrophy of liver cells. Also *waxy liver.* **biliary cirrhotic l.** A cirrhotic liver resulting from disease of the biliary tract. It is characteristically deeply bile-stained and nodular, and it may be caused by obstruction due to cancer or stone or by autoimmune damage to the small intrahepatic bile ducts, as in primary biliary cirrhosis. **brimstone l.** The enlarged, bright yellow liver often seen in an individual with congenital syphilis or fulminant hepatitis. **bronze l.** A liver that is bronze colored due to deposits of malarial pigment, mainly within Kupfer cells. **cirrhotic l.** A liver affected by cirrhosis, a characteristic nodular transformation and scarring of the hepatic parenchyma. Externally, the normally smooth capsule shows multiple nodular protuberances which gives it the so-called hobnail appearance. Cirrhotic nodules range from 2 to 10 mm in diameter. Although not infrequently cirrhotic livers are of cryptogenic origin, alcoholism and viral hepatitis are common etiologies. Also *hobnail liver.* **desiccated l.** Dried powder prepared from whole mammalian livers. It is a good source of riboflavin, nicotinic acid, choline, vitamin $B_{12}$, and iron, hence it is used as a nutritional supplement and is sometimes given in the treatment of macrocytic anemia. **fatty l.** A liver with increased amounts of neutral fat in the cytoplasms of hepatocytes. This change results in a yellow, soft, and greasy liver. Microscopically, cytoplasmic fat vacuoles distend the hepatocyes. Although this condition may be caused by several systemic disorders such as diabetes mellitus, the most common cause is alcoholism. Also *hepar adiposum.* **fatty l. of Brahmin children** An Indian term for KWASHIORKOR. **foamy l.** A putrefying liver commonly found in decomposing bodies and filled with variously sized gaseous cysts imparting a foamy or bubbly appearance to the capsular and cut surfaces. The cysts are formed by the putrefactive action of anaerobic bacilli, particularly *Clostridia* species. **frosted l.** A liver with hyaline thickening of its capsule, resulting in a white appearance that resembles cake icing. This is a non-specific and functionally unimportant change that is probably due to the organization of proteinaceous peritoneal exudates on the liver capsule. Also *perihepatitis chronica hyperplastica.* **hobnail l.** CIRRHOTIC LIVER. **iron l.** A liver loaded with hemosiderin deposits. It is grossly chocolate brown and microscopically the pigment is found within hepatocytes, Kupfer cells, bile duct epithelium, and scar tissue. It may be caused by any disorder that results in excess iron in the body, such as hemolytic disorders, multiple transfusions, and hemochromatosis. **nutmeg l.** A liver affected by chronic vascular congestion that produces a characteristic alternating pattern of dark red centrilobular areas and paler peripheral lobular regions. This color pattern is reminiscent of the spice nutmeg. The condition is caused most often by right-sided heart failure. Also *stasis liver.* **polycystic l.** A liver affected with multiple congenital cysts, most often subcapsular in location. These cysts do not impair hepatic function. The condition is probably the result of defective formation of bile ducts, and may be associated with polycystic kidneys of the adult type. **stasis l.** NUTMEG LIVER. **waxy l.** AMYLOID LIVER.

**livid** \liv′id\ [L *livid(us)* leaden in color, bluish, black and blue] Bluish black or deep purplish red, as a bruise; black-and-blue.

**lividity** \livid′itē\ [LIVID + -ITY] **1** A black and blue discoloration of the skin, such as that caused by a contusion. **2** A leaden or ashen hue, as occurring in cyanosis. Also *livor.* **cadaveric l.** LIVOR MORTIS. **postmortem l.** LIVOR MORTIS.

**livor** \lī′vər\ [L, a bluish color, lividness, a blue or livid spot] LIVIDITY. **l. mortis** The reddish blue to purple postmortem discoloration of the dependent, noncompressed skin surfaces, caused by the gravitational accumulation of reduced hemoglobin containing erythrocytes in subcutaneous capillaries. It begins forming immediately after death and is usually perceptible within two hours following the cessation of circulation. It is fully established after four hours but is absent in those areas where pressure, exerted by body weight on the supporting surface, compresses the capillary bed. Within 8 to 12 hours livor mortis becomes fixed, i.e., no blanching occurs when the skin surface is pressed. The fixation is caused by capillary obstruction, due to postmortem blood clotting, and by capillary constriction due to congealed adipose tissue. Therefore, finding fixed nondependent livor mortis may indicate that a body was moved following death. Also *postmortem lividity, cadaveric lividity, livor.*

**LLL** left lower lobe (of lung).

**Lloyd** [Putnam C. *Lloyd,* U.S. physician, flourished early 20th century] Lloyd syndrome. See under MULTIPLE ENDOCRINE NEOPLASIA.

**LLQ** left lower quadrant (of abdomen).

**LM** **1** linguomesial. **2** light minimum.

**LMA** left mentoanterior position (of a fetus). See under MENTUM ANTERIOR POSITION.

**LMF** lymphocyte mitogenic factor.

**LMP** left mentoposterior position (of a fetus). See under MENTUM POSTERIOR POSITION.

**LMT** left mentotransverse position (of a fetus). See under MENTUM TRANSVERSE POSITION.

**LNPF** lymph node permeability factor.

**LOA** left occipitoanterior position (of a fetus). See under OCCIPUT ANTERIOR POSITION.

***Loa*** \lō′ə\ A genus of filarial nematodes (family Onchocercidae) transmitted by blood-sucking flies. The adult nematodes wander in the subdermal spaces and the microfilariae are found in the bloodstream. ***L. loa*** A filarial worm, the African eye worm, found in western equatorial Africa, and the etiologic agent of loiasis. Males average 25–35 mm long, females 50–60 mm. The sheathed microfilariae, which have nuclei that extend to the tip of the tail, can be found in peripheral blood primarily during the day, unlike *Wuchereria bancrofti.* Humans are the only known definitive hosts, with tabanid flies (genus *Chrysops*) serving as vectors. Infective larvae require from three years to mature following transmission, and the adults may live as long as 17 years in the subcutaneous connective tissues. Moving freely, they can sometimes be observed wriggling across the eye under the conjunctiva, hence the name eye worm. They are also responsible for Calabar swellings. Also *Filaria diurna, Filaria loa.*

**load** [Old English *lād*] **1** The deviation from normal body content, as of salt, heat, or water. **2** The mechanical force, energy, or power a subject must expend during a stress test. **3** The impedance seen by the output of an electronic generator such as a pacemaker or defibrillator. **4** To enter data into the memory of a computer. **filtered l.** The amount of a substance that appears in the glomerular urinary space via filtration across the glomerular capillary wall per unit time. The load is calculated by multiplying the glomerular filtration rate by the concentration of the substance in glomerular filtrate. **genetic l.** **1** The reduction in health, longevity, or fitness of an individual or a population because of deleterious genes. Also *mutational load.* **2** A formal genetic concept, developed by H.J. Muller in 1950. It specifies for any locus the proportion by which the genetic fitness of the individual or population is reduced because of deleterious alleles, when compared to the optimal genotype. **mutational l.** GENETIC LOAD.

**loading** The administration of a substance either in a quantity sufficient to saturate binding sites in the body or as a prelude to maintaining a constant plasma concentration. It facilitates measurement of the rate of metabolism or excretion of the substance.

**loaiasis** \lō′ə·ī′əsis\ LOIASIS.

**lobar** \lō′bər, lō′bär\ Relating to or involving a lobe.

**lobate** \lō′bāt\ Provided with or arranged in lobes. Also *lobose.*

**lobation** \lōbā′shən\ **1** The formation of lobes. **2** A lobe or lobate structure.

**lobe** \lōb\ [New L *lobus.* See LOBUS.] **1** A rounded projection or subdivision of an organ or structure demarcated by fissures, sulci, constrictions, or connective tissue septa; lobus. **2** A cusp on the crown of a tooth. An outmoded usage. **ansiform l.** That portion of the cerebellar hemisphere lying between the posterior superior fissure anteriorly and the gracile lobule posteriorly. The horizontal fissure divides it into the superior and inferior semilunar lobules (crus I and crus II, respectively). **anterior l. of hypophysis** ADENOHYPOPHYSIS. **anterior l. of pituitary gland** ADENOHYPOPHYSIS. **appendicular l.** A tongue-shaped downward extension of the right lobe of the liver. Also *linguiform lobe, Riedel's lobe.* **azygos l.** A small accessory lobe at the apex of the right lung, marked off by a groove made by the azygos vein. **caudate l. of cerebrum** *Obs.* INSULA. **caudate l. of liver** LOBUS CAUDATUS HEPATIS. **l.'s of cerebrum** LOBI CEREBRI. **cuneate l.** CUNEUS. **cuneiform l.** LOBULUS CUNEIFORMIS. **digastric l.** LOBULUS BIVENTER. **falciform l.** *Outmoded* LIMBIC LOBE. **flocculonodular l.** The smallest and phylogenetically oldest division of the cerebellum, made up of a midline nodulus and two stalklike flocculi located on the posterior and ventral surface of the remainder of the cerebellum, from which it is almost entirely separated by the posterolateral fissure. It is functionally related to the vestibular nerve and nuclei. Also *archicerebellum, flocculonodular complex.* **frontal l.** LOBUS FRONTALIS. **grand l. limbique of Broca** LIMBIC LOBE. **hepatic l.'s** LOBI HEPATIS. **Home's l.** SUBTRIGONAL GLAND. **inferior crescentic l. of cerebellum** *Outmoded* LOBULUS SEMILUNARIS INFERIOR. **inferior l. of lung** LOBUS INFERIOR PULMONIS. **inferior semilunar l.** LOBULUS SEMILUNARIS INFERIOR. **lateral l.'s of prostate gland** LOBUS PROSTATAE DEXTER ET SINISTER. **left l. of liver** LOBUS HEPATIS SINISTER. **limbic l.** The part of the brain situated on the medial surface of the hemisphere, surrounding the rostral brainstem and the interhemispheric commissures, and including the subcallosal, cingulate, and parahippocampal gyri, as well as the underlying hippocampal formation and dentate gyrus. It comprises the phylogenetically oldest portions of the cerebral cortex, and has maintained a remarkable constancy of gross and microscopic organization during the course of phylogeny. Also *gyrus fornicatus, grand lobe limbique of Broca, circumvolutio cristata, gyrus limbicus, lobus falciformis* (outmoded), *falciform lobe* (outmoded). • The term *limbic lobe* was introduced in 1878 by the French neurologist, Paul Broca. **linguiform l.** APPENDICULAR LOBE. **l.'s of liver** LOBI HEPATIS. **lower l. of lung** LOBUS INFERIOR PULMONIS. **l.'s of lung** Major divisions of the lung, separated by fissures. The right lung has superior, middle, and inferior lobes, and the left lung has superior and inferior lobes. **l.'s of mammary gland** LOBI GLANDULAE MAMMARIAE. **median l. of prostate** LOBUS MEDIUS PROSTATAE. **middle l. of cerebellum** VERMIS CEREBELLI. **middle l. of right lung** LOBUS MEDIUS PULMONIS DEXTRI. **occipital l.** LOBUS OCCIPITALIS. **olfactory l.** LOBUS OLFACTORIUS. **parietal l.** LOBUS PARIETALIS. **piriform l.** A portion of the anterior and ventromedial face of the temporal lobe composed of the terminal extensions of the lateral olfactory stria, the uncus, and the anterior part of the parahippocampal gyrus. It is demarcated laterally by the rhinal sulcus. Also *pyriform lobe.* **l.'s of the placenta** PLACENTAL COTYLEDON. **posterior l. of hypophysis** NEUROHYPOPHYSIS. **posterior l. of pituitary gland** NEUROHYPOPHYSIS. **prefrontal l.** The part of the frontal lobe of the cerebral hemispheres anterior to Brodmann's areas 6 and 8 (the motor and premotor zones), representing one of the latest phylogenetic developments of the brain. It is well developed only in primates, especially man. **l.'s of prostate** Lobus prostatae (dexter et sinister) and lobus medius prostatae. **pulmonary l.'s** See under LOBES OF LUNG. **pyramidal l. of thyroid gland** LOBUS PYRAMIDALIS GLANDULAE THYROIDEAE. **pyriform l.** PIRIFORM LOBE. **quadrangular l. of cerebellum** LOBULUS QUADRANGULARIS CEREBELLI. **quadrate l. of cerebral hemisphere** PRECUNEUS. **quadrate l. of liver** LOBUS QUADRATUS HEPATIS. **renal l.'s** LOBI RENALES. **Riedel's l.** APPENDICULAR LOBE. **right l. of liver** LOBUS HEPATIS DEXTER. **side l.** An undesired minor beam of sound traveling out in directions not included in the primary beam. **spigelian l.** LOBUS CAUDATUS HEPATIS. **superior crescentic l. of cerebellum** LOBULUS SEMILUNARIS SUPERIOR. **superior l. of lung** LOBUS SUPERIOR PULMONIS. **superior semilunar l.** LOBULUS SEMILUNARIS SUPERIOR. **temporal l.** LOBUS TEMPORALIS. **l.'s of thyroid gland** LOBI GLANDULAE THYROIDEAE DEXTER ET SINISTER. **upper l. of lung** LOBUS SUPERIOR PULMONIS. **vermiform l.** VERMIS CEREBELLI.

**lobectomy** \lōbek′təmē\ [*lob(e)* + -ECTOMY] The excision of a lobe, as of the brain, lung, or thyroid.

**lobelism** \lō′bəlizm\ Poisoning from overdosage of lobeline, the chief alkaloid extracted from *Lobelia inflata,* Indian tobacco. Symptoms are increased respiration and blood pressure, and muscular fasciculations mimicking the nicotinic effects of acetylcholine.

**lobi** \lō′bī\ Plural of LOBUS.

**lobite** \lō′bit\ Designating or limited to a single lobe.

**Lobo** [Jorge *Lobo,* Brazilian physician, flourished early 20th century] Lobo's disease. See under LOBOMYCOSIS.

**lobocyte** \lō′bəsīt\ POLYMORPHONUCLEAR LEUKOCYTE.

**lobomycosis** \lō′bəmīkō′sis\ [after Jorge *Lobo,* Brazilian physician, flourished 1931 + MYCOSIS] A localized, chronic, subepidermal fungal disease caused by *Loboa loboi.* It consists of keloidal, verrucoid, or nodular lesions. Also *Lobo's disease.*

**lobopodium** \lō′bəpō′dē·əm\ [Gk *lobo(s)* lobe + PODIUM] (*pl.* lobopodia) A thick, lobed, pseudopodium of amebas containing ectoplasm and endoplasm, or only endoplasm. Also *lobopod.* See also AXOPODIUM, FILOPODIUM, RHIZOPODIUM.

**lobose** \lō′bōs\ LOBATE.

**lobotomy** \lōbät′əmē\ [*lob(e)* + *-o-* + -TOMY] The incision of a lobe, as of the brain or of a lung. **frontal l.** Lobotomy of the frontal lobe of the cerebrum in psychosurgery to sever the white connecting fibers. Also *prefrontal lobotomy, leukotomy* (chiefly British). **prefrontal l.** FRONTAL LOBOTOMY. **transorbital l.** Division of the white fibers of the cerebrum by an instrument introduced through the orbit. Also *transorbital leukotomy* (used especially in the U.K.).

**Lobstein** [Johann Georg C. F. M. *Lobstein,* German pathologist, 1777–1835] **1** Splanchnic ganglion of Lobstein, Lobstein's ganglion. See under GANGLION SPLANCHNICUM. **2** Lobstein's disease. See under SYNDROME.

**lobular** \läb′yələr\ Pertaining to or resembling a lobule; composed of lobules.

**lobulated** \läb′yəlā′tid\ Composed of or characterized by lobules.

**lobulation** \läb′yəlā′shən\ The process of forming lobules or the state of being lobulated. **fetal l.** A superficial lobular appearance on the surface of kidneys in postnatal life due to persistent shallow linear indentations characteristic of fetal kidneys. The lobulation may persist into adulthood. On roentgenograms the cortical indentations are seen to correspond to the regions of the renal columns. The lobulations are usually smooth and regular but at times may be confused with renal masses. **portal l.** A pattern of regeneration seen in the liver following hepatic vein obstruction, characterized by periportal regenerative nodules.

**lobule** \läb′yool\ [*lob(e)* + -ULE] LOBULUS. **ansiform l.** That portion of the lateral lobe (hemisphere) of the cerebellum between the posterior superior fissure and the gracile lobule. **anterior lunate l.** LOBULUS SEMILUNARIS SUPERIOR. **anterior quadrangular l.** PARS ANTERIOR LOBULI QUADRANGULARIS. **l. of auricle** LOBULUS AURICULAE. **biventral l.** LOBULUS BIVENTER. **caudal semilunar l.** LOBULUS SEMILUNARIS INFERIOR. **central l. of cerebellum** LOBULUS CENTRALIS CEREBELLI. **cerebellar l.** A subdivision of a cerebellar lobus, examples of which include the lobulus simplex, the paramedian lobule, and the superior and inferior semilunar lobules. **cortical l.'s** LOBULI CORTICALES RENIS. **cortical l.'s of kidney** LOBULI CORTICALES RENIS. **cranial semilunar l.** LOBULUS SEMILUNARIS SUPERIOR. **digastric l.** LOBULUS BIVENTER. **ear l.** LOBULUS AURICULAE. **l.'s of epididymis** LOBULI EPIDIDYMIDIS. **floccular l.** A small structure on the inferior ventral aspect of the cerebellum just above the roof of the fourth ventricle. With the adjacent nodulus, it comprises the flocculonodular complex or archicerebellum. **fusiform l.** GYRUS FUSIFORMIS. **glandular l.** A unit of glandular tissue that is supplied by a single duct and demarcated from adjacent glandular tissue by a connective tissue layer. **glomerular l.** One of several similar lobules of the renal glomerulus, formed by a peripheral capillary loop and its attached endothelial, epithelial, and mesangial structures. Normally, glomerular lobules are barely apparent, but in glomerular diseases a distinct lobular pattern often develops. **gracile l.** That portion of the cerebellar hemisphere situated anterior to the biventral lobule and posterior to the inferior semilunar lobule. **hepatic l.'s** LOBULI HEPATIS. **inferior parietal l.** LOBULUS PARIETALIS INFERIOR. **inferior semilunar l.** LOBULUS SEMILUNARIS INFERIOR. **l.'s of lung** LOBULI PULMONUM. **l.'s of mammary gland** LOBULI GLANDULAE MAMMARIAE. **olfactory l.** LOBUS OLFACTORIUS. **paracentral l.** LOBULUS PARACENTRALIS. **portal l. of liver** A unit of liver tissue centering on one portal canal. In this concept, interlobular vessels are intra-acinar and several veins are at the periphery of the unit. Compare LOBULI HEPATIS. **posterior lunate l.** LOBULUS SEMILUNARIS INFERIOR. **posterior quadrangular l.** LOBULUS SIMPLEX. **primary l. of lung** LOBULUS PULMONIS PRIMARIUS. **pulmonary l.'s** LOBULI PULMONUM. **quadrangular l. of cerebellum** LOBULUS QUADRANGULARIS CEREBELLI. **quadrate l.** PRECUNEUS. **renal l.** Any of several medullary rays of collecting ducts of the kidney, surrounded by the nephrons which drain into these ducts. Interlobular arteries demarcate the individual lobules. **secondary l. of lung** LOBULUS PULMONIS SECUNDARIUS. **spermatic l.'s** LOBULI TESTIS. **superior parietal l.** LOBULUS PARIETALIS SUPERIOR. **superior semilunar l.** LOBULUS SEMILUNARIS SUPERIOR. **l.'s of testis** LOBULI TESTIS. **l.'s of thyroid gland** LOBULI GLANDULAE THYROIDEAE.

**lobulette** \läb′yəlet′\ A tiny lobule or a primary subdivision of a lobule.

**lobuli** \läb′yəlī\ Plural of LOBULUS.

**lobulization** \läb′yəlīzā′shən\ The process by which homogeneous tissue is changed into a lobulated state.

**lobulose** \läb′yəlōs\ Organized into, or having, lobules. Also *lobulous.*

**lobulus** \läb′yələs\ [New L (from French or English *lobule*), a little lobe] (*pl.* lobuli) A small lobe, or one of the parts into which a lobe is subdivided. Also *lobule.* **l. auriculae** [NA] The soft, lowest part of the auricle of the ear, situated below the antitragus, devoid of cartilage and consisting of fatty and fibrous tissue; earlobe. Also *lobule of auricle, ear lobule.* **l. biventer** [NA] A lobule on the posterior and inferior surface of the cerebellum, situated between the tonsilla of the cerebellum and the gracile lobule. Also *digastric lobule, biventral lobule, digastric lobe.* **l. centralis cerebelli** [NA] An anterior portion of the vermis situated between the culmen and lingula and overlapping the anterior medullary velum. Also *central lobule of cerebellum.* **l. clivi** DECLIVE. **lobuli corticales renis** [NA] Imperfectly separated portions of the renal cortex, each of which extends from the base of a renal pyramid to the fibrous capsule and comprises a pars radiata and a pars convoluta. Interlobular blood vessels may partially demarcate the units. Also *cortical lobules of kidney, cortical lobules, cortical arches of the kidney.* **l. culminis** CULMEN. **l. cuneiformis** The medial aspect of the occipital lobe bounded rostrally by the parieto-occipital sulcus, and inferiorly by the calcarine sulcus. Also *cuneiform lobe.* **lobuli epididymidis** [NA] The conical masses forming the head of the epididymis and composed of dilated and highly convoluted efferent ductules of the testis. Also *lobules of epididymis, coni epididymidis, vascular cones, Haller's cones.* **l. folii** That portion of the vermis cerebelli lying in front of the lobus clivi and behind the fissura prima. **lobuli glandulae mammariae** [NA] The small glandular units forming the lobes of the mammary gland and consisting of clusters of saccular or tubulosaccular alveoli connected by areolar tissue and blood vessels. Each unit is drained by a duct which joins with adjacent ducts to form larger ducts which eventually terminate as the lactiferous duct draining each lobe of the gland. Also *lobules of mammary gland.* **lobuli glandulae thyroideae** [NA] Irregular subdivisions of each lobe of the thyroid gland formed by inward extensions of the investing connective tissue and composed of spherical follicles of varying size and number surrounded by very vascular connective tissue. Also *lobules of thyroid gland.* **lobuli hepatis** [NA] Microscopic functional units of the liver tissue which comprise a central vein from which rows or plates of liver cells with intervening sinusoids radiate to the periphery of the units where the portal canals are situated. Also *hepatic lobules.* Compare PORTAL LOBULE OF LIVER. **l. paracentralis** [NA] A group of gyri on the superior part of the medial surface of the cerebral hemisphere, more or less continuous with the precentral and postcentral gyri of the frontal and parietal lobes, and bounded inferiorly by the cingulate sulcus. It surrounds the medial termination of the central sulcus of Rolando, and is composed of both sensory and motor cortex representing the lower leg and foot. Also *paracentral lobule.* **l. parietalis inferior** [NA] That portion of the parietal lobe on the lateral surface of the cerebral hemisphere lying below the intraparietal sulcus, above the posterior ramus of the lateral cerebral fissure, and behind the postcentral sulcus. It includes the supramarginal and angular gyri, and in the dominant hemisphere is concerned with speech mechanisms. It overlaps but is not entirely congruent with the sensory speech area (Wernicke's center). Also *inferior parietal lobule.* **l. parietalis superior** [NA] That portion of the parietal lobe on the lateral surface of the cerebral hemisphere situated between the postcentral sulcus anteriorly and the parieto-occipital fissure posteriorly, and above the intraparietal sulcus. It includes a group of association areas for somesthesia. Also *superior parietal lobule.* **l. pulmonis primarius** [NA] A microscopic subdivision of the lung consisting of a respiratory bronchiole together with its associated alveolar ducts, alveolar sacs and alveoli. Also *primary lobule of lung.* **l. pulmonis secundarius** [NA] A microscopic subdivision of the lung consisting of about fifty primary lobules and delineated by fibrous interlobular septa. Also *secondary lobule of lung.* **lobuli pulmonum** Either primary or secondary lobules of the lung. *Outmoded.* Also *lobules of lung, pulmonary lobules.* See also LOBULUS PULMONIS PRIMARIUS, LOBULUS PULMONIS SECUNDARIUS. **l. quadrangularis cerebelli** [NA] The quadrangular lobule of the cerebellum; those portions of the cerebellar hemisphere that appear as lateral continuations of the culmen and declive and lie on both sides of the primary fissure. Also *quadrangular lobule of cerebellum, quadrangular lobe of cerebellum.* **l. semilunaris inferior** [NA] That portion of the cerebellar hemisphere appearing as the lateral continuation of the tuber vermis. Also *crus II, inferior crescentic lobe of cerebellum, area lunata* (obs.)*, inferior semilunar lobule, inferior semilunar lobe, caudal semilunar lobule, posterior lunate lobule.* **l. semilunaris superior** [NA] That portion of the cerebellar hemisphere appearing as a lateral continuation of the folium vermis. Also *crus I, superior crescentic lobe of cerebellum, superior semilunar lobule, anterior lunate lobule, cranial semilunar lobule, superior semilunar lobe.* **l. simplex** [NA] That portion of the cerebellar hemisphere continuous with the declive of the vermis. Also *posterior quadrangular lobule, pars posterior lobuli quadrangularis.* **lobuli testis** [NA] The cone-shaped subdivisions or units of the glandular structure of the testis, numbering more than two hundred and each containing up to four convoluted seminiferous tubules supported by loose connective tissue with scattered groups of interstitial cells. The units are incompletely separated from each other by the septula testis, their apices converging on the mediastinum testis while their bases are on the surface of the testis. Also *lobules of testis, spermatic lobules.*

**lobus** \lō′bəs\ [New L (from Gk *lobos* the lobe of the ear, of the liver), a lobe] (*pl.* lobi) Any rounded projection or subdivision of an organ or structure demarcated by fissures, sulci, constrictions, or connective tissue septa; a lobe. **l. anterior hypophyseos** ADENOHYPOPHYSIS. **l. caudatus hepatis** [NA] A small elongated lobe situated on the posterior part of the diaphragmatic surface and the visceral surface of the liver between the fissure for the ligamentum venosum on the left and the groove for the inferior vena cava on the right. It is bounded anteroinferiorly by the porta hepatis just posterior to which the caudate process connects it to the right lobe. Also *caudate lobe of liver, spigelian lobe.* **l. centralis** That portion of the anterior cerebellar vermis between the lingula and culmen. **lobi cerebri** [NA] The major subdivisions of the cerebral pallium, defined by fissures, sulci, or arbitrary boundaries, and named for the bones of the skull which overlie them. They include frontal, parietal, occipital, and temporal lobes. Some include the limbic lobe, an arc of pallium on the medial surface of the hemisphere surrounding the corpus callosum, and continuations of the upper brainstem to the cerebrum. Also *lobes of cerebrum.* **l. clivi** The posterior crescent-shaped lobes of the cerebellum. *Outmoded.* **l. falciformis** *Outmoded* LIMBIC LOBE. **l. frontalis** [NA] The anterior portion of the cerebral hemisphere, extending from the anterior pole to the sulcus centralis. Also *frontal lobe.* **lobi glandulae mammariae** [NA] The fifteen to twenty major subdivisions or lobes of the glandular substance of the breast. They are distributed in a radial fashion around the nipple as the central point. Each constitutes a separate modified sweat gland of the apocrine type consisting of lobules and each is drained by a lactiferous duct opening on the surface of the nipple. The lobes are surrounded and held together by connective tissue, fibrous strands of which attach them to the skin and to the underlying pectoral fascia. Also *lobes of mammary gland.* **lobi glandulae thyroideae dexter et sinister** The right and left cone-shaped lateral lobes of the thyroid gland, which are connected across the midline by the narrow isthmus, surrounded by the pretracheal fascia. They are in contact medially with the thyroid cartilage, cricothyroid muscle, cricoid cartilage, and the upper four or five tracheal cartilages, while laterally they are in contact with the carotid sheath on each side. Also *lobes of thyroid gland.* **l. glandularis of hypophysis** ADENOHYPOPHYSIS. **lobi hepatis** [NA] The morphological divisions of the liver which, according to surface markings, are named lobus hepatis dexter and lobus hepatis sinister, of which the former has two further subdivisions, lobus caudatus and lobus quadratus. Their internal structure is divided into segments according to the distribution of the hepatic ducts, portal vein, and hepatic arteries. Also *lobes of liver, hepatic lobes.* **l. hepatis dexter** [NA] Morphologically, the right five-sixths of the liver, separated from the left lobe anteriorly and superiorly by the line of attachment of the falciform ligament, and on the posterior and visceral surfaces by the fissure for ligamentum venosum and the fissure for ligamentum teres. On the visceral surface and the posterior part of the diaphragmatic surface it has two subdivisions, the caudate and quadrate lobes. Its substance is divided into anterior and posterior segments. Also *right lobe of liver.* **l. hepatis sinister** [NA] Morphologically, the left one sixth of the liver separated from the right lobe anteriorly and superiorly by the line of attachment of the falciform ligament and on the posterior and visceral surfaces by the fissure for ligamentum venosum and the fissure for ligamentum teres. It is thin and flattened superoinferiorly. Its substance is divided into medial and lateral segments. Also *left lobe of liver.* **l. inferior pulmonis** [NA] The large lobe of the lung situated below and behind the oblique fissure which separates it from the superior lobe in the left lung and from the superior and middle lobes in the right lung. In both lungs it comprises five bronchopulmonary segments (VI through X). Its inferior surface forms the base of the lung. Also *inferior lobe of lung, lower lobe of lung.* **l. insularis** [NA] INSULA. **l. medius prostatae** [NA] The slightly elevated portion of the prostate, between the ejaculatory ducts and the urethra, which forms the superior part of the posterior surface of the prostate. Its size varies considerably and it usually only becomes obvious when enlarged. Also *median lobe of prostate, Morgagni's caruncle, morgagnian caruncle.* **l. medius pulmonis dextri** [NA] The small, wedge-shaped lobe of the right lung which is separated from the superior lobe by the horizontal fissure and from the inferior lobe by the oblique fissure. It varies in size and comprises the lateral (IV) and medial (V) bronchopulmonary segments. Also *middle lobe of right lung.* **l. nervosus neurohypophyseos** [NA] The body of the neurohypophysis, the site of storage and release of oxytocin and vasopressin. Along with the infundibulum (hypophysial stalk), it constitutes the neurohypophysis. Also *neural lobe, pars nervosa hypophyseos.* **l. occipitalis** [NA] The posterior portion of the cerebral hemisphere, extending from the posterior pole to an imaginary line connecting the parieto-occipital fissure superiorly and medially with the preoccipital notch inferiorly. Also *occipital lobe.* **l. olfactorius** Those structures on the inferior surface of the frontal lobe of the cerebral hemisphere directly concerned with olfaction. It comprises the olfactory bulb, tract, trigone, and striae, and is maximally developed in macrosmatic animals. Also *olfactory lobule, olfactory lobe.* **l. parietalis** [NA] The upper and central portion of the cerebral hemisphere, primarily on the lateral surface. It is separated anteriorly from the frontal lobe by the central sulcus, and inferiorly from the temporal lobe by the lateral sulcus, though there is some confluence at the posterior end of both lobes. It appears continuous behind with the occipital lobe on the lateral surface, but is separated from it on the medial surface by the parieto-occipital sulcus. For topographical purposes, division is made between the parietal and occipital lobes on the lateral surface by means of an imaginary line connecting the parieto-occipital sulcus (just visible at the vertex) with the preoccipital notch on the inferior surface. Also *parietal lobe.* **l. posterior hypophyseos** NEUROHYPOPHYSIS. **l. prostatae dexter et sinister** [NA] The lateral portions, right and left, of the prostate below the transverse groove on the posterior surface, which is formed by the two ejaculatory ducts penetrating the gland and from which a median vertical furrow extends downward to demarcate the two lateral portions. They occupy the main mass of the gland, and are continuous behind the urethra and are connected in front of it by the isthmus. Also *lateral lobes of prostate gland.* **l. pyramidalis glandulae thyroideae** [NA] A conical third lobe, present in about forty percent of thyroid glands, extending upwards from either the isthmus or the left lobe, and occasionally becoming continuous with a fibrous or fibromuscular band that attaches to the hyoid bone. It represents the distal remnant of the thyroglossal duct. Also *pyramidal lobe of thyroid gland.* **l. quadratus hepatis** [NA] A quadrilateral-shaped lobe on the visceral surface of the liver, structurally a part of the right lobe and bounded on the left by the fissure for ligamentum teres, on the right by the fossa of the gallbladder, anteriorly by the inferior margin of the liver, and posteriorly by the porta hepatis. Also *quadrate lobe of liver.* **lobi renales** [NA] The functional units of the kidney, each being a segment that drains through a renal papilla and containing several lobules. Up to six pyramids may be connected to a single papilla. In the normal human adult these units are not demarcated and the renal surface is smooth, but in fetuses and infants the surface is irregular and lobated. Also *renal lobes.* **l. superior pulmonis** [NA] The large lobe of the lung situated above and in front of the oblique fissure in the left lung and the oblique and horizontal fissures in the right lung. Its upper limit forms the apex of the lung. In the right lung it contains bronchopulmonary segments I–III while in the left it includes I through V. Also *superior lobe of lung, upper lobe of lung.* **l. temporalis** [NA] The ventral and lateral portion of the cerebral hemisphere. It lies below the lateral cerebral fissure lateral to the collateral fissure and merges with the occipital lobe posteriorly. Also *temporal lobe.*

**local** Confined to a particular site or region of the body; limited in distribution or effect.

**localization** \lō′kəlīzā′shən\ **1** The determination of the position of an object. **2** The determination of the confines of a phenomenon. **3** The process of confining to a limited area of extent. **cerebral l.** The concept that different regions of the cerebral cortex are specialized to express specific functional attributes. **pneumotaxic l.** Localization of cerebral structures as revealed by ventriculography. Modern noninvasive methods of visualization such as nuclear magnetic resonance radiography have replaced the method. **selective l.** The specific accumulation of a radionuclide in an organ or tissue. **spatial l.** The ability to recognize the positioning of a stimulus on the body surface.

**localized** \lō′kəlīzd\ Confined to a particular region, as an infection.

**localizer** \lō′kəlī′zər\ COLLIMATOR.

**loc. dol.** *loco dolenti* (L, to the painful spot).

**lochia** \lō′kē·ə\ [neut. pl. of Gk *lochios* (from *lochos* the act of lying in wait, an ambush, a lying-in, childbirth) pertaining to childbirth; as substantive *ta lochia* the discharge after childbirth] The uterine discharge that issues from the vagina postpartum. Adj. lochial. **l. alba** A uterine discharge of a light color, usually the last of several uterine discharges after delivery. Lochia alba consists primarily of leukocytes. Also *lochia purulenta.* **l. cruenta** LOCHIA RUBRA. **l. purulenta** LOCHIA ALBA. **l. rubra** A bright red uterine discharge that appears immediately after delivery. It consists primarily of blood. Also *lochia cruenta.*

**lochiocyte** \lo′kē-ōsīt′\ A decidual cell contained in the lochia.

**lochiometritis** \lō′kē·ōmētrī′tis\ [Gk *lochio(s)* pertaining to childbirth + METRITIS] PUERPERAL ENDOMETRITIS.

**lochometritis** \lō′kōmētrī′tis\ [Gk *locho(s)* a lying in, childbirth + METRITIS] PUERPERAL ENDOMETRITIS.

**loci** \lō′sī\ Plural of LOCUS.

**lock** / **friction l.** A lower extremity prosthetic knee mechanism that dampens the swing phase of gait and provides increased stability when the prosthesis is extended during the stance phase. **transfer l.** In a controlled environment, opening in a laminar air flow tent that permits passage of materials to the patient.

**Locke** [Frank Spiller *Locke*, English physiologist, 1871–1949] **1** Citrated Locke solution. See under SOLUTION. **2** Locke-Ringer solution. See under SOLUTION.

**locking** / **head l.** INTERLOCKING.

**lockjaw** **1** Trismus, especially as a manifestation of tetanus. *Popular.* **2** *Popular* TETANUS.

**Lockwood** [Charles Barrett *Lockwood*, English surgeon, 1858–1914] **1** See under SIGN. **2** Lockwood suspensory ligament. See under SUSPENSORY LIGAMENT OF EYEBALL.

**locomotion** \lō′kəmō′shən\ [L *loc(us)* place + *o* + MOTION] Movement from place to place effected or controlled by means of some mechanism within the moving object. **fictive l.** Essentially normal locomotor activity produced through electric or pharmacologic stimulation of a central nervous structure.

**locomotive** Relating to movement from one place to another. Also *locomotory.*

**locomotor** \lō′kəmō′tər\ Relating to locomotion or to the locomotive apparatus of the body.

**locomotorial** \lō′kəmōtôr′ē·əl\ Describing or pertaining to the locomotor system.

**locular** \läk′yələr\ Pertaining to a loculus or loculi.

**loculate** \läk′yəlāt\ Possessing or divided into a number of loculi.

**loculation** \läk′yəlā′shən\ The process of forming loculi or the state of having loculi.

**loculus** \läk′yələs\ [L (dim. of *locus* a place) a small space, compartment] (*pl.* loculi) A small chamber or cavity.

**locus** \lō′kəs\ [L, a place, position] (*pl.* loci) **1** A particular site or position, as of an anatomic part. **2** In genetics, the position in the linkage map or in the chromosome of a gene, of a cluster of genes, or of a regulatory region that does not yield a product but that influences nearby genes. **l. ceruleus** [NA] A deeply pigmented group of neurons in the superior angle of the floor of the fourth ventricle. The 3000–4000 cells in the paired nuclear complex generate a widespread axonal system that constitutes the major norepinephrine pathway of the central nervous system. Also *locus* *cinereus, locus ferrugineus, nucleus pigmentosus pontis, substantia ferruginea.* **l. cinereus** LOCUS CERULEUS. **complex l.** A locus on a chromosome having more than one site at which recombination can occur. **l. ferrugineus** LOCUS CERULEUS. **H-2 l.** One of the principal components, along with the Ir gene, of the major histocompatibility complex in the mouse. It is comparable to the HLA loci in humans. **histocompatibility l.** One of the genes located within the major histocompatibility complex that specifies transplantation antigens or immune response functions. **l. niger** SUBSTANTIA NIGRA. **operator l.** A regulator locus that governs the transcription of adjacent structural genes through interaction with specific regulatory proteins. In bacterial genetics, the operator is proximal to the structural genes of the operon and is the binding site of a repressor protein molecule. Also *operator.* **l. perforatus anticus** SUBSTANTIA PERFORATA ANTERIOR. **l. perforatus posticus** SUBSTANTIA PERFORATA POSTERIOR. **PTC l.** A human gene which, by an unknown mechanism, determines whether the substance phenylthiocarbamide can be tasted or not. Also *taster gene.* **l. ruber** NUCLEUS RUBER.

**Loeb** [Leo *Loeb,* U.S. pathologist, 1869–1959] Loeb's decidual reaction. See under REACTION.

**Loeffler** See under LÖFFLER.

**loeffleria** \lefler′ē·ə\ [after Friedrich August Johannes *Loeffler* (or *Löffler*), German bacteriologist, 1852–1915 + -IA] A condition in which *Corynebacterium diphtheriae* are present but the characteristic symptoms of diphtheria are not. Also *löffleria.*

**loempe** \lem′pē\ BERIBERI.

**Loenen** [Johannes Jacobus Guilielmus van *Loenen,* Dutch physician, flourished 19th century] Loenen sign. See under HEGAR SIGN.

**Loewenstein** [Ludwig W. *Loewenstein,* German-born dermatologist, active in the United States, flourished 20th century] Tumor of Buschke-Loewenstein. See under TUMOR.

**Löffler** [Friedrich August Johannes *Löffler,* German bacteriologist, 1852–1915] **1** Klebs-Löffler bacillus. See under *CORYNEBACTERIUM DIPHTHERIAE.* **2** Löffler serum agar, Löffler serum, Löffler medium. See under LÖFFLER'S BLOOD CULTURE MEDIUM (at CULTURE MEDIUM) **3** See under METHYLENE BLUE.

**Löffler** [Wilhelm *Löffler,* Swiss physician, born 1887] **1** Löffler's parietal fibroplastic endocarditis, Löffler's disease. See under LÖFFLER'S ENDOCARDITIS. **2** Löffler's eosinophilia, Löffler's pneumonia, Löffler's disease. See under LÖFFLER SYNDROME.

**löffleria** \lefler′ē·ə\ LOEFFLERIA.

**log-** \läg-\ LOGO-.

**logadectomy** \läg′ədek′təmē\ [Gk *logad(es)* the whites of the eyes + -ECTOMY] Excision of a part of the conjunctiva.

**logaditis** \läg′ədī′tis\ [Gk *logad(es)* the whites of the eyes + -ITIS] SCLERITIS.

**logagnosia** \läg′agnō′zhə\ [LOG- + Gk *agnosia* ignorance, a not knowing] Inability to recognize spoken or written words. *Obs.* Also *alogognosia, asemognosia.*

**logagraphia** \läg′əgraf′ē·ə\ Agraphia with particular inability to express meaning by the written word. Adj. logographic.

**logamnesia** \läg′amnē′zhə\ [LOG- + AMNESIA] Word deafness or word blindness.

**Logan** [William H. G. *Logan,* U.S. plastic surgeon, flourished 20th century] See under BOW.

**logaphasia** \läg′əfā′zhə\ [LOG- + APHASIA] BROCA'S APHASIA.

**logasthenia** \läg′asthē′nē·ə\ *Outmoded* WERNICKE'S APHASIA.

**Log Etronics** A process for reproducing x-ray or photographic images with the use of electronic methods to change contrast or density or both. Also *logetronography.*

**-logia** \-lō′jə\ -LOGY.

**logic** [Gk *logikē,* fem. of *logikos* (from *logos* word, reason + *-ikos* -IC) pertaining to speech or reason] **1** A discipline embodying sets of rules for determining the validity of an argument or a chain of reasoning without regard to empirical content. **2** In a logic circuit, the physical realization of a particular type or principle of logic, as in *binary logic,* or *AND gate logic.*

**-logist** \-ləjist\ [Gk *log(os)* word, speech, reason + -IST] A combining form designating one who specializes in a science or study or adheres to a particular doctrine.

**logit** \läj′it\ **1** In statistics, the natural logarithm of the odds corresponding to the probability *P* of a specified outcome given the existence of a stated attribute, for example, of a coronary attack given a diastolic blood pressure of 95 mmHg. Logit $P = \log_e\left(\frac{P}{1-P}\right)$. The logarithm of the odds ratio is conveniently expressed as the difference of two logits. **2** In bioassay, a transformation based on a logistic model of the dose-response relationship such that the logit of the response is linearly dependent on the dose.

**logo-** \läg′ə-\ [Gk *logos* word, speech, reason] A combining form meaning word or speech. Also *log-.*

**logoclonia** \-klō′nē·ə\ [LOGO- + Gk *klon(os)* confusion, tumult + -IA] Rhythmic and meaningless repetition of a word or of the last few syllables of a word, as seen particularly in presenile or senile dementia and in general paresis. Also *logoklony.*

**logokophosis** \-kōfō′sis\ [LOGO- + Gk *kōphōsis* dumbness, deafness, dullness] *Outmoded* WERNICKE'S APHASIA.

**logomania** \-mā′nē·ə\ [LOGO- + -MANIA] Excessive, rapid speech, as in mania. Also *lalorrhea, logorrhea, tachylogia, verbomania, tachyphemia, tachyphrasia, tachyphasia.*

**logopaedics** *Brit.* LOGOPEDICS.

**logopathy** \lägäp′əthē\ [LOGO- + -PATHY] Any disorder of speech caused by disease of the central nervous system.

**logopedics** \-pē′diks\ [LOGO- + English *(ortho)pedics,* from ORTHO- + Gk *pais,* gen. *paidos,* a child] The study and treatment of speech disorders. Also *logopedia.*

**logorrhea** \läg′ôrē′ə\ [LOGO- + -RRHEA] LOGOMANIA. **jargonaphasic l.** JARGON APHASIA.

**-logy** \-ləjē\ [Gk *logos* word, speech, reason] A combining form designating a (specified) science, study, doctrine, or treatise. Also *-logia.*

**Lohmann** [Karl *Lohmann,* German biochemist, born 1898] **1** See under REACTION. **2** Lohmann's enzyme. See under CREATINE KINASE.

**loiasis** \lō·ī′əsis\ [*Lo(a)* + -IASIS] Filariasis caused by *Loa loa,* a nematode parasite widely distributed in western and central Africa. Calabar swellings are a classic manifestation caused by local inflammatory response to migration of adult worms in subcutaneous tissues. Adult worms occasionally migrate across the eye surface, hence the name eye worm. Microfilariae are found in the peripheral blood. Treatment is with diethylcarbamazine. Also *loaiasis.*

**loin** \loin\ LUMBUS.

**loliism** \lō′lē·izm\ [*Loli(um temulentum)* + -ISM] Poisoning by seeds of *Lolium temulentum,* darnel ryegrass, which may contaminate grain made into flour and used for bread. Symptoms are tremors, blurred vision, vomiting and prostration. Also *lolism.*

**Lombard** [Etienne *Lombard,* French physician, 1869–1920] See under TEST.

**Londe** [P. F. L. *Londe,* French neurologist, 1864–1944] 1 Fazio-Londe atrophy. See under ATROPHY. 2 Fazio-Londe syndrome, Fazio-Londe disease. See under INFANTILE PROGRESSIVE BULBAR PALSY.

**longevity** \länjevʹitē\ Length of life.

**longitudinal** \länʹjitʸooʹdinəl\ Lying or directed lengthwise; parallel to the long axis of the body or of one of its organs or parts.

**longitypical** \länʹjitipʹikəl\ DOLICHOMORPHIC.

**longsightedness** HYPEROPIA.

**loop** [Middle English *loupe*] 1 ANSA. 2 The characteristic shape of the arched dermal ridges in dermatoglyphics. 3 A curvature, varying from a gentle arch to an acute bend, in an anatomical structure. **Axenfeld's nerve l.** An intrascleral nerve commonly associated with a small cuff of uveal pigment, usually occurring several millimeters above the upper limbus in heavily pigmented persons. Its clinical significance is that it may be mistaken for an imbedded foreign body. **capillary l.'s** The capillaries in the dermal papillae. **closed l.** In an automatic control system, a signal path which includes a feedback path, which compares the controlled value with the desired value, and a forward path, which reduces any difference between the controlled value and the desired value. Also *feedback mechanism, regulatory feedback loop.* **gamma l.** The reflex arc involving the gamma efferent fibers arising in the anterior horns and the sensory afferent fibers arising in the muscle spindles. It is involved in the control of muscle tone. **l. of Henle** A U-shaped portion of the nephron, the descending limb of which extends from the straight portion of the proximal convoluted tubule in the cortex to the medulla where it makes a U-turn into the ascending limb which extends towards the glomerulus to form the distal convoluted tubule. The lower parts of the limbs and the U-turn are often attenuated to form the thin segment, and are known as the tubulus attenuatus. The limbs run radially and are parallel in the medullary rays. There are numerous variations including loops of juxtaglomerular nephrons being long and thin and extending to the apex of the renal papilla, while loops of subcapsular nephrons are short, with the U-turn formed by a thick descending limb and extending only to the outer part of the medulla. Also *nephronic loop, Henle's ansa, ansa nephroni, Henle's canal.* **l. of hypoglossal nerve** ANSA CERVICALIS. **Hyrtl's l.** An occasional communication between the right and left hypoglossal nerves in the geniohyoid or genioglossus muscle. Also *Hyrtl's anastomosis.* **intestinal l.** One of several U-shaped flexures formed by the jejunum and ileum, the convex surface of which is free while the concave surface is attached to the mesentery through which the gut receives its vessels and nerves. The free surfaces of the flexures are in contact with each other or with the anterior abdominal wall. **lenticular l.** ANSA LENTICULARIS. **Lippes l.** An S-shaped intrauterine contraceptive device. **Meyer's l.** The portion of the geniculocalcarine radiation that runs anterolaterally before looping around the inferior horn of the lateral ventricle and turning posteriorly. Due to its relatively widesweeping trajectory through the temporal lobe, it is a sensitive indicator of temporal lobe pathology, particularly for space-occupying lesions. **nephronic l.** LOOP OF HENLE. **P l.** The loop formed by atrial activity in the vectorcardiogram. **l. of the pectoral nerves** A common anastomotic loop between the medial pectoral and lateral pectoral nerves in front of the axillary artery and usually just below the origin of the thoracoacromial artery. **peduncular l.** ANSA PEDUNCULARIS. **platinum l.** A ring of platinum wire, mounted in a heat-resistant handle, that is used to transfer microbiologic material. Because it is highly resistant to solution and withstands very high temperatures, platinum can undergo repeated exposure to harsh sterilizing conditions. **primitive intestinal l.** The simple intestinal tube of a four-week human embryo. It lies in the median plane, loops ventrally from the stomach to the cloaca, and is continuous at midpoint with the stalk of the yolk sac. The segment above the midpoint is the cranial limb of the intestinal loop, that below is the caudal limb. **QRS l.** The loop formed by ventricular depolarization in the vectorcardiogram. **l. of recurrent laryngeal nerve** The anteroposterior loop formed by the recurrent laryngeal nerve after arising from the vagus nerve. The one on the right hooks around the front, lower, and posterior surfaces of the first part of the right subclavian artery, while that on the left hooks below the arch of the aorta and behind the attachment of the ligamentum arteriosum and then up the left side of the trachea. Developmentally the nerve turns under the sixth pair of aortic arches, the distal part of which on the left side forms the ligamentum arteriosum while on the right side this part and the fifth arch disappear so that the nerve ascends to the fourth arch, the right subclavian artery. **regulatory feedback l.** CLOSED LOOP. **Roux en Y l.** The structure that results from a surgical procedure in which a nonfunctioning loop of jejunum is anastomosed to the remaining proximal small bowel about 40 cm downstream. The procedure is undertaken to drain the pancreatic and/or biliary secretions following procedures. **Silastic l.'s** Silicon rubber fashioned into loops that, when passed once or twice around a vessel, can be used to occlude blood flow during surgery. **l.'s of spinal nerves** ANSAE NERVORUM SPINALIUM. **subclavian l.** ANSA SUBCLAVIA. **vector l.** The loop inscribed on a vectorcardiogram by cardiac electrical activity. **ventricular l.** A U-shaped loop resulting from the early bending on itself of the embryonic cardiac tube. The ventricle develops at the bottom of the loop. **l. of Vieussens** ANSA SUBCLAVIA.

**loopful** The amount of fluid held by a platinum loop during the transfer of materials for microbiologic examination. It is used for estimating the concentration of organisms.

**loosening** A disturbance of mental associations that renders thinking vague, diffuse, imprecise, and unfocused.

**Looser** [Emil *Looser,* Swiss physician, 1877–1936] 1 Looser's transformation zones. See under ZONE. 2 Looser-Milkman syndrome. See under MILKMAN SYNDROME.

**LOP** left occipitoposterior position (of a fetus). See under OCCIPUT POSTERIOR POSITION.

**lophodont** \läfʹōdänt\ [Gk *loph(os)* a ridge of ground + -ODONT] Denoting a dentition in which the molar cusps fuse to form ridges, characteristic of horses and other grazing animals.

**lophophorine** \lōfäfʹərin\ $C_{13}H_{17}NO_3$. An extremely toxic alkaloid found in the cactus *Lophophora williamsii.* It has strychninelike effects if ingested.

**lophotrichous** \lōfätʹrikəs\ In bacteria, possessing multiple flagella at one pole only. Compare PERITRICHOUS.

**Lorain** [Paul Joseph *Lorain,* French physician, 1827–1875] 1 Lévi-Lorain infantilism, Lorain's infantilism, Lorain-Lévi syndrome, Lévi-Lorain type, Lorain type. See under HYPOPHYSIAL DWARFISM. 2 Lévi-Lorain dwarf, Lorain-Lévi dwarf. See under HYPOPHYSIAL DWARF.

**Lorand** [Lazlo *Lorand,* Hungarian-born U.S. physiologist, born 1923] Laki-Lorand factor. See under FACTOR XIII.

**lorazepam** $C_{15}H_{10}Cl_2N_2O_2$. 7-Chloro-5-(2-chloro-phenyl)-1,3-dihydro-3-hydroxy-2*H*-1,4-benzodiazopin-2-one. A benzodiazepine drug with actions and uses like those of diazepam.

**lorbamate** $C_{12}H_{22}N_2O_4$. 2-(Hydroxymethyl)-2-methylpentyl cyclopropanecarbamate ester. It has been used as a muscle-relaxant drug.

**lordoscoliosis** \lôr′dōskō′lē·ō′sis\ Increased lordosis in association with the lateral deviation of a scoliosis in the lumbar vertebrae.

**lordosis** \lôrdō′sis\ [Gk *lordōsis* (from *lordoun* to bend the body forward and inward + *-ōsis* -OSIS) a bending forward and inward] **1** The anatomical anterior concavity of the cervical and lumbar vertebrae. **2** An abnormally increased anatomical anterior concavity of the cervical and lumbar vertebrae. Also *dorsal lordosis, cervical lordosis, hollow-back, backward curvature, saddle back, sway back.* **compensatory l.** An increased anterior concave curvature of the lumbar spine taken up to balance the rest of the proximal spine or a pelvic obliquity deformity. **dorsal l.** LORDOSIS.

**lordotic** \lôrdät′ik\ **1** Of or relating to lordosis. **2** Exhibiting lordosis.

**Lorenz** [Adolf *Lorenz,* Austrian orthopedic surgeon, 1854–1946] **1** Hoffa-Lorenz operation. See under LORENZ OPERATION. **2** See under METHOD, SIGN, OSTEOTOMY.

**loss / anaphase lag l.** SOMATIC NONDISJUNCTION. **autoimmune sensorineural hearing l.** Bilateral sensorineural hearing loss due to inflammatory changes produced by the deposition in the ear of autoimmune antigen-antibody complexes. It is usually confined to the inner ear and is progressive over weeks or months. Vestibular responses are diminished or lost and facial paralysis may occur. Consistent improvement has been reported with dexamethasone and cyclophosphamide therapy. Also *immune complex associated deafness.* **birth l.** REPRODUCTIVE WASTAGE. **coincidence l.** Undercounting in a radiation detector due to the occurrence of ionizing events at a rate faster than the resolution time of the counting system. **conductive hearing l.** Hearing loss arising from causes in the external meatus or in the middle-ear cleft and its contained structures. Also *conductive hearing impairment, transmission deafness.* **congenital hearing l.** Hearing loss present from birth or occurring in the perinatal period. It may arise from genetic or intrauterine causes. **dissociated sensory l.** Sensory impairment with one form of sensation, such as touch, pain or temperature, or position and joint sense, being affected more severely than the other forms. **evaporative water l.** Water that is lost through the skin when the vapor pressure of the skin exceeds that of the ambient air. Such loss is about 500 ml per day in normal adults, and may be ten times greater in patients with severe burns. **hearing l.** **1** An increased auditory threshold above normal resulting in a diminished sense or acuity of hearing. The pure tone audiogram may show a raised threshold for one or two frequencies, or there may be a greatly increased threshold across the whole range of hearing. Also *hearing impairment, amblyacusis, amblykusis, surdity.* **2** DEAFNESS. **noise-induced hearing l.** Hearing loss resulting from exposure to high ambient noise levels. Also *noise-induced deafness, acoustic-trauma deafness.* **nonorganic hearing l.** Hearing loss for which there is no structural or neurologic basis. It usually arises out of an acute or repeatedly stressful situation in which hearing plays an important role. It is to be distinguished from the assumed deafness of malingering. Also *hysterical deafness.* **ototoxic hearing l.** Hearing loss arising from exposure to therapeutic agents which cause damage to the organ of Corti or related structures. Such agents include certain alkaloids and diuretics and the aminoglycoside antibiotics. Also *ototoxic deafness, toxic deafness* (older term). **profound hearing l.** Hearing loss to such a degree that there may be no sensation of hearing for even the loudest environmental sounds. The pure tone audiogram is usually considered as showing a profound loss when the threshold is 90 dB HL or worse. **saddle sensory l.** Loss or impairment of sensation in the perineum and medial aspect of the buttocks, resulting usually from a low cauda equina lesion. The area affected is the part of the body which would come into contact with a saddle. **sensorineural hearing l.** Hearing loss arising out of pathologic changes affecting the biochemistry, electric potential, vascular supply and end organ structures within the cochlea, or its neural connections with the brainstem and the cochlear nuclei. Also *sensorineural deafness, neural deafness, perceptive deafness* (outmoded). **water l.** Loss of water from the body in urine and stools, by insensible losses from the skin and expired air, and by sweating.

**LOT** left occipitotransverse position (of a fetus). See under OCCIPUT TRANSVERSE POSITION.

**lot.** *lotio* (L, lotion).

**lota** \lō′tə\ PINTA.

**Lotheissen** [Georg *Lotheissen,* German surgeon, 1868–1941] See under OPERATION.

**lotio** [L (from *lotus,* a past part. of *lavare* to wash, bathe), a washing, lotion] LOTION. **l. alba** WHITE LOTION. **l. calaminae oleosa** OILY LOTION OF CALAMINE. **l. evaporans** EVAPORATING LOTION. **l. potassae sulphuratae cum zinco** WHITE LOTION. **l. zinci sulphatis** LOTION OF ZINC SULFATE.

**lotion** [L *lotio.* See LOTIO.] A liquid preparation for external application containing suspended or emulsified medicinal ingredients. Also *lotio.* **benzyl benzoate l.** A lotion containing a dilute aqueous solution of benzoyl benzoate. **calamine l.** A lotion containing calamine, zinc oxide, glycerin, bentonite, and calcium hydroxide. **evaporating l.** A lotion containing alcohol, ammonium chloride, and water. Also *lotio evaporans.* **oily l. of calamine** A lotion consisting of an oily emulsion of calamine, oleic acid, wool fat, arachis oil, and a solution of calcium hydroxide. Also *lotio calaminae oleosa.* **phenolated calamine l.** A modified preparation of calamine lotion containing 1% phenol. **white l.** A lotion containing potassium sulfate and zinc sulfate in water. Also *lotio alba, lotio potassae sulphuratae cum zinco.* **l. of zinc sulfate** A lotion containing zinc sulfate and amaranth in water. Also *lotio zinci sulphatis.*

**loudness** **1** The intensity of a sound or noise. It may be expressed in phons. **2** The attribute of sound which enables the hearer to classify it by intensity of effect, one of the fundamental psychological qualities of auditory sensation. It has a nonlinear relation to the physical intensity of a sound, the relation being partly dependent on frequency.

**Louis** [Pierre-Charles-Alexandre *Louis,* French physician, 1787–1872] **1** See under LAW. **2** Angle of Louis. See under ANGULUS STERNI.

**Louis-Bar** [Denise *Louis-Bar,* European physician, flourished mid-20th century] Louis-Bar disease, Louis-Bar syndrome. See under ATAXIA-TELANGIECTASIA.

**loupe** \loop\ [French, a lens of biconvex glass for magnifying] A small magnifying lens.

**louse** [Old English *lūs*] (*pl.* lice) A small, dorsoventrally flattened insect that is ectoparasitic on mammals or birds, belonging to the order Anoplura (sucking lice) or Malloph-

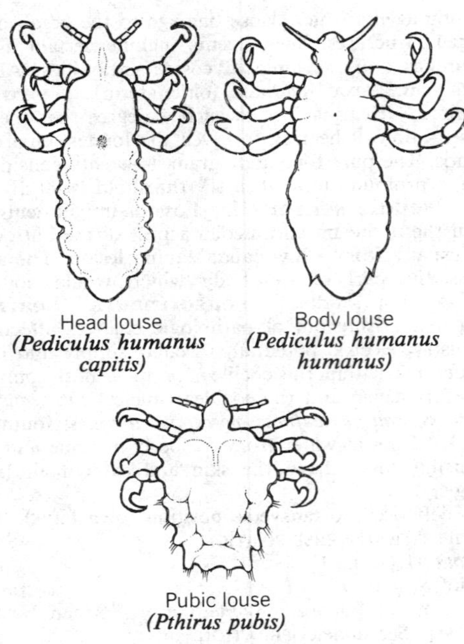


**Common lice of humans**

aga (biting or chewing lice). **biting l.** A member of the insect order Mallophaga. Also *chewing louse.* **body l.** A louse of the subspecies *Pediculus humanus humanus.* Also *clothes louse.* **crab l.** PUBIC LOUSE. **head l.** A louse of the subspecies *Pediculus humanus capitis.* **pubic l.** A louse of the species *Pthirus pubis.* Also *crab louse, crab* (popular). **sucking l.** A member of the insect order Anoplura.

**lousicide** \lou′sisīd\ [*lous(e)* + *i* + -CIDE ] PEDICULICIDE.

**lovastatin** $C_{24}H_{36}O_5$. 2-Methylbutanoic acid 1,2,3,7,8,8a-hexahydro-3,7-dimethyl-8-[2-(tetrahydro-4-hydroxy-6-oxo-2*H*-pyran-2-yl)ethyl]-1-naphthalenyl ester. The precursor of the β-hydroxy acid form that inhibits the enzyme 3-hydroxy-3-methylglutaryl-CoA reductase, a rate-limiting step in the synthesis of cholesterol. Lovastatin is obtained from the fungus *Monascus ruber.* It is administered orally and is used in the treatment of hypercholesterolemia, where it has been shown to be effective in lowering low-density lipoprotein. Induction of LDL receptors on the hepatocyte, which may lower LDL, is associated with its administration. It has been associated with hepatotoxicity. Also *mevinolin, monacolin K, 6-α-methyl compactin.*

**love / smother l.** Overprotectiveness, overpossessiveness, and total control that is exhibited under the guise of love and concern but which deprives the object of any possibility of achieving independence. Also *maternal overprotection.*

**Lovelace** [William Randolph *Lovelace* II, U.S. surgeon, 1907–1965] See under BLB MASK.

**Loven** [Otto Christian *Loven,* Swedish physician, 1835–1904] See under REFLEX.

**Løvset** [Jorgen *Løvset,* Norwegian obstetrician, flourished 20th century] Løvset's method. See under MANEUVER.

**Low** [George C. *Low,* English physician, 1872–1952] Castellani-Low symptom. See under SYMPTOM.

**low-cervical** Denoting animal preparations in which a cervical transection of the neuraxis is made at the $C_6$ level or lower (i.e., with retention of diaphragmatic breathing). Attention is usually centered on nervous functions below the transection.

**Lowe** [Charles Upton *Lowe,* U.S. pediatrician, born 1921] Lowe's disease, Lowe syndrome. See under OCULOCEREBRORENAL SYNDROME.

**Löwe** [Karl F. *Löwe,* German optician, 1874–1955] See under RING.

**Löwenberg** [Benjamin Benno *Löwenberg,* German-born French laryngologist, 1836–1905] Löwenburg's canal. See under DUCTUS COCHLEARIS.

**Löwenstein** [Ernst *Löwenstein,* Austrian-born U.S. pathologist, 1878–1950] Löwenstein-Jensen agar, Löwenstein-Jensen medium. See under AGAR.

**Löwenthal** [Wilhelm *Lowenthal,* German physician, 1850–1894] Löwenthal's tract. See under TRACTUS TECTOSPINALIS.

**Lower** [Richard *Lower,* English physiologist, 1631–1691] **1** Lower's rings. See under ANNULI FIBROSI CORDIS. **2** See under SAC. **3** Lower's tubercle. See under TUBERCULUM INTERVENOSUM.

**Lown** [Bernard *Lown,* U.S. cardiologist, born 1921] Lown-Ganong-Levine syndrome. See under SHORT PR SYNDROME.

**low-spin** Denoting the state of a transition metal in which the electrons have as few unpaired spins as possible. They therefore leave some orbitals empty, and this is energetically favored if those orbitals are raised in energy by interaction with electrons of ligands. The iron of oxyhemoglobin is in the low-spin state, because the oxygen ligand raises the energy of one of its orbitals. The change in spin state on oxygenation allows the iron atom to fit more closely into the plane of the porphyrin, and this movement triggers the change of conformation that facilitates binding of oxygen molecules to the other heme groups of the molecule.

**loxapine** $C_{18}H_{18}ClN_3O$. 2-Chloro-11-(4-methylpiperazinlyl)dibenz[*b,f*][1,4]oxazepine. A tricyclic antipsychotic drug, also used for its tranquilizing properties.

**loxapine succinate** $C_{18}H_{18}ClN_3O{\cdot}C_4H_6O_4$. A dibenzoxazepine drug with antipsychotic actions like the phenothiazines. It is used as a minor tranquilizer.

**loxia** \läk′sē·ə\ TORTICOLLIS.

**loxophthalmus** \läk′säfthal′məs\ [Gk *lox(os)* slanting, crosswise + *ophthalmos* the eye] MANIFEST DEVIATION.

***Loxosceles*** \läksäs′əlēz\ [Gk *loxo(s)* slanting, crosswise, oblique + *skelos* the leg] A genus of spiders in the family Loxoscelidae (or in some classifications, Scytodidae); the brown or fiddleback spiders. They are characterized by having six eyes (instead of the usual eight), tawny color, and a flattened, heavily sclerotized carapace, on which some species have a pattern suggestive of a violin. Certain species of the western hemisphere are often found in human dwellings and have a bite that can be seriously poisonous. See also LOXOSCELISM. ***L. laeta*** The Chilean brown spider, which has a cytotoxic venom, medically important as a cause of loxoscelism in South America. The venom causes localized cellulitis and necrosis, hemorrhage, and a strong leukocytic and eosinophilic response. Some consider this severe clinical reaction to indicate an autopharmacologic response as well. About 5 percent of reported cases have resulted in death. ***L. reclusa*** A species found principally in the south central United States; the brown recluse or violin spider. Its bite commonly results in local cutaneous necrosis and sometimes persistent ulceration. A number of deaths following systemic complications have been reported.

**loxoscelism** \läksäs′əlizm\ [*Loxoscel(es)* + -ISM] Poisoning from the bite of a spider of the genus *Loxosceles*, such as the South American *L. laeta* or the North American *L. reclusa*, the brown recluse. The hemolytic and necrotizing venom produces a long-lasting ulcerative lesion that often leaves a disfiguring scar at the site of the bite. Fever, muscle weakness, nausea, and vomiting are commonly observed.

***Loxotrema ovatum*** \läk′sətrē′mə ōvā′təm\ *METAGONIMUS YOKOGAWAI.*

**lozenge** [Middle English *losenge*, from Middle French *losange* a diamond-shaped heraldic figure, prob. from Old French *lauze* a flat stone] A tablet containing a medication in a flavored and sweetened base. It is designed for local treatment of the mouth and throat by the steady release of the medicine while the mass slowly dissolves in the mouth. Also *troche, trochiscus, morsulus, rotula.*

**LP** lumbar puncture.

**LPF** lymphocytosis-promoting factor.

**LPH** lipotropic hormone.

**LPS** lipopolysaccharide.

**Lr** **1** Symbol for the element, lawrencium. **2** Immunological symbol for limit of reaction. **3** Symbol for the Limes reacting dose of diphtheria toxin.

**LRF** luteinizing hormone releasing factor (gonadotropin releasing hormone).

**LSA** left sacroanterior position (of a fetus). See under SACRUM ANTERIOR POSITION.

**LSD** lysergic acid diethylamide.

**LSH** lutein-stimulating hormone.

**LSP** left sacroposterior position (of a fetus). See under SACRUM POSTERIOR POSITION.

**LST** left sacrotransverse position (of a fetus). See under SACRUM TRANSVERSE POSITION.

**LT** **1** labile toxin. **2** lymphotoxin

**LTH** luteotropic hormone.

**Lu** Symbol for the element, lutetium.

**lubb** An onomatopoeic term used to represent the first heart sound on auscultation.

**lubb-dupp** The onomatopoeic syllables allegedly made during the first and second heart sounds on auscultation.

**lubricant** \loo′brəkənt\ An agent used to reduce friction between two surfaces in contact.

**Luc** [Henri *Luc*, French laryngologist, 1855–1925] See under FORCEPS.

**lucanthone hydrochloride** $C_{20}H_{25}ClN_2OS$. 1-(2-Diethylaminoethylamino)-4-methylthiaxanthone hydrochloride. An antischistosomal drug used in the treatment of both urinary tract and intestinal schistosomiasis.

**Lucas** [Richard Clement *Lucas*, English anatomist and surgeon, 1846–1915] Groove of Lucas. See under STRIA SPINOSA.

**lucent** \loo′sənt\ [L *lucens*, gen. *lucentis*, pres. part. of *lucere* to shine, light] **1** RADIOLUCENT. **2** TRANSLUCENT.

**lucid** \loo′sid\ **1** Easily understood; clear. **2** Able to think clearly.

**luciferase** \loosif′ərās\ An enzyme which catalyzes, in the presence of adenosine triphosphate, the transfer of an electron from luciferin to oxygen, with the emission of light. The reaction is the basis of the bioluminescence which occurs in fireflies, glowworms, certain bacteria, and some fungi.

**luciferin** Any of several substances involved in the emission of light by a living organism. Luciferins are chemically diverse, according to the organism. They are oxidized enzymically (with luciferase) by molecular oxygen to form a product in an electronically excited state. This product can lose its excitation with emission of light.

***Lucilia*** \loosil′yə\ A genus of blowflies (Calliphoridae) known popularly as greenbottle flies. ***L. caesar*** An Old World species of blowfly which normally breeds in decaying meat or carrion. The larvae were formerly used in treatment of septic wounds. Larvae sometimes cause traumatic and cutaneous myiasis in humans, while the adult, like *Musca domestica* and other filth flies, has been implicated as a carrier of the cholera vibrio. Accidental intestinal myiasis has also been reported. ***L. regina*** *PHORMIA REGINA.* ***L. sericata*** *PHAENICIA SERICATA.*

**Lucio** [R. *Lucio*, Mexican physician, 1819–1866] See under PHENOMENON.

**Lucké** [Balduin *Lucké*, German-born U.S. pathologist, 1889–1954] See under VIRUS.

**lückenschädel** \lik′ənshā′dəl\ [German *Lücken* gaps, breaches + *Schädel* skull] CRANIOFENESTRIA.

**Luckett** [William Henry *Luckett*, U.S. surgeon, born 1872] See under OPERATION.

**lucotherapy** \loo′kōther′əpē\ PHOTOTHERAPY.

**Luder** [Joseph *Luder*, English pediatrician, flourished 20th century] Luder-Sheldon syndrome. See under SYNDROME.

**Ludloff** [Karl *Ludloff*, German orthopedic surgeon, 1864–1945] See under SIGN, OPERATION.

**Ludwig** [Carl Friedrich Wilhelm *Ludwig*, German anatomist and physiologist, 1816–1895] **1** See under GANGLION. **2** Isaacs-Ludwig arteriole. See under ARTERIOLE. **3** Ludwig's labyrinths. See under LABYRINTH. **4** Ludwig's nerve, depressor nerve of Ludwig. See under AORTIC NERVE.

**Ludwig** [Daniel *Ludwig*, German anatomist, 1625–1680] Angle of Ludwig. See under ANGULUS STERNI.

**Ludwig** [Wilhelm Friedrich von *Ludwig*, German surgeon, 1790–1865] Aryvocalis muscle of Ludwig, Ludwig's muscle. See under ARYVOCALIS.

**lues** \loo′ēz\ [L (akin to Gk *lysis* dissolution) a plague, pestilence, corruption; orig. dissolution, rot] SYPHILIS. Adj. luetic. **l. nervosa** NEUROSYPHILIS. **l. tarda** LATE SYPHILIS. **l. venerea** SYPHILIS.

**luette** \loo·et′\ [French, from *l(a)* the + *uette*, from Vulgar L *uvitta*, dim. of *uva* grape(s), uvula] UVULA. **Lieutaud's l.** UVULA VESICAE.

**Luft** [Rolf *Luft*, Swedish endocrinologist, born 1914] **1** Luft syndrome. See under HYPERMETABOLIC MYOPATHY. **2** See under DISEASE.

**lug** A projection from a dental casting. **occlusal l.** OCCLUSAL REST. **retention l.** A lug fixed to a tooth in order to provide an undercut for the retention of an appliance.

**LUL** left upper lobe (of lung).

**luliberin** \loolib′ərin\ GONADOTROPIN RELEASING HORMONE.

**lumbago** \lumbā′gō\ [L, from *lumbus* loin] Pain in the lumbar, or loin, region. Also *lumbar rheumatism, lumbodynia.*

**lumbar** \lum′bər, lum′bär\ Pertaining to the loin, or lumbus.

**lumbarization** \lum′bərīzā′shən\ [LUMBAR + *-iz(e)* + -ATION] A condition in which the last thoracic vertebra or the first vertebral segment of the sacrum displays anatomic characteristics similar to or identical with those of lumbar vertebrae. The change is particularly striking with the first sacral segment, which may exhibit a degree of independent movement.

**lumbo-** \lum′bō-\ [L *lumbus* the loins] A combining form meaning the loins, lumbar.

**lumbocostal** \-käs′təl\ Pertaining to the lumbar region, particularly the vertebrae, and the ribs. Also *costolumbar.*

**lumbocrural** \-kroo′rəl\ 1 Pertaining to the lumbar and the crural regions. 2 LUMBOINGUINAL.
**lumbodynia** \-din′ē·ə\ LUMBAGO.
**lumboiliac** \lum′bō·il′ē·ak\ Pertaining to the lumbar and iliac regions.
**lumboinguinal** \lum′bō·ing′gwinəl\ Pertaining to the lumbar and inguinal regions. Also *lumboiliac, lumbocrural.*
**lumbrical** \lum′brikəl\ 1 Any one of the musculi lumbricales. 2 Vermiform; earthwormlike; lumbricoid.
**lumbrici** \lumbrī′sē\ Plural of LUMBRICUS.
**lumbricide** *Obs.* ASCARICIDE.
**lumbricoid** \lum′brikoid\ [L *lumbric(us)* earthworm + -OID] Earthworm or ascaridlike in appearanceor form.
**lumbricus** \lum′brikəs\ A worm of the genus *Ascaris.*
**lumbus** \lum′bəs\ [L, loin] The lower part of the back, between the lowest rib and the iliac crest on either side of the vertebral column. Also *loin.*
**lumen** \loo′mən\ [L (akin to *lux* light) a light, source of light, an aperture for admission of light, an orifice] (*pl.* lumina, lumens) 1 The cavity within a tubular structure, either natural or artificial. 2 The SI derived unit of luminous flux; the luminous flux emitted within the solid angle of one steradian by a point source having a uniform intensity of one candela. Also *candela steradian.* Symbol: lm **l. per square meter** 1 The SI derived unit of illuminance, more commonly referred to by the special name lux. 2 The SI derived unit of luminous exitance. Also *luminous emittance* (outmoded). Symbol: $lm/m^2$, $lm{\cdot}m^{-2}$ **l. per watt** The SI derived unit of luminous efficacy and spectral luminous efficacy. Symbol: lm/W, $lm{\cdot}W^{-1}$
**lumen-second** The SI derived unit of quantity of light; the time integral of luminous flux. Symbol: lm·s
**lumina** \loo′minə\ Plural of LUMEN.
**luminal** \loo′minəl\ Of or pertaining to a lumen.
**luminescence** \loo′mines′əns\ [L *lumen,* gen. *luminis,* light, daylight + -ESCENCE] The emission of infrared, visible, or ultraviolet light by matter from any cause other than incandescence.
**luminiferous** \loo′minif′ərəs\ [L *lumen,* gen. *luminis,* light + -FEROUS] Capable of transmitting light.
**luminoscope** \loo′minəskōp′\ An instrument which scans the surface of coal-gasification workers suspected of contamination with toxic polycyclic aromatic hydrocarbons. Ultraviolet light at 365 nanometers is transmitted by fiberoptics and resultant fluorescent light is detected by a photomultiplier tube.
**lumirhodopsin** \loo′mirōdäp′sin\ An intermediate photopigment in the degradation of rhodopsin.
**lumisome** \loo′misōm\ [*lumi(nescent)* + -SOME] One of the membrane-enclosed cytoplasmic vesicles, 0.1–0.2 μm in diameter, within which the bioluminescent reactions of certain cells occur.
**lumpectomy** \lumpek′təmē\ [English *lump* + -ECTOMY] A localized, surgical excision of a breast mass, usually cancer, and the surrounding tissue; a tylectomy used especially in the treatment of breast cancer.
**Lumsden** [Thomas William *Lumsden,* English physician, 1874–1953] Lumsden center. See under PNEUMOTAXIC CENTER.
**lunar** \loo′nər\ [L *lunar(is)* (from *lun(a)* the moon + *-aris* -AR) lunar] 1 Of or relating to the moon. 2 Crescent in shape.
**lunate** \loo′nāt\ 1 Crescent-shaped or moon-shaped; semilunar. 2 OS LUNATUM.
**lunatomalacia** \loonā′tōməlā′shə\ KIENBÖCK'S DISEASE.
**lung** [Old English *lungen*] One of a pair of highly elastic cone-shaped organs of respiration occupying the thoracic cavity, where each is surrounded by a pleural sac and separated from the other by the heart and other contents of the mediastinum; pulmo. **bird-breeders' l.** BIRD-BREEDERS' DISEASE. **bird-fanciers' l.** BIRD-BREEDERS' DISEASE. **black l.** COAL WORKERS' PNEUMOCONIOSIS. **coal miners' l.** COAL WORKERS' PNEUMOCONIOSIS. **colliers' l.** COAL WORKERS' PNEUMOCONIOSIS. **eosinophilic l.** TROPICAL PULMONARY EOSINOPHILIA. **farmers' l.** A common form of extrinsic allergic alveolitis, occurring among farmers from the inhalation of moldy hay. In its acute stage it is characterized by general malaise, slight fever, and dyspnea. Repeated exposure causes pulmonary fibrosis with emphysema. Also *harvesters' lung, threshers' lung.* **fluid l.** WET LUNG. **harvesters' l.** FARMERS' LUNG. **honeycomb l.** A roentgenographic appearance of the lung, consisting of multiple small areas of radiolucency with intervening borders of soft-tissue density, seen in interstitial pulmonary disease with fibrosis. **hyperlucent l.** A lung which casts abnormally few shadows on chest radiograph, usually due to emphysema, overinflation, or reduction of blood flow. **iron l.** *Popular* TANK VENTILATOR. **mushroom workers' l.** MUSHROOM WORKERS' DISEASE. **postperfusion l.** A condition of atelectasis, pulmonary arterial venous shunting, and consolidation of the lung that is seen following cardiopulmonary bypass. Also *pump lung.* **shock l.** ADULT RESPIRATORY DISTRESS SYNDROME. **threshers' l.** FARMERS' LUNG. **traumatic wet l.** ADULT RESPIRATORY DISTRESS SYNDROME. **uremic l.** A complication of both acute and chronic renal failure characterized by dyspnea, orthopnea, and a perihilar vascular congestion and pulmonary edema yielding a "butterfly" pattern on roentgenograms. The etiology is controversial. Some believe it is due to uremic toxins, but most authorities believe it is due to circulatory overload. Also *uremic pneumonitis* (imprecise). **vanishing l.** Any condition in which the lung appears radiographically to become smaller or less opaque. **Vietnam l.** ADULT RESPIRATORY DISTRESS SYNDROME. **wet l.** An edematous lung; pulmonary edema. Also *fluid lung.* **white l.** PNEUMONIA ALBA.
**lunula** \loo′nyələ\ [L (from *luna* moon) a crescent-shaped ornament] (*pl.* lunulae) 1 A small or narrow crescent-shaped or moon-shaped marking or structure; half-moon; demilune. Also *lunule.* 2 [NA] An opaque white semilunar area at the proximal end of the body and the root of the nail where the papillae are less vascular. It is partially covered by the eponychium. Also *lunula unguis, lunule of nail, selene unguium.* **lunulae of semilunar valves of aorta** LUNULAE VALVULARUM SEMILUNARIUM AORTAE. **lunulae of semilunar valves of pulmonary trunk** LUNULAE VALVULARUM SEMILUNARIUM TRUNCI PULMONALIS. **l. unguis** LUNULA. **lunulae valvularum semilunarium aortae** [NA] Crescentic areas of thinning of the free edges of the three semilunar cusps, or valvules, of the aortic valve, one thin area being on each side of the thick nodule in the center of the margin of each cusp. Also *lunulae of semilunar valves of aorta.* **lunulae valvularum semilunarium trunci pulmonalis** [NA] Crescentic areas of thinning of the free edges of the three semilunar cusps, or valvules, of the pulmonary valve, one thin area being on each side of the thick nodule in the center of the margin of each cusp. Also *lunulae of semilunar valves of pulmonary trunk.*
**lunulae** \loo′nyəlē\ Plural of LUNULA.
**lunule** \loo′nʸool\ LUNULA. **l. of nail** LUNULA.
**lupiform** \loo′pifôrm\ LUPOID.
**lupinine** \loo′pinin\ $C_{10}H_{19}NO$. Octahydroquinolizine-1-methanol, a solid alkaloid obtained from *Lupinus luteus* and other species.

**lupoid** \loo′poid\ Resembling lupus vulgaris. Also *lupiform.*

**lupoma** \loopō′mə\ [ *lup(us)* + -OMA] A small granulomatous nodule characteristic of lupus vulgaris.

**lupus** \loo′pəs\ [Med L (from L *lupus* a wolf) a "voracious" cutaneous ulcer] **1** *Popular* LUPUS VULGARIS. **2** *Popular* LUPUS ERYTHEMATOSUS. ● The term is used in combination with the designation of a specific disease and of itself has no specific meaning. **butterfly l.** Lupus erythematosus that appears in a butterfly-shaped patch on the nose and cheeks. **discoid l. erythematosus** A form of lupus erythematosus in which only the skin is involved, with a characteristic rash but with no visceral involvement. It presents as plaques of erythema and telangiectasis with follicular plugging. Also *cutaneous lupus erythematosus, lupus erythematosus discoides.* **disseminated l. erythematosus** SYSTEMIC LUPUS ERYTHEMATOSUS. **disseminated follicular l.** ACNE AGMINATA. **drug-induced l. erythematosus** An illness similar to spontaneous systemic lupus erythematosus, but occurring after exposure to any one of several drugs, such as procaine amide, which are capable of inducing this illness. The symptoms remit upon withdrawal of the offending drug. **l. endemicus** CUTANEOUS LEISHMANIASIS. **l. erythematosus** Either of two diseases that have similar cutaneous manifestations: discoid lupus erythematosus and systemic lupus erythematosus. Also *Cazenave's disease* (obs.), *lupus* (popular). **l. erythematosus discoides** DISCOID LUPUS ERYTHEMATOSUS. **l. erythematosus hypertrophicus** Chronic lupus erythematosus in which dense scarring and deep involvement of the dermis is evident. **l. erythematosus migrans** Lupus erythematosus marked by transitory lesions. **l. erythematosus profundus** An uncommon lupus erythematosus in which warty thickened plaques extend deep into the dermis and subcutis. **l. erythematosus tumidus** Lupus erythematosus marked by raised, indurated lesions. **l. fibrosus** LUPUS SCLEROSUS. **hydralazine l.** A disorder resembling systemic lupus erythematosus provoked in a proportion of subjects by the prolonged administration of the drug hydralazine and disappearing with its discontinuance. Hydralazine lupus, however, usually does not include nephritis or antidouble-stranded DNA antibodies. Also *hydralazine lupus syndrome.* **laryngeal l.** Lupus vulgaris spreading from the nose by way of the pharynx to reach the supraglottic larynx. This is a rare site, the epiglottis being more commonly involved. **l. lymphaticus** *Obs.* LYMPHANGIOMA CIRCUMSCRIPTUM. **l. miliaris disseminatus faciei** ACNE AGMINATA. **l. pernio** A form of sarcoidosis in which soft, bluish red plaques appear on the nose, cheeks, ears, fingers, and hands. **photosensitive l. erythematosus** Lupus erythematosus exacerbated by exposure to sunlight. **postexanthematic l.** A disseminated form of lupus vulgaris occurring after acute specific fevers in children. **l. sclerosus** Thickened scars complicating lupus vulgaris. Also *lupus fibrosus, lupus vulgaris fibromatosus.* **l. serpiginosus** A spreading form of tuberculous lupus. **systemic l. erythematosus** A multisystem disease of unknown etiology characterized by vasculitis, serositis, synovitis, and involvement of the kidneys, skin, and nervous system. Women are affected much more frequently than men. There are a wide variety of autoantibodies in the serum of affected subjects, particularly to nonorgan-specific intracellular components. Antinuclear antibodies to double-stranded DNA and to native DNA nucleohistone are diagnostic. Immune complexes of autoantibodies and autoantigens play an important role in the pathogenesis of the disease. Certain species other than man, including dogs and several strains of inbred mice, are also susceptible to the disease. Also *disseminated lupus erythematosus.* Abbr. SLE **l. tumidus** Lupus vulgaris manifested as a soft, raised nodule. **l. verrucosus** WARTY LUPUS. **l. vulgaris** A progressive chronic form of cutaneous tuberculosis that occurs as a postprimary infection in a subject with a moderate or high degree of immunity. Also *lupus* (popular), *tuberculosis luposa.* **l. vulgaris fibromatosus** LUPUS SCLEROSUS. **warty l.** Lupus vulgaris characterized by wartlike eruptions. Also *lupus verrucosus.*

**LUQ** left upper quadrant (of abdomen).

**lura** \loo′rə\ The constricted termination of the pituitary stalk or infundibulum. *Outmoded.*

**Luschka** [Hubert von *Luschka,* German anatomist, 1820–1875] **1** Luschka's body, Luschka's gland, Luschka's ganglion. See under GLOMUS COCCYGEUM. **2** Luschka's ducts. See under LUSCHKA'S CRYPTS. **3** Luschka sinus. See under SINUS PETROSQUAMOSUS. **4** Luschka's tubercle. See under CARINA URETHRALIS VAGINAE. **5** Luschka's crypts. See under ROKITANSKY-ASCHOFF SINUSES OF THE GALLBLADDER. **6** Joints of Luschka. See under JOINT. **7** Cricotracheal ligament of Luschka. See under LIGAMENT. **8** Luschka's fossa. See under RECESSUS ILEOCECALIS SUPERIOR. **9** Luschka's tonsil. See under TONSILLA PHARYNGEALIS. **10** Nerve of Luschka. See under RAMUS MENINGEUS NERVORUM SPINALIUM. **11** Nerve of Luschka. See under NERVUS ETHMOIDALIS POSTERIOR. **12** Laryngeal cartilage of Luschka, Luschka's cartilage. See under CARTILAGO SESAMOIDEA. **13** Ligaments of Luschka. See under LIGAMENTA STERNOPERICARDIACA. **14** Luschka's muscles. See under MUSCULUS RECTOUTERINUS.

**Lust** [Franz Alexander *Lust,* German pediatrician, born 1880] Lust's phenomenon, Lust's reflex. See under SIGN.

**Lustig** [Alessandro *Lustig,* Italian pathologist and bacteriologist, 1857–1937] Lustig-Galeotti vaccine. See under VACCINE.

**luteal** \loo′tē·əl\ [*lute(o)-* + -AL] Pertaining to, arising from, having the characteristics of, or involving the corpus luteum. Also *luteinic.*

**luteectomy** \loo′tē·ek′təmē\ [*(corpus) lute(um)* + -ECTOMY] The surgical removal of the corpus luteum.

**lutein** \loo′tē·in\ A yellow pigment, closely related to xanthophyll, occurring in the luteal cells of the corpus luteum.

**luteinic** \loo′tē·in′ik\ LUTEAL.

**luteinization** \loo′tē·in′īzā′shən\ The transformation of granulosa cells into lutein cells in the formation of the corpus luteum of the ovary. Other cells may undergo luteinization, including theca cells, and coelomic and cervical cells.

**luteinize** \loo′tē·inīz′\ To subject to the process of or undergo luteinization.

**Lutembacher** [René *Lutembacher,* French cardiologist, 1884–1916] Lutembacher's complex, Lutembacher's disease. See under SYNDROME.

**luteo-** \loo′tē·ō-\ [L *luteus* (from *lutum* yellow dye) golden yellow, saffron yellow] A combining form meaning (1) yellow, yellowish; (2) the corpus luteum.

**luteogenic** \-jen′ik\ [LUTEO- + -GENIC] Inducing the growth, development, or hormonal secretion of the corpus luteum; luteinizing.

**luteohormone** \-hôr′mōn\ [LUTEO- + HORMONE] *Older term* PROGESTERONE.

**luteoid** \loo′tē·oid\ **1** Like or acting like progesterone. **2** A luteoid substance.

**luteolysis** \loo′tē·äl′isis\ Destruction or natural involution of the corpus luteum.

**luteoma** \loo′tē·ō′mə\ [*lute(o)-* + -OMA] **1** A growth of hyperplastic nodules made up of lutein cells of the ovary, sometimes found in the third trimester of pregnancy, occurring most commonly in black women, and in some cases having the property of secreting androgenic hormones. They are not true tumors and they regress after parturition. Also *luteoma of pregnancy.* **2** LIPOID CELL TUMOR OF OVARY.

**luteotrophic** \-träf′ik\ LUTEOTROPIC.

**luteotrophin** \-träf′in\ PROLACTIN.

**luteotropic** \-träp′ik\ [LUTEO- + -TROPIC[2]] Promoting or stimulating the development, maturation, or hormonal secretion of the corpus luteum. Also *luteotrophic.*

**luteotropin** \-träp′in\ PROLACTIN.

**lutetium** Element number 71, having atomic weight 174.967. It is a silvery white metal of the lanthanide series. There are two natural isotopes, the stable lutetium 175 (97.4% natural abundance) and radioactive lutetium 176 (2.6%), having a half-life of $3 \times 10^{10}$ years. Many synthetic unstable isotopes have been identified. Symbol: Lu

**lututrin** A water soluble, relaxinlike factor from the corpus luteum of sow ovaries. It has been used as a uterine relaxant.

**Lutz** [Adolfo *Lutz,* Brazilian bacteriologist, 1855–1940] Lutz-Splendore-Almeida disease. See under SOUTH AMERICAN BLASTOMYCOSIS.

**Lutz** [Wilhelm *Lutz,* Swiss dermatologist, 1888–1958] Lewandowsky-Lutz disease. See under EPIDERMODYSPLASIA VERRUCIFORMIS.

***Lutzomyia*** \lut′sōmī′yə\ [after Adolfo *Lutz,* Brazilian bacteriologist, 1855–1940, + Gk *myia* a fly] A New World genus of sandflies, family Psychodidae, subfamily Phlebotominae, that includes a number of vectors of American cutaneous and visceral leishmaniasis (*Leishmania mexicana* and *L. brasiliensis* complexes and *L chagasi*). Sandflies of this genus play a role in New World leishmaniasis comparable to that of *Phlebotomus* species in the Old World disease. ***L. flaviscutellata*** The vector of *Leishmania mexicana amazonensis,* agent of a mild, nonulcerating form of cutaneous leishmaniasis in the Amazon basin and the state of Mato Grosso in Brazil. In this same area and in Venezuela, this sandfly has also been implicated as the probable vector of *L. pifanoi,* agent of diffuse cutaneous leishmaniasis. In Trinidad it has been implicated in the transmission of a subspecies of *L. mexicana,* causing a local form of cutaneous leishmaniasis. Also *Phlebotomus flaviscutellatus.* ***L. intermedia*** A vector of *Leishmania braziliensis braziliensis,* agent of mucocutaneous leishmaniasis in the rainforests of Brazil, Peru, Ecuador, Bolivia, Venezuela, Paraguay, and Colombia. The role of this sandfly has been demonstrated by inoculating hamsters. Also *Phlebotomus intermedius.* ***L. longipalpis*** The principal sandfly vector of *Leishmania chagasi* (or *L. donovani chagasi*), agent of kala-azar in northern Argentina, Paraguay, Bolivia, Brazil, Venezuela, Colombia, Guatemala, El Salvador, and Mexico. ***L. olmeca*** A sandfly vector of *Leishmania mexicana mexicana,* agent of chiclero ulcer, a form of cutaneous leishmaniasis found among woodcutters of the Yucatan and Guatemala. A different subspecies (*L. olmeca bicolor*) has been implicated as the probable intermediate host of *Leishmania mexicana aristedesi,* agent of Herrer's cutaneous leishmaniasis, occurring in Panama. ***L. peruensis*** The probable sandfly vector of *Leishmania peruviana,* agent of uta, a mild form of cutaneous leishmaniasis found in the mountains of Peru, along the arid western open slopes of the Andes. ***L. pessoai*** A vector of *Leishmania braziliensis braziliensis,* agent of Brazilian mucocutaneous leishmaniasis or espundia in the rainforests of central and northern South America. Also *Phlebotomus pessoai.* ***L. verrucarum*** A species in Peru that transmits *Bartonella bacilliformis,* causal agent of Carrion's disease or bartonellosis in the Andes. Also *Phlebotomus verrucarum.*

**lux** \luks\ [L, the light, daylight] (*pl.* lux) A special name for the SI derived unit of illuminance, an illuminance of one lumen per square meter. Symbol: lx

**luxatio** \luksā′shō\ [L (from *luxatus,* past part. of *luxare* to dislocate, disjoint), a dislocating] DISLOCATION. **l. erecta** DISLOCATIO ERECTA.

**luxation** \luksā′shən\ [L *luxatio.* See LUXATIO.] DISLOCATION. **Malgaigne's l.** The dislocation of the radial head out of the annular ligament.

**luxon** \luk′sän\ [LUX + -ON] TROLAND.

**luxus** \luk′səs\ [L, luxury, voluptuousness, splendor] An excess.

**Luys** [Jules Bernard *Luys,* French physician, 1828–1895] **1** Syndrome of the corpus Luysii, body of Luys syndrome. See under HEMIBALLISMUS. **2** Nucleus of Luys. See under NUCLEUS SUBTHALAMICUS. **3** Centrum medianum of Luys. See under NUCLEUS MEDIALIS CENTRALIS THALAMI.

**LVH** left ventricular hypertrophy.

**Lw** Former symbol for the element, lawrencium.

**Ly** See under LY ANTIGENS.

**lyapolate sodium** A synthetic heparinlike anticoagulant that has had limited use in ointments for the resolution of hematomas. Also *ethenesulfonic acid homopolymer sodium salt, sodium polyethylene sulfonate.*

**lyase** \lī′ās\ Any enzyme that catalyzes the elimination of one molecule from another with formation of a double bond. Examples include isocitrate lyase, which catalyzes elimination of succinate from isocitrate and leaves glyoxylate, and fumarate hydratase, which catalyzes elimination of water from malate to leave fumarate.

**Lyb** See under LY ANTIGENS.

**lycoperdonosis** \lī′kōpur′dənō′sis\ A respiratory disease resulting from inhalation of the spores of puffballs (*Lycoperdon* sp.).

**lycopersicin** TOMATINE.

**lycorexia** \lī′kôrek′sē·ə\ BULIMIA.

***Lycosa*** \līkō′sə\ A genus of large wolf spiders (family Lycosidae), including *L. tarentula,* the European tarantula.

**lydimycin** \lī′dimī′sin\ $C_{10}H_{14}N_2O_3S$. An antibiotic from *Streptomyces lydicus* with antifungal activity.

**Lyell** [Alan *Lyell,* English dermatologist, flourished 20th century] Lyell's disease. See under TOXIC EPIDERMAL NECROLYSIS.

**Lygranum** Antigens derived from *Chlamydia trachomatis* grown on chick embryos and used in the complement-fixation test and the Frei test for lymphogranuloma venereum. A proprietary name.

**lying / pathologic l.** Lying usually with the intent to defraud or deceive others but sometimes as a way of denying to oneself one's true value, worth, achievements, or status. It is often an aspect of the antisocial personality. Also *mendacity, mythomania, pseudoreminiscence.*

**lying-in** The period or state following childbirth; the postpartum period or state.

***Lymnaea*** \lim′nē·ə\ [irreg. from Gk *limnaios* (from *limnē* a large body of standing water, lake, esp. a marshy lake, a basin or reservoir for water) marshy, stagnant] A widespread genus of freshwater pulmonate snails, species of which are intermediate hosts for various trematodes, such as *Fasciola gigantica* and *F. hepatica.*

**lymph** \limf\ [L *lymph(a)* (prob. variant of *nympha,* from Gk *nymphē* a maiden, nymph, water nymph) a water nymph, water (poetic)] A collection of tissue fluids which passes through the lymphatic vessels into the venous system. It is usually pale yellow and contains lymphocytes. When rich in fat it looks opalescent, and may be rose colored if red blood corpuscles are present. Also *lympha*. **intercellular l.** INTERSTITIAL FLUID. **intravascular l.** Fluid within the lymphatic vessels. **Koch's l.** OLD TUBERCULIN. **plastic l.** BRAWNY EDEMA. **tissue l.** *Outmoded* INTERSTITIAL FLUID. **vaccine l.** Lymph containing vaccinia virus taken from vaccinial vesicles of a calf and used to immunize against smallpox.

**lymph-** \limf-\ LYMPHO-.

**lympha** \lim′fə\ LYMPH.

**lymphaden** \lim′fəden\ [LYMPH + Gk *adēn* gland] NODUS LYMPHATICUS.

**lymphadenectomy** \limfad′ənek′təmē\ The surgical removal of one or more lymph nodes.

**lymphadenitis** \limfad′ənī′tis\ [LYMPHADEN + -ITIS] Inflammation of lymph nodes. Also *adenolymphitis*. **acute mesenteric l.** Inflammation of the lymph nodes of the mesentery of the large intestine or the vermiform appendix that may clinically resemble acute appendicitis. **acute suppurative l.** Acute inflammation of lymph nodes, accompanied by pus formation and usually due to bacterial infections. Occasionally the overlying skin may become involved, resulting in draining sinuses. **caseous l.** Caseating granulomatous inflammation of lymph nodes, usually due to tuberculosis. **mesenteric l.** MESENTERIC ADENITIS. **nonbacterial regional l.** CAT-SCRATCH DISEASE. **regional l.** 1 The inflammation of lymph nodes draining a nearby site of infection. 2 An imprecise and outmoded term for CAT-SCRATCH DISEASE. **tuberculoid l.** An inflammation of the lymph nodes which resembles that occurring in tuberculosis but which results from other diseases such as sarcoidosis, leprosy, syphilis, or regional enteritis. **tuberculous l.** Tuberculosis of the lymph nodes, occurring either as a result of lymphatic spread from a primary focus of infection or as an aspect of the disseminated disease. Cervical and mediastinal nodes are the most commonly affected. See also SCROFULA. **venereal suppurative benign l.** An inflammation accompanied by a discharge of pus from the inguinal lymph glands that is caused by venereal disease, most often chancroid or lymphogranuloma venereum.

**lymphadenocele** \limfad′ənōsēl′\ A cyst of a lymph node.

**lymphadenocyst** \limfad′ənōsist′\ A degenerating lymph node caused by obstruction or occlusion of the afferent lymphatic.

**lymphadenography** \limfad′ənäg′rəfē\ LYMPHANGIOGRAPHY.

**lymphadenoid** \limfad′ənoid\ Resembling lymph node or lymphatic tissue.

**lymphadenoma** \limfad′ənō′mə\ [LYMPHADEN + -OMA] LYMPHOMA. **malignant l.** LYMPHOMA. **multiple l.** 1 LYMPHOMA. 2 HODGKIN'S DISEASE.

**lymphadenomatosis** \limfad′ənōmətō′sis\ LYMPHOMA.

**lymphadenomatous** \limfad′ənō′mətəs\ Pertaining to lymphadenoma.

**lymphadenopathy** \limfad′ənäp′əthē\ [LYMPHADEN + *o* + -PATHY] Enlargement of lymph nodes due to uncertain or nonspecific causes. Also *adenopathy, lymphadenosis*. **dermatopathic l.** A reactive benign enlargement of the local draining lymph nodes that is secondary to a cutaneous disease. Also *dermopathic lymphadenopathy*. **giant follicular l.** NODULAR LYMPHOMA.

**lymphadenosis** \limfad′ənō′sis\ [LYMPHADEN + -OSIS] LYMPHADENOPATHY. **acute epidemic l.** INFECTIOUS MONONUCLEOSIS. **benign l.** BENIGN LYMPHOCYTOMA CUTIS. **leukemic l.** Infiltration of lymph nodes by leukemic cells. *Rare*. **malignant l.** LYMPHOMA.

**lymphadenotomy** \limfad′ənät′əmē\ [LYMPHADEN +*o* + -TOMY] A surgical incision into one or more lymph nodes.

**lymphadenovarix** \limfad′ənōver′iks\ Enlargement and varicose deformity of a lymph node resulting from lymphangiectasis. Also *adenovarix*.

**lymphagogue** \lim′fəgäg\ [LYMPH + -AGOGUE] A stimulant of lymph formation.

**lymphangeitis** \lim′fanjē·ī′tis\ LYMPHANGITIS.

**lymphangial** \limfan′jē·əl\ Pertaining to a lymph vessel.

**lymphangiectasia** \limfan′jē·ektā′zhə\ LYMPHANGIECTASIS. **intestinal l.** Dilatation of the intestinal lymphatics with subsequent protein-losing enteropathy, steatorrhea and diarrhea. It may be congenital, due to hypoplasia of the thoracic duct, or acquired, due to inflammation or neoplasm of the lymphatics. Small bowel biopsy is characteristic, with dilated lacteals in intestinal villi.

**lymphangiectasis** \limfan′jē·ek′təsis\ [*lymphangi(o)-* + ECTASIS] Dilatation of lymphatic vessels. Also *lymphangiectasia*. Adj. lymphangiectatic. **cystic l.** CYSTIC LYMPHANGIOMA. **pericaliceal l.** Dilated lymph channels along the principal renal lymph ducts resulting in single or multiple cysts around the calices. **pulmonary l.** A congenital condition of the lung in which there are multiple small cystic dilatations in the lymphatic network, associated with neonatal respiratory distress and death. **l. of the scrotum** Idiopathic dilatation of the scrotal lymphatics probably due to a congenital or postinflammatory defect in the lymphatic system of the scrotum.

**lymphangiectodes** \limfan′jē·ektō′dēz\ [*lymphangiect(asis)* + Gk *-ōdēs*, combining form denoting resembling] LYMPHANGIOMA CIRCUMSCRIPTUM.

**lymphangiectomy** \limfan′jē·ek′təmē\ [*lymphangi(o)-* + -ECTOMY] The surgical removal of one or more lymphatic vessels.

**lymphangiitis** \limfan′jē·ī′tis\ LYMPHANGITIS.

**lymphangio-** \limfan′jē·ō-\ [LYMPH- + ANGIO-] A combining form denoting lymphatic vessel.

**lymphangioadenography** \-ad′ənäg′rəfē\ LYMPHANGIOGRAPHY.

**lymphangioendothelioma** \-en′dəthē′lē·ō′mə\ [LYMPHANGIO- + ENDOTHELIOMA] A tumor of the lymphatic endothelium. These cells may form layers within the vascular channels. The tumor is considered malignant (lymphangiosarcoma) when cellular atypia is present. Also *lymphangioendothelioblastoma, lymphendothelioma*. **malignant l.** LYMPHANGIOSARCOMA.

**lymphangiography** \limfan′jē·äg′rəfē\ [LYMPHANGIO- + -GRAPHY] Radiographic study of the lymphatic channels and lymph nodes after their opacification by the injection of an oily radiopaque material into one or more small lymph channels in the foot, or, less commonly, in the hand. Also *lymphography, lymphadenography, lymphangioadenography, hydrangiography* (rare).

**lymphangioleiomyomatosis** \-lī′ōmī′ōmətō′sis\ A proliferation of lymphatic vessels and smooth muscle. It typically affects the lungs and lymph nodes. It is a lesion of women of the reproductive age. Large cysts and a honeycomb appearance of the lung can occur, which leads to respiratory insufficiency.

**lymphangiology** \limfan′je·äl′əjē\ The study of the lymphatic vessels. Also *hydrangiology, lymphology*.

**lymphangioma** \limfan′jē·ō′mə\ [*lymphangi(o)-* + -OMA]

A benign growth composed exclusively of lymph vessels of various size lined by a single layer of endothelial cells. The lesion is often congenital. Lymphangiomas can be subtyped as capillary, cavernous, or cystic. The cavernous and cystic forms (hygroma) are most frequent in the cervical, mediastinal, and retroperitoneal regions of infants and children. Capillary lymphangiomas are exceedingly rare and are difficult to distinguish from capillary hemangiomas. **l. capsulare varicosum** LYMPHANGIOMA CIRCUMSCRIPTUM. **cavernous l.** A lymphangioma with large, dilated, thin-walled channels. Also *lymphangioma cavernosum, cavernoma lymphaticum.* **l. circumscriptum** A circumscribed developmental defect of cutaneous and subcutaneous lymphatics presenting clinically as a yellowish cluster of thick-walled vesicles. Also *lymphangiectodes, lymphangioma capsulare varicosum, lymphangioma xanthelasoideum, lupus lymphaticus* (obs.). **cystic l.** A lymphangioma characterized by large, lymph-filled cysts. It is seen most commonly in the regions of the neck and groin in children. Also *cystic lymphangiectasis.* **fissural l.** A lymphangioma at the site of a fetal skin fissure. **l. xanthelasmoideum** LYMPHANGIOMA CIRCUMSCRIPTUM.

**lymphangiomatous** \limfan′jē·ō′mətəs\ Pertaining to lymphangioma.

**lymphangiomyoma** \-mī·ō′mə\ [LYMPHANGIO- + MYOMA] A growth composed of bundles of smooth muscle tissue about cavernous or slitlike, endothelium-lined lymph spaces. Aggregates of lymphocytes may be found in association with the smooth muscle tissue. The tumor has been observed only in the mediastinum and retroperitoneum in close association with the thoracic duct and its tributaries. Chylothorax and pulmonary complications are common.

**lymphangion** \limfan′jē·än\ VAS LYMPHATICUM.

**lymphangiophlebitis** \-flebī′tis\ Inflammation of both lymph vessels and blood vessels.

**lymphangioplasty** \limfan′jē·əplas′tē\ The surgical replacement or repair of damaged or destroyed lymphatic vessels. Also *lymphoplasty.* **Handley's l.** A surgical treatment for elephantiasis in which cotton wicks are inserted into the tissues to allow for external lymphatic drainage.

**lymphangiosarcoma** \-särkō′mə\ [LYMPHANGIO- + SARCOMA] A malignant tumor of lymphatic tissue, mainly associated with chronic lymph stasis, usually secondary to radical mastectomy. Also *malignant lymphangioendothelioma, lymphangioendothelial sarcoma.*

**lymphangiotomy** \limfan′jē·ät′əmē\ [LYMPHANGIO- + -TOMY] A surgical incision into one or more lymphatic ducts.

**lymphangitis** \lim′fanjī′tis\ [*lymphang(io)-* + -ITIS] Inflammation of lymphatic vessels, usually as a result of extension of an adjacent bacterial infection into or through their wall. Also *angioleukitis, angiolymphitis, lymphangeitis, lymphangiitis.* **l. carcinomatosa** 1 The growth of carcinoma in lymphatics. 2 The obstruction of lymphatics by carcinoma. **carcinomatous l.** The filling of lymphatic channels by metastatic cancer cells, particularly those of the lungs where the distended tumor-filled lymphatics are visible to the naked eye as whitish streaks or cords extending from the pleura to the hilum. **nonvenereal sclerosing l.** Inflammation and sclerosis of the lymphatics arising from or around the coronal sulcus of the penis.

**lymphatic** \limfat′ik\ 1 Relating to lymph. 2 A lymph vessel; vas lymphaticum. **afferent l.** A vessel carrying lymph to a lymph node. **efferent l.** A vessel conducting lymph away from a lymph node. **gluteal l.'s** Lymphatic vessels draining the gluteal region, the superficial group draining to the superficial inguinal lymph nodes while the deep vessels drain along the gluteal arteries and veins to the pelvic nodes along the internal iliac artery and vein. **ischial l.'s** Deep lymph vessels of the ischial region following the course of corresponding arteries and veins. **obturator l.'s** Deep lymphatic vessels along the obturator vessels which drain to the external and internal iliac lymph nodes either directly or through the obturator lymph nodes.

**lymphaticosplenic** \limfat′ikōsplē′nik\ Pertaining to lymph nodes and the spleen.

**lymphaticostomy** \limfat′ikäs′təmē\ [*lymphatic* + *o* + -STOMY] The surgical creation of an opening that establishes drainage from a large lymphatic duct, such as the thoracic duct.

**lymphatism** \lim′fətizm\ STATUS LYMPHATICUS.

**lymphatology** \limfətäl′əjē\ The study of the lymphatic system.

**lymphedema** \lim′fədē′mə\ [LYMPH- + EDEMA] The accumulation of interstitial fluid as a result of obstruction of lymphatic vessels, disorders of lymph nodes, or surgical removal of lymph nodes for cancer. Also *lymphatic edema.* **filarial l.** Chronic edema and associated lymphangitis caused by the blockage by filariae of major lymphatics, such as those of the scrotum or lower extremities. Eventually fibrosis develops, leading to elephantiasis. *Wuchereria bancrofti* and *Brugia malayi* are the species usually responsible for these deformities. **hereditary l. type I** Congenital edema, predominantly affecting the legs, that is inherited as an autosomal dominant trait. It may be associated with intestinal protein loss and pleural effusion. Also *Milroy's disease, Nonne-Milroy disease, hereditary lymphedema, early-onset type.* **hereditary l. type II** An autosomal dominant, variable, slowly progressive form of lymphedema with onset around puberty. Also *Meige lymphedema, late-onset lymphedema, Meige's disease, trophoedema of Meige.* **l. praecox** Lymphedema occurring in girls approaching puberty, and characterized by puffiness and swelling of the lower extremities. **secondary l.** Lymphedema due to radiotherapy, surgery, or other cause obstructing lymphatic drainage from a part.

**lymphendothelioma** \lim′fendōthē′lē·ō′mə\ LYMPHANGIOENDOTHELIOMA.

**lymphepithelioma** \lim′fepithē′lē·ō′mə\ LYMPHOEPITHELIOMA.

**lymphization** \lim′fīzā′shən\ LYMPHOPOIESIS.

# lymph node

**lymph node** NODUS LYMPHATICUS. **anterior cecal l.'s** NODI LYMPHATICI PRECECALES. **anterior cervical l.'s** NODI LYMPHATICI CERVICALES ANTERIORES. **anterior jugular l.'s** NODI LYMPHATICI JUGULARES ANTERIORES. **anterior mediastinal l.'s** NODI LYMPHATICI MEDIASTINALES ANTERIORES. **anterior tibial l.** NODUS TIBIALIS ANTERIOR. **anterior vesical l.'s** Nodes of the nodi lymphatici vesicales laterales which are situated on the middle and inferior parts of the anterior wall of the urinary bladder. **apical l.'s** NODI LYMPHATICI APICALES. **l. of arch of azygos vein** NODUS ARCUS VENAE AZYGOS. **axillary l.'s** NODI LYMPHATICI AXILLARES. **biliary l.'s** Lymph nodes situated along the extrahepatic biliary ducts, including nodi lymphatici hepatici, nodus cysticus, and nodus foraminalis. **brachial l.'s** NODI LYMPHATICI BRACHIALES. **bronchopulmonary l.'s** NODI LYMPHATICI BRONCHOPULMONALES. **buccal l.'s** See under NODI LYMPHATICI FACIALES. **buccal group of facial l.'s** NODUS BUCCINATORIUS. **cecoappendicular l.'s** The nodi lymphatici prececales, nodi lymphatici retrocecales, and nodi lymphatici appendiculares considered together. **celiac l.'s** NODI LYMPHATICI COELIACI. **central l.'s** NODI LYMPHATICI CENTRALES. **common iliac l.'s** NODI LYMPHATICI ILIACI COMMUNES. **cubital l.'s** NODI LYMPHATICI CUBITALES. **l.'s of cubital fossa** NODI LYMPHATICI CUBITALES. **deep cervical l.'s** NODI LYMPHATICI CERVICALES PROFUNDI. **deep inguinal l.'s** NODI LYMPHATICI INGUINALES PROFUNDI. **deep parotid l.'s** NODI LYMPHATICI PAROTIDEI PROFUNDI. **l.'s of deltopectoral groove** Small lymph nodes along the course of the cephalic vein between the deltoid and pectoralis major muscles which drain into the infraclavicular nodes or the apical nodes. **epitrochlear l.'s** NODI LYMPHATICI CUBITALES. **external iliac l.'s** NODI LYMPHATICI ILIACI EXTERNI. **facial l.'s** NODI LYMPHATICI FACIALES. **femoral l.'s** Inconstant lymph nodes along the course of the femoral vein in the lower and middle parts of the thigh which receive the efferents of the popliteal nodes and send their lymph to the deep inguinal nodes. **l.'s of gastroduodenal artery** NODI LYMPHATICI PYLORICI. **gastroepiploic l.'s** The nodi lymphatici gastro-omentales dextri and nodi lymphatici gastro-omentales sinistri. **hemal l.** A lymph node in which blood flows through the sinusoidal system. Such structures have been identified in a number of experimental animals, particularly in the retroperitoneal position. **hepatic l.'s** NODI LYMPHATICI HEPATICI. **ileocolic l.'s** NODI LYMPHATICI ILEOCOLICI. **inferior auricular parotid l.'s** NODI LYMPHATICI INFRA-AURICULARES. **inferior diaphragmatic l.'s** NODI LYMPHATICI PHRENICI INFERIORES. **inferior epigastric l.'s** NODI LYMPHATICI EPIGASTRICI INFERIORES. **inferior gastric l.'s** NODI LYMPHATICI GASTRO-OMENTALES DEXTRI. **inferior mesenteric l.'s** NODI LYMPHATICI MESENTERICI INFERIORES. **inferior tracheobronchial l.'s** NODI LYMPHATICI TRACHEOBRONCHIALES INFERIORES. **infraclavicular l.'s** 1 NODI LYMPHATICI APICALES. 2 One or two lymph nodes along the cephalic vein in the infraclavicular fossa at the upper end of the deltopectoral groove. Their efferents pierce the clavipectoral fascia to end in the apical group of axillary nodes. **infrahyoid l.'s** A group of lymph nodes situated on the front of the thyrohyoid membrane and deep to the investing layer of the deep cervical fascia. They receive afferents from the anterior cervical nodes and their efferents end in the deep lateral cervical nodes. **inguinal l.'s** Nodi lymphatici inguinales superficiales and nodi lymphatici inguinales profundi. **intercostal l.'s** NODI LYMPHATICI INTERCOSTALES. **internal iliac l.'s** NODI LYMPHATICI ILIACI INTERNI. **internal jugular l.'s** The nodi lymphatici jugulares laterales and nodi lymphatici jugulares anteriores. **internal thoracic l.'s** NODI LYMPHATICI PARASTERNALES. **jugulodigastric l.** NODUS JUGULODIGASTRICUS. **jugulo-omohyoid l.** NODUS JUGULO-OMOHYOIDEUS. **lateral aortic l.'s** NODI LYMPHATICI AORTICI LATERALES. **lateral axillary l.'s** NODI LYMPHATICI LATERALES. **lateral cervical l.'s** NODI LYMPHATICI CERVICALES LATERALES. **lateral jugular l.'s** NODI LYMPHATICI JUGULARES LATERALES. **lateral tracheal group of deep anterior cervical l.'s** NODI LYMPHATICI PARATRACHEALES. **lateral vesical l.'s** NODI LYMPHATICI VESICALES LATERALES. **left colic l.'s** NODI LYMPHATICI COLICI SINISTRI. **left gastric l.'s** NODI LYMPHATICI GASTRICI SINISTRI. **left gastroepiploic l.'s** NODI LYMPHATICI GASTRO-OMENTALES SINISTRI. **l.'s of lesser curvature** NODI LYMPHATICI GASTRICI SINISTRI. **lingual l.'s** Small inconstant lymph nodes which lie along the lymph vessels draining the tongue on the external surfaces of the hyoglossus and genioglossus muscles and between the latter muscles. **lumbar l.'s** NODI LYMPHATICI LUMBALES. **mandibular l.'s** See under NODI LYMPHATICI FACIALES. **mastoid l.'s** NODI LYMPHATICI MASTOIDEI. **mesenteric l.'s** NODI LYMPHATICI MESENTERICI. **middle colic l.'s** NODI LYMPHATICI COLICI MEDII. **obturator l.'s** NODI LYMPHATICI OBTURATORII. **occipital l.'s** NODI LYMPHATICI OCCIPITALES. **pancreaticolienal l.'s** Nodi lymphatici splenici and nodi lymphatici pancreatici considered together. **pancreaticosplenic l.'s** NODI LYMPHATICI PANCREATICOLIENALES. **paracolic l.'s** NODI LYMPHATICI PARACOLICI. **parasternal l.'s** NODI LYMPHATICI PARASTERNALES. **paratracheal l.'s** NODI LYMPHATICI PARATRACHEALES. **parotid l.'s** Nodi lymphatici parotidei superficiales and nodi lymphatici parotidei profundi. **pectoral l.'s** NODI LYMPHATICI PECTORALES. **peritracheal l.'s** NODI LYMPHATICI PARATRACHEALES. **popliteal l.'s** NODI LYMPHATICI POPLITEALES. **posterior auricular l.'s** NODI LYMPHATICI MASTOIDEI. **posterior cecal l.'s** NODI LYMPHATICI RETROCECALES. **posterior intercostal l.'s** NODI LYMPHATICI INTERCOSTALES. **posterior mediastinal l.'s** NODI LYMPHATICI MEDIASTINALES POSTERIORES. **posterior tibial l.'s** Inconstant lymph nodes situated along the lymphatic vessels accompanying the posterior tibial vessels, mainly in the middle of the leg. **preaortic l.'s** NODI LYMPHATICI PREAORTICI. **preauricular l.'s** NODI LYMPHATICI PREAURICULARES. **precaval l.'s** NODI LYMPHATICI PRECAVALES. **prelaryngeal l.'s** NODI LYMPHATICI PRELARYNGEALES. **prepericardiac l.'s** NODI LYMPHATICI PREPERICARDIALES. **pretracheal l.'s** NODI LYMPHATICI PRETRACHEALES. **pulmonary l.'s** NODI LYMPHATICI PULMONALES. **pyloric l.'s** NODI LYMPHATICI PYLORICI. **retroaortic l.'s** NODI LYMPHATICI POSTAORTICI. **retroauricular l.'s** NODI LYMPHATICI MASTOIDEI. **retrocaval l.'s** NODI LYMPHATICI POSTCAVALES. **retropharyngeal l.'s** NODI LYMPHATICI RETROPHARYNGEALES. **right colic l.'s** NODI LYMPHATICI COLICI DEXTRI. **right gastric l.'s** NODI LYMPHATICI GASTRICI DEXTRI. **right gastroepiploic l.'s** NODI LYMPHATICI GASTRO-OMENTALES DEXTRI. **sacral l.'s** NODI LYMPHATICI SACRALES. **sternal l.'s** NODI LYMPHATICI PARASTERNALES. **submandibular l.'s** NODI LYMPHATICI SUBMANDIBULARES. **submental l.'s** NODI LYMPHATICI SUBMENTALES. **subscapular l.'s** NODI LYMPHATICI SUBSCAPULARES. **superficial cervical l.'s** NODI LYMPHATICI CERVICALES SUPERFICIALES. **superficial inguinal l.'s** NODI LYMPHATICI INGUINALES SUPERFICIALES. **superficial parotid l.'s** NODI LYMPHATICI PAROTIDEI SUPERFICIALES. **superior gastric l.'s** NODI LYMPHATICI GASTRICI SINISTRI. **superior mesenteric l.'s** NODI LYMPHATICI MESENTERICI SUPERIORES. **superior tracheobronchial l.'s** NODI LYMPHATICI TRACHEOBRONCHIALES SUPERIORES. **supraclavicular l.'s** NODI LYMPHATICI SUPRACLAVICULAR[illegible] **supratrochlear l.'s** NODI LYMPHATICI CUBITA[illegible] **thyroid l.'s** NODI LYMPHATICI THYROIDEI. **tra**[illegible] **l.'s** NODI LYMPHATICI PARATRACHEALES. **tr**[illegible] **bronchial l.'s** NODI LYMPHATICI TRACHEOBRO[illegible]

**l. of Troisier** SENTINEL NODE. **uterovaginal l.** A lymph node situated at the junction of the uterus and vagina on each side. *Outmoded.* **visceral l.'s of abdomen** NODI VISCERALES ABDOMINIS.

**lympho-** \lim′fō-\ [LYMPH + *-o-*] A combining form denoting lymph or lymphatic tissue. Also *lymph-*.

**lymphoblast** \lim′fəblast\ An immature cell of the lymphocytic series that is 15–20 microns in diameter, with a nucleus that has a diffuse chromatin pattern and usually one or two nucleoli, and with rather scanty cytoplasm devoid of granules. The lymphoblast was formerly conceived as the precursor cell of the mature lymphocyte, but now is considered to be a lymphocyte that has been transformed from a resting state to a proliferating state by antigenic stimulation. Lymphoblasts occur in the blood in large numbers in acute lymphocytic leukemia. Also *lymphocytoblast, lymphogone.*

**lymphoblasthemia** \-blas·thē′mē·ə\ LYMPHOBLASTOSIS.

**lymphoblastic** \-blas′tik\ Of or relating to lymphoblasts.

**lymphoblastoma** \-blastō′mə\ A lymphoblastic lymphoma. See under LYMPHOCYTIC LYMPHOMA. **giant follicular l.** NODULAR LYMPHOMA.

**lymphoblastosis** \-blastō′sis\ The presence of lymphoblasts in blood, as in acute lymphocytic leukemia. Also *lymphoblasthemia.*

**lymphocele** \lim′fəsēl\ [LYMPHO- + -CELE[2]] Any cystic structure that contains lymph.

**lymphocinesia** \-sinē′zhə\ LYMPHOKINESIS.

**lymphocystosis** \-sistō′sis\ The development of multiple cystic lymphangiomas.

**lymphocyte** \lim′fəsīt\ [LYMPHO- + -CYTE] A leukocyte of blood, bone marrow, and lymphatic tissue that characteristically has a round nucleus with well-condensed chromatin, no identifiable nucleolus, and usually agranular cytoplasm that stains pale blue with Romanowsky dyes. A narrow lighter halo, or perinuclear clear zone, may surround the nucleus, and a few azurophilic granules may be seen in the cytoplasm. Lymphocytes play a major role in both cellular and humoral immunity, and thus several different functional and morphologic types must be recognized, i.e. the small, large, B-, and T-lymphocytes, with further morphologic distinctions being made among the B-lymphocytes. These distinctions are important in the classification of lymphocytic malignancies. Also *lymphoid leukocyte, lymphoid corpuscle, lymphoid cell, lymph cell.* **atypical l.** A large lymphocyte which by Romanowsky stain has abundant basophilic cytoplasm that often exhibits distinct paler cytoplasmic zones and an oval nucleus resembling that of a monocyte. Atypical lymphocytes, when numerous in blood, are characteristic of infectious mononucleosis, cytomegalovirus infection, viral hepatitis, and other viral infections. Also *Downey cell, variant lymphocyte, virocyte.* **B l.** One of the two major classes of lymphocytes having important immune regulatory functions. In birds, B lymphocytes pass through the bursa of Fabricius during their development. In mammals, the fetal liver is believed to be the equivalent of the bursa of Fabricius. B lymphocytes carry certain characteristic surface markers such as membrane-bound immunoglobulin. They recognize antigen independent of MHC molecules. When stimulated by antigens, they enlarge, develop very basophilic cytoplasm (from increase in RNA), and transform into plasma cells that secrete antibody. Also *B cell, thymus-independent lymphocyte.* Compare T LYMPHOCYTE. **educated T l.** A thymus-derived lymphocyte that has been exposed to antigen on an antigen-presenting cell and thus may be used in experiments of T lymphocyte-B lymphocyte cooperation to cause splenocytes from irradiated animals to respond to the antigen. **helper T l.** HELPER CELL. **killer l.** NATURAL KILLER CELL. **large l.** A common lymphocyte in normal blood and lymph nodes. It is approximately 15 microns in diameter, having more cytoplasm than small lymphocytes. The nucleus occupies approximately one third of the cell volume. **NUL l.** A lymphocyte which possesses neither T nor B cell markers on its surface. Also *null cell.* **primed l.** A lymphocyte which has been exposed to antigen and has thereby become more immunologically responsive. Upon further antigen exposure, it is capable of dividing rapidly, synthesizing antibody, or taking part in a cell-mediated immune reaction. **small l.** The predominant lymphocyte in normal blood and lymph nodes. It is approximately 10 microns in diameter, with a nucleus that is more than half the cell volume. **suppressor T l.** SUPPRESSOR CELL. **T l.** One of the two major classes of lymphocyte having important immune regulatory and effector functions. T lymphocytes must pass through the thymus during their development. T lymphocytes carry certain characteristic surface markers such as thy 1 and T3 antigens. They recognize antigen only in the context of MHC molecules, and they are responsible for the phenomena of cell-mediated immunity. Also *T cell, thymus-dependent lymphocyte, thymus-dependent cell, thymus-derived cell.* Compare B LYMPHOCYTE. **thymus-dependent l.** T LYMPHOCYTE. **thymus-independent l.** B LYMPHOCYTE. **variant l.** ATYPICAL LYMPHOCYTE.

**lymphocythemia** \-sīthē′mē·ə\ LYMPHOCYTOSIS.

**lymphocytic** \-sit′ik\ Of or relating to lymphocytes.

**lymphocytoblast** \-sī′təblast\ LYMPHOBLAST.

**lymphocytoma** \-sītō′mə\ *Obs.* LYMPHOCYTIC LYMPHOMA. **benign cutaneous l.** BENIGN LYMPHOCYTOMA CUTIS. **benign l. cutis** A nonmalignant aggregate of lymphoid cells in the dermis. On occastion it is found in follicular form. Also *benign cutaneous lymphadenosis, Bäfverstedt syndrome, benign lymphocytic reticulosis, benign lymphadenosis.*

**lymphocytopenia** \sī′təpē′nē·ə\ A fewer than normal number of lymphocytes in blood. Also *lymphopenia, sublymphemia, lymphocytic leukopenia, hypolymphemia.*

**lymphocytopoiesis** \-sī′təpoi·ē′sis\ LYMPHOPOIESIS.

**lymphocytopoietic** \-sī′təpoi·et′ik\ Characteristic of lymphocyte production.

**lymphocytosis** \-sītō′sis\ [*lymphocyt(e)* + -OSIS] A greater than normal number of lymphocytes in blood. Also *lymphocythemia.* **acute infectious l.** An acute, benign, infectious disease of obscure, but presumably viral, etiology affecting children. Symptoms are mild, with fever, headache, and upper respiratory symptoms seen in most cases and abdominal pain and central nervous system involvement reported in some cases. Multiple cases occur in families and in institutional populations. The significant feature is a leukocytosis of one to two months duration in which small, mature lymphocytes account for 60–90 percent of the differential count. The heterophile antibody test is negative in all cases, and the illness is not associated with a rise in Epstein-Barr virus antibody. **relative l.** An increase in the proportion of lymphocytes in the blood compared with other leukocytes, often the result of a decrease in the number of neutrophils.

**lymphocytotoxin** \-sī′tətäk′sin\ A complement-fixing antilymphocyte antibody.

**lymphodermia** \-dur′mē·ə\ [LYMPHO- + -DERMIA] An abnormality in the lymphatic vessels in the skin. *Obs.* **l. perniciosa** *Obs.* LEUKEMIA CUTIS.

**lymphoduct** \lim′fədukt\ VAS LYMPHATICUM.

**lymphoedema** *Brit.* LYMPHEDEMA.

**lymphoepithelioma** \-ep′ithē′lē·ō′mə\ A carcinoma of the nasopharynx or oropharynx infiltrated by large numbers of lymphoid cells. The lymphoid cells are not neoplastic. Also *lymphoepithelial carcinoma, lymphepithelioma.*

**lymphogenesis** \-jen′əsis\ LYMPHOPOIESIS.

**lymphogenous** \limfäj′ənəs\ **1** LYMPHOPOIETIC. **2** Originating in the lymphatic system.

**lymphogone** \limf′əgōn\ LYMPHOBLAST.

**lymphogranuloma** \-gran′yəlō′mə\ Any of several conditions characterized by lymphadenopathy and multiple granulomas in lymph nodes, such as sarcoidosis, lymphogranuloma venereum, and Hodgkin's disease. **l. benignum** *Outmoded* SARCOIDOSIS. **l. inguinale** LYMPHOGRANULOMA VENEREUM. **l. malignum** HODGKIN'S DISEASE. **l. venereum** A disease caused by microorganisms of the *Chlamydia trachomatis* group, transmitted by sexual contact, and characterized by transient genital ulcerations, systemic symptoms, and subsequent inguinal lymphadenopathy (bubo). Late complications include urethral and rectal strictures, genital lymphedema, and rectovaginal fistulas. Also *strumous bubo, tropical bubo, Frei's disease, Nicolas-Favre disease, lymphogranuloma inguinale, lymphyogranulomatosis inguinalis, poradenolymphitis, groin ulcer.*

**lymphogranulomatosis** \-gran′yəlōmətō′sis\ [LYMPHOGRANULOMA + *t* + -OSIS] A term used in Europe, but rarely in the U.S., for HODGKIN'S DISEASE. • Although this term might logically be used to embrace other conditions of lymphogranuloma, such as sarcoidosis, it is not, in practice, used that way. **benign l.** *Outmoded* SARCOIDOSIS. **l. inguinalis** LYMPHOGRANULOMA VENEREUM. **malignant l.** HODGKIN'S DISEASE.

**lymphography** \limfäg′rəfē\ LYMPHANGIOGRAPHY.

**lymphoid** \lim′foid\ Pertaining to or resembling lymph or lymphatic tissue. Also *adenoid.*

**lymphoidocyte** \limfoi′dəsīt\ HEMOCYTOBLAST.

**lymphokentric** \-ken′trik\ Stimulating the production of lymphocytes.

**lymphokine** \lim′fəkīn\ Any of several soluble mediators produced by lymphocytes, usually in response to reaction with lectins or specific antigens, and which participate in inflammatory reactions or in the growth and differentiation of other lymphocytes.

**lymphokinesis** \-kīnē′sis\ **1** The movement of lymph in the body. **2** The movement of endolymph within the membraneous labyrinth of the ear. For defs. 1 and 2 *Rare.* also *lymphocinesia.*

**lymphology** \limfäl′əjē\ LYMPHANGIOLOGY.

**lymphoma** \limfō′mə\ [LYMPH- + -OMA] Any of various malignant neoplasms primarily affecting lymph nodes, including the lymphocytic lymphomas, histiocytic lymphoma, and Hodgkin's disease. All but the last are known as non-Hodgkin's lymphomas. Also *malignant lymphoma, hematosarcoma* (rare), *lymphadenomatosis, malignant lymphadenoma, lymphadenoma, malignant lymphadenosis, lymphomatosis.* • Lymphomas have been variously classified over the years. For descriptions of the major classifications see under CLASSIFICATION. **African l.** BURKITT'S LYMPHOMA. **B cell l.** A lymphoma of B lymphocytes. **Burkitt's l.** A malignant lymphoma involving extranodal sites such as the jaws, orbit, abdominal viscera, and ovaries. The tumor contains lymphoid cells with considerable cytoplasmic basophilia and lipid-containing vacuoles. Macrophages with pale cytoplasm are interspersed among the tumor cells to give a "starry sky" effect. It is the most common childhood tumor in parts of tropical Africa, usually affecting children between five and nine years of age. It also occurs in other tropical and, to a lesser extent, temperate countries, most commonly where mean monthly temperature is over 15.5°C and relative humidity is high. It is possibly caused by the Epstein-Barr virus, but is also associated with stable falciparum malaria. Also *Burkitt's tumor, African lymphoma.* **centroblastic l.** FOLLICULAR CENTER CELL LYMPHOMA. **centrocytic l.** FOLLICULAR CENTER CELL LYMPHOMA. **convoluted cell l.** A lymphoma with cells having pronounced nuclear convolutions. **cutaneous T cell l.** SÉZARY SYNDROME. **diffuse l.** A lymphoma in which the histologic pattern is one of diffuse rather than of nodular growth. **fascicular l.** A lymphoma whose cells are arranged in rows separated by fine stromal fibers. **follicular l.** NODULAR LYMPHOMA. **follicular center cell l.** A lymphoma with cells derived from the follicular centers of lymphoid tissue. Also *centroblastic lymphoma, centrocytic lymphoma, germinoblastic lymphoma.* **giant follicular l.** NODULAR LYMPHOMA. **granulomatous l.** HODGKIN'S DISEASE. **histiocytic l.** A form of malignant lymphoma that appears to be composed of histiocytes. Most of these cases are actually poorly differentiated lymphocytic lymphomas. Also *histiocytic sarcoma, reticulum cell sarcoma, reticulosarcoma* (obs.), *clasmocytoma* (obs.). **immunoblastic l.** A diffuse lymphoma composed of large cells with basophilic cytoplasm and a single prominent nucleolus. **intestinal l.** A form of lymphoma typically arising in the small intestines. It may be associated with alpha heavy-chain disease. **Lennert's l.** LYMPHOEPITHELIOID CELL LYMPHOMA. **lymphoblastic l.** See under LYMPHOCYTIC LYMPHOMA. **lymphocytic l.** A malignant lymphoma composed of lymphocytes. The pattern may be either nodular or diffuse, and the cells may be either well-differentiated small lymphocytes or poorly differentiated lymphocytes that are larger and have less-condensed nuclear chromatin and nucleoli. Poorly differentiated lymphocytic lymphoma has also been called lymphoblastic lymphoma in earlier classifications. Also *lymphosarcoma* (obs.), *lymphocytoma* (obs.). **lymphocytic l. of intermediate differentiation** PROLYMPHOCYTIC LYMPHOMA. **lymphoepithelioid cell l.** A rare form of lymphoma characterized by replacement of lymph nodes by lymphocytes and aggregates of epithelioid cells. The condition as originally described was thought to be a form of Hodgkin's disease, but it is now thought to be a separate entity. It has poor prognosis, with median survival of one year. Also *Lennert's lymphoma.* **lymphoplasmacytic l.** *Rare* WALDENSTRÖM'S MACROGLOBULINEMIA. **malignant l.** LYMPHOMA. **nodular l.** A lymphoma composed of cells arranged in groups somewhat like lymphoid follicles. Also *Brill-Symmers disease, Symmers disease, giant follicular lymphadenopathy, giant follicular lymphoma, nodular malignant lymphoma, follicular lymphoma, giant follicular lymphoblastoma.* **non-Hodgkin's l.** Any malignant lymphoma other than Hodgkin's disease. **poorly differentiated lymphocytic l.** A lymphoma composed of immature lymphocytes. Also *poorly differentiated lymphosarcoma.* **prolymphocytic l.** A malignant lymphoma composed of lymphocytes that are slightly larger and that have less condensed nuclear chromatin than the cells of well-differentiated lymphocytic lymphoma. Also *lymphocytic lymphoma of intermediate differentiation.* **sclerosing l.** A lymphoma with a prominent stromal component. **signet-ring cell l.** A rare form of malignant lymphoma consisting of cells with a large cytoplasmic vacuole of immunoglobulin which displaces the nucleus to the periphery. It thus simulates signet-ring cell carcinoma and may be positive with the periodic acid-Schiff reaction. It gives negative results for mucin content with stains such as Alcian blue and mucicarmine. **stem cell l.** A lymphoma composed of large blastlike cells. Also *undifferentiated malignant lymphoma.* **T cell l.** A lymphoma of T lymphocytes. **undifferentiated malignant l.** STEM CELL LYMPHOMA.

**lymphomatoid** \limfō′mətoid\ [*lymphomat(a),* pl of LYMPHOMA + -OID] Resembling lymphoma.

**lymphomatosis** \-mətō′sis\ [*lymphomat(a),* pl. of LYMPHOMA + -OSIS] LYMPHOMA. **osteopetrotic l.** A neoplastic disease of poultry characterized by thickening of bones, particularly the long bones of the legs. It belongs to the leukosis-sarcoma group of the avian leukosis complex. Also *thick leg disease, osteopetrosis gallinarum.*

**lymphomatous** \limfō′mətəs\ Pertaining to lymphoma.

**lymphonodi** \-nō′dī\ Plural of LYMPHONODUS.

**lymphonodus** \-nō′dəs\ [LYMPHO- + NODUS] (*pl.* lymphonodi) NODUS LYMPHATICUS.

**lymphopathy** \limfäp′əthē\ Any disorder of the lymphatic system. *Seldom used.* **ataxic l.** Swelling of the lymph nodes which may occur during a pain crisis of locomotor ataxia.

**lymphopenia** \-pē′nē·ə\ LYMPHOCYTOPENIA.

**lymphoplasty** \lim′fəplas′tē\ LYMPHANGIOPLASTY.

**lymphopoiesis** \-poi·ē′sis\ The production of lymphocytes. Also *lymphocytopoiesis, lymphogenesis, lymphization.*

**lymphopoietic** \-poi·et′ik\ Characterized by lymphopoiesis. Also *lymphogenous.*

**lymphopoietin** \-poi′ətin\ A soluble factor required for the maturation of lymphocytes. Recent advances in the study of the growth and differentiation factors needed by lymphocytes make it clear that there are a substantial number of lymphopoietic molecules.

**lymphoproliferative** \-prōlif′ərā′tiv\ Pertaining to the proliferation of lymphoid cells.

**lymphoreticular** \-retik′yələr\ Of or relating to the lymphoid tissues and organs and their associated reticuloendothelial framework.

**lymphoreticulosis** \-retik′yəlō′sis\ Any proliferation of the constituent cells of lymphoid tissues. **benign l.** CAT-SCRATCH DISEASE.

**lymphorrhage** \lim′fôrij\ The escape of lymph from a ruptured lymphatic vessel.

**lymphorrhea** \lim′fôrē′ə\ [LYMPHO- + -RRHEA] The flow of lymph from a disrupted lymphatic channel. Also *lymphorrhagia.*

**lymphorrhoid** \lim′fôroid\ [LYMPHO- + *-rrh(ea)* + -OID] A local dilatation of perianal lymphatics, occurring in lymphogranuloma venereum. It is similar in appearance to a hemorrhoid.

**lymphosarcoleukemia** \-sär′kəlookē′mē·ə\ LYMPHOSARCOMA CELL LEUKEMIA.

**lymphosarcoma** \-särkō′mə\ [LYMPHO- + SARCOMA] *Obs.* LYMPHOCYTIC LYMPHOMA. **Murphy-Sturm l.** A chemically induced, transplantable lymphocytic lymphoma of rats. Lymphoid leukemia also occurs. **poorly differentiated l.** POORLY DIFFERENTIATED LYMPHOCYTIC LYMPHOMA.

**lymphosarcomatous** \-särkō′mətəs\ Related to or describing lymphosarcoma.

**lymphoscrotum** \-skrō′təm\ [LYMPHO- + SCROTUM] ELEPHANTIASIS SCROTI.

**lymphostasis** \limfäs′təsis\ The absence of flow within lymphatic vessels.

**lymphotaxis** \-tak′sis\ [LYMPHO- + Gk *taxis* an arranging, ordering] The induction of lymphocyte movement.

**lymphotoxic** \-täk′sik\ Pertaining to any substance that is toxic to lymphoid tissue.

**lymphotoxin** \-täk′sin\ **1** A substance which is toxic or destructive to lymphocytes. **2** A toxin produced by T lymphocytes during an immune response which causes membrane damage and death of certain target cells.

**lymphotrophic** \-träf′ik\ **1** Relating to lymphotrophy. **2** Attracted to the lymphatic system. • Although widely used, in this sense it is linguistically incorrect.

**lymphotrophy** \limfät′rəfē\ The carrying of nutrients by the lymphatic system to tissues which have a defective blood supply.

**lymphous** \lim′fəs\ Pertaining to or containing lymph.

**lymphuria** \limfoo′rē·ə\ [LYMPH + -URIA] CHYLURIA. **filarial l.** The presence of lymph in the urine due to lymphatic obstruction around a kidney, ureter, or bladder in some cases of filariasis. If chyle is present the urine appears milky. *Wuchereria bancrofti* and *Brugia malayi* are usually responsible.

**lymph-vascular** \limf-vas′kyələr\ Pertaining to or having lymphatic vessels.

**lynestrenol** \lines′trənôl\ $C_{20}H_{28}O$. 19-Nor-pregn-4-en-20-yn-17α-ol. A semisynthetic progestin or progestogen.

**lyo-** \lī′ō-\ [Gk *lyein* to loosen, dissolve, wash] A combining form meaning dispersed, dissolved, loosened.

**Lyon** [Bethuel Boyd Vincent *Lyon,* U.S. physician, 1880–1953] Meltzer-Lyon test. See under TEST.

**Lyon** [Mary Frances *Lyon,* English geneticist, born 1925] Lyon-Russell hypothesis, Lyon hypothesis. See under LYON PHENOMENON.

**lyonization** \lī′ōnīzā′shən\ LYON PHENOMENON.

**lyophilic** \-fil′ik\ [LYO- + -PHILIC] Dispersing or dissolving easily because of having an affinity for the solvent: said of colloidal particles or macromolecules.

**lyophilization** \lī·äf′il īzā′shən\ [LYO- + -PHIL + *-iz(e)* + -ATION] The process of drying a sample by submitting it to a vacuum while frozen, so that ice sublimes out of it. Also *freeze-drying.* • The term is somewhat misleading, as the process does not render materials lyophilic, but merely keeps them lyophilic to the extent that it avoids denaturing proteins.

**lyophobic** \-fō′bik\ [LYO- + PHOBIC] Difficult to disperse because of having little affinity for the solvent: said of a colloidal material.

**lyotropic** \-träp′ik\ Concerning the relative ability of ions to influence the medium in which they are dissolved. Hence ions high in a lyotropic series have great effect on solvent properties, particularly for colloidal substances, e.g. they are especially effective in salting out proteins.

***Lyponyssus*** \lī′pōnis′əs\ *ORNITHONYSSUS.*

**lypressin** Vasopressin with lysine in place of arginine at position 8, found in the supraopticoneurohypophysial unit of members of the pig family. The hippopotamus and domestic pig have lysine vasopressin only; the wart hog and peccary have both lysine and arginine vasopressin. The peptide is arranged into a five-member S-S bonded ring with a three-member side chain in which lysine occupies the position next to the terminal glycinamide. It is an antidiuretic and a vasopressor hormone, and is used as a nasal spray in the treatment of diabetes insipidus of central origin. Also *vasopressin 8-lysine, lysine vasopressin.*

**lyra** \lī′rə\ [L (Gk *lyra*), a lyre, lute, harp] An anatomic structure suggestive of the shape of a lyre or lute. Also *lyre.*

**Lys** Symbol for lysine.

**lys-** \lis-, līs-\ LYSO-.

**lysate** \lī′sāt\ The product of lysis.

**lyse** \līz\ [back-formation from LYSIS] To subject to lysis; to break up or rupture (a cell membrane).

**lysemia** \līsē′mē·ə\ Intravascular hemolysis with hemoglobinemia. *Rare.*

**lysenkoism** \līseng′kō·izm\ A doctrine of genetics that embraced inheritance of acquired characteristics and denied the central role of genes and chromosomes. It was promulgated by T.D. Lysenko (1898–1976) and was the official position of the U.S.S.R. in the mid-twentieth century, but it wrought disastrous consquences on agronomy and the biological sciences in that country.

**lysergic acid** One of the ergot alkaloids, a component of the ergotamine molecule. Its molecule contains four rings, two of them containing nitrogen, and it is derived biosynthetically from tryptophan and dimethylallyl pyrophosphate.

**lysergic acid diethylamide** A hallucinogenic indole amine that is highly subject to abuse. Unlike the ergot alkaloids, this compound directly affects the central nervous system with effects resembling those of mescaline. It can induce temporary manifestations of schizophrenia, and it is suspected of causing chromosomal damage. Abbr. LSD, LSD-25

**lysin** \lī′sin\ [LYS- + -IN] Any substance capable of causing lysis, especially a complement-fixing antibody: often used in combination to indicate the type of cell to which the action of the lysin is specifically directed, as hemolysin or bacteriolysin. **hot-cold l.** Any of those lysins that are activated only following incubation at 37°C followed by refrigeration, as $\beta$-hemolysin. **immune l.** An antibody detected by giving rise to complement-mediated cell lysis. *Outmoded.*

**lysine** $NH_2—[CH_2]_4—CH(NH_2)COOH$. One of the twenty amino acids that are incorporated into proteins. It is important in human nutrition because it is essential. Diets may be deficient in it because, in general, plant proteins contain less lysine than do animal proteins. Lysine residues in proteins are usually on the outside of the molecules, providing positive charges, and lysine residues in enzymes sometimes form imines with carbonyl substrates or cofactors.

**lysine vasopressin** LYPRESSIN.

**lysis** \lī′sis\ [Gk *lysis* (from *lyein* to loosen, dissolve, slacken, set free, weaken) a loosing, release] **1** Any form of dissolution, particularly the breaking of membrane-bound structures such as cells. **2** A gradual reduction in strength of the symptoms of a disease, leading to its eventual disappearance. Compare CRISIS. Adj. lytic. **bone l.** OSTEOLYSIS. **immune l.** The destruction of cells by immunologic mechanisms. These include lysis of antibody-sensitized cells by complement or killer cells and lysis of specific target cells by cytotoxic T lympyhocytes. **osmotic l.** Rupture of the plasma membrane of a cell following immersion in a hypotonic solution.

**lyso-** \lī′sō-\ [Gk *lysis* (from *lyein* to loosen, dissolve, wash) dissolution, loosing, decomposition] A combining form meaning lysis or dissolution. When applied to lipids, it signifies that one of the two acyl groups has been removed from the glycerol part of the molecule. Also *lys-*.

**lysochrome** \lī′səkrōm\ A lipid-soluble pigment that is suitable for staining fats.

**lysocythin** \-sī′thin\ A cytolytic substance formed by the reaction of body tissues to an animal venom.

**lysogenic** \-jen′ik\ [LYSO- + -GENIC] Denoting a strain of bacterium that perpetuates a bacteriophage in the prophage state. The lysogenic condition usually renders the bacteria immune to further infection by particles of the bacteriophage they carry, but not to particles of different phages.

**lysogenization** \līsäj′ənīzā′shən\ The process whereby a bacterium is rendered lysogenic by bacteriophage infection.

**lysogeny** \līsäj′ənē\ [LYSO- + -GEN + -Y] A process whereby viral nucleic acid that has entered a cell does not initiate the synthesis of more viral material but becomes attached to specific sites in the chromosome, and is then both reproduced together with the chromosome and transmitted to daughter cells at each cell division: used particularly of viruses that infect bacteria (bacteriophages) and which, when in lysogeny, are described as being in the prophage state.

**lysokinase** \-kī′nās\ TISSUE PLASMINOGEN ACTIVATOR.

**lysolecithin** \-les′ithin\ LYSOPHOSPHATIDYLCHOLINE.

**lysophosphatidylcholine** A lipid in which phosphoric acid forms an ester link between a monoacylglycerol and choline. Also *lysolecithin.*

**lysosomal** \-sō′məl\ Pertaining to or derived from a lysosome.

**lysosome** \lī′səsōm\ [LYSO- + -SOME] A membrane-limited cytoplasmic organelle containing hydrolytic enzymes which have a pH optimum in the acid range. Also *cytolysome.* **primary l.** A newly formed lysosome as it separates from the Golgi membranes. **secondary l.** A cytoplasmic sac formed by the fusion of a primary lysosome and a phagosome containing material to be digested. Also *digestive vacuole.*

**lysostaphin** An enzyme produced by *Staphylococcus staphylolyticus* that has antibacterial activity. The enzyme has specific action against staphylococci.

**lysotype** \lī′sətīp\ A type within a bacterial species as determined by its pattern of sensitivity to a set of test phages.

**lysozyme** \lī′səzīm\ [*lys(ing) (en)zyme*] An enzyme found in tears, saliva, milk, and many other secretions that hydrolyzes the muramic acid linkages in the peptidoglycan of some bacterial cell walls.

**lysozymuria** \-zīmoo′rē·ə\ Excretion of lysozyme in the urine. Greater than normal lysozymuria is characteristic of myeloproliferative disorders, especially chronic granulocytic leukemia and myelomonocytic leukemia.

**lyssa** \lis′ə\ [Gk *lyssa* rage, frenzy] *Obs.* RABIES.

***Lyssavirus*** \lis′əvī′rəs\ A genus of the Rhabdoviridae family that includes rabies virus.

**lysyl oxidase** PROTEIN-LYSINE 6-OXIDASE.

**Lyt** See under LY ANTIGENS.

**lytic** \lit′ik\ Related to or capable of producing lysis.

***Lytta*** \lit′ə\ A genus of blister beetles. ***L. vesicatoria*** *CANTHARIS VESICATORIA.*

# M

**M** 1 A symbol widely used in chemistry to denote concentration in moles per liter. 2 Symbol for methionine. 3 Symbol for mega-: used with SI units.

**M.** 1 *mille* (L, thousand). 2 *misce* (L, mix). 3 *mistura* (L, mixture). 4 myopia. 5 mucoid (colony).

**m** 1 Symbol for milli-: used with SI units. 2 Symbol for the unit, meter.

**$m^{-1}$** Symbol for the unit, reciprocal meter.

**$m^2$** Symbol for the unit, square meter.

**$m^3$** Symbol for the unit, cubic meter.

**μ** 1 Symbol for micro-: used with SI units. 2 Symbol for the unit, micrometer. An incorrect symbol. 3 Symbol for magnetic permeability.

**MA** 1 mental age. 2 meter angle.

**Ma** Mach number.

**mA** Symbol for the unit, milliampere.

**mÅ** Symbol for the unit, milliångström.

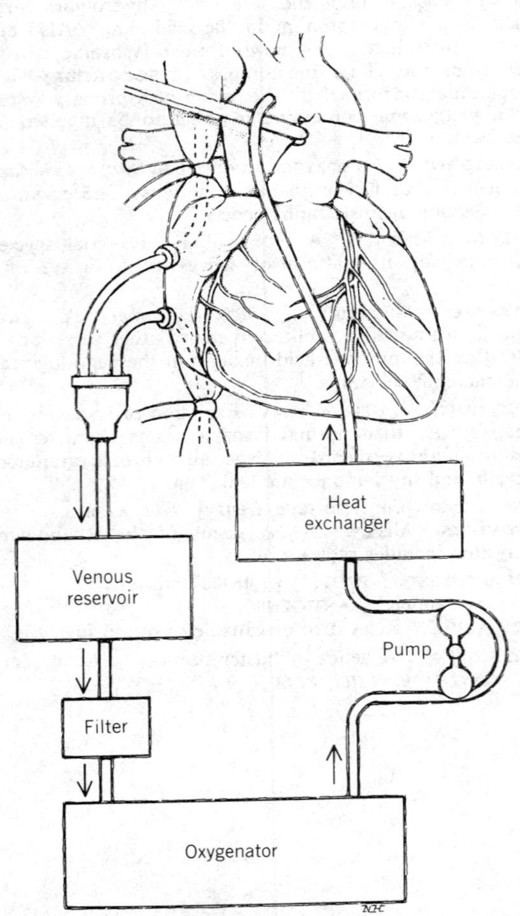


**Heart–lung machine**

**MAC** 1 maximum allowable concentration. 2 minimum alveolar concentration.

**mac.** *macerare* (L, macerate).

***Macaca*** \məkä′kə\ [New L, fem. of Portuguese *macaco* a monkey] A genus of the primate family Cercopithecidae; the macaques. They are characterized by stout bodies, powerful limbs, and a somewhat elongate snout. There are about 12 species distributed from Gibraltar to eastern Asia. Several species of macaques are important subjects in medical and space research. ***M. mulatta*** The rhesus monkey. It is widely used in medical and biological research.

**macaque** \məkak′\ [French. See *MACACA*.] Any monkey of the genus *Macaca*. **crab-eating m.** CYNOMOLGUS.

**MacCallum** [William George *MacCallum*, Canadian pathologist active in the United States, 1874–1944] See under PATCH.

**MacConkey** [Alfred Theodore *MacConkey*, English bacteriologist, 1861–1931] See under AGAR.

**Macdonald** [George *Macdonald*, English malariologist, born 1903] See under INDEX.

**Macdowel** [Benjamin George *Macdowel*, Irish anatomist and surgeon, 1820–1885] Macdowel's frenum. See under FRENULUM.

**Mace** [contraction of *m(ethylchloroform chloro)ace(tophenone)*] $C_8H_7ClO$. A form of tear gas. It causes coughing, lacrimation, and vomiting, thus incapacitating its target. A proprietary name. Also *Chemical Mace*.

**maceration** \mas′ərā′shən\ [L *macer(are)* to soak, soften by steeping + -ATION] 1 In histology, the softening and disintegration of a mass of tissue by soaking in acids or enzymes. 2 The autolysis of fetal tissues, which develops when death occurs *in utero* and the fetus is retained.

**Macewen** [Sir William *Macewen*, Scottish surgeon, 1848–1924] 1 See under SIGN. 2 Tibial spine of Macewen. See under SPINE. 3 Macewen's osteotomy. See under OPERATION.

**Mache** [Heinrich *Mache*, Austrian physicist, 1876–1954] See under UNIT.

**machine** / **anesthesia m.** An apparatus used to supply anesthetic gases and vapors plus oxygen. It is capable of quantifying the volumes delivered, as well as delivering mixtures to a patient's breathing circuit for the inducement of general anesthesia. Also *gas machine*. **gas m.** ANESTHESIA MACHINE. **heart-lung m.** A combination of pump and oxygenator to effect extracorporeal circulation and oxygenation of blood during open-heart surgery. **Holtz m.** An early form of high-voltage electrostatic generator. **panoramic rotating m.** A type of x-ray equipment for dental pantomography, producing images of all the teeth and surrounding structures on one film. Its principle is the use of a reciprocating motion of the x-ray tube and a curved extraoral film. **static m.** ELECTROSTATIC GENERATOR. **Van de Graaff m.** VAN DE GRAAFF GENERATOR.

**Machover** [Karen Alper *Machover*, U.S. psychologist, born 1902] Machover test. See under DRAW-A-PERSON TEST.

**macies** \mā′shi·ēz\ [L, leanness] WASTING.

**MacKay** [Ralph Stuart *MacKay*, U.S. biophysicist, born 1924] MacKay-Marg electronic tonometer. See under TONOMETER.

**Mackenrodt** [Alwin Karl *Mackenrodt*, German gynecologist, 1859–1925] See under OPERATION.

**Mackenzie** [Sir James *Mackenzie,* Scottish physician, 1853–1925] Mackenzie's disease. See under X DISEASE.

**Mackenzie** [Sir Stephen *Mackenzie,* English physician, 1844–1909] **1** Jackson-Mackenzie syndrome, Mackenzie syndrome. See under JACKSON'S PARALYSIS. **2** See under AMPUTATION.

**Macleod** [William Mathieson *Macleod,* English pneumologist, 1911–1977] Swyer-James-Macleod syndrome. See under SYNDROME.

**macr-** \makr-\ MACRO-.

***Macracanthorhynchus*** \mak′rəkan′thôring′kəs\ A genus of giant, thorny-headed, intestinal worms of the phylum Acanthocephala, order Archiacanthocephala. ***M. hirudinaceus*** A common species of extremely large worms found in the small intestine of the pig and, rarely, in humans. The female is 25–60 cm long and the male, 5–10 cm. It is pink, pseudosegmented (transversely wrinkled), with a long, tapering, flattened body and a knoblike proboscis armed with five or six rows of thorns. The spiny proboscis induces development of nodules at the point of attachment. Soil-dwelling grubs of May beetles (*Cotinus*) and June beetles (*Phyllophaga*) serve as intermediate hosts, infecting pigs that root in the soil. Also *Echinorhynchus gigas, Echinorhynchus hominis, Gigantorhynchus hirudinaceus.*

**macro-** \mak′rō-, mak′rə-\ [Gk *makros* long, large] A combining form meaning (1) large or long; (2) abnormally or excessively large. Also *macr-, makro-.*

**macroamylasemia** \-am′ilāsē′mē·ə\ [MACRO- + *amylas(e)* + -EMIA] The elevation of measured serum amylase due to the presence of macroamylase, a complex of amylase and globulin with a high molecular weight that does not pass through the glomerular filter. It may occur as a nonspecific laboratory abnormality in subjects with alcoholism, malabsorption, or other disorders of the digestive tract.

***Macrobdella decora*** \mak′rōdel′ə dekôr′ə\ The American leech, a species found in the United States and Canada and formerly used for drawing blood in place of the European medicinal leech, *Hirudo medicinalis..*

**macrobiote** \-bī′ōt\ [MACRO- + Gk *biotē,* also *biotos* life, means of life] A long-lived organism, with special reference to prolonged survival in a dormant, resistant state, such as clostridial spores, eggs of *Ascaris,* or the survival qualities of certain ticks.

**macroblast** \mak′rəblast\ [MACRO- + -BLAST] Any unusually large normoblast. *Rare.* **m. of Naegeli** PRONORMOBLAST.

**macrobrachia** \-brā′kē·ə\ [MACRO- + *brach(ium)* + -IA] Excessive length or size in one or both arms.

**macrocardia** \-kär′dē·ə\ [MACRO- + -CARDIA] **1** Abnormal largeness of the heart in an infant or child with congenital cardiac disease. The increased size is usually the result of attempted functional compensation for circulatory inefficiency secondary to developmental defects. Also *megalocardia.* **2** CARDIOMEGALY.

**macrocardius** \-kär′dē·əs\ [MACRO- + *cardi(a)* + New L *-us,* masc. noun suffix] An individual possessing an enlarged heart.

**macrocephaly** \-sef′əlē\ [MACRO- + CEPHAL- + -Y ] A disproportionate largeness of the head, either a general enlargement of the entire head or an increase in particular dimensions or parts. Also *megacephaly, megalocephaly.*

**macrocheilia** \-kī′lē·ə\ [MACRO- + CHEIL- + -IA ] An abnormal largeness of a lip, usually owing to a cavernous lymphangioma. Also *macrolabia.*

**macrochylomicron** \-kī′lōmī′krän\ [MACRO- + CHYLOMICRON] A chylomicron of unusually large size.

**macrochylomicronemia** \-kī′lōmī′krənē′mē·ə\ The presence of unusually large chylomicrons in blood.

**macroclitoris** \-klit′əris\ [MACRO- + CLITORIS] Pathologic hypertrophy of the clitoris occurring in any virilizing disorder. Also *clitorimegaly, megaloclitoris.*

**macrocrania** \-krā′nē·ə\ [MACRO- + *cran(i)-* + -IA] Disproportionate enlargement of the cranium compared to the face. It is seen in hydrocephalus. Compare MACROPROSOPIA.

**macrocryoglobulinemia** \-krī′ōgläb′yəlinē′mē·ə\ CRYOGLOBULINEMIA.

**macrocytase** \-sī′tās\ A cytase or complement which destroys tissue cells or blood cells and which is formed in large mononuclear leukocytes. *Obs.*

**macrocyte** \mak′rəsīt\ A large erythrocyte, usually more than nine micrometers in diameter or 100 femtoliters in volume, observed in the peripheral blood following recent hemorrhage, in hemolytic disorders, or as a result of deficiency of vitamin $B_{12}$ or folic acid. Also *macroerythrocyte, megalocyte.*

**macrocytosis** \-sītō′sis\ A greater than normal mean corpuscular volume of erythrocytes in blood, generally greater than 100 femtoliters. It is observed whenever there is accelerated formation of erythrocytes, as in hemolytic disorders or following hemorrhage. It is also characteristic of vitamin $B_{12}$ or folate deficiency. Also *macrocythemia, megalocythemia, megalocytosis.*

**macrodactyly** \-dak′tilē\ [MACRO- + DACTYL- + -Y ] The abnormal largeness of one or more digits. Also *digital gigantism, megadactyly, dactomegaly.*

**macrodont** \makr′ədänt\ [MACR- + -ODONT] **1** Having abnormally large teeth. Also *megadontic, macrodontic.* **2** An abnormally large tooth, often bilateral. Its occurrence often follows familial or hereditary tendencies. Also *megadont, megalodont.*

**macrodystrophia** \-distrō′fē·ə\ [MACRO- + DYSTROPHIA] The disproportionate overgrowth of any part. **m. lipomatosa progressiva** An overgrowth of adipose tissue in a part or a region resulting in partial or localized gigantism of the affected part.

**macroencephaly** \-ensef′əlē\ [MACRO- + ENCEPHAL- + -Y] The condition of having an excessively large brain. Also *megaloencephaly.*

**macroerythroblast** \-irith′rəblast\ MACRONORMOBLAST.

**macroerythrocyte** \-irith′rəsīt\ MACROCYTE.

**macroesthesia** \-esthē′zhə\ [MACRO- + -ESTHESIA] A defect of tactile perception, in which objects felt or handled appear to be larger than they are. Also *macrostereognosis.*

**macroevolution** \-ev′əloo′shən\ [MACRO- + EVOLUTION] Evolution which gives rise to new species or other categories of organisms.

**macrogamete** \-gam′ēt\ The larger, or egglike, gamete produced in anisogamy. It fuses with the microgamete, leading to zygote formation. Also *megagamete.*

**macrogametocyte** \-gəmē′təsīt\ The mother cell that produces macrogametes in anisogametic reproduction. Also *macrogamont.*

**macrogenesis** \-jen′əsis\ [MACRO- + GENESIS] The excessive growth of a part.

**macrogenitosomia** \-jen′itōsō′mē·ə\ [MACRO- + GENITO- + Gk *sōm(a)* the body + -IA] Excessive and untimely somatic and genital growth and development. **m. praecox** A pathologic increase in growth and development of the body and genitals, occurring in early childhood, caused by untimely secretion of the sex steroids by the gonads or adrenal cortex. • The term is sometimes incorrectly used to denote specifically the premature somatic and genital development associated with certain tumors of the pineal body, such as those associated with the Pellizzi syndrome. **m. praecox suprarenalis** Premature somatic and genital growth and development, often occurring from infancy, in congenital adrenocortical hyperplasia with virilism in males and females.

**macroglia** \makräg′lē·ə\ [MACRO- + GLIA] The large neuroglial cells derived from neurectoderm, including astrocytes and oligodendrocytes. • The term is sometimes incorrectly used exclusively for astrocytes.

**macroglial** \-glī′əl\ Of or pertaining to macroglia.

**macroglobulin** \-gläb′yəlin\ [MACRO- + GLOBULIN] Any globulin in serum of molecular mass above about 400 kDa. One of the most important is the versatile proteinase inhibitor called $\alpha_2$-macroglobulin. **γ m.** *Obs.* IMMUNOGLOBULIN M.

**macroglobulinemia** \-gläb′yəlinē′mē·ə\ [MACROGLOBULIN + -EMIA] A greater than normal concentration in plasma of macroglobulin. **Waldenström's m.** A lymphocytic lymphoma characterized by proliferation of lymphocytes, plasma cells, and cells that resemble both lymphocytes and plasma cells ("plasmacytoid lymphocytes") in association with high serum concentration of a monoclonal macroglobulin, or IgM. Also *primary macroglobulinemia, lymphoplasmacytic lymphoma.*

**macroglossia** \-gläs′ē·ə\ [MACRO- + GLOSS- + -IA ] Diffuse enlargement of the tongue. It may be due, for example, to congenital muscular hypertrophy or lymphangioma, and occurs in certain endocrinopathies. Also *megaloglossia.*

**macrognathia** \mak′rənā′thē·ə\ [MACRO- + GNATH- + -IA ] An abnormally large jaw. Either the upper or lower jaw may be or may become abnormally large in a variety of conditions ranging from acromegaly to mandibular prognathism. Also *megagnathia.* Adj. macrognathic.

**macrogol** A spectrum of polyethylene glycols, including both liquid and solid forms. The types are designated by numbers relating to the solidity of the substance; the higher the number, the harder the preparation. They are used as ointment bases and have many industrial uses.

**macrogol 400** Polyethylene glycol with an average molecular weight of 380 to 420. It is a clear, hygroscopic, viscous liquid, used as a constituent of ointments and to stabilize emulsions.

**macrogol 4000** Polyethylene glycol with an average molecular weight between 3100 and 3700. It is a solid, creamy-white, waxlike flaky material or a white powder. It is practically insoluble in water and not absorbed at all from the intestinal tract, but it is used as a vehicle of drugs to give a sustained release and slow absorption.

**macrogyria** \-jī′rē·ə\ [MACRO- + *gyr(us)* + -IA] Enlargement of the cerebral gyri.

**macrolabia** \-lā′bē·ə\ [MACRO- + *lab(ium)* + -IA] MACROCHEILIA.

**macrolecithal** \-les′ithəl\ [MACRO- + LECITH- + -AL] MEGALECITHAL.

**macrolide** A natural lactone, whose ring is large, usually of about 14–20 atoms. Several antibiotics, including erythromycin, are macrolides. These inhibit protein biosynthesis.

**macromastia** \-mas′tē·ə\ [MACRO- + MAST- + -IA] Excessive size of the breasts, usually not due to hormonal cause. Also *megalomastia, macromazia* (rare).

**macromelia** \-mē′lyə\ [MACRO- + MEL-[1] + -IA] An excessive size of one or more limbs. Also *megalomelia.*

**macromere** \mak′rəmir\ [MACRO- + -MERE] A large blastomere, as opposed to a micromere. In the eggs of batrachians, the macromeres situated at the inferior pole are well supplied with yolk and will supply especially the entoblastic elements. In mammals, provided that cleavage results in differences between the blastomeres, there exists at a certain time four micromeres and four macromeres. These last, after they have multiplied, become indistinct and form the inner cell mass.

**macromethod** \mak′rəmeth′əd\ Any analytical technique that uses standard quantities of reagents and of the specimen to be tested.

**macromolecular** \-məlek′yələr\ Concerned with or possessing large molecules: in biology used especially of protein or nucleic acid.

**macromolecule** \-mäl′əkyool\ [MACRO- + MOLECULE] A very large molecule, such as a protein, nucleic acid, or polysaccharide molecule. **informational m.** A macromolecule which stores information for cellular structure and function, as the molecule of deoxyribonucleic acid or ribonucleic acid.

**macronodular** \-näd′yələr\ Characterized by the presence of large nodules, as in macronodular cirrhosis.

**macronormoblast** \-nôr′məblast\ A large normoblast. Also *macroerythroblast, macronormochromoblast.*

**macronucleus** \-n^y^oo′klē·əs\ [MACRO- + NUCLEUS] The larger of the two nuclei in ciliated protozoans, the smaller being the micronucleus. Macronuclei divide amitotically during fission and disappear during conjugation. They govern the metabolic functions of the vegetative cell. Also *meganucleus, nutrition nucleus, somatic nucleus, trophic nucleus, vegetative nucleus.*

**macronutrients** \-n^y^oo′trē·ənts\ [MACRO- + *nutrients,* pl. of NUTRIENT] **1** The fat, protein, and carbohydrate contents of the diet. **2** All nutrients required by the body in more than trace amounts, including the above plus the major minerals (calcium, magnesium, sodium, and potassium).

**macronychia** \-nik′ē·ə\ [MACR- + ONYCH- + -IA] A condition marked by excessive size or thickness of fingernails or toenails. Also *megalonychosis, macronychosis.*

**macroparasite** \-par′əsīt\ [MACRO- + PARASITE] A parasite visible to the naked eye, such as a tick or an intestinal worm.

**macropenis** \mak′rəpē′nis\ An excessive size or length of the penis. Also *macrophallus, megalopenis, megalophallus.*

**macrophage** \mak′rəfāj\ [MACRO- + -PHAGE] A cell found in many tissues in the body which is derived from the blood monocyte and which has an important role in host defense mechanisms. It phagocytizes and kills many bacteria and is the site of infection for a number of intracellular parasites. Also *macrophagocyte, clasmatocyte* (older term), *endothelial leukocyte, rhagiocrine cell.* **alveolar m.** A phagocytic cell found in the alveoli of the lungs. It serves to eliminate foreign particles brought into the lungs in inspired air. Also *alveolar phagocyte, dust cell.* **fixed m.** A mononuclear phagocytic cell that is resident in one of several possible tissues of the body and does not migrate to various sites in response to stimuli. Also *resting wandering cell.* **free m.** A mononuclear phagocytic cell, primarily found in the vascular system, which moves to various parts of the body, often in response to a chemotactic stimulus. **inflammatory m.** A mononuclear phagocytic cell found as one of the cellular components of inflammatory response, often as a result of bacterial invasion of the tissues. **tingible-body m.** A macrophage that has engulfed residual nuclear material from multiplying follicular center cells. The presence of tingible-body macrophages indicates follicular reactivity and distinguishes reactive follicles from the rounded cell masses of nodular lymphoma.

**macrophagocyte** \-fag′əsīt\ MACROPHAGE.

**macrophagocytosis** \-fag′əsītō′sis\ The ingestion of foreign bodies by macrophages of the reticuloendothelial system.

**macrophallus** \mak′rəfal′əs\ MACROPENIS.

**macrophthalmia** \mak′räfthal′mē·ə\ [MACR- + OPHTHALMIA] An excessive size of the eyeball. Also *megalophthalmia, megalophthalmus, megalophthalmos, megophthalmos, ophthalmacrosis.*

**macropia** \makrō′pē·ə\ MACROPSIA.

**macroplasia** \-plā′zhə\ [MACRO- + -PLASIA] Excessive growth of a tissue or organ.

**macropodia** \-pō′dē·ə\ [MACRO- + -POD + -IA] Abnormal largeness of the feet. Also *megalopodia.*

**macropolycyte** \-päl′isīt\ An abnormally large, hypersegmented polymorphonuclear leukocyte characteristic of pernicious anemia.

**macropromyelocyte** \-prōmī′ələsīt′\ An abnormally large promyelocyte, sometimes seen in pernicious anemia.

**macroprosopia** \-prōsō′pē·ə\ [MACRO- + PROSOP- + -IA] A disproportionate largeness of the face, usually relative to the cranium. Also *megaprosopia.* Compare MACROCRANIA.

**macropsia** \makräp′sē·ə\ [MACR- + -OPSIA] A visual fault which causes objects to appear magnified in size. Also *macropia, megalopia, megalopsia.*

**macroscelia** \-sē′lyə\ [MACRO- + Gk *skel(os)* the leg + -IA] An abnormal girth or length of the legs.

**macroscopic** \-skäp′ik\ Of ore relating to structures that are of sufficient size so as to be visible for study without the use of a microscope.

**macroscopy** \makräs′kəpē\ [MACRO- + -SCOPY] The study of structures by direct vision.

**macrosis** \makrō′sis\ [MACR- + -OSIS] An increase in size.

**macrosomatia** \-sōmā′shə\ [MACRO- + SOMAT- + -IA] GIGANTISM.

**macrosomia** \-sō′mē·ə\ [MACRO- + Gk *sōm(a)* body + -IA] GIGANTISM.

**macrostereognosis** \-ster′ē·ägnō′sis\ [MACRO- + STEREO- + Gk *gnōsis* knowledge] MACROESTHESIA.

**macrostomia** \-stō′mē·ə\ [MACRO- + STOM- + -IA] A rare congenital defect resulting in abnormal elongation of the mouth. The defect may be unilateral or bilateral, partial or complete. In complete cases, the oral fissure extends as far as the ear. See also GENAL CLEFT.

**macrostructural** \-struk′chərəl\ Pertaining to gross structure, as opposed to microscopic structure.

**macrotia** \makrō′shə\ [MACR- + OT- + -IA] Abnormally large external ears occurring as a rare congenital malformation.

**macrotome** \makr′ətōm\ [MACRO- + -TOME] A slicing device for cutting large tissue sections for gross anatomic study.

**macula** \mak′yələ\ [L, a spot, stain, blemish] (*pl.* maculae) **1** A small spot perceptibly different from the surrounding tissue. **2** MACULA RETINAE. **maculae acusticae** The macula sacculi and macula utriculi considered together. *Outmoded.* Also *acoustic maculae.* **m. acustica sacculi** MACULA SACCULI. **m. acustica utriculi** MACULA UTRICULI. **m. adherens** DESMOSOME. **maculae caeruleae** Blue-gray macules sometimes seen on the abdominal wall and the thighs in pthiriasis pubis. Also *blue spot.* **m. communis** The epithelial ridge on the medial wall of the otocyst from which the maculae of the saccule and utricle and the ampullary cristae differentiate in the seventh week of embryonic life. *Outmoded.* **m. corneae** A circular white scar of the cornea. **m. cribrosa inferior** [NA] The perforated area on the medial wall of the vestibule through which the branches of the vestibular division of the eighth cranial nerve pass to the posterior semicircular canal. Also *inferior macula cribosa.* **m. cribrosa media** [NA] The perforated area on the wall of the vestibule through which branches of the vestibular division of the eighth cranial nerve pass to the sacculus. Also *middle macula cribrosa.* **m. cribrosa superior** [NA] The perforated area on the wall of the vestibule through which branches of the vestibular division of the eighth cranial nerve pass to the utricle and to the anterior and lateral semicircular canals. Also *superior macula cribrosa.* **m. densa** A short section of the distal tubule of the kidney in which the nuclei are larger and more closely packed than normal. It forms part of the juxtaglomerular apparatus. **false m.** The nonfoveal portion of the retina that has a straight-ahead directional value during binocular vision by a strabismic patient with abnormal retinal correspondence. **m. flava laryngis** A yellowish, occasionally cartilaginous, nodule at the anterior end of each vocal ligament in the larynx. *Outmoded.* **m. flava retinae** *Outmoded* MACULA RETINAE. **m. folliculi** The point on the surface of an ovary at which a mature follicle ruptures and an ovum is extruded. **inferior m. cribrosa** MACULA CRIBROSA INFERIOR. **m. lutea** MACULA RETINAE. **m. lutea retinae** MACULA RETINAE. **middle m. cribrosa** MACULA CRIBROSA MEDIA. **mongolian m.** MONGOLIAN SPOT. **m. neglecta** A region of the embryonic saccule which has only a temporary existence. **m. occludens** See under TIGHT JUNCTION. **m. retinae** [NA] An oval area, with the long axis placed horizontally, near the center of the posterior part of the retina. It is below and lateral to the optic disk and is characterized by a yellow pigment in the inner layers. In its center is the fovea centralis, an area modified for acute vision. Also *macula lutea retinae, macula flava retinae* (outmoded), *macula lutea, yellow spot, punctum luteum* (outmoded), *neuroepithelium macularum, neuroepithelium of maculae, Soemmering spot.* **m. sacculi** [NA] An oval-shaped thickening of the epithelium of the anterior wall of the saccule which receives the saccular fibers of the vestibulocochlear nerve. Its plane is at right angles to that of the macula utriculi. The elongated columnar epithelium contains supporting cells and hair cells which project into the membrana statoconiorum and are concerned with equilibratory vestibular reflexes and possibly the reception of certain auditory stimuli. Also *saccular spot, macula acustica sacculi.* **m. solaris** FRECKLE. **superior m. cribrosa** MACULA CRIBROSA SUPERIOR. **m. utriculi** [NA] A thickening of the epithelium of the lateral part of the floor and adjoining lateral wall of the portion of the utricle that occupies the elliptical recess of the vestibule. It receives the utricular fibers of the vestibulocochlear nerve. Its plane is at right angles to that of the macula sacculi. The elongated columnar epithelium contains supporting cells and hair cells which project into the membrana statoconiorum and are concerned with equilibratory vestibular reflexes. Also *macula acustica utriculi.*

**maculae** \mak′yəlē\ Plural of MACULA.

**macular** \mak′yələr\ [*macul(a)* + -AR] **1** Of, characterized by, or consisting of a macule or macules. Also *maculate* (seldom used). **2** Relating to or denoting the macula retinae.

**macule** \mak′yool\ [L *macula* a spot, blemish] A small circumscribed area of discolored skin that is neither depressed nor elevated.

**maculocerebral** \mak′yəlōser′əbrəl\ Pertaining to disease affecting the macula lutea retinae and the brain. Also *cerebromacular.*

**Maddox** [Ernest Edmund *Maddox,* English ophthalmologist, 1860–1933] **1** See under PRISM. **2** Maddox rods. See under ROD.

**Madelung** [Otto Wilhelm *Madelung,* German surgeon, 1846–1926] **1** Madelung syndrome. See under DEFORMITY. **2** Madelung's disease. See under DIFFUSE SYMMETRICAL LIPOMAS OF THE NECK.

**Madlener** [Max *Madlener,* German gynecologist, 1868–1951] See under OPERATION.

**madness** *Imprecise* INSANITY. **myxedema m.** Psychosis due to hypothyroidism, usually responsive to appropriate hormone replacement therapy. Also *myxedematous madness, myxedematous dementia.*

***Madurella*** \madʸərel′ə\ A genus of fungi implicated in maduromycosis.

**maduromycosis** \mədʸoo′rōmīkō′sis\ [*Madur(a foot)* (after the city of Madura in southern India) + MYCOSIS] MYCETOMA.

**MAF** macrophage activating factor.

**mafenide** \mā′fənīd\ $C_7H_{10}N_2O_2S$. An antibacterial sulfonamide used in the topical treatment of superficial infections, burns, and wounds.

**Maffucci** [Angelo *Maffucci,* Italian physician, 1847–1903] See under SYNDROME.

**mag.** *magnus* (L, large).

**magaldrate** $Al_2H_{14}Mg_4O_{14}{\cdot}2H_2O$. Aluminum magnesium hydroxide. A compound mixture of aluminum hydroxide and magnesium hydroxide. It is used as an oral antacid medication.

**magenblase** \mä′gənblä′zə\ [German *Magen* the stomach + *Blase* bubble] The stomach bubble, seen on erect roentgenogram of the abdomen as a radiolucency in the proximal stomach above the density of fluid in the stomach.

**Magendie** [François *Magendie,* French physiologist, 1783–1855] **1** Magendie symptom, Magendie-Hertwig sign, Magendie sign, Hertwig-Magendie sign, Hertwig-Magendie syndrome, Hertwig-Magendie phenomenon. See under SKEW DEVIATION. **2** Magendie's law. See under BELL-MAGENDIE LAW. **3** Magendie space. See under CAVITAS SUBARACHNOIDEA.

**magenstrasse** \mä′gənshträ′sə\ [German (from *Magen* stomach + *Strasse* street, way) gastric canal] CANALIS GASTRICUS.

**magenta** \məjen′tə\ [named for its color suggestive of the blood spilled in the battle of *Magenta* in Italy, 1859, fought shortly before the discovery of the dye] BASIC FUCHSIN.

**maggot** \mag′ət\ [Middle English *maddock, magotte, mathek* grub, worm, maggot, akin to or from Old English *matha* maggot, worm, from the Scandinavian] The larva of a fly (order Diptera), a wormlike feeding stage. Blowfly maggots, for example, develop in carrion, flesh fly maggots, in necrotic or normal tissues of living hosts, and filth fly maggots live on excrement and decaying organic matter. **cheese m.** CHEESE SKIPPER. **rat-tail m.** The larva of a fly of the genus *Eristalis* or the genus *Helophilus,* so called because of their long filiform, flexible and extendable respiratory process. These maggots may cause accidental nasal and intestinal myiasis in domestic animals and humans. Their presence in feces may also suggest intestinal parasitism, but the feces may also have been contaminated after passage. Also *rat-tailed larva.* **surgical m.** The larva of a myiasis fly used in World War I to remove putrifying or necrotic tissue from battle wounds. The use of such maggots was discontinued after it was discovered that some normal flesh was also attacked.

**magistery** **1** An unusual remedy or prescription. **2** A chemical precipitate. An outmoded usage.

**magistral** Prepared under the guidelines of a physician's prescription: used of medicines. Compare OFFICINAL.

**magma** [L (from Gk *magma,* from *magm-,* perf. inf. root of *massein* to touch, handle, knead), a thin or soft mass or paste] **1** Finely divided material suspended in a small quantity of water. **2** A pastelike preparation of any organic substance. **m. reticularis** The primary mesenchyme present in the cavity of the blastocyst of certain primates, including man, filling the space between the trophoblast externally, the amnion and the primary yolk sac. It forms a loose reticulum of cells, the origin and fate of which has been much discussed. Later, small cavities appear in it to form the extraembryonic coelom. Also *magma reticulare.*

**Magnan** [Valentin J. J. *Magnan,* French psychiatrist, 1835–1916] **1** Magnan's trombone movement. See under TROMBONE TONGUE. **2** Magnan sign, Magnan symptom. See under FORMICATION.

**magnesemia** \mag′nəsē′mē·ə\ HYPERMAGNESEMIA.

**magnesia** MgO. The oxide of magnesium. It is a solid of low solubility in water, but it neutralizes acids to give soluble magnesium salts. **citrate of m.** MAGNESIUM CITRATE. **cream of m.** An aqueous suspension of hydrated magnesium oxide containing the equivalent of 7.45–8.35% weight for weight of magnesium hydroxide. It is used as an antacid in small doses and as a laxative in high doses. Also *magnesium hydroxide mixture.* **heavy m.** MgO. A fine, white powder of magnesium oxide that is practically insoluble in water. It is used in powders and tablets as an antacid and mild laxative. **milk of m.** A suspension of 7–8.5% weight for weight of magnesium hydroxide. It may also contain 0.1% citric acid and up to 0.05% of one or more essential oils as flavoring agents. Also *magnesia magma.*

**magnesium** \magnē′zē·əm\ Element number 12, having atomic weight 24.312. There are three stable natural isotopes. Five radioactive isotopes have been identified, the longest lived being magnesium 28 with a half-life of 21 hours. Magnesium is the eighth most abundant element in the lithosphere. It is a silvery white metal, never found naturally in the free state. The valence is 2. The magnesium ion is one of the principal cations governing the electrochemical properties of living systems. Magnesium is a constituent of the chlorophyll molecule, and it is required for the activity of many enzymes. Symbol: Mg

**magnesium carbonate** $Mg(OH)_2{\cdot}3MgCO_3{\cdot}XH_2O$ ($X$=3 or 4). A white, almost tasteless powder used as an antacid and laxative, often with other ingredients.

**magnesium chloride** $MgCl_2{\cdot}6H_2O$. Colorless flakes or a crystalline salt. It is used to replace electrolytes lost in peritoneal dialysis and blood dialysis.

**magnesium citrate** $C_{12}H_{10}Mg_3O_{14}$. A white, odorless, crystalline powder, used in solution as a mild cathartic. Also *citrate of magnesia.* **effervescent m.** A powder containing a mixture of magnesium carbonate, citric acid, sodium bicarbonate, and sugar. It is used as a laxative.

**magnesium hydroxide** $Mg(OH)_2$. A white, amorphous, odorless, and tasteless powder almost insoluble in water. It is used as an antacid in the treatment of peptic ulcers, and it has mild laxative properties. It is used in tablets alone or in combination with other antacids, or as an aqueous suspension.

**magnesium peroxide** $MgO_2$. A white, tasteless powder, practically insoluble in water. It gradually decomposes, releasing oxygen. It is utilized medically as an antacid and anti-infective agent.

**magnesium phosphate** TRIBASIC MAGNESIUM PHOSPHATE. **tribasic m.** $Mg_3(PO_4)_2 \cdot 5H_2O$. A white, odorless, tasteless powder, practically insoluble in water. It is an antacid and mild laxative, much like magnesium trisilicate, which has largely replaced it. Also *magnesium phosphate, trimagnesium phosphate.*

**magnesium stearate** Magnesium compounded with stearic acid and palmitic acid in various proportions. It is insoluble in water and employed as a tablet lubricant in pharmaceutical preparations and dusting powders.

**magnesium sulfate** $MgSO_4 \cdot 7H_2O$. The heptahydrate, colorless crystals have been employed as an anticonvulsant agent, but its main medical uses are as a cathartic and as a local anti-inflammatory treatment. Also *Epsom salts.* **effervescent m.** A powder mixture of magnesium sulfate, sodium bicarbonate, tartaric acid, and citric acid, used as a laxative. **exsiccated m.** Hydrated magnesium sulfate that has been dried at 100°C to reduce the weight by 25%. It is used as a paste for boils.

**magnesium trisilicate** A combination in various proportions of magnesium oxide, silicon dioxide, and water. It is used as a pharmaceutical aid and as an antacid.

**magnetocardiograph** \mag′nətōkär′dē·əgraf′\ An instrument for recording the magnetic field of the heart, produced by the same ionic currents that generate the electrocardiogram.

**magnetoencephalograph** \mag′nətō·ensef′əlōgraf′\ An instrument for recording the magnetic field of the brain, produced by the same ionic currents that generate the electroencephalogram.

**magnicellular** \mag′nisel′yələr\ Composed of large cells. Also *magnocellular.*

**magnification** \mag′nifikā′shən\ Apparent increase of the image size of an object examined with a light or electron microscope. **biologic m.** BIOACCUMULATION.

**magnify** To increase the apparent image size of.

**magnocellular** \mag′nəsel′yələr\ MAGNICELLULAR.

**Magnus** [Rudolf *Magnus,* German physiologist, 1873–1927] Magnus and de Kleijn neck reflex. See under REFLEX.

**Maier** [Rudolf Robert *Maier,* German physician, 1824–1888] 1 Kussmaul-Maier disease. See under POLYARTERITIS NODOSA. 2 See under SINUS.

**maim** \mām\ [Middle English *maymen,* from Old French *mahaigner* to disable] To seriously wound, injure, disfigure, dismember, or disable.

**main** \maN\ [French, the hand] Hand.

**maintainer** / **space m.** SPACE RETAINER.

**maintenance** 1 The act or process of maintaining. 2 Designed to maintain stable function or condition, as distinguished from remedial or prophylactic effect, as in *a maintenance dose of methadone, a maintenance ration to a laboratory animal.* **space m.** The provision of an appliance in orthodontics or pedodontics, where a tooth is missing or unerupted, to prevent the movement of adjacent teeth into the space.

**Maissiat** [Jacques Henri *Maissiat,* French anatomist, 1805–1878] Iliotibial ligament of Maissiat, ligament of Maissiat, Maissiat's band, Maissiat's tract. See under TRACTUS ILIOTIBIALIS.

**maize** \māz\ [Spanish *maíz,* from Taino (West Indies) *mahiz* Indian corn] A cereal grass of the species *Zea mays,* widely used in human diets. Maize, or corn, oil, which is refined from the embryo of *Zea mays,* is used a solvent for injections and in the preparation of food. Also *corn, Indian corn.* Adj. zeistic.

**Majocchi** [Domenico *Majocchi,* Italian dermatologist, 1849–1929] Majocchi's disease. See under PURPURA ANNULARIS TELANGIECTODES.

**majority** The age at which a person becomes legally entitled to the full civil rights of an adult. The age varies by jurisdiction. In the United States, the age of 21 is most commonly used. • In Canada and India, the age of majority is 21. In Japan, it is 20 (although the term *majority* is not used), and there is a national day to celebrate it, January 15. The age of majority is 18 in the United Kingdom, South Africa, Australia, and New Zealand.

**Makeham** [William Matthew *Makeham,* English statistician, died 1892] See under HYPOTHESIS.

**makeshift** Denoting a shunt constructed from a large variceal collateral vessel to a systemic vein when a standard shunt cannot be employed. It is used in operations for portal hypertension.

**Makkas** [M. *Makkas,* German surgeon, flourished 20th century] See under OPERATION.

**makro-** \mak′rō-, mak′rə-\ MACRO-.

**mal** \mal\ [French and Spanish (from L *malum* an evil, harm) an evil, pain, ache, illness] 1 Disease; illness. 2 Pain. **m. comitial** MAJOR EPILEPSY. **m. de Cayenne** FILARIAL ELEPHANTIASIS. **m. de los pintos** PINTA. **m. del pinto** PINTA. **grand m.** MAJOR EPILEPSY. • This term was once used to identify any convulsive epileptic attack with major manifestations, as opposed to petit mal. **haut m.** MAJOR EPILEPSY. **m. morado** ONCHOCERCIASIS. **m. perforant** PERFORATING ULCER OF THE FOOT. **petit m.** See under PETIT MAL. **m. rouge** A condition brought about by the ingestion of any substance which blocks the enzyme system responsible for conversion of ethanol to carbon dioxide and water, thus allowing the accumulation of acetaldehyde. Symptoms are nausea, vomiting, headache, flushing, palpitation, and marked fall in blood pressure.

**mal-** \mal-\ [Old French, from L *male* badly, poorly, adv. from *malus* bad] A combining form meaning (1) bad, badly; (2) abnormally, defectively.

**mala** \mā′lə\ [L, cheekbone, jawbone, cheek, jaw] 1 BUCCA. 2 OS ZYGOMATICUM.

**malabsorption** \mal′absôrp′shən\ [MAL- + ABSORPTION] Impaired or incomplete absorption of nutrients by the intestine. **lactose m.** A reduced capacity to absorb lactose arising as a result of lactase deficiency. This is the most frequently reported isolated enzyme deficiency in both children and adults, but is more common in adults. It is believed to be an inherited enzyme deficiency, but it can also be acquired secondary to diseases that result in mucosal damage. It does not seem to be induced in man through abstinence from milk. Estimates of lactase deficiency in North America range from 16–55% with the higher level found in blacks. In children under 11 years, 10% of Caucasians suffer and 35% of blacks. The frequency in children gradually increases with age due to a gradual decline in lactase activity. The majority of adults in the world have lower lactase activity than do children. Unhydrolyzed lactose is not absorbed, and remains in the gut lumen where it exerts a hyperosmolar effect. Large volumes of water are pulled into the gut lumen causing abdominal distension and discomfort. The flora of the lower bowel and colon metabolize the lactose to produce lactic, butyric, and other acids, causing cramps and diarrhea. A flat glucose curve is obtained in lactose intolerance when a 100 g load of lactose is ingested. However, the same patient when given equimolar amounts of glucose or galactose will show a rise of 20 mg of glucose per 100 ml of serum. Treatment involves the exclusion of lactose from the diet.

**malacia** \mәlā′shә\ [Gk *malakia* (from *malakos* soft) softness] The pathologic softening of any tissue. Often used in combination to designate specific conditions, such as osteomalacia. **m. cordis** Morbid softening of the heart. **metaplastic m.** OSTEITIS FIBROSA CYSTICA.

**malacic** \mәlā′sik\ Characterized by softening.

**malaco-** \mal′әkō-\ [Gk *malakos* soft, gentle] A combining form meaning soft, softness.

**malacosteon** \mal′әkäs′tē·än\ OSTEOMALACIA.

**malacotic** \mal′әkät′ik\ [MALACO- + *t* + -IC] Softer than normal: said of teeth.

**malacotomy** \mal′әkät′әmē\ [MALACO- + -TOMY] A surgical incision into soft tissue, such as the anterior abdominal wall.

**malactic** EMOLLIENT.

**maladie** \maladē′\ [French, a disease, illness. See MALADY.] Disease. **m. de Roger** ROGER'S DISEASE. **m. des tics** GILLES DE LA TOURETTE SYNDROME.

**malady** \mal′әdē\ [Old French *maladie* (from *malade* ill, sick, from L *male habitus* "keeping poorly," from *male* poorly + past part. of *habere* to have) illness] A disease; illness.

**malagma** \mәlag′mә\ [Gk *malagma*, a plaster, emollient, poultice] An emollient or medicated poultice.

**malaise** \malāz′\ [French (from *mal* bad + *aise* ease, comfort, from L *adjacens*, pres. part. of *adjacere* to lie near) discomfort, uneasiness] A feeling of untoward weakness, lethargy, or discomfort, as of impending illness.

**malakoplakia** \mal′әkōplā′kē·ә\ [Gk *malako(s)* soft + *plax*, gen. *plak(os)* flat object + -IA ] A form of chronic inflammation principally involving the urinary bladder and characterized by soft, pale or yellow plaques on its mucosa. The plaques are composed of macrophages and lymphocytes and an occasional multinucleated giant cell. Mineralized, laminated concretions (Michaelis-Gutmann bodies) and altered bacteria may be present within the macrophages. A localized defect in macrophage function or an abnormal response to coliform bacteria is believed to be the cause.

**malalignment** \-әlīn′mәnt\ **1** The healing of a fractured jaw with the parts incorrectly aligned. **2** The state of having a tooth or teeth not in the normal position in the dental arch.

**malar** \mā′lәr\ [L *mala* cheek] **1** Pertaining to the cheek. **2** Of or relating to the zygomatic bone.

**malaria** \mәler′ē·ә\ [Italian (from *mal(a)* bad + *aria* air) lit., bad air; the disease was attributed to noxious atmospheric emanations from marshy ground] A febrile disease caused by infection with haemosporidian protozoa of the genus *Plasmodium* transmitted by the bites of infected female mosquitoes of the genus *Anopheles*. The four species in human malaria are *P. falciparum* (malignant tertian, subtertian), *P. vivax* (tertian), *P. ovale* (tertian), and *P. malariae* (quartan). The disease accounts for very great morbidity and mortality in tropical countries. Children are particularly vulnerable. The parasite is inoculated into the human host as a sporozoite and undergoes an asymptomatic exoerythrocytic developmental cycle in the liver before large numbers of merozoites invade red blood cells, establishing the erythrocytic cycle which produces the characteristic symptoms of disease, including chills followed by rapid onset of high fever and sweating at regular intervals, varying with the species of parasite. Hemolytic anemia, jaundice, and splenomegaly may result. Severe cases of *P. falciparum* infection may be complicated by renal failure and cerebral involvement. Gametocytes produced during the erythrocytic cycle are ingested by mosquitoes with the blood meal, initiating the sexual developmental cycle. The sporozoites ultimately produced by nuclear division in the oocyst accumulate in the salivary glands of the mosquito, and are ready to infect a new host when the mosquito feeds, usually within 8–21 days. Diagnosis is made by demonstration of malaria parasites in blood films. Serodiagnosis is also of value. Although chloroquine has been the drug of choice in prophylaxis and treatment, malaria parasites in some regions have become resistant to this drug and others, and therapy of the disease has become complex. Also *fever and ague* (obs.), *marsh fever, malarial fever, paludal fever, paludism.* **acute m.** Malaria characterized by intermittent, remittent, or irregular but frequent paroxysms of chills, fever, and sweating, caused by the synchronous release of merozoites from red blood cells. The frequency of acute symptoms varies with the species of parasite. *Plasmodium falciparum* is responsible for the most severe disease, which if accompanied by renal and cerebral complications often leads to death. The acute disease is especially serious in children and during pregnancy. Rapid diagnosis and urgent treatment are vital if mortality is to be avoided. Compare CHRONIC MALARIA. **algid m.** *Plasmodium falciparum* malaria with shock, cold skin, prostration, and visceral involvement, especially of the vessels of the gastrointestinal tract. **autochthonous m.** Endemic malaria acquired from sporozoites transmitted by local mosquitoes. Imported malarial organisms, passed to endemic mosquitoes in a new region, become a cause of autochthonous malaria when the parasites are transmitted within the newly invaded population. **benign subtertian m.** A form of vivax malaria in which the 48-hour pattern of chills, fever, and sweats is irregular or modified. **benign tertian m.** VIVAX MALARIA. **cerebral m.** A serious complication of *Plasmodium falciparum* infection, usually occurring in nonimmune subjects, frequently children. It is characterized by headache, irritability, hyperpyrexia, convulsions, and coma. Electroencephalographic abnormalities are also present. There is gross congestion with stasis in cerebral blood vessels as well as numerous petechial hemorrhages and intravascular coagulation. Although there is often a heavy parasitemia in the peripheral blood, that is not always the case. Even with adequate treatment, the condition carries a significant death rate. Also *plasmodial meningitis.* **chronic m.** Prolonged human infection with malaria parasites, *Plasmodium vivax, P. ovale,* and especially *P. malariae*. Serum globulin and IgG component are usually raised and malaria serology is usually positive. Chronic anemia and splenomegaly are usual, and there may be severe constitutional abnormaiities. Chronic renal involvement (nephrotic syndrome) has been associated especially with *P. malariae* infections. An immune-complex basis seems likely, and treatment is unsatisfactory. Massive splenomegaly occasionally results from an aberrant immune mechanism, especially in tropical Africa and Papua New Guinea (tropical splenomegaly syndrome). Serum IgM concentration is high and hepatic sinusoidal lymphocytosis common. There is some evidence that chronic malaria increases the potential of the Epstein-Barr virus to cause Burkitt's lymphoma and to produce high $HB_sAg$ carrier rates. Compare ACUTE MALARIA. **double tertian m.** QUOTIDIAN MALARIA. **dysenteric m.** Falciparum malaria marked by bloody diarrhea. **estivoautumnal m.** Falciparum malaria with a summer-autumn onset, linked to the behavior of the *Anopheles* vectors. It was formerly endemic in parts of the United States. Also *estivoautumnal fever.* **falciparum m.** A form of malaria caused by *Plasmodium falciparum,* often characterized by paroxysms of fever occurring at 48-hour intervals and in severe cases sometimes by acute cerebral or renal manifestations attributable to the large number of red blood cells involved and by the tendency of infected cells to clump together or to adhere to the endothelial lining of blood vessels, resulting in blocked capillaries. The incubation period is 10–14 days but may be longer. Pyrexia of 40°C or more, hepatospenomegaly, tachycardia, hypotension, pallor, and sometimes hemolytic jaundice occur, especially in those with a high parasitemia. If untreated, mortality rates are high. Special clinical forms are called cerebral, algid, gastric, hemorrhagic, dysenteric, and comatose malaria, blackwater fever, and other descriptive terms. Also *malignant tertian malaria, malignant tertian fever, subtertian malaria.* **gastric m.** Falciparum malaria marked by continual vomiting. **hemolytic m.** BLACKWATER FEVER. **induced m.** MALARIOTHERAPY. **intermittent m.** Malaria in which there is a complete absence of fever and other symptoms in intervals between paroxysms, usually seen in the tertian (vivax) or quartan (malariae) types. **latent m.** Malarial infection in which there is a balance between the parasite and the body's defense mechanisms, so that no symptoms of the disease are produced. **malariae m.** A form of malaria in which febrile paroxysms recur every 72 hours, caused by the release of merozoites of the parasite *Plasmodium malariae.* Also *quartan malaria, quartan fever.* **malignant tertian m.** FALCIPARUM MALARIA. **nonan m.** A form of malaria in which febrile paroxysms occur every ninth day. **ovale m.** A usually mild form of malaria caused by *Plasmodium ovale* which causes a benign tertian type of disease. Infection in conjunction with *P. falciparum* is not uncommon. Most cases occur in tropical Africa. latent periods of up to four years after infection have been documented. Relapses tend to occur after intervals of about three months. Treatment is with chloroquine and primaquine. Also *ovale tertian malaria, tertian malaria.* **pernicious m.** Falciparum malaria characterized by severe symptoms accompanied by cerebral, hemorrhagic, or gastroenteric complications. **quartan m.** MALARIAE MALARIA. **quintan m.** A form of malaria in which febrile paroxysms recur every fifth day. **quotidian m.** A form of malaria characterized by daily febrile paroxysms. It is commonly due to simultaneous infection with two distinct groups of *Plasmodium vivax* parasites, but possibly with two species (e.g., *P. falciparum* and *P. vivax*), or with two forms of *P. falciparum.* Also *double tertian malaria.* **recrudescent m.** A form of malarial resurgence, usually in disease caused by *Plasmodium malariae,* in which a latent or repressed erythrocytic infection begins to multiply rapidly and induces a clinical infection. This form of quartan malarial resurgence can continue for a long period, 30 years or more. In contrast, the shorter-lived relapsing malaria from *P. vivax* or *P. ovale* originates in the liver and rarely occurs more than five years after the initial mosquito-borne infection. **relapsing m.** Malaria characterized by the resurgence of clinical symptoms from a latent or delayed hepatic infection at an interval following the primary attack, usually within five years. The causative agent is usually *Plasmodium vivax* or *P. ovale.* **remittent m.** Malaria, usually of the falciparum type, in which the elevated body temperature falls somewhat but does not drop to normal in the interval between febrile attacks. **subtertian m.** FALCIPARUM MALARIA. **tertian m.** 1 VIVAX MALARIA. 2 OVALE MALARIA. **therapeutic m.** MALARIOTHERAPY. **vivax m.** A form of malaria in which paroxysms recur every 48 hours due to the release of merozoites from red blood cells infected by the parasite *Plasmodium vivax.* It is the most common and widespread form of human malaria, although it has been largely eradicated from temperate zone areas. It does not occur in most of tropical west Africa, being replaced there by ovale malaria. Also *benign tertian malaria, tertian malaria.*

**malarial** \məler′ē·əl\ Of or pertaining to malaria.

**malaricidal** \məler′isī′dəl\ [*malari(a)* + *-cid(e)* + -AL] Destructive to malarial parasites. Also *malariacidal.*

**malariology** \məler′ē·äl′əjē\ [*malari(a)* + *o* + -LOGY] The systematic study of malaria.

**malariotherapy** \məler′ē·əther′əpē\ Malaria produced through human agency, usually by inoculation with infective material, formerly a treatment for neurosyphilis and certain other conditions. Also *therapeutic malaria, induced malaria, malarial therapy, malarization therapy.*

**malarious** \məler′ē·əs\ Affected by or marked by the presence of malaria.

**malarticulation** \-ärtik′yəlā′shən\ Impaired speech articulation.

**Malassez** [Louis Charles *Malassez,* French physiologist, 1842–1909] Debris of Malassez, rests of Malassez. See under REST.

***Malassezia*** \mal′əsē′zē·ə\ [after Louis Charles *Malassez,* French physiologist, 1842–1910 + -IA] A form-genus of lipophilic yeasts of the normal skin flora. Also *Pityrosporum.* ***M. furfur*** The form-species of fungus that causes pityriasis versicolor. ***M. ovale*** A form-species that is characteristically thick-walled and ovoid in form and that buds from a broad base. In man it is found especially on the scalp, face, and upper trunk. It may be identical to *M. furfur.*

**malate dehydrogenase** Any of several enzymes that catalyze the dehydrogenation of malate with the concomitant reduction of $NAD^+$ or $NADP^+$. The most important (EC 1.1.1.37) is one that forms oxaloacetate in a step that is part of the citric acid cycle. Some enzymes of the group, designated "oxaloacetate decarboxylating," form pyruvate and carbon dioxide in place of oxaloacetate.

**malate dehydrogenase (oxaloacetate decarboxylating)** An enzyme that catalyzes the reaction of malate and $NADP^+$ to yield pyruvate, carbon dioxide, NADPH, and $H^+$. It is important in the supply of NADPH for fat synthesis, as well as in the cycle that allows acetyl groups to be exported from mitochondria as citrate for this purpose. Also *malic enzyme.*

**malathion** \malā′thē·än, mal′əthī′än\ $C_{10}H_{19}O_6PS_2$. An organophosphate compound used to control a wide variety of insects, including aphids, spider mites, scale insects, houseflies, and mosquitoes, by inhibiting cholinesterase, thus interfering with nerve conduction.

**malaxate** To compound into a single mass; to mix up a medicinal preparation, as in the production of pharmaceuticals.

**malaxation** [Gk *malax(is)* a softening + -ATION] The act of working a mixture into a single mass; the process of mixing.

**maldevelopment** \-divel′əpmənt\ [MAL- + DEVELOPMENT] TERATISM.

**maldigestion** \-dijes′chən\ The impaired digestion of nutrients in the gastrointestinal tract.

**male** [Old French, from earlier *masle,* from L *masculus* (dim. of *mas* the male of humans, animals, and plants) male, masculine] 1 Of or belonging to the sex that in animals produces spermatozoa and begets young. 2 An individual of the male sex, as a man. **genetic m.** 1 A human possessing a normal male karyotype, 46,XY. 2 In any species, an individual possessing the karyotype that is usually present in the male.

**maleic hydrazide** 1,2-dihydro-3,6-pyridazine dione. Maleic acid hydrazide. A compound resulting from the reaction of maleic anhydride with hydrazine hydrate in alcohol.

The compound is believed to selectively damage mitochondria in the cell. It also inhibits plant growth.

**maleruption** \-irup′shən\ The eruption of a tooth into a position of malalignment.

**malethamer** A polymer of maleic anhydride and ethylene, crosslinked with one or two percent vinyl crotonate. It is an antiperistalic agent.

**maleylacetoacetate isomerase** The enzyme (EC 5.2.1.2) that catalyzes the interconversion of the *cis* and *trans* isomers of HOOC—CH═CH—CO—$CH_2$—CO—$CH_2$—COOH, a reaction in the pathway of breakdown of phenylalanine and tyrosine in mammals and other organisms.

**malformation** \-fôrmā′shən\ [MAL- + FORMATION] **1** Any product of abnormal development, particularly a structural defect. **2** MALFORMATION SEQUENCE. **3** TERATISM. **arteriovenous m.** A congenital failure of development of capillaries, resulting in a localized congeries of arteries and veins, the latter containing arterial blood. Also *vascular malformation.* **Ebstein's m.** EBSTEIN'S ANOMALY. **Ebstein-like m. of the mitral valve** A lesion of the morphologically mitral valve in which the annular attachment of the mural (posterior) leaflet is displaced into the left ventricular cavity. **Klippel-Feil m.** The dominant feature of the Klippel-Feil syndrome in which malformation of the cervical spine results in a short, webbed neck. **major m.** A life-threatening malformation or one likely to cause significant impairment of health, longevity, or functional capacity. Malformations causing clinical disease or significant cosmetic problems are usually included. *Imprecise.* **minor m.** A malformation not likely to cause clinical disease or significant cosmetic problem. *Imprecise.* **Mondini m.** An abnormality of the cochlea present in a small proportion of congenitally deaf children. Only the first one and a half turns of the cochlea are normal, the remainder showing severe hypoplasia. **Taussig-Bing m.** A congenital malformation characterized by the aorta arising from the morphologically right ventricle and the pulmonary trunk overriding an anterior interventricular communication. The ventriculoarterial connection is usually double-outlet right ventricle but may be discordant (complete transposition). Also *Taussig-Bing disease, Taussig-Bing syndrome.* **vascular m.** ARTERIOVENOUS MALFORMATION.

**malfunction** \-fungk′shən\ Disordered or impaired function. **eustachian tube m.** Failure of the eustachian tube to maintain normal middle-ear ventilation. This tends to produce middle-ear effusion and atelectasis.

**Malgaigne** [Joseph François *Malgaigne*, French surgeon, 1806–1865] **1** Malgaigne's triangle. See under TRIGONUM CAROTICUM. **2** See under LUXATION.

**Malherbe** [Albert *Malherbe*, French surgeon, 1845–1915] Malherbe's epithelioma, Malherbe's tumor. See under PILOMATRIXOMA.

**malic acid** HOOC—$CH_2$—CHOH—COOH. The *S*-isomer of this compound, known as L-malic acid, is an intermediate in the citric acid cycle, being formed by hydration of fumarate, and being converted into oxaloacetate by malate dehydrogenase. It also has other metabolic roles, especially in plants.

**malignancy** \məlig′nənsē\ The state of being malignant.

**malignant** \məlig′nənt\ [Late L *malignans*, gen. *malignantis*, pres. part. of *malignare* (from L *malignus* wicked, malicious) to act wickedly or with malice] Tending to destroy, harm, or kill, particularly the last, as *malignant tumor, malignant hypertension.*

**malingering** \məling′gəring\ [*malinger*, from French *malingre* (from *mal* bad + Old French *haingre, heingre* thin, haggard) sickly + -ING] Simulation of illness or injury with conscious intent to deceive. Also *pathomimesis, pathomimia, pathomimicry.*

**Mall** [Franklin P. *Mall*, U.S. anatomist, 1862–1917] Periportal space of Mall. See under SPACE.

**malleal** \mal′ē·əl\ Pertaining to the malleus. Also *mallear.*

**malleiform** \malē′ifôrm\ Hammer-shaped.

**malleoidosis** \mal′ē·oidō′sis\ MELIOIDOSIS.

**malleoincudal** \mal′ē·ō·ing′kyədəl\ Of the malleus and incus. Also *incudomalleal.*

**malleolus** \malē′ōləs\ [L (dim. of *malleus* a hammer, mallet), a little hammer] (*pl.* malleoli) A rounded bony projection, as on either side of the ankle joint. Adj. malleolar. **m. lateralis** [NA] The triangular, projecting lower end of the fibula. It presents four surfaces, the lateral being subcutaneous and the medial having an articular facet for the talus in the ankle joint. Its apex reaches a lower level than that of the medial malleolus. Also *lateral malleolus, lateral malleolus of fibula.* **m. medialis** [NA] The short, expanded medial part of the lower end of the tibia that projects medially and downwards. Its lateral surface articulates with the medial aspect of the talus in the ankle joint, the medial surface is subcutaneous, while the posterior surface is grooved by the tendon of the tibialis posterior muscle. Also *medial malleolus, medial malleolus of tibia.*

***Malleomyces*** \mal′ē·ōmī′sēz\ [L *malleus* glanders + Gk *mykēs* a mushroom, fungus] *PSEUDOMONAS.* ***M. whitmori*** *PSEUDOMONAS PSEUDOMALLEI.*

**malleus** \mal′ē·əs\ [L, a hammer, mallet] (*pl.* mallei) [NA] The largest of the auditory ossicles in the tympanic cavity resembling a club and consisting of a head, or caput; neck, or collum; handle, or manubrium; and two processes, anterior and lateral. It is attached to the tympanic membrane, and its head articulates posteriorly with the incus. Also *hammer, plectrum* (outmoded).

**Mallory** [Frank Burr *Mallory*, U.S. pathologist, 1862–1941] **1** Mallory's acid fuchsin. See under MALLORY'S TRIPLE STAIN. **2** Mallory's phosphotungstic acid hematoxylin stain. See under STAIN. **3** Mallory's bodies. See under BODY.

**Mallory** [George Kenneth *Mallory*, U.S. pathologist, born 1900] Mallory-Weiss syndrome. See under SYNDROME.

**malnutrition** \-n^y^ootrish′ən\ [MAL- + NUTRITION] Any disorder resulting from a deficiency or an excess of one or more essential nutrients. This may arise as a result of an unbalanced diet or an inability to absorb or metabolize any nutrient. **malignant m.** KWASHIORKOR. **protein m.** KWASHIORKOR. **protein-calorie m.** Malnutrition resulting from an inadequate intake of sources of energy and/or protein which usually occurs in children under five years who are consuming a diet insufficient in these substances. People of any age may suffer from this disorder but in adults it is less common and the clinical symptoms less severe, because after growth ceases, the protein and energy needs are diminished. The spectrum of clinical manifestations range from marasmus, due to a chronic restriction of all nutrients, to kwashiorkor, due to a deficiency of protein without an accompanying inadequate intake of energy sources. Between these two extremes are a host of forms in which the clinical features are due to a combination of protein and energy deficiencies as well as deficiencies of vitamins and minerals and related infections. Also *nutritional marasmus.*

**malocclusion** \-əkloo′zhən\ [MAL- + OCCLUSION] Any deviation from normal occlusion. Also *patho-occlusion, odontoparallaxis.*

**malomaxillary** \mā′lōmak′siler′ē\ Of the malar bone and maxilla.

**malonal** BARBITAL.
**malonic acid** HOOC—$CH_2$—COOH. Propanedioic acid. It competitively inhibits the oxidation of succinate to fumarate by succinate dehydrogenase.
**malonyl** The univalent 2-carboxyacetyl group, HOOC—$CH_2$—CO—. • In strict chemical nomenclature this is the bivalent acyl group formed from malonic acid, namely —CO—$CH_2$—CO—.
**malonyl-ACP** The thiol ester of malonic acid with acyl carrier protein, an intermediate in the biosynthesis of fatty acids in bacteria.
**malonyl-coenzyme A** The thiol ester of malonic acid with coenzyme A, it is formed from acetyl-CoA by carboxylation in a reaction catalyzed by a biotinyl enzyme that hydrolyzes ATP and uses carbon dioxide. This is a step in the biosynthesis of fatty acids. The malonyl group is transferred onto the synthetic enzyme before condensation with another thiol ester group and release of carbon dioxide in the chain-lengthening step.
**malonylurea** BARBITURIC ACID. • This name is sometimes used because it is urea acylated on its nitrogen atoms with the two carboxyl groups of malonic acid.
**Malpighi** [Marcello *Malpighi,* Italian anatomist and physiologist, 1628–1694] **1** Malpighian tubes. See under MALPIGHIAN TUBULES. **2** Pyramid of Malpighi. See under RENAL PYRAMID. **3** Malpighi's vesicles. See under ALVEOLI PULMONIS.
**malposition** \-pəzish′ən\ An abnormal position, as of teeth.
**malpractice** \-prak′tis\ [MAL- + PRACTICE] Misconduct on the part of a professional practitioner while rendering a professional service, which results in injury or loss to the recipient of the service. See also NEGLIGENCE. **medical m.** Negligent conduct on the part of a medical practitioner or health facility resulting in injury, loss, or damage to a patient. All of the following elements must be established to prove medical malpractice: a voluntary professional relationship must exist between the two parties, thereby obligating the physician or other provider of care to a duty of care to the patient; the provider of care must breach that duty of care by virtue of negligence; and the negligent act must be the proximate cause of the injury or loss sustained by the patient. In addition, the injury of loss must be compensable in monetary terms.
**malpresentation** \-pres′əntā′shən\ [MAL- + PRESENTATION] An abnormal lie of the fetus during or preceding labor: commonly used in reference to all presentations other than the vertex presentation.
**malrotation** \-rōtā′shən\ A developmental failure of rotation in the normal direction or to the normal degree. Such failure is seen mostly in the digestive tract, but sometimes in other structures that undergo a degree of rotation during embryogenesis, such as the heart, kidneys, and limbs.
**Malthus** [Thomas Robert *Malthus,* English economist and demographer, 1766–1834] Malthusian theory. See under MALTHUSIANISM.
**malthusianism** \malthoo′zē·ənizm\ [after Thomas Robert *Malthus,* English economist and demographer, 1766–1834 + *-ian,* adjectival suffix + -ISM] **1** Originally a social doctrine based on the theory that population increases by geometric progression while food production increases arithmetically, and leading to the conclusion that the number of births must be restricted by sexual continence or other means. Contrary to a widely held view, the theory is not based on any scientific analysis, but flows from *a priori* speculations. Also *malthusian theory.* **2** NEOMALTHUSIANISM.

**maltose** The disaccharide of glucose containing an $\alpha$1-4 linkage. It is a hydrolysis product of starch and glycogen.
**malum** \mal′əm\ [L, an evil, harm, disease] A disease. **m. coxae** Arthritis of the hip, usually osteoarthritis.
**malunion** \-yoo′nyən\ Union of a fracture in an abnormal position.
**malvaria** \malvar′ē·ə\ [L *malva* mallow + *r* + -IA] The presumed disorder of subjects whose urine showed a mauve factor when analyzed chromatographically.
**mamanpian** \məmän′pē·än′\ [French *maman* mother + *pian* yaw. See PIAN.] MOTHER YAW.
**mamba** \mam′bə\ [Zulu *imamba* mamba] Any venomous snake of the genus *Dendraspis* of the Elapidae family.
**mamelon** \mam′əlän\ [French (dim. of *mamelle* woman's breast, from L *mamilla* a breast, teat), nipple, any round protuberance] A small tubercle on the incisal edge of an unworn incisor tooth.
**mamelonated** \mam′ələnā′tid\ *Outmoded* MAMILLATED.
**mamilla** \məmil′ə\ [L (dim. of *mamma* breast), breast, teat, nipple] (*pl.* mamillae) **1** PAPILLA MAMMARIA. **2** Any nipplelike structure. Also *mammilla.*
**mamillary** \mam′iler′ē\ Pertaining to or resembling a nipple. Also *mammillary.*
**mamillated** \mam′ilā′tid\ Covered with nipplelike protuberances. Also *mammillated, mamelonated* (outmoded), *mammillate.*
**mamillation** \mam′ilā′shən\ **1** A mamilliform protuberance. **2** The state of possessing nipples. For defs. 1 and 2 also *mammillation.*
**mamilliform** \məmil′ifôrm\ Nipple-shaped. Also *mammilliform, mamilloid.*
**mamilliplasty** \məmil′iplas′tē\ [*mamill(a)* + *i* + -PLASTY] THELEPLASTY.
**mamillitis** \mam′ilī′tis\ [*mamill(a)* + -ITIS] Inflammation of the nipple or teat. Also *mammillitis, thelitis.*
**mamillopeduncular** \məmil′ōpidungk′yələr\ Denoting the peduncles entering and exiting the mamillary bodies of the hypothalamus. These include the mamillary peduncle bringing afferent fibers from the reticular formation, and the mamillothalamic tract carrying efferents to the anterior mamillary nuclear complex.
**mamma** \mam′ə\ [L, the breast, a female breast, teat] (*pl.* mammae) [NA] One of a pair of rounded subcutaneous protuberances on each side of the front of the chest. They are functional and developed in the female and rudimentary in the male, extending from the second to the sixth ribs vertically and from the side of the sternum to the midaxillary line horizontally. Protruding from approximately the center is the nipple, on which open 15–20 lactiferous ducts from the mammary gland proper; surrounding the nipple is the areola. The glandular portion comprises lobes, made up of lobules and acini, between and around which are connective tissue, blood vessels, lymphatics, nerves, and fat, which gives the organ its rounded contour. In the female it undergoes considerable development after puberty and during pregnancy, secreting milk during lactation after parturition. It alters in shape and size with aging. Also *breast.* **accessory mammae** SUPERNUMERARY MAMMAE. **m. areolata** An unusual degree of protuberance of the areola of the breast. **m. erratica** Supernumerary mammae present at locations other than those corresponding to the embryonic milk line. **m. masculina** [NA] A mamma in a male, usually rudimentary throughout life and comprising only ducts that are usually solid, with some connective tissue and fat. The areola is developed but the papilla is small. In the adult male, it rarely develops beyond the female prepubertal stage. Also *mamma virilis, male breast.*

**supernumerary mammae** Mammary glands at sites other than the usual location of the breasts. They are most often along the embryonic milk lines extending from the axillae to the groin. Also *accessory mammae, accesory mammary glands.* **m. virilis** MAMMA MASCULINA.

**mammae** \mam′ē\ Plural of MAMMA.

**mammal** [Late L *mammal(is)* (from L *mamm(a)* a woman's breast + *-alis* -AL) pertaining to the breasts] Any member of the vertebrate class Mammalia.

**mammalgia** \məmal′jə\ [*mamm(o)-* + -ALGIA] MASTODYNIA.

**Mammalia** \məmā′lyə\ [New L, from Late L *mammalis* pertaining to the breasts, from L *mamma* breast, teat] The class of homeothermic vertebrates characterized by hair and by milk-secreting mammary glands that nourish the young. The diaphragm is muscular, the heart four-chambered. The ramus of the mandible is composed of a single bone, the dentary, and the jaw articulates directly with the squamosal bone. There are three ear ossicles. Except for the egg-laying monotremes, all mammals are viviparous.

**mammaplasty** \mam′əplas′tē\ MAMMOPLASTY.

**mammary** \mam′ərē\ Pertaining to the mamma or breast.

**mammectomy** \məmek′təmē\ [*mamm(o)-* + -ECTOMY] MASTECTOMY.

**mammiform** \mam′ifôrm\ Shaped like a mamma. Also *mammose.*

**mammilla** \məmil′ə\ **1** MAMILLA. **2** PAPILLA MAMMARIA.

**mammillary** \mam′iler′ē\ MAMILLARY.

**mammillate** \mam′ilāt\ MAMILLATED.

**mammillated** \mam′ilā′tid\ MAMILLATED.

**mammillation** \mam′ilā′shən\ MAMILLATION.

**mammilliform** \məmil′ifôrm\ MAMILLIFORM.

**mammilliplasty** \məmil′iplas′tē\ [See MAMILLIPLASTY.] THELEPLASTY.

**mammillitis** \mam′ilī′tis\ MAMILLITIS.

**mammitis** \mamī′tis\ MASTITIS.

**mammo-** \mam′ə-, mam′ō-\ [L *mamma* mother's breast] A combining form denoting the breasts.

**mammogen** \mam′əjən\ [MAMMO- + -GEN] Any agent promoting or stimulating development of the breast.

**mammogram** \mam′əgram\ A roentgenogram obtained during mammography.

**mammography** \mamäg′rəfē\ [MAMMO- + -GRAPHY] Radiographic examination of the breast.

**mammoplasia** \-plā′zhə\ [MAMMO- + -PLASIA] The growth and development of the breast. **adolescent m.** The growth and development of the breast during puberty, especially the moderate development that often occurs transiently in the adolescent male.

**mammoplasty** \mam′ōplas′tē\ [MAMMO- + -PLASTY] Any plastic operation on the breast. Also *mammaplasty, mastoplasty.* **augmentation m.** A mammoplasty performed to increase breast size, generally using alloplastic materials. **reduction m.** A mammoplasty performed to reduce breast size, yet preserve a natural contour and a normal relationship of the nipple to the breast.

**mammose** \mamōs′\ **1** Having full or large breasts. **2** MAMMIFORM.

**mammotomy** \məmät′əmē\ [MAMMO- + -TOMY] Incision into the breast.

**mammotropic** \-träp′ik\ [MAMMO- + -TROPIC[1]] **1** Stimulating the mammary gland. **2** Pertaining to the development, milk production, and milk secretion of the mammary gland.

**mammotropin** \-trō′pin\ [*mammotrop(ic)* + -IN] PROLACTIN.

**man** [Old English] **1** A male adult human being. **2** Humanity or mankind including especially the species *Homo sapiens* but extended also to include other species of the genus *Homo* known from the fossil record. • Some human fossils, Peking man, for example, were originally assigned to other genera of the family Hominidae but have mostly been reclassified as species of *Homo.* Hominids currently classified in other genera are usually not called "man" or "human." **Cro-Magnon m.** An upper Pleistocene, European "race" of man typified by a group of skeletons found at Cro-Magnon in France by L. Lartet in 1868. The cranium is sometimes described as dolichopentagonal: large, long, and five-sided as seen from above. The postcranial skeleton is that of modern humans in all respects and indicates tall, slender, and muscular people. **Heidelberg m.** A human fossil represented by a mandible recovered in 1908 from a sand pit near the village of Mauer near Heidelberg, West Germany. The deposits contain a fauna that suggest the climate was warm-temperate, perhaps during the first European interglacial period. Initially attributed to a separate human species, *Homo heidelbergensis,* it is now more commonly regarded as a European pre-Neandertal form. **Java m.** Any of a group of fossil human remains recovered in Java since 1891 from various sites all of which are probably less than 1 000 000 but more than 500 000 years old. Initially assigned to a new genus and species of "ape-man," *Pithecanthropus erectus,* the Java fossils are now widely regarded as belonging to an archaic species of man known as *Homo erectus.* **Neandertal m.** See under *HOMO NEANDERTHALENSIS.* **Peking m.** An extinct human population represented by a group of fossil remains recovered from Choukoutien (Zhoukoudian), near Peking, China, since 1927. The fossils consist of skulls, jaws, teeth, and a few postcranial bones. Initially regarded as a new genus and species, *Sinanthropus pekinensis,* it was later recognized as belonging to *Homo erectus.* **reference m.** A hypothetical man whose anatomy, physiology, biochemistry, clinical chemistry, and hematologic values are within normal limits, and with whom all other men may be compared. Also *standard man.* **Rhodesian m.** An extinct human population represented by a group of fossil remains recovered from Broken Hill, Zambia (formerly Northern Rhodesia), comprising a skull and postcranial remains from several individuals. The remains are dated as more than 100 000 years old. Initially assigned to a separate species, *Homo rhodesiensis,* they were later classified as belonging to an archaic subspecies of modern man, *Homo sapiens rhodesiensis.* **spinal m.** A patient with complete transection of the spinal cord at any level. **standard m.** REFERENCE MAN.

**man.** *manipulus* (L, a handful).

**mandible** \man′dibəl\ [L *mandibula.* See MANDIBULA.] **1** The bone of the lower jaw of mammals; mandibula. **2** A member of the anterior pair of mouthparts in some invertebrates.

**mandibula** \mandib′yələ\ [Late L (from L *mandere* to chew, akin to Gk *masasthai* to chew and to English *mouth*) the lower jaw] [NA] The large, arched, movable bone of the lower part of the face, consisting of a curved horizontal body on each side, fused in the midline at the symphysis menti. It is continuous posteriorly with a vertical ramus, the upper border of which ends posteriorly in a condyle that articulates with the temporal bone at the temporomandibular joint. The upper, or alveolar, border of the body supports the lower teeth. Its functions include protection of the tongue, and involvement in mastication and speech. Also *mandible, lower jaw, inferior jaw, jaw bone, submaxilla* (outmoded), *inferior maxilla* (outmoded), *lower jaw bone.* Adj. mandibular.

**mandibulae** \mandib′yəlē\ Plural of MANDIBULA.

**mandibulectomy** \məndib′yəlek′təmē\ The excision of the lower jaw.

**mandibulofacial** \məndib′yəlōfā′shəl\ Pertaining to the mandible and the facial bones.

**mandibuloglossus** \məndib′yəlōgläs′əs\ An occasional muscle bundle that extends from the posterior border of the mandible, above the angle, to the side of the tongue.

**mandibulomarginalis** \məndib′yəlōmär′jənā′lis\ One of the accessory slips of the platysma muscle, extending forward from the mastoid process over the angle of the mandible to the main body of the muscle.

**mandibulopharyngeal** \məndib′yəlōfərin′jē·əl\ Of or relating to the mandible and the pharynx: used especially of the anatomic area between them.

**mandrake** \man′drāk\ [Middle English; Old English *mandragora* (from L and Gk *mandragoras* mandrake) the mandrake] A plant of the species *Posophyllum peltatum*, the roots of which are used to make podophyllum resin. Also *May apple, mayapple, Indian apple.*

**mandrel** \man′drəl\ [prob. from French *mandrin* mandrel, from Provençal, from L *mamphur* bow-drill, prob. from Oscan] A rotating shaft used in a dental handpiece to hold abrasive instruments by means of a screw, chuck, or pin. Also *mandril.*

**mandrin** \man′drin\ [prob. French. See MANDREL.] A stylet used to help introduce soft catheters.

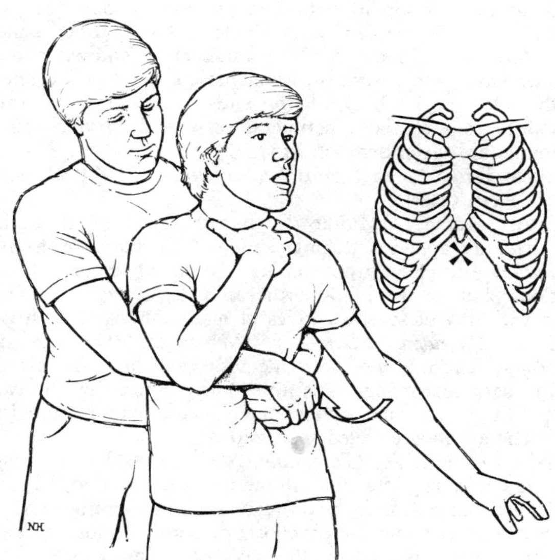

Heimlich maneuver

**maneuver** [French *manoeuvre* (from L *manu* by hand + *opera*, pl. of *opus* work) an operation, maneuver] A manual procedure, especially a skillful one. **Adson m.** See under ADSON'S TEST. **Allen m.** A maneuver to confirm the presence of the scalenus anterior syndrome by testing for the obliteration of the radial pulse when compressing the subclavicular artery against the scalenus muscle as the head is rotated to the opposite shoulder and the arm is extended and externally rotated. **Bracht m.** A procedure used in assisting a breech delivery. The fetus is allowed to be delivered to the umbilicus. Then, while the fetal arms are held against the sides, the fetal body is elevated anteriorly toward the symphysis pubis. The maneuver usually results in delivery of the vertex. **Brandt-Andrews m.** A procedure used in assisting delivery of the placenta. While exerting traction on the umbilical cord with one hand, the other is placed on the abdomen to displace the uterus upwards. Also *Brandt-Andrews method.* **Chassard-Lapiné m.** A special roentgenographic projection in which the patient sits at the edge of the table, bending far forward with the head near the knees, and the x-ray beam is directed from above, centered to the pelvis, penetrating the spine. This projection is used to demonstrate the pelvic inlet and also during barium enema examination to display the loops of the sigmoid with diminished overlapping. **Credé's m.** **1** Placenta expulsion by manual pressure on the uterus by the abdominal wall. **2** The instillation of a solution of 0.1 percent silver nitrate in the eyes of newborns. **3** Urine expulsion by pressure on the bladder through the abdominal wall. For defs. 1, 2, and 3 also *Credé's method.* **DeLee's m.** A procedure used in obstetrics of converting a face presentation to a brow presentation. **Fowler m.** A test for contracted intrinsic musculature with ulnar deviation at the metacarpophalangeal joint. The test is performed by flexing the wrists. In normal subjects the fingers can be extended. In intrinsic muscle contraction the fingers remain in flexion at the proximal interphalangeal joint. **Halstead m.** A maneuver to confirm the presence of the scalenus anterior syndrome by the obliteration of the radial pulse when the head is rotated contralaterally and and examiner applies downward pressure on the extended limb of the involved side. **Hampton m.** A radiographic technique during gastrointestinal series, designed to demonstrate the duodenal cap with a combination of barium coating and air distention, as in an air-contrast examination. The supine patient is placed in the left posterior oblique position. This maneuver is helpful for the roentgenographic demonstration of a posterior-wall ulcer. **Heimlich m.** A procedure designed to clear the airway of a bolus, especially food, in an emergency by exerting a sudden, intense pressure inward on the abdomen immediately below the diaphragm, thus forcing the victim to expel air from the lungs. If the victim is standing, the rescuer places his or her arms around the victim, placing a fist just below the sternum, and, with the other open hand around the fist, thrusts the fist inward and upward. This forces an explosive release of air which, it is hoped, will dislodge the blockage. Variations of the maneuver can accommodate victims who are sitting or supine. **Hippocratic m.** A maneuver used to restore to proper position a dislocated shoulder. The operator's foot is placed in the patient's axilla and the patient's arm is pulled downward. **Hodge m.** A means of assisting vaginal delivery of a fetus. The obstetrician aids flexion of the fetal head by exerting pressure on the fetal brow with each uterine contraction. **Hoguet's m.** A surgical procedure in which the sac of an inguinal hernia is passed beneath the deep epigastric vessels to facilitate its removal. **Jendrassik's m.** A procedure for facilitation or reinforcement of the patellar reflex: the patient is asked to pull on his hands which are clasped together in claw fashion, while the patellar tendon is percussed. Also *reinforcement of tendon reflexes.* **key-in-lock m.** A method of rotating the fetal head using obstetric forceps. After an initial arc of rotation, the forceps are reapplied in order to complete the rotation. Most frequently, this method is utilized to convert a fetal head from a transverse or posterior position to an anterior position. **Kocher's m.** A method of reducing a dislocated shoulder by internally rotating and adducting the flexed involved limb across the trunk. **Kristeller's m.** An obstetric procedure in which pressure is maintained on the uterine fundus in an effort to express the infant. The procedure is not always successful and carries a risk of uterine rupture. Also *Kristeller's method, Kristeller's technique.* **Lasègue's m.** NERI SIGN. **Leadbetter m.** A method of reducing a fractured femoral neck by applying a vertical force on the flexed femur and then extending it into abduction. **Leopold's m.'s** A series of four steps in palpating the abdomen of a pregnant woman in order to ascertain the position and presentation of the fetus. **Levret m.** A type of internal fetal version utilizing rotation in an effort to disimpact a fetus from the pelvic brim. **Løvset's m.** A method of extracting the arms in a breech delivery by rotating the trunk of the fetus after it has delivered to the level of the umbilicus. Also *Løvset's method.* **Mauriceau m.** A method of delivering the head in a breech delivery. **Mauriceau-Smellie-Veit m.** A modified Mariceau maneuver utilized to deliver the head in a breech delivery. **McDonald m.** A method of estimating the duration of a pregnancy by measuring the distance from the symphysis pubis to the top of the gravid uterus with a tape measure. **McMurray's circumduction m.** A test for a tear in a knee meniscus in which the acutely flexed knee is extended and a varus or valgus strain is applied. The examiner will feel a click or catch, and the subject will experience pain, if a tear is present. **modified Ritgen m.** A procedure to assist delivery of the head in a vertex presentation by producing extension through pressure on the brow, maxilla, and chin in succession, using the tips of the fingers placed on the perineum just behind the anus. **Müller's m.** MÜLLER'S EXPERIMENT. **Müller-Hillis m.** A means of assessing the size of the fetal head in relation to the maternal pelvis in order to determine whether or not there is cephalopelvic disproportion. **Munro Kerr m.** A means of assessing the size of the fetal head in relation to the maternal pelvis in order to determine whether or not there is cephalopelvic disproportion. **Pajot m.** The application of traction with both hands to facilitate vaginal delivery of a fetus with forceps. Also *Saxtorph's maneuver.* **Phalen's m.** A method of bringing out or accentuating the symptoms of a carpal tunnel syndrome by forced flexion of the affected wrist for 30–60 seconds or by applying a sphygnomanometer cuff to the arm at above arterial pressure for one minute. **Pinard m.** A procedure to identify and deliver a foot during a breech delivery. **Prague m.** A procedure used in a breech delivery in which a finger is hooked over the shoulder of the fetus to exert traction and allow engagement of the head, facilitating subsequent delivery. **Proust-Lichtheim m.** A way to demonstrate that an aphasic patient knows and recognizes a word he is unable to say, by having him gesture or tap out with a finger the number of letters or syllables the word contains. **Ritgen m.** A means of facilitating delivery of the fetal head in a vertex presentation. Originally described in 1855, the initial method has been replaced by the modified Ritgen maneuver. Also *Ritgen's method.* **Saxtorph's m.** PAJOT MANEUVER. **Scanzoni m.** A method of midforceps rotation of the fetal head from a posterior to an anterior position. **Schatz m.** A method of converting a face presentation to a brow presentation in order to facilitate vaginal delivery. **Sellick's m.** The application of pressure on the cricoid cartilage to occlude the esophagus posteriorly, thereby preventing regurgitation and aspiration of gastric contents. It is used for a patient with a full stomach during rapid induction of anesthesia and tracheal intubation. **Thorn m.** A method of converting a face presentation to a vertex presentation in order to facilitate vaginal delivery. **Toynbee's m.** The production of alterations in intratympanic pressure by swallowing with the mouth closed and the nose pinched. These alterations are assessed by listening to the sounds produced using an auscultation tube. **Valsalva m.** **1** The forcible inflation of the middle ear by a strong expiratory effort made with the mouth closed and the nostrils pinched. It is frequently adopted by patients to gain relief from the discomfort in the ears and impaired hearing caused by negative pressure consequent on obstruction of the eustachian tubes. It is used by otologists as a test of tubal patency. Also *Valsalva's procedure, Valsalva's experiment, auto inflation.* **2** A forceable exhalation against a closed glottis. The increased pressure which develops within the thorax causes a change in venous return and in heart rate. Compare MÜLLER'S EXPERIMENT. **Van Hoorn m.** A modification of the Prague maneuver in which transabdominal pressure is appled to the fetal brow with one hand in order to facilitate engagement of the fetal head. **Westphal m.** The use of movements of the head and/or the eyes by dyslexic patients to trace out the outline of letters or symbols which they cannot read at a glance. **Wigand's m.** An external transabdominal palpatory maneuver to convert a transverse lie of a fetus to a vertex presentation. Also *Wigand-Martin maneuver.* **Wigand-Martin m.** WIGAND'S MANEUVER.

**manganese** \mang′gənēs\ Element number 25, having atomic weight 54.9380. It is a hard, brittle metal resembling iron. Its compounds are widely distributed in the lithosphere and the ocean floor in spots is strewn with nodules containing about 24% manganese. A single stable isotope, manganese 55, occurs in nature. Nine radioactive isotopes and an isomer have been described. Manganese is a reactive element, with valences 1, 2, 3, 4, 6, and 7. Biologically, small amounts are essential constituents of several enzymes. Large amounts are toxic. Symbol: Mn

**manganism** \mang′gənizm\ [*mangan(ese)* + -ISM] MANGANESE POISONING.

**mange** \mānj\ [Middle English *manjewe*; Old French *mangeue* an appetite, itching, eating, from *mangier* (from L *manducare* to chew, from *mandere* to chew) to eat] A contagious skin disease of domestic animals, caused by infestation with any of several species of mange mites of such genera as *Chorioptes, Demodex, Notoedres, Psoroptes,* and *Sarcoptes,* causing chorioptic, demodectic, notoedric, psoroptic, or sarcoptic mange. The mites burrow into the skin causing multiple vesicular and papular lesions and intense itching. The agents are called scab mites.

**mania** \mā′nē·ə\ [Gk *mania.* See -MANIA.] **1** A syndrome consisting of elated although unstable mood, hyperactivity, and mental overactivity expressed in garrulousness. As part of manic-depressive psychosis or bipolar disorder, mania is sometimes classified on the basis of intensity as hypomania, acute mania, or delirious mania. Also *psycheclampsia* (obs.), *psychlampsia* (obs.). **2** Any type of mental disorder, especially if symptoms have an impulsive, compulsive, or repetitive quality. **alcoholic m.** PATHOLOGIC INTOXICATION. **m. a potu** PATHOLOGIC INTOXICATION. **Bell's m.** DELIRIOUS MANIA. **dancing m.** CHOREOMANIA. **delirious m.** The most severe form of mania, seen in manic-depressive psychosis, with such intense psychomotor excitement that physical collapse and death may ensue. Partial or complete disorientation is usually a prominent feature. Also *Bell's mania, collapse delirium, delirium grave, hypermania, Bell's delirium.* **doubting m.** FOLIE DU DOUTE.

**-mania** \-mā′nē·ə\ [Gk *mania* (from *mainesthai* to rage in war, rave with anger, be mad with wine) madness, frenzy, rage, enthusiasm] A combining form meaning a morbid preference or irresistible impulse for behaving (in a specified way), a morbid fondness for or attachment to (something specified).

**manic** \man′ik, mā′nik\ Of, characterized by, or suffering from mania.

**manic-depressive** \-dipres′iv\ See under MANIC-DEPRESSIVE PSYCHOSIS.

**manifestation** \man′əfestā′shən\ [Late L *manifestatio* (from *manifestatus,* past part. of *manifestare* to make evident, make clear, from L *manus* the hand + *-festus* as in *infestus* hostile, aggressive) a making clear, revealing] Something manifested, especially an observable sign or symptom of disease. **ictal epileptic m.'s** Electroencephalographic or clinical manifestations indicative of an epileptic attack. Also *critical epileptic phenomena.* **interictal epileptic m.'s** Electroencephalographic or clinical manifestations occurring in epileptic patients between clinically overt attacks. Also *intercritical epileptic phenomena, interictal epileptic phenomena.* **postictal epileptic m.'s** Electroencephalographic or clinical manifestations which may occur in epileptic patients immediately after an attack. Electroencephalographically, they usually comprise focal or diffuse slow waves. Clinical features include coma, confusion, and automatism. Also *postcritical epileptic phenomena.* **preictal epileptic m.'s** Electroencephalographic or clinical manifestations which occur in epileptic patients and may presage an impending attack. These symptoms can often be carefully differentiated from those which herald the onset of the attack (the aura). Electroencephalographically, there are usually more and more frequent generalized or focal subclinical epileptic discharges. Clinically, the precritical epileptic symptoms are generally vague and ill-defined and are sometimes called prodromal epileptic symptoms. Also *precritical epileptic phenomena.*

**manikin** \man′ikin\ [Dutch *manneken* a little man, dim. of *man* man] An anatomical model of the human body, usually with movable and detachable parts. It is made of plastic, plaster of Paris, ceramic, or other materials, and used for various teaching purposes.

**maniphalanx** \man′ifā′langks\ A phalanx of any finger. Compare PEDIPHALANX.

**maniple** MANIPULUS.

**manipulation** \mənip′yəlā′shən\ [French (from *manipul(e)* an apothecary's handful, from L *manipul(us)* handful + *-ation* -ATION) a performing of manual operations in chemistry or pharmaceutics] **1** Any manual operation. **2** The application of a passive change in position by a skillful hand maneuver.

**manipulus** [L, a handful] A handful. Also *maniple.*

**Mann** [Frank Charles *Mann,* U.S. surgeon and physiologist, 1887–1962] Mann-Bollman fistula. See under FISTULA.

**Mann** [Gustav *Mann,* German physiologist active in England and the United States, born 1864] Mann stain. See under METHOD.

**Mann** [Henry Berthold *Mann,* Austrian-born U.S. mathematician, born 1905] Mann-Whitney U test. See under TEST.

**manner of death** In forensic pathology, one of the means by which death occurs. There are four etiologic categories of manner of death relating to the circumstances and events surrounding death. The four categories are natural, suicide, homicide, and accident. In instances where accurate, unequivocal determination of manner of death cannot be made, a fifth category, undetermined, is used.

**mannitol** $CH_2OH—[CHOH]_4—CH_2OH$. The alcohol formed by chemical reduction of mannose. It may also be formed by enzymatic reduction of fructose, or, together with sorbitol, by chemical reduction of fructose.

**mannitol hexanitrate** $C_6H_8N_6O_{18}$. It is a vasodilator, prepared by the nitration of mannitol. It is slower in its actions than nitroglycerin.

**mannose** One of the aldohexose sugars, the 2-epimer of glucose. Its residues occur widely in glycolipids and glycoproteins.

**mannosidase** \man′ōsī′dās\ An enzyme that catalyzes the hydrolysis of the glycoside mannoside to form an alcohol and D-mannoside. There are two forms, $\alpha$- and $\beta$-mannosidase, which are responsible for degrading $\alpha$-D mannoside and $\beta$-D mannoside.

**mannosidostreptomycin** A naturally occurring derivative of streptomycin in which the latter is combined in glycosidal linkage to a *D*-mannose molecule.

**manoeuvre** *Brit.* MANEUVER.

**manometer** \mənäm′ətər\ [Gk *manos* thin, scanty + -METER] An instrument for measuring pressures of liquids and gases. Also *pressometer.* **airway pressure m.** An apparatus for measuring the pressure of gas in the airways. **aneroid m.** A manometer comprising a pointer attached to a diaphragm which forms the end of an evacuated box. Changes of pressure may be recorded directly by movement of the pointer. **Koenig's m.** An instrument for detecting pressure variations associated with sound waves of different frequency.

**manometry** \mənäm′ətrē\ [Gk *mano(s)* thin, scanty + -METRY] The measurement of pressure of fluids and gases. **Cartesian diver m.** A gasometric technique for measuring the metabolic activity of small quantities of respiring tissue.

**man. pr.** *mane primo* (L, early in the morning).

**manslaughter** The unlawful killing of one human being by another under circumstances devoid of premeditation, deliberation, and express or implied malice. **involuntary m.** **1** The unintentional killing of another by an individual committing an unlawful but not felonious act or an unlawful act not usually associated with potentially lethal injury, such as striking and killing a pedestrian while operating a vehicle in excess of the speed limit. **2** The unintentional killing of another by an individual committing a lawful act in which the requisite skills or necessary precautions associated with the act have not been employed, such as the intraoperative or postoperative death of a patient undergoing surgery performed by an intoxicated surgeon or one under the influence of drugs, if no extenuating circumstances existed. **voluntary m.** The unpremeditated killing of one individual by another in a sudden heat of passion, as when a quarrel between two individuals leads to a fight resulting in one person's death. A lack of previous intent to kill must be proven.

**Manson** [Sir Patrick *Manson,* British physician and parasitologist 1844–1922] **1** See under TAPEWORM. **2** Manson's disease, Manson schistosomiasis. See under SCHISTOSOMIASIS MANSONI. **3** Pyosis of Manson. See under PEMPHIGUS CONTAGIOSUS.

***Mansonella*** \man′sənel′ə\ [after Sir Patrick *Manson,* British parasitologist, 1844–1922] A genus of filiarial parasites of primates, characterized by unsheathed microfilariae, a narrow, poorly formed esophagus (as contrasted with the well-developed muscular and glandular esophagus of *Dipetalonema*), and four terminal lobes in the female (contrasted with two in *Dipetalonema*). The human parasites *Mansonella* *perstans* and *M. streptocerca* have been transferred to this genus from *Dipetalonema* and from the synonymized genus *Tetrapetalonema*. ***M. ozzardi*** A filarial nematode occurring in the visceral fat and mesentery of humans and found in Panama, Colombia, Argentina, Guyana, Surinam, and Yucatan. The microfilariae are unsheathed, and nuclei are absent in the tail. Humans are the only known definitive host, punkies or midges (*Culicoides* spp.) serving as intermediate hosts. The parasite is not known to cause any serious disease. Also *Filaria demarquayi, Filaria juncea, Filaria ozzardi.* ***M. perstans*** A species found in humans and other primates in Africa and Central and South America, transmitted by biting midges of the genus *Culicoides* and chiefly of the species *C. austeni.* Generally considered nonpathogenic, the adult worms live in pleural and peritoneal cavities, the pericardium, or on mesenteries and retroperitoneal tissues. Also *Acanthocheilonema perstans.* ***M. streptocerca*** A filarial nematode found in the corium of the skin of humans in west Africa; the cause of streptocerciasis. Nonhuman primates probably serve as reservoir hosts. The microfilariae are sometimes confused with those of *Onchocerca volvulus,* which are also found in the skin. The vector of *M. streptocerca* is the biting midge, *Culicoides grahami.* Also *Acanthocheilonema streptocerca, Filaria streptocerca, Agamofilaria streptocerca.*

**mansonelliasis** \man′sənelī′əsis\ [*Mansonell(a)* + -IASIS] A usually asymptomatic infection with the filarial worm *Mansonella ozzardi,* infecting human mesenteries and visceral fat in the American tropics.

***Mansonia*** \mansō′nē·ə\ A genus of mosquitoes whose larvae obtain air from the roots or stems of aquatic plants. They are important as vectors of *Brugia malayi,* and also transmit viral equine encephalomyelitis in the Orient. Also *Taeniorhynchus.* ***M. annulifera*** An important vector of *Brugia malayi* in India.

**mantle** \man′tl\ [L *mantel(um),* also *mantellum* a cloak, mantle, cover] **1** A covering or surrounding layer. **2** *Popular* CORTEX CEREBRI. **blue m.'s of Manasse** Basophilic bone deposited in the perivascular spaces produced by the resorption of enchondral bone in otosclerosis. It is one of the principal histologic features of the disease. **brain m.** CORTEX CEREBRI. **chordomesodermal m.** The continuous epithelial sheet of notochordal and mesodermal material which forms on the dorsal side of the amphibian embryo during gastrulation. **myoepicardial m.** The mesodermal wall of the embryonic pericardial cavity. It later surrounds the heart tube and gives rise to the myocardium and epicardium of the heart. Also *epimyocardium.*

**Mantoux** [Charles *Mantoux,* French physician, 1887–1947] **1** See under CONVERSION. **2** Mantoux reaction. See under TEST.

**manubrial** \mənʸoo′brē·əl\ **1** Pertaining to the manubrium sterni. **2** Shaped like the manubrium sterni.

**manubriosternal** \mənʸoo′br·ōstur′nəl\ Pertaining to the manubrium and the corpus of the sternum.

**manubrium** \mənʸoo′brē·əm\ [L (from *manus* hand) a handle, haft] (*pl.* manubria) **1** A structure or part resembling a handle or hilt. **2** MANUBRIUM STERNI. **m. mallei** [NA] The large, elongated process that extends downward, posteriorly, and medially below the neck of the malleus and is attached to the inner surface of the tympanic membrane by its lateral margin. The tensor tympani muscle is inserted into its upper end. Also *manubrium of malleus, handle of malleus.* **m. sterni** [NA] A flattened, irregularly shaped bone that is broader superiorly than inferiorly where it joins the body of the sternum and the second costal cartilages at the sternal angle. Superolaterally it articulates with the clavicles and the first costal cartilages. The notched and thick superior border forms the lower limit of the neck in the midline, and its anterior surface is subcutaneous. Also *manubrium of sternum, presternum* (outmoded), *manubrium.*

**manuduction** \manʸooduk′shən\ [L *manu,* ablative of *manus* hand + *ductio* a conveying, pulling, or drawing] Any surgical or obstetrical procedure in which the unaided hands are used.

**manus** \man′əs\ [L, the hand] [NA] The extremity of the upper limb distal to the forearm; hand. It comprises a bony skeleton of eight carpal bones forming the wrist; five metacarpal bones forming the palm and the dorsum; and three phalanges for each finger except the thumb, which only has two; as well as a series of intrinsic and extrinsic muscles. It is a prehensile organ capable of grasping, precise and/or coarse manipulation by the fingers, and a variety of movements. • In naming the different deformities of the hand, reference is given to the deviation from the general plane of the forearm. **m. cava** Excessive concavity of the palm of the hand. **m. extensa** A club hand with deviation or fixation in the direction of extension, particularly at the wrist. **m. flexa** A club hand with deviation or fixation in the direction of flexion. **m. valga** A club hand with deviation toward the ulna and adduction at the wrist. **m. vara** A club hand with deviation toward the radius and adduction at the wrist.

**Manzullo** [Alfredo *Manzullo,* Argentinian immunologist, born 1909] Manzullo's test. See under TELLURITE TEST.

**MAO** monoamine oxidase.

**MAOI** monoamine oxidase inhibitor.

**map** [Med L *mappa* (from L, a napkin, supposedly of Punic origin) a map] A graphic representation on a flat surface of the relative positions of particular units or parts; chart for locating position in a configuration or in three-dimensional space. **chromosome m.** The linear arrangement of genes along the chromosomes of an organism. It is usually presented graphically, with the location of each gene determined by one or more of a variety of mapping techniques. Also *cytogenetic map, genetic map.* **cognitive m.** A hypothesized representation in the mind of the environment, which serves as an organizing schema for establishing relationships between the events that occur in a learning situation. Once a mental picture of this kind is complete, responses quite different from those made during the original learning can be initiated in order to attain the goal. **cytogenetic m.** CHROMOSOME MAP. **fate m.** A plan which shows areas of prospective fate in normal embryonic development, principally applied to regional localization at the blastula or early gastrula stage. **genetic m.** CHROMOSOME MAP. **linkage m.** The linear arrangement of genetic loci as determined by linkage analysis. Loci within linkage groups are ordered by a variety of family, biochemical, and cytogenetic techniques and, similarly, are ordered into syntenic groups that correspond to individual chromosomes. The linkage map is most often represented graphically as the linear array of loci along each chromosome, and genes close together will recombine less frequently than those further apart. Also *genetic map.*

**Mapharsen** A proprietary name for oxophenarsine hydrochloride.

**mapping** / **cytologic m.** The process by which identifiable chromosome changes, such as deletions and inversions, are used to order genes on the chromosome map. The technique is used to particular advantage in organisms with polytene chromosomes. **deletion m.** The process by which spontaneous or induced deletions of portions of a chromosome are used in cytologic, linkage, or biochemical analysis to order genes in the chromosome map. Also *deletion method.* **fine structure genetic m.** The process of determining the order of nucleotide sequences around individual genes, especially those of functional significance such as introns, exons, promoters, and enhancers. It may be achieved by a variety of methods including restriction enzyme analysis, deletion mapping, and direct nucleotide sequencing. **genetic m.** The process by which a chromosome map is constructed. It involves a variety of techniques, such as cytologic, deletion, complementation, and linkage mapping; *in situ* hybridization; pedigree analysis; recombinant DNA studies; and somatic cell genetics.

**maprotiline** $C_{20}H_{23}N$. *N*-Methyl-9,10-ethananthracene-9(10*H*)-propylamine. It is used clinically as an antidepressant agent.

**Maraglas** An epoxy resin that is used as an embedding medium in electron microscopy. A proprietary name.

**Maragliano** [Edoardo *Maragliano,* Italian physician, 1849–1940] See under TUBERCULIN.

**Marañón** [Gregorio *Marañón,* Spanish endocrinologist, 1887–1960] Marañón sign. See under REACTION.

**marasmic** \məraz′mik\ Of or relating to marasmus. Also *marantic, marasmatic.*

**marasmoid** \məraz′moid\ Resembling marasmus.

**marasmus** \məraz′məs\ [Late L, from Gk *marasmos* (from *marainesthai* to wither) a wasting, withering] Starvation occurring in children. It occurs most frequently in infants under one year of age and is more often found in urban populations. In this environment, there may be a rapid succession of pregnancies and early and abrupt weaning followed by dirty and inadequate bottle feeding consisting of very small amounts of dilute milk serving as a low source of energy and protein. The unsterile foods cause repeated infections, especially of the gastrointestinal tract, which the mother treats by long periods of fasting. The clinical symptoms are growth retardation (weight more so than height), abnormal behavior (irritability), dehydration, diarrhea, extreme hunger or anorexia, weak musculature, dry and atrophic skin and mucous membranes, absence of subcutaneous fat, and presence of vitamin deficiencies. If a child is exposed to marasmus for only a short period, complete recovery is possible. If the disease is severe and of long duration, the prognosis is often poor and the child may become mentally retarded and growth retarded. Also *athrepsia, marcor, infantile atrophy, Parrot's atrophy of the newborn, pedatrophia.* **nutritional m.** PROTEIN-CALORIE MALNUTRITION.

**Marburg** [Otto *Marburg,* German neurologist, born 1878] See under TRIAD.

**march** [French *marche* (from *marcher* to walk, march, progress) progression] The progressive spread of abnormal electrical discharge to contiguous areas of the motor cortex in patients with focal motor epilepsy. **jacksonian m.** The spread of focal convulsive phenomena, whether motor or sensory, from one part of the body to another, in the order in which these areas are represented in those parts of the cerebral motor and/or sensory cortex contiguous with the area in which the discharge originates. Also *jacksonism* (seldom used), *protospasm* (outmoded).

**Marchant** [Gerard T. Joseph *Marchant,* French surgeon, 1850–1903] Marchant's detachable zone. See under ZONE.

**marche à petits pas** \märsh′ äpətē′ pä′\ A slow, shuffling gait with very short steps, as seen in parkinsonism. Also *Petren gait.*

**Marchesani** [Oswald *Marchesani,* German ophthalmologist, 1900–1952] Marchesani syndrome. See under WEILL-MARCHESANI SYNDROME.

**Marchetti** [Andrew A. *Marchetti,* U.S. obstetrician and gynecologist, 1901–1970] Marshall-Marchetti operation. See under OPERATION.

**Marchi** [Vittorio *Marchi,* Italian physiologist, 1851–1908] **1** Marchi's tract. See under TRACTUS TECTOSPINALIS. **2** See under REACTION, METHOD.

**Marchiafava** [Ettore *Marchiafava,* Italian pathologist, 1847–1935] **1** Marchiafava's disease, Marchiafava-Bignami disease. See under MARCHIAFAVA-BIGNAMI SYNDROME. **2** Marchiafava-Micheli syndrome. See under PAROXYSMAL NOCTURNAL HEMOGLOBINURIA.

**marcid** \mär′sid\ [L *marcid(us)* withered, languid, feeble] Wasted; emaciated.

**marcor** \mär′kôr\ MARASMUS.

**Marcus Gunn** [Robert *Marcus Gunn,* English ophthalmologist, 1850–1909] **1** Marcus Gunn phenomenon, Gunn's phenomenon, Gunn syndrome. See under MARCUS GUNN SYNDROME. **2** Marcus Gunn inverse syndrome, inverse Marcus Gunn phenomenon, inverted Marcus Gunn phenomenon. See under MARIN AMAT SYNDROME. **3** Gunn's pupillary phenomenon, Gunn's pupillary sign, Marcus Gunn pupillary sign. See under MARCUS GUNN PUPILLARY PHENOMENON. **4** Gunn's dots. See under DOT.

**Marey** [Etienne Jules *Marey,* French physiologist, 1830–1904] See under REFLEX.

**Marfan** [Antonin Bernard Jean *Marfan,* French pediatrician, 1858–1942] **1** Marfan's epigastric puncture. See under EPIGASTRIC PUNCTURE. **2** See under METHOD. **3** See under MARFAN SYNDROME.

**Marg** [Elwin *Marg,* U.S. scientist, born 1918] MacKay-Marg electronic tonometer. See under TONOMETER.

# margin

**margin** [L *margo,* gen. *marginis,* a brink, brim, edge, border, margin] The edge or border of a structure or organ. **alveolar m. of mandible** ARCUS ALVEOLARIS MANDIBULAE. **alveolar m. of maxilla** ARCUS ALVEOLARIS MAXILLAE. **anterior m. of fibula** MARGO ANTERIOR FIBULAE. **anterior m. of lung** MARGO ANTERIOR PULMONIS. **anterior m. of pancreas** MARGO ANTERIOR PANCREATIS. **anterior m. of parietal bone** MARGO FRONTALIS OSSIS PARIETALIS. **anterior m. of spleen** MARGO SUPERIOR SPLENIS. **anterior m. of testis** MARGO ANTERIOR TESTIS. **anterior m. of tibia** MARGO ANTERIOR TIBIAE. **anterior m. of ulna** MARGO ANTERIOR ULNAE. **axillary m. of scapula** MARGO LATERALIS SCAPULAE. **cervical m.** The part of a cavity margin adjacent to the gingiva. **ciliary m. of iris** MARGO CILIARIS IRIDIS. **crenate m. of spleen** MARGO SUPERIOR SPLENIS. **dentate m.** PECTINATE LINE. **dorsal m. of radius** MARGO POSTERIOR RADII. **dorsal m. of ulna** MARGO POSTERIOR ULNAE. **external m. of scapula** MARGO LATERALIS SCAPULAE. **falciform m. of saphenus hiatus** MARGO FALCIFORMIS HIATUS SAPHENUS. **free m. of eyelid** The anterior margin of each eyelid where the anterior and posterior surfaces meet. Each margin bears eyelashes and has a rounded anterior edge and a sharp posterior edge. **free gingival m.** GINGIVAL MARGIN. **free m. of nail** MARGO LIBER UNGUIS. **free m. of**

**ovary** MARGO LIBER OVARII. **frontal m. of greater wing of sphenoid bone** MARGO FRONTALIS ALAE MAJORIS. **frontal m. of parietal bone** MARGO FRONTALIS OSSIS PARIETALIS. **gingival m.** The edge of the gingiva which is not directly attached to tooth or bone. Also *free gingival margin, gum margin.* **gum m.** GINGIVAL MARGIN. **hidden m. of nail** MARGO OCCULTUS UNGUIS. **inferior m. of liver** MARGO INFERIOR HEPATIS. **inferior m. of lung** MARGO INFERIOR PULMONIS. **inferior m. of suprarenal gland** FACIES RENALIS GLANDULAE SUPRARENALIS. **infraorbital m. of maxilla** MARGO INFRAORBITALIS MAXILLAE. **infraorbital m. of orbit** MARGO INFRAORBITALIS ORBITAE. **interosseous m. of fibula** MARGO INTEROSSEUS FIBULAE. **interosseous m. of tibia** MARGO INTEROSSEUS TIBIAE. **interosseous m. of ulna** MARGO INTEROSSEUS ULNAE. **lacrimal m. of maxilla** MARGO LACRIMALIS MAXILLAE. **lambdoid m. of occipital bone** MARGO LAMBDOIDEUS SQUAMAE OCCIPITALIS. **lateral m. of foot** MARGO LATERALIS PEDIS. **lateral m. of humerus** MARGO LATERALIS HUMERI. **lateral m. of kidney** MARGO LATERALIS RENIS. **lateral m. of nail** MARGO LATERALIS UNGUIS. **lateral m. of scapula** MARGO LATERALIS SCAPULAE. **lateral m. of tongue** MARGO LINGUAE. **lateral m. of uterus** MARGO UTERI DEXTER ET SINISTER. **left m. of heart** *Outmoded* FACIES PULMONALIS CORDIS. **mastoid m. of occipital bone** MARGO MASTOIDEUS SQUAMAE OCCIPITALIS. **mastoid m. of parietal bone** ANGULUS MASTOIDEUS OSSIS PARIETALIS. **medial m. of foot** MARGO MEDIALIS PEDIS. **medial m. of forearm** MARGO MEDIALIS ANTEBRACHII. **medial m. of humerus** MARGO MEDIALIS HUMERI. **medial m. of kidney** MARGO MEDIALIS RENIS. **medial m. of suprarenal gland** MARGO MEDIALIS GLANDULAE SUPRARENALIS. **medial m. of tibia** MARGO MEDIALIS TIBIAE. **mesovarial m. of ovary** MARGO MESOVARICUS OVARII. **mesovarian m. of ovary** MARGO MESOVARICUS OVARII. **nasal m. of frontal bone** MARGO NASALIS OSSIS FRONTALIS. **occipital m. of parietal bone** MARGO OCCIPITALIS OSSIS PARIETALIS. **occipital m. of temporal bone** MARGO OCCIPITALIS OSSIS TEMPORALIS. **orbital m.** MARGO ORBITALIS. **parietal m. of frontal bone** MARGO PARIETALIS OSSIS FRONTALIS. **parietal m. of great wing of sphenoid bone** MARGO PARIETALIS ALAE MAJORIS. **parietal m. of occipital bone** MARGO LAMBDOIDEUS SQUAMAE OCCIPITALIS. **parietal m. of parietal bone** MARGO SAGITTALIS OSSIS PARIETALIS. **parietal m. of temporal bone** MARGO PARIETALIS OSSIS TEMPORALIS. **parietofrontal m. of great wing of sphenoid bone** MARGO FRONTALIS ALAE MAJORIS. **posterior m. of fibula** MARGO POSTERIOR FIBULAE. **posterior m. of testis** MARGO POSTERIOR TESTIS. **posterior m. of ulna** MARGO POSTERIOR ULNAE. **pupillary m. of iris** MARGO PUPILLARIS IRIDIS. **radial m. of forearm** MARGO LATERALIS ANTEBRACHII. **red m.** VERMILION BORDER. **m. of safety** A measure of drug safety based upon the dose required to produce an effective, therapeutic response in most people, versus the dose required to produce toxic effects in a few individuals. The $LD_1/ED_{99}$, rather than the $LD_{50}/ED_{50}$ is preferred for this purpose. The margin of safety is similar to, but not the same as, the therapeutic index. See also EFFECTIVE DOSE. **sagittal m. of parietal bone** MARGO SAGITTALIS OSSIS PARIETALIS. **sphenoidal m. of parietal bone** ANGULUS SPHENOIDALIS OSSIS PARIETALIS. **sphenoidal m. of temporal bone** MARGO SPHENOIDALIS OSSIS TEMPORALIS. **sphenotemporal m. of parietal bone** MARGO SQUAMOSUS OSSIS PARIETALIS. **squamous m. of greater wing of sphenoid bone** MARGO SQUAMOSUS ALAE MAJORIS. **squamous m. of parietal bone** MARGO SQUAMOSUS OSSIS PARIETALIS. **superior m. of pancreas** MARGO SUPERIOR PANCREATIS. **superior m. of parietal bone** MARGO SAGITTALIS OSSIS PARIETALIS. **superior m. of scapula** MARGO SUPERIOR SCAPULAE. **superior m. of spleen** MARGO SUPERIOR SPLENIS. **superior m. of suprarenal gland** MARGO SUPERIOR GLANDULAE SUPRARENALIS. **supraorbital m. of frontal bone** MARGO SUPRAORBITALIS OSSIS FRONTALIS. **supraorbital m. of orbit** MARGO SUPRAORBITALIS ORBITAE. **temporal m. of parietal bone** MARGO SQUAMOSUS OSSIS PARIETALIS. **tibial m. of foot** MARGO MEDIALIS PEDIS. **m. of tongue** MARGO LINGUAE. **ulnar m.'s of fingers** FACIES MEDIALES DIGITORUM MANUS. **ulnar m. of forearm** MARGO MEDIALIS ANTEBRACHII. **vertebral m. of scapula** MARGO MEDIALIS SCAPULAE. **zygomatic m. of greater wing of sphenoid bone** MARGO ZYGOMATICUS ALAE MAJORIS.

**margination** \mär′jinā′shən\ The collection of leukocytes on blood vessel walls early in the injury response.

**margines** \mär′jinēz\ Plural of MARGO.

**marginoplasty** \mär′jinōplas′tē\ Any plastic operation on an anatomic border or margin.

# margo

**margo** \mär′gō\ [L, a brink, brim, edge, border, margin] (*pl.* margines) The edge or border of an organ or a structure; margin. **m. anterior fibulae** [NA] The anterior border of the fibula extending from the head down to a point proximal to the lateral malleolus where it divides into two, surrounding a triangular subcutaneous area. The anterior intermuscular septum of the leg is attached to it. Also *anterior margin of fibula, anterior crest of fibula.* **m. anterior pancreatis** [NA] The border of the pancreas that separates the anterior from the inferior surface and over which the transverse mesocolon separates onto the two surfaces. Also *anterior margin of pancreas, anterior border of pancreas.* **m. anterior pulmonis** [NA] The thin anterior border of the lung that overlaps the pericardium and separates the costal and mediastinal surfaces. Also *anterior margin of lung.* **m. anterior radii** [NA] A ridge of bone that extends inferolaterally from the radial tuberosity to the lateral margin of the anterior surface, along which it runs to the anterior margin of the styloid process, separating the anterior from the lateral surfaces. Also *anterior border of radius.* **m. anterior testis** [NA] The convex anterior border, between the medial and lateral surfaces, of the testis. Also *anterior margin of testis.* **m. anterior tibiae** [NA] The subcutaneous sinuous crest extending from the lateral edge of the tuberosity of the tibia to the anterior border of the medial malleolus; shin. It provides attachment for the deep fascia of the leg. Also *anterior margin of tibia, anterior border of tibia, tibial crest, anterior crest of tibia.* **m. anterior ulnae** [NA] The rounded anterior border of the ulna extending downward and posteriorly from the medial side of the ulnar tuberosity to the base of the styloid process. It provides origin for the flexor digitorum profundus and pronator quadratus muscles. Also *anterior margin of ulna.* **m. ciliaris iridis** [NA] The peripheral border of the iris, where it becomes continuous with the ciliary body and also connected to the cornea by the pectinate ligament. Also *ciliary margin of iris, peripheral border of iris, base of iris, iridociliary junction.* **m. dexter cordis** [NA] The rounded, vertical right surface of the heart formed by the right atrium and extending from the termination of the superior vena cava to the point of entry of the inferior vena cava into the right atrium. Also *right border of heart.* **m. falciformis hiatus saphenus** [NA] The sharp, arched, well-defined lateral margin of the saphenous opening in the fascia lata of the upper thigh. The cribriform fascia is attached to it. Also *falciform margin of saphenus hiatus, Hey's ligament, Burns ligament, falciform fold of fascia lata.* **m. fibularis pedis** MARGO LATERALIS PEDIS. **m. frontalis alae majoris** [NA] A triangular sutural edge formed by the superior margins of the cerebral, orbital and temporal surfaces of the greater wing of the sphenoid bone and articulating with the orbital plate of the frontal bone. Also *frontal margin of greater wing of sphenoid bone, parietofrontal margin of great wing of sphenoid bone.* **m. frontalis ossis parietalis** [NA] The markedly serrated and beveled anterior border of the parietal bone articulating with the frontal bone and forming one half of the coronal suture on each side. Also *frontal margin of parietal bone, anterior margin of parietal bone coronal margi.* **m. inferior hepatis** [NA] The sharp border of the liver that separates the diaphragmatic surface and visceral surface anteriorly. Also *inferior border of liver, inferior margin of liver, anterior border of liver.* **m. inferior pancreatis** [NA] The inferior border of the pancreas which separates the inferior from the posterior surface. Also *inferior border of pancreas.* **m. inferior pulmonis** [NA] The lower border of the lung, which is thin and sharp between the costal and the diaphragmatic surfaces and rounded between the mediastinal and the diaphragmatic surfaces. Also *inferior margin of lung.* **m. inferior splenis** [NA] The straight and rounded margin of the spleen which separates the renal impression of the visceral surface from the diaphragmatic surface. Normally it lies at the level of the lower margin of the left eleventh rib. Also *inferior border of spleen.* **m. infraorbitalis maxillae** [NA] The rounded anterior margin of the orbital surface of the maxilla, forming a portion of the circumference of the orbit at its junction with the anterior surface of the body of the maxilla and being continuous medially with the lacrimal crest on the frontal process. Also *infraorbital margin of maxilla.* **m. infraorbitalis orbitae** [NA] The sharp lower margin of the circumference of the orbital opening. It is formed medially by the infraorbital margin of maxilla meeting the orbital margin of the zygomatic bone laterally. Also *infraorbital margin of orbit.* **m. interosseus fibulae** [NA] A sharp ridge medial to the anterior margin of the fibula for the attachment of the interosseous membrane. Also *interosseous margin of fibula, interosseous border of fibula, interosseous ridge of fibula.* **m. interosseus radii** [NA] The conspicuous ridge on the medial side of the radius, between the anterior and the posterior surfaces. It commences proximally at the posterior part of the radial tuberosity, where it is rounded, and terminates distally by dividing and becoming continuous with the anterior and posterior borders of the ulnar notch. Also *interosseous border of radius, interosseous ridge of radius.* **m. interosseus tibiae** [NA] A prominent longitudinal ridge on the lateral side of the tibia extending from the front of the fibular articular surface proximally to the fibular notch, above which it divides around a rough triangular area for the interosseous ligament. Also *interosseous margin of tibia, interosseous border of tibia, interosseous ridge of tibia.* **m. interosseus ulnae** [NA] The prominent, sharp, middle two fourths of the lateral margin of the ulna. Also *interosseous border of ulna, interosseous margin of ulna, interosseous ridge of ulna.* **m. lacrimalis maxillae** [NA] The posterior border of the upper end of the frontal process of the maxilla that articulates with the lacrimal bone. Also *lacrimal border of maxilla, lacrimal margin of maxilla.* **m. lambdoideus squamae occipitalis** [NA] The serrated superolateral border on either side of the squamous part of the occipital bone, extending from the superior to the lateral angle and articulating with the occipital border of the parietal bone to form one half of the lambdoid suture. Also *lambdoid margin of occipital bone, lambdoid border of occipital bone, parietal margin of occipital bone.* **m. lateralis antebrachii** [NA] The outer, or radial, border of the forearm. Also *radial margin of forearm, margo radialis antebrachii.* **m. lateralis humeri** [NA] The outer border of the humerus, extending from the posteroinferior part of the greater tubercle to the lateral epicondyle. It is prominent only in its distal third where it provides attachment for the lateral intermuscular septum. Also *lateral margin of humerus, lateral border of humerus.* **m. lateralis pedis** [NA] The outer, or fibular, border of the foot, extending from the heel to the fifth toe. Also *lateral margin of foot, margo fibularis pedis.* **m. lateralis renis** [NA] The narrow convex outer border of the kidney separating the anterior or visceral surface from the posterior or parietal surface. Also *lateral margin of kidney.* **m. lateralis scapulae** [NA] The thick outer border of the scapula, extending from the lower margin of the glenoid cavity to the inferior angle. Also *lateral border of scapula, axillary margin of scapula, external margin of scapula, lateral margin of scapula.* **m. lateralis unguis** [NA] The edge on either side of a nail, extending from the proximal edge to the free border and partially covered by the nail wall. Also *lateral margin of nail.* **m. liber ovarii** [NA] The rounded, free border of the ovary directed into the rectouterine pouch of peritoneum and towards the ureter. Also *free margin of ovary.* **m. liber unguis** [NA] The distal free border of a nail that overlaps the tip of a digit. Also *free margin of nail.* **m. linguae** [NA] The free lateral border on each side of the tongue that separates the dorsum from the inferior surface and meets the opposite border at the apex. It is in contact with the gums and the teeth. Also *margin of tongue, lateral margin of tongue.* **m. mastoideus squamae occipitalis** [NA] The margin of the squamous part of the occipital bone. It extends from the lateral angle to the jugular process and articulates with the occipital margin of the petrous part of the temporal bone to form the occipitomastoid suture. Also *mastoid margin of occipital bone.* **m. medialis antebrachii** [NA] The inner, or ulnar, border of the forearm. Also *medial margin of forearm, ulnar margin of forearm, medial border of forearm.* **m. medialis glandulae suprarenalis** [NA] The paravertebral border of the suprarenal gland. Also *medial margin of suprarenal gland.* **m. medialis humeri** [NA] The inner border of the humerus. It commences at the lesser tubercle, continuing as the medial lip of the intertubercular sulcus for the attachment of the teres major muscle, and extends to the medial epicondyle. Also *medial margin of humerus, medial border of humerus.* **m. medialis pedis** [NA] The inner, or tibial, border of the foot, extending from the heel to the great toe. Also *medial margin of foot, medial border of foot, tibial margin of foot.* **m. medialis renis** [NA] The medial border of each kidney. It is concave in the center and convex over each pole above and below. Also *medial margin of kidney.* **m. medialis scapulae** [NA] The medial, and longest, border of the scapula, extending from the superior to the inferior angle. Also *vertebral margin of scapula.* **m. medialis tibiae** [NA] The inner border of the tibia. It is rounded proximally and distally but sharp in the middle, extending from the posterior part of the medial condyle to the posterior margin of the medial malleolus. The soleus muscle is attached to its middle third. Also *medial margin of tibia, medial border of tibia.* **m. mesovaricus ovarii** [NA] The straight border of the ovary which is attached to the back of the broad ligament of the uterus by the mesovarium and is directed towards the obliterated umbilical artery. Also *mesovarian margin of ovary, mesovarial margin of ovary.* **m. nasalis** [NA] The curved margin of the frontal bone that articulates with the nasal bones at the frontonasal suture. **m. nasalis ossis frontalis** [NA] The curved inferior edge of the nasal part of the frontal bone, on either side of the nasal spine, that articulates with the nasal bones and the frontal process of the maxilla. Also *nasal margin of frontal bone, nasal incisure of frontal bone.* **m. occipitalis ossis parietalis** [NA] The serrated posterior border of the parietal bone. It extends from the occipital angle to the mastoid angle and articulates with the parietal margin of the occipital bone to form one half of the lambdoid suture. Also *occipital margin of parietal bone.* **m. occipitalis ossis temporalis** [NA] A portion of the inferior margin of the posterior surface of the petrous part of the temporal bone that articulates with the occipital squama along the occipitomastoid suture. Also *occipital margin of temporal bone.* **m. occultus unguis** [NA] The irregular, thin proximal edge of a nail that is completely covered by the nail wall. Also *hidden margin of nail.* **m. orbitalis** The quadrangular base, or anterior boundary, of the orbital cavity. It comprises four margins, namely, margo supraorbitalis, margo infraorbitalis, margo lateralis, and margo medialis. Also *orbital margin.* **m. parietalis alae majoris** [NA] The superior extremity of the greater wing of the sphenoid bone that articulates with the sphenoidal angle of the parietal bone. Also *parietal margin of great wing of sphenoid bone, parietal angle of sphenoid bone.* **m. parietalis ossis frontalis** [NA] The thick, serrated posterior border of the frontal bone, semicircular in shape and beveled on its inner aspect. It articulates with the parietal bone. Also *parietal margin of frontal bone.* **m. parietalis ossis temporalis** [NA] The arched superior border of the squamous part of the temporal bone, beveled internally and overlapping the inferior border of the parietal bone to form the squamosal suture. Also *parietal margin of temporal bone.* **m. posterior fibulae** [NA] A ridge, ill-defined proximally, that extends from the back of the head of the fibula to the medial margin of the peroneal groove on the distal extremity. Also *posterior margin of fibula, crista lateralis fibulae, posterior border of fibula, lateral crest of fibula.* **m. posterior partis petrosae ossis temporalis** The border or margin on the petrous portion of the temporal bone that separates the inferior from the posterior surfaces. It is intermediate in length between the superior border and anterior angle. Its medial half helps to form the sulcus for the anterior petrosal sinus behind which and laterally is the jugular fossa that helps to form the jugular foramen. Also *posterior border of petrous portion of temporal bone, posterior angle of petrous portion of temporal bone.* **m. posterior radii** [NA] A ridge on the posterior aspect of the radius, extending from the posteroinferior part of the radial tuberosity to the region of the dorsal tubercle on the posterior aspect of the distal end of the radius. Also *posterior border of radius, dorsal margin of radius.* **m. posterior testis** [NA] The flattened posterior border of the testis, separating the medial and lateral surfaces and attached to the epididymis and spermatic cord laterally. In its upper two thirds is the mediastinum testis for the blood vessels and lymphatics of the testis. Also *posterior margin of testis, dorsum of testis.* **m. posterior ulnae** [NA] A thick, rounded crest that extends in a sinuous course from the apex of the posterior aspect of the subcutaneous olecranon to the styloid process and separates the posterior from the medial surface of the ulna. Also *posterior margin of ulna, dorsal margin of ulna.* **m. pupillaris iridis** [NA] The inner margin of the iris which surrounds the circular aperture of the pupil. It rests upon the front surface of the lens, which elevates it slightly, and it is edged by a finely notched, dark seam. Also *pupillary margin of iris.* **m. radialis antebrachii** MARGO LATERALIS ANTEBRACHII. **m. sagittalis ossis parietalis** [NA] The markedly serrated, thick medial edge of the parietal bone that articulates with the corresponding border of the opposite bone to form the sagittal suture. Also *sagittal margin of parietal bone, superior margin of parietal bone, parietal margin of parietal bone.* **m. sphenoidalis ossis temporalis** [NA] The anterior, serrated border of the squamous part of the temporal bone that articulates with the posterior margin of the greater wing of the sphenoid bone. Also *sphenoidal margin of temporal bone.* **m. squamosus alae majoris** [NA] The border of the greater wing of the sphenoid bone that extends forwards from the sphenoidal spine and is serrated and thinned to articulate with the squamous part of the temporal bone. Also *squamous margin of greater wing of sphenoid bone.* **m. squamosus ossis parietalis** [NA] The lateral or inferior edge of the parietal bone that is divided into three portions: a thin, short anterior portion that is overlapped by the parietal margin of the greater wing of the sphenoid bone; an arched, beveled middle portion overlapped by the squamous part of the temporal bone; and a short, thick and serrated posterior part that articulates with the mastoid portion of the temporal bone. Also *squamous margin of parietal bone, sphenotemporal margin of parietal bone, temporal margin of parietal bone.* **m. superior glandulae suprarenalis** [NA] The curved superolateral border of the suprarenal gland which joins the upper extremities of the medial border and the renal surface and separates the anterior from the posterior surface. Also *superior margin of suprarenal gland, superior border of suprarenal gland.* **m. superior pancreatis** [NA] The upper border of the pancreas which separates the anterior from the posterior surface. Also *superior border of pancreas, superior margin of pancreas.* **m. superior partis petrosae ossis temporalis** [NA] The border or margin that separates the anterior and posterior surfaces of the petrous portion of the temporal bone, of which it is the longest border. Also *superior border of petrous portion of temporal bone, superior angle of petrous portion of temporal bone, angulus superior pyramidis ossis temporalis.* **m. superior scapulae** [NA] The short, thin, upper border of the scapula extending from the coracoid process to the superior angle. Also *superior margin of scapula, superior border of scapula.* **m. superior splenis** [NA] The rounded, upper border of the spleen which separates the diaphragmatic surface from the gastric impression of the visceral surface. Also *superior margin of spleen, superior border of spleen, anterior margin of spleen, crenate margin of spleen.* **m. supraorbitalis orbitae** [NA] The sharp, arched upper margin of the circumference of the orbital opening formed by the supraorbital margin of the frontal bone and extending from its nasal margin to the zygomatic process. Also *supraorbital margin of orbit.* **m. supraorbitalis ossis frontalis** [NA] The curved anterior edge of the frontal bone at the junction of its external and orbital surfaces, articulating medially at its nasal margin with the frontal process of the maxilla and laterally at its zygomatic process with the zygomatic bone. It is interrupted by the supraorbital notch. Also *supraorbital margin of frontal bone, supraorbital arch of frontal bone, orbital arch of frontal bone.* **m. uteri dexter et sinister** [NA] The convex junction between the anterior and posterior surfaces on each side of the body of the uterus. It extends as far as the lateral angles where the uterine tubes enter the uterine wall, below which the broad ligament is attached as well as the round ligament of the uterus and the ligament of the ovary between its folds on each side. Also *lateral margin of uterus.* **m. zygomaticus alae majoris** [NA] The anterior border of the greater wing of the sphenoid bone. It separates its orbital and temporal surfaces and articulates inferiorly with the free edge of the orbital surface of the zygomatic bone, and often with the maxilla. Also *zygomatic margin of greater wing of sphenoid bone, zygomatic crest of great wing of sphenoid bone, malar crest of great wing of sphenoid bone.*

**Marie** [Pierre *Marie,* French physician, 1853–1940] **1** Bamberger-Marie disease, Marie-Bamberger disease, Marie-Bamberger syndrome. See under HYPERTROPHIC PULMONARY OSTEOARTHROPATHY. **2** Marie-Strümpell arthritis, Marie-Strümpell spondylitis, Marie-Strümpell disease, Strümpell-Marie disease. See under ANKYLOSING SPONDYLITIS. **3** Marie-Strümpell disease, Strümpell-Marie disease. See under ACUTE INFANTILE HEMIPLEGIA. **4** Quadrilateral space of Marie. See under SPACE. **5** See under HYPERTROPHY. **6** Nonne-Marie syndrome, Marie sclerosis. See under MARIE'S HEREDITARY CEREBELLAR ATAXIA. **7** Marie-Foix sign. See under SIGN. **8** Marie-Tooth disease, Charcot-Marie atrophy, Charcot-Marie-Tooth atrophy, Charcot-Marie-Tooth-Hoffmann syndrome. See under CHARCOT-MARIE-TOOTH DISEASE. **9** Marie syndrome. See under ACROMEGALY.

**marihuana** \mar′əʰwä′nə\ [Mexican Spanish *marihuana,* also *mariguana*] The dried leaves, stems, and flowers of *Cannabis sativa.* It is smoked or used in foods. It produces distorted perception and sometimes hallucinogenic effects. Also *ganja, subjee, churganja.* Also *marijuana.*

**Marin Amat** [Manuel *Marin Amat,* Spanish ophthalmologist, born 1879] Marin Amat phenomenon. See under SYNDROME.

**Marinesco** [Georges *Marinesco,* Rumanian pathologist, 1863–1938] Marinesco-Garland syndrome, Marinesco-Sjögren-Garland syndrome. See under MARINESCO-SJÖGREN SYNDROME.

**marinobufagin** A toxin produced by the skin glands of *Bufo marinus,* a marine toad, which secretes an extremely toxic venom. Its action is similar to that of the cardiac glycosides.

**Marion** [Georges *Marion,* French urologist, 1869–1932] See under DISEASE.

**Mariotte** [Edmé *Mariotte,* French physicist, 1620–1684] **1** See under EXPERIMENT. **2** Mariotte's law. See under BOYLE'S LAW.

**Marjolin** [Jean Nicolas *Marjolin,* French physician, 1780–1850] Marjolin's ulcer. See under BURN SCAR CARCINOMA.

**mark** [Old English *mearc;* akin to L *margo* margin] A sign or spot on a surface, as a circumscribed area of skin visibly different from the surrounding skin. **birth m.** See under BIRTHMARK. **current m.** A cutaneous lesion produced by the passage of electrical current through the skin, a sign that may be useful in forensic pathology. However, current marks may or may not cause death and cannot be uniformly distinguished from similar appearing lesions produced by other causes. Not all contacts with electrical current produce current marks. They do not appear in circumstances in which the current contacts a large surface area of the body, lasts only a few seconds, and is of low amperage. **hesitation m.'s** See under HESITATION WOUNDS. **lightning m.** An erythematous line, usually 2–8 cm wide, and extending continuously or discontinuously in a craniocaudal direction on the skin surface of a person struck by lightning. It is essentially identical to a first degree thermal burn except for the pattern which is fernlike and arborescent. It may not be visible until several hours after the lightning strikes. **mulberry m.** A dark-colored variety of strawberry nevus. Also *nevus morus.* **pock m.** See under POCKMARK. **quillon m.** An abrasion adjacent to a stab wound which is produced by the impact of the quillon or guard separating the blade from the handle of the knife. **raspberry m.** STRAWBERRY NEVUS. **strawberry m.** STRAWBERRY NEVUS.

**marker** [MARK + -ER] **1** Something used to mark. **2** ANTIGENIC DETERMINANT. **Crane-Kaplan pocket m.** A modified form of dental tweezer for marking the depth of a pocket on the oral surface of the gingiva prior to gingivectomy. **genetic m.** Any distinct phenotype, determined by a single gene or mutant allele, that can be used in experimental genetics for such purposes as estimating the linkage distance between two loci in recombination analysis. **time m.** On a graphic recorder, an instrument that marks the time at regular intervals such as every second.

**marking** / **Fontana's m.'s** Fine, superficial, transverse indentations seen on branching peripheral nerves.

**Maroteaux** [Pierre *Maroteaux,* French physician, born 1926] **1** Maroteaux-Lamy disease. See under DISEASE. **2** Maroteaux-Lamy syndrome. See under MUCOPOLYSACCHARIDOSIS VI.

**Marriott** [Williams McKim *Marriott,* U.S. physician, 1885–1936] Levy, Rowntree, and Marriott method. See under METHOD.

**marrow** \mar′ō\ [Old English *maerg* (akin to German *Mark* marrow and Russian *mozg* marrow, medulla, brain) bone marrow] MEDULLA. **bone m.** The soft mesenchymal tissue occupying the cavities within bone, consisting of a reticular meshwork filled with fat, blood cells, and their precursors; medulla ossium. Also *medulla of bone, medullary substance of bone.* **depressed m.** Bone marrow with abnormally decreased production of blood cells. **fat m.** YELLOW BONE MARROW. **gelatinous m.** Marrow that has lost its normal cellular elements and fat. It resembles gelatin in gross appearance, due to a relative increase in glycosaminoglycan-rich ground substance. **red bone m.** Bone marrow that produces formed blood elements. Also *red marrow, primary marrow, hemopoietic marrow, medulla ossium rubra.* **spinal m.** MEDULLA SPINALIS. **yellow bone m.** Adipose tissue in which the connective tissue supports predominantly fat cells and only a few primitive blood cells. It is found mostly in long bones. Also *yellow marrow, fat marrow, medulla ossium flava, yellow medullary substance of bones.*

**marrowbrain** \mar′ōbrān\ *Older term* MYELENCEPHALON.

**Marshall** [Don *Marshall,* U.S. ophthalmologist, born 1905] See under SYNDROME.

**Marshall** [John *Marshall,* English anatomist, 1818–1891] **1** Accompanying artery of vein of Marshall. See under ARTERY. **2** Vein of Marshall, Marshall's oblique vein. See under VENA OBLIQUA ATRII SINISTRI.

**Marshall** [Victor F. *Marshall,* U.S. urologist, born 1913] Marshall-Marchetti operation. See under OPERATION.

**Marshall Hall** [*Marshall Hall,* English physiologist, 1790–1857] Marshall Hall's facies. See under FACIES.

**marsupia** \märsooʹpē·ə\ Plural of MARSUPIUM.

**marsupialization** \märsooʹpē·əlīzāʹshən\ [*marsupi(um)* + -AL + *-iz(e)* + -ATION] A method of treating a dental or other large cyst when complete removal of the cyst lining is not possible. A wide opening is made and it is maintained by the use of an obturator which is gradually reduced in depth as the cyst cavity becomes shallower. Also *Partsch's operation.*

**marsupium** \märsooʹpē·əm\ [L (from Gk *marsipion, marsypion* a small bag or pouch, dim. of *marsipos, marsypos* a bag or pouch), a purse, pouch] (*pl.* marsupia) **1** The abdominal pouch of a female marsupial. It contains the teats and is the site of extensive postgestation development of the young. **2** SCROTUM.

**Martin** [August E. *Martin,* German gynecologist, 1847–1933] See under PELVIMETER.

**Martin** [Henry Austin *Martin,* U.S. surgeon, 1824–1884] See under DISEASE.

**Martinotti** [Giovanni *Martinotti,* Italian physician, 1857–1928] See under CELL, NEURON.

**Martius** [Karl Alexander *Martius,* German chemist, 1838–1920] See under YELLOW.

**Martorell** [Fernando *Martorell,* Spanish physician, born 1906] Martorell syndrome. See under TAKAYASU'S ARTERITIS.

**maschale** \masʹkəlē\ [Gk *maschalē* armpit] FOSSA AXILLARIS.

**masculine** [L *masculinus* (from *masculus* male, masculine, from *mas* the male of humans, animals, and plants) masculine, manly, male] Of or relating to the male sex; having the qualities characteristic of men.

**masculinity** \masʹkyəlinʹitē\ The state of being masculine; possession of the normal characteristics of men. Also *virilism.*

**masculinization** \masʹkyəlinīzāʹshən\ [*masculiniz(e)* + -ATION] **1** VIRILIZATION. **2** Normal development of secondary sex characters in the male.

**masculinize** \masʹkyəlinīzʹ\ [L *masculin(us)* pertaining to the male + -IZE] **1** To induce the development in the male of male secondary sex characters. **2** VIRILIZE.

**masculinizing** \masʹkyəlinīzʹing\ VIRILIZING.

**masculinovoblastoma** \masʹkyəlinōʹvəblastōʹmə\ [*masculin(e)* + OVO- + BLASTOMA] An ovarian tumor causing masculinization.

**masculonucleus** \masʹkyəlōnʸooʹklē·əs\ [L *mascul(inus)* male, masculine + *o* + NUCLEUS] MALE PRONUCLEUS.

**MASH** mobile army surgical hospital.

**mask** [French *masque* (from Italian *máschera* a mask, cover, from Med L *masca* a witch) a false face with cartoon painting] **1** A gauze covering for the nose and mouth to preserve antiseptic conditions or to prevent the spread of infection. **2** A patient's facial expression or characteristic facial appearance as affected by disease, such as Parkinson's facies. **3** A metal frame covered with gauze placed over the face of a patient for the administration of inhalation anesthesia. **4** To cover metal parts of (a denture) with an opaque material. **BLB m.** An oxygen mask used at high altitudes, having a combined inspiratory and expiratory valve in a rebreathing bag. • The mask is named after its designers, Boothby, Lovelace, and Bulbulian. **full-face m.** A device fitting tightly over the nose and mouth and used for general inhalation anesthesia or respiratory assistance. **Hutchinson's m.** TABETIC MASK. **luetic m.** A masklike pigmentation and depigmentation of the upper face that is associated with the late stages of syphilis. **nonrebreathing m.** A tight-fitting mask placed over the nose and mouth in order to permit the inhalation of fresh gas during general anesthesia or respiratory assistance, while allowing for the elimination of expired gas without rebreathing. **Parkinson's m.** The expressionless face that is characteristic of parkinsonism. **partial rebreathing m.** An oxygen mask which permits some of the exhaled air to be rebreathed. **m. of pregnancy** MELASMA GRAVIDARUM. **tabetic m.** A sense of tightness of the skin of the face experienced by some patients with tabes dorsalis. Also *Hutchinson's mask.* **tracheostomy m.** A mask placed over a tracheostomy for delivery of oxygen or humidity. **Venturi m.** A mask that delivers a constant concentration of oxygen, using the Venturi principle of entrainment of air to dilute the flow of pure oxygen.

**masked** \maskt\ Disguised or hidden by unrelated symptoms or organisms, as when a reducing diet conceals signs of a wasting disease.

**masker** \masʹkər\ **tinnitus m.** A device, resembling an ear-level hearing aid, for use in the treatment of tinnitus. An extraneous noise is produced by the instrument and adjusted with the aim of masking the subjective noise experienced by the patient.

**masking** \masʹking\ The process by which one perceptible event or activity is rendered imperceptible by another. In audiology it refers to the process by which a sound of a particular frequency is rendered inaudible by a louder sound the frequency spectrum of which includes the frequency of the occluded or masked sound. It is of special importance in determining the auditory threshold of a deafened ear in the presence of normal hearing in the other ear: the normal ear must be exposed to an appropriate level of masking noise of the appropriate frequency spectrum in order to avoid a spurious result. That is, the level of hearing in the deafened ear might be assessed as better than it should be, owing to the test sound's being picked up by the better hearing ear. **central m.** The masking effect on heard sounds that is induced by the central, neural interaction between the two ears.

**masochism** \masʹəkizm\ [after Leopold von Sacher-*Masoch,* 1835–1895, Austrian novelist, who introduced masochism into his stories, + -ISM] **1** A paraphilia in which the individual has a preference for or need to be humiliated, beaten, or otherwise subjected to suffering in order to achieve sexual arousal. Also *algophilia* (obs.), *passive algolagnia.* **2** A general pattern of self-destructive behavior that invites abuse, exploitation, or mistreatment by others.

**masochist** \masʹəkist\ A person having an inclination toward masochism.

**mas. pil.** *massa pilularum* (L, pill mass).

**mass** [L *massa.* See MASSA.] **1** The quantitative measure of inertia, that is, of resistance to acceleration. **2** A collection of tissue; body; massa. **achromatic m.** A nonstaining mass of protoplasm which surrounds the chromosomes during mitosis and meiosis. **atomic m.** The mass of a neutral atom of a given species, categorized as physical or chemical. Also *atomic weight* (imprecise but customary). Symbol: m, $m_a$ • The International Organization for Standardization (ISO) recommends that the term *atomic mass* be applied only to the value in SI units, i.e., kilograms. A separate term, *relative atomic mass,* is to be used for the dimensionless number obtained by dividing the mass of an atom in atomic mass units. This distinction, however, is rarely observed. **blue m.** MERCURY MASS. **cell m.**

The active metabolizing tissue in the body. In an active lean healthy individual, it represents approximately 55% of the total body weight. In an obese person, the figure is much less. It may be calculated by multiplying cell water by 100/70. Since 70% of the whole cell mass is water, cell water is calculated by subtracting extracellular water from total body water. Cell mass may also be measured from an assessment of total potassium 40 in the body using a whole-body counter. **chemical atomic m.** The average atomic mass of the naturally occurring isotopes of an atom, weighted according to their relative abundances. **critical m.** The minimum mass of fissionable material capable of maintaining a chain reaction. **electronic m.** The mass of an electron, $9.1 \times 10^{-28}$ gram. **injection m.** A solution that is injected into vascular or other spaces of a tissue or organ to form a permanent cast of that structure. The surrounding tissue is subsequently either dissolved or rendered transparent. **inner cell m.** The initial small group of cells which segregates within the enveloping trophoblast at one pole of the hollow mammalian blastocyst and which is destined to develop into the embryo. **intermediate m.** ADHESIO INTERTHALAMICA. **intermediate cell m.** A mass of mesoderm in early embryos situated between the medially placed paraxial mesoderm and the lateral plate mesoderm. In human embryos it becomes fused from the eighth somite caudally into an unsegmented column, termed the nephrogenic cord. The nephrotomes develop in the metameric segments of the cord to give rise to three embryonic kidney systems: pronephros, mesonephros, and metanephros. **lateral m. of atlas** MASSA LATERALIS ATLANTIS. **lateral m. of ethmoid bone** LABYRINTHUS ETHMOIDALIS. **lateral m. of occipital bone** PARS LATERALIS OSSIS OCCIPITALIS. **lateral m. of sacrum** PARS LATERALIS OSSIS SACRI. **lean body m.** The weight of the fat-free component of the body. **mercury m.** A mixture of mercury oleate, mercury, honey, glycerin, and other ingredients formerly used for the treatment of pediculosis pubis. Also *blue mass, massa hydrargyri.* **molecular m.** The mass of a molecule of given chemical species, equal to the sum of the masses of the atoms of which the molecule is composed. The numerical value of the molecular mass in atomic mass units (or daltons) is equal to the relative molecular mass. **muscle m.** The total amount of muscle found in the body of a human or other animal. Urinary excretion of creatinine is often used as an estimate of muscle mass in the presence of normal renal function. However, this is subject to a twofold error as muscle creatine concentrations vary from 0.3%–0.5%. **physical atomic m.** Atomic mass of a single isotope. Its value in atomic mass units is very nearly equal to the mass number of the isotope. Also *isotopic mass, isotopic weight* (rare and imprecise). **pilular m.** A soft, solid drug of a consistency suitable for being made into pills. Also *pill mass.* **relative atomic m.** The mass of a nuclide in atomic mass units, where the atomic mass unit is defined as 1/12 the mass of the nuclide carbon 12. **relative molecular m.** The quantity characteristic of a substance obtained by dividing the mass of its molecule by the atomic mass unit or dalton. It is therefore a dimensionless number, equal to the numerical part of the molar mass of the substance in g/mol and to that of the molecular mass in daltons. Symbol: $M_r$ • *Molecular weight* is the common usage, although *relative molecular mass* is more accurate. See note at MOLECULAR MASS. **relativistic m.** The increased mass of a body due to its velocity. Change in mass is negligible until the velocity approaches that of light. **sarcoplasmic m.'es** Masses of undifferentiated sarcoplasm not containing myofibrils as seen in transverse sections of skeletal muscle in the periphery of some muscle fibers, especially in patients with dystrophia myotonica. **Stent's m.** STENT DRESSING. **total red cell m.** The total volume of erythrocytes in the blood. **ventrolateral m.** A ventrolateral, hypaxial, division of the myotome which gives rise to the ventral and lateral trunk muscles, supplied by the anterior primary rami of the spinal nerves. Also *hypomere.*

**massa** \mas′ə\ [L (from Gk *maza* barley bread, barley cake, from *massein* to knead), a lump, mass] [NA] A cohesion of tissue. **m. hydrargyri** MERCURY MASS. **m. innominata** PARADIDYMIS. **m. intermedia** ADHESIO INTERTHALAMICA. **m. lateralis atlantis** One of two bulky portions of the atlas, each with superior and inferior articular facets. They are connected to each other by the anterior and the posterior arches. On the medial aspect of each is a small tubercle for the transverse ligament and on the lateral aspect is the transverse process. Also *lateral mass of atlas.* **m. mollis** *Obs.* ADHESIO INTERTHALAMICA.

**massae** \mas′ē\ Plural of MASSA.

**massage** [French (from *masser* to massage, from Arabic *mass* to touch, palpate) the act of massaging] Therapeutic stimulation of soft tissue by manual or mechanical means. **cardiac m.** Rhythmic manual compression of the heart either through a thoracotomy (open cardiac massage) or by pressure applied to the sternum (closed cardiac massage), used as a means of resuscitation when the heart has stopped beating or is beating very feebly. Also *cardiac compression, heart massage.* **carotid sinus m.** Massage of the carotid sinus by firm stroking in the region of the sinus, a technique used to cause reflex slowing of the heart, particularly for the identification or correction of supraventricular tachycardias. **electrovibratory m.** Superficial stimulation of the skin and underlying muscles by use of an electrical device that produces mechanical vibration. **heart m.** CARDIAC MASSAGE. **nerve-point m.** Deep friction massage localized to points of tenderness as described by Alfons Cornelius in Berlin in 1909. It might be considered a precursor of modern trigger point massage. **spray m.** Spray application of a vapo-coolant such as ethyl chloride for the relief of muscle spasm and myofascial pain. **trigger point m.** Focal massage directed to the "breaking up" of trigger points, that is, local diminution of pain probably related to vasodilation. See also NERVE-POINT MASSAGE.

**massc.** mass concentration.

**masseter** \masē′tər\ [irreg. from Gk *masētēr* (from *masasthai* to chew) a chewer, muscle of the lower jaw used in chewing] MUSCULUS MASSETER.

**masseteric** \mas′əter′ik\ Of or relating to the masseter muscle.

**masseur** \məsur′, masœr′\ [French, from *mass(er)* to knead, massage + *-eur* -ER] A person trained in, or who practices, the art and techniques of massage. • In current usage *masseur* may refer either to a man or a woman, and usually designates a lay practitioner or one whose profession is limited to massage.

**masseuse** \məsoos′, masœz′\ [French, fem. of MASSEUR] A female masseur.

**massfr.** mass fraction.

**Masson** [Claude Laurent Pierre *Masson*, French-born Canadian pathologist, 1880–1959] Masson stain, Masson's trichrome method. See under MASSON'S TRICHROME STAIN.

**mast-** \mast-\ MASTO-.

**mastadenitis** \mas′tadənī′tis\ [MAST- + ADENITIS] MASTITIS.

**mastadenovirus** \mastad′ənōvī′rəs\ A member of the genus *Mastadenovirus* in the family Adenoviridae, which includes all adenovirus species isolated from mammalian hosts. Most viruses of the genus, except some bovine strains, share a common antigen absent in the aviadenoviruses. Over 50 serotypes have been described. The virions are naked, ether-resistant, icosahedral particles, 70–80 nm in diameter. They contain a linear, double-stranded DNA genome with a mass of 20–25 million daltons.

**mastalgia** \mastal′jə\ [MAST- + -ALGIA] MASTODYNIA.

**mastecchymosis** \mastek′imō′sis\ [MAST- + ECCHYMOSIS] Subcutaneous hemorrhage in the breast, which creates a blue or purple patch.

**mastectomy** \mastek′təmē\ [MAST- + -ECTOMY] Removal of the breast. Also *mammectomy.* **radical m.** A mastectomy involving the pectoral muscles, axillary lymph nodes, and associated skin and subcutaneous tissue, in breast cancer. Also *Halsted radical mastectomy, Meyer's operation, Halsted's operation.* **simple m.** Removal of the breast only. **subcutaneous m.** A mastectomy wherein the areola and sufficient skin are preserved in preparation for reconstruction of the breast by means of a mammary implant. It is used for mastodynia and for the prophylaxis of breast cancer, but not in the treatment of breast cancer.

**Master** [Arthur Matthew *Master,* U.S. cardiologist, 1895–1973] See under TEST.

**mastic** \mas′tik\ [Gk *mastichē* (akin to *mastichan* to gnash the teeth) mastic gum] A resinous exudate from *Pistacia lentiscus,* composed primarily of mastichic acid and masticin. It has been used as a carminative, as an ingredient in temporary dental fillings and cavity varnishes, and in commercial varnishes and perfumes.

**masticate** \mas′tikāt\ [Late L *masticat(us),* past part. of *masticare* (from Gk *mastichan* to gnash the teeth, from *mastax* the jaws, a mouthful) to chew] To chew (food) in preparation for swallowing.

**Mastigophora** \mas′tigäf′ərə\ [New L, from Gk *mastigophoros* (from *mastix* whip, scourge + *pherein* to bear, carry) whip-bearing] A subphylum of protozoa characterized by having one or more flagella, particularly in the trophozoite stage of development. Most species are free-living but many are found as parasites of invertebrates and vertebrates, including humans. The taxon includes the classes Phytomastigophorea and Zoomastigophorea. Also *Euflagellata* (former name).

**mastigophoran** \mas′tigäf′ərən\ **1** Pertaining or belonging to the subphylum Mastigophora. **2** A member of the subphylum Mastigophora; a mastigote or flagellate.

**mastigote** \mas′tigōt\ [irreg. from Gk *mastix,* gen. *mastigos,* a whip, scourge] A member of the subphylum Mastigophora; a flagellate.

**mastitis** \mastī′tis\ [MAST- + -ITIS] Inflammation of the mammary gland or breast. Also *mastadenitis, mammitis.* **acute m.** Inflammation or infection of the breast with rapid onset. **chronic cystic m.** CYSTIC MASTOPATHY. **glandular m.** Inflammatory disease of the breast that involves the lactiferous tubules. Also *parenchymatous mastitis.* **interstitial m.** An inflammatory disease of the breast in which bacteria gain access to the connective tissue through a crack or deep fissure. Also *phlegmonous mastitis.* **m. neonatorum** **1** An infection of the breast tissue in neonates. **2** The enlargement and secretory activity of the breasts (witch's milk) which is common in infants of both sexes in the first days of life. **parenchymatous m.** GLANDULAR MASTITIS. **periductal m.** Inflammation of tissues about the ducts of the breast. **phlegmonous m.** INTERSTITIAL MASTITIS. **plasma cell m.** Mastitis in which inspissation and stasis are present, making this a chemical rather than a bacterial inflammation. Those affected are usually multiparas. **puerperal m.** Postpartum inflammation of the breast. **stagnation m.** Inflammation or local engorgement in a galactocele in a lactating woman. **submammary m.** SUBMAMMARY ABSCESS. **suppurative m.** Inflammation of the breast due to infection by pyogenic bacteria.

**masto-** \mas′tō-, mas′tə-\ [Gk *mastos* a woman's breast] A combining form denoting (1) the breast or mammary glands; (2) the mastoid process. Also *mast-*.

**mastoccipital** \mas′täksip′itəl\ MASTO-OCCIPITAL.

**mastocyte** \mas′təsīt\ MAST CELL.

**mastocytogenesis** \-sī′təjen′əsis\ The development and maturation of mast cells.

**mastocytoma** \-sītō′mə\ A tumor of mast cells. **solitary m.** An isolated cutaneous tumor that consists of an aggregate of mast cells.

**mastocytosis** \-sītō′sis\ [*mastocyt(e)* + -OSIS] **1** Infiltration of tissues by mast cells. **2** An increased number of mast cells in bone marrow. For defs. 1 and 2 also *mast cell disease.* See also URTICARIA PIGMENTOSA. **diffuse cutaneous m.** A benign but widespread increase in the number of mast cells in the dermis. Thickening and pigmentation of the overlying epidermis is common. **malignant m.** MAST CELL LEUKEMIA. **systemic m.** A widespread form of mast cell proliferation with involvement of skin (urticaria pigmentosa), liver, lymph nodes, intestinal tract, bone, and bone marrow.

**mastodynia** \-din′ē·ə\ [MAST- + -ODYNIA] Pain in the breast. Also *mammalgia, mastalgia, mazodynia.*

**mastoid** \mas′toid\ [MAST- + -OID] **1** Resembling a nipple or breast in shape. **2** PROCESSUS MASTOIDEUS OSSIS TEMPORALIS. **3** Of or relating to the mastoid process, the mastoid antrum, or the mastoid cells. Also *mastoidal.* **acellular m.** SCLEROTIC MASTOID. **diploic m.** The mastoid process of the temporal bone in the early stage of development, when it is occupied by bone marrow, that is, before pneumatization has occurred. In some individuals this diploic pattern persists into adult life. **ivory m.** SCLEROTIC MASTOID. **pneumatized m.** The mastoid process of the temporal bone in its normal cellular state, that is, honeycombed with air cells of variable size. Also *pneumatic mastoid.* **sclerotic m.** The mastoid process of the temporal bone when neither air cells nor marrow spaces are found and the process throughout is of the consistency of ivory. Also *acellular mastoid, ivory mastoid.*

**mastoidal** \mastoi′dəl\ MASTOID.

**mastoidale** \mas′toidā′lē\ In craniometry, the lowest point of the mastoid process.

**mastoidectomy** \mas′toidek′təmē\ [MASTOID + -ECTOMY] Any operation requiring removal of part of the mastoid process of the temporal bone, with the object of eradicating disease and/or gaining access to deeper parts, especially the middle-ear spaces. Also *mastoid operation.* **Bondy m.** MODIFIED RADICAL MASTOIDECTOMY. **combined approach m.** Radical or modified radical mastoidectomy in which access is gained to the sites of disease by both the transmastoid and transmeatal routes, leaving intact the posterosuperior bony canal wall so as to facilitate subsequent tympanoplasty. **conservative m.** SIMPLE MASTOIDECTOMY. • The operation is conservative in the sense that it avoids interference with the sound-conduction apparatus of the middle ear, thus conserving the potential for normal hearing. **cortical m.** SIMPLE MASTOIDECTOMY. • The operation was designed to provide access to the diseased air cells by removal of a portion of the cortical bone of the mastoid process. **modified radical m.** An operation undertaken as an alternative to radical mastoidectomy, when it is judged that certain middle-ear structures may be safely and advantageously conserved, for example the pars tensa of the tympanic membrane and the attached malleus handle. Also *Bondy mastoidectomy, Bondy operation.* **radical m.** The excision of all diseased tissues in the tympanic portion (tympanectomy) as well as the mastoid portion of the middle-ear cleft. Access to the tympanum is gained by removing a large part of the bone of the posterior meatal and outer attic walls and preserved by creating suitable flaps of the posterior meatal skin. The usual indication is cholesteatoma. Currently, intact canal wall techniques are often preferred. Also *mastoidotympanectomy.* **Schwartze m.** SIMPLE MASTOIDECTOMY. **simple m.** The classical operation for the relief of acute mastoiditis, intended to achieve exenteration of all infected mastoid air cells, to exclude spread of disease to important adjacent structures, such as the meninges, and to restore normal hearing. Also *Schwartze mastoidectomy, Schwartze's operation, cortical mastoidectomy, conservative mastoidectomy.*

**mastoiditis** \mas′toidī′tis\ [MASTOID + -ITIS] Inflammation of the mastoid process of the temporal bone involving at first the mucoendosteum of the air cells but in more severe cases resulting in osteitis and sometimes a subperiosteal abscess behind or beneath the ear. It occurs as a complication of acute suppurative otitis media. **Bezold's m.** Mastoiditis leading to destruction of the mastoid tip on its medial aspect, and abscess formation (Bezold's abscess) deep to the upper fibers of the sternomastoid muscle. **coalescent m.** Mastoiditis in a cellular mastoid process where destruction of the cell walls results in more or less extensive cavitation. **masked m.** Mastoiditis in the absence of overt physical signs such as swelling and tenderness over the mastoid process. It is a potentially dangerous condition, usually occurring as a consequence of inadequate antibiotic treatment. Also *silent mastoiditis.* **silent m.** MASKED MASTOIDITIS. **tuberculous m.** A rare manifestation of tuberculous otitis media, with its highest incidence in childhood. It is usually diagnosed only after laboratory reports on granulation tissue are obtained at mastoidectomy. **zygomatic m.** Acute mastoiditis spreading forward into zygomatic air cells and presenting as a swelling in front of the ear over the zygomatic process of the temporal bone.

**mastoidotympanectomy** \mastoi′dōtim′pənek′təmē \ RADICAL MASTOIDECTOMY.

**mastomenia** \-mē′nē·ə\ [MASTO- + Gk *mēn* month + -IA] Vicarious menstruation from the breast.

***Mastomys natalensis*** \mas′təmis nā′təlen′sis\ A species of rat which is widely distributed in Africa. In west Africa it is a host of Lassa virus.

**masto-occipital** \-äksip′itəl\ Of or relating to the mastoid process of the temporal bone and the occipital bone. Also *mastoccipital.*

**mastoparietal** \mas′tōpərī′ətəl\ PARIETOMASTOID.

**mastopathia** \-path′ē·ə\ [MASTO- + -PATHIA] MASTOPATHY. **m. cystica** CYSTIC MASTOPATHY.

**mastopathy** \mastäp′əthē\ [MASTO- + -PATHY] Any disease of the mammary glands. Also *mastopathia.* **cystic m.** A breast condition in which cysts are formed and the breast has an indurated consistency primarily in the upper quadrants. Also *shotty breast, cystic breast, adenocystic disease, Bloodgood's disease, cystic disease of breast, fibrocystic disease of breast, Schimmelbusch disease, mammary dysplasia, cystic hyperplasia of the breasts, chronic cystic mastitis, mastopathia cystica, mastosis.*

**mastopexy** \mas′təpek′sē\ [MASTO- + -PEXY] A plastic operation on the breast to eliminate ptosis and restore a youthful contour. This usually requires relocation of the nipple. Also *mazopexy.*

***Mastophora gasteracanthoides*** \mastäf′ərə gas′tərak′anthoi′dēz\ The cat-headed spider of Argentina, Chile, and Peru, whose bite causes necrotic sores among vineyard workers.

**mastoplastia** \-plas′tē·ə\ [MASTO- + *-plast(y)* + -IA] Hyperplasia and hypertrophy of the breast.

**mastoplasty** \mas′təplas′tē\ [MASTO- + -PLASTY] MAMMOPLASTY.

**mastoptosis** \mas′tōtō′sis\ [MASTO- + PTOSIS] Dropping of the breasts.

**mastorrhagia** \mas′tôrā′jə\ [MASTO- + -RRHAGIA] Hemorrhage from a breast.

**mastoscirrhus** \-skir′əs\ [MASTO- + SCIRRHUS] Hardening of the breast, usually as the effect of a carcinoma.

**mastosis** \mastō′sis\ [MASTO- + -SIS] CYSTIC MASTOPATHY.

**mastosquamous** \-skwā′məs\ Of or relating to the mastoid and squamous parts of the temporal bone.

**mastostomy** \mastäs′təmē\ [MASTO- + -STOMY] Incision of the breast for drainage of blood or pus. Also *mastotomy.*

**mastosyrinx** \-sir′ingks\ [MASTO- + Gk *syrinx* a pipe, windpipe, fistula, nostrils, trachea] A fistula of the breast.

**mastotomy** \mastät′əmē\ [MASTO- + -TOMY] MASTOSTOMY.

**masturbation** \mas′tərbā′shən\ [L *masturbatus,* past part. of *masturbari* (prob. from *ma(nus)* hand + *stuprare* to defile, deflower) to masturbate] Self-manipulation of the genitals to achieve sexual gratification. In the adolescent and adult, masturbation is usually accompanied by frankly sexual fantasies.

**Masugi** [Matazo *Masugi,* Japanese pathologist, flourished 20th century] See under NEPHRITIS.

**masurium** [New L (after *Masuria,* a region in northern Poland + suffix *-ium*), former name of chemical element 43] *Outmoded* TECHNETIUM.

**Matas** [Rudolph *Matas,* U.S. surgeon, 1860–1957] See under TREATMENT, OPERATION.

**matching** 1 Comparison, selection, or adjustment for compatibility or similarity. 2 A reduction in the effects of an impedance difference at a boundary by inserting a material of intermediate impedance value. **impedance m.** Assistance to the passage of sound waves across an interface between media of different acoustic impedance such as is provided by the transformer mechanism of the middle ear to the passage of sound waves from air to the inner ear fluids.

**Mátéfy** [Ladislaus *Mátéfy,* Hungarian physician, born 1889] Mátéfy's reaction. See under TEST.

**materia** \mətir′ē·ə\ [L (from *mater* mother, source + *-ia,* derivative noun suffix) substance, material] Matter; substance. **m. alba** A soft whitish deposit on the teeth consisting of food debris, desquamated cells, and unorganized microorganisms. It is easily washed away with a water spray. This deposit has been confused with dental plaque. **m. medica** The medical science that deals with the origin and preparation of drugs, their administration, and mode of action; pharmacology.

**material** [MATERIA + L *-alis* -AL] The substance of which something is made or composed. **air-equivalent m.** In radiology, any material having the same effective atomic number as air in respect to the absorption of x rays. **cross-reacting m.** A mutated form of an enzyme or other biologically active molecule that has lost biological activity but can be detected and quantitated by antibody to the native molecule. Such products have been very important in relating biological function to protein structure. Abbr. CRM **fissionable m.** Material containing, as a major component, one or more elements whose nuclei are capable of dividing into two very roughly equal fragments, or of being stimulated to do so by bombardment with suitable subatomic projectiles (usually neutrons). The process entails conversion of some mass into a relatively huge amount of energy. The most important of the fissionable nuclides are uranium 235 and plutonium 239. **genetic m.** The molecules that constitute genes; principally deoxyribonucleic acid. **impression m.** One of the many substances used for taking impressions, such as plaster of Paris, alginate, hydrocolloid, compound, or elastomeric. **target m.** That material which is the object of bombardment by high energy subatomic particles for the purpose of producing nuclear reactions within the material. **tissue equivalent m.** A material whose properties are similar in some manner, as in radiation absorption, to average human tissue. **trace m.** An element which exists in extremely minute amounts in tissues or other materials.

**materialization** \mətir′ē·əlīzā′shən\ PAIR PRODUCTION.

**materies** \mətir′i·ēz\ [see MATERIA.] Substance.

**maternal** \mətur′nəl\ [Med L *maternal(is)* (from L *matern(us)* pertaining to a mother + *-alis* -AL) maternal] **1** Of or pertaining to a mother; motherly. **2** Derived or received from a mother.

**maternity** [Med L *maternitas* (from L *maternus* maternal, motherly, from *mater* mother; Gk *mētēr* mother; + L *-itas* -ITY) maternity, motherhood] **1** The condition of being a mother; motherhood. **2** An obstetric hospital.

**maternohemotherapy** \mətur′nōhē′mōther′əpē\ [*matern(al)* + *o* + HEMO- + THERAPY] The injection of infants with blood from their mothers, with the intention of transferring immunity to such diseases as tetanus, measles, or poliomyelitis.

**Mathieu** [Albert *Mathieu*, French physician, 1855–1917] Lancereaux-Mathieu disease, Mathieu's disease. See under ICTERIC LEPTOSPIROSIS.

**mating** **1** The union of a pair of individuals for the purpose of sexual reproduction. Mating usually involves individuals of different sex, but it may involve pairs of hermaphroditic forms. **2** In bacteriology, the process in which a plasmid transfers part of the bacterial chromosome from donor to recipient cell; bacterial conjugation. **backcross m.** BACKCROSS.

**matrical** \mat′rikəl\ Of or relating to a matrix. Also *matricial.*

**matrices** \mā′trisēz\ Plural of MATRIX.

**matricial** \mətrish′əl\ MATRICAL.

**matrilineal** \mā′trilin′ē·əl\ Pertaining to or limited to the female line, as in cytoplasmic inheritance.

**matrix** \mā′triks\ [L (from *mater* mother, source) a breeding female animal; later, a womb, roll, list] (*pl.* matrices) **1** The intercellular substance in a tissue. **2** A mold, for a dental restoration, in the form of a thin steel or plastic strip surrounding a tooth. **3** In dentistry, the female component of a precision attachment. Adj. matrical, matricial. **bone m.** The ground substance of bony tissue, which is composed of protein and mucopolysaccharide. As the bony tissue matures the content of collagen fibers and bone salt increases. **cartilaginous m.** A basic, homogeneous basophil substance of embryonic skeletal tissue in the center of which articular cartilage develops. **cytoplasmic m.** The fluid portion of the cytoplasm interspersed between the organelles, filaments, and tubules. **hair m.** The germinative layer of the epithelium of the hair follicles. **mesangial m.** A mesh in the space between the renal glomerular capillary loops, formed from material similar to that of the capillary basement membrane. Mesangial cells are scattered in the matrix, which is made up of a homogeneous substance probably composed of mucopolysaccharides and glycoproteins. The matrix also contains filaments related to collagen. The mesangial cells are phagocytic, while the matrix is permeable to substances of large molecular size or to aggregates which may become localized in the matrix as deposits. **mitochondrial m.** The contents of the inner compartment of the mitochondrion. The cristae of the inner membrane partially divide the matrix into compartments. The composition of the matrix is maintained by selective pumps in the inner membrane. Soluble enzymes of the citric acid cycle are contained within the matrix. **nail m.** MATRIX UNGUIS. **nuclear m.** The translucent material between the various chromatin granules and filaments within the nucleus. **sarcoplasmic m.** The fluid portion of the cytoplasm of a muscle cell, containing the soluble enzymes. **m. unguis** [NA] The modified corium and the germinative zone upon which the body and root of the nail rest. It has longitudinal vascular ridges homologous to dermal papillae. Also *nail matrix, nail bed, lactulum unguis, keratogenous membrane* (outmoded), *onychostroma.*

**matrocliny** \mā′trōklī′nē\ Any mode of inheritance in which the offspring predictably resemble the female parent more than the male parent, as in hologynic inheritance. Compare PATROCLINY.

**matron** \mā′trən\ [L *matron(a)* (from *mater*, gen. *matris*, a mother) a wife, matron] The chief nursing officer in a small hospital with total responsibility for nursing services and supervisory responsibility for services other than medical services which directly affect patient care, such as catering and domestic services.

**Matson** [Donald Darrow *Matson*, U.S. neurosurgeon, 1913–1969] See under OPERATION.

**matter** [Old French *matere* or *matiere* (from L *materia* matter, stuff, wood, timber, source, from *mater* mother) substance] **1** Material; substance. **2** Pus. **gelatinous m.** SUBSTANTIA GELATINOSA. See under SUBSTANTIA GELATINOSA MEDULLAE SPINALIS ROLANDI. **gray m.** SUBSTANTIA GRISEA. **gray m. of spinal cord** SUBSTANTIA GRISEA MEDULLAE SPINALIS. **medullary white m.** SUBSTANTIA ALBA. **white m.** SUBSTANTIA ALBA.

**mattress** / **alternating pressure m.** RIPPLE MATTRESS. **divided m.** A mattress that is split, generally in the perineal area, so that excrement can be collected and removed. **ripple m.** A mattress consisting of transverse, inflatable tubes which are usually 5–12 cm in diameter. Alternate tubes are linked in series to a pump working on a fixed cycle so that each alternate tube is inflating while the tube next to it is deflating. Thus the area of compression between skin and mattress changes on a regular cycle, helping to prevent the formation of decubitus ulcers or bed sores. Also *alternating pressure mattress.*

**maturant** An agent that brings about a maturation, or ripening, of a boil or an ovarian follicle.

**maturate** \mach′ərāt\ To suppurate or to come close to the point of spontaneous drainage of pus.

**maturation** \mach′ərā′shən\ [L *maturatio* (from *maturare* to ripen, hasten) anticipation, hastening. See MATURE.] **1** The division of gonadal cells to produce an ovum or sperm cells, which have half the chromosome number characteristic of the somatic cells of the species. **2** The process of reaching full development or maturity. See also MATURATION-DEVELOPMENT. **m. of the fetus** The morphologic and physiologic development of the fetus up to the time of birth. A fetus is called "mature" when all such processes have reached certain stages in their completion compatible with the independent existence of the neonate, and "immature" when they have not. Immaturity of the neonate should be related to its age, but certain adverse conditions may also affect development.

**maturation-development** The process by which children, concomitant with the biologic maturation of the body, pass by stages, at predictable times, from the condition of newborn helplessness to independence, with socialization and the power of abstract reasoning. The infant moves in one year from primitive type of motor response when newly born to the complex pattern required for upright posture, and then to highly complex skills in the next three years, acquiring at the same time fluent use of language, control of bowel and bladder, control of aggression, use of memory, and ability to solve problems. Developmental attainment can be assessed at any age by tests and reference to norms. Brain-damaged children mature at a much slower rate and cease developing earlier than normal children. Also *postnatal development.*

**mature** [L *maturus* ripe, mature, developed, timely] **1** Fully developed, as an ovum following meiosis; ripe. **2** To reach full development; ripen. **3** Having reached puberty.

**maturity** [L *maturitas* ripeness, maturity] **1** Puberty. **2** The state of completed growth. **3** The gestational age or stage of development of a fetus or newborn infant.

**matut.** *matutinus* (L, in the morning).

**Mauchart** [Burkhard David *Mauchart,* German anatomist, 1696–1751] Mauchart's ligaments. See under LIGAMENTA ALARIA.

**Maurer** [Georg *Maurer,* German physician active in Sumatra] Maurer's clefts, Maurer spots, Maurer stippling. See under MAURER'S DOTS.

**Mauriceau** [François *Mauriceau,* French obstetrician, 1637–1709] **1** See under MANEUVER. **2** Mauriceau-Smellie-Veit maneuver. See under MANEUVER.

**Mauthner** [Ludwig *Mauthner,* Austrian ophthalmologist, 1840–1894] **1** See under FIBER. **2** Mauthner's membrane, Mauthner sheath. See under AXOLEMMA.

**MAVIS** mobile artery and vein imaging system.

**max** maximum.

**maxilla** \maksil′ə\ [L (dim. of *mala* the cheekbone, jawbone), the jawbone, jaw (upper and lower)] (*pl.* maxillae) [NA] One of a pair of facial bones that is irregular in shape, supports the upper teeth, and takes part in the formation of the orbit, nasal cavity and hard palate, as well as the infratemporal and pterygopalatine fossae. The central body contains a sinus. Superiorly, the frontal and zygomatic processes project; inferiorly are the palatine and alveolar processes. Also *upper jaw, upper jaw bone, maxillary bone, supermaxilla* (outmoded), *supramaxilla* (outmoded). **inferior m.** *Outmoded* MANDIBULA.

**maxillae** \maksil′ē\ Plural of MAXILLA.

**maxillary** \mak′siler′ē\ Pertaining to the maxilla.

**maxillectomy** \mak′silek′təmē\ [*maxill(a)* + -ECTOMY] The surgical removal of the maxilla or part of it.

**maxillofacial** \maksil′ōfā′shəl\ [*maxill(a)* + *o* + FACIAL] Relating to both the face and the jaws, but more particularly to the face and upper jaw.

**maxima** \mak′simə\ Plural of MAXIMUM.

**maximal** Being or related to a maximum; greatest or most.

**Maximow** [Alexander Alexandrovich *Maximow,* Russian-born histologist active in Germany and the United States, 1874–1928] Maximow's method. See under HEMATOXYLIN-EOSIN-AZURE II STAIN.

**maximum** [L (neut. of *maximus* the greatest, most; superl. of *magnus* great), the largest amount] (*pl.* maximums, maxima) **1** The greatest or greatest possible degree or quantity. Abbr. max **2** MAXIMAL. **excretory tubular transport m.** The greatest quantity of a substance that can be excreted in unit time by the renal tubular excretory mass. **glucose transport m.** The greatest quantity of glucose that can be transported across a biological membrane in unit time. **reabsorptive tubular transport m.** The greatest quantity of a substance that can be reabsorbed in unit time by the total of the renal tubules. **transport m.** The maximum rate at which the renal tubules can secrete or reabsorb a substance. Symbol: Tm **tubular m.** The greatest rate at which the renal tubules can excrete or reabsorb substances. **tubular reabsorption m.** The maximum rate in milligrams per minute at which a substance filtered by the glomerulus can be actively reabsorbed by the renal tubules. For example, as the plasma glucose level increases so does the filtered glucose load, and the rate of tubular glucose reabsorption is exceeded. The reabsorption maximum is calculated by the difference between glucose filtered per minute and the amount excreted into the bladder urine per minute. The reabsorption maximum for glucose reflects the proximal convoluted tubular mass. Inorganic sulfate, inorganic phosphate, and some amino acids also have reabsorption maxima.

**Maxwell** [Patrick William *Maxwell,* Irish ophthalmologist, 1856–1917] See under RING, SPOT.

**maxwell** \maks′wəl\ [after James Clerk *Maxwell,* Scottish physicist, 1831–1879] A CGS electromagnetic unit of magnetic flux, equal to $10^{-8}$ weber. An obsolete unit. Symbol: Mx

**May** [Richard *May,* German physician, 1863–1936] **1** May-Hegglin anomaly. See under ANOMALY. **2** May-Grünwald stain. See under STAIN.

**mayapple** \mā′ap′əl\ MANDRAKE.

**Mayer** [Carl *Mayer,* Austrian neurologist, 1862–1932] Mayer's reflex. See under FINGER-THUMB REFLEX.

**Mayer** [Karl Wilhelm *Mayer,* German gynecologist, 1795–1868] See under PESSARY.

**Mayer** [Paul *Mayer,* German chemist, 1848–1923] **1** Mayer solution. See under MAYER'S HEMALUM. **2** See under MUCIHEMATEIN. **3** Mayer mucicarmine stain. See under STAIN. **4** Mayer's mucicarmine. See under MUCICARMINE.

**mayhem** \mā′em, mā′hem\ [Middle English *maym, mayme, maheym,* from Middle French *mahaing, main, mahaim* a disabling, maiming] An act resulting in disfigurement of survivors of violence or postmortem mutilation of nonsurvivors.

**mayidism** \mā′idizm\ [irreg. from Spanish *maíz* maize + ISM] *Obs.* PELLAGRA.

**Mayo** [William James *Mayo,* U.S. surgeon, 1861–1939] **1** Mayo's operation. See under OPERATION. **2** Mayo's vein. See under VENA PREPYLORICA.

**Mayor** [Mathias Louis *Mayor,* Swiss surgeon, 1775–1847] See under SCARF.

**Mayo-Robson** [Sir Arthur William *Mayo-Robson,* English surgeon, 1853–1933] Mayo-Robson position. See under ROBSON'S POSITION.

**maze** \māz\ [Middle English *maze, mase*] A labyrinth for observing learning in human or animal subjects. It consists of a series of pathways between a starting point and a goal, usually with only one path leading from the start to the finish, all alternate branches being blind alleys. Learning is measured by the time needed to reach the goal, or by the number of errors made, or by some combination of those two over a series of trials until performance becomes error-free. **radiation m.** An arrangement of protective walls and corridors leading to a room containing a radiation source.

**mazindol** $C_{16}H_{13}ClN_2O$. 5-(4-Chlorophenyl)-2,5-dihydro-3*H*-imidazo[2,1-*a*]isoindol-5-ol. A compound that stimulates the central nervous system and has properties similar to those of amphetamine. It is used as an anorexic drug in the treatment of obesity.

**mazo-** \maz′ō-\ [Gk *mazos* a woman's breast] A combining form denoting the breast.

**mazodynia** \-din′ē·ə\ [*maz(o)-* + -ODYNIA] MASTODYNIA.

**mazopexy** \maz′əpek′sē\ MASTOPEXY.

**Mazzoni** [Vittorio *Mazzoni*, Italian physiologist, 1880–1940] **1** Golgi-Mazzoni corpuscles. See under GOLGI-MAZZONI ENDINGS. **2** See under CORPUSCLE.

**M.B.** *Medicinae Baccalaureus* (L, Bachelor of Medicine).

**m.b.** *misce bene* (L, mix well).

**MBC** maximum breathing capacity.

**MBD** minimal brain dysfunction.

**MBP** mean blood pressure.

**McBurney** [Charles *McBurney*, U.S. surgeon, 1845–1913] See under OPERATION, SIGN, INCISION, POINT.

**McCarthy** [Daniel J. *McCarthy*, U.S. neurologist, 1874–1958] **1** McCarthy's reflex. See under SUPRAORBITAL REFLEX. **2** See under SIGN.

**McClintock** [Alfred Henry *McClintock*, Irish physician, 1822–1881] See under SIGN.

**McCune** [Donovan James *McCune*, U.S. pediatrician, born 1902] McCune-Albright syndrome, Albright-McCune-Sternberg syndrome. See under ALBRIGHT'S DISEASE.

**McDonald** [Ellice *McDonald*, U.S. gynecologist, 1876–1955] See under MANEUVER, RULE.

**MCF** macrophage chemotactic factor.

**McGoon** [Dwight Charles *McGoon*, U.S. heart surgeon, born 1925] See under TECHNIQUE.

**MCH** mean corpuscular hemoglobin.

**MCHC** mean corpuscular hemoglobin concentration.

**MCHg** mean corpuscular hemoglobin.

**McKee** [George Kenneth *McKee*, British orthopedic surgeon, born 1930] See under LINE.

**McKinnon** [Neil E. *McKinnon*, Canadian physician, born 1894] See under TEST.

**MCL** midclavicular line.

**McLean** [Malcolm *McLean*, U.S. obstetrician, 1848–1924] Tucker-McLean forceps. See under FORCEPS.

**McMurray** [Thomas Porter *McMurray*, English orthopedic surgeon, 1887–1949] **1** McMurray's circumduction maneuver. See under MANEUVER. **2** McMurray's test. See under SIGN.

**McNeal** [Ward J. *McNeal*, U.S. bacteriologist, 1881–1946] Novy, McNeal and Nicolle medium. See under MEDIUM.

**McNemar** [Quinn *McNemar*, U.S. psychologist and statistician, born 1900] See under TEST.

**MCR** metabolic clearance rate.

**MCT** mean circulation time.

**MCV** mean corpuscular volume.

**McVay** [Chester Bidwell *McVay*, U.S. surgeon, born 1911] See under OPERATION.

**M.D.** *Medicinae Doctor* (L, Doctor of Medicine).

**Md** Symbol for the element, mendelevium.

**MDA** **1** mentum dexter anterior (a fetal position). **2** methylenedioxyamphetamine

**MDR** minimum daily requirement.

**Me** methyl.

**MEA** multiple endocrine adenomatosis (multiple endocrine neoplasia).

**meal** / **barium m.** An emulsion or suspension of barium sulfate taken orally by a patient undergoing roentgenography of the upper gastrointestinal tract. **motor m.** A test meal administered to determine the progress of substances through some part of the digestive tract. It usually contains radiopaque material for roentgenographic observation. **opaque m.** A light solid or liquid meal containing a radiopaque contrast medium, usually barium sulfate, for roentgenographic examination of the stomach and intestinal tract. **test m.** A meal containing specified amounts of specified substances which is used in the diagnostic evaluation of the stomach or small intestine, either radiographically or by later analysis of the gastric or intestinal contents obtained by peroral intubation and aspiration.

**mean** An average of a set of values. • Without qualification, the term always refers to the arithmetic mean. **arithmetic m.** The ratio of the sum of the terms in a statistical series to their number. Also *average*. **geometric m.** A value indicating the central tendency of a statistical series of *n* terms, equal to the positive *n*th root of their product. The geometric mean cannot be calculated if the series contains a negative or a zero term. The geometric mean is less than the arithmetic mean. **harmonic m.** For a given set of values, the reciprocal of the mean of the reciprocals of the individual values. Thus, the harmonic mean of the set 10, 20, 50 is

$$\frac{1}{\frac{1}{3}\left(\frac{1}{10}+\frac{1}{20}+\frac{1}{50}\right)} = 17.65.$$

**measle** \mē′zəl\ [See MEASLES.] CYSTICERCUS.

**measles** [Middle English *meseles*, pl. of *mesel* measles; Dutch *maselen*, dim. of *masa* a spot] A highly contagious viral disease caused by a paramyxovirus (measle virus) and occurring chiefly in young children. An incubation period of 10–14 days precedes the prodrome in which fever, coryza, cough, conjunctivitis, and malaise occur. Koplik spots, blue-gray spots with a red areola, appear on the buccal membranes at the end of the prodrome and are virtually pathognomonic of measles. An erythematous, maculopapular rash spreading downward from the head and face to the trunk and limbs then erupts and lasts about five days. Complications include pneumonia, otitis media, and subacute sclerosing panencephalitis. The disease is especially severe in tropical regions of west Africa and Central and South America, and malnourished children living in these areas may be most seriously affected. Recovery from measles confers immunity. A live measles vaccine is available. Also *rubeola, morbilli*. **bastard m.** RUBELLA. **black m.** HEMORRHAGIC MEASLES. **confluent m.** Measles in which the lesions of the rash merge. **French m.** RUBELLA. **German m.** RUBELLA. **hemorrhagic m.** A severe form of measles in which the rash is extremely dark and petechial due to hemorrhages into the skin. Also *black measles*. **three-day m.** RUBELLA.

**measly** \mēz′lē\ [*measl(e)* + -Y] Infected with cysticerci, the larval stage of the cestode *Taenia*, as in *measly pork* (infected with *T. solium* larvae) and *measly beef* (with *T. saginata*).

**measure** [L *mensura* (from *mensus*, past part. of *metiri* to measure, akin to Gk *metron* a measure, rule) a measuring, amount] **1** To ascertain the magnitude of (a physical quantity) by comparison to some accepted standard or by calculation. 2 A specified or standard magnitude of a physical quantity. 3 A graduated instrument used to measure an object or substance.

**measurement** 1 The act or process of measuring. 2 A result of measuring, as a dimension of something measured. **end-point m.** The quantitation of a substance performed by measuring the change in a variable after the completion of the chemical reaction. Compare KINETIC MEASUREMENT. **kinetic m.** The quantitation of a substance, usually an enzyme, performed by monitoring the changes in absorbance over time, either continuously or at frequent intervals. Compare END-POINT MEASUREMENT. **mental m.** The measurement of mental phenomena, or the externally observable behavior representing such events, by an application either of mental tests or of psychophysical methods. It is used most often to describe individual differences, with responses of different subjects assigned a position on a common quantitative scale. **real-time m.** 1 A measurement made at the actual time that a physical process takes place. This is required in a control system so that no delay occurs in supplying corrective action. 2 A measurement made at normal system operating speed or frequency as distinguished from slowed down operation. **skinfold m.'s** Determinations of the thickness of a fold of skin using calipers. Measurements are used to assess body fat content. Standard tables are available relating skinfold thickness to body fat as a percentage of body weight according to age and sex.

**meatal** \mē·ā′təl\ Of or relating to a meatus.

**meatitis** \mē′ətī′tis\ Inflammation of the tissues of a meatus. **ulcerative m.** A common affection of the urinary meatus caused by various microorganisms, resulting in reddening of the meatus with vesiculation.

**meato-** \mē·at′ō-, mē′ətō-\ [L *meatus* a going, passage, passing] A combining form denoting meatus.

**meatome** \mē′ətōm\ MEATOTOME.

**meatometer** \mē′ətäm′ətər\ [MEATO- + -METER] An apparatus devised to measure a meatus, especially the urinary meatus.

**meatoplasty** \mē·ā′tōplas′tē\ [MEATO- + -PLASTY] Reconstructive surgery of a meatus, usually the external auditory meatus. The procedure requires the use of flaps of meatal skin. **Stacke's m.** A type of meatoplasty used as the final stage of the radical mastoidectomy operation. A large rectangular flap of meatal skin, hinged inferiorly, is turned back to line the floor of the mastoid cavity.

**meatorrhaphy** \me′ətôr′əfē\ [MEATO- + -RRHAPHY] The suturing of the urethral membrane to the glans penis following surgery to enlarge the urinary meatus.

**meatotome** \mē·at′ətōm\ [MEATO- + -TOME] A surgical instrument used to incise and enlarge the urinary meatus. Also *meatome.*

**meatotomy** \mē′ətät′əmē\ [MEATO- + -TOMY] An incision of a meatus, as the urinary meatus, to increase its diameter. Also *porotomy.*

**meatus** \mē·ā′təs\ [L (from *meatus,* past part. of *meare* to go, pass), a going, motion, path, way] An opening to a canal or passage in the body. **acoustic m.** 1 MEATUS ACUSTICUS EXTERNUS. 2 MEATUS ACUSTICUS INTERNUS. **m. acusticus externus** [NA] The S-shaped canal of the external ear leading from the concha of the auricle to the tympanic membrane. It comprises an outer cartilaginous portion and an inner bony portion, and it has constrictions about midway and near the membrane. It is lined by skin which continues on to the tympanic membrane. Also *external acoustic meatus, external auditory meatus, auricular canal, acoustic meatus, external auditory foramen, external auditory canal, external acoustic canal.* **m. acusticus externus cartilagineus** [NA] The outer one third of the external acoustic meatus, composed of fibrocartilage and shaped like a trough, the deficient posterosuperior part being filled by collagen and the anterior part having two or more fissures. Laterally it is continuous with the auricular cartilage and medially it is attached to the bony part by fibrous tissue. The lining skin contains fine hairs and sebaceous and ceruminous glands. Also *cartilaginous external acoustic meatus, cartilaginous external auditory meatus.* **m. acusticus externus osseus** The medial two thirds of the external acoustic meatus, located in the temporal bone and connecting the cartilaginous portion, to which it is attached by fibrous tissue, to the tympanic cavity. At its narrow, oblique, medial end is the incomplete tympanic sulcus to which the circumference of the tympanic membrane is attached. The adherent lining skin is devoid of hair and glands. Also *bony external acoustic meatus, bony external auditory meatus.* **m. acusticus internus** [NA] A short canal above the anterior part of the jugular foramen in the petrous part of the temporal bone transmitting the facial, intermediate and vestibulocochlear nerves and the labyrinthine vessels, and extending from the internal acoustic opening near the apex of the posterior surface of the bone to the fundus, where a plate of bone pierced by foramina separates the meatus from the internal ear. Also *internal acoustic meatus, internal auditory meatus, acoustic meatus, internal auditory canal, internal acoustic canal.* **bony external acoustic m.** MEATUS ACUSTICUS EXTERNUS OSSEUS. **bony external auditory m.** MEATUS ACUSTICUS EXTERNUS OSSEUS. **cartilaginous external acoustic m.** MEATUS ACUSTICUS EXTERNUS CARTILAGINEUS. **cartilaginous external auditory m.** MEATUS ACUSTICUS EXTERNUS CARTILAGINEUS. **external acoustic m.** MEATUS ACUSTICUS EXTERNUS. **external auditory m.** MEATUS ACUSTICUS EXTERNUS. **fish-mouth m.** An inflamed and everted urinary meatus evident in gonorrhea. **inferior nasal m.** MEATUS NASI INFERIOR. **internal acoustic m.** MEATUS ACUSTICUS INTERNUS. **internal auditory m.** MEATUS ACUSTICUS INTERNUS. **middle nasal m.** MEATUS NASI MEDIUS. **m. nasi inferior** [NA] The space between the arched inferior nasal concha superiorly and the floor of the nose inferiorly. The nasolacrimal duct opens into the anterior portion of its lateral wall. Also *inferior nasal meatus.* **m. nasi medius** [NA] The passage under cover of the middle nasal concha, deeper anteriorly than posteriorly and continuous anteriorly with the atrium. On its lateral wall is the rounded bulla ethmoidalis, anterior and inferior to which is the curved hiatus semilunaris and the openings of the anterior and middle ethmoidal sinuses. Into the anterior end, or infundibulum, the frontonasal duct opens while near the roof is the opening of the maxillary sinus. Also *middle nasal meatus.* **m. nasi superior** [NA] A short, narrow passage located partly under the superior nasal concha and extending above the middle nasal concha for about half its length. The posterior ethmoidal sinuses open into the anterior end, usually by way of a single aperture. Also *superior nasal meatus.* **m. nasopharyngeus** [NA] The posterior part of the nasal cavity, extending from the posterior ends of the middle and inferior nasal conchae to the choanae and situated between the adjacent lateral and medial walls of the nasal fossa. Also *nasopharyngeal meatus.* **m. of nose** The passages in the lateral wall of the nose, such as meatus nasi superior, meatus nasi medius, and meatus nasi inferior. **superior nasal m.** MEATUS NASI SUPERIOR. **m. of urethra** OSTIUM URETHRAE EXTERNUM. **urinary m.** OSTIUM URETHRAE EXTERNUM.

**mebendazole** $C_{16}H_{13}N_3O_3$. 5-Benzoyl-2-benzimidazole-carbamic acid methyl ester. An agent given by oral administration as an anthelmintic in the treatment of trichuriasis, enterobiasis, hookworm, and ascariasis.

**mebeverine hydrochloride** $C_{25}H_{35}NO_5 \cdot HCl$. 4-[Ethyl-(*p*-methoxy-α-methylphenethyl)amino]butyl veratrate hydrochloride. A smooth muscle relaxant agent used to treat disorders affecting the gastrointestinal tract.

**mebutamate** $C_{10}H_{20}N_2O_4$. 2-Methyl-2-(1-methylpropyl)-1,3-propanediol dicarbamate. A drug used to treat hypertension, often in combination with diuretics or other hypotensive agents. It is given orally.

**mecamine** Mecamylamine. See under MECAMYLAMINE HYDROCHLORIDE.

**mecamylamine hydrochloride** $C_{11}H_{22}ClN$. *N*,2,3,3-Tetramethylbicyclo[2.2.1]-heptan-2-amine hydrochloride. A ganglionic blocking agent which has been used orally for the treatment of severe hypertension.

**mechanical** 1 Done or assisted by machine. 2 Referring to a process or mechanism that does not involve chemical or cellular changes.

**mechanicoreceptor** \məkan′ikōrisep′tər\ MECHANORECEPTOR.

**mechanics** The branch of physics concerned with the interaction of force and matter. **animal m.** BIOMECHANICS. **body m.** Kinesiologic principles of body movement and posture. **developmental m.** The mechanisms of development as revealed principally by the techniques of experimental embryology.

**mechanism** 1 A contrivance or machinelike device. 2 A process or technique by which some result is achieved. **coping m.** Any of the conscious or unconscious ways that a person uses to adjust to environmental demands. **countercurrent multiplier m.** The mechanism by which the loop of Henle contributes to the production of a concentrated urine. Small osmolar concentration differences established between the fluid contents of the two limbs at each level of the loop are enhanced by the flow of fluid in opposite directions in the descending and ascending limbs. The gradient of increasing osmolarity in the renal medulla between the corticomedullary junction and the tips of the renal papillae is established by the active pumping of sodium chloride out of the ascending limb of the loop of Henle which is believed to be water impermeable. **defense m.** Any of the mechanisms developed by the ego to control impulses that if left unchecked would cause conflict between the ego and id. Various defenses have been described, including repression, displacement, identification, dissociation, introjection, isolation, postponement of affect, projection, reaction formation, regression, undoing, and sublimation. **Douglas m.** The spontaneous movement of a fetus from a transverse lie to a vertex presentation. **Duncan m.** Delivery of the placenta with the maternal surface appearing first at the vaginal introitus. **feedback m.** CLOSED LOOP. **Frank-Starling m.** The alteration of the energy of cardiac muscle contraction that accompanies changes in the fiber length at the start of contraction. See also STARLING'S LAW. **immunological m.'s of tissue damage** A system for classifying immunological reactions that can produce damage to host tissues, in which the initiating immunological event provides the basis of the classification. It was devised by R. R. A. Coombs and P. G. H. Gell. Four types of reactions are distinguished. Type 1 reactions (anaphylactic reactions, immediate hypersensitivity) are initiated by antigens reacting with cell-bound antibody, usually IgE. Release of mediators, mainly from basophils and mast cells, provide the pathogenic mechanism. Type 2 reactions (cytotoxic reactions) are initiated by antibody reacting with cell-bound antigen. Type 3 reactions are initiated by antigen-antibody complexes formed either at the site of tissue damage (Arthus reactions) or localizing from the circulation (soluble immune complex reactions). Type 4 reactions (delayed hypersensitivity) are initiated by antigen-reactive T cells reacting with specific antigen. These four types of reactions are also referred to as Type 1–4 hypersensitivity reactions. **ion-exchange m.** 1 A mechanism affecting passive or active transport of ions across a biologic membrane in such a way that the movements of ions in opposite directions are related quantitatively. 2 The replacement of ions in solution by ions of similar charge present in materials such as synthetic resins with which the solution is brought into contact. This technique has been used in water softening and in the removal of unwanted ions from the body. **middle-ear transformer m.** The mechanism provided by the tympanic membrane acting together with the ossicular chain which, by reason of the ossicular lever ratio along with the middle-ear areal ratio, greatly increases the force of the sound arriving at the oval window compared with the force incident on the tympanic membrane. **mote-beam m.** A mechanism by which an individual becomes oblivious to the presence of an undesirable trait in himself but is acutely aware of its existence in others. **pressoreceptive m.** A mechanism sensitive to blood pressure changes, such as a carotid sinus receptor. **reentrant m.** A fundamental mechanism of arrhythmogenesis in which cardiac tissue is reexcited by the same impulse for one or more cycles. The prerequisites for this arrhythmia mechanism are: an area, anatomic or functional, of unidirectional conduction; a pathway, anatomic or functional, with a conduction time long enough to permit reexcitation; and an initiating impulse. See also REENTRY. **scapegoat m.** 1 A method of rationalizing for one's failures by blaming them on another. 2 A mechanism by which all the emotions that a family cannot accept as originating from themselves are attributed to one member of the family, typically the one identified as sick or disturbed. **Schultze m.** Delivery of the placenta with the smooth fetal surface appearing first at the vaginal opening. **somatic m.** The structures and tissues that form the framework or walls of the body, excluding the viscera, and that are considered to be a functional entity. **splanchnic m.** The internal organs of the body considered as a functional entity. **suspensory m.** An arrangement of collagen fibers in the periodontal membrane which appears to suspend a tooth in its socket.

**mechano-** \mek′ənō-\ [Gk *mēchanē* instrument, machine] A combining form meaning machine, mechanical.

**mechanoreceptor** \-risep′tər\ Any of a variety of tactile end organs responsive to low-amplitude cutaneous displacement. Also *tactile receptor, touch receptor, contact receptor, contact ceptor, mechanicoreceptor.*

**mecism** \mē′sizm\ [Gk *mēk(os)* length, height + -ISM] The abnormal length of a part of the body or of the body as a whole.

**Meckel** [Johann Friedrich *Meckel,* the elder, German anatomist, 1724–1774] 1 Meckel's ganglion. See under GANGLION PTERYGOPALATINUM. 2 Lesser ganglion of Meckel. See under GANGLION SUBMANDIBULARE. 3 Meckel's cavity, Meckel's space. See under CAVUM TRIGEMINALE. 4 Meckel's ligament. See under BAND.

**Meckel** [Johann Friedrich *Meckel,* the younger, German anatomist and surgeon, 1781–1833] 1 See under DIVERTICULUM. 2 Meckel-Gruber syndrome. See under MECKEL SYNDROME.

**meclizine dihydrochloride** $C_{25}H_{29}Cl_3N_2$. 1-(*p*-Chloro-α-phenylbenzyl)-4-(*m*-methylbenzyl)piperazine dihydrochloride. It is an antihistaminic agent used in the management of nausea and vomiting caused by motion sickness. It may also be effective in the treatment of vertigo caused by diseases affecting the vestibular apparatus. It is given orally.

**meclocycline** $C_{22}H_{21}ClN_2O_8$. 7-Chloro-6-methylene-5-hydroxy-tetracycline. A topically applied antibiotic closely related to chlortetracycline. It is used as a dermatologic anti-infective agent.

**mecloqualone** $C_{15}H_{11}ClN_2O$. 3-(2-Chlorophenyl)-2-methyl-4(3*H*)-quinazolinone. A compound with hypnotic and sedative properties.

**meconalgia** \mek'ənal'jə\ [Gk *mēkōn* the poppy + -ALGIA] Spontaneous neuralgic pain occurring after the withdrawal of opiate remedies to which the individual has become addicted.

**meconic acid** A plant acid whose molecules possess a 6-membered ring which contains an oxygen atom, two double bonds, and a carbonyl group, and which also possess a hydroxyl group and two carboxyl groups. Alkaloids are often found as their salts with meconic acid.

**meconism** \mē'kənizm\ Opium addiction or opium poisoning.

**meconium** \mēkō'nē·əm\ [L, from Gk *mēkōnion* juice of the poppy, opium, discharge from the bowels of newborn children] The black or greenish black, odorless, sticky, semisolid material that fills the lower bowel of the newborn infant. Meconium stools are replaced by feces within the first two or three days of life.

**mecystasis** \məsis'təsis\ A state in which muscle shows unchanged characteristics of tension contraction and relaxation despite an increase in initial length.

**MED** 1 minimal effective dose. 2 minimal erythema dose.

**medallion** [French *médaillon* (from Italian *medaglione* a medallion, augmentative of *medaglia* a medal, coin, from Late L *medialis* middle, from L *medi(us)* middle + *-alis* -AL) a medallion, locket] The circumscribed red scaly patch that is the characteristic lesion of pityriasis rosea.

**medazepam hydrochloride** $C_{16}H_{15}ClN_2 \cdot HCl$. 7-Chloro-2,3-dihydro-1-methyl-5-phenyl-1*H*-1,4-benzodiazepine monohydrochloride. It is used as a weak tranquilizer and antianxiety medication.

**Medex** [shortened form of French *médecin extension* physician extension] A physician assistant training program used in the United States, originally developed to adapt former military corpsmen for civilian duty but more recently expanded to train other individuals for medical care duties under the supervision of a physician.

**medi-** \mē'dē-\ MEDIO-.

**media** \mē'dē·ə\ 1 Plural of MEDIUM. 2 A middle layer; tunica media.

**mediad** \mē'dē·ad\ Toward a median line or plane.

**medial** \mē'dē·əl\ 1 Of, at, or toward the middle. 2 Relatively near the midline or median plane of the body, as compared with other structures or parts situated farther to the right or left. Compare LATERAL. 3 Relating to a tunica media or any middle layer.

**medialecithal** \mē'dē·əles'ithəl\ [L *media*, fem. of *medius* middle, middling + LECITH- + -AL] Having a moderate quantity of yolk: said of an ovum. Also *mesolecithal.*

**medialis** \mē'dē·ā'lis\ [NA] Medial.

**median** \mē'dē·ən\ 1 The term in an ordered statistical series such that the number of observations which are less than it is the same as the number that exceed it. 2 Lying in the middle or in the vertical plane at the midline dividing a structure bilaterally.

**mediastina** \mē'dē·astī'nə\ Plural of MEDIASTINUM.

**mediastinal** \mē'dē·astī'nəl\ Pertaining to the mediastinum.

**mediastinitis** \mē'dē·as'tīnī'tis\ [*mediastin(um)* + -ITIS] Inflammation of the mediastinum. **fibrous m.** MEDIASTINAL FIBROSIS. **indurative m.** MEDIASTINAL FIBROSIS.

**mediastinography** \mē'dē·as'tinäg'rəfē\ Roentgenography of the mediastinal structures. **gas m.** Radiographic study of the mediastinum after injection of a gas, such as nitrous oxide, into the mediastinum via a needle introduced behind the sternum or behind the trachea. Also *pneumomediastinography.* **opaque m.** Radiographic study of the mediastinum after injection of an opaque medium into the mediastinum.

**mediastinopericarditis** \mē'dē·astī'nōper'ikärdī'tis\ Inflammation of the pericardium and adjacent mediastinal tissues that usually results in the formation of fibrous adhesions between the parietal pericardium and surrounding structures.

**mediastinoscope** \mē'dē·astī'nəskōp\ [*mediastin(um)* + *o* + -SCOPE] An endoscope used to visualize structures in the superior mediastinum. It is usually inserted through a small suprasternal cervical incision.

**mediastinoscopy** \mē'dē·as'tinäs'kəpē\ The examination of structures of the superior mediastinum by the use of a mediastinoscope.

**mediastinum** \mē'dē·əstī'nəm\ [New L, short for *septum mediastinum* a median partition, from Med L *mediastinus* intervening, intermediary, from L *mediast(r)inus* a general-duty servant, prob. from *medius* middle, intermediate] (*pl.* mediastina) 1 A median septum or partition between two parts of a cavity or an organ. 2 [NA] The interval between the right and left pleural sacs, extending from the thoracic inlet above to the diaphragm below, and from the sternum in front to the thoracic vertebrae behind. It contains the heart, pericardium, great vessels, and all other thoracic viscera lying between the pleural sacs. It is divided into superior, anterior, middle, and posterior mediastina. Also *mediastinal septum, interpleural space.* **m. anterius** [NA] A shallow space between the pericardium and the body of the sternum above the level of the fourth costal cartilages. It is narrow because of the close approximation near the midline of the left and the right mediastinal pleurae, and contains loose connective tissue, the lower part of the thymus gland, the sternopericardial ligaments, lymph nodes and vessels, and a few mediastinal branches of the internal thoracic vessels. Also *anterior mediastinum, cavum mediastinale anterius, anterior mediastinal cavity.* **m. medium** [NA] The large central portion of the lower part of the mediastinal space occupied by the pericardium, heart, ascending aorta, the pulmonary trunk dividing into left and right pulmonary arteries, the bifurcation of the trachea and the bronchi, the arch of the azygos vein, the lower part of the superior vena cava, the left and right pulmonary veins, the phrenic nerves and accompanying vessels, tracheobronchial lymph nodes, and the deep part of the cardiac plexus. Also *middle mediastinum.* **m. posterius** [NA] The mediastinal space bounded by the lower eight thoracic vertebrae posteriorly; the mediastinal pleura on each side; and the pericardium, bifurcation of trachea, pulmonary vessels, and the upper surface of the diaphragm anteriorly. It is continuous superiorly with the posterior part of the superior mediastinum, and it contains the esophagus, descending thoracic aorta, azygos and hemiazygos veins, thoracic duct, vagus and splanchnic nerves, and lymph nodes. Also *posterior mediastinum, cavum mediastinale posterius, posterior mediastinal cavity, postmediastinum.*

**m. superius** [NA] The mediastinal space bounded posteriorly by the upper four thoracic vertebrae and longus colli muscles, anteriorly by the manubrium sterni and sternohyoid and sternothyroid muscles, laterally by the mediastinal pleurae, superiorly by the thoracic inlet, and inferiorly by the plane between the sternal angle and the lower border of the body of the fourth thoracic vertebra, below which its posterior part is continuous with the posterior mediastinum. It contains connective tissue; part of the thymus gland; the arch of the aorta and its branches; the brachiocephalic veins; the upper part of the superior vena cava; lymph nodes; and the vagus, cardiac, phrenic and left recurrent laryngeal nerves. Also *superior mediastinum.* **m. testis** [NA] The incomplete vertical septum formed by the projection of the tunica albuginea into the testis through its posterior border along its upper two thirds. Through it pass the blood vessels and lymphatics of the testis. It also contains the rete testis. Also *septum of testis, body of Highmore, corpus highmori.*

**mediate** \mē′dē·āt\ [L *mediat(us),* past part. of *mediare* to be in the middle, from *medi(us)* middle] **1** Acting or occurring indirectly through an agent. **2** To be such an agent for effecting (a result). **3** Intermediate; intervening.

**mediation** \mē′dē·ā′shən\ The act or result of mediating. **chemical m.** The linking of related functions by a chemical intermediary, especially used of the transmission of nerve impulses between presynaptic and postsynaptic elements.

**mediator** \mē′dē·ā′tər\ Something that mediates; an agent that effects a result. **chemical m.** An intermediary agent which is chemical in nature.

**medicable** \med′ikəbəl\ Capable of being treated medically and with the expectation of effective cure.

**Medicaid** A federally aided, state-operated and administered program in the United States which provides medical care benefits for certain low-income, medically indigent individuals through a governmental insurance type of entitlement program.

**medical** [Late L *medicalis* (from L *medicus* healing, curative, a healer, physician, from *mederi* to heal, cure, treat, from the Indo-European root *med-/mod-* as in *meditate, moderate, mete* to measure) pertaining to healing or medicine] Of or relating to medicine or to the practice of medicine. **major m.** Insurance designed to offset high medical expenses resulting from catastrophic or prolonged illness or injury.

**medicament** \med′ikəmənt, mədik′əmənt\ [French *médicament* (from L *medicament(um)* medicine, remedy, from *medica(ri)* to heal, cure + *-mentum* -MENT) substance used for curing illness] A medicinal agent or any substance used as a therapeutic material. Adj. medicamentous.

**medicamentous** Referring to a medication, or related to the use of a therapeutic agent. Also *medicamentosus.*

**Medicare** A nationwide, federally funded and administered insurance program in the United States for individuals aged 65 and over and certain others, which provides funding for a number of specified health care services, but is not all-inclusive. • A similar national program of health insurance of the same name exists in Australia.

**medicate** \med′ikāt\ **1** To impregnate or permeate with a medicinal substance. **2** To treat by administering a drug.

**medicated** \med′ikā′tid\ Treated or impregnated with a medicinal substance.

**medication** **1** A medicinal substance; a medicine. **2** Treatment by the administration of medicines. **3** Impregnation or permeation with a medicinal substance. **preanesthetic m.** Medication administered prior to local or general anesthesia, as sedatives or tranquilizers for anxiety, analgesics (such as opioids), and vagolytic agents (such as atropine and scopolamine) to block vagal-induced, excessive airway secretion or bradycardia. Also *preanesthesia, premedication.*

**medicator** \med′ikā′tər\ An instrument for applying a medicine locally, especially within a body cavity.

**medicerebral** \mē′dēser′əbrəl\ Denoting to the central portion of the cerebrum.

**medicinal** \mədis′ənəl\ **1** Having healing properties. **2** Of or relating to medicine.

**medicine** [Old French, from L *medicina* (short for *ars medicina* the healing art, from *medicinus* pertaining to healing, from *medicus* curative, healing, healer; see MEDICAL) the practice of medicine, a cure, remedy] **1** The art and science dealing with the maintenance and restoration of health, including the prevention and treatment of disease. **2** The branch of medicine that employs nonsurgical methods of treatment. **3** Any substance used to treat disease or alleviate pain. **adolescent m.** The branch of medicine dealing with the care and treatment of individuals from the onset of puberty to about age 19. Also *ephebiatrics.* **aerospace m.** SPACE MEDICINE. **aviation m.** A specialized branch of medicine dealing with the physiologic, pathologic, and psychologic conditions which occur in professional fliers and people transported by air. It includes the selection, maintenance, and treatment of aircraft personnel, advising on the design of aircraft and related equipment, and dealing with the transport of the sick and wounded. Also *aeromedicine.* **behavioral m.** The application of the principles of learning and learning theory to treat those disorders, caused at least in part by psychologic factors, as if they were behaviors. Specific techniques are applied to reverse the expressions of maladaptive functioning, whether purely psychologic, as in a phobia, or partly physiologic, as in faulty patterns of learned autonomic nervous system response leading to cardiovascular disease. **clinical m.** Medical practice or instruction involving and based on direct observation of patients as opposed to theoretical study, laboratory investigation, or classroom teaching. **community m.** The practice of medicine or the study of health care services focusing on community needs and care rather than on the individual. Examples include public health services and preventive medicine. **domestic m.** The treatment of illness or injury in the home, without the advice or assistance of a physician. **dosimetric m.** The administration of drugs or medicines by an exact and standardized system of dosages. **emergency m.** A branch of medicine that specializes in providing immediate diagnosis and treatment of those who are acutely and often suddenly ill or severely injured, such that any considerable delay would likely result in deterioration or death. **environmental m.** The study of the environmental aspects related to the etiology and prevention of disease as well as specific environmental aspects of the promotion of good health. **experimental m.** Medical research based on experimentation with animals, especially for the study of disease processes and therapies. **family m.** *Popular* FAMILY PRACTICE. **fetal-maternal m.** A subspecialty of obstetrics and gynecology dealing with the care of the pregnant mother and her fetus with particular emphasis on managing high-risk situations. **folk m.** The treatment of illness or injury based on tradition, especially an oral tradition passed from one generation to the next, rather than on scientific practice. It often utilizes indigenous flora as remedies. **forensic m.** The application of theoretical and practical medical knowledge and skill to the solution of problems encountered in the administration of justice. Also *legal medicine, medical jurisprudence.* • The term was first used in Scotland and England. **geographical m.** A branch of medicine concerned with geographical differences in the clinical manifestations and pathology of diseases, their incidence, and their economic impact. **geriatric m.** A medical specialty concerned with the diagnosis, prevention, and treatment of physical and mental disorders and diseases of the elderly. Also *geriatrics* (popular), *gerontotherapy* (seldom used), *presbyatrics.* **holistic m.** An approach to health care based on the theory that health is the result of harmony between body, mind, and spirit and that stress of any kind, including physical, psychological, and social pressure, is inimical to health. Also *whole person medicine.* **hyperbaric m.** Medical treatment under conditions exceeding normal atmospheric pressure. ⟨"Hyperbaric medicine's origin as a therapy for divers with decompression sickness still hasn't been left behind, though. The field's professional association is named the Undersea Medical Society." —*Medical World News,* 28 Feb. 1983, 29.⟩ **industrial m.** *Outmoded* OCCUPATIONAL MEDICINE. **internal m.** The branch of medicine which deals with the diagnosis and nonsurgical treatment of diseases and disorders affecting internal parts or systems of the body. • The English term was apparently borrowed from the German, *Innere Medizin,* which became common in Germany in the early 1880s. (William B. Bean, *New England Journal of Medicine,* 21 Jan. 1982, 182–183). *Internal medicine* is used in the U.S., Canada, India, New Zealand, the United Kingdom (where *general medicine* is preferred), and Japan, where *Innere Medizin* is also used. The corresponding term in South Africa is simply *medicine*; *internal medicine* is not used. **legal m.** FORENSIC MEDICINE. **manipulative m.** Medical practice based on manipulative therapy; chiropractic. **neonatal m.** NEONATOLOGY. **nuclear m.** The branch of medicine dealing with the diagnostic, therapeutic (exclusive of sealed radiation sources), and investigative use of radionuclides. Also *nuclear radiology.* **occupational m.** A branch of medicine dealing with prevention of disease and injury among people at work. It has two main functions: to ensure the suitability of an individual for particular kinds of work in order to protect the health and safety of that individual, fellow workers, and, where appropriate, the public; and to identify and control health and safety hazards in the workplace. Also *industrial medicine* (outmoded). **oral m.** The study and treatment of diseases of the soft tissues of the mouth. **osteopathic m.** OSTEOPATHY. **patent m.** A medicine protected by a trademark, often with the composition not completely made known. **perinatal m.** A specialized branch of medicine dealing with the management of mother and fetus during pregnancy and of the infant immediately after delivery. In contrast to general obstetrics, special emphasis is placed on managing high-risk pregnancies. **physical m. and rehabilitation** The branch of medicine concerned with the use of physical agents and modalities including electricity, light, heat, sound, mechanical devices, and physical activity in the diagnosis, treatment, and prevention of disease. In the last several decades this medical specialty has been increasingly focused on the diagnosis, treatment, and prevention of physical disabilities, including pain. Also *physiatrics* (used chiefly in the U.S. and Canada), *physiatry* (used chiefly in the U.S. and Canada). • Originally and still known in many countries as *physical medicine,* the specialty was broadened in the United States in 1949 to include *rehabilitation* as part of its formal name. *Physical medicine* is the term by which this specialty is known in the United Kingdom, South Africa, India, New Zealand, and Australia, although in Australia *rehabilitation medicine* appears to be gaining ground. In Japan, *rehabilitation* is preferred. *Physiatrics* and *physiatry* are widely used only in the United States and Canada. **preclinical m.** **1** Medical science and practice that deals with the prevention or treatment of illness prior to the point at which clinical measures become necessary or advisable. **2** The part of the medical curriculum that precedes, and prepares the student for, clinical instruction and training, and which typically includes the study of biology, anatomy, physiology, pharmacology, and related sciences. **preventive m.** The branch of medicine concerned with the prevention of disease, injury, and disability, and with the promotion of safety and of practices aimed at lessening the probability of disease, with regard to individuals and whole populations, as distinguished from remedial or curative measures. **proprietary m.** A drug or medicine the manufacture or composition of which is controlled by an owner through patent rights or copyrights previously obtained. **psychological m.** PSYCHIATRY. **psychosomatic m.** The branch of medicine devoted to psychosomatic disorders. Also *psychopneumatology* (obs.). **rehabilitation m.** The branch of medicine specializing in the treatment of the disabled to restore normal function. When applied to the restoration of physical function, it is generally identified with the specialty known as physical medicine and rehabilitation. • See note at PHYSICAL MEDICINE AND REHABILITATION, under MEDICINE. **socialized m.** **1** STATE MEDICINE. **2** Any medical care system which is administered or controlled predominantly by government or other public agencies and in which private practice is limited in scope or significance. **space m.** A special branch of aviation medicine which deals with the stresses imposed on man by projection through and beyond the earth's atmosphere, flight in interplanetary space, and return to earth. Such stresses include the agravic state, exposure to radiation, and isolation. Also *aerospace medicine.* **state m.** A medical care system in which the organization and provision of care is under the direct control of government and in which the providers are employed directly or through contractual arrangements by the government. Also *socialized medicine.* **tropical m.** The medical specialty concerned with those diseases and disorders that are contracted chiefly in a hot or warm climate, or which exhibit unique characteristics in tropical countries. See also TROPICAL DISEASE. **veterinary m.** The branch of medicine that deals with the diagnosis and treatment of disease in all animals other than man. **whole person m.** HOLISTIC MEDICINE.

**medico-** \med′ikō-\ [L *medicus* physician, surgeon] A combining form meaning medical.

**medicolegal** \-lē′gəl\ [MEDICO- + LEGAL] Pertaining to forensic medicine or to that which involves both medicine and law.

**medicopsychology** \-sīkäl′əjē\ [MEDICO- + PSYCHOLOGY] PSYCHIATRY.

**medifrontal** \mē′dēfrun′təl\ MIDFRONTAL.

**Medin** [Oskar *Medin,* Swedish physician, 1847–1927] Medin's disease, Heine-Medin disease. See under ACUTE ANTERIOR POLIOMYELITIS.

**medio-** \mē′dē·ō-\ [L *medius* middle] A combining form meaning middle. Also *medi-*.

**mediocarpal** \-kär′pəl\ MIDCARPAL.

**medioccipital** \mē′dē·äksip′itəl\ MIDOCCIPITAL.

**mediofrontal** \-frun′təl\ MIDFRONTAL.

**medionecrosis** \-nekrō′sis\ Necrosis of the tunica media of an artery, usually the aorta. **m. of the aorta** CYSTIC MEDIAL NECROSIS.

**mediopontine** \-pän′tīn\ Denoting the central portion of the pons.

**mediosylvian** \-sil′vē·ən\ Denoting that portion of the lateral cerebral fissure of Sylvius which is closer to midline.

**mediotarsal** \-tär′səl\ MIDTARSAL.

**mediotemporal** \-tem′pərəl\ Denoting the central portion of the temporal lobe of the cerebrum.

**mediotrusion** \-troo′zhən\ [MEDIO- + *(trans)trusion*] Inward transtrusion.

**mediscalenus** \mē′dēskālē′nəs\ *Outmoded* MUSCULUS SCALENUS MEDIUS.

**medium** [L (substantive from *medium,* neut. of *medius* middle, midmost, akin to Gk *mesos* middle), the middle] (*pl.* media) **1** A material in which a substance, an impulse, or information is transported. **2** A material in which interactions take place. **3** CULTURE MEDIUM. See also AGAR, BROTH, CULTURE, CULTURE MEDIUM. **Apathy's m.** An aqueous medium for mounting slide preparations directly from water. It is used when dehydration with alcohol and xylene would be detrimental. **Bavister's m.** A simple culture medium in which hamster and human eggs may be fertilized *in vitro* in the laboratory. The medium, a modification of the Tyrode solution, contains bovine serum albumin. Also *Tyrode-B.* **brain-heart infusion m.** **1** A liquid culture medium containing peptone and infusion solids of calf brain and beef heart. It is used in cultivating many microorganisms, especially fastidious bacteria. **2** BRAIN-HEART INFUSION AGAR. **Cary-Blair transport m.** A medium used for the collection and transport of clinical specimens intended for microbiologic examination. **clearing m.** A medium used to make histologic specimens transparent or translucent. **complete m.** Any medium for the *in vitro* culture of cells, tissues, or organisms that contains, in addition to basic nutrients, supplemental nutrients to support growth of fastidious or mutant cells or organisms. **contrast m.** In radiology, a substance of different radiopacity from that of the organ or tissues being studied, to allow roentgenographic demonstration of the contours of a lumen or structure. When the substance is more radiopaque than the tissues, it is called a positive contrast medium, for example, a substance containing barium or iodine. When the substance is less radiopaque than the tissues, it is called a negative contrast medium, for example, air. Also *radiopaque medium.* **culture m.** See under CULTURE MEDIUM. **deoxycholate-citrate m.** DEOXYCHOLATE-CITRATE AGAR. **dioptric media** REFRACTING MEDIA. **Dubos m.** A culture medium containing oleic acid and albumin for growing the tubercle bacillus. **Löffler m.** LÖFFLER'S BLOOD CULTURE MEDIUM. **Löwenstein-Jensen m.** LÖWENSTEIN-JENSEN AGAR. **marking m.** A material used for marking occlusal contacts or pressure points on the fitting surface of a denture. **minimal m.** Any medium for the *in vitro* culture of cells, tissues, or organisms that contains only those nutrients needed for growth of wild types or otherwise normal cells or organisms, the only carbon and nitrogen sources being salts and pure and defined chemicals. **motility test m.** A nutrient medium prepared with a low concentration of agar so that the consistency is less solid than usual and allows motile organisms to establish growth in parts of the medium away from the line of inoculation. It is used in differentiating species of bacteria. Also *semisolid culture medium.* **mounting m.** Any substance used to mount objects on slides for microscopic study, usually a resin, glycerol, or polymer. Also *mountant.* **Novy, McNeal and Nicolle m.** A saline rabbit's blood medium suitable for the culturing of *Leishmania donovani.* Also *NNN medium, N.N.N. culture medium.* **radiopaque m.** CONTRAST MEDIUM. **refracting media** The portions of the eye able to change the vergence of light. Also *dioptric media.* **separating m.** In dentistry, a material such as oil, petroleum jelly, soft soap, or alginate solution, used to prevent the adhesion of one surface to another, as of freshly mixed plaster of Paris to the surface of a set mix. **Stuart transport m.** A non-nutritive medium of soft consistency containing thioglycollate, glycerophosphate, and cysteine, used to transport specimens and prevent the death of fastidious organisms before the specimen is planted on appropriate culture media. Also *Stuart broth.* **Thayer-Martin m.** THAYER-MARTIN AGAR. **transparent media of the eye** The cornea, lens, aqueous humor, and vitreous body.

**MEDLARS** [Acronym formed from *Med(ical) L(iterature) A(nalysis and) R(etrieval) S(ystem)*] A computerized system providing on-line search and retrieval services to the extensive medical bibliography of the U.S. National Library of Medicine by means of various databases, including MEDLINE, the database devoted to worldwide coverage of recent biomedical literature.

**MEDLINE** [Acronym formed from *MED(LARS) (on)-line*] See under MEDLARS.

**medphalan** D-3-[*p*[Bis(2-chloroethyl)amino]-phenyl]-alanine. A mustard-type antineoplastic drug.

**medroxyprogesterone acetate** $C_{24}H_{34}O_4$. 17α-Hydroxy- 6α-methylpregn-4-ene-3,20-dione 17-acetate, a progestin widely used as a contraceptive and to treat precocious puberty in the female, functional uterine bleeding, dysmenorrhea, endometriosis, and threatened abortion, and to suppress postpartum lactation.

**medulla** \midul′ə\ [L (prob. altered by influence of *medius* middle, from earlier *merulla,* akin to Old English *(s)meoru* fat, grease and *smierwan* to smear) marrow, pulp, pith, inner part] (*pl.* medullae) **1** [NA] The innermost or middle part of an organ or structure. Also *marrow, medullary substance.* **2** MEDULLA OBLONGATA. **adrenal m.** MEDULLA GLANDULAE SUPRARENALIS. **m. of bone** BONE MARROW. **m. glandulae suprarenalis** The internal reddish or reddish brown layer of the suprarenal, or adrenal, gland that is composed of groups of nerve cells and a network of cords and groups of chromaffin cells with large anastomosing venous sinusoids between them. Also *adrenal medulla, medulla of suprarenal gland, suprarenal medulla, substantia medullaris glandulae suprarenalis.* **m. of hair shaft** The central core of the hair shaft, present in all but the finest hairs. Also *hair pulp.* **m. of kidney** MEDULLA RENALIS. **m. nodi lymphatici** The darker central portion of a lymph node that extends to the surface at the hilum where it is continuous with the efferent lymph vessels. It has a trabecular meshwork containing a well defined fibrocellular reticulum and cords of cells, such as lymphocytes, and lymph sinuses around the cords. Also *medulla of lymph node, substantia medullaris lymphoglandulae.* **m. oblongata** [NA] The caudal portion of the brainstem that extends between the pons and the most rostral part of the cervical spinal cord. It lies anterior to the cerebellum, and its upper posterior part forms the floor of the lower half of the fourth ventricle. The medulla oblongata contains large cellular groups of neurons that form the central nuclei of the glossopharyngeal, vagus, accessory, and hypoglossal nerves, and it is importantly related to the reflex functions of the pharynx, larynx, and tongue and in the regulation of life-sustaining respiratory and cardiovascular reflexes as well as consciousness. Through the medulla oblongata course the long ascending afferent tracts to the cerebellum and thalamus and the descending pathways from higher brain centers that control motor activity. Also *spinal bulb, medulla, oblongata* (seldom used). **m. ossium** [NA] The soft tissue found in the cavities of bones; bone marrow. It differs in composition in different bones and at different ages, and usually as two types, red marrow and yellow marrow. The basic meshwork of connective tissue contains blood vessels and cells, such as fat cells and various blood cells. See also CAVITAS MEDULLARIS OSSIUM. **m. ossium flava** YELLOW BONE MARROW. **m. ossium rubra** RED BONE MARROW. **m. ovarii** [NA] The central, vascular portion of the ovary which consists of loose connective tissue with elastin fibers, smooth muscle fibers, and a mass of contorted blood vessels. It is surrounded by the thick cortex except at the hilum where strands of smooth muscle fibers extend into it from the mesovarium. Also *zona vasculosa, zona vasculosa of Waldeyer, medulla of ovary.* **m. renalis** [NA] The inner part of the kidney, comprising a number of striated pyramidal masses (the renal pyramids), the bases of which face outward abutting on the cortex while their apices are directed to the renal sinus, where they appear as the renal papillae projecting into the minor calices. Each pyramid is composed of renal tubules. Also *medulla of kidney, substantia medullaris renis* (outmoded), *medullary zone, medullary substance of kidney.* **m. spinalis** [NA] The elongated cylindrical part of the central nervous system, located in the vertebral canal and covered by three membranes. It extends from the upper border of the atlas, where it is continuous with the medulla oblongata, to the first or second lumbar vertebra (in the adult human), where it forms the tapered conus medullaris from which the filum terminale extends downward. The vertebral level of the conus medullaris varies with species and developmental age. Also *spinal cord, spinal medulla, spinal marrow, chorda spinalis* (obs.), *funis argenteus* (obs.). **suprarenal m.** MEDULLA GLANDULAE SUPRARENALIS. **m. of suprarenal gland** MEDULLA GLANDULAE SUPRARENALIS.

**medullae** \medul′ē\ Plural of MEDULLA.

**medullary** \med′yəler′ē\ **1** Pertaining to a medulla. **2** Resembling marrow. For defs. 1 and 2 also *medullar.*

**medullated** \med′yəlā′tid\ **1** Having a lipoprotein (myelin) sheath; myelinated: said of a nerve fiber. **2** Having a medulla.

**medullectomy** \med′yəlek′təmē\ [*medull(a)* + -ECTOMY] A surgical procedure in which the medulla, or most central portion of a body part, is removed.

**medulliadrenal** \medul′ē·adrē′nəl\ MEDULLOADRENAL.

**medullispinal** \medul′ispī′nəl\ Pertaining to the spinal cord.

**medullitis** \med′yəlī′tis\ [*medull(a)* + -ITIS] **1** MYELITIS. **2** Inflammation of the medulla oblongata. **3** OSTEOMYELITIS.

**medulloadrenal** \medul′ō·adrē′nəl\ Pertaining to the medulla of the adrenal gland. Also *medulliadrenal.*

**medulloblast** \medul′əblast\ A cell derived from a germinal cell of the inner ependymal layer, rounded, poor in cytoplasm and without processes, found in the middle (mantle) layer of the embryonic neural tube. According to some embryologists, it will be bipotent and able to differentiate into either a glioblast or a neuroblast. Others maintain this bipotentiality does not exist except for medulloblasts of the cerebellum. Elsewhere, the medulloblasts will already correspond to two cell types, apolar neuroblasts and apolar glioblasts.

**medulloblastoma** \medul′ōblastō′mə\ [*medull(a)* + *o* + BLASTOMA] A malignant brain tumor composed of small, poorly differentiated cells which tend to form pseudorosettes. The main site of growth is the midline of the cerebellum and in the roof of the fourth ventricle. Children are affected mostly. **desmoplastic m.** A variant form of medulloblastoma, with similar tumor cells but with an abundant network of reticulin fibers in a fibrous stroma. It affects older patients, and is often lateral on the cerebellar surface. Also *circumscribed cerebellar arachnoidal sarcoma.*

**medulloepithelioma** \medul′ō·ep′ithē′lē·ō′mə\ [*medull(a)* + *o* + *epitheli(o)* + -OMA] **1** A tumor of the eye, primarily of children, characterized by the formation of multilayered sheets of undifferentiated cells resembling the primitive medullary epithelium of the optic vesicle. Benign and malignant forms occur. The latter resemble retinoblastoma. Medulloepitheliomas are mainly found at the ciliary body and rarely in the retina. Also *dictyoma, diktyoma.* **2** A very rare malignant tumor of the central nervous system composed of undifferentiated columnar cells forming tubular or papillary patterns resembling primitive neural epithelium. Also *embryonal medulloepithelioma, neurocytoma.*

**medullosis** \med′yəlō′sis\ *Obs.* LEUKEMIA.

**medullosuprarenoma** \medul′ōsoo′prərēnō′mə\ [*medull(a)* + *o* + SUPRA- + REN + -OMA] PHEOCHROMOCYTOMA.

**medullotherapy** \medul′ōther′əpē\ A prophylactic treatment for rabies introduced by Pasteur, utilizing emulsions of fixed virus from the spinal medulla of rabbits.

**medusocongestin** A toxic agent obtained from the tentacles of the jellyfish *Rhizostoma cuvieri* and causing intense congestion of the splanchnic vessels. It is thought to be identical to congestin.

**mefenamic acid** $C_{15}H_{15}NO_2$. 2-[2,3-Dimethylphenyl)-amino]benzoic acid. An agent with analgesic, anti-inflammatory, and antipyretic properties. It is administered orally to relieve mild pain.

**mefexamide** $C_{15}H_{24}N_2O_3$. *N*-[2-(Diethylamino)ethyl]-2-(4-methoxyphenoxy)-acetamide. A stimulant having specific actions on the central nervous system. It has been used to treat fatigue and depression.

**mefruside** $C_{13}H_{19}ClN_2O_5S_2$. 4-Chloro-*N′*-methyl-*N′*-(tetrahydro-2-methyl-furfuryl)-*m*-benzenedisulfonamide. A substance with uses similar to those of chlorothiazide.

**MEG** magnetoencephalograph.

**mega-** \meg′ə-\ [Gk *megas* great, large] **1** A prefix denoting $10^6$, one million: used with SI units. Symbol: M **2** MEGALO-.

**megabecquerel** \meg′əbekərel′\ [MEGA- + BECQUEREL] A unit of activity of a radionuclide equal to $10^6$ becquerel. Symbol: MBq

**megabladder** \meg′əblad′ər\ MEGALOCYSTIS.

**megacardia** \-kär′dē·ə\ CARDIOMEGALY.

**megacephaly** \-sef′əlē\ [MEGA- + CEPHAL- + -Y] MACROCEPHALY.

**megacolon** \meg′əkō′lən\ [MEGA- + COLON] Enlargement of the colon, either segmental or total, marked by clinical manifestations of constipation or obstipation. Also *giant colon* (seldom used). **acquired m.** Enlargement of the colon either secondary to an associated disease or of psychogenic origin. There is neither aganglionosis nor any other congenital motor abnormality. **acute m.** TOXIC MEGACOLON. **aganglionic m.** The absence of ganglion cells in the myenteric plexus. It results in dilatation of the affected bowel segment, which is most often the distal colon and rectum. It is the major feature of congenital megacolon, and it is also found in the Down syndrome, Waardenburg syndrome, familial piebaldness, and Chagas disease. **congenital m.** An autosomal recessive condition characterized by a marked dilatation of the colon proximal to a "narrowed" segment in which intramural ganglion cells are absent (aganglionosis) in the submucosal (Meissner's) and myenteric (Auerbach's) plexuses. This aganglionic intestine does not enter into normal propulsion of colonic contents, and the dilatation of the normally innervated areas is secondary to the distal obstruction. The condition is more common in males, and it is usually a multifactorial trait. Also *Hirschsprung's disease, Ruysch disease, congenital aganglionic megacolon.* **idiopathic constitutional m.** Megacolon of unknown etiology thought to be related to chronic laxative abuse. **toxic m.** Gross distention of the colon not due to mechanical obstruction and associated with systemic signs of illness such as fever, tachycardia, or hypotension. Usually associated with severe ulcerative colitis, it has been seen with granulomatous colitis, infectious colitis, colitis related to antibiotics, and even to lymphoma of the colon. It is thought to be due at least in part to impairment of muscular or neuromuscular function in the colon wall, leading to progressive dilatation. Also *acute megacolon.*

**megacurie** \meg′əkyoo′rē\ [MEGA- + CURIE] A unit of activity of a radionuclide or of a radioactive source equal to $10^6$ curies; $3.7 \times 10^{16}$ becquerels exactly. Symbol: MCi

**megacycle per second** A unit of frequency equal to $10^6$ cycles per second; $10^6$ hertz or one megahertz. Also *megacycle* (popular but incorrect). Symbol: Mc/s ● The term *megahertz* is now commonly employed.

**megacystis** \-sis′tis\ MEGALOCYSTIS.

**megadactyl** \-dak′til\ MEGALODACTYLOUS.

**megadactyly** \-dak′tilē\ MACRODACTYLY.

**megadont** \meg′ədänt\ MACRODONT.

**megadontic** \-dän′tik\ MACRODONT.

**megaelectronvolt** \-ilek′tränvōlt′\ A unit of energy equal to $10^6$ electronvolts; $1.602\ 19 \times 10^{-13}$ joule; 160.219 petajoules. Symbol: MeV

**megaesophagus** \meg′ə·ēsäf′əgəs\ Enlarged esophagus as commonly found in achalasia. Also *megaloesophagus.*

**megagamete** \-gam′ēt\ MACROGAMETE.

**megagnathia** \meg′ənā′thē·ə\ MACROGNATHIA.

**megahertz** \meg′əhurts\ A unit of frequency equal to $10^6$ hertz. Symbol: MHz

**megakaryoblast** \-kar′ē·əblast′\ A large bone-marrow cell with an unsegmented nucleus and abundant, usually granular, cytoplasm. It is the precursor of the megakaryocyte.

**megakaryocyte** \-kar′ē·əsīt′\ [MEGA- + KARYO- + -CYTE] A very large bone-marrow cell, usually with multiple nuclear lobes and copious granular cytoplasm, which releases membrane-enclosed fragments of its cytoplasm as platelets. Also *megalokaryocyte.* **basophilic m.** PROMEGAKARYOCYTE. **lymphoid m.** PROMEGAKARYOCYTE. **stage II m.** PROMEGAKARYOCYTE.

**megakaryocytopenia** \-kar′ē·əsī′təpē′nē·ə\ An abnormal decrease in the number of megakaryocytes in the bone marrow.

**megakaryocytosis** \-ker′ē·əsītō′sis\ **1** An increase in the number of megakaryocytes in the bone marrow. **2** The occurrence of megakaryocytes in the peripheral blood.

**megalecithal** \-les′ithəl\ [MEGA- + LECITH- + -AL] Full of yolk: said of an ovum. Also *macrolecithal, polylecithal.*

**megalerythema** \meg′əler′ithē′mə\ ERYTHEMA INFECTIOSUM.

**megalo-** \meg′əlō-\ [Gk *megas,* gen. *megalou* large, big] A combining form meaning of abnormally large size. Also *mega-.*

**megaloblast** \meg′əlōblast′\ [MEGALO- + -BLAST] Any of a series of abnormally large, nucleated erythrocyte precursors seen in the bone marrow in pernicious anemia or other disorders of vitamin $B_{12}$ or folic acid metabolism. **m. of Sabin** PRONORMOBLAST.

**megaloblastic** \-blas′tik\ Exhibiting the morphologic features of megaloblasts: said of erythrocyte precursors. Compare NORMOBLASTIC.

**megaloblastoid** \-blas′toid\ Having some features resembling megaloblastic maturation of the erythrocytic series. An erythrocyte precursor is said to be megaloblastoid when nuclear chromatin condensation is in clumps, as it is normally, but parachromatin is prominent: i.e., open, transparent, unstained clefts are prominent in the nucleus and the contours of the nucleus are irregular.

**megaloblastosis** \-blastō′sis\ The presence of megaloblasts in the bone marrow.

**megalocardia** \-kär′dē·ə\ CARDIOMEGALY.

**megalocephalia** \-səfā′lyə\ MACROCEPHALY.

**megalocheiria** \-kī′rē·ə\ CHEIROMEGALY.

**megaloclitoris** \-klit′əris\ [MEGALO- + CLITORIS] MACROCLITORIS.

**megalocornea** \-kôr′nē·ə\ [MEGALO- + CORNEA] A sex-linked recessive condition in which the corneal diameter is enlarged, without increased intraocular pressure. Also *keratoglobus, cornea globata, macrocornea.*

**megalocystis** \-sis′tis\ An abnormally enlarged or distended bladder. Also *megacystis, megabladder.*

**megalocyte** \meg′əlōsīt′\ MACROCYTE.

**megalocythemia** \-sīthē′mē·ə\ MACROCYTOSIS.

**megalocytosis** \-sītō′sis\ MACROCYTOSIS.

**megalodactylous** \-dak′tiləs\ Exhibiting macrodactyly. Also *megadactyl.*

**megalodont** \meg′əlōdänt′\ MACRODONT.

**megaloencephalic** \-ensəfal′ik\ Exhibiting macroencephaly.

**megaloencephaly** \-ensef′əlē\ MACROENCEPHALY.

**megaloenteron** \-en′tərän\ Abnormal largeness of the intestinal tract or segment thereof; enteromegaly.

**megaloesophagus** \meg′əlō·isäf′əgəs\ MEGAESOPHAGUS.

**megalogastria** \-gas′trē·ə\ [MEGALO- + GASTR- + -IA] Abnormal enlargement or distention of the stomach.

**megaloglossia** \-gläs′ē·ə\ MACROGLOSSIA.

**megalokaryocyte** \-kar′ē·əsīt′\ MEGAKARYOCYTE.

**megalomania** \-mā′nē·ə\ [MEGALO- + -MANIA] A delusion of grandeur characterized by belief in one's unsurpassed power, greatness, or eminence, as in some field of endeavor.

**megalomastia** \-mas′tē·ə\ MACROMASTIA.

**megalomelia** \-mē′lyə\ MACROMELIA.

**megalonychosis** \-nikō′sis\ MACRONYCHIA.

**megalopenis** \meg′əlōpē′nis\ MACROPENIS.

**megalophallus** \meg′əlōfal′əs\ MACROPENIS.

**megalophthalmia** \meg′əläfthal′mē·ə\ MACROPHTHALMIA.

**megalophthalmos** \meg′əläfthal′məs\ MACROPHTHALMIA.

**megalophthalmus** \meg′əläfthal′məs\ MACROPHTHALMIA.

**megalopia** \meg′əlō′pē·ə\ MACROPSIA.

**megaloplastocyte** \-plas′təsīt\ GIANT PLATELET.

**megalopodia** \-pō′dē·ə\ [MEGALO- + -POD + -IA] MACROPODIA.

**megalopsia** \meg′əläp′sē·ə\ MACROPSIA.

***Megalopyge opercularis*** \meg′əläp′ijē ōpur′kyəler′is\ A species of flannel moth whose larvae have hairs that carry an urticating toxic substance and can pierce the skin, causing caterpillar dermatitis.

**megalosplenia** \-splē′nē·ə\ SPLENOMEGALY.

***Megalosporon*** \meg′əläs′pərän\ *Obs.* TRICHOPHYTON.

**megalosyndactyly** \-sindak′tilē\ [MEGALO- + SYNDACTYLY] A condition characterized by the abnormally large size and fusion of two or more digits.

**megaloureter** \meg′əlōyoorē′tər\ In an infant, an abnormally large size of a ureter occurring in the absence of evident obstruction or infection. It is presumed to be of developmental origin.
**megalourethra** \meg′əlōyoorē′thrə\ [MEGALO- + URETHRA] In an infant, an abnormally large urethra occurring in the absence of obstruction or infection. It is presumed to be of developmental origin.
**-megaly** \-meg′əlē\ [Gk *megaleios* (from *megas,* feminine *megalē,* large, big) magnificent] A combining form meaning of abnormally large size.
***Meganthropus palaeojavanicus*** \megan′thrəpəs pā′lē·ōjavan′ikəs\ A taxonomic designation that has been applied to some fossil hominids of Java represented by mandibular fragments. They are now commonly classified as early *Homo erectus.*
**meganucleus** \-nʸoo′klē·əs\ [MEGA- + NUCLEUS] MACRONUCLEUS.
**megaprosopia** \-prōsō′pē·ə\ [MEGA- + PROSOP- + -IA ] MACROPROSOPIA.
**megarectum** \meg′ərek′təm\ Marked distension of the rectum.
***Megarhinus*** \-rī′nəs\ *TOXORHYNCHITES.*
**megaroentgen** \-rent′gen\ [MEGA- + ROENTGEN] A unit of ionization exposure equal to $10^6$ roentgen; $2.58 \times 10^2$ coulomb per kilogram. Symbol: MR
***Megaselia*** \-sē′lyə\ A genus of flies some species of which have produced myiasis in humans from larvae in wounds. *M. scalaris (Apiochaeta ferruginea)* has also been reported as a cause of human intestinal myiasis.
**megasigmoid** \-sig′moid\ Marked distension and elongation of the sigmoid colon.
**megasoma** \-sō′mə\ GIGANTISM.
**megasome** \meg′əsōm\ [MEGA- + Gk *sōm(a)* body] An individual with gigantism. Also *giant.*
**megasomia** \-sō′mē·ə\ [MEGA- + Gk *sōm(a)* body + -IA] GIGANTISM.
**megavoltage** \meg′əvōltij\ Voltage of more than a million volts. Megavoltage radiation may refer to x rays or gamma rays having photon energies greater than a million electron volts.
**megestrol acetate** $C_{25}H_{32}O_4$. 17-(Acetyloxy)-6-methyl-16-methylene-pregna-4,6-diene-3,20-dione. A synthetic progentin used as an antineoplastic agent in the palliative management of metastatic endometrial carcinoma. It is given orally.
**Méglin** [Jean Antoine *Méglin,* French physician, 1756–1824] See under POINT.
**meglumine diatrizoate** A methylglucamine salt of diatrizoic acid, used as a water-soluble positive contrast medium for intravascular administration, as in angiography and urography.
**meglumine iothalamate** A methylglucamine salt of iodothalamic acid, used as a radiopaque medium administered intravascularly, as in angiography and urography.
**megophthalmos** \meg′äfthal′məs\ MACROPHTHALMIA.
**Meibom** [Heinrich *Meibom,* German anatomist, 1638–1700] **1** Meibomian glands. See under GLANDULAE TARSALES. **2** Meibomian stye. See under STYE.
**meibomianitis** \mībō′mē·ənī′tis\ Inflammation of the tarsal glands (meibomian glands).
**Meigs** [Arthur Vincent *Meigs,* U.S. physiologist, 1850–1912] Meigs capillaries. See under CAPILLARY.
**Meigs** [Joe Vincent *Meigs,* U.S. gynecologist, 1892–1963] See under SYNDROME.
**meio-** \mī′ō-, mī′ə-\ MIO-.
**meiogenic** \-jen′ik\ [MEIO- + -GENIC] Promoting or causing meiosis.
**meiosis** \mī·ō′sis\ [Gk *meiōsis* (from *meioun* to lessen) a lessening, diminution] The process of genetic recombination and division of diploid germ cells to produce haploid gametes occurring in gonadal tissue. The functional steps are DNA replication; pairing of homologous chromosomes; crossing-over (recombination); meiotic division I, in which each diploid daughter cell receives one duplicated homologue (two sister chromatids); and meiotic division II, in which each haploid gamete receives one sister chromatid of each chromosome of the set. Adj. meiotic.
**meiospore** \mī′əspôr\ A spore formed as a result of meiosis.
**meiotic** \mī·ät′ik\ Pertaining to or resulting from meiosis.
**Meirowsky** [Emil *Meirowsky,* U.S. dermatologist, 1876–1960] See under PHENOMENON.
**Meissner** [Georg *Meissner,* German histologist, 1829–1905] **1** See under GANGLION. **2** Meissner's plexus. See under PLEXUS SUBMUCOSUS. **3** Meissner's corpuscles. See under CORPUSCULA TACTUS.
**mel** [Gk *mel(i)* honey] Honey, especially the refined, clarified honey used in pharmaceutical preparations.
**mel-**[1] \mēl-, mel-\ [Gk *melos* limb] A combining form meaning limb. Also *melo-*[1].
**mel-**[2] \mel-\ MELO-[2].
**mel-**[3] \mel-, mēl-\ MELI-.
**melan-** \mel′ən-\ MELANO-.
**melancholia** \mel′ənkō′lyə\ [Gk (from *melaina cholē* black bile) an excess of black bile in the system, melancholy] **1** DEPRESSION. **2** ENDOGENOUS DEPRESSION. **3** A condition characterized by severe depression as manifested by loss of pleasure in all activities, early morning awakening, marked agitation or retardation, severe anorexia with weight loss, intensification of symptoms in the morning, and excessive or inappropriate guilt feelings. Also *athymia* (obs.), *cafard, tristimania.* **involutional m.** A major depression occurring for the first time in the involutional period, between 40 and 55 years in females and 50 to 65 years in males. Its characteristic triad of symptoms are delusions of guilt or poverty, obsession with death, and delusional fixation on gastrointestinal functioning all within a setting of agitation and depression. In some, paranoid delusions of persecution also occur. Also *climacteric psychosis, agitated depression, involutional depression, involutional psychosis, climacteric melancholia, agitated melancholia, melancholia agitata, involutional psychotic reaction, involutional paraphrenia.* **stuporous m.** DEPRESSIVE STUPOR.
**melanedema** \-ēdē′mə\ [MELAN- + EDEMA] COAL WORKERS' PNEUMOCONIOSIS.
**melanemia** \mel′ənē′mē·ə\ The presence of melanin in blood.
**melanin** \mel′ənin\ [MELAN- + -IN] The natural pigment of hair and skin, also found in other parts of the body. It is formed by the oxidation of tyrosine via dopa and dopaquinone to a complex polymeric material.
**melanism** \mel′ənizm\ [MELAN- + -ISM] Excessive melanin pigmentation.
**melano-** \mel′ənō-\ [Gk *melas* (genitive *melanos*) black, dark] A combining form meaning black, dark. Also *melan-.*
**melanoacanthoma** \-ak′ənthō′mə\ A seborrheic keratosis in which a high melanin content is present within melanocytes.
**melanoblast** \-mel′ənōblast′\ A derivative of the neural crest which differentiates in an embryo into a melanocyte. **amelanotic m.** A precursor of the melanocyte that does not contain demonstrable melanin.

**melanocyte** \mel′ənōsīt′\ A cell bearing or capable of forming melanin. Also *pigment cell of skin, Merkel-Ranvier cell.*

**melanocytoma** \-sītō′mə\ [MELANO- + CYT- + -OMA ] A benign pigment deposit upon the optic disk, occurring especially in black persons. **compound m.** A benign tumor that arises from epidermal melanocytes and is characterized both by junctional activity and nevus cells in the dermis. **dermal m.** A cutaneous lesion arising from a proliferation of dermal melanocytes.

**melanoderma** \-dur′mə\ [MELANO- + DERMA] An excess of melanin pigmentation in the skin. **parasitic m.** VAGRANTS' DISEASE. **senile m.** Hyperpigmentation of the skin that appears with advancing age.

**melanogen** \mel′ənəjən\ A colorless intermediate in the metabolic pathway of tyrosine to melanin that may be nonenzymatically converted to melanin under certain circumstances.

**melanogenemia** \-jənē′mē·ə\ [MELANO- + -GEN + -EMIA] The presence of melanin precursors, such as 3,4-dihydroxyphenylalanine, or related substances, in the blood. This phenomenon may occur in persons with disseminated malignant melanoma.

**melanogenesis** \-jen′əsis\ [*melan(in)* + *o* + GENESIS] The process of melanin formation. Adj. melanogenic.

**melanoid** \mel′ənoid\ **1** Dark in color. **2** A pigment resembling melanin.

***Melanoides*** \mel′ənoi′dēz\ *THIARA.*

***Melanolestes picipes*** \mel′ənōles′tēz pī′sipes\ A species of kissing bug, the black corsair, common in parts of the United States. Its bite is said to have an effect like that of a wasp's sting.

**melanoleukoderma** \-loo′kədur′mə\ Patchy and irregular increased and decreased melanosis. It is usually postinflammatory. Also *leukomelanoderma.*

**melanoma** \mel′ənō′mə\ [MELAN- + -OMA] Any benign or malignant melanocytic tumor. **acral lentiginous m.** A malignant melanoma occurring on the palms, soles, or nailbeds and characterized by a lentiginous growth of atypical melanocytes in the epidermis, elongated rete ridges, and acanthosis. **amelanotic m.** A melanoma without pigment. • This term is usually applied to a malignant melanoma and not to a nonpigmented nevus. **benign m.** NEVUS. **benign juvenile m.** EPITHELIAL AND/OR SPINDLE CELL NEVUS. **juvenile m.** EPITHELIAL AND/OR SPINDLE CELL NEVUS. **malignant m.** A highly malignant tumor of melanocytic cells. The tumor most often occurs in the skin. It may arise de novo, from a preexisting nevus or from a precancerous melanosis (Hutchinson's melanotic freckle). It appears to be more frequent in light-skinned people than in the heavily pigmented races. It is rare in children. The eye is the second most frequent site. Here melanoma typically arises from uveal structures. As in skin, darkly pigmented peoples are not commonly affected. Among other sites for primary malignant melanoma are the oral mucosa, nose, vagina, lung, and meninges. All are rare and highly malignant. Metastases are typically widespread, at unusual sites, for example, the heart and small bowel, and may appear after long quiesecent periods. **spindle cell m.** A malignant melanoma with fusiform tumor cells: used more for ocular than dermal melanomas. Spindle cell melanomas of the eye are often less aggressive than epithelioid cell melanomas. **subungual m.** A malignant melanoma arising under a fingernail. Also *melanotic whitlow.*

**melanonychia** \-nik′ē·ə\ [MELAN- + ONYCH- + -IA ] Black or brown discoloration of the nails. It may appear as diffuse, longitudinal, or transverse streaking.

**melanophage** \mel′ənōfāj′\ A cell which contains melanin pigment due to phagocytosis but which is unable to synthesize melanin.

**melanophore** \mel′ənōfôr′\ A pigment cell containing melanin. Melanophores contribute to rapid color changes in some organisms due to the movement of melanosomes within the melanophores.

**melanophorin** \-fôr′in\ A chemical which can cause the dispersion of the pigment in a melanophore.

**melanoplakia** \-plā′kē·ə\ The presence of pigmented patches on the oral or genital mucous membrane.

**melanoptysis** \mel′ənäp′tisis\ The expectoration of black-tinged sputum containing carbon pigment due to the repeated inhalation of great amounts of coal dust, as in coal mining.

**melanorrhagia** \mel′ənôrā′jə\ [MELANO- + -RRHAGIA] The passage of melenic and bloody stool.

**melanosis** \mel′ənō′sis\ [MELAN- + -OSIS] The abnormal black-brown pigmentation of tissues due to the deposition of melanin or melaninlike substances. Adj. melanotic. **m. coli** The presence of a brown to black mucosal discoloration in the colon or a segment thereof that has no clinical significance and is due to the accumulation of macrophages within the lamina propria containing a melanin-like pigment. The pigment is histochemically similar to melanin and lipofuscin. **oculocutaneous m.** OTA'S NEVUS. **precancerous m. of Dubreuilh** HUTCHINSON'S MELANOTIC FRECKLE. **Riehl's m.** Melanosis that affects primarily the forehead and temples and is possibly caused by external contact with photodynamic agents. **m. sclerae** Congenital pigmented flecks in the sclera.

**melanosome** \mel′ənōsōm′\ [MELANO- + Gk *sōm(a)* body] A discrete melanin-containing organelle, usually located near a Golgi body. The melanosome appears uniformly electron-dense and without demonstrable tyrosinase activity. Also *melanin granule.* **compound m.** The precursor of the mature melanin granule. It has a spiral or laminar structure contained within an oval vesicle.

**melanotic** \mel′ənät′ik\ Affected with melanosis.

**melanotrichia** \-trik′ē·ə\ [MELANO- + TRICH- + -IA] A darkness of the hair. **m. linguae** BLACK HAIRY TONGUE.

**melanotropin** \-trō′pin\ The pituitary hormone that stimulates melanin-granule dispersion in amphibian and fish melanocytes, as well as melanin synthesis in mammalian melanocytes. Two forms exist, $\alpha$-melanotropin, an *N*-acylated tridecapeptide amide, and $\beta$-melanotropin, a peptide of 18 residues. Both are formed by proteolysis of larger molecules. The sequence of $\alpha$-melanotropin is included within the corticotropin molecule, and $\beta$-melanotropin has several residues in common with it.

**melanuria** \mel′ənʸoo′rē·ə\ [MELAN- + -URIA] The excretion of melanin in the urine as seen in patients with widely metastatic malignant melanoma. Melanin is excreted as a colorless precursor that becomes dark when the urine stands at room temperature for several hours. Also *melanuresis.* Adj. melanuric.

**melarsoprol** \melär′səprôl\ $C_{12}H_{15}AsN_6OS_2$. A narrow-spectrum antiprotozoal drug containing trivalent arsenic (melarsen oxide) and dimercaprol. It is used for treating advanced African trypanosomiasis with central nervous system involvement. Also *Mel B.*

**melasma** \məlaz′mə\ [Gk *melasma* (from *melas* black) a black spot] Hypermelanosis affecting the cheeks, forehead, and chin. Also *chloasma.* **m. gravidarum** Melasma associated with pregnancy. Also *mask of pregnancy, chloasma gravidarum.*

**melatonin** \mel′ətō′nin\ *N*-Acetyl-5-methoxytryptamine. A natural substance formed by methylation and acetylation of serotonin. It is nearly uniquely synthesized in and secreted by the pineal gland, and in amphibia it has an action opposite to that of melanocyte stimulating hormone. It stimulates the aggregation of melanosomes in melanophores, thus lightening the skin. Postulated to be the pineal hormone, its physiologic role in man is unknown. Also *melanocyte inhibiting factor.*

**Mel B** MELARSOPROL.

**melena** \məlē′nə\ [Gk *melaina,* fem. of *melas* black] The passage of dark or blackish, tarry stools stained with altered blood. Compare HEMATOCHEZIA. **m. spuria** Melena produced from blood resulting from bleeding other than in the gastrointestinal tract, such as deglutition from a nose bleed, or produced by ingestion of other substances that can cause black stools, such as bismuth. **m. vera** True melena; dark stool due to the presence of blood derived from bleeding into the intestinal tract.

**melenemesis** \mel′ənem′əsis\ [Gk *melain(a),* fem. of *melas* black + *emesis* a vomiting] COFFEE-GROUND VOMIT.

**Meleney** [Frank Lamont *Meleney,* U.S. surgeon, 1889–1963] **1** Meleney synergistic gangrene. See under PROGRESSIVE POSTOPERATIVE GANGRENE. **2** See under ULCER.

**melenic** \melē′nik\ Relating to or characterized by melena. Also *melenotic.*

**melenotic** \mel′ənät′ik\ MELENIC.

**meli-** \mel′ē-, mē′lē-\ [Gk *meli* (genitive *melitos*) honey] A combining form meaning honey, sweet. Also *mel-* .

**melibiose** The disaccharide consisting of galactose bearing an α-glucosyl group on O-6. It occurs naturally as a digestion product of raffinose.

**melicera** \mel′əsir′ə\ [Gk *melikēra* (from *meli* honey + *kēros* wax) a virulent eruption on the head] A cyst containing viscous, sticky, semisolid material.

**melilotoxin** \mel′ilōtäk′sin\ DICUMAROL.

**melioidosis** \mē′lē-oidō′sis\ [Gk *mēli(s)* glanders + -OID + -OSIS] An infectious disease primarily affecting rodents that occurs occasionally in farm and pet animals and humans. It resembles equine glanders and is caused by *Pseudomonas pseudomallei.* The portal of entry is probably via open skin lesions and by inhalation. The severity of illness ranges from inapparent infection to overwhelming septicemia. The disease has a protean clinical spectrum, including acute or chronic localized suppurative infection, acute pneumonitis with abscess formation, and septicemia. Hepatic and splenic abscesses may also be present. It occurs most commonly in India, Malaysia, Burma, Thailand, and Indonesia. Isolation of the organism from urine, blood, or skin pustules is the best method of diagnosis in the acute disease. In the chronic form, serologic tests are of value. *P. pseudomallei* is usually sensitive to chloramphenicol, tetracycline, sulfadiazine, and novobiocin. Also *pseudoglanders, malleoidosis, Whitmore's fever, Stanton's disease.*

**melissotherapy** \melis′ōther′əpē\ APIOTHERAPY.

**melitensis** \mel′iten′sis\ [after *Melit(a),* ancient L name of Malta + L *-ensis* English *-ese*] MALTA FEVER.

**melitin** A preparation of soluble antigen of *Brucella melitensis,* used in the diagnosis of undulant fever. When injected intradermally in the arm a skin reaction may develop, indicating that a *Brucella* infection has occurred previously.

**melituria** \mel′itʸoo′rē·ə\ [Gk *meli* (gen. *melitos*) honey + -URIA] The presence of sugar in the urine. Also *mellituria.* Adj. melituric.

**Melkersson** [Ernst Gustaf *Melkersson,* Swedish physician, 1898–1932] Melkersson syndrome. See under MELKERSSON-ROSENTHAL SYNDROME.

**mellitum** \melī′təm\ [L, substantive from *mellitum,* neut. sing. of *mellitus* pertaining to honey] Any sweet pharmaceutical preparation containing honey.

**mellituria** \mel′itʸoo′rē·ə\ MELITURIA.

**Melnick** [John Charles *Melnick,* U.S. roentgenologist, born 1928] Melnick-Needles syndrome. See under SYNDROME.

**melo-¹** MEL-¹.

**melo-²** \mel′ō-\ [Gk *mēlon* apple, fruit of a tree, cheek] A combining form meaning cheek. Also *mel-* .

**melocervicoplasty** \-sur′vikōplas′tē\ [MELO- + CERVICO- + -PLASTY] FACE-LIFT.

**melomelia** \-mē′lyə\ [MELO-¹ + MEL-¹ + -IA] A condition of unequal conjoined twins in which both normal limbs and rudimentary accessory limbs are present.

**melonoplasty** \mel′ənōplas′tē\ MELOPLASTY.

**meloplastic** \-plas′tik\ Pertaining to meloplasty.

**meloplasty** \mel′əplas′tē\ [MELO- + -PLASTY] Any plastic operation on the cheeks. Also *melonoplasty.*

**melorheostosis** \mē′lôrē′ästō′sis\ [Gk *melo(s)* limb + *rhe(o)-* + OST- + -OSIS] A rare abnormality of long bone growth in which the cortex becomes thickened and irregular to resemble the appearance of a candle with melted wax that has flowed down the sides. Also *Leri's disease, candle wax disease, rheostosis, flowing hyperostosis, osteopathia hyperostotica congenita.*

**meloschisis** \məläs′kəsis\ [MELO- + -SCHISIS] A congenital facial cleft in which a groove or fissure crosses the cheek. It may run obliquely upward toward the lower eyelid (oblique facial cleft) or it may cross the face transversely from the corner of the mouth (genal cleft).

**melotia** \melō′shə\ [MEL-² + OT- + -IA] The congenital displacement of the external ears, as in low-set ears.

**Melotte** [George W. *Melotte,* U.S. dentist, 1835–1915] See under METAL.

**melphalan** \mel′fəlan\ $C_{13}H_{18}Cl_2N_2O_2$. 4-[Bis(2-chloroethyl)amino]-L-phenylalanine. A phenylalanine analogue of the nitrogen mustards, used as an antineoplastic agent. It is given orally.

**melting** **1** The transition of solid to liquid, in which ions or molecules leave ordered positions and acquire random motions. **2** Any of several processes in which molecules or parts of molecules acquire greater random movement, such as the tumbling motion of lipid hydrocarbon chains within a biologic membrane and the disruption of base stacking in nucleic acid on heating.

**Meltzer** [Samuel James *Meltzer,* U.S. physiologist, 1851–1920] **1** Meltzer's law. See under LAW OF CONTRARY INNERVATION. **2** Meltzer-Lyon test. See under TEST.

**member** A constituent or part of a body; a limb or appendage; membrum. **inferior m.** MEMBRUM INFERIUS. **virile m.** PENIS.

**membra** \mem′brə\ Plural of MEMBRUM.

**membrana** \membrā′nə\ [L (from *membrum* a member, part; akin to Gk *mēninx* a membrane) skin, integument, membrane] (*pl.* membranae) [NA] A thin layer of tissue that covers a surface of a part, cavity, or organ; that connects two structures; or that divides a space or an organ. Also *membrane.* **m. atlanto-occipitalis anterior** [NA] A sheet of dense fibers extending from the anterior surface and upper margin of the anterior arch of the atlas to the anterior margin of the foramen magnum and the inferior aspect of the basilar part of the occipital bone. The thicker central fibers, attached to the anterior tubercle, are continuous inferiorly with the anterior longitudinal ligament. Also *anterior atlanto-occipital membrane, anterior atlanto-occipital* *ligament, deep atlanto-occipital ligament.* **m. atlanto-occipitalis posterior** [NA] A broad, flaccid sheet extending from the posterior surface and upper margin of the posterior arch of the atlas to the posterior margin of the foramen magnum between the two condyles. It corresponds to the position of the ligamenta flava and is adherent to the dura mater anteriorly. It forms part of the floor of the suboccipital triangle and is pierced by the vertebral artery and the posterior ramus of the first cervical nerve. Also *posterior atlanto-occipital membrane, posterior atlanto-occipital ligament.* **m. basalis ductus semicircularis** [NA] The homogeneous basement membrane contained in the internal lining of the simple epithelium of the internal ear's semicircular duct. Also *basal membrane of semicircular duct.* **m. capsulopupillaris** The segment of the embryonic membrana pupillaris that extends sideways between the pupil and the anterior surface of the lens. **m. choriocapillaris** LAMINA CHOROIDOCAPILLARIS. **m. cricovocalis** CONUS ELASTICUS LARYNGIS. **membranae deciduae** [NA] The layers of the altered endometrium, or decidua, of the uterus that become continuous with the placenta and are shed after parturition. Also *deciduous membranes, decidual membranes.* **m. fibroelastica laryngis** [NA] A layer of fibrous and elastic tissue beneath the mucous membrane of the larynx that is interrupted on each side by the gap between the vocal and the vestibular ligaments. Thus it consists of an upper part, the quadrangular membrane, and a lower part, the conus elasticus. A middle portion lies opposite the ventricle of the larynx. Also *fibroelastic membrane of larynx.* **m. fibrosa capsulae articularis** [NA] The outer layer of the articular capsule of a synovial joint. It is composed of white fibrous tissue and some elastic fibers, varying in thickness and often strengthened either by fiber bundles forming ligaments or by incorporation of tendons of muscles. It attaches to bone by blending with the periosteum. Also *fibrous membrane of articular capsule, fibrous articular capsule, fibrous layer of articular capsule.* **m. fusca** LAMINA FUSCA SCLERAE. **m. germinativa** BLASTODERM. **m. gliae superficialis** The fine, closely adherent outer membrane of the brain and spinal cord made up of the pia arachnoid and adherent neuroglial end feet. Also *pial-glial membrane.* **m. intercostalis externa** [NA] An aponeurotic layer that replaces the anterior portion of an external intercostal muscle between the costal cartilages as far as the sternum. It is usually absent in the tenth and eleventh spaces and occasionally in the first. Also *external intercostal membrane, external intercostal ligament, anterior intercostal membrane.* **m. intercostalis interna** [NA] An aponeurotic layer that replaces the posterior portion of an internal intercostal muscle. It extends backward from the posterior costal angle, where it is continuous anteriorly with the fascia between the external and internal intercostal muscles and posteriorly with the superior costotransverse ligaments and the subcostal muscle. Also *internal intercostal membrane, internal intercostal ligament.* **m. interossea antebrachii** [NA] A thin fibrous sheet, the fibers of which run obliquely downward and medially from the interosseous border of the radius to that of the ulna. It holds the two bones together and increases the surface area for the attachment of the deep muscles of the forearm. Also *interosseous membrane of forearm.* **m. interossea cruris** [NA] A thin aponeurotic layer, the fibers of which run obliquely connecting the interosseous borders of the tibia and fibula. It separates the deep muscles on the front and on the back of the leg and serves as an attachment for some muscles. The anterior tibial artery pierces it proximally while the perforating branch of the peroneal artery pierces it distally. It is continuous inferiorly with the interosseous ligament of the tibiofibular syndesmosis. Also *interosseous membrane of leg, crural interosseous membrane.* **m. obturatoria** [NA] A fibrous sheet attached to the pelvic aspect of the bony margin of the obturator foramen, closing it except superiorly where the membrane is deficient, forming the lower boundary of the obturator canal. The obturator externus and internus muscles arise partly from its external and pelvic surfaces, respectively. Also *obturator membrane.* **m. perinei** [NA] A strong, somewhat triangular fibrous sheet that spans the pubic arch between the ischiopubic rami. The posteriorly directed base is attached centrally to the perineal body, while it is attached superiorly to the endopelvic fascia and inferiorly to the membranous layer of the superficial fascia of the perineum behind the superficial transverse perineal muscle. The anteriorly directed apex is flattened and thickened to form the transverse perineal ligament. Also *perineal aponeurosis, superficial layer of triangular ligament, perineal ligament of Carcassonne, fascia diaphragmatis urogenitalis inferior, Carcassonne's ligament, superficial layer of urogenital diaphragm, perineal membrane, inferior layer of urogenital diaphragm, triangular ligament of Colles.* **m. preformativa** An apparent thickening of the basement membrane between the inner enamel epithelium and the dental papilla which precedes the initial formation of dentin. Also *membrana preformata, dentinoenamel membrane.* **m. propria ductus semicircularis** [NA] The layer of fibrous tissue, which contains blood vessels and pigment cells, that forms the outer of the three layers of the membranous semicircular ducts of the internal ear. It lines the endosteum of the bony labyrinth and may be adherent to it. Also *proper membrane of semicircular duct.* **m. quadrangularis** [NA] The upper portion of the fibroelastic membrane of the larynx, extending between the side of the epiglottic cartilage anteriorly and the arytenoid cartilage posteriorly. Its upper edge is within the aryepiglottic fold, which it supports, and anteroinferiorly it is attached in the angle of the thyroid cartilage, the inferior free margin forming the vestibular ligament within the vestibular fold. Also *quadrangular membrane.* **m. reticularis ductus cochlearis** [NA] In the organ of Corti, a delicate layer of cytoplasmic processes that extend from the cells of Deiters and the outer rod or pillar cells. This membrane is perforated by the stereocilia of the hair cells. Also *lamina reticularis, reticular lamina of the spiral organ, Kölliker's membrane, reticular membrane of organ of Corti, reticulated membrane.* **m. serosa** **1** TUNICA SEROSA. **2** CHORION. **m. serotina** *Outmoded* DECIDUA BASALIS. **m. stapedis** [NA] A thin mucosal lamina filling the space between the two crura and the base of the stapes. Also *stapedial membrane, membrane of stapes.* **m. statoconiorum macularum** [NA] A flattened gelatinous layer between and upon the projecting sensory hairs of the maculae of the utricle and the saccule. It contains, superficially, numerous minute granules of calcite and protein, called otoconia, otoliths, or statoconia. The gelatinous material is secreted by the supporting cells. Also *statoconic membrane of maculae, otolithic membrane.* **m. sterni** [NA] A dense fibrous layer investing the sternum. It is formed by interweaving of the periosteum with fibers of the radiate sternocostal ligaments and, anteriorly, tendinous fibers of the pectoralis major muscle. Also *sternal membrane.* **m. suprapleuralis** [NA] A domelike expansion of endothoracic fascia that is attached anteriorly to the inner border of the first rib and posteriorly to the transverse process of the seventh cervical vertebra. It strengthens the cervical pleura over the apex of the lung. On its superior surface are strengthening muscle fibers from the scalene muscles. Also *suprapleural membrane, Sibson's fascia, Sibson's aponeurosis, scalene fascia.* **m. synovialis capsulae articularis** The inner layer of the articular capsule of synovial joints, consisting of loose connective tissue, elastic fibers, and a varying amount of fat. It is coextensive with the outer fibrous layer and usually attached to bone at or near the peripheral border of the articular cartilage. Occasionally it forms folds or pouches or is continuous with the lining of bursae. It produces synovial fluid, and its inner smooth surface faces the joint cavity. Also *synovial membrane of articular capsule, synovial layer of articular capsule, synovial capsule, synovium* (outmoded), *synovial membrane.* **m. tectoria** [NA] The cranial prolongation of the anterior layer of the posterior longitudinal ligament inside the vertebral canal, extending from the posterior surfaces of the bodies of the third and second cervical vertebrae to the inner aspect of the basilar part of the occipital bone where it blends with dura mater. Also *tectorial membrane, long occipitoaxial membrane, occipitoaxial ligament.* **m. tectoria ductus cochlearis** [NA] A flexible gelatinous membrane that is attached to the limbus laminae spiralis osseae and that covers the sensory receptive mechanism of the spiral organ of Corti, including the inner and outer hair cells and rods. Also *tectorial membrane of cochlear duct, Corti's membrane.* **m. thyrohyoidea** [NA] A broad fibroelastic sheet that extends from the upper margin of the thyroid cartilage and the front of the superior cornua to the upper margin of the posterior surface of the body and greater cornua of the hyoid bone, being separated from the hyoid body by a bursa. Also *thyrohyoid membrane, hyothyroid membrane.* **m. tympani** [NA] The thin, ellipsoid, semitransparent membranous partition between the external acoustic meatus and the tympanic cavity. The thick border of the larger inferior portion, the pars tensa, is attached by a fibrocartilaginous ring to the tympanic sulcus of the temporal bone, while the triangular anterosuperior portion, the pars flaccida, is attached directly to the bone at the tympanic notch. It is obliquely set and comprises three layers: an outer stratum corneum, an intermediate fibrous layer having outer radiate fibers and inner circular fibers, and an inner stratum mucosum. The manubrium of malleus is attached to its inner surface. Also *tympanic membrane, eardrum, drum membrane, drumhead, myrinx, myringa, drum head, drum.* **m. tympani secundaria** [NA] The fibrous mucosa-covered sheet that closes the fenestra cochleae. It is situated posteroinferior to the promontory on the medial wall of the tympanic cavity. Also *secondary tympanic membrane, Scarpa's membrane.* **m. vitellina** VITELLINE MEMBRANE. **m. vitrea** [NA] The condensation of the gel and fibrillar framework at the periphery of the vitreous body of the eyeball. It is attached to the ciliary epithelium and processes and to the margin of the optic disk. Also *vitreous membrane, hyaloid membrane.*

**membranaceous** \mem′brənā′shəs\ MEMBRANOUS.

**membranae** \membrā′nē\ Plural of MEMBRANA.

**membranate** \mem′brənāt\ Having the properties of a membrane.

# membrane

**membrane** \mem′brān\ [L *membrana.* See MEMBRANA.] MEMBRANA. **adamantine m.** NASMYTH'S MEMBRANE. **allantoid m.** ALLANTOIS. **alveolocapillary m.** The composite structure of an alveolar lining cell, basement membrane, and pulmonary capillary wall through which respiratory exchange takes place. **alveolodental m.** PERIODONTIUM. **anal m.** In the embryo, the posterior part of the cloacal membrane after the transverse division of the latter into two portions by the urorectal (cloacal) septum at about the seventh week. The membrane breaks down during the ninth week and the anal canal comes to open into the amniotic cavity. **anterior atlanto-occipital m.** MEMBRANA ATLANTO-OCCIPITALIS ANTERIOR. **anterior intercostal m.** MEMBRANA INTERCOSTALIS EXTERNA. **aponeurotic m.** APONEUROSIS. **arachnoid m.** ARACHNOIDEA. **basal m.** BASEMENT MEMBRANE. **basal m. of semicircular duct** MEMBRANA BASALIS DUCTUS SEMICIRCULARIS. **basement m.** A condensation of glycoprotein and tropocollagen that is formed by and closely applied to the surfaces of Schwann cells, muscle cells, endothelial cells, and all epithelial cells. In the latter case, the basement membrane is most apparent at the interface with the underlying connective tissue. Also *basement tissue, basement layer, basement lamina, basilemma, basal membrane.* **basilar m. of cochlear duct** LAMINA BASILARIS DUCTUS COCHLEARIS. **Bichat's m.** HENLE'S FENESTRATED MEMBRANE. **black lipid m.** An artificial bimolecular lipid membrane made between two liquid compartments for the study of membrane phenomena, e.g. the effects of ionophores on electrical conductance. It is called black because it is too thin to show interference effects with light in the visible wavelength range. **Bogros serous m.** A serous membrane that lines the space of Tenon and separates it from the posterior pole of the eyeball. **Bowman's m.** LAMINA LIMITANS ANTERIOR CORNEAE. **brood m.** The germinal layer of the hydatid cyst of *Echinococcus granulosus.*. **Bruch's m.** COMPLEXUS BASALIS CHOROIDEAE. **Brunn's m.** The epithelium of the nasal olfactory region. **bucconasal m.** In the embryo, the membrane which separates the olfactory pit from the primitive buccal cavity towards the sixth week of development. It then breaks down to mark the position of the primitive posterior naris. Also *bucconasal septum.* **buccopharyngeal m.** A transitory membrane in the embryo formed where the anterior part of the primitive intestine makes contact with the outer wall of the body. Composed of ectoderm, it separates the external depression of the stomodeum from the future pharynx. It breaks down in man in the middle of the fourth week to establish communication between these cavities. No trace of the membrane is found in the adult. Also *oral membrane.* **capsulopupillary m.** PUPILLARY MEMBRANE. **cell m.** PLASMA MEMBRANE. **chorioallantoic m.** CHORIOALLANTOIS. **cloacal m.** A transitory membrane in the embryo where the posterior part of the primitive intestine makes contact with the caudal region of the body. Endoderm of the intestine becomes opposed to ectoderm with no intervening mesoderm. The membrane breaks down to form the urogenital and anal orifices. **compound m.** A membrane that is formed from two or more differing tissue layers. Also *complex membrane.* **Corti's m.** MEMBRANA TECTORIA DUCTUS COCHLEARIS. **costocoracoid m.** FASCIA CLAVIPECTORALIS. **cribriform m.** FASCIA CRIBROSA. **cricothyroid m.** CONUS ELASTICUS LARYNGIS. **cricotracheal m.** LIGAMENTUM CRICOTRACHEALE. **cricovocal m.** CONUS ELASTICUS LARYNGIS. **crural interosseous m.** MEMBRANA INTEROSSEA CRURIS. **cytoplasmic m.** PLASMA MEMBRANE. **decidual m.'s** MEMBRANAE DECIDUAE. **deciduous m.'s** MEMBRANAE DECIDUAE. **Demours m.** LAMINA LIMITANS POSTERIOR CORNEAE. **dentino-**

enamel m. MEMBRANA PREFORMATIVA. **Descemet's m.** LAMINA LIMITANS POSTERIOR CORNEAE. **dialysis m.** A semipermeable membrane which separates the blood compartment from the dialysate compartment of the hemodialyzer. The membrane usually is made of cellulose but a large variety of other substances with differing permeability to substances of varying molecular weights has been used. In general, a membrane is most permeable to substances of small molecular weight, such as water, electrolytes, urea, and creatinine, and decreasingly permeable to substances of greater molecular weight, becoming impermeable, or almost so, to large molecules such as protein molecules and the formed elements of blood. Diffusion of substances across the semipermeable membrane according to the concentration gradient between blood and dialysate is the fundamental principle underlying hemodialysis. **diphtheritic m.** The characteristic pseudomembrane of diphtheria that covers the mucous membranes of the nasopharynx, oropharynx, and laryngopharynx. **drum m.** MEMBRANA TYMPANI. **Duddell's m.** LAMINA LIMITANS POSTERIOR CORNEAE. **egg m.'s** Coverings, varying in structure and number and additional to the vitelline membrane, that can be demonstrated in all eggs. Primary membranes are created by the ovum, secondary ones by the cells of the corona radiata, and tertiary ones are added on the outside of the ovum from secretions of the uterine tube or the uterus. The zona pellucida is an example of a mammalian egg membrane, probably of the secondary type, and an avian eggshell is a tertiary membrane. Also *egg envelopes.* **elastic m.** ELASTIC LAMELLA. **enamel m.** NASMYTH'S MEMBRANE. **endoneural m.** NEURILEMMA. **excitable m.** A cell membrane which can generate action potentials and transmit them along its surface. Membranes on nerve and muscle cells are excitable. **exocoelomic m.** A thin layer of cells, possibly delaminated from the inner surface of the cytotrophoblast, that lies between the cytotrophoblast and the primary yolk sac in early human embryos. Other sites of origin, such as extraembryonic mesoderm and disk endoderm, have been suggested for various primate species. The layer soon disappears as the yolk sac develops. Also *Heuser's membrane.* **external elastic m.** EXTERNAL ELASTIC LAMINA. **external intercostal m.** MEMBRANA INTERCOSTALIS EXTERNA. **external limiting m.** An ill-defined layer formed by the outermost terminations of the glial cells in the retina between the rod and cone processes and their cell bodies. Also *stratum limitans externum.* **extraembryonic m.** Any of the membranous structures surrounding or pertaining to an embryo which protect it, provide it with oxygen and nutritive substances, and remove waste, and some of which may produce hormones. They are the chorion, amnion, yolk sac, and allantois. At a later stage in development, they are called fetal membranes. **false m.** PSEUDOMEMBRANE. **fetal m.** Any of the extraembryonic structures that provide protection, nutrition, respiration, excretion, or hormonal secretion to aid or affect the fetus. They include the chorion, amnion, yolk sac, allantois, and all parts of the functional placenta. **fibroelastic m. of larynx** MEMBRANA FIBROELASTICA LARYNGIS. **fibrous m. of articular capsule** MEMBRANA FIBROSA CAPSULAE ARTICULARIS. **Fielding's m.** *Obs.* TAPETUM. **flaccid m. of Shrapnell** PARS FLACCIDA MEMBRANAE TYMPANI. **filtration slit m. of glomerulus** A fine membranous layer between the glomerular basement membrane and the slit pores of the epithelial cell foot processes. This membrane is covered by material continuous with the surface of the foot processes, a material which has the staining characteristics of polysaccharides and which represents glycoproteins. Also *filtration slit diaphragm of glomerulus.* **glomerular basement m.** The thick basal membrane that separates the podocytes of the visceral wall of the renal glomerulus from the endothelium of the glomerular capillaries. It is involved with selective filtration between these structures. Also *lamina densa* (outmoded), *glomerular capillary basement membrane, dense layer.* **gradocol m.'s** Thin films of collodion that are made with pore sizes of controlled diameter, usually 3–10 μm. They are used in ultrafiltration to determine the size of particulate elements, especially viruses. **Haller's m.** LAMINA VASCULOSA CHOROIDEAE. **Held's limiting m.** BLOOD-BRAIN BARRIER. **Henle's m.** COMPLEXUS BASALIS CHOROIDEAE. **Henle's elastic m.** EXTERNAL ELASTIC LAMINA. **Henle's fenestrated m.** The thick membrana elastica interna beneath the endothelium. It is characterized by a number of irregular, rounded openings and is found in the wall of large arteries. Also *Bichat's membrane.* **Heuser's m.** EXOCOELOMIC MEMBRANE. **homogeneous m.** A thin layer or deposits of fibrinoid found in the boundary zone between fetal and maternal tissues from early in human pregnancy. It is also found on the surface of the syncytiotrophoblast of the chorionic villi. **Hovius m.** COMPLEXUS BASALIS CHOROIDEAE. **Huxley's m.** HUXLEY'S LAYER. **hyaline m.** Any membrane with a relatively clear, untextured appearance, particularly the membrane lining the pulmonary alveoli implicated in the respiratory distress syndrome of newborn. **hyaloid m.** MEMBRANA VITREA. **hymenal m.** HYMEN. **hyoepiglottic m.** LIGAMENTUM HYOEPIGLOTTICUM. **hyoglossal m.** A strong fibrous sheet that extends from the body of the hyoid bone to the undersurface of the root of the tongue. It receives some fibers of the genioglossus muscle anteriorly. **hyothyroid m.** MEMBRANA THYROHYOIDEA. **inner nuclear m.** The inner layer of a double-walled sac that encloses the nucleus of a cell. **internal intercostal m.** MEMBRANA INTERCOSTALIS INTERNA. **internal limiting m.** The innermost layer of the retina that separates the nerve fiber layer from the vitreous body. It is formed by the innermost terminations of the retinal glial cells. Also *stratum limitans internum.* **interosseous m. of forearm** MEMBRANA INTEROSSEA ANTEBRACHII. **interosseous m. of leg** MEMBRANA INTEROSSEA CRURIS. **intersutural m.** SUTURAL LIGAMENT. **ion-selective m.** A cell membrane that impedes the transmission of certain ions and facilitates the passage of others. **Jacob's m.** STRATUM NEUROEPITHELIALE RETINAE. **keratogenous m.** *Outmoded* MATRIX UNGUIS. **Kölliker's m.** MEMBRANA RETICULARIS DUCTUS COCHLEARIS. **limiting m.** A membrane that forms the boundary, or limit, of a tissue or structure. **long occipitoaxial m.** MEMBRANA TECTORIA. **Mauthner's m.** AXOLEMMA. **meconic m.** A desquamated epithelial film covered with mucus and stained with bile. It is formed in the fetal intestine and voided shortly after birth. **medullary m.** ENDOSTEUM. **mucocutaneous m.** A compound membrane with a modified cutaneous layer on one side and a mucous membrane on the other. **mucous m.** TUNICA MUCOSA. **Nasmyth's m.** An integument consisting of the primary enamel cuticle and the reduced enamel epithelium which covers the completed enamel of an unerupted tooth. Also *enamel cuticle, enamel membrane, adamantine membrane.* **m. of Nitabuch** A fibrinoid layer which, from the third or fourth month of gestation, separates the decidual from the trophoblastic elements within the basal plate of the placenta. The layer is thought by some to originate from degenerating cytotrophoblast. It tends to thicken as pregnancy advances and, near term, the trophoblast cells only make contact with it as discontinuous islands. This fibrinoid material is actually present elsewhere in the placenta. It unites the anchoring villi to the basal plate, and is encountered in many places in the intervillous spaces (fibrinoid substance of Rohr) or forms islands on the chorionic plate (fibrinoid substance of Langhans). Also *striae of Nitabuch, layer of Nitabuch.* **nuclear m.** The inner membrane of the nuclear envelope. **obturator m.** MEMBRANA OBTURATORIA. **olfactory m.** TUNICA MUCOSA OLFACTORIA. **olfactory mucous m.** TUNICA MUCOSA OLFACTORIA. **oral m.** BUCCOPHARYNGEAL MEMBRANE. **otolithic m.** MEMBRANA STATOCONIORUM MACULARUM. **outer m.** A membrane outside the peptidoglycan layer in Gram-negative bacteria, and connected to the inner membrane at intervals by localized junctions through gaps in the peptidoglycan. The inner leaflet contains phospholipids and the lipid termini of lipoproteins. In the outer leaflet the lipid A portion of lipopolysaccharide may be the only lipid. The number of different proteins is much smaller than in the inner membrane; the matrix protein provides a molecular sieve whose pores exclude molecules larger than 800–900 daltons. Abbr. OM **outer nuclear m.** The outer layer of a double-walled sac that encloses the nucleus of a cell. It is this outer layer that is contiguous with the rough-surfaced endoplasmic reticulum of the cell cytoplasm. **peridental m.** PERIODONTIUM. **perineal m.** MEMBRANA PERINEI. **periodontal m.** PERIODONTIUM. **periorbital m.** PERIORBITA. **pharyngobasilar m.** FASCIA PHARYNGOBASILARIS. **pial-glial m.** MEMBRANA GLIAE SUPERFICIALIS. **placental m.** The anatomic barrier in the placenta which lies between the fetal and maternal bloodstreams. It varies in thickness and in the number of layers of which it is composed, depending on the order, or even the species, involved. Terms such as epitheliochorial, endotheliochorial, and hemochorial indicate the layers present respectively in ungulates, Carnivora, and man. **plasma m.** The three-layered membrane surrounding the cytoplasm. It is composed of a phospholipid layer coated with proteins on the outer and inner surfaces, the outer surface also having associated glycoproteins which form the glycocalyx. Also *cytoplasmic membrane, cell membrane, plasmalemma, cytomembrane, cytolemma, ectosarc.* **platelet demarcation m.** The membrane that outlines a newly-formed platelet as it buds from a megakaryocyte. **pleuropericardial m.** A membrane on each side of the embryo which helps to separate the pericardial and pleural cavities. Within its substance are the common cardinal vein and the phrenic nerve. Also *pericardiopleural septum.* **posterior atlanto-occipital m.** MEMBRANA ATLANTO-OCCIPITALIS POSTERIOR. **postsynaptic m.** That portion of the plasma membrane of a neuron in closest apposition to an impinging afferent presynaptic terminal, from which it is separated only by a synaptic cleft. It represents the target structure upon which neurotransmitter molecules (in a chemogenic synapse) or current fluxes (in an electrogenic synapse) are directed. **presynaptic m.** The portion of the plasma membrane of a neuron in closest apposition to its target element, from which it is separated only by a synaptic cleft. In chemogenic synapses its highly complex molecular substructure allows for the selective release of neurotransmitter molecules, usually by discharge of synaptic vesicles, and the subsequent uptake of inactivated neurotransmitter fragments following termination of the synaptic process. **proper mucous m.** LAMINA PROPRIA MUCOSAE. **proper m. of semicircular duct** MEMBRANA PROPRIA DUCTUS SEMICIRCULARIS. **pupillary m.** The delicate, vascular mesodermal membrane, part of the embryonic lens capsule, on the anterior surface of the lens epithelium which closes the pupil until about the sixth month of human development. If the capsule is not completely resorbed it can persist to give rise to congenital atresia of the pupil. Also *capsulopupillary membrane.* **purple m.** The membrane of halophilic bacteria containing rhodopsin and capable of pumping hydrogen ions in response to illumination. **quadrangular m.** MEMBRANA QUADRANGULARIS. **Ranvier's m.** A hyaline membrane at the dermoepidermal junction. **Reichert's m.** LAMINA LIMITANS ANTERIOR CORNEAE. **Reissner's m.** PARIES VESTIBULARIS DUCTUS COCHLEARIS. **respiratory m.** The alveolar membrane through which gas exchange in the lung takes place. **reticular m. of organ of Corti** MEMBRANA RETICULARIS DUCTUS COCHLEARIS. **reticulated m.** MEMBRANA RETICULARIS DUCTUS COCHLEARIS. **Rivinus m.** PARS FLACCIDA MEMBRANAE TYMPANI. **ruffle m.** A thin cytoplasmic fold that extends out from a macrophage and is capable of engulfing large particulate matter. **Ruysch m.** LAMINA CHOROIDOCAPILLARIS. **ruyschian m.** LAMINA CHOROIDOCAPILLARIS. **Scarpa's m.** MEMBRANA TYMPANI SECUNDARIA. **schneiderian m.** TUNICA MUCOSA NASI. **Schwann's m.** NEURILEMMA. **secondary tympanic m.** MEMBRANA TYMPANI SECUNDARIA. **semipermeable m.** A membrane that allows the free passage of water or other solvent but restricts the movement of certain solutes or colloidally dispersed material. **serous m.** TUNICA SEROSA. **serous m. of epididymis** TUNICA VAGINALIS TESTIS. **Shrapnell's m.** PARS FLACCIDA MEMBRANAE TYMPANI. **spiral m. of cochlear duct** PARIES TYMPANICUS DUCTUS COCHLEARIS. **stapedial m.** MEMBRANA STAPEDIS. **m. of stapes** MEMBRANA STAPEDIS. **statoconic m. of maculae** MEMBRANA STATOCONIORUM MACULARUM. **sternal m.** MEMBRANA STERNI. **subepithelial m.** A basement membrane on the deep surface of an epithelium. **submucous m.** TELA SUBMUCOSA. **submucous m. of stomach** TELA SUBMUCOSA GASTRICA. **subzonal m.** The outermost layer of the amnion. **suprapleural m.** MEMBRANA SUPRAPLEURALIS. **sutural m.** SUTURAL LIGAMENT. **synaptic m.** The portion of plasma membrane separating one neuron from another at a point of synapse. **synovial m.** MEMBRANA SYNOVIALIS CAPSULAE ARTICULARIS. **synovial m. of articular capsule** MEMBRANA SYNOVIALIS CAPSULAE ARTICULARIS. **tarsal m.** SEPTUM ORBITALE. **tectorial m.** MEMBRANA TECTORIA. **tectorial m. of cochlear duct** MEMBRANA TECTORIA DUCTUS COCHLEARIS. **Tenon's m.** VAGINA BULBI. **thyrohyoid m.** MEMBRANA THYROHYOIDEA. **Toldt's m.** The anterior layer of the fascia of the kidney. **tympanic m.** MEMBRANA TYMPANI. **undulating m.** 1 A membrane that runs, finlike, along the body of certain flagellate parasites such as trypanosomes and trichomonads. The margin of the membrane is formed by the flagellum, which in some cases extends free beyond the membrane. A rippling movement is characteristic of the undulating membrane and serves to propel the organism. 2 An organelle found in the oral groove of some ciliates (protozoan phylum Ciliophora), formed by the fusion of one or more longitudinal rows of cilia. For defs. 1 and 2 also *undulatory membrane.* **unit m.** A model of membrane structure in which a phospholipid layer is coated on its outer and inner surfaces by proteins in the extended $\beta$-configuration. This membrane shows a trilaminar (dark-light-dark) pattern of electron density. **urogenital m.** The anterior part of the cloacal membrane in the embryo, formed by the transverse division of the membrane into two parts by the downgrowth of the cloacal (urorectal) septum at about the seventh week in man. It closes off the end of the urogenital sinus and is prolonged forwards in forming a temporary cover (until the ninth week) for the urogenital groove on the inferior aspect of the genital tubercle, later to form the penis in the male. **urorectal m.** CLOACAL SEPTUM. **vestibular m. of cochlear duct** PARIES VESTIBULARIS DUCTUS COCHLEARIS. **vitelline m.** The cell membrane of an ovum, produced by the cytoplasm of the ovum. Also *membrana vitellina.* **vitreous m.** 1 LAMINA LIMITANS POSTERIOR CORNEAE. 2 MEMBRANA VITREA. 3 COMPLEXUS BASALIS CHOROIDEAE. **Zinn's m.** The anterior layer of the iris, comprising a layer of flattened endothelial cells.

**membranectomy** \mem′brənek′təmē\ [*membran(e)* + -ECTOMY] The surgical removal of part or all of a membrane.

**membraniform** \membrā′nifôrm\ Having the appearance of a membrane.

**membranocartilaginous** \mem′brənōkär′tilaj′inəs\ Of or relating to both membranous and cartilaginous tissue.

**membranocranium** \mem′brənōkrā′nē·əm\ [*membran(e)* + *o* + CRANIUM] The primitive precursor of the skull in the embryo. It is made of membranous material and precedes the bony and other elements which eventually form the fetal skull proper.

**membranoid** \mem′brənoid\ Like a membrane, as in appearance or quality.

**membranous** \mem′brənəs\ Being or having the properties of a membrane. Also *membranaceous.*

**membroid** A capsule of membranous composition which is resistant to the actions of gastric secretions but dissolves in the lumen of the small intestine. It is a type of enteric coating for drugs to be delivered to the intestinal portion of the gastrointestinal tract.

**membrum** \mem′brəm\ [L (akin to Gk *mēros* the thigh) a member, limb, part] (*pl.* membra) A limb or appendage. **m. inferius** The lower limb of the human body, including the hip, thigh, leg and foot. Also *inferior limb, lower extremity, inferior extremity, extremitas inferior, inferior member, pelvic limb, lower limb.* **m. superius** [NA] The upper limb of the human body, including the shoulder, arm, forearm, wrist and hand. Also *superior limb, extremitas superior* (outmoded), *superior extremity, upper extremity, thoracic limb, upper limb.*

**memory** [Middle French *memorie* (from L *memori(a)* memory, from *memor* mindful, from *meminisse* to remember) memory] 1 The persistence of the effects of experience on the behavior of living organisms. Memory includes several stages; learning, retaining, recognizing, and recalling. 2 The recall of one's past or of a particular object or event. 3 Equipment or media in which information for a computer can be stored and retrieved. 4 That portion of a computer in which instructions and data are stored. 5 A tendency to retain effects as a result of past treatment, as a permanent deformation in a plastic after a load is removed. **iconic m.** The hypothesized first stage of visual memory formation, in which a faint copy of a visual input persists very briefly in the sensory register, allowing a longer interval for the extraction of information. **immediate m.** SHORT-TERM MEMORY. **immunologic m.** The capacity of the immune system to mount an increased and more sustained response to a subsequent exposure to a particular antigen than was mounted to the initial exposure. Immunologic memory is produced by the expansion of clones of antigen-reactive lymphocytes as a result of the first contact with antigen. These cells (memory cells) can then be stimulated to proliferate and differentiate when antigen is encountered again. **kinesthetic m.** Memory for movements rather than events. **long-term m.** The hypothesized substage of the memory process in which information is stored in a relatively permanent way, possibly for the lifetime of the organism, and which can be retrieved for use as required. **random access m.** A computer memory, usually using a semiconductor, that permits immediate access for writing data into any storage location or reading data from any storage location. Also *read/write memory.* Abbr. RAM **read-only m.** A computer memory, usually using a semiconductor, that contains unalterable programs or data. Like a dictionary, data are easily accessed, cannot be changed, and are not lost when the power turns off. Abbr. ROM **recent m.** In clinical usage, the ability to recall events that have occurred within the past hours, days, or weeks. **remote m.** In clinical usage, the ability to recall events that occurred several years, or many years, ago. Also *palinmnesis.* **retrograde m.** The memory for events prior to a trauma or other incident that has affected one's memory. **rote m.** The memorizing or learning of a body of material without regard to understanding its meaning but only with the intent to reproduce it later in the exact form in which it has been memorized. **screen m.** The memory of a real event that covers or blurs the memory of an allied event. **short-term m.** A hypothesized substage of the memory process assumed to be of short duration, and in any event not exceeding 25 minutes, and to possess a distinctly limited capacity, possibly of five to nine items. Although material is thought to be held only very briefly in the short-term memory stage, this may suffice to allow processing of the information into the long-term memory store for later use. Also *immediate memory.* **virtual m.** A computer technique that permits the programmer to treat external memory, such as a floppy disk, as an extension of random access memory, thus giving the virtual appearance of a larger random access memory.

**MEN** multiple endocrine neoplasia.

**menacme** \menak′mē\ [Gk *mēn* month + *akmē* a point, the highest point, bloom] 1 The height of menstrual activity. 2 The years between menarche and menopause.

**menadiol** 2-Methylnaphthalene-1,2-diol. The reduced form of menadione.

**menadiol sodium diphosphate** 2-Methyl-1,4-naphthalenediol bis(dihydrogen phosphate) tetra-sodium salt hexahydrate. A synthetic derivative of menadione (vitamin $K_3$) that is biologically transformed into an active metabolite with vitamin K activity. It is used for the same indications as menadione and is given orally, intravenously, or subcutaneously.

**menadione** 2-Methyl-1,4-naphthoquinone. It is the parent substance of the various forms of vitamin K, which differ in the nature of the substituent at C-3. 3-Substituted menadiones are collectively called menaquinones, and the substituent is a chain of isoprene units. Also *vitamin* $K_3$.

**menadione sodium bisulfite** The water-soluble, sodium bisulfite form of menadione, used as a source of vitamin K in the treatment of hemorrhagic conditions associated with hypoprothrombinemic states. It has the same actions and uses as menadione.

**menalgia** \menal′jə\ [*men(o)-* + -ALGIA] DYSMENORRHEA.

**menaquinone** Any of several 3-substituted manadiones, which vary in the length of the polyisoprenoid substituent. All have vitamin K activity. Also *vitamin* $K_2$, *farnoquinone* (obs.).

**menarche** \men′ärkē\ [*men(o)-* + Gk *archē* a beginning, origin] The appearance of the first menstrual period. Adj. menarchal, menarcheal, menarchial. **delayed m.** PRIMARY AMENORRHEA.

**mendacity** \mendas′itē\ [Late L *mendacitas* (from L *mendax*, deceitful, lying + *-itas* -ITY) mendacity] PATHOLOGIC LYING.

**Mendel** [Felix *Mendel*, German physician, 1862–1912] Mendel's test. See under MANTOUX TEST.

**Mendel** [Johann Gregor *Mendel*, Austrian botanist, 1822–1884] **1** Mendelian inheritance. See under INHERITANCE. **2** Mendelian law. See under MENDEL'S LAWS. **3** Mendelian disorder. See under DISORDER. **4** Mendelism. See under MENDELIAN THEORY. **5** Mendelian rate. See under MENDELIAN RATIO.

**Mendel** [Kurt *Mendel*, German neurologist, 1874–1946] Bekhterev-Mendel reflex, Mendel's reflex, Mendel's dorsal reflex of foot. See under MENDEL-BEKHTEREV REFLEX.

**mendelevium** A synthetic element of the actinide series, having atomic number 101. Mendelevium 256 was discovered in 1952, produced by bombarding einsteinium with alpha particles. Its half-life is approximately 1.25 hours. Four isotopes are recognized. The longest lived, mendelevium 258, has a half-life of 2 months. Symbol: Md

**mendelian** \mendē′lē·ən\ Associated with the work of or developed by Gregor Mendel, as *mendelian theory*.

**mendelism** \men′dəlizm\ MENDELIAN THEORY.

**Mendelson** [Curtis Lester *Mendelson*, U.S. obstetrician and gynecologist, born 1913] See under SYNDROME.

**Ménétrier** [Pierre *Ménétrier*, French physician, 1859–1935] See under DISEASE.

**Menge** [Karl *Menge*, German gynecologist, 1864–1945] See under PESSARY.

**mengovirus** \meng′gōvī′rəs\ MENGO VIRUS.

**menhidrosis** \men′hīdrō′sis\ [Gk *mēn* month + HIDROSIS ] A form of vicarious menstruation characterized by monthly extrusion of sweat, sometimes bloody, at the expected time of menses. Also *menidrosis*.

**Menière** [Prosper *Menière*, French physician, 1799–1862] Menière syndrome. See under DISEASE.

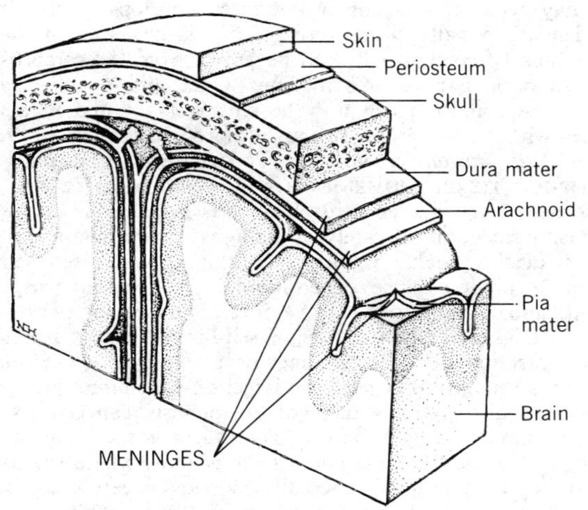


**Meninges and surrounding structures**

**mening-** \məning-, məninj-\ MENINGO-.

**meningeal** \menin′jē·əl\ Describing, pertaining to, or affecting the meninges.

**meningematoma** \menin′jēmətō′mə\ A hematoma involving the dura mater. Also *meninghematoma*.

**meningeocortical** \menin′jē·ōkôr′tikəl\ MENINGOCORTICAL.

**meningeorrhaphy** \menin′jē·ôr′əfē\ [*meninge(al)* + *o* + -RRHAPHY] Suture of the dura mater.

**meninges** \menin′jēz\ [See MENINX.] (*sing.* meninx) [NA] The three membranes that envelop the brain and spinal cord, comprising a dense, fibrous outer cover (dura mater), a thin inner layer adhering closely to the underlying neural tissue (pia mater), and a trabeculated middle layer (the arachnoidea). The last two are usually grouped together as the leptomeninges.

**meninghematoma** \menin′gēmətō′mə\ MENINGEMATOMA.

**meningi-** \mənin′jē-, men′injī′-\ MENINGO-.

**meninginitis** \menin′jinī′tis\ [*meningin(a)* (term coined by François Chaussier, French physician, 1746–1828, for the pia-arachnoid; irreg. from Gk *mēninx*, gen. *mēningos*, membrane) + -ITIS] LEPTOMENINGITIS.

**meningioma** \mənin′jē·ō′mə\ [MENINGI- + -OMA] A tumor of the cellular elements of the meninges. It is most often attached to the dura, especially where arachnoid villi are numerous. It is typically benign, but may compress the brain, erode and extend into bone and, on rare occasions, become malignant through transformation into a sarcoma. A number of morphologic subtypes are recognized, but their behavior does not seem to differ greatly from one another. **anaplastic m.** A recognizable meningioma with anaplastic features. This differs from a meningeal sarcoma, which does not contain features of a meningioma. **angiomatous m.** A meningioma with many large and small vascular channels predominating. **arachnotheliomatous m.** MENINGOTHELIOMATOUS MENINGIOMA. **endotheliomatous m.** MENINGOTHELIOMATOUS MENINGIOMA. **fibrous m.** A meningioma in which fibroblastlike cells predominate. Collagen and reticulin are abundant. **hemangioblastic m.** A meningioma which closely resembles a capillary hemangioblastoma of the cerebellum. **hemangiopericytic m.** A meningioma with the histologic appearance of a hemangiopericytoma. **meningothelial m.** MENINGOTHELIOMATOUS MENINGIOMA. **meningotheliomatous m.** A meningioma composed of cells with poorly defined cell membranes, which result in a syncytial appearance. Also *arachnotheliomatous meningioma, endotheliomatous meningioma, meningothelial meningioma, syncytial meningioma.* **mixed m.** TRANSITIONAL MENINGIOMA. **myxomatous m.** A meningioma with a myxomatous appearance histologically. **m. of olfactory groove** A meningioma developing in the olfactory groove in relation to the undersurface of one frontal lobe, usually giving rise to unilateral anosmia and other variable neurologic symptoms and signs. **parasagittal m.** A meningioma arising in the parasagittal region between the two cerebral hemispheres and often becoming evident first with spastic weakness of both legs and feet. **psammomatous m.** A meningioma, usually spinal, in which psammoma bodies are a predominant feature. **syncytial m.** MENINGOTHELIOMATOUS MENINGIOMA. **transitional m.** A meningioma composed of a mixture of syncytial and fibroblastic elements. Also *mixed meningioma*.

**meningiomatosis** \menin′jē·ōmətō′sis\ [MENINGIOMA + *t* + -OSIS] The presence of multiple meningiomas.

**meningion** \menin′jē·än\ *Obs.* ARACHNOIDEA.
**meningism** \menin′jizm\ [*mening(itis)* + -ISM] A group of symptoms and signs suggesting meningitis which may occur in the absence of any identifiable pathologic lesion of the meninges. The major manifestations are headache and neck stiffness. The syndrome usually occurs in children suffering from febrile infections such as pneumonia, tonsillitis, and systemic viral infections. Also *pseudomeningitis Dupré syndrome* (obs.), *meningismus, Dupré's disease.*
**meningitic** \men′injit′ik\ [*meningit(is)* + -IC] Describing or pertaining to meningitis.
**meningitides** \men′injit′idēz\ Plural of MENINGITIS.

## meningitis

**meningitis** \men′injī′tis\ [MENING- + -ITIS] (*pl.* meningitides) Any inflammation of the meninges. Meningitis has been termed cerebral, spinal, or cerebrospinal, according to whether the inflammation affects principally the meninges over the brain alone, those investing the spinal cord alone, or the whole cerebrospinal complex. This distinction has little validity in clinical practice, since there is usually though not invariably some spread of inflammation from one compartment to the other. Two principal forms can be distinguished on pathologic grounds, pachymeningitis, which involves the dura mater, and leptomeningitis, which affects the arachnoid and the pia mater. The latter is much commoner, and by common usage meningitis is usually taken to mean leptomeningitis. The major manifestations include headache, vomiting, fever, and neck stiffness. The condition can result from many kinds of microorganism, including bacteria, fungi, spirochetes, viruses, and parasites. It can also be aseptic, due to irritation of the meninges by chemical or physical agents, or to tumor metastasizing in the meninges. Adj. meningitic. **acute aseptic m.** Acute meningitis, usually with a lymphocytic pleocytosis and usually viral in origin. **acute benign lymphocytic m.** LYMPHOCYTIC CHORIOMENINGITIS. **acute septic m.** Any form of bacterial meningitis resulting in pus formation in the subarachnoid space, whether due to a primary meningitic illness, as in most cases of meningococcal or pneumococcal meningitis, or due to spread of infection from the brain, in cerebral abscess, from the ears or paranasal sinuses, or from some other more distant infective focus, as from the lungs in bronchiectasis. Also *acute purulent meningitis.* **aseptic m.** Inflammation of the meninges resulting from aseptic processes, and resulting from a variety of infectious, toxic, chemical, or physical agents, including, for example, that secondary inflammatory process which may result from bleeding or from the injection or release of air, drugs, or other foreign substances into the subarachnoid space. No bacterial organisms can be identified in or isolated from the cerebrospinal fluid, but studies often reveal viral etiology. Also *sterile meningitis.* • *Aseptic meningitis* is sometimes used to refer to meningitides of viral origin, but *viral meningitis* is preferred in this sense. ***Bacteroides* m.** Meningitis due to anaerobic fusiform bacilli of the genus *Bacteroides.* **basal m.** Meningitis largely restricted to the meninges over the base of the brain. This may occur in subacute, chronic, or inadequately treated bacterial meningitis, or in granulomatous processes such as tuberculosis or sarcoidosis. Also *basilar meningitis, meningitis of the base.* **benign lymphocytic m.** See under LYMPHOCYTIC MENINGITIS. **benign recurrent endothelioleukocytic m.** A form of acute meningitis of undetermined etiology characterized by an abrupt onset, a marked pleocytosis in the cerebrospinal fluid with initially a high proportion of endothelial cells in the fluid, rapid spontaneous remission, and frequent relapses. A virus has been isolated in one case. Also *Mollaret's meningitis.* **brucellar m.** Meningitis which may arise as a complication of brucellosis. It is seen either as a typical meningeal syndrome or else as a simple pleocytosis in the cerebrospinal fluid. Many and various neurologic syndromes have been attributed to infection with *Brucella* species. **m. carcinomatosa** Widespread or diffuse metastatic carcinoma in the meninges. **cerebrospinal m.** An infectious and at times epidemic disease caused by a variety of microorganisms, but usually meningococci, transmitted by direct human contact, often with asymptomatic carriers who harbor the organisms in the nasopharynx. The onset is typically abrupt, with fever, headache, and vomiting, followed almost immediately by neck stiffness, and leading to drowsiness, delirium, and ultimately coma if untreated. The Kernig and Brudzinski signs are positive in about 50% of cases. In acute cases, especially in childhood, there may be a purpuric rash on the skin, and in some cases there is an associated septicemia. The pressure of the cerebrospinal fluid is raised, and it is purulent at this time, containing many abnormal polymorphonuclear leukocytes and bacteria, which are often surprisingly scanty. The protein level is raised and the glucose content reduced or absent. With appropriate antibiotics the prognosis is usually good in adults and older children, but the condition can still be more serious in young children. Also *epidemic meningitis, petechial fever, tetanoid fever, spotted sickness, cerebrospinal fever, stiffneck fever.* **chemical m.** Aseptic meningitis due to irritation of the meninges resulting from the presence of any foreign chemical substance in the subarachnoid space. **chronic posterior basic m.** A form of indolent meningitis largely confined to the basal meninges. The usual cause is inadequate resolution or treatment of pyogenic meningitis due to the meningococcus or pneumococcus. Since the introduction of antibiotics this condition has become very rare. Also *posterior meningitis, posterior basic meningitis.* **m. circumscripta spinalis** Localized spinal meningitis due to any cause. **cryptococcal m.** A form of meningitis, sometimes occurring acutely but much more often in a subacute or chronic form, due to *Cryptococcus neoformans.* It may occur spontaneously but often develops in cachectic patients, especially those with reticulosis or carcinomatosis. The causal fungus usually can be grown from the cerebrospinal fluid on Sabouraud's medium. Once almost universally fatal, the condition can now be effectively treated in many cases with amphotericin B and 5-fluorocytosine. Also *torula meningitis, torular meningitis.* **curable serous m.** LYMPHOCYTIC CHORIOMENINGITIS. **eosinophilic m.** A disorder of the human central nervous system due either to parasitic infection or, rarely, to malignancy and characterized by headache, nuchal rigidity, vomiting or decreased sensorium, a predominance of eosinophils in the cerebrospinal fluid, and, possibly, low-grade fever and cranial nerve defects. It is most often a benign, self-limited illness resulting from infection with the rat lungworm, *Angiostrongylus cantonensis,* although other parasitic infections, including paragonimiasis, schistosomiasis, and gnathostomiasis, can give rise to a very similar clinical picture. The illness is seen almost exclusively in the Far East and Pacific islands, where the parasites may be ingested accidentally by persons eating contaminated raw vegetables, snails, or shellfish. While human angiostrongyliasis is usually a subclinical illness, in some cases the larvae migrate to the central nervous system where they provoke eosinophilic meningitis. Rarely, eosinophilic meningitis develops in persons with malignancies, especially Hodgkin's disease and other lymphomas. In these instances, the illness, if untreated, is associated with high mortality. Also *eosinophilic meningoencephalitis.* **epidemic m.** CEREBROSPINAL MENINGITIS. **epidemic serous m.** LYMPHOCYTIC CHORIOMENINGITIS. **external m.** PACHYMENINGITIS. **gonococcal m.** A rare form of purulent meningitis complicating gonococcal septicemia, occasionally confused with meningococcal meningitis after examination of the cerebrospinal fluid because of the resemblance between meningococci and gonococci on Gram stain. The course is less acute than that of meningococcal meningitis, and there is a marked tendency towards loculation of the infection in the meninges. **granulomatous m.** Any form of meningitis producing granulomatous changes in the subarachnoid space. The commonest causes include tuberculosis, syphilis, and sarcoidosis. **gummatous m.** Meningitis occurring in the tertiary stage of syphilis, marked pathologically by gummata scattered either in the pia mater or alternatively in the dura mater. These are particularly abundant over the base of the skull. Clinically the condition produces either signs of increased intracranial pressure or a picture of subacute meningitis. **herpetic m.** Meningitis caused by infection with any of the human herpes viruses, such as herpes simplex virus or herpes zoster virus, complicating the skin rash or preceding it by a few hours or days. It produces a meningeal syndrome, with clear cerebrospinal fluid containing abundant lymphocytes and an increased protein content. The meningeal signs usually disappear within a few days, and recovery is generally complete. *Imprecise.* **influenzal m.** Meningitis due to *Haemophilus influenzae.* **leptospiral m.** Meningitis due to *Leptospira* species. **localized tuberculous m.** A form or stage of tuberculous meningitis in which the inflammation is or becomes localized to some part of the subarachnoid space such as the basal meninges, the fourth ventricle and basal cisterns, or the spinal canal. **lymphocytic m.** Any form of meningitis in which the cerebrospinal fluid shows lymphocytic pleocytosis. • The term *benign lymphocytic meningitis* is often used to identify a group of self-limiting viral meningitides which usually recover spontaneously. **meningococcal m.** Cerebrospinal meningitis caused by meningococci (*Neisseria meningitidis*). Also *meningococcic meningitis.* **Mollaret's m.** BENIGN RECURRENT ENDOTHELIOLEUKOCYTIC MENINGITIS. **mumps m.** Meningitis complicating mumps, resulting from the invasion of the subarachnoid space by the virus, and sometimes preceding involvement of the parotid glands, or even being the sole manifestation of the infection. The onset is typically abrupt, but the course of the condition is usually short, the meningeal signs disappearing towards the end of the first week. In some cases the meningeal symptoms are associated with manifestations of encephalitis. The cerebrospinal fluid is often under increased pressure. It shows a lymphocytic pleocytosis and contains a modest increase in protein content, and the mumps virus can usually be isolated. **mycotic m.** Meningitis complicating any mycotic infection, such as cryptococcosis, aspergillosis, and others, and the bacterial infection, actinomycosis. **neonatal m.** Meningitis in the newborn infant. The infecting agent is commonly Gram-negative bacteria such as *Escherichia coli.* The illness is frequently fatal, especially if infection develops within the first three days of life. **m. ossificans** Ossification or calcification in the meninges in chronic meningitis. **otogenic m.** Any type of meningitis complicating acute or chronic otitis media. Also *otitic meningitis.* **plague m.** Meningitis caused by *Yersinia pestis.* **plasmodial m.** CEREBRAL MALARIA. **pneumococcal m.** A severe purulent form of meningitis, occurring at any age but commoner in young children. It sometimes complicates infection in some other part of the body, such as sinusitis, otitis, pneumonia, empyema, endocarditis, or peritonitis, but more often develops in the absence of any evident focus elsewhere of pneumococcal infection. Modern chemotherapy and antibiotic treatment have improved the prognosis, but unless treatment is started early prognosis is still poor. **posterior m.** CHRONIC POSTERIOR BASIC MENINGITIS. **posterior basic m.** CHRONIC POSTERIOR BASIC MENINGITIS. **post-traumatic m.** Meningitis following head injury due usually to skull fracture involving the middle ear or paranasal sinuses thus allowing organisms to enter the cranial cavity. **purulent m.** Meningitis caused by pyogenic bacteria, such as meningococci, pneumococci, staphylococci, streptococci, *Haemophilus influenzae,* or coliforms, and characterized by large numbers of polymorphonuclear leukocytes in the cerebrospinal fluid. Also *pyogenic meningitis, suppurative meningitis.* **pyogenic m.** PURULENT MENINGITIS. **rheumatic m.** Meningitis complicating any rheumatic illness, such as systemic lupus erythematosus, the Behçet syndrome, and, rarely, rheumatoid arthritis. **sarcoid m.** Granulomatous meningitis due to sarcoidosis. **saturnine m.** The meningeal reaction which may occur as a manifestation of lead encephalopathy. *Obs.* **septicemic m.** An acute inflammation of the meninges following an episode of septicemia. **m. serosa circumscripta cystica** Localized arachnoiditis with arachnoidal cyst formation. **serum m.** A meningeal reaction occurring as one manifestation of serum sickness, usually developing about seven or eight days after the injection of foreign serum. • The term is a misnomer, as the cerebrospinal fluid is usually normal, or else it shows a minimal pleocytosis with a modest increase in protein content. The clinical manifestations are those of an encephalopathy and not of a true meningitis. **spinal m.** Inflammation of the spinal meninges. This may occur as a result of loculation of an inflammatory process in the spinal canal in any form of meningitis, but rare forms of staphylococcal and tuberculous meningitis largely restricted to the spinal meninges have been described. Also *spinitis* (obs.). **staphylococcal m.** A severe type of purulent meningitis which can arise as a complication of staphylococcal septicemia, or by infection of the meninges, either as a result of a compound skull fracture or through spread of infection from a staphylococcal cranial or spinal osteomyelitis. A rare variety of primary spinal staphylococcal meningitis has been described. **sterile m.** ASEPTIC MENINGITIS. **streptococcal m.** A severe type of purulent meningitis, usually resulting from the introduction of streptococci into the subarachnoid space either as a consequence of trauma, of otitis media or sinusitis, or through metastatic spread from a distant septic focus in septicemia or acute endocarditis. **suppurative m.** PURULENT MENINGITIS. **syphilitic m.** Meningitis occurring as a manifestation of either secondary syphilis, in which case it is an acute, self-limiting lymphocytic type, or in meningovascular syphilis, in which case the meningitis is usually subacute and granulomatous in type. **torula m.** CRYPTOCOCCAL MENINGITIS. **torular m.** CRYPTOCOCCAL MENINGITIS. **trypanosomal m.** Meningitis complicating African trypanosomiasis. An acute meningitis may occur in the course of the disease, with lymphocytosis and a moderately raised albumen level in the cerebrospinal fluid. In advanced disease, high IgM concentrations are present in cerebrospinal fluid. Lymphocytes, mononuclear cells, eosinophils, morula cells, and trypanosomes may also be present. In the later states, meningoencephalomyelitis may occur. **tuberculous m.** Meningitis due to the tubercle bacillus. This usually complicates primary or miliary tuberculosis but can develop in patients with tuberculosis at any stage and is generally due to the rupture of a cortical tuberculoma into the subarachnoid space. The onset may be acute but more often the illness runs a subacute or chronic course, and a few days or weeks of general malaise, mild fever, and headache may presage the development of more typical symptoms of meningitis. This form of meningitis is often complicated by variable manifestations of encephalomyelopathy, by cranial nerve palsies, by neurologic signs resulting from cerebral ischemia due to endarteritis of basal vessels, and by communicating hydrocephalus or by other manifestations resulting from the formation of adhesions in the subarachnoid space with consequent loculation of the inflammatory process. A chronic spinal form has been described, often giving rise to paraparesis. The cerebrospinal fluid is under increased pressure and is often clear or only faintly turbid, but a fine fibrin web often forms after the specimen has been allowed to stand overnight. The fluid invariably contains an increase in cells (polymorphonuclear in the early stages, lymphocytes and other mononuclears later), the cell count usually varying from 50–1000 white cells per cubic millimeter. Its protein content is raised and its sugar content moderately reduced. Tubercle bacilli may be isolated by culture or, rarely, identified in the cerebrospinal fluid by microscopy. Also *tubercular meningitis, cerebral tuberculosis.* **typhoid m.** 1 A clinical meningeal syndrome sometimes seen in typhoid fever as a manifestation of an aseptic meningeal reaction or a secondary infection. 2 An unusual form of meningitis due to invasion of the subarachnoid space by *Salmonella typhi.* In most cases this complication develops towards the end of the course of typhoid fever. **viral m.** Meningitis caused by a virus infection and characterized by fever, headache, stiffness of the neck, nausea, malaise, and the presence of lymphocytes in the cerebrospinal fluid. Viruses that commonly produce this disorder include enteroviruses, mumps virus, lymphocytic choriomeningitis virus, and herpes simplex virus type 2. See also LYMPHOCYTIC MENINGITIS. **Wallgren's aseptic m.** LYMPHOCYTIC CHORIOMENINGITIS. **yeast m.** Meningitis due to yeasts such as *Cryptococcus* or *Blastomyces.*

**meningium** \mənin′jē·əm\ *Obs.* ARACHNOIDEA.

**meningo-** \məning′gō-\ [Gk *mēninx* (gen. *mēningos*) membrane] A combining form denoting the meninges. Also *mening-, meningi-.*

**meningoblast** \məning′gəblast\ [MENINGO- + -BLAST] A primitive or precursor cell that contributes toward the formation of the meninges.

**meningocele** \məning′gōsēl\ [MENINGO- + -CELE[1]] The protrusion of the dura mater and the arachnoid meningeal layers surrounding the brain or the spinal cord through a developmental defect in the osseoligamentous coverings of these organs. It is usually manifested as a fluid-filled sac covered by modified skin on the midline of the cranium or back. Rarely, an acquired meningocele can follow trauma or surgery. **cerebral m.** A meningocele involving cranial meninges and appearing on the surface of the head or, rarely, in the orbital, nasal, or nasopharyngeal cavities. **spurious m.** TRAUMATIC MENINGOCELE. **traumatic m.** The protrusion of a fluid-filled sac through an acquired defect in the cranial cavity or spinal canal as a result of trauma. Also *Billroth's disease.*

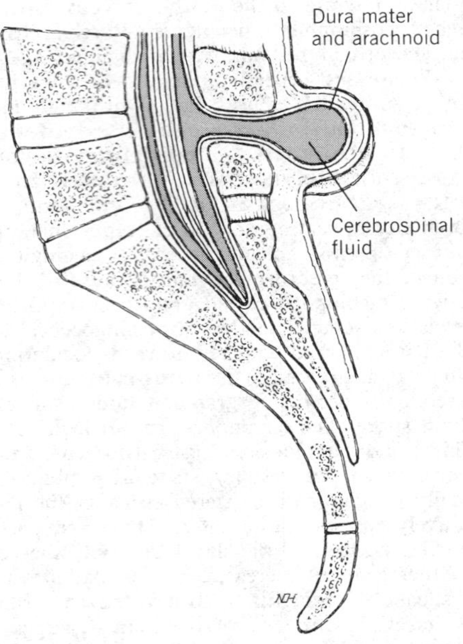


**Meningocele** (occurring between L4 and L5)

**meningocephalitis** \-sef′əlī′tis\ MENINGOENCEPHALITIS.

**meningocerebritis** \-ser′əbrī′tis\ MENINGOENCEPHALITIS.

**meningococcemia** \-käksē′mē·ə\ [*meningococc(us)* + -EMIA] The presence of meningococci in the bloodstream. It is often associated with a diffuse petechial rash and, at times, disseminated intravascular coagulation, shock, and death. **acute fulminating m.** Severe meningococcal sepsis with or without meningitis and often associated with purpura, disseminated intravascular coagulation, bilateral adrenal hemorrhages, collapse, and death. See also WATERHOUSE-FRIDERICHSEN SYNDROME. **chronic m.** A syndrome of persistent or recurrent meningococcal bacteremia and low-grade fever which may be associated with rash and arthritis.

**meningococci** \-käk′sī\ Plural of MENINGOCOCCUS.

**meningococcosis** \-käkō′sis\ [*meningococc(us)* + -OSIS] Any meningococcal infection or disease.

**meningococcus** \-käk′əs\ [MENINGO- + COCCUS] (*pl.* meningococci) A microorganism of the species *Neisseria meningitidis.*

**meningocortical** \-kôr′tikəl\ Of or pertaining to the meninges and the cerebral cortex. Also *meningeocortical.*

**meningoencephalitis** \-ensef′əlī′tis\ [MENINGO- + ENCEPHAL- + -ITIS] Inflammation of the brain and meninges. Also *cerebromeningitis, encephalomeningitis, meningocephalitis, meningocerebritis, periencephalitis, periencephalomeningitis, cephalomeningitis* (seldom used). Adj. meningoencephalitic. **biundulant m.** The central European subtype of tick-borne encephalitis. See under TICK-BORNE ENCEPHALITIS. **chronic m.** 1 Any meningoencephalitis running a chronic course. 2 GENERAL PARESIS. **eosinophilic m.** EOSINOPHILIC MENINGITIS. **mumps m.** Meningoencephalitis due to mumps virus. **primary amebic m.** Meningoencephalitis caused by free-living soil or freshwater pathogenic strains of *Naegleria* or *Acanthamoeba* species. Infection usually is via the cribriform plate, death occurring in three to five days following onset. **syphilitic m.** 1 Acute or subacute meningoencephalitis in meningovascular syphilis. 2 GENERAL PARESIS. **trypanosomal m.** A subacute or chronic meningoencephalitis involving the base of the brain predominantly, caused by the highly pathogenic flagellate protozoa *Trypanosoma gambiense* or *T. rhodesiense.* The complications occur in weeks to a few months with *T. rhodesiense* and in months or years with *T. gambiense.* Onset is insidious in most cases. The condition leads to progressive mental deterioration and classic sleeping sickness. See also TRYPANOSOMIASIS. **Tüga's m.** A rickettsial disease of the Far East, transmitted by the tick *Haemaphysalis cincinna,* and giving rise to meningoencephalitic symptoms and benign recurrent fever.

**meningoencephalocele** \-ensef′əlōsēl′\ ENCEPHALOCELE.

**meningoencephalomyelitis** \-ensef′əlōmī′əlī′tis\ [MENINGO- + ENCEPHALOMYELITIS] Inflammation of the meninges and of the brain and spinal cord.

**meningoencephalomyelopathy** \-ensef′əlōmī′əläp′əthē\ [MENINGO- + ENCEPHALO- + MYELOPATHY] Any disease involving the brain, meninges, and spinal cord.

**meningoencephalomyeloradiculoneuritis** \-ensef′əlōmī′əlōrədik′yəlōnʸurī′tis\ [MENINGO- + ENCEPHALO- + MYELO- + RADICULONEURITIS] Inflammation of the brain, meninges, spinal cord, nerve roots, and peripheral nerves.

**meningoencephalopathy** \-ensef′əläp′əthē\ [MENINGO- + ENCEPHALOPATHY] Any of a large group of diffuse disorders of function of the brain and meninges not due to inflammation. • The term is somewhat imprecise and is used infrequently, but many varieties of toxic and metabolic encephalopathy have been described.

**meningomyelitis** \-mī′əlī′tis\ [MENINGO- + MYELITIS] Inflammation of the spinal cord and of its covering membranes, usually of the arachnoid and pia mater, less frequently of the dura mater. **blastomycotic m.** Meningomyelitis due to one of the several known systemic, human, pathogenic, blastomycotic fungi, *Paracoccidioides brasiliensis, Histoplasma capsulatum, H. capsulatum* var. *duboisii, Coccidioides immitis,* and *Blastomyces dermatitidis..* **sporotrichotic m.** Meningomyelitis due to *Sporothrix schenkii.* **torular m.** Meningomyelitis due to *Cryptococcus neoformans..* • *Torular* refers to the genus *Torula,* an earlier name for *Cryptococcus.*

**meningomyelocele** \-mī′əlōsēl′\ A protrusion of the spinal cord and associated meninges through a developmental defect in the spinal canal, resulting in exposure at the surface along the midline of the back. Also *myelomeningocele.* • This is a nonspecific term that is often used regardless of the presence or absence of a cystlike lesion or of demonstrated cord tissue in the herniated parts.

**meningomyeloradiculitis** \-mī′əlōrədik′yəlī′tis\ [MENINGO- + MYELO- + RADICULITIS] Inflammation of the meninges, of the spinal cord, and of the spinal nerve roots. Also *meningoradiculomyelitis.*

**meningo-osteophlebitis** \-äs′tē-ōflebī′tis\ Periostitis that is associated with inflammation of the venous sinuses of a bone.

**meningopathy** \men′ing·gäp′əthē\ [MENINGO- + -PATHY] Any disease or disorder affecting the meninges.

**meningoradiculitis** \-rədik′yəlī′tis\ [MENINGO- + RADICULITIS] Inflammation of the spinal meninges and of the spinal nerve roots.

**meningoradiculomyelitis** \-rədik′yəlōmī′əlī′tis\ MENINGOMYELORADICULITIS. **progressive m.** 1 A rare and late spinal complication of cerebrospinal meningitis, resulting in progressive paraparesis. 2 Any of several distinct varieties of progressive myelitis, such as subacute necrotic myelitis.

**meningorrhagia** \məning′gôrā′jə\ [MENINGO- + -RRHAGIA] Extravasation of blood within the cerebral or spinal meninges. Also *meningorrhea.*

**meningothelium** \-thē′lē·əm\ [MENINGO- + *(epi)-thelium*] Epithelium-like cells of the arachnoidea that line the inner aspect of the dura mater.

**meningotropism** \-trō′pizm\ [MENINGO- + TROPISM] An affinity for the meninges.

**meninx** \mē′ningks\ [Gk *mēninx* membrane] 1 A membrane. 2 Singular of MENINGES. **m. primitiva** ECTOMENINX.

**meniscal** \mənis′kəl\ Pertaining to a meniscus.

**meniscectomy** \men′isek′təmē\ [*menisc(us)* + -ECTOMY] The surgical excision of a semilunar cartilage of the knee. **arthroscopic m.** The removal of all or part of a damaged semilunar cartilage of the knee through an arthroscope.

**menischesis** \men′iskē′sis\ MENOSCHESIS.

**menisci** \mənis′ī, -kī\ Plural of MENISCUS.

**meniscitis** \men′isī′tis\ Inflammation of a meniscus.

**meniscocyte** \mənis′kəsīt\ SICKLE CELL.

**meniscocytosis** \mənis′kəsītō′sis\ SICKLE CELL ANEMIA.

**meniscopathy** \men′iskäp′əthē\ [*menisc(us)* + *o* + -PATHY] Any abnormality of a meniscus.

**meniscopexy** \mənis′kōpek′sē\ The surgical repositioning of a displaced meniscus.

**meniscotomy** \men′iskät′əmē\ An incision of semilunar cartilage in the knee.

**meniscus** \menis′kəs\ [New L, from Gk *mēniskos* (dim. of *meis,* gen. *mēnos* crescent moon) a crescent] (*pl.* menisci) 1 A crescent-shaped structure, or one that is crescent-shaped in cross-section. 2 The upper surface of a liquid column, which assumes a concave shape (if the liquid wets the container) due to capillarity. Measurements are taken from the bottom of a concave meniscus. 3 A concavoconvex or convexoconcave lens. 4 One of the semilunar fibrocartilaginous disks (lateral or medial) in the knee joint. **m. articularis** [NA] A crescentic wedge of fibrocartilage or dense fibrous tissue found in certain synovial joints, such as the knee. Its broad convex base is usually attached to the articular capsule, while the two sides are in contact with apposing articular surfaces of the bones, deepening a flat or shallow articular surface and usually adding to the stability of the joint. Also *articular meniscus, articular crescent, intra-articular disk.* **converging m.** A concavoconvex lens, oriented with the convex side away from the eye. Also *positive meniscus.* **discoid m.** A congenital abnormality in which the semilunar cartilage of the knee is rounded in shape. **discoid lateral m.** A congenital abnormality of a disk-shaped lateral meniscus. It is seen more frequently than a similar abnormality in the medial compartment of the knee joint. **diverging m.** A convexoconcave lens, oriented with the concave side away from the eye. Also *negative meniscus.* **Kuhnt's m.** The neuroglial layer on the anterior surface of the optic disk. **m. lateralis articulationis genus** [NA] A near-complete ring of fibrocartilage situated on the circumferential part of the superior articular surface of the tibia. Its anterior end is attached anterior to the lateral intercondylar tubercle of the tibia behind the anterior cruciate ligament, and its posterior end is attached behind the tubercle where it blends with the posterior cruciate ligament behind it. It is less firmly attached to the articular capsule than the medial meniscus. The popliteus tendon lies between it and the fibular collateral ligament. The transverse ligament is attached to its anterior portion. Also *lateral meniscus of knee joint, external semilunar fibrocartilage, external* *semilunar cartilage of knee joint, lateral meniscus.* **m. medialis articulationis genus** [NA] An oval crescent of fibrocartilage situated on the circumferential part of the superior articular surface of the tibia. Its broad anterior end is attached to the anterior intercondylar area of the tibia in front of the anterior cruciate ligament and continuous with the transverse ligament, while its posterior end is attached to the posterior intercondylar area between the posterior end of lateral meniscus and posterior cruciate ligament. Its outer margin is adherent to the fibrous articular capsule and the tibial collateral ligament. Also *medial meniscus of knee joint, internal semilunar fibrocartilage, internal semilunar cartilage of knee joint, medial meniscus.* **negative m.** DIVERGING MENISCUS. **positive m.** CONVERGING MENISCUS. **m. tactus** Any of the concave neurofibrillar disks forming the terminal expansions of nerve fiber in the deeper portions of the germinative layers of the skin. Each disk is closely applied to a modified epithelial cell and acts as a touch receptor. Also *Merkel cell, Merkel's disk, tactile disk, tactile meniscus.* **m. of temporomandibular joint** DISCUS ARTICULARIS ARTICULATIONIS TEMPOROMANDIBULARIS.

**Menkes** [John H *Menkes,* Austrian-born U.S. pediatric neurologist, born 1928] Menkes disease. See under SYNDROME.

**meno-** \men′ō-\ [Gk *mēn* (genitive *mēnos*) month] A combining form denoting the menses.

**menolipsis** \-lip′sis\ [MENO- + Gk *leipsis* a ceasing, failing] *Seldom used* AMENORRHEA.

**menometrorrhagia** \-mē′trôrā′jə\ [MENO- + METRO- + -RRHAGIA] Abnormal uterine bleeding characterized both by occurrence between menstrual periods and increased flow during menstrual periods. Also *metromenorrhagia.*

**menopause** \men′əpôz\ [French *ménopause* (from MENO- + Gk *pausis* a cessation, from *pauein* to cease, bring to an end) the menopause] The immediate postreproductive phase of a woman's life, when menstrual function ceases due to failure to form ovarian follicles and ova. It is usually of several years' duration, with onset usually between age 45–50, and is accompanied by a variety of physiologic alterations. Irregularity of the menses usually occurs at the onset of menopause, leading to cessation. Symptoms include sudden sensations of heat and flushing (known popularly as hot flashes) of the face and torso, and vaginal dryness. Osteoporosis is a common postmenopausal symptom. Also *menostasis.* **artifical m.** Menopause caused by hypophysectomy, ovariectomy, radiation, or chemotherapy. **male m.** CLIMACTERIC. **premature m.** Premature failure of cyclic ovarian function. In the United States and other countries, ovarian failure before the age of 38 is considered premature menopause. When not due to systemic illness, severe malnutrition, or discernible endocrine cause, as a destructive pituitary tumor, the etiology is unknown. Also *menopause praecox, climacterium praecox.*

**menoplania** \-plā′nē·ə\ [MENO- + Gk *plan(ē)* a wandering, error + -IA] VICARIOUS MENSTRUATION.

**menorrhagia** \men′ôrā′jə\ [MENO- + -RRHAGIA] Excessive or prolonged menstruation. **functional m.** Menorrhagia not due to detectable organic cause, but the result of disordered ovarian function involving the normal cyclic secretion of estrogen and progesterone. Also *primary menorrhagia.*

**menorrhalgia** \men′ôral′jə\ [*menorrh(ea)* + -ALGIA] DYSMENORRHEA.

**menorrhea** \men′ôrē′ə\ [MENO- + -RRHEA] Normal menstruation.

**menoschesis** \men′äskē′sis\ [MENO- + Gk *schesis* a holding, retention] Suppression of menstruation. Also *menischesis.*

**menostasis** \mənäs′təsis, men′əstā′sis\ MENOPAUSE.

**menostaxis** \-stak′sis\ [MENO- + Gk *staxis* a dripping] AMENORRHEA.

**menses** \men′sēz\ [L, pl. of *mensis* month] **1** The flow or discharge occurring at menstruation. Also *catamenia.* **2** MENSTRUATION.

**mens rea** \menz rē′ə\ [L *mens* the mind, intention + *rea,* fem. of *reus* answerable for, guilty] CRIMINAL INTENT.

**menstrual** \men′stroo·əl\ Of, relating to, or characteristic of menstruation; pertaining to the menses. Also *menstruous.*

**menstruation** [Late L *menstru(ari)* (from L *menstrua,* neut. pl. of *menstruus* monthly, from *mensis* month) to menstruate + -ATION] The physiologic cyclic shedding of the uterine endometrium at a mean interval of 28 days, unless pregnancy intervenes, and characterized by vaginal bleeding of three to seven days' duration in the mature human female and in other higher primates. The hormonal basis is cyclic hypothalamic-adenohypophysial secretion of gonadotropic hormones, including a sharp midcycle surge of luteinizing hormone releasing hormone and of luteinizing hormone, resulting normally in ovulation. These hormonal rhythms are reflected in cyclic variations of ovarian secretion of estrogen and progesterone with consequent formation of first proliferative, then secretory endometrium. Also *menses, menstrual period, monthly period.* **anovulatory m.** Periodic uterine bleeding occurring in the absence of ovulation. Also *nonovulational menstruation, anovulatory cycle.* **infrequent m.** OLIGOMENORRHEA. **nonovulational m.** ANOVULATORY MENSTRUATION. **regurgitant m.** RETROGRADE MENSTRUATION. **retained m.** HEMATOCOLPOS. **retrograde m.** A flow of menstrual blood through the fallopian tubes. Also *regurgitant menstruation.* **vicarious m.** Bleeding from any surface other than the endometrium occurring periodically at the time when normal menstruation takes place. It is usually caused by endometriosis. Also *menoplania.*

**menstruous** \men′stroo·əs\ MENSTRUAL.

**menstruum** \men′stroo·əm\ [Med. L (from neut. sing. of L *menstruus* monthly, menstruous), menses] **1** The menstrual blood. **2** The liquid vehicle used to extract the active ingredients from a crude source of a drug and prepare an official tincture of the drug. **Pitkin m.** A mixture of gelatin, dextrose, glacial acetic acid, and water, that has been used as a medium for certain drugs, such as heparin, to delay diffusion of the drug and prolong the drug action.

**mensuration** \men′sərā′shən\ [Late L *mensuratio* (from *mensuratus,* past part. of *mensurare* to measure, from L *mensus,* past part. of *metiri* to measure) a measuring] The act or process of measuring.

**-ment** \-mənt\ [French (from L *-mentum,* noun suffix), suffix forming nouns from verbs signifying action, concrete result, state, or condition] A noun suffix denoting action, state, or result.

**mental¹** [Late L *mental(is)* (from L *mens,* gen. *mentis,* the mind + *-alis* -AL) pertaining to the mind] Pertaining to mind or to the activities or processes of the mind.

**mental²** [L *ment(um)* chin, beard + -AL] Of or pertaining to the chin; genial.

**Menten** [Maud Lenore *Menten,* U.S. physician, 1879–1960] **1** Michaelis-Menten equation. See under EQUATION. **2** Michaelis-Menten kinetics. See under MICHAELIS KINETICS.

**menthol** \men′thəl\ 2-Isopropyl-5-methylcyclohexanol, with the isopropyl group *trans* and the methyl group *cis* to the hydroxyl group. It is a terpene alcohol, found in *Mentha piperita* and other mint species and also produced synthetically. It is used as a nasal decongestant, antiseptic, anesthetic, counterirritant, and topical antipruritic. Also *peppermint camphor.*

**menti-** \men′ti-\ [L *mens,* gen. *mentis,* the mind] A combining form meaning the mind.

**mento-** \men′tō-, men′tə-\ [New L, from L *mentum* the chin] A combining form denoting the chin.

**mentoanterior** \-antir′ē·ər\ [MENTO- + ANTERIOR] In a face presentation, having the fetal chin pointing anteriorly in relation to the maternal pelvis.

**mentoplasty** \men′təplas′tē\ [MENTO- + -PLASTY] Any plastic operation performed on the chin.

**mentoposterior** \-pästir′ē·ər\ [MENTO- + POSTERIOR] In a face presentation, having the fetal chin pointing posteriorly in relation to the maternal pelvis.

**mentotransverse** \-trans′vurs\ [MENTO- + TRANSVERSE] In a face presentation, having the fetal chin pointing laterally in relation to the maternal pelvis.

**mentula** \men′tʸələ\ [L, penis] *Outmoded* PENIS.

**mentulagra** \men′tʸəlag′rə\ [*mentul(a)* + -AGRA] PRIAPISM.

**mentum** \men′təm\ [L, the chin] The anterior prominence of the mandible that is produced by the mental protuberance; chin. The fleshy muscles and connective tissues covering it are separated from the lower lip by a groove.

**mepacrine hydrochloride** QUINACRINE HYDROCHLORIDE.

**meparfynol** $C_6H_{10}O$. A colorless or pale yellow liquid with an unpleasant burning taste. It is used as a short-acting hypnotic.

**mepazine** $C_{19}H_{22}N_2S$. 10-[(-methyl-3-piperidinyl)methyl]-10*H* phenothiazine. A tranquilizer employed as a sedative in the treatment of a variety of anxiety states. It is also used as a preoperative or postoperative sedative. It is administered orally or intramuscularly. Also *pecazine.*

**mepenzolate bromide** $C_{21}H_{26}BrNO_3$. 3-[(Hydroxydiphenylacetyl)oxy]-1,1-dimethyl-piperidinium bromide. An anticholinergic agent used in the treatment of disorders where hypermotility of the colon is of concern. It is given orally.

**meperidine hydrochloride** $C_{15}H_{21}NO_2$·HCl. Ethyl-1-methyl-4-phenylpiperidine-4-carboxylate hydrochloride. A synthetic white, odorless powder, soluble in water and alcohol. It is a narcotic analgesic with spasmolytic properties. Its continued use may lead to addiction. It is usually given orally or intramuscularly. Also *pethidine hydrochloride, isonipecaine.*

**mephenamine** ORPHENADRINE.

**mephenesin** $C_{10}H_{14}O_3$. 3-(2-Methylphenoxy)-1,2-propanediol. It is a white, crystalline powder employed as a skeletal muscle relaxant agent. It is given orally. Also *stilalgin, cresoxypropanediol, cresoxydiol.*

**mephenoxalone** $C_{11}H_{13}NO_4$. 5-[(*o*-Methoxyphenoxy)methyl]-2-oxazolidinone. It possesses mild tranquilizing properties, and is used as a skeletal muscle relaxant.

**mephentermine sulfate** $(C_{11}H_{17}N)2·H_2SO_4$. *N*α,α-Trimethylbenzeneethanamine. A white, crystalline powder with adrenergic properties. It is used for its vasopressor effects in the treatment of certain hypotensive states. It can be given orally, intramuscularly, or intravenously, and may be applied topically to the nasal mucosa as a decongestant drug.

**mephenytoin** $C_{12}H_{14}N_2O_2$. 5-Ethyl-3-methyl-5-phenyl-2,4-imidazolidenedione. It is used as an anticonvulsant drug in the control of focal, jacksonian, grand mal, and psychomotor seizures that are not responsive to other drugs. It is given orally.

**mephobarbital** $C_{13}H_{14}N_2O_3$. 5-Ethyl-1-methyl-5-phenyl-2,4,6(1*H*,3*H*,5*H*)-pyrimidinetrione. A barbiturate with prolonged actions, used as a sedative in the treatment of anxiety. It is also employed as an anticonvulsant in the treatment of grand mal and petit mal epilepsy. It is given orally. Also *phemitone.*

**mepivacaine** $C_{15}H_{22}N_2O$. *N*-(2,6-Dimethylphenyl)-1-methyl-2-piperidine-carboxamide. A white, crystalline powder which is administered as the hydrochloride salt. It is an analogue of lidocaine, used to produce local anesthesia by infiltration injection, peripheral nerve block, and epidural block.

**meprednisone** $C_{22}H_{28}O_5$. 17-α,21-Dihydroxy-16β-methyl-pregna-1,4-diene-3,11,20-trione. A synthetic glucocorticoid which occurs as a white powder. It is used in the treatment of inflammatory, rheumatic, and allergic conditions, and is also used to treat corticosteroid-responsive diseases, such as certain connective tissue disorders and some neoplastic diseases. It is given orally.

**meprobamate** $C_9H_{18}N_2O_4$. 2-Methyl-2-propyl-1,3-propanediol dicarbamate. A white powder with activity as a tranquilizer and muscle relaxant, and with anticonvulsant properties. It is used orally as a sedative and antianxiety medication, and to promote sleep in tense patients. It is used intramuscularly as an adjunct treatment for tetanus.

**meprylcaine hydrochloride** $C_{14}H_{21}NO_2$·HCl. 2-Methyl-2-(propylamino)-1-propanol benzoate (ester) hydrochloride. A white, crystalline powder, used as a local anesthetic for infiltration and nerve block anesthesia.

**mepyramine maleate** PYRILAMINE MALEATE.

**mepyrapone** METYRAPONE.

**mEq** Symbol for the quantity, milliequivalent.

**mequidox** $C_{10}H_{10}N_2O_3$. 3-Methyl-2-quinoxalinemethanol 1,4-dioxide. It is employed as an antibacterial agent.

**meractinomycin** ACTINOMYCIN D.

**meralein sodium** $C_{19}H_9HgI_2NaO_7S$. 2,7-Diiodo-4-hydroxymercuriresorcinsulfonphthalein monosodium salt. A water-soluble, topically applied, anti-infective agent.

**meralgia** \meral′jə\ [*mer(o)-*[2] + -ALGIA] A pain in the thigh. **m. paresthetica** A benign but troublesome syndrome resulting from compression of the lateral cutaneous nerve of the thigh as it passes beneath or through the fibers of the inguinal ligament just medial to the anterior superior iliac spine. It may develop spontaneously, often in obese subjects, but sometimes first appears in pregnancy. Pain and paresthesiae are felt, particularly on standing for long periods, on the outer aspect of the thigh, and blunting of cutaneous sensation is usually noted in this area. Also *Bernhardt's disease, Bernhardt-Roth syndrome, Bernhardt's paresthesiae, Rot's disease, Roth's disease, Roth syndrome.*

**meralluride** $C_{16}H_{22}HgN_6O_7$. *N*-[[2-Methoxy-3-[(1,2,3,6-tetrahydro-1,3-dimethyl-2,6-dioxopurin- 7-yl)mercuri]propyl]-carbamoyl]succinamic acid. A diuretic agent used in the treatment of edema secondary to congestive heart failure, nephrosis, and ascites of liver disease. It is given intramuscularly or subcutaneously.

**merbromin** $C_{20}H_8Br_2HgNa_2O_6$. (2′7′-Dibromo-3′,6′-dihydroxy-3-oxospiro[isobenzofuran-1(3*H*),9′[9*H*]xanthene]-4′-yl)-hydroxomercury disodium salt. It is used clinically as a topical antibacterial drug.

**mercaptalbumin** The form of serum albumin that has one thiol group per molecule, in distinction from the form in which this group exists as the mixed disulfide with a thiol of low molecular mass. *Seldom used.*

**mercaptan** *Obs.* THIOL.

**mercaptide** *Obs.* THIOLATE.

**mercapto-** \mərkap′tō-\ [Med L *mer(curium),* accus. of *mercurius* mercury + L *capt(ans),* pres. part. of *captare* to seize + *o*] A combining form denoting substitution of a hydrogen atom by a thiol group. See also SULFHYDRYL.

**mercaptoethanol** HS—$CH_2$—$CH_2OH$. One of the most commonly used reagents containing a thiol group, often added to cell extracts to prevent or reverse the formation of —S—S— bonds from thiol groups by materials in these extracts. It is of particular utility because the hydroxyl group lowers its volatility and gives it considerable solubility in water.

**mercaptoethylamine** $C_2H_7NS$. A compound prepared from ethanolamine and carbon disulfide via 2-mercaptothiazoline. It has been used in treating radiation sickness and chronic leukemia. It is a component of the coenzyme A molecule. Also *cysteamine.*

**2-mercaptoimidazole** An antithyroid agent of the thiouricil family. It is considered to be about five times more potent than methylthiouricil.

**mercaptomerin sodium** $C_{16}H_{25}HgNNa_2O_6S$. *N*-[3-(Carboxymethylthiomercuri)-2-methoxypropyl]-α-camphoramate. A mercurial diuretic drug that is given subcutaneously or intramuscularly.

**mercaptopurine** 6-Purinethiol. A hypoxanthine and adenine analogue that serves as a purine antagonist. It is utilized primarily as an antineoplastic agent since it is a potent inhibitor of DNA synthesis.

**mercapturic acid** An *S*-aryl-*N*-acetylcysteine. It is found in the urine after ingestion of aromatic halogen compounds.

**Mercier** [Louis Auguste *Mercier,* French urologist, 1811–1882] **1** See under VALVE. **2** Mercier's barrier, Mercier's bar. See under PLICA INTERURETERICA. **3** Mercier's barrier. See under MEDIAN BAR.

**mercupurin** *Outmoded* MERCUROPHYLLINE.

**mercuramide** MERSALYL SODIUM.

**mercurial** **1** Of, relating to, or resembling mercury. **2** Denoting a preparation of mercury or one containing mercury, as in *mercurial diuretic.*

**mercurialentis** \mərkyoo′rē·əlen′tis\ [English *mercuria(l)* + L *lens,* gen. *lentis,* a lentil] A bilateral and symmetric, light gray or brownish discoloration of the anterior capsule of the crystalline lens due to the deposition of mercury. It is a sign of chronic exposure to low levels of inorganic mercury or its compounds.

**mercurialism** \mərkyoo′rē·əlizm\ MERCURY POISONING.

***p*-mercuribenzoate** The substance formed from the anion of benzoic acid by substitution of the *p*-hydrogen by $Hg^+$—. The mercury atom normally bears an anionic ligand such as $Cl^-$ or $OH^-$, but this is exchangeable, and easily replaced by a thiolate. This gives mercuribenzoate a high affinity for thiols, and its use in titrating thiol groups and as an inhibitor of enzymes depends on this property.

**mercuric** \mərkyoo′rik\ [*mercur(y)* + -IC] Concerning mercury in its Hg(II) form. Mercuric salts are toxic because of their high affinity for the thiol groups of proteins.

**mercuric chloride** $HgCl_2$. A water-soluble salt of mercury. It is highly toxic owing to the $Hg^{2+}$ ions it contains. It is used as a secondary fixative where preservation of proteins is particularly important. Also *corrosive sublimate* (obs.).

**mercuric sulfide** HgS. A bright red powder that has been used in an ointment base as a treatment for chronic skin diseases. Also *cinnabar.*

**Mercurochrome** A proprietary name for merbromin

**mercurophylline** An organic mercurial diuretic agent in combination with theophylline in approximately equimolecular amounts. It is given by intramuscular or intravenous injection. Also *mercupurin* (outmoded).

**mercurous** \mərkyoo′rəs\ Concerning the ion $Hg^+$—$Hg^+$. Its chloride, calomel, has very low solubility in water.

**mercurous chloride** CALOMEL.

**mercury** \mur′kyərē\ [after *Mercurius* (Mercury) son of Jupiter and Maia, and messenger of the gods; his name was given to the planet and later to the metal, possibly because his swiftness was deemed characteristic of mercury (quicksilver)] A metallic element of atomic number 80, atomic weight 200.59, specific gravity 13.5, and boiling point −38.842°C. It is the only common metal that is liquid (and volatile) at ordinary temperatures. It does not occur in the free state but is readily freed from its principal ore, cinnabar, by heat. Natural mercury consists of seven stable isotopes. Numerous radioactive isotopes have been identified, all of them relatively short lived. Valences are 1 and 2. In an electric discharge, mercury combines with the so-called inert gases argon, krypton, neon, and xenon. Though relatively rare in the lithosphere, mercury is universally familiar through its use in thermometers, barometers, and the like. It is indispensable in many industrial and research operations. It is commonly used in dental amalgams and has several other medical applications. But its vapor and some of its compounds are virulent poisons. The vapor is readily absorbed through mucous membrane or unbroken skin. Methyl mercury is a dangerous environmental pollutant. It is elaborated by anaerobic bacteria in many rivers and streams where mercury-containing waste has been discharged, and thence it can enter the food chain via fishes, insects, and birds. Also *quicksilver, hydrargyrum.* Symbol: Hg See also MERCURY POISONING. **ammoniated m.** $HgNH_2Cl$. A substance occurring as a white, amorphous powder or as small, white granules. It is applied topically in an ointment base as an anti-infective medication. Also *hydrargyrum ammoniatum.*

**-mere** \-mir\ [Gk *meros* a part] A combining form meaning a part.

**Merendino** [Alvin Aurelius *Merendino,* U.S. surgeon, born 1914] See under TECHNIQUE.

**merethoxylline** Dehydro-2-[*n*-(3″-hydroxymercuri-2″-methoxyethoxy)propylcarbamoyl]phenoxyacetic acid.

**merethoxylline procaine** A combination of merethoxylline, theophylline, and procaine. It is used in the treatment of edema secondary to congestive heart failure and the nephrotic syndrome. It is given intramuscularly or subcutaneously.

**meridian** \mərid′ē·ən\ [L *meridianus.* See MERIDIANUS.] MERIDIANUS. **m.'s of eyeball** MERIDIANI BULBI OCULI. **horizontal m.** An imaginary line that passes through the point of visual fixation and is oriented horizontally in the frontal plane. **vertical m.** A line that passes through the point of visual fixation and is oriented vertically in the frontal plane.

**meridiani** \mərid′ē·ā′nī\ Plural of MERIDIANUS.

**meridianus** \mərid′ē·a′nəs\ [L (from *meri-,* alteration of *medi- mid-,* from *medius* middle + *dies* day + *-anus* adjectival suffix), of or at midday] [NA] An imaginary line on the surface of a spherical body passing along the plane of its axis. Also *meridian.* **meridiani bulbi oculi** Circumferential lines joining the poles of the eyeball. Also *meridians of eyeball.*

**meridional** \mərid′ē·ənəl\ Pertaining to a meridian.

**merispore** \mer′əspôr\ A secondary spore resulting from the segmentation of a compound or septate spore.

**Merkel** [Friedrich S. *Merkel* German anatomist and physiologist, 1845–1919] **1** Merkel's disk, Merkel cell. See under MENISCUS TACTUS. **2** Merkel cell carcinoma. See under CARCINOMA. **3** Merkel's corpuscles. See under CORPUSCLE. **4** Merkel-Ranvier cell. See under MELANOCYTE.

**Merkel** [Karl Ludwig *Merkel*, German anatomist and laryngologist, 1812–1876] **1** Merkel's filtrum, Merkel's fossa. See under FILTRUM VENTRICULI. **2** Merkel's muscle. See under MUSCULUS CERATOCRICOIDEUS.

**mero-**[1] \mer′ō-\ [Gk *meros* part] A combining form meaning part, partial.

**mero-**[2] [Gk *mēros* upper part of the thigh, the ham] A combining form denoting the thigh.

**meroanencephaly** \-an′ensef′əlē\ [MERO-[1] + ANENCEPHALY] Anencephaly in which less than the usual erosion of cerebral tissue has occurred during intrauterine life and identifiable parts of the cerebrum such as peduncles and thalamus may remain.

**meroblastic** \-blas′tik\ [MERO-[1] + BLAST- + -IC] See under MEROBLASTIC CLEAVAGE.

**merocele** \mir′əsēl\ [MERO-[2] + -CELE[2]] FEMORAL HERNIA.

**merocrine** \mer′əkrin\ [MERO-[1] + Gk *krin(ein)* to separate, put apart] Denoting or characterized by secretion that involves the discharge of the secretory product from an intact cell. Compare HOLOCRINE.

**merocyte** \mer′əsīt\ [MERO-[1] + -CYTE] An incompletely isolated cell found in the vicinity of the yolk of a fertilized ovum during segmentation. Its nucleus is generally derived from accessory spermatozoa. Ova with abundant yolk often manifest this phenomenon (physiologic polyspermy).

**meroencephaly** \-ensef′əlē\ [MERO-[1] + ENCEPHAL- + -Y] The developmental absence of a part of the brain, such as the cerebellum or the corpus callosum.

**meroergasia** \mir′ō-ərgā′zhə\ NEUROSIS.

**merogony** \mirāg′ənē\ [MERO-[1] + -GONY] **1** The development of only a portion of an egg. If the egg contains only the male pronucleus, the development is termed andromerogony, and if only the female pronucleus, gynomerogony. **2** SCHIZOGONY. **diploid m.** Development of a portion of an egg containing the combined products of the male and female pronuclei.

**merology** \miräl′əjē\ [MERO-[1] + -OLOGY] The study of the rudimentary tissues.

**meromelia** \-mē′lyə\ [MERO-[1] + MEL-[1] + -IA] The developmental absence of a part of one or more limbs. Also *limb reduction defect*. See also HEMIMELIA, PEROMELIA, MICROMELIA, ECTRODACTYLY, AMELIA.

**meromicrosomia** \-mīk′rəsō′mē-ə\ [MERO-[1] + MICRO- + *som(ato)-* + -IA] The developmental smallness of a part of the body. • The term is used in reference to a part not readily described by the prefix *micro*, as with specific organs or regions.

**meromyosin** [MERO-[1] + MYOSIN] One of two proteins, heavy meromyosin and light meromyosin, formed by enzymatic digestion of myosin. The region of myosin susceptible to the proteolysis lies near the "head" of the molecule, i.e. the region that protrudes from the fibril and interacts with actin. Heavy meromyosin molecules contain these heads and have the ability to interact with actin and to hydrolyze ATP. Light meromyosin molecules interact with each other to form fibrils. The separation of these substances and the characterization of their properties led to increased understanding of the mechanism of muscular contraction.

**merorachischisis** \-rəkis′kisis\ [MERO-[1] + RACHISCHISIS] Rachischisis limited to a short segment of the spinal cord.

**meros** \mir′əs\ [Gk *mēros* upper part of the thigh, the ham] **1** The femur. **2** The thigh.

**merotomy** \mirät′əmē\ [MERO-[1] + -TOMY] Dissection into parts, particularly the dissection of a cell, in order to study the capacity for growth and development of the separate parts.

**merozoite** \-zō′īt\ [MERO-[1] + *zo(o)-* + -ITE] A motile form of a sporozoan that results from the asexual division of the schizont during schizogony. In the life cycle of the malarial plasmodium in man, the merozoite is released into the blood from the exoerythrocytic stage in the liver or from the erythrocytic stages in infected red cells, from which it invades new erythrocytes. Also *schizozoite, zoite*.

**merozygote** \-zī′gōt\ A bacterium that is diploid for a portion of its genome through transduction, F-duction, or some other process that introduces exogenous DNA. Processes that introduce a DNA fragment rather than a replicon (conjugation, transformation) yield a transient merozygote.

**merphalan** A racemic mixture of melphalan and medphalan. It is used as an antineoplastic drug.

**Merritt** [Katharine Krom *Merritt*, U.S. pediatrician, born 1886] Kasabach-Merritt syndrome. See under SYNDROME.

**mersalyl acid** A mixture of *o*-carboxymethylsalicyl-(3-hydroxymercuric-2-methoxypropyl)-amide and its anhydride. It is used for the same indications as mersalyl sodium.

**mersalyl sodium** $C_{13}H_{16}HgNNaO_6$. [3-[[2-Carboxymethoxy)-benzoyl]amino]-2-methoxy-propyl] hydroxymercury monosodium salt. A diuretic used in combination with theophylline in the treatment of edema secondary to such conditions as cardiorenal disease, nephrosis, and hepatic cirrhosis. It is given intramuscularly or intravenously. Also *mercuramide*.

**mersalyl sodium and theophylline** Mersalyl sodium mixed with theophylline for administration together to lessen the degree of decomposition of the former.

**Merthiolate** A proprietary name for thimerosal

**Merzbacher** [Ludwig *Merzbacher*, German neurologist active in Argentina, born 1875] Merzbacher-Pelizaeus disease, Pelizaeus-Merzbacher sclerosis, Pelizaeus-Merzbacher type diffuse sclerosis. See under PELIZAEUS-MERZBACHER DISEASE.

**mes-** \mez-, mes-\ MESO-.

**mesad** \mē′sad\ MESIAD.

**mesal** \mē′səl\ MESIAL.

**mesangiolysis** \-an′jē-äl′isis\ Degeneration of mesangial cells and matrix secondary to radiation and some snake toxins.

**mesangium** \-an′jē-əm\ [New L, from MES- + Gk *angeion* vessel] The framework of the glomerulus, which arises from the vascular pole and extends into the intercapillary spaces, forming lobule centers. The mesangium contains matrix and mesangial cells in communication with the capillary lumen. The mesangial cells are phagocytic, while large molecules and aggregates may accumulate in the matrix. Adj. mesangial.

**mesaortitis** \mes′ā-ôrtī′tis\ MESOAORTITIS.

**mesarteritis** \mes′ärtərī′tis\ Inflammation localized to the media, or muscular layer, of an artery. **Mönckeberg's m.** MÖNCKEBERG SCLEROSIS.

**mesaxon** \-äk′sän\ The contact interface between pairs of parallel membranes formed by the concentric growth of the Schwann cell enfolding an axon. **internal m.** The innermost portion of the mesaxon which is adjacent to the axon itself. Also *inaxon*.

**mescal** \meskal′\ PEYOTE.

**mescaline** \mes′kəlin\ 3,4,5-Trimethoxyphenethylamine. It is a hallucinogenic alkaloid found in the peyote cactus (mescal button).

**mesectoderm** \-ek'tədurm\ [MES- + ECTODERM] The part of the middle layer of the embryo arising from the ectoderm through the intermediary of the neural plate, or more specifically, directly from the neural crest. It is sometimes contrasted with mesentoderm and with mesentoblast, but it is more properly distinguished from true mesoderm.

**mesencephalic** \-en'səfal'ik\ Pertaining to the mesencephalon.

**mesencephalitis** \-ensef'əlī'tis\ [MES- + ENCEPHALITIS] Encephalitis affecting the midbrain especially severely.

**mesencephalon** \-ensef'əlän\ [MES- + ENCEPHALON] 1 That portion of the brainstem that lies between the pons and the diencephalon in the fully developed brain. 2 The middle of the three expansions which develop in the early embryo at the front of the primitive neural tube. These expansions are called the primitive brain vesicles. It gives rise to the colliculi, the tegmentum, and the crura cerebri. Also *midbrain vesicle.* For defs. 1 and 2 also *midbrain.*

**mesencephalotomy** \-ensef'əlät'əmē\ [*mesencephalo(n)* + -TOMY] An incision into the mesencephalon, such as division of pain tracts for the relief of intractable pain.

**mesenchyme** \mez'ənkīm\ [MES- + Gk *enchyma* infusion, juice, from EN- + Gk *chymos* juice, from *cheein* to pour, spill] Primitive embryonic connective or packing tissue originating from mesoderm and developing into the supporting tissues. It consists of widely separated stellate cells surrounded by ground substance and some reticular fibers. Also *mesenchyma, embryonal connective tissue, mesenchymal tissue, desmohemoblast.* Adj. mesenchymal, mesenchymatous. **interzonal m.** A plate of homogenous mesenchymatous tissue which separates the centers of chondrification at the joints formed from the fifth week of human embryonic development. In the synovial joints, this zone includes three regions: two chondrogenic layers, each in continuity with the perichondrium of the future skeletal elements, and an intermediate avascular layer continuous at the periphery with the synovial mesenchyme. It is within this intermediate layer that a cleft will appear to become the future joint cavity. **primary m.** Mesenchyme appearing at an early stage between the trophoblast on one side, and the amnion and the yolk sac on the other, while the embryo is still two-layered. Its origin is still not certain. **secondary m.** Intraembryonic mesenchyme essentially derived from dissociation of the mesoblast.

**mesenchymoma** \-eng'kīmō'mə\ [MESENCHYME + -OMA] A rare, benign or malignant tumor consisting of two or more clearly identifiable mesenchymal elements in addition to fibrous tissue. The mixed mesodermal tumors of the genitourinary tract are not included in this group. **benign m.** A mesenchymoma whose component tissues are mature and without evidence of aggressive growth. **malignant m.** A mesenchymoma one or more of whose component tissues shows malignant characteristics. This may appear as a fibrosarcoma, liposarcoma, leiomyosarcoma, osteosarcoma, etc.

**mesenterectomy** \-en'tərek'təmē\ [*mesenter(y)* + ECTOMY] The surgical removal of part or all of a mesenteric attachment.

**mesenteric** \-enter'ik\ Pertaining to mesentery.

**mesenteriolum** \-en'terī'ələm\ [dim. of *mesenterium.* See MESENTERIUM.] A mesentery of small size.

**mesenteriopexy** \-enter'ē-əpek'sē\ A surgical procedure in which a torn or ptotic redundant mesentery is resuspended and repaired. Also *mesopexy.*

**mesenteriorrhaphy** \-enter'ē-ôr'əfē\ A surgical procedure in which sutures are used to repair or resuspend a damaged or redundant mesentery. Also *mesorrhaphy, mesentorrhaphy.*

**mesenteriplication** \-enter'ēplikā'shən\ A surgical procedure in which a redundant mesentery is shortened by folding it upon itself and then suturing the folds into place.

**mesenteritis** \mes'enterī'tis\ Mesenteric inflammation. Adj. mesenteritic. **retractile m.** A chronic inflammation of the mesentery resulting in progressive fibrosis and nodular thickening with retraction and distortion of the intestinal loops. A condition of uncertain etiology, it is believed to be similar to and related to retroperitoneal fibrosis.

**mesenterium** \mes'enter'ē-əm\ [New L (from Gk *mesenterion* or *mesenteron* mesentery, from MES- + Gk *enteron* a piece of gut, pl. *entera* the intestines), mesentery] 1 A fold of peritoneum that encloses an abdominal viscus while anchoring it to the abdominal wall, and that carries between its two layers blood vessels, lymphatics, and nerves to and from the viscus. 2 [NA] The extensive peritoneal fold attaching the jejunum and ileum to the posterior abdominal wall and extending obliquely from the duodenojejunal junction to the ileocecal junction. For defs. 1 and 2 also *mesentery, mesostenium* (outmoded).

**mesenteron** \-en'terän\ [MES- + Gk *enteron* a piece of gut] MIDGUT.

**mesentery** \mez'ənter'ē\ [New L *mesenterium.* See MESENTERIUM.] MESENTERIUM. **caval m.** A fold of dorsal body wall tissue, just to the right of the main dorsal mesentery, bridging the cephalic pole of the right mesonephros and the liver. Vessels in this fold differentiate to form the infrahepatic segment of the interior vena cava. Also *caval fold.* **common dorsal m.** A double-layered partition of visceral splanchnic mesoderm which divides the embryonic coelom into halves, suspends the primitive digestive tube from the posterior body wall, and carries the blood supply to the tube. The covering coelomic epithelium is continuous with the parietal splanchnic mesoderm, and together they will form the future peritoneum, its folds, ligaments, and mesenteries. Initially, there is also a ventral mesentery related to the gastroduodenal portion of the tube from which the lesser omentum is derived. The common dorsal mesentery, at first called the primitive mesentery, applies to all of the embryonic dorsal mesentery. It stretches the entire length of the primitive digestive tube and takes part in the complex development of the latter. Also *common mesentery, dorsal mesentery.* See also PERSISTENT COMMON MESENTERY. **dorsal m.** COMMON DORSAL MESENTERY. **persistent common m.** A condition in which the embryonic dorsal mesentery or parts thereof retain the primitive attachments between the mid-dorsal body wall and the gastrointestinal tract. During normal embryogenesis the dorsal mesentery is either lost by fusion with the body wall or by repositioning, as the various segments of the gastrointestinal tract undergo rotation while the midgut is withdrawn from the umbilical stalk. In malrotation or incomplete rotation of the tract the mesentery retains some of its embryonic relationships. **primitive m.** Double-layered embryonic membrane formed by the union of the two opposing splanchnopleuric layers when the abdominal wall closes off and the peritoneal cavity develops. It has dorsal and ventral parts in relation to the gut which it encloses. The dorsal part of the primitive mesentery will become the common dorsal mesentery. **m. of rectum** MESORECTUM. **m. of sigmoid colon** MESOCOLON SIGMOIDEUM. **ventral m.** A fold of peritoneum which extends from the ventral wall of the foregut toward the diaphragm and anterior abdominal wall as far down as the umbilicus. It is probably derived from the septum transversum and it contributes to the definitive lesser omentum and the falciform ligament. **m. of vermi-**

**form appendix** MESOAPPENDIX.
**mesentorrhaphy** \-entôr′əfē\ MESENTERIORRHAPHY.
**mesepithelium** \mez′epithē′lē·əm\ MESOTHELIUM.
**mesh** One of the spaces in a screen or sieve, or the intersecting wires which form such spaces.
**meshwork** NETWORK. **trabecular m.** RETICULUM TRABECULARE SCLERAE.
**mesiad** \mē′sē·ad\ Directed or proceeding toward the median sagittal plane of the body or, specifically, following the dental arch toward the center line. Also *mesad.*
**mesial** \mē′sē·əl\ [MESI(O)- + -AL] Nearer or nearest the midline in the dental arch: used especially of the surface of a tooth. Also *mesal.* Compare DISTAL.
**mesio-** \mē′zē·ō-\ [Gk *mesos* (adjective) middle, in the middle, between] A combining form meaning mesial.
**mesioclusion** \mē′zē·əkloo′zhən\ [MESIO- + *oc(c)lusion*] MANDIBULAR PROGNATHISM.
**mesiodens** \mē′zē·ədenz\ [MESIO- + L *dens* tooth] A centrally placed upper supernumerary tooth.
**mesion** \mē′zē·än\ MEDIAN PLANE.
**mesio-occlusal** \-əkloo′zəl\ [MESIO- + OCCLUSAL] Relating to both the mesial and occlusal surfaces of a tooth: said of cavities and restorations involving these surfaces. Abbr. MO
**mesio-occlusion** \-əkloo′zhən\ MANDIBULAR PROGNATHISM.
**mesio-occlusodistal** \-əkloo′zōdis′təl\ [MESIO- + OCCLUSODISTAL] Relating to all the mesial, occlusal, and distal surfaces of a tooth: said of cavities and restorations involving these surfaces. Abbr. MOD
**mesioversion** \-vur′zhən\ [MESIO- + VERSION] **1** A position of a tooth nearer the median line than normal. **2** A more than normally anterior position of a jaw. Also *mesial displacement, mesioplacement.*
**mesiris** \mesī′ris\ STROMA IRIDIS.
**meso-** \mez′ō-\ [Gk *mesos* (adjective) middle, in the middle, between] **1** A prefix meaning intermediate or connective, or denoting a means of attachment to a designated organ. Also *mes-.* **2** In stereochemistry, a prefix denoting an isomer of dissymmetric compounds that possesses dissymmetric carbon atoms but is not itself dissymmetric because of internal compensation. **3** In chemistry, a prefix denoting substitution of a bridging atom.
**mesoaortitis** \-ā′ôrtī′tis\ Inflammation localized to the middle, or muscular, layer of the aorta. Also *mesaortitis.* **m. syphilitica** Inflammation of the media of the ascending aorta due to syphilitic infection. It is a chronic process characterized by loss of elastic fibers and their replacement by fibrous scars that cause the aorta to dilate and even rupture.
**mesoappendix** \-əpen′diks\ [NA] A triangular fold of peritoneum around the vermiform appendix, one side being attached for varying distances along the appendix and the other side attaching the latter to the posterior surface of the mesentery of the ileum. The artery to the appendix runs along the free margin of the fold. Also *mesentery of vermiform appendix.*
**mesoarial** \-er′ē·əl\ Pertaining to the mesovarium. *Outmoded.*
**mesoblast** \mez′əblast\ [MESO- + -BLAST] MESODERM.
**mesocardium** \-kär′dē·əm\ [New L, from MESO- + Gk *kardia* the heart] A double-layered dorsal or posterior serous membrane which suspends the embyronic heart tube from the dorsal wall of the pericardial cavity. It fenestrates very soon, leaving a gap (the transverse pericardial sinus). There is also a ventral or anterior mesocardium but it disappears immediately after its appearance. Also *dorsal mesocardium.* **arterial m.** The tube of visceral pericardium reflected along the pulmonary trunk and the ascending aorta. *Outmoded.* **dorsal m.** MESOCARDIUM. **venous m.** The serous pericardium reflected over the roots of the pulmonary veins and of the venae cavae. *Outmoded.*
**mesocarpal** \-kär′pəl\ MIDCARPAL.
**mesocephalic** \-səfal′ik\ Having head proportions intermediate between dolichocephalic and brachycephalic, with a cephalic index between 76 and 80.9.
**mesocephaly** \-sef′əlē\ [MESO- + CEPHAL- + -Y] Intermediate length-breadth proportions of the head, with a cephalic index between 76 and 80.9.
**mesochord** \mez′əkôrd\ MESOCORD.
**mesochoroidea** \-kôroi′dē·ə\ *Outmoded* LAMINA CHOROIDOCAPILLARIS.
**mesocoelia** \-sē′lyə\ *Obs.* AQUEDUCTUS CEREBRI.
**mesocolic** \-kō′lik\ Of or relating to the mesocolon.
**mesocolon** \-kō′lən\ [MESO- + COLON] [NA] The peritoneal fold attaching the various parts of the colon to the posterior abdominal wall. Only the transverse colon and the sigmoid colon usually have actual mesenteries connecting them to the abdominal wall. **m. ascendens** [NA] The short peritoneal fold that, in about one in four adults, surrounds the ascending colon and attaches it to the posterior abdominal wall. Usually the ascending colon is covered by peritoneum only anteriorly and on the sides. Also *ascending mesocolon, right mesocolon* (outmoded). **m. descendens** The short peritoneal fold that, in approximately one in three adults, surrounds the descending colon and attaches it to the posterior abdominal wall. Usually the descending colon is covered by peritoneum only anteriorly and on the sides. Also *descending mesocolon, left mesocolon* (outmoded) . **descending m.** MESOCOLON DESCENDENS. **iliac m.** *Outmoded* MESOCOLON SIGMOIDEUM. **left m.** *Outmoded* MESOCOLON DESCENDENS. **pelvic m.** MESOCOLON SIGMOIDEUM. **right m.** *Outmoded* MESOCOLON ASCENDENS. **sigmoid m.** MESOCOLON SIGMOIDEUM. **m. sigmoideum** [NA] A peritoneal fold securing the sigmoid colon to the pelvic wall in the shape of an inverted V. Also *pelvic mesocolon, iliac mesocolon* (outmoded), *mesentery of sigmoid colon, mesosigmoid* (outmoded), *sigmoid mesocolon.* **transverse m.** MESOCOLON TRANSVERSUM. **m. transversum** [NA] A broad peritoneal fold that connects the transverse colon to the structures on the posterior abdominal wall, especially the head of pancreas and the anterior border of the body of the pancreas. Also *transverse mesocolon.*
**mesocolopexy** \-kō′ləpek′sē\ A surgical procedure in which the mesocolon is fixed or resuspended to prevent ptosis or torsion of the transverse colon.
**mesocoloplication** \-kō′ləplikā′shən\ A surgical procedure in which the mesocolon is folded back on itself and then sutured into place in order to control the mobility of the transverse colon.
**mesocord** \mez′əkôrd\ [MESO- + CORD] An umbilical cord, a segment of which is bound to the placenta by an accessory fold. Also *mesochord.*
**mesocornea** \-kôr′nē·ə\ *Outmoded* SUBSTANTIA PROPRIA CORNEAE.
**mesocortex** \-kôr′teks\ [MESO- + CORTEX] **1** The cerebral cortex of the cingulate and retrospenial gyri that does not pass through a six-layered developmental stage, but approximates the appearance of isocortex in the adult. **2** GYRUS CINGULI.
**mesocranium** \-krā′nē·əm\ VERTEX.
**mesocuneiform** \-kyoonē′ifôrm\ OS CUNEIFORME INTERMEDIUM.

**mesocyst** \mezʹəsist\ A rare peritoneal fold that suspends the gallbladder from its fossa on the liver. Usually only its posteroinferior surface and sides are covered by peritoneum.

**mesoderm** \mezʹədurm\ [MESO- + -DERM] One of the three primary germ layers, formed between the ectoderm (outermost layer) and endoderm (innermost layer) of the embryo. From this layer are derived the majority of the skeletal system, the circulatory system, the musculature, the excretory system and most of the reproductive system of vertebrates. Also *mesoblast.* **extraembryonic m.** The mesoderm that develops outside the embryo and separates the primary yolk sac from the trophoblast. In human embryos, it appears to be derived from trophoblast. It increases in amount and forms the loose magma reticulare. Also *primary mesoderm.* **head m.** Mesoderm situated cranially to the somites. **intermediate m.** A continuous longitudinal tract of mesoderm in the embryo, lying between the paraxial and the lateral plate mesoderm from which the nephrogenic cord will develop. Also *intermediate cell mass, mesomere.* **intraembryonic m.** Mesoderm formed within the boundaries of the early embryo almost entirely from the primitive streak. **lateral plate m.** That part of the intraembryonic, or secondary, mesoderm which develops lateral to the paraxial mesoderm of the embryo. It is continuous with the extraembryonic, or primary, mesoderm beyond the margins of the embryonic disk. Also *lateral mesoderm.* **paraxial m.** The part of the mesoblast forming a thickened mass of tissue at the level of the head region of the embryo in the immediate neighborhood of and at each side of the neural groove. **peristomal m.** Mesoderm that develops from the ventral aspect of the blastoporal lips. **primary m.** EXTRAEMBRYONIC MESODERM. **prochordal m.** The part of the mesoderm derived from division of the cells of the prochordal plate. It plays an inductive role in causing formation of various structures anteriorly in the head and gives rise, probably conjointly with ectomesenchyme, to several facial skeletal elements. **secondary m.** Mesoderm formed from the primitive streak of the embryonic disk which spreads laterally and forward between the ectoderm and underlying endoderm. Secondary mesoderm for the head region is contributed from the prochordal plate and, at least in lower vertebrates, from the cranial end of the neural crest. This type of mesoderm gives rise to connective and supporting tissue, muscle, blood, and lymphatic tissues, part of the urogenital system, and the mesothelium lining the serous cavities. **somatic m.** The outer layer formed as a result of the splitting of the lateral plate mesoderm when the intraembryonic coelom is formed. Together with the overlying ectoderm, it becomes the somatopleure. **splanchnic m.** The inner layer formed as a result of the splitting of the lateral plate mesoderm when the intraembryonic coelom appears. Together with the underlying endoderm, it becomes the splanchnopleure. Also *visceral plate.*

**mesoduodenitis** \-dʸooʹədənīʹtis\ Inflammation of the mesentery of the duodenum.

**mesoduodenum** \-dʸooʹədēʹnəm\ A part of the primitive midline dorsal mesentery in relation to the embryonic duodenum. After the rotation of the gut and the development of the pancreas between the two layers of the mesoduodenum, the latter becomes adherent on its posterior surface to the primitive posterior parietal peritoneum. Later, both layers are absorbed, and so the duodenum becomes retroperitoneal. The suspensory muscle (of Treitz) and its fascia develop in this region, and extend from the right crus of the diaphragm retroperitoneally to the terminal part of the duodenum. Adj. mesoduodenal.

**mesoepididymis** \-epʹididʹimis\ An occasional fold of tunica vaginalis that connects the testis to the epididymis.

**mesoesophagus** \-esäfʹəgəs\ [MESO- + ESOPHAGUS] That part of the primitive dorsal mesentery attached to the esophagus. It persists in the adult only at the lower end near its junction with the stomach below the diaphragm.

**mesogastrium** \-gasʹtrē·əm\ [MESO- + GASTR- + *-ium,* New L noun suffix] That part of the primitive dorsal mesentery which is related to the developing stomach in an embryo and which becomes the greater omentum. Also *mesogaster.* Adj. mesogastric. **dorsal m.** The part of the primitive midline dorsal mesentery which connects the embryonic stomach to the posterior abdominal wall. It is concerned with development of a large sacculation, the omental bursa, or lesser sac of peritoneum, and finally forms the greater omentum. The body of the pancreas and the spleen develop in its thickened portions. **ventral m.** The primitive midline mesentery which in the embryo connects the stomach and the superior part of the loop of the duodenum to the anterior abdominal wall as far as the umbilicus. The liver develops between the two layers of this mesentery and the ligamentum teres. The falciform ligament and the lesser omentum of the adult are derived from it.

**mesoglia** \mesägʹlē·ə\ [MESO- + *(neuro)glia*] Nonastrocytic neuroglia, i.e., oligodendroglia and microglia. *Seldom used.*

**mesogluteal** \-glooʹtē·əl\ Of or relating to the gluteus medius muscle.

**mesognathic** \mezʹənāʹthik\ Having an average jaws-to-head relationship or a gnathic index of between 98 and 103. Also *mesognathous.*

**mesognathion** \mezʹənāʹthē·än\ The lateral segment of the os incisivum, or premaxilla, bearing the lateral incisor. It is located lateral to the medial segment, or endognathion, and considered to derive from a separate center of ossification.

***Mesogonimus heterophyes*** \-gänʹiməs hetʹəräfʹi·ēz\ *HETEROPHYES HETEROPHYES.*

**mesoileum** \-ilʹē·əm\ That portion of the mesentery that attaches the ileum to the posterior abdominal wall.

**mesojejunum** \-jəjooʹnəm\ That portion of the mesentery attaching the jejunum to the posterior abdominal wall.

**mesolecithal** \-lesʹithəl\ [MESO- + LECITH- + -AL] MEDIALECITHAL.

**mesomelia** \-mēʹlyə\ **1** The relative shortening of the middle segment of the limbs. **2** MESOMELIC DWARFISM.

**mesomelic** \-mēʹlik\ [MESO- + MEL-¹ + -IC] Pertaining to the midportion of the upper or lower limb.

**mesomere** \mezʹəmir\ [MESO- + -MERE] **1** INTERMEDIATE MESODERM. **2** SOMITE.

**mesometrium** \-mēʹtrē·əm\ [NA] The portion of the broad ligament below the mesovarium.

**mesomorph** \mezʹəmôrf\ [MESO- + -MORPH] An individual with the characteristics of mesomorphy.

**mesomorphy** \mezʹəmôrʹfē\ [MESOMORPH + -Y] A type of human body conformation with characteristics between those of the ectomorph and the endomorph. In contrast to these the physique is usually muscular and well proportioned. Compare ENDOMORPHY, ECTOMORPHY. Adj. mesomorphic.

**meson** \mēʹzän, mesʹän\ [MES- + *-on,* suffix denoting an elementary particle] Any of several kinds of short-lived elementary particles belonging to the class that takes part in the strong nuclear interaction, and having intrinsic angular momentum (spin) equal to the integral multiple of Planck's constant divided by $2\pi$. They may be positively or negatively charged or neutral. Their masses range from about 275 times the mass of the electron to as much as about 10 times the mass of the proton. Also *mesotron, barytron* (outmoded).

**mesonasal** \-nā′zəl\ Located in or pertaining to the middle of the nose.

**mesonephroi** \-nef′roi\ Plural of MESONEPHROS.

**mesonephros** \-nef′räs\ [MESO- + Gk *nephros* a kidney] The part of renal tissue situated between the pronephros anteriorly and the metanephros posteriorly. It appears just after the first month of embryonic development. It consists of a series of nephrotomes communicating through nephric tubules with the wolffian duct. In mammals the mesonephros is functional for part of the fetal period but eventually it involutes, leaving some vestigial remnants. In the male these remnants include the efferent ductules of the testis while in the female they form tubules of the epoöphoron. Also *wolffian body.* **caudal m.** The caudal part of the mesonephros, which forms the tubules of the paroöphoron. **cranial m.** A part of the mesonephros anterior of the gonad. It atrophies as development advances. **genital m.** That part of the mesonephros which gives rise to the ductuli efferentes and is opposite to the gonad.

**mesopallium** \-pal′ē·əm\ *Obs.* PALEOPALLIUM.

**mesopexy** \mez′əpek′sē\ MESENTERIOPEXY.

**mesopic** \mesō′pik\ Pertaining to vision in the twilight range, between photopic and scotopic.

**mesopneumon** \mez′ən$^y$oo′män\ The visceral pleura that covers the root of the lung proximally, anteriorly, and posteriorly where it becomes continuous with the mediastinal pleura. Also *mesopneumonium.*

**mesoporphyrin** The porphyrin whose ring substituents are: methyl, ethyl, methyl, ethyl, methyl, 2-carboxyethyl, 2-carboxyethyl, methyl. It differs from the protoporphyrin that is found in hemoglobin by hydrogenation of the two vinyl groups to form ethyl groups.

**mesoprosopic** \-prəsō′pik\ Having a face of medium width, the facial index being about 90.

**mesopulmonon** \-pulmō′nän\ [MESO- + PULMON- + -ON] The root of the mesentery for each developing lung, derived from the dorsal thoracic mesentery or mediastinum, The tissue is drawn outwards as the lung grows and forms the visceral pleura.

**mesorchium** \mesôr′kē·əm\ [MES- + *orch(i)-* + L *-ium,* neut. noun suffix] A thick fold of peritoneum which in the male embryo connects the developing testis to the mesonephric fold. It contains the testicular vessels and nerves and some undifferentiated mesenchyme. Also *mesotestis.*

**mesorectum** \-rek′təm\ The peritoneum that almost surrounds the upper portion of the rectum. The middle portion of the rectum has peritoneum on the front and sides, and the lower portion in front only. Also *mesentery of rectum.* ● The term is a misnomer in that the rectum has no mesentery.

**mesoridazine** $C_{21}H_{26}N_2OS_2$. 10-[2-(1-Methyl-2-piperidinyl)ethyl]-2-(methylsulfinyl)-10*H*-phenothiazine. A metabolite of thioridazine that has activity as an antipsychotic agent.

**mesorrhaphy** \mesôr′əfē\ MESENTERIORRHAPHY.

**mesosalpinx** \-sal′pingks\ [NA] The portion of the broad ligament of the uterus that lies above the mesovarium and the ligament of the ovary, and extends to the free border. The uterine tube is located in it.

**mesosigmoid** \-sig′moid\ *Outmoded* MESOCOLON SIGMOIDEUM.

**mesosigmoidopexy** \-sigmoi′dəpek′sē\ A surgical procedure in which the mesocolon of the sigmoid colon is suspended from the abdominal wall in order to prevent sigmoid volvulus or rectal prolapse.

**mesosome** \mez′əsōm\ [MESO- + Gk *sōm(a)* body] A convoluted membranous body formed by involution of the bacterial plasma membrane. It functions in cellular respiration and septum formation.

**mesostenium** \-stē′nē·əm\ *Outmoded* MESENTERIUM.

**mesosyphilis** \-sif′əlis\ SECONDARY SYPHILIS.

**mesotarsal** \-tär′səl\ MIDTARSAL.

**mesotendineum** \-tendin′ē·əm\ A threadlike band of vascular connective tissue covered by synovial membrane that extends between a tendon within its synovial sheath and an osseous groove or adjacent connective tissue structure. It is located at the point of invagination of a tendon into its sheath and is essentially the junction of the visceral and parietal layers. It is homologous to a mesentery and conveys blood vessels and nerve fibers, and it may be quite extensive. Specialized cordlike forms are called vincula tendinum. Also *mesotendon, mesotenon.*

**mesotestis** \-tes′tis\ [MESO- + TESTIS] MESORCHIUM.

**mesothelioma** \-thē′lē·ō′mə\ [*mesotheli(um)* + -OMA] A benign or malignant tumor arising from the mesothelial lining of one of the coelomic cavities, usually the pleura or peritoneum, and consisting of epitheloid and spindle cell elements. It is usually subtyped by predominance as epithelioid, fibrous (spindle cell), or biphasic. Benign mesotheliomas are usually localized. Malignant mesotheliomas grow in a diffuse manner. Epithelioid tumors show tubular and/or papillary growth patterns. The fibrous type may resemble a fibroma or fibrosarcoma. Mesotheliomas associated with exposure to asbestos fibers are invariably malignant. **pleural m.** A mesothelioma arising from the pleura. Localized forms are usually benign. Diffuse growth indicates malignancy but widespread metastases are not common. The tumor may encase the lung. Malignant mesotheliomas of the pleura are associated with exposure to asbestos.

**mesothelium** \-thē′lē·əm\ Epithelial cells of mesodermal origin which come to line the serous cavities such as the peritoneal, pleural, and pericardial cavities, and are also found as the secretory epithelium in the kidney and the mesothelium of the anterior chamber of the eye. Also *celothel, coelothel, celothelium, coelothelium, coelarium, mesepithelium.* See also COELOMIC EPITHELIUM. Adj. mesothelial.

**mesothenar** \-thē′när\ *Outmoded* MUSCULUS ADDUCTOR POLLICIS.

**mesotron** \mez′əträn\ MESON.

**mesotropic** \-träp′ik\ Located toward the median plane of a cavity, as the abdomen.

**mesoturbinal** \-tur′binəl\ CONCHA NASALIS MEDIA.

**mesoturbinate** \-tur′bināt\ CONCHA NASALIS MEDIA.

**mesovarium** \mes′ōver′ē·əm\ [NA] A short, thick, peritoneal fold that attaches the straight mesovarian border of the ovary to the posterior layer of the broad ligament just below its superior border. Between its two layers blood vessels and nerves pass to the hilum of the ovary.

**mesoxalyl urea** ALLOXAN.

**messenger** 1 Designating the RNA that carries the information encoded in a DNA sequence to the site of protein biosynthesis, where it specifies the order of amino-acid residues. 2 The mediator of an effect, e.g. a hormone secreted in one part of an organism and having an effect on distant cells, sometimes operating via a second messenger. **second m.** A substance produced when a hormone acts on a cell and mediating the response of the cell to that hormone. The hormone itself is regarded as the first messenger. An example is cAMP produced in response to epinephrine.

**mestranol** 3-Methoxy-19-nor-17$\alpha$-pregna-1,3,5(10)-triene-20-yne-17$\alpha$-ol. An estradiol derivative used as an estrogenic component in some progestin-estrogenic oral contraceptives.

**mesurpine hydrochloride** $C_{19}H_{26}N_2O_5S\cdot HCl$. 2″-Hydroxy-5′-[1-hydroxy-2-[*p*-methoxyphenethyl)amino]propyl]-methanesulfonanilide monohydrochloride. A compound used as a vasodilator and as a smooth muscle relaxant agent.

**Met** Symbol for methionine.

**met-** \met-\ META-.

**meta-** \met′ə-\ [Gk *meta* (*meth-* as prefix before Gk aspirated vowel) after, among, between, with, by means of, during, back again, over] **1** A prefix meaning changed in form or position, transformed. **2** A prefix meaning after, behind, following. **3** A prefix meaning with, next to. **4** A prefix meaning above, beyond, transcending. For defs. 1–4 also *met-*. **5** A prefix indicating the position of a substituent in benzene as being on C-3 when the numbering is defined in relation to a reference substituent on C-1. Symbol: *m-*

**metabolic** \met′əbäl′ik\ Of or related to metabolism.

**metabolism** \mətab′əlizm\ [Gk *metabolē* (from META- + Gk *bolē* a throw, from *ballein* to throw) a change + -ISM] The totality of the chemical processes occurring in a living organism, especially those associated with the exchange of matter and energy between a cell and its environment. Adj. metabolic. **acid-base m.** The processes influencing the hydrogen ion concentration in the body. **aerobic m.** Metabolic activity that is dependent upon the presence of gaseous oxygen. **basal m.** The state of minimal metabolic activity associated with the maintenance of body function at its normal temperature in the postabsorptive state at mental and physical rest. **endergonic m.** Metabolic activity associated with a positive standard free-energy change. **endogenous m.** **1** The chemical changes associated with the nitrogenous components of the body tissues. **2** The chemical changes associated with the turnover of body tissues as distinct from the turnover of ingested food materials. **exergonic m.** Metabolic activity associated with a negative standard free-energy charge. **exogenous m.** The chemical changes associated with ingested food materials not incorporated as constituents of body tissues. **intermediary m.** The chemical changes associated with the synthesis of cellular components from food materials and their degradation.

**metabolite** \mətab′əlīt\ A substance taking part in or produced by metabolic activity. **essential m.** An indispensable component of a metabolic process. **secondary m.** Any of the compounds produced by many microorganisms under conditions (idiophase) in which foodstuffs are no longer converted into the primary metabolites of growth but are converted into other products, which vary widely in different organisms. The antibiotics are a subclass.

**metabolize** \mətab′əlīz\ [Gk *metabol(ē)* a change, changing + -IZE] To subject to metabolic change.

**metabutethamine hydrochloride** $C_{13}H_{21}ClN_2O_2\cdot HCl$. 2-[(2-Methylpropyl)amino]ethanol 3-aminobenzoate (ester)monohydrochloride. It is used in dentistry as a local anesthetic, producing infiltration and nerve block anesthesia.

**metacarpal** \-kär′pəl\ **1** Pertaining to the metacarpus. **2** Any one of ossa metacarpi I–V.

**metacarpectomy** \-kärpek′təmē\ [*metacarp(al)* + -ECTOMY] The surgical removal of a part or all of one or more metacarpal bones.

**metacarpophalangeal** \-kär′pōfəlan′jē·əl\ Of or relating to the metacarpus and the phalanges.

**metacarpus** \-kär′pəs\ [NA] A series of five cylindrical bones articulating with the carpus proximally and with the proximal phalanges distally. See also OSSA METACARPI I-V.

**metacentric** \-sen′trik\ In cytogenetics, having the centromere near the middle of a chromosome, resulting in nearly equal lengths of the arms. In humans, this is characteristic of chromosomes of groups A and F.

**metacercaria** \-sərker′ē·ə\ [META- + CERCARIA] (*pl.* metacercariae) The encysted stage of a digenetic trematode, which occurs in the tissues or on the surface of its intermediate host, such as a snail, aquatic arthropod, amphibian, or fish, or on vegetation. This stage is the usual infective or transfer stage to the definitive host.

**metachromasia** \-krōmā′zhə\ [New L (from META- + *chroma(t)-* + *-ia,* derivative noun suffix) color change] A phenomenon in which a histologic stain reacts with certain tissue elements, such as sulfated polysaccharides and sialic acid mucins, to give a different color from that of surrounding structures. The color change is normally toward the shorter wavelength of the visual spectrum and is thought to be due to polymerization of dye molecules. Also *metachromia, metachromatism*. Adj. metachromatic.

**metachromatism** \-krō′mətizm\ METACHROMASIA.

**metachromatophil** \-krōmat′əfil\ METACHROMOPHIL.

**metachromia** \-krō′mē·ə\ METACHROMASIA.

**metachromophil** \-krō′məfil\ A cell that contains substances exhibiting metachromasia. Also *metachromophile, metachromatophil.*

**metacoele** \met′əsēl\ [META- + -COELE] The cavity of the metencephalon in the embryo, which eventually contributes to the fourth ventricle.

**metacone** \met′əkōn\ [META- + CONE] The distobuccal cusp of the trigonid; the outer posterior of the mammalian upper molar tooth.

**metaconid** \-kō′nid\ [*metacon(e)* + -ID[2]] The distolingual cusp of the trigonid; the inner anterior cusp of the mammalian lower molar tooth.

**metacortandracin** PREDNISONE.

**metacortandralone** PREDNISOLONE.

**metacryptozoite** \-krip′təzō′īt\ [META- + CRYPTO- + *zo(o)-* + -ITE] A merozoite of the second generation of the exoerythrocytic cycle in the development of malarial parasites in the liver. Also *metacryptomerozoite.*

**metaduodenum** \-d[y]oo′ədē′nəm\ [META- + DUODENUM] That part of the embryonic duodenum which is derived from the midgut. It is the distal part beyond the entry of the papilla.

**metaerythrocytic** \met′ə·irith′rəsit′ik\ EXOERYTHROCYTIC.

**metafemale** \-fē′māl\ Any genetic female possessing one or more extra female sex-determining chromosomes in addition to the normal diploid set of autosomes. The most common example of a human metafemale is the triple-X syndrome associated with a 47,XXX karyotype. Also *superfemale* (outmoded).

**metaglobulin** \-gläb′yəlin\ A derived protein resulting from the partial degradation of albumin, usually due to action of an acid or an alkali (acid or alkali albuminate).

**metagonimiasis** \-gän′imī′əsis\ Infection with trematodes of the genus *Metagonimus.*

***Metagonimus*** \-gän′iməs\ [New L, from META- + Gk *gonimos* fruitful] A genus of heterophyid trematodes that encyst on fish, infecting fish-eating animals, including humans. ***M. yokogawai*** An intestinal heterophyid fluke found in the Far East, the Balkans, and the Near East. It occurs in the small intestine, the smallest trematode infecting man (1 to 2.5 mm in length), transmitted by snails of the genus *Semisulcospira* to various fish, and subsequently to fish-eating mammals and birds, as well as to humans eating raw or undercooked fresh or brackish-water fish. Also *Loxotrema ovatum, Metagonimus ovatus.*

**metagranulocyte** \-gran′yəlōsīt′\ METAMYELOCYTE.

**metainfective** \-infek′tiv\ [META- + INFECTIVE] Occurring as a sequel to infection or during the convalescent stage of an infectious disease: said especially of a fever.

**metakentrin** \-ken′trin\ *Older term* LUTEINIZING HORMONE.

**metal** [L *metallum* a metal, mineral, mine, from Gk *metallon* a mine, quarry] Any of several chemical elements that share, more or less, a group of characteristic properties: they are good conductors of electricity or heat, are malleable, often have a shiny appearance, are generally basic, form oxides, and liberate cations. **Babbitt's m.** An alloy composed of tin, copper, and antimony, used in dental technology. **heavy m.** A metal which is at least five times denser than water. Some heavy metals, such as mercury, copper, lead, and cadmium, are toxic, but the degree of toxicity varies. The toxicity of their cations is often due to their tight binding to essential proteins of the body. **Melotte's m.** An alloy composed of bismuth, lead, and tin, used in dental technology. Also *Newton's alloy.* **noble m.** A metal difficult to oxidize to its salts, and easily produced from them. Examples are gold, silver, and platinum.

**metalloenzyme** \mətal′ō·en′zīm\ Any enzyme which has metal atoms as its prosthetic group, such as the cytochromes ($Fe^{2+}$ or $Fe^{3+}$), cytochrome oxidase ($Cu^{2+}$ or $Cu^{+}$), or alcohol dehydrogenase ($Zn^{2+}$).

**metalloflavodehydrogenase** Any of a class of dehydrogenase enzymes which are active only if a flavin nucleotide, as a coenzyme, and metal ions, as iron or copper, are available.

**metallophil** \mətal′əfil\ A cell or tissue which stains with metallic salts, such as silver salts, generally the reticular cells.

**metallophilic** \mətal′ōfil′ik\ Having an affinity for metallic stains: said of cells or tissues.

**metalloprotein** A protein with a metal ion bound to it. Normally this ion is a bi- or tervalent ion that is chelated by the protein and hence fairly firmly bound. Many enzymes are metalloproteins.

**metallothionein** \mətal′ōthī′ōnē′in\ A cadmium-binding protein originally isolated from equine kidney. Its major distinctive features are the absence of aromatic amino acids, high cysteine content, and a high affinity for certain metals, especially cadmium, zinc, mercury, silver, and tin. It is found in many tissues of both man and animals, having been isolated from kidney, spleen, liver, intestine, heart, brain, lung, and skin.

**metamale** \-māl\ In *Drosophila,* a fly with one X chromosome and 3 sets of autosomes.

**metamere** \met′əmir\ [META- + -MERE] Any one of a series of similarly constructed segments forming the body of an animal. Metameres are seen best in segmented forms such as the annelid earthworm, but they are a feature of all vertebrate embryos. In most terrestrial vertebrates and in man metameric segmentation is obscured. Also *body segment.* See also SOMITE.

**metameric** \-mer′ik\ 1 Pertaining to or characterized by metamerism. 2 Arising from a metamere.

**metamerism** \mətam′ərizm\ [META- + *mer(o)-*[1] + -ISM] The repetition of similar parts or segments in the body of an animal. Also *metameric segmentation.* **cutaneous m.** An area of the skin surface corresponding to a primitive spinal segment or neurotome.

**metamorphopsia** \-môrfäp′sē·ə\ [META- + MORPH- + -OPSIA] Distortion of the visual image, which may be due to physical displacement of the macular portion of the retina, usually by small amounts of subretinal fluid, or which may result from central lesions such as parietal lobe disorders or from intoxication with drugs such as mescaline or lysergic acid. Also *anorthopia, visus defiguratus.*

**metamorphosis** \-môr′fəsis\ [Gk *metamorphōsis* (from *metamorphoun* to transform, from META- + Gk *morphē* form, shape + *-ōsis* -OSIS) a transformation] The transformation of shape or structure: used especially in relation to the forms an organism passes through during its various stages of development from egg to adult, as illustrated, for example, by the life cycle of the holometabolous orders of insects. Adj. metamorphic. **fatty m.** FATTY CHANGE. **retrograde m.** 1 A degenerative change in which cells or tissues seem to revert to an earlier or less differentiated type. 2 Metamorphosis of insects or other life forms which reverses the normal course of development; retromorphosis. For defs 1 and 2 also *retrogressive metamorphosis.*

**metamorphotic** \-môrfät′ik\ Relating to, or characterized by, metamorphosis.

**metamyelocyte** \-mī′əlōsīt′\ An intermediate form in neutrophil maturation, between myelocyte and band neutrophil, that has an indented or "kidney-bean" nucleus with condensed chromatin, no identifiable nucleoli, and neutrophilic cytoplasmic granules. Also *metagranulocyte, juvenile cell.*

**metamyxovirus** \-mik′səvī′rəs\ Any of a subgroup of viruses of the Paramyxoviridae family that includes respiratory syncytial virus and pneumonia virus of mice.

**metanephrogenic** \-nef′rəjen′ik\ Having to do with the formation of the metanephros.

**metanephroi** \-nef′roi\ Plural of METANEPHROS.

**metanephros** \-nef′räs\ [META- + Gk *nephros* a kidney] The tubular system in the embryo, caudal to the mesonephros and developing after it, which gives rise to the definitive kidney of reptiles, birds, and mammals. The metanephros is formed from two parts: from mesenchymatous tissue corresponding to fused nephrotomes of the sacral region, and from an outgrowth of the mesonephric duct called the ureteric bud or diverticulum. Also *definitive kidney, hind-kidney.*

**metanil yellow** An acid dye that is used as a pH indicator, changing from red at a pH of 1.2 to yellow at pH 2.3. Also *metaniline yellow, tropaeolin G.*

**metaphase** \met′əfāz\ The stage of mitosis or meiosis during which the chromosomes are aligned on the equatorial plate.

**metaphosphate** Any of several phosphate species, notionally formed from orthophosphate by loss of water. The highly reactive ion $PO_3^{2-}$, transferred from ATP when it phosphorylates compounds, is monomeric metaphosphate. Trimetaphosphate refers to the cyclic triphosphate ion, $P_3O_9^{3-}$.

**metaphrenon** \-frē′nän\ The dorsum, especially the region associated with the kidneys. *Outmoded.*

**metaphyseal** \-fiz′ē·əl\ Pertaining to the metaphysis. Also *metaphysial.*

**metaphysis** \mətaf′isis\ (*pl.* metaphyses) [NA] The actively growing zone at each end of the diaphysis adjacent to the epiphysial cartilage in a growing long bone. In the adult, with the cessation of growth, the bony metaphysis is indistinguishably fused to the epiphysis and diaphysis.

**metaphysitis** \-fisī′tis\ [*metaphys(is)* + -ITIS] Inflammation, usually with infection, of a metaphysis of a long bone.

**metaplasia** \-plā′zhə\ [META- + -PLASIA] The abnormal transformation from one differentiated, adult tissue form to another type of adult tissue within a given organ. It is an acquired condition, usually representing an adaptative response of tissues to many forms of injury. **agnogenic myeloid m.** Extramedullary hematopoiesis, especially of the spleen, associated with myelofibrosis. It presents insidiously or in the context of one of the myeloproliferative syndromes. The spleen is markedly enlarged and may weigh several pounds. The extramedullary hematopoiesis affects primarily the red pulp with erythroid, myeloid, and megakaryocytic precursors being represented. The liver and, rarely, the lymph nodes also show metaplasia. Also *myeloid metaplasia, primary myeloid metaplasia, nonleukemic myelosis, chronic nonleukemic myelosis.* **apocrine m.** A metaplasia of the epithelium of the breast to apocrine sweat gland epithelium, commonly seen in fibrocystic disease. **intestinal m.** The transformation of gastric mucosa into a glandular epithelium reminiscent of that of the small intestines. It contains goblet and Paneth cells, and is typically seen in chronic atrophic gastritis. **myeloid m.** AGNOGENIC MYELOID METAPLASIA. **primary myeloid m.** AGNOGENIC MYELOID METAPLASIA. **pseudopyloric m.** A histologic variant of atrophic gastritis characterized by replacement of acid and pepsinogen-secreting glands by simple glands of the pyloric type. It does not carry an increased incidence of malignant change. **m. of pulp** A change in the dental pulp to nonspecialized connective tissue incapable of producing dentin. **squamous m.** The transformation of an epithelium, usually mucosal or glandular, to a stratified squamous epithelium. It is a common adaptation to injury such as occurs to the ciliated, columnar, respiratory epithelium under the prolonged effect of cigarette smoking.

**metaplasis** \mətap′ləsis\ [Gk *metaplasis* transformation] The state of completed growth or development.

**metaplastic** \-plas′tik\ Characterized by metaplasia.

**metaplexus** \-plek′səs\ The choroid plexus of the fourth ventricle of the medulla oblongata. *Obs.* Also *metatela.*

**metapneumonic** \met′ənʸoomän′ik\ Subsequent to, or secondary to, pneumonia or pneumococcal infection.

**metapophysis** \-päf′isis\ [MET- + APOPHYSIS] PROCESSUS MAMMILLARIS VERTEBRARUM LUMBALIUM.

**metaprotein** \-prō′tēn\ A protein obtained when an acid or a base acts upon a natural protein. Metaproteins are generally soluble in weak acids or bases but insoluble at a neutral pH.

**metaproterenol sulfate** $C_{22}H_{36}N_2O_{10}S$. A potent $\beta$-adrenergic stimulant with a rapid onset of action and a longer duration than isoproterenol. It is used as a bronchodilator in the treatment of bronchial asthma, bronchitis, and emphysema.

**metapyretic** \-pīret′ik\ POSTFEBRILE.

**metapyrone** METYRAPONE.

**metaraminol** $C_9H_{13}NO_2$. *m*-Hydroxyphenylpropanolamine. A compound with vasopressor activity that is given parenterally to elevate the blood pressure, usually in the form of the bitartrate salt.

**metaraminol bitartrate** $C_{13}H_{19}NO_8$. The bitartrate salt of metaraminol, freely soluble in water. It is a potent sympathomimetic amine that increases the systolic and diastolic pressures. It is used to prevent or treat acute hypotension due to spinal anesthesia, surgical complications, and hemorrhage or brain damage.

**metarhodopsin** \-rōdäp′sin\ An intermediate formed in the retina of the eye as the unstable lumirhodopsin degrades. Metarhodopsin is also unstable and degrades to scotopsin and *trans*-retinene.

**metarteriole** \met′ärtir′ē-ōl\ That part of the terminal arteriole that is surrounded by an additional layer of smooth muscle cells and acts as the final control of blood flow into the capillary bed. Also *central channel* (outmoded), *arteriola precapillaris, junctional capillary, arterial capillary, precapillary, arteriolar capillary, precapillary arteriole.*

**metarubricyte** \-roo′brisīt\ ORTHOCHROMATIC NORMOBLAST.

**metastable** \met′əstābəl\ Denoting a substance that has a negligible rate of breakdown to a specified product, but for which the Gibbs energy change for such breakdown is negative. It is therefore unstable from a thermodynamic viewpoint, but stable kinetically, since there is no facile pathway for the breakdown.

**metastasectomy** \-stəsek′təmē\ [*metastas(is)* + -ECTOMY] The resection of a metastatic lesion, such as a metastasized malignant tumor.

**metastasis** \mətas′təsis\ [Gk (from *methistanai* to change position or location, from *met(a)-* TRANS- + *histanai* to stand, be situated) transfer, removal, migration] (*pl.* metastases) **1** The transfer of a disease from one body site to another: said especially of cancers and infectious diseases. **2** A secondary growth of a malignant tumor at a site separate from the primary from which it was derived. It is usually the result of blood-borne or lymphatic spread, although it may occur through the cerebrospinal fluid circulation or along other channels. The metastasis usually shows histologic features similar to that of the primary growth. Also *metastatic cancer, metastatic tumor.* **3** The process of developing metastases. **cannonball m.** Metastatic cancer in the lung producing a round radiographic image similar in appearance to a cannonball. Also *cotton-ball metastasis.* **cotton-ball m.** CANNONBALL METASTASIS. **implantation m.** A form of metastasis in which the tumor cells are brought to the site by fluid, usually along a serosal surface. **osteoblastic m.** An osseous metastasis in which an increase in bone formation is associated with the tumor cells. It is most typical of carcinoma of the prostate. Also *osteoplastic metastasis.* **osteolytic m.** An osseous metastasis which produces destruction of the invaded bone. **osteoplastic m.** OSTEOBLASTIC METASTASIS. **paradoxical m.** Metastasis in a direction other than that of the expected flow of blood or lymph. It may be due to reflux from obstruction of lymphatics, lymph nodes, or blood vessels. Also *retrograde metastasis.* **retrograde m.** PARADOXICAL METASTASIS.

**metastasize** \mətas′təsīz\ To spread by metastasis.

**metastatic** \-stat′ik\ [Gk *metastatikos* concerning transfer or migration] Pertaining to or resulting from metastasis.

**metasynapsis** \-sinap′sis\ The abnormal end-to-end joining of homologous chromosomes during meiosis. Also *metasyndesis.*

**metasyphilitic** \-sif′ilit′ik\ Pertaining to manifestations associated with syphilis.

**metatarsal** \-tär′səl\ **1** Pertaining to the metatarsus. **2** Any one of the five bones of the metatarsus.

**metatarsalgia** \-tärsal′jə\ Pain in the metatarsal region. It usually arises beneath the metatarsal heads in the transverse plantar arch.

**metatarsectomy** \-tärsek′təmē\ The surgical removal of one or more metatarsal bones.

**metatarsometatarsal** \-tär′sōmet′ətär′səl\ Pertaining to the relationships of the metatarsal bones to each other.

**metatarsophalangeal** \-tär′sōfəlan′jē-əl\ Pertaining to the metatarsal bones and the phalanges of the foot.

**metatarsus** \-tär′səs\ [META- + Gk *tarsos* flat of the foot, the foot] [NA] A series of five cylindrical bones in the distal part of the foot articulating with the tarsus proximally and with the phalanges distally. They lie almost parallel to each other and are numbered from the medial side. Each bone is a miniature long bone with a base, shaft, and head. **m. adductocavus** Talipes varus associated with talipes cavus; talipes with abnormal adduction at the ankle and excessive curvature of the arch. **m. adductovarus** Talipes varus in which the distal foot is rotated in extreme adduction. **m. adductus** A fixed deformity in which the distal foot is bent on the longitudinal axis of the foot as a whole so that the digits to a degree turn inward toward the midsagittal plane of the body. **m. atavicus** An abnormal degree of shortness of the first metatarsal bone. **m. latus** BROAD FOOT. **m. primus varus** An abnormal angulation of the first metatarsal bone toward the sagittal plane of the body. Hallux valgus and bunion formation inevitably result from the malformation. **m. varus** A fixed deformity in which the distal part of the foot is rotated on the longitudinal axis of the foot so that the plantar surfaces of the ball and toes tend to face the sagittal plane of the body.

**metatela** \-tē′lə\ METAPLEXUS.

**metathalamus** \-thal′əməs\ [META- + THALAMUS] [NA] That portion of the thalamus composed of the medial and lateral geniculate bodies.

**metathesis** \mətath′əsis\ The deliberate moving of a pathologic process to a site where it will be less troublesome.

**metathrombin** \-thräm′bən\ A thrombin-antithrombin complex that is formed during clotting and is inactive.

**metatroph** \met′əträf\ HETEROTROPH.

**metatrophic** \-träf′ik\ HETEROTROPHIC.

**metatypical** \-tip′ikəl\ Characterized by tissue that is typical of its site with respect to its component elements, but atypical in the way those elements are arranged: used in reference to tumors. Also *metatypic.*

**metaxalone** $C_{12}H_{15}NO_3$. 5-[(3,5-Dimethylphenoxy)methyl]-2-oxazolidinone. It is used therapeutically as a skeletal muscle relaxant in the treatment of severe musculoskeletal conditions. It is given orally.

**metaxeny** \mətak′sənē\ HETERECISM.

**Metazoa** \-zō′ə\ [META- + Gk *zōa*, pl. of *zōon*, a living being, animal] A subkingdom of the kingdom Animalia comprising all multicellular organisms having specialized cells arranged in tissues and, in the higher forms, into organ systems. The Metazoa include all phyla except those in the subkingdom Protozoa.

**metazoan** \-zō′ən\ (*pl.* metazoa, metazoans) **1** Any member of the Metazoa; any multicellular animal. **2** Of or pertaining to members of the Metazoa.

**metazonal** \-zō′nəl\ Located after or distal to a sclerozone.

**metazoonosis** \-zō′ənō′sis\ [META- + ZOONOSIS] A type of zoonosis requiring both an invertebrate and a vertebrate host stage in the life cycle of the causative organism, as, for example, human helminth infections that involve a snail intermediate host or an insect vector.

**Metchnikoff** [Elie *Metchnikoff*, Russian-born bacteriologist and zoologist active in France, 1845–1916] See under THEORY.

**metecious** \metē′shəs\ HETERECIOUS.

**metencephalic** \met′ensəfal′ik\ Of or pertaining to the metencephalon.

**metencephalon** \met′ensef′əlän\ [*met(a)-* + ENCEPHALON] The more rostral of the two parts that develop from the rhombencephalon in the embryo. It develops into the cerebellum and pons. Also *afterbrain.*

**meteorism** \mē′tē·ərizm\ TYMPANITES.

**meteoropathology** \mē′tē·ərōpəthäl′əjē\ The study of ill effects on the body caused by climatic conditions.

**meteorotropic** \mē′tē·ərōträp′ik\ **1** Affected by meteorologic conditions or events: said especially of certain diseases. **2** Pertaining to meteorotropism.

**meteorotropism** \mē′tē·ərōtrō′pizm\ The innate or involuntary tendency of an organism to be influenced by meteorologic factors.

**meter** [French *mètre* (from Gk *metron* a measure, rule, standard) unit of length equaling one ten-millionth of a quarter of a terrestrial meridian] **1** The SI base unit of length, approximately equal to 39.37 inches, 3.28 feet, or 1.09 yards. The meter is equal to the distance traveled by electromagnetic radiation through a vacuum in 1/299 792 458 second, a measure based on the speed of light. Between 1960 and 1983, the meter was defined as being equal to 1 650 763.73 wavelengths in vacuum of the radiation corresponding to the transition between the levels $2p_{10}$ and $5d_5$ of the krypton-86 atom. Symbol: m • In Great Britain and in international usage, the spelling *metre* is preferred, but in the United States *meter* is the usual spelling. **2** An instrument for measuring. **counting-rate m.** A device that indicates the average rate of arrival of random pulses put out by a radiation detector. The usual readout is by milliammeter, whose reading may be unsteady if the pulse rate is low. **dosage m.** DOSIMETER. **dose-rate m.** In radiology, an instrument which displays the radiation dose rate. **electronic pH m.** A device that determines the pH of a solution by measuring the voltage differences generated at the surface of a pH-responsive electrode. **flicker m.** FLICKER PHOTOMETER. **Geiger-Müller survey m.** A portable instrument used for the detection of radiation, commonly used for radiation protection. The instrument is based on the Geiger-Müller counter principle. **integrating dose m.** Any dose meter that displays the total dose received rather than the dose rate. **peak flow m.** A device for measuring peak expiratory flow. **potential acuity m.** An optical system for measuring the acuity of a cataract patient. It focuses the standard visual-acuity letter chart down to a diameter of 150 nm and beams it through a clear window in the cataract to the retina. **rate m.** Any instrument designed to show or measure the speed of some function or phenomenon, as a radiation detector which continually shows radiation intensity. **sound level m.** An acoustic instrument which measures the very small oscillations of atmospheric air pressure induced by sound producing activity. The result is displayed in dB SPL. See also WEIGHTING NETWORK. **survey m.** A portable device used for the detection and measurement of radiation. **zero-crossing m.** A component of Doppler devices that produces an analog waveform by converting into voltage the number of flow directional changes within an artery.

**-meter** \-mē′tər (1), -mətər (2)\ [Gk *metron* measure, rule, standard] A combining form meaning (1) measure, measurement; (2) instrument for measuring.

**metestrus** \metes′trəs\ The period intermediate between estrus and diestrus in the estrous cycle. Also *metestrum.*

**metformin** $C_4H_{11}N_5$. 1,1-Dimethylbiguanide. It is a structural analogue of phenformin and is also an oral hypoglycemic agent that has been used in the treatment of diabetes.

**meth-** \meth-\ A combining form denoting a relationship to the methyl group, —$CH_3$.

**methacetin** ACETANISIDINE.

**methacholine** The $\beta$-methyl derivative of acetylcholine, usually administered in the form of its chlorine or bromide salt. It is much more stable than acetylcholine and has only muscarinic actions. It has some clinical use in the treatment of paroxysmal tachycarditis. Also *methylacetylcholine, acetyl-β-methylcholine.*

**methacholine bromide** $C_8H_{18}BrNO_2$. A white, crystalline powder with the same pharmacological properties as methacholine chloride. It is very hygroscopic.

**methacholine chloride** $C_8H_{18}ClNO_2$. A colorless, crystalline powder that has been used as a cholinergic drug, particularly for its muscarinic properties on the cardiovascular system. Also *acetyl-β-methylcholine chloride.*

**methacrylate** \methak′rilāt\ METHYL METHACRYLATE.

**methacycline** $C_{22}H_{22}N_2O_8$. 6-Methyleneoxytetracycline. A semisynthetic antibiotic of the tetracycline family of drugs. It is effective against a wide spectrum of bacterial species. It is given orally as the hydrochloride.

**methadone** \meth′ədōn\ $C_{21}H_{27}NO$. 6-Dimethylamino 4,4-diphenyl-3-heptanone. A synthetic narcotic analgesic with morphinelike effects. It is used in opiate withdrawal and as maintenance treatment of heroin addicts, and is a drug of abuse. It is usually given as the hydrochloride.

**methadyl acetate** ACETYLMETHADOL.

**methaemalbumin** *Brit.* METHEMALBUMIN.

**methaemoglobin** *Brit.* METHEMOGLOBIN.

**methallenestril** $C_{18}H_{22}O_3$. β-Ethyl-6-methoxy-χ,χ-dimethyl-2-naphthalenepropionic acid. A synthetic, nonsteroidal estrogenic agent used orally for its estrogenic activity.

**methallibure** $C_7H_{14}N_4S_2$. 1-Methyl-6-(1-methylallyl)-2,5-dithiobiurea. This compound has the ability to activate the anterior pituitary gland and stimulate the production of hormones in swine.

**methamphetamine** $C_{10}H_{15}N$. (*S*)-*N*,α-Dimethylbenzeneethanamine. A sympathomimetic amine that is a structural analogue of amphetamine. It is used as a general central nervous system stimulant.

**methamphetamine hydrochloride** $C_{10}H_{16}ClN$. The hydrochloride salt of methamphetamine, having the same actions and uses as the parent compound.

**methandriol** $C_{20}H_{32}O_2$. 17α-Methyl-5-androstene-3β,17β-diol. A steroid with anabolic activity. It is used therapeutically for this purpose. Also *5,6-dehydroandrosterone.*

**methandrostenolone** Δ′-17α-Methyltesterone. A steroid with strong anabolic and androgenic properties.

**methane** \meth′ān\ $CH_4$. The simplest hydrocarbon, it is a constituent of natural gas. It is sometimes known as marsh gas, because it is formed by anaerobic microorganisms that live in marshes.

**methanol** \meth′ənôl\ $CH_3$—OH. A colorless, inflammable liquid, miscible with water, ethanol, ether, and gasoline. Its freezing point is −97.8°C, and the boiling point is 64.65°C. Once prepared by distillation of wood, it is now obtained synthetically. It is toxic, and can quite often cause damage to the eyes if drunk. It is a general solvent. Also *methyl alcohol, wood alcohol, carbinol* (obs.).

**methantheline bromide** $C_{21}H_{26}BrNO_3$. β-Diethylaminoethyl-9-xanthenecarboxylate bromide. An anticholinergic agent used to supress gastric motility and secretions.

**methapyrilene** $C_{14}H_{19}N_3S$. *N,N*-Dimethyl-*N′*-2-pyridinyl-N′-(2-thienylmethyl)-1,2-ethanediamine, an antihistaminic agent of relatively short duration and moderate potency. It has some sedative activity. It is given orally, and it is also available as the fumarate and hydrochloride salts.

**methapyrilene fumarate** $(C_{14}H_{19}N_3S)_2 \cdot 3C_4H_4O_4$. The fumarate salt of methapyrilene, having the same properties and uses as the parent drug. It is given orally.

**methapyrilene hydrochloride** $C_{14}H_{20}ClN_3S$. *N,N*-Dimethyl-*N′*-2-pyridinyl-*N′*-(2-thienylmethyl)-1,2-ethanediamine hydrochloride. An effective antihistaminic agent, used therapeutically for that purpose. It is given orally or parenterally.

**methaqualone** $C_{16}H_{14}N_2O$. 2-Methyl-3-(2-methylphenyl)-4(3*H*)-quinazolinone. An agent used therapeutically as a sedative and a hypnotic. Chronic use has been reported to lead to psychological and physical dependence.

**metharbital** $C_9H_{14}N_2O_3$. 5,5-Diethyl-1-methyl-2,4,6-(1*H*,3*H*,5*H*)pyridinetrione. A barbiturate employed as an anticonvulsant drug in the treatment of various forms of seizures, as of grand mal, petit mal, or myoclonic seizure. It is given orally.

**methazolamide** $C_5H_8N_4O_3S_2$. *N*-[5-(Aminosulfonyl)-3-methyl-1,3,4-thiadiazol-2(3*H*)-ylidene]-acetamide. A white, crystalline powder used as a carbonic anhydrase inhibitor to reduce intraocular pressure for the treatment of glaucoma. It is given orally.

**MetHb** methemoglobin.

**methdilazine** $C_{18}H_{20}N_2S$. 10-[(1-Methyl-3-pyrrolidinyl)-methyl]-phenothiazine, an antihistaminic agent used to treat pruritus of allergic or nonallergic origin. It is given orally as tablets or a syrup. It is also available as the hydrochloride salt.

**methemalbumin** \met′hēmalbyoo′min\ A complex of plasma albumin with heme, in the Fe(III) state, released from hemoglobin. It occurs in small amounts in plasma when there is intravascular hemolysis.

**metheme** \met′hēm\ Heme that has its iron in the Fe-(III) state.

**methemoglobin** \met·hē′məglō′bin\ [*met(a)-* + HEMOGLOBIN] A derivative of hemoglobin in which the iron component has been oxidized from the Fe(II) to the Fe(III) state. Methemoglobin imparts a brownish color to blood and is unable to transport oxygen. Also *oxidized hemoglobin, ferrihemoglobin.*

**methemoglobinemia** \met′hēməglō′binē′mē·ə\ [METHEMOGLOBIN + -EMIA] The presence of methemoglobin in blood in greater than normal concentration, i.e. greater than 1% of the total hemoglobin pigments. Methemoglobinemia is a cause of cyanosis. **congenital m.** HEREDITARY METHEMOGLOBINEMIA. **enterogenous m.** Methemoglobinemia that results from intestinal absorption of nitrite following reduction of ingested nitrate to nitrite by bacteria of the intestinal tract. Nitrite rapidly oxidizes hemoglobin to methemoglobin. **hereditary m.** A rare type of methemoglobinemia that is life-long in duration and of genetic transmission. The principal manifestation is cyanosis, which may be very slight or quite marked. Most often, hereditary methemoglobinemia is an autosomal recessive disorder due to deficiency of erythrocyte methemoglobin reductase. Autosomal dominant hereditary methemoglobinemia may be due to inheritance of one of several very rare hemoglobinopathies, such as Hb M-Saskatoon, Hb M-Boston, Hb M-Iwate, among others. Also *congenital methemoglobinemia, primary methemoglobinemia.* **secondary m.** Methemoglobinemia that is induced rather than due to an intrinsic abnormality of the erythrocyte or of hemoglobin. **toxic m.** Methemoglobinemia that results from exposure of hemoglobin to drugs or their metabolites or to nitrites. The drugs most commonly responsible are phenacetin, sulfones (especially dapsone), and chemically related substances such as acetanilid and phenazopyridine.

**methemoglobinemic** \met·hē′məglō′binē′mik\ Having methemoglobinemia.

**methemoglobin reductase** An erythrocyte enzyme that converts methemoglobin to hemoglobin while oxidizing NADPH. Also *NADPH diaphorase.*

**methemoglobinuria** \met·hē′məglō′binoo′rē·ə\ HEMOGLOBINURIA. • Hemoglobin in the urine is usually methemoglobin. The distinction is not made in practice, so the term is redundant.

**methenamine** $C_6H_{12}N_4$. Hexamethylenetetramine. A colorless or white crystalline solid that is soluble in water and alcohol and very slightly soluble in ether. Its molecules contain four nitrogen atoms arranged in a tetrahedron and bridged by methylene groups. It is a mild disinfectant, probably because of its slow hydrolysis to formaldehyde, and it was formerly used in treating bacterial infections of the urinary tract. Also *hexamine, acetoform, hexamethylenaminesalicylsulfonic acid.*

**methenamine hippurate** $C_6H_{12}N_4,C_9H_9NO_3$. Hexamethylenetetramine hippurate. A white crystalline powder, soluble in water and alcohol. It has the same antimicrobial action as methenamine, though hippuric acid, a bacteriostatic agent, may contribute to the effect. It is used to treat urinary tract infections. Also *hexamine hippurate.*

**methenamine mandelate** $C_6H_{12}N_4,C_8H_8O_3$. Hexamethylenetetramine mandelate. A white crystalline solid, very soluble in water and alcohol. It is used to treat urinary tract infections. The salt has the same antimicrobial spectrum of activity as methenamine, plus the bacteriostatic contribution of mandelic acid. Also *hexamine mandelate.*

**methestrol** PROMETHESTROL.

**methetoin** $C_{12}H_{14}N_2O_2$. 5-Ethyl-1-methyl-5-phenyl-2,4-imidazoleidinedione. An analogue of phenytoin used as an anticonvulsant agent in the treatment of various forms of epileptic seizures. It is given orally.

**methexenyl** HEXOBARBITAL.

**methicillin sodium** $C_{17}H_{19}N_2NaO_6S$. 6-(2,6-Dimethoxybenzamido)-3,3-dimethyl-7-oxo-4-thia- 1-azabicyclo [3.2.0]-heptane-2-carboxylic acid sodium salt. A semisynthetic antibiotic derived from penicillin. It is used in the treatment of infections due to organisms resistant to penicillin G, due to penicillinase production. It is given intramuscularly or intravenously. Also *dimethoxyphenyl penicillin sodium, sodium methicillin.*

**methimazole** \methim′əzōl\ $C_4H_6N_25$. 1-Methyl-2-mercaptoimidazole, a potent and widely used antithyroid agent, used in the treatment of hyperthyroidism (Graves disease). It acts by interfering with the incorporation of iodine into an organic form, thus inhibiting the biosynthesis of the thyroid hormones.

**methiodal sodium** $CH_2INaO_3S$. Iodomethanesulfonic acid sodium salt. An iodine-containing compound used as a contrast medium to visualize the urinary-tract structures by intravenous urography and retrograde pyelography.

**methionine** $CH_3—S—CH_2—CH_2—CH(NH_3^+)—COO^-$. One of the twenty amino acids that can be incorporated into proteins. It is essential in mammalian diet. It is converted by methionine adenosyltransferase into the sulfonium salt *S*-adenosylmethionine, which is the main biologic donor of methyl groups. Symbol: Met, M **active m.** *Outmoded* *S*-ADENOSYLMETHIONINE.

**methionine adenosyltransferase** The enzyme (EC 2.5.1.6) that converts methionine into *S*-adenosylmethionine using ATP, and forming also orthophosphate and pyrophosphate (diphosphate). This reaction activates methionine for methyl donation.

**methionine sulfoximine** The compound formed by changing the group —S— in methionine into —S(O)(NH)—. It is formed from methionine residues in flour when this is treated with nitrogen trichloride, as was once done to bleach it. The compound is highly toxic.

**methisazone** 2-(1,2-Dihydro-1-methyl-2-oxo-3*H*-indol-3-ylidene)hydrazinecarbothioamide. A synthetic antiviral agent of little clinical use. It has been reported to confer short-term protection against smallpox, but is ineffective once the disease has developed. Also *thiosemicarbazone.*

**methixene hydrochloride** $C_{20}H_{23}N_5HCl{\cdot}H_2O$. 1-Methyl-3-(9*H*-thioxanthen-9-yl-methyl)piperidine hydrochloride. An anticholinergic agent utilized therapeutically in the treatment of gastrointestinal hypermotility and spasm. It is given orally.

**methocarbamol** $C_{11}H_{15}NO_5$. 3-(*o*-Methoxyphenoxy)-1,2-propanediol-1-carbamate. A muscle relaxant agent administered orally, intramuscularly, or intravenously.

# method

**method** [Gk *methodos* (from *met(a)-* after, pursuing + *hodos* a way, road) a way to go after something] A way or manner of performing an action or of accomplishing a result. For terms not found under *method,* see also under *procedure, technique, stain,* and *test.* **Abbott's m.** A technique for the correction of scoliosis in which the patient is placed on a special frame and a plaster body jacket is applied while the patient is undergoing traction. **Abell-Kendall m.** An analytical technique for quantifying total serum cholesterol. The cholesterol and cholesteryl esters are first extracted from the serum and hydrolyzed, thus avoiding interferences from protein and nonspecific chromogens. Acetic anhydride and sulfuric acid are then combined with the serum to obtain the final color reaction. **agar diffusion m.** A method of estimating drug sensitivity or concentration by determining the diameter of the area of growth inhibition around a deposit of the drug on a heavily seeded plate. The method is also used for bioassay of a nutrient required by an auxotrophic test organism. Also *auxanographic method.* **Altmann-Gersh m.** A method of freeze-drying tissue in a vacuum for histologic examination. **aniline-fuchsin-methyl green m.** A staining method for mitochondria utilizing acid fuchsin dissolved in aniline water, followed by a methyl green counterstain. **Ashby m.** A technique for measuring the survival of transfused red cells without using radionuclide labeling. Compatible cells that possess a surface antigen absent from the host's cells are injected into the host. An agglutinating antibody specific for that surface antigen is then added. The proportion of transfused cells present in an aliquot of blood is determined by counting cell agglutinates. Also *differential agglutination method.* **auxanographic m.** AGAR DIFFUSION METHOD. **Bangerter's m.** PLEOPTICS. **Bass m.** A vibratory toothbrushing technique in which an attempt is made to clean the gingival sulcus. The bristles of a soft brush are directed at 45° into the gingival sulcus, and the brush head vibrated with a very small circular movement. **bathophenanthroline m.** An analytical technique for measuring iron in serum. Ferric iron is dissociated from serum proteins, reduced to the ferrous state, and reacted with the disodium salt of bathophenanthroline (4,7-diphenyl-1,10-phenanthroline) sulfonate to yield a red-colored complex which can be measured spectrophotometrically. **Beck's m.** BECK'S GASTROSTOMY. **Bell m.** A vertical toothbrushing technique in which the bristles of a soft multituft brush are swept from the teeth to gums. **Benedict's m.** A method for detecting glucose and other reducing substances in urine, based on the reduction of copper (II) ions to the copper (I) state. **Benedict and Newton m.** Preparation of a protein-free filtrate following precipitation of blood proteins by use of a tungstomolybdic acid reagent. **Bielschowsky's m.** BIELSCHOWSKY STAIN. **Bliss m.** The transformation into probits of the relative frequency of responses obtained in a bioassay. Also

*Bliss transformation.* **Bloch's m. for dopa oxidase** A histochemical method used to demonstrate dopa oxidase activity in cells, usually undertaken to identify melanoblasts. A dark brown pigment localizes the sites where dopa oxidase acts upon the substrate L-dopa. **Bodian m.** A method of staining nerve cells and fibers with silver in paraffin sections. **Born m. of wax plate reconstruction** The construction of a series of wax plates of equal thickness cut out according to the scaled enlargements of serial sections of the part or structure being reconstructed. The plates are placed on top of each other to produce a three-dimensional model of the part or structure. **Brandt-Andrews m.** BRANDT-ANDREWS MANEUVER. **breath alcohol m.** A method for measuring the alcohol concentration in expired alveolar air, as of a motor vehicle operator suspected of being impaired by the influence of alcohol. Various tests are used, but all are based on an equation derived from Henry's law: the weight of alcohol in 2100 mls of expired alveolar air equals the weight of alcohol in one ml of blood. **bromcresol green m.** A dye-binding method for quantification of serum albumin. A bromcresol green solution buffered to pH 4.2 is mixed with the serum sample, and the absorbance change is read at 628 nm. The method may conveniently be automated and is not subject to bilirubin or salicylate interference. It may, however, give erroneously high readings at very low albumin concentrations. **C m.** A chromosome banding technique which stains the centric regions and other constitutive heterochromatic regions of the chromosome. Also *centric heterochromatin method.* **Cajal m.** A histologic technique for demonstrating the presence of astrocytes in nervous tissue that uses gold chloride impregnation. **caliper m.** A method for estimating body fat content by using calipers to measure the skin fold thickness at selected points on the body surface. **Callahan's m.** CHLOROPERCHA METHOD. **Castañeda's m.** A procedure for visualizing rickettsiae and viral inclusion bodies in smears. A thin smear is made in a phosphate buffer, then is stained with methylene blue solution and counterstained with safranine solution. Rickettsiae and inclusion bodies stain pale blue while tissue cells stain red. **Castel m.** **1** A histochemical method to demonstrate arsenic in tissue, which is fixed in formalin containing 2.5% cupric acetate. Arsenic, if present, produces bright green cupric acetoarsenite. **2** A histochemical method to demonstrate the presence of bismuth in frozen sections of formalin-fixed tissue. A positive reaction is the formation of red quinine iodobismuthate. **centric heterochromatin m.** C METHOD. **Charter's m.** A vibratory toothbrushing technique in which the bristles of a hard two-rowed brush are applied at 45° to the long axes of the teeth directed toward the biting surfaces. The head of the brush is rotated in small circles with the bristles forced between the teeth and exerts a massaging action on the gingiva. **Chervin's m.** CHERVIN'S TREATMENT. **chloropercha m.** A method of filling a root canal with gutta percha cones partially dissolved in chloroform. Also *Callahan's method, Johnston's method.* **Clark-Collip m.** A classic reference method, now seldom used, for measuring serum calcium. Calcium is precipitated as calcium oxalate, which is converted to oxalic acid by solution in sulfuric acid. The oxalic acid is measured by titration against potassium permanganate. **Conway m.** A diffusion technique for the measurement of volatile materials or substances that can be converted quantitatively to volatile analytes. The material to be volatized is placed in the outer ring of a sealed chamber; a central chamber contains material that will both trap and quantify or titrate the diffused analyte. The technique was used originally for determination of ammonia and urea nitrogen, and it is still employed for analysis of volatile toxic substances. **Coons fluorescent antibody m.** The use of fluoresence labeling to identify the location of antibody on a slide. An antibody conjugated to a fluorochrome can be used in direct immunofluorescent techniques, in which a labeled antibody reacts with its specific antigen, or in indirect immunofluorescent techniques, in which a fluorochrome-labeled antiglobulin serum attaches to and allows visualization of an unlabeled antibody that has reacted with an antigen in cells or tissues. **Copenhagen m.** A technique of artificial respiration developed in the Danish army. With the patient in prone position, inspiration is produced by extension of the arms and expiration by pressure on the scapulae. Also *Holger Nielsen method.* **copper sulfate m.** Determination of the specific gravity of blood or plasma by observing the rise, fall, or motionless suspension of drops of blood or other assay fluid in a series of copper sulfate solutions having specific gravity increments of 0.004. **coupling m.** A technique used in transmitting ultrasound from the transducer surface into the body without significant loss of ultrasonic energy. Typically a gel fills the space between the transducer and the skin to exclude the film of air that would cause large reflections. **Coutard's m.** A method of roentgentherapy consisting of the administration of small doses of irradiation at intervals over a prolonged time. **Cox modification of Golgi's corrosive sublimate m.** A modern variant of Golgi's method for staining nervous tissue that uses mercuric chloride. **Crane m.** The use of a skin flap to transfer tissue to a distant recipient site, after which the flap is returned to its original location. **Credé's m.** CREDÉ'S MANEUVER. **Credé m. of expressing placenta** Application to the uterus of pressure down into the pelvis while massaging the uterine fundus. **cross-sectional m.** A method of research in psychology which focuses on a given process, such as intelligence or psychomotor coordination. This may be measured in two or more groups of subjects at different stages of development, but at a given time. Contrasts between the groups can then be made and some inferences attempted about the form and development that particular process would have taken if the same individuals could have been followed at intervals over a lifetime. Also *cross-sectional study.* **cyanmethemoglobin m.** Determination of hemoglobin concentration of blood by conversion of all forms of hemoglobin (except sulfhemoglobin) to cyanmethemoglobin and measuring absorbence at 540 nm relative to known standards. **Davenport's alcoholic silver nitrate m.** A silver impregnation technique for the differential staining of nerve cells and nerve fibers. Also *Davenport stain.* **definitive m.** An analytic method whose precision, specificity, and freedom from systematic error have been studied and expressed in an uncertainty statement, which shows the method to be optimally compatible with the goals of the analysis. The midpoint of the overall bounds of error can be taken as the true value. **deletion m.** DELETION MAPPING. **Dick's m.** DICK TEST. **Dickinson m.** A technique to control postpartum hemorrhage. The uterus is lifted superiorly out of the pelvis and compressed against the vertebral column. **differential agglutination m.** ASHBY METHOD. **direct centrifugal flotation m.** A method of concentrating nonoperculated helminth eggs and protozoan cysts by suspending filtered fecal matter in a saturated saline solution, which is then centrifuged. The supernatant is picked up with a bacterial loop or by touching it with a coverslip. This suspension is then examined microscopically for parasites. Also *Lane* *method.* **disk sensitivity m.** The antimicrobial susceptibility test performed with drug-impregnated disks placed on an agar culture medium. **Douglas m.** The spontaneous conversion of a fetal transverse lie to a breech presentation through intrauterine rotation. **Duke's m.** DUKE BLEEDING TIME TEST. **Erlangen m.** A method of radiation therapy consisting of the delivery of a large dose of irradiation through multiple portals at one treatment session. **Esbach's m.** A method for semiquantitative measurement of protein in the urine. It involves precipitation with picric acid, followed by measuring the volume of the precipitate. Although rarely used now, for many years this was one of the useful methods for estimating the degree of proteinuria. **falling-drop m.** A means of determining specific gravity by adding drops of a liquid to cylinders containing solutions of known specific gravity. By observing the specific gravity of the solutions in which the drop falls, remains stationary, or rises, one can infer the specific gravity of the test material, precision being dependent upon the gradations of known specific gravities used. This method is most often used as a rapid means of ascertaining acceptable hemoglobin levels in the blood of prospective blood donors. **Faust's m.** A centrifugal concentration method for detecting helminth eggs or larvae or protozoan cysts, in which zinc sulfate solution (relative density 1.18) is the suspending medium. **Feulgen m.** A histologic technique used to demonstrate the presence of DNA. Mild acid hydrolysis releases aldehyde groups which can then be demonstrated using the periodic acid-Schiff stain. The appearance of a purple color indicates a positive reaction, or the presence of DNA. Also *Feulgen procedure, Feulgen's test.* **Fick's m.** A technique for measuring cardiac output using the Fick principle. **Fiske and Subbarow m.** **1** Determination of acid-soluble phosphorus by heating with nitric and sulfuric acids to denature organic matter, precipitating phosphorus as magnesium ammonium phosphate, reducing precipitate with *p*-aminonaphthylsulfonic acid, and colorimetric comparison with known phosphate standards. **2** Determination of inorganic phosphate by precipitating as ammonium phosphomolybdate, followed by reduction and colorimetric assay as above. **flash m.** A process used for pasteurizing milk in which the temperature of the milk is raised to 74°C for a few seconds and then quickly cooled. In the normal pasteurization procedure a temperature of 60°C is used. However, in the flash method, the length of time of heating is much reduced below the 30 seconds normally used. This leads to less development of a "cooked" flavor. **flotation m.** Any of a number of methods for separating helminth ova and protozoan cysts from other components of feces, based on using a solution of a density (specific gravity usually 1.180) intermediate between that of parasitic ova and cysts, which float, and the remainder of the stool that is heavier and is deposited as sediment following centrifugation or direct flotation. **Folin and Svedberg m.** The determination of blood urea by urease conversion to ammonium carbonate, addition of Nessler's reagent, distillation of ammonia, and colorimetric measurement. **Fones m.** A toothbrushing technique with the teeth in occlusion and the head of the brush describing large circles over the teeth and gums. With the teeth apart smaller circles are used for lingual surfaces and an anteroposterior scrub for the occlusal aspects. Also *Fones technique.* **Fülleborn's m.** A flotation method for detecting parasite eggs in feces that involves grinding 1 gm of stool, mixing it with 20 ml of a saturated solution of salt and, after an hour, placing a coverglass on the surface of the mixture, transferring the adherent liquid and parasitic material directly to a slide for microscopic examination. Also *Hung's method, Wilson's method.* **G m.** GIEMSA METHOD. **Gerota's m.** A technique of injecting lymphatics for anatomical purposes with prussian blue dissolved in chloroform, ether, or alcohol. **Giemsa m.** A method of chromosome banding in which chromosomes are treated with trypsin, which denatures chromosomal protein, and are then stained with Giemsa stain. The chromosomes take the stain in a pattern of dark and light bands (G bands). Also *G method.* **Girard's m.** GIRARD'S TREATMENT. **glucose oxidase m.** A highly specific analytical method for the detection of glucose in which the enzyme glucose oxidase acts on glucose to yield gluconic acid and hydrogen peroxide. The attendant oxygen consumption may be measured directly, or a second peroxidase step may be added to yield a colored end product. **Golgi's m.** A histologic technique for differentiating nervous tissue that uses potassium dichromate followed by silver nitrate impregnation. It is used to demonstrate a selection of neurons and neuroglial cells. **Gomori's m.** **1** A histologic silver impregnation technique for reticulin fibers. **2** An aldehyde fuchsin method for distinguishing elastic fibers. **3** Any of several histochemical techniques for identifying acid and alkaline phosphatase. For defs. 1, 2, and 3 also *Gomori stain.* **Gordon and Sweet m.** A histologic silver impregnation technique for the demonstration of reticulin fibers. **Graff m.** INDOPHENOL TEST. **Gram's m.** GRAM STAIN. **Greenwood-Yule m.** A statistical technique to test whether the occurrence of a disease or abnormality is dependent on birth order. The procedure is not subject to bias due to associations between risk and sibship size and is therefore less subject to disturbance from factors influencing the latter. It has the disadvantage that sibships must be complete before the analysis can be undertaken. **Habel's m.** A test for potency of rabies vaccines made from inactivated rabies virus, in which lethality of a standard virus preparation is compared in vaccinated and nonvaccinated mice. **Hamilton's m.** A technique to control postpartum hemorrhage. One hand maintains pressure on the uterine fundus while the other hand is placed as a fist in the vagina. **Handley's m.** HANDLEY'S LYMPHANGIOPLASTY. **Hartel's m.** A technique of injecting the gasserian ganglion which involves approaching the foramen ovale from inside the mouth. **hematoxylin-safranin m.** A double stain that uses the metachromatic property of safranin to demonstrate the presence of mucin and cartilage. **Heublein m.** A method of whole-body irradiation using low doses for many hours each day for several days. **hexokinase m.** An analytical method for detecting the presence of glucose in which the enzyme hexokinase acts on glucose and ATP to yield glucose 6-phosphate and ADP. A second enzyme, glucose-6-phosphate dehydrogenase, converts the glucose 6-phosphate and NADP to 6-phosphogluconate and NADPH, which can be measured spectrophotometrically. **Hirschfeld's m.** A vibratory toothbrushing technique with the bristles approximately at right angles to the teeth. For the inner aspects of the dental arches, the brush is held as nearly vertical as possible. **Holger Nielsen m.** COPENHAGEN METHOD. **horizontal scrub m.** A toothbrushing technique in which the teeth and gums are brushed with short horizontal strokes. **Hortega m.** A histologic technique that uses silver carbonate impregnation of nervous tissue to demonstrate the presence of glial cells. **Hotchkiss m.** SCHIFF'S TEST. **Howard's m.** An artificial respiration technique in which the patient is prone with the head lower than the abdomen and the hands under the head. Respiration is effected by pressure applied to both sides of the thoracic cage. **Hung's m.** FÜLLEBORN'S METHOD. **Hunt's m.** A bioassay using mice that was developed to measure the activity of thyroid preparations, based upon the reduction in toxicity of a test dose of acetonitrile after a 10-day administration of the test material (thyroid preparation). **impedance m.** The use of electrical impedance measurements for localizing brain structures. **India ink m.** A method for visualizing spirochetes and yeasts or other fungi. A smear is made using a loopful of the material to be examined with a loopful of India ink. The organisms appear white against a black background. Also *India ink stain, negative stain.* **indirect m.** A method of making a gold inlay or other gold casting by first taking an impression of the prepared tooth and making a die from it. A wax pattern is built up on the die, and after removal from the die it is invested, heated and cast in gold. It is returned to the die for finishing and polishing and is then ready to be cemented to the prepared tooth. **introspective m.** A technique of psychological experimentation making use of systematic self-observation. The subject gives a verbal report on all conscious experience or feelings that may be related to a stimulus situation, usually without any attempt at discovering meaning or interpretation but only to provide an objective report on the contents, elements, or processes of consciousness. **Italian m.** ITALIAN RHINOPLASTY. **Ivy's m.** IVY BLEEDING TIME TEST. **Japanese m.** A technique to improve adherence of tissue sections to glass slides by using Mayer's albumin. **Johnston's m.** CHLOROPERCHA METHOD. **Karr's m.** Determination of urea in blood by enzymatic conversion to ammonium carbonate, treatment with Nessler's reagent, and colorimetric comparison with known standards similarly prepared. **Kenny's m.** A poliomyelitis rehabilitation technique extensively used in the early twentieth century. Hot wet packs and passive range-of-motion exercises and muscle reeducation are utilized in the acute stage of the disease. **Kety-Schmidt m.** A method of measuring cerebral blood flow using inhalation of nitrous oxide. **Kittrich m.** A straining method for detecting epidermal cells of fetal origin in amniotic fluid discharged per vaginam. They stain red after application of dilute Nile blue sulfate. **Kjeldahl's m.** KJELDAHL'S TEST. **Korotkoff's m.** The determination of blood pressure using auscultation. See also KOROTKOFF SOUNDS. **Kristeller's m.** KRISTELLER'S MANEUVER **Lamaze m.** A technique utilized by women in labor in which concentration is shifted from the discomfort of uterine contractions to relaxing maneuvers in order to reduce or eliminate the need for analgesia. In addition, the method requires antenatal practice of exercises and provides detailed information about labor and delivery so that couples are fully prepared for childbirth. **Lane m.** DIRECT CENTRIFUGAL FLOTATION METHOD. **Langendorff's m.** LANGENDORFF PREPARATION. **lateral condensation m.** A method of filling a root canal with a number of gutta percha cones one after the other, space being made for each addition by spreading the others apart with a special instrument called a root canal spreader. Also *multiple cone method.* **m. of least squares** A statistical procedure involving the substitution of some function of the variable from each observed value such that the sum of the squares of the differences between the pairs of observed and calculated values is a minimum. The technique is used for calculating a line of best fit in linear regression. **Leboyer m.** A method of conducting labor and delivery in which the newborn is handled as gently as possible by avoiding obstetric forceps, not using bright lights, and by placing the infant in a warm bath immediately after delivery. **Letonoff and Reinhold m.** A colorimetric method for determination of inorganic sulfate in serum after deproteinization, precipitation and redissolution. **Levaditi's m.** A histologic staining method for detecting spirochetes in which a block of tissue is impregnated with silver nitrate and sectioned after reducing the silver with pyrogallol. **Levy, Rowntree, and Marriott m.** Determination of the hydrogen ion concentration of blood by dialysis against physiologic saline, addition of phenolsulfonphthalein to the dialysate, and colorimetric comparison with known standards. **Lewisohn's m.** A technique of treating blood with sodium citrate, thereby making indirect transfusion possible. **Lindemann's m.** An obsolete but historical technique of direct blood transfusion utilizing a system of cannula and syringe connecting the venous circulations of the donor and recipient. **Ling's m.** SWEDISH GYMNASTICS. **Linser's m.** The injection of mercuric chloride into varicose veins to obliterate the varices. *Obs.* **Lister's m.** LISTERISM. **longitudinal m.** A method of research in psychology which studies the same individual, or group of individuals, over a considerable period of time, making periodic measurements of a given process at critical stages of developmental change or over the entire life span. Also *longitudinal study.* **Looney and Dyer m. for potassium in blood** A colorimetric method for determination of serum potassium after deproteinization, precipitation as a metallic nitrite complex, and redissolution. **Lorenz m.** A manipulation technique for the reduction of a congenitally dislocated hip. **Løvset's m.** LØVSET'S MANEUVER. **macro-Kjeldahl m.** KJELDAHL'S TEST. **Majorström m.** The use of a vacuum extractor, a suction device applied to the fetal head, to effect vaginal delivery of an infant. **Malloy-Evelyn m.** A diazo reaction used to measure bilirubin. Conjugated bilirubin reacts directly with diazotized sulfanilic acid, forming purple azobilirubin. The addition of methanol to the specimen allows unconjugated bilirubin to react. **Manchester m.** A method of repairing a bilateral congenital cleft lip. **Mann's m.** A histologic staining technique that uses a mixture of methyl blue and eosin to distinguish nerve cells, Negri bodies, and amebas. Also *Mann stain.* **Mantel-Haenszel m.** A method of statistical analysis of data from case-control studies to estimate the odds ratio and its standard error both when matched pairs are compared and when there is more than one matched control per case. ⟨Mantel, M. and Haenszel, W. *Journal of the National Cancer Institute* 22:719, 1959⟩ **Marchi's m.** A histologic technique that uses osmium tetroxide and potassium chlorate to differentiate normal from degenerating myelin. **Marfan's m.** The technique of aspirating a pericardial effusion by epigastric puncture. **Masson's trichrome m.** MASSON'S TRICHROME STAIN. **Maximow's m.** HEMATOXYLIN-EOSIN-AZURE II STAIN. **micro-Astrup m.** A technique to determine partial pressure of carbon dioxide ($P_{CO_2}$) in the blood by extrapolation from pH measurements. The measured pH of the specimen is plotted on a line constructed from the pH values determined on reference specimens of known $P_{CO_2}$. **micro-Kjeldahl m.** A modification of Kjeldahl's test that is designed to measure quantities of protein nitrogen in the range of a few milligrams. **Millard m.** A method of repairing a bilateral congenital cleft lip. Also *Millard operation.* **Minkowski's m.** A technique of kidney palpation following gas dilatation of the colon. Also *Naunyn-Minkowski method.* **multiple cone m.** LATERAL CONDENSATION METHOD. **Murphy m.** An obsolete method of vascular suture in which the vessel ends are invaginated over a small metal tube. **Myers m.** Estimation of the urea concentration of blood by conversion of urea to ammonium carbonate through the action of uricase. Ammonium is converted to ammonia, which is collected and measured by reaction with Nessler's reagent. **Naunyn-Minkowski m.** MINKOWSKI'S METHOD. **Nègre and Bretey m.** BCG vaccination by means of cutaneous scarifications, the number and dimension of which vary with the age of the subject. **nigrosin m.** The use of the dye nigrosin as a negative stain to delineate microorganisms in a smear of unstained material, especially spirochetes or diphtheria bacilli. Organisms appear clear against a black background. **Nimeh's m.** A radiological technique of evaluating liver and spleen size by appropriate flat plates of the abdomen with or without carbon dioxide gas insufflation of the retroperitoneal space. **Nissl's m.** A histologic technique that demonstrates the presence of aggregated RNA or Nissl granules in the cytoplasm of neurons. **no-touch m.** 1 A technique used in cancer surgery for excision of a tumor whereby the blood and lymph supply is divided before the tumor itself is touched. This method is said to decrease the likelihood of disseminating tumor cells. 2 In a surgical procedure or in the treatment of wounds, a method of cleaning and dressing without the introduction of the sterile gloved hand or fingers into the wound or incision, all manipulation being performed by the use of sterile instruments. **nutritional table m.** The calculation of food intake using food composition tables. **Ogino-Knaus m.** A modification of the rhythm birth control method. **Ombrédanne m.** A method of correcting hypospadias by reconstructing the urethra with a long rectangular turnover flap based at the receded urethral meatus. The resultant skin defect on the ventral shaft of the penis is then covered with another turnover flap fashioned from the prepuce. This second turnover flap must have a small slit incised in its center to accommodate the glans. **Orr m.** ORR TREATMENT. **ovulation m.** A method of contraception in which intercourse is avoided during the fertile midmenstrual cycle time period, which is identified by monitoring changes in the cervical or vaginal mucus. **Pachon's m.** An oscillometric method for assessing the patency of arteries. *Obs.* **Paracelsian m.** The treatment of diseases only by chemicals. **parallax m.** A radiologic method of localization, as of a radiopaque foreign structure within the body, by measuring the shift in position of the structure caused by a predetermined shift in the position of the x-ray tube. **Pavlov's m.** The technique for studying conditioned reflex activity by measuring gastric or salivary secretion in awake dogs. **Payr's m.** An archaic method of vascular anastomosis that uses absorbable magnesium cylinders. **Perdrau's m.** A silver impregnation technique for the demonstration of reticulin fibers in tissue. **point source m.** A method of radiation therapy to the wall of the urinary bladder, consisting of a point source of radiation at the center of a Foley catheter bag, which is then distended with a solution, such as water, saline, or contrast medium. **Price-Jones m.** Determination of the distribution of erythrocyte diameters in a blood specimen. **probit m.** A statistical method of displaying the distribution of responses in biological assays that is based upon normal equivalent deviation units. The resulting plot of cumulative probability units versus the logarithm of the dose can be used to calculate the $ED_{50}$ value and the dispersion of the population about the mean. **projective m.** A psychological assessment technique utilizing unstructured tests that give minimal clues as to the appropriate responses and thus elicit interpretations based on the subject's needs, impulses, defenses, and drives. The Rorschach inkblot test and the ambiguous pictures of the thematic apperception test are examples of the use of the projective method. **Pryce slide-culture m.** A microculture technique to demonstrate *Mycobacterium tuberculosis.* The material is placed on a slide, dried, treated with acid, then washed and incubated with hemolyzed blood for seven days. It is then examined directly for the presence of acid-fast bacilli. **psychometric m.** The application of standardized tests for measuring one or more aspects of the mental ability of an individual, such as intelligence, aptitudes, interests, or personality characteristics. **psychophysical m.** Any of several standard procedures devised for investigating the relation between systematic variations in physical energies and the experience reported, or behavior evoked, in an experimental subject. **pulse reflection m.** PULSE ECHO TECHNIQUE. **Purmann's m.** A method of obliterating an aneurysmal sac. **quinacrine fluorescent m.** A chromosome banding technique in which chromosomes are treated with quinacrine mustard compounds which produce fluorescent bands, or Q bands, across the chromosomes. Also *Q method.* **R m.** REVERSE GIEMSA METHOD. **radioactive balloon m.** A method of radiation therapy applied to the wall of the urinary bladder, consisting of the intravesical placement of a Foley catheter, the bag of which is then filled with a radioactive solution or suspension. **recall m.** A method employed in the quantitative study of memory: the number of items learned, to an agreed-upon criterion of mastery, that can be successfully reproduced following an elapsed interval of time provides a measure of the degree of retention. **recognition m.** A method employed in the quantitative study of memory: the subject is required to select those items to which he has been previously exposed in the experiment from among several other items to which he has not been exposed. **Reed and Muench m.** A method for determining the median lethal dose by interpolation. **reference m.** An analytic technique that is used as a standard against which other measurement procedures are compared or that is used to define reference materials that can be used to standardize other procedures. It is highly accurate but usually is too tedious or demanding for routine analysis. **Regaud m.** A radiotherapy technique for cancer of the cervix, using intracavitary irradiation by probe and irradiation of the parametria by colpostat. **Reichert's m.** The crystallization of oxyhemoglobin in ammonium oxalate. **retrofilling m.** A method of filling the apical part of a root canal or its equivalent after apicoectomy from the apical end, usually with dental amalgam. **Reverdin's m.** REVERDIN GRAFT. **reverse Giemsa m.** A chromosome banding technique in which the chromosomes are pretreated with heat followed by Giemsa staining. The resulting dark and light bands (R bands) are the reverse of the G and Q bands. Also *R method.* **rhythm m.** A means of contraception by avoiding sexual intercourse just prior to and after ovulation in the middle of the menstrual cycle. Also *rhythm contraception, periodic abstinence.* **Ritchie's formol-ether m.** A method for detecting parasitic cysts and ova in fecal material. The specimen is fixed in formol-saline solution and extracted with ether. The washed residue is then examined microscopically. **Ritgen's m.** RITGEN MANEUVER. **roll m.** A toothbrushing technique in which the bristles are placed on the gums and swept toward the biting surfaces of the teeth by rotation of the toothbrush. **Roughton-Scholander m.** SYRINGE-CAPILLARY METHOD. **savings m.** A method used for the quantitative study of memory. A body of material is first learned, then an interval is allowed to elapse that is sufficient to assure partial or complete forgetting, followed by an opportunity to relearn the same material. The difference between the time, or the number of trials, needed to achieve the same degree of mastery provides an index of the amount of the original material that has been retained. Also *relearning*. **Sayre's m.** SAYRE'S OPERATION. **sectional m.** SEGMENTATION METHOD. **segmentation m.** A method of filling a root canal with gutta percha cones in stages, with a short segment starting at the apex. Also *sectional method*. **Sippy m.** See under SIPPY DIET. **Skoog's m.** A method of repairing a bilateral congenital cleft lip. Also *Skoog's operation*. **Sluder's m.** **1** Treatment of sphenopalatine neuralgia by injecting the ganglion, via the sphenopalatine foramen, with local anesthetic. **2** A method of guillotine enucleation of the tonsils used in the early part of the 20th century. *Obs*. **Smellie's m.** A technique of delivering the aftercoming head in a breech presentation by resting the baby's trunk on the obstetrician's forearm. **Somogyi m.** **1** A copper reduction method for demonstrating the presence of glucose and other reducing sugars in body fluids. **2** A saccharogenic method for measuring serum amylase. A copper reduction test is applied to the reducing substances released from starch by action of the amylase. **split cast m.** SPLIT CAST MOUNTING. **Staffieri's m.** An operation to create a phonatory neoglottis to enable the patient to speak after total laryngectomy. A low tracheostome is established and the larynx is removed so as to conserve several tracheal rings above this level. A fistulous opening into the hypopharynx is created just above the laryngeal stump and the hypopharyngeal musculature surrounding the fistula is sutured to the top of the trachea so that the fistula becomes the neoglottis. **Stillman's m.** A vibratory toothbrushing technique with the bristles at a 45° angle to the long axis of the teeth, directed toward the apices. A modified version of the method adds a vertical sweep toward the biting surfaces at the end of each vibratory phase. **Stoll's m.** A method for quantifying helminth ova in feces, calculated by counting the eggs in a known volume of feces diluted and suspended in 0.1 normal solution of sodium hydroxide and then multiplying to determine the number present per gram of feces. A correction factor is used to relate fecal consistency to weight. **m. of successive approximations** SHAPING. **suction m.** A gynecologic procedure in which the uterine contents are removed by aspiration through a cannula, using a device to produce negative pressure. Most commonly the procedure is used to carry out abortion during the first one-third of pregnancy. **suspension m.** A method of radiation therapy to the wall of the urinary bladder, consisting of the instillation of a radioactive solution or suspension into the vesical lumen, usually via a urethral catheter. **symptothermal m.** A method of contraception in which intercourse is avoided during the fertile midmenstrual cycle time period, which is identified by monitoring changes in the cervical or vaginal mucus and symptoms suggesting ovulation, including a plot of basal body temperatures. **syringe-capillary m.** A micromethod for measurement of the volume of gases in blood, in which a graduated capillary tube serves as the manometer. Also *Roughton-Scholander method*. **Thane's m.** The locating of the upper end of the central sulcus of the brain by finding the midpoint of a line that is drawn between the glabella and the inion. **thick-film m.** An examination of several drops of hemolyzed blood (fixed in methyl alcohol and stained in Giemsa's or other Romanowski-type blood stains) for the gross detection of intraerythrocytic parasites, as the malarial parasites. Species diagnosis is based on a subsequent study of a standard thin blood smear, which can conveniently be placed on the same slide. **turbidity m.** The demonstration of the presence of protein in a body fluid by precipitating the fluid with sulfosalicylic acid or other additives. **urease m.** Any of several methods for measuring urea that is based on the quantity of ammonia produced following hydrolysis of urea by urease. **Van Slyke and Neill m.** The measurement of the volume of oxygen or other gases in blood or other fluids by use of a manometer. **Wade's m.** A method of detecting *Mycobacterium leprae*. A small sample of tissue pulp and lymph from a leprosy lesion are obtained by pinching a fold of skin, inserting a scalpel, and rotating the blade to scrape the sides of the incision. The sample is stained with carbolfuchsin and examined for the presence of *M. leprae*. **Wade-Fite m.** A staining method to demonstrate acid-fast bacilli in paraffin tissue sections which are dewaxed in rectified turpentine and heavy paraffin oil, stained with carbolfuchsin, decolorized in sulfuric acid, and stained with picric acid and acid fuchsin. Acid-fast organisms appear dark blue to blue-black. **Wade-Fite-Faraco m.** A staining method to demonstrate acid-fast bacilli in paraffin tissue sections after the sections are dewaxed with a mixture of paraffin oil and rectified turpentine or paraffin oil and aviation gasoline. They are then stained with carbolfuchsin, decolorized with hydrochloride and ethanol, and counterstained with methylene blue. The acid-fast organisms appear red against a light blue background. **Walgren's m.** Intradermal vaccination with bacille Calmette-Guérin. **Wardill four-flap m.** A method of closing a cleft palate using four mucoperiosteal flaps. **Wardill two-flap m.** A method of closing clefts of the palate utilizing two mucoperiosteal flaps. This procedure is used if the defect involves less than half of the hard palate. **Weed-McKibben m.** Treatment of increased intracranial pressure by the parenteral injection or oral ingestion of hypertonic solutions such as sucrose or magnesium sulfate. **Weigert-Pal m.** A modification of Weigert's myelin sheath stain that is particularly useful for demonstrating large areas of demyelination within the nervous system. An oxalic acid-potassium sulfite mixture is used for differentiation. Also *Weigert-Pal technique*. **Weil-Hallé m.** Subcutaneous vaccination with bacille Calmette-Guérin in which half of the 0.05 mg dose is injected into the loose skin under each armpit. The vaccination usually gives rise to a cutaneous reaction within one to two months. **Welcker's m.** A measurement of purines, in which phosphates are first removed with magnesium oxides, then the purine bases are precipitated with ammonium hydroxide and silver nitrate, and then the nitrogen content of the precipitate is determined by the Kjeldahl method. **Westergren m.** A procedure for measurement of erythrocyte sedimentation rate that employs a column 20 cm long, with 2 mm internal diameter, graduated in millimeters. Anticoagulated blood is introduced into this "Westergren tube," which is then supported in a vertical position, and at one hour, the number of millimeters between the upper level of plasma and the upper level of erythrocytes is recorded. The normal erythrocyte sedimentation rate for men is 0–15 mm/hr, for women 0–20 mm/hr. **Wilson's m.** **1** A technique used in experimental teratology to diagnose soft tissue and other internal malformations in fetal and newborn laboratory animals. A fixed specimen is cut transversely into 1 mm sections with a razor blade and examined with a dissecting microscope. **2** FÜLLEBORN'S METHOD. **Wintrobe m.** The determination of hematocrit, using a glass tube, called a Wintrobe tube, with $2.5 \times 115$ nm bore. The tube is calibrated from 0 to 100 nm. **Wintrobe and**

**Landsberg m.** The determination of erythrocyte sedimentation rate by measurement of sedimentation at one hour and correction for hematocrit value by a standard table. **Wynn m.** A method of repairing a cleft lip by lengthening the prolabium on the side of the cleft by means of a superiorly based triangular transposition flap taken from a segment of the lateral part of the lip.

**methodology** \meth′ədäl′əjē\ The methods used in a particular field.

**methohexital** A methyl-substituted barbiturate used for intravenous induction of general anesthesia characterized by rapid onset and recovery.

**methohexital sodium** $C_{14}H_{17}N_2NaO_3$. 5-Allyl-1-methyl-5-(1-methyl-2-pentynyl)barbituric acid sodium salt. A very short-acting barbiturate used intravenously to produce anesthesia of short duration or for induction of general anesthesia. It is used like sodium thiopental.

**methopromazine** METHOXYPROMAZINE.

**methotrexate** $C_{20}H_{22}N_8O_5$. 4-Amino-10-methylfolic acid. A very potent folic acid antagonist which has been used as a cytotoxic drug in the treatment of neoplastic diseases and as an immunosuppressant agent. Also *amethopterin.*

**methotrimeprazine** 10-(3-Dimethylamino-2-methyl-propyl)2-methoxyphenothiazine. A phenothiazine with potent analgesic properties. It is used as an analgesic for severe pain, for obstetric analgesic effects without respiratory depression, and as a preanesthetic medication.

**methoxamine hydrochloride** $C_{11}H_{17}NO_3{\cdot}HCl$. $\alpha$-(1-Aminoethyl)-2,5-dimethoxybenzoyl alcohol hydrochloride. A white crystalline compound, used as an adrenergic vasopressor in hypotensive states and to end attacks of paroxysmal atrial tachycardia.

**methoxsalen** $C_{12}H_8O_4$. 9-Methoxy-7*H*-furo[3,2-*g*][1]benzopyran-7-one. A psoralen compound occurring in the plant, *Amni majus.* This agent may be used in association with ultraviolet light exposure to enhance repigmentation after idiopathic vitiligo. It is also used to precipitate a phototoxic response in treatment of psoriasis. It has the capacity to accelerate suntan and functions as a sun screen. It is used both topically and orally. Also *xanthotoxin, 8-methoxypsoralen.*

**methoxy-** \meth′äksē-\ A combining form indicating the presence of a methoxyl radical ($CH_3$—O—) in a molecule.

**methoxy acetanilide** ACETANISIDINE.

**methoxychlor** $Cl_3CCH(C_6H_4OCH_3)_2$. 2,2-bis(*p*-Methoxyphenyl)-1,1,1-trichloroethane. An insecticide that is used to control mosquito larvae and flies.

**methoxyindoles** Indoles containing a methoxy group of the class of melatonin, the secretory product of the pineal, having in experimental animals actions on sodium balance, light-dark adaptation, dermal melanin pigmentation and possibly upon gonadotropin release by the adenohypophysis. Their physiologic role and their importance in man are not known.

**methoxyl** The univalent group $CH_3$—O—.

**methoxyphenamine** $C_{11}H_{17}NO{\cdot}HCl$. 2-Methoxy-*N*,$\alpha$-dimethylbenzeneethanamine hydrochloride. An adrenergic agent with actions pharmacologically as a bronchodilator. It is used chiefly in the treatment of bronchial asthma and given orally.

**methoxypromazine** $C_{18}H_{22}N_2OS$. 2-Methoxy-*N,N*-dimethyl-10*H*-phenothiazine-10-propanamine. A phenothiazine with actions typical of that class of compounds. It is usually used clinically as the maleate salt as a tranquilizer. Also *methopromazine.*

**8-methoxypsoralen** METHOXSALEN.

**methscopolamine bromide** $C_{18}H_{24}BrNO_4$. 6$\beta$-7$\beta$-Epoxy-3$\alpha$-hydroxy-8-methyl-1$\alpha$*H*,5$\alpha$*H*-tropanium tropate (ester). A quaternary derivative of scopolamine with anticholinergic actions like scopolamine but absorbed less rapidly and having less effect on the central nervous system. It is used for gastrointestinal spasm and as a preoperative medication. Also *hyoscine methobromide, epoxymethamine bromide.*

**methsuximide** $C_{12}H_{13}NO_2$. 1,3-Dimethyl-3-phenyl-2,5-pyrrolidinedione. An anticonvulsant agent employed therapeutically in the treatment of psychomotor and petit mal epilepsy. It is given orally.

**methyclothiazide** $C_9H_{11}Cl_2N_3O_4S_2$. 6-Chloro-3-(chloromethyl)-3,4-dihydro-2-methyl-2*H*-1,2,4-benzothiadiazine-7-sulfonamide 1,1-dioxide. A thiazide antihypertensive, diuretic agent. It is employed in the treatment of edema secondary to congestive heart failure, chronic renal disease, pregnancy, premenstrual syndrome, cirrhosis, and obesity and in steroid therapy. It is given orally for edema and hypertension.

**methyl** \meth′əl\ The univalent group $CH_3$-. **angular m.** A methyl group attached to the atom that forms the junction between two rings in a molecule. There are two such groups in cholesterol.

**methyl-** \meth′əl-\ [English *methyl,* back formation from French *methyl(ène)* methylene, from Gk *meth(y)* wine + *(h)yl(ē)* wood, matter + *-ēnē,* fem. patronymic suffix] A combining form denoting the presence of the methyl (—$CH_3$) group in a chemical compound.

**methylacetylcholine** METHACHOLINE.

**methylal** $CH_2(OCH_3)_2$. Dimethoxymethane. A colorless liquid used as an anesthetic and hypnotic drug. It is also used as a reagent in some organic syntheses and as an ingredient in perfumes.

**methyl alcohol** METHANOL.

**methylaspartate ammonia-lyase** An enzyme (EC 4.3.1.2) which catalyzes the removal of ammonia from 3-methylaspartate with the formation of a double bond. The reaction is a step in the fermentation of glutamate by some bacteria.

**methylated** \meth′əlā′tid\ Containing the methyl group or having it attached.

**methylation** \meth′əlā′shən\ The reaction of introducing a methyl group into a substance, either in replacement of a hydrogen atom or with gain of a positive charge. Hydroxyl groups of sugars are methylated, often with methyl sulfate, in determining which are free and which masked by ring formation or intersugar bonds. In living beings methylation is usually by transmethylation from the $CH_3$—$S^+R_1R_2$ group of *S*-adenosylmethionine. Methylation determines the susceptibility of certain nucleotide sequences to restriction by site-specific nucleases and influences or even controls gene activity.

**methylatropine hydrobromide** $C_{18}H_{25}O_3NHBr$. An anticholinergic agent with actions similar to those of atropine. It is employed as a mydriatic drug as well as in the treatment of pyloric stenosis in infants. Also *atropine methylbromide.*

**methylatropine nitrate** ATROPINE METHYL NITRATE.

**methylbenzenethonium chloride** $C_{28}H_{44}ClNO_2$. Benzyldimethyl-[2-[2-(*p*-1,1,3,3-tetramethylbutylcresoxy)-ethoxy]-ethyl]ammonium chloride. It is used as a topical anti-infective medication to decrease bacterial proliferation in preparations to treat diaper rash and ammonia dermatitis.

**methyl bromide** $CH_3Br$. A highly toxic, colorless gas, usually odorless, with a sweetish, chloroformlike odor. Its principal uses are as an insect fumigant in mills, ships, and freight cars, and as a soil fumigant. It is also used in fire extinguishers, but because of its toxicity, this use is being discouraged in smaller devices. It is dangerous because symptoms of illness from exposure are delayed. After inhalation convulsions may occur without warning or may be preceded by giddiness, numbness of limbs, weakness, drowsiness, and headache. Patients who survive the convulsions may suffer permanent brain damage. Also *bromomethane.*

**(24S)-methylcalciol** VITAMIN $D_4$.

**methylcatechol** GUAIACOL.

**methylcellulose** A methyl ether of cellulose prepared from wood pulp or cotton. It is a white, odorless, tasteless granular material which forms a colorless liquid after being dissolved in water or other solvents. It is used as a bulk laxative and as a colloidal constituent in emulsions and as a suspending agent.

**methylcholanthrene** One of the carcinogenic polycyclic hydrocarbons found in coal tar.

**6-α-methyl compactin** LOVASTATIN.

**methyl cyanide** ACETONITRILE.

**methyldopa** $C_{10}H_{13}NO_4$. 3-Hydroxy-α-methyl-L-tyrosine. An antihypertensive agent used to treat essential hypertension. It acts centrally via α-methylnorepinephrine on α-adrenergic receptors to inhibit sympathetic activity. The drug is given orally.

**methylene** \meth′ilēn\ A bivalent radical of the formula —$CH_2$—.

**methylene blue** A blue dyestuff, once widely used in biochemical investigations of dehydrogenases, which is easily reduced to a colorless compound. It is a thiazine. Its reduced form is related to bis(*p*-dimethylaminophenyl)amine by fusion of the two benzene rings through a sulfur atom at the position *ortho* to the bridging nitrogen and *meta* to the dimethylamino groups. On oxidation, one ring becomes quinonoid. **Löffler's m.** A stain used to detect polymetaphosphate granules, particularly in corynebacteria. **polychrome m.** A mixture of methylene blue, methylene green, methylene azure, and methylene violet.

**methylene green** A synthetic metachromatic dye that can be used to distinguish mast cell granules.

**methylene iodide** An alcohol-soluble yellow liquid with a relative density of 3.33. It is insoluble in water and used in separation procedures and density determinations. Also *diiodomethane.*

**methylenetetrahydrofolate dehydrogenase** One of two enzymes that catalyze the dehydrogenation of 5,10-methylenetetrahydrofolate, a complex of formaldehyde with tetrahydrofolate, to form 5,10-methenyltetrahydrofolate. One of them (EC 1.5.1.5) uses $NADP^+$ as the hydrogen acceptor, and the other (EC 1.5.1.15) uses $NAD^+$.

**methylergonovine maleate** $C_{24}H_{29}N_3O_6$. *N*-[α-(Hydroxymethyl)propyl]-D-lysergamide maleate. It is an oxytocic agent used to induce uterine contractions to shorten the third stage of labor. It is also used after delivery to combat postpartum atony and hemorrhage from the uterus. The drug can be given orally, intramuscularly, or intravenously.

**methylglucamine** 1-Deoxy-1-(methylamino)-D-glucitol. A compound used in the synthesis of certain pharmaceuticals. It is prepared from methylamine and D-glucose.

**methylguanosine** A type of nucleoside found in tRNA, consisting of guanosine methylated on N-1 or on N-7.

**methylhexaneamine** $C_7H_{17}N$. 1,3-Dimethylamylamine. It is an adrenergic agent used primarily in inhalers to relieve congestion of the nasal airways.

**methylidyne** The tervalent group CH.

**methylinosine** A nucleoside sometimes present in a tRNA molecule. It is a rare base.

**ε-*N*-methyllysine** Lysine methylated on its side-chain nitrogen. This amino acid occurs in many proteins, such as myosin, and is produced by methylation of lysine residues already incorporated into the protein. It is subject to further methylation, which may give di- and trimethyllysines. The same compounds can also be produced by treating proteins with formaldehyde and a reducing agent such as borohydride. Since the residues remain positively charged, the modification does not usually alter protein conformation, but it prevents the lysine from entering some chemical reactions.

**methylmalonicaciduria** \-məlän′ikas′idʸoo′rē·ə\ An abnormal elevation of methylmalonic acid in the blood. It may be caused by inborn errors in the metabolism of methylmalonic acid which have varying clinical presentations and therapeutic responses to vitamin $B_{12}$. Enzyme defects that produce the condition include methymalonyl-CoA racemase, methylmalonyl-CoA mutase, and several enzymes involved in $B_{12}$ metabolism. The condition also occurs in the dietary $B_{12}$ deficiency caused by the reduced activity of methylmalonyl-CoA mutase.

**methylmalonyl-CoA mutase** The enzyme (EC 5.4.99.2) that isomerizes (*R*)-methylmalonyl-CoA to form succinyl-CoA. This exchange of hydrogen and carboxyl groups requires a cobamide coenzyme, and probably the reversible breaking of a carbon-cobalt bond. It is the one well-characterized reaction in mammals that involves coenzyme $B_{12}$, and it is part of the pathway by which propionyl-CoA can be metabolized.

**methylmalonyl-coenzyme A** The substance formed from propionyl-CoA by the enzyme methylmalonyl-CoA carboxyltransferase, which forms the *S*-isomer. This is then epimerized to the *R*-isomer before isomerization to give succinyl-CoA. These reactions place it on the pathway of utilization of fatty acids with an odd number of carbon atoms.

**methyl mercury** An alkyl mercury compound formed by aquatic anaerobes in the presence of metallic mercury. Used as a fungicide, it has seen limited production and use in the United States because of its adverse effects on the central nervous system.

**methyl methacrylate** $CH_2{:}C(CH_3)COOCH_3$. An acrylic resin derived from methyl acrylic acid. It occurs as a monomer, which is a liquid, and a polymer, which is a solid. The two forms are mixed to make a plastic substance which sets into a rigid material by virtue of the polymerization of the monomer. It is used to make denture bases, artificial teeth, crowns, and restorations. Also *methacrylate.*

**methyl orange** A weakly acidic aminobenzene dye that is widely used as a pH indicator, turning from red to yellow at pH 3.0 to 4.4. Also *helianthin, tropaeolin D, orange III.*

**methylpentose** Any of the 6-deoxyhexoses, such as rhamnose or fucose.

**methylphenidate hydrochloride** $C_{14}H_{19}NO_2{\cdot}HCl$. Methyl-α-phenyl-2-piperidineacetate hydrochloride salt. It is used in the treatment of hyperkinetic children because of its actions as a mild central nervous system psycomotor stimulant. It is given orally.

**methylprednisolone** $C_{20}H_{30}O_5$. 11β,17α,21-Trihydroxy-6α-methyl-1,4-pregnadiene-3,20-dione. It is a methylated analogue of prednisolone, maintaining the same actions and uses as the parent compound. It is given orally.

**methylpurine** Any methylated purine, especially one formed from adenine and guanine by methylation in tRNA.

**methyl salicylate** $C_8H_8O_3$. 2-Hydroxybenzoic acid methylester. An ester naturally present in leaves of *Gaultheria procumbens* and in *Betula lenta.* It is a colorless, oily liquid with a strong, pleasant odor. It is used in perfumes and as a flavoring for candies, and it is applied in preparations externally as a counterirritant. Also *wintergreen oil, sweet birch oil, teaberry oil.*

**methyltestosterone** $C_{25}H_{38}O_2$. 17α-Methyl-4-androstene-17(β)-ol-one. An androgenic steroidal agent generally used as a replacement therapy for androgen-deficiency disease states. It is given orally.

**$N^5$-methyltetrahydrofolic acid** An intermediate in the conversion of formaldehyde and its donors into methyl groups. It is formed under the action of 5,10-methylenetetrahydrofolate reductase, and it transfers its methyl group e.g. to homocysteine under the action of the cobamide-containing enzyme tetrahydropteroylglutamate methyltransferase to form methionine, and, in some anaerobic bacteria, to a $C_1$-unit to form acetate.

**methylthio-** \meth′ilthī′ō-\ [METHYL- + THIO-] A combining form denoting the group $CH_3$—S—, which may substitute for either hydrogen or hydroxyl in the compound whose name follows, since the term *thio* can mean either the bivalent group —S—, or substitution of sulfur for oxygen.

**methyltransferase** Any of many enzymes, classified as EC 2.1.1, that transfer methyl groups. Most of them use *S*-adenosylmethionine as donor. Also *transmethylase.*

**5-methyluracil** THYMINE.

**methyl violet** A synthetic metachromatic basic dye composed of crystal violet and two other pararosanilins with lesser degrees of methylation and correspondingly redder shades of violet. Methyl violet is used as a stain for amyloid. Also *Paris violet.*

**methysergide** $C_{21}H_{27}N_3O_2$. 1-Methyl-*d*-lysergic acid butanolamide. It is a serotonin receptor antagonist used therapeutically as a vasoconstrictor in the treatment of severe vascular headaches, such as migraine. It is given orally.

**methysergide maleate** $C_{21}H_{27}N_3O_2 \cdot C_4H_4O_4$. *N*-[1-(Hydroxymethyl)propyl]-4-methyl-(+)-lysergamide hydrogen maleate. A serotonin antagonist that, like the parent drug, is used to prevent severe migraine headaches. It is given orally.

**MetMb** metmyoglobin.

**metmyoglobin** \metmī′əglō′bin\ Myoglobin oxidized to the iron(III) state.

**metocurine iodide** $C_{39}H_{46}I_2N_2O_6$. *d*-Tubocurarine iodine dimethyl ether. A derivative of tubocurarine that is more potent and longer acting than tubocurarine. Also *dimethyltubocurarine iodide.*

**metoecious** \metē′shəs\ HETERECIOUS.

**metonymy** \mətän′imē\ [Gk *metōnymia* (from *meta* over + *onym(a)* name + *-ia* -IA) change of name] A disorder in which the patient uses an approximate but related term in place of the specific or idiomatic term, a form of loosening.

**metopagus** \mətäp′əgəs\ [New L (from Gk *metō(pon)* the forehead, from *meta* between + *ōps* the eye, + *pagos* a thing fixed)] Equal conjoined twins with union at the forehead.

**metopic** \metäp′ik\ Pertaining to the forehead.

**metopion** \metō′pē·än\ The craniometric point at which a line joining the frontal eminences intersects the median sagittal plane.

**metopism** \met′əpizm\ The persistence in the adult of the frontal, or metopic, suture.

**metopoplasty** \met′əpōplas′tē\ [Gk *metōpo(n)* the forehead + -PLASTY] Any plastic operation on the forehead.

**metoxenous** \metäk′sənəs\ HETERECIOUS.

**metoxeny** \metäk′sənē\ HETERECISM.

**metr-** \metr-, mətr-\ METRO-.

**metra** \mē′trə\ [Gk *mētra* uterus] *Outmoded* UTERUS.

**metra-** \met′rə-\ METRO-.

**metranastrophe** \mē′tranas′trəfē\ [METR- + Gk *anastrophē* a turning about] INVERSION OF UTERUS.

**metratomy** \mētrat′əmē\ [METRA- + -TOMY] HYSTEROTOMY.

**metratonia** \mē′trətō′nē·ə\ [METR- + ATONIA] Atony of the uterus.

**metratrophia** \mē′trətrō′fē·ə\ [METR- + ATROPHIA] Uterine atrophy. Also *metratresia.*

**metre** \mē′tər\ *Brit.* METER.

**metrectasia** \mē′trektā′zhə\ [METR- + ECTASIA] Dilatation of a nonpregnant uterus.

**metrectomy** \mētrek′təmē\ [METR- + -ECTOMY] HYSTERECTOMY.

**metrectopia** \mē′trektō′pē·ə\ [METR- + ECTOPIA] Any type of uterine displacement. *Older term.*

**metreurynter** \mē′troorin′tər\ [METR- + Gk *euryn(ein)* to dilate + *-tēr,* agentive suffix] A soft bag that is inserted into the cervix and inflated in order to dilate the cervical canal. Also *colpeurynter, hysteurynter.*

**metreurysis** \mētroo′risis\ [METR- + EURY- + -SIS] Dilatation of the cervical canal by means of an inflatable bag which is inserted through the cervical os.

**metrifonate** \met′rifō′nāt\ $C_4H_8Cl_3O_4P$. A schistosomicidal drug that is particularly effective against the bladder blood fluke, *Schistosoma haematobium.*

**metriocephalic** \met′rē·ōsəfal′ik\ Having a moderately vaulted skull, the altitudinal index being between 72 and 77.

**metritic** \mētrit′ik\ Pertaining to or characteristic of metritis.

**metritis** \metrī′tis\ [METR- + -ITIS] An inflammation of the uterus. **dissecting m.** An acute inflammatory process of the uterus that extends along interstitial planes in the myometrium. **puerperal m.** Any postpartum infection of the uterus.

**metrizamide** \met′rizam′īd\ A nonionic radiographic contrast agent found to be significantly less toxic than standard contrast media.

**metrizoate sodium** The sodium salt of metrizoic acid. It is used as a contrast medium for diagnostic purposes such as coronary arteriography.

**metrizoic acid** $C_{12}H_{11}I_3N_2O_4$. 3-(Acetylamino)-5-(acetylmethylamino)-2,4,6-triiodobenzoic acid, a compound used as a contrast medium in diagnostic procedures. It is most often used in its sodium or *N*-methylglucamine salt form.

**metro-** \mē′trō-, met′rō-\ [Gk *mētra* uterus] A combining form denoting the uterus. Also *metr-, metra-.*

**metroendometritis** \-en′dōmētrī′tis\ ENDOMYOMETRITIS.

**metrogenous** \mēträj′ənəs\ Arising from the uterus.

**metromalacia** \-məlā′shə\ Necrosis and softening of the uterus, especially the myometrium.

**metromenorrhagia** \-men′ôrā′jə\ [METRO- + MENORRHAGIA] MENOMETRORRHAGIA.

**metronania** \-nā′nē·ə\ [METRO- + *nan(o)-* + -IA] Unusually small size of the uterus.

**metronidazole** $C_6H_9N_3O_3$. 1-(β-Hydroxyethyl)-2-methyl-5-nitroimidazole. It has trichomonacidal and amebicidal activity against *Trichomonas vaginalis* and *Endomoeba histolytica.* It is used to treat acute intestinal amebiasis and amebic liver abscess. It is also used to treat trichomoniasis in males and females. It is given orally and it is well absorbed. The drug has been reported to be carcinogenic in rodents, and it should be reserved for those special conditions in which it is particularly effective.

**metropathia** \-path′ē·ə\ METROPATHY.

**metropathy** \mēträp′əthē\ [METRO- + -PATHY] Any disease of the uterus. Also *metropathia, hysteropathy.* Adj. metropathic.

**metroperitoneal** \-per′itənē′əl\ Of or relating to the uterus and the peritoneum.

**metropexy** \mē′trəpek′sē\ [METRO- + -PEXY] HYSTEROPEXY.
**metrophlebitis** \-flebī′tis\ Inflammation of the veins of the uterus.
**metroplasty** \mē′trəplas′tē\ [METRO- + -PLASTY] UTEROPLASTY.
**metroptosis** \mē′trətō′sis\ [METRO- + PTOSIS] PROLAPSE OF UTERUS.
**metrorrhagia** \mē′trôrā′jə\ [METRO- + -RRHAGIA] Uterine bleeding occurring at times other than the expected menses. Also *endometrorrhagia.*
**metrosalpinx** \-sal′pingks\ TUBA UTERINA.
**metroscope** \mē′trəskōp\ [METRO- + -SCOPE] HYSTEROSCOPE.
**metrostenosis** \-stenō′sis\ Stenosis of the uterine cavity, as may occur in synechiae of the uterus.
**metrotomy** \mēträt′əmē\ [METRO- + -TOMY] HYSTEROTOMY.
**-metry** \-mətrē\ [Gk *metrein* to measure] A combining form meaning the act or process of measuring.
**m. et sig.** *misce et signa* (L, mix and write a label).
**metyrapone** $C_{14}H_{14}N_2O$. 2-Methyl-1,2-di-3-pyridyl-1-propanone. It is used as a diagnostic aid in the detection of abnormalities in pituitary function. It reduces the levels of cortisol by inhibition of adrenal 11-$\beta$-hydroxylase. In normal individuals this is followed by an increase in ACTH release from the pituitary, followed by an increase in the release of 17-hydroxycorticoids. Also *metapyrone, mepyrapone.*
**Meunier** [Leon *Meunier,* French physician, born 1856] See under SIGN.
**mevalonate kinase** The enzyme (EC 2.7.1.36) that catalyzes the phosphorylation of the 5-hydroxyl group of mevalonic acid, with ATP acting as the phosphate donor. This is the first step in the biosynthetic pathway from mevalonic acid to steroids and terpenes.
**mevalonic acid** (3*R*)-3,5-Dihydroxy-3-methylvaleric acid. It is produced by reduction of 3-hydroxy-3-methylglutaryl-CoA in the pathway of biosynthesis of sterols and isoprenoids in plants and animals.
**mevinolin** LOVASTATIN.
**Meyenburg** [Hans von *Meyenburg,* Swiss pathologist, born 1877] Meyenburg's complexes. See under COMPLEX.
**Meyer** [Adolf *Meyer,* Swiss-born U.S. psychiatrist and neurologist, 1866–1950] **1** See under LOOP. **2** Meyer system, Meyer's theory. See under PSYCHOBIOLOGY.
**Meyer** [Georg Hermann von *Meyer,* German anatomist, 1815–1892] **1** See under LINE. **2** Meyer sinus. See under SINUS MEYERI.
**Meyer** [Hans Horst *Meyer,* German pharmacologist, 1853–1939] Meyer-Overton theory. See under LIPOID THEORY OF NARCOSIS.
**Meyer** [Victor *Meyer,* German chemist, 1848–1897] See under LAW.
**Meyer** [Willy *Meyer,* U.S. surgeon, 1859–1932] Meyer's operation. See under RADICAL MASTECTOMY.
**Meyer-Betz** [Friedrich *Meyer-Betz,* German physician, flourished early 20th century] Meyer-Betz disease. See under FAMILIAL MYOGLOBINURIA.
**Meyerhof** [Otto Fritz *Meyerhof,* German biochemist, 1884–1951] Embden-Meyerhof cycle. See under EMBDEN-MEYERHOF PATHWAY.
**Meynert** [Theodor Hermann *Meynert,* German-born physician active in Austria, 1833–1892] **1** Meynert's bundle, Meynert's fasciculus, Meynert's tract, fibers of Meynert. See under FASCICULUS RETROFLEXUS. **2** Meynert's commissure. See under VENTRAL SUPRAOPTIC COMMISSURE. **3** Meynert's cells. See under CELL. **4** See under NUCLEUS. **5** Meynert's layer. See under INTERNAL PYRAMIDAL LAYER.
**MF** **1** microscopic factor. **2** mitotic figure. **3** multiplying factor. **4** mycosis fungoides.
**MFD** minimal fatal dose.
**m. ft.** *mistura fiat* (L, let a mixture be made).
**Mg** Symbol for the element, magnesium.
**mg** Symbol for the unit, milligram.
**μg** Symbol for the unit, microgram.
**MGUS** monoclonal gammopathy of undetermined significance.
**mGy** Symbol for the unit, milligray.
**μGy** Symbol for the unit, microgray.
**MHC** major histocompatibility complex.
**μHg** Symbol for the unit, micron of mercury.
**MHz** Symbol for the unit, megahertz.
**Mibelli** [Vittorio *Mibelli,* Italian dermatologist, 1860–1910] See under POROKERATOSIS.
**mication** \mīkā′shən\ [L *micatus,* past part. of *micare* to move quickly, flicker, glance] A rapid motion, such as blinking.
**micelle** \mīsel′\ [French (from L *mica* crumb, morsel, particle), a particle formed from an aggregate of similar molecules] **1** A submicroscopic unit of protoplasm. **2** A molecular aggregate as that of a colloid, often formed by the action of detergents on a hydrocarbon in water. It usually has a hydrocarbon interior and a surface of charged groups.
**Michaelis** [Gustav Adolph *Michaelis,* German obstetrician, 1798–1848] See under RHOMBOID.
**Michaelis** [Leonor *Michaelis,* German-born U.S. chemist, 1875–1949] **1** See under CONSTANT. **2** Michaelis equation. See under MICHAELIS-MENTEN EQUATION. **3** Michaelis-Menton kinetics. See under MICHAELIS KINETICS. **4** Michaelis-Gutmann bodies. See under BODY.
**Micheli** [Ferdinando *Micheli,* Italian physician, 1872–1937] **1** Marchiafava-Micheli syndrome. See under PAROXYSMAL NOCTURNAL HEMOGLOBINURIA. **2** Microelliptopoikilocytic anemia of Rietti, Greppi, and Micheli. See under ANEMIA.
**miconazole** $C_{18}H_{14}Cl_4N_2O{\cdot}HNO_3$. 1-[2,4-Dichloro-$\beta$-[(2,4-dichlorobenzyl)oxy]phenethyl]imidazole mononitrate. An antifungal agent.
**micr-** \mīkr-\ MICRO-.
**micra** \mī′krə\ Plural of MICRON.
**micranatomy** \mī′kranat′əmē\ HISTOLOGY.
**micrangiopathy** \mīkran′jē·äp′əthē\ MICROANGIOPATHY.
**micrangium** \mīkran′jē·əm\ [MICR- + *ang(i)-* + L *-ium,* neut. sing. noun termination] A group of small blood vessels, such as capillaries and arterioles.
**micrencephalon** \mī′krensef′əlän\ [MICR- + ENCEPHALON] *Obs.* CEREBELLUM.
**micro-** \mī′krō-\ [Gk *mikros* small, little] A combining form meaning (1) very small, minute; (2) abnormally small; (3) acting to enlarge an image; (4) depending on or relating to microscopy, microscopic; (5) $10^{-6}$, one millionth: used with SI units. Also *micr-, mikro-.* Symbol: μ
**microabscess** \-ab′ses\ [MICRO- + ABSCESS] A small abscess, usually a millimeter or less in diameter and often multiple, seen in multiple organs during septicemia. **Munro's m.'es** One of the characteristic lesions of psoriasis, consisting of focal accumulations of polymorphonuclear leukocytes in the upper layer of the epidermis. Also *Munro's abscesses.* **Pautrier's m.'es** Focal collections of atypical T lymphocytes in the epidermis of patients with mycosis fungoides. Also *Pautrier's abscesses.*
**microadenoma** \-ad′ənō′mə\ [MICRO- + ADENOMA] A

small, nonmalignant, glandular tumor, such as those associated with Cushing's disease.

**microaerophil** \-er′əfil\ An anaerobe that can tolerate or requires a low oxygen tension. Adj. microaerophilic.

**microaerosol** \-er′əsôl\ A suspension in the air of minute particles, the maximum diameter of which is variously taken as 1 to 10 μm.

**microalbuminuria** \-albyoo′minoo′rē·ə\ Excretion in the urine of less than 100 μg per minute of albumin but more than 15 μg per minute. A sensitive radioimmunoassay technique is necessary to measure albumin in this range. Microalbuminuria is an early sign of diabetic glomerulopathy.

**microampere** \mī′krō·am′pir\ [MICRO- + AMPERE] A unit of electric current equal to $10^{-6}$ ampere. Symbol: μA

**microanalysis** Analysis using small amounts of material, particularly by modern methods that are much more sensitive than the classical methods of chemical analysis that involved weighing precipitated material.

**microanatomist** \-ənat′əmist\ HISTOLOGIST.

**microanatomy** \-ənat′əmē\ HISTOLOGY.

**microaneurysm** \-an′yərizm\ An aneurysmal dilitation affecting small arteries, arterioles, or capillaries. Capillary microaneurysms in the retina are a feature of diabetes mellitus. Microaneurysms also occur in other disorders, including thrombotic thrombocytopenic purpura. **diabetic m.** Multiple, small (10–200 μm in diameter) aneurysms arising from retinal capillaries, a sign that is virtually diagnostic of diabetic mellitus and, together with the associated exudates and hemorrhage, constitute the characteristic feature of diabetic retinopathy.

**microangiography** \-an′jē·äg′rəfē\ [MICRO- + ANGIOGRAPHY] Magnification roentgenography of small blood vessels which have been opacified by the injection of a contrast medium.

**microangiopathy** \-an′jē·äp′əthē\ [MICRO- + ANGIO- + -PATHY] A disease process affecting small blood vessels. Also *micrangiopathy.* **diabetic m.** Thickening of the basement membrane in capillaries at many sites in diabetes mellitus, as in the retina and kidney. It is a major cause of severe pathologic complications contributing to disability. The pathogenesis is poorly understood, but appears to be related to poor control of hyperglycemia. **diabetic renal m.** Disease of the small blood vessels of the kidney, including the afferent and efferent arterioles, in long-standing diabetes mellitus, characterized by thickening of the basement membrane and, often, associated microaneurysms. It is associated with the Kimmelstiel-Wilson syndrome. **thrombotic m.** Microangiopathy associated with or due to clots in arterioles and capillaries.

**microangioscopy** \-an′jē·äs′kəpē\ CAPILLARIOSCOPY.

**microbalance** \mī′krəbal′əns\ An analytical balance used for weighing in increments as small as 1 μg.

**microbe** \mī′krōb\ [French, irreg. coinage from MICRO- + Gk *bios* life] MICROORGANISM.

**microbemia** \mī′krōbē′mē·ə\ SEPTICEMIA.

**microbial** \mīkrō′bē·əl\ Pertaining to or caused by a microbe or microbes. Also *microbic.*

**microbicidal** \mīkrō′bisī′dəl\ Lethal to microbes.

**microbicide** \mīkrō′bisīd\ [*microb(e)* + *i* + -CIDE] An agent that kills microbes.

**microbid** \mī′krōbid\ A widespread eruption in a sensitized subject that is attributed to the dissemination of bacterial allergens from a focus of infection.

**microbiemia** \mī′krōbē·ē′mē·ə\ SEPTICEMIA.

**microbioassay** \-bī′ō·as′ā\ A nonquantitative analytical technique for demonstrating the presence of biologically active materials, based on the effect exerted on the growth of cultured microorganisms.

**microbiology** \-bī·äl′əjē\ [MICRO- + BIOLOGY] The branch of science concerned with microorganisms. It can be divided variously into branches, either by content (bacteriology, virology, mycology, protozoology, phycology) or by area of application (medical, soil, etc.). Adj. microbiologic.

**microbism** \mī′krəbizm\ The state of being infected with microbes. **latent m.** The asymptomatic presence of certain pathogenic microorganisms in the body; a carrier state.

**microblephary** \-blef′ərē\ [MICRO- + BLEPHAR- + -Y] An abnormal smallness of the eyelids, often associated with smallness of the palpebral fissure.

**microbody** \mī′krəbäd′ē\ [MICRO- + BODY] A membrane-bound cytoplasmic particle, approximately 0.5–1.0 μm in diameter, containing enzymes. See also PEROXISOME, GLYOXISOME.

**microbrachia** \-brā′kē·ə\ [MICRO- + L *brachia* arms] Abnormal smallness of one or both arms.

**microbrenner** \mī′krōbren′ər\ [MICRO- + German *Brenner* burner] An electric cautery with a needlelike point.

**microcalculus** \-kal′kyələs\ [MICRO- + CALCULUS] A very small calculus formed in the lumen of a renal tubule and which may serve as a focus for calcification of the tubule. Also *microlith.*

**microcalorie** \-kal′ərē\ *Outmoded* 15°C CALORIE.

**microcalorimetry** \-kal′ərim′ətrē\ The measurement of heat absorption or production in minute systems.

**microcapsule** \-kap′s$^y$əl\ A layer too thin to be visualized but providing a bacterium with the surface antigen characteristic of a capsule.

**microcardia** \-kär′dē·ə\ [MICRO- + -CARDIA] An abnormal small size of the heart.

**microcarriers** \-kar′ē·ərs\ Miniature beads that multiply the surface area and hence the yield for anchorage-dependent cells during cell culture.

**microcaulia** \-kô′lē·ə\ [MICRO- + Gk *kaul(os)* stem, stalk, penis + -IA] An abnormal smallness of the penis.

**microcephaly** \-sef′əlē\ [MICRO- + Gk *kephalē* the head + -Y] Abnormal smallness of the brain case specifically, or of the head as a whole. Also *microcrania.* **encephaloclastic m.** Microcephaly associated with congenital growth deficiencies in localized parts of the brain. **schizencephalic m.** Microcephaly associated with specific developmental defects of the brain, particularly those of an aplastic nature.

**microcheilia** \-kī′lē·ə\ [MICRO- + CHEIL- + -IA] The abnormal smallness of one or both lips.

**microcheiria** \-kī′rē·ə\ [MICRO- + CHEIR- + -IA] An abnormal smallness of one or both hands.

**microcirculation** \-sur′kyəlā′shən\ [MICRO- + CIRCULATION] The circulation in the small vessels (arterioles, capillaries, and venules).

**Micrococcaceae** \-käkā′si·ē\ [*Micrococc(us)* + -ACEAE] A family of Gram-positive spherical bacteria that characteristically divide in more than one plane to yield irregular clusters. The family includes the aerobic micrococci found in the environment and the facultative staphylococci found on animals. However, the two are biologically distant, the G + C content being 65–70% and 30–35%, respectively.

**micrococci** \-käk′sī\ Plural of MICROCOCCUS.

**micrococcin** \-käk′sin\ A naturally occurring antibiotic obtained from a particular strain of *Micrococcus.* It has antitubercular activity.

***Micrococcus*** \-käk′əs\ [New L, from MICRO- + COCCUS] A genus of the family Micrococcaceae that is found in the environment. They resemble staphylococci morphologically but differ in other fundamental respects.

**micrococcus** (*pl.* micrococci) Any organism of the genus *Micrococcus.*

**microcolony** \-käl′ənē\ A colony so small as to require magnification for ready observation.

**microcoria** \-kôr′ē·ə\ [MICRO- + *cor(e)-* + -IA] An abnormal smallness of the pupil, particularly as seen in congenital constriction of the pupil.

**microcornea** \-kôr′nē·ə\ [MICRO- + CORNEA] An abnormally small cornea, associated with relatively normal size of the rest of the eye.

**microcrania** \-krā′nē·ə\ MICROCEPHALY.

**microcurie** \mī′rəkyoo′rē\ A unit of activity of a radionuclide or of a radioactive source equal to $10^{-6}$ curie; $3.7 \times 10^4$ becquerels exactly. Symbol: μCi

**microcurie-hour** A unit of total number of nuclear transformations or transitions, equal to $10^{-6}$ curie-hour; $1.332 \times 10^8$ transformations. Symbol: μCi·h

**microcystometer** \-sistäm′ətər\ [MICRO- + CYSTO- + -METER] A small device to measure pressure in the urinary bladder.

**microcytosis** \-sītō′sis\ A predominance of microcytes in the blood. Also *microcythemia.*

**microdactyly** \-dak′tilē\ [MICRO- + DACTYL- + -Y] An abnormal smallness of one or more fingers or toes.

**microdentism** \-den′tizm\ MICRODONTIA.

**microdissection** \-disek′shən\ The dissection of tissue using a dissecting microscope for visualization and very fine instruments for manipulation.

**microdontia** \-dän′shə\ [MICR- + -ODONTIA] The condition of having abnormally small teeth. Also *microdentism, microdontism.*

**microdrepanocytic** \-drep′ənōsit′ik\ Pertaining to hemoglobin S-β-thalassemia.

**microdrepanocytosis** \-drep′ənōsītō′sis\ HEMOGLOBIN S-β-THALASSEMIA. Adj. microdrepanocytic.

**microecology** \-ikäl′əjē\ That aspect of parasite ecology that deals with the mutual effects of the host-parasite relationship.

**microelectrode** \-ilek′trōd\ In electroencephalography, an electrode with a very small tip diameter (less than 100 μm) which is placed in direct contact with the surface of the brain, or which is inserted into the brain substance in an attempt to record the activity of a single neuron.

**microelectrophoresis** \-ilek′trōfôrē′sis\ An analytic technique in which the direction and velocity of electrophoretic migration of charged particles is observed and measured microscopically.

**microembolus** \-em′bələs\ (*pl.* microemboli) An embolus which occludes a small vessel.

**microesthesia** \-esthē′zhə\ [MICRO- + ESTHESIA] A defect of sensation in which the patient underestimates the weight and volume of an object held in the hand.

**microfibril** \-fī′bril\ FIBRIL.

**microfilament** \-fil′əmənt\ A cytoplasmic filament 4–6 nm in diameter, composed of the protein actin and often associated with cellular movement. Microfilaments are present in most eukaryotic cells.

**microfilaremia** \-fī′lerē′mē·ə\ [*microfilar(ia)* + -EMIA] The presence of microfilariae in the peripheral blood.

**microfilaria** \-filer′ē·ə\ [MICRO- + FILARIA] (*pl.* microfilariae) A prelarval parasite of the superfamily Filarioidea, family Onchocercidae, found extracellularly in the blood or tissue fluids of the human host and in the tissues of the vector. • The term has sometimes been used as a pseudogenus name, but it has no taxonomic significance, and when combined with species epithets as in the subentries below, it is better not capitalized or italicized. **m. bancrofti** The sheathed, blood-inhabiting microfilaria of *Wuchereria bancrofti,* found only at night in the peripheral blood of the nocturnally periodic strains. **m. loa** The sheathed microfilaria of *Loa loa,* found diurnally in the peripheral blood of its human or other primate host. Also *microfilaria diurna* (obs.). **m. malaya** The sheathed microfilaria of *Brugia malayi* found in peripheral blood, appearing at night in the nocturnally periodic strains. **sheathed m.** A microfilaria encased in a stretched vitelline membrane that extends beyond either end of the organism. Species that have sheathed microfilariae found in human blood include *Wuchereria bancrofti, Brugia malayi,* and *Loa loa.* **m. streptocerca** The skin-inhabiting, unsheathed microfilaria of *Mansonella streptocerca.* **m. volvulus** The unsheathed microfilaria of *Onchocerca volvulus,* found in dermal tissue fluids.

**microfilariasis** \-fil′ərī′əsis\ The presence of microfilariae in the blood or tissue fluids of the host.

**microfilm** \mī′krəfilm\ **1** A photographic film bearing greatly reduced images of printed records. **2** To record on microfilm.

**microfollicular** \-fəlik′yələr\ Composed of very small follicles.

**microfracture** \mī′krəfrak′chər\ HAIRLINE FRACTURE.

**microfungus** \-fung′gəs\ [MICRO- + FUNGUS] A small fungus, usually best observed using a microscope. The majority of fungi other than some Ascomycetes and Basidiomycetes fall into this category.

**microgamete** \-gam′ēt\ The smaller, or spermlike, motile gamete produced in anisogamy. It fuses with the macrogamete, leading to zygote formation.

**microgametocyte** \-gəmē′təsīt\ The mother cell that produces microgametes in anisogametic reproduction. Also *microgamont.*

**microgamy** \mīkräg′əmē\ [MICRO- + GAM- + -Y] ISOGAMY.

**microgastria** \-gas′trē·ə\ [MICRO- + GASTR- + -IA ] An abnormal smallness of the stomach.

**microgenesis** \-jen′əsis\ HYPOPLASIA.

**microgenia** \-jē′nē·ə\ [MICRO- + Gk *gen(eion)* the chin + -IA] An abnormal smallness of the chin.

**microgenitalism** \-jen′ətəlizm\ [MICRO- + GENITAL + -ISM] **1** The occurrence of abnormally small genitalia in relation to the overall developmental stage. **2** The presence of infantile genitalia in an adolescent or adult individual.

**microglia** \mīkräg′lē·ə\ [MICRO- + GLIA] Small cells of nonectodermal origin that form the third of the three major families of neuroglia in the central nervous system. Microglia are believed to be of mesodermal origin and may have several sources, such as circulating monocytes and perivascular pericytes. Following infection or damage to brain tissue, they become actively phagocytic (gitter cells), rounded with phagocytized material, and are usually carried away and destroyed. Also *microglial cells, perivascular glial cells, Hortega cells.*

**microglial** \mīkräg′lē·əl\ Of or pertaining to microglia.

**microglioma** \mīkräg′lē·ō′mə\ [MICRO- + GLIOMA] A primary lymphoma of the central nervous system.

**microgliomatosis cerebri** \mīkräg′lē·ōmətō′sis ser′əbrī\ A diffuse neoplastic process originating in the microglial cells and spreading widely through the brain. Also *cerebral reticulum cell sarcoma.*

**microgliosis** \mīkräg′lē·ō′sis\ [*microgli(a)* + -OSIS] An excess or proliferation of microglia.

**microglobulin** \-gläb′ʸəlin\ [MICRO- + GLOBULIN] Any serum or urinary globulin of molecular mass below about 40

kDa, including especially Bence-Jones proteins.
**β-microglobulin** A polypeptide of 11 600 daltons that forms the light chain of class 1 major histocompatibility antigens and can therefore be detected on all cells bearing these antigens. Free β2-microglobulin is found in the blood and in particular the urine of patients with certain diseases, such as Wilson's disease, cadmium poisoning, and renal tubular acidosis.
**microglossia** \-gläs′ē·ə\ [MICRO- + GLOSS- + -IA ] An abnormally small tongue. It is often seen in hypomicrognathus and agnathia.
**microglossic** \-gläs′ik\ Having a short tongue: said particularly of certain insects.
**micrognathia** \mīk′rənā′thē·ə\ [MICRO- + GNATH- + -IA ] Abnormal smallness of either the upper or lower jaw, particularly the lower. Congenital or acquired varieties occur. The condition may be apparent only, due to the abnormal position of the jaws.
**microgram** \mī′krəgram\ [MICRO- + GRAM] A unit of mass or weight equal to $10^{-6}$ gram, or $10^{-9}$ kilogram. Symbol: μg **m. per liter** A unit of mass concentration equal to $10^{-6}$ gram per liter. Symbol: μg/l, μg·$l^{-1}$
**micrograph** \mī′krəgraf\ [MICRO- + -GRAPH] **1** PHOTOMICROGRAPH. **2** An instrument that converts pressure fluctuations, such as those from the arterial pulse, to minute deviations of a diaphragm. The deviations are magnified by a reflected light beam and recorded on moving film. **acoustic m.** The image produced by an acoustic microscope. **electron m.** The photographic image that is produced by an electron microscope.
**micrographia** \-graf′ē·ə\ [MICRO- + GRAPH- + -IA ] Writing in very small letters, often decreasing progressively in size, as often seen in patients with Parkinson's disease.
**micrography** \mīkräg′rəfē\ **1** MICROSCOPY. **2** A description of materials observed by microscopic examination.
**microgray** \mī′krəgrā\ [MICRO- + GRAY] A unit of absorbed dose in the field of ionizing radiation equal to $10^{-6}$ gray. Symbol: μGy
**microgyria** \-jī′rē·ə\ [MICRO- + GYR- + -IA] The abnormal smallness or narrowness of cerebral convolutions, usually associated with polygyria.
**microhematocrit** \-hēmat′ōkrit\ Use of a capillary tube to determine by centrifugation the packed cell volume of a small sample of blood.
**microhepatia** \-hepā′shə\ [MICRO- + HEPAT- + -IA ] An abnormal smallness of the liver. It can result from developmental or pathologic causes.
**microheterogeneity** \-het′ərōjənē′itē\ The occurrence of molecules that are not identical, but whose differences are very limited. A glycoprotein, for example, might have molecules all of which possessed the same polypeptide chain, glycosylated on the same amino-acid residues, but by oligosaccharides that differed slightly in numbers of monosaccharide residues.
**microhistology** \-histäl′əjē\ HISTOLOGY.
**microincineration** \-insin′ərā′shən\ The reduction to ashes of very small pieces of tissue or other material prior to the identification of their constituent elements.
**microincision** \-insizh′ən\ [MICRO- + INCISION] A small opening into a cell, usually made to remove or destroy a cellular organelle. Microincisions can be made with a laser beam.
**microinfarct** \-in′färkt\ An infarct resulting from occlusion of a small vessel.
**microinjection** \-injek′shən\ [MICRO- + INJECTION] The injection of small quantities of material into a cell, usually using a micromanipulator and a microneedle.
**microinjector** A device permitting the delivery, by infusion, of a very small quantity of drug or other medicinal agent.
**microinvasion** \-invā′zhən\ [MICRO- + INVASION] Invasion by a cancer too short a distance to be detected without a microscope. The term usually applies to squamous cell carcinoma of the cervix invading the underlying stroma.
**microkatal** \mī′krəkatal′\ [MICRO- + KATAL] A unit of catalytic activity equal to $10^{-6}$ katal; $10^{-6}$ mole per second. Symbol: μkat
**microlaryngoscopy** \-lar′ing·gäs′kəpē\ Suspension laryngoscopy using a specially designed laryngoscope through which the surgeon may inspect a magnified image of the interior of the larynx with the operating microscope and carry out any necessary surgery with correspondingly greater precision.
**microlecithal** \-les′ithəl\ [MICRO- + LECITH- + -AL] MIOLECITHAL.
**microlentia** \-len′shə\ SPHEROPHAKIA.
**microleukoblast** \-loo′kəblast\ MYELOBLAST.
**microliter** \mī′krəlē′tər\ [MICRO- + LITER] A unit of volume or capacity equal to $10^{-6}$ liter, $10^{-9}$ cubic meter, or $10^{-3}$ cubic centimeter. Symbol: μl
**microlith** \mī′krəlith\ [MICRO- + Gk *lith(os)* a stone] MICROCALCULUS.
**microlithiasis** \-lithī′əsis\ [MICRO- + LITHIASIS] Small mineral concretions present within an organ, such as those seen in pulmonary alveoli and prostatic glands. **pulmonary alveolar m.** A condition of unknown cause in which innumerable small hard calcium-containing nodules are present in the alveoli of both lungs. Also *microlithiasis alveolaris pulmonum*.
**micromandible** \-man′dibəl\ An abnormal shortness of the mandible. Also *brachygnathia*.
**micromanipulation** \-mənip′yəlā′shən\ The handling or management of extremely small pieces of tissue or cells or parts of cells, as in removing a defective gene from a cell and replacing it with a normal gene.
**micromanometer** \-mənäm′ətər\ A device for measuring pressure of minute amounts of gas or vapor. It is used especially in measuring gas generated by metabolic activity of small tissue specimens.
**micromelia** \-mē′lyə\ [MICRO- + MEL-[1] + -IA] A disproportionate shortness or smallness of one or more limbs. **rhizomelic m.** A developmental deformity of a limb in which the limb is shortened because of the absence or deficient development of the proximal segments.
**micromere** \mī′krəmir\ [MICRO- + -MERE] A small blastomere resulting from unequal cleavage of a developing zygote.
**micrometastasis** \-mətas′təsis\ [MICRO- + METASTASIS] (*pl.* micrometastases) A metastatic deposit of cancer of microscopic size.
**micrometer¹** \mī′krəmē′tər\ [MICRO- + METER] A unit of length equal to $10^{-6}$ meter. Also *micron* (older term). Symbol: μm
**micrometer²** \mīkräm′ətər\ [French *micromètre,* from *micro-* MICRO- + *-mètre* -METER] **1** An instrument containing a microscope for accurate linear measurement of very small units of length. **2** A caliper having a spindle moved by a screw for measuring minute distances. **caliper m.** A caliper that is driven by a finely threaded screw (micrometer screw) and used to measure extremely thin objects. **eyepiece m.** A calibrated scale for linear measurement that is inserted into the eyepiece of a compound microscope and used for direct determination of the size of objects viewed. Also *ocular micrometer.* **filar m.** An eyepiece

micrometer consisting of two parallel wires and a graduated distance scale. Measurement is made by moving one of the two wires across the graduated scale away from the fixed wire. **ocular m.** EYEPIECE MICROMETER. **slide m.** A measuring scale marked on a glass slide and intended for use in a microscope field of view. **stage m.** A micrometer ruled on a microscope stage, which is usually movable. It is often in the form of a vernier to allow accurate measurement of very small movements of the viewing field.

**micromethod** \mīʹkrəmethʹəd\ Any laboratory procedure that uses much smaller quantities of test materials and reagents than a standard method.

**micrometre** *Brit.* MICROMETER.

**micrometry** \mīkrämʹətrē\ The use of a micrometer and microscope to measure minute objects.

**micromicro-** \mīʹkrōmīʹkrə-\ [MICRO- + MICRO-] A combining form denoting $10^{-12}$: formerly used with SI units, now replaced by *pico-*. Symbol: μμ

**micromicrogram** \mīʹkrōmīʹkrəgram\ [MICROMICRO- + GRAM] *Outmoded* PICOGRAM. Symbol: μμg

**micromilli-** \mīʹkrōmilʹē-\ [MICRO- + MILLI-] A combining form denoting $10^{-9}$: formerly used with SI units, now replaced by *nano-*. Symbol: μm

**micromilligram** \mīʹkrəmilʹigram\ [MICROMILLI- + GRAM] *Outmoded* NANOGRAM. Symbol: μmg

**micromillimeter** \mīʹkrəmilʹimēʹtər\ [MICROMILLI- + METER] *Outmoded* NANOMETER. Symbol: μmm

**micromolar** \mīʹkrəmōʹlər\ A unit of concentration equal to $10^{-6}$ molecular weight in grams ($10^{-6}$ mole) dissolved in one liter of solution. An obsolete unit. Symbol: μM

***Micromonospora*** \-mōnäsʹpərə\ A genus of actinomycete that has yielded a few antibiotics, designated by the suffix *-micin*.

**micromotor** \-mōʹtər\ [MICRO- + MOTOR] A miniaturized high-speed electric motor attached directly to the handpiece of a dental drill.

**micromyelia** \-mī·ēʹlyə\ [MICRO- + MYEL- + -IA] A disproportionate smallness or shortness of the spinal cord.

**micromyeloblast** \-mīʹəlōblastʹ\ A small myeloblast sometimes seen in acute myelogenous leukemia. Because of its small size, the micromyeloblast may be mistaken for a lymphocyte or lymphoblast.

**micromyelolymphocyte** \-mīʹəlōlimʹfəsīt\ *Obs.* MYELOBLAST.

**micron** \mīʹkrän\ [neut. of Gk *mikros* small] *Older term* MICROMETER¹. Symbol: μ

**microneedle** \mīʹkrənēʹdəl\ A thin glass needle used in microdissection or microsurgery.

**microneme** \mīʹkrənēm\ [MICRO- + *-neme,* combining form from Gk *nēma* thread, yarn, tissue] A small, rod-shaped organelle in the anterior portion of certain stages of sporozoa of the phylum Apicomplexa. It is a characteristic structure of merozoites and sporozoites and helps to define the phylum Apicomplexa. Also *sarconeme, toxoneme.*

**micronize** \mīʹkrənīz\ [MICRON + -IZE] To pulverize or reduce material to particles of very small size, often to size that will pass through mesh of 400 to 1000 gauge.

**micronormoblast** \-nôrʹməblast\ An erythrocyte precursor that is smaller than normal. The nucleus is pyknotic, and the cytoplasm contains some hemoglobin and forms a small rim around the nucleus. Micronormoblasts are present in the bone marrow in iron deficiency anemia.

**micronucleus** \-nʸooʹklē·əs\ **1** The smaller of the two types of nuclei found in ciliate protozoa, the one involved in sexual or genetic exchange rather than in the vegetative functions of the macronucleus. Also *reproductive nucleus, karyogonad, gonad nucleus, gametic nucleus.* **2** NUCLEOLUS.

**micronutrient** \-nʸooʹtrē·ənt\ [MICRO- + NUTRIENT] Any essential dietary constituent, such as the vitamins and trace minerals, required by the body in small quantities.

**micronychia** \-nikʹē·ə\ [MICR- + ONYCH- + -IA] An abnormal smallness of one or more nails.

**micronystagmus** \-nistagʹməs\ Very small spontaneous movements of the eye, occurring normally in all persons.

**micro-orchidia** \-ôrkidʹē·ə\ MICRORCHIDIA.

**microorganism** \-ôrʹgənizm\ Any single-celled organism, formally assigned to the kingdom Protista. Also *microbe.*

**microparasite** \-parʹəsīt\ A parasitic microorganism.

**micropenis** \mīʹkrəpēʹnis\ [MICRO- + PENIS] A disproportionate smallness or shortness of the penis.

**microphage** \mīʹkrəfāj\ A small phagocyte, specifically a polymorphonuclear leukocyte. Microphages engulf and digest bacteria, whereas macrophages, such as monocytes, engulf and digest dead or senescent cells and cellular debris. Also *microphagocyte, microphagus.*

**microphakia** \-fāʹkē·ə\ SPHEROPHAKIA.

**microphonia** \-fōʹnē·ə\ LEPTOPHONIA.

**microphonics** \-fänʹiks\ **cochlear m.** Electrical potentials generated in the cochlea by the passage of sound waves across the middle ear. Also *electrophonic effect* (seldom used), *Wever-Bray phenomenon.*

**microphonograph** \-fōʹnəgraf\ A device to amplify and simultaneously to record, used in speech therapy for the hearing-impaired.

**microphotograph** \-fōʹtəgraf\ PHOTOMICROGRAPH.

**microphthalmia** \mīʹkräfthalʹmē·ə\ [MICR- + OPHTHALMIA] Abnormal smallness of one or both eyeballs. This is a recessive trait in humans. Also *microphthalmos, microphthalmus.*

**microphthalmic** \mīʹkräf·thalʹmik\ [MICR- + OPHTHALMIC] Having abnormally small eyes.

**microphthalmos** \mīʹkräf·thalʹməs\ MICROPHTHALMIA.

**microphthalmus** MICROPHTHALMIA.

**micropia** \mīkrōʹpē·ə\ MICROPSIA.

**micropipet** \-pipetʹ\ **1** A pipet calibrated for accurate delivery of very small quantities, usually less than 0.5 ml. **2** A pipet with a fine tip used in microinjection.

**microplasia** \-plāʹzhə\ [MICRO- + -PLASIA] Abnormally limited growth, as in dwarfism.

**microplicae** \-plīʹsē\ (*sing.* microplica) Ridgelike folds on the surface of a cell. They are especially evident on epithelial cells from the inner cheek.

**micropodia** \-pōʹdē·ə\ [MICRO- + POD- + -IA ] An abnormal smallness of one or both feet.

**micropolygyria** \-pälʹijīʹrē·ə\ POLYGYRIA.

**micropore** \mīʹkrəpôr\ [MICRO- + PORE] A submicroscopic break in the membrane of a protozoan cell or microbe through which exchange of material, pinocytosis or other minute forms of flow may occur. It is seen in electron micrographs of *Eimeria* and *Plasmodium.*

**microprobe** \mīʹkrəprōb\ An ultrafine probe used for exploration and fixation of tissues in microsurgical procedures. **laser m.** A diagnostic device consisting of a very fine laser beam that vaporizes a small region of tissue. The vapor is then analyzed by emission spectroscopy. Also *laser microscope.*

**microprojection** \-prəjekʹshən\ A projection upon a screen of the visual field of a microscope.

**microprosopus** \-prōsōʹpəs, -präsʹəpəs\ [MICRO- + New L *prosopus* face, irreg. from Gk *prosōpon* face] A fetus or postnatal individual with small or underdeveloped facial region.

**micropsia** \mīkräp′sē·ə\ [MICR- + -OPSIA] Perception of objects as being much smaller than they would normally appear. It may result from stretching of the retina, as in retinal detachment, or occur as a visual hallucination in temporal lobe epilepsy, in intoxication from drugs, in febrile deliriums, and in other systemic or central nervous system disorders. Also *visual diminutus, micropia, lilliputian hallucination, microptic hallucination*. Adj. microptic.

**micropuncture** \-pungk′chər\ [MICRO- + PUNCTURE] An experimental technique involving the insertion of a micropipet into the lumen of a renal tubule to collect tubular fluid in order to analyze functions of specific portions of the tubule.

**micropyknometer** \-piknäm′ətər\ A device used to measure the relative density of very small quantities of liquid.

**microquantity** A very small quantity, expressed in microgram units.

**microradiograph** \-rā′dē·əgraf′\ A recorded image obtained by microradiography, used for high-resolution imaging of thin objects such as tissue sections. Also *microradiogram*.

**microradiography** \-rā′dē·äg′rəfē\ A technique by which a radiograph of a thin object, as a tissue section, is produced on fine-grained film and can be examined microscopically or enlarged with a resolution approaching the resolution of the photographic emulsion.

**microrchidia** \mī′krôrkid′ē·ə\ [MICR- + *orchid(o)*- + -IA] An abnormal smallness of one or both testicles. Also *micro-orchidia*.

**microrefractometer** \-rē′fraktäm′ətər\ An instrument for studying the fine structure of cells as indicated by variations in optical properties of cell components.

**microrhinia** \-rī′nē·ə\ [MICRO- + RHIN- + -IA] The disproportionate smallness of the nose.

**microroentgen** \-rent′gən\ [MICRO- + ROENTGEN] A unit of ionization exposure equal to $10^{-6}$ roentgen; $2.58 \times 10^{-10}$ coulomb per kilogram. Symbol: μR, μr

**microscope** \mī′krəskōp\ [MICRO- + -SCOPE] An optical instrument having one or more lenses, used to view magnified images of small objects. **acoustic m.** A device in which ultrasound distorts a reflective surface, which is then optically scanned to produce an image. Also *ultrasonic microscope*. **binocular m.** A microscope with two eyepieces, intended for binocular viewing. **capillary m.** A microscope used for examining the capillaries, particularly those of the nail bed. **centrifuge m.** An optical device located within a centrifuge that permits observation of material undergoing high-speed centrifugation. The objective rotates and projects the image onto a stationary ocular located at the axis. **comparison m.** An optical device that allows the simultaneous viewing, through a single set of eyepieces, of images transmitted by two different objectives. Also *comparator microscope*. **compound m.** A microscope with more than one lens system. The magnified image transmitted by the system nearest the object is further magnified by passage through lenses near the eye of the viewer. **corneal m.** SLIT LAMP. **dark-field m.** A microscope that employs dark-field illumination. Unstained objects appear bright against a dark background. **dissecting m.** A compound microscope with two sets of eyepieces and objectives, constructed to present a nonreversed, stereoscopic image of three-dimensional objects. The distance between the objective lenses and the object stage is great enough to allow manipulation of the object examined. **electron m.** A microscope that uses a beam of electrons to visualize particles too small to be resolved by a light microscope. Also *ultramicroscope, supermicroscope*. **fluorescence m.** A compound microscope in which ultraviolet or violet-blue visible light is used to produce a fluorescence of the examined object, which may have natural fluorescence or may have been treated with a fluorochrome. **flying spot m.** A microscope in which the object is subjected to light from an optical scanning device. **hypodermic m.** A system for examining the microscopic detail of tissues that uses a fiberoptic probe which can be passed through a hollow needle. **infrared m.** A microscope used for examining opaque, particulate objects in which the image is obtained by observing or measuring the absorption of infrared light waves. **interference m.** A microscope used to examine unstained, transparent, or reflecting specimens. Incident and diffracted waves from a single light source are recombined at the plane of image, where their interference effects cause the differences in refraction and light transmission to become visible. **ion m.** A device that is used to etch surfaces, using a beam of atoms passing through a vacuum. The final preparation is then examined in an electron microscope. **laser m.** LASER MICROPROBE. **light m.** A device used to obtain a magnified image of very small objects, viewed with light in the visible range. Also *optical microscope*. **ocular m.** A microscope with a single lens system. **operating m.** A microscope specially designed to be used by surgeons when operating on very small structures. It helps to improve visibility and precision. Its essential features are an adequate working distance between objective lens and operative field, brilliant illumination and ease of adjustment. Also *surgical microscope*. **optical m.** LIGHT MICROSCOPE. **phase m.** A microscope in which light is transmitted at slightly different phases, so that differences in refraction within the object examined become visible as contrasting areas of different intensity. It is used especially to examine living cells or unstained material. Also *phase-contrast microscope*. **polarizing m.** A microscope in which the specimen is illuminated by polarized light. It is used to examine birefringent specimens, which cause the refractive index to vary with the direction of light transmission. **reflecting m.** A compound microscope in which the objective lens system is replaced by a concave and a convex mirror, creating an image system free of chromatic aberration at any wavelength of visible light. **scanning electron m.** A microscope that produces a detailed surface view of an object by scanning a narrow electron beam over its surface. The secondary electrons given off from the surface are then used to build up a composite picture in an image analyzer. **schlieren m.** A microscope that uses schlieren optics so that differences in the density of the examined object become visible as differences in the refraction of transmitted light. **simple m.** A magnifying device consisting of a single lens. **slit lamp m.** SLIT LAMP. **stereoscopic m.** A microscope with dual eyepieces and objectives, arranged so that the separate images combine to give a stereoscopic or three-dimensional image. **surgical m.** OPERATING MICROSCOPE. **ultrapaque m.** A microscope that is designed to examine the surface structure of opaque organs by using an incident light source instead of a transmitted light source. **ultrasonic m.** ACOUSTIC MICROSCOPE. **ultraviolet m.** A microscope whose energy source is electromagnetic radiation with a wavelength of 180–400 nm. The image is visualized by reflecting optics, fluorescence optics, or crystal objectives that transmit ultraviolet wavelengths. **x-ray m.** A microscope which uses a beam of x rays instead of light, with the image usually being recorded on photographic film.

**microscopic** \mi′krəskäp′ik\ **1** Extremely small; specifically, of a size that can be seen only with the aid of a microscope. 2 Of or relating to microscopes or their use.

**microscopy** \mīkräs′kəpē\ [MICRO- + -SCOPY] The study of both animate and inanimate objects using the magnifying power of a microscope. Also *micrography*. **bright-field m.** Microscopy in which there is direct, vertical illumination. **dark-field m.** Microscopy that uses a condenser, resulting in a dark background and illumination from the side so that microorganisms appear light in a dark field. **electron m.** The preparation of material and the subsequent examination in an electron microscope. Also *ultramicroscopy*. **immersion m.** A microscopic examination in which the objective lens and the cover glass are both immersed in a liquid with the same refractive index as glass. **immune electron m.** The use of an electron microscope to study a specimen that has been stained with a labeled specific antibody capable of identifying a particular protein. Abbr. IEM **immunofluorescent m.** Fluorescence microscopy in which antigens are identified by use of antibodies to which are attached fluorescent dyes. **phase-contrast m.** The use of a microscope which changes the phase relationships of light passing through and around an object so that staining and other special preparations are not necessary for visualization of the object. **scanning transmission electron m.** The process of examining a specimen by both transmission and scanning electron microscopy within the same instrument. **transmission electron m.** The use of a microscope in which an electron beam is passed through an ultrathin section of tissue to provide a detailed image of cell and tissue components according to their capacity to permit or obstruct the flow of electrons.

**microsecond** \mī′krəsek′ənd\ [MICRO- + SECOND] A unit of time equal to $10^{-6}$ second. Symbol: μs

**microsection** \-sek′shən\ A thin slice of tissue that is prepared for examination with a microscope.

**microsomatia** \-sōmā′shə\ MICROSOMIA.

**microsome** \mī′krəsōm\ [MICRO- + Gk *sōm(a)* body] A fragment of endoplasmic reticulum with associated ribosomes. Such fragments are usually obtained by homogenizing cells and centrifuging them at high speed. Also *cytomicrosome*. Adj. microsomal.

**microsomia** \-sō′mē·ə\ [MICRO- + Gk *sōma* body + -IA] A general smallness of the body, as seen in dwarfism. Also *microsomatia*. **m. fetalis** An abnormally small-sized fetus in relation to fetal age.

**microspectrography** \-spekträg′rəfē\ The study of the composition of an object, especially of cellular constituents, using a spectroscope that makes a photographic record of the spectrum.

**microspectrophotometer** \-spek′trōfōtäm′ətər\ An instrument used to measure the absorption, reflection, or emission of light by objects under a microscope. It is used especially for spectral analysis of constituents of individual cells.

**microspectrophotometry** \-spek′trōfōtäm′ətrē\ The analysis of the absorption spectrum of a single cell's constituents, a process used especially for characterizing nucleoproteins.

**microspectroscope** \-spek′trəskōp\ A spectroscope designed for use in the eyepiece of a compound microscope. It is used especially to analyze the spectrum of living cells.

**microspherocyte** \-sfir′əsīt\ SPHEROCYTE.

**microspherocytosis** \-sfir′əsītō′sis\ SPHEROCYTOSIS.

**microspherulation** \-sfir′əlā′shən\ ERYTHROCYTORRHEXIS.

**microsplanchnia** \-splangk′nē·ə\ Abnormal smallness of a viscus or viscera, particularly abdominal viscera.

**microsplanchnic** \-splangk′nik\ 1 Possessing small abdominal viscera. 2 Of or relating to a body constitution in which the horizontal diameters are less developed than the vertical ones and in which the abdominal portion is relatively smaller than the thoracic. For defs. 1 and 2 also *microsplanchnous*.

**microsplenia** \-splē′nē·ə\ [MICRO- + SPLEN- + -IA ] The abnormal smallness of the spleen, as is often seen in the presence of accessory splenic tissue.

**microsporid** \mīkräs′pərid\ A dermatophytid that is provoked by a *Microsporum* species. Also *microsporide*.

**microsporide** \mīkräs′pərīd\ MICROSPORID.

**microsporosis** \-spôrō′sis\ Ringworm, especially ringworm of the scalp, that is caused by a *Microsporum* species.

***Microsporum*** \mīkräs′pôrəm\ [New L (from MICRO- + New L *-sporum*, combining form denoting spore, from Gk *spora* a sowing, seed)] A genus of fungi that causes various dermatophytoses, including tinea corpus and tinea capitis.

**microstereognosia** \-ster′ē·ägnō′zhə\ [MICRO- + STEREO- + Gk *-gnōsia*, combining form from *gnōs(is)* knowledge + *-ia* -IA] An abnormality of tactile sensation in which objects seem abnormally small when touched or felt.

**microstethophone** \-steth′əfōn\ [MICRO- + STETHO- + Gk *phōnē* sound, voice] A stethoscope utilizing an amplifying device which may be electronic.

**microstomia** \-stō′mē·ə\ [MICRO- + STOM- + -IA] A disproportionate smallness of the oral orifice.

**microstrabismus** \-strəbiz′məs\ [MICRO- + STRABISMUS] A very small angle of manifest ocular deviation.

**microsurgery** \-sur′jərē\ [MICRO- + SURGERY] Surgery performed with the aid of an enlarging lens or dissecting microscope.

**microsuture** \-soo′chər\ A very fine monofilament used in microsurgery. The diameter of the suture is usually 40 μm or less.

**microtia** \mīkrō′shē·ə\ [MICR- + OT- + -IA] The abnormal smallness of the pinna or auricle of the ear. The external auditory meatus may be reduced in bore, end blindly, or be absent.

**microtome** \mī′krətōm\ [MICRO- + -TOME] A mechanical device used for preparing histologic sections for microscopic examination. Also *histotome, section cutter*. **freezing m.** A mechanical device for cutting frozen sections of tissue without a temperature control cabinet. It usually includes a device for quick freezing of unfixed or unprocessed tissue. Also *cryotome*. **rotary m.** A microtome in which the block of tissue to be sectioned is moved up and down against a horizontal knife blade, using a rotary hand action.

**microtomization** \-tō′mīzā′shən\ The use of a microtome to obtain a section for examination.

**microtomography** \-tōmäg′rəfē\ A technique for rotating a small sample in an electron microscope through 90 degrees, processing the data by computer, and displaying three-dimensional images, as of the changes within living cells.

**microtomy** \mīkrät′əmē\ [MICRO- + -TOMY] The cutting of tissue sections so as to make them suitable for examination with a microscope.

**microtonometer** \-tōnäm′ətər\ An instrument for measuring the partial pressure of gases in minute quantities of material.

**microtrichia** \-trik′ē·ə\ [MICRO- + TRICH- + -IA ] An unusual fineness of the hair, with a reduced mean diameter of the individual hairs.

***Microtrombidium akamushi*** \-trämbid′ē·əm ak′əmoo′shē\ See under *LEPTOTROMBIDIUM*.

**microtubule** \-t$^y$oo′byəl\ [MICRO- + TUBULE] A small,

hollow, cylindrical structure found in the cytoplasm of nearly all eukaryotic cells. It has an outside diameter of 250 Å, with a wall thickness of 50 Å, and hence an inside diameter of 150 Å. The wall is a polymer composed of equal numbers of units of α-tubulin and β-tubulin. Microtubles function as a cellular skeleton and are also involved in the phenomena of cell movement. **chromosomal m.** CHROMOSOMAL SPINDLE FIBER. **kinetochore m.** CHROMOSOMAL SPINDLE FIBER. **spindle m.** Any of the microtubules which form the mitotic spindle. The spindle fibers are composed of bundles of microtubules.

**microvasculature** \-vas′kyələchər\ The total of all arterioles, capillaries, and venules in the body.

**microvilli** \-vil′ī\ Plural of MICROVILLUS.

**microvillus** \-vil′əs\ [MICRO- + L *villus* a long hair, shaggy hair] A minute fingerlike process from a cell surface that is visible under an electron microscope. Microvilli are often arranged together in a closely packed form to provide a brush border. **placental m.** A minute extension from a trophoblastic cell of the placenta.

**microvoltometer** \-vōltäm′ətər\ A device for measuring the very small changes in electric potential that occur in cellular physiology and pathology.

**microwave** \mī′krəwāv\ An electromagnetic wave of short wavelength, especially between 100 and 1 cm. Sources of emission include radar, cathode-ray tubes, induction furnaces, and electrotherapy devices. There is evidence that microwave exposure can cause cataract and thermal damage to the eye. Also *microelectric wave.*

***Micruroides*** \mī′kroorοi′dēz\ A genus of venomous snakes of the Elapidae family; coral snakes.

***Micrurus*** \mīkroo′rəs\ A genus of venomous snakes of the Elapidae family; coral snakes. Also *Elaps.*

**miction** \mik′shən\ [Late L *mictio,* from L *mictus,* past part. of *meiere,* later *mingere* to urinate] URINATION.

**micturate** \mik′chərāt\ [L *mictur(ire)* to urinate + -ATE] URINATE.

**micturition** \mik′chərish′ən\ [L *micturitus,* past part. of *micturire,* desiderative verb from *mictus,* past part. of *meiere,* later *mingere* to urinate] URINATION.

**MID** 1 minimal infective dose. 2 minimal inhibiting dose.

**midbody** An accumulation of electron-dense material at the peripheral spindle fibers associated with the process of furrowing during cytokinesis. As constriction proceeds to pinch the cell in two, the midbody becomes smaller, usually disappearing before cleavage is complete.

**midbrain** MESENCEPHALON.

**midcarpal** \mid′kär′pəl\ 1 Pertaining to the center of the carpus. 2 Between the proximal and distal rows of the carpal bones. For defs. 1 and 2 also *mediocarpal, mesocarpal.*

**midclavicular** \mid′kləvik′yələr\ Pertaining to the central point or portion of the clavicle.

**middlepiece** MIDDLE PIECE.

**midepigastric** \mid′epigas′trik\ Pertaining to the middle of the epigastrium in the transverse plane.

**midfoot** The central portion of the foot in the region of the cuboid, navicular, and cuneiform bones.

**midfrontal** \midfrun′təl\ 1 Of or relating to the middle of the frontal bone, or forehead. 2 Both median and frontal. For defs. 1 and 2 also *mediofrontal, medifrontal.*

**midge** \mij\ [Middle English *migge,* from Old English *mycg,* akin to Gk *myia* a fly and L *musca* a fly] Any of the small flies of the families Chironomidae, Ceratopogonidae, and others. They often appear in great numbers and the Ceratopogonidae give painful bites. Some species are vectors of the filarial worms *Mansonella ozzardi, Dipetalonema perstans, D. streptocerca,* and other parasites.

**midget** [dim. of *midge,* from Middle English *migge,* from Old English *mycg*] An abnormally small but normally proportioned individual. *Popular.*

**midgut** 1 The middle segment of the embryonic intestine, precursor of the stomach, of the small intestine, and of the colon with the exception of the sigmoid colon and the rectum. It connects with the yolk sac through the vitellointestinal duct at the level of the umbilical ring. 2 The region of the arthropod gut derived from endoderm, between the ectodermal, chitin-lined foregut and hindgut. Also *mesenteron.*

**midhead** CENTRICIPUT.

**midline** 1 MEDIAN PLANE. 2 The central axis of a part or organ. 3 Any line that bisects a structure along its axis.

**midoccipital** \mid′äksip′itəl\ Pertaining to the central portion or point of the occiput. Also *medioccipital.*

**midphalangeal** \mid′fəlan′jē·əl\ 1 Of or relating to the middle phalanx. 2 Of or relating to the middle of a phalanx.

**mid-piece** 1 A globulin fraction of complement which precipitates when electrolytes are removed from serum. It unites with sensitized erythrocytes but produces hemolysis only if another complement fraction, the end-piece, is also present. 2 MIDDLE PIECE.

**midplane** PELVIC PLANE OF LEAST DIMENSIONS.

**midriff** DIAPHRAGMA.

**midsection** A slice or cut through the middle of an organ or a structure.

**midsternum** \midstur′nəm\ CORPUS STERNI.

**midtarsal** \midtär′səl\ 1 Pertaining to the center of the tarsus. 2 Between the calcaneus and talus proximally and the cuboid and navicular bone distally. For defs. 1 and 2 also *mediotarsal, mesotarsal.*

**midventral** \midven′trəl\ Pertaining to the middle part of a ventral surface.

**midvesical** \midves′ikəl\ Of or relating to the middle of a bladder.

**midwife** [Middle English *midwif, midwyf,* from Middle and Old English *mid* with + Middle English *wif* a woman, from Old English *wif, wīf* a woman] A health care worker, who may or may not be formally trained and is not a physician, that delivers babies and provides associated maternal care.

**midwifery** \mid′wifrē, mid′wīfərē\ The practice of obstetrics by a midwife.

**Mierzejewski** [Johann Lucian *Mierzejewski,* Russian neurologist and psychiatrist, 1839–1908] See under EFFECT.

**Miescher** [Johann Friedrich *Miescher,* Swiss pathologist, 1811–1887] Miescher's tube, Miescher's tubule. See under SARCOCYST.

***Miescheria*** \mēshē′rē·ə\ *SARCOCYSTIS.*

**MIF** 1 migration inhibition factor (of macrophages). 2 melanocyte stimulating hormone inhibiting factor.

**migraine** \mī′grān\ [French (from Gk *hēmikrania* headache on one side of the head, from *hēmi-* half + *kranion* the upper part of the head, skull, a headache) hemicrania, migraine] A common syndrome characterized by recurrent paroxysmal attacks of headache, often throbbing in character and sometimes, but not invariably, unilateral in distribution. The attacks, which often last for hours, less commonly for several days, are often preceded by visual phenomena, such as hemianopia, scotoma, teichopsia, or fortification spectra, or by sensory phenomena such as paresthesiae, and are usually accompanied by nausea or vomiting, and photophobia. The aura or warning is due to arterial constriction, the headache to extracranial and intracranial dilatation. Often the headache occurs without an aura, less commonly the aura is not followed by headache. Also *hemicrania*. **abdominal m.** Episodic abdominal symptoms such as pain and nausea or vomiting occurring in migraine sufferers. They are believed to represent migrainous equivalents. **complicated m.** An attack of migraine in which the manifestations of the aura, such as hemianopia, hemiplegia, aphasia, etc., are unusually severe or long-lasting or in which the attack is accompanied by exceptional manifestations such as syncope or epilepsy. **epileptic m.** 1 The concurrence of epilepsy and migraine in the same individual. 2 Headache resembling that of migraine preceding or following an attack of epilepsy. An obsolete and imprecise term. **facioplegic m.** Unilateral and transient facial palsy occurring in an attack of migraine. **hemiplegic m.** Migraine in which recurrent episodes of hemiplegia occur during the attacks. This disorder is often familial and probably of dominant inheritance. **menstrual m.** Migraine in which the attacks occur at or about the time of the menstrual periods. **ophthalmic m.** Any of several visual symptoms, such as transient amblyopia, hemianopia, photophobia, scintillating scotomata, and teichopsia, occurring as manifestations of the aura of migraine. In rare cases visual field defects may remain permanent, due to occlusion of retinal arteries or of one posterior cerebral artery. **ophthalmoplegic m.** Paresis or paralysis of one of the cranial nerves which innervate the external ocular muscles (usually the oculomotor, less often the abducens or trochlear) occurring during an attack of migraine. Some afflicted patients are found to have an intracranial aneurysm of the internal carotid artery, but in the majority, who suffer recurrent attacks, no such physical cause is demonstrated. Also *Charcot's disease, Möbius disease, Möbius syndrome, relapsing ophthalmoplegia*.

**migrainous** \mī′grānəs\ Relating to migraine.

**migrate** To move from place to place, as cells, parasitic organisms, large populations of animals, or individually perceived sensations.

**migration** [L *migratio* (from *migratus*, past part. of *migrare* to leave a place), a removal, changing of habitation] Movement from one place to another. **external m. of ovum** TRANSPERITONEAL MIGRATION. **internal m. of ovum** The passage of an ovum to the contralateral fallopian tube following ovulation. The ovum passes through the oviduct on the same side as ovulation and into the uterus, followed by entry into the other tube. **m. of ovum** The passage of the ovum through the fallopian tube following ovulation. **tooth m.** DRIFTING. **transperitoneal m.** The passage of an ovum to the contralateral fallopian tube following ovulation without passing through the uterus. Also *external migration of ovum*.

**Mikity** [Victor G. *Mikity*, U.S. radiologist, born 1919] Wilson-Mikity syndrome. See under SYNDROME.

**mikro-** \mī′krō-\ MICRO-.

**Mikulicz** [Johannes von *Mikulicz*-Radecki, Polish surgeon active in Germany, 1850–1905] 1 See under PROCEDURE, RESECTION, CELL, OPERATION. 2 Heineke-Mikulicz operation. See under HEINEKE-MIKULICZ PYLOROPLASTY. 3 Mikulicz aphthae. See under PERIADENITIS MUCOSA NECROTICA RECURRENS. 4 Mikulicz-Sjögren syndrome, Mikulicz-Radecki syndrome, Mikulicz syndrome. See under VON MIKULICZ SYNDROME.

**mil** [L *mil(le)* a thousand] A unit of volume, used epecially in pharmaceutical work, equal to one milliliter. An obsolete, popular unit.

**Miles** [William Ernest *Miles*, English surgeon, 1869–1947] See under OPERATION.

**milia** \mil′ē·ə\ Plural of MILIUM.

**miliaria** \mil′ē·er′ē·ə\ [L, fem. of *miliarius* (from *milium* millet) pertaining to millet] An eruption of minute vesicles, papules, or nodules, each of which is related to a sweat duct. It results from the obstruction of the duct at various levels and is associated with prolonged sweating. Also *sweat fever, summer eruption*. **m. crystallina** An eruption of minute, very superficial vesicles, each related to a sweat pore. It is caused by the obstruction of the sweat duct within the stratum corneum and is associated with profuse sweating. Also *sudamina, miliaria alba*. **m. papulosa** Miliaria characterized mainly by papules. Also *miliary papulosis*. **m. profunda** Miliaria marked by an eruption of skin-colored dermal papules or nodules due to the obstruction of the sweat duct within the dermis. It is often not itchy but may lead to anhidrosis and anhidrotic heat exhaustion. **m. propria** MILIARIA RUBRA. **pustular m.** Miliaria rubra or miliaria profunda in which the vesicles are purulent and are the result of bacterial infection. Also *miliary impetigo*. **m. rubra** Miliaria caused by the obliteration of the sweat duct within the epidermis. It manifests itself as minute erythematous papules or vesicles. Also *prickly heat, summer rash, miliaria propria, lichen tropicus*. **m. vesiculosa** Miliaria rubra or miliaria crystallina that is clinically evidenced by vesicle formation.

**miliary** \mil′ē·er′ē\ [L *milarius* (from *milium* millet) pertaining to millet] 1 Of a size roughly that of a millet seed (about 2 mm in diameter or somewhat less) and commonly multiple, as *miliary embolism, miliary tubercle*. 2 Characterized by miliary lesions, as *miliary tuberculosis*.

**milieu** \milyoo′, mēlyœ′\ [French (from *mi* middle, from L *medius* middle + French *lieu* place, from L *locus* place), center, middle, environment] Surroundings; environment. **m. extérieur** EXTERNAL ENVIRONMENT. **m. intérieur** INTERNAL ENVIRONMENT.

**milium** \mil′ē·əm\ [L (akin to Gk *melinē* millet) millet] (*pl.* milia) A white nodule in the skin, composed of densely packed keratin which forms a globular lesion. Also *whitehead, closed comedo, sebaceous tubercle*. **colloid m.** A degenerative disorder of the dermal connective tissue, characterized clinically by the development of yellowish translucent plaques or papules on skin exposed to light. Also *colloid acne, Wagner's disease, pseudomilium*. **milia neonatorum** Minute yellowish dots visible on a newborn infant's face, marking the orifices of sebaceous glands. Also *milium of the newborn*.

**milk** [Old English *milc, meolc, meoluc*] 1 The secretion of the mammary glands used for feeding infants. Milk from different animals varies in composition. All types contain water, protein, carbohydrate, and fats. Buffalo, goat, ass, mare, and ewe milks are often used as food, but bovine milk is most frequently used. 2 An aqueous suspension resembling milk in appearance, as *milk of magnesia*. **acidophilus m.** A milk soured by *Lactobacillus acidophilus*. It contains 0.1–2.0% fat with increased quantities of the other milk constituents. It is similar to soured buttermilk with a slightly acid flavor. It is used therapeutically in patients with gastrointestinal disorders as a means of changing the composition of the bacterial flora existing in the gastrointestinal tract. Also *lactic acid milk*. **adapted m.** Cows' milk which has been adapted to make it more similar to human milk. This usually involves reducing the proportion of protein, particularly casein, and increasing the ration of unsaturated to saturated fatty acid in the fat. **after-m.** The milk taken from the breast at the end of a feed. It has been suggested that the fat content of breast milk increases during a feed. Thus the after-milk should contain more fat than the milk removed from the breast at the beginning of a feed. Also *hind milk.* **breast m.** Milk produced by the mammary gland, especially that from a mother used to nourish an infant. Between 600–800 ml of milk can be produced by a woman daily for a period after she has given birth. The composition and daily output are little influenced by maternal diet except in starvation situations. However, the type of fat present in the milk and its quantitative content of water-soluble vitamins are affected by maternal food intake. The initial milk produced (colostrum) is rich in certain antibodies such as IgA. **certified m.** Milk that has been designated as being pure by a board of physicians or a medical milk commission. **condensed m.** Milk that has been evaporated to one third of its original volume and sweetened with sugar. The sugar acts as a preservative. Condensed milk is available as full cream or skimmed milk. Also *lactein, lactolin.* **diabetic m.** Milk that has had most of its lactose removed. **dried m.** Milk in a state of dryness resulting from evaporation of its water content using either spray-drying or roller-drying. **evaporated m.** Milk that has been reduced to approximately 45% of its original volume through evaporation of its water content. It contains not less than 7–8% fat and 25.5% total solids. **fore-m.** The first milk produced by the mammary gland at any one milking. It usually has a lower fat content than the after-milk. **fortified m.** Milk which has been supplemented with some nutrient such as vitamin D, cream, or egg-white and so has a higher nutrient content than in the natural state. **fortified vitamin D m.** Milk that contains 400 IU per quart or liter. It is obtained by adding vitamin D directly to the milk. **hind m.** AFTER-MILK. **homogenized m.** Milk treated mechanically after pasteurization to break down the fat globules into very small droplets of approximately equal size, which are evenly distributed throughout the milk. These globules absorb much of the milk protein, which stabilizes the emulsion and prevents the cream from rising to the top. **humanized m.** Cow's milk that has been modified to resemble human milk. The main changes are a reduction in the protein content from 3–4% to 0.9–1.0% and an increase in the lactose content from 5% to 7%. Also *modified milk.* **kefir m.** See under KEFIR FUNGUS. **lactic acid m.** ACIDOPHILUS MILK. **m. of magnesia** See under MAGNESIA. **modified m.** HUMANIZED MILK. **pasteurized m.** Milk that has been heated at low temperatures in order to destroy all its inherent pathogens. However, it still contains benign bacteria, such as the lactic acid bacteria and so sours within a few days. **roller-dried m.** Milk that has been dried by pouring it over the surface of internally heated rollers. The milk is spread over the rollers in a very thin layer and dries in a few seconds. It is then scraped off by rotating the rollers against a blade. The milk is subject to minimal damage but greater losses of vitamins B and C result than in the spray-drying procedure. **skimmed m.** Milk that has had the cream removed. In all other respects it is the same as whole milk. **sterilized m.** Milk that has been homogenized and maintained at a temperature of 104–116°C for 20–40 minutes to precipitate all the albumin contained in it. The albumin is filtered off and the milk is tested for turbidity before it is certified as sterilized. Ammonium sulfate is added to the milk and if any albumin is present it will be precipitated and the milk will become cloudy. If it has been properly sterilized no albumin remains and the milk will stay clear. **tuberculin-tested m.** Milk from cows that have been examined by a veterinary inspector and have been found free from tuberculin. **uterine m.** A whitish liquid, resembling milk, containing nutritious substances (proteins, fats, and carbohydrates have been identified) derived from secretion of uterine glands and by transudation through the uterine wall. It is present in the uterine cavity before implantation and is a source of nutrition for the blastocyst. It is also found between the chorion and the uterine epithelium in pigs and ruminants exhibiting epitheliochorial placentas. See also EMBRYOTROPH. **vegetable m.** Artificial milk made out of vegetables such as soya. It is sometimes used to feed infants who are allergic to milk or suffer from lactose intolerance. **vitamin D m.** Cow's milk that has been supplemented with vitamin D through irradiation by ultraviolet light, direct addition of the vitamin, or feeding of the cows with irradiated yeast. **witch's m.** A few drops of milk that may be expressed from a newborn infant's nipples during the first few days of life. Also *hexenmilch.*

**milking** A manual or mechanical technique for removing fluid from a body part. It can be used for reduction of local edema, or to obtain specimens of secretions such as might accumulate in the urethra.

**Milkman** [Louis Arthur *Milkman,* U.S. physician, 1895–1951] Looser-Milkman syndrome. See under MILKMAN SYNDROME.

**milkpox** \milk′päks\ ALASTRIM.

**Millard** [Auguste *Millard,* French internist, 1830–1915] Millard-Gubler paralysis, Gubler-Millard paralysis. See under MILLARD-GUBLER SYNDROME.

**Miller** [Thomas Grier *Miller,* U.S. physician, born 1886] Abbott-Miller tube. See under MILLER-ABBOTT TUBE.

**Miller Fisher** See under FISHER.

**milli-** \mil′ē-\ [L *mille* a thousand] A combining form denoting $10^{-3}$, one thousandth: used with SI units. Symbol: m

**milliampere-hour** In radiotherapy, the product of tube current in milliamperes and the exposure time in hours.

**millibar** \-bär\ [MILLI- + BAR] A unit of pressure equal to $10^{-3}$ bar; 100 pascals. A popular unit. Symbol: mbar, mb • The symbol *mb* is used especially in meteorology.

**millicurie** \-kyoo′rē\ [MILLI- + CURIE] A unit of activity of a radionuclide or of a radioactive source equal to $10^{-3}$ curie; $3.7 \times 10^6$ becquerels exactly. Symbol: mCi, mc. (outmoded) **m. destroyed** A unit of x-ray dosage; a dose equivalent to a drop of one millicurie in the radioactivity of a brachytherapy source. An obsolete unit. Symbol: mCiδ **intensity m.** The intensity of gamma radiation existing one centimeter from a one milligram point source of radium filtered by 0.5 millimeter of platinum, equal to 8.4 roentgens per hour; $3.612 \times 10^{-5}$ coulomb per kilogram second. An obsolete unit.

**millicurie-hour** A unit of total number of nuclear transformations or transitions equal to $10^{-3}$ curie hour; $1.332 \times 10^{11}$ transformations. Symbol: mCi·h, mc.h. (outmoded), mc-h (outmoded)

**milliequivalent** \-ikwiv′ələnt\ **1** A quantity equal to $10^{-3}$ of the equivalent weight of an element or compound. **2** The amount of substance in one milliliter of normal solution. Symbol: mEq

**milligram** \-gram\ [MILLI- + GRAM] A unit of mass or weight equal to $10^{-3}$ gram or $10^{-6}$ kilogram; 0.0154 grain. Symbol: mg **m.'s percent** The concentration of a solution expressed in milligrams per 100 milliliters. Also *milligram-percent.* Symbol: mg% **m. per liter** A unit of mass concentration equal to $10^{-3}$ gram per liter. Symbol: mg/l, $mg{\cdot}l^{-1}$

**milligram-hour** A unit of radiation dose equal to the radiation emission in one hour from a source having an equivalent radium content of one milligram. An obsolete unit. Also *milligramage.* Symbol: mg·h

**milligram-percent** MILLIGRAMS PERCENT. See under MILLIGRAM.

**milligray** \-grā\ [MILLI- + GRAY] A unit of absorbed dose in the field of ionizing radiation equal to $10^{-3}$ gray. Symbol: mGy

**Millikan** [Robert Andrews *Millikan,* U.S. physicist, 1868–1954] Millikan rays. See under COSMIC RAYS.

**millikatal** \-katal'\ [MILLI- + KATAL] A unit of catalytic activity equal to $10^{-3}$ katal; $10^{-3}$ mole per second. Symbol: mkat **m. per liter** A unit of catalytic concentration or concentration of enzymic activity equal to $10^{-3}$ katal per liter; one mole per meter cubed second. Symbol: mkat/l, mkat·$l^{-1}$

**milliliter** \-lē'tər\ [MILLI- + LITER] A unit of volume or capacity equal to $10^{-3}$ liter, $10^{-6}$ cubic meter, or one cubic centimeter; 0.034 fluid ounce. Symbol: ml

**millilitre** \-lē'tər\ *Brit.* MILLILITER.

**millimeter** \-mē'tər\ [MILLI- + METER] A unit of length equal to $10^{-3}$ meter; 0.039 37 inch. Symbol: mm **conventional m. of mercury** A unit of pressure equal to 13.5951 conventional millimeters of water; 133.322 pascals. Symbol: mmHg **conventional m. of mercury minute per liter** A unit of vascular resistance to flow; $79.9934 \times 10^6$ pascals second per meter cubed; 79.9934 kilopascals second per liter. Symbol: mmHg·min/l, mmHg·min·$l^{-1}$ **conventional m. of water** A unit of pressure, the pressure due to an ideal column of water of height one millimeter, of uniform density one gram per cubic centimeter, and under the action of the standard acceleration of 9.806 65 meters per second squared; 9.806 65 pascals. Symbol: $mmH_2O$ **cubic m.** A unit of volume equal to $10^{-9}$ cubic meter, or one microliter. Symbol: $mm^3$ **m. of mercury** See under CONVENTIONAL MILLIMETER OF MERCURY. **m. of mercury minute per liter** See under CONVENTIONAL MILLIMETER OF MERCURY MINUTE PER LITER. **square m.** A unit of area equal to $10^{-6}$ square meter; $10^{-2}$ square centimeter. Symbol: $mm^2$ **m. of water** See under CONVENTIONAL MILLIMETER OF WATER.

**millimetre** \-mē'tər\ *Brit.* MILLIMETER.

**millimicro-** \mil'ēmī'krə-\ [MILLI- + MICRO-] A combining form denoting $10^{-9}$: formerly used with SI units, now replaced by *nano-*. Symbol: mμ

**millimicrocurie** \-mī'krəkyoo'rē\ [MILLIMICRO- + CURIE] *Outmoded* NANOCURIE. Symbol: mμCi

**millimicrogram** \-mī'krəgram\ [MILLIMICRO- + GRAM] *Outmoded* NANOGRAM. Symbol: mμg

**millimicrometer** \-mī'krəmē'tər\ [MILLIMICRO- + METER] *Outmoded* NANOMETER.

**millimicron** \-mī'krän\ [MILLI- + Gk *mikron,* neut. of *mikros* little, small] *Outmoded* NANOMETER.

**millimole** \-mōl\ [MILLI- + MOLE[3]] A unit of amount of substance equal to $10^{-3}$ mole. Symbol: mmol **m. per liter** A unit of substance concentration equal to $10^{-3}$ mole per liter; one mole per cubic meter. Symbol: mmol/l, mmol·$l^{-1}$

**millirad** \-rad\ A unit of absorbed dose of ionizing radiation equal to $10^{-3}$rad; $10^{-5}$ gray. Symbol: mrad

**millirem** \-rem\ A unit of radiation dose equal to $10^{-3}$ rem; $10^{-5}$ joule per kilogram; $10^{-5}$ sievert or 10 microsievert. Symbol: mrem

**milliroentgen** \-rent'gən\ A unit of ionization exposure equal to $10^{-3}$ roentgen; $2.58 \times 10^{-7}$ coulomb per kilogram. Symbol: mR

**millisecond** \-sek'ənd\ [MILLI- + SECOND] A unit of time equal to $10^{-3}$ second. Symbol: ms

**Mills** [Charles Karsner *Mills,* U.S. neurologist, 1845–1931] See under TEST.

**Milroy** [William Forsyth *Milroy,* U.S. physician, 1855–1942] Milroy's disease. See under HEREDITARY LYMPHEDEMA TYPE I.

**milzbrand** \milts'bränt\ [German, anthrax, from *Milz* spleen + *Brand* a burning, fire, gangrene, necrosis] ANTHRAX.

***Mima*** \mī'mə\ A former genus of aerobic Gram-negative diplococci, now included in *Acinetobacter.*

**mimesis** \mimē'sis, mī-\ [Gk *mimēsis* imitation] The resemblance of one disease or condition to another. Also *mimosis.*

**mimetic** \mimet'ik, mī-\ **1** Of or relating to mimesis. **2** An agent that affects mimesis. Also *mimic.*

**mimic** \mim'ik\ **1** To imitate. **2** MIMETIC. **genetic m.** **1** A species that exhibits, through evolution of a genetically determined phenotype, a resemblance to selectively advantageous characteristics of another species. **2** GENOCOPY.

**mimicry** \mim'ikrē\ The imitation of one species by another in an adaptation tending to improve its survival chances. **antigenic m.** The antigenic similarity seen between unrelated macromolecules, especially with respect to the antigenic cross-reaction between components of group A streptococci and tissue-specific mammalian antigens. Such antigenic mimicry is believed to play a part in the pathogenesis of diseases such as rheumatic fever. Also *molecular mimicry.* **molecular m.** ANTIGENIC MIMICRY.

**mimosis** \mimō'sis\ MIMESIS.

**min** **1** Symbol for the unit, minute (of time). **2** In Great Britain, symbol for the obsolete unit, minim. **3** minimum.

**mind** [Middle English *minde, mynde,* from Old English *(ge)mynd* memory, akin to L *mens* mind and Gk *mania* madness] The organized total of psychological processes and contents that allow the individual to respond to external and internal stimuli in an integrated and dynamic way, relating response of the present to both the past and the future of the individual. The processes of perceiving, learning, thinking, remembering, feeling, and behaving with intelligence are its principal processes. The contents of the mind vary with experience. Adj. mental.

**Minderer** [Raymond *Minderer* (Mindererus), German physician, 1570–1621] Spirit of Mindererus. See under AMMONIUM ACETATE SOLUTION.

**mineral** [Med L *mineralis* (from *miner(a)* ore, a mine, from Old French *miniere* pertaining to mines, from *mine* a mine, + *-alis* -AL) pertaining to mines] Any substance of nonbiologic origin, including inorganic constituents of living matter. The meaning is extended to include petroleum, as its biologic origin is only remote. **trace m.'s** Minerals needed by the body in very small amounts. These include iodine, copper, manganese, magnesium, iron, cobalt, zinc, and chromium. Iodine is usually the only one lacking in the diet, although zinc deficiency is sometimes encountered in the United States, especially in children.

**mineralization** \min'ərəlīzā'shən\ The conversion of organic material into inorganic material. Examples include the deposition of salts in living organisms, e.g. calcium phosphate in bone formation, and the complete oxidation of organic compounds, so that their carbon and hydrogen are oxidized to carbon dioxide and water, and other elements present to inorganic oxidation products, whose amounts may be measured comparatively easily.

**mineralocorticoid** \min'ərəlōkôr'tikoid\ Any of the

class of corticosteroids that act principally on the renal retention of sodium and the excretion of potassium, such as aldosterone.

**minicell** \min′isel\ [*mini(ature)* + CELL] A small cell, produced frequently by some mutants by an abnormal cell division, that lacks a chromosome but contains all the constituents of the cytoplasm. The inclusion of plasmids makes these cells useful for obtaining the products of their transcription and translation.

**minifilm** \min′ifilm\ A small-sized radiographic film, usually of the chest, used for economy in large surveys.

**minim** \min′im\ [L *minim(us)* least, smallest] **1** In the United States, a unit of capacity for liquid measure only, equal to $^1/_{480}$ (US) fluid ounce or 0.0616115 milliliter. Symbol: minim **2** In Great Britain, a unit of capacity equal to $^1/_{480}$ (UK) fluid ounce or 0.0591939 milliliter. An obsolete unit. Symbol: min

**minimum** [L (neut. sing. of *minimus*, least, smallest, superl. of *parvus* little, small), the smallest amount or size; as adv., very little] (*pl.* minimums, minima) **1** The least or least possible degree or quantity. Abbr. min Adj. minimal. **2** Least in quantity, range, or extent.

**minipill** \min′ipil\ An oral contraceptive consisting of progestin only or progestin and very low doses of estrogen.

**minipolymyoclonus** \min′ipäl′imī′əklō′nəs\ [L *mini-(mus)* least, smallest + POLY- + MYO- + CLONUS] A type of action tremor of the limbs described in some patients with spinal muscular atrophy.

**Minkowski** [Oskar *Minkowski*, Russian pathologist active in Germany, 1858–1931] **1** Naunyn-Minkowski method. See under MINKOWSKI'S METHOD. **2** Minkowski-Chauffard syndrome. See under HEREDITARY SPHEROCYTOSIS.

**minocycline** $C_{23}H_{27}N_3O_7$. 4,7-Bis(dimethylamino)-1,4α, 4aα, 5α, 5aα, 6, 11, 12aα-octahydro-3, 10, 12, 12a-tetrahydroxy-1, 11-dioxo-2-naphthacenecarboxamide. A semisynthetic antibiotic belonging to the tetracycline group of agents. It has a wide range of actions and uses. The hydrochloride salt may be given orally or by intravenous infusion for infections, chiefly staphylococcal, that are responsive to tetracyclines as well as others that do not respond to them.

**minor** \mī′nər\ **1** Lesser or smaller: usually denoting the lesser of two similar structures. **2** One who has not yet reached the legal age (the age of majority) for being accorded the full civil rights of an adult. The age varies by jurisdiction. • See note at MAJORITY.

**minute** [L *minut(us)* (past part. of *minuere* to lessen) small, minute] **1** A unit of time equal to 60 seconds. Symbol: min **2** A unit of plane angle equal to $^1/_{60}$ degree; $\pi/_{10\,800}$ radian. Symbol: ′

**MIO** minimal identifiable odor.

**mio-** \mī′ō-\ [Gk *meiōn* (comparative of *mikros* small, little and of *oligos* few, little) smaller, less, fewer] A combining form meaning (1) little, smaller; (2) reduction, constriction. Also *meio-*.

**miocardia** \-kär′dē·ə\ SYSTOLE.

**miodidymus** \-did′iməs\ [MIO- + -DIDYMUS] CRANIOPAGUS PARASITICUS.

**miolecithal** \-les′ithəl\ [MIO- + LECITH- + -AL] Having little or no yolk, as the ova of placental mammals. Also *alecithal, isolecithal, oligolecithal, microlecithal.*

**miopus** \mī′əpəs\ [New L, from *mi(o)-* + Gk *ōps*, gen. *ōpos* eye, face] Unequal conjoined twins united at the head in such fashion that the face of one member is rudimentary.

**miosis** \mī·ō′sis\ [Gk *meiōsis* (from *meiōn*, comparative of *mikros* small and *oligos* small) a lessening, diminishing] Marked constriction of the pupil. Also *myosis.* Adj. miotic. **paralytic m.** Smallness of the pupil due to paralysis of the dilator muscle of the iris. **spastic m.** Smallness of the pupil due to excessive contraction of the iris sphincter.

**miotic** \mī·ät′ik\ **1** Pertaining to or causing miosis. **2** A medication, such as a parasympathomimetic drug or morphine, that causes constriction of the pupil. Also *myotic.*

**miracidium** \mir′əsid′ē·əm\ [New L (from Gk *meirax* boy, girl + New L *-idium*, diminishing suffix)] (*pl.* miracidia) The first-stage ciliated larva that emerges from the egg of a trematode. After hatching it moves rapidly in search of a specific snail intermediate host, which it must penetrate to continue its life cycle. In some groups (families Opisthorchiidae, Heterophyidae) the minute eggs are eaten by the snail. When they hatch, the larvae penetrate the snail's tissues from within to initiate the sporocyst-rediacercaria series of ontogenetic and multiplicative stages.

**Miracil D** A proprietary name for lucanthone hydrochloride

**mire** \mir\ [French (from *mirer* to reflect, see in a mirror) a sighting device] A luminous pattern used to measure curvature by reflection.

**mirror** [Middle English *mirour* (from Old French *mireour* mirror, from *mirer* to gaze at one's reflection in, from L *mirari* to wonder at, admire) mirror] A polished surface, as of glass, capable of reflecting images under illumination. **head m.** A concave mirror, worn on a headband or spectacle frame, used for focusing a beam of light from an outside source onto a small area to be examined. The observer looks through a hole in the center of the mirror into a well-illuminated, shadow-free field. Also *frontal mirror.* **laryngeal m.** A circular plane mirror used to examine the interior of the larynx and hypopharynx. It is around 2.5 cm in diameter, mounted at an angle of about 120 degrees on a slender shank and handle, and altogether some 22 cm in length. **nasopharyngeal m.** A small laryngeal mirror, around 1 cm in diameter, used to examine the nasopharynx. Also *postnasal mirror.* **van Helmont's m.** *Outmoded* CENTRUM TENDINEUM.

**mis-** \mis-\ MISO-.

**miscarriage** \miskar′ij\ [English *mis-*, prefix denoting badly + *carriage* (from Middle English *cariage* carriage, from Old North French *carier* to transport)] *Popular* SPONTANEOUS ABORTION.

**misce** [L, 2nd person sing. imperative of *miscere* to mix] Mix: a direction used in pharmacy.

**miscible** \mis′əbəl\ [Med L *miscibilis* (from L *misc(ere)* to mix + *-ibilis* English *-ible*) capable of being mixed] Capable of being mixed, without forming separate phases, as ethanol and water.

**mismatch** / **acoustic m.** A significant difference in acoustic impedance between two materials at the interface between them, which increases reflections and decreases transmission.

**miso-** \mis′ō-, mis′ə-\ [Gk *misos* hatred] A combining form meaning hatred. Also *mis-*.

**mist.** *mistura* (L, a mixture).

**mister** In the United Kingdom, a title of address prefixed to the name of a surgeon. Abbr. Mr. • Usage in Australia accords with that of Britain. In South Africa the usage is obsolescent, with *doctor* replacing it. *Mister* is still used of surgeons in New Zealand but is regarded by some as pretentious and is not used in universities. The title is never used in the United States, Canada, or Japan.

**mistura** [L (from *mistus*, also *mixtus*, past part. of *miscere* to mix; Gk *mixai*, first aorist inf. of *mignynai* to mix, mingle), a mixture] Mixture: used in pharmacy.

**mit.** *mitte* (L, send).

**Mitchell** See under WEIR MITCHELL.

**mite** [Old English *mīte* a small insect] A very small arachnid of the subclass Acari. The mites are an extremely large and varied group and occupy many different habitats. Most are under 1 mm long and many are microscopic. Most kinds of mite are free-living, predatory soil dwellers, feeding on various invertebrates, soil microbes, insect eggs, and other organisms. Many are parasitic for at least part of their life cycles, feeding on skin and blood of vertebrates. Others are permanent obligate parasites living within the skin. The abdomen and the cephalothorax are broadly joined, and segmentation is often difficult to discern. Four pairs of legs are present in nymphs and adults, but are reduced in follicular and scabies mites. Larvae have three pairs of legs. The tick-like mesostigmatic mites possess a hypostome while the others do not. Some 200 families are recognized. The current classification places the mesostigmatic mites and ticks in the order Parasitiformes, and the other mites in the order Acariformes and Opilioacariformes. Also *acarus*. **burrowing m.** A mite that forms burrows in the skin, as the female of the human scabies mite. **cheese m.** A mite of the species *Tyrophagus longior*. **chigger m.** A trombiculid mite; a chigger. **copra m.** A meal or grain mite causing copra itch, usually *Tyrophagus putrescentiae*. **face m.** A mite of the species *Demodex folliculorum*. **follicle m.** A mite of the genus *Demodex*. **grain m.** Any of various mites that are pests on grain crops. Many of them can cause dermatitis among workers handling these crops or their products. Also *meal mite*. See also TYROPHAGUS. **grain itch m.** A mite of the genus *Pyemotes*. **hair follicle m.** A mite of the genus *Demodex*. **harvest m.** A mite of the species *Trombicula autumnalis*. Also *harvest bug*. **mange m.** Any mite that causes mange, such as those of the genera *Chorioptes, Knemidokoptes, Psoroptes,* and *Sarcoptes*. **meal m.** GRAIN MITE. **red m.** An adult mite of the family Trombiculidae, the chigger mites. The mature mites, oval or figure eight in shape, are usually covered with a dense coat of bright red, velvety hairlike setae. Also *red bug*. **spider m.** A web-spinning mite of the family Tetranychidae that is a pest on various crops. A temporary itching dermatitis may develop in hop-pickers and other harvesters who become sensitized to the mites. Also *spinning mite*. **straw m.** A mite belonging to any of several genera of the family Pyemotidae, which is commonly found as a predator of insects, and which may produce skin lesions in humans associated with straw, hay, grains, or grasses.

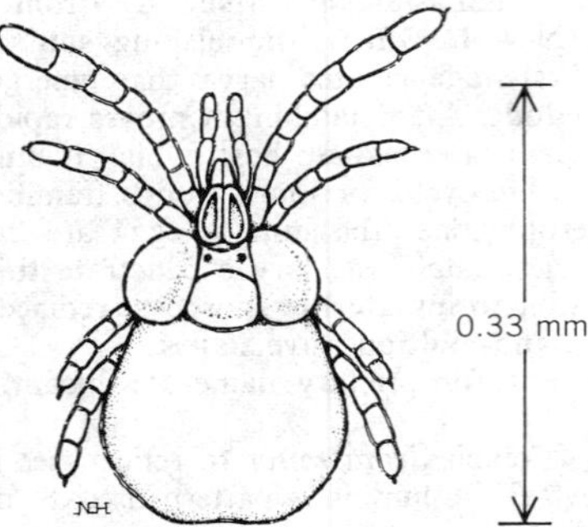

**Red mite** *(Trombicula)*

**mithramycin** \mith′rəmī′sin\ $C_{52}H_{72}O_{24}$. An antibiotic used chiefly as an antineoplastic agent. It is produced by *Streptomyces argillaceus, S. tanashiensis,* and *S. plicatus,* and is a yellow, crystalline powder. It is used therapeutically in the treatment of various testicular carcinomas which cannot be removed surgically. The agent is also used in the treatment of various forms of hypercalcemia secondary to carcinomas. It is given intravenously.

**miticidal** \mī′tisī′dəl\ [*mit(e)* + *i* + *-cid(e)* + -AL] Destructive to mites.

**mitigate** \mit′igāt\ To make or become milder; moderate.

**mitis** \mī′tis\ [L, sweet, soft, mild] Mild: used in prescription writing to denote the weaker of two available preparations.

**mito-** \mī′tō-\ [Gk *mitos* thread, web of the loom] A combining form meaning (1) thread, threadlike; (2) mitosis.

**mitochondrion** \-kän′drē·än\ [MITO- + Gk *chondrion* (dim. of *chondron,* also *chondros* a grain) a small grain, granule] (*pl.* mitochondria) A cytoplasmic organelle of eukaryotic cells, enclosed by a double membrane. The inner membrane infolds to form cristae which partially divide the inner compartment. Mitochondria may be rod-shaped, branched, spherical, or donut-shaped. The mitochondria represent the site of aerobic respiration in the cell. Mitochondria contain ribosomes and possess extranuclear genes. Division is by binary fission. Also *Altmann's granule, electrosome*. **giant m.** An unusually large mitochondrion, which is produced as a consequence of nutritional deficiencies, toxic influences, or the effects of electromagnetic fields. **m. of hemoflagellates** The single, extremely large mitochondrion characteristic of hemoflagellates, extending through much of the length of the body. Its structure varies with the biochemical activity at different developmental stages of the flagellate, being most elaborate in the midgut stage of the insect vector, and relatively simple, with few short and tubular cristae, in the blood-inhabiting, elongate stages in which the energy sources of the vertebrate host are utilized and the biochemical independence of the parasite is minimal.

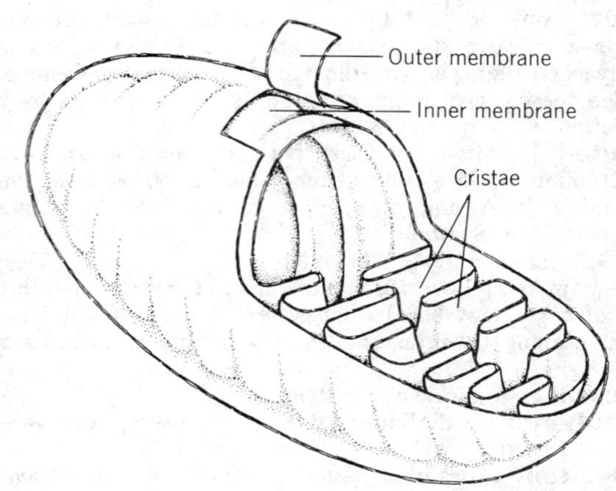

**Mitochondrion**

**mitocromin** An antibiotic employed chiefly as an antineoplastic agent. It is produced by the species *Streptomyces viridochromogenes*.

**mitogen** \mī′təjən\ [MITO- + -GEN] An agent which promotes mitosis. **pokeweed m.** A mitogen acting mainly on B cells derived from the plant *Phytolacca americana*.

**mitogenesis** \-jen′əsis\ [MITO- + GENESIS] **1** The initiation of mitosis. **2** Formation as a result of division by mitosis. For defs. 1 and 2 also *mitogenesia*.

**mitogenic** \-jen′ik\ Stimulating or promoting mitosis. Also *mitogenetic*.

**mitomalcin** An antibiotic agent used chiefly for its antineoplastic activity. It is a product of the species *Streptomyces malayensis*.

**mitomycin** \-mī′sin\ A group of antibiotic substances produced by species of *Streptomyces* and differentiated as mitomycin A, B, and C. Mitomycin C inhibits cell division by blocking the cross-linking of DNA strands, thus preventing DNA synthesis. It is used as an antineoplastic agent.

**mitoschisis** \mitäs′kisis\ [MITO- + Gk *schisis* a cleaving, division] KARYOKINESIS.

**mitosis** \mītō′sis\ [MITO- + -OSIS] (*pl.* mitoses) The division of the nucleus of a cell to produce two daughter nuclei, each having a genome identical with that of the parent nucleus. Mitosis is a genetically controlled process and is usually followed by cytokinesis. Mitosis is divided into four phases beginning with prophase during which the reduplicated chromosomes appear in species-specific number. At the beginning of prophase the chromosomes appear as long threads consisting of two chromatids each. During prophase the chromosomes become progressively shorter and more compact. Prophase ends with the disruption of the nuclear envelope, the formation of the spindle, and the movement of chromosomes toward the metaphase plate. During metaphase, the second phase of mitosis, the chromosomes reach the metaphase plate with all centromers aligned at the spindle equator. Anaphase follows metaphase with the separation of the sister chromatids and their movement toward the opposite poles of the spindle. During telophase, which commences as the chromatids arrive at the poles, the nuclear envelope is reformed, and the chromatin is uncoiled. Also *karyomitosis, mitotic cycle, indirect nuclear division* (older term). **anastral m.** Mitosis in which asters are not present. **astral m.** Mitosis characterized by the presence of centrioles, asters, and a spindle, as generally observed in animal cells. **asymmetrical m.** A mitotic division in which the two daughter cells have unequal chromosome numbers, a result of an irregular chromosome distribution or a reduction in chromosome number in one nucleus. **heterotypic m.** Mitosis in which the sister chromatids are united at their ends, forming ring structures. **homeotypic m.** Mitosis in which two asters are present, daughter chromosomes separate, and one daughter chromosome of each type moves to each aster. This is the typical mitotic sequence. **multipolar m.** Mitosis in which three or more asters are present at the poles of the spindle resulting in the formation of a nucleus at each aster. The result is an aberrant chromosome distribution. It is a mechanism by which polyploid cells reduce ploidy. Also *multicentric mitosis*.

**mitotic** \mītät′ik\ Of or pertaining to mitosis. Also *karyomitotic*.

**mitral** \mī′trəl\ **1** Denoting a structure in the shape of a turban or of a bishop's miter. **2** Pertaining to the mitral valve of the heart.

**mitralization** \mī′trəlīzā′shən\ A configuration of the heart shadow, consisting of straightening of the left cardiac border, often resulting from stenosis of the mitral valve with enlargement of the left atrial appendage and the pulmonary artery.

**mitroid** \mī′troid\ Having the shape of a miter.

**Mitsuda** [Kensuke *Mitsuda*, Japanese physician, born 1876] **1** Mitsuda reaction, Mitsuda test. See under LEPROMIN TEST. **2** Mitsuda antigen. See under LEPROMIN.

**mittelschmerz** \mit′əlshmerts\ [German *mittel* middle + *Schmerz* pain] Pain in the lower abdomen at the time of ovulation. Also *dysmenorrhea intermenstrualis, intermenstrual pain*.

**Mittendorf** [William F. *Mittendorf*, U.S. physician, flourished late 19th century] See under DOT.

**mix** / **case m.** The composition of the practice of a health care provider, program, or organization according to types of case, as specified by diagnoses. Also *case-mix*. **patient m.** The composition of the practice of a health care provider, program, or organization according to the number and types of patients served.

**mixer** / **amalgam m.** A machine for mixing dental alloy and mercury. The components are placed in a capsule with a steel ball and vigorously vibrated.

**mixing** / **vacuum m.** The mixing of plaster of Paris and water in a state of partial vacuum in order to reduce the size of air bubbles in the final mixture.

**mixotrophic** \miks′ōträf′ik\ Able to oxidize inorganic substrates, and therefore lithotrophic, but also able to use organic substrates and often showing enhanced growth with them.

**Mixter** [Samuel Jason *Mixter*, U.S. surgeon, 1855–1926] See under DILATOR.

**mixture** [L *mistura*. See MISTURA.] A combining or blending of two or more substances without chemical reaction, so that the properties of the components are retained. Pharmaceutical mixtures usually contain a solid component dispersed as a suspension in a liquid containing gum acacia, sugar, or some other viscid substance. Also *admixture*. **ACE m.** A mixture of alcohol, chloroform, and ether, formerly used as an inhalation anesthetic. **compound m. of senna** A liquid extract of senna, magnesium sulfate, extract of licorice, tincture of cardamom, and aromatic spirit of ammonia. It has been used as a laxative. Also *black draft, haustus niger*. **expectorant m.** A mixture of ammonium carbonate, fluid extract of senega and squill, camphorated tincture of opium, syrup of tolu, and water. It is used to loosen and increase bronchial secretions. Also *pectoral mixture*. **extemporaneous m.** A mixture prepared at the time ordered from a prescription, rather than from a stock supply. **kaolin m. with pectin** A mixture containing kaolin, pectin, tragacanth, benzoic acid, saccharin, glycerin, and peppermint oil in purified water. It is used as an adsorbant medication and as a lenitive agent. **magnesium hydroxide m.** CREAM OF MAGNESIA. **pectoral m.** EXPECTORANT MIXTURE. **Ringer's m.** RINGER SOLUTION. **toxin-antitoxin m.** See under TOXIN-ANTITOXIN. **Vincent's m.** A combination of sodium hypochlorite and boric acid that has been used to cover surgical or traumatic wounds.

**Miyagawa** [Yoneji *Miyagawa*, Japanese bacteriologist, 1885–1959] Miyagawa bodies. See under BODY.

***Miyagawanella*** \mē′yəgä′wənel′ə\ *Obs.* CHLAMYDIA.

**MK** monkey lung cells (as used in tissue culture).

**MKS** meter-kilogram-second (system).

**ML** midline.

**ml** Symbol for the unit, milliliter.

**μl** Symbol for the unit, microliter.

**MLA** mentolaeva anterior (a fetal position).

**MLC** mixed lymphocyte culture.

**MLD** **1** median lethal dose. **2** minimal lethal dose.

**MLP** mentolaeva posterior (a fetal position).

**MLT** mentolaeva transversa (a fetal position).

**MM** 1 mucous membrane. 2 myeloid metaplasia (agnogenic myeloid metaplasia).

**mm** 1 Symbol for the unit, millimeter. 2 muscles, musculi.

**mμ** 1 Symbol for millimicro-. 2 Symbol for the obsolete unit, millimicron.

**μm** 1 Symbol for the unit, micrometer. 2 Symbol for micromilli-.

**mμg** Symbol for the unit, millimicrogram (nanogram).

**μmg** Symbol for the unit, micromilligram (nanogram).

**μμg** Symbol for the unit, micromicrogram (picogram).

**mmHg** Symbol for the unit, conventional millimeter of mercury.

**MMI** methylmercaptoimidazole.

**μmm** Symbol for the unit, micromillimeter (nanometer).

**mmol** Symbol for the unit, millimole.

**μmol** Symbol for the unit, micromole.

**MMPI** Minnesota multiphasic personality inventory.

**mmpp** millimeters partial pressure (partial pressure as expressed in conventional millimeters of mercury).

**MMTV** mouse mammary tumor virus.

**Mn** Symbol for the element, manganese.

**M'Naghten** [Daniel *M'Naghten*, British criminal, died 1865] M'Naghten test. See under M'NAGHTEN RULE.

**mnemonic** \nēmän′ik\ [Gk *mnēmonik(os)* (from *mnēmōn* remembering, from *mnasthai* to remember, + *-ikos* -IC) pertaining to memory] Aiding the recall of verbal or numerical materials from memory.

**mnemonics** \nēmän′iks\ [Gk *mnēmon(ika)*, neut. pl. of *mnēmon(ikos)* (from *mnēmōn* mindful + *-ikos* -IC) pertaining to memory + -ICS] The use, or devising, of techniques to facilitate memory and rote learning. Also *mnemotechnics*.

**MO** mesio-occlusal.

**Mo** Symbol for the element, molybdenum.

**mobility** \mōbil′itē\ [L *mobilitas* (from *mobilis* movable, from *movere* to move + *-itas* -ITY) mobility] The capacity for movement. **electrophoretic m.** The velocity at which ions of a substance migrate in an electric field. It has the dimensions of velocity divided by potential gradient. Relative values are often stated rather than absolute ones.

**mobilization** \mō′bilīzā′shən\ A process or an operation whereby an object or a substance is freed or made mobile, as, for example, a physical therapy technique to restore the normal range of motion to a joint or body part whose movement has become restricted. **chromosome m.** The conjugative transfer of part or all of a bacterial chromosome, resulting from integration of a plasmid that codes for transfer of itself. **stapes m.** The transmeatal operative mobilization of the stapes ankylosed by otosclerosis. It is intended to restore the impaired hearing. It has been almost entirely superseded by stapedectomy. Also *stapediolysis, stapes mobilization operation.*

**mobilizer** \mō′bilī′zər\ **patient m.** An electric device for transferring an immobile patient from a bed to a gurney. A thin sheet of rollers moves under the patient and, in conveyer belt fashion, retracts back to the gurney, bringing the patient along with it.

**Mobitz** [Woldemar *Mobitz*, German cardiologist, born 1889] Mobitz-type atrioventricular dissociation. See under BLOCK.

**Möbius** [Paul Julius *Möbius*, German neurologist, 1853–1907] 1 See under SIGN, SYNDROME. 2 Möbius disease, Möbius syndrome. See under OPHTHALMOPLEGIC MIGRAINE. 3 Ledyen-Möbius dystrophy. See under LIMB-GIRDLE MUSCULAR DYSTROPHY.

**moccasin** \mäk′əsən\ [from the Algonquian] Any venomous snake of the crotaline genus *Agkistrodon*. **water m.** A semiaquatic venomous snake of the species *Agkistrodon piscivorous.* Also *cottonmouth.*

**MOD** mesio-occlusodistal.

**modality** \mōdal′itē\ [French *modalité* (from Med L *modal(is)* modal + French *-ité* -ITY, from L *mod(us)* measure + *-alis* -AL) form, mode] A major functional category: sight and hearing, for example, are sensory modalities; chemotherapy and radiotherapy are therapeutic modalities.

**mode** \mōd\ [L *modus* a measure, standard, manner, mode] 1 The most frequent value of the variable in a frequency distribution. 2 A specific manner of operation or presentation. Adj. modal. **A m.** A mode of ultrasonic imaging in which the horizontal axis in the display represents depth and the vertical axis represents echo amplitude. **B m.** A mode of ultrasonic imaging in which the display presents a two-dimensional image of a slice through the body with brightness contours determined by echo amplitude. **isocontour m.** In radiation therapy, a display mode in which contours are plotted, each representing the locus in space of a preselected level of radiation intensity, often defined by count rate. **list m.** A data collection technique in nuclear medicine in which the position information of each detected radioactive event is recorded, together with its time of collection relative to other pulses collected during the study. It is a particularly helpful method of collecting dynamic data since images and activity curves in time mode can be constructed. **M m.** A mode of ultrasonic imaging in which the display records a spot brightening for each echo received, producing a one-dimensional display of reflector position and motion versus time. Also *TM mode.* **radial m.** Oscillation of an ultrasound transducer in the radial direction. **TM m.** M MODE.

**model** [French *modèle* (from Italian *modello* a model, pattern, from L *modus* a measure, standard + *-ulus* -ULE) an object that is reproduced by imitation] A means by which something else can be visualized or represented, as an object fashioned on the same or a smaller scale after something else (as of anatomic parts) or a representation in a different form, as in mathematical symbols or computer codes, to provide a basis for analysis or experimentation. **animal m.** A pathologic condition or physiologic event occurring in an animal species but analogous to or illuminative of an event occurring in humans. **Danielli-Davson m.** A representation of the molecular arrangement of the components of the cellular membranes in which a lipid layer separates two protein layers. The lipids are phospholipids and are arranged in two monomolecular layers with their hydrophobic tails toward the inside of the membrane and their hydrophilic phosphates toward the surface protein. **Hassell-Varley m.** A mathematical model found useful in describing certain host-parasite and predator-prey population interactions. **Watson-Crick m.** A molecular model which represents the structure of deoxyribonucleic acid as a double helix with a right-handed coiling. The two strands of the helix are composed of antiparallel strands of polynucleotides. See also DEOXYRIBONUCLEIC ACID.

**modeling** The normal process by which a child comes to acquire appropriate social and cognitive behaviors by observing and imitating the behavior observed by significant others, such as parents or older sibs. This copying is in its turn rewarded and positively reinforced by members of the social group. Modeling thus serves as an important mechanism for the socialization of new members.

**modelling** *Brit.* MODELING.

**modification** \mäd′əfikā′shən\ [L *modificatio* (from *modus* a measure, standard + *-ficatio* -FICATION) the measuring of a thing] A change in an organism that is acquired or learned and does not involve heredity.

**modifier** \mäd′əfī′ər\ MODIFYING GENE.

**modiolus** \mōdī′ələs\ [L (dim. of *modius* a measuring vessel), a drinking vessel, hub of a wheel, instrument for cutting out bone] 1 [NA] The conical central bony axis of the cochlea which is tunneled by longitudinal canals and a spiral canal for the conduction of nerves and vessels, while projecting outward throughout its length is the osseous spiral lamina. Its broad base is at the lateral end of the internal acoustic meatus. 2 MODIOLUS LABII. **m. labii** A nodular mass just lateral to the angle of the mouth where muscle fibers of the upper and lower lips decussate with each other and with those of several other facial muscles, such as the zygomaticus major and minor, levator anguli oris, depressor anguli oris, and buccinator muscles. Also *modiolus.*

**mod. praesc.** *modo praescripto* (L, in the manner prescribed).

**modulation** \mäj′əlā′shən\ [L *modulatio* (from *modulatus,* past part. of *modulari* to measure, modulate) a rhythmical measure] 1 The functional and morphologic adaptation of cells to changes in environment. 2 The change in amplitude or pitch of the voice. 3 Variation of the amplitude, frequency, or phase of a single-frequency wave (carrier wave) in order to transmit a message such as in radio. **amplitude m.** Modulation of the amplitude, usually of a carrier radio wave by an audio signal wave. Abbr. AM **frequency m.** Modulation of the frequency, usually of a radio carrier wave by an audio signal wave. Abbr. FM **intensity m.** Variation of the electron beam current in a cathode ray tube to achieve variation in brightness of the image, as for example in a television or ultrasonic monitor.

**modulator** \mäj′əlā′tər\ In embryology, an inductor that specifically produces features related to definite regions during development.

**modulus** \mäj′ələs\ [L (dim. of *modus* a measure), a small measure] The ratio between the logarithm of a number to one base (especially the Naperian logarithm) and the logarithm of that number to another base. **m. of elasticity** The factor of proportionality in the mathematical equation expressing the experimental law that when a body is subjected to a mechanical stress, the resulting fractional deformation (called strain) is up to a point, proportional to the applied stress. **Young's m.** A coefficient of elasticity of a substance, as a bone, pertaining to the change in dimension under unidirectional tension or compression, expressed in pascals. It is defined as the ratio of the tensile or compressional stress (force per unit cross-sectional area) to the fractional change in dimension parallel to the stress. Symbol: *E*

**Moeller** [Julius Otto Ludwig *Moeller,* German physician, 1819–1887] Moeller's glossitis. See under CHRONIC SUPERFICIAL GLOSSITIS.

**Moersch** [Frederick Paul *Moersch,* U.S. neurologist, born 1889] Moersch-Woltman syndrome. See under STIFF-MAN SYNDROME.

**mogi-** \mäj′ē-\ [Gk *mogis* with difficulty] A combining form meaning with difficulty.

**mogiarthria** \-är′thrē-ə\ [MOGI- + ARTHR- + -IA] A form of dysarthria in which spasm, similar to that of writer's cramp in the hand, involves the muscles of articulation.

**Mohs** [Frederic Edward *Mohs,* U.S. surgeon, born 1910] See under CHEMOSURGERY.

**moiety** \moi′itē\ [Middle English *moite* (from Middle French *moité,* also *moitié* a half, from L *medietas* the middle, mean, from *medius* middle) half] 1 An approximate half; either of two parts of equal status. 2 One of two or more main components, such as the groups of atoms in a complex molecule.

**mol** Symbol for the unit, mole.

**molality** \mōlal′itē\ The amount of substance of a solute divided by the mass of the solvent, expressed in moles per kilogram. Abbr. molal

**molar**[1] \mō′lər\ 1 Divided by amount of substance: divided by mole. 2 Having a concentration of one mole per liter. See also MOLE[3].

**molar**[2] [L *molar(is)* (from *mola* a mill, millstone) pertaining to a mill, millstone; as substantive, a millstone, huge stone, grinding tooth, molar] Any of the most posterior teeth in each jaw, two per quadrant in the human deciduous dentition and three per quadrant in the human permanent dentition. Also *molar tooth, multicuspid tooth, multicuspidate.* **dome-shaped m.** See under SYPHILITIC TOOTH. **Moon's m.** See under SYPHILITIC TOOTH. **mulberry m.** See under SYPHILITIC TOOTH. **third m.** The third tooth from the front of the molar series; the most posterior tooth of the human permanent dentition. Also *wisdom tooth.*

**molarity** \mōlar′itē\ The concentration of a substance expressed in moles per liter.

**mold**[1] [Middle English *moulde,* past part. of *moulen* to become moldy; prob. akin to Gk *mykēs* fungus and *myxa* mucus, L *mucus* mucus] Any fungus having a cottony appearance, abundant in damp, dark locations, that is highly destructive to stored materials though an essential element of recycling of organic material and soil formation. Also *mould* (British spelling). **slime m.** Any of a heterogeneous group of eukaryotic organisms, with both ameboid and moldlike phases in their life cycles. They include the acellular slime molds (myxomycetes) and the cellular slime molds (acrasiae).

**mold**[2] [Old French *modle,* from L *modulus* a measure] 1 A hollow form in which a plastic material is shaped or cast. 2 To shape or cast in a mold. 3 That which is cast in a mold. 4 The shape of a molded object, such as an artificial tooth. For defs. 1–4 also *mould* (British spelling). **ear m.** A plastic fitting molded to the contours of the entrance to the external auditory meatus, forming part of an electrical hearing aid. **refractory m.** A mold for dental casting that can withstand high temperature.

**molding** 1 A process whereby an object or a mass is caused by surrounding objects or pressures to assume a certain shape. 2 The shaping of the fetal head during labor and delivery that facilitates passage through the birth canal. **border m.** The shaping of the borders of a dental impression by the action of the adjacent soft tissues in function or by manipulation. Also *tissue molding, muscle-trimming.* **compression m.** Forming a cast by using a mold of which the two parts are first separated and a mass of plastic material, such as acrylic resin in the "dough" stage of setting, is placed between them. They are then forced together and the material sets, usually with the application of heat, to the shape of the mold. This is the method used most frequently in the making of dentures. **injection m.** Forming a cast by injecting a fluid material into a mold through tunnels. The material then sets, usually by the cooling of previously heated thermoplastic material, to the shape of the mold. **tissue m.** BORDER MOLDING.

**mole**[1] [Old Englih *māl* (possibly akin to Gk *miainein* to stain, defile) a blemish, spot] A circumscribed, pigmented lesion of the skin, often slightly elevated; nevus pigmentosus. Also *soft nevus, nevocytic nevus.* **hairy m.** NEVUS PILOSUS. **pigmented m.** A benign cutaneous nevus derived from the melanocyte system. **warty m.** A raised cutaneous lesion that is usually derived from the melanocyte system and that bears a superficial resemblance to a viral wart.

**mole²** [L *mola* (akin to Gk *mylē* mill) salt cake, a mill, millstone, mooncalf, mole, false conception] An amorphous mass or tumor that forms in the uterus after degeneration of the conceptus. It usually consists of blood clots and remnants of the placenta and fetal membranes, but it may be calcified or develop cysts, as a hydatidiform mole. **carneous m.** A spontaneous abortion in which the ovum is surrounded by a capsule of clotted blood. Also *blood mole, hemorrhagic mole.* **cystic m.** HYDATIDIFORM MOLE. **fleshy m.** A degenerated retained placenta having a fleshy appearance. Also *maternal mole.* **grape m.** HYDATIDIFORM MOLE. **hemorrhagic m.** CARNEOUS MOLE. **hydatid m.** HYDATIDIFORM MOLE. **hydatidiform m.** A trophoblastic lesion characterized by large grapelike, edematous, avascular chorionic villi. Trophoblastic cells may show signs of proliferation, but the lesion is benign. Also *grape mole, cystic mole, hydatid mole, vesicular mole.* **invasive m.** CHORIOADENOMA DESTRUENS. **invasive hydatidiform m.** CHORIOADENOMA DESTRUENS. **malignant m.** CHORIOADENOMA DESTRUENS. **malignant hydatidiform m.** CHORIOADENOMA DESTRUENS. **maternal m.** FLESHY MOLE. **metastasizing m.** CHORIOADENOMA DESTRUENS. **placental m.** Degeneration of the placenta to form a variety of intrauterine mole. **true m.** A mole derived from a degenerating ovum. **tubal m.** The residue of a conceptus, comprising clotted blood and degenerating chorionic villi, in a tubal pregnancy. **tuberous m.** A type of missed abortion in which only chorionic vesicles surrounded by blood clot, placenta, and decidua are expelled. Also *tuberous subchorial hematoma, subchorial tuberous hematoma of the placenta, hematomole.* **vesicular m.** HYDATIDIFORM MOLE.

**mole³** [*(gram) mole(cule)* or German *Mole(kulargewicht)* molecular weight] The SI base unit of amount of substance, equal to that amount of substance of a system which contains as many elementary entities as there are atoms in 0.012 kilogram of carbon 12. When the mole is used, the elementary entities must be specified and may be atoms, molecules, ions, electrons, other particles, or specified groups of such particles. Also *gram molecular weight* (obs.). Symbol: mol **m. per cubic meter** The SI derived unit of substance concentration. Symbol: $mol/m^3$, $mol{\cdot}m^{-3}$ **m. per kilogram** The SI derived unit of molality, or of substance content. Symbol: mol/kg, $mol{\cdot}kg^{-1}$ **m. per liter** A unit of substance concentration equal to $10^3$ mole per cubic meter. Symbol: mol/l, $mol{\cdot}l^{-1}$ **m. per second** The SI derived unit of catalytic (or enzymatic) activity. Symbol: mol/s, $mol{\cdot}s^{-1}$

**molecular** \məlek′yələr\ **1** Concerned with molecules, as with the mass or structure of a single molecule. **2** Relating to the study of structures and processes occurring at the molecular level, especially of the macromolecules that are components of living matter, as in *molecular biology.*

**molecule** \mäl′ikyool\ [Late L *molecula*, dim. of L *moles* a mass, shapeless mass, trouble, burden] The smallest entity of a substance. It is composed of atoms. **effector m.** **1** A cell or organ that responds to a stimulus, such as a nervous impulse, by an active process, such as secretion or contraction. **2** In the operon model of genetic regulation, a molecule that interacts with and either enhances or inhibits the action of the repressor. **3** A metabolite of a biochemical pathway that interacts with and modifies the activity of an enzyme catalyzing a reaction in the pathway.

**molimen** \mōlī′mən\ [L (from *moliri* to struggle, labor), a great exertion] The effort exerted in the performance of a bodily function: sometimes applied to the discomfort associated with menstruation. **menstrual m.** Perimenstrual symptoms, such as swelling and cramps.

**Molisch** [Hans *Molisch*, Austrian botanist and chemist, 1836–1937] See under REACTION, TEST.

**Moll** [Jakob Anthoni *Moll*, Dutch anatomist and ophthalmologist, 1832–1914] Moll's glands. See under GLANDULAE CILIARES PALPEBRARUM.

**Mollaret** [Pierre *Mollaret*, French neurologist, born 1898] Mollaret's meningitis. See under BENIGN RECURRENT ENDOTHELIOLEUKOCYTIC MENINGITIS.

**Mollicutes** \mäl′ikyoo′tēz\ [L *mollis* soft + *cutis* skin] The class of bacteria commonly referred to as mycoplasmas. It has two families, Mycoplasmataceae, which require sterols for growth, and Acholeplasmataceae, which do not. Genera include *Mycoplasma, Acholeplasma, Ureaplasma, Spiroplasma, Thermoplasma*, and *Anaeroplasma*.

**mollities** \mōlish′i·ēz, mōlī′ti·ēz\ [L (from *mollis* soft, tender, pliant, mild), softness, pliancy, flexibility, weakness, effeminacy. Also *mollitia*.] Abnormal softening, denoting a portion of an organ or part of the body softened by necrosis. *Obs.* **m. ossium** OSTEOMALACIA. **m. unguium** A softness of the nail. *Rare.*

**mollusc** \mäl′əsk\ MOLLUSK.

**Mollusca** \mälus′kə\ [New L, from neut. pl. of L *molluscus* rather soft. See MOLLUSCUM.] A major phylum of invertebrate animals constituting some 45 000 extant species in seven classes, and including a variety of marine, freshwater and terrestrial types, ranging from microscopic specimens to those quite large in size. Examples include snails, slugs, clams, whelks, limpets, octopuses, and squids.

**molluscicidal** \mälus′isī′dəl\ [MOLLUSC + *i* + *-cid(e)* + -AL] Toxic to mollusks.

**molluscum** \məlus′kəm\ [L (from *mollis* soft) an excrescence or gall that grows on trees] An eruption of soft cutaneous nodules. **m. contagiosum** A benign infectious disease of the skin caused by a poxvirus and characterized by small, rounded, pearly white, umbilicated papules which yield basophilic, Feulgen-positive, intracytoplasmic inclusion bodies. The lesions appear most often on the trunk and anogenital area. Infection is transmitted by direct contact and by fomites. Venereal spread has been suggested. Also *molluscum epitheliale, molluscum verrucosum, condyloma subcutaneum, molluscum.* **m. giganteum** Molluscum contagiosum with large lesions. **m. verrucosum** MOLLUSCUM CONTAGIOSUM.

**mollusk** \mäl′əsk\ A member of the phylum Mollusca. Also *mollusc*. Adj. molluscan.

**Moloney** [Paul Joseph *Moloney*, Canadian physician, 1870–1939] Moloney reaction. See under TEST.

**Moloy** [Howard Carman *Moloy*, U.S. obstetrician and gynecologist, 1903–1953] Caldwell-Moloy classification. See under CLASSIFICATION.

**mol wt** molecular weight.

**molybdate** Any anion with a central molybdenum atom, especially $MoO_4^{2-}$, or a salt containing such an anion. Molybdate is used in biochemistry to test for phosphate and to test for reducing agents, especially tyrosine residues in proteins, in the Folin test. Phosphate and molybdate can react to form the ion $PMo_{12}O_{40}^{3-}$, and its partial reduction to a mixture of Mo(V) and Mo(VI) gives an intensely blue complex.

**molybdenum** \mōlib′dənəm\ Element number 42, having atomic weight 95.94. A silvery white, very hard metal, which is never found native but is widely distributed in various ores of other metals. It is an important alloying element in steel and has other technologic applications. Biologically, it is an essential trace element in plant nutrition and is required for activity of several animal enzymes. Symbol: Mo

**moment of death** That point in time when an individual is declared dead. This determination is based upon criteria which are defined by law and which differ according to the situation. For autopsy or burial purposes, criteria include the clinical judgment that respiration and circulation have ceased as well as the appearance of a secondary indication of death, such as livor or algor mortis. If tissues are to be obtained for organ transplantation, a criterion such as brain death is employed even though functional circulatory and respiratory activities may persist.

**momentum** \məmen′təm\ [L, that which moves the balance, weight, movement, motion] The product of the mass and velocity of a body, an index of the "quantity of motion." In a collision, total momentum is conserved. **angular m.** A vector quantity expressing the quantity of angular motion, depending on the rotational speed and the distribution of mass relative to the axis of rotation.

**mon-** \män-, mən-\ MONO-.

**monacolin K** LOVASTATIN.

**monad** \män′ad, mō′nad\ **1** A solitary unicellular organism, especially a free-swimming flagellate such as one of the genus *Monas*. **2** A single chromatid or member of a tetrad in meiosis. **springing m.** A flagellate protozoan of the species *Bodo saltans*.

**Monakow** [Constantin von *Monakow*, Russian-born Swiss neurologist, 1853–1930] **1** Striae of Monakow. See under STRIAE MEDULLARES VENTRICULI QUARTI. **2** See under SYNDROME. **3** Monakow's bundle, fasciculus aberrans of Monakow, Monakow's fasciculus, Monakow's fibers, Monakow's tract, von Monakow's fibers. See under TRACTUS RUBROSPINALIS. **4** Clarke-Monakow nucleus, Monakow's nucleus. See under NUCLEUS CUNEATUS ACCESSORIUS.

**monarthric** \-ärth′rik\ MONOARTICULAR.

**monarthritis** \-ärthrī′tis\ [MON- + ARTHRITIS] Arthritis of a single joint. Compare OLIGOARTHRITIS, POLYARTHRITIS. **traumatic deforming m.** Degenerative osteoarthrosis affecting a joint that was previously damaged by injury.

**monarticular** \-ärtik′yələr\ MONOARTICULAR.

**monaster** \-as′tər\ An aberrant spindle apparatus which may arise by the suppression of centriole division. When a monaster forms, the chromosomes fail to separate.

**monauchenos** \-ôk′ənəs\ [MON- + Gk *auchēn*, gen. *auchenos*, the neck] Equal conjoined twins with complete union in all parts except the head, resulting in a single trunk with two heads on a single neck. Also *dicephalus monauchenos*.

**monaural** \-ôr′əl\ Using only one ear or, in sound amplification, only one channel of transmission.

**monaxial** \-ak′sē·əl\ **1** Of or denoting a neuron possessing only one axon. **2** Denoting a structure organized around a single axis, as a monaxial filament.

**Mönckeberg** [Johann Georg *Mönckeberg*, German pathologist, 1877–1925] Mönckeberg's arteriosclerosis, Mönckeberg's degeneration, Mönckeberg's mesarteritis, Mönckeberg's medial sclerosis. See under MÖNCKEBERG SCLEROSIS.

**Mondor** [Henri Jean Justin *Mondor*, French surgeon, 1885–1962] See under DISEASE.

**monellin** A two-chain, 94-residue protein found in the fruit of an African shrub, *Dioscoreophyllum cumminsii*, and exhibiting a sweetness $10^5$ times greater than that of sucrose on a molar basis. It is temperature-sensitive and easily spoiled.

**monesthetic** \-esthet′ik\ [MON- + ESTHETIC] Describing, relating to, or affecting a single sense or variety of sensation.

**monestrous** \-es′trəs\ Characterized by the occurrence of estrus once each year; having one mating period a year.

**Monge** [Carlos *Monge*, Peruvian physician, 1884–1970] Monge's disease. See under MOUNTAIN SICKNESS.

**mongol** \mäng′gəl\ A person with the Down syndrome. An imprecise and outmoded term.

**mongolism** \mäng′gəlizm\ *Outmoded* DOWN SYNDROME. **translocation m.** *Outmoded* TRANSLOCATION DOWN SYNDROME.

**Mongoloid** \mäng′gəloid\ **1** Characterized by or similar to the physical features of the peoples of eastern Asia. **2** An individual having such physical features. • The term *mongoloid* (not capitalized in this sense) was formerly much used in reference to the Down syndrome. This usage is not recommended.

**monilated** \män′ilā′tid\ MONILIFORM.

**monilethrix** \mōnil′əthriks\ [L *monile* a necklace, collar + Gk *thrix* hair] A developmental defect of the hair shaft in which it becomes beaded and brittle. Elliptical nodes, 0.7–1 mm apart, are separated by internodes at which the medulla is lacking.

***Monilia*** \mōnil′ē·ə\ [L, pl. of *monile* a collar, necklace] *Obs. CANDIDA.*

**Moniliaceae** \mōnil′ē·ā′si·ē\ [*monili(a)* + -ACEAE] A form-family of fungi which includes many saprobes, but in addition has included numerous plant and animal parasites, including human pathogens. Also *Perisporiaceae* (obs.).

**monilial** \mōnil′i·əl\ **1** Pertaining to the form-family Moniliaceae. **2** *Incorrect* CANDIDAL.

**moniliasis** \män′ilī′əsis, mōn′-\ [*Monil(ia)* + -IASIS] *Older term* CANDIDIASIS. **oral m.** THRUSH.

**moniliform** \mōnil′ifôrm\ [L *monili(a)*, pl. of *monile* collar, necklace + -FORM] Having a structure suggestive of a string of beads. Also *monilated*.

**monitor** [L (from *monitus*, past part. of *monere* to remind, warn, foretell, chastise, akin to *monstrare* to show, demonstrate and to *meminisse* to remember; + *-or* OR), an adviser, admonisher] **1** To keep close watch over; check carefully and continually. **2** An apparatus used to record or display data, as of physiologic signs of a patient under continuous surveillance. See also under MONITORING. **apnea m.** An alarm system for alerting attendants to the occurrence of apnea, usually in a premature infant. Two types are in common use. One consists of an air mattress in which the breathing or any other slight movement causes a flow of air across a thermistor, producing resistance changes which can operate an electrical alarm if they cease. The other type is an impedance pneumograph which detects changes in electrical impedance through the chest during breathing.

**monitoring** [MONITOR + -ING] **1** The maintenance of close and sometimes continuous supervision, especially over patients considered at risk, often utilizing electronic equipment to monitor vital functions. **2** Periodic or continuous surveillance of a radioactive source or area, including the people in it, to provide early warning of adverse changes. The instruments used are designed to detect low-level ionizing radiation of various kinds, especially neutrons and gamma rays. **biological m.** BIOASSAY. **cardiac m.** The continuing observation of the functions of the heart, notably the electrocardiogram and vascular pressures. **electronic fetal m.** A method whereby patterns of fetal heart rate and uterine contractions are recorded utilizing an electronic instrument. Prolonged depression of heart rate following a contraction is predictive of an increased likelihood of fetal death. **wound m.** A periodic surveillance of a burn or other open wound using bacterial cultures. Increasing colony counts predict impending infection. High colony counts (generally considered greater than 100 000 organisms per gram of tissue) make successful wound closure

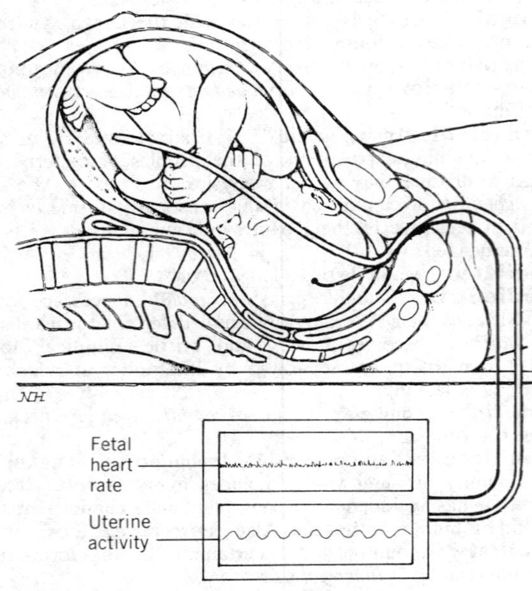


**Electronic fetal monitoring**

less likely. See also QUANTITATIVE CULTURE.

**monkey** [prob. of Germanic origin, akin to Old Spanish *mona* monkey] Any member of the families Cebidae and Cercopithecidae. **rhesus m.** A large macaque, *Macaca mulatta*, distributed over a large area including northern India, southern China, and all of southeast Asia. Because it is plentiful and easily raised in captivity, it is widely used in medical and biological research.

**mono-** \män′ə-, män′ō-\ [Gk *monos* single, only, standing alone] **1** A combining form meaning one, single. **2** A combining form denoting the presence of a single atom of a specified element in a molecule or a single grouping within a molecule. Also *mon-*.

**monoamine** Any amine containing only one amino group.

**monoamine oxidase** The flavin-containing amine oxidase (EC 1.4.3.4). It oxidizes primary amines with dioxygen, and forms an aldehyde, hydrogen peroxide and ammonia. It also acts on secondary and tertiary amines with small substituents. It is important in the catabolism of epinephrine and tyramine. The traditional name. Also *tyraminase* (obs.), *tyramine oxidase*.

**monoamino acid** An amino acid with only one amino group, usually an amino acid without a basic group in its side chain.

**monoamniotic** \-am′nē·ät′ik\ [MONO- + AMNIOTIC] Possessing a single amnion, as in a certain type of twinning. See also MONOZYGOTIC TWINS.

**monoarticular** \-ärtik′yələr\ [MONO- + ARTICULAR] Pertaining to a single joint. Also *monarthric, monarticular, uniarticular, uniarticulate*.

**monoauricular** \-ôrik′yələr\ Of or relating to only one auricle.

**monobacterial** \-baktir′ē·əl\ Pertaining to or caused by a single species of bacteria: said especially of an infection.

**monoballism** \-bal′izm\ [MONO- + BALLISM] Hemiballismus confined to either the upper or the lower limb.

**monobasic** Having only one acidic group in its molecule: said of an acid.

**monobenzone** $C_{13}H_{12}O_2$. 4-(Phenylmethoxy)phenol, the monobenzyl ether of hydroquinone. It has been used in ointment form to produce irreversible depigmentation of skin areas.

**monoblast** \män′əblast\ The precursor of mature monocytes. It is not normally present in blood or bone marrow.

**monoblastoma** \-blastō′mə\ MONOCYTIC LEUKEMIA.

**monobrachia** \-brā′kē·ə\ [MONO- + *brach(i)-* + -IA ] A condition marked by having one arm or forelimb. Also *unilateral brachial amelia*.

**monocarboxylic** Having only one carboxyl group in its molecule: used of a compound.

**monocellular** \-sel′yələr\ UNICELLULAR.

**monocentric** \-sen′trik\ **1** Having one center. **2** Of or relating to a chromosome that has one centromere.

**monocephalus** \-sef′ələs\ CEPHALOPAGUS.

**monochord** \män′əkôrd\ An instrument with a single string stretched over a sounding board, used at one time for the study of musical intervals but subsequently adapted for testing hearing. **Schultze m.** A monochord designed for testing high tone hearing, particularly the upper limit thereof. It has been rendered obsolete by electrical audiometers.

**monochorea** \-kôrē′ə\ [MONO- + CHOREA] Choreic movements restricted to a single limb.

**monochorionic** \-kôr′ē·än′ik\ [MONO- + CHORIONIC] Possessing a single chorion, as in a certain type of twinning. Also *monochorial*.

**monochroic** \-krō′ik\ MONOCHROMATIC.

**monochromasy** \-krō′məsē\ [MONO- + Gk *chrōma* color + *s* + -Y] COMPLETE COLOR BLINDNESS.

**monochromat** \-krō′mat\ [MONO- + Gk *chrōma* (gen. *chrōmatos*) color] A subject affected with total color blindness.

**monochromatic** \-krōmat′ik\ **1** Having or producing a single color. **2** Pertaining to total color blindness. For defs. 1 and 2 also *monochroic, monochromic*.

**monochromatism** \-krō′mətizm\ [MONO- + CHROMAT- + -ISM] COMPLETE COLOR BLINDNESS.

**monochromatophil** \-krōmat′əfil\ **1** A cell or a tissue element that readily combines with a single stain. **2** The property of combining with only one stain.

**monochromatophilic** \-krōmat′əfil′ik\ Capable of combining with or being stained by only a single dye: said of cells present in tissue sections. Also *monochromophilic*.

**monochromator** \-krō′mətər\ A spectograph that is adapted to allow isolation of a specific band of wavelengths for analysis or manipulation.

**monochromic** \-krō′mik\ MONOCHROMATIC.

**monochromophilic** \-krō′məfil′ik\ MONOCHROMATOPHILIC.

**monoclonal** \-klō′nəl\ Pertaining to or originating in a single clone of cells. All of the cells in such a clone would have identical products, such as specific antibodies or proteins. Compare POLYCLONAL.

**monocontaminated** \-kəntam′inā′tid\ Infected by or contaminated with a single species of organism: said of an animal that is otherwise germ-free. Also *monoxenic*.

**monocranius** \-krā′nē·əs\ CEPHALOPAGUS.

**monocrotic** \-krät′ik\ Characterized by a single wave uninterrupted by notches: said of a pulse. Compare DICROTIC, TRICROTIC.

**monocular** \mänäk′yələr\ [MON- + OCULAR] Pertaining to one eye only.

**monoculus** \mänäk′yələs\ [MON- + L *oculus* the eye] 1 CYCLOPS. 2 A bandage over one eye.

**monocyte** \män′əsīt\ [MONO- + -CYTE] A leukocyte which differs from the granular leukocytes by its larger size (12–20μm in diameter), and by a round or indented (kidney-shaped) nucleus. Its cytoplasm has no granules and on staining has a blue-gray frosted glass appearance. It is related to the tissue macrophages. Monocytes make up 3–6% of the circulating leukocyte population and are also found in marrow, lymphatic tissues, lung, and liver. Also *hyaline leukocyte* (obs.), *endothelial phagocyte.*

**monocytic** \-sit′ik\ Relating to monocytes.

**monocytoid** \-sī′toid\ Resembling a monocyte.

**monocytoma** \-sītō′mə\ MONOCYTIC LEUKEMIA.

**monocytopenia** \-sī′təpē′nē·ə\ A less than normal number of monocytes in the circulating blood. Also *monopenia, monocytic leukopenia.*

**monocytopoiesis** \-sī′təpoi·ē′sis\ The formation of monocytes in the bone marrow.

**monocytosis** \-sītō′sis\ [*monocyt(e)* + -OSIS] A greater than normal number of monocytes in blood.

**monodactyly** \-dak′tilē\ [MONO- + DACTYL- + -Y] The occurrence of a single digit on a hand or a foot.

**monodal** \mänō′dəl\ Connected to one terminal of a coil of wire so that high-frequency resonating current passes through the capacitance formed by the patient and ground.

**monodidymus** \-did′iməs\ [MONO- + -DIDYMUS] An individual that is one of twins.

**monodisperse** Occurring as suspended particles of uniform size.

**monoesterase** Any enzyme that catalyzes the hydrolysis of a monoester of an acid, usually phosphoric acid, that can form diesters.

**monofactorial** \-faktôr′ē·əl\ Relating to a single factor.

**monofilament** \-fil′əmənt\ A single filament, as of a synthetic material, used as a suture.

**monofilm** \män′əfilm\ MONOLAYER.

**monogenesis** \-jen′əsis\ 1 The production of offspring that are all of one type, or all of one sex, in each generation. 2 The production of uniparental progeny, as in nonsexual generation or in parthenogenesis. 3 MONOXENY.

**monogenetic** \-jənet′ik\ Pertaining to or characterized by monogenesis. Also *monogenous.*

**monogenic** \-gen′ik\ Pertaining to a phenotype or biologic process that is determined primarily by a single gene.

**monogenous** \mänäj′ənəs\ [MONO- + -GENOUS] 1 Derived from a single source. 2 MONOGENETIC.

**monoglyceride** A glycerol molecule acylated on one of its hydroxyl groups; a monoacylglycerol. *Outmoded.*

**monohybrid** \-hī′brid\ An offspring of two parents differing only in that each is homozygous for a different allele at a specific locus. The offspring is thus heterozygous at that locus.

**monohydrate** A substance with one molecule of water added per molecule of substance. This water may be bound, or may have crystallized together with the substance.

**monoinfection** \-infek′shən\ [MONO- + INFECTION] An infection caused by a single kind of organism.

**monoiodotyrosine** Tyrosine that is iodinated, usually on C-3, in distinction from tyrosine doubly iodinated, on C-3 and C-5, which is also a precursor in the biosynthesis of thyroxin.

**monolayer** \män′əlā′ər\ 1 A layer of molecules a single molecule thick. Such layers may form through the attraction of nonpolar parts of the molecules for each other, and the attraction of a polar end of each for the solvent. They are commonly encountered in studies of phospholipids. Also *monofilm, monomolecular layer.* 2 A cell culture preparation in which a single layer of uniformly contiguous cells completely covers the surface.

**monolepsis** \-lep′sis\ The appearance in offspring of the characteristics of one, but not the other, parent. *Seldom used.*

**monolobular** \-läb′yələr\ Pertaining to or possessing one lobule.

**monolocular** \-läk′yələr\ Composed of a single cavity.

**monomastigote** \-mas′tigōt\ [MONO- + MASTIGOTE] A mastigote with a single flagellum.

**monomelic** \-mē′lik\ Pertaining to, affecting, or possessing one limb.

**monomer** \män′əmər\ [MONO- + Gk *mer(os)* part] A single unit or molecule which can polymerize with similar units to form a chain or polymer. **fibrin m.** The monomer that results at the instant that fibrinogen loses its fibrinopeptides A and B. Such monomers promptly polymerize.

**monomeric** \-mer′ik\ Containing a single unit in its molecule, in contrast with substances in which two or more such units are joined.

**monomethylmorphine** CODEINE.

**monomicrobic** \-mīkrō′bik\ Pertaining to or characterized by the presence of a single species of a microorganism.

**monomorphic** \-môr′fik\ [MONO- + MORPH- + -IC] Having one form only; unchangable in form throughout development.

**monomorphism** \-môr′fizm\ [MONO- + MORPH- + -ISM] Possession of a single body form throughout the life cycle.

**monomorphous** \-môr′fəs\ Composed of cells or lesions of the same type.

**monomphalus** \mänäm′fələs\ [New L (from MON- + Gk *omphalos* navel)] OMPHALOPAGUS.

**mononeuralgia** \-n[y]Ural′jə\ [MONO- + NEURALGIA] Neuralgia in the region supplied by a single nerve.

**mononeuritis** \-n[y]Urī′tis\ [MONO- + NEURITIS] Neuritis affecting a single peripheral nerve. **m. multiplex** A syndrome of concurrent lesions of several individual peripheral nerves, as distinct from the syndrome of polyneuritis or polyneuropathy in which various components of the peripheral nervous system are diffusely involved in a disease process. Multiple involvement of peripheral nerves is usually of vascular origin, as in polyarteritis nodosa or the other collagen or connective tissue disorders, or due to inflammatory processes such as leprosy. • *Multiple neuritis* can also be used, but is better avoided as it has been used by some authors as a synonym of polyneuropathy.

**mononeuropathy** \-n[y]Uräp′əthē\ [MONO- + NEUROPATHY] Disease or dysfunction of a single nerve, as in the neuropathy of diabetes mellitus or carcinoma. **cranial m.** Disease or dysfunction of a single cranial nerve.

**monont** \män′änt\ [MON- + Gk *-ont,* combining form from *ōn,* gen. *ontos,* pres. part. of *einai* to be] *Obs.* SCHIZONT.

**mononuclear** \-n[y]oo′klē·ər\ Having a single nucleus: used especially of a cell. Also *mononucleate, uninuclear, uninucleate.*

**mononucleosis** \-n[y]oo′klē·ō′sis\ [*mononucle(ar cell)* + -OSIS] A greater than normal number of mononuclear leukocytes in the blood. Lymphocytes, monocytes, metamyelocytes, and more immature cells of the granulocytic, lymphocytic, and monocytic series are all mononuclear cells. **infectious m.** An acute infectious disease caused by the Epstein-Barr virus and most often affecting adolescents and young adults. It is usually characterized by fever, sore throat, malaise, fatigue, weakness, lymphadenopathy, hepatosplenomegaly, a mononuclear leukocytosis, atypical lymphocytes, and high titers of sheep erythrocyte agglutinins. The acute and convalescent phases of the disease may persist for months, and, rarely, the disease follows a chronic, relapsing course. An illness resembling infectious mononucleosis may be caused by other microbial agents, including *Toxoplasma gondii* and cytomegalovirus. Also *glandular fever, acute epidemic lymphadenosis, acute infectious adenitis, kissing disease* (popular), *Pfeiffer's disease, Filatov's disease.* **post-transfusion m.** An acute febrile illness that may follow transfusion, accompanied by lymphadenopathy, often by splenomegaly, and by the presence of numerous atypical lymphocytes in the blood. The condition is due to transmission of a virus, such as Epstein-Barr virus or cytomegalovirus. Also *postperfusion syndrome, post-transfusion syndrome.*

**mononucleotide** A nucleotide composed of a phosphorylated nucleoside, in distinction from one in which two or more such units are combined, as in nucleic acids.

**mono-osteitic** \-äs′tē·it′ik\ Denoting inflammation localized to a single bone.

**monoparesis** \-pərē′sis\ [MONO- + PARESIS] Paresis of a single limb or part of a limb.

**monoparesthesia** \-par′esthē′zhə\ [MONO- + PARESTHESIA] Paresthesia involving a single limb.

**monopenia** \-pē′nē·ə\ MONOCYTOPENIA.

**monophasic** \-fā′zik\ **1** Presenting only one phase or variation. **2** In electroencephalography, denoting a deflection of the trace to one side of the baseline only. **3** Exhibiting or characterized by monophasia.

**monophenol monooxygenase** A group of copper-containing enzymes (EC 1.14.18.1) that oxidize phenols such as tyrosine using dioxygen as oxidant, forming an *o*-quinone. They can use benzene-1,2-diols as substrates. Also *tyrosinase, monophenol oxidase* (outmoded).

**monophosphate** A compound bearing one phosphate group, in distinction from a diphosphate, which bears one residue of diphosphoric acid, or from a bisphosphate, which bears two separate phosphate groups.

**monophyletic** \-fīlet′ik\ Originating from a single ancestral type.

**monophyletism** \-fī′lətizm\ [MONO- + Gk *phylet(ēs)* one of the same tribe + -ISM] **1** The hypothesis that all blood cells originate from a common ancestral cell type. **2** The hypothesis that all living organisms are descended from a common ancestor.

**monophyletist** \-fī′lətist\ An individual who holds to the theory of the monophyletic origin of living organisms or of cells, such as blood cells.

**monoplastic** \-plas′tik\ UNICELLULAR.

**monoplegia** \-plē′jə\ [MONO- + -PLEGIA] Paralysis restricted to a single limb or part of a limb. Adj. monoplegic.

**monoploid** \män′əploid\ HAPLOID.

**monopodia** \-pō′dē·ə\ **1** The presence of a single foot, as in those forms of sirenomelus in which a symmetrical footlike structure is present at the distal end of the fused lower extremity. Also *sirenoid monopodia.* **2** A limb reduction deformity in which one foot is present and one missing, as in unilateral transverse hemimelia or unilateral apodia.

**monopus** \män′əpəs\ [New L (from MONO- + New L *-pus*, combining form denoting foot, from Gk *pous* foot)] SYMPUS MONOPUS.

**monorchidism** \mänôr′kidizm\ [MON- + *orchid(o)-* + -ISM] The condition of having one testis or the appearance of one testis when the other is undescended, as in cryptorchidism. Also *monorchia.*

**monosaccharide** \-sak′ərīd\ A simple sugar, in contrast with carbohydrates formed by glycosylation of one sugar by another.

**monosexual** \-sek′shoo·əl\ [MONO- + SEXUAL] Displaying the characteristics of a single sex.

**monosodium glutamate** The sodium salt of glutamic acid, with only one sodium ion per molecule of glutamic acid. Its solutions are neutral. It is used for enhancing the flavor of food, and in large doses it may cause discomfort to some people (Chinese restaurant syndrome).

**monosome** \män′əsōm\ [MONO- + Gk *sōma* body] **1** In a normally diploid cell or organism, any chromosome of the usual set lacking a homologue. This routinely occurs in the sex chromosomes of the heterogametic sex. For example, in the human male, the X and the Y chromosomes are monosomes. It also occurs whenever an aberrant meiosis or mitosis results in loss of an autosome. **2** A single ribosome bound to mRNA. Compare POLYSOME.

**monosomic** \-sō′mik\ Pertaining to or characterized by monosomy.

**monosomy** \män′əsō′mē, män′əsō′mē\ **1** Aneuploidy in which a normally diploid cell or organism lacks one chromosome of a homologous pair. **2** The chromosome complement of the heterogametic sex in which neither sex chromosome has a complete homologue. Each sex chromosome can be considered a monosome. *Seldom used.*

**monospermy** \-spur′mē\ [MONO- + SPERM + -Y] Fertilization effected by a single spermatozoon.

***Monosporium*** \-spôr′ē·əm\ A genus of ascomycetous fungi that causes mycetoma. Its perfect (sexual) stage is *Allescheria.*

**monostotic** \män′ästät′ik\ Pertaining to or involving a single bone. Compare POLYOSTOTIC.

**monostratified** \-strat′ifīd\ Arranged in a single layer or sheet. Also *monostratal.*

**monosymptom** \-simp′təm\ A symptom occurring in isolation.

**monosynaptic** \-sinap′tik\ Denoting or pertaining to a neuronal pathway, such as a reflex arc, containing only a single synapse.

**monoterpene** A substance whose molecules are composed of two isoprene residues, and have the general formula $C_{10}H_{16}$. It is found in plant oils.

**monotic** \mänō′tik\ Pertaining to one ear only. Also *uniaural.*

**monotrichous** \mänät′rikəs\ [MONO- + TRICH- + -OUS] Possessing a single flagellum. Also *monotrichate.*

**monovalent** \-vā′lənt\ UNIVALENT.

**monovular** \mänäv′yələr\ [MON- + OVULAR] Developed from a single ovum, as monozygotic twins.

**monovulatory** \mänäv′yələtôr′ē\ [MON- + OVULATORY] Liberating a single ovum at each ovulation in the reproductive cycle. This is usually characteristic of the human female.

**monoxenic** \män′äksē′nik\ MONOCONTAMINATED.

**monoxenous** \mänäk′sənəs\ [MONO- + *xen(o)-* + -OUS] Requiring only one host to complete the life cycle; autecious.

**monoxeny** \mänäk′sənē\ [MONO- + *xen(o)-* + -Y] A life cycle pattern, characteristic of many parasites, in which only one host is required for the organism to complete the cycle. Also *monogenesis.*

**monoxide** \mänäk′sīd\ Signifying the addition of one atom of oxygen per atom, or specified number of atoms, of another element, as in *carbon monoxide*, CO.

**monozygosity** \-zīgäs′itē\ [MONO- + ZYGOSITY] Development from a single fertilized ovum, as in certain twins.

**monozygotic** \-zīgät′ik\ [MONO- + ZYGOTIC] Developed from a single fertilized ovum, as in *monozygotic twins.* Also *enzygotic.*

**Monro** [Alexander *Monro,* Secundus, Scottish anatomist, 1733–1817] **1** Foramen of Monro. See under FORAMEN INTERVENTRICULARE. **2** Monro-Kellie doctrine. See under DOCTRINE. **3** Fissure of Monro, sulcus of Monro. See under SULCUS HYPOTHALAMICUS. **4** Monro's line. See under MONRO-RICHTER LINE.

**mons** \mänz\ [L, gen. *montis,* mountain] In anatomy, a prominence or an elevation. **m. pubis** [NA] The rounded prominence in front of the symphysis pubis formed by a varying mass of subcutaneous fatty tissue and covered by coarse hair at puberty. It is continuous inferiorly with the commissura labiorum anterior. Also *mons veneris.*

**Monson** [George S. *Monson,* U.S. dentist, 1869–1933] See under CURVE.

**monster** [L *monstrum* (from *monere* to warn, foretell) a thing shown, omen, monster] A congenitally deformed individual, particularly one whose malformations are severe. • This is a popular but archaic term that has much of the connotation of "sideshow freak."

**montage** \mäntäzh′, môNtäzh′\ [French (from *mont(er)* to mount, from L *mons,* gen. *montis,* a mountain, + French *-age* -AGE), a combining of various pictures, an assembling, mounting] In electroencephalography, an arrangement of electrodes applied to the scalp in such a way that the electrical activity of the entire brain or of a particular area of the brain can be recorded simultaneously. When using the bipolar technique, there is usually one electrode common to two successive leads, the three electrodes being in series, that is, connected in pairs to two amplifying channels, the common electrode being linked in opposite polarity to the two channels.

**Monteggia** [Giovanni Battista *Monteggia,* Italian surgeon, 1762–1815] Monteggia's fracture, Monteggia's dislocation. See under FRACTURE-DISLOCATION.

**Montgomery** [William Fetherston *Montgomery,* Irish gynecologist, 1797–1859] **1** Montgomery's tubercles. See under TUBERCLE. **2** Montgomery's follicles. See under FOLLICLE. **3** Montgomery's cups. See under NABOTHIAN CYSTS.

**monticulus** \mäntik′yələs\ A small eminence or elevation. **m. cerebelli** The eminence formed by the central portion of the cerebellar vermis.

**mood** [Middle English *mod, mood,* from Old English *mōd* spirit, akin to L *mos,* gen. *moris,* manner, custom, whence English *morae*] An enduring but not permanent emotional predisposition to react in a certain way, as with sadness or anger.

**mood-congruent** \-käng′groo·ənt\ In harmony with the prevailing affect, as are delusions or hallucinations whose content is consistent with the manic's ideas of inflated worth, or with the depressive subject's feelings of worthlessness, guilt, and need for retribution.

**Moon** [Henry *Moon,* English dental surgeon, 1845–1892] Moon's tooth. See under SYPHILITIC TOOTH.

**Moon** [Robert Charles *Moon,* U.S. ophthalmologist, 1844–1914] Laurence-Moon syndrome. See under SYNDROME.

**Moore** [Edward Mott *Moore,* U.S. surgeon, 1814–1902] See under FRACTURE.

**Moore** [Matthew Thibaud *Moore,* U.S. neuropsychiatrist, born 1901] Moore syndrome. See under ABDOMINAL EPILEPSY.

**Mooren** [Albert *Mooren,* German oculist, 1828–1899] See under ULCER.

**Mooser** [Hermann *Mooser,* Swiss pathologist active in Mexico, born 1891] Neill-Mooser reaction. See under SCROTAL REACTION.

**MOPP** The anticancer chemotherapeutic combination of nitrogen mustard (mechlorethamine), vincristine (Oncovin), procarbazine, and prednisone. It is especially effective in Hodgkin's disease.

**Morand** [Sauveur François *Morand,* French surgeon, 1697–1773] Vein of calcar avis of Morand. See under VEIN.

**Morawitz** [Paul Oskar *Morawitz,* German physiologist, 1879–1936] See under THEORY.

**Morax** [Victor *Morax,* French ophthalmologist, 1866–1935] **1** Morax-Axenfeld bacillus. See under BACILLUS. **2** Morax-Axenfeld conjunctivitis. See under ANGULAR CONJUNCTIVITIS.

***Moraxella lacunata*** \môr′aksel′ə lak′ʸoonā′tə\ A Gram-negative coccobacillus (family Neisseriaceae) that is parasitic on mucous membranes and occasionally causes conjunctivitis.

**morbid** \môr′bid\ [L *morbidus* (from *morbus* disease) diseased, disease-causing] **1** Affected by disease; in a diseased state; pathologic. **2** Causing or capable of causing disease; pathogenic.

**morbidity** \môrbid′itē\ [MORBID + -ITY] **1** A diseased state or character; ill health. **2** The result of exposing a person or group of persons to the causes of disease. **3** Within a given population, the number of sick persons or cases of disease recorded as of a stated point in time or over a stated period. Thus, morbidity may be expressed as the number of new cases arising (incidence) or the number of cases existing whether old or newly arisen (prevalence). **puerperal m.** A temperature of 100.4°F (38°C) occurring on any two of the first 10 postpartum days with the exception of the first 24 hours. The temperature must be taken by a standard oral technique at least four times a day.

**morbigenous** \môrbij′ənəs\ *Obs.* PATHOGENIC.

**morbilli** \môrbil′ī\ [Med L, pl. of *morbillus* pustule, dim. of L *morbus* disease] MEASLES.

**morbilliform** \môrbil′ifôrm\ [MORBILLI + -FORM] Resembling the eruption characteristic of measles.

***Morbillivirus*** \môrbil′ivī′rəs\ A genus of the Paramyxoviridae family that includes measles virus.

**morbus** \môr′bəs\ [L, a disease, sickness, grief] A disease. **m. basedowii** GRAVES DISEASE. **m. coxae senilis** Degenerative arthritis of the hip joint, especially of the aged. **m. dormitivus** **1** GAMBIAN TRYPANOSOMIASIS. **2** RHODESIAN TRYPANOSOMIASIS. **m. errorum** VAGRANTS' DISEASE. **m. maculosus neonatorum** HEMORRHAGIC DISEASE OF THE NEWBORN. **m. morsus muris** RAT-BITE FEVER. **m. saltatorius** CHOREA. **m. strangulatorius** DIPHTHERIA. **m. vagabondus** VAGRANTS' DISEASE.

**morcel** \môrsel′\ [French *morcel(er)* (from L *morsus* a bite, biting) to divide into pieces or parts] To remove in section rather than en bloc, as a tissue mass.

**morcellation** \môr′selā′shən\ [French *morcel(er)* (from *morceau* a piece, from L *morsus* a bite) to divide into parts + *l* + English -ATION] The division of a mass into many small sections in order to facilitate its surgical removal. Also *morcellement.*

**morcellement** \môrselmäN′\ MORCELLATION.

**mordant** \môr′dənt\ [French, pres. part. of *mordre* (from L *mordere* to bite) to bite] **1** An agent that combines with dye to form an insoluble compound. It is used to fix and intensify stains in tissue or cell preparations, or dyestuffs in textiles. Alum, anilines, and phenol are the most common histologic mordants. **2** To subject to the action of a mordant.

**mor. dict.** *more dicto* (L, in the manner directed).

**Morel** [Augustin Benoit *Morel,* French psychiatrist, 1809–1873] See under EAR.

**Morel** [Ferdinand *Morel,* Swiss psychiatrist and neurologist, 1888–1957] **1** Morel-Wildi syndrome. See under SYNDROME. **2** Stewart-Morel syndrome, Morgagni-Stewart-Morel syndrome, Morel syndrome. See under HYPEROSTOSIS FRONTALIS INTERNA.

**Morelli** [F. *Morelli,* Italian physician, died 1918] See under TEST.

***Morerastrongylus costaricensis*** \môr′ərasträn′jiləs käs′tərisen′sis\ A nematode that ordinarily infects the mesenteric arteries of wild rodents in tropical America. Human infection, reported usually in children, probably results from accidental ingestion of infected snails or slugs. Thickening of the wall of the cecum and appendix, with necrosis and heavy eosinophilic infiltration, is caused by blockage of arterioles by juvenile worms and eggs. Symptoms include intestinal pain and high fever. Also *Angiostrongylus costaricensis.*

**Morgagni** [Giovanni Battista *Morgagni,* Italian physician, 1682–1771] **1** See under CATARACT, CRYPT, FORAMEN. **2** Morgagni-Adams-Stokes syndrome. See under ADAMS-STOKES SYNDROME. **3** Morgagni's globules. See under GLOBULE. **4** Morgagni spheres. See under SPHERE. **5** Morgagni's glands. See under GLANDULAE URETHRALES URETHRAE MASCULINAE. **6** Fovea of Morgagni, crypt of Morgagni. See under FOSSA NAVICULARIS URETHRAE. **7** Morgagni's tubercle. See under MONTGOMERY'S TUBERCLE. **8** Morgagni's tubercle. See under BULBUS OLFACTORIUS. **9** Morgagnian cysts. See under APPENDICES VESICULOSAE EPOÖPHORI. **10** Columns of Morgagni. See under COLUMNAE ANALES. **11** Pedunculated hydatid of Morgagni. See under HYDATID. **12** Pedunculated hydatid of Morgagni. See under APPENDIX OF THE EPIDIDYMIS. **13** Morgagni's disease, Morgagni's hyperostosis, Morgagni-Stewart-Morel syndrome, Morgagni syndrome. See under HYPEROSTOSIS FRONTALIS INTERNA. **14** Cartilage of Morgagni. See under CARTILAGO CUNEIFORMIS. **15** Morgagni's caruncle. See under LOBUS MEDIUS PROSTATAE. **16** Hydatid of Morgagni. See under APPENDIX MORGAGNII. **17** Hydatid of Morgagni. See under APPENDIX TESTIS. **18** Frenulum of Morgagni, frenum of Morgagni. See under FRENULUM VALVAE ILEALIS. **19** Morgagni's nodules. See under NODULI VALVULARUM SEMILUNARIUM VALVAE AORTAE. **20** Morgagni's ventricle, sinus of Morgagni. See under VENTRICULUS LARYNGIS. **21** Morgagni's valves. See under VALVULAE ANALES. **22** Sinus of Morgagni. See under PROSTATIC UTRICLE. **23** Papilla of Morgagni. See under ANAL PAPILLA.

**Morgan** [Thomas Hunt *Morgan, U.S. geneticist, 1866–1945*] Morgan unit. See under MORGAN.

**morgan** \môr′gən\ [after Thomas Hunt *Morgan,* U.S. geneticist, 1866–1945] The standard unit of genetic map length, equal to the map distance between two loci that experience, on average, one cross-over during each meiosis. Distances between loci are usually expressed in centimorgans and are determined by the recombination fraction. Also *morgan unit.* Abbr. M

**morgue** \môrg\ [French] **1** A building or a room designated for the purpose of retaining unidentified or unclaimed bodies pending identification and disposition of the remains. **2** A building or room where dead bodies are retained for the purpose of autopsy and subsequent burial or cremation. For defs. 1 and 2 also *mortuary.*

**moria** \môr′ē·ə\ [Gk *mōria* (from *mōr(os)* silly + *-ia* -IA) silliness, folly] WITZELSUCHT.

**moribund** \môr′ibənd\ [L *moribund(us)* (from *mori* to die) about to die] Dying; close to death.

**Morison** [James Rutherford *Morison,* English surgeon, 1853–1939] Morison's pouch. See under RECESSUS HEPATORENALIS.

**Moro** [Ernst *Moro,* German pediatrician, 1874–1951] **1** Moro's reagent. See under TUBERCULIN. **2** See under TEST. **3** Moro's embrace reflex. See under MORO'S REFLEX.

**morph-** \môrf-\ MORPHO-.

**-morph** \-môrf\ [Gk *morphē* form, appearance] A combining form meaning an organism or part characterized by a specified form.

**morphea** \môrfē′ə\ [Med L] A circumscribed form of scleroderma, presenting as a central atrophic lesion with a pigmented border. It does not progress to systemic scleroderma. Also *localized scleroderma, kelis* (obs.), *Addison's keloid.* **acroteric m.** SCLERODACTYLY. **guttate m.** Morphea with small discrete lesions. This condition may be confused with lichen sclerosus. Also *white spot disease.* **linear m.** LINEAR SCLERODERMA. **m. pigmentosa** The pigmented component of a morphea lesion.

**morphine** \môr′fēn\ [L *Morph(eus),* god of dreams (in Ovid's *Metamorphoses*) + -INE] $C_{17}H_{19}NO_3 \cdot H_2O$. The white, crystalline, principle alkaloid of opium. Morphine is almost insoluble in water, alcohol, or ether, and it is levorotatory. It is a potent narcotic analgesic. It also causes drowsiness, respiratory depression, decreased gastrointestinal motility, nausea, vomiting, and changes in mood, including euphoria. Repeated use leads to tolerance, physical dependence, and addiction. Also *morphinium, morphina, morphia, morphium.*

**morphine sulfate** $(C_{17}H_{19}NO_3)_2 \cdot H_2SO_4 \cdot H_2O$. A white, crystalline salt of morphine soluble in water. This form of morphine is commonly used for various parenteral preparations.

**morphine tartrate** $(C_{17}H_{19}NO_3)_2 \cdot C_4H_6O_6 \cdot 3H_2O$. A white, crystalline powder form of morphine, much more soluble in water than morphine base and used for various parenteral preparations.

**morphinic** \môrfin′ik\ Relating to morphine.

**morphinism** \môr′finizm\ [*morphin(e)* + -ISM] **1** A diseased state brought on by the prolonged use of morphine. **2** Addiction to morphine.

**morphinium** \môrfin′ē·əm\ MORPHINE.

**morphinization** \môr′finīzā′shən\ Subjection to the effects of morphine.

**morphium** \môr′fē·əm\ MORPHINE.

**morpho-** \môr′fō-, môr′fə-\ [Gk *morphē* form, appearance] A combining form meaning form, structure. Also *morph-.*

**morphocytology** \-sītäl′əjē\ The science dealing with the morphology of the cell.

**morphodifferentiation** \-dif′əren′shē·ā′shən\ [MORPHO- + DIFFERENTIATION] The emergence of shape and form in a developing embryo, or in any of its parts or organs.

**morphogenesis** \-jen′əsis\ [MORPHO- + GENESIS] The development or evolutionary appearance of structural form or shape in an organism. It can be considered from both phylogenetic and ontogenetic viewpoints. It involves differentiation of cells and tissues coordinated spatially and at specific times in a definite order, and results in all parts and organs reaching specific relationships with one another and attaining the right cellular constitution and cell number and thus overall size.

**morphogenetic** \-jənet′ik\ Relating to or effecting morphogenesis, as *morphogenetic hormone.*

**morphology** \môrfäl′əjē\ [MORPHO- + -LOGY] The study of the form, shape, and structure of animals and plants. Also *tectology.* **colonial m.** The form of a bacterial colony, including such important features as size, shape, color, surface texture, opacity, and friability. These features are of considerable diagnostic significance. Observation requires well-isolated colonies in order to avoid changes due to inadequate nutrition or to interaction with products of neighboring colonies.

**morphoplasm** \môr′fəplazm\ The protoplasm which makes up the cellular reticulum.

**morphosynthesis** \-sin′thəsis\ [MORPHO- + SYNTHESIS] The activity performed in the cerebral cortex of the parietal lobes in integrating concepts of shapes, sizes, and interrelationships of parts of the body so as to produce a body image.

**-morphous** \môr′fəs, -môr′fəs, -mərfəs\ [Gk *morphē* form, appearance + English suffix *-ous*] A combining form meaning characterized by a specified form.

**Morquio** [Luis *Morquio,* Uruguayan physician, 1867–1935] Morquio's disease, Morquio syndrome, Morquio-Ullrich syndrome, Morquio-Brailsford syndrome. See under MUCOPOLYSACCHARIDOSIS IV.

**morrhuate sodium** The sodium salt of morrhuic acid, the oily yellow liquid that represents the fatty acids of cod-liver oil. The salt is used as a sclerosing material and is injected into varicose veins.

**Morris** [John McLean *Morris,* U.S. surgeon, born 1914] Morris syndrome. See under TESTICULAR FEMINIZATION.

**Morrison** [Ashton B. *Morrison,* U.S. pathologist, born 1922] Verner-Morrison syndrome. See under SYNDROME.

**morsal** [L *mors(us)* a bite, biting + -AL] OCCLUSAL.

**morselize** \môr′səlīz\ [*morsel* + -IZE] To divide into small bits or pieces, such as is done with larger fragments of bone or cartilage used to reshape an area of the skeleton. It is also used in treating premature closure of skull sutures.

**mor. sol.** *more solito* (L, in the usual way).

**morsulus** LOZENGE.

**mortal** [L *mortal(is)* (from *mors,* gen. *mortis,* death + *-alis* -AL) subject to death, causing death] **1** Subject to death. **2** Resulting in or causing death.

**mortality** \môrtal′itē\ [L, *mortalitas* (from *mortalis* subject to death, mortal, from *mors* death; + *-itas* -ITY) mortality, mankind] **1** The fact of being subject to death. **2** DEATH RATE. **fetal m.** STILLBIRTH RATE. **neonatal m.** Mortality during the first month or four weeks of life. **perinatal m.** The combined mortality from stillbirths and deaths in the first week of life. **postnatal m.** *Incorrect* POSTNEONATAL MORTALITY. **postneonatal m.** Mortality occurring between the end of the first month (neonatal period) and the age of one year. Also *postnatal mortality* (incorrect). **proportionate m.** PROPORTIONATE MORTALITY RATIO. **reproductive m.** The total mortality related to the reproductive function, including, in addition to deaths directly attributable to the complications of pregnancy, confinement, and the puerperium, associated deaths of pregnant or parturient women from other diseases such as diabetes and chest disease as well as deaths connected with the use of any form of contraception, temporary or permanent.

**mortar** A vessel with a rounded interior that is used for the crushing of drugs and other substances with a pestle.

**mortification** \môr′tifikā′shən\ [Late L *mortificatio* (from *mortificatus,* past part. of *mortificare* to kill, mortify, from L *mors,* gen. *mortis,* death + *-ficare* -FY) a killing, mortification] Gangrene or necrosis; death of a part.

**Mortimer** [Mrs. *Mortimer,* English patient of Sir Jonathan Hutchinson, flourished 19th century] Mortimer's disease. See under SARCOIDOSIS.

**mortinatality** \môr′tēnātal′itē\ [L *mors,* gen. *mortis* death + NATALITY] STILLBIRTH RATE.

**mortise** \môr′tis\ **ankle m.** The space occupied by the talus in the talocrural joint.

**Morton** [Dudley J. *Morton,* U.S. orthopedic surgeon, 1884–1960] See under SYNDROME.

**Morton** [Thomas George *Morton,* U.S. surgeon, 1835–1903] **1** Morton's neuralgia, Morton's toe. See under NEUROMA. **2** See under TEST.

**mortuary** \môr′choo·er′ē\ [L *mortuar(ius)* (from *mortu(us),* past part. of *mori,* also *moriri* to die, + *-arius* -ARY) pertaining to burial] **1** Pertaining to death. **2** MORGUE.

**morula** \môr′yələ, môr′oolə\ [New L (dim. of L *morum* a mulberry) a small mulberrylike object] A solid mass of cells formed by the cleavage of the fertilized egg. The arrangement of the blastomeres in the morula varies in different groups, the arrangement being orderly in some groups, such as batrachians, but more complex in others, such as mammals.

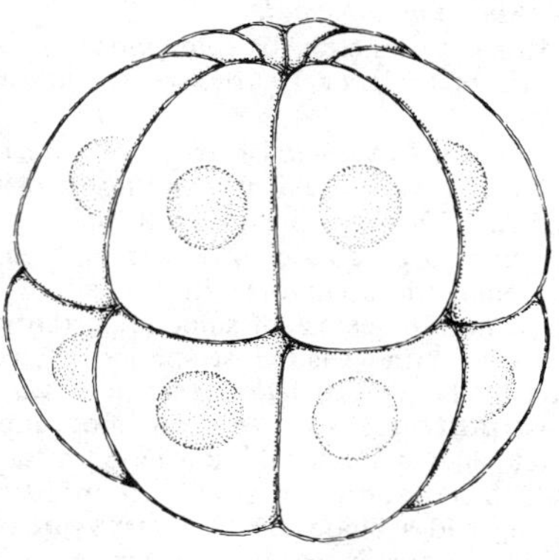

Morula

**morulation** \môr′yəlā′shən\ [MORULA + *-(a)tion*] The formation of a morula.

**morulus** \môr′yələs, môr′ooləs\ [See MORULA.] The lesion characteristic of yaws, resembling a mulberry or raspberry.

**Morvan** [Augustin Marie *Morvan,* French physician, 1819–1897] Morvan's disease. See under SYNDROME.

**mosaic** \mōzā′ik\ [French *mosaïque* (from Late L *musaicus* (adj.) mosaic, from L *musæum (opus)* mosaic (work), from Gk *mouseion,* neut. sing. of *mouseios* pertaining to the muses, from Gk *mousa* a muse) mosaic work] **1** In genetics, an individual whose cells consist of at least two genotypically distinct populations that arose after fertilization through somatic mutation or somatic nondisjunction. **2** Of or pertaining to such an individual. **3** A protein that contains multiple domains, some of which are shared with other proteins. It arises through gene duplication, exon shuffling, or other mechanisms that are obscure. **chromosomal m.** The state of being mosaic for a morphologic variation in karyotype. A common example in humans is an individual with one chromosomally normal cell line and another lacking (or having an additional) sex chromosome, such as 46,XY/45,X.

**mosaicism** \mōzā′isizm\ The state or situation of being mosaic. **erythrocyte m.** The presence of two distinct populations of erythrocytes in the blood of one individual, when not the result of blood transfusion or chimerism. Mosaicism usually occurs in erythrocytes (and all other cells) of women who are heterozygous for an X-chromosome-linked genetic trait such as glucose-6-phosphate dehydrogenase deficiency. Males, who have but one X-chromosome, do not exhibit mosaicism. **gonadal m.** In genetics, the presence in a gonad of a germ-cell line that is genotypically distinct from that comprising the rest of the individual. One potential result is the appearance in multiple offspring of a dominant phenotype not present in the parent. **haploid-diploid m.** A situation in which some of the component cells of an originally haploid individual have diploidized while others have remained haploid, so that both haploid and diploid cells of a genetically identical pedigree are present within the same individual. Compare HAPLODIPLOIDY.

**Mosher** [Harris Payton *Mosher,* U.S. surgeon and laryngologist, 1867–1954] Air cells of Mosher. See under CELL.

**Mosler** [Karl Friedrich *Mosler,* German physician, 1831–1911] See under SIGN.

**mosquiticidal** \məskē′təsī′dəl\ Lethal or destructive to mosquitoes. Also *mosquitocidal.*

**mosquiticide** \məskē′təsīd\ [*mosquit(o)* + *i* + -CIDE] An agent that is toxic or destructive to mosquitoes. Also *mosquitocide.*

**mosquito** \məskē′tō\ [Spanish (dim. of *mosca* a fly, from L *musca* a fly) a gnat, mosquito] Any insect of the dipteran family Culicidae. The eggs are generally laid on water, and larvae and pupae are aquatic. Most larvae feed on organic debris but some are predators. In the adult, females are bloodsuckers and are vectors of some important viral, protozoan, and filarial pathogens. Most species of medical importance belong to the genera *Aedes, Anopheles, Culex,* and *Stegomyia.* **anautogenous m.** A mosquito unable to produce viable eggs without taking a blood meal. **autogenous m.** A mosquito that is able to produce viable eggs without having had a blood meal. **eurygamous m.** A mosquito that requires extensive outdoor space for breeding. **house m.** Any of the abundant and widespread mosquitoes, such as *Culex pipiens,* that are commonly found living and feeding in human dwellings. **stenogamous m.** A mosquito able to breed in captivity or in limited space. **tiger m.** A mosquito of the species *Aedes aegypti.*

**mosquitocidal** \məskē′təsī′dəl\ MOSQUITICIDAL.

**mosquitocide** \məskē′təsīd\ MOSQUITICIDE.

**Mosso** [Angelo *Mosso,* Italian, physiologist, 1846–1910] See under ERGOGRAPH.

**moth** [Old English *moththe*] Any of numerous lepidopteran insects characterized by filamentous, often plumate antennae and usually nocturnal habits, in contrast with butterflies, which have smooth, knobbed antennae and are usually diurnal. **brown-tail m.** A moth of the species *Euproctis chrysorrhoea.* **flannel m.** A moth of the family Megalopygidae, especially one of the genus *Megalopyge.* The stout, hairy caterpillars have stinging hairs that can cause a painful urticaria. **Io m.** A moth of the species *Automeris io.* **tussock m.** A moth of the genus *Hemerocampa.*

**mother** [Old English *mōdor,* akin to L *mater* a mother and Gk *mētēr* a mother] **1** A woman who has borne a child; a female parent. **2** A pregnant woman, considered as distinct from her developing fetus. • This sense is commonly used in obstetrics, where a distinction between the fetus and the woman carrying it is often important. In such contexts, *mother* is equivalent to *expectant mother.* **3** The original model or central source from which similar units are derived. **4** A cell which divides to give rise to two daughter cells. Adj. maternal. **Colles m.** A clinically asymptomatic mother of a child with congenital syphilis. **expectant m.** A pregnant woman. **phallic m.** The male child's belief that his mother possesses a penis. **schizophrenogenic m.** A mother whose own psychopathology and handling of her child is a basic determinant in the subsequent development of schizophrenia in that child. **surrogate m.** **1** A woman who bears the offspring of another, typically infertile woman, whose partner's sperm is utilized, usually by artificial insemination, to achieve conception. *In vitro* development of the conceptus followed by early implantation in the uterus of the surrogate mother has also been successfully employed. **2** MOTHER SURROGATE. See under MOTHER SURROGATE.

**mothering / surrogate m.** The medicolegal practice by which a surrogate mother bears offspring for another woman and her male partner, by whose sperm she is impregnated, usually by artificial insemination, and relinquishes the offspring to the father and his partner following parturition. See also SURROGATE MOTHER.

**mother surrogate** An object or animal that performs or is perceived as performing one or more of the functions normally executed by the natural mother of a young animal, as a person acting as a substitute or deputy mother for an infant or child, or an animal of one species acting as a substitute for the offspring of an animal of a different species. Objects identified with warmth have also been used in experimental studies as mothers surrogate. Also *surrogate mother.* See also SURROGATE MOTHER.

**motile** \mō′til\ [L *mot(us)* (past part. of *movere* to move, stir, put in motion) + *-ilis,* -ILE[1]] Capable of self-generated movement, an important diagnostic criterion in bacteria.

**motilin** \mōtil′in\ A gastrointestinal polypeptide of 22 amino acids and molecular weight 2700, located in the enterochromaffin cells, chiefly of the duodenum and upper jejunum, having the effects of increasing gastric and colonic motility. It is released by changes in the pH of small intestinal contents.

**motility** \mōtil′itē\ [MOTILE + -ITY] The capacity for spontaneous movement. **automatic m.** SPONTANEOUS MOVEMENT. **segmental m.** Regularly spaced ring-like contractions of the small intestine that, as they disappear, are replaced by similar contractions in the segments of the intestine between those previously contracted. Also *segmentation movement, pendular movement.* **voluntary m.** VOLUNTARY MOVEMENT.

**motion** [L *motio* (from *movere* to move, impel) movement] **1** The act or process of moving; movement. **2** The process of defecation. **3** Matter defecated. **active m.** ACTIVE MOVEMENT.

**motivation** \mō′tivā′shən\ [*motiv(e)* + -ATION] The hypothesized inner state of a person or animal that serves to arouse, maintain, and guide behavior toward a goal.

**motoceptor** \mō′təsep′tər\ [*moto(r)* + *(re)ceptor*] A muscle sense receptor, such as a muscle spindle or Golgi tendon organ, located in muscle. *Seldom used.*

**motofacient** \mō′təfā′shənt\ Causing movement.

**motoneuron** \mō′tōn[y]oo′rän\ [*moto(r)* + NEURON] A central neuron whose target organ is an effector structure such as a muscle or gland; an efferent neuron conveying motor impulses. Also *motor neuron, motor cell, exciter neuron, peripheral motor neuron.* **$\alpha$-m.'s** Neurons of the anterior horn of the spinal cord which give rise to $\alpha$-efferents innervating skeletal muscles. Neuron soma sizes vary from about 20–100 $\mu$m, the larger ones innervating large pale muscle fibers, and the smaller supplying red muscle fibers. **$\beta$-m.'s** Neurons which give rise to $\beta$-efferents innervating both extrafusal and intrafusal fibers of muscle spindles. The axons are of the size of smaller $\alpha$-motoneuron axons and contribute to the $\alpha$-wave of an evoked neurogram recorded from the ventral root. **heteronymous m.'s** Motor cells supplying muscles which do not directly supply them with afferent impulses. **lower m.'s** Motor cell bodies in the anterior horn of the spinal cord or in the cranial nuclei whose axons terminate in skeletal muscles. **upper m.'s** Cerebral cortical nerve cells whose axons project upon motor nuclei of cranial nerves or the anterior horn of the spinal cord. Most of these cells are found in the posterior portion of the frontal lobe along the anterior wall of the central sulcus.

**motor** [L (from *movere* to move, set in motion) mover, one who imparts motion] 1 Carrying or transmitting an impulse to a peripheral effector organ of the nervous system, either to elicit a response or to inhibit it. 2 A mechanism that imparts motion. **air m.** An air-driven, medium-speed motor attached directly to the handpiece of a dental drill. **club m.** A plastic motor in which the attachment is by means of a knob or club of tissue. **loop m.** A plastic motor in which the attachment is by means of a loop of tissue. **plastic m.** An arrangement of muscles and tendons used in kineplasty whereby muscle tissue of the stump is used to provide power to the prosthetic limb.

**motorogerminative** \mō′tərōjur′minətiv\ [MOTOR + *o* + *germinative*] Giving rise to muscle, as does the myotome of an embryo.

**Mouchet** [Albert *Mouchet*, French surgeon, born 1869] See under DISEASE.

**mould** \mōld\ *Brit.* MOLD.

**mound** / **anal m.** A small, midline swelling in front of the anal opening of an embryo. It is formed by the union of the anal tubercles.

**Mount** [Lester Adran *Mount*, U.S. neurosurgeon, born 1910] Mount-Reback syndrome. See under MOUNT SYNDROME.

**mount** 1 To prepare for microscopic or gross examination. 2 A material prepared for microscopic or gross examination.

**mountant** \moun′tənt\ MOUNTING MEDIUM.

**mounting** 1 The preparation of slides or specimens for examination. 2 The attachment to an an articulator of casts of the jaws. **split cast m.** A method of mounting in dentistry which permits accurate remounting of the cast on the same articulator. Grooves are cut in the base of the cast before mounting, or special metal plates may be used. Also *split cast method*.

**mouse** [Old English *mūs*, akin to L *mus* a mouse, rat and to Gk *mys* a mouse, muscle] A small rodent, *Mus musculus*, which weighs about 30 g and has a sleek body, smooth hair coat, long hairless tail, and erect rounded ears. Vast numbers are used throughout the world in laboratory research for which numerous defined strains have been developed. **B m.** A mouse subjected to an experimental procedure that destroys both T and B lymphocytes, followed by a second procedure replacing the B lymphocytes. Also *deprived mouse*. **BALB/c m.** An inbred strain of white mice commonly used in experimental immunology. It has a low incidence of mammary tumors and leukemia and is extremely sensitive to radiation. Arteriosclerosis is common in both males and females and amyloidosis of the spleen is usual in males by 20 months. **CBA m.** An inbred strain of white mice of which one substrain carries an easily recognizable chromosomal marker. **deprived m.** B MOUSE. **joint m.** A free cartilaginous fragment within the joint space. **New Zealand black m.** An inbred strain of mouse characterized by autoimmune hemolytic anemia, extramedullary hematopoiesis, and lupuslike nephritis with glomerular and tubular damage. Also *NZB mouse*. **nude m.** A hairless mouse with a mutant gene on chromosome 11 characterized by congenital absence of the thymus, reduction in number of T cells, inability to reject allogeneic or xenogeneic skin grafts, a deficient supply of immunoglobulins, antinuclear autoantibody, and glomerulonephritis. Such mice have proved a valuable tool for investigating the role of the thymus in the development of immune responses. Also *nu nu mouse*. **NZB m.** NEW ZEALAND BLACK MOUSE. **peritoneal m.** A discrete, small, calcific density seen on an abdominal roentgenogram, representing an appendix epiploica or small piece of omentum which has twisted, become necrotic, and, lying free in the peritoneal cavity, has been encrusted with calcium. **pleural m.** A soft-tissue density, usually round, seen on a chest roentgenogram, representing a fibrin body in the pleural space. Such a fibrin body may be secondary to pneumothorax, pleural fluid, or other pleural disease. **Snell-Bagg m.** An inbred strain of mice, some of which have abnormalities of the pituitary and thymus with resultant lack of thymic tissue and depressed cell-mediated immunity. A recessive gene causes a deficiency of pituitary hormones and thus the appearance of dwarf mice in Snell-Bagg litters. Such mice have a life-span of about five months, one quarter that of normal littermates.

**mouth** [Old English *mūth*, akin to L *mandere* to chew, eat and to Gk *masasthai* to touch, chew] 1 OS[1]. 2 OSTIUM. **denture sore m.** DENTURE STOMATITIS. **dry m.** XEROSTOMIA. **tapir m.** The characteristic pouting appearance of the lips seen in facioscapulohumeral muscular dystrophy. Also *tapir lips*. **trench m.** NECROTIZING ULCERATIVE GINGIVITIS.

**mouthwash** A solution for rinsing the mouth, having antibacterial, palliative, astringent, or deodorant properties.

**movement** The act or process of moving; activity causing a change in position. **active m.** A movement produced by a subject's own action; a voluntary action. Also *active motion*. **adversive m.** A turning or beginning or progression to the side on which a sensory or electrical stimulus to a central nervous structure has been applied or which a lesion has been made. **ameboid m.** Locomotion of cells such as leukocytes or amebas resulting from protoplasmic streaming into pseudopodia. The relative degree of protoplasmic rigidity determines the rate and direction of flow, and the presence of microtubules is required for the movement to take place. Also *streaming movement*. **apparent m.** The subjective impression that physically stationary stimuli, when exposed in quick succession, are actually moving, as, for example, in cinematic motion pictures. The illusion is most often perceived in response to visual stimuli, but it can occur in other sensory modes as well. Also *delta movement, phi phenomenon*. **associated m.** The involuntary movement of one part of the body that accompanies movement of another part of the body. **associated contralateral m.** In a hemiplegic patient, an involuntary movement occurring on the affected side that is induced by a corresponding voluntary movement on the normal side. **athetoid m.'s** Movements resembling those seen in athetosis. **automatic m.'s** Movements occurring in a state of automatism. **Bennett m.** A lateral shift of the head of the condyle of the mandible towards the working side as the mandible is lowered and swung outwards in preparation for chewing on that side. **bodily m.** The lateral movement of a tooth without tipping. **brownian m.** The rapid random motion of small particles suspended in a liquid that is caused by the unequal impact of the molecules of the liquid on the particles. Also *molecular movement, brunonian movement, Brownian-Zsigmondy movement*. **cardinal m.'s** The six cardinal positions of the eye: up lateral, straight lateral, and down lateral, to each side. **choreiform m.'s** Movements occurring in or resembling those of chorea. They are involuntary, abrupt, rapid, arrhythmic, and variable in location, often involving the whole body but sometimes predominating on one side. They are more marked in the face and arms. They are increased by fatigue, emotion, and effort, and cease when the patient is asleep. They take the form of aimless, wild gestures. In the arms they comprise flexion, extension, and abduction movements, adduction of the hands and fingers, flinging out the arms, and shrugging of the shoulders. The facial movements cause the patient to grimace and he may protrude his tongue intermittently. The movements may be transient or persistent. **circus m.** 1 A gait involving circumduction of both legs, as in bilateral hemiparesis. 2 Electrical activation of part of the heart occurring over a circular pathway, thought to be responsible for atrial flutter. **curtain m.** The sideways movement of the posterior pharyngeal wall seen in cases of unilateral paralysis of the superior constrictor muscle of the pharynx when the patient gags, says "Ah," etc. The movement, like the pulling aside of a curtain, is in a direction away from the paralyzed side. **cytoplasmic m.** PROTOPLASMIC MOVEMENT. **delta m.** APPARENT MOVEMENT. **dystonic m.** A slow and often bizarre involuntary movement, resembling in some respects those of athetosis but generally associated with a fixed alteration in posture of the affected part of the body. **forced m.** INVOLUNTARY MOVEMENT. **free mandibular m.** A movement of the mandible not affected by occlusion or by food. **Frenkel's m.'s** A system of exercises used in the treatment of parkinsonism and ataxia to increase precision and spontaneity of movement by cortical reinforcement. Footprints are painted or pasted on the floor at appropriate intervals and the patient is encouraged to walk on them. **gliding m. of the mandible** MANDIBULAR GLIDE. **index m.** Cephalic movement about the fixed caudal part of a body. **involuntary m.** Involuntary contraction of one or more muscle groups or rarely of a single muscle, producing movement of a limb or of some other part of the body. This may be due to a variety of neurologic disorders, including principally focal motor seizures, clonus and myoclonus, tremor, chorea, athetosis, dystonia, hemiballismus, and facial dyskinesia. Involuntary contraction of bundles of muscle fibers not producing movement at a joint (fasciculation) is not usually so classified, nor are tics (habit spasm), as the latter are initially under voluntary control. Also *forced movement.* Compare VOLUNTARY MOVEMENT. **Magnan's trombone m.** TROMBONE TONGUE. **mirror m.** ALLOKINESIS. **molecular m.** BROWNIAN MOVEMENT. **morphogenetic m.** The changes in position and displacements of cells and groups of cells, the folding and rearrangement of layers of cells, and any alteration in position of structures or organs during the development of the embryo. Gastrulation eventually establishes the three germ layers, ectoderm, endoderm and mesoderm which move into the positions where they will subsequently develop into particular parts and features of the embryo. **opening m.** Any mandibular movement increasing the distance between the upper and lower anterior teeth. **pedal m.** A type of repetitive movement of the feet, which make pedaling or paddling movements. In rare cases, this is seen in Parkinson's disease, but it may be a result of treatment with levodopa. **pendular m.** SEGMENTAL MOTILITY. **percussion m.'s** Rapid, short blows used in massage. Various methods involve the fingertips or the side of the hand in different positions. Also *tapotement.* **protoplasmic m.** Movement of a mass of protoplasm, usually effected by the action of microtubules or microfilaments. Also *cytoplasmic movement.* **rapid eye m.** 1 The jerky ocular movements observed in deep sleep. Abbr. REM. 2 SACCADE. **resistive m.** Movement in which a muscle or limb is obliged to work against external weight or resistance, as used, for example, in progressive resistive exercises. **running m.'s** STEPPING. **saccadic m.** SACCADE. **segmentation m.** SEGMENTAL MOTILITY. **spontaneous m.** Movement occurring without voluntary or apparent external stimulation. Also *automatic motility.* **stepping m.'s** STEPPING. **streaming m.** AMEBOID MOVEMENT. **Swedish m.** SWEDISH GYMNASTICS. **synkinetic m.** An involuntary movement that accompanies more gross voluntary activity, such as the grimace associated with physical exertion. **tipping m.** The lateral movement which occurs when a force is applied to one point of a crown. The tooth rotates in the vertical plane about an imaginary fulcrum near the apex, which moves in the opposite direction to the crown. **voluntary m.** Activity that occurs as a consequence of a conscious decision. Also *voluntary motility.* Compare INVOLUNTARY MOVEMENT.

**mover** / **prime m.** A muscle that constantly initiates and maintains a particular movement of a part, such as the brachialis muscle in flexion of the elbow joint; an agonist.

**moxalactam** $C_{20}H_{20}N_6O_9S$. 7-[[Carboxy(4-hydroxyphenyl)acetyl]amino]-7-methoxy-3-[[(1-methyl-1*H*-tetrazol-5-yl)thio]-methyl]-8-oxo-5-oxal-azabicyclo[4.2.0]oct-2-ene-2-carboxylic acid. An anti-infective agent like the cephalosporins, with a broad antibiotic spectrum much like that of cefotaxime. It is given parenterally, usually as the sodium salt (latamoxef sodium).

**moyamoya** \moiʹəmoiʹə\ [Japanese, misty, foggy, hazy, gloomy, from duplicated *moya* a mist, fog, haze] See under MOYAMOYA DISEASE.

**Mozart** [Wolfgang Amadeus *Mozart*, Austrian composer, 1756–1791] See under EAR.

**mp** melting point.

**MPD** maximum permissible dose.

**MPO** minimum perceptible odor.

**MPS** 1 mucopolysaccharidosis. 2 multiphasic screening.

**MPV** mean platelet volume.

**MR** Symbol for the unit, megaroentgen.

**Mr.** mister (used as a title of address prefixed to a name). • See note at MISTER.

**mR** Symbol for the unit, milliroentgen.

**μR** Symbol for the unit, microroentgen.

**mrad** Symbol for the unit, millirad.

**MRD** minimal reacting dose.

**mrem** Symbol for the unit, millirem.

**MRI** magnetic resonance imaging.

**mRNA** messenger ribonucleic acid.

**MRO** minimum recognizable odor (minimal identifiable odor).

**MS** 1 multiple sclerosis. 2 mitral stenosis.

**ms** Symbol for the unit, millisecond.

**μs** Symbol for the unit, microsecond.

**μsec** Symbol for the unit, microsecond. An incorrect symbol.

**MSH** melanocyte stimulating hormone.

**MSH/ACTH 4–10** Met-Glu-His-Phe-Arg-Trp-Gly. An amino acid common to the adrenocorticotropic hormone (ACTH) and β-melanocyte stimulating hormone (MSH) molecules, which functions as an endogenous psychoactive drug in having anti-anxiety effects in normal subjects and in improving visual memory in senile patients.

**MSHRF** melanocyte stimulating hormone releasing factor (melanocyte stimulating hormone releasing hormone).

**MSHRH** melanocyte stimulating hormone releasing hormone.

**MSL** midsternal line.

**MT** **1** empty. **2** medical technologist. **3** membrana tympani. **4** metatarsal.

**MTF** modulation transfer function.

**MTU** methylthiouracil.

**MTX** methotrexate.

**MU** In medicine, mouse unit.

**M.u.** Mache unit.

**mu** The name of the twelfth letter of the Greek alphabet. Symbol: $\mu$

**Mucha** [Viktor *Mucha,* Austrian dermatologist, 1877–1919] Mucha's disease, Mucha-Habermann disease, Mucha-Habermann syndrome. See under PITYRIASIS LICHENOIDES.

**mucicarmine** \myoo'sikär'mīn\ A staining solution containing carmine and aluminum chloride or aluminum hydroxide in water or alcohol. It is used in tissue sections to demonstrate mucin and as a stain for fungi. Also *Mayer's mucicarmine.*

**muciform** \myoo'sifôrm\ Like mucus in appearance and consistency.

**mucigenous** \myoosij'ənəs\ Mucus-producing. Also *muciparous, blennogenic, blennogenous.*

**mucigogue** \myoo'sigäg\ [*muc(us)* + *i* + *-(a)gogue*] **1** An agent that stimulates the secretion of mucus. **2** Provoking the secretion of mucus.

**mucihematein** \myoo'sihē'mətē·in\ **Mayer's m.** A staining solution that is based on hematein, the oxidized form of hematoxylin, and is used to demonstrate the presence of the connective tissue mucin.

**mucilage** \myoo'siləj\ [Late L *mucilago.* See MUCILAGO.] **1** A gumlike plant cell product composed of sulfate esters of complex polysaccharides. **2** An aqueous solution of a gum utilized for suspending rather insoluble substances in mixtures. Another use is to increase the viscosity of oil-in-water emulsions, such as those used for dermatologic preparations and lubricating medications. For defs. 1 and 2 also *mucilago.*

**mucilaginous** \myoo'silaj'ənəs\ Having a viscous, mucoid, or slimy consistency.

**mucilago** \myoo'silāgō\ [Late L (from L *mucus* mucus) a musty fluid, gelatinous substance] MUCILAGE. **m. tragacanthae** GUM TRAGACANTH.

**mucilloid** \myoo'siloid\ A thick, sticky, gluelike preparation resembling mucilage.

**mucin** \myoo'sin\ Any mucoprotein secreted by cells which raises the viscosity of the medium around them.

**mucinase** \myoo'sinās\ Any of several enzymes that break down glycosaminoglycans. They break glycoside bonds either by hydrolysis or by elimination reactions.

**mucinemia** \myoo'sinē'mē·ə\ The presence of mucin in blood, a condition that may occur in metastatic malignancies of the gastrointestinal tract or the ovaries. Also *myxemia.*

**mucinoblast** \myoosin'əblast\ A precursor of a mucin-secreting cell.

**mucinolytic** \myoo'sinəlit'ik\ Capable of breaking down mucoproteins or glycosaminoglycans.

**mucinosis** \myoo'sinō'sis\ [MUCIN + -OSIS] An abnormal accumulation of mucopolysaccharides in the skin. **follicular m.** An inflammatory disorder characterized clinically by infiltrated cutaneous plaques, with scaling and loss of hair. Histologically it is manifested by the accumulation of acid mucopolysaccharides in the sebaceous glands and the outer root sheath of the hair follicle.

**mucinuria** \myoo'sinoo'rē·ə\ [MUCIN + -URIA] The presence of mucin in the urine, a condition which may reflect contamination from the vagina.

**muciparous** \myoosip'ərəs\ MUCIGENOUS.

**mucivorous** \myoosiv'ərəs\ [*muc(o)-* + *i* + L *vor(are)* to devour, swallow + -OUS] Subsisting on mucus, as microbes.

**Muckle** [Thomas James *Muckle,* Canadian pediatrician, flourished 20th century] Muckle-Wells syndrome. See under SYNDROME.

**muco-** \myoo'kō-\ [L *mucus*] A combining form meaning mucus, mucous.

**mucoalbuminous** \-albyoo'minəs\ Having both a watery and mucoid consistency.

**mucoantibody** \-an'tibäd'ē\ Antibody present on a mucous surface, as of the bronchial tree or in the intestinal lumen. These antibodies are predominantly secretory IgA and are found mixed with the mucous secretion of the membrane concerned. They form the immunologic component of the mucosal barrier protecting the mucosal surfaces from infectious agents. *Seldom used.*

**mucobuccal** \-buk'əl\ Pertaining to the mucous membrane lining the cheek.

**mucocartilage** \-kär'təlij\ Cartilaginous tissue with a soft mucoid matrix, as is found in the central nucleus pulposus of the intervertebral disk.

**mucocele** \myoo'kəsēl\ [MUCO- + -CELE[1]] **1** A retention cyst of a mucous gland. **2** Distension with mucus of a mucous membrane-lined organ or compartment of the body (for example, the gallbladder, appendix, frontal sinus) as the result of acquired atresia of its duct or lumen. **ethmoid sinus m.** A mucocele seeming to have its origin in the ethmoid air cells. It is among the more common paranasal sinus mucoceles. **frontal sinus m.** A mucocele of the frontal sinus. It is the most common of the paranasal sinus mucoceles and, in neglected cases, liable to reach such a size as to displace an eye or even destroy the function of that eye. **frontoethmoid m.** A large mucocele occupying both the frontal sinus and the anterior part of the ethmoid labyrinth. It probably arises in the frontal sinus and expands into the adjacent ethmoid cells by destroying the intervening bony walls. The majority of large mucoceles in the frontal region, particularly those which displace the orbital contents, fall into this category. **lacrimal m.** A mucocele of the lacrimal sac, presenting as a swelling at the inner canthus of the eye under the medial palpebral ligament. It must be distinguished from a mucocele of the anterior ethmoidal cells which presents above the medial palpebral ligament. **maxillary sinus m.** Mucocele of the maxillary sinus, a rare variety of paranasal sinus mucocele. **paranasal sinus m.** A mucocele arising in any one of the paranasal sinuses. It is a rare occurrence of uncertain cause, and includes the frontal sinus and frontoethmoidal mucoceles as the more common varieties, in which acquired atresia of the frontonasal duct is a constant finding. Also *serous sinusitis* (incorrect).

**mucoclasis** \myookäk'ləsis\ [MUCO- + -CLASIS] The surgical removal or destruction of the inner lining of any hollow organ.

**mucocolpos** \-käl'pəs\ [MUCO- + Gk *kolpos* bosom, uterus, fold] The accumulation of mucus in the vagina.

**mucocutaneous** \-kyootā'nē·əs\ [MUCO- + CUTANEOUS] Pertaining to the skin and mucous membranes.

**mucocyte** \myoo'kəsīt\ [MUCO- + -CYTE] An amorphous extracellular basophilic, metachromatic mass averaging 100 $\mu$m in diameter found in the white matter of normal and abnormal brains. It is believed to be artefactual and derived from precipitation of a component of myelin in the process of tissue fixation.

**mucoderm** \myoo′kədurm\ [MUCO- + -DERM] LAMINA PROPRIA MUCOSAE.

**mucoepidermoid** \myoo′kō·ep′idur′moid\ Showing characteristics of both a mucus-secreting and an epidermal cell type of epithelial structure: used especially in describing tumor differentiation.

**mucofibrous** \-fī′brəs\ MYXOID.

**mucogingival** \-jin′jivəl\ [MUCO- + GINGIVAL] Pertaining to the junction between the gingival mucosa and the alveolar mucosa.

**mucohemorrhagic** \-hem′ôraj′ik\ MUCOSANGUINEOUS.

**mucoid** \myoo′koid\ **1** Resembling or having the characteristics of mucus. **2** Describing the glistening appearance of a bacterial colony, often associated with excessive uptake of water by the polysaccharides in the cell envelope. **3** An acid-soluble glycoprotein. *Obs.*

**mucolipidosis** \-lip′idō′sis\ [MUCO- + LIPIDOSIS] Any inborn error of metabolism that has clinical and cytologic characteristics of both the mucopolysaccharidoses and the sphingolipidoses. Four distinct conditions, designated mucolipidoses I through IV, have been labeled on the basis of a classification first proposed by Spranger and Wiedemann in 1970. The distinctions have limited utility, however, because of extensive biochemical and pathogenic diversity. Also *lipomucopolysaccharidosis.* Abbr. ML **m. I** A now largely abandoned entity based on disorders of glycoprotein metabolism that were seen in patients who had clinical features of both mucopolysaccharide and glycolipid storage disease. **m. II** An inborn error of post-translational modification of lysosomal enzymes. The autosomal recessive phenotype is obvious in infancy and is characterized by coarse facies, severe growth and mental retardation, dysostosis multiplex, and death by age 5 years. The basic defect involves UDP-*N*-acetylglucosamine:lysosomal enzyme *N*-acetylglucosaminylphosphotransferase, an enzyme that attaches sugar groups to enzymes stored in lysosomes. Also *I-cell disease.* **m. III** An inborn error in the post-translational modification of multiple lysosomal enzymes. The phenotype is similar to but milder than those of mucopolysaccharidosis IH and mucolipidosis II (ML II). Patients have an intracellular deficit and an increased serum level of most lysosomal hydrolases. The basic defect in some patients is the same as in ML II, suggesting that the defects are allelic. Genetic heterogeneity has been found *in vitro* among patients with this condition. Also *pseudo-Hurler polydystrophy, pseudo-Hurler's disease.* **m. IV** A diverse group of conditions that share features of mucopolysaccharide and glycolipid storage diseases, often accompanied by an autosomal recessive defect in a ganglioside-specific, nonlysosomal neuraminidase. *Imprecise.*

**mucolytic** \-lit′ik\ Having the property of liquifying or breaking down mucus.

**mucopeptide** Any glycosylated peptide derived from a mucoprotein. Its carbohydrate component normally has alternate residues of aminosugars and uronic acids.

**mucoperiosteum** \-per′ē·äs′tē·əm\ A mucous membrane that is applied directly to a layer of periosteum, as is seen in the petrous temporal bone, nasal cavities, and air sinuses. Adj. mucoperiosteal.

**mucopoiesis** \-poi·ē′sis\ [MUCO- + -POIESIS] The formation of mucus. Also *myxopoiesis.*

**mucopolysaccharide** \-päl′ēsak′ərīd\ GLYCOSAMINOGLYCAN.

**mucopolysaccharidoses** \-päl′ēsak′əridō′sēz\ Plural of MUCOPOLYSACCHARIDOSIS.

**mucopolysaccharidosis** \-päl′ēsak′əridō′sis\ [*mucopolysaccharid(e)* + -OSIS] Any of the inborn errors of mucopolysaccharide metabolism, each of which is due to deficiency of a specific degradative, lysosomal enzyme and characterized by mucopolysacchariduria, short stature, and dysostosis multiplex. Also *polydystrophic dwarfism.* **m. I** An autosomal recessive inborn error of mucopolysaccharide metabolism due to a deficiency of α-iduronidase. Depending on the severity of the symptoms, the syndrome is designated mucopolysaccharidosis IH, mucopolysaccharidosis IH/S, or mucopolysaccharidosis IS. **m. IH** An autosomal recessive inborn error of mucopolysaccharide metabolism due to a deficiency of α-iduronidase and characterized by progressive mental retardation and physical deterioration, short stature, coarse facies, corneal clouding, dysostosis multiplex, restricted joint mobility, and death by the mid-second decade as a result of pulmonary or cardiac complications. Also *Hurler syndrome, gargoylism* (outmoded). Abbr. MPS IH **m. IH/S** An autosomal recessive inborn error of mucopolysaccharide metabolism caused by a deficiency of α-iduronidase and characterized by a phenotype intermediate to those of MPS IH and MPS IS. Intelligence is usually subnormal and death due to pulmonary complications occurs in the third or fourth decade. Some cases may represent genetic compounds between MPS IH and MPS IS alleles while others are homozygotes for other alleles at the α-iduronidase locus on chromosome 22. Also *Hurler-Scheie syndrome, Hurler-Scheie compound.* Abbr. MPS IH/S **m. IS** An autosomal recessive inborn error of mucopolysaccharide metabolism due to deficiency of α-iduronidase and characterized by corneal clouding, progressive arthropathy that particularly affects the hip, mild dysostosis multiplex, and aortic valvular disease. Although biochemically indistinguishable from MPS IH, its features are much milder and intelligence is often normal. Also *Scheie syndrome.* Abbr. MPS IS **m. II** An X-linked recessive inborn error of mucopolysaccharide metabolism caused by a deficiency of iduronate-sulfate sulfatase, with a phenotype distinguishable from MPS IH only by the absence of affected females and the absence of corneal clouding. There is a mild form, with normal intelligence, which is presumably due to an allelic mutation. Also *Hunter syndrome, X-linked recessive gargoylism* (outmoded). **m. III** A group of autosomal recessive inborn errors of mucopolysaccharide metabolism that are all characterized by coarse facies, hirsutism, mild dysostosis multiplex, and profound mental retardation. The four types, which can be distinguished only by enzyme assay, are: IIIA, a deficiency of heparan sulfate sulfatase; IIIB, a deficiency of *N*-acetyl-α-D-glucosaminidase; IIIC, a deficiency of acetyl-CoA:α-glucosaminidase *N*-acetyltransferase; and IIID, a deficiency of *N*-acetyl-glucosamine-6-sulfate sulfatase. Also *Sanfilippo syndrome.* **m. IV** An autosomal recessive inborn error of mucopolysaccharide metabolism characterized by corneal clouding, short stature particularly involving the vertebral column, keratosulfaturia, odontoid hypoplasia, and aortic valvular disease. At least two distinct enzyme deficiencies produce this phenotype: galactosamine-6-sulfatase deficiency results in enamel hypoplasia, and β-galactosidase deficiency results in a milder phenotype with normal enamel. Also *Morquio syndrome, Morquio-Ullrich syndrome, Morquio-Brailsford syndrome, Morquio's disease.* **m. V** A mucopolysaccharidosis that is no longer considered to be a distinct entity. See under MUCOPOLYSACCHARIDOSIS IS. **m. VI** An autosomal recessive inborn error of mucopolysaccharide metabolism due to deficiency of arylsulfatase B, characterized by severe dysostosis multiplex, corneal clouding, aortic valvular disease, and urinary excretion of chondroitin sulfate. Severe, mild, and intermediate forms occur, presumably due to allelic variation at the arylsulfatase locus on chromosome 5. Also *Maroteaux-Lamy syndrome, Maroteaux-Lamy disease.* **m. VII** An autosomal recessive inborn error of mucopolysaccharide metabolism due to deficiency of β-glucuronidase. The phenotype is variable, but dysostosis multiplex, hepatosplenomegaly, mental retardation, and granular inclusions in polymorphonuclear leukocytes have been consistent features. Also *Sly syndrome.*

**mucopolysacchariduria** \-päl′ēsak′əridoo′rē·ə\ [*mucopolysaccharid(e)* + -URIA] The excretion of mucopolysaccharides in the urine, a feature of mucopolysaccharidosis.

**mucoprotein** One of several substances whose solutions are highly viscous and which often have lubricant function. They are glycoproteins, more specifically proteoglycans, i.e. ones whose carbohydrate parts are polysaccharides, usually composed of alternate resides of hexosamine and of uronic acid, and often esterified with sulfate. **Tamm-Horsfall m.** A large glycoprotein produced by the renal epithelial cells lining Henle's loop, the distal convoluted tubule, and the collecting ducts. A normal constituent of urine, it precipitates in conditions of retarded flow, high urine concentration, and abnormal concentrations of albumin, and it constitutes the matrix of most urinary casts.

**mucopurulent** \-pyoo′rʸələnt\ Denoting an exudate composed of pus and mucus.

**mucopus** \myoo′kōpus′\ An exudate composed of pus and mucus.

***Mucor*** \myoo′kôr\ [L (from *mucere* to be moldy), mold] A genus of zygomycetous fungi which grow saprophytically on a variety of substrates, including foodstuffs and soil, and some of which are human pathogens that cause mucormycosis.

**Mucoraceae** \myoo′kôrā′si·ē\ [*MUCOR* + -ACEAE] A family of fungi, some of which are causal agents of mucormycosis and otomycosis. Important genera include *Mucor, Chlamydomucor, Actinomucor, Absidia, Zygorhynchus, Rhizopus, Circinella,* and *Phycomyces.*.

**mucormycosis** \myoo′kôrmīkō′sis\ [*MUCOR* + MYCOSIS] An infection by one of several genera of fungi, notably *Rhizopus, Mucor,* and *Absidia.* The disease is most often manifested in the head including the nose and sinuses, and in the facial and cranial areas. Also *zygomycosis, phycomycosis, phycomycetosis, phycomycotic infection.*

**mucosa** \myookō′sə\ [L (fem. of *mucosus* mucous, from *mucus* mucus), alone or with *membrana* membrane: mucous membrane] TUNICA MUCOSA. **alveolar m.** The nonkeratinized mucosa which covers the alveolar process of the mandible or maxilla apical to the attached gingiva. **buccal m.** The stratified squamous epithelium and underlying connective tissue layer that lines the inner aspect of the cheek. **endocervical m.** The mucus-secreting columnar epithelium and underlying connective tissue layer that lines the cervical canal of the uterus. **labial m.** The stratified squamous epithelium and underlying connective tissue layer that covers the inner surface of both lips and extends as far forward as the vermilion border. **laryngeal m.** A respiratory epithelium and underlying connective tissue layer that lines the larynx. **masticatory m.** Mucous membrane involved in masticatory activity, comprising the hard palate, gingivae, edentulous ridges, and the dorsum of the tongue. **muscular m.** A thin layer of smooth muscle that marks the deep margin of the mucosa in the stomach, small intestine, and large intestine. **olfactory m.** The mucous membrane that lines the roof of the nasal cavity and contains the olfactory cells and their supporting cells. **oral m.** The moist integument lining of the oral cavity. **pharyngeal m.** A nonkeratinizing stratified squamous epithelium and underlying connective tissue layer that lines the pharynx. **respiratory m.** A ciliated columnar cell epithelium, which contains goblet cells, and an underlying connective tissue layer that line the respiratory tract. **tracheal m.** A respiratory epithelium and its underlying connective tissue layer that line the trachea.

**mucosal** \myookō′səl\ Pertaining to the tunica mucosa.

**mucosalpinx** \-sal′pingks\ [MUCO- + Gk *salpinx* tube] A dilated, closed fallopian tube containing mucus.

**mucosanguineous** \-sang·gwin′ē·əs\ Containing both mucus and blood. Also *mucohemorrhagic.*

**mucosedative** A drug or therapeutic agent that produces a soothing effect on mucus-bearing surfaces.

**mucoserous** \-sir′əs\ Of or relating to the production of both mucin and proteinaceous secretions.

**mucosin** \myookō′sin\ Mucus of a particularly sticky or tenacious variety that is found especially in the upper respiratory tract and uterine cervix.

**mucostatic** \-stat′ik\ Having the effect of reducing or arresting the secretion of mucus.

**mucotome** \myoo′kətōm\ [MUCO- + -TOME] An instrument similar to a dermatome, used to harvest mucous membrane for transplantation.

**mucous** \myoo′kəs\ Of or relating to mucus or to the production of mucin. Also *muculent.*

**mucoviscidosis** \-vis′idō′sis\ CYSTIC FIBROSIS.

**mucro** \myoo′krō\ [L (gen. *mucronis,* akin to Gk *amyssein* to tear, wound), a sharp point, point or edge of a sword, sword] In anatomy, the pointed end, or tip, of a structure or an organ.

**mucronate** \myoo′krənāt\ Possessing or pertaining to a sharp pointed tip or end.

**muculent** \myoo′kyələnt\ MUCOUS.

**mucus** \myoo′kəs\ [L (akin to *emunctus,* past part. of *emungere* to blow the nose, and to Gk *myxa* mucus, phlegm), mucus] A viscid secretion of mucous membranes. Also *blenna.* **cervical m.** The secretion from the columnar epithelium lining the upper portion of the uterine cervical canal.

**Muench** [Hugo *Muench,* U.S. physician and statistician, 1894–1972] Reed and Muench method. See under METHOD.

**muliebria** \myoo′lē·eb′rē·ə\ [L (substantive from *muliebria,* neut. pl. of *muliebris* female, pertaining to women), female genitalia] The female genitalia. *Outmoded.*

**muliebris** \myoo′lē·eb′ris\ Pertaining to a female; feminine.

**mull** [Short for *mulmul,* an Indian term for muslin, from Hindi *malmal* muslin, probably from Persian] A thin cloth made of cotton or similar material and impregnated with ointment or other medication for dressings. **plaster m.** A sheet of muslin coated with gutta-percha. It is used as a dressing in the treatment of skin conditions.

**Müller** [Fritz *Müller,* German naturalist, 1821–1897] Müller-Haeckel law. See under RECAPITULATION THEORY.

**Müller** [Heinrich *Müller,* German anatomist, 1820–1864] **1** See under MUSCLE. **2** Müller's fibers. See under FIBER. **3** Müller cells. See under SUSTENTACULAR CELLS.

**Müller** [Hermann F. *Müller,* German histologist, 1866–1898] Formol-Müller fluid. See under ORTH SOLUTION.

**Müller** [Johannes Peter *Müller,* German anatomist, physiologist, and pathologist, 1801–1858] **1** Ganglion of Müller. See under GANGLION SUPERIUS NERVI GLOSSOPHARYNGEI. **2** Müllerian duct. See under PARAMESONEPHRIC DUCT. **3** Müllerian mixed tumor. See under TUMOR. **4** Müller's law. See under LAW OF SPECIFIC IRRITABILITY. **5** Vieth-Müller horopter. See under HOROPTER. **6** Müller's maneuver. See under EXPERIMENT.

**Müller** [Peter *Müller*, German obstetrician, 1836–1922] Müller-Hillis maneuver. See under MANEUVER.
**Müller** [Walther *Müller*, German physicist, flourished 20th century] **1** Geiger-Müller counter. See under COUNTER. **2** Geiger-Müller survey meter. See under METER. **3** Geiger-Müller tube. See under TUBE.
**mulling** \mul′ing\ The kneading of a dental amalgam to complete the mixing process after the dental alloy and mercury have been ground in a mortar. It is not necessary if an amalgam mixer is used.
**multi-** \mul′tē-, mul′ti\ [L *multus* many, much] A combining form meaning many, more than one, much.
**multiallelic** \-alē′lik\ Characterized by multiple allelic variants, as a genetic locus.
**multiarticular** \-ärtik′yələr\ Of or pertaining to many joints. Also *polyarticular.*
**multicapsular** \-kap′s^yələr\ Encased by many layers of outer coat.
***Multiceps*** \mul′tiseps\ [MULTI- + L *-ceps,* combining form of *caput* the head] A genus of tapeworms of the family Taeniidae. The larval forms (coenuri) are found in herbivores, and those of some species occasionally infect humans. The mature worms generally inhabit the intestines of carnivores.
**multicipital** \-sip′itəl\ Possessing many heads, as of origins of a muscle.
**multiclonal** \-klō′nəl\ POLYCLONAL.
**multicore** \mul′tēkôr\ **m.'s in muscle** A variant of central core disease of muscle in which many skeletal muscle fibers contain several cores. See also CENTRAL CORE DISEASE OF MUSCLE.
**multicostate** \-käs′tāt\ Possessing many ribs.
**multicuspidate** \-kus′pidāt\ **1** Possessing more than two cusps. **2** MOLAR².
**multidentate** \-den′tāt\ Possessing many teeth or tooth-like processes.
**multideterminaton** \-ditur′minā′shən\ OVERDETERMINATION.
**multidigitate** \-dij′itāt\ Possessing many digits or digitate processes.
**multifetation** \-fētā′shən\ [MULTI- + FETATION] The development of more than one fetus within the uterus.
**multifid** \mul′tifid\ Divided into many parts or segments.
**multiflagellate** \-flaj′əlāt\ Having more than two flagella.
**multifocal** \-fō′kəl\ Pertaining to or arising from many foci. Also *plurifocal.*
**multiganglionate** \-gang′glē·ənāt′\ Having many ganglia.
**multiganglionic** \-gang′glē·än′ik\ Relating to, characterized by, or affecting many ganglia.
**multigesta** \-jes′tə\ [MULTI- + L *gesta,* fem. of *gestus,* past part. of *gerere* to produce, bear] MULTIGRAVIDA.
**multiglandular** \-glan′dyələr\ PLURIGLANDULAR.
**multigravida** \-grav′idə\ [MULTI- + GRAVIDA] A woman who has been pregnant more than once. Also *multigesta, plurigravida.* **grand m.** A woman who has been pregnant six or more times.
**multihallucism** \-hal′^yoosizm\ A form of polydactyly characterized by the presence of more than one great toe on one or both feet.
**multihematinic** \-hē′mətin′ik\ A medication promoting formation of red blood cells and containing several components effective for this purpose, such as various iron salts, certain vitamins, and trace metals that facilitate iron absorption.
**multi-infarct** \-in′färkt\ A number of areas of cell death resulting directly from impairment of blood supply, usually due to vascular disease.
**multi-infection** \-infek′shən\ An infection caused by more than one kind of organism; mixed infection.
**multilobar** \-lō′bər\ Possessing many lobes.
**multilobular** \-läb′yələr\ Possessing many lobules. Also *polylobular.*
**multilocular** \-läk′yələr\ Possessing many compartments or cells. Also *plurilocular, multiloculate.*
**multimammae** \-mam′ē\ POLYMASTIA.
**multimer** \mul′timər\ [MULTI- + Gk *mer(os)* part] A substance whose molecule consists of many identical units.
**multinodal** \-nō′dəl\ Possessing many nodes.
**multinodular** \-näd′yələr\ Possessing many nodules.
**multinuclear** \-n^yoo′klē·ər\ [MULTI- + NUCLEAR] Having two or more nuclei in a common protoplasmic mass. Also *multinucleated, plurinuclear, polynuclear, polynucleated.*
**multipara** \multip′ərə\ [MULTI- + L *par(ere)* to bear or bring forth young + *a*] A woman who has carried more than one pregnancy to a stage of viability, regardless of whether all gestations resulted in a live-born infant. Also *pluripara.* **grand m.** A woman who has carried at least six pregnancies to a viable stage.
**multiparity** \-par′itē\ [*multipar(a)* + -ITY] The condition of being multiparous. Also *pluriparity.*
**multiparous** \multip′ərəs\ [*multipar(a)* + -OUS] **1** Having carried more than one pregnancy to a viable stage. **2** Producing more than one offspring during the same gestation.
**multipartite** \-pär′tīt\ Composed of or having many parts or lobes; multilobar. Also *pluripartite.*
**multipennate** \-pen′āt\ [MULTI- + PENNATE] Having several tendons between which the fasciculi run obliquely in a featherlike fashion: said of certain muscles. Also *multipenniform.*
**multipenniform** \-pen′ifôrm\ MULTIPENNATE.
**multiphasic** \-fā′zik\ Composed of or performed in several separate phases.
**multiple** \mul′təpəl\ **1** Involving more than one, as *multiple birth.* **2** Existing concurrently in several or numerous parts of the body.
**multiplexer** \mul′tiplek′sər\ A device which permits transmission of two or more signals over one line. A time-division multiplexer uses a multiposition electronic switch for time-sharing by alternating the signals. A frequency-division multiplexer transmits signals simultaneously in different frequency bands.
**multiplicitas** \-plis′itas\ [Late L (from L *multiplex,* gen. *multiplicis,* manifold + *-itas* -ITY), multiplicity] A developmental defect characterized by supernumerary organs or parts. **m. cordis** The presence of one or more accessory or supernumerary hearts.
**multipolar** \-pō′lər\ **1** Denoting a cell having a mitotic spindle with more than two poles. This may result from polyspermy and usually results in aberrant chromosome distribution. **2** Denoting a cell having a number of cytoplasmic processes, as a neuron with an axon and numerous dendrites. For defs. 1 and 2 also *pluripolar.*
**multipollicism** \-päl′isizm\ [MULTI- + L *pollex,* gen. *pollicis,* the thumb, great toe + -ISM] A form of polydactyly characterized by the presence of more than one thumb on one or both hands.
**multisynaptic** \-sinap′tik\ Denoting a physiological event or neuroanatomical pathway involving more than two neurons.

**multisystem** \mul′tēsis′təm\ Involving more than one bodily system, as a disease.

**multituberculate** \-t$^y$ubur′kyəlāt\ Possessing many tubercles.

**multivalent** \-vā′lənt\ **1** Possessing a valence of a fairly high value, at least two. **2** Denoting the repression of the biosynthesis of a protein by several substances, all of which are needed for maximal repression. For defs. 1 and 2 also *polyvalent.*

**mu-meson** \m$^y$oo′-\ A subatomic particle having a mass equal to 207 times the mass of the electron, and a charge of either plus or minus one. Also *muon.*

**mummification** \mum′ifikā′shən\ Dessication of the whole or a part such that it resembles a mummy, as in dry gangrene. **fetal m.** The process of absorption of fluid from a dead fetus and its conversion to a dried state suggesting mummification. **m. of pulp** **1** Dry gangrene of the pulp of a tooth. **2** A method of endodontic treatment in teeth of which the radicular pulp cannot be completely removed because of extreme curvature or other obstruction. The parts of the pulp which cannot be removed are treated with paraformaldehyde or other mummifying agents.

**mumps** [pl. of English dialect *mump* a grimace] An acute generalized infection with a paramyxovirus, which occurs most frequently in school-age children and is characterized by fever, malaise, and parotitis. Complications include aseptic meningitis, encephalitis, pancreatitis, and in postpubertal patients, epididymo-orchitis or oophoritis. The disease is endemic world-wide and often occurs epidemically, especially in closed communities. A live attenuated mumps vaccine is available. Also *epidemic parotitis, angina parotidea* (obs.). **iodine m.** A toxic hypersensitivity or idiosyncratic reaction to iodine therapy resulting in enlargement of salivary and lacrimal glands. **metastatic m.** A complication of mumps in which the virus infects various glands and organs of the body, particularly the meninges, testes, ovaries, pancreas, or mammary glands.

**Münchhausen** [Baron Karl Friedrich Hieronymus Freiherr von *Münchhausen,* German hunter and soldier, 1720–1797] See under MÜNCHAUSEN SYNDROME.

**Münchmeyer** [Ernst *Münchmeyer,* German physician, 1846–1880] Münchmeyer's disease, Münchmeyer syndrome. See under FIBRODYSPLASIA OSSIFICANS PROGRESSIVA.

**munity** \myoo′nitē\ [back-formation from IMMUNITY] A condition of particular susceptibility to infection.

**Munro** [William John *Munro,* Australian dermatologist, flourished late 19th century] Munro's abscesses. See under MUNRO'S MICROABSCESSES.

**Munro Kerr** [John Martin *Munro Kerr,* U.S. gynecologist and obstetrician, born 1868] See under MANEUVER.

**muon** \myoo′än\ [contraction of *mu-(mes)on*] MU-MESON.

**mural** \myoo′rəl\ [L *mural(is)* (from *mur(us)* wall + *-alis* -AL) pertaining to a wall] In anatomy, of or relating to the wall of a cavity.

**muramic acid** 2-Amino-3-](1*R*)-1-carboxyethyl]-2-deoxyglucose. An ether formed between lactic acid and glucosamine. It occurs in bacterial cell walls, usually *N*-acetylated, in a $\beta$1-4-linked structure alternating with residues of *N*-acetylglucosamine, and cross-linked through peptides attached to the carboxyl group of the lactic acid residue.

**muramidase** \myooram′idās\ *Obs.* LYSOZYME.

**Murat** [Louis *Murat,* French physician, born 1874] See under SIGN.

**Murchison** [Charles *Murchison,* English physician, 1830–1879] Murchison-Pel-Ebstein fever. See under PEL-EBSTEIN FEVER.

**murein** \myoo′rē·in\ The rigid layer of the bacterial cell wall, consisting of a sacculus in which the peptidoglycan chains are covalently cross-linked both within a layer and between layers, forming a single giant molecule. In some Gram-negative organisms a lipoprotein of the outer membrane is also covalently linked to peptidoglycan. Also *basal wall* (outmoded).

**murein hydrolase** An enzyme that hydrolyzes the bond between the lactyl carboxyl of muramic acid and the N terminus of the tetrapeptide in murein. The enzyme has been useful in analyzing peptidoglycan structure, and it plays a role in shaping the cell.

**murexide** The purple-red ammonium salt of purpuric acid, a pyrimidine dimer formed by the action of nitric acid on purines, especially uric acid. *Seldom used.* See also MUREXIDE TEST.

**muriatic acid** HYDROCHLORIC ACID.

**murine** \myoo′rēn, -rīn\ [L *murinus* (from *mus,* gen. *muris* mouse) pertaining to mice] Of or pertaining to the rodent family Muridae, comprising rats and mice, as in *murine pneumonia.*

# murmur

**murmur** [L, a murmur] A prolonged or continuous auscultatory sound, particularly one deriving from the heart or cardiovascular system. Also *susurrus, susurration.* **anemic m.** Cardiac murmur heard in anemia, usually a pulmonary midsystolic murmur. Also *blood murmur, hemic murmur.* **aortic m.** A murmur arising from a disorder of the aortic valve or aorta. **apical m.** A murmur heard in the apical region of the heart. **apical diastolic m.** A diastolic murmur in the apical region of the heart. **arterial m.** A murmur or bruit heard over an artery, often associated with stenosis or aneurysm. **atriosystolic m.** A murmur caused by atrial systole, usually presystolic in timing. **attrition m.** PERICARDIAL RUB. **Austin Flint m.** An apical mid-diastolic or presystolic murmur in aortic regurgitation. Austin Flint originally described the murmur as presystolic and "blubbering." Also *Flint's murmur.* **basal diastolic m.'s** Murmurs heard at the base of the heart due to aortic or pulmonary regurgitation. **blood m.** ANEMIC MURMUR. **bronchial m.** See under BRONCHIAL BREATHING. **cardiac m.** A murmur arising from the heart. **cardiopulmonary m.** A sound heard during auscultation of the chest which is related to breathing but is modified by the beating of the heart. Also *cardiorespiratory murmur.* **Carey Coombs m.** An apical mid-diastolic murmur occurring in the acute phase of rheumatic fever but disappearing thereafter and not due to mitral stenosis. **continuous m.** A murmur which continues from a systole into diastole. Most characteristic of persistent ductus arteriosus, it occurs in other disorders in which there is an arteriovenous shunt, such as arteriovenous fistulae and aortopulmonary septal defect, and also when there is prolonged flow through a stenosis as in some cases of coarctation of the aorta and pulmonary arterial stenosis. **cooing m.** A murmur resembling the cooing of a dove. **crescendo m.** A murmur which increases in loudness and is then abruptly terminated, such as the presystolic murmur of mitral stenosis which terminates with the onset of the first heart sound. **Cruveilhier-Baumgarten m.** A venous murmur heard over the veins in the abdominal wall when there are anastomoses between the veins of the portal and caval systems. **diamond-shaped m.** A murmur of the ejection type which increases and decreases in such a way as to produce a diamond-shaped appearance on the phonocardiogram. **diastolic m.** A murmur occurring at some time in the interval between the second heart sound and the first heart sound. **Duroziez m.** A to-and-fro murmur heard over a major peripheral artery, particularly the femoral, in cases of aortic regurgitation. Also *double murmur of Duroziez.* **ejection m.** A murmur caused by the ejection of blood from one or the other ventricle into the related great artery. **exocardial m.** EXTRACARDIAC MURMUR. **expiratory m.** A sound heard during exhalation in auscultation of the lungs. **extracardiac m.** A murmur arising outside the heart, as in a pericardial murmur or cardiorespiratory murmur. Also *exocardial murmur.* **Flint's m.** AUSTIN FLINT MURMUR. **friction m.** PERICARDIAL RUB. **functional m.** A murmur occurring in a structurally normal heart, either in the absence of any abnormality or as a result of such conditions as anemia, thyrotoxicosis, or pregnancy. Also *physiologic murmur.* **Gibson's m.** The continuous murmur of a persistent ductus arteriosus. **Graham Steell's m.** The murmur of pulmonary regurgitation, usually associated with pulmonary hypertension, particularly as a consequence of mitral stenosis. Also *Steell's murmur.* **hemic m.** ANEMIC MURMUR. **holodiastolic m.** A murmur occupying the whole of diastole. **holosystolic m.** A murmur lasting the whole of systole, that is, from the first heart sound to the second heart sound. Also *pansystolic murmur.* **hourglass m.** A murmur which on a phonocardiographic record has an hourglass appearance, being loud at onset and at termination but softer in between. **humming-top m.** VENOUS HUM. **innocent m.** Murmur occurring in the absence of organic heart disease. Also *inorganic murmur.* **late systolic m.** A murmur occurring in the latter part of systole, often associated with a click and due to mitral valve prolapse. **machinery m.** A continuous, machinelike, rumbling murmur such as is encountered in persistent ductus arteriosus. **mid-diastolic m.** A murmur occurring in the mid-portion of diastole, characteristically appearing in mitral stenois immediately after the opening snap. It may also occur in atrial myxoma and in conditions in which there is a high flow through the mitral valve shortly after its opening, as in some cases of mitral regurgitation and ventricular septal defect. **mill wheel m.** A splashing auscultatory sound heard in the chest, suggestive of that made by a mill wheel. It may be of cardiac, pericardial, or pleural origin. Also *waterwheel murmur, waterwheel sound, bruit de moulin.* **mitral m.** A murmur heard in the mitral area. **musical m.** A cardiac murmur having a musical quality. **organic m.** A murmur resulting from organic disease of the heart or a blood vessel. **pansystolic m.** HOLOSYSTOLIC MURMUR. **pericardial m.** PERICARDIAL RUB. **physiologic m.** FUNCTIONAL MURMUR. **presystolic m.** A murmur occurring immediately before the first heart sound, that is, during atrial systole but immediately prior to ventricular systole. It is particularly associated with mitral stenosis and tricuspid stenosis. **pulmonic m.** A murmur occurring as a consequence of a disorder of the pulmonary valve or pulmonary artery. Also *pulmonary murmur.* **regurgitant m.** A murmur occurring in association with regurgitation through a valvular orifice. **Roger's m.** A murmur occurring in Roger's disease; a holosystolic murmur at the left sternal edge due to a small ventricular septal defect. **sea gull m.** A murmur suggesting the raucous call of a gull, occurring in some cases of aortic regurgitation associated with prolapse or rupture of an aortic cusp. **seesaw m.** A to-and-fro murmur, likened to the sound of a seesaw. **short systolic m.** A murmur occurring in only a small part of systole. **Steell's m.** GRAHAM STEELL'S MURMUR. **Still's m.** An innocent murmur of twanging quality, heard to the left of the sternum in children. **systolic m.** A murmur occurring during a part or the whole of systole. Also *systolic bruit.* **transmitted m.** A sound conducted to a location remote from the site of production. **Traube's m.** GALLOP RHYTHM. **tricuspid m.** A murmur deriving from disease at the tricuspid valve. **vascular m.** A murmur heard over a blood vessel. **venous m.** A murmur heard over a vein. **vesicular m.** The normal sound of breathing heard during auscultation of the chest. **waterwheel m.** MILL WHEEL MURMUR.

**Murphy** [James Bumgardner *Murphy,* U.S. pathologist, 1884–1950] Murphy-Sturm lymphosarcoma. See under LYMPHOSARCOMA.

**Murphy** [John Benjamin *Murphy,* U.S. surgeon, 1857–1916] See under PUNCH, SIGN, TREATMENT.

***Musca*** \mus′kə\ [L, a fly; akin to Gk *myia* a fly] A genus of flies of the family Muscidae in which the mouth parts are adapted for sponging and lapping. They are generally dull in color and of small to medium size. They are synanthropic in habits and noxious as filth feeders and as mechanical spreaders of bacterial and other infectious agents of human and animal disease. They include the houseflies. ***M. domestica*** The common housefly, which is predominantly gray, has four dark stripes on the dorsal thorax and is 6 to 9 mm long. It occurs wherever humans congregate and human waste and debris are found. Breeding in organic waste and filth, it is a mechanical vector of many pathogens. ***M. vomitoria*** *CALLIPHORA VOMITORIA.*

**musca** (*pl.* muscae) A fly; a housefly. A Latin term. **muscae hispanicae** CANTHARIDES. **muscae volitantes** Entoptic floating spots perceived visually due to opacities, suspended within the vitreous humor, which cast shadows on the retina. Also *opplotentes.*

**muscarine** \mus′kərin\ [*(Amanita) muscar(ia)* + -INE] A toxic alkaloid derived from *Amanita muscaria* and other fungi. Its molecules consist of a tetrahydrofuran ring carrying methyl, hydroxyl, and trimethylammoniomethyl substituents. It binds to some of the receptors for acetylcholine in the nervous system (muscarinic receptors), mainly in the autonomic nervous system.

**muscarinic** \mus′kərin′ik\ Denoting the biologic actions of acetylcholine that mimic those of muscarine.

**muscarinism** \mus′kərənizm\ [*muscarin(e)* + -ISM] Poisoning from ingestion of muscarine, a poisonous alkaloid present in *Amanita muscaria* in minute amounts, and in *Inocybe* and *Clitocybe* in larger amounts. It causes nausea, vomiting, lacrimation, bradycardia, circulatory collapse, coma, and occasionally death.

**muscicide** \mus′isid\ [*Musci(dae)* + -CIDE] An agent destructive to flies.

**Muscidae** \mus′idē\ [*Musc(a)* + -IDAE] A family of flies (order Diptera) that includes the genera *Musca* (houseflies), *Stomoxys* (stable flies), *Fannia* (lesser house flies, latrine flies), *Muscina* (false stable flies), *Hydrotaea, Atherigona, Ophyra, Morella* (sweat flies), and others.

***Muscina*** \musī′nə\ A genus of dung-breeding, nonbiting stable flies in the family Muscidae, related to the houseflies (*Musca*) and having similar habits.

# muscle

**muscle** [French, from L *musculus* muscle. See MUSCULUS.] 1 A basic tissue of the body, the cells of which are characteristically contractile, enabling movement to take place; muscular tissue. Three types are usually described: striated muscle, cardiac muscle, and nonstriated muscle. See also MUSCULUS SKELETI, CARDIAC MUSCLE, SMOOTH MUSCLE. 2 One of the individual organs composed of muscular tissue; musculus. **abductor m. of great toe** MUSCULUS ABDUCTOR HALLUCIS. **abductor m. of little finger** MUSCULUS ABDUCTOR DIGITI MINIMI MANUS. **abductor m. of little toe** MUSCULUS ABDUCTOR DIGITI MINIMI PEDIS. **accessory m.** An additional muscle slip not usually present, often being a variant of the usual attachments of a muscle. Occasionally it represents a muscle better developed in animals other than humans. **accessory flexor m.** MUSCULUS QUADRATUS PLANTAE. **adductor m. of great toe** MUSCULUS ADDUCTOR HALLUCIS. **adductor m. of thumb** MUSCULUS ADDUCTOR POLLICIS. **Aeby's m.** 1 A muscle located in the lips of the mouth and composed of fibers passing obliquely between the skin and the mucous membrane of the inner margin and somewhat at right angles to the fibers of musculus orbicularis oris. It is better developed in infants than in adults. 2 MUSCULUS DEPRESSOR LABII INFERIORIS. **agonistic m.** AGONIST. **Albinus m.** 1 MUSCULUS RISORIUS. 2 MUSCULUS SCALENUS MINIMUS. 3 A triangular muscle band extending between the side of the nose and the nasolabial furrow. **anconeus m.** MUSCULUS ANCONEUS. **antagonistic m.** A muscle that either opposes the action of a prime mover or initiates and maintains an opposite movement, thereby either controlling the action of the prime mover, neutralizing its contraction, or stabilizing or fixating a joint so that other prime movers may act on it. Also *antagonist.* **anterior auricular m.** MUSCULUS AURICULARIS ANTERIOR. **anterior intertransverse m.'s of neck** MUSCULI INTERTRANSVERSARII ANTERIORES CERVICIS. **anterior papillary m. of left ventricle** MUSCULUS PAPILLARIS ANTERIOR VENTRICULI SINISTRI. **anterior papillary m. of right ventricle** MUSCULUS PAPILLARIS ANTERIOR VENTRICULI DEXTRI. **anterior sacrococcygeal m.** MUSCULUS SACROCOCCYGEUS VENTRALIS. **anterior scalene m.** MUSCULUS SCALENUS ANTERIOR. **anterior serratus m.** MUSCULUS SERRATUS ANTERIOR. **anterior tibial m.** MUSCULUS TIBIALIS ANTERIOR. **antigravity m.'s** Muscles whose tonic state opposes the force of gravity and maintains the posture of an animal. Also *postural muscles.* **m. of antitragus** MUSCULUS ANTITRAGICUS. **appendicular m.** Any one of the skeletal muscles of a limb. **arrector m.'s of hair** MUSCULI ARRECTORES PILORUM. **articular m.** MUSCULUS ARTICULARIS. **articular m. of elbow** MUSCULUS ARTICULARIS CUBITI. **articular m. of knee** MUSCULUS ARTICULARIS GENUS. **aryepiglottic m.** MUSCULUS ARYEPIGLOTTICUS. **aryvocalis m. of Ludwig** ARYVOCALIS. **m.'s of auditory ossicles** MUSCULI OSSICULORUM AUDITUS. **axial m.** Any one of the skeletal muscles of the trunk or head. **Bell's m.** A band of oblique muscle fibers arising behind each ostium ureteris in the base of the bladder, descending along each side of the trigone towards the dorsum of the prostate, and inserting into the median lobe of the prostate by a fibrous band. **biceps m. of arm** MUSCULUS BICEPS BRACHII. **biceps m. of thigh** MUSCULUS BICEPS FEMORIS. **bicipital m.** A muscle with two heads of origin, such as the biceps brachii. **bipennate m.** MUSCULUS BIPENNATUS. **bipenniform m.** MUSCULUS BIPENNATUS. **Bowman's m.** MUSCULUS CILIARIS. **brachial m.** MUSCULUS BRACHIALIS. **brachioradial m.** MUSCULUS BRACHIORADIALIS. **Braune's m.** MUSCULUS PUBORECTALIS. **bronchoesophageal m.** MUSCULUS BRONCHOESOPHAGEUS. **Brücke's m.** The external part of the ciliary muscle, composed of meridional, or longitudinal, fibers. Also *Crampton's muscle.* **buccinator m.** MUSCULUS BUCCINATOR. **buccopharyngeal m.** PARS BUCCOPHARYNGEA MUSCULI CONSTRICTORIS PHARYNGIS SUPERIORIS. **bulbar m.'s** MUSCULI BULBI. **bulbocavernous m.** MUSCULUS BULBOSPONGIOSUS. **canine m.** MUSCULUS LEVATOR ANGULI ORIS. **cardiac m.** The involuntary but striated muscle constituting the myocardium of the heart and situated in all its walls and in those of the pulmonary veins and superior vena cava. The muscle fibers are composed of several individual cells joined end to end by cell junctions, or intercalated disks, and usually containing a single nucleus. In addition, they consist of myofibrils, sarcoplasm, and sarcolemma. Between the fibers is the endomysium, containing small blood vessels and lymphatics. The fibers contract rhythmically and automatically. Also *textus muscularis striatus cardiacus.* **Casser's m.** LIGAMENTUM MALLEI ANTERIUS. **casserian m.** LIGAMENTUM MALLEI ANTERIUS. **Casser's perforated m.** MUSCULUS CORACOBRACHIALIS. **ceratocricoid m.** MUSCULUS CERATOCRICOIDEUS. **ceratopharyngeal m.** PARS CERATOPHARYNGEA MUSCULI CONSTRICTORIS PHARYNGIS MEDII. **cheek m.** MUSCULUS BUCCINATOR. **chondroglossus m.** MUSCULUS CHONDROGLOSSUS. **chondropharyngeal m.** PARS CHONDROPHARYNGEA MUSCULI CONSTRICTORIS PHARYNGIS MEDII. **ciliary m.** 1 MUSCULUS CILIARIS. 2 RIOLAN'S MUSCLE. **circumpennate m.** A muscle in which the fasciculi arise from surrounding bones and fasciae and converge obliquely towards a centrally situated tendon in a fanlike fashion. Also *circumpennate.* **coccygeal m.** MUSCULUS COCCYGEUS. **coccygeal m.'s** MUSCULI COCCYGEI. **Coiter's m.** MUSCULUS CORRUGATOR SUPERCILII. **compressor m. of naris** PARS TRANSVERSA MUSCULI NASALIS. **congenerous m.'s** Muscles that perform the same function. **coracobrachial m.** MUSCULUS CORACOBRACHIALIS. **costocervicalis m.** MUSCULUS ILIOCOSTALIS CERVICIS. **Crampton's m.** BRÜCKE'S MUSCLE. **cremaster m.** MUSCULUS CREMASTER. **cricopharyngeal m.** PARS CRICOPHARYNGEA MUSCULI CONSTRICTORIS PHARYNGIS INFERIORIS. **cricothyroid m.** MUSCULUS CRICOTHYROIDEUS. **cutaneous m.** MUSCULUS CUTANEUS. **dartos m. of scrotum** MUSCULUS DARTOS. **deep flexor m. of fingers** MUSCULUS FLEXOR DIGITORUM PROFUNDUS. **deep transverse m. of perineum** MUSCULUS TRANSVERSUS PERINEI PROFUNDUS. **deltoid m.** MUSCULUS DELTOIDEUS. **depressor m. of angle of mouth** MUSCULUS DEPRESSOR ANGULI ORIS. **depressor m. of lower lip** MUSCULUS DEPRESSOR LABII INFERIORIS. **depressor m. of nasal septum** MUSCULUS DEPRESSOR SEPTI NASI. **dermal m.** MUSCULUS CUTANEUS. **detrusor urinae m.** MUSCULUS DETRUSOR VESICAE. **detrusor m. of urinary bladder** MUSCULUS DETRUSOR VESICAE. **diaphragmatic m.** DIAPHRAGMA. **digastric m.** MUSCULUS DIGASTRICUS. **dilator m. of nose** PARS ALARIS MUSCULI NASALIS.

**dilator m. of pupil** MUSCULUS DILATOR PUPILLAE. **dorsal m.'s** MUSCULI DORSI. **dorsal interosseous m.'s of foot** MUSCULI INTEROSSEI DORSALES PEDIS. **dorsal interosseous m.'s of hand** MUSCULI INTEROSSEI DORSALES MANUS. **dorsal sacrococcygeal m.** MUSCULUS SACROCOCCYGEUS DORSALIS. **Dupré's m.** MUSCULUS ARTICULARIS GENUS. **Duverney's m.** PARS LACRIMALIS MUSCULI ORBICULARIS OCULI. **emergency m.'s** Muscles that contract to assist prime movers when considerable force is needed. **epicranial m.** MUSCULUS EPICRANIUS. **epimeric m.** A muscle derived from the dorsal part of a myotome, or epimere, and innervated by the dorsal ramus of a spinal nerve. **erector m. of spine** MUSCULUS ERECTOR SPINAE. **extensor m. of fingers** MUSCULUS EXTENSOR DIGITORUM. **extensor m. of index finger** MUSCULUS EXTENSOR INDICIS. **extensor m. of little finger** MUSCULUS EXTENSOR DIGITI MINIMI. **external intercostal m.'s** MUSCULI INTERCOSTALES EXTERNI. **external oblique m. of abdomen** MUSCULUS OBLIQUUS EXTERNUS ABDOMINIS. **external obturator m.** MUSCULUS OBTURATORIUS EXTERNUS. **external pterygoid m.** *Outmoded* MUSCULUS PTERYGOIDEUS LATERALIS. **external sphincter m. of anus** MUSCULUS SPHINCTER ANI EXTERNUS. **extraocular m.'s** MUSCULI BULBI. **extrinsic m.** A muscle inserted into a structure, part, or organ from without. **m.'s of eye** MUSCULI BULBI. **facial m.** Any one of the several muscles of the face and scalp that affect the movements of the eyelids, nose, lips, ears, and scalp and are able to produce the various expressions of the face. **m.'s of fauces** MUSCULI PALATI ET FAUCIUM. **fixator m.'s** Prime movers and antagonistic muscles acting together either to stabilize the position of a joint or part or to permit other prime movers to act on the joint or part. Also *fixation muscles.* **frontal m.** VENTER FRONTALIS MUSCULI OCCIPITOFRONTALIS. **frontalis m.** VENTER FRONTALIS MUSCULI OCCIPITOFRONTALIS. **fusiform m.** MUSCULUS FUSIFORMIS. **gastrocnemius m.** MUSCULUS GASTROCNEMIUS. **Gavard's m.** FIBRAE OBLIQUAE GASTRICAE. **genioglossus m.** MUSCULUS GENIOGLOSSUS. **geniohyoid m.** MUSCULUS GENIOHYOIDEUS. **glossopalatine m.** MUSCULUS PALATOGLOSSUS. **glossopharyngeal m.** PARS GLOSSOPHARYNGEA MUSCULI CONSTRICTORIS PHARYNGIS SUPERIORIS. **gracilis m.** MUSCULUS GRACILIS. **great adductor m.** MUSCULUS ADDUCTOR MAGNUS. **greater pectoral m.** MUSCULUS PECTORALIS MAJOR. **greater psoas m.** MUSCULUS PSOAS MAJOR. **greater rhomboid m.** MUSCULUS RHOMBOIDEUS MAJOR. **greater zygomatic m.** MUSCULUS ZYGOMATICUS MAJOR. **greatest gluteal m.** MUSCULUS GLUTEUS MAXIMUS. **Guthrie's m.** MUSCULUS SPHINCTER URETHRAE. **hamstring m.** One of the muscles at the back of the thigh: the semimembranosus, semitendinosus, or biceps femoris. **m. of Henle** MUSCULUS AURICULARIS ANTERIOR. **Hilton's m.** MUSCULUS ARYEPIGLOTTICUS. **Horner's m.** PARS LACRIMALIS MUSCULI ORBICULARIS OCULI. **Houston's m.** 1 Compressor venae dorsalis of the penis. 2 A fasciculus of the ischiocavernosus muscle that occasionally is inserted into the fascia on the dorsum of the penis. **hyoglossal m.** MUSCULUS HYOGLOSSUS. **hyoglossus m.** MUSCULUS HYOGLOSSUS. **hypaxial m.'s** The muscles ventral to the vertebral column, such as longus capitis, longus colli, the vertebral portion of the diaphragm, and sacrococcygeus anterior. Also *subvertebral muscles.* **hypomeric m.** A muscle derived from the ventral, or hypaxial, region of a myotome that migrates anteriorly in the body wall, or somatopleure, and is innervated by a ventral ramus of a spinal nerve. **iliac m.** MUSCULUS ILIACUS. **iliococcygeal m.** MUSCULUS ILIOCOCCYGEUS. **iliocostal m.** MUSCULUS ILIOCOSTALIS. **iliocostal m. of loins** MUSCULUS ILIOCOSTALIS LUMBORUM. **iliocostal m. of neck** MUSCULUS ILIOCOSTALIS CERVICIS. **iliocostal m. of thorax** MUSCULUS ILIOCOSTALIS THORACIS. **iliopsoas m.** MUSCULUS ILIOPSOAS. **incisive m.'s of lower lip** MUSCULI INCISIVI LABII INFERIORIS. **incisive m.'s of upper lip** MUSCULI INCISIVI LABII SUPERIORIS. **m. of incisure of helix** MUSCULUS INCISURAE HELICIS. **inferior constrictor m. of pharynx** MUSCULUS CONSTRICTOR PHARYNGIS INFERIOR. **inferior gemellus m.** MUSCULUS GEMELLUS INFERIOR. **inferior longitudinal m. of tongue** MUSCULUS LONGITUDINALIS INFERIOR LINGUAE. **inferior oblique m. of eyeball** MUSCULUS OBLIQUUS INFERIOR BULBI. **inferior oblique m. of head** MUSCULUS OBLIQUUS CAPITIS INFERIOR. **inferior pharyngeal constrictor m.** MUSCULUS CONSTRICTOR PHARYNGIS INFERIOR. **inferior posterior serratus m.** MUSCULUS SERRATUS POSTERIOR INFERIOR. **inferior rectus m. of bulb** MUSCULUS RECTUS INFERIOR BULBI. **inferior straight m.** MUSCULUS RECTUS INFERIOR BULBI. **inferior tarsal m.** MUSCULUS TARSALIS INFERIOR. **infrahyoid m.'s** MUSCULI INFRAHYOIDEI. **infraspinous m.** MUSCULUS INFRASPINATUS. **innermost intercostal m.'s** MUSCULI INTERCOSTALES INTIMI. **inspiratory m.'s** The muscles taking part in quiet, deep and forced inspiration, including the diaphragm, intercostal, scalene, pectoral, and erector spinae muscles. **interarytenoid m.'s** The musculus arytenoideus obliquus and the musculus arytenoideus transversus. **intercostal m.** Any of the short voluntary muscles between adjacent ribs. **internal intercostal m.'s** MUSCULI INTERCOSTALES INTERNI. **internal oblique m. of abdomen** MUSCULUS OBLIQUUS INTERNUS ABDOMINIS. **internal obturator m.** MUSCULUS OBTURATORIUS INTERNUS. **internal pterygoid m.** *Outmoded* MUSCULUS PTERYGOIDEUS MEDIALIS. **internal sphincter m. of anus** MUSCULUS SPHINCTER ANI INTERNUS. **interspinal m.'s** MUSCULI INTERSPINALES. **interspinal m.'s of loins** MUSCULI INTERSPINALES LUMBORUM. **interspinal m.'s of neck** MUSCULI INTERSPINALES CERVICIS. **interspinal m.'s of thorax** MUSCULI INTERSPINALES THORACIS. **intertransverse m.'s** MUSCULI INTERTRANSVERSARII. **intertransverse m.'s of thorax** MUSCULI INTERTRANSVERSARII THORACIS. **intraocular m.'s** The intrinsic muscles of the eyeball, such as the musculus ciliaris, musculus dilator pupillae, and musculus sphincter pupillae. **intratympanic m.** Either musculus tensor tympani or musculus stapedius. **intrinsic m.** A muscle in which both origin and insertion are contained within the same part or organ. **involuntary m.** Collectively, muscles that are not usually under the direct control of the will, such as those in the walls of the alimentary and urogenital tracts and blood vessels. Although cardiac muscle is involuntary it is different in structure from both skeletal and nonstriated muscle. Also *nonstriated muscle, smooth muscle, textus muscularis nonstriatus, unstriated muscle.* **iridic m.'s** The muscles that regulate the iris, namely the musculus dilator pupillae and the musculus sphincter pupillae. **ischiocavernous m.** MUSCULUS ISCHIOCAVERNOSUS. **Jung's m.** MUSCULUS PYRAMIDALIS AURICULAE. **Landström's m.** Minute peribulbar smooth muscle bundles around the anterior aspect of the eyeball that are attached to the orbital septum and the palpebral muscles. **m.'s of larynx** MUSCULI LARYNGIS. **lateral cricoaryte-**

**noid m.** MUSCULUS CRICOARYTENOIDEUS LATERALIS. **lateral intertransverse m.'s of loins** MUSCULI INTERTRANSVERSARII LATERALES LUMBORUM. **lateral pterygoid m.** MUSCULUS PTERYGOIDEUS LATERALIS. **lateral rectus m. of bulb** MUSCULUS RECTUS LATERALIS BULBI. **lateral straight m.** MUSCULUS RECTUS LATERALIS BULBI. **latissimus dorsi m.** MUSCULUS LATISSIMUS DORSI. **least gluteal m.** MUSCULUS GLUTEUS MINIMUS. **lesser rhomboid m.** MUSCULUS RHOMBOIDEUS MINOR. **lesser zygomatic m.** MUSCULUS ZYGOMATICUS MINOR. **levator m. of angle of mouth** MUSCULUS LEVATOR ANGULI ORIS. **levator ani m.** MUSCULUS LEVATOR ANI. **levator m. of prostate** MUSCULUS LEVATOR PROSTATAE. **levator m.'s of ribs** MUSCULI LEVATORES COSTARUM. **levator m. of scapula** MUSCULUS LEVATOR SCAPULAE. **levator m. of thyroid gland** MUSCULUS LEVATOR GLANDULAE THYROIDEAE. **levator m. of upper eyelid** MUSCULUS LEVATOR PALPEBRAE SUPERIORIS. **levator m. of upper lip** MUSCULUS LEVATOR LABII SUPERIORIS. **levator m. of upper lip and ala of nose** MUSCULUS LEVATOR LABII SUPERIORIS ALAEQUE NASI. **levator m. of velum palatinum** MUSCULUS LEVATOR VELI PALATINI. **long abductor m. of thumb** MUSCULUS ABDUCTOR POLLICIS LONGUS. **long adductor m.** MUSCULUS ADDUCTOR LONGUS. **long extensor m. of great toe** MUSCULUS EXTENSOR HALLUCIS LONGUS. **long extensor m. of thumb** MUSCULUS EXTENSOR POLLICIS LONGUS. **long extensor m. of toes** MUSCULUS EXTENSOR DIGITORUM LONGUS. **long fibular m.** MUSCULUS PERONEUS LONGUS. **long flexor m. of great toe** MUSCULUS FLEXOR HALLUCIS LONGUS. **long flexor m. of thumb** MUSCULUS FLEXOR POLLICIS LONGUS. **long flexor m. of toes** MUSCULUS FLEXOR DIGITORUM LONGUS. **long m. of head** MUSCULUS LONGUS CAPITIS. **longissimus m.** MUSCULUS LONGISSIMUS. **longissimus m. of head** MUSCULUS LONGISSIMUS CAPITIS. **longissimus m. of neck** MUSCULUS LONGISSIMUS CERVICIS. **longissimus m. of thorax** MUSCULUS LONGISSIMUS THORACIS. **longitudinal m.** A muscle or muscle mass in which the fibers extend in a lengthwise direction. **long levator m.'s of ribs** MUSCULI LEVATORES COSTARUM LONGI. **long m. of neck** MUSCULUS LONGUS COLLI. **long palmar m.** MUSCULUS PALMARIS LONGUS. **long peroneal m.** MUSCULUS PERONEUS LONGUS. **Ludwig's m.** ARYVOCALIS. **lumbrical m.'s of foot** MUSCULI LUMBRICALES PEDIS. **lumbrical m.'s of hand** MUSCULI LUMBRICALES MANUS. **Luschka's m.'s** MUSCULUS RECTOUTERINUS. **masseter m.** MUSCULUS MASSETER. **medial intertransverse m.'s of loins** MUSCULI INTERTRANSVERSARII MEDIALES LUMBORUM. **medial pterygoid m.** MUSCULUS PTERYGOIDEUS MEDIALIS. **medial rectus m. of bulb** MUSCULUS RECTUS MEDIALIS BULBI. **medial straight m.** MUSCULUS RECTUS MEDIALIS BULBI. **Merkel's m.** MUSCULUS CERATOCRICOIDEUS. **middle constrictor m. of pharynx** MUSCULUS CONSTRICTOR PHARYNGIS MEDIUS. **middle gluteal m.** MUSCULUS GLUTEUS MEDIUS. **middle pharyngeal constrictor m.** MUSCULUS CONSTRICTOR PHARYNGIS MEDIUS. **middle scalene m.** MUSCULUS SCALENUS MEDIUS. **Müller's m.** 1 FIBRAE CIRCULARES MUSCULI CILIARIS. 2 MUSCULUS TARSALIS SUPERIOR. 3 MUSCULUS ORBITALIS. **multicipital m.** A muscle with several heads of origin. **multifidus m.'s** MUSCULI MULTIFIDI. **multipennate m.** A muscle with several tendons between which the fasciculi run obliquely in featherlike fashion, as in the deltoid muscle. **multi-unit m.** A type of smooth muscle in which many cells receive motor terminals from nerve plexuses that initiate contraction, such as in the muscle of the iris and the walls of larger arteries. Compare UNITARY MUSCLE. **mylohyoid m.** MUSCULUS MYLOHYOIDEUS. **mylopharyngeal m.** PARS MYLOPHARYNGEA MUSCULI CONSTRICTORIS PHARYNGIS SUPERIORIS. **nasal m.** MUSCULUS NASALIS. **m.'s of neck** MUSCULI COLLI. **nonstriated m.** INVOLUNTARY MUSCLE. **oblique arytenoid m.** MUSCULUS ARYTENOIDEUS OBLIQUUS. **oblique m. of auricle** MUSCULUS OBLIQUUS AURICULAE. **obturator externus m.** MUSCULUS OBTURATORIUS EXTERNUS. **obturator internus m.** MUSCULUS OBTURATORIUS INTERNUS. **occipital m.** VENTER OCCIPITALIS MUSCULI OCCIPITOFRONTALIS. **occipitofrontal m.** MUSCULUS OCCIPITOFRONTALIS. **ocular m.'s** MUSCULI BULBI. **Oddi's m.** MUSCULUS SPHINCTER AMPULLAE HEPATOPANCREATICAE. **omohyoid m.** MUSCULUS OMOHYOIDEUS. **opposing m. of little finger** MUSCULUS OPPONENS DIGITI MINIMI. **opposing m. of thumb** MUSCULUS OPPONENS POLLICIS. **orbicular m.** MUSCULUS ORBICULARIS. **orbicular m. of eye** MUSCULUS ORBICULARIS OCULI. **orbicular m. of mouth** MUSCULUS ORBICULARIS ORIS. **orbital m.** MUSCULUS ORBITALIS. **m.'s of ossicles** MUSCULI OSSICULORUM AUDITUS. **m.'s of palate and fauces** MUSCULI PALATI ET FAUCIUM. **palatoglossus m.** MUSCULUS PALATOGLOSSUS. **palatopharyngeal m.** MUSCULUS PALATOPHARYNGEUS. **palmar interosseous m.'s** MUSCULI INTEROSSEI PALMARES. **papillary m.'s** MUSCULI PAPILLARES. **pectinate m.'s** MUSCULI PECTINATI. **pectineal m.** MUSCULUS PECTINEUS. **pectorodorsalis m.** One of the accessory muscles of the pectoral region. It consists of a slip from the pectoralis major muscle that may either fuse with either the latissimus dorsi or teres major muscle, or extend from latissimus dorsi either to the long tendon of the biceps brachii muscle, to the axillary fascia, or to the coracoid process. Also *axillary arch, Langer's axillary arch.* **pennate m.** A muscle in which the fasciculi are oblique to the line of pull of the tendon in featherlike patterns that are categorized as unipennate, bipennate, circumpennate, or multipennate. Also *penniform muscle.* **perineal m.'s** MUSCULI PERINEI. **m.'s of perineum** MUSCULI PERINEI. **piriform m.** MUSCULUS PIRIFORMIS. **plantar m.** MUSCULUS PLANTARIS. **plantar interosseous m.'s** MUSCULI INTEROSSEI PLANTARES. **platysma m.** PLATYSMA. **pleuroesophageal m.** MUSCULUS PLEUROESOPHAGEUS. **popliteal m.** MUSCULUS POPLITEUS. **postaxial m.** A muscle located caudal to the axial line of an extremity. **posterior auricular m.** MUSCULUS AURICULARIS POSTERIOR. **posterior cricoarytenoid m.** MUSCULUS CRICOARYTENOIDEUS POSTERIOR. **posterior intertransverse m.'s of neck** MUSCULI INTERTRANSVERSARII POSTERIORES CERVICIS. **posterior papillary m. of left ventricle** MUSCULUS PAPILLARIS POSTERIOR VENTRICULI SINISTRI. **posterior papillary m. of right ventricle** MUSCULUS PAPILLARIS POSTERIOR VENTRICULI DEXTRI. **posterior sacrococcygeal m.** MUSCULUS SACROCOCCYGEUS DORSALIS. **posterior scalene m.** MUSCULUS SCALENUS POSTERIOR. **posterior tibial m.** MUSCULUS TIBIALIS POSTERIOR. **postural m.'s** ANTIGRAVITY MUSCLES. **preaxial m.** A muscle located cranial to the axial line of an extremity. **prevertebral m.'s** A deep group of muscles situated on the anterior surface of the cervical and first three thoracic vertebrae. They are symmetrically placed on each side of the median plane and comprise the musculus longus capitis, musculus longus colli, musculus rectus capitis anterior, and musculus rectus capitis lateralis. Together they flex the head and the neck. They are innervated by the ventral rami of the cervical nerves. Some authorities also include the scalene muscles in this group. **procerus m.** MUSCULUS PROCERUS. **pterygopharyngeal m.** PARS PTERYGOPHARYNGEA MUSCULI CONSTRICTORIS PHARYNGIS SUPERIORIS. **pubococcygeal m.** MUSCULUS PUBOCOCCYGEUS. **puboprostatic m.** MUSCULUS PUBOPROSTATICUS. **puborectal m.** MUSCULUS PUBORECTALIS. **puborectalis m.** MUSCULUS PUBORECTALIS. **pubovaginal m.** MUSCULUS PUBOVAGINALIS. **pubovesical m.** MUSCULUS PUBOVESICALIS. **pyramidal m.** MUSCULUS PYRAMIDALIS. **pyramidal m. of auricle** MUSCULUS PYRAMIDALIS AURICULAE. **quadrate pronator m.** MUSCULUS PRONATOR QUADRATUS. **quadrate m. of sole** MUSCULUS QUADRATUS PLANTAE. **quadrate m. of thigh** MUSCULUS QUADRATUS FEMORIS. **quadriceps femoris m.** MUSCULUS QUADRICEPS FEMORIS. **quadriceps m. of thigh** MUSCULUS QUADRICEPS FEMORIS. **radial flexor m. of wrist** MUSCULUS FLEXOR CARPI RADIALIS. **rectococcygeus m.** MUSCULUS RECTOCOCCYGEUS. **rectourethral m.** MUSCULUS RECTOURETHRALIS. **rectouterine m.** MUSCULUS RECTOUTERINUS. **rectovesical m.** MUSCULUS RECTOVESICALIS. **red m.** Skeletal muscle of dark color, rich in myoglobin and containing numerous mitochondria, characterized by slow contractability. Compare WHITE MUSCLE. **Reisseisen's m.'s** The smooth muscle fibers of the smallest bronchi and the bronchioles. **ribbon m.'s** MUSCULI INFRAHYOIDEI. **riders' m.'s** The adductor muscles of the thigh, used to grip the saddle during horseback riding. **Riolan's m.** **1** The portion of the orbicularis oculi nearest to the eyelid margin. Also *ciliary muscle.* **2** MUSCULUS CREMASTER. **risorius m.** MUSCULUS RISORIUS. **rotator m.'s** MUSCULI ROTATORES. **rotator m.'s of neck** MUSCULI ROTATORES CERVICIS. **rotator m.'s of thorax** MUSCULI ROTATORES THORACIS. **Rouget's m.** FIBRAE CIRCULARES MUSCULI CILIARIS. **round pronator m.** MUSCULUS PRONATOR TERES. **sacrospinal m.** *Outmoded* MUSCULUS ERECTOR SPINAE. **salpingopharyngeal m.** MUSCULUS SALPINGOPHARYNGEUS. **Santorini's m.** **1** MUSCULUS RISORIUS. **2** MUSCULUS INCISURAE HELICIS. **3** A partial band of smooth muscle fibers under the sphincter urethrae. **m. of Sappey** MUSCULUS TEMPOROPARIETALIS. **sartorius m.** MUSCULUS SARTORIUS. **scalene m.'s** Those muscles that pass from cervical vertebral transverse processes to the first rib. **Sebileau's m.** The deeper fibers of the tunica dartos that bend inward at the raphe of the scrotum to help form the septum of the scrotum. **semimembranous m.** MUSCULUS SEMIMEMBRANOSUS. **semispinal m.** MUSCULUS SEMISPINALIS. **semispinal m. of head** MUSCULUS SEMISPINALIS CAPITIS. **semispinal m. of neck** MUSCULUS SEMISPINALIS CERVICIS. **semispinal m. of thorax** MUSCULUS SEMISPINALIS THORACIS. **semitendinous m.** MUSCULUS SEMITENDINOSUS. **short abductor m. of thumb** MUSCULUS ABDUCTOR POLLICIS BREVIS. **short adductor m.** MUSCULUS ADDUCTOR BREVIS. **short extensor m. of great toe** MUSCULUS EXTENSOR HALLUCIS BREVIS. **short extensor m. of thumb** MUSCULUS EXTENSOR POLLICIS BREVIS. **short extensor m. of toes** MUSCULUS EXTENSOR DIGITORUM BREVIS. **short flexor m. of great toe** MUSCULUS FLEXOR HALLUCIS BREVIS. **short flexor m. of little finger** MUSCULUS FLEXOR DIGITI MINIMI BREVIS MANUS. **short flexor m. of little toe** MUSCULUS FLEXOR DIGITI MINIMI BREVIS PEDIS. **short flexor m. of thumb** MUSCULUS FLEXOR POLLICIS BREVIS. **short flexor m. of toes** MUSCULUS FLEXOR DIGITORUM BREVIS. **short levator m.'s of ribs** MUSCULI LEVATORES COSTARUM BREVES. **short palmar m.** MUSCULUS PALMARIS BREVIS. **short peroneal m.** MUSCULUS PERONEUS BREVIS. **short radial extensor m. of wrist** MUSCULUS EXTENSOR CARPI RADIALIS BREVIS. **shunt m.'s** See under SHUNT MUSCLE THEORY. **Sibson's m.** MUSCULUS SCALENUS MINIMUS. **skeletal m.** MUSCULUS SKELETI. **smaller pectoral m.** MUSCULUS PECTORALIS MINOR. **smaller psoas m.** MUSCULUS PSOAS MINOR. **smallest adductor m.** MUSCULUS ADDUCTOR MINIMUS. **smallest scalene m.** MUSCULUS SCALENUS MINIMUS. **smooth m.** INVOLUNTARY MUSCLE. **Soemmering's m.** MUSCULUS LEVATOR GLANDULAE THYROIDEAE. **soleus m.** MUSCULUS SOLEUS. **sphincter m.** MUSCULUS SPHINCTER. **sphincter m. of bile duct** MUSCULUS SPHINCTER DUCTUS CHOLEDOCHI. **sphincter m. of hepatopancreatic ampulla** MUSCULUS SPHINCTER AMPULLAE HEPATOPANCREATICAE. **sphincter m. of membranous urethra** MUSCULUS SPHINCTER URETHRAE. **sphincter m. of pancreatic duct** MUSCULUS SPHINCTER DUCTUS PANCREATICI. **sphincter m. of pupil** MUSCULUS SPHINCTER PUPILLAE. **sphincter m. of pylorus** MUSCULUS SPHINCTER PYLORICUS. **sphincter m. of urethra** MUSCULUS SPHINCTER URETHRAE. **sphincter m. of urinary bladder** MUSCULUS SPHINCTER VESICAE URINARIAE. **spinal m.** MUSCULUS SPINALIS. **splenius m. of head** MUSCULUS SPLENIUS CAPITIS. **splenius m. of neck** MUSCULUS SPLENIUS CERVICIS. **spurt m.'s** See under SHUNT MUSCLE THEORY. **stapedius m.** MUSCULUS STAPEDIUS. **sternal m.** MUSCULUS STERNALIS. **sternocleidomastoid m.** MUSCULUS STERNOCLEIDOMASTOIDEUS. **sternohyoid m.** MUSCULUS STERNOHYOIDEUS. **sternomastoid m.** MUSCULUS STERNOCLEIDOMASTOIDEUS. **sternothyroid m.** MUSCULUS STERNOTHYROIDEUS. **strap m.'s** MUSCULI INFRAHYOIDEI. **striated m.** MUSCULUS SKELETI. • Cardiac muscle, though involuntary, is also striated. **striped m.** MUSCULUS SKELETI. **styloglossus m.** MUSCULUS STYLOGLOSSUS. **stylohyoid m.** MUSCULUS STYLOHYOIDEUS. **stylopharyngeus m.** MUSCULUS STYLOPHARYNGEUS. **subanconeus m.** MUSCULUS ARTICULARIS CUBITI. **subclavius m.** MUSCULUS SUBCLAVIUS. **subcostal m.'s** MUSCULI SUBCOSTALES. **subscapular m.** MUSCULUS SUBSCAPULARIS. **subvertebral m.'s** HYPAXIAL MUSCLES. **superciliary corrugator m.** MUSCULUS CORRUGATOR SUPERCILII. **superciliary depressor m.** MUSCULUS DEPRESSOR SUPERCILII. **superficial flexor m. of fingers** MUSCULUS FLEXOR DIGITORUM SUPERFICIALIS. **superficial transverse m. of perineum** MUSCULUS TRANSVERSUS PERINEI SUPERFICIALIS. **superior auricular m.** MUSCULUS AURICULARIS SUPERIOR. **superior constrictor m. of pharynx** MUSCULUS CONSTRICTOR PHARYNGIS SUPERIOR. **superior gemellus m.** MUSCULUS GEMELLUS SUPERIOR. **superior longitudinal m. of tongue** MUSCULUS LONGITUDINALIS SUPERIOR LINGUAE. **superior oblique m. of eyeball** MUSCULUS OBLIQUUS SUPERIOR BULBI. **superior oblique m. of head** MUSCULUS OBLIQUUS CAPITIS SUPERIOR. **superior pharyngeal constrictor m.** MUSCULUS CONSTRICTOR PHARYNGIS SUPERIOR. **superior posterior serratus m.** MUSCULUS SERRATUS POSTERIOR SUPERIOR. **superior rectus m. of bulb** MUSCULUS RECTUS SUPERIOR BULBI. **superior tarsal m.** MUSCULUS TARSALIS SUPE-

RIOR. **supinator m.** MUSCULUS SUPINATOR. **suprahyoid m.'s** MUSCULI SUPRAHYOIDEI. **supraspinous m.** MUSCULUS SUPRASPINATUS. **suspensory m. of duodenum** MUSCULUS SUSPENSORIUS DUODENI. **synergistic m.** A muscle that complements a prime mover acting across a multiaxial joint or a number of joints by serving as a partial antagonist and permitting the prime mover to maximize its action. Also *synergic muscle.* **temporal m.** MUSCULUS TEMPORALIS. **temporoparietal m.** MUSCULUS TEMPOROPARIETALIS. **tensor m. of fascia lata** MUSCULUS TENSOR FASCIAE LATAE. **tensor tympani m.** MUSCULUS TENSOR TYMPANI. **tensor m. of tympanic membrane** MUSCULUS TENSOR TYMPANI. **tensor m. of tympanum** MUSCULUS TENSOR TYMPANI. **tensor m. of velum palatinum** MUSCULUS TENSOR VELI PALATINI. **teres major m.** MUSCULUS TERES MAJOR. **teres minor m.** MUSCULUS TERES MINOR. **thenar m.'s** The muscles forming the thenar eminence, namely, abductor pollicis brevis, flexor pollicis brevis, and opponens pollicis. **third peroneal m.** MUSCULUS PERONEUS TERTIUS. **thyroarytenoid m.** MUSCULUS THYROARYTENOIDEUS. **thyroepiglottic m.** MUSCULUS THYROEPIGLOTTICUS. **thyrohyoid m.** MUSCULUS THYROHYOIDEUS. **thyropharyngeal m.** PARS THYROPHARYNGEA MUSCULI CONSTRICTORIS PHARYNGIS INFERIORIS. **Tod's m.** MUSCULUS OBLIQUUS AURICULAE. **m.'s of the tongue** MUSCULI LINGUAE. **tracheal m.** MUSCULUS TRACHEALIS. **m. of tragus** MUSCULUS TRAGICUS. **transverse m. of abdomen** MUSCULUS TRANSVERSUS ABDOMINIS. **transverse arytenoid m.** MUSCULUS ARYTENOIDEUS TRANSVERSUS. **transverse m. of auricle** MUSCULUS TRANSVERSUS AURICULAE. **transverse m. of chin** MUSCULUS TRANSVERSUS MENTI. **transverse m. of thorax** MUSCULUS TRANSVERSUS THORACIS. **transverse m. of tongue** MUSCULUS TRANSVERSUS LINGUAE. **transversospinal m.'s** MUSCULI TRANSVERSOSPINALES. **transversus abdominis m.** MUSCULUS TRANSVERSUS ABDOMINIS. **trapezius m.** MUSCULUS TRAPEZIUS. **m. of Treitz** MUSCULUS SUSPENSORIUS DUODENI. **triangular m.** MUSCULUS DEPRESSOR ANGULI ORIS. **triceps m. of arm** MUSCULUS TRICEPS BRACHII. **triceps m. of calf** MUSCULUS TRICEPS SURAE. **tricipital m.** A muscle with three heads of origin, as the triceps brachii. **ulnar flexor m. of wrist** MUSCULUS FLEXOR CARPI ULNARIS. **unipennate m.** MUSCULUS UNIPENNATUS. **unitary m.** A smooth muscle with relatively scanty motor innervation, so that its rhythmic contraction is myogenic in origin, such as in the walls of the uterus, intestines, stomach, and ureter. Compare MULTI-UNIT MUSCLE. **unstriated m.** INVOLUNTARY MUSCLE. **m. of uvula** MUSCULUS UVULAE. **Valsalva's m.** MUSCULUS TRAGICUS. **ventral sacrococcygeal m.** MUSCULUS SACROCOCCYGEUS VENTRALIS. **vertical m. of tongue** MUSCULUS VERTICALIS LINGUAE. **vestigial m.** A muscle that is rudimentary or incompletely developed in humans but fully developed and functional in some lower mammals. **vocal m.** MUSCULUS VOCALIS. **voluntary m.** A muscle that is usually under the direct control of the will. This type of muscle is usually skeletal, and its myofibrils are striated, except for cardiac muscle which, though striated, is involuntary. **white m.** Skeletal muscle of pale color, having little myoglobin and few mitochondria, characterized by fast contractability. Compare RED MUSCLE.

**muscle-trimming** BORDER MOLDING.

**muscoid** \mus′koid\ Of or belonging to the dipteran superfamily Muscoidea, suborder Cyclorrhapha, which includes the many disease-bearing and pestiferous flies of the family Muscidae.

**muscular** \mus′kyələr\ [*muscul(us)* + -AR] **1** Of or pertaining to muscles. **2** Characterized by or consisting of muscles. **3** Having well-developed musculature.

**muscularis** \mus′kyəlar′is\ [New L] Muscular: applied especially to a tunica muscularis, or muscular coat, of a tubular structure or hollow organ.

**muscularity** \mus′kyəlar′itē\ The state of being muscular or of possessing strong muscles.

**musculation** \mus′kyəlā′shən\ The contraction of a muscle.

**musculature** \mus′kyəlā′chər\ **1** The muscle system as a whole or of a part. **2** The arrangement of muscles in a part or an organ.

**musculi** \mus′kyəlī\ Plural of MUSCULUS.

**musculo-** \mus′kyəlō-\ [L *musculus* muscle] A combining form meaning muscle or muscular.

**musculoaponeurotic** \-ap′ōnʸůrät′ik\ Pertaining to a structure that is composed of both muscle and an aponeurosis.

**musculocutaneous** \-kyootā′nē·əs\ Pertaining to muscles and skin, especially in reference to certain nerves supplying both muscle and skin. Also *musculodermic* (outmoded), *myocutaneous.*

**musculoelastic** \-ilas′tik\ Pertaining to or possessing both muscle and elastic tissues.

**musculofascial** \-fash′ē·əl\ Composed of both muscular and fascial tissues.

**musculofibrous** \-fī′brəs\ Pertaining to tissue that is both muscular and fibrous.

**musculomembranous** \-mem′brənəs\ Pertaining to or possessing both muscle fibers and membrane.

**musculophrenic** \-fren′ik\ Pertaining to or supplying muscles and the diaphragm.

**musculorachidian** \-rəkid′ē·ən\ Pertaining to the spinal muscles.

**musculoskeletal** \-skel′ətəl\ Pertaining to muscles and the skeleton, as *musculoskeletal system.*

**musculospiral** \-spī′rəl\ Pertaining to muscles and a spiral direction, especially with reference to nervus radialis.

**musculospiralis** \-spirā′lis\ *Seldom used* NERVUS RADIALIS.

**musculotegumentary** \-teg′yəmen′tərē\ Pertaining to muscle and the integument.

**musculotendinous** \-ten′dinəs\ Pertaining to or comprising both muscle and tendinous fibers.

**musculotonic** \-tän′ik\ Denoting the sustained contraction and active tension of a muscle.

**musculotropic** \-träp′ik\ Directed to or attracted by muscle tissue.

# musculus

**musculus** \mus′kyələs\ [L (dim. of *mus* a mouse, rat; akin to Gk *mys* a mouse, muscle), a little mouse, a muscle] (*pl.* musculi) An organ of the body composed of tissue the contraction of which produces motion; muscle. See also MUSCULUS SKELETI, CARDIAC MUSCLE, SMOOTH MUSCLE. **musculi abdominis** [NA] The muscles forming the walls, roof, and floor of the abdominal cavity. **m. abductor digiti minimi manus** [NA] A muscle originating from the pisiform bone, pisohamate ligament and the tendon of the flexor carpi ulnaris muscle. It is inserted onto the medial side of proximal phalanx of little finger and the medial border of dorsal expansion of extensor digiti minimi. It is supplied by the ulnar nerve, and abducts the extended little finger. Also *abductor muscle of little finger.* **m. abductor digiti minimi pedis** [NA] A muscle originating from the medial and lateral processes of the calcanean tuberosity and the bone between them, the central portion of plantar aponeurosis, and the lateral intermuscular septum. It is inserted onto the lateral surface of the proximal phalanx of fifth toe. It is supplied by the lateral plantar nerve and abducts and flexes the proximal phalanx of little toe. Also *abductor muscle of little toe.* **m. abductor hallucis** [NA] A muscle originating from flexor retinaculum, medial process of calcaneal tuberosity, plantar aponeurosis, and medial intermuscular septum. It is inserted with tendon of flexor hallucis brevis into the base of the proximal phalanx of the great toe. It is supplied by the medial plantar nerve, abducts and flexes the proximal phalanx of hallux, and helps to maintain the medial longitudinal arch. Also *abductor muscle of great toe.* **m. abductor pollicis brevis** [NA] A muscle originating from flexor retinaculum, and from the tubercles of the trapezium and scaphoid bones. Its medial fibers are inserted into the lateral side of the base of the proximal phalanx of thumb, and its lateral fibers into the dorsal expansion of the extensor pollicis longus muscle. Supplied by the median nerve, it abducts the thumb, rotating it medially; flexes the proximal phalanx; and extends the terminal phalanx. Also *short abductor muscle of thumb.* **m. abductor pollicis longus** [NA] A muscle originating from the upper middle portion of the lateral part of the posterior surface of the ulna, the adjacent interosseous membrane, and the middle third of the posterior surface of the radius. It is inserted into the lateral side of the base of the first metacarpal bone and the trapezium, and supplied by the posterior interosseous nerve. It abducts the thumb; helps to extend the thumb; and helps to abduct the hand. Also *long abductor muscle of thumb.* **m. adductor brevis** [NA] A muscle originating from the medial part of the outer aspect of the body and inferior ramus of pubis. It is inserted by aponeurotic bands into the lower part of the pectineal line and upper third of the linea aspera of femur. It is supplied by the obturator nerve, and adducts and helps to flex and laterally rotate the thigh. Also *short adductor muscle.* **m. adductor hallucis** [NA] A muscle of which the caput obliquum originates from the bases of the second, third, and fourth metatarsals, and from the sheath of the tendon of the peroneus longus muscle; and caput transversum from the plantar metatarsophalangeal ligaments of the lateral three toes and deep transverse metatarsal ligaments between them. It is inserted into the lateral part of base of proximal phalanx of hallux and onto the lateral sesamoid bone. It is supplied by the lateral plantar nerve, and adducts and flexes the proximal phalanx of the great toe. Also *adductor muscle of great toe.* **m. adductor longus** [NA] A muscle originating at the front of the pubis in the angle between the crest and the symphysis pubis. It is inserted into the middle third of linea aspera of femur, fused with the medial intermuscular septum. It is supplied by the anterior division of the obturator nerve, and adducts, flexes, and medially rotates the thigh. Also *long adductor muscle.* **m. adductor magnus** [NA] A muscle originating from the inferior pubic ramus, the ramus of the ischium, and the inferolateral portion of the ischial tuberosity. It is inserted into the medial margin of the gluteal ridge, the distal three-fourths of the linea aspera, the proximal portion of the medial supracondylar line, and the adductor tubercle. It is supplied by the posterior division of the obturator nerve and the tibial division of the sciatic nerve. It adducts, extends, and medially rotates the thigh; and acts synergistically with the other adductors in locomotion and in controlling erect posture. Also *great adductor muscle.* **m. adductor minimus** The superior portion of the adductor magnus muscle that arises from the inferior pubic ramus and inserts into the medial margin of the gluteal ridge and the upper part of linea aspera. It is supplied by the nerve to quadratus femoris or the obturator nerve. Also *smallest adductor muscle.* **m. adductor pollicis** [NA] A muscle of which the caput obliquum originates from the bases of the second and third metacarpal bones, the capitate, and the palmar ligaments of the carpus; and caput transversum from the distal two-thirds of the palmar ridge of the third metacarpal bone. It is inserted onto the ulnar side of the palmar surface of the base of the proximal phalanx of thumb. It is supplied by the deep branch of the ulnar nerve, adducts and flexes the first metacarpal bone, and flexes the proximal phalanx of the thumb, especially in gripping movements. Also *adductor muscle of thumb.* **m. anconeus** [NA] A muscle originating from the posterior surface of the lateral epicondyle of humerus and the adjacent capsule of the elbow joint. It is inserted into the lateral side of the olecranon and the adjacent posterior surface of the shaft of the ulna. It is supplied by the radial nerve, helps the triceps brachii muscle to extend the elbow joint, and may abduct the ulna in pronation. Also *anconeus muscle.* **m. antitragicus** [NA] A muscle originating from the outer part of the antitragus and inserted into the cauda helicis and antihelix. It is supplied by the temporal and posterior auricular branches of the facial nerve, and produces very slight, if any, modification of the shape and position of the ear in humans. Also *muscle of antitragus, antitragicus.* **musculi arrectores pilorum** [NA] The muscles that cause the erection of the hairs. Also *arrector muscles of hair, arrectores pilorum.* **m. articularis** [NA] A muscle that inserts, either partly or completely, into the capsule of a joint, usually in order to lift the capsule in certain movements. Also *articular muscle.* **m. articularis cubiti** [NA] A muscle that originates by a slip of muscle from the deep surface of the lower part of the triceps brachii muscle. It is inserted into the back of the fibrous capsule of the elbow joint. It is supplied by the radial nerve, and lifts up the back of the capsule of the elbow joint during extension of the forearm. Also *articular muscle of elbow, subanconeus muscle.* **m. articularis genus** [NA] A muscle originating from the anterior surface of the lower part of the shaft of the femur, and inserted into the upper portion of the synovial membrane of the knee joint. It is supplied by the femoral nerve, and draws up the synovial membrane during extension of the knee joint. Also *articular muscle of knee, Dupré's muscle.* **m. aryepiglotticus** [NA] Some fibers of musculus arytenoideus obliquus that extend beyond the lateral side of the apex of the arytenoid cartilage and insert into the aryepiglottic fold. It assists the oblique arytenoid muscle as a sphincter of the inlet of the larynx. It is innervated by the recurrent laryngeal nerve. Also *aryepiglottic muscle, Hilton's muscle.* **m. arytenoideus obliquus** [NA] Two bands of muscle fibers, each arising from the posterior aspect of the muscular process of an arytenoid cartilage and inserting into the apex of the adjacent arytenoid cartilage. It is supplied by the recurrent laryngeal nerve, and serves as a sphincter of the inlet of the larynx. Also *oblique arytenoid muscle.* **m. arytenoideus transversus** [NA] A single muscle arising from the posterior aspect of the muscular process and lateral margin of one arytenoid cartilage and inserting into corresponding parts of the other arytenoid cartilage. It is supplied by the recurrent laryngeal nerve, and by bringing the two arytenoid cartilages together it helps to close the rima glottidis. Also *transverse arytenoid muscle.* **m. auricularis anterior** [NA] A muscle originating from the lateral margin of the epicranial aponeurosis, and inserted into the spine of the helix of external ear. It is supplied by the temporal branch of the facial nerve, and pulls the auricle forwards and upwards. Also *anterior auricular muscle, muscle of Henle.* **m. auricularis posterior** [NA] A muscle originating from the mastoid process of the temporal bone and inserted into the ponticulus of eminentia conchae. It is supplied by the posterior auricular branch of the facial nerve, and pulls back the auricle. Also *posterior auricular muscle.* **m. auricularis superior** [NA] A muscle originating from the epicranial aponeurosis and inserted into the upper part of the cartilage of the auricle. It is supplied by the temporal branch of the facial nerve, and pulls the auricle upward. Also *superior auricular muscle.* **m. biceps brachii** [NA] A muscle of which the caput breve originates from the tip of the coracoid process of scapula, and caput longum from the supraglenoid tubercle and the glenoid labrum within the fibrous capsule. It is inserted into the posterior half of the tuberosity of the radius and, by the bicipital aponeurosis, into the deep fascia on the upper medial side of the forearm. It is supplied by the musculocutaneous nerve, supinates and flexes the forearm, and slightly flexes the shoulder joint. Also *biceps muscle of arm, biceps brachii.* **m. biceps femoris** [NA] A muscle of which the caput longum originates from the superomedial aspect of the ischial tuberosity and the sacrotuberous ligament, and caput breve from the lower half of the lateral lip of linea aspera, the upper two-thirds of the lateral supracondylar line of the femur, and the lateral intermuscular septum. It is inserted into the head of the fibula, the lateral condyle of the tibia, and the fibular collateral ligament. Its caput longum is supplied by the tibial part of the sciatic nerve, and caput breve by the common peroneal. It laterally rotates the leg when the knee is partly flexed, laterally rotates the thigh when the hip is extended, and together with the semitendinosus and semimembranosus it flexes the leg and extends the hip joint. Also *biceps muscle of thigh, biceps femoris.* **m. bipennatus** [NA] A muscle in which the fasciculi converge obliquely on a central tendon from two sides in a featherlike pattern, as in the rectus femoris and the dorsal interossei. Also *bipennate muscle, bipenniform muscle.* **m. brachialis** [NA] A muscle originating from the lower half of the front of the humerus, and from the intermuscular septa. It is inserted onto the tuberosity of the ulna and the front of the coronoid process of the ulna. It is supplied by the musculocutaneous and radial nerves, and flexes the forearm. Also *brachial muscle.* **m. brachioradialis** [NA] A muscle originating from the upper two-thirds of the lateral supracondylar ridge of the humerus and the front of the lateral intermuscular septum. It is inserted into the lateral aspect of the base of the styloid process of the radius and supplied by a branch of the radial nerve containing fibers of the fifth and sixth cervical nerves. It flexes the forearm, especially in the semiprone position, is active in rapid extension of the forearm, and helps in pronation when the forearm is supine and flexed. Also *brachioradial muscle.* **m. bronchoesophageus** [NA] Inconstant muscle fasciculi extending from the back of the left bronchus to the esophagus. Also *bronchoesophageal muscle.* **m. buccinator** [NA] A muscle originating from the outer surface of the molar area of the alveolar process of the maxilla and of the mandible, and from the anterior aspect of the pterygomandibular raphe. It is inserted into the orbicularis oris muscle at the angle of the mouth. It is supplied by buccal branches of the facial nerve, flattens the cheeks, and pulls the angle of the mouth laterally. Also *buccinator muscle, cheek muscle, buccinator.* **musculi bulbi** [NA] The muscles inside the orbit that move the eyeball. They include the superior rectus, inferior rectus, lateral rectus, medial rectus, orbital, superior oblique, inferior oblique, and levator palpebrae superioris muscles. Also *extraocular muscles, muscles of eye, ocular muscles, bulbar muscles.* **m. bulbospongiosus** [NA] A muscle that is located anterior to the anus and composed of symmetrical right and left halves. In the male, it originates from a median raphe that joins the two halves and the central tendon of the perineum, and is inserted into the perineal membrane and the sides of corpus spongiosum penis. It is supplied by the perineal branch of the pudendal nerve. It compresses the urethra, expelling urine at the end of micturition, and assists in erection of the penis and in ejaculation. In the female, it originates from the central tendon of perineum, blending with the external anal sphincter. It is inserted into the perineal membrane on each side of the vagina lateral to the vestibular bulbs and the sides of corpora cavernosa clitoridis. It is supplied by the perineal branch of the pudendal nerve, compresses the orifice of the vagina, and helps in erection of the clitoris. Also *bulbospongiosus, bulbocavernosus, bulbocavernous muscle.* **musculi capitis** [NA] The muscles of the head, including the muscles of mastication, muscles of expression, and the suboccipital muscles. **m. ceratocricoideus** [NA] An occasional band of the lower margin of the posterior cricoarytenoid muscle that attaches to the inferior horn of the thyroid cartilage and the adjacent cricoid lamina. Also *ceratocricoid muscle, Merkel's muscle, ceratocricoideus.* **m. chondroglossus** [NA] A muscle originating from the medial side and base of the lesser horn and the adjacent part of the body of the hyoid bone, and inserted into the intrinsic muscles of the tongue between the genioglossus and hyoglossus muscles. It is supplied by the hypoglossal nerve, and assists in depressing the tongue. Also *chondroglossus muscle, chondroglossus.* **m. ciliaris** [NA] The nonstriated muscle mass that forms the bulk of the ciliary body of the eye and comprises three portions which are mostly attached to the scleral spur from which they run in various directions. They are the outermost fibrae meridionales (also called meridional or longitudinal fibers, Brücke's muscle, or tensor muscle of choroid); the innermost fibrae circulares (also called circular fibers, Rouget's muscle, or Müller's muscle); and the intermediate fibrae radiales (also called radiating fibers). It is innervated by the short ciliary nerves and its action produces changes in the shape of the lens in the process of accommodation. Also *ciliary muscle, Bowman's muscle, ciliaris.* **m. cleidomastoideus** The lateral, or clavicular, portion of the sternocleidomastoid muscle. **musculi coccygei** [NA] The muscles attached to the coccyx, including the coccygeus and the dorsal and ventral sacrococcygeal muscles. Also *coccygeal muscles.* **m. coccygeus** [NA] A muscle originating from the pelvic aspect of the ischial spine and from the sacrospinous ligament, and inserted onto the lateral margin of the coccyx and of the fourth and fifth sacral vertebrae. It is supplied by the third and fourth or fourth and fifth sacral nerves, flexes the coccyx, and supports it, especially after defecation and parturition. Also *coccygeal muscle, ischiococcygeus.* **musculi colli** [NA] The anterolateral muscles of the neck, including the sternocleidomastoid, suprahyoid, infrahyoid, scalene, longus colli, and platysma muscles. Also *muscles of neck.* **m. compressor naris** PARS TRANSVERSA MUSCULI NASALIS.

**m. compressor urethrae** [NA] Some deep fibers of musculus sphincter urethrae arising from the ramus of the ischium. **m. constrictor pharyngis inferior** [NA] The lowest of the three constrictor muscles of the pharynx that consists of two parts, pars cricopharyngea and pars thyropharyngea, arising from the cricoid and thyroid cartilages. Their fibers run posteriorly and medially to be inserted with the fibers from the opposite side into a fibrous raphe in the midline posteriorly. It is supplied by the pharyngeal plexus and branches of the external and recurrent laryngeal nerves, and takes part in constriction of the pharynx and propulsion of its contents during swallowing. Also *inferior constrictor muscle of pharynx, inferior pharyngeal constrictor muscle.* **m. constrictor pharyngis medius** [NA] The middle of the three constrictor muscles of the pharynx that consists of two parts, pars chondropharyngea and pars ceratopharyngea, arising from the lesser and greater horns of the hyoid bone and the stylohyoid ligament. Their fibers run posteriorly and medially and are inserted with the fibers of the opposite side in a fibrous raphe in the midline posteriorly. It is supplied by the pharyngeal plexus, and constricts the pharynx during swallowing. Also *middle constrictor muscle of pharynx, middle pharyngeal constrictor muscle.* **m. constrictor pharyngis superior** [NA] The highest of the three constrictor muscles of the pharynx that consists of four parts, namely, pars pterygopharyngea from the medial pterygoid plate, pars buccopharyngea from the pterygomandibular raphe, pars mylopharyngea from the back of the mylohyoid line of the mandible, and pars glossopharyngea from the side of the tongue. Their fibers run posteriorly and medially to be inserted with the fibers from the opposite side into the fibrous raphe in the midline posteriorly as well as in the pharyngeal tubercle on the basilar part of the occipital bone. It is supplied by the pharyngeal plexus, and constricts the pharynx during swallowing. Also *superior constrictor muscle of pharynx, superior pharyngeal constrictor muscle.* **m. coracobrachialis** [NA] A muscle originating from the tip of the coracoid process of the scapula with the tendon of the short head of biceps brachii muscle, and inserted onto the middle of the medial surface of the humerus. It is supplied by the musculocutaneous nerve, and flexes and adducts the arm. Also *coracobrachial muscle, coracobrachialis, Casser's perforated muscle.* **m. corrugator supercilii** [NA] A muscle originating from the medial end of the superciliary arch of the frontal bone, and inserted into the skin above the medial part of the supraorbital margin. It is supplied by temporal branches of the facial nerve, and pulls the eyebrow downward and medially producing the vertical furrows above the nasal bridge, as in frowning. Also *superciliary corrugator muscle, Coiter's muscle.* **m. cremaster** [NA] A muscle well developed in the male, arising from the inguinal ligament and the lower part of the internal oblique and transversus abdominis muscles. It forms loosely arranged loops around the spermatic cord as far as the tunica vaginalis, helps to form the cremasteric fascia, and is inserted into the pubic tubercle. It is supplied by the genital branch of the genitofemoral nerve, and lifts the testis towards the superficial inguinal ring. Also *cremaster muscle, Riolan's muscle, cremaster.* **m. cricoarytenoideus lateralis** [NA] A muscle originating from the superior margin of the arch of the cricoid cartilage and the adjacent conus elasticus, and inserted into the anterior surface of the muscular process of the arytenoid cartilage. It is supplied by the recurrent laryngeal nerve, and approximates the vocal processes and closes the rima glottidis. Also *lateral cricoarytenoid muscle.* **m. cricoarytenoideus posterior** [NA] A muscle originating from the posterior surface of the cricoid lamina on each side of the median crest, and inserted into the posterior surface and tip of the muscular process of the arytenoid cartilage. It is supplied by the recurrent laryngeal nerve, widens the rima glottidis, and tenses the vocal ligaments. Also *posterior cricoarytenoid muscle.* **m. cricothyroideus** [NA] A muscle originating from the anterior and lateral surfaces of the cricoid cartilage. Its pars obliqua is inserted into the anterior margin of the inferior horn of the thyroid cartilage, and pars recta into the posterior part of the lower margin of the lamina of the thyroid cartilage. It is supplied by the external laryngeal branch of the superior laryngeal nerve, and tenses and elongates the vocal ligaments. Also *cricothyroid muscle.* **m. cutaneus** [NA] A striated muscle inserted into the skin. Also *dermal muscle, cutaneous muscle.* **m. dartos** [NA] A thin layer of smooth muscle fibers in the superficial fascia of the scrotum, the more superficial fibers being attached to the skin, while the deeper fibers in the sagittal plane take part in the formation of a septum that divides the scrotum into two cavities by attaching to the inferior surface of the radix of the penis. The fibers produce the transverse ridges on the surface of the scrotum. It is innervated by the genitofemoral nerve. When it contracts, it wrinkles and tightens the scrotum. Also *dartos muscle of scrotum, dartos.* **m. deltoideus** [NA] A muscle originating from the anterior margin and superior surface of the lateral third of the clavicle, the lateral margin and superior surface of the acromion, and the inferior border of the crest of the spine of the scapula. It is inserted onto the deltoid tuberosity on the lateral side of the shaft of the humerus. It is supplied by the axillary nerve and abducts the arm 90°. The anterior fibers can flex and medially rotate the arm, while the posterior fibers can extend and laterally rotate it. Also *deltoid muscle, deltoid.* **m. depressor anguli oris** [NA] A muscle originating from the oblique line of the mandible, and inserted into the skin of the angle of the mouth, and into the orbicularis oris muscle and other muscles at the angle of mouth. It is supplied by the buccal branch or mandibular branch of the facial nerve, and pulls the angle of the mouth downwards and laterally. Also *depressor muscle of angle of mouth, triangular muscle, depressor anguli oris, triangularis.* **m. depressor labii inferioris** [NA] A muscle originating from the oblique line of the mandible between the mental protuberance and the mental foramen, and inserted into the orbicularis oris muscle, the depressor muscle from the opposite side, and the skin and mucosa of the lower lip. It is supplied by the mandibular branch of the facial nerve, and pulls down and everts the lower lip. Also *depressor muscle of lower lip, Aeby's muscle, depressor labii inferioris.* **m. depressor septi nasi** [NA] A muscle originating from the incisive fossa of the maxilla, and inserted into the cartilaginous part of the nasal septum and the ala of the nose. It is supplied by the buccal branch of the facial nerve, pulls the ala of nose downward, and helps the nasalis in widening the nostrils in deep inspiration. Some consider the muscle to be a portion of the alar part of the nasalis muscle. Also *depressor muscle of nasal septum.* **m. depressor supercilii** [NA] The upper fasciculi of the orbital part of the orbicularis oculi muscle that insert into the skin and subcutaneous tissue of the eyebrow. Also *superciliary depressor muscle.* **m. detrusor vesicae** [NA] The three layers of the tunica muscularis vesicae urinariae considered as a single functional unit. The term has been applied, incorrectly, to either the external longitudinal layer alone or the musculus pubovesicalis. Also *detrusor muscle of urinary bladder, detrusor urinae, musculus detrusor urinae, detrusor urinae muscle, detrusor vesicae.* **m. digastricus** [NA] A muscle of which the venter anterior originates from the digastric fossa on each side of the midline on the base of the mandible; and venter posterior from the mastoid notch of the temporal bone. Its intermediate tendon is attached by a fibrous loop to the body and greater cornu of the hyoid bone. Its venter anterior is supplied by the mylohyoid branch of the inferior alveolar nerve, and venter posterior by the facial nerve. It depresses the mandible and elevates the hyoid bone. Also *digastric muscle.* **m. dilator** A muscle that expands or opens the orifice or lumen of an organ, tube, or space. **m. dilator naris** PARS ALARIS MUSCULI NASALIS. **m. dilator pupillae** [NA] A thin layer of radially arranged nonstriated muscle fibers with myoepithelial cells that extends from the sphincter pupillae almost to the base of the iris. Superficial and posterior to this layer are the pigmented cells of the posterior epithelium. It is innervated by the short and long ciliary nerves and its function is to dilate the pupil. Also *dilator muscle of pupil, iridodilator.* **musculi dorsi** [NA] The muscles of the back, including the trapezius, latissimus dorsi, rhomboid, serratus posterior, levator scapulae, erector spinae, transversospinalis, interspinal, and intertransverse muscles. Also *dorsal muscles.* **m. epicranius** [NA] The muscular layer of the scalp, comprising musculus occipitofrontalis, musculus temporoparietalis, and the galea aponeurotica. Also *epicranial muscle.* **m. erector spinae** [NA] The superficial longitudinal muscle mass on either side of the spines of the vertebral column that splits in the upper lumbar region into three columns, namely, a medial, or spinalis, group; an intermediate, or longissimus, group; and a lateral, iliocostalis or iliocostocervicalis group. Its tendinous origin attaches to the median sacral crest, the spines and supraspinous ligaments of all the lumbar and the twelfth and eleventh thoracic vertebrae, the medial surface of the posterior part of the iliac crest, and the adjacent sacrotuberous and dorsal sacroiliac ligaments. It is supplied by the dorsal rami of the lumbar, thoracic, and cervical spinal nerves, and is a powerful extensor as well as a lateral flexor of the vertebral column. Also *sacrospinal muscle, erector muscle of spine.* **m. extensor carpi radialis brevis** [NA] A muscle originating from the lateral epicondyle of the humerus, the radial collateral ligament of the elbow joint, and the intermuscular septa; and inserted onto the posterior surface of the base of the third metacarpal bone and the adjacent part of the second metacarpal bone. It is supplied by the posterior interosseous nerve, extends the wrist, abducts the hand and, acting synergistically with the finger flexors, steadies the wrist when they act. Also *short radial extensor muscle of wrist.* **m. extensor carpi radialis longus** [NA] A muscle originating from the lower third of the lateral supracondylar ridge of the humerus and the lateral intermuscular septum, and inserted into the lateral aspect of the posterior surface of the base of the second metacarpal bone. It is supplied by the radial nerve; extends the wrist, abducts the hand and, acting synergistically with the finger flexors, steadies the wrist when they act. Also *long radial extensor of wrist.* **m. extensor carpi ulnaris** [NA] A muscle of which the caput humerale originates from the lateral epicondyle of the humerus and the antebrachial fascia, and caput ulnare from the proximal three fourths of the posterior margin of the ulna. It is inserted into the medial side of the base of the fifth metacarpal bone, supplied by the posterior interosseous nerve, and adducts the hand medially and extends it. Also *ulnar extensor of wrist.* **m. extensor digiti minimi** [NA] A muscle originating from the lateral epicondyle of the humerus with the common extensor tendon and the intermuscular septa, and inserted into the dorsal digital expansion of the fifth digit. It is supplied by the posterior interosseous nerve, extends the little finger and, with musculus extensor digitorum, extends the wrist. Also *extensor muscle of little finger.* **m. extensor digitorum** [NA] A muscle originating from the lateral epicondyle of the humerus by the common extensor tendon, the intermuscular septa, and the antebrachial fascia. It is inserted by four tendons into the dorsal digital expansion of each of the medial four fingers, the intermediate slip of which attaches to the base of the middle phalanx while the two collateral slips reunite to attach to the back of the base of the distal phalanx. It is supplied by the posterior interosseous nerve, extends the fingers at the metacarpophalangeal and interphalangeal joints, and then extends the wrist. Also *extensor muscle of fingers.* **m. extensor digitorum brevis** [NA] A muscle originating from the anterior part of the superolateral surface of the calcaneus and the stem of the inferior extensor retinaculum. It is inserted by four tendons, the most medial being the extensor hallucis brevis, while the lateral three are attached to the lateral margins of the tendons of the extensor digitorum longus with slips to the bases of the proximal phalanges. It is supplied by the deep peroneal nerve, and extends the phalanges of the middle three toes. Also *short extensor muscle of toes.* **m. extensor digitorum longus** [NA] A muscle originating from the lateral condyle of the tibia, the upper three fourths of the medial surface of the fibula, the upper anterior surface of the interosseous membrane, the anterior crural intermuscular septum, and the fascia cruris. It is inserted by four tendons into the dorsal digital expansion of each of the lateral four toes, the intermediate slip of which attaches to the base of the middle phalanx, while the two collateral slips reunite and attach to the dorsum of the base of the distal phalanx. It is supplied by the deep peroneal nerve, extends the toes, and dorsiflexes the foot. Also *long extensor muscle of toes.* **m. extensor hallucis brevis** [NA] The large, medial belly of musculus extensor digitorum brevis that is inserted into the dorsum of the base of the proximal phalanx of the great toe. It is supplied by the deep peroneal nerve, and extends the proximal phalanx of the great toe. Also *short extensor muscle of great toe.* **m. extensor hallucis longus** [NA] A muscle originating from the middle two fourths of the medial surface of the fibula and the front of the interosseous membrane. It is inserted onto the dorsum of the base of the distal phalanx of the great toe. It is supplied by the deep peroneal nerve, dorsiflexes the foot, and extends the phalanges of the great toe. Also *long extensor muscle of great toe.* **m. extensor indicis** [NA] A muscle originating from the proximal part of the distal third of the posterior surface of the ulna and from the interosseous membrane. It is inserted into the medial side of the tendon of the extensor digitorum muscle to the index finger. It is supplied by the posterior interosseous nerve, and helps to extend the index finger and the wrist. Also *extensor muscle of index finger, indicator.* **m. extensor pollicis brevis** [NA] A muscle originating from the distal part of the middle third of the posterior surface of the radius, and from the interosseous membrane; and inserted into the dorsal surface of the base of the proximal phalanx of the thumb. It is supplied by the posterior interosseous nerve, and extends the thumb. Also *short extensor muscle of thumb.* **m. extensor pollicis longus** [NA] A muscle originating from the middle third of the lateral part of the posterior surface of the ulna and from the interosseous membrane, and inserted into the dorsum of the base of the distal phalanx of the thumb. It is supplied by the posterior interosseous nerve; extends the thumb; adducts the extended thumb, rotating it laterally; and helps to adduct the hand. Also *long extensor muscle of* *thumb.* **m. fibularis brevis** MUSCULUS PERONEUS BREVIS. **m. fibularis longus** MUSCULUS PERONEUS LONGUS. **m. fibularis tertius** MUSCULUS PERONEUS TERTIUS. **m. flexor carpi radialis** [NA] A muscle originating from the medial epicondyle of humerus by the common flexor tendon, the antebrachial fascia, and the intermuscular septa; and inserted onto the base of the second metacarpal and usually by a slip to the third metacarpal. It is supplied by the median nerve, and helps to flex and abduct the hand. Also *radial flexor muscle of wrist.* **m. flexor carpi ulnaris** [NA] A muscle of which the caput humerale originates from the medial epicondyle of humerus by the common flexor tendon; and caput ulnare from the medial side of the olecranon and the upper two thirds of the posterior margin of the ulna. It is inserted onto the pisiform bone and by the pisohamate and pisometacarpal ligaments to the hamate bone and the base of fifth metacarpal bone respectively. It is supplied by the ulnar nerve, and helps to flex and adduct the hand. Also *ulnar flexor muscle of wrist.* **m. flexor digiti minimi brevis manus** [NA] A muscle originating from the hook of the hamate bone and the flexor retinaculum, and inserted onto the medial side of the base of the proximal phalanx of the little finger. It is supplied by the deep branch of the ulnar nerve, and flexes the proximal phalanx of the little finger. Also *short flexor muscle of little finger.* **m. flexor digiti minimi brevis pedis** [NA] A muscle originating from the sheath of the peroneus longus muscle and from the plantar aspect of the base of the fifth metatarsal bone, and inserted onto the lateral side of the base of the proximal phalanx of the little toe. It is supplied by the superficial branch of the lateral plantar nerve, and flexes the proximal phalanx of the little toe. Also *short flexor muscle of little toe.* **m. flexor digitorum brevis** [NA] A muscle originating from the medial process of the calcaneal tuberosity, the central part of the plantar aponeurosis, and the medial and lateral intermuscular septa. It is inserted by four tendons into the sides of the middle phalanges of the lateral four toes after splitting to allow the corresponding long flexor tendons through, then rejoining, decussating, and dividing again. It is supplied by the medial plantar nerve, and flexes the middle and proximal phalanges of the lateral four toes. Also *short flexor muscle of toes.* **m. flexor digitorum longus** [NA] A muscle originating from the medial part of the posterior surface of the tibia below the soleal line. It is inserted by four tendons into the base of the terminal phalanx of the lateral four toes after passing through a gap in the corresponding tendon of flexor digitorum brevis. It is supplied by the tibial nerve, flexes the toes and foot when the foot is off the ground, and acts synergistically with other plantar muscles to stabilize the foot when it is on the ground. Also *long flexor muscle of toes.* **m. flexor digitorum profundus** [NA] A muscle originating from the upper three fourths of the posterior margin and of the medial and anterior surfaces of the ulna, and from the anterior surface of the adjacent interosseous membrane. It is inserted by four tendons into the base of the distal phalanx of the medial four fingers after passing through an opening in the corresponding tendon of flexor digitorum superficialis. It is supplied by the ulnar nerve and the anterior interosseous branch of the median nerve, flexes the distal phalanges, and helps to flex the wrist. Also *deep flexor muscle of fingers.* **m. flexor digitorum superficialis** [NA] A muscle of which the caput humeroulnare originates from the medial epicondyle of humerus by the common flexor tendon, and from the ulnar collateral ligament of the elbow joint, the medial margin of the coronoid process of ulna, and the intermuscular septum between it and overlying muscles; and caput radiale from the oblique line of radius and the anterior margin below it. It is inserted by four tendons that divide over the proximal phalanges of the medial four fingers to allow passage of the corresponding tendons of flexor digitorum profundus, and then reunite, decussate and divide again to attach to the sides of the middle phalanges. It is supplied by the median nerve, flexes the middle and proximal phalanges, and helps to flex the wrist. Also *superficial flexor muscle of fingers.* **m. flexor hallucis brevis** [NA] A muscle originating from the medial side of the plantar surface of the cuboid bone and the lateral cuneiform bone, and inserted by medial and lateral parts into corresponding sides of the base of the proximal phalanx of the great toe, each containing a sesamoid bone and each blending with adjacent muscles. It is supplied by the medial plantar nerve, and flexes the proximal phalanx of the great toe. Also *short flexor muscle of great toe.* **m. flexor hallucis longus** [NA] A muscle originating from the distal two thirds of the posterior surface of the fibula, the adjacent interosseous membrane, and posterior crural intermuscular septum; and inserted into the base of the terminal phalanx of great toe. It is supplied by the tibial nerve, flexes the great toe, and helps to invert the foot and to plantiflex the ankle joint. Also *long flexor muscle of great toe.* **m. flexor pollicis brevis** [NA] A muscle of which the caput superficiale originates from the tubercle of trapezium and the adjacent part of flexor retinaculum; and caput profundum from the trapezoid and capitate bones and palmar ligaments. It is inserted onto the lateral side of the base of proximal phalanx of thumb. It is supplied by the recurrent branch of the median nerve and the deep branch of the ulnar nerve, flexes the proximal phalanx of thumb, and flexes and medially rotates the first metacarpal bone. Also *short flexor muscle of thumb.* **m. flexor pollicis longus** [NA] A muscle originating from the anterior surface of the radius from the radial tuberosity to the upper margin of attachment of the pronator quadratus muscle; and from the adjacent interosseous membrane; and inserted onto the anterior aspect of the base of the distal phalanx of thumb. It is supplied by the anterior interosseous branch of the median nerve, flexes the thumb, and helps to flex the wrist. Also *long flexor muscle of thumb.* **m. fusiformis** [NA] A spindle-shaped muscle in which the longitudinal fasciculi of its fleshy belly are parallel and taper to a tendon at one or both ends. Also *fusiform muscle.* **m. gastrocnemius** [NA] A muscle of which the caput laterale originates from the posterolateral surface of the lateral condyle of femur, the lower part of the lateral supracondylar line, and the capsule of the knee joint; and caput mediale from the posterosuperior part of the medial condyle of femur behind the adductor tubercle, the popliteal surface superolateral to this, and the capsule of the knee joint. It is inserted with the soleus muscle by the tendo calcaneus into the middle of the posterior surface of the calcaneus. It is supplied by the tibial nerve; plantiflexes the foot, raising the heel off the ground; and flexes the knee. Also *gastrocnemius muscle, gastrocnemius.* **m. gemellus inferior** [NA] A muscle originating from the upper part of the inner surface of the ischial tuberosity and sacrotuberous ligament, and inserted into the tendon of the obturator internus muscle and the medial aspect of the greater trochanter of the femur.It is supplied by the nerve to the quadratus femoris and, with the obturator internus and superior gemellus muscles, laterally rotates the extended thigh and abducts the flexed thigh. Also *inferior gemellus muscle.* **m. gemellus superior** [NA] A muscle originating from the posterior surface of the ischial spine and the adjacent part of the lesser sciatic notch and inserted into the tendon of the obturator internus muscle and the medial surface of the greater trochanter of femur. It is supplied by the nerve to obturator internus and, with the obturator internus and inferior gemellus muscles, it laterally rotates the extended thigh and abducts the flexed thigh. Also *superior gemellus muscle.* **m. genioglossus** [NA] A muscle originating from the upper genial tubercle of the mental spine on the lingual surface of the symphysis menti, and inserted onto the anterior surface of the body of the hyoid bone and the inferior surface of the tongue. It is supplied by the hypoglossal nerve, pulls forward the tongue and protrudes the apex, and depresses the tongue. Also *genioglossus muscle, genioglossus, geniohyoglossus.* **m. geniohyoideus** [NA] A muscle originating from the lower genial tubercle of the mental spine behind the symphysis menti, and inserted onto the anterior surface of the body of the hyoid bone. It is supplied by the first cervical spinal nerve via the hypoglossal nerve, elevates and draws forward the hyoid bone, and depresses the mandible when the hyoid is fixed. Also *geniohyoid muscle, geniohyoideus.* **m. gluteus maximus** [NA] A muscle originating from the outer surface of the ilium posterior to the posterior gluteal line and the adjacent iliac crest, the aponeurosis of the erector spinae muscle, the posterior surface of the fourth and fifth sacral vertebrae, the coccyx and the sacrotuberous ligament, and the gluteal fascia, and inserted into the gluteal tuberosity of femur and the iliotibial tract. It is supplied by the inferior gluteal nerve, extends and laterally rotates the thigh, tenses the fascia lata and steadies the knee joint, abducts the thigh, steadies the trunk during locomotion, and rotates the pelvis backwards on the femur. Also *greatest gluteal muscle.* **m. gluteus medius** [NA] A muscle originating from the outer surface of the ilium between the anterior and posterior gluteal lines and the iliac crest above this area, and from the gluteal fascia; and inserted into the posterosuperior angle and oblique ridge on the outer surface of the greater trochanter of femur. It is supplied by the superior gluteal nerve. It abducts the thigh, anterior fibers medially rotate and flex the thigh, posterior fibers laterally rotate and extend the thigh, and it tends to pull down and stabilize the pelvis when the opposite leg is off the ground, thereby maintaining the trunk upright. Also *middle gluteal muscle.* **m. gluteus minimus** [NA] A muscle originating from the outer surface of the ilium between the anterior and inferior gluteal lines, and from the margin of the greater sciatic notch; and inserted onto the anterolateral surface of the greater trochanter of femur. It is supplied by the superior gluteal nerve, and agrees with the gluteus medius in all of its actions. Also *least gluteal muscle.* **m. gracilis** [NA] A muscle originating from the medial margin of the inferior pubic ramus and the adjoining ischial ramus and inserted onto the upper part of the medial surface of the tibia, below the condyle and behind the insertion of the sartorius muscle. It is supplied by the obturator nerve, flexes and medially rotates the leg, and adducts the thigh. Also *gracilis muscle.* **m. helicis major** [NA] A muscle originating from the spine of the helix of the pinna and inserted into the anterosuperior margin of the helix, where it turns posteriorly. It is supplied by the temporal branch of the facial nerve. **m. helicis minor** [NA] A slender muscle fasciculus extending from the anterior margin of the helix to the concha of the pinna and covering the crus helicis. **m. hyoglossus** [NA] A muscle originating from the greater horn and lateral part of the body of the hyoid bone, and inserted into the side of the tongue between the inferior longitudinal and styloglossus muscles. It is supplied by the hypoglossal nerve. It depresses the tongue. Also *hyoglossal muscle, hyoglossus muscle.* **m. iliacus** [NA] A muscle originating from the upper two thirds of the iliac fossa, the adjacent inner lip of the iliac crest, the iliolumbar ligament, the ventral sacroiliac ligaments, and the ala of sacrum; and inserted into the tendon of the psoas major muscle and the femur below the lesser trochanter. It is supplied by the femoral nerve and, with the psoas major muscle, it flexes the thigh and also flexes the pelvis on the thigh. Also *iliac muscle.* See also MUSCULUS PSOAS MAJOR, MUSCULUS ILIOPSOAS. **m. iliococcygeus** [NA] A morphological subdivision of the levator ani muscle that arises from the ischial spine and the posterior part of the tendinous arch of the obturator fascia and inserts into the coccyx and the median raphe behind the anus. For nerve supply and action, see musculus levator ani. Also *iliococcygeal muscle, iliococcygeus.* **m. iliocostalis** [NA] The lateral column of the erector spinae muscle that separates in the upper lumbar region into iliocostalis lumborum, iliocostalis thoracis, and iliocostalis cervicis. It is supplied by dorsal rami of lower cervical, thoracic, and upper lumbar spinal nerves; and extends and laterally flexes the vertebral column. Also *iliocostal muscle.* **m. iliocostalis cervicis** [NA] A muscle originating from the angles of the third to sixth ribs, and inserted onto posterior tubercles of the transverse processes of the fourth, fifth, and sixth cervical vertebrae. It is supplied by dorsal rami of the lower cervical spinal nerves. Also *iliocostal muscle of neck, costocervicalis muscle, costocervicalis.* **m. iliocostalis lumborum** [NA] A muscle originating from the erector spinae muscle in the upper lumbar region and inserted onto the inferior margins of the angles of the lower six or seven ribs. It is supplied by dorsal rami of the upper lumbar spinal nerves. Also *iliocostal muscle of loins.* **m. iliocostalis thoracis** [NA] A muscle originating from the superior margins of the angles of the lower six or seven ribs, and inserted onto the superior margins of the angles of the upper six ribs and the transverse process of the seventh cervical vertebra. It is supplied by dorsal rami of the thoracic spinal nerves. Also *iliocostal muscle of thorax.* **m. iliopsoas** [NA] A compound muscle comprising musculus iliacus and musculus psoas major. It is a powerful flexor of the thigh. When the muscles on both sides act together from below, they pull the trunk and pelvis forward against resistance, as on rising from the supine position to a sitting position. Also *iliopsoas muscle, iliopsoas.* **musculi incisivi labii inferioris** Fibers of the orbicularis oris muscle that arise on either side of the midline from the mandible, lateral to the mentalis muscle, and then curve to the angle of the mouth where it intermingles with other muscle fibers. Also *incisive muscles of lower lip.* **musculi incisivi labii superioris** Fibers of the orbicularis oris muscle that arise from the alveolar border of the maxilla above the lateral incisor tooth on either side and curve to the lateral angle of the mouth, where they intermingle with other muscle fibers. Also *incisive muscles of upper lip.* **m. incisurae helicis** [NA] A small muscle occasionally present in the auricle extending anteriorly from the musculus tragicus across the incisure of the cartilaginous meatus. It is supplied by the temporal branch of the facial nerve. Also *muscle of incisure of helix, Santorini's muscle.* **musculi infrahyoidei** [NA] The group of muscles attached to the hyoid bone from below and serving as antagonists to the suprahyoid muscles in depressing the hyoid bone. They include the sternohyoid, omohyoid, sternothyroid, and thyrohyoid muscles. Also *infrahyoid muscles, strap muscles, ribbon muscles.* **m. infraspinatus** [NA] A muscle originating from the medial three fourths of the infraspinous fossa of the scapula, the inferior surface of the spine of scapula, and the infraspinous fascia, and inserted onto the middle facet on the greater tubercle of humerus. It is supplied by the suprascapular nerve, laterally rotates the arm, and helps adjacent muscles to steady the head of the humerus, especially in abduction. Also *infraspinous muscle.* **musculi intercostales externi** [NA] Muscles, eleven on each side, originating from the inferior border of the rib between the tubercle posteriorly and the costal cartilage anteriorly, and inserted onto the superior border of the rib below between the tubercle and the costal cartilage. They are supplied by the intercostal nerves, elevate the ribs during inspiration, and may act with internal intercostals during forced respiration. Also *external intercostal muscles.* **musculi intercostales interni** [NA] Muscles, eleven on each side, originating from the floor of the costal groove and the corresponding costal cartilage, and inserted onto the superior border of the rib below. They are supplied by the intercostal nerves, draw adjacent ribs together, may depress the ribs during expiration, and act with external intercostals during forced inspiration. Also *internal intercostal muscles.* **musculi intercostales intimi** [NA] The deepest layer of the internal intercostal muscles, separated from the latter by the intercostal vessels and nerves. Their innervation and action are identical to those of the internal intercostal muscles. Also *innermost intercostal muscles.* **musculi interossei dorsales manus** [NA] Four bipennate muscles in each hand, originating from the adjacent sides of two metacarpal bones and inserted onto the bases of proximal phalanges and dorsal digital expansions, the first on the radial side of the index finger, the second and third on radial and ulnar sides, respectively, of the middle finger, and the fourth on the ulnar side of the ring finger. They are supplied by the ulnar nerve; abduct the second, third and fourth fingers from the midline axis of the middle finger; flex the proximal phalanges; and extend the middle and distal phalanges. Also *dorsal interosseous muscles of hand.* **musculi interossei dorsales pedis** [NA] Four bipennate muscles, originating from the adjacent sides of two metacarpal bones and inserted onto the bases of the proximal phalanges and dorsal digital expansions, the first on the medial side of the second toe, and the second, third, and fourth on the lateral sides of the second, third, and fourth toes. They are supplied by the deep branch of the lateral plantar nerve; abduct the second, third, and fourth toes from the midline axis of the second toe; flex the proximal phalanges; and extend the middle and distal phalanges. Also *dorsal interosseous muscles of foot.* **musculi interossei palmares** [NA] Four muscles, though often only three are recognized, the first being considered a part of either flexor pollicis brevis or adductor pollicis. The first originates from the medial side of the palmar surface of the first metacarpal bone near the base, the second from the medial side of the second metacarpal, the third from the lateral side of the fourth metacarpal, and the fourth from the lateral side of the fifth metacarpal. The first is inserted onto the medial side of the base of the proximal phalanx and the dorsal digital expansion of thumb, the second into the medial side of the digital expansion of the index finger, the third into the lateral side of the digital expansion of the ring finger, and the fourth into the lateral side of the digital expansion and base of the proximal phalanx of the little finger. They are supplied by the deep branch of the ulnar nerve; adduct the fingers toward the axial midline of the middle finger; and flex the proximal phalanges and extend the middle and distal phalanges of the medial four fingers, while the first flexes and adducts the proximal phalanx of thumb. Also *palmar interosseous muscles.* **musculi interossei plantares** [NA] Three muscles originating from the bases and medial surfaces of the third, fourth, and fifth metatarsal bones, inserted onto the medial sides of the bases of the proximal phalanges of the third, fourth, and fifth toes and their dorsal digital expansions. They are supplied by the deep branch of lateral plantar nerve, adduct the lateral three toes towards the axial midline of the second toe, flex proximal phalanges, and extend the middle and distal phalanges. Also *plantar interosseous muscles.* **musculi interspinales** [NA] Short muscle bundles between the spines of adjacent vertebrae, one on each side of the interspinous ligaments, divided into three groups for the cervical, thoracic, and lumbar regions. They are innervated by dorsal rami of spinal nerves, and extend the vertebral column. Also *interspinal muscles.* **musculi interspinales cervicis** [NA] Six pairs of distinct muscle bundles extending between the adjacent bifid spines of the seven cervical and first thoracic vertebrae. They are supplied by dorsal rami of the cervical spinal nerves. Also *interspinal muscles of neck.* **musculi interspinales lumborum** [NA] Four pairs of short muscle bundles extending between the spines of adjacent lumbar vertebrae on either side of the interspinous ligaments. They are supplied by dorsal rami of the lumbar spinal nerves. Also *interspinal muscles of loins.* **musculi interspinales thoracis** [NA] Short muscle bundles extending between the spines of adjacent thoracic vertebrae, usually poorly developed except between the first two, the second and third, and the last two thoracic vertebrae. They are supplied by dorsal rami of the thoracic spinal nerves. Also *interspinal muscles of thorax.* **musculi intertransversarii** [NA] A deep group of small muscle bundles extending between the transverse processes of the vertebrae in the lumbar, thoracic, and cervical regions, and subdivided into anterior and posterior groups in the neck, and lateral and medial groups in the lumbar region. They act with other muscles to produce lateral flexion of the vertebral column and serve as postural muscles. Also *intertransverse muscles.* **musculi intertransversarii anteriores cervicis** [NA] Seven pairs of small muscle bundles extending between the anterior tubercles of contiguous cervical vertebrae, and separated from the posterior intertransverse muscles by the ventral rami of the spinal nerves, which innervate the former. Also *anterior intertransverse muscles of neck.* **musculi intertransversarii laterales lumborum** [NA] The lateral set of intertransverse muscles of the lumbar region that are subdivided into anterior and posterior parts, the anterior bundles extending between the transverse processes of adjacent lumbar vertebrae, while each posterior bundle extends between the accessory process of one vertebra and the transverse process of the next. They are homologous with the intercostal muscles, and supplied by anterior primary rami of lumbar spinal nerves. Also *lateral intertransverse muscles of loins.* **musculi intertransversarii mediales lumborum** [NA] The medial set of intertransverse muscles of the lumbar region, each extending between the accessory process of one lumbar vertebra and the mamillary process of the next on each side. They are homologous with the levatores costarum, and represent the true intrinsic musculature of the back. They are supplied by medial divisions of posterior primary rami of lumbar spinal nerves. Also *medial intertransverse muscles of loins.* **musculi intertransversarii posteriores cervicis** [NA] Seven pairs of small muscle bundles extending between the posterior tubercles of contiguous cervical vertebrae and separated from the anterior intertransverse muscles by the ventral rami of the spinal nerves. They are subdivided into medial and lateral parts, supplied by the dorsal and ventral rami of the cervical spinal nerves respectively. Also *posterior intertransverse muscles of neck.* **musculi intertransversa-**

**rii thoracis** [NA] Single muscle bundles extending between the adjacent transverse processes of the lowest three thoracic and first lumbar vertebrae. In the remaining thoracic region they are poorly developed or represented by ligamentous bands. They are supplied by dorsal rami of thoracic spinal nerves. Also *intertransverse muscles of thorax.* **m. ischiocavernosus** [NA] A muscle originating from the medial surface of the ischial tuberosity behind the crus penis or crus clitoridis and the ramus of the ischium, and inserted into the sides and inferior surface of crus penis or crus clitoridis. It is supplied by the perineal branch of the pudendal nerve, and compresses the crus penis or crus clitoridis. Also *ischiocavernous muscle.* **musculi laryngis** [NA] The intrinsic muscles of the larynx that act on the vocal cords, including the cricothyroid, posterior and lateral cricoarytenoid, transverse and oblique arytenoid, aryepiglottic, thyroarytenoid, vocalis, and thyroepiglottic muscles. All except the transverse arytenoid muscle are paired, and all except the cricothyroid muscle are innervated by the recurrent laryngeal nerve. Also *muscles of larynx.* **m. latissimus dorsi** [NA] A muscle originating from the spines and interspinous ligaments of the lower six thoracic and upper lumbar vertebrae, the thoracolumbar fascia, the posterior third of the outer lip of iliac crest, and the outer surface of the lower three or four ribs; and inserted onto the floor of the intertubercular sulcus of humerus. It is supplied by the thoracodorsal nerve; adducts, extends, and medially rotates the arm; and pulls the trunk up and forwards when the arms are fixed, as in climbing. Also *latissimus dorsi muscle.* **m. levator anguli oris** [NA] A muscle originating from the canine fossa of maxilla, inferior to the infraorbital foramen; and inserted into the skin and muscles of the angle of the mouth. It is supplied by the zygomatic branch of the facial nerve, and raises the angle of the mouth, pulling it medially and accentuating the nasolabial furrow. Also *levator muscle of angle of mouth, canine muscle, caninus.* **m. levator ani** [NA] A broad muscle sheet attached to the inner aspect of the wall of the true pelvis and meeting the opposite muscle centrally to form most of the pelvic diaphragm, or floor, of the pelvis. Morphologically it is divisible into musculus pubococcygeus, musculus levator prostatae, musculus puborectalis, and musculus iliococcygeus. It originates from the inner surface of the body of the pubis lateral to the symphysis, and from the arcus tendineus of the obturator fascia and the inner aspect of the ischial spine. It inserts onto the lateral margin of the lower two coccygeal segments, the anococcygeal raphe, sphincter ani externus, and the perineal body; and is supplied by the fourth sacral nerve and the inferior rectal, or perineal, branch of the pudendal nerve. It supports and raises the pelvic floor, resisting increased intra-abdominal pressure, and constricts the anorectal junction and vagina. Also *levator ani muscle.* **musculi levatores costarum** [NA] Twelve small muscle bundles on each side of the thorax. They originate from the tip and lower margin of a transverse process of the seventh cervical and upper eleven thoracic vertebrae, and are inserted onto the upper margin and posterior surface of the rib below the vertebra from which it takes origin, from the tubercle to the angle. The lower four muscles have two fasciculi of insertion, the one attaching as above and the other missing the rib below and attaching to the second rib below the vertebra of origin. They are supplied by the intercostal nerves, and elevate the ribs. Also *levator muscles of ribs.* **musculi levatores costarum breves** [NA] The levatores costarum muscles, each of which inserts on the upper margin and external surface of the rib, between the tubercle and the angle, below the vertebra from which it takes origin. Also *short levator muscles of ribs.* **musculi levatores costarum longi** [NA] One of the two fasciculi of insertion of the lower four levatores costarum muscles that misses the rib below and attaches to the second rib below the vertebra from which it takes origin. Also *long levator muscles of ribs.* **m. levator glandulae thyroideae** [NA] A muscular or fibromuscular band that occasionally extends from the body of the hyoid bone to either the isthmus of the thyroid gland or its pyramidal lobe, when present. It is located more often on the left side of the midline. Also *levator muscle of thyroid gland, Soemmering's muscle.* **m. levator labii superioris** [NA] A muscle originating from the infraorbital margin of the maxilla and from the zygomatic bone just above the infraorbital foramen. It is inserted into the skin and muscles of the upper lip medial to the angle of the mouth. It is supplied by the facial nerve, and raises and everts the upper lip. Also *levator muscle of upper lip.* **m. levator labii superioris alaeque nasi** [NA] A muscle originating from the middle of the frontal process of the maxilla. Its medial fasciculus is inserted into the skin and alar cartilage of the nose, and its lateral fasciculus into the skin and muscles of the lateral part of the upper lip. It is supplied by the facial nerve. Its medial fasciculus dilates the nostril, and its lateral fasciculus raises and everts the upper lip, elevating the nasolabial furrow. Also *levator muscle of upper lip and ala of nose.* **m. levator palpebrae superioris** [NA] A muscle originating from the inferior surface of the lesser wing of the sphenoid bone, above and in front of the optic canal. Its lamina superficialis is inserted into the anterior surface of the superior tarsus and the skin of the upper eyelid, and lamina profunda (superior tarsal muscle) onto the upper margin of the superior tarsus, and by fascia to the superior conjunctival fornix. It is supplied by the oculomotor and cervical sympathetic nerves, and raises the upper eyelid. Also *levator muscle of upper eyelid.* **m. levator prostatae** [NA] The most anterior fibers of the levator ani muscle that pass backwards, downwards, and medially across the side of the prostate to insert into the central tendon of the perineum in the male. Also *levator muscle of prostate, elevator of prostate.* **m. levator scapulae** [NA] A muscle that originates from the posterior tubercles of transverse processes of the first four cervical vertebrae and is inserted onto the medial margin of scapula between the superior angle and the medial end of the spine. It is supplied by the third and fourth cervical and the dorsal scapular nerves, helps to elevate and retract the scapula, and helps to rotate and depress the scapula. Also *levator muscle of scapula.* **m. levator veli palatini** [NA] A muscle originating from the inferior surface of the petrous part of the temporal bone and the inferior surface of the cartilaginous part of the auditory tube, and inserted onto the upper surface of the palatine aponeurosis. It is supplied by the pharyngeal plexus, and elevates the soft palate. Also *levator muscle of velum palatinum.* **musculi linguae** [NA] The extrinsic and intrinsic muscles that form and move the tongue and change its shape, the former including the genioglossus, hyoglossus, chondroglossus, and styloglossus muscles, and the latter including the superior and the inferior longitudinal, the transverse, and the vertical muscles. Also *muscles of tongue.* **m. longissimus** [NA] The intermediate, and largest, column of the musculus erector spinae, extending from the sacral region to the mastoid process of the temporal bone and divided into musculus longissimus capitis, musculus longissimus cervicis, and musculus longissimus thoracis. Also *longissimus muscle.* **m. longissimus capitis** [NA] A muscle originating from the transverse processes of the upper three or four thoracic vertebrae and from the articular processes of the lower three or four cervical vertebrae, and inserted onto the posterior margin of the mastoid process. It is supplied by the dorsal rami of the lower cervical spinal nerves, extends the head, and rotates the head to the same side. Also *longissimus muscle of head.* **m. longissimus cervicis** [NA] A muscle originating from the transverse processes of the upper four or five thoracic vertebrae, and inserted onto the posterior tubercles of the transverse processes of the middle cervical vertebrae. It is supplied by the dorsal rami of the lower cervical and upper thoracic spinal nerves, and helps to extend and laterally flex the vertebral column. Also *longissimus muscle of neck.* **m. longissimus thoracis** [NA] A muscle that, blended with the iliocostalis lumborum, originates from the posterior surfaces of the transverse processes and accessory processes of the lumbar vertebrae, and from the thoracolumbar fascia; and is inserted onto the tips of the transverse processes of all the thoracic vertebrae, and onto the lower eight or nine ribs lateral to the tubercles. It is supplied by the dorsal rami of the lumbar and thoracic spinal nerves, and helps to extend the vertebral column and to bend and rotate the trunk to one side. Also *longissimus muscle of thorax.* **m. longitudinalis inferior linguae** [NA] A narrow intrinsic muscle of the tongue extending on each side along the inferior surface from the base to the apex. Some posterior fibers may be attached to the body of the hyoid bone. It is supplied by the hypoglossal nerve, helps to shorten the tongue, and pulls the apex downward. Also *inferior longitudinal muscle of tongue.* **m. longitudinalis superior linguae** [NA] A thin, superficial intrinsic muscle of the tongue extending along the dorsum from the base to the apex just deep to the lingual aponeurosis, to which some fibers are attached. It is supplied by the hypoglossal nerve, helps to shorten the tongue, and turns the margins and apex upwards, making the dorsum concave. Also *superior longitudinal muscle of tongue.* **m. longus capitis** [NA] A muscle originating from the anterior tubercles of the transverse processes of the third to sixth cervical vertebrae and inserted onto the inferior surface of the basilar portion of the occipital bone, anterolateral to the pharyngeal tubercle. It is supplied by the ventral rami of the first to fourth cervical nerves, flexes the head, and rotates the head to the same side. Also *long muscle of head.* **m. longus colli** [NA] A triangular muscle comprising three parts: the superior oblique, or superolateral, part, originating from the anterior tubercles of the transverse processes of the third to sixth cervical vertebrae, and inserted onto the anterior tubercle of atlas; the inferior oblique, or inferolateral, part, originating from the anterolateral parts of the bodies of the first three thoracic vertebrae, and inserted onto the anterior tubercles of the transverse processes of the fifth and sixth cervical vertebrae; and the vertical, or medial, part, originating from the anterolateral parts of the bodies of the first three thoracic and last three cervical vertebrae, and inserted onto the anterolateral surfaces of the bodies of the second to fourth cervical vertebrae. It is supplied by the ventral rami of the second to sixth cervical nerves. It flexes the neck; the superior oblique part flexes the neck laterally and rotates it to the same side; and the inferior oblique part rotates the neck to the opposite side. Also *long muscle of neck.* **musculi lumbricales manus** [NA] Four small muscles in each hand, of which the first and second originate from the lateral sides and palmar surfaces of the flexor digitorum profundus tendons to the index and middle fingers, and the medial two originate from adjacent sides of the deep flexor tendons to the middle and ring fingers and ring and little fingers respectively. They are inserted onto the lateral margin of the dorsal digital expansions of the extensor digitorum tendons to the medial four fingers. The lateral two are supplied by the median nerve, and the medial two by the deep branch of the ulnar nerve. They help to flex the proximal phalanges and extend the middle and distal phalanges of the medial four fingers. Also *lumbrical muscles of hand.* **musculi lumbricales pedis** [NA] Four small muscles in each foot, of which the first originates from the medial margin of the flexor digitorum longus tendon to the second toe, and the lateral three from adjacent sides of the long flexor tendons to the third, fourth, and fifth toes. They are inserted into the medial sides of the dorsal digital expansions of the lateral four toes. The first is supplied by the medial plantar nerve, and the lateral three by the deep branch of the lateral plantar nerve. They flex the proximal phalanges of the lateral four toes, and slightly extend the other phalanges of those toes. Also *lumbrical muscles of foot.* **m. masseter** [NA] A muscle of which pars superficialis originates from the anterior two thirds of the inferior margin of zygomatic arch and from the zygomatic process of maxilla, and pars profunda from the inferior margin and deep surface of the zygomatic arch. Pars superficialis is inserted onto the lower half of the lateral surface of the ramus, and onto the angle and the adjacent part of the body of mandible; and pars profunda onto the upper half of the lateral surface of the ramus and the coronoid process of the mandible. It is supplied by the mandibular nerve, elevates the mandible, and participates in protraction and retraction and side-to-side movements of the mandible. Also *masseter muscle, masseter.* **musculi membri inferioris** [NA] The muscles of the various segments of the lower limb, namely, thigh, leg, and foot. **musculi membri superioris** [NA] The muscles of the various segments of the upper limb, namely, shoulder, arm, forearm, and hand. **m. mentalis** [NA] A muscle originating from the incisive fossa of mandible; inserted into the skin of the chin, fusing with the muscle of the opposite side; and supplied by the mandibular branch of the facial nerve. It draws up and wrinkles the skin of the chin, protruding the lower lip. **musculi multifidi** [NA] The second layer of the transversospinalis group of muscles of the back. They originate from the back of the sacrum, the aponeurosis of erector spinae muscle, the posterior superior iliac spine, dorsal sacroiliac ligaments, mamillary processes of lumbar vertebrae, transverse processes of thoracic vertebrae, and articular processes of the lower four cervical vertebrae. They are inserted onto the spines of vertebrae from fifth lumbar to axis, either onto the contiguous one above or spanning two to four vertebrae. They are supplied by the dorsal rami of the spinal nerves. They extend, laterally flex, and rotate the vertebral column; and participate in general control of posture. Also *multifidus muscles.* **m. mylohyoideus** [NA] A muscle originating from the mylohyoid line on the inner surface of the body of the mandible. It is inserted onto the front of the body of the hyoid bone and into a median fibrous raphe between it and its opposite fellow. It is supplied by the mylohyoid branch of the inferior alveolar nerve, elevates the floor of the mouth at the beginning of the act of swallowing, elevates the hyoid bone, and depresses the mandible. Also *mylohyoid muscle, diaphragm of mouth, oral diaphragm.* **m. nasalis** A muscle of which pars transversa originates from the maxilla lateral to the lower part of the nasal notch, and pars alaris from the maxilla, medial to pars transversa. Pars transversa is inserted into an aponeurosis across the bridge of the nose in common with the part of the opposite side; and pars alaris is inserted into the cartilage of the ala nasi. It is supplied by the buccal branch of the facial nerve. Pars transversa compresses the nasal aperture, and pars alaris pulls the ala downwards and laterally, dilating the anterior nasal opening. Also *nasal muscle.* **m. obliquus auriculae** [NA] A muscle originating from the posterosuperior aspect of eminentia conchae of the auricle of the external ear, inserted onto the eminentia triangularis, and supplied by the posterior auricular branch of the facial nerve. It helps to modify the shape and position of the ear. Also *Tod's muscle, oblique muscle of auricle.* **m. obliquus capitis inferior** [NA] A muscle originating from the spine and adjacent lamina of the axis, inserted onto the back of the tip of transverse process of atlas, and supplied by the dorsal ramus of the first cervical nerve. It pulls the head to the same side. Also *inferior oblique muscle of head.* **m. obliquus capitis superior** [NA] A muscle originating from the upper surface of the transverse process of atlas, inserted onto the lateral part of the area between the superior and inferior nuchal lines of the occipital bone, and supplied by the dorsal ramus of the first cervical nerve. It extends the head and rotates it to the same side. Also *superior oblique muscle of head.* **m. obliquus externus abdominis** [NA] A muscle originating on the outer surfaces of the lower eight ribs lateral to the costal cartilages. It inserts onto the anterior two thirds of the outer lip of the iliac crest; by an aponeurosis into linea alba, upper border of pubic symphysis, and pubic crest; by the inguinal ligament to pubic tubercle and anterior superior iliac spine; and by the lacunar ligament to the pecten pubis. It is supplied by the ventral rami of the lower six thoracic spinal nerves. It supports and compresses abdominal viscera, depresses and compresses the lower part of the thorax during expiration, flexes the trunk when the pelvis is fixed, rotates the trunk to the opposite side, and flexes and rotates the pelvis when the thorax is fixed. Also *external oblique muscle of abdomen.* **m. obliquus inferior bulbi** [NA] A muscle that originates on the orbital surface of the maxilla lateral to the nasolacrimal groove. It is inserted onto the outer surface of the sclera behind the equator of the eyeball, between the insertions of the superior rectus and lateral rectus muscles. It is supplied by the oculomotor nerve, and serves to rotate the eyeball so as to turn the cornea upward and outward. When the cornea is deviated medially, it elevates the cornea. Also *inferior oblique muscle of eyeball.* **m. obliquus internus abdominis** A muscle that originates in the lateral two thirds of the inguinal ligament, the anterior two thirds of the intermediate line of the iliac crest, and the thoracolumbar fascia. It inserts onto the lower three or four ribs, the conjoint tendon, and the linea alba and seventh, eighth, and ninth costal cartilages through the rectus sheath. It is supplied by the ventral rami of the lower six thoracic and first lumbar spinal nerves. It supports and compresses the abdominal viscera, depresses the lower thorax during expiration, flexes the trunk forwards and laterally, rotates the trunk to the same side, and flexes and rotates the pelvis when the thorax is fixed. Also *internal oblique muscle of the abdomen.* **m. obliquus superior bulbi** [NA] A muscle of the eyeball that originates on the body of the sphenoid bone above and medial to the optic canal within the orbit. It is inserted onto the outer surface of the sclera behind the equator of the eyeball and between the insertions of the superior rectus and lateral rectus muscles. It is supplied by the trochlear nerve, and it rotates the eyeball so as to turn the cornea downward and outward. When the cornea is deviated medially, it turns the cornea downward. Also *superior oblique muscle of eyeball.* **m. obturatorius externus** [NA] A muscle that arises from the lateral surface of the pubic and ischial rami adjacent to the obturator foramen and of the obturator membrane. It is inserted onto the trochanteris fossa of the femur. Supplied by the posterior branch of the obturator nerve, it rotates the thigh laterally and serves as a postural muscle in steadying the hip joint. Also *external obturator muscle, obturator externus muscle.* **m. obturatorius internus** [NA] A leg muscle that arises from the medial part of the pelvic surface of the obturator membrane, and the pubic rami and ischial ramus adjacent to the obturator foramen. It is inserted onto the anterior part of the medial surface of the greater trochanter of the femur. Supplied by the nerve to the obturator internus, it laterally rotates the extended thigh and abducts the flexed thigh. Also *internal obturator muscle, obturator internus muscle.* **m. occipitofrontalis** [NA] A muscle of the scalp with two venters, or bellies. Its venter occipitalis originates from the lateral two thirds of the supreme nuchal line and mastoid process on each side. Its venter frontalis originates from the galea aponeurotica. The venter occipitalis inserts onto the galea aponeurotica, whereas the venter frontalis inserts onto the skin and muscles of the eyebrows and the root of the nose. The venter occipitalis is supplied by the posterior auricular branch of the facial nerve; and the venter frontalis, the temporal branches of the facial nerve. The venter frontalis raises the eyebrows and skin above the nose and wrinkles the forehead, and the venter occipitalis pulls the scalp back and tenses the galea aponeurotica. Also *occipitofrontal muscle, occipitofrontalis.* **m. omohyoideus** [NA] A muscle that consists of an inferior and a superior belly, united at an angle by an intermediate tendon that is encircled by deep cervical fascia that attaches it to the clavicle and first rib. Its origin, by the inferior belly, is at the superior margin of the scapula adjacent to the scapular notch. It inserts, by the superior belly, onto the inferior margin of the body of the hyoid bone. The inferior belly is innervated by the ansa cervicalis, and the superior belly is innervated by the superior ramus of the ansa cervicalis. The muscle helps to pull down and steady the hyoid bone, as during swallowing and phonation. Also *omohyoid muscle, omohyoid.* **m. opponens digiti minimi** [NA] A muscle of the little finger that originates at the distal margin of the hook of the hamate bone and its adjacent flexor retinaculum. It is inserted onto the medial margin of the fifth metacarpal bone. It is supplied by the deep branch of the ulnar nerve and serves to pull the fifth metacarpal anteriorly and rotate it laterally, helping to cup the hand. Also *opposing muscle of little finger.* **m. opponens pollicis** [NA] A muscle of the thumb that originates at the flexor retinaculum and tubercle of the trapezium and inserts onto the whole lateral half of the anterior surface of the first metacarpal bone. It is supplied by the median nerve and serves to flex, abduct, and medially rotate the first metacarpal in opposition. Also *opposing muscle of thumb.* **m. orbicularis** [NA] A muscle in which the fibers are arranged in a circular fashion around an opening, such as the mouth or orbit. Also *orbicular muscle, orbicularis.* **m. orbicularis oculi** [NA] A muscle of which the pars orbitalis originates from the frontal process of maxilla, the nasal portion of the frontal bone, and the medial palpebral ligament; pars palpebralis from the medial palpebral ligament and adjacent bone; and pars lacrimalis from the posterior lacrimal crest and lacrimal fascia. Of pars orbitalis, many fibers are inserted into the skin of the eyebrows and others blend with the venter frontalis musculi occipitofrontalis; pars palpebralis is inserted into the lateral palpebral raphe; and pars lacrimalis into the tarsi of eyelids and lateral palpebral raphe. It is supplied by the temporal and zygomatic branches of the facial nerve and closes the eyelids tightly when all parts act together, as well as pulling the skin of the forehead and the skin lateral to the eye towards the inner canthus of eye. The pars palpebralis alone can close the eyelids, while the pars lacrimalis pulls the eyelids and lacrimal papillae medially. Also *orbicular muscle of eye, sphincter of eye.* **m. orbicularis oris** [NA] A composite, sphincterlike muscle surrounding the oral orifice and comprising two superficial layers, pars marginalis and pars labialis, and a deep layer composed of some fibers of musculus buccinator, musculus incisivus labii superioris, and musculus incisivus labii inferioris. The fibers of pars marginalis blend with eight or nine surrounding muscles that converge and interlace in the modiolus at each angle of the mouth. The fibers of pars labialis are those confined to the lips, and include oblique fibers of the compressor muscle of lip extending between the skin and the mucous membrane. It is supplied by the buccal, and mandibular branches of the facial nerve. It closes the mouth, compresses the lips against the teeth, and protrudes the lips. Also *orbicular muscle of mouth, orbicularis oris.* **m. orbitalis** [NA] A thin layer of nonstriated muscle that bridges the inferior orbital fissure and the infraorbital groove posteriorly. It is innervated by sympathetic nerves. The actions are obscure. Also *orbital muscle, Müller's muscle.* **musculi ossiculorum auditus** [NA] The muscles attached to and acting on the ossicles in the middle ear, namely, musculus tensor tympani and musculus stapedius. Also *muscles of auditory ossicles, muscles of ossicles.* **musculi palati et faucium** [NA] The muscles of the soft palate and the palatoglossal and palatopharyngeal arches, namely, musculus levator veli palatini, musculus tensor veli palatini, musculus uvulae, musculus palatoglossus, and musculus palatopharyngeus. Also *muscles of palate and fauces, muscles of fauces.* **m. palatoglossus** [NA] A muscle that originates on the inferior surface of the palatine aponeurosis of the soft palate and inserts onto the side of the tongue. It is innervated by the pharyngeal plexus, and it serves to elevate the root of the tongue and pull the palatoglossal arch medially, closing off the oral cavity from the oropharynx. Also *palatoglossus muscle, glossopalatine muscle.* **m. palatopharyngeus** [NA] A muscle that originates on the superior surface of the palatine aponeurosis of the soft palate and the posterior margin of the osseous palate. It inserts onto the posterior margin of the thyroid cartilage and the pharyngobasilar fascia of the pharyngeal wall. Supplied by the pharyngeal plexus, it elevates the pharynx during swallowing. Acting with the opposite side it brings together the arches narrowing the pharyngeal isthmus. It also depresses the soft palate. Also *palatopharyngeal muscle.* **m. palmaris brevis** [NA] A muscle that originates on the medial edge of the palmar aponeurosis and flexor retinaculum. It inserts onto the skin on the medial margin of the hand. Supplied by the superficial branch of the ulnar nerve, it pulls the skin on the medial side of the hand toward the hollow of the palm, deepening the palm. Also *short palmar muscle.* **m. palmaris longus** A muscle that originates on the common flexor tendon on the medial epicondyle of the humerus, and on the antebrachial fascia. It is inserted onto the distal part of the flexor retinaculum and the palmar aponeurosis, and it is supplied by the medial nerve. It flexes the hand and tenses the palmar aponeurosis. Also *long palmar muscle.* **musculi papillares** [NA] Conical portions of the trabeculae carneae that are attached by their bases to the ventricular walls while their apices project inward and are continuous with the chordae tendineae, which are attached to the triangular cusps of the atrioventricular valves. In each ventricle there are two papillary muscles, anterior and posterior, while in the right ventricle there are also some small septal papillary muscles. Each papillary muscle is usually attached by chordae tendineae to more than one cusp. Also *papillary muscles.* **m. papillaris anterior ventriculi dextri** [NA] The anterior and larger of the two papillary muscles in the right ventricle, the chordae tendineae of which connect it to the anterior and posterior cusps of the tricuspid valve. It is attached to the sternocostal wall of the ventricle. Also *anterior papillary muscle of right ventricle.* **m. papillaris anterior ventriculi sinistri** [NA] The large anterior papillary muscle attached to the sternocostal wall of the left ventricle and connected by chordae tendineae to both cusps of the mitral valve. Also *anterior papillary muscle of left ventricle.* **m. papillaris posterior ventriculi dextri** [NA] The posterior and smaller of the two papillary muscles in the right ventricle which is attached to the diaphragmatic wall. Occasionally it consists of several parts and its chordae tendineae connect it to the posterior and septal cusps of the tricuspid valve. Also *posterior papillary muscle of right ventricle.* **m. papillaris posterior ventriculi sinistri** [NA] One of the two papillary muscles of the left ventricle of the heart which arises from the diaphragmatic wall of the ventricle. Its rounded free extremity gives attachment to chordae tendineae which extend to both cusps of the mitral valve. Also *posterior papillary muscle of left ventricle.* **musculi pectinati** [NA] Prominent ridges of myocardium forming a network on the internal walls of the auricles of the heart. In the right auricle they extend into a portion of the right atrium as parallel ridges on the lateral side of the crista terminalis. Also *pectinate muscles.* **m. pectineus** [NA] A muscle that originates from the pecten of the pubis and the bone in front of it, and from the pectineal fascia. It is inserted onto the upper part of the pectineal line behind and below the lesser trochanter of the femur. The femoral or, occasionally, the obturator nerve supplies the muscle, which adducts and flexes the thigh. Also *pectineal muscle.* **m. pectoralis major** [NA] A muscle of which pars clavicularis originates from the medial half of anterior surface of the clavicle; pars sternocostalis from the anterior surface of sternum down to sixth costal cartilage and the anterior surface of second to sixth costal cartilages; and pars abdominalis from the aponeurosis of obliquus externus abdominis. It is inserted onto the lateral lip of intertubercular sulcus of humerus, and is supplied by the medial and lateral pectoral nerves. It flexes, adducts, and medially rotates the arm when the thorax is fixed; and pulls the chest upwards when arms are fixed, as in climbing or in forced inspiration. Also *greater pectoral muscle.* **m. pectoralis minor** [NA] A muscle originating from the second to fifth ribs near the costal cartilages. It is inserted onto the medial margin and upper surface of the coracoid process of scapula, and supplied by the medial and lateral pectoral nerves. It helps serratus anterior to pull the scapula forwards, and depresses and rotates the scapula. Also *smaller pectoral muscle.* **musculi perinei** [NA] The muscles occupying the inferior pelvic aperture, including those of the pelvic diaphragm, urogenital diaphragm, and external genitals. Also *muscles of perineum, perineal muscles.* **m. peroneus brevis** [NA] A muscle that originates from the distal two thirds of the lateral surface of the fibula, and the anterior and posterior crural intermuscular septa. It inserts onto the lateral aspect of the base of the fifth metatarsal bone. Supplied by the superficial peroneal nerve, it everts and plantar flexes the foot. Also *short peroneal muscle, musculus fibularis brevis.* **m. peroneus longus** [NA] A leg muscle that originates at the head and proximal two thirds of the lateral surface of the fibula, the anterior and posterior crural intermuscular septa, and lateral condyle of the tibia. It is inserted on the inferior surface of the medial cuneiform bone and lateral side of the base of the first metatarsal bone. Supplied by the superficial peroneal nerve, it everts and plantarflexes the foot as well as supports the transversearch of the foot. Also *long peroneal muscle, musculus fibularis longus, long fibular muscle.* **m. peroneus tertius** [NA] A muscle of the leg that originates at the distal third of the medial surface of the fibula and adjacent interosseous membrane. It is inserted onto the dorsal surface of the base and part of the medial margin of the shaft of the fifth metatarsal bone. Supplied by the deep peroneal nerve, it dorsiflexes and everts the foot. Also *third peroneal muscle, musculus fibularis tertius.* **m. piriformis** [NA] A muscle that originates from the lateral part of the anterior surface of the second, third, and fourth sacral vertebrae, the areas between the pelvic sacral foramina, and the posterior margin of the greater sciatic notch. It is inserted onto the anteromedial part of the upper margin of the greater trochanter of the femur. It is innervated by the fifth lumbar and first and second sacral nerves. It serves to laterally rotate the extended thigh and abduct the flexed thigh. Also *piriform muscle.* **m. plantaris** [NA] A muscle that originates from the distal part of the lateral supracondylar line and oblique popliteal ligament. It is inserted onto the middle of the posterior surface of the calcaneus with the tendo calcaneus. Supplied by the tibial nerve, it plantarflexes the foot. Also *plantar muscle, plantaris.* **m. pleuroesophageus** [NA] An accessory slip of smooth muscle fibers that occasionally connects the left mediastinal pleura to the esophagus, helping to fix it. Also *pleuroesophageal muscle.* **m. popliteus** [NA] A muscle that originates from a facet at the anterior end of the groove on the lateral aspect of the lateral condyle of the femur and arcuate popliteal ligament. It is inserted onto the posterior surface of the shaft of the tibia above the soleal line, and it is supplied by the tibial nerve. It rotates the tibia medially and flexes it, and laterally rotates the femur when the tibia is fixed. Also *popliteal muscle, popliteus.* **m. procerus** [NA] A muscle of the face that originates from the upper part of the lateral nasal cartilage and the fascia over the nasal bone. It is inserted into the skin just above the root of the nose and the frontal part of the occipitofrontalis muscle. It is supplied by the buccal branches of the facial nerve. It pulls down the medial end of the eyebrows and skin of the forehead, producing transverse wrinkles above the root of the nose. Also *procerus muscle, procerus.* **m. pronator quadratus** [NA] A muscle of the forearm that originates from the medial side of the anterior surface of the distal fourth of the ulna. It is inserted onto the lower fourth of the anterior surface and anterior margin of the radius and into a small area above the ulnar notch of radius. It is innervated by the anterior interosseous branch of the median nerve, and it serves to pronate the forearm and hand. Also *quadrate pronator muscle.* **m. pronator teres** [NA] A muscle of the forearm that has two heads. The caput humerale originates from the upper part of the anterior surface of the medial epicondyle and the common flexor tendon, whereas the caput ulnare originates from the medial margin of the coronoid process of the ulna. The muscle is inserted onto the middle third of the lateral surface of the radius. It is supplied by the median nerve, and it serves to pronate the forearm and hand as well as to help flex the forearm. Also *round pronator muscle.* **m. psoas major** [NA] A muscle of the back that originates from the intervertebral disks between the twelfth thoracic and fifth lumbar vertebrae and adjacent margins of the bodies of these vertebrae, the anterior surfaces and lower borders of the transverse processes of the lumbar vertebrae, and the fibrous arches over the lateral aspects of the bodies of the lumbar vertebrae. It inserts onto the lesser trochanter of the femur, and it is supplied by the ventral rami of the first, second, and third lumbar nerves. It acts with the iliacus muscle to flex the thigh upon the pelvis, to flex the pelvis and trunk on the thigh, to laterally flex the vertebral column, and medially rotate the free lower limb. Also *greater psoas muscle.* **m. psoas minor** [NA] A muscle that originates from the sides of the bodies of the twelfth thoracic and first lumbar vertebrae and the disk between them. It is inserted onto the iliopectineal eminence and pecten pubis. It is supplied by the first lumbar nerve, and it weakly flexes the trunk. Also *smaller psoas muscle.* **m. pterygoideus lateralis** [NA] A muscle whose upper head originates from the infratemporal crest and infratemporal surface of the greater wing of the sphenoid bone and whose lower head originates from the lateral surface of the lateral pterygoid plate. It is inserted onto the front of the neck of the mandibular condyle and the articular disk and capsule of the temperomandibular joint. It is innervated by the mandibular nerve, and it serves to open the mouth and protrude the mandible when both sides act with the medial pterygoids. It can also rotate the jaw to the opposite side. Also *lateral pterygoid muscle, external pyerygoid muscle* (outmoded). **m. pterygoideus medialis** [NA] A muscle of the jaw that originates from the medial surface of the lateral pterygoid plate, the pyramidal process of the palatine bone, and the tuberosity of the maxilla. It is inserted onto the lower half of the medial surface of the ramus and the angle of the mandible. Supplied by the mandibular nerve, it elevates the mandible, protrudes the mandible when acting with both lateral pterygoids, and produces side-to-side movements of the mandible when the two sides act alternately. Also *medial pterygoid muscle, internal pterygoid muscle* (outmoded). **m. pubococcygeus** [NA] A morphologic subdivision of the levator ani muscle that originates from the pelvic surface of the pubis and anterior part of the arcus tendineus. It is inserted onto the anterior sacrococcygeal ligament, the anococcygeal ligament, and the rectum. Also *pubococcygeal muscle, pubococcygeus.* **m. puboprostaticus** [NA] Smooth muscle fibers of the external longitudinal layer of the urinary bladder that are located in the medial puboprostatic ligament. Also *puboprostatic muscle.* **m. puborectalis** [NA] A thick portion of musculus levator ani that arises from the back of the pubis below the origin of pubococcygeus, the obturator fascia, and the pelvic surface of the urogenital diaphragm. It then extends on each side of the rectum, where some fibers blend with its longitudinal layer of muscle and descend to the anal canal between the internal and external sphincters of the anus, even extending to the skin. Other fibers loop behind the anorectal junction to end in the anococcygeal ligament. Also *puborectal muscle, Braune's muscle, puborectalis muscle.* **m. pubovaginalis** [NA] The most anterior fibers of the levator ani muscle in the female that pass backwards and medially across the sides of the vagina to end in the central tendon of the perineum, serving as a sphincter of the vagina. It is homologous to the levator prostatae in the male. Also *pubovaginal muscle.* **m. pubovesicalis** [NA] Some smooth muscle fibers of the external longitudinal layer of the urinary bladder that extend into the pubovesical ligaments in the female. It is homologous to musculus puboprostaticus in the male. Also *pubovesical muscle.* **m. pyramidalis** [NA] A muscle that originates from the front of the body of the pubis and pubic symphysis. It is inserted onto the linea alba about midway between the pubis and the umbilicus. Supplied by the subcostal nerve, it tenses the linea alba. Also *pyramidal muscle, pyramidalis.* **m. pyramidalis auriculae** [NA] A small muscle of the external ear that is occasionally present as an upward extension of some fibers of musculus tragicus to the spine of the helix. Also *pyramidal muscle of auricle, Jung's muscle.* **m. quadratus femoris** [NA] A muscle that originates from the upper part of the lateral margin and adjacent surface of the ischial tuberosity. It is inserted onto a tubercle about midway along the intertrochanteric crest of the femur and a short distance below. It is supplied by a branch from the fifth lumbar and first sacral nerves, and serves to rotate the thigh laterally. Also *quadrate muscle of thigh.* **m. quadratus lumborum** [NA] A muscle that originates from the iliolumbar ligament and adjacent inner lip of the iliac crest and the transverse processes of the lower three or four lumbar vertebrae. It is inserted onto the medial part of the lower margin of the twelfth rib and the transverse processes of the upper three or four lumbar vertebrae. It is innervated by the ventral rami of the twelfth thoracic and upper three or four lumbar nerves. It acts to depress and fix the twelfth rib, especially in inspiration; flex the trunk laterally; and, when both sides act together, to assist in the extension of the vertebral column. **m. quadratus plantae** [NA] A muscle of the foot that originates by lateral and medial heads from the inferior surface of the calcaneus anterior to the lateral and medial processes, respectively. It is inserted onto the tendon or tendons of the musculus flexor digitorum longus, and it is supplied by the lateral plantar nerve. It exerts traction on the tendon of the flexor digitorum longus so as to flex the toes along their axes and helps to maintain the longitudinal arches of the foot. Also *quadrate muscle of sole, accessory flexor muscle.* **m. quadriceps femoris** [NA] A muscle that originates by four heads: musculus rectus femoris, musculus vastus medialis, musculus vastus intermedius, and musculus vastus lateralis. It is inserted onto the base of the patella by a common tendon, the tuberosity of the tibia by the ligamentum patellae, and the medial and lateral patellar retinacula. Supplied by the femoral nerve, it extends the leg. Also *quadriceps muscle of thigh, quadriceps femoris muscle, quadriceps femoris.* **m. rectococcygeus** [NA] Two nonstriated muscle bundles that arise from the front of the second and third coccygeal vertebrae where they blend with fibers of the levator ani muscle and extend anteriorly to join the longitudinal muscle fibers on the posterior wall of the anal canal and the perirectal fascia. It helps to elevate and retract the lower part of the rectum and the anal canal. Also *rectococcygeal muscle.* **m. rectourethralis** [NA] Some fasciculi of the anterior longitudinal muscle of the rectal ampulla that extend anteriorly to the central tendon of the perineum and the membranous urethra in the male. Also *rectourethral muscle.* **m. rectouterinus** [NA] A band of longitudinal muscle fibers of the uterus that passes backwards from the cervix in the rectouterine fold, helping to form the uterosacral ligament, to blend with longitudinal muscle fibers of the rectum. Also *rectouterine muscle, Luschka's muscles.* **m. rectovesicalis** [NA] Some muscle fibers of the external longitudinal layer of the urinary bladder that extend from the base to the front of the rectum. Also *rectovesical muscle.* **m. rectus abdominis** [NA] A muscle that originates from the crest of the pubis, the front of the pubic symphysis, and the lower part of the linea alba. It is inserted onto the fifth, sixth, and seventh costal cartilages and the xiphoid process. It is supplied by the ventral rami of the lower six or seven thoracic spinal nerves. The muscle serves to flex the trunk forward when the pelvis is fixed, helps to compress the abdominal viscera, and acts to flex the pelvis when the thorax is fixed. **m. rectus capitis anterior** [NA] A muscle that originates from the anterior surface of the lateral mass and part of the transverse process of the atlas. It is inserted onto the inferior surface of the basilar part of the occipital bone in front of the condyle. Supplied by the first and second cervical nerve, it serves to flex the head forward and rotate the head toward the same side. **m. rectus capitis lateralis** [NA] A muscle that originates from the upper surface of the transverse part of the atlas and is inserted onto the inferior surface of the jugular process of the occipital bone. Supplied by the first and second cervical nerves, it serves to bend the head to the same side. **m. rectus capitis posterior major** [NA] A muscle whose origin is on the spine of the axis and whose insertion is located on the lateral half of the inferior nuchal line of the occipital bone. It is supplied by the dorsal ramus of the first cervical nerve, and it serves to extend the head and rotate the head to the same side. **m. rectus capitis posterior minor** [NA] A muscle that originates from the tubercle on the posterior arch of the atlas. It is inserted onto and below the medial third of the inferior nuchal line of the occipital bone. Supplied by the dorsal ramus of the first cervical nerve, it serves to extend the head. **m. rectus femoris** [NA] A muscle of which the straight head originates from the anterior inferior iliac spine and the reflected head from the groove above the acetabulum. It is inserted onto the upper margin of the patella, the tendon of the quadriceps femoris muscle, and onto the tuberosity of tibia by the ligamentum patellae. It is supplied by the femoral nerve, extends the leg, and flexes the thigh. **m. rectus inferior bulbi** [NA] A muscle that originates from the lower part of the annulus tendineus communis and is inserted onto the lower aspect of the outer surface of the sclera behind the corneal margin. Supplied by the oculomotor nerve, it rotates the visual axis, downward about the transverse axis and medially about the vertical axis. It also extorts the eye. Also *inferior straight muscle, inferior rectus muscle of bulb.* **m. rectus lateralis bulbi** [NA] A muscle that originates from the lateral side of the annulus tendineus communis and the orbital surface of the greater wing of the sphenoid bone, just lateral to the tendon. It is inserted onto the lateral aspect of the sclera behind the corneal margin. Supplied by the abducent nerve, the muscle rotates the eyeball laterally. Also *lateral straight muscle, lateral rectus muscle of bulb.* **m. rectus medialis bulbi** [NA] A muscle that originates from the medial aspect of the annulus tendineus communis and is inserted onto the medial aspect of the scleral surface behind the corneal margin. Supplied by the oculomotor nerve, it rotates the eyeball medially. With the lateral rectus, it can act on both eyes together to produce convergence or divergence. Also *medial straight muscle, medial rectus muscle of bulb.* **m. rectus superior bulbi** [NA] A muscle of the eye that originates from the upper part of the annulus tendineus communis and is inserted onto the upper part of the sclera behind the corneal margin. Supplied by the oculomotor nerve, it acts in the elevation, medial rotation, and intorsion of the eyeball. Also *superior rectus muscle of bulb.* **m. rhomboideus major** [NA] A muscle that originates from the spines of the second to fifth thoracic vertebrae and their supraspinous ligaments. It is inserted onto the medial margin of the scapula from the root of the spine to the inferior angle. Supplied by the dorsal scapular nerve, it elevates and retracts the scapula and helps to rotate the scapula and depress the point of the scapula. Also *greater rhomboid muscle.* **m. rhomboideus minor** [NA] A muscle originating from the lower part of the ligamentum nuchae and the spines of the seventh cervical and first thoracic vertebrae. It is inserted onto the medial margin of the scapula opposite the root of the spine. Supplied by the dorsal scapular nerve, it elevates and retracts the scapula and helps to rotate and depress the point of the scapula. Also *lesser rhomboid muscle.* **m. risorius** [NA] A muscle of the face that originates from the parotid fascia and is inserted into the skin and mucosa at the angle of the mouth. Supplied by the buccal branches of the facial nerve, it pulls the angle of the mouth laterally. Also *risorius muscle, Santorini's muscle, Albinus muscle.* **musculi rotatores** [NA] The deepest layer of transversospinal muscles comprising small muscles between the transverse and spinous processes of the vertebrae and extending from the sacrum to the spinous process of the axis. They are divided into three morphologic units: the musculi rotatores cervicis, musculi rotatores thoracis, and musculi rotatores lumborum. They are supplied by the dorsal rami of the spinal nerves in their respective regions. They rotate the vertebral column, help to laterally flex and extend the vertebral column, and help to control posture, especially in steadying the vertebral column during body movements. Also *rotator muscles.* **musculi rotatores cervicis** [NA] Variable muscle bundles that connect the transverse process of a cervical vertebra to the lamina of the vertebra next above, extending as far as the root of its spine. Also *rotator muscles of neck.* **musculi rotatores lumborum** [NA] Variable and irregular muscle bundles that each connect the transverse process of a lumbar vertebra to the lamina of the vertebra next above, extending as far as the root of its spine. **musculi rotatores thoracis** [NA] A series of eleven muscles on each side that each connects the upper part of a transverse process of a thoracic vertebra to the outer surface of the lamina of the vertebra next above, extending as far as the root of its spine. Also *rotator muscles of thorax.* **m. sacrococcygeus dorsalis** [NA] An inconstant accessory muscle composed of a few fasciculi extending behind the sacrococcygeal joint, from the posterior surface of lower sacral vertebrae or from the posterior inferior iliac spine to the posterior aspect of the coccyx. Also *dorsal sacrococcygeal muscle, posterior sacrococcygeal muscle.* **m. sacrococcygeus ventralis** [NA] An inconstant muscle that arises from the sides of the fourth and fifth sacral vertebrae, the front of the first coccygeal vertebra, and the sacrospinous ligament, and that is inserted into the second to fourth coccygeal vertebrae and anterior sacrococcygeal ligament. Also *ventral sacrococcygeal muscle, anterior sacrococcygeal muscle.* **m. salpingopharyngeus** [NA] A muscle that originates from the inferior surface of the cartilage of the auditory tube near its opening in the pharynx and fuses with the palatopharyngeus muscle in the wall of the pharynx. Supplied by the pharyngeal plexus, it elevates the upper part of the pharynx and aids in opening the auditory tube during swallowing. Also *salpingopharyngeal muscle.* **m. sartorius** [NA] A muscle that originates from the anterior superior iliac spine and the surface just below it. It is inserted onto the upper end of the medial surface of the tibia and into the fascia cruris. It is supplied by the femoral nerve, and it flexes, abducts, and laterally rotates the thigh as well as flexes and medially rotates the leg. Also *sartorius muscle.* **m. scalenus anterior** [NA] A muscle that originates from the anterior tubercles of the transverse process of the third to sixth cervical vertebrae and is inserted onto the scalene tubercle and the upper surface of the first rib. It is supplied by the ventral rami of the third to sixth cervical nerves. Acting from above, it elevates the first rib; acting from below, it flexes the cervical vertebrae forward and sideways and rotates them to the opposite side. Also *anterior scalene muscle, scalenus anticus* (outmoded). **m. scalenus medius** [NA] A muscle that originates from the transverse process of the axis, and often of the atlas, and the posterior tubercles of the transverse processes of the lower five cervical vertebrae. It is inserted onto the upper surface of the first rib behind the subclavian groove. It is supplied by the ventral rami of the third to eighth cervical nerves. Acting from above, it raises the first rib. Acting from below it flexes the cervical vertebrae to the same side. Also *middle scalene muscle, mediscalenus.* **m. scalenus minimus** [NA] A separate muscle band occasionally present between the scalenus anterior and medius muscles. It arises from the anterior tubercles of the transverse processes of the sixth and seventh cervical vertebrae and is inserted on the inner border of first rib and to the dome of the pleura, which it tenses on contraction. Also *smallest scalene muscle, Sibson's muscle, Albinus muscle.* **m. scalenus posterior** [NA] A muscle that arises from the posterior tubercles of the transverse processes of the fourth, fifth, and sixth cervical vertebrae. It is inserted onto the lateral surface of the second rib, and it is supplied by the ventral rami of the sixth, seventh, and eighth cervical spinal nerves. Acting from above, it elevates the second rib; acting from below, it flexes the lower cervical vertebrae to the same side. Also *posterior scalene muscle.* **m. semimembranosus** [NA] A muscle that arises from the superolateral impression on the upper part of the ischial tuberosity. It is inserted onto the back of the medial condyle of the tibia, the lateral femoral condyle by the oblique popliteal ligament, and the capsule of the knee joint. Supplied by the tibial nerve, it flexes the leg and medially rotates the flexed leg as well as extends the thigh and medially rotates the extended thigh. Also *semimembranous muscle.* **m. semispinalis** [NA] The superficial mass of the transversospinal group of muscles, extending from the thorax to the occipital bone and divided into three morphological units: the musculus semispinalis capitis, musculus semispinalis cervicis, and musculus semispinalis thoracis. It is supplied by the dorsal rami of the cervical and thoracic spinal nerves. Also *semispinal muscle, semispinalis.* **m. semispinalis capitis** [NA] A muscle that arises from the transverse processes of the upper six or seven thoracic and seventh cervical vertebrae and the articular processes of the lower four cervical vertebrae. It is inserted onto the medial part of the area between the superior and inferior nuchal lines of the occipital bone. Supplied by the dorsal rami of the cervical spinal nerves, it extends the head and rotates it to the opposite side. Also *semispinal muscle of the head, complexus.* **m. semispinalis cervicis** [NA] A muscle that arises from the transverse processes of the upper five or six thoracic vertebrae. It is inserted onto the spines of the second to sixth cervical vertebrae, and it is supplied by the dorsal rami of the cervical and thoracic spinal nerves. It extends the cervical and thoracic vertebrae and rotates the vertebral column to the opposite side. Also *semispinal muscle of neck.* **m. semispinalis dorsi** *Outmoded* MUSCULUS SEMISPINALIS THORACIS. **m. semispinalis thoracis** [NA] A muscle of the back that arises from the transverse processes of the sixth to tenth thoracic vertebrae and is inserted onto the spines of the upper four thoracic and lower two cervical vertebrae. It is supplied by the dorsal rami of the cervical and thoracic spinal nerves. It extends the cervical and thoracic vertebrae and rotates them to the opposite side. Also *semispinal muscle of thorax.* **m. semitendinosus** [NA] A muscle that arises from the inferomedial impression on the upper part of the ischial tuberosity. It is inserted onto the upper part of the medial surface of the tibia behind and below the insertion of the gracilis muscle. Supplied by the tibial nerve, it flexes the leg and medially rotates the flexed leg. It also extends the thigh and medially rotates the extended thigh. Also *semitendinous muscle.* **m. serratus anterior** [NA] A muscle that arises by digitations from the outer surfaces of the anterior angles of the upper eight or nine ribs. It is inserted onto the costal surface of the superior and inferior angles and intervening medial margin of the scapula. Supplied by the long thoracic nerve, it draws the shoulder girdle forward and laterally and helps to rotate the scapula, especially in lifting the arm above shoulder level. The upper part helps to pull the scapula downward and forward. Also *anterior serratus muscle.* **m. serratus posterior inferior** [NA] A muscle that arises from the spines of the lower two thoracic and first two lumbar vertebrae and the supraspinous ligament. It is inserted onto the lower margins of the last four ribs lateral to their angles. Supplied by the ventral rami of the ninth to twelfth thoracic spinal nerves, it depresses the ribs. Also *inferior posterior serratus muscle.* **m. serratus posterior superior** [NA] A muscle that arises from the lower part of the ligamentum nuchae, the spines of the lower two cervical and upper two thoracic vertebrae, and the supraspinous ligament. It is inserted onto the outer surfaces of the second to fifth ribs lateral to their angles. Supplied by the second to fifth intercostal nerves, it elevates the ribs. Also *superior posterior serratus muscle.* **m. skeleti** A muscle attached to the axial and appendicular skeleton and crossing at least one joint on which it acts. It consists of long, thin multinucleated fibers containing myofibrils with regularly spaced alternate dark and light striations, lying in semifluid sarcoplasm and enclosed in a sheath, the sarcolemma. The fibers are organized in bundles, or fasciculi. Also *skeletal muscle, striated muscle, striped muscle, textus muscularis striatus.* **m. soleus** [NA] A muscle that arises from the upper fourth of the posterior surface of the shaft and back of the head of the fibula, the soleal line and middle third of the medial margin of the tibia, and the fibrous arch between the tibia and fibula. It is inserted onto the middle of the posterior surface of the calcaneus by the tendo calcaneus. Supplied by the tibial nerve, it plantarflexes and inverts the foot and raises the heel off the ground. Also *soleus muscle.* **m. sphincter** [NA] A ring of muscle fibers that surround a tube, duct, or orifice which is diminished or closed by their contraction. Also *sphincter, sphincter muscle.* **m. sphincter ampullae hepatopancreaticae** [NA] The thickened circular muscle of the wall of the descending part of the duodenum that forms a compound sphincter comprising the circular muscle around the terminal part of the common bile duct (the musculus sphincter ductus choledochus), of the pancreatic duct (the musculus sphincter ductus pancreatici), and around the ampulla hepatopancreatica. They are continuous with one another but one or both of the latter two may be absent or weakly formed. Also *Oddi sphincter, Oddi's muscle, Glisson sphincter, sphincter muscle of hepatopancreatic ampulla, sphincter of hepatopancreatic ampulla, duodenal sphincter.* **m. sphincter ani externus** [NA] A voluntary muscle which surrounds the anal canal and extends from the central tendon of the perineum and the skin to the coccyx. It is divided into three parts that are imperfectly separated, namely, pars profunda, pars subcutanea, and pars superficialis. It is innervated by the inferior rectal branch of the pudendal nerve and the perineal branch of the fourth sacral nerve. Also *external sphincter muscle of the anus, external sphincter of anus.* **m. sphincter ani internus** [NA] The annular thickening of the circular fibers of the tunica muscularis recti. It extends from the anorectal junction to the intersphincteric groove just above the anal orifice. Also *internal sphincter muscle of the anus, internal sphincter of anus.* **m. sphincter ductus choledochi** [NA] A thickening of the circular muscle fibers of the wall of the descending part of the duodenum around the lower part of the common bile duct just before it joins the pancreatic duct. Also *choledochal sphincter, sphincter muscle of bile duct, sphincter of common bile duct, sphincter of Boyden, Giordano sphincter, sphincter of bile duct.* **m. sphincter ductus pancreatici** [NA] An inconstant thickening of the circular muscle fibers of the wall of the descending part of the duodenum around the terminal part of the pancreatic duct just before it joins the common bile duct in the ampulla. Also *sphincter muscle of pancreatic duct, sphincter of duct of Wirsung.* **m. sphincter pupillae** [NA] A circular flattened band of nonstriated muscle fibers in the stroma iridis, near the periphery of the pupil to which they run parallel. Posteriorly it is attached by collagen fibers to the dilator pupillae. It is innervated by the short ciliary nerves. Also *sphincter muscle of pupil, sphincter pupillae.* **m. sphincter pyloricus** [NA] A ring of thickened circular muscle fibers of the tunica muscularis around the pyloric canal of the stomach. Also *sphincter muscle of pylorus, pyloric sphincter.* **m. sphincter urethrae** [NA] A group of striated muscle fibers that surrounds the membranous urethra and rises on the prostate almost to the base of the bladder. It arises from the transverse perineal ligament and the fascial sheath of the pudendal vessels and is inserted onto the central tendon of the perineum and around the membranous urethra. It is supplied by the perineal branch of the pudendal nerve. In the male it compresses the membranous urethra and takes part in ejaculation. In the female it encircles the lower end of the urethra, and some fibers end

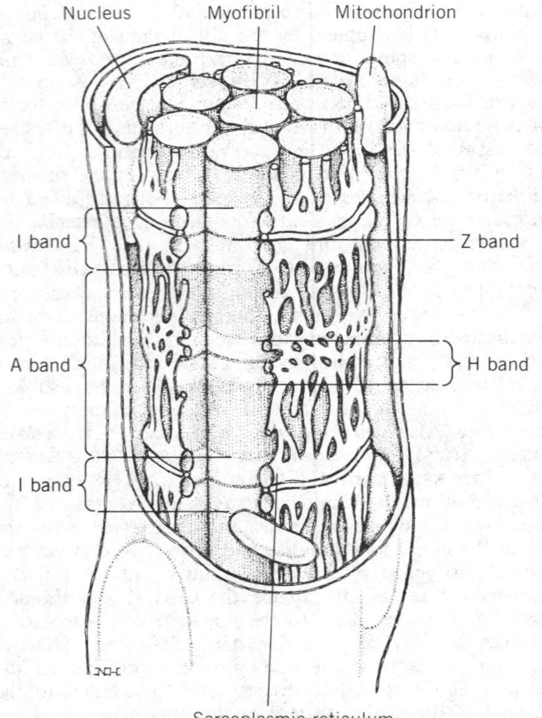


**Skeletal muscle**

in the vaginal wall. Also *sphincter muscle of membranous urethra, sphincter muscle of urethra, Guthrie's muscle, sphincter urethrae.* **m. sphincter vesicae urinariae** A group of smooth muscle fibers of the circular layer of the urinary bladder that encircle the internal urethral orifice and are continuous with the levator prostatae muscle surrounding the proximal part of the urethra. It is innervated by the vesical plexus and it helps in controlling micturition. Also *sphincter muscle of urinary bladder.* **m. spinalis** [NA] The medial column of the musculus erector spinae, comprising the musculus spinalis capitis, musculus spinalis cervicis, and musculus spinalis thoracis. It is supplied by the dorsal rami of the lower cervical and thoracic spinal nerves, and it extends the vertebral column. Also *spinal muscle.* **m. spinalis capitis** [NA] An inconstant prolongation of musculus spinalis cervicis to the medial part of the area between the superior and inferior nuchal lines of the occipital bone, and usually blended with the musculus semispinalis capitis. Also *biventer cervicis.* **m. spinalis cervicis** [NA] An inconstant muscle, often absent, that arises from the spines of the lower two cervical and upper two thoracic vertebrae. It is inserted onto the spines of the second and third cervical vertebrae. **m. spinalis thoracis** [NA] A muscle that arises from the tips of the spines of the two upper lumbar and lower two thoracic vertebrae and is inserted onto the spines of the upper thoracic vertebrae. It is usually fused to the musculus semispinalis thoracis. **m. splenius capitis** [NA] A muscle that arises from the lower part of the ligamentum nuchae and the spines of the seventh cervical and upper three or four thoracic vertebrae. It is inserted onto the mastoid process and the lateral part of the superior nuchal line of the occipital bone. It is supplied by the dorsal rami of the middle cervical spinal nerves, and it helps to extend the head, pull it to one side, and rotate it to the same side. Also *splenius muscle of head.* **m. splenius cervicis** [NA] A muscle that arises from the spines of the lower cervical and upper thoracic vertebrae. It is inserted onto the posterior tubercles of the transverse processes of the upper two or three cervical vertebrae. Supplied by the dorsal rami of the lower cervical spinal nerves, it helps to extend the head and neck as well as rotate the head to the same side. Also *splenius muscle of neck.* **m. stapedius** [NA] A muscle that arises from within the pyramidal eminence on the posterior wall of the middle ear. It is inserted onto the posterior surface of the neck of the stapes and is supplied by the facial nerve. It reflexly aids the tensor tympani muscle in dampening the intensity of sounds reaching the internal ear. Also *stapedius muscle.* **m. sternalis** [NA] An inconstant muscle slip on the surface of the musculus pectoralis major, running parallel to the sternum and extending from the rectus sheath and lower costal cartilages to either the sternal origin of the musculus sternocleidomastoideus or the pectoral fascia. It is innervated by nerves to the sternocleidomastoid or pectoral muscles. Also *sternal muscle, sternalis.* **m. sternocleidomastoideus** [NA] A muscle of the neck that has a sternal or medial head arising from the upper anterior surface of the manubrium sterni below the clavicular notch and a clavicular or lateral head arising from the medial third of the upper surface of the clavicle. It is inserted onto the anterior margin and lateral surface of the mastoid process and the lateral part of the superior nuchal line of the occipital bone. It is supplied by the accessory nerve and the ventral rami of the second and third cervical nerves. It flexes the head laterally and rotates it to the opposite side, flexes the head forward when both sides act together, and, when both sides act together from above, helps to elevate the thorax in forced inspiration. Also *sternomastoid muscle, sternocleidomastoid muscle.* **m. sternohyoideus** [NA] A muscle that arises from the posterosuperior aspect of the manubrium sterni and the posterior surface of the medial end of the clavicle. It is inserted onto the inferior margin of the body of the hyoid bone. Supplied by the ansa cervicalis, it depresses the hyoid bone. Also *sternohyoid muscle.* **m. sternothyroideus** [NA] A muscle that arises from the posterior surface of the manubrium sterni and the first costal cartilage. It is inserted onto the oblique line on the lamina of the thyroid cartilage. Supplied by the ansa cervicalis, it pulls the thyroid cartilage downward after it has been elevated. Also *sternothyroid muscle, sternothyreoideus.* **m. styloglossus** [NA] A muscle originating from the anterolateral surface of the styloid process of the temporal bone near its apex and from the contiguous part of the stylomandibular ligament. It is inserted into the side of the tongue, is supplied by the hypoglossal nerve, and pulls the tongue backwards and upwards. Also *styloglossus muscle, styloglossus.* **m. stylohyoideus** [NA] A muscle that arises from the posterior surface of the styloid process of the temporal bone near its base and is inserted onto the body of the hyoid bone at the junction with the greater cornu. Supplied by the facial nerve, it elevates and pulls back the hyoid bone. Also *stylohyoid muscle, stylohyoid.* **m. stylopharyngeus** [NA] A muscle that originates from the medial side of the base of the styloid process of the temporal bone. It is inserted onto the posterior margin of the thyroid cartilage with the palatopharyngeus muscle, the lateral glossoepiglottic fold, and the pharyngeal constrictor muscles. Supplied by the glossopharyngeal nerve, it elevates the pharynx. Also *stylopharyngeus muscle.* **m. subclavius** [NA] A muscle that arises from the upper surface of the junction of the first rib and its cartilage. It is inserted onto the inferior surface of the middle third of the clavicle and is supplied by the fifth and sixth cervical nerve. It acts to depress the clavicle and point of the shoulder when the first rib is fixed. It also helps in forced inspiration when the clavicle is fixed and steadies the clavicle against the sternum in movements of the shoulder. Also *subclavius muscle.* **musculi subcostales** [NA] A series of muscle fibers on the internal aspect of the thoracic wall that are closely associated with the lower internal intercostal muscles, each one extending from the inner surface of a rib near its angle to the inner surface of the second or third rib below. The lateral margin of each is continuous with the posterior margin of adjacent intercostales intimi. They depress the ribs. Also *subcostal muscles.* **m. subscapularis** [NA] A muscle that arises from the medial two thirds of the subscapular fossa of the scapula and the intermuscular septa. It is inserted onto the capsule of the shoulder joint and lesser tubercle of the humerus. Supplied by the upper and lower subscapular nerves, it medially rotates the arm and helps to steady the head of the humerus in the glenoid cavity during movements of the shoulder joint. Also *subscapular muscle.* **m. supinator** [NA] A muscle that arises from the lower part of the posterior surface of the lateral epicondyle of the humerus, the radial collateral ligament of the elbow joint, the area below the radial notch and supinator crest of the ulna. It is inserted onto the proximal third of the lateral surface of the radius. Supplied by the posterior interosseous nerve, it laterally rotates the forearm to turn the palm of the hand to face forward. Also *supinator muscle, supinator.* **musculi suprahyoidei** [NA] The muscles that connect the upper margin of the hyoid bone to the base of the skull and the mandible, namely, the stylohyoid, digastric, mylohyoid, and geniohyoid muscles. They elevate the hyoid bone and the larynx, and the latter three also depress the mandible. Also *suprahyoid muscles.* **m. supraspinatus** [NA] A muscle of the scapula that arises from the medial two thirds of the supraspinous fossa of the scapula and the supraspinous fascia. It is inserted onto the highest of three facets on the greater tubercle of the humerus. Supplied by the suprascapular nerve, it helps to initiate abduction of the arm and helps to steady the head of the humerus and to prevent downward sliding in the glenoid cavity. Also *supraspinous muscle.* **m. suspensorius duodeni** [NA] A fibromuscular band that extends from the right crus of the diaphragm near the esophageal hiatus to the back of the upper part of the duodenojejunal flexure as well as to the horizontal and ascending portions of the duodenum. Its contraction maintains and increases the angle of the flexure, tending to prevent obstruction. Also *suspensory muscle of duodenum, muscle of Treitz, ligament of Treitz, retention band, suspensory ligament of duodenum.* **m. tarsalis inferior** [NA] A layer of smooth muscle extending between the fascial sheath of the inferior rectus muscle and the inferior tarsus, and serving to depress the lower eyelid. It is innervated by sympathetic fibers. Also *inferior tarsal muscle.* **m. tarsalis superior** [NA] A layer of smooth muscle in the inferior lamella of the musculus levator palpebrae superioris that is attached to the upper anterior margin of the superior tarsus and serves to elevate the upper eyelid. It is innervated by sympathetic fibers. Also *superior tarsal muscle, Müller's muscle.* **m. temporalis** [NA] A muscle that originates from the temporal fossa and fascia. It is inserted onto the apex, margins, and medial surface of the coronoid process of the mandible and the anterior margin of the ramus of the mandible, and supplied by deep temporal branches of the mandibular nerve. It elevates the mandible and closes the mouth, its posterior fibers retract the mandible, and it helps in side-to-side movements of the mandible. Also *temporal muscle, temporalis.* **m. temporoparietalis** [NA] A variable sheet of muscle extending between the frontal part of the musculus occipitofrontalis and the anterior and superior auricular muscles. It is supplied by the temporal branches of the facial nerve. Also *temporoparietal muscle, muscle of Sappey.* **m. tensor fasciae latae** [NA] A muscle that arises from the anterior part of the outer lip of the iliac crest, on the outer surface of the anterior superior iliac spine and the area below it. It is inserted into the upper anterior part of the iliotibial tract and supplied by the superior gluteal nerve. It extends and laterally rotates the leg, medially rotates the thigh when the foot is off the ground, and helps to steady and flex the pelvis when the foot is on the ground and the leg is fixed. Also *tensor muscle of fascia lata.* **m. tensor tympani** [NA] A muscle that arises from the cartilaginous part of the auditory tube, the adjacent part of the greater wing of the sphenoid bone, and the bony semicanal in which it lies. It is inserted onto the manubrium of the malleus, and it is supplied by the nerve to the medial pterygoid. The muscle tenses the tympanic membrane and helps to dampen sound vibrations. Also *tensor tympani muscle, tensor muscle of tympanic membrane, tensor muscle of tympanum.* **m. tensor veli palatini** [NA] A muscle that arises from the scaphoid fossa of the pterygoid process, the spine of the sphenoid bone, and the lateral lamina of the cartilage of the auditory tube. It is inserted into the palatine aponeurosis of the soft palate and the transverse ridge on the inferior surface of the horizontal plate of the palatine bone. Supplied by the mandibular nerve, it tightens the soft palate and opens the auditory tube. Also *tensor muscle of velum palatinum.* **m. teres major** [NA] A muscle that originates from the posterior surface of the inferior angle of the scapula and from the intermuscular septa, is inserted into the medial lip of the intertubercular groove of the humerus and supplied by the lower subscapular nerve. It adducts, medially rotates, and extends the arm. Also *teres major muscle.* **m. teres minor** [NA] A muscle that arises from the upper two thirds of the posterior surface of the lateral margin of the scapula. It is inserted onto the lowest of the three facets on the greater tubercle of the humerus and about one inch below it. Supplied by the axillary nerve, it helps to rotate the arm laterally, adducts the arm, and helps to steady the head of the humerus in the glenoid cavity during movements of the shoulder joint. Also *teres minor muscle.* **musculi thoracis** [NA] The muscles of the walls of the thorax, including the pectoral, subclavius, serratus anterior, levatores costarum, intercostal, subcostal, and transversus thoracis muscles. **m. thyroarytenoideus** [NA] A muscle that arises from the lower part of the inner surface of the angle of the thyroid cartilage and is inserted onto the lateral margin of the arytenoid cartilage. Supplied by the recurrent laryngeal nerve, it pulls forward and rotates the arytenoid cartilage to relax the vocal ligament. Also *thyroarytenoid muscle.* **m. thyroepiglotticus** [NA] A muscle that arises from the inner surface of the angle of the thyroid cartilage at the upper margin of the thyroarytenoid muscle. It is inserted onto the lateral margin of the epiglottis. Supplied by the recurrent laryngeal nerve, it widens the inlet of the larynx. Also *thyroepiglottic muscle.* **m. thyrohyoideus** [NA] A muscle that arises from the oblique line on the lamina of the thyroid cartilage. It is inserted onto the inferior margin of the lateral third of the body and the lateral surface of the greater cornu of the hyoid bone. It is supplied by the first cervical spinal nerve via the hypoglossal nerve, and it serves to depress the hyoid bone and elevate the larynx. Also *thyrohyoid muscle.* **m. tibialis anterior** [NA] A muscle that arises from the lower part of the lateral condyle and the upper two thirds of the lateral surface of the tibia, the interosseous membrane, and the fascia cruris. It is inserted onto the medial surface of the medial cuneiform bone and the base of the first metatarsal bone. Supplied by the deep peroneal nerve, it dorsiflexes and inverts the foot, increases the medial longitudinal arch, and pulls the leg forward when acting from below. Also *anterior tibial muscle.* **m. tibialis posterior** [NA] A muscle that arises from the lateral part of the middle third of the posterior surface of the tibia below the soleal line, from the interosseous membrane, and from the medial part of the upper two thirds of the posterior surface of the fibula. Its superficial or medial division is inserted onto the tuberosity of the navicular bone and the inferior surface of the medial cuneiform bone, and its deep or lateral division is inserted onto the intermediate and lateral cuneiform and cuboid bones and the plantar surface of the bases of the second, third, and fourth metatarsal bones. Supplied by the tibial nerve, it inverts and plantarflexes the foot. Also *posterior tibial muscle.* **m. trachealis** [NA] The tunica muscularis of the trachea, extending transversely between the free ends of the tracheal cartilages in the posterior wall of the trachea. It pulls together the ends and diminishes the lumen of the trachea. Also *tracheal muscle.* **m. tragicus** [NA] A short, flattened band of muscle fibers running vertically on the outer surface of the tragus of the external ear. It is innervated by temporal branches of the facial nerve. Also *muscle of tragus, Valsalva's muscle.* **musculi transversospinales** [NA] A system of deep muscles of the back whose fibers run obliquely upward and medially from the transverse process of a vertebra to the spine or lamina of a vertebra at a higher level, spanning up to six vertebrae. The system is subdivided according to the number of vertebrae crossed, the semispinalis group spanning more than four vertebrae, the multifidus group spanning two to four vertebrae. The short and long rotators, the deepest group, attach to the next vertebra or the one above that. Also *transversospinal muscles.* **m. transversus abdominis** [NA] A muscle that arises from the inner surfaces of the lower six costal cartilages, the thoracolumbar fascia, the inner lip of the anterior two thirds of the iliac crest, and the lateral third of the inguinal ligament. It is inserted into the upper two thirds of the linea alba through the posterior lamella of the rectus sheath, the lower third of the linea alba through the anterior lamella of the rectus sheath, the crest and pecten of the pubis by the conjoint tendon, and the superior pubic ramus by the interfoveolar ligament. Supplied by the ventral rami of the lower six thoracic and first lumbar spinal nerves, it supports and compresses the abdominal viscera and helps to compress the thorax during expiration. Also *transverse muscle of abdomen, transversus abdominis muscle.* **m. transversus auriculae** [NA] A small group of muscle and tendinous fibers on the cranial aspect of the auricle connecting the eminentia conchae to the eminentia scaphae. It is supplied by the posterior auricular branch of the facial nerve. Also *transverse muscle of auricle.* **m. transversus linguae** [NA] An intrinsic muscle of the tongue arising from the septum linguae and inserted into the lingual aponeurosis at the lateral margins of the tongue. Supplied by the hypoglossal nerve, it narrows and elongates the tongue. Also *transverse muscle of tongue.* **m. transversus menti** [NA] An occasional fibromuscular band of the musculus depressor anguli oris that crosses the midline to interdigitate with the muscle of the other side below the chin. Also *transverse muscle of chin.* **m. transversus perinei profundus** [NA] A muscle that arises from the inner aspect of the ramus of the ischium and is inserted into the medial raphe and perineal body. Supplied by the perineal branch of the pudendal nerve, it pulls back and stabilizes the perineal body. Also *deep transverse muscle of perineum.* **m. transversus perinei superficialis** [NA] A poorly developed and occasionally absent thin muscular slip that arises from the anteromedial part of the ischial tuberosity and is inserted into the perineal body. Supplied by the perineal branch of the pudendal nerve, it pulls back and stabilizes the perineal body. Also *superficial transverse muscle of perineum.* **m. transversus thoracis** [NA] A muscle that arises from the lower part of the posterior surface of the body of the sternum and the posterior surface of the xiphoid process. It is inserted onto the posterior surface of the cartilages of the second to sixth ribs. Supplied by the second to sixth intercostal nerves, it pulls down the costal cartilages, especially in expiration. Also *transverse muscle of thorax, sternocostalis.* **m. trapezius** [NA] A muscle that arises from the medial part of the superior nuchal line of the occipital bone, the external occipital protuberance, the ligamentum nuchae, and the spines of the seventh cervical and all thoracic vertebrae and their supraspinous ligaments. It is inserted onto the posterosuperior aspect of the lateral third of the clavicle, the medial margin of the acromion, the upper margin of the spine of the scapula, and the tubercle at the medial end of the spine of the scapula. It is supplied by the accessory nerve and the ventral rami of the third and fourth cervical nerves. It elevates the scapula and point of the shoulder, helps to rotate the scapula forward and the glenoid cavity upward, retracts the scapula, extends the head and bends it to the same side when the shoulder is fixed, and helps to control the scapula in movements of the upper limb. Also *trapezius muscle.* **m. triceps brachii** [NA] A muscle of the arm. Its caput longum arises from the infraglenoid tubercle of the scapula; its caput laterale arises from the upper lateral part of the posterior surface of the humerus, the lateral margin of the humerus, and the lateral intermuscular septum; and its caput mediale arises from the posterior surface of the humerus below the radial groove and the medial and lateral intermuscular septa. It is inserted onto the upper surface of the olecranon, and the antebrachial fascia posterolaterally. Supplied by the radial nerve, it extends the forearm. Its caput longum helps to extend and adduct the arm. Also *triceps muscle of arm.* **m. triceps surae** [NA] The gastrocnemius and soleus muscles considered as one muscle mass, inserting by the tendo calcaneus into the middle of the posterior surface of the calcaneus. Also *triceps muscle of calf, triceps surae.* **m. unipennatus** [NA] A muscle in which the fibers attach obliquely to the long axis of the muscle along one side of the tendon, as in the flexor pollicis longus. Also *unipennate muscle.* **m. uvulae** [NA] A muscle that arises from the posterior nasal spine of the palatine bone and the palatine aponeurosis of the soft palate. It is inserted into the mucous membrane of the uvula and is supplied by the pharyngeal plexus. It raises and contracts the uvula. Also *muscle of uvula.* **m. vastus intermedius** [NA] A muscle that arises from the upper two thirds of the anterior and lateral surfaces of the shaft of the femur and the lateral intermuscular septum. It is inserted onto the tendon of the quadriceps femoris muscle, the upper and lateral margins of the patella, and the tuberosity of the tibia by the ligamentum patellae. Supplied by the femoral nerve, it extends the leg. Also *crureus.* **m. vastus lateralis** [NA] A muscle that arises from the upper part of the intertrochanteric line of the femur, the anteroinferior margin of the greater trochanter, the gluteal tuberosity, the upper part of the lateral lip of the linea aspera, and the lateral intermuscular septum. It is inserted onto the tendon of the quadriceps femoris muscle, the upper and lateral margins of the patella, the tibial tuberosity by the ligamentum patellae, and the lateral condyle of the tibia by an expansion. Supplied by the femoral nerve, it extends the leg and helps to stabilize the knee joint. **m. vastus medialis** [NA] A muscle that arises from the lower part of the intertrochanteric line, the spiral line, the medial lip of the linea aspera, the upper part of the medial supracondylar line, and the medial intermuscular septum. It is inserted onto the tendon of the quadriceps femoris muscle, the upper and medial margins of the patella, the tibial tuberosity by the ligamentum patellae, and the medial condyle of the tibia by an expansion. Supplied by the femoral nerve, it extends the leg and stabilizes the patella on the patellar surface of the femur during extension of the knee joint. **m. verticalis linguae** [NA] A group of muscle fibers that extends vertically from the aponeurosis of the dorsum to the inferior surface of the front part of the tongue and decussates with the transverse muscle fibers. Supplied by the hypoglossal nerve, it flattens and widens the tongue. Also *vertical muscle of tongue.* **m. vocalis** [NA] The upper and deeper fibers of the thyroarytenoid muscle that lie parallel and lateral to the vocal ligament and extend from the angle of the thyroid cartilage to the vocal process and oblong fovea of the arytenoid cartilage. Many fibers are attached to the vocal ligament. Supplied by the recurrent laryngeal nerve, it draws forward the arytenoid cartilage and relaxes the ligament, as well as helping to control the tension of the vocal ligament. Also *vocal muscle.* **m. zygomaticus major** [NA] A muscle that arises from the lateral surface of the zygomatic bone behind the inferolateral margin of the orbit. It is inserted into the muscles, skin, and mucosa at the angle of the mouth. Supplied by the buccal branches of the facial nerves, it pulls the angle of the mouth upward and laterally. Also *greater zygomatic muscle*. **m. zygomaticus minor** A muscle that arises from the lateral surface of the zygomatic bone just behind the zygomaticomaxillary suture. It is inserted into the skin and muscle of the upper lip medial to the angle of the mouth. Supplied by the buccal branches of the facial nerve, it raises the outer part of the upper lip and accentuates the nasolabial furrow. Also *lesser zygomatic muscle*.

**musicogenic** \myoo′zikōjen′ik\ Caused or triggered by music, as *musicogenic epilepsy*.

**musicolepsy** \myooz′ikōlep′sē\ MUSICOGENIC EPILEPSY.

**Musset** [Alfred de *Musset*, French poet, 1810–1857] Musset sign. See under DE MUSSET SIGN.

**mussitation** \mus′itā′shən\ [L *mussitatio* (from *mussitare* to mutter, murmur) muttering, subdued noise] Movement of the lips as in speaking, but without the production of sounds, as seen in some patients with various types of severe brain disease.

**mustard** [Old French *moustarde* (from *moust* must, from L *mustum* new wine, from L *mustum*, neut. sing of *mustus* juicy, wet, new) mustard] A plant of the genus *Brassica*, which includes asparagus, broccoli, Brussels sprouts, cabbage, cauliflower, kale, kohlrabi, and mustard. The crushed seeds of many species are used as a pungent condiment, rubefacient, and counterirritant. Volatile mustard oil, from the dried ripe seeds of *B. nigra*, black mustard, is a strong irritant that can blister the skin. Expressed mustard oil is obtained by pressure from the seeds of *B. nigra* as a by-product in the manufacture of volatile mustard oil.

**mutafacient** \myoo′təfā′shənt\ *Outmoded* MUTAGENIC.

**mutagen** \myoo′təjən\ [*muta(tion)* + -GEN] Any physical or chemical agent that acts on chromosomes to alter their genetic information.

**mutagenesis** \myoo′təjen′əsis\ The process by which a change in genetic information either occurs in nature or is induced experimentally. **directed m.** In experimental genetics, the creation of genetic change at a specific nucleotide sequence by means of recombinant DNA techniques. **insertional m.** The creation of genetic change and, as a result, altered expression of a host cell's genome, by insertion of a foreign segment of DNA.

**mutagenic** \myoo′təjen′ik\ Of or relating to a mutagen. Also *mutafacient* (outmoded).

**mutagenicity** \myoo′təjənis′itē\ The effectiveness of an agent in inducing mutation, usually relative to other agents.

**mutagenize** \myootaj′ənīz\ To experimentally treat an organism or colony with a mutagen.

**mutant** \myoo′tənt\ [L *mutans*, gen. *mutantis*, pres. part. of *mutare* to move, shift, change] **1** In classical genetics, an organism that carries an alteration in its genotype capable of exerting a detectable effect on its phenotype. **2** In molecular genetics, an organism or cell with an alteration in its genotype that is detectable by analysis of protein or nucleic acid sequence, but that may not grossly alter the phenotype. **3** Designating an organism or the part of the genome (chromosome, locus, gene) so altered. **amber m.** See under AMBER CODON. **auxotrophic m.** A mutant with an additional growth requirement, resulting from loss of a biosynthetic enzyme. Such mutants are conveniently selected by exposure of growing bacteria, in minimal medium, to an agent (e.g., penicillin) that kills only growing cells. They have been useful in analyzing biosynthetic pathways and as markers in genetic studies. **cryptic m.** An organism or cell line that contains a nucleotide alteration from the wild type in one or more of its chromosomes not expressed in the phenotype. **leaky m.** An incompletely blocked auxotrophic mutation, whose growth is stimulated by but does not require a particular nutrient. **polarity m.** POLAR MUTATION. **R m.** ROUGH MUTANT. **rough m.** A mutant that forms a rough colony, because it no longer makes a surface constituent, such as lipopolysaccharide side chains in Gram-negative bacteria or certain lipids in mycobacteria, required for forming a smooth colony. Also *R mutant*. **temperature-sensitive m.** A mutant strain of bacteria or viruses unable to grow at certain temperatures that permit growth of the parent. The term is usually applied to strains that can grow at 34°C or less but not at 37°C, those exhibiting the reverse effect being designated "cold-sensitive." Also *ts mutant*.

**mutase** \myoo′tās\ Any enzyme that catalyzes an isomerization involving the transfer of a group from one part of a molecule to another.

**mutation** \myootā′shən\ [L *mutatio* (from *mutare* to change) a change, alteration] **1** In classical genetics, any change within a genotype that can be detected by its effect on the phenotype. **2** Any change in the nucleotide sequence of the DNA in a chromosome, which may or may not affect the phenotype. **3** A change in chromosomes that is recognized as morphologically abnormal. **amber m.** A nonsense mutation which results in production of an amber codon (UAG) in the reading frame of messenger RNA, causing premature termination of transcription. In prokaryotes this process is suppressible by amber suppressors. **back m.** Any change in nucleotide sequence of the DNA of a chromosome that results in re-establishing a function of a phenotype that had been lost through a forward mutation. A true back mutation exactly reverses the original mutation. Compare FORWARD MUTATION. See also REVERSION. **cold sensitive m.** A genetic mutation that expresses a wild-type phenotype on the culture or growth of the cells or organism at a permissive temperature and a mutant phenotype at a lower, restrictive, temperature. **conditional lethal m.** Any mutation which is lethal under only certain environmental or genetic conditions. **constitutive m.** Any change in the genome resulting in the loss of metabolic regulation of a gene product, such as a mutation that results in the synthesis of constant amounts of an enzyme which is, in the wild type, inducible. **forward m.** Any mutation that is subsequently completely or partially corrected at the level of the phenotype by another mutation. Compare BACK MUTATION. **frame-shift m.** An insertion or deletion of nucleotides that results in an alteration in the sequence in which nucleotides are grouped, or read, as codons (the reading frame). The sequence distal to the mutation contains missense, nonsense, and sense codons. The resulting polypeptide chain will therefore have an altered amino acid sequence and be either too short or too long. **genomic m.** An alteration in the number of complete chromosomes in a genome, giving rise to aneuploidy or polyploidy. **heat sensitive m.** Any change in the genome that causes no change in wild-type phenotype at one range of temperatures, known as the permissive temperatures, but results in an altered phenotype at a higher temperature, the restrictive temperature. **homeotic m.** A genetic change recognized by the appearance of homeosis. Identification of the mutation suggests that the nucleotide sequence involved is part of a gene that participates in development. **induced m.** A mutation caused by an external mutagen. It often occurs by design in experimental genetics. Compare NATURAL MUTATION. **lethal m.** Any alteration in the genotype, such as a point mutation or a chromosome aberration, that prevents reproduction of the affected organism. For example, the organism may die before reproducing, never become sexually mature, or be infertile. **missense m.** A change in DNA nucleotide sequence that alters one or more codons such that different amino acids are inserted in a polypeptide. • The term was coined on the analogy of *nonsense mutation* (with *mis-* as in *miscode*). **natural m.** A change in DNA nucleotide sequence that occurs spontaneously (as through a mistake by a polymerase, or because of ultraviolet light). Also *spontaneous mutation*. Compare INDUCED MUTATION. **neutral m.** A mutation that has no effect on the adaptability of the organism and does not alter selection. **nonsense m.** A mutation that alters the sequence of a codon such that no amino acid is encoded; the polypeptide chain therefore prematurely terminates. The three nonsense codons in mRNA are UAG (amber codon), UAA (ochre codon), and UGA (umber codon). **ochre m.** A nonsense mutation which results in production of an ochre codon (UAA) in the reading frame of messenger RNA, causing premature termination of transcription. **opal m.** UMBER MUTATION. **point m.** 1 A change in a single nucleotide in the DNA of the genome. 2 In classical genetics, a small alteration in the genome, recognized phenotypically but not cytogenetically, which is capable of recombining with many other small mutations in the same region of the genome. **polar m.** Any mutation that affects the expression of genes distal to the altered nucleotide sequence. Also *polarity mutant*. **silent m.** 1 A mutation that has no effect on phenotype. 2 A mutation that has no effect on the amino acid sequence of the gene product because of redundancy of the genetic code. **somatic m.** Any change in the genome of a nongerm line cell. If the mutation is perpetuated in a clone of cells, the organism becomes a mosaic with respect to the altered locus, loci, or chromosome. Somatic mutations can be transmitted to progeny if the change occurs early enough in embryogenesis and occurs in a cell destined to be a progenitor of the gonads, in which case germinal mosaicism occurs. **spontaneous m.** NATURAL MUTATION. **suppressor m.** A change in the genome that reverses or mitigates the phenotype produced by a mutation at another gene (intergenic suppressor mutation) or within the same gene (intragenic or intracistronic suppressor mutation). The suppressor mutation thus serves phenotypically as a back mutation. Examples are a frameshift mutation that re-establishes the correct reading frame distal to a primary frameshift mutation, and a mutation that generates a suppressor tRNA that misreads the primary mutation. **temperature sensitive m.** Any change in the genome that is expressed as an altered phenotype only at certain temperatures. Also *TS mutation*. **umber m.** A nonsense mutation which results in production of an umber codon (UGA) in the reading frame of messenger RNA, causing premature termination of transcription. Also *opal mutation*.

**mutational** \myootā′shənəl\ Pertaining to or characterized by a mutation.

**mute** [Old French *muet* (from *mu*, from L *mutus* speechless, inarticulate) dumb, mute] 1 Unable to speak. Also *dumb*. 2 One who cannot talk. The cause may be deafness or severe, primary expressive disorder or it may be a deliberate cessation as the result of psychogenic disorder. **deaf m.** One who has such a severe degree of hearing impairment that he is unable to hear the sounds of speech and therefore cannot learn to talk normally, without special help. The deafness is usually congenital or arises in early childhood before the full development of speech and language has taken place. Also *deaf-mute*.

**mutilate** \myoo′tilāt\ [L *mutilare* (from *mutilus* lacking a part, truncated) to truncate, mutilate] 1 In criminal law, to subject to any injury that totally destroys or removes an organ, limb, or other essential body part, thus rendering less capable of fighting. 2 To subject to such extreme injury as to render grotesque or, in death, often unidentifiable.

**mutism** \myoo′tizm\ [*mut(e)* + -ISM] The state of being mute. **akinetic m.** A state of severely disordered consciousness, usually due to a midbrain lesion, in which the subject is mute and immobile although the eyes are open and may move randomly. Also *Cairns stupor*. **deaf m.** The condition of being a deaf mute. Also *deaf-mutism*. **elective m.** Self-imposed silence by a child in all his interpersonal contacts except for a few close friends and family members. At times it may constitute a symptom of a school phobia and be related to actual or threatened separation from the family.

**muton** \myoo′tän\ The smallest unit of deoxyribonucleic acid which is capable of undergoing a mutation.

**MV** Symbol for the unit, megavolt.

**Mv** Symbol for the element, mendelevium.

**MVV** maximum voluntary ventilation.

**MW** molecular weight.

**My.** myopia.

**my-** \mī-\ MYO-.

**myalgia** \mī·al′jə\ [MY- + -ALGIA] Pain in the muscles. Also *myosalgia*. Adj. myalgic. **m. capitis** Pain in the muscles attached to the scalp. **epidemic m.** EPIDEMIC PLEURODYNIA. **spastic m.** Pain in muscles affected by spasticity.

**myasis** \mī·əsis\ MYIASIS.

**myasthenia** \mī′asthē′nē·ə\ [MY- + ASTHENIA] Abnormal muscle fatigue; reduction of muscle power. Also *amyosthenia, muscle asthenia, myoasthenia*. Adj. myasthenic. **angiosclerotic paroxysmal m.** INTERMITTENT CLAUDICATION. **carcinomatous m.** LAMBERT-EATON SYNDROME. **m. gravis** A neuromuscular disorder of autoimmune origin in which weakness occurs in certain muscle groups or, less often, throughout the skeletal musculature and is greatly increased by exertion or repeated contraction of the affected muscles. In some cases the disease is limited to the external ocular muscles, resulting in ptosis, diplopia, and variable strabismus, but more often the weakness is evident in the muscles of swallowing and chewing and to a variable extent in those of the limbs and trunk. In some patients there is thymic enlargement or even a thymoma, and there is an association with hyperthyroidism and to a lesser extent with other autoimmune disorders. Myasthenic crises may occur and may be fatal if untreated, due to respiratory paralysis. There is evidence of a defect of neuromuscular transmission due to the formation of autoantibodies against the acetylcholine receptors on the surface of the muscle fibers. Diagnosis is made by noting the improvement in muscle power produced by intravenous edrophonium. Spontaneous remissions may occur. Treatment with pyridostigmine, with thymectomy, or with steroids is effective, depending upon the circumstances of the individual case. Also *Erb-Goldflam syndrome, bulbospinal paralysis, myasthenia gravis pseudoparalytica, Hoppe-Goldflam syndrome, Erb syndrome, Erb-Oppenheim-Goldflam syndrome, Erb-Goldflam disease, Wilks symptom complex, Wilks syndrome, Goldflam's disease, Goldflam-Erb disease, asthenobulbospinal paralysis* (incorrect), *asthenic bulbar paralysis* (incorrect), *bulbospinal asthenia* (incorrect). **m. gravis pseudoparalytica** MYASTHENIA GRAVIS. **m. laryngis** Weakness of the muscles of phonation, particularly the thyroarytenoid and interarytenoid muscles. It occurs chiefly as the result of excessive use of the voice as is seen in professional singers, actors, etc. The condition often occurs as a complication in other laryngeal disorders. It manifests itself in weak and unreliable vocalization. Also *phonasthenia.* **neonatal m.** Myasthenia gravis in the newborn infant of a myasthenic mother.

**myasthenic** \mī′asthen′ik\ Pertaining to or suffering from myasthenia. Also *amyosthenic.*

**myatonia** \mī′ətō′nē·ə\ [MY- + ATONIA] Reduction in or absence of muscle tone. Also *muscle atony, amyotonia, myatony.* Adj. myatonic. **m. congenita** A syndrome of severe congenital hypotonia of the skeletal musculature. Also *Oppenheim's disease, amyotonia congenita, Oppenheim's amyotonia, congenital atonic pseudoparalysis, Oppenheim syndrome.* • The condition was once thought to represent a disorder in which the infantile hypotonia was benign and was generally followed by improvement or even recovery, but subsequently it became apparent that most such patients were suffering from acute infantile spinal muscular atrophy (Werdnig-Hoffmann disease). Hence the term is now obsolete in this sense, though there are many other disease processes which cause infantile hypotonia, some of which are benign, and these may still sometimes be described as *myatonia congenita* or *myatonia congenita syndrome.* **periodic m.** *Outmoded* PERIODIC PARALYSIS.

**myatony** \mī·at′ənē\ MYATONIA.

**myatrophy** \mī·at′rəfē\ AMYOTROPHY.

**myautonomy** \mī′ôtän′əmē\ [MY- + AUTONOMY] A state of a muscle characterized by abnormally protracted delay in contraction following excitation.

**myc-** \mīs-, mis-, mīk-\ MYCO-.

**mycelium** \mīsē′lyəm\ [MYC- + Gk *hēl(os)* nail, wart, callus, corn + New L noun suffix *-ium*] (*pl.* mycelia) The mass of hyphae that constitutes the body of a fungus. Adj. mycelial.

**-myces** \-mī′sēz\ [Gk *mykēs* a mushroom, fungus] A combining form meaning fungus or funguslike.

**mycet-** \mīsēt′-\ MYCO-.

**-mycetes** \-mīsē′tēz\ [Gk *mykētes,* pl. of *mykēs* mushroom, fungus] A combining form designating fungal classes.

**mycethemia** \mī′səthē′mē·ə\ [MYCET- + -HEMIA] The presence of fungi in blood. Also *mycohemia, fungemia.*

**mycetism** \mī′sətizm\ [MYCET- + -ISM] *Older term* MUSHROOM POISONING.

**mycetismus** \mī′sətiz′məs\ [New L (MYCET- + New L *-ismus* -ISM)] *Older term* MUSHROOM POISONING. **m. cerebris** Mushroom intoxication characterized by hallucinations. Mushrooms in the genera *Psilocybe, Paneolus,* and *Conocybe* are known to be hallucinogenic. **m. choleriformis** A form of mushroom poisoning following the ingestion of *Amanita phalloides, A. verna, A. virosa,* or *A. bisporagera,* or several species of *Galerina.* The chief toxicologic effect is severe gastroenteritis, as evidenced by bloody diarrhea and persistent vomiting which may be so severe as to result in shock, coma, and death. The onset of symptoms is usually delayed for several hours. **m. gastrointestinalis** A mild form of poisoning marked by nausea, vomiting, and diarrhea, due to the ingestion of certain species of mushroom such as *Clitocybe illudens..* **m. nervosus** Poisoning caused by the ingestion of any of several species of *Amanita,* especially *A. muscaria,* a mushroom containing muscarine. The signs are characteristic of stimulation of the parasympathetic nervous system and include salivation, lacrimation, miosis, nausea, vomiting, defecation, and bradycardia, terminating in convulsions. The effects can be completely reversed by atropine. **m. sanguinarius** Poisoning resulting from the ingestion of mushrooms of the *Gyromitra* species, especially *Gyromitra esculenta.* The toxin, gyromitrin (monomethyl hydrazine), may cause symptoms of nausea, vomiting, diarrhea, cramps, weakness, headaches, and develop to convulsions, coma, and even death.

**myceto-** \mī′sətō-, mīsē′tō-\ MYCO-.

**mycetogenic** \mī′sətōjen′ik\ [MYCETO- + -GENIC] Produced or brought about by a fungus or fungi, as a disease. Also *mycetogenous.*

**mycetoid** \mī′sətoid\ [MYCET- + -OID] FUNGOID.

**mycetoma** \mī′sətō′mə\ [*mycet(o)-* + -OMA] **1** A chronic infection of the subcutaneous and deeper tissues caused by any of various fungi (*Eumycetes*) such as *Madurella* or by actinomycetes such as *Nocardia* and *Streptomyces.* It is characterized by local swelling, necrosis, sinus formation, and suppuration. Infection is usually by puncture of the skin by infected thorns. Mycetoma occurs worldwide but is seen most often in tropical and subtropical areas of northwest and central Africa, Asia, and Central and South America. Mycetoma of the foot (the most common site) is called Madura foot or foot fungus. Historically, some types of mycetoma were named according to the color of the granules in the pus. Staining affinities are of value in differentiation. Also *maduromycosis, Madura boil, Ballingall's disease.* **2** A nodule or non-neoplastic tumor made up largely of mycelial elements, such as an aspergilloma. **Carter's black m.** A mycetoma containing black granules, caused by *Madurella mycetomatis,* and found in tropical Africa, India, southeast Asia, and parts of North and South America.

**mycid** \mī′sid\ [MYC- + -ID[2]] *Obs.* DERMATOPHYTID.

**-mycin** \-mī′sin\ [MYC- + -IN] A combining form meaning something derived from a fungus.

**myco-** \mī′kō-\ [Gk *mykēs* (genitive *mykētos*) fungus, mushroom] A combining form meaning fungus or funguslike. Also *myc-, mycet-, myceto-, myko-.*

**mycobacidin** ACTITHIAZIC ACID.

**mycobacteria** \-baktir′ē·ə\ Plural of MYCOBACTERIUM.

**mycobacteriosis** \-baktir′ē·ō′sis\ Any infection caused by mycobacteria.

***Mycobacterium*** \-baktir′ē·əm\ [MYCO- + BACTERIUM] A genus of bacteria of the family Mycobacteriaceae, order Actinomycetales. The cardinal characteristic is acid-fast staining, due to the large amount of lipid in the outer layer of the wall. Corynebacteria and nocardiae share some of the same special lipids, such as mycolic acids. Growth is slow. They are obligate aerobes, and are straight or curved, slender rods, occasionally mycelial. ***M. avium*** A bacillus that produces tuberculosis in birds and pigs and occasionally in humans. It forms smooth colonies and has a higher temperature optimum (41°C) than *M. tuberculosis.* It closely resembles *M. intracellulare* immunologically. Also *Mycobacterium tuberculosis avium.* ***M. bovis*** A species that is the cause of bovine tuberculosis and of milk-borne tuberculosis in humans. More microaerophilic than *M. tuberculosis,* it differs slightly immunologically, and is more pathogenic in rabbits. Also *Mycobacterium tuberculosis bovis.* ***M. fortuitum*** A relatively fast-growing mycobacterium that is abundant in soil and occasionally causes abscesses in humans. It includes the former species *M. ranae.* No pigment has been found in this species. ***M. intracellulare*** A species closely related immunologically to *Mycobacterium avium* but less pathogenic for birds and having a lower temperature optimum. It is considered by some to be an intermediate form of *M. avium.* It has been isolated from human lesions, but is also found in the soil. Also *Battey bacillus.* ***M. kansasii*** A photochromogen that is a common cause of human mycobacterial disease other than that due to *M. tuberculosis.* ***M. leprae*** The species that causes human leprosy. Though found in great numbers in lesions and morphologically almost indistinguishable from *M. tuberculosis,* it has not been cultivated and experimental transmission to man has been unsuccessful. It can be propagated in the foot pads of mice and in the nine-banded armadillo. Generation time is 12 to 13 days. ***M. marinum*** A photochromogen that causes disease in fish and chronic human skin lesions which are acquired through abrasions in a marine environment. The optimum growth temperature is 33°C. ***M. microti*** A mycobacterium that causes natural tuberculosis in voles. It is similar immunologically to *M. tuberculosis* and *M. bovis.* ***M. paratuberculosis*** An obligate parasite that causes a chronic enteritis (paratuberculosis) in cattle and sheep. The tuberculin, johnin, cross-reacts with that of *M. tuberculosis.* It requires mycobactin for growth in artificial culture. Also *Johne's bacillus.* ***M. scrofulaceum*** A scotochromogenic species that is a common cause of lymphadenitis in children. It has some antigens in common with *M. avium* and *M. intracellulare.* ***M. tuberculosis*** A very slow-growing mycobacterium species (generation time at least 12 hours) that causes granulomatous lesions in man; the tubercle bacillus. There is no reservoir in nature. Cells are hydrophobic and disperse poorly in liquid media. They form rough colonies, virulent strains aggregating more than avirulent strains and growing as serpentine cords. Growth requirements are simple. A heat-stable protein (tuberculin) from culture filtrates is used in a delayed reaction skin test. Also *Mycobacterium tuberculosis hominis.* ***M. tuberculosis avium*** *MYCOBACTERIUM AVIUM.* ***M. tuberculosis bovis*** *MYCOBACTERIUM BOVIS.* ***M. tuberculosis hominis*** *MYCOBACTERIUM TUBERCULOSIS.* ***M. ulcerans*** A mycobacterium that causes cutaneous ulcers in humans. It grows only below 33°C. ***M. xenopi*** A thermophilic scotochromogen, first isolated from a toad and then also from water storage tanks and from chronic human pulmonary lesions.

**mycobacterium** [MYCO- + BACTERIUM] (*pl.* mycobacteria) Any of a group of bacteria characterized by a hydrophobic waxy coat that results in acid-fast staining. **atypical mycobacteria** A wide variety of mycobacteria, with reservoirs in soil and water or in lower animals, that may cause disease in humans, usually less severe than classical tuberculosis. The importance of these agents has been recognized increasingly as infection with *Mycobacterium tuberculosis* and *M. bovis* has waned. Also *anonymous mycobacteria* (outmoded).

**mycobactin** \-bak′tin\ A siderophore containing hydroxamic acid, formed by most mycobacteria and required for growth by *Mycobacterium paratuberculosis.*

**mycocide** \mī′kəsīd\ *Seldom used* FUNGICIDE.

**mycohemia** \-hē′mē·ə\ MYCETHEMIA.

**mycoid** \mī′koid\ [MYC- + -OID] FUNGOID.

**mycologist** \mīkäl′əjist\ A specialist in mycology.

**mycology** \mīkäl′əjē\ [MYCO- + -LOGY] The science or study of fungi. Adj. mycologic.

**mycopathogen** \-path′əjən\ [MYCO- + PATHOGEN] Any fungus that causes disease.

**mycopathology** \-pəthäl′əjē\ The study of fungal diseases.

**mycophage** \mī′kəfāj\ [MYCO- + PHAGE] Any phage which causes lysis of fungi.

**mycophenolic acid** $C_{17}H_{20}O_6$. A bacteriostatic and fungostatic antibiotic derived from cultures of *Penicillium brevi-compactum* and related species.

***Mycoplasma*** \-plaz′mə\ A major genus in the group of mycoplasma. Unlike *Acholeplasma,* it requires a sterol for growth. ***M. hominis*** A commensal species of mycoplasma found occasionally in the mouth and frequently in the genital tract. It may be responsible for some cases of salpingitis. ***M. hyorhinis*** A species of mycoplasma that often contaminates tissue cultures. It may grow on artificial media and is usually identified by immunofluorescence. ***M. mycoides*** The organism that causes contagious bovine pleuropneumonia. This was the first of the mycoplasmas to be recognized. ***M. orale*** An anaerobic mycoplasma widely present as a commensal in the human mouth. ***M. pneumoniae*** The agent of mycoplasmal pneumonia (primary atypical pneumonia), long thought to be a virus because it is filterable.

**mycoplasma** [MYCO- + PLASMA] Any of the bacteria of the class Mollicutes, which lack a rigid cell wall. This feature and their small size permit them to pass through 450 nm filters. They slowly form very small colonies, which tend to burrow into the agar. They are found widely in nature and also cause human mycoplasmal pneumonia and a wide variety of serious diseases in animals. Some mycoplasmas have a specialized terminal structure that plays a role in attachment and in gliding motility. Also *pleuropneumonialike organism* (outmoded). **T m.** A group of mycoplasmas that cause nonspecific urethritis.

**mycoses** \mīkō′sēz\ Plural of MYCOSIS.

**mycosis** \mīkō′sis\ [MYC- + -OSIS] (*pl.* mycoses) Any disease brought on by a fungus. Adj. mycotic. **cutaneous m.** TINEA. **m. fungoides** A malignant neoplasm of lymphoid cells that arises in the upper dermis. The cells spread to the epidermis as aggregates. Lymph nodes and viscera may subsequently be involved. **m. fungoides en plaques** A skin condition that is characterized by the appearance of erythematous pruritic plaques on the skin. Histologically, a lymphoid infiltrate in the epidermis develops into small dermal papillae. It may present with large fungating tumors, but it is more often preceded, sometimes by several years, by plaques of erythema and fine scaling which later show poikilodermatous atrophy. This precedes the onset of mycosis fungoides. Despite its name, the condition is not fungal. **Gilchrist's m.** BLASTOMYCOSIS.

**mycostat** \mī′kəstat\ FUNGISTAT.

**mycotic** \mīkät′ik\ Pertaining to mycosis.

**mycotoxicology** \-täk′sikäl′əjē\ [MYCO- + TOXICOLOGY] The study of the actions, detection, and treatment of fungal poisons.

**mycotoxicosis** \-täk′sikō′sis\ [MYCO- + TOXICOSIS] Poisoning caused by the ingestion of any fungal toxin such as, for example, aflatoxin.

**mycotoxin** \-täk′sin\ A toxin produced by a fungus under special conditions of moisture and temperature.

**mydesis** *Obs.* PUTREFACTION.

**Mydriacyl** A proprietary name for tropicamide

**mydriasis** \midrī′əsis\ [Gk, dilatation of the pupil] Enlargement of pupil size. Adj. mydriatic. **alternating m.** Dilatation of first one pupil, then the other. Also *springing mydriasis, bounding mydriasis.* **paralytic m.** Dilatation of the pupil because of paralysis of the iris sphincter muscle. **spastic m.** Dilatation of the pupil due to excessive activity of the iris dilator muscle. Also *spasmodic mydriasis.* **springing m.** ALTERNATING MYDRIASIS.

**mydriatic** \mid′rē·at′ik\ **1** Pertaining to or causing mydriasis. **2** A sympathomimetic drug capable of dilating the pupil, but without cycloplegic effect.

**myectomy** \mī·ek′təmē\ [MY- + -ECTOMY] The surgical removal of part or all of a muscle or a group of muscles.

**myectopy** \mī·ek′təpē\ Displacement of a muscle from its usual position. Also *myectopia.*

**myel-** \mī′əl-, mī·el′-\ MYELO-.

**myelanalosis** \mīʹəlanʹəlōʹsis\ *Outmoded* TABES DORSALIS.

**myelencephalitis** \mīʹəlensefʹəlīʹtis\ ENCEPHALOMYELITIS.

**myelencephalon** \mīʹəlensefʹəlän\ [MYEL- + ENCEPHALON] **1** The posterior of the two brain vesicles formed in the developing embryo by the maturative division of the primitive hindbrain, or rhombencephalon. **2** [NA] The most posterior portion of the brainstem, including the medulla oblongata and the caudal half of the fourth vesicle. Also *marrowbrain* (older term).

**myelic** \mī·elʹik\ [MYEL- + -IC] Pertaining to or affecting the spinal cord.

**myelin** \mīʹəlin\ [German (from Gk *myelinos* marrowlike, from *myelos* marrow) medullary (substance), a soft, white substance] A substance formed from the compacted layers of cell membranes of either oligodendroglial or Schwann cells and which forms an insulating sheath around the axons of some nerve fibers.

**myelinated** \mīʹəlināʹtid\ Having a myelin sheath: said of a nerve fiber.

**myelination** \mīʹəlināʹshən\ [MYELIN + -ATION] The process by which the nerve fibers acquire myelin sheaths, which enhance the conduction of nerve impulses. For peripheral axons, myelinization is brought about by neurilemmal, or Schwann, cells and for central nervous system axons by oligodendrocytes. It commences during fetal life and in humans continues through the first two or three years after birth. Also *myelinization, myelogenesis, myelinogenesis.*

**myelinic** \mīʹəlinʹik\ Of or relating to myelin.

**myelinization** \mīʹəlinʹīzāʹshən\ MYELINATION.

**myelinogenesis** \mīʹəlinʹōjenʹəsis\ MYELINATION. **dystopic cortical m.** The appearance of the cerebral cortex in the Alpers syndrome. Also *driftwood cortex.*

**myelinogenetic** \mīʹəlinʹōjənetʹik\ Forming myelin by the process of myelinization.

**myelinogeny** \mīʹəlinäjʹənē\ MYELOGENY.

**myelinolysis** \mīʹəlinälʹisis\ DEMYELINATION. **central pontine m.** Massive demyelination of the central part of the pons, giving rise to progressive dysarthria and spastic quadriplegia. This disorder may complicate alcoholism, liver disease, or uremia. Also *pontine myelinosis.*

**myelinopathy** \mīʹəlinäpʹəthē\ [MYELIN + *o* + -PATHY ] Any disease or dysfunction of myelin.

**myelinosis** \mīʹəlinōʹsis\ Fat necrosis with formation of myelin. **pontine m.** CENTRAL PONTINE MYELINOLYSIS.

**myelitis** \mīʹəlīʹtis\ [MYEL- + -ITIS] **1** Inflammation of the spinal cord. • The term is also used in certain contexts to denote chronic and noninflammatory changes in the spinal cord. Also *medullitis, notomyelitis* (obs.). **2** An inflammatory condition of the bone marrow. Rarely used in this sense. Adj. myelitic. **acute syphilitic m.** Transverse myelitis occurring in meningovascular syphilis, partly as a result of inflammation but more often due to endarteritis and vascular occlusion, and giving rise to flaccid paraplegia, often of abrupt onset, and associated with a well-defined upper level of sensory loss on the trunk and with sphincter paralysis. **acute transverse m.** Acute inflammation of the spinal cord usually due to a postinfective demyelinating process and giving rise either to a clinical picture suggesting a transverse cord lesion or to acute ascending paralysis. **amyotrophic syphilitic m.** Syphilitic meningomyelitis giving rise to a clinical picture resembling that of amyotrophic lateral sclerosis. **angiohypertrophic spinal m.** SUBACUTE NECROTIC MYELITIS. **ascending m.** Myelitis which extends progressively upwards from the lower part of the spinal cord. There are many different causes of such a process, including multiple sclerosis, syphilis, and subacute necrotic myelitis. **cavitary m.** SYRINGOMYELIA. **cavitating m.** *Obs.* SYRINGOMYELIA. **central m.** Inflammation of the spinal cord restricted chiefly to the gray matter. *Seldom used.* **cervical m.** Myelitis restricted to the cervical region of the spinal cord. **compression m.** *Outmoded* COMPRESSION MYELOPATHY. **cornual m.** Myelitis principally involving the horns of gray matter. **descending m.** Myelitis which extends progressively downwards from the upper part of the spinal cord to the conus. *Seldom used.* **disseminated m.** Myelitis in which many discrete affected areas are found in different parts of the spinal cord. Multiple sclerosis is the commonest cause. Also *diffuse myelitis.* **focal m.** Myelitis localized to one part of the spinal cord. **metastatic m.** Myelitis caused by microorganisms derived from a distant site of infection. Also *intramedullary spinal abscess.* **neuro-optic m.** NEUROMYELITIS OPTICA. **parenchymatous m.** PARENCHYMATOUS MYELOPATHY. **postvaccinal m.** Myelitis of the postinfectious demyelinating type following smallpox vaccination. **pressure m.** COMPRESSION MYELOPATHY. **pseudotumoral m.** Myelitis in which there is severe edema of the inflamed segments of the spinal cord giving a myelographic appearance which simulates that of intramedullary tumor. **radiation m.** RADIATION MYELOPATHY. **subacute necrotic m.** Myelitis progressing gradually over the course of about two years, and resulting in paraplegia, sensory loss, and sphincter disturbance of increasing severity. Generally, there is a marked increase in the protein content of the cerebrospinal fluid. The condition may be associated with cor pulmonale or other chronic respiratory disease. In most cases occluded and distended veins are found over and within the cord at autopsy, and many authorities believe that the primary cause is a venous angioma. A different form of subacute necrotizing myelitis has been described as a remote manifestation of malignant disease. Also *Foix-Alajouanine disease, Foix-Alajouanine syndrome, angiodysgenetic myelomalacia, angiohypertrophic spinal myelitis, Spiller syndrome.* **transverse m.** Myelitis in which the inflammatory process principally involves one or more restricted spinal cord segments, showing the manifestations of a transverse cord lesion which usually develops acutely. Initially there is a flaccid paraplegia with sphincter paralysis and total loss of sensation below the level of the lesion, but as the acute spinal shock passes off the paraplegia later becomes spastic. Acute multiple sclerosis and postinfective myelitis are among the commonest causes of this syndrome, which must be distinguished from spinal cord infarction due to anterior spinal artery occlusion. In the latter, posterior column sensibility is usually comparatively spared. **traumatic m.** Myelitis following injury to the spinal cord, usually following fracture dislocation of the spine. Direct physical injury to the cord does not produce a myelitis. **tuberculous m.** Myelitis due to tuberculosis, usually developing as a complication of spinal tuberculous meningitis. Also *caseous osteitis.*

**myelo-** \mīʹəlō-\ [Gk *myelos* marrow, medulla] A combining form meaning (1) bone marrow; (2) the spinal cord; (3) myelin, myelin sheath. Also *myel-.*

**myeloarchitecture** \-ärʹkitekʹchər\ The organization of nerve fibers and fiber tracts in the cerebral hemispheres, brainstem, cerebellum, and spinal cord, as revealed by staining techniques selective for myelin sheaths.

**myeloblast** \mīʹəlōblastʹ\ [MYELO- + -BLAST] The earliest precursor of granulocytes. The cell is usually 15–20 μm diameter, with a nucleus that has fine, nonaggregated chromatin and 2–5 pale nucleoli, and with absence of granules in the cytoplasm. Myeloblasts normally comprise 1–3% of bone marrow cells. When present in blood they usually signify acute myelogenous leukemia. Also *microleukoblast, micromyelolymphocyte* (obs.), *type I myeloblast, premyeloblast.* **type I m.** MYELOBLAST. **type II m.** A cell that is intermediate in maturation between a typical myeloblast (type I myeloblast) without cytoplasmic granules and a typical progranulocyte with numerous prominent primary granules. The type II myeloblast has a small number of primary granules. Also *early progranulocyte.*

**myeloblastemia** \-blastē′mē·ə\ The presence of myeloblasts in blood, as in acute myelogenous leukemia. Also *myeloblastosis.*

**myeloblastic** \-blas′tik\ Having to do with, or characterized by an excessive number of myeloblasts.

**myeloblastosis** \-blastō′sis\ MYELOBLASTEMIA.

**myelocele** \mī′əlōsēl′\ [MYELO- + -CELE[1]] A neural tube defect in which the embryonic neural plate fails to close in some part of the spinal cord, with the result that the persisting neural plate is not subsequently covered by cutaneous and mesodermal structures. The unclosed neural tissue and the laterally continuous epidermis enclose a sac of cerebrospinal fluid that protrudes on the back as fluid pressure rises.

**myeloclast** \mī′əlōklast′\ [MYELO- + -CLAST] A cell which lyses or degrades the coverings of medullated nerve fibers.

**myelocoele** \mī′əlōsēl′\ [MYELO- + -COELE] The central canal of the spinal cord, especially in the embryo.

**myelocyst** \mī′əlōsist′\ A malformation of the spinal cord characterized by dilatation of the central canal which is lined by ependymal cells. It is caused by defective lamination of the posterior vertebral arches. Adj. myelocystic.

**myelocystocele** \-sis′təsēl\ [MYELO- + CYSTO- + -CELE[1]] A myelocele which becomes a prominent cystlike protrusion on the back.

**myelocystography** \-sistäg′rəfē\ [MYELO- + CYSTO- + -GRAPHY] The examination to demonstrate an intramedullary spinal cord cyst, either by roentgenography after percutaneous injection of air or contrast material into the cyst, or by scanning after injection of a radionuclide into the cyst.

**myelocystomeningocele** \-sis′təməning′gōsēl\ A myelocystocele in which meninges are thought to be or are demonstrated to be present in association with the protruding neural plate. If the sac of neural tissue and modified skin remain intact, meninges only line the underlying fluid-filled cyst.

**myelocyte** \mī′əlōsīt′\ [MYELO- + -CYTE] A polymorphonuclear leukocyte at the earliest recognizable stage of differentiation, with a nucleus that exhibits chromatin condensation, that contains no recognizable nucleoli, and is round, oval or slightly indented, and a cytoplasm that contains secondary (specific) granules which permit the myelocyte to be identified as belonging to the neutrophilic, eosinophilic, or basophilic series.

**myelocytosis** \-sītō′sis\ The presence in blood of a much greater than normal number of myelocytes. Also *myelocythemia.*

**myelodiastasis** \-dī·as′təsis\ [MYELO- + DIASTASIS] Necrosis of the spinal cord. Also *myelodiastema.*

**myelodysplasia** \-displā′zhə\ [MYELO- + DYSPLASIA] **1** Any developmental defect of the spinal cord. **2** Abnormal formation of blood cell precursors in bone marrow. Adj. myelodysplastic.

**myeloencephalic** \-en′səfal′ik\ Denoting the spinal cord and brain.

**myeloencephalitis** \-ensef′əlī′tis\ ENCEPHALOMYELITIS. **epidemic m.** ACUTE ANTERIOR POLIOMYELITIS.

**myelofibrosis** \-fībrō′sis\ The presence of fibrous tissue in bone marrow, as may occur following radiotherapy to adjacent structures, in some cases of Hodgkin's disease, as a late stage of polycythemia vera, or in the absence of any known cause. Also *myelosclerosis* (ambiguous), *osteomyelofibrotic syndrome, osteomyelosclerosis.* See also AGNOGENIC MYELOID METAPLASIA. **acute m.** A malignant disorder characterized by rapidly progressing pancytopenia and fibrosis of the bone marrow. The disorder appears to be the result of a malignant transformation of megakaryocytes analogous to an acute leukemia. **osteosclerosis m.** An obliteration of the bone marrow by new bone formation, seen in some advanced myeloproliferative syndromes. Also *centro-osteosclerosis, centrosclerosis.*

**myelogenesis** \-jen′əsis\ MYELINATION.

**myelogenous** \mī′əläj′ənəs\ [MYELO- + -GENOUS] Originating in bone marrow. Also *myelogenic.*

**myelogeny** \mī′əläj′ənē\ [MYELO- + -GEN + -Y] The development of myelin sheaths throughout the central nervous system to their final state. Also *myelinogeny.*

**myelogone** \mī′əlōgōn′\ HEMATOGONE.

**myelography** \mī′əläg′rəfē\ [MYELO- + -GRAPHY] Roentgenography of the spinal canal after injection of a contrast medium into the subarachnoid space, usually of the lumbar spine. Also *perimyelography.* **air m.** Myelography with the use of air as the contrast medium.

**myeloid** \mī′əloid\ [MYEL- + -OID] **1** Resembling or pertaining to the spinal cord. **2** Resembling or pertaining to the bone marrow. **3** Pertaining to granulocytes.

**myelokentric** \-ken′trik\ Stimulatory to the formation of leukocytes of the granulocytic series.

**myeloleukemia** \-lookē′mē·ə\ GRANULOCYTIC LEUKEMIA.

**myelolipoma** \-lipō′mə\ [MYELO- + LIPOMA] A benign tumor composed of hematopoietic and adipose tissues. It occurs in the adrenal gland and, less frequently, in the retroperitoneum and pelvis. It is not associated with hematopoietic abnormalities.

**myelolymphangioma** \-limfan′jē·ō′mə\ FILARIAL ELEPHANTIASIS.

**myelolysis** \mī′əläl′isis\ The degradation and dissolution of myelin.

**myeloma** \mī′əlō′mə\ [MYEL- + -OMA] A neoplastic proliferation of plasma cells, characterized by bone tumors and often complicated by pathologic fractures. Diffuse infiltration as well as tumors may also occur in the bone marrow and viscera. Uncommonly, solitary myeloma tumors of bone may show very slow progression and only become generalized after several years. The generalized disease is usually associated with IgA, or light-chain (Bence-Jones) monoclonal immunoglobulin production, and a monoclonal protein is detectable in the serum and/or urine by immunochemical techniques. Occasionally the anomalous immunoglobulin is IgD or very rarely IgE. Such protein abnormalities are not a feature of solitary myelomas. Also *multiple myeloma, myelomatosis, plasma cell myeloma, peripheral plasmacytoma, solitary plasmocytoma, plasmoma.* **endothelial m.** EWING SARCOMA. **extramedullary m.** An extraskeletal plasmacytoma. **multiple m.** MYELOMA. **plasma cell m.** MYELOMA.

**myelomalacia** \-məlā′shə\ Pathologic softening of the spinal cord, usually resulting from recent infarction. **angiodysgenetic m.** SUBACUTE NECROTIC MYELITIS.

**myelomatoid** \mī′əlō′mətoid\ [MYELOMA + *t* + -OID] Resembling myeloma.

**myelomatosis** \-mətō′sis\ [MYELOMA + *t* + -OSIS] MYELOMA.

**myelomenia** \-mē′nē·ə\ [MYELO- + *men(o)-* + -IA] Endometriosis involving the spinal cord.

**myelomeningocele** \-məning′gōsēl\ MENINGOMYELOCELE.

**myelomere** \mī′əlōmir′\ [MYELO- + -MERE] A segmental portion of the developing central nervous system.

**myelomonocyte** \-män′əsīt\ A leukocyte that appears to resemble both myelocytes and monocytes, in that nuclear chromatin is less condensed than in the myelocyte, and the cytoplasm has few neutrophilic granules. Enzyme cytochemistry may also identify the cell as being of either monocytic or neutrophilic lineage. Such cells represent aberrant maturation, as occurs in myelomonocytic leukemia.

**myeloneuritis** \-nʸUrī′tis\ [MYELO- + NEURITIS] Inflammation of the spinal cord and peripheral nerves.

**myelo-opticoneuropathy** \-äp′tikōnʸUräp′əthē\ [MYELO- + OPTICO- + NEUROPATHY] Any disease or dysfunction of the spinal cord and the optic and peripheral nerves. Also *myelopticoneuropathy.* **subacute m.** A syndrome characterized by a sensorimotor polyneuropathy involving the arms and legs and sometimes the oculomotor nerves, combined often with signs of optic atrophy and of corticospinal tract dysfunction, indicative of spinal cord involvement. It is the result of excessive and long-continued self-medication with clioquinol and its derivatives, taken for prophylaxis or treatment of intestinal affections, especially chronic diarrhea. Withdrawal of the causative drug is generally followed by recovery in one to two years, but occasional fatal cases have been described, and some patients have shown evidence of permanent neurologic sequelae. Abbr. SMON

**myelopathy** \mī′əläp′əthē\ [MYELO- + -PATHY] Any disease or dysfunction of the spinal cord. Adj. myelopathic. **arteriosclerotic m.** Ischemic myelopathy resulting from arteriosclerosis. **ascending m.** Any myelopathy in which symptoms and signs begin in the lower limbs and later spread upwards. **cervical m.** Compression myelopathy in the cervical region due to spondylosis or other causes. **compression m.** Any myelopathy resulting from compression of the spinal cord. Also *compression myelitis* (outmoded), *pressure myelitis.* **descending m.** Any myelopathy in which symptoms and signs begin in the upper limbs and later spread to the lower limbs. **diabetic m.** Damage to the spinal cord in diabetes mellitus, consisting of segmentally localized degeneration in the posterior columns and localized necrosis and degenerative changes in the lateral columns. This is a rare complication, possibly due to diabetic angiopathy of arterioles in the affected areas. **focal m.** The clinical syndrome produced by any focal lesion of the spinal cord. **ischemic m.** NEUMAYER'S AMYOTROPHIC LATERAL PSEUDOSCLEROSIS. **necrotic m.** SUBACUTE NECROTIC MYELOPATHY. **parenchymatous m.** Any myelopathy predominantly involving the neurons of the spinal cord. *Outmoded.* Also *parenchymatous myelitis.* **radiation m.** A progressive myelopathy which usually begins from six months to two years after inadvertent exposure to excessive doses of ionizing radiation incidental to radiotherapy for neoplastic lesions in the neck, thorax, or abdomen. Also *radiation myelitis.* **subacute necrotic m.** A progressive ascending myelopathy in which there is necrosis of the lower spinal cord segments with slow upward extension. It may occur in subjects with malignant disease outside the nervous system or in those with cor pulmonale in whom there is venous infarction of the spinal cord. Also *necrotic myelopathy.* **toxic m.** Myelopathy due to exogenous or endogenous toxins. **transverse m.** Any myelopathy producing a transverse lesion of the spinal cord. Transverse myelitis is one example.

**myeloperoxidase** \-pəräk′sidās\ A peroxidase obtained from human leukocytes. Also *verdoperoxidase.*

**myelopetal** \mī′əläp′ətəl\ Traveling towards the spinal cord, as a nerve impulse.

**myelophage** \mī′əlōfāj′\ A macrophage which phagocytoses myelin. Adj. myelophagous.

**myeloplasm** \mī′əlōplazm′\ [MYELO- + PLASM] Material of which the wall of the primitive neural tube in the embryo is composed. It is derived from neurectoderm and is similar to a primitive syncytium either lacking, or with very thin, plasma membranes.

**myelopoiesis** \-poi·ē′sis\ [MYELO- + -POIESIS] The formation, growth, and maturation of blood cells in the bone marrow. Adj. myelopoietic. **ectopic m.** Formation of granulocytes in a location other than bone marrow. Also *extramedullary myelopoiesis.*

**myeloproliferative** \-prəlif′ərətiv\ Characterized by an increased rate of formation of leukocytes of the granulocytic series. Any of several neoplastic conditions affecting principally granulocytes, megakaryocytes, and erythroblasts are myeloproliferative disorders, including chronic granulocytic leukemia, polycythemia vera, myelofibrosis, erythroleukemia, and essential thrombocythemia.

**myelopticoneuropathy** \mī′əläp′tikōnʸUräp′əthē\ MYELO-OPTICONEUROPATHY.

**myeloradiculitis** \-rədik′yəlī′tis\ Inflammation of the spinal cord and the spinal nerve roots.

**myeloradiculodysplasia** \-rədik′yəlōdisplā′zhə\ [MYELO- + RADICULO- + DYSPLASIA] Any developmental defect of the spinal cord and spinal nerve roots.

**myeloradiculopathy** \-rədik′yəläp′əthē\ Any disease affecting the spinal cord and spinal nerve roots.

**myeloradiculopolyneuronitis** \-rədik′yəlōpäl′ēnʸUr′-ōnī′tis\ [MYELO- + RADICULO- + POLYNEURONITIS] Inflammation of the spinal cord, spinal roots, and peripheral nerves.

**myelorrhagia** \mī′əlôrā′jə\ [MYELO- + -RRHAGIA] Hemorrhage into the spinal cord.

**myelosarcoma** \-särkō′mə\ *Seldom used* GRANULOCYTIC SARCOMA. **erythroblastic m.** A rare form of myeloid sarcoma containing a preponderant number of cells of the erythroid series. Also *erythrosarcoma.*

**myeloschisis** \mī′əläs′kisis\ [MYELO- + Gk *schisis* a cleaving, division] Any developmental defect of the spinal cord in which the embryonic neural tube fails to close, in part or in toto, or in which the neural tube reopens after having closed, if indeed such ever occurs.

**myelosclerosis** \-sklirō′sis\ **1** Sclerosis of the spinal cord. **2** Multiple sclerosis restricted to the spinal cord. **3** *Ambiguous* MYELOFIBROSIS. Adj. myelosclerotic.

**myelosis** \mī′əlō′sis\ [MYEL- + -OSIS] **1** Any kind of abnormal proliferation of cells in the bone marrow, including various leukemias, myelofibrosis, and myeloma. **2** Abnormal proliferation of medullary cells in the spinal cord. **aplastic m.** APLASTIC ANEMIA. **chronic nonleukemic m.** AGNOGENIC MYELOID METAPLASIA. **erythremic m.** A neoplastic disorder of erythropoiesis, characterized by megaloblastoid and dyserythropoietic erythroid hyperplasia, varying myeloid dysplasia, anemia with immature erythrocytes in the circulating blood, and hepatosplenomegaly. The acute form is erythroleukemia, and there is also a chronic form. **nonleukemic m.** AGNOGENIC MYELOID METAPLASIA.

**myelospongium** \-spän′jē·əm\ [MYELO- + SPONGI- + New L noun suffix *-um*] A network made by the interconnections of spongioblasts in the neural tube of the embryo.

**myelosyringocele** \-siring′gəsēl\ SYRINGOMYELIA.

**myelosyringosis** \-sir′ing·gō′sis\ SYRINGOMYELIA.

**myelotome** \mī′əlōtōm′\ A knife for making incisions in the spinal cord.

**myelotomy** \mī′əlät′əmē\ [MYELO- + -TOMY] **1** Incision into the spinal cord or into the medulla oblongata. **2** Division of a tract as the spinothalamic tract for relief of pain. **Bischof's m.** COMMISSURAL MYELOTOMY. **commissural m.** A longitudinal incision through the midline of the spinal cord in order to divide pain fibers. Also *midline myelotomy, Bischof's myelotomy, commissurotomy.* **midline m.** COMMISSURAL MYELOTOMY.

**myelotoxicity** \-täksis′itē\ The capability to destroy bone marrow.

**myelotoxin** \-täk′sin\ Any substance that causes the death of bone marrow cells. Adj. myelotoxic.

**myelotropic** \-träp′ik\ Showing a selective affinity for the spinal cord.

**myentasis** \mī·en′təsis\ MYOTASIS.

**myenteric** \mī′enter′ik\ [MY- + ENTERIC] Relating to the muscular coat of the intestine.

**myenteron** \mī·en′təran\ TUNICA MUSCULARIS INTESTINI TENUIS.

**Myers** [Victor Caryl *Myers,* U.S. biochemist, born 1883] See under METHOD.

**myesthesia** \mī′esthē′zhə\ [MY- + ESTHESIA] Sensations, exclusive of pain, that arise in a muscle, particularly during contraction. Also *mesoblastic sensibility.* Also *myoesthesia.*

**myiasis** \mī·ī′əsis\ [Gk *my(ia)* a fly + -IASIS ] Infection, usually of the skin and subcutis, by fly larvae. Also *myiosis, myasis.* **aural m.** Infestation of the external ear by the larvae of various species of fly, a disease becoming increasingly rare. **creeping m.** CUTANEOUS LARVA MIGRANS. **creeping cutaneous m.** CUTANEOUS LARVA MIGRANS. **cutaneous m.** Infestation of the skin by the larvae of dipterous flies. Also *dermal myiasis, myiasis dermatosa.* **intestinal m.** Infestation of the intestine by fly maggots. Also *enteromyiasis.* **m. linearis** CUTANEOUS LARVA MIGRANS. **nasal m.** Infestation of one or both nasal cavities with larvae of flies of the species *Musca domestica* and the genera *Calliphora, Lucilia* and others. Also *peenash* (Indian). **ocular m.** Invasion of the conjunctival sac or eyeball by larvae of any of various species of flies, such as warble flies (*Hypoderma bovis, H. lineata),* blow flies (*Sarcophaga* species), and bot flies (*Gasterophilus intestinalis* and others). Also *ophthalmomyiasis.* **subcutaneous m.** CUTANEOUS LARVA MIGRANS. **traumatic m.** An infection of a necrotic lesion by fly larvae that normally breed in carrion or rotting meat. Blowflies of various species (family Calliphoridae) are usually involved, including *Calliphora vicina, Phaenicia sericata, P. cuprina, Lucilia illustris, L. caesar, Phormia regina, Cochliomyia macellaria,* and *Chrysomyia* species. Flies of other families also may be involved, such as *Sarcophaga haemorrhoidalis,* the phorid *Megaselia scalaris,* or even the housefly, *Musca domestica.* Also *wound myiasis.*

**myiocephalon** \mī′yōsef′əlän\ *Outmoded* IRIDOCELE.

**myiocephalum** \mī′yōsef′ələm\ *Outmoded* IRIDOCELE.

**myiosis** \mīyō′sis\ MYIASIS.

**myitis** \mī·ī′tis\ MYOSITIS.

**myko-** \mī′kō-\ MYCO-.

**mylohyoid** \mī′lōhī′oid\ [Gk *myl(ē)* a millstone, molar + *o* + HYOID] Pertaining to the molar teeth, or the bony region related to them, and the hyoid bone.

**myo-** \mī′ō-\ [Gk *mys,* gen. *myo(s)* a mouse, muscle] A combining form denoting muscle. Also *my-.*

**myoasthenia** \-asthē′nē·ə\ MYASTHENIA.

**myoatrophy** \-at′rəfē\ AMYOTROPHY.

**myoblast** \mī′əblast\ [MYO- + -BLAST] Each of the primitive cells forming the mass of a muscle (myotome) during development. The myoblasts multiply by mitosis and then elongate to become multinucleated myocytes. Myofibrils develop as rows of granules which fuse and eventually exhibit cross-striation. Also *myogenic cell, sarcoblast.*

**myoblastoma** \-blastō′mə\ [MYOBLAST + -OMA] GRANULAR CELL TUMOR. **granular cell m.** GRANULAR CELL TUMOR.

**myoblastomyoma** \-blas′təmī·ō′mə\ [MYO- + BLASTO- + MYOMA] GRANULAR CELL TUMOR.

**myocardial** \-kär′dē·əl\ Pertaining to the myocardium. Also *myocardiac.*

**myocardiopathy** \-kär′dē·äp′əthē\ CARDIOMYOPATHY. **alcoholic m.** ALCOHOLIC CARDIOMYOPATHY. **chagasic m.** A myocardiopathy induced by Chagas disease, characterized in its severe form by saccular apical ventricular aneurysm.

**myocardiorrhaphy** \-kär′dē·ôr′əfē\ Suture of the myocardium.

**myocardiosis** \-kär′dē·ō′sis\ CARDIOMYOPATHY.

**myocarditis** \-kärdī′tis\ [*myocard(ium)* + -ITIS] Inflammation of the muscle of the heart. **acute bacterial m.** Myocarditis due to infection by bacteria, usually pyogenic. **acute isolated m.** Interstitial myocarditis, without associated endo- or pericarditis. It is an acute illness of unknown cause, sometimes fatal. Also *Fiedler's myocarditis, idiopathic myocarditis.* **acute rheumatic m.** Myocarditis occurring as a complication of rheumatic fever, characterized by foci of inflammation (Aschoff's bodies) with accumulation of multinucleate giant cells and mononuclear leucocytes and swelling of collagen fibrils. **Chagas m.** Subacute or chronic interstitial myocarditis occurring in Chagas disease. **chronic m.** Chronic myocardial damage or destruction from any cause with replacement by collagen. **chronic interstitial m.** Chronic inflammation of heart muscle with collections of leucocytes and some collagen between the often damaged muscle fibers, as may occur following acute rheumatic fever or in Chagas disease. Also *fibrous myocarditis.* **Coxsackie m.** Acute or chronic myocarditis due to infection with coxsackievirus, especially group B. **diphtheritic m.** An acute cardiomyopathy, often leading to necrosis, with reactive inflammation, due to toxin absorbed from a diphtheria infection elsewhere. It is often fatal, but recovery is usually complete in survivors. Also *diphtherial myocarditis.* **fibrous m.** CHRONIC INTERSTITIAL MYOCARDITIS. **Fiedler's m.** ACUTE ISOLATED MYOCARDITIS. **giant cell m.** Myocarditis with multinucleated giant cells as well as leukocytes, as in rheumatic fever, granulomatous diseases, and immunoreactive diseases. **idiopathic m.** ACUTE ISOLATED MYOCARDITIS. **interstitial m.** Myocarditis with exudate, diffuse or focal, between the muscle fibers, which are damaged secondarily. There are many causes, including rheumatic fever. **local m.** Myocarditis confined to one or to relatively few areas, usually due to bacterial infection, adjacent or blood-borne. **nutritional m.** A cardiomyopathy due to undernutrition, including protein deficiency as in kwashiorkor, or thiamin deficiency as in beriberi. **parenchymatous m.** A cardiomyopathy with inflammatory changes secondary to heart muscle fiber damage, especially by bacterial toxins as in diphtheria, typhoid fever, or pneumonia. **rheumatic m.** Interstitial myocarditis due to rheumatic fever. It may be acute, subacute, or chronic. **suppurative m.** A focal form of myocarditis with abscesses, usually due to infection by pyogenic bacteria. **syphilitic m.** Myocarditis due to syphilis giving rise usually to one or more gummas, or more rarely, to diffuse inflammation. **toxic m.** Myocarditis caused by toxicity from exogenous sources such as drugs, or from bacterial toxins such as that of diphtheria. **tuberculous m.** Myocarditis associated with foci of tuberculous infection of the myocardium. **virus m.** Myocarditis due to infection by a virus, such as type B coxsackievirus.

**myocardium** \-kär′dē·əm\ [New L, from MYO- + Gk *kardia* the heart] [NA] The intermediate, contractile muscular layer of the heart wall, constituting cardiac muscle, and comprising atrial and ventricular fibers separated by fibrous rings.

**myocardosis** \-kärdō′sis\ CARDIOMYOPATHY.

**myocele** \mī′əsēl\ [MYO- + -CELE[1]] A muscle hernia whereby the fleshy belly protrudes through a gap in its fascial covering.

**myoceptor** \mī′əsep′tər\ MOTOR ENDPLATE.

**myocinesimeter** \-sin′əsim′ətər\ MYOKINESIMETER.

**myoclonia** \-klō′nē·ə\ MYOCLONUS. **m. epileptica** EPILEPTIC MYOCLONUS. **m. fibrillaris multiplex** PARAMYOCLONUS MULTIPLEX. **fibrillary m.** PARAMYOCLONUS MULTIPLEX. **infectious m.** SYDENHAM'S CHOREA. **Unverricht's m.** PROGRESSIVE MYOCLONIC EPILEPSY.

**myoclonic** \-klä′nik\ Characterized by myoclonus.

**myoclonus** \-klō′nəs, mī·äk′lənəs\ [MYO- + CLONUS] A brief, shocklike contraction of a single muscle or of one or more muscle groups, rarely of part of a muscle. The phenomenon may be physiologic, as in nocturnal myoclonus, or pathologic, as a manifestation of many brain diseases, in which it can occur sporadically but repetitively. Myoclonus may also occur repetitively in many widespread muscle groups throughout the body in response to startle, in hereditary essential myoclonus (paramyoclonus multiplex). Also *myoclonic attack, myoclonic contraction, myoclonia, myoclonic jerk*. Adj. myoclonic. **action m.** Myoclonus of one part of the body, particularly of one limb, which does not occur when the patient is completely relaxed, but which appears when he undertakes muscular activity, such as maintaining a position or attitude (postural or attitudinal myoclonus), the automatic execution of a movement, or, in particular, purposive voluntary movement (intention myoclonus). This is an important sequel of diffuse cerebral anoxia. Also *intention myoclonus, postural myoclonus*. **diaphragmatic m.** EPIDEMIC HICCUP. **encephalitic m.** Myoclonic jerking in encephalitis lethargica. **epileptic m.** Myoclonus occurring in association with generalized epilepsy, with progressive myoclonic epilepsy, and with a variety of inflammatory or degenerative brain diseases. Also *myoclonia epileptica*. **facial m.** FACIAL HEMISPASM. **focal m.** Myoclonus involving one limb, part of a limb, or some other restricted part of the body, as the lips, eyeball, palate, or tongue. Usually such myoclonus is an epileptic phenomenon (focal epileptic myoclonus) but in rare cases it is physiologic, occurring in patients who demonstrate no other manifestations of epilepsy, or else it results from a focal cerebral or spinal lesion, in which event its epileptic character is uncertain. **hereditary essential m.** An uncommon and benign disorder of dominant inheritance in which there are frequent myoclonic jerks of the extremities, often elicited by a sudden noise or other sensory stimulus, but there is no association with epilepsy or other neurologic manifestation. See also PARAMYOCLONUS MULTIPLEX. **intention m.** ACTION MYOCLONUS. **massive epileptic m.** Epileptic myoclonus involving virtually the entire body and resulting from a hypersynchronous neuronal discharge arising in the brainstem. In the EEG there is usually simultaneous discharge of multispikes, or of multispike-waves, less frequently of spike-wave or spike-slow wave complexes. **m. multiplex** PARAMYOCLONUS MULTIPLEX. **nocturnal m.** Transient myoclonic jerks of the limbs and trunk which commonly occur in normal people during the early or slow wave stage of sleep, less often at other times in sleep. **palatal m.** Myoclonus of the soft palate, either unilateral or bilateral, a variety of palatopharyngeal myoclonus where only the palatal muscles are seen to be involved; often responsible for a clicking tinnitus, audible in some cases to others close to the patient. Also *palatal nystagmus*. **palatopharyngolaryngeal m.** Myoclonus of the soft palate, pharynx, and larynx, which may also involve the tongue, facial muscles, and diaphragm. The myoclonus is rhythmic (100 to 200 per minute) and does not stop when the patient is asleep. It is usually associated with a lesion of unknown etiology in the olivary bodies, the dentate nucleus, and sometimes in the central tegmental tract of the midbrain. Also *velopalatine myoclonic syndrome*. **petit mal m.** Transient generalized myoclonus occurring during attacks of petit mal or in patients who also suffer from petit mal. **postural m.** ACTION MYOCLONUS. **spinal m.** Myoclonic jerking limited to the muscles of the abdominal wall and trunk or less often of the legs and resulting from spinal cord disease. **startle m.** Myoclonic jerks elicited by startle.

**myocoele** \mī′əsēl\ [MYO- + -COELE] The cavity inside a myotome. Also *somite cavity*.

**myocolpitis** \-kälpī′tis\ Inflammation of the uterus and vagina.

**myoculator** \mīyäk′yəlā′tər\ [MY- + *ocul(o)-* + *-at(e)* + -OR] An orthoptic device that presents a target that moves laterally, vertically, and in rotation and also permits fusion.

**myocutaneous** \-kyootā′nē·əs\ MUSCULOCUTANEOUS.

**myocyst** \mī′əsist\ A cystic tumor in muscle tissue.

**myocyte** \mī′əsīt\ [MYO- + -CYTE] MUSCLE CELL. **Anichkov's m.** CARDIAC HISTIOCYTE.

**myocytolysis** \-sītäl′isis\ The absence of myofibrils and concomitant vacuolar change of the cytoplasm of cardiac muscle cells. It commonly occurs in the subendocardial region of the myocardium and at the periphery of old scars. Although a nonspecific change, it is believed by some to result from and be indicative of chronic ischemia. **focal m. of heart** A form of chronic, principally ischemic damage to the myocardial cells characterized by almost complete disappearance of sarcomeres with preservation of sarcolemmal membranes and nuclei. Because this change is typically found next to old infarcts and subendocardially, it is thought to represent a state of adaptation of myocardial cells to chronic ischemia, and the cells so affected to be viable though not capable of contraction.

**myocytoma** \-sītō′mə\ A rare benign tumor consisting of bundles of myocytes.

**myodegeneration** \-dijen′ərā′shən\ A deteriorating of muscle, either due to prior muscle disease or secondary to interruption of the nerve supply to the muscles.

**myodiastasis** \-dī·as′təsis\ The separation of a muscle from its bony origin.

**myodiopter** \-dī·äp′tər\ The force of ciliary muscle contraction required to produce one diopter of accommodation.

**myodynamics** \-dīnam′iks\ The subject concerned with the production and translation of force within a muscle.

**myodysplasia** \-displā′zhə\ [MYO- + DYSPLASIA] Impaired development of skeletal muscle. **m. fibrosa multiplex** PROGRESSIVE MYOSCLEROSIS.

**myodystonia** \-distō′nē·ə\ Any disorder that gives rise to abnormal muscle tone. Also *myodystony.*

**myodystrophia** \-distrō′fē·ə\ MUSCULAR DYSTROPHY. **m. fetalis** CONGENITAL MULTIPLE ARTHROGRYPOSIS.

**myodystrophy** \-dis′trəfē\ MUSCULAR DYSTROPHY.

**myoedema** \mī′ō·idē′mə\ Edema of a muscle.

**myoelastic** \mī′ō·ilas′tik\ Pertaining to a combination of smooth muscle fibers with elastic fibers, as is seen in the walls of blood vessels.

**myoepithelioma** \mī′ō·ep′ithē′lē·ō′mə\ [MYO- + EPITHELIOMA] A tumor of myoepithelial cells.

**myoepithelium** \mī′ō·ep′ithē′lē·əm\ Epithelial tissue possessing contractile properties. Also *muscle epithelium.*

**myoesthesia** \mī′ō·esthē′zhə\ MYESTHESIA.

**myofascial** \-fash′ē·əl\ Of or relating to the connective tissue that is associated with muscle.

**myofascitis** \-fasī′tis\ The inflammation of a muscle and its fascia. It often leads to interstitial fibrosis and induration of the muscle.

**myofiber** \mī′əfī′bər\ *Seldom used* MUSCLE FIBER.

**myofibril** \-fī′bril\ One of the parallel bundles of myofilaments running longitudinally in a muscle fiber. The myofibrils are one to two micrometers in diameter. Also *myofibrilla, muscle rod, muscle fibril.*

**myofibroblast** \-fī′brəblast\ A fibroblast which, when viewed in electron microscopy, has certain features characteristic of a smooth muscle cell. Believed to be caused by myofibroblasts, wound contraction can be inhibited experimentally by the administration of smooth muscle antagonists. Also *contractile fibroblast.*

**myofibroma** \-fībrō′mə\ [MYO- + FIBROMA] LEIOMYOMA.

**myofibrosis** \-fībrō′sis\ Fibrous replacement, focal or interstitial, of muscle.

**myofibrositis** \-fī′brəsī′tis\ Interstitial inflammation and fibrosis of skeletal muscle.

**myofilament** \-fil′əmənt\ Any of the individual thick or thin filaments of the myofibril. The thick filaments are composed of the protein myosin, the thin filaments of actin associated with tropomyosin and troponin.

**myogaster** \-gas′tər\ VENTER MUSCULI.

**myogenesis** \-jen′əsis\ [MYO- + GENESIS] Formation of muscular tissue in the embryo.

**myogenic** \-jen′ik\ [MYO- + -GENIC] **1** Having the property of forming muscle tissue: said of undifferentiated cells. **2** Originating in muscle tissue. For defs. 1 and 2 also *myogenous.* **3** Describing muscle tissue that is capable of generating spontaneous electrical activity and movement. Compare NEUROGENIC.

**myogenous** \mī·äj′ənəs\ MYOGENIC.

**myoglia** \mī·äg′lē·ə\ Fine connective tissue fibrils attached to the external aspects of a muscle cell.

**myoglobin** \-glō′bin\ [MYO- + GLOBIN] A respiratory pigment which is seen in muscle cells. It binds reversibly with molecular oxygen, thus functioning in oxygen storage. Myoglobin contains a globular protein of molecular weight 16 900, containing 153 amino-acid residues and a prosthetic (heme) group. Also *myohemoglobin.*

**myoglobinemia** \-glō′binē′mē·ə\ The presence of myoglobin in the blood plasma or serum.

**myoglobinuria** \-glō′binoo′rē·ə\ [MYOGLOBIN + -URIA] Excretion of myoglobin in the urine. It may follow muscle trauma or severe muscular exercise, extreme hyperthermia, extensive infarction when the main artery of a limb is occluded, or it may be associated with polymyositis, Haff disease, alcoholic polymyopathy, or McArdle disease. Some cases are familial, usually of unknown pathogenesis. Large amounts of myoglobin impart a burgundy red color to the urine, but since myoglobin is cleared rapidly by the kidneys, the serum usually is normal, in contrast to the early phases of hemoglobinuria where the serum is pink. Severe myoglobinuria may result in acute renal failure. Myoglobin and hemoglobin in urine are distinguished by differential absorption. Ammonium sulfate precipitates out hemoglobin and does not affect myoglobin. **familial m.** Any heritable condition that results in abnormal skeletal muscle lysis and myoglobinuria. It is a feature of acute recurrent rhabdomyolysis, carnitine palmityltransferase deficiency, and muscle phosphorylase deficiency. Also *Meyer-Betz disease.* **paroxysmal m.** IDIOPATHIC RHABDOMYOLYSIS. **traumatic m.** The presence of myoglobin in the urine resulting from disruption of muscle cells following a crush injury, overly strenuous exercise, or deep thermal burn. Acute renal failure is a common consequence.

**myognathus** \mī·äg′nəthəs\ [New L (from MYO- + Gk *gnathos* jaw, esp. the lower jaw)] Unequal conjoined twins in which the parasitic member is attached to the lower jaw of the host.

**myogram** \mī′əgram\ [MYO- + -GRAM] A record of muscular contraction.

**myograph** \mī′əgraf\ [MYO- + -GRAPH] An apparatus for recording muscular contraction.

**myography** \mī·äg′rəfē\ **1** The recording of the activity of a muscle during rest or contraction by means of a special apparatus. **2** The detailed description of muscles.

**myohemoglobin** MYOGLOBIN.

**myohypertrophia** \-hī′pərtrō′fē·ə\ Hypertrophy of muscle.

**myoid** \mī′oid\ [MY- + -OID] **1** Resembling muscle; musclelike. **2** A substance resembling muscle.

**myoidema** \mī′oidē′mə\ [MY- + Gk *oidēma* a swelling] A phenomenon in which a sharp tap upon the belly of a voluntary muscle, especially deltoid, biceps brachii, or gastrocnemius, produces a localized linear ridge which is electrically silent on electromyography and which gradually disappears within a few seconds. The cause of the phenomenon is unknown. It usually occurs in malnourished or cachectic patients, occasionally in hypothyroidism.

**myoideum** \mī·oi′dē·əm\ MUSCULAR TISSUE.

**myoidism** \mī′ō·id′izm\ [MY- + -OID + -ISM] A state of unusual responsiveness of muscles to mechanical stimulation.

**myoischemia** \mī′ō·iskē′mē·ə\ A localized loss of the blood supply to muscle tissue.

**myokinase** *Older term* ADENYLATE KINASE.

**myokinesimeter** \-kī′nēsim′ətər\ A device for measuring, and usually recording, the time course and amplitude of a muscle's contraction. *Seldom used.* Also *myocinesimeter.*

**myokinesiogram** \-kīnē′zē·əgram′\ A record of muscle contraction, expressed either as change in tension or angular excursion of a joint, as recorded by a myokinesimeter.

**myokymia** \-kim′ē·ə\ [MYO- + Gk *kym(a)* anything swollen, a wave + -IA] **1** Any of several syndromes characterized by involuntary contraction of skeletal muscle, such as facial myokymia. *Ambiguous.* **2** A syndrome of widespread, benign, coarse fasciculation of the voluntary muscles, often associated with hyperhidrosis and anxiety symptoms. **3** A rare syndrome of widespread muscular fasciculation with manifestations of myotonia, spasm of muscles, and contractures in the extremities. Also *neuromyotonia, live flesh, Isaacs syndrome, kymatism.* **facial m.** A continuous or intermittent, wavelike or rippling movement of the facial muscles, usually unilateral and often of unknown cause though it may occur in multiple sclerosis. **hereditary m.** A rare inherited disorder in which myokymia, hypoglycemia, and hypothyroidism occur.

**myolemma** \-lem′ə\ SARCOLEMMA.

**myologia** \-lō′jə\ [MYO- + -LOGIA] [NA] The nomenclature dealing with muscles, bursae, and synovial sheaths.

**myology** \mī·äl′əjē\ [MYO- + -LOGY] The study of muscles and associated structures.

**myolysis** \mī·äl′isis\ [MYO- + LYSIS] The disintegration and liquifaction of muscle tissue. It may follow atrophy or fatty degeneration.

**myoma** \mī·ō′mə\ [MY- + -OMA] A benign tumor of muscle tissue. Also *muscular tumor.* **myoblastic m.** GRANULAR CELL TUMOR. **m. previum** A myoma which obstructs the uterine canal in pregnancy. **m. striocellulare** RHABDOMYOMA.

**myomalacia** \-məlā′shə\ An abnormal softening of muscle tissue. **m. cordis** Necrosis and softening of heart muscle, most often due to coronary artery occlusion, sometimes to severe poisoning.

**myomata** \mī·ō′mətə\ Plural of MYOMA.

**myomatectomy** \-mətek′təmē\ MYOMECTOMY.

**myomatous** \mī·ō′mətəs\ Pertaining to myomas.

**myomectomy** \-mek′təmē\ [*myom(a)* + -ECTOMY] The surgical excision of a uterine fibromyoma or leiomyoma. Also *myomatectomy.* **abdominal m.** The surgical removal of one or more tumors of muscular tissue from within or about the abdominal cavity. Also *celiomyomectomy, laparomyomectomy.* **vaginal m.** The surgical removal of a leiomyoma of the cervix or uterus via the vagina. Also *colpomyomotomy, colpomyomectomy.*

**myomelanosis** \-mel′ənō′sis\ An abnormal black pigmentation of muscle.

**myomere** \mī′əmir\ [MYO- + -MERE] The part of a somite which forms the elements of the musculature after other elements have differentiated to form the sclerotome. Together they demonstrate metameric segmentation (metamerism) in that the two elements establish the somites.

**myometritis** \-mētrī′tis\ Inflammation of the myometrium usually secondary to endometritis. Also *idiometritis.* **acute m.** Abrupt onset of or the first episode of an inflammatory condition of the myometrium.

**myometrium** \-mē′trē·əm\ [New L, from MYO- + Gk *mētra* uterus] TUNICA MUSCULARIS UTERI.

**myomitochondrion** \-mī′təkän′drē·än\ (*pl.* myomitochondria) SARCOSOME.

**myomotomy** \mī′ōmät′əmē\ [*myom(a)* + *o* + -TOMY ] An incision into one or more muscular tumors. *Seldom used.*

**myon** \mī′än\ [MY- + *-on,* suffix denoting a unit] A group of muscle cells that together form a single, functional, contractile unit.

**myonecrosis** \-nekrō′sis\ [MYO- + NECROSIS] Necrosis of muscular tissue.

**myonephropexy** \-nef′rəpek′sē\ [MYO- + NEPHRO- + -PEXY] Surgical fixation of a movable kidney to muscle tissue to prevent its movement.

**myoneural** \-n^y^ur′əl\ [MYO- + NEURAL] **1** Of or denoting both muscle and nerve. **2** Denoting the highly specialized junction between motor nerve terminals and muscle fibers.

**myoneurasthenia** \-n^y^ur′asthē′nē·ə\ Muscle weakness occurring in conjunction with neurasthenia.

**myoneure** \mī′ən^y^ur\ [MYO- + *neur(on)*] A nerve cell that communicates with a muscle cell.

**myoneuroma** \-n^y^urō′mə\ A tumor that consists of proliferating Schwann cells together with myocytes.

**myonitis** \-nī′tis\ MYOSITIS.

**myonosus** \-nō′səs\ MYOPATHY.

**myopathia** \-path′ē·ə\ [MYO- + -PATHIA] MYOPATHY. **Biemond's m. distalis juvenilis hereditaria** A disease with clinical manifestations similar to those of Welander's myopathia distalis tarda hereditaria, but with an earlier onset. This condition is not a myopathy but a neuropathy, almost certainly one form of peroneal muscular atrophy. **m. cordis** CARDIOMYOPATHY.

**myopathic** \-path′ik\ Pertaining to or characteristic of myopathy.

**myopathy** \mī·äp′əthē\ [MYO- + -PATHY] Any disease of skeletal or voluntary muscle. Also *myopathia, myonosus.* Adj. myopathic. • In clinical parlance, this term has often been used in the past as a synonym of muscular dystrophy, but this incorrect usage is becoming less frequent. **acromegalic m.** A presumably specific weakness and wasting of skeletal muscles occurring late in the course of acromegaly, due to some deleterious effect of growth hormone on muscle. **ACTH m.** A myopathy associated with increased levels of circulating ACTH following bilateral adrenalectomy for Cushing's disease. **acute thyrotoxic m.** Myopathy occurring acutely during the course of Graves disease. **alcoholic m.** Myopathy due to the toxic effects of alcohol occurring in alcoholic subjects. Both acute and subacute forms occur. Also *alcoholic paralysis.* **arachnodactyly nemaline m.** Nemaline myopathy occurring in subjects showing some features of arachnodactyly. **carcinomatous m.** A myopathy associated with a carcinoma. It is a paraneoplastic phenomenon. **centronuclear m.** A benign congenital myopathy in which many muscle fibers show central nuclei and resemble fetal myotubes. Also *myotubular myopathy.* **corticosteroid-induced m.** Myopathy due to prolonged treatment with corticosteroid drugs, involving first the limb girdle muscles and later the distal musculature. It also occurs in spontaneously occurring Cushing syndrome. It is characterized histochemically by type II fiber atrophy. Removal of the excessive corticosteroid restores muscular structure and function to normal. Also *steroid myopathy.* **Cushing's disease m.** Myopathy complicating Cushing's disease. **diabetic m.** Proximal muscular weakness in association with diabetes mellitus. The nature of the relation between diabetes and the myopathy is not clear. **distal m.** Myopathy beginning in the distal muscles of the upper and lower limbs, especially in the small muscles of the hands. **Duchenne's m.** DUCHENNE TYPE MUSCULAR DYSTROPHY. **fingerprint body m.** A benign congenital myopathy in which electron microscopy of sections of skeletal muscle reveals structures resembling fingerprints. **granulomatous m.** A subacute inflammatory myopathy in which there are large collections of inflammatory cells, often with giant cells resembling multiple granulomas, in sections of affected skeletal muscle. **hypermetabolic m.** A rare form of mitochondrial myopathy in which there is a greatly increased basal metabolic rate but without hyperthyroidism. Also *Luft syndrome.* **hyperparathyroid m.** A mild disorder of proximal limb muscles in primary and secondary hyperparathyroidism, characterized by muscular weakness and fatigue, atrophy of muscles, and pressure tenderness of bones. The exact relation of muscle involvement to hypercalcemia is not clear. **hypothyroid m.** MYXEDEMATOUS MYOPATHY. **Landouzy-Dejerine m.** FACIOSCAPULOHUMERAL MUSCULAR DYSTROPHY. **late distal hereditary m.** A dominantly inherited form of muscular dystrophy beginning in middle or late life and involving first the muscles of the hands and of the forearms and later the distal muscles of the legs. Many cases have been described in Sweden, few in other countries. The course of the disease is indolent. Also *slow hereditary distal myop-*

*athy, Welander's myopathy.* **megaconial m.** A form of mitochondrial myopathy in which the mitochondria in skeletal muscle are greatly enlarged and many contain paracrystalline inclusions. **metabolic m.** Any myopathy resulting from a metabolic disorder. **mitochondrial m.** Any of a group of metabolic myopathies in which the mitochondria are structurally and biochemically abnormal. The attendant biochemical abnormalities include in different cases impaired oxidative phosphorylation, hypermetabolism, metabolic acidosis, and disorders of the electron transport chain. **myogranular m.** *Obs.* NEMALINE MYOPATHY. **myotonic m.** DYSTROPHIA MYOTONICA. **myotubular m.** CENTRONUCLEAR MYOPATHY. **myxedematous m.** Weakness, myxedema, and slowed speed of contractility and relaxation of proximal limb muscles in hypothyroidism with myxedema. Serum values of creatine phosphokinase are greatly elevated, but muscle biopsies are often normal with the occasional presence of a mucoid substance within muscle fibers; the clinical picture is reversed with thyroid hormone. Also *hypothyroid myopathy.* **nemaline m.** A rare benign congenital myopathy in which the clinical features sometimes suggest arachnodactyly and in which muscle fibers often show collections of structures like rods or threads lying beneath the sarcolemma. Also *rod myopathy.* **ocular m.** Progressive muscular dystrophy of the external ocular muscles. Also *Kiloh-Nevin syndrome.* **pleoconial m.** A mitochondrial myopathy in which an abnormally large number of mitochondria are seen in sections of skeletal muscle. **primary progressive m.** MUSCULAR DYSTROPHY. **progressive atrophic m.** MUSCULAR DYSTROPHY. **rod m.** NEMALINE MYOPATHY. **sarcoid m.** Granulomatous myopathy due to sarcoidosis. **scapuloperoneal m.** Progressive muscular dystrophy beginning in the peroneal and anterior tibial muscles of the lower limbs and in serratus and other muscles around the scapulae in the upper limbs. **slow hereditary distal m.** LATE DISTAL HEREDITARY MYOPATHY. **steroid m.** CORTICOSTEROID-INDUCED MYOPATHY. **thyrotoxic m.** A disorder of skeletal muscle in hyperthyroidism or Graves disease, affecting more than half of patients. The shoulder and pelvic girdle are commonly weak and atrophied, and, less often, the extraocular muscles and the bulbar musculature are afflicted. The disorder is reversible when a euthyroid state is restored. **uremic m.** Myopathy of the proximal limb muscles resulting from chronic uremia, usually in cases of renal failure. **Welander's m.** LATE DISTAL HEREDITARY MYOPATHY.

**myope** \mī′ōp\ A nearsighted individual.

**myopericarditis** \-per′ikärdī′tis\ [MYO- + PERICARDITIS] Inflammation of both myocardium and pericardium. Also *cardiopericarditis.*

**myophage** \mī′əfāj\ A phagocyte which destroys muscle tissue.

**myophagia** \-fā′jə\ MUSCULAR ATROPHY.

**myophagism** \mī·äf′əjizm\ MUSCULAR ATROPHY.

**myopia** \mī·ō′pē·ə\ [Gk *myōp(s)* (from *my(ein)* to close, squint + *ōps* eye) nearsighted + -IA] The refractive error requiring correction with a concave lens in order to see clearly in the distance. Also *nearsightedness, shortsightedness, brachymetropia, near sight, short sight, hypometropia* (seldom used), *plesiopia, visus brevior.* Adj. myopic. **curvature m.** Myopia due to a steeper than normal contour of the cornea or lens. **index m.** Myopia due to denser optical media. Also *indicial myopia.*

**myopic** \mī·äp′ik\ Pertaining to or affected by myopia. Also *nearsighted, brachymetropic, shortsighted.*

**myoplasm** \mī′əplazm\ SARCOPLASM.

**myoplastic** \-plas′tik\ Pertaining to myoplasty.

**myoplasty** \mī′əplas′tē\ [MYO- + -PLASTY] Any plastic operation on muscle. **mastoid m.** A variety of the mastoid obliteration operation in which a pedicled flap of temporalis muscle is turned down to occupy the mastoid excavation.

**myoplegia** \-plē′jə\ [MYO- + -PLEGIA] Muscular paralysis. *Obs.* **familial m.** PERIODIC PARALYSIS.

**myoprotein** \-prō′tēn\ Any protein found within muscle cells.

**myoreceptor** \-risep′tər\ *Obs.* MUSCLE RECEPTOR.

**myorrhaphy** \mī·ôr′əfē\ [MYO- + -RRHAPHY] The rejoining of transected muscle, usually with suture material. Also *myosuture.*

**myorrhexis** \mī′ôrek′sis\ [MYO- + -RRHEXIS] The rupture of a muscle.

**myorrhythmia** \mī′ôriTH′mē·ə\ Slow, regular, involuntary contraction of the limb muscles, giving rise to rhythmic movements as one sees particularly in patients with postencephalitic parkinsonism.

**myosalgia** \-sal′jə\ MYALGIA.

**myosalpinx** \-sal′pingks\ TUNICA MUSCULARIS TUBAE UTERINAE.

**myosarcoma** \-särkō′mə\ A malignant tumor of muscle tissue.

**myoschwannoma** \-shwanō′mə\ [MYO- + SCHWANNOMA] GRANULAR CELL TUMOR.

**myosclerosis** \-sklirō′sis\ An abnormal hardening of muscle tissue. **progressive m.** A neuromuscular disorder which is sometimes sporadic, sometimes familial, in which progressive muscular weakness and wasting is accompanied by marked intramuscular proliferation of connective tissue leading to increasingly severe contractures. This is probably a syndrome of multiple etiology. In many reported cases the individuals have been found to be suffering from spinal muscular atrophy. Also *myodysplasia fibrosa multiplex.*

**myoseptum** \-sep′təm\ [MYO- + SEPTUM] (*pl.* myosepta) A thin mesenchymatous septum which in the embryo separates the muscular masses derived from myotomes. Myosepta are also common in fishes.

**myoserum** \-sir′əm\ SARCOPLASM.

**myosin** \mī′əsin\ [MYO- + *s* + -IN] The component of muscle that forms the thicker fibrils. Myosin molecules have two components: heads, which stick out from the fibril, have ATPase activity, and are responsible for interaction with the actin fibrils; and tails, which associate together and are responsible for fibril formation.

**myosis** \mī·ō′sis\ **1** MIOSIS. **2** A condition affecting muscular tissue. **endolymphatic stromal m.** A uterine tumor resembling endometrial stroma which permeates the myometrium, usually by way of vascular spaces. It is typically of low-grade malignancy. Also *interstitial endometriosis.*

**myositis** \-sī′tis\ [MYO- + *s* + -ITIS] The inflammation of a muscle. Also *myonitis, myitis, sarcitis* (obs.). **acute disseminated m.** PRIMARY MULTIPLE MYOSITIS. **acute progressive m.** A rare inflammatory disease of the muscle in which all muscle groups become involved and result ultimately in death from respiratory failure. **Coxsackie m.** Myositis resulting from infection with one of the Coxsackie group of viruses. Epidemic pleurodynia is one example. **epidemic m.** EPIDEMIC PLEURODYNIA. **m. fibrosa** A syndrome of widespread muscular contractures with proliferation of connective tissue in the affected muscles, developing usually in childhood in a subject with polymyositis. **generalized m. ossificans** A rare progressive disorder, often familial, in which there is progressive calcification and sometimes ossification within certain skeletal muscles, often beginning in those around the scapula and in the back and cervical region. **infectious m.** An inflammation of skeletal muscle that is characterized by pain and swelling. It is most commonly seen in the upper limbs and shoulders. **multiple m.** POLYMYOSITIS. **orbital m.** Myositis limited to the external ocular muscles, usually resulting in pain, proptosis, and ophthalmoplegia. The process is generally autoimmune and steroid-responsive. Also *ocular myositis.* **m. ossificans** Bone formation in muscle, whether localized or generalized. **m. ossificans circumscripta** Localized dystrophic calcification and ossification occurring within a muscle, most often associated with persistent trauma. **m. ossificans progressiva** FIBRODYSPLASIA OSSIFICANS PROGRESSIVA. **m. ossificans traumatica** The presence of bonelike calcium deposits within muscle following injury, as in the triceps tendon at the elbow following a severe burn. The metabolic cause is unknown, and it can occur in muscles remote from the injury. **primary multiple m.** An inflammatory disease of acute onset that is characterized by foci of inflammation of muscles and overlying skin. The condition appears identical to dermatomyositis. Also *acute disseminated myositis.* **m. purulenta** SUPPURATIVE MYOSITIS. **m. purulenta tropica** TROPICAL PYOMYOSITIS. **rheumatoid m.** FIBROSITIS. **suppurative m.** Inflammation and suppuration in muscles resulting from infection with pyogenic microorganisms such as streptococci and staphylococci. The inflammation may be diffuse, spreading, localized, or abscess-forming, and general symptoms of septic infection may be apparent. Also *myositis purulenta.* See also TROPICAL PYOMYOSITIS. **trichinous m.** The changes occurring in skeletal muscle following hematogenous dissemination of *Trichinella spirallis.* Initially there are acute inflammatory changes with eosinophilic infiltrates followed by encapsulation and formation of cysts containing the microorganisms. **tropical m.** TROPICAL PYOMYOSITIS.

**myospasia** \-spā′zhə\ PARAMYOCLONUS MULTIPLEX.

**myospasm** \mī′əspazm\ A condition that gives rise to spasmodic contraction, which may be prolonged, in the voluntary muscles. **facial m.** FACIAL HEMISPASM.

**myostasis** \-stā′sis\ A fixed muscle length, as occurs after prolonged splintage.

**myostatic** \-stat′ik\ **1** Related to the resting tension of a muscle. **2** Generated by the stretching of a muscle at rest as in myostatic reflex. For defs. 1 and 2 also *myotatic.*

**myosteoma** \mī·ös′tē·ō′mə\ A benign tumor of muscle containing bony elements.

**myosthenic** \mī′ästhen′ik\ Of or relating to the strength of a muscle.

**myosuture** \-soo′chər\ MYORRHAPHY.

**myotactic** \-tak′tik\ Denoting any reflex or phenomenon evoked by tapping the belly or tendon of a skeletal muscle; related to proprioceptive function.

**myotasis** \mī·ät′əsis\ [MYO- + Gk *tasis* a stretching] The stretching of muscle. Also *myentasis.*

**myotatic** \-tat′ik\ [MYO- + Gk *tatik(os)* (from *teinein* to stretch) exerting tension] MYOSTATIC.

**myotendinitis** \-ten′dinī′tis\ [MYO- + TENDINITIS] Inflammation of a muscle and its attached tendon. Also *myotenositis.*

**myotendinous** \-ten′dinəs\ Of or relating to a muscle and tendon unit.

**myotenontoplasty** \-tenän′təplas′tē\ TENOMYOPLASTY.

**myotenositis** \-ten′ōsī′tis\ MYOTENDINITIS.

**myotenotomy** \-tenät′əmē\ The surgical excision of part of a muscle and its tendon. Also *tenomyotomy, tenontomyotomy.*

**myotic** \mī·ät′ik\ MIOTIC.

**myotome** \mī′ətōm\ [MYO- + -TOME] **1** That part of a somite in an embryo that is formed from paraxial mesoderm and gives rise to skeletal muscle. It appears to be derived from the edges of the dermatome and is at first made up of closely packed, flattened cells. Also *muscle segment.* **2** All of the voluntary or striated muscles that are supplied by neurons within a single segment of the spinal cord. **3** A surgical instrument for performing myotomy; a knife.

**myotomy** \mī·ät′əmē\ [MYO- + -TOMY] An incision into muscle tissue. **cricopharyngeal m.** The surgical division of the fibers of the cricopharyngeal muscle, indicated in three unrelated conditions: (1) for the symptomatic relief of dysphagia in certain pharyngeal palsies, (2) as a step towards preventing recurrence after the excision of hypopharyngeal diverticula, and (3) to assist voice production in certain cases after laryngectomy.

**myotonia** \-tō′nē·ə\ [MYO- + Gk *ton(os)* tension, stretching, tightening + -IA] A phenomenon characterized by an apparent delay in relaxation after a muscular contraction, accompanied by an electrical afterdischarge in the electromyogram after voluntary innervation ceases. The condition is due to an abnormality of the muscular fiber membrane, and the diagnosis can be confirmed by the occurrence of typical spontaneous discharges in the electromyogram. When an affected patient grasps an object there is difficulty in letting go, and the fingers uncurl slowly. A brisk tap upon a muscle belly evokes either a contraction of the whole muscle, if small, followed by slow relaxation, or else formation of a dimple, which slowly disappears (mechanical myotonia). This phenomenon is seen in three dominantly inherited disorders, myotonia congenita, paramyotonia congenita, and dystrophia myotonica. Also *myotony.* Adj. myotonic. **m. atrophica** DYSTROPHIA MYOTONICA. **chondrodystrophic m.** A rare disorder of infancy characterized by generalized myotonia, dwarfism, a typical appearance of the face with puckered lips and narrow palpebral fissures, as well as widespread skeletal abnormalities. Also *Schwartz-Jampel syndrome.* **m. congenita** A dominantly inherited myotonia that is generalized throughout the skeletal muscles from birth, often causing difficulty in feeding and a "strangled" cry. The myotonia is temporarily relieved by exercise and worsened by cold. A gradual improvement takes place as the subject ages, widespread muscular hypertrophy is common, and dystrophic features do not develop. Also *Thomsen's disease, congenital myotonia, myotonia hereditaria.* **m. congenita intermittens** PARAMYOTONIA CONGENITA. **congenital m.** MYOTONIA CONGENITA. **m. dystrophica** DYSTROPHIA MYOTONICA. **m. hereditaria** MYOTONIA CONGENITA. **m. paradoxa** Myotonia which appears to be worsened rather than relieved by repeated contraction of the affected muscle.

**myotonic** \-tän′ik\ Characterized by or pertaining to myotonia.

**myotonus** \-tō′nəs\ MUSCLE SPASM.

**myotony** \mī·ät′ənē\ MYOTONIA.

**myotrophic** \-träf′ik\ [MYO- + -TROPHIC] **1** Concerning the stimulation of muscle growth. **2** Of or relating to muscle nutrition.

**myotropic** \-trō′pik\ [MYO- + -TROPIC[1]] Directed toward or acting upon a muscle.

**myotube** \mī′ət$^y$oob\ A developing skeletal muscle cell in which the centrally positioned nuclei cause the sarcoplasm to assume a tubular appearance. Also *myotubule.*

**myovascular** \-vas′kyələr\ Pertaining to the anatomical

unit that consists of a muscle and its blood supply.

**myria-** \mir′ē·ə-\ [Gk *myrios* countless, huge in size, endless in time; pl. *myrioi* as substantive, ten thousand] A combining form denoting $10^4$, 10 000. An obsolete form. Symbol: ma

**myricin** **1** $C_{30}H_{61}·C_{16}H_{31}O_2$. Myricyl palmitate. A substance extracted from beeswax by crystallization. **2** A medicinal agent prepared by concentration of the principle of the dried bark of the root *Myrica cerifera*. It was formerly used as an emetic and astringent and in the treatment of indolent ulcers.

**myring-** \miring-\ MYRINGO-.

**myringa** \miring′gə\ [New L (alteration of Med. L *miringa* membrane, alteration of Late L *mininga*, also *meninga* membrane, from Gk *mēninx*, gen. *mēningos*, membrane] MEMBRANA TYMPANI.

**myringitis** \mir′injī′tis\ [MYRING- + -ITIS] Inflammation of the tympanic membrane. • The tympanic membrane, serving as the wall separating the external ear from the middle ear, will usually share in inflammatory processes affecting either compartment. However, it is unusual to describe the inflamed membrane typical, for example, of acute suppurative otitis media as an example of myringitis. **m. bullosa hemorrhagica** Otitis externa hemorrhagica in which the bullae are confined to the surface of the tympanic membrane. Also *bullous myringitis, myringitis bullosa*.

**myringo-** \miring′gō-\ [New L *myringa* tympanic membrane, from late L *meninga* membrane, from Gk *mēninx* (genitive *mēningos*) membrane] A combining form denoting the membrana tympani. Also *myring-*.

**myringoplasty** \miring′gōplas′tē\ [MYRINGO- + -PLASTY] The surgical repair of a perforated tympanic membrane. It may be performed as part of a tympanoplasty. **inlay m.** A variation of underlay myringoplasty. **onlay m.** A technique of myringoplasty in which a fascial graft is applied to the outer surface of the tympanic membrane after the surface epithelium has been removed. **underlay m.** A method of performing myringoplasty in which a fascial graft is applied to the inner aspect of the perforated tympanic membrane.

**myringostapediopexy** \-stāpē′dē·əpek′sē\ A variety of tympanoplasty in which the tympanic membrane, or the graft needed to repair it, is applied directly to the stapes, because the incus has been destroyed or so damaged by disease that its removal is unavoidable.

**myringotome** \miring′gətōm\ [MYRINGO- + -TOME] The fine lancet used for myringotomy.

**myringotomy** \mir′ing·gät′əmē\ [MYRINGO- + -TOMY] Incision of the tympanic membrane. Before the advent of chemotherapy and antibiotics, it was the obligatory treatment for acute suppurative otitis media with a bulging drumhead. At present, it is frequently employed to treat cases, usually in children, of secretory otitis media. In most instances it is performed in order to insert ventilation tubes. Also *paracentesis tympani, tympanotomy*.

**myrinx** \mir′ingks, mī′ringks\ [See MYRINGA.] MEMBRANA TYMPANI.

**myristicin** \miris′tisin\ A toxic, crystalline, safrole derivative present in star anise, parsley seed oil, and nutmeg oil. When ingested in large quantities, it can cause convulsions, hallucinations, tachycardia, and possibly death.

**myrrh** \mur\ [Gk *myrrha* (from Semitic, akin to Hebrew *mōr* myrrh, from root of *mar* bitter) myrrh] A gum resin obtained from cuts made in the bark of trees of the genus *Commiphora*, especially *C. myrrha*, the common myrrh tree. It is widely used in incense, perfume, salves, medicines, disinfectants, and embalming mixtures and has carminative, tonic, and astringent properties. It has been compounded in mouthwashes and also used as a local stimulant to the mucous membranes.

**mysophilia** \mī′sōfil′yə\ [Gk *myso(s)* filth, defilement + -PHILIA] A paraphilia in which dirt or filth is essential for sexual arousal. It is often associated with coprophilia and urophilia.

**mysophobia** \mī′sōfō′bē·ə\ [Gk *myso(s)* filth, defilement + -PHOBIA] Pathologic fear of dirt, uncleanliness, or contamination, often manifested as compulsive handwashing.

**mythomania** \mith′ōmā′nē·ə\ PATHOLOGIC LYING.

**myx-** \miks-\ MYXO-.

**myxadenitis** \mik′sadənī′tis\ Inflammation of mucous glands. **m. labialis** CHEILITIS GLANDULARIS.

**myxedema** \miks′ədē′mə\ [MYX- + EDEMA] The condition that accompanies severe hypothyroidism characterized by yellowish pallor and nonpitting edema, especially obvious in the face, with scanty hair in the eyebrows, periorbital puffiness, and thick lips. The tongue is large, movements are sluggish, and the voice is hoarse. Anemia is usually present, and the heart may be seriously affected. The mucoid deposits that constitute the edema and the clinical syndrome are both corrected by thyroid hormone. Also *mucous edema* (outmoded), *solid edema* (rare). Adj. myxedematous. **circumscribed m.** Myxedema associated with the thyrotoxicosis of Graves disease and almost invariably accompanied by exophthalmos. The edematous lesions are localized, typically in the pretibial region, less often on the face or the dorsa of the feet or hands. The lesions appear as subcutaneous swellings, the overlying skin being shiny, violaceous, and resembling orange peel in texture. **circumscribed plane m.** *Rare* PRETIBIAL MYXEDEMA. **congenital m.** CRETINISM. **hypothalamic m.** HYPOTHALAMIC HYPOTHYROIDISM. **juvenile m.** Hypothyroidism in a child or adolescent. The thyroid deficiency is usually of mild degree. The effects develop insidiously and are characterized by marked stunting of growth, a sallow complexion, supraclavicular pads of fat, potbelly, placidity, and often little or no impairment of intelligence. The condition is rare in countries with adequate diagnostic services. **nodular m.** TUBEROUS MYXEDEMA. **operative m.** POSTOPERATIVE MYXEDEMA. **pituitary m.** Myxedema associated with thyroprivic hypothyroidism. **postoperative m.** Myxedema resulting from removal of all or part of the thyroid gland and the consequent loss of thyroid function. Also *surgical myxedema, operative myxedema*. **pretibial m.** Circumscribed myxedema occurring in the pretibial region. Also *circumscribed plane myxedema* (rare). See under CIRCUMSCRIBED MYXEDEMA. **surgical m.** POSTOPERATIVE MYXEDEMA. **tertiary m.** HYPOTHALAMIC HYPOTHYROIDISM. **tuberous m.** A nodular form of circumscribed myxedema. The mucin-containing nodules are about the size of a bean or a pea. They may be isolated or in bunches and occur in reddish or waxy plaques, especially on hairy skin, in the prepatellar region, the forearm, or in the intergluteal crease. Also *nodular myxedema*.

**myxedematous** \mik′sədem′ətəs\ Of, relating to, or characterized by myxedema.

**myxemia** \miksē′mē·ə\ MUCINEMIA.

**myxo-** \mik′sō-, mik′sə-\ [Gk *myxa* discharge from the nose, mucus, phlegm] A combining form meaning mucus or slime. Also *myx-*.

**myxoblastoma** \-blastō′mə\ **1** MYXOMA. **2** MYXOSARCOMA.

**myxocystitis** \-sistī′tis\ [MYXO- + CYSTITIS] Inflammation of the mucous membrane of the urinary bladder.

**myxocystoma** \-sistō′mə\ MUCINOUS CYSTADENOMA.

**myxocyte** \mik′səsīt\ [MYXO- + -CYTE] An angulated or stellate connective tissue cell that is responsible for the production of myxoid connective tissue.
**myxofibroma** \-fībrō′mə\ FIBROMYXOMA.
**myxoid** \mik′soid\ [MYX- + -OID] Having the consistency and appearance of mucus: used especially of a connective tissue with a high content of mucoproteins and mucopolysaccharides. Also *mucofibrous.*
**myxolipofibrosarcoma** \-lip′ōfī′brōsärkō′mə\ [MYXO- + LIPO- + FIBROSARCOMA] MYXOID LIPOSARCOMA.
**myxolipoma** \-lipō′mə\ A lipoma with myxoid components. This must be distinguished from a well-differentiated myxoid liposarcoma. Also *fibromyxolipoma, lipomyxoma, lipoma myxomatodes, lipomatous myxoma.*
**myxoliposarcoma** \-lip′ōsärkō′mə\ MYXOID LIPOSARCOMA.
**myxoma** \miksō′mə\ [MYX- + -OMA] A benign but often infiltrating growth of unknown histogenesis, characterized by rather small, inconspicuous, round, spindle, or stellate cells within a matrix containing abundant mucoid material, chiefly hyaluronic acid, a loose meshwork of reticulin and collagen fibrils, and scant vascularity. The large muscles of the shoulder and thigh are the most common sites. Except in the jaws true myxomas of bone rarely occur. **atrial m.** A soft gelatinous mobile tumor, more often found in the left then the right atrium of the heart, usually tethered by a narrow stalk to the interatrial septum. The symptoms and signs often mimic those of mitral stenosis, but vary more from time to time. **giant mammary m.** CYSTOSARCOMA PHYLLODES. **m. of the heart** A benign gelatinous tumor of the heart occurring especially in the cavity of the left atrium, and derived from primitive mucoid connective tissue (mesenchyme) with scanty polyhedral cells. See also ATRIAL MYXOMA. **lipomatous m.** MYXOLIPOMA.
**myxomatosis** \-mətō′sis\ [MYXOMA + *t* + -OSIS] The presence of multiple myxomas.
**myxomatous** \miksō′mətəs\ Pertaining to myxoma.
**myxopoiesis** \-poi·ē′sis\ MUCOPOIESIS.
**myxorrhea** \mik′sôrē′ə\ [MYXO- + -RRHEA] Mucinous discharge. *Seldom used.*
**myxosarcoma** \-särkō′mə\ [MYXO- + SARCOMA] The malignant counterpart of a myxoma. Most so-called myxosarcomas are probably myxoid liposarcomas. Adj. myxosarcomatous.
**myxovirus** \mik′səvī′rəs\ [MYXO- + VIRUS] **1** ORTHOMYXOVIRUS. **2** Any virus of the Orthomyxoviridae or Paramyxoviridae families.

# N

**N** **1** Symbol for the unit, newton. **2** Symbol for the element, nitrogen. **3** Symbol for normal. **4** Symbol for asparagine. **5** Symbol for radiance.
**n** **1** Symbol for nano-: used with SI units. **2** Symbol for normal. **3** refractive index.
$\mathbf{n_d}$ refractive index.
$\nu$ Symbol for the quantity, kinematic viscosity, expressed in meters squared per second.
**NA** **1** Nomina Anatomica. **2** numerical aperture.
**Na** Symbol for sodium.
**Naboth** [Martin *Naboth,* German anatomist and physician, 1675–1721] Naboth's ovules, Naboth's vesicles, nabothian glands, ovula nabothi, nabothian follicles, vesiculae nabothi. See under NABOTHIAN CYSTS.
**NAD** **1** Symbol for nicotinamide adenine dinucleotide. **2** no appreciable disease, nothing abnormal detected.
**NADH** Symbol for the reduced form of nicotinamide adenine dinucleotide.
**nadide** NICOTINAMIDE ADENINE DINUCLEOTIDE.
**NAD kinase** An enzyme (EC 2.7.1.23) which catalyzes the transfer of a phosphate in the following reaction: ATP + $NAD^+ \rightleftharpoons$ ADP + $NADP^+$.
**NADP** Symbol for nicotinamide adenine dinucleotide phosphate. It usually represents both oxidized and reduced forms of the compound, which are distinguished by the symbols $NADP^+$and NADPH, respectively. Occasionally, however, it is used for the oxidized form, with the reduced form being represented as $NADPH_2$.
**NADPH** Symbol for the reduced form of NADP.
**NADPH diaphorase** METHEMOGLOBIN REDUCTASE.
**Naegeli** [Otto *Naegeli,* Swiss hematologist, 1871–1938] **1** See under LAW. **2** Macroblast of Naegeli. See under PRONORMOBLAST.
***Naegleria*** \nāgler′ē·ə\ A genus of free-living amebas having both an ameboid and a flagellate stage. They are found primarily in stagnant waters, and as coprozoites in feces. Also *Dimastigamoeba.* ***N. fowleri*** A species of ameba that has been isolated and cultured from cerebrospinal fluid and brain tissue suspensions of patients who died of an acute meningoencephalitis. Infection has been associated with swimming in stagnant, warm freshwater lakes or ponds, with entry of amebas via the olfactory mucosa and cribriform plate.It now appears that exposure is frequent but penetration leading to the disease is extremely rare.
**naevus** \nē′vəs\ *Brit.* NEVUS.
**nafcillin sodium** $C_{21}H_{21}N_2NaO_5S \cdot H_2O$. Sodium 6-(2-ethoxy-1-naphthamido)penicillanate monohydrate. A penicillin with antimicrobial activity like that of cloxacillin. It is used intramuscularly to treat severe infections by organisms resistant to benzylpenicillin, or orally for less serious infections.
**Naffziger** [Howard Christian *Naffziger,* U.S. surgeon, 1884–1961] **1** See under DECOMPRESSION, OPERATION, TEST. **2** Naffziger syndrome. See under SCALENUS ANTERIOR SYNDROME.
**Nägele** [Franz Karl *Nägele,* German obstetrician, 1777–1851] **1** Nägele's obliquity. See under ANTERIOR ASYNCLITISM. **2** See under RULE.
**Nageotte** [Jean *Nageotte,* French histologist, 1866–1948] Babinski-Nageotte syndrome. See under SYNDROME.
**Nagler** [F. P. O. *Nagler,* Australian bacteriologist, flourished 20th century] See under REACTION.
**nail** [Old English *nægl, nægel* ] **1** A rigid, wirelike piece of metal or other substance often with a pointed end that can be driven into bone fragments to fix them in place. **2** A horny keratin structure that covers the dorsal aspect of the terminal phalanx of each digit; unguis. **cloverleaf n.** An orthopedic device, shaped like a cloverleaf when

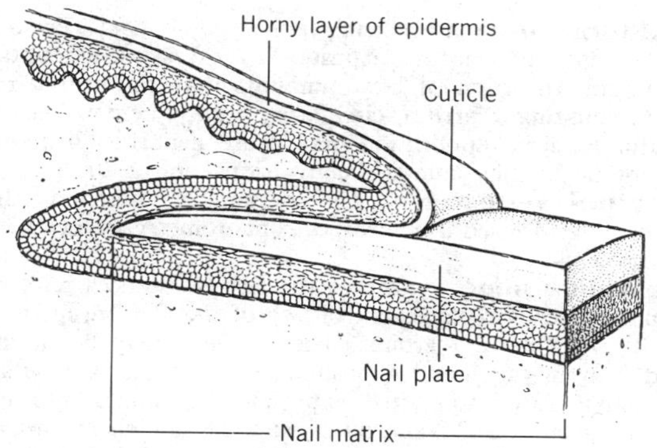


**Structure of the nail (unguis)**

viewed in cross-section, that is used for internal fixation of fractures. **eggshell n.** A thin nail that assumes a semitransparent, bluish white hue resembling the color of an egg. It is sometimes seen in vitamin A deficiencies. **n. en raquette** A congenital abnormality of the thumb, inherited as an autosomal dominant trait, that is characterized by one or both distal phalanges and their nails being shorter and wider than normal. The lateral curvature of the nail is lost, so that the nail resembles a tennis racket. It is more common among women. Also *racket nail.* **fracture n.** A rod of metal or other rigid material that is used to provide internal fixation to one or more fracture fragments. **hippocratic n.** A loss of the normal angle between the nail and the posterior nail fold that is characteristic of clubbed fingers. **ingrowing n.** A painful inflammation of the perionychial area that is caused by the overlapping of the nail by adjacent tissues, producing granulation and ulceration. It usually affects the great toe. Also *incarnatio, unguis incarnatus.* **Jewett n.** A rod of metal and attached plate that are used to provide internal fixation for an intratrochanteric femoral fracture. **Küntscher n.** A long, metal, hollow nail, trefoil-shaped in cross section, that is passed down the medullary cavity of a large long bone such as a femur. **pitted n.'s** Nails marked by small depressions in the surface of the nail plate. The condition is seen in psoriasis and alopecia areata. Occasionally, pits are seen in normal nails. **racket n.** NAIL EN RAQUETTE. **reedy n.** A nail that is marked by longitudinal ridges. **Smith-Petersen n.** A rigid rod with a large flange that is used to provide internal fixation in fractures of the neck of the femur. **Thornton n.** A metallic orthopedic nail used to provide internal fixation of intertrochanteric femoral fractures.

**nailing** The internal fixation of fractured bone by insertion of a rigid rodlike device to stabilize the fragments. **intramedullary n.** A surgical procedure in which a rigid nail or rod is placed in the marrow cavity of a fractured bone in order to provide internal fixation following an open reduction. Also *marrow nailing, medullary nailing.* **marrow n.** INTRAMEDULLARY NAILING. **medullary n.** INTRAMEDULLARY NAILING.

***Naja*** \näʹjə\ A genus of venomous snakes of the Elapidae family; the cobras. The venom is neurotoxic and the teeth are proteroglyphic. Six species are distributed in Africa and Asia.

**Najjar** [Victor Assad *Najjar,* Lebanese-born U.S. pediatrician, born 1914] Crigler-Najjar disease. See under SYNDROME.

**naked** [Old English *nacod,* akin to Old High German *nackot,* L *nudus,* Gk *gymnos,* all meaning naked, unclad] Without a lipid envelope: said of certain viruses.

**nalidixic acid** $C_{12}H_{12}N_2O_3$. 1-Ethyl-1,4-dihydro-7-methyl-4-oxo-1,8-naphthyridine-3-carboxylic acid. An antibiotic with antibacterial activity against Gram-negative bacteria. It is used orally against urinary-tract infections caused by susceptible microorganisms such as *Proteus* strains, *Klebsiella, Enterobacter,* and *Escherichia coli.*

**Nalline** A proprietary name for nalorphine.

**nalorphine hydrochloride** $C_{19}H_{21}NO_3 \cdot HCl$. *N*-Allylnormorphine hydrochloride. A narcotic antagonist given intravenously to reverse the respiratory depression produced by narcotics, such as morphine, methadone, and meperidine. Also *allorphine hydrochloride.*

**naloxone hydrochloride** $C_{19}H_{21}NO_4 \cdot HCl$. 17-Allyl-4,5-epoxy-3,14-dihydroxymorphinan-6-one hydrochloride. The prototype narcotic antagonist. It is structurally related to morphine, and is used parenterally as an antidote to narcotic overdosage, or for an overdose of pentazocine.

**name / nonproprietary n.** A shortened, commonly used name of a chemical or drug, which is not protected by trademark rights. It is not identical to the generic name of a drug. **scientific n.** The name of an organism which includes the generic name and the specific epithet. The first letter of the generic name is capitalized; the species name is in lower-case letters. Both names are italicized. A subspecies name may also be included. See also BINOMIAL NOMENCLATURE. **semisystematic n.** The name of a chemical which is partly a systematic designation and partly a trivial name. For example, *benzoylcholine* includes the systematic *benzoyl* for $C_6H_5CO$, and the trivial *choline* for (2-hydroxyethyl)trimethylammonium. Many generic and nonproprietary drug names are semisystematic but are said to be trivial names even if not entirely so. Also *semitrivial name.* **semitrivial n.** SEMISYSTEMATIC NAME. **systematic n.** The name for a chemical based upon the structure and substituents present so that the chemical structure can be deduced from the name using specific, conventional rules. **trivial n.** A chemical name that gives no systematic indication of the structural components present in the molecule. Examples are *aspirin, insulin,* and *quinine.* The assignment of trivial names is often arbitrary, and usually rather short, for convenience. **vernacular n.** Any name, other than the official taxonomic designation, that is used to identify an organism.

**naming** An association disorder seen in schizophrenia in which the subject's only response and contact with the outside world consists of naming and touching objects, or stating the action he is performing, such as saying "now he is standing up."

**nandrolone decanoate** $C_{28}H_{44}O_3$. 17$\beta$-[(1-Oxodecyl)-oxy]-estr-4-en-3-one, an ester with anabolic properties that is administered by intramuscular injection.

**nanism** \nāʹnizm, nanʹizm\ [*nan(o)-* + -ISM] DWARFISM.

**nano-** \(1) nanʹō-; (2) nanʹə-\ [Gk *nanos* dwarf] **1** A combining form meaning dwarf, dwarfish. **2** A combining form denoting $10^{-9}$, one billionth: used with SI units. Symbol: n

**nanocephaly** \-sefʹəlē\ [NANO- + CEPHAL- + -Y] **1** Extreme smallness of the head, often accompanied by specific malformations of the face or cranium. Also *nanocephalia.* **2** An inexact and outmoded term for SECKEL SYNDROME. Adj. nanocephalic.

**nanocormia** \-kôrʹmē·ə\ [NANO- + Gk *korm(os)* trunk of a tree, log + -IA] An abnormal smallness of the trunk as compared with the head and limbs.

**nanocurie** \-kyoo′rē\ [NANO- + CURIE] A unit of activity of a radionuclide or of a radioactive source equal to $10^{-9}$ curie; 37 becquerels exactly. Also *millimicrocurie* (outmoded). Symbol: nCi

**nanogram** [NANO- + GRAM] A unit of mass or weight equal to $10^{-9}$ gram. Also *micromilligram* (outmoded), *millimicrogram* (outmoded). Symbol: ng

**nanomelia** \-mē′lyə\ [NANO- + MEL-$^{1}$ + -IA ] A disproportionate smallness of the limbs compared with the head and trunk.

**nanometer** \-mē′tər\ [NANO- + METER] A unit of length equal to $10^{-9}$ meter. Also *micromillimeter* (outmoded), *millimicrometer* (outmoded), *millimicron* (outmoded). Symbol: nm

**nanometre** *Brit.* NANOMETER.

***Nanophyetus*** \nanō′fē·ətəs\ A genus of digenetic flukes of the family Nanophyetidae (formerly placed in the family Troglotrematidae) that parasitize fish-eating mammals, including man. It was formerly included in the genus *Troglotrema.*

**nanosoma** \-sō′mə\ [NANO- + Gk *sōma* body] DWARFISM.

**nanosomia** \-sō′mē·ə\ [NANO- + Gk *sōm(a)* body + -IA] DWARFISM.

**nanosomus** \-sō′məs\ DWARF.

**nanous** \nā′nəs\ [Gk *nan(os)* dwarf + -OUS] Dwarfish; undersized.

**Nanta** [A. *Nanta*, French physician, flourished early 20th century] Gandy-Nanta disease. See under SIDEROTIC SPLENOMEGALY.

**nanukayami** \nä′nookäyä′mē\ [Japanese *nanu-*, combining form denoting seven + *-ka*, combining form denoting day + *-yami*, combining form denoting illness] A form of leptospirosis of man caused by *Leptospira hebdomadis* and transmitted by the field vole. First reported in Japan, the disease is characterized by fever and jaundice. Also *seven-day fever, nanukayami fever, leptospirosis hebdomadis, akiyami, autumn fever.*

**nanus** \nā′nəs\ [Gk *nanos* dwarf] DWARF.

**NAP** nasion, point A, pogonion. (The three points forming the angle of convexity, used as a measure of prognathism).

**nape** \nāp\ [of obscure origin; possibly akin to Old English *cnæp* top of a hill] NUCHA.

**napex** \nā′peks\ [the *apex* of the *nape*] That part of the scalp just below the external occipital protuberance.

**naphazoline hydrochloride** $C_{14}H_{14}N_2HCl$. 4,5-Dihydro-2-(1-naphthalenyl methyl)-1*H*-imidazole monohydrochloride. A white, crystalline powder utilized as an adrenergic agent to produce vasoconstriction. It may be applied topically to the nasal or ocular surfaces.

**naphthalene** \naf′thəlēn\ $C_{10}H_8$. The compound whose molecule consists of two benzene rings fused together. It is a white solid obtained from coal tar, and is used for chemical syntheses and, domestically, as moth balls. **chlorinated n.** Any of the compounds of naphthalene in which the hydrogenations in the naphthalene are replaced by chlorine. Some of these compounds are waxes which have special insulating and water-resistant properties. Occupational exposure causes a severe form of pruritic acne, which itches, and toxic jaundice. Chlorinated naphthalenes are also used in combination with chlorinated diphenyls, which have similar toxic effects. Also *perna, perchloronaphthalene*.

**naphthol** \naf′thôl\ Either of the two isomeric phenols derived from naphthalene by substitution of a hydroxyl group for a hydrogen atom.

**naphtholism** \naf′thəlizm\ [*naphthol* + -ISM] Poisoning from acute or chronic exposure to excessive amounts of naphthol. Ingestion of large amounts may cause abdominal pain, vomiting, diarrhea, circulatory failure, convulsions, and death. External application may cause nephritis, hematuria, hemolytic anemia, jaundice, convulsions, and death.

**naphthol yellow S** The sodium or potassium salt of flavianic acid, used in microspectrophotometry to localize basic proteins.

**naphthoquinone** One of the two substances related to naphthalene by replacement of two of the CH groups in one of its rings by CO groups. These groups may be in the 1 and 2 or in the 1 and 4 positions. Substances with vitamin K activity are substituted naphtho-1,4-quinones, bearing a methyl group on C-2 and a polyisoprene side chain on C-3.

**naphthyl** The group formed from naphthalene by removal of one hydrogen atom. It may be $\alpha$ or $\beta$, according to whether H-1 or H-2 is removed.

**naphthylamine** One of two amines formed by replacing H-1 or H-2 of naphthalene with an amino group. When H-2 is so replaced, the compound, which may be designated $\beta$-naphthylamine, is carcinogenic.

**naproxen** $C_{14}H_{14}O_3$. (+)-6-Methoxy-$\alpha$-methyl-2-naphthaleneacetic acid. A white, crystalline powder employed as an anti-inflammatory, antipyretic agent, and as an analgesic. It can be given orally for the treatment of rheumatoid arthritis.

**narcism** \när′sizm\ NARCISSISM.

**narcissism** \när′sisizm\ [L *Narciss(us)* (from Gk *Narkissos*) a youth in Gk myth who fell in love with his own reflection + -ISM] **1** The stage in development of object relationships that follows the autoerotic or somatogenic stage. The child does not differentiate between self and nonself and believes he is omnipotent. **2** As applied to the adult, hypercathexis of the self or self-love. Also *autophilia.* **3** Genital love of the self, sometimes expressed as a need to watch oneself masturbating in front of a mirror. For defs. 1, 2, and 3 also *narcism.* **primary n.** The most primitive type of object relationship, where all available libido is stored in the ego and has not yet been directed onto representations of objects external to oneself. *Imprecise.* **secondary n.** Narcissism in which the psychic force involved is directed toward the ego after having been attached to objects. Somatic overconcern that develops in association with diminution in object relationships is an example.

**narco-** \när′kō-\ [Gk *narkē* numbness, stupor] A combining form meaning stupor, numbness, narcosis.

**narcohypnia** \-hip′nē·ə\ [NARCO- + HYPN- + -IA] SLEEP PARALYSIS.

**narcolepsy** \när′kōlep′sē\ [NARCO- + -LEPSY] A disorder characterized by an irresistible tendency to fall asleep in circumstances which would be normally conducive to relaxation, as during a lecture or during the performance of a semiautomatic, monotonous task, such as driving a car. The sufferer can be aroused as from physiologic sleep, and the attacks may last for minutes or for hours. The etiology is unknown. The pattern of sleep in narcoleptic subjects is immediately of the paradoxical (REM) type. Most narcoleptic subjects also suffer from cataplexy, and some also experience sleep paralysis and hypnagogic hallucinations. Also *Gélineau syndrome, sleeping disease, hypnolepsy, pyknolepsy, paroxysmal sleep, Friedmann's disease.* Adj. narcoleptic.

**narcosine** NOSCAPINE.

**narcosis** \närkō′sis\ [Gk *narkōsis* (from *narkoun* to benumb) an act of benumbing] An alteration in consciousness, ranging from mere sleep to deep, unresponsive coma. It can be produced by sedatives, narcotics, anesthetics, or physical means. **basal n.** BASAL ANESTHESIA. **basis n.** BASAL ANESTHESIA. **carbon dioxide n.** Coma or stupor due to abnormally high levels of carbon dioxide in arterial blood. **nitrogen n.** Confusion, stupefaction, or unconsciousness resulting from breathing the nitrogen of atmospheric air at increased barometric pressures, as during depth diving. **prolonged n.** CONTINUOUS SLEEP TREATMENT.

**narcostimulant** An agent with both narcotic and stimulant properties.

**narcotic** \närkät′ik\ [Gk *narkōtikos* benumbing, narcotic] **1** Relating to or producing narcosis. **2** A sleep-producing or pain-relieving agent, commonly an opioid. • Because almost all known agents capable of relieving severe pain also tend to induce sleep, they are often called narcotics even when their primary purpose is relief from pain. Such drugs are usually addictive. See also the note at HYPNOTIC.

**narcoticoirritant** **1** Having both narcotic and irritant properties. **2** A narcoticoirritant drug or agent.

**narcotine** NOSCAPINE.

**narcotize** \när′kətīz\ [*narcot(ic)* + -IZE] To subject to the effect of a narcotic agent to diminish consciousness, as in the administration of general anesthesia or sedation.

**nares** \ner′ēz, nar′ēz\ [L, the nostrils] (*sing.* naris) [NA] The rounded external openings of the nasus externus, on either side of the septal cartilage and bounded laterally by the alae. Also *nostrils, prenares.*

**naris** \ner′is, nar′is\ Singular of NARES. **anterior n.** Either of the two external openings of the nasal cavity. Also *external naris.* **internal n.** *Outmoded* CHOANA. **posterior n.** CHOANA.

**narrowing** / **aortic n. of esophagus** A normal constriction of the esophagus produced by the right side of the arch of the aorta at the level of the fourth thoracic vertebra. Also *aortic indentation of esophagus.* **bronchial n. of esophagus** A normal constriction of the esophagus that is produced by the left principal bronchus crossing in front of it at the level of the fifth thoracic vertebra. **cardiac n. of esophagus** A ventral concavity of the esophagus due to its passage behind the left atrium of the heart. **cricoid n. of esophagus** A normal constriction of the commencement of the esophagus at the distal border of the cricoid cartilage opposite the sixth cervical vertebra. **diaphragmatic n. of esophagus** A normal constriction of the esophagus at the site of its passage through the diaphragm into the abdominal cavity and at the level of the tenth thoracic vertebra. **iliac n. of ureter** A normal narrowing of the lumen of the ureter at the level where it crosses the brim of the pelvis anterior to either the common or the external iliac vessels.

**nasal** \nā′zəl\ [Late L *nasalis* (from L *nasus* nose) pertaining to the nose] **1** Of or relating to the nose. Also *rhinal.* **2** Nearer or toward the nose; medial: applied to positions and directions in the eye or the visual field. Compare TEMPORAL.

**nasality** \nāzal′itē\ [NASAL + -ITY] The quality of speech associated with nasal emission.

**nasion** \nā′zē·än\ [L *nas(us)* the nose + Gk *-ion,* dim. suffix] A craniometric point situated at the midpoint of the nasofrontal suture.

**Nasmyth** [Alexander *Nasmyth,* Scottish dentist and anatomist, died 1847] See under MEMBRANE.

**naso-** \nā′zō-\ [L *nasus* nose, sense of smell] A combining form meaning nose, nasal.

**nasoalveolar** \-alvē′ələr\ Pertaining to or joining nasion and prosthion.

**nasoantral** \-an′trəl\ Pertaining to the nose and the maxillary sinus. Also *nasomaxillary.*

**nasobronchial** \-brang′kē·əl\ Pertaining to the nasal cavity and the bronchi.

**nasobuccal** \-buk′əl\ Pertaining to the nose and the cheek.

**nasobuccopharyngeal** \-buk′ōfərin′jē·əl\ Pertaining to the nose, cheek, and pharynx.

**nasociliary** \-sil′ē·er′ē\ Pertaining to the nose and the eyelids, as the nasociliary nerve.

**nasocular** \nāzäk′yələr\ Pertaining to the nose and the eye.

**nasoendoscope** \-en′dəskōp\ An instrument inserted through one of the nostrils to examine the nasal cavity.

**nasoendoscopy** \-endäs′kəpē\ Examination of the interior of the nose, nasopharynx, or larynx using an endoscope passed through one of the anterior nares.

**nasofacial** \-fā′shəl\ Pertaining to the nose and the face.

**nasogastric** \-gas′trik\ [NASO- + GASTRIC] Relating to the nose and the stomach: applied principally to stomach tubes inserted via the nose and esophagus.

**nasolabial** \-lā′bē·əl\ Of or relating to the nose and the upper lip.

**nasolacrimal** \-lak′rəməl\ **1** Pertaining to the nasal cavity and the lacrimal apparatus. **2** Of or relating to the nasal and lacrimal bones.

**nasomanometer** \-mənäm′ətər\ RHINOMANOMETER.

**nasomaxillary** \-mak′siler′ē\ **1** Of or relating to the nasal and maxillary bones. **2** NASOANTRAL.

**naso-occipital** \-äksip′itəl\ Pertaining to the nose and the occiput: said especially of craniometric dimensions.

**nasopharyngeal** \-fərin′jē·əl\ Pertaining to the nasopharynx. Also *epipharyngeal, pharyngonasal.*

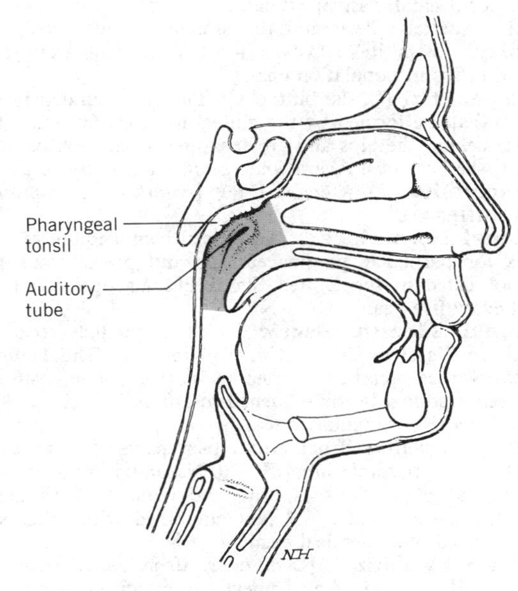


**Nasopharynx**

**nasopharyngitis** \-far′ənjī′tis\ Postnasal pharyngitis, a common accompaniment of many upper respiratory infections including the common cold. Also *epipharyngitis, rhinopharyngitis.*

**nasopharyngoscope** \-fəring′gəskōp\ Any optical instrument used for nasopharyngoscopy, rhinoscopy, or laryngoscopy. For these purposes, flexible fiberscopes with controllable tips have replaced rigid electrical endoscopes that used distal illumination.

**nasopharyngoscopy** \-far′əng·gas′kəpē\ Examination of the nasopharynx either indirectly through the mouth using a nasopharyngeal mirror or directly through the nose using a nasopharyngoscope. Also *posterior rhinoscopy.*

**nasopharynx** \-far′ingks\ PARS NASALIS PHARYNGIS.

**nasorostral** \-räs′trəl\ Of or relating to the nasal cavity and the rostrum of the sphenoid bone.

**nasoscope** \nā′zōskōp\ [NASO- + -SCOPE] RHINOSCOPE.

**nasoseptal** \-sep′təl\ Pertaining to the septum of the nose.

**nasus** \nā′səs\ [L, the nose] The centrally located facial structure that serves as the peripheral organ of smell and a part of the respiratory system; nose. It is located above the roof of the mouth and comprises the external nose and the nasal cavity. **n. externus** [NA] The external, projecting portion of the nose. It is formed above by bones attached to the forehead between the eyes and below by hyaline cartilages on each side which are covered by muscles and skin. Internally it is lined by periosteum and perichondrium covered by mucous membrane. It is divided into two compartments by a median cartilaginous septum that is attached posteriorly to the bony septum of the nasal cavity. It extends from the root, where the bones form the bridge, to the apex or tip. The intervening portion constitutes the dorsum and is continuous on either side with the alae, the distal openings of which being the nostrils. Also *external nose, nose.* **n. osseus** The bony framework of the nose.

**natal**[1] \nā′təl\ [L *natalis* (from *natus,* past part. of *(g)nasci* to be born) natal, native] Relating to birth.

**natal**[2] \nā′təl\ Pertaining to the nates, or buttocks.

**natality** \nātal′itē\ [NATAL[1] + -ITY] In demography, the role of births in population change.

**nates** \nā′tēz\ [L, the buttocks] The two rounded prominences that are formed by the gluteal muscles, fat, and other tissues behind the hips and are separated from each other by a cleft; the buttocks. Also *clunes, natiform protuberance.*

**natimortality** \nā′tēmôrtal′itē\ [*nat(ality)* + *mortality*] STILLBIRTH RATE.

**National Formulary** An official compendium of standards for particular pharmaceuticals and preparations that are not listed in the United States Pharmacopeia. It is revised every five years. Abbr. NF

**National Health Service** The publicly operated health care system in the United Kingdom. The National Health Service Act was enacted by Parliament in 1946 and has been modified by subsequent legislation.

**natis** \nā′tis\ Singular of NATES.

**native** [L *nativus* (from *natus,* past part. of *nasci* to be born) native, natural, inborn] **1** Naturally originating in an area, as populations of flora and fauna. **2** Unaltered from the natural state. **3** Not combined with other substances: used of a chemical element.

**nativism** \nā′tivizm\ [L *nativ(us)* (from *natus* born) native, inbred + -ISM] Any tendency to attach greater importance to the influence of heredity as opposed to environment on the expression of abilities, such as intelligence.

**natriuresis** \nā′trēyoorē′sis\ [New L *natri(um)* sodium + -URESIS] Increased excretion of sodium in the urine. It occurs in tubulointerstitial disease and cystic renal disease, the Bartter syndrome, the diuretic recovery phase of acute renal failure, and during spontaneous or diuretic-induced reduction of edema. Also *natruresis.* Adj. natriuretic.

**natriuretic** \nā′trēyooret′ik\ **1** Pertaining to or causing increased urinary excretion of sodium. **2** A drug that promotes urinary excretion of sodium. Also *natruretic.*

**natural** Not dependent on prior experience, as in *natural immunity.*

**nature-nurture** \nā′chər-nur′chər\ The controversial problem of determing the relative contribution made by hereditary factors (nature), as opposed to that made by environmental factors (nurture), to the development and expression of adult characteristics or abilities, as in an attempt to account for individual differences in intelligence or personality.

**naturopathy** \nā′chəräp′əthē\ A system of folk medicine utilizing the forces of nature such as air, light, water, heat, cold, physical activity, and massage, and eschewing all drugs.

**Naunyn** [Bernard *Naunyn,* German physician, 1839–1925] Naunyn-Minkowski method. See under MINKOWSKI'S METHOD.

**nausea** \nô′zē·ə, nô′zhə\ [L (from Gk *nausia* seasickness, retching, from *naus* a ship + -IA), seasickness] An unpleasant sensation of needing to vomit. **n. gravidarum** MORNING SICKNESS. **n. marina** SEASICKNESS.

**nauseant** An agent that induces or precipitates nausea.

**nauseous** \nô′shəs, nô′zē·əs\ **1** Causing an urge to vomit. **2** Feeling an urge to vomit; nauseated.

**navel** [Old English *nafela*] UMBILICUS. **blue n.** CULLEN SIGN.

**navicular** \nəvik′yələr\ [Late L *navicularis* (from *navicula* a small ship, boat, from *navis* a ship) like or pertaining to a boat] **1** SCAPHOID. **2** Designating the os naviculare.

**naviculocuboid** \nəvik′yəlōkyoo′boid\ CUBOIDEONAVICULAR.

**Nb** Symbol for the element, niobium.

**NBS** National Bureau of Standards.

**NCA** **1** neurocirculatory asthenia. **2** nonspecific cross-reacting antigen.

**NCF** neutrophil chemotactic factor.

**NCI** National Cancer Institute.

**NCV** **1** noncholera vibrios. **2** nerve conduction velocity.

**Nd** Symbol for the element, neodymium.

**Ne** Symbol for the element, neon.

**neanderthaloid** \nē·an′dərthô′loid\ Exhibiting characteristics of Neandertal man. See also *HOMO NEANDERTHALENSIS.*

**nearsighted** MYOPIC.

**nearsightedness** MYOPIA.

**nearthrosis** \nē′ärthrō′sis\ NEOARTHROSIS.

**nebenkern** \nā′bənkern\ [German *neben* near + *Kern* kernel, grain] A mitochondrial mass formed by the coalescence of numerous smaller mitochondria, located near the nucleus in the spermatid and around the axial filament of the flagellum in the spermatozoon.

**nebramycin** \neb′rəmī′sin\ A mixture of semisynthetic aminoglycoside antibiotics closely related to kanamycin B.

**nebula** \neb′yələ\ [L, mist, fog, vapor, cloud] **1** A minimal corneal opacity. **2** A liquid preparation for use in atomizer sprays. **n. epinephrinae hydrochloridi** A preparation of epinephrine hydrochloride in an aqueous or alcoholic solution containing sodium metabisulfite in an atomizer, suitable for spraying the throat or intranasally.

**nebulizer** \neb′yəlīzər\ A device for converting liquid into a mist or cloud, used primarily for permeating the atmosphere of an enclosed space or for direct inhalation. **ultrasonic n.** A nebulizer in which a high-frequency oscillator drives a piezoelectric transducer. The high-frequency vibrations at the air-water surface break the water into droplets 0.5 to 3 micrometers in diameter for inhalation therapy.

***Necator*** \nēkā′tər\ [L (from *necare* to kill) a murderer] A genus of hookworms of the family Ancylostomatidae, subfamily Necatorinae, characterized by cutting plates rather than teeth in the buccal cavity and by fused copulatory spicules in the male. ***N. americanus*** The New World or tropical hookworm, a species common in humans in tropical areas of Central and South America, central and southern Africa, southern Asia, and Polynesia. Adult worms live in the small intestine, causing disease through their blood-sucking activities. In heavy, long-term infections, severe weight loss and hypochromic microcytic anemia may result. Infection occurs through penetration of the skin by third-stage filariform larvae, that migrate via blood vessels into the alveoli, where they molt and move, a week later, into the bronchioles, up the ciliated air passages to the trachea, and downward to the jejunum where they mature. Also *Ancylostoma americanum, Uncinaria americana.*

**necatoriasis** \nēkā′tərī′əsis\ [*Necator* + -IASIS] Infection by hookworms of the genus *Necator,* especially *N. americanus.* The symptoms are similar to those of ancylostomiasis.

**necessity / pharmaceutic n.** A substance having little or no therapeutic value, but used in the preparation of various drugs or medicinals. Examples are preservatives, solvents, ointments, flavorings, colorings, emulsifying agents, and suspending agents. Also *pharmaceutic aid.*

**neck** [Old English *hnecca*] **1** A narrowing or constriction. **2** COLLUM. **3** CERVIX. **anatomical n. of humerus** COLLUM ANATOMICUM HUMERI. **n. of ankle bone** COLLUM TALI. **buffalo n.** BUFFALO HUMP. **bull n.** Massive swelling of the upper cervical lymph nodes, particularly as seen in cases of pharyngeal diphtheria. **n. of condylar process of mandible** COLLUM MANDIBULAE. **n. of femur** COLLUM OSSIS FEMORIS. **n. of gallbladder** COLLUM VESICAE BILIARIS. **n. of glans penis** COLLUM GLANDIS PENIS. **n. of hair follicle** The part of the hair follicle between the hair bulb and the follicular orifice. Also *collum folliculi pili.* **n. of humerus** COLLUM ANATOMICUM HUMERI. **n. of implant substructure** The vertical projection, from the framework, which carries the abutment and is surrounded by oral mucosa. Also *implant post.* **Madelung's n.** Multiple symmetrical lipomatosis affecting the neck. **n. of malleus** COLLUM MALLEI. **n. of mandible** COLLUM MANDIBULAE. **n. of pancreas** An ill-defined constricted area between the head and the body of the pancreas. It corresponds to a groove on its posterior surface that is formed by the termination of the superior mesenteric vein and the portal vein. **n. of penis** COLLUM GLANDIS PENIS. **n. of radius** COLLUM RADII. **n. of rib** COLLUM COSTAE. **n. of scapula** COLLUM SCAPULAE. **stiff n.** *Popular* MYOGENIC TORTICOLLIS. **surgical n. of humerus** COLLUM CHIRURGICUM HUMERI. **n. of talus** COLLUM TALI. **n. of tooth** A region of a tooth, often slightly constricted, where the crown and the root unite. Also *cervix dentis.* **true n. of humerus** COLLUM ANATOMICUM HUMERI. **n. of urinary bladder** CERVIX VESICAE. **uterine n.** CERVIX UTERI. **n. of uterus** CERVIX UTERI. **webbed n.** A neck that appears to be unusually broad because of bilateral folds of skin extending from the regions of the clavicles to the lower lateral parts of the head. **wry n.** TORTICOLLIS.

**necklace** A band, usually rashlike in character, that surrounds the neck. **Casal's n.** The erythema and pigmentation that characteristically encircles the neck in pellagra. Also *Casal's collar.*

**necr-** \nekr-\ NECRO-.

**necrectomy** \nekrek′təmē\ NECRONECTOMY.

**necro-** \nek′rō-, nek′rə-\ [Gk *nekros* (adjective) dead, (noun) dead body] A combining form meaning (1) dead body, corpse; (2) death; (3) dead, necrotic. Also *necr-, nekro-.*

**necrobacillosis** \-bas′ilō′sis\ [NECRO- + *bacill(us)* + -OSIS] Infection with *Fusobacterium necrophorum,* an anaerobic microorganism which occurs in the normal flora of man and animals and is implicated in a variety of infections in them. It is always associated with necrosis of the affected tissue by virtue of its necrotizing endotoxin. Also *bacillary necrosis.*

**necrobiosis** \-bī·ō′sis\ [NECRO- + BIOSIS] **1** Physiologic, or normal, cell death in the midst of living tissue. Also *bionecrosis.* **2** A pathologic process of incomplete or circumscribed tissue necrosis, especially of the dermis. Adj. necrobiotic. **n. lipoidica** An inflammatory disorder characterized by necrobiosis and chronic inflammation. It usually appears on the lower legs and arises as a rounded, firm, dull red papule which may slowly spread to form large areas with an atrophic, waxy yellow center. It is classically but uncommonly associated with diabetes mellitus, and atypical forms do occur. Also *Urbach-Oppenheim disease, necrobiosis lipoidica diabeticorum.*

**necrocytotoxin** \-sī′tətäk′sin\ A toxin that causes cellular necrosis.

**necrogenic** \-jen′ik\ **1** Capable of causing cell or tissue death. **2** Caused by contact with infective necrotic tissue. For defs. 1 and 2 also *necrogenous.*

**necrologist** \nekräl′əjist\ A specialist in necrology.

**necrology** \nekräl′əjē\ [NECRO- + -LOGY] **1** A list of dead persons, especially the recent dead; an obituary. **2** The study of death statistics. Adj. necrologic.

**necrolysis** \nekräl′isis\ [NECRO- + LYSIS] Dissolution, separation, or exfoliation of dead tissue. *Seldom used.* **toxic epidermal n.** A syndrome in which most of the body surface becomes erythematous and the inflamed and necrotic epidermis strips off. The appearance resembles scalding. In infancy and childhood staphylococci, phage type 71 (Group 2), are often the causative organisms. In adults most cases are due to drug reactions, although staphylococci are occasionally incriminated and in some the etiology is unknown. Also *scalded skin syndrome, Lyell's disease, epidemic exfoliative dermatitis, exfoliative dermatitis of the newborn.*

**necronectomy** \-nek′təmē\ [NECRO- + *n* + -ECTOMY] A surgical procedure in which necrotic tissue is removed or débrided. Also *necrectomy.*

**necrophilia** \-fil′yə\ [NECRO- + -PHILIA] A paraphilia in which sexual arousal is possible only if the sexual object, whether of the same or opposite sex, is dead.

**necrophilous** \nekräf′iləs\ [NECRO- + -PHIL + -OUS ] Growing on dead tissue.

**necropsy** \nek′räpsē\ [NECR- + *-opsy* as in AUTOPSY] AUTOPSY.

**necrose** \nek′rōs\ To undergo or to cause necrosis.

**necroses** \nekrō′sēz\ Plural of NECROSIS.

**necrosis** \nekrō′sis\ [Gk *nekrōsis* (from *nekroun* to mortify, necrose, from *nekros* dead, a corpse) mortification, necrosis] The morphologic changes that follow cell death, characterized most frequently by nuclear changes. These include pyknosis, karyolysis, and karyorrhexis. Cytoplasmic changes that may be seen include increased eosinophilia, vacuolated cytoplasm, and increased cytoplasmic homogeneity. The changes seen are variable and depend on the tissues involved, the causative factors, and the magnitude of the accompanying inflammatory response. **acute tubular n.** Severe damage to the epithelial cells of renal tubules, especially those of the proximal convoluted tubules, characterized by loss of microvilli, endoplasmic reticulum, and often by disruption of the tubular basement membrane. Clinically the condition is characterized by acute renal failure and may follow severe trauma or major surgery, hemorrhagic shock, or toxic drugs or chemicals. In ischemic tubular necrosis, tubular damage may be represented by scattered foci of tubular necrosis. Also *tubular necrosis, Bywaters syndrome, lower nephron nephrosis* (outmoded and imprecise). **arteriolar n.** Necrosis of arterioles as seen in malignant hypertension. The lesion is accompanied by fibrinoid necrosis and characteristically affects the afferent glomerular arterioles. **aseptic n.** Tissue death that is secondary to any pathologic process other than infection. It is most commonly due to ischemia. Also *spontaneous necrosis, quiet necrosis, bland necrosis.* **avascular n.** Necrosis due to inadequate blood supply, frequently used in the context of infarction of the head of the femur. **bacillary n.** NECROBACILLOSIS. **bilateral renal cortical n.** Diffuse ischemic necrosis of both renal cortices due to disseminated intravascular coagulation. Microscopically, fibrin thrombi occlude glomerular capillaries and afferent arterioles, resulting in confluent microinfarcts. Also *cortical necrosis.* **bland n.** ASEPTIC NECROSIS. **caseous n.** The characteristic lesion of tuberculosis, it appears grossly as friable, gray-white areas that resemble cheese. Microscopically, the necrotic cells are not totally liquefied, resulting in eosinophilic, amorphous, granular debris seen within confluent granulomas. Also *cheesy degeneration, caseation.* **central n.** Coagulation necrosis of the central part of an organ or tissue. This term is almost exclusively used to describe necrosis of the liver cells adjacent to the central vein of a lobule, most often due to ischemia resulting from cardiac failure or shock. **chemical n.** Tissue destruction caused by a chemical substance. **coagulation n.** Necrosis in which coagulation of proteins preserves the general shape of cells and solidity of tissue for a time after cell death. It presumably results from denaturation of the proteins, including the enzymes that accomplish the necrotic process itself, but the cause of such denaturation is not well understood. Coagulation necrosis is typical of infarcts in tissues other than those of the brain. Also *coagulative necrosis.* Compare LIQUEFACTION NECROSIS. **colliquative n.** LIQUEFACTION NECROSIS. **cortical n.** BILATERAL RENAL CORTICAL NECROSIS. **coumarin n.** A rare and often lethal form of disseminated intravascular coagulation that occurs following ingestion of a coumarin anticoagulant drug such as warfarin. Gangrene of extremities, breasts, genitalia, or large areas of skin is characteristic. **cystic medial n.** A degenerative condition of the media of the aorta of unknown cause. It tends to give rise to dissecting aneurysm. Also *mucoid medial degeneration, medionecrosis of the aorta, Erdheim's cystic medial necrosis, Erdheim syndrome.* **diphtheritic n.** Local epithelial necrosis caused by infection with *Corynebacterium diphtheriae* and resulting from the inhibition of the normal inflammatory response by the exotoxin produced by the organism. The necrotic tissue, along with an exudate rich in fibrin and a great many bacteria, forms the characteristic pseudomembrane. **embolic n.** Ischemic necrosis due to embolic occlusion of an artery. **epiphysial ischemic n.** Necrosis due to inadequate blood supply of the articular end of a long bone, such as the femoral head. Also *epiphysial aseptic necrosis.* **Erdheim's cystic medial n.** CYSTIC MEDIAL NECROSIS. **fat n.** Abnormal destruction of fat cells due to extracellular lipases as in acute pancreatitis. The enzymes convert the adipose cells' triglycerides into free fatty acids which then complex with calcium to form calcium soaps. Thus, foci of fat necrosis appear chalky white grossly. Also *adiponecrosis.* **fibrinoid n.** Necrosis in which the affected tissue stains deeply eosinophilic, homogeneous, and refractile, resembling fibrin. Most often used in referring to necrosis of blood vessel walls, as in immune complex vasculitis. Here the fibrinoid material represents fibrinogen and other plasma proteins that accumulate due to increased permeability of the damaged vessel wall. Also *fibrinous degeneration.* **gangrenous n.** A clinical term for the combination of coagulation and liquefaction necrosis, most often seen in a lower limb that has become ischemic and secondarily infected. Either coagulation necrosis (dry gangrene) or liquefaction necrosis (wet gangrene) may predominate. **glomerular n.** Necrosis of all or part of a glomerulus, characterized by karyorrhexis and the presence of debris. Total necrosis of a glomerulus follows occlusion of the afferent arteriole, and is characterized by glomerular hemorrhage. **gummatous n.** Coagulative necrosis within the granulomatous inflammatory lesions of tertiary syphilis (gummas). Also *syphilitic necrosis.* **hyaline n.** Segmental necrosis of muscle cells characterized by the eosinophilic, glassy, homogeneous appearance of the affected fibers. It may be seen in prolonged infections such as typhoid fever and hepatitis. This change can be artificially induced by mechanical injury such as that caused by handling of live muscle with dissecting tools. Also *Zenker's necrosis, Zenker's degeneration.* **ischemic n.** Coagulative necrosis due to interruption of blood flow. **laminar cortical n.** Necrosis localized to one or more specific layers of the cerebral cortex, as seen in anoxia. **liquefaction n.** Necrosis characterized by softening and liquefaction of the affected tissue as the result of the action of hydrolytic enzymes released by polymorphonuclear leukocytes in the course of pyogenic bacterial infections. It is also the characteristic type of necrosis seen in brain infarcts. Also *colliquative necrosis.* Compare COAGULATION NECROSIS. **mandibular n.** PHOSSY JAW. **massive hepatic n.** Necrosis of confluent areas of hepatocytes involving entire lobules, usually due to fulminant acute viral hepatitis, hepatotoxins, or drug hypersensitivity. It is accompanied by acute hepatic failure and is almost always fatal. **mechanical n.** Tissue destruction by the forceful disruption of cells or of the blood supply to the tissue. Also *physical necrosis.* **medial n.** Necrosis of the media of an artery. It may lead to rupture. **nephrotoxic tubule n.** Acute tubular necrosis due to a toxic agent. **papillary n.** RENAL PAPILLARY NECROSIS. **peripheral n.** Necrosis of the outer aspect of an organ or structure. • This term may be used to describe necrosis of the periportal areas of the liver lobule, as it occurs in eclampsia and phosphorus poisoning. **phosphorus n.** PHOSSY JAW. **physical n.** MECHANICAL NECROSIS. **postpartum pituitary n.** The adenohypophysial lesion causing the Sheehan syndrome. **pressure n.** Necrosis of a tissue due to interference with its blood supply by external pressure. It is seen especially in decubitus ulcers. **progressive emphysematous n.** GAS GANGRENE. **quiet n.** ASEPTIC NECROSIS. **renal coagulation n.** Coalescing areas of opacification and condensation of cytoplasm with nuclear pyknosis, karyolysis, or karyorrhexis. The cells may desquamate resulting in denuded basement membrane, which is often thickened and sometimes fragmented. Coagulation necrosis may follow renal ischemia or severe trauma. **renal papillary n.** Necrosis of one or more pyramids, characterized clinically by renal colic, pyuria, and acute or chronic renal failure. Roentgenography may show a characteristic appearance. Papillary necrosis may result from pyelonephritis, diabetes mellitus, excessive analgesic drug intake, obstructive uropathy, sickle cell disease, or cyclophosphamide toxicity. Renal papillae may be passed in the urine. Also *papillary necrosis.* **septic n.** Necrosis occurring as a result of infection, usually bacterial. **simple n.** Coagulative necrosis in an aseptic area of the body. **spontaneous n.** ASEPTIC NECROSIS. **subcutaneous fat n.** Ischemic damage to the subcutaneous fat cells in the newborn by trauma, such as pressure of a forceps blade on the cheek or pressure on other parts, resulting in cell necrosis with release of the fat, at first in a solid state. Indurated plaques can be felt in the skin. Later the fat may liquefy or calcify. It is finally dispersed and absorbed. Also *subcutaneous adiponecrosis in infants, pseudosclerema* (obs.), *cytosteatonecrosis.* **subendocardial n.** Diffuse, laminar necrosis of the myocardium subjacent to the endocardial lining. It occurs primarily in the left ventricle, and is due to either hypoperfusion, as in shock, or partial stenosis of a coronary artery. **syphilitic n.** GUMMATOUS NECROSIS. **transmural n.** Necrosis through the entire wall of a hollow viscus, a blood vessel, or the heart, as the necrosis following a transmural myocardial infarct. **tubular n.** ACUTE TUBULAR NECROSIS. **Zenker's n.** HYALINE NECROSIS.

**necrospermia** \-spur′mē·ə\ [NECRO- + SPERM + -IA] A condition in which the sperm in the seminal fluid are nonliving. Also *necrozoospermia.* Compare ZOOSPERMIA.

**necrosteosis** \nekräs′tē·ō′sis\ The pathological processes involved in bone necrosis.

**necrotic** \nekrät′ik\ [Gk *nekrōtikos* causing mortification, necrotizing] Characterized by or pertaining to necrosis.

**necrotize** \nek′rətīz\ To cause necrosis.

**necrotomy** \nekrät′əmē\ [NECRO- + -TOMY] An operative procedure in which a bone sequestrum is removed.

**necrozoospermia** \-zō′əspur′mē·ə\ [NECRO- + ZOOSPERMIA] NECROSPERMIA.

**needle** [Old English *nædl* akin to L *nere* to spin and to Gk *nēn* or *nein* to spin] **1** Any of various long, thin, surgical instruments, hollow or solid, used for aspiration, injection, or suturing. **2** To pierce with a needle, as for the diagnostic or therapeutic aspiration. **aneurysm n.** A large tapered needle that once was used to oversew aneurysms on large blood vessels. **aspirating n.** A long, thin, hollow instrument designed to permit safe removal of fluid or gas from a body cavity. **atraumatic n.** A surgical needle that permits suturing with minimal damage to the tissues being sutured. Its diameter in cross section is smaller than that of the suture material, thus minimizing tissue damage. **biopsy n.** A long, thin, hollow instrument with a sharp point designed to obtain small cores of tissue for diagnostic purposes. **butterfly n.** A small-gauge, thin-walled metal needle with flanges, used for introduction into small veins such as a scalp vein in an infant. **cataract n.** KNIFE NEEDLE. **cutting n.** A long, thin, sharp instrument with triangular or honed edges to permit easy penetration of firm structures. **discission n.** KNIFE NEEDLE. **electrosurgical n.** A needle equipped with a handle and attached to an electric cautery for incising, destroying, or coagulating tissue by means of an electric current. **fascia n.** A large suturing needle with a large eye which can accommodate strips of fascia for use as suture material. **Hagedorn's n.** A curved surgical needle with two cutting edges and a sharp point that was formerly used for suturing. **hypodermic n.** A needle suitable for an injection under the skin. **knife n.** A thin and small surgical knife for incision of the lens capsule. Also *cataract needle, discission needle.* **lumbar puncture n.** A hollow needle used principally for introduction into the spinal subarachnoid space for the purpose of measuring pressure, withdrawing fluid, or injecting a liquid. Also *spinal needle.* **Menghini n.** A long, thin, hollow surgical instrument that is designed to take core samples for biopsy, specifically of the liver, without the need of rotating the device. **radium n.** A needle-pointed tube, 1–2 mm in diameter and 1–5 cm in length, in which is sealed a few milligrams of radium. It is used for interstitial radiation treatments. **Silverman n.** A long, thin, hollow surgical instrument with two moving parts. It is used to take core samples of tissue for biopsy without the need to rotate the device. **spinal n.** LUMBAR PUNCTURE NEEDLE. **stop n.** A long, thin, sharp surgical instrument with a flange that prevents insertion beyond the flange. **swaged n.** A sharp, thin, rodlike surgical device to which suture material is permanently attached for use during an operative procedure. **ventriculopuncture n.** A semisharp, calibrated needle designed for introduction into the cerebral ventricle. **vicat n.** A device used to determine the time required for plaster or other materials to set. **Vim-Silverman n.** A split hollow needle used to obtain a core of tissue from the liver for histologic study.

**Needles** [Carl F. *Needles,* U.S. pediatrician, born 1935] Melnick-Needles syndrome. See under SYNDROME.

**needling** Incision of the lens capsule with a knife needle.

**Neel** [Axel Valdemar *Neel,* Danish physician, 1878–1952] Bing-Neel syndrome. See under SYNDROME.

**Neelsen** [Friedrich Carl Adolf *Neelsen,* German pathologist, 1854–1894] Ziehl-Neelsen carbolfuschin, Ziehl-Neelsen technique. See under ZIEHL-NEELSEN STAIN.

**neencephalon** \nē′ensef′əlän\ [*ne(o)-* + ENCEPHALON] The phylogenetically newer parts of the brain, especially the cerebral cortices. *Seldom used.* Also *neoencephalon* (seldom used).

**NEEP** negative end-expiratory pressure.

**NEFA** nonesterified fatty acids.

**negation** \nega′shən\ The act of denying; denial.

**negative** [L *negativ(us)* (from *negare* to deny + *-ivus* -IVE) expressing a negation, inhibiting] **1** Lacking positive or affirmative character. **2** Characterized by or signifying the absence of a condition, especially one being tested, or the failure of a particular response to occur. **3** A negative finding or result. **false n.** A test result that is negative when the correct result would be positive. **n. G** The pull of gravity toward the head when one is in an upside-down position.

**negatol** A colloidal product obtained from the reaction of metacresolsulfonic acid with formaldehyde. It is applied topically to the cervix as a germicidal, antiparasital, or bacteriostatic agent.

**neglect / senile n.** DIOGENES SYNDROME.

**negligence** [L *neglegentia* (from *neglegere* to disregard, neglect from *nec-* not + *legere* to select) carelessness, neglect] **1** An unintentional failure to perform a legally recognized duty, causing foreseeable injury or loss to another. **2** In medical practice, the failure of a physician to exercise the degree of skill, prudence, and care that would usually and customarily be exercised by other reputable physicians treating the patient in question or a similar patient. Negligence is the basis for most claims of medical malpractice. It includes both acts of commission and omission. **comparative n.** In negligence law, the practice of comparing proven contributory negligence with proven professional negligence to assess degrees of responsibility and determine the proportion of damages. In medical malpractice cases involving proven negligence by both physician and patient, percentages are used to express the relative degree of each party's responsibility. If contributory negligence is responsible for 60% of the injury or loss, then the physician would be responsible for paying 40% of the total assessed damages. **contributory n.** In negligence law as it pertains to medical malpractice, the negligent conduct on the part of the patient concurrent with that of the physician's negligence and constituting a part of the proximate cause of the injury or loss for which damages are being sought.

**Negri** [Adelchi *Negri*, Italian pathologist, 1876–1912] Negri bodies. See under BODY.

**Negri** [Silvio *Negri*, Italian physician, flourished 20th century] Jacod-Negri syndrome. See under PETROSPHENOID SYNDROME.

**Negro** [Camillo *Negro*, Italian neurologist, 1861–1927] **1** Negro's phenomenon. See under COGWHEEL SIGN. **2** See under SIGN.

**Negroid** \nē′groid\ Characterized by or similar to the physical features of the "black" races of man. • The term is usually applied to the major race of Africa but on occasion has been applied to both Africans and to the spiral-haired peoples of southern Asia and Oceania.

**Negus** [Victor Ewings *Negus*, English otorhinolaryngologist, born 1887] **1** See under TUBE, ESOPHAGOSCOPE. **2** Negus hydrostatic dilator. See under DILATOR.

**neighborwise** \nā′bərwīz\ In embryology, in a manner similar to that prevailing locally: said of the development of transplanted cells when they adopt the behavior prevalent in their new surroundings.

**Neill** [James Maffett *Neill*, U.S. bacteriologist, born 1894] Van Slyke and Neill method. See under METHOD.

**Neill** [Mather Humphrey *Neill*, U.S. physician, 1882–1930] Neill-Mooser reaction. See under SCROTAL REACTION.

**Neisser** [Max *Neisser*, German bacteriologist, 1869–1938] Neisser-Wechsberg phenomenon. See under COMPLEMENT DEVIATION.

***Neisseria*** \nīsir′ē·ə\ [after Albert Ludwig Siegmund *Neisser*, German bacteriologist and physician, 1855–1916 + -IA] A genus of aerobic, fastidious, small, Gram-negative diplococci whose cultivation requires elevated concentrations of carbon dioxide and protection (by serum, starch, or charcoal) against inhibitory traces of detergents and ions of heavy metals. The major pathogens are *N. gonorrhoeae* and *N. meningitidis*. Related nonpathogens or rare pathogens, also in the family Neisseriaceae, include species of *Acinetobacter, Moraxella*, and *Veillonella*. ***N. catarrhalis*** A frequent and nonpathogenic inhabitant of the nasopharynx, easily mistaken for the meningococcus. ***N. gonorrhoeae*** The species that causes gonorrhea; the gonococcus. There are many types based on heterogeneity in the outer membrane proteins, pili, and lipopolysaccharide. Piliated strains enter and multiply in cells of the epithelial mucosae. In purulent discharges the organisms are directly recognized as Gram-negative intracellular diplococci, in leukocytes. ***N. lactamica*** A nonpathogenic species often found in the nasopharynx of children. It closely resembles *N. meningitidis* except that it ferments lactose. ***N. meningitidis*** A species of a Gram-negative diplococci frequently present in the normal nasopharynx; the meningococci. There are several groups based on a polysaccharide capsule, and several types based on a surface protein. Group A is the main cause of epidemics of meningitis. Groups B and C cause endemic cases.

**neisseria** \nīser′ē·ə\ (*pl.* neisseriae) Any organism of the genus *Neisseria*.

**neisseriology** \nīser′ē·äl′əjē\ [*Neisseri(a)* + *o* + -LOGY] The scientific study of gonorrhea.

**nekro-** \nek′rō-, nek′rə-\ NECRO-.

**Nélaton** [Auguste *Nélaton*, French surgeon, 1807–1873] **1** Nélaton's catheter. See under FLEXIBLE CATHETER. **2** See under TUMOR, DISLOCATION, LINE. **3** Nélaton sphincter. See under FOLD.

**nelavane** \nel′əvān\ **1** GAMBIAN TRYPANOSOMIASIS. **2** RHODESIAN TRYPANOSOMIASIS.

**Nelson** [Don H. *Nelson*, U.S. internist, born 1925] See under SYNDROME.

**nem** \nem\ [German *Nahrungs Einheit Milch* nutritional unit milk] A unit of nutrition; the amount of an infant food equivalent in nutritional value to 1 gram of breast milk.

**nemat-** \nem′ət-\ NEMATO-.

**nemathelminth** \nem′əthel′minth\ [NEMAT- + HELMINTH] NEMATODE.

**Nemathelminthes** \nem′əthelmin′thēz\ [NEMAT- + Gk *helminthes*, pl. of *helmins* worm] NEMATODA.

**nematicide** \nəmat′isīd\ NEMATOCIDE.

**nemato-** \nem′ətō-\ [Gk *nēma* (genitive *nematos*) thread, yarn, tissue] A combining form meaning (1) thread, threadlike; (2) nematode. Also *nemat-*.

**nematoblast** \nem′ətōblast′\ [NEMATO- + -BLAST] SPERMATID.

**Nematocera** \nem′ətäs′ərə\ [NEMATO- + Gk *kera(s)* horn] A suborder of the order Diptera comprising the most primitive flies, characterized by antennae with numerous segments. It includes gnats, mosquitoes, midges, blackflies, crane flies, and gallflies.

**nematocide** \nəmat′əsīd\ [NEMATO- + -CIDE] An agent that kills nematodes. Also *nematicide*.

**Nematoda** \nem′ətō′də\ [See NEMATODE.] A phylum of helminths characterized by an extremely protective cuticular wall, a tapered cylindrical shape, muscles oriented longitudinally, and a triradiate esophagus. It includes both parasitic and nonparasitic species, the latter being the more common and including both soil and aquatic forms. The two major taxonomic groups are based on the presence or absence of olfactory caudal organs called phasmids. Roundworms such as *Ancylostoma, Ascaris, Enterobius*, and the blood and tissue filarial roundworms are placed in the phasmidial class Secernentea (formerly called Phasmidia) while the nonphasmidial nematodes, which include *Trichinella, Trichuris, Capillaria*, and *Dioctophyma*, are in the class Adenophorea (formerly called Aphasmidia). Also *Nemathelminthes*.

**nematode** \nem′ətōd\ [Gk *nēmatōdēs* (from *nēma*, gen. *nēmatos* thread) filamentous, threadlike] **1** Of or belonging to the phylum Nematoda. **2** A member of the phylum Nematoda; a roundworm. Also *nemathelminth*.

**nematodiasis** \nem′ətōdī′əsis\ [*nematod(e)* + -IASIS] Infection by a nematode. Also *nematodosis, nematosis*. **nonpatent n.** VISCERAL LARVA MIGRANS.

**nematodosis** \nem′ətōdō′sis\ NEMATODIASIS.

**nematoid** \nem′ətoid\ [*nemat(ode)* + -OID] **1** Resembling a nematode. **2** A nematode; a member of the Nematoidea (Nematoda).

**nematologist** \nem′ətäl′əjist\ A specialist in nematology.

**nematology** \nem′ətäl′əjē\ [NEMATO- + -LOGY] The scientific study of nematode worms, including subspecialties related to agriculture, medicine, genetics, and biological control.

**nematosis** \nem′ətō′sis\ NEMATODIASIS.

**nematospermia** \nem′ətōspur′mē·ə\ [NEMATO- + SPERM- + -IA] A trait, possessed by man, of producing spermatozoa with long, slender tails.

**Nembutal** A proprietary name for pentobarbital sodium.

**neo-** \nē′ō-\ [Gk *neos* new, youthful] A combining form meaning new.
**neoantigen** \-an′təjən\ Antigenic determinants that are produced when a protein (or other antigenic substance) is chemically attached to another protein (or to a cell) but that are not found in either of the two components of the reaction when not chemically combined.
**neoantimosan** STIBOPHEN.
**neoarsphenamine** $C_{13}H_{13}As_2N_2NaO_4S$. [5-[(3-Amino-4 hydroxy-phenol)arseno]-2-hydroxyanilino]methonol sulfoxylate sodium. A soluble compound containing arsphenamine, formerly used as a major antisyphilitic medication. Also *novarsenobenzene, novarsenobenzol.*
**neoarthrosis** \-ärthrō′sis\ A new joint, as a pseudarthrosis or a surgically placed artificial joint. Also *nearthrosis.*
**neoblastic** \-blas′tik\ [Gk *neoblast(os)* (from *neo-* new + *blastos* a shoot, sprout) sprouting anew + -IC] Of or relating to the development of new tissue.
**neocerebellum** \-ser′əbel′əm\ [NA] The largest and phylogenetically newest part of the cerebellum, including all of the cerebellum between the primary fissure anteriorly and the posterolateral fissure posteriorly. • Although the midline vermis is included, the term is used most often in reference to the cerebellar hemispheres, which are especially related to the coordination of skilled movements initiated at cortical levels.
**neocinetic** \-sinet′ik\ NEOKINETIC.
**neocortex** \-kôr′teks\ ISOCORTEX. Adj. neocortical.
**neocystostomy** \-sistäs′təmē\ [NEO- + CYSTOSTOMY] The creation of a new opening in the urinary bladder to permit drainage. **ureteral n.** The creation of a new connection between a ureter and the urinary bladder. **ureteroileal n.** A surgically created opening between the urinary bladder and one or both ureters, utilizing a segment of defunctionalized ileum for drainage from the bladder.
**neocyte** \nē′əsīt\ An immature erythrocyte, especially a reticulocyte.
**neocytosis** \-sītō′sis\ The presence of immature erythrocytes, especially reticulocytes, in the circulating blood.
**neodarwinism** \-där′winizm\ A blending of the darwinian concept of the survival of the fittest and mendelian laws of heredity. This is a modern view of natural selection and survival of the fittest.
**neodentatum** \-dentā′təm\ That portion of the dentate nucleus of the cerebellum which exclusively receives fibers from the cerebellar hemisphere.
**neodymium** An element of the lanthanide series, having atomic number 60 and atomic weight 144.24. It has limited use, chiefly in manufacturing colored glass. Its compounds are moderately toxic. Symbol: Nd
**neoencephalon** \-ensef′əlän\ *Seldom used* NEENCEPHALON.
**neofetus** \-fē′təs\ The fetus when it has just been formed at the end of the embryonic period at about the eighth week of human intrauterine development. Adj. neofetal.
**neoformation** \-fôrmā′shən\ [NEO- + FORMATION] NEOPLASM.
**neoformative** \-fôr′mətiv\ Pertaining to a newly formed structure or to a neoplasm.
**Neofrakt** A system of pouring polyurethane foam into a cotton stocking to produce casts, splints, braces, and temporary artificial limbs. A proprietary name.
**neogala** \nē·äg′ələ\ [NEO- + Gk *gala* milk] COLOSTRUM.
**neogenesis** \-jen′əsis\ [NEO- + GENESIS] New formation or growth; regeneration. Adj. neogenetic.
**neoglottis** \-glät′is\ PHONATORY NEOGLOTTIS. **phonatory n.** A hypopharyngeal fistula constructed at the upper end of the trachea after total laryngectomy and serving as a new glottis. Also *neoglottis.*
**neokinetic** \-kinet′ik\ [*neo(cortical)* + KINETIC] Describing or pertaining to the pyramidal (corticospinal) motor system which controls voluntary movement. Also *neocinetic.*
**neologism** \nē·äl′əjizm\ [NEO- + LOG- + -ISM] **1** A newly coined word or phrase. **2** In psychiatry, the practice of using neologisms that are typically obscure or incomprehensible to others, thus constituting an impediment to communication.
**neomalthusianism** \-malthoo′sē·ənizm\ [NEO- + MALTHUSIANISM] A doctrine which advocates birth control, abortion, and sterilization, together or separately, in order to curb population growth. Also *malthusianism.*
**neomembrane** \-mem′brān\ PSEUDOMEMBRANE.
**neomin** \nē′ōmin\ NEOMYCIN.
**neomorph** \nē′ōmôrf\ [NEO- + -MORPH] An entirely new feature or characteristic that has recently appeared in the course of evolutionary development.
**neomycin** \-mī′sin\ An antibacterial substance obtained from the metabolic products of *Streptomyces fradiae* and active against a variety of Gram-negative and Gram-positive microorganisms. The sulfate salt is administered orally and applied topically. The drug may produce ototoxicity and nephrotoxicity. Also *nyacyne, neomin.*
**neomycin palmitate** The palmitate salt of neomycin. It is applied topically as an antibacterial agent in the treatment of skin infections, burns, wounds, and ulcers.
**neomycin sulfate** The sulfate salt of neomycin. It is a white or slightly yellow powder, used as an anti-infective agent for the treatment of urinary tract, skin, eye, ear, and enteric infections. It is also used for preoperative disinfection. It may be administered orally, topically, or intramuscularly.
**neomycin undecenoate** The undecenoic acid derivative of neomycin. It has the same properties and uses as the sulfate, and it is used primarily in ear drops for the treatment of otitis externa. Also *neomycin undecylenate.*
**neon** Element number 10, having atomic weight 20.179. Neon is a colorless, odorless gas, occurring uncombined in the atmosphere in a ratio of about 15 parts per million. Three stable isotopes occur, and five radioactive isotopes have been described. The valence is 0. Symbol: Ne
**neonatal** \-nā′təl\ [NEO- + NATAL] Of or relating to a newborn infant from birth to the 28th day, or to this period of life.
**neonate** \nē′ōnāt\ [New L *neonatus,* from NEO- + L *natus* born] An infant during the first four weeks of postnatal life. Also *newborn.* • Although the first 28 days of life comprise the usual period designating a *neonate* or *newborn,* for statistical purposes some have reckoned the period as the first 7 days. The term *early neonate* has been used to describe the first week of life.
**neonatologist** \-nātäl′əjist\ A physician specializing in neonatology.
**neonatology** \-nātäl′əjē\ [*neonat(e)* + *o* + -LOGY] The branch of medicine dealing with the newborn infant and its diseases, as well as its physical and psychological care, assessment, and development. Also *neonatal medicine.*
**neo-olive** \-äl′iv\ The largest and phylogenetically newest portion of the inferior olivary nucleus of the medulla oblongata, comprising the lateral two thirds of the principal olivary nucleus.
**neopallium** \-pal′ē·əm\ ISOCORTEX.
**neophasia** \-fā′zhə\ The invention of one or more new languages by a subject who alone knows the grammar, syn-

tax, or vocabulary of the invented tongue. It is a rare phenomenon that has been reported in expansive paranoia and mania.

**neoplasia** \-plā′zhə\ [NEO- + -PLASIA] The process of tumor formation. **multiple endocrine n.** Any of a group of uncommon syndromes characterized by benign or malignant tumors of more than one endocrine gland. Type I (MEN I, sometimes called Lloyd syndrome) includes lesions of the parathyroids, the adenohypophysis (hypopituitarism or acromegaly), the pancreas ($\beta$ cells and non-$\beta$ cells, hypoglycemia, hypergastrinemia) and, less commonly, the adrenal cortex and thyroid. Zollinger-Ellison syndrome is often associated. The familial form of MEN I is known as the Wermer syndrome. Type II (MEN II) comprises tumors of the thyroid (medullary carcinoma) and the adrenal medulla (pheochromocytoma) and chief cell hyperplasia of the parathyroids. The familial form of MEN II is known as the Sipple syndrome. Type III, sometimes considered part of Type II, includes thyroid carcinoma (medullary), pheochromocytoma, and associated neurologic abnormalities, mucosal neuromas, and hyperplastic corneal nerves. Also *multiple endocrine adenomatosis, polyendocrine adenomatosis, pluriglandular adenomatosis, pluriglandular syndrome, endocrine adenomatosis, familial polyendocrine adenomatosis, multiple endocrine adenomas, polyendocrinoma, endocrine polyglandular syndrome, polyglandular syndrome.* Abbr. MEN

**neoplasm** \nē′ōplazm\ [NEO- + -PLASM] A benign or malignant expanding lesion composed of proliferating cells; a tumor. Also *neoformation, new growth, histioma* (obs.), *histoma* (obs.), *true tumor, oncoma.* **benign n.** A neoplasm that cannot metastasize. It typically grows in an expansile manner, displacing or compressing surrounding tissues rather than invading them. **malignant n.** CANCER. **metastatic n.** **1** A primary neoplasm which has metastasized. **2** A neoplasm at a secondary (metastatic) site. **trophoblastic n.** Any of a group of biologically and morphologically interrelated tumors of trophoblastic tissue that arise either from pregnancy (gestational) or from ovary, testes, or extragonadal tissues (nongestational).

**neoplastic** \-plas′tik\ [Gk *neoplast(ēs)* (from *neo-* new + *plas(sein)* to form) newly formed + -IC] Pertaining to a tumor or tumor formation.

**neoplastigenic** \-plas′tijen′ik\ [NEO- + -PLAST + *i* + -GENIC] ONCOGENIC.

***Neorickettsia helminthoeca*** \-riket′sē·ə hel′minthē′kə\ A rickettsial species responsible for poisoning dogs and other mammals that eat raw salmon infected with the metacercariae of a nanophyetid fluke *(Nanophyetes salmincola)* that harbors the rickettsial organisms. About 90 percent of infected dogs die, but those that recover usually have a lifelong immunity.

**neostigmine bromide** The bromide salt of neostigmine. It is a white, crystalline powder, used as a cholinergic drug in the symptomatic treatment of myasthenia gravis. It is also used as a miotic, and may be given orally or applied topically to the conjunctiva.

**neostigmine methylsulfate** The methylsulfate salt of neostigmine. It is a white, crystalline powder, used as a reversible cholinesterase inhibitor in the symptomatic treatment of myasthenia gravis. It is also used for urinary retention and as an antidote for excessive treatment with curare. It is given either intravenously or subcutaneously.

**neostomy** \nē·äs′təmē\ [NEO- + -STOMY] The creation of an artificial opening into any organ or body cavity.

**neostriatum** \-strī·ā′təm\ The phylogenetically newest parts of the corpus striatum that share a common origin, including the caudate nucleus and the putamen. Also *striatum.*

**neostrophingic** \-strōfin′jik\ [NEO- + Gk *stroph(ē)* a turning + English *(h)ing(e)* + -IC] Of or relating to the surgical relief of mitral stenosis by rehinging the septal leaflet. The procedure is performed by extending the arcuate line of valve closure.

**neotenin** \nē·ät′ənin\ JUVENILE HORMONE.

**neoteny** \nē·ät′ənē\ [NEO- + New L *-ten(ia)*, combining form from Gk *teinein* to extend + -Y] The extension of the larval state, such as occurs in certain termite castes which hold larvae as future replacements of the queen. This condition can be induced under laboratory conditions by injection of the juvenile hormone neotenin into developing insects, which inhibits the maturation process stimulated by the opposing growth and differentiation hormone, ecdysone. Compare PEDOGENESIS.

**neothalamus** \-thal′əməs\ The phylogenetically newest part of the thalamus, especially the ventrolateral and dorsolateral nuclei. • These were formerly contrasted with the so-called paleothalamus, or medial and midline nuclei, which were not believed to project to the neocortex. Reciprocal connections between these medial thalamic structures and the neocortex are now known to exist, so that the term has essentially lost its significance.

**neovascular** \-vas′kyələr\ Pertaining to or characterized by newly formed vessels.

**neovascularization** \-vas′kyəler′īzā′shən\ The formation of new blood vessels in abnormal locations, as in diabetic retinopathy, or in abnormal tissues, as in tumors.

**nepenthic** \nipen′thik\ [Gk *nēpenth(es)* (from *nē-*, negative prefix + *penthos* grief, misery) a drug that alleviates grief and misery + -IC] **1** Producing peace, tranquility, or forgetfulness. **2** A nepenthic drug or agent.

**nephelometer** \nef′əläm′ətər\ [Gk *nephel(ē)* a cloud + *o* + -METER] A photometer designed to estimate the amount of particulate matter in a turbid medium, measuring light-scattering properties to make comparisons with a series of standard suspensions. Also *suspensiometer.* **photoelectric n.** A nephelometer in which the scattered light falls upon and is measured by a photoelectric cell.

**nephr-** \nefr-\ NEPHRO-.

**nephralgia** \nefral′jə\ [NEPHR- + -ALGIA] Pain in the renal area.

**nephrectasia** \nef′rektā′zhə\ [NEPHR- + ECTASIA] Distension of the renal pelvis, usually secondary to obstruction.

**nephrectomy** \nəfrek′təmē\ [NEPHR- + -ECTOMY] The resection of one or both kidneys. **abdominal n.** A nephrectomy using an anterior, transperitoneal approach. Also *anterior nephrectomy.* **lumbar n.** A nephrectomy using a posterior, retroperitoneal approach through a flank incision. Also *paraperitoneal nephrectomy, posterior nephrectomy.* **radical n.** Total removal of the kidney and surrounding tissues, usually as a surgical treatment of cancer of the kidney. **simple n.** Surgical removal of the kidney without the removal of surrounding tissues characteristic of radical nephrectomy. **transthoracic n.** The resection of one or both kidneys by making an incision in the chest and exposing the kidneys through the diaphragm.

**nephric** \nef′rik\ [NEPHR- + -IC] Of or relating to the kidney; renal.

**nephritic** \nefrit′ik\ Of, relating to, or affected by nephritis.

**nephritides** \nefrit′idēz\ Plural of NEPHRITIS.

# nephritis

**nephritis** \nəfrī′tis\ [Gk, short for *nephritis nosos*, kidney disease, from adj. *nephritis*, fem. of *nephrītēs* renal (from *nephros* kidney) + *nosos* disease] Inflammation of the kidney, involving the parenchyma, interstitium, or vascular system of the organ. **acute n.** ACUTE DIFFUSE GLOMERULONEPHRITIS. **acute focal n.** An acute process involving the glomeruli or the renal interstitium in a focal distribution. **acute serum sickness n.** Acute nephritis occurring in the course of serum sickness. It is characterized clinically by the acute nephritic syndrome with oliguria and hematuria; and pathologically by acute diffuse proliferative glomerulonephritis, with immunofluorescent and electromicroscopic evidence of immune complex pathogenesis. Serum complement is reduced. This form of nephritis can be readily produced in experimental animals by two appropriately spaced injections of a foreign protein. Immune complex reaction to penicillin may be a close approximation of serum sickness nephritis. **acute suppurative n.** RENAL ABSCESS. **allergic n.** **1** Acute renal parenchymal, interstitial, or vascular hypersensitivity reaction to a drug or food. **2** An inflammatory reaction produced in the kidney by an immunologic mechanism. **anaphylactoid purpura n.** SCHÖNLEIN-HENOCH PURPURA NEPHRITIS. **antiglomerular basement membrane antibody n.** GOODPASTURE SYNDROME. **antitubular basement membrane tubulointerstitial n.** Tubulointerstitial nephritis due to antibodies directed against tubular basement membrane material. Such antibodies and disease may be produced in experimental animals. Antitubular basement membrane antibodies have been demonstrated in association with antiglomerular basement membrane antibodies in the Goodpasture syndrome, methicillin poisoning, and renal transplant rejection, or alone in some instances of tubulointerstitial nephritis. **arteriosclerotic n.** ARTERIONEPHROSCLEROSIS. **bacterial n.** PYELONEPHRITIS. **Balkan n.** A chronic progressive interstitial nephritis characterized by focal tubular atrophy, and interstitial edema and infiltration leading to interstitial fibrosis and contracted kidneys. The disease occurs only in the area where Yugoslavia, Rumania, and Bulgaria meet. The geographical distribution suggests some toxin but the etiology remains unknown. Clinically, the disease is characterized by impaired concentrating ability, mild proteinuria, tubular acidosis, and progressive renal failure, along with high incidence of papillary transition cell carcinoma in the renal pelvis and upper ureter. Also *Balkan nephropathy*. **chronic n.** Slowly progressive nephritis with persistent proteinuria and often microscopic hematuria and cylinduria. Progressive renal insufficiency eventually is complicated by uremia, hypertension, edema, and visual disturbances. Renal functions are decreased. Anatomically, the kidneys usually are small with a granular surface. Microscopically, hyalinized glomeruli are associated with vascular sclerosis, interstitial fibrosis, and tubule degeneration. Chronic nephritis may follow acute nephritis or a number of other renal diseases, or may be idiopathic. Most instances of chronic nephritis are glomerular or vascular in origin. **chronic interstitial n.** Renal insterstitial cellular infiltration, fibrosis, and tubular damage. Glomerular involvement occurs only in the late stages. Clinical manifestations include little or no proteinuria, minimal pyuria, impaired concentrating ability, and slowly progressive renal failure with acidosis and inability to conserve sodium. The condition may occur in infections, ischemia, analgesic abuse, sickle cell anemia, urinary tract obstruction, and Balkan nephritis. **chronic suppurative n.** Chronic abscesses in one or both kidneys. **congenital n.** Nephritis present at birth. It is often a result of congenital syphilis. **degenerative n.** *Obs.* LIPOID NEPHROSIS. **diffuse n.** Nephritis characterized by lesions involving all nephrons. **diffuse suppurative n.** Multiple abscesses in one or both kidneys. **embolic n.** FOCAL EMBOLIC GLOMERULONEPHRITIS. **epidemic n.** Acute nephritis which occurs in epidemics. Former epidemics were of unknown etiology, but in recent years epidemics of poststreptococcal acute glomerulonephritis have been associated with nephritogenic group A hemolytic streptococcal infections of the skin or pharynx. **exudative n.** Any renal lesion with leukocytic infiltration. **familial n.** HEREDITARY NEPHRITIS. **familial hemorrhagic n.** HEREDITARY NEPHRITIS. **focal embolic n.** FOCAL EMBOLIC GLOMERULONEPHRITIS. **glomerular n.** GLOMERULONEPHRITIS. **n. gravidarum** NEPHRITIS OF PREGNANCY. **hemorrhagic n.** Nephritis in which the predominant symptom is hematuria. **hereditary n.** A genetically heterogenous group of disorders characterized by familial nephropathy of various types, with or without other organ involvement. It includes the Alport syndrome and familial nephropathy with and without gout. Also *familial nephritis, familial hemorrhagic nephritis, familial nephropathy, hereditary hematuria*. **hereditary n. and nerve deafness** A genetically heterogenous group of disorders characterized by progressive nephritis, variable sensorineural deafness, and variable ocular abnormalities. X-linked and, perhaps, autosomal recessive forms occur, as well as an autosomal dominant form known as the Alport syndrome. **Heymann's n.** An experimental disease in rats produced by injection of homologous kidney extract and Freund's adjuvant. The disease is due to deposition of circulating complexes of autoantibodies and autologous antigens from renal tubular epithelial cells. Also *Heymann's nephrosis*. **interstitial n.** **1** Acute or chronic nephritis characterized by primary or secondary inflammation of the renal interstitium. The acute form can be due to an adverse reaction to a drug, acute deposition of uric acid, a remote reaction to an infection, or to direct pyogenic suppuration. The chronic form involves variable degrees of interstitial cellular infiltration and fibrosis with early damage to the lower tubules and late glomerular damage. Proteinuria is usually minimal. Hypertension may be a late development. The chronic form is common in many conditions including analgesic abuse, drug hypersensitivities, infections, ischemia, sickle-cell anemia, hypokalemia, hyperkalemia, and urinary-tract obstruction. Also *tubulointerstitial nephritis*. **2** NEPHROSCLEROSIS. **interstitial granulomatous n.** Nephritis characterized by focal distribution of granulomas in the renal interstitium. It may be caused by a variety of chronic infections such as tuberculosis, syphilis, brucellosis, or mycoses, by accumulations of urate crystals, or by surrounding casts in distal tubules in multiple myeloma. Granulomas are characterized by giant cells, mononuclear cells, and increased fibrous tissue. **interstitial nonsuppurative n.** Nephritis characterized by infiltration of the renal interstitium by inflammatory cells and edema fluid in the acute stage. Later, interstitial fibrosis may develop. The disease may develop acutely in the course of an infection or as a reaction to a drug. The chronic form may follow as the acute phase subsides or may develop insidiously. Differentiation from chronic pyelonephritis is difficult if not impossible. **interstitial scarlatinal n.** An acute, nonsuppurative, interstitial nephritis, once a common complication of scarlet fever. It has almost disappeared since the advent of antibiotic therapy. **interstitial suppurative n.** Infection of the renal parenchyma, either of hematogenous origin or secondary to ascending extension of a urinary tract infection. **interstitial syphilitic n.** **1** Nephritis of congenital syphilis characterized by periglomerular and periarterial fibrosis. **2** Nephritis of syphilis in infants, characterized by gummas in the renal interstitium. **latent n.** The asymptomatic phase of chronic glomerulonephritis. **leptospiral n.** Leptospirosis involving the kidney with distal convoluted tubule dilatation, necrosis, and basement membrane rupture in the early stages, and later with interstitial edema and infiltration with lymphocytes, neutrophils, plasma cells and histiocytes. Glomerular lesions occur late and are nonspecific. Hemorrhages into the renal parenchyma characterize the later phases of severe cases, and acute tubular necrosis is a serious complication. Clinically, renal involvement is manifested by proteinuria, hematuria, pyuria, and rapidly progressive renal failure. Recovery of renal function in survivors is the rule, although some permanent impairment of concentrating ability is common. Leptospira may be recovered from the blood and urine in the acute phase. **Löhlein's n.** FOCAL EMBOLIC GLOMERULONEPHRITIS. **lupus n.** Any of the several forms of glomerulonephritis that may occur during the course of systemic lupus erythematosus. Focal glomerulonephritis is associated with little proteinuria, microscopic hematuria, and little impairment of renal function. The prognosis usually is good, but the condition may become more diffuse and lead to renal failure. Diffuse proliferative glomerulonephritis is more serious and is characterized by more proteinuria, hematuria, cylinduria, and renal functional impairment. A third variety of lupus nephritis is diffuse membranous glomerulopathy and a fourth is membranoproliferative glomerulonephritis. Both have an intermediate prognosis. These forms are mesangial IgA/IgG glomerulonephritis and arteritis. The pathogenesis of all forms of lupus nephritis is assumed to be related to circulating immune complexes. IgG, other immunoglobulins, and complement components are easily demonstrable in glomeruli by immunofluorescent techniques. Serum complement fractions are reduced in active forms of proliferative lupus nephritis. Treatment with steroid hormones and immunosuppressive agents appears to be effective. Recently, plasmapheresis plus immunosuppression have appeared promising. **Masugi n.** An experimental glomerulonephritis produced in rats by injections of heterologous antibodies against glomerular basement membrane material. The lesion is characterized by continuous accumulation of immunoglobulins and complement components along the glomerular capillary basement membranes. This was the original model for immunologically produced glomerulonephritis. Also *nephrotoxic nephritis.* **pneumococcal n.** Acute nephritis following a pneumococcal infection. It has been described clinically in a few cases but only rarely has concomitant group A hemolytic streptococcal infection been ruled out. **poststreptococcal n.** POSTSTREPTOCOCCAL ACUTE GLOMERULONEPHRITIS. **potassium-losing n.** Any chronic nephritis in which deficient tubular reabsorption of potassium leads to a negative potassium balance. Only moderate impairment of renal function may be present, proteinuria usually is minimal, and muscle weakness and characteristic electrocardiographic changes reflect potassium deficiency. **n. of pregnancy** Any nephritic condition occuring during pregnancy, excluding toxemia of pregnancy. Also *nephritis gravidarum.* **radiation n.** Interstitial nephritis and arteriolar lesions with chronic progressive renal failure and often hypertension resulting from irradiation of a kidney exceeding 2300 rads. **salt-losing n.** A syndrome in patients with chronic nephritis who lose excess amounts of sodium chloride in the urine, characterized by polyuria, hyponatremia, dehydration, asthenia, muscle cramps, nausea, and vomiting. Diagnostic criteria include appearance of symptoms of dehydration on normal salt intake, and control of symptoms by saline administration. Also *salt-wasting nephritis.* **saturnine n.** Nephritis due to chronic lead poisoning. **scarlatinal n.** Acute glomerulonephritis secondary to scarlet fever. **Schönlein-Henoch purpura n.** Glomerulonephritis in the form of glomerular lesions associated with Schönlein-Henoch purpura. The disease is commoner and usually less severe in young persons than in adults. By immunofluorescent techniques IgA and C3, and sometimes IgG, can be demonstrated in a granular pattern in the mesangium. The lesions are similar to those of IgA nephropathy. Also *anaphylactoid purpura nephritis.* **shunt n.** A glomerulonephritis probably of immune complex pathogenesis secondary to infection of a ventriculoatrial, ventriculojugular, or ventriculoperitoneal shunt established in a child, or sometimes an adult, to correct internal hydrocephalus, and usually consisting of diffuse proliferative, membranous or mesangiocapillary lesions. The clinical findings include proteinuria, microhematuria, and renal function impairment. Serum C3 levels usually are low and rheumatoid factor and cryoglobulins often are present. The infecting organism most frequently is a coagulase-negative staphylococcus, but numerous other organisms have been implicated. Early recognition and appropriate antibiotic therapy are important and may lead to healing of the glomerular lesions. **Steblay n.** AUTOIMMUNE GLOMERULONEPHRITIS. **subacute n.** RAPIDLY PROGRESSIVE GLOMERULONEPHRITIS. **suppurative n.** Abscesses in one or both kidneys. **suppurative cortical n.** Multiple abscesses in the renal cortex, usually due to staphylococci. **syphilitic n.** Glomerular lesions which may develop with or without the nephrotic syndrome in both congenital and secondary syphilis. The lesions usually are membranous, often with some degree of proliferation. Granular deposits of IgG and complement suggest an immune-complex pathogenesis. Elution of antitreponemal antibody from the glomeruli of a man with acquired syphilis supports this hypothesis. The lesions have been reported to resolve after penicillin therapy. However, spontaneous resolution also has been reported. Gummas of the kidney may develop in tertiary syphilis. **transfusion n.** Acute tubular necrosis and renal failure secondary to intravascular hemolysis in a mismatched blood transfusion. **trench n.** WAR NEPHRITIS. **tubular n.** Renal disease affecting the renal tubules. It occurs in renal tubular acidosis, the Fanconi syndrome, acute renal failure, and tubulointerstitial nephritis. **tubulointerstitial n.** INTERSTITIAL NEPHRITIS. **war n.** Acute epidemic nephritis occurring under war conditions as in the American Civil War and in World War I, presumably due to group A hemolytic streptococci. Also *trench nephritis.* **water-losing n.** NEPHROGENIC DIABETES INSIPIDUS.

**nephritogenic** \nef′ritōjen′ik\ [*nephrit(is)* + *o* + -GENIC] Causing nephritis: said of conditions, or of agents such as strains of group A hemolytic streptococci that cause acute glomerulonephritis.

**nephro-** \nef′rō-, nef′rə-\ [Gk *nephros* kidney] A combining form denoting the kidney. Also *nephr-*.

**nephroblastoma** \-blastō′mə\ [NEPHRO- + BLASTOMA] A malignant renal tumor of nephroblastic tissue forming structures which resemble embryonic kidney. It is typically a tumor of childhood. Also *Wilms tumor, adenosarcoma, embryonal adenosarcoma* (outmoded), *embryonal nephroma, malignant nephroma.*

**nephrocapsulectomy** \-kap′s$^y$əlek′təmē\ The removal of the renal capsule from one or both kidneys; decapsulation of the kidney. Also *nephrocapsectomy.*

**nephrocapsulotomy** \-kap′s$^y$əlät′əmē\ An incision into the renal capsule of one or both kidneys for the purpose of exploration or decompression.

**nephrocele** \nef′rəsēl\ [NEPHRO- + -CELE[1]] A hernia containing a kidney.

**nephrocoele** \nef′rəsēl\ [NEPHRO- + -COELE] The cavity of the nephrotome in an embryo.

**nephrocolopexy** \-kō′ləpek′sē\ A surgical procedure in which the kidney and colon are sutured to the nephrocolic ligament for the purpose of suspension or prevention of ptosis.

**nephrogenesis** \-jen′əsis\ [NEPHRO- + GENESIS] The formation of a kidney or of renal tissue.

**nephrogenic** \-jen′ik\ [NEPHRO- + -GENIC] Developing kidney tissue. Also *renogenic, nephropoietic.*

**nephrogenous** \nefräj′ənəs\ [NEPHRO- + -GENOUS] Pertaining to or originating in the kidneys.

**nephrogram** \nef′rəgram\ [NEPHRO- + -GRAM] The appearance of renal parenchymal opacification during intravenous urography or renal angiography.

**nephrography** \nefräg′rəfē\ [NEPHRO- + -GRAPHY] Radiography of the kidney whose parenchyma has been opacified by appropriate iodinated contrast medium intravascularly administered. **isotope n.** An inaccurate term for RADIORENOGRAPHY.

**nephroid** \nef′roid\ Resembling the shape or nature of a kidney. Also *reniform.*

**nephrolith** \nef′rəlith\ [NEPHRO- + -LITH] RENAL CALCULUS.

**nephrolithiasis** \-lithī′əsis\ The presence of renal calculi. Calcarous stones account for approximately 90 percent of cases, and usually are secondary to hypercalciuria due to excess resorption of bone, increased intestinal absorption of calcium, or impaired renal tubule reabsorption of calcium. Hyperuricemia hyperoxaluria also may lead formation of calcarous stones. Noncalcarous stones may be formed by uric acid, cystine, or xanthine. Also *renal lithiasis.* **uric acid n.** Nephrolithiasis caused by uric acid stones, usually a consequence of hyperuricemia.

**nephrolithotomy** \-lithät′əmē\ An incision into the renal parenchyma for the purpose of removing one of more renal calculi. Also *lithonephrotomy.*

**nephrologic** \-läj′ik\ **1** Pertaining to the kidneys. **2** Related to nephrology.

**nephrologist** \nefräl′əjist\ A specialist in nephrology.

**nephrology** \nefräl′əjē\ [NEPHRO- + -LOGY] A subspecialty of internal medicine comprising the study of the kidney, its structure, function, and diseases, and of hypertensive and fluid electrolyte disorders.

**nephrolysis** \nefräl′isis\ [NEPHRO- + LYSIS] Surgical separation of a kidney from perinephric adhesions. Adj. nephrolytic.

**nephroma** \nəfrō′mə\ [NEPHR- + -OMA] A tumor of the kidney. **embryonal n.** NEPHROBLASTOMA. **malignant n.** NEPHROBLASTOMA. **mesoblastic n.** A tumor of the kidney composed of tissue resembling smooth muscle. Cartilage and cysts may be present. It is typically present in infants and is considered benign. Also *leiomyomatous hamartoma, fetal hamartoma.* **multilocular cystic n.** A rare congenital and benign unilateral multilocular lesion which contains dysontogenetic mesenchymatous tissues including cartilage and smooth and striated muscle. It is enclosed in a capsule.

**nephromegaly** \-meg′əlē\ [NEPHRO- + -MEGALY] Enlargement of a kidney, usually as a result of compensatory hypertrophy after surgical removal or disease of the other kidney.

**nephromere** \nef′rəmir\ [NEPHRO- + -MERE] NEPHROTOME.

**nephron** \nef′rän\ [German, from Gk *nephros* kidney] The functional unit of the kidney, consisting of a glomerulus and attached tubule. A human kidney has approximately one million nephrons. **lower n.** The distal convuluted tubule and collecting ducts of the nephron.

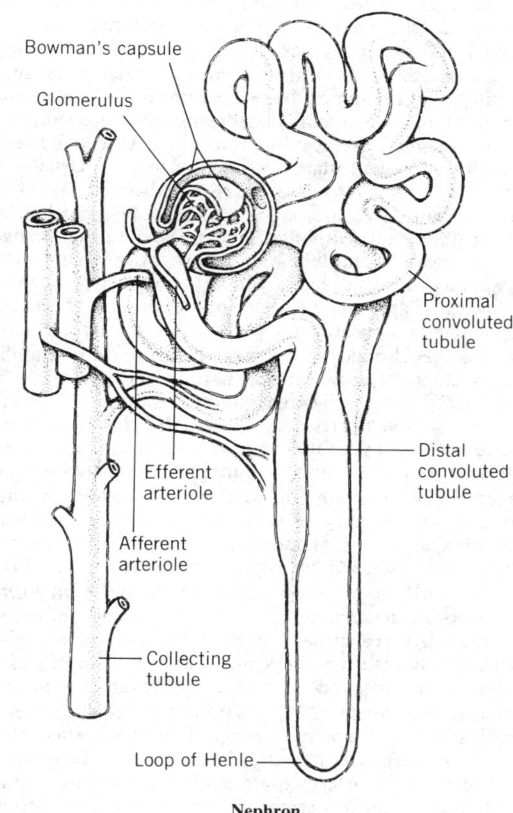


**Nephron**

**nephronophthisis** \-näf′thisis\ [NEPHRON + *o* + PHTHISIS] MEDULLARY CYSTIC DISEASE. **familial juvenile n.** Medullary cystic disease inherited as an autosomal recessive. It is usually fatal during childhood.

**nephro-omentopexy** \-ōmen′təpek′sē\ An antiquated surgical procedure in which the greater omentum is used to cover a decapsulated ischemic kidney or kidneys. It was originally proposed as a means of establishing a new blood supply and thus treat hypertension.

**nephropathia** \-path′ē·ə\ NEPHROPATHY. **n. epidemica** EPIDEMIC NEPHROPATHY.

**nephropathic** \-path′ik\ [NEPHRO- + -PATH + -IC] Causing organic renal disease or impairment of renal function.

**nephropathy** \nəfräp′əthē\ [NEPHRO- + -PATHY] Any organic disease of the kidneys. Also *renopathy, nephropathia.* **acute hypokalemic n.** Reversible histologic changes in the kidney, including vacuolization of proximal convoluted tubule cells and expansion of the subbasilar extracellular compartments, due to short-term potassium deficiency. **acute urate n.** Rapid deposition of urates in the interstitium and collecting tubules of the kidneys characterized clinically by acute renal failure. It usually follows effective chemotherapy of certain malignant disease such as leukemias and lymphomas when large amounts of nucleoprotein are released and converted to uric acid. **amphotericin B n.** The primary reaction to the toxicity of amphotericin B, with cylindruria as the first sign, soon followed by proteinuria, microhematuria, renal tubular acidosis with increasing urine pH, and then decrease of glomerular filtration rate to less than half of the pretreatment level. Focal necrosis of both proximal and distal tubules is interspersed with regenerative foci of epithelial cells. Calcification of tubule casts and the interstitium is a common feature. Diuresis and alkali administration should be maintained during amphotericin B therapy. If azotemia develops amphotericin B should be reduced or discontinued, and mannitol may be helpful. Usually renal function will return to normal. **analgesic n.** Kidney damage resulting from long-term analgesic ingestion, especially of phenacetin, although salicylates and other analgesics also have been implicated. The nephropathy is characterized by papillary necrosis and secondary obstructive changes in the cortex. Papillary necrosis may have a characteristic roentgenologic appearance, and sloughed necrotic papillae may cause renal colic. Impairment of concentrating ability is an early clinical feature, and hematuria and pyuria are common. Slowly progressive renal failure is usual. **Balkan n.** BALKAN NEPHRITIS. **bismuth n.** Renal tubule damage, caused by soluble bismuth salts and characterized by proteinuria, glycosuria, cylindruria, desquamation of tubule epithelial cells, and hyposthenuria. Anuria or the nephrotic syndrome may develop. This condition has become uncommon since the abandonment of bismuth therapy for syphilis. Also *bismuth toxicity.* **cadmium n.** Proteinuria with little or no histologic changes following ingestion of or exposure to cadmium. It may also be accompanied by glycosuria, hypercalciuria, aminoaciduria, and increased uric acid excretion with hypouricemia. Characteristic of cadmium toxicity in humans and animals is excretion of a protein of low molecular weight (20 000–30 000) which differs electrophoretically from protein excreted in other metal intoxications. Also *cadmium toxicity.* **carbon tetrachloride n.** Acute tubular necrosis and acute renal failure due to ingestion, inhalation, or dermal absorption of carbon tetrachloride. **chronic hypokalemic n.** Progressive chronic interstitial nephritis characterized by hyposthenuria and nocturia and renal failure, which are reversible in the early stages, due to prolonged potassium deficiency. **chronic urate n.** Very slowly progressive renal failure associated with chronic hyperuricemia. Even after focal changes in the medulla and interstitium develop, renal function may remain normal. Proteinuria and impaired concentrating ability are the first signs of chronic urate nephropathy, followed by decreasing glomerular filtration rate. The passage of urate stones or gravel may occur, but is not necessary to make the diagnosis. **copper n.** Intravascular hemolysis and acute tubular necrosis, especially of the ascending limb of the loop of Henle and the distal convoluted tubules, due to acute copper poisoning, usually from ingestion of copper sulfate. **diabetic n.** Any renal disease related to diabetes mellitus, including diabetic glomerulosclerosis, arterionephrosclerosis, arteriolonephrosclerosis, and papillary necrosis and pyelonephritis. **epidemic n.** A febrile illness, found in northern Scandinavia and Finland, which is followed by heavy proteinuria, oliguria, and moderate renal failure. Recovery is prompt and complete. It has been established that this disease is caused by a virus either identical to or closely related to that responsible for epidemic hemorrhagic fever (Hantaan virus). Clinically, however, it is considerably milder and carries a lower mortality. Also *nephropathia epidemica.* See also EPIDEMIC HEMORRHAGIC FEVER. **familial n.** HEREDITARY NEPHRITIS. **gold n.** Proteinuria followed by the nephrotic syndrome developing in a small percentage of cases of rheumatoid arthritis treated with organic gold salts. Immune deposits or gold deposits or both may appear in the lysosomes of the proximal tubules, and immune subendothelial deposits may occur in the glomeruli. The lesions and clinical manifestations usually disappear when gold therapy is discontinued. **gouty n.** Urate nephropathy or nephrosclerosis developing during the course of gout. Also *gouty kidney.* **hypercalcemic n.** Functional and histologic abnormalities of the kidneys due to hypercalcemia from any cause, the severity being related to the duration of the hypercalcemia. Impairment of renal concentrating ability is an early sign which may be followed rapidly by decreased glomerular filtration rate and renal failure. **hypokalemic n.** Renal functional impairment and renal lesions due to potassium deficiency. Also *kaliopenic nephropathy, nephropathy of potassium depletion.* **iodide n.** Nephropathy related to the iodide in contrast media used in radiography of vasculature and of urinary or biliary tracts. Nephrotoxicity may result in direct cellular toxicity, decreased renal blood flow, obstructive uric acid crystalluria, or an idiosyncratic reaction. Dose-related decrease in renal function or acute tubular, medullary, or cortical necrosis may develop. Dehydration prior to radiography and excessive contrast dosage should be avoided. **iron n.** Acute tubular necrosis and acute renal failure in children as a result of large doses of ferrous sulfate. Hemochromatosis and severe hemosiderosis may result in iron pigment deposition, interstitial fibrosis, and chronic renal failure. **kaliopenic n.** HYPOKALEMIC NEPHROPATHY. **kanamycin n.** Proteinuria, microscopic hematuria, and cylindruria resulting from kanamycin therapy. At a dosage of 25–50 mg·kg/day it develops in 10–20 percent of patients. Two to three weeks on this dose causes significant decrease in glomerular filtration rate and concentrating ability in half the patients. The incidence of kanamycin nephropathy is greater in cases of preexisting renal disease and of concomitant streptomycin or viomicin therapy. **lead n.** An interstitial nephritis resulting from chronic ingestion of lead. Two types of renal effects have been observed in man: damage to the proximal tubules with a decrease in the tubular reabsorption of glucose, amino acids, and phosphate; and interstitial fibrosis, sclerosis of blood vessels, and glomerular atrophy. **malarial n.** Clinical or histopathologic renal disorders associated with *Plasmodium malariae* malarial infections, sometimes leading to the nephrotic syndrome and progressive renal failure. Glomerular lesions may be proliferative, membranous, or mesangiocapillary. Most commonly found in Africa, especially among adolescents. In all varieties, response to steroid and other therapies has been poor or absent. Falciparum malaria is a rare cause of proliferative glomerulonephritis, in addition to being associated with blackwater fever and acute renal failure. **membranous n.** MEMBRANOUS GLOMERULONEPHRITIS. **mesangial n.** MESANGIAL IGA/IGG GLOMERULONEPHRITIS. **ob-**

**structive n.** Nephropathy due to obstruction of the urinary tract. **oxalate n.** Any of variety of renal diseases possibly related to excess oxalate production or gastrointestinal absorption, which may result in oxalate deposition, calcium oxalate calculi, or nephrocalcinosis. Causes of oxalate nephropathy include excess intake of foods high in oxalic acid, such as rhubarb and beets, ethylene and other glycol exposure, and primary or acquired increases of oxalate excretion, as in primary or secondary hyperoxaluria. **phenacetin n.** See under ANALGESIC NEPHROPATHY. **polymyxin n.** Renal tubular necrosis, with proteinuria and decreased concentrating ability, related to dosage in polymixin therapy. **n. of potassium depletion** HYPOKALEMIC NEPHROPATHY. **salt-losing n.** Any renal disease that results in excess salt excretion in the urine, usually related to tubulointerstitial disease or advanced renal failure. Salt-losing nephropathy is characterized by polyuria, hypovolemia and often hyponatremia. Dehydration and postural hypotension are common clinical features. The condition responds to salt and water replacement. **silver n.** Acute renal failure due to silver salts. The condition has been reported in photo developers. In rabbits intraperitoneal silver salts cause tubular degeneration and silver deposits and edema in the renal interstitium. **streptomycin n.** Proteinuria and cylindruria consequent to streptomycin therapy. The condition occurs in up to 20 percent of patients on streptomycin. Only a few have decreased glomerular filtration rate and acute tubular necrosis is rare. **sulfonamide n.** Renal complications following sulfonamide therapy, usually caused by precipitation of insoluble crystals of such compounds as sulfapyridine, sulfadiazine, and sulfathiazole in the renal tubules and urinary tract. Symptoms are flank pain, hematuria, cylindruria, crystalluria, and renal failure. Although such side effects were common and serious in the first decade of sulfonamide therapy, they have been greatly reduced by the use of sulfonamide mixtures and more soluble congeners, and more effective antibiotics. The few instances of sulfonamide crystallization at present are due to overdosage. Hypersensitivity reaction to a sulfonamide may cause an acute interstitial nephritis and renal failure. Steroid therapy may be effective, and complete recovery is possible. **tetracycline n.** A toxic nephropathy due to degradation products of outdated tetracycline which appears after three or four days of administration as a reversible Fanconi syndrome or as Bence Jones proteinuria, transient hyperglycemia, and a maculopapular skin rash. Histopathologically, there may be tubular necrosis, desquamated epithelial cells and regenerative foci. Both new and outdated tetracyclines block protein synthesis and thus cause increased azotemia in persons whose renal function is already impaired. **toxic n.** Any disease of the kidney resulting from a toxic agent or from an adverse reaction to a drug. The primary damage usually is to the tubules. In severe instances either acute or chronic renal failure may develop. **tubular n.** Any disease of the renal tubules. **urate n.** Renal impairment consequent to the progressive decrease in glomerular filtration rate and tubule function which occurs in hyperuricemia as urate is deposited in the distal convoluted and collecting tubules where concentration and acidification are greatest. Resultant obstruction, dilatation, and subsequent atrophy of renal tubules proximal to the obstruction lead to necrosis and fibrosis. Urate deposits also occur in the interstitium, where they initiate an inflammatory reaction with lymphocytic infiltration and fibrosis. Large interstitial crystalline deposits distinguish urate from other forms of interstitial nephritis. Hyalinization and thickening of the intima and media of the renal arterioles and small arteries contribute to the renal ischemia of urate nephropathy. **vascular n.** Any nephropathy associated with vasculitis, such as arteriolonephrosclerosis or arterionephrosclerosis.

**nephropexy** \nef′rəpek′sē\ [NEPHRO- + -PEXY] A surgical procedure in which one or both floating kidneys are sutured to the abdominal wall for the purposes of suspension and prevention of ptosis.

**nephropoietic** \-poi·et′ik\ [NEPHRO- + Gk *poiētikos* productive, creative] NEPHROGENIC.

**nephroptosis** \nef′räptō′sis\ [NEPHRO- + PTOSIS] Abnormal mobility of a kidney, usually asymptomatic but occasionally responsible for renal colic. The kidneys are displaced toward the pelvis. Also *movable kidney, floating kidney* (popular).

**nephropyelolithotomy** \-pī′əlōlithät′əmē\ A surgical incision into the renal parenchyma for the purpose of removing one or more stones from the renal pelvis.

**nephropyeloplasty** \-pī′əlōplas′tē\ [NEPHRO- + PYELO- + -PLASTY] The surgical reconstruction of a deformed or injured renal pelvis.

**nephrorrhaphy** \nefrôr′əfē\ [NEPHRO- + -RRHAPHY] The insertion of single or multiple sutures in the kidney for the purpose of reconstruction after surgical intervention or trauma.

**nephrosclerosis** \-sklerō′sis\ [NEPHRO- + SCLEROSIS] Interstitial fibrosis of the renal cortex and glomerulosclerosis due to renal arterial or arteriolar disease. Also *sclerotic kidney.* Adj. nephrosclerotic. **arterial n.** ARTERIONEPHROSCLEROSIS. **benign n.** ARTERIONEPHROSCLEROSIS. **congenital n.** FOCAL GLOMERULOSCLEROSIS. **hyaline arteriolar n.** Nephrosclerosis associated with hyaline thickening of the walls of the afferent arterioles in hypertension or diabetes. **hyperplastic arteriolar n.** A marked thickening of the intima of interlobular and arcuate renal arteries in malignant hypertension, often associated with fibrinoid necrosis and an "onion skin" appearance of the arterioles and rapidly progressive renal failure. **malignant n.** Nephrosclerosis associated with malignant hypertension and rapidly progressive renal failure.

**nephrosclerotic** \-sklerät′ik\ [NEPHRO- + SCLEROTIC] Related to or pertaining to nephrosclerosis.

**nephroses** \nefrō′sēz\ Plural of NEPHROSIS.

**nephrosis** \nəfrō′sis\ [NEPHR- + -OSIS] NEPHROTIC SYNDROME. Adj. nephrotic. **acute n.** Nephrotic syndrome of sudden onset. In severe cases it may cause hypovolemia, hypotension, and decreased glomerular filtration rate. **amyloid n.** Renal amyloidosis associated with the nephrotic syndrome. **congenital n.** Nephrotic syndrome developing in infancy in association with hematuria, cylinduria, hypertension, and progressive renal failure. Immunoglobulins and complement components may be demonstrated along the glomerular capillary basement membranes. Therapy is almost always ineffective, with death before age two. **glycogen n.** The presence of glycogen inclusions (Armanni-Ebstein lesions) in the pars recta of the proximal convoluted tubules in poorly controlled diabetes. **hemoglobinuric n.** Acute tubular necrosis and acute renal failure associated with acute intravascular hemolysis and hemoglobinuria. *Outmoded.* **Heymann's n.** HEYMANN'S NEPHRITIS **lipoid n.** A primary glomerular disease characterized by heavy proteinuria and the nephrotic syndrome. The disease is most common in children but may occur at any age. The glomeruli appear normal by light and immunofluorescent microscopy but on electron microscopy the foot processes of the epithelial cells appear smudged. The proteinuria usually is highly selective and renal function remains normal. Remissions occur spontaneously or may be induced by steroid hormones or immunosuppressive agents. However, relapses may occur. Also *glomerular epithelial cell disease, lipid nephrosis, foot process disease, minimal change disease, minimum change glomerulopathy, pure nephrosis, nil disease, minimal lesion disease, degenerative nephritis.* **lower nephron n.** An outmoded and imprecise term for ACUTE TUBULAR NECROSIS. • This term was introduced during World War II to describe the renal lesions noted in soldiers suffering from acute renal failure due to crush and other severe trauma. **mercurial n.** Membranous nephropathy and the nephrotic syndrome due to prolonged exposure to mercurial diuretics or to ingestion or absorption through the skin of small amounts of mercury. **osmotic n.** Marked dilatation of renal tubules with vacuolization of the pars recta of the proximal tubule. The condition may develop in severe glycosuria due to diabetes mellitus. Similar lesions may develop in patients given intravenous hypertonic sucrose to treat cerebral edema or mannitol to induce diuresis. The renal cortex is congested after administration of mannitol and the diameter of the tubule lumen is decreased. The lesions are reversible within 96 hours. No functional disorders accompany the histologic lesions. However, the infusion of dextrons of low molecular weight to treat peripheral vascular disorders has been followed by florid osmotic nephrosis, and oliguria secondary either to toxic effects on tubule cell function or to narrowing of the tubule lumens by swollen cells. **pure n.** LIPOID NEPHROSIS. **toxic n.** Acute tubular necrosis following ingestion, inhalation, or skin absorption of toxic agents, such as bichloride of mercury.

**nephrosonephritis** \nefrō'sənəfrī'tis\ [*nephros(is)* + *o* + NEPHRITIS] **1** The renal syndrome characteristic of epidemic hemorrhagic fever. *Rare.* **2** *Rare* EPIDEMIC HEMORRHAGIC FEVER. **hemorrhagic n.** EPIDEMIC HEMORRHAGIC FEVER.

**nephrosplenopexy** \-splē'nəplek'sē\ The suspension of the left kidney and the spleen from the abdominal wall in order to prevent ptosis of a floating kidney or spleen.

**nephrostogram** \nefräs'təgram\ [*nephrosto(my)* + -GRAM] A roentgenogram of the kidney after its pelvis has been opacified by instillation of contrast medium via a nephrostomy tube.

**nephrostomy** \nefräs'təmē\ [NEPHRO- + -STOMY] A form of urinary diversion involving placement of a tube within the kidney pelvis or calyces in order to provide urinary drainage directly to an external urinary collection appliance. The nephrostomy tube may be temporary or permanent, and is used to provide urinary drainage in a kidney which has become obstructed. A nephrostomy tube may be established by open surgical exposure of the kidney, or by use of a technique wherein the tube is passed directly through the skin in to the kidney (percutaneous nephrostomy).

**nephrotic** \nefrät'ik\ [NEPHR- + -OTIC[1]] Related to or associated with the nephrotic syndrome (nephrosis).

**nephrotome** \nef'rətōm\ [NEPHRO- + -TOME] One of a series of segmental units in the intermediate mesoderm from which the nephric tubules differentiate. They comprise the three successive renal organs during development: pronephros, mesonephros, and metanephros. Also *nephromere.*

**nephrotomography** \-tomäg'rəfē\ [NEPHRO- + TOMOGRAPHY] Body section roentgenography of the kidney whose parenchyma has been opacified by intravascularly administered appropriate iodinated contrast medium.

**nephrotomy** \nefrät'əmē\ [NEPHRO- + -TOMY] A surgical incision into one or both kidneys. **abdominal n.** An incision into the kidney, utilizing a transperitoneal or anterior approach. **lumbar n.** An incision into one or both kidneys utilizing a retroperitoneal flank approach.

**nephrotoxic** \-täk'sik\ [NEPHRO- + TOXIC] Causing renal lesions or impairing renal function.

**nephrotoxicity** \-täksis'itē\ [NEPHRO- + TOXICITY] The ability of an agent or drug to produce renal lesions or functional impairment. **salicylate n.** See under ANALGESIC NEPHROPATHY.

**nephrotoxin** \-täk'sin\ [NEPHRO- + TOXIN] Any agent or substance that causes renal lesions or impairment of renal function.

**nephrotresis** \-trē'sis\ [NEPHRO- + Gk *trēsis* a boring, piercing, hole] The surgical creation of a fistula by suturing the edges of a nephrostomy to the muscles of the abdominal wall.

**nephrotrophic** \-träf'ik\ Having an effect on the kidneys: said of a substance. Also *nephrotropic, renotrophic, renotropic.*

**nephroureterectomy** \nef'rōyur'ətərek'təmē\ The resection of one or both kidneys and ureters.

**nephroureterocystectomy** \nef'rōyoorē'tərōsistek'təmē\ Surgical extirpation of the kidney, the ureter, and all or part of the bladder wall.

**neptunium** \neptyoo'nē·əm\ Element number 93, having atomic weight 237.0482. First discovered as a synthetic product of neutron bombardment of uranium 238, traces also exist in uranium ores. Thirteen isotopes are known, of which the most stable is neptunium 237, an energetic emitter of alpha radiation with a half-life of $2.4 \times 10^6$ years. This isotope is produced in gram quantities in nuclear reactors as a by-product of plutonium production. Symbol: Np

**Neri** [Vincenzo *Neri,* Italian neurologist, born 1882] See under SIGN.

**Nernst** [Walther Hermann *Nernst,* German chemist, 1864–1941] See under POTENTIAL, LAW, EQUATION.

**nerol** $(CH_3)_2C{=}CH{-}[CH_2]_2{-}C(CH_3){=}CH{-}CH_2OH$. A terpene alcohol formed from two isoprene units. It is the *cis*-isomer of geraniol. Its diphosphate is formed from geranyl diphosphate as an intermediate in the biosynthesis of several terpenes.

# nerve

**nerve** [L *nervus.* See NERVUS.] A cordlike structure, visible to the naked eye, made up of nerve fibers conveying impulses between a part of the central nervous system and some other region of the body. A nerve is made up of individual nerve fibers with their sheaths and supporting cells, small blood vessels, and a surrounding connective tissue sheath. Each nerve fiber (axon) is surrounded by a cellular sheath (neurilemma) from which it may or may not be separated by a laminated lipoprotein layer (myelin sheath) derived from the neurilemma (Schwann) cells. A number of such nerve fibers, making up a fasciculus, are surrounded by a sheet of connective tissue (perineurium), leaflets of which also surround each individual nerve fiber (endoneurium). All of the fasciculi and the nourishing blood vessels are bound together by a thicker investment of connective tissue (epineurium). Also *nervus.* **abducent n.** NERVUS ABDUCENS. **accelerator n.'s** The cardiac sympathetic nerves, whose stimulation increases the rate of cardiac contraction. **accessory n.** NERVUS ACCESSORIUS. **accessory obturator n.** NERVUS OBTURATORIUS ACCESSORIUS.

**accessory phrenic n.'s** NERVI PHRENICI ACCESSORII. **acoustic n.** NERVUS VESTIBULOCOCHLEARIS. **n. to adductor brevis muscle** A branch of the anterior ramus of the obturator nerve. When this branch is absent, the muscle receives a branch from the posterior ramus. **n. to adductor longus muscle** A branch of the anterior ramus of the obturator nerve. Occasionally the muscle may receive a branch from the accessory obturator nerve when present. **n. to adductor magnus muscle** **1** A branch of the posterior ramus of the obturator nerve. **2** Any of the branches ($L_{2-4}$) of the tibial division of the sciatic nerve. **adrenergic n.** The sympathetic postganglionic axons that liberate epinephrine or norepinephrine at their terminals. **afferent n.** A nerve fiber or bundle that conducts towards the central nervous system or to a given neuron. Also *centripetal nerve.* ● See note at AFFERENT. **ampullary n.'s** The branches of the vestibular nerve that convey afferent impulses from the ampullae of the semicircular ducts of the internal ear to the brain, namely, the nervus ampullaris anterior, nervus ampullaris lateralis, and nervus ampullaris posterior. **Andersch n.** NERVUS TYMPANICUS. **anococcygeal n.'s** NERVI ANOCOCCYGEI. **anterior ampullary n.** NERVUS AMPULLARIS ANTERIOR. **anterior auricular n.'s** NERVI AURICULARES ANTERIORES. **anterior crural n.** NERVUS FEMORALIS. **anterior cutaneous n. of abdomen** RAMUS CUTANEUS ANTERIOR PECTORALIS ET ABDOMINALIS NERVORUM INTERCOSTALIUM. **anterior cutaneous n. of neck** NERVUS TRANSVERSUS COLLI. **anterior ethmoidal n.** NERVUS ETHMOIDALIS ANTERIOR. **anterior gastric n.** TRUNCUS VAGALIS ANTERIOR. **anterior interosseous n. of forearm** NERVUS INTEROSSEUS ANTEBRACHII ANTERIOR. **anterior labial n.'s** NERVI LABIALES ANTERIORES. **anterior palatine n.** NERVUS PALATINUS MAJOR. **anterior scrotal n.'s** NERVI SCROTALES ANTERIORES. **anterior superior alveolar n.'s** RAMI ALVEOLARES SUPERIORES ANTERIORES NERVI INFRAORBITALIS. **anterior supraclavicular n.'s** NERVI SUPRACLAVICULARES MEDIALES. **anterior thoracic n.** The medial and lateral pectoral nerves. *Obs.* **anterior vagal n.** TRUNCUS VAGALIS ANTERIOR. **aortic n.** A branch of the vagus nerve which supplies afferent fibers to the aortic arch and base of the heart. Its stimulation results in cardiac slowing, peripheral vascular dilatation, and a fall in blood pressure. Also *Ludwig's nerve, depressor nerve of Ludwig, Cyon's nerve.* **Arnold's n.** RAMUS AURICULARIS NERVI VAGI. **n. to articularis genus muscle** A filament of one of the muscular branches of the femoral nerve to the vastus intermedius muscle that pierces the latter to reach the articularis genus muscle. **auditory n.** NERVUS VESTIBULOCOCHLEARIS. **augmentor n.'s** Nerve fibers of sympathetic origin which increase the rate and force of contraction of the heart. **auricular n. of vagus** RAMUS AURICULARIS NERVI VAGI. **auriculotemporal n.** NERVUS AURICULOTEMPORALIS. **autonomic n.'s** Any of the peripheral nerves of the sympathetic and parasympathetic nervous systems. **axillary n.** NERVUS AXILLARIS. **Bell's n.** NERVUS THORACICUS LONGUS. **Bock's n.** RAMUS PHARYNGEUS GANGLII PTERYGOPALATINI. **n. to brachioradialis muscle** A branch of the radial nerve given off in front of the lateral intermuscular septum of the arm. **buccal n.** NERVUS BUCCALIS. **buccinator n.** NERVUS BUCCALIS. ● The term is misleading, since the nervus buccalis has no direct connection with the buccinator muscle. **caroticotympanic n.'s** NERVI CAROTICOTYMPANICI. **cavernous n.'s of clitoris** NERVI CAVERNOSI CLITORIDIS. **cavernous n.'s of penis** NERVI CAVERNOSI PENIS. **celiac n.'s** RAMI CELIACI NERVI VAGI. **centrifugal n.** EFFERENT NERVE. **centripetal n.** AFFERENT NERVE. **cerebral n.'s** *Outmoded* NERVI CRANIALES. **cervical n.'s** NERVI CERVICALES. **cholinergic n.'s** Nerves that release the neurotransmitter acetylcholine at their terminations, including all autonomic preganglionic nerves, parasympathetic postganglionic nerves, and somatic motor nerves. **circumflex humeral n.** NERVUS AXILLARIS. **coccygeal n.** NERVUS COCCYGEUS. **cochlear n.** **1** PARS COCHLEARIS NERVI OCTAVI. **2** RADIX INFERIOR NERVI VESTIBULOCOCHLEARIS. **common digital n.** NERVUS DIGITALIS COMMUNIS. **common fibular n.** NERVUS PERONEUS COMMUNIS. **common peroneal n.** NERVUS PERONEUS COMMUNIS. **n. of Cotunnius** NERVUS NASOPALATINUS. **cranial n.'s** NERVI CRANIALES. **crotaphitic n.** *Outmoded* NERVUS MAXILLARIS. **cubital n.** NERVUS ULNARIS. **cutaneous n.** NERVUS CUTANEUS. **Cyon's n.** AORTIC NERVE. **deep fibular n.** NERVUS PERONEUS PROFUNDUS. **deep peroneal n.** NERVUS PERONEUS PROFUNDUS. **deep petrosal n.** NERVUS PETROSUS PROFUNDUS. **deep radial n.** NERVUS INTEROSSEUS ANTEBRACHII POSTERIOR. **deep temporal n.'s** NERVI TEMPORALES PROFUNDI. **deep vidian n.** NERVUS PETROSUS PROFUNDUS. **dental n.** Either nervus alveolaris inferior or one of the nervi alveolares superiores. **depressor n.** A nerve which upon stimulation lowers the blood pressure, especially the carotid sinus nerve. **depressor n. of Ludwig** AORTIC NERVE. **descending cervical n.** RADIX INFERIOR ANSAE CERVICALIS. **diaphragmatic n.** NERVUS PHRENICUS. **digastric n.** RAMUS DIGASTRICUS NERVI FACIALIS. **digital n.'s** NERVI DIGITALES. **dorsal n. of clitoris** NERVUS DORSALIS CLITORIDIS. **dorsal cutaneous n. of forearm** NERVUS CUTANEUS ANTEBRACHII POSTERIOR. **dorsal digital n.'s** NERVI DIGITALES DORSALES. **dorsal digital n.'s of foot** NERVI DIGITALES DORSALES PEDIS. **dorsal n. of penis** NERVUS DORSALIS PENIS. **dorsal n. of scapula** NERVUS DORSALIS SCAPULAE. **dorsal scapular n.** NERVUS DORSALIS SCAPULAE. **efferent n.** A nerve conducting away from a central neuronal aggregate, mainly to muscles and glands. Also *centrifugal nerve.* **eighth cranial n.** NERVUS VESTIBULOCOCHLEARIS. **eleventh cranial n.** NERVUS ACCESSORIUS. **ethmoidal n.** Either nervus ethmoidalis anterior or nervus ethmoidalis posterior. **n. to extensor carpi radialis brevis muscle** A branch of the deep terminal branch of the radial nerve that occasionally arises from the beginning of the superficial branch of the radial nerve. **n. to extensor carpi radialis longus muscle** A branch of the radial nerve that arises in front of the lateral intermuscular septum of the arm. **n. of external acoustic meatus** NERVUS MEATUS ACUSTICI EXTERNI. **external carotid n.'s** NERVI CAROTICI EXTERNI. **external laryngeal n.** RAMUS EXTERNUS NERVI LARYNGEI SUPERIORIS. **external palatine n.** NERVUS PALATINUS MEDIUS. **external pterygoid n.** NERVUS PTERYGOIDEUS LATERALIS. **external respiratory n. of Bell** *Imprecise* NERVUS THORACICUS LONGUS. **external saphenous n.** NERVUS SURALIS. **external spermatic n.** RAMUS GENITALIS NERVI GENITOFEMORALIS. **external superficial petrosal n.** A twig leaving the sympathetic plexus on the middle meningeal artery to pass along the auriculotemporal nerve and up the facial canal as far as the geniculate ganglion. **facial n.** NERVUS FACIALIS. **femoral n.** NERVUS FEMORALIS. **fifth cra-**

**nial n.** NERVUS TRIGEMINUS. **first cranial n.** NERVI OLFACTORII. **n. to flexor digitorum longus muscle** A muscular branch of the tibial nerve that arises deep to the soleus muscle in the leg and supplies the flexor digitorus longus muscle. **n. to flexor hallucis longus muscle** A muscular branch of the tibial nerve that arises deep to the soleus muscle and accompanies the peroneal vessels to supply the flexor hallucis longus muscle. **fourth cranial n.** NERVUS TROCHLEARIS. **frontal n.** NERVUS FRONTALIS. **furcal n.** NERVUS FURCALIS. **Galen's n.** RAMUS COMMUNICANS NERVI LARYNGEI SUPERIORIS CUM NERVO LARYNGEO INFERIORI. **gastric n.'s** Truncus vagalis anterior and truncus vagalis posterior. **n. to gemellus inferior and quadratus femoris muscles** NERVUS MUSCULI QUADRATI FEMORIS. **n. to gemellus superior muscle** A branch of the nerve to the obturator internus muscle that is given off below the piriformis muscle in the gluteal region and enters the posterior surface of the gemellus superior muscle. **n. to geniohyoid muscle** A branch of the hypoglossal nerve that consists of fibers of the first cervical spinal nerve destined for the geniohyoid muscle. **genitofemoral n.** NERVUS GENITOFEMORALIS. **glossopalatine n.** That portion of the seventh cranial (facial) nerve made up of the nervus intermedius and including the geniculate ganglion, chorda tympani and greater superficial petrosal nerve, in addition to the parasympathetic part including the submaxillary and sphenopalatine ganglia and their branches. **glossopharyngeal n.** NERVUS GLOSSOPHARYNGEUS. **n. to gracilis muscle** A branch of the anterior branch of the obturator nerve that is given off behind the pectineus muscle and in front of the adductor longus muscle. It proceeds medially to innervate the gracilis muscle. **great auricular n.** NERVUS AURICULARIS MAGNUS. **greater occipital n.** NERVUS OCCIPITALIS MAJOR. **greater palatine n.** NERVUS PALATINUS MAJOR. **greater petrosal n.** NERVUS PETROSUS MAJOR. **greater splanchnic n.** NERVUS SPLANCHNICUS MAJOR. **greater superficial petrosal n.** NERVUS PETROSUS MAJOR. **great sciatic n.** NERVUS ISCHIADICUS. **Hering's n.** RAMUS SINUS CAROTICI NERVI GLOSSOPHARYNGEI. **n.'s to hyoglossus and styloglossus muscles** Lingual branches of the hypoglossal nerve which arise on the lateral surface of the hyoglossus muscle and supply the hyoglossus and styloglossus muscles. **hypogastric n.** NERVUS HYPOGASTRICUS DEXTER ET SINISTER. **hypogastric n. of Latarjet** NERVUS HYPOGASTRICUS DEXTER ET SINISTER. **hypoglossal n.** NERVUS HYPOGLOSSUS. **iliohypogastric n.** NERVUS ILIOHYPOGASTRICUS. **ilioinguinal n.** NERVUS ILIOINGUINALIS. **n.'s to iliopsoas muscle** Branches to the iliacus muscle and the psoas major muscle that arise from the second and third, and occasionally the fourth, lumbar nerves of the lumbar plexus. **inferior alveolar n.** NERVUS ALVEOLARIS INFERIOR. **inferior ampullar n.** NERVUS AMPULLARIS POSTERIOR. **inferior cardiac n.** NERVUS CARDIACUS CERVICALIS INFERIOR. **inferior cervical cardiac n.** NERVUS CARDIACUS CERVICALIS INFERIOR. **inferior clunial n.'s** NERVI CLUNIUM INFERIORES. **inferior dental n.** NERVUS ALVEOLARIS INFERIOR. **inferior gluteal n.** NERVUS GLUTEUS INFERIOR. **inferior hemorrhoidal n.'s** NERVI RECTALES INFERIORES. **inferior laryngeal n.** NERVUS LARYNGEUS INFERIOR. **inferior lateral brachial cutaneous n.** NERVUS CUTANEUS BRACHII LATERALIS INFERIOR. **inferior lateral cutaneous n. of arm** NERVUS CUTANEUS BRACHII LATERALIS INFERIOR. **inferior rectal n.'s** NERVI RECTALES INFERIORES. **inferior splanchnic n.** NERVUS SPLANCHNICUS MINOR. **inferior vesical n.'s of pudendal plexus** NERVI VESICALES INFERIORES PLEXUS PUDENDI. **inferior vesical n.'s of vesical plexus** NERVI VESICALES INFERIORES PLEXUS VESICALIS. **infraoccipital n.** NERVUS SUBOCCIPITALIS. **infraorbital n.** NERVUS INFRAORBITALIS. **infratrochlear n.** NERVUS INFRATROCHLEARIS. **intercostal n.'s** See under RAMI VENTRALES NERVORUM THORACICORUM. **intercostobrachial n.'s** NERVI INTERCOSTOBRACHIALES. **intermediary n.** NERVUS INTERMEDIUS. **intermediate dorsal cutaneous n.** NERVUS CUTANEUS DORSALIS INTERMEDIUS. **intermediate supraclavicular n.'s** NERVI SUPRACLAVICULARES INTERMEDII. **intermediate n. of Wrisberg** NERVUS INTERMEDIUS. **internal auricular n.** RAMUS POSTERIOR NERVI AURICULARIS MAGNI. **internal carotid n.** NERVUS CAROTICUS INTERNUS. **internal cutaneous n.** NERVUS CUTANEUS BRACHII MEDIALIS. **internal laryngeal n.** RAMUS INTERNUS NERVI LARYNGEI SUPERIORIS. **internal occipital n.** NERVUS OCCIPITALIS MAJOR. **internal popliteal n.** NERVUS TIBIALIS. **internal pterygoid n.** NERVUS PTERYGOIDEUS MEDIALIS. **internal superior laryngeal n.** RAMUS INTERNUS NERVI LARYNGEI SUPERIORIS. **interosseous n. of leg** NERVUS INTEROSSEUS CRURIS. **ischiadic n.** NERVUS ISCHIADICUS. **Jacobson's n.** NERVUS TYMPANICUS. **jugular n.** NERVUS JUGULARIS. **jugular n. of Arnold** NERVUS JUGULARIS. **lacrimal n.** NERVUS LACRIMALIS. **n.'s of Lancisi** Stria longitudinalis lateralis corporis callosi and stria longitudinalis medialis corporis callosi. Also *longitudinal nerves of Lancisi*. **Langley's n.'s** PILOMOTOR NERVES. **laryngeal n.** Any one of several nerves that supply portions of the intrinsic musculature and/or lining of the larynx. They include external, internal, inferior, and superior components. **lateral ampullary n.** NERVUS AMPULLARIS LATERALIS. **lateral antebrachial cutaneous n.** NERVUS CUTANEUS ANTEBRACHII LATERALIS. **lateral cutaneous n. of calf** NERVUS CUTANEUS SURAE LATERALIS. **lateral cutaneous n. of forearm** NERVUS CUTANEUS ANTEBRACHII LATERALIS. **lateral cutaneous n. of thigh** NERVUS CUTANEUS FEMORIS LATERALIS. **lateral dorsal cutaneous n. of foot** NERVUS CUTANEUS DORSALIS LATERALIS. **lateral femoral cutaneous n.** NERVUS CUTANEUS FEMORIS LATERALIS. **lateral pectoral n.** NERVUS PECTORALIS LATERALIS. **lateral plantar n.** NERVUS PLANTARIS LATERALIS. **lateral popliteal n.** NERVUS PERONEUS COMMUNIS. **lateral pterygoid n.** NERVUS PTERYGOIDEUS LATERALIS. **lateral superior cutaneous n. of arm** NERVUS CUTANEUS BRACHII LATERALIS SUPERIOR. **lateral supraclavicular n.'s** NERVI SUPRACLAVICULARES LATERALES. **lateral sural n.** A general sensory nerve formed by union of the medial sural cutaneous branch of the tibial nerve and the peroneal communicating branch of the common peroneal nerve. Distribution includes skin on back of leg and side of foot. **lateral n.'s of uterus** Branches of the uterovaginal plexus that enter the base of the broad ligament of the uterus and accompany the uterine arteries on either side of the uterus, supplying branches to the body of the uterus and the uterine tubes and communicating with tubal nerves of the inferior hypogastric plexus and branches of the ovarian plexus. The branches to the body of the uterus end in the myometrium and endometrium. **least occipital n.** NERVUS OCCIPITALIS TERTIUS. **least splanchnic n.** NERVUS SPLANCHNICUS IMUS. **lesser occipital n.** NERVUS OCCIPITALIS MINOR. **lesser palatine n.'s**

NERVI PALATINI MINORES. **lesser petrosal n.** NERVUS PETROSUS MINOR. **lesser splanchnic n.** NERVUS SPLANCHNICUS MINOR. **lesser superficial n.** NERVUS PETROSUS MINOR. **lesser superficial petrosal n.** NERVUS PETROSUS MINOR. **n.'s to levator ani muscle** A branch from the fourth sacral spinal nerve and a branch from the perineal division of the pudendal nerve that supply the levator ani muscle on each side. It may also receive a branch from the inferior rectal nerve. **lingual n.** NERVUS LINGUALIS. **long buccal n.** NERVUS BUCCALIS. **long ciliary n.'s** NERVI CILIARES LONGI. **n. to long head of biceps brachii muscle** A branch of the musculocutaneous nerve that arises after the nerve has pierced the coracobrachialis muscle. It supplies the long head of the biceps brachii muscle. **n. to long head of triceps muscle** One of the medial muscular branches of the radial nerve that innervates the long head of the triceps muscle before the nerve enters the radial sulcus behind the humerus. **longitudinal n.'s of Lancisi** NERVES OF LANCISI. **long thoracic n.** NERVUS THORACICUS LONGUS. **lowest splanchnic n.** NERVUS SPLANCHNICUS IMUS. **Ludwig's n.** AORTIC NERVE. **lumbar n.'s** NERVI LUMBALES. **lumbar splanchnic n.'s** NERVI SPLANCHNICI LUMBALES. **lumboinguinal n.** RAMUS FEMORALIS NERVI GENITOFEMORALIS. **n. of Luschka** 1 RAMUS MENINGEUS NERVORUM SPINALIUM. 2 NERVUS ETHMOIDALIS POSTERIOR. **major splanchnic n.** NERVUS SPLANCHNICUS MAJOR. **mandibular n.** NERVUS MANDIBULARIS. **masseteric n.** NERVUS MASSETERICUS. **maxillary n.** NERVUS MAXILLARIS. **medial antebrachial cutaneous n.** NERVUS CUTANEUS ANTEBRACHII MEDIALIS. **medial cutaneous n. of arm** NERVUS CUTANEUS BRACHII MEDIALIS. **medial cutaneous n. of calf** NERVUS CUTANEUS SURAE MEDIALIS. **medial cutaneous n. of forearm** NERVUS CUTANEUS ANTEBRACHII MEDIALIS. **medial dorsal cutaneous n. of foot** NERVUS CUTANEUS DORSALIS MEDIALIS. **n. to medial head of triceps and anconeus** A long branch of the radial nerve that is given off in the radial sulcus behind the humerus and descends through the medial head of the triceps muscle, supplying it, and ending in the anconeus muscle after crossing behind the elbow joint. It is accompanied by the middle collateral branch of the profunda brachii artery. **medial pectoral n.** NERVUS PECTORALIS MEDIALIS. **medial plantar n.** NERVUS PLANTARIS MEDIALIS. **medial popliteal n.** NERVUS TIBIALIS. **n. to medial pterygoid muscle** NERVUS PTERYGOIDEUS MEDIALIS. **medial supraclavicular n.'s** NERVI SUPRACLAVICULARES MEDIALES. **medial sural cutaneous n.** NERVUS CUTANEUS SURAE MEDIALIS. **median n.** NERVUS MEDIANUS. **meningeal n.** RAMUS MENINGEUS NERVI VAGI. **mental n.** NERVUS MENTALIS. **middle alveolar n.** RAMUS ALVEOLARIS SUPERIOR MEDIUS NERVI INFRAORBITALIS. **middle cardiac n.** NERVUS CARDIACUS CERVICALIS MEDIUS. **middle cervical cardiac n.** NERVUS CARDIACUS CERVICALIS MEDIUS. **middle clunial n.'s** NERVI CLUNIUM MEDII. **middle deep temporal n.** The middle branch of the nervi temporales profundi of the mandibular nerve which traverses the porus crotaphiticobuccinatorius behind the nerve to the masseter muscle and passes between the lateral pterygoid muscle and the greater wing of the sphenoid bone to end in the middle part of the temporalis muscle. It is occasionally absent. **middle gluteal n.'s** NERVI CLUNIUM MEDII. **middle palatine n.** NERVUS PALATINUS MEDIUS. **middle subscapular n.** NERVUS THORACODORSALIS. **middle superficial petrosal n.** NERVUS PETROSUS MINOR. **middle supraclavicular n.'s** NERVI SUPRACLAVICULARES INTERMEDII. **minor splanchnic n.** NERVUS SPLANCHNICUS MINOR. **mixed n.** A peripheral nerve containing both afferent and efferent axons. Also *sensorimotor nerve*. **motor n.** An efferent nerve to skeletal muscle. **motor n. of tongue** NERVUS HYPOGLOSSUS. **n. to muscle of malleus** NERVUS MUSCULI TENSORIS TYMPANI. **musculocutaneous n.** NERVUS MUSCULOCUTANEUS. **musculocutaneous n. of arm** NERVUS MUSCULOCUTANEUS. **musculocutaneous n. of foot** NERVUS PERONEUS SUPERFICIALIS. **musculocutaneous n. of leg** NERVUS PERONEUS PROFUNDUS. **musculospiral n.** NERVUS RADIALIS. **mylohyoid n.** NERVUS MYLOHYOIDEUS. **nasociliary n.** NERVUS NASOCILIARIS. **nasopalatine n.** NERVUS NASOPALATINUS. **ninth cranial n.** NERVUS GLOSSOPHARYNGEUS. **obturator n.** NERVUS OBTURATORIUS. **n. to obturator externus** A branch of the posterior branch of the obturator nerve. The posterior branch pierces and supplies the obturator externus muscle at the upper part of the obturator foramen before it continues between the adductor brevis and adductor magnus muscles. *Outmoded.* **oculomotor n.** NERVUS OCULOMOTORIUS. **olfactory n.'s** NERVI OLFACTORII. **ophthalmic n.** NERVUS OPHTHALMICUS. **ophthalmic recurrent n.** RAMUS TENTORII NERVI OPHTHALMICI. **ophthalmic n. of Willis** NERVUS OPHTHALMICUS. **optic n.** NERVUS OPTICUS. **orbital n.'s** RAMI ORBITALES GANGLII PTERYGOPALATINI. **palatine n.'s** NERVI PALATINI. **palmar digital n.'s** NERVI DIGITALES PALMARES. **parasympathetic n.** Any of the nerves of the parasympathetic division of the autonomic nervous system. **parotid n.'s** RAMI PAROTIDEI NERVI AURICULOTEMPORALIS. **pathetic n.** NERVUS TROCHLEARIS. **n. to pectineus muscle** The nerve supplying the pectineus muscle that arises from the femoral nerve above the inguinal ligament and passes behind the femoral sheath to enter the muscle. **n.'s to pectoralis major muscle** The nervus pectoralis lateralis and nervus pectoralis medialis. **pelvic splanchnic n.'s** NERVI SPLANCHNICI PELVICI. **perineal n.'s** NERVI PERINEALES. **peripheral n.'s** 1 All nerves whose distribution is to the skin or peripheral parts of the body. 2 Any nerves that enter or leave the central nervous system. **peroneal communicating n.** RAMUS COMMUNICANS PERONEUS NERVI PERONEI COMMUNIS. **peroneal cutaneous n.** *Outmoded* NERVUS CUTANEUS SURAE LATERALIS. **n.'s to peroneus longus muscle** Muscular branches of the superficial peroneal nerve that supply the peroneus longus muscle as the nerve descends deep to the muscle in the lateral compartment of the leg. **n. to peroneus tertius** A branch of the deep peroneal nerve that is given off in the lower part of the leg. **petrosal n.** The nervus petrosus major, nervus petrosus minor, nervus petrosus profundus, or nervus petrosus superficialis. **phrenic n.** NERVUS PHRENICUS. **phrenicoabdominal n.'s** RAMI PHRENICOABDOMINALES NERVI PHRENICI. **pilomotor n.'s** Peripheral axons innervating the arrectores pilorum muscles of cutaneous hairs. Also *Langley's nerves*. **n. to piriformis muscle** NERVUS PIRIFORMIS. **plantar digital n.'s** NERVI DIGITALES PLANTARES. **n. to plantaris muscle** A branch to the plantaris muscle that is given off by the tibial nerve as it passes between the two heads of the gastrocnemius muscle. **pneumogastric n.** NERVUS VAGUS. **n. to popliteus muscle** A branch of the tibial nerve that is given off between the two heads of the gastrocnemius muscle and then descends laterally and obliquely across the popliteal vessels to the lower margin of the popliteus muscle. Around the popliteus muscle it bends to enter the anterior surface of the muscle. **posterior ampullary n.** NERVUS AMPULLARIS POSTERIOR. **posterior antebrachial cutaneous n.** NERVUS CUTANEUS ANTEBRACHII POSTERIOR. **posterior auricular n.** NERVUS AURICULARIS POSTERIOR. **posterior brachial cutaneous n.** NERVUS CUTANEUS BRACHII POSTERIOR. **posterior cutaneous n. of arm** NERVUS CUTANEUS BRACHII POSTERIOR. **posterior cutaneous n. of forearm** NERVUS CUTANEUS ANTEBRACHII POSTERIOR. **posterior cutaneous n. of thigh** NERVUS CUTANEUS FEMORIS POSTERIOR. **posterior ethmoidal n.** NERVUS ETHMOIDALIS POSTERIOR. **posterior femoral cutaneous n.** NERVUS CUTANEUS FEMORIS POSTERIOR. **posterior gastric n.** TRUNCUS VAGALIS POSTERIOR. **posterior interosseous n. of forearm** NERVUS INTEROSSEUS ANTEBRACHII POSTERIOR. **posterior labial n.'s** NERVI LABIALES POSTERIORES. **posterior palatine n.** NERVUS PALATINUS POSTERIOR. **posterior scrotal n.'s** NERVI SCROTALES POSTERIORES. **posterior supraclavicular n.'s** NERVI SUPRACLAVICULARES LATERALES. **posterior thoracic n.** NERVUS THORACICUS LONGUS. **posterior vagal n.** TRUNCUS VAGALIS POSTERIOR. **post-trematic n.** The main nerve of a branchial (pharyngeal) arch. It lies just behind the preceding pharyngeal pouch and in some instances gives off a pretrematic branch which contributes to the innervation of the preceding arch. **presacral n.** PLEXUS HYPOGASTRICUS SUPERIOR. **pressor n.** An afferent nerve which upon stimulation elevates blood pressure. **pretrematic n.** The branch of the main post-trematic nerve in each pharyngeal arch which loops over the adjacent pouch to supply part of the preceding arch. **proper digital n.** NERVUS DIGITALIS PROPRIUS. **proper palmar digital n.'s** NERVI DIGITALES PALMARES PROPRII. **n. of pterygoid canal** NERVUS CANALIS PTERYGOIDEI. **pterygopalatine n.'s** NERVI PTERYGOPALATINI. **pudendal n.** NERVUS PUDENDUS. **pudic n.** NERVUS PUDENDUS. **n. to quadratus femoris muscle** NERVUS MUSCULI QUADRATI FEMORIS. **n.'s to quadratus lumborum** The ventral rami of the twelfth thoracic and the upper third and fourth lumbar spinal nerves. **radial n.** NERVUS RADIALIS. **n.'s to rectus capitis anterior muscle** Branches from the loop between the ventral rami of the first and second cervical spinal nerves. **recurrent n.** NERVUS LARYNGEUS RECURRENS. **recurrent laryngeal n.** NERVUS LARYNGEUS RECURRENS. **renal n.** NERVUS SPLANCHNICUS IMUS. **n. to rhomboids** NERVUS DORSALIS SCAPULAE. **saccular n.** NERVUS SACCULARIS. **sacral n.'s** NERVI SACRALES. **sacral splanchnic n.'s** NERVI SPLANCHNICI SACRALES. **saphenous n.** NERVUS SAPHENUS. **Scarpa's n.** NERVUS NASOPALATINUS. **sciatic n.** NERVUS ISCHIADICUS. **second cranial n.** NERVUS OPTICUS. **secretomotor n.'s** SECRETOMOTORIC FIBERS. **secretory n.'s** SECRETOMOTORIC FIBERS. **segmental n.** Any nerve supplying structures from one of the original body somites, as an intercostal nerve. **n. to semimembranosus** A branch of the tibial portion of the sciatic nerve that arises in common with the branch to the ischial head of the adductor magnus muscle in the upper portion of the back of the thigh and supplies the semimembranosus muscle. **sensorimotor n.** MIXED NERVE. **sensory n.** A peripheral axon or bundle of axons conveying activity from sense organs to the central nervous system. ● See note at AFFERENT. **n. to serratus anterior** NERVUS THORACICUS LONGUS. **seventh cranial n.** NERVUS FACIALIS. **short ciliary n.'s** NERVI CILIARES BREVES. **short saphenous n.** NERVUS SURALIS. **sinus n.** RAMUS SINUS CAROTICI NERVI GLOSSOPHARYNGEI. **sinuvertebral n.** RAMUS MENINGEUS NERVORUM SPINALIUM. **sixth cranial n.** NERVUS ABDUCENS. **small deep petrosal n.'s** NERVI CAROTICOTYMPANICI. **small sciatic n.** NERVUS CUTANEUS FEMORIS POSTERIOR. **Soemmering's n.** NERVUS PUDENDUS. **n. to soleus muscle** A branch that arises from the tibial nerve as it passes between the two heads of the gastrocnemius muscle. It enters the posterior surface of the soleus muscle. **somatic n.'s** Nerves that supply muscle and somatic tissue with motor and sensory fibers. **somitic n.** 1 Each of the nerves which in the embryo corresponds with a somite. They are the evidence of the original metamerism and conserve their primitive theoretical disposition in the region of the spinal cord, where the nerve roots have a typical segmental arrangement. The intercostal nerves in the thoracic region are the most characteristic. 2 Any of certain cranial nerves developing in the somitic territories of the head (muscles of the eye and the tongue), as opposed to the branchial nerves corresponding to each of the branchial arches which take part in the construction of the head and the neck. The somitic cranial nerves are: the oculomotor (third cranial nerve), the trochlear (fourth cranial nerve), the abducent (sixth cranial nerve) and the hypoglossal (twelfth cranial nerve). **space n.** A branch of the auditory nerve which innervates the semicircular canals. **sphenoid-palatine n.** *Outmoded* NERVUS NASOPALATINUS. **spinal n.'s** NERVI SPINALES. **spinal accessory n.** NERVUS ACCESSORIUS. **splanchnic n.'s** The nerves supplying viscera and blood vessels, especially the visceral branches of the thoracic, lumbar, and pelvic portions of the sympathetic trunks. They represent axons of preganglionic neurons that pass through the paravertebral ganglion and the sympathetic trunk en route to the celiac and mesenteric ganglia. **stapedial n.** NERVUS STAPEDIUS. **stylohyoid n.** RAMUS STYLOHYOIDEUS NERVI FACIALIS. **stylopharyngeal n.** RAMUS MUSCULI STYLOPHARYNGEI NERVI GLOSSOPHARYNGEI. **subclavian n.** NERVUS SUBCLAVIUS. **n. to subclavius muscle** NERVUS SUBCLAVIUS. **subcostal n.** NERVUS SUBCOSTALIS. **subcutaneous temporal n.'s** RAMI TEMPORALES SUPERFICIALES NERVI AURICULOTEMPORALIS. **sublingual n.** NERVUS SUBLINGUALIS. **submaxillary n.'s** RAMI GLANDULARES GANGLII SUBMANDIBULARIS. **suboccipital n.** NERVUS SUBOCCIPITALIS. **subscapular n.'s** NERVUS SUBSCAPULARIS. **sudomotor n.'s** Autonomic nerves controlling the activity of sweat glands. **superficial cervical n.** NERVUS TRANSVERSUS COLLI. **superficial ciliary n.'s** Sensory fibers of the ophthalmic and long ciliary nerves that participate in the annular plexus at the periphery of the cornea from which filaments enter the substantia propria and radiate towards the center. *Outmoded.* **superficial fibular n.** NERVUS PERONEUS SUPERFICIALIS. **superficial peroneal n.** NERVUS PERONEUS SUPERFICIALIS. **superficial radial n.** RAMUS SUPERFICIALIS NERVI RADIALIS. **superior alveolar n.'s** NERVI ALVEOLARES SUPERIORES. **superior ampullary n.** NERVUS AMPULLARIS ANTERIOR. **superior cardiac n.** NERVUS CARDIACUS CERVICALIS SUPERIOR. **superior cervical cardiac n.** NERVUS CARDIACUS CERVICALIS SUPERIOR. **superior clunial n.'s** NERVI CLUNIUM SUPERIORES. **superior dental n.'s** NERVI ALVEOLARES SUPERIORES. **superior gluteal n.** NERVUS GLUTEUS SUPERIOR. **superior laryngeal n.** NERVUS LARYNGEUS SUPERIOR.

**superior lateral cutaneous n. of arm** NERVUS CUTANEUS BRACHII LATERALIS SUPERIOR. **superior vesical n.'s of vesical plexus** NERVI VESICALES SUPERIORES PLEXUS VESICALIS. **supraclavicular n.'s** NERVI SUPRACLAVICULARES. **supraorbital n.** NERVUS SUPRAORBITALIS. **suprascapular n.** NERVUS SUPRASCAPULARIS. **supratrochlear n.** NERVUS SUPRATROCHLEARIS. **supreme cardiac n.'s** RAMI CARDIACI CERVICALES SUPERIORES NERVI VAGI. **sural n.** NERVUS SURALIS. **sympathetic n.** 1 One of the nerves of the sympathetic division of the autonomic nervous system. 2 TRUNCUS SYMPATHICUS. See also SYSTEMA NERVOSUM AUTONOMICUM. **temporal facial n.** RAMI TEMPORALES NERVI FACIALIS. **n. of tensor tympani muscle** NERVUS MUSCULI TENSORIS TYMPANI. **n. of tensor veli palatini** NERVUS TENSORIS VELI PALATINI. **tenth cranial n.** NERVUS VAGUS. **tentorial n.** RAMUS TENTORII NERVI OPHTHALMICI. **n. to teres minor muscle** A branch of the posterior branch of the axillary nerve that arises as the nerve passes through the quadrangular space where it enters the teres minor muscle. It often possesses a pseudoganglion. **terminal n.** NERVUS TERMINALIS. **third cranial n.** NERVUS OCULOMOTORIUS. **third occipital n.** NERVUS OCCIPITALIS TERTIUS. **thoracic n.'s** NERVI THORACICI. **thoracic cardiac n.'s** NERVI CARDIACI THORACICI. **thoracodorsal n.** NERVUS THORACODORSALIS. **n. to thyrohyoid muscle** RAMUS THYROHYOIDEUS ANSAE CERVICALIS. **tibial n.** NERVUS TIBIALIS. **n.'s to tibialis anterior muscle** Branches of the deep peroneal nerve that enter the tibialis anterior muscle near the middle of the leg. Occasionally a branch from the common peroneal nerve enters the proximal portion of the muscle. **n.'s to tibialis posterior muscle** Small branches of the tibial nerve that supply the tibialis posterior muscle near the middle of the leg. **tonsillar n.'s** RAMI TONSILLARES NERVI GLOSSOPHARYNGEI. **transverse cervical n.** NERVUS TRANSVERSUS COLLI. **transverse cutaneous n. of neck** NERVUS TRANSVERSUS COLLI. **transverse n. of neck** NERVUS TRANSVERSUS COLLI. **n.'s to trapezius** Branches from a plexus formed by the termination of the accessory nerve and the ventral rami of the third and fourth cervical spinal nerves that is situated deep to the trapezius muscle. **trifacial n.** NERVUS TRIGEMINUS. **trigeminal n.** NERVUS TRIGEMINUS. **trochlear n.** NERVUS TROCHLEARIS. **trophic n.** Any nerve concerned with the control of nutrition, digestion, and growth. **twelfth cranial n.** NERVUS HYPOGLOSSUS. **twelfth thoracic n.** NERVUS SUBCOSTALIS. **tympanic n.** NERVUS TYMPANICUS. **tympanic n. of Jacobson** NERVUS TYMPANICUS. **ulnar n.** NERVUS ULNARIS. **ulnar collateral n. of Krause** The muscular branch of the radial nerve to the medial head of the triceps that arises on the medial side of the arm at the base of the axilla. It is accompanied by the ulnar nerve and superior ulnar collateral artery as far as the distal third of the arm. **upper lateral cutaneous n. of arm** NERVUS CUTANEUS BRACHII LATERALIS SUPERIOR. **uterine n.'s** PLEXUS UTERINUS. **utricular n.** NERVUS UTRICULARIS. **utriculoampullar n.** NERVUS UTRICULOAMPULLARIS. **vagal accessory n.** RADICES CRANIALES NERVI ACCESSORII. **vaginal n.'s** NERVI VAGINALES. **vagus n.** NERVUS VAGUS. **vasoconstrictor n.** Any autonomic nerve which upon stimulation causes constriction of blood vessel walls. **vasodilator n.** Any autonomic nerve which upon stimulation causes increased lumen size and flow in blood vessels. **vasomotor n.'s** The autonomic nerves that control the smooth muscle walls of blood vessels. Also *nervi vasorum*. **n. to vastus lateralis muscle** A large branch of the posterior division of the femoral nerve that runs laterally and downwards with the descending branch of the lateral circumflex femoral artery deep to the rectus femoris muscle. It ends in the lower part of the vastus lateralis muscle. It sends a branch to the knee joint. **n. to vastus medialis muscle** A large branch of the posterior division of the femoral nerve that descends along the surface of the vastus medialis muscle in the upper part of the adductor canal to end in the middle of the muscle. It sends a branch to the knee joint. **vertebral n.** NERVUS VERTEBRALIS. **vestibular n.** NERVUS VESTIBULARIS. **vestibulocochlear n.** NERVUS VESTIBULOCOCHLEARIS. **volar interosseous n.** NERVUS INTEROSSEUS ANTEBRACHII ANTERIOR. **n. of Willis** NERVUS ACCESSORIUS. **n. of Wrisberg** 1 NERVUS INTERMEDIUS. 2 NERVUS CUTANEUS BRACHII MEDIALIS. **zygomatic n.** NERVUS ZYGOMATICUS. **zygomaticofacial n.** RAMUS ZYGOMATICOFACIALIS NERVI ZYGOMATICI. **zygomaticotemporal n.** RAMUS ZYGOMATICOTEMPORALIS NERVI ZYGOMATICI.

**nerve-plate / terminal n. of Rouget** *Obs.* MOTOR ENDPLATE.

**nervi** \nur′vī\ Plural of NERVUS.

**nervimotility** \nur′vēmōtil′itē\ NEURIMOTILITY.

**nervimotor** \nur′vēmō′tər\ NEURIMOTOR.

**nervone** The cerebroside formed from sphingosine by acylation of its amino group with nervonic acid and glycosylation of its hydroxyl group with galactose.

**nervonic acid** The $C_{24}$ unsaturated acid of structure $CH_3—[CH_2]_7—CH{=}CH—[CH_2]_{13}—COOH$. It is found in the cerebroside nervone, in which it acylates the amino group of the sphingosine part of the molecule.

**nervosism** \nur′vōsizm\ NEURASTHENIA.

**nervous** 1 Of or relating to a nerve or nerves, as *nervous tissue, central nervous system.* 2 Marked by a feeling of acute and agitated sensitivity. *Popular.*

# nervus

**nervus** \nur′vəs\ [L (akin to Gk *neuron* sinew, tendon, nerve) a sinew, tendon, nerve] (*pl.* nervi) [NA] NERVE. **n. abducens** [NA] The sixth cranial nerve, originating in the caudal pons beneath the floor of the fourth ventricle, emerging anteriorly at the junction of the medulla and pons, and supplying the lateral rectus muscle of the eye. Also *abducent nerve, sixth cranial nerve, abducens.* **n. accessorius** [NA] The eleventh cranial nerve which arises from cranial roots emerging from the ventrolateral surface of the medulla and from spinal roots emerging from the upper 3–5 cervical segments. The roots unite, forming a nerve which divides into a cranial or internal branch and a spinal or external branch. The cranial portion runs with the vagus nerve and innervates the palate, pharynx, larynx, and thoracic viscera. The spinal branch supplies the sternocleidomastoid and trapezius muscles. The nerves include general somatic efferent and general visceral efferent (parasympathetic) components. Also *accessory nerve, eleventh cranial nerve, spinal accessory nerve, nerve of Willis.* **n. acusticus** NERVUS VESTIBULOCOCHLEARIS. **nervi alveolares superiores** [NA] Branches arising from the maxillary nerve in the pterygopalatine fossa or infraorbital canal that supply innervation to the teeth and gingiva of the upper jaw. Posterior, middle and anterior nerves are recognized. Also *superior alveolar nerves, superior dental nerves.* **n. alveolaris inferior** [NA] The direct continuation of the posterior division of the mandibular nerve that descends deep to the lateral pterygoid muscle to pass between the sphenomandibular ligament and ramus of the mandible, where, after giving off the mylohyoid nerve, it enters the mandibular foramen. Within the mandibular canal, branches supply motor and premolar teeth and the adjacent gum, and at the mental foramen gives rise to the mental nerve to the cutaneous and mucosal surfaces of the lower lip. Also *inferior alveolar nerve, inferior dental nerve.* **n. ampullaris anterior** [NA] Fibers of the vestibular nerve that supply the crista ampullaris of the anterior semicircular canal. They travel in the utriculoampullary division of the nerve. Also *anterior ampullary nerve, superior ampullary nerve, nervus ampullaris superior.* **n. ampullaris inferior** NERVUS AMPULLARIS POSTERIOR. **n. ampullaris lateralis** [NA] Component of the utriculoampullary nerve leading from the ampulla of the lateral semicircular canal. Also *lateral ampullary nerve.* **n. ampullaris posterior** [NA] A branch of the vestibular nerve that runs through the foramen singulare at the bottom of the internal auditory meatus and divides into filaments supplying the posterior semicircular canal. Also *posterior ampullary nerve, nervus ampullaris inferior, inferior ampullary nerve.* **n. ampullaris superior** NERVUS AMPULLARIS ANTERIOR. **nervi anococcygei** [NA] An offshoot of the coccygeal plexus ($S_{4,7}$Co) which, after piercing the sacrotuberous ligament, supplies the coccyx and overlying skin. Also *anococcygeal nerve.* **nervi auriculares anteriores** [NA] Two small branches of the auriculotemporal nerve which supply the skin over the tragus of the ear. Also *anterior auricular nerves.* **n. auricularis magnus** [NA] A sensory branch of the cervical plexus that passes around the posterior margin of the sternocleidomastoid muscle and ascends beneath the platysma to the level of the parotid gland, where it divides into an anterior branch distributed to skin over the gland and a posterior branch to skin over the mastoid process, back of the auricle, and ear lobe. A filament pierces the cartilage of the auricle to innervate the concha. It carries fibers from $C_2$ and $_3$ segmental levels. Also *great auricular nerve.* **n. auricularis posterior** [NA] A branch of the facial nerve that ascends between the external acoustic meatus and mastoid process to supply the auricularis posterior and intrinsic auricular muscles via an auricular branch, and the occipitalis muscle through its occipital branch. Also *posterior auricular nerve.* **n. auriculotemporalis** [NA] A sensory branch from the posterior trunk of the mandibular nerve, arising from two roots that embrace the middle meningeal artery. It supplies anterior auricular branches to the tragus, external meatus, and tympanic membrane; temporal branches to the temple and scalp; twigs to the temporomandibular joint; and relays otic ganglion and sympathetic fibers to the parotid gland. Also *auriculotemporal nerve.* **n. axillaris** [NA] One of the five major terminal branches of the brachial plexus. Composed of $C_5$ and $C_6$ axons from the posterior cord, it winds around the humerus by passing backward through the quadrangular space. Its branches supply the deltoid and teres minor muscles, and form the upper lateral cutaneous nerve of the arm. Also *axillary nerve, circumflex humeral nerve.* **n. buccalis** [NA] A branch of the anterior trunk of the mandibular nerve. After passing forward between the two heads of the lateral pterygoid, it courses downward to cross the pterygomandibular raphe and join with branches of the facial nerve that ramify on the buccinator muscle. It supplies the skin and mucosa of the cheek near the mouth and the buccal surface of the gums, and sends a motor branch to the lateral pterygoid. Also *buccal nerve, long buccal nerve, buccinator nerve, nervus buccinatorius.* **n. canalis pterygoidei** [NA] A nerve formed in the foramen lacerum by the joining of parasympathetic and sensory fibers of the greater petrosal nerve (from the facial nerve) with sympathetic fibers of the deep petrosal nerve. It passes through the pterygoid canal, at the rostral end of which it enters the pterygopalatine fossa. The parasympathetic fibers synapse in the pterygopalatine ganglion, while sympathetic and sensory axons simply pass through for distribution over the ganglion's branches. Also *nerve of pterygoid canal.* **nervi cardiaci cervicale** Nerves that arise at three levels along the cervical sympathetic trunk and descend through the thoracic inlet to end in the cardiac plexuses. Their sympathetic fibers ultimately reach the lungs and other thoracic viscera, as well as the heart. Afferent fibers mediating pain travel in the middle and inferior cervical cardiac nerves, but not in the superior one. **nervi cardiaci thoracici** [NA] Filaments that arise from the second to fourth thoracic sympathetic ganglia and end in the deep cardiac plexus. They have an acceleratory influence on the heart equal to that of the cervical cardiac nerves, and carry visceral afferent fibers. Also *thoracic cardiac nerves.* **n. cardiacus cervicalis inferior** [NA] A nerve that arises from the cervicothoracic ganglion of the sympathetic trunk to descend behind the subclavian artery and join the deep cardiac plexus. Also *nervus cardiacus inferior, inferior cardiac nerve, inferior cervical cardiac nerve.* **n. cardiacus cervicalis medius** [NA] The largest of the sympathetic nerves to the heart. It arises from the middle cervical sympathetic ganglion or nearby trunk, and ends in the deep cardiac plexus. Also *middle cervical cardiac nerve, middle cardiac nerve, nervus cardiacus medius.* **n. cardiacus cervicalis superior** [NA] A cardiac nerve arising from the lower pole of the superior cervical sympathetic ganglion. On the right side it enters the deep cardiac plexus and, on the left, the superficial part of the plexus. Also *nervus cardiacus superior, superior cardiac nerve, superior cervical cardiac nerve.* **n. cardiacus inferior** NERVUS CARDIACUS CERVICALIS INFERIOR. **n. cardiacus medius** NERVUS CARDIACUS CERVICALIS MEDIUS. **n. cardiacus superior** NERVUS CARDIACUS CERVICALIS SUPERIOR. **nervi carotici externi** [NA] Twigs bridging over to the superior cervical sympathetic ganglion from the external carotid plexus. Their axons are distributed via branches of the artery. Also *external carotid nerves.* **nervi caroticotympanici** [NA] Two tiny filaments that leave the internal carotid sympathetic plexus to pass through openings in the posterior wall of the carotid canal and enter the middle ear, where they join the tympanic plexus. Inferior and superior nerves are distinguished. Also *caroticotympanic nerves, small deep petrosal nerves.* **n. caroticus internus** [NA] A fine nerve passing upward from the superior cervical sympathetic ganglion to join the internal carotid plexus. Also *internal carotid nerve.* **nervi cavernosi clitoridis** [NA] Bundles, composed of sympathetic, parasympathetic, and sensory fibers, that supply the erectile tissue of the clitoris. They are forward continuations of the uterovaginal plexus. Also *cavernous nerves of clitoris.* **nervi cavernosi penis** [NA] Nerves that supply the erectile tissue of the corpora cavernosa and corpus spongiosum. They arise as offshoots from the front of the prostatic plexus, are joined by branches of the pudendal nerve, and carry postganglionic sympathetic, parasympathetic, and sensory fibers. Also *cavernous nerves of penis.* **nervi celiaci** RAMI CELIACI NERVI VAGI. **nervi cerebrales** *Outmoded* NERVI CRA-

NIALES. **nervi cervicales** [NA] Spinal nerves arising from cervical segments of the spinal cord. There are eight, including the suboccipital nerve ($C_1$) and the nerve ($C_8$) passing through the foramen between the last cervical and first thoracic vertebrae. Each divides into a dorsal and ventral primary ramus. The ventral primary rami at levels $C_1$–$C_4$ form the cervical plexus, and at levels $C_5$–$C_8$ contribute to the brachial plexus. Also *cervical nerves.* **n. cervicalis superficialis** NERVUS TRANSVERSUS COLLI. **nervi ciliares breves** [NA] Filaments that leave the ciliary ganglion carrying postganglionic parasympathetic fibers as well as transient sympathetic and general sensory axons to the eyeball. Ten to twelve nerves leave the ganglion, and subdivide into 15–20 strands that pierce the sclera around the optic nerve and travel forward in impressions on the sclera to supply the sphincter pupillae and ciliaris muscles and blood vessels and sensory endings of the choroid and iris. Also *short ciliary nerves.* **nervi ciliares longi** [NA] Two or three slender branches of the nasociliary nerve that penetrate the sclera near the optic nerve and run forwards between the sclera and choroid to terminals in the ciliary body, iris, and cornea. They carry superior cervical sympathetic post-ganglionic fibers to the dilator pupillae and the sensory innervation of the cornea. Also *long ciliary nerves.* **nervi clunium inferiores** [NA] Several branches of the posterior femoral cutaneous nerve that round the inferior border of the gluteus maximus to supply the skin over the lower part of that muscle. Also *inferior clunial nerves.* **nervi clunium medii** [NA] Two or three branches of the lateral divisions of the dorsal primary rami that pierce the gluteus maximus to innervate the skin over the adjacent gluteal and sacral area. A gap separates the segmental representation, $S_{1-3}$, of these nerves from that of the superior gluteal nerves, $L_{1-3}$. Also *middle clunial nerves, middle gluteal nerves.* **nervi clunium superiores** [NA] Lateral branches of the $L_{1-3}$ dorsal primary rami that appear at the outer border of the erector spinae and cross the iliac crest to supply the skin over the upper and lateral gluteal region.

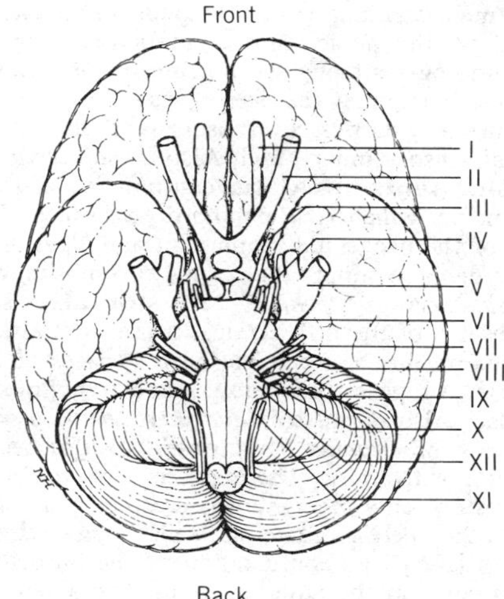


**Cranial nerves** (bottom view) (I) Olfactory; (II) optic; (III) oculomotor; (IV) trochlear; (V) trigeminal; (VI) abducens; (VII) facial; (VIII) vestibulocochlear; (IX) glossopharyngeal; (X) vagus; (XI) accessory; (XII) hypoglossal.

Also *superior clunial nerves.* **n. coccygeus** [NA] One of the pair of nerves that emerge from the coccygeal segment of the spinal cord to supply the region of the coccyx. Also *coccygeal nerve.* **n. cochleae** PARS COCHLEARIS NERVI OCTAVI. **nervi craniales** The twelve pairs of nerves which are connected with the intracranial portion of the central nervous system. Also *cranial nerves, nervi cerebrales* (outmoded), *cerebral nerves* (outmoded). **n. cutaneus** [NA] A nerve supplying an area of skin and its underlying fascia. It carries sympathetic fibers to the glands, blood vessels, and arrectores pili and other smooth muscle, as well as sensory axons. Also *cutaneous nerve.* **n. cutaneus antebrachii dorsalis** NERVUS CUTANEUS ANTEBRACHII POSTERIOR. **n. cutaneus antebrachii lateralis** [NA] The cutaneous component ($C_{5,6}$) of the musculocutaneous nerve. It sends an anterior branch along the volar aspect of the forearm and a posterior branch down the dorsal surface, both reaching as far as the thenar eminence. Also *lateral antebrachial cutaneous nerve, lateral cutaneous nerve of forearm.* **n. cutaneus antebrachii medialis** [NA] A nerve ($C_8$, $T_1$) arising from the medial cord of the brachial plexus. It supplies the skin over the anteromedial aspect of the elbow and forearm to the wrist, and an adjoining strip on the dorsal aspect of the forearm. Also *medial antebrachial cutaneous nerve, medial cutaneous nerve of forearm.* **n. cutaneus antebrachii posterior** [NA] A branch ($C_{5,6,7,8}$) of the radial nerve that pierces the lateral head of the triceps to supply an extensive area of skin along the dorsolateral side of the arm, elbow, and forearm down to the wrist. Also *posterior antebrachial cutaneous nerve, posterior cutaneous nerve of forearm, nervus cutaneus antebrachii dorsalis, dorsal cutaneous nerve of forearm.* **n. cutaneus brachii lateralis inferior** [NA] A branch ($C_{5,6}$) of the radial nerve that pierces the lateral head of the triceps to supply the skin over the lateral part of the lower half of the arm. Anteriorly the distribution adjoins that of the medial brachial cutaneous nerve. Also *inferior lateral brachial cutaneous nerve, inferior lateral cutaneous nerve of arm.* **n. cutaneus brachii lateralis superior** [NA] A branch of the axillary nerve that passes around the posterior margin of the deltoid muscle to supply the skin over the insertion of that muscle and the adjacent triceps. Also *upper lateral cutaneous nerve of arm, superior lateral cutaneous nerve of arm, lateral superior cutaneous nerve of arm.* **n. cutaneus brachii medialis** [NA] A small offshoot ($C_8$, $T_1$) of the medial cord of the brachial plexus that supplies the skin over the medial side of the lower third of the arm. It is usually joined by the intercostobrachial nerve ($T_2$), or may be replaced by that nerve. Also *medial cutaneous nerve of arm, internal cutaneous nerve, nerve of Wrisberg.* **n. cutaneus brachii posterior** [NA] A nerve ($C_{5,6,7,8}$) that, in the axilla, leaves the radial nerve to supply a small area of skin over the dorsum of the middle third of the arm. Also *posterior brachial cutaneous nerve, posterior cutaneous nerve of arm.* **n. cutaneus colli** NERVUS TRANSVERSUS COLLI. **n. cutaneus dorsalis intermedius** [NA] The smaller of two terminal branches of the superficial peroneal nerve. It supplies the skin on the lateral aspect of the ankle and on contiguous sides of the lateral three toes, as well as nearby joints. Also *intermediate dorsal cutaneous nerve.* **n. cutaneus dorsalis lateralis** [NA] The continuation of the sural nerve along the lateral border of the foot ($L_5$, $S_{1,2}$). Also *lateral dorsal cutaneous nerve of foot.* **n. cutaneus dorsalis medialis** [NA] The branch of the superficial peroneal nerve supplying the skin and joints along the medial side of the great toe and the cleft between the second and third toes. Also *medial dor-*

*sal cutaneous nerve of foot.* **n. cutaneus femoris lateralis** [NA] A nerve supplying the skin over the lateral and anterior aspects of the thigh from the inguinal ligament to the knee. It arises from posterior divisions of the $L_2$ and $L_3$ anterior primary rami, and leaves the pelvis by passing beneath the inguinal ligament near the anterior superior iliac spine. Also *lateral femoral cutaneous nerve, lateral cutaneous nerve of thigh.* **n. cutaneus femoris posterior** [NA] A large contribution of the sacral plexus to cutaneous innervation of the thigh. Arising from $S_{1-3}$ levels, it lies dorsomedial to the sciatic nerve as the latter passes out the infrapiriform aperture of the sciatic foramen. Below the gluteus maximus it becomes cutaneous and runs down the middle of the thigh and onto the calf. It supplies the skin along this zone, and sends inferior cluneal branches over the lower portion of the gluteus maximus and a long perineal branch to the lateral extent of the perineum. Also *posterior femoral cutaneous nerve, small sciatic nerve, posterior cutaneous nerve of thigh.* **n. cutaneus surae lateralis** [NA] A branch ($L_{4,5}$ $S_1$) of the common peroneal nerve that supplies the skin over the anterior, posterior, and lateral surfaces of the proximal leg. It gives rise to the sural communicating branch. Also *lateral cutaneous nerve of calf, peroneal cutaneous nerve* (outmoded). **n. cutaneus surae medialis** [NA] The tibial nerve component of the sural nerve. It descends between the heads of the gastrocnemius and is then joined by the communicating branch of the lateral sural to form the sural nerve. Also *medial sural cutaneous nerve, medial cutaneous nerve of calf.* **n. descendens cervicalis** RADIX INFERIOR ANSAE CERVICALIS. **nervi digitales** One of the four nerves that course along the dorsolateral and ventrolateral aspects of a digit to supply its joints, skin, and nailbed. It may arise directly from a major parent nerve, e.g., ulnar, or through bifurcation of a common digital nerve. Also *digital nerves.* **nervi digitales dorsales** [NA] Small nerves that extend varying distances along the dorsolateral surfaces of a digit to give cutaneous and articular innervation. In the human hand those to the radial $2^1/_2$ fingers arise from common or proper digital branches of the superficial radial nerve (nervi digitales dorsales nervi radiales) while nerves to the remaining fingers arise from comparable branches of the dorsal carpal branch of the ulnar nerve (nervi digitales dorsales nervi ulnaris). Also *dorsal digital nerves.* **nervi digitales dorsales pedis** [NA] Branches of the deep and superficial peroneal nerves that supply a single side of toe, i.e., proper digital nerves, or split to supply adjacent sides of two toes, i.e., common digital nerves. Also *dorsal digital nerves of foot.* **nervi digitales palmares** Digital nerves that course along the ventral aspect of a finger. They arise from the ulnar and median nerves. Also *palmar digital nerves.* **nervi digitales palmares communes** [NA] Sensory nerves of the palmar surface of the hand which, as they approach the cleft between two fingers, divide into proper digital nerves supplying adjacent surfaces of the digits. Two arise from the median nerve and one from the ulnar nerve. **nervi digitales palmares proprii** [NA] Small nerves coursing along the two sides of a digit on its volar aspect. In the human hand six usually arise through bifurcation of common digital nerves, while single branches arising directly from the ulnar and median nerve trunks travel along the ulnar side of the little finger, radial side of the index finger, and both sides of the thumb. They innervate the joints, the skin over the volar surfaces, the nail bed, and generally, via dorsal branches, the skin over the middle and distal phalanges. Also *proper palmar digital nerves, nervi digitales volares proprii.* **nervi digitales plantares** Digital nerves that course along the ventral aspect of a toe. They arise from the medial and later plantar nerves. Also *plantar digital nerves.* **nervi digitales plantares communes nervi plantaris lateralis** [NA] The two digital nerves into which the superficial branch of the lateral plantar nerve divides. The lateral of these supplies the flexor digiti minimi brevis muscle and two interosseous muscles in the fourth intermetatarsal space, and then continues along the lateral aspect of the little toe as the sensory nerve to that region. The more medial nerve divides into two proper branches that serve as the sensory nerves, each supplying one of the adjacent surfaces of the fourth and fifth toes. Also *common plantar digital nerves of lateral plantar nerve.* **nervi digitales plantares communes nervi plantaris medialis** [NA] The three digital nerves into which themedial plantar nerve divides. Each splits into two proper digital nerves that supply cutaneous innervation to the four medial toes. The most medial of these supplies proper plantar digital nerves to the adjacent sides of the great toe and the second toe; the intermediate nerve supplies the adjacent sides of the second and third toes; and the most lateral supplies the adjacent sides of the third and fourth toes. Also *common plantar digital nerves of medial plantar nerve.* **nervi digitales plantares proprii nervi plantaris lateralis** [NA] Proper digital branches of the lateral plantar nerve. They are distributed to adjacent sides of the digits IV and V, and to the lateral side of the fifth digit. **nervi digitales plantares proprii nervi plantaris medialis** [NA] Proper digital branches of the medial plantar nerve. They are distributed to the medial three toes and one side of the fourth toe, each branch supplying one side of a toe. Several arise through bifurcation of common digital nerves destined for adjacent sides of two toes. **nervi digitales volares proprii** NERVI DIGITALES PALMARES PROPRII. **n. digitalis communis** A digital nerve which as it approaches the cleft between two fingers divides into two proper digital nerves supplying the adjacent surfaces of the digits. Also *common digital nerve.* **n. digitalis proprius** A digital nerve which arises directly from a major nerve without being associated with nerves to other digits. Also *proper digital nerve.* **n. dorsalis clitoridis** [NA] The main continuation of the pudendal nerve. It passes forward along the pubic ramus, enters the urogenital diaphragm, and courses along the dorsum of the clitoris to end in the glans. It supplies the deep transverse perineal muscle, sphincter urethra, corpus cavernosum, and glans with motor and general sensory innervation. Also *dorsal nerve of clitoris.* **n. dorsalis penis** [NA] The continuation of the internal pudendal nerve, which runs on the deep surface of the inferior layer of the urogenital diaphragm and then on the dorsum of the penis to supply the corpus cavernosum and glans. Also *dorsal nerve of penis.* **n. dorsalis scapulae** [NA] A branch of the fifth cervical nerve that, after piercing the scalenus medius to reach the deep surfaces of the rhomboid muscles, supplies these muscles and sometimes the levator scapulae. Also *dorsal scapular nerve, nerve to rhomboids, dorsal nerve of scapula.* **nervi erigentes** NERVI SPLANCHNICI PELVICI. • The term is not preferred, since these nerves not only innervate the erectile tissue of the genitalia, but other pelvic organs as well. **n. ethmoidalis anterior** [NA] The continuation of the nasociliary nerve beyond its entry in the anterior ethmoid foramen and canal. It supplies internal nasal branches to the septum and lateral wall of the nasal cavity, and then emerges at the distal border of the nasal bone as the external nasal branch supplying the skin over the bridge, apex, ala, and vestibule of the nose. Also *anterior ethmoidal nerve.* **n. ethmoidalis poste-**

**rior** [NA] A twig of the nasociliary nerve that exits the orbit through the posterior ethmoid foramen to supply posterior ethmoidal air cells and the sphenoid sinus. Also *posterior ethmoidal nerve, nerve of Luschka.* **n. facialis** [NA] The seventh cranial nerve and a derivative of the second branchial arch. Arising anteriorly to the inferior cerebellar peduncle at the caudal border of the pons as a motor root and a distinct nervus intermedius bearing sensory and parasympathetic preganglionic fibers, it traverses the internal acoustic meatus and enters the facial canal, where the geniculate ganglion of its sensory fibers is located. The main nerve leaves the canal at the stylomastoid foramen and in the parotid gland separates into branches distributed to muscles of the scalp, auricle and face, the platysma, stylohyoid muscles and posterior belly of the digastric. Also *seventh cranial nerve, facial nerve, portio dura paris septimi* (outmoded). **n. femoralis** [NA] The sensorimotor nerve to an extensive anteromedial region of the lower leg. Contributions from $L_{2-4}$ spinal nerves join within the belly of the psoas muscle to form the nerve trunk which, still resting on the muscle surface, leaves the abdomen by passing beneath the inguinal ligament. Within the femoral trigone it splits into several muscular and cutaneous branches, of which the saphenous nerve is the direct continuation. The nerve supplies the sartorius, quadriceps femoris, and pectineus muscles, the skin over the anterior and medial surfaces of the limb from the inguinal ligament to the big toe, and nearby sectors of joints. Also *femoral nerve, anterior crural nerve.* **n. fibularis communis** NERVUS PERONEUS COMMUNIS. **n. fibularis profundus** NERVUS PERONEUS PROFUNDUS. **n. fibularis superficialis** NERVUS PERONEUS SUPERFICIALIS. **n. frontalis** [NA] The largest branch of the ophthalmic nerve. It enters the orbit through the superior orbital fissure, and coursing between the levator palpebrae and periorbita separates into a supraorbital nerve and a smaller, more medially located supratrochlear nerve. Also *frontal nerve.* **n. furcalis** The lumbar spinal nerve whose anterior primary ramus bifurcates to contribute to both the lumbar and sacral plexuses. Generally it is the $L_4$ nerve, but it may be $L_3$ or $L_5$. Also *furcal nerve.* **n. genitofemoralis** [NA] A mixed nerve arising from $L_1$ and $_2$ levels of the lumbar plexus. It passes obliquely downwards through and on the psoas major muscle to divide above the inguinal ligament into an external spermatic nerve that enters the deep inguinal ring and a femoral branch that descends beneath the inguinal ligament to the femoral trigone. Also *genitofemoral nerve, nervus genitocruralis.* **n. glossopharyngeus** [NA] The ninth cranial nerve, innervating structures derived from the third branchial arch, including the mucosa of the oropharynx, tonsil, and the postsulcal part of the tongue, as well as one muscle, the stylopharyngeus. All the general and the special sensory fibers have their cell bodies in the inferior and superior ganglia located in the jugular foramen. Centrally the fibers of general sensibility synapse in the nucleus of the spinal tract of the trigeminal nerve, while the taste fibers end in the nucleus of the tractus solitarius. The motor fibers arise in the nucleus ambiguus. The nerve's parasympathetic fibers come from the inferior salivatory nucleus, and pass through the lesser petrosal branch to the otic ganglion, which gives off postsynaptic fibers to the parotid gland. Also *glossopharyngeal nerve, glossopharyngeus, ninth cranial nerve.* **n. gluteus inferior** [NA] A nerve arising from ventral rami of the $L_5$, $S_{1,2}$ nerves that leaves the pelvis below the piriformis muscle to supply the gluteus maximus. Also *inferior gluteal nerve.* **n. gluteus superior** [NA] The superior ($L_{4,5}$ $S_1$) of two nerves supplying the main gluteal muscles. It leaves the pelvis through the suprapiriform portion of the greater sciatic foramen to enter the gluteal region. A superior branch ends in the gluteus medius, and an inferior branch supplies this muscle, the gluteus minimus, and farther anteriorly the tensor fasciae latae. The latter branch also supplies the hip joint. Also *superior gluteal nerve.* **nervi haemorrhoidales inferiores** NERVI RECTALES INFERIORES. **nervi haemorrhoidales medii** *Obs.* PLEXUS RECTALES MEDII. **n. hypogastricus dexter et sinister** [NA] The bundle of nerve filaments between the point of bifurcation of the superior hypogastric plexus and the more expanded inferior hypogastric plexus of one side. Also *hypogastric nerve, hypogastric nerve of Latarjet.* **n. hypoglossus** [NA] The twelfth cranial nerve, providing innervation to all the muscles of the tongue except the palatoglossus. The fibers arise in cell columns of the medulla homologous in position with the anterior column in the cord at lower levels, an indication of their origin from four occipitocervical somites. Rootlets surface in the centerolateral sulcus between the pyramid and olive and, after gathering into one or more bundles, pass forward through the hypoglossal canal. A recurrent branch passes to meninges of the posterior fossa. Fibers from the first cervical nerve join the true hypoglossal fibers, to pass on to the geniohyoid and thyrohyoid muscles and, via the descendens hypoglossi branch, to strap muscles of the neck. Also *hypoglossal nerve, hypoglossus, motor nerve of tongue, twelfth cranial nerve.* **n. iliohypogastricus** [NA] The main trunk of the first lumbar nerve. In its course between the transversalis abdominis and internal oblique muscles above the iliac crest, it divides into a lateral cutaneous branch that supplies the skin over the posterolateral gluteal region, and an anterior trunk that sends branches to the two muscles and then perforates the external oblique aponeurosis to supply the skin above the pubis. Also *iliohypogastric nerve.* **n. ilioinguinalis** [NA] The major continuation of the first lumbar spinal nerve which, in an oblique course across the abdomen, supplies the abdominal muscles, the skin and peritoneum over the pubis symphysis, and the anterior scrotum or labia. It is homologous with the collateral branch of an intercostal nerve. The nerve emerges from behind the psoas major muscle, and crosses the posterior abdominal wall to pass through the deep inguinal ring and inguinal canal. A lateral branch supplies the skin over a superomedial area of the thigh. Also *ilioinguinal nerve.* **n. infraorbitalis** [NA] The continuation of the maxillary nerve beyond its entry into the infraorbital groove and canal. After exiting from the infraorbital foramen, it divides into branches spreading to the alae of the nose, the lower eyelid, and the skin and mucous membrane of the cheek and upper lip. Also *infraorbital nerve.* **n. infratrochlearis** [NA] A branch of the nasociliary nerve. It runs forward along the upper border of the medial rectus muscle, and just below the trochlea pierces the orbital septum to supply the skin of the eyelids, conjunctiva, lacrymal sac, duct and caruncle, and an adjacent portion of the nose. Also *infratrochlear nerve.* **nervi intercostobrachiales** [NA] The particularly large lateral cutaneous branch of the second intercostal nerve. It crosses the axilla to supply the skin over medial and posterior aspects of the upper arm. The homologous third intercostal branch supplying the axilla and medial aspect of the arm is sometimes distinguished as a second intercostobrachial nerve. Also *intercostobrachial nerves.* **n. intermedius** The smaller root of the seventh cranial (facial) nerve which contains special sensory fibers for taste to the anterior two thirds of the tongue and parasympathetic fibers supplying secretomotor impulses to the submaxillary, sublingual, lacrimal, nasal, and palatine glands. Also *intermediate nerve of*

*Wrisberg, nerve of Wrisberg, nervus intermedius of Wrisberg, intermediary nerve, portio intermedia nervi acustici* (outmoded). **n. interosseus antebrachii anterior** [NA] A major branch of the median nerve that courses along the interosseous membrane deep to the flexor pollicis longus, flexor digitorum profundus, and pronator quadratus muscles, supplying these muscles, sensory receptors on the interosseous membrane, and distally the radioulnar, radiocarpal, and carpal joints. Also *anterior interosseous nerve of forearm, volar interosseous nerve, nervus interosseus antebrachii volaris.* **n. interosseus antebrachii posterior** [NA] A motor branch of the radial nerve that innervates the majority of muscles on the dorsal aspect of the forearm. It separates from the superficial radial nerve in the lateral part of the cubital fossa, sends branches to the extensor carpi radialis brevis and supinator; short branches to the extensores digitorum, digiti minimi and carpi ulnaris; a lateral branch to the abductor pollicis longus and extensor pollicis brevis; and a medial branch ot the extensores pollicis longus and indicis. Also *posterior interosseous nerve of forearm, ramus profundus nervi radialis, deep radial nerve, deep branch of radial nerve.* **n. interosseus antebrachii volaris** NERVUS INTEROSSEUS ANTEBRACHII ANTERIOR. **n. interosseus cruris** [NA] A branch of the popliteus muscle nerve (from the tibial nerve) that descends alongside the fibula as far as the inferior tibiofibular joint. It supplies this joint and sensory receptors on the interosseous membrane. Also *interosseous nerve of leg.* **n. ischiadicus** [NA] The major contribution of the sacral plexus ($L_4$-$S_3$) to innervation of the lower extremity. The largest nerve in the body, it typically enters the gluteal region through the infrapiriform aperture of the greater sciatic foramen, though its peroneal (dorsal) division often pierces the piriformis, or may be separated by the entire muscle from the tibial (ventral) division. The latter gives rise to branches to the hamstring muscles, including the ischial head of the adductor magnus, while the peroneal division supplies the short head of the biceps femoris. A sprig is sent to the hip joint. The nerve divides at the upper limit of the popliteal fossa into the tibial and common peroneal nerves. Also *sciatic nerve, great sciatic nerve, ischiadic nerve.* **n. jugularis** [NA] A nerve that leaves the superior cervical sympathetic ganglion to ascend toward the base of the skull, where it sends branches to the inferior ganglion of the glossopharyngeal nerve and the superior ganglion of the vagus, as well as filaments to the jugular bulb and meninges. Also *jugular nerve, jugular nerve of Arnold.* **nervi labiales anteriores** [NA] Sensory branches of the ilioinguinal nerve supplying the anterior extent of the labium major. Its segmental supply, $L_{1,2}$, contrasts sharply with that of the adjoining posterior labial branches of the pudendal nerve, $S_{3,4}$. Also *anterior labial nerves.* **nervi labiales posteriores** [NA] Medial and lateral branches of the perineal nerve that, after piercing the inferior fascia of the urogenital diaphragm, innervate a major portion of the labia majora. Also *posterior labial nerves.* **n. lacrimalis** [NA] The smallest branch of the ophthalmic nerve. It enters the orbit through the superior orbital fissure, runs along the upper border of the rectus lateralis, and after piercing the orbital septum supplies the skin of the upper eyelid. It is joined by secretomotor fibers from the zygomaticotemporal nerve, which are given off to the lacrimal gland and nearby conjunctiva. Also *lacrimal nerve.* **n. laryngeus inferior** [NA] The continuation of the recurrent laryngeal nerve beyond its point of entrance into the larynx deep to the inferior constrictor muscle and posterior to the cricothyroid articulation. It is distributed to the mucosa and glands of the larynx below the vocal cord, and the laryngeal musculature except for the cricothyroid. Also *inferior laryngeal nerve.* **n. laryngeus recurrens** [NA] A branch of the vagus nerve distributed to portions of the larynx, trachea, and esophagus. It supplies sensory and autonomic innervation to the cervical esophagus, the trachea, and the larynx up as far as the vocal cords, as well as motor fibers to all the skeletal muscles of the larynx except the cricothyroid. At its origin from the vagus, it sends branches to the deep cardiac plexus that are distributed to thoracic viscera. After leaving the main vagus trunk on the right side it winds around the subclavian artery, and on the left side winds around the arch of the aorta just distal to the ligamentum arteriosum. Thereafter it travels up the groove between esophagus and trachea to enter the larynx. Also *recurrent laryngeal nerve, recurrent nerve, ramus laryngeus recurrens nervi vagi, nervus recurrens, ramus laryngei inferior nervi vagi.* **n. laryngeus superior** [NA] A branch of the vagus nerve that, after arising from the inferior vagal ganglion, splits into the internal and external laryngeal nerves, which give sensory and autonomic innervation to the hypopharynx and the larynx above the vocal cord, as well as motor fibers to the inferior constrictor and cricothyroid muscles. Also *superior laryngeal nerve.* **n. lingualis** [NA] The sensory nerve to the mucous membrane of the floor of the mouth, the lingual aspect of the mandibular gums, and the two-thirds of the tongue anterior to the terminal sulcus, exclusive of the taste receptors. It arises from the posterior division of the mandibular nerve, and is joined by the chorda tympani for distribution to sublingual and lingual salivary glands. Also *lingual nerve.* **nervi lumbales** [NA] The five anterior primary rami of spinal nerves that appear through intervertebral foraminae below respective lumbar vertebrae. The four more cranial rami join the lumbar plexus and two join the sacral plexus, the fourth nerve (the furcal nerve) generally contributing to both plexuses. They also connect with the sympathetic trunk by gray and, at the upper first or second levels, white rami. Also *lumbar nerves.* **n. lumboinguinalis** RAMUS FEMORALIS NERVI GENITOFEMORALIS. **n. mandibularis** [NA] The largest division of the trigeminal nerve. It is formed from a sensory root from the lateral third of the semilunar ganglion and a motor root, which join after passing through the foramen ovale. The nerve divides into anterior and posterior trunks whose branches supply the skin of the temporal region, the auricle, the lower lip and face, the mucosa of the pre-sulcal part of the tongue and floor of the mouth, and the teeth and gums of the mandible. The motor component supplies all the muscles of mastication. Sprigs from the main trunk reach the internal pterygoid nerve and the meninges. Also *mandibular nerve.* **n. massetericus** [NA] The nerve supply of the masseter muscle. It arises from the anterior trunk of the mandibular nerve and passes through the mandibular notch, giving a twig en route to the temporomandibular joint. Also *masseteric nerve.* **n. masticatorius** *Obs.* RADIX MOTORIA NERVI TRIGEMINI. **n. maxillaris** [NA] The intermediate division of the trigeminal nerve, supplying derivatives of the embryonic maxillary and frontonasal processes. Arising in the semilunar ganglion, it passes through the cavernous sinus, exits the foramen rotundum, crosses the pterygopalatine fossa, and continues as the infraorbital nerve after entering the inferior orbital fissure. Branches go to the meninges of the middle fossa, the teeth, skin and mucosal linings of the upper jaw, and the palate, lip, cheek, lower lid, and nasal and sinus cavities. Also *maxillary nerve, crotaphitic nerve* (outmoded). **n. meatus acustici externi** [NA] The sensory branch of the auriculotemporal nerve supplying the tympanic membrane and the skin lining the external auditory meatus. Also *nerve of external acoustic meatus, nervus meatus auditorii externi.* **n. medianus** [NA] The major nerve ($C_5$-$T_1$) to flexor aspects of the forearm and hand. It arises as two roots springing from lateral and medial cords of the brachial plexus, and courses deep within the medial bicipital furrow to the cubital fossa, where it passes between two heads of the pronator teres. It then descends deep to the flexor digitorum superficialis and flexor retinaculum, finally dividing into palmar digital nerves to the radial $3^1/_2$ digits and a stout muscular branch. The latter is of major functional importance, since it innervates the flexor pollicis brevis, abductor pollicis brevis, and opponens pollicis. In the forearm the median nerve gives rise to the nervus interosseous antebrachii. Also *median nerve.* **n. meningeus medius** RAMUS MENINGEUS MEDIUS NERVI MAXILLARIS. **n. mentalis** [NA] The continuation of the inferior alveolar nerve after it emerges from the mental foramen. It sends separate branches to the skin over the chin, the skin of the lip, and the mucosa. Also *mental nerve.* **n. musculi quadrati femoris** [NA] A nerve arising from the ventral branches of the ventral rami of the fourth and fifth lumbar and first sacral nerves and passing through the greater sciatic foramen below the piriform muscle to run deep to the sciatic nerve, obturator internus, and gemelli muscles. It supplies branches to the anterior surface of the gemellus inferior muscle and the hip joint, and it ends in the quadratus femoris muscle. Also *nerve to gemellus inferior and quadratus femoris muscles, nerve to quadratus femoris muscle.* **n. musculi tensoris tympani** [NA] Fibers of the nerve to medial pterygoid muscle which pass through the otic ganglion without synapsing with its cells and run posteriorly to provide motor and proprioceptive innervation to the tensor tympani muscle. Also *nervus tensoris tympani* (outmoded), *nerve of tensor tympani muscle, nerve to muscle of malleus.* **n. musculocutaneus** [NA] A major terminal branch ($C_{5-7}$) of the lateral cord of the brachial plexus, innervating flexor aspects of the upper limb. It perforates and supplies the coracobrachialis, sends branches to the brachialis and biceps as it courses distalward between these muscles, and emerges as the lateral cutaneous nerve supplying the skin along the radial forearm as far as the thenar eminence. Branches are sent into the elbow joint and nutrient foramen of the humerus. Also *musculocutaneous nerve, musculocutaneous nerve of arm.* **n. mylohyoideus** [NA] A branch of the inferior alveolar nerve that descends along the medial aspect of the mandible to reach the inferior surface of the mylohyoid muscle. It innervates this muscle and the anterior belly of the digastric. Also *mylohyoid nerve.* **n. nasociliaris** A branch of the ophthalmic division of the fifth cranial (trigeminal) nerve. It supplies sensory innervation to the mucous membrane of the nasal cavity and sinuses and to the skin of the ala and apex of the nose. Also *nasociliary nerve.* **n. nasopalatinus** A branch of the maxillary division of the fifth cranial (trigeminal) nerve, supplying sensory innervation to the roof of the nasal cavity and septum. Also *nasopalatine nerve, nerve of Cotunnius, Scarpa's nerve, sphenoidpalatine nerve* (outmoded). **nervi nervorum** Filaments supplying sensory and sympathetic innervation to the sheath and endoneurium of a peripheral nerve. **n. obturatorius** [NA] The major nerve to the adductor group of leg muscles. It arises from anterior divisions of the $L_{2-4}$ anterior primary rami, assembles in the belly of the psoas major muscle, and passes along the lateral pelvic wall to the entrance of the obturator canal. Within the canal it splits into an anterior branch that sends branches to the gracilis, adductores longus and brevis, and often the pectineus; and a posterior branch deep to the brevis that supplies this muscle and more anterior portions of the adductor magnus. Filaments are sent to the hip and knee joints. Also *obturator nerve.* **n. obturatorius accessorius** [NA] A fairly constant nerve that arises from the ventral branches of the ventral rami of the third and fourth lumbar nerves and accompanies the obturator nerve along the medial border of the psoas major muscle into the pelvis. There it crosses the superior pubic ramus behind the pectineus muscle and divides into branches that supply the pectineus, the hip joint, and the adductor longus muscle. Also *accessory obturator nerve.* **n. obturatorius internus** [NA] A nerve that is formed by the ventral branches of the ventral rami of the fifth lumbar and first and second sacral nerves. It leaves the pelvis through the greater sciatic foramen below the piriformis muscle, and, after crossing the ischial spine, it re-enters the pelvis through the lesser sciatic foramen and ends in the pelvic surface of the obturator internus muscle. Above the ischial spine it also gives a branch to the gemellus superior muscle. **n. occipitalis major** [NA] A nerve which, passing upward around the inferior oblique muscle (i.e., outside the occipital triangle) and semispinalis capitis, pierces the latter and fibers of the trapezius to ramify in the scalp as far forward as the vertex. A motor branch is given to the semispinalis. It represents the medial branch of the dorsal primary ramus of the $C_2$ spinal nerve. Also *greater occipital nerve, internal occipital nerve.* **n. occipitalis minor** [NA] A branch arising from the anterior primary ramus of the second cervical nerve and sometimes the third, that supplies the scalp between the territories of the greater occipital and great auricular nerves, and through an auricular branch the skin over the cranial surface of the upper third of the pinna. Also *lesser occipital nerve, mastoid branch of cervical plexus* (outmoded). **n. occipitalis tertius** [NA] A nerve that pierces the trapezius to supply the skin of the suboccipital and low occipital areas medial to the zone supplied by the greater occipital nerve. It represents the medial branch of the posterior primary ramus at $C_3$. Also *third occipital nerve, least occipital nerve.* **n. octavus** NERVUS VESTIBULOCOCHLEARIS. **n. oculomotorius** [NA] The third cranial nerve, originating in the cell groups of the oculomotor nucleus in the rostral two thirds of the midbrain, containing somatic efferent fibers for the ocular muscles and parasympathetic fibers for the ciliary ganglion, and innervating the medial, inferior, and superior rectus muscles, the levator palpebrae superioris, and the sphincter muscles of the pupil and the muscles of accommodation in the iris. Also *oculomotor nerve, third cranial nerve.* **nervi olfactorii** [NA] The first cranial nerve, consisting of approximately ten million very fine, slowly conducting fibers which are the central processes of the olfactory receptors. They run from the upper part of the nasal cavity through the cribriform plate of the ethmoid bone, enter the ventral surface of the olfactory bulb, and terminate in axodendritic tufts (glomeruli). Also *olfactory nerve, first cranial nerve, olfactory fibers, fila olfactoria.* **n. ophthalmicus** [NA] The superior division of the trigeminal nerve, providing sensory supply to the forehead, the eyes and orbit, the nasal cavity, and the skin over the nose. Commencing in the anteromedial part of the trigeminal ganglion, the nerve passes through the cavernous sinus, enters the orbit through the superior orbital fissure, and divides into three branches, the lacrimal, frontal, and nasociliary. Also *ophthalmic nerve, ophthalmic nerve of Willis.* **n. opticus** [NA] The cranial nerve mediating vision. Forming through concentration at the optic disc of axons from retinal ganglion cells, it takes a sinuous course through the orbit to the optic foramen. At the intracranial end of the optic canal it separates at the optic chiasma into bundles of fibers that cross to the opposite optic tract and those that remain ipsilateral. Also *optic nerve, second cranial nerve, opticus.* **nervi palatini** Two, or sometimes three, maxillary nerve branches that supply the palate and posterior portions of the nasal cavity. They arise from the pterygopalatine ganglion and descend in the greater and lesser palatine canals to exit through foramina on the inferior surface of the bony palate. Included are general sensory fibers from the maxillary nerve, postganglionic parasympathetic fibers from the pterygopalatine ganglion, and postganglionic sympathetic and facial nerve taste fibers. Also *palatine nerves.* **nervi palatini minores** [NA] Palatine nerves that, after leaving the lesser palatine canal and foramen, supply the soft palate, uvula, and tonsil. They carry some taste fibers. Also *lesser palatine nerves.* **n. palatinus major** [NA] The larger of the palatine nerves. A branch of the maxillary nerve, it descends in the palatine canal and exits through the greater palatine foramen to appear on the inferior surface of the bony palate. It then runs forward, supplying in its course the gums, mucosa, and glands of the hard palate and a small zone of the soft palate. Also *greater palatine nerve, anterior palatine nerve, nervus palatinus anterior.* **n. palatinus medius** A nerve containing fibers of the maxillary nerve and sphenopalatine ganglion that descends in the pterygopalatine canal and emerges from a lesser palatine foramen to supply the tonsil and soft palate. Also *middle palatine nerve, external palatine nerve.* **n. palatinus posterior** The more posterior and larger of the nervi palatini minores. Also *posterior palatine nerve.* **n. patheticus** NERVUS TROCHLEARIS. **n. pectoralis lateralis** [NA] A branch ($C_{5-7}$) arising from the lateral cord or upper and medial trunks of the brachial plexus that innervates clavicular and upper sternal sections of the pectoralis major. Some of its fibers reach the pectoralis minor through a communication with the nervus pectoralis medialis. Also *lateral pectoral nerve.* **n. pectoralis medialis** [NA] A branch ($C_8$, $T_1$) of the medial cord of the brachial plexus that, after entering and supplying the pectoralis minor, continues on to innervate costal and lower sternal portions of the pectoralis major. Also *medial pectoral nerve.* **nervi perineales** [NA] Branches of the perineal nerve that supply muscles in the superficial perineal pouch, portions of the external anal sphincter and levator ani, the bulb and bulbar urethra of the penis and, through posterior scrotal and labial nerves, posterior portions of the scrotum and labia major. Also *perineal nerves, nervi perinei.* **n. peroneus communis** [NA] The terminal component of the sciatic nerve arising from the posterior divisions of the lumbosacral plexus ($L_4$–$S_2$) and destined to supply extensor aspects of the embryonic limb bud. Separating from the tibial division of the sciatic nerve high in the popliteal fossa, it descends obliquely to the head of the fibula, where it divides into the superficial and deep peroneal nerves. In the fossa it gives rise to the lateral cutaneous nerve of the calf and a communicating branch to the sural nerve, as well as branches to the knee and tibiofibular joints. The nerve to the short head of the biceps arises from the peroneal division of the sciatic before it separates from the tibial division. Also *common peroneal nerve, nervus fibularis communis, common fibular nerve, lateral popliteal nerve.* **n. peroneus profundus** [NA] A nerve supplying the muscles of the peroneal compartment, deep structures on the dorsum of the ankle, and a small area of skin on the toes. Arising from the common peroneal nerve lateral to the fibula, it sends branches to the peroneus longus, extensor digitorum longus, extensor hallucis longus, and peroneus tertius, and then continues down the interosseous membrane and across the tarsus before bifurcating. The lateral branch supplies the extensor digitorum brevis, tarsal and metatarsal joints of digits II and III. The medial branch supplies the metatarsophalangeal joint of the hallux, and the skin on adjacent sides of the great and second toes. Also *deep peroneal nerve, nervus fibularis profundus, deep fibular nerve, musculocutaneous nerve of leg.* **n. peroneus superficialis** [NA] A branch of the common peroneal nerve that, as it descends in the lateral compartment of the leg, supplies the peroneus longus and brevis muscles, then sends medial and lateral branches to the skin and joints of the dorsal surfaces of the ankle, tarsus, and most toes. It does not supply the cleft between the great and second toes or the lateral surface of the little toe. The medial branch ($L_{4,5}$) communicates with the saphenous nerve, and the lateral ($L_5$ $S_1$) with the sural nerve. Also *nervus fibularis superficialis, superficial fibular nerve, superficial peroneal nerve, musculocutaneous nerve of foot.* **n. petrosus major** [NA] An intracranial derivative of the nervus intermedius portion of the cranial nerve carrying sensory and parasympathetic innervation destined for orbital, nasal, nasopharyngeal, and palatine areas. It arises from the genicular ganglion, appears along a groove on the anterior side of the petrous pyramid, and crosses the foramen lacerum beneath the trigeminal ganglion. There it is joined by the deep petrosal nerve to form the nerve of the pterygoid canal for eventual distribution by branches of the pterygopalatine ganglion to the lacrimal gland, nasal and palatine glands, and taste receptors on the soft palate. Also *greater petrosal nerve, greater superficial petrosal nerve, nervus petrosus superficialis major.* **n. petrosus minor** [NA] A branch of the ninth cranial nerve bringing preganglionic parasympathetic fibers to the otic ganglion. Arising in the tympanic plexus, it travels along a canal inferior to the tensor tympani to enter the middle cranial fossa, and then passes out of the cranium via the foramen ovale or innominatus to reach the ganglion. Also *lesser petrosal nerve, lesser superficial petrosal nerve, nervus petrosus superficialis minor, middle superficial petrosal nerve, lesser superficial nerve.* **n. petrosus profundus** [NA] A bundle of nerve fibers that leave the internal carotid artery plexus in the vicinity of the foramen lacerum to join the greater petrosal nerve and form the nerve of the pterygoid canal. It carries postganglionic fibers from the superior cervical sympathetic ganglion destined for lacrimal, nasal, and palatine glands and vessels. Also *deep petrosal nerve, deep vidian nerve.* **n. petrosus superficialis major** NERVUS PETROSUS MAJOR. **n. petrosus superficialis minor** NERVUS PETROSUS MINOR. **nervi phrenici accessorii** [NA] The contribution made by the $C_5$ spinal nerve to the phrenic nerve when at cervical levels it courses at a distance from the main nerve. It is usually associated with the subclavian nerve. Also *accessory phrenic nerves.* **n. phrenicus** [NA] The motor nerve to the diaphragm. It arises from branches of the $C_3$, $C_4$ and $C_5$ levels of the cervical plexus which joining in front of the anterior scalene muscle, enter the thoracic inlet, pass anterior to the root of the lung, and pierce the diaphragm to innervate it on its inferior surface. Sprigs are sent to the pericardium (ramus pericardiacus) and celiac plexus (ramus phrenicoabdominalis). Also *phrenic nerve, diaphragmatic nerve.* **n. piriformis** [NA] A nerve that is formed by the dorsal branches of the ventral rami of the first and second sacral nerves. It ends in the anterior surface of the piriformis muscle. Also *nerve to piriformis muscle.* **n. plantaris lateralis** [NA] The smaller of two terminal branches of the tibial nerve. It innervates the quadratus plantae, abductor and flexor digitorum minimi, adductor hallucis, all the interossei and the lateral three lumbrical muscles. Branches also go to the joints and skin of the lateral sole, little toe, and adjacent surface of the fourth toe. Also *lateral plantar nerve.* **n. plantaris medialis** [NA] The more medial of the two branches into which the posterior tibial nerve splits deep to the flexor retinaculum. It supplies the abductor pollicis muscle, the flexores hallucis and digitorum brevis, the first lumbrical muscle, and the joints and skin of the instep and medial $3^1/_2$ toes. Also *medial plantar nerve.* **n. presacralis** PLEXUS HYPOGASTRICUS SUPERIOR. **n. pterygoideus externus** NERVUS PTERYGOIDEUS LATERALIS. **n. pterygoideus internus** NERVUS PTERYGOIDEUS MEDIALIS. **n. pterygoideus lateralis** [NA] A branch to the lateral pterygoid muscle arising from the anterior division of the mandibular nerve. Also *lateral pterygoid nerve, nervus pterygoideus externus, external pterygoid nerve.* **n. pterygoideus medialis** [NA] A slender branch that separates from the mandibular nerve just below the foramen ovale to innervate the medial pterygoid muscle. Other sprigs, after passing through the otic ganglion, supply the tensor tympani and tensor veli palatini. Also *nerve to medial pterygoid muscle, nervus pterygoideus internus, internal pterygoid nerve.* **nervi pterygopalatini** Two short nerves passing between the maxillary nerve and the pterygopalatine ganglion lying beneath it. They carry sensory axons passing through the ganglion and postganglionic axons traveling to destinations of the maxillary nerve. Also *pterygopalatine nerves, nervi sphenopalatini.* **n. pudendus** [NA] The principal nerve to the skin and muscles of the anal and perineal regions. Derived from $S_{2\text{-}4}$ levels, it leaves the pelvis through the infrapiriform aperture to enter the gluteal region, and immediately passes through the lesser sciatic foramen to enter the pudendal canal on the wall of the ischiorectal fossa. After giving off inferior rectal nerves, it ends at the posterior margin of the urogenital diaphragm by dividing into a perineal nerve and a dorsal nerve of the penis or clitoris. Also *pudendal nerve, pudic nerve, Soemmering's nerve, pudendal plexus.* **n. radialis** [NA] The major nerve ($C_{5\text{-}8}$) supplying extensor aspects of the upper limb. The largest terminal branch of the brachial plexus, it arises from the posterior cord and winds posteriorly around the humerus in the radial groove to appear along the lateral side of the cubital fossa, where it separates into the deep and superficial radial nerves. In the arm, it supplies the heads of the triceps, anconeus, brachioradialis, and extensor digitorum longus, and sends sprigs to the brachialis and the elbow joint. Arising above the level of the elbow are also the posterior and lower lateral cutaneous nerves of the arm and the posterior cutaneous nerve to the forearm. Together these branches provide sensibility over the dorsal surface from the level of the deltoid insertion to the dorsum of the wrist. Also *radial nerve, musculospiral nerve, musculospiralis* (seldom used). **nervi rectales inferiores** [NA] Several branches of the pudendal nerve that pierce the wall of the pudendal canal and cross the ischiorectal fossa to innervate the external anal sphincter, ectodermal mucosa of the anal canal, and perianal skin. The latter area ($S_{3,4}$) dorsally adjoins that of the anococcygeal nerve ($S_5C_1$). Also *inferior rectal nerves, nervi haemorrhoidales inferiores, inferior hemorrhoidal nerves.* **n. recurrens** NERVUS LARYNGEUS RECURRENS. **n. saccularis** [NA] The inferior branch of the vestibular nerve which as filaments traverses foramina in the inferior vestibular area of the internal acustic meatus to end on receptors of the macula in the saccule. Also *saccular nerve.* **nervi sacrales** **1** [NA] The five anterior primary rami that pass through anterior sacral foramina and between the sacrum and coccyx to join the sacral and coccygeal plexuses. **2** The nerve of this sacral series, usually the fourth nerve, that splits to contribute to both plexuses. Also *sacral nerves.* **n. saphenus** [NA] The largest cutaneous branch ($L_{3,4}$) of the femoral nerve. It descends in the adductor canal, emerging at the lower end to take a subcutaneous course on the medial aspect of the knee and leg, where it splits into two branches. One of these ends at the ankle, while the other passes in front of the ankle to reach the base of the big toe. An infrapatellar branch runs in front of the patella, where it joins in the patellar plexus. Also *saphenous nerve.* **nervi scrotales anteriores** [NA] Branches of the ilioinguinal nerve that supply the skin over the root of the penis and anterosuperior portions of the scrotum. The segmental levels represented ($L_{1,2}$) contrast sharply with those of the adjacent territory of the posterior scrotal nerve ($S_{2\text{-}4}$). Also *anterior scrotal nerves.* **nervi scrotales posteriores** [NA] Two branches of the perineal nerve, medial and lateral, that pierce the inferior fascia of the urogenital diaphragm and pass forward to innervate posterior aspects of the scrotum. Also *posterior scrotal nerves.* **n. spermaticus externus** RAMUS GENITALIS NERVI GENITOFEMORALIS. **nervi sphenopalatini** NERVI PTERYGOPALATINI. **nervi spinales** [NA] The nerves on each side of the spinal column formed by the union of dorsal (posterior) and ventral (anterior) spinal roots. Shortly after emerging from an intervertebral foramen, each nerve splits into dorsal and ventral primary rami that bring sensory and motor innervation to the trunk, limbs, and viscera. Also *spinal nerves.* **n. spinosus** *Obs.* RAMUS MENINGEUS NERVI MANDIBULARIS. **nervi splanchnici lumbales** [NA] Four branches leaving the sympathetic chain to join respectively the celiac, renal, and intermesenteric plexuses; the lower part of the intermesenteric plexus; the superior mesenteric plexus via a route anterior to the common iliac vessels; and the superior mesenteric plexus via a route deep to these vessels. Also *lumbar splanchnic nerves.* **nervi splanchnici pelvici** [NA] Branches of the anterior primary rami of sacral nerves 2, 3 and 4 that, joining the inferior hypogastric plexus, bring preganglionic sympathetic innervation to pelvic viscera and, via the superior hypogastric plexus, to the rectum and descending colon. The ganglia are located both in the plexuses and in walls of the viscera. The nerves also carry sensory fibers from the viscera. Also *pelvic splanchnic nerves, nervi erigentes.* **nervi splanchnici sacrales** [NA] Branches passing between the sacral sympathetic trunk and the superior and inferior hypogastric plexuses. They contain pre– and postganglionic sympathetic fibers and sensory axons from pelvic viscera. Also *sacral splanchnic nerves.* **n. splanchnicus imus** [NA] The lowermost of visceral branches given off by the thoracic sympathetic trunk. Recognizable in 50% of bodies, it enters the abdomen alongside the sympathetic trunk and ends in the renal plexus. Also *lowest splanchnic nerve, renal nerve, least splanchnic nerve, minor splanchnic nerve, nervus splanchnicus minimus* (outmoded). **n. splanchnicus major** [NA] The largest of the nerves to abdominal viscera formed by the joining of offshoots from the thoracic sympathetic trunk. It arises from the fifth to ninth or tenth thoracic ganglia, perforates the crus of the diaphragm, and ends in the celiac and aorticorenal ganglia and in the medulla of the suprarenal gland. A splanchnic ganglion of variable size is present on the nerve above the diaphragm, and at this level a few filaments pass to the aorta. The nerve carries preganglionic myelinated sympathetic axons from roots T1 to 8, especially T4, and afferent fibers from the viscera. Also *greater splanchnic nerve, major splanchnic nerve.* **n. splanchnicus minimus** *Outmoded* NERVUS SPLANCHNICUS IMUS. **n. splanchnicus**

**minor** [NA] A nerve formed by filaments leading off from the 9th and 10th, or 10th and 11th ganglia of the thoracic sympathetic trunk. It perforates the crus of the diaphragm to join the aorticorenal ganglion. Also *lesser splanchnic nerve, inferior splanchnic nerve.* **n. stapedius** [NA] The motor nerve to the stapedius muscle. It arises from the facial nerve in the facial canal to pass forward and sharply upward in a minute canal leading to the pyramidal eminence and muscle. Also *stapedius nerve, stapedial nerve.* **n. statoacusticus** NERVUS VESTIBULOCOCHLEARIS. **n. subclavius** [NA] A branch ($C_{5,6}$) from the superior trunk of the brachial plexus that supplies the subclavius muscle. It is often accompanied by the $C_5$ contribution to the phrenic nerve. Also *subclavian nerve, nerve to subclavius muscle.* **n. subcostalis** [NA] The anterior primary ramus of the spinal nerve that passes between the last thoracic and first lumbar vertebrae. In man, it ravels below the 12th rib and beyond to supply lower portions of the abdominal musculature, including the pyramidalis muscle, and a strip of skin and mucosa culminating above the pubis. A gluteal branch homologous to a lateral cutaneous branch of an intercostal nerve supplies the skin over the anterolateral aspect of the thigh. Also *subcostal nerve, twelfth thoracic nerve.* **n. sublingualis** [NA] A branch of the lingual nerve supplying parasympathetic fibers to the sublingual glands and sensory fibers to adjacent mucosa in the floor of the mouth. Also *sublingual nerve.* **n. suboccipitalis** [NA] A nerve representing the posterior primary ramus of the first spinal nerve. Leaving the spinal canal between the skull and the neural arch of the atlas vertebra, it enters the suboccipital triangle where branches pass to the rectus capitis major and minor muscles, the obliquus superior and inferior, and a sector of the semispinalis capitis. Also *suboccipital nerve, infraoccipital nerve.* **n. subscapularis** [NA] The nervous contributions of the posterior cord to innervation of the subscapularis and teres major muscles. The NA recognizes only a single nerve, but a superior subscapular nerve to the cranial portion of the subscapular muscle, and an inferior subscapular nerve supplying the caudal portion and teres major are always distinguishable. Also *subscapular nerves.* **nervi supraclaviculares** [NA] Three nerves or nerve bundles that arise by a common trunk from $C_3$ and $C_4$ cervical nerves to supply the skin over the lower neck, uppermost thorax, and shoulder. Also *supraclavicular nerves.* **nervi supraclaviculares anteriores** NERVI SUPRACLAVICULARES MEDIALES. **nervi supraclaviculares intermedii** [NA] The middle of the three supraclavicular nerve bundles. It supplies the skin over the clavicle, pectoralis major, and deltoid to the level of the second rib. Also *intermediate supraclavicular nerves, middle supraclavicular nerves.* **nervi supraclaviculares laterales** [NA] A nerve bundle supplying the skin over the lateral and posterior aspects of the shoulder and upper arm. Also *lateral supraclavicular nerves, nervi supraclaviculares posteriores, posterior supraclavicular nerves.* **nervi supraclaviculares mediales** [NA] A nerve bundle supplying the skin over the insertion of the sternocleidomastoid muscle, the first intercostal space, and the manubrium. A twig goes to the sternoclavicular joint. Also *nervi supraclaviculares anteriores, anterior supraclavicular nerves, medial supraclavicular nerves.* **nervi supraclaviculares posteriores** NERVI SUPRACLAVICULARES LATERALES. **n. supraorbitalis** [NA] The major continuation of the frontal nerve. Separating from the supratrochlear nerve between the levator palpebrae and the roof of the orbit, it passes through the supraorbital notch and, via medial and lateral branches, extends backwards nearly to the lambdoid suture. Branches are given to the frontal sinus, conjunctiva and eyelid, pericranium, and scalp. Also *supraorbital nerve.* **n. suprascapularis** [NA] A branch ($C_{5,6}$) of the superior trunk of the brachial plexus that innervates the supraspinatus and infraspinatus muscles, and gives twigs to the shoulder and acromioclavicular joints. It passes beneath the ligament that bridges the suprascapular notch. Also *suprascapular nerve.* **n. supratrochlearis** [NA] A branch of the frontal nerve that passes forward above the trochlea of the superior oblique and then curves around the orbital margin to continue upward deep to the corrugator and frontalis muscles. Branches are given off to the conjunctiva and skin of the upper eyelid, the root of the nose, and the skin over the forehead near the midline. Also *supratrochlear nerve.* **n. suralis** [NA] A nerve formed midway down the calf by the union of the medial sural cutaneous nerve and the communicating branch of the common peroneal nerve. Accompanying the small saphenous vein, it descends along the tendo calcaneus to round the lateral malleolus and continue along the side of the foot and little toe. Named branches are the rami calcanei laterales to the heel and sole, and the nervus cutaneus dorsalis lateralis. Also *sural nerve, short saphenous nerve, external saphenous nerve.* **nervi temporales profundi** [NA] Branches of the anterior trunk of the mandibular nerve that supply the temporalis muscle. Two, often three, branches round the infratemporal crest of the skull, above the lateral pterygoid, to enter the deep surface of the muscle. Also *deep temporal nerves.* **n. tensoris tympani** *Outmoded* NERVUS MUSCULI TENSORIS TYMPANI. **n. tensoris veli palatini** A branch of the mandibular nerve that supplies the tensor of the palate. Below the foramen ovale, it is included in the nerve to the medial pterygoid, but shortly separates, passing through the otic ganglion en route to the muscle. Also *nerve of tensor veli palatini.* **n. tentorii** RAMUS TENTORII NERVI OPHTHALMICI. **n. terminalis** [NA] A small nerve lying between the olfactory bulb and crista galli that receives unmyelinated filaments from the nasal mucous membrane, and caudally enters the anterior perforated substance where its fibers pass into the lamina terminalis and anterior hypothalamus. A ganglion terminal is located along the nerve. It has been suggested that it mediates special osmoreception or supplies blood vessels and glands of the nasal mucosa. Also *terminal nerve.* **n. thoracalis longus** NERVUS THORACICUS LONGUS. **nervi thoracici** [NA] The thoracic spinal nerves, including eleven pairs of intercostal nerves and one pair of subcostal nerves. Each is designated by the number of the vertebra beneath which it appears. Also *thoracic nerves, nervi thoracales.* **n. thoracicus longus** [NA] The nerve supplying the serratus anterior. It originates from branches of the $C_5$ and $C_6$ nerves that pierce the scalenus medius and pass behind the axillary artery and brachial plexus to descend near the midaxillary line. Twigs are given off to each digitation of the serratus. In 40 percent of bodies it receives a $C_7$ contribution. Also *long thoracic nerve, posterior thoracic nerve, nerve to serratus anterior, external respiratory nerve of Bell* (imprecise), *nervus thoracalis longus, Bell's nerve.* **n. thoracodorsalis** [NA] The nerve to the latissimus dorsi. Carrying $C_{6,7,8}$ fibers, it arises from the posterior cord between the upper and lower subscapular nerves. Also *the thoracodorsal nerve, middle subscapular nerve.* **n. tibialis** [NA] The larger terminal branch of the sciatic nerve. Representing dorsal divisions of $L_4$-$S_3$ components of the lumbosacral plexus, it supplies muscles of the dorsal aspect of the thigh (except the short head of the biceps femoris), the calf, and the plantar aspect of the foot, as well as the skin over the calf and sole of the foot and a number of joints. After giving rise to muscle, crural interosseous, medial sural cutaneous, and medial calcaneal branches, the tibial nerve terminates by bifurcating into the medial and lateral plantar nerves. Also *tibial nerve, medial popliteal nerve, internal popliteal nerve.* **n. transversus colli** [NA] A cutaneous nerve that, arising from $C_2$ and $C_3$ cervical nerves, turns around the sternocleidomastoid to supply anterolateral regions of the neck extending from mandible to sternum. Also *transverse cervical nerve, transverse cutaneous nerve of neck, anterior cutaneous nerve of neck, transverse nerve of neck, nervus cervicalis superficialis, superficial cervical nerve, nervus cutaneus colli.* **n. trigeminus** [NA] The largest of the cranial nerves, emerging from the lateral surface of the pons and containing both sensory and motor components, together with some intermediate fibers. Cell bodies of origin of the sensory root are located in the trigeminal ganglion of Gasser, from which the three divisions of the nerve (n. ophthalmicus, n. maxillaris, and n. mandibularis) arise. The sensory components supply the face, teeth, mouth, and nasal cavity, and the motor components supply the muscles of mastication. Also *trigeminal nerve, fifth cranial nerve, trifacial nerve.* **n. trochlearis** [NA] The motor nerve to the superior oblique muscle of the eyeball, taking origin from a cell cluster in the ventral part of the central gray substance just lateral to the midline and dorsal to the medial longitudinal fasciculus. The fibers run dorsally and laterally, then cross the midline in the superior medullary velum to emerge from the dorsolateral aspect of the midbrain below the inferior colliculi. The nerve runs forward in the lateral wall of the cavernous sinus and traverses the superior orbital fissure. Also *trochlear nerve, fourth cranial nerve, nervus patheticus, pathetic nerve.* **n. tympanicus** [NA] A nerve arising from the inferior, or petrosal, ganglion of the glossopharyngeal nerve and ascending via the inferior tympanic canaliculus to the tympanic cavity, where it divides into the tympanic plexus, which supplies branches to the mucous membrane of the tympanic cavity, the auditory tube, and the mastoid air cells; the lesser petrosal nerve; and the greater petrosal nerve. It is thought to be general sensory and parasympathetic in function. Also *tympanic nerve, Jacobson's nerve, Andersch nerve, tympanic nerve of Jacobson.* **n. ulnaris** [NA] A mixed peripheral nerve that originates in the medial cord of the brachial plexus, ($C_8$ and $T_1$, though often receiving fibers from $C_7$). Descending through the axilla and along the medial side of the brachial artery, it then traverses a groove on the dorsum of the medial epicondyle and reaches the wrist along the medial surface of the forearm. Its branches are articular, muscular, palmer cutaneous, dorsal, superficial terminal, and deep terminal. Its distribution is largely to the skin on the front and back of the medial portion of the hand, some flexor muscles on the front of the forearm, and many short muscles of the hand, elbow joint, and joints of the hand. Also *ulnar nerve, cubital nerve.* **n. utricularis** [NA] The branch of the vestibular portion of the eighth cranial nerve that innervates the macula of the utricle. Also *utricular nerve.* **n. utriculoampullaris** [NA] A nerve that arises from the vestibular portion of the eighth cranial nerve and supplies the utricle and ampullae of the semicircular canals. Also *utriculoampullar nerve.* **nervi vaginales** [NA] Nerves arising from the lower parts of the inferior hypogastric and uterovaginal plexuses and following the vaginal arteries to be distributed to the vaginal walls, the clitoris, and the urethra. The nerves contain many parasympathetic fibers that facilitate the vasodilation of erectile tissue. Also *vaginal nerves, plexus vaginalis.* **n. vagus** [NA] The tenth cranial nerve, a mixed nerve emerging from the lateral aspect of the medulla oblongata between the inferior olive and the inferior cerebellar peduncle. It exits the skull via the jugular foramen and continues through the neck and thorax into the abdomen. It supplies sensory fibers to the ear, tongue, pharynx, and larynx; motor fibers to the pharynx, larynx, and esophagus; and parasympathetic and visceral afferent fibers to thoracic and abdominal viscera as far as the splenic flexure of the colon. Its major branches include the superior and recurrent laryngeal nerves; the meningeal, auricular, pharyngeal, cardiac, bronchial, gastric, hepatic, celiac, and renal rami; and the pharyngeal, pulmonary, and esophageal plexuses. Also *vagus nerve, tenth cranial nerve, pneumogastric nerve.* **nervi vasorum** VASOMOTOR NERVES. **n. vertebralis** [NA] A nerve originating from cervicothoracic and vertebral ganglia. Each component ascends along the vertebral artery, forming part of a sympathetic plexus that supplies the spinal meninges, cervical nerves, and the posterior cranial fossa. Also *vertebral nerve.* **nervi vesicales inferiores plexus pudendi** A small group of nerve fibers thought to arise from the pudendal plexus and innervating the bladder. *Obs.* Also *inferior vesical nerves of pudendal plexus.* **nervi vesicales inferiores plexus vesicalis** The nerve fibers reaching the vesical plexus by way of the inferior vesical artery. *Obs.* Also *inferior vesical nerves of vesical plexus.* **nervi vesicales superiores plexus vesicalis** The nerve fibers reaching the vesical plexus via the superior vesical artery. *Obs.* Also *superior vesical nerves of vesical plexus.* **n. vestibularis** [NA] The vestibular part of the eighth cranial nerve; the nerve of equilibrium, arising from bipolar cells in the vestibular ganglion. Its peripheral fibers divide into three branches: a superior branch ends in the utricle and ampullae of the superior and lateral semicircular canals, an inferior branch ends in the saccule, and the posterior branch ends in the ampulla of the posterior semicircular canal. Central fibers enter the medulla oblongata and bifurcate, descending fibers form the spinal root, and ascending fibers end in the vestibular nuclei. Also *pars vestibularis nervi octavi, vestibular nerve, vestibular branch of eighth nerve.* **n. vestibulocochlearis** [NA] The eighth cranial nerve, emerging in the groove between pons and medulla behind the facial nerve and in front of the inferior cerebellar peduncle. It consists of two components, both of which are concerned with transmission of afferent impulses from the inner ear. The vestibular root arises from cells of the vestibular ganglion and conveys information about position and movement in space from the semicircular canals, utricle, and saccule. The cochlear root originates from cells of the spinal ganglion and transmits auditory information from the cochlea. Also *vestibulocochlear nerve, eighth cranial nerve, auditory nerve, acoustic nerve, nervus acusticus, nervus statoacusticus, auditorius, portio mollis paris septimi* (outmoded), *nervus octavus.* **n. zygomaticus** [NA] A nerve originating in the maxillary branch of the fifth cranial nerve in the pterygopalatine fossa, entering the orbit via the inferior orbital fissure, and dividing into the zygomaticotemporal and zygomaticofacial nerves. It supplies the skin on the temple and the prominence of the cheek. Also *zygomatic nerve.*

**nesidiectomy** \nēsid′ē·ek′təmē\ [Gk *nēsidi(on)* an islet, dim. of *nēsos* an island + -ECTOMY] The excision of the pancreatic islands of Langerhans.

**nesidioblastoma** \nēsid′ē·ōblastō′mə\ [Gk *nēsidio(n)* (dim. of *nēsos* an island) an islet + BLASTOMA] ISLET CELL TUMOR. **malignant n.** ISLET CELL CARCINOMA.

**nesidioblastosis** \nēsid′ē·ōblastō′sis\ [Gk *nēsidio(n)* (dim. of *nēsos* an island) an islet + -BLAST + -OSIS] Hyperplasia of the pancreatic islet cells.

**-ness** \-nis\ [Old English suffix denoting condition, quality, or degree] A noun suffix denoting state or quality.

**Nessler** [Julius *Nessler,* German chemist, 1827–1905] Nessler solution. See under REAGENT.

**nest** [Old English, akin to L *nidus* a nest] A small group or collection, as of cells within a tissue. **Brunn's epithelial n.'s** Cell clusters found in the normal ureter. **cell n.** A collection of densely packed cells, usually epithelial, surrounded by connective tissue, such as those seen in carcinomas. **egg n.** The envelope of epithelial granulosa cells and the enclosed oogonium or primary oocyte. See also PRIMORDIAL OVARIAN FOLLICLE. **Walthard's cell n.'s** Nests of epithelial cells found in the subserosal region of the ovary or fallopian tubes. They are thought to originate from squamous metaplasia of mesothelial cells, and may be a factor in the development of Brenner's tumor of the ovary. Also *Walthard's inclusions.*

**nesteostomy** \nes′tē·äs′təmē\ [See NESTIOSTOMY.] JEJUNOSTOMY.

**nestiostomy** \nes′tē·äs′təmē\ [Gk *nēsti(s)* fasting; the jejunum + *o* + -STOMY] JEJUNOSTOMY.

**net** [Old English *net, nett,* akin to L *nodus* a knot] NETWORK. **achromatic n.** The part of a cell structure that does not take up histologic stains. **Chiari's n.** An embryonic vestige consisting of anastomosing strands of fibrous tissue in the right atrium that are a result of incomplete or less than the usual resorption of the embryonic septum spurium. **chromidial n.** A network of material within the cell cytoplasm that stains with basic dyes and corresponds to cytoplasmic RNA. **nerve n.** A loose, intersecting assemblage of fine nerves arranged for the most part in a plane. They may or may not be functionally interconnected by synaptic or electrically inductive contacts. **Trolard's n.** *Seldom used* PLEXUS VENOSUS CANALIS HYPOGLOSSI.

**Netherton** [Earl Weldon *Netherton,* U.S. dermatologist, born 1893] See under SYNDROME.

**network** An arrangement of interconnecting fibers or vessels that resembles a meshed fabric in a reticulum, rete, plexus, or anastomosis. Also *net, meshwork.* **acromial n.** An arterial anastomosis on the superior surface of the acromion process of the scapula that is formed by the acromial branches of the thoracoacromial artery and the suprascapular artery and the posterior circumflex humeral artery. Also *acromial rete.* **arterial n.** RETE ARTERIOSUM. **calcanean n.** RETE CALCANEUM. **cell n.** CYTORETICULUM. **lateral malleolar n.** RETE MALLEOLARE LATERALE. **medial malleolar n.** RETE MALLEOLARE MEDIALE. **neurofibrillar n.** A plexus of the fine, threadlike structures running throughout the cell body, axon, and dendrites of a neuron. They were originally discovered during examination of reduced silver sections with the light microscope, but they are studied to best advantage with the electron microscope, which shows that they are composed of much finer, tubelike structures, the neurotubules, microtubules, and microfilaments. **peritarsal n.** A deep plexus of lymphatic vessels in front of and behind the tarsal plates of the eyelids, most of which drain to the superficial and deep parotid lymph nodes. Those of the medial half of the lower eyelid and of the medial angle drain to the submandibular nodes. **Purkinje's n.** JUNCTIONAL TISSUE. **subpapillary n.** RETE ARTERIOSUM SUBPAPILLARE. **trabecular n.** RETICULUM TRABECULARE SCLERAE. **venous n.** RETE VENOSUM. **weighting n.** The electronic circuitry in a sound level meter which filters the acoustic input and shapes it so that usually the response is no longer linear but gives greater emphasis to the range of frequencies at which human hearing is most sensitive.

**Neubauer** [Johann Ernst *Neubauer,* German anatomist, 1742–1777] Neubauer's artery. See under ARTERIA THYROIDEA IMA.

**Neufeld** [Fred *Neufeld,* German bacteriologist, 1861–1945] **1** See under PHENOMENON. **2** Neufeld reaction. See under QUELLUNG REACTION.

**Neumann** [Ernst F. C. *Neumann,* German pathologist, 1834–1918] **1** Neumann syndrome. See under PEMPHIGUS VEGETANS. **2** See under SHEATH.

**neur-** \n$^y$ur-\ NEURO-.

**neuradynamia** \n$^y$ur′ədīnā′mē·ə\ NEURASTHENIA.

**neural** \n$^y$ur′əl\ [NEUR- + -AL] **1** Denoting or pertaining to the structure or function of nerves and their connections. **2** Denoting or pertaining to the nervous system or any part of it.

**neuralgia** \n$^y$ural′jə\ [NEUR- + -ALGIA] Pain occurring in the area served by a sensory nerve, either because of compression or disease of that nerve, or else occurring without any apparent organic cause. Neuralgia is often paroxysmal and, in some cases, attacks may be precipitated by various stimuli applied over the course of the nerve or in its area of cutaneous innervation. Adj. neuralgic. **atypical facial n.** A type of chronic facial pain, occurring most often in young and middle-aged women. The pain is constant, dull, and aching in character and often affects predominantly the upper jaw region, though it may spread to other parts of the head and neck, and it may persist for months or years. While local physical disease, as of the teeth, sinuses, etc., must not be excluded, in most cases the pain is a manifestation of chronic tension and anxiety and/or depression. Also *atypical facial pain.* **auriculotemporal n.** Neuralgic pain involving the region of the ear and temple, sometimes resulting from temporomandibular joint dysfunction. **brachial n.** Recurrent neuralgic pain in the arm. See also CERVICOBRACHIAL NEURALGIA. **cervical n.** Recurrent neuralgic pain in the neck, corresponding to the distribution of the sensory cervical neurons. **cervicobrachial n.** Recurrent pain in the arm. This symptom has many causes, cervical radiculopathy due to spondylosis being one of the commonest. **ciliary n.** Periodic migrainous neuralgia in which the pain is located behind the eye. **facial n.** Any form of facial pain, including trigeminal neuralgia (tic douloureux), supraorbital neuralgia, and sometimes pain of dental or other origin. *Outmoded.* **n. facialis vera** TRIGEMINAL NEURALGIA. **femoral n.** Neuralgic pain over the anteromedial aspect of the thigh and knee, usually caused by irritation of the femoral nerve from various causes, such as compression by hernia or tumor, injury to the pelvis, or uterine disease, but also occurring commonly in diabetes mellitus, along with atrophy of the quadriceps (diabetic amyotrophy). **glossopharyngeal n.** A paroxysmal episode of neuralgic pain, similar to that of trigeminal neuralgia, but involving the back of the throat on one side and sometimes the ear and precipitated by swallowing. Surgical division of the glossopharyngeal nerve may be required to afford relief in the more severe cases. Also *pharyngotympanic cephalalgia, Legal's disease.* **herpetic n.** POSTHERPETIC NEURALGIA. **intercostal n.** Recurrent neuralgic pain, often in girdle distribution, following the course of an intercostal nerve. Also *intercostal neuropathy.* **mandibular joint n.** Neuralgic pain in or around the temporomandibular joint or considered to arise from a disorder of this joint, as in temporomandibular joint syndrome. **migrainous n.** An attack of severe burning pain occurring in or around one eye, and lasting from half an hour up to two hours, usually recurring once or twice in each twenty-four hour period, often at the same time of the day or night. Often there is ipsilateral lacrimation and blockage of the nose. The attacks usually occur in bouts lasting for a few weeks or months, separated by intervals of freedom. Also *cluster headache, vasculosympathetic facial pain, histamine headache, Horton's vascular headache, histamine cephalalgia.* **Morton's n.** MORTON'S NEUROMA. **nasociliary n.** Migrainous neuralgia in which the pain is located in the nose and behind the eye. **obturator n.** Neuralgic pain radiating down the upper and medial aspect of the thigh and resulting from compression or irritation of the obturator nerve due to lesions in the pelvis or in the region of the obturator foramen, where an obturator hernia may be the cause. **Parsonage and Turner amyotrophic n.** SHOULDER GIRDLE SYNDROME. **phrenic n.** A rare type of neuralgia described as radiating along the course of the phrenic nerve from the diaphragm to the cervical region and exacerbated by diaphragmatic movement, as coughing or breathing, and by swallowing hot or cold liquids. It is unlikely that the so-called idiopathic type exists, even though pain resembling that described may occur in patients with pericarditis, pleurisy, and aortitis, but more especially in cases of hiatus hernia. *Obs.* **posterior auricular n.** Neuralgic pain behind the ear, following the distribution of the posterior auricular nerve. **postherpetic n.** Continuous neuralgic pain in the distributions of the affected sensory roots (dermatomes) following an attack of herpes zoster. Also *herpetic neuralgia.* **pudendal plexus n.** Neuralgic pain in the perineum, scrotum, penis, and/or testes. **sciatic n.** SCIATICA. **Sluder's n.** SPHENOPALATINE NEURALGIA. **sphenopalatine n.** Periodic migrainous neuralgia in which pain occurs in the nose and pharynx, and sometimes also in the tongue, side of the neck, and upper jaw. The cause is unknown and the connection with the sphenopalatine ganglion debatable. Also *Sluder's neuralgia, vidian neuralgia, Sluder syndrome, sphenopalatine ganglion neurosis.* **stump n.** Recurrent neuralgic pain in an amputation stump. **supraorbital n.** Neuralgia in the distribution of the supraorbital nerve. **symptomatic n.** Any neuralgic pain resulting from, or associated with a disease not primarily involving the nervous system. **symptomatic trigeminal n.** Trigeminal neuralgia occurring as a symptom of a structural lesion such as posterior fossa tumor or multiple sclerosis. The possibility that the syndrome may be symptomatic may be suspected if there is sensory loss in the distribution of the affected trigeminal nerve or diminution of the appropriate corneal reflex. **trigeminal n.** A common form of paroxysmal facial neuralgia, usually occurring in late middle life or old age, but occasionally seen in young people, when it may be associated with multiple sclerosis. The pain is confined to the skin areas supplied by the trigeminal nerve and never crosses the midline. It is momentary, sharp, and lancinating, but a faint, dull ache may be present between paroxysms and it is often provoked by more than one trigger, such as touching or washing the face, especially in a "trigger" zone, or speaking, laughing, or chewing. The pain is so severe that it often appears to elicit an involuntary contraction of facial muscles on the affected side (which is why the condition is also called tic douloureux). Physical signs are generally absent. The cause is uncertain but is believed to be due to pressure on the nerve root by an adjacent artery or by an organic lesion such as a posterior fossa tumor or multiple sclerosis. Spontaneous remissions lasting weeks or months sometimes occur. Also *tic douloureux, trismus dolorificus, neuralgia facialis vera, trifacial neuralgia, prosopalgia.* **vidian n.** SPHENOPALATINE NEURALGIA. **Wartenberg's paresthetic n.** CHEIRALGIA PARESTHETICA.

**neuralgic** \nʸUral′jik\ Denoting, pertaining to, or affected by neuralgia.

**neuralgiform** \nʸUral′jifôrm\ [*neuralgi(a)* + -FORM] Resembling neuralgia.

**neuraminic acid** 5-Amino-4,6,8,9-pentahydroxy-2-oxononanoic acid. Its *N*-acetyl derivative is formed by reaction of *N*-acetylmannosamine, i.e. 2-acetamido-2-deoxymannose, which provides C-4 to C-9 of the product, with phosphoenolpyruvate, which provides C-1 to C-3, with splitting off of orthophosphate. It normally occurs in the pyranose form, with C-2 linked to O-6. Its acylated derivatives are known as sialic acids, and they occur in both glycoproteins (including those of the cell surface) and glycolipids.

**neuraminidase** SIALIDASE.

**neuranagenesis** \nʸUr′anəjen′əsis\ [NEUR- + ANA- + GENESIS] Regeneration in the nervous system.

**neurangiosis** \nʸUr′anjē·ō′sis\ [NEUR- + ANGIO- + -SIS] Blood vessel proliferation in the nervous system.

**neurapraxia** \nʸUr′əprak′sē·ə\ [NEUR- + APRAXIA] A peripheral nerve lesion in which there is temporary failure of conduction in the affected nerve fibers, often resulting from compression, but without actual division of axons. Also *axonapraxis.*

**neurarchy** \nʸUr′ärkē\ [NEUR- + Gk *arch(ē)* sovereignty, dominion + -Y] The dominant, controlling influence of the nervous system over other bodily systems.

**neurarthropathy** \nʸUr′ärthräp′əthē\ NEUROGENIC ARTHROPATHY.

**neurasthenia** \nʸUr′əsthē′nē·ə \ [NEUR- + ASTHENIA] A condition characterized by fatigability, weakness, multiple aches and pains, and insomnia, often with symptoms focused on a particular organ or body system. Because the accompanying affect is typically one of disaffection or unhappiness, current classifications group such syndromes among the affective disorders as a form of neurotic depressive disorder. Also *neurotic asthenia, Beard's disease, nervosism, neuradynamia, neurasthenic neurosis.* **traumatic n.** Anxiety or emotional distress following an emotional crisis or an injury. *Outmoded.*

**neuraxis** \nʸUrak′sis\ [NEUR- + AXIS] **1** SYSTEMA NERVOSUM CENTRALE. **2** *Seldom used* AXON. Adj. neuraxial.

**neuraxitis** \nʸUr′aksī′tis\ [*neurax(is)* + -ITIS] Inflammation of the neuraxis. Adj. neuraxitic. **epidemic n.** ENCEPHALITIS LETHARGICA. **multilocular n.** MULTIPLE SCLEROSIS.

**neuraxon** \nʸUrak′sän\ AXON.

**neurectoderm** \nʸUrek′tədurm\ NEUROBLAST.

**neurectomy** \nʸUrek′təmē\ [NEUR- + -ECTOMY] Excision of a nerve. **gastric n.** Resection of the vagus nerve. Also *vagectomy, vagotomy.* **presacral n.** Excision of the unpaired hypogastric sympathetic nerve plexus lying retroperitoneally at the promontory of the sacrum. **retrogasserian n.** Excision of the root of the trigeminal nerve, usually by avulsion. **tympanic n.** Surgical excision of part of the tympanic nerve, where it passes across the promontory as a component of the plexus tympanicus, with the object of interrupting the secretomotor nerve supply of the parotid gland. Tympanic neurectomy is used as a means of diminishing parotid secretion when ligating the parotid duct for chronic or recurrent parotid sialadenitis and for the relief of the crocodile tear syndrome.

**neurectopy** \nʸUrek′təpē\ [NEUR- + ECTOPY] The occurrence of neural tissue which is displaced from its normal position, is found in an abnormal anatomical situation, or is abnormally distributed as a nerve or nerve trunk. Also *neurectopia.*

**neurenteric** \nʸUr′enter′ik\ [NEUR- + ENTERIC] Pertaining to the neural tube and the archenteron, or primitive gut.

**neurepithelial** \nʸʊr′epithē′lē·əl\ NEUROEPITHELIAL.

**neurepithelium** \nʸʊr′epithē′lē·əm\ NERVE EPITHELIUM.

**neurexeresis** \nʸʊr′ekser′əsis\ [NEUR- + EXERESIS] NERVE AVULSION.

**neuricity** \nʸʊris′itē\ Nervous energy; the excitable property found in all neural tissue.

**neurilemma** \nʸʊr′ilem′ə\ [orig. *neurilema,* from NEUR- + Gk *(e)ilēma* veil, covering, wrapper; re-formed by assimilation to LEMMA] A sheath of flattened cells whose plasma membranes and accompanying basement membrane invest the myelin of larger peripheral nerve fibers. It also provides a thin layer surrounding the axoplasm of unmyelinated nerves. Also *Schwann's membrane, sheath of Schwann, endoneural membrane, neurilemmal sheath, nucleated sheath, neurolemma.*

**neurilemmitis** \nʸʊr′ilemī′tis\ [*neurilemm(a)* + -ITIS] Inflammation of the neurilemma. Also *neurolemmitis.*

**neurilemmoma** \nʸʊr′ilemō′mə\ [*neurilemm(a)* + -OMA] A benign and usually well-demarcated or encapsulated tumor, arising from the Schwann cells of the neurilemma. Hemorrhage, thrombosis, hemosiderin, and perivascular hyalinization are common within the tumor. There are two typical growth patterns: Antoni type A with organized cell arrangements, and Antoni type B with loosely structured tissue. Also *schwannoma, neurinoma, schwannoglioma, peripheral glioma* (outmoded), *lemmocytoma, neurolemmoma, Schwann cell tumor, neurilemoma.* **acoustic n.** A neurilemmoma of the acoustic nerve. Also *acoustic neuroma, acoustic neurofibroma.* **malignant n.** MALIGNANT SCHWANNOMA.

**neurilemmosarcoma** \nʸʊr′ilem′ōsärkō′mə\ [*neurilemm(a)* + *o* + SARCOMA] MALIGNANT SCHWANNOMA.

**neurilemoma** \nʸʊr′ilemō′mə\ NEURILEMMOMA.

**neurility** \nʸʊril′itē\ [NEUR- + -ILITY] The inherent electrical conductive property of nervous tissue.

**neurimotility** \nʸʊr′imōtil′itē\ Neuromuscular activity. Also *nervimotility.*

**neurimotor** \nʸʊr′imō′tər\ Pertaining to motor nerves. Also *nervimotor.*

**neurinoma** \nʸʊr′inō′mə\ [NEUR- + INO- + -OMA ] NEURILEMMOMA. **malignant n.** MALIGNANT SCHWANNOMA.

**neurite** \nʸʊr′īt\ A long process of a neuron. • The term usually denotes the axon, but is occasionally used collectively to include dendritic processes.

**neuritic** \nʸʊrit′ik\ **1** Relating to nerves, or acting upon the nervous system, as *neuritic poison.* **2** Relating to neuritis.

**neuritis** \nʸʊrī′tis\ [NEUR- + -ITIS] **1** Inflammation of a nerve. **2** A disease characterized by or attributed to nerve inflammation. • Many disorders so classified in the past are now more properly referred to as *neuropathy,* since the dysfunction of the nerve, previously attributed to inflammation, is now known to be due to a noninflammatory process, often of traumatic, toxic, or metabolic origin. Adj. neuritic. **alcoholic n.** Neuritis, or more correctly neuropathy or polyneuropathy, complicating chronic alcoholism. **amyloid n.** AMYLOID NEUROPATHY. **arsenical n.** Peripheral neuritis following acute or chronic exposure to arsenic. **brachial n.** SHOULDER GIRDLE SYNDROME. **compression n.** Neuropathy or neuritis caused by pressure on a nerve from circumferential swelling, swelling of a compartment, or wrapping applied too tightly. Also *pressure neuritis.* **degenerative n.** Degeneration and progressive fragmentation of the axon and myelin sheath of a peripheral nerve. **diphtheritic n.** Neuritis caused by the effects of the toxins produced by *Corynebacterium diphtheriae* and affecting the cranial nerves or any of the peripheral nerves. Neuritis may occur during the course of diphtheria or it may appear two to six weeks or more after the onset of diphtheria, and usually first or exclusively affects muscles supplied by nerves adjacent to the site of infection. In some cases the neuritis is localized from the outset, while in other cases it begins as a generalized polyneuritis. **experimental allergic n.** An autoimmune disease produced in various animal species following injection of preparations of peripheral nerve incorporated in complete Freund's adjuvant. The disease is characterized by focal perivascular accumulation of mononuclear cells and by demyelination of peripheral nerves and resembles the human Guillain-Barré syndrome. **exudative n.** The combined pathologic changes of edema of the myelin sheaths with leukocytic infiltration of peripheral nerves, as sometimes seen in the Guillain-Barré syndrome. *Obs.* **facial n.** *Outmoded* BELL'S PALSY. **femoral n.** An isolated neuropathy of the femoral nerve. **influenzal n.** A peripheral neuritis attributed to influenza virus infection. **interstitial n.** Neuritis or neuropathy thought to be due to inflammation in and around the peripheral nerves, giving rise to degeneration of the myelin sheath. Many cases of compression neuropathy and of inflammatory and demyelinating neuropathy were probably included under this title in the past. *Obs.* **ischemic n.** Nerve damage causing pain, numbness, or paralysis due to impairment of a nerve's blood supply. **jake n.** JAMAICA JAKE PARALYSIS. **lead n.** NEURITIS SATURNINA. **leprous n.** Any one of the forms of neuritis due to leprosy. **malarial n.** Mononeuropathy or polyneuropathy occurring as a complication of malaria. **migrating n.** Mononeuritis multiplex spreading from one nerve to another. Also *neuritis migrans.* **multiple n.** **1** POLYNEUROPATHY. **2** See under MONONEURITIS MULTIPLEX. **n. multiplex endemica** BERIBERI. **optic n.** Inflammation of the second cranial nerve. Also *postocular neuritis, retrobulbar neuritis, fasciculitis optica* (outmoded), *ophthalmoneuritis.* **paralytic brachial n.** SHOULDER GIRDLE SYNDROME. **peripheral n.** Polyneuritis or polyneuropathy. **porphyric n.** Polyneuropathy in acute porphyria. **postfebrile n.** Polyneuropathy following any acute febrile disorder. **postocular n.** OPTIC NEURITIS. **pressure n.** COMPRESSION NEURITIS. **n. puerperalis traumatica** Obstetric pressure palsy of the lumbosacral plexus. **radiation n.** Neuropathy due to ionizing radiation. **radicular n.** RADICULITIS. **retrobulbar n.** OPTIC NEURITIS. **rheumatic n.** Neuritis associated with musculoskeletal complaints. This term has no precise diagnostic implications. **n. saturnina** Neuropathy or neuritis due to chronic exposure to lead. Also *lead neuritis.* **sciatic n.** SCIATICA. **serum n.** SERUM NEUROPATHY. **shoulder girdle n.** SHOULDER GIRDLE SYNDROME. **syphilitic n.** Any form of neuropathy due to syphilis. Also *tabetic neuritis* (obs.). **tabetic n.** *Obs.* SYPHILITIC NEURITIS. **terminal n.** *Outmoded* ERYTHROMELALGIA. **toxic n.** Neuritis or neuropathy due to endogenous or exogenous toxic agents, including bacterial and chemical toxins. **traumatic n.** Neuropathy due to physical injury or compression of a nerve trunk. *Obs.*

**neuro-** \nʸʊr′ō-, nʸʊr′ə-\ [Gk *neuron* nerve, sinew, tendon] A combining form meaning (1) nerve, neural; (2) relating to the nervous system. Also *neur-.*

**neuroallergy** \-al′ərjē\ Allergy manifested in nervous tissue.

**neuroanastomosis** \-ənas′tōmō′sis\ [NEURO- + ANASTO-

MOSIS] A surgical joining of the cut ends of two nerves.

**neuroanatomy** \-ənat′əmē\ [NEURO- + ANATOMY] The science concerned with the anatomy of the nervous system. With the development of new research techniques, the field now includes gross descriptive anatomy; the study of tracts and pathways, i.e., tractology or hodology; the microscopic and ultramicroscopic study of neural tissue, i.e., histology; the study and identification of cell fiber systems on the basis of contained transmitter substances, i.e., histofluorescence; and the examination of living neural tissue *in vivo* or *in vitro,* i.e., tissue culture, among others.

**neuroanemia** \-anē′mē·ə\ *Obs.* PERNICIOUS ANEMIA.

**neuroarthropathy** \-ärthräp′əthē\ NEUROGENIC ARTHROPATHY.

**neuroastrocytoma** \-as′trōsītō′mə\ [NEURO- + ASTROCYTOMA] GANGLIOGLIOMA.

**neuroavitaminosis** \-āvī′təminō′sis\ [NEURO- + AVITAMINOSIS] Any neurologic disorder resulting from vitamin deficiency.

**neurobiology** \-bī·äl′əjē\ [NEURO- + BIOLOGY] The study of the biology of the nervous system; cellular neuroscience.

**neurobiotaxis** \-bī′ətak′sis\ [NEURO- + BIOTAXIS] The migration of a nerve cell in the direction from which it habitually receives stimuli. A nerve cell tends to remain close to its source of stimulation but development of neighboring structures may prevent the maintenance of such proximity and migration follows. Examples of such shifting in position of groups of nerve cells in the embryo are furnished by the lateral migration of the visceral motor nuclei of the cranial nerves, and in particular by the curious course of the fibers arising from the facial nucleus.

**neuroblast** \nʸUr′əblast\ [NEURO- + -BLAST] **1** That part of the ectoderm which invaginates and then differentiates into the neural tube and neural crest with their derivatives. Also *neurectoderm.* **2** An embryonic nerve cell which will give rise to a neuron. **sympathetic n.** SYMPATHOBLAST.

**neuroblastoma** \-blastō′mə\ [NEUROBLAST + -OMA] A highly malignant tumor of undifferentiated neuroblasts. The cells are small with dark-staining nuclei and indistinct cytoplasm. Arrangement of the cells in spheroid groups about a central tangle of fibrillary material (Homer Wright rosettes) is a characteristic feature. The tumor occurs predominantly in children under the age of four years, usually in close association with the adrenal medulla or the sympathetic chain. Also *sympathoblastoma, sympathicoblastoma, neurocytoma, sympathogonioma.* **olfactory n.** A malignant nasal tumor of olfactory neural tissue with cells showing pleomorphism and only scant amounts of neurofibrillar matrix. **Pepper type n.** Neuroblastoma of the right adrenal gland with metastases mostly confined to the liver.

**neurocardiac** \-kär′dē·ak\ Denoting, pertaining to, or affecting the nervous system and the heart.

**neurocentrum** \-sen′trəm\ [NEURO- + CENTRUM] A relatively dense part of the vertebral primordium in an embryo. It gives rise to the centrum of a vertebra and the neural arch. Adj. neurocentral.

**neuroceptor** \-sep′tər\ **1** A terminal element of a neuron that is specialized to receive stimuli. Peripherally, neuroceptors act as transducers, converting physical or chemical stimuli of many types into discrete electrical signals (action potentials) which then enter the central nervous system. **2** A dendrite within the central nervous system serving as a receptive structure that is postsynaptic to impinging presynaptic axons from other neurons.

**neuroceratin** \-ser′ətin\ NEUROKERATIN.

**neurochemistry** \-kem′istrē\ The chemistry of the nervous system, including that of the passage of the nervous system and its transmission across synapses.

**neurochitin** \-kī′tin\ A fibrous substance thought to form the supportive framework for nerve fibers. *Obs.*

**neurocirculatory** \-sur′kyələtôr′ē\ Denoting, pertaining to, or affecting the nervous and circulatory systems.

**neurocladism** \nʸUräk′lədizm\ [NEURO- + Gk *klad(os)* a young branch, slip, or shoot + -ISM] Regeneration of axons in peripheral nerves following division, and the process by which these regenerating axons eventually become connected to the peripheral end organ. Also *odogenesis.*

**neurocranium** \-krā′nē·əm\ The part of the embryonic skull that surrounds the brain; braincase. Constituted initially of a dense mesenchyme, it includes the base of the skull (chondrocranium), which undergoes endochondral ossification, and the cranial vault of flat bones, which undergoes intramembranous ossification. Compare SPLANCHNOCRANIUM. Adj. neurocranial.

**neurocrine** \nʸUr′əkrīn\ NEUROENDOCRINE.

**neurocutaneous** \-kyootā′nē·əs\ **1** Of or relating to nerves and the skin. **2** Pertaining to nerves of the skin.

**neurocyte** \nʸUr′əsīt\ [NEURO- + -CYTE] NEURON.

**neurocytology** \-sītäl′əjē\ The study of the cellular components of the nervous system.

**neurocytolysin** \-sītäl′isin\ A toxin that destroys nerve cell membranes, occurring especially in snake venoms, usually in low concentrations. Higher concentrations are found in venoms of North American coral snakes and in the water moccasin (cottonmouth) of the eastern United States.

**neurocytolysis** \-sītäl′isis\ [*neurocyt(e)* + *o* + LYSIS] Destruction, or lysis, of the cells of the nervous system.

**neurocytoma** \-sītō′mə\ [*neurocyt(e)* + -OMA] **1** NEUROEPITHELIOMA. **2** MEDULLOEPITHELIOMA. **3** NEUROBLASTOMA. **olfactory n.** A rare nasal tumor, corresponding clinically to the olfactory neuroblastoma but displaying histologic differences, the cells appearing uniform with prominent neurofibrillar matrix. Pseudorosettes are frequent. Also *esthesioneurocytoma* (rare).

**neurodegenerative** \-dijen′ərətiv\ Characterized by or relating to degeneration of the nervous tissue.

**neurodendrite** \-den′drīt\ DENDRITE.

**neurodendron** \-den′drän\ DENDRITE.

**neuroderm** \nʸUr′ədurm\ NEURAL TUBE.

**neurodermatitis** \-dur′mətī′tis\ [NEURO- + DERMATITIS] A skin disorder of psychosomatic genesis or in which psychological factors play an important part, as when rubbing and scratching induce circumbscribed patches of thickened skin. • In some countries the term is applied more generally to atopic dermatitis. This use is imprecise, since it falsely implies that nervous factors are always present. **circumscribed n.** LICHEN SIMPLEX.

**neurodermatomyositis** \-dur′mətōmī′əsī′tis\ Neuromyositis with skin involvement.

**neurodiagnosis** \-dī′əgnō′sis\ [NEURO- + DIAGNOSIS] Diagnosis of disorders of the nervous system.

**neuroectoderm** \-ek′tədurm\ [NEURO- + ECTODERM] Ectodermal cells which become neuroepithelial cells. Adj. neuroectodermal.

**neuroelectricity** \-ēlektris′itē\ The electrical activity generated in nervous system tissues.

**neuroencephalomyelopathy** \-ensef′əlōmī′əläp′əthē\ ENCEPHALOMYELOPATHY. **optic n.** NEUROMYELITIS OPTICA.

**neuroendocrine** \-en′dəkrin\ Of or relating to neuroendocrinology; relating to the interactions between the nervous and endocrine systems. Also *neurocrine.*

**neuroendocrinology** \-en′dəkrinäl′əjē\ [NEURO- + ENDOCRINOLOGY] The study of the interactions between the nervous and endocrine systems.

**neuroenteric** \-enter′ik\ NEURENTERIC.

**neuroepidermal** \-ep′idur′məl\ Giving rise to or pertaining to neural and epidermal cells.

**neuroepithelial** \-ep′ithē′lēəl\ Of or relating to the neuroepithelium. Also *neurepithelial.*

**neuroepithelioma** \-ep′ithē′lē·ō′mə\ [NEURO- + EPITHELIOMA] **1** A tumor of primitive neural tissue arising in the central nervous system. **2** A form of olfactory neurogenic tumor; olfactory neuroepithelioma. Also *esthesioneuroepithelioma, neurocytoma, neuroepithelial tumor.*

**neuroepithelium** \-ep′ithē′lyəm\ [NEURO- + EPITHELIUM] NERVE EPITHELIUM. **n. of ampullary crest** The sensory epithelium that covers the ampullary crests of the semicircular canals in the membranous labyrinth of the inner ear. **n. of maculae** MACULA RETINAE. **n. macularum** MACULA RETINAE.

**neurofibril** \-fī′bril\ A fine, threadlike structure visible within the cytoplasm of a neuron with light microscopy. Electron microscopy reveals that it corresponds to a bundle of neurofilaments. Also *nerve fibril, neurofibrilla.* Adj. neurofibrillar.

**neurofibroma** \-fībrō′mə\ [NEURO- + FIBROMA] (*pl.* neurofibromas, neurofibromata) A benign localized or diffuse tumor, consisting of a mixture of Schwann cells and fibroblasts accompanied by loosely arranged collagen fibers and mucinous material. Plexiform neurofibromas are the result of growth within and about a preformed nerve, giving the nerve trunk a tortuous, thickened, and plexiform appearance. Neurites can be frequently demonstrated within these tumors. Malignant transformation of neurofibromas may occur. Also *endoneural fibroma, neurofibromyxoma.* **acoustic n.** ACOUSTIC NEURILEMMOMA. **dumbbell n.** HOURGLASS TUMOR. **n. gangliocellulare** GANGLIONEUROMA. **n. ganglionare** GANGLIONEUROMA. **granular cell n.** GRANULAR CELL TUMOR. **malignant n.** MALIGNANT SCHWANNOMA. **symmetrical bundle n.'s** HEREDITARY HYPERTROPHIC INTERSTITIAL NEUROPATHY.

**neurofibromatosis** \-fī′brōmətō′sis\ **1** The presence of numerous neurofibromas. **2** Any of various clinically and genetically heterogeneous disorders associated with multiple neurofibromas. The vast majority of cases are von Recklinghausen's disease, and are characterized by café-au-lait skin macules, axillary freckling, fibromatous tumors, Lisch nodules of the iris, scoliosis, and autosomal dominant inheritance. The severity of the condition is extremely variable, and a predisposition of malignancy exists. Other neurofibromatosis syndromes involve acoustic neuromas with rare or nonexistent cutaneous signs, or multiple intestinal neurofibromas.

**neurofibromyxoma** \-fī′brōmiksō′mə\ [NEURO- + FIBRO- + MYXOMA] NEUROFIBROMA.

**neurofibrosarcoma** \-fī′brōsärkō′mə\ [NEURO- + FIBROSARCOMA] MALIGNANT SCHWANNOMA.

**neurofilament** \-fil′əmənt\ An elongate, tubular protein chain of indefinite length and approximately 100 Å in diameter observed in the soma, dendrites, and axons of neurons with the electron microscope. Bundles of neurofilaments can be impregnated with metallic salts to form the neurofibrils of light microscopy.

**neuroganglioma** \-gang′glē·ō′mə\ GANGLIONEUROMA.

**neuroganglion** \-gang′glē·än\ GANGLION.

**neuroganglionitis** \-gang′glē·ənī′tis\ [NEURO- + GANGLIONITIS] Inflammation of nerves and ganglia. Also *neuroganglitis.*

**neurogastric** \-gas′trik\ Of or involving the nervous system and the stomach; relating to the innervation of the stomach.

**neurogen** \n^yŭr′əjən\ [NEURO- + -GEN] A chemical substance essential to neural plate formation.

**neurogenesis** \-jen′əsis\ [NEURO- + GENESIS] The development of a nervous system.

**neurogenetics** \-jənet′iks\ The field of knowledge concerned with genetic mechanisms underlying early embryonic development, as well as cell differentiation, patterns of neural organization, and genetic disorders of the nervous system.

**neurogenic** \-jen′ik\ [NEURO- + -GENIC] **1** In embryology, having the property of forming neural tissue: said of undifferentiated cells. **2** Originating in the nervous system. For defs. 1 and 2 also *neurogenous.* **3** Describing muscle tissue that is quiescent unless activated by transmitter substances released from motor nerves. Compare MYOGENIC.

**neuroglia** \n^yŭräg′lē·ə\ [NEURO- + GLIA] Collectively, the non-neuronal cellular components of the central nervous system that, together with the fine tissue web they generate, make up the structural and functional support system of the brain and spinal cord. Neuroglial cells are usually divided into two major categories, macroglia and microglia. The macroglia consists of astrocytes and oligodendrocytes (oligodendroglia), which are of ectodermal origin. Astrocytes may be of protoplasmic or fibrillary type, the latter developing particularly in later life or in response to neural tissue injury. Oligodendrocytes frequently surround neurons closely as satellite cells or lie among myelinated axon bundles as interfascicular oligodendroglia. All of these types may be involved in the control of the ionic and molecular medium and in the synthesis of important neurally active materials. Interfascicular oligoglia are also concerned with the formation and maintenance of myelin. The microglia, of mesodermal origin, are believed to be derived from blood vessels, and they form wandering phagocytes. Also *glia, Kölliker's reticulum.* Adj. neuroglial, neurogliar. **interfascicular n.** Collectively, oligodendrocytes of white matter found along the myelin sheaths and concerned with the formation and maintenance of myelin. See also OLIGODENDROGLIA. **protoplasmic n.** PROTOPLASMIC ASTROCYTE.

**neurogliocytoma** \n^yŭräg′lē·əsītō′mə\ [*neurogli(a)* + *o* + CYT- + -OMA] GLIOMA.

**neuroglioma** \-glī·ō′mə\ GLIOMA. **n. ganglionare** GANGLIOGLIOMA.

**neurogliosis** \-glī·ō′sis\ [*neurogli(a)* + -OSIS] Diffuse hyperplasia of neuroglial tissue.

**neurohemal** \-hē′məl\ Denoting or relating to systems of axon terminals of neurons in contact with small blood vessels which characteristically synthesize, store, and release their secretions (neurohormones) into the circulation.

**neurohistology** \-histäl′əjē\ The study of the microscopic structure of the nervous system.

**neurohormonal** \-hôr′mōnəl\ Designating or pertaining to hormones originating in the nervous system.

**neurohormone** \n^yŭr′ōhôr′mōn\ [NEURO- + HORMONE] A secretory product of a neuron which enters the bloodstream and acts as a hormone, such as vasopressin or thyrotropin-releasing hormone. Also *neurohumor* (older term).

**neurohumoral** \-hyoo′mərəl\ *Older term* NEUROHORMONAL.

**neurohumoralism** \-hyoo′mərəlizm\ The theory that autonomic nervous system effects are mediated by the release of specific neurotransmitters.

**neurohypnology** \-hipnäl′əjē\ [NEURO- + HYPNO- + -LOGY] The study of hypnotism. Also *neurypnology.*

**neurohypophyseal** \-hī′pōfiz′ē·əl\ NEUROHYPOPHYSIAL.

**neurohypophysectomy** \-hī′pōfizek′təmē\ [*neurohypophys(is)* + -ECTOMY] The surgical removal of the posterior lobe of the hypophysis.

**neurohypophysial** \-hī′pōfiz′ē·əl\ Describing or pertaining to the neurohypophysis. Also *neurohypophyseal.*

**neurohypophysis** \-hīpäf′isis\ [NEURO- + HYPOPHYSIS] [NA] The posterior lobe of the pituitary gland (hypophysis), which develops in the embryo as an evagination from the floor of the diencephalon. Its major afferent nerve supply is the supraoptico-hypophysial tract. Also *lobus posterior hypophyseos, posterior lobe of hypophysis, posterior lobe of pituitary gland, pituitarium posterius, infundibular body.* See also PITUITARY GLAND.

**neuroid** \n$^y$ur′oid\ Resembling neural tissue.

**neurokeratin** \-ker′ətin\ The artifactitious network of pseudokeratin seen in histologic sections of nerve in which myelin is inadequately preserved. Also *neuroceratin.*

**neurolabyrinthitis** \-lab′ərinthī′tis\ [NEURO- + LABYRINTH + -ITIS] Inflammation of the vestibular sense organs and the vestibular nerve. It has been postulated as the cause in certain cases of epidemic vertigo when a viral agent is suspected.

**neurolathyrism** \-lath′irizm\ [NEURO- + LATHYRISM] LATHYRISM.

**neurolemma** \-lem′ə\ NEURILEMMA.

**neurolemmitis** \-lemī′tis\ NEURILEMMITIS.

**neurolemmoma** \-lemō′mə\ NEURILEMMOMA.

**neuroleptanalgesia** \-lept′analjē′zē·ə\ The effects achieved by the combined administration of a neuroleptic and of an analgesic drug. Also *ataralgesia.*

**neuroleptanalgesic** \-lept′analjē′sik\ **1** Denoting, pertaining to, or producing neuroleptanalgesia. **2** A neuroleptanalgesic agent.

**neuroleptanesthesia** \-lept′anesthē′zhə\ A technique in which the pain relief of neuroleptanalgesia is combined with general anesthesia induced by nitrous oxide and oxygen. It is stress-free, causes relative hypotension, and requires neuromuscular blockers for relaxation of muscles during surgery.

**neuroleptanesthetic** \-lept′anesthet′ik\ **1** Relating to neuroleptanesthesia. **2** Any substance resulting in the state characterizing neuroleptanesthesia.

**neuroleptic** \-lep′tik\ [NEURO- + Gk *lēptikos* (from *lambanein* to take hold) taking hold, assimilative] **1** Acting to prevent or alleviate mental disorders, as a drug. **2** A neuroleptic chemical or drug. For defs. 1 and 2 also *antipsychotic.*

**neurolipomatosis** \-lip′ōmətō′sis\ [NEURO- + *lipomat(a),* pl. of *lipoma* + -OSIS] NEUROLIPOMATOSIS DOLOROSA. **n. dolorosa** A disorder largely restricted to females which produces localized painful accumulations of subcutaneous fat. Also *Dercum's disease, neurolipomatosis, adiposis dolorosa.*

**neurologic** \-läj′ik\ Pertaining to neurology.

**neurologist** \n$^y$uräl′əjist\ A physician who specializes in neurology.

**neurology** \n$^y$uräl′əjē\ [NEURO- + -LOGY] That branch of medicine dealing with diseases of the nervous system. **clinical n.** The study of the clinical manifestations of neurologic disorders.

**neurolymph** \n$^y$ur′əlimf\ [NEURO- + LYMPH] *Seldom used* LIQUOR CEREBROSPINALIS.

**neurolymphomatosis** \-lim′fōmətō′sis\ [NEURO- + LYMPHOMATOSIS] Invasion of nerves by malignant lymphoma. **peripheral n.** Involvement of peripheral nerves by deposits of lymphoma or other reticuloses or by leukemic infiltrations.

**neurolysis** \n$^y$uräl′isis\ [NEURO- + LYSIS] **1** Destruction or dissolution of nervous tissue. **2** A surgical procedure in which a nerve is freed from compression by scar tissue or other compressive agents. **3** Destruction of a nerve by injecting alcohol or phenol into it. Adj. neurolytic.

**neuroma** \n$^y$urō′mə\ [NEUR- + -OMA] A benign tumor or tumorlike lesion composed of a mass of nerve fibers. It may be congenital or arise after trauma. The nerve fibers may be myelinated or unmyelinated, and cyst formation may occur. **acoustic n.** ACOUSTIC NEURILEMMOMA. **amputation n.** TRAUMATIC NEUROMA. **appendiceal n.** A tumorlike lesion composed of proliferated nerve fibers in a chronically inflammed vermiform appendix. Also *appendical neuroma.* **false n.** TRAUMATIC NEUROMA. **ganglionic n.** **1** A neuroma containing nerve cells. **2** GANGLIONEUROMA. **3** GANGLIONEUROFIBROMA. **malignant n.** MALIGNANT SCHWANNOMA. **Morton's n.** A painful tumorlike lesion of an interdigital plantar nerve, usually between the second and third toes, that is characterized by the proliferation of perineural tissues with the degeneration of axons and myelin. It is caused by pressure on the nerve at the metatarsophalangeal joint. Also *Morton's neuralgia, Morton's toe.* **plexiform n.** A neuroma in which there are interlacing neural elements resembling a plexus. Also *Verneuil's neuroma.* **post-traumatic n.** TRAUMATIC NEUROMA. **traumatic n.** A benign, nonneoplastic overgrowth of nerve fibers, Schwann cells, and scar tissue occurring at the proximal end of a severed nerve trunk. Also *amputation neuroma, post-traumatic neuroma, false neuroma.* **Verneuil's n.** PLEXIFORM NEUROMA. **n. verum** GANGLIONEUROMA.

**neuromalacia** \-məlā′shə\ Softening and cavitation in the nervous system. Also *neuromalakia.*

**neuromatous** \n$^y$uräm′ətəs\ Pertaining to a neuroma.

**neuromechanism** \-mek′ənizm\ A functional property dependent upon the nervous system.

**neuromelanin** \-mel′ənin\ [NEURO- + MELANIN] Pigment granules within the cytoplasm of neurons in the substantia nigra.

**neuromeningeal** \-menin′jē·əl\ Denoting, pertaining to, or affecting the central nervous system and meninges.

**neuromere** \n$^y$ur′əmir\ [NEURO- + -MERE] Each of the segments of the neural tube. Also *neural segment, neurotome.*

**neuromery** \n$^y$uräm′ərē\ [NEURO- + *mer(o)-*[1] + -Y] Segmentation of the embryonic neural tube exhibited by localized enlargments (neuromeres) separated from one another by constrictions.

**neuromodulator** \-mäd′yəlā′tər\ One of the numerous substances contained in neurons that do not serve as neurotransmitters at synapses but modulate neuronal membrane events, including hormones, nucleotides, and a variety of peptides.

**neuromuscular** \-mus′kyələr\ [NEURO- + MUSCULAR] Denoting, pertaining to, or affecting the lower motor neurons and muscles. Also *neuromyal, neuromotor.*

**neuromyasthenia** \-mī′asthē′nē·ə\ Neurasthenia in which emotional lability and muscular weakness are the predominant symptoms. *Older term.* **epidemic n.** BENIGN MYALGIC ENCEPHALOMYELITIS.

**neuromyelitis** \-mī′əlī′tis\ [NEURO- + MYELITIS] Myelitis associated with neuritis, especially that form of demyelinating myelitis occurring in neuromyelitis optica (Devic's disease). **n. hyperalbuminotica** GUILLAIN-BARRÉ SYNDROME. **n. optica** Demyelination involving one or both optic nerves and the spinal cord. Some such cases ultimately prove to be suffering from multiple sclerosis. Also

*Devic's disease, neuro-optic myelitis, ophthalmoneuromyelitis, optic neuroencephalomyelopathy.*

**neuromyocardium** \\-mī′əkär′dē·əm\\ The myocardial tissues that constitute the conduction system of the heart.

**neuromyopathy** \\-mī·äp′əthē\\ Any disease process which involves both the peripheral or central nervous system and the voluntary muscles. Adj. neuromyopathic. **carcinomatous n.** Any paraneoplastic syndrome giving rise to disease of the central nervous system but more often of the peripheral nerves in association with a myopathy. Often the causative neoplasm is an oat cell bronchial carcinoma.

**neuromyositis** \\-mī′əsī′tis\\ [NEURO- + MYOSITIS] **1** Polymyositis and polyneuritis occurring together in the same patient. *Imprecise.* **2** POLYNEUROMYOSITIS.

**neuromyotonia** \\-mī′ətō′nē·ə\\ MYOKYMIA.

**neuron** \\n$^y$ʊr′än\\ [Gk *neuron* a sinew, tendon, nerve, string] **1** The basic cellular conducting element of the central and peripheral nervous systems. A typical neuron consists of a cell body, or perikaryon, containing a nucleus and cytoplasm, and several radiating processes of varying shape and length. The axon, usually a long, thin cytoplasmic structure, conducts impulses away from the cell body. Dendrites, ordinarily consisting of multiple branching protoplasmic extensions that greatly extend the surface area of the receptive membrane of the cell body, generally serve as the receptive pole of the neuron. The cell body cytoplasm in most cases contains a dense, multilaminate, membranous system, the endoplasmic reticulum, which is concerned with protein synthesis and helps to maintain the extended structure of the cell. The neuron also contains an extensive endocellular skeleton of microtubules and microfilaments, the neurofibrillar network, which may be involved in structural support and transport roles throughout the nerve cell. Also *nerve cell, neurocyte, nerve unit.* **2** *Obs.* AXON. **alpha motor n.** A central neuron whose peripheral axon innervates skeletal muscle fibers and conducts at the highest velocities. **bipolar n.** A neuron with two major neurofibril-containing processes. During maturation, one process usually becomes the axon, or central process, and the other becomes the dendrite, or peripheral process. Bipolar neurons are usually sensory in function and subserve impulses generated by olfactory, visual, auditory, and vestibular receptor endings. **central n.** A neuron whose cell body lies within the central nervous system. **connector n.** INTERNEURON. **effector n.** A neuron that carries impulses toward an effector. **exciter n.** MOTONEURON. **first-order n.** PRIMARY NEURON. **gamma motor n.** A central neuron whose peripheral axon innervates the intrafusal muscle fibers of muscle spindles and conducts impulses at velocities in the range of gamma efferent nerve fibers. Also *gamma neuron, fusimotor neuron.* **Golgi type I n.'s** Nerve cells having long axons that leave the local neuropil area of the parent cell body, enter the white matter, and project to other parts of the nervous system. Compare GOLGI TYPE II NEURONS. • The two major neuronal types were originally distinguished by Camillo Golgi on the basis of axonal length. **Golgi type II n.'s** Nerve cells having axons with short trajectories, typified by the stellate cells of the cerebral and cerebellar cortex. Axonal length and trajectory may vary. In some cases, the axon system is contained entirely within the confines of the dendrite system of the parent cell. In others, such as the cerebellar granules cell, the axon may run for 1–3 mm. Many authorities include all neurons whose axons do not enter the white matter, thereby remaining within the local neuropil. Also *cells of van Gehuchten.* Compare GOLGI TYPE I NEURONS. **horizontal n.'s** HORIZONTAL CELLS. **intercalary n.** INTERNEURON. **internuncial n.** INTERNEURON. **Martinotti n.** Small local circuit neurons of the cerebral cortex whose axons characteristically ascend toward the cortical surface. **motor n.** MOTONEURON. **multiform n.** POLYMORPHIC NEURON. **peripheral motor n.** MOTONEURON. **peripheral sensory n.** PRIMARY SENSORY NEURON. **phasic motor n.** An alpha motor neuron whose peripheral axon controls skeletal muscles initiating rapid movements. **polymorphic n.** A nerve call of irregular shape usually characterized by multipolar configuration with dendrites emerging at many points along the cell body. Also *multiform neuron.* **premotor n.** UPPER MOTOR NEURON. **primary n.** In a neural pathway, a neuron, as a sensory receptor, whose axon forms a synapse with another neuron (second-order neuron) for the transmission of an impulse. Also *first-order neuron.* **primary sensory n.** A dorsal root ganglion cell possessing one neurite extending to a peripheral sense organ and a neurite entering the central nervous system. Also *sensory neuron, peripheral sensory neuron.* **projection n.** A neuron that transmits activity from the cerebral cortex to motor neurons. **pyramidal n.** PYRAMIDAL CELL. **second-order n.** In a neural pathway, the neuron on which the axon of a primary (first-order) neuron synapses, as for example the spinothalamic neurons serving to relay impulses from axons of sensory receptors, or in sympathetic ganglia, the postganglionic neuron contacted by the sympathetic motoneuron whose cell body is the spinal cord. **sensory n.** PRIMARY SENSORY NEURON. **superior motor n.** UPPER MOTOR NEURON. **tonic motor n.** An alpha motor neuron whose peripheral axon controls postural muscle tone. **unipolar n.** A neuron with only one process, usually the axon. Such cells are unusual in the central nervous system, where the best-known examples, the cells of the dorsal root spinal ganglia and of the mesencephalic root of the fifth nerve, are actually of bipolar derivation, having become unipolar through subsequent fusion of the two processes. Such neurons are also called T-shaped unipolar cells. Also *unipolar cell.* **upper motor n.** A neuron that controls activity in motor neurons. Also *superior motor neuron, premotor neuron.*

**neuronagenesis** \\n$^y$ʊr′änəjen′əsis\\ [NEURON + Gk *a*-priv. + GENESIS] A failure of neuron development.

**neuronal** \\n$^y$ʊr′ənəl, n$^y$ʊrō′nəl\\ Of, pertaining to, or affecting a neuron.

**neurone** \\n$^y$ʊr′ōn\\ *Brit.* NEURON.

**neuronevus** \\-nē′vəs\\ A nevus composed of cells that exhibit neural characteristics.

**neuronitis** \\n$^y$ʊr′ənī′tis\\ [NEURON + -ITIS] CELLULONEURITIS. **infective n.** *Outmoded* GUILLAIN-BARRÉ SYNDROME. **myoclonic spinal n.** A rare and poorly understood syndrome in which spinal myoclonus occurs and inclusion bodies may be found in the anterior horn cells of the spinal cord. **vestibular n.** A form of vertigo of acute onset, causing prostration, nausea, and vomiting, and lasting often for several days during which any movement of the head induces severe vertigo. Recovery is eventually complete. The condition may occur in epidemics and is believed to be due to a viral infection involving the vestibular nuclei of the brainstem. Also *Gerlier's disease, Gerlier syndrome, paralytic vertigo, paralyzing vertigo.*

**neuronography** \\-näg′rəfē\\ [NEURON + *o* + -GRAPHY] **1** The study of connections among neurons, originally used with reference to microanatomic techniques that allowed for visual tracing of connections. **2** A physiologic method of mapping connections within the cerebral cortex by recording electrical discharges elicited in various cortical zones following the local application of strychnine. **strychnine n.**

An electrophysiological technique for tracing connections in the central nervous system based on the capability of strychnine to synchronize neuronal firing patterns.

**neuronophage** \n$^y$Urän′əfāj\ Any phagocytic, usually microglial, cell which has ingested dead neurons or neuronal debris.

**neuronophagia** \-nōfā′jə\ The ingestion of dead neurons or neuronal debris by phagocytes.

**neuronosis** \-nō′sis\ *Seldom used* NEUROPATHY.

**neuronotropic** \n$^y$Urän′ōträp′ik\ Possessing a selective affinity for neurons.

**neuro-ophthalmology** \-äf′thalmäl′əjē\ [NEURO- + OPHTHALMOLOGY] The science or study of relationships between the central nervous system and the eyes, including the nervous control of vision and ocular movement. Also *neurophthalmology.*

**neuro-otology** \-ōtäl′əjē\ The study of phenomena, particularly diseases, of concern both to neurologists and otologists; the mutual management of patients with such diseases. Also *neurotology, otoneurology.*

**neuropacemaker** \-pās′mākər\ [NEURO- + PACEMAKER] An implanted electrical nerve stimulator that helps to relieve intractable pain.

**neuropapillitis** \-pap′ilī′tis\ [NEURO- + PAPILLITIS] PAPILLEDEMA.

**neuroparasite** \-par′əsīt\ **1** A parasite whose development takes place exclusively in the nervous system of the host. **2** A parasite of the nervous system. Adj. neuroparasitic.

**neuropathic** \-path′ik\ Pertaining to, inducing, or caused by neuropathy.

**neuropathology** \-pathäl′əjē\ The study of pathologic changes in the nervous system.

**neuropathy** \n$^y$Uräp′əthē\ [NEURO- + -PATHY] **1** Any disease of the central or peripheral nervous system. **2** A disorder of the peripheral nerves, as distinct from myelopathy or encephalopathy in which the central nervous system is involved. Also *neuronosis* (seldom used). **abetalipoproteinemic n.** ABETALIPOPROTEINEMIA. **acrodystrophic n.** Any peripheral neuropathy producing severe trophic changes, including sometimes painless ulceration or destruction of tissue in the extremities. **acute autonomic n.** A rare syndrome of sudden onset in children and adults, characterized by postural hypotension, paralysis of accommodation, anhidrosis, loss of lacrimation, and urinary and fecal retention. Spontaneous recovery is usual in a few weeks or months. Also *pandysautonomia.* **alcoholic n.** Polyneuropathy complicating alcoholism and resulting as a rule from associated thiamine deficiency. Also *alcoholic paralysis, alcoholic polyneuritis, alcoholic polyneuropathy.* **amyloid n.** Polyneuropathy due to deposition of amyloid (amyloidosis) in peripheral nerves. Portuguese, Iowa, and Indiana types have been described. See under AMYLOIDOSIS. Also *amyloid neuritis, amyloid polyneuropathy.* **Andrade type amyloid n.** PORTUGUESE TYPE AMYLOIDOSIS. **ascending n.** Polyneuropathy first affecting the feet and legs and only later the trunk and upper limbs. **autonomic n.** Polyneuropathy principally or wholly involving autonomic nerves. Also *vasoneuropathy.* **axonal n.** Any neuropathy in which the primary pathologic change is one involving axons rather than their myelin sheaths. **carcinomatous n.** Polyneuropathy developing as a complication of carcinoma without direct invasion of peripheral nerves by malignant cells. **Denny-Brown sensory n.** A paraneoplastic disorder, usually associated with oat cell carcinoma of the bronchus, giving rise to paresthesiae and sensory loss in the distal parts of the limbs and progressive sensory ataxia, resulting from progressive degeneration of posterior root ganglia, sensory fibers in peripheral nerves and secondary degeneration in ascending sensory tracts in the spinal cord. Motor function is unaffected. Also *Denny-Brown syndrome.* **descending n.** Polyneuropathy first affecting the upper limbs and later spreading to the trunk, legs, and feet. **diabetic n.** The distal, bilateral, usually symmetrical, and predominantly sensory polyneuropathy associated with diabetes mellitus. The chief symptoms are hyperesthesia of hands and feet with signs of trophic changes in the extremities, such as coldness, loss of hair, thinness of skin, and disorders of sweating. **dying-back n.** Polyneuropathy in which the degeneration of axons begins at the periphery and spreads centripetally. **entrapment n.** Neuropathy, usually limited to a single peripheral nerve, in which the nerve is entrapped or compressed within a bony or fibrous canal. Also *pressure neuropathy.* **giant axonal n.** Neuropathy in which the principal pathologic finding is a massive swelling or enlargement of affected axons. **glue-sniffers' n.** Polyneuropathy due to the accidental or more often deliberate sniffing of the vapor given off by certain glues used, for example, in plastic modeling kits. The toxic agent appears to be *n*-hexane. **hereditary hypertrophic interstitial n.** A disease, often familial, with onset in infancy, marked by symmetrical muscular atrophy of the extremities, with severe sensory disorders and ataxia, arising from ascending neuritis with an associated spinal cord lesion. This form of familial hypertrophic neuropathy, sometimes dominantly inherited, sometimes due to an autosomal recessive trait, is characterized clinically by distal muscular weakness and sensory loss in the limbs and pathologically by demyelination of peripheral nerves with Schwann cell proliferation giving rise to concentric "onion bulb" formation. Spinal cord compression may result from massive hypertrophy of motor and sensory roots within the spinal canal. Pupillary abnormalities, resembling the Argyll Robertson pupil, and/or optic atrophy have been described in some affected individuals and families. It is closely related to peroneal muscular atrophy (Charcot-Marie-Tooth disease) and must be distinguished from the non-familial forms of hypertrophic neuropathy, some of which are due to autoimmunity and may be steroid-responsive. Also *neuritic amyotrophy, hypertrophic interstitial radiculoneuropathy, symmetrical bundle neurofibromas, Schwann hyperplasia, Dejerine-Sottas syndrome, Dejerine disease, Gombault's degeneration, progressive hypertrophic interstitial neuropathy, progressive hypertrophic polyneuritis.* **hereditary sensorimotor n. types I-III** CHARCOT-MARIE-TOOTH DISEASE. **hereditary sensory n.** A form of genetically determined neuropathy of autosomal recessive inheritance characterized histologically by degeneration of posterior root ganglia and clinically by severe sensory impairment, usually with painless ulceration, in the extremities. Also *hereditary sensory radicular neuropathy.* **hypertrophic n.** Any neuropathy associated with hypertrophy of peripheral nerves. Some forms are inherited, others inflammatory, with repeated cycles of demyelination and remyelination giving the so-called onion-bulb hypertrophy of the affected nerves. Also *hypertrophic interstitial neuropathy.* **Indiana type amyloid n.** INDIANA TYPE AMYLOIDOSIS. **intercostal n.** INTERCOSTAL NEURALGIA. **Iowa type amyloid n.** IOWA TYPE OF AMYLOIDOSIS. **ischemic n.** Local or diffuse lesions of peripheral nerves resulting either from restriction of blood supply to a single peripheral nerve, often due to compression or from diffuse arterial disease. **isoniazid n.** ISONIAZID POLYNEUROPATHY. **Jamaican n.** JAMAICA JAKE PARALYSIS. **lead**

**n.** Mononeuropathy or polyneuropathy due to exposure to lead. Principal symptoms are wristdrop and weakness of the extensor muscles. Hyperesthesia and analgesia may also occur. Also *lead paralysis, lead palsy.* **myxedematous n.** Polyneuropathy developing in patients with hypothyroidism. **peripheral n.** POLYNEUROPATHY. **plexus n.** Neuropathy of nerves which form part of either the brachial or sacral plexus. **Portuguese type amyloid n.** PORTUGUESE TYPE AMYLOIDOSIS. **pressure n.** ENTRAPMENT NEUROPATHY. **radiation n.** Damage to nerves, especially peripheral nerves, caused by radiation. **sensorimotor n.** Any neuropathy or polyneuropathy involving motor and sensory nerves or fibers. **sensory n.** Any neuropathy or polyneuropathy involving only sensory nerves or fibers. **serum n.** Mononeuropathy or polyneuropathy following the injection of foreign serum. Also *serum neuritis, serum paralysis.* **trigeminal n.** A neuropathy restricted to one or both trigeminal nerves. **triorthocresyl phosphate n.** The severe and irreversible sensorimotor axonal neuropathy which may result from intoxication with triorthocresyl phosphate. An outbreak of Jamaica jake paralysis in 1930 was caused by contamination of ginger extract with cresyl phosphates. Other incidents have occurred since then due to unintentional contamination of food by triorthocresyl phosphate or contaminated fuel oil improperly sold for cooking purposes. Also *triorthocresyl phosphate polyneuritis.* **tropical ataxic n.** Neuropathy due to cyanide intoxication and giving rise to optic atrophy, ataxia, and polyneuropathy in varying combinations. It is endemic in Nigeria and in other parts of Africa, where it results from the dietary ingestion of cassava root. Also *nutritional spinal ataxia.* **uremic n.** UREMIC POLYNEUROPATHY.

**neuropharmacology** The branch of pharmacology dealing with the action of drugs on the nervous system and its functions.

**neurophil** \nʸur′əfil\ NEUROSPONGIUM.

**neurophilic** \-fil′ik\ NEUROTROPIC.

**neurophonia** \-fō′nē·ə\ Attacks in which the subject produces abrupt harsh or high-pitched cries as the result of intermittent spasm of the laryngeal and respiratory musculature. *Seldom used.*

**neurophrenia** \-frē′nē·ə\ [NEURO- + -PHRENIA] *Seldom used* MINIMAL BRAIN DYSFUNCTION.

**neurophthalmology** \nʸur′äfthalmäl′əjē\ NEURO-OPHTHALMOLOGY.

**neurophysin** One of two proteins of low molecular mass (10 kDa) of the neurohypophysis. It is capable of binding oxytocin or vasopressin. It is believed to be a carrier protein for the hormones and may play a role in their storage in the posterior pituitary.

**neurophysiology** \-fiz′ē·äl′əjē\ [NEURO- + PHYSIOLOGY] The study of the relation of structure and function in the nervous system.

**neuropil** \nʸur′əpil\ [NEURO- + Gk *pil(os)* wool or hair wrought into felt] The dense feltwork of cytoplasmic processes of nerve cells and neuroglia that constitutes the basic stroma of the central nervous system. It generally corresponds to the gray matter, and includes virtually all zones where synaptic interactions may occur, in contradistinction to the long tracts, or white matter (substantia alba). Also *neuropilem* (obs.), *neuropile* (a chiefly British spelling).

**neuroplasm** \nʸur′əplazm\ The unstructured cytoplasm of a nerve cell of neuron. Adj. neuroplasmic.

**neuropodia** \-pō′dē·ə\ Plural of NEUROPODIUM.

**neuropodium** \-pō′dē·əm\ END FOOT.

**neuropore** \nʸur′əpôr\ [NEURO- + Gk *poros* a passage, way through, pore] An opening which temporarily allows communication between the canal within the neural tube of an embryo of protochordates and vertebrates with the outside. An anterior neuropore is always present, but the existence of the posterior neuropore in every form is debatable. **anterior n.** An opening at the cranial end of the embryonic neural tube leading into the amniotic cavity. Its closure occurs at the 20-somite stage, about the 26th day of intrauterine life in man. **posterior n.** An opening at the caudal end of the embryonic neural tube communicating with the amniotic cavity. Its closure occurs at about the 25-somite stage, around the 28th day of intrauterine life in man.

**neuroprobasia** \-prōbā′zhə\ [NEURO- + Gk *probas(is)* (from *probainein* to step forward) a stepping forward + -IA] Progression along nerves, a characteristic of certain viral disease processes.

**neuroprosthesis** \-prōsthē′sis\ Any prosthetic device applied to a peripheral nerve or implanted in a central nervous structure for purposes of chronic stimulation.

**neuropsychiatrist** \-sīkī′ətrist\ A specialist in neuropsychiatry.

**neuropsychiatry** \-sīkī′ətrē\ That branch of medicine which embraces both neurology and psychiatry.

**neuropsychology** \-sīkäl′əjē\ [NEURO- + PSYCHOLOGY] The study of the relationship between the central nervous system and behavior, centering on the integrative functioning of the brain as principal mediator of all mental processes and behavioral reactions.

**neuropsychopathy** \-sīkäp′əthē\ [NEURO- + PSYCHO- + -PATHY] Any disorder which affects the nervous system and the mind.

**neuropsychopharmacology** The branch of pharmacology dealing with the effects of drugs on psychiatric illnesses and the mechanism of action of these agents.

**neuroradiology** \-rā′dē·äl′əjē\ A subspecialty of radiology dealing with the diagnosis of diseases of the nervous system.

**neuroregulation** \-reg′yəlā′shən\ The control of physiological processes by the nervous system.

**neuroretinitis** \-ret′inī′tis\ [NEURO- + RETINITIS] Inflammation of optic disk and retina. Also *papilloretinitis, retinopapillitis.*

**neuroretinopathy** \-ret′inäp′əthē\ [NEURO- + RETINOPATHY] A disorder of the optic disk and retina.

**neurorrhaphy** \nʸurôr′əfē\ [NEURO- + -RRHAPHY] Approximation by suture of a divided nerve. Also *neurosuture, nerve suture.*

**neurosarcoma** \-särkō′mə\ [NEURO- + SARCOMA] MALIGNANT SCHWANNOMA.

**neurosecretion** \-sikrē′shən\ **1** The sum of the processes by which neurons elaborate substances that are released or secreted into the bloodstream and act as hormones. **2** A substance so produced and having an effect or influence on other cells.

**neurosecretory** \-sikrē′tərē, -sē′krətôr′ē\ Of or relating to neurosecretion.

**neurosegmental** \-segmen′təl\ Denoting a spinal division or segment served by a dorsal and ventral root pair.

**neurosensory** \-sen′sərē\ Describing, pertaining to, or affecting sensory components of the nervous system.

**neuroses** \nʸurō′sēz\ Plural of NEUROSIS.

**neurosis** \nʸurō′sis\ [NEUR- + -OSIS] Any of various functional disorders of behavior characterized by excessive anxiety or by behavior distorted by an exaggerated use of avoidance behaviors or by other recognized mechanisms for defending against anxiety. In psychoanalytic usage, neurosis is the symptomatic expression of conflict between the id's sexual and aggressive impulses and the ego's need to cope with and adapt to reality. One or more distressing and ego-dystonic symptoms develop as a result of the ego's attempt to defend itself against the id. Also *psychoneurosis, neurotic disorder, defense neurosis, meroergasia, defense psychoneurosis.* • Although DSM-III has discarded *neurosis* in favor of *neurotic disorder,* the former term is still widely used. **accident n.** COMPENSATION NEUROSIS. **actual n.** According to Freud, those symptoms arising from present-day disturbances of sexuality in contrast to neuroses which arise from infantile conflicts. Neurasthenia, hypochondriasis, and anxiety neurosis were considered actual neuroses. Also *true neurosis, physioneurosis.* **anankastic n.** OBSESSIVE-COMPULSIVE NEUROSIS. **anxiety n.** According to Freud, an actual neurosis manifested in general irritability, anxious expectation and excessive free-floating anxiety, pangs of conscience, and exaggerated fear of common dangers such as snakes, mice, or vermin. Also *anxiety syndrome.* **artificial n.** EXPERIMENTAL NEUROSIS. **association n.** SHARED DELUSION. **character n.** CHARACTER DISORDER. **compensation n.** A neurosis that develops or persists in a person who has suffered injury from an accident while a tort claim is pending. It tends to prolong the illness (a manifestation of epinosic gain) and delay recovery. Also *pension neurosis, accident neurosis.* **compulsion n.** OBSESSIVE-COMPULSIVE NEUROSIS. **conversion n.** CONVERSION HYSTERIA. **craft n.** OCCUPATIONAL CRAMP. **defense n.** NEUROSIS. **depressive n.** NEUROTIC DEPRESSIVE DISORDER. **expectation n.** A neurosis characterized by the fear that one will be inadequate in performing the anticipated task. It is often a symptom of agoraphobia. **experimental n.** A neurosis created in animals by altering the experimental conditions to which they have adapted. They can no longer discriminate between the different stimuli presented and therefore cannot supply what has been learned as the correct response to a specific stimulus. Also *artificial neurosis.* **fright n.** *Older term* TRAUMATIC NEUROSIS. **housewife's n.** 1 An obsessive-compulsive neurosis characterized by preoccupation with cleanliness and orderliness of the household. Also *housewife's psychosis.* 2 A syndrome of homemakers characterized by chronic dissatisfaction and feelings of stagnation and emptiness because marriage and parenthood have eliminated the stimulation of employment and freedom of movement among active and accomplishing adults. Also *tired housewife syndrome.* **hysterical n.** HYSTERIA. **neurasthenic n.** NEURASTHENIA. **obsessional n.** OBSESSIVE-COMPULSIVE NEUROSIS. **obsessive-compulsive n.** A neurosis characterized by intruding, ego-dystonic, anxiety-provoking thoughts and repetitive impulses to perform actions that are often distasteful or unwanted but are the only way to achieve a temporary surcease of the anxiety. Also *obsessional neurosis, compulsion neurosis, anankastic neurosis, substitution neurosis, obsessive-ruminative state, compulsive-obsessive psychoneurosis, obsessive-compulsive reaction, compulsive state.* **occupational n.** OCCUPATIONAL CRAMP. **organ n.** PSYCHOSOMATIC DISORDER. **pension n.** COMPENSATION NEUROSIS. **phobic n.** ANXIETY HYSTERIA. **phobic anxiety-depersonalization n.** A state in which the individual feels symptoms of both anxiety and depersonalization. It is characterized by giddiness, mood changes, and other symptoms of depersonalization as well as fear of collapse or loss of control in public. Also *pseudoschizophrenic neurosis.* **professional n.** OCCUPATIONAL CRAMP. **pseudoschizophrenic n.** PHOBIC ANXIETY-DEPERSONALIZATION NEUROSIS. **sphenopalatine ganglion n.** SPHENOPALATINE NEURALGIA. **substitution n.** OBSESSIVE-COMPULSIVE NEUROSIS. **traumatic n.** A neurosis brought on by physical injury and triggered by the threat of subsequent harm or actual physical injury. This leads to intrusive recollections of the stressful event, recurrent frightening dreams about it, contraction of the general level of functioning, general irritability, and proclivity to explosive aggressive reactions. Also *fright neurosis* (older term). **true n.** ACTUAL NEUROSIS. **vagabond n.** WANDERLUST. **vegetative n.** PINK DISEASE.

**neuroskeletal** \-skel′ətəl\ 1 Pertaining to the neuroskeleton. 2 Pertaining to nervous and skeletal muscle tissues.

**neuroskeleton** \-skel′ətən\ 1 The bony parts surrounding the brain, or neurocranium, and spinal cord, or vertebral column. 2 ENDOSKELETON.

**neurosonology** \-sōnäl′əjē\ ECHOENCEPHALOGRAPHY.

**neurosplanchnic** \-splangk′nik\ [NEURO- + SPLANCHNIC] Of, pertaining to, or affecting the autonomic nerves innervating the viscera. Also *neurovisceral.*

**neurospongioma** \-spän′jē·ō′mə\ [NEURO- + SPONGI- + -OMA] GLIOMA.

**neurospongium** \-spän′jē·əm\ [NEURO- + New L *-spongium,* combining form from L *spongia* sponge] An intricate meshwork of axons, dendrites, and neuroglial processes within the central nervous system. Also *neurophil.*

**neurostimulator** \-stim′yəlā′tər\ An implantable electric stimulator similar to a pacemaker with output electrodes that encircle a nerve to effect muscle contraction or block pain.

**neurosurgeon** \-sur′jən\ [NEURO- + SURGEON] One who performs surgery on the nervous system.

**neurosurgery** \-sur′jərē\ [NEURO- + SURGERY] Surgery of the nervous system and its supporting structures, as the vascular supply to the brain and spine.

**neurosuture** \-soo′chər\ NEURORRHAPHY.

**neurosyphilid** \-sif′ilid\ CIRCINATE SYPHILITIC ERYTHEMA.

**neurosyphilis** \-sif′əlis\ Any of the forms of syphilis of the central nervous system, including secondary syphilis, late syphilis, and tabes dorsalis. Also *lues nervosa.* **juvenile n.** Neurosyphilis occurring in early adolescence with symptoms similar to general paresis in adults except that delusions are more puerile, the dementia is more complete, and the course is more prolonged. It is a subtype occurring in not more than one percent of congenital syphilitics. **latent n.** Asymptomatic neurosyphilis that is revealed only by examination of the cerebrospinal fluid. **meningeal n.** Syphilis of the coverings of the brain and spinal cord. **meningovascular n.** Syphilitic involvement of the meninges and cerebral blood vessels, frequently with involvement of cranial nerves. **paretic n.** GENERAL PARESIS. **tabetic n.** TABES DORSALIS.

**neurotabes** \-tā′bēz\ TABES DORSALIS.

**neurotendinous** \-ten′dinəs\ Of, pertaining to, or affecting nerves and tendons.

**neuroterminal** \-tur′minəl\ END ORGAN.

**neurothele** \-thē′lē, -thēl′\ [NEURO- + Gk *thēlē* a nipple] NERVE PAPILLA.

**neurothelion** \-thē′lē·än\ [*neurothel(e)* + *-ion,* New L dim. suffix] A small nerve papilla.

**neurotic** \n^yUrät′ik\ 1 Relating to or characterized by neurosis. 2 A patient suffering from neurosis. • In popular usage, the term in this sense is often used perjoratively to indicate that the subject does not act consistently in the way others expect or want, or that the subject's complaints are imaginary and without foundation.

**neuroticism** \nʸŏŏrät′isizm\ [*neurotic* + -ISM] The state of suffering from neurosis.
**neurotization** \nʸŏŏr′ätīzā′shən\ [NEURO- + *t* + *-iz(e)* + -ATION] **1** Implantation of nerve into muscle. **2** Regeneration of a nerve.
**neurotmesis** \nʸŏŏr′ätmē′sis\ [NEURO- + Gk *tmēsis* (from *temnein* to cut) a cutting, division] A lesion of a peripheral nerve in which there is actual division of axons, so that regeneration will be needed for recovery to take place.
**neurotology** \-täl′əjē\ NEURO-OTOLOGY.
**neurotome** \nʸŏŏr′ətōm\ [NEURO- + -TOME] **1** A narrow-bladed knife for cutting nerves. **2** NEUROMERE.
**neurotomy** \nʸŏŏrät′əmē\ [NEURO- + -TOMY] **1** The dissection of nerves. **2** Division of a nerve. **retrogasserian n.** TRIGEMINAL RHIZOTOMY.
**neurotoxic** \-täk′sik\ Having a toxic effect on the nervous system.
**neurotoxicity** \-täksis′itē\ [NEURO- + TOXICITY] The quality of having a toxic effect upon the nervous system.
**neurotoxin** \-täk′sin\ Any toxin which acts directly upon neurons, sometimes affecting the cell body but more often acting at synapses, whether excitatory or inhibitory, and thus giving rise to disordered neuronal function. For example, some neurotoxins act at the neuromuscular junction, causing paralysis, while others, such as tetanus toxin, act upon interneuronal connections in the spinal cord causing hyperexcitability of neurons.
**neurotransmitter** \-transmit′ər\ Any chemical substance released at a nerve terminal as a result of the nerve impulse and capable of transmitting that impulse across a synapse by binding to receptors in another cell, thereby exciting it. Also *transmitter substance.*
**neurotrauma** \-trô′mə\ [NEURO- + TRAUMA] Any injury to a nerve. Also *neurotrosis.*
**neurotrophic** \-träf′ik\ [NEURO- + -TROPHIC] **1** Relating to neurotrophy. **2** Describing trophic disorders of nervous origin.
**neurotrophy** \nʸŏŏrät′rəfē\ The maintenance of the nutrition and of the structural and functional integrity of nervous tissue.
**neurotropic** \-träp′ik\ Having an affinity or attraction for nervous tissue. Also *neurophilic.*
**neurotropism** \nʸŏŏrät′rəpizm\ The possession of neurotropic qualities. Also *neurotropy, neutropism.*
**neurotrosis** \-trō′sis\ [NEURO- + Gk *trōsis* (from *titrōskein* to wound) a wound] NEUROTRAUMA.
**neurotubule** \-tʸōōb′yōōl\ Long microtubules of fixed ≈20–30 nm diameter seen in the axons of neurons with the electron microscope. The long axes of the microtubules are parallel to the long axis of the axon. The neurotubules are involved in growth and axonal transport of intracellular materials.
**neurovaccine** \-vak′sin\ A vaccine prepared by utilizing the brain of a rabbit for the growth of the virus.
**neurovascular** \-vas′kyələr\ Of, pertaining to, or affecting the nervous and vascular systems.
**neurovegetative** \-vej′itā′tiv\ Pertaining to or affecting the autonomic nervous system.
**neurovirulence** \-vir′ʸələns\ [NEURO- + VIRULENCE] Pathogenicity of an infective agent for tissue of the central nervous system.
**neurovirulent** \-vir′ʸələnt\ Pathogenic for nerve tissue of the central nervous system: said of infective agents.
**neurovirus** \-vī′rəs\ NEUROTROPIC VIRUS.
**neurovisceral** \-vis′ərəl\ NEUROSPLANCHNIC.
**neurula** \nʸŏŏr′ōōlə\ [New L, from NEUR- + *-ula* as in *gastrula*] The embryonic stage following that of the gastrula during which a portion of the ectoderm forms the neural plate, from which the neural tube, the precursor of the central nervous system, will be fashioned.
**neurulation** \nʸŏŏr′ōōlā′shən\ [*neurul(a)* + -ATION] The development of the embryonic neural plate, the neural folds, and then the neural tube from which the central nervous system arises.
**neurypnology** \nʸŏŏr′ipnäl′əjē\ NEUROHYPNOLOGY.
**neutral** [L *neutralis* (from *neuter* neither, from *ne-* negative + *uter* either) neutral, neuter] **1** Being neither acidic nor basic, but having a pH near 7: used of a solution. **2** Having neither acidic nor basic properties: used of a substance.
**neutrality** \nʸōōtral′itē\ The state of being neutral, especially the acidity of water when the concentrations of $H^+$ and $OH^-$ ions are equal, i.e. pH 7.
**neutralization** \nʸōō′trəlīzā′shən\ **1** The addition of an acid to a base in solution, or vice-versa, so as to obtain a neutral solution. **2** The addition to water of chemical substances in order to adjust the pH to 7.
**neutralized** \nʸōō′trəlīzd\ **1** Describing an acid which has been converted into a salt by adding a base, or a base converted into a salt by adding an acid. **2** Rendered ineffective by combination with a reagent: said of a property of a group or molecule. **3** In crystallography and geology, describing mineral acids, rich in silica, that have been more or less completely converted into their salts.
**neutrino** \nʸōōtrē′nō\ A subatomic particle postulated to account for energy discrepancies in beta decay. It has no charge and, at most, one percent of the mass of an electron. It takes part in only the weak nuclear interaction (and possibly gravitation), and so has enormous penetrating power.
**neutroclusion** \nʸōō′träklōō′zhən\ [L *neuter,* gen. *neutri,* neutral, neuter + *o* + *(oc)clusion*] Normal anatomic relation between the dental arches.
**neutrocyte** \nʸōō′trəsīt\ NEUTROPHIL.
**neutrocytopenia** \nʸōō′trəsī′tōpē′nē·ə\ NEUTROPENIA.
**neutrocytophilia** \nʸōō′trəsī′tōfil′yə\ NEUTROPHILIA.
**neutrocytosis** \nʸōō′trəsitō′sis\ NEUTROPHILIA.
**neutron** \nʸōō′trän\ [*neutr(al)* + *-on,* suffix denoting an elementary particle] A nuclear particle with no electric charge, with a mass about 1.0014 times that of a proton and with $^1/_2$ unit of spin. Apart from the lighter elements, neutrons contribute roughly 40% to a typical nuclear mass. A free neutron decays (with a half-life of 15 minutes) into a proton, an electron, and an antineutrino. **fast n.** Any neutron having a high kinetic energy, of the order of 1 MeV or more. • Some authorities call any neutron "fast" if its energy is greater than 100 KeV. **fission n.** Any neutron emitted during nuclear fission in a nuclear reactor. **high-energy n.** A neutron that has an energy exceeding $10^5$ eV. **prompt n.** A neutron emitted no more than a few milliseconds after the fission event that produced it. More than 99% of fission neutrons are prompt. Also *instant neutron.* **slow n.** A neutron having kinetic energy of 1 eV or less. **thermal n.** Any neutron in thermal equilibrium with the environment, thus having low kinetic energy, about 0.025 eV.
**neutrontherapy** \nʸōō′tränther′əpē\ Radiotherapy using either fast or slow neutrons.
**neutropenia** \nʸōō′trəpē′nē·ə\ [*neutro(phil)* + -PENIA] A decreased number of neutrophils in the circulating blood. Also *neutrocytopenia, neutrophilopenia, neutrophilic leukopenia.* **chronic benign n.** An uncommon condition of unknown cause in which neutrophils are much lower than normal in the blood and all other blood elements are normal. The bone marrow is usually normal. Mouth ulcers or

respiratory infections may occur when the number of neutrophils is very low. **chronic hypoplastic n.** A rare syndrome of granulocytic hypoplasia in the marrow, chronic neutropenia in the circulating blood, mild to moderate splenomegaly, and recurrent infections especially involving the skin and oral cavity. **congenital n.** A rare and usually lethal disorder that is probably of autosomal recessive genetic transmission, characterized by onset in infancy of recurrent cutaneous infections, aphthous ulcers, severe neutropenia of blood, hyperplasia of early granulocyte precursors in bone marrow, and paucity of later stages of granulocyte maturation. Also *infantile genetic agranulocytosis, infantile lethal agranulocytosis, Kostmann's disease, congenital aleukia, congenital leukopenia.* **cyclic n.** A syndrome of neutropenia regularly recurring at intervals of 12–35 days and lasting 4–10 days, accompanied by fever, malaise, infections, and arthralgias. Also *periodic neutropenia.* **familial benign chronic n.** A rare syndrome of autosomal-dominant inheritance, characterized by mild neutropenia and impaired granulocytic maturation beyond the myelocyte, but with few infections or symptoms. **hypersplenic n.** A condition marked by neutropenia, myeloid hyperplasia of the marrow, splenomegaly, and frequent bacterial infections, and which responds to splenectomy. Also *primary splenic neutropenia.* **malignant n.** AGRANULOCYTOSIS. **periodic n.** CYCLIC NEUTROPENIA. **primary splenic n.** HYPERSPLENIC NEUTROPENIA. **toxic n.** Neutropenia resulting from exposure to drugs, chemicals or physical agents which decrease neutrophil production by the bone marrow. **transitory neonatal n.** Severe neutropenia in infants born of mothers with neutropenia of autoimmune origin, attributed to the passage of maternal antibody against neutrophils across the placenta. Neutropenia abates as antibody titre declines after delivery, and it seldom lasts over 21 days.

**neutrophil** \nʸoo′trəfil\ [*neutr(al)* + -PHIL] **1** A polymorphonuclear leukocyte that has numerous minute cytoplasmic granules that are "neutral" in their tinctorial properties, i.e. that stain a pale pink or rose color with Romanowsky dyes. An increase in the number of neutrophils in blood is commonly observed in systemic bacterial infections or inflammatory disorders. Also *neutrophil leukocyte, heterophil leukocyte, heterophil granulocyte, neutrophil granulocyte, neutrophilic cell, neutrocyte, orthoneutrophil.* **2** Any cell or histologic structure that is stainable by neutral dyes or by both acid and basic dyes. **3** Readily stainable by both acid and basic dyes; neutrophilic. **band n.** A neutrophil in which the nucleus is elongated but not segmented into distinct lobes. Band neutrophils are intermediate in maturation between metamyelocytes and mature neutrophils. Also *juvenile neutrophil, stab neutrophil, stab, stab cell, staff cell, band cell, rod neutrophil, nonfilamented neutrophil.* **filamented n.** SEGMENTED NEUTROPHIL. **giant n.** An abnormally large, hypersegmented neutrophil; a macropolycyte. It is seen in deficiency of vitamin $B_{12}$ or folic acid. **hypersegmented n.** Any neutrophil having six or more nuclear lobes, seen in deficiencies of vitamin $B_{12}$ or folic acid, in some chronic myeloproliferative disorders, and, rarely, through inheritance. **immature n.** A neutrophilic granulocyte which has not matured sufficiently to have a segmented nucleus. **juvenile n.** BAND NEUTROPHIL. **mature n.** SEGMENTED NEUTROPHIL. **nonfilamented n.** BAND NEUTROPHIL. **rod n.** BAND NEUTROPHIL. **segmented n.** A mature granular neutrophil displaying a nucleus of two to five lobes joined by fine chromatin threads and a cytoplasm containing fine granules and displaying chemotaxis, phagocytosis, and immune complex binding. Also *mature neutrophil, filamented neutrophil, polymorphonuclear granulocyte, polymorph, poly, segmented cell.* **stab n.** BAND NEUTROPHIL.

**neutrophilia** \nʸoo′trəfil′yə\ An increased number of neutrophils in the peripheral blood. Also *neutrocytophilia, neutrocytosis.*

**neutrophilic** \nʸoo′trəfil′ik\ **1** Having the property of staining equally with acid and basic stains, or of staining with neutral dyes. **2** Characterized by the presence of neutrophilic granulocytes.

**neutrophilopenia** \nʸoo′trəfil′ōpē′nē·ə\ NEUTROPENIA.

**neutropism** \nʸoo′trəpizm\ NEUROTROPISM.

**neutrotaxis** \nʸoo′trətak′sis\ The phenomenon of neutrophil movement toward (positive neutrotaxis) or away from (negative neutrotaxis) various substances.

**nevi** \nē′vī\ Plural of NEVUS.

**Nevin** [Samuel *Nevin,* English neurologist, born 1905] Kiloh-Nevin syndrome. See under SYNDROME.

**nevocytic** \nē′vōsit′ik\ Of or relating to a nevus cell.

**nevolipoma** \nē′vōlipō′mə\ [*nev(us)* + *o* + LIPOMA] A deposit of fatty tissue in the dermis with characteristics of a nevus. Also *nevus molluscum.*

# nevus

**nevus** \nē′vəs\ [L *naevus* a mole or mark on the body] **1** A localized cutaneous malformation of the skin or mucous membranes, congenital in origin, and involving either an excess or relative deficiency of any one of the normal cutaneous structures. Also *spilus.* **2** A benign proliferation of melanocytic cells. Also *benign melanoma.* **achromic n.** A pale nevus characterized by the relative absence or poor functional capacity of cutaneous capillaries. **n. acneiformis** An epidermal nevus characterized by the presence of dilated pilar sebaceous follicles and comedones, or blackheads. **n. acneiformis unilateris** A linear epidermal nevus distinguished by the presence of comedones. Also *nevus unilateralis comedonicus.* **amelanotic n.** A nevus characterized by the presence of melanocytic nevus cells that do not produce normal quantities of melanin pigment. Also *nonpigmented nevus.* **n. anemicus** A nevus characterized by the presence of pale macules on the skin surface. It is caused by a relative absence of local capillary vessels or by the inability of the vessels to dilate. **angiomatous n.** VASCULAR NEVUS. **n. arachnoideus** SPIDER TELANGIECTASIS. **n. araneosus** SPIDER TELANGIECTASIS. **n. araneus** SPIDER TELANGIECTASIS. **balloon cell n.** A nevus many of whose cells have abundant amounts of clear cytoplasm. **basal-cell n.** BASAL CELL NEVUS SYNDROME. **bathing trunk n.** A large congenital melanocytic nevus that frequently contains terminal hairs and is characterized by a tendency to malignant change. It is usually located on skin of the pelvic and thigh regions, areas formerly covered by bathing trunks. **Becker's n.** A nevus that comprises a large number of tan macules. It is frequently seen on the shoulder area or the hips and forms after prolonged sun exposure. Onset commonly occurs during childhood or adolescence as one or more brown patches. As they enlarge, new patches develop beyond the spreading edge, to which they eventually become attached. At puberty, hypertrichosis develops in the same region as the pigmentation but is not coextensive with it. The increase in pigment is caused by an increase in melanocyte activity without an increase in the number of melanocytes. Also *nevus spilus tar-*

*dus.* **blue n.** A circumscribed intradermal nevus of blue-black color composed of dermal melanocytes that are bipolar dendritic cells and that usually contain large quantities of melanin pigment. The nevi develop as discrete nodular growths 2–15 mm in diameter on the face, forearms, and hands during childhood. Also *Jadassohn-Tièche nevus.* **blue rubber bleb n.** The presence of multiple bluish cutaneous hemangiomas resembling nevi on the skin surface. It is usually inherited by the autosomal dominant transmission pattern. **capillary n.** CAPILLARY HEMANGIOMA. **cellular n.** A nevus characterized by the presence of melanocytic nevus cells. **cellular blue n.** A rare blue nevus that is most often found on the wrists or buttocks and is characterized by interlacing foils of bipolar dendritic cells. **comedo n.** An epidermal nevus characterized by the presence of comedones or blackheads. **compound n.** A melanocytic nevus characterized by the presence of both junctional activity and melanocytic nevus cells within the dermis. **connective tissue n.** A nevus comprising only dermal elements and characterized by changes in the normal elastic tissue, collagen, or other structures within the dermis. **n. elasticus** A connective tissue nevus characterized by excessive amounts of elastic tissue. **n. elasticus of Lewandowsky** A dermal nevus composed of connective tissue elements and characterized by smooth white papules. It is usually seen on the trunk. **epidermal n.** A nevus comprising only abnormalities of epidermal tissue. **epithelial and/or spindle cell n.** A compound nevus with abundant elongated and/or epithelioid cells. Melanin is usually minimal or absent. It is benign and commonly occurs on the face, mostly in children. Also *benign juvenile melanoma, Spitz nevus, spindle cell and/or epithelioid nevus, juvenile melanoma.* **n. epitheliomatocylindromatosus** ECCRINE DERMAL CYLINDROMA. **erectile n.** STRAWBERRY NEVUS. **fatty n.** NEVUS LIPOMATOSUS. **n. follicularis** HAIR FOLLICLE NEVUS. **n. fragarius** STRAWBERRY NEVUS. **n. fuscoceruleus acromiodeltoideus** NEVUS OF ITO. **n. fuscoceruleus ophthalmomaxillaris** OTA'S NEVUS. **giant pigmented n.** A large, congenital skin lesion, usually darkly pigmented, which contains both superficial and deep components. The deep part extends into the subcutaneous tissue. The meninges may also be affected by melanocytic lesions in affected patients. Malignant melanoma develops in a significant number of affected patients. **hair follicle n.** A nevus characterized by the presence of excessive numbers of hair follicles. Also *nevus follicularis.* **hairy n.** A nevus marked by excessive growth of body hair. It is usually associated with excessive pigmentation and the presence of melanocytic nevus cells in the dermis and epidermis. Most hairy nevi are congenital in origin. **halo n.** A nevus characterized by the presence of melanocytic cells in the center and surrounded by a depigmented white halo. Also *Sutton's nevus.* **hard n.** An epidermal nevus that appears as an overgrowth. It may form in infancy. **honeycomb n.** ULERYTHEMA OPHRYOGENES. **intradermal n.** A nevus characterized by the presence of melanocytic nevus cells in the dermis. **n. of Ito** A dermal nevus composed of excessive numbers of bipolar dendritic pigment-containing nevus cells. Such nevi are found in those areas innervated by the posterior supraclavicular and lateral cutaneous brachial nerves. Also *nevus fuscoceruleus acromiodeltoideus.* **Jadassohn-Tièche n.** BLUE NEVUS. **junctional n.** A melanocytic nevus characterized by the presence of large numbers of melanocytes at the dermoepidermal junction. Also *marginal nevus.* **n. lipomatodes superficialis** A cutaneous nevus that arises from a proliferation of fat cells. Clinically it is seen most often on the buttocks and appears as a large yellowish plaque. **n. lipomatosus** A nevus characterized by excessive amounts of fatty tissue and fat cells in the dermis. Also *fatty nevus.* **lymphatic n.** A nevus characterizd by an excessive number of lymphatic vessels in the dermis. Also *nevus lymphangiectodes.* **n. maculosus** A flat, macular, melanocytic nevus. **malignant blue n.** A malignant melanoma arising in a blue nevus. These appear to be less aggressive than the usual malignant melanomas despite the fact that they lie deeply in the skin. **marginal n.** JUNCTIONAL NEVUS. **melanocytic n.** A nevus characterized by an excessive number of melanocytes in the dermis or epidermis. **mixed n.** A nevus formed by more than one type of cell, such as an epidermal nevus derived in part from apocrine sweat glands and in part from sebaceous glands. **n. molluscum** NEVOLIPOMA. **n. morus** MULBERRY MARK. **multiplex n.** SEBACEOUS NEVUS. **n. nervosus** NEVUS UNIUS LATERIS. **nevocytic n.** **1** MOLE[1]. **2** A melanocytic nevus composed of melanocytic nevus cells that are found at the dermoepidermal junction and in the dermis. Also *nevus-cell nevus.* **nodular connective tissue n.** A nevus, commonly seen in children, that is clinically composed of raised yellow nodules on the trunk and histologically evidenced by a thickening of collagen fibers and abnormalities in the quantity of elastic tissue. **nonpigmented n.** AMELANOTIC NEVUS. **oral epithelial n.** WHITE SPONGE NEVUS. **Ota's n.** A dermal nevus comprising dermal melanocytes that involve the ocular tissues and the facial skin in a unilateral pattern. Also *nevus fuscoceruleus ophthalmomaxillaris, oculocutaneous melanosis.* **pigmented n.** NEVUS PIGMENTOSUS. **pigmented hairy epidermal n.** An epidermal nevus marked by an increase in melanin pigmentation and some terminal hair growth. **n. pigmentosus** A nevus containing excessive melanin that arises as a result of proliferation of melanocytes or nevus cells; in common usage, a mole. Also *pigmented nevus.* **n. pilosus** A nevus characterized by the outgrowth of terminal hair from the lesion. Also *hairy mole.* **plane n.** A nevus that does not protrude above the level of the surrounding tissue. Also *nevus planus.* **port-wine n.** PORT-WINE STAIN. **n. profundus** A vascular nevus that extends deeply into the underlying dermis. **raspberry n.** STRAWBERRY NEVUS. **n. sanguineus** VASCULAR NEVUS. **sebaceous n.** An epidermal nevus characterized by an excessive number of sebaceous glands. These lesions are most commonly seen on the scalp. Throughout childhood they appear as slightly raised yellow areas with hypotrichosis. At puberty the sebaceous component enlarges in response to the circulating androgen. Transformation to basal cell carcinoma may occur in adult life. Also *congenital sebaceous gland hyperplasia, multiplex nevus, sebaceous nevus of Jadassohn.* **segmental n.** A cutaneous nevus following the distribution of one or more dermotomes. Also *zoniform nevus.* **soft n.** MOLE[1]. **spider n.** SPIDER TELANGIECTASIS. **n. spilus** A flat, congenital melanocytic nevus that is spotted with areas of darker pigmentation. **n. spilus tardus** BECKER'S NEVUS. **spindle cell and/or epithelioid n.** EPITHELIAL AND/OR SPINDLE CELL NEVUS. **Spitz n.** EPITHELIAL AND/OR SPINDLE CELL NEVUS. **n. spongiosus albus mucosae** WHITE SPONGE NEVUS. **stellar n.** SPIDER TELANGIECTASIS. **straight-hair n.** A circumscribed area of the scalp in which straight hair replaces the type of hair normal for that site. **strawberry n.** A superficial type of cavernous hemangioma consisting of a red, raised lesion appearing in the newborn period, and often growing rapidly at first before starting to regress. Spontaneous and complete healing occurs in five years or less. Also *strawberry angioma, strawberry mark, strawberry birthmark, nevus fragarius, raspberry nevus, raspberry mark, erectile nevus.* **subcutaneous n.** A vascular nevus, most often a cavernous angioma, comprising abnormalities of the deeper capillary plexus. The overlying epidermis is relatively normal. **Sutton's n.** HALO NEVUS. **n. syringocystadenosus papilliferus** A nevus arising from the apocrine sweat gland apparatus. **n. tardus** A nevus that is not present at birth. It may develop after prolonged exposure to the sun, as a Becker's nevus. **n. unilateralis comedonicus** NEVUS ACNEIFORMIS UNILATERIS. **n. unius lateris** An epidermal nevus having a linear distribution and commonly involving a limb. Also *nevus nervosus.* **Unna's n.** *Obs.* PORT-WINE STAIN. **vascular n.** A nevus that arises as a result of an excess of dermal capillaries. Also *nevus sanguineus, angiomatous nevus.* **n. vascularis fungosus** A pedunculated cavernous angioma, which is usually red or purple in color. **n. vasculosus** Any cutaneous nevus characterized by the presence of excessive capillaries in the skin and subcutis. **n. venosus** A nevus comprising a circumscribed area of excessive cutaneous venules. **venous n.** A superficial venous hemangioma. **verrucous n.** A nevus with an irregular, superficial brown warty appearance. **white sponge n.** A nevus arising on the oral mucous membrane. It is frequently a familial condition that is believed to be inherited by autosomal dominant transmission. Also *white folded gingivostomatitis, nevus spongiosus albus mucosae, oral epithelial nevus.* **zoniform n.** SEGMENTAL NEVUS.

**newborn** 1 NEONATE. 2 Born recently.

**Newton** [Isaac *Newton,* English mathematician and astronomer, 1642–1727] 1 See under DISK. 2 Newton's rings. See under RING. 3 Newton's alloy. See under MELOTTE'S METAL. 4 Newtonian constant. See under GRAVITATIONAL CONSTANT. 5 Non-newtonian fluid. See under FLUID. 6 Newton's law of gravitation. See under LAW.

**newton** \n$^y$oo′tän\ [after Sir Isaac *Newton,* English mathematician and physicist, 1642–1727] Special name for the SI derived unit of force, equal to the force which, applied to a mass of one kilogram, gives to it an acceleration of one meter per second squared; one newton equals one kilogram times one meter per second squared. Symbol: N **n. per square meter** The SI derived unit of pressure or stress, equal to the pressure or stress produced by a force of one newton applied uniformly distributed over an area of one square meter, more commonly referred to by the special name pascal. Symbol: $N/m^2$, $N{\cdot}m^{-2}$

**newton-meter** 1 The SI derived unit of work generally known by the special name joule. Symbol: N·m 2 The SI derived unit of moment of a force or torque. Symbol: N·m **n. per second** The SI derived unit of power, generally known by the special name watt. Symbol: N·m/s, $N{\cdot}m{\cdot}s^{-1}$

**nexus** \nek′səs\ [L (from *nexus,* past part. of *nectere* to tie, bind, fasten), a binding, tying together] 1 A bond or an interlacing. 2 GAP JUNCTION.

**Neyman** [Jerzy *Neyman,* Rumanian-born U.S. statistician, born 1894] See under BIAS.

**Nezelof** [C. *Nezelof,* French pathologist, born 1922] See under SYNDROME.

**NF** *National Formulary.*

**ng** Symbol for the unit, nanogram.

**NGF** nerve growth factors.

**NHC** 1 National Health Council. 2 neonatal hypocalcemia.

**NHL** non-Hodgkin's lymphoma.

**NHS** 1 National Health Service (United Kingdom). 2 normal human serum.

**Ni** Symbol for the element, nickel.

**niacin** \nī′əsin\ Nicotinic acid: used especially in nutritional contexts. Niacin is a member of the B complex vitamins and is needed for the synthesis of the coenzyme nicotinamide adenine dinucleotide, which is the hydrogen acceptor for many dehydrogenases. It can be made in the body from tryptophan, 60 mg of tryptophan being equivalent to 1 mg of niacin. A deficiency of niacin gives rise to pellagra. The dietary requirement is 6.6 mg per 1000 dietary kcals. Also *antipellagra vitamin, pellagramin, anti-blacktongue factor, antipellagra factor.*

**niacinamide** NICOTINAMIDE.

**niacinamidosis** \nī′əsin′əmidō′sis\ PELLAGRA.

**nialamide** $C_{16}H_{18}N_4O_2$. 4-Pyridinecarboxylic acid 2-[3-oxo-3-[(phenylmethyl)amino]propyl]hydrazine. An antidepressant drug that acts as an inhibitor of monoamine oxidase. It is given orally.

**nib** [Old English *neb, nebb* beak] The tip of a dental condenser. The face of the tip which compresses the amalgam or foil is flat and may be smooth or serrated. Also *condenser point.*

**niche** \nich, nēsh\ [French (from *nicher* to nest from L *nidificare* to nest, from *nidus* a nest), recess in a wall for a statue] In radiology, a depression in the wall of a hollow organ, best demonstrated as a localized projection when the lumen of the organ is filled with contrast medium, as *the niche of a peptic ulcer.* **Barclay's n.** A small ulcer projection of the duodenal cap as seen on gastrointestinal series. **Haudek's n.** A crater of a penetrating gastric ulcer which, on the erect projection during gastrointestinal series, has triple layering consisting of barium at the bottom, gastric fluid above it, and air at the top. Also *Haudek sign, niche sign.*

**nick** 1 A break in a protein chain that permits subsequent separation of the resulting polypeptides (e.g., polypeptides A and B of diphtheria toxin, whose separation is important for its action). Also *single chain break, single strand break.* 2 To cause such a break.

**nickel** Element number 28, having atomic weight 58.71. It is a hard, malleable metal used chiefly as a constituent of stainless steel and other alloys. Symbol: Ni

**nickel carbonyl** $C_4NiO_4$. A colorless, volatile liquid with high vapor pressure at room temperature, used to refine impure nickel powder. It is highly poisonous, causing acute symptoms of headache, giddiness, shortness of breath, and vomiting. The highly insoluble vapor penetrates to the alveoli, causing pulmonary edema.

**nicking** AV NICKING. **AV n.** Apparent indentation of a retinal vein by the overlying arteriole, due to opacity of the arteriolar wall. Also *nicking.*

**nickkrampf** \nik′krämpf\ [German *Nick* a nod + *Krampf* a cramp, spasm] INFANTILE MASSIVE SPASM.

**niclosamide** $C_{13}H_8Cl_2N_2O_4$. 2′,5-Dichloro-4′-nitrosalicylanilide, an antiparasitic agent effective against tapeworm infections. It is incapable of destroying tapeworm ova, however, and cysticercosis may follow inadequate treatment to remove the tapeworm segments.

**Nicolas** [Joseph *Nicolas,* French physician, born 1868] Nicolas-Favre disease. See under LYMPHOGRANULOMA VENEREUM.

**Nicolle** [Charles Jules Henri *Nicolle,* French bacteriologist, 1866–1936] Novy, McNeal and Nicolle medium. See under MEDIUM.

**nicotinamide** \nik′ətin′əmīd\ A biologically active amide of nicotinic acid that forms needlelike, white, bitter crystals, soluble in water and alcohol. It is a member of the vitamin B complex, differing from niacin in that it lacks vasodilator action. It occurs naturally in the body and is interconvertible with niacin. It is used in the treatment of pellagra. Also *nicotinic acid amide, niacinamide.*

**nicotinamide adenine dinucleotide** A hydrogen acceptor for many dehydrogenases. Its molecule consists of *N*-(5-phosphoribosyl)nicotinamide joined by a pyrophosphate bond to the phosphate group of adenosine 5′-phosphate. In the course of its reduction, a hydride ion is accepted by the pyridine ring of the nicotinamide, on C-4, to give a dihydropyridine derivative. The respiratory chain of mitochondria, aerobic microorganisms, etc. can reoxidize the reduced form at the expense of molecular oxygen. Also *factor V* (the letter V), *coenzyme I* (obs.), *cozymase* (obs.), *diphosphopyridine nucleotide* (obs.), *nadide.* Symbol: NAD

**nicotinamide adenine dinucleotide phosphate** Nicotinamide adenine dinucleotide phosphorylated on O-2′ of the adenosine group. It is hydrogen acceptor for some dehydrogenases. Its reduced form is the hydrogen donor for many biosyntheses, including fat synthesis. Also *coenzyme II* (obs.), *phosphocozymase* (obs.). Symbol: NADP

**nicotinamide mononucleotide** Nicotinamide bearing a 5-phosphoribosyl group on its ring nitrogen atom; an intermediate in NAD formation.

**nicotine** \nik′ətēn\ $C_{10}H_{14}N_2$. 1-Methyl-2-(3-pyridyl)pyrrolidine, a colorless, toxic liquid obtained from leaves of the tobacco plant. It is responsible for many of the effects derived from the smoking or chewing of tobacco and is also used as a botanical insecticide.

**nicotinehydroxamic acid methiodide** An agent with the capacity to reactivate cholinesterase inhibited by organophosphates. Its actions are like those of pralidoxime.

**nicotinic** Of or relating to nicotine or to effects resembling those produced by nicotine.

**nicotinic acid** Pyridine-3-carboxylic acid. It is a vitamin, being needed for the formation of NAD and NADP. It can be made by oxidizing 3-methylpyridine, which is a constituent of coal tar.

**nicotinic acid amide** NICOTINAMIDE.

**nicotinism** \nik′ətinizm\ [*nicotin(e)* + -ISM] Poisoning due to chronic exposure to excessive amounts of nicotine through inhalation or ingestion. The smoking or chewing of tobacco causes stimulation, followed by depression, of the central and autonomic nervous systems, vasoconstriction in the hands and feet, and a slight rise in blood pressure and heart rate. In middle age, chronic smokers often develop slowly progressive fogginess of vision and inability to do fine work.

**nicotinolytic** \nik′ətinōlit′ik\ Blocking the action of nicotine.

**nicotinomimetic** \nik′ətin′ōmimet′ik\ Mimicking the action of nicotine; nicotinic.

**nicotinuric acid** The amide formed by acylation of glycine with nicotinic acid. It is a minor metabolite of nicotinic acid and is found in urine.

**nictatio spastica** \niktā′shō spas′tikə\ SPASMUS NUTANS.

**nictitate** \nik′titāt\ [Med L *nictitat(us),* past part. of *nictitare,* alteration of L *nictare* to wink, blink] To blink.

**nidal** \nī′dəl\ Pertaining to a nidus.

**nidation** \nīdā′shən\ [L *nid(us)* nest + English -ATION] IMPLANTATION.

**NIDDM** non-insulin-dependent diabetes mellitus.

**nidi** \nī′dī\ Plural of NIDUS.

**nidus** \nī′dəs\ [L, nest] **1** A focus of origin, such as a collection of bacteria in infections or the point of precipitation in calculus formation. **2** The nucleus of a nerve in the central nervous system.

**Niemann** [Albert *Niemann,* German surgeon, 1880–1921] **1** Niemann-Pick lipid. See under SPHINGOMYELIN. **2** Niemann-Pick disease. See under DISEASE. **3** Niemann-Pick cell. See under CELL.

**nightmare** [*night* + Middle English *mare,* from Old English *maere* an incubus] A reaction of fright or a terrifying dream occurring during REM sleep, usually within an hour or two after falling asleep. It is much more frequent in children than adults.

**nightshade** \nīt′shād\ **deadly n.** BELLADONNA.

**nigral** \nī′grəl\ [L *nigr(a),* fem. sing. of *niger* black, dusky, dark + -AL] Pertaining to the substantia nigra.

**nigrostriatal** \nī′grōstrī·ā′təl\ Denoting the substantia nigra and corpus striatum, especially the fine-fibered but functionally significant dopaminergic tract between them (strionigral tract), now known to be causally involved in Parkinson's disease.

**NIH** National Institutes of Health.

**nihilism** \nī′hilizm\ [L *nihil* nothing + -ISM] In psychiatry, the delusion of nonexistence of the self or the world, in whole or in part. **therapeutic n.** Disbelief in or extreme skepticism about the curative powers of drugs or other therapies.

**nikethamide** $C_{10}H_{14}N_2O$. *N,N*-Diethyl-3-pyridinecarboxamide, a centrally acting stimulant of the respiratory and cardiovascular centers. The margin between the dose required to obtain stimulation of these centers and the dose producing convulsions is narrow. Other, safer stimulants have supplanted such older stimulants.

**Nikolsky** [Pyotr Vasilyevich *Nikolsky,* Russian dermatologist, 1858–1940] See under SIGN.

**nimazone** $C_{11}H_9ClN_4O$. 3-(4-Chlorophenyl)-4-imino-2-oxo-1-imidazolideneacetonitrile. A compound with anti-inflammatory activity.

**Nimeh** [William *Nimeh,* Lebanese gastroenterologist, born 1891] See under METHOD.

**NIMH** National Institute of Mental Health.

**ninhydrin** The substance whose molecule consists of the group —CO—C(OH)$_2$—CO— substituted for hydrogen on adjacent atoms of a benzene ring. It is essentially a triketone, but the central carbonyl group is rendered so reactive by the electron attraction of the others that it normally exists in the hydrated state. Ninhydrin is used to detect and determine amino acids and peptides. When it is heated with an amino acid R—CH(NH$_2$)COOH in an appropriate medium, imine formation leads to decarboxylation of the amino acid, and release of the aldehyde R—CHO leaves the triketone group of the ninhydrin in the form —C(—O$^-$)═C(NH$_2$)—CO—. The compound so produced forms an imine with a second molecule of ninhydrin, whose delocalized charges give it a deep purple color, absorbing maximally at 570 nm. When the reaction is applied to peptides, it is largely the N-terminus that reacts, and the color is roughly proportional to the total peptide concentration, irrespective of the lengths of the peptides present. Also *triketohydrindene hydrate* (obs.).

**niobium** \nī·ō′bē·əm\ Element number 41, having atomic weight 92.9064. It is a soft, lustrous white metal with numerous technologic applications, most notably as an alloying element. Also *columbium* (a term used mostly in commerce and technology). Symbol: Nb

**niphablepsia** \nif′əblep′sē·ə\ [Gk *niph(a)* snow + *ablepsia* blindness] SNOW BLINDNESS.

**nippers** \nip′ərs\ [Middle English *nipp(en)* to nip + -ER + *s*] A surgical instrument in the form of pliers with cutting beaks used for cutting small amounts of either soft tissue or bone.

**nipple** [prob. dim. of Middle English *neb* beak, nose] The pigmented, blunted, conical projection at the apex of the breast. The lactiferous ducts open into it; papilla mammaria. Also *papillula*. **cracked n.** The superficial fissuring of the skin of the nipple, a problem sometimes noted in breast-feeding mothers. **crater n.** A nipple that has remained in the fetal state. Its lactiferous ducts open normally on its surface, which is, however, invaginated below the level of the areola. **herniated n.** A deformity of the breast wherein the nipple and areola bulge out from the surface of the breast. **inverted n.** A nipple that has retracted behind the areola, leaving a pucker where the nipple usually presents. It is usually a benign condition, but if it occurs in a previously normal nipple it may be a sign of underlying breast cancer. **retracted n.** A nipple whose contour is deformed due to scarring or to an underlying carcinoma.

***Nippostrongylus*** \nip′ōstrăn′jələs\ [New L (from *Nippo(n)* + Gk *strongylos* round)] A monotypic genus of hookworms (subfamily Viannaiinae, family Trichostrongylidae). Its single species, the rat hookworm, *N. brasiliensis*, occurs in the anterior portion of the small intestine of domiciliated rats and the house mouse throughout the world. It is far commoner in rats than in mice, in which the more common hookworm is *Nematospiroides dubius*). *N. brasiliensis* is widely used as a model for parasite immunologic research.

**nisin** \nī′sin\ A 34-residue peptide antibiotic produced by *Streptococcus lactis*. It contains residues of lanthionine and 3-methyllanthionine, which provide thioether cross-linking between different parts of the chain. They are derived by reaction of cysteine residues with residues of 2-aminoacrylic acid (derived by dehydration of serine) and 2-aminocrotonic acid (derived by dehydration of threonine), respectively. The peptide also contains unreacted residues of 2-aminoacrylic and 2-aminocrotonic acids.

**Nissl** [Franz *Nissl*, German neurologist, 1860–1919] **1** Primary reaction of Nissl. See under AXON REACTION. **2** Nissl's degeneration. See under AXONAL DEGENERATION. **3** See under METHOD. **4** Nissl bodies, Nissl granules. See under SUBSTANCE.

**nit** [Old English *hnitu*] The egg of a louse, especially of the human louse (*Pediculus humanus*) or the pubic louse (*Pthirus pubis*). The lice secrete a gluelike chitinous substance which they use to attach the nits to the base of hairs or to clothing.

**Nitabuch** [Raissa *Nitabuch*, German physician, flourished 19th century] Striae of Nitabuch, layer of Nitabuch. See under MEMBRANE.

**nitr-** \nītr-\ NITRO-.

**nitrate** **1** The anion $NO_3^-$ derived from nitric acid, or a salt containing it, or an ester of nitric acid. Nitrate is one of the main sources of nitrogen available to plants. Plants and many microorganisms can reduce it to ammonia, which they can incorporate into amino acids for protein biosynthesis. **2** To substitute with a nitro group.

**nitrate reductase** Any of several enzymes that catalyze the reduction of nitrate to nitrite. They use various reductants and they vary in chemical nature, some containing molybdenum. The reaction allows some bacteria to use nitrate as a terminal electron acceptor, and it allows plants to use nitrate as a source of nitrogen for protein synthesis, since the nitrite formed can be further reduced. Also *nitratase* (obs.).

**nitrazepam** $C_{15}H_{11}N_3O_3$. 1,3-Dihydro-7-nitro-5-phenyl-2*H*-1,4-benzodiazepin-2-one, an antianxiety drug used to produce hypnosis and sedation. It is also used as an anticonvulsant drug. It is given orally.

**nitremia** \nītrē′mē·ə\ AZOTEMIA.

**nitric acid** $HNO_3$. An acid obtained industrially by catalytic oxidation of ammonia. It is a colorless liquid which fumes in air. The anhydrous acid boils at 83°C, with decomposition, particularly if illuminated. With water it gives a negative azeotrope, 68% acid, boiling at 120.5°C. It is a strong acid and a strong oxidizing agent, and its salts (nitrates) are almost all soluble in water. It is used for preparing nitrated derivatives which contain the $NO_2$ group. It is dangerous to breathe and colors the skin yellow (xanthoproteic reaction) by nitrating tyrosine residues. *o*-Nitrophenols are appreciably dissociated at neutral pH and their anions are yellow. Also *spirit of nitre, aqua fortis*.

**nitrification** The oxidation of ammonia to nitrite and nitrate. This reaction is an essential part of the nitrogen cycle, preserving fixed nitrogen in the soil in a nonvolatile form. The main nitrifying organisms are *Nitrosomonas*, which oxidizes only to nitrite, and *Nitrobacter*.

**nitrile** Any compound of general formula R—C≡N. It can be considered as derived from the ammonium salts of carboxylic acids by loss of two molecules of water.

**nitrilo-** \nī′trilō-\ [from *nitrile* from Gk *nitron* soda, carbonate of soda + *-ile* English suffix used in making certain names, especially diketones] A combining form signifying the tervalent nitrogen atom, as in nitrilotriacetic acid, $N(—CH_2—COOH)_3$.

**nitrite** \nī′trīt\ The ion $NO_2^-$ derived from nitrous acid, or a salt containing it, or an ester of nitrous acid. Nitrites are added as preservatives to foods, such as cooked meats. Since, however, they react slowly with secondary amines to form nitrosamines, some of which are carcinogenic, this practice may not be without danger.

**nitrituria** \nī′tritoo′rē·ə\ The excretion of nitrites in the urine, usually an index of bacterial proliferation. *Rare*.

**nitro-** \nī′trə-, nī′trō-\ [L *nitrum* from Gk *nitron*] A combining form denoting the presence of the nitro group, $—NO_2$, in a molecule. It is a strongly electron-withdrawing group. Also *nitr-*.

**nitrofuran** Any of a group of antibacterial agents such as furazolidone, nitrofurazone, and nitrofurantoin, each having actions on a wide variety of bacteria.

**nitrofurantoin** $C_8H_6N_4O_5$. 1-[[(5-Nitro-2-furanyl)methylene]amino]-2,4-imidazolidinedione, a synthetic antibacterial agent. It is effective against some Gram-negative and Gram-positive organisms, including *Escherichia coli, Staphylococcus pyogenes, S. aureus*, and some strains of *Proteus* and *Pseudomonas*. It is given orally to treat urinary tract infections.

**nitrofurazone** 5-Nitro-2-furaldehyde semicarbazone. An antibacterial agent used in the treatment of burns and infections of the skin, otitis, and ophthalmic conditions. It is also used in the treatment of trypanosomiasis.

**nitrogen** \nī′trəjən\ [French *nitrogène* (from L *nitrum* natron, natural soda, niter, saltpeter + French *-gène*, noun suffix from Gk *-gen*, noun suffix from *gennan* to beget, produce, bring forth) nitrogen, azote] Element number 7, having atomic weight 14.0067. It is a colorless, odorless gas forming 78% of the volume of the atmosphere. It is obtained from liquid air by fractional distillation. There are two natural isotopes, having mass numbers 14 and 15, the former comprising over 99.6% of the total. Five radioactive isotopes are known. Valences are 3 and 5. Elemental nitrogen is fairly inert but its compounds are very reactive and are a constituent of food, fertilizers, and many explosives and poisons. It is a key element in the substance of all living organisms. See also NITROGEN CYCLE. Symbol: N **blood urea n.** The amount of nitrogen in plasma or serum deriving from the urea molecule, expressed in mg/dl or mmol/l. The two atoms of nitrogen per molecule of urea constitute 46.64% of urea mass. Normal levels depend somewhat upon the analytical method used, but approximate 7–18 mg/dl or 5–13 mmol/l. Abbr. BUN **Kjeldahl n.** See under KJELDAHL'S TEST. **n. fixation** See under FIXATION. **nonprotein n.** The amount of nitrogen in a sample that does not belong to protein. It was once commonly determined by nitrogen analysis after protein precipitation, often as a check on the individual components of blood, such as urea, creatinine, amino acids, and ammonia. Also *rest nitrogen* (seldom used). **urea n.** The portion of urea composed of nitrogen, representing approximately half the urea molecule. In the United States blood or serum levels are reported in terms of urea nitrogen, but in the United Kingdom urea levels are reported. In the past, urea nitrogen was usually measured in whole blood, but with currently available automatic analyzers urea nitrogen is measured in serum. Since urea is distributed throughout body water, the results in blood and serum are very close.

**nitrogen 13** A cyclotron-produced radioisotope of nitrogen, decaying by positron emission. It can be used for study of the metabolism of many nitrogen-containing compounds. Physical half-life is 10 minutes. Symbol: $^{13}N$

**nitrogen 15** A stable isotope of nitrogen comprising 0.37 percent of natural nitrogen. It may be separated by mass spectrography and used as a metabolic tracer. Symbol: $^{15}N$

**nitrogenous** \nīträj′ənəs\ Containing nitrogen, usually in combined form.

**nitroglycerin** Any ester of glycerol with nitric acid, particularly glycerol trinitrate, which is used as an explosive. Nitroglycerin is also used medicinally as a vasodilator for treating angina pectoris. Exposed workers in factories manufacturing explosives may suffer headaches, nausea, vomiting, and lowered pulse pressures. They usually develop a tolerance, which may be lost during weekends. Such workers may have a higher than expected sudden death rate from coronary heart disease. Nitroglycerin is also a skin irritant. Also *trinitrin, trinitroglycerol, trinitroglycerin.* See also DYNAMITE HEADACHE.

**nitromersol** $C_7H_5HgNO_3$. 5-Methyl-2-nitro-7-oxa-8-mercurabicyclo[4.2.0]octa-1,3,5-triene, a synthetic organic mercurial compound used as an antiseptic for the skin and mucous membranes.

**nitrophenol** Any of the disubstituted benzene compounds in which a nitro group and a hydroxyl group may be in the ortho-, para-, or meta- configuration. They are used as pH indicators and as intermediates in organic synthesis.

***p*-nitrophenyl phosphate** An ester of *p*-nitrophenol with phosphoric acid, or any of its salts. It is used as a substrate for phosphatases, because the release of *p*-nitrophenol is easily followed due to the bright yellow color of its quinonoid anion.

**nitrosamine** Any nitrosylated secondary amine, of general formula RR′N—NO. Many are carcinogenic and mutagenic, especially if R or R′ is acyl, because they can decompose to form alkylating agents.

**nitroso-** \nītrō′sō-\ [L *nitrosus* (from Gk *nitron* soda, carbonate of soda) nitrous] A combining form denoting the presence of the univalent radical —N═O in a molecule. Also *nitros-*.

***p*-nitrosulfathiazole** $C_9H_7N_3O_4S_2$. *p*-Nitro-*N*-2-thiazolylbenzenesulfonamide. A very insoluble sulfonamide antibacterial agent used in the treatment of ulcerative colitis.

**nitrous oxide** $N_2O$. A fairly inert gas, used as an anesthetic. Also *dinitrogen monoxide, laughing gas.*

**njovera** \njōver′ə\ A Zimbabwean term for BEJEL.

**NK** Nomenklatur Kommission. (A Committee of the Anatomical Society in Germany appointed to revise and supplement the Basle Nomina Anatomica.).

**NM** **1** nuclear medicine. **2** neuromuscular.

**nm** Symbol for the unit, nanometer.

**NMN** nicotinamide mononucleotide.

**NMR** nuclear magnetic resonance.

**nn.** *nervi* (L, nerves).

**NND** neonatal death.

**No** Symbol for the element, nobelium.

**no** number.

**nobelium** \nōbel′ē·əm\ A synthetic element of the actinide series, having atomic number 102. Seven isotopes are recognized, the longest lived having atomic mass 255. Half-lives range from 2.3 seconds to 3 minutes. Symbol: No

**nocardamin** $C_{27}H_{48}N_6O_9$. An antibiotic substance produced by a strain of *Nocardia*. It is bacteriostatic against mycobacteria, and bacteriocidal only at very high concentrations.

***Nocardia*** \nōkär′dē·ə\ [after Edmond Isidore Étienne *Nocard*, French veterinarian and biologist, 1850–1903 + -IA] A genus of Gram-positive, weakly acid-fast, aerobic actinomycetes of the family Nocardiaceae. These organisms are found in the soil. Two species, *N. asteroides* and *N. brasiliensis*, may cause severe pulmonary lesions (pulmonary nocardiosis), or spreading subcutaneous abscesses (mycetomas), much like those caused by *Actinomyces* species. The presence of mycolic acids in the cell wall relates the organisms to mycobacteria. ***N. asteroides*** An aerobic actinomycete, found in soil, and intermediate in staining between Gram-positive and acid-fast bacilli. It forms granulating and suppurative pulmonary lesions, and chronic subcutaneous abscesses (mycetomas). ***N. brasiliensis*** An actinomycete closely resembling *N. asteroides*, found mostly in Mexico.

**nocardiasis** \nō′kärdī′əsis\ NOCARDIOSIS.

**nocardin** An antibiotic substance derived from *Nocardia coeliaca*. It has activity against tubercle bacilli.

**nocardiosis** \nōkär′dē·ō′sis\ [*Nocardi(a)* + -OSIS] Infection with microorganisms of the genus *Nocardia*. Also *nocardiasis.* **granulomatous n.** An atypical inflammatory response to Nocardia, characterized by ill-defined granulomas instead of the usual abscesses.

**noci-** \nō′sē-\ [L *nocere* to injure] A combining form meaning pain or injury.

**nociception** \-sep′shən\ [NOCI- + *(per)ception*] PAIN SENSE.

**nociceptive** \-sep′tiv\ [NOCI- + *(per)ceptive*] Denoting responsiveness or sensitivity to noxious stimuli capable of eliciting pain.

**nociceptor** \-sep′tər\ [NOCI- + *(re)ceptor*] A class of sense organs uniquely excited by noxious stimuli that threaten or produce frank tissue damage. Also *pain ending, pain receptor, algoceptor, nocifensor.*

**nocifensor** \-fen′sər\ NOCICEPTOR. • The term is used from the point of view of its role in protecting tissue from injury.

**noci-influence** \-in′floo·əns\ Anything having a damaging effect, or the effect itself.

**nociperception** \-pərsep′shən\ [NOCI- + PERCEPTION] The recognition by the nervous system or organism of a traumatic or hurtful stimulus.

**noct.** *nocte* (L, at night).

**noctambulation** \näk′tambyəlā′shən\ SOMNAMBULISM.

**noctambulic** \näk′tambyoo′lik\ [French *noctambule* (from L *nox*, gen. *noctis*, night + *ambulare* to walk) one who goes about at night + -IC] Pertaining to somnambulism.

**noct. maneq.** *nocte maneque* (L, at night and in the morning).

**nocturia** \näktoo′rē·ə\ [L *nox* (gen. *noctis*) night + -URIA] Urination during normal sleeping hours. The interruption of sleep to urinate may reflect a large fluid intake before retiring, decreased concentrating ability, or bladder overflow in obstructive disease such as prostatic hypertrophy. Also *nycturia.*

**nocturnal** \näktur′nəl\ Pertaining to night, especially to a night-time period of animal activity. Also *nycterine.* Compare DIURNAL.

**nocuous** [L *nocu(us)* hurtful + -OUS] Injurious; poisonous; harmful.

**nodal** \nō′dəl\ **1** Like, consisting of, or having a node. **2** Pertaining to or originating in the atrioventricular node of the heart, as *nodal rhythm.* Compare SINUS.

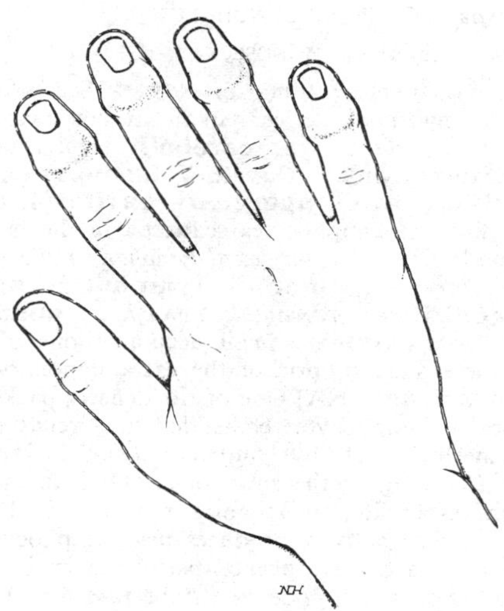

Heberden's nodes

**node** \nōd\ [L *nodus.* See NODUS.] NODUS. **anterior auricular n.'s** NODI LYMPHATICI PAROTIDEI SUPERFICIALES. **n. of anterior border of epiploic foramen** NODUS FORAMINALIS. **Aschoff's n.** NODUS ATRIOVENTRICULARIS. **n. of Aschoff and Tawara** NODUS ATRIOVENTRICULARIS. **atrioventricular n.** NODUS ATRIOVENTRICULARIS. **Auerbach's n.** AUERBACH'S GANGLION. **A-V n.** NODUS ATRIOVENTRICULARIS. **Babès n.'s** BABÈS TUBERCLES. **Bouchard's n.'s** Osteophytic swellings around the proximal interphalangeal joints of the fingers in osteoarthrosis. Also *Bouchard's nodules.* **Cloquet's n.** The highest of the deep inguinal lymph nodes, situated either in the femoral canal or the femoral ring. Also *Cloquet's gland, Rosenmüller's gland, Rosenmüller's node.* **coronary n.** The highest part or extension of the atrioventricular node, closest to the orifice of the coronary sinus in the right atrium of the heart. **cystic n.** NODUS CYSTICUS. **Delphian n.** A lymph node situated in the pretracheal fascia in the midline in front of either the isthmus or the pyramidal lobe of the thyroid gland. **epitrochlear n.'s** NODI LYMPHATICI CUBITALES. **Ewald's n.** SENTINEL NODE. **Féréol's n.'s** RHEUMATIC NODULES. **Flack's n.** NODUS SINUATRIALIS. **gouty n.** Palpable swelling due to tophus. **Heberden's n.'s** Bony swellings of the distal interphalangeal joints of the hands, characteristic of osteoarthritis. Also *Heberden sign, Heberden's arthropathy.* **hemolymph n.** A lymph node that contains erythrocytes in its sinuses due to hemorrhage in its tributary field. Also *hemolymph gland.* **Hensen's n.** A specialized area at the cephalic extremity of the primitive streak present in embryos of higher vertebrates. An invagination or pit (blastopore) forms in the region of the node and the invaginating cord of cells migrates forwards to give origin to the notochordal or head process. This is essentially the precursor of the notochord which is itself the primary organizer and precursor of the axial skeleton. Also *primitive node, primitive knot, node of Hensen.* **His-Tawara n.** NODUS ATRIOVENTRICULARIS. **juxta-articular n.** A lymph node near a joint, usually an abnormally enlarged node, as the epitrochlear node. Also *juxta-articular nodule.* **Keith's n.** NODUS SINUATRIALIS. **Keith-Flack n.** NODUS SINUATRIALIS. **Koch's n.** NODUS ATRIOVENTRICULARIS. **lymph n.** NODUS LYMPHATICUS. **lymphatic n.** NODUS LYMPHATICUS. **n. of neck of gallbladder** NODUS CYSTICUS. **Osler n.'s** Tender, swollen, erythematous areas that are 2–15 mm in size. They may be seen on the pads of the fingers or toes, the palms of the hands, or the soles of the feet and are associated with infective endocarditis. **pectoral axillary n.'s** NODI LYMPHATICI PECTORALES. **preauricular n.'s** NODI LYMPHATICI PAROTIDEI SUPERFICIALES. **primitive n.** HENSEN'S NODE. **n.'s of Ranvier** The periodic constrictions of the myelin sheath surrounding large axons. They demarcate the junctions between adjacent Schwann cells, and are the sites for impulse generation. **Rosenmüller's n.** **1** PARS PALPEBRALIS GLANDULAE LACRIMALIS. **2** CLOQUET'S NODE. **Rotter's n.'s** Lymph nodes between the pectoralis major and pectoralis minor muscles which may contain metastatic cancer from a primary carcinoma of the breast. **n. of Rouviere** The lateral retropharyngeal node of the retropharyngeal group, which drains the auditory tube. **S-A n.** NODUS SINUATRIALIS. **Schmorl's n.** SCHMORL'S NODULE. **sentinel n.** A palpable, usually left, supraclavicular lymph node containing metastatic cancer from a frequently undisclosed deep-seated primary site. Also *signal node, Troisier's node, Virchow's node, Virchow's gland, Ewald's node, Troisier sign, lymph node of Troisier.* **singers' n.'s** VOCAL NODULES. **sinoatrial n.** NODUS SINUATRIALIS. **sinuatrial n.** NODUS SINUATRIALIS. **sinuatrial n. of Keith and Flack** NODUS SINUATRIALIS. **syphilitic n.** A subcutaneous, hard, fibrous swelling occurring around the joints or on tendon sheaths, especially on the fingers, during late syphilis. The condition is only rarely seen. **n. of Tawara** NODUS ATRIOVENTRICULARIS. **triticeous n.** CARTILAGO TRITICEA. **Troisier's n.** SENTINEL NODE. **Virchow's n.** SENTINEL NODE. **vital n.** NOEUD VITAL. **vocal n.'s** VOCAL NODULES.

**nodi** \nō′dī\ Plural of NODUS.

**nodose** \nō′dōs\ Characterized by nodes or localized swellings. Also *nodulated, nodulous.*

**nodosity** \nōdäs′itē\ A knoblike swelling or node.

**nodular** \näj′ələr\ **1** Pertaining to or resembling a node or a nodule. **2** Characterized by nodules. For defs. 1 and 2 also *toruloid.*

**nodulated** \näj′əlā′tid\ NODOSE.

**nodulation** \näj′əlā′shən\ The formation of nodules.

**nodule** \näd′yool\ [L *nodulus.* See NODULUS.] **1** A

small node. • This term is commonly used in referring to circumscribed, solid, elevated skin lesions greater than 5 mm in diameter, as compared to papules, which are less than 5 mm in diameter. 2 NODULUS. **accessory thymic n.'s** Minute aggregations of thymic tissue left behind during the migration of the thymus from the primitive pharyngeal region to its adult position within the upper thoracic region. Also *noduli thymici accessorii.* **aggregate n.'s** FOLLICULI LYMPHATICI AGGREGATI. **Albini's n.'s** Small gray nodules occasionally seen on the free margins of atrioventricular valvular cusps. Also *Cruveilhier's nodule.* **n.'s of aortic valve** NODULI VALVULARUM SEMILUNARIUM VALVAE AORTAE. **apple jelly n.'s** The epithelioid tubercles characteristic of lupus vulgaris. They are best displayed by diascopic examination. **n.'s of Arantius** NODULI VALVULARUM SEMILUNARIUM VALVAE AORTAE. **Aschoff's n.'s** ASCHOFF BODIES. **Babès n.'s** BABÈS TUBERCLES. **Bianchi's n.'s** NODULI VALVULARUM SEMILUNARIUM VALVAE AORTAE. **Bouchard's n.'s** BOUCHARD'S NODES. **Caplan's n.'s** See under CAPLAN SYNDROME. **cold n.** Any space-occupying lesion in the substance of the thyroid gland that fails to take up administered radiotracer, usually iodine or technetium. It is generally held to be compatible with but not diagnostic of a malignant neoplasm. **cortical n.** NODULUS LYMPHATICUS. **Cruveilhier's n.** ALBINI'S NODULES. **enamel n.** ENAMEL PEARL. **Fraenkel's n.'s** Nodules forming on the cutaneous blood vessels as a result of vascular endothelial proliferation. They are characteristic lesions of typhus. **Gamna n.'s** GAMNA-GANDY BODIES. **Gandy-Gamna n.'s** GAMNA-GANDY BODIES. **hot n.** Any space-occupying lesion in the substance of the thyroid gland that takes up administered radiotracer, usually iodine or technetium. It is generally held to indicate the presence of a benign thyroidal lesion rather than a malignant neoplasm. Also *warm nodule.* **juxta-articular n.** JUXTA-ARTICULAR NODE. **n.'s of Kerckring** NODULI VALVULARUM SEMILUNARIUM VALVAE AORTAE. **Koester's n.** A granuloma consisting of a double layer of cells enclosing a single giant cell, as seen in granulomatous inflammation. **Leishman's n.'s** Pinkish nodules seen in cutaneous leishmaniasis. **lumbar-sacral n.'s** Nodules composed of subcutaneous adipose tissue herniated through the fascia of the lumbar-sacral region. They are believed by some to explain the pain associated with non-articular rheumatism in this part of the body. **lymphatic n.** NODULUS LYMPHATICUS. **malpighian n.'s** FOLLICULI LYMPHATICI SPLENICI. **Morgagni's n.'s** NODULI VALVULARUM SEMILUNARIUM VALVAE AORTAE. **periosteal n.'s** Palpable swellings along a bony prominence, occurring between periosteum in bone. **primary n.** NODULUS PRIMARIUS. **pulmonary n.'s** Small solid lumps within the lung substance, or small opacities seen on the chest radiograph. **n.'s of pulmonary trunk valves** NODULI VALVULARUM SEMILUNARIUM VALVAE TRUNCI PULMONALIS. **rabic n.'s** BABÈS TUBERCLES. **rheumatic n.'s** Cutaneous nodules present in the skin in rheumatic disease that consist of noncaseating, pallisading granulomata. Also *Féréol's nodes.* **Schmorl's n.** A localized depression of a vertebral plate due to herniation of the nucleus pulposus into the bone. The appearance is most easily seen on a lateral roentgenogram of the spine. Also *Schmorl body, Schmorl's node.* **siderotic n.'s** GAMNA-GANDY BODIES. **singers' n.'s** VOCAL NODULES. **splenic lymph n.'s** FOLLICULI LYMPHATICI SPLENICI. **subcutaneous n.** Any of several different types of swellings that occur beneath skin and are not attached to underlying bone. Subcutaneous nodules are commonly found in rheumatic diseases, such as rheumatoid arthritis, rheumatic fever, and gout. **triticeous n.** CARTILAGO TRITICEA. **tubal lymphatic n.'s** TONSILLA TUBARIA. **typhus n.** A focal collection of mononuclear cells surrounding the small vessel lesions of ricksettsial diseases, especially typhus fever. Although they may occur in any tissue, they are most commonly seen in skin and brain. **n. of vermis** NODULUS VERMIS. **vestigial n.** TUBERCULUM AURICULAE. **vocal n.'s** Small, white, symmetrically placed nodules, somewhat pyramidal in shape, occurring at the junction of the anterior with the middle one-third of the vocal cords. They occur as the result of misuse or overuse of the voice, particularly in susceptible individuals such as singers, preachers, and teachers. The early complaint is slight huskiness and, in soprano singers, difficulty in singing high notes softly. Surgical treatment should be the last resort. Also *vocal nodes, singers' nodules, singers' nodes, nodules of the vocal cords, chorditis nodosa.* **warm n.** HOT NODULE.

**noduli** \näj′əlī\ Plural of NODULUS.

**nodulous** \näj′ələs\ NODOSE.

**nodulus** \näd′yələs\ [dim. of NODUS. See NODUS.] (*pl.* noduli) A small nodus; a very small knotlike mass of tissue or cells. Also *nodule.* **n. cerebelli** NODULUS VERMIS. **n. intercaroticus** *Outmoded* GLOMUS CAROTICUM. **noduli lymphatici aggregati cavitatis laryngis** Accumulations of lymphocytes scattered in the lamina propria of the larynx. Also *laryngeal lymphatic follicles, folliculi lymphatici laryngei.* **noduli lymphatici aggregati tubae auditivae** TONSILLA TUBARIA. **noduli lymphatici bronchiales** Small accumulations of lymphocytes in the lamina propria of the extrapulmonary bronchi. **n. lymphaticus** [NA] One of the densely packed spherical masses of lymphocytes embedded in a relatively scanty reticular meshwork of any lymphatic tissue. It varies in appearance according to the stage of lymphocytopoietic activity. When responding to an antigen its germinal center or secondary nodule actively produces new lymphocytes and is surrounded by a densely packed peripheral zone or corona. In the cortex of lymph nodes the trabeculae tend to separate these masses from each other. They are also located in the tonsils and spleen. Solitary masses are found in the walls of the alimentary canal, although in the intestine they may aggregate into loosely organized structures or Peyer's patches. Also *lymphatic nodule, folliculus lymphaticus, cortical nodule, lymphatic follicle.* **n. primarius** A lymphatic nodule, such as in the cortex of a lymph node, in which the secondary nodule or germinal center either has not yet appeared, as in the first few months after birth, or has become mitotically inactive. Also *primary nodule.* **noduli thymici accessorii** ACCESSORY THYMIC NODULES. **noduli valvularum semilunarium valvae aortae** The small, dense fibrous tubercle at the center of the free margins of the three semilunar valvules or cusps of the aortic valve from which tendinous fibers radiate to the attached margins. Also *Morgagni's nodules, nodules of Kerckring, Bianchi's nodules, nodules of Arantius, nodules of aortic valve.* **noduli valvularum semilunarium valvae trunci pulmonalis** The small, dense fibrous tubercle at the center of the free margins of the three semilunar valvules or cusps of the valve of the pulmonary trunk from which tendinous fibers radiate to the attached margins. Also *nodules of pulmonary trunk valves.* **n. vermis** **1** That portion of the cerebellar vermis on the ventral surface, to which the inferior medullary velum is attached. **2** The midline portion of the archicerebellum whose afferent and efferent connections are primarily with the vestibular nuclei. Also *nodule of vermis, nodulus cerebelli.*

# nodus

**nodus** \nō′dəs\ [L (akin to *nectere* to tie, bind, fasten), a knot, knob, bond] (*pl.* nodi) **1** A knotlike mass of tissue or cells. **2** A small knoblike protuberance or organ. **3** A swelling. For defs. 1, 2, and 3 also *node.* **n. arcus venae azygos** [NA] A large lymph node that belongs either to the superior tracheobronchial or to the paratracheal nodes of the right side. It is related to the arch of the azygos vein anterior to the origin of the right principal bronchus. Also *lymph node of arch of azygos vein.* **n. atrioventricularis** [NA] A collection of specialized cardiac muscle fibers located in the atrial septum just above the coronary sinus of the right atrium. It is composed of a dense network of Purkinje fibers enmeshed with connective tissue. The fibers are continuous with the surrounding atrial muscle fibers and the atrioventricular bundle. It is supplied by the right coronary artery. Also *atrioventricular node, Aschoff's node, node of Aschoff and Tawara, node of Tawara, A-V node, His-Tawara node, Koch's node.* **n. buccinatorius** [NA] Any of the one or more lymph nodes that are part of the nodi lymphatici faciales and are situated along the facial vein overlying the buccinator muscle. Also *buccal group of facial lymph nodes.* **n. cysticus** [NA] A constant constituent of the nodi lymphatici hepatici that is situated at the junction of the cystic and common hepatic ducts. Also *cystic node, node of neck of gallbladder.* **n. foraminalis** [NA] A constant constituent of the nodi lymphatici hepatici which is situated along the upper part of the common bile duct in the lesser omentum. Also *node of anterior border of epiploic foramen.* **n. jugulodigastricus** [NA] A large node in a group of superior deep cervical lymph nodes that is situated between the internal jugular vein, the facial vein, and the posterior belly of the digastric muscle, just below the angle of the mandible and at the level of the greater cornu of the hyoid bone. It receives lymph from the posterior third of the tongue and the palatine tonsil. Also *jugulodigastric lymph node.* **n. jugulo-omohyoideus** [NA] One of the inferior deep cervical lymph nodes that is situated on or above the intermediate tendon of the omohyoid muscle where it crosses the internal jugular vein. It receives lymph from the tongue both directly and indirectly. Also *jugulo-omohyoid lymph node.* **n. ligamentis arteriosi** [NA] The most inferior node of the left group of anterior mediastinal lymph nodes which is situated in front of the ligamentum arteriosum and below the left pulmonary artery. Also *ganglion of duct of Botallo.* **nodi lymphatici aortici laterales** [NA] The group of nodi lymphatici lumbales sinistri that are situated along the left side of the abdominal aorta. They drain the viscera and other structures, mainly on the left side, that are supplied by the lateral and posterior branches of the aorta, such as the left suprarenal gland, kidney, ureter, testis, ovary, and some pelvic viscera. Also *lateral aortic lymph nodes.* **nodi lymphatici apicales** The apical group of six to twelve axillary lymph nodes situated in the apex of the axilla medial to the axillary vein and behind the clavipectoral fascia. They drain all the lymph nodes in the axilla, the infraclavicular nodes along the cephalic vein, and lymphatics directly from the upper outer quadrant of the breast. Most of the efferents drain into the subclavian lymph trunk. Also *apical lymph nodes, infraclavicular lymph nodes.* **nodi lymphatici axillares** A large group of 20 to 30 lymph nodes situated in and along the walls of the axilla, draining the whole upper limb, most of the breast, and part of the side and back of the trunk. It is subdivided into five groups: a lateral group (nodi lymphatici laterales), an anterior or pectoral group (nodi lymphatici pectorales), a posterior or subscapular group (nodi lymphatici subscapulares), a central group (nodi lymphatici centrales), and an apical group (nodi lymphatici apicales). Also *axillary lymph nodes, pectoral glands, axillary glands.* **nodi lymphatici brachiales** [NA] A few lymph nodes situated along the brachial vessels in the arm. They receive lymph from the deep nodes in the forearm as well as from the supratrochlear lymph nodes that are situated superficial to the deep fascia above the medial epicondyle of the humerus. They drain into the axillary lymph nodes, specifically the lateral group. Also *brachial glands, brachial lymph nodes.* **nodi lymphatici bronchopulmonales** One of the five main groups of tracheobronchial lymph nodes situated in the hilum of each lung. It drains and is continuous with the pulmonary nodes on the one side and continuous with the superior and inferior tracheobronchial nodes on the other. Also *bronchopulmonary lymph nodes.* **nodi lymphatici buccales** See under NODI LYMPHATICI FACIALES. **nodi lymphatici centrales** The central group of four or five axillary lymph nodes through which the intercostobrachial nerve passes. Its afferents come mainly from the pectoral, lateral, and subscapular groups of nodes as well as the cubital nodes, while the efferents end in

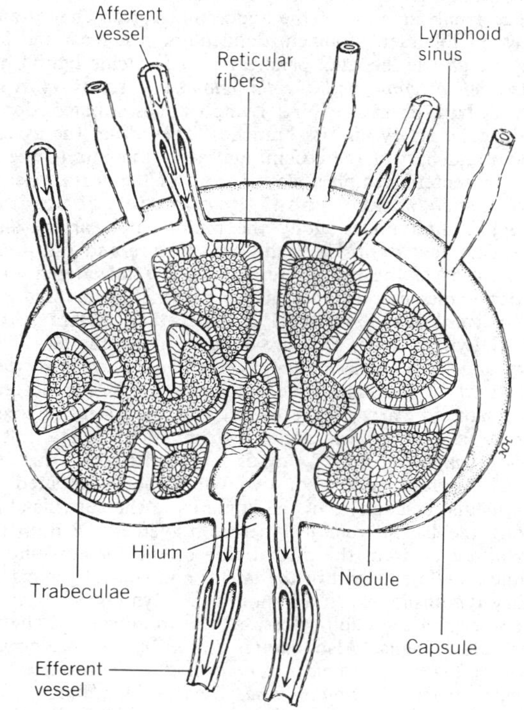


**Lymph node**

the apical group of axillary nodes. Also *central lymph nodes.* **nodi lymphatici cervicales anteriores** [NA] An inconstant group of lymph nodes situated in the midline of the neck anteriorly and divided into a superficial and a deep series. They drain the lower part of the larynx, thyroid gland and the upper part of the trachea and their efferents end in adjacent superior deep cervical nodes. Also *anterior cervical lymph nodes.* **nodi lymphatici cervicales laterales** [NA] The vertical chains of lymph nodes that are situated on the lateral side of the neck and that can be divided into superficial, deep, and retropharyngeal groups. The superficial group includes the submandibular nodes and a few nodes along the external jugular vein. Their lymph drains into the upper nodes of the deep group. The deep group includes the nodi lymphatici jugulares laterales, nodi lymphatici jugulares anteriores, nodi lymphatici supraclaviculares, nodus jugulodigastricus, and nodus jugulo-omohyoideus. The retropharyngeal group comprises the nodi lymphatici retropharyngeales and drains the nasal cavity, paranasal sinuses, soft and hard palate, nasopharynx, oropharynx, and middle ear. Also *lateral cervical lymph nodes.* **nodi lymphatici cervicales profundi** [NA] A large chain of lymph nodes situated along the internal jugular vein and the subclavian vein, draining all the lymphatics of the head and neck either directly or through intermediate groups of nodes. Their efferents form the jugular trunk. Also *deep cervical lymph nodes.* **nodi lymphatici cervicales superficiales** [NA] A few lymph nodes along the external jugular vein superficial to the sternocleidomastoid muscle. They drain part of the external ear, the lower parotid area, and the skin over the angle of the mandible. The efferents end either in the superior or the inferior deep cervical nodes. Also *superficial cervical lymph nodes.* **nodi lymphatici coeliaci** [NA] A group of lymph nodes adjacent to the celiac trunk in front of the abdominal aorta. They drain the liver, gallbladder, stomach, duodenum, pancreas, and spleen via the gastric, hepatic, pancreatic, and splenic lymph nodes. Also *celiac lymph nodes, celiac glands.* **nodi lymphatici colici dextri** [NA] Lymph nodes situated along the right colic artery and its branches. They drain the ascending colon and part of the cecum, and send efferents to the superior mesenteric lymph nodes in front of the aorta. Also *right colic lymph nodes.* **nodi lymphatici colici medii** [NA] Lymph nodes along the middle colic artery and its branches that drain the right colic flexure and the proximal two thirds of the transverse colon and send efferents to the superior mesenteric nodes in front of the aorta. Also *middle colic lymph nodes.* **nodi lymphatici colici sinistri** [NA] Lymph nodes that are situated along the left colic artery and its branches. They receive lymphatics from the distal third of the transverse colon and from the descending and sigmoid parts of the colon, and they send efferents to the inferior mesenteric nodes in front of the aorta. Also *left colic lymph nodes.* **nodi lymphatici cubitales** [NA] A group of one or two lymph nodes situated above the medial epicondyle of the humerus in the superficial fascia along the basilic vein just before it pierces the deep fascia. Its afferents drain the medial side of the forearm and hand while its efferents end in the lateral and central groups of axillary lymph nodes. In addition, a few lymph nodes are situated deep in the cubital fossa at the confluence of the radial and ulnar veins. Also *cubital lymph nodes, supratrochlear lymph nodes, epitrochlear lymph nodes, epitrochlear nodes, lymph nodes of cubital fossa, Sigmund's glands.* **nodi lymphatici epigastrici inferiores** [NA] A few small lymph nodes, situated along the inferior epigastric vessels, that receive afferents from the lower anterior abdominal wall and send efferents to the external iliac lymph nodes. Also *inferior epigastric lymph nodes.* **nodi lymphatici faciales** [NA] The nodi lymphatici buccales (buccal lymph nodes) and the nodi lymphatici mandibulares (mandibular lymph nodes) considered together. These nodes are situated along the facial vein and comprise the nodus buccinatorius, nodus nasolabialis, nodus malaris, and nodus mandibularis, and are located on the buccinator muscle, in the nasolabial furrow, in the infraorbital area, and on the lower margin of the mandible, respectively. They receive afferents from some of the skin and mucous membrane of the nose, cheek, and lips; from the medial part of the eyelids and conjunctiva, and also from some parotid nodes. The efferents drain to the submandibular nodes. Also *facial lymph nodes.* **nodi lymphatici gastrici dextri** [NA] Two or three lymph nodes along the right gastric artery that drain the pyloric portion adjacent to the lesser curvature of the stomach and send efferents to the hepatic nodes around the common hepatic artery. Also *right gastric lymph nodes.* **nodi lymphatici gastrici sinistri** [NA] A chain of lymph nodes situated along the left gastric artery and divided into three groups: an upper, on the stem of the artery; a lower, in the lesser omentum along the cardiac half of the lesser curvature; and a paracardial group around the esophagogastric junction. They drain the cardia, the lesser curvature and adjacent half of the stomach, and the abdominal part of the esophagus, while their efferents follow the course of the artery to end in the celiac lymph nodes. Also *left gastric lymph nodes, superior gastric lymph nodes, lymph nodes of lesser curvature.* **nodi lymphatici gastroepiploici dextri** NODI LYMPHATICI GASTRO-OMENTALES DEXTRI. **nodi lymphatici gastroepiploici sinistri** NODI LYMPHATICI GASTRO-OMENTALES SINISTRI. **nodi lymphatici gastro-omentales dextri** [NA] A short chain of about six lymph nodes that are situated along the right gastro-omental artery in the greater omentum along the pyloric part of the greater curvature of the stomach. They receive afferents from the lower part of the left half of the stomach and send efferents to the pyloric nodes. Also *right gastroepiploic lymph nodes, inferior gastric lymph nodes, nodi lymphatici gastroepiploici dextri.* **nodi lymphatici gastro-omentales sinistri** [NA] A few lymph nodes that are situated along the greater curvature of the stomach in the greater omentum along the left gastro-omental artery. They drain the adjacent surfaces of the stomach and greater omentum. They are usually associated with and included among the nodi lymphatici pancreatici. Also *nodi lymphatici gastroepiploici sinistri, left gastroepiploic lymph nodes.* **nodi lymphatici hepatici** [NA] A small chain of lymph nodes extending along the hepatic artery between the layers of the lesser omentum to the porta hepatis. Afferents are received from some deep lymphatics of the liver, parts of the visceral surface and lower anterior part of the diaphragmatic surface of the liver, the gallbladder, the right gastroepiploic lymph nodes, and part of the pyloric portion of the stomach. Efferents proceed to the celiac lymph nodes. Also *hepatic lymph nodes.* **nodi lymphatici ileocolici** [NA] Clumps of lymph nodes situated along the ileocolic artery and its branches. They receive lymph from the cecal nodes along the anterior and posterior cecal arteries and the appendicular nodes along the appendicular artery, as well as afferents from the terminal ileum via the ileal node and from the commencement of the ascending colon. Efferents end in the superior mesenteric lymph nodes. Also *ileocolic lymph nodes.* **nodi lymphatici iliaci communes** [NA] A group of lymph nodes situated around the common iliac vessels and below the bifurcation of the aorta, the afferents being lymphatics from the external and internal iliac lymph nodes while the efferents proceed to the lumbar lymph nodes. Also *common iliac lymph nodes.* **nodi lymphatici iliaci externi** [NA] Several lymph nodes, located lateral, medial, and anterior to the external iliac vessels, that receive lymphatics from the inguinal nodes; the deep layers of the anterior abdominal wall below the umbilicus, including efferents from the inferior epigastric and circumflex iliac nodes; as well as lymphatics from the prostate gland, fundus of the bladder, the membranous urethra, the cervix, and part of the uterus and vagina. Efferents run to the common iliac nodes but lymphatics also connect with the internal iliac nodes. Also *external iliac lymph nodes.* **nodi lymphatici iliaci interni** [NA] Lymph nodes located around the internal iliac vessels and the junctions of their branches, receiving afferents either directly or via intermediate nodes, from all the pelvic viscera, the deeper aspects of the perineum, the gluteal region, and back of the thigh. The efferents proceed to the common iliac lymph nodes and connect with the external iliac nodes. Also *internal iliac lymph nodes.* **nodi lymphatici infra-auriculares** [NA] One or two nodes of the nodi lymphatici parotidei superficiales that are situated below the ear and outside the parotid gland but deep to its fascia in the region of the commencement of the external jugular vein. Also *inferior auricular parotid lymph nodes.* **nodi lymphatici inguinales profundi** [NA] One to three lymph nodes medial to the femoral vein at the base of the femoral triangle. They receive deep lymphatics of the lower limb that accompany the femoral vein, some lymphatics from the superficial inguinal nodes, and those from the glans penis or clitoridis. Their efferents pass through the femoral canal to end in the external iliac lymph nodes. Also *deep inguinal lymph nodes.* **nodi lymphatici inguinales superficiales** [NA] A large number of lymph nodes, arranged in a T shape, superficial to the deep fascia below the inguinal ligament and divided into upper and lower groups. The upper group is parallel to the inguinal ligament and receives lymphatics from the anterior abdominal wall below the umbilicus, the gluteal region, the external genitalia, the perianal area, and lower part of anal canal. The lower group lies vertically along the terminal part of the great saphenous vein and receives superficial lymphatics from the whole limb except the back and lateral side of the leg. Most of the efferents pass through the femoral sheath directly to the external iliac lymph nodes, but a few end in the deep inguinal nodes. Also *superficial inguinal lymph nodes.* **nodi lymphatici intercostales** [NA] One or two lymph nodes at the back of each intercostal space near the heads of the ribs that drain the posterolateral parts of the thoracic wall and parietal pleura. The efferents of the nodes in the upper spaces end in the thoracic duct on the left and the right lymphatic duct on the right, whereas those of the lower spaces unite to form a trunk that ends either in the cisterna chyli or into the commencement of the thoracic duct. Also *intercostal lymph nodes, posterior intercostal lymph nodes.* **nodi lymphatici jugulares anteriores** [NA] Lymph nodes of the deep group of nodi lymphatici cervicales laterales that are situated anterior to the internal jugular vein, especially above the level where it is crossed by the omohyoid muscle. The jugulodigastric node may be included in this group. Also *anterior jugular lymph nodes.* **nodi lymphatici jugulares laterales** [NA] Lymph nodes of the deep group of nodi lymphatici cervicales laterales that lie lateral to the internal jugular vein. Their drainage pattern cannot be separated from that of the deep group as a whole. Also *lateral jugular lymph nodes.* **nodi lymphatici laterales** Three to six lymph nodes around the axillary vein, the afferents of which drain most of the upper limb and the efferents end in the central and apical groups of axillary lymph nodes. Also *lateral axillary lymph nodes.* **nodi lymphatici lumbales** [NA] A large number of prominent lymph nodes situated around the whole length of the abdominal aorta and part of the inferior vena cava. They are divided into right, left, and intermediate groups. The left group includes the lateral aortic, pre-aortic, and postaortic nodes lying lateral, anterior, and posterior to the aorta respectively. The right group includes the left caval, precaval, and postcaval nodes in relation to the inferior vena cava. Afferents are received from the common iliac nodes, the organs and tissues supplied by the paired branches of the aorta, and by the inferior mesenteric artery. The efferents of the uppermost nodes form a lumbar trunk on each side that terminates in the cisterna chyli. Also *lumbar lymph nodes.* **nodi lymphatici mandibulares** See under NODI LYMPHATICI FACIALES. **nodi lymphatici mastoidei** [NA] A few lymph nodes behind the auricle on the mastoid insertion of the sternocleidomastoid muscle and deep to the posterior auricular muscle. They receive afferents from the scalp above the ear, the cranial surface of the upper part of the auricle, and the posterior wall of the external acoustic meatus, and they send efferents to the superior deep cervical nodes. Also *retroauricular lymph nodes, posterior auricular lymph nodes, subauricular glands, mastoid lymph nodes.* **nodi lymphatici mediastinales anteriores** [NA] A number of small lymph nodes located in the superior mediastinum in front of the brachiocephalic veins and the arch of the aorta. They receive lymphatics from the thymus and thyroid glands, the upper part of the pericardium and pleura, superior lobe of left lung, and the right side of the heart. The efferents unite with those of the tracheobronchial and parasternal lymph nodes to form the bronchomediastinal lymph trunks. Also *anterior mediastinal lymph nodes.* **nodi lymphatici mediastinales posteriores** [NA] A number of lymph nodes located behind the pericardium and adjacent to the esophagus and thoracic aorta. They receive afferents from the esophagus, the back of the pericardium and diaphragm, and some intercostal spaces. Most of the efferents end in the thoracic duct, whereas a few end in the tracheobronchial lymph nodes. Also *posterior mediastinal lymph nodes.* **nodi lymphatici mesenterici** [NA] A large number of small lymph nodes situated between the two layers of the mesentery in three groups: a peripheral group along the vasa recta close to the wall of the intestine; an intermediate group among the primary arcades and intestinal arteries; and a third group along the upper part of the stem of the superior mesenteric artery. Also *mesenteric lymph nodes, mesocolic glands.* **nodi lymphatici mesenterici inferiores** [NA] Lymph nodes situated in front of the abdominal aorta around the main trunk of the inferior mesenteric artery, draining the distal third of the transverse colon, the descending colon, the sigmoid colon, and upper part of the rectum via the left colic, sigmoid, and superior rectal nodes, respectively. The efferents end in the superior mesenteric and left lateral aortic groups of lymph nodes. Also *inferior mesenteric lymph nodes.* **nodi lymphatici mesenterici superiores** [NA] Lymph nodes situated in front of the duodenum and head of pancreas around the main trunk of the superior mesenteric artery and its origin from the aorta. They receive afferents from the mesenteric, ileocolic, right colic, and middle colic nodes that drain the jejunum, ileum, cecum, appendix, ascending colon, and proximal two thirds of the transverse colon, as well as afferents from some of the pyloric nodes and part of the duodenum and the head of the pancreas. Efferents pass to the celiac lymph nodes and intestinal lymph trunks. Also *superior mesenteric lymph nodes.* **nodi lymphatici mesocolici** [NA] Lymph nodes that drain the ascending, transverse, and descending colon. They are divided into paracolic nodes, which lie along the mesenteric border of the colon, and colic nodes, which lie along the right, middle, and left colic arteries. Their efferents drain into nodes lying around the trunks of the superior and inferior mesenteric arteries that are continuous with the corresponding preaortic lymph nodes. Also *mesocolic glands.* **nodi lymphatici obturatorii** [NA] Lymph nodes along the obturator vessels that drain the lymphatics of the adductor region of the thigh. A constant node is present on the obturator nerve in the sulcus of the obturator foramen. Their efferents end in the external iliac nodes. Also *obturator lymph nodes.* **nodi lymphatici occipitales** [NA] A small group of lymph nodes located along the occipital artery at the apex of the posterior triangle of the neck, between the proximal attachments of the trapezius and sternocleidomastoid muscles. They drain the occipital region of the scalp and the superficial tissues of the upper part of the neck. Some efferents drain to the superior deep cervical nodes while most end in nodes along the accessory nerve in the posterior triangle of the neck. Also *occipital lymph nodes.* **nodi lymphatici pancreatici** [NA] Lymph nodes, including the nodi lymphatici gastro-omentales, that are situated along the splenic artery on the posterosuperior surface of the pancreas. They receive afferents from the fundus and upper part of the body of the stomach and the pancreas. The efferents end in the celiac group of nodes. **nodi lymphatici pancreaticolienales** The nodi lymphatici pancreatici and nodi lymphatici splenici. Also *pancreaticosplenic lymph nodes.* **nodi lymphatici paracolici** [NA] Lymph nodes situated along the medial borders of the ascending and descending colon and the mesenteric borders of the transverse and sigmoid colon. They drain the epicolic nodes in the wall of the gut and their efferents pass to the intermediate colic nodes. Also *paracolic lymph nodes.* **nodi lymphatici pararectales** [NA] Numerous lymph nodes that lie in the wall of the rectum next to the muscular coat. Most drain to the superior rectal nodes and then to the preaortic nodes at the origin of the inferior mesenteric artery. Others drain to the internal iliac and common iliac lymph nodes. **nodi lymphatici parasternales** [NA] Lymph nodes situated along the internal thoracic artery at the anterior ends of the upper three or four intercostal spaces. They receive lymphatics from the medial part of the mammary gland, the deeper part of the anterior thoracic wall and the anterior abdominal wall above the umbilicus, and the upper surface of the liver. The efferents may join those of the tracheobronchial and brachiocephalic nodes to form the bronchomediastinal lymph trunk. Also *parasternal lymph nodes, sternal lymph nodes, internal thoracic lymph nodes.* **nodi lymphatici paratracheales** **1** [NA] One of the five groups of tracheobronchial lymph nodes that is located on each side of the thoracic part of the trachea and receives afferents from the superior tracheobronchial nodes. Its efferents terminate in the bronchomediastinal lymph trunks. Also *peritracheal lymph nodes, tracheal lymph nodes.* **2** [NA] A group of deep anterior cervical lymph nodes that is situated along the recurrent laryngeal nerve on each side between the trachea and the esophagus. Their efferents end either in the lowest deep cervical nodes, in the jugular trunk, or in the thoracic duct. Also *lateral tracheal group of deep anterior cervical lymph nodes, paratracheal lymph nodes.* For defs. 1 and 2 also *nodi lymphatici tracheales.* **nodi lymphatici parotidei profundi** [NA] Intraglandular lymph nodes embedded in the substance of the parotid gland and deep to the gland on the lateral wall of the pharynx. Some of the lymph from the external acoustic meatus and eyelids draining to the superficial parotid nodes also reaches the deep nodes, as well as lymph from the gland, the middle ear, auditory tube, soft palate, and the posterior part of the floor of the nasal cavity. Their efferents join the adjacent upper deep cervical nodes. Also *deep parotid lymph nodes.* **nodi lymphatici parotidei superficiales** [NA] Lymph nodes superficial or deep to the parotid fascia that include the preauricular group in front of the tragus of the ear, draining the temporal and frontal regions of the scalp, the lateral surface of the auricle, the external wall of the external acoustic meatus and the lateral parts of the eyelids and conjunctiva. Their efferents end in the upper deep cervical nodes. Also *superficial parotid lymph nodes, preauricular nodes, anterior auricular nodes.* **nodi lymphatici pectorales** Three to five lymph nodes lying along the lateral thoracic artery at the junction of the anterior and medial walls of the axilla. The efferents join the central and apical groups of axillary nodes. Also *pectoral lymph nodes, pectoral axillary nodes.* **nodi lymphatici phrenici inferiores** [NA] A series of lymph nodes located on the abdominal surface of the diaphragm along the right inferior phrenic artery. They receive lymphatics from the posterior surface of the right lobe of the liver and adjacent diaphragm, and their efferents end in the right lateral caval nodes. Also *inferior diaphragmatic lymph nodes.* **nodi lymphatici phrenici superiores** [NA] A series of lymph nodes located on the thoracic surface of the diaphragm and comprising three sets. The anterior nodes are situated behind the xiphisternal joint and seventh costal cartilages, receiving afferents from the diaphragmatic surface of the liver, the adjacent diaphragm, and anterior abdominal wall. They send efferents to the parasternal nodes. The middle nodes are adjacent to the phrenic nerves, receiving lymphatics from the middle part of the diaphragm and part of the liver surface and sending efferents to the anterior phrenic nodes. The posterior nodes lie behind the crura of the diaphragm, draining that area and connecting with the lumbar and posterior mediastinal nodes. **nodi lymphatici popliteales** [NA] A number of lymph nodes located in the fat of the popliteal fossa and divided into superficial and deep groups. A superficial node is situated at the termination of the small saphenous vein, receiving lymphatics from the superficial region at the back and lateral side of the leg. A deep group is related to the popliteal vessels, receiving lymphatics from the knee joint as well as deep lymphatics accompanying the anterior tibial, posterior tibial, and peroneal vessels. Their efferents end in the deep inguinal nodes. Also *popliteal lymph nodes.* **nodi lymphatici postaortici** [NA] Lumbar lymph nodes that are situated behind the abdominal aorta and are essentially members of both the right and the left lumbar groups of nodes, as they have no defined area of drainage. Also *retroaortic lymph nodes.* **nodi lymphatici postcavales** [NA] Lumbar lymph nodes that are situated behind the inferior vena cava along the medial border of the psoas major muscle and on the right crus of the diaphragm. Also *retrocaval lymph nodes.* **nodi lymphatici preaortici** [NA] Lymph nodes that are situated immediately in front of the abdominal aorta and drain outlying intermediate nodes of the gastrointestinal tract, liver, spleen, and pancreas. Their efferents end in the intestinal trunks that help to form the cisterna chyli. Also *preaortic lymph nodes.* **nodi lymphatici preauriculares** [NA] Some nodes of the nodi lymphatici parotidei profundi that are located deep to the fascia of the parotid gland in front of the tragus of the auricle. Some authorities include them in the nodi lymphatici parotidei superficiales. They receive efferents from the latter nodes or directly from the external acoustic meatus, the lateral portions of the eyelids, the auricle, and skin of the temporal and frontal regions. Also *preauricular lymph nodes.* **nodi lymphatici precavales** [NA] Those right lateral aortic lymph nodes that are situated in front of the inferior vena cava from its origin as far as the renal veins. One constant node is situated at the level of the bifurcation of the aorta. They receive afferents from structures supplied by lateral and posterior branches of the aorta and from outlying nodes of the iliac arteries. Also *precaval lymph nodes.* **nodi lymphatici prececales** [NA] Several lymph nodes that lie along the anterior cecal arteries and drain lymphatics on the front of the cecum and root of the vermiform appendix. Their efferents pass to the ileocolic nodes. Also *anterior cecal lymph nodes.* **nodi lymphatici prelaryngeales** [NA] A group of deep cervical lymph nodes lying on the conus elasticus and the median cricothyroid ligament and deep to the investing layer of deep fascia. They receive afferents from the walls of the larynx and from the thyroid gland. Their efferents pass to lower deep cervical nodes. Also *prelaryngeal lymph nodes.* **nodi lymphatici prepericardiales** [NA] Lymph nodes situated behind the xiphoid process and the sixth and seventh costal cartilages on each side. They constitute the anterior group of the superior phrenic nodes and receive afferents from the liver and the front of the diaphragm. The efferents end in the parasternal nodes. Also *prepericardiac lymph nodes.* **nodi lymphatici pretracheales** [NA] One of the deep groups of the anterior cervical lymph nodes lying anterior to the trachea and along the inferior thyroid vessels. They receive afferents from the upper, cervical part of the trachea and the thyroid gland, and send efferents to the inferior deep cervical nodes. Also *pretracheal lymph nodes.* **nodi lymphatici pulmonales** One of the five groups of tracheobronchial lymph nodes that is situated along the larger branches of the principal bronchi in the lung substance. It receives the lymphatics draining the deep plexus in the bronchial submucosa and the peribronchial connective tissue, and its efferents pass to the contiguous bronchopulmonary nodes. Also *pulmonary lymph nodes.* ● Some authorities combine this group with the bronchopulmonary nodes under the single latter term. **nodi lymphatici pylorici** [NA] Some lymph nodes around the termination of the gastroduodenal artery in front and behind the groove between the junction of the first and second parts of the duodenum and the head of pancreas. They receive lymphatics from the right gastroepiploic nodes, the duodenum, and the pyloric part of the stomach, and they send efferents up to the hepatic nodes and down to the superior mesenteric nodes of the preaortic group. Also *pyloric lymph nodes, lymph nodes of gastroduodenal artery.* **nodi lymphatici retrocecales** [NA] Several lymph nodes that lie along the posterior cecal arteries and drain lymphatics on the back of the cecum and root of the vermiform appendix. Their efferents pass to the ileocolic nodes. Also *posterior cecal lymph nodes.* **nodi lymphatici retropharyngeales** [NA] A few lymph nodes of each deep cervical lymph chain situated between the fascia of the pharynx and the prevertebral fascia along the lateral margin of the longus capitis muscle. They receive afferents from the nasal fossae, paranasal sinuses, nasopharynx, auditory tube, oropharynx, and adjacent vertebral joints. The efferents end in the superior deep cervical nodes. Also *retropharyngeal lymph nodes.* **nodi lymphatici sacrales** [NA] Two or three peripheral nodes of the internal iliac lymph nodes located along the median and lateral sacral vessels in front of the second and third sacral foramina. They receive afferents from the rectum, uterus, vagina, prostate gland, and posterior pelvic wall. Also *sacral lymph nodes.* **nodi lymphatici splenici** [NA] Lymph nodes situated along the terminal part of the splenic artery and in the gastrosplenic ligament. Afferents derive from the spleen and efferents pass to the celiac lymph nodes. **nodi lymphatici submandibulares** [NA] Three or more lymph nodes deep to the deep cervical fascia in or around the submandibular salivary gland and related to the facial artery below the inferior margin of the mandible. They receive afferents from the facial and submental lymph nodes, thereby receiving much of the lymph from the central portion of the face, as well as lymphatics from the submandibular and sublingual salivary glands. The efferents pass to both the superior and the inferior deep cervical nodes. Also *submandibular lymph nodes.* **nodi lymphatici submentales** [NA] Two to four lymph nodes situated on the external surface of the mylohyoid muscle. They receive afferents from the middle portion of the lower lip and gums, floor of the mouth, and tip of the tongue. The efferents end in both the submandibular and jugulo-omohyoid lymph nodes. Also *submental lymph nodes.* **nodi lymphatici subscapulares** The posterior group of axillary lymph nodes located along the subscapular vessels and their branches. Their efferents drain to the central and apical groups of axillary nodes. Also *subscapular lymph nodes.* **nodi lymphatici supraclaviculares** [NA] A group of inferior deep cervical lymph nodes situated above the clavicle just behind the clavicular attachment of the sternocleidomastoid muscle and in close relation to the junction of the internal jugular and subclavian veins. They receive lymph from the superior deep cervical nodes as well as from nodes and lymphatics along the subclavian vessels. Their efferents enter the jugular trunk. Also *jugular glands, supraclavicular lymph nodes.* **nodi lymphatici thyroidei** [NA] Small lymph nodes on the course of the lymphatics draining the thyroid gland, which tend to follow the blood vessels of the gland, as well as a large node occasionally located in front of the middle of the thyroid cartilage. Also *thyroid lymph nodes.* **nodi lymphatici tracheales** NODI LYMPHATICI PARATRACHEALES. **nodi lymphatici tracheobronchiales** [NA] A large number of lymph nodes forming a continuous chain along the bronchi, both inside and ouside the lungs, and the trachea, and divided into five groups; paratracheal, superior tracheobronchial, inferior tracheobronchial, bronchopulmonary, and pulmonary. The afferents drain the lungs, visceral pleura, bronchi, the thoracic part of trachea, the heart, and the posterior mediastinal lymph nodes. The efferents unite with those of the parasternal and anterior mediastinal nodes to form the left and right bronchomediastinal trunks. Also *tracheobronchial lymph nodes.* **nodi lymphatici tracheobronchiales inferiores** [NA] One of the five groups of tracheobronchial lymph nodes that is situated in the angle between the two bronchi just below the bifurcation of the trachea. They receive afferents from the bronchopulmonary nodes and send efferents to the superior tracheobronchial nodes. Also *inferior tracheobronchial lymph nodes.* **nodi lymphatici tracheobronchiales superiores** [NA] One of the five groups of tracheobronchial lymph nodes, situated in the angle between the trachea and the brochus on each side just above the bifurcation of the trachea. They receive afferents from the inferior tracheobronchial nodes and send efferents to the paratracheal lymph nodes. Also *superior tracheobronchial lymph nodes.* **nodi lymphatici vesicales laterales** [NA] Small lymph nodes that are located along the lymph vessels running upward on each lateral aspect of the urinary bladder. They drain the region of the trigone and base as well as the sides of the bladder. Most of their efferents end in the external iliac nodes, but a few may pass directly to the internal or common iliac nodes. Also *lateral vesical lymph nodes.* **n. lymphaticus** [NA] Any of the small rounded or oval masses of lymphoid tissue that are irregularly placed along the course of lymphatic vessels and through which the lymph of those vessels passes. Also *lymph node, lymphatic node, lymphonodus, lymphatic gland, lymph gland, lymphaden.* **n. malaris** [NA] One of the nodi lymphatici faciales that is situated along the facial vein anterior to the zygomatic bone near the nasal bridge. **n. mandibularis** [NA] One of the nodi lymphatici faciales that is situated along the facial vein at the inferior margin of the body of the mandible just anterior to its angle. There are usually more than one node. **n. nasolabialis** [NA] One of the nodi lymphatici faciales that is situated along the facial vein in the nasolabial furrow. **n. sinuatrialis** [NA] A narrow, U-shaped collection of specialized cardiac muscle situated at the upper end of the sulcus terminalis of the right atrium near the junction of the entrance of the superior vena cava and the right auricle. It comprises slender fusiform fibers that contract more rapidly than the surrounding cardiac muscle and it is considered to initiate the cardiac cycle of contraction. Hence it is called the pacemaker of the heart. Also *S-A node, sinoatrial node, sinuatrial node, Keith's node, sinuatrial node of Keith and Flack, Keith-Flack node, Flack's node, Keith's bundle, atrionector.* **n. tibialis anterior** [NA] An inconstant lymph node that drains some of the deep lymphatics accompanying the anterior tibial vessels and is located along their upper third. Its efferents end in the deep group of popliteal nodes. Also *anterior tibial lymph node.* **nodi viscerales abdominis** Lymph nodes situated along the efferent lymphatics of the abdominal viscera. They lie along the celiac artery and its branches, the superior mesenteric artery, the inferior mesenteric artery, and the biliary tract. Also *visceral lymph nodes of abdomen.*

**noeud vital** \nœ vētäl′\ The respiratory centers of the brain. *Obs.* Also *vital node.*

**no-fault** Referring to insurance compensation to the insured for specified damages regardless of who caused the loss.

**nogalamycin** An anticancer antibiotic, the product of *Streptomyces nogalater.*

**noise** [Middle English, from Old French, hubbub, disturbance, from L *nausea* seasickness] **1** Sound usually of a random nature the spectrum of which does not exhibit any clearly defined frequency components. **2** An unpleasant or undesired sound. **3** Electric oscillations of an undesired or random nature such as the 60-cycle frequency wave in an electrocardiogram. **transient n.** Sounds of extremely short duration such as clicks and impulse noise and certain speech sounds. **white n.** Nonperiodic sound in which there is an equal distribution of acoustic energy throughout the audible range of frequencies and beyond. It is used in otology for masking one ear while the other is being tested. Also *white sound.*

**noma** \nō′mə\ [Gk *nomē* (from *nemein* to devour, pasture, feed on; of ulcers, to spread) a pasture, feeding on, spreading, spreading ulcer] Spreading gangrene, usually of the facial tissues in and around the mouth (cancrum oris) but sometimes of the female external genitalia, (noma vulvae) occurring in the severely malnourished, chiefly children, and as a complication of the exanthemata.

**nomadic** \nōmad′ik\ Not fixed or stabilized; moving or apt to move freely.

**nomen** \nō′mən\ [L, a name] (*pl.* nomina) A name.

**nomenclature** \nō′mənklā′chər\ [L *nomenclatura* (from *nomen* a name + *calare* to call, call out, summon) a naming, listing of names, terminology] A system for naming or the names assigned to particular types that can be usefully distinguished from others in a science or other discipline, as of animals or plants or their structures. **binomial n.** The system developed by Linnaeus for naming flora and fauna. A species is designated by a unique combination of two names, a generic name and a specific epithet.

**Nomina Anatomica** \näm′inə an′ətäm′ikə\ The standard anatomical terminology, which was adopted by the German Anatomical Society at Basle (later *Basel,* abbreviated *BNA*), Switzerland, in 1895. It was revised in 1933 (Birmingham Revision) and in 1936 (Jena Nomina Anatomica). In 1955 a completely revised Nomina Anatomica, First Edition (abbreviated *NA*), was published, and since then several revisions have been issued. The fourth edition, published in 1977, also included a Nomina Histologica and a Nomina Embryologica, as have subsequent editions. Abbr. NA

**nomo-** \näm′ə-, nō′mō-\ [Gk *nomos* law, usage, custom] A combining form meaning law, custom, usage.

**nomogram** \nō′məgram\ [NOMO- + -GRAM] A diagram representing the relationships between variables in a given system. For example, if the system consists of three variables, the value taken by one of them is represented in the nomogram for each pair of values taken by the other two, in a graphical manner. Also *nomograph.* **blood volume n.** A nomogram that indicates the normal blood volume for a person's height and weight.

**nomograph** \näm′əgraf\ [NOMO- + -GRAPH] NOMOGRAM.

**nomothetic** \näm′əthet′ik\ Relating to general or universal laws based on the observation of many cases.

**nomotopic** \näm′ətäp′ik\ Occurring in the normal place.

**non-** \nän-\ [L *non* (from early *noenum, noenu* none, no one, from *ne* not + *unum* one) not] A prefix meaning not.

**nona-** \nō′nə-\ [L *nonus* (feminine *nona*) ninth] A combining form meaning nine.

**nonaccess** \nänak′ses\ The lack of an opportunity to engage in sexual intercourse or the absence of sexual intercourse. In cases of disputed paternity, nonaccess is a common defense used by a putative father.

**nonadherent** \-adhir′ənt\ Not attached to or connected with contiguous structures.

**nonan** \nō′nən\ [L *nonan(us) (from nonus* ninth) pertaining to the ninth] Recurring or characterized by attacks every ninth day, as *nonan malaria.*

**nonarticular** \-ärtik′yələr\ Not occurring in a joint: used especially with reference to periarticular complaints.

**nonchromaffin** \-krōmaf′in\ [NON- + CHROMAFFIN] Not staining with chromium salts: said especially of cells of the adrenal medulla, carotid body, or paraganglia that do not secrete epinephrine.

**noncomitance** \-kō′mitəns\ [NON- + COMITANCE] A misalignment of the eyes in which theangle of the deviation changes with different directions of gaze. Adj. noncomitant.

**non compos mentis** \nän käm′pōs men′tis\ [L *non* not + *compos* master of + *mentis,* gen. of *mens* reason] Not of sound mind; in legal usage, not competent to manage one's affairs or to execute specified actions or judgments independently. Compare COMPOS MENTIS.

**nondepolarizer** A muscle relaxant agent that causes striatal muscular paralysis by competitively blocking neurotransmission at the myoneural junction. An example is *d*-tubocurarine.

**nondisjunction** \nän′disjungk′shən\ The failure of normal segregation of chromosomes to daughter cells during cell division. **primary n.** Nondisjunction that occurs during the first meiotic division in which both chromosomes of a homologous pair segregate to a secondary gametocyte. **secondary n.** Nondisjunction occurring during the second stage of meiosis, in which both chromatids of a chromosome segregate to a gamete during anaphase. **somatic n.** Nondisjunction occurring during mitosis in which one daughter cell receives both, and the other cell receives neither, chromosome of an homologous pair. Also *anaphase lag loss.*

**nonencapsulated** \-enkap′səlā′tid\ Not surrounded by a containing capsule: used of a swelling, such as a tumor or abscess.

**nongranulocyte** \-gran′yəlōsīt′\ A blood leukocyte that does not contain granules in its cytoplasm. Lymphocytes and monocytes are nongranulocytes.

**nonhomogeneity** \-häm′əjənē′itē\ A lack of uniformity in a structure or population.

**nonhomologues** \-hōmäl′əgəs\ NONHOMOLOGOUS CHROMOSOMES.

**noninvasive** \-invā′siv\ Not involving the penetration of a body cavity or the skin: used especially of a therapeutic or diagnostic procedure.

**nonionic** \nän′ī-än′ik\ Not containing charges in its molecule, as in detergents whose hydrophilic groups are not ionized.

**nonlamellar** \-ləmel′ər\ Not arranged in layers: said of immature bony tissue in which the collagen bundles are not arranged in regular layers and consequently do not give a lamellar pattern with polarized light microscopy.

**nonmedullated** \-med′yəlā′tid\ UNMYELINATED.

**nonmetal** \-met′əl\ **1** Not possessing the properties of a metal. **2** An electronegative element.

**nonmyelinated** \-mī′əlinā′tid\ UNMYELINATED.

**Nonne** [Max *Nonne,* German neurologist, 1861–1939] **1** Nonne-Froin syndrome. See under FROIN SYNDROME. **2** Nonne-Marie syndrome. See under MARIE'S HEREDITARY CEREBELLAR ATAXIA. **3** Nonne-Milroy disease. See under HEREDITARY LYMPHEDEMA TYPE I. **4** Nonne syndrome. See under SCALENUS ANTERIOR SYNDROME.

**non-nucleated** \-n$^y$oo′klē-ā′tid\ ANUCLEAR.

**nonoliguric** \-äl′igoo′rik\ [NON- + OLIGURIC] Producing urine in normal volume: usually said of acute renal failure that is without the usual oliguria.

**nononcogenic** \-äng′kəjen′ik\ [NON- + ONCOGENIC] Not capable of causing tumors.

**nonovulatory** \-äv′yələtôr′ē\ Characterized by the absence of ovulation, usually associated with absence of menstruation.

**nonoxynol-9** Nonylphenoxypolyethoxyethanol, with 9 oxyethylene groups in the polyoxyethylene, $(OCH_2CH_2)n$, chain. It is used as a spermicidal component in some contraceptive materials, including aerosol foams.

**nonparous** \-par′əs\ [NON- + PAROUS] NULLIPAROUS.

**nonpenetrant** \-pen′ətrənt\ In genetics, pertaining to a trait which is not apparent or evident on assay despite the presence of a particular genotype capable of determining the trait. It usually refers to monogenic traits, such as a heterozygote for a completely recessive trait.

**nonpermissive** \-pərmis′iv\ Allowing a conditionally lethal mutation to block formation of a required gene product: said of environmental conditions, such as temperature.

**nonpolar** \-pō′lər\ Having molecules that possess no charges or dipole moments: used of substances such as paraffins. When applied to solvents it suggests that they will not dissolve polar compounds and will not favor chemical reactions whose mechanism involves charge separation. The term is also applied to an environment without charges or dipoles.

**non rep.** *non repetatur* (L, do not repeat; no refill).

**nonrotation** \-rōtā′shən\ Failure of a structure during embryonic life to rotate to its normal position. **n. of the intestine** Lack of rotation of the embryonic intestine when normally it should rotate from a sagittally aligned loop to take up its adult relationships in the abdominal cavity.

**nonsecretor** \-sikrē′tər\ An individual who lacks the inherited ability to secrete A, B, and H antigens in his body fluids while being able to express these substances on his tissue cells.

**nonself** \nän′self\ Those antigens that are not a normal constituent of the body of a given individual and to which antibodies can be formed. Being foreign to the self, such antigens are recognized by the immune system. Also *not-self.* Compare SELF.

**nonspecific** **1** Not caused by one particular microorganism: said of an infection or disease. **2** Denoting a general effect of a drug, in contrast to its effect from specific interaction at a designated site of action or receptor.

**nonsurgical** \-sur′jikəl\ Not requiring operative intervention: used especially of a therapeutic or diagnostic procedure.

**nontaster** \-tā′stər\ **1** In a linkage between loci, an individual incapable of tasting a specific substance when the ability to taste is a mendelian trait. **2** An individual incapable of tasting phenylthiocarbamide (PTC), due to homozygosity of an allele at the PTC locus. Such an inability is an autosomal recessive trait.

**nonunion** \-yoo′nyən\ The failure of a fractured bone to heal with new bone formation. Also *faulty union.* **established n.** Stabilization of the healing process of a fracture without evidence that eventual union will take place.

**nonviable** \-vī′əbl\ [NON- + VIABLE] Describing a fetus that has not yet reached that stage of intrauterine development at which it could survive birth. A fetus of less than five months' gestation is generally regarded as being nonviable.

**nonvisualization** \-vizh′oo-əlīzā′shən\ [NON- + VISUALIZATION] In radiology, the failure to demonstrate in an organ an administered radiopaque contrast medium normally excreted by that organ, as during intravenous urography.

**Noonan** [Jacqueline Anne *Noonan,* U.S. cardiologist, born 1921] See under SYNDROME.

**nootropic** \nō′əträp′ik\ Activating or stimulating to mental activity; causing cerebral or intellectual activity.

**nopalin G** An eosin dye which has a bluish color.

**nor-** [shortened from *normal.* See NORMA.] **1** A prefix signifying the removal of a methylene group, —$CH_2$—, from a named compound. Thus for example, norepinephrine contains —NH— where epinephrine contains —N(—$CH_3$)—. **2** A prefix denoting the isomer of the amino acid that has an unbranched chain: used in this sense only in the names *norvaline* and *norleucine.*

**noradrenalin** \nôr′adren′əlin\ NOREPINEPHRINE.

**noradrenaline** \nôr′adren′əlin\ The British term for NOREPINEPHRINE.

**noradrenalin *N*-methyltransferase** The enzyme (EC 2.1.1.28) responsible for the conversion of norepinephrine into epinephrine. The donor of the methyl group is *S*-adenosylmethionine.

**norepinephrine** \nôr′epinef′rin\ A catecholamine, *l*-$\beta$-[3,4-dihydroxyphenyl]-$\alpha$-aminoethanol, a major adrenergic neurotransmitter liberated by postganglionic adrenergic nerve endings, and secreted also by the chromaffin granules of the adrenal medulla in response to splanchnic stimulation. Acting chiefly upon the α adrenergic receptors of effector organs, its chief property is to induce arteriolar constriction with raised systolic and diastolic arterial blood pressure, venoconstriction, and increased peripheral resistance. Also *arterenol, levarterenol, arterenol, noradrenalin, noradrenaline* (British usage), *sympathin E* (outmoded).

**norethandrolone** $C_{20}H_{30}O_2$. 17-Hydroxy-19-norpregn-4-en-3-one. A synthetic androgenic steroid similar in structure to testosterone. It has similar pharmacologic effects and is used primarily as an anabolic steroid.

**norethindrone** $C_{20}H_{26}O_2$. 17-Hydroxy-19-nor-17α-pregn-4-en-20-yn-3-one. A progestational steroid with some estrogenic and androgenic activity. It is used as a substitute for progesterone and it is combined with an estrogenic agent as an oral contraceptive medication.

**norethindrone acetate** $C_{22}H_{28}O_3$. The acetate salt of norethindrone. It has the same actions and uses as the parent compound.

**norethynodrel** $C_{20}H_{26}O_2$. 17-Hydroxy-19-nor-17α-pregn-5(10)-en-20-yn-3-one. A progestational steroid used in combination with ethynylestradiol 3-methyl eter as an oral contraceptive agent.

**norfloxacin** $C_{16}H_{18}FN_3O_3$. 1-Ethyl-6-fluoro-1,4-dihydro-4-oxo-7-(1-piperazinyl)-3-quinolinecarboxylic acid, a synthetic quinolone antibiotic. Its best activity is against Gram-negative bacteria, and it is used in the treatment of urinary tract infections. It is administered orally.

**norleucine** $CH_3—[CH_2]_3—CH(NH_3{}^+)—COO^-$. 2-Aminohexanoic acid, the isomer of leucine with an unbranched carbon chain. It is somewhat misleading as a name, because the prefix *nor-* does not have its usual meaning of removal of a methylene group. It is used as a standard in amino-acid analysis, as it does not normally occur in biologic material. Symbol: Nle

**norm** \nôrm\ [L *norm(a)*. See NORMA.] A statistical measure of usual observed performance.

**norma** \nôr′mə\ [L (prob. from Etruscan, from Gk *gnōmōn*, accus. *gnōmona* carpenter's square, rule, pointer, index) a carpenter's square, right angle, standard, pattern] In anatomy, an aspect of the cranium or skull from a particular viewpoint, often as seen in outline. **n. anterior** NORMA FACIALIS. **n. basilaris** The outline of the inferior surface of the base of the skull. It extends from the front of the dental arch to the superior nuchal lines of the occipital bone. Also *norma inferior* (outmoded), *norma ventralis* (outmoded), *norma basalis, basis cranii externa* (imprecise). **n. facialis** [NA] The outline of the skull as viewed from the front. Also *norma frontalis, norma anterior.* **n. inferior** *Outmoded* NORMA BASILARIS. **n. lateralis** [NA] The outline of the skull as viewed from either side. Also *norma temporalis* (outmoded). **n. occipitalis** [NA] The outline of the skull as viewed from behind. It resembles a broad arch with a flat base. Its features include the external occipital protuberance, the nuchal lines, and the lambdoid suture. Also *norma posterior* (outmoded). **n. sagittalis** The outline of a sagittal section through the skull. *Outmoded.* **n. superior** *Outmoded* NORMA VERTICALIS. **n. temporalis** *Outmoded* NORMA LATERALIS. **n. ventralis** *Outmoded* NORMA BASILARIS. **n. verticalis** [NA] The outline of the skull as viewed from above. Anteriorly it is continuous with the norma facialis. It varies considerably, and the coronal, sagittal, and lambdoid sutures are exposed. Also *norma superior* (outmoded).

**normal** [L *normal(is)* (from *norm(a)* a carpenter's square, rule of any kind, standard + *-alis* -AL) according to rule] **1** Conforming to a standard or norm; specifically, considered to be substantially free from defect, such that no intervention or correction is warranted, as *normal pulse, normal hearing.* **2** Being of satisfactory or average health. **3** Having a linear carbon chain: used of an alcohol or alkyl radical. **4** Describing the concentration of a solution one liter of which yields or reacts with one mole of the unitary entities involved in a specified reaction, usually a titration, such as protons in acidimetry, or electrons in oxidation-reduction reactions. **5** Referring to standard conditions of temperature, 0°C (273.15K exactly), or of pressure, one atmosphere (101.325 kPa exactly).

**normalize** \nôr′məlīz\ To adjust the values in a determination to an arbitrary standard, usually by multiplying them all by the same factor so that their total comes to a value known by an independent determination.

**Norman** [Ronald Melville *Norman*, English physician, flourished mid-20th century] Norman-Wood syndrome. See under SYNDROME.

**normergic** \nôrmur′jik\ Concerning normal responsiveness to stimulation.

**normetanephrine** An intermediate in the catabolism of norepinephrine, from which it is produced by methylation of the phenolic hydroxyl *meta* to the carbon side chain.

**normo-** \nôr′mə-\ [L *norma* rule, law, standard] A combining form meaning normal.

**normoblast** \nôr′məblast\ [NORMO- + -BLAST] Any erythrocyte precursor that exhibits normal characteristics of nuclear chromatin and cytoplasm, in contradistinction to the megaloblast. Several stages of maturation of the normoblast are recognized: pronormoblast, basophilic normoblast, polychromatophilic normoblast, and the penultimate stage, orthochromatic normoblast. Also *hemonormoblast.* **acidophilic n.** ORTHOCHROMATIC NORMOBLAST. **basophilic n.** A stage of maturation of erythrocyte precursors in which the nucleus exhibits slight chromatin condensation, no nucleolus is identifiable, the nucleus occupies about half the volume of the cell, and the cytoplasm is free of granules and is a deep blue color when stained by Romanowsky dyes. Also *basophilic erythroblast, early erythroblast, early normoblast, prorubricyte.* **eosinophilic n.** ORTHOCHROMATIC NORMOBLAST. **intermediate n.** POLYCHROMATOPHILIC NORMOBLAST. **orthochromatic n.** The final stage in maturation of erythrocyte precursors before extrusion of the nucleus and release of the cell from bone marrow to blood. The cell is slightly larger than an erythrocyte, and the nucleus is small, about one fourth of the cell volume or less, with dense chromatin. The cytoplasm is red-orange, tinctorially identical with a mature erythrocyte, when stained with Romanowsky dyes. Also *acidophilic erythroblast, eosinophilic erythroblast, late erythroblast, orthochromatic erythroblast, oxyphilic erythroblast, metarubricyte, acidophilic normoblast, eosinophilic normoblast, late normoblast, oxyphilic normoblast.* **polychromatophilic n.** A stage of maturation of erythrocyte precursors, following the basophilic stage and preceding the orthochromatic stage, in which the nucleus exhibits prominent chromatin condensation and parachromatin, often resembling a checkerboard, and no nucleoli are identifiable. The nucleus occupies approximately one-third of the cell volume, and the cytoplasm is slate gray to lavender when stained by Romanowsky dyes. The color of the cytoplasm reflects the presence of both hemoglobin and abundant RNA in the cytoplasm. This is the last maturation stage at which cell division still occurs. Also *intermediate erythroblast, polychromatophilic erythroblast, intermediate normoblast, rubricyte.*

**normoblastic** \-blas′tik\ Having the morphologic characteristics of the normal maturation of erythrocyte precursors. Also *erythroblastic.* Compare MEGALOBLASTIC.

**normoblastosis** \-blastō′sis\ The presence of nucleated erythrocyte precursors (normoblasts) in blood.

**normocalcemia** \-kalsē′mē·ə\ A normal concentration of calcium in blood or serum.

**normocalcemic** \-kalsē′mik\ Exhibiting normocalcemia.

**normocapnia** \-kap′nē·ə\ A normal concentration of carbon dioxide (and carbonic acid) in blood. Also *eucapnia.*

**normocapnic** \-kap′nik\ Exhibiting normocapnia.

**normocholesterolemia** \-kōles′tərōlē′mē·ə\ A normal concentration of cholesterol in blood plasma or serum.

**normocholesterolemic** \-kōles′tərōlē′mik\ Exhibiting normocholesterolemia.

**normochromasia** \-krōmā′zhə\ NORMOCHROMIA.

**normochromatic** \-krōmat′ik\ Having normal color in stained blood films: used of erythrocytes or erythrocyte precursors. In Wright-stained blood films the cytoplasm exhibits no bluish tinge.

**normochromia** \-krō′mē·ə\ A normal concentration of hemoglobin in erythrocytes. Also *normochromasia.*

**normochromic** \-krō′mik\ Having normal concentration of hemoglobin in erythrocytes. Also *orthochromatic.*

**normocyte** \nôr′məsīt\ An erythrocyte of normal volume, usually 82–99 fl. Also *normoerythrocyte.*

**normocytic** \-sit′ik\ Having erythrocytes of normal volume.

**normocytosis** \-sītō′sis\ The state of having erythrocytes of normal volume. Also *normo-orthocytosis.*

**normoerythrocyte** \-irith′rəsīt\ NORMOCYTE.

**normoglycemia** \-glīsē′mē·ə\ [NORMO- + GLYC- + -EMIA] The presence of glucose in normal concentration in the blood.

**normoglycemic** \-glīsē′mik\ Characterized by or having blood glucose concentration within the accepted normal range.

**normokalemia** \-kəlē′mē·ə\ A normal concentration of plasma or serum potassium. ● As used, this term is not meant to apply to whole blood. Red cell $K^+$ concentration is much higher than that of serum.

**normokalemic** \-kəlē′mik\ Having normal plasma or serum potassium concentration.

**normo-orthocytosis** \-ôr′thəsītō′sis\ NORMOCYTOSIS.

**normoreflexia** \-riflek′sē·ə\ [NORMO- + REFLEX + -IA] Reflexes within the range of normal variation.

**normosthenuria** \-sthenoo′rē·ə\ The state of normal urine production.

**normotension** \-ten′shən\ [NORMO- + TENSION] Normal arterial blood pressure.

**normotensive** \-ten′siv\ [NORMO- + *tens(ion)* + -IVE] Characterized by normal arterial blood pressure.

**normotonia** \-tō′nē·ə\ [NORMO- + *ton(o)-* + -IA] Normal blood pressure; normotension.

**normotonic** \-tän′ik\ Characterized by normal blood pressure; normotensive.

**normotrophic** \-träf′ik\ [NORMO- + -TROPHIC] Concerning normal growth and development.

**normovolemia** \-vōlē′mē·ə\ Normal blood volume.

**normovolemic** \-vōlē′mik\ Having a normal blood volume.

**nornicotine** \nôrnik′ətēn\ $C_9H_{12}N_2$. A toxic pyridine alkaloid present in plant species of the genera *Duboisia, Nicotiana, Salpiglossis* and *Zinnia.* It is used in agriculture as an insecticide.

**norophthalmic acid** The tripeptide γ-glutamylalanylglycine, found in the lens of the eye. It differs from ophthalmic acid, which occurs with it, in having $—CH_3$ rather than $—CH_2—CH_3$ as the side chain of its central residue, where glutathione has $—CH_2SH$.

**norpseudoephedrine** $C_9H_{13}NO$. A central nervous system stimulant present in the dried leaves of *Catha edulis.* It has had limited use as an anorectic agent. Also *cathine.*

**nortriptyline** $C_{19}H_{21}N$. 3-(10,11-Dihydro-5*H*-dibenzo[*a,d*]cyclohepten-5-ylidene)-*N*-methyl-1-propanamine. A tricyclic antidepressant drug. The mechanism by which these agents exert their mood elevation effect is not known. It is generally given orally as the hydrochloride salt.

**noscapine** $C_{22}H_{22}NO_7$. An isoquinoline alkaloid which has cough-suppressing properties and aids respiration. It occurs in the capsules of *Papaver somniferum* and hence in opium. It is used in treating whooping cough and bronchitis. Also *narcotine, narcosine, opian, opianine.*

**nose** [Old English *nosu,* akin to L *nasus* the nose] **1** NASUS EXTERNUS. **2** The nasus externus and cavitas nasi considered together; nasus. **cleft n.** The appearance as of duplicated nose due to persistence of the embryonic frontonasal groove or improper union of the medial nasal processes. Various degrees of this congenital deformity are seen. Rarely it is associated with other anomalies such as optic hypertelorism or hypotelorism, cleft lip and cleft palate. **copper n.** RHINOPHYMA. **external n.** NASUS EXTERNUS. **familial hump n.** A condition of the nose where there is a conspicuous hump in the bridge line, usually a familial trait. **potato n.** RHINOPHYMA. **saddle n.** A nose deformed by the collapse of the support of the dorsum between the tip and the nasal bones normally provided by the cartilage of the nasal septum. The resultant deformity is characterized by a saddle-shaped depression of the nasal dorsum. The causes are many and include trauma (accidental or surgical), septal infection (abscess, syphilis, etc.), and congenital deformity. **strawberry n.** RHINOPHYMA. **Swedish n.** A device for helping to maintain the humidity of the lower airways in cases of tracheostomy. It consists of wire mesh disks in a plastic container fitted to the tracheostomy tube. During expiration water vapor condenses on the wire mesh, which acts as a humidifier when the patient breathes in. **telescope n.** Atrophy of the septum and vomer causing a depression below the root of the nose. This condition is seen in leprosy. **whisky n.** RHINOPHYMA.

**nosebleed** EPISTAXIS.

**nosebrain** *Obs.* RHINENCEPHALON.

**nosegay** \nōz′gā\ In anatomy, a structure or structures resembling a small bunch of flowers. *Rare.* **Riolan's n.** The group of muscles and ligaments attached to the styloid process of the temporal bone. Also *bouquet of Riolan.*

**nosepiece** In a compound microscope, the mounting to which the objective lens is attached. It is often in the form of a pivoting plate on which are mounted several interchangeable objectives.

**noso-** \näs′ō-\ [Gk *nosos* sickness, disease] A combining form meaning disease.

**nosocomial** \-kō′mē·əl\ [Gk *nosokomei(on)* (from *noso(s)* sickness + *komeein* to attend, take care of) infirmary, hospital + -AL] Pertaining to or acquired in a hospital or other health facility: used especially in reference to hospital-acquired infections and diseases.

**nosogenic** \-jen′ik\ *Obs.* PATHOGENIC.

**nosology** \nōsäl′əjē\ [NOSO- + -LOGY] **1** The science of the systematic classification of diseases. **2** A systematic classification or list of diseases. **psychiatric n.** The study of mental disorders from the point of view of their classification, grouping, ordering, and relationship to one another.

**nosomania** \-mā′nē·ə\ [NOSO- + -MANIA] *Obs.* HYPOCHONDRIASIS.

**nosomycosis** \-mīkō′sis\ [NOSO- + MYCOSIS] Any fungal disease or infection.

**nosoparasite** \-par′əsīt\ [NOSO- + PARASITE] **1** An organism associated with a particular disease and able to modify its course, but not serving as the actual causal agent. **2** A pathogenic parasite that attacks only already diseased tissues.

**nosophilia** \-fil′yə\ [NOSO- + -PHILIA] *Obs.* HYPOCHONDRIASIS.

**nosopoietic** \-poi·et′ik\ *Obs.* PATHOGENIC.

***Nosopsyllus fasciatus*** \nä′sōsil′əs fash′ē·ā′təs\ The northern or European rat flea, a species that transmits the plague bacillus between rats and rarely to man. It is also a suspected vector of murine typhus. Also *Ceratophyllus fasciatus, Pulex fasciatus.*

**nosotherapy** \-ther′əpē\ [NOSO- + THERAPY] The use of one disease to treat another, such as malaria-induced fever for the treatment of central nervous system syphilis.

**nosotoxicosis** \-täk′sikō′sis\ TOXICOSIS.

**nosotoxin** \-täk′sin\ Any toxin causing or associated with a disease.

**nosotropic** \-träp′ik\ [NOSO- + -TROPIC[1]] Directed against the manifestations or symptoms of a disease: said of a treatment or medication. Compare ETIOTROPIC.

**nostology** \nästäl′əjē\ [Gk *nosto(s)* a return home + -LOGY] *Obs.* GERONTOLOGY.

**nostrate** \näs′trāt\ [L *nostras*, gen. *nostratis* (from *noster* ours) pertaining to our own country or nation, indigenous] *Older term* ENDEMIC.

**nostrils** NARES.

**nostrum** [L, neut. sing. of *noster* our, ours] A quack medication, usually a preparation made with a private, secret formula and promoted with exaggerated claims about its healing powers for a variety of diseases.

**notal** \nō′təl\ Pertaining to the back; dorsal.

**notalgia** \nōtal′jə\ DORSALGIA. **n. paresthetica** Pain and paresthesiae in the back following the distribution of the posterior primary rami of the lumbar nerves. It is thought to be due to entrapment of one or more of these nerves.

**notancephalia** \nō′tansəfā′lyə\ [*not(o)-* + Gk *an-* priv. + *kephal(ē)* the head + -IA] A congenital deficiency in the posterior part of the skull.

**notanencephalia** \nō′tanen′səfā′lyə\ [*not(o)-* + Gk *an-* priv. + ENCEPHAL- + -IA] A congenital absence or deficiency of the cerebellum. *Seldom used.*

**notatin** *Obs.* GLUCOSE OXIDASE.

# notch

**notch** INCISURA. **acetabular n.** INCISURA ACETABULI. **anacrotic n.** A notch on the upstroke of an arterial pulse tracing. Also *anacrotic incisura.* **angular n.** INCISURA ANGULARIS GASTRICA. **anterior cerebellar n.** INCISURA CEREBELLI ANTERIOR. **anterior n. of ear** INCISURA ANTERIOR AURIS. **aortic n.** DICROTIC NOTCH. **n. of apex of heart** INCISURA APICIS CORDIS. **cardiac n. of left lung** INCISURA CARDIACA PULMONIS SINISTRI. **cardiac n. of stomach** INCISURA CARDIACA GASTRICA. **catacrotic n.** A notch, or one of the notches, additional to the dicrotic notch on the downstroke of an arterial pulse tracing. **clavicular n. of sternum** INCISURA CLAVICULARIS STERNI. **costal n.'es of sternum** INCISURAE COSTALES STERNI. **cotyloid n.** INCISURA ACETABULI. **craniofacial n.** An occasional defect in the bony partition separating the orbital and nasal cavities. **dicrotic n.** The notch preceding the dicrotic wave in the downstroke of an arterial pulse tracing, marking the closure of the semilunar valve. Also *aortic notch.* **digastric n.** INCISURA MASTOIDEA OSSIS TEMPORALIS. **n. of ethmoid** INCISURA ETHMOIDALIS OSSIS FRONTALIS. **ethmoidal n. of frontal bone** INCISURA ETHMOIDALIS OSSIS FRONTALIS.. **fibular n. of tibia** INCISURA FIBULARIS TIBIAE. **frontal n.** INCISURA FRONTALIS. **n. of frontal bone** INCISURA FRONTALIS. **gastric n.** INCISURA ANGULARIS GASTRICA. **greater ischiatic n.** INCISURA ISCHIADICA MAJOR. **greater sciatic n.** INCISURA ISCHIADICA MAJOR. **hamular n.** SULCUS HAMULI PTERYGOIDEI. **Hutchinson's crescentic n.** A notch in the incisal edge of a permanent incisor tooth, caused by congenital syphilis. **inferior n. of neck of pancreas** INCISURA PANCREATIS. **inferior thyroid n.** INCISURA THYROIDEA INFERIOR. **inferior vertebral n.** INCISURA VERTEBRALIS INFERIOR. **interarytenoid n.** INCISURA INTERARYTENOIDEA LARYNGIS. **interclavicular n.** INCISURA JUGULARIS STERNI. **intercondylar n.** FOSSA INTERCONDYLARIS FEMORIS. **intercondylar n. of femur** FOSSA INTERCONDYLARIS FEMORIS. **interlobar n.** INCISURA LIGAMENTI TERETIS. **intertragic n.** INCISURA INTERTRAGICA. **jugular n. of occipital bone** INCISURA JUGULARIS OSSIS OCCIPITALIS. **jugular n. of sternum** INCISURA JUGULARIS STERNI. **jugular n. of temporal bone** INCISURA JUGULARIS OSSIS TEMPORALIS. **lacrimal n. of maxilla** INCISURA LACRIMALIS MAXILLAE. **lesser ischiatic n.** INCISURA ISCHIADICA MINOR. **lesser sciatic n.** INCISURA ISCHIADICA MINOR. **n. of ligamentum teres** INCISURA LIGAMENTI TERETIS. **mandibular n.** INCISURA MANDIBULAE. **marsupial n.** *Obs.* INCISURA CEREBELLI POSTERIOR. **mastoid n.** INCISURA MASTOIDEA OSSIS TEMPORALIS. **median prostatic n.** A well marked notch at the terminal end of the vertical median sulcus. It is located on the posterior border of the base of the prostate, just anterior to which is a deep depression for the entrance of the ejaculatory ducts. **nasal n. of maxilla** INCISURA NASALIS MAXILLAE. **palatine n. of palatine bone** INCISURA SPHENOPALATINA OSSIS PALATINI. **pancreatic n.** INCISURA PANCREATIS. **parietal n. of temporal bone** INCISURA PARIETALIS OSSIS TEMPORALIS. **parotid n.** The space occupied by the parotid gland, between the ramus of the mandible and the mastoid process of the temporal bone. **popliteal n.** A groove in the extreme posterior part of the area intercondylaris posterior on the tibia where the posterior cruciate ligament is attached. **posterior cerebellar n.** INCISURA CEREBELLI POSTERIOR. **preoccipital n.** INCISURA PREOCCIPITALIS. **presternal n.** INCISURA JUGULARIS STERNI. **pterygoid n.** INCISURA PTERYGOIDEA. **radial n. of ulna** INCISURA RADIALIS ULNAE. **rivinian n.** INCISURA TYMPANICA. **n. of Rivinus** INCISURA TYMPANICA. **scapular n.** INCISURA SCAPULAE. **sphenopalatine n. of palatine bone** INCISURA SPHENOPALATINA OSSIS PALATINI. **spinoglenoid n.** The arched gap between the concave lateral margin of the spine of the scapula and the dorsal surface of the neck of the scapula. **sternal n.** INCISURA JUGULARIS STERNI. **superior thyroid n.** INCISURA THYROIDEA SUPERIOR. **superior vertebral**

**n.** INCISURA VERTEBRALIS SUPERIOR. **supraorbital n.** 1 INCISURA SUPRAORBITALIS. 2 INCISURA FRONTALIS. **suprascapular n.** INCISURA SCAPULAE. **suprasternal n.** INCISURA JUGULARIS STERNI. **tentorial n.** INCISURA TENTORII. **terminal n. of auricle** INCISURA TERMINALIS AURIS. **trochlear n. of ulna** INCISURA TROCHLEARIS ULNAE. **tympanic n.** INCISURA TYMPANICA. **ulnar n. of radius** INCISURA ULNARIS RADII. **umbilical n.** INCISURA LIGAMENTI TERETIS.

**notching / rib n.** Localized erosions of the undersurfaces of ribs by enlarged and tortuous intercostal arteries, most commonly demonstrated radiologically and typically seen in patients with coarctation of the aorta.

**note** A sound, as one heard on auscultation. **bell n.** COIN SOUND. **cracked-pot n.** See under CRACKED-POT SOUND. **percussion n.** A sound produced by percussion, as of the chest.

***Notechis*** \nōtē′kis\ A genus of active, aggressive, and fast-moving venomous snakes of the Elapidae family, occurring in Australia. They are considered extremely dangerous.

**notencephalocele** \nō′tensef′əlōsēl′\ [*not(o)-* + ENCEPHALOCELE] A protrusion of the brain through a developmental defect in the posterior part of the skull.

**Nothnagel** [Carl Wilhelm Hermann *Nothnagel*, Austrian physician, 1841–1905] See under SIGN, SYNDROME, ACROPARESTHESIA.

**notifiable** \nō′tifī′əbl\ Requiring notification by statute or regulation to a competent authority, as a government health department or local health officer, of a newly diagnosed case of a specified disease, an industrial injury, or other specified event.

**notification of birth** The legal requirement to inform a competent authority, usually a local health officer, of the occurrence of a birth. In some countries, notification of birth is required by law in addition to a legal obligation to register the birth with a registration officer.

**noto-** \nō′tə-\ [Gk *nōton* the back] A combining form denoting the back.

**notochord** \nō′tōkôrd\ [NOTO- + CHORD] A rod-shaped body composed of cells derived from the mesoblast, below the primitive groove of the embryo, found in all species of the phylum Chordata. It extends from the tail region cranially to the caudal edge of the thickened prochordal plate. In adult mammals it probably only persists as the nucleus pulposus, within the intervertebral disk. The notochord probably acts as the inductor for the axial nervous system. Also *chorda dorsalis.*

**notochordoma** \-kôrdō′mə\ [NOTO- + CHORDOMA] CHORDOMA.

**notogenesis** \-jen′əsis\ [NOTO- + GENESIS] The formation of the notochord in the early embryo.

**notomyelitis** \-mī′əlī′tis\ [NOTO- + MYELITIS] *Obs.* MYELITIS.

**not-self** NONSELF.

**novarsenobenzene** NEOARSPHENAMINE.

**novarsenobenzol** NEOARSPHENAMINE.

**novaurantia** \nō′vəyooran′shə\ ORANGE G.

**novobiocin** \nō′vəbī′əsin\ A toxic antibiotic with a narrow spectrum of activity. It is no longer used, but it is of value in research because it inhibits DNA gyrase. Also *cardelmycin.*

**Novocain** A proprietary name for procaine hydrochloride.

**Novy** [Frederick George *Novy*, U.S. bacteriologist, 1864–1957] Novy, McNeal and Nicolle medium. See under MEDIUM.

**noxious** \näk′shəs\ [L *noxius* (from *noxa* harm, injury, akin to *nocere* to injure) hurtful, injurious] Harmful or injurious to health.

**noxious thing** In forensic medicine, a substance unlawfully administered to another or taken by oneself with a deliberate intent to cause ill effects or death. It may be a poison or any substance capable of producing injury. The amount administered, the form of administration, and an individual's response must be considered before a substance can be designated a noxious thing.

**noy** \noi\ A unit of perceived noisiness equal to the perceived noisiness of random noise in the frequency band 910–1090 Hz at a sound pressure level of 40 dB above 0.0002 microbar.

**Np** Symbol for the element, neptunium.

**NPH** neutral protamine Hagedorn (insulin).

**NPH Iletin** A proprietary name for isophane insulin suspension.

**NPN** nonprotein nitrogen.

**NRC** normal retinal correspondence.

**n.s.** not significant (i.e., statistically, or, in common usage, having a P value greater than 0.05).

**NSHD** nodular sclerosing Hodgkin's disease.

**NSILA** nonsuppressible insulinlike activity.

**NSR** normal sinus rhythm.

**N-terminal** Denoting the end of a polypeptide chain in which the amino acid has a free $NH_2$ group. Also *amino-terminal.*

**NTP** Symbol for normal temperature and pressure (usually 0°C and 1 standard atmosphere).

**nucha** \noo′kə\ [Med. L, perhaps orig. a scribal error for *nucra*, from Arabic *nuqra* the nape, by confusion with Arabic *nukhāʻ* spinal marrow] The back of the neck. It extends vertically between a horizontal line through the external occipital protuberance and one through the spine of the seventh cervical vertebra, and is bounded laterally approximately by the lateral margin of trapezius muscle on each side. Also *nape.*

**Nuck** [Anton *Nuck*, Dutch anatomist, 1650–1692] Canal of Nuck. See under PERITONEOVAGINAL CANAL.

**nuclear** \n$^y$oo′klē·ər\ [*nucle(us)* + -AR] Pertaining to a nucleus.

**nuclease** \n$^y$oo′klē·ās\ Any enzyme that catalyzes the hydrolysis of nucleic acid. **micrococcal n.** An enzyme (EC 3.1.31.1) from *Micrococcus* which hydrolyzes a polynucleotide, by endonucleolytic cleavage, to 3′-phosphomono- and oligonucleotide products.

**nucleated** \n$^y$oo′klē·ā′tid\ Having a nucleus, as a eukaryotic cell.

**nucleation** \n$^y$oo′klē·ā′shən\ [*nucle(us)* + -ATION] The process of formation of nuclei; specifically, the formation of small crystals in a saturated solution, a process necessary before crystal growth can occur.

**nuclei** \n$^y$oo′klē·ī\ Plural of NUCLEUS.

**nucleic acid** A nucleotide polymer composed of subunits which are either deoxyribonucleotides or ribonucleotides, joined to each other by phosphodiester bridges between (usually) the 5′-hydroxyl group of one nucleotide and the 3′-hydroxyl group of another. It is one of a group of long linear molecules found in chromosomes, mitochondria, ribosomes, bacteria, and viruses. The molecule may be DNA or various types of RNA. Upon hydrolysis it yields purine and pyrimidine bases, phosphoric acid, and a pentose sugar. Also *nucleinic acid.* **yeast n.** RIBONUCLEIC ACID.

**nucleiform** \n$^y$ooklē′ifôrm\ Having the general form of a cell nucleus.

**nucleinic acid** NUCLEIC ACID.

**nucleo-** \nʸoo′klē·ō-\ [L *nucleus* (for *nuculeus*; from *nux*, gen. *nucis*, nut) kernel of a nut, stone of a fruit] A combining form meaning nucleus, nuclear.

**nucleocapsid** \-kap′sid\ A unit of viral structure which consists of a nucleic acid encapsulated in a protein coat. A simple virus may be a single nucleocapsid, or nucleocapsids may be only part of the structure of a more complex virus.

**nucleography** \nʸoo′klē·äg′rəfē\ DISKOGRAPHY.

**nucleohistone** \-his′tōn\ [NUCLEO- + HIST- + Gk -*ōnē*, fem. patronymic suffix] A complex of histone proteins and deoxyribonucleic acid found in the cell nucleus.

**nucleoid** \nʸoo′klē·oid\ [*nucle(us)* + -OID] **1** Having the appearance of a nucleus; resembling a nucleus. **2** A structure of variable shape in prokaryotes, containing the genetic material of the cell. Unlike the eukaryotic nucleus, the prokaryotic nucleoid does not have a membrane.

**nucleoli** \nʸooklē′əlī\ Plural of NUCLEOLUS.

**nucleolonema** \-lōnē′mə\ A threadlike network composed of granules arranged in irregular rows in the nucleolus of the cell. The network is composed of nucleolar genes involved in the transcription of ribosomal RNA. **reticular n.** A pattern of nucleolar structure in which the pars granulosa forms an open framework.

**nucleolus** \nʸooklē′ələs\ [dim. of NUCLEUS. See NUCLEUS.] (*pl.* nucleoli) A dense spherical accumulation of fibers and granules found in the nucleus of most eukaryotic cells. It is the site of transcription of ribosomal ribonucleic acid and of the production of ribosomes. The size of the nucleolus and the number of nucleoli varies with the requirement of a given cell for ribosomes and protein synthesis. Also *nucleolonucleus, micronucleus, plasmosome* (obs.). Adj. nucleolar. **chromatin n.** KARYOSOME. **false n.** KARYOSOME. **secondary n.** A small granular mass located near and resembling the nucleolus.

**nucleolymph** \nʸoo′klē·əlimf′\ [NUCLEO- + LYMPH] KARYOLYMPH.

**nucleomicrosome** NUCLEOSOME.

**nucleon** \nʸoo′klē·än\ [*nucle(us)* + *(prot)on*] One of the building blocks of an atomic nucleus, especially a proton or a neutron.

**nucleophilic** \-fil′ik\ Having an affinity for the nucleus of a cell, as a stain.

**nucleoplasm** \nʸoo′klē·əplazm′\ The protoplasm of the cell nucleus. Also *karyoplasm*.

**nucleoprotein** \-prō′tēn\ A complex of protein and nucleic acid, such as chromatin.

**nucleorrhexis** \nʸoo′klē·ôrek′sis\ [NUCLEO- + -RRHEXIS] Degradation of a cell nucleus in which the nuclear material forms irregular cytoplasmic granules which are excreted from the cell. Also *karyorrhexis, karyoclasis*.

**nucleosidase** **1** The enzyme (EC 3.2.2.1) that hydrolyzes an *N*-ribosylpurine to ribose and a purine. **2** Any enzyme that catalyzes the hydrolysis of a nucleoside.

**nucleoside** \nʸoo′klē·əsīd′\ A molecule formed by bonding a purine or pyrimidine base with a pentose sugar, with an *N*-glycoside bond.

**nucleoside deaminase** An enzyme which catalyzes the deamination of the purine of a nucleoside, adenosine forming inosine, and guanosine forming xanthosine.

**nucleosidediphosphatase** The enzyme (EC 3.6.1.6) that catalyzes the hydrolysis of a nucleoside 5′-diphosphate to orthophosphate and a nucleoside 5′-phosphate. It is found preferentially at the forming face of the Golgi body in the cell cytoplasm and serves as an indicator of the inner face. Also *thiamin pyrophosphatase*.

**nucleoside diphosphate** A nucleoside esterified on one of its hydroxyl groups, nearly always on O-5′, with diphosphoric acid. Such compounds are formed by transfer of phosphate groups from nucleoside triphosphates, which are common biologic phosphate donors.

**nucleoside diphosphate kinase** Any of a class of enzymes (EC 2.7.4.6) which catalyze the conversion of adenosine triphosphate and a nucleoside diphosphate to adenosine diphosphate and a nucleotide triphosphate. Also *nucleoside diphosphokinase*.

**nucleoside diphosphate sugars** Any of the compounds consisting of nucleoside diphosphate with a simple, or complex, sugar bonded to the 5′-diphosphate group. Examples are uridine diphosphoglucose, and guanosine diphosphomannose.

**nucleoside diphosphokinase** NUCLEOSIDE DIPHOSPHATE KINASE.

**nucleoside monophosphate** Any nucleoside esterified with phosphoric acid on one of its hydroxyl groups. Unless otherwise indicated, the position of substitution is usually O-5′.

**nucleosidemonophosphate kinase** The enzyme (EC 2.7.4.4) that catalyzes the transfer of a group from ATP to a nucleoside 5′-phosphate to form ADP and a nucleoside 5′-diphosphate. This is usually a prelude to the building of a nucleoside 5′-triphosphate.

**nucleoside phosphate** PENTOSE NUCLEOTIDE.

**nucleoside triphosphate** A nucleoside esterified, usually on O-5′, with triphosphoric acid. Nucleoside triphosphates are the precursors of nucleic acids, and they also act as phosphate donors and as the precursors of cyclic nucleotides.

**nucleosin** \nʸoo′klē·əsin′\ THYMOPOIETIN.

**nucleosis** \nʸoo′klē·ō′sis\ The proliferation of nuclei within a single cell, such as that occurring in subsarcolemmal nuclei during regeneration of injured skeletal muscle cells. *Seldom used.*

**nucleosome** The fundamental packing unit of chromatin. It is composed of a core particle and a unit of linker DNA for a total of about 200 base pairs of DNA. Also called *nucleomicrosome*.

**nucleospindle** \-spin′dl\ The achromatic mitotic spindle formed during division of a cell nucleus.

**nucleotidase** **1** Any enzyme that catalyzes the hydrolysis of a nucleotide. **2** The enzyme (EC 3.1.3.31) that catalyzes the hydrolysis of many nucleoside 2′-, 3′- and 5′-phosphates to the nucleoside and orthophosphate. Also *phosphonuclease*.

**nucleotide** \nʸoo′klē·ətīd′\ A molecule formed from the combination of one nitrogenous base (purine or pyrimidine), a sugar (ribose or deoxyribose), and a phosphate group. It is a hydrolysis product of a nucleic acid.

**nucleotide pyrophosphatase** The enzyme (EC 3.6.1.9) that catalyzes the hydrolysis of a dinucleotide in which there is a residue of diphosphate (pyrophosphate) with breakage of the anhydride bond in this group, so that two molecules of mononucleotide are formed.

**nucleotidyl** The group formed by removing hydroxyl from the phosphorus atom of a nucleotide.

**nucleotidyltransferase** Any enzyme transferring a nucleotidyl group, usually using a nucleoside 5′-triphosphate as the donor. Such enzymes include DNA and RNA polymerases.

**nucleotoxin** \-täk′sin\ [NUCLEO- + TOXIN] **1** Any substance which is toxic to the cell nucleus. **2** A toxic material which is produced by the cell nucleus.

**nucleotropic** \-träp′ik\ Denoting antimicrobial or antiviral agents that alter nucleic acids.

# nucleus

**nucleus** \nʸoo′klē·əs\ [L (for *nuculeus;* from *nux,* gen. *nucis,* nut, akin to Old English *hnutu* nut), kernel of a nut, stone of a fruit] (*pl.* nuclei) **1** A membrane-bounded compartment in a eukaryotic cell which contains the genetic material and the nucleoli. The nucleus represents the control center of the cell. The nucleus divides by mitosis or meiosis. **2** The inner or central part of any structure; core. **3** In neuroanatomy, an aggregate of neurons. **4** The positively charged central core of the atom, consisting of protons and neutrons, except in the ordinary hydrogen atom, where there is a proton only. Over 99.9% of an atom's mass is in the nucleus. **abducens n.** NUCLEUS NERVI ABDUCENTIS. **n. of abducens nerve** NUCLEUS NERVI ABDUCENTIS. **n. abducentis** NUCLEUS NERVI ABDUCENTIS. **n. accessorius** NUCLEUS OCULOMOTORIUS ACCESSORIUS. **accessory n.** NUCLEUS OCULOMOTORIUS ACCESSORIUS. **accessory n. of auditory nerve** NUCLEI COCHLEARES VENTRALIS ET DORSALIS. **accessory cuneate n.** NUCLEUS CUNEATUS ACCESSORIUS. **n. of accessory nerve** NUCLEUS NERVI ACCESSORII. **accessory oculomotor n.** NUCLEUS OCULOMOTORIUS ACCESSORIUS. **n. accumbens septi** A nucleus in the floor of the anterior horn of the lateral ventricle of the brain between the head of the caudate nucleus and the anterior perforated substance. It is closely associated with the inferior part of the septal gray matter and is believed to be an extension of the corpus striatum. **acetabular n.** OS ACETABULI. ULI. **nuclei of acoustic nerve** NUCLEI NERVI VESTIBULOCOCHLEARIS. **n. acusticus** Any of the nuclei comprising the nuclei nervi vestibulocochlearis. **n. acusticus inferior et lateralis** NUCLEI COCHLEARES VENTRALIS ET DORSALIS. **n. acusticus superior** NUCLEUS VESTIBULARIS SUPERIOR. **n. alae cinereae** NUCLEUS DORSALIS NERVI VAGI. **n. ambiguus** [NA] A column of cells in the lower half of the medulla oblongata, approximately halfway between the spinal nucleus of the trigeminal nerve and the inferior olivary complex. The nucleus receives afferents from the corticobulbar system and from the pharyngeal and laryngeal muscles and mucosa via the vagal, glossopharyngeal, and trigeminal nerves. Efferent fibers join the vagal, glossopharyngeal, and cranial part of the spinal accessory nerves. Also *ambiguous nucleus, laryngeal nucleus, vagoglossopharyngeal nucleus* (seldom used). **n. amygdalae** CORPUS AMYGDALOIDEUM. **n. amygdaliformis of J. Stilling** NUCLEUS SUBTHALAMICUS. **amygdaloid n.** CORPUS AMYGDALOIDEUM. **n. angularis** NUCLEUS VESTIBULARIS SUPERIOR. **n. of the ansa lenticularis** Small groups of neurons scattered along the course of the ansa lenticularis in the subthalamus. **anterior cochlear n.** See under NUCLEI COCHLEARES VENTRALIS ET DORSALIS. **nuclei anteriores thalami** [NA] Three groups of neurons lying beneath the dorsal surface of the rostral pole of the thalamus, where they form a distinct swelling, the tuberculum anterius thalami. The cell complex comprises a large principle nucleus, the anteroventral, and two accessory cell groups, the anterodorsal and anteromedial. The major afferent fiber source is the mamillary body, and all of the nuclei appear to project to the cingulate gyrus, Brodmann's areas 23, 24 and 32. These cell groups and their input and output connections form the thalamic portion of the Papez circuit. Also *anterior nuclei of thalamus.* **anterior median n.** The most rostral cell contingent of the paired visceral nuclei collectively referred to as the Edinger-Westphal nucleus. This portion of the oculomotor nerve nucleus lies on each side of the raphe and gives rise to uncrossed preganglionic parasympathetic fibers that emerge with the somatic root fibers. **anterior olfactory n.** NUCLEUS NERVI OLFACTORII. **anterior nuclei of thalamus** NUCLEI ANTERIORES THALAMI. **anterior ventral n. of thalamus** NUCLEUS ANTEROVENTRALIS. **n. anterodorsalis** [NA] One of three components of the nuclei anteriores thalami. It contains small round cell bodies that receive afferents from the lateral mamillary nucleus and send efferents to the cingulate gyrus via the anterior limb of the internal capsule. **anterolateral ventral n.** NUCLEUS VENTRALIS ANTEROLATERALIS. **n. anteromedialis** [NA] One of the three components of the nuclei anteriores thalami. It contains small round cells that receive afferents from the medial mamillary nucleus and send efferents to the cingulate gyrus. **n. anteroventralis** [NA] One of the three components of the nuclei anteriores thalami. It contains small round cells that receive afferents from the medial mamillary nucleus and fornix and send efferents to the cingulate gyrus. Also *anterior ventral nucleus of thalamus.* **nuclei arciformes** NUCLEI ARCUATI. **arcuate n.** NUCLEUS VENTRALIS POSTEROMEDIALIS. **nuclei arcuati** [NA] Small irregular masses of grey matter found along the ventromedial aspect of the pyramid of the medulla oblongata. Afferent fibers are derived from the cerebral cortex, while efferent fibers project to the cerebellum as the crossed external arcuate fibers. Also *arcuate nuclei of medulla oblongata, nuclei arciformes.* **auditory nuclei** NUCLEI NERVI VESTIBULOCOCHLEARIS. **nuclei of auditory nerve** NUCLEI NERVI VESTIBULOCOCHLEARIS. **autonomic n. of oculomotor nerve** NUCLEUS OCULOMOTORIUS ACCESSORIUS. **basal n.** **1** *Seldom used* NUCLEUS OLIVARIS. **2** Basal ganglia: used in the plural. **n. basalis** *Seldom used* NUCLEUS OLIVARIS. **basal olfactory nuclei** Cell masses on the ventral and medial aspects of the cerebral hemisphere related to olfactory function. They include the nucleus of the olfactory tract, olfactory trigone, olfactory area, gyrus paraterminalis, and parolfactory area. **Bekhterev's n.** NUCLEUS VESTIBULARIS SUPERIOR. **n. of Burdach's column** NUCLEUS CUNEATUS. **n. caudalis centralis** [NA] A midline group of cells in the caudal third of the oculomotor nucleus. It gives rise to fibers, both crossed and uncrossed, that innervate the levator palpebrae muscle. Also *central caudal nucleus.* **caudal vestibular n.** NUCLEUS VESTIBULARIS INFERIOR. **n. caudatus** [NA] An elongated, arched mass of gray matter that forms one of the basal ganglia located deep to the cerebral cortex and bordering the lateral ventricle. It consists of a pear-shaped head lying rostral and lateral to the thalamus, a more slender body extending along the dorsolateral border of the thalamus, and a long curved tail that tapers around the roof of the ventricular temporal horn as far as the central nucleus of the amygdaloid body. The caudate nucleus, together with the putamen, from which it is separated by the internal capsule, form a functional unit known as the neostriatum of the basal ganglia. Major sources of afferent fibers are the cerebral cortex, medial thalamic nuclei, and substantia nigra. Most of its efferent fibers project to the putamen and globus pallidus. The caudate and lentiform nuclei are usually grouped together as the corpus striatum, and they help form the extrapyramidal system that influences the motor functions of the cerebral cortex, brainstem, and spinal cord. Also *caudate nucleus, caudate, caudatum* (seldom used), *intraventricular nucleus of corpus striatum* (outmoded). **central caudal n.** NUCLEUS CAUDALIS CENTRALIS. **n. centralis thalami** A group of small and medium-sized neurons lying close to the wall of the third ventricle between the medial and posterior ventral complex of nuclei. They occupy the medial half of the intralaminar nuclei and are considered part of the intralaminar or nonspecific nuclei of the thalamus. Their connections are not completely understood, but they are believed to receive afferents from various cortical areas, the basal ganglia, more laterally-lying thalamic nuclei, and the brainstem. Efferent fibers probably project back upon most of these sites. Also *central nucleus of thalamus.* **centrodorsal n.** NUCLEUS PROPRIUS OF POSTERIOR HORN. **n. centromedianus thalami** NUCLEUS MEDIALIS CENTRALIS THALAMI. **n. cerebelli** NUCLEUS DENTATUS CEREBELLI. **cervical n.** NUCLEUS LATERALIS CERVICALIS. **n. cinereum** The central gray substance of the spinal cord. *Obs.* **n. of circumolivary bundle of the pyramid** See under CIRCUMOLIVARY BUNDLE OF THE PYRAMID. **Clarke's n.** NUCLEUS THORACICUS. **n. of Clarke's column** NUCLEUS THORACICUS. **clavate n.** NUCLEUS GRACILIS. **Clarke-Monakow n.** NUCLEUS CUNEATUS ACCESSORIUS. **nuclei cochleares ventralis et dorsalis** [NA] The ventral, or anterior, and dorsal, or posterior, nuclei of the cochlear division of the eighth cranial nerve. These structures form a more or less continuous cell mass lateral and dorsolateral to the inferior cerebellar peduncle near the pontomedullary junction, but each contains distinctive cell types and cytoarchitectural organization. The dorsal cochlear nucleus forms an eminence (the acoustic tubercle) on the most lateral portion of the ventricular floor. Both nuclei receive axons that are the central processes of cells in the spiral ganglion. Efferent fibers from both nuclei are grouped into three acoustic striae, which are distributed bilaterally to several auditory processing centers in the brainstem, including the superior olive, the internal and external preolivary nuclei, the nucleus of the trapezoid body, and the nucleus of the lateral lemniscus. Also *accessory nucleus of auditory nerve, nucleus acusticus inferior et lateralis, nuclei nervi cochlearis, nuclei of cochlear nerve, cochlear nuclei.* **n. colliculi inferioris** [NA] A mass of nerve cell bodies comprising most of the substance of the inferior colliculus. They are divided into three groups: an ovoid cell mass, the central nucleus; a thin dorsal layer of cells, or cortex; and a pericollicular tegmentum surrounding the central nucleus on its ventral, lateral, and medial aspects and containing most of the myelinated fibers entering and leaving the colliculus. Afferent fibers come from the lateral lemniscus, the opposite inferior colliculus, the reticular formation, the ipsilateral medial geniculate body, and the auditory cortex. Efferent fibers project to the medial geniculate body, the contralateral inferior colliculus, the superior colliculus, and to more caudal relay nuclei in the auditory system. Also *nucleus of inferior colliculus.* **commissural n.** The right and left dorsal motor nuclei, when they merge at the midline to form a single cell cluster. **conjugation n.** ZYGOTE NUCLEUS. **n. corporis geniculati lateralis** [NA] The nucleus of the lateral geniculate body, composed of a large, horseshoe-shaped, laminated mass of cells dorsally and a less defined ventral component. The dorsal complex consists of six concentric cell layers separated by intervening fiber bands. Crossed fibers from the optic tract terminate in laminae 1, 4, and 6, and uncrossed fibers end in laminae 2, 3, and 5. Corticogeniculate afferents arise from visual area 18. Efferent fibers project mainly to the primary visual cortex (area 17). The ventral nucleus is believed to represent a subthalamic structure related to the zona incerta. Also *nucleus of lateral geniculate body.* **n. corporis geniculati medialis** [NA] A neuron complex composed of small cells dorsally and large cells ventrally. Afferent fibers originate in a number of secondary auditory nuclei and the inferior colliculus, entering via the brachium of the inferior colliculus. Efferent fibers project to the superior temporal convolution via the auditory (geniculotemporal) radiation. Also *nucleus of medial geniculate body, medial geniculate nucleus, nucleus of internal geniculate body.* **nuclei corporis mamillaris** [NA] The nuclei of the mamillary body, which is located on the ventral surface of the posterior hypothalamus. There are three major cell groups: medial, intermediate, and lateral, of which the medial group is largest in man. The nuclei receive fibers from basal olfactory areas, septum, and fornix, and project to the anterior thalamus and mesencephalic tegmentum via mamillothalamic and mamillotegmental fasciculi. Also *nuclei of mamillary body.* **nuclei corporis trapezoidei** [NA] Several groups of nerve cells scattered among the fibers of the trapezoid body, medial to the superior olive in the tegmentum of the lower pons. These large, globular neurons receive thick axons from the contralateral cochlear nuclei that terminate on the trapezoidal cell bodies by means of large calixes in a one-to-one relationship. The cells project to the lateral superior olive on the same side. **cortical n. of amygdala** PERIAMYGDALOID CORTEX. **nuclei of cranial nerves** NUCLEI NERVORUM CRANIALIUM. **n. cuneatus** [NA] A wedge-shaped mass of neurons on the dorsolateral aspect of the posterior medulla oblongata just above the spinobulbar junction. It is one of two major nuclei of the posterior funiculi and receives the ascending, heavily myelinated axonal branches of dorsal root ganglia, which transmit sensory impulses from the upper six thoracic and all cervical dermatomes. These fibers ascend in the fasciculus cuneatus and end in oblique serial laminae on the cells of the nucleus cuneatus. Efferent axons project ventromedially as internal arcuate fibers, cross the midline, and continue rostrally toward the thalamus as the medial lemnisci. Also *cuneate nucleus, nucleus of Burdach's column, nucleus funiculi cuneati.* **n. cuneatus accessorius** A group of nerve cells lying lateral to the nucleus cuneatus on the dorsolateral aspect of the caudal medulla oblongata. It receives heavily myelinated axons from dorsal root ganglia transmitting impulses from the first cervical through first thoracic dermatomes. It relays information from muscle spindles, group II fibers, and cutaneous afferents, and gives rise to cuneocerebellar fibers which enter the cerebellum via the inferior cerebellar peduncle. This nucleus is the medullary equivalent of the dorsal nucleus of Clarke. Also *lateral cuneate nucleus, accessory cuneate nucleus, external cuneate nucleus, Monakow's nucleus, Clarke-Monakow nucleus.* **n. of Darkschewitsch** One of three accessory oculomotor nuclei lying inside the ventrolateral border of the periaqueductal gray matter and lateral to the somatic cell columns of the oculomotor (III) complex. It is believed to receive fibers from the medial longitudinal fasciculus and superior colliculus. Its efferent fibers enter the posterior commissure, but do not reach the oculomotor complex or lower brain stem. Also *Darkschewitsch's ganglion.* **daughter n.** Either of the two nuclei resulting from mitosis. Each daughter nucleus has the same genetic information as the mother nucleus. **n. of Deiters** NUCLEUS VESTIBULARIS LATERALIS. **dental n.** DENTAL PULP. **n. dentatus cerebelli** [NA] The largest of the deep, or roof, nuclei of the cerebellum, situated in the cerebellar white matter just lateral to the nucleus emboliformis. It receives axons from the Purkinje cells of the neocerebellum and collaterals from cerebellopetal mossy fibers. Its efferent fibers form most of the superior cerebellar peduncle and project mainly to the contralateral red nucleus and the ventrolateral nucleus of the thalamus. Also *dentate* *nucleus, dentate nucleus of cerebellum, nucleus cerebelli, dentatum, nucleus oliva cerebellaris, corpus dentatum cerebelli* (obs.). **n. of descending fifth nerve** NUCLEUS TRACTUS SPINALIS NERVI TRIGEMINI. **descending vestibular n.** NUCLEUS VESTIBULARIS INFERIOR. **diploid n.** A nucleus which contains two haploid sets of chromosomes, typical of the somatic cells of most animals. **dorsal accessory olivary n.** NUCLEUS OLIVARIS ACCESSORIUS DORSALIS. **dorsal n. of Clarke** NUCLEUS DORSALIS CLARKII. **dorsal cochlear n.** See under NUCLEI COCHLEARES VENTRALIS ET DORSALIS. **dorsal n. of glossopharyngeal nerve** NUCLEUS DORSALIS NERVI GLOSSOPHARYNGEI. **n. dorsalis clarkii** A column of neurons located in the medial part of spinal cord lamina VII at the base of the dorsal horn, and extending from $C_8$ through $L_2$ or $L_3$. Afferent fibers convey impulses from stretch, touch, and pressure receptors located in the lower extremities, abdomen, and trunk. Efferent fibers constitute the posterior spinocerebellar tract and project rostrally to the cerebellum. Also *dorsal nucleus of Clarke, Clarke's column of spinal cord, nucleus dorsalis stillingi.* **n. dorsalis corporis trapezoidei** *Seldom used* NUCLEUS OLIVARIS SUPERIOR. **n. dorsalis nervi glossopharyngei** The rostral portion of the cell column forming the dorsal nucleus of the vagus (X) nerve. It is believed to contribute some fibers to the glossopharyngeal nerve. Also *dorsal nucleus of glossopharyngeal nerve.* **n. dorsalis nervi vagi** [NA] The dorsal motor nucleus of the vagus nerve, situated dorsal or dorsolateral to the nucleus intercalatus. It receives afferents from sensory nuclei of the glossopharyngeal and vagus nerves and gives origin to parasympathetic fibers, many of which are secretomotor in function. Also *nucleus alae cinereae, dorsal nucleus of vagus nerve.* **n. dorsalis stillingi** NUCLEUS DORSALIS CLARKII. **dorsal lateral n.** NUCLEUS DORSOLATERALIS. **dorsal tegmental nuclei** NUCLEI TEGMENTI MESENCEPHALICI. **dorsal n. of trapezoid body** NUCLEUS OLIVARIS SUPERIOR. **dorsal n. of vagus nerve** NUCLEUS DORSALIS NERVI VAGI. **n. dorsolateralis** [NA] A dorsally situated cell group in the lateral part of the oculomotor nuclear complex that innervates the inferior rectus muscle. Also *dorsolateral nucleus, dorsal lateral nucleus.* **n. dorsomedialis hypothalami** The more dorsal of two cell groups in the medial part of the tuberal region of the hypothalamus. Also *nucleus hypothalamicus dorsomedialis, dorsomedial nucleus of hypothalamus.* **dorsomedial n. of thalamus** A prominent nuclear mass lying between the periventricular gray matter and the internal medullary lamina. It is composed of a magnocellular zone lying medially and a larger, more lateral, parvicellular zone. Extensive two-way connections exist with the cortex, basal forebrain, and amygdala, hypothalamus, and other areas of the thalamus. Connections between the parvicellular area and the prefrontal cortex are especially prominent in man. Also *medial nucleus of thalamus, nucleus medialis thalami* (seldom used). **droplet n.** The dried or partially dried residue, 0.1–3μm in diameter, of an air-borne droplet that results from coughing, sneezing, or spraying. **Edinger's n.** NUCLEUS OCULOMOTORIUS ACCESSORIUS. **Edinger-Westphal n.** NUCLEUS OCULOMOTORIUS ACCESSORIUS. **n. of the eleventh cranial nerve** NUCLEUS NERVI ACCESSORII. **n. emboliformis cerebelli** [NA] A deep cerebellar (roof) nucleus found in great apes and man, lying between the nucleus globosus medially and the nucleus dentatus laterally. It receives fibers from Purkinje cells in the cerebellar hemispheres, and collaterals from cerebellopetal afferents. Its efferents project to the mesencephalon and thalamus via the superior cerebellar peduncle. Also *embolus, emboliform nucleus of cerebellum.* **entopeduncular n.** NUCLEUS INTERPEDUNCULARIS. **external cuneate n.** NUCLEUS CUNEATUS ACCESSORIUS. **n. facialis** NUCLEUS NERVI FACIALIS. **n. of facial nerve** NUCLEUS NERVI FACIALIS. **n. fastigii cerebelli** [NA] The most medial and phylogenetically oldest of the deep cerebellar nuclei, near the midline in the roof of the fourth ventricle. It receives fibers from Purkinje cells in the cerebellar vermis, and collaterals from olivocerebellar afferents. Efferent fibers reach the brainstem via the uncinate bundle (of Russell) and the juxtarestiform body. Also *fastigial nucleus of cerebellum, nucleus tecti, nucleus of roof of cerebellum.* **fertilization n.** ZYGOTE NUCLEUS. **n. funiculi cuneati** NUCLEUS CUNEATUS. **n. funiculi gracilis** NUCLEUS GRACILIS. **gametic n.** MICRONUCLEUS. **n. gelatinosus** NUCLEUS PULPOSUS DISCI INTERVERTEBRALIS. **gingival n.** A cerebellar nucleus appearing during the fourth month of fetal life. **n. globosus cerebelli** [NA] A deep cerebellar nucleus peculiar to the great apes and man, located between the emboliform nucleus laterally and the fastigial nucleus medially. It receives afferents from Purkinje cells of the paravermal cerebellar cortex, and collaterals from many cerebellar afferent fiber systems. Its axons leave the cerebellum primarily via the superior cerebellar peduncle, and project to various brainstem and thalamic nuclei. Also *globose nucleus, spherical nucleus* (seldom used). **n. of Goll's column** NUCLEUS GRACILIS. **gonad n.** MICRONUCLEUS. **n. gracilis** [NA] A column of neurons in the caudal portion of the medulla oblongata at the rostral end of the fasciculus gracilis of the spinal cord. This nucleus, which serves as the site of the initial synapse for the long ascending branches of cells in the dorsal root ganglia, also receives collaterals from the brainstem reticular formation and the pyramidal tract. Its efferent fibers exit the nucleus ventromedially, decussate, and turn rostrally to form the medial lemniscus, which projects to the nucleus ventrobasolateralis of the thalamus. Also *gracile nucleus, clavate nucleus, nucleus funiculi gracilis, nucleus of Goll's column.* **gray n.** SUBSTANTIA GRISEA MEDULLAE SPINALIS. **nuclei habenulae** [NA] Two cell groups within the habenular trigone of the epithalamus that receive terminals from the stria medullaris thalami and give rise to the habenulointerpeduncular tract (fasciculus retroflexus). Also *nuclei of habenula, habenular nuclei.* **haploid n.** A nucleus containing only a single set of chromosomes, as the nucleus of a gamete. **hypoglossal n.** NUCLEUS NERVI HYPOGLOSSI. **n. hypoglossalis** NUCLEUS NERVI HYPOGLOSSI. **n. of hypoglossal nerve** NUCLEUS NERVI HYPOGLOSSI. **hypothalamic n.** NUCLEUS SUBTHALAMICUS. **n. hypothalamicus dorsomedialis** NUCLEUS DORSOMEDIALIS HYPOTHALAMI. **n. of inferior colliculus** NUCLEUS COLLICULI INFERIORIS. **inferior olivary n.** NUCLEUS OLIVARIS. **inferior salivatory n.** NUCLEUS SALIVATORIUS INFERIOR. **inferior vestibular n.** NUCLEUS VESTIBULARIS INFERIOR. **infundibular n.** INFUNDIBULUM HYPOTHALAMI. **n. intercalatus** [NA] A group of neurons lying between the hypoglossal nucleus and the dorsal nucleus of the vagus nerve and forming part of the perihypoglossal nuclear complex. The cerebellum constitutes a primary source of afferent fibers, and efferents have been traced to several portions of cerebellum including the flocculus, nodulus, vermis, and anterior lobe. Also *nucleus of Staderini.* **intermediate ventral n. of thalamus** NUCLEUS VENTRALIS INTERMEDIUS. **n. intermediolateralis** COLUMNA INTERMEDIOLATERALIS. **n. intermediomedialis** A column of small and medium-sized neurons lying in the most medial portion of lamina VII of the spinal cord, lateral to the central canal. The nucleus, which extends throughout almost the entire length of the spinal cord, receives small numbers of dorsal root fibers at all levels and may serve as a relay in the transmission of impulses to visceral motor neurons. **n. of internal geniculate body** NUCLEUS CORPORIS GENICULATI MEDIALIS. **n. interpeduncularis** [NA] An unpaired nuclear mass in the raphe of the ventral mesencephalic tegmentum, dorsal to the interpeduncular fossa and between the cerebral peduncles. It receives afferents from the stria medullaris thalami and habenular nuclei via the fasciculus retroflexus. Efferents project into the adjacent dorsal tegmental nucleus. Also *entopeduncular nucleus, interpeduncular ganglion, intercrural ganglion, ganglion isthmi* (obs.). **n. interstitialis** [NA] A small collection of multipolar neurons near the rostral end of the medial longitudinal fasciculus in the mesencephalon. Afferent fibers come from various sources, largely via the medial longitudinal fasciculus. Efferent fibers are distributed to several nuclei of the oculomotor complex, the trochlear nuclei, the ipsilateral medial vestibular nucleus, and the spinal cord. **nuclei intralaminares** [NA] The nuclei within the internal medullary lamina of the thalamus. They include the centromedian and parafascicular nuclei and a group of smaller, more rostrally situated cell groups, such as the paracentral, central lateral, and central median nuclei. The connections of this system are not fully understood. Afferent fibers come from the spinal cord, brainstem, basal ganglia, and cortex, and efferents may be equally broadly distributed. Also *intralaminar nuclei of thalamus.* **intraventricular n. of corpus striatum** *Outmoded* NUCLEUS CAUDATUS. **Kölliker's n.** SUBSTANTIA INTERMEDIA CENTRALIS MEDULLAE SPINALIS. **n. lacrimalis** [NA] A poorly delineated group of neurons near the superior salivatory nucleus thought to project through the facial nerve to the pterygopalatine ganglion, where they synapse with neurons that then supply the lacrimal gland. Also *lacrimatory nucleus.* **large cell auditory n.** NUCLEUS VESTIBULARIS LATERALIS. **laryngeal n.** NUCLEUS AMBIGUUS. **lateral cervical n.** NUCLEUS LATERALIS CERVICALIS. **lateral cuneate n.** NUCLEUS CUNEATUS ACCESSORIUS. **nuclei laterales thalami** A complex nuclear mass occupying the lateral half of the thalamus between the internal medullary lamina and the internal capsule, dorsal to the ventral nuclear group. Constituent cell masses include, from anterior to posterior, the lateral dorsal, lateral posterior, and pulvinar nuclei. Afferent connections are poorly understood, and efferent fibers project mainly to parieto-occipital neocortex. **n. of lateral geniculate body** NUCLEUS CORPORIS GENICULATI LATERALIS. **n. lateralis** NUCLEUS LATERALIS THALAMI. **n. lateralis cervicalis** The lateral cervical nucleus of the spinal cord. A small longitudinal column of neurons in the lateral funiculus of the first and second cervical segments, serving as a relay center in the spinocervicothalamic pathway. Uncrossed afferent fibers come from cells in the posterior horn, reach the nucleus via the spinocervical tract, and transmit low-threshold cutaneous stimuli. Efferent fibers cross to the opposite side of the spinal cord, ascend in association with the contralateral medial lemniscus and terminate in the ventral posterolateral nucleus of the thalamus. Also *lateral cervical nucleus, cervical nucleus.* **n. lateralis dorsalis** [NA] A group of neurons located in the dorsolateral aspect of the thalamus that forms one of the nuclei in the lateral thalamic nuclear complex. In addition to having connections with other thalamic nuclei, this nuclear group appears to project to the cingulate gyrus as well as to the supralimbic cortex of the parietal lobe above that gyrus. **n. lateralis medullae oblongatae** [NA] A small group of neurons in the ventrolateral portion of the medulla oblongata, dorsal to the inferior olive. It receives afferents from cerebral cortex, red nucleus, and spinal cord. Efferent fibers project almost exclusively to the anterior lobe and vermis of the cerebellum. Also *lateral reticular nucleus.* **n. lateralis thalami** [NA] The cell masses occupying the lateral half of the thalamus. Also *nucleus lateralis, lateral nucleus of thalamus.* See also NUCLEI LATERALES THALAMI. ● Because of the complexity of the area, the term is seldom used in its singular form. **n. of lateral lemniscus** NUCLEUS LEMNISCI LATERALIS. **lateral posterior n.** A large, thalamic association nucleus in the dorsolateral portion of the posterior thalamus. **lateral reticular n.** NUCLEUS LATERALIS MEDULLAE OBLONGATAE. **lateral sympathetic n.** COLUMNA INTERMEDIOLATERALIS. **lateral n. of thalamus** NUCLEUS LATERALIS THALAMI. **lateral tuberal nuclei** NUCLEI TUBERALES. **lateral vestibular n.** NUCLEUS VESTIBULARIS LATERALIS. **n. lemnisci lateralis** Diffuse groups of cells situated along the medial face of the lateral lemniscus during its course through the pons and caudal mesencephalon. Also *nucleus of lateral lemniscus.* **n. of lens** NUCLEUS LENTIS. **n. lentiformis** [NA] That portion of the corpus striatum consisting of the globus pallidus and putamen. In frontal sections it appears wedge-shaped, and is located adjacent to the inferolateral border of the internal capsule, which separates it from the caudate nucleus rostrally and the thalamus caudally. Also *nucleus lenticularis, lenticular body* (obs.), *lenticula, lentiform nucleus, lentiform.* ● Though considered an anatomical entity because of its roughly lens-shaped configuration, the embryological derivation and connections of its two component nuclei differ. **n. lentis** [NA] The hard central core of the substance of the lens of the eye. Also *nucleus of lens, central cartilage* (outmoded). **lower sensory n. of trigeminal nerve** *Obs.* NUCLEUS TRACTUS SPINALIS NERVI TRIGEMINI. **n. of Luys** NUCLEUS SUBTHALAMICUS. **n. magnocellularis** *Obs.* NUCLEUS VESTIBULARIS LATERALIS. **magnocellular vestibular n.** NUCLEUS VESTIBULARIS LATERALIS. **nuclei of mamillary body** NUCLEI CORPORIS MAMILLARIS. **medial accessory olivary n.** NUCLEUS OLIVARIS ACCESSORIUS MEDIALIS. **medial geniculate n.** NUCLEUS CORPORIS GENICULATI MEDIALIS. **n. of medial geniculate body** NUCLEUS CORPORIS GENICULATI MEDIALIS. **n. medialis centralis thalami** [NA] The largest, most caudal, and most easily defined of the thalamic intralaminar nuclei, lying between the dorsomedial nucleus above and the ventral posteromedial nucleus below, and composed of several cell types, both large and small. Its medial border interfaces with the parafascicular nucleus, and its edges are swept by fibers of the internal medullary lamina. Its connections are not fully understood, but it is known to receive afferent fibers from a number of sites, including Brodmann's area 4 of the cerebral cortex, the basal ganglia, thalamus, brainstem reticular formation, spinothalamic tract, globus pallidus, and spinal cord. Efferent fibers project to more lateral thalamic nuclei, the caudate nucleus, putamen, and cerebral cortex. Also *nucleus centromedianus thalami, centrum medianum of Luys.* **n. medialis dorsalis** [NA] A thalamic nucleus consisting of a rostral magnocellular and a caudal parvocellular part. It has interconnecting fibers with many other thalamic nuclei and receives input from the amygdaloid nuclei and the piriform cortex; this nucleus sends fibers to the corpus striatum, the hypothalamus, and the frontal cortex. Also *nucleus mediodorsalis.* **n. medialis thalami** [NA] *Seldom used*

DORSOMEDIAL NUCLEUS OF THALAMUS. **n. medialis ventralis** [NA] Part of the thalamic midline nuclei, or central commissural system. Also *nucleus reuniens.* **medial mamillary n.** The largest component of the nuclei corporis mamillaris containing the neurons contributing axons principally to the mamillothalamic and mamillotegmental tracts. **medial thalamic nuclei** An ambiguous term for the nuclei of the medial, but not midline, thalamus, the largest component of which in man is the huge nucleus medialis dorsalis, the neurons of which project to frontal lobe association cortex. **medial n. of thalamus** NUCLEUS MEDIALIS THALAMI. **medial vestibular n.** NUCLEUS VESTIBULARIS MEDIALIS. **n. mediodorsalis** NUCLEUS MEDIALIS DORSALIS. **n. medullaris cerebelli** *Obs.* CORPUS MEDULLARE CEREBELLI. **n. of mesencephalic tract of trigeminal nerve** NUCLEUS TRACTUS MESENCEPHALICI NERVI TRIGEMINI. **n. mesencephalicus nervi trigemini** NUCLEUS TRACTUS MESENCEPHALICI NERVI TRIGEMINI. **metastable n.** An atomic nucleus between the stable and unstable state, in a state of excitation but unable to release energy and return to the normal state until it is involved in another collision or other influence. **n. of Meynert** Groups of neurons located in the basal forebrain surrounding the diagonal band, anterior commissure, and the ventral border of the anterior half of the globus pallidus. These cells, which are rich in acetylcholine and choline acetyltransferase, project widely upon cerebral neocortex and undergo extensive degenerative changes in Alzheimer's disease. **Monakow's n.** NUCLEUS CUNEATUS ACCESSORIUS. **mother n.** The cell nucleus prior to mitosis, which generally divides to produce two daughter nuclei. **motion n.** KINETOPLAST. **motor n.** Any collection of nerve cells of the central nervous system giving rise to the motor fibers of a nerve. **n. motorius nervi trigemini** [NA] The nucleus of origin of the motor fibers of the fifth cranial nerve, located in the dorsolateral portion of the pons just medial to the entering sensory root and the main sensory nucleus. Efferent fibers innervate the muscles of mastication, the tensor tympani, and the tensor veli palatini. Also *motor nucleus of trigeminal nerve.* **motor n. of spinal cord** A group of somatic motor cells located in the anterior horn whose axons project to striated voluntary muscles. It includes large alpha motor neurons (40–100 mm) and small gamma motor neurons (10–25 mm). **motor n. of trigeminal nerve** NUCLEUS MOTORIUS NERVI TRIGEMINI. **n. nervi abducentis** [NA] The nucleus of the abducens of the sixth cranial nerve, lying in the caudal part of the pontine tegmentum, forming the lateral portion of the facial colliculus in the floor of the fourth ventricle. Efferent fibers innervate the lateral rectus muscle of the eye. Discrete unilateral lesions there characteristally produce conjugate weakness or paralysis of lateral gaze toward the side of the lesion. Also *nucleus abducentis, abducens nucleus, nucleus of abducens nerve, nucleus of the sixth cranial nerve.* **n. nervi accessorii** [NA] The nucleus of the eleventh cranial nerve, the most caudal of all the cranial nerves. It is divided into cranial and spinal portions, which form, respectively, the internal and external branches of the nerve. The cranial root arises from neurons in the caudal portion of the nucleus ambiguus. The spinal portion arises from a cell column in the anterior horn extending from the fifth cervical segment to the level of the pyramidal decussation. The cranial root joins the vagus nerve and, as motor fibers of the inferior (recurrent) laryngeal nerve, supplies the intrinsic muscles of the larynx. The spinal root supplies the sternocleidomastoid and upper parts of the trapezius muscles. Also *nucleus of accessory nerve, nucleus of the eleventh cranial nerve.* **nuclei nervi acustici** NUCLEI NERVI VESTIBULOCOCHLEARIS. **nuclei nervi cochlearis** NUCLEI COCHLEARES VENTRALIS ET DORSALIS. **n. nervi facialis** **1** [NA] A collection of multipolar neurons in the ventrolateral tegmentum of the caudal pons dorsal to the superior olivary nucleus. Its efferent fibers innervate the muscles of facial expression, the platysma, the buccinator, and the posterior belly of the digastric and stapedius muscles. The emergent fibers first ascend into the dorsomedial portion of the tegmentum, where they turn sharply from medial to lateral around the rostral pole of the abducens nucleus, forming the internal genu of the facial nerve. They then descend to emerge from the ventrolateral aspect of the pons. Also *nucleus of facial nerve, nucleus facialis.* **2** Collectively, the superior salivatory nucleus and the nucleus of the tractus solitarius, in conjunction with the motor nucleus. **n. nervi glossopharyngei** The nuclear complex serving as origin and termination of the glossopharyngeal or ninth cranial nerve. Located in the medulla oblongata, it consists of sensory and motor, somatic and visceral elements served by the inferior salivatory nucleus, the rostral part of the nucleus ambiguus, and the rostrolateral, or gustatory, portion of the nucleus of the tractus solitarius. **n. nervi hypoglossi** [NA] The nucleus of origin of the hypoglossal or twelfth cranial nerve, consisting of a column of large somatic motor cells in the dorsomedial portion of the caudal half of the medulla oblongata. The fibers supply the extrinsic muscles of the tongue. Also *nucleus hypoglossalis, nucleus of hypoglossal nerve, hypoglossal nucleus.* **n. nervi oculomotorii** [NA] Several cell masses located in the dorsal part of the mesencephalic tegmentum immediately ventral to the central gray matter and lying between the medial longitudinal fasciculi. The nuclear complex is made up of lateral paired somatic cell groups, a median, unpaired somatic nucleus found only in the caudal third of the complex, and paired visceral cell masses (nucleus oculomotorius accessorius, also known as the Edinger-Westphal nucleus), which is parasympathetic in function. The somatic groups innervate the levator palpebrae superioris and all of the extraocular muscles except the lateral rectus and superior oblique. The visceral nuclei supply the sphincter pupillae and ciliary muscle via the ciliary ganglion and the short ciliary nerves. Also *nucleus of oculomotor nerve.* **n. nervi olfactorii** The neuronal region at the caudal end of the olfactory bulb, embedded in the olfactory tract to which it contributes axons. Also *anterior olfactory nucleus, nucleus of olfactory tract.* **n. nervi pneumogastrici** *Obs.* FLOCCULUS. **nuclei nervi trigemini** [NA] The complex of nuclei serving as origin and termination of the trigeminal nerve. The component nuclei extend from high cervical spinal cord levels to the mesencephalon, and include the spinal (descending) tract of the trigeminal nerve, the motor nucleus, the main sensory nucleus, and the mesencephalic root. Also *nuclei of trigeminal nerve.* **n. nervi trochlearis** [NA] A small compact group of cells constituting the nucleus of origin of the fourth cranial nerve. It lies close to the midline in the ventral part of the central grey matter of the caudal mesencephalon, indenting the dorsal surface of the medial longitudinal fasciculus. The emergent fibers have a long intracranial course, decussating dorsally in the superior medullary vellum, and innervate the superior oblique muscle of the eye. Also *nucleus of trochlear nerve.* **n. nervi vagi** [NA] The nuclear complex constituting the origin and termination of the vagus nerve. Situated in the floor of the fourth ventricle and in the dorsal third of the medulla oblongata, it includes the nucleus dorsalis, the nucleus ambiguus and the nucleus of the tractus solitarius. Also *nuclei of vagus nerve, vagal nuclei.* **nuclei nervi vestibularis** VESTIBULAR NUCLEI. **nuclei nervi vestibulocochlearis** The nuclei of termination of the sensory fibers of the vestibular and cochlear divisions of the eighth cranial nerve, located in the dorsolateral portion of the medulla oblongata, and comprising the ventral and dorsal cochlear nuclei and the four vestibular nuclei, medial, lateral, inferior, and superior. Also *vestibulocochlear nuclei* (seldom used), *nuclei of acoustic nerve, nuclei nervi acustici, nuclei of auditory nerve, auditory nuclei.* **nuclei nervorum cranialium** [NA] Those nerve cell groups whose axons form the twelve pairs of cranial nerves. With the exception of the spinal portion of the nucleus accessorius (XI), all are located within the cranial cavity. They include the nucleus nervi olfactorii (I), optici (II), oculomotorii (III), trochlearis (IV), trigemini (V), abducentis (VI), facialis (VII), vestibulocochlearis (VIII), glossopharyngei (IX), vagi (X), accessorii (XI), and hypoglossi (XII). Also *nuclei of cranial nerves, nuclei nervorum cerebralium.* **nutrition n.** MACRONUCLEUS. **n. oculomotorius accessorius** [NA] A cluster of neurons located dorsal to the rostral part of the main oculomotor nucleus in the midbrain. It contains the preganglionic neuron cell bodies of the parasympathetic visceromotor nerve fibers that course in the oculomotor nerve and synapse in the ciliary ganglion. Also *accessory oculomotor nucleus, nucleus accessorius, autonomic nucleus of oculomotor nerve, accessory nucleus, Edinger-Westphal nucleus, Westphal's nucleus, Edinger's nucleus.* **n. of oculomotor nerve** NUCLEUS NERVI OCULOMOTORII. **n. of olfactory tract** NUCLEUS NERVI OLFACTORII. **n. oliva cerebellaris** NUCLEUS DENTATUS CEREBELLI. **n. olivaris** [NA] A folded and convoluted band of gray matter enclosing a white core (the hilum nuclei olivaris), located in the ventral portion of the medulla oblongata just lateral and dorsal to the pyramidal tract. The largest nuclear mass of the medulla, it receives afferents from the spinal cord, mesencephalon, subthalamus, and cerebral cortex, and sends all of its efferents to the contralateral cerebellum, both vermis and hemisphere, via the inferior cerebellar peduncle. Also *olivary nucleus, inferior olivary nucleus, nucleus olivaris inferior, nucleus basalis* (seldom used), *basal nucleus* (seldom used), *corpus dentatum olivae* (obs.), *inferior olive, dentoliva* (obs.). **n. olivaris accessorius dorsalis** [NA] The band of cells lying dorsal to the primary nucleus of the inferior olive. It receives afferents mainly from the spinal cord, and sends efferents to the contralateral cerebellum, particularly the vermis. Also *dorsal accessory olivary nucleus.* **n. olivaris accessorius medialis** [NA] The band of gray matter lying between the olivary nucleus and the midline that projects fibers to the contralateral portion of the cerebellum, mainly the vermis. Also *medial accessory olivary nucleus, pyramidal nucleus.* **n. olivaris inferior** NUCLEUS OLIVARIS. **n. olivaris superior** [NA] A column of nerve cells in the caudal portion of the ventrolateral pontile tegmentum, just dorsal to the trapezoid body. It receives afferents from the cochlear nuclei and sends efferents to the trapezoid body and lateral lemniscus. Also *superior olivary nucleus, nucleus dorsalis corporis trapezoidei* (seldom used), *dorsal nucleus of trapezoid body* (seldom used), *superior olive.* **olivary n.** NUCLEUS OLIVARIS. **ootid n.** Any one of the four haploid nuclei that are produced by oocyte maturation through meiosis. In humans, three of the nuclei are polar bodies which degenerate. **Pander's n.** *Outmoded* NUCLEUS SUBTHALAMICUS. **parabducent n.** A group of neurons believed to lie in the reticular formation adjacent to or within the abducens nucleus that may give rise to efferents directed to the oculomotor nucleus for controlling horizontal eye movements. Also *pontine center for lateral gaze.* **parabigeminal n.** A group of cells lying between the lateral lemniscus and the periphery in the caudal half of the mesencephalon. Its connections are still obscure but it is believed to send efferents to the lateral nuclei of the pons. **paracentral n. of the thalamus** A small cell group associated with the internal medullary lamina and constituting one of the intralaminar nuclei. It lies along the lateral border of the dorsomedial nucleus, fusing with the lateral central nucleus dorsolaterally and the medial central nucleus ventromedially. Its connections are uncertain, but it probably receives afferents from the brainstem reticular formation and frontal cortex, and sends efferents to the caudate nucleus. **parafascicular n. of the thalamus** A group of cells in the caudal third of the thalamus lying medial to the centromedian nucleus and ventral to the dorsomedial nucleus. The fasciculus retroflexus of Meynert almost bisects it from dorsal to ventral. Its connections are not yet clear, but it appears to receive afferents from the spinothalamic tract, the brainstem reticular formation, and Brodmann's area 6 of cerebral cortex, and send efferents to the striatum, cerebral cortex, and possibly the mesencephalic tegmentum. **paramedian reticular nuclei** Cell clusters located in the medullary reticular formation, dorsal to the inferior olive. Their major axonal projection is to the cerebellum. **nuclei paraventriculares antepriores et posteriores** [NA] Rather distinct clusters of neurons located in the dorsomedial ventricular wall of the thalamus that are classified as belonging to the median or midline group of thalamic nuclei. **n. paraventricularis hypothalami** A well-defined cell group in the wall of the third ventricle in the supraoptic portion of the hypothalamus. Many of the cells are neurosecretory in function and send efferent fibers to the posterior lobe of the hypophysis. Also *paraventricular nucleus of hypothalamus.* **perihypoglossal nuclei** The nuclei adjacent to the hypoglossal nucleus, including the nucleus intercalatus, nucleus prepositus, and nucleus of Roller. **n. of Perlia** A group of cells in the midline of the oculomotor nuclear complex. It is believed to be associated with ocular convergence. See also CONVERGENCE CENTER. **n. pigmentosus pontis** LOCUS CERULEUS. **polymorphic n.** A nucleus with an irregular shape and having a number of lobes connected by strands of nucleoplasm. **nuclei pontis** [NA] Groups of nerve cells among the fiber bundles of the pyramidal tract in the ventral portion of the pons upon which the fibers of the corticopontine system synapse. Efferent axons project largely, though not completely, upon the contralateral brachium pontis and thence to the cerebellum. Also *pontine nuclei.* **pontobulbar n.** A cell column located along the lateral and ventral aspects of the inferior cerebellar peduncle. It is believed to be a caudal continuation of the ventral pontine nuclei. **posterior cochlear n.** See under NUCLEI COCHLEARES VENTRALIS ET DORSALIS. **n. posterior hypothalami** [NA] A group of nerve cells in the posterior portion of the hypothalamus dorsal to the mamillary bodies. The nucleus has a number of afferent and efferent connections with the brainstem via the periventricular fibers and the dorsal longitudinal bundle. The area is sensitive to conditions of decreasing body temperature, and controls mechanisms for conservation and increased production of heat. Also *posterior nucleus of hypothalamus.* **n. posterior thalami** [NA] The large, caudal, pillowlike expansion constituting the posterior pole of the thalamus, generally divided, in man, into three main nuclei. Although its connections are not fully understood, it is known to receive afferents from the upper brainstem, thalamus, and cortex and to send efferents to occipital, parietal, and temporal parts of the cerebral cortex. Parts of this nucleus receiving tectothalamic projections may transmit visual information to the extrastriate visual cortex. Also *pulvinar, pulvinar thalami, gibber inferior thalami, posterior nucleus of thalamus, posterior tubercle of thalamus, tuberculum posterius thalami.* **posterior ventral n. of thalamus** NUCLEUS VENTRALIS THALAMI POSTERIOR. **posterolateral ventral n. of thalamus** NUCLEUS VENTRALIS POSTEROLATERALIS. **posteromarginal n.** A thin layer of large nerve cells covering the tip of the dorsal horn and constituting lamina 1 of the spinal gray matter. Afferent fibers probably include many pain-transmitting axons from the lateral division of the dorsal root. Efferents enter the lateral white funiculus as ascending and descending fibers of the propriospinal system. They are known to be activated by stimuli causing tissue injury, and to be inhibited by descending serotonergic fibers from the raphe nuclei of the brainstem. **premamillary n.** A small group of hypothalamic cells lying near the anterosuperior surface of the medial mamillary nucleus. **preolivary nuclei** Small groups of nerve cells lying ventromedial and ventrolateral to the superior olive. They probably serve as intercalated nuclei in the secondary auditory pathways. **nuclei preoptici medialis et lateralis** [NA] Groups of small and medium-sized neurons located in the preoptic region of the basal forebrain, rostral to the anterior hypothalamic nuclei and dorsal to the supraoptic and suprachiasmatic nuclei. The medial preoptic nucleus lies immediately lateral to the preoptic periventricular nucleus, and the lateral preoptic nucleus is located adjacent but lateral to the medial preoptic nucleus. **n. prepositus** An elongated group of nerve cells in the medulla oblongata extending from the oral pole of the hypoglossal nucleus almost to the abducens nucleus, and constituting one of the perihypoglossal nuclei. Afferent fibers come principally from the cerebellum, with smaller numbers from the midbrain and the face region of the sensorimotor cortex. Efferent fibers project to the cerebellum and to the ocular motor nuclei. **n. pretectalis** [NA] A group of cells with indistinct boundaries lying rostral to the superior colliculi at the level of the posterior commissure. It receives afferents from the optic tract, the lateral geniculate body, several cortical areas, and the posterior thalamic nuclei, and sends efferents to the visceral nuclei of the oculomotor complex. It is thought to function as the principal midbrain center involved in the pupillary light reflex. **principal sensory n. of trigeminal nerve** NUCLEUS SENSORIUS SUPERIOR NERVI TRIGEMINI. **n. proprius of posterior horn** A rather poorly defined column of cells of diverse morphology located in laminae III, IV, and V of the dorsal horn of the spinal cord. It is found at all levels of the cord, but the cells are most numerous in the lumbosacral area. Also *centrodorsal nucleus.* **n. pulposus disci intervertebralis** [NA] The inner, semifluid core of the intervertebral disks, composed at birth of soft, gelatinous mucoid material that is gradually replaced by fibrocartilage as it loses its elasticity and water-binding property with age, so that it merges with the surrounding annulus fibrosus. It is better developed in the cervical and lumbar regions than in the thoracic, and it is situated nearer the posterior than the anterior part of the disk. It is derived from the embryonic notochord, but all the notochordal cells disappear by the end of the second decade of life. Also *pulpy nucleus, nucleus gelatinosus.* **pulvinar n.** The thalamic nucleus that forms a caudal bulge (or "pillow") adjacent to the lateral geniculate nucleus. In the human brain it is a nuclear complex with its several nuclei comprising the largest thalamic region dominating the posterolateral thalamus. **pyknotic n.** The shrunken, deeply basophilic appearance of the nucleus following cell death, due to clumping of the chromatin. **pyramidal n.** NUCLEUS OLIVARIS ACCESSORIUS MEDIALIS. **n. radicis descendentis nervi trigemini** NUCLEUS TRACTUS MESENCEPHALICI NERVI TRIGEMINI. **red n.** NUCLEUS RUBER. **reproductive n.** MICRONUCLEUS. **n. reticularis tegmenti** A medial tegmental extension of pontine nuclear cells receiving afferents from the frontal and parietal cortex and from the cerebellum via the brachium conjunctivum, and sending efferents to the cerebellum via the middle cerebellar peduncle. Also *reticulotegmental nucleus.* **n. reticularis thalami** [NA] A thin sheet of multipolar nerve cells on the lateral surface of the thalamus within the external medullary lamina. Afferents are received from almost all of the thalamic specific nuclei, mesencephalic reticular cells, and the cerebral cortex. Virtually all of the efferents project back upon the thalamus, thereby providing powerful inhibitory modulation of thalamocortical activity. Also *reticular nucleus of thalamus.* **reticular n. of subthalamus** Groups of neurons scattered along the thalamic and lenticular fasciculi and the tegmental field of Forel and probably functioning as bed nuclei for these largely thalamopetal tracts. *Seldom used.* Also *nucleus of tegmental field.* **reticular n. of thalamus** NUCLEUS RETICULARIS THALAMI. **reticulotegmental n.** NUCLEUS RETICULARIS TEGMENTI. **n. reuniens** NUCLEUS MEDIALIS VENTRALIS. **Roller's n.** A group of large nerve cells in the medulla oblongata lying ventral to the rostral pole of the hypoglossal nucleus and adjacent to its root fibers. Like the other perihypoglossal nuclei of which it is considered part, its principal connections are with the cerebellum. Also *sublingual nucleus.* **n. of roof of cerebellum** NUCLEUS FASTIGII CEREBELLI. **roof nuclei of cerebellum** The deep nuclei of the cerebellum, lying in the roof of the fourth ventricle and comprising the dentate, emboliform, globose, and fastigial nuclei. **n. ruber** [NA] A paired, red ovoid mass in the anterior part of the midbrain, forming a part of the extrapyramidal system. Also *red nucleus, tectorial nucleus, locus ruber, nucleus of Sappey* (seldom used). **sacral n.** The extension into the lumbosacral spinal cord of the nucleus thoracicus. Also *Stilling's nucleus.* **n. salivatorius caudalis** NUCLEUS SALIVATORIUS INFERIOR. **n. salivatorius cranialis** NUCLEUS SALIVATORIUS SUPERIOR. **n. salivatorius inferior** [NA] The caudal portion of the column of scattered cells in the dorsolateral part of the reticular formation in the upper pons and lower medulla oblongata whose axons constitute the general visceral efferent (parasympathetic) outflow of the glossopharyngeal nerve which, via the otic ganglion, supplies the parotid gland. Also *inferior salivatory nucleus, nucleus salivatorius caudalis.* **n. salivatorius superior** [NA] A group of scattered visceral neurons in the dorsolateral reticular formation of the upper medulla oblongata and the lower pons that constitutes the general visceral efferent (parasympathetic) outflow of the facial nerve (via the nervus intermedius), supplying the lacrimal, nasal, palatine, submandibular, and sublingual glands. The more caudal elements of this cell group constitute the nucleus salivatorius interior. Also *superior salivatory nucleus, nucleus salivatorius cranialis.* **n. of Sappey** *Seldom used* NUCLEUS RUBER. **Schwalbe's n.** NUCLEUS VESTIBULARIS MEDIALIS. **secondary n.** SUBNUCLEUS. **semilunar n.** NUCLEUS VENTRALIS POSTEROMEDIALIS. **n. sensorius inferior nervi trigemini** NUCLEUS TRACTUS SPINALIS NERVI TRIGEMINI. **n. sensorius superior nervi trigemini** [NA] The primary receptive nucleus for afferent fibers carrying impulses for sensations of touch and pressure from all three divisions of the trigeminal nerve, located in the dorsolateral part of the medial pons. The neurons are characterized by large receptive fields, show high levels of spontaneous activity, and respond to a wide range of pressure stimuli with little adaptation. Also *principal sensory nucleus of trigeminal nerve, superior sensory nucleus of trigeminal nerve, nucleus sensorius principalis nervi trigemini.* **sensory n.** Any aggregate of neurons which receives the terminals of afferent (sensory) fibers entering the nervous system via a peripheral (spinal or cranial) nerve. **septal nuclei** The paired medial and lateral nuclei continuous with septum pellucidum, near the base of the pillars of the fornix and overlying the nucleus of the diagonal band. Its connections are diverse but principally with the hippocampal formation via the fornix. **shadow n.** A cell nucleus in a stage of dissolution where it has lost its chromatin and does not stain with a nuclear stain. **n. of the sixth cranial nerve** NUCLEUS NERVI ABDUCENTIS. **n. solitarius** [NA] NUCLEUS TRACTUS SOLITARII. **n. of solitary tract** NUCLEUS TRACTUS SOLITARII. **somatic n.** MACRONUCLEUS. **sperm n.** MALE PRONUCLEUS. **spherical n.** *Seldom used* NUCLEUS GLOBOSUS CEREBELLI. **n. spinalis nervi accessorii** The groups of nerve cells in the anterior horn of the spinal cord at levels $C_1$ through $C_5$ or $C_6$ that contribute to the formation of the spinal roots of the accessory nerve. Also *spinal nucleus of accessory nerve.* **n. of spinal tract of trigeminal nerve** NUCLEUS TRACTUS SPINALIS NERVI TRIGEMINI. **spinal n. of trigeminal nerve** NUCLEUS TRACTUS SPINALIS NERVI TRIGEMINI. **spinal vestibular n.** NUCLEUS VESTIBULARIS INFERIOR. **spinocerebellar n.** NUCLEUS THORACICUS. **n. of Staderini** NUCLEUS INTERCALATUS. **Stilling's n.** 1 NUCLEUS THORACICUS. 2 SACRAL NUCLEUS. **sublingual n.** ROLLER'S NUCLEUS. **submedial n. of thalamus** Nucleus submedius: a small cell group lying along the internal medullary lamina in the anterior portion of the thalamus, ventral to the paracentral nucleus and dorsal to the nucleus medialis ventralis. It is considered part of the nonspecific or diffusely projecting nuclei of the medial thalamus. **n. subthalamicus** [NA] A lens-shaped mass of gray matter on the inner surface of the peduncular portion of the internal capsule. Afferent fibers come primarily from the lateral segment of the globus pallidus via the subthalamic fasciculus, and efferents traverse the internal capsule and project primarily to the caudal portions of the medial segment of the globus pallidus. In man, discrete lesions of the nucleus result in forceful chorealike movements (hemiballismus). Also *hypothalamic nucleus, corpus subthalamicum, nucleus of Luys, body of Luys* (outmoded), *corpus luysii, nucleus amygdaliformis of J. Stilling, Pander's nucleus* (outmoded). **superior n.** NUCLEUS VESTIBULARIS SUPERIOR. **superior olivary n.** NUCLEUS OLIVARIS SUPERIOR. **superior salivatory n.** NUCLEUS SALIVATORIUS SUPERIOR. **superior sensory n. of trigeminal nerve** NUCLEUS SENSORIUS SUPERIOR NERVI TRIGEMINI. **superior vestibular n.** NUCLEUS VESTIBULARIS SUPERIOR. **suprachiasmatic n.** The small hypothalamic nucleus lying on the optic chiasm. It receives optic nerve fibers and it has been implicated in the control of circadian rhythms. **suprageniculate n.** A triangular-shaped group of neurons extending dorsomedially from the medial geniculate nucleus between the pretectal area and the pulvinar. *Seldom used.* **supramamillary n.** A group of cells lying dorsal to the mamillary nucleus and thought to be a rostral extension of the tegmental gray matter. **n. supraopticus hypothalami** [NA] A sharply defined group of hypothalamic cells lying just above the optic chiasm that send their axons to the posterior lobe of the hypothalamus in the supraopticohypophysial tract. The cells are clearly neurosecretory in function and probably produce both vasopressin and oxytocin. Also *nucleus supraopticus, supraoptic nucleus of hypothalamus.* **supraspinal n.** Small clusters of somatic motor neurons in the ventral horn of the first cervical segment of spinal cord that extend a short distance into the lower medulla. Also *nucleus supraspinalis of Jacobson.* **n. sympathicus lateralis** COLUMNA INTERMEDIOLATERALIS. **n. tecti** NUCLEUS FASTIGII CEREBELLI. **tectorial n.** NUCLEUS RUBER. **tegmental nuclei** NUCLEI TEGMENTI MESENCEPHALICI. **n. of tegmental field** RETICULAR NUCLEUS OF SUBTHALAMUS. **tegmental nuclei of Gudden** NUCLEI TEGMENTI MESENCEPHALICI. **nuclei tegmenti mesencephalici** [NA] Several cell groups in the rostral pons and caudal mesencephalon that lie close to the course of the superior cerebellar peduncle. Afferent fibers probably come from the precentral gyrus and the globus pallidus, while efferent projections are still uncertain. Also *tegmental nuclei, dorsal tegmental nuclei, tegmental nuclei of Gudden.* **n. thoracicus** [NA] A column of large nerve cells found in the medial part of the base of the dorsal horn of the spinal cord just lateral to the central canal, extending from the seventh or eighth cervical to the second or third lumbar segment. The cells receive large-caliber primary afferent fibers primarily from muscle spindles, and efferents give rise to the ipsilateral dorsal spinocerebellar tract, which terminates ipsilaterally in the cerebellar vermal cortex as mossy fibers. Also *nucleus of Clarke's column, Clarke's nucleus, Stilling's nucleus, spinocerebellar nucleus, posterovesicular column of Clarke.* **n. tractus mesencephalici nervi trigemini** [NA] A slender cell column in the dorsolateral portion of the rostral pons and caudal mesencephalon. The cell bodies are unique in being monopolar primary sensory neurons, and resemble dorsal root ganglion cells. The peripheral processes of the cells form the mesencephalic tract, and carry proprioceptive impulses from the muscles of mastication. The central processes have widespread connections with brainstem and cerebellum, including the motor nucleus of the trigeminal nerve. Also *nucleus of mesencephalic tract of trigeminal nerve, nucleus radicis descendentis nervi trigemini, nucleus mesencephalicus nervi trigemini.* **n. tractus solitarii** A column of nerve cells lying in the dorsolateral aspect of the medulla oblongata to which course primary visceral afferent fibers from the facial, glossopharyngeal, and vagus nerves. These fibers include special sensory afferents conveying taste impulses from the tongue and palate, as well as general visceral afferents from the pharynx, esophagus, and gastrointestinal organs. Prior to entering the nucleus, the primary afferent fibers course longitudinally in the adjacent tractus solitarius. Neurons in the nucleus of the tractus solitarius project rostrally to the pons and to diencephalic levels. Also *nucleus of solitary tract, nucleus solitarius.* **n. tractus spinalis nervi trigemini** A column of nerve cells that extends from the site of entry of the trigeminal nerve in the pons caudally through the medulla oblongata to about the second cervical level of the spinal cord. It lies along the medial border of the descending or spinal tract of the trigeminal nerve, and primary afferent nerve fibers from this tract terminate within the nucleus throughout its extent. It is usually divided into an oral part, an interpolar part, and a caudal part and pain impulses and thermal and tactile sensations from most of the head and face are relayed from this nucleus to the reticular formation and the thalamus by way of secondary trigeminal tracts. Also *spinal nucleus of tri-*

*geminal nerve, nucleus of descending fifth nerve, nucleus of spinal tract of trigeminal nerve, nucleus sensorius inferior nervi trigemini, lower sensory nucleus of trigeminal nerve.* **n. of trapezoid body** NUCLEUS VENTRALIS CORPORIS TRAPEZOIDEI. **n. triangularis** NUCLEUS VESTIBULARIS MEDIALIS. **nuclei of trigeminal nerve** NUCLEI NERVI TRIGEMINI. **n. of trochlear nerve** NUCLEUS NERVI TROCHLEARIS. **trophic n.** MACRONUCLEUS. **nuclei tuberales** [NA] Two or three well-delimited cell groups in the middle part of the lateral hypothalamus near the tuber cinereum. They contain small multipolar neurons arranged in round or oval clusters surrounded by a delicate fiber capsule. They often produce small elevations on the basal surface of the hypothalamus. Their functions and connections are unknown. Also *nuclei tuberis, lateral tuberal nuclei, tuberal nuclei.* **vagal nuclei** NUCLEUS NERVI VAGI. **vagoglossopharyngeal n.** *Seldom used* NUCLEUS AMBIGUUS. **nuclei of vagus nerve** NUCLEUS NERVI VAGI. **vegetative n.** MACRONUCLEUS. **ventral cochlear n.** See under NUCLEI COCHLEARES VENTRALIS ET DORSALIS. **n. ventralis anterolateralis** The rostral subdivision of the ventral nucleus of the thalamus. It contains clusters of multipolar neurons arranged in distinct magnocellular and parvocellular portions. It receives input from the substantia nigra and globus pallidus, and projects to the cerebral cortex. Also *nucleus ventralis thalami anterior, anterolateral ventral nucleus.* **n. ventralis corporis trapezoidei** [NA] A group of nerve cells situated among the transverse auditory fibers crossing the pontine tegmentum as the trapezoid body. It acts as a relay for some fibers from the opposite cochlear nuclei, and contributes fibers to the lateral lemniscus. Also *ventral nucleus of trapezoid body, nucleus of trapezoid body.* **n. ventralis intermedius** The median subdivision of the ventral nucleus of the thalamus. It is subdivided into pars oralis, medialis, and caudalis, and receives projections from the contralateral half of the cerebellum and from the ipsilateral substantia nigra and globus pallidus. It projects to Brodmann's areas 4 and 6 of the precentral cortex. Also *nucleus ventralis lateralis, nucleus ventralis thalami intermedius, intermediate ventral nucleus of thalamus.* **n. ventralis posterolateralis** [NA] The lateral portion of the nucleus ventralis thalami posterior, subdivided into pars oralis and caudalis. It receives sensory fibers of the spinothalamic tract and medial lemniscus, and projects to the postcentral cortex. Also *posterolateral ventral nucleus of thalamus.* **n. ventralis posteromedialis** [NA] The medial portion of the nucleus ventralis thalami posterior, receiving sensory data from the head via secondary trigeminal fibers and projecting to the postcentral cortex. Also *arcuate nucleus, semilunar nucleus, posterior ventral nucleus of thalamus.* **n. ventralis thalami** The ventral portion of the lateral nuclear mass of the thalamus, containing specific relay nuclei that project to motor and sensory areas of cerebral cortex. It is subdivided into a rostral nucleus ventralis anterolateralis, an intermediate nucleus ventralis intermedius, and a caudal nucleus ventralis thalami posterior. Also *ventral nucleus of thalamus.* **n. ventralis thalami anterior** NUCLEUS VENTRALIS ANTEROLATERALIS. **n. ventralis thalami intermedius** NUCLEUS VENTRALIS INTERMEDIUS. **n. ventralis thalami posterior** The largest and most caudal part of the nucleus ventralis thalami. It is subdivided into nucleus ventralis posterolateralis and nucleus ventralis posteromedialis, which relay sensory data to the postcentral gyrus. **ventral n. of thalamus** NUCLEUS VENTRALIS THALAMI. **ventral n. of trapezoid body** NUCLEUS VENTRALIS CORPORIS TRAPEZOIDEI. **n. ventrobasolateralis** The lateral segment of the thalamic ventrobasal nuclear complex, receiving its principal lemniscal input from the nucleus gracilis; nucleus ventrobasalis, pars externa; and nucleus ventralis posterolateralis. **ventromedial n. of hypothalamus** NUCLEUS VENTROMEDIALIS HYPOTHALAMI. **n. ventromedialis** [NA] Neurons in the ventral part of the oculomotor (III) nucleus. *Seldom used.* **n. ventromedialis hypothalami** A cluster of small neurons situated ventrally in the tuberal region of the medial hypothalamus. It functions in the regulation of food and water intake. Also *ventromedial nucleus of hypothalamus.* **vestibular nuclei** A group of four relay nuclei found in the floor of the fourth ventricle. They receive primary vestibular fibers from the cristae of the semicircular canals and maculae of the saccule and utricle. They give rise to secondary vestibular projections to cerebellum, spinal cord, and motor nuclei of cranial nerves III, IV, and VI. The nuclei comprise the nucleus vestibularis inferior, lateralis, medialis, and superior. Also *nuclei nervi vestibularis.* **n. vestibularis caudalis** NUCLEUS VESTIBULARIS INFERIOR. **n. vestibularis cranialis** NUCLEUS VESTIBULARIS SUPERIOR. **n. vestibularis inferior** [NA] A group of neurons located in the dorsolateral aspect of the medulla oblongata that extends from the rostral limit of the nucleus gracilis to the pontomedullary junction adjacent to the point of entrance of the vestibular nerve. It receives fibers from the descending root of the vestibular nerve and gives rise to vestibulocerebellar fibers that project to the cerebellum, and descending fibers that join the medial longitudinal fasciculus. Also *spinal vestibular nucleus, descending vestibular nucleus, caudal vestibular nucleus, nucleus vestibularis caudalis, inferior vestibular nucleus.* **n. vestibularis lateralis** [NA] A group of nerve cells located laterally in the floor of the fourth ventricle at the caudal border of the pons, immediately rostral to the nucleus vestibularis inferior. It receives incoming primary afferent nerve fibers from the vestibular division of the vestibulocochlear nerve and axons from the cerebellar cortex and the fastigial nucleus of the cerebellum, and it gives rise to fibers that form the vestibulospinal tract, which exerts important facilitating influences on extensor muscle tone and spinal reflex activity. Also *nucleus of Deiters, magnocellular vestibular nucleus, lateral vestibular nucleus, large cell auditory nucleus, nucleus magnocellularis* (obs.). **n. vestibularis medialis** [NA] A group of nerve cells located in the floor of the fourth ventricle medial to the lateral and inferior vestibular nuclei. The rostral part of the nucleus receives ascending branches of the bifurcated primary vestibular afferent fibers, while the more caudal part receives primary vestibular fibers by way of the descending root of the vestibular nerve. Also *Schwalbe's nucleus, nucleus triangularis, medial vestibular nucleus.* **n. vestibularis superior** [NA] A small aggregate of nerve cell bodies, the most rostrally located of the vestibular nuclei, lying in the pons at the angle formed by the floor and lateral wall of the fourth ventricle, cranial to the medial and lateral vestibular nuclei. Primary vestibular afferent fibers terminate in its central region. Also *nucleus vestibularis cranialis, superior vestibular nucleus, nucleus angularis, Bekhterev's nucleus, nucleus acusticus superior, superior nucleus.* **vestibulocochlear nuclei** *Seldom used* NUCLEI NERVI VESTIBULOCOCHLEARIS. **Westphal's n.** NUCLEUS OCULOMOTORIUS ACCESSORIUS. **zygote n.** The nucleus of the fertilized ovum when the male and female pronuclei first unite. Also *conjugation nucleus, fertilization nucleus, synkaryon.*

**nuclide** \n$^y$oo′klīd\ [*nucl(eo)-* + *-ide,* irreg. from Gk *eid(os)* form, shape, species] A nuclear species as characterized by its atomic number (number of protons) and either its mass number or (less commonly) the number of neutrons. **radioactive n.** RADIONUCLIDE.

**Nuel** [Jean-Pierre *Nuel,* Belgian physician, 1847–1920] See under SPACE.

**NUG** necrotizing ulcerative gingivitis.

**Nuhn** [Anton *Nuhn,* German anatomist, 1814–1899] Nuhn's gland, Blandin and Nuhn gland, anterior lingual gland of Blandin and Nuhn. See under GLANDULA LINGUALIS ANTERIOR.

**nuisance** In forensic medicine, any activity or condition caused by one or more individuals, that potentially or in fact offends public or private sensibilities, violates precepts of common decency, or endangers life and health. The resulting discomfort, annoyance, or inconvenience must be of sufficient magnitude that the law will presume resulting damage.

**nulligravid** \nul′igrav′id\ [*null(us)* no one, none, no + *i* + *gravid(a)* pregnant] Having never been pregnant.

**nulligravida** \nul′igrav′idə\ [L *null(us)* no one, none, no + *i* + GRAVIDA] A woman who has never been pregnant.

**nullipara** \nulip′ərə\ [L *null(us)* no one, none, no + *i* + PARA] A woman who has never given birth to a viable infant.

**nulliparous** \nulip′ərəs\ Having never given birth to a viable infant. Also *nonparous.*

**nullisomic** \nul′isō′mik\ Lacking both members of a particular pair of homologous chromosomes.

**numb** [Middle English *nomen,* past part. of *nimen* to seize, take] Being without sensation.

**number** [French *nombre* (from L *numerus* a number, measure, akin to *nomen* a name and to Gk *nemein* to deal out, distribute) a number] **1** The sum total of a collection of units. **2** Relative place in a sequence of units determined by assigning a unique designation to each unit according to a system of counting. **3** A symbol or word used to designate number. **atomic n.** The number of protons in an atomic nucleus. This number determines the normal number of orbiting electrons, and therefore the chemical properties of the atom and its position in the periodic table. Symbol: Z **Avogadro's n.** The number of specified particles in one mole of substance. It is about $6.023 \times 10^{23}$. **basic n.** HAPLOID NUMBER. **chromosome n.** The number of chromosomes normally present in the somatic cell of an organism. This number is the diploid or $2n$ chromosome number. One set of chromosomes ($n$) is contributed by each gamete in the formation of a zygote ($2n$). The chromosome number in human somatic cells is 46. **dibucaine n.** A figure indicating the extent to which the enzyme pseudocholinesterase can be inhibited by dibucaine. Normal forms of the enzyme are inhibited to 75% or above. The variant form of the enzyme, associated with clinical conditions of excessive susceptibility to the effects of succinyl choline, is resistant to dibucaine. Homozygotes for the atypical enzyme have inhibition levels below 25%, and heterozygotes for the gene determining atypical enzyme activity usually have 40 to 60% inhibition. **haploid n.** The number of chromosomes that comprise a set. Also *basic number, monoploid number, gametic number.* **iodine n.** An expression of the degree of unsaturation of fatty acids in a fat. It is derived from the quantity of iodine, in grams, that combine with 100 grams of the fat. Also *iodine value.* **linking n.** The number of superhelical turns present in a topographically constrained piece or region of DNA; designated $\alpha$. The relaxed linking number ($\alpha_0$) is the number of turns present in a topographically defined, but unconstrained, piece or region of DNA. A "+" sign indicates right-hand winding. Also *linkage number, winding number.* **mass n.** The sum of the number of protons and the number of neutrons in the nucleus of a nuclide. It is the integer closest to the physical atomic mass of the nuclide. Symbol: A **monoploid n.** HAPLOID NUMBER. **neutron n.** The number of neutrons in a nucleus, obtained by subtracting the number of protons from the mass number. Symbol: *N* **random n.** In statistics, a number expressed by a sequence of randomly chosen digits, from 0 to 9, each digit being such that any other might have been chosen with equal probability. Such numbers may be generated either by resort to irrational mathematical functions or to a mechanism that operates in an essentially random fashion. Tables of random numbers are available, and by their use an unbiased selection of a sample is assured, resulting in a random sample. **turnover n.** A measure of enzyme activity equal to the number of molecules of substrate modified by one molecule of enzyme per unit time, usually when the enzyme is saturated with substrate. It is therefore equal to the rate constant for breakdown to products of the enzyme-substrate complex. **viable n.** The number of bacteria in a preparation that are capable of forming colonies when placed on an adequate culture medium. With bacteria that do not separate regularly on cell division, such as streptococci, the usual procedure measures the number of clumps and not of cells. **winding n.** LINKING NUMBER.

**numbering** The assignment of numbers, as to atoms in a molecule, for identifying position, sequence, or quantity.

**numbness** The condition of being numb. **waking n.** Transient numbness of the extremities on awakening.

**nummular** \num′yələr\ [French *nummulaire* (from L *nummul(us),* dim. of *nummus* a coin, from Gk *nomimos* legal, + French *-aire* -AR) a plant with coin-shaped leaves] Having or tending to assume the shape of a coin; discoid. See also NUMMULAR SPUTUM.

**Numorphan** A proprietary name for oxymorphone hydrochloride.

**nunnation** \nunā′shən\ [New L *nunnatio* (from Arabic *nūn,* the letter *n* + L *-atio* -ATION) the adding of a final *n* in the declining of Arabic nouns] **1** Undue use of the sound of the letter "n" during speech. **2** The faulty production of the sound of the letter "n" which leads to the substitution of another sound such as that of the letter "d." *Imprecise.*

**nuptiality** \nupshal′itē\ [L *nuptial(is)* (from *nupti(ae)* nuptials, from *nuptus,* past part. of *nubere* to be wedded; + *-alis* -AL) pertaining to marriage + English -ITY] The frequency of marriages in a given population. The nuptiality rate is usually expressed as the number of marriages per 1000 population. Also *marriage rate.*

**nurse** [French *nourrice* (from L *nutricia,* fem. of *nutricius* nourishing, akin to *nutrix,* gen. *nutricis,* a nurse, foster mother and to *nutrire* or *nutriri* to suckle, nourish, bring up) a wet nurse] **1** A health care professional trained to perform the duties and to assume the responsibilities of assisting the sick or disabled and of maintaining health; a practitioner of nursing. See also NURSING CARE. **2** A person charged with the duties of taking care of an infant or small child; a nursemaid. **charge n.** The nurse in charge of patient care for an individual or an organizational unit. **licensed practical n.** A nurse who is licensed by the government as a practical nurse. **occupational health n.** A nurse who has been trained in occupational health to promote and maintain health, to prevent disease and injury, and to provide treatment for injury and disease where necessary, for industrial workers. **operating room n.** OR NURSE. **OR n.** A member of the operating room nursing staff specially trained to provide assistance to the operating team of surgeons. Also *operating room nurse, theater nurse* (used in India). **practical n.** A nurse who performs certain nursing functions but is not a graduate of a degree program in nursing and who may or may not be licensed. **private n.** PRIVATE DUTY NURSE. **private duty n.** A nurse who is employed by or for a private patient. Also *private nurse.* **public health n.** A nurse who is employed by a public health agency or is involved in the provision of public health services. **registered n.** A nurse who has graduated from a formal training program and has been licensed by the appropriate governmental authority to practice nursing. Abbr. RN **scrub n.** A member of the operating room nursing staff who is in attendance at the operating table, having completed a surgical scrub and donned gown and gloves. **theater n.** 1 In Britain, the first assistant to the operating theater sister. 2 A term used in India for OR NURSE. • The sense of def. 1 is also found in South Africa and New Zealand. **visiting n.** A nurse who visits and cares for patients in their homes or in other residential facilities. **wet n.** A woman engaged to breast-feed the infant of another.

**nurse aide** NURSE'S AIDE. See under AIDE.

**nurse-anesthetist** A trained nurse who administers anesthetic agents to patients.

**nurse-midwife** A nurse who provides care to pregnant women including performing deliveries and associated services.

**nurse-practitioner** A nurse who usually has additional specialty training and who provides primary care or specialized services, usually under the supervision of a physician.

**nursery** [Middle English *norserie,* from *norse* (from Old French *norice* a nurse, from Late L *nutricia* a nurse, from L *nutrix,* gen. *nutricis,* a wet nurse, from *nutrire* to nourish) a nurse + *-rie* -RY] An area in a hospital where newborn infants are cared for. **day n.** A place where preschool children may be left under supervision during the day.

**nursing** The health care profession devoted to the provision of nursing care and the training of nurses. Most training takes the form of a four-year degree program or a three-year diploma program. Nurses with additional training beyond the minimum requirements may assume a greater independent clinical role in providing health care. See also NURSING CARE. **foster n.** The nursing of a young animal by one other than the natural mother.

**Nussbaum** [Moritz *Nussbaum,* German histologist, 1850–1915] See under EXPERIMENT.

**nutation** \n^y^ootā′shən\ [L *nutatio* (from *nutatus,* past part. of *nutare* to nod, wag the head) a nodding] Involuntary or repetitive nodding of the head. Adj. nutatory.

**nutatory** \n^y^oo′tətôr′ē\ Denoting or pertaining to nutation.

**nutrient** \n^y^oo′trē·ənt\ [L *nutriens,* gen. *nutrientis,* pres. part. of *nutrire* or *nutriri* to suckle, nourish, bring up] Any substance in the diet which furnishes nourishment to the body. **essential n.'s** Essential dietary substances that cannot be made in the body, such as vitamins, minerals, carbohydrate, some amino acids, and some fatty acids. **secondary n.** A substance that stimulates the gut flora to produce other nutrients. **trace n.** Any nutrient that is required by the body in quantities of a few milligrams or less.

**nutriment** \n^y^oo′trəmənt\ [L *nutriment(um)* food, nutriment] That which gives nourishment; food.

**nutrition** [Late L *nutritio* (from L *nutritus,* past part. of *nutrire* or *nutriri* to suckle, nourish, bring up) nourishment, the act of nourishing or being nourished] 1 The process by which animals and plants assimilate and utilize exogenous substances for synthesis of new tissue and production of energy. Also *threpsis.* 2 The study of the dietary requirements of human beings and other animals in a variety of normal and pathologic states. **adequate n.** Nutrition which supplies the body with all the essential nutrients in adequate amounts to maintain functioning. **parenteral n.** The provision of nutritional requirements by a parenteral route. It is usually done intravenously, by means of a peripheral vein cannula or a central vein catheter. **total parenteral n.** The provision of all nutritional requirements by a parenteral route, usually by infusion of a solution containing all the essential nutrients by way of a central or peripheral venous catheter. This method is used when oral or tube feeding is inadequate to prevent starvation or for hyperalimentation of a malnourished patient.

**nutritional** \n^y^ootrish′ənəl\ Pertaining or contributing to nutrition. Also *nutritive, nutritory.*

**nutritiongram** \n^y^ootrish′əngram\ [NUTRITION + -GRAM] Five tests sometimes used to assess nutritional status. Total lymphocyte count, serum albumin analysis, and delayed hypersensitivity skin tests are used to measure visceral proteins and immune response. Triceps skinfold and midarm circumference measurements are used to assess body fat and muscle mass respectively.

**nutritionist** \n^y^ootrish′ənist\ One who has specialized knowledge in the professional study of the effects of food on the body in health and disease.

**nutritious** \n^y^ootrish′əs\ Having nutritional value.

**nutritive** \n^y^oo′tritiv\ NUTRITIONAL.

**nutritory** \n^y^oo′tritôr′ē\ NUTRITIONAL.

**nutriture** \n^y^oo′trichər\ [*nutrit(ion)* + -URE] The nutritional status of the body with regard to all nutrients or just one, such as a specific vitamin.

**Nuttall** [John Michael *Nuttall,* English physicist, died 1958] Geiger-Nuttall law. See under LAW.

***Nuttallia*** \nutal′ē·ə\ [after George Henry Falkiner *Nuttall,* American-born English biologist, 1862–1937 + -IA] *BABESIA.*

**nux vomica** \nuks väm′ikə\ The poisonous dried ripe fruit of *Strychnos nux-vomica.* The cell wall and cell contents contain alkaloids, including strychnine and brucine. It is used as a bitter tonic and a central nervous system stimulant.

**nyacyne** \nī′əsīn\ NEOMYCIN.

**nychthemeral** \nik·thē′mərəl\ [Gk *nychthēmer(os)* (from *nyx,* gen. *nykt(os)* night + *hēmera* day) lasting a night and a day + -AL] Of or relating to the alternation of day and night, particularly a single night followed by day. Also *nycterohemeral, nyctohemeral.*

**nyct-** \nikt-\ NYCTO-.

**nyctalgia** \niktal′jə\ [NYCT- + -ALGIA] Any recurrent nocturnal pain. *Outmoded.*

**nyctalope** \nik′təlōp\ [Gk *nyktalōp(s)* (from *nyx,* gen. *nyktos,* night + *al(aos)* blind + *ōps* eye) one afflicted with night blindness] An individual who is unable to see under scotopic (dark) conditions; one affected by nyctalopia.

**nyctalopia** \nik′təlō′pē·ə\ [Gk *nyktalōp(s)* (see NYCTALOPE) + *-ia* -Y] The inability to see well under scotopic (dark) conditions, due to faulty rod function. Also *night blindness.*

**nycterine** \nik′tərīn\ NOCTURNAL.

**nycterohemeral** \nik′tərōhē′mərəl\ NYCHTHEMERAL.

**nycto-** \nik′tə-, nik′tō-\ [Gk *nyx,* gen. *nyktos* night] A combining form meaning night, nocturnal. Also *nyct-.*

**nyctohemeral** \nik′təhē′mərəl\ NYCHTHEMERAL.

**nyctotyphlosis** \nik′tətiflō′sis\ [NYCTO- + TYPHLO-^2^ + -SIS] NYCTALOPIA.

**nycturia** \niktoo′rē·ə\ [NYCT- + -URIA] NOCTURIA.

**NYD** not yet diagnosed.

**Nyhan** [William Leo *Nyhan*, U.S. physician, born 1926] Lesch-Nyhan syndrome. See under SYNDROME.

**nymph** \nimf\ [Gk *nymph(ē)* a bride, wife, marriageable young woman] A developmental stage in certain acarines and hemimetabolous insects, in which the developing juvenile resembles the adult, lacking mature genitalia and (in insects) fully developed wings, and in which growth occurs without any intermediate stages into the adult form.

**nymph-** \nimf-\ NYMPHO-.

**nympha** \nim′fə\ [Gk *nymphē* bride, chrysalis; in pl. *nymphai* part of the female genitalia.] (*pl.* nymphae) LABIUM MINUS PUDENDI.

**nymphae** \nim′fē\ Plural of NYMPHA.

**nymphal** \nim′fəl\ **1** Relating to a nymph. **2** Relating to the nymphae or labia minora.

**nymphectomy** \nimfek′təmē\ [NYMPH- + -ECTOMY] The excision of one or both labia minora.

**nymphitis** \nimfī′tis\ [NYMPH- + -ITIS] An inflammation of the labia minora. *Obs.*

**nympho-** \nim′fō-, nim′fə-\ [Gk *nymphē* bride, married woman] A combining form denoting the nymphae (labia minora). Also *nymph-*.

**nymphoid** \nim′foid\ [NYMPH + -OID] Resembling a nymph; nymphlike.

**nymphotomy** \nimfät′əmē\ [NYMPHO- + -TOMY] An incision into one or both of the labia minora.

**Nyssen** [René *Nyssen*, Belgian neurologist, flourished 20th century] Van Bogaert-Nyssen-Peiffer disease. See under METACHROMATIC LEUKODYSTROPHY.

**nystagmic** \nistag′mik\ Pertaining to or having the characteristics of nystagmus.

**nystagmography** \nis′tagmäg′rəfē\ The recording of eye movements in nystagmus.

**nystagmus** \nistag′məs\ [Gk *nystagmos* (akin to *nystazein* to nod, esp. in sleep, to slumber, sleep, to be sleepy) a nodding, esp. in sleep, drowsiness] Spontaneous, rapid, rhythmic movement of the eyes, occurring either on fixation or on ocular movement, and often due to faulty supranuclear or internuclear innervation. It may, however, be oscillatory or pendular due to poor fixation resulting from impaired visual acuity and is sometimes congenital. Also *nystaxis, talantropia, ocular ataxia*. Adj. nystagmic. **ataxic n.** Internuclear ophthalmoplegia due to a lesion of the medial longitudinal fasciculus, giving rise to nystagmus in the abducting eye appearing on lateral movement of the eyes, associated with impairment of medial movement of the adducting eye. Also *anterior internuclear ophthalmoplegia, Harris sign, medial longitudinal fasciculus syndrome*. **aural n.** VESTIBULAR NYSTAGMUS. **benign positional n.** The nystagmus accompanying paroxysms of benign positional vertigo. **caloric n.** Nystagmus occurring as the result of chilling or warming the inner ear by way of the external auditory meatus as in the caloric test. **cervical torsion n.** A form of vestibular nystagmus induced by asymmetric impairment of arterial blood flow to the inner ears by rotation of the head and neck causing distortion of a vestibular artery. **congenital n.** Nystagmus that is present at or soon after birth. It may be the result of a birth injury or of a sex-linked inheritance without associated neurologic lesions. **deviational n.** NYSTAGMOID JERKS. **disjunctive n.** Repetitive ocular movements consisting of recurring convergence and divergence of the eyes. **dissociated n.** Any nystagmus in which the range of movement is different in the two eyes. Also *incongruent nystagmus*. **down-beat n.** Vertical nystagmus occurring on downward gaze. **end-point n.** NYSTAGMOID JERKS. **end-position n.** NYSTAGMOID JERKS. **fixation n.** Nystagmus occurring when attention is directed towards an object. **incongruent n.** DISSOCIATED NYSTAGMUS. **jerking n.** PHASIC NYSTAGMUS. **labyrinthine n.** VESTIBULAR NYSTAGMUS. **latent n.** Nystagmus that occurs only when one eye is covered or receives reduced illumination. **lateral n.** Nystagmus in which the rhythmic movements are in a side to side direction. **miners' n.** Nystagmus caused by inefficient lighting which prevents stimulation of the macula sufficient to support reflex macular fixation. Movements of the eyeball are undulatory or rotary. This condition used to occur among coal miners, but with improved lighting in coal mines it is now rarely found. The condition is presently associated with psychoneurotic symptoms. **monocular n.** Nystagmus occurring in only one eye. **occupational n.** A condition resulting from prolonged deficient illumination and retinal fatigue. It used to be common among coal miners, but it has also been described among sewermen, ceiling plasterers, train dispatchers, and telegraphers. **optokinetic n.** Nystagmus induced by looking at a moving pattern, such as houses observed from the window of a train or vertical stripes on a rotating drum. This can be induced on examination to test the integrity of ocular and vestibular mechanisms. Also *opticokinetic nystagmus, railroad nystagmus, train-dispatchers' nystagmus, optomotor nystagmus*. **oscillating n.** Any nystagmus in which the movements of the eyes in each direction are similar in speed and amplitude. Also *undulatory nystagmus, vibratory nystagmus*. **palatal n.** PALATAL MYOCLONUS. **pendular n.** Oscillating nystagmus with slow, smooth, to-and-fro movements of the eyes like the swing of a long pendulum. **phasic n.** Nystagmus evoked by ocular movement in which there is a rapid repetitive movement of the eyes towards the direction of gaze followed each time by a slow recoil. Also *jerking nystagmus, resilient nystagmus, rhythmic nystagmus*. **positional n.** Nystagmus induced by movement of the head in a particular direction or by any change in position of the head. It is often associated with positional vertigo. Also *postural nystagmus*. **postrotational n.** The nystagmus observed in a subject immediately following rotation, as for example, after pirouetting or, in test conditions, rotating in the Bárány chair. It is due to the inertia of the endolymph in the semicircular canals resulting in a continuing flow relative to the now static fixed labyrinthine structure. Also *secondary nystagmus*. **postural n.** POSITIONAL NYSTAGMUS. **provocation n.** Nystagmus provoked either by rapid side-to-side movements of the head or by the variety of cervical posture tests. The condition is best observed if the subject wears Frenzel glasses. **railroad n.** OPTOKINETIC NYSTAGMUS. **rebound n.** An uncommon variety of nystagmus seen in some patients with cerebellar degeneration in whom phasic nystagmus occurs on lateral gaze but fatigues in about 20 seconds. When the eyes return to the midline, phasic nystagmus to the opposite side develops but also fatigues rapidly. **resilient n.** PHASIC NYSTAGMUS. **retraction n.** Retraction of the globe of the eyes toward the orbit with each voluntary or spontaneous movement of the eyes. It is a sign of disease in the midbrain. Also *nystagmus retractorius*. **rhythmic n.** PHASIC NYSTAGMUS. **rotatory n.** Nystagmus in which the rhythmic ocular movements show a rotatory component rather than to-and-fro movement in a horizontal or vertical plane. **secondary n.** POSTROTATIONAL NYSTAGMUS. **seesaw n.** A rare form of nystagmus in which one eye moves upward while the other moves downward repetitively. It usually results from lesions in the third ventricle or the pons. **train-dispatchers' n.** OPTOKINETIC NYSTAGMUS. **undulatory n.** OSCILLAT-

ING NYSTAGMUS. **unilateral n.** Nystagmus evoked by movement of the eyes to one side only and not to the other. **up-beat n.** Nystagmus in which the rhythmic movements are in an up and down direction. **vertical n.** Nystagmus occurring only in a vertical as distinct from a horizontal direction. **vestibular n.** Nystagmus arising from disturbance of function of the vestibular end organs subserving the various balance mechanisms located within the bony labyrinth. Also *aural nystagmus, labyrinthine nystagmus.* **vibratory n.** OSCILLATING NYSTAGMUS. **visual n.** Pendular nystagmus due to poor vision and impaired ocular fixation, as in albinism.

**nystagmus-myoclonus** A rare form of congenital nystagmus that is associated with abnormal involuntary movements of the limbs and trunk.

**nystatin** $C_{46}H_{77}NO_{19}$. An antibiotic produced by *Streptomyces nowsei.* Specific actions on *Candida albicans* account for its use in the treatment of vaginal, intestinal, oral, and dermatologic infections by the latter. It is given orally or by topical application. Also *fungicidin.*

**nystaxis** \nistak′sis\ NYSTAGMUS.

**Nysten** [Pierre Humbert *Nysten,* Belgian physician active in France, 1771–1818] See under LAW.

**nyxis** \nik′sis\ [Gk *nyxis* a puncture, piercing] PARACENTESIS.

# O

**O** Symbol for the element, oxygen.

**O.** **1** Symbol for the nonmotile strain of an organism. **2** oculus. **3** occiput.

**$O_2$** oxygen (diatomic form).

**$O_3$** ozone.

***o-*** *ortho-.*

**Ω** Symbol for the unit, ohm.

**OAF** osteoclast activating factor.

**oak** [Old English *āc*] Any deciduous, semi-evergreen or evergreen tree or shrub of the genus *Quercus.* **poison o.** **1** Either of two species of *Toxicodendron* shrub or vine. *T. diversilobum,* western poison oak, and *T. quercifolium,* eastern poison oak, can cause contact dermatitis as well as severe reactions in the oral cavity and gastrointestinal tract if ingested. An extract of the plant is used as an inhibitor of allergic reactions. **2** Dermatitis resulting from contact or exposure to the toxin of the poison oak plant.

**oario-** \ō·er′ē·ō-\ OOPHORO-.

**oath** [Old English *āth*] A solemn assertion, declaration, or affirmation. **hippocratic o.** See under HIPPOCRATES.

**OB** obstetrics.

**ob-** \äb-, əb-\ [L *ob* (assimilated before *c, f, g,* and *p* as *oc-, of-, og-,* and *op-*) against, in front of, before, on account of] A prefix meaning (1) towards, facing; (2) against, opposed to; (3) inverse, opposite. Also *oc-, of-, og-, op-.*

**obedience** / **automatic o.** The execution of another person's order blindly without regard for possible harmful consequences to oneself. It is particularly likely to occur in catatonic states and in mental retardation.

**O'Beirne** [James *O'Beirne,* Irish surgeon, 1786–1862] **1** See under EXPERIMENT. **2** O'Beirne's valve. See under SPHINCTER.

**Ober** [Frank Roberts *Ober,* U.S. surgeon, 1881–1960] **1** Ober's test. See under SIGN. **2** See under OPERATION.

**Obersteiner** [Heinrich *Obersteiner,* Austrian neurologist, 1847–1922] Obersteiner-Redlich line. See under OBERSTEINER-REDLICH SPACE.

**obese** \ōbēs′\ [L *obesus* (from OB- + L *esus,* past part. of *edere* to eat) fat, gross] Characterized by an excess accumulation of body fat; marked by or relating to obesity.

**obesity** \ōbē′sitē\ [L *obesitas* (from *obesus* fat) fatness] A state of excess accumulation of body fat. Obesity is often defined specifically as an increase in body weight of more than 20% above the standard weight for a person's height, adjusted for age, sex, and race, although some authorities recommend that an excess of 10% is cause for treatment. Obesity has been associated etiologically with genetic, hypothalamic, and endocrine factors, and physical and psychologic trauma. Obese individuals have increased morbidity and mortality from respiratory diseases, hypertension, and endocrine and metabolic disorders. The usual treatment consists of diet therapy and behavior modification. Also *hyperadiposis, hyperadiposity, adiposis.* **adrenocortical o.** The obesity characteristic of Cushing syndrome. There is a typical distribution of fat deposits in the cheeks, the nape of the neck, the supraclavicular fossae, and the trunk, the extremities being spared. Also *centripetal obesity, hyperinterrenal obesity.* **alimentary o.** EXOGENOUS OBESITY. **centripetal o.** ADRENOCORTICAL OBESITY. **endocrine o.** Obesity associated with any of several endocrine diseases, such as Cushing syndrome with hypercortisolism, eunuchoidism, and hyperinsulinism. **exogenous o.** Obesity resulting from overindulgence in food. Also *alimentary obesity, simple obesity.* **o. of hyperinsulinism** Obesity due to excessive secretion of insulin, with hypoglycemia and gross increase of appetite. It is frequently observed in cases of islet cell adenoma of the pancreas. Also *hyperinsulinar obesity.* **hyperinterrenal o.** *Older term* ADRENOCORTICAL OBESITY. **hypogonadal o.** Obesity associated with deficient secretion of sex hormones. It is especially notable in cases of male hypogonadism. Also *hypogonad obesity.* **hypothalamic o.** Adiposity due to any lesion affecting those centers of the hypothalamus that are involved in the control of appetite. Also *pituitary obesity* (incorrect). **hypothyroid o.** A condition associated with myxedema, in which the accumulation of mucoid material and water subcutaneously and elsewhere gives a misleading appearance of obesity, whereas fat synthesis is actually diminished. Also *myxedematous obesity.* **pituitary o.** *Incorrect* HYPOTHALAMIC OBESITY. **plethoric o.** Adrenocortical obesity with associated florid facies resulting from thin facial skin and polycythemia. **simple o.** EXOGENOUS OBESITY.

**obesogenous** \ō′bēsäj′ənəs\ Conducive to obesity.

**obex** \ō′beks\ [L (for *objex* a barrier, from *objectus,* past part. of *objicere* to put before), what is put before, hindrance, barrier] [NA] The midline apex of the V-shaped inferior boundaries of the fourth ventricle.

**object** / **transitional o.** Any material thing such as a sheet or security blanket that soothes and reduces anxiety in the infant under stress, and particularly when going to sleep. Attachment to the object is made directly by the infant rather than by passive acceptance of a pacifier thrust upon him.

**objective** \əbjek′tiv\ [L *objectus* (from *objectus,* past part. of *objicere* to throw or put before, proffer, offer) a placing before, an object + *-ivus* -IVE] **1** Verifiably perceptible to the senses. **2** In a compound microscope, the lens system nearest the object to be viewed, functioning to focus the rays coming from or through the viewed object. Also *object glass.* **achromatic o.** An objective lens system that is corrected for axial (chromatic) aberration for two colors. **apochromatic o.** A combination of fluorite lenses that allows correction for chromatic aberration in three wavelengths and for spherical aberration in two wavelengths. Also *apochromat.* **binocular o.'s** A pair of objectives used to provide a stereoscopic image in dissecting microscopes. **dry o.** Any microscope objective intended for use with air alone between the lens and the object examined. **immersion o.** Any microscope objective intended for use with a liquid that bathes both the lens and the object examined. **oil-immersion o.** An objective lens intended for use with immersion oil in contact with the lens and the cover glass over the object examined. **semiapochromatic o.** A system of fluorite and optical glass lenses in which chromatic aberration is corrected for three wavelengths, but correction of spherical aberration is less than that possible with apochromatic objectives. Also *semiapochromat.*

**obligate** \äb′ligit\ [L *obligat(us),* past part. of *obligare* (from *ob* against + *ligare* to bind) to tie to, bind] Having no alternative way of living, as, for example, an obligate parasite, an organism that can live only as a parasite. Compare FACULTATIVE.

**obliquity** \əblik′witē\ Oblique character or condition; inclination from the vertical or horizontal. **biparietal o.** ASYNCLITISM. **Litzmann's o.** POSTERIOR ASYNCLITISM. **Nägele's o.** ANTERIOR ASYNCLITISM. **o. of pelvis** An abnormal tilt of the pelvis in relation to the vertebral column, as seen in structural scoliosis of the lumbar spine. **Roederer's o.** A fetal position in normal labor such that the occiput presents and flexion of the head will be likely.

**obliquus** \əblī′kwəs\ Oblique.

**obliteration** \əblit′ərā′shən\ The complete loss of a space or solid part of the body, by disease, irradiation, or surgery. **percutaneous transhepatic o. of varices** An embolization of the coronary vein to halt bleeding from gastroesophageal varices. A catheter is inserted percutaneously into a portal vein radicle within the liver, then into the main portal vein, and finally into the coronary vein.

**oblongata** \äb′läng·gā′tə\ [New L, fem. of *oblongatus,* past part. of *oblongare* (from L *oblongus* oblong, rather long) to lengthen] *Seldom used* MEDULLA OBLONGATA.

**obnubilation** \əbnʸoo′bilā′shən\ [Late L *obnubilatio* (from L *obnubilatus,* past part. of *obnubilare* to make cloudy or obscure) a making clouded, darkened, obscure] STUPOR.

**obsession** \əbsesh′ən\ [L *obsessio* (from *obsessus,* past part. of *obsidere* to beset, sit down near, blockade, from OB- + L *sedere* to sit, stay fixed) a blockade, a besetting] An idea or sensory image, usually experienced as senseless or repugnant, that repetitively and insistently forces itself into consciousness even though the subject tries his best to ignore or suppress it. Obsessions are a prominent feature of obsessive-compulsive neurosis. Also *imperative idea, ruminative idea.*

**obsolescence** \äb′sōles′əns\ [English *obsolesc(ent),* from L *obsolescens,* gen. *obsolescentis,* pres. part. of *obsolescere* to become antiquated + -ENCE] A process of becoming or the state of being useless, as a physiologic function; otioseness. **glomerular o.** Loss of glomerular function due to sclerosis, hyalinization, or fibrosis.

**obsolete** \äb′sōlēt\ No longer used, as a procedure or a word.

**obstetric** \əbstet′rik\ [L *obstetricius* pertaining to midwifery, from *obstetrix,* gen. *obstetricis* a midwife, from *obst(are)* to stand facing (the parturient woman), (from OB- + *stare* to stand) + *-trix,* fem. agentive suffix] Relating to the care of women during pregnancy, labor, delivery, and postpartum. Also *obstetrical.*

**obstetrician** \äb′stətrish′ən\ A physician who specializes in obstetrics. Also *accoucheur, obstetrist.*

**obstetrics** \əbstet′riks\ [L *obstetr(ix)* a midwife + -ICS. See OBSTETRIC.] The field of medicine dealing with the care of women during pregnancy, labor and delivery, and the postpartum period. Also *maieutics* (older term), *tictology* (older term), *tocology* (older term). Adj. obstetric, obstetrical.

**obstipation** \äb′stipā′shən\ [Late L *obstipatio* (from L *obstipatus,* past part. of *obstipare* to press against) close pressure] An extreme degree of constipation.

**obstruction** \əbstruk′shən\ [L *obstructio* (from *obstructus,* past part. of *obstruere* to build against, block, stop, from OB- + *struere* to put together, build, devise, akin to Gk *storennynai* to spread, make level) a hindrance, a closing up by building] Blockage to the normal flow of a hollow viscus, a duct, or a blood vessel. **false colonic o.** OGILVIE SYNDROME. **female prostatic o.** Obstruction of the bladder neck due to inflammation and/or hypertrophy of the proximal urethral glands which surround the posterior neck of the female urethra. **idiopathic ureteropelvic junction o.** Obstruction of the renal pelvis outlet by extrinsic fibrous bands, intrinsic stenosis, or high insertion of the ureter in the renal pelvis. The conditions usually are congenital, and may or may not cause hydronephrosis. **renal pelvic o.** Obstruction of the renal pelvis by calculi, tumor, or idiopathic ureteropelvic junction obstruction. Hydronephritis and secondary infections with loss of renal function are common. **ureteral o.** Obstruction of the ureter by a calculus, tumor, extrinsic fibrous bands, localized intrinsic stenosis, or retroperitoneal fibrosis. One or both ureters may be involved. Calculi may be associated with renal colic, and hydronephrosis and secondary infections are common. **ureteropelvic o.** Obstruction of the renal pelvic outlet by a calculus, tumor, or idiopathic ureteropelvic junction obstruction. Hydronephrosis and secondary infections are common. **ureterovesical o.** Obstruction of the ureter at the ureterovesical junction due to calculus or tumor. Hydronephrosis and secondary infection are common. **urinary tract o.** Obstruction due to calculi, tumor, or other abnormalities anywhere in the urinary tract, including the renal pelvis, ureter, bladder, and urethra. **uteropelvic o.** A stenosis or a blockage at the renal pelvis and ureteral junction.

**obstructive** \əbstruk′tiv\ Tending or acting to obstruct; causing or apt to cause obstruction.

**obstruent** \äb′stroo·ənt\ [L *obstruens,* gen. *obstruentis,* pres. part. of *obstruere* to build against, block or wall up, hinder. The past part. is *obstructus.*] **1** Causing obstruction. **2** An agent causing obstruction.

**obtundation** \äb′tundā′shən\ [L *obtund(ere)* (from *ob* against + *tundere* to beat or strike repeatedly, stun) to beat, belabor, blunt, dull + -ATION] Any general depression of cerebral function ranging from sedation to coma; a clouding of consciousness.

**obtundity** \əbtun′ditē\ [L *obtund(ere)* to beat, blunt, dull + -ITY] A state of dulled or blunted consciousness.

**obturation** \äb′tʸərā′shən\ [from L *obturatus,* past part.

of *obturare* to stop or close up] Closure or occlusion of an opening or cleft.

**obturator** \äb′tʸərā′tər\ [New L (from L *obturat(us),* past part. of *obturare* to stop or close up + *-or* -OR)] **1** A device for closing or occluding an opening or cavity. **2** A prosthetic appliance closing a congenital or acquired opening in the palate. **3** Describing an anatomic structure, e.g., the obturator membrane, that occludes an opening. **4** Pertaining to or associated with the obturator membrane, as *obturator foramen, obturator hernia.* **buccofacial o.** A mechanical device for closing a pathological opening of the cheek to facilitate speech and feeding.

**obtusion** \əbtʸoo′zhən\ [L *obtusus* (past part. of *obtundere* to beat, blunt) blunt, dull, weakened] A state of diminished sensibility or consciousness.

**oc-** \äk-, ək-\ OB-.

**Occam** [William of *Occam,* English philosopher, c. 1285–c. 1349] See under RAZOR.

**occipital** \äksip′itəl\ Of or relating to the occiput.

**occipitalization** \äksip′itəlīzā′shən\ The fusion of the atlas with the occiput by synostosis.

**occipito-** \äksip′itō-\ [L *occiput* (genitive *occipitis)* back of the head] A combining form meaning occiput, occipital.

**occipitoanterior** \-antir′ē·ər\ [OCCIPITO- + ANTERIOR] Having the occiput directed towards the mother's symphysis pubis: said of a fetal position.

**occipitobasilar** \-bas′ilər\ Pertaining to the occiput and the base of the skull.

**occipitocalcarine** \-kal′kərīn\ Denoting axons of the occipital cerebral cortex traced to the calcarine sulcus.

**occipitocervical** \-sur′vikəl\ Pertaining to the occiput and the neck.

**occipitofrontal** \-frun′təl\ Pertaining to the occiput and the forehead or frontal bone.

**occipitofrontalis** \-fruntā′lis\ MUSCULUS OCCIPITOFRONTALIS.

**occipitomastoid** \-mas′toid\ Pertaining to the occipital bone and the mastoid process.

**occipitomental** \-men′təl\ Pertaining to the occiput and the chin.

**occipitoparietal** \-pərī′ətəl\ PARIETO-OCCIPITAL.

**occipitopontine** \-pän′tīn\ Denoting the occipital cortex and pons, or connections between them.

**occipitoposterior** \-pästir′ē·ər\ [OCCIPITO- + POSTERIOR] Having the occiput directed towards the mother's sacrum: said of a fetal position.

**occipitotemporal** \-tem′pərəl\ Pertaining to the occipital and the temporal bones or lobes of the cerebrum. Also *temporo-occipital.*

**occipitothalamic** \-thəlam′ik\ Denoting the nerve fibers between the caudal thalamus (lateral geniculate body) and occipital lobe cerebral cortex.

**occiput** \äk′siput\ [L, from *oc-* OC- + *caput* head] The back part of the skull or head. Compare SINCIPUT.

**occlude** \əklood′\ **1** To close off or stop up; obstruct. **2** To bring or come into a state of occlusion, as upper and lower teeth.

**occluder** \əkloo′dər\ ARTICULATOR.

**occlusal** \əkloo′səl\ [L *occlus(us)* (past part. of *occludere* to shut) closed, shut + -AL] Describing the surface of a tooth which faces or contacts a tooth in the opposite jaw. Also *morsal.*

**occlusion** \əkloo′zhən\ [L *occlusus* (past part. of *occludere* to shut, close, from OC- + *claudere* to shut; Gk *kleiein* to shut) closed, shut + *-io* -ION] **1** The act of occluding or the condition of being occluded. **2** The relation between upper and lower antagonistic teeth in contact with each other. **3** The spacial overlap of central neural excitation in a reflex event where the sum of two or more inputs together is less than the sum of their effects individually. **acentric o.** ECCENTRIC OCCLUSION. **acquired eccentric o.** Eccentric occlusion with maximum contact of teeth. It is caused by a deflecting premature contact. Also *convenience occlusion, convenience bite, habitual occlusion.* **anatomic o.** An occlusion with the teeth arranged in their correct positions in the arches and occluding correctly in centric occlusion. **anterior o.** MANDIBULAR PROGNATHISM. **balanced o.** An occlusion that provides even contact throughout the dental arch in centric and eccentric positions. Also *balanced articulation, balanced bite.* **centric o.** Occlusion with maximal tooth contacts and the mandible in centric position. Also *normal occlusion, centric relation occlusion, central occlusion, centric contact.* **convenience o.** ACQUIRED ECCENTRIC OCCLUSION. **coronary o.** Occlusion of a coronary artery or its branches, most often due to thrombosis, less often to spasm or embolism, and often causing myocardial infarction. **distal o.** DISTOCLUSION. **dynamic o.** DENTAL ARTICULATION. **eccentric o.** The occlusion when the mandible is in any eccentric position. Also *acentric occlusion.* **edge-to-edge o.** An occlusion in which the tips of the upper and lower anterior teeth meet instead of overlapping. Also *edge-to-edge bite.* **equilibrated o.** An occlusion which has been brought into balance. **gliding o.** DENTAL ARTICULATION. **habitual o.** ACQUIRED ECCENTRIC OCCLUSION. **hepatic vein o.** Occlusion of one or both hepatic veins, most often due to thrombosis and giving rise to the Budd-Chiari syndrome. **ideal o.** An anatomic occlusion which is also balanced. **locked o.** An occlusion with very limited eccentric movements, as a deep overbite or scissors crossbite. Also *locked bite.* **mesenteric artery o.** Cessation of flow in the mesenteric artery, especially of the superior mesenteric artery, due to embolism or thrombosis. **mesial o.** An occlusion in which a lower tooth is positioned mesial to its equivalent in the upper jaw. Also *prenormal occlusion.* **normal o.** **1** CENTRIC OCCLUSION. **2** Normal anatomic relation of dental arches and of teeth within each arch. Also *normal bite, neutral occlusion.* **posterior o.** MANDIBULAR RETRUSION. **postnormal o.** DISTOCLUSION. **prenormal o.** MESIAL OCCLUSION. **protrusive o.** MANDIBULAR PROGNATHISM. **o. of the renal artery** Complete obliteration of the lumen of the renal artery or one of its branches due to embolism or thrombosis. It may cause hypertension, and if bilateral, may produce renal failure. **retrusive o.** MANDIBULAR RETRUSION. **spherical form of o.** A pattern of occlusion corresponding to the surface of a sphere. **traumatic o.** An occlusion causing injury to the periodontium, to an edentulous ridge, or to the teeth. **traumatogenic o.** An occlusion considered to be capable of causing injury to the periodontium, the teeth, the temporomandibular joints, or the residual ridge.

**occlusive** \əkloo′siv\ Sealing against exposure to air, as a dressing.

**occlusometer** \äk′loosäm′ətər\ [*occlus(ion)* + *o* + -METER] GNATHODYNAMOMETER.

**occult** \əkult′\ [L *occult(us),* past part. of *occulare* to cover, hide] Not readily apparent or detectable; hidden or disguised, as an infection, the presence of blood, or a tumor, as, for example, a cancer whose primary site is hidden but whose metastases are evident.

**occupancy** The period during which a unit quantity of a substance, administered in a particular fashion, is present in a specific part of the body or at certain sites, before it is excreted or metabolized.

**ocellus** \ōsel′əs\ [L, a little eye, an eye] (*pl.* ocelli) **1** EYESPOT. **2** The simple eye found in some insects and other arthropods. **3** One of the units of a compound eye of an insect. **4** An eyelike color patch.

***Ochrogaster contraria*** \ō′krōgas′tər kəntrer′ē·ə\ A species of caterpillar whose hairs cause an allergic reaction characterized by urticaria and a papular pruritic eruption in susceptible individuals.

**ochronosis** \ō′krōnō′sis\ [New L *ochronosus,* from Gk *ōchro(s)* pale, ocher-colored + *nosos* disease, with ending assimilated to the suffix -OSIS; so called because of the ocher-colored microscopic appearance of the deposited pigments] Chronic joint disease associated with the deposition of pigment within articular cartilage and found in patients with alkaptonuria. Also *ochronosus.* Adj. ochronotic. **ocular o.** Scleral pigmentation associated with alkaptonuria.

**ochronosus** \ō′krōnō′səs\ OCHRONOSIS.

**Ochsner** [Albert John *Ochsner*, U.S. surgeon, 1858–1925] See under RING.

**oct-** \äkt-, əkt-\ OCTA-.

**octa-** \äk′tə-\ [Gk *oktō* eight] A combining form meaning eight. Also *oct-, octi-, octo-.*

**octahedral** \-hē′drəl\ **1** Having the symmetry of an octahedron. **2** Denoting a molecular configuration in which six ligands are regularly arranged around a center.

**octahedron** \-hē′drän\ [Gk *oktaedron* (from neut. of *oktaedros* eight-sided, from *oct(ō)* eight + *a* + *(h)edra* a seat, base) an octahedron] The regular polyhedron with eight faces, which are equilateral triangles, and six vertices.

**octan** \äk′tən\ [L *oct(o)* eight + English *-an,* as in *quartan*] Recurring every eighth day, as certain febrile paroxysms.

**octanoic acid** $CH_3$—$[CH_2]_6$—COOH. One of the fatty acids, occurring in butter as its esters. Also *caprylic acid* (outmoded).

**octarius** [L *octo* eight] A measure of volume equal to a pint, or one-eighth of a gallon.

**octi-** \äk′ti-\ OCTA-.

**octo-** \äk′tə-, äk′tō-\ OCTA-.

***Octomitus hominis*** \äk′təmī′təs häm′ənis\ *PENTATRICHOMONAS HOMINIS.*

**Octoson** \äk′təsän\ An automatic ultrasound imaging system employing a series of eight transducers mounted in a water bath in such a way that the image lies in the focal zone of each transducer. The transducers are moved mechanically in an arc, each producing a scan which is integrated into a single picture.

**octyl gallate** Octyl 3,4,5-trihydroxybenzoate. It has been employed as an antioxidizing agent in pharmaceutic preparations, particularly fat-soluble compounds.

**ocular** \äk′yələr\ [*ocul(o)-* + -AR] **1** Pertaining to the eye. **2** EYEPIECE. **Huygen's o.** HUYGENIAN EYEPIECE. **wide-field o.** WIDEFIELD EYEPIECE.

**oculentum** \äk′yəlen′təm\ [L *ocul(us)* eye + *-entum* English *-ent*] An ointment for use in or around the eye.

**oculi** \äk′yəlī\ Plural of OCULUS.

**oculist** \äk′yəlist\ [*ocul(o)-* + -IST] OPHTHALMOLOGIST.

**oculo-** \äk′ʸəlō-\ [L *oculus* the eye] A combining form denoting the eye.

**oculocephalic** \-səfal′ik\ [OCULO- + CEPHALIC] Pertaining to or affecting the eyes and brain.

**oculocephalogyric** \-sef′əlōjī′rik\ [OCULO- + CEPHALO- + GYR- + -IC] Pertaining to abnormal movements of both head and eyes, as in the oculogyric crises of Parkinson's disease.

**oculocutaneous** \-kyootā′nē·əs\ [OCULO- + CUTANEOUS] Pertaining to conditions affecting both skin and eyes.

**oculogyric** \-jī′rik\ [OCULO- + GYR- + -IC] Describing, pertaining to, or producing spontaneous and sustained ocular movements, usually in an upward direction as in parkinsonism. Also *ophthalmogyric.*

**oculometroscope** \-met′rəskōp\ [OCULO- + *-metr(y)* + *o* + -SCOPE] A retinoscope in which the trial lenses are rotated automatically by the instrument.

**oculomotor** \-mō′tər\ [OCULO- + MOTOR] Pertaining to or affecting ocular movement.

**oculomycosis** \-mīkō′sis\ [OCULO- + MYCOSIS] Any fungous disease of the eye.

**oculopathy** \äk′yəläp′əthē\ [OCULO- + -PATHY] Any disorder of the eye.

**oculoplethysmography** \-pleth′ismäg′rəfē\ A diagnostic technique whereby the presence of critical internal carotid artery stenosis or occlusion is indirectly inferred by demonstrating an ipsilateral delay in the arrival of ocular pressures transmitted from branches of the ophthalmic artery, when compared with arrival of the ipsilateral external carotid artery pulse as manifested by an ear lobe photocell.

**oculopneumoplethysmography** \-nʸoo′mōpleth′ismäg′rəfē\ An indirect test for demonstrating the presence of a critical carotid artery stenosis or occlusion by measuring the negative pressure, when applied to the eye, that is required to obliterate pulsations due to the pulse pressure in branches of the ophthalmic artery. Also *pneumoplethysmography.*

**oculosensory** \-sen′sərē\ [OCULO- + SENSORY] Pertaining to or affected by stimuli to the eye.

**oculus** \äk′yələs\ [L (akin to Gk *ōps*), the eye] (*pl.* oculi) [NA] The organ of vision comprising bulbus oculi and nervus opticus; eye. **o. caesius** GLAUCOMA. **o. dexter** The right eye. Abbr. OD **o. laevus** The left eye. Abbr. OL **o. leporinus** LAGOPHTHALMOS. **o. sinister** The left eye. Abbr. OS

**ocyodinic** \ō′sē·ōdin′ik\ OXYTOCIC.

**OD** **1** oculus dexter. **2** optical density (absorbance). **3** (drug) overdose *Popular.* **4** outside diameter.

**odaxetic** \ō′dakset′ik\ [Gk *odax(ein)* to bite, sting + *-etik(os)* adjectival suffix] Producing a sense of itching or of being bitten.

**Oddi** [Ruggero *Oddi*, Italian physician, 1864–1913] Oddi's muscle. See under MUSCULUS SPHINCTER AMPULLAE HEPATOPANCREATICAE.

**odds / relative o.** ODDS RATIO.

**odiferous** \ōdif′ərəs\ ODORIFEROUS.

**odogenesis** \äd′ōjen′əsis\ [Gk *(h)odo(s)* a way, path + GENESIS] NEUROCLADISM.

**odont-** \ōdänt′-\ ODONTO-.

**-odont** \-ədänt\ [Gk *odous* or Ionic variant *odōn* (gen. of both, *odontos*) tooth] A combining form meaning having teeth (of a specified kind). Also *-dont.*

**odontalgia** \ō′däntal′jə\ [ODONT- + -ALGIA] TOOTHACHE.

**odonterism** \ōdän′tərizm\ [ODONT- + Gk *erism(a)* a quarreling] Chattering of the teeth. *Seldom used.*

**odontexesis** \ōdän′teksē′sis\ [ODONT- + *e* + Gk *xesis* a polishing by scraping or planing] Scaling and polishing of the teeth.

**-odontia** \-ōdän′shə\ [Gk *odous,* gen. *odont(os)* tooth + *-ia,* derivative noun suffix] A combining form meaning (1) state or condition of the teeth; (2) study or treatment of the teeth.

**odontic** \ōdän′tik\ [ODONT- + -IC] Relating to the teeth.

**odonto-** \ōdän′tō-\ [Gk *odous* (genitive *odontos*) tooth] A combining form denoting tooth or teeth. Also *odont-.*

**odontoameloblastoma** \-am′əlōblastō′mə\ [ODONTO- + AMELOBLASTOMA] A very rare neoplasm characterized by the presence of enamel, dentin, and an odontogenic epithelium resembling that of an ameloblastoma both in structure and behavior.
**odontoatlantal** \-ətlan′təl\ ATLANTOAXIAL.
**odontoblast** \ōdän′təblast\ [ODONTO- + -BLAST] One of the specialized connective tissue cells which take part in the formation of the dentin of a tooth. They form a layer of columnar cells on the outer part of the dental pulp and each cell leaves a dentinal fiber within a dentinal tubule as the dentin is deposited on the outer aspect of the odontoblast layer. Odontoblasts persist throughout the life of a tooth. Also *dentinoblast.*
**odontoblastoma** \-blastō′mə\ [ODONTO- + BLASTOMA] A tumor of odontoblasts.
**odontoclamis** \-klā′mis\ [ODONTO- + Gk *chlamys* a horseman's short cloak or mantle] DENTAL OPERCULUM.
**odontoclast** \ōdän′təklast\ [ODONTO- + -CLAST] A cell, indistinguishable from an osteoclast, which is involved in the resorption of the roots of deciduous teeth.
**odontodysplasia** \-displā′zhə\ [ODONTO- + DYSPLASIA] A developmental anomaly affecting both dentin and enamel production. Also *ghost teeth.*
**odontogenesis** \-jen′əsis\ [ODONTO- + GENESIS] The initiation and development of teeth. Also *odontogeny.* Adj. odontogenetic. **o. imperfecta** DENTINOGENESIS IMPERFECTA.
**odontogeny** \ō′däntäj′ənē\ ODONTOGENESIS.
**odontologist** \ō′däntäl′əjist\ [*odontolog(y)* + -IST] DENTIST.
**odontology** \ō′däntäl′əjē\ [ODONTO- + -LOGY] DENTISTRY. **forensic o.** FORENSIC DENTISTRY.
**odontoma** \ō′däntō′mə\ [ODONT- + -OMA] A malformative odontogenic tumorlike lesion in which a mixture of dental tissues, particularly enamel and dentin, is present. Also *odontome.* **ameloblastic o.** An odontoma with ameloblastic epithelium. **calcified o.** A calcified tumor arising from odontogenic cells, such as cementoma, complex odontoma, compound odontoma, dentinoma, and enameloma. **complex o.** A tumorlike malformative lesion of the jaw in which all dental tissues are present. The components are well formed, but arranged in a disorderly manner. Also *composite odontoma.* **compound o.** A tumorlike malformative lesion of the jaw in which all dental tissues are present and in a more orderly manner than in a complex odontoma, so that the relations between the components resemble that seen in the normal tooth. Also *composite odontoma.* **cystic o.** An odontoma with an associated follicular cyst. **dilated o.** DENS INVAGINATUS. **dilated composite o.** DENS INVAGINATUS. **epithelial o.** An odontoma of ectodermal origin, such as ameloblastoma, adenoameloblastoma, calcifying epithelial odontogenic tumor, and calcifying epithelial odontogenic cyst. **fibrous o.** ODONTOGENIC FIBROMA. **gestant o.** DENS INVAGINATUS.
**odontome** \ōdän′tōm\ ODONTOMA.
**odontoparallaxis** \-par′əlak′sis\ [ODONTO- + PARALLAXIS] MALOCCLUSION.
**odontoperiosteum** \-per′ē·äs′tē·əm\ PERIODONTIUM.
**odontoplasty** \ōdän′təplas′tē\ [ODONTO- + -PLASTY] Reshaping the crown and/or root surface of teeth, mainly to improve accessibility for oral hygiene.
**odontosarcoma** \-särkō′mə\ [ODONTO- + SARCOMA] AMELOBLASTIC ODONTOSARCOMA. **ameloblastic o.** A very rare malignant tumor similar to the ameloblastic fibrosarcoma but containing dysplastic dentine and enamel.
**odontotheca** \-thē′kə\ DENTAL FOLLICLE.
**odor** [L (akin to *olere* to emit an odor, and to Gk *ozein* to have a smell and *odmē* a smell, scent, sweet or bad odor), an odor] The property of something that excites the sense of smell.
**odorant** \ō′dərənt\ **1** Producing an odor; odoriferous. **2** Any substance producing an odor.
**odoriferous** \ō′dôrif′ərəs\ Characterized by or disseminating an odor, particularly an agreeable odor. Also *odorous, odiferous* (seldom used).
**odorogram** \ōdôr′əgram\ OLFACTORY SPECTROGRAM.
**odorous** \ō′dərəs\ ODORIFEROUS.
**odynacusis** \ō′dinək$^y$oo′sis\ [*odyn(o)-* + -ACUSIS] Pain in the ear induced by sound. Also *odynacousis.*
**-odynia** \-ōdin′ē·ə\ [Gk *odynē* pain, distress] A combining form meaning pain.
**odyno-** \äd′inō-, ō′dinō-\ [Gk *odynē* pain, distress] A combining form meaning pain.
**odynometer** \ō′dinäm′ətər\ [ODYNO- + -METER] An instrument designed to measure pain.
**odynophagia** \ō′dinōfā′jə\ [ODYNO- + -PHAGIA] Pain on swallowing.
**odynuria** \ō′dinoo′rē·ə\ [ODYN- + -URIA] Pain while urinating.
**oe-** \ē-\ For words beginning *oe-*, see also under E-.
**oeco-** \ēk′ō-, ek′ə-\ ECO-.
**oedema** \idē′mə\ *Brit.* EDEMA.
**oedematous** \idē′mətəs\ *Brit.* EDEMATOUS.
**oedipism** \ed′ipizm\ [after *Oedip(us),* legendary king of Thebes, who mistakenly killed his father, married his mother, and tore out his own eyes in anguish + -ISM] The act of inflicting injury upon one's own eyes. *Older term.*
**Oehl** [Eusebio *Oehl,* Italian anatomist, 1827–1903] Oehl's layer. See under STRATUM LUCIDUM EPIDERMIDIS.
**oesophagitis** *Brit.* ESOPHAGITIS.
**oesophago-** \esäf′əgō-\ *Brit.* ESOPHAGO-.
**oesophagocele** \esäf′əgōsēl′\ *Brit.* ESOPHAGOCELE.
**oesophagoscope** \esäf′əgōskōp′\ *Brit.* ESOPHAGOSCOPE.
**oesophagoscopy** \esäf′əgäs′kəpē\ *Brit.* ESOPHAGOSCOPY.
***Oesophagostomum apiostomum*** \ēsäf′əgäs′təməm ā′pē·äs′təməm\ A species of nematode commonly parasitic in monkeys and apes in central Africa, India, the Philippines, China, and Brazil. The larvae can encyst in the human intestine, sometimes causing a form of dysentery. Tumorlike lesions of the ileocecal region with eosinophilic infiltration have been reported in Uganda. The worms leave the nodules to become adults in the lumen of the large intestine. Treatment is with intestinal anthelmintics. Also *Oesophagostomum brumpti.*
**oesophagostomy** *Brit.* ESOPHAGOSTOMY.
**oesophagotomy** *Brit.* ESOPHAGOTOMY.
**oesophagus** \esäf′əgəs\ *Brit.* ESOPHAGUS.
**oestradiol** \es′trədī′ôl\ *Brit.* ESTRADIOL.
**oestriasis** \estrī′əsis\ [*Oestr(us)* + -IASIS] Infestation of sheep by maggots of the genus *Oestrus..* Also *estriasis.*
**oestriol** *Brit.* ESTRIOL.
**oestrogen** *Brit.* ESTROGEN.
**oestrone** *Brit.* ESTRONE.
**oestrous** \es′trəs\ *Brit.* ESTROUS.
***Oestrus ovis*** \es′trəs ō′vis\ The sheep botfly or head maggot, a now cosmopolitan species of botfly that was originally imported into North America from Europe. The adult deposits larvae in the sheep's nostrils. The larvae develop in the nasal cavities and sinuses, disrupting feeding and causing irritation and a mucous discharge. They can cause serious problems, if present in large numbers, particularly in weak, old, or very young animals. Occasionally they cause myiasis

in humans, especially ocular myiasis.

**oestrus** \es′trəs\ *Brit.* ESTRUS.

**of-** \äf-, əf-\ OB-.

**OFD I** OROFACIODIGITAL SYNDROME I.

**OFD II** OROFACIODIGITAL SYNDROME II.

**office** A room or suite of rooms in which a medical or other health professional regularly receives patients and treats them insofar as more extensive facilities are not required. • This usage of *office* is established in the United States and to some extent in Canada and New Zealand. In the United Kingdom and elsewhere, *surgery* is preferred, though it is somewhat more specific and is distinguished, for example, from *consulting room.*

**officer / house o.** A health care professional, usually a physician, who is in training in a hospital; a member of the house staff.

**official** Recognized by, and meeting the requirements of, an authoritative body such as the National Formulary, the U.S. Pharmacopeia, or the British Pharmaceutical Codex.

**officinal** Denoting a chemical or drug kept regularly in stock in a pharmacy, as opposed to those preparations compounded as requested, as specified by a prescription. Compare MAGISTRAL.

**off-line** 1 Not under the direct control of a central computer processing unit: used of equipment such as a printer. 2 Designating the operative of input/output devices not under direct control of a system. 3 Designating a system in which an aliquot is withdrawn from the stream and conveyed to the detector.

**og-** \äg-, əg-\ OB-.

**Ogilvie** [Sir William Heneage *Ogilvie,* English physician, flourished 20th century] See under SYNDROME.

**Ogino** [Kyusaka *Ogino,* Japanese physician, born 1881] Ogino-Knaus method. See under METHOD.

**ogo** \ō′gō\ GANGOSA.

**Ogston** [Sir Alexander *Ogston,* Scottish surgeon, 1844–1929] See under LINE.

**Oguchi** [Chuta *Oguchi,* Japanese ophthalmologist, 1875–1945] See under DISEASE.

**Ohara** [Hachiro *Ohara,* Japanese physician, born 1882] Ohara's disease. See under TULAREMIA.

**Ohlmacher** [Albert Philip *Ohlmacher,* U.S. physician, 1865–1916] See under SOLUTION.

**Ohm** [Georg Simon *Ohm,* German physicist, 1787–1854] See under LAW.

**ohm** \ōm\ [after Georg Simon *Ohm,* German physicist, 1787–1854] The special name for the SI derived unit of electric resistance; the electric resistance between two points of a conductor when a constant potential difference of one volt, applied at those points, produces in the conductor a current of one ampere, the conductor not being the seat of any electromotive force; 1 ohm = 1 volt/1 ampere. Symbol: Ω **reciprocal o.** A unit of electrical conductance, now generally referred to by the special name siemens. Symbol: $\Omega^{-1}$

**-oic** [*o* + -IC] A suffix replacing the final -e of the suffix *-ane* of a hydrocarbon to convert its name into that of a carboxylic acid.

**-oid** \-oid\ [Gk stem vowel *-o-* + *-eid(ēs)* -like, akin to *eidos* form, shape, kind] A suffix meaning having the form of, like, resembling.

**oiko-** \oi′kō-\ ECO-.

**oikosite** \oi′kōsīt\ [OIKO- + Gk *sit(os)* food] ECOSITE.

**oil** [Old French *oile* (from L *oleum* olive oil, oil, from Gk *elaion* olive oil, oil) oil] Any viscous, combustible liquid, often a petroleum fraction, insoluble in water and soluble in ether. Also *oleum.* **ajowan o.** An essential oil extracted from the dried, ripe fruits of *Trachyspermum ammi.* It is used as a carminative and antispasmodic agent. **o. of amber** A pale yellow or brownish yellow oil with a penetrating odor and a sharp, burning taste, obtained by the destructive distillation of certain resins. It was formerly obtained from amber. It has properties like those of turpentine oil and is used in liniments. Also *oleum succini.* **aromatic castor o.** A mixture of castor oil with cinnamon oil, clove oil, saccharin, vanilla, and alcohol. It is used as a laxative. Also *oleum ricini aromaticum.* **artificial essential o. of almond** BENZALDEHYDE. **cade o.** JUNIPER TAR. **camphorated o.** CAMPHOR LINIMENT. **carbolic o.** PHENOLATED OIL. **castor o.** A fixed oil cold-pressed from the kernel of the seeds of *Ricinus communis.* Its principal constituent is triricinolein. It also contains isoricinolein, palmitin, and dihydroxystearin. The mild purgative property of ricinoleic acid and its isomer is produced in the duodenum by hydrolysis. It has been used in the treatment of hemorrhoids, during pregnancy, as an ointment for irritated skin, a solvent for alkaloids in treating the conjunctiva, and as an ingredient of soaps. The seeds also contain a highly toxic substance. Also *oleum ricini, ricinus oil, oil of Palma Christi.* **cedar o.** A volatile oil obtained from the distillation of the wood of various species of cedar, principally *Juniperus virginiana.* The oil consists almost entirely of cedrene, a liquid sesquiterpene, and cedral. It is used in microscopy as a clearing agent and immersion medium with oil-immersion objectives, and also in perfumery. **clove o.** An oil obtained by the distillation of the dried, highly aromatic, unopened flower buds and twig tips of the clove tree, *Eugenia caryophyllata.* Its chief constituent is eugenol. Taken internally, it is used as an antispasmodic and a carminative. It is used externally as a rubefacient, counterirritant, and a mild analgesic, and it is used in histology as a clearing agent. **distilled o.** VOLATILE OIL. **essential o.** VOLATILE OIL. **ethereal o.** VOLATILE OIL. **eucalyptus o.** A volatile oil from the oil distilled from the fresh leaves of various *Eucalyptus* species. It is used as an antiseptic, deodorant, diaphoretic, expectorant, and in the synthesis of menthol. **Haarlem o.** JUNIPER TAR. **halibut liver o.** Oil obtained from the liver of the halibut, *Hippoglossus hippoglossus.* The oil is used as a convenient way of administering vitamins A and D, as it contains 100 times as much vitamin A as cod liver oil and 250 times as much vitamin D. It has only a slight fishy odor and taste. Also *oleum hippoglossi.* **immersion o.** In immersion microscopy, the oil that is interposed between the objective lens and the cover slip over the object being examined. Cedarwood or cedar oil, from *Juniperus virginiana,* is often used. **Indian melissa o.** LEMON GRASS OIL. **Indian o. of verbena** LEMON GRASS OIL. **iodized o.** A vegetable oil containing organically combined iodine and used as a contrast medium in radiologic examinations, such as bronchography, hysterosalpingography and laryngography. **jojoba o.** A liquid derived from the crushed seeds of *Simmindsia chinensis* and *S. californica,* shrubs indigenous to the Southwestern U.S. and Northern Mexico. It is used mainly as a lubricant. **juniper tar o.** JUNIPER TAR. **lemon grass o.** An oil obtained by distillation from the grasses *Cymbopogon flexuosus* and *C. citratus* from India. It was formerly used as a flavoring agent and carminative, but is now primarily used as a source of citral, which is important in vitamin A synthesis, and in perfumery. It also contains traces of geraniol, citronellal, and dipentene. Also *Indian oil of verbena, Indian melissa oil.* **mineral o.** 1 A petroleum fraction of fairly high boiling point, usually purified to the standards necessary for medicinal use.

It is not absorbed from the gut and is therefore sometimes used as a laxative. Also *liquid paraffin.* 2 PETROLEUM. **o. of Palma Christi** CASTOR OIL. **phenolated o.** A 5% weight per volume solution of phenol in arachis oil. It was formerly used as local anesthetic on the skin, but dizziness and fever sometimes followed its use. Dilution of phenolic solutions with water are caustic, and glycerine should be used instead. Also *carbolic oil.* **rectified camphor o.** A volatile, colorless or yellow oil that is formed as a by-product in the manufacture of camphor from *Cinnamomum camphora.* It consists of safrol, acetaldehyde, camphor, terpineol, eugenol, cineol, *d*-pinene, phellandrene, dipentene, and cadinene. It is used as a counterirritant, rubefacient, and parasiticide, and it is applied topically to rheumatic and inflamed joints. Also *oleum camphorae essentiale, oleum camphorae rectificatum.* **ricinus o.** CASTOR OIL. **sweet birch o.** METHYL SALICYLATE. **teaberry o.** METHYL SALICYLATE. **volatile o.** An odorous principle found in different parts of plants which evaporates when exposed to air at ordinary temperatures. Volatile oils represent the essences or active principle in plants. Although differing greatly in their chemical composition, they have several physical properties in common. They have characteristic odors due to the presence of oxygenated derivatives of terpenes and sesquiterpenes. They have high refractive indices. Most are optically active. Generally, they are not miscible with water but are soluble in alcohol, ether, and most organic solvents. The oils are obtained by steam distillation, enzymatic hydrolysis, expression, enfleurage, and destructive distillation. Also *distilled oil, essential oil, ethereal oil.* **wintergreen o.** METHYL SALICYLATE.

# ointment

**ointment** [Old French *oignement* (irreg. from L *unguentum* an ointment, perfume, akin to *unctus,* past part. of *ungere* to wet, anoint, smear; Gk *hygros* wet, soft) an ointment] A semisolid preparation of one or more medicinal substances in a suitable base. There are hydrocarbon bases for emollient effects, water-in-oil emulsion bases for good absorption, creams that can be washed off for cosmetic reasons, and greaseless ointment bases. Also *salve, unction, unguent, unguentum, uncture, aliptic.* **ammoniated mercury o.** An ointment containing ammoniated mercury, usually at about a 5% concentration, in a suitable oily base. It has been used in the past for external application for some skin conditions but has been generally replaced with other medications. The danger of mercury poisoning is too serious to use such mercurial agents. Also *white precipitate ointment, unguentum hydrargyri ammoniati.* **anthralin o.** An ointment containing anthralin in a soft paraffin or other suitable base, used for the treatment of psoriasis and a number of other chronic dermatoses. **benzoic and salicylic acid o.** An ointment containing 6% benzoic acid and 3% salicylic acid. Also *Whitfield's ointment, unguentum acidi benzoici compositum.* **boric acid o.** An ointment containing 1% boric acid in white petrolatum. Also *unguentum acidi borici.* **calamine o.** An ointment containing 15% calamine in white petrolatum. Also *Turner cerate, unguentum calaminae.* **carbolic acid o.** PHENOL OINTMENT. **chloramphenicol ophthalmic o.** A sterile eye ointment containing 1% chloramphenicol. **chrysarobin o.** An ointment containing 4% chrysarobin. Also *unguentum chrysarobini.* **coal tar o.** An ointment containing coal tar, polysorbate 80, and zinc paste. It is used in the treatment of eczema. Also *unguentum picis carbonis.* **compound o. of calamine** An ointment containing calamine and zinc oxide in white petrolatum combined in solution with coal tar in hydrous wool fat. Also *unguentum calaminae compositum, unguentum sedativum.* **compound o. of capsicum** An ointment containing capsicum oleoresin, menthol, chloral hydrate, camphor, and petrolatum. Also *chillie paste, unguentum capsici compositum, unguentum oleoresinae capsici compositum.* **compound resorcinol o.** An ointment containing resorcinol, bismuth subnitrate and zinc oxide. It is used to treat certain skin diseases. Also *unguentum resorcini compositum, unguentum resorcinolis compositum.* **compound undecylenic acid o.** An ointment containing 20% zinc undecylenate and 5% undecylenic acid. It is used topically as an antifungal agent in the treatment or prevention of dermatophytoses. Also *unguentum acidi undecylenici compositum.* **dexamethasone sodium phosphate ophthalmic o.** A sterile ointment containing 0.05% of dexamethasone phosphate. It is applied to the conjunctiva as an anti-inflammatory medication. **dimethisoquin hydrochloride o.** An ointment containing 0.5% dimethisoquin hydrochloride. It is used as a surface anesthetic agent. **emulsifying o.** An ointment composed of emulsifying wax, white petrolatum, and mineral oil. Also *unguentum emulsificans.* **epinephrine bitartrate ophthalmic o.** An eye ointment containing approximately 1% epinephrine bitartrate in a hydrophilic petrolatum base. Also *unguentum epinephrinae bitartratis ophthalmicum.* **eserine o.** PHYSOSTIGMINE OINTMENT. **flurandrenolide o.** An ointment containing 0.025 or 0.05% flurandrenolide. It is used as a topical preparation to provide glucocorticoid therapy in certain dermatoses as an anti-inflammatory agent. **gentamicin sulfate o.** A preparation containing 0.1% gentamicin in a suitable ointment base. It is applied topically to the conjunctiva as an antibacterial medication. **golden o.** YELLOW MERCURIC OXIDE OPHTHALMIC OINTMENT. **hydrocortisone o.** A preparation of hydrocortisone in an ointment base, containing 90–110% of the labeled 0.5, 1.0, or 2.5% hydrocortisone. These products are employed as anti-inflammatory corticosteroid medications. Also *unguentum hydrocortisoni.* **hydrocortisone acetate o.** A 1.0–1.25% preparation of hydrocortisone acetate in a suitable ointment base. It is used topically as an adrenocortical steroid. Also *unguentum hydrocortisoni acetatis.* **hydrocortisone acetate ophthalmic o.** An ointment base containing 90–110% of the labeled 0.5% hydrocortisone acetate. It is utilized as an anti-inflammatory remedy and is applied topically to the conjunctiva. **hydrophilic o.** An emulsion of water in oil containing methylparaben, propylparaben, sodium lauryl sulfate, propylene glycol, stearyl alcohol, white petrolatum, and purified water. It is used as a base for ointments. Also *unguentum hydrophilicum.* **hydroquinone o.** A preparation of 2% or 4% hydroquinone in a suitable ointment base. It is used as a depigmenting agent on the skin to inhibit the formation of melanin. **o. of hydrous wool fat** An ointment composed of equal parts of lanolin and petrolatum. Also *unguentum adipis lanae hydrosi.* **idoxuridine ophthalmic o.** A preparation containing 0.45–0.55% idoxuridine in a suitable petrolatum base. It is applied topically to the conjunctivae as an antiviral agent, and is used in the treatment of herpes simplex keratitis. **iodine o.** Iodine in arachis oil and yellow soft paraffin in ointment form. It is used externally for its potent microbicidal actions. Also *unguentum iodi.* **iodochlorhydroxy-**

**quin o.** Iodochlorhydroxyquin in a suitable ointment base, containing 90–110% of the labeled 3% iodochlorhydroxyquin. It is used in the treatment of some dermatoses, such as eczema, as an anti-infective medication. **iodochlorhydroxyquin and hydrocortisone o.** An ointment preparation containing 90–110% of the labeled 3 and 5% or 3 and 1% of iodochlorhydroxyquin and hydrocortisone. It is used as a local anti-infective agent and a glucocorticoid medication. **isoflurophate ophthalmic o.** A 0.0225–0.0275% preparation of isoflurophate in a suitable anhydrous base. It is used in the treatment of glaucoma, and is applied to the conjunctiva as a cholinergic agent that acts by inhibition of acetylcholinesterase. **o. of kaolin** An ointment containing kaolin in a hard paraffin base. It has been used to protect abraded skin. Also *unguentum kaolini.* **lanolin o.** An ointment containing a mixture of lanolin and soft paraffin. It is used as a skin emollient and as a general ointment base. Also *unguentum lanolini.* **lidocaine o.** A preparation of lidocaine in a hydrophilic base containing 95–105% of the labeled 5% lidocaine hydrochloride. It is applied topically as a local anesthetic. **methyl salicylate o.** An ointment containing 50 g methyl salicylate, 25 g white beeswax, and 25 g of lanolin. It has been used as a skin dressing to relieve pain of rheumatic and deep muscle origin. Also *wintergreen ointment.* **monobenzone o.** An ointment preparation containing 94–106% of the labeled 20% monobenzone in a water-soluble base. It has been used as a depigmenting agent on the skin. **neomycin sulfate o.** A suitable ointment base containing 3.5 mg of neomycin per gram. It is applied topically as an antibacterial medication. **nitrofurazone o.** An ointment containing 0.2% nitrofurazone in a suitable water-miscible base. It is used as an antibacterial treatment in the care of burns, but is not applied for more than a few days, as sensitization and allergic reactions are then likely to be encountered. Also *unguentum nitrofurazoni.* **nystatin o.** A suitable ointment base containing in each gram 90–130% of the labeled 100 000 units of nystatin activity. It is applied topically as an antifungal medication. **o. of oil of cade** An ointment composed of 25 g of cade oil, 12.5 g of yellow beeswax, and 62.5 g of yellow soft paraffin. It is used in the treatment of eczema and psoriasis. **oily cream hydrous o.** An ointment consisting of 50 g of wood alcohol ointment, 1 g of phenoxyethanol, 500 mg of dried magnesium phosphate, and 48.5 g of water. It is used as a base for water-and-oil emulsions. **paraffin o.** An ointment composed of beeswax, paraffin wax, and white and yellow soft paraffin. It is used mainly as a stable base for emulsions and creams. Also *unguentum paraffini.* **penicillin o.** An ointment base containing calcium penicillin, crystalline penicillin, or procaine penicillin. Also *unguentum penicillini.* **petrolatum rose water o.** An ointment containing spermaceti, white wax, mineral oil, sodium borate, rose water, and rose oil, an emollient and ointment base. Also *unguentum aquae rosae petrolatum.* **phenol o.** An ointment of phenol in lard and paraffin. It is used topically for its antipruritic action. Also *carbolic acid ointment, unguentum acidi carbolici, unguentum phenolis.* **physostigmine o.** A preparation containing physostigmine salicylate and chloroform in a yellow soft paraffin base. It is used in the eye as a miotic medication. Also *eserine ointment, unguentum physostigminae.* **pine tar o.** An ointment containing pine tar, yellow wax, and yellow ointment. Also *unguentum picis pini.* **polyethylene glycol o.** A water-soluble ointment base containing a mixture of polyethylene glycol 4000 and polyethylene glycol 400. Also *unguentum glycolis polyethyleni.* **polymyxin B sulfate o.** A topical antibacterial medication composed of polymyxin B sulfate in an anhydrous petrolatum base. It contains 90–120% of the labeled 20 000 polymyxin B sulfate units per gram. **o. of resorcinol** $C_6H_6O_2$. Benzene-1,3-diol. 2–5% resorcinol in a suitable ointment base, utilized as a keratolytic agent in the treatment of acne and seborrheic dermatitis. It is also applied to the skin for its antipruretic and exfoliative properties. Also *unguentum resorcini, unguentum resorcinolis.* **rose water o.** An ointment containing rose water, beeswax, borax, almond oil, and rose oil. Also *unguentum aquae rosae.* **simple o.** An ointment composed primarily of white petrolatum with various amounts of lanolin and white beeswax. Also *unguentum simplex.* **sodium sulfacetamide ophthalmic o.** A sterile ointment of sodium sulfacetamide in a suitable base, which can be applied topically to the conjunctiva as an antibacterial medication for sulfonamide-responsive eye infections. Also *unguentum sulfacetamidi sodici.* **sulfur o.** Precipitated sulfur mixed with mineral oil and white ointment. It is used as a scabicide. Also *unguentum sulfuris.* **o. of tar** An ointment consisting of tar, lard, and yellow beeswax. It has been used on the skin for antipruritic effects in treating chronic skin diseases. Also *unguentum picis liquidae.* **tetracaine ophthalmic o.** A white petrolatum ointment base containing 0.45–0.55% added tetracaine. It is used as a local anesthetic agent. **triamcinolone acetonide o.** $C_{24}H_{31}FO_6$. A suitable ointment base containing triamcinolone acetonide. It is a corticosteroid preparation that is applied topically in the treatment of diseases of the skin. **triclobisonium chloride o.** A suitable ointment base containing triclobisonium chloride that is applied topically as an anti-infective agent, mainly in combating gynecologic infections. **white o.** An ointment containing 5% white beeswax and 95% white petrolatum. Also *unguentum album.* **white precipitate o.** AMMONIATED MERCURY OINTMENT. **Whitfield's o.** BENZOIC AND SALICYLIC ACID OINTMENT. **wintergreen o.** METHYL SALICYLATE OINTMENT. **yellow o.** An ointment base containing yellow wax and petrolatum. Also *unguentum flavum.* **yellow mercuric oxide ophthalmic o.** An ointment containing finely powdered yellow mercuric oxide, liquid petrolatum, and white ointment, the concentration of mercuric oxide being 0.9–1.1%. It is used as a topical anti-infective agent in the eye. Also *golden ointment, Pagenstecher's ointment, unguentum hydrargyri oxidi flavi.* **zinc oxide o.** A medication containing zinc oxide and mineral oil in a white ointment base. It is used topically as an astringent and protective product. Also *zinc ointment, unguentum zinci oxidi.* **o. of zinc oxide with benzoin** An ointment containing tincture of benzoin in zinc oxide ointment. It is used to aid in the healing of minor injuries to the skin. Also *unguentum zinci oxidi cum benzoino.* **zinc undecenoate o.** A mixture of zinc undecenoate and undecenoic acid in an emulsifying ointment base. It is used primarily in the treatment of mycotic infections. Also *unguentum undecylenati.*

**OL** oculus laevus.

**ol.** *oleum* (L, oil).

**-ol** [*(alcoh)ol.* See ALCOHOL.] A suffix designating the presence of a hydroxyl group, —OH. It replaces the final -e in the name of an alkane, e.g., *ethane* yields *ethanol.*

**-ole** \\-ōl\\ [L *-olus* suffix diminishing nouns] A suffix meaning a small or little one.

**oleaginous** \\ō′lē·aj′inəs\\ Having the consistency of oil; oily.

**oleandomycin** $C_{35}H_{61}NO_{12}$. A macrolide antibiotic produced by *Streptomyces antibioticus* no. ATCC 11891. Its structure is like that of erythromycin, and it is given parenterally for the treatment of staphylococci and some other Gram-positive bacteria. It is usually administered as its phosphate, or triacetyl derivative, troleandomycin.

**oleandrin** \ō′lē·an′drin\ $C_{32}H_{48}O_9$. A cardiac glycoside obtained from *Nerium oleander*, oleander. In therapeutic amounts it is used to treat cardiac insufficiency, but in cases of excess ingestion, it may be fatal.

**oleandrism** \ō′lē·an′drizm\ [*oleand(e)r* + -ISM] Poisoning from ingestion of a cardiac glycoside contained in the roots, flowers, seeds, or bark of oleander, *Nerium oleander*. It may result in nausea, vomiting, bradycardia, heart block, cardiac arrhythmia, and cardiac arrest.

**olecranal** \ōlek′rənəl\ Of or relating to the olecranon.

**olecranarthrocace** \ōlek′rānärthrāk′əsē\ [*olecran(on)* + ARTHROCACE] An inflammation, often tuberculous in nature, of the elbow joint. *Older term.*

**olecranarthropathy** \ōlek′rānärthrāp′əthē\ [*olecran(on)* + ARTHROPATHY] Abnormality of the olecranon bursa, olecranon, and elbow joint.

**olecranoid** \ōlek′rənoid\ Resembling or shaped like the olecranon.

**olecranon** \ōlek′rənän, ō′ləkrā′nən\ [Gk *ōlekranon* (from *ōle(nē)* elbow, forearm + *kran(i)on* cranium, head, top) head of the ulna, tip of the elbow] [NA] The proximal part of the upper end of the ulna, bent forward at its highest point so that its concave anterior surface forms the upper part of the trochlear notch. The quadrangular-shaped superior surface has a rough posterior part for the insertion of the tendon of the triceps muscle and a smooth anterior part related to the subtendinous bursa. The junction of the superior and posterior surfaces forms the angular tip of the elbow. The latter surface is triangular and subcutaneous, its apex being continuous distally with the posterior margin of the shaft of the ulna. The anterior margins provide attachment for the capsule of the elbow joint. Also *olecranon process of ulna, gibber ulnae* (outmoded).

**olefin** A hydrocarbon containing a double bond.

**oleic acid** $CH_3$—$[CH_2]_7$—CH=CH—$[CH_2]_7$—COOH. The *cis* form of octadec-9-enoic acid. It occurs in fats and phospholipids. Its compounds in membranes increase their fluidity in comparison with saturated fatty acids. Unlike some other unsaturated fatty acids, it can be made in the mammalian body.

**oleo-** \ō′lē-ō-, ō′lē-ə-\ [L *oleum* olive oil, oil] A combining form denoting oil.

**oleochrysotherapy** \-kris′ōther′əpē\ [OLEO- + CHRYSOTHERAPY] Treatment with gold salts in a fat or oily base.

**oleoetherization** \-ē′thərīzā′shən\ Etherization involving the use of oil as a conduit for the ether.

**oleogranuloma** \-gran′yəlō′mə\ [OLEO- + GRANULOMA] PARAFFINOMA.

**oleoinfusion** \-infyoo′zhən\ A medicinal preparation obtained by extraction of the active components of a crude drug into an oil.

**oleoma** \ō′lē·ō′mə\ LIPOGRANULOMA.

**oleoresin** \-rez′in\ **1** A combination of a resin and a volatile oil present in some plants. **2** A semisolid pharmaceutical product obtained by removing the volatile oils and resins from a plant or plant part with a solvent and then evaporating the solvent. **aspidium o.** An extract made from aspidium. It has been used in the treatment of tapeworm infection. Also *aspidum oleoresin*. **capsicum o.** A thick, dark, reddish brown liquid containing not less than 8% capsicin, obtained by extraction of capsicum with hot acetone or alcohol, evaporating the solvent, and extracting the residue with cold 90% alcohol, followed by evaporation of the alcohol. It is used as a carminative agent in very dilute solutions and externally as an irritant.

**oleum** \ō′lē·əm\ **1** OIL. **2** Fuming sulfuric acid. **o. camphorae essentiale** RECTIFIED CAMPHOR OIL. **o. camphorae rectificatum** RECTIFIED CAMPHOR OIL. **o. hippoglossi** HALIBUT LIVER OIL. **o. iodisatum** IODIZED OIL. **o. ricini** CASTOR OIL. **o. ricini aromaticum** AROMATIC CASTOR OIL. **o. succini** OIL OF AMBER.

**olfact** \äl′fakt\ [L *olfact(us)*, past part. of *olfacere* (from *ol(ere)* to emit an odor + *facere* to make) to smell] The mean minimal perceptible odor as measured by the Proetz olfactometer.

**olfactie** \älfak′tē\ The unit of olfactory acuity measured by the olfactometer of Zwaardemaker, expressed as the distance on the centimeter scale at which the subject just perceives the test odor.

**olfaction** \älfak′shən\ [OLFACT + -ION] **1** The process of smelling. Also *osmesis* (seldom used). **2** The sense of smell. Also *osphresis* (seldom used).

**olfactism** \älfak′tizm\ [L *olfact(us)*, past part. of *olfacere* (from *ol(ere)* to smell, scent + *facere* to make) to smell, scent + -ISM] A sensation of smell produced by a sensory stimulus which is not normally olfactory.

**olfactometer** \äl′faktäm′ətər\ [OLFACT + *o* + -METER] An instrument or arrangement, as of various odorants, for assessing the acuity of the sense of smell or for measuring the olfactory threshold for a selected range of odors. **blast o.** An olfactometer for injecting into the nose a measured volume of air containing a constant concentration of the odorant under test. **Proetz o.** An olfactometer consisting of a rack of one-hundred small bottles arranged in ten rows. Each row across is concerned with one particular odorant, the concentration of which increases from left to right. The results are recorded in units called "olfacts," corresponding to the concentration in grams of the odorant per liter of the diluent. **o. of Zwaardemaker** An olfactometer consisting of two tubes, one sliding within the other, the outer one being impregnated with one of a variety of odorants. The inner tube of glass, calibrated in centimeters, was designed to enable the subject to breathe through it, using one side of the nose or the other. According to the length of outer tube exposed, by sliding out the inner tube, the intensity of the odor in the inspired air could be varied and represented as so many centimeters. It is no longer used.

**olfactory** \älfak′tərē\ [L *olfactori(us)*, from *olfact(us)*, past part. of *olfacere* (from *ol(ere)* to emit a smell + *facere* to make, do) to smell (a thing); + *-orius* -ORY] **1** Of or relating to the sense of smell. **2** Possessing a sense of smell. For defs. 1 and 2 also *osmatic, osphretic*.

**olig-** \äl′ig-\ OLIGO-.

**oligergasia** \äl′igərgā′zhə\ *Outmoded* MENTAL RETARDATION.

**oligo-** \äl′igō-\ [Gk *oligos* few, little] A combining form meaning (1) small, few; (2) abnormally small or few. Also *olig-*.

**oligoamnios** \-am′nē·əs\ The presence of a less than normal amount of amniotic fluid.

**oligoarthritis** \-ärthrī′tis\ [OLIGO- + ARTHRITIS] Arthritis of a few joints. Compare MONARTHRITIS, POLYARTHRITIS.

**oligoastrocytoma** \-as′trəsītō′mə\ [OLIGO- + ASTROCYTOMA] A glioma with a conspicuous mixture of oligodendroglial and astrocytic components.

**oligoblast** \äl′igōblast′\ [OLIGO- + -BLAST] A primitive macroglial cell that differentiates into an oligodendrocyte. Also *oligodendroblast*.

**Oligochaeta** \-kē′tə\ [OLIGO- + Gk *chaitē* long flowing hair] An order of worms in the phylum Annelida that includes the common earthworm, *Lumbricus,* and related forms, as well as many freshwater annelids.
**oligochromasia** \-krōmā′zhə\ HYPOCHROMIA.
**oligocythemia** \-sīthē′mē·ə\ *Obs.* ANEMIA.
**oligodactyly** \-dak′tilē\ ECTRODACTYLY.
**oligodendria** \-den′drē·ə\ *Seldom used* OLIGODENDROGLIA.
**oligodendroblast** \-den′drəblast\ [OLIGO- + DENDRO- + -BLAST] OLIGOBLAST.
**oligodendrocyte** \-den′drəsīt\ Any cell of the oligodendroglia.
**oligodendroglia** \-dendräg′lē·ə\ [OLIGO- + DENDRO- + GLIA] A group of macroglial cells that is subdivided into perineuronal, interfascicular, and juxtavascular types. Most cells are characterized by thin, flat processes that envelop axons to form segments of their myelin sheaths. Also *oligodendria* (seldom used), *oligoglia* (seldom used), *interfascicular oligoglia.*
**oligodendroglioma** \-den′drōglī·ō′mə\ [*oligodendrogli(a)* + -OMA] A tumor composed predominantly of oligodendroglial cells. The cells are usually uniform, with round nuclei, clear cytoplasm and well-defined cell membranes giving a halo appearance. Calcification is often present. This is typically a slow-growing tumor but an anaplastic form is recognized.
**oligodendrogliomatosis** \-den′drōglī′ōmətō′sis\ Diffuse neoplastic growth of oligodendroglia. **o. cerebri** GLIOMATOSIS CEREBRI.
**oligodipsia** \-dip′sē·ə\ [OLIGO- + -DIPSIA] HYPODIPSIA.
**oligodontia** \-dän′shə\ [*olig(o)-* + -ODONTIA] HYPODONTIA.
**oligoencephalon** \-ensef′əlän\ MICRENCEPHALON.
**oligogalactia** \-gəlak′shə\ [OLIGO- + GALACT- + -IA] Abnormally low secretion of breast milk.
**oligoglia** \äl′igäg′lē·ə\ *Seldom used* OLIGODENDROGLIA. **interfascicular o.** OLIGODENDROGLIA.
**oligohidrosis** \-hidrō′sis\ HYPOHIDROSIS.
**oligohydramnios** \-hīdram′nē·əs\ [OLIGO- + HYDR- + *amnio(n)* + *s*] A deficiency in the amount of amniotic fluid.
**oligohypermenorrhea** \-hī′pərmen′ôrē′ə\ [OLIGO- + HYPER- + MENORRHEA] Infrequent episodes of menstrual bleeding characterized by a heavy flow.
**oligohypomenorrhea** \-hī′pōmen′ôrē′ə\ [OLIGO- + HYPO- + MENORRHEA] Infrequent episodes of menstrual bleeding associated with scant flow.
**oligolecithal** \-les′ithəl\ [OLIGO- + LECITHAL] MIOLECITHAL.
**oligoleukocythemia** \-loo′kəsīthē′mē·ə\ LEUKOPENIA.
**oligoleukocytosis** \-loo′kəsītō′sis\ LEUKOPENIA.
**oligomenorrhea** \-men′ôrē′ə\ [OLIGO- + MENORRHEA] A reduction in the frequency of menstruation, with cycle lengths usually exceeding 40 days. Also *infrequent menstruation.*
**oligomer** \äl′igōmir′\ [*oligo-* + *-mer(e)*] A substance whose molecules are formed by combination of a few simpler molecules, usually identical.
**oligomeric** \-mir′ik\ Containing two or more polypeptides, which may be the same or different: used of a protein.
**oligomycin** Any of several macrolide antibiotics produced by an actinomycete similar to *Streptomyces* and having specific actions against fungi. Oligomycin A shows activity against fungi such as *Blastomyces dermatitides,* and oligomycin B is a potent inhibitor of mitochondrial oxidative phosphorylation.
**oligonucleotide** A compound whose molecules consist of a few nucleoside-phosphate residues joined together. Such compounds are obtained on partial hydrolysis of nucleic acids.
**oligo-ovulation** \-äv′yəlā′shən\ [OLIGO- + OVULATION] A reduction in the number of oocytes maturing or in the frequency of ovulation.
**oligopeptide** A peptide whose molecule contains a few amino-acid residues, up to about 20.
**oligophrenia** \-frē′nē·ə\ [OLIGO- + -PHRENIA] *Older term* MENTAL RETARDATION.
**oligoplasmia** \-plaz′mē·ə\ An abnormal reduction in the amount of plasma in the blood. See also HEMOCONCENTRATION.
**oligoplastic** \-plas′tik\ Possessing an abnormally reduced capacity for repair.
**oligopnea** \äl′igäp·nē′ə\ HYPOPNEA.
**oligopyrene** \-pī′rēn\ Having a reduced chromosome complement, especially in a sperm. Also *oligopyrous.*
**oligopyrous** \-pī′rəs\ OLIGOPYRENE.
**oligosaccharide** A compound whose molecule consists of a few sugar residues joined by glycoside links.
**oligosideremia** \-sid′ərē′mē·ə\ HYPOFERREMIA.
**oligospermatic** \-spərmat′ik\ [OLIGO- + SPERMATIC] Characterized by an abnormally low number of sperm in semen.
**oligospermia** An abnormally low number of sperm in semen. Also *oligozoospermia.*
**oligosteatosis** \äl′igäs′tē·ətō′sis\ Dryness of the skin caused by insufficient sebum excretion. Also *asteatosis, hyposteatosis.*
**oligosymptomatic** \-simp′təmat′ik\ Having or producing few symptoms.
**oligosynaptic** \-sinap′tik\ Denoting a neural pathway that includes only one or two interneurons, i.e., a di- or trisynaptic connection.
**oligotrichy** \äl′igät′rikē\ HYPOTRICHOSIS.
**oligozoospermia** \-zō′əspur′mē·ə\ OLIGOSPERMIA.
**oliguria** \äl′igoo′rē·ə\ [OLIG- + -URIA] Scanty urine excretion. It may occur in acute renal failure, dehydration, shock, congestive heart failure, and urinary tract obstruction in the urethra, in bilateral ureteral obstruction, or in unilateral renal obstruction if only one kidney is functional. Adj. oliguric.
**olisthe** \ōlis′thē\ OLISTHY.
**olistherochromatin** \ōlis′thərōkrō′matin\ The components of the constricted region of a chromosome.
**olisthy** \ōlis′thē\ [Gk *olisthan(ein)* to slip, slide + -Y] A slipping of the bones of a joint so that they remain in an abnormal relationship to each other. Also *olisthe.*
**oliva** \ōlī′və\ [L, olive, olive tree] [NA] A prominent oval elevation, located on the ventrolateral aspect of the medulla oblongata and produced by the underlying inferior olivary nucleus. Also *olivary body, olivary eminence, olive, medullary olive.*
**olivae** \ōlī′vē\ Plural of OLIVA.
**olive** [L *oliv(a)* (from Gk *elaia* the olive tree, olive) the olive tree, olive] **1** OLIVA. **2** The smooth, rounded, elliptical tip on the end of an internal vein stripper, so placed to avoid piercing the vein wall while the stripper is passed through the vein. **inferior o.** NUCLEUS OLIVARIS. **medullary o.** OLIVA. **superior o.** NUCLEUS OLIVARIS SUPERIOR.
**olivifugal** \äl′ivif′ʸəgəl\ Originating in and projecting from the inferior olive.
**olivipetal** \äl′ivip′ətəl\ Converging upon the inferior olive.

**olivocerebellar** \äl′ivōser′əbel′ər\ Denoting the inferior olive and cerebellum, as the olivocerebellar fibers connecting them, which form the largest component of the restiform body projecting to the cerebellar cortex.

**olivocortical** \äl′ivōkôr′tikəl\ Pertaining to nerve fibers that arise in the inferior olive and terminate in the cerebellar cortex.

**olivonuclear** \äl′ivōn$^y$oo′klē·ər\ Pertaining to nerve fibers passing from the inferior olive to the deep cerebellar nuclei.

**olivopontocerebellar** \äl′ivōpän′təser′əbel′ər\ Denoting the inferior olivary nucleus, ventral pons, and the cerebellar cortex, and especially denoting the course of fibers entering the middle cerebellar peduncle, as well as olivopontocerebellar atrophy, ataxia, or degeneration, which is a heredodegenerative disease involving the middle cerebellar peduncles and pontine, arcuate, and olivary nuclei.

**olivospinal** \äl′ivōspī′nəl\ Denoting the inferior olivary nucleus and the spinal cord, and especially denoting fibers that originate in the olivary nucleus and descend in a tract located near the anterolateral surface of the spinal cord.

**Ollendorff** [Helene *Ollendorff,* German dermatologist, flourished early 20th century] Buschke-Ollendorff syndrome. See under DISSEMINATED LENTICULAR DERMATOFIBROSIS.

**Ollier** [Léopold *Ollier,* French surgeon, 1830–1900] **1** Ollier's layer. See under STRATUM OSTEOGENETICUM. **2** Ollier's osteochondromatosis. See under UNILATERAL CHONDRODYSPLASIA.

**Ollier** [Louis Xavier Edouard *Ollier,* French surgeon, 1830–1900] **1** See under OPERATION. **2** Ollier's disease. See under UNILATERAL CHONDRODYSPLASIA.

**olophonia** \äl′ōfō′nē·ə\ [Gk *olo(os)* destroyed, undone + PHON- + -IA] An impediment of speech due to maldevelopment of any of the organs of speech. *Rare.*

**Olszewski** [Jerzy *Olszewski,* Polish-born Canadian neurologist, 1913–1966] Steele-Richardson-Olszewski syndrome. See under PROGRESSIVE SUPRANUCLEAR PALSY.

**oltipraz** \äl′tipraz\ A 1,2-dithiole synthetic antischistosomal compound effective against *Schistosoma mansona* and *S. haematobium.*

**OM** **1** outer membrane. **2** otitis media.

**o.m.** *omni mane* (L, every morning).

**-oma** \-ō′mə\ [Gk stem vowel *-ō-* + noun-forming suffix *-ma*] A suffix meaning tumor or neoplasm. • In Greek the ending *-ōma* had no specialized meaning; note *symptōma* (symptom), *strōma* (bed), *skotōma* (dizziness), etc. The modern oncological use developed chiefly by analogy from Gk *karkinōma, sarkōma,* and a few others that happened to share this meaning. There is a small but important group of modern medical words that end in *-oma* but do not designate neoplasms, e.g., *hematoma, glaucoma, trachoma, scotoma, atheroma,* and others.

**Ombrédanne** [Louis *Ombrédanne,* French physician, 1871–1956] See under OPERATION, METHOD.

**-ome** \-ōm\ [Gk *-ōma* as in *rhizōma* a mass of roots. See also -OMA.] A suffix denoting an aggregation, set, group, or community, as in *genome* (a set of genes), *biome* (a community of life forms).

**omega** \ōmē′gə, ō′megə\ The name of the 24th and last letter of the Greek alphabet. Symbol: $\omega$

**omenta** \ōmen′tə\ Plural of OMENTUM.

**omental** \ōmen′təl\ Of or relating to the omentum.

**omentectomy** \ō′məntek′təmē\ The partial or complete removal of the greater omentum and sometimes the lesser omentum, either partially or completely, as well. Also *epiploectomy, omentumectomy.*

**omentitis** \ō′məntī′tis\ [*oment(um)* + -ITIS] Inflammation of the omentum. Also *epiploitis.*

**omentopexy** \ōmen′təpek′sē\ [*oment(um)* + *o* + -PEXY] **1** A surgical procedure in which the greater omentum is used as a graft to serve either as a mechanical patch or as a vascular supply to damaged tissues. **2** The surgical fixation of the omentum. Also *epiplopexy, omentofixation, epiplopexia.*

**omentoplasty** \ōmen′təplas′tē\ [*oment(um)* + *o* + -PLASTY] Any plastic operation on omentum. Also *epiploplasty.*

**omentoportography** \ōmen′təpôrtäg′rəfē\ [*oment(um)* + *o* + *port(al)* + *o* + -GRAPHY] Roentgenography of the portal veins in the liver after the injection of a radiopaque, water-soluble contrast medium into an omental vein.

**omentorrhaphy** \ō′məntôr′əfē\ [*oment(um)* + *o* + -RRHAPHY] The rejoining, by suture, of lacerated or transected omentum. Also *epiplorrhaphy.*

**omentosplenopexy** \ōmen′təsplē′nəpek′sē \ A surgical procedure in which the omentum and the spleen are suspended from the abdominal wall to prevent ptosis or torsion.

**omentotomy** \ō′məntät′əmē\ [*oment(um)* + *o* + -TOMY] A surgical incision into the omentum.

**omentovolvulus** \ōmen′təväl′vyələs\ A volvulus involving torsion of the omentum.

**omentum** \ōmen′təm\ [L, fat skin, fat, the caul of the entrails, the bowels] A double layer of peritoneum that connects the stomach to another abdominal organ. Also *epiploon.* **colic o.** *Outmoded* OMENTUM MAJUS. **gastric o.** OMENTUM MAJUS. **gastrocolic o.** OMENTUM MAJUS. **gastrohepatic o.** *Outmoded* OMENTUM MINUS. **greater o.** OMENTUM MAJUS. **lesser o.** OMENTUM MINUS. **o. majus** [NA] A double layer of peritoneum that is folded on itself in front of the small intestine to form four layers. Two layers are attached to the greater curvature of the stomach and the beginning of the duodenum, which, after descending and forming a fold, ascend to the anterosuperior margin of the transverse colon to fuse with the anterior layer of the transverse mesocolon. Also *greater omentum, colic omentum* (outmoded), *gastrocolic omentum, gastric omentum, great epiploon* (outmoded). **o. minus** [NA] The double layer of peritoneum that extends, on the one side, from the abdominal portion of the esophagus, the lesser curvature of the stomach, and the commencement of the duodenum to the porta hepatis and the bottom of the fissure for the ligamentum venosum on the other side. Also *lesser omentum, gastrohepatic omentum* (outmoded), *hepatogastroduodenal ligament, lesser epiploon* (outmoded), *Willis pouch* (outmoded). **pancreaticosplenic o.** A portion of the ligamentum splenorenale that occasionally unites the tail of the pancreas with the lower part of the visceral surface of the spleen. *Outmoded.*

**omentumectomy** \ōmen′təmek′təmē\ OMENTECTOMY.

**omn. bih.** *omni bihora* (L, every two hours).

**omn. hor.** *omni hora* (L, every hour).

**omnipotence of thought** The conviction that one's thoughts control the outside world, that wishing does in fact make it so. It is normal in the infant, usually expressed only symbolically in the adult neurotic, but may appear as a delusion in the psychotic.

**omn. noct.** *omni nocte* (L, every night).

**omo-** \ō′mō-\ [Gk *ōmos* shoulder, shoulder with upper part of arm] A combining form denoting the shoulder.

**omocephalus** \-sef′ələs\ [OMO- + -CEPHALUS] An embryo, fetus, or newborn infant with severe malformation of the head associated with agenesis of the upper extremities.

**omocervicalis** \-sur′vikā′lis\ LEVATOR CLAVICULAE.

**omohyoid** \-hī′oid\ MUSCULUS OMOHYOIDEUS.

**omophagia** \ō′mōfā′jə\ [Gk *ōmo(s)* raw, undressed + -PHAGIA] The consumption of uncooked food.

**omoplata** \-plā′tə\ *Outmoded* SCAPULA.

**omosternum** \-stur′nəm\ The articular disk of the sternoclavicular joint.

**omothyroid** \-thī′roid\ An occasional muscle slip that extends between the omohyoid muscle and the superior horn of the thyroid cartilage.

**omphal-** \äm′fəl-\ OMPHALO-.

**omphalectomy** \äm′fəlek′təmē\ [OMPHAL- + -ECTOMY] A partial or total resection of the umbilicus.

**omphalic** \ämfal′ik\ UMBILICAL.

**omphalitis** \äm′fəlī′tis\ [OMPHAL- + -ITIS] Inflammation of the umbilicus.

**omphalo-** \äm′fəlō-\ [Gk *omphalos* navel] A combining form denoting the umbilicus. Also *omphal-*.

**omphalocele** \ämfal′əsēl\ [OMPHALO- + -CELE[1]] Herniation of intra-abdominal viscera into the umbilical cord. The herniated viscera are contained in a thin translucent sac of peritoneum and amnion. The condition may present with membranes (peritoneum and amnion) ruptured. Also *exomphalos, exomphalos hernia*. Compare UMBILICAL HERNIA.

**omphalodidymus** \-did′iməs\ [OMPHALO- + Gk *didymos* a twin] OMPHALOPAGUS.

**omphalogenesis** \-jen′əsis\ [OMPHALO- + GENESIS] Development of the umbilicus in the embryo.

**omphaloma** \äm′fəlō′mə\ [OMPHAL- + -OMA] A tumor of the umbilicus. Also *omphaloncus*.

**omphalopagus** \äm′fəläp′əgəs\ [OMPHALO- + Gk *pagos* a thing fixed or hardened] Conjoined twins linked at the umbilicus. Also *monomphalus, omphalodidymus*.

**omphalophlebitis** \-flebī′tis\ [OMPHALO- + PHLEBITIS] Inflammation or infection of the umbilical veins.

**omphalos** \äm′fələs\ UMBILICUS.

**omphalosite** \äm′fəlōsīt′\ [OMPHALO- + Gk *sit(os)* food] The parasitic member of unequal monochorial twins that derives its blood supply from the placental vessels of the autosite. The omphalosite is not capable of independent existence after birth. Also *placental parasitic twin, chorioangiopagus parasiticus*.

**omphalus** \äm′fələs\ UMBILICUS.

**om. quar. hor.** *omni quadrante hora* (L, every quarter of an hour).

**-on** [Gk, neuter noun suffix] A suffix designating an elementary particle or basic unit, as in *electron, codon*.

**onanism** \ō′nənizm\ [after Judah's son *Onan*, who spilled his seed on the ground so as not to give it to his dead brother's wife (Genesis 38:9) + -ISM] COITUS INTERRUPTUS.

**onc-**[1] \ängk-\ ONCO-[1].

**onc-**[2] \ängk-\ ONCO-[2].

**oncho-** \äng′kō-\ ONCO-[2].

***Onchocerca*** \äng′kōsur′kə\ [properly *Oncocerca*. See *ONCOCERCA*. A genus of long, threadlike filarial nematodes of the family Onchocercidae. They are found in subcutaneous and connective tissue, or confined within tough, fibrous cysts. The most important species, *O. volvulus*, is the cause of human onchocerciasis. Other species cause cutaneous diseases among domestic and wild herbivores. Also *Oncocerca*. ***O. volvulus*** A species of filarial worm that causes human onchocerciasis. It is widely distributed in western, central, and, less commonly, eastern Africa, and in Guatemala and the Yucatan peninsula. It is transmitted by the bite of blackflies of the genus *Simulium*, such as *S. damnosum* and *S. neavei* in Africa and *S. ochraceum, S. metallicum, S. callidum*, and *S. exiguum* in Central America. Also *Onchocerca caecutiens, Filaria volvulus*.

**onchocerciasis** \-sərkī′əsis, -sərsī′əsis\ [*Onchocerc(a)* + -IASIS] A disease caused by infection with filarial worms of the genus *Onchocerca*, primarily *O. volvulus*, transmitted by the bite of female blackflies of the genus *Simulium*. The disease is characterized by nodular swellings formed by fibrous cysts containing the worms. Microfilariae are found both in the nodules and in intercellular lymph in the skin. Onchocerciasis often results in blindness after a long period, because lesions occur in all parts of the eye as a result of the presence of microfilariae. The passage of microfilariae through the dermal tissues causes breakdown of elastic fibers resulting in conditions known by such descriptive names as elephant skin and hanging groin. Other dermatologic manifestations are known as lizard skin and leopard skin. There may be an eosinophilia. Filarial serology is positive; histological examination of the skin samples (skin-snips) is diagnostic. Treatment is with diethylcarbamazine and suramin, both of which cause serious systemic and ocular side effects. Mebendazole is an alternative. The disease is common near fast-flowing rivers in western, central, and, less commonly, eastern Africa and in Guatemala and the Yucatan peninsula. Twenty to fifty million people are affected. In some areas 15 percent of the population is rendered blind by the parasite. Also *onchocercosis, volvulosis, blinding disease, Robles disease, mal morado*. Also *oncocerciasis*. **ocular o.** Ocular complication of chronic onchocerciasis, including iridocyclitis, retrobulbar neuritis, keratitis, choroiditis, glaucoma, and blindness (river blindness) due to prolonged presence of microfilariae of *Onchocerca volvulus*.

**onchocercid** \-sur′sid, -sur′kid\ **1** Of or belonging to the family Onchocercidae. **2** A member of the family Onchocercidae.

**Onchocercidae** \-sur′sidē\ [*Onchocerc(a)* + -IDAE] A family of filarial worms in the superfamily Onchocercoidea, suborder Filarina. It includes most of the important filarial parasites of humans and domestic animals, including such genera as *Wuchereria, Brugia, Loa, Onchocerca, Dipetalonema, Elaeophora*, and *Litomosoides*..

**onchocercoma** \-sərkō′mə\ [*Onchocerc(a)* + -OMA] A subcutaneous nodule or lesion, usually situated near a bony prominence, that contains the adult worms in infections caused by *Onchocerca* species, especially *O. volvulus*. It is composed of a dense mass of connective tissue with cystic areas containing adult worms and microfilariae.

**onchocercosis** \-sərkō′sis\ ONCHOCERCIASIS.

**onchodermatitis** \-dur′mətī′tis\ [*Oncho(cerca)* + DERMATITIS] The skin lesions in onchocerciasis, caused by migratory movements of the *Onchocerca* microfilariae.

***Oncicola*** \änsik′ələ\ A genus of the phylum Acanthocephala, order Archiacanthocephala, parasitic in mammals. As is the case with most acanthocephalans, the first intermediate host is undoubtedly an arthropod and probably an insect.

**onco-**[1] \äng′kō-\ [Gk *onkos* mass, bulk] A combining form meaning (1) tumor; (2) mass, bulk, volume. Also *onc-*.

**onco-**[2] \ang′kō-\ [Gk *onkos* the barb of an arrow, a hook] A combining form meaning barb, hook, hooklike. Also *onc-, oncho-*.

***Oncocerca*** \-sur′kə\ [New L (from ONCO-[2] + Gk *kerkos* tail) barb-tailed] ONCHOCERCA.

**oncocerciasis** \-sərkī′əsis, -sərsī′əsis\ ONCHOCERCIASIS.

**oncocyte** \äng′kəsīt\ [ONCO-[1] + -CYTE] A large cell with abundant, granular, eosinophilic cytoplasm, found in a variety of glandular tissues, such as salivary glands, thyroid, and parathyroids. By electron microscopy the cells are shown to contain large numbers of mitochondria. The significance of the cell is unknown, and some consider it to be involuted. In the thyroid, oncocytes are known as Hürthle cells, and may be components of follicular adenomas or follicular carcinomas (Hürthle-cell carcinoma). Adj. oncocytic.

**oncocytoma** \-sītō′mə\ ONCOCYTIC ADENOMA.

**oncocytosis** \-sītō′sis\ [*oncocyt(e)* + -OSIS] Extensive oncocytic metaplasia.

**oncogene** \äng′kəjēn\ [ONCO-[1] + GENE] Any gene involved in the causation of cancer or cellular transformation. Oncogenes arise from mutation of loci (proto-oncogenes) present in all normal cells, and usually have similar or identical counterparts in viruses (viral oncogenes) that are capable of transforming eukaryotic cells. The products of proto-oncogenes include growth factors, membrane receptors, and DNA-binding proteins, all of which may function in cell division or differentiation. More than one oncogene may be necessary to change a normal cell to a cancer cell.

**oncogenesis** \-jen′əsis\ [ONCO-[1] + GENESIS] The formation of tumors.

**oncogenetic** \-jənet′ik\ [ONCO-[1] + GENETIC] Pertaining to the cause, origin, or formation of tumors.

**oncogenic** \-jen′ik\ [ONCO-[1] + -GENIC] Pertaining to the causation of a tumor, as *oncogenic virus*. Also *neoplastigenic*. • *Carcinogenic* and *cancerogenic* refer to malignant tumors, whereas *oncogenic* refers to both benign and malignant tumors.

**oncogenicity** \-jənis′itē\ The ability to cause the formation of tumors.

**oncologic** \-läj′ik\ Related to oncology.

**oncologist** \ängkäl′əjist\ A specialist in oncology.

**oncology** \ängkäl′əjē\ [ONCO-[1] + -LOGY] The study of tumors.

**oncolysis** \ängkäl′isis\ [ONCO-[1] + LYSIS] Destruction of tumors or tumor cells.

**oncolytic** \-lit′ik\ [ONCO-[1] + LYTIC] Able to destroy tumors or tumor cells.

**oncoma** \ängkō′mə\ [Gk *onkōma* (from *onkos* bulk, mass) a swelling] NEOPLASM.

***Oncomelania*** \-məlā′nē·ə\ [ONCO-[2] + *Melania*, another snail genus] A monotypic genus of prosobranch (operculated) snails that are important in the transmission of schistosomiasis japonica. The genus has been transferred from the family Hydrobiidae to the family Pomatiopsidae along with *Tricula* and other genera of importance as hosts of trematodes of medical interest. Snails of the genus are amphibious, small, dextrally coiled, with conical shells. They are found along moist weedy banks, often in large numbers, their small size and conical form rendering them inconspicuous. Control of these snails is made difficult by their amphibious habit, which allows them to escape molluscicides placed in the water. Also *Katayama*.

**oncometer** \ängkäm′ətər\ [ONCO-[1] + -METER] An apparatus used to encapsulate an organ for the purpose of determining changes in its size.

**Oncornavirinae** \ängkôr′nəvir′inē\ A subfamily of the Retroviridae family which includes the oncoviruses.

**oncornavirus** \ängkôr′nəvī′rəs\ [ONCO-[1] + *RNA* + VIRUS] ONCOVIRUS.

**oncosis** \ängkō′sis\ [ONC-[1] + -OSIS] The development of tumors.

**oncosphere** \äng′kəsfir\ [ONCO-[2] + SPHERE] The six-hooked embryo formed within the eggshell of cestodes of the subclass Eucestoda, which usually penetrates the gut wall of its host and forms the infective larval stage (procercoid, cysticercus, cysticercoid, strobilicercus, coenurus, or hydatid, depending on the kind of tapeworm). Also *hexacanth*.

**oncotherapy** \-ther′əpē\ Treatment of tumors.

**oncotic** \ängkät′ik\ [ONC-[1] + -OTIC[1] (by analogy to *osmotic*)] **1** Capable of causing volume changes across a membrane. **2** Pertaining to or caused by a neoplasm.

**oncotomy** \ängkät′əmē\ [ONCO-[1] + -TOMY] A surgical incision into a tumor.

**oncotropic** \-träp′ik\ Having an affinity for neoplastic cells.

**oncovirus** \-vī′rəs\ [ONCO-[1] + VIRUS] Any of various tumor-producing viruses of the Retroviridae family. They are grouped into three genera or types. Type B includes mouse mammary tumor viruses. Type C viruses produce leukemias and sarcomas in various birds, mammals, and reptiles. Type D viruses produce tumors in primates. Also *oncornavirus*.

**-oncus** \-äng′kəs\ [New L (from Gk *onkos* mass, bulk)] A combining form meaning a tumor, mass.

**-one** [Gk suffix *-ōnē* denoting female descendant; chemical suffix] A combining form indicating replacement of $CH_2$ by CO in a molecule so that the substance is a ketone. Thus propane, $CH_3—CH_2—CH_3$, gives propanone, $CH_3—CO—CH_3$, the systematic name for acetone.

**oneiric** \ōnī′rik\ [*oneir(o)* + -IC] Pertaining to or resembling a dream. Also *oniric*.

**oneiro-** \ōnī′rō-\ [Gk *oneiros* dream] A combining form meaning dream. Also *onir-*, *oniro-*.

**oneirodelirium** \-dilir′ē·əm\ [ONEIRO- + DELIRIUM] SOMNAMBULISM.

**oneirophrenia** \-frē′nē·ə\ [ONEIRO- + PHREN- + -IA] Schizophreniform psychosis with clouding of the sensorium.

**onir-** \ōnīr-, ōnir-\ ONEIRO-.

**oniric** \ōnī′rik\ ONEIRIC.

**oniro-** \ōnī′rō-\ ONEIRO-.

**-onium** [*(amm)onium*. See AMMONIUM.] A suffix indicating that an atom has acquired a positive charge by addition of a hydrogen ion. It is frequently used for substituted derivatives, thus $R_3S^+$is a sulfonium cation.

**onlay** \än′lā\ [*on* + *lay*] **1** ONLAY GRAFT. **2** A cast metal restoration covering the cusps of a tooth, but not the entire crown.

**onomatopoiesis** \än′əmat′əpoi·ē′sis\ [Gk *onomatopoiēsis* (from *onoma*, gen. *onomato(s)* name + -POIESIS) word-coinage] The practice of forming words (as *swish* or *fizz*) whose meanings represent the sounds made in pronouncing the words. It is sometimes seen in schizophrenics.

**onset of labor** See under LABOR.

***Onthophagus*** \änthäf′əgəs\ A genus of beetles of the family Scarabeidae (scarabs). Some species, such as *O. bifasciatus* and *O. unifasciatus*, are occasionally found in the rectum of children in India, Sri Lanka and South Africa, causing diarrhea and debilitation. *O. granulatus* perforates the stomach of horses and calves in Australia in cases of scarabiasis.

**ontogenesis** \än′təjen′əsis\ [Gk *ōn*, gen. *onto(s)* being (pres. part. of *einai* to be) + GENESIS] ONTOGENY.

**ontogeny** \äntäj′ənē\ [See ONTOGENESIS.] The development of an individual member of a species. Also *ontogenesis*, *henogenesis*. Compare PHYLOGENY.

**onyalai** \ō′nē·al′ā\ A form of thrombocytopenic purpura encountered in East, Central, and South Africa, characterized by bloody vesicles affecting oral mucous membranes. Also *chilopa*, *kafindo*, *akembe*.

**onych-** \än′ik-\ ONYCHO-.

**onychatrophia** \ō′nikətrō′fē·ə\ A congenital or acquired reduction in the size and thickness of the nail plate, often accompanied by fragmentation and splitting. The nail may be replaced by scar tissue.

**onychectomy** \än′ikek′təmē\ [ONYCH- + -ECTOMY] The partial or complete removal of a nail and/or a nail bed.

**onychia** \ōnik′ē·ə\ [ONYCH- + -IA] An inflammation of

the nail matrix, either following trauma or accompanying paronychia. Also *onyxitis, onychitis.* **o. lateralis** PARONYCHIA. **monilial o.** An inflammation of the nail matrix that is caused by a *Monilia* or *Candida albicans* infection. It may be associated with paronychia. **o. periungualis** PARONYCHIA. **o. sicca** A dry brittleness of the nails. **syphilitic o.** A syphilitic inflammation of the nail matrix.

**onychitis** \än′ikī′tis\ ONYCHIA.

**onycho-** \än′ikō-\ [Gk *onyx* (genitive *onychos*) talon, claw, nail] A combining form denoting nail or claw. Also *onych-*.

**onychodystrophy** \-dis′trəfē\ Any disorder of the nails.

**onychography** \än′ikäg′rəfē\ [ONYCHO- + -GRAPHY] The procedure of recording the blood pressure in the capillaries beneath the nails.

**onychogryposis** \-gripō′sis\ [ONYCHO- + Late Gk *grypōsis* (from Gk *gryp(ousthai)* to become bent or hooked + *-ōsis* -OSIS) excessive curvature] A thickening and curvature of the nail which is associated with an increase in length such that the nail resembles a ram's horn. Also *gryposis unguium, gryposis, gryphosis.*

**onychology** \än′ikäl′əjē\ [ONYCHO- + -LOGY] A study of the nails and their disorders.

**onycholysis** \än′əkäl′isis\ [ONYCHO- + LYSIS] A separation of the nail plate from the nail bed.

**onychomadesis** \-mədē′sis\ [ONYCHO- + Gk *madēsis* a becoming bald] A spontaneous shedding of the nail, starting at the base and extending forward. Also *piptonychia, defluvium unguium.*

**onychomycosis** \-mīkō′sis\ [ONYCHO- + MYCOSIS] Any fungal infection of the nails. Usually, invasion of the nail plate rather than just the nail fold is implied, but the distinction between damage caused by the fungus, as in ringworm, and harmless colonization of an already damaged nail, as occurs with aspergilli, is often unclear.

**onycho-osteodysplasia** \-äs′tē·ədisplā′zhə\ NAIL-PATELLA SYNDROME.

**onychopacity** \-pas′itē\ LEUKONYCHIA.

**onychophosis** \-fō′sis\ [ONYCHO- + PHOSIS] A condition marked by a horny epithelial growth in the nailbed.

**onychorrhexis** \än′ikôrek′sis\ [ONYCHO- + -RRHEXIS] The presence of longitudinal striations in the nail plate.

**onychoschizia** \-skiz′ē·ə\ [ONYCHO- + SCHIZ- + -IA] The splitting of the nail plate into layers.

**onychostroma** \-strō′mə\ MATRIX UNGUIS.

**onychotomy** \än′ikät′əmē\ [ONYCHO- + -TOMY] Incision through a fingernail, usually for the release of pus or blood.

**onyxitis** \än′iksī′tis\ ONYCHIA.

**oo-** \ō′ə-\ [Gk *ōon* egg] A combining form denoting egg or ovum.

**oocinete** \ō′əsī′nēt\ OOKINETE.

**oocyst** \ō′əsist\ [OO- + CYST] The encysted form of the zygote in the sporozoan life cycle, in which multiplication occurs by sporogony, resulting in the formation of sporozoites. In some forms, as among the coccidia, the oocyst contents first form sporocysts within which the sporozoites form. Examples are seen in *Eimeria, Isospora, Toxoplasma,* and *Sarcocystis.*

**oocyte** \ō′əsīt\ [OO- + -CYTE] A female germ cell situated in the thickened ovarian cortex, resulting from the transformation of an oogonium at the end of the multiplicative phase of the primordial oogonia. Also *ovocyte.* **primary o.** A female germ cell resulting from the proliferation of the primordial oogonia before the phases of growth and maturation in oogenesis. Its essential characteristic is the presence, centered in the nucleus, of changes related to the process of meiosis and thus a reduction by half in the number of chromosomes of each species. Proliferation before, at, and just after birth results in female neonates possessing a definitive stock of primary oocytes. In each human ovary this stock consists of 300 000–400 000 oocytes. **secondary o.** A female germ cell arising from a primary oocyte during the second phase of maturation in oogenesis, which starts at puberty.

**oogamous** \ō·äg′əməs\ Of or characterized by oogamy.

**oogamy** \ō·äg′əmē\ Fertilization of a nonmotile oocyte by a motile gamete.

**oogenesis** \ō′əjen′əsis\ [OO- + GENESIS] The formation and development of the female germ cells. Oogenesis comprises three phases: a phase of proliferation, in which the oogonia in the ovarian cortex divide several times, usually during fetal life or just after birth to produce numerous primary oocytes; a phase of growth, in which the oocytes increase in size and accumulate yolk as a food reserve; and a phase of maturation, in which the primary oocyte undergoes a reduction division which results in two daughter cells, one very small (the first polar body), destined to degenerate, the other (the secondary oocyte) which may grow to a size larger than the parent cell but with a haploid chromosome number. The secondary oocyte divides into two unequal cells, the second polar body, which degenerates, and the ovum (ootid) ready for fertilization. However, in most mammals it is a secondary oocyte which is shed at ovulation, and the final maturation division occurs only after penetration of the secondary oocyte by a spermatozoon. The final maturation division results, therefore, in the extrusion of the second polocyte (polar body) and the formation of the female pronucleus within an ovum already containing a spermatozoon. Also *ovogenesis.*

**oogenetic** \ō′əjənet′ik\ Pertaining to oogenesis.

**oogenic** \ō′əgen′ik\ [OO- + -GENIC] Producing ova. Also *oogenous, ovigenic, ovigenous.*

**oogonium** \ō′əgō′nē·əm\ [OO- + New L *gonium* (from GON- suffix denoting seed + L *-ium,* neut. sing. noun suffix)] (*pl.* oogonia) The precursor in the ovary of an oocyte. It is derived from a primordial female germ cell, which in mammals probably arises from the primitive endoderm and in man has been identified in the endoderm of the yolk sac. The primordial cells migrate into the embryo and pass via the dorsal mesentery to reach the genital ridge from which the ovary will develop. They proliferate in the ovarian cortex by mitosis to form oogonia, and the full number for each individual is reached just before or shortly after parturition.

**ookinete** \ō′əkī′nēt\ [OO- + Gk *kinēt(os)* moving] The motile, fertilized macrogamete, or zygote, of a malarial parasite. It moves to the outer lining of the gut wall of the vector mosquito and there forms the oocyst, in which masses of sporozoites are produced. Also *oocinete, pseudovermicule, pseudovermiculus, traveling vermicule.*

**oophor-** \ō′əfôr-\ OOPHORO-.

**oophoralgia** \ō′əfôral′jə\ [OOPHOR- + -ALGIA] OVARIALGIA.

**oophorectomy** \ō′əfôrek′təmē\ [*oophor(o)-* + -ECTOMY] Removal of one or both ovaries. Also *ovariectomy, ovariosteresis, oothecectomy, oothectomy.* **bilateral partial o.** Removal of tissue from each ovary.

**oophoritis** \ō′əfôrī′tis\ [OOPHOR- + -ITIS] Inflammation of an ovary, usually associated with salpingitis. Also *ovaritis.* **o. parotidea** Oophoritis resulting from infection with the mumps virus and occurring during, before, or as the only manifestation of mumps.

**oophoro-** \ō′əfôr′ō-\ [Gk *ōophoron* (from *ōon* egg +

-*phoros* bearing) ovary] A combining form denoting the ovary. Also *oario-*, *oophor-*.

**oophoroma** \ō′əfôrō′mə\ [OOPHOR- + -OMA] A tumor of the ovary. **o. folliculare** BRENNER TUMOR.

**oophoron** \ō·äf′ərän\ [Gk noun from *ōophoros* egg-carrying; see OOPHORO-.] OVARIUM.

**oophoropathy** \ō·äf′əräp′əthē\ [OOPHORO- + -PATHY] Any disease of the ovary. Also *ovariopathy*.

**oophoropexy** \ō·äf′ərōpek′sē\ [OOPHORO- + -PEXY] The surgical attachment of the ovary to the lateral pelvic wall, sometimes carried out to protect the ovary when pelvic radiation therapy is needed. Also *ovariopexy*.

**oophoroplasty** \ō·äf′ərōplas′tē\ [OOPHORO- + -PLASTY] Any plastic operation on an ovary.

**oophorosalpingectomy** \ō·äf′ərōsal′pinjek′təmē\ SALPINGO-OOPHORECTOMY.

**oophorosalpingitis** \ō·äf′ərōsal′pinjī′tis\ SALPINGO-OOPHORITIS.

**oophorostomy** \ō·äf′əräs′təmē\ [OOPHORO- + -STOMY] A surgical opening into an ovary or an ovarian cyst to permit drainage. Also *oothecostomy, ovariostomy*.

**oophorotomy** \ō·äf′ərät′əmē\ [OOPHORO- + -TOMY] A surgical incision into one or both ovaries. Also *ovariotomy*.

**oophorrhagia** \ō·äf′ôrā′jə\ [*oopho(r)-* + -RRHAGIA] Bleeding from an ovary.

**ooplasm** \ō′əplazm\ [OO- + -PLASM] The cytoplasm of the egg. Also *ovoplasm*.

**oosome** \ō′əsōm\ [OO- + *-some*, suffix denoting body, from Gk *sōma* body] GERM-CELL DETERMINANT.

**oothec-** \ō′əthēk-\ OOTHECO-.

**oothecectomy** \ō′əthēsek′təmē\ OOPHORECTOMY.

**ootheco-** \ō′əthē′kō-\ [Modern L *ootheca* (from Gk *ōon* egg + *thēkē* case, box) egg case, ovary] A combining form denoting the ovary. Also *oothec-*.

**oothecosalpingectomy** \-sal′pinjek′təmē\ SALPINGO-OOPHORECTOMY.

**oothecostomy** \ō′əthēkäs′təmē\ OOPHOROSTOMY.

**oothectomy** \ō′əthek′təmē\ OOPHORECTOMY.

**ootid** \ō′ətid\ [OO- + *t* + -ID[1]] A mature ovum, a product of meiosis in the ovary. In most mammals fertilization occurs prior to the completion of meiosis, thus the ootid contains male and female pronuclei.

**ootomy** \ō·ät′əmē\ [OO- + -TOMY] Incision in a fertilized ovum, carried out for experimental reasons, particularly in order to study the development of its various parts.

**ootype** \ō′ətīp\ [OO- + TYPE] An egg-processing structure in the center of the female reproductive system of cestodes and trematodes. It is the site of fertilization, after which yolk material is compressed around the ovum and shell material is laid down. Then the egg is passed into the uterus and the shell is tanned and hardened.

**oozooid** \ō′əzō′oid\ Any individual developed from an ovum.

**op-** \äp-, əp-\ OB-.

**opacify** \ōpas′ifī\ To lose transparency; be in the process of becoming opaque.

**opacity** \ōpas′itē\ [L *opacitas* shadiness] The condition of being opaque, as that resulting from the loss of transparency.

**opalescent** \ō′pəles′ənt\ Pertaining to the scattering of light through translucent media. Also *opaline*.

**opaline** \ō′pəlēn\ OPALESCENT.

**Opalski** [Adam *Opalski*, Polish physician, 1897–1963] See under CELL.

**OPD** outpatient department.

**-ope** \-ōp\ [Gk *ōps*, gen. *ōpos*, eye] One having a (specified) visual characteristic or condition.

**open** Not covered with intact skin, as an injury to deeper tissues.

**opening** An orifice, aperture or entrance in or to a structure, organ, cavity, or tube. **anterior o. of aqueduct of Sylvius** The orifice of the aqueductus mesencephali in the posteroinferior wall of the third ventricle below the posterior commissure. Also *opening of Vieussens, orifice of Vieussens*. **anterior o. of orbital cavity** ADITUS ORBITAE. **aortic o.** 1 OSTIUM AORTAE. 2 HIATUS AORTICUS. **aortic o. in diaphragm** HIATUS AORTICUS. **bite o.** Increasing of the vertical relation when the teeth are in occlusion. **cardiac o.** OSTIUM CARDIACUM. **o. of coronary sinus** OSTIUM SINUS CORONARII. **esophageal o. in diaphragm** HIATUS ESOPHAGEUS. **external o. of aqueduct of cochlea** APERTURA EXTERNA CANALICULI COCHLEAE. **ileocecal o.** OSTIUM ILEOCAECALE. **ileocolic o.** OSTIUM ILEOCAECALE. **o. in adductor magnus muscle** HIATUS TENDINEUS. **inferior o.'s of caroticotympanic canaliculi** The tiny openings in the carotid canal in the petrous part of the temporal bone through which filaments of the carotid sympathetic plexus and branches of the internal carotid artery enter the canaliculi caroticotympanici. **inferior o. of pelvis** APERTURA PELVIS INFERIOR. **inferior o. of sacral canal** HIATUS SACRALIS. **inferior thoracic o.** APERTURA THORACIS INFERIOR. **o. of inferior vena cava** 1 OSTIUM VENAE CAVAE INFERIORIS. 2 FORAMEN VENAE CAVAE. **internal urethral o.** OSTIUM URETHRAE INTERNUM. **interventricular o.** FORAMEN INTERVENTRICULARE. **o. to lesser sac of peritoneum** FORAMEN OMENTALE. **o. for lesser superficial petrosal nerve** HIATUS CANALIS NERVI PETROSI MINORIS. **lower thoracic o.** APERTURA THORACIS INFERIOR. **nasal o. of facial skeleton** APERTURA PIRIFORMIS. **o. of omental bursa** FORAMEN OMENTALE. **orbital o.** ADITUS ORBITAE. **ovarian o. of uterine tube** OSTIUM ABDOMINALE TUBAE UTERINAE. **o. of parotid duct** The opening in the tip of the papilla parotidea in the oral vestibule opposite the upper second molar tooth. **pharyngeal o. of auditory tube** OSTIUM PHARYNGEUM TUBAE AUDITIVAE. **pharyngeal o. of eustachian tube** OSTIUM PHARYNGEUM TUBAE AUDITIVAE. **piriform o.** APERTURA PIRIFORMIS. **o. of pulmonary trunk** OSTIUM TRUNCI PULMONALIS. **pyloric o.** OSTIUM PYLORICUM. **saphenous o.** HIATUS SAPHENUS. **semilunar o. of ethmoid bone** HIATUS SEMILUNARIS. **o. for smaller superficial petrosal nerve** HIATUS CANALIS NERVI PETROSI MINORIS. **o. of sphenoidal sinus** APERTURA SINUS SPHENOIDALIS. **superior o. of pelvis** APERTURA PELVIS SUPERIOR. **superior thoracic o.** APERTURA THORACIS SUPERIOR. **superior o. of tympanic canal** The upper opening of the tympanic canaliculus through which the tympanic branch of the glossopharyngeal nerve enters the tympanic cavity. **tendinous o.** HIATUS TENDINEUS. **tympanic o. of auditory tube** OSTIUM TYMPANICUM TUBAE AUDITIVAE. **o. for tympanic branch of glossopharyngeal nerve** The inferior opening of the tympanic canaliculus, located on the ridge between the jugular fossa and the opening of the carotid canal on the inferior surface of the petrous part of the temporal bone. It transmits the tympanic branch of the glossopharyngeal nerve. **upper thoracic o.** APERTURA THORACIS SUPERIOR. **uterine o. of uterine tube** OSTIUM UTERINUM TUBAE UTERINAE. **o. for vena cava** FORAMEN VENAE CAVAE. **o. of vermiform appendix** OSTIUM APPENDICIS VERMIFORMIS. **vertical o.** VERTI-

CAL RELATION. **vesicourethral o.** OSTIUM URETHRAE INTERNUM. **o. of Vieussens** ANTERIOR OPENING OF AQUEDUCT OF SYLVIUS.

**operability** \äp′ərəbil′itē\ The state of susceptibility to successful surgical treatment.

**operable** \äp′ərəbl\ [L *oper(ari)* to work, take pains with + *-abilis* English *-able*] Susceptible to treatment by surgical means with a significant degree of safety and success.

**operant** \äp′ərənt\ [L *operans,* gen. *operantis,* pres. part. of *operari* to work, take pains with] **1** Describing a response or pattern of responses defined by its effects on the environment, and by its effectiveness in achieving reward or reinforcement. An operant response is identified by its known consequences in a definable situation rather than in terms of the stimulus which may have given rise to that behavior. **2** An operant response considered as a unit of behavior. **3** Designating a method of conditioning based on the control of operant responses.

**operate** [L *operat(us),* past part. of *operari* to work, labor, operate. See OPERATION.] To perform a surgical procedure.

# operation

**operation** [L *operatio* (from *operatus,* past part. of *operari* to work, labor, from *opus,* gen. *operis,* work, labor) a working, laboring, operation] **1** A surgical procedure. **2** The act of carrying out a task, especially in an orderly way according to established practice. **Abbe's o.** The repair of a lip defect making use of an Abbe flap. **Abbe-Estlander o.** An operation utilizing a cross-lip flap of either the Abbe or Estlander type. **Adams o.** **1** Excision of a wedge of tissue from the eyelid margin, used to treat ectropion. **2** An operation once performed for the correction of traumatic deformitites of the nose and nasal septum by forcibly refracturing and repositioning the septum and, if necessary, the nasal bones, using a special forceps (Adams forceps). It was superseded by such procedures as submucous resection of the nasal septum and, more recently, septorhinoplasty. **Adelmann's o.** The disarticulation of a finger together with the metacarpal head. **Albee's o.** A spinal fusion procedure that uses a tibial bone graft. The graft is keyed into the split spinous processes of the vertebrae. **Aldridge o.** The use of a fascial sling to elevate the posterior urethrovesical angle to correct urinary stress incontinence. **Allarton's o.** MEDIAN LITHOTOMY. **Ammon's o.** DACRYOCYSTOTOMY. **anastomotic o.** A surgical procedure which consists, at least in part, of the creation of a connection between two vessels or organs. **Anderson's o.** **1** The longitudinal splitting of a tendon, followed by a pulling along one of the cut edges in order to gain length. **2** A method of lengthening a limb, using an external fixation device along with the gradual distraction of a step osteotomy. For defs. 1 and 2 also *Anderson's amputation.* **Annandale's o.** A method of suturing displaced menisci in the knee. **Arlt's o.** Surgical fracture of the tarsus for trachomatous entropion. **Babcock's o.** The stripping of varicose veins by the use of olive-tipped sounds that are passed through the veins via a small skin incision. Also *Jackson-Babcock operation.* **Barkan's o.** GONIOTOMY. **Barraquer's o.** A technique of intracapsular cataract extraction utilizing a suction device to grasp the capsular surface. **Barsky's o.** A method of repairing a congenital cleft hand. **Barton's o.** A method of achieving an arthrodesis of a joint by removing V-shaped segments of bone and cartilage from either side of the joint, thus creating an interlocking continuity. **Barwell's o.** A method of correcting a genu valgum deformity in children by dividing the upper tibia below its proximal epiphysis and the lower tibia above its distal epiphysis. **Bassini's o.** A surgical repair of an inguinal hernia in which the entire length of the posterior wall of the inguinal canal is incised and reconstructed by suturing the medial structures—the transverse fascia and aponeurosis, the transverse abdominal muscle, and the internal oblique muscle—laterally to the reflected edge of the inguinal ligament. This procedure is often performed today without incising the posterior wall. **Battle's o.** A surgical procedure in which normal ovaries are removed to treat certain hormone-dependent conditions, such as uterine fibroids. **Beck I o.** An obsolete operation to revascularize the ischemic heart in which the collateral blood supply is stimulated by pericardial poudrage, epicardial abrasion, and partial occlusion of the coronary sinus. **Beck II o.** An obsolete operation once used to revascularize the ischemic heart. It is performed to two stages, the first of which creates an anastomosis between the coronary sinus and the descending thoracic aorta. The second procedure forms a partial occlusion of the coronary sinus to direct aortic blood retrograde into the coronary veins. **Belfield's o.** VASOTOMY. **Bent's o.** An excision of the arm at the shoulder using a flap from the deltoid region. **Berger's o.** An interscapulothoracic amputation of the upper limb. Also *Berger's amputation.* **Bernard's o.** A method of reconstructing the lower lip utilizing sliding flaps taken from the cheeks. **Bevan's o.** A surgical procedure in which an undescended testicle is brought into the scrotum. **Billroth's o.** A surgical procedure in which a gastroenterostomy or gastroduodenostomy is performed following a distal gastric resection. Also *Billroth anastomosis.* **Blalock's o.** An operation to palliate diminished pulmonary artery blood flow secondary to valvular or infundibular pulmonary stenosis by anastomosing the subclavian or innominate artery to the ipsilateral pulmonary artery; a form of systemic-pulmonary artery shunt for palliation of diminished pulmonary artery blood flow. Also *Blalock-Taussig operation.* **Blalock-Hanlon o.** An operation in which a portion of the atrial septum is excised to enable more adequate mixing of left and right atrial blood to palliate transposition of the great arteries. The operation is done employing vascular occlusion techniques rather than using cardiopulmonary bypass. **Blalock-Taussig o.** BLALOCK'S OPERATION. **bloodless o.** A surgical procedure in which little or no blood is lost. **Boari's o.** Implantation of the ureter into a tube of bladder tissue to obtain more length when the ureter is short. **Bondy o.** MODIFIED RADICAL MASTOIDECTOMY. **Bozeman's o.** HYSTEROCYSTOCLEISIS. **Bricker's o.** A surgical procedure in which an ileal conduit for urine is created as a substitute for the bladder. **Brock's o.** TRANSVENTRICULAR CLOSED VALVOTOMY. **Brunschwig's o.** TOTAL PELVIC EXENTERATION. **Buck's o.** An operation for repairing the defect in spondylolysis in which a compression screw is passed across the defect in the pars interarticularis. **buttonhole o.** A small surgical incision or counterincision usually made to provide drainage through a separate wound. **Caldwell-Luc o.** An operation for the relief of chronic maxillary sinusitis. The maxillary sinus is opened by a sublabial incision, diseased sinus mucosa is removed, and a counter-opening is made from the interior of the sinus into the inferior meatus of the nose. Also *radical maxillary antrostomy.* **Calot's o.** The forcible manipulation and correction of tuberculous kyphosis followed by immobilization of the spine in a plaster cast. **capital o.** Any surgical procedure of such magnitude that it may represent a significant threat to the patient's life. **Carnochan's o.** An operation on the gasserian ganglion and nerve through an opening in the maxillary antrum, for the relief of facial pain. **Carpue's o.** INDIAN RHINOPLASTY. **Cecil's o.** An operation for urethral stricture which is performed in three stages. **celsian o.** PERINEAL LITHOTOMY. **Charles o.** A surgical procedure for lymphedema in which lymphedematous skin and subcutaneous tissue are excised and the operative site is covered by skin grafts. **Chopart's o.** 1 CHOPART'S AMPUTATION. 2 MEDIOTARSAL AMPUTATION. **cinch o.** A shortening of the extraocular muscles for strabismus correction by means of a form of tucking. **Civiale's o.** LITHOLAPAXY. **Codivilla's o.** 1 A method of treating a pseudarthrosis by surrounding the region with slivers of osteoperiosteal bone taken from the anteromedial surface of the tibia. 2 The original surgical method of obtaining an increase in limb length by cutting the bone and applying traction. **Colonna's o.** An arthroplasty of the hip joint used in neglected cases of congenital dysplasia or dislocation of the hip. **commando o.** An operation in which resection of a primary malignant tumor of the floor of the mouth, cheek, tongue, tonsillar area, pharynx, or larynx is combined with radical dissection of the lymph nodes in the neck. • It was named after the Allied commando raid on Dieppe, a famous combined operation undertaken in 1942. **cosmetic o.** An operation designed to correct an undesirable bodily feature so that the feature will more closely match that which is generally considered normal. Also *esthetic surgery, featural surgery.* **Cotte's o.** The excision of presacral nerves. **Cotting's o.** An operation for the removal of the nail fold and the side of the nail. It is performed to treat an ingrowing toenail. **crescent o.** Surgical repair of a lacerated perineum, secondary to an obstetrical delivery. **Cushing's o.** SUBTEMPORAL DECOMPRESSION. **Dana's o.** POSTERIOR RHIZOTOMY. **decompression o.** The surgical removal of structures confining an organ that is under pressure, as in subtemporal decompression of the brain or decompression laminectomy of the spinal cord. **Denis Brown o.** 1 A method of correction of hypospadias, in which a strip of skin is separated, extending from the urethral meatus to the end of the penis, the adjacent skin is closed, and then a catheter is placed between the skin strip and the closed skin. The skin strip then becomes a tube by epithelialization. 2 A variation of the Swenson anal pull-through procedure used for primary resection and anastomosis in the treatment of congenital megacolon. This procedure varies in that the rectosigmoid is completely mobilized and pulled through before the bowel is divided. **Denker's o.** A modification of the Caldwell-Luc operation intended to afford easier postoperative access from the nose to the interior of the maxillary antrum by bringing the antrostome further forward. **Dohlman's o.** An endoscopic operation to relieve the symptoms of hypopharyngeal diverticulum. The wall separating the diverticulum from the esophagus is exposed with a special speculum and divided using diathermy. **Doléris o.** A surgical operation to treat uterine retroversion by shortening the round ligaments by fixing them to the rectus sheath. **Dorrance o.** PALATAL PUSHBACK OPERATION. **Doyen's o.** Relief of hydrocele by eversion of the sac. **Dührssen's o.** A seldom-used obstetrical operation in which one or more radial incisions are made into the cervix to expedite delivery of the fetal head. **Dupuy-Dutemps o.** Repair of an eyelid defect by transplantation of tissue from the opposing eyelid. **Eagleton's o.** An operation designed to drain infected air cells in cases of petrositis. It utilizes an extrapetrosal approach to the apex of the petrous portion of the temporal bone, with the site of disease being reached by elevating the dura mater of the middle fossa. **Emmet's o.** TRACHELORRHAPHY. **equilibrating o.** Correction of an ocular imbalance due to muscle paralysis by severing the opposite muscle tendon from the sclera. **Estes o.** A procedure for infertility in which the ovary is placed into the interstitial portion of the uterine tube. **Estlander's o.** An operation in which a cross-lip flap is transferred from the lateral portion of one lip to a defect in the ipsilateral side of the other lip. Its pedicle receives its blood supply from the coronary artery and vein at the new corner of the mouth. The pedicle need not be severed, and the mouth can be opened and closed immediately. **face-lift o.** FACE-LIFT. **Fasanella-Servat o.** An operation for correcting minor degrees of ptosis of the upper eyelid. The lid is everted and then up to three millimeters is excised of the tarsus, conjunctiva, Müller's muscle and levator muscle. **fenestration o.** An operation for the relief of deafness due to ankylosis of the stapes, in which a fistula from the middle ear into the inner ear is made at the site of the lateral semicircular canal in order to provide alternative sound access. The procedure is now outmoded. Also *fenestration.* **Fick o.** SACCULOTOMY. **filtering o.** A procedure for glaucoma that creates a passage permitting the aqueous humor to escape from the anterior chamber into the subconjunctival space. **Finney's o.** FINNEY PYLOROPLASTY. **Finzi-Harmer o.** An operation once regularly employed for carcinoma of the larynx, involving the use of a palisade of radium needles inserted into a window created by resection of part of the ala of the thyroid cartilage adjacent to the tumor. It is now largely superseded by teletherapy. **flap o.** A periodontal surgical procedure in which mucoperiosteal flaps are reflected to allow better access for root planing and bone reshaping. **Fontan o.** A surgical procedure designed to treat tricuspid valve atresia, in which right atrial blood is shunted through a valved conduit to the pulmonary artery. **forceps o.** Any manipulation with obstetric forceps to effect the delivery of an infant. **Förster's o.** Posterior spinal rhizotomy for the treatment of spastic paralysis. **Fothergill o.** A surgical operation to correct uterine prolapse by amputation of the cervix followed by attachment of the cardinal ligaments to the anterior uterus. **Fothergill-Donald o.** MANCHESTER OPERATION. **Franco's o.** SUPRAPUBIC CYSTOTOMY. **Frank's o.** The creation of a gastrostomy by utilizing a mushroom-shaped section of anterior gastric wall that is sutured to the abdominal wall. Also *Ssabanejew-Frank operation.* **Frazier-Spiller o.** Selective trigeminal rhizotomy for the relief of trigeminal neuralgia. **Freckner's o.** An operation designed to drain infected air cells for relief of petrositis, utilizing an intrapetrosal surgical approach working inward under the arch of the superior semicircular canal. **Fredet-Ramstedt o.** PYLOROMYOTOMY. **Freyer's o.** Suprapubic enucleation of an enlarged prostate. **Fuller's o.** An incision of the seminal vesicles to effect drainage. **Gifford's o.** An attempt to prevent progression of a corneal ulcer by cutting the stroma at the border of the ulcer. **Gill o.** An operative procedure to relieve the symptoms of spondylolisthesis in which the loose lamina and spinous processes are removed. **Gilliam's o.** A surgical operation used to suspend the uterus and correct retrodisplacement, whereby the round ligaments are shortened by suturing a loop of the ligament which has been brought through the anterior peritoneum to the rectus fascia. **Glenn's o.** An anastomosis of the superior vena cava to the right pulmonary artery for palliation of cyanotic congenital cardiac defects such as tricuspid atresia, certain tetralogy of Fallot lesions, and pulmonary atresia. **Graefe's o.** Peripheral iridectomy for angle-closure glaucoma. **Gritti's o.** GRITTI'S AMPUTATION. **Guyon's o.** GUYON'S AMPUTATION. **Hajek's o.** A radical osteoplastic operation for the relief of chronic frontal sinusitis. Through an L-shaped incision above the eye, a triangular osteoplastic flap is created from the front wall of the sinus and hinged above so as to provide good access to the interior of the sinus and the upper end of the frontonasal duct. It has been superseded by the modern osteoplastic frontal sinus operation. **Halsted's o.** **1** RADICAL MASTECTOMY. **2** A type of inguinal hernioplasty. **Hartley-Krause o.** Excision of the gasserian ganglion, using an extradural temporal approach, for the relief of facial neuralgia. An outdated procedure. **Haultaim's o.** A modification of the Küstner operation for chronic inversion of the uterus. **Heath's o.** Mastoidectomy in which drainage of the mastoid cavity was provided by the creation of a fistula between the cavity and the external auditory meatus adjacent to the tympanic annulus. This operation is no longer practiced. **Heineke's o.** A surgical type of pyloroplasty, similar to a Heineke-Mikulicz pyloroplasty. **Heineke-Mikulicz o.** HEINEKE-MIKULICZ PYLOROPLASTY. **Heller's o.** CARDIOMYOTOMY. **Herbert's o.** A transscleral filtering operation for glaucoma. **high forceps o.** The application of obstetric forceps before the fetal head is engaged. This procedure is condemned by modern obstetricians. **Hoffa's o.** LORENZ OPERATION. **Hoffa-Lorenz o.** LORENZ OPERATION. **Hofmeister o.** A method of anastomosing the stomach to the jejunum. It involves the closure of a portion of the lesser curvature side of the divided stomach and the implantation of the greater curvature side of the divided stomach into the side of the jejunum. **Hoke's o.** Arthrodesis of the hindfoot that involves both the talocalcaneal and talonavicular junctures. **Holmes o.** A method of excising the os calcis via an incision on the upper outer border of the foot and another across the plantar surface of the heel. **Holth's o.** Sclerocorneal excision for open-angle glaucoma. **Horgan's o.** TRANSANTRAL ETHMOIDECTOMY. **Horton-Devine o.** A method of correcting hypospadias, utilizing a tube-shaped full-thickness skin graft taken from the prepuce to provide the additional length needed for the urethra. **Huntington's o.** A gynecologic operation for chronic inversion of the uterus. From the abdominal approach, the operator successively grasps the walls of the inverted uterus with tenacula and exerts traction in an effort to reverse the uterus to its normal position. **Indian o.** INDIAN RHINOPLASTY. **interposition o.** WATKINS OPERATION. **interval o.** A surgical procedure performed in the period between the cessation and expected recurrence of an acute attack, as in appendicitis. **iris inclusion o.** A procedure for relief of glaucoma, consisting of incarceration of a piece of iris within a limbal incision, so as to maintain an open leak of aqueous humor to the subconjunctival space. **Irving sterilization o.** A surgical sterilization procedure in which the medial cut end of the oviduct is buried in the myometrium posteriorly and the distal cut end is buried in the mesosalpinx. **Italian o.** ITALIAN RHINOPLASTY. **Jaboulay's o.** INTERPELVIABDOMINAL AMPUTATION. **Jackson-Babcock o.** BABCOCK'S OPERATION. **Jacobaeus o.** The division of pleural adhesions by cauterization using a thoracoscope. **Jewett o.** A form of surgical anastomosis between the ureter and the sigmoid colon. **Jonnesco's o.** Cervical sympathectomy for the relief of exophthalmos. **Joseph's o.** A reduction rhinoplasty performed subcutaneously through intranasal incisions. **Kelly's o.** **1** A surgical procedure to correct urinary incontinence in women. **2** A variety of arytenoidectomy for the relief of bilateral abductor paralysis of the larynx. A square window was excised in the posterior part of the thyroid ala, through which the arytenoid cartilage was removed. It was soon superseded by Woodman's operation. *Outmoded.* **Killian frontal sinus o.** An operation for the relief of chronic frontal sinusitis requiring the removal of most of the front wall and floor of the sinus but the preservation of the upper orbital arch to avoid deformity. Also *Killian's operation.* **King's o.** An arytenoidopexy utilized to improve the airway in cases of bilateral abductor paralysis of the larynx. The object is to abduct one of the paralyzed cords by fixing the arytenoid with the vocal process rotated outward. **Kocks o.** A gynecologic vaginal operation to treat uterine prolapse by shortening the cardinal ligaments. **Kondoleon o.** A procedure to relieve elephantiasis by removing strips of subcutaneous connective tissue. **König's o.** An acetabuloplasty performed to correct congenital dislocation of the hip whereby an osteoperiosteal flap is created from the outer border of the ilium to deepen the floor of the acetabulum. Also *shelving operation, shelf procedure.* **Kraske's o.** A rectal resection following freeing of the coccyx and left sacral wing to provide posterior exposure. **Krönlein o.** Removal of the outer wall of the orbit to provide operative access to the orbital contents. **Kuhnt-Szymanowski o.** A method of correcting ectropion of the lower eyelid wherein the lid is split along its free margin into a tarsoconjunctival layer and a skin-muscle layer. Sections of tissue that are offset one from the other are then removed from each layer and the layers are closed independently. Also *Kuhnt-Szymanowski procedure.* **Küstner o.** A gynecologic operation to correct chronic inversion of the uterus. The myometrium is incised posteriorly to expose the fundus and traction is then applied to restore the uterus to its normal position. **Landolt's o.** Reconstruction of the lower eyelid with a bridge flap of skin brought down from the upper lid. **laryngeal drop o.** LARYNGEAL RELEASE. **Latzko's o.** A gynecologic operation to repair genital tract fistulas. A flap of vaginal mucosa is utilized to cover the fistula tract. **Laurens o.** An operation for the repair of postauricular fistulas persisting after mastoidectomy. The cicatricial circumference of the fistula is excised, vertical extensions are incised upwards and downwards from the opening, and the skin widely elevated as anterior and posterior flaps are carefully sutured together. **Lawson's o.** A submucous resection of the vocal cord performed by way of the laryngofissure approach. Through a mucosal incision along the cord, the arytenoid cartilage along with the thyroarytenoid and cricoarytenoid muscles are removed. **Le Fort's o.** A gynecologic operation to treat uterine prolapse whereby the anterior and posterior walls of the vagina are sutured together, obliterating most of the vagina. Also *Le Fort-Neugebauer operation.* **lip adhesion o.** The first of two operations to repair a congenital cleft lip and palate where the width of the cleft in the palate is great. A temporary incomplete closure of the lip is carried out with the object of providing continuous traction by the joined muscles of the lip on the components of the cleft palate in the hope of narrowing the cleft ahead of a later definitive operation. **Lisfranc's o.** LISFRANC'S AMPUTATION. **Lorenz o.** An operation for congenital dislocation of the hip in which the head of the femur is fixed against the rudimentary acetabulum until a socket is formed. Also *Hoffa-Lorenz operation, Hoffa's operation.* **Lotheissen's o.** MCVAY'S OPERATION. **low forceps o.** The application of obstetric forceps when the head of the fetus is on the pelvic floor and the sagittal suture lies in the anteroposterior diameter of the pelvic outlet. **Luckett o.** An operation for the correction of congenital lop ears in which excisions are made of a crescent-shaped portion of skin from the posteromedial aspect of the pinna and a smaller subjacent strip of cartilage, to restore the antihelical fold. It was the basis of subsequent procedures to correct this defect. **Ludloff's o.** An oblique osteotomy of the first metatarsal bone for the correction of the metatarsus primus varus deformity of hallux valgus. **Macewen's o.** A supracondylar osteotomy of the femur for correction of a genu valgum deformity. Also *Macewen's osteotomy.* **Mackenrodt's o.** An old-fashioned gynecologic operation whereby the round ligaments are fixed to the vagina in an effort to correct a retroflexed uterus. **Madlener o.** A surgical sterilization procedure in which a knuckle of the oviduct is crushed and then ligated without resection. **Makkas o.** An operation for treatment of ectopia of the bladder. **Manchester o.** A gynecologic operation to correct uterine prolapse whereby the cervix is amputated, the cardinal ligaments are attached anteriorly to the upper cervix, and an anterior colporrhaphy is performed. Also *Fothergill-Donald operation, Manchester-Fothergill operation.* **Marshall-Marchetti o.** An operation for the correction of stress incontinence in which the urethra and bladder are attached to the pubic bone. **mastoid o.** MASTOIDECTOMY. **mastoid obliteration o.** Any operation for obliterating the cavity remaining after mastoidectomy, especially after radical mastoidectomy and, before it became outmoded, the fenestration operation. A number of techniques have been employed using cancellous bone, bone paste, acrylic resin, fat and, particularly, pedicled fascia and muscle flaps. In general, such operations have fallen out of favor. **Matas o.** Any of several types of endoaneurysmorrhaphy. **Matson's o.** Anastomosis between the proximal end of a ureter and the spinal arachnoid. The operation is performed for relief of increased intracranial pressure such as in the communicating type of hydrocephalus. The subarachnoid ureterostomy requires the sacrifice of a kidney and mobilization of its ureter. **Mayo's o.** **1** A surgical repair of an umbilical hernia, utilizing a two-layer, overlapping closure. **2** A surgical procedure in which the duodenum is excluded by pyloric excision and a posterior gastrojejunostomy performed. **3** Removal of varicose veins of the lower extremity, using an external stripper. **McBurney's o.** A surgical procedure to treat inguinal hernias by excising the sac and securing the overlying imbricated skin to underlying musculature. **McKissock's o.** A reduction mammoplasty in which the blood supply to the nipple is preserved by means of a bipedicled vertical de-epithelized skin flap. **McVay's o.** A groin hernioplasty in which the repair involves the pectineal ligament. Also *Lotheissen's operation, Cooper's ligament hernioplasty.* **Meyer's o.** RADICAL MASTECTOMY. **midforceps o.** The application of obstetric forceps after the fetal head has become engaged but is not on the pelvic floor and/or the sagittal suture is not in the anteroposterior diameter of the pelvic outlet. **mika o.** Creation of a fistula in the male urethra in order to prevent reproduction. **Mikulicz o.** **1** An excision of the sternocleidomastoid muscle for the correction of congenital torticollis. **2** An excision of the hindfoot in which the talus and the os calcis are excised together with the articular surfaces of the tibia, fibula, and the cuboid and navicular bones. The foot is then brought into alignment with the leg. **Miles o.** Abdominoperineal resection of rectal carcinoma. **Millard o.** MILLARD METHOD. **Millard rotation-advancement o.** A popular method for the repair of unilateral congenital cleft lip wherein the cupid's bow on the medial side of the cleft is rotated into anatomic position by means of a curved convex incision along the medial border of the cleft, usually with the assistance of a back cut at the superior end. The lateral lip segment is then formed onto an advancement flap and joined to the repositioned medial segment. Many modifications and refinements have been described. Also *Millard operation.* **Millin-Read o.** An operation for the correction of urinary stress incontinence in which fascial strips from the anterior abdominal wall are used for a suprapubic sling which passes around the urethra. **Müller's o.** A method of completing vaginal hysterectomy by splitting the uterus in the midline into halves and then resecting each half separately. **Mustard's o.** MUSTARD PROCEDURE. **Naffziger o.** Intracranial decompression of the orbit for the relief of exophthalmos. **Ober's o.** The division of a joint capsule for the correction of contractures. **Ollier's o.** **1** The transfer of a thin split-skin graft. **2** An operation for the repair of a defect in the lower lip with a flap obtained from the submental region. **3** Decortication of the nose in cases of rhinophyma. **Ombrédanne's o.** A surgical procedure for correction of hypospadias, wherein the preputial skin is opened upon itself, leaving a dorsal attachment. The flap thus created is then folded onto the ventral surface of the penis, and the glans penis passed through a small incision in the center of the flap. **open o.** A surgical procedure by which, as a result of the incision, internal organs and tissues become exposed to view. **osteoplastic frontal sinus o.** An operation for the relief of chronic frontal sinusitis. The principal feature is the turning down, as an osteoplastic flap, of the anterior wall of the frontal sinuses, previously marked out using an x-ray template. With access to the interior of the sinuses so afforded, the lining mucosa is meticulously removed and drainage established into the nose by creating a passage through the ethmoidal air cells from above. **palatal pushback o.** **1** An operation for the repair of cleft palate, now superseded by the Wardill V-Y pushback operation. Palatal pushback is a two-stage operation in which the palatal soft tissues are raised and the anterior palatine arteries ligated and, two or three weeks later, the delayed flap is moved backwards and the repair completed. Also *Dorrance operation.* **2** An operation to correct velopharyngeal insufficiency by the posterior repositioning of the soft palate. For defs. 1 and 2 also *pushback procedure.* **Partsch's o.** MARSUPIALIZATION. **Peet's o.** A supradiaphragmatic sympathectomy for vascular hypertension. **Phelps o.** A soft tissue release operation through the medial aspect of the foot to correct a talipes deformity. **Phemister o.** The insertion of a cancellous bone graft for a delayed union or nonunion of a stable fracture. **plastic o.** An operation to improve form or function, primarily by molding, shifting, or adding tissues. Also *plastic surgery.* **Pollock's o.** An amputation of the lower limb through the knee joint using a long anterior flap and retaining the patella. **Polya's o.** A surgical reconstruction following a distal gastrectomy in which a retrocolic gastrojejunostomy is not preceded by a Hofmeister operation. **Pomeroy's o.** A simple method of achieving sterilization whereby a loop of fallopian tube is ligated with catgut suture without crushing it and the loop is then resected. **Portmann interposition o.**

A variety of stapedectomy in which the stapes superstructure is left intact and attached to the incus while only the foot-plate is removed. A vein graft is interposed between the stapedial crura and the patent oval window. No prosthesis is required. Also *platinectomy*. **Potts o.** The creation of an anastomosis between the descending aorta and pulmonary artery in patients with severe pulmonary stenosis, as seen especially in the tetralogy of Fallot. Also *Potts-Smith-Gibson operation*. **Puussepp's o.** A posterior longitudinal incision in the spinal cord, for the treatment of syringomyelia. **Ramadier's o.** An operation for the relief of petrositis involving an intrapetrosal surgical approach to the apex of the petrous portion of the temporal bone. The procedure entails retraction of the carotid artery forward to gain access to the site of infection through the posterior wall of the bony carotid canal. **Ramstedt o.** PYLOROMYOTOMY. **Rastelli's o.** The correction of various forms of cyanotic congenital cardiac anomalies, such as truncus arteriosus, pulmonary artery atresia, and transposition of the great arteries with pulmonary stenosis by the use of a valved prosthetic or allograft conduit between the right ventricle and the pulmonary artery. **reconstructive o.** RECONSTRUCTIVE SURGERY. **Reverdin's o.** REVERDIN GRAFT. **Rose-Thompson o.** A method of repairing minimal degrees of congenital cleft lip, wherein the additional length required on the medial side of the cleft is obtained by means of curved concave incisions on either side. When the curved edges are approximated as a straight line, the necessary extra length is automatically provided. **Roux en Y o.** A surgical procedure in which a defunctionalized limb of the small bowel is created by an end-to-end enteroenterostomy. The end of this loop may be used for a number of types of biliary, enteric, gastric, or pancreatic anastomoses. **Royle's o.** Lumbar sympathectomy, for improving the blood supply to the lower limb. **saccus o.** Any one of several operations intended to relieve the symptoms of Menière's disease by decompressing the saccus endolymphaticus. Over the years, this has included incision of the saccus, the use of an endolymphatic shunt, and the exposing of the saccus without opening it. **Sayre's o.** A nonsurgical treatment of spondylitis or Pott's disease by use of a plaster body cast. Also *Sayre's method*. **Scanzoni's o.** An operation utilizing obstetrical forceps to rotate a fetal head from the posterior to the anterior position. After the fetus is rotated, the forceps are reapplied so that they are aligned with the pelvic axis. **Schauta-Amreich vaginal o.** A method of treating carcinoma of the uterine cervix by performing a radical or extended vaginal hysterectomy whereby the uterus is removed close to its attachments to the pelvic wall. Also *Schauta's operation*. **Schauta-Wertheim o.** WERTHEIM-SCHAUTA OPERATION. **Scheie's o.** A thermal shrinkage of the scleral edge of a limbal incision to permit aqueous drainage to the subconjunctival space as a treatment for glaucoma. **Schwartze's o.** SIMPLE MASTOIDECTOMY. **seton o.** A filtering operation for glaucoma in which the drain site is kept open by the presence of a foreign substance. **shelving o.** KÖNIG'S OPERATION. **Sistrunk o.** A method for removal of thyroglossal cysts and sinuses. Because the thyroglossal tract is intimately related to the body of the hyoid bone and may be identified as far as the foramen cecum, it was advocated that the central portion of the hyoid bone together with a core of lingual muscle should be excised to ensure against recurrence. **Sjöquist's o.** Medullary section of the tract of the trigeminal nerve, for the relief of trigeminal neuralgia. **Skoog's o.** **1** A technique of repairing unilateral congenital cleft lip wherein the additional length needed is obtained on the medial side of the cleft by the interposition of two small triangular flaps from the lateral side. **2** SKOOG'S METHOD. **Smith's o.** Intracapsular delivery of a cataract by pressure applied to the inferior sclera. **Smith-Robinson o.** A cervical spine fusion using an anterior approach that is effected by the removal of an intervertebral disk and the grafting of bone. **Smithwick's o.** LUMBODORSAL SPLANCHNICECTOMY. **Socin's o.** Enucleation of a thyroid tumor to preserve functioning thyroid tissue. **Spinelli's o.** An operation to correct chronic uterine inversion in which the anterior myometrium is incised and traction is exerted on the exposed fundus in order to restore the uterus to its normal status. **Ssabanejew-Frank o.** FRANK'S OPERATION. **Stacke's o.** A variety of radical mastoidectomy advocated in cases where the mastoid is sclerotic and the mastoid antrum hard to find. A tympanectomy is performed first and then the antrum is opened working upwards and backwards from the meatus. **stapes mobilization o.** STAPES MOBILIZATION. **Steindler's o.** **1** An arthrodesis of the elbow performed by using a cortical bone graft extending from the lower end of the humerus to the olecranon. **2** A method of correcting talipes cavus by stripping all muscle and fascia from the plantar surface of the heel. **Stokes o.** GRITTI-STOKES AMPUTATION. **Stookey-Scarff o.** The creation of an opening between the third ventricle and the pontine cistern for a cerebrospinal fluid shunt. This operation is used in the treatment of a ventricular obstruction at a point distal to the third ventricle. **string o.** The dilatation of an esophageal stricture in which the patient swallows a string and esophageal dilatators are then passed, using the string as a guide. **Strombeck's o.** A reduction mammoplasty wherein the blood supply to the nipple is preserved by means of a bipedicled horizontal de-epithelized skin flap. **Sturmdorf's o.** Excision of the squamocolumnar junction of the uterine cervix by making a conical incision to excise the tissue and then suturing flaps of adjacent vaginal mucosa into the area of excision to control bleeding and encourage healing. **Swenson's o.** A surgical treatment for congenital megacolon in which the normal colon is pulled through the aganglionic rectum and sutured into place. **Syme's o.** SYME AMPUTATION. **Szymanowski o.** An operation for the repair of a defect of the upper lip by using a rotation flap from the cheek, which is brought as far as the midline. **Taarnhøj's o.** Decompression of the ganglion and root of the trigeminal nerve, for the relief of trigeminal neuralgia. **tack o.** An operation for the relief of the symptoms of Menière's disease by intermittent decompression of the saccule. It is a modification of sacculotomy. A stainless steel tack is inserted through the stapes foot-plate so as to puncture the saccule whenever it should become distended. **tagliacotian o.** *Outmoded* ITALIAN RHINOPLASTY. **Tanner's o.** The surgical ligation of the portal azygos connections and the division and resuturing of the stomach immediately below the gastroesophageal junction to correct bleeding esophageal varices. **Tansini's o.** Mastectomy followed by use of a skin flap from the back to cover the defect. **Tanzer's o.** A method of reconstructing a congenitally absent external ear, utilizing costal cartilage grafts for the framework and skin grafts and local skin flaps for the integument. **Teale's o.** TEALE'S AMPUTATION. **Tennison-Randall o.** A method for repairing congenital cleft lip deformities wherein a triangular flap from the lateral segment affords additional vertical height necessary for correction. **Tessier's o.** The surgical repositioning of the frontal bone, the bony orbits, and sometimes the maxilla and zygomata, in the treatment of craniofacial anomalies. **Thiersch o.** OLLIER-THIERSCH GRAFT. **Torkildsen's o.** TORKILDSEN SHUNT. **Toti's o.** A variety of external dacryocystorhinostomy, no longer used. After removing the inner wall of the lacrimal sac, bone was resected to expose the nasal lining adjacent to the front end of the middle concha. A portion of nasal mucosa was then removed to encourage fistula formation between the sac and the nasal cavity. **Trendelenburg's o.** **1** Pulmonary embolectomy, especially without the use of cardiopulmonary bypass. **2** The surgical removal of a varicose vein. **3** The ligation of a saphenous vein. **4** SYNCHONDROSEOTOMY. **uterine suspension o.** Any operative procedure utilized to reposition the uterus from retroversion to anteversion. **vacuum extraction o.** The use of a suction cup placed on the fetal head to facilitate vaginal delivery. The suction device takes the place of obstetric forceps and is used for the same indications. **van Hook's o.** URETEROURETEROSTOMY. **Verhoeff's o.** A technique for management of expulsive hemorrhage during cataract surgery, in which the blood is released via a posterior sclerotomy. **Vineberg's o.** An operation to revascularize an ischemic heart by implanting a divided internal mammary artery into a myocardial tunnel. **von Langenbeck's o.** An operation for the closure of a cleft palate utilizing von Langenbeck's bipedicled mucoperiosteal flaps. Flaps are raised on each side of the cleft and then sutured together near the midline. **Watkins o.** A vaginal operation used to treat uterine and vaginal prolapse. The uterine fundus is brought forward and is transposed to lie against the base of the bladder in order to prevent futher prolapse. Also *interposition operation.* **Weir's o.** APPENDICOSTOMY. **Wertheim's o.** A hysterectomy consisting of excision at the origin of the uterine attachments and removal of the upper portion of the vagina. This operation is employed in treating carcinoma of the cervix and is often performed in conjunction with a pelvic lymphadenectomy. **Wertheim-Schauta o.** Radical hysterectomy carried out through a primary vaginal incision. Also *Schauta-Wertheim operation.* **Whipple's o.** PANCREATICODUODENECTOMY. **Whitehead's o.** The treatment of severe rectal hemorrhoids by excising a ring of abnormal mucosa and closing the defect with normal rectal mucosa drawn down from above. **Witzel's o.** A surgical procedure in which a tube jejunostomy is created for enteric feeding by way of a jejunal tunnel. **Woodman's o.** A variety of arytenoidectomy and cordopexy used for the relief of bilateral abductor paralysis of the larynx. Through a skin incision along the anterior border of the sternomastoid muscle, the inferior constrictor muscle is separated from the thyroid cartilage, permitting elevation of the thyroid ala and exposure of the arytenoid cartilage where it articulates with the cricoid cartilage. The arytenoid cartilage is removed and the posterior end of the vocal cord stitched to the inferior horn of thyroid cartilage. **Ziegler's o.** A cautery of the eyelid to correct malposition by shrinking the tissue. **Z-plastic relaxing o.** Z-PLASTY.

**operative** \äp′ərətiv\ [Middle French *operatif* (from L *operat(us),* past part. of *operari* to work, take pains with) pertaining to a work] **1** Pertaining to surgical procedures. **2** Active or effective; not passive or inert.

**operator** **1** One who performs an operation. **2** One who operates equipment. **3** OPERATOR LOCUS. **gene o.** A segment of a chromosome which is located adjacent to a structural gene and which controls transcription of the structural gene.

**opercle** \ōpur′kl\ OPERCULUM.

**opercula** \ōpur′kyələ\ Plural of OPERCULUM.

**operculated** Possessing an operculum, or lid. Also *operculate.*

**operculitis** \ōpur′kyəlī′tis\ [*opercul(um)* + -ITIS] PERICORONITIS.

**operculum** \ōper′kyələm\ [L (from *opertus,* past part. of *operiri* to cover, from OP- + L *partus,* past part. of *parere* to bring forth, bear), a lid, cover] (*pl.* opercula) **1** A covering membrane or lid, such as occurs in a wide variety of vertebrate and invertebrate animals. It varies in form from a membranous flap to a horny lid, and generally serves as a movable, protective covering that can seal off an internal organ or system. Also *opercle.* **2** The cortical lid or cover on the insula, formed by those portions of the frontal, parietal, and temporal lobes bordering the lateral (sylvian) fissue. • The plural form *opercula insulae* is often used when referring to the folds comprising this cover. **cortical o.** **1** Generically, the "apron" of cortex hidden within a deep cerebral fissure. **2** Specifically, the operculum of the lateral sulcus overlying the insula. **dental o.** The flap of oral mucosa partially or completely covering an erupting or impacted tooth. **o. frontale** [NA] The part of the inferior frontal gyrus that forms the anterior part of the cortical covering of the insula. It borders the lateral sulcus, and is subdivided into orbital, triangular, and opercular portions. In the left (or dominant) hemisphere, the triangular and opercular portions constitute Broca's motor speech area. Also *frontal operculum, operculum orbitale, pars frontalis operculi, pars triangularis.* **o. frontoparietale** [NA] The part of the cortical covering of the insula lying along the superior border of the lateral sulcus between the ascending and posterior branches of that sulcus. It includes the opercular portion of the inferior frontal gyrus, the lower ends of the precentral and postcentral gyri, and the supramarginal gyrus of the inferior parietal lobule. Also *frontoparietal operculum, pars parietalis operculi.* **opercula insulae** See under OPERCULUM. **occipital o.** The portion of the occipital lobe forming the posterior wall of the simian fissure, or sulcus lunatus, when this fissure is present in the human brain. **o. orbitale** OPERCULUM FRONTALE. **parietal o.** The inferior portions of the precentral, postcentral, and supramarginal gyri bordering the lateral sulcus and overlying the insula. Stimulation of the parietal operculum produces gustatory sensations. **o. temporale** [NA] The part of the superior temporal gyrus forming the lower margin of the lateral sulcus and overlying the insula. The transverse gyri of Heschel lie on its superior surface, and the most anterior of these gyri is the auditory area. Also *temporal operculum, pars temporalis operculi.* **trophoblastic o.** The lid of trophoblast which closes over the point of implantation on the endometrial surface.

**operon** \äp′ərän\ A functional unit of DNA that includes one or more structural genes, an adjacent promoter that can initiate transcription, and an operator locus whose interaction with regulatory molecules modulates the activity of the promoter. **lac o.** A region of the chromosome of *Escherichia coli* consisting of three adjacent structural genes plus an operator and a promoter, the promoter being the site to which ribonucleic acid polymerase first binds. The structural genes of the lac operon code for the enzymes $\beta$-galactosidase, galactoside permease, and galactoside transacetylase, which allow utilization of the sugar lactose.

**ophi-** \ō′fē-\ OPHIO-.

**ophiasis** \ōfī′əsis\ [Gk *ophiasis* a bald place on the head, winding in form] OPHIASIC ALOPECIA AREATA.

**ophidism** \ō′fidizm\ [OPHI- + *d* + -ISM] Poisoning from snake venom.

**ophio-** \ō′fē·ō-\ [Gk *ophis* a serpent, snake] A combining form meaning snake, snakelike. Also *ophi-*.

***Ophiophagus hannah*** \ō′fē·äf′əgəs han′ə\ A venomous snake of the Elapidae family; the king cobra.

**ophthalm-** \äfthalm-\ OPHTHALMO-.

**ophthalmacrosis** \äfthal′məkrō′sis\ MACROPHTHALMIA.

**ophthalmatrophia** \äfthal′mətrō′fē·ə\ [OPHTHALM- + ATROPHIA] PHTHISIS BULBI.

**ophthalmectomy** \äf′thalmek′təmē\ [OPHTHALM- + -ECTOMY] The surgical enucleation of the eye.

**ophthalmia** \äfthal′mē·ə\ [OPHTHALM- + -IA] Inflammation of the eye. Also *ophthalmitis*. **actinic ray o.** ACTINIC CONJUNCTIVITIS. **caterpillar o.** CATERPILLAR CONJUNCTIVITIS. **Egyptian o.** TRACHOMA. **electric o.** ACTINIC CONJUNCTIVITIS. **gonococcal o. of newborn** Purulent conjunctivitis due to *Neisseria gonorrhoeae*. The infection is derived from the mother's birth canal, and generally becomes evident about the third day of life. It may be unilateral or bilateral. Infant-to-infant infection may also occur in an infant nursery. Because the conjunctival infection can spread to other structures within the eye, the condition was at one time a major cause of blindness. Prophylactic treatment of the eyes at birth with drops (for example, one percent silver nitrate) has therefore often been routinely applied. **gonorrheal o.** GONOCOCCAL CONJUNCTIVITIS. **jequirity o.** Severe inflammation of the eye and its deeper structures due to self-mutilation by placing the toxic seeds of jequirity, *Arbus precatorius*, in the conjunctival sac. **o. neonatorum** INFANTILE PURULENT CONJUNCTIVITIS. **neuroparalytic o.** NEUROPARALYTIC KERATITIS. **o. nivialis** SNOW BLINDNESS. **o. nodosa** CONJUNCTIVITIS NODOSA. **phlyctenular o.** PHLYCTENULAR KERATOCONJUNCTIVITIS. **solar o.** GLARE CONJUNCTIVITIS. **spring o.** VERNAL KERATOCONJUNCTIVITIS. **sympathetic o.** A severe posttraumatic uveitis due to autoimmunity to uveal pigment, affecting both eyes even if the original injury damaged only one eye. Also *sympathetic uveitis, sympathetic ophthalmitis*. **ultraviolet ray o.** ACTINIC CONJUNCTIVITIS. **varicose o.** Ophthalmia associated with a varicose condition of the conjunctival veins.

**ophthalmic** \äfthal′mik\ [OPHTHALM- + -IC] Pertaining to the eye.

**ophthalmic acid** A tripeptide first isolated from the eye. It is the analogue of glutathione in which the thiol group is replaced by a methyl group.

**ophthalmitis** \äf′thalmī′tis\ [OPHTHALM- + -ITIS] OPHTHALMIA. Adj. ophthalmitic. **sympathetic o.** SYMPATHETIC OPHTHALMIA.

**ophthalmo-** \äfthal′mō-\ [Gk *ophthalmos* eye] A combining form denoting the eye. Also *ophthalm-*.

**ophthalmocopia** \-kō′pē·ə\ [OPHTHALMO- + Gk *kop(os)* weariness + -IA] ASTHENOPIA.

**ophthalmodiaphanoscope** \-dī′əfan′əskōp\ A device using transillumination to view the ocular fundus.

**ophthalmodonesis** \-dōnē′sis\ [OPHTHALMO- + Gk *donēsis* a trembling] Flickering or trembling of the eyes and eyelids.

**ophthalmodynamometer** \-dī′nəmäm′ətər\ A device that measures the intraocular blood pressure by measuring the external pressure required to stop the circulation of blood.

**ophthalmodynamometry** \-dī′nəmäm′ətrē\ [OPHTHALMO- + Gk *dynam(is)* + *o* + -METRY] A technique of measuring the blood pressure in the ophthalmic artery by applying an ophthalmodynamometer to the globe of the eye.

**ophthalmograph** \äfthal′məgraf\ [OPHTHALMO- + -GRAPH] A device to record eye movements during reading.

**ophthalmography** \äf′thalmäg′rəfē\ [OPHTHALMO- + -GRAPHY] The recording of eye movements during reading.

**ophthalmogyric** \-jī′rik\ OCULOGYRIC.

**ophthalmologic** \-läj′ik\ Pertaining to ophthalmology.

**ophthalmologist** \äf′thalmäl′əjist\ A physician specializing in the care and treatment of the eye; a specialist in ophthalmology. Also *oculist*.

**ophthalmology** \äf′thalmäl′əjē\ [OPHTHALMO- + -LOGY] The medical and surgical specialty of eye care, including treatment of diseases of the eye and the correction of refractive error. Adj. ophthalmologic, ophthalmological.

**ophthalmomalacia** \-məlā′shə\ Infarction or necrosis of the eye. Also *ophthalmophthisis*.

**ophthalmometer** \äf′thalmäm′ətər\ KERATOMETER.

**ophthalmometry** \äf′thalmäm′ətrē\ [OPHTHALMO- + -METRY] KERATOMETRY.

**ophthalmomyiasis** \-mī′yəsis\ [OPHTHALMO- + MYIASIS] OCULAR MYIASIS.

**ophthalmomyotomy** \-mī·ät′əmē\ [OPHTHALMO- + MYOTOMY] A surgical severing of an extraocular muscle.

**ophthalmoneuritis** \-n^y^urī′tis\ [OPHTHALMO- + NEURITIS] OPTIC NEURITIS.

**ophthalmoneuromyelitis** \-n^y^ur′ōmī′əlī′tis\ NEUROMYELITIS OPTICA.

**ophthalmoparalysis** \-pəral′isis\ OPHTHALMOPLEGIA.

**ophthalmopathy** \äf′thalmäp′əthē\ [OPHTHALMO- + -PATHY] Any disorder of the eye or its adnexa. **endocrine o.** EXOPHTHALMIC OPHTHALMOPLEGIA. **hyperthyroid o.** EXOPHTHALMIC OPHTHALMOPLEGIA. **infiltrative o.** EXOPHTHALMIC OPHTHALMOPLEGIA. **thyrotoxic o.** EXOPHTHALMIC OPHTHALMOPLEGIA.

**ophthalmophacometer** \-fākäm′ətər\ A device for measuring the curvatures of the lens and cornea and the distances separating these surfaces.

**ophthalmophthisis** \äf′thalmäf′thisis\ OPHTHALMOMALACIA.

**ophthalmoplasty** \äfthal′mōplas′tē\ A plastic operation on the eye or its adnexa.

**ophthalmoplegia** \-plē′jə\ [OPHTHALMO- + -PLEGIA] Paralysis of ocular muscles. Also *ophthalmoparalysis*. Adj. ophthalmoplegic. **anterior internuclear o.** ATAXIC NYSTAGMUS. **basal o.** Ophthalmoplegia due to any pathologic process, such as meningitis or arachnoiditis, involving the meninges at the base of the brain. **congenital o.** The paralysis of one or more motor nerves of the eye from birth. **diabetic o.** Ocular palsy associated with diabetes mellitus, particularly, involvement of the third cranial nerve by diabetic neuropathy with resulting paresis of extraocular muscle. **exophthalmic o.** Swelling of the external ocular muscles and orbital contents in Graves disease, usually presenting with diplopia (often due initially to weakness of one superior rectus muscle) and with exophthalmos, either unilateral or bilateral. The latter may become very severe. Also *ophthalmic Graves disease, infiltrative ophthalmopathy, thyrotoxic ophthalmopathy, thyrotoxic ophthalmoplegia, hyperthyroid ophthalmopathy, hyperthyroid ophthalmoplegia, endocrine ophthalmopathy*. **external o.** Paralysis of the extraocular muscles. Also *ophthalmoplegia externa, Ballet's disease*. **hyperthyroid o.** EXOPHTHALMIC OPHTHALMOPLEGIA. **internal o.** Ophthalmoplegia of the iris or ciliary body. Also *ophthalmoplegia interna*. **internuclear o.** Ophthalmoplegia due to a lesion of any of the nerve fiber tracts, such as the medial longitudinal bundle, which connect the nuclei of the third, fourth, and sixth cranial nerves. Also *internuclear paralysis*. **nuclear o.** Ophthalmoplegia due to a lesion or lesions of one or more of the nuclei of the third, fourth, and sixth cranial nerves. **orbital o.** Paralysis of the extraocular muscles caused by a condition within the orbit. **painful o.** 1 SUPERIOR ORBITAL FISSURE SYNDROME. 2 TOLOSA-HUNT SYNDROME. **Parinaud's o.** PARINAUD SYNDROME. **posterior internuclear o.** Paralysis of lateral movement of one eye with normal adduction of the other due to a lesion immediately rostral to the sixth nerve nucleus on the affected side. **progressive o.** Progressive paralysis of the external ocular muscles causing bilateral ptosis and ultimately inability to move the eyes in any direction. Some cases may be due to nuclear degeneration, but most result from a progressive myopathy of the external ocular muscles. Also *Graefe's disease.* **relapsing o.** OPHTHALMOPLEGIC MIGRAINE. **Sauvineau's o.** Paralysis of the medial rectus of one eye and overaction of the lateral rectus of the other eye, as may occur when the paretic eye is used for fixation. **sensorimotor o.** *Seldom used* ORBITAL APEX SYNDROME. **thyrotoxic o.** EXOPHTHALMIC OPHTHALMOPLEGIA.

**ophthalmoplegic** \-plē′jik\ Pertaining to ophthalmoplegia.

**ophthalmoptosis** \äfthal′mäptō′sis\ EXOPHTHALMOS.

**ophthalmoreaction** \-rē·ak′shən\ CALMETTE'S REACTION.

**ophthalmoscope** \äfthal′məskōp\ [OPHTHALMO- + -SCOPE] A device for viewing the fundus of the eye. Also *funduscope* (imprecise). **direct o.** An ophthalmoscope that causes the retinas of subject and observer to be directly conjugate with each other without an intervening real image. **indirect o.** An ophthalmoscope that forms an inverted real image between the fundus and the observer.

**ophthalmoscopy** \äf′thalmäs′kəpe\ [OPHTHALMO- + -SCOPY] The clinical examination of the interior of the eye by means of an ophthalmoscope. Also *funduscopy* (imprecise), *fundoscopy* (imprecise). Adj. opthalmoscopic. **direct o.** Observation of the retina with an ophthalmoscope that images the retina directly upon the observer's retina, without the interposition of an inverted aerial real image. **indirect o.** Observation of the retina with an ophthalmoscope that projects an inverted real image between the patient's retina and the observer.

**ophthalmostat** \äfthal′mōstat\ EXOPHTHALMOMETER.

**ophthalmostatometer** \-stətäm′ətər\ EXOPHTHALMOMETER.

**ophthalmotoxin** \-täk′sin\ [OPHTHALMO- + TOXIN] Any toxin exerting a deleterious effect upon the eye.

**ophthalmotrope** \äfthal′mōtrōp\ [OPHTHALMO- + -TROPE] A model of the eye and attached muscles for the demonstration of ocular movements resulting from contraction of the extraocular muscles.

**ophthalmovascular** \-vas′kyələr\ Concerning the blood vessels of the eye.

**-opia** \-ō′pē·ə\ [Gk *ōps,* gen. *ōpos,* eye + -IA] A combining form meaning having vision (of a specified kind). Also *-opsia.*

**opian** NOSCAPINE.

**opianine** NOSCAPINE.

**opiate** A medicinal agent containing opium or an alkaloid obtained from opium.

**opinion / second o.** A judgment independently arrived at by a practitioner not previously consulted on a case as to the correctness of a diagnosis or, especially, as to the advisability of a proposed medical or surgical treatment.

**opisth-** \ōpisth-\ OPISTHO-.

**opisthenar** \ōpis′thənär\ The dorsum of the hand.

**opisthencephalon** \ōpis′thensef′əlän\ *Rare* CEREBELLUM.

**opisthiobasial** \ōpis′thē·ōbā′sē·əl\ Pertaining to the opisthion and the basion, especially the line or distance between them as used in craniometry.

**opisthionasial** \ōpis′thē·ōnā′zē·əl\ Pertaining to the opisthion and the nasion, especially the distance between them as measured in craniometry.

**opistho-** \ōpis′thō-\ [Gk *opisthe* (*opisthen* before vowel) to the rear, backward] A combining form meaning backward, posterior, dorsal. Also *opisth-.*

**opisthocranion** \-krā′nē·än\ [Late Gk *opisthokranion* (from Gk *opisth(e)* (adverb) behind + *o* + *kranion* the skull)] A craniometric point situated on the occipital bone at its most posterior point in the midline when the skull is orientated in the Frankfort horizontal plane. Also *occipital point.*

**opisthoglyphic** \-glif′ik\ [OPISTHO- + Gk *glyph(ein)* to carve + -IC] Having two to three pairs of grooved poison fangs at the rear of the upper jaw: used of snakes. The fangs are held in the wound after striking to permit the infusion of venom. Because this mechanism for delivering venom is relatively inefficient, opisthoglyphic snakes are generally less dangerous than other venomous snakes. Compare SOLENOGLYPHIC, PROTEROGLYPHIC.

**opisthoporeia** \-pôrī′ə\ [OPISTHO- + Gk *poreia* a walking, going] RETROPULSION.

**opisthorchiasis** \ō′pisthôrkī′əsis\ Infection with flukes of the genus *Opisthorchis. O. viverrini* is a normal parasite of dogs and cats, and *O. felineus* of dogs, cats, and pigs. Human infection is common in northern Thailand, eastern Europe, and the USSR. Eggs are passed in feces by the definitive host into water. Following development in intermediate snail hosts, metacercariae encyst in the flesh of fish which if eaten raw infects man. They are free in the small intestine and travel up the biliary system, where they become adult flukes. Biliary obstruction, abscess formation, and adenocarcinoma of the biliary system result. Treatment is with praziquantel. Also *opisthorchosis.*

**opisthorchid** \ō′pisthôr′kid\ [OPISTH- + *orch(i)-* + -ID[1]] 1 Of or belonging to the genus *Opisthorchis* or the family Opisthorchiidae. 2 A member of the genus *Opisthorchis* or the family Opisthorchiidae.

***Opisthorchis*** \ō′pisthôr′kis\ [OPISTH- + Gk *orchis* a testicle] A genus of digenetic flukes of the family Opisthorchiidae, species of which are parasitic in the livers of fish-eating carnivores, including cats, dogs, foxes, pigs, and man. ***O. tenuicollis*** A species of fluke that is parasitic in the gallbladder and bile ducts of cats, dogs, pigs, and humans in India, Japan, southeast Asia, Siberia, and Europe; the cat liver fluke. The eggs are ingested by snails of the genus *Bithynia,* which release cercariae that encyst in fish. Human infection is acquired by eating raw or undercooked fish. Infection without clinical disease is common, but biliary cirrhosis, chronic pancreatitis, and cholangitis have been reported. Also *Opisthorchis felineus, Distoma felineum* (obs.).

**opisthorchosis** \ō′pisthôrkō′sis\ OPISTHORCHIASIS.

**opisthotic** \ō′pisthät′ik\ Located behind the ear.

**opisthotonoid** \ō′pisthät′ənoid\ Resembling opisthotonos.

**opisthotonos** \ō′pisthät′ənəs\ [Gk (from *opisthe* backwards + *tonos* tension) drawn tensely back] Spasmodic contraction of the muscles of the neck and back with arching of the body. When severe, the subject may rest only on his head and heels. This may occur in tetanus, in some brainstem lesions, or in far-advanced meningitis in infants and children. Also *opisthotonus.* Compare EMPROSTHOTONOS. Adj. opisthotonic. **o. fetalis** A hyperextended position of the fetus during labor in which the head is bent backward and the back is arched.

**opisthotonus** \ō′pisthät′ənəs\ OPISTHOTONOS.

**Opitz** [John Marius *Opitz,* German-born U.S. pediatrician, born 1935] Smith-Lemli-Opitz syndrome. See under SYNDROME.

**opium** [L (from Gk *opion* poppy juice, opium, from *opos* juice, esp. of trees or plants; milky juice, resin, gum), the dried juice of the poppy] A gummy exudate of the poppy *Papaver album* or *P. somniferum.* It yields various alkaloids, of which morphine is the most important and abundant. Other significant alkaloids isolated are codeine, narcotine, thebaine, narceine, and papaverine. Opium is primarily a narcotic, but preparations have been used as aphrodisiacs, as diaphoretics, and as sedatives. Also *gum opium.* **denarcotized o.** Opium powder that has been extracted with pure petroleum benzene in order to remove certain constituents that cause nausea. Also *opium deodoratum, deodorized opium.* **granulated o.** Opium pulverized to a coarse powder form. Also *opium granulatum.* **powdered o.** Opium that has been dried and reduced to a fine powder at a temperature not in excess of 70°C. This product contains not less than 10% nor more that 10.5% anhydrous morphine, and may be used in the composition of products with any of the dilutants of powdered extracts, except for starch. Also *opium pulveratum.*

**opocephalus** \ō′pōsef′ələs\ [Gk *ōps,* gen. *ōpos,* eye, face + -CEPHALUS] An embryo, fetus, or newborn infant with various serious malformations of the head including agenesis of mouth and nose, a rudimentary jaw, fused ears, and a single eye.

**opodidymus** \ō′pōdid′iməs\ [Gk *ōps,* gen. *ōpos,* eye, face + *didymos* double, a twin] Equal conjoined twins with a single body, a normal complement of limbs, and two heads united in the neck and occipital regions but more or less separate in the facial regions. Also *opodymus.*

**Oppenheim** [Hermann *Oppenheim,* German neurologist, 1858–1919] **1** Oppenheim's reflex. See under SIGN. **2** Erb-Oppenheim-Goldflam syndrome. See under MYASTHENIA GRAVIS. **3** Oppenheim syndrome, Oppenheim's amyotonia, Oppenheim's disease. See under MYOTONIA CONGENITA. **4** Ziehen-Oppenheim disease. See under DYSTONIA MUSCULORUM DEFORMANS.

**Oppenheim** [Maurice Oppenheim, U.S. dermatologist, 1876–1949] Urbach-Oppenheim disease. See under NECROBIOSIS LIPOIDICA.

**opplotentes** \äp′lōten′tēz\ [Gk *ōps,* gen. *ōpos,* the eye + *plōtos* sailing, floating, swimming] MUSCAE VOLITANTES.

**opponens** \əpō′nənz\ [L, pres. part. of *opponere* to place against] Opposing or placing against: in anatomy, designating those muscles of the thumb and little finger that move these digits so as to touch each other or other digits.

**opportunist** \äp′ərt^y^oo′nist\ A normally harmless organism that becomes pathogenic in a host with reduced resistance.

**opportunistic** \äp′ərt^y^oonis′tik\ [L *opportun(us)* (from *op-* against + *portus* a port, place of refuge) + -IST + -IC] **1** Denoting a microorganism which produces disease only in a host whose immunological status has been compromised by other infections, disease processes, or drugs. In a host with normal immune function, the organism may be present but does not cause disease. **2** Denoting a disease or infection produced by an opportunistic pathogen.

**-opsia** \-äp′sē·ə\ -OPIA.

**opsin** \äp′sin\ The protein that combines with retinal to form a visual pigment.

**opsiometer** \äp′sē·äm′ətər\ OPTOMETER.

**-opsis** \-äp′sis\ [Gk *opsis* sight, vision, appearance] A combining form denoting an organism or part likened to or resembling (something specified).

**opsoclonus** \äp′sōklō′nəs\ [Gk *ōps* the eye + *o* + CLONUS] A sudden, shocklike, clonic movement of the eyes. Such movements are sometimes irregularly repetitive. They may occur as a manifestation of myoclonic encephalopathy in childhood. Also *opsoclonia.*

**opsomania** \äp′sōmā′nē·ə\ [Gk *opso(n)* rich or dainty food + -MANIA] A great desire for a specific food, especially sweets. *Seldom used.*

**opsone** \äp′sōn\ OPSONIN.

**opsonic** \äpsän′ik\ Relating to or having the action of an opsonin; inducing opsonization.

**opsonification** \äpsän′ifikā′shən\ OPSONIZATION.

**opsonin** \äpsō′nin\ [Gk *opson* (akin to *epsein* to boil, seethe, and to *opsōnion* provisions and *opsōnein* to buy fish or victuals) boiled meat, flesh, meat, sauce, seasoning + -IN] Any of various substances capable of binding to the surfaces of bacteria or other cells to make them more susceptible to phagocytosis. Opsonins occur in blood plasma and may be antibodies, fragments of complement components, or enzymes such as lysozyme. Also *opsone.* **immune o.** OPSONIZING ANTIBODY. **normal o.** The opsonin normally present in blood. It is more easily denatured by heat than is the specific opsonin that appears in response to bacterial infection. Also *thermolabile opsonin.*

**opsonization** \äp′sənīzā′shən\ The modification of bacteria and other cells, most usually by coating them with antibody and/or complement, to make them more susceptible to phagocytosis. Also *opsonification.*

**opsonocytophagic** \äp′sənōsī′təfā′jik\ Relating to phagocytosis of bacteria coated with opsonin.

**-opsy** \-əpsē\ -OPIA.

**opt-** \äpt-, əpt-\ OPTO-.

**optic** [Gk *optikos* (akin to *ōps* eye) pertaining to the eye or to vision] Of or relating to the eye.

**optical** [OPTIC + -AL] Of or relating to vision or to means of enhancing vision, especially lenses.

**optician** [OPTIC + *-ian,* suffix meaning practitioner] One who practices opticianry; one who fills ophthalmic prescriptions for spectacles and dispenses them. Also *dispensing optician* (British and South African usage). • See note at OPTOMETRIST. **ophthalmic o.** In Great Britain, an optician who also tests vision and prescribes corrective lenses. • See note at OPTOMETRIST.

**opticianry** \äptish′ənrē\ The science or practice of preparing ophthalmic prescriptions, such as spectacle lenses and contact lenses, and fitting them.

**optico-** \äp′tikō-\ [Gk *optikos* (akin to *ōps* eye) pertaining to the eye or to vision] A combining form meaning optic, especially in reference to the optic nerve. See also OPTO-.

**opticoagnosia** \-agnō′zhə\ VISUAL AGNOSIA. **Wernicke subcortical o.** PURE WORD BLINDNESS.

**opticokinetic** \-kinet′ik\ [OPTICO- + KINETIC] Pertaining to eye movements mediated through the cerebral cortex as part of the following reflex.

**opticonasion** \-nā′zhən\ A cephalometric measure of the linear distance from the posterior margin of the optic canal to the nasion.

**opticopupillary** \-pyoo′piler′ē\ Relating to or affecting the optic nerve and the pupil.

**optics** [Gk *optika* (neut. pl. of *optikos* optical, akin to *optos* visible and to *ōps* the eye) the science of vision] The science that deals with light, including its origin, propagation, and use. **electron o.** The physical principles that influence the passage of an electron beam through an electron microscope and the formation of an image on a fluorescent screen

or photographic plate. **physiological o.** The science of visual perception.
**opticus** \äp′tikəs\ NERVUS OPTICUS.
**optimeter** \äptim′ətər\ OPTOMETER.
**optimism** A cheerful habit of mind characterized by an inclination to believe that the uncertainties of the present will be resolved favorably. **therapeutic o.** An inclination to believe that a particular method of treatment will be successful. Compare THERAPEUTIC PESSIMISM.
**optimization** \äp′timīzā′shər\ [*optim(um)* + *-iz(e)* + -ATION] **1** The selection of principles or components during the design of a system to maximize or minimize some performance index. **2** The adjustment of parameters during the operation of a system to obtain the best operating conditions.
**optimum** \äp′timəm\ The best set of conditions for a particular activity or function, as for obtaining the best or most reliable results. Adj. optimal.
**optist** \äp′tist\ OPTOMETRIST.
**opto-** \äp′tə-, äp′tō-\ [Gk *optos* seen or *optikos* (from *ōps,* gen. *ōpos,* eye) pertaining to the eye] A combining form meaning sight, vision, optical. Also *opt-*.
**optoacoustic** \äp′tō·əkoo′stik\ Perceived by or relating to both vision and hearing.
**optoblast** \äp′təblast\ A retinal ganglion cell, with a large cell body suggestive of a primitive or blast cell.
**Optochin** A proprietary name for ethyl hydrocuprein chloride.
**optogram** \äp′təgram\ [OPTO- + -GRAM] The retinal image produced by a visual stimulus.
**optokinetic** \äp′tōkinet′ik\ [OPTO- + KINETIC] Pertaining to movement of the eye.
**optomeninx** \äp′tōmē′ningks\ RETINA.
**optometer** \äptäm′ətər\ [OPTO- + -METER] A device for measurement of the refractive error of the eye. Also *opsiometer, optimeter.*
**optometrist** \äptäm′ətrist\ [*optometr(y)* + -IST] One who practices optometry; a practitioner skilled in the measurement of visual defect and in the prescription and fitting of corrective lenses. Also *optist.* ● The term is used in the U.S., Australia, New Zealand, and India. In the United Kingdom and South Africa, the equivalent term is *optician* (also sometimes used in New Zealand). In Britain, *optician* is often qualified by *ophthalmic* if used in the sense described above, and by *dispensing* if used in the sense of one who fills prescriptions for spectacles. In the U.S., such a person is simply called an optician.
**optometry** \äptäm′ətrē\ [OPTO- + -METRY] **1** The practice of nonmedical eye care, dealing primarily with the testing of vision for refractive error and with the prescription and fitting of corrective lenses. **2** The measurement of refractive error by means of an optometer. ● *Optometry* (def. 1) is used throughout the English-speaking world, in spite of the variety of terms applying to the sense of optometrist. See the note at OPTOMETRIST.
**optomyometer** \äp′tōmī·äm′ətər\ A device for measuring eye muscle balance and vergence.
**optophone** \äp′təphōn\ [OPTO- + Gk *phōnē* sound, voice] An assistive device for the blind which converts variations in light intensity to variations in sound.
**optotype** \äp′tətīp\ [OPTO- + TYPE] TEST TYPE.
**OR** operating room.
**-or** \-ər, -ôr\ [L noun suffix, agentive or abstract] A suffix denoting a person or thing performing an action.
**ora[1]** \ôr′ə\ [L, edge, border] Margin; edge. **o. serrata retinae** [NA] The anterior crenated margin of the pars optica retinae that marks the junction between the posterior periphery of the ciliary body and the choroid and the site where the sensory part of the retina is abruptly reduced to two layers of epithelial cells. The cell layers continue anteriorly as the pars ciliaris retinae. The serrated appearance is produced by dentate processes extending from the retina along grooves in the orbiculus ciliaris.
**ora[2]** Plural of os[1].
**orad** \ôr′ad\ Toward the mouth.
**orae** \ôr′ē\ Plural of ORA[1].
**oral** \ôr′əl\ [L *os,* gen. *oris,* mouth + -AL] Of, for, or with the mouth. Also *stomatic, stomal.*
**orale** \ôrā′lē\ [L *os,* gen. *oris,* mouth + *-ale,* neut. sing. of *-alis* -AL] In craniometry, the midpoint of a line drawn tangential to the posterior margins of the sockets of the upper central incisor teeth.
**orality** \ôral′itē\ The oral components of psychic development, including signs of their persistence into adult life. See also PSYCHOSEXUAL DEVELOPMENT.
**Oram** [Samuel *Oram,* English cardiologist, born 1913] Holt-Oram syndrome. See under SYNDROME.
**orange** / **o. II** An orange acid dye of the monoazo group that is sometimes used as a pH indicator, turning from yellow at a pH of 11.0 to red at 13.0. It is used occasionally to stain sections of plant or animal tissue. Also *gold orange.* **o. III** METHYL ORANGE. **o. G** An acid azo dye often used as a cytoplasmic counterstain in histologic preparations, particularly in Mallory's triple stain. It is also used in the Papanicolaou stain for cytology preparations. Also *wool orange, novaurantia.* **gold o.** ORANGE II. **wool o.** ORANGE G.
**orb** \ôrb\ [French *orbe* (from L *orb(is)* a ring, disk, circle, socket of the eye, the eye) orbit] **1** A sphere. **2** *Outmoded* BULBUS OCULI.
**Orbeli** [Leon Abgarovich *Orbeli,* Russian physiologist, 1882–1958] Orbeli phenomenon. See under EFFECT.
**orbicular** \ôrbik′yələr\ Circular; spherical. Also *orbicularis.*
**orbicularis** \ôrbik′yəler′is\ **1** ORBICULAR. **2** MUSCULUS ORBICULARIS. **o. oris** MUSCULUS ORBICULARIS ORIS.
**orbiculi** \ôrbik′yəlī\ Plural of ORBICULUS.
**orbiculus** \ôrbik′yələs\ [L (dim. of *orbis* a ring, disk, coil, wheel), a small disk] A small, disk-shaped structure. **o. ciliaris** [NA] The smooth, annular posterior two thirds of the internal aspect of the ciliary body. It is continuous anteriorly with the corona ciliaris and ends posteriorly at the ora serrata. The dentate processes of the ora serrata extend along it to meet the striae of the ciliary zonule, producing meridional grooves in it. Also *ciliary disk, annulus ciliaris* (outmoded), *ciliary ring.*
**orbit** [L *orbit(a).* See ORBITA.] ORBITA.
**orbita** \ôr′bitə\ [L (from *orbis* a ring, disk, coil, wheel) the track of a wheel, path, course] (*pl.* orbitae) [NA] The pyramidal bony cavity in the skull that contains the eyeball and its accessory organs and comprises a roof, a floor, medial and lateral walls, and the orbital opening which forms the base anteriorly. The apex is directed posteromedially and leads into the middle cranial fossa. Also *orbit, orbital cavity, eye socket, arcula* (outmoded).
**orbitae** \ôr′bitē\ Plural of ORBITA.
**orbital** \ôr′bitəl\ **1** Pertaining to the orbit or its contents. **2** Denoting an electron confined to its orbit in an atom, as distinguished from a free electron.
**orbitalis** \ôr′bitā′lis\ Referring to one or both orbits.
**orbitonometer** \ôr′bitōnäm′ətər\ [*orbi(t)* + TONOMETER] A device for measuring the ease of displacement of the eye into the orbital tissue, of value in the study of exophthalmos.

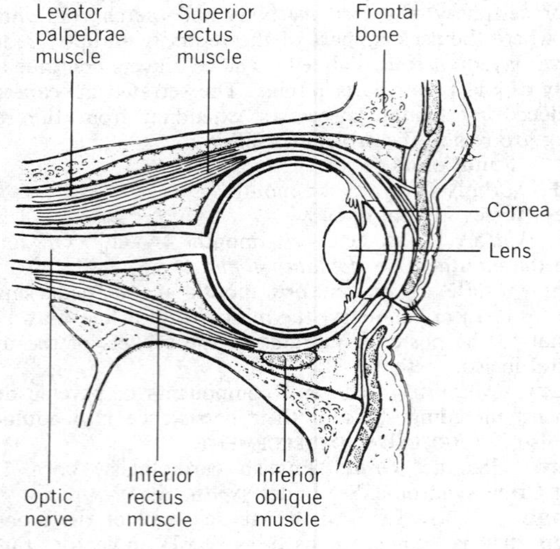


**Orbit**

**orbitonometry** \ôr′bitōnäm′ətrē\ [*orbi(t)* + TONOMETRY] Measurement of the ease of displacement of the eye into the orbital tissue. This is of value in the study of exophthalmos.

**orbitopagus** \ôr′bitäp′əgəs\ [English *orbit* + *o* + Gk *pagos* anything fixed or hardened] Unequal conjoined twins in which the parasitic member, usually very poorly formed, is attached in the orbital region of the host. Also *teratoma orbitae.*

**orbitotomy** \ôr′bität′əmē\ [ORBIT + *o* + -TOMY] Any operation creating an opening into the orbit. The approach may be either anterior or lateral.

**orbivirus** \ôr′bivī′rəs\ A member of the *Orbivirus* genus of the Reoviridae family. Viruses of this genus have two protein capsids and double-stranded RNA. They include bluetongue virus and Colorado tick fever virus.

**orcein** \ôr′sē·in\ A brown stain that is used to demonstrate the presence of elastic fibers. Originally obtained from lichens, it is now prepared synthetically.

**orchectomy** \ôrkek′təmē\ ORCHIDECTOMY.

**orchi-** \ôr′kē-\ ORCHIO-.

**orchialgia** \ôr′kē·al′jə\ [ORCHI- + -ALGIA] Pain affecting the testis. Also *orchidalgia, orchiodynia, orchioneuralgia, testalgia.*

**orchiatrophy** \ôr′kē·at′rəfē\ [ORCHI- + ATROPHY] TESTICULAR ATROPHY.

**orchic** \ôr′kik\ ORCHIDIC.

**orchidalgia** \ôr′kidal′jə\ ORCHIALGIA.

**orchidatrophia** \ôr′kidətrō′fē·ə\ [*orchid(o)-* + ATROPHIA] TESTICULAR ATROPHY.

**orchidatrophy** \ôr′kidat′rəfē\ [*orchid(o)-* + ATROPHY] TESTICULAR ATROPHY.

**orchidectomy** \ôr′kidek′təmē\ [*orchid(o)-* + -ECTOMY] Surgical excision of one testis. The operation may be performed through an incision in the scrotal wall (simple orchidectomy), or through an inguinal approach (inguinal orchidectomy). When the testis is found to have a tumor, both the testis and the spermatic cord are removed through an inguinal incision (radical orchidectomy). Also *orchiectomy, orchectomy, testectomy.*

**orchidic** \ôrkid′ik\ Referring to one or both testes. Also *orchic.*

**orchiditis** \ôr′kidī′tis\ ORCHITIS.

**orchido-** \ôr′kidō-\ [erroneous form for genitive of Gk *orchis* testicle] ORCHIO-.

**orchidoepididymectomy** \-ep′idid′imek′təmē\ Surgical excision of a testis and the epididymis. Operative removal of the testis (orchidectomy), either simple or radical, implies simultaneous excision of the epididymis.

**orchidoepididymitis** \-ep′idid′imī′tis\ ORCHIEPIDIDYMITIS.

**orchidometer** \ôr′kidäm′ətər\ [ORCHIDO- + -METER] Any device for measuring the size of a testicle, especially the Prader orchidometer. **Prader o.** Plastic beads, graded in size, which enable an examiner to gauge by comparison the size of a testicle.

**orchidopathy** \ôr′kidäp′əthē\ ORCHIOPATHY.

**orchidopexy** \ôr′kidōpek′sē\ ORCHIOPEXY.

**orchidoplasty** \ôr′kidōplas′tē\ [ORCHIDO- + -PLASTY] A plastic operation on the testicle. Also *orchioplasty.*

**orchidoptosis** \ôr′kidäptō′sis\ [ORCHIDO- + PTOSIS] Testicular prolapse due to either a lax scrotum or a varicocele.

**orchidorrhaphy** \ôr′kidôr′əfē\ ORCHIOPEXY.

**orchidotherapy** \-ther′əpē\ Therapeutic administration of testicular extracts.

**orchidotomy** \ôr′kidät′əmē\ ORCHIOTOMY.

**orchiectomy** \ôr′kē·ek′təmē\ ORCHIDECTOMY.

**orchiepididymitis** \ôr′kē·ep′idid′imī′tis\ [ORCHI- + EPIDIDYMITIS] Inflammation of the testis and epididymis. Also *orchidoepididymitis.*

**orchil** CUDBEAR.

**orchio-** \ôr′kē·ō-\ [Gk *orchis* (genitive *orchios*) testicle] A combining form denoting the testes. Also *orchi-, orchido-.*

**orchiocatabasis** \-kətab′əsis\ The descent of the testes.

**orchiocele** \ôr′kē·əsēl′\ [ORCHIO- + -CELE[1]] **1** Herniation of a testis. **2** SCROTAL HERNIA.

**orchiodynia** \-din′ē·ə\ [ORCHI- + -ODYNIA] ORCHIALGIA.

**orchioneuralgia** \-n$^y$Ural′jə\ [ORCHIO- + NEURALGIA] ORCHIALGIA.

**orchiopathy** \ôr′kē·äp′əthē\ [ORCHIO- + -PATHY] Disease of the testes. Also *orchidopathy, testopathy.*

**orchiopexy** \ôr′kē·əpek′sē\ [ORCHIO- + -PEXY] The surgical repositioning of a testicle usually performed to place an undescended testicle within the scrotum. Also *orchidopexy, orchiorrhaphy, orchidorrhaphy, cryptorchidopexy.*

**orchioplasty** \ôr′kē·əplas′tē\ ORCHIDOPLASTY.

**orchiorrhaphy** \ôr′kē·ôr′əfē\ ORCHIOPEXY.

**orchiotomy** \ôr′kē·ät′əmē\ [ORCHIO- + -TOMY] Incision into a testis, as to allow drainage. Also *orchotomy, orchidotomy.*

**orchis** \ôr′kis\ [Gk *orchis* a testicle, the testicles] TESTIS.

**orchitis** \ôrkī′tis\ [*orch(i)-* + -ITIS] Inflammation of the testis, manifested by swelling and tenderness and usually of infectious origin, as in tuberculosis, mumps, syphilis, or certain fungal diseases. Also *testitis, didymitis, orchiditis.* **acute pyogenic o.** Acute purulent inflammation of the testes. **acute syphilitic o.** An acute, rare form of testicular infection usually occurring during the second stage of syphilis and clinically resembling acute pyogenic orchitis. **metastatic o.** The spread of infection to the testis via the bloodstream, as may occur in mumps in postpubertal males. **mumps o.** ORCHITIS PAROTIDEA. **o. parotidea** Orchitis resulting from infection with the mumps virus and occurring before, during, or as the only manifestation of mumps. Also *mumps orchitis.* **spermatogenic**

**granulomatous o.** Nontuberculous granulomatous inflammation of a testis, most often seen in middle-aged men after trauma to the testis. It is believed to be due to an autoimmune response to the extravasation of sperm. **traumatic o.** Inflammation of a testicle following injury to the testicle or other part of the male genital system. It can follow surgical procedures as well as direct mechanical trauma. **o. variolosa** Orchitis occurring as a complication of smallpox.

**orchotomy** \ôrkät′əmē\ ORCHIOTOMY.

**ORD** optical rotatory dispersion.

**order** 1 A hierarchical rank or category. 2 A taxonomic group ranking between class and family. **birth o.** 1 In demography, the number of children born alive to the mother, including the present child. 2 The serial ranking of the members of a sibship according to date of birth. **form-o.** See under FORM.

**orderly** An assistant or health worker who performs a wide range of services in a hospital, generally involving patient care or institutional operations, but not at the level of nursing care.

**orectic** \ôrek′tik\ [Gk *orektik(os)* (from *orekt(os)* stretched out, from *oregein* to reach or stretch out, desire, + *-ikos* -IC) having an appetite] 1 Having an appetite. 2 A substance that enhances the appetite.

**orexia** \ôrek′sē·ə\ [*orex(is)* + -IA] APPETITE.

**orexigenic** \ôrek′sējen′ik\ [Gk *orexi(s)* a yearning after, desire for + -GENIC] Serving to stimulate the appetite.

**oreximania** \ôrek′sēmā′nē·ə\ [Gk *orexi(s)* a yearning for a thing + -MANIA] The consumption of enormous quantities of food motivated by a fear of losing weight. *Older term.*

**orexis** \ôrek′sis\ [Gk (from *oregein* to reach for) appetency, yearning] APPETITE.

**organ** [L *organum* (Gk *organon* an instrument, tool, engine, musical instrument, work) an implement, instrument, esp. a musical instrument] Any differentiated part or structure that is adapted for one or more special functions of an organism; organum. **absorbent o.** The tissue, containing odontoclasts, which resorbs the root of a deciduous tooth as the successor erupts. **accessory o.'s of eye** ORGANA OCULI ACCESSORIA. **acoustic o.** ORGANUM SPIRALE. **adipose o.** A localized collection of adipose tissue, such as the greater omentum. **cell o.** ORGANELLE. **cement o.** A tissue composed of cementoblasts, which gives rise to the cement substance of a tooth. **o. of Chievitz** An ectodermal outgrowth from embryonic cheek epithelium behind the site of origin of the parotid salivary gland. Although it can give rise to a tumor, it usually disappears completely. **o. of Corti** ORGANUM SPIRALE. **critical o.** The organ showing adverse effects at the lowest dose, with no reference to the severity of the effects. Other organs may be markedly affected but only at higher doses. **cutaneous sense o.'s** The variety of mechanical, thermal, and nociceptive afferent organs in the skin, most terminating in the dermal papillary layer and overlying basal epidermis. **digestive o.'s** APPARATUS DIGESTORIUS. **effector o.** EFFECTOR. **enamel o.** One of the series of knoblike thickenings which develop from the dental lamina and which produce the enamel of the teeth. The enamel organ forms an invaginated bell-shaped cap over the dental papilla. It has an inner enamel layer composed of ameloblasts, which produce enamel at the surfaces situated against the dental papilla. It also plays an important part in molding the final shape of a tooth. **end o.** The encapsulated ending of the peripheral part of a sensory nerve fiber. These comprise exteroceptors, enteroceptors, and proprioceptors. Also *neuroterminal.* **external genital o.'s** The labia majora, labia minora, and clitoris in the female, and the penis and scrotum in the male. **female genital o.'s** The organa genitalia feminina externa and organa genitalia feminina interna. **female reproductive o.'s** The various structures in the female related to reproduction, including the external genital organs, the vagina, the uterus, the fallopian tubes, and the ovaries. Also *organa genitalia muliebria.* **genital o.'s** ORGANA GENITALIA. **Golgi tendon o.** TENDON ORGAN. Abbr. GTO **gustatory o.** ORGANUM GUSTUS. **internal reproductive o.'s** The vagina, uterus, fallopian tubes, and ovaries in the female, and the prostate, seminal vesicles, and testes in the male. **o. of Jacobson** VOMERONASAL ORGAN. **male genital o.'s** ORGANA GENITALIA MASCULINA. **male reproductive o.'s** The testes, epididymis, ductus deferens, seminal vesicles, ejaculatory duct, prostate, bulbourethral gland, and penis. **motorial end o.** *Obs.* MOTOR ENDPLATE. **neurotendinous o.** TENDON ORGAN. **olfactory o.** ORGANUM OLFACTUS. **pineal o.** CORPUS PINEALE. **primitive fat o.** INTERSCAPULAR GLAND. **reproductive o.'s** GENITALIA. **Rosenmüller's o.** EPOÖPHORON. **rudimentary o.** An undeveloped or uncompleted organ. **o. of Ruffini** BRUSHES OF RUFFINI. **segmental o.** HOLONEPHROS. **sex o.** One of the reproductive organs. **o. of smell** ORGANUM OLFACTUS. **spiral o.** ORGANUM SPIRALE. **subcommissural o.** A group of specialized columnar ciliated ependymal cells that line the dorsal aspect of the cerebral aqueduct just caudal to the posterior commissure. The function of these cells is uncertain. **subfornical o.** A glomoid neurosecretory structure in the third ventricle, attached below the descending columns of the fornix, that has been described in various mammals. It is believed by some researchers to play a role in electrolyte balance. **taste o.** ORGANUM GUSTUS. **tendon o.** An encapsulated recep-

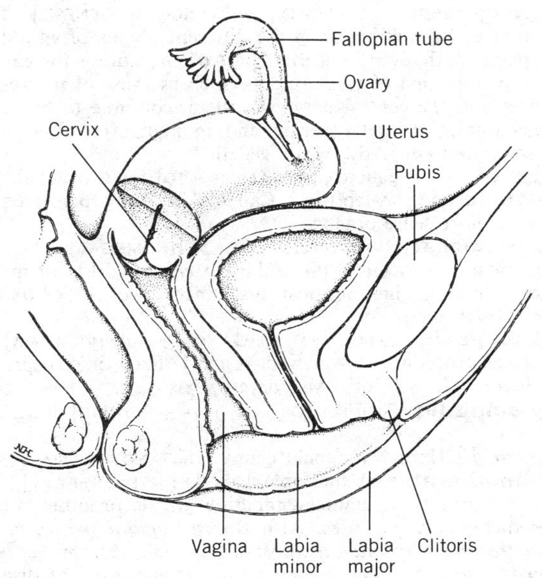


**Female reproductive organs**

tor lying at the musculotendinous junction or within the tendon, hence in series with the muscle fibers and sensitive to tension developed either during contraction or passive stretch of the muscle. The discharge elicits the lengthening reaction. Also *Golgi tendon organ, Golgi corpuscle, neurotendinous organ, tendon spindle, fusus neurotendineus, neurotendinous spindle.* **terminal o.** A sense organ or muscle; the organ at either end of a neural reflex arc. **touch o.'s** 1 CORPUSCULA TACTUS. 2 PINKUS-IGGO RECEPTOR. **vestibular o.** LABYRINTHUS VESTIBULARIS. **vestibular end o.** *Outmoded* GANGLION VESTIBULARE. **vestibulocochlear o.** ORGANUM VESTIBULOCOCHLEARE. **vestigial o.** Any organ which today is seen only in undeveloped or rudimentary form but which in the evolutionary past was well developed and functional. **o. of vision** ORGANUM VISUS. **visual o.** ORGANUM VISUS. **vomeronasal o.** A rudimentary diverticulum on the median wall of each nasal fossa in higher vertebrates. At 8 mm stage in man it forms a groove, supported by special cartilages and supplying nerve fibers to join the olfactory nerve. It begins to regress after the sixth month of intrauterine life but may persist into adult life. In many tetrapods it functions as a supplementary olfactory organ. Also *organ of Jacobson, organum vomeronasale.* **o.'s of Zuckerkandl** CORPORA PARA-AORTICA.

**organa** \ôrgan′ə\ Plural of ORGANUM.

**organella** \ôr′gənel′ə\ (*pl.* organellae) ORGANELLE.

**organellae** \ôr′gənel′ē\ Plural of ORGANELLA.

**organelle** \ôr′gənel′\ [New L *organell(a)* (from L *organ(um)* organ + *-ella,* diminishing suffix] An intracellular structure having a specialized function, such as a mitochondrion, lysosome, or chloroplast. Also *cell organ, organoid, organella.* **paired o.** RHOPTRY.

**organic** \ôrgan′ik\ 1 Relating to or of the nature of animals and plants. 2 Of or relating to an organ. 3 Structural in nature or origin, as *organic defect.* ⟨"His condition [paralysis] was not organic (*i.e.*, it must have been learned) because under pentothal narcosis he was able to move his arm in all directions with ease." —John Dollard and Neal E. Miller, *Personality and Psychotherapy,* 1950, p. 165.⟩ 4 Containing carbon other than that occurring in carbon dioxide or its salts or in carbon monoxide: used of a chemical compound. 5 Derived from or relating to the use of fertilizer of plant or animal origin rather than that of artificially produced substances.

**organicism** \ôrgan′isizm\ 1 The belief that each organ of the body has a unique constitution. 2 The theory that all symptoms are due to organic disease, whether physical or psychologic in nature.

**organism** [ORGAN + -ISM] Any living individual considered as a whole, whether plant or animal, viral or microbial. **pleuropneumonialike o.** *Outmoded* MYCOPLASMA.

**organization** [Med L *organizatio* (from *organizatus,* past part. of *organizare* to organize, from L *organum* an implement, instrument; + *-io* -ION) an act of organizing] 1 A group of individuals functioning as a system in a collective enterprise or of things contributing to a result that depends on their participation. 2 The transformation of a pathological state into vascularized connective tissue by the ingrowth of fibroblasts and capillary buds. • This sense is most often applied to the resolution of a thrombus or of a fibrinous exudate. **health maintenance o.** An organization that provides prepaid health care services to an enrolled clientele, using its own facilities or those contracted for in the community in which it operates. It generally offers comprehensive coverage including preventive care. There are usually few if any copayments on the part of the enrollee beyond a contribution to the premium that is required in some plans. Abbr. HMO • The term *health maintenance organization* was originally used in United States federal legislation passed in the early 1970s to promote prepaid forms of practice, and has been more extensively used in recent years. The term is also used in Australia. **preferred provider o.** In the United States, a health-care insurer that offers benefits through an arrangement of contractual commitments by community-based providers who usually agree to a preferential negotiated rate of payment for specific services offered to individuals enrolled in the insurance. Abbr. PPO

**organizer** 1 A part or region of an embryo which is capable of evoking and controlling the morphologic differentiation of other groups of cells within the embryo. The groups of cells therefore act as an evocator which is capable of determining the fate of other cell groups with which it comes into contact. Also *activating agent, inductor, organizer zone.* 2 See under PRIMARY ORGANIZER. 3 INDUCTOR. **mesodermic o.** The early notochord in its capacity to act as an inductor region which stimulates the differentiation of the adjacent mesoderm into somites. **nucleolar o.** A site on the chromosome containing multiple copies of ribosomal ribonucleic acid genes where the nucleolus originates. Also *nucleololus.* **primary o.** The region of the dorsal lip of the blastopore in lower vertebrates and Hensen's node in higher vertebrates that differentiates without prior induction. This region acts as an inductor and is capable of evoking the formation of the medullary plate and adjacent ectoderm. **secondary o.** A part previously formed as a result of induction, that is in turn capable of providing a morphogenetic stimulus on an adjacent part or parts of the embryo. An example is the induction of the lens by the underlying optic vesicle. **tertiary o.** A part of the embryo that has developed as a result of induction by a secondary organizer, which is in turn capable of providing morphogenetic stimulus on an adjacent part or parts. An example is the tympanic ring which exerts influences on the tympanic membrane.

**organo-** \ôr′gənō-\ [Gk *organon* organ] A combining form meaning organ.

**organogenesis** \-jen′əsis\ [ORGANO- + GENESIS] Formation and development of the different organs of an animal or plant. Although the greater part occurs during the embryonic period, that of some organs, such as those of the special senses and the central nervous system, continue to be developed during the fetal period and in man even after birth. Also *organogeny.* Adj. organogenetic.

**organoid** \ôr′gənoid\ [ORGAN + -OID] ORGANELLE.

**organoleptic** \-lep′tik\ Capable of being perceived by one or more sense organs.

**organomegaly** \-meg′əlē\ SPLANCHNOMEGALY.

**organon** \ôr′gənän\ [Gk (akin to *ergon* work), an instrument, tool, engine, musical instrument, work] *Outmoded* ORGANUM.

**organopexia** \-pek′sē·ə\ [ORGANO- + *-pex(y)* + -IA] A surgical procedure in which an organ is fixed or resuspended to increase its support. Also *organopexy.*

**organophilic** \-fil′ik\ [ORGAN + *o* + -PHILIC] ORGANOTROPIC.

**organophilism** \ôr′gənäf′ilizm\ ORGANOTROPISM.

**organotherapy** \-ther′əpē\ [ORGANO- + THERAPY] The use of extracts of animal endocrine glands or other organs for therapeutic purposes. Also *Brown-Séquard treatment, organ treatment, cellular therapeutics, organic therapy.* **heterologous o.** The use of organ extracts to treat diseases of a different or unrelated organ. **homologous o.** The use of animal organ extracts to treat human diseases of the same organ system.

**organotrope** \ôrgan′ōtrōp\ [ORGANO- + -TROPE] An agent or substance that has an affinity for a particular organ or organ system.

**organotrophic** \-träf′ik\ Pertaining to the nutrition of an organ or organs of the body.

**organotropic** \-träp′ik\ [ORGAN + *o* + -TROPIC[2]] Having an affinity for or an effect on particular organs or organ systems; characterized by organotropism. Also *organophilic.*

**organotropism** \ôr′gənät′rəpizm\ [ORGANO- + TROPISM] An affinity for particular organs or organ systems, such as that exhibited by certain chemical agents, drugs, and pathogens. Also *organotropy, organophilism.*

**organ-specific** \-spəsif′ik\ Found in or having an action directed to a particular organ, as that of certain antigens or antibodies.

**organum** \ôr′gənəm\ [L (Gk *organon* an instrument, tool, engine, musical instrument, work), an implement, instrument, esp. a musical instrument] (*pl.* organa) Any differentiated part or structure that is adapted for one or more special functions of an organism; organ. Also *organon* (outmoded). **organa genitalia** The reproductive organs of the urogenital apparatus, subdivided into organa genitalia masculina interna, organa genitalia masculina externa, organa genitalia feminina interna, and organa genitalia feminina externa. Also *genital organs.* **organa genitalia feminina externa** The external genital organs of the female, including the pudendum feminum, or vulva, the clitoris, and the urethra feminina. **organa genitalia feminina interna** [NA] The internal genital or reproductive organs and ducts of the female, including ovarium, tuba uterina, uterus, and vagina. **organa genitalia masculina** The organa genitalia masculina externa and organa genitalia masculina interna. Also *male genital organs.* **organa genitalia masculina externa** [NA] The external genital organs of the male, including penis, scrotum and urethra masculina. Also *partes genitales masculinae externae* (outmoded). **organa genitalia masculina interna** [NA] The internal genital or reproductive organs and ducts of the male, including the testis, epididymis, ductus deferens, vesicula seminalis, funiculus spermaticus, prostata, and glandula bulbourethralis. **organa genitalia muliebria** FEMALE REPRODUCTIVE ORGANS. **o. gustus** [NA] A number of microscopic taste buds, or caliculi gustatorii, that comprise the organ of taste. They are located mostly in the tongue epithelium of the vallate papillae or fungiform papillae and in the surface between them, whereas a few are found in the lingual surface of the soft palate and on the epiglottis. Also *taste organ, gustatory organ.* **organa oculi accessoria** [NA] The structures associated with the eyeball in the orbit, namely, the bulbar muscles, orbital fasciae, eyebrows, eyelids, conjunctiva, and lacrimal apparatus. Also *accessory organs of the eye, appendages of the eye.* **o. olfactus** [NA] The organ of smell which comprises the specialized epithelium on the superior nasal concha, the opposing part of the nasal septum, and the roof of the nasal cavity as well as its nervous connections. Also *olfactory organ, organ of smell.* **o. spirale** [NA] The specialized structures in the internal ear subserving the function of hearing and comprising a series of epithelial structures that rest upon the zona arcuata of the basilar membrane in the cochlear duct. In the center are the inner and outer rods of Corti, or pillar cells, separated from each other by the inner tunnel of Corti. On the medial side of the tunnel of Corti is a single row of inner hair cells. On the lateral side of the outer rods are four rows of outer hair cells and supporting cells, namely, the phalangeal cells of Deiters and the cells of Hensen and of Claudius. The free ends of the outer hair cells protrude through the netlike reticular membrane, and the whole complex is covered by the tectorial membrane. The basal ends of the hair cells are in synaptic contact with the fibers of the cochlear nerve. Also *spiral organ, acoustic organ, organ of Corti.* **o. vestibulocochleare** [NA] The anatomical structures outside the central nervous system that serve the functions of hearing and balance and that comprise the external, middle, and internal ear. Also *vestibulocochlear organ.* **o. visus** [NA] The organ that controls vision and conducts visual stimuli to and from the central nervous system. It comprises the optic nerve; the bulbus oculi, including its fibrous, vascular, and internal coats; blood vessels, chambers, and the lens, as well as the organa oculi accessoria. Also *organ of vision, visual organ.* **o. vomeronasale** VOMERONASAL ORGAN.

**orgasm** \ôr′gazm\ [Gk *orgasm(os)* (from *organ* to swell, be lustful or passionate, akin to *orgē* a violent passion, anger) luxuriant fullness, appetite] The peak of genital excitation; sexual climax. **inhibited male o.** EJACULATIO RETARDATA.

**orgasmolepsy** \ôrgas′mōlep′sē\ [ORGASM + *o* + -LEPSY] An attack of epilepsy resulting from a discharge arising in the lobulus paracentralis or, more frequently, in the temporal lobe, producing erotic sensations simulating orgasm.

**orientation** \ôr′ē-entā′shən\ [L *oriens* (gen. *orientis,* pres. part. of *oriri* to rise) rising + -ATION] **1** The conscious mental ability to determine one's position in time and space. **2** In psychiatry, one's philosophy or point of view, as the body of theory to which one subscribes, as *psychoanalytic orientation, behavioristic orientation.* **double o.** The maintenance of two attitudes about the self that would logically appear to be mutually exclusive, such as the bus driver who has worked dutifully for many years even as he is convinced that he is a prime minister. **reality o.** A form of therapy intended to promote awareness of time, space, person, and identity in persons who are confused or disoriented from any cause. It is most often used with severely regressed schizophrenics and patients with organic dementia.

**orifice** \ôr′əfis, är′-\ [L *orificium.* See ORIFICIUM.] Any opening to or from an organ, cavity, tube, or structure, including any foramen, meatus, or ostium. Also *orificium.* **abdominal o. of uterine tube** OSTIUM ABDOMINALE TUBAE UTERINAE. **aortic o.** **1** OSTIUM AORTAE. **2** HIATUS AORTICUS. **buccal o.** RIMA ORIS. **cardiac o.** OSTIUM CARDIACUM. **duodenal o. of stomach** OSTIUM PYLORICUM. **epiploic o.** FORAMEN OMENTALE. **esophagogastric o.** OSTIUM CARDIACUM. **o. of external acoustic meatus** PORUS ACUSTICUS EXTERNUS. **external o. of aqueduct of vestibule** APERTURA EXTERNA AQUEDUCTUS VESTIBULI. **external o. of female urethra** OSTIUM URETHRAE EXTERNUM FEMININAE. **external o. of male urethra** OSTIUM URETHRAE EXTERNUM MASCULINAE. **external o. of uterus** OSTIUM UTERI. **gastroduodenal o.** OSTIUM PYLORICUM. **golf-hole ureteral o.** A ureteral orifice (the ostium ureteris) which has taken on a funnel shape, commonly associated with vesicoureteral reflux. **hymenal o.** OSTIUM VAGINAE. **internal o. of urethra** OSTIUM URETHRAE INTERNUM. **left atrioventricular o.** OSTIUM ATRIOVENTRICULARE SINISTRUM. **o. of maxillary sinus** HIATUS MAXILLARIS. **mitral o.** OSTIUM ATRIOVENTRICULARE SINISTRUM. **pharyngeal o.** OSTIUM PHARYNGEUM TUBAE AUDITIVAE. **pilosebaceous o.** The opening at the skin surface of the pilosebaceous follicle. **pulmonary o.** OSTIUM TRUNCI PULMONALIS. **pyloric o.** OSTIUM PYLORICUM. **right atrioventricular o.** OSTIUM ATRIOVENTRICULARE DEX-

TRUM. **tricuspid o.** OSTIUM ATRIOVENTRICULARE DEXTRUM. **o. of ureter** OSTIUM URETERIS. **uterine o. of uterine tube** OSTIUM UTERINUM TUBAE UTERINAE. **vaginal o.** OSTIUM VAGINAE. **vesicourethral o.** OSTIUM URETHRAE INTERNUM. **o. of Vieussens** 1 ANTERIOR OPENING OF AQUEDUCT OF SYLVIUS. 2 One of the foramina venarum minimarum cordis.

**orificia** \ôr′ifish′ē·ə\ Plural of ORIFICIUM.

**orificium** \ôr′əfish′ē·əm\ [L (from *os*, gen. *oris*, mouth + *-ficium*, noun suffix from *facere* to make), orifice] ORIFICE.

**oriform** Shaped like a mouth.

**origin** [L *origo* (gen. *originis*; from *oriri* to rise, akin to Gk *ornynai* to make to arise, rouse) origin] 1 The more fixed attachment of a muscle from which it exerts its action on the more mobile part on which it is inserted. Under certain circumstances this direction of action may be reversed. 2 The parent stem from which a nerve or vessel arises or branches off. 3 The first site or manifestation in the embryo or fetus of a structure, tissue, or organ.

**Orinase** A proprietary name for tolbutamide.

**ormetoprim** \ôrmet′ōprim\ $C_{14}H_{18}N_4O_2$. 2,4-Diamino-5-(6-methylveratryl)pyrimidine, an antibacterial agent.

**Ormond** [John Kelso *Ormond*, U.S. urologist, born 1886] Ormond's disease. See under IDIOPATHIC RETROPERITONEAL FIBROSIS.

**Orn** Symbol for ornithine.

**ornithine** $NH_2$—$[CH_2]_3$—$CH(NH_2)$—COOH. An amino acid not incorporated into proteins, it is an intermediate in the urea cycle. It is formed together with urea on hydrolysis of arginine by arginase, and it is converted into citrulline by the action of ornithine carbamoyltransferase. It is present in blood. Birds excrete aromatic (benzoic, nicotinic) acids as diacyl ornithines. Symbol: Orn

**ornithine carbamoyltransferase** The enzyme (EC 2.1.3.3) that catalyzes the transfer of the carbamoyl group from carbamoyl phosphate to ornithine in the synthesis of citrulline. This is a step in urea synthesis in the liver.

**ornithine decarboxylase** An enzyme (EC 4.1.1.17) which catalyzes the decarboxylation of ornithine to form putrescine.

**ornithinemia** \ôr′nithinē′mē·ə\ A rare inherited deficiency of ornithine aminotransferase resulting in greatly elevated blood ornithine levels. It is usually accompanied by gyrate atrophy of the choroid and retina. It is not associated with hyperammonemia or any other known disturbances.

***Ornithodoros*** \ôr′nithäd′ôrəs\ [Gk *ornis* (gen. *ornithos*) a bird + *doros* a leather bag] A genus of soft-bodied ticks of the family Argasidae. They are characterized by a subterminal capitulum hidden by the dorsum, a well-developed hypostome, and a patterned integument. About 90 species, placed in seven subgenera, are known, some of which infest mammals and some, birds. Many species are involved in transmission of pathogenic agents, the most important of which are spirochetes that cause relapsing fever. ***O. coriaceus*** A species found in the mountains and coastal areas of California and Mexico; the pajaroello or tlalaja tick. The adults are parasitic on cattle and deer and will also attack humans. Their bite is painful and irritating. ***O. hermsi*** A species found on rodents and an important vector of spirochetes such as *Borrelia hermsii*, a cause of relapsing fever. The geographic distribution includes the western United States and parts of Canada. ***O. moubata*** A group of African ticks originally considered a single species, now recognized as including four species and one subspecies, which transmit agents of relapsing fever. *O. moubata* proper, the tampan tick, is found on a variety of hosts domestic and wild, and is widely distributed in arid regions of Africa. *O. compactus* is a parasite of South African tortoises. *O. apertus*, a large and rare tick, is found in the burrows of porcupines. *O. porcinus*, an ectoparasite of warthogs, carries African swine fever virus. *O. porcinus domesticus* is common in human dwellings in east Africa. Distinct races are described that feed on humans and fowls in different ecotypes. ***O. parkeri*** A species found in the western United States that transmits *Borrelia parkeri*, an agent of relapsing fever. ***O. rudis*** A species important as a vector of *Borrelia venezuelensis*, an agent of relapsing fever in Central and South America. It is thought to form a species complex similar to that of *O. moubata* and to include the form known as *O. venezuelensis*. ***O. savigni*** A species that is a vector of *Borrelia kochii*, an agent of relapsing fever in eastern Africa, the south of Egypt, Ethiopia, and southwestern Asia. In addition, the bite itself can be toxic. Bovines have been reported to die overnight from attacks of the tick, which has proteinlike toxins in the saliva. ***O. talaje*** A species found on wild rodents and domestic animals in Mexico, Central America, and South America. It also attacks humans, causing extreme pain and irritation by its bite, and transmitting *Borrelia mazzottii*, a spirochete that causes relapsing fever. ***O. tholozani*** A species that transmits *Borrelia persica*, an agent of relapsing fever. Records kept for 16 to 30 years of tick-borne spirochetosis in uninhabited areas of Turkmenistan suggest long periods of transovarial transmission. ***O. turicata*** A species found in the western United States and Mexico that transmits *Borrelia turicatae*, an agent of relapsing fever.

***Ornithonyssus*** \ôr′nithōnis′əs\ [New L (from Gk *ornis*, gen. *ornithos*, a bird + *nyssa* a starting post or turning post on a racetrack or *nyssein* to spur, pierce, prick)] A genus of mites in the family Macronyssidae (formerly listed in the family Dermanyssidae). They are morphologically homogeneous and chiefly tropical in distribution. Also *Liponyssus, Lyponyssus*. ***O. bacoti*** The tropical rat mite, a cosmopolitan species particularly closely associated with the roof rat, *Rattus rattus*. Its bite may cause a painful form of dermatitis known as rat-mite dermatitis. It is the intermediate host of the cotton rat filaria *Litomosoides carinii* in a host-vector-filaria system widely used for testing antifilarial drugs. There are no reports of natural transmission of human disease, though experimental transmission of various pathogens has taken place in the laboratory (murine typhus, plague, rickettsialpox). Also *Leiognathus bacoti*. ***O. sylviarum*** The northern fowl mite, found on many species of domestic and wild fowl. It causes itching and annoyance in humans, especially among poultry and egg handlers. It can survive away from an avian host for three to six weeks.

**ornithosis** \ôr′nithō′sis\ PSITTACOSIS.

**oro-**[1] \ôr′ō-, ôr′ə-\ [L *os* (genitive *oris*) mouth] A combining form meaning mouth, oral.

**oro-**[2] \ôr′ō-, ôr′ə\ ORRHO-.

**oroantral** \-an′trəl\ Situated between the inside of the mouth and the interior of the maxillary antrum: applied particularly to fistulas.

**oronasal** \-nā′zəl\ Relating to both the mouth and the nose.

**oropharynx** \-far′ingks\ PARS ORALIS PHARYNGIS.

***Oropsylla*** \-sil′ə\ [Gk *oros* a mountain or L *os* (gen. *oris*) mouth + Gk *psylla* a flea] A genus of fleas that infest rodents. ***O. idahoensis*** A species found on rodents in the western United States that is involved in the transmission of sylvatic plague. ***O. silantiewi*** A species found on *Marmota sibirica*, the Manchuria marmot, or tarabagan, that can transmit plague from animal to animal. Trappers of these valuable fur animals suffered from a plague outbreak in the Transbaikalian region of Siberia, initiating the last major pandemic of plague reported. The pathogens were spread from humans to commensal rat fleas along trade routes, causing the Hong Kong epidemic of 1894, and thence over much of the globe.

**orotate** The salt of orotic acid. It is the biological precursor of orotidylic acid.

**orotate phosphoribosyltransferase** An enzyme (EC 2.4.2.10) which catalyzes the conversion of orotidine-5′-phosphate and pyrophosphate to orotate and 5-phospho-α-D-ribose 1-diphosphate.

**orotic acid** 6-Carboxyuracil. A pyrimidine synthesized in the cell from carbamoyl phosphate and aspartic acid via condensation, dehydration, and oxidation. It reacts with 5-phosphoribosylpyrophosphate to form inorganic pyrophosphate and orotidine 5′-phosphate, whose decarboxylation leads to the pyrimidine nucleotides uridylic acid, UTP, and (after its amination) CTP.

**oroticaciduria** \ôrät′ikas′idoo′rē·ə\ OROTIC ACIDURIA.

**orotidine** $N^1$-Ribosylorotic acid, the nucleoside of orotic acid. Its 5′-phosphate, is an intermediate in pyrimidine biosynthesis.

**orotidylic acid** Orotidine 5′-phosphate. Its decarboxylation to uridylic acid is the final step in pyrmidine biosynthesis. It is made biologically from orotate and 5-phosphoribose 1-diphosphate by transfer of the 5-phosphoribosyl group.

**orphenadrine** $C_{18}H_{23}NO$. *N,N*-Dimethyl-2-(*o*-methyl-α-phenylbenzyl)oxy-ethylamine. An antispasmodic, antitremor agent that has antihistaminic properties. It is used in the treatment of painful musculoskeletal disorders. Also *mephenamine.*

**orphenadrine citrate** $C_{18}H_{23}NO{\cdot}C_6H_8O_7$. The citrate salt form of orphenadrine. It is used as a skeletal muscle relaxant in treating acute spasms of voluntary muscles, regardless of location. Post-traumatic and tension muscle spasms also respond to this drug. It can be given intramuscularly, intravenously, or orally.

**orphenadrine hydrochloride** $C_{18}H_{23}NO{\cdot}HCl$. The hydrochloride salt form of orphenadrine. It serves as a muscle relaxant agent and antispasmodic drug in the treatment of parkinsonism and drug-induced extrapyramidal tract diseases.

**Orr** [Hiram Winnett *Orr,* U.S. orthopedic surgeon, 1877–1956] Orr method, Orr technique. See under TREATMENT.

**orrho-** \ôr′ō-\ [Gk *orrhos* whey, serum] A combining form meaning serum. Also *oro-* .

**Orth** [Johannes J. *Orth,* German pathologist, 1847–1923] Orth stain. See under SOLUTION.

**orth-** \ôrth-\ ORTHO-.

**orthergasia** \ôr′thərgā′zhə\ EUERGASIA.

**orthesis** \ôrthē′sis\ ORTHOSIS.

**orthetic** \ôrthet′ik\ ORTHOTIC.

**orthetics** \ôrthet′iks\ ORTHOTICS.

**orthetist** \ôr′thətist\ ORTHOTIST.

**ortho-** \ôr′thə-, ôr′thō-\ [Gk *orthos* straight, upright] **1** A combining form meaning (1) straight; (2) upright, erect; (3) normal, standard, correct; (4) corrective, straightening. Also *orth-*. **2** A prefix signifying substitution on the atom of a benzene ring adjacent to the reference atom, which is usually one already substituted. This prefix is italicized and joined to what follows by a hyphen. Abbr. *o-* **3** A combining form signifying an ester of the structure R—C(—OR′)$_3$, where R—CO—OR′ would be the normal ester of the same acid R—COOH. **4** A combining form signifying a particular state of hydration of an inorganic oxoacid, e.g. $H_3PO_4$ rather than $HPO_3$.

**orthocardiac** \-kär′dē·ak\ Concerning the effects on the heart from assuming an upright posture.

**orthochromatic** \-krōmat′ik\ NORMOCHROMIC.

**orthochromia** \-krō′mē·ə\ The tinctorial characteristic of a mature erythrocyte, in staining red with Romanowsky dyes and exhibiting no degree of basophilia.

**orthochromic** \-krō′mik\ Having the expected affinity for histochemical reagents.

**orthodactylous** \-dak′tiləs\ Characterized by straight fingers or toes.

**orthodentin** \-den′tin\ Dentin containing tubules within which are extensions of the odontoblasts.

**orthodiagraph** \-dī′əgraf\ [ORTHO- + DIA- + -GRAPH] A radiographic device for recording the size and shape of internal organs without the distortion of ordinary roentgenography. Also *orthodiascope.*

**orthodiagraphy** \-dī·ag′rəfē\ [ORTHO- + DIA- + -GRAPHY] A method by which the exact outlines of an organ, especially the heart, can be measured by using a fluoroscopic image. Also *orthoroentgenography, orthodiascopy, orthoradioscopy, orthoskiagraphy.*

**orthodiascope** \-dī′əskōp\ ORTHODIAGRAPH.

**orthodiascopy** \-dī·as′kəpē\ ORTHODIAGRAPHY.

**orthodontia** \-dän′shə\ [ORTH- + -ODONTIA] The study of irregularities in position of the teeth and of malocclusion, and their treatment.

**orthodontics** \-dän′tiks\ [ORTH- + -ODONT + -ICS] The putting into practice of orthodontia. Also *orthodontology, dental orthopedics, dentofacial orthopedics.* **interceptive o.** Early orthodontic treatment to the primary or mixed dentitions. **preventive o.** The prevention of tooth migration by space maintenance. Also *prophylactic orthodontics.* **surgical o.** Correction of malocclusion by the surgical repositioning of the jaw, or segments of the jaw.

**orthodontist** \-dän′tist\ A dentist who specializes in orthodontics.

**orthodontology** \-däntäl′əjē\ ORTHODONTICS.

**orthodromic** \-dräm′ik\ Concerning movement of impulses in their normal direction.

**orthoglycemic** \-glīsē′mik\ Denoting the state of normal blood sugar concentration.

**orthogonal** \ôrthäg′ənəl\ Situated at right angles; intersecting in perpendicular planes.

**orthograde** \ôr′thəgrād\ Characterized by walking in a direction perpendicular to the long axis of the body; walking upright. Compare PRONOGRADE.

**orthokeratosis** \-ker′ətō′sis\ [ORTHO- + KERATOSIS] Normal keratinization of tissue.

**orthokinetics** \-kinet′iks\ The dynamic use of an orthotic device to facilitate movement of one muscle while inhibiting its antagonist, as a treatment for spasticity.

**orthomelic** \-mē′lik\ Relating to the correction of limb deformities.

**orthometer** \ôrthäm′ətər\ EXOPHTHALMOMETER.

**orthomolecular** \-mōlek′yələr\ Concerning the maintenance of optimal quantities of bodily substances.

**Orthomyxoviridae** \-mik′sōvir′idē\ [ORTHO- + MYXO- + *vir(us)* + -IDAE] A family of RNA-containing enveloped viruses which includes the influenza viruses.

**orthomyxovirus** \-mik′sōvī′rəs\ Any virus of the Orthomyxoviridae family. Also *myxovirus.*

**orthoneutrophil** \-nʸoo′trəfil\ NEUTROPHIL.

**orthopaedic** \-pē′dik\ ORTHOPEDIC.

**orthopaedics** \-pē′diks\ ORTHOPEDICS.

**Orthopantomograph** \-pantäm′əgraf\ [ORTHO- + PAN- + TOMO- + -GRAPH] A proprietary type of x-ray apparatus used in dental radiology to make orbiting panoramic radiographs.

**orthopedic** Of or relating to orthopedics. Also *orthopaedic*.

**orthopedics** \-pē′diks\ [ORTHO- + Gk *pais* (gen. *paidos*) a child + -ICS] A branch of surgery which deals with the preservation and restoration of function in the musculoskeletal system, particularly the joints and bones, including the alleviation of pain in these structures. Also *orthopaedics*. **dental o.** ORTHODONTICS. **dentofacial o.** ORTHODONTICS.

**orthopedist** \-pē′dist\ ORTHOPEDIC SURGEON.

**orthophoria** \-fôr′ē·ə\ [ORTHO- + -PHORIA] Spontaneous accurate alignment of the eyes for a given distance of fixation, without the aid of fusion stimuli. Adj. orthophoric.

**orthophosphate** Any of the anions, or a salt containing one of them, of orthophosphoric acid, $H_3PO_4$, or of its esters: used to distinguish the phosphate from those derived from other phosphoric acids, e.g. from diphosphoric acid, $H_4P_2O_7$.

**orthophosphoric acid** PHOSPHORIC ACID. ● This term is used to distinguish $H_3PO_4$, the commonest form, from its condensed forms, such as diphosphoric acid, $H_4P_2O_7$, or from its dehydrated form, $HPO_3$, which is very unstable and exists only as a reaction intermediate.

**orthoplast** \ôr′thəplast\ [ORTHO- + -PLAST] A plastic that becomes flexible when heated and rigid when cooled. It is used to make splints that conform to the affected part.

**orthopnea** \ôr′thäp·nē′ə\ [ORTHO- + -PNEA] Shortness of breath experienced when lying down. Compare PLATYPNEA.

**orthopneic** \ôr′thäp·nē′ik\ Affected by or relating to orthopnea.

**orthopnoea** *Brit.* ORTHOPNEA.

**orthopoxvirus** \-päks′vī′rəs\ A virus of the *Orthopoxvirus* genus of the Poxviridae. Viruses of this genus infect mammals and most of them cause generalized infection with rash. Variola, vaccinia, cowpox, ectromelia, rabbitpox, and monkeypox viruses are included in the genus. The virions are large, enveloped, and brick-shaped. They contain double-stranded DNA and are 90 percent protein with at least 30 recognized polypeptides, including a numer of enzymes. Suspensions of virus agglutinate erythrocytes. The different viruses of the genus are serologically closely related but fine discrimination between species and strains can be made. Vaccinia virus is the type species.

**orthopraxy** \ôr′thəprak′sē\ [ORTHO- + Gk *prax(is)* a doing, action + -Y] Correction of body and limb deformities by mechanical means. Also *orthopraxis*.

**orthopsychiatry** \-sīkī′ətrē\ The division of psychiatry concerned with mental hygiene, prevention of mental disorder, and early detection of developmental deviations.

**Orthoptera** \ôrthäp′tərə\ [ORTHO- + Gk *ptera* (pl. of *pteron* feather) feathers, wings] A major order of hemimetabolous insects that includes grasshoppers, locusts, katydids, crickets, mantises, and the like.

**orthoptic** \ôrthäp′tik\ Designed to improve ocular motility and binocular function; pertaining to orthoptics.

**orthoptics** \ôrthäp′tiks\ [ORTH- + OPTICS] A method of therapy intended to train the eyes to achieve improved muscle balance and binocular vision.

**orthoptist** \ôrthäp′tist\ [ORTH- + OPT- + -IST] A technician who measures ocular motility and binocular function and provides therapy to improve them.

**orthoradioscopy** \-rā′dē·äs′kəpē\ ORTHODIAGRAPHY.

**orthoroentgenography** \-rent′genäg′rəfē\ ORTHODIAGRAPHY.

**orthoscope** \ôr′thəskōp\ [ORTHO- + -SCOPE] A stereoscope used for evaluation of relative image size of the two eyes.

**orthoscopic** \ôr′thəskäp′ik\ Pertaining to a distortion-free optical system.

**orthoscopy** \ôrthäs′kəpē\ [ORTHO- + -SCOPY] Examination of the eye for visual distortion.

**orthosis** \ôrthō′sis\ [Gk *orthōsis* (from *orthoun* to straighten, guide, from *orthos* straight) guidance, straightening] (*pl.* orthoses) A device or appliance worn on the body to correct or prevent joint deformity, provide support for ambulation, reduce pain, diminish weight-bearing force, or assist motion. Also *orthesis, orthotic*. Adj. orthotic. **balanced forearm o.** An orthosis that facilitates motion of a weakened shoulder or elbow. It supports the forearm and is attached to a wheelchair through a swivel mechanism. **dynamic o.** An orthosis that includes movable components activated by the patient or by external power. Also *lively orthosis*. **inductive o.** An orthosis used to correct postural problems by causing the patient to assume a better posture. **lively o.** DYNAMIC ORTHOSIS.

**orthoskiagraphy** \-skī·ag′rəfē\ ORTHODIAGRAPHY.

**orthostatic** \-stat′ik\ Relating to the erect posture.

**orthostatism** \ôr′thəstat′izm\ The erect position of the torso when standing.

**orthostereoscope** \-ster′ē·əskōp′\ [ORTHO- + STEREOSCOPE] An apparatus for viewing stereograms.

**orthosympathetic** \-sim′pəthet′ik\ Pertaining to the sympathetic or thoracolumbar division of the autonomic nervous system as distinct from the parasympathetic or craniosacral division. *Outmoded*.

**orthothanasia** \-thanā′zhə\ PASSIVE EUTHANASIA.

**orthotherapy** \-ther′əpē\ Treatment aimed at correcting postural abnormalities.

**orthotic** \ôrthät′ik\ **1** Relating to the use of orthoses or other devices for improving or restoring function in the musculoskeletal system. Also *orthetic*. **2** ORTHOSIS.

**orthotics** \ôrthät′iks\ The speciality relating to orthoses and their use. Also *orthetics*.

**orthotist** \ôr′thətist\ A practitioner of orthotics. Also *orthetist*.

**orthotonos** \ôrthät′ənəs\ [ORTHO- + *-tonos* as in *opisthotonos*] A spasmodic or tetanic contraction of axial muscles causing the body to be held rigid in a straight line. Also *orthotonus*.

**orthotopic** \-täp′ik\ **1** Occurring in the normal or usual place; not heterotopic or ectopic. **2** Describing a graft of tissue of a type normally found in the recipient site.

**orthovoltage** \-vōl′tij\ [ORTHO- + VOLTAGE] High voltage, as used for x-ray production, in the range of 200 to 300 kilovolts.

**orthuria** \ôrthoo′rē·ə\ [ORTH- + -URIA] Urination at normal, regular intervals.

**Ortolani** [Marius *Ortolani*, Italian orthopedic surgeon, flourished 20th century] See under SIGN.

**-ory** \-ərē, -ôr′ē\ [L *-orium*, neut. of *-orius*, suffix denoting a place for] A suffix meaning a place or instrument for (performing an action).

**OS** oculus sinister (left eye).

**Os** Symbol for the element, osmium.

**os**[1] \ōs, äs\ [L (gen. *oris*), the mouth, an opening, the face, speech] (*pl.* ora) **1** [NA] The proximal end of the digestive tract, comprising the oral cavity (cavitas oris), teeth, tongue and palate and communicating externally through the space or fissure between the lips and internally with the oropharynx through the isthmus of the fauces. **2** [NA] The lips and the space between them. For defs. 1 and 2 also *mouth*. **3** [NA] OSTIUM. **external o. of uterus** OSTIUM

UTERI. **incompetent cervical o.** An acquired or congenital weakness of the uterine cervix such that a pregnancy cannot be carried beyond the second trimester. **Scanzoni second o.** PATHOLOGIC RETRACTION RING. **o. uteri externum** OSTIUM UTERI.

# OS

**os²** \äs\ [L, gen. *ossis* (akin to Gk *osteon* bone) a bone] (*pl.* ossa) [NA] One of the constituent units of the skeleton, composed of a specialized connective tissue in which lamellae of helically arranged collagen fibers are held together by a ground substance impregnated with inorganic salts, providing hardness and rigidity to the tissue, which yet remains plastic; bone. Bones form the skeletal framework of the body, supporting and protecting vital organs, serving as a store for calcium, and providing attachment to muscles and ligaments involved in locomotion. They consist of an outer compact layer and an inner spongy layer containing marrow and are surrounded by a vascular layer, or periosteum. Bones are classified as long, short, flat, and irregular. **o. acetabuli** Either of two secondary centers of ossification appearing in the triradiate cartilage of the acetabulum of the hip bone at about the twelfth year. Also *cotyloid bone, Krause's bone, acetabular nucleus, acetabular bone.* **o. acromiale** An acromion separated from the spine of the scapula due to failure of fusion, occurring in about five percent of individuals. Also *acromiale os.* **o. acromiale secundarium** A rounded structure seen on x ray above the greater tubercle of the humerus. Also *acromiale os secundarium.* **o. basilare** The basisphenoid and basioccipital bones considered together. **o. breve** [NA] A type of bone the three dimensions of which are approximately equal and that is characterized by compactness, many articular surfaces, and limited mobility, as those of the carpus and tarsus. Also *short bone.* **o. calcis** CALCANEUS. **o. capitatum** [NA] The largest bone of the carpus, situated in the distal row between the trapezoid and hamate bones and presenting a rounded proximal and lateral portion, or head, for articulation with the lunate and scaphoid bones, and a distal cubical portion for the bases of the second, third, and fourth metacarpal bones. Also *capitate, capitate bone.* **ossa carpi** [NA] The eight bones of the carpus, or wrist, arranged in two rows and including os scaphoideum, os lunatum, os triquetrum, os pisiforme, os trapezium, os trapezoideum, os capitatum, and os hamatum. Also *carpal bones.* **o. centrale** [NA] An additional cartilaginous nodule occasionally found in the wrist of a two month old fetus that usually fuses with the cartilaginous scaphoid but may remain separate as a bony nodule on the dorsum of the wrist between the trapezoid, capitate, and scaphoid bones. It occurs normally in many mammals. Also *accessory multangular bone, central carpal bone.* **o. coccygis** [NA] A small triangular bone, the base of which articulates with the apex of the sacrum at the distal end of the vertebral column. It comprises four, and sometimes five, rudimentary vertebrae fused in the adult to form a curved bone, the apex of which is directed distally and anteriorly. It represents the skeleton of the tail in humans. Also *coccyx, coccygeal bone, cuckoo bone.* **o. costale** [NA] One of the 24 curved, narrow bones that are arranged in 12 pairs on either side of the thoracic vertebrae; rib. Each comprises a head, neck, and body, the latter presenting a tubercle at its junction with the neck, an angle posteriorly, and a groove along its inferior margin internally. They extend anteriorly from the thoracic vertebrae to the sternum to form the skeletal thorax. Also *costal bone, costa.* **o. coxae** [NA] A large irregularly-shaped bone articulating posteriorly with the sacrum and anteriorly with its opposite fellow to form the bony walls of the pelvis. It is composed of three bones, the pubis, ilium, and ischium that are fused in the adult at a central constriction, the acetabulum, which articulates with the head of the femur in the hip joint. Also *hip bone, innominate bone* (outmoded), *pelvic bone, innominatum.* **ossa cranii** [NA] The eight bones of the cerebral cranium, comprising an occipital, two parietal, two temporal, a frontal, a sphenoid, and an ethmoid bone. Also *cranial bones, bones of cranium, bones of cerebral cranium, bones of skull.* **o. cuboideum** [NA] An irregular cubical bone on the lateral side of the distal row of the tarsus, articulating with the calcaneus proximally, the fourth and fifth metatarsal bones distally, and the lateral cuneiform and navicular bones medially. Also *cuboid bone, cuboides.* **o. cuneiforme intermedium** [NA] A wedge-shaped bone of the distal row of the tarsus, possessing a square dorsal surface and lying between the medial and the lateral cuneiform bones while it articulates proximally with the navicular bone and distally with the base of the second metatarsal bone. Also *intermediate cuneiform bone, mesocuneiform bone, middle cuneiform bone, second cuneiform bone, mesocuneiform.* **o. cuneiforme laterale** [NA] A wedge-shaped bone in the distal row of the tarsus situated between the intermediate cuneiform and cuboid bones while it articulates proximally with the navicular bone and distally with the base of the third metatarsal bone. Its dorsal surface is rectangular, and the plantar surface forms a narrow edge. Also *lateral cuneiform bone, third cuneiform bone, external cuneiform bone.* **o. cuneiforme mediale** [NA] The medial bone of the distal row of the tarsus, shaped like a large wedge with its base plantarward and its apex dorsal and situated between the navicular bone proximally and the base of the first metatarsal bone distally. Lateral to it is the intermediate cuneiform bone. Also *medial cuneiform bone, first cuneiform bone, internal cuneiform bone, entocuneiform.* **ossa digitorum manus** [NA] The fourteen bones, or phalanges, that constitute the skeleton of the digits of the hand. Each finger has a proximal, middle, and distal phalanx, except the thumb, which only has a proximal and a distal phalanx. Also *phalanges of fingers, phalangeal bones of hand, bones of fingers.* **ossa digitorum pedis** [NA] The fourteen bones, or phalanges, that constitute the skeleton of the digits of the foot. Each toe has a proximal, middle, and distal phalanx, except the great toe, which only has a proximal and a distal phalanx. Also *phalanges of toes, bones of toes, phalangeal bones of foot.* **o. ethmoidale** [NA] A cube-shaped bone situated in the base of the skull anteriorly between the orbital parts of the frontal bone below the ethmoidal notch, which is occupied by the cribriform plate that roofs the ethmoid bone. It takes part in the formation of the medial walls of the orbits, as well as of the roof, lateral walls, and septum of the nasal cavity and the anterior cranial fossa. It comprises the cribriform plate, the perpendicular plate, and two lateral masses, or labyrinths, enclosing air cells. Also *ethmoid bone, cribriform bone, ethmoid.* **ossa faciei** The bones forming the skeleton of the facial part of the skull or visceral cranium and surrounding the orbits (in part), the nose, and the mouth. They include the paired maxilla, zygomatic, lacrimal, palatine, nasal, and inferior nasal concha and the unpaired mandible and vomer, as well as the hyoid bone and the malleus, incus, and stapes of the tympanic cavity. Also *facial bones, bones of* *face.* **ossa fonticulorum** Sutural bones located at the sites of fetal fontanels or fonticuli. **o. frontale** [NA] The large, curved bone that has a vertical portion, or squama, forming the forehead above the skeleton of the face while its horizontal, or orbital, portion extends posteriorly from the inferior or supraorbital margin of the squama on each side to form most of the roof of each orbital cavity. The central part of the inferior margin is the nasal portion that articulates with the nasal bones and forms part of the roof of the nasal cavity. The posterior, or parietal, margin of the squama articulates with the parietal bones and the greater wings of the sphenoid bone, while the posterior margin of the orbital portion articulates with the lesser wings of the sphenoid bone. Between the orbital portions and behind the nasal portion is the ethmoidal notch. Also *frontal bone.* **o. hamatum** [NA] A wedge-shaped carpal bone with a hooklike process, or hamulus, projecting from its palmar surface. It is located at the medial side of the distal row of carpal bones, its triangular proximal aspect lying between the triquetrum medially and the capitate laterally, while the apex articulates with the lunate. The broad distal surface articulates with the bases of the fourth and fifth metacarpal bones. The laterally directed concave surface of the hamulus bounds the carpal tunnel, while the deep branch of the ulnar nerve grooves its base distally. Also *hamate bone, unciform bone, uncinate bone, hamatum, hamate, unciform.* **o. hyoideum** [NA] A U-shaped bone situated in the anterior part of the neck between the base of the tongue and the larynx and suspended from the styloid processes of the temporal bones by the stylohyoid ligaments. Below, it is connected to the thyroid cartilage by the thyrohyoid membrane. It is divided into a body and two pairs of processes, the greater and lesser cornua. Also *hyoid bone, lingual bone, hyoid.* **o. ilii** [NA] The quadrangular upper blade of the hip bone that is divided into an upper curved and flattened wing, or ala, and a body, or corpus, inferiorly, forming the upper two-fifths of the acetabulum. The ala presents three surfaces, namely, gluteal, sacropelvic, and the iliac fossa. It is a separate bone at birth but later fuses with the pubis and the ischium. Also *ilium, iliac bone, flank bone.* **o. incisivum** [NA] A paired and separate bone anterior to the maxilla in most vertebrates, but in humans one secondary center of ossification appears above the incisor tooth germs and becomes overgrown by bone from the rest of the maxilla that fuses anteriorly with the alveolar process so that no separate bone is apparent after the third month of fetal life. Also *incisive bone, premaxilla, premaxillary bone, intermaxillary bone, Goethe's bone, intermaxilla.* **o. interfrontale** An occasional sutural bone located in the lower part of the metopic suture. **o. intermetatarseum** An occasional additional bone occurring on the dorsum of the foot in the angle between the medial cuneiform and the first and second metatarsal bones. **o. interparietale** [NA] The interparietal portion of the occipital squama above the highest nuchal line when it remains separated from the rest of the occipital bone throughout life. Also *interparietal bone, incarial bone, inca bone.* **o. ischii** [NA] The posteroinferior portion of the hip bone, comprising a body, or corpus, and a ramus. It is a separate bone at birth but later fuses with the pubis and the ilium. Also *ischium, ischial bone, chancebone.* **o. japonicum** A zygomatic bone that is divided into two or three parts, a condition stated to occur more commonly (about 7%) among Japanese than other populations. **o. lacrimale** [NA] One of two delicate bones, the smallest in the face, which is quadrilateral in shape and situated at the front end of the medial wall of each orbit. It articulates with the frontal process of the maxilla, the orbital plate of the ethmoid bone, the frontal bone, and the orbital surface of the maxilla. Also *lacrimal bone.* **o. longum** [NA] Any of the elongated bones of the limbs in which the length exceeds the breadth, reflecting the degree of power and speed in movement. It consists of a tubular shaft, or diaphysis, containing a medullary cavity, and two expanded ends, or epiphyses, which develop from separate centers of ossification and are usually articular. Also *long bone.* **o. lunatum** [NA] A crescent-shaped bone in the middle of the proximal row of the carpal bones lying between the scaphoid on the lateral side and the triquetral on its medial side. Its convex proximal surface articulates with the radius and the articular disk of the inferior radioulnar joint, while its concave distal surface articulates with the head of the capitate bone. Also *lunate bone, semilunar bone, lunate.* **ossa membri inferioris** [NA] The skeleton of the lower limb including the pelvic girdle, composed of the hip bones, and the bones of the free inferior limb, namely, os femoris, patella, tibia, fibula, tarsals, metatarsals, and the phalanges of the digits. Also *bones of lower limb.* **ossa membri superioris** [NA] The skeleton of the upper limb, composed of the pectoral girdle, comprising the clavicle and the scapula, and the bones of the free superior limb, namely, humerus, radius, ulna, carpals, metacarpals, and phalanges of digits. Also *bones of upper limb.* **ossa metacarpi I–V** [NA] The five cylindrical miniature long bones forming the skeleton of the palm of the hand, numbered from lateral to medial side, each having a rounded head or caput at the distal extremity, a shaft, or corpus, and an expanded base, or basis, at the proximal extremity. The bases articulate with the carpal bones, while each head articulates with the base of a proximal phalanx. The heads produce the prominent knuckles when the hand is clenched. Also *metacarpal bones.* **ossa metatarsi I–V** [NA] The five cylindrical miniature long bones at the front end of the foot, numbered from medial to lateral side, each having a rounded head, or caput, at the distal extremity, a shaft, or corpus, and an expanded base at the proximal extremity. The heads articulate with the proximal phalanges of their respective digits, while the bases articulate with each other and with the distal row of tarsal bones. Also *metatarsal bones.* **o. nasale** [NA] One of two small oblong bones that lie parallel to each other contiguously between the frontal processes of the maxillae and below the nasal part of the frontal bone to form the bridge of the nose. Inferiorly each is attached to the lateral nasal cartilage. Also *nasal bone.* **o. naviculare** [NA] A flattened, oval bone interposed on the medial side between the proximal and distal rows of tarsal bones, that is, between the head of talus proximally and the cuneiform bones distally. The dorsal surface is convex from side to side, while the plantar surface is concave and ends in the enlarged prolongation or tuberosity of the medial surface. Also *navicular bone, navicular bone of foot.* **o. naviculare pedis retardatum** KÖHLER'S DISEASE. **o. novum** New bone formed from implanted periosteum. **o. occipitale** [NA] A curved, trapezoidal bone forming a large part of the back and base of the cranium and comprising four parts, namely, the squamous part above and behind the foramen magnum, the basilar part in front of the foramen magnum, and a lateral part on each side of the foramen magnum. The external surface is convex and the internal surface is concave. It articulates with the two parietal and the two temporal bones on either side, with the sphenoid bone anteriorly, and by its condyles with the atlas inferiorly. Also *occipital bone.* **o. odontoideum** The dens of the axis that does not fuse with and remains separated from the body of the axis. **o. palatinum** [NA] One of a pair of L-shaped bones that helps to form the back of the hard palate and floor of the nasal cavity with its horizontal plate, the lateral wall of the nasal cavity with its perpendicular plate that lies between the maxilla and the medial plate of pterygoid process, and the back of the floor of the orbit with its orbital process. At the junction of the horizontal and the perpendicular plates is the pyramidal process, while at the top of the perpendicular plate are the orbital and sphenoidal processes with the sphenopalatine notch between them. Also *palatine bone, palate bone.* **o. parietale** [NA] One of two irregularly quadrangular bones forming a large part of the vault and sides of the cranium, each having a convex external surface and a concave internal surface. There are four margins, namely, sagittal, frontal, occipital, and squamosal; and four angles, namely, frontal, sphenoidal, occipital, and mastoid. Also *parietal bone, bregmatic bone.* **o. pisiforme** [NA] A small pea-shaped bone with a flattened dorsal surface with which it articulates with the triquetral bone. Its rough palmar surface provides attachment for the flexor retinaculum and abductor digiti minimi muscles and the tendon of flexor carpi ulnaris and its extensions, the pisohamate and pisometacarpal ligaments of which give it the appearance of being a sesamoid bone. Also *pisiform bone, pisiform.* **o. planum** **1** [NA] A type of bone that is platelike, such as some of the bones of the cranium that comprise an inner and an outer compact layer, or table, between which is a layer of trabecular bone, the diploë. However, in the scapula, sternum, and ribs the two layers of compact bone enclose a thin marrow space. Also *flat bone, tabular bone.* **2** *Outmoded* LAMINA ORBITALIS OSSIS ETHMOIDALIS. **o. pneumaticum** Any bone containing air-filled cavities or sinuses. Also *pneumatic bone.* **o. pubis** [NA] The anteroinferior portion of the hip bone, comprising a body, or corpus, from which the superior ramus extends backward and upward and the inferior ramus extends backward and downward. The medial surface of the body meets that of the opposite side at the symphysis pubis. It is a separate bone at birth but later becomes fused with os ilium and os ischii. Also *pubic bone, pubis.* **o. purum** Bone detached from surrounding connective tissue suitable for bone grafting. **o. sacrum** [NA] A large triangular bone formed by the fusion of the five sacral vertebrae at the base of the vertebral column and lying between the hip bones at the posterosuperior aspect of the pelvic cavity. Its broad base articulates superiorly with the fifth lumbar vertebra, while its apex articulates inferiorly with the coccyx. The auricular surface at the anterosuperior end of the lateral surface articulates with the ilium at the sacroiliac joint. In the erect posture it is directed posteroinferiorly and its convex posterior surface provides attachment for powerful muscles and ligaments, while its concave pelvic surface has four pairs of pelvic sacral foramina that communicate with the sacral canal. Also *sacrum, sacral bone, resurrection bone.* **o. scaphoideum** [NA] The largest bone in the proximal row of the carpal bones, situated on the lateral side with its convex proximal surface articulating with the radius and its convex distal surface articulating with the trapezium and trapezoid bones. The medial surface has a concave facet for the capitate bone as well as a crescentic facet for the lunate bone. The palmar surface has a tubercle for the attachment of the flexor retinaculum and abductor pollicis brevis muscle. The radial collateral ligament of the wrist is attached to its lateral surface. Also *scaphoid bone, navicular bone of hand, scaphoid bone of hand, radial carpal bone, scaphoid.* **ossa sesamoidea** [NA] Ovoid nodules of varying sizes and shapes that are partly or completely ossified and found usually in tendons passing over either articular surfaces or sharply angulated bones. The surface of the nodule in relation to these surfaces is covered by articular cartilage, thereby modifying pressure, diminishing friction and possibly affecting the direction of action of the muscle. These nodules may also occur in the capsule of a joint or in a tendon unrelated to a joint or bony surface. They tend to ossify late, often only postpubertally. Also *sesamoid bones.* **ossa sesamoidea manus** [NA] Sesamoid bones in the hand that are usually limited to tendons passing over the palmar aspects of joints, as in the adductor pollicis and flexor pollicis brevis muscles over the head of the first metacarpal bone, where nodules are also present in the capsule. They may also be encountered in front of the metacarpophalangeal joints of the other fingers. Also *sesamoid bones of hand.* **ossa sesamoidea pedis** [NA] Sesamoid bones that are usually found, analogously to those in the hand, articulating with the plantar aspect of the head of a metatarsal or, less commonly, of a phalanx, such as the pair of nodules in the tendons of the flexor hallucis brevis muscle on the plantar aspect of the metatarsophalangeal joint of the great toe, as well as in the capsules over the other metatarsophalangeal joints and the interphalangeal joint of the great toe. Sesamoid bones may also occur in the tendons of peroneus longus adjacent to the calcaneus and the cuboid bones, of the tibialis anterior muscle over the medial cuneiform bone, and of tibialis posterior over the medial surface of the head of the talus. Also *sesamoid bones of foot.* **o. sphenoidale** [NA] An irregular bone occupying a central position in the base of the skull in front of the temporal bones and the basilar part of the occipital bone and taking part in the formation of the floor of the anterior, middle, and posterior cranial fossae, as well as of the nasal cavity and orbit and of the infratemporal and temporal fossae. It consists of a central portion or body, two greater and two lesser wings, which extend outward from the sides of the body, and two pterygoid processes that hang down from the junctions of the body and the greater wings. Also *sphenoid bone, alar bone, azyges, sphenoid.* **o. styloideum** The prominent styloid process of the third metacarpal bone when it occasionally develops a separate center of ossification and persists as a distinct ossicle not fusing with the base of the metacarpal bone. **ossa suprasternalia** [NA] Ossicles that occasionally develop in the ligaments of the sternoclavicular articulation along the upper margin of the manubrium sterni. Also *suprasternal bones, Breschet's bones, episternal bones, episternal ossicles.* **ossa suturalia** [NA] Irregular, isolated bones or ossicles situated in the course of the sutures of the skull, the lambdoid suture being the most commonly involved, and over the sites of fetal fontanels. They develop from extra centers of ossification, and are often symmetrical on the two sides. Also *ossa suturarum, sutural bones, epactal bones, wormian bones, wormian bones of the sutures.* **ossa tarsi** [NA] The bones of the ankle, or tarsus, that are grouped in a proximal row consisting of talus and calcaneus, and a distal row consisting of the medial, intermediate, and lateral cuneiform bones and the cuboid bone, while interposed between the rows on the medial side is the navicular bone. Their shapes vary greatly, partly dependent on their functions in weight bearing and maintenance of the arches of the foot. Also *tarsal bones.* **o. temporale** [NA] One of a pair of bones located at the side and the base of the cranium and composed of three parts: the anterosuperior thin squamous part (pars squamosa) forming part of the lateral wall of the cranium; the dense pyramidal petrous part (pars petrosa) wedged between the sphenoid and occipital bones at the base of the skull; and the curved quadrilateral platelike tympanic part (pars tympanica) situated below the squamous part and in front of the mastoid process and contributing to the wall of the tympanic cavity and the external acoustic meatus. In addition, the styloid process develops from the back of the hyoid bone in association with the petrous part and fuses with the floor of the tympanic cavity. The three parts are distinct at birth but fuse later to form one bone. Also *temporal bone.* **o. tibiale posterius** A sesamoid bone that may occur in the tendon of the tibialis posterior muscle, where it plays over the medial side of the head of the talus. It usually occurs late in life and may fuse with the tuberosity of the navicular. Also *tibiale externum.* **o. trapezium** [NA] An irregular oblong bone situated laterally in the distal row of the carpal bones and articulating proximally with the scaphoid and distally by a saddle-shaped facet with the base of the first metacarpal. Its medial surface articulates with the trapezoid bone. It is characterized by a tubercle for the attachment of muscles and the flexor retinaculum and by a groove for the flexor carpi radialis tendon on its palmar surface. Also *greater multangular bone, trapezoid bone of Lyser, trapezium.* **o. trapezoideum** [NA] A small triangular bone in the distal row of the carpal bones wedged between the trapezium laterally, the capitate medially, the base of the second metacarpal distally and the scaphoid proximally. Also *lesser multangular bone* (outmoded), *trapezium bone of Lyser, lesser trapezium bone, trapezoid.* **o. triangulare** OS TRIGONUM. **o. tribasilare** A synostotic bone resulting from fusion of the occipital, temporal, and sphenoid bones at the base of the skull in infancy, which may eventuate in shortening of the base. **o. trigonum** [NA] A small accessory bone in the foot that occasionally develops when an additional primary center of ossification forms in the lateral tubercle of the posterior process of the talus and remains separate from the rest of the talus or joined to it by cartilage. Also *triangular bone of tarsus, os triangulare.* **o. triquetrum** [NA] A pyramidal bone on the medial side of the proximal row of the carpal bones, the base of which is directed proximally to articulate with the lunate, while the distal apex is rough for the attachment of the ulnar collateral ligament of the wrist joint. The medial surface moves against the articular disk in full adduction, and the lateral surface articulates with the hamate. On its palmar surface is the characteristic oval facet for articulation with the pisiform bone. Also *triquetral bone, triangular bone, cubital bone, cuneiform bone of carpus, pyramidal bone, ulnar carpal bone, triquetrum.* **o. zygomaticum** [NA] A roughly quadrilateral bone forming the prominence of the cheek and completing the zygomatic arch. Its frontal process articulates with the zygomatic process of the frontal bone, thereby completing part of the margin, floor, and wall of the orbit. Besides an orbital surface, it also presents a convex external, or lateral, and a temporal surface. Also *zygomatic bone, jugal bone, mala, malar bone, zygoma, cheek bone, cheekbone.*

**osazone** A compound formed by reaction of a reducing sugar, aldose or ulose, with phenylhydrazine. In the reaction C-2 of the aldose and C-1 of the ulose are oxidized to give a second carbonyl group, and both carbonyl groups then form hydrazones, so that the product contains the grouping —C(=N—NH—Ph)—CH=N—NH—Ph. Osazones have characteristic crystal forms and were previously much used in identifying particular sugars.

**osch-** \äsk-\ OSCHEO-.

**oschea** \äs′kē·ə\ SCROTUM.

**oscheal** \äs′kē·əl\ Referring to the scrotum.

**oscheitis** \äs′kē·ī′tis\ [Gk *osche(o)-* + -ITIS] Inflammation of the scrotum. Also *oschitis.*

**oscheo-** \äs′kē·ō-\ [Gk *oscheon* scrotum] A combining form denoting the scrotum. Also *osch-.*

**oscheocele** \äs′kē·əsēl′\ [OSCHEO- + -CELE[1]] **1** A tumor affecting the scrotum. **2** SCROTAL HERNIA. **3** OSCHEOMA.

**oscheolith** \äs′kē·əlith′\ [OSCHEO- + -LITH] A calculous mass in the sebaceous glands of the scrotum.

**oscheoma** \äs′kē·ō′mə\ [*osche(o)-* + -OMA] A tumor of the scrotum. Also *oscheocele, oscheoncus.*

**oscheoplasty** \äs′kē·əplas′tē\ [OSCHEO- + -PLASTY] A reconstructive, reparative, or plastic operation of the scrotum.

**oschitis** \äskī′tis\ OSCHEITIS.

**oscillation** \äs′ilā′shən\ [L *oscillatio* (from *oscillatus,* past part. of *oscillare* to swing) a swinging] **1** A regular back and forth movement, as of a pendulum, in a periodic sequence. Also *vibration.* **2** A variance between extremes which might be periodic, as in an electric oscillator. See also CYCLE. **damped o.** An oscillation whose amplitude decreases with time because of dissipation of energy in the system.

**oscillator** \äs′ilā′tər\ An electrical circuit for producing alternating current, especially at audio and radio frequencies.

**oscillograph** \äsil′əgraf\ [L *oscill(are)* (from *oscillum* a swing) to swing + *o* + -GRAPH] A measuring instrument that permanently records voltage variations as a function of time. It usually contains a galvanometer, which deflects a light beam or a direct-writing pen, and moving paper, as in an electrocardiograph.

**oscillometer** \äs′iläm′ətər\ [L *oscill(um)* a swing + *o* + -METER] An instrument for measuring oscillations, especially those recorded from blood-pressure fluctuations during sphygmomanometry.

**oscillometric** \äs′ilōmet′rik\ Relating to oscillometry or to the use of an oscillometer.

**oscillometry** \äs′iläm′ətrē\ [L *oscill(are)* to swing + *o* + -METRY] The measurement of oscillations.

**oscillopsia** \äs′iläp′sē·ə\ [*oscill(ating)* + -OPSIA] A condition in which the visual image is seen to move rapidly from side to side or vertically.

**oscilloscope** \äsil′ōskōp\ [L *oscill(are)* (from *oscillum* a swing) to swing + *o* + -SCOPE] A measuring instrument that transiently displays voltage variations, usually as a function of time. The voltage deflects a cathode-ray beam, which causes illumination of the fluorescent screen.

**oscitate** \äs′itāt\ YAWN.

**oscitation** \äs′itā′shən\ [L *oscitatio* (from *oscitatus,* past part. of *oscitare* to yawn) a yawning] YAWNING.

**osculum** \äs′kyələm\ [L (dim. of *os* mouth) an orifice] A small aperture or pore.

**-ose[1]** \-ōs\ [L *-osus,* a combining form meaning full of, possessing] A suffix meaning having, characterized by, or full of.

**-ose[2]** \-ōs\ [by analogy from *glucose,* the prototype of sugars. See GLUCOSE.] A combining form designating a sugar. If applied directly to a numerical prefix, as in *octose,* it signifies the aldose sugar with the specified number of carbon atoms. The ending is modified to indicate various derivatives; for example, its replacement with *-itol* signifies the sugar alcohol obtained by reduction of the —CHO group in an aldose to —$CH_2$OH, or the —CO— group in a ketose to —CHOH—. Thus D-mannitol can be formed by the reduction of D-mannose or of D-fructose.

**Osgood** [Robert Bayley *Osgood,* U.S. orthopedic surgeon, 1873–1956] Osgood-Schlatter disease. See under DISEASE.

**Osiander** [Johann Friedrich *Osiander,* German obstetrician, flourished early 19th century] See under SIGN.

**-osis** \-ō′sis\ [Gk stem vowel *-ō-* + noun-forming suffix *-sis*] A suffix designating (1) a process or activity, as in *mei-*

*osis, leukocytosis, diagnosis*; (2) a pathologic process or the condition resulting from it, as in *sclerosis, necrosis*; (3) a disease of specified etiology or pathology, as in *trichinosis, tuberculosis*; (4) a disease affecting a specified organ or system, as in *nephrosis, psychosis*. • With a combining form indicating the organ or system affected, *-osis* often implies a noninflammatory process, as contrasted with *-itis*: *nephrosis* (noninflammatory) distinguished from *nephritis* (inflammatory).

**osladin** \äs′lədin\ A steroid saponin occurring in the rhizomes of *Polypodium vulgare* that is a sugar substitute.

**Osler** [Sir William *Osler*, Canadian-born physician active in the United States and England, 1849–1919] **1** Osler nodes, Osler sign. See under NODE. **2** Rendu-Osler-Weber syndrome, Rendu-Osler-Weber disease, Osler's disease, Osler-Weber-Rendu disease. See under HEREDITARY HEMORRHAGIC TELANGIECTASIA. **3** Osler's disease, Osler-Vaquez disease. See under POLYCYTHEMIA VERA.

**osmatic** \äzmat′ik\ OLFACTORY.

**osmesis** \äzmē′sis\ *Seldom used* OLFACTION.

**osmesthesia** \äz′mesthē′zhə\ [*osm(o)-*[2] + -ESTHESIA] The sense of smell.

**osmic acid** $OsO_4$. Osmium tetroxide, which can form salts with alkali. It is used to oxidize alkenes to 1,2-diols in organic chemistry.

**osmicate** \äz′mikāt\ To treat with osmium tetroxide, as in preparation for electron microscopy.

**osmication** \äz′mikā′shən\ The process of treating with osmium tetroxide. Also *osmification*.

**osmidrosis** \äz′midrō′sis\ BROMHIDROSIS.

**osmification** \äz′mifikā′shən\ OSMICATION.

**osmiophilic** \äz′mē·əfil′ik\ Having the property of reducing osmium tetroxide to its black, lower oxide.

**osmium** \äz′mē·əm\ Element number 76, having atomic weight 190.2. Found associated with platinum and other metals, osmium is one of the heaviest elements known (relative density, 22.61). The metal in solid form is not affected by air, but the powdered and sintered metal gives off exceedingly toxic fumes of osmium tetroxide. Symbol: Os

**osmium tetroxide** An expensive, toxic chemical that is used for both its staining and fixative properties in electron microscopy. It is reduced to the black lower oxide by both protein and lipid substances.

**osmo-**[1] \äz′mō-\ [Gk *ōsmos* (from *ōthein* push) impulsion] A combining form denoting osmosis.

**osmo-**[2] \äz′mō-\ [Gk *osmē* odor, smell, scent] A combining form meaning smell, scent.

**osmoceptor** \-sep′tər\ OSMORECEPTOR.

**osmoconformer** \-kənfôr′mər\ A cell having an internal osmotic pressure that varies with the osmotic pressure of its environment. Compare OSMOREGULATOR.

**osmol** Symbol for osmole.

**osmolal** \äzmō′ləl\ [*osmol(e)* + -AL] Having a concentration of one osmole per kilogram of solution.

**osmolality** \äz′mōlal′itē\ [OSMOLAL + -ITY] The concentration of a solution in osmolal units. **calculated serum o.** A figure for serum osmolality derived from the measured levels of solutes which determine osmolality, especially the electrolytes, glucose, urea, and the serum proteins. Different formulas can be used according to the degree of accuracy desired and the number of measurements available.

**osmolar** \äzmō′lər\ Having a concentration of one osmole per liter.

**osmolarity** The concentration of a solution in osmolar units.

**osmole** \äz′mōl\ [*os(mo)-*[1] + MOLE[3]] **1** A mole of particles that exist as separate entitites in solution. Hence one osmole of sodium chloride is half a mole of NaCl, since 0.5 mol of $Na^+$ and 0.5 mol of $Cl^-$ summate to 1 mol of total particles, which is what determines the osmotic pressure of the solution. **2** The amount of ideal solute that has the same effect on osmotic pressure as the actual amount of solute present. Symbol: osmol

**osmology** \äzmäl′əjē\ [OSMO-[1] + -LOGY] *Rare* OSPHRESIOLOGY.

**osmometer** \äzmäm′ətər\ [OSMO-[1] + -METER] **1** An instrument used to determine the osmolal concentration of a solution. **2** An instrument used to determine osmotic pressure.

**osmometry** \äzmäm′ətrē\ [OSMO-[1] + -METRY] A process of measuring molecular weights based on the osmotic pressure derived when molecules diffuse through a semipermeable membrane.

**osmophilic** \-fil′ik\ Having an affinity for osmium, and thus having a black appearance under the light microscope, or being electron dense when examined electronmicroscopically. Osmium tetroxide is used both as a fixative and stain in the preparation of tissues for electron microscopy.

**osmophore** \äz′məfôr\ [OSMO-[2] + -PHORE] The group of atoms in a compound whose arrangement is responsible for its characteristic odor.

**osmoreceptor** \-risep′tər\ **1** A specialized peripheral sense organ or a neuron in the brain whose electrical activity is altered by local changes in fluid ionic concentration. Also *osmoceptor*. **2** *Outmoded* OLFACTORY RECEPTOR.

**osmoregulator** \-reg′yəlā′tər\ A cell that can utilize energy to control the concentration of salts in the intracellular fluid and therefore maintain an osmotic pressure independent of the environment. Compare OSMOCONFORMER.

**osmose** \äz′mōs\ [back-formation from OSMOSIS] To move in consequence of osmotic forces.

**osmosis** \äzmō′sis\ [Gk *ōsm(os)* (from *ōthein* to push) impulsion + -OSIS] The movement of solvent through a membrane from a lower solute concentration to a higher solute concentration. The membrane is impermeable or semipermeable to the solute but permeable to the solvent. **reverse o.** The passage of solvent across a semipermeable membrane from an area of higher solute concentration to an area of lower solute concentration, the reverse of usual osmotic flow. The direction of flow is reversed by application of hydrostatic pressure to the compartment with higher solute concentration.

**osmotaxis** \-tak′sis\ [OSMO-[1] + Gk *taxis* an arranging] Cell movement induced by the density of its fluid environment.

**osmotherapy** \-ther′əpē\ The use of hypertonic solutions by intravenous injection to reduce edema and dehydrate body tissues.

**osmotic** \äzmät′ik\ Of or relating to osmosis.

**osphresiology** \äsfrē′zē·äl′əjē\ [Gk *osphrēsi(s)* a smelling, smell + *o* + -LOGY] The study of the nature and associations of odorants and of the sense of smell. Also *osmology* (rare).

**osphresiometer** \äsfrē′zē·äm′ətər\ *Rare* OLFACTOMETER.

**osphresis** \äsfrē′sis\ *Seldom used* OLFACTION.

**osphretic** \äsfret′ik\ OLFACTORY.

**osphyotomy** \äs′fē·ät′əmē\ [Gk *osphys*, gen. *osphyos*, hip, loin + -TOMY] A surgical incision into the loin.

**ossa** \äs′ə\ Plural of OS[2].

**ossature** \äs′əchər\ [L *ossa*, pl. of *os* bone + *t* + -URE] The bony arrangement of the body or parts thereof.

**ossein** \äs′ē·in\ Bone collagen. Also *ostein*.

**osseo-** \äs′ē·ō-\ [L *osseus* of bone, bony] A combining form meaning bone, osseous.

**osseoaponeurotic** \-ap′ōnʸʊrät′ik\ Relating both to bone and to muscle fascial covering.
**osseocartilaginous** \-kär′tilaj′ənəs\ Relating to or consisting of bone and cartilage. Also *osteocartilaginous.*
**osseofibrous** \-fī′brəs\ Pertaining to or composed of bone and fibrous tissue.
**osseoligamentous** \-lig′əmen′təs\ Relating to ligament and bone.
**osseomucin** \-myoo′sin\ The ground substance of bone that is present between the fibrous and cellular elements.
**osseomucoid** \-myoo′koid\ A mucin that is present within bone. Also *osteomucoid.*
**osseosonometer** \-sōnäm′ətər\ An instrument used to measure the conduction of sound through bone.
**osseosonometry** \-sōnäm′ətrē\ The measurement of sound waves conducted through bone.
**osseous** \äs′ē·əs\ [L *osseus* (from *os,* gen. *ossis,* bone + *-eus* English *-eous*) bony] Consisting of or resembling bone; bony.
**ossicle** \äs′ikl\ [L *ossiculum.* See OSSICULUM.] OSSICULUM. **auditory o.'s** OSSICULA AUDITUS. **Bertin's o.'s** CONCHA SPHENOIDALIS. **episternal o.'s** OSSA SUPRASTERNALIA. **Kerckring's o.** An occasional center of ossification that appears in the posterior margin of the foramen magnum about the sixteenth week of embryonic life and usually unites with the adjacent squamous parts before birth. **pterion o.** EPIPTERIC BONE. **Riolan's o.'s** Small sutural bones occasionally located between the occipital bone and the petrous part of the temporal bone. Also *Riolan's bones.* **sphenoturbinal o.'s** CONCHA SPHENOIDALIS.
**ossicula** \äsik′yələ\ Plural of OSSICULUM.
**ossicular** \äsik′yələr\ Pertaining to an ossicle or ossicles.
**ossiculectomy** \äsik′yəlek′təmē\ [L *ossicul(um)* an ossicle, dim. of *os,* gen. *ossis,* a bone + -ECTOMY] The surgical removal of one or more of the auditory ossicles, usually in the course of mastoidectomy and because of damage by cholesteatoma. It is often followed by attempts at repair, employing one of the various tympanoplasty techniques.
**ossiculoplasty** \äsik′yəlōplas′tē\ [L *ossicul(um)* a little bone, dim. of *os* a bone + *o* + -PLASTY] The surgical reconstruction of the ossicular chain when this is congenitally deficient or has been damaged or destroyed by injury or disease. The operation is usually undertaken in the course of tympanoplasty with the aim of improving the hearing. A number of techniques have been favored, including the use of autograft or allograft bone, cartilage or remodeled ossicle and, more recently, prostheses made from a range of alloplastic materials such as high density polyethylene sponge, aluminum or calcium phosphate, or special glass.
**ossiculum** \äsik′yələm\ [L (dim. of *os,* gen. *ossis,* a bone), a small bone] (*pl.* ossicula) [NA] A small bone or bony nodule, especially one of the small bones in the tympanic cavity. Also *ossicle.* **ossicula auditus** [NA] The three small movable bones in the middle ear, namely, malleus, incus, and stapes, stretching chainlike from the tympanic membrane, to which the handle of the malleus is attached, to the fenestra vestibuli, to the circumference of which the base of the stapes is attached. Because of the synovial joints between the bones, they act collectively like a bent lever, converting the vibrations of the tympanic membrane into thrusts of the stapes against the perilymph, which in turn affects the secondary tympanic membrane occupying the fenestra cochleae. Also *auditory ossicles, ear bones, ossicular chain, phonophores* (outmoded).
**ossidesmosis** \äs′idezmō′sis\ OSTEODESMOSIS.

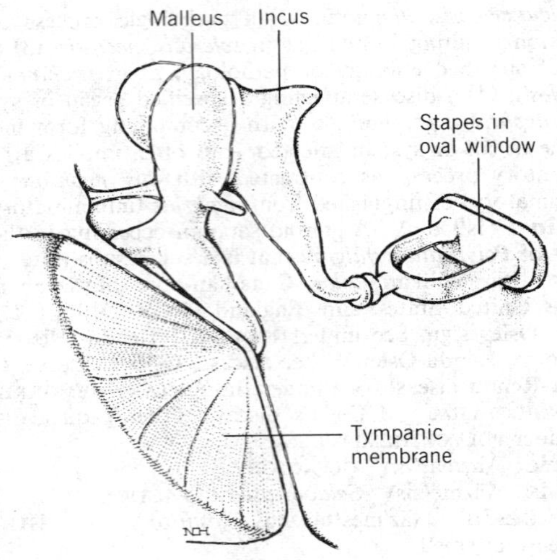


**Auditory ossicles**

**ossiferous** \äsif′ərəs\ Possessing the ability to produce bone.
**ossific** \äsif′ik\ Pertaining to the formation of bone.
**ossification** \äs′əfəkā′shən\ [L *os* (gen. *ossis*) a bone + *-ficatio* -FICATION] The process by which other tissues are converted to bone. **cartilaginous o.** Ossification that takes place in a cartilage model. **endochondral o.** Ossification that occurs at the metaphyseal side of the cartilaginous growth plate. Also *endochondral bone formation.* **heterotopic o.** The formation of bone in a site where bone does not normally occur. **intramembranous o.** The development of bone from connective tissue, as distinct from a cartilage model. Such a process is seen in the skull. **membranous o.** The formation of bony tissue directly within fibrocellular, vascular connective tissue without the development of a cartilage precursor. **metaplastic o.** The formation of bone in pathological tissues such as those of heart valves, blood vessels, and old scars. **perichondral o.** Bone that is formed on the surface of cartilage beneath the perichondrium.
**ossiform** \äs′ifôrm\ Resembling bone. Also *osteoid.*
**ossify** \äs′ifī\ To convert to bony tissue.
**ost-** \äst-\ OSTEO-.
**ostalgia** \ästal′jə\ OSTEALGIA.
**ostarthritis** \äs′tärthrī′tis\ OSTEOARTHRITIS.
**oste-** \äs′tē-\ OSTEO-.
**osteal** \äs′tē·əl\ Bony; osseous.
**ostealgia** \äs′tē·al′jə\ [OSTE- + -ALGIA] Pain arising from bone. Also *ostalgia, osteodynia.* Adj. ostealgic.
**osteanabrosis** \äs′tē·an′əbrō′sis\ OSTEOPOROSIS.
**ostearthritis** \äs′tē·ärthrī′tis\ OSTEOARTHRITIS.
**ostearthrotomy** \äs′tē·ärthrät′əmē\ The excision of an articular surface of bone. Also *osteoarthrotomy.*
**ostectomy** \ästek′təmē\ [OST- + -ECTOMY] Removal of bone around a tooth in the treatment of chronic periodontitis. Also *osteectomy, osteoectomy.*
**osteectopia** \äs′tē·ektō′pē·ə\ The state of having a bone in an abnormal position within the body. Also *osteectopy, osteoectopia.*
**ostein** \äs′tē·in\ OSSEIN.

**osteite** \äs′tē·īt\ An isolated center of ossification.
**osteitic** \äs′tē·it′ik\ 1 Relating to an osteite. 2 Of or relating to osteitis.
**osteitis** \äs′tē·ī′tis\ [OSTE- + -ITIS] An inflammation of bone that is characterized by bone enlargement, with local tenderness and continuous pain. Also *ostitis.* **alveolar o.** Osteomyelitis of a tooth socket, which may occur after a tooth extraction. **apical o.** Osteitis adjacent to the apex of a tooth. **benign necrotizing o. of the external auditory meatus** An uncommon infection of the external auditory meatus characterized by the insidious occurrence of shallow ulceration of the deep meatal floor, where bone becomes exposed. A small sequestrum may separate before healing takes place. The pathogenesis is uncertain, but some cases follow exposure to irradiation. **carious o.** OSTEOMYELITIS. **caseous o.** TUBERCULOUS MYELITIS. **central o.** Osteomyelitis affecting chiefly the medullary cavity. **chronic o.** Chronic inflammation of a bone, most commonly due to infection. **chronic nonsuppurative o.** SCLEROSING OSTEITIS. **o. condensans** CONDENSING OSTEITIS. **o. condensans generalisata** OSTEOPOIKILOSIS. **o. condensans ilii** Pain in the sacroiliac joint that is caused by a thickening of the iliac bone adjacent to the joint. **condensing o.** Chronic osteitis in the alveolar bone manifested by reduction of bone marrow space and increase in radiopacity. Also *osteitis condensans, productive osteitis, chronic sclerosing osteomyelitis.* **cortical o.** PERIOSTITIS. **o. deformans** A bone disease of unknown etiology marked by episodes of bone resorption followed by repair, resulting in excessive bone turnover. The subsequent destruction of the normal bony architecture can cause weakness, which can lead to bowing of the long bones and pathologic fractures. Also *Paget's disease, Paget's disease of bone, pagetoid osteitis.* **fibrocystic o.** OSTEITIS FIBROSA CYSTICA. **o. fibrosa circumscripta** Monostotic fibrous dysplasia. See under FIBROUS DYSPLASIA. **o. fibrosa cystica** A radiographically visible lesion of long bones, marked by large bone cysts filled with fibrous tissue. It is characteristic and virtually pathognomonic of the excessive secretion of parathyroid hormone in primary hyperparathyroidism. Also *osteitis fibrosa osteoplastica, parathyroid osteitis, necrotic osteitis, osteodystrophia fibrosa, osteodystrophia cystica, metaplastic malacia, osteoplastica, fibrocystic osteitis, chronic hemorrhagic osteomyelitis, hemorrhagic osteomyelitis, Recklinghausen's disease of bone, fibrocystic disease of bone, Engel-Recklinghausen disease.* **o. fibrosa disseminata** MULTIFOCAL OSTEITIS FIBROSA. **o. fibrosa osteoplastica** OSTEITIS FIBROSA CYSTICA. **formative o.** *Obs.* SCLEROSING OSTEITIS. **o. fragilitans** *Obs.* OSTEOGENESIS IMPERFECTA. **Garré's o.** NONSUPPURATIVE OSTEOMYELITIS. **gummatous o.** A chronic form of osteitis that is seen in syphilitic infections. **hematogenous o.** Hematogenous osteitis that is seen as a complication of septicemia. It usually occurs in children and is typically located in the metaphyses of the long bones. **multifocal o. fibrosa** The polyostotic form of fibrous dysplasia. Also *osteitis fibrosa disseminata.* **necrotic o.** OSTEITIS FIBROSA CYSTICA. **pagetoid o.** OSTEITIS DEFORMANS. **parathyroid o.** OSTEITIS FIBROSA CYSTICA. **polycystic o.** An inflammatory condition of bone that is characterized by the development of cystic cavities. It is symptomatic of sarcoidosis and hyperparathyroidism. **productive o.** CONDENSING OSTEITIS. **o. pubis** 1 A painful inflammatory condition of the pubic symphysis which may follow genitourinary surgery, urinary tract infection, rheumatoid arthritis, or pregnancy. It is characterized by lytic areas with surrounding bony sclerosis. 2 Sclerosis of bone adjacent in the pubic symphysis which may be seen as an incidental finding on radiographs. **sclerosing o.** 1 Any osteitis that causes a condensation of bony tissue as is seen in osteitis condensans ilii. Also *chronic nonsuppurative osteitis, formative osteitis* (obs.). 2 NONSUPPURATIVE OSTEOMYELITIS. **secondary hyperplastic o.** HYPERTROPHIC PULMONARY OSTEOARTHROPATHY. **typhoid o.** TYPHOID OSTEOMYELITIS. **o. tuberculosa cystica** SARCOIDOSIS. **o. tuberculosa multiplex cystoides** SARCOIDOSIS.
**ostemia** \äste′mē·ə\ OSTEOPOROSIS.
**ostempyesis** \äs′tempī·ē′sis\ Suppurative osteomyelitis.
**osteo-** \äs′tē·ō-, äs′tē·ə-\ [Gk *osteon* a bone] A combining form denoting bone. Also *ost-, oste-.*
**osteoanabrosis** \-an′əbrō′sis\ OSTEOPOROSIS.
**osteoanesthesia** \-an′esthē′zhə\ The insensitivity to pain that is seen in bone.
**osteoaneurysm** \-an′yŭrizm\ An aneurysm within a bone.
**osteoarthrectomy** \-ärthrek′təmē\ Excision of a joint including the adjacent bone.
**osteoarthritis** \-ärthrī′tis\ [OSTEO- + ARTHRITIS] A form of chronic arthritis characterized by cartilage degradation, mildly inflammatory or noninflammatory joint fluid, joint-space narrowing and bone sclerosis, and absence of abnormalities in blood tests of the sedimentation rate or in tests for rheumatoid factor. Osteoarthritis generally occurs in an older age group, or in those whose joints have been previously deformed for any reason. Also *osteoarthrosis, atrophic arthritis, degenerative arthritis, senescent arthritis, arthrosis deformans, degenerative joint disease, ostarthritis, ostearthritis, Heberden's rheumatism.* **o. deformans** Osteoarthritis of a severe degree causing deformity, especially of the knees or back. **endemic o.** Osteoarthritis occurring at a high frequency in a given population. **erosive o.** A subset of osteoarthritis, in which the onset is often inflammatory, and x rays demonstrate erosive changes as well as the typical features of osteoarthritis. **hypertrophic o.** Osteoarthritis marked by osteophyte formation. **ochronotic o.** Secondary osteoarthritis due to and associated with ochronosis. **primary generalized hypertrophic o.** A form of osteoarthritis in which the onset is primarily inflammatory and involves multiple joints within a short period of time. It usually occurs in middle-aged women with a positive family history.
**osteoarthropathy** \-ärthräp′əthē\ [OSTEO- + ARTHROPATHY] Any abnormality involving both bones and joints. **familial o. of fingers** THIEMANN'S DISEASE. **hypertrophic pulmonary o.** A condition caused by chronic lung or heart disease that is marked by arthritis, subperiosteal new bone formation, an often malignant pulmonary lesion, and, occasionally, skin changes. Localized swellings of the terminal phalanges and the long bones of the forearm and leg result from symmetrical osteitis that appears secondarily. The condition may also be associated with nonpulmonary diseases. Also *tuberculous polyarthritis, pneumogenic osteoarthropathy, Marie-Bamberger syndrome, Marie-Bamberger disease, Bamberger-Marie disease, osteopulmonary arthropathy, secondary hyperplastic osteitis, secondary hypertrophic osteoarthropathy.* **idiopathic hypertrophic o.** A condition similar to hypertrophic pulmonary osteoarthropathy but occurring in the absence of a defined primary cause. It is often familial. **pneumogenic o.** HYPERTROPHIC PULMONARY OSTEOARTHROPATHY. **secondary hypertrophic o.** HYPERTROPHIC PULMONARY OSTEOARTHROPATHY. **tabetic o.** TABETIC ARTHROPATHY.

**osteoarthrosis** \-ärthrō′sis\ OSTEOARTHRITIS.

**osteoarthrotomy** \-ärthrät′əmē\ OSTEARTHROTOMY.

**osteoarticular** \-ärtik′yələr\ Pertaining to both bones and joints.

**osteoblast** \äs′tē·əblast′\ [OSTEO- + -BLAST] A cell capable of forming bone and located on the surface of bony trabeculae and within lacunae. Also *osteogenic cell.*

**osteoblastic** \-blas′tik\ [OSTEO- + -BLAST + -IC] Forming bone: used especially of radiographically visible bone sclerosis, as seen in certain types of tumors. Also *osteoplastic.*

**osteoblastoma** \-blastō′mə\ [OSTEO- + BLASTOMA] A benign lesion with a histologic structure similar to that of osteoid osteoma, but characterized by its large size, usually more than 1 cm, and by the usual absence of any surrounding zone of reactive bone formation. Osteoblastomas are less frequent than osteoid osteomas. They usually occur in the vertebrae, ilium, ribs, and the bones of the hand or foot. Also *giant osteoid osteoma.*

**osteocampsia** \-kamp′sē·ə\ The abnormal curvature of a bone. Also *osteocampsis.*

**osteocartilaginous** \-kär′tilaj′ənəs\ OSSEOCARTILAGINOUS.

**osteocele** \äs′tē·əsēl′\ [OSTEO- + -CELE[1]] A bony nodule in a hernia sac.

**osteocementum** \-simen′təm\ CELLULAR CEMENTUM.

**osteochondral** \-kän′drəl\ Of or relating to a bone and its articular cartilage or growth plate.

**osteochondritis** \-kändrī′tis\ [OSTEO- + CHONDR- + -ITIS] An inflammatory process affecting bone and its cartilage simultaneously. **adolescent o.** Osteochondritis dissecans of the medial femoral condyle occurring in adolescents. It is similar to the osteochondrosis of the proximal femoral epiphysis (Perthes disease) seen in children, and is of unknown etiology. **calcaneal o.** 1 ACHILLES BURSITIS. 2 SEVER'S DISEASE. **o. deformans juvenilis** PERTHES DISEASE. **o. deformans juvenilis dorsi** SCHEUERMANN'S KYPHOSIS. **o. dissecans** An osteochondritic process resulting in the separation of pieces of cartilage and the underlying bone into a joint cavity. It most often affects the convex surfaces of the knee, shoulder, or ankle joints. Also *König's disease, osteochondrosis dissecans, osteochondrolysis.* **o. ischiopubica** A radiographic feature sometimes seen in children, that appears to be fragmentation of the junction of the pubis and ischium. **syphilitic o.** WEGNER'S DISEASE. **o. of the tarsal navicular** KÖHLER'S DISEASE.

**osteochondroarthropathy** \-kän′drō·ärthräp′əthē\ A joint disease brought on by the disease of its associated bone and cartilage.

**osteochondrodysplasia** \-kän′drōdisplā′zhə\ A developmental disorder of cartilage and bone. More than 100 heritable disorders have been so labeled, and most are characterized by skeletal deformities and short stature. Also *osteochondrodystrophy, skeletal dysplasia, hereditary bone dysplasia, chondro-osteodystrophy.*

**osteochondrolysis** \-kändräl′isis\ OSTEOCHONDRITIS DISSECANS.

**osteochondroma** \-kändrō′mə\ [OSTEO- + CHONDROMA] A cartilage-capped, bony projection on the external surface of a bone. This is a frequent type of bone lesion. It may be solitary or part of a generalized condition, as in hereditary multiple exostoses. Osteochondromas are commonly located in the metaphyseal regions of long bones, particularly the lower femur, upper tibia, and upper humerus, but may also be found in other bones, such as the scapula or ilium. Solitary lesions may have either a broad or a narrow base, that is, they may be either sessile or pedunculated, while in the multiple lesions the whole metaphysis of a bone may be involved. They occur most frequently in children, and their growth usually ceases at the time of skeletal maturation. They are probably disorders of growth rather than true neoplasms. Malignant change is rare in solitary osteochondromas, but it occurs more frequently in cases of hereditary multiple exostoses. Also *cartilaginous exostosis, ecchondroma, enchondroma petrificum, osteocartilaginous exostosis, osteochondrophyte.*

**osteochondromatosis** \-kän′drōmətō′sis\ The presence of multiple osteochondromas. **Ollier's o.** UNILATERAL CHONDRODYSPLASIA. **synovial o.** SYNOVIAL CHONDROMATOSIS.

**osteochondropathia** \-kän′drōpath′ē·ə\ OSTEOCHONDROPATHY. **o. cretinoidea** LÄWEN-ROTH SYNDROME.

**osteochondropathy** \-kändräp′əthē\ Any disease or injury affecting both bone and articular or growth plate cartilage. Also *osteochondropathia.*

**osteochondrophyte** \-kän′drōfīt\ OSTEOCHONDROMA.

**osteochondrosis** \-kändrō′sis\ [OSTEO- + CHONDROSIS] A disease of growth cartilage in children involving secondary centers of ossification which become necrotic and fragmented. **o. deformans tibiae** An osteochondrotic process of the medial tibial condyle that leads to tibia vara deformity. Also *Blount's disease, nonrachitic bowleg.* **o. dissecans** OSTEOCHONDRITIS DISSECANS.

**osteochondrous** \-kän′drəs\ Consisting of cartilage and bone.

**osteoclasia** \-klā′zhə\ The absorption of bone tissue by osteoclasts.

**osteoclasis** \äs′tē·äk′ləsis\ [OSTEO- + -CLASIS] The controlled surgical fracture of bone, a procedure used to correct bony deformity. Also *diaclasis, osteoclasty.*

**osteoclast** \äs′tē·əklast′\ [OSTEO- + Gk *klastos* broken in pieces, from *klan* to break, break in pieces] 1 A multinuclear giant cell responsible for bone absorption and destruction. Also *osteophage.* 2 An instrument once used to perform osteoclasis.

**osteoclastic** \-klas′tik\ Capable of bone destruction as exhibited by an osteoclast.

**osteoclastoma** \-klastō′mə\ GIANT CELL TUMOR OF BONE.

**osteoclasty** \äs′tē·əklas′tē\ OSTEOCLASIS.

**osteocranium** \-krā′nē·əm\ [OSTEO- + CRANIUM] The fetal skull after its ossification has begun.

**osteocystoma** \-sistō′mə\ BONE CYST.

**osteocyte** \äs′tē·əsīt′\ [OSTEO- + -CYTE] An effete osteoblast that has become embedded in a bone lacuna. It forms a contact with other osteocytes via canaliculi that contain fine cytoplasmic processes. Also *bone corpuscle, osseous cell, bone cell.*

**osteodentin** \-den′tin\ Dentin that resembles bone histologically. It is the normal dentin of some fish, but may occur pathologically in many species, including man. It may be the result of rapid secondary dentin formation with the inclusion of cells.

**osteodermia** \-dur′mē·ə\ [OSTEO- + -DERMIA] OSTEOSIS CUTIS.

**osteodesmosis** \-dezmō′sis\ The formation of bone within a tendon. Also *ossidesmosis.*

**osteodiastasis** \-dī·as′təsis\ The separation of two bones that normally lie adjacent to each other.

**osteodynia** \-din′ē·ə\ OSTEALGIA.

**osteodysplasia** \-displā′zhə\ Any disorder characterized by abnormal bone development.

**osteodysplasty** \-dis′plas′tē\ MELNICK-NEEDLES SYNDROME.

**osteodystrophia** \-distrō′fē·ə\ [OSTEO- + DYSTROPHIA] OSTEODYSTROPHY. **o. cystica** OSTEITIS FIBROSA CYSTICA. **o. fibrosa** OSTEITIS FIBROSA CYSTICA.

**osteodystrophy** \-dis′trəfē\ [OSTEO- + DYSTROPHY] Abnormal bone formation. Also *osteodystrophia*. **Albright's hereditary o.** An inherited disease in which patients evince, at about age 8, the clinical features of pseudohypoparathyroidsm with nonresponse to parathyroid hormone, or of pseudopseudohypoparathyroidism with the skeletal characteristics but not the biochemical abnormalities of pseudohypoparathyroidism. Manifestations are any combination of mental retardation, short stature, round face, ectopic bone formation, and short metacarpals. The basic abnormality may be a defective parathyroid hormone receptor-adenyl cyclase system in bone, kidney and elsewhere. Inheritance is thought to be sex-influenced autosomal dominance or genetic heterogeneity. Also *Albright syndrome, Albright's dystrophy*. **azotemic o.** RENAL OSTEODYSTROPHY. **parathyroid o.** A condition consisting of bone demineralization, paracortical erosions, fractures, and, occasionally, brown tumors, which occurs in states of prolonged and severe parathyroid hormone excess. The most common cause is chronic renal failure. **renal o.** Skeletal pathology secondary to chronic renal failure, including osteomalacia, osteitis fibrosa, osteosclerosis, osteoporosis, or any combination of these. Associated calcification of soft tissue is common. Etiologies include secondary or tertiary hyperparathyroidism, acidosis, and defects in vitamin D metabolism. Renal osteodystrophy may exist for several years before becoming symptomatic. Also *azotemic osteodystrophy, pseudorickets, renal rickets, renal osteosis*.

**osteoectomy** \-ek′təmē\ OSTECTOMY.

**osteoectopia** \-ektō′pē·ə\ OSTEECTOPIA.

**osteoepiphysis** \-epif′isis\ EPIPHYSIS.

**osteofibroma** \-fībrō′mə\ [OSTEO- + FIBROMA] OSSIFYING FIBROMA.

**osteofibromatosis** \-fī′brōmətō′sis\ The presence of multiple ossifying fibromas. **cystic o.** Polyostotic fibrous dysplasia having a cystic appearance due to a thin cortical shell of bone and a cavity filled with fibrous tissue containing trabeculae of immature bone.

**osteofibrosis** \-fībrō′sis\ Fibrosis of the bone, principally entailing the red bone marrow.

**osteofluorosis** \-flôrō′sis\ A metabolic disorder of the bone, manifested as osteosclerosis and osteomalacia, that is caused by excess consumption of fluoride.

**osteogenesis** \-jen′əsis\ [OSTEO- + GENESIS] The process by which bone tissue and the bones of the skeleton are formed, including all stages of bone formation, not just mineralization. Also *ostosis, osteogeny*. Adj. osteogenic, osteogenetic. **endochondral o.** The process of forming bone from cartilage through osteoblastic activity. Also *intracartilaginous bone formation*. **o. imperfecta** Any of the several heritable disorders of connective tissue that are marked by bone fragility. Individual syndromes are distinguishable clinically by the presence or absence of blue sclerae, opalescent teeth, and hearing loss; by mode of inheritance; and by biochemical definition of defects in collagen. One classification scheme includes four major types (osteogenesis imperfecta types I, II, III, and IV), whereas older schemes include the designations *tarda* and *congenita*. Also *osteitis fragilitans* (obs.), *brittle bone syndrome*. **o. imperfecta congenita** The severest form of osteogenesis imperfecta in which intrauterine fractures of long bones are manifested at birth. Also *Vrolik's disease*. **o. imperfecta cystica** A condition characterized by growths of myxomatous fibroid tissue within the marrow spaces. On x rays the growths appear to be cysts. **periosteal o.** The formation of new bony tissue on the surface of a bone by the deeper layer of periosteal tissue.

**osteogeny** \äs′tē·äj′ənē\ OSTEOGENESIS.

**osteohalisteresis** \-həlis′tərē′sis\ OSTEOMALACIA.

**osteohydatidosis** \-hī′dətidō′sis\ A hydatid disease affecting bone.

**osteohypertrophic** \-hī′pərträf′ik\ Pertaining to any condition in which bony overgrowth is a feature.

**osteoid** \äs′tē·oid\ [OSTE- + -OID] **1** The collagenous matrix of bone that precedes mineralization. **2** OSSIFORM.

**osteolith** \äs′tē·əlith′\ [OSTEO- + -LITH] A stonelike osseous fragment found in an ectopic (nonbony) site.

**osteologia** \äs′tē·əlō′jə\ [NA] The nomenclature dealing with bones.

**osteologist** \äs′tē·äl′əjist\ A person professionally involved in the study of bone and bones.

**osteology** \äs′tē·äl′əjē\ The study of bones including the morphological, physical, and chemical properties and functions of bone.

**osteolysis** \äs′tē·äl′isis\ [OSTEO- + LYSIS] The resorption of bone, especially its mineralized component. Also *bone lysis*.

**osteolytic** \-lit′ik\ Of or relating to osteolysis.

**osteoma** \äs′tē·ō′mə\ [OSTE- + -OMA] A benign lesion consisting of well-differentiated mature bone tissue with a predominantly lamellar structure, and showing very slow growth. These lesions are regarded by some as hamartomas rather than true neoplasms. They are almost entirely restricted to the skull and the mandible and sometimes grow into paranasal sinuses as dense, ivorylike, bony masses. **compact o.** An osteoma made of dense bone with little medullary space. Also *osteoma eburneum, osteoma durum, ivory osteosis, ivorylike tumor*. **o. cutis** An osteoma in the dermis. **o. durum** COMPACT OSTEOMA. **o. eburneum** COMPACT OSTEOMA. **ethmoid sinus o.** An osteoma arising from the ethmoid bone, usually from the ethmoidal labyrinth. It is the site of some 25% of osteomas involving the paranasal sinuses. **frontal sinus o.** An osteoma within the frontal sinus. Approximately 70% of paranasal sinus osteomas occur in this location where they are usually discovered on routine radiology. They may reach a large size, making their removal difficult. **giant osteoid o.** OSTEOBLASTOMA. **ivory o.** An osteoma with a dense structure simulating ivory. It is typically found in paranasal sinuses. **maxillary o.** An osteoma arising from the maxilla, a rare site but significant since a proportion of these tumors are cancellous, in contrast with the commoner ivory osteomas of the frontal and ethmoidal bones. **osteoid o.** A benign osteoblastic lesion characterized by its small size, usually less than 1 cm, its clearly demarcated outline, and the usual presence of a surrounding zone of reactive bone formation. Histologically, it consists of cellular, highly vascularized tissue made up of immature bone and osteoid tissue. Osteoid osteomas mostly occur in the shafts of long bones, particularly the tibia and femur. The patient is usually an adolescent or young adult, and males are more frequently affected than females. The lesions are generally painful. They do not appear to enlarge, as judged by clinical observation. See also OSTEOBLASTOMA. **sphenoidal sinus o.** A variety of paranasal sinus osteoma occurring in the sphenoidal sinus. It is extremely rare but important as a sometimes unsuspected cause of headache and because orbital involvement may be an eventual consequence.

**osteomalacia** \-məlā′shə\ [OSTEO- + MALACIA] An impairment of bone mineralization that is characterized by the excess deposition of osteoid tissue. It leads to a gradual softening and deformation of the bones, particularly those that are weight-bearing. Also symptomatic are muscle weakness and poor appetite. It is caused by a vitamin D and/or calcium deficiency or by renal tubular dysfunction. The condition is seen more often in females than in males. Also *osteohalisteresis, tardy rickets, mollities ossium, avitaminosis D, late rickets, adult rickets, malacosteon, rachitis tarda, Miller's disease, halisteresis* (obs.), *acute adolescent osteomalacia, halisteretic atrophy, halosteresis.* **anticonvulsant o.** Osteomalacia developing in patients under treatment with anticonvulsant drugs. **familial hypophosphatemic o.** FAMILIAL HYPOPHOSPHATEMIC BONE DISEASE. **infantile o.** RICKETS. **juvenile o.** RICKETS. **puerperal o.** Osteomalacia that follows repeated pregnancies and periods of lactation, with marked depletion of the calcium phosphate complexes of the skeleton. **renal tubular o.** Osteomalacia that results from a deficiency in the production of ammonia by the renal tubules, with consequent acidosis and hypercalciuria.

**osteomatoid** \äs′tē·ō′mətoid\ Having the appearance of an osteoma.

**osteomatosis** \-mətō′sis\ HEREDITARY MULTIPLE EXOSTOSES.

**osteomere** \äs′tē·əmir′\ One of a series of similarly formed segments of bone, as the vertebrae.

**osteometric** \-met′rik\ Relating to osteometry.

**osteometry** \äs′tē·äm′ətrē\ [OSTEO- + -METRY] The measurements of bones.

**osteomucoid** \-myoo′koid\ OSSEOMUCOID.

**osteomyelitic** \-mī′əlit′ik\ Relating to or characteristic of osteomyelitis.

**osteomyelitis** \-mī·əlī′tis\ [OSTEO- + MYELITIS] An inflammation of bone that is caused by a pathogenic organism, such as staphylococci, and that involves all elements of bone from the periosteum to the marrow. Also *medullitis, bone abscess, ossifluent abscess* (seldom used), *carious osteitis.* **chronic hemorrhagic o.** OSTEITIS FIBROSA CYSTICA. **chronic sclerosing o.** CONDENSING OSTEITIS. **Garré's o.** NONSUPPURATIVE OSTEOMYELITIS. **hemorrhagic o.** OSTEITIS FIBROSA CYSTICA. **nonsuppurative o.** Chronic osteomyelitis that is not accompanied by suppuration but is evidenced by a marked thickening of the cortices of the long bones. Also *sclerosing nonsuppurative osteomyelitis, Garré's osteomyelitis, Garré's disease, sclerosing osteitis, Garré's osteitis.* **tuberculous spinal o.** TUBERCULOUS SPONDYLITIS. **typhoid o.** Osteomyelitis due to *Salmonella typhi* and occurring during the course of or consequent to typhoid fever. Also *typhoid osteitis.*

**osteomyelodysplasia** \-mī′əlōdisplā′zhə\ An inflammatory disease marked by intermittent fever, leukopenia, vascular enlargement of the marrow spaces, and thinning of the overlying cortices.

**osteomyelosclerosis** \-mī′əlōsklerō′sis\ MYELOFIBROSIS.

**osteon** \äs′tē·än\ [OSTE- + -ON] The basic unit of compact bone. It is composed of a central core (the haversian canal) containing blood vessels and nerve endings, surrounded by a variable number (approximately six) of concentric osseous lamellae, which are each 3–7 mm thick. The osteons are arranged longitudinally to follow the axis of the bone and communicate with one another. Also *haversian system, osteone.*

**osteonecrosis** \-nekrō′sis\ Death of the mass of bone.

**osteoneuralgia** \-n$^y$Ural′jə\ Bone pain.

**osteonosus** \äs′tē·än′əsəs\ OSTEOPATHY.

**osteopath** \äs′tē·əpath′\ [OSTEO- + -PATH] A practitioner who specializes in osteopathy.

**osteopathia** \-path′ē·ə\ [OSTEO- + -PATHIA] OSTEOPATHY. **o. condensans** OSTEOPOIKILOSIS. **o. condensans disseminata** OSTEOPOIKILOSIS. **o. condensans generalisata** OSTEOPOIKILOSIS. **o. hyperostotica congenita** MELORHEOSTOSIS. **o. hyperostotica multiplex infantilis** PROGRESSIVE DIAPHYSEAL DYSPLASIA. **o. striata** A developmental, asymptomatic condition in which segmental lines of condensed bone form as a result of the failure of remodeling in the metaphyseal-diaphyseal cancellous areas. Also *Voorhoeve's disease.*

**osteopathic** \-path′ik\ Relating to osteopathy.

**osteopathy** \äs′tē·äp′əthē\ [OSTEO- + -PATHY] **1** Any disease or pathology of bone. Also *osteonosus, osteopathia.* **2** A system or method of medical practice in which accepted diagnostic and therapeutic measures of treatment are used with emphasis placed on the importance of maintaining normal body mechanics and posture and the use of manipulative methods to detect and correct faulty physical structure. This system was postulated by A.T. Still (1828–1917), who stated that the body, when "in correct adjustment" with its own structural relationship, normal nutrition, and favorable environment, has the capacity to make its own remedies against disease and other toxic conditions. Also *osteopathic medicine.* **alimentary o.** HUNGER OSTEOPATHY. **disseminated condensing o.** OSTEOPOIKILOSIS. **hunger o.** Any disease of the bones arising as a result of inadequate nutrition, and frequently found in populations subject to famine. It is characterized by impaired bone calcification usually resulting from inadequate intakes of vitamin D. Also *alimentary osteopathy.* See also RICKETS, OSTEOMALACIA. **scorbutic o.** INFANTILE SCURVY. **starvation o.** Any disease of bones resulting from starvation. Such diseases include rickets and osteomalacia both of which result from vitamin D and/or calcium deprivation.

**osteopedion** \-pē′dē·än\ [OSTEO- + Gk *paidion* a young child, dim. of *pais* a child] LITHOPEDION.

**osteopenia** \-pē′nē·ə\ [OSTEO- + -PENIA] **1** A reduction in bone mass that is caused by decreased osteoid formation in the presence of normal bone resorption. **2** Any decrease in bone density or mass below normal amounts. **hyperthyroid o.** Osteoporosis and high rate of bone turnover associated with thyrotoxicosis. Radiographic evidence of generalized bone demineralization is often best seen in the skull. Osteitis fibrosa and wide osteoid seams are frequently found histologically.

**osteoperiostitis** \-per′i·ästī′tis\ [OSTEO- + PERIOSTITIS] An inflammation of bone and adjacent periosteum. Also *periostosteitis.* **alveolodental o.** PERIODONTITIS.

**osteopetrosis** \-pētrō′sis\ A heterogeneous group of hereditary disorders that share generalized sclerosis and fragility of the skeleton and elevated serum acid phosphatase. In the autosomal dominant form, cranial nerve palsies and "bone-within-bone" radiologic appearance occur, and longevity is usually unimpaired. In one autosomal recessive form, macrocephaly, blindness, and severely impaired hematopoiesis occur in infancy and cause early death. Bone marrow transplantation to provide normal osteoclasts has been successful in treating the condition. A mild recessive form and one with renal tubular acidosis also occur. Also *Albers-Schönberg disease, marble bone disease, osteosclerosis fragilis generalisata, osteosclerosis fragilis.* **o. gallinarum** OSTEOPETROTIC LYMPHOMATOSIS.

**osteophage** \äs′tē·əfāj′\ OSTEOCLAST.

**osteophagia** \-fā′jə\ The osteoclastic erosion of bone.

**osteophlebitis** \-flebī′tis\ An inflammation of osseous veins.

**osteophyte** \äs′tē·əfīt′\ A bony outgrowth, seen most often in osteoarthrosis of a joint, that forms at a location adjacent to the eroded articular cartilage. It can arise either by endochondral or intramembranous ossification.

**osteophytosis** \-fītō′sis\ [OSTEO- + PHYTOSIS] A condition characterized by the formation of osteophytes. **spinal o.** The presence of osteophytes around the intervertebral joints, as is seen in degenerative spondylosis. **subperiosteal o.** A bone outgrowth arising from intramembranous ossification.

**osteoplasia** \-plā′zhə\ Bone formation that results from osteoblastic activity.

**osteoplastic** \-plas′tik\ OSTEOBLASTIC.

**osteoplastica** \-plas′tikə\ OSTEITIS FIBROSA CYSTICA.

**osteoplasty** \äs′tē·əplas′tē\ [OSTEO- + -PLASTY] The reshaping of marginal alveolar bone in periodontal surgery in order to improve the gingival contour, and not necessarily to eliminate pockets.

**osteopoikilosis** \-poi′kilō′sis\ [OSTEO- + *poikil(o)-* + -OSIS] An autosomal dominant condition marked by mottled or spotted bones. It is seen most often in compact bones and the ends of the long bones as multiple sclerotic foci or stippled areas of dense bone. The condition is benign. Also *osteopathia condensans disseminata, osteopathia condensans generalisata, osteopathia condensans, disseminated condensing osteopathy, osteitis condensans generalisata.* Adj. osteopoikilotic.

**osteoporosis** \-pôrō′sis\ [OSTEO- + POROSIS] A reduction in the quantity and quality of bone by the loss of both bone mineral and protein content. It can be primary, as is seen in postmenopausal women or elderly men, or secondary, as a consequence of thyrotoxicosis, hypersteroidism, or prolonged immobilization. Also *bone atrophy, osteoanabrosis, osteanabrosis, ostemia.* Adj. osteoporotic. **o. circumscripta cranii** Circumscribed lytic lesions of the skull that occur in osteitis deformans (Paget's disease of bone). Also *Schüller's disease* (seldom used). **postmenopausal o.** Primary osteoporosis that is seen in postmenopausal women. It most often involves the thoracolumbar spine and causes pain, the crushing of vertebral bodies, and pathologic fractures. **post-traumatic o.** Demineralization of bone that is caused by disuse resulting from injury. The disease may result either from direct damage to the area or from disuse because of severe pain. Also *traumatic osteoporosis, post-traumatic atrophy of bone, Sudeck's disease, Sudeck's atrophy, Leriche's disease, fracture disease, Sudeck-Leriche syndrome.* **o. with renal diabetes** GLUCOPHOSPHATEMIC DIABETES. **traumatic o.** POST-TRAUMATIC OSTEOPOROSIS.

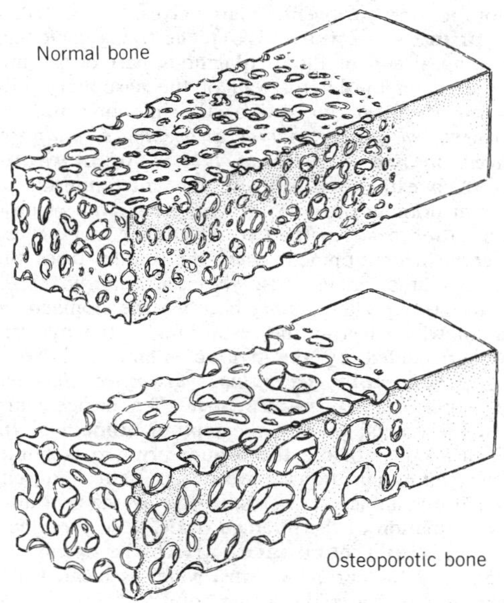


**Osteoporosis**

**osteoradionecrosis** \-rā′dē·ōnekrō′sis\ The destruction of bone tissue following irradiation.

**osteosarcoma** \-särkō′mə\ [OSTEO- + SARCOMA] A highly malignant tumor characterized by the direct formation of bone or osteoid tissue by the tumor cells. Osteosarcoma is the most common of the primary malignant tumors of bone. Most of them occur in patients between the ages of 10 and 20 years, and males are more frequently affected than females. Many of the tumors developing after middle age are associated with Paget's disease. The metaphyses of the long bones, particularly the lower end of the femur, the upper end of the tibia, and the upper end of the humerus, are common sites. The usual osteosarcoma, in contrast to the juxtacortical variety, arises centrally and expands and invades the surrounding tissue as it grows. Also *osteogenic sarcoma.* **juxtacortical o.** A distinct type of osteosarcoma, characterized by an origin on the external surface of a bone and a high degree of structural differentiation. This tumor grows relatively slowly, and has a better prognosis than the ordinary type of osteosarcoma. It usually occurs in young adults, and involves the shafts of long bones, most commonly the lower part of the femur and the upper part of the humerus. It is a circumscribed and sometimes lobulated lesion, adherent to or surrounding the cortex of the bone. The central marrow cavity is involved only at a late stage. It is relatively infrequent compared with the usual type of osteosarcoma. Histologically, the tumor tissue is often mature, merging with the adjacent cortical bone. The cells of the tumor usually show little anaplasia or mitotic activity, except when there is invasion of adjacent tissues. The distinction from myositis ossificans may be difficult, especially when a juxtacortical osteosarcoma is at an early stage of development. Also *parosteal osteosarcoma.* **parosteal o.** JUXTACORTICAL OSTEOSARCOMA. **telangiectatic o.** A highly vascularized osteosarcoma. Also *osteotelangiectasia* (outmoded).

**osteosarcomatous** \-särkō′mətəs\ Pertaining to osteosarcoma.

**osteosclerosis** \-sklerō′sis\ [OSTEO- + SCLEROSIS] Any abnormal thickening of bone that results in increased density on radiography. It may take the form of eburnation or condensing osteitis. Also *centrosclerosis* (obs.). Adj. osteosclerotic. **o. congenita** ACHONDROPLASIA. **o. fragilis** OSTEOPETROSIS. **o. fragilis generalisata** OSTEOPETROSIS. **myelofibrosis o.** See under MYELOFIBROSIS.

**osteoseptum** \-sep′təm\ The bony part of the nasal septum, formed almost entirely by the vomer and the perpendicular plate of the ethmoid. *Seldom used.*

**osteosis** \äs′tē·ō′sis\ [OSTE- + -OSIS] The abnormal deposition of bone salt complexes in connective tissues. Also *ostosis.* **o. cutis** The presence of bony deposits in the skin.

Also *osteodermia*. **ivory o.** COMPACT OSTEOMA. **parathyroid o.** Any of several bone abnormalities due to hyperfunction or hypofunction of the parathyroid gland. **renal o.** RENAL OSTEODYSTROPHY.

**osteosynthesis** \-sin′thəsis\ A closing up and apposing of bony fragments by surgical, mechanical means. Also *synthetism*.

**osteotelangiectasia** \-təlan′jē·ektā′zhə\ *Outmoded* TELANGIECTATIC OSTEOSARCOMA.

**osteothrombophlebitis** \-thräm′bōflebī′tis\ A spreading thrombosis of small veins or venules in a bone that has become infected. It is frequently seen in the mastoid. Also *osteothrombosis*.

**osteotome** \äs′tē·ətōm′\ A surgical instrument that is used to cut bone.

**osteotomy** \äs′tē·ät′əmē\ [OSTEO- + -TOMY] The sectioning, cutting, or perforation of bone. **block o.** An osteotomy performed to remove a segment of bone. **cuneiform o.** An osteotomy in which a wedge of bone is removed. **cup-and-ball o.** An osteotomy in which the end of one bone fragment is rounded and recessed and the end of the other bone fragment is curved to fit into the rounded, recessed end. **dome o.** The surgical division of bone in which the distal fragment is pointed and the proximal fragment is recessed, thus permitting long bone realignment without a reduction in length. **hinge o.** A curved osteotomy combined with bending of the bone. **innominate o.** A division of the innominate bone joint, with its downward displacement. It is usually performed over a dysplastic or shallow hip joint. **intertrochanteric o.** The division of the femur between the lesser and greater trochanter to allow reorientation of the hip joint. It is most commonly performed to relieve osteoarthrosis of the hip joint. **Le Fort I o.** An operation in which the tooth-bearing portion of the maxilla is separated from its bony attachments by cutting transversely with saw or chisel in order to reposition the maxilla. **Le Fort II o.** An operation in which the entire maxilla and the contiguous nasal bones are freed *en bloc* from their bony attachments in order to reposition them. **Le Fort III o.** An operation in which the maxilla, the nasal bones, and both zygomata are freed *en bloc* from their bony attachments for the purpose of repositioning. **linear o.** A straight cut through bone. **Lorenz o.** A V-shaped osteotomy through the neck of the femur to provide weight bearing support around the hip joint. **Macewen's o.** MACEWEN'S OPERATION. **Mitchell's o.** An osteotomy of the first metatarsal to correct metatarsus primus varus. **pelvic o.** An osteotomy performed through the innominate or pubic bones. **segmental alveolar o.** The separation of blocks of alveolar bone and teeth, as a preliminary to repositioning them. **step o.** A surgical division of bone in which a lateral shift of the two fragments obliterates all cortical continuity. **subtrochanteric o.** The correction of a deformity of the upper femur by dividing the femur below the level of the lesser trochanter. **transtrochanteric o.** An osteotomy between the trochanters of the upper femur.

**ostia** \äs′tē·ə\ Plural of OSTIUM.

**ostial** \äs′tē·əl\ Pertaining to an ostium or orifice. Also *ostiary* (obs.).

**ostiary** \äs′tē·er′ē\ *Obs.* OSTIAL.

**ostitis** \ästī′tis\ [OST- + -ITIS] OSTEITIS.

**ostium** \äs′tē·əm\ [L (from *os* the mouth), a door, entrance] (*pl.* ostia) A small orifice or opening, especially into a cavity or a tubular organ or structure. Also *os, mouth.* Adj. ostial. **o. abdominale tubae uterinae** [NA] The narrow lateral opening of the uterine tube situated at the bottom of the expanded infundibulum, the margins of which extend out to form the fingerlike branching fimbriae. The opening communicates with the pelvic peritoneal cavity adjacent to the ovary. Also *abdominal orifice of uterine tube, ovarian opening of uterine tube.* **o. aortae** [NA] The circular opening in the left ventricle that lies immediately in front and to the right of the left atrioventricular orifice, from which it is separated by the anterior cusp of the mitral valve. It is guarded by the aortic valve, which separates it from the ascending aorta. Also *aortic orifice, aortic opening.* **o. appendicis vermiformis** [NA] The orifice between the vermiform appendix and the cecum. Also *opening of vermiform appendix.* **o. atrioventriculare dextrum** [NA] The large rounded orifice situated between the right atrium and the right ventricle of the heart. It is surrounded by a fibrous ring to which is attached the right atrioventricular, or tricuspid, valve which closes the orifice during systole. Also *right atrioventricular orifice, tricuspid orifice.* **o. atrioventriculare sinistrum** [NA] The oval orifice, smaller than the tricuspid orifice, situated between the left atrium and the left ventricle of the heart a little below and to the left of the aortic orifice. It is surrounded by a fibrous ring to which the left atrioventricular, or mitral, valve is attached. Also *left atrioventricular orifice, mitral orifice.* **o. cardiacum** [NA] The opening leading from the esophagus into the cardiac part of the stomach, situated on the left of the median plane behind the seventh costal cartilage. Also *cardiac opening, esophagogastric orifice, cardia, cardiac orifice.* **o. commune** The single atrioventricular canal in the embryo. It may persist in certain cardiac abnormalities such as hemicardia. **o. ileocaecale** [NA] The opening between the terminal part of the ileum and the large intestine at the junction of the cecum and the ascending colon. Also *ileocecal opening, ileocolic opening.* **o. maxillare** HIATUS MAXILLARIS. **persistent o. primum** A persistence of the embryonic interatrial foramen primum that results in an abnormal communication between the cardiac atria through the interatrial septum immediately above and posterior to the atrioventricular valves. **o. pharyngeum tubae auditivae** [NA] The triangular opening of the pharyngeal end of the cartilaginous part of the auditory tube, located on the lateral wall of the nasopharynx behind and below the posterior end of the inferior nasal concha. Also *pharyngeal orifice, pharyngeal opening of auditory tube, pharyngeal opening of eustachian tube.* **o. primum** An orifice which exits transitorily in the anteroinferior part of the septum primum of the embryonic heart and which allows communication between the two developing atria. It is obliterated early in development when the septum fuses with the atrioventricular cushions. Also *foramen primum.* **o. pyloricum** [NA] The opening between the stomach and the duodenum which lies at the distal end of the pyloric canal and is surrounded by the pyloric sphincter. Also *pyloric opening, pyloric orifice, gastroduodenal orifice, duodenal orifice of stomach.* **o. secundum** An orifice which appears in the cranial part of the septum primum of the embryonic heart just before the ostium primum is obliterated. It allows communication between the right and left atria even when overlapped on its right side by the septum secundum on formation of the foramen ovale. Also *foramen secundum.* **o. sinus coronarii** [NA] The opening for the termination of the coronary sinus, which is located in the sinus venarum of the right atrium of the heart between the orifice of the inferior vena cava and the atrioventricular orifice. It is guarded by the valve of the coronary sinus which covers its lower part. Also *opening of coronary sinus.* **o.**

**trunci pulmonalis** [NA] The circular opening between the right ventricle and the origin of the pulmonary trunk, located at the top of the infundibulum of the right ventricle of the heart near the ventricular septum and guarded by the pulmonary valve, which is closed during diastole. Also *opening of pulmonary trunk, pulmonary orifice.* **o. tympanicum tubae auditivae** The opening of the bony part of the auditory tube in the superior part of the anterior wall of the tympanic cavity just below the orifice of the canal for the tensor tympani muscle. Also *tympanic opening of auditory tube.* **o. ureteris** [NA] The ureteral opening into the bladder, situated at each posterolateral angle of the trigone and connected to each other by the interureteric crest. Also *orifice of ureter.* **o. urethrae externum** Either the ostium urethrae externum femininae or the ostium urethrae externum masculinae. Also *urinary meatus, meatus of urethra.* **o. urethrae externum femininae** [NA] The external orifice of the female urethra in the vestibule, located posteroinferior to the glans clitoridis and anterior to the orifice of the vagina. Usually it has raised margins and it is very distensible. Also *external orifice of female urethra.* **o. urethrae externum masculinae** [NA] A vertical slitlike opening at the tip of the glans penis that is the narrowest part of the urethra. It is bounded on each side by a small elevated lip. Also *external orifice of male urethra.* **o. urethrae internum** [NA] The crescentic internal orifice of the urethra, situated at the apex of the trigone of the bladder. Also *internal orifice of urethra, internal urethral opening, vesicourethral orifice, vesicourethral opening.* **o. uteri** [NA] The opening in the center of the vaginal part of the cervix uteri through which the cavity of the uterus communicates with that of the vagina. It is placed transversely, with thick anterior and posterior lips. Also *external orifice of uterus, external os of uterus, os uteri externum.* **o. uterinum tubae uterinae** [NA] The small opening of the uterine tube in the anterolateral part of the uterine cavity. Also *uterine orifice of uterine tube, uterine opening of uterine tube.* **o. vaginae** [NA] The external orifice of the vagina, partly or totally closed in the virgin by the hymen and located in the midline below and behind the external orifice of the urethra in the vestibule. Also *hymenal orifice, vaginal orifice.* **o. venae cavae inferioris** [NA] The orifice of the inferior vena cava in the lowest part of the right atrium of the heart near the interatrial septum. It is partly protected by a valve. Also *opening of inferior vena cava.* **o. venae cavae superioris** [NA] The orifice of the superior vena cava in the posterosuperior part of the right atrium of the heart. It has no valve. **ostia venarum pulmonalium** [NA] The openings of the pulmonary veins in the upper part of the posterior surface of the left atrium of the heart, two on each side of the midline and devoid of valves. The two on the left often open into a single orifice.

**ostomy** \äs′təmē\ [back-formation from *colostomy, ileostomy,* etc. See -STOMY.] **1** The surgical creation of an artificial opening through which a body fluid may flow. **2** The opening surgically created for the purpose of fluid passage.

**ostosis** \ästō′sis\ [OST- + -OSIS] **1** OSTEOGENESIS. **2** OSTEOSIS.

**ostraceous** \ästrā′shəs\ Shaped like or resembling the appearance of an oyster shell.

**ostreotoxism** \äs′trē-ōtäk′sizm\ [Gk *ostreo(n)* oyster + TOX- + -ISM] Poisoning from ingestion of contaminated oysters.

**Ostrum** [Herman William *Ostrum,* Russian-born U.S. roentgenologist, born 1893] Ostrum-Furst syndrome. See under KLIPPEL-FEIL SYNDROME.

**Ostwald** [Wilhelm *Ostwald,* German chemist, 1853–1932] See under COEFFICIENT.

**OT** **1** old tuberculin. **2** original tuberculin (new tuberculin). **3** occupational therapy.

**ot-** \ät-, ət-\ OTO-.

**Ota** [Masao T. *Ota,* Japanese dermatopathologist, 1885–1945] See under NEVUS.

**otalgia** \ōtal′jə\ [OT- + -ALGIA] Pain in the ear. Also *otodynia* (seldom used). Adj. otalgic. ● In some parts of the world, the term is taken to mean only neuralgic pain, either trigeminal or referred. **geniculate o.** Pain in the ear as a feature of the Ramsay Hunt syndrome. **referred o.** Pain referred to the ear from some site of disease elsewhere but within the areas innervated by the fifth, ninth, and tenth cranial nerves and the second and third cervical nerves. Also *reflex otalgia, secondary otalgia.* **tabetic o.** Otalgia in tabes dorsalis due to involvement of the nervus intermedius root of the facial nerve.

**otalgic** \ōtal′jik\ **1** Referring to or resembling otalgia. **2** An earache remedy.

**OTC** over the counter (designating drugs that may be purchased from stores without a prescription from a physician).

**otic** \ō′tik\ [Gk *ōtikos* (from *ous,* gen. *ōtos* ear) of or for the ear] Relating to the ear.

**-otic[1]** \-ät′ik\ [adjectival suffix formed from noun suffix -OSIS] A suffix meaning (1) of the nature of a state, condition, or process; (2) of or characterized by a diseased or abnormal condition; (3) marked by formation, production, or increase.

**-otic[2]** \-ō′tik\ [See OTIC.] A combining form meaning of or relating to the ear.

**oticodinia** \ō′tikōdin′ē·ə\ [OTIC + *o* + Gk *din(os)* whirling, vertigo + -IA] *Obs.* AURAL VERTIGO.

**otitis** \ōtī′tis\ [OT- + -ITIS] Inflammation of the ear. Adj. otitic. **adhesive o. media** A condition of the middle ear in which fibrous adhesions have formed as the result of past inflammation. Also *adhesive otitis* (popular). ● The term is inaccurate because the inflammation is no longer active. **aviation o.** AEROTITIS. **barotraumatic o.** OTITIC BAROTRAUMA. **barotraumatic o. media** Otitic barotrauma as it affects the middle ear. Also *barotitis media.* **catarrhal o.** SECRETORY OTITIS MEDIA. **catarrhal o. media** *Older term* SECRETORY OTITIS MEDIA. **o. externa** Inflammation of the external ear. The auricle or the external auditory meatus or both may be involved. **o. externa hemorrhagica** A painful variety of otitis externa in which bullae or blisters, containing blood-stained fluid, appear in the external auditory meatus, on the surface of the tympanic membrane, or in both localities. It is thought to be due to virus infection, particularly influenza. Also *influenzal otitis.* **o. externa mycotica** MYCOTIC OTITIS EXTERNA. **exudative o.** SECRETORY OTITIS MEDIA. **exudative o. media** SECRETORY OTITIS MEDIA. **furuncular o. externa** Circumscribed inflammation of the external ear characterized by the presence of a furuncle or furuncles. **influenzal o.** OTITIS EXTERNA HEMORRHAGICA. **o. interna** *Rare* LABYRINTHITIS. **malignant o. externa** A grave, frequently fatal variety of external otitis occurring in elderly diabetics and due to infection with *Pseudomonas aeruginosa.* Commencing with pain and purulent otorrhea, the condition spreads rapidly to involve cartilage and bone and even cranial nerves, particularly the facial nerve. Treatment includes the intravenous use of the appropriate antibiotic and sometimes radical surgery. Also *necrotizing otitis externa.* **o. media** Inflammation of the middle ear. **o. media with effusion** SECRETORY OTITIS MEDIA. **o. media sclerotica** *Older term* TYMPANOSCLEROSIS. **o. mycotica** *Older term* OTOMYCOSIS. **mycotic o. externa** Otomycosis confined to the skin of the external ear, a common variety of external otitis in tropical climates and increasingly seen in temperate climates since the introduction of topical antibiotic treatment for external otitis. *Aspergillus niger* and *Candida albicans* are most frequently responsible. Also *otitis externa mycotica.* **necrotizing o.** NECROTIZING OTITIS MEDIA. **necrotizing o. externa** MALIGNANT OTITIS EXTERNA. **necrotizing o. media** A variety of severe otitis media in which the whole or a major part of the pars tensa of the tympanic membrane is destroyed. It was once common as a complication of the exanthematous fevers of childhood and still occurs where these diseases coincide with malnutrition. Also *necrotizing otitis.* **parasitic o.** Inflammation of the ear caused by a parasite. Such disease is almost unknown in man although infestation of the external ear of certain animals with mites (otoacariasis) is not rare. • In older texts, the fungus diseases of the ear will be found included as examples of parasitic otitis. **pneumococcal o. media** Otitis media caused by the pneumococcus (*Streptococcus pneumoniae*) recognized, prior to the advent of antibiotics, as a deceptively silent disease in which middle ear suppuration would sometimes exist in the presence of an intact and relatively normal tympanic membrane, or abscess formation would occur in the mastoid process in the course of acute otitis media after discharge had dried up and the tympanic membrane healed. **secretory o. media** Nonsuppurative otitis media in which seromucous secretions collect in the middle ear probably as the result of malfunction of the eustachian tube. Most of the cases occur in children, in whom it is a common disease. It is widely treated by the insertion of ventilation tubes to correct negative pressure in the middle ear. Also *secretory otitis, serous otitis, exudative otitis, seromucous otitis, catarrhal otitis, serous otitis media, exudative otitis media, seromucous otitis media, catarrhal otitis media* (older term), *tympanic hydrops, hydrotympanum, middle-ear effusion, glue ear* (popular), *otitis media with effusion.* **traumatic o.** Otitis following an injury to the ear. This includes both traumatic external otitis and traumatic otitis media but is usually taken to mean traumatic otitis media. **tuberculous o. media** Otitis media due to infection with species of *Mycobacterium,* especially *M. tuberculosis.* In almost every case, it presents secondary to pulmonary tuberculosis. Also *tuberculous otitis.*

**oto-** \ō′tō-\ [Gk *ous,* gen. *ōtos* ear] A combining form denoting the ear. Also *ot-.*

**otocephaly** \-sef′əlē\ [OTO- + CEPHAL- + -Y ] A developmental defect characterized by extreme underdevelopment of the lower jaw (agnathia), permitting close approximation or union of the ears on the anterior aspect of the neck (synotia).

**otoconia** \-kō′nē·ə\ STATOCONIA.

**otoconites** \-kōnī′tis\ STATOCONIA.

**otoconium** \-kō′nē·əm\ Singular of OTOCONIA.

**otocrane** \ō′təkrān\ OTOCRANIUM.

**otocranial** \-krā′nē·əl\ Pertaining to the otocranium.

**otocranium** \-krā′nē·əm\ **1** The portion of the petrous part of the temporal bone that houses the internal ear. **2** The petrous part and the mastoid process of the temporal bone, containing the hearing apparatus. Also *petromastoid, otocrane.*

**otocyst** \ō′təsist\ The precursor of the membranous labyrinth of the internal ear. It is formed when the otic placode invaginates and closes off. It then becomes surrounded by mesoderm which forms the otic capsule. Also *otic vesicle, acoustic vesicle, auditory vesicle.*

**otodynia** \-din′ē·ə\ *Seldom used* OTALGIA.

**otoencephalitis** \-ensef′əlī′tis\ Encephalitis due to otitis media.

**otoganglion** \-gang′glē·än\ *Seldom used* GANGLION OTICUM.

**otogenous** \ōtäj′ənəs\ Originating in the ear; in particular, caused by ear disease. Also *otogenic.*

**otolaryngologist** \-lar′ing·gäl′əjist\ OTORHINOLARYNGOLOGIST.

**otolaryngology** \-lar′ing·gäl′əjē\ OTORHINOLARYNGOLOGY.

**otolites** \ō′təlīts\ STATOCONIA.

**otolith** \ō′təlith\ See under STATOCONIA.

**otologist** \ōtäl′əjist\ A specialist in otology, usually a medical practitioner trained in otorhinolaryngology with a special interest in otology. Also *aurist* (older term).

**otology** \ōtäl′əjē\ [OTO- + -LOGY] The study of the ears, in particular their diseases and disorders and their treatment. Otology is a branch of otorhinolaryngology.

***Otomyces*** \ō′təmī′sēz\ [OTO- + Gk *mykēs* mushroom, fungus] An invalid genus of fungi implicated in outer ear infections. It is currently included in the genus *Aspergillus.*

**otomycosis** \-mīkō′sis\ Infection of the ear, usually the external ear, with a fungus though not necessarily a pathogenic fungus. Frequently the fungus is a saprophyte growing on the dead wax-keratin shed into the external auditory meatus. Also *otitis mycotica* (older term).

**otomyiasis** \-mī·ī′əsis\ [OTO- + MYIASIS] Infestation of the ear by the larvae of any myiasis-producing fly.

**otopathy** \ōtäp′əthē\ [OTO- + -PATHY] Any disease of the ear. *Rare.*

**otophone** \ō′təfōn\ *Obs.* AUSCULTATION TUBE.

**otoplasty** \ō′təplas′tē\ [OTO- + -PLASTY] Any plastic operation on the ear.

**otorhinolaryngologist** \-rī′nōlar′ing·gäl′əjist\ A practitioner of otorhinolaryngology. Also *otolaryngologist.*

**otorhinolaryngology** \-rī′nōlar′ing·gäl′əjē\ [OTO- + RHINO- + LARYNGO- + -LOGY] The study of the ears, nose, and throat, in particular the diseases and disorders of these parts and their treatment. Also *ENT, otolaryngology.*

**otorrhea** \ō′tôrē′ə\ [OTO- + -RRHEA] Discharge from the ear. **cerebrospinal fluid o.** Drainage of cerebrospinal fluid from the ear, usually evidence of fracture of the petrous bone with laceration of the dura-archnoid and perforation of the tympanic membrane, but also, rarely, of injury to the dura-arachnoid in the course of surgery on the ear.

**otosclerosis** \-sklerō′sis\ [OTO- + SCLEROSIS] A disease of the bone surrounding the inner ear, leading in approximately 15% of affected cases to impaired hearing, usually of the conductive kind. The hereditary pattern, probably autosomal dominant, is obscured by the high incidence of symptomless cases. The usual lesion, responsible for the characteristic slow deterioration of hearing, is ankylosis of the stapes. It is common among Caucasian peoples but rare among the Negro races. Surgery on the stapes has been used to improve the hearing of an increasing proportion of patients. Also *otospongiosis.* **clinical o.** Otosclerosis when it causes hearing impairment, either as the result of ankylosis of the stapes or, less commonly, cochlear involvement. **cochlear o.** Otosclerosis producing sensorineural deafness as a result of involvement of the endosteal bone adjacent to the spiral ligament and, eventually, degenerative changes in the cochlear hair cells. **obliterative o.** Otosclerosis at an advanced stage with otosclerotic bone obliterating the oval window and involving the crura, so that the margins of the footplate are no longer discernible. It is associated with a relatively severe degree of hearing loss.

**otoscope** \ō′təskōp′\ [OTO- + -SCOPE] An instrument for examining parts of the external and middle ear by way of the external auditory meatus. Also *auriscope*. See also AUSCULTATION TUBE. **Siegle's o.** An otoscope for observing the effect on the tympanic membrane of air-pressure changes induced in the external ear. It consists of an ear speculum closed at the broad end by a lens and connected to a rubber bulb for producing the pressure changes. Also *Siegle's pneumatic ear speculum*. **Toynbee's o.** AUSCULTATION TUBE.

**otoscopy** \ōtäs′kəpē\ [OTO- + -SCOPY] Examination of the ear by means of an otoscope.

**otospongiosis** \-spän′jē·ō′sis\ OTOSCLEROSIS.

**otosteons** \ōtäs′tē·äns\ STATOCONIA.

**ototoxic** \-täk′sik\ [OTO- + TOXIC] Poisonous to the ear: applied particularly to drugs liable to be so.

**ototoxicity** \-täksis′itē\ The quality of being ototoxic.

**Otto** [Adolph Wilhelm *Otto*, German surgeon, 1786–1845] Otto's disease, Otto pelvis. See under PROTRUSIO ACETABULI.

**OU** 1 oculi unitas (both eyes together). 2 oculus uterque (each eye).

**ouabain** \wäbā′in\ [French *ouaba(ïo)*, from Somali *wabayo*, a name of a tree of the genus *Acocanthera* + -IN] $C_{29}H_{44}O_{12}$. 3-[(6-Deoxy-α-L-mannopyranosyl)oxy]-1,5,11α,-14,19-pentahydroxycard-20(22)-enolide, a cardiac glycoside obtained from the seeds of *Strophanthus gratus* or the wood or root of *Acocanthera schimperi*. It is a crystalline solid, soluble in water and alcohol and slightly soluble in ether The pharmacological action of ouabain is similar to that of digitalis but it acts more rapidly and has shorter duration. It is used in the treatment of congestive heart failure. Also *acocantherin, acokantherin, ouabaio*.

**Ouchterlony** [Orjan Thomas Gunnarsson *Ouchterlony*, Swedish bacteriologist, born 1914] 1 See under LINE. 2 Ouchterlony test. See under TECHNIQUE.

**Oudin** [Paul *Oudin*, French physician, 1851–1923] See under CURRENT.

**oula** \oo′lə\ [Gk, the gum] *Outmoded* GINGIVA.

**ounce** [L *unica* the twelfth part of any whole, an ounce, inch] 1 A unit of mass or weight equal to 0.0625 pound avoirdupois and 0.0833 pound troy. See under OUNCE AVOIRDUPOIS, OUNCE TROY. • When *ounce* is used without qualification it is usually taken to mean *ounce avoirdupois*. 2 See under FLUID OUNCE. **apothecaries' o.** A unit of mass or weight, used especially in pharmacy, equal to 480 grains 31.1035 grams. Also *ounce apothecary*. Symbol: oz ap (in the United States), oz apoth (in Great Britain) **o. apothecary** APOTHECARIES' OUNCE. **o. avoirdupois** An avoirdupois unit of mass or weight equal to $^{1}/_{16}$ or 0.0625 pound; 437.5 grains; 28.3495 grams. Symbol: oz **fluid o.** 1 In the United States, a unit of capacity equal to $^{1}/_{128}$ (US) gallon, $^{1}/_{16}$ (US) pint or 29.5735 milliliters. Also *liquid ounce*. Symbol: fl oz 2 In Great Britain, a unit of capacity equal to $^{1}/_{160}$ (UK) gallon, $^{1}/_{20}$ (UK) pint, or 28.4131 milliliters. Symbol: fl oz **imperial o.** A unit of mass or weight equal to $^{1}/_{16}$ imperial pound; 28.3495 grams, approximately. **liquid o.** FLUID OUNCE. Symbol: liq oz **o. troy** A troy unit of mass or weight equal to $^{1}/_{12}$ or 0.0833 pound troy; 480 grains; 31.103 grams. Symbol: oz t (in the United States), oz tr (in Great Britain)

**-ous** \-əs\ [L *-os(us)*, adj. suffix meaning full of, rich in] 1 A suffix meaning possessing or characterized by. 2 In chemistry, a suffix applied to the names of elements to indicate that they are in their lower oxidation state. Compare -IC.

**outbreak** The sudden appearance or increased incidence of a disease in a community. An outbreak may or may not spread more broadly to become an epidemic. • The term is usually restricted to infectious diseases but may apply to disease or injury due to other causes such as drug abuse or industrial or other toxins.

**outbreeding** 1 The mating of individuals who are less closely related than the average mating pair from the population. Compare INBREEDING. 2 In experimental genetics or animal or plant breeding, the purposeful mating of individuals who share as few alleles as possible, or who are different at selected loci, for the purpose of improving fitness or growth in the offspring through genetic diversity.

**outcross** 1 The product of outbreeding. 2 To engage in outbreeding.

**outflow** / **craniosacral o.** Preganglionic parasympathetic fibers in the oculomotor (III), facial (VII), glossopharyngeal (IX) and vagus (X) cranial nerves and in the second, third, and fourth sacral spinal nerves. **thoracolumbar o.** SYSTEMA NERVOSUM AUTONOMICUM, PARS SYMPATHICA.

**outfracture** \-frak′chər\ The surgical repositioning of a medially displaced nasal bone.

**outgrowth** / **spore o.** The final stage in germination, in which the vegetative genes of the spore are selectively activated, their products convert the spore into a vegetative cell, and the disrupted spore integument is discarded.

**outlay** ONLAY GRAFT.

**outlet** In anatomy, an opening that permits escape or outward movement of some of the contents of a walled area or space, such as the pelvis and thorax. **pelvic o.** APERTURA PELVIS INFERIOR. **thoracic o.** APERTURA THORACIS INFERIOR.

**outlier** \out′lī′ər\ [*out* + *li(e)* + -ER ] An observation so far removed from the others in a set of observations as to suggest that it belongs to a different population or is the result of faulty technique of sampling or measurement.

**outlimb** The distal part of a limb.

**outpatient** \out′pā′shənt\ A patient receiving care from a health care institution but not admitted for a stay in a facility of that institution. Compare INPATIENT.

**outpocket** The protuberance of a tissue or organ as a result of evagination.

**outpocketing** EVAGINATION.

**outpouching** EVAGINATION.

**output** 1 The quantity produced by a system. 2 The power delivered by a mechanical machine or an electric circuit. 3 In digital computers, the computed results delivered by the computer. 4 In a computer or a circuit, the terminals which deliver the output. **average acoustic power o.** The acoustic power emitted, as from an ultrasound transducer, averaged over the pulse repetition period. **cardiac o.** The volume of blood ejected by the heart in a unit of time, usually one minute. Also *kinemia* (outmoded). **stroke o.** The volume of blood ejected in each ventricular systole. **urinary o.** The amount of water or solutes excreted by the kidneys per unit of time.

**ov-** \äv-, ōv-\ OVO-.

**ova** \ō′və\ Plural of OVUM.

**oval** \ō′vəl\ 1 Having the shape of an egg. 2 Of or relating to an ovum.

**ovalbumin** \äv′albyoo′mən\ A major protein of egg white. It is a glycoprotein, carrying one oligosaccharide chain, and has a molecular mass of about 44 kDa.

**ovalocytary** \ō′vəlōsī′tərē\ ELLIPTOCYTIC.

**ovalocyte** \ō′vəlōsīt′\ ELLIPTOCYTE.

**ovalocytosis** \ō′vəlōsītō′sis\ ELLIPTOCYTOSIS.

**ovarialgia** \ōver′ē·al′jə\ [*ovari(o)-* + -ALGIA] Pain in an ovary. Also *oophoralgia.*

**ovarian** \ōver′ē·ən\ Of, relating to, or having the characteristics of an ovary or ovaries.

**ovariectomy** \ō′verē·ek′təmē\ [*ovari(o)-* + -ECTOMY] OOPHORECTOMY.

**ovario-** \ōver′ē·ə-, ōver′ē·ō-\ [L *ovarium* ovary] A combining form denoting the ovary.

**ovariocele** \ōver′ē·əsēl′\ [OVARIO- + -CELE[1]] A hernia of an ovary, usually into the inguinal canal. **vaginal o.** Hernia of the ovary into the vagina. The condition is usually seen after hysterectomy.

**ovariocentesis** \-sentē′sis\ [OVARIO- + -CENTESIS] Puncture of an ovarian cyst or follicle in order to aspirate follicular fluid or oocytes. Also *paracentesis ovarii.*

**ovariocyesis** \-sī·ē′sis\ [OVARIO- + CYESIS] OVARIAN PREGNANCY.

**ovarioepilepsy** \-ep′əlep′sē\ [OVARIO- + EPILEPSY] CATAMENIAL EPILEPSY.

**ovariolytic** \-lit′ik\ [OVARIO- + LYTIC] Having the property of destroying the ovary. *Seldom used.*

**ovariopathy** \ōver′ē·äp′əthē\ [OVARIO- + -PATHY] OOPHOROPATHY.

**ovariopexy** \ōver′e·əpek′sē\ OOPHOROPEXY.

**ovariorrhexis** \-rek′sis\ [OVARIO- + -RRHEXIS] Rupture of an ovary.

**ovariosteresis** \-stērē′sis\ [OVARIO- + Gk *sterēsis* (from *sterein* to deprive) privation, loss] OOPHORECTOMY.

**ovariostomy** \ōver′ē·äs′təmē\ [OVARIO- + -STOMY] OOPHOROSTOMY.

**ovariotestis** \-tes′tis\ OVOTESTIS.

**ovariotomy** \ōver′ē·ät′əmē\ [OVARIO- + -TOMY] OOPHOROTOMY.

**ovaritis** \ō′verī′tis\ [*ovari(o)-* + -ITIS] OOPHORITIS.

**ovarium** \ōver′ē·əm\ [New L (from L *ov(um)* egg + -ARIUM *-ary*), ovary] (*pl.* ovaria) [NA] One of the paired internal genital organs of the female, located on each side of the uterus near the lateral wall of the pelvis, attached by the mesovarium to the posterosuperior surface of the broad ligament of the uterus. It is covered by peritoneum adhering to a layer of germinal epithelium deep to which is a thick cortex which, after puberty, contains the follicles and corpora lutea and encloses a vascular medulla. The organ produces hormones including estrogens and progesterone, and it may interact with the hypophyseal gonadotrophic hormones and others. With increasing age it becomes more fibrotic and after the menopause most of its activities, such as forming follicles and corpora lutea, cease; ovary. Also *oophoron.* **o. bipartitum** An ovary whose shape is such that it resembles two connecting structures. Also *ovarium disjunctum, ovarium lobatum.* **o. gyratum** An ovary whose surface has irregular convolutions or grooves. **o. lobatum** OVARIUM BIPARTITUM.

**ovary** \ō′vərē\ [New L *ovarium.* See OVARIUM.] One of the paired internal genital organs of the female; ovarium. **adenocystic o.** An ovary which has numerous small cysts, thus resembling a glandular structure. **embryonic o.** An ovary located in an embryo. **oyster ovaries** Large, edematous ovaries containing multiple theca-lutein cysts, often associated with gestational trophoblastic disease. **polycystic o.** An ovary containing multiple follicular cysts and often excessive fibrous tissue, sometimes associated with excessive secretion of androgenic hormone and varying degrees of virilization and ovarian dysfunction. Also *sclerocystic disease of the ovary.*

**overbite** VERTICAL OVERLAP. **deep o.** Excessive vertical overlap. **horizontal o.** HORIZONTAL OVERLAP. **vertical o.** VERTICAL OVERLAP.

**overbreathing** *Popular* HYPERVENTILATION.

**overclosure** \-klō′zhər\ An abnormally small vertical relation with the teeth, natural or artificial, in occlusion. It is often accompanied by an abnormally large interocclusal distance. Also *closed bite.*

**overdenture** \-den′chər\ A denture constructed over deliberately retained roots which may be either exposed or covered with mucous membrane. If exposed the roots are root-filled and sometimes capped. Compare OVERLAY DENTURE.

**overdetermination** \-ditur′mənā′shən\ In psychiatry, the state of having a multiplicity of factors, motives, causes, or reasons upon which the final form of a symptom or neurosis depends. Also *multidetermination.*

**overdominance** \-däm′inəns\ A property of a phenotype by which, when the genotype at a locus is heterozygous, the quality or fitness of the phenotype is superior to that present when either allele is homozygous.

**overdrive** The device of purposely increasing heart rate, as by an artificial pacemaker, in order to eliminate undesirable rhythms.

**overeruption** \-irup′shən\ The vertical extrusion of a tooth beyond its normal position in the dental arch. It occurs when there is no opposing tooth at the time of eruption. At other times, overeruption is caused by periodontitis and in extreme cases it can prevent proper closure of the jaws. Artificial overeruption, by means of springs, may be used in the treatment of periodontitis to reduce pocket depth.

**overflexion** \-flek′shən\ HYPERFLEXION.

**overgraft** **1** To reinforce (a skin graft or other area from which epithelium has been stripped) by overgrafting. **2** A graft so reinforced.

**overgrowth** An increase in size of a body part due to either hypertrophy or hyperplasia.

**overjet** HORIZONTAL OVERLAP.

**overlap** The relation between the upper incisors and the opposing teeth. In normal arrangement of the teeth there is a slight overlap of the upper incisors over the lowers when all the teeth are in contact, with the jaws in centric occlusion. **horizontal o.** The projection in the horizontal plane of the upper incisor teeth beyond the lowers so that there is a space between the upper and lower incisors when the jaws are in centric occlusion. Also *horizontal overbite, overjet.* **vertical o.** The overlap in the vertical plane of the upper incisors over the lowers with the jaws in centric occlusion. The opposing incisor teeth may be in contact with each other or there may also be a horizontal overlap. Also *overbite, vertical overbite.*

**overlay** **1** An additional component to an existing condition. **2** A cast inlay or crown that covers one or more cusps of a tooth. See also OVERLAY DENTURE.

**overload** A load greater than the rated load of an electronic device and which can cause damage or waveform distortion. **aortic o.** Increased or excessive requirement of left ventricular work resulting from conditions in the aorta such as hypertension. **circulatory o. in renal failure** CIRCULATORY CONGESTION IN RENAL FAILURE. **iron o.** An excessive accumulation of iron in the body due to a greater than normal absorption of iron from the gastrointestinal tract or from parenteral injection. This may arise from idiopathic hemochromatosis, excessive iron intake, chronic alcoholism, certain types of refractory anemia, or transfusional hemosiderosis. The excess iron is deposited as hemosiderin in reticuloendothelial cells or parenchymal cells of various organs. Plasma iron and transferrin saturation are increased. Total iron-binding capacity is depressed. This disorder can lead to cirrhosis, diabetes, hyperpigmentation of the skin, cardiac failure, and hypofunction of the endocrine glands.

**overnutrition** \-n^y^ootrish′ən\ The consumption of more food than is required by the body to sustain normal functions and maintain body weight. It is often used in reference to obesity (overconsumption of calories) and other pathologic states arising from overeating.

**overprotection** Oversolicitousness and inhibition of independence in the guise of preventing harm or evil. **maternal o.** SMOTHER LOVE.

**overriding** **1** A malposition of toes in which one digit lies wholly or in part on another. Also *overtoe.* **2** The slipping of one fragment of a fractured bone over the other fragment.

**overstain** To apply an excess of histologic stain such that subsequent removal of the excess provides maximal differentiation of structural detail.

**overstimulation** \-stim′yəlā′shən\ Traumatization occurring when there is a flooding of the organism with more stimuli than it can master, either because its coping mechanisms are not adequate or because the stimulus intensity is so great that it would constitute a significant stressor to anyone.

**overt** \ōvurt′, ō′vurt\ Apparent, as a sign of an illness; plainly demonstrable.

**overtoe** \ō′vərtō\ OVERRIDING.

**Overton** [Charles Ernst *Overton,* German anesthesiologist, born 1865] Meyer-Overton theory. See under LIPOID THEORY OF NARCOSIS.

**overtone** \ō′vərtōn\ An additional tone emitted by a resonant musical instrument, the voice, and other sound-producing devices, which is higher in frequency than the fundamental tone and to which it bears a simple numerical relationship. It is usually one of a series of overtones or harmonics.

**overventilation** \-ven′təlā′shən\ HYPERVENTILATION.

**overweight** Having a body weight in excess of that stipulated by standard height-weight tables, which may be due to an excess accumulation of adipose tissue or of lean body mass.

**ovi** \ō′vī\ Of an ovum, as *vitellus ovi.*

**ovi-** \ō′vē-\ OVO-.

**oviduct** \ō′vidukt\ **1** TUBA UTERINA. **2** In zoology, the duct along which ova pass to the exterior of the body of the female.

**oviferous** \ōvif′ərəs\ Bearing ova.

**ovification** \ō′vifikā′shən\ OVULATION.

**oviform** \ō′vifôrm\ [OVI- + -FORM] OVOID.

**ovigenic** \ō′vijen′ik\ [OVI- + -GENIC] OOGENIC.

**ovigenous** \ōvij′ənəs\ OOGENIC.

**oviparous** \ōvip′ərəs\ [L *oviparus* (from *ov(um)* egg + *i* + *par(ere)* to bear young + *-us* -OUS) egg-laying] Producing eggs that hatch outside the body. Compare OVOVIVIPAROUS, VIVIPAROUS.

**oviposit** \ō′vipäz′it\ [OVI- + L *posit(us),* past part. of *ponere* to place, set, lay] To lay eggs, especially if associated with specialized organs or behavior, as in many insects, such as the grasshoppers and cockroaches.

**oviposition** \ō′vipəzish′ən\ The deposition or laying of eggs, as by insects.

**ovisac** \ō′visak\ VESICULAR OVARIAN FOLLICLE.

**ovium** \ō′vē·əm\ [New L, from L *ov(um)* egg + *-ium,* New L noun suffix] The mature female germ cell, or ovum.

**ovo-** \ō′və-, ō′vō-\ [L *ovum* egg] A combining form denoting egg or ovum. Also *ovi-.*

**ovocyte** \ō′vəsīt\ OOCYTE.

**ovogenesis** \-jen′əsis\ [OVO- + GENESIS] OOGENESIS.

**ovoid** \ō′void\ [OV- + -OID] Resembling a hen's egg in shape. Also *oviform.* **fetal o.** The ovoid intrauterine shape of the fetus. **Manchester o.** An egg-shaped radium applicator with a diameter of 2–3 cm, used in the treatment of cancer of the cervix.

**ovolarviparous** \-lärvip′ərəs\ [OVO- + *larv(a)* + *i* + *-parous,* combining form from L *par(ere)* to beget or bear young + -OUS] Producing eggs that hatch within the female, the larvae being held within the uterus and later deposited in the host organism: said of certain myiasis flies, nematodes, and other invertebrates.

**ovomucoid** \-myoo′koid\ A glycoprotein of the white of birds' eggs, having a molecular mass of about 28 kDa. It is an inhibitor of trypsin.

**ovoplasm** \ō′vəplazm\ [OVO- + -PLASM] OOPLASM.

**ovotestis** \-tes′tis\ [OVO- + TESTIS] A gonad containing both ovarian and testicular elements, as seen in one form of true hermaphroditism. Also *ovariotestis.*

**ovotransferrin** \-transfer′in\ CONALBUMIN.

**ovovitellin** \-vītel′in\ [OVO- + L *vitell(us)* the yolk of an egg + -IN] A protein in the yolk, or vitellus, of an ovum.

**ovoviviparous** \-vīvip′ərəs\ [OVO- + VIVIPAROUS] Characterized by the production of large, yolky, shell-protected eggs which are retained and develop within the reproductive tract of the female. The young receive nourishment only from the yolk. Hatching is internal, and the young are then released to the outside. Some insects, sharks, fish, snakes, and lizards are ovoviviparous. Compare OVIPAROUS, VIVIPAROUS.

**ovula** \äv′yələ\ Plural of OVULUM.

**ovulation** \ō′vyəlā′shən, äv′yə-\ [New L *ovul(um)* (dim. of L *ovum* an egg) a little egg + -ATION] The expulsion of a secondary oocyte from a mature graafian follicle. Also *ovification.* **anestrous o.** Ovulation in animals in the absence of other features of the estrous cycle. **paracyclic o.** An additional ovulation during an estrous cycle, occurring at a time different from that of the regular ovulation in that cycle. Also *supplementary ovulation.*

**ovule** \ō′vyool\ [New L *ovul(um),* dim. of *ovum* egg] An ovum lying within a follicle. **Naboth's o.'s** NABOTHIAN CYSTS. **primitive o.** An anlage of an ovum contained within the ovary. Also *primordial ovule.*

**ovulo-** \äv′yəlō-\ [New L *ovulum* (dim. of L *ovum* egg) a small egg, ovule] A combining form denoting ovule or ovum.

**ovulum** \äv′yələm\ [New L (dim. of L *ovum* egg), a little egg] **1** OVUM. **2** Any small egglike structure resembling an ovum. **ovula nabothi** NABOTHIAN CYSTS.

**ovum** \ō′vəm\ [L, an egg] (*pl.* ova) The unfertilized reproductive cell produced by the ovary in the female, appearing initially as an oogonium, then as a primary oocyte in the ovarian follicle where it matures into the secondary oocyte, which is surrounded by the zona pellucida or cells of the cumulus. When the follicle ruptures, the liberated oocyte enters the uterine tube and reaches the uterus surrounded by the cells of the corona radiata in a matrix containing hyaluronic acid, where it is either fertilized by a sperm or discharged during the next menstrual period. The oocyte undergoes a number of changes during maturation and when it is discharged from the ovarian follicle it contains half the number of chromosomes originally present in the primary oocyte. The term is applied to any or all of the above stages. Also *ovulum.* **blighted o.** An ovum whose development is arrested. Frequently, all that is seen is a fluid-filled sac either without a trace of a fetus or with a small amount of amor-

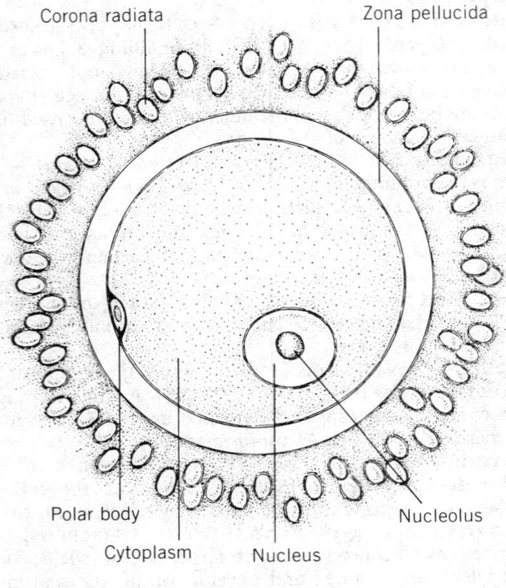


**Ovum**

phous tissue where the fetus is usually located. **centrolecithal o.** An egg in which the relatively abundant yolk is concentrated in the interior with the cytoplasm distributed as a thin coat on the external surface. An island of cytoplasm is also present in the center of the egg. It occurs in arthropods, especially insects. **ectolecithal o.** An egg in which the yolk is distributed around the periphery with the cytoplasm in the center. It occurs in Platyhelminthes. **fertilized o.** ZYGOTE. **Hertig-Rock ova** A series of specimens of fertilized human ova and embryos ranging in estimated age from one to 17 days. Some were abnormal or blighted, but over 20 were considered normal and were described in detail. The series is unique in size and range. **holoblastic o.** An ovum that has undergone holoblastic cleavage. **macrolecithal o.** MEGALECITHAL OVUM. **medialecithal o.** An ovum possessing a moderate amount of yolk or deutoplasm, as in amphibians. Also *mesolecithal ovum.* **megalecithal o.** An ovum containing much yolk or deutoplasm, as in bony fishes, reptiles, and birds. Also *macrolethical ovum.* **meroblastic o.** An ovum rich in yolk (megalecithal), with partial segmentation, of which the part richest in yolk, having little or no contribution to make in segmentation, does not participate in the constitution of the embryo and only provides nutritive material. The other part, poor in yolk and rich in cytoplasm, and which contains the nucleus, is alone segmented into blastomeres, then in cells. It is the only region which participates in the formation of the embryo. **mesolecithal o.** MEDIALECITHAL OVUM. **miolecithal o.** An ovum having a small quantity of yoke evenly distributed throughout its cytoplasm, as found in many invertebrates, mammals, and man. Also *microlecithal ovum, oligolecithal ovum.* **oligolecithal o.** MIOLECITHAL OVUM. **telolecithal o.** An ovum possessing moderate or much yolk. • The term has been used for both medialecithal and megalecithal eggs, and thus some authorities suggest it should not be used except as a synonym. **unfertilized o.** The haploid female germ cell which has not been fertilized.

**Owen** [Sir Richard *Owen,* English anatomist, 1804–1892] Lines of Owen. See under LINE.

**Owren** [Paul A. *Owren,* Norwegian hematologist, born 1905] Owren's disease. See under FACTOR V DEFICIENCY.

**oxacillin** $C_{19}H_{18}N_3O_5S$. An antibiotic with actions and uses similar to those of nafcillin. Its sodium salt is used for treatment of infections from staphylococci that are resistant to penicillin G or for mixed infections in which resistant staphylococci are present.

**oxalate** An ion, salt, or ester derived from oxalic acid. The dianion binds calcium ions strongly and precipitates them. **balanced o.** A mixture of two parts potassium oxalate, which causes erythrocytes to shrink, and three parts ammonium oxalate, which causes erythrocytes to swell. It is used as an anticoagulant for blood specimens that are to be subjected to hematologic examination. Also *double oxalate.*

**oxalated** \äk′səlā′tid\ Having oxalate dianion added, usually in order to remove calcium ions. This treatment inhibits the clotting of blood.

**oxalemia** \äk′səlē′mē·ə\ The presence of abnormally large amounts of oxalates in the blood.

**oxalic acid** HOOC—COOH. Ethanedioic acid. It occurs in some plants and is toxic because it binds calcium ions tightly.

**oxalism** \äk′səlizm\ Poisoning by oxalic acid or its salts. Ingestion of oxalic acid (about 5 g) can be fatal. It causes corrosive damage to the gastrointestinal tract, shock, convulsions, and renal damage. Kidney damage results from the formation of insoluble calcium oxalate deposited in the kidney.

**oxaloacetate** $^{-}$OOC—CO—$CH_2$—COO$^{-}$. The dianion of oxaloacetic acid, the form in which it exists in neutral solution. In the tricarboxylic acid cycle, it reacts with acetyl-CoA to form citrate; this is oxidized ultimately to regenerate oxaloacetate, the final step being the dehydrogenation of malate. It is also formed reversibly from aspartate by transamination and decarboxylated, both enzymically and spontaneously, to pyruvate.

**oxaloacetic acid** The acid corresponding to oxaloacetate.

**oxalosis** \äk′səlō′sis\ The deposition of calcium oxalate crystals in many tissues and organs. The condition is associated with hyperoxaluria, but tests for oxalates in the urine are difficult. The diagnosis may be established by demonstration of birefractile crystals in polarized light that do not take up von Kossa's stain. The crystals have characteristic appearances on polarography and x-ray diffraction. On crystallographic analysis, renal oxalate calculi consist mostly of calcium oxalate monohydrate. **o. I** A heritable error of oxalic acid metabolism that results in markedly increased urinary excretion of the salts of oxalic, glycolic, and glyoxylic acids. The basic defect is deficient activity of alphaketoglutarate:glyoxylate carboligase. The clinical syndrome is autosomal recessive and consists of progressive nephrocalcinosis and kidney accumulation of oxalate stones. Renal failure occurs in the second to third decades. Also *primary hyperoxaluria type I, glycolic aciduria.* **o. II** A heritable error of oxalic acid metabolism that results in increased urinary excretion of oxalate but normal amounts of glyoxylic and glycolic acids. The basic defect is a deficiency of D-glycerate dehydrogenase. Also *primary hyperoxaluria type II, glyceric aciduria.*

**oxalosuccinate** An enzyme-bound intermediate in the oxidative decarboxylation of isocitrate by isocitrate dehydrogenase to give 2-oxoglutarate. The enzyme can bind and decarboxylate free oxalosuccinate.

**oxalosuccinic acid** HOOC—$CH_2$—CH(COOH)—CO—COOH. The undissociated form of oxalosuccinate.

**oxaluria** \äk′səloo′rē·ə\ [*oxal(ate)* + -URIA] The excretion of oxalates in the urine. See also OXALOSIS.

**oxamniquine** $C_{14}H_{21}N_3O_3$. A tetrahydroquinoline compound effective against *Schistosoma mansoni.* It is well absorbed from the gastrointestinal tract and its metabolites are excreted in the urine. The mechanism of action on the adult parasite is unknown.

**oxanamide** $C_8H_{15}NO_2$. 2,3-Epoxy-2-ethyl-hexanamide. A tasteless, odorless, white crystalline compound used as a tranquilizer and sedative.

**oxandrolone** A cyclic and rogenic steroid 17$\beta$-hydroxy-17$\alpha$-methyl-2oxa-5$\alpha$-androstan-3-one, an anabolic steroid.

**oxethazaine** $C_{28}H_{41}N_3O_3$. 2,2′-[(2-Hydroxyethyl)imino]-bis[*N*-(1,1-dimethyl-2-phenylethyl)-*N*-methylacetamide]. A crystalline white powder with a bitter taste. It is a surface anesthetic that is poorly absorbed from mucous membranes. It has been given with antacids by mouth to relieve indigestion and gastric discomfort.

**oxidant** \äk′sədənt\ A reactant that oxidizes another and is thereby reduced.

**oxidase** \äk′sədās\ Any enzyme that uses dioxygen as an oxidant, reducing it to hydrogen peroxide, superoxide, or water. Also *aerobic dehydrogenase* (obs.). **xanthine o.** The enzyme (EC 1.2.3.2) that catalyzes the oxidation of xanthine to uric acid, using dioxygen as second substrate. The other product is superoxide, which decomposes, enzymatically or spontaneously, to hydrogen peroxide. The enzyme also acts on hypoxanthine, and is important in purine catabolism. It is a flavoprotein. Also *hypoxanthine oxidase* (outmoded), *Schardinger enzyme.*

**oxidation** \äk′sədā′shən\ [French (now *oxydation*; from *oxider*, now *oxyder*, to become oxidized, from Gk *oxys* sharp, + *-ation* -ATION), a combining with oxygen] The addition of oxygen in a chemical reaction, or any other process deemed to be equivalent, such as addition of an electronegative element, removal of hydrogen or of an electropositive element, removal of electrons. **aerobic o.** Oxidation in the presence of air, usually with dioxygen of the air as oxidant. **anaerobic o.** Oxidation in the absence of air, often with nitrate, sulfate, or other inorganic anion as electron acceptor. The process is of importance to many obligate and facultative anaerobic microorganisms. **beta-o.** The process of degradation of fatty acids, so called because C-3 of the fatty acid, its $\beta$-carbon, is the point of oxidation in the sense that 3-hydroxy and 3-oxo acids are formed as their coenzyme-A derivatives. **omega-o.** A pathway of metabolism, of some importance in plants, by which a fatty acid is converted into a molecule with a carboxyl group at each end. The $\omega$-carbon is the carbon atom furthest from the original carboxyl group.

**oxide** \äk′sīd\ A compound with oxygen, usually a binary compound.

**oxidizable** \äk′sədīz′əbəl\ Capable of being oxidized.

**oxidize** \äk′sədīz\ To bring about the oxidation of.

**oxidoreductase** Any enzyme that catalyzes the oxidation of one substrate and the reduction of another.

**oxidoreduction** \äk′sədōriduk′shən\ A chemical reaction in which oxidation and reduction occurs. Such reactions are more commonly called oxidations or reductions, according to whether it is the oxidation of one reactant or the reduction of another that is to be emphasized. This term is used to emphasize the fact that both processes are occurring. See also OXIDATION-REDUCTION POTENTIAL.

**oximeter** \äksim′ətər\ [*ox(ygen)* + *i* + -METER] A photoelectric instrument used to measure the oxygen saturation of blood. Also *whole blood oximeter.*

**oxo-** [French *ox(ygène)* oxygen + *o*] **1** The prefix used in organic nomenclature to indicate replacement of a methylene group, —$CH_2$—, by the carbonyl group, —CO—, as in 2-oxoglutarate. **2** In inorganic nomenclature, a prefix indicating the binding of oxygen.

**oxoacid** **1** In organic chemistry, an acid, usually carboxylic, containing a carbonyl group. **2** In inorganic chemistry an acid with one or more oxygen atoms bound to a central atom, e.g. phosphoric acid, $(HO—)_3P{=}O$.

**3-oxoacyl-ACP reductase** The enzyme (EC 1.1.1.100), 3-oxoacyl-[acyl-carrier-protein] reductase, responsible for one step in fatty-acid biosynthesis in bacteria. A similar enzyme, which also reduces the carbonyl group to —CHOH—, is present in other organisms, but the carrier of the acyl group differs. Also *$\beta$-ketoacyl-ACP reductase.*

**3-oxoacyl-ACP synthase** The enzyme (EC 2.3.1.41) that catalyzes the transfer of an acyl group from acyl-carrier protein onto a malonyl group that is also an acyl-carrier protein, with formation of a 2-oxoacyl group and release of carbon dioxide. This is the chain-lengthening reaction in fatty-acid biosynthesis.

**oxogestone phenpropionate** 20$\beta$-Hydroxy-19-norpregn-4-en-3-one, a progestin.

**oxoglutarate dehydrogenase** The first component of the multienzyme complex by which 2-oxoglutarate is oxidized to carbon dioxide and succinyl-CoA, with concomitant uptake of coenzyme A and reduction of $NAD^+$ to NAD + $H^+$. It is the component (EC 1.2.4.2) that catalyzes the decarboxylation of 2-oxoglutarate with combination of the residual 4-carbon compound, at the oxidation level of succinic semialdehyde, to the thiamin diphosphate molecule the enzyme contains. Also *$\alpha$-ketoglutarate dehydrogenase* (outmoded).

**2-oxoglutaric acid** HOOC—$CH_2$—$CH_2$—CO—COOH. An intermediate in the citric acid cycle, formed by the oxidative decarboxylation of isocitrate, and converted into succinyl-CoA by the action of the multienzyme oxoglutarate dehydrogenase complex. It may also be formed reversibly from glutamate, either by the action of glutamate dehydrogenase, which uses $NADP^+$ or $NAD^+$ as cosubstrate, or by the action of an aminotransferase, which uses another 2-oxoacid as cosubstrate. Also *$\alpha$-ketoglutaric acid.*

**oxoisomerase** *Outmoded* GLUCOSEPHOSPHATE ISOMERASE.

**oxolinic acid** $C_{13}H_{11}NO_5$. 5-Ethyl-5,8-dihydro-8-oxo-1,3-dioxolo-[4,5-*g*]quinoline-7-carboxylic acid. A synthetic antibiotic specific for Gram-negative organisms and used mainly in the treatment of urinary-tract infections.

**oxonium** \äksō′nē·əm\ The ion $H_3O^+$. Since the name still applies to this ion when substituted, it generally means any compound containing a tervalent, positively charged, oxygen atom, e.g. triethyloxonium, $Et_3O^+$. Also *hydronium* (outmoded).

**oxonuria** \äk′sənoo′rē·ə\ *Seldom used* KETONURIA.

**oxophenarsine** $C_6H_6AsNO_2$·HCl. An odorless white hygroscopic powder, the hydrochloride of 2-amino-4-arsenosophenol. It is employed as an antitrypanosomal compound.

**oxtriphylline** $C_{12}H_{21}N_5O_3$. 1-Hydroxy-*N,N,N*-trimethylethanaminium salt with 3,7-dihydro-1,3-dimethyl-1*H*-purine-2,6-dione. A compound of choline and theophylline used orally as a bronchodilator. Also *theophylline cholinate.*

**oxy-¹** \äk′si-\ [*oxy(gen)*. See OXYGEN.] A combining form denoting the presence of oxygen in a compound.

**oxy-²** \äk′si-\ [Gk *oxys* sharp, pointed] A combining

form meaning (1) pointed, sharp; (2) keen, acute; (3) quick, hastening; (4) acid, sour.

**oxybenzoic acid** SALICYLIC ACID.

**oxycalorimeter** \-kal′ôrim′ətər\ An apparatus in which food is burned in the presence of oxygen, the carbon dioxide produced is absorbed, and the oxygen consumed is measured to enable the indirect determination of the calorific value of the food.

**oxycephaly** \-sef′əlē\ [OXY-$^2$ + CEPHAL- + -Y] A form of craniostenosis characterized by an abnormally peaked or conical configuration of the cranium, resulting from premature closure of the lambdoidal and coronal sutures. Also *acrocephaly, tower head.*

**oxychromatin** \-krō′mətin\ The chromatin which has an affinity for acid stains.

**oxyesthesia** \-esthē′zhə\ HYPERESTHESIA.

**oxygen** \äk′səjən\ [French *oxygène* (from Gk *oxy(s)* sharp, sour + French *-gène* -GEN) lit., acid-generator] Element number 8, having atomic weight 15.9994. It is a colorless, odorless, tasteless gas making up about 21% of the volume of the atmosphere and, in various compounds (water is the most familiar), comprising about 49% by weight of the lithosphere. It is obtained in pure form by fractional distillation of liquid air. An allotropic form of oxygen, ozone, is formed by the action on ordinary oxygen of ultraviolet light or by an electric discharge. Ordinary oxygen combines with most elements. The valence is 2. It is a component of countless organic compounds. Roughly one fourth of the atoms in the human body are oxygen atoms. Oxygen is required for respiration in plants and animals. Besides the three naturally occurring stable isotopes, there are five short-lived radioactive isotopes, the least unstable having a half-life of 122 seconds. Symbol: O **o. carrier** Any substance that carries oxygen, usually in the bloodstream of animals. It combines with oxygen at relatively high oxygen pressures and releases it at relatively low ones. Hemoglobin is the mammalian oxygen carrier.

**oxygenase** Any enzyme that catalyzes the incorporation of oxygen from dioxygen into a single substrate. Oxygenases are divided into dioxygenases, which incorporate both atoms from the dioxygen, and monooxygenases, with which one atom is incorporated, and the other accepts hydrogen to form water.

**oxygenate** \äkəsəjənāt′\ [French *oxygène* oxygen + English suffix *-ate*] To add or supply oxygen to. This may be done to a solution, by dissolving oxygen in it from a stream of air bubbles, or to substances, e.g., by reversible binding of a dioxygen molecule, as with hemoglobin.

**oxygenated** **1** Containing oxygen or capable of yielding it. **2** Treated with oxygen or with a substance that can yield it.

**oxygenation** \-jənā′shən\ **1** A reversible addition of molecular oxygen to a compound, in contrast with oxidation by oxygen in which the oxygen molecule is more profoundly changed, as by reduction to water. **2** Treatment of a substance with oxygen, especially passage of oxygen gas through a liquid to achieve a solution of oxygen. **apneic o.** DIFFUSION RESPIRATION. **hyperbaric o.** Administration of oxygen at pressure greater than one atmosphere.

**oxygenator** \äk′sijənā′tər\ [*oxygenat(e)* + -OR] A mechanical device for oxygenating venous blood extracorporeally during cardiopulmonary bypass. **membrane o.** A device, generally consisting of a semipermeable silicone rubber or cellophane membrane encased in a container of oxygen, used for oxygenization of blood during cardiopulmonary bypass. **pump o.** See under PUMP-OXYGENATOR.

**oxygeusia** \-joo′sē·ə\ [OXY-$^2$ + Gk *geus(is)* a tasting, sense of taste + -IA] **1** Exceptionally keen taste perception. **2** A variety of dysgeusia in which everything tastes sour.

**oxyhaemoglobin** A British spelling for OXYHEMOGLOBIN.

**oxyhematin** \-hē′mətin\ HEME.

**oxyheme** \äk′sihēm\ HEME.

**oxyhemochromogen** \-hē′mōkrō′məjən\ HEME.

**oxyhemocyanin** \-hē′məsī′ənin\ The oxygenated form of hemocyanin.

**oxyhemoglobin** \-hē′məglō′bin\ The oxygenated form of hemoglobin, in which the iron atom has reversibly bound a molecule of dioxygen. It is bright scarlet. Also *oxidized hemoglobin.*

**oxyhydrocephalus** \-hī′drəsef′ələs\ [OXY-$^2$ + HYDROCEPHALUS] Hydrocephalus in which the enlarged cranium assumes a peaked or conical configuration instead of the usual spheroidal contour.

**oxykrinin** \-krin′in\ *Obs.* SECRETIN.

**oxylalia** \-lā′lyə\ [OXY-$^2$ + -LALIA] Fast speech, usually excessively fast.

**oxymetazoline hydrochloride** $C_{16}H_{24}N_2O$. 6-*tert*-Butyl-3-(2-imidazolin-2-ylmethyl)-2,4-dimethylphenol hydrochloride. A drug that is used as a nasal decongestant.

**oxymorphone hydrochloride** $C_{17}H_{20}ClNO_4$. 4,5-Epoxy-3,14-dihydroxy-17-methylmorphinan-6-one hydrochloride, a semisynthetic derivative of morphine with actions and properties like morphine, except that is has no significant antitussive activity. It is used for relief of severe pain and it is given parenterally.

**oxymyoglobin** \-mī′əglō′bin\ The oxygenated form of myoglobin, in which the iron atom has reversibly bound a molecule of dioxygen.

**oxyntic** \äksin′tik\ [Gk *oxyn(ein)* to sharpen, make acid + *t* + -IC] Acid-producing: used primarily in reference to the parietal cells of the stomach.

**oxyopter** \-äp′tər\ [OXY-$^2$ + OPT- + -ER] The reciprocal of the visual angle, used as a measure of visual acuity.

**oxyosmia** \-äz′mē·ə\ [OXY-$^2$ + *osm(o)*-$^2$ + -IA] Heightened olfactory acuity.

**oxypathia** \-path′ē·ə\ [OXY-$^2$ + -PATHIA] HYPERPATHIA.

**oxypathy** \äksip′əthē\ [OXY-$^2$ + -PATHY] HYPERPATHIA.

**oxypertine** $C_{23}H_{29}N_3O_2$. 5,6-Dimethoxy-2-methyl-3-[2-(4-phenyl-1-piperazinyl)ethyl]indole. An antidepressant drug of the indole family with psychotropic activity.

**oxyphenbutazone** $C_{19}H_{20}N_2O_3$. 4-Butyl-1-(4-hydroxyphenyl)-2-phenyl-3,5-pyrazolidinedione. A metabolite of phenylbutazone, occurring as a water-soluble sodium salt, also soluble in alcohol and organic solvents. It is an anti-inflammatory drug often used in the treatment of acute forms of arthritis, such as gout.

**oxyphencyclimine** $C_{20}H_{28}N_2O_3$. $\alpha$-Cyclohexyl-$\alpha$-hydroxybenzeneacetic acid (1,4,5,6-tetrahydro-1-methyl-2-pyrimidinyl)-methyl ester, an anticholinergic agent with antispasmodic, antisecretory, and antimotility activities on the gastrointestinal tract. It is used orally to treat peptic ulcer and spasms of the gastrointestinal tract.

**oxyphil** \äk′səfil\ ACIDOPHILIC.

**oxyphilic** \-fil′ik\ ACIDOPHILIC.

**oxyphilous** \äksif′ələs\ ACIDOPHILIC.

**oxyplasm** \äk′səplazm\ The portion of the cytoplasm which has an affinity for acid stains.

**oxyquinoline sulfate** 8-HYDROXYQUINOLINE SULFATE.

**oxyspore** \äk′səspôr\ [OXY-$^2$ + SPORE] SPOROZOITE.

**oxytalan** \-tal′ən\ A periodontal fiber found in man and some other animals. After oxidation, it can be stained with aldehyde fuchsin.

**oxytetracycline** $C_{22}H_{24}N_2O_9$. 4-(Dimethylamino)-1,4,4$\alpha$,-

5,5α,6,11,12α-octahydro-3, 5, 6, 10, 12, 12a-hexahydro-6-methyl-1,11-dioxo-2-naphthacenecarboxamide. An antibiotic substance obtained from *Streptomyces rimosus.* It is a broad-spectrum antibiotic, acting by the inhibition of protein synthesis in a wide range of Gram-negative and Gram-positive organisms. Susceptible organisms include rickettsiae, mycoplasmas, and species of *Pasteurella* and *Vibrio.* It is usually given intramuscularly. Also *hydroxytetracycline, riomitsin.*

**oxytetracycline hydrochloride** The monohydrochloride salt of oxytetracycline. It has the same properties and uses as the parent drug, and it is given orally or by intravenous injection.

**oxytocic** \-tō′sik\ [OXY-[2] + *toc(o)-* + -IC] **1** Inducing or stimulating uterine contractions. Also *ecbolic, ocyodinic, parturifacient.* **2** An oxytocic agent, as oxytocin, prostaglandins, or ergot compounds.

**oxytocin** \-tō′sin\ [OXY-[2] + *toc(o)-* + -IN] One of the two major neurohormones secreted by the supraoptic nuclei of the hypothalamus and stored in the neurohypophysis. The other is vasopressin. Oxytocin is an octapeptide with an essential pentapeptide ring and a terminal glycine amide, differing structurally from vasopressin only in positions 3 and 8. Stimuli for release of the two hormones, such as sucking by the newborn, are similar. Actions are to stimulate milk ejection, uterine contraction, and vasodepression, antidiuretic and vasopressor actions being minimal. Its exact role in mammalian parturition is not known. It is used in man and animals to induce parturition and postpartum contraction of the uterus. Also *oxytocic hormone, α-hypophamine* (seldom used).

**oxytocinase** \-tō′sinās\ A glycoprotein aminopeptidase, probably of uterine and placental origin, that appears in plasma during pregnancy, reaching greatest concentration before term and decreasing after parturition. The enzyme cleaves the 1-cysteine to 2-tyrosine peptide bonds of oxytocin and vasopressin, inactivating both hormones. Also *vasopressinase.*

**oxyuria** \äk′siyoo′rē·ə\ OXYURIASIS.

**oxyuriasis** \äk′siyoorī′əsis\ [*oxyur(id)* + -IASIS] Infection with oxyurid worms, especially *Enterobius vermicularis*; enterobiasis. Also *oxyurosis, oyxuria, oxyuriosis.*

**oxyuricide** \äk′siyoo′risīd\ [*oxyuri(d)* + -CIDE] An agent destructive to oxyurids.

**oxyurid** \äk′siyoo′rid\ **1** Of or belonging to the family Oxyuridae. **2** A member of the family Oxyuridae.

**Oxyuridae** \äk′siyoo′ridē\ [OXY-[2] + Gk *our(a)* tail + -IDAE] A large family of pinworms (superfamily Oxyuroidea) that are parasitic in the large intestine and cecum of many mammals, especially rodents. Among the important genera are *Aspicularis* (in rodents), *Enterobius* (primates and rodents), *Oxyuris* (equids, ruminants, rodents, and primates), *Passalurus* (rabbits and rodents), and *Syphacia* (rodents). *Enterobius vermicularis* is the only species normally found in humans.

**oxyuriosis** \äk′siyoo′rē·ō′sis\ OXYURIASIS.

***Oxyuris vermicularis*** \äk′siyoo′ris vur′mik$^y$əler′is\ *Older term* *ENTEROBIUS VERMICULARIS.*

**oxyurosis** \äk′siyoorō′sis\ OXYURIASIS.

**oz** Symbol for the unit, ounce.

**ozaena** *Brit.* OZENA.

**ozamin** \äz′əmin\ BENZOPURPURINE.

**oz ap** In the United States, symbol for the unit, apothecaries' ounce.

**oz apoth** In Great Britain, symbol for the unit apothecaries' ounce.

**ozena** \ōzē′nə\ [Gk *ozaina* (from *ozein* to have a smell) a fetid polyp in the nose] **1** Rhinitis of whatever kind that imparts a foul smell to the breath. **2** ATROPHIC RHINITIS.

**o. laryngis** Advanced atrophic laryngitis, with foul-smelling crusting, secondary to ozena of the nose. It was once regarded as a separate clinical entity. Nowadays its occurrence is extremely rare.

**ozone** $O_3$. The triatomic allotrope of oxygen, formed from dioxygen subjected to an electric discharge. It is used for chemical oxidations, particularly that of carbon-carbon double bonds to form ozonides. Since ozonides react with water to form two carbonyl groups, the molecule attacked is normally split into two, so that analysis of the products allows the original double bond to be located. Ozone is toxic, but is removed by reaction fairly rapidly from air. It may be concentrated by liquefaction to a blue, explosive liquid. Oxygen containing ozone has been used as a disinfectant. The presence of ozone in the stratosphere sustains life by stopping ultraviolet radiation from the sun and preventing it from reaching the earth in lethal amounts.

**oz t** In the United States, symbol for the unit, ounce troy.

**oz tr** In Great Britain, symbol for the unit, ounce troy.

# P

**P** **1** Symbol for the element, phosphorus. **2** Symbol for peta-: used with SI units. **3** plasma. **4** Symbol for proline. **5** Symbol for properdin. • Though P is frequently used, the correct symbol for properdin is FP. **6** P value.

**P.** **1** position. **2** presbyopia.

**$P_1$** Symbol for first parental generation. In genetics, the generation which gives rise to the first filial ($F_1$) generation.

**p** Symbol for pico-: used with SI units.

***p-*** *para-.*

**$p_{CO_2}$** Symbol for partial pressure of carbon dioxide in the blood, expressed in kilopascals.

**$p_{O_2}$** Symbol for partial pressure of oxygen in the blood, expressed in kilopascals.

**$\pi$** The sum to infinity of the series $4(1 - 1/3 + 1/5 - 1/7 + 1/9 \ldots)$.

**PA** **1** physician assistant. **2** paralysis agitans. **3** pulmonary artery. **4** pernicious anemia.

**P-A** posteroanterior.

**P&A** percussion and auscultation.

**Pa** **1** Symbol for the element, protactinium. **2** Symbol for the unit, pascal.

**Paas** [Hermann *Paas,* German physician, born 1900] See under DISEASE.

**PAB** *p*-aminobenzoate.

**PABA** *p*-aminobenzoic acid.

**pabular** Relating to food.

**pabulin** \pab′yəlin\ [L *pabul(um)* pasturage, food + -IN] The products of protein and fat digestion that are found in blood.

**pabulum** \pab′yələm\ [L (akin to *panis* bread, *pascere* to feed, lead to pasture), food, pasture] Food; nutrient; aliment.

**PAC** premature atrial contraction.

**Pacchioni** [Antonio *Pacchioni,* Italian anatomist, 1665–1726] **1** Pacchionian granulations, granulationes arachnoideales Pacchioni, granulationes pacchioni. See under GRANULATIONES ARACHNOIDEALES. **2** Pacchionian foramen, foramen of Pacchioni. See under FORAMEN DIAPHRAGMATIS SELLAE. **3** Foramen ovale of Pacchioni. See under INCISURA TENTORII. **4** Fossae of Pacchioni. See under FOVEOLAE GRANULARES.

**pacemaker** A specialized tissue, substance, or device that establishes and maintains the rate or the rhythm of a process. **artificial cardiac p.** An electrical pulse generator that controls and stimulates the heart beat, used

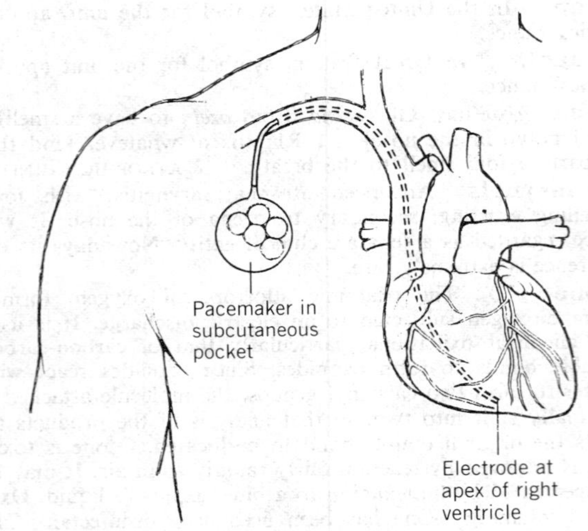

**Artificial cardiac pacemaker**

especially when sinuatrial or atrioventricular block has damaged the normal conduction pathways. **asynchronous p.** An artificial cardiac pacemaker which stimulates the heart, most often the right ventricle, at a fixed rate and is unaffected by spontaneous atrial or ventricular activity. Also *fixed-rate pacemaker.* **cardiac p.** The group of cells, normally in the sinuatrial node, which determine the rate of the heartbeat. If the sinuatrial node fails, other groups of cells elsewhere, as in the atrioventricular node, will act as cardiac pacemaker. **catheter p.** A flexible rod or tube, or group of them, containing conducting wires and with one or more electrodes at the tip. Inserted into a vessel and passed under x-ray control into the heart, it can be used for diagnostic or treatment purposes to control its rate of contraction. **demand p.** An artificial cardiac pacemaker which is inhibited from generating impulses by the patient's own heart beats and only functions in their absence. **ectopic p.** A cardiac pacemaker located elsewhere than in the sinuatrial node. **external p.** An artificial cardiac pacemaker in which the impulse generator lies outside the body. The stimulating electrodes are either sewn onto the myocardium and connected to the pacemaker by wires through the chest wall, or lie in a ventricle at the end of an intravenous catheter. **fixed-rate p.** ASYNCHRONOUS PACEMAKER. **implanted p.** An artificial cardiac pacemaker whose impulse generator is designed to be placed beneath the skin. **radio-frequency p.** An artificial cardiac pacemaker in which an external pulse generator transmits impulses to a subcutaneous radio receiver, which in turn transmits them to electrodes sewn into the heart muscle. This generator is activated by an external antenna coil which in turn responds to an external portable radio transmitter. **shifting p.** WANDERING PACEMAKER. **synchronous p.** An artificial cardiac pacemaker in which the patient's own atrial impulses stimulates the electronic pacemaker to generate impulses which then stimulate a ventricle through electrodes placed there. **transvenous catheter p.** A catheter pacemaker passed through the venous circulation into the heart. The impulse generator may be either external or implanted. **uterine p.** One of two regions of the uterus near the uterine horns, or cornu, where the uterine contractile waves of labor originate. **ventricular p.** **1** An ectopic pacemaker located in a ventricle. **2** An artificial cardiac pacemaker whose active electrode is placed in a ventricle. **wandering p.** A cardiac pacemaker which from time to time alters its position from the normal to an abnormal one, such as the atrioventricular node, or from one abnormal position to another. Also *shifting pacemaker.*

**Pachon** [Michel Victor *Pachon,* French physiologist, 1867–1938] See under METHOD.

**pachonychia** \pak′ənik′ē·ə\ PACHYONYCHIA.

**pachy-** \pak′i-\ [Gk *pachys* thick, large, curdled] A combining form meaning thick.

**pachycephaly** \-sef′əlē\ [PACHY- + CEPHAL- + -Y] An abnormal thickness of the calvaria, or of the skull as a whole.

**pachyderma** \-dur′mə\ [PACHY- + -DERMA] PACHYDERMIA. **p. oralis** Leukoplakia of the mouth with focal keratosis as the predominant lesion. *Outmoded.* **p. vesicae** Plaque present on the mucous membrane of the bladder.

**pachydermatocele** \-dərmat′əsēl\ [*pachydermato(us)* + -CELE] Neurofibromatosis producing an elephantiasislike appearance.

**pachydermatous** \-dur′mətəs\ [PACHYDERMA + *t* + -OUS] Characterized by thick skin. Also *pachydermic.*

**pachydermia** \-dur′mē·ə\ [Gk (from *pachydermos* thick-skinned, from *pachys* thick + *derma* skin) thickness of the skin] An increased thickness of the skin. Also *pachyderma.* **laryngeal contact p.** A rare variety of chronic hyperplastic laryngitis, characterized by severe hoarseness due to annular epithelial overgrowth centered on the vocal processes of the arytenoid cartilages. It results from long-standing vocal abuse. Also *contact ulcer of the larynx, pachydermia verrucosa laryngis, posterior hypertrophic pachydermia of the larynx.* **p. laryngis** Any variety of chronic laryngitis characterized by areas of gross hyperplastic thickening of the laryngeal lining, particularly that of the vocal folds. **lymphangiectatic p.** A thickening of the skin that accompanies chronic lymphedema. **posterior hypertrophic p. of the larynx** LARYNGEAL CONTACT PACHYDERMIA. **p. verrucosa laryngis** LARYNGEAL CONTACT PACHYDERMIA.

**pachydermic** \-dur′mik\ PACHYDERMATOUS.

**pachydermoperiostosis** \-dur′məper′i·ästō′sis\ The complete syndrome of hypertrophic osteoarthropathy, including the characteristic thickened skin, especially over the forehead and anterior shins. This is more often seen in idiopathic hypertrophic osteoarthropathy than in hypertrophic pulmonary osteoarthropathy. Also *pachyperiosteoderma, Touraine-Solente-Golé syndrome.*

**pachygyria** \-jī′rē·ə\ [PACHY- + GYR- + -IA] An abnormal coarseness or breadth of the cerebral convolutions.
**pachyleptomeningitis** \-lep′təmen′injī′tis\ [PACHY- + LEPTO- + MENINGITIS] Inflammation of the pachymeninges and leptomeninges.
**pachymeninges** \-mənin′jēz\ Plural of PACHYMENINX.
**pachymeningitis** \-men′injī′tis\ [PACHY- + MENINGITIS] Inflammation and thickening of the dura mater. Also *external meningitis, perimeningitis* (seldom used) . **acute spinal p.** The prodromal phase of acute spinal epidural abscess in which there may be poorly localized inflammation in the epidural space. Fever, pain in the back and limbs, and local tenderness followed by progressive paraplegia are the usual manifestations unless treatment is instituted early. *Obs.* Also *acute epiduritis.* **cerebral p.** Inflammation of the dura mater of the cranial vault. **p. cervicalis hypertrophica** Chronic proliferative meningitis of the spinal pachymeninges in the cervical region, usually due to tertiary syphilis. Also *syphilitic hyperplastic pachymeningitis, hypertrophic spinal pachymeningitis, syphilitic hypertrophic pachymeningitis, syphilitic spinal pachymeningitis.* **fibrinohemorrhagic p.** Acute suppurative pachymeningitis due to compound fracture of the skull, to septic thrombosis of intracranial venous sinuses, or to cranial osteomyelitis. Also *suppurative pachymeningitis.* **hemorrhagic p.** *Obs.* SUBDURAL HEMATOMA. **hypertrophic spinal p.** PACHYMENINGITIS CERVICALIS HYPERTROPHICA. **p. intralamellaris** SUBDURAL ABSCESS. **purulent p.** 1 EXTRADURAL ABSCESS. 2 SUBDURAL ABSCESS. **pyogenic p.** 1 EXTRADURAL ABSCESS. 2 SUBDURAL ABSCESS. **serous internal p.** *Obs.* COMMUNICATING HYDROCEPHALUS. **spinal p.** Inflammation of the spinal dura mater. **suppurative p.** FIBRINOHEMORRHAGIC PACHYMENINGITIS. **syphilitic hyperplastic p.** PACHYMENINGITIS CERVICALIS HYPERTROPHICA. **syphilitic hypertrophic p.** PACHYMENINGITIS CERVICALIS HYPERTROPHICA. **syphilitic spinal p.** PACHYMENINGITIS CERVICALIS HYPERTROPHICA.
**pachymeninx** \-mē′ningks\ DURA MATER.
**pachynema** \-nē′mə\ PACHYTENE.
**pachyonychia** \-ōnik′ē·ə\ [PACHY- + ONYCH- + -IA ] An abnormal thickness of one or more nails. This may be acquired as a result of a fungus infection of the nail plate and the hyponychium, or it may be present as a developmental defect alone or associated with the other epidermal defects. Also *pachonychia, pachonychosis.* **p. congenita** An ectodermal disorder characterized by abnormal thickness of the nails at birth associated with palmar and plantar hyperkeratosis, bullae on the soles, thickening of the ends of the nails, and a glazed appearance of the tongue due to papillary atrophy. Verrucosis and diffusely disseminated epidermal steatomas are also present. It is inherited as an autosomal dominant trait and affects males more often than females. Also *Jadassohn-Lewandowsky syndrome, Schafer syndrome.*
**pachyonychosis** \-ō′nikō′sis\ PACHYONYCHIA.
**pachypelviperitonitis** \-pel′viper′itənī′tis\ Chronic pelvic peritonitis accompanied by thickening of the inflamed serosa.
**pachyperiosteoderma** \-per′i·äs′tē·ədur′mə\ PACHYDERMOPERIOSTOSIS.
**pachyperitonitis** \-per′itənī′tis\ Chronic peritonitis accompanied by thickening of the serosal membrane.
**pachypleuritis** \-plUrī′tis\ FIBROTHORAX.
**pachysalpingitis** \-sal′pinjī′tis\ [PACHY- + SALPINGITIS] Inflammation of the oviducts with swelling or thickening. Also *parenchymatous salpingitis, hypertrophic salpingitis, mural salpingitis.*
**pachysalpingo-ovaritis** \-salping′gō-ō′verī′tis\ [PACHY- + SALPINGO- + OVARITIS] CHRONIC SALPINGO-OOPHORITIS.
**pachytene** \-tēn′\ The middle stage of meiosis, during which the homologous chromosomes separate, except at their centromeres, into chromatids, forming tetrads. At this point, crossing over can occur. Pachytene ends with separation of paired sister chromatids. Also *pachynema, strepsitene* (obs.).
**pachyvaginitis** \-vaj′inī′tis\ Chronic vaginitis accompanied by thickening and induration of the vaginal walls. This condition is rarely seen today.
**pacifier** A rubber or plastic nipple given to infants to suck. Also *dummy* (British and New Zealand usage). • *Pacifier* is used chiefly in the U.S. and Canada.
**pacing** A determination of the speed at which some specified activity or repeated action is to be carried out over time. The rate chosen may relate to efficiency or to the satisfaction of the performer, or both. **atrial p.** Artificial electric stimulation of the atrium of the heart, used therapeutically to increase heart rate or as a diagnostic test for angina pectoris or arrhythmias. **cardiac p.** Controlling the rate of contraction of the heart by an electronic impulse-making apparatus. **endocardial p.** Electrical stimulation of the heart with an electrode positioned against its endocardial surface. **epicardial p.** Electrical stimulation of the epicardial surface of the ventricles in order to control the heart rate in heart block or to suppress arrhythmias. **overdrive p.** The use of rapid stimulation from an artificial cardiac pacemaker to suppress an arrhythmia. **paired p.** Pacing with two closely associated impulses, which has the effect of slowing the heart. **programed p.** Pacing by means of a programable pacemaker, in which it is possible to change the characteristics of the output of the pacemaker as required. **sequential p.** Electrical stimulation of one part of the heart after another, as in sequential atrioventricular pacing, in which the atrium is stimulated first and the ventricle afterwards. **ventricular p.** Cardiac pacing using a ventricular stimulus.
**Pacini** [Filippo *Pacini,* Italian anatomist, 1812–1883] 1 Pacinian tumor. See under TUMOR. 2 Pacini's corpuscles, Vater-Pacini corpuscles. See under PACINIAN CORPUSCLES.
**pacinitis** \pas′inī′tis\ Inflammation of the pacinian corpuscles of the skin.
**pack** 1 Envelopment of the body or an extremity in a substance or material to achieve a therapeutic purpose. This may be done with towels or blankets that may be dry or moist and of variable temperature, with substances such as mud, clay, or packed ice, or with specially designed pliable containers having a capacity to retain heat or cold and adapt to body contours. These are commonly made of cloth filled with polyurethane foam or synthetic jell substances. 2 Something used to occlude a wound or body orifice, as to control hemorrhage. 3 To apply a pack to. **cold p.** A pliable container filled with a cold-retaining substance which may be applied to a part of the body for cooling purposes, conforming to the shape of the part. **hot p.** A pliable container filled with a heat-retaining substance which may be liquid, semisolid, or a gel, to be applied to a part of the body for warming purposes, conforming to the shape of the part. **periodontal p.** A surgical dressing applied after periodontal surgery. It is applied around the necks of the teeth to cover the whole of any raw area and left for approximately one week. Many different formulas have been used, but most dressings set sufficiently hard to protect the area from trauma and they may include antiseptics and astringents. **surgical p.** An absorbent pad that is used

to collect blood so as to provide exposure during surgery and to fill cavities or potential cavities in the postoperative period.

**packing** 1 The process of filling a wound or cavity with gauze or other material. 2 Material of whatever kind that is used to fill a wound or cavity. **denture p.** The filling of a two-part mold with plastic material, such as acrylic resin, and the compression of this material by squeezing the two halves of the mold together in the making of a plastic denture.

**pad** 1 Any soft material that can be used to protect a tender or vulnerable surface or be used as a wedge or filler, as to hold a dressing securely in place. 2 Any of the collections of fleshy tissue, usually fat, that cushion certain structures which are subject to pressure or are weight-bearing, as the toes of an animal. **abdominal p.** 1 A large sheet of soft, absorbent material used to cover a surgical or traumatic wound in the abdominal wall. 2 An absorbent pad used during surgical procedures to absorb blood and to provide exposure. **Bichat's fat p.** CORPUS ADIPOSUM BUCCAE. **buccal fat p.** CORPUS ADIPOSUM BUCCAE. **butterfly p.** A hemispherical pad that is attached to the pelvic band of a lower limb brace to push the buttocks forward. **fat p.** A mass of adipose tissue often partly encapsulated and cushioning a small space. **infrapatellar fat p.** CORPUS ADIPOSUM INFRAPATELLARE. **knuckle p.'s** Fibrous nodules on the dorsal aspects of the fingers, usually a normal variant. **occlusal p.** DENTAL OPERCULUM. **Passavant's p.** PASSAVANT'S BAR. **periarterial p.** *Obs.* JUXTAGLOMERULAR APPARATUS. **retrodiscal p.** SAPPEY'S LIGAMENT. **retromolar p.** A mound of soft tissue behind the lower third molar tooth or at the distal extremity of the mandibular residual alveolar ridge. **retropatellar fat p.** CORPUS ADIPOSUM INFRAPATELLARE. **sucking p.** CORPUS ADIPOSUM BUCCAE. **suctorial p.** CORPUS ADIPOSUM BUCCAE. **synovial fat p.** A collection of fat tissue found within the joint space underlying the synovium.

**Padgett** [Earl C. *Padgett*, U.S. surgeon, 1893–1946] See under DERMATOME.

**padimate A** $C_{14}H_{21}NO_2$. Amyl dimethylaminobenzoate, a yellow liquid used as a constituent in skin creams and lotions as a sunscreen.

**p. ae.** *partes aequales* (L, equal parts).

***Paecilomyces*** \pē′siləmī′sēz\ A form-genus of a fungus found in abundance in soil, formerly included in the genus *Penicillium*. Several species are pathogenic for a number of cold-blooded animals (sea turtles, tortoises, chameleons), and two, *P. lilacinum* and *P. variotii*, cause human disease. The most common type of human infection due to *P. lilacinum* has been a mycotic keratitis presenting as an opportunistic infection following implantation of plastic prosthetic lenses.

**paed-** \pēd-\ PEDO-[1].

***Paederus*** \pē′dərəs\ A widespread genus of blister beetles. They produce the vesicant pederin.

**paedi-** \pē′dē-\ PEDO-[1].

**paediatrician** *Brit.* PEDIATRICIAN.

**paediatrics** *Brit.* PEDIATRICS.

**paedo-** \pē′dō-, pē′də-\ PEDO-[1].

**paedogenesis** PEDOGENESIS.

**paedophilia** *Brit.* PEDOPHILIA.

**Paget** [Sir James *Paget*, English surgeon and pathologist, 1814–1899] 1 Paget's disease of the skin. See under DISEASE. 2 Paget's disease of the nipple. See under MAMMARY PAGET'S DISEASE. 3 Extramammary Paget's disease. See under DISEASE. 4 Paget-von Schroetter syndrome. See under EFFORT THROMBOSIS. 5 Juvenile Paget's disease. See under HYPERPHOSPHATASIA. 6 Paget's disease, Paget's disease of bone. 7 Paget cells. See under CELL.

**pagetoid** \paj′ətoid\ Of or relating to Paget's disease (osteitis deformans). Also *pagetic*.

**-pagus** \-pəgəs\ [Gk *pagos* anything fixed or hardened or stiffened] A combining form denoting the region or extent of union of conjoined twins. It follows the name or names of the regions united, as in *craniopagus* or *thoracogastropagus*. Also *-didymus*.

**PAH** *p*-aminohippuric acid.

**PAHA** *p*-aminohippuric acid.

**paidonyx** \pēdän′iks\ [Gk *pais* (gen. *paidos*) a child + *onyx* a nail, claw, talon] A rudimentary nail of a finger or toe.

**pain** [Old French *peine* (from L *poena* punishment, penalty, from Gk *poinē* fine, compensation) penalty, suffering] A distressing sensation due either to irritation of sensory nerves by injury or inflammation, or to emotional suffering. **atypical facial p.** ATYPICAL FACIAL NEURALGIA. **bearing-down p.** The uterine contractions during the second stage of labor. Also *expulsive pains.* **boring p.** Pain which feels as if the affected part were being pierced with a drill or other boring instrument. Also *terebrant pain, terebrating pain.* **central p.** Pain resulting from a lesion in the central nervous system. **cross-referred p.** EVOKED CONTRALATERAL PAIN. **dilating p.'s** The uterine contractions of the first stage of labor. **eccentric p.** REFERRED PAIN. **evoked contralateral p.** Sciatic pain induced in the affected lower limb by flexion and adduction of the opposite leg, or by flexion of the opposite lower limb at the hip with the leg extended at the knee. Also *Lasègue's contralateral sign, Moutard-Martin sign, cross-referred pain.* **expulsive p.'s** BEARING-DOWN PAIN. **fulgurant p.'s** LIGHTNING PAINS. **girdle p.** Pain which spreads around the trunk that often follows the distribution of a single sensory root or intercostal nerve. **growing p.'s** Any musculoskeletal complaint occurring in adolescence. It has no medical standing as an entity. *Popular.* **heterotopic p.** REFERRED PAIN. **intermenstrual p.** MITTELSCHMERZ. **lancinating p.** Sharp, shooting, transient pain, as if stabbed with a sharp point. **lightning p.'s** Spontaneous sharp, shooting pains in the limbs which occur repeatedly in many subjects with tabes dorsalis. Also *fulgurant pains.* **nerve p.** Any pain resulting from disease, compression, or injury of a nerve. **phantom limb p.** See under PHANTOM LIMB. **precordial p.** Pain felt over the heart. It is not necessarily indicative of disease of the heart. **premonitory p.'s** Uterine contractions during the latent phase of labor. **referred p.** Pain originating in an organ or viscus and felt in a part of the body not obviously related anatomically to the organ or viscus. Pain in the left arm due to heart disease is one example. Also *eccentric pain, heterotopic pain, synalgia, telalgia.* **rest p.** A symptom, diagnostic of severe, far-advanced arterial insufficiency, that is characterized by excruciating pain of the distal foot. The pain may be relieved, at least in its early stages, by placing the foot below the rest of the body. Rest pain has significant prognostic implications, since its presence means that basal metabolic requirements are not being served and presages tissue death. **root p.** Pain radiating along the cutaneous area or dermatome corresponding to one or more spinal roots and resulting from disease, compression, or injury of the affected root, roots, or spinal nerve. **shooting p.'s** Pains which start or shoot from one part of the body to another, such as lightning pains. **terebrant p.** BORING PAIN. **terebrating p.** BORING PAIN. **thalamic p.** Spontaneous pain occurring as a predominant part of the thalamic syndrome. There is a rise in the sensory threshold, but if a sensation is perceived at all it is felt as disagreeable and unpleasant. Also *thalamic hyperpathia.* **vasculosympathetic facial p.** MIGRAINOUS NEURALGIA.

**paint** 1 To apply a liquid, as a medication, by brushing or swabbing. 2 A liquid preparation for application to a body surface.

**pair** [L *paria* (neut. pl. of *par* a match, an equal) a pair] Two similar or identical things regarded as a structural or functional unit. **base p.** See under BASE. **electron p.** The pair of electrons of opposite spin that can fill a single atomic or molecular orbital. They may form a chemical bond, or they may be a "lone pair" not directly involved in bonding. **ion p.** Two ions of equal charge, one positive, the other negative, produced by the action of ionizing radiation on a neutral atom or molecule.

**pairing** 1 SYNAPSIS. 2 The formation of hydrogen bonds between complementary nucleotides of polynucleotide chains. **base p.** A structural characteristic of DNA and RNA, the purine and pyrimidine bases of the nucleotides of the complementary strands of the nucleic acid double helix being joined with hydrogen bonds around the axis of the helix. See also BASE PAIR under BASE. **distributive p.** During metaphase of the first meiotic division, the pairing of maternal chromatids and of paternal chromatids just before separation into the daughter gametocytes. **exchange p.** During prophase of the first meiotic division, the pairing of homologous chromosomes (maternally derived with paternally derived) that permits crossing over. It is mediated by the synaptonemal complex. **somatic p.** The colinear association of homologous chromosomes, as is seen in the somatic cells of dipterans.

**pajaroello** \pəhär′ō·el′yō\ [Origin unknown. Possibly in part from Spanish *pájaro* bird.] A tick of the species *Ornithodoros coriaceus.*

**Pajot** [Charles *Pajot,* French obstetrician, 1816–1896] See under LAW, MANEUVER.

**Pal** [Jacob *Pal,* Hungarian-born Austrian physician, 1863–1936] Weigert-Pal technique. See under WEIGERT-PAL METHOD.

**Palade** [George Emil *Palade,* Rumanian cytologist active in the United States, born 1912] Palade granule. See under RIBOSOME.

**palae-** \pal′ē-\ *Brit.* PALE-. See under PALEO-.

**palaeo-** \pal′ē·ō-\ *Brit.* PALEO-.

**palat-** \palət-\ PALATO-.

**palata** \pəlā′tə\ Plural of PALATUM.

**palatal** \pal′ətəl\ Pertaining to or directed toward the palate.

**palate** \pal′it\ [L *palatum.* See PALATUM.] PALATUM. **artificial p.** A palatal prosthesis for use in cases of cleft palate or following excision of the soft palate. Also *artificial velum.* **bony p.** PALATUM OSSEUM. **cleft p.** A congenital defect along the midline of the soft palate, or the hard and soft palates, that permits abnormal communication between the oral and nasal cavities. It results from failure of the embryonic palatal shelves to unite with each other and with the nasal septum. It sometimes extends anteriorly to form clefts of the alveolar process and lip. Cleft palate is more frequent in females than in males, and from surveys, heredity is a factor in between 10 and 14 percent of reported cases. Also *palatoschisis, uranoschisis, palatum fissum.* **gothic p.** An unusually high, arched palate. Also *palatum ogivale.* **hard p.** PALATUM DURUM. **osseous p.** PALATUM OSSEUM. **pendulous p.** *Outmoded* UVULA PALATINA. **primary p.** The first incomplete closure, triangular in shape, between the buccal and nasal cavities, formed at the end of the sixth week of human development and arising from the internal nasal (maxillary) processes which fuse in the midline. These processes are called the median palatine processes and they unite in the midline in front of the future incisive foramen. Also *premaxillary palate.* **secondary p.** The second closure developing between the buccal and nasal cavities towards the eighth week of human development by fusion in the midline of the secondary palatal (internal maxillary) processes. The secondary palate fuses in front with the primary palate (the incisive foramen marks the point of fusion) to form the definitive palate. **smokers' p.** The condition of the palate, chiefly the hard palate, seen in cases of stomatitis nicotina. Advanced cases develop a nodular, keratinized appearance, the nodules being marked by a central red depression, the site of a mucous gland. **soft p.** PALATUM MOLLE. **submucous cleft p.** A cleft palate in which the bone and/or muscles of the palate are not united but the overlying mucosa is intact.

**palatine** \pal′ətīn\ Of or relating to the palate.

**palato-** \pal′ətō\ [L *palatum* or *palatus* roof of the mouth, palate] A combining form denoting the palate. Also *palat-*.

**palatoglossal** \-gläs′əl\ 1 Of or relating to the palate and the tongue. 2 Of or relating to the musculus palatoglossus.

**palatognathous** \pal′ətäg′nəthəs\ [PALATO- + GNATH- + -OUS] Characterized by a congenitally defective palate.

**palatograph** \pal′ətōgraf′\ [PALATO- + -GRAPH] A device used to indicate, measure, or record the movements of the soft palate. Modern devices usually incorporate electronic sensors and are frequently made as individual palatal prostheses, their function being extended to monitor patterns of contact between the tongue and hard palate during speech.

**palatography** \pal′ətäg′rəfē\ [PALATO- + -GRAPHY] The procedure by which movement of the soft palate is identified and assessed. This may be effected by using an individually worn palatograph, or by specialized radiographic and cineradiographic techniques with or without contrast media.

**palatomyograph** \-mī′əgraf\ An electromyographic recording from the palatal muscles. It is used as a means of studying palatal function during such activities as swallowing, speech, and respiration.

**palatopagus** \pal′ətäp′əgəs\ [PALATO- + Gk *pagos* anything fixed or hardened] Conjoined twins united in the palatal region. It is doubtful that equal conjoined twins are united in this way, but instances of unequal twins with the parasitic member attached to the host in the palatal region are on record. The latter condition should be designated *palatopagus parasiticus.*.

**palatopharyngoplasty** \-fering′gōplas′tē\ 1 An operation to narrow the nasopharyngeal isthmus by suturing a flap raised from the posterior pharyngeal wall to the posterior edge of the soft palate. It is used for the symptomatic relief of various kinds of velopharyngeal insufficiency. 2 The removal of redundant tissue from the posterior edge of the soft palate in an attempt to relieve severe snoring.

**palatoplasty** \pal′ətōplas′tē\ [PALATO- + -PLASTY] A plastic operation performed on the palate. Also *palatorrhaphy, uraniscoplasty, uraniscorrhaphy, uranoplasty, uranorrhaphy, uranostaphyloplasty.*

**palatoplegia** \-plē′jə\ [PALATO- + -PLEGIA] PALATAL PARALYSIS.

**palatorrhaphy** \pal′ətôr′əfē\ [PALATO- + -RRHAPHY] PALATOPLASTY.

**palatoschisis** \pal′ətäs′kisis\ [PALATO- + -SCHISIS] CLEFT PALATE.

**palatum** \pəlā′təm\ [L, the roof of the mouth, palate] [NA] The structure that forms the roof of the mouth cavity proper and consists of the hard palate anteriorly and the soft palate posteriorly. The former separates the oral cavity from the nasal cavity and the latter separates the oral cavity and oropharynx from the nasopharynx. Also *palate, uraniscus, roof of mouth.* **p. durum** [NA] The anterior two thirds of the palate, continuous anteriorly and at the sides with the gums, covering the alveolar processes of the maxillae, and posteriorly with the soft palate. It is formed by the osseous palate covered by periosteum which is adherent to the overlying mucous membrane, and it is related superiorly to the nasal cavity and inferiorly to the oral cavity. The inferior surface is lined by keratinized stratified squamous epithelium, whereas the nasal surface has ciliated epithelium. Also *hard palate.* **p. durum osseum** *Outmoded* PALATUM OSSEUM. **p. fissum** CLEFT PALATE. **p. molle** [NA] The soft, mobile, posterior one third of the palate. It is attached anteriorly to the posterior margin of the hard palate and laterally to the pharyngeal wall, and it extends backwards and downwards into and between the nasal and oral parts of the pharynx. It comprises a fold of mucous membrane containing the palatine aponeurosis, muscle fibers, vessels, nerves, lymphoid tissue, and glands. Its pendulous free margin projects posteriorly as the uvula in the midline, from the base of which the palatoglossal and palatopharyngeal arches extend inferiorly. Also *soft palate, velum palatinum, claustrum gutturis* (outmoded), *claustrum oris* (outmoded). **p. ogivale** GOTHIC PALATE. **p. osseum** [NA] The skeleton of the hard palate, formed by the meeting in the midline of the palatine processes of the maxillae anteriorly and the horizontal plates of the palatine bones posteriorly. Anteriorly and laterally it is continuous with the alveolar processes of the maxillae while posteriorly it has a sharp free margin with the nasal spine in the midline. It separates the nasal from the oral cavity and its inferior surface is marked by grooves, such as for the greater palatine vessels and nerves posterolaterally, and by pits for the palatine glands. In the midline behind the incisor teeth are the orifices of the incisive canals occupying a deep fossa. Also *bony palate, osseous palate, palatum durum osseum* (outmoded).

**pale-** \pal′ē-\ PALEO-.

**paleo-** \pal′ē·ō-\ [Gk *palaios* old] A combining form meaning (1) old; (2) primitive. Also *pale-, palaeo-* (British spelling), *palae-* (British spelling).

**paleocerebellar** \-ser′əbel′ər\ Denoting the paleocerebellum, or the anterior lobe of the cerebellum and its connections.

**paleocerebellum** \-ser′əbel′əm\ [NA] The phylogenetically older parts of the cerebellum, represented in man by the anterior lobe, situated rostral to the primary fissure and composed of the lingula, the central and anterior quadrangular lobules, and the culmen. It receives spinocerebellar and cuneocerebellar projections, and is concerned with the regulation of muscle tone.

**paleocinetic** \-sinet′ik\ PALEOKINETIC.

**paleocortex** \-kôr′teks\ PALEOPALLIUM.

**paleogenesis** \-jen′əsis\ The appearance of characters in recent descendants that were present in remote ancestors, theoretically as a result of hereditary transmission and latency or nonpenetrance in intervening generations. Also *palingenesis.*

**paleokinetic** \-kinet′ik\ Denoting movements believed to be primitive and of early appearance in development: used especially of movements controlled by the basal ganglia. *Outmoded.* Also *paleocinetic.*

**paleo-olive** \-äl′iv\ The accessory olivary nuclei and the most medial part of the main olivary nucleus, which are the phylogenetically oldest part of the inferior olivary nuclear complex and which project to the cerebellar vermis.

**paleopallium** \-pal′ē·əm\ The phylogenetically primitive olfactory lobe, which in man denotes the rhinencephalon. Also *paleocortex, mesopallium* (obs.).

**paleopathology** \-pəthäl′əjē\ The study of disease in ancient and prehistoric times by examination of skeletons, other preserved bodily remains, or fossils.

**paleophrenia** \-frē′nē·ə\ [PALEO- + -PHRENIA] *Obs.* SCHIZOPHRENIA.

**paleorubrum** \-roo′brəm\ The phylogenetically older or magnocellular portion of the red nucleus. Also *magnocellular part of red nucleus.*

**paleosensation** \-sensā′shən\ Sensation such as pain, crude touch, and temperature sensibility which is phylogenetically older than the finer and more discriminative aspects of somatic sensibility.

**paleosensibilities** \-sen′səbil′itēs\ Sensations derived from phylogenetically older senses. *Outmoded.*

**paleostriatal** \-strī·ā′təl\ PALLIDAL.

**paleostriatum** \-strī·ā′təm\ [PALEO- + STRIATUM; because phylogenetically it is the oldest part of the corpus striatum] GLOBUS PALLIDUS.

**paleothalamus** \-thal′əməs\ The medial portion of the thalamus, which is the phylogenetically older part that lacks connections with the neocortex.

**pali-** \pal′ē-\ PALIN-.

**palicinesia** \-sīnē′zhə\ PALIKINESIA.

**paligraphia** \-graf′ē·ə\ [PALI- + -GRAPH + -IA] Incessant repetition of the same words or fragments of phrases in writing, seen particularly in some patients with pseudobulbar palsy, Parkinson's disease, and presenile or senile dementia. Also *palingraphia.*

**palikinesia** \-kīnē′zhə\ [PALI- + KINESIA] Incessant, involuntary repetition of the same movement. Also *palicinesia.*

**palilalia** \-lā′lyə\ [PALI- + -LALIA] A state in which there is a repetition of a phrase with increasing rapidity, usually occurring as a sign of organic brain disorder. Also *palinphrasia, paliphrasia.*

**palin-** \pal′in-\ [Gk *palin* back, backward] A combining form signifying repetition of a (specified) pathologic condition. Also *pali-.*

**palindrome** \pal′indrōm\ A sequence of the double-stranded deoxyribonucleic acid molecule in which the code reads the same in either direction.

**palindromia** \pal′indrō′mē·ə\ [Gk *palindromia* (from *palin* back + *drom(os)* a race, running, course + *-ia* -IA) a running back, recurrence] The recurrence of or return to a former worse state of a disease. Also *palinodia.* Adj. palindromic.

**palingenesis** \-jen′əsis\ PALEOGENESIS.

**palingraphia** \-graf′ē·ə\ PALIGRAPHIA.

**palinmnesis** \pal′inē′sis\ [PALIN- + Gk *mnesis* memory] REMOTE MEMORY.

**palinodia** \-ō′dē·ə\ PALINDROMIA.

**palinphrasia** \-frā′zhə\ PALILALIA.

**paliphrasia** \pal′ifrā′zhə\ PALILALIA.

**palisade** \pal′isād, pal′isād′\ The arrangement of cells or nuclei into an elongated row, reminiscent of a picket fence. Such palisading gives a characteristic appearance to certain lesions, e.g., the rheumatoid nodule.

**palladium** \pəlā′dē·əm\ Element number 46, having atomic weight 106.4. Palladium is a metal similar to platinum. It is used in alloys for dentistry and surgical instruments. Finely divided palladium is a catalyst in hydrogenation and dehydrogenation reactions. Symbol: Pd

**pallanesthesia** \pal′anesthē′zhə\ [Gk *pall(ein)* to sway, vibrate + ANESTHESIA] Loss or impairment of vibration sense such as the inability to perceive the vibrations of a tuning fork. Also *palmanesthesia, apallesthesia.*
**pallesthesia** \pal′esthē′zhə\ [Gk *pall(ein)* to sway, vibrate + ESTHESIA] VIBRATORY SENSIBILITY.
**pallesthetic** \pal′esthet′ik\ Pertaining to vibratory sensibility. Also *palmesthetic.*
**pallial** \pal′e·əl\ Denoting the pallium or cerebral cortex.
**palliate** \pal′ē·āt\ [Late L *palliat(us),* past part. of *palliare* (back-formation from L *palliatus* cloaked, from *pallium* a cloak) to conceal, hide] To moderate the severity of; relieve some symptoms of.
**palliative** \pal′ē·ətiv\ [*palliat(e)* + -IVE] **1** Serving to relieve the severity of symptoms without acting to cure the disease: used especially of a medication or treatment. **2** A palliative agent or treatment.
**pallid-** \pal′id-\ PALLIDO-.
**pallidal** \pal′idəl\ Pertaining to the globus pallidus. Also *paleostriatal.*
**pallidectomy** \pal′idek′təmē\ [PALLID- + -ECTOMY] Excision or destruction of the globus pallidus.
**pallido-** \pal′idō-\ [L *pallidus* pale] A combining form denoting the globus pallidus.
**pallidofugal** \pal′idäf′yəgəl\ Projecting away from the globus pallidus: used of impulse conduction or efferent axons.
**pallidohypothalamic** \-hī′pōthəlam′ik\ Denoting the globus pallidus and the hypothalamus.
**pallidotomy** \pal′idät′əmē\ [*(globus) pallid(us)* + *o* + -TOMY] Incision or partial destruction of the globus pallidus.
**pallidus** \pal′idəs\ GLOBUS PALLIDUS.
**Pallister** [Richard Alan *Pallister,* English physician, flourished 20th century] Hawes-Pallister-Landor syndrome. See under STRACHAN-SCOTT SYNDROME.
**pallium** \pal′ē·əm\ [L, a cloak, mantle] CORTEX CEREBRI.
**pallor** \pal′ər\ [L, paleness] Paleness, due to lack of melanin or of blood in the skin. **elevational p.** The marblelike, waxy appearance of the feet of patients with far-advanced arterial insufficiency, seen when the lower extremities are raised above the level of the heart. Dependent rubor will appear in such extremities when placed below the level of the heart. **temporal p.** Pallor of the temporal part of the optic disk, usually seen as a sequel to optic neuritis in multiple sclerosis.
**palm** [Middle English and Middle French *paume* palm of the hand, from L *palma* palm of the hand] PALMA MANUS. **p. of hand** PALMA MANUS. **liver p.** Erythema of the palm attributable to liver disease.
**palma** \pal′mə\ (*pl.* palmae) PALMA MANUS. **p. manus** [NA] The anterior, slightly hollowed surface of the hand, stretching between the distal crease of the wrist and the bases of the fingers. Its surface is grooved by characteristic flexion creases. Also *palma, palm, palm of hand, volar region of hand* (outmoded), *vola manus* (outmoded).
**palmanesthesia** \pal′manesthē′zhə\ PALLANESTHESIA.
**palmar** \pal′mər\ Pertaining to the palm.
**palmaris** \palmar′is\ Of or relating to the palm of the hand. Also *volaris.*
**palmate** \pal′māt\ Resembling the shape of a hand with outspread fingers.
**palmature** \pal′məchər\ WEBBED FINGERS.
**palmesthesia** \pal′mesthē′zhə\ VIBRATORY SENSIBILITY.
**palmesthetic** \pal′mesthet′ik\ PALLESTHETIC.
**palmitic acid** $CH_3—[CH_2]_{14}—COOH$. Hexadecanoic acid, one of the major natural fatty acids.
**palmitoleic acid** $CH_3—[CH_2]_5—CH{=}CH—[CH_2]_7—COOH$. 9-Hexdecenoic acid. It is one of the main unsaturated fatty acids.
**palmitoyl-CoA** The thioester of coenzyme A with palmitic acid. It is the main product of fatty-acid biosynthesis and is the donor of palmitoyl groups for fat and phospholipid formation. Also *palmityl-CoA.*
**palmitoyl-CoA hydrolase** The enzyme (EC 3.1.2.2) that catalyzes the hydrolysis of palmitoyl-CoA to palmitic acid and coenzyme A.
**palmityl-CoA** PALMITOYL-CoA.
**palmprint** The dermatoglyphic pattern and secondary folds and creases of a palmar surface. Palmprints have the same individual specificity as fingerprints and are often used for supplemental identification of newborns.
**palmus** \pal′məs\ [New L (from Gk *palmos* a swinging, quivering, palpitation] Pulsation of the heart; palpitation.
**palpable** \pal′pəbl\ **1** Readily perceived; evident. **2** Capable of being perceived by palpation.
**palpate** \pal′pāt\ [L *palpare* to stroke, caress] To explore or examine by touching and probing with the hands and fingers.
**palpation** \palpā′shən\ [*palpat(e)* + -ION] Examination performed by touching and probing with the hands and fingers.
**palpatometry** \pal′pətäm′ətrē\ [*palpat(e)* + *o* + -METRY] Measurement of the pressure threshold for pain.
**palpatopercussion** \pal′pətōpərkush′ən\ Palpation and percussion used together in examining a patient.
**palpebra** \pal′pəbrə\ [L (akin to *palpitare* to throb, palpitate, and to *palpare* and *palpari* to touch softly, caress) an eyelid] (*pl.* palpebrae) [NA] Either of the two loose, movable, and reinforced skin folds that cover and protect the anterior parts of the eyeballs; eyelid. They are separated from each other by a fissure and they are united at the angles at each end by the commissures. Eyelashes are embedded in their free margins where openings of ciliary, sebaceous, and tarsal glands are located. Each fold has an anterior and a posterior surface that meet at a free margin and consists of (from without interiorward) skin, areolar tissue, orbicularis oculi muscle, tarsus, orbital septum, tarsal glands, and conjunctiva. Also *blepharon.* **p. inferior** [NA] The lower, less mobile and smaller of the two reinforced folds of skin that protect each eyeball anteriorly. It contains the palpebral part of the orbicularis oculi muscle which produces blinking, and its posterior surface is lined by conjunctiva. The punctum lacrimale near the medial end of its free margin is larger and nearer the medial angle than that on the upper fold. Also *lower eyelid.* **p. superior** [NA] The upper, more mobile, and larger of the two reinforced folds of skin that protect each eyeball anteriorly. It extends superiorly as far as the eyebrow. Its tarsus is larger than that of the lower fold, and fibers of the superficial lamella of the aponeurosis of the levator palpebrae superioris muscle are attached to its anterior surface so that it can be elevated. It contains more tarsal glands than does the lower fold. The palpebral part of the lacrimal gland projects into its lateral part. Also *upper eyelid.*
**palpebrae** \pal′pəbrē\ Plural of PALPEBRA.
**palpebral** \pal′pəbrəl\ [L *palpebralis,* from *palpebra* eyelid] Of or relating to one or both eyelids.
**palpebritis** *Obs.* BLEPHARITIS.
**palpiform** \pal′pifôrm\ Having the form of a palp; resembling the segmented tactile or sensory process of an insect.
**palpitate** \pal′pitāt\ [L *palpitat(us),* past part. of *palpitare*

to throb, palpitate, beat quickly] To beat rapidly, forcefully, or irregularly: used most commonly with reference to the heart.

**palpitation** \pal′pitā′shən\ [*palpit(ate)* + -ATION] The sensation produced by rapid, forceful, or irregular beating of the heart. Also *tremor cordis, trepidatio cordis, tumultus cordis.*

**palsy** \pôl′zē\ [Middle English *palesie, parlesie,* from Old French *paralisie* palsy, from Gk *paralysis.*] PARALYSIS. **acute thyrotoxic bulbar p.** Weakness or paralysis of swallowing and articulation in thyrotoxicosis. It is of acute onset and is usually due to associated myasthenia gravis. Also *thyrotoxic bulbar palsy.* **atonic cerebral p.** Cerebral palsy in which the affected limbs are hypotonic and not spastic. **Bell's p.** Unilateral, peripheral, facial paralysis resulting from paralysis of the seventh cranial nerve, of unknown etiology and acute onset. The fully established case is characterized by ipsilateral paralysis of all the muscles of facial expression, including inadequate closure of the eyelids (orbicularis oculi paralysis). Dysarthria is a common complaint. Full, spontaneous recovery occurs in all but 25 percent of cases. Also *idiopathic facial paralysis, Bell's paralysis, facial palsy, facial neuritis* (outmoded). **bilateral cord p.** 1 Bilateral vocal cord paralysis. 2 BILATERAL LARYNGEAL ABDUCTOR PARALYSIS. **birth p.** OBSTETRICAL PARALYSIS. **brachial p.** BRACHIAL PLEXUS PARALYSIS. **brachial birth p.** A partial or sometimes extensive paralysis of muscles in the upper extremity owing to a birth injury to the brachial plexus or one of its major derivative nerves such as the radial, median, or ulnar nerves. **bulbar p.** Paralysis of bulbar muscles, such as those of the soft palate, tongue, pharynx, and larynx. **cerebral p.** Any of a number of chronic, nonprogressive disorders of the brain which impair motor function, occurring in young children. The brain lesion may be developmental or acquired as the result of prenatal infection, birth injury or asphyxia, or kernicterus, often due to Rh factor incompatibility. Occasionally it results from postnatal infection or trauma. The typical picture is one of spastic tetraplegia, diplegia, or hemiplegia, often combined with athetosis or ataxia. In addition, both convulsions and mental retardation are common. Also *infantile cerebral palsy.* See also LITTLE'S DISEASE. **craft p.** OCCUPATIONAL CRAMP. **cranial nerve p.** Paralysis of the muscles supplied by any of the cranial nerves. **creeping p.** PROGRESSIVE MUSCULAR ATROPHY. **crossed leg p.** Transient paralysis caused by compression of the common peroneal nerve at the neck of the fibula when sitting with the legs crossed. **divers' p.** DIVERS' PARALYSIS. **epidemic infantile p.** ACUTE ANTERIOR POLIOMYELITIS. **Erb's p.** 1 DUCHENNE-ERB SYNDROME. 2 LIMB-GIRDLE MUSCULAR DYSTROPHY. 3 SYPHILITIC SPASTIC PARAPLEGIA. **facial p.** BELL'S PALSY. **hod-carriers' p.** Winging of the scapula due to pressure upon the nerve to serratus anterior resulting from carrying over the shoulder a hod containing bricks. **hypotonic cerebral p.** FÖRSTER'S DIPLEGIA. **infantile cerebral p.** CEREBRAL PALSY. **infantile progressive bulbar p.** A rare form of genetically determined progressive bulbar palsy beginning in infancy. Also *Fazio-Londe disease, Fazio-Londe syndrome, familial infantile bulbar paralysis.* **inherited bulbar p.** Genetically determined progressive bulbar palsy. Dominant, autosomal, recessive, and X-linked varieties have been described. **ischemic p.** ISCHEMIC PARALYSIS. **jake p.** JAMAICA JAKE PARALYSIS. **Klumpke's p.** DEJERINE-KLUMPKE SYNDROME. **lateral popliteal p.** COMMON PERONEAL NERVE PARALYSIS. **lead p.** LEAD NEUROPATHY. **minimal cerebral p.** MINIMAL BRAIN DYSFUNCTION. **night p.** SLEEP PARALYSIS. **occupational p.** Muscular weakness or atrophy resulting from activities peculiar to a particular occupation. It may follow the excessive use of certain muscles, as in printers' palsy or writers' cramp; the compression of a nerve, as in hod-carriers' palsy, toxic exposures causing peripheral neuropathy, as in lead palsy; and other factors such as decompression, as in divers' paralysis. Also *occupational paralysis.* **ocular p.** Paralysis of external ocular muscles due to a lesion of one of the cranial nerves which innervate them. **painters' p.** Lead palsy from exposure to paint containing lead. **palate p.** PALATAL PARALYSIS. **pharyngeal p.** Paralysis, either unilateral or bilateral, of the constrictor muscles of the pharynx, occurring in such diseases as thrombosis of the posterior inferior cerebellar artery, bulbar poliomyelitis, and motor neuron disease. It is a cause of dysphagia. Also *pharyngeal paralysis, pharyngoparalysis, pharynoplegia.* **posticus p.** *Older term* LARYNGEAL ABDUCTOR PARALYSIS. **pressure p.** A lesion of any spinal root or peripheral nerve resulting from compression. **printers' p.** Polyneuropathy due to the toxic effects of antimony occurring in printers. **progressive bulbar p.** A motor neuron disease resulting from degeneration of the motor nuclei of the brainstem and marked by paralysis of the bulbar muscles, often associated with spastic weakness and hyperreflexia in the limbs. Also *glossolabial paralysis, glossopharyngolabial paralysis, labial paralysis, labioglossolaryngeal paralysis, labioglossopharyngeal paralysis, progressive bulbar paralysis, Duchenne syndrome.* **progressive supranuclear p.** A rare degenerative disorder in which progressive bilateral ptosis and impairment of conjugate gaze in a vertical and often in a horizontal direction occur in association with features resembling parkinsonism. Also *Steele-Richardson-Olszewski syndrome.* **pseudobulbar p.** PSEUDOBULBAR PARALYSIS. **radial p.** RADIAL NERVE PARALYSIS. **Saturday night p.** SATURDAY NIGHT PARALYSIS. **scriveners' p.** WRITERS' CRAMP. **shaking p.** PARALYSIS AGITANS. **spastic bulbar p.** PSEUDOBULBAR PARALYSIS. **supranuclear p.** Impairment of movement in muscles innervated by cranial nerves due to a lesion of the motor pathway above the nucleus or nuclei of the nerves concerned. Also *supranuclear paralysis.* **tardy median p.** CARPAL TUNNEL SYNDROME. **tardy ulnar p.** CUBITAL TUNNEL SYNDROME. **thyrotoxic bulbar p.** ACUTE THYROTOXIC BULBAR PALSY. **Todd's p.** POSTEPILEPTIC PARALYSIS. **transverse p.** CROSSED PARALYSIS. **unilateral cord p.** UNILATERAL VOCAL CORD PARALYSIS.

**Paltauf** [Arnold *Paltauf,* German physician, 1860–1893] Paltauf's dwarf. See under HYPOPHYSIAL DWARF.

**Paltauf** [Richard *Paltauf,* Austrian pathologist, 1858–1924] See under STAIN.

**paludism** \pal′ədizm\ [L *palus,* gen. *paludis,* a marsh, swamp + -ISM] MALARIA.

**pamabrom** $C_{11}H_{18}BrN_5O_3$. 8-Bromotheophylline compound with 2-amino-2-methyl-1-propanol (1:1), a mild diuretic medication used to reduce premenstrual tension and pain. It is given orally.

**pamaquine** \pam′əkwin\ A toxic antimalarial now superseded by primaquine.

**pampiniform** \pampin′ifôrm\ [L *pampin(us)* the tender shoot of a vine with its leaves + *i* + -FORM] Having a form suggestive of vine shoots or tendrils.

**pampinocele** \pam′pinəsēl′\ VARICOCELE.

**pamplegia** \pamplē′jə\ [PAN- + Gk *plēg(ē)* a stroke + -IA] PARAPLEGIA.

***Pan*** \pan\ A genus of anthropoid apes comprising the

chimpanzees. There are two species: *Pan troglodytes*, the common chimpanzee, and *P. paniscus*, the pygmy chimpanzee.

**pan-** \pan-\ [Gk *pas* (feminine *pasa*, neuter *pan*, masculine and neuter genitive *pantos*) all, whole] A combining form meaning all, whole, complete. Also *pant-, panto-*.

**panacinar** \-as′ənär\ Involving the whole of a pulmonary acinus.

**panagglutinable** \-əgloo′tənəbl\ Capable of agglutinating upon contact with serum from any member of a particular species: said of erythrocytes.

**panagglutination** \-əgloo′tənā′shən\ **1** Agglutination of erythrocytes from an individual of a species following contact with serum from any member of that species. **2** Agglutination by a single serum of erythrocytes from all members of a particular species.

**panagglutinin** \-əgloo′tinin\ An agglutinin that agglutinates the erythrocytes from all members of a particular species.

**pananxiety** \-angzī′itē\ Anxiety that intrudes into every aspect of the subject's life, seen in some subjects with early schizophrenia, borderline psychosis, or latent schizophrenia.

**panaris** \pan′əris\ PARONYCHIA. **analgesic p.** SYRINGOMYELIA.

**panaritium** \-ərī′tē·əm, -ərish′ē·əm\ PARONYCHIA.

**panarteritis** \-är′tərī′tis\ POLYARTERITIS.

**panarthritis** \-ärthrī′tis\ An inflammation of numerous joints or of all the structures making up a joint.

**panatrophy** \-at′rəfē\ Atrophy affecting the entire body, or all the constituents of a specific organ or body structure. Also *pantatrophy, pantatrophia*. **p. of Gowers** A rare disorder in which sharply defined areas of atrophy of the skin and subcutis develop without being preceded by inflammatory changes.

**pancarditis** \-kärdī′tis\ [PAN- + CARDITIS] Inflammation of endocardium, myocardium, and pericardium. **rheumatic p.** Pancarditis due to rheumatic fever.

**pancavernositis** \-kav′ərnōsī′tis\ [PAN- + CAVERNOSITIS] CAVERNITIS.

**panchromatic** \-krōmat′ik\ Sensitive to all colors, as photographic film.

**Pancoast** [Henry Khunrath *Pancoast*, U.S. radiologist, 1875–1939] See under TUMOR, SYNDROME.

**pancolectomy** \-kōlek′təmē\ Resection of the entire large intestine accompanied by the creation of a permanent end ileostomy.

**pancreas** \pan′krē·əs\ [Gk *pankreas* (from *pan*, neut. of *pas* all, + *kreas* flesh) the sweetbread] [NA] A soft, fleshy, mallet-shaped organ that is situated transversely behind the stomach across the posterior abdominal wall in the epigastric and left hypochondriac regions at the level of the first and second lumbar vertebrae. It extends from right to left, its head and uncinate process lying within the loop of the duodenum, linked to the triangular body by a neck, and terminating at its narrow tail in the splenorenal ligament in contact with the spleen. It is composed of two different glandular elements, the main mass forming a lobulated, racemose acinar exocrine gland within which are scattered clumps of endocrine cells forming the pancreatic islets. The exocrine secretion or pancreatic juice passes along the main and accessory pancreatic ducts into the duodenum. The internal secretions, including insulin and glucagon, are elaborated by the islets and enter the bloodstream to serve as an important agent in carbohydrate metabolism. **accessory p.** A detached nodule of pancreatic tissue sometimes found in the vicinity of the duodenum but usually near the head of the pancreas and corresponding more or less in position to the uncinate process. Sometimes accessory pancreatic tissue is found within the wall of the stomach, the duodenum, or a Meckel's diverticulum. Also *pancreas accessorium*. **annular p.** A developmental defect in which pancreatic tissue and/or ducts completely encircle the duodenum in such manner as to form a confining ring about the intestine. It is thought to result from an abnormal rotation of the embryonic ventral pancreas around the ventral aspect of the duodenum and fusion with the dorsal pancreas. **divided p.** A developmental defect in which the pancreas consists of two separate glands, one corresponding to the body of the pancreas and draining directly into the duodenum, and the other corresponding to the head of the pancreas and draining into the common duct. The two glands are derived from the dorsal and ventral embryonic pancreatic lobes, respectively. Also *pancreas divisum*. **dorsal p.** One of two embryonic rudiments of the pancreas. It grows out from the concavity of the duodenum into the dorsal mesentery. It gives origin to the neck, body, and tail of the definitive pancreas. The duodenal end of its duct either atrophies or forms the accessory pancreatic duct. **lesser p.** PROCESSUS UNCINATUS PANCREATIS. **unciform p.** PROCESSUS UNCINATUS PANCREATIS. **ventral p.** One of two embryonic pancreatic rudiments. It grows from the convexity of the duodenum, together with the hepatic rudiment, into the ventral mesentery. Owing to differential growth, the ventral pancreas subsequently lies dorsal to the dorsal pancreas and forms part of the head and uncinate process of the definitive pancreas. Its duct contributes the duodenal end of the main pancreatic duct. **Willis p.** PROCESSUS UNCINATUS PANCREATIS. **Winslow's p.** PROCESSUS UNCINATUS PANCREATIS.

**pancreat-** \pan′krē·at-\ PANCREATO-.

**pancreata** \pan′krē·ā′tə\ Plural of PANCREAS.

**pancreatectomy** \pan′krē·ətek′təmē\ The resection of part or all of the pancreas. Also *pancreectomy*.

**pancreatic** \pan′krē·at′ik\ Of or relating to the pancreas.

**pancreatico-** \pan′krē·at′ikō-\ PANCREATO-.

**pancreaticoduodenal** \-d$^y$oo′ədē′nəl\ Relating to or involving both the pancreas and the duodenum.

**pancreaticoduodenectomy** \-d$^y$oo′ədənek′təmē\ The surgical removal of all or part of the pancreas, the duodenum, and the most distal parts of the common bile duct and stomach. This operation is usually done for periampullary malignancy but it may be performed following trauma or because of inflammatory disease. Also *pancreatoduodenectomy, Whipple's operation*.

**pancreaticoduodenostomy** \-d$^y$oo′ədənäs′təmē\ A surgical procedure to create an opening between the pancreatic duct and the duodenum, usually following a partial pancreatic resection. Rarely, such an opening may result spontaneously from trauma, a neoplasm, or inflammation. Also *pancreatoduodenostomy*.

**pancreaticoenterostomy** \-en′təräs′təmē\ A surgically created opening between the pancreatic ductal system and the small bowel, usually made following partial pancreatic resection or for ductal obstruction. Such an opening may also occur spontaneously, but rarely, as a result of neoplastic, inflammatory, or traumatic disease processes. Also *pancreatoenterostomy*.

**pancreaticogastrostomy** \-gasträs′təmē\ An opening between some portion of the pancreatic ductal system and the stomach, usually created surgically. Such an opening may rarely occur spontaneously as a result of neoplasm, trauma, or inflammatory disease.

**pancreaticojejunostomy** \-jē′joonäs′təmē\ An opening between some part of the pancreatic ductal system and the proximal small bowel, usually created surgically. Such an opening may rarely occur spontaneously following trauma or in cases of neoplastic or inflammatory disease.

**pancreaticosplenic** \-splen′ik\ Relating to or involving both the pancreas and the spleen.

**pancreatin** A product derived from hog or ox pancreas and containing enzymes such as amylase, protease, and lipase. These enzymes have the same actions as pancreatic juice, and when administered to patients with pancreatic insufficiency improve the ability to metabolize starches, proteins, and fats.

**pancreatitis** \pan′krē·ətī′tis\ Inflammation of the pancreas. **acute p.** Inflammation of the pancreas of rapid onset, characterized by varying amounts of morphologic change in the gland, from edema to hemorrhage and necrosis. Clinical manifestations include abdominal pain, nausea, vomiting, and in severe cases circulatory failure. Although often associated with gallstones and alcohol intake, the cause of many cases is unknown. **acute hemorrhagic p.** Acute pancreatitis with variable amounts of interstitial hemorrhage, the clinical signs being those of severe acute pancreatitis, with the pancreatic hemorrhage occasionally manifest by the spread of blood throughout the abdominal cavity and the retroperitoneum. **edematous p.** An inflammatory process involving the pancreas and adjacent retroperitoneal tissue, characterized by edema and marked increase in size of the pancreas. There is little hemorrhage or tissue necrosis. The process is most commonly due to alcohol or biliary tract disease. **mumps p.** An inflammatory process of the pancreas which may complicate the course of mumps parotitis. The disease is characterized by abdominal pain, nausea, and vomiting but generally subsides without complications.

**pancreato-** \pan′krē·ətō-, pankrē′ətō-\ [Gk *pancreas* (from *pan* neuter of *pas* all + *kreas* flesh) pancreas] A combining form denoting the pancreas. Also *pancreat-, pancreatico-*.

**pancreatoduodenectomy** \-d$^y$oo′ədənek′təmē\ PANCREATICODUODENECTOMY.

**pancreatoduodenostomy** \-d$^y$oo′ədənäs′təmē\ PANCREATICODUODENOSTOMY.

**pancreatoenterostomy** \-en′təräs′təmē\ PANCREATICOENTEROSTOMY.

**pancreatogenous** \pan′krē·ətäj′ənəs\ Originating in the pancreas or resulting from pancreatic function or malfunction. Also *pancreatogenic.*

**pancreatography** \pan′krē·ətäg′rəfē\ [PANCREATO- + -GRAPHY] Radiographic examination of the pancreas after the injection of contrast material into the duct of Wirsung during endoscopic examination of the duodenum.

**pancreatolipase** \-lip′ās\ PANCREATIC LIPASE.

**pancreatolith** \pan′krē·at′əlith\ [PANCREATO- + -LITH] PANCREATIC CALCULUS.

**pancreatolithectomy** \-lithek′təmē\ [*pancreat(ic duct)* + *o* + LITHECTOMY] The removal of a stone from a pancreatic duct.

**pancreatolithiasis** \-lithī′əsis\ The presence of calculi in the pancreatic duct.

**pancreatolithotomy** \-lithät′əmē\ An incision into the pancreas or a pancreatic duct for the purpose of removing a stone or stones. Also *pancreolithotomy.*

**pancreatolysis** \pan′krē·ətäl′isis\ PANCREOLYSIS.

**pancreatolytic** \-lit′ik\ PANCREOLYTIC.

**pancreatomegaly** \-meg′əlē\ Pathologic enlargement of the pancreas due to any cause.

**pancreatomy** \pan′krē·ät′əmē\ PANCREATOTOMY.

**pancreatotomy** \pan′krē·ətät′əmē\ [PANCREATO- + -TOMY] A surgical incision into the pancreas. Also *pancreatomy.*

**pancreatotropic** \-träp′ik\ [PANCREATO- + -TROPIC[1]] Directed toward or acting on the pancreas. Also *pancreatropic, pancreatotrophic, pancreotropic.*

**pancreectomy** \pan′krē·ek′təmē\ PANCREATECTOMY.

**pancreolith** \pan′krē·əlith′\ PANCREATIC CALCULUS.

**pancreolithotomy** \pan′krē·əlithät′əmē\ PANCREATOLITHOTOMY.

**pancreolysis** \pan′krē·äl′isis\ [*pancre(as)* + *o* + -LYSIS] Destruction of the pancreas by pancreatic enzymes, as in severe acute pancreatitis. Also *pancreatolysis.*

**pancreolytic** \pan′krē·əlit′ik\ Of or relating to pancreolysis; destructive to the pancreas. Also *pancreatolytic.*

**pancreotropic** \pan′krē·əträp′ik\ PANCREATOTROPIC.

**pancreozymin** \pan′krē·əzī′min\ CHOLECYSTOKININ.

**pancuronium bromide** $C_{35}H_{60}Br_2N_2O_4$. 1,1′[2β,3α,5α,16β,17β)-3,17-Bis(acetyloxy)-androstane-2,16-dihyl]-bis[1-methyl]piperidinium bromide. A nondepolarizing muscle relaxant agent with curare-type actions. It is used as an adjunct to anesthesia, and is given intravenously.

**pancytolysis** \-sītäl′isis\ The destruction of all formed elements in the blood.

**pancytopenia** \pan′sītəpē′nē·ə\ [PAN- + CYTOPENIA] A decrease in number of all formed elements of the blood. Also *panhematopenia.* **congenital p.** FANCONI'S ANEMIA. **Fanconi's p.** FANCONI'S ANEMIA.

**pancytosis** \-sītō′sis\ An increase in number of all formed elements of the blood.

**pandemic** \-dem′ik\ [Gk *pandēm(os)* (from *pan*, neut. sing. of *pas* all + *dēmos* the people) pertaining to all the people + -IC] **1** An epidemic affecting a very high proportion of the population of a major geographic region. • This term is customarily restricted to diseases such as cholera, plague, and influenza. **2** Relating to a pandemic.

**Pander** [Heinrich C. von *Pander*, German anatomist, 1794–1865] **1** Pander's island. See under BLOOD ISLAND. **2** Pander's nucleus. See under NUCLEUS SUBTHALAMICUS.

**pandiculation** \pan′dikyəlā′shən\ [L *pandiculat(us)*, past part. of *pandiculari* to stretch as when awakening + -ION] The stretching of trunk and limbs, as might occur with yawning.

**pandysautonomia** \-dis′ôtənō′mē·ə\ [PAN- + DYSAUTONOMIA] ACUTE AUTONOMIC NEUROPATHY.

**panel** **1** In the United States and Canada, a group of patients or survey respondents who are examined or questioned several times in a prospective study. **2** In Great Britain, a list of physicians prepared to provide medical care under a governmentally supervised insurance plan. **3** A list of persons assigned to a physician under a prepaid health care plan or a governmentally supervised insurance plan. **4** REGISTRY. **closed p.** Characterizing a health care plan, system, or provider organization in which patients must use the facilities and providers of that plan, system, or organization. **open p.** Characterizing a health care plan in which any beneficiary can select from among any eligible provider and any provider is eligible to offer services. **patch p.** A concentrated assembly of computer-circuit inputs and outputs that enables circuit reconfiguration by plugging jumper wires between receptacles.

**panelectroscope** \-ilek′trəskōp\ An instrument which utilizes an electric light to facilitate examination of such internal organs as the esophagus, stomach, urethra, and rectum.

**panencephalitis** \pan′ensef′əlī′tis\ [PAN- + ENCEPHALITIS] Encephalitis involving all cellular components and white matter of the brain. **subacute sclerosing p.**

A rare, progressive, inflammatory brain disease affecting children and adolescents and caused by a measleslike virus which is probably a defective variant of the measles virus. The pathogenesis of this noncontagious slow infection remains unexplained. The disease begins insidiously with character disturbance and intellectual decline. Seizures, rhythmic myoclonus, hypertonia, and progressive decline into a decorticate state follow, with death occurring almost invariably within months (in children) or years (in adolescents). Intranuclear inclusion bodies are generally demonstrable in neurons and glial cells in the gray matter. The incidence of the disease seems to be declining because of widespread use of the live measles virus vaccine. Also *subacute sclerosing leukoencephalitis, van Bogaert's encephalitis, van Bogaert sclerosing leukoencephalitis, subacute inclusion body encephalitis, Bodechtel-Guttmann disease, subacute sclerosing leukoencephalopathy, diffuse sclerosing encephalitis, Dawson's encephalitis, inclusion encephalitis, inclusion body encephalitis.*

**panendoscope** \-en′dəskōp\ [PAN- + ENDOSCOPE] A modified cystoscope with an optic system that permits visualization of the urethra and bladder at the same time.

**panendoscopy** \-endäs′kəpē\ [PAN- + ENDOSCOPY] Visualization through a panendoscope.

**panesthesia** \-esthē′zhə\ The totality of all sensations simultaneously perceived.

**Paneth** [Josef *Paneth,* Austrian physiologist, 1857–1890] See under CELL.

**pang** A sudden shooting, piercing, or stabbing pain.

**pangenesis** \-jen′əsis\ [PAN- + GENESIS] The hypothesis, proposed by Charles Darwin in 1868, that representative "germs" of protoplasm from all parts of an organism circulate, reproduce themselves, and aggregate to form the germ plasm, thus explaining how the germ cells could reproduce a whole organism and carry all its hereditary traits.

***Pangonia*** \pang·gō′nē·ə\ A genus of particularly annoying tabanid biting flies of Africa, affecting both humans and animals.

**panhematopenia** \-hem′ətōpē′nē·ə\ PANCYTOPENIA.

**panhidrosis** \-hidrō′sis\ [PAN- + HIDROSIS] Excessive sweating over the whole body surface. Also *panidrosis.*

**panhyperemia** \-hī′pərē′mē·ə\ PLETHORA.

**panhypopituitarism** \-hī′pōpit^y^oo′itərizm\ [PAN- + HYPOPITUITARISM] Total anterior pituitary insufficiency, in the adult characterized by deficient or absent secretion of gonadotropins, thyrotropins, and adrenocorticotropin, in the child by tropic hormone failure and absence of growth hormone secretion with dwarfism. Clinical features include lassitude, pallor, loss of body hair, loss of sexual function, intolerance of cold, myxedema, hypotension, hypoglycemia, intolerance of minor illnesses, and mental aberrations. Also *Simmonds disease* (outmoded). **prepubertal p.** HYPOPHYSIAL DWARFISM.

**panhysterectomy** \-his′tərek′təmē\ [PAN- + HYSTERECTOMY] COMPLETE HYSTERECTOMY.

**panhysterocolpectomy** \-his′tərōkälpek′təmē\ HYSTEROCOLPECTOMY.

**panhysterosalpingectomy** \-his′tərōsal′pinjek′təmē\ HYSTEROSALPINGECTOMY.

**panhysterosalpingo-oophorectomy** \-his′tərōsalping′gō-ō′əfôrek′təmē\ HYSTEROSALPINGO-OOPHORECTOMY.

**panic** [Gk *panik(on)* (after *Pan,* the god who inspired fear + *-ikon,* neut. sing. of *-ikos* -IC) Pan-inspired fear, panic] Overwhelming anxiety sometimes accompanied by intense physiologic manifestations such as dyspnea, palpitations, chest pain, vertigo, paresthesia, sweating, faintness, tremors, and feelings of unreality and fear of impending death or of losing one's mind.

**paniculus** \pənik′yələs\ [See PANNICULUS.] A layer or sheet of membranous tissue, such as superficial fascia. Also *panniculus.* **p. adiposus** [NA] Subcutaneous tissue that contains a thick layer of fat. Also *subcutaneous fatty tissue.* **p. carnosus** A thin sheet of striated muscle that is embedded in the tela subcutanea in many parts of the body in lower animals. In humans the platysma muscle is the chief remnant.

**panidrosis** \-idrō′sis\ PANHIDROSIS.

**panimmunity** \-imyoo′nitē\ [PAN- + IMMUNITY] A general immunity to infectious diseases.

**Panizza** [Bartolomeo *Panizza,* Italian anatomist, 1785–1867] See under PLEXUS.

**panlobular** \-läb′yələr\ Involving the whole of a lobule; panacinar.

**panmyeloid** \-mī′əloid\ Relating to or affecting all bone marrow cell lines.

**panmyelopathy** \-mī′əläp′əthē\ A proliferative disorder involving all elements of the bone marrow. Also *panmyelopathia.* **constitutional infantile p.** FANCONI'S ANEMIA.

**panmyelophthisis** \-mī′əläf′thisis\ Pancytopenia due to replacement of bone marrow by infection, neoplasm, or other disease.

**panmyelosis** \-mī′əlō′sis\ Hyperplasia of all the normal cells of the bone marrow, especially those of the erythroid and granulocytic series and megakaryocytes.

**Panner** [Hans Jessen *Panner,* Danish roentgenologist, 1871–1930] See under DISEASE.

**panneuritis** \-n^y^ŪRī′tis\ [PAN- + NEURITIS] Neuritis in which all components of the affected peripheral nerve or nerves are inflamed. **p. epidemica** BERIBERI.

**panniculalgia** \pənik′yəlal′jə\ [*panniculus(us)* + -ALGIA] A state of pain in areas of subcutaneous fat. *Seldom used.* Also *adiposalgia* (seldom used).

**panniculitis** \pənik′yəlī′tis\ [*panniculus(us)* + -ITIS] An inflammatory change in the subcutaneous fat. Also *adipositis.* **LE p.** In lupus erythematosus profundus, the involvement of the subcutaneous fat as a result of the downward extension of the disease process. **relapsing febrile nonsuppurative p.** A disease characterized by the successive development, over a long period, of inflammatory nodules of panniculitis in the subcutaneous and sometimes also the visceral fat. Also *Christian-Weber disease, Christian's disease, Weber-Christian disease, nodular nonsuppurative panniculitis, Weber-Christian syndrome.* **subacute nodular migratory p.** One or more nodules of panniculitis that change in configuration over a period of weeks or months. It is sometimes associated with chronic pancreatic disease.

**panniculus** \pənik′yələs\ [dim. of PANNUS. See PANNUS.] PANICULUS.

**pannus** \pan′əs\ [L, web, cloth] A fibrovascular inflammatory membrane superficial to a joint or to Bowman's membrane of the cornea; superficial vascularization of the cornea resulting in opacification. **p. carateus** *Seldom used* PINTA. **p. siccus** A dry, glistening, superficial corneal opacification.

**panodic** \pənō′dik\ PANTHODIC.

**panophobia** \pan′əfō′bē·ə\ PANPHOBIA.

**panophthalmitis** \-äfthalmī′tis\ [PAN- + OPHTHALMITIS] Inflammation of the entire eyeball. Also *panophthalmia.*

**panosteitis** \-ästē·ī′tis\ An inflammation of all tissues that make up a bone, including the periosteum and the medullary cavity cells. Also *panostitis.*

**panphobia** \-fō′bē·ə\ [PAN- + -PHOBIA] Pathologic fear or dread of everything. Also *panophobia, pantophobia.*

**panproctocolectomy** \-präk′əkōlek′təmē\ The resection of the entire large intestine and the rectum with the creation of a permanent end ileostomy.

**Pansch** [Adolf *Pansch,* German anatomist, 1841–1887] Pansch's fissure. See under SULCUS INTRAPARIETALIS.

**pansclerosis** \-skliroˈsis\ Complete and diffuse hardening of an organ, tissue, or part of the body.

**panseptum** \-sepˈtəm\ The nasal septum in its entirety, including both cartilaginous and bony elements.

**pansinusitis** \-sīnəsīˈtis\ Inflammation of all the paranasal sinuses on one or, rarely, both sides of the head.

***Panstrongylus*** \panstränˈjiləs\ [New L, from PAN- + Gk *strongylos* round, rounded] A genus of South American reduviid bugs in the subfamily Triatominae. ***P. geniculatus*** An important vector of *Trypanosoma cruzi* in Panama and Brazil. ***P. infestans*** See under TRIATOMA. ***P. megistus*** A vector of *Trypanosoma cruzi* in Brazil. It frequently bites the face of sleeping persons and is therefore given the colloquial name barbeiro (barber). Also *Triatoma megista.*

**pansystolic** \-sistälˈik\ Lasting throughout the whole of cardiac systole, that is, from first to second heart sound; holosystolic.

**pant** To take rapid, shallow breaths.

**pant-** \pant-\ PAN-.

**pantachromatic** \panˈtəkrōmatˈik\ Exhibiting a complete lack of chromatic aberration: said of a lens.

**pantamorphia** \panˈtəmôrˈfē·ə\ [PANT- + Gk *a-* priv. + -MORPH + -IA] A complete absence of the usual form or shape.

**pantanencephaly** \pantanˈensefˈəlē\ [PANT- + ANENCEPHALY] Extreme or total anencephaly.

**pantatrophia** \panˈtətrōˈfē·ə\ PANATROPHY.

**pantatrophy** \pantatˈrəfē\ PANATROPHY.

**pantetheine** *N*-(*N*-Pantoyl-*β*-alanyl)2-mercaptoethylamine. It occurs in coenzyme A, linked through a diphosphate group on its pantoic residue to adenosine 3′-phosphate. It also occurs linked through phosphate to a serine residue in the fatty-acid synthase complex. Its thiol group carries fatty acids during their biosynthesis and catabolism.

**pantherine** \panˈthərīn\ A toxic fungal compound produced by several species of *Amanita.*

**panthodic** \panthädˈik\ [PANT- + Gk *hod(os)* road, path, way + -IC] Radiating in all directions: used especially of nerve impulses. Also *panodic, pollodic.*

**panto-** \panˈtə-\ PAN-.

**pantograph** \panˈtəgraf\ [PANTO- + -GRAPH] An arrangement of face-bows, one attached to each jaw, for the purpose of recording movements of the mandible in three planes.

**pantoic acid** $CH_2OH—C(CH_3)_2—CHOH—COOH$. 2,4-Dihydroxy-3,3-dimethylbutyric acid. It is found as a constituent of pantetheine, e.g. in coenzyme A, and is a growth factor for some bacteria. The natural enantiomer is the *R* compound.

**pantomography** \-mägˈrəfē\ [PAN- + *tom(e)-* + *o* + -GRAPHY] A technique of body section roentgenography of curved surfaces at any depth of the body. Adj. pantomographic.

**pantomorphic** \-môrˈfik\ Capable of assuming a variety of shapes; variable and indefinite in shape, as an ameboid or phagocytic cell.

**pantophobia** \-fōˈbēə\ PANPHOBIA.

**pantoscopic** \-skäpˈik\ [PANTO- + *-scop(e)* + -IC] Pertaining to a lens that affords a wide viewing angle.

**pantothenate synthase** The enzyme (EC 6.3.2.1) that catalyzes the formation of pantothenic acid from pantoic acid and *β*-alanine, with concomitant hydrolysis of ATP to AMP and pyrophosphate (diphosphate). This reaction is a step in the biosynthesis of coenzyme A.

**pantothenic acid** $HO—CH_2—C(CH_3)_2—CHOH—CO—NH—CH_2—CH_2—COOH$. *N*-Pantoyl-*β*-alanine. It is a constituent of coenzyme A, and a constituent of the bacterial acyl carrier protein. Good dietary sources include liver, kidney, yeast, and fresh vegetables. It is found in all human cells, and signs of deficiency do not appear in man. In rats deficiency can cause dermatitis, graying of hair, and adrenal damage, while chicks show dermatitis and dogs show gastrointestinal disturbances. Also *anticanities factor, antidermatitis factor of chicks, chick antipellagra factor, filtrate factor, liver filtrate factor, yeast filtrate factor.*

**pantoyl taurine** THIOPANIC ACID.

**pantropic** \-träpˈik\ [PAN- + -TROPIC[1]] Having an affinity for all tissues: said especially of certain viruses.

**panturbinate** \-turˈbināt\ Any of the nasal conchae in its entirety, which comprises the bone and the overlying soft tissues.

**Panum** [Peter Ludwig *Panum,* Danish physiologist, 1820–1885] See under AREA.

**panuveitis** \-yooˈvē·īˈtis\ [PAN- + UVEITIS] Inflammation of the entire uveal tract.

**panzerherz** \punˈtsərherts\ [German *Panzer* coat of mail + *Herz* the heart] ARMORED HEART.

**pap** \pap\ [Middle English *pape,* prob. from L *pappa* soft food of bread and water for infants] Any food that is soft.

**papain** \papāˈin, papˈān\ The cysteine proteinase (EC 3.4.22.2) found in papaya latex. It has a single polypeptide chain of molecular mass 21 kDa, containing disulfide cross-links. The thiol group of its cysteine residue attacks the carbonyl group of the peptide bond it splits in its substrates.

**Papanicolaou** [George Nicholas *Papanicolaou,* Greek-born U.S. anatomist and cytologist, 1883–1962] **1** See under CLASSIFICATION, STAIN. **2** Pap test. See under PAPANICOLAOU TEST. **3** Pap smear. See under PAPANICOLAOU SMEAR.

**papaverine hydrochloride** $C_{20}H_{21}NO_4·HCl$. 1-[(3,4-Dimethoxyphenyl)methyl]-6,7-dimethoxyisoquinoline hydrochloride. A synthesized or unsynthesized hydrochloride form of an opium alkaloid. It is used therapeutically as a smooth muscle relaxant in the treatment of cerebral and peripheral ischemia associated with arterial spasm, and for myocardial ischemia complicated by arrhythmias. It is given intramuscularly or orally.

**papaverine sulfate** The sulfate form of papaverine, which is more soluble in aqueous media than the hydrochloride salt. Its actions and uses are similar to those of the hydrochloride salt.

**Papez** [James Wenceslas *Papez,* U.S. anatomist, 1883–1958] **1** See under CIRCUIT. **2** Papez theory of emotion. See under THEORY.

**paper** / **articulating p.** Paper coated with pressure-sensitive colored material. It is placed between opposing teeth to register points of contact when the teeth meet. Also *occluding paper.* **bibulous p.** A coarsely textured paper of highly absorbent fibers that is used to absorb water. **filter p.** Unglazed, absorbent paper that is made in varying pore sizes. It is used to filter solutions and as a support medium for chromatography and electrophoresis. **indicator p.** Paper strips impregnated with any material that changes color to indicate a change in pH or in oxidation potential. Also *test paper.* **litmus p.** See under LITMUS. **occluding p.** ARTICULATING PAPER. **test p.** INDICATOR PAPER.

**Papez** [James Wenceslas *Papez,* U.S. anatomist,

1883–1958] **1** See under CIRCUIT. **2** Papez theory of emotion. See under THEORY.

**papill-** \papil-\ PAPILLO-.

**papilla** \pəpil′ə\ [L (dim. or variant of *papula* a pimple, pustule), a nipple, teat] (*pl.* papillae) **1** A small nipplelike projection or elevation. **2** DISCUS NERVI OPTICI. **acoustic p.** The evagination from the ventral part of the embryonic utriculosaccular chamber which gives rise to the cochlear duct. **anal p.** One of the small epithelial elevations occasionally situated on either the free edges of the anal valves or at their junctions with the bases of the anal columns. They are most prominent posteriorly in the anal canal and are thought to be the remnants of the anal membrane. Also *papilla of Morgagni.* **Bergmeister's p.** The embryonic mesodermal tissue associated with the posterior portion of the hyaloid artery. Harmless remnants of this tissue commonly persist upon the optic disk and must be distinguished from diseased conditions during ophthalmoscopy. **circumvallate papillae** PAPILLAE VALLATAE. **papillae conicae** [NA] Occasional modified short filiform papillae that are scattered among the rows of taller filiform papillae on the dorsum of the tongue, parallel and anterior to the sulcus terminalis. Also *conical papillae.* **papillae corii** [NA] DERMAL PAPILLAE. **dental p.** A localized mass of mesenchyme found on the inner aspect of a tooth germ and representing the precursor of the pulp of a tooth. Also *dentinal papilla.* **dermal papillae** The connective tissue elevations of the dermis that interdigitate with the rete ridging of the overlying epidermis. Also *skin papillae, papillae corii.* **p. duodeni major** [NA] A small, rounded mucosal elevation near the lower end of the junction of the medial and posterior walls of the descending part of the duodenum. On its summit is the opening of either the narrow distal end of the hepatopancreatic ampulla or the common bile duct and pancreatic duct separately. Also *major duodenal papilla, papilla of Vater, papilla of Santorini.* **p. duodeni minor** [NA] A small, rounded, mucosal elevation that is situated in the descending part of the duodenum about 2 cm proximal and anterior to the major duodenal papilla. The accessory pancreatic duct opens on it. Also *minor duodenal papilla.* **papillae filiformes** [NA] Tall conical papillae set in rows on the dorsum of the tongue anterior and parallel to sulcus terminalis. Each has a conical primary core of connective tissue of the lamina propria with secondary papillae and is covered with hard squamous cells at its apex. Also *filiform papillae, lingual villi.* **papillae foliatae** [NA] Approximately five vertical mucosal folds that are studded with taste buds and are located on the margins of the tongue immediately in front of the attachment of the palatoglossal arches. Also *foliate papillae.* **papillae fungiformes** [NA] Round mushroomlike papillae with short stalks and broad caps that are scattered irregularly over the dorsum of the oral part of the tongue. They also may be numerous at the apex and sides of the tongue. The connective tissue core of each has secondary papillae over which the epithelium may be thin and reddish in color. Also *fungiform papillae.* **gingival p.** INTERDENTAL PAPILLA. **hair p.** The connective tissue enclosed within the hair bulb and in contact with the hair matrix. Also *papilla pili.* **p. ileocecalis** [NA] The elevation produced by the terminal ileum opening into the large intestine at the junction of the cecum and the ascending colon. It is formed by two semilunar folds or lips of mucous membrane which overlie the muscle of the valve; produce an oval, circular, or slitlike opening; and coalesce laterally to become prolonged as the frenula of the valve. Also *ileocecal papilla.* **p. incisiva** [NA] A small mucosal elevation at the anterior end of the median raphe of the hard palate that overlies the incisive fossa. Also *incisive papilla.* **interdental p.** A pyramidal projection of the gingiva which is situated in the embrasure between the proximal surfaces of adjacent teeth. Also *gingival papilla, interproximal papilla.* **p. lacrimalis** [NA] A small conical elevation on the posterior part of the free margin of each eyelid near the medial angle of the eye. The punctum lacrimale is at its apex. Also *lacrimal papilla, lacrimal tubercle* (outmoded) . **lagenar p.** A small embryonic organ situated temporarily at the bottom of the saccule. **papillae lentiformes** [NA] Small, flattened varieties of papillae fungiformes. Also *lenticular papillae, lentiform papillae, papillae lenticulares* (outmoded). **papillae linguales** [NA] Numerous projections of the epithelium of the mucous membrane of the dorsum of the tongue, produced by elevations of the underlying corium and giving the dorsum its characteristic rough appearance. Several varieties are distinguished with some intermediate forms occurring, namely, filiform, fungiform, vallate, conical, lentiform and foliate papillae. Also *lingual papillae.* **major duodenal p.** PAPILLA DUODENI MAJOR. **p. mammaria** [NA] The pigmented, blunted, conical projection at the apex of the breast on the surface of which the lactiferous ducts open; nipple. Its position relative to the thoracic cage varies with size, age, and activity of the breast. Occasionally it is discoid and even invaginated. Its corium is devoid of fat and has a loose texture and numerous smooth muscle fibers. Also *papilla mammae, mammary papilla, mamilla, mammilla, teat, thele.* **minor duodenal p.** PAPILLA DUODENI MINOR. **p. of Morgagni** ANAL PAPILLA. **nerve p.** A dermal indentation of the epidermis containing a cutaneous sense organ. Also *neurothele.* **p. nervi optici** *Outmoded* DISCUS NERVI OPTICI. **optic p.** DISCUS NERVI OPTICI. **p. parotidea** [NA] The small conical elevation of the buccal mucosa on which the parotid duct opens opposite the crown of the second upper molar tooth. Also *parotid papilla.* **p. pili** [NA] HAIR PAPILLA. **papillae renales** [NA] The prominent conical apices of the renal pyramids that project into the minor calices and are perforated by the openings of the papillary ducts of Bellini, forming the area cribrosa. Also *renal papillae.* **p. of Santorini** PAPILLA DUODENI MAJOR. **skin papillae** DERMAL PAPILLAE. **sublingual p.** CARUNCULA SUBLINGUALIS. **tactile papillae** CORPUSCULA TACTUS. **urethral p.** The raised margins of the external urethral orifice, posteroinferior to the glans clitoridis and anterior to the orifice of the vagina. **papillae vallatae** [NA] Eight to twelve large papillae on the dorsum of the tongue lying anterior and parallel to the sulcus terminalis. Each is attached by a narrow stalk within a circular depression and separated by a sulcus from the surrounding wall. The free surface is broad and round, extending above the surface of the tongue and having many small secondary papillae under the stratified squamous epithelium covering it. They contain numerous taste buds. Also *vallate papillae, circumvallate papillae.* **vascular p.** A connective tissue papilla that projects upwards from the dermis and that contains prominent capillary loops. **p. of Vater** PAPILLA DUODENI MAJOR.

**papillae** \pəpil′ē\ Plural of PAPILLA.

**papillary** \pap′iler′ē\ Pertaining to, belonging to, or resembling a papilla.

**papillate** \pap′ilāt\ PAPILLIFEROUS.

**papilledema** \pap′ilədē′mə\ [PAPILL- + EDEMA] Swelling of the optic disk due to increased pressure in and engorgement of the veins of the disk itself, and resulting from increased intracranial pressure. Also *choked disk, ophthalmo-*

*vascular choke, neuropapillitis, papillary stasis.*

**papilliferous** \pap′ilif′ərəs\ Bearing papillae. Also *papillate, papillose.*

**papilliform** \pəpil′ifôrm\ Resembling a papilla.

**papillitis** \pap′ilī′tis\ [PAPILL- + -ITIS] **1** Inflammation of the optic disk from any cause. **2** Inflamation of the papillae renales.

**papillo-** \pap′ilō-, pəpil′ō-\ [L *papilla* (dim. or variant of *papula* a pimple, pustule) a nipple, teat] A combining form meaning papilla, papillary. Also *papill-*.

**papillocarcinoma** \-kär′sinō′mə\ [PAPILLO- + CARCINOMA] PAPILLARY CARCINOMA.

**papilloedema** \pap′ilēdē′mə\ *Brit.* PAPILLEDEMA.

**papilloma** \pap′əlō′mə\ [PAPILL- + -OMA] A benign tumor of skin, mucous membranes and ducts composed of epithelium covering a fibrous stalk. The growth may be broad-based (sessile), or pedunculated with fingerlike processes. Common sites are the skin, bladder, nasal cavity, larynx, and breast. The type of epithelium can be further designated, such as squamous cell papilloma or transitional cell papilloma. Adj. papillomatous. **p. of the bladder** A villous growth of the bladder mucosa, typically of transitional cell type, in which case it is called *transitional cell papilloma.* Recurrence is frequent, and although histologically benign, it is potentially malignant. **p. canaliculum** **1** INTRADUCTAL PAPILLOMA. **2** INTRACANALICULAR PAPILLOMA. **p. choroideum** A papilloma of the choroid plexus. **p. of choroid plexus** A papilloma arising in the choroid plexus of one of the cerebral ventricles and usually giving rise to hydrocephalus or recurrent subarachnoid hemorrhage. **cockscomb p.** A cockscomb appearance to the uterine cervix which occasionally occurs during pregnancy but which regresses following delivery. **ductal p.** INTRADUCTAL PAPILLOMA. **fibroepithelial p.** A papilloma with a prominent fibrous core. **hirsutoid p.'s of the penis** Dome-shaped or filiform angiofibromatous papules of the corona penis that arise in young adults as a developmental defect. Also *pearly penile papules, hirsuties papillaris penis.* **intracanalicular p.** A papilloma growing in a small duct. Also *papilloma canaliculum.* **intracystic p.** A papilloma growing into a cystic space. **intraductal p.** A benign tumor of mammary ductal epithelium which grows in a papillary manner within dilated ducts. It may cause bleeding from the nipple. Also *ductal papilloma, papilloma canaliculum, duct adenoma.* **inverted p.** A papilloma in which the epithelial cells grow in an endophytic rather than an exophytic manner. The cells therefore appear to grow into the stroma rather than covering stromal cores. The nasal cavity is a common site. **inverted nasal p.** RINGERTZ TUMOR. **p. molle** A soft papilloma. **p. of the renal pelvis** A papillomatous growth deriving from transitional epithelium of the renal pelvis. Though histologically benign, it may become malignant. **Shope p.** A naturally occurring, virus induced, transplantable squamous cell papilloma of the skin of rabbits. **transitional cell p.** A papilloma composed of transitional epithelium. It is typically found in the urinary bladder. **p. venereum** CONDYLOMA ACUMINATUM. **villous p.** VILLOUS ADENOMA. **warty p.** A benign, projecting, warty tumor of the skin.

**papillomatosis** \pap′əlō′mətō′sis\ The presence of numerous papillomas. The bladder, respiratory tract, and breast are sites where this more commonly occurs. **confluent and reticulate p.** A rare syndrome characterized by the development, usually in the second decade, of an irregular network of warty papules around the midline of the chest and back. Also *Gougerot-Carteaud syndrome.* **malignant p. of Degos** A disseminated vasculitis with distinctive cutaneous papular lesions. Also *malignant papulosis.*

**papillomatous** \pap′ilō′mətəs\ Pertaining to a papilloma.

**papillomavirus** \pap′əlō′məvī′rəs\ [PAPILLOMA + VIRUS] Any virus of the *Papillomavirus* genus and Papovaviridae family, consisting of small, ether-resistant, icosahedral viruses with double-stranded circular DNA which causes warts, or papillomas, in various species of animals including humans, rabbits, and dogs. **human p.** A papillomavirus that causes plain warts and common plantar warts in humans. Transmission appears to be by both direct and indirect contact. The virus causes proliferation of the malpighian layer of the skin and both eosinophilic and basophilic intranuclear inclusions. At least three serologic types have been distinguished. Also *wart virus, human wart virus.* **rabbit p.** SHOPE PAPILLOMAVIRUS. **Shope p.** A papillomavirus which produces papilloma in wild rabbits. This is of historical importance because it is one of the first viruses to be shown to produce tumors in animals. Also *rabbit papillomavirus, Shope papilloma virus.*

**Papillon** [M. M. *Papillon,* French dermatologist, flourished 20th century] Papillon-Lefèvre syndrome. See under SYNDROME.

**papillopathy** \pap′iläp′əthē\ **ischemic p.** Ischemia of the optic disk and retina, often producing low-tension glaucoma.

**papilloretinitis** \-ret′inī′tis\ [PAPILLO- + RETINITIS] NEURORETINITIS.

**papillose** \pap′ilōs\ PAPILLIFEROUS.

**papillosphincterotomy** \-sfingk′tərät′əmē\ An incision into the ampulla hepatopancreatica so as to relieve a relative or absolute stricture or to permit passage of a common bile duct stone.

**papillula** \pəpil′yələ\ **1** A small papilla. **2** NIPPLE.

**Papovaviridae** \pəpō′vəvir′idē\ [*pa(pilloma)* + *po(lyoma)* + *va(cuolating agent)* + *vir(us)* + -IDAE] A family of DNA viruses associated with the production of tumors. It includes papillomaviruses, polyomaviruses, and the SV40-like human viruses.

**papovavirus** \pəpō′vəvī′rəs\ Any member of the family Papovaviridae.

**Pappenheim** [Arthur *Pappenheim,* German internist, 1870–1916] **1** Unna-Pappenheim stain. See under STAIN. **2** Pappenheim's reagent. See under STAIN. **3** Lymphoid hemoblast of Pappenheim. See under HEMATOGONE.

**papular** \pap′yələr\ [*papul(e)* + -AR] Consisting of or pertaining to a papule.

**papule** \pap′yool\ [L *papula* a pimple, pustule, tubercle] A small palpable elevation of the skin. Also *pimple* (popular). **mucous p.** FLAT CONDYLOMA. **pearly penile p.'s** HIRSUTOID PAPILLOMAS OF THE PENIS. **piezogenic pedal p.'s** Soft, skin-colored papules that form on the part of the heel that does not bear weight. They are caused by a herniation of fat into the dermis and can be painful when the subject is standing. **prurigo p.** An intensely irritable papule in any of the forms of prurigo.

**papulopustule** \pap′yəlōpus′tyool\ [*papul(e)* + *o* + PUSTULE] A papule that becomes a pustule.

**papulosis** \pap′yəlō′sis\ [*papul(a)* + -OSIS] A condition characterized by the development of papules. **lymphomatoid p.** A skin condition that is characterized by the appearance of crops of pruritic papules. Histologic features are suggestive of a lymphoma, but the clinical course is benign though chronic. **miliary p.** MILIARIA PAPULOSA.

**par** \pär\ [L, equal, a pair] A pair.

**par-** \par-\ PARA-.

**para** \par′ə\ [back-formation from the word-ending *-para* (as in *primipara*), from L *parere* to give birth] A woman who has borne a viable offspring, regardless of whether the child was stillborn. • The term is often used in conjunction with numerals to designate the number of pregnancies that have produced viable offspring. Thus, a woman who has borne no viable offspring is designated *para 0* (or *nullipara*); one viable offspring, *para I* (or *primipara*); two offspring, *para II* (or *secundipara*); three offspring, *para III* (or *tripara*), and so forth. The number refers to the number of viable pregnancies, not necessarily to the number of offspring; a multiple birth counts as one.

**para-** \par′ə-\ [Gk *para* beside, alongside of] **1** A prefix meaning (1) beside, bordering; (2) beyond, apart from; (3) resembling but not identical to (a specified condition or disease); (4) secondary, ancillary; (5) diverging from the normal or regular; disordered or diseased. Also *par-*. **2** In chemistry, a prefix indicating that the substituent prefixed is on ring atom number 4 of a benzene derivative, i.e., on the opposite side of the ring to the reference substituent. Symbol: *p-*

**para-actinomycosis** \-ak′tinōmīkō′sis\ PSEUDOACTINOMYCOSIS.

**para-albuminemia** \-albyoo′mənē′mē·ə\ BISALBUMINEMIA.

**para-aortic** \-ā·ôr′tik\ Situated beside the aorta. Also *paraortic*.

**parabigeminal** \-bījem′inəl\ Adjacent to the superior and inferior colliculi of the midbrain.

**parabiosis** \-bī·ō′sis\ [PARA- + BIOSIS] The joining of two animals by their major blood vessels to form artificial Siamese twins. Adj. parabiotic.

***Parabuthus*** \-boo′thəs\ A genus of dangerous scorpions found in arid regions of Africa from South Africa to the Sudan.

**paracardiac** \-kär′dē·ak\ [PARA- + CARDIAC] By the side of the heart.

**paracasein** The product of partial digestion of casein with chymosin. *Obs.*

**paracele** \par′əsēl\ [PARA- + -CELE[2]] *Obs.* VENTRICULUS LATERALIS CEREBRI.

**Paracelsus** [Philippus Aureolus *Paracelsus*, Swiss alchemist and physician, 1493–1541] Paracelsian method. See under METHOD.

**paracentesis** \-sentē′sis\ [PARA- + -CENTESIS] The insertion of a fine hollow needle into a body cavity for the purpose of aspirating fluid. This may be done for either diagnostic or therapeutic reasons. Also *nyxis*. **abdominal p.** ABDOMINOCENTESIS. **p. abdominis** ABDOMINOCENTESIS. **p. of the chest** THORACENTESIS. **p. cordis** Surgical puncture of the heart. Also *cardiopuncture, cardiocentesis*. **p. ovarii** OVARIOCENTESIS. **p. pericardii** A puncture of the pericardial cavity for removal of fluid. It is usually performed with a needle. **p. pulmonis** Surgical puncture of a lung to drain fluid from an abscess or cyst. **p. thoracis** THORACENTESIS. **p. tunicae vaginalis** Surgical puncture of the tunica vaginalis testis. **p. tympani** MYRINGOTOMY. **p. vesicae** Surgical puncture of the urinary bladder, as for relief of obstruction.

**paracerebellar** \-ser′əbel′ər\ Denoting the lateral portions of the cerebellum.

**paracetaldehyde** PARALDEHYDE.

**paracetamol** ACETAMINOPHEN.

**parachlorometaxylenol** $C_8H_9ClO$. 4-Chloro-3,5-dimethylphenol, a halogenated phenolic disinfectant used most often on skin surfaces. It is formulated in a cream, lotion, and solution for topical application.

**parachlorophenol** $C_6H_5ClO$. A topical antibacterial agent specific for most Gram-negative organisms. Also *p-chlorophenol*. **camphorated p.** A preparation of 33–37% parachlorophenol and 63–67% camphor. It is used in dentistry as an anti-infective agent for endodontic procedures. It is applied topically to root canals and the periapical region.

**paracholera** \-käl′ərə\ A disease which resembles cholera clinically but is caused by a microorganism other than *Vibrio cholerae*.

**parachordal** \-kôr′dəl\ Situated alongside the notochord.

**paraclonus** \-klō′nəs\ PARAMYOCLONUS MULTIPLEX.

**paracnemidion** \par′ak·nēmid′ē·än\ *Outmoded* FIBULA.

**paracnemis** \par′ak·nē′mis\ *Outmoded* FIBULA.

**paracoccidioidomycosis** \-käksid′ē·oi′dōmīkō′sis\ [PARA- + COCCIDIOIDOMYCOSIS] SOUTH AMERICAN BLASTOMYCOSIS.

**paracoele** \par′əsēl\ [PARA- + -COELE] *Obs.* VENTRICULUS LATERALIS CEREBRI.

**paracolpitis** \-kälpī′tis\ [PARA- + COLPITIS] Inflammation of tissue around the vagina. Also *paravaginitis, pericolpitis, perivaginitis*.

**paracolpium** \-käl′pē·əm\ The tissues that surround the vagina.

**paracone** \par′əkōn\ [PARA- + CONE] The mesiobuccal cusp of the trigon; the outer anterior cusp of the mammalian upper molar tooth.

**paracoxalgia** \-käksal′jə\ A pain similar to that caused by a hip joint disease.

**paracusia** \-kyoo′sē·ə\ [*paracus(is)* + -IA] A hearing disorder. **p. loci** Difficulty in sound localization.

**paracusis** \-k[y]oo′sis\ [Gk *parakousis* (from *par(a)-* mis- + *akousis* hearing) a mishearing] An additional, sometimes intrusive auditory phenomenon noticed by the subject, often in specific and identifiable circumstances. **p. of Willis** The auditory phenomenon in which the hearing-impaired subject finds he can hear speech better in noisy surroundings.

**paracystic** \-sis′tik\ Located alongside or around the urinary bladder. Also *paravesical*.

**paracystitis** \-sistī′tis\ [PARA- + CYSTITIS] Inflammation of the connective and other tissues surrounding the urinary bladder.

**paracystium** \-sis′tē·əm\ The tissue around or near the urinary bladder.

**paradental** \-den′təl\ [PARA- + DENTAL] PERIODONTAL.

**paradentitis** \-dentī′tis\ PERIODONTITIS.

**paradentium** \-den′shē·əm\ PERIODONTIUM.

**paraderm** \par′ədurm\ [PARA- + -DERM] That part of the vitellus where cells develop to produce those forming the body of an embryo.

**paradidymis** \-did′imis\ [PARA- + *(epi)didymis*] A small collection of convoluted tubules lined with ciliated columnar epithelium and situated above the head of the epididymis in the lower part of the spermatic cord. They are formed from the caudal tubules of the mesonephros of the male embryo.

**paradontosis** \-däntō′sis\ PERIODONTOSIS.

**paradox** \par′ədäks\ [Gk *paradoxos* (from PARA- + Gk *doxa* a notion, opinion, judgment, from *dokein* to think, expect, imagine) contrary to opinion, strange, unexpected] A statement that apparently cannot be true, as because of its incompatibility with known facts or its contradiction of widely held opinion, but that may nevertheless be true. **neurotic p.** The persistence of neurotic symptoms even though they bring distress, pain, and harm to the subject. At least superficially such persistence is contrary to all learning theory in that the pain of the symptoms should extinguish the symptoms rather than maintain them.

**paradoxical** \-däk′siəkəl\ Of the nature of a paradox; possibly true but appearing to contradict facts or confirmed opinion.

**paradysentery** \-dis′ənter′ē\ **1** A diarrheal illness resembling mild dysentery. **2** Bacillary dysentery caused by *Shigella flexneri (S. paradysenteriae).*

**paraendocrine** \par′ə·en′dəkrīn\ **1** Capable of secreting polypeptides or amines foreign to the specific cells but normally secreted by other APUD cells: used especially of a kind of apudoma. **2** Describing an endocrine function of an organ not conventionally regarded as an endocrine gland. Activation of angiotensin I by normal lung tissue and secretion of adrenocorticotropin by a thymic tumor are paraendocrine activities.

**paraenteric** \par′ə·enter′ik\ PARENTERIC.

**paraepilepsy** \par′ə·ep′ilep′sē\ MINOR FOCAL EPILEPSY.

**paraesophageal** \par′ə·ē′sōfā′jē·əl\ Adjacent to the esophagus.

**paraesthesia** *Brit.* PARESTHESIA.

**parafascicular** \-fasik′yələr\ Adjacent to a fascicle, or bundle of nerve fibers.

**par. aff.** *pars affecta* (L, the part affected).

**paraffin** \par′əfin\ [German, from L *par(um)* insufficient, insignificant and L *affin(itas)* affinity; so called for its neutral properties.] ALKANE. **liquid p.** MINERAL OIL. **pliable p.** A mixture of paraffin and other substances formerly used to make a flexible dressing for burns and wounds. It is currently used as a liquid in a tank designed to allow exercise of the extremities under a decreased influence of gravity.

**paraffinoma** \-finō′mə\ A tumorlike chronic inflammatory reaction due to continuous exposure to paraffin. Also *paraffin tumor, oleogranuloma.*

**paraflagellate** \-flaj′əlāt\ PARAMASTIGOTE.

**paraflocculus** \-fläk′yələs\ [NA] ACCESSORY FLOCCULUS.

**paraformaldehyde** Polymeric material reversibly formed from formaldehyde, which it can slowly form by depolymerization.

***Parafossarulus*** \-fäser′ələs\ A genus of small, conical freshwater snails in the family Hydrobiidae. ***P. manchouricus*** A species that is the principal intermediate host of the liver fluke *Clonorchis sinensis* in Japan and an important host in China as well. It also harbors *Opisthorchis tenuicollis (O. felineus)* and *Echinochasmus perfoliatus.*.

**parafoveal** \-fō′vē·əl\ Pertaining to the macular area immediately surrounding the fovea centralis.

**parafunction** \par′əfungk′shən\ Abnormal or disordered function.

**paragammacism** \-gam′əsizm\ [PARA- + Gk *gamma,* third letter of the alphabet + *c* + -ISM] Inability to pronounce *g* and *k* correctly.

**paraganglia** \-gang′glē·ə\ Plural of PARAGANGLION.

**paraganglioma** \-gang′glē·ō′mə\ [*paragangli(a)* + -OMA] A tumor of paraganglia or of a chemoreceptor organ, such as a glomus jugulare tumor. Also *receptoma, chemoreceptor tumor, chemodectoma.* **medullary p.** PHEOCHROMOCYTOMA. **nonchromaffin p.** A paraganglioma whose cells do not give a positive chromaffin reaction.

**paraganglion** \-gang′glē·än\ (*pl.* paraganglia) **1** In embryology, a structure derived from the neural crest and composed of cells secreting substances analogous to those secreted by nerve cells at the periphery. Also *chromaffin body, Zuckerkandl's body.* **2** A collection of chromaffin or nonchromaffin cells situated along the aorta, its major branches, or associated with autonomic ganglia. **adrenergic p.** A paraganglion which secretes epinephrine and norepinephrine. The most important example is the suprarenal medulla which arises from several ganglionic primordia derived from the neural crest. The constituent cells migrate more or less in isolation, become mixed together and invade the medial side of the cortical primordium, and then form the tissue mass (medulla) in the center of the suprarenal. The presence of epinephrine can be recognized fairly early (twelfth week in man), but the histochemical reactions for chromaffin tissue only become obvious later. It is only after birth that epinephrine is present in high concentration. **aortic paraganglia** CORPORA PARA-AORTICA. **cardiac paraganglia** **1** The corpora para-aortica situated within the cardiac plexus. **2** Paraganglia that are associated with sympathetic ganglia of the cardiac plexus. **cholinergic p.** A paraganglion which, unlike the adrenergic paraganglion, will not give the chromaffin reaction for epinephrine but secretes acetylcholine.

**paragenesis** \-jen′əsis\ **1** Modification of embryonic development brought about artificially by experimental means. **2** Production in an animal or plant of characteristics belonging to two different species, as in hybridism.

**paragenetic** \-jənet′ik\ Of or pertaining to an alteration in the expression of one or more syntenic genes by a change in the chromosome that does not occur within any of the affected loci.

**paragenitalis** \-jen′itā′lis\ [PARA- + L *genitalis* genital] The paradidymis in the male or the paroöphoron in the female.

**parageusia** \-joo′sē·ə\ [PARA- + Gk *geus(is)* taste + -IA] Distortion or perversion of the sense of taste, usually giving an unpleasant taste in the mouth. Adj. parageusic.

**paragglutination** \par′əgloo′tinā′shən\ GROUP AGGLUTINATION.

**paraglobulin** *Obs.* THROMBIN.

**paragnathus** \pərag′nəthəs, par′agnath′əs\ [PARA- + Gk *gnathos* jaw, esp. the lower jaw] An embryo, fetus, or postnatal individual with an accessory jaw or parts thereof.

**paragnosis** \par′agnō′sis\ [PARA- + Gk *gnōsis* inquiry, knowledge] A posthumous analysis of a person's physical disabilities and diseases based on descriptions of physical signs and symptoms left by the individual or his contemporaries, a method used to surmise the cause of death of historical personages who lived in eras before modern medicine.

**paragomphosis** \-gämfō′sis\ [PARA- + Gk *gomph(oun)* (from *gomphos* a large nail or bolt) to nail or bolt + -OSIS] Impaction of the fetal head in the birth canal.

**paragonimiasis** \-gō′nimī′əsis\ Infection with flukes of the genus *Paragonimus,* most commonly *P. westermani.* Distributed throughout southeast Asia and the Pacific, it is also present in India, Sri Lanka, and west Africa. Human infection is caused by ingestion of crayfish or crabs eaten raw, salted, or pickled. Most infections are asymptomatic, but chest infections with fever and blood-stained sputum may occur. Chronic bronchitis, bronchiectasis, pleural effusions, and fibrosis are complications. Also *parasitic hemoptysis, pulmonary diastomiasis, endemic hemoptysis, lung fluke disease, oriental lung fluke disease, oriental hemoptysis, paragonimosis.*

***Paragonimus*** \-gän′əməs\ A genus of flukes in the family Troglotrematidae (sometimes given family rank, Paragonimidae), parasitic in the lungs of humans and many other mammals. The best known is *Paragonimus westermani* (lung fluke) although several species are pathogenic in man. ***P. kellicotti*** A species similar to *P. westermani* that is found in the lungs of dogs, cats, hogs, man, and a wide variety of carnivores in the eastern United States, particularly in the Great Lakes region. It is transmitted by pomatiopsid snails as an initial host and freshwater crustaceans, such as crayfish, as second host. ***P. ringeri*** *PARAGONIMUS WESTERMANI*. ***P. westermani*** A species that is distributed throughout Korea, Japan, China, Thailand, and the Philippines. Commonly known as the human lung fluke, it is the cause of paragonimiasis. Adult worms usually are found paired in cysts in the lungs and occasionally in the pleura, abdominal cavity, liver, or brain. They are oval, reddish-brown, and heavily encapsulated, 8 to 12 by 4 to 6 mm by 3 mm thick. The ova, passed in feces or sputum, hatch, releasing miracidia that invade pomatiopsid snails such as *Melania* or *Semisulcospira*. After larval mutiplication in the snail, the short-tailed cercariae leave and crawl to crabs or crayfish, entering muscles and viscera. Infection is acquired by ingesting undercooked or raw crustacea or uncooked foods contaminated with material from infected crustacea. Metacercaria excyst in the duodenum and migrate through the gut wall and diaphragm and enter the lungs. The flukes cause inflammation and form fibrous pulmonary nodules. Also *Distoma ringeri* (obs.), *Distoma westermani* (obs.), *Paragonimus ringeri*.

**paragrammatism** \-gram′ətizm\ [PARA- + *grammat(ic)* + -ISM] Inability to construct a phrase correctly or to recognize grammatical errors in test phrases.

**paragranuloma** \-gran′yəlō′mə\ A subdivision in the now obsolete Jackson and Parker classification of Hodgkin's disease. It corresponds to lymphocyte-predominant Hodgkin's disease in current classifications, and is of relatively favorable prognosis.

**paragraphia** \-graf′ē·ə\ A variant of agraphia, related to receptive aphasia, in which the patient substitutes incorrect or nonexistent words for the correct ones.

**parahemophilia** \-hē′mōfil′yə\ FACTOR V DEFICIENCY.

**parahepatitis** \-hep′ətī′tis\ PERIHEPATITIS.

**paraheredity** \-həred′itē\ The transmission of hereditary information from mother cell to daughter cells by a medium other than nuclear DNA.

**parahexyl** SYNHEXYL.

**parahormone** \-hôr′mōn\ A substance resembling a hormone in its effects but not recognized as a true hormone.

**parahypophysis** \-hīpäf′isis\ [PARA- + HYPOPHYSIS] An accessory or ectopic pituitary gland.

**parainfluenza** \-in′floo·en′zə\ **1** A disease caused by a parainfluenza virus. Most commonly, parainfluenza viruses produce a common cold with bronchitis, but they may cause severe illnesses, the most common of which are the croup syndrome, bronchiolitis, and pneumonia. **2** Any disease clinically resembling influenza but caused by an organism other than the influenza viruses. *Imprecise*.

**parainfluenzal** \-in′floo·en′zəl\ Pertaining to parainfluenza.

**parakeratosis** \-ker′ətō′sis\ [PARA- + KERATOSIS] An abnormality of keratinization in which the cells of the stratum corneum retain their nuclei. Clinically, parakeratosis usually manifests as scaling. **p. ostracea** PARAKERATOSIS SCUTULARIS. **p. psoriasiformis** An eruption characterized by thick scales resembling those of psoriasis. **p. scutularis** An eruption of hard, shieldlike, crusted scaly lesions that affect mainly the legs and sometimes the scalp. The hair follicles are involved and the emerging hairs are enveloped by the crusted scales. The condition is rare and may be an unusual form of psoriasis. Also *parakeratosis ostracea, parakeratosis scutularis of Unna*. **p. variegata** POIKILODERMA ATROPHICANS VASCULARE.

**paralambdacism** \-lam′dəsizm\ A speech defect in which there is difficulty in articulating the sounds represented by the letter *l*.

**paraldehyde** $C_6H_{12}O$. 2,4,6-Trimethyl-1,3,5-trioxane. A polymeric form of acetaldehyde with rapidly acting sedative and hypnotic properties. It is used therapeutically in the control of agitation, delirium, excitement, convulsions, and insomnia. It is a colorless liquid, and is given rectally, intramuscularly, or by intravenous infusion. Also *paracetaldehyde*.

**paraldehydism** \pəral′dəhī′dizm\ A condition produced by excessive use of paraldehyde, which has been used as a hypnotic and anticonvulsant. Prolonged administration may result in mental deterioration along with other symptoms resembling those of chronic alcoholism. See also PARALDEHYDE POISONING.

**paralexia** \-lek′sē·ə\ [PAR- + ALEXIA] A form of alexia, causing difficulty in reading aloud and marked by the substitution of meaningless words for some of those in the text. Adj. paralexic.

**paralgesia** \par′aljē′sē·ə\ Painful paresthesiae. Also *paralgia*. Adj. paralgesic.

**parallax** \par′əlaks\ [Gk *parallax* (from PARA- + Gk *allos* other, another) alternately, in alternating rows] The apparent displacement of the background some distance behind an object when the observer changes his position of view. Parallactic displacement observed during ophthalmoscopy establishes the fact that the object under examination is elevated above the fundus background. Adj. parallactic. **crossed p.** The displacement of images found in exotropia when seen alternately with each eye. Also *heteronymous parallax*. **heteronymous p.** CROSSED PARALLAX. **homonymous p.** UNCROSSED PARALLAX. **uncrossed p.** The apparent movement of the most distant of two objects when the position of the observer is changed. In relation to the nearer object, the distant object moves the same direction as does the observer. Also *homonymous parallax*. **vertical p.** The apparent vertical movement of images seen when changing fixation from one eye to the other in strabismus in which one eye is higher than the other.

**paralyses** \pəral′isēz\ Plural of PARALYSIS.

# paralysis

**paralysis** \pəral′isis\ [Gk (from *paralyesthai* to be disengaged, disabled, paralyzed, from *para-* beside, off, amiss + *lyein* to loose, undo) disablement, paralysis] Transient or permanent loss of motor function, generally caused by disease or dysfunction of the central nervous system or of the peripheral neuromuscular system. Also *palsy*. Adj. paralytic. **abducens p.** Paralysis of the lateral rectus muscle due to a lesion of the sixth cranial (abducens) nerve which supplies it. **p. of accommodation** CYCLOPLEGIA. **acute ascending p.** LANDRY'S PARALYSIS. **acute ascending spinal p.** LANDRY'S PARALYSIS. **acute atrophic p.** PARALYTIC POLIOMYELITIS. **acute infectious p.** ACUTE ANTERIOR POLIOMYELITIS. **acute spinal p.** ACUTE ANTERIOR POLIOMYELITIS. **acute wasting p.** ACUTE ANTERIOR POLIOMYELITIS. **p. agitans** The idiopathic variety of Parkinson's disease, which usually begins in middle or late life. Characteristic symptoms are a masklike facial expression, a progressive stoop, tremor, rigidity, and akinesia in varying combinations with a shuffling or a festinating gait. The voice becomes slow and monotonous, and there may be associated autonomic disturbances, such as excessive salivation and sweating. The principal pathologic abnormalities are in the substantia nigra, where the content of dopamine is smaller than normal. Also *chorea festinans* (obs.), *shaking palsy, basal-ganglionic paralysis, pseudoparalysis agitans* (obs.), *locus niger snydrome, paleostriatal syndrome, paralysis agitans syndrome.* **alcoholic p.** 1 ALCOHOLIC NEUROPATHY. 2 ALCOHOLIC MYOPATHY. **alternate p.** CROSSED PARALYSIS. **alternating p.** CROSSED PARALYSIS. **ambiguoaccessorius-hypoglossal p.** JACKSON'S PARALYSIS. **ambiguospinothalamic p.** AVELLIS PARALYSIS. **anterior spinal p.** ACUTE ANTERIOR POLIOMYELITIS. **ascending p.** Any form of paralysis marked by weakness which progresses upwards from the feet and legs, as caused by some spinal cord lesions and in some forms of polyneuropathy. **ascending tick p.** Ascending myelitis due to the bite of a tick, often attributed to *Ixodes pilosus,* the paralysis tick, or to species of *Dermacentor.* The precise cause is unknown, but the ticks are found attached in the occipital region, often for a prolonged period. It has been reported in children in western North America, and in dogs, sheep, and calves. Also *tick paralysis.* **association p.** BULBAR PARALYSIS. **asthenic bulbar p.** *Incorrect* MYASTHENIA GRAVIS. **asthenobulbospinal p.** *Incorrect* MYASTHENIA GRAVIS. **atrophic muscular p.** PROGRESSIVE MUSCULAR ATROPHY. **atrophic spinal p.** ACUTE ANTERIOR POLIOMYELITIS. **Avellis p.** Unilateral paralysis of the soft palate, pharynx, and vocal cords due to a lesion of the vagal nucleus in brainstem infarction. Also *Avellis hemiplegia, Avellis syndrome, Avellis-Longhi syndrome, ambiguospinothalamic paralysis, syndrome of the nucleus ambiguus and spinal fillet.* **axillary nerve p.** A syndrome resulting from a lesion of the axillary nerve leading to paralysis of the deltoid muscle with impairment of flexion and abduction of the arm at the shoulder, with a patch of sensory loss over the upper outer aspect of the arm near the insertion of the deltoid. This may be caused by fracture of the neck of the humerus, dislocation of the shoulder, or neuralgic amyotrophy (shoulder-girdle neuritis). Also *axillary paralysis, circumflex paralysis.* **basal-ganglionic p.** PARALYSIS AGITANS. **Bell's p.** BELL'S PALSY. **bifacial p.** FACIAL DIPLEGIA. **bilateral laryngeal abductor p.** Laryngeal abductor paralysis where both vocal cords are involved so that the glottis is seriously narrowed and fails to open on inspiration. When the onset is sudden, as when both recurrent laryngeal nerves are injured during neck surgery, respiratory obstruction may occur and urgent tracheostomy or intubation may be necessary. Also *bilateral cord palsy.* **birth p.** Paralysis due to birth injury to the spinal cord, roots, or plexuses. **brachial plexus p.** Paralysis of various upper limb muscles caused by damage to one or more components of the brachial plexus, in which the symptoms and signs vary according to the site of the damage. Two principal forms of birth injury to the plexus due to difficult delivery, Erb's paralysis and Klumpke's paralysis have been described. In later life physical injury, as in road accidents, is the commonest cause. Also *brachial paralysis, brachial palsy.* **brachiofacial p.** Paralysis of one side of the face and of the arm on the same side. **Brown-Séquard p.** BROWN-SÉQUARD SYNDROME. **bulbar p.** Paralysis of muscles supplied by the lower motor cranial nerves (the bulbar muscles). Also *association paralysis.* **bulbospinal p.** MYASTHENIA GRAVIS. **central p.** Any form of paralysis attributable to damage to the central nervous system. . *Obs.* **central facial p.** The type of facial muscle weakness which is seen as a consequence of contralateral supranuclear upper motor neuron lesions, as in hemiplegia. Weakness is most evident in the lower facial muscles around the angle of the mouth, while those of the forehead and around the eye may contract almost normally. **cerebral spastic infantile p.** SPASTIC DIPLEGIA. **cervical sympathetic p.** Any lesion of the cervical sympathetic ganglia or trunk giving rise to the Horner syndrome. **circumflex p.** AXILLARY NERVE PARALYSIS. **common peroneal nerve p.** Loss of dorsiflexion of the foot and of the proximal toe joints, with loss of abduction of the foot, leading to footdrop. This is caused by a lesion of the lateral popliteal or common peroneal branch of the sciatic nerve near the head of the fibula (fracture or compression or irritation) and is usually associated with anesthesia over the posterolateral aspect of the foot and over the anterolateral aspect of the leg, together with atrophy of the anterior tibial and peroneal muscles. Also *Zenker's paralysis, lateral popliteal palsy.* **congenital abducens-facial p.** MÖBIUS SYNDROME. **congenital p. of horizontal gaze** MÖBIUS SYNDROME. **congenital oculofacial p.** MÖBIUS SYNDROME. **conjugate p.** Paralysis of simultaneous movements of both eyes in the same direction due to a disorder of supranuclear innervation. **creeping p.** PROGRESSIVE MUSCULAR ATROPHY. **crossed p.** 1 Paralysis caused by damage to the corticospinal (pyramidal) tract above the bulbar decussation. 2 Paralysis affecting one side of the face and the opposite side of the trunk and limbs and resulting from a pontine lesion involving the facial nerve nucleus and the corticospinal tract. Also *alternate paralysis, alternating paralysis, cruciate paralysis, transverse palsy.* **crossed hypoglossal p.** MEDIAN MEDULLARY SYNDROME. **cruciate p.** CROSSED PARALYSIS. **crural p.** FEMORAL NERVE PARALYSIS. **crutch p.** Radial nerve palsy or other manifestations of pressure upon the nerves arising from the brachial plexus, sometimes with associated features of limb ischemia, due to pressure of an axillary crutch on the brachial artery. **Cruveilhier's p.** PROGRESSIVE MUSCULAR ATROPHY. **cubital p.** ULNAR NERVE PARALYSIS. **decubitus p.** Compression paralysis of one or more peripheral nerves in bedridden subjects. **Dejerine-Klumpke p.** DEJERINE-KLUMPKE SYNDROME. **divers' p.** Spastic paraplegia or monoplegia involving the lower extremities and resulting from bubble formation in the blood vessels and in the tissues of the spinal cord. It is a serious complication of decompression sickness. Also *divers' palsy.* **drunkards'-arm p.** SATURDAY NIGHT PARALYSIS. **Duchenne's p.** 1 DUCHENNE-ERB SYNDROME. 2 DUCHENNE TYPE MUSCULAR DYSTROPHY. **Duchenne-Erb p.** DUCHENNE-ERB SYNDROME. **epidemic infantile p.** ACUTE ANTERIOR POLIOMYELITIS. **epidural ascending spinal p.** Ascending paraparesis due either to spinal pachymeningitis or to spinal epidural abscess. **Erb's p.** 1 DUCHENNE-ERB SYNDROME. 2 LIMB-GIRDLE MUSCULAR DYSTROPHY. 3 SYPHILITIC SPASTIC PARAPLEGIA. **Erb-Duchenne p.** DUCHENNE-ERB SYNDROME. **Erb syphilitic spinal p.** SYPHILITIC SPASTIC PARAPLEGIA. **esophageal p.** Paralysis of esophageal movements, however produced. Also *lemoparalysis.* **essential p.** Paralysis of unknown cause. **extraocular p.** Paralysis of any of the extraocular muscles. **facial p.** Weakness or paralysis of facial muscles resulting from paralysis of the facial nerve (seventh cranial nerve), as in Bell's palsy. Also *facioplegia.* **false p.** PSEUDOPARALYSIS. **familial hyperkalemic periodic**

**p.** PERIODIC PARALYSIS II. **familial hypokalemic periodic p.** PERIODIC PARALYSIS I. **familial infantile bulbar p.** INFANTILE PROGRESSIVE BULBAR PALSY. **familial periodic p.** PERIODIC PARALYSIS. **familial recurrent p.** PERIODIC PARALYSIS. **familial spastic p.** HEREDITARY SPASTIC PARAPLEGIA. **faucial p.** Paralysis of the muscles of the faucial arches, the palatoglossus, and palatopharyngeal muscles, occurring as an element of palatal paralysis. **Felton's p.** A form of specific immunologic unresponsiveness produced by a large dose of pneumococcal polysaccharide. Since the antigen cannot be degraded *in vivo*, the unresponsiveness was attributed to a continuous process of the antibody formed reacting with antigen and being catabolized, the antigen being then available for further reaction. Also *treadmill phenomenon.* **femoral nerve p.** Paralysis of the quadriceps with impaired hip flexion and virtual paralysis of knee extension, caused by a lesion of the femoral nerve (intrapelvic compression, pelvic fracture, femoral fracture, infarction, diabetic amyotrophy, etc.), and accompanied by anesthesia over the anterior aspect of the thigh, the internal aspect of the leg, and the inner edge of the foot. Also *crural paralysis.* **flaccid p.** Paralysis with complete loss of muscle tone and absence of deep tendon reflexes. **functional p.** Any type of paralysis due to emotional causes and not resulting from organic disease of the central or peripheral nervous system. **p. of gaze** Paralysis of conjugate ocular movement in any direction. **general p.** GENERAL PARESIS. **ginger p.** JAMAICA JAKE PARALYSIS. **glossolabial p.** PROGRESSIVE BULBAR PALSY. **glossopharyngolabial p.** PROGRESSIVE BULBAR PALSY. **Gubler's p.** MILLARD-GUBLER SYNDROME. **Gubler-Millard p.** MILLARD-GUBLER SYNDROME. **hereditary cerebrospinal p.** HEREDITARY SPASTIC PARAPLEGIA. **hyperkalemic periodic p.** PERIODIC PARALYSIS II. **hypoglossal p.** Paralysis of the muscles of one half of the tongue due to a lesion of the hypoglossal nucleus in the medulla oblongata or of the trunk of the nerve in its peripheral course. When the tongue is protruded it deviates to the paralyzed side, and there may be consequent slight dysarthria. Eventually wasting of the muscles of the tongue on the affected side becomes conspicuous. **hypokalemic periodic p.** PERIODIC PARALYSIS I. **idiopathic facial p.** BELL'S PALSY. **immune p.** The loss of immune reactivity to a specific antigen following exposure to massive doses of that antigen. Also *immunologic paralysis.* **incomplete p.** PARESIS. **infantile p.** ACUTE ANTERIOR POLIOMYELITIS. **infantile cerebral ataxic p.** Ataxic cerebral palsy. See under CEREBRAL PALSY. **infantile flaccid and atrophic spinal p.** ACUTE ANTERIOR POLIOMYELITIS. **infantile nuclear p.** *Incorrect* MÖBIUS SYNDROME. **infantile spastic p.** LITTLE'S DISEASE. **infantile spinal p.** ACUTE ANTERIOR POLIOMYELITIS. **inferior alternate p.** MILLARD-GUBLER SYNDROME. **infranuclear p.** Paralysis of any of the motor cranial nerves due to a lesion at some point in the course of the nerve distal to its nucleus in the brainstem. **internuclear p.** INTERNUCLEAR OPHTHALMOPLEGIA. **ischemic p.** Paralysis due to lack of blood supply to nerve or muscle. Also *ischemic palsy.* **Jackson's p.** A rare brainstem syndrome, usually due to infarction, comprising damage to the nuclei of the ninth, tenth, eleventh, and twelfth cranial nerves on one side of the medulla oblongata, and giving rise to unilateral paralysis of the pharyngeal and laryngeal muscles and soft palate, unilateral paralysis of the sternomastoid and trapezius muscles, and of the muscles of one side of the tongue. These signs, involving muscles on the same side as the lesion, are usually accompanied by variable contralateral motor and sensory changes in the trunk and limbs due to the involvement of long ascending and descending tracts. Also *Jackson-Mackenzie syndrome, Mackenzie syndrome, Jackson syndrome, ambiguoaccessorius-hypoglossal paralysis, vagoaccessory hypoglossal paralysis.* **Jamaica jake p.** Neuropathy due to bootleg alcohol contaminated with triorthocresylphosphate. Also *jake neuritis, jake palsy, ginger paralysis, jake paralysis, Jamaica ginger paralysis, Jamaica ginger polyneuritis, Jamaican neuropathy.* See also TRIORTHOCRESYL PHOSPHATE NEUROPATHY. **juvenile p.** JUVENILE PARESIS. **juvenile p. agitans** Paralysis agitans developing in early life, due to degeneration of the globus pallidus and substantia nigra. This condition may be familial. Also *Ramsay Hunt syndrome, Ramsay Hunt paralysis, Hunt's disease, pallidal atrophy, juvenile parkinsonism,Hunt striatal syndrome, Winkelman's disease,.* **juvenile distal atrophic p.** CHARCOT-MARIE-TOOTH DISEASE. **juvenile general p.** JUVENILE PARESIS. **Klumpke's p.** DEJERINE-KLUMPKE SYNDROME. **Klumpke-Dejerine p.** DEJERINE-KLUMPKE SYNDROME. **Kussmaul's p.** LANDRY'S PARALYSIS. **Kussmaul-Landry p.** LANDRY'S PARALYSIS. **labial p.** PROGRESSIVE BULBAR PALSY. **labioglossolaryngeal p.** PROGRESSIVE BULBAR PALSY. **labioglossopharyngeal p.** PROGRESSIVE BULBAR PALSY. **Landry's p.** A syndrome of acute ascending flaccid paralysis, beginning in the legs and spreading to involve the trunk and upper limbs and often the respiratory and bulbar muscles. This is a syndrome of multiple etiology, in rare cases resulting from poliomyelitis but more often due to either transverse myelitis or the Guillain-Barré syndrome. *Obs.* Also *acute ascending paralysis, Landry's disease, Kussmaul's paralysis, Kussmaul-Landry paralysis, acute ascending spinal paralysis, Landry syndrome.* **laryngeal p.** Partial or complete loss of laryngeal muscular function, laryngeal sensation, or both, due to some lesion of the recurrent or superior laryngeal nerves, of the vagus nerves, or of their central connections. It may exist alone or as part of a symptom complex. **laryngeal abductor p.** Laryngeal paralysis affecting only or chiefly one or both posterior cricothyroid muscles. Also *posticus palsy* (older term). **lead p.** LEAD NEUROPATHY. **Little's p.** *Seldom used* ACUTE ANTERIOR POLIOMYELITIS. **lovers' p.** Saturday night paralysis produced by the partner's head resting on the arm. **lower brachial plexus p.** Paralysis due to a lesion of the medial (or lower) cord of the brachial plexus that results in the loss of ulnar nerve function, as in Dejerine-Klumpke syndrome. **masticatory p.** Paralysis of the muscles of mastication. It almost always occurs unilaterally. It is symptomatic of lesions involving the corresponding motor division of the trigeminal nerve. **medial popliteal nerve p.** Paralysis marked by loss of plantar flexion of the foot and of the proximal toe joints, and also by loss of adduction of the foot. This makes it impossible to stand on tiptoe (the Chiray sign) and may lead to walking on the heel and contracture of the anterior tibial muscle. The ankle jerk is abolished and the calf muscles are atrophic. There is anesthesia of the sole of the foot and of the toes. The nerve may be compressed by lesions in the popliteal fossa, or damaged by direct injury. **median p.** Paralysis caused by a lesion of the median nerve. If the lesion is situated in the arm, at the elbow, or in the upper forearm, there is impaired pronation of the forearm, flexion of the fingers (especially of the thumb, index, and middle fingers) and impaired opposition of the thumb to the other fingers with sensory loss over the palmar surface of all of the digits except the little finger and the ulnar half of the ring finger. A lesion at the wrist, as in the carpal tunnel syndrome, produces atrophy and weakness of the muscles of the lateral half of the thenar eminence and similar sensory loss. Also *paralysis of the median nerve.* **medullary tegmental paralyses** A series of syndromes resulting from infarction of the medullary tegmentum due to vertebrobasilar insufficiency. They include crossed hemiplegia and the syndromes of Tapia, Babinski-Nageotte, and Cestan. **mesencephalic p.** Crossed hemiplegia due to a midbrain lesion as in the Weber syndrome. **Millard-Gubler p.** MILLARD-GUBLER SYNDROME. **mimetic p.** Paralysis of facial muscles. **morning p.** SLEEP PARALYSIS. **motor p.** The loss of voluntary movement due to any lesion in the motor pathways. **motor trigeminal p.** TRIGEMINAL MASTICATOR PARALYSIS. **musculocutaneous nerve p.** Paralysis of flexion of the forearm at the elbow, caused by a lesion of the musculocutaneous nerve (which innervates the coracobrachialis, biceps brachii, and brachialis muscles), resulting most commonly from injury. This movement may still be possible in pronation due to the action of the brachioradialis. There may be a band of anesthesia on the anterior aspect of the forearm, but this is often only slight. **myogenic p.** Any type of paralysis caused by a primary muscle disease. **neurogenic p.** Any type of paralysis which is caused by a disease of the anterior horn cells or peripheral nerves. Compare MYOGENIC PARALYSIS. **normokalemic periodic p.** PERIODIC PARALYSIS III. **p. notariorum** WRITERS' CRAMP. **nuclear p.** Any type of paralysis caused by damage to nuclei in the central nervous system, especially paralysis of muscles innervated by cranial nerves that results from lesions involving the appropriate brainstem nuclei. **obstetrical p.** 1 Any form of paralysis in the newborn infant resulting from physical injury during delivery. Lesions include pressure on a nerve, as a facial nerve, damage to nerve roots, rarely to the spinal cord, or fracture of bones, as the clavicle, humerus, or femur. The commonest lesions involve the arm (Erb's paralysis). Also *birth palsy.* 2 Partial paralysis of one or both lower limbs in a mother following delivery, as from injury to the lumbosacral plexus caused by the fetal head or by obstetric forceps. **obturator nerve p.** A rare type of paralysis characterized by impaired adduction of the thigh, often with marked atrophy of the adductor muscles. There is a triangular zone of anesthesia on the internal aspect of the thigh. **occupational p.** OCCUPATIONAL PALSY. **oculofacial p.** MÖBIUS SYNDROME. **palatal p.** Paralysis of the muscles of the soft palate, either on one side or both. The cause may be peripheral as in diphtheritic paralysis, or central as in bulbar poliomyelitis or pseudobulbar palsy. Rhinolalia aperta and regurgitation, particularly of fluids, through the nose on swallowing are features of bilateral cases. Also *palate palsy, palatoplegia.* **periodic p.** A group of disorders that are characterized by periodic attacks of muscle weakness or paralysis. Three forms have been described, each inherited as an autosomal dominant trait. Two are associated with alterations in the serum potassium concentration that promote the muscle effects. Also *familial myoplegia, familial recurrent paralysis, familial periodic paralysis.* **periodic p. I** Periodic paralysis in which the muscle weakness is associated with hypokalemia. It is usually inherited as an autosomal dominant trait, but penetrance is markedly reduced in females. It may also occur as a complication of thyrotoxicosis, particularly in Orientals. Also *familial hypokalemic periodic paralysis, hypokalemic periodic paralysis.* **periodic p. II** Periodic paralysis in which the muscle weakness is associated with hyperkalemia. Inheritance of the disorder is autosomal dominant. Also *familial hyperkalemic periodic paralysis, hyperkalemic periodic paralysis, Gamstorp's disease.* **periodic p. III** Periodic paralysis in which the serum potassium remains normal during an episode of muscle weakness. Some authorities doubt that this type is distinct from periodic paralysis II. Also *normokalemic periodic paralysis, sodium-responsive periodic paralysis* (imprecise). **peripheral facial p.** Unilateral paralysis of the facial muscles caused by damage to the facial nerve, at any point from its nucleus in the pons to its termination. This makes the face lopsided at rest and more particularly when it moves. Food may trickle from the paralyzed corner of the mouth, and it may be difficult to articulate labial sounds and to whistle. Sometimes there is loss of taste on the anterior two thirds of the tongue, and unilateral hyperacusis on the same side if the lesion responsible is proximal to the geniculate ganglion. The orbitofacial, nasopalpebral, and cochleopalpebral reflexes are abolished. Keratitis may be a complication due to trauma to the exposed cornea. The condition may result from many different lesions and disease processes including fracture of the petrous temporal bone, otitis media, poliomyelitis, herpes zoster of the geniculate ganglion, leukemia, cerebellopontine angle tumors, and many more. The commonest cause is Bell's palsy (idiopathic facial paralysis), presumed to be due to swelling of the nerve in its bony canal, of unknown etiology, though many causes including viral infection (especially with herpes simplex) and allergy have been postulated. In many such cases the lesion is neurapraxial and rapid recovery may occur, but if there is actual division of nerve fibers, recovery through regeneration may be slow or incomplete. In such cases facial hemispasm may be a late complication. **peroneal p.** Pressure palsy of the common peroneal nerve or its superficial or deep peroneal branches. **pharyngeal p.** PHARYNGEAL PALSY. **phrenic p.** A lesion of the phrenic nerve, causing paralysis of the corresponding hemidiaphragm. On radiologic examination the damaged hemidiaphragm is seen to be abnormally raised, and takes no active part in respiration. It undergoes passive movement in a direction opposite to that of the unaffected hemidiaphragm (Kienböck's phenomenon). Phrenic paralysis was sometimes induced therapeutically in the past for treatment of cavitary pulmonary tuberculosis. **postdormital p.** SLEEP PARALYSIS. **postepileptic p.** 1 Transient paralysis immediately following certain types of convulsive epileptic attack. The commonest variety is transient hemiplegia following attacks of unilateral or jacksonian epilepsy. 2 Persistent paralysis, such as spastic hemiplegia following unilateral epilepsy. Almost invariably this indicates a focal cerebral lesion causing both the epilepsy and the paralysis. Also *critical epileptic paralysis* (outmoded). **Pott's p.** POTT'S PARAPLEGIA. **progressive bulbar p.** PROGRESSIVE BULBAR PALSY. **pseudobulbar p.** A syndrome of bilateral spasticity of the muscles of articulation and swallowing, causing explosive speech, dysphagia with a brisk jaw jerk, and hyperreflexia in the limbs. Often there is associated emotional lability (pathological or inappropriate laughing and crying) and the gait is often slow and shuffling (arteriosclerotic parkinsonism). There is an associated dementia in many cases. The syndrome results from any disease process giving rise to bilateral lesions of the corticospinal tracts about the pontomedullary junction. Thus features of the condition may be seen in true progressive bulbar palsy (motor neuron disease) but are then associated with signs of lower motor neuron lesions. The commonest cause is diffuse multifocal infarction (often a lacunar state) due to hypertension and associated arterial disease. Also *pseudobulbar palsy, Henneberg's disease, spastic bulbar palsy, laughing sickness.* **psychic gaze p.** BALINT SYNDROME. **radial nerve**

**p.** Paralysis of the long extensors of the wrist and fingers resulting in wristdrop and fingerdrop with impaired abduction of the hand at the wrist and of the thumb. If the lesion of the radial nerve is situated high in the upper arm, there may also be paralysis of the triceps with impaired extension at the elbow. The usual cause is injury to or compression of the nerve as it lies in the spiral groove of the humerus, caused by humeral fracture, or by compression as when the arm is rested for a long period over the back of a chair. Pressure from a crutch may have a similar effect. Also *radial paralysis, radial palsy, radial syndrome.* **Ramsay Hunt p.** JUVENILE PARALYSIS AGITANS. **recurrent laryngeal nerve p.** Vocal cord paralysis due to a lesion of the recurrent laryngeal nerve on the same side, the lesion responsible for the great majority of cases. The clinical features depend on whether the lesion is unilateral or bilateral, partial or complete, but include dysphonia, sometimes minimal, or respiratory obstruction or both. Similar clinical features may result from a lesion of the vagus nerve proximal to the point of origin of the recurrent laryngeal nerve. The left recurrent laryngeal nerve is involved twice as often as the right due to its long mediastinal course. Common causes include surgical trauma and neoplasia occurring in the neck or upper mediastinum. **Rieder's p.** RIEDER SYNDROME. **Saturday night p.** Paralysis of muscles supplied by one radial nerve. This condition was originally described in individuals who went to sleep in a drunken stupor on a Saturday night with one arm over the back of a chair so that the nerve was compressed in its spiral groove. Also *Saturday night palsy, Sunday morning paralysis, drunkards'-arm paralysis.* **sensory p.** An inaccurate term for PSEUDOPARALYSIS. **serratus anterior p.** Paralysis of the serratus anterior muscle, causing winging of the scapula on pushing forwards with the hand and impairment of full abduction of the arm. This muscle is often involved early in muscular dystrophy but isolated paralysis more often results from a lesion of the nerve to serratus anterior (the long nerve of Bell) due to trauma or neuralgic amyotrophy (shoulder-girdle neuritis). **serum p.** SERUM NEUROPATHY. **sleep p.** A benign disorder, presumably involving the reticular substance, in which the subject on waking is alert but unable to move for a few seconds or longer. Ability to move is quickly established if the individual is touched, but in any event movement is soon established spontaneously without stimulation. It may be associated with narcolepsy and cataplexy. Also *waking paralysis, morning paralysis, postdormital paralysis, night palsy, narcohypnia, cataplexie du réveil, delayed awakening.* **sodium-responsive periodic p.** *Imprecise* PERIODIC PARALYSIS III. **spastic p.** Paralysis accompanied by increased muscle tone and exaggerated tendon reflexes (spasticity). **spinal accessory nerve p.** Paralysis of one sternocleidomastoid and of the trapezius muscle on the same side due to a lesion of the spinal accessory (eleventh cranial) nerve. The lesion may involve the nucleus of the nerve in the brainstem or the trunk of the nerve on leaving the brainstem, as in the jugular foramen. **Sunday morning p.** SATURDAY NIGHT PARALYSIS. **superior laryngeal nerve p.** Paralysis of the superior laryngeal branch of the vagus nerve, a rare lesion, sometimes due to surgical injury, resulting in anesthesia of the corresponding half of the larynx above the vocal folds along with adjacent parts of the pharynx, and also paralysis of the ipsilateral cricothyroid muscle. **supranuclear p.** SUPRANUCLEAR PALSY. **suxamethonium p.** Prolonged paralysis after the administration of suxamethonium due to a congenital deficiency of pseudocholinesterase. **syphilitic spastic spinal p.** SYPHILITIC SPASTIC PARAPLEGIA. **tegmental mesencephalic p.** BENEDIKT SYNDROME. **tensor p. of the larynx** Paralysis of the thyroarytenoid muscles, the internal tensors of the vocal cords, producing a bowed appearance of the glottis on phonation. A rare lesion in isolation, it commonly occurs only in association with abductor paralysis. **thyrotoxic periodic p.** Attacks of hypokalemic periodic paralysis occurring in thyrotoxic subjects. The condition is resolved by effective treatment of the hyperthyroidism. It is commonest in Chinese and Japanese subjects. **tick p.** ASCENDING TICK PARALYSIS. **Todd's p.** POSTEPILEPTIC PARALYSIS. **tourniquet p.** Transient paralysis due to compression of peripheral nerves by a tourniquet. **trigeminal masticator p.** Paralysis caused by a lesion of the motor nucleus or root of the trigeminal nerve, causing displacement of the lower jaw towards the paralyzed side on opening the mouth, unilateral weakness and atrophy of the temporal and masseter muscles, and inability to move the jaw towards the affected side due to paralysis of the external pterygoid muscle. Also *motor trigeminal paralysis.* **trochlear p.** Paralysis of the superior oblique muscle due to a lesion of the fourth cranial (trochlear) nerve. **ulnar nerve p.** The syndrome resulting from a lesion of the ulnar nerve. A lesion in the upper arm causes weakness of flexion of the little and ring fingers and atrophy and weakness of all of the small hand muscles except those of the lateral half of the thenar eminence, with sensory loss on the medial aspect of the lower forearm and on the palmar aspect of the hand, extending one third of the way across the palm from its ulnar border and involving the little finger and one half of the ring finger. A lesion at the elbow due to compression behind the medial epicondyle, sometimes due to previous injury or fracture (tardy ulnar palsy) or to compression as the nerve passes between the two heads of the flexor carpi ulnaris (the cubital tunnel syndrome), gives a similar clinical picture with a claw hand, except that the long flexors of the little and ring fingers are less often involved and sensory loss is usually confined to the hand. A lesion of the deep branch of the nerve in the palm causes atrophy of the ulnar-innervated small hand muscles without sensory loss. Also *cubital paralysis, cubital syndrome.* **unilateral p.** **1** Total hemiplegia; hemiplegia affecting equally half the face, the arm, and the leg on the same side of the body. **2** Paralysis of half an organ, as *unilateral paralysis of the tongue.* **unilateral vocal cord p.** Partial or complete paralysis of one vocal cord only, the left being involved twice as often as the right. The relatively long intrathoracic course of the left recurrent laryngeal nerve, supplying the muscles concerned, exposes it to risk from such pathology as carcinoma of the bronchus. The greatest hazard to either nerve is from thyroid gland surgery. Also *unilateral cord palsy.* **upper brachial plexus p.** Paralysis due to a lesion of the upper cord of the brachial plexus as in Duchenne-Erb paralysis. **p. vacillans** CHOREA. **vagal p.** Paralysis resulting from damage to the vagus nerve, the symptoms and signs varying according to the site of the lesion. When the paralysis is complete it includes ipsilateral paralysis of the soft palate with abolition of the palatal reflex, unilateral paralysis of laryngeal muscles, hemianesthesia of the soft palate, tachycardia, and sometimes breathing difficulty, with frequent coughing. **vagoaccessory hypoglossal p.** JACKSON'S PARALYSIS. **vasomotor p.** Vasodilatation due to a lesion of vasoconstrictor nerves. Also *angioparalysis, vasoparalysis.* **Vernet's p.** Damage to the ninth, tenth, and eleventh cranial nerves due to a lesion in or near the jugular foramen, causing unilateral paralysis of the muscles of the soft palate, larynx, and pharynx, loss of taste over the posterior third of the tongue, and ipsilateral paralysis of the sternomastoid and trapezius muscles. The usual causes are basal carcinoma, meningioma, or a glomus tumor. Also *jugular foramen syndrome, Vernet syndrome.* **vestibular p.** Impairment of vestibular function as a consequence of damage to the vestibular apparatus resulting from drugs, such as streptomycin, or other toxins or pathologic processes the least rare of which is suppurative labyrinthitis. The severity and duration of the consequent vertigo will depend on whether the lesion is unilateral or bilateral and the age of the patient, the prognosis being bad in the elderly. **p. of the vocal cords** Complete or partial paralysis of the intrinsic laryngeal muscles which abduct and adduct the vocal cords and maintain their tension. Complete paralysis involves all the muscles and leaves the vocal cords in the cadaveric position preventing phonation (phonetic paralysis). The most important partial lesion affecting both cords is bilateral laryngeal abductor paralysis. The causes are many and varied. **Volkmann's p.** VOLKMANN'S ISCHEMIC CONTRACTURE. **Volkmann's ischemic p.** VOLKMANN'S ISCHEMIC CONTRACTURE. **waking p.** SLEEP PARALYSIS. **wasting p.** PROGRESSIVE MUSCULAR ATROPHY. **Weber's p.** WEBER SYNDROME. **Werdnig-Hoffmann p.** WERDNIG-HOFFMANN DISEASE. **writers' p.** WRITERS' CRAMP. **Zenker's p.** COMMON PERONEAL NERVE PARALYSIS.

**paralyssa** \-lis′ə\ [PARA- + LYSSA] A form of paralytic rabies caused by the bite of a vampire bat (*Desmodus*) found in Trinidad and Brazil. Also *Trinidad disease.*

**paralytic** \-lit′ik\ Of or relating to paralysis.

**paralyzant** \par′əlī′zənt\ [*paralyz(e)* + *-ant,* suffix denoting causing or being] **1** Resulting in paralysis. **2** Any substance or agent that causes paralysis. For defs. 1 and 2 also *paralysant* (British spelling).

**paralyze** \par′əlīz\ To put into a state of paralysis.

**paramagnetic** \-magnet′ik\ Possessing permanent magnetism, which tends to align with an applied magnetic field so that the field is reinforced. Substances with unpaired electrons, e.g. transition metal ions, are paramagnetic. Such ions are useful in conjunction with nuclear magnetic resonance methods, because their proximity to a nucleus under investigation can be detected by their line-broadening effect on its spectrum.

**paramastigote** \-mas′tigōt\ [PARA- + MASTIGOTE] A mastigote with one long and one short flagellum. Also *paraflagellate.*

**paramastitis** \-mastī′tis\ [PARA- + MASTITIS] Inflammation of the tissues around the breast.

**paramecia** \-mē′shə\ Plural of PARAMECIUM.

***Paramecium*** \-mē′shē·əm\ [New L (from Gk *para-* beside + *mēk(ēs)* oval, oblong + L *-ium,* neut. sing. suffix)] A genus of free-living ciliates of the order Hymenostomatida, class Oligohymenophorea, phylum Ciliophora. Members are large, monomorphic, freshwater microphagous forms. Many species and strains have been used in laboratory studies in genetics, morphogenesis, physiology, host-predator studies (with *Didinium*), population dynamics, and ecology.

**paramecium** [New L (from Gk *paramēk(ēs)* oblong, from *para-* beside + *mēkos* length, + New L *-ium,* noun suffix)] (*pl.* paramecia) A member of the genus *Paramecium.*

**paramedial** \-mē′dē·əl\ Alongside a medially situated structure.

**paramedian** \-mē′dē·ən\ Alongside the median plane. Also *parasagittal, paramesial.*

**paramedic** \-med′ik\ A health-care worker who provides services that are associated with and complement those of medical practitioners; a paramedical worker. *Popular.* • See note at PARAMEDICAL.

**paramedical** \-med′ikəl\ **1** Ancillary to the medical profession; designating or relating to health workers and health professionals whose work is associated with and complements that of medical practitioners, as occupational therapists, physiotherapists, laboratory technicians, and emergency medical technicians. **2** A paramedical worker. • The specific range of application of *paramedical* varies from country to country. In the United States, *paramedical personnel* is often considered synonymous with *allied health personnel.* In South Africa, paramedical personnel are called *ancillary workers.*

**paramenia** \-mē′nē·ə\ [PARA- + Gk *mēn* month + -IA] Menstruation which is difficult or abnormal.

**paramesial** \-mē′shəl\ PARAMEDIAN.

**parameter** \pəram′ətər\ [PARA- + -METER] In statistics, a magnitude characterizing a frequency distribution or a stochastic model. For example, a normal distribution is uniquely defined by two parameters, the mean and the standard deviation. The estimation of population parameters from observed sample values is a fundamental objective of statistical method. **malthusian p.** The rate of change in size of a breeding population, with age distribution, birth rate, and death rate specified.

**paramethadione** $C_7H_{11}NO_3$. 5-Ethyl-3,5-dimethyl-2,4-oxazolidinedione. An anticonvulsant drug utilized in the treatment of petit mal epilepsy. It is given orally.

**paramethasone acetate** $C_{24}H_{31}FO_6$. 21-(Acetyloxy)-6α-fluoro-11β,17-dihydroxy-16α-methyl-pregna-1,4-diene-3,20-dione. A glucocorticoid used as an anti-inflammatory and antiallergic agent. It occurs as a fluffy white crystalline powder, and is administered orally.

**parametrial** \-mē′trē·əl\ Relating to the parametrium.

**parametric¹** \-mē′trik\ [PARA- + METR- + -IC ] Located adjacent to the uterus.

**parametric²** \-met′rik\ Of or pertaining to a parameter.

**parametrismus** \-mētriz′məs\ [*parametr(ium)* + New L *-ismus* -ISM] A painful spasm located in muscle fibers in the base of the broad ligament.

**parametritic** \-mētrit′ik\ Relating to parametritis.

**parametritis** \-mētrī′tis\ [*parametr(ium)* + -ITIS] Inflammation or infection located in the parametrium. Also *pelvic cellulitis, pelvicellulitis.* **anterior p.** Parametritis located above or anterior to the uterosacral ligaments. **posterior p.** Parametritis located at the uterosacral ligaments.

**parametrium** \-mē′trē·əm\ [NA] The connective tissue that is lateral to the uterus between the two layers of the broad ligament and that separates the supravaginal part of the cervix anteriorly from the bladder. The uterine vessels are located in this tissue lateral to the cervix.

**parametropathy** \-mēträp′əthē\ [*parametr(ium)* + *o* + -PATHY] A pathologic condition of the parametrium.

**paramnesia** \par′amnē′zhə\ A disturbance of memory entailing the acceptance of a dream or fantasy as a memory of a real event, or the incorrect and often uncanny feeling that a totally novel experience has been lived through at some earlier time, as in déjà vu or déjà fait.

**paramolar** \-mō′lər\ [PARA- + MOLAR] A supernumerary tooth in the molar area.

**paramorph** \par′əmôrf\ An individual or part in which an unusual or atypical structure has been induced by environmental influences, such as occupational or behavioral factors, without a corresponding genetic change.

**paramorphia** \-môr′fē·ə\ Any abnormality of structure not the result of teratogenesis or abnormal embryogenesis.

**paramorphine** THEBAINE.

**paramusia** \-myoo′zē·ə\ [PARA- + Gk *mous(a)* music, song + -IA] Impairment or loss of the ability to read or play music.

**paramutable** \-myoo′təbl\ Susceptible to paramutation.

**paramutagenic** \-myoo′təjen′ik\ Of or relating to an allele that causes paramutation in another allele at the same locus when the two are present heterozygously.

**paramutation** \-myootā′shən\ The alteration of the action of a paramutable allele in diploid organisms by a change in local chromosome organization, such as heterochromatization, or by the presence of a separate allele, which is paramutagenic, at the same locus.

**paramyoclonus multiplex** \par′əmī′əklō′nəs mul′tipleks, -mī·äk′lənəs\ A chronic but benign disorder characterized by widespread and irregular myoclonic jerks of the skeletal musculature occurring from 10 to 50 times a minute but without associated epilepsy, dementia, or ataxia or the other features seen in progressive myoclonic epilepsy. Sometimes the condition is familial and is then known as hereditary essential myoclonus. Also *Friedreich's disease, fibrillary myoclonia, myoclonia fibrillaris multiplex, myoclonus multiplex, paraclonus, paramyoclonus, convulsive tremor, myospasia, tetanilla* (seldom used).

**paramyosinogen** \-mī′əsin′əjən\ A muscle protein which comprises about 20% of the muscle and which coagulates at about 47°C.

**paramyotone** \-mī′ətōn\ PARAMYOTONUS.

**paramyotonia** \-mī′ətō′nē·ə\ [PARA- + MYOTONIA] **1** Myotonia occurring only on exposure to cold. **2** *Incorrect* MYOTONIA PARADOXA. **p. congenita** A dominantly inherited syndrome which resembles myotonia congenita, but in which the myotonia occurs only on exposure to cold and the affected individuals also suffer episodes of periodic paralysis usually associated with hyperkalemia. So-called myotonic periodic paralysis is clearly related to, if not identical with, this syndrome, which is also related to hyperkalemic periodic paralysis. Also *Eulenberg's disease, congenital paramyotonia, myotonia congenita intermittens.*

**paramyotonus** \-mī·ät′ənəs\ [PARA- + MYO- + TONUS] Increased muscle tone with tonic spasms. *Obs.* Also *paramyotone.*

**Paramyxoviridae** \-mik′səvir′idē\ A family of RNA viruses that includes the genera *Paramyxovirus, Morbillivirus,* and *Pneumovirus.*

**paramyxovirus** \-mik′səvī′rəs\ [PARA- + MYXOVIRUS] Any of a genus (*Paramyxovirus*) in the Paramyxoviridae family, including parainfluenza virus types 1–4, Newcastle disease virus, and mumps virus. They are single-stranded RNA viruses with a helical nucleocapsid surrounded by an envelope.

**paranasal** \-nā′zəl\ Alongside or near the nasal cavity.

**paranea** \-nē′ə\ *Obs.* PARANOIA.

**paraneoplasia** \-nē′ōplā′zhə\ [PARA- + NEOPLASIA] Indirect and remote phenomena associated with the presence of a neoplasm. These can serve as signs and symptoms of the neoplasm.

**paraneoplastic** \-nē′əplas′tik\ [PARA- + NEOPLASTIC] Referring to indirect or remote effects produced by tumor metabolites or other substances associated with tumors, such as ectopic hormone production or neurologic and dermal changes.

**paraneoxenous** \-nē′äk′sənəs\ HYPERPARASITIC.

**paranephric** \-nef′rik\ **1** Near the kidneys. **2** Pertaining to the paranephros.

**paranephritis** \-nefrī′tis\ PERINEPHRITIS.

**paranephros** \-nef′rəs\ [PARA- + Gk *nephros* kidney] *Outmoded* GLANDULA SUPRARENALIS.

**paraneural** \-nʸʊr′əl\ Situated close to or alongside a nerve.

**parangi** \pəran′jē\ A Sri Lankan term for YAWS.

**paranoia** \par′ənoi′ə\ [Gk (from *paranoein* to think amiss or wrongly), derangement, madness] A gradually developing delusional state or fixed delusional system with preservation of intelligence and orderly thinking. Most commonly the delusions are persecutory in nature, although they may also be of grandiose, religious, erotomanical, or of other content. Also *intellectual monomania, paranea, paranoiac psychosis, paranoid psychosis.* **alcoholic p.** A state of paranoia manifested in infidelity delusions and associated with alcoholism. Also *alcoholic paranoid state.* **amorous p.** EROTOMANIA. **heboid p.** *Obs.* PARANOID SCHIZOPHRENIA. **p. querulans** Paranoia characterized by incessant quarrelsomeness and a seeking of redress for imagined injustices at the hands of the law. Also *litigious paranoia, querulant paranoia, querulous paranoia.*

**paranoid** \par′ənoid\ **1** Manifesting paranoia or paranoialike symptoms. **2** Resembling paranoia.

**paranomia** \-nō′mē·ə\ [PARA- + Gk *(o)nom(a)* a name + -IA] Aphasia in which objects or people are incorrectly named. **visual p.** A syndrome with features of visual agnosia and receptive aphasia in which objects which are seen are incorrectly named.

**paranormal** \-nôr′məl\ [PARA- + NORMAL] Not explicable in terms of known scientific principles.

**paranosic** \-nō′sik\ [PARA- + *nos(o)-* + -IC] Relating to the primary advantage derived from an illness, as in *paranosic gain.*

**paranosis** \-nō′sis\ [PARA- + *no(so)-* + -SIS] PARANOSIC GAIN.

**paranucleolus** \-nʸooklē′ələs\ [PARA- + NUCLEOLUS] (*pl.* paranucleoli) A basophilic mass located in the nucleus near the nucleolus.

**paranucleus** \-nʸoo′klē·əs\ (*pl.* paranuclei) **1** A micronucleus, as present in certain protozoa. **2** A spherical body or mass located in the cytoplasm near the nucleus, as an aggregation of mitochondria.

**paraomphalic** \-ämfal′ik\ Adjacent to the umbilicus.

**paraoperative** \-äp′ərətiv\ Necessary to or accompanying a surgical procedure, as techniques or materials.

**paraoral** \par′ə·ôr′əl\ Parenteral: used especially of the administration of medications.

**paraortic** \par′ā·ôr′tik\ PARA-AORTIC.

**parapancreatic** \-pan′krē·at′ik\ Adjacent to the pancreas.

**paraparesis** \-pərē′sis\ Paresis restricted to the lower limbs and lower half of the trunk. Adj. paraparetic. **spastic p.** Paraparesis with spasticity of the legs.

**paraparetic** \-pəret′ik\ Pertaining to or affected by paraparesis.

**paraperitoneal** \-per′itənē′əl\ Adjacent to the peritoneum.

**parapertussis** \-pərtus′is\ An acute respiratory tract infection resembling pertussis and caused by *Bordetella parapertussis.*

**paraphasia** \-fā′zhə\ **1** A condition typified by disordered speech. **2** Aphasia in which the subject comprehends speech but cannot speak correctly and words are incorrectly formed. Also *paraphemia.* **choreic p.** *Obs.* JARGON APHASIA. **literal p.** JARGON APHASIA.

**paraphemia** \-fē′mē·ə\ PARAPHASIA.

**paraphilia** \-fil′yə\ [PARA- + -PHILIA] Any psychosexual disorder consisting of deviance from what is considered normal heterosexuality in that certain conditions must be met before full sexual arousal or gratification can occur.

DSM-III lists eight paraphilias: fetishism, transvestism, bestiality, pedophilia, exhibitionism, voyeurism, sexual masochism, and sexual sadism. Other classifications include homosexuality as well.

**paraphimosis** \-fīmō′sis\ [PARA- + PHIMOSIS] Constriction of the glans penis caused by retraction and inflammatory swelling of the retracted foreskin. Compression of the dorsal veins and lymphatics results in an edematous swelling of the glans penis and prepuce.

**paraphrenia** \-frē′nē·ə\ [PARA- + -PHRENIA] A group of paranoid disturbances in which systematization is not complete enough to justify a diagnosis of paranoia, and in which thinking and reality testing are not disturbed enough to justify a diagnosis of paranoid schizophrenia. **involutional p.** INVOLUTIONAL MELANCHOLIA. **late p.** Paraphrenia with symptoms of paranoia but without symptoms of degenerative dementia. It appears for the first time after the age of 65 years.

**paraphysis** \pəraf′isis\ [PARA- + PHYSIS] (*pl.* paraphyses) An evagination of the roof of the diencephalon in front of the pineal and near the interventricular foramina. It usually disappears during fetal life in man but may persist to form cysts in postnatal life. Also *paraphyseal body*. Adj. paraphyseal.

**paraplectic** \-plek′tik\ PARAPLEGIC.

**paraplegia** \-plē′jə\ [PARA- + Gk *plēgē* a blow, stroke, from *plēssein* to strike, smite, + -IA] Flaccid or spastic paralysis of the lower limbs. If caused by a spinal cord lesion there is also associated paralysis of the lower trunk and sphincters. Also *pamplegia*. Adj. paraplegic, paraplectic. **alcoholic p.** Paraplegia due to alcoholic polyneuropathy. **ataxic p.** Paraplegia associated with sensory ataxia, attributable to damage to the posterior columns of the cord. **cerebral p.** Paraplegia due to a lesion or lesions involving the leg and foot areas of the motor cortex in both cerebral hemispheres. **cervical p.** Paraplegia due to a lesion of the lower cervical cord. **congenital spastic p.** Cerebral palsy characterized by spastic weakness of both lower limbs, due to meningeal hemorrhage following birth injury. Also *infantile spastic paraplegia*. **Erb's p.** SYPHILITIC SPASTIC PARAPLEGIA. **familial spastic p.** HEREDITARY SPASTIC PARAPLEGIA. **flaccid p.** Paraplegia with complete loss of tone. **functional p.** Pseudoparalysis of the lower limbs due to emotional rather than physical causes. Also *hysterical paraplegia*. **hereditary spastic p.** One of the degenerative diseases of the hereditary ataxia group, usually of early onset and dominant inheritance, but sometimes recessive, marked by slowly progressive spastic paraplegia and pes cavus, sometimes associated with minimal cerebellar signs. Also *familial spastic paralysis, familial spastic paraplegia, hereditary cerebrospinal paralysis, progressive spastic paraplegia* (imprecise). **hysterical p.** FUNCTIONAL PARAPLEGIA. **infantile spastic p.** CONGENITAL SPASTIC PARAPLEGIA. **Jamaican p.** JAMAICAN SPASTIC PARAPLEGIA. **Jamaican spastic p.** A form of progressive spastic paraplegia of unknown cause endemic in Jamaica and sometimes but not invariably associated with optic atrophy and posterior column dysfunction. It has been variously attributed to yaws, syphilis, the consumption of bush tea, or to unknown nutritional factors. Also *Jamaican paraplegia*. **Pott's p.** Paraplegia following Pott's disease (tuberculous spinal osteomyelitis). Also *Pott's paralysis*. **primary spastic p.** PRIMARY LATERAL SCLEROSIS. **progressive spastic p.** *Imprecise* HEREDITARY SPASTIC PARAPLEGIA. **senile myopathic p.** Paraplegia occurring in elderly patients, once wrongly attributed to myopathy. While progressive denervation of lower limb muscles has been shown to occur in extreme old age due to progressive fallout of anterior horn cells, there are many other causes of paraplegia occurring in elderly individuals. *Obs.* **South Indian p.** A form of progressive spastic paraplegia presumed to be of dietary origin but at present of unknown cause, described in South India and resembling Jamaican spastic paraplegia. **spastic p.** Paraplegia associated with increased tone of the affected muscles and with increased tendon reflexes. **syphilitic p.** SYPHILITIC SPASTIC PARAPLEGIA. **syphilitic spastic p.** Spastic paraplegia due to meningomyelitis occurring in the tertiary stage of syphilis. Also *Erb's paralysis, Erb's palsy, Erb syphilitic spinal paralysis, syphilitic spastic spinal paralysis, syphilitic paraplegia, Erb's paraplegia, Erb spastic paraplegia, Erb-Charcot disease*.

**paraplegia-in-extension** Paraplegia accompanied by severe spasticity of the leg extensor muscles, usually due to partial interruption of the corticospinal tracts in the spinal cord.

**paraplegia-in-flexion** Paraplegia accompanied by severe spasticity of the flexor muscles of the lower limbs, attributable to complete interruption of the corticospinal tracts in the spinal cord.

**paraplegic** \-plē′jik\ **1** Relating to or characterized by paraplegia. **2** One who is suffering from paraplegia. For defs. 1 and 2 also *paraplectic*.

**paraplexus** \-plek′səs\ *Obs.* PLEXUS CHOROIDEUS VENTRICULI LATERALIS.

**parapoxvirus** \-päks′vīrəs\ Any virus of a genus (*Parapoxvirus*) in the Poxviridae family. They generally produce vesiculopustular lesions in ungulates and may occasionally be transmitted to humans. The virion is an enveloped prolate 220–330 nm long with a characteristic spiral appearance when seen by negative staining. It contains double-stranded DNA and is inactivated by both ether and chloroform. Species show considerable serologic cross-reactivity. Orf (contagious ecthyma) virus is the type species. Bovine papular stomatitis and pseudocowpox are caused by parapoxviruses.

**paraproctium** \-präk′shē·əm, -präk′tē·əm\ The connective tissues around the rectum and the anal canal.

**paraprofessional** **1** Ancillary to but outside of a given profession. **2** A trained worker who assists a health-care professional or whose work is ancillary to that of professionals. ● The term is used variously and imprecisely, and is sometimes applied to any worker in the field of allied health.

**paraprostatitis** \-präs′tətī′tis\ [PARA- + PROSTATITIS] Inflammation of the tissues around the prostate gland.

**paraprotein** \-prō′tē·in\ An immunoglobulin produced in greatly excessive quantity, particularly in certain diseases. Originally believed to be abnormal proteins because when seen in protein electrophoresis of plasma in certain diseases, they were identified by abnormal peaks of sharply restricted electrophoretic mobility, paraproteins are most usually monoclonal immunoglobulins of normal structure, as in multiple myeloma, Waldenström's macroglobulinemia (IgM only), and not infrequently in the elderly without obviously related disease (monoclonal gammopathy of undetermined significance). Paraproteins of abnormal structure do sometimes occur, however, as in heavy chain disease.

**paraproteinemia** \-prō′tē·inē′mē·ə\ The presence in blood of monoclonal protein in a greater than normal amount.

**parapsoriasis** \-sôrī′əsis\ [PARA- + PSORIASIS] Any of a group of scaly, erythmatous eruptions. *Ambiguous.* **p. acuta** PARAPSORIASIS VARIOLIFORMIS. **acute p.** PARAPSORIASIS VARIOLIFORMIS. **p. en plaques** **1** An eruption of sharply marginated plaques of erythema and fine scaling. Also *resistant maculopapular scaly erythroderma, parapsoriasis maculata.* 2 POIKILODERMA ATROPHICANS VASCULARE. **guttate p.** PITYRIASIS LICHENOIDES. **p. lichenoides chronica** The chronic form of pityriasis lichenoides. Also *parapsoriasis varioliformis chronica.* **p. maculata** PARAPSORIASIS EN PLAQUES. **retiform p.** Parapsoriasis manifested as scaly papules that are distributed in an irregular network. Also *parapsoriasis papulata.* **p. varioliformis** An acute form of pityriasis lichenoides that leaves scars. Also *pityriasis lichenoides et varioliformis acuta.* **p. varioliformis chronica** PARAPSORIASIS LICHENOIDES CHRONICA.

**parapsychology** \-sīkäl′əjē\ [PARA- + PSYCHOLOGY] The attempt to apply systematic or scientific research methods to the study of those relationships between a person and the external world that are not explicable by known natural laws or principles. Among the kinds of paranormal phenomena investigated are telepathy, clairvoyance, precognition, and telekinesis.

***Parapsyllus*** \pərap′siləs\ A genus of rodent fleas, some species of which are vectors of plague.

**parapyramidal** \-pīram′idəl\ Situated beside the pyramids of the medulla oblongata.

**paraquat** \par′əkwät\ $C_{12}H_{14}N_2$. 1,1′-Dimethyl-4,4′-bipyridinium. A compound used to control weeds, produced in the form of dichloride, dibromide, or dimethosulfate. Accidental or intentional ingestion produces lung, liver, and kidney damage, and may be fatal. The principal toxic effect is pulmonary fibrosis even when the lung is the secondary route of exposure.

**paraqueduct** \parak′widukt\ HYLA.

**pararectal** \-rek′təl\ 1 In the region of the rectum. 2 Adjacent to a rectus muscle.

**parareflex** \-rē′fleks\ A reflex evoked by a stimulus which normally induces a different type of reflex. *Obs.*

**parareflexia** \-riflek′sē·ə\ Any abnormality of reflexes.

**pararenal** \-rē′nəl\ Related to the area immediately surrounding a kidney.

**pararrhythmia** \par′əriTH′mē·ə\ [PAR- + ARRHYTHMIA] Abnormal rhythm of the heart in which rhythms from two different foci compete. It includes both parasystole and partial atrioventricular dissociation.

**pararthria** \pərär′thrē·ə\ [*par(a)-* + ARTHR- + -IA] Abnormal articulation of speech. *Seldom used.*

**parasagittal** \-saj′itəl\ PARAMEDIAN.

**parasalpingeal** \-salpin′jē·əl\ Located adjacent to or in the wall of the fallopian tube.

**parasalpingitis** \-sal′pinjī′tis\ [PARA- + SALPINGITIS] Inflammation or infection adjacent to the fallopian tube.

**parascarlatina** \-skär′lətē′nə\ EXANTHEM SUBITUM.

**parasecretion** \-sikrē′shən\ [PARA- + SECRETION] Any abnormality of secretion especially hypersecretion. *Seldom used.*

**parasellar** \-sel′ər\ Situated beside the sella turcica of the sphenoid bone.

**parasexual** \-sek′shoo·əl\ Of or relating to a genetic system in which the recombination of genomes from different individuals occurs by mechanisms other than the formation of a zygote following meiosis. Examples are heterokaryon formation in fungi; the multiple infecting of a host cell with genetically distinct viruses; and bacterial conjugation, transduction, and transformation.

**parasexuality** \-sek′shoo·al′itē\ PARAPHILIA.

**parasinoidal** \-sīnoi′dəl\ Adjacent to a sinus, especially a cerebral sinus.

**parasite** \par′əsīt\ [L *parasitus* (from Gk *parasitos* one who lives at another's table, a parasite, from PARA- + Gk *sitos* grain, wheat, food) a guest, parasite] 1 An animal, plant, or microbe that lives within or on another organism, the host, and depends upon it for energy or sustenance. 2 The less complete or smaller of conjoined twins, which is dependent on the larger or more normal member (the autosite). **accidental p.** An organism found parasitizing another organism that is not its usual kind of host. Also *incidental parasite.* **animal p.** Any parasitic member of the animal kingdom, including species of protozoa, annelids, helminths, arthropods, or others. Also *parazoon.* **autistic p.** A parasite that is derived from the host's tissues; a host-originated parasite. Also *autochthonous parasite.* **autochthonous p.** An endemic parasite; one that is locally derived, or native. **coelozoic p.** A parasite that lives in a cavity of the host's body. **cytozoic p.** INTRACELLULAR PARASITE. **digenetic p.** A parasite characterized by a life cycle in which alternate generations inhabit different hosts; a two-stage heterogenetic parasite. **ectozoic p.** An animal ectoparasite. **entozoic p.** A parasite that lives in the lumen of the host's intestine. **euroxenous p.** A parasite that has a broad range of hosts or lacks host specificity. **eurytrophic p.** An ectoparasite that can obtain nourishment from a variety of hosts. **facultative p.** An organism capable of living either independently or as a parasite. Also *optimal parasite.* Compare OBLIGATE PARASITE. **false p.** PSEUDOPARASITE. **hematozoic p.** A parasite that lives in blood. **heterogenetic p.** A parasite that requires more than one host to complete its life cycle; a heterecious parasite. **incidental p.** ACCIDENTAL PARASITE. **intracellular p.** Any parasitic organism that can grow or sustain itself, usually with multiplication, within a host eukaryotic cell. Examples are chlamydiae, rickettsiae, tubercle bacilli, leishmaniae, toxoplasmas, even some multicellular parasites such as certain larval filarial worms developing in their insect vector. Also *cytozoic parasite.* **karyozoic p.** A parasite located within the nucleus of a cell. **obligate p.** A parasite that cannot live independently of its host. Also *obligatory parasite.* Compare FACULTATIVE PARASITE. **optimal p.** 1 A well-adapted parasite, causing little pathological change, or disease, in its host. 2 FACULTATIVE PARASITE. **periodic p.** A parasite that lives in its host for short periods only. **specific p.** A parasite that is limited to a particular host species. **spurious p.** PSEUDOPARASITE. **stenotrophic p.** A parasite limited to a single or narrow range of hosts; a host-specific parasite. Also *stenoxenous parasite.* **teratoid p.** TERATOMA.

**parasitemia** \-sītē′mē·ə\ [*parasit(e)* + -EMIA] The presence of parasites in the blood, for example, malarial parasites or microfilariae.

**parasitic** \-sit′ik\ Characteristic of or caused by parasites.

**parasiticidal** \-sit′isī′dəl\ Destructive to parasites.

**parasiticide** \-sit′isīd\ [*parasit(e)* + *i* + -CIDE] An agent that kills parasites.

**parasiticus** \-sit′ikəs\ [L (from Gk *parasitikos* pertaining to a parasite, from *para* beside + *sit(os)* food + *-ikos* -IC), parasitic] The smaller, usually more poorly developed of unequal conjoined twins. • The word follows the suffix *-pagus,* compounded with the name of the region in which union occurs, as in *thoracopagus parasiticus.*

**parasitiferous** \-sitif′ərəs\ Containing a parasite; carrying parasites.

**parasitism** \par′əsitizm\ [*parasit(e)* + -ISM] A symbiotic process in which one individual or population lives at the expense of another. **extracellular p.** Infection by microorganisms that grow outside host cells. **intracellular p.** Infection by microorganisms that grow inside host cells, either obligatorily, as do rickettsiae or chlamydiae, or facultatively, as the tubercle bacillus. **multiple p.** A state in which two or more different species of parasites are living in a single host. Also *polyparasitism*.

**parasitization** \-sī′tīzā′shən\ Invasion of, or subsistence in or on (a host) by a parasite.

**parasitize** \par′əsitīz′\ [*parasit(e)* + -IZE] To invade (a host) or to subsist in or on (a host) in the manner of a parasite.

**parasitocenose** \-sī′tōsənōz′\ [*parasit(e)* + Gk *koinōsis* a sharing] The host-parasite ecosystem; the total complex of species and individual parasites found in a specific host.

**parasitogenesis** \-sī′təjen′əsis\ The origin or evolution of a parasite or parasitocenose.

**parasitogenic** \-sī′təjen′ik\ [*parasit(e)* + *o* + -GENIC] Caused by, or derived from, a parasite.

**parasitoid** \par′əsī′toid\ **1** Intermediate between parasitic and predatory. **2** An organism that is intermediate in its way of life between a parasite and a predator, for example, a wasp that deposits its eggs in the body of an arthropod host, which is fed upon and finally killed by the wasp larvae that hatch from the eggs.

**parasitoidism** \par′əsī′toidizm\ A predatory form of parasitism, such as that seen in parasitic wasps, in which the parasitized host usually dies.

**parasitologist** \-sītäl′əjist\ A specialist in the science of parasitology.

**parasitology** \-sītäl′əjē\ [*parasit(e)* + *o* + -LOGY] The branch of biology and of medicine that focuses on various aspects of parasitism, parasitic disease, and host-parasite relationships.

**parasitome** \par′əsītōm\ [*parasit(e)* + -OME] All individuals of one species of parasite located in or on a specific host, including all developmental stages.

**parasitotropic** \-sī′tətrāp′ik\ Having an affinity for parasites: said of antiparasitic drugs or other agents.

**parasitotropism** \-sītät′rəpizm\ [*parasit(e)* + *o* + TROPISM] The affinity of certain drugs or other agents for parasites rather than for their hosts. Also *parasitotropy*.

**parasmallpox** \-smôl′päks\ ALASTRIM.

**parasomnia** \-säm′nē·ə\ [PARA- + L *somn(us)* sleep + -IA] Any disorder of sleep rhythm caused by disease of the central nervous system.

**paraspadias** \-spā′dē·as\ A rare developmental defect of the penis in which the urethra appears to open on the lateral aspect. Usually the defect is a distortion of hypospadias or epispadias.

**parasplenic** \-splen′ik\ Adjacent to the spleen.

**parastriate** \-strī′āt\ Situated next to the striate area or visual projection area of the occipital cortex.

**parasympathetic** \-sim′pəthet′ik\ Denoting the craniosacral portions of the autonomic nervous system.

**parasympathicotonia** \-simpath′ikōtō′nē·ə\ VAGOTONIA.

**parasympathin** \-sim′pəthin\ A hypothetical substance, thought to be released by activity or stimulation of any cranial or sacral nerve containing parasympathetic fibers, possessing the property of stimulating parasympathetic ganglia.

**parasympatholytic** \-simpath′əlit′ik\ Denoting an effect or chemical agent that interferes with or interrupts the action of parasympathetic nerves. Also *parasympathoparalytic*.

**parasympathomimetic** \-sim′pəthōmimet′ik\ Denoting an effect or chemical agent that is similar to the result of parasympathetic nerve excitation, especially cholinergic drugs.

**parasympathoparalytic** \-sim′pəthōpar′əlit′ik\ PARASYMPATHOLYTIC.

**parasympathotonia** \-sim′pəthōtō′nē·ə\ VAGOTONIA.

**parasynapsis** \-sinap′sis\ The longitudinal pairing of homologous chromosomes during meiosis. Also *parasyndesis*.

**parasynovitis** \-sin′əvī′tis\ [PARA- + SYNOVITIS] Inflammation of extra-articular structures.

**parasyphilis** \-sif′əlis\ Collectively, the effects of tertiary syphilis, such as generalized paresis and tabes dorsalis, which were once thought to be not directly related to syphilis. *Obs.* Adj. parasyphilitic.

**parasystole** \-sis′təlē\ [PARA- + SYSTOLE] An abnormal rhythm of the heart in which a second focus of impulse generation, usually in a ventricle, operating at a slower rate than the sinuatrial node and protected from the latter by unidirectional block, excites ventricular contractions at predictable intervals.

**parataenial** \-tē′nē·əl\ Next to a taenia, or bandlike structure.

**paratarsium** \-tär′sē·əm\ The side of the tarsus of the foot. . *Outmoded.*

**paratenesis** \-tənē′sis\ [*para(site)* + L *ten(ere)* to hold, keep, possess, support, maintain, nourish + -ESIS] The conveyance of a parasite by a transport host, in which the parasite does not undergo maturation or cyclic development, to another host.

**paratenic** \-ten′ik\ Relating to or characterized by paratenesis. See also TRANSPORT HOST.

**paratenon** \-ten′än\ The loose areolar and fatty tissue surrounding tendons and their sheaths in fascial compartments such as the palmar spaces. *Outmoded.*

**paratereseomania** \-terē′sē·ōmā′nē·ə\ [Gk *paratērēseo(s)*, gen. of *paratērēsis* an observing closely + -MANIA] *Obs.* VOYEURISM.

**paraterminal** \-tur′minəl\ Adjoining or near an ending or termination.

**parathion** \-thī′än\ $C_{10}H_{14}NO_5PS$. Diethyl-*p*-nitrophenylthiophosphate, a pale yellow liquid used as an agricultural insecticide that acts as a cholinesterase inhibitor.

**parathormone** PARATHYRIN.

**parathymia** \-thī′mē·ə\ [PARA- + -THYMIA] Inappropriate or incongruent expression of feeling; expression that is out of harmony with the expected mood or with the subject's own words.

**parathyrin** A peptide hormone of 84 residues produced by the parathyroid gland in response to lowered blood concentrations of calcium, whose intestinal absorption and mobilization from bone it increases. Also *parathyroid hormone, parathormone*.

**parathyroid** \-thī′roid\ [PARA- + THYROID] **1** Situated alongside the thyroid gland. **2** Any of the four parathyroid glands. See under GLAND.

**parathyroidal** \-thīroi′dəl\ Of or relating to the parathyroid glands.

**parathyroidectomy** \-thī′roidek′təmē\ [PARATHYROID + -ECTOMY] Surgical removal of one or more parathyroid glands.

**parathyroprival** \-thī′rōprī′vəl\ Of, pertaining to, or resulting from the absence of the parathyroid glands. Also *parathyroprivic*.

**parathyroprivia** \-thī′rōprī′vē·ə\ [PARA- + THYRO- + L *priv(us)* deprived of + -IA] Absence of the parathyroid glands, or the physiologic condition resulting from such absence.

**parathyroprivic** \-thī′rōpriv′ik\ PARATHYROPRIVAL.

**parathyrotropic** \-thī′rōträp′ik\ [*parathyro(id)* + -TRO-

PIC[1]] Directed toward or acting on the parathyroid glands. Also *parathyrotrophic.*

**paratoloid** \-tō′loid\ OLD TUBERCULIN.

**paratoloidin** \-tōloi′din\ OLD TUBERCULIN.

**paratonia** \-tō′nē·ə\ [PARA- + *ton(o)-* + -IA] A defect of muscle contraction in which the contraction tends to persist and the part of the limb involved is momentarily frozen in the position which it has just taken up.

**paratonic** \-tän′ik\ Pertaining to or exhibiting paratonia.

**paratonsillar** \-tän′silər\ Situated near or beside the tonsil.

**paratope** \par′ətōp\ [PARA- + Gk *top(os)* a place, position] ANTIBODY COMBINING SITE.

**paratose** \par′ətōs\ 3,6-Dideoxy-D-glucose. A component of the O antigen in group A salmonellae. It was first isolated from *Salmonella paratyphi A.*

**paratrachoma** \-trəkō′mə\ INCLUSION CONJUNCTIVITIS.

**paratrophy** \pərat′trəfē\ *Obs.* DYSTROPHY.

**paratubal** \-t$^y$oo′bəl\ Surrounding or located near a fallopian tube.

**paratuberculosis** \-t$^y$ubur′kyəlō′sis\ [PARA- + TUBERCULOSIS] A disease resembling tuberculosis but not caused by *Mycobacterium tuberculosis..*

**paratyphoid** \-tī′foid\ PARATYPHOID FEVER.

**paratypical** \-tip′ikəl\ Differing from the normal type; atypical. Also *paratypic.*

**paraungual** \par′ə·ung′gwəl\ Close or adjacent to a nail.

**paraureteric** \par′əyoo′rəter′ik\ Related to the area immediately surrounding a ureter or a portion thereof.

**paraurethra** \par′əyoorē′thrə\ An accessory urethra.

**paraurethritis** \par′əyoo′rəthrī′tis\ [PARA- + URETHRITIS] Inflammation of the tissues near or alongside the urethra.

**parauterine** \par′əyoo′tərin\ Located adjacent to the uterus.

**paravaginal** \-vaj′ənəl\ Adjacent to the vagina.

**paravaginitis** \-vaj′ənī′tis\ [PARA- + VAGINITIS] PARACOLPITIS.

**paravalvular** \-val′vyələr\ By the side of a valve.

**paravenous** \-vē′nəs\ By the side of a vein.

**paraventricular** \-ventrik′yələr\ Beside or near a ventricle.

**paravesical** \-ves′ikəl\ PARACYSTIC.

**paraxial** \pərak′sē·əl\ Alongside or near the axis of a body or part.

**parazone** \par′əzōn\ [PARA- + ZONE] One of the white bands which alternate with dark bands (diazones) seen in cross-sections of tooth enamel.

**parazoon** \-zō′än\ [PARA- + Gk *zōon* living being, animal] (*pl.* parazoa) ANIMAL PARASITE.

**Paré** [Ambroise *Paré,* French surgeon, 1510–1590] See under SUTURE.

**paregoric** \par′əgôr′ik\ A liquid preparation containing powdered opium, anise oil, benzoic acid, camphor, dilute alcohol, and glycerin. It contains 35–40 mg of anhydrous morphine in every 100 ml, and is used orally as an antiperistaltic agent in the treatment of diarrhea. Also *camphorated opium tincture.*

**parelectronomy** \par′ilekträn′əmē\ [PAR- + ELECTRO- + *nom(o)-* + -Y] The state of defying the rules of electrical excitability. *Seldom used.*

**parencephalitis** \par′ensef′əlī′tis\ [*par(a)-* + ENCEPHALITIS] CEREBELLAR ENCEPHALITIS.

**parencephalocele** \par′ensef′əlōsēl′\ An encephalocele involving protrusion of the cerebellum.

**parencephalon** \par′ensef′əlän\ *Seldom used* CEREBELLUM.

**parenchyma** \pəreng′kimə\ [Gk (from *parenchein* to pour in alongside, from PAR- + *enchein* to pour in) the characteristic substance of any of the viscera (thought by the ancient Greeks to be infused into the organs via their extrinsic blood vessels)] The characteristic or functional tissue or cells of a gland or an organ. Also *parenchyme, parenchymatous tissue.* Compare STROMA. **p. of lens** SUBSTANTIA LENTIS. **p. prostatae** [NA] The glandular tissue of the prostate comprising many follicles of small compound tubuloalveolar glands that drain into the urethra by small excretory ducts. They are embedded in a dense stroma containing muscle fibers, areolar tissue continuous with the fibrous capsule at the periphery and a capillary plexus. The glandular tissue is distributed in two concentric zones that partially envelop the urethra, namely, a peripheral zone and an internal zone. Also *substantia glandularis prostatae* (outmoded), *glandular substance of prostate, corpus glandulare prostatae.* **p. testis** [NA] The spermatazoa-producing seminiferous tubules within the lobules of the testis. Also *parenchyma of testis.*

**parenchymal** \pəreng′kiməl\ Pertaining to or resembling parenchyma. Also *parenchymatous.*

**parenchyme** \pəreng′kim\ PARENCHYMA.

**parent** [L *parens,* gen. *parentis* (from *parere* to bear young) a parent] **1** An individual who has produced at least one offspring through sexual reproduction. **2** A radionuclide whose decay product is referred to as a daughter, often used in connection with a series of radionuclides. For example, molybdenum 99 is the parent of technetium 99m, which in turn is the parent of technetium 99, the parent of ruthenium 99. **3** Any source or basis, as for the elaboration of a substance.

**parental** Pertaining to or derived from a parent.

**parenteral** \pəren′tərəl\ [PAR- + ENTER- + -AL ] By some means other than the alimentary canal; specifically, using a muscle, vein, or any pathway other than the mouth to introduce a substance into the body.

**parenteric** \par′enter′ik\ Typhoid- or paratyphoidlike but not caused by *Salmonella* organisms; entericoid. Also *paraenteric.*

**parenting** \per′ənting\ **1** The care and bringing up of a child or children; the skills required of a parent. **2** The act of reproducing; the attainment of parenthood.

**parepicoele** \pərep′isēl\ [PAR- + EPI- + -COELE] *Obs.* RECESSUS LATERALIS VENTRICULI QUARTI.

**parepididymal** \pərep′idid′iməl\ Situated alongside the epididymis.

**parepididymis** \pərep′idid′imis\ PARADIDYMIS.

**parergasia** \par′ərgā′zhə\ [PAR- + Gk *ergasia* work, occupation] **1** *Obs.* SCHIZOPHRENIA. **2** *Obs.* SCHIZOPHRENIFORM PSYCHOSIS.

**paresis** \pərē′sis, par′isis\ [Gk *paresis* (from *parienai* to let fall, unloose, relax, allow) a letting go, letting pass, remission, weakening] Weakness as distinct from total paralysis, with reduction in muscle power. Also *incomplete paralysis.* Adj. paretic. **canal p.** One of the two principal patterns of response to the caloric test for vestibular function: one or both ears fail, partially or completely, to respond to both the warm and cold stimulus. Also *vestibular canal paresis.* **galloping p.** Rapidly progressive general paresis. **general p.** Syphilis of the parenchymatous cerebrum, developing in the quaternary stage of the disease. The major manifestations include progressive dementia, epileptiform attacks in some cases, variable spastic paresis of the limbs, dysarthria, tremor of the tongue, and Argyll-Robertson pupils. In some cases so-called congestive attacks (transient episodes of confusion, epilepsy, and/or paresis) occur, and fatuous euphoria and/or hypomania are sometimes seen. The cerebrospinal fluid usually contains an increase in cells, protein and gamma globulin, the Lange curve is paretic in type, and serologic tests for syphilis (the Wassermann reaction and more specific tests such as the treponema immobilization test) are generally positive in both the blood and cerebrospinal fluid. Also *general paralysis, paralytic dementia, Bayle's disease, cerebral tabes, psychomotor ataxia, paretic neurosyphilis, chronic meningoencephalitis, syphilitic meningoencephalitis, holoplexia, paretic dementia, parenchymatous syphilis, softening of the brain* (popular). **juvenile p.** General paresis developing in childhood, adolescence, or early adult life and due to congenital syphilis. There may be associated features of tabes dorsalis (taboparesis) and the pupils, though not reacting to light, are often dilated rather than small, irregular, and unequal as in the typical Argyll Robertson pupil. Also *juvenile paralysis, juvenile general paralysis.* **vestibular canal p.** CANAL PARESIS.

**paresoanalgesia** \par′əsō·an′aljē′sē·ə\ [*pares(is)* + *o* + ANALGESIA] Paresis accompanied by loss of pain sensation in the affected part or parts.

**paresoanesthesia** \par′əsō·an′esthē′zhə\ Paresis accompanied by loss of sensation, especially to touch, in the affected part or parts. **whitlow p. of the upper extremities** MORVAN SYNDROME.

**paresthesia** \par′esthē′zhə\ [PAR- + -ESTHESIA] (*pl.* paresthesiae, paresthesias) Any sensation, such as pins and needles, burning, prickling, etc., which occurs spontaneously without external cause in disease or dysfunction of the central or peripheral nervous system. Adj. paresthetic. **Bernhardt's paresthesiae** MERALGIA PARESTHETICA.

**paresthetic** \par′esthet′ik\ Relating to or characterized by paresthesiae.

**paretic** \pəret′ik\ Of or relating to paresis.

**pareunia** \pəroo′nē·ə\ COITUS.

**parfocal** \pärfō′kl\ [L *par* equal + FOCAL] Pertaining to eyepieces or objectives that may be interchanged without altering the focal length of the optical system. Also *confocal.*

**pargyline hydrochloride** $C_{11}H_{13}N{\cdot}HCl$. *N*-Methyl-*N*-2-propylbenzylamine hydrochloride. An antihypertensive agent that is given orally.

**Parham** [Frederick William *Parham*, U.S. surgeon, 1856–1927] See under BAND.

**paries** \par′i·ēz\ [L, a wall, fence, hedge] (*pl.* parietes) The wall or boundary of an organ or cavity. **p. anterior gastris** [NA] The anterosuperior surface of the stomach that is covered by the peritoneum of the greater sac. The left half is separated by the diaphragm from the left pleura and the sixth to ninth ribs, while the right half abuts the left lobe and the quadrate lobe of the liver. Also *anterior surface of stomach.* **p. anterior vaginae** [NA] The anterior wall of the vagina. It is closely related to the base of the bladder and the urethra which is embedded in it, and it is shorter than the posterior wall. **p. caroticus cavitatis tympanicae** [NA] The narrow anterior or carotid wall of the tympanic cavity. At its upper part is the semicanal for the tensor tympani muscle lying above and parallel to the orifice of the bony part of the auditory tube. The part below them forms the thin posterior wall of the carotid canal and is pierced by the caroticotympanic nerves and the tympanic branches of the internal carotid artery. **p. externus ductus cochlearis** [NA] The outer or peripheral wall of the cochlear duct. Its endosteum is thickened below to form the spiral ligament that projects inwards for the attachment of the outer edge of the basilar membrane. Just above is the highly vascular thickening, the spiral prominence, which continues upward to line the wall as the stria vascularis as far as the attachment of the vestibular membrane. **p. inferior orbitae** [NA] The almost horizontal thin floor or inferior wall of the pyramid-shaped orbit which also forms most of the roof of the underlying maxillary sinus. It is formed by the orbital surfaces of the zygoma and maxilla and the orbital process of the palatine bone. It is grooved longitudinally by the infraorbital nerve which enters a canal anteriorly. Also *floor of orbit.* **p. jugularis cavitatis tympanicae** [NA] The thin bony floor of the tympanic cavity which separates it from the superior bulb of the internal jugular vein and contains the canaliculus for the tympanic branch of the glossopharyngeal nerve. Also *jugular wall of middle ear, inferior wall of tympanic cavity, paries jugularis cavi tympani, jugular wall of tympanic cavity, jugular floor of tympanic cavity.* **p. labyrinthicus cavitatis tympanicae** [NA] The bony medial wall of the tympanic cavity that separates it from the internal ear. In the center is the rounded promontory. Posterosuperior to it is the fenestra vestibuli and posteroinferior is the fenestra cochleae. Above the fenestra vestibuli the prominence of the facial canal extends anteroposteriorly. Also *labyrinthine wall of middle ear, medial wall of middle ear, paries labyrinthicus cavi tympani.* **p. lateralis orbitae** [NA] The oblique lateral wall of the pyramid-shaped orbit that is formed by the orbital surfaces of the zygomatic process of the frontal bone, the zygomatic bone, and the greater wing of the sphenoid bone. It is separated posteriorly from the roof by the superior orbital fissure and from the floor by the inferior orbital fissure. **p. mastoideus cavitatis tympanicae** [NA] The posterior or mastoid wall of the tympanic cavity, which has the aditus to the mastoid antrum passing backwards from the epitympanic recess at its upper end. **p. medialis orbitae** [NA] The thin, sloping, medial wall of the pyramid-shaped orbit, formed by the frontal process of the maxilla, the lacrimal bone, the orbital plate of the ethmoid bone, and the body of the sphenoid bone. Anteriorly is the lacrimal groove, the floor of which also forms part of the lateral wall of the nasal cavity, and behind which the ethmoid separates the orbit from the ethmoidal sinuses. Posteriorly the medial wall also forms the lateral wall of the sphenoidal sinus. **p. membranaceus bronchi** [NA] The membranous wall of the bronchi. It is continuous with that of the trachea and is also composed mainly of collagen, some elastin, and nonstriated muscle fibers, joining the ends of the incomplete cartilaginous rings posteriorly. **p. membranaceus cavitatis tympanicae** [NA] The lateral or membranous wall of the tympanic cavity, formed mainly by the tympanic membrane and the osseous tympanic ring to which it is attached. **p. membranaceus tracheae** [NA] The membranous wall of the trachea, composed mainly of collagen, some elastin and nonstriated muscle fibers and joining the ends of the incomplete cartilaginous rings posteriorly. Also *posterior membranous lamina of trachea.* **p. posterior gastris** [NA] The posteroinferior surface of the stomach, which is covered by peritoneum and separated by the omental bursa from the stomach bed and by the transverse mesocolon and greater omentum from the small intestine. Also *posterior surface of stomach.* **p. posterior vaginae** [NA] The posterior wall of the vagina, the upper part of which is covered by the peritoneum of the rectouterine pouch which separates it from the rectum. The rectal ampulla is separated from the middle part by the rectovaginal septum of the pelvic fascia, while the lower part is separated from the anal canal by the perineal body. **p. superior orbitae** [NA] The slightly arched superior wall or roof of the orbit. It is composed mainly of the orbital surface of the frontal bone containing the frontal sinus between its tables anteriorly. At its posterior end is the lesser wing of the sphenoid bone, which is separated from the lateral wall of the orbit by the superior orbital fissure and from the medial wall by the optic canal and foramen. The thin roof separates the orbit from the anterior cranial fossa, and anterolaterally it is hollowed for the orbital part of the lacrimal gland. Also *roof of orbit, superior wall of orbit.* **p. tegmentalis cavitatis tympanicae** [NA] The roof of the middle ear, formed by the tegmen tympani which separates the cranial cavity from the tympanic cavity. Also *tegmental wall of middle ear.* **p. tympanicus ductus cochlearis** [NA] The wall of the cochlear duct separating it from the scala tympani and comprising the basilar membrane and the osseous spiral lamina. Also *tympanic wall of cochlear duct, spiral membrane of cochlear duct.* **p. vestibularis ductus cochlearis** [NA] The wall of the cochlear duct that separates it from the scala vestibuli and comprises the vestibular membrane which stretches from the thickened endosteum covering the osseous spiral lamina to the outer wall of the cochlea. It consists of two layers of flattened epithelial cells with a basal lamina between them. Also *vestibular wall of cochlear duct, vestibular membrane of cochlear duct, Reissner's membrane.*

**parietal** \pərī′ətəl\ [L *parietalis* (from *paries,* gen. *parietis* a wall) pertaining to walls] **1** Pertaining to any wall limiting a cavity or organ. **2** Pertaining to the wall or outer framework of the body, especially where it bounds the thoracic and abdominal cavities. Compare VISCERAL. **3** Pertaining to or near the lateral walls of the cranium, as *parietal bone, parietal lobe.*

**parietes** \pərī′ətēz\ Plural of PARIES.

**parieto-** \pərī′ətō-\ [L *paries,* gen. *parietis* a wall] A combining form denoting (1) the wall of an organ or of a cavity; (2) the parietal bone or lobe.

**parietofrontal** \-frun′təl\ Pertaining to the parietal and the frontal bones or lobes of the cerebrum. Also *frontoparietal.*

**parietography** \pərī′ətäg′rəfē\ [L *paries,* gen. *parietis,* a partition wall + *o* + -GRAPHY ] Radiography of the wall of a hollow organ by filling the lumen with air and injecting air into the surrounding space. Most often it is used to study the stomach, where it combines pneumoperitoneum with air study of the gastric antrum. **gastric p.** Roentgenography of the stomach by special techniques to demonstrate the thickness of the gastric wall, as by injecting air around the stomach and filling its lumen with a contrast medium.

**parietomastoid** \-mas′toid\ Pertaining to the parietal bone and the mastoid process of the temporal bone. Also *mastoparietal.*

**parieto-occipital** \-äksip′ətəl\ Pertaining to the parietal and the occipital bones or lobes of the cerebrum. Also *occipitoparietal.*

**parietosphenoid** \-sfē′noid\ SPHENOPARIETAL.

**parietosplanchnic** \-splangk′nik\ PARIETOVISCERAL.

**parietosquamosal** \-skwāmō′səl\ SQUAMOPARIETAL.

**parietotemporal** \-tem′pərəl\ TEMPOROPARIETAL.

**parietovisceral** \-vis′ərəl\ **1** Both parietal and visceral. **2** Pertaining to the wall or walls of a cavity and the viscera contained therein. For defs. 1 and 2 also *parietosplanchnic.*

**pari passu** \par′ē pas′oo\ [L *pari,* ablative of *par* equal + *passu,* ablative of *passus* pace, step] At a like pace, i.e., at the same time, or to the same proportion or degree.

**parity** \par′itē\ [L *par(ere)* to bear young + -ITY] The parous state of a woman, i.e., the number of times she has borne children, counting a multiple birth as one and usually including stillbirths. In some demographic studies, however, stillbirths are not counted.

**Park** [Henry *Park,* English surgeon, 1744–1831] See under ANEURYSM.

**Parker** [Edward Mason *Parker,* U.S. surgeon, 1860–1941] Parker-Kerr suture. See under SUTURE.

**Parker** [Ralph Robinson *Parker,* U.S. zoologist, 1888–1949] Spencer-Parker vaccine. See under VACCINE.

**Parkinson** [James *Parkinson,* English physician, 1755–1824] **1** Parkinsonian crisis. See under OCULOGYRIC CRISIS. **2** See under COMPLEX, SIGN, MASK. **3** Parkinsonian tremor. See under TREMOR. **4** Parkinson's facies. See under MASKLIKE FACE. **5** Parkinson syndrome, parkinsonian syndrome. See under DISEASE. **6** Parkinsonian rigidity. See under RIGIDITY.

**Parkinson** [Sir John *Parkinson,* English cardiologist, born 1885] Wolff-Parkinson-White syndrome. See under SYNDROME.

**parkinsonian** \pär′kinsō′nē·ən\ [*parkinson(ism)* + *-ian,* adjectival suffix] Relating to or characteristic of Parkinson's disease.

**parkinsonism** \pär′kinsənizm\ [after James *Parkinson,* English physician, 1755–1824 + -ISM] **1** PARKINSON'S DISEASE. **2** A neurologic syndrome resembling Parkinson's disease and developing as a side effect of some antipsychotic drugs. **atherosclerotic p.** A syndrome of rigidity of the limbs with a slow, shuffling gait, hyperreflexia, and (usually) extensor plantar responses, often associated with features of pseudobulbar palsy but without parkinsonian facies, superficially resembling paralysis agitans but due to diffuse cerebral softening resulting from atherosclerosis and usually associated arterial hypertension. Also *arteriosclerotic parkinsonism, vascular parkinsonism.* **drug-induced p.** A neurologic syndrome resembling Parkinson's disease but developing as a side-effect of some psychotropic drugs, especially the phenothiazines. **hemiplegic p.** Paralysis agitans involving one arm and leg much more severely than the contralateral limbs and at first sight suggesting a hemiparesis. **intoxication p.** A parkinsonian syndrome resulting from cerebral anoxia, as in carbon monoxide poisoning, manganese intoxication, or following use of drugs such as the phenothiazines. **juvenile p.** JUVENILE PARALYSIS AGITANS. **postencephalitic p.** Parkinsonism developing as a sequel to encephalitis lethargica, often many years after the acute illness. **symptomatic p.** A parkinsonian syndrome symptomatic of drug intoxication or of a brain disease other than paralysis agitans or postencephalitic parkinsonism. **traumatic p.** BOXERS' ENCEPHALOPATHY. **vascular p.** ATHEROSCLEROTIC PARKINSONISM.

**parodontal** \par′ōdän′təl\ PERIODONTAL.

**parodontitis** \par′ōdänti′tis\ PERIODONTITIS.

**parodontium** \par′ōdän′shē·əm\ PERIODONTIUM.

**parodontopathy** \par′ōdäntäp′əthē\ [PAR- + -ODONTO + -PATHY] PERIODONTAL DISEASE.

**parolfactory** \par′älfak′tərē\ Situated adjacent to the olfactory area of the cerebral cortex.

**parolivary** \pəräl′iver′ē\ Located beside or near the olivary nuclei.

**paromomycin** $C_{23}H_{45}N_5O_{14}$. An aminoglycoside antibiotic produced by *Streptomyces rimosus* var. *paromomycinus.* It is effective against Gram-negative, Gram-positive, and acid-fast bacteria. Its actions are like those of neomycin, and it is also effective against intestinal amebiasis. Also *crestomycin.*

**paromphalocele** \par′ämfal′əsēl\ A hernia located near the navel.

**Parona** [Francesco *Parona,* Italian surgeon, flourished late 19th century] See under SPACE.

**paronychia** \par′ənik′ē·ə\ [Gk *parōnychia* (from PARA- + Gk *onyx*, gen. *onychos*, a claw, talon, in humans a nail) a felon, whitlow] An inflammation of the proximal or lateral nail folds. It may be acute or chronic, and it can be an occupational hazard of hairdressers, fishmongers, caterers, or bartenders. Also *panaritium, panaris, whitlow, perionychial whitlow, onychia lateralis, onychia periungualis.* **herpetic p.** A suppurative inflammation of the nail fold that is due to a herpes simplex infection. It may be seen in dentists and dental nurses. **p. tendinosa** Inflammation and infection of a tendon sheath of the fingers.

**paronychomycosis** \par′ōnik′əmīkō′sis\ [PAR- + ONYCHO- + MYCOSIS] Any fungal infection around the nails.

**paroophoric** \par′ə·ōfôr′ik\ PAROVARIAN.

**paroophoritis** \par′ō·äf′ôrī′tis\ [PAR- + OOPHORITIS] Inflammation adjacent to the ovary. Also *perioophoritis, periovaritis.*

**paroöphoron** \par′ō·äf′ərän\ [PAR- + OOPHORON] A small collection of coiled tubules, more often present in the child, found in the broad ligament between the epoöphoron and the uterus. They are the remnants of the caudal tubules of the mesonephros in the female. Also *parovarium.*

**parorchis** \parôr′kis\ *Outmoded* EPIDIDYMIS.

**parorexia** \par′ōrek′sē·ə\ [PAR- + Gk *orex(is)* a longing for + -IA] EATING DISORDER.

**parosteal** \paräs′tē·əl\ Of or relating to the superficial layer of the periosteum.

**parosteitis** \par′ästē·ī′tis\ An inflammation of tissues that are adjacent to bone. Also *parostitis.*

**parosteosis** \par′ästē·ō′sis\ The ossification of soft tissues outside the periosteum. Also *parostosis.*

**parostitis** \par′ästī′tis\ PAROSTEITIS.

**parostosis** \par′ästō′sis\ PAROSTEOSIS.

**parotic** \pərät′ik\ Adjacent to or near the ear. Also *parotid.*

**parotid** \pərät′id\ [L *parotis*, gen. *parotidis* (from Gk *parōtis*, gen. *parōtidos*, the gland beside and behind the ear, tumor of the parotid gland, from *par(a)-* beside + *ous*, gen. *ōtos*, the ear) a tumor near the ear, swelling of the parotid gland] **1** GLANDULA PAROTIDEA. **2** PAROTIC.

**parotidectomy** \pərät′idek′təmē\ [PAROTID + -ECTOMY] Excision of part or of the whole parotid gland but often only of the portion superficial to the facial nerve. Such action is indicated for certain parotid tumors and, occasionally, for recurrent parotitis. The preservation of the facial nerve, ramifying between the superficial and deep portions of the gland, is a critical feature of the operation.

**parotidoauricularis** \pərät′idō·ôrik′yəler′is\ An occasional slip of the posterior auricular muscle that runs beneath the ear and attaches to the parotid fascia.

**parotitis** \par′ətī′tis\ Any kind of inflammation of the parotid gland or glands. **celiac p.** An inflammation of the parotid gland that occurs as a complication of abdominal surgery. It is usually caused by poor oral hygiene or by a decrease in salivary secretions. **epidemic p.** MUMPS. **postoperative p.** Acute parotitis, usually staphylococcal, occurring postoperatively particularly in debilitated or elderly patients. Dehydration and lack of oral hygiene are predisposing factors. **tropical suppurative p.** An acute infective condition of the parotid glands, usually unilateral, which commonly occurs in tropical countries, especially in debilitated people. Poor oral hygiene is one predisposing factor. The presence of staphylococci and streptococci can often be demonstrated, but a coxsackievirus has also been suggested as an etiologic agent. In Uganda, the disease is most common during the rainy season.

**parous** \par′əs\ [L *par(ere)* to bear or bring forth young + -OUS] Having borne at least one viable offspring.

**parovarian** \par′ōver′ē·ən\ [PAR- + New L *ovarian(us)* ovarian] Located adjacent to the ovary. Also *paroophoric.*

**parovarium** \par′ōver′ē·əm\ **1** EPOÖPHORON. **2** PAROÖPHORON.

**paroxia** \pəräk′sē·ə\ PICA.

**paroxysm** \par′əksizm\ [Gk *paroxysmos* (from *paroxynein* to irritate, provoke, from *par(a)-* beyond, amiss + *oxynein* to sharpen, from *oxys* sharp, acute) exasperation, aggravation, paroxysm] **1** A sudden attack, as a convulsion or spasm. **2** A sharp intensification of the symptoms of a disorder. **3** In electroencephalography, an electrical discharge or waveform which stands out abruptly from the background rhythm.

**paroxysmal** \par′əksiz′məl\ **1** Of or resembling a paroxysm; having the character of a paroxysm. **2** Characterized by paroxysms, as a disease.

**Parrot** [Joseph Marie Jules *Parrot*, French physician, 1829–1883] **1** Parrot's pseudoparalysis, Parrot's disease. See under SYPHILITIC PSEUDOPARALYSIS. **2** Parrot's atrophy of the newborn. See under MARASMUS. **3** See under ULCER. **4** Parrot's disease. See under ACHONDROPLASIA.

**Parry** [Caleb Hillier *Parry*, English physician, 1755–1822] **1** Parry's disease. See under GRAVES DISEASE. **2** Parry-Romberg syndrome. See under ROMBERG'S PROGRESSIVE FACIAL HEMIATROPHY.

# pars

**pars** \pärs\ [L (gen. *partis*), a part, portion] (*pl.* partes) A portion of an organ, a structure, or a surface; a part. **p. abdominalis aortae** [NA] The distal part of the descending aorta, which commences as the continuation of the thoracic aorta in the opening in the diaphragm in the median plane at the level of the lower margin of the twelfth thoracic vertebra. It descends in front of the lumbar vertebrae to the level of the fourth, where it divides into two common iliac arteries at the left of the midline. Its branches may be grouped into anterior and lateral supplying viscera, posterior supplying the abdominal wall, and terminal branches that proceed to the pelvis and lower limbs. Also *abdominal aorta, abdominal part of aorta, aorta abdominalis.* **p. abdominalis esophagi** [NA] The portion of the esophagus that extends from the diaphragm to its termination at the cardiac notch of the stomach and that lies behind the left lobe of the liver. It is covered in front and on its left side by the peritoneum of the upper left part of the lesser omentum. Also *abdominal part of esophagus, cardiac antrum.* Also *pars abdominalis oesophagi.* **p. abdominalis musculi pectoralis majoris** [NA] The part of the pectoralis major muscle that arises from the aponeurosis of the musculus obliquus externus abdominis and curves around the lower border to the posterior and upper aspects of the pectoralis major muscle. **p. abdominalis oesophagi** PARS ABDOMINALIS ESOPHAGI. **p. abdominalis ureteris** [NA] The part of the ureter that extends from the renal pelvis to the brim of the pelvis, lying behind peritoneum and in front of the medial margin of the psoas major muscle. Also *abdominal part of ureter.* **p. alaris musculi nasalis** The part of the nasalis muscle that lies below the nasal aperture and arises from the maxilla above the upper lateral incisor and canine teeth. Also *alar part of nasalis muscle, musculus dilatator naris, dilator muscle of* *nose.* **p. alveolaris mandibulae** [NA] The upper margin of the body of the mandible that forms the alveolar arch with the opposite side. It contains sixteen hollowed sockets on each side for the roots of the lower teeth. Also *alveolar part of mandible, alveolar process of mandible.* **p. amorpha** The distinct component of extremely fine, electron-dense filaments densely packed together within the nucleolonema of a nucleolus. *Outmoded.* Also *pars filamentosa nucleolonemae, pars fibrosa nucleolonemae.* **p. annularis vaginae fibrosae digitorum manus** The thick band of transverse fibers that strengthens the digital fibrous sheaths anteriorly opposite the middle of the proximal and of the middle phalanges of the fingers. Each is attached to the margins of the phalanges. Also *annular ligaments of fingers, annular ligaments of digits of hand, annular ligaments of tendon sheaths of fingers.* **p. annularis vaginae fibrosae digitorum pedis** [NA] The thick band of transverse fibers that strengthens the digital fibrous sheaths anteriorly opposite the middle of the proximal end of the middle phalanges of the toes. Each is attached to the margins of the phalanges. Also *annular ligaments of digits of foot.* **p. anterior commissurae anterioris cerebri** The anterior part of the anterior cerebral commissure, greatly reduced in man, that interconnects the anterior olfactory nuclei. **p. anterior faciei diaphragmaticae hepatis** [NA] The anterior subdivision of the diaphragmatic surface of the liver. It is related anteriorly through the diaphragm to the costal arches and xiphisternum above and to the anterior abdominal wall lower down. The falciform ligament is attached to it. Also *anterior part of diaphragmatic surface of liver.* **p. anterior fornicis vaginae** [NA] The anterior part of the continuous circular recess in the vagina between the cervix uteri and the anterior wall of the vagina. Also *anterior fornix.* **p. anterior lobuli quadrangularis** [NA] Anterior part of quadrangular lobule; the portion of the cerebellar hemispheres situated in front of the primary fissure and within the anterior lobe of the cerebellum. Also *anterior quadrangular lobule.* **p. ascendens aortae** [NA] The proximal part of the aorta. At its origin the right and left coronary arteries arise from the upper part of or above the aortic sinuses. Also *ascending aorta, ascending part of aorta, aorta ascendens.* **p. ascendens duodeni** [NA] The fourth or terminal part of the duodenum that ascends in front and to the left of the abdominal aorta for about one inch to end at the duodenojejunal flexure. Also *fourth part of duodenum.* **p. basilaris ossis occipitalis** [NA] A platelike rectangular portion of the occipital bone that extends forward and upward from the foramen magnum to fuse with the sphenoid bone at the sphenoccipital synchondrosis by about the twenty-fifth year. Also *basilar apophysis, basilar bone, basioccipital bone, basilar part of occipital bone, basilar process.* **p. basilaris pontis** PARS VENTRALIS PONTIS. **p. buccopharyngea** PARS BUCCOPHARYNGEA MUSCULI CONSTRICTORIS PHARYNGIS SUPERIORIS. **p. buccopharyngea musculi constrictoris pharyngis superioris** [NA] The part of the superior pharyngeal constrictor muscle that arises from the pterygomandibular raphe. Also *buccopharyngeal muscle, buccopharyngeal part of superior constrictor muscle of pharynx, pars buccopharyngea.* **p. cardiaca gastris** [NA] An ill-defined area about 3-4 cm in breadth that is adjacent to and includes the cardiac orifice of the stomach. The cardiac glands are situated in it. Also *cardiac part of stomach, pars cardiaca ventriculi, cardiac stomach, cardia of stomach.* **p. cartilaginea tubae auditivae** [NA] That part of the auditory tube formed by a triangular plate of cartilage composed of medial and lateral laminae forming a hook-shaped groove, the open ends of which are connected by a fibrous membrane. The part is joined at its apex to the medial end of the bony part of the tube by fibrous tissue, whereas its base is covered by mucous membrane of the lateral wall of the nasopharynx to form the tubal elevation behind the orifice of the tube. Also *cartilaginous part of auditory tube.* **p. centralis ventriculi lateralis cerebri** [NA] The curved part of the lateral ventricle located within the parietal lobe and extending from the interventricular foramen to the splenium of the corpus callosum. **p. ceratopharyngea musculi constrictoris pharyngis medii** [NA] The part of the middle pharyngeal constrictor muscle arising from the superior margin of the greater cornu of the hyoid bone. Also *ceratopharyngeal muscle, ceratopharyngeal part of middle constrictor muscle of pharynx, ceratopharyngeus.* **p. cervicalis esophagi** [NA] The part of the esophagus that is situated in the neck, extending from its continuation of the pharynx at the lower margin of the cricoid cartilage opposite the sixth cervical vertebra to the superior mediastinum of the thorax at the oblique plane of the first ribs. **p. cervicalis medullae spinalis** The cervical portion of the spinal cord, contained within the upper part of the vertebral canal. It is expanded as the cervical enlargement, and gives rise to eight pairs of cervical spinal nerves. **p. cervicalis systematis sympathici** [NA] The cervical portion of the sympathetic nervous system. **p. cervicalis tracheae** [NA] The upper portion of the trachea, which is situated in the midline of the neck. It is continuous with the larynx superiorly, extending from the lower border of the cricoid cartilage at the level of the sixth cervical vertebra to the superior mediastinum at the level of the upper border of the manubrium sterni where it continues into the thoracic cavity. Also *cervical part of trachea, cervical trachea.* **p. chondropharyngea musculi constrictoris pharyngis medii** [NA] The part of the middle pharyngeal constrictor muscle that arises from the lesser cornu of the hyoid bone and the lower part of the stylohyoid ligament. Also *chondropharyngeal part of the middle constrictor muscle of the pharynx, chondropharyngeal muscle.* **p. ciliaris retinae** [NA] The epithelium that lines the internal surface of the ciliary body. It is formed by the two layers of epithelial cells of the retina extending anteriorly from the ora serrata and ending as the pars iridica retinae. Also *ciliary part of retina.* **p. clavicularis musculi pectoralis majoris** [NA] The part of the pectoralis major muscle that arises from the medial half of the anterior surface of the clavicle. **p. cochlearis nervi octavi** The cochlear part of the nervus vestibulocochlearis (eighth cranial nerve), arising from bipolar cells of the spiral ganglion of the cochlea. Also *nervus cochleae, cochlear nerve, pars cochlearis of eighth nerve.* **p. convoluta** PARS CONVOLUTA LOBULI CORTICALIS RENALIS. **p. convoluta lobuli corticalis renalis** [NA] The portion of the renal cortex that lies between the medullary rays and contains renal corpuscles and the proximal and distal convoluted tubules. Also *convoluted part of kidney lobule, cortical labyrinth, renal labyrinth, pars convoluta.* **p. costalis diaphragmatis** [NA] The part of the diaphragm that arises from the internal surfaces of the cartilages and adjacent parts of the lower six ribs on each side. Also *costal part of diaphragm, sternocostal part of diaphragm.* **p. cricopharyngea musculi constrictoris pharyngis inferioris** [NA] The more distal part of the inferior pharyngeal constrictor muscle. It arises from the lateral side of the cricoid cartilage, and its lower fibers are continuous with the circular fibers of the esophagus. Its tonic contraction keeps the upper end of the esophagus closed, serving as a sphincter during swallowing and relaxing when the thyropharyngeus part contracts. Also *cricopharyngeal muscle, cricopharyngeal part of inferior constrictor muscle of the pharynx, cricopharyngeal sphincter, Killian's bundle, cricopharyngeus.* **p. cruciformis vaginae fibrosae digitorum manus** [NA] The oblique fibers of the fibrous sheaths of the digits of the hand that criss-cross anterior to the interphalangeal joints, producing strong but thin portions of the sheaths that do not interfere with flexion of the fingers. Also *cruciform part of fibrous sheaths of digits of hand, cruciate ligaments of fingers, crucial ligaments of fingers.* **p. cruciformis vaginae fibrosae digitorum pedis** [NA] The oblique fibers of the fibrous sheaths of the toes that criss-cross on the plantar aspects of the interphalangeal joints, producing strong but thin portions of the sheaths that do not interfere with flexion of the joints. Also *cruciform part of fibrous sheaths of digits of toes, cruciate ligaments of toes.* **p. cupularis recessus epitympanici** [NA] The lateral part of the epitympanic recess that is incompletely separated by the head of the malleus, the body and short limb of the incus, and the incudal fold. Also *cupular part of epitympanic recess, cupulate part of epitympanic recess, cupola space.* **p. descendens aortae** [NA] The part of the aorta distal to the aortic arch which is divided into the pars thoracica aortae and the pars abdominalis aortae. Also *descending part of aorta, descending aorta, aorta descendens, dorsal aorta.* **p. descendens duodeni** [NA] The vertical portion of the duodenum which extends downward in front of the anteromedial part of the right kidney and medial to the right lateral line from the superior duodenal flexure at the level of the first lumbar vertebra to the inferior duodenal flexure at the level of the third lumbar vertebra. Also *descending part of duodenum, second part of duodenum.* **p. dextra faciei diaphragmaticae hepatis** [NA] The portion of the diaphragmatic surface of the liver that is deep to the seventh to eleventh costal arches on the right side and separated from them by the diaphragm, pleura, and a piece of the base of the right lung. Also *right part of diaphragmatic surface of liver.* **p. distalis adenohypophyseos** [NA] The main body of the adenohypophysis. See under PITUITARY GLAND. **p. dorsalis pontis** [NA] The dorsal, or posterior, part of the pons representing, with the exception of the pyramids, a direct rostral continuation of the structures in the medulla oblongata. Also *tegmentum pontis, tegmentum of pons, pontile tegmentum, tegmentum rhombencephali.* **p. fibrillaris** The part of the nucleolus that is composed of fine filaments and within which RNA synthesis commences. The DNA template for this also exists within the pars fibrillaris. **p. fibrosa nucleolonemae** PARS AMORPHA. **p. filamentosa nucleolonemae** PARS AMORPHA. **p. flaccida membranae tympani** [NA] The thin, triangular, slack part of the tympanic membrane, located above the anterior and posterior mallear folds. Also *flaccid part of tympanic membrane, Shrapnell's membrane, Rivinus membrane, flaccid membrane of Shrapnell.* **p. frontalis capsulae internae** CRUS ANTERIUS CAPSULAE INTERNAE. **p. frontalis coronae radiatae** The frontal part of the corona radiata, composed of projection fibers that connect the frontal lobes of the cerebral cortex with the lower brain and spinal cord. **p. frontalis corporis callosi** PARS FRONTALIS RADIATIONIS CORPORIS CALLOSI. **p. frontalis operculi** OPERCULUM FRONTALE. **p. frontalis radiationis corporis callosi** Frontal radiations of the corpus callosum, composed of commissural fibers that radiate from the genu at the anterior end of the corpus callosum into the frontal poles of the cerebral cortex. Also *pars frontalis corporis callosi.* **partes genitales masculinae externae** *Outmoded* ORGANA GENITALIA MASCULINA EXTERNA. **p. glabra** The smooth, hairless part of the developing lip. **p. glandularis** *Outmoded* ADENOHYPOPHYSIS. **p. glossopharyngea musculi constrictoris pharyngis superioris** [NA] A few fibers of the superior constrictor muscle of the pharynx that arise from the side of the root of the tongue deep to the hyoglossus muscle. Also *glossopharyngeal part of superior constrictor muscle of pharynx, glossopharyngeal muscle, glossopharyngeus.* **p. granulosa** The part of the nucleolus that has a granular structure and represents stored RNA prior to its transfer to the cell cytoplasm. **p. grisea hypothalami** The gray matter of the hypothalamus, comprising the various hypothalamic nuclei. **p. horizontalis duodeni** [NA] The horizontal part of the duodenum. It extends transversely from the inferior duodenal flexure, across the level of the third lumbar vertebra in front of the inferior vena cava, to the front of the abdominal aorta, where it becomes the ascending part. Also *horizontal part of duodenum, third part of duodenum, inferior part of duodenum.* **p. inferior fossae rhomboideae** The inferior part of the rhomboid fossa. **p. inferior gyri frontalis medii** The inferior part of the middle frontal gyrus, lying beneath the middle frontal sulcus. **p. inferior partis vestibularis nervi octavi** The inferior part of the vestibular portion of the eighth cranial nerve, consisting of saccular and posterior ampullar fibers. **p. infraclavicularis plexus brachialis** [NA] The portion of the brachial plexus below the level of the clavicle. It comprises the three cords and the branches arising in the axilla. Also *infraclavicular part of brachial plexus.* **p. infrasegmentalis** PARS INTERSEGMENTALIS. **p. infundibularis adenohypophyseos** PARS TUBERALIS ADENOHYPOPHYSEOS. **p. interarticularis** The part of the vertebral arch on each side between the superior and inferior articular processes: applied chiefly to the lumbar vertebrae. **p. intercartilaginea rimae glottidis** [NA] The posterior two fifths of the rima glottidis, located between the vocal processes of the arytenoid cartilages. Also *intercartilaginous part of glottis, respiratory glottis, intercartilaginous glottis, interarytenoid space, rima glottidis cartilaginea* (outmoded). **p. intermedia bulborum** [NA] A narrow median band of erectile tissue that unites the anterior ends of the two bulbs of the vestibule and attaches to the clitoris. Also *commissure of the bulb, commissure of the vestibule.* **p. intermedia fossae rhomboideae** Intermediate part of the rhomboid fossa; the middle part of the floor of the fourth ventricle extending from an imaginary line at the level of the superior foveae to the horizontal sections of the taeniae of the ventricle and prolonged into the lateral recesses. **p. intermedia adenohypophyseos** [NA] The intermediate part of the adenohypophysis, vaguely delimited in man. See under PITUITARY GLAND. **p. intermembranacea rimae glottidis** [NA] The anterior three fifths of the rima glottidis situated between the vocal folds. Also *intermembranous part of glottis.* **p. intersegmentalis** [NA] The tributary of a pulmonary vein that runs in the connective tissue between two adjacent bronchopulmonary segments and may drain segments or portions of them. It joins similar and intrasegmental tributaries to form a single vein for each lobe. Also *pars infrasegmentalis, intersegmental vein, infrasegmental vein.* **p. intersegmentalis rami anterioris venae pulmonalis dextrae superioris** [NA] An intersegmental tributary of the anterior branch of the right superior pulmonary vein that helps to drain the anterior bronchopulmonary segment (B III) of the superior lobe of the right lung. **p. intersegmentalis rami anterioris venae pulmonalis sinistrae superioris** [NA] An intersegmental tributary of the anterior branch of the left superior pulmonary vein that helps to drain the anterior bronchopulmonary segment (B III) of the superior lobe of the left lung. **p. intersegmentalis rami apicalis venae pulmonalis dextrae superioris** [NA] An intersegmental tributary of the apical branch of the right superior pulmonary vein that helps to drain the apical bronchopulmonary segment (B I) of the superior lobe of the right lung. **p. intersegmentalis rami apicoposterioris venae pulmonalis sinistrae superioris** [NA] An intersegmental tributary of the apicoposterior branch of the left superior pulmonary vein that helps to drain the apicoposterior bronchopulmonary segment (B I + II) of the superior lobe of the left lung. **p. intrasegmentalis** [NA] A tributary of a pulmonary vein that lies within and drains a single bronchopulmonary segment of a lung. It joins similar tributaries and intersegmental veins to form a single vein for each pulmonary lobe. Also *intrasegmental vein.* **p. intrasegmentalis rami anterioris venae pulmonalis dextrae superioris** [NA] The intrasegmental tributary of the anterior branch of the right superior pulmonary vein. It helps to drain the anterior bronchopulmonary segment (B III) of the superior lobe of the right lung. **p. intrasegmentalis rami anterioris venae pulmonalis sinistrae superioris** [NA] The intrasegmental tributary of the anterior branch of the left superior pulmonary vein that helps to drain the anterior bronchopulmonary segment (B III) of the superior lobe of the left lung. **p. intrasegmentalis rami apicalis venae pulmonalis dextrae superioris** [NA] The intrasegmental tributary of the apical branch of the right superior pulmonary vein that helps to drain the apical bronchopulmonary segment (B I) of the superior lobe of the right lung. **p. intrasegmentalis rami apicoposterioris venae pulmonalis sinistrae superioris** [NA] The intrasegmental tributary of the apicoposterior branch of the left superior pulmonary vein that helps to drain the apicoposterior bronchopulmonary segment (B I + II) of the superior lobe of the left lung. **p. iridica retinae** [NA] The thin part of the retina that extends over the posterior surface of the iris and comprises two layers of pigmented, cubical cells, which become continuous at the pupillary border. Also *iridial part of retina.* **p. labialis musculi orbicularis oris** [NA] The part of the orbicularis oris muscle that is limited to the lips, comprising mostly fibers of the buccinator muscle. **p. lacrimalis musculi orbicularis oculi** [NA] The part of the orbicularis oculi muscle that lies behind the lacrimal sac and arises from the posterior crest and adjacent lateral surface of the lacrimal bone as well as the lacrimal fascia. After passing laterally, it divides into upper and lower slips that are inserted into the medial parts of the upper and lower tarsal plates respectively, as well as into the lateral palpebral raphe. Also *lacrimal part of orbicularis oculi muscle, Duverney's muscle, Horner's muscle.* **p. laryngea pharyngis** [NA] The lower part of the pharynx, lying posterior to the larynx and extending from the upper margin of the epiglottis to the lower margin of the cricoid cartilage, where it continues as the esophagus. Its anterior wall comprises the laryngeal inlet and the posterior surfaces of the arytenoid and cricoid cartilages. Posteriorly are the bodies of the third to sixth cervical vertebrae. Also *laryngeal part of pharynx, laryngopharynx, hypopharynx, laryngeal pharynx, pharyngolaryngeal cavity, laryngopharyngeal cavity, pharyngoesophagus.* **p. lateralis arcus longitudinalis pedis** The lateral part of the longitudinal arch of the foot that is formed by the calcaneus, cuboid, and the lateral two metatarsals. It steadies the foot on the ground in standing and during locomotion. It is maintained by ligaments, the intrinsic muscles of the foot, and the long muscles of the leg. **p. lateralis fornicis vaginae** [NA] The lateral part of the continuous circular recess in the vagina between the cervix uteri and the lateral wall of the vagina. The domelike roof is related to the terminal part of the ureter, being crossed by the uterine artery on each side. Also *lateral fornix.* **p. lateralis musculorum intertransversariorum posteriorum cervicis** [NA] The lateral portion of the posterior intertransverse muscles of the cervical region that is supplied by the ventral rami of cervical nerves. **p. lateralis ossis occipitalis** [NA] The portion of the occipital bone that forms the lateral boundary of the foramen magnum and has the articular condyle on its inferior surface for the atlas. Also *lateral part of occipital bone, condylar part of occipital bone, exoccipital bone, exoccipital part of occipital bone, jugular part of occipital bone, lateral mass of occipital bone.* **p. lateralis ossis sacri** [NA] The bars of bone between the pelvic sacral foramina and between the dorsal sacral foramina, representing the costal elements of other vertebrae, that fuse with each other and with the base lateral to these foramina and, posteriorly, with the transverse processes. Also *lateral part of sacrum, lateral mass of sacrum, ala sacralis, ala of sacrum.* **p. libera columnae fornicis** COLUMNA FORNICIS. **p. lumbalis diaphragmatis** [NA] The posterior origin of the diaphragm from the lumbar vertebrae by two crura, the right crus from the first three vertebrae and the left crus from the first two; and from two fibrous arches, the medial and lateral arcuate ligaments. Also *lumbar part of diaphragm, vertebral part of diaphragm.* **p. lumbalis medullae spinalis** [NA] The lumbar part of the spinal cord, situated in the lumbar part of the vertebral canal. It is expanded as the lumbar enlargement, and gives rise to five pairs of lumbar spinal nerves. **p. mamillaris hypothalami** CORPUS MAMILLARE. **p. marginalis musculi orbicularis oris** [NA] A complex arrangement of muscle fibers around the outer margin of the lips. It comprises fibers prolonged from surrounding facial muscles decussating at the corners of the mouth. **p. marginalis sulci cinguli** The marginal part of the cingulate sulcus; the posterior portion of the cingulate sulcus, extending dorsally between the paracentral lobule and the precuneus, or quadrate lobule. **p. medialis arcus longitudinalis pedis** The medial part of the longitudinal arch of the foot, comprising the calcaneus, talus, navicular, three cuneiform, and three medial metatarsal bones. It provides a very arched and elastic support for the body weight during such activities as walking, jumping, and running. **p. medialis musculorum intertransversariorum posteriorum cervicis** [NA] The medial slips of the posterior intertransverse muscles of the neck, considered to be the proper intertransverse muscle which, in turn, is subdivided by the pathway through it of the dorsal ramus of the cervical nerve. **p. membranacea septi interventricularis cordis** [NA] The thin, fibrous upper portion of the interventricular septum of the heart. It is small and oval and located immediately below the junction of the right and anterior valvules of the aortic valve. Also *membranous part of interventricular septum of heart.* **p. membranacea septi nasi** [NA] The thickened skin and subcutaneous tissue below the medial crura of the major alar cartilages at the anteroinferior margin of the nasal septum. It is part of the pars mobilis septi nasi. Also *membranous part of nasal septum, membranous septum of nose.* **p. membranacea urethrae mascu-**

**linae** [NA] The shortest and least dilatable part, except for the external orifice, of the male urethra. It extends from the apex of the prostate to the bulb of the penis and passes through the perineal membrane between them. Also *membranous part of male urethra, membranous urethra.* **p. mobilis septi nasi** [NA] The movable anteroinferior part of the nasal septum, composed of the medial crura or septal processes of the two major alar cartilages, thickened skin, and subcutaneous tissue. The crura are attached by fibrous tissue to the distal end of the septal cartilage. Also *mobile part of nasal septum, mobile septum of nose.* **p. muscularis septi interventricularis cordis** [NA] The thick, muscular portion of the interventricular septum of the heart. It occupies most of the septum. **p. mylopharyngea musculi constrictoris pharyngis superioris** [NA] The part of the superior pharyngeal constrictor muscle that arises from the posterior fifth of the mylohyoid line on the inner surface of the body of the mandible adjacent to the ramus. Also *mylopharyngeal part of superior constrictor muscle of pharynx, mylopharyngeal muscle.* **p. nasalis ossis frontalis** [NA] The part of the frontal bone that projects inferiorly between the orbital margins, lying in front of the ethmoidal notch and ending anteroinferiorly at the curved nasal margin, behind which the nasal spine projects downwards in the median line into the nasal septum behind the nasal bones. Extending back on each side of the spine is a groove that forms part of the roof of the nasal cavity. Also *prefrontal bone, nasal process of frontal bone, nasal part of frontal bone.* **p. nasalis pharyngis** [NA] The part of the pharynx that lies behind the nasal cavity and and above the level of the soft palate, communicating anteriorly with the nose through the choanae and inferiorly with the oral pharynx through the pharyngeal isthmus. Also *nasopharynx, nasal part of pharynx, pharyngonasal cavity, rhinopharynx, postnasal space, throat.* **p. nervosa hypophyseos** LOBUS NERVOSUS NEUROHYPOPHYSEOS. **p. obliqua musculi cricothyroidei** [NA] The lower fibers of the cricothyroid muscle, which extend posteriorly and laterally to be inserted into the anterior margin of the inferior horn and the inner surface of the thyroid cartilage. **p. occipitalis capsulae internae** CRUS POSTERIUS CAPSULAE INTERNAE. **p. occipitalis coronae radiatae** The occipital part of the corona radiata, containing projection fibers that connect the occipital lobes of the cerebral cortex with the lower brain and spinal cord. **p. occipitalis radiationis corporis callosi** Commissural fibers extending posteriorly from the splenium of the corpus callosum into the occipital lobes of the cerebral cortex. Also *occipital radiations of corpus callosum.* **p. opercularis gyri frontalis inferioris** The opercular part of the inferior frontal gyrus, a subdivision of the inferior frontal gyrus lying posterior to the ascending ramus of the lateral sulcus and continuous with the precentral gyrus. **p. optica hypothalami** The rostral part of the hypothalamus, which lies above the optic chiasma. *Outmoded.* **p. optica retinae** [NA] The region of the retina between the ora serrata and the optic disk which contains the visual photosensitive receptors. It comprises the stratum, or pars, pigmentosum and the multilayer stratum, or pars, nervosum. Also *optic part of retina.* **p. oralis pharyngis** [NA] The part of the pharynx extending from the soft palate to the upper border of the epiglottis and opening anteriorly into the mouth through the oropharyngeal isthmus between the palatoglossal folds. It is continuous above with the nasopharynx and below with the laryngeal part of the pharynx. Also *oral part of pharynx, oral pharynx, oropharynx, pharyngo-oral cavity.* **p. orbitalis glandulae lacrimalis** [NA] The upper and larger part of the lacrimal gland, situated in the lacrimal fossa just within the superolateral margin of the orbit, where it is bound to the periosteum by fibrous tissue. Also *orbital part of lacrimal gland, principal lacrimal gland.* **p. orbitalis gyri frontalis inferioris** The orbital part of the inferior frontal gyrus, a subdivision of the inferior frontal gyrus located below the anterior ramus of the lateral sulcus and curving on to the orbital surface of the frontal lobe. **p. orbitalis musculi orbicularis oculi** [NA] The outer part of the orbicularis oculi muscle that arises from the medial palpebral ligament, the nasal part of the frontal bone, and the anterior lacrimal crest of the maxilla. It forms a flat ring surrounding the orbit, some of its fibers blending with muscles of the forehead and cheeks and others inserting into the skin of the eyebrow. Also *orbital part of orbicularis oculi muscle.* **p. orbitalis ossis frontalis** [NA] One of two triangular plates of bone that extend posteriorly at right angles to the squama of the frontal bone to form the roofs of the orbits and the floor of the anterior cranial fossa. The two are separated from each other by the ethmoid notch. Also *orbital part of frontal bone, orbital plate of frontal bone.* **p. ossea septi nasi** [NA] The bony part of the medial wall or septum of the nasal cavity. Also *bony part of nasal septum.* **p. ossea tubae auditivae** [NA] The part of the auditory tube that extends from the anterior wall of the middle ear to the angle of junction of the petrous and squamous parts of the temporal bone. There the cartilaginous part of the tube is attached to it by fibrous tissue. Also *bony part of auditory tube.* **p. palpebralis glandulae lacrimalis** [NA] The lower and smaller part of the lacrimal gland. It is continuous with the orbital part around the lateral margin of the aponeurosis of the levator palpebrae superioris muscle, and it extends below the aponeurosis into the lateral part of the upper eyelid. It is attached to the superior fornix of the conjunctiva where its ducts open. Also *palpebral part of lacrimal gland, Rosenmüller's gland, Rosenmüller's node.* **p. palpebralis musculi orbicularis oculi** [NA] The collection of fibers of the orbicularis oculi muscle that arises from the medial palpebral ligament and from the adjacent bone. The fibers then extend across the upper and lower eyelids in front of the orbital septum to interdigitate at the lateral commissure to form the lateral palpebral raphe. It is innervated by the facial nerve and its function is to close the eyelids either voluntarily or reflexly. Also *palpebral part of orbicularis oculi muscle.* **p. parasympathica systematis nervosi autonomici** SYSTEMA NERVOSUM AUTONOMICUM, PARS PARASYMPATHICA. **p. parietalis coronae radiatae** The parietal part of the corona radiata, composed of projection fibers connecting the parietal lobes of the cerebral cortex with the lower brain and spinal cord. **p. parietalis operculi** OPERCULUM FRONTOPARIETALE. **p. parietalis radiationis corporis callosi** Commissural fibers that project from the trunk of the corpus callosum into the parietal lobes of the cerebral cortex. Also *parietal radiations of corpus callosum.* **p. pelvica ureteris** [NA] The part of the ureter that passes through the pelvis from the pelvic brim to the base of the urinary bladder. Also *pelvic part of ureter.* **p. pelvina systematis sympathici** The pelvic portion of the sympathetic nervous system. **p. petrosa ossis temporalis** [NA] The pyramid-shaped dense part of the temporal bone that projects medially and anteriorly between the occipital and sphenoid bones at the base of the skull and houses the middle and internal ears. It has an apex, a base, three margins, and three surfaces. Its posterior portion forms the mastoid process. Also *petrous part of temporal bone, pet-*

*romastoid, petrosal bone, petrous bone, petrosa.* **p. pharyngea lobi anterioris hypophyseos** ADENOHYPOPHYSIS. **p. postcommunicalis** [NA] The part beyond the junction of the communicating artery, such as the portion of the anterior cerebral artery beyond or distal to the junction of the anterior communicating artery, or that portion of the posterior cerebral artery beyond or distal to the junction of the posterior communicating artery. Also *postcommunical segment.* **p. posterior commissurae anterioris cerebri** The posterior part of the anterior cerebral commissure, forming the bulk of the anterior commissure. **p. posterior faciei diaphragmaticae hepatis** [NA] The triangular and smallest part of the diaphragmatic surface of the liver that comprises the bare area of the right lobe of the liver and the caudate lobe. Also *posterior part of diaphragmatic surface of liver.* **p. posterior fornicis vaginae** [NA] The posterior part of the continuous circular recess in the vagina between the cervix uteri and the wall of the vagina. It is deeper than the anterior part and has its dome covered externally by the peritoneum of the rectouterine pouch. Also *posterior fornix.* **p. posterior lobuli quadrangularis** LOBULUS SIMPLEX. **p. profunda glandulae parotideae** [NA] The part of the parotid salivary gland that is usually deep to the anterior branches of the facial nerve. Its anteromedial aspect extends forward between the ramus of the mandible and the medial pterygoid muscle, whereas its posteromedial aspect is related posteriorly to the mastoid process and inferiorly to the anterior border of the sternocleidomastoid muscle. Also *deep part of parotid gland.* **p. profunda musculi masseteris** [NA] The deep part of the masseter muscle, arising from the posterior third of the inferior margin and the whole inner surface of the zygomatic arch. It is inserted into the upper two thirds of the outer surface of the ramus of the mandible and into the coronoid process. **p. profunda musculi sphincteris ani externi** [NA] The ringlike deep part of the external anal sphincter, lying above the superficial part and surrounding the internal sphincter. **p. prostatica urethrae masculinae** [NA] The most dilatable and widest part of the male urethra, descending through the prostate from the base to the apex. Also *prostatic urethra.* **p. pterygopharyngea musculi constrictoris pharyngis superioris** [NA] The part of the superior pharyngeal constrictor muscle that arises from the lower part of the posterior margin of the medial pterygoid plate and the pterygoid hamulus. Also *pterygopharyngeal muscle, pterygopharyngeal part of superior constrictor muscle of pharynx.* **p. pylorica gastris** [NA] The small portion of the stomach distal to a plane through the angular incisure and the greater curvature opposite. It consists of the pyloric antrum, canal and sphincter. Also *pyloric part of stomach.* **p. quadrata** [NA] The portion of the medial segment of the left lobe of the liver that is included in the quadrate lobe. **p. radiata lobuli corticalis renis** [NA] The portion of the renal cortex that is composed of a series of pale conical areas that extend outward radially from the base of each renal pyramid, tapering towards the capsule and consisting of straight tubules, including the ascending and descending limbs of the loops of Henle and collecting tubules, which lie between the intervening strips of the pars convoluta. Also *medullary ray, pyramid of Ferrein, cortical ray.* **p. recta musculi cricothyroidei** [NA] The anterosuperior part of the cricothyroid muscle that passes upward posteriorly. It is inserted into the inferior margin of the lamina of the thyroid cartilage. Also *straight part of cricothyroid muscle.* **p. retrolentiformis capsulae internae** [NA] The retrolentiform part of the internal capsule, lying behind the lentiform nucleus and consisting of parietopontine and occipitopontine fibers, occipital projections to the superior colliculus and pretectal area, and the posterior thalamic radiation. **p. spongiosa urethrae masculinae** [NA] The part of the male urethra within the corpus spongiosum penis that extends from the end of the membranous urethra where it enters the bulb of penis to the external urethral orifice at the tip of the glans penis. It is surrounded by erectile tissue throughout its length, and it contains two dilated parts, namely, the intrabulbar fossa at its commencement in the bulb and the fossa navicularis in the glans. The ducts of the bulbourethral glands enter it just beyond the perineal membrane. Also *spongiose part of male urethra, spongy urethra, penile urethra, anterior urethra, cavernous urethra.* **p. squamosa ossis temporalis** [NA] The upper and front part of the temporal bone that is flat, scalelike, and thin, forming part of the lateral wall of the cranium. The uneven upper border forms about two thirds of a circle, and from the lower part of the temporal surface the zygomatic process projects anteriorly. Posteriorly it fuses with the mastoid process of the petrous part behind the external acoustic meatus. On the inferior aspect of the root of the zygomatic process is the mandibular fossa. Also *squama temporalis* (outmoded). **p. sternalis diaphragmatis** [NA] The part of the diaphragm that arises by two fleshy slips from the posterior aspect of the xiphoid process. Also *sternal part of diaphragm.* **p. sternocostalis musculi pectoralis majoris** [NA] The part of the pectoralis major muscle that arises from the front and side of the sternum as far as the sixth costal cartilage and from the front of the cartilages of the second to sixth ribs. **p. subcutanea musculi sphincteris ani externi** [NA] The small bandlike part of the external anal sphincter muscle that lies deep to the skin around the anal orifice. It also surrounds the lower part of the anal canal below the lower margin of the superficial part of the external sphincter and of the internal sphincter muscle. **p. subfrontalis sulci cinguli** The subfrontal part of the cingulate sulcus; the anterior portion of the cingulate sulcus lying beneath the superior frontal gyrus. **p. sublentiformis capsulae internae** [NA] The sublentiform part of the internal capsule, lying behind and beneath the lentiform nucleus and containing temporopontine and parietopontine fibers and the acoustic radiation. **p. superficialis glandulae parotideae** [NA] The part of the parotid salivary gland that is usually superficial to the anterior branches of the facial nerve. It extends forward superficial to the masseter muscle and backward to the mastoid process and the anterior border of the sternocleidomastoid muscle. The parotid duct emerges from its anterior border, and small lymph nodes are located on the surface of this part. Also *superficial part of parotid gland.* **p. superficialis musculi masseteris** [NA] The superficial part of the masseter muscle that arises by an aponeurosis from the anterior two thirds of the lower border of the zygomatic bone and is inserted into the lower half of the lateral surface of the ramus, the angle, and the adjacent part of the body of the mandible. **p. superficialis musculi sphincteris ani externi** [NA] The elliptical superficial part of the external anal sphincter that lies deep to the subcutaneous part and superficial to the internal sphincter. It arises from the posterior aspect of the lowest segment of the coccyx by the anococcygeal raphe and inserts into the perineal body. **p. superior duodeni** [NA] The most movable part of the duodenum, commencing at the pylorus and passing backward, upward and to the right to the neck of the gallbladder. There it turns downwards to form the descending part. It is covered anteriorly by peritoneum but is bare posteriorly except where adjacent to the pylorus. There the right margin of the lesser omentum splits around it. The portion adjacent to the pylorus is prominent in roentgenograms and referred to as the ampulla duodeni. Also *first part of duodenum, superior part of duodenum, duodenal bulb.* **p. superior faciei diaphragmaticae hepatis** [NA] The convex upper part of the diaphragmatic surface of the liver on which the shallow cardiac impression is situated and which is divided by the falciform ligament into a smaller left portion and a larger right portion. Through the diaphragm it is related to the base of the right lung and its pleura, the pericardium and heart, and, to a small extent, the base of the left lung and its pleura. **p. superior fossae rhomboideae** Superior part of the rhomboid fossa; the triangular part of the floor of the fourth ventricle limited laterally by the superior cerebellar peduncles. **p. superior gyri frontalis medii** The superior part of the middle frontal gyrus, situated above the middle frontal sulcus. **p. superior partis vestibularis nervi octavi** The superior part of the vestibular portion of the eighth cranial nerve, consisting of utricular and anterior and posterior ampullar fibers. **p. supraclavicularis plexus brachialis** [NA] The part of the brachial plexus that lies above the clavicle in the neck. It comprises the roots and trunks and their branches, namely, branches to the scalene and longus colli muscles, to the phrenic nerve, the dorsal scapular nerve and the long thoracic nerve from the roots, as well as the nerve to the subclavius and the suprascapular nerve from the superior trunk. **p. supraoptica** The most rostral or anterior region of the hypothalamus, lying dorsal to the optic nerves and between the preoptic region rostrally, and dorsal to the infundibular or tuberal region of the hypothalamus. **p. tecta columnae fornicis** CRUS FORNICIS. **p. temporalis coronae radiatae** The temporal part of the corona radiata; the projection fibers that connect the temporal lobe of the cerebral cortex with the brainstem and spinal cord. **p. temporalis operculi** OPERCULUM TEMPORALE. **p. temporalis radiationis corporis callosi** The temporal part of the radiations of the corpus callosum; fibers of the trunk and splenium of the corpus callosum that project into the temporal lobes of the cerebral cortex and form the lateral walls of the inferior horns of the lateral ventricles. **p. tensa membranae tympani** [NA] The lower, major part of the tympanic membrane below the triangular pars flaccida which is thicker and firmer than the pars flaccida. The handle of the malleus is attached to its inner surface. Also *tense part of tympanic membrane.* **p. thoracalis medullae spinalis** PARS THORACICA MEDULLAE SPINALIS. **p. thoracalis systematis autonomici** The thoracic part of the autonomic nervous system, consisting of the sympathetic trunk in the thorax with each ganglion connected by white and gray rami communicantes to its corresponding thoracic spinal nerve, the greater, lesser and lowest splanchnic nerves, and the cardiac, pulmonary, and esophageal plexuses. Also *pars thoracalis systematis sympathici.* **p. thoracica aortae** [NA] The proximal part of the descending aorta, situated in the posterior mediastinum and extending from the arch of the aorta at the level of the lower margin of the fourth thoracic vertebra to end as the abdominal aorta at the level of the lower margin of the twelfth thoracic vertebra. There it passes through the diaphragm. It supplies parietal branches to the walls of the thoracic cavity and visceral branches to the bronchi, lungs, esophagus, and pericardium. Also *thoracic part of aorta, thoracic aorta, aorta thoracica, descending thoracic aorta.* **p. thoracica esophagi** [NA] The part of the esophagus that extends through the superior and then the posterior mediastinum from the inlet of the thorax to the hiatus in the right crus of the diaphragm at the level of the tenth thoracic vertebra. There it enters the abdominal cavity. It lies posterior to the trachea, left bronchus, and pericardium, especially the left atrium of the heart; and anterior to the vertebral column and descending thoracic aorta. As the thoracic duct passes upwards it crosses behind the esophagus from the right to the left side. **p. thoracica medullae spinalis** [NA] The thoracic part of the spinal cord; the narrowed part of the spinal cord between the cervical and lumbar enlargements that gives rise to twelve pairs of thoracic spinal nerves. Also *pars thoracalis medullae spinalis.* **p. thyropharyngea musculi constrictoris pharyngis inferioris** [NA] The part of the inferior pharyngeal constrictor muscle that arises from the oblique line of the thyroid cartilage and a part posterior to it, and from a fibrous arch over the cricothyroid muscle, extending from the inferior thyroid tubercle to the cricoid cartilage. It inserts into the pharyngeal raphe. Also *thyropharyngeal part of inferior constrictor muscle of pharynx, thyropharyngeal muscle.* **p. tibiocalcaneus ligamenti medialis** [NA] The superficial central fibers of the medial or deltoid ligament of the talocrural joint that extend straight down from the medial malleolus to the upper and medial margin of the sustentaculum tali of the calcaneus. Also *calcaneotibial ligament.* **p. tibionavicularis ligamenti medialis** [NA] The superficial anterior band of the medial or deltoid ligament of the talocrural joint that extends from the front of the medial malleolus to be attached to the navicular bone and the medial margin of the plantar calcaneonavicular ligament. Also *tibionavicular ligament.* **p. tibiotalaris anterior ligamenti medialis** [NA] The deep anterior fibers of the medial or deltoid ligament of the talocrural joint that extend from the anterior margin of the medial malleolus to the nonarticular part of the medial surface of the talus. Also *anterior talotibial ligament.* **p. tibiotalaris posterior ligamenti medialis** [NA] The posterior band of the medial or deltoid ligament of the talocrural joint that extends posteriorly from the medial malleolus to the medial surface of the body of the talus and its medial tubercle. Also *posterior talotibial ligament.* **p. transversa musculi nasalis** [NA] The transverse part of the nasalis muscle that arises from the upper part of the canine eminence of the maxilla and ascends upwards and medially. It ends in an aponeurosis that meets its fellow of the opposite side over the bridge of the nose. Also *constrictor naris, compressor naris, musculus compressor naris, compressor muscle of naris.* **p. transversa rami sinistri venae portae hepatis** [NA] The long proximal portion of the left branch of the portal vein that runs transversely into the left lobe of the liver from its origin from the portal vein in the right end of the porta hepatis. It terminates by making a 90° turn anteriorly at the point of attachment of the ligamentum venosum to it. It then continues as the pars umbilicalis. It gives branches to the caudate lobe. It represents the original left branch of the fetal portal vein which anastomoses with the left umbilical vein and ductus venosus. Also *transverse part of left portal vein.* **p. triangularis** OPERCULUM FRONTALE. **p. triangularis gyri frontalis inferioris** [NA] The triangular part of the inferior frontal gyrus, a subdivision of the inferior frontal gyrus situated between the ascending and anterior rami of the lateral sulcus. **p. tuberalis adenohypophyseos** [NA] That part of the adenohypophysis comprised of a thin mantle of glandular cells covering the anterior and lateral surfaces of the proximal end of the hypophysial stalk (infundibulum hypothalami). Also *pars infundibularis adenohypophyseos.* **p. tympanica ossis temporalis** [NA] The curved, triangular plate of the temporal bone that has the squamous part above and anterior to it and the petrous part behind and medial to it. Its concave upper surface forms most of the three walls of the external acoustic meatus, while its anterior surface forms the posterior wall of the mandibular fossa. Also *tympanic part of temporal bone, tympanic bone.* **p. umbilicalis rami sinistri venae portae hepatis** [NA] The terminal portion of the left branch of the portal vein that arises in the left lobe of the liver as the continuation of the pars transversa where the latter turns sharply forward at 90°C. It is attached posteriorly to the ligamentum venosum and anteriorly to the ligamentum teres, and it gives many branches to the left and quadrate lobes of the liver. It represents the persistence of part of the fetal left umbilical vein which carried blood through the liver to the ductus venosus and anastomosed with the fetal left portal vein. Also *umbilical part of left portal vein, sagittal part of left portal vein.* **p. uterina placentae** UTERINE PLACENTA. **p. uterina tubae uterinae** [NA] The interstitial portion of the fallopian tube. **p. ventralis pontis** [NA] The ventral part of the pons, consisting of bundles of longitudinally directed corticopontine and corticospinal fibers, transversely directed pontocerebellar fibers constituting the brachium pontis, and small masses of neurons, the nuclei pontis, scattered among the transverse fibers. These are parts of the corticopontocerebellar path. Also *pars basilaris pontis.* **p. vertebralis faciei costalis pulmonis** [NA] The rounded posterior part of the costal surface of each lung that is related medially to the sides of the vertebral column. **p. vestibularis nervi octavi** NERVUS VESTIBULARIS. **p. villosa** The villus-bearing area on the inner aspect of the embryonic lip. The villi disappear at birth or soon after. Also *labial villi.*

**Parsonage** [Maurice John *Parsonage,* English neurologist, flourished 20th century] Parsonage-Turner syndrome, Parsonage and Turner amyotrophic neuralgia. See under SHOULDER GIRDLE SYNDROME.

# part

**part** / **abdominal p. of aorta** PARS ABDOMINALIS AORTAE. **abdominal p. of esophagus** PARS ABDOMINALIS ESOPHAGI. **abdominal p. of ureter** PARS ABDOMINALIS URETERIS. **accessory p. of parotid gland** GLANDULA PAROTIDEA ACCESSORIA. **alar p. of nasalis muscle** PARS ALARIS MUSCULI NASALIS. **alveolar p. of mandible** PARS ALVEOLARIS MANDIBULAE. **anterior p. of diaphragmatic surface of liver** PARS ANTERIOR FACIEI DIAPHRAGMATICAE HEPATIS. **ascending p. of aorta** PARS ASCENDENS AORTAE. **basilar p. of occipital bone** PARS BASILARIS OSSIS OCCIPITALIS. **bony p. of auditory tube** PARS OSSEA TUBAE AUDITIVAE. **bony p. of nasal septum** PARS OSSEA SEPTI NASI. **buccopharyngeal p. of superior constrictor muscle of pharynx** PARS BUCCOPHARYNGEA MUSCULI CONSTRICTORIS PHARYNGIS SUPERIORIS. **calcaneonavicular p. of bifurcated ligament** LIGAMENTUM CALCANEONAVICULARE. **cardiac p. of stomach** PARS CARDIACA GASTRIS. **cartilaginous p. of auditory tube** PARS CARTILAGINEA TUBAE AUDITIVAE. **ceratopharyngeal p. of middle constrictor muscle of pharynx** PARS CERATOPHARYNGEA MUSCULI CONSTRICTORIS PHARYNGIS MEDII. **cervical p. of trachea** PARS CERVICALIS TRACHEAE. **chondropharyngeal p. of middle constrictor muscle of pharynx** PARS CHONDROPHARYNGEA MUSCULI CONSTRICTORIS PHARYNGIS MEDII. **ciliary p. of retina** PARS CILIARIS RETINAE. **condylar p. of occipital bone** PARS LATERALIS OSSIS OCCIPITALIS. **convoluted p. of kidney lobule** PARS CONVOLUTA LOBULI CORTICALIS RENALIS. **costal p. of diaphragm** PARS COSTALIS DIAPHRAGMATIS. **cranial p. of accessory nerve** RADICES CRANIALES NERVI ACCESSORII. **cricopharyngeal p. of inferior constrictor muscle of pharynx** PARS CRICOPHARYNGEA MUSCULI CONSTRICTORIS PHARYNGIS INFERIORIS. **cruciform p. of fibrous sheaths of digits of hand** PARS CRUCIFORMIS VAGINAE FIBROSAE DIGITORUM MANUS. **cruciform p. of fibrous sheaths of digits of toes** PARS CRUCIFORMIS VAGINAE FIBROSAE DIGITORUM PEDIS. **cupular p. of epitympanic recess** PARS CUPULARIS RECESSUS EPITYMPANICI. **cupulate p. of epitympanic recess** PARS CUPULARIS RECESSUS EPITYMPANICI. **deep p. of parotid gland** PARS PROFUNDA GLANDULAE PAROTIDEAE. **descending p. of aorta** PARS DESCENDENS AORTAE. **descending p. of duodenum** PARS DESCENDENS DUODENI. **exoccipital p. of occipital bone** PARS LATERALIS OSSIS OCCIPITALIS. **first p. of duodenum** PARS SUPERIOR DUODENI. **flaccid p. of tympanic membrane** PARS FLACCIDA MEMBRANAE TYMPANI. **fourth p. of duodenum** PARS ASCENDENS DUODENI. **glossopharyngeal p. of superior constrictor muscle of pharynx** PARS GLOSSOPHARYNGEA MUSCULI CONSTRICTORIS PHARYNGIS SUPERIORIS. **horizontal p. of duodenum** PARS HORIZONTALIS DUODENI. **inferior p. of duodenum** PARS HORIZONTALIS DUODENI. **infraclavicular p. of brachial plexus** PARS INFRACLAVICULARIS PLEXUS BRACHIALIS. **intercartilaginous p. of glottis** PARS INTERCARTILAGINEA RIMAE GLOTTIDIS. **intermembranous p. of glottis** PARS INTERMEMBRANACEA RIMAE GLOTTIDIS. **intravaginal p. of cervix** PORTIO VAGINALIS CERVICIS. **iridial p. of retina** PARS IRIDICA RETINAE. **jugular p. of occipital bone** PARS LATERALIS OSSIS OCCIPITALIS. **lacrimal p. of orbicularis oculi muscle** PARS LACRIMALIS MUSCULI ORBICULARIS OCULI. **laryngeal p. of pharynx** PARS LARYNGEA PHARYNGIS. **lateral p. of cricothyroid ligament** CONUS ELASTICUS LARYNGIS. **lateral p. of occipital bone** PARS LATERALIS OSSIS OCCIPITALIS. **lateral p. of sacrum** PARS LATERALIS OSSIS SACRI. **lumbar p. of diaphragm** PARS LUMBALIS DIAPHRAGMATIS. **magnocellular p. of red nucleus** PALEORUBRUM. **membranous p. of interventricular septum of heart** PARS MEMBRANACEA SEPTI INTERVENTRICULARIS CORDIS. **membranous p. of male urethra** PARS MEMBRANACEA URETHRAE MASCULINAE. **membranous p. of nasal septum** PARS MEMBRANACEA SEPTI NASI. **mobile p. of nasal septum** PARS MOBILIS SEPTI NASI. **mylopharyngeal p. of superior constrictor muscle of pharynx** PARS MYLOPHARYNGEA MUSCULI CONSTRICTORIS PHARYNGIS SUPERIORIS. **nasal p. of frontal bone** PARS NASALIS OSSIS FRONTALIS. **nasal p. of pharynx** PARS NASALIS PHARYNGIS. **occipital p. of occipital bone** SQUAMA OCCIPITALIS. **optic p. of retina** PARS OPTICA RETINAE. **oral p. of pharynx** PARS ORALIS PHARYNGIS. **orbital p. of frontal bone** PARS ORBITALIS OSSIS FRONTALIS. **orbital p. of lacrimal gland** PARS

ORBITALIS GLANDULAE LACRIMALIS. **orbital p. of orbicularis oculi muscle** PARS ORBITALIS MUSCULI ORBICULARIS OCULI. **palpebral p. of lacrimal gland** PARS PALPEBRALIS GLANDULAE LACRIMALIS. **palpebral p. of orbicularis oculi muscle** PARS PALPEBRALIS MUSCULI ORBICULARIS OCULI. **parietal p. of pelvic fascia** FASCIA PELVIS PARIETALIS. **pectineal p. of inguinal ligament** LIGAMENTUM LACUNARE. **petrous p. of temporal bone** PARS PETROSA OSSIS TEMPORALIS. **pelvic p. of ureter** PARS PELVICA URETERIS. **posterior p. of diaphragmatic surface of liver** PARS POSTERIOR FACIEI DIAPHRAGMATICAE HEPATIS. **presenting p.** The lowermost part of the fetus in the birth canal just prior to or during labor. Also *presentation.* **pterygopharyngeal p. of superior constrictor muscle of pharynx** PARS PTERYGOPHARYNGEA MUSCULI CONSTRICTORIS PHARYNGIS SUPERIORIS. **pyloric p. of stomach** PARS PYLORICA GASTRIS. **right p. of diaphragmatic surface of liver** PARS DEXTRA FACIEI DIAPHRAGMATICAE HEPATIS. **sagittal p. of left portal vein** PARS UMBILICALIS RAMI SINISTRI VENAE PORTAE HEPATIS. **second p. of duodenum** PARS DESCENDENS DUODENI. **spinal p. of accessory nerve** RAMUS EXTERNUS NERVI ACCESSORII. **spongiose p. of male urethra** PARS SPONGIOSA URETHRAE MASCULINAE. **squamous p. of occipital bone** SQUAMA OCCIPITALIS. **squamous p. of temporal bone** PARS SQUAMOSA OSSIS TEMPORALIS. **sternal p. of diaphragm** PARS STERNALIS DIAPHRAGMATIS. **sternocostal p. of diaphragm** PARS COSTALIS DIAPHRAGMATIS. **straight p. of cricothyroid muscle** PARS RECTA MUSCULI CRICOTHYROIDEI. **superficial p. of parotid gland** PARS SUPERFICIALIS GLANDULAE PAROTIDEAE. **superior p. of duodenum** PARS SUPERIOR DUODENI. **tendinous p. of epicranius muscle** GALEA APONEUROTICA. **tense p. of tympanic membrane** PARS TENSA MEMBRANAE TYMPANI. **third p. of duodenum** PARS HORIZONTALIS DUODENI. **thoracic p. of aorta** PARS THORACICA AORTAE. **thyropharyngeal p. of inferior constrictor muscle of pharynx** PARS THYROPHARYNGEA MUSCULI CONSTRICTORIS PHARYNGIS INFERIORIS. **transverse p. of left portal vein** PARS TRANSVERSA RAMI SINISTRI VENAE PORTAE HEPATIS. **tympanic p. of temporal bone** PARS TYMPANICA OSSIS TEMPORALIS. **umbilical p. of left portal vein** PARS UMBILICALIS RAMI SINISTRI VENAE PORTAE HEPATIS. **vaginal p. of cervix** PORTIO VAGINALIS CERVICIS. **vertebral p. of diaphragm** PARS LUMBALIS DIAPHRAGMATIS. **visceral p. of pelvic fascia** FASCIA PELVIS VISCERALIS.

**part. aeq.** *partes aequales* (L, equal parts): used in prescription writing.

**partal** \pär′təl\ [L *part(us)* childbirth (from *parere* to give birth) + -AL] Relating to labor and delivery.

**partes** \pär′tēz\ Plural of PARS.

**parthenogenesis** \pär′thənōjen′əsis\ [Gk *partheno(s)* a virgin, maiden + GENESIS] A form of nonsexual reproduction in which the female produces offspring without a genetic contribution from the male. Also *virgin generation, unisexual reproduction, parthogenesis.* **artificial p.** The development of an unfertilized egg, initiated by chemical or mechanical stimulation or other artificial means.

**parthogenesis** \pär′thōjen′əsis\ PARTHENOGENESIS.

**partialism** \pär′shəlizm\ A type of paraphilia in which a part of the partner's body is the actual excitant to sexual gratification.

**participant-observer** \pärtis′əpənt-\ An analyst or psychotherapist who takes active part in the interpersonal process of therapy.

**particle** [L *particula* (dim. of PARS) a small part, a particle] **1** An extremely small object or portion of matter. **2** Any of the constituents of the atom, such as protons, neutrons, or electrons, or a quantum of electromagnetic energy when its wave aspects are unimportant. **alpha p.** A helium-4 ion; a positively charged particle formed by two protons and two neutrons. Alpha particles are emitted with characteristic energies from the nuclei of certain radionuclides, in which case they are sometimes referred to as alpha rays. In living tissues, alpha particles have a short range and do much damage. **beta p.** A high-speed electron or positron emitted by a radionuclide. Beta particles constitute one form of ionizing radiation. They are emitted in a range of energies varying from zero to a maximum determined by the difference in mass between the initial and final nuclei. They tend to be more penetrating than alpha particles, but less so than gamma photons. **C p.** A structure associated with sarcoma or leukemia virus characterized by a centrally placed and spherical nucleoid containing the RNA genome enclosed by a lipid membrane envelope. • This term, along with *A particle* and *B particle*, was coined to designate one or the several types of particles associated with tumor viruses. **chromatin p.'s** HOWELL-JOLLY BODIES. **collodion p.'s** Immunologically inert particles of cellulose tetranitrate. They are sometimes used as a solid-phase carrier for soluble antigens or antibodies in an agglutination system. **core p.** The globular or disk-shaped structure of nucleoprotein that is visible in electron micrographs of decondensed chromatin as the bead of the "beads-on-a-string" configuration. Each is 11–12.5 nm in diameter and is composed of 2 molecules of histones H2A, H2B, H3, and H4, and about 146 base pairs of DNA. Together with linker DNA, it comprises the nucleosome. **Dane p.** The complete virion of hepatitis B virus. It is a complex double-layered sphere, 42 nm in diameter, composed of an outer layer or envelope surrounding a central core. **elementary p.** The knob, stalk, and base plate which extends as a unit from the inner surface of the inner mitochondrial membrane. It functions in the transport of electrons. **kappa p.'s** Inheritable cytoplasmic symbionts occurring in some strains of *Paramecium*, which produce an element that is destructive to other host strains. **lens p.'s** A few tiny fragments of the membrana pupillaris of the fetus that remain on the anterior surface of the lens capsule and, exceptionally, may persist into adult life. **nuclear p.'s** HOWELL-JOLLY BODIES. **viral p.** VIRION.

**particulate** \pärtik′yələt\ Consisting of discrete tiny particles.

**partition** \pärtish′ən\ In anatomy, a wall-like structure that separates or divides two parts of an organ, such as a septum.

**Partsch** [Carl *Partsch*, German physician, born 1855] Partsch's operation. See under MARSUPIALIZATION.

**parturient** \pärt$^y$oo′rē·ənt\ [L *parturiens*, gen. *parturientis*, pres. part. of *parturire* to be in labor, bring forth] **1** A woman in labor. **2** Relating to parturition.

**parturifacient** \pär′t$^y$ərifā′shənt\ OXYTOCIC.

**parturiometer** \pär′t$^y$ərē·äm′ətər\ [L *parturi(re)* to be in labor, bring forth + *o* + -METER] A device to measure the strength of uterine contractions during labor.

**parturition** \pär′t$^y$ərish′ən\ [Late L *parturitio* (from L *parturire* to be in labor, from *part(us)* giving birth, delivery + *-urire*, desiderative verb ending) parturition, labor] The process of giving birth; labor. Also *partus, accouchement* (older term). **double p.** The process of giving birth to twins.

**partus** \pär′təs\ [L (from *partus,* past part. of *parere* to bear or bring forth young) a bringing forth or bearing of young] PARTURITION. **p. maturus** Labor and delivery at full term. **p. preparator** Any measure or procedure designed to facilitate an approaching labor.

**part. vic.** *partitis vicibus* (L, in divided doses), used in prescription writing.

**party / third p.** Any organization, including a governmental entity, that pays, insures, or otherwise assumes financial responsibility to reimburse beneficiaries for health care services. Also *third party payer.*

**parulis** \pəroo′lis\ [Gk *paroulis* (from *par(a)-* beside + *oul(on)* a gum) gumboil] ALVEOLAR ABSCESS.

**paruria** \pəroo′rē·ə\ [PAR- + -URIA] Any abnormality of urine or urination.

**parvicellular** \pär′visel′yələr\ Composed of small cells.

**parvilocular** \pär′vilō′kyələr\ Containing only a few spaces or vacuoles.

**Parvoviridae** \pär′vōvir′idē\ [L *parv(us)* little + *o* + *vir(us)* + -IDAE] A family of small, icosahedral viruses containing single-stranded DNA of either negative or positive polarity. Members are grouped as defective or autonomous depending on their requirement for a helper virus for growth.

**parvovirus** \pär′vōvī′rəs\ [L *parvus* little, small + VIRUS] Any of a genus (*Parvovirus*) in the Parvoviridae family of small (18–26 nm), ether-resistant viruses containing single-stranded, linear, infectious DNA. They include adeno-associated virus, mink enteritis virus, Kilham rat virus, and densonucleosis virus. **bovine p.** A virus, widely distributed in the United States, which naturally infects the intestinal and genitourinary tract of cattle. **porcine p.** A worldwide virus of pigs which has been associated with infertility and abortion.

**parvule** \pär′vyool\ A small tablet, pill, or granule of medicine.

**Pascal** [Blaise *Pascal,* French mathematician and physicist, 1623–1662] Pascal distribution. See under NEGATIVE BINOMIAL DISTRIBUTION.

**pascal** \pas′kəl\ [after Blaise *Pascal,* French mathematician and philosopher, 1623–1662] Special name for the SI derived unit of pressure or stress, newton per square meter, equal to the pressure or stress produced by a force of one newton applied, uniformly distributed over an area of one square meter. Symbol: Pa

**Pascheff** [Constantin *Pascheff,* Bulgarian ophthalmologist, 1873–1961] Pascheff's conjunctivitis. See under CONJUNCTIVITIS NECROTICANS INFECTIOSA.

**Paschen** [Enrique *Paschen,* German physician, 1860–1936] Paschen's granules, Paschen's corpuscles. See under GUARNIERI BODIES.

**Pasini** [Agostino *Pasini,* Italian dermatologist, flourished 20th century] Pasini-Pierini syndrome. See under IDIOPATHIC ATROPHODERMA OF PASINI AND PIERINI.

**passage** A channel, meatus, duct, or any opening or gap between two structures or organs. **blind p.** In a serial transfer of infectious material, the inoculation of later members of the series with material taken from earlier cultures or experimental animals in which there is no evidence of disease or of pathogenic activity. **cloacal p.** A communication beneath the cloacal septum in 8 mm human embryos between the allantois and the hindgut. When the cloacal septum reaches the cloacal membrane, the passage is closed to form the urogenital sinus and the rectum. **false p.** An unnatural channel or communication in the body. **serial p.** The inoculation of a series of cultures, experimental animals, or other growth media, using material from the initially infected examples in a progressive sequence to infect later examples.

**Passavant** [Gustav *Passavant,* German surgeon, 1815–1893] Passavant's cushion, Passavant's pad, Passavant's ridge. See under BAR.

**passband** The band of frequencies that pass through an electrical filter with little attenuation.

**passenger** The fetus during labor.

**passive** [L *passiv(us)* (from *pass(us),* past part. of *pandere* to spread out, extend + *-ivus* -IVE) passive] **1** Acted upon by external agents; receptive rather than initiating activity. **2** Submissive or unresponsive. **3** Effective automatically without the need for voluntary action: said of safety devices, as a *passive automobile restraint.*

**Past.** *Pasteurella.*

**paste** [Late L *pasta* (prob. from Gk *pastē* barley sauce) dough, paste] An oily or gelatinous medicinal preparation for external use. The active ingredients may confer the oily or pasty nature to the preparation, or this may come from the addition of a suitable base, such as soft paraffin. **aluminum p.** A mixture of powdered aluminum, zinc oxide ointment, and petrolatum. It is used to prevent excoriation of the skin around intestinal stomata or fistulas. **arsenical p.** A devitalizing paste containing compounds of arsenic. **chillie p.** COMPOUND OINTMENT OF CAPSICUM. **desensitizing p.** A paste used to reduce the sensitivity of exposed dentin. It may contain a high concentration of sodium fluoride. **impression p.** A dental impression material produced by mixing two pastes. One paste contains zinc oxide and oil, such as liquid paraffin, with an accelerator. The other is a resin, such as colophony, dissolved in eugenol. Also *zinc oxide and eugenol paste.* **Leunbach's p.** A substance which was formerly injected into the endometrial cavity in order to induce abortion. Due to the high rate of associated complications, this practice is condemned by modern obstetricians. **zinc oxide and eugenol p.** IMPRESSION PASTE.

**paster** \pā′stər\ The segment of a bifocal lens for near vision.

**Pasteur** [Louis *Pasteur,* French chemist, 1822–1895] **1** See under TREATMENT. **2** Pasteur's reaction. See under EFFECT. **3** Pasteur vaccine. See under ANTIRABIES VACCINE OF PASTEUR.

***Pasteurella*** \pas′tərel′ə\ [after Louis *Pasteur,* French chemist and bacteriologist, 1822–1895 + *-ella,* L fem. diminishing suffix] A genus of zoonotic bacteria. It formerly included organisms now designated as *Yersinia* and *Francisella.* ***P. multocida*** A species of small, Gram-negative, bipolar staining, nonmotile, facultatively anaerobic coccobacilli. They are pathogenic for many animals and occasionally for humans, especially after an animal bite. ***P. pestis*** A former name for *YERSINIA PESTIS.* ***P. pneumotropica*** A species closely related to *P. multocida,* often pathogenic in laboratory rodents and occasionally acquired by humans through dog bites. ***P. pseudotuberculosis*** A former name of *YERSINIA PSEUDOTUBERCULOSIS.* ***P. tularensis*** A former name of *FRANCISELLA TULARENSIS.*

**pasteurism** \pas′tərizm, pas′chər-\ [after Louis *Pasteur,* French chemist and bacteriologist, 1822–1895 + -ISM] The method of active immunization developed by Louis Pasteur using attenuated cultures.

**pasteurization** \pas′tərīzā′shən, pas′chər-\ [after Louis *Pasteur,* French chemist and bacteriologist, 1822–1895 + *-iz(e)* + -ATION] The process originated by Pasteur in which milk or another liquid is heated to a specified moderate temperature for a set period of time, for example, to

60°C for 30 minutes, in order to kill pathogenic bacteria and delay the growth of other bacteria. The process does not cause major alteration in the character of the liquid.

**Pastia** [C. *Pastia,* Rumanian physician, flourished 20th century] Pastia sign, Pastia's lines. See under LINE.

**pastille** A lozenge with a gelatin base. Also *pastil.*

**past-pointing** One of the clinical signs of cerebellar ataxia due to a lesion or disease of the cerebellar hemisphere as distinct from the vermis: the pointing finger overshoots the target.

**PAT** paroxysmal atrial tachycardia.

**Patau** [Klaus *Patau,* U.S. geneticist, flourished 20th century] Patau syndrome. See under TRISOMY 13 SYNDROME.

**patch** 1 A circumscribed area that differs in some respect from the surrounding area. 2 A small piece of material used to repair a worn or torn place. **Bayer p.** ZONE OF ADHESION. **Bitot's p.'es** BITOT SPOTS. **butterfly p.** BUTTERFLY ERUPTION. **Carrel p.** A technique for facilitating reimplantation of small arterial branches by excising and using as an anastomotic cuff a portion of the wall of the larger artery from which the branch vessel arises. **cotton wool p.'es** Microinfarctions of the retina, appearing as fluffy, light-colored areas somewhat less than a disk diameter in size. Also *cotton wool exudates, cotton wool spots.* **herald p.** The initial lesion of pityriasis rosea. **Hutchinson's p.** SALMON PATCH. **MacCallum's p.** Irregular thickening of the mural endocardium of the left atrium found in acute rheumatic carditis. These lesions are subendocardial aggregations of Aschoff bodies. They progress to fibrosis over time, resulting in an irregular plaquelike area of endocardial scarring. **milk p.'es** MILK SPOTS. **mucous p.** The gray desquamating epithelium that overlies a mucous membrane lesion of syphilis. Also *mucous plaque, opaline patch, opaline plaque.* **opaline p.** MUCOUS PATCH. **Peyer's p.'es** Aggregates of lymphoid follicles in the lamina propria and submucosa of the terminal ileum, which may be visible macroscopically as raised nodules in the mucosa. Also *Peyer's plaques, aggregated lymphatic follicles of Peyer.* **salmon p.** A reddish discoloration of part of the cornea due to the deep vascularization of syphilis. Also *Hutchinson's patch.* **shagreen p.** SHAGREEN SKIN. **smokers' p.** LEUKOPLAKIA. **soldiers' p.'es** MILK SPOTS. **white p.'es** MILK SPOTS.

**patching** The redistribution of antigenically active components of cell membranes following their interaction with antibody molecules such that determinants evenly distributed over the cell surface cluster together in discrete patches, separated by membrane areas without determinants. The process is distinct from capping in that it does not require the active participation of cell membrane and is not inhibited by low temperature or inhibitors of membrane mobility.

**patefaction** \pā'tēfak'shən\ [L *patefactio* (from *patefactus,* past part. of *patefacere* to lay open, from *pate(re)* to be open + *facere* to make) a laying open] The surgical procedure of laying wide open.

**patella** \pətel'ə\ [L (dim. of *patina* a plate, shallow dish, from Gk *patanē* a flat dish) a small dish, the kneecap] [NA] A large triangular-shaped sesamoid bone in the back of the tendon of the quadriceps femoris muscle, located anteriorly in the knee joint and articulating with the distal extremity of the femur. It has anterior and posterior surfaces, three margins, and an apex that is directed downward. Also *kneecap, knee cap, rotula* (outmoded), *whirl bone, whirlbone.* **bipartite p.** A patella consisting of two pieces of bone joined by fibrous tissue. Also *patella bipartita.* **p. cubiti** A sesamoid bone in one of the tendons or fascial sheets on the extensor surface of the elbow joint, most often in the tendon of the triceps brachii. **floating p.** A patella that is separated from the underlying femoral condyle by an effusion within the knee joint. **p. partita** A patella that consists of two or more bony parts.

**patellectomy** \pat'əlek'təmē\ The surgical removal of the patella.

**patency** \pā'tənsē\ The state of being patent.

**patent** \pā'tənt\ [L *patens,* gen. *patentis* (from *patens,* pres. part. of *patere* to be open) open, lying open] Open; unobstructed, as a duct.

**Paterson** [Donald Rose *Paterson,* English otolaryngologist, 1863–1939] Paterson syndrome, Paterson-Brown Kelly syndrome, Paterson-Kelly syndrome. See under PLUMMER-VINSON SYNDROME.

**path** [Old English *pæth*] 1 A route or course. 2 The direction of movement of a nerve impulse. **mean free p.** The average distance that a radiated particle, or a photon, travels between collisions of a specified type in the absorbing material. **occlusal p.** The track taken by a point on the occlusal surface of a mandibular tooth in relation to the maxilla.

**path-** \path-, pəth-\ PATHO-.

**-path** \-path\ [back-formation from -PATHY] A combining form meaning (1) one having a (specified) disease; (2) a practitioner of a (specified) system for the treatment of disease.

**pathema** \pəthē'mə\ [Gk *pathēma* a suffering, attack of sickness, state of mind] Any disease or pathologic condition.

**pathematology** \path'ēmətäl'əjē\ [Gk *pathēma,* gen. *pathēmatos,* a suffering + -LOGY] *Obs.* PSYCHOPATHOLOGY.

**pathetic** \pəthet'ik\ [Gk *pathētik(os)* sensitive, capable of feeling] Denoting the nervus trochlearis, or nervus patheticus.

**-pathia** \-path'ē·ə\ -PATHY.

**patho-** \path'ō-, path'ə-\ [Gk *pathos* (from *paschein* to undergo, be affected) an incident, experience, sensation, emotion, mishap, trouble, suffering] A combining form meaning disease, pathologic. Also *path-.*

**pathoanatomy** \-ənat'əmē\ ANATOMIC PATHOLOGY.

**pathobiology** \-bī·äl'əjē\ PATHOLOGY.

**pathoclisis** \-klis'is\ [PATHO- + -CLISIS] The affinity of certain toxins for specific organs or organ systems. Also *pathoklisis.*

**pathocure** \path'əkyoor\ Elimination of neurotic symptoms upon the appearance of an organic disorder.

**pathogen** \path'əjən\ [PATHO- + -GEN] A microorganism capable of causing disease. It may be a primary pathogen, often or regularly associated with disease, or it may be an opportunist, becoming pathogenic in weakened hosts.

**pathogenesis** \-jen'əsis\ The mechanisms involved in the development of disease. Also *pathogenesy, pathogeny.* **drug p.** The provocation of disease symptoms by using therapeutic agents; iatrogenic conditions brought about by using drugs.

**pathogenesy** \-jen'əsē\ PATHOGENESIS.

**pathogenetic** \-jənet'ik\ Pertaining to pathogenesis.

**pathogenic** \-jen'ik\ [PATHO- + -GENIC] Able to cause disease. Also *morbific, morbigenous* (obs.), *nosogenic* (obs.), *nosopoietic* (obs.).

**pathogenicity** \-jənis'itē\ 1 The ability to cause disease. 2 The degree of virulence of a microorganism, which depends upon its communicability, invasiveness, and toxigenicity.

**pathogeny** \pəthäj'ənē\ PATHOGENESIS.

**pathognomonic** \path'əgnōmän'ik\ [Gk *pathognōmonikos* (from *patho(s)* condition, affection + *gnōmōn,* gen. *gnōmonos* discerner, indicator, from *(gi)gnō(skein)* to recognize, perceive) indicating a particular disease or condition] Specific and characteristic of a given disease or condition, as Aschoff bodies are of rheumatic carditis. Also *pathognostic.*

**pathognomy** \pəthäg′nəmē\ Disease diagnosis based on the patient's signs and symptoms.

**pathognostic** \path′əgnäs′tik\ PATHOGNOMONIC.

**pathography** \pəthäg′rəfē\ [PATHO- + -GRAPHY] A treatise on disease.

**pathoklisis** \-klis′is\ PATHOCLISIS.

**pathologic** \-läj′ik\ PATHOLOGICAL.

**pathological** \-läj′ikəl\ **1** Denoting an abnormal finding, particularly a morphological alteration. **2** Pertaining to pathology; resulting from disease. For defs. 1 and 2 also *pathologic.*

**pathologist** \pəthäl′əjist\ A physician trained and experienced in anatomic, clinical, and/or experimental pathology. **speech p.** An individual trained in the speech sciences who undertakes the analysis and the assessment of the causes of the disorders of speech and language, both developmental and acquired.

**pathology** \pəthäl′əjē\ [PATHO- + -LOGY] The biomedical science and medical specialty that studies the causes, development, and effects of disease as well as the structural and functional changes that are produced by disease. It is concerned with these issues at all levels, ranging from individual biochemical and molecular events to gross morphologic alterations visible to the naked eye. Also *pathobiology.* **anatomic p.** The subspecialty of pathology that studies the gross and microscopic changes in the body caused by disease. It includes postmortem examinations and interpretation of biopsies and surgical specimens. Also *morbid anatomy, pathological anatomy, pathoanatomy.* **cellular p.** The study of disease as a manifestation of alterations in the structure or function of individual cells, as initiated by Virchow in 1858. **chemical p.** The field of clinical pathology that studies chemical alterations induced by disease. **clinical p.** The subspecialty of pathology that comprises the measurement and identification of substances, cells, and microorganisms in body fluids. It utilizes methods and procedures of bacteriology, chemistry, mycology, parasitology, virology, immunology, hematology, biophysics, and other, related disciplines. Also *clinicopathology.* **experimental p.** The subspecialty of pathology that investigates and elucidates previously unknown disease processes and their causes through laboratory experimentation. **forensic p.** The application of the principles and practice of pathology to problems of law and the administration of justice. It is primarily concerned with the determination of the cause and manner of death of individuals who die suddenly or under suspicious, unusual, unexplained, or violent circumstances. **functional p.** PHYSIOPATHOLOGY. **general p.** The study of the general mechanisms of disease such as cell injury and repair, inflammation, thrombosis, hyperplasia and neoplasia, etc. **medical p.** The study of diseases that are not surgically treatable. Also *internal pathology.* **molecular p.** The study of the molecular events that produce disease or that occur in the course of disease. **speech p.** The assessment and study of abnormal voice, speech, and language. It may be subdivided into disturbances of the development of spoken language in the child, and the acquired deficits of the adult and elderly. The primary classifications for each are the receptive disorders affecting speech perception and verbal comprehension, and those conditions, structural or neurologic in origin, which impair the expressive aspects of speech and language. **surgical p.** The field of anatomical pathology that studies the gross and microscopic changes observed in biopsy and surgical specimens for living patients, with special emphasis on precise diagnosis of the patient's disease.

**pathomimesis** \-mimē′sis\ MALINGERING.

**pathomimia** \-mim′ē·ə\ MALINGERING.

**pathomimicry** \-mim′ikrē\ MALINGERING.

**pathomorphism** \-môr′fizm\ [PATHO- + MORPH- + -ISM] Deviant or abnormal morphology.

**pathomorphology** \-môrfäl′əjē\ The study of pathomorphism.

**pathonomy** \pəthän′əmē\ [PATHO- + *nom(o)-* + -Y] The study or scientific knowledge of the laws of disease processes. Also *pathonomia.*

**patho-occlusion** \-äkloo′zhən\ [PATHO- + OCCLUSION] MALOCCLUSION.

**pathophoresis** \-fôrē′sis\ [PATHO- + -PHORESIS] The spread of disease.

**pathophysiology** \-fiz′ē·äl′əjē\ [PATHO- + PHYSIOLOGY] **1** The study of disordered physiology. **2** Disordered physiology.

**pathopoiesis** \-poi·ē′sis\ [PATHO- + -POIESIS] The etiology of disease.

**pathway** **1** A structural course leading from one place to another, as of nerve fibers. **2** A sequence of reactions by which one substance is converted into another. **afferent p.** **1** The course of an aggregate or series of axonal bundles conducting toward central neurons, especially the central relay paths from sense organs to the brain. Also *afferent tract.* **2** A neural pathway that conducts impulses towards a specific region in the central nervous system. Compare EFFERENT PATHWAY. **alternative complement p.** The pathway of complement activation that is recruited by particulate polysaccharides and by many parasites, usually in an antibody independent manner. The alternative pathway requires only magnesium ions (and not calcium ions) for the generation of $\overline{C3_1B}$, and is active only at low dilutions of serum. C1, C4, and C2 are not required by the alternative pathway. Factor B, factor D, and properdin are the components peculiar to the alternative pathway. Compare CLASSICAL COMPLEMENT PATHWAY. **anabolic p.** BIOSYNTHETIC PATHWAY. **auditory p.'s** The series of axons excited by acoustic nerve stimulation and coursing

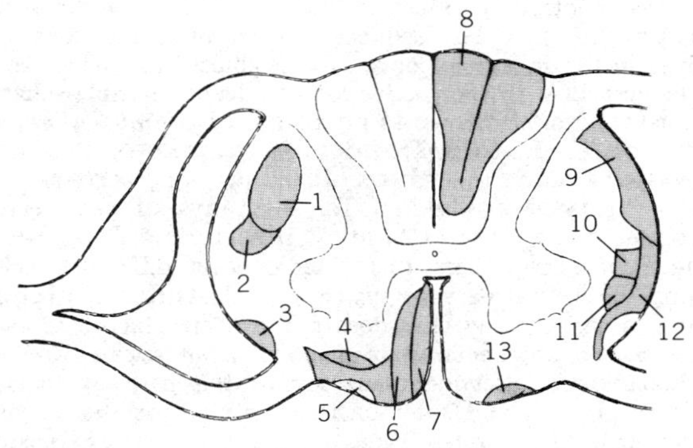


**Neural pathways** *Efferent:* (1) Lateral corticospinal tract; (2) rubrospinal tract; (3) olivospinal tract; (4) tectospinal tract; (5) vestibulospinal tract; (6) ventral corticospinal tract; (7) sulcomarginal fasciculus. *Afferent:* (8) Fasciculus gracilis; (9) dorsal spinocerebellar tract; (10) lateral spinothalamic tract; (11) spinotectal tract; (12) ventral spinocerebellar tract; (13) ventral spinothalamic tract.

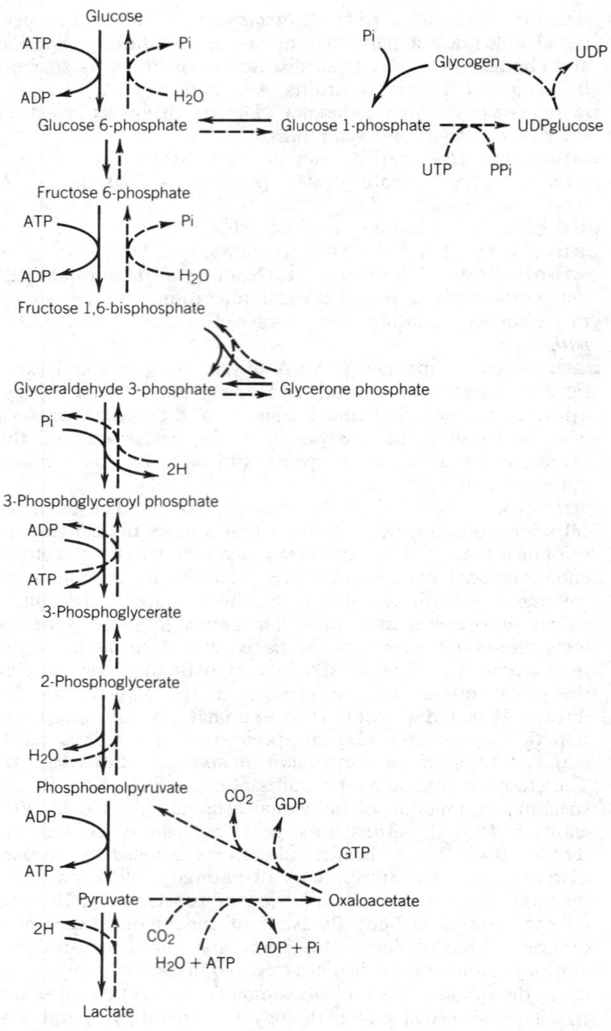

from the ear to the cerebral cortex. **biosynthetic p.** A sequence of chemical reactions in a living organism leading to the formation of a more complex compound from simpler components. Also *anabolic pathway.* **cerebellorubral p.** TRACTUS CEREBELLORUBRALIS. **classical complement p.** The pathway of complement activation that brings about the lysis of sheep erythrocytes sensitized with rabbit or horse antibody when heated with guinea-pig or human serum as source of complement. This was the classical model system on which complement activation was analyzed. The classical pathway requires both calcium ions (for $\overline{C1}$ activation) and magnesium ions (for the generation of $\overline{C42}$, and is active at high dilutions of serum. C1, C4, and C2 are the components peculiar to the classical complement pathway. Compare ALTERNATIVE COMPLEMENT PATHWAY. **corticopontocerebellar p.'s** CORTICOPONTOCEREBELLAR SYSTEM. **corticostrionigral p.** CORTICOSTRIONIGRAL SYSTEM. **distribution p.** **1** The course taken by a peripheral nerve or artery to the region or structures that it innervates or supplies. **2** The course followed by a group of nerve fibers in the central nervous system coursing from one region to a projection field in another region, such as the distribution pathway of thalamocortical projection fibers. **efferent p.** **1** The course of axons leaving a central neuronal aggregate. **2** A neural pathway that conducts impulses away from a specific region in the central nervous system. Compare AFFERENT PATHWAY. **3** A bundle of axons innervating effector organs or the series of neurons controlling muscles and glands. **Embden-Meyerhof p.** The sequence of chemical reactions involved in the anaerobic conversion of glucose to pyruvic acid or lactic acid with the production of adenosine triphosphate, the pathway often known as glycolysis. Also *Embden-Meyerhof cycle.* **Entner-Doudoroff p.** KETODEOXYGLUCONATE PATHWAY. **glyoxylate p.** GLYOXYLATE CYCLE. **gustatory p.'s** The pathways of the nerves involved in the sense of taste. **internuncial p.** Any bundle of nerve fibers that interconnects different nuclei within the central nervous system. **ketodeoxygluconate p.** A pathway that does not convert glucose to two three-carbon fragments, as in glycolysis, but releases C-1 as carbon dioxide. Pseudomonads employ this pathway to metabolize glucose, and enterobacteria only to metabolize gluconic acid. Also *Entner-Doudoroff pathway.* **membrane attack complement p.** See under COMPLEMENT. **metabolic p.** The series of consecutive reactions by which a substance is transformed in a living organism, such as the glycolytic pathway from carbohydrate to lactate or ethanol. **olfactory p.'s** The course of the nerves involved in the sense of smell. **optical p.'s** The pathways of the nerves involved in vision. **pallidofugal p.'s** PALLIDAL SYSTEM. **pentose phosphate p.** The sequence of chemical reactions in which glucose 6-phosphate is converted into ribose 5-phosphate with the formation of the reduced form of nicotinamide adenine dinucleotide. In animals, it occurs in liver and some other tissues, and it allows NADPH to be formed for fat synthesis and ribose 5-phosphate for nucleotide synthesis. It is also widespread in plants and microorganisms. Also *phosphogluconate pathway* (ambiguous). **phosphogluconate p.** *Ambiguous* PENTOSE PHOSPHATE PATHWAY. • This name has been used because this pathway goes through phosphogluconate on the way to pentose phosphates. However, another pathway, the ketodeoxygluconate pathway, also goes via 6-phosphogluconate. **reaction p.** The route by which a chemical reaction occurs. The term may be applied both to a series of discrete reactions to indicate what these are, and to a single reaction, to indicate the nature of intermediates and transition states through which the reacting substance passes. **reentrant p.** The track of a single cardiac impulse which, having once activated a segment of heart muscle and passed on, is able to do so again after that segment has ceased to be refractory. **spinocervicothalamic p.** The ascending projection system from dorsal horn to the lateral cervical nucleus containing both tactile and nociceptive input which is conveyed to the thalamus together with the anterolateral tract termination. This is prominent in cats but negligible in man and other primates. **thalamostriate p.'s** THALAMOSTRIATE RADIATION.

**The Embden-Meyerhof pathway** Dotted arrows show the route for reversal of the pathway in mammals (the conversion of pyruvate into phosphoenolpyruvate goes by different reactions in microorganisms).

**-pathy** \-pəthē\ [PATH- + -Y] A combining form meaning

(1) disease or abnormal condition; (2) treatment of disease. Also *-pathia.*

**patient** [L *patiens,* gen. *patientis* (pres. part. of *pati* to undergo, suffer) suffering, tolerant] A recipient of health care services, especially medical services. **private p.** 1 A patient under the care of a health care provider who is paid for that care by the patient or by a nongovernmental third party. 2 A patient in a private room of an inpatient facility. **public p.** A patient under the care of a health care provider or organization within a governmental program. Also *service patient.*

**patient-day** A measure of inpatient health care utilization reflecting the number of days of care used by a patient or a group of patients.

**patricide** \pat′risīd\ [Late L *patricidium,* from L *pater,* gen. *patris,* father + *-cidium* -CIDE)] Murder of one's own father.

**Patrick** [Hugh Talbot *Patrick,* U.S. neurologist, 1860–1938] Patrick's trigger areas. See under AREA.

**patrilineal** \pat′rilin′ē·əl\ 1 Pertaining to or derived from the father. Also *patroclinous.* 2 Descended through the male line.

**patroclinous** \pat′rəklī′nəs\ Pertaining to an offspring who has characters more closely resembling those of the father than the mother.

**patrocliny** \pat′rəklī′nē\ Any mode of inheritance in which the offspring predictably resemble the male parent more than the female parent. Compare MATROCLINY.

**patrogenesis** \pat′rəjen′əsis\ ANDROGENESIS.

**PAT-SED** PSEUDOACHONDROPLASTIC DYSPLASIA.

**patten** \pat′ən\ [Middle French *patin (from pate, patte* paw, hoof, from presumed Vulgar L *patta* paw) shoe sole] A metal support worn under the foot and usually fixed to a leg caliper. It relieves weight-bearing forces through the hip joint.

**pattern** A model or design, or a set of facts or conditions considered as composing an integrated design. **action p.** The repeatable behavior, consisting of both congenital and acquired reflex responses, which an individual exhibits to a particular situation or stimulus pattern. **arch p.** The simplest of the three basic fingerprint patterns, consisting of arches formed by epidermal ridges that enter from one side of the fingertip and flow to the opposite margin. **A-V p.'s** Motility fields in which the amount of strabismus is different on upward and downward gaze. **beam p.** The intensity of an ultrasonic or electromagnetic beam plotted as a function of distance and angle from the axis. **cloverleaf p.** A postulated two-dimensional outline of the transfer ribonucleic acid molecule, formed by loops and folds of the incompletely base-paired polynucleotide chain. **dicing p.** DICING ABRASIONS. **diffraction p.** A pattern observed as a spot of light, or electrons, is diffracted as it passes through a specimen, producing a specific pattern composed of a series of concentric light and dark circles, which can be used to identify the chemical structure of the specimen. **fingerprint p.** The dermatoglyphic pattern of the distal volar surface of the fingers and thumbs, as in arch, loop, and whorl patterns and their variations and composite forms. **honeycomb p.** An ultrasound echo pattern consisting of interlacing echo lines surrounding anechoic, clear areas of uniform size. **interference p.** Any graphic pattern indicative of interference. **juvenile p.** The pattern of T wave inversion in right-sided ECG chest leads other than $V_1$, seen normally in childhood and occasionally in adults, especially black adults. **loop p.** A basic fingerprint pattern, consisting of loops formed by epidermal ridges entering on one side of the fingertip and curving to flow back to exit (recurrent ridges) on the same side. Loops are designated as radial or ulnar depending on the side from which they enter and exit. **occlusal p.** The shape of the occlusal surfaces of artificial teeth or prostheses. **sedimentation p.** The configuration that particles assume in an antigen-antibody test performed by sedimentation in a test tube or multi-well plate. The reaction of the antigen on the particle surface with an agglutinating antibody causes the particles to settle on the bottom in a pattern distinctly different from that of particles that are not agglutinated. **skeletal p.** The anteroposterior relationship of the mandible to the maxilla, in connection with orthodontic prognosis. The main classes of Angle's classification of malocclusion of the teeth have been applied to this relationship. **startle p.** STARTLE RESPONSE. ● The term is used especially of those features visually observable. **stimulus p.** 1 The total set of sensory stimuli surrounding or impinging on a subject in a particular situation. 2 The pattern in timing and amplitude of a sequence of stimuli of one sort, such as electrical impulses, light flashes, etc. **wax p.** A construction in wax which when reproduced in metal or resin will become a crown, denture, or other appliance or part thereof. It is invested in plaster of Paris or a refractory material to make a mold. Also *wax form.* **wear p.** The position, size, and angle of wear facets on the teeth produced by both masticatory and nonmasticatory movements of the mandible. **whorl p.** The most complex of the three basic fingerprint patterns, consisting of whorls formed by epidermal ridges arranged in concentric spiral or ellipse patterns. Whorls require at least two triradii.

**patterning** \pat′ərning\ 1 The manipulation of body parts or the entire subject so as to activate reflex patterns with the therapeutic objective of reinforcing related voluntary neuromuscular control. 2 The repeated exposure of an experimental animal to a set of stimuli so as to instill a desired behavioral response.

**patulous** \pat′yələs\ [L *patulus* (from *patere* to be open) standing open, spreading] Spreading wide apart, as the branches of a tree; wide open.

**Paul** [Gustav *Paul,* Austrian physician, 1859–1935] See under TREATMENT, TEST.

**Paul** [John Rodman *Paul,* U.S. physician, 1893–1971] 1 Paul-Bunnell reaction. See under PAUL-BUNNELL TEST. 2 Paul-Bunnell-Davidsohn test. See under TEST.

**Pauling** [Linus Carl *Pauling,* U.S. chemist and physicist, born 1901] Pauling-Corey helix. See under ALPHA HELIX.

**pause** [L *pausa* (Gk *pausis* a cessation) an end, cessation] An interval of inaction. **cardiac p.** A long interval between heart beats. **compensatory p.** The pause which follows a premature ventricular ectopic beat. Its length compensates for the short interval which preceded that beat, so that the total heart rate is unchanged. **post-extrasystolic p.** The pause which follows any kind of extrasystole. **sinus p.** A pause in the regular discharge of the sinuatrial node which lasts for a length of time that is not an exact multiple of its usual interval.

**Pautrier** [Lucien Marius Adolphe *Pautrier,* French dermatologist, 1876–1959] Pautrier's abscesses. See under PAUTRIER'S MICROABSCESSES.

**pavementing** \pāv′mənting\ The characteristic appearance, due to leukocyte adherence, of the endothelium of an inflamed blood vessel.

**pavex** \pā′veks\ [*pa(ssive) v(ascular) ex(ercise)*] An apparatus used in the treatment of peripheral vascular diseases which, by alternating positive and negative pressure on a muscle, simulates the effect of exercise on the blood vessels of that muscle.

**pavilion** \pəvil′yən\ [L *papilio* (gen. *papilionis*) a butterfly, tent] Any expanded or dilated end of a canal. **p. of the oviduct** The fimbriated end of the fallopian tube.

**Pavlov** [Ivan Petrovich *Pavlov*, Russian physiologist, 1849–1936] **1** Pavlov stomach. See under POUCH. **2** See under METHOD. **3** Pavlov's reflex. See under AURICULOPRESSOR REFLEX.

**pavor** \pā′vər\ [L, fear, terror] Fear; terror. **p. diurnus** A sleep disorder marked by terror occurring during a child's daytime nap, similar in symptoms to pavor nocturnus. Also *day terrors.* **p. nocturnus** A sleep disorder of children, marked by terror and similar to but more serious and distressing than a nightmare. The child awakes abruptly in a state of semiconsciousness characterized by autonomic arousal and disorientation. The episode usually lasts 1–10 minutes. Also *angor nocturnus, night terrors.*

**payer** / **third party p.** THIRD PARTY.

**Payr** [Erwin *Payr*, German surgeon, 1871–1946] **1** Payr's disease. See under SPLENIC FLEXURE SYNDROME. **2** See under CLAMP, METHOD.

**PB** **1** *Pharmacopoeia Britannica* (British Pharmacopoeia). **2** pressure breathing.

**Pb** Symbol for the element, lead.

**PBC** **1** point of basal convergence. **2** primary biliary cirrhosis.

**PBE** perlsucht bacillen emulsion.

**PBI** protein-bound iodine.

**PC** professional corporation.

**p.c.** **1** *post cibum* (L, after meals). **2** *pondus civile* (L, civil, i.e., avoirdupois weight).

**PCA** passive cutaneous anaphylaxis.

**PCB** polychlorinated biphenyl.

**PcB** punctum convergens basalis.

**PCG** phonocardiogram.

**pCi** Symbol for the unit, picocurie.

**PCM** protein-calorie malnutrition.

**$P_{CO_2}$** Symbol for carbon dioxide partial pressure.

**pcs** preconscious.

**PCV** packed-cell volume.

**Pd** Symbol for the element, palladium.

**PDA** patent ductus arteriosus.

**pd** **1** pupillary distance. **2** potential difference. **3** prism diopter.

**PDGF** platelet derived growth factor.

**PDI** periodontal disease index.

**PDLL** poorly differentiated lymphocytic lymphoma.

**PE** **1** physical examination. **2** pulmonary edema. **3** pulmonary embolism. **4** potential energy.

**peak** **1** Maximum point; highest level. **2** The highest point on a curve or in the graphic record of a fluctuating quantity. **biclonal p.** A notched or biphasic upward deflection of the densitometer tracing of serum electrophoresis on serum from an individual with increased levels of globulins that are derived from two different abnormally proliferating clones of B lymphocytes. **Bragg p.** The peak in the relative ionization which occurs near the end of the path of a charged particle as it travels through an absorber. **kilovolt p.** The maximum value of the voltage applied to an x-ray tube. Abbr. kVp **monoclonal p.** A single, sharply defined upward deflection of the densitometer tracing obtained in the electrophoresis of serum proteins from an individual with excessive globulins produced by a single clone of proliferating B lymphocytes. Also *M spike.*

**peak-to-peak** Describing the amplitude of an alternating current or voltage measured from the positive maximum to the negative maximum.

**pearl** [French *perle* (from Vulgar L *pernula*, dim. of L *perna* a sea mussel) pearl] **1** A concretion of calcium carbonate from various mollusks, once believed to have beneficial medicinal powers. **2** A small globule of a medicine, or a glass bulb containing a volatile medicine released by pressure, such as amyl nitrite. **3** A rounded, firm pellet of mucoid or cellular exudate, seen in attacks of bronchial asthma. **Elschnig's p.'s** ELSCHNIG BODIES. **enamel p.** An ectopic nodule of enamel, sometimes containing dentin and even pulp, situated at the cementoenamel junction of molar teeth, particularly in furcation areas. Also *enameloma, enamel nodule, enamel drop.* **epithelial p.'s** A rounded or oval, compact, whorled aggregate of squamous epithelial cells and keratin found in some well-differentiated squamous cell carcinomas. Also *pearly bodies, epidermic pearls.* **Epstein's p.'s** Small yellowish masses seen on the hard palate of newborn infants. **gouty p.** TOPHUS. **parakeratotic p.** A small round mass of squamous cells arranged in concentric layers and showing increasing keratinization towards the center. Parakeratotic pearls are a feature of squamous cells carcinoma of the skin, especially in more differentiated tumors.

**Pearson** [Karl *Pearson*, English scientist, 1857–1936] Poisson-Pearson formula. See under FORMULA.

**peau** \pō\ [French, skin] **p. d'orange** A dimpled appearance to the skin, simulating orange peel. It is produced by lymphedema and characteristic of certain carcinomas of the breast and other conditions.

**pecazine** MEPAZINE.

**peccant** \pek′ənt\ [L *peccans*, gen. *peccantis*, pres. part. of *peccare* to do wrong, injure, sin. Old French *peccant* means diseased or causing disease.] Unhealthy; diseased.

**pecilo-** \pəsil′ō-\ POIKILO-.

**Pecquet** [Jean *Pecquet*, French physician and anatomist, 1622–1674] **1** Receptaculum pecqueti, cistern of Pecquet. See under CISTERNA CHYLI. **2** Duct of Pecquet. See under DUCTUS THORACICUS.

**pecten** \pek′tən\ [L (from *pectere* to comb; akin to Gk *pekein* to comb or card wool), a comb] **1** Any structure with a toothed, comblike appearance. **2** PECTEN ANALIS. **p. analis** [NA] A narrow zone just distal to the anal valves, comprising stratified epithelium intermediate in thickness between the epithelium above the valves and the skin that lines the lower part of the anal canal. Deep to it is the internal rectal venous plexus. Also *transitional zone, pecten.* **p. ossis pubis** [NA] The sharp ridge that forms the superior border of the superior ramus of the pubis and its pectineal surface. It extends from the pubic tubercle to the iliopubic eminence, providing attachment for the conjoint tendon, the lacunar ligament, the pectineal ligament, and the iliopectineal arch. Also *pectineal line.*

**pectenosis** \pek′tənō′sis\ [L *pecten* a comb, scallop + -OSIS] Stenosis of the anal canal, between the anal groove and anal crypts, due to a rigid ring of tissue, and manifest by anal irritation, bleeding, and pain on defecation.

**pectenotomy** \pek′tənek′təmē\ [L *pecten* a comb, scallop + *o* + -TOMY] The incision and subsequent release of the tight, inelastic ring of tissue (pecten analis) within the anal canal.

**pectinate** \pek′tināt\ [L *pecten*, gen. *pectinis*, a comb + -ATE. See PECTEN.] Having toothlike projections; comblike. Also *pectiniform.*

**pectineal** \pektin′ē·əl\ **1** Of or pertaining to the os pubis. **2** Of or relating to any comblike structure.

**pectiniform** \pektin′ifôrm\ PECTINATE.

**pectoral** \pek′tərəl\ [L *pectoralis* (from *pectus*, gen. *pecto-*

*ris* chest, breast) of the breast] Pertaining to the chest.
**pectoralis** \pek'tərā'lis\ Pectoral: applied chiefly to chest muscles.
**pectoriloquy** \pek'təril'əkwē\ [L *pectus,* gen. *pectoris,* chest + *loqui* to speak] Abnormal clearness of voice sounds heard on auscultation over parts of the chest where they are not normally heard, in cases of consolidated or cavitated lung. **whispering p.** A marked degree of pectoriloquy such that whispered speech can be clearly heard on auscultation of the chest.
**pectus** \pek'təs\ [L (gen. *pectoris*), the breast, the breast as the seat of the affections] The anterior part of the thorax or chest; the breast. **p. carinatum** An unusual prominence of the sternum with flattening of the thoracic cage on either side, creating the appearance of a keel of a boat. The deformity occurs in infancy or childhood, when the rib cage and cartilages are more pliant, by unbalanced action of the muscles of respiration. The pull of the muscle of inspiration is exaggerated when there is chronic impedance of the airway at any level. This forces the sternum upwards and forwards. Also *pigeon breast, chicken breast, keeled breast, pigeon chest, keeled chest.* **p. excavatum** Backward displacement of the xiphoid process and often the lower part of the body of the sternum, creating a depression in the middle of the surface of the chest. Also *pectus recurvatum, funnel chest.*
**ped-**[1] \pēd-, ped-\ PEDO-[1].
**ped-**[2] \ped-, pēd-\ PEDO-[2].
**pedal** \ped'əl\ [L *pes,* gen. *pedis,* foot + -AL] **1** Pertaining to the foot or feet. **2** Pertaining to any pes.
**pedatrophia** \pē'dətrō'fē·ə\ [PED-[1] + ATROPHIA] MARASMUS.
**pederasty** \pē'dəras'tē, ped'-\ [Gk *paiderastia* (from *pais,* gen. *paid(os)* a boy + *erasthai* to love, lust after) love of boys] Anal intercourse with a boy as the passive, receptive partner. Also *pedication.*
**pedes** \pē'dēz\ Plural of PES.
**pedi-**[1] \pē'dē-, ped'ē-\ PEDO-[1].
**pedi-**[2] \ped'ē-, pē'dē-\ PEDO-[2].
**pediadontia** \pē'dē·ədän'shə\ [misspelling of *pediodontia*] PEDODONTIA.
**pedialgia** \pēd'ē·al'jə\ A pain in the foot.
**pediatric** \pē'dē·at'rik\ Of or relating to pediatrics. Also *pedologic.*
**pediatrician** \pē'dē·ətrish'ən\ A physician specializing in pediatrics. Also *pediatrist, pedologist.*
**pediatrics** \pē'dē·at'riks\ [PED-[1] + -IATRICS] The branch of medical science dealing with the disorders and normal physical and mental development of children and young adolescents. Also *pediatry, pedology.*
**pediatrist** \pē'dē·at'rist\ PEDIATRICIAN.
**pediatry** \pē'dē·at'rē\ PEDIATRICS.
**pedication** \ped'ikā'shən\ PEDERASTY.
**pedicel** \ped'isel\ A cytoplasmic process that is expanded where it makes contact with a basement membrane, as is seen in the epithelial cells of the renal glomerulus. Also *foot plate, footplate, foot process.*
**pedicellate** \pedis'əlāt\ Possessing a pedicel. Also *pedicellated.*
**pedicle** \ped'ikl\ PEDICULUS. **cone p.** The furrowed invagination of retinal cones forming the synaptic region contacted by bipolar and horizontal cells. **Filatov-Gillies tubed p.** A tubular bipedicle flap constructed by making two parallel incisions several centimeters apart through skin and subcutaneous tissue, elevating these structures from the underlying bed except at each extremity and then suturing the cut edges of the elevated flap together to create a tube receiving its blood supply from each end which has been left intact. The original bed from which the flap was raised may be closed beneath the pedicle primarily or the area may be covered with a split-thickness skin graft. **p. of vertebral arch** Each of two bony columns of the neural arch, one right and one left, extending from front to back on each side of the vertebral foramen, from the vertebral body as far as the bony mass which gives rise to the lamina, to the transverse process and to the articular processes of a vertebra. Each develops from a cartilaginous center in each neural arch, which for the first few years in man is connected to the vertebral body by a synchondrosis called the neurocentral joint. The upper and lower borders of the pedicle, together with those of adjacent vertebrae, form the boundaries of the intervertebral foramina. Also *pedicle of neural arch, pediculus arcus vertebrae.*
**pedicled** \ped'ikəld\ Provided with a pedicle.
**pedicular** \pēdik'yələr\ [*pedicul(us)* a louse + -AR] Relating to, or caused by, lice.
**pediculate** \pēdik'yəlāt\ PEDICULATED.
**pediculated** \pēdik'yəlā'tid\ Having a pedicle; pedunculated; stalked. Also *pediculate.*
**pediculation** \pēdik'yəlā'shən\ **1** PEDICULOSIS. **2** The development of a pedicle.
**pediculi** \pēdik'yəlī\ Plural of PEDICULUS.
**pediculicide** \pēdik'yəlisīd'\ [L *pedicul(us)* a louse + *i* + -CIDE] An agent destructive to lice. Also *lousicide.*
***Pediculoides*** \pēdik'yəloi'dēz\ *PYEMOTES.*
**pediculosis** \pədik'yəlō'sis\ [*pedicul(us)* + -OSIS] An infestation of the body with *Pediculus* or *Pthirus*; an infestation of lice. Also *lousiness.* **p. capitis** An infestation of the head hair with *Pediculus humanus capitis.* Also *phthiriasis capitis.* **p. corporis** Infestation with the body louse *Pediculus humanus corporis.* Also *phthiriasis corporis.* **p. inguinalis** PTHIRIASIS. **p. pubis** PTHIRIASIS. **p. vestimenti** The presence of body lice in clothing. Also *pediculosis vestimentorum.*
**pediculous** \pēdik'yələs\ [L *pediculus* (dim. of *pedis,* gen. *pedis,* a louse) a louse] Infested with lice; lousy.
***Pediculus*** \pədik'yələs\ [L (dim. of *pedis,* gen. *pedis,* a louse), a louse] A genus of sucking lice of humans and other primates (order Anoplura, family Pediculidae). ***P. humanus capitis*** The head louse, a variant or subspecies of the body louse. It is usually confined to the fine hair of the head. Though it may occasionally wander to the body, it seldom infests clothing. The species is cosmopolitan, among all peoples, and recently has occurred in urban foci in western nations in heavy outbreaks, especially among school children or confined persons in close quarters. No disease has been associated with head lice, probably because they are less frequently passed from person to person than body lice are. ***P. humanus humanus*** The body louse, clothes louse, or cootie, which usually stays in clothing except to feed (by sucking blood). In wintertime when several layers of clothing are worn, lousiness becomes most acute. Eggs (nits) are deposited with a gluelike material in the seams of clothing, perhaps 100 eggs per female. Heavy infestation causes intense discomfort and skin sensitization with red papules at feeding sites which may weep and become swollen. Epidemic typhus results from transmission of *Rickettsia prowazekii* to humans. Body lice also transmit the spirochete that causes relapsing fever, *Borrelia recurrentis,* and the rickettsial agent of trench fever, *Rochalimaea quintana,* especially common during World War I. Also *Pediculus humanus vestimentorum, Pediculus humanus corporis, Pediculus vestimenti.* ***P. pubis*** A former name of *PTHIRUS PUBIS.* ***P. vestimenti*** *PEDICULUS HUMANUS HUMANUS.*
**pediculus** [L (dim of *pes,* gen. *pedis* foot) a small foot,

base, pedicle] (*pl.* pediculi) A part or structure resembling a short stem or base. Also *pedicle.* **p. arcus vertebrae** [NA] PEDICLE OF VERTEBRAL ARCH.

**pedigree** \ped′əgrē\ [Middle English *pee de grue* (from Old French *pee* foot, from L *pes* foot + *de* from + *grus* crane) crane's foot, from the form sketched by genealogical lines] In genetics, a diagrammatic representation of a family. Each generation occupies a separate horizontal array, and the line of descent is arranged vertically. Usually square symbols represent males and circles, females, and details within the symbols indicate phenotypic features of interest. See also diagram at MENDELIAN INHERITANCE.

**pediodontia** \pē′dē·ōdän′shə\ [PEDI-[1] + -ODONTIA] PEDODONTIA.

**pedion** \pē′dē·än\ The plantar surface or sole of the foot. Also *pedium.*

**pedipalpus** \ped′ipal′pəs\ [PEDI-[2] + L *palpus,* also *palpum* a gentle stroke, soft blow or pat] (*pl.* pedipalpi) A postoral jointed appendage variously modified for sensory and manipulative functions, occurring in certain arthropods. In spiders, the pedipalpi may resemble an additional pair of legs. In spiders and allies they are chelate, the terminal segment being jointed to permit grasping. Also *pedipalp.*

**pediphalanx** \ped′ifā′langks\ A phalanx of a toe. Compare MANIPHALANX.

**pedistibulum** \ped′istib′yələm\ *Outmoded* STAPES.

**pedium** \pē′dē·əm\ PEDION.

**pedo-[1]** \pē′dō-, ped′ō-\ [Gk *pais,* gen. *paidos* child] A combining form meaning child. Also *ped-, pedi-, paed-, paedi, paedo-.*

**pedo-[2]** \ped′ō-, pē′dō-\ [L *pes,* gen. *pedis* foot] A combining form meaning foot, pedal. Also *ped-, pedi-.*

**pedobaromacrometer** \-bar′ōməkräm′ətər\ [PEDO-[1] + BARO- + MACRO- + -METER] A scale for weighing and measuring the length of a baby.

**pedobarometer** \-bəräm′ətər\ [PEDO-[1] + BARO- + -METER] A scale for weighing a baby.

**pedodontia** \ped′ōdän′shə\ [PED-[1] + -ODONTIA] The study of dentistry as applied to children. Also *pediodontia.*

**pedodontics** \pē′dōdon′tiks\ [PED-[1] + ODONT- + -ICS] The practice of dentistry for children.

**pedodynamometer** \-dī′nəmäm′ətər\ An instrument for measuring the muscle power of a leg.

**pedogenesis** \-jen′əsis\ [PEDO-[1] + GENESIS] The sexual development and production of offspring by larval forms, as in certain midges of the genus *Miastor.* Also *paedogenesis.* Compare NEOTENY.

**pedologic** \-läj′ik\ PEDIATRIC.

**pedologist** \pēdäl′əjist\ PEDIATRICIAN.

**pedology** \pēdäl′əjē\ [PEDO-[1] + -LOGY] PEDIATRICS.

**pedometer** \pēdäm′ətər\ [PEDO-[2] + -METER] An instrument that records the number of steps taken in order to calculate the distance walked. Also *podometer.*

**pedophilia** \-fil′yə\ [PEDO-[1] + -PHILIA] A paraphilia in which a prepubertal child is essential to sexual gratification.

**peduncle** \pədung′kl\ PEDUNCULUS. **anterior p. of thalamus** A collection of nerve fibers in which are located the anterior thalamic radiation and corticothalamic pathways that serve to interconnect the anterior and medial nuclei of the thalamus with the cerebral cortex of the frontal lobe. The anterior thalamic peduncle courses in the anterior limb of the internal capsule and contains thalamofrontal fibers from the dorsomedial thalamic nucleus, frontothalamic fibers from the prefrontal cortex, thalamocingulate fibers from the anterior thalamic nuclear group, and cingulothalamic fibers from the cingulate gyrus. Also *frontal thalamic peduncle, pedunculus thalami frontalis, pedunculus thalami anterior.* **cerebellar p.'s** Six large bundles of white fibers that interconnect the cerebellum with the brainstem. They are arranged in three pairs and named the superior (cranial), middle, and inferior (caudal) cerebellar peduncles. The superior cerebellar peduncles interconnect the cerebellum with the midbrain, while the middle and inferior peduncles attach the cerebellum to the pons and medulla oblongata respectively. Also *brachia cerebelli.* See also PEDUNCULUS CEREBELLARIS INFERIOR, PEDUNCULUS CEREBELLARIS MEDIUS, PEDUNCULUS CEREBELLARIS SUPERIOR. **cerebral p.** PEDUNCULUS CEREBRI. **p. of corpus callosum** The anterior extensions of the medial and lateral longitudinal striae (of Lancici), where these narrow bundles of white fibers curve around the genu and rostrum of the corpus callosum to reach the paraterminal gyrus. *Seldom used.* **p. of flocculus** PEDUNCULUS FLOCCULI. **frontal thalamic p.** ANTERIOR PEDUNCLE OF THALAMUS. **p. of hypophysis** *Obs.* INFUNDIBULUM HYPOTHALAMI. **inferior cerebellar p.** PEDUNCULUS CEREBELLARIS INFERIOR. **inferior p. of thalamus** PEDUNCULUS THALAMI INFERIOR. **p. of lentiform nucleus** The band of gray substance that fuses the anterior end of the caudate nucleus with the putamen of the lentiform nucleus just above the anterior perforated substance. *Seldom used.* **mamillary p.** PEDUNCULUS CORPORIS MAMILLARIS. **p. of mamillary body** PEDUNCULUS CORPORIS MAMILLARIS. **middle cerebellar p.** PEDUNCULUS CEREBELLARIS MEDIUS. **olfactory p.** In comparative neuroanatomy, the region of attachment of the olfactory tract to the cerebral cortex. **pineal p.** PEDUNCULUS CORPORIS PINEALIS. **p. of pineal body** PEDUNCULUS CORPORIS PINEALIS. **posterior cerebellar p.** *Seldom used* PEDUNCULUS CEREBELLARIS INFERIOR. **posterior thalamic p.** PEDUNCULUS THALAMI SUPERIOR. **superior cerebellar p.** PEDUNCULUS CEREBELLARIS SUPERIOR. **superior thalamic p.** PEDUNCULUS THALAMI SUPERIOR.

**pedunculated** \pidungk′yəlā′tid\ Having a peduncle; pediculated; stalked. Also *polypoid, pedunculate.*

**pedunculotomy** \pidungk′yəlät′əmē\ [*peduncul(us)* + *o* + -TOMY] Incision of the cerebral peduncle.

**pedunculus** \pədung′kyələs\ [New L, dim. of L *pes* (gen. *pedis*) a foot] A stalk- or stemlike connecting part, usually denoting a bundle of nerve fibers, such as the cerebral peduncle containing corticospinal axons. Also *peduncle.* **p. cerebellaris inferior** [NA] A bundle of afferent and efferent fibers connecting the cerebellum to a variety of nuclei in the spinal cord and medulla oblongata. Also *corpus restiforme, restiform body, inferior cerebellar peduncle, processus e cerebello ad medullam, posterior cerebellar peduncle* (seldom used), *restibrachium, restis, restiform process of Henle* (outmoded). **p. cerebellaris medius** [NA] A compact bundle composed almost entirely of the axons from the nuclei pontis that cross the midline to reach the cortex of the contralateral cerebellar hemisphere. These are second-order fibers of the extensive corticopontocerebellar pathway. Also *brachium pontis, crus cerebelli ad pontem* (obs.), *pontibrachium, middle cerebellar peduncle, pontocerebellar tract, processus e cerebello ad pontem.* **p. cerebellaris superior** [NA] The largest cerebellar efferent bundle, containing fibers from the dentate, emboliform, and globose nuclei that enter the midbrain, decussate, and project to the opposite red nucleus and ventrolateral and intralaminar nuclei of the thalamus. Also *brachium conjunctivum cerebelli, superior cerebellar peduncle, superior crus of cerebellum, processus e cerebello ad testes.* **p. cerebri** [NA] A massive band of descending corticospinal and corticolbulbar fibers situated in the most ventral part of the midbrain. Also *pes pedunculi,* *cerebral peduncle, caudex cerebri* (obs.). See also CRUS CEREBRI. **p. corporis callosi** *Obs.* GYRUS SUBCALLOSUS. **p. corporis mamillaris** A discrete bundle, formed by the convergence of several ascending sensory pathways in the midbrain tegmentum, that ends in the mamillary body. Also *mamillary peduncle, peduncle of mamillary body.* **p. corporis pinealis** The region of attachment of the pineal body to the dorsal diencephalon, divided into superior and inferior laminae separated by the pineal recess of the third ventricle. The inferior lamina contains the posterior commissure, and the superior lamina contains the habenular commissure. Also *pineal stalk, peduncle of pineal body, pineal peduncle.* **p. flocculi** [NA] A portion of the flocculonodular lobe of the cerebellum that forms the wall of each lateral recess of the fourth ventricle. Also *peduncle of flocculus.* **p. thalami anterior** ANTERIOR PEDUNCLE OF THALAMUS. **p. thalami frontalis** ANTERIOR PEDUNCLE OF THALAMUS. **p. thalami inferior** [NA] The reciprocal connections of the posterior thalamus and medial geniculate nucleus with the temporal lobe cortex. Also *inferior peduncle of thalamus.* **p. thalami posterior** A fiber bundle that joins the pulvinar and lateral geniculate nuclei with the posterior parietal and occipital cortex. Also *posterior thalamic peduncle.* **p. thalami superior** The region of attachment between the precentral and postcentral gyri of the frontal and parietal lobes with ventral and lateral thalamic nuclear groups. Also *superior thalamic peduncle.* **p. vitellinus** YOLK STALK.

**peel** [Middle French *peler* (from L *pilare* to deprive of hair, from *pilus* a single hair) to remove the hair from, peel] **lip p.** LIP SHAVE.

**peeling** The desquamation of the cutaneous epidermis that usually occurs from three to seven days after a first-degree burn, as from exposure to the sun or a toxic substance that produces erythema.

**peenash** \pē′nash\ An Indian term for NASAL MYIASIS.

**PEEP** positive end-expiratory pressure.

**Peet** [Max Minor *Peet,* U.S. neurosurgeon, born 1885] See under OPERATION.

**peg** A projecting structure that is more or less circular in cross-section. **bone p.** A strut of bone that is used to stabilize a pseudarthrosis or to support an area of bone collapse. **cortical bone p.** A bone peg consisting entirely of cortical bone that is used to add structural support to an area of bone loss or destruction. **epithelial p.'s** RETE RIDGES. **rete p.'s** RETE RIDGES.

**Pel** [Pieter Klaases *Pel,* Dutch physician, 1852–1919] Murchison-Pel-Ebstein fever, Pel-Ebstein pyrexia, Pel-Ebstein symptom. See under PEL-EBSTEIN FEVER.

**pelage** \pel′ij, pelähzh′\ [French (from Middle French *poil* hair, from L *pilus* hair + French *-age* -AGE), the hair covering of an animal] The hair coat in its entirety.

**Pelger** [Karel *Pelger,* Dutch physician, 1885–1931] Pelger-Huët nuclear anomaly. See under PELGER-HUËT ANOMALY.

**pelidisi** \pel′idē′sē\ [L *p(ondus)* a weight + *(d)e(cies)* ten times + *li(nearis)* linear + *di(visus)* divided + *si(dentis)* sitting + *(altitudo)* height] The unit of Pirquet's index: the cube root of ten times the weight (in grams) divided by the sitting height (in centimeters).

**peliosis** \pē′lē·ō′sis\ [Gk *peliōsis* (from *pel(os),* also *pell(os)* dark-colored + *i* + *-ōsis* -OSIS) extravasation of the blood] *Obs.* PURPURA. **p. hepatis** A rare condition characterized by the presence of multiple microscopic pods of blood, often lined with endothelium, in the hepatic lobules. It is thought to stem from congestion of the liver and subsequent necrosis. Also *peliosis of the liver, hepatic angiomatosis.*

**pellagra** \pəlā′grə, pəlag′rə\ [Italian *pelle* (from L *pellis* the skin of an animal, hide) skin, hide + *agra* sour, sharp, rough, prob. from Gk *agra* a hunting, catching, seizure] A disease caused by a dietary deficiency of nicotinic acid and characterized by cutaneous, gastrointestinal, and psychiatric symptoms. It is marked by a bilateral, symmetric, scaly rash on skin surfaces exposed to the sun, as the face and extremities, with associated polyneuropathy, confusion, and irritability progressing to psychotic symptoms such as delirium. Other symptoms are diarrhea and loss of surface features of the tongue, accompanied by swelling of the tongue and edema. Also *alpine scurvy, psilosis pigmentosa, niacinamidosis, erythema endemicum.* **p. sine p.** The syndrome of pellagra without the typical skin changes.

**pellagragenic** \pelag′rəjen′ik\ Giving rise to pellagra.

**pellagramin** \pelag′rəmin\ NIACIN.

**pellant** \pel′ənt\ DEPURATIVE.

**Pellegrini** [Augusto *Pellegrini,* Italian surgeon, born 1877] Pellegrini's disease, Köhler-Pellegrini-Stieda disease. See under PELLEGRINI-STIEDA DISEASE.

**pellet** A small granule or pill composed of steroid hormones which can be implanted subcutaneously to allow slow, prolonged release of the steroid. **foil p.** A small piece of gold foil, loosely rolled, used in building up a gold foil restoration by the process of cold-welding.

**pellicle** \pel′ikl\ [L *pellicul(a)* (dim. of *pellis* skin, hide) a little skin or hide] **1** A skin or thin membrane. **2** A skinlike film of coagulated material on the surface of a liquid. **3** A bacterial growth in a liquid medium that forms a surface film or sheet. **dental p.** A thin mucinous integument formed from the saliva on the surface of erupted teeth.

**Pellizzi** [G. B. *Pellizzi,* Italian physician, flourished early 20th century] See under SYNDROME.

**pellote** \pāyō′tə\ PEYOTE.

**pelmatic** \pelmat′ik\ PLANTAR.

**pelo-** \pē′lō-\ [Gk *pēlos* clay, mud] A combining form meaning mud.

**pelotherapy** \pē′lōther′əpē\ [PELO- + THERAPY] Application of mud for therapeutic purposes, commonly in the form of hot mud packs in conjunction with mineral spa therapy, or by beauticians for purported effects on the skin. Also *pelopathy.*

**pelta** \pel′tə\ [L, a short buckler or target in the shape of a half-moon] A crescent-shaped membranous organelle present in certain flagellates related to *Trichomonas.* It stains with silver and is found near the base of the anterior flagella.

**peltatin** \peltā′tin\ Either of two lignans, α-peltatin or β-peltatin, which occurs in podophyllum resin. β-pelatin, $C_{22}H_{22}O_8$, contains a methoxyl group in place of the hydroxyl group in α-peltatin, $C_{21}H_{20}O_8$. Both forms are active against wartlike neoplasms and show tumor-damaging activity in mice.

**pelves** \pel′vēz\ Plural of PELVIS.

**pelvi-** \pel′vi-\ [L *pelvis* bowl, basin] A combining form denoting the pelvis. Also *pelvio-, pelvo-.*

**pelvic** \pel′vik\ Of or relating to the pelvis.

**pelvicellulitis** \-sel′yəlī′tis\ PARAMETRITIS.

**pelvicephalometry** \-sef′əläm′ətrē\ [PELVI- + CEPHALO- + -METRY] Comparative measurement of the fetal head and maternal pelvis in order to assess the presence of cephalopelvic disproportion.

**pelvifemoral** \-fem′ərəl\ Pertaining to the pelvis and the femur or thigh.

**pelvifixation** \-fiksā′shən\ [PELVI- + FIXATION] A surgical procedure in which a floating or poorly fixed pelvic organ is suspended to prevent further ptosis or torsion.

**pelvilithotomy** \-lithät′əmē\ PYELOLITHOTOMY.

**pelvimeter** \pelvim′ətər\ [PELVI- + -METER] A device used to measure the pelvic dimensions. **Budin's p.** A caliper-shaped pelvimeter. **Martin's p.** A caliper-shaped pelvimeter with a reversed curve on its arms.

**pelvimetry** \pelvim′ətrē\ [PELVI- + -METRY] Measurement of the diameters of the female pelvis in pregnancy and of the size of the fetal head. **combined p.** Measurement of the pelvic dimensions made both internally and externally. **digital p.** Pelvimetry performed with the examiner's fingers. Also *manual pelvimetry.* **external p.** Pelvic measurements made outside the body. **internal p.** Measurement of the internal dimensions of the pelvis. **manual p.** DIGITAL PELVIMETRY. **x-ray p.** The measurement of the dimensions of the pelvis by roentgenographic methods.

**pelvio-** \pel′vē·ō-\ PELVI-.

**pelvioileoneocystostomy** \-il′ē·ōnē′·ōsistäs′təmē\ A surgical procedure in which the renal pelvis is anastomosed to a defunctionalized loop of ileum which in turn is anastomosed to the urinary bladder, in order to bypass a damaged or obstructed ureter.

**pelviolithotomy** \-lithät′əmē\ PYELOLITHOTOMY.

**pelvioneocystostomy** \-nē′ōsistäs′təmē\ The surgical establishment of a new connection between the renal pelvis and the urinary bladder in order to bypass a damaged or obstructed ureter.

**pelvioneostomy** \-nē·äs′təmē\ [PELVIO- + NEOSTOMY] URETERONEOPYELOSTOMY.

**pelvioperitonitis** \-per′itənī′tis\ PELVIC PERITONITIS.

**pelvioplasty** \pel′vē·əplas′tē\ [PELVIO- + -PLASTY] PYELOPLASTY.

**pelvioscopy** \pel′vē·äs′kəpē\ [PELVIO- + -SCOPY] The visual inspection of the pelvis or the pelvic viscera.

**pelviostomy** \pel′vē·äs′təmē\ PYELOSTOMY.

**pelviotomy** \pel′vē·ät′əmē\ [PELVIO- + -TOMY] PYELOTOMY.

**pelviperitonitis** \-per′itənī′tis\ Peritonitis of the pelvic cavity.

# pelvis

**pelvis** \pel′vis\ [L (akin to Gk *pellis* the pelvis, to *pyelos* a tub, trough, or vessel for feeding animals, bathtub, and to *pella* a wooden bowl, milk pail), a bowl, basin] (*pl.* pelves) **1** [NA] The large, circular, basin-shaped region at the junction of the trunk and the lower limbs. It is composed of the two hip bones, the sacrum, and the coccyx that enclose the pelvic cavity and its contents. It is divided into the major pelvis and the minor pelvis by an oblique plane formed by the terminal lines at the sides and in front and the sacral promonotory behind. This plane also limits the superior aperture, or inlet, of the minor, or true, pelvis, which communicates with the exterior through its inferior aperture or outlet. The major pelvis also forms the lower portion of the abdomen. **2** Any basin-shaped or funnel-shaped structure, such as the renal pelvis. Adj. pelvic. **achondroplastic p.** The broad, flattened pelvis that is characteristic of achondroplasia. **p. aequabiliter justo major** GIANT PELVIS. **p. aequabiliter justo minor** PELVIS JUSTO MINOR. **android p.** A female pelvis shape hav-

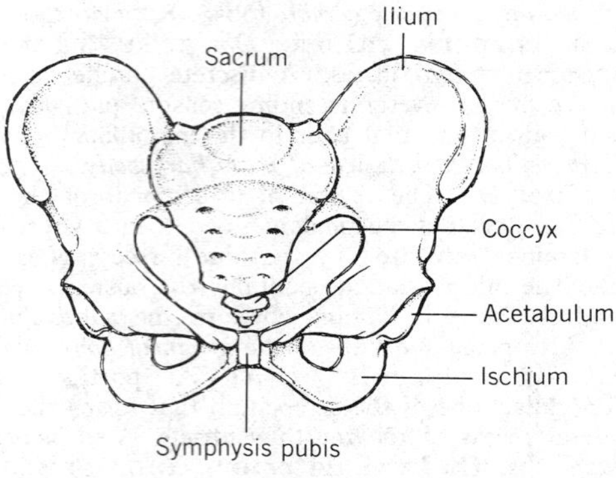


**Pelvis**

ing certain characteristics of the typical male pelvis. The inlet is wedge-shaped, the side walls converge, and the retropubic angle and the subpubic arch are both narrow. Also *funnel-shaped pelvis.* **anthropoid p.** A pelvis with a long, narrow inlet in which the anterior-posterior diameter is greater than usual. **assimilation p.** A pelvic girdle in which the sacrum has become fused, either with the lowest lumbar vertebra (high-assimilation pelvis) or with the highest coccygeal segment (low-assimilation pelvis). **asymmetrical p.** Pelvic obliquity caused by either a discrepancy in leg length or fixed lumbar scoliosis. **beaked p.** A pelvis in which the bones are compressed laterally and tilted anteriorly. **bifid p.** A renal pelvis in which there are two rather than the usual single major calix. **blunderbuss p.** A pelvis with divergent side walls. **bony p.** PELVIS OSSEA. **brachypellic p.** A pelvis which is flat and oval and in which the anteroposterior diameter of the inlet is shorter than the transverse diameter. **caoutchouc p.** OSTEOMALACIC PELVIS. **contracted p.** A pelvis in which one or more diameters are shorter than normal. **cordate p.** A heart-shaped pelvis due to an anterior projection of the sacrum. Also *cordiform pelvis.* **coxarthrolisthetic p.** A pelvis in which one or both femoral heads project into the pelvic cavity as a result of softening near the acetabulum. **Deventer's p.** A pelvis that is flat, with a short anteroposterior diameter. **dolichopellic p.** A pelvis in which the anteroposterior diameter of the inlet is longer than the transverse diameter. **dwarf p.** A pelvis that is very small, with the bones united by cartilage as in infants. **elastic p.** OSTEOMALACIC PELVIS. **extrarenal p.** Extension of renal pelvis beyond the renal substance. **false p.** PELVIS MAJOR. **flat p.** A pelvis in which the anteroposterior dimensions are abnormally shortened. **frozen p.** Fixation of the uterus and its adenexae in the pelvis due to pathologic conditions such as carcinoma, endometriosis, or pelvic inflammatory disease. Also *hardened pelvis.* **funnel-shaped p.** ANDROID PELVIS. **generally contracted p.** A pelvis with more than one abnormally short dimension. **generally enlarged p.** A pelvis with dimensions which are longer than normal. **giant p.** A pelvis that is symmetric but unusually large. Also *justomajor pelvis, pelvis justo major, pelvis aequabiliter justo major, justo major.* **greater p.** PELVIS MAJOR. **gynecoid p.** The normal female pelvis, having a well-rounded oval shape to the inlet. **hardened p.** FROZEN PELVIS. **high-assimilation p.** See under ASSIMILATION PELVIS. **infantile p.** A contracted pelvis having an oval inlet, marked inclination of the walls, and a high, prominent sacrum. Also *juvenile pelvis.* **inverted p.** SPLIT PELVIS. **justomajor p.** GIANT PELVIS. **p. justo major** GIANT PELVIS. **justominor p.** PELVIS JUSTO MINOR. **p. justo minor** A pelvis which is small yet symmetrical in shape. Also *justominor pelvis, pelvis aequabiliter justo minor, justo minor.* **juvenile p.** INFANTILE PELVIS. **kyphorachitic p.** A deformed pelvis in which the combined effects of kyphosis, which leads to lengthening of the true conjugate, and rachitis, which shortens the conjugate, result in minimal changes. **kyphoscoliorachitic p.** A pelvis that is contracted due to kyphosis, scoliosis, and rachitis. The superior strait may be quite deformed, but in general the pelvis is more favorable from an obstetric standpoint than some of the other types of rachitic deformity. **kyphoscoliotic p.** An evenly contracted pelvis secondary to rachitis. **kyphotic p.** A pelvis that, due to kyphoscoliosis, is contracted transversely. The sacral promontory is rotated up and backward, the coccyx is rotated forward and inward, and the entire pelvis has a marked inclination. **large p.** *Outmoded* PELVIS MAJOR. **lesser p.** PELVIS MINOR. **lordotic p.** A pelvis that is deformed by an anterior curvature of the lumbar vertebrae. **low-assimilation p.** See under ASSIMILATION PELVIS. **p. major** [NA] The upper part of the pelvis, which is above the lineae terminales on the sides and in front and the sacral promontory behind. It is bounded by the iliac bones at the sides. It is also the skeleton and cavity of the lower part of the abdomen proper. Also *false pelvis, greater pelvis, large pelvis* (outmoded), *pelvis spuria* (outmoded). **mesatipellic p.** A pelvis in which the inlet is almost perfectly round, the anteroposterior and transverse dimensions being approximately equal. Also *round pelvis.* **p. minor** [NA] The part of the pelvis that lies below the lineae terminales at the sides and in front and the sacral promontory behind. The cavity is short, wide, and curved, and it is continuous with the abdominal cavity at the superior aperture of the pelvis. Also *lesser pelvis, small pelvis, true pelvis, pelvic region.* **Nägele's p.** A pelvis in which the distortion is such that the conjugate diameter has an oblique orientation. The deformity results from incomplete development of the sacrum and the innominate bone on one side. Also *oblique pelvis.* **obliquely contracted p.** A pelvis that is asymmetrically deformed such that vaginal delivery of a fetus at term is not possible. **p. obtecta** A kyphotic pelvis in which the vertebral column extends into the anteroposterior diameter of the inlet. **p. ossea** The ring-shaped skeleton of the pelvis, formed by the two innominate bones anteriorly and laterally and the sacrum and the coccyx posteriorly. The weight of the trunk is transmitted from the vertebral column through it to the lower limbs. Also *bony pelvis.* **osteomalacic p.** A triradiate pelvis that results from the reduction of mineralized tissue within the bone. Also *rubber pelvis, caoutchouc pelvis, elastic pelvis.* **Otto p.** PROTRUSIO ACETABULI. **platypelloid p.** A pelvis in which the transverse diameter of the inlet markedly exceeds the anteroposterior diameter, thus giving a flattened shape to the inlet. Also *platypellic pelvis, pelvis plana.* **Prague p.** SPONDYLOLISTHETIC PELVIS. **rachitic p.** The triradiate pelvis seen in rickets. **p. renalis** [NA] The funnel-shaped, saccular continuation of the upper end of the ureter. Its broad part lies within the renal sinus and the smaller truncated apical portion extends outside the hilum to continue as the ureter. Within the sinus it divides into two or three major calices which, in turn, divide into several short minor calices. Occasionally the major part of the sac may extend outside the hilum. Also *renal pelvis, pelvis of ureter.* **Robert's p.** A pelvis that is transversely contracted secondary to osteoarthritis. The inlet has a shape of a narrow wedge due to involvement of the sacroiliac joints. **Rokitansky's p.** SPONDYLOLISTHETIC PELVIS. **round p.** MESATIPELLIC PELVIS. **rubber p.** OSTEOMALACIC PELVIS. **scoliotic p.** A fixed, oblique, and deformed pelvis seen in association with scoliosis. **simple flat p.** A pelvis in which the anteroposterior diameter of the inlet is shorter than normal. **small p.** PELVIS MINOR. **split p.** A pelvis with a congenital separation of the symphysis pubis, usually seen in exstrophy of the bladder. Also *inverted pelvis.* **spondylolisthetic p.** A pelvis that is tilted posteriorly, with the fifth or, less commonly, the fourth or third, lumbar vertebra lying in front of the body of the sacrum. Also *Prague pelvis, Rokitansky's pelvis.* **p. spuria** *Outmoded* PELVIS MAJOR. **stove-in p.** A pelvis in which, as a result of a major injury, the bones are imploded into the pelvic cavity. **triangular p.** A pelvis in which the inlet is triangular. **triradiate p.** A deformed pelvis in which the acetabulae are protruded centrally. It is seen in osteomalacia or osteogenesis imperfecta as a result of weakened or easily deformed bones. Also *pelvis triradiata.* **true p.** PELVIS MINOR. **p. of ureter** PELVIS RENALIS.

**pelvisacrum** \-sā′krəm\ The pelvis and the sacrum considered as a single unit.

**pelvitherm** \-thurm′\ A device inserted into the vagina for the purpose of applying heat to the pelvic organs.

**pelvitomy** \pelvit′əmē\ [PELVI- + -TOMY] A seldom-used obstetric operation in which a portion of the bony pelvis is severed in order to facilitate vaginal delivery.

**pelvo-** \pel′vō-\ PELVI-.

**pelvocaliectasis** \-kal′ē·ek′təsis\ [PELVO- + CALIECTASIS] Dilatation of the renal pelvis and calices due to hydronephrosis.

**pelvocaliceal** \-kal′isē′əl\ Related to the lower collecting system within the kidney and renal pelvis.

**pelvospondylitis** \-spän′dilī′tis\ Ankylosing spondylitis affecting the sacroiliac joint. **p. ossificans** Anklyosing spondylitis involving the sacroiliac joints and distal lumbar vertebrae.

**pelycephalometry** \pel′isef′əläm′ətrē\ [*pely(co)-* + CEPHALO- + -METRY] Measurement of the pelvic dimensions and fetal head in order to determine the degree of cephalopelvic disproportion.

**pelyco-** \pel′ikō-\ [Gk *pelyx* (genitive *pelikos*) wooden bowl] A combining form denoting the pelvis. • This form is seldom used, having largely been superseded by *pelvi-*.

**pelycology** \pel′ikäl′əjē\ [PELYCO- + -LOGY] The study of the pelvis, particularly in relation to pregnancy and labor.

**pemoline** $C_9H_8N_2O_2$. 2-Amino-5-phenyl-4(5*H*)-oxazolone. A central nervous system stimulant used in the treatment of depression and of hyperactivity in children. Its chronic use may lead to tolerance and physical dependence.

**pemphigoid** \pem′figoid\ [PEMPHIGUS + -OID] A blistering disease of the elderly that often starts with urticarial or pruritic erythematous lesions which later develop large tense blisters. The bullae are subepidermal, and intact epidermis forms the roof. Immunoglobulin and complement are found in the basement membrane zone in perilesional skin and circulating antibodies specific for this site are found in the majority of subjects. Treatment with corticosteroids and immunosuppressive drugs results in permanent remission in as many as half the patients. Also *bullous pemphigoid.* **benign mucosal p.** A rare and distinctive disorder in which recurrent bullae of the conjunctiva, orificial mucous membranes, and, less often, limited areas of skin, result in scarring. If the eyes are involved, it can lead to blindness.

The aged are most often affected. **bullous p.** PEMPHIGOID. **chronic localized p.** Pemphigoid that remains stable for long periods of time in a confined area but that may eventually spread and affect the mucous membranes.

**pemphigus** \pem′figəs\ [New L (from Gk *pemphix*, gen. *pemphigos*, air, breath, a thing filled with air, pustule, blister, akin to *pomphos* a bubble, blister)] **1** A group of rare, chronic, blistering diseases with a number of distinctive variants. Histologically, there is ancantholysis and blister formation within the epidermis. Immunoglobulins and complement are found in the intercellular area in perilesional skin, and circulating antibodies against this site can be detected in the majority of patients. **2** PEMPHIGUS VULGARIS. **benign familial p.** A rare inherited disorder characterized by recurrent vesicles and bullae and later by erosions usually occurring in sites of friction such as the neck, axillae, and groin. The histologic changes resemble pemphigus vulgaris and show acantholysis of epidermal cells with suprabasal splitting. However, immunoglobulins and complement are not found in perilesional skin. Also *Hailey-Hailey disease, Darier's disease, recurrent herpetiform dermatitis repens.* **p. contagiosus** Staphylococcal bullous impetigo. Also *pyosis of Manson.* **p. erythematosus** Pemphigus characterized by erythematous, scaly, hyperkeratotic, crusted lesions on the face, chest, and intertriginous areas. The acantholysis and epidermal splitting occurs either in the stratum granulosum or subcorneally. In addition, patients show clinical and immunological signs of chronic lupus erythematosus. Also *Senear-Usher syndrome.* **p. foliaceus** Pemphigus characterized by small flaccid blisters that may resemble dermatitis herpetiformis. The blistered areas are soon replaced by scaling and crusting and may give rise to exfoliative erythroderma. The acantholysis and epidermal splitting occurs either in the stratum granulosum or subcorneally. Also *Cazenave's disease.* **p. solitarius** A solitary blister which may be due to bacterial infection or pemphigus. *Obs.* **syphilitic p.** The bullous skin lesions of infantile congenital syphilis. **p. vegetans** Pemphigus vulgaris in which the eroded areas rapidly develop hypertrophic granulation at their edges. Later these vegetations develop small pustules and in time become dry, elevated, hyperkeratotic, and fissured. The treatment and prognosis are the same as in pemphigus vulgaris. Also *Neumann syndrome.* **p. vegetans (Hallopeau type)** A chronic pustular and vegetating condition of the axilla and groin with a benign prognosis. It is now thought to be a tissue response rather than a pemphigus variant. **p. vulgaris** Pemphigus characterized by flaccid blister formation that often initially involves only the mucous membranes. Later the skin is affected and, if untreated, steady deterioration and death results. The blisters occur in the suprabasal layers of the epidermis. Autoantibodies to the intercellular "prickles" of the prickle cell layer are highly characteristic of pemphigus vulgaris and believed to be involved in the pathogenesis of the blisters. Treatment with high dose corticosteroids and immunosuppressive drugs may result in long-term remission. Also *pemphigus.*

**pen** STYLUS. **light p.** A photosensor mounted in the tip of a pen for sensing the cathode-ray tube beam from a computer terminal. It permits the operator to enter, delete, and modify lines and characters displayed.

**pendelluft** \pen′dəluft\ [German *Pendel*, also *Pendul* pendulum + *Luft* air, vent] Nonsynchronous ventilation in which one part of a lung fills while other parts empty. See also FLAIL CHEST.

**Pendred** [Vaughan *Pendred*, English physician, 1869–1946] Pendred syndrome. See under FAMILIAL GOITER WITH DEAF-MUTISM.

**pendulum** \pen′dələm, pen′jələm\ **Pulfrich p.** An instrument which can be used to assess whether conduction is delayed in the visual pathways.

**penectomy** \pēnek′təmē\ PEOTOMY.

**penetrance** \pen′ətrəns\ [L *penetr(are)* to set or put into, penetrate (akin to *penitus* inward, internal) + -ANCE] The frequency of appearance of a dominant or recessive monogenic trait in individuals who are either heterozygous or homozygous, respectively, for the allele which determines the trait. In a given individual, a monogenic trait is either penetrant or not. In a population, the detection of the extent of penetrance depends on the sensitivity of methods for assaying the trait and ranges between zero (in heterozygotes for a completely recessive trait) and 100 percent. Also *genetic penetrance.* **complete p.** A condition in which all individuals in a population who have a particular genotype capable of specifying a particular trait actually express the trait. It usually refers to monogenic traits. **genetic p.** PENETRANCE.

**penetrant** \pen′ətrənt\ Pertaining to a trait that is apparent or evident on assay. It usually refers to monogenic traits, for example, a heterozygote for a completely dominant trait. Compare NONPENETRANT.

**penetration** \pen′ətrā′shən\ The act or extent of penetrating or piercing, as of a deep wound.

**penetrometer** \pen′əträm′ətər\ [*penetr(ation)* + *o* + -METER] An instrument to measure the penetrating ability of an x-ray beam. Also *qualimeter.*

**Penfield** [Wilder Graves *Penfield*, U.S.-born Canadian surgeon, born 1891] Penfield syndrome. See under DIENCEPHALIC AUTONOMIC EPILEPSY.

**penfluridol** $C_{28}H_{27}ClF_5NO$. 1-[4,4-Bis(4-fluorophenyl) butyl]-4-[4-chloro-3-(trifluoromethyl)phenyl]-4-piperidinol. A white, crystalline powder used as a tranquilizer, with actions similar to those of haloperidol. It is given orally.

**-penia** \-pē′nē·ə\ [Gk *penia* poverty, need] A combining form meaning an abnormal decrease or deficiency of (something specified).

**penial** \pē′nē·əl\ PENILE.

**D-penicillamine** D-3,3-Dimethylcysteine. A chelating agent used to remove some toxic metals from the body tissues. It is prepared by degradation of penicillin, and has been used to remove copper in patients with Wilson's disease and in the treatment of lead poisoning. The L- and DL-forms are not used because the L- form is toxic and inhibits enzymes requiring pyridoxal. Also *penicillamine.*

**penicillanic acid** A derivative of penicillin lacking a substituent in position 6 of the β-lactam ring. It has no antibacterial activity.

**penicilli** \pen′isil′ī\ Plural of PENICILLUS.

**penicillin** \pen′isil′in\ [*Penicill(ium)* + -IN] A group of β-lactam antibiotics in which the β-lactam ring is fused with a 5-membered thiazolidine ring. The fused rings are derived from L-cysteine and D-valine. The naturally occurring penicillins (such as penicillin G, or benzylpenicillin), from *Penicillium notatum*, are active chiefly on Gram-positive organisms. The antibacterial spectrum has been broadened, and sensitivity to penicillinase has been decreased, by the development of semisynthetic penicillins with various substituents on the fused rings. **p. I** PENICILLIN F. **p. II** PENICILLIN G. **p. III** PENICILLIN X. **p. IV** PENICILLIN K. **p. V** A semisynthetic penicillin with a phenoxymethyl group in place of the benzyl group of penicillin G. It has properties like those of penicillin G, except that it is more stable in acid and better absorbed from the gastrointestinal tract. Also *phenoxymethylpenicillin.* **p. B** *Obs.* GLUCOSE

OXIDASE. **buffered crystalline p. G** A preparation of crystalline potassium or sodium penicillin G buffered with not less than 4% or more than 5% sodium citrate. **depot p.** A preparation that releases penicillin slowly from the site of injection. Examples are the suspension of penicillin in oils, and the use of a procaine salt of penicillin. Also *repository penicillin.* **p. F** A natural penicillin from *Pencillium notatum.* It has an *n*-amyl group in place of the benzyl group of penicillin G, and properties similar to the latter. Also *2-pentenylpenicillin, penicillin I.* • This was the form of penicillin originally isolated by British workers. **p. G** Probably the most commonly used form of penicillin. It is a natural product of *Penicillium notatum* and other *Penicillium* species. It is an effective antibiotic against Gram-positive organisms, and it can be given by oral and parenteral routes of administration. It is susceptible to hydrolysis by the penicillinase of *Staphylococcus aureus.* Also *benzylpenicillin, penicillin II.* **p. K** One of the natural penicillins of *Penicillium notatum.* It has an *n*-heptyl group in place of the benzyl group of penicillin G, and resembles the latter in its properties. Also *penicillin IV, heptylpenicillin.* **p. N** CEPHALOSPORIN N. **p. O** A type of penicillin produced by growing the *Penicillium* mold in a medium containing allylmercaptomethylacetic acid. The side chain is an allylmercaptomethyl group in place of the benzoyl group of penicillin G. Its actions and properties are like those of penicillin G. **repository p.** DEPOT PENICILLIN. **p. X** One of the natural penicillins of *Penicillium notatum.* It has a *p*-hydroxy-benzyl group in place of the benzyl group of penicillin G. It has no advantages over penicillin G but resembles the latter in its properties. Also *penicillin III.*

**penicillinase** \pen′isil′inās\ A bacterial enzyme that inactivates penicillin by hydrolyzing the β-lactam bond. It is an important factor in resistance to penicillins, especially in staphylococci. See also β-LACTAMASE.

**penicillin dihydro F sodium** AMYLPENICILLIN SODIUM.

**penicillin G benzathine** The penicillin G salt of benzathine (N,N′-dibenzylethylene-diamine). The intramuscular injection of benzathine penicillin forms a depot so that effective concentrations of penicillin are maintained in the blood for a week. By oral administration, the penicillin levels are also prolonged over those from a soluble penicillin salt.

**penicillin G potassium** $C_{16}H_{17}KN_2O_4S$. 3,3-Dimeth-7-oxo-6-[(phenylacetyl)amino]-4-thia-1-azabicyclo-[3.2.0]heptane-2-carboxylic acid potassium salt. A widely used form of penicillin and a natural product of fermentation by *Penicillium notatum.* It is a broad-spectrum antibiotic but not resistant to acid hydrolysis or penicillinase degradation. It is thus less effective by oral administration than by intramuscular injection, and it is not as useful as other penicillins against staphylococcal infections. Also *benzylpenicillin potassium, potassium penicillin G.*

**penicillin G sodium** $C_{16}H_{17}N_2NaO_4S$. Benzylpenicillinic acid sodium salt. The properties and uses are essentially the same as described for the potassium salt. Also *benzylpenicillin sodium, sodium penicillin G.*

**penicillinic acid** The basic structure common to the penicillins, with or without any substitutions on the 6-carbamido group of the β-lactam ring.

**penicillin V potassium** $C_{16}H_{17}KN_2O_5S$. Phenoxymethylene penicillinic acid potassium salt. A semisynthetic penicillin which is more resistant to acid hydrolysis than penicilllin G, but it is also susceptible to hydrolysis by penicillinases. It is used orally for many conditions responding to penicillin treatment. Also *potassium phenoxymethyl penicillin.*

***Penicillium*** \pen′əsil′yəm\ [New L, from L *penicillum,* also *penicillus* an artist's brush. See also PENICILLUS.] A form-genus of widely distributed fungi, of the class Ascomycetes, order Aspergillales, which are common agents of food spoilage. Several species are useful as antibiotic sources and organic acid producers. A few are troublesome human pathogens. ***P. chrysogenum*** A form-species of fungus from which penicillin is obtained.

**penicilloic acid** The acid formed by hydrolysis of the amide bond in the four-membered ring of penicillin. The strain in this ring makes penicillin highly reactive in substituting with a penicilloyl group, and this is part of the mechanism by which it can inhibit enzymes of bacterial wall synthesis. Penicilloic acid is the product of breakdown of penicillin by penicillinases.

**penicilloyl-polylysine** An agent used for intradermal skin testing for penicillin allergy. It is composed of polylysine units and penicilloic acid.

**penicillus** \pen′isil′əs\ [L (dim. of *penis* a tail) an artist's brush, a swab] (*pl.* penicilli) **1** A small tuft or brushlike structure. **2** One of the penicilli splenis. **penicilli splenis** [NA] The terminal small straight branches of the splenic artery in the red pulp of the spleen. Each branch has three successive parts, namely, the artery of the pulp, the sheathed artery, and the short third portion that is a simple arterial capillary which usually does not divide. Some authorities believe that the latter capillaries become continuous with venous sinusoids in the red pulp, whereas others consider them to open directly into the interstices of the reticular tissue. Also *penicilli arteriae lienalis, penicilli arteries.*

**penile** \pē′nīl\ Pertaining or belonging to the penis. Also *penial.*

**penis** \pē′nis\ [L (akin to Gk *peos* the penis), a tail, the penis] [NA] The male organ of copulation that contains the third portion of the urethra for excretion of urine and seminal fluid. It is cylindrical in shape and composed of the root, or radix, attached to the pubic arch; the body or corpus completely enclosed in skin; and the conical glans at the extremity. The crura of the root are continuous with the two corpora cavernosa that lie side by side in front of the corpus spongiosum through which passes the urethra. These three structures are capable of enlargement when they are engorged with blood during erection of the organ. The glans is the cup-shaped terminal enlargement of the corpus spongiosum, at the distal end of which is the external orifice of the urethra. Also *phallus, priapus, mentula* (outmoded), *virile member.* **p. captivus** Inability to withdraw the erect penis during sexual intercourse as a result of vaginismus. **chordeic p.** CHORDEE. **cleft p.** DIPHALLIA. **clubbed p.** Curvature of the penis when erect. **p. femineus** *Outmoded* CLITORIS. **p. muliebris** *Outmoded* CLITORIS. **p. palmatus** A penis that is partially or largely enclosed by the scrotum, as in extreme degrees of hypospadias. **webbed p.** A penis the undersurface of which is connected by a prominent fold of skin to the anterior aspect of the scrotum.

**penischisis** \pēnis′kisis\ [*peni(s)* + -SCHISIS] Any cleft of the penis through which the urethra opens to the exterior at a site other than at the usual meatus, as in hypospadias or epispadias.

**penitis** \pēnī′tis\ [*pen(is)* + -ITIS] Inflammation of the penis. Also *phallitis.*

**pennate** \pen′āt\ [L *pennatus* (from *penna* a wing, feather) winged or feathered] Resembling a feather in structure: said especially of muscles in which the fasciculi converge on a tendon like barbs on the shaft of a feather. Also *penniform.* See also BIPENNATE, UNIPENNATE.

**penniform** \pen′ifôrm\ PENNATE.

**Penrose** [Charles Bingham *Penrose,* U.S. gynecologist, 1862–1925] Penrose drain. See under CIGARETTE DRAIN.
**pent-** \pent-, pənt-\ PENTA-.
**penta** \pen′tə\ *Popular* PENTACHLOROPHENOL.
**penta-** \pen′tə-\ [Gk *pente* five] A combining form meaning five. Also *pent-*.
**pentachlorophenol** $C_6HCl_5O$. Needlelike crystals with a pungent odor when hot. It is used as an insecticide for termite control, preharvest defoliant, herbicide, and wood preservative. It is highly toxic, particularly the technical grade. Ingestion causes damage to the central nervous system, lungs, liver, and kidneys. Also *penta* (popular).
**pentachromic** \-krō′mik\ [Gk *penta-*, combining form from *pente* five + CHROM- + -IC] **1** Capable of distinguishing five of the spectral colors. **2** Of or relating to five of the seven spectral colors.
**pentadactyl** \-dak′til\ Possessing five fingers on the hand or five toes on the foot.
**pentaerythritol tetranitrate** $C_5H_8N_4O_{12}$. 2,2-Bis-[(nitrooxy)methyl]-1,3-propanediol dinitrate (ester). A nitric acid ester of a tetrahydric alcohol. It is used to relieve the pain of angina pectoris attacks and may be useful also in preventing attacks. It is given orally, in regular or sustained-release preparations.
**pentagastrin** \-gas′trin\ A synthetic derivative of gastrin that is used as a stimulus for acid production in a test of gastric acid secretion.,
**pentalogy** \pental′əjē\ [PENTA- + -LOGY] Five components, elements, or symptoms that may characterize a condition or disease. **p. of Fallot** The tetralogy of Fallot with the addition of an interatrial communication.
**pentamer** \pen′təmər\ [Gk *penta-*, combining form from *pente* five + *mer(os)* a part] A structure consisting of five subunits, such as a pentagonal capsomere of viruses.
**pentamethazene** A chemical sometimes used to produce ganglionic blockade for deliberate hypotension in anesthesia. Also *azamethonium.*
**pentamidine** $C_{19}H_{24}N_4O_2$. A diamidine used in the treatment of African trypanosomiasis, especially arsenic-resistant strains of the disease, and antimony-resistant kala-azar.
**1,5-pentanediol** GLUTARALDEHYDE.
***Pentastoma*** \pentas′təmə\ [Gk *penta-*, combining form from *pente* five + *stoma* mouth] *LINGUATULA.*
**pentastome** \pen′təstōm\ [Gk *penta-*, combining form from *pente* five + *stom(a)* mouth] A member of the phylum Pentastomida; a tongue worm.
**pentastomiasis** \-stōmī′əsis\ Infection with pentastomid larvae. Lesions resembling those of tuberculosis occur in the lymph nodes of the digestive tract.
**pentastomid** \-stō′mid\ **1** Of or belonging to the phylum Pentastomida. **2** A member of the phylum Pentastomida.
**Pentastomida** \-stäm′idə\ A phylum, or a class in some taxonomic systems, of cylindrical or flattened parasitic worms externally ringed with pseudosegments; the tongue worms. They are found as adults in the respiratory tract of vertebrates, and as larvae in viscera (liver and mesenteric nodes) of mammals or other intermediate hosts. The larvae have four to six minute clawlike feet, thought by some to ally them to arthropods, perhaps mites. Other investigators have allied them to annelids, but most workers consider them far enough removed from any original stock to warrant placing them in a distinct phylum. Some 60 species, in two orders, have been described. Most pentastomids of medical and veterinary importance belong to the families Porocephalidae and Linguatulidae of the order Porocephalida.
***Pentatrichomonas*** \-trikäm′ənas\ [Gk *penta-* for *pente-*, prefix denoting five + TRICHOMONAS] A genus of flagellate protozoan parasites previously considered part of the genus *Trichomonas.* It is now considered a separate genus because of a granular parabasal body and the presence of five anterior flagella. ***P. hominis*** A species found as a commensal in the colon of dogs, cats, oxen, rodents, man, and other primates. Also *Trichomonas hominis, Pentatrichomonas ardin delteili, Trichomonas intestinalis, Cercomonas hominis, Octomitus hominis.*
**pentazocine** $C_{19}H_{27}NO$. 1,2,3,4,5,6-Hexahydro-8-hydroxy-6,11-dimethyl-3-(3-methylbut-2-enyl)-2,6-methano-3-benzazocine. A synthetic analgesic with actions and uses like those of morphine. It has less propensity for dependence than morphine, but chronic use may lead to dependence and addiction. It is given orally as the hydrochloride and parenterally as the lactate for relief of moderate to severe pain.
**2-pentenylpenicillin** PENICILLIN F.
**penthienate bromide** $C_{18}H_{30}BrNO_3S$. 2-(2-Cyclopentyl-2-thien-2ylglycoloyloxy)ethyldiethylmethylammonium bromide. An anticholinergic, quaternary ammonium compound. It is given orally in the treatment of peptic ulcers and pylorospasm.
**pentobarbital sodium** $C_{11}H_{17}N_2O_3$. 5-Ethyl-5-(1-methylbutyl)-2,4,6-(1*H*,3*H*,5*H*)-pyrimidinetrione monosodium salt. A prototype short-to-intermediate acting barbiturate used as a sedative and hypnotic. It is given orally, or parenterallyfor its anticonvulsant effects. Also *pentobarbitone sodium, sodium pentobarbital.*
**penton** \pen′tän\ [PENT- + -ON] A capsomere of the virus capsid surrounded by five nearest neighbors.
**pentose** [PENT- + -OSE[2]] Any sugar containing five carbon atoms, such as ribose.
**pentosemia** \pen′təsē′mē·ə\ The presence of any of the pentoses in the blood.
**pentose nucleotide** A nucleotide in which the phosphate ester of a pentose (ribose or deoxyribose) is united to a purine or pyrimidine base through a $\beta$-*N*-glycosyl bond between C-1 of the pentose and either N-9 of the purine or N-1 of the pyrimidine. Also *nucleoside phosphate.*
**pentose phosphate** Any of the phosphates of pentoses, especially ribose 5-phosphate, ribulose 5-phosphate, and xylulose 5-phosphate, which are intermediates in the pentose phosphate pathway.
**pentoside** \pen′təsīd\ A glycoside in which the sugar component is a pentose, as a nucleoside in which the pentose sugar, ribose, is linked to a pyrimidine or purine base.
**pentosuria** \pen′təsoo′rē·ə\ [*pentos(e)* + -URIA] A benign, autosomal recessive condition characterized by the daily urinary excretion of more than 1 g of L-xylulose, a 5-carbon sugar. It occurs predominantly in Ashkenazi Jews due to a defect in NADP-xylitol dehydrogenase. Also *L-xylulosuria, primary pentosuria* (outmoded), *xylitol dehydrogenase deficiency, essential pentosuria, L-xyulose reductase deficiency.*
**pentosyl** The group formed by removing hydroxyl from the anomeric carbon atom of the hemiacetal ring form of a pentose sugar, e.g. the ribosyl group in a nucleoside.
**pentosyltransferase** Any enzyme that catalyzes the transfer of a pentosyl group.
**Pentothal** A proprietary name for thiopental
**Pentothal sodium** A proprietary name for thiopental sodium.
**pentoxifylline** A methylxanthine-derived agent that renders cell membranes less rigid and permits red blood cells to pass through capillaries more easily, thereby improving tissue perfusion.
**pentyl** \pen′til\ The group $CH_3$—$[CH_2]_4$—.

**pentylenetetrazole** $C_6H_{10}N_4$. 6,7,8,9-Tetrahydro-5*H*-tetrazolo[1,5-*a*]azepine. A central nervous system stimulant of use in laboratory experiments to evaluate the effectiveness of anticonvulsant agents. It has been used in the past as a cardiovascular stimulant, for shock treatment, and to treat depressed geriatric patients, but it is either ineffective or much less effective than other agents for these uses. It is of value as a diagnostic aid in epilepsy. Also *leptazol*.

**penumbra** \pənum′brə\ [New L (from L *paen(e)* nearly, almost + *umbra* shadow, shade)] That portion of the shadow of an object illuminated by an extended source into which light from part, but not all, of the source can propagate.

**peotomy** \pē·ät′əmē\ [Gk *peo(s)* the penis + -TOMY] Partial or total amputation of the penis, an operation utilized primarily for treatment of penile cancer. Also *phallectomy, penectomy*.

**peplomer** \pep′ləmər\ [Gk *peplo(s)* a woven cloth used for a covering, a robe + *mer(os)* a part] A component of the envelope (peplos) of a virus.

**peplos** \pep′lōs\ [Gk *peplos* any woven cloth used for a covering, a woman's large robe] ENVELOPE.

**Pepper** [William *Pepper*, Jr., U.S. physician, 1874–1947] See under NEUROBLASTOMA, SYNDROME.

**pepsic** \pep′sik\ PEPTIC.

**pepsigogue** \pep′sigäg\ An agent capable of stimulating pepsin secretion.

**pepsin** \pep′sin\ [Gk *pepsis* (from *pessein*, later also *peptein*, to soften, boil, cook) digestion, a cooking + -IN] Any of a species of proteases found in gastric juice and active only at low pH. They are derived from the proenzyme pepsinogen which is completely inactive, but which is converted to pepsin in solutions more acid than pH 6.0. Pepsin owes its stability in acid and instability in neutral solution to its unusual composition: its 300 residues contain only four basic residues but many carboxyl groups. Also *pepsinase, pepsinum*.

**pepsiniferous** \pep′sinif′ərəs\ PEPSINOGENOUS.

**pepsinogen** \pepsin′əjən\ The inactive precursor of pepsin. Its sequence of about 340 residues includes that of pepsin as its C-terminal 300. Most of the basic residues are in the N-terminal 40, which are split off on activation, allowing pepsin to have litt net charge in the acidic medium of the stomach, which enhances the stability of its folding. Also *propepsin*.

**pepsinogenous** \pep′sinäj′ənəs\ Pepsin producing. Also *pepsiniferous*.

**pepsinum** \pep′sinəum\ PEPSIN.

**pepsinuria** \pep′sinoo′rē·ə\ [PEPSIN + -URIA] The presence of pepsin in the urine.

**peptase** PEPTIDASE.

**peptic** \pep′tik\ [Gk *peptik(os)* (from *pessein* or *peptein* to cook, concoct, digest) digestive] Pertaining to or associated with gastric secretion, particularly the secretion of pepsin and acid. Also *pepsic*.

**peptidase** Any enzyme that catalyzes the hydrolysis of peptide bonds. Also *peptase*.

**peptide** \pep′tīd\ [*pept(one)* + *-ide* as in *oxide*] Any substance composed of amino-acid residues joined by amide bonds. Some natural peptides are the products of enzymatic synthesis, while others are derived by hydrolysis of proteins synthesized on ribosomes. **adrenocorticotropic p.** *Outmoded* ADRENOCORTICOTROPIC HORMONE. **p. bond** The amide bond between two amino-acid residues in a peptide or protein. Such bonds are usually between C-1 of one residue and N-2 of another, when they may be called eupeptide bonds, but may be between other carboxyl and other amino groups, when they may be called isopeptide bonds. **C-p.** A metabolically inactive polypeptide chain connecting proinsulin and insulin, produced by the pancreatic $\beta$ cells in equimolar amounts with insulin as a result of proinsulin cleavage. C-peptide levels are low when insulin production is low. Measurement is useful in distinguishing insulinoma, which is characterized by high C-peptide levels, from factitious hypoglycemia, in which exogenous insulin injections produce high insulin levels but low C-peptide levels. Also *connecting peptide*. **leader p.** The signal peptide involved in the secretion of many proteins. **signal p.** A peptide of 20–30 residues at the N-terminus of the intracellular precursor of many secreted proteins, in eukaryotes and in bacteria. This peptide, predominantly hydrophobic but with a basic amino acid near its beginning, evidently initiates cotranslational secretion and is cleaved in the process by a membrane protease.

**peptidoglycan** A substance found in bacterial cell walls, consisting of a polysaccharide of alternate *N*-acylated residues of glucosamine and muramic acid, with the muramic acid carrying a peptide. The peptide contains both L- and D-amino-acid residues and is cross-linked. In Gram-positive bacterial cell walls the peptidoglycan extends throughout the wall and makes up 40–90% by weight of the wall. In Gram-negative bacteria the peptidoglycan is limited to a thin layer between the plasma membrane and the outer surface. Penicillin acts by interfering with the cross-linking process.

**peptidolytic** PROTEOLYTIC.

**peptidyl** \pep′tidil\ The acyl group formed by removing hydroxyl from the carboxyl group of a peptide. It is by transfer of a peptidyl group onto the amino group of aminoacyl-tRNA that a peptide chain grows during protein biosynthesis. **p. site** One of the two sites for tRNA in the ribosomes. It is the one to which the newly made peptidyl-tRNA is transferred before an aminoacyl-tRNA binds at the site where the peptidyl-tRNA had been formed. This allows transfer of the peptidyl group onto the aminoacyl group with lengthening of the peptide chain as a new peptidyl-tRNA is formed. The liberated tRNA then dissociates from the peptidyl site.

**peptidyltransferase** Any enzyme or its activity that catalyzes transfer of a peptidyl group, especially the transfer of the group from peptidyl-tRNA in protein biosynthesis.

**peptidyl-tRNA** Transfer RNA with a peptidyl group acylating its terminal adenosine. Such compounds are intermediates of protein biosynthesis, being formed by transfer of a peptidyl or aminoacyl group from its compound with tRNA onto the amino group of aminoacyl-tRNA, and in turn serving as donor of the peptidyl group for the next step of chain elongation.

***Peptococcus*** \pep′təkäk′əs\ [Gk *pept(ein)* to digest + COCCUS] A genus of anaerobic, Gram-positive cocci, often forming pairs, chains or packets. They can ferment peptone and carbohydrates, yielding mixed acids rather than the lactic fermentation of streptococci. They are indigenous flora, opportunistically pathogenic.

**peptogenic** \pep′təjen′ik\ Peptide-producing. Also *peptogenous*.

**peptolysis** PROTEOLYSIS.

**peptolytic** PROTEOLYTIC.

**peptone** \pep′tōn\ A mixture of peptides formed by the action of proteinases on protein. It is used as a medium for bacterial growth. • The word is obsolete in its original meaning, which specified a definite degree of breakdown, as judged by the precipitation properties of the peptides.

**peptonize** \pep′təniz\ To hydrolyze protein partially.

***Peptostreptococcus*** \pep′tōstrep′təkäk′əs\ [Gk *pept(ein)*, earlier *pessein,* to soften, boil, cook + *o* + STREPTOCOCCUS] A genus of organisms resembling *Peptococcus* but characteristically forming chains.

**peptotoxin** \pep′tətäk′sin\ A toxin produced during the acid or enzymatic hydrolysis of a native protein to form a peptone.

**per-** \per-, pur-, pər-\ [L *per* through] **1** A prefix meaning (1) through, by way of; (2) throughout. **2** A prefix indicating (1) the presence of elements, bodies, or groups in amounts larger than is considered normal; (2) an element in its highest valence.

**peracephalus** \pur′əsef′ələs\ [PER- + ACEPHALUS] An omphalositic unequal twin consisting of little more than a pelvis and lower limbs attached to the placenta or umbilical cord of the larger, more normal twin.

**peracid** \pərasʹid\ In organic chemistry, a substance containing the group —CO—O—OH, which may be formed by reaction of a carboxylic acid with hydrogen peroxide.

**peracidity** \pur′asid′itē\ HYPERACIDITY.

**per anum** \pur ā′nəm\ [PER- + *anum,* accus. of ANUS] By way of the anus.

**perarticulation** \pur′ärtik′yəlā′shən\ ARTICULATIO SYNOVIALIS.

**peraxillary** \pərak′siler′ē\ Through the axilla.

**perborax** \pərbôr′aks\ $NaBo_3 4H_2O$. Sodium perborate, a compound that has been used in dentifrices and as a mouthwash.

**perc** TETRACHLOROETHYLENE.

**percentile** \pərsen′tīl, -til\ [*percent* (from PER- + L *centum* one hundred) + *-ile* as in *quartile*] Any of the 99 values in an ordered series of statistical data which divide the series into 100 equal groups. Thus, the ninetieth percentile is that value which equals or exceeds 90% of the items in the series.

**perception** \pərsep′shən\ [L *perceptio* (from *perceptus,* past part. of *percipere* lay hold of, feel, receive mentally, grasp, from PER- + L *capere* to take, seize) a receiving, comprehension] The combined processes of selection, organization, and interpretation of the sensory data available to a human observer. Through these processes one becomes aware of the existence of objects, of an object's qualities, or of events or relationships existing in the external world and giving rise to one's experience of the world. While perception always contains purely sensory elements, it is also influenced by learning, by mental sets, and by the prior experience of the perceiver. **abstract p.** BLANK HALLUCINATION. **depth p.** A direct awareness of the distance between an observer and an object within the field of view, or of the solidity and three dimensional quality of that object. **subliminal p.** Any response or behavior by an experimental subject that can be demonstrably linked to the presentation of sensory stimuli that are too weak to be apprehended in a specific way, but which may influence behavior or affect conscious processes indirectly.

**perceptorium** \pur′septôr′ē·əm\ SENSORIUM.

**perceptuomotor** \pərsep′too·əmō′tər\ Requiring the simultaneous learning of new perceptual and new motor relationships, as in the pursuit movements needed to track a visual target moving in a pattern not immediately discernible. Perceptuomotor behavior combines continuously modified skeletomuscular action with discrimination, memory, or other cognitive processes.

**perchlorate** The ion $ClO_4^-$ or a salt that contains it. Perchlorates are used in chemistry when it is desired to have an anion with very low nucleophilic tendency or tendency to bind to metal ions.

**perchloric acid** $HClO_4$. An acid obtained from its potassium salt. It is a colorless hygroscopic liquid, having a melting point of −112°C and a boiling point of 19°C at 11 mmHg. It can decompose explosively if distilled at atmospheric pressure. It is commercially available as its azeotrope with water, containing 71.6% of the acid. It is one of the strongest acids known. Its anion does not associate with metal ions so its salts are largely ionic. It is a strong oxidizing agent and a widely used analytic reagent, particularly to precipitate protein from biologic material, from which it is then removed by precipitation as $KClO_4$. There is always some risk when it is manipulated in contact with organic matter because the evaporated fumes may combine in the apparatus with organic matter to form an explosive mixture.

**perchlormethylformate** DIPHOSGENE.

**perchloroethylene** TETRACHLOROETHYLENE.

**perchloronaphthalene** CHLORINATED NAPHTHALENE.

**percolate** \pur′kəlāt\ [L *percolatus,* past part. of *percolare* (from *per-* PER- + *colare* to strain liquid through a cloth or sieve) to strain through] **1** To filter or cause to filter through a porous medium, as surface water into the subsoil. **2** To extract the soluble component of a powdered drug by filtering a solvent down through it, allowing that component time to dissolve, and then collecting the resulting solution at the bottom.

**percolator** A container having a straining component suitable for extracting drugs from their source materials by percolation.

**per contiguum** \pur kəntig′yoo·əm\ Contiguous, or arranged so that the edges touch each other.

**per continuum** \pur kəntin′yoo·əm\ Continuous; without breaks or interruptions.

**percuss** \pərkus′\ To strike or tap (a part of the body); to perform percussion on (a part of the body) for diagnosis or in massage.

**percussible** \pərkus′ibl\ Capable of detection by means of percussion.

**percussion** \pərkush′ən\ [L *percussio* (from *percussus,* past part. of *percutere* to strike hard, pierce, from PER- + L *quatere* to shake, shatter) a striking, beating] The delivery of quick, light blows or taps on a part of the body, for diagnostic or therapeutic purposes. In clinical examination of the chest or other hollow structure, the surface of the body is struck sharply and the character of the sound produced is noted. In physical therapy, percussion movements are used in various massage techniques. **bimanual p.** The usual technique of percussion, in which the fingers of the left hand, placed in contact with the chest, are struck sharply by a finger of the right hand. **chest wall p.** Percussion in which the chest wall is struck directly. **comparative p.** Percussion over corresponding areas on both sides of the chest for comparing the condition of the two lungs. **direct p.** Percussion in which the chest is struck directly by the percussing finger. Also *immediate percussion.* **finger p.** Percussion in which the fingers of one hand strike those of the other hand which lie on the area being examined. **immediate p.** DIRECT PERCUSSION. **mediate p.** Percussion utilizing a pleximeter.

**percussor** \pərkus′ər\ **1** Any instrument, such as a hammer, used in percussion. **2** A device used in massage to apply low-frequency percussion. For defs. 1 and 2 also *percuteur.*

**percutaneous** \pur′kyootā′nē·əs\ Through the skin: used especially of penetration of the skin by absorption, as by inunction. Also *per cutem, diadermic, transcutaneous, transdermic.*

**percuteur** \pur′kootyoor′, perkootœr′\ PERCUSSOR.

**perencephaly** \pur′ensef′əlē\ PORENCEPHALY.

**perforans** \pur′fôranz\ Penetrating: said of certain muscles, vessels, and nerves that penetrate or perforate other structures.

**perforate** \pur′fərāt\ [L *perforare* (from *per-* through + *forare* to bore, pierce) to make a hole through] To transgress the full thickness of a wall: used especially of injuries or lesions.

**perforation** \pur′fərā′shən\ 1 Penetration through the full thickness of a wall. 2 A hole through the full thickness of a wall. **p. of nasal septum** The condition where a perforation has formed through the whole thickness of the nasal septum creating a communication between one nasal cavity and the other, both layers of mucosa and the intervening cartilage or bone having been destroyed. The causes are many including, in order of frequency, trauma (particularly nose picking and surgical trauma), the inhaling of irritants (particularly compounds of chrome, mercury, arsenic, and copper), ritualistic practices (in parts of the world where ornaments are worn through the nose), chronic inflammation (such as leprosy, late syphilis and lupus) and neoplastic disease. When drug addicts use cocaine as snuff, septal perforation sometimes occurs. The site and size of the perforation is determined by the nature and severity of the causative pathology. **radicular p.** Lateral perforation of a tooth root occurring after the formation of the root, unlike an accessory root canal, which is formed during root growth.

**perforator** \pur′fərā′tər\ An instrument used to perforate the fetal skull and thus reduce its size in order to facilitate vaginal delivery in cases of hydrocephalus.

**perfrication** \pur′frikā′shən\ INUNCTION.

**perfrigeration** \pərfrij′ərā′shən\ FROSTBITE.

**perfusate** \pərfyoo′zāt\ [L *perfus(us),* past part. of *perfundere* to wet, moisten, sprinkle + -ATE] A liquid which has been passed through or over a structure such as a membrane or a body tissue or organ.

**perfuse** \pərfyooz′\ [L *perfus(us),* past part. of *perfundere* to wet, moisten, sprinkle] To pour into or through.

**perfusion** \pərfyoo′zhən\ The passage of blood or other fluid through the blood or lymph vessels of the body or of part of it. **regional p.** Selective perfusion of a localized site, organ, or limb to expose to higher concentration of a drug or substance than the remaining tissues.

**peri-** \per′i-, per′ē-\ [Gk *peri* around, about, near] A prefix meaning around, about, near.

**periacinal** \-as′inəl\ Located around an acinus. Also *periacinar, periacinous.*

**periadenitis** \-ad′ənī′tis\ [PERI- + ADENITIS] Inflammation of the tissues around a gland. **p. mucosa necrotica recurrens** A severe form of recurrent aphthous stomatitis that tends to heal with atrophic scars which may become numerous. Clinically it may be difficult to differentiate from the Behçet syndrome. Also *Mikulicz aphthae, recurrent scarring aphthae, Sutton's disease.*

**periadventitial** \-ad′ventish′əl\ Of or relating to the area around the tunica adventitia of a blood vessel.

**perianal** \per′i·ā′nəl\ [PERI- + ANAL] CIRCUMANAL.

**periangiitis** \-an′jē·ī′tis\ Inflammation of the outer coat of or the tissues around a blood or lymph vessel.

**periangioma** \-an′jē·ō′mə\ [PERI- + ANGIOMA] HEMANGIOPERICYTOMA.

**periaortic** \per′i·ā·ôr′tik\ Around the aorta.

**periapex** \-ā′peks\ [PERI- + APEX] The part of the periodontal ligament and alveolar bone surrounding the apex of a tooth.

**periapical** \-ap′ikəl, -ā′pikəl\ Situated near or around the apex of a tooth root.

**periappendicitis** \-əpen′disī′tis\ Inflammation of the tissue adjacent to the vermiform appendix.

**periappendicular** \-ap′endik′yələr\ Adjacent to or surrounding an appendix.

**periaqueductal** \-ak′wēduk′təl\ Located around the cerebral aqueduct.

**periarteriolar** \-ärtir′ē·ō′lər\ Situated around arterioles.

**periarteritis** \-är′tərī′tis\ [PERI- + ARTERITIS] Inflammation of the outer coat of an artery and sometimes also of surrounding structures. **disseminated necrotizing p.** POLYARTERITIS NODOSA. **p. nodosa** POLYARTERITIS NODOSA.

**periarthric** \-ärth′rik\ Adjacent to or around a joint.

**periarthritis** \-ärthrī′tis\ [PERI- + ARTHRITIS] An inflammation of the tissues near a joint. Also *perisynovitis.* **p. calcarea** CALCIFIC TENDINITIS.

**periarticular** \-ärtik′yələr\ Situated near a joint. Also *perisynovial.*

**periatrial** \-ā′trē·əl\ [PERI- + ATRIAL] Around one or both atria of the heart.

**periblast** \per′iblast\ [PERI- + -BLAST] 1 A syncytial layer peripheral to the cytoplasmic cap (germinal disk) of blastomeres in meroblastic cleavage which adheres closely to the yolk. The layer does not take part in the formation of the embryo but is supposed to break down yolk and make it available to the embryo. 2 A thin outer stratum of platelike cells in embryonic skin which undergoes a form of desquamation. Adj. periblastic.

**peribronchial** \-brăng′kē·əl\ Adjacent to or surrounding a bronchus.

**peribronchiolar** \-brăng′kē·ō′lər\ Adjacent to or surrounding a bronchiole.

**peribronchitis** \-brăngkī′tis\ Inflammation of the tissues surrounding bronchi.

**peribulbar** \-bul′bər\ [PERI- + BULBAR] Surrounding the eye; pertaining to the tissues immediately surrounding the eye.

**peribursal** \-bur′səl\ Pertaining to the space about a bursa.

**pericapillary** \-kap′iler′ē\ Around a capillary; surrounding capillaries.

**pericapsular** \-kap′s$^y$ələr\ Located near or around a renal glomerulus or the external renal capsule.

**pericardectomy** \-kärdek′təmē\ [PERI- + CARD- + -ECTOMY] PERICARDIECTOMY.

**pericardiac** \-kär′dē·ak\ PERICARDIAL.

**pericardial** \-kär′dē·əl\ Pertaining to the pericardium; around the heart. Also *pericardiac.*

**pericardicentesis** \-kär′disentē′sis\ PERICARDIOCENTESIS.

**pericardiectomy** \-kär′dē·ek′təmē\ [PERI- + CARDI- + -ECTOMY] Surgical excision of the pericardium. Also *pericardectomy.*

**pericardiocentesis** \-kär′dē·ōsentē′sis\ The procedure of removing fluid from the pericardium by puncture of its wall and aspiration. Also *pericardicentesis.*

**pericardiolysis** \-kär′dē·äl′isis\ The procedure of removing adhesions between the two layers of the pericardium or between the pericardium and surrounding structures.

**pericardiomediastinitis** \-kär′dē·ōmē′dē·as′tinī′tis\ Inflammation of both the pericardium and adjoinng structures in the mediastinum. **adhesive p.** Inflammation leading to adhesions between the pericardium and structures in the mediastinum.

**pericardiopleural** \-kär′dē·ōplŭr′əl\ Pertaining to or involving pericardium and pleura; pleuropericardial.

**pericardiorrhaphy** \-kär′dē·ôr′əfē\ [PERI- + CARDIOR-

RHAPHY] A suturing of the pericardium.

**pericardiostomy** \-kär′dē·äs′təmē\ PERICARDIOTOMY.

**pericardiotomy** \-kär′dē·ät′əmē\ [PERI- + CARDIOTOMY] A surgical incision of the pericardium. Also *pericardiostomy.*

**pericarditic** \-kärdit′ik\ Pertaining to or characterized by pericarditis.

**pericarditis** \-kärdī′tis\ [*pericard(ium)* + -ITIS] Inflammation of the pericardium. **acute benign p.** Pericarditis with or without serous effusion and sometimes followed by adhesions occurring as a short-term illness with good prognosis. **acute exudative p.** Acute pericarditis with fluid in the pericardial sac. **adhesive p.** Fibrous adhesions resulting from previous inflammation, obliterating some or all of the pericardial sac and sometimes involving surrounding structures. Also *synechia pericardii.* **amebic p.** Pericarditis with a purulent exudate in the pericardial sac due to an *Entamoeba histolytica* abscess in the liver rupturing through the diaphragm. **bread-and-butter p.** Pericarditis villosa in which the deposits of fibrin on the serosal surfaces have an appearance suggestive of the parted surfaces of a bread and butter sandwich. **carcinomatous p.** Pericarditis due to infiltration of carcinomatous cells, usually from surrounding structures. **constrictive p.** Chronic pericarditis which has enclosed the heart in a fibrous bag, so that both filling and emptying are impeded. Dense calcification is usually present. **fibrinous p.** Pericarditis with relatively little fluid formation and with deposits of fibrin on the serosal surfaces of the sac. **fibrous p.** Pericarditis of the outer, fibrous layer of the pericardium; external pericarditis. **hemorrhagic p.** Pericarditis with blood-stained effusion, often due to malignant or tuberculous disease, sometimes to uremia. **leukemic p.** Pericarditis as a complication of leukemia. **malignant p.** Pericarditis, often with effusion, which may be blood-stained. It is usually due to infiltration by adjacent cancer tissue. **purulent p.** Pericarditis, usually bacterial, with pus in the sac. **rheumatic p.** Pericarditis occurring in the course of rheumatic disease, as rheumatic fever, often with associated endocarditis and myocarditis. **septic p.** Bacterial pericarditis, especially that due to pyogenic organisms. **serofibrinous p.** Pericarditis with serous fluid in the sac and fibrin deposits on the walls. **uremic p.** Pericarditis complicating and due to renal failure. **p. villosa** Fibrinous pericarditis with shaggy deposits of fibrin on the serosal surfaces. Also *hairy heart.* **viral p.** Pericarditis due to infection by a virus.

**pericardium** \-kär′dē·əm\ [Gk *perikardion* (from PERI- + Gk *kardia* the heart) the sac around the heart] [NA] A fibroserous sac that contains the heart and the roots of the aorta and pulmonary trunk. It consists of an outer sac (fibrous pericardium) and an inner, double-layered closed sac (serous pericardium), comprising visceral and parietal layers. Between the two is a protected space, lined with endothelium and containing a small amount of pericardial fluid between them. It is located in the mediastinum behind the body of the sternum and the cartilages of the second through sixth ribs and its base is adherent to the upper surface of the central tendon of the diaphragm. Also *capsula cordis, capsule of heart, pericardial sac, heart sac, theca cordis* (outmoded), *vagina cordis* (outmoded). **adherent p.** The pericardium as seen in adhesive pericarditis, in which postinflammatory fibrous bands connect some or all of its two layers, and/or the outer layer and surrounding structures. **calcified p.** A pericardium with deposits of calcium salts in the fibrous tissue, resulting from previous, often suppurative, inflammation. **p. fibrosum** [NA] The outer sac of strengthening fibrous tissue that surrounds the closed double-layered serous pericardium. It has an apex continuous with the external coats of the great vessels and a base attached to the central tendon of the diaphragm. Superiorly it is also continuous with the pretracheal fascia while anteriorly the superior and inferior sternopericardial ligaments anchor it to the sternum. It maintains the heart in the middle mediastinum, and its shape changes with respiration. Also *fibrous pericardium.* **parietal p.** LAMINA PARIETALIS PERICARDII. **p. serosum** [NA] A double-layered membranous sac invaginated by the heart and comprising a visceral layer, or epicardium, which covers the surface of the heart and the origin of the great vessels, from which it is reflected to form the parietal layer lining the inside of the fibrous pericardium. It is formed by loose connective tissue covered by a single layer of mesothelium. Between the two layers is the pericardial cavity. Also *serous pericardium.* **visceral p.** LAMINA VISCERALIS PERICARDII.

**pericaryon** \-kar′ē·än\ PERIKARYON.

**pericaval** \-kā′vəl\ Around the superior or inferior vena cava.

**pericecal** \-sē′kəl\ Surrounding or near the cecum. Also *perityphlic.*

**pericellular** \-sel′yələr\ Surrounding a cell, as a net of glial origin surrounding a neuron.

**pericementitis** \-sē′mentī′tis\ [*pericement(um)* + -ITIS] Inflammation of the periodontal membrane. **apical p.** ALVEOLAR ABSCESS.

**pericementum** \-simen′təm\ PERIODONTIUM.

**pericholangitis** \-kō′lanjī′tis\ An inflammatory process involving the portal tracts of the liver, characterized pathologically by increased numbers of leukocytes and edema. The inflammation may complicate biliary tract infections or chronic ulcerative colitis.

**pericholecystitis** \-kō′lēsistī′tis\ Inflammation of the tissue near the gallbladder. **gaseous p.** EMPHYSEMATOUS CHOLECYSTITIS.

**perichondral** \-kän′drəl\ Of or pertaining to perichondrium. Also *perichondrial.*

**perichondritis** \-kəndrī′tis\ [PERI- + CHONDRITIS] An inflammation of the perichondrium. **p. of the auricle** PERICHONDRITIS OF THE PINNA. **p. of the larynx** Inflammation of the perichondrium of the cartilages of the larynx due to pyogenic infection consequent on surgical or accidental trauma, complicating ulceration of the soft tissues from various causes or where interference with the blood supply predisposes, as with ionizing radiation. Chondral necrosis, abscess formation, and laryngeal stenosis may ensue. **p. of the pinna** Inflammation of the perichondrium of the pinna due to infection introduced by an accidental or surgical injury. It is liable to lead to necrosis of the subjacent cartilage resulting in deformity of the pinna. Also *perichondritis of the auricle.*

**perichondrium** \-kän′drē·əm\ [NA] The fibrous connective tissue that covers all cartilage surfaces, other than articular cartilage.

**perichondroma** \-kändrō′mə\ A benign cartilaginous tumor arising from the perichondrium.

**perichord** \per′ikôrd\ [PERI- + *(noto)chord*] A membranous investing sheath of the notochord in embryos.

**perichoroidal** \-kôroi′dəl\ Surrounding the choroid; pertaining to the tissues immediately external to the choroid of the eye. Also *perichorioidal.*

**pericision** \-sizh′ən\ [PERI- + *(in)cision*] The sectioning of the free gingival fibers of the periodontal ligament. It is undertaken to prevent relapse of a tooth that has been rotated orthodontically.

**pericolic** \-kō′lik\ Surrounding or adjacent to the colon.

**pericolitis** \-kōlī′tis\ [PERI- + COLITIS] Inflammation of the tissues adjacent to the colon, usually due to colonic disease. Also *pericolonitis.*
**pericolpitis** \-kälpī′tis\ PARACOLPITIS.
**periconchal** \-käng′kəl\ PERIORBITAL.
**pericorneal** \-kôr′nē·əl\ Surrounding or encircling the cornea; pertaining to the limbus corneae.
**pericoronal** \-kôr′ənəl\ [PERI- + CORONAL] Surrounding the crown of a tooth.
**pericoronitis** \-kôr′ənī′tis\ [PERI- + *coron(a)* + -ITIS] Inflammation of the tissue surrounding or covering the crown of a partially erupted or impacted tooth. Also *operculitis.*
**pericranial** \-krā′nē·əl\ **1** Of or relating to the pericraniuim. **2** Around the skull.
**pericranium** \-krā′nē·əm\ [NA] The periosteum adherent to the outer surface of the skull. Also *periosteum cranii.*
**pericystic** \-sis′tik\ Located near or around a cyst.
**pericystitis** \-sistī′tis\ [PERI- + CYSTITIS] Inflammation affecting the tissues surrounding the urinary bladder.
**pericyte** \per′isīt\ [PERI- + -CYTE] An occasional contractile cell that is found in the connective tissue layer around capillaries and that also forms the precapillary sphincters of metarterioles. Also *perivascular satellite, hemangiopericyte, perivascular cell, pericapillary cell, Rouget cell, spider cell, adventitial cell.*
**pericytoma** \-sītō′mə\ [*pericyt(e)* + -OMA] HEMANGIOPERICYTOMA.
**peridectomy** \-dek′təmē\ [PERI- + *d* + -ECTOMY ] A limbal conjunctival excision.
**perideferentitis** \-def′ərentī′tis\ [PERI- + DEFERENT + -ITIS] Inflammation involving the structures near the vas deferens.
**peridendritic** \-dendrit′ik\ Situated around the dendrites of a nerve cell.
**peridens** \per′idenz′\ [PERI- + L *dens* tooth] An accessory tooth on the outer side of the dental arch.
**peridental** \-den′təl\ PERIODONTAL.
**peridentitis** \-dentī′tis\ PERIODONTITIS.
**peridentium** \-den′shē·əm\ PERIODONTIUM.
**periderm** \per′idurm\ [PERI- + -DERM] The outer stratum of flattened cells lying on the basal cubical cells of the epiblast (stratum germinativum) in the developing skin of mammalian embryos.
**perididymis** \-did′imis\ TUNICA ALBUGINEA TESTIS.
**perididymitis** \-did′imī′tis\ [*perididym(is)* + -ITIS] Inflammation affecting the perididymis. Also *vaginitis testis.*
**peridiverticulitis** \-dī′vərtik′yəlī′tis\ [PERI- + DIVERTICULITIS] Inflammation involving the tissues near an intestinal diverticulum.
**periductal** \-duk′təl\ Around a duct, particularly a duct of the mammary gland. Also *periductile.*
**periduodenitis** \-d$^{y}$oo′ədenī′tis\ An inflammation in tissues adjacent to the duodenum, most commonly due to a pathologic process originating in the duodenum.
**peridurogram** \-d$^{y}$oo′rəgram\ The radiographic record, or picture, obtained in peridurography.
**peridurography** \-d$^{y}$ooräg′rəfē\ [PERI- + *(epi)dur(al)* + *o* + -GRAPHY] A radiologic technique of visualizing the spinal canal and its contents by injecting contrast medium into the spinal epidural space.
**periencephalitis** \-ensef′əlī′tis\ MENINGOENCEPHALITIS.
**periencephalography** \-ensef′əläg′rəfē\ Radiologic demonstration of the intracranial subarachnoid space and its cisterns using gas, air, or contrast medium.
**periencephalomeningitis** \-ensef′əlōmen′injī′tis\ MENINGOENCEPHALITIS.
**periependymal** \per′i·ēpen′diməl\ Being in close relationship to the ependyma; specifically, referring to the microscopic zone of loose texture between the ependyma and adjacent neuropil along the walls of the ventricular system and central canal of the nervous system.
**periesophageal** \per′i·ēsäf′əjē′əl\ Surrounding the esophagus.
**periesophagitis** \per′i·ēsäf′əjī′tis\ Inflammation of the tissues surrounding the esophagus.
**perifocal** \-fō′kəl\ Surrounding a focus, especially the focus of an infection.
**perifolliculitis** \-fōlik′yəlī′tis\ [PERI + FOLLICULITIS] An inflammation of a follicle and the connective tissue surrounding it. **p. capitis abscedens et suffodiens** A chronic inflammatory disorder of the scalp in which tender nodules coalesce to form roughly cerebriform ridges, the follicles in which discharge pus. **superficial pustular p.** BOCKHART'S IMPETIGO.
**perigangliitis** \-gang′glē·ī′tis\ [PERI- + *gangli(on)* + -ITIS] Inflammation of the tissues covering or around a ganglion.
**periganglionic** \-gang′glē·än′ik\ Lying around a ganglion.
**perigastritis** \-gastrī′tis\ Inflammation of the peritoneal coat of the stomach.
**periglottis** \-glät′is\ The mucous membrane of the tongue. *Outmoded.*
**perihepatic** \-hepat′ik\ Surrounding the liver.
**perihepatitis** \-hep′ətī′tis\ [PERI- + HEPATITIS] Inflammation of the fibrous tunic of the liver (tunica fibrosa hepatis). It may result from infection, trauma, or systemic inflammatory disease. Also *hepatic capsulitis, glissonitis, hepatitis externa, parahepatitis.* **p. chronica hyperplastica** FROSTED LIVER. **gonococcal p.** Perihepatitis in women with antecedent gonorrheal salpingitis. See also FITZ-HUGH AND CURTIS SYNDROME.
**perihilar** \-hī′lər\ Adjacent to or surrounding a hilum.
**perihypophysial** \-hī′pōfiz′ē·əl\ Surrounding or near the pituitary gland.
**perikaryon** \-kar′ē·än\ **1** The protoplasm surrounding the nucleus of a cell. **2** The cell body of a neuron. For defs. 1 and 2 also *pericaryon.*
**perikymata** \-kī′mətə\ [PERI- + Gk *kymata,* pl. of *kyma* a wave, billow] Transverse ridges on the enamel surface of a tooth, especially numerous towards the neck of the tooth.
**perilabyrinth** \-lab′ərinth\ The tissues of and around the perilymphatic space of the labyrinth of the internal ear.
**perilabyrinthitis** \-lab′ərinthī′tis\ *Imprecise* CIRCUMSCRIBED LABYRINTHITIS.
**perilenticular** \-lentik′yələr\ Pertaining to the area surrounding the crystalline lens.
**periligamentous** \-lig′əmen′təs\ Of or relating to the loose connective tissue layer around ligaments.
**perilimbal** \-lim′bəl\ [PERI- + LIMBAL] Oriented circumferentially about the periphery of the cornea.
**perilymph** \per′ilimf\ PERILYMPHA.
**perilympha** \-lim′fə\ [NA] The clear fluid in the perilymphatic spaces surrounding the membranous labyrinth within the bony labyrinth of the internal ear. It resembles cerebrospinal fluid but its source, mode of circulation, absorption, and removal are uncertain. Also *perilymph, Cotunnius liquid* (obs.), *aqua labyrinthi* (outmoded), *labyrinthine fluid* (outmoded).
**perilymphadenitis** \-lim′fadenī′tis\ Inflammation of tissues adjoining a lymph node.
**perilymphangial** \-limfan′jē·əl\ Surrounding a lymph vessel; around lymphatic channels. Also *perilymphangeal.*

**perilymphangitis** \-lim′fanjī′tis\ Inflammation of tissue around a lymph vessel.
**perilymphatic** \-limfat′ik\ **1** Pertaining to the perilympha. **2** Around a lymph vessel or node.
**perimacular** \-mak′yələr\ Pertaining to the retinal area adjacent to the macula.
**perimastitis** \-mastī′tis\ [PERI- + MASTITIS] Inflammation surrounding the breast.
**perimeningitis** \-men′injī′tis\ *Seldom used* PACHYMENINGITIS.
**perimeter** \pərim′ətər\ [PERI- + -METER] **1** A device for measuring the visual field. **2** A line defining the extent of a plane figure. **arc p.** A flat strip surface, curved 180°, upon which the peripheral field of vision can be measured. **projection p.** A device for measuring the visual field in which the test stimulus is a spot of light.
**perimetric** \-met′rik\ Pertaining to a perimeter or to measurement of the visual field.
**perimetritis** \-mētrī′tis\ [PERI- + METRITIS] Inflammation of the serosa of the uterus. Adj. perimetritic.
**perimetrium** \-mē′trē·əm\ [PERI- + METR- + L *-ium*, neut. sing. noun termination] TUNICA SEROSA UTERI.
**perimetry** \perim′ətrē\ [PERI- + -METRY] Examination and measurement of the visual field. This is of value in documenting and diagnosing lesions of the visual pathways. **flicker p.** A technique of perimetry using the measurement of critical flicker fusion frequency. **quantitative p.** A technique of perimetry in which the visual fields are charted in isopters of equal sensitivity of retinal perception.
**perimycin** FUNGIMYCIN.
**perimyelis** \-mī′əlis\ ENDOSTEUM.
**perimyocarditis** \-mī′əkärdī′tis\ Combined inflammation of myocardium and pericardium.
**perimyoendocarditis** \-mī′ə·en′dōkärdī′tis\ Inflammation affecting the pericardium, myocardium, and endocardium.
**perimyometrium** \-mī′əmē′trē·əm\ [PERI- + MYOMETRIUM] A layer of connective tissue which in an embryo surrounds the developing muscular walls of the uterus.
**perimysial** \-mis′ē·əl\ Describing or pertaining to the perimysium.
**perimysium** \-mis′ē·əm\ [PERI- + Gk *mys* a mouse, muscle + New L *-ium* noun suffix] (*pl.* perimysia) [NA] A connective tissue that separates adjacent fasciculi of muscle fibers. **external p.** EPIMYSIUM. **p. externum** EPIMYSIUM. **internal p.** ENDOMYSIUM.
**perinatal** \-nā′təl\ [PERI- + NATAL[1]] Pertaining to the period extending from the 28th week of gestation to the 28th day after birth.
**perinatologist** \-nātäl′əjist\ A physician who specializes in perinatology.
**perinatology** \-nātäl′əjē\ [PERI- + *nat(al)*[1] + *o* + -LOGY] The medical field or specialty dealing with the care of the pregnant woman, the developing fetus, and the newborn infant.
**perineal** \per′inē′əl\ Pertaining to the perineum.
**perineo-** \per′inē′ō-\ [See PERINEUM.] A combining form meaning perineum, perineal.
**perineocele** \per′inē′əsēl\ A perineal hernia between the rectum and either the bladder, vagina, or prostate.
**perineometer** \per′inē·äm′ətər\ An instrument for measuring the strength of perineal contraction.
**perineoplasty** \per′inē′əplas′tē\ [PERINEO- + -PLASTY] Any plastic operation on the perineum.
**perineorectal** \-rek′təl\ Relating to the perineal and rectal areas.
**perineorrhaphy** \per′inē·ôr′əfē\ [PERINEO- + -RRHAPHY] The repair of a perineal injury.
**perineoscrotal** \-skrō′təl\ Relating to the perineum and scrotum.
**perineosynthesis** \-sin′thəsis\ [PERINEO- + SYNTHESIS] The repair of a perineal laceration extending from the vaginal introitus to the rectum. *Older term.*
**perineotomy** \per′inē·ät′əmē\ [PERINEO- + -TOMY] An incision into the perineum.
**perineovaginal** \-vaj′ənəl\ Relating to the perineum and vagina.
**perineovaginorectal** \-vaj′ənôrek′təl\ Relating to the perineum, vagina, and rectum.
**perineovulvar** \-vul′vər\ Relating to the perineum and vulva.
**perinephric** \-nef′rik\ Located near or around a kidney. Also *perirenal.*
**perinephritis** \-nefrī′tis\ [PERI- + NEPHRITIS] Bacterial infection of the perirenal fat usually due to secondary extension of infection from the kidney, or occasionally to bacterial metastasis from infection elsewhere. Also *paranephritis.*
**perinephrium** \-nef′rē·əm\ The peritoneal envelope and other tissues surrounding the kidneys.
**perineum** \per′inē′əm\ [New L, from Gk *perineon*, also *perinaion*, of uncertain source, the space between the anal opening and the scrotum] [NA] The diamond-shaped area superficial to the inferior pelvic aperture. On the surface of the male it is bounded by the scrotum anteriorly, the buttocks posteriorly, and the inner sides of the thighs laterally. In the female the vulva is included anteriorly. A line drawn transversely in front of the ischial tuberosities divides the area into an anterior urogenital region and a posterior anal region. It includes the diaphragma pelvis, spatium perinei profundum, spatium perinei superficiale, and fossa ischioanalis and their contents. **anterior p.** REGIO UROGENITALIS. **posterior p.** REGIO ANALIS. **watering-can p.** A perineum containing multiple fistulas or sinus tracts. Also *watering-pot perineum, shot-gun perineum.*
**perineural** \-n$^y$ur′əl\ Covering or lying in close relationship to a nerve.
**perineuritic** \-n$^y$urit′ik\ Pertaining to perineuritis.
**perineuritis** \-n$^y$urī′tis\ [PERI- + NEURITIS] Inflammation of the tissues covering or surrounding a nerve.
**perineurium** \-n$^y$ur′e·əm\ The connective tissue sheath that encircles a bundle of nerve fibers in a peripheral nerve. Also *lamellar sheath, vagina cellulosa* (seldom used).
**perinuclear** \-n$^y$oo′klē·ər\ Surrounding the nucleus. Also *circumnuclear.*
**periocular** \-äk′yələr\ [PERI- + OCULAR] Pertaining to the area immediately surrounding the eye. Also *perioptic.*
**period** \pir′ē·əd\ [Gk *periodos* (from PERI- + *(h)odos* way) a circuit, cycle] **1** A portion of time. **2** An episode of menstrual discharge. *Popular.* **absolute refractory p.** The period just after nerve or muscle excitation when it is totally inexcitable regardless of stimulus strength. **acceleration p.** The time during the active phase of labor when the rate of cervical dilatation is continuously increasing. **antepartum p.** The period in a pregnancy from conception until the onset of labor. **child-bearing p.** The reproductive years in a woman's life usually extending from menarche to the menopause. **critical p.** **1** In embryology, a period of time during development of tissues and organs when they are particularly susceptible to the effects of any factor causing abnormality. The critical period is usually of short duration and always covers important morphogenetic events, such as occur in the heart, nervous system and special senses. **2** That point in growth during which a particular environment, or a class of stimuli within that envi-

ronment, will exert the greatest influence on the acquisition of a specific behavioral response, such as the following behavior seen in chicks. **D p.** M PERIOD. **deceleration p.** The time during the active phase of labor, just prior to full cervical dilatation, when the rate of cervical dilatation decreases. **early neonatal p.** The first seven days of life. **eclipse p.** ECLIPSE. **p. of emptying** The time during the lactation cycle when the breast is emptied of milk. **fertile p.** The time in the midportion of a menstrual cycle when ovulation occurs and sexual intercourse can lead to conception. **p. of filling** The time during the lactation cycle when the breast fills with milk. **$G_1$ p.** A period or phase in the cell cycle immediately following division, designated the pre-DNA synthesis period. Noncycling cells generally are in the $G_1$ period. **$G_2$ p.** The period or phase of the cell cycle following the S period and preceding the M period. Cells in the $G_2$ period generally contain twice the normal amount of DNA. **p. of gestation** The duration of a pregnancy, conventionally measured from the first day of the last menstrual period until delivery. For humans, the average gestational period is 40 weeks. **incubation p.** The interval between the time an infection is acquired by a person and the time it becomes clinically manifest. Also *incubative stage, stage of invasion, stage of latency.* **induction p.** INDUCTIVE PHASE. **intrapartum p.** The time in a pregnancy from the onset of labor until the delivery of the placenta. **isoelectric p.** A period of time, as during the cycle of the heart beat, when there is no difference in potential between two electrodes, so that a galvanometer shows no deflection. During ventricular systole, it is represented in the electrocardiogram by a horizontal line between the end of the S wave and the beginning of the T. **isometric p. of the cardiac cycle** See under ISOVOLUMETRIC INTERVAL. **lag p.** LAG PHASE. **latent p.** 1 The time elapsing between the presentation of a discrete sensory stimulus or a change in internal or environmental status and the resulting response. 2 The interval between any insult to an organism, as by radiation, infection, poison, etc., and the appearance of symptoms referable to the injury or infection. Also *latency period.* **M p.** The period or phase of the mitotic cell cycle during which cell division occurs. Also *D period.* **menstrual p.** MENSTRUATION. **monthly p.** MENSTRUATION. **neonatal p.** The time interval from birth to the 28th day of life. **Oedipus p.** OEDIPAL PHASE. **oral p.** ORAL PHASE. **patent p.** The period in an infectious disease, especially a parasitic disease, during which the causative organisms can be found in the body. **perinatal p.** The period extending from the 28th week of gestation to the seventh day after birth. **postneonatal p.** The period from the end of the first month of life, or the first 28 days, to the age of one year. **postpartum p.** The period occurring just after delivery and measured from the delivery of the placenta until about six weeks later. Also *postpregnancy period, pueperal period, puerperium.* **prefunctional p.** In development, the interval between the first appearance of an organ or structure and the time it starts to function. **prenatal p.** The time in a pregnancy from conception until the onset of labor. **prepatent p.** PREPATENCY. **puerperal p.** POSTPARTUM PERIOD. **quarantine p.** The interval which must elapse before a person exposed to any given infectious disease may be regarded as being incapable of either developing or transmitting the disease. **reaction p.** The time between stimulus application and response. **refractory p.** That period following a stimulus during which a tissue, as a nerve, is unresponsive either partially or completely to a subsequent stimulus. Also *inertia time.* **relative refractory p.** The time period following nerve or muscle response during which the tissue requires a stronger stimulus to be re-excited. **reproductive p.** The portion of her life during which a woman is fecund, extending from puberty to menopause. For statistical purposes, unless otherwise stated, the period is by convention taken to extend from age 15 to age 44. **S p.** The period or phase of the mitotic cell cycle, between the $G_1$ and $G_2$ periods, during which the chromosomes (including DNA and histones) are synthesized. **safe p.** The time during the menstrual cycle when conception is least likely. It lasts from about ten days before menstruation to about ten days after menstruation. **silent p.** 1 An interval in the course of a disease in which the symptoms are absent or nearly absent. 2 A pause or lessening of electromyographic activity after initial reflex excitation of the muscle by a tendon tap. Contributing factors are inhibition from discharge of tendon organs in the muscle and spindle afferents in antagonist muscles, Renshaw cell excitation, and disfacilitation due to unloading of the muscle's spindles. **steady p.** The time during the active phase of labor when the cervix dilates at a uniform rate. **waiting p.** The period of time that must elapse after the writing of a health insurance policy before the subscriber becomes eligible for coverage or for special benefits after overall coverage has commenced. **Wenckebach p.** The progressively prolonged P-R interval seen in a Wenckebach block.

**periodic** \pir′ē·äd′ik\ Recurring at regular intervals.

**periodicity** \pir′ē·ədis′itē\ Recurrence at regular time intervals. **diurnal p.** The increase of microfilariae in the peripheral blood during the daylight hours, as in *Loa loa* infection. **lunar p.** Recurrence at intervals that are synchronous with phases of the moon, such as reproductive cycles in certain annelids and other invertebrates. **nocturnal p.** An increase of microfilariae in the peripheral blood at night, as in certain strains of *Wuchereria bancrofti* or *Brugia malayi.* In other strains, a subperiodic microfilaremia is noted. Specific periodicity patterns of microfilaremia in peripheral blood is generally associated with biting habits of the particular vector of that strain. **subperiodic p.** Microfilarial periodicity in filariasis that is not strictly nocturnal, tending to range from evening through early morning. This is usually associated with the less regular biting times of the particular mosquito hosts involved.

**periodontal** \-ōdän′təl\ Pertaining to the periodontium. Also *paradental, parodontal, peridental.*

**periodontia** \-ōdän′shə\ 1 PERIODONTICS. 2 Plural of PERIODONTIUM.

**periodontics** \-ōdän′tiks\ The dental specialty dealing with the science and treatment of periodontal diseases. Also *periodontia.*

**periodontist** \-ōdän′tist\ A dentist specializing in periodontics.

**periodontitis** \-ō′däntī′tis\ [*periodont(ium)* + -ITIS] An inflammatory condition of the periodontium. Usually only a portion of the periodontium is involved, as in chronic periodontitis. An infected dental pulp may cause an apical periodontitis. Also *paradentitis, parodontitis, peridentitis, alveolodental osteoperiostitis.* **acute local p.** Acute inflammation of part of the periodontium around a single tooth, rendering it sensitive to percussion. Also *dental periostitis* (outmoded). **apical p.** Inflammation of the periodontium around the apex or apices of a tooth, the result of infection in the pulp. **chronic p.** Chronic periodontal disease where the inflammatory process has extended beyond the gingival tissues. Lysis of gingival fiber apparatus, resorption of alveolar bone, loss of crestal fibers of the periodontal ligament, and downgrowth of junctional epithelium lead to the formation of periodontal pockets. Clinically, the differential diagnosis between gingivitis and chronic periodontitis is made on the finding of (true) pockets on the roots of the teeth. Also *marginal periodontitis.* **chronic suppurative p.** Chronic periodontitis with a purulent exudate that can be expressed from the pockets. Also *pyorrhea* (popular). **p. complex** Chronic periodontitis in which systemic factors in addition to dental plaque are considered of importance in the etiology. The alveolar bone resorption is of a "vertical" type. *Outmoded.* Also *complex periodontitis.* **juvenile p.** See under PERIODONTOSIS. **marginal p.** CHRONIC PERIODONTITIS. **simple p.** PERIODONTITIS SIMPLEX. **p. simplex** Chronic periodontitis caused by local factors only. Loss of alveolar bone is "horizontal." Also *simple periodontitis.* **suppurative p.** See under CHRONIC SUPPURATIVE PERIODONTITIS.

**periodontium** \-ōdän′shē·əm\ [New L (from PERI- + ODONT- + New L *-ium*, noun suffix] (*pl.* periodontia) [NA] A well-vascularized layer of fibrous connective tissue between the root of a tooth and the bone of its socket. Also *periodontal ligament, alveolodental ligament, cemental ligament, circular ligament, dental capsule, alveolodental membrane, peridental membrane, periodontal membrane, odontoperiosteum, paradentium, parodontium, pericementum, peridentium, alveolar periosteum* (outmoded), *periosteum alveolare* (outmoded). ● In dentistry, *periodontium* is used more broadly to include not only the periodontium itself (termed *periodontal ligament*), but also the gingiva, the cementum, and the alveolar bone.

**periodontology** \-ō′däntäl′əjē\ [PERI- + ODONTO- + -LOGY] The science and study of the periodontium and periodontal diseases.

**periodontosis** \-ō′däntō′sis\ [PERIODONT(IUM) + -OSIS] Loss of attachment and destruction of bone adjacent to permanent first molars and/or incisors in children, adolescents, and young adults. Other teeth may also be affected. Clinically, there is migration of the affected teeth, with loosening and pocketing of irregular depth. Also *paradontosis.* ● It was once described as a degenerative condition but the evidence for this is scanty and the term *juvenile periodontitis* has been suggested as an alternative.

**periodoscope** \pir′ē·äd′əskōp\ [*(menstrual) period* + *o* + -SCOPE] A chart used to estimate the date of birth based on the date of the last menstrual period.

**periomphalic** \-ämfal′ik\ Being in the region of the umbilicus. Also *periumbilical.*

**perionychia** \-ōnik′ē·ə\ [PERI- + ONYCHIA] An inflammation around the nail. Also *perionyxis.*

**perionyx** \-ō′niks\ [PERI- + Gk *onyx* talon, claw, nail] [NA] The skin around the nail. Also *perionychium.*

**perionyxis** \-ōnik′sis\ PERIONYCHIA.

**perioophoritis** \-ō′əfôrī′tis\ PAROOPHORITIS.

**perioophorosalpingitis** \-ō′əfôr′ōsal′pinjī′tis\ PERISALPINGOOPHORITIS.

**perioptic** \-äp′tik\ PERIOCULAR.

**periorbita** \-ôr′bitə\ [NA] The periosteum attached closely to the bony walls of the orbit. It is continuous posteriorly with the dura mater at the optic foramen and the superior orbital fissure. Also *periorbital membrane, periorbit.*

**periorbital** \-ôr′bitəl\ Surrounding the ocular orbit; pertaining to the tissues immediately surrounding the contents of the bony eye socket. Also *periconchal.*

**periorchitis** \-ôrkī′tis\ [PERI- + ORCHITIS] Inflammation of the tunica vaginalis testis.

**periost** \per′ē·äst\ PERIOSTEUM.

**periosteal** \-äs′tē·əl\ Of or related to the periosteum.

**periosteitis** \-äs′tē·ī′tis\ PERIOSTITIS.

**periosteoma** \-äs′tē·ō′mə\ A bony outgrowth that arises from the periosteum and surrounds the bone. Also *periostoma.*

**periosteomedullitis** \-äs′tē·ōmed′yəlī′tis\ An inflammation of the bone marrow cavity together with its periosteal covering.

**periosteomyelitis** \-äs′tē·ōmī′əlī′tis\ An inflammation of all bony structures, including the periosteum.

**periosteophyte** \-äs′tē·əfīt′\ A bony outgrowth that arises from the periosteum. Also *periosteophyma.*

**periosteorrhaphy** \-äs′tē·ôr′əfē\ The surgical repair of the margins of divided periosteum.

**periosteosis** \-äs′tē·ō′sis\ PERIOSTOSIS.

**periosteotome** \-äs′tē·ətōm′\ A strong, curved surgical knife that is used to divide the periosteum or elevate it from the underlying bone. Also *periostotome.*

**periosteotomy** \-äs′tē·ät′əmē\ The surgical division of the periosteum.

**periosteous** \-äs′tē·əs\ Of or related to the nature of periosteum.

**periosteum** \-äs′tē·əm\ [New L, from Gk *periosteon,* neut. of *periosteos* around the bone, from PERI- + Gk *osteon* bone] [NA] The tissue that envelopes bone. It consists of an inner osteoblastic layer, a middle fibrous layer, and an outer adventitial layer. Also *periost.* **alveolar p.** *Outmoded* PERIODONTIUM. **p. alveolare** *Outmoded* PERIODONTIUM. **p. cranii** PERICRANIUM.

**periostitis** \-ästī′tis\ [*periost(eum)* + -ITIS] An inflammatory condition of the periosteum. Also *periosteitis, cortical osteitis.* **albuminous p.** Periostitis with a collection of serous fluid between the periosteum and the bone. It occurs in cases of subacute bone inflammation. **dental p.** *Outmoded* ACUTE LOCAL PERIODONTITIS. **diffuse p.** A generalized inflammation of the periosteum of the long bones. **hemorrhagic p.** Periosteal inflammation in which blood collects beneath the periosteal surface, as may be seen in scurvy. **orbital p.** An inflammation of the soft tissues within the orbit.

**periostoma** \-ästō′mə\ PERIOSTEOMA.

**periostosis** \-ästō′sis\ **1** The development of one or more periosteomas. **2** The abnormal deposition of periosteal bone. For defs. 1 and 2 also *periosteosis.*

**periostosteitis** \-äs′tästē·ī′tis\ OSTEOPERIOSTITIS.

**periostotome** \-äs′tətōm\ PERIOSTEOTOME.

**periotic** \-ō′tik\ [PERI- + -OTIC²] Around the otic vesicle: said of the osseous labyrinth in the petrous part of the temporal bone that is derived from the cartilaginous ear, or otic, capsule.

**periovaritis** \-ō′verī′tis\ [PERI- + OVARITIS] PAROOPHORITIS.

**periovular** \-äv′yələr\ [PERI- + OVULAR] Around the ovum.

**peripancreatitis** \-pan′krē·ətī′tis\ Inflammation of the tissues surrounding the pancreas.

**peripatetic** \-pətet′ik\ Ambulatory: used especially of cases of typhoid fever in which the patient is not bedridden.

**periphakus** \-fā′kəs\ LENS CAPSULE.

**peripherad** \pərif′ərad\ In a peripheral direction.

**peripheral** \pərif′ərəl\ **1** Relating to or located at the periphery. Also *peripheric.* **2** Any auxiliary unit attached to the central processor of a digital computer, such as a printer, terminal, or memory.

**periphery** \pərif′ərē\ The part of the body or a system outside the central region, such as the limbs or skin.

**periphlebitic** \-flebit′ik\ Relating to or characterized by periphlebitis.

**periphlebitis** \-flebī′tis\ Inflammation of the outer coat of a vein, or of adjoining structures, or both. Also *periveni-tis.*
**periphoria** \-fôr′ē·ə\ [PERI- + -PHORIA] STRABISMUS.
***Periplaneta*** \-plənē′tə\ A genus of cockroaches in the family Blattidae, order Dictyoptera. ***P. americana*** The American cockroach. Actually a native of Africa, it is very large (30–40 mm), chestnut brown, domiciliated, and often the dominant cockroach in tropical or warmer temperate zones. It is found in sewer systems, restaurants, and sheltered warm areas including large buildings. ***P. australasiae*** The Australian cockroach, a cosmopolitan domiciliated species in tropical and warm, humid regions. Like the American cockroach, it was originally native to Africa.
**periplasm** \per′iplazm\ [PERI- + -PLASM] The thin aqueous space, containing specific proteins, between the inner and the outer membranes of Gram-negative bacteria. It contains various hydrolytic enzymes, as well as binding proteins involved in transport of small molecules and in chemotaxis.
**periplasmic** \-plas′tik\ Of or relating to the space in Gram-negative bacteria that is outside their plasma membrane but inside their peptidoglycan wall.
**peripolesis** \-pōlē′sis\ [Gk *peripolēsis* (from *peripolein* to go around, circumambulate, from *peri-* around + *polein* to range over, haunt, from *polos* a pole, pivot) movement around] The migration of one type of cell around cells of some other type: said especially of the adherence of lymphocytes around macrophages in cell cultures made from immunologically stimulated lymphoid tissue.
**periporitis** \-pôrī′tis\ [PERI- + *por(e)* + -ITIS] Miliaria complicated by infection, usually staphylococcal, so that inflammation develops around the sweat pores. The condition is seen most frequently in infants.
**periportal** \-pôr′təl\ Surrounding or adjacent to the portal vein or the portal canals in the liver. Also *peripylic.*
**periproctal** \-präk′təl\ Situated near the anus and rectum. Also *periproctic.*
**periproctitis** \-präktī′tis\ Inflammation of tissues adjacent to the rectum and anus.
**periprostatitis** \-präs′tətī′tis\ [PERI- + *prostat(e)* + -ITIS] Inflammation affecting the tissues located around the prostate.
**peripyelitis** \-pī′əlī′tis\ [PERI- + PYELITIS] Inflammation or infection around the renal pelvis.
**peripylephlebitis** \-pī′ləflebī′tis\ Inflammation of the tissues around the portal vein.
**peripylic** \-pī′lik\ [PERI- + PYLIC] PERIPORTAL.
**perirectal** \-rek′təl\ Surrounding the rectum.
**perirenal** \-rē′nəl\ [PERI- + RENAL] PERINEPHRIC.
**perisalpingitis** \-sal′pinjī′tis\ [PERI- + SALPINGITIS] Inflammation around the oviduct.
**perisalpingoophoritis** \-salping′gō·əfôrī′tis\ [PERI- + SALPING- + OOPHORITIS] Inflammation around the fallopian tube and ovary. Also *perioophorosalpingitis, perisalpingo-ovaritis.*
**periscopic** \-skō′pik\ Having a wide field, as a lens.
**perispermatitis** \-spur′mətī′tis\ [PERI- + SPERMAT- + -ITIS] Inflammation affecting the tissues surrounding the spermatic cord.
**perisplanchnic** \-splangk′nik\ Surrounding viscera; surrounding any viscus.
**perisplenic** \-splen′ik\ Surrounding the spleen.
**perisplenitis** \-splēnī′tis\ Inflammation of the peritoneal covering of the spleen.
**perispondylic** \-spändil′ik\ Around the posterior facet joints of the vertebrae.
**perispondylitis** \-spän′dilī′tis\ An inflammation of the tissues that surround the vertebral joints.
**Perisporiaceae** \-spôr′ē·ā′si·ē\ *Obs.* MONILIACEAE.
**peristalsis** \-stal′sis\ [New L, from the adjective PERISTALTIC] Successive waves of contraction passing for shorter or longer distances along tubular muscular organs such as the alimentary tract. **mass p.** Strong bursts of peristalsis that occur over long stretches of the colon and are usually associated with defecation. **retrograde p.** Peristaltic contractions reversed in direction from the normal, tending to propel the contents cephalad. Also *antiperistalsis, reversed peristalsis, retrostalsis.*
**peristaltic** \-stal′tik\ [Gk *peristaltikos* (from *peristellein* to wrap up, compress round, from *peri-* around + *stellein* to put on) surrounding and compressing] Of or relating to peristalsis.
**perisynovial** \-sinō′vē·əl\ PERIARTICULAR.
**perisynovitis** \-sin′əvī′tis\ PERIARTHRITIS.
**peritectomy** \-tek′təmē\ [PERI- + *t* + -ECTOMY ] Removal of limbal conjunctiva.
**peritendineum** \-tendin′ē·əm\ (*pl.* peritendinea) [NA] The fibrous connective tissue sheath around a tendon. Its intercepting membranes between the fibers make up the tendon.
**peritendinitis** \-ten′dənī′tis\ [PERI- + TENDINITIS] An inflammation of the tendon sheath. **adhesive p.** Peritendinitis characterized by adhesions between the sheath and its tendon. **p. crepitans** An adhesive inflammation of the tendon sheath accompanied by an audible noise on movement. **p. serosa** GANGLION.
**peritendinous** \-ten′dinəs\ Surrounding a tendon.
**peritenon** \-tē′nän\ The connective tissues that surround the tendon structure.
**perithelial** \-thē′lē·əl\ Of or relating to a perithelium.
**perithelioma** \-thē′lē·ō′mə\ [*peritheli(um)* + -OMA] HEMANGIOPERICYTOMA.
**perithelium** \-thē′lē·əm\ [*peri(cyte)* + *(endo)thelium*] A layer of connective tissue around capillaries and other small vessels in which pericytes may be identified. Also *pericyte layer.*
**peritomize** \pərit′əmīz\ To perform peritomy on.
**peritomy** \pərit′əmē\ [PERI- + -TOMY] The cutting free of the conjunctiva at the limbus as a preparatory step in surgical exposure of the deeper ocular structures.
**peritoneal** \-tənē·′əl\ Relating to the peritoneum.
**peritonealgia** \-tō′nē·al′jə\ [*peritone(um)* + -ALGIA] Pain in the peritoneum.
**peritonealize** \-tənē′əlīz\ To cover a hollow or solid organ with peritoneum. Also *peritonize.*
**peritoneocentesis** \-tənē′əsentē′sis\ ABDOMINOCENTESIS.
**peritoneoclysis** \-tō′nē·äk′lisis\ Injection of fluid into the peritoneal cavity.
**peritoneography** \-tō′nē·äg′rəfē\ Radiographic examination of the contents of the peritoneal cavity following the instillation of an opaque contrast medium or gas into it.
**peritoneopathy** \-tō′nē·äp′əthē\ Disease of the peritoneum.
**peritoneopexy** \-tō′nē·əpek′sē\ [*peritone(um)* + *o* + -PEXY] The transvaginal surgical fixation of the uterus.
**peritoneoplasty** \-tō′nē·əplas′tē\ [*peritone(um)* + *o* + -PLASTY] **1** A surgical procedure in which adhesions are lysed and raw surfaces are imbricated or covered to prevent the reformation of adhesions. **2** Any plastic operation on the peritoneum.
**peritoneoscope** \-tənē′əskōp\ LAPAROSCOPE.

**peritoneoscopy** \-tō′nē·äs′kəpē\ LAPAROSCOPY.

**peritoneotome** \-tənē′ətōm\ The area of peritoneum supplied by a single posterior nerve root.

**peritoneotomy** \-tō′nē·ät′əmē\ [*peritone(um)* + *o* + -TOMY] An incision into the peritoneum.

**peritoneum** \-tənē′əm\ [Late L (from Gk *peritonaion* a thing that is stretched over, from PERI- + Gk *tonos* tension, from *teinein* to stretch, strain), the membrane containing the abdominal viscera] [NA] An extensive serous membrane that lines the walls of the abdominal and pelvic cavities from which it is reflected to invest or cover, to a varying degree, the viscera of those cavities. Peritoneal duplications supporting or tethering certain viscera and organs constitute their mesenteries, omenta, and ligaments. In the male it forms a closed sac surrounding the peritoneal cavity, while in the female the free ends of the uterine tubes open into the cavity. The free internal surface of the membrane is lined by a single layer of flattened mesothelial cells, and it secretes serous fluid permitting free movement of the viscera against each other and against the parietal layer. **abdominal p.** *Outmoded* PERITONEUM PARIETALE. **intestinal p.** *Outmoded* PERITONEUM VISCERALE. **p. parietale** [NA] The layer of peritoneum that lines the inner surface of the walls of the abdomen and pelvis. It is continuous with the visceral peritoneum. Also *parietal peritoneum, abdominal peritoneum* (outmoded). **p. viscerale** [NA] The layer of peritoneum that covers, partly or almost completely, the viscera of the abdomen and pelvis. It is continuous with the parietal peritoneum. Also *visceral peritoneum, intestinal peritoneum* (outmoded).

**peritonism** \per′itənizm\ [*periton(eum)* + -ISM] A condition characterized by abdominal pain and shock which simulates peritonitis, without actual inflammation of the peritoneum.

**peritonitis** \-tənī′tis\ [*periton(eum)* + -ITIS] Inflammation of the visceral and parietal peritoneal membrane of the abdomen, usually a result of bacterial infection of the peritoneal cavity or of chemical irritation, as in bile peritonitis. It is characterized by severe abdominal pains, vomiting, abdominal tenderness, and muscle wall rigidity. **acute sterile p.** Acute peritonitis of a noninfectious nature, usually chemical peritonitis. **adhesive p.** Peritonitis in which fibrinous exudation causes matting together of intestines and other organs. **benign paroxysmal p.** Episodic noninfectious peritonitis, usually occurring in the setting of recurrent polyserositis. **bile p.** Inflammation of the peritoneum caused by the presence of bile in the peritoneal cavity. Also *choleperitonitis, biliary peritonitis.* **chemical p.** Peritonitis due to rupture of a hollow abdominal viscus with release of its contents, e.g. bile or gastric acid, and subsequent chemical irritation of the peritoneum. This may lead to severe abdominal pain and circulatory collapse, and when generalized has a high mortality rate. **chyle p.** Peritonitis due to free chyle in the peritoneal cavity. **familial paroxysmal p.** FAMILIAL MEDITERRANEAN FEVER. **meconium p.** Inflammation of the peritoneum due to perforation of the gut *in utero,* with extravasation of meconium into the peritoneal cavity causing a sterile (chemical) peritonitis. As a result of the inflammatory reaction, intestinal obstruction may result from adhesions or atresia. On an x ray of the abdomen, calcification may be evident. It is usually a complication of cystic fibrosis. **pelvic p.** Inflammation or infection of the peritoneal surfaces within the pelvic cavity. Also *pelvioperitonitis.* **serous p.** Peritonitis characterized by the exudation of large amounts of fluid.

**peritonization** \-tō′nīzā′shən\ The surgical process by which hollow or solid organs within the abdominal cavity are covered by a layer of peritoneum.

**peritonize** \per′itəniz\ PERITONEALIZE.

**peritrichous** \pərit′rikəs\ Having flagella on the entire surface of a cell: used especially of bacteria. Also *peritrichal, peritrichic, peritrichate.* Compare LOPHOTRICHOUS.

**peritrochanteric** \-trō′kanter′ik\ Surrounding a trochanter.

**perityphlic** \-tif′lik\ PERICECAL.

**periumbilical** \-umbil′ikəl\ PERIOMPHALIC.

**periungual** \per′i·ung′gwəl\ [PERI- + L *ungu(is)* fingernail or toenail + -AL] Around the nail.

**periureteritis** \per′iyur′ətərī′tis\ [PERI- + URETERITIS] Inflammation of the connective tissue surrounding the ureter, often secondary to inflammation within the ureter itself (ureteritis). In conjunction with the inflammation in the surrounding adventitia, the ureteral wall may become thickened and peristalsis of the ureter reduced. **p. plastica** IDIOPATHIC RETROPERITONEAL FIBROSIS.

**periurethritis** \per′iyur′əthrī′tis\ [PERI- + URETHRITIS] Inflammation of the tissues surrounding the urethra, as in periurethral abscess, a complication of gonorrheal urethritis, or in periurethral urinary extravasation, seen in the presence of urethral trauma or urethral fistula formation.

**periuterine** \per′iyoo′tərīn\ Being in the region of the uterus.

**perivaginal** \-vaj′ənəl\ Being in the region of the vagina.

**perivaginitis** \-vaj′ənī′tis\ PARACOLPITIS.

**perivascular** \-vas′kyələr\ [PERI- + VASCULAR] Around a blood or lymph vessel. Also *circumvascular.*

**perivasculitis** \-vas′kyəlī′tis\ Inflammation of the connective tissue sheath surrounding a blood or lymph vessel.

**perivenitis** \-vēnī′tis\ PERIPHLEBITIS.

**perivenous** \-vē′nəs\ [PERI- + VENOUS] Around a vein.

**perivertebral** \-vur′təbrəl\ Surrounding one or more vertebrae.

**perivesiculitis** \-vesik′yəlī′tis\ [PERI- + VESICULITIS] Inflammation of the tissues surrounding the seminal vesicles. Diagnosis is infrequent since the condition is difficult to document or identify clinically.

**perivisceral** \-vis′ərəl\ Situated around a viscus or the viscera; perisplanchnic.

**perivitelline** \-vītel′īn\ Surrounding the yolk, or vitellus.

**perivulvar** \-vul′vər\ [PERI- + VULV- + -AR ] Being in the region of the vulva.

**perlèche** \perlesh′\ [French, poor condition of the corners of the mouth] ANGULAR CHEILITIS.

**Perlia** [Richard *Perlia,* German ophthalmologist, flourished late 19th century] See under NUCLEUS.

**perlsucht** \purl′sookt\ [German *Perle* pearl, bead + *Sucht* malady, disease] See under SPENGLER'S TUBERCULIN.

**permanganate** The ion $MnO_4^-$, or a salt containing it. It is used as an oxidizing agent, and is colored purple.

**permeability** \pur′mē·əbil′itē\ [L *perme(are)* (from PER- + L *meare* to go, pass) to go through, pass through + *-abilitas* -ABILITY] **1** The state of being permeable. **2** The specific measurement of a porous material based on the rate by volume at which a fluid of unit viscosity passes through a unit cross section of the material under the influence of unit pressure gradient. **differential p.** The attribute of maintaining selective permeability characteristics, as a membrane through which some substances but not others can pass. **magnetic p.** The ratio of the magnetism induced in a body to the strength of the magnetic field of induction. Symbol: $\mu$

**permeable** \pur′mē·əbl\ Permitting passage or penetration, as of fluids through a membrane. Also *pervious.*
**permeant** \pur′mē·ənt\ Able to pass through specified biologic membranes: used of substances or ions.
**permease** A membrane protein that specifically effects the passage of a substance through the membrane. • The word contains the suffix *-ase,* normally applied to enzymes, because such proteins show many of the characteristics of enzymes, particularly Michaelis kinetics.
**permeatal** \pur′mē·ā′təl\ TRANSMEATAL.
**permeation** \pur′mē·ā′shən\ The process of penetrating or spreading through, especially that of cancer cells invading lymphatic and blood vessels.
**permissive** \pərmis′iv\ Allowing expression of a conditionally lethal mutant gene and hence multiplication of a cell or virus. Depending on the nature of the mutation, the permissive condition may be low temperature, high temperature, or the presence of a codon-specific suppressor tRNA.
**perna** \pur′nə\ CHLORINATED NAPHTHALENE.
**pernasal** \pərnā′zəl\ Through the nose.
**perneiras** \pernā′rəs \ A Brazilian term for BERIBERI.
**perniciosiform** \pərnish′ē·ō′sifôrm\ Having the appearance of a fatal or malignant disorder, although in fact benign.
**pernicious** \pərnish′əs\ Having a severe progressive course with fatal outcome. • In *pernicious anemia,* the adjective is retained for historical reasons, although this disease, formerly fatal (therefore pernicious) is easily and effectively treated with vitamin $B_{12}$.
**perniosis** \pur′nē·ō′sis\ [L *pernio* chilblain + -SIS] 1 CHILBLAIN. 2 A cold injury.
**pero-** \per′ō-, per′ə-\ [Gk *pēros* disabled in a limb, maimed] A combining form meaning deformed, malformed.
**perobrachius** \-brā′kē·əs\ [New L, from PERO- + L *brachium* arm] A fetus or postnatal individual with congenitally malformed hands or hands and forearms.
**perocephaly** \-sef′əlē\ [PERO- + Gk *kephalē* the head] A developmental abnormality of the face and head.
**perochirus** \-kī′rəs\ [New L, from PERO- + Gk *cheir* hand] A fetus or postnatal individual with congenitally malformed hands.
**perodactyly** \-dak′tilē\ [PERO- + DACTYL + -Y ] A congenital deformity of the fingers and/or toes.
**peromelia** \-mē′lyə\ [PERO- + MEL-[1] + -IA] A congenital malformation of any or all extremities, usually of severe degree. A nonspecific designation.
**peroneal** \per′ənē′əl\ [Gk *peronē* pin or tongue of a buckle, fibula + -AL] 1 Pertaining to the lateral side of the leg. 2 FIBULAR.
**peroneocuboideus** \perō′nē·ōkyooboi′dē·əs\ An occasional slip of either the peroneus longus or peroneus brevis muscle that is inserted into the cuboid bone.
**peroneus** \per′ōnē′əs\ [New L, peroneal] 1 Peroneal, fibular. 2 Any of several muscles that originate from the fibula, as musculus peroneus brevis, musculus peroneus longus. **p. accessorius** An occasional accessory muscular slip arising from the fibula between the peroneus longus and brevis muscles and joining the tendon of the peroneus longus in the sole of the foot. **p. accessorius digiti minimi** A rare muscular slip in humans that arises from the lower fourth of the fibula deep to the peroneus brevis muscle. It inserts into the dorsal digital expansion of the fifth toe. It occurs normally in many nonhuman primates. Also *peroneus digiti quinti* (outmoded). **p. accessorius quartus** An occasional muscular slip from either the peroneus brevis muscle or the fibula between the peroneus brevis and flexor hallucis muscles. It is inserted into either the peroneal spine of calcaneus or the tuberosity of the cuboid. **p. digiti quinti** *Outmoded* PERONEUS ACCESSORIUS DIGITI MINIMI.
**per. op. emet.** *peracta operatione emetici* (L, when the emetic action is finished).
**peropus** \pir′ōpəs\ [PERO- + New L *-pus* (from Gk *pous* foot), combining form denoting foot] A fetus or postnatal individual with congenitally malformed lower limbs.
**peroral** \pərôr′əl\ Through the mouth.
**per os** \pur äs′, ōs′\ [L *per* by, through + *os* the mouth] By mouth.
**perosomy** \-sō′mē\ [PERO- + Gk *sōm(a)* the body + -Y] A developmental malformation of the trunk.
**perosplanchnia** \-splangk′nē·ə\ [PERO- + SPLANCHN- + -IA] A developmental malformation of several viscera within the same individual.
**peroxidase** The enzyme (EC 1.11.1.7) that catalyzes the oxidation of a wide range of substances using hydrogen peroxide as oxidant. It is a heme protein. Similar forms occur in both plants and animals.
**peroxidatic** Related to peroxidase.
**peroxide** \per′əksīd\ 1 The ion $O_2^{2-}$, or the group —O—O—, or any substance containing either. 2 HYDROGEN PEROXIDE.
**peroxisome** \pəräk′sisōm\ [*peroxi(de)* + Gk *sōm(a)* body] A membrane-bound cytoplasmic vesicle found in most cells. It is rich in enzymes that form and utilize hydrogen peroxide, such as glycolate oxidase, which catalyzes the reaction of glycolate with dioxygen to form glyoxylate and hydrogen peroxide. It is similar to a lysosome in appearance though slightly larger.
**peroxyacylnitrate** Any of a group of organic compounds that causes eye irritation and respiratory distress and occurs as a secondary product of air pollution by the internal combustion engine.
**per primam intentionem** [L, by first intention] See under HEALING BY FIRST INTENTION.
**per rectum** \pur rek′təm\ [L *per* by, through + RECTUM] Through the rectum.
**Perrin** [Maurice *Perrin,* French surgeon, 1826–1889] Perrin-Ferraton disease. See under SNAPPING HIP.
**PERRLA** pupils equal, round, and react to light and accommodation.
**Perroncito** [Aldo *Perroncito,* Italian histologist, 1882–1929] Apparatus of Perroncito, Perroncito spirals. See under PHENOMENON.
**per secundam intentionem** [L, by second intention] See under HEALING BY SECOND INTENTION.
**perseveration** \pur′sevərā′shən\ [L *perseveratio* (from *perseveratus,* past part. of *perseverare* to persist, from *perseverus* very strict, from *per-* intensive + *severus* grave, strict) a persisting] The involuntary continuation of an activity or response even though it is no longer appropriate or relevant to the situation.
**persio** CUDBEAR.
**persistence** \pərsis′təns\ **hereditary p. of fetal hemoglobin** The persistence, beyond the first year of life, of an increased proportion of hemoglobin F in erythrocytes without associated anemia or thalassemia. The condition is hereditary, of autosomal transmission, and is the result of deletion of the δ and β gene loci. Several types of this condition are recognized. In blacks with heterozygous HPFH, hemoglobin F is about 15–30% of total hemoglobin, and its distribution is usually nearly uniform from cell to cell. A similar condition occurs in some Greeks and other Mediterranean people, and is known as Greek type HPFH. Swiss and British types exhibit, in heterozygotes, 3–10% hemoglo-

bin F, which has a nonuniform or heterocellular distribution. Abbr. HPFH

**persisters** \pərsis′tərs\ The very small fraction of phenotypically resistant cells in a bacterial population that remain viable much longer than would be expected from the exponential curve of killing by a bactericidal agent. On subculture their progeny show normal sensitivity. The mechanism is not well understood, but the phenomenon is one reason why chemotherapy must be continued for several days.

**person / disabled p.** A person who on account of impaired physical or mental health, injury, or congenital deformity is substantially handicapped in obtaining or keeping employment or in independently undertaking work of a kind which, were it not for such disease, injury, or deformity, would have been suited to his or her age, experience, and qualifications. • In many countries there are legal definitions of *disabled person* which, while differing in detail, generally resemble the above.

**persona** \pərsō′nə\ [L, an actor's mask, a role, person, character] In jungian psychology, the attitude, visage, or mode of self-presentation adopted and assumed by a person to meet the demands of the immediate environment, and the person's momentary conscious intentions as means of ignoring or disguising more deeply rooted personality components.

**personality** [L *persona* an actor's mask, a role, person, character + *-alis* -AL + *-itas* -ITY] CHARACTER. **affective p.** CYCLOTHYMIC PERSONALITY. **aggressive p.** 1 A subtype of the passive-aggressive personality characterized by strivings to dominate, control, compete with, succeed over, or overpower others. 2 A type of antisocial personality characterized by extractive manipulativeness, cruelty, and wanton disregard of others' needs or rights. **alternating p.** MULTIPLE PERSONALITY. **amoral p.** A subtype of the antisocial personality believed to result from being reared in a criminal or lawless environment and without adequate social role models, as a result of which no enduring value system or sense of right and wrong develops. Also *dyssocial personality*. **anancastic p.** COMPULSIVE PERSONALITY. **antisocial p.** A personality characterized by a life pattern of truancy, delinquency, running away from home, lying, promiscuity, vandalism, excessive fighting, etc., before the age of 15 years, with persisting social difficulties in adulthood that may include an inconsistent work record, irresponsibility as a parent, defiance of the law, multiple arrests, impulsivity, and disregard of others and of others' property. Also *psychopathic personality*. **as-if p.** A personality type reflecting a severely damaged ego resulting from early loss of the mother. Such a personality is characterized by a lack of genuineness in object relationships, formal and unconvincing emotional display, passive attitude toward the social environment, readiness to adopt expected attitudes and behavior, and mimicry of and identification with the chance object to which the subject is attached at the moment (pseudoidentification). **borderline p.** A personality characterized by an unstable sense of self, peculiarly subject to feelings of abandonment, rage, and aloneness. Manifestations include emotional lability, impulsivity, chronic feelings of boredom, and self-damaging actions such as substance abuse, gambling, shoplifting, or self-mutilation. • The term is variously used by different writers and is often used to refer to the character structure of patients who do not respond well to conventional therapy. Originally, *borderline personality* referred to patients whose illnesses were diagnosed as intermediate between psychosis and neurosis. This sense is no longer current. **compulsive p.** A personality characterized by order, parsimony, obstinacy, conformity, perfectionism, scrupulosity, overconscientiousness, lack of spontaneity and need to maintain rigid control over impulses and affectivity, stubbornness, passiveness, and obstructionistic resistance to change. Also *anal character, anancastic personality, obsessive personality, obsessive-compulsive personality*. **cycloid p.** CYCLOTHYMIC PERSONALITY. **cyclothymic p.** A personality type characterized by recurring or alternating mood variations ranging from highs of elation, ambition, energy, warmth, enthusiasm, optimism, and self-assurance to lows of dejection, pessimism, worrying, low levels of energy, feelings of uselessness, and lack of self-confidence. Also *affective personality, cycloid personality, cycloid type*. **dependent p.** PASSIVE-DEPENDENT PERSONALITY. **dissociated p.** 1 MULTIPLE PERSONALITY. 2 Any one of the different personalities differentiated in a person with multiple personality. Also *split-off personality*. **double p.** MULTIPLE PERSONALITY. **dual p.** MULTIPLE PERSONALITY. **dyssocial p.** AMORAL PERSONALITY. **epileptoid p.** EPILEPTIC CHARACTER. **explosive p.** EPILEPTIC CHARACTER. **kolytic p.** *Seldom used* SCHIZOID PERSONALITY. **multiple p.** A personality type marked by two or more relatively distinct and separate subpersonalities or coconscious personalities existing in one person. The original personality is called primary while the dissociated personalities are termed secondary, tertiary, etc. Also *alternating personality, dissociated personality, split personality, double personality, dual personality*. **obsessive p.** COMPULSIVE PERSONALITY. **obsessive-compulsive p.** COMPULSIVE PERSONALITY. **passive p.** PASSIVE-DEPENDENT PERSONALITY. **passive-aggressive p.** A personality type characterized by resistance to conformity to the usual occupational or social performance standards, expressed indirectly through such habitual behavior as procrastination, dawdling, stubbornness, inefficiency, and forgetfulness. **passive-dependent p.** A personality type characterized by an inability to perform independently, accept responsibility, or take the initiative. An individual with such a personality has low self-esteem, a lack of self-confidence, an intolerance of being alone, a tendency to parasitize others, and a need for help, protection, and guidance from others as signaled through helplessness. Also *dependent personality, passive personality*. **psychopathic p.** ANTISOCIAL PERSONALITY. **schizoid p.** A personality characterized by shyness, aloofness, insensitivity to others' feelings because of preoccupation with one's own, seclusiveness, and difficulty in initiating or maintaining close emotional relationships. Also *seclusive personality, shut-in personality, schiothymic personality, schizoid type*. **schizothymic p.** SCHIZOID PERSONALITY. **seclusive p.** SCHIZOID PERSONALITY. **shut-in p.** SCHIZOID PERSONALITY. **split p.** MULTIPLE PERSONALITY. **split-off p.** DISSOCIATED PERSONALITY.

**personnel** \pur′sənel′\ **allied health p.** Health care workers who are trained to assist physicians, dentists, nurses, or other practitioners in the fields of patient care and public health. Allied health personnel work under the general supervision of such practitioners, but often exercise independent judgment within their areas of competence. See also PARAMEDICAL, PARAPROFESSIONAL.

**perspiration** SWEATING. **insensible p.** INSENSIBLE SWEATING. **sensible p.** SENSIBLE SWEATING.

**perspire** [L *perspir(are)* (from *per-* through + *spirare* to breathe) to breathe through; later, to pass out or escape as vapor through pores or by evaporation, to perspire] SWEAT.

**pertechnetate** \pərtek′nətāt\ The monovalent radical —$TcO_4^-$, or its salts; especially the generator-produced sodium salt, $Na^{99m}TcO_4$. The pertechnetates are widely used in diagnostic and other medical work. The $—TcO_4^-$ ion becomes concentrated in the thyroid gland (where, unlike iodide, it remains an ion) and in the salivary and gastric glands. It also diffuses readily into cerebral and other neoplasms, making gamma imaging possible. Pertechnetate technetium is easily reduced chemically, permitting the formation of technetium complexes with many organic compounds, useful as tracers. See also TECHNETIUM.

**Perthes** [Georg Clemens *Perthes*, German surgeon, 1869–1927] **1** See under TEST. **2** Calvé-Perthes disease, Legg-Calvé-Perthes disease. See under PERTHES DISEASE.

**Pertik** [Otto *Pertik*, Hungarian pathologist, 1852–1913] See under DIVERTICULUM.

**pertubation** \pur′tʸəbā′shən\ [PER- + *tub(a)* + -ATION] The injection of fluid or gas into an oviduct to demonstrate or maintain tubal patency.

**perturbation** \pur′tərbā′shən\ The effect on a dynamic system of an external influence. Usually the term is applied to a situation in which the force or energy provided by the external influence is small relative to the forces or energy internal to the system.

**pertussal** \pərtus′əl\ Pertaining to pertussis.

**pertussis** \pərtus′is\ [L *per-* intensive + *tussis* a cough] An acute, highly contagious disease caused by *Bordetella pertussis* or, less frequently, *B. bronchiseptica* and *B. parapertussis.* Although atypical disease occurs in adults, the illness is most commonly seen in children under five years of age, in which case it is characterized by paroxysms of coughing which end in whooping inspiration. After an incubation period of 7–14 days, the disease begins as a catarrhal infection, then progresses to the paroxysmal stage which may last 3–4 weeks or occasionally much longer. A relatively toxic, killed, whole cell vaccine is available and is usually given beginning in infancy. Also *whooping cough, tussis convulsiva, bex convulsiva.*

**per vaginam** \pur vajī′nəm\ Via the vagina.

**pervenous** \pərvē′nəs\ Inserted or administered by way of a vein or veins; transvenous.

**perversion** \pərvur′zhən\ [L *perversio* (from *pervertere* to upset, reverse, invert, corrupt, from *per-* thoroughly + *vertere* to turn) an upset, reversal, inversion, corruption] Any deviation from the correct, expected, or normal range. **polymorphous p.** Perversion involving diverse forms of sexual gratification that include any or all of the pregenital aspects of sexual development, which are normal in the child, but classified as aberrations in the adult.

**per vias naturales** [L *per* through, by means of + *vias*, accus. pl. of *via* way + *naturales*, fem. pl. of *naturalis* natural] **1** By natural ways; by natural means. **2** Through the natural or normal passages.

**pervious** \pur′vē·əs\ PERMEABLE.

**pes** \pēz, pās\ [L (gen. *pedis*; akin to Gk *pous*, gen. *podos*, a foot) the foot] **1** [NA] The distal end of the lower limb; foot. It is joined to the leg at the talocrural joint and is composed of tarsal, metatarsal, and phalangeal bones, which are held together by joints and supported and acted on by ligaments and by muscles, both intrinsic and extrinsic. It presents dorsal and plantar surfaces and a medial and a lateral margin. Its architecture serves to support the weight of the body and to propel it during locomotion. **2** Any part or structure resembling a foot. **p. abductus** TALIPES VALGUS. **p. adductus** TALIPES VARUS. **p. anserinus** PLEXUS INTRAPAROTIDEUS. **p. calcaneus** TALIPES CALCANEUS. **p. cavus** An abnormally high longitudinal arch of the foot. It may be a congenital condition or may result from muscular weakness, imbalance, or contracture. **p. cerebri** CRUS CEREBRI. **congenital convex p. valgus** TALIPES VALGUS. **p. equinovalgus** TALIPES EQUINOVALGUS. **p. equinovarus** TALIPES EQUINOVARUS. **p. febricitans** FILARIAL ELEPHANTIASIS. **p. hippocampi** [NA] Two or three shallow grooves with intervening elevations giving a pawlike appearance to the anterior end of the hippocampus. **p. hippocampi major** HIPPOCAMPUS. **p. hippocampi minor** CALCAR AVIS. **p. pedunculi** PEDUNCULUS CEREBRI. **p. planovalgus** TALIPES PLANOVALGUS. **p. planus** TALIPES PLANUS. **p. pronatus** TALIPES VALGUS. **p. valgus** TALIPES VALGUS. **p. varus** TALIPES VARUS.

**pessary** \pes′ərē\ [Late L *pessarium* (from *pessus* a pessary, from Gk *pessos* an oval stone used in playing checkers) a pessary] A device that is placed intravaginally to support the uterus or other pelvic structures. It is used to treat pelvic relaxation or prolapse, to correct retrodisplacement of the uterus, or to prevent sperm from reaching the uterus. Also *pessulum, pessum, pessus.* **air-ball p.** A pessary which is filled with air following intravaginal placement. **check p.** DIAPHRAGM PESSARY. **contraceptive p.** DIAPHRAGM PESSARY. **cup p.** A pessary whose upper portion is shaped like a cup to fit over the uterine cervix. **diaphragm p.** A membranelike device inserted intravaginally and utilized as a barrier in order to prevent conception. Also *contraceptive pessary, check pessary.* **doughnut p.** A ring-shaped rubber pessary which is inflated with air following intravaginal placement. **Hodge's p.** A pessary utilized to treat retrodisplacement of the uterus. It is shaped like a double horseshoe with equidistant levers. **Mayer's p.** A pessary consisting of an elastic ring. **Menge's p.** A pessary consisting of a ring, a crossbar, and a detachable stem. **prolapse p.** A pessary used to treat uterine prolapse. **retroversion p.** A pessary used to treat uterine retroversion. **ring p.** A pessary whose basic shape is that of a ring, used for uterine prolapse. **Smith's p.** A pessary utilized to treat retrodisplacement of the uterus. **stem p.** A pessary with a small projection, or stem, which is inserted into the cervical canal of the uterus. **Thomas p.** A type of vaginal pessary designed for women who have never been pregnant.

**pessimism** [L *pessim(us)* (superl. of *pejor* worse) the worst, very bad + -ISM] A melancholy habit of mind characterized by an inclination to believe that the uncertainties of the present will end badly. It is a common manifestation of depression. **therapeutic p.** An inclination to believe that a particular method of treatment will not produce any effective improvement. Compare THERAPEUTIC OPTIMISM.

**pessulum** \pes′ʸələm\ [Late L (dim. of *pessum* or *pessus* a pessary, from Gk *pessos* an oval stone used in playing checkers, possibly also a pessary), a pessary] PESSARY.

**pessum** \pes′əm\ [Late L, a pessary. See PESSULUM.] PESSARY.

**pessus** \pes′əs\ [Late L, a pessary. See PESSULUM.] PESSARY.

**pest** [L *pestis.* See PESTIS.] **1** Plague; pestilence. **2** Any harmful or annoying organism, especially an infestive animal.

**pesticemia** \pes′tisē′mē·ə\ [L *pesti(s)* plague, epidemic + *c* + -EMIA] The presence of *Yersinia pestis* in the bloodstream.

**pesticide** \pes′tisīd\ [PEST + *i* + -CIDE] Any substance or mixture of substances intended to kill or control pests such as insects, fungi, rodents, weeds, or nematodes. Pesticides include plant regulators, defoliants, and substances used for the control of germs except those in or on the human body. **hard p.** PERSISTENT PESTICIDE. **nonper-**

**sistent p.** A pesticide compound that is rapidly biodegradable with a half life of a few days. Also *soft pesticide.* **persistent p.** A pesticide compound that remains in the environment for relatively long periods of time. The extent of its persistence depends on several factors, such as the type of soil, its moisture, temperature, and pH, and the extent of cultivation and cover crops. Also *hard pesticide.* **soft p.** NONPERSISTENT PESTICIDE.

**pestis** \pes′tis\ [L, a pest, pestilence, plague, infectious disease] PLAGUE. **p. ambulans** AMBULATORY PLAGUE. **p. bubonica** BUBONIC PLAGUE. **p. major** Bubonic plague or pneumonic plague; the typical severe form of plague. **p. minor** AMBULATORY PLAGUE. **p. siderans** SEPTICEMIC PLAGUE. **p. variolosa** SMALLPOX.

**pestivirus** \pes′tivī′rəs\ Any of a genus (*Pestivirus*) of viruses in the Togaviridae family that includes, among others, the agents of hog cholera and bovine viral diarrhea.

**pestle** \pes′əl\ [Middle English *pestel,* from L *pistillum* (dim. of *pistum,* neut. sing. of *pistus,* past part. of *pinsere* to bray) pestle] A weighted cylindrical implement, often with an enlarged and rounded end, which is used to crush, grind, or pulverize material in a mortar.

**PET** 1 positron emission tomography. 2 preeclamptic toxemia.

**peta-** \pet′ə-\ [Gk *pe(n)ta-,* combining form of *pente* five] A combining form denoting $10^{15}$: used with SI units.

**-petal** \-pətəl\ [L *pet(ere)* to seek + -AL] A combining form meaning seeking, tending toward.

**petechia** \pētē′kē·ə\ [Italian *petecchia* a red or purple spot on the skin] (*pl.* petechiae) A small spot of discoloration in the skin or a mucous membrane that arises from an extravasation of blood; a small ecchymosis.

**petechiae** \pētē′ki·ē\ Plural of PETECHIA.

**petechiometer** \pētē′kē·äm′ətər\ A suction-cup device to expose the skin to a negative pressure for evaluating capillary fragility. Positive-pressure methods, such as the tourniquet test, are more popular.

**Peters** [Albert *Peters,* German ophthalmologist, 1862–1938] Peters anomaly. See under ANTERIOR CHAMBER CLEAVAGE SYNDROME.

**Petersen** [C. F. *Petersen,* German surgeon, 1845–1908] See under BAG.

**pethidine hydrochloride** MEPERIDINE HYDROCHLORIDE.

**petiole** \pet′ē·ōl\ [L *petiol(us),* misspelling of *peciolus* (for *pediciolus,* dim. of *pediculus,* dim. of *pes* foot) a little foot, the stalk of a fruit] The stem (petiolus) of a leaf. **epiglottic p.** PETIOLUS EPIGLOTTIDIS.

**petiolus epiglottidis** \petī′ələs ep′iglät′idis\ [NA] The long, tapered stalk at the lower end of the epiglottis to the anterior surface of which the thyroepiglottic ligament is attached. Also *epiglottic petiole, stalk of the epiglottis.*

**Petit** See under POURFOUR DU PETIT.

**Petit** [Antoine *Petit,* French surgeon and anatomist, 1718–1794] Petit's ligament. See under UTEROSACRAL LIGAMENT.

**Petit** [Jean Louis *Petit,* French surgeon, 1674–1750] Petit's triangle, Petit's lumbar triangle. See under TRIGONUM LUMBALE.

**petit mal** \pətē′ mäl′, pet′ē mäl′\ [French *petit* small + MAL] 1 An attack of transient impairment of consciousness without motor accompaniments other than brief myoclonus, beginning invariably in childhood, often occurring frequently, and associated with bilateral, synchronous, and symmetrical spike-wave 3 Hz rhythm in the EEG. 2 Any minor form of epilepsy in which rhythmic 3 Hz spike-wave complexes are seen in the electroencephalogram during or between attacks. 3 Formerly, any minor form of epilepsy. Also *petit mal epilepsy, epilepsia mitis, sphagiasmus, absence seizure.* See also ABSENCE. **atonic p.** An attack of atonic epilepsy in which there is sudden loss of postural tone during the transient episode of loss of consciousness, but of such brief duration that the patient does not fall. Such attacks are associated with rhythmic, generalized 3 Hz spike-wave discharge. When falling occurs (akinetic epilepsy) this should not be classified as petit mal. **intellectual p.** *Incorrect* PETIT MAL STATUS. **myoclonic p.** Petit mal in which transient myoclonus consistently accompanies the attacks.

**petits maux** \pətē′ mō′, pet′ē mō′\ Contractions that occur during the prodromal stage of labor.

**Pétrequin** [Theodore Joseph Eleonord *Pétrequin,* French surgeon, 1810–1876] See under LIGAMENT.

**Petri** [Julius Richard *Petri,* German bacteriologist, 1852–1921] See under DISH.

**petrifaction** \pet′rifak′shən\ Conversion to stone or to a stony substance.

**pétrissage** \pā′trēsäzh′\ [French (from *pétriss-,* stem of *pétrir* to make dough, form with clay + *-age* -AGE), kneading dough, kneading muscles in massage] KNEADING.

**petrobasilar** \pet′rəbas′ilər\ Pertaining to the petrous part of the temporal bone and the basilar part of the occipital bone.

**petrogenous** \pəträj′ənəs\ [L *petr(a)* a stone, rock + *o* + -GENOUS] Contributing to the formation of calculi.

**petrolatum** A mixture of high boiling petroleum fractions, often highly purified, too viscous to flow at ambient temperatures. It is used as an emollient and lubricant, and as the basis for ointments and salves. Also *petroleum jelly, mineral jelly.*

**petroleum** [Med L, from L *petr(a)* rock + *oleum* oil] A substance consisting of natural hydrocarbon deposits found in the earth. Also *mineral oil.* **p. ether** A light petroleum consisting of a mixture of hydrocarbons of specified range of boiling points, usually within the limits of 60°C and 120°C, from pentanes upwards. **p. jelly** PETROLATUM.

**petromastoid** \pet′rəmas′toid\ 1 PARS PETROSA OSSIS TEMPORALIS. 2 OTOCRANIUM.

**petropharyngeus** \pet′rōfərin′jē·əs\ A small slip of the salpingopharyngeus muscle that occasionally arises from the lower surface of the petrous part of the temporal bone and blends with the pharyngeal constrictor muscles.

**petrosa** \pətrō′sə\ PARS PETROSA OSSIS TEMPORALIS.

**petrosectomy** \pet′rəsek′təmē\ [L *petros(us)* (from *petr(a)* a rock, stone + *-osus* -OSE) rocky, stony + -ECTOMY] Excision of the petrous portion of the temporal bone. It is the principal feature of the radical operation for malignancy of the middle ear. The sacrifice of important adjacent parts, including the parotid gland with the facial nerve and the temporomandibular joint as well as the middle ear contents and, usually, the external ear, is implicit.

**petrositis** \pet′rəsī′tis\ [L *petros(us)* (from *petr(a)* a rock, stone + *-osus* -OSE) + -ITIS] Inflammation of the petrous part of the temporal bone as results from infection of its air cells. It is a rare complication of acute mastoiditis and the cause of the Gradenigo syndrome. Treatment is surgical drainage by one of a number of approaches.

**petrous** \pet′rəs\ 1 Having the consistency of a rock. 2 Referring to the petrosa.

**Petruschky** [Johannes *Petruschky,* German bacteriologist, born 1863] See under SIGN.

**PETT** 1 positron emission transaxial tomography (positron emission tomography). 2 pendular eye-tracking test.

**Petzetaki** [M. *Petzetaki,* Greek physician, flourished 20th century] Petzetaki's reaction. See under TEST.

**Petzval** [Josef Miksa *Petzval*, Hungarian mathematician, 1807–1891] See under CURVATURE.

***Peucetia*** \pʸoosē′tē·ə\ A genus of spiders in the family Gnathophosidae that are responsible for bites of moderate severity reported in the United States. ***P. viridans*** A species of lynx spider that produces a painful burn in the eye by spraying a corrosive liquid.

**Peutz** [J. L. A. *Peutz*, Dutch physician, flourished early 20th century] Peutz-Jeghers syndrome. See under SYNDROME.

**pexia** \pek′sē·ə\ PEXIS.

**pexin** CHYMOSIN.

**pexis** \pek′sis\ [Gk *pēxis* a fixing, making fast] The holding or suspension of organs and structure, either by their natural attachments or by surgical reparative techniques. Also *pexia*. Adj. pexic.

**-pexy** \-pek′sē\ [Gk *pēxis* (from *pēxō* future of *pēgnynai* to fix in, fasten upon) a fixing, a making fast] A combining form meaning fixation.

**Peyer** [Johann Konrad *Peyer*, Swiss anatomist, 1653–1712] **1** Aggregated lymphatic follicles of Peyer, Peyer's plaques. See under PEYER'S PATCHES. **2** Peyer's glands. See under FOLLICULI LYMPHATICI AGGREGATI.

**peyote** \pā·ō′tē\ A cactus of the species *Lophophora williamsii*. Mescaline, a hallucinogen, is prepared from the flowering heads (mescal buttons) of the plant. Also *mescal*. Also *pellote*.

**Peyronie** [Françǫis de la *Peyronie*, French surgeon, 1678–1747] See under DISEASE.

**Pfannenstiel** [Hermann Johann *Pfannenstiel*, German gynecologist, 1862–1909] See under INCISION.

**PFC** plaque-forming cells.

**Pfeiffer** [Emil *Pfeiffer*, German physician, 1846–1921] Pfeiffer's disease. See under INFECTIOUS MONONUCLEOSIS.

**Pfeiffer** [R. A. *Pfeiffer*, German physician, flourished 20th century] Pfeiffer syndrome. See under ACROCEPHALOSYNDACTYLY TYPE IV.

**Pfeiffer** [Richard Friedrich Johann *Pfeiffer*, German bacteriologist, 1858–1945] **1** Pfeiffer's bacillus. See under *HAEMOPHILUS INFLUENZAE*. **2** Pfeiffer reaction. See under PHENOMENON.

**Pflüger** [Eduard Friedrich Wilhelm *Pflüger*, German physiologist, 1829–1910] Pflüger's cords. See under CORD.

**PFU** plaque-forming unit.

**PGY** postgraduate year (qualified as PGY-1, PGY-2, etc., to indicate year of medical residency).

**Ph** **1** Symbol for phenyl. **2** pharmacopeia.

**pH** [potential of hydrogen ions] An expression of the acidity or alkalinity of a solution. It represents minus the logarithm (to base 10) of the concentration of free hydrogen ions in moles per liter. Thus $pH = -\log[H^+]$ where $[H^+]$ is the hydrogen-ion concentration. Since in a normal solution of completely dissociated acid $[H^+] = 1$ M, $pH = 0$. Since in water $[H^+][OH^-] = 10^{-14}M^2$, when $[H^+] = [OH^-]$, $[H^+] = 10^{-7}M$, and the $pH = 7$. This is known as neutrality. **isoelectric p.** ISOELECTRIC POINT. **optimum p.** The pH at which a process, often an enzyme-catalyzed reaction, proceeds fastest.

**PHA** phytohemagglutinin.

**phacitis** \fəsī′tis\ [*phac(o)-* + -ITIS] PHAKITIS.

**phaco-** \fak′ō-, fak′ə-\ [Gk *phakos* a lentil, lentil-shaped object, a freckle or mole] A combining form denoting (1) lens, especially the crystalline lens of the eye; (2) a lentil-shaped lesion. For words beginning *phaco-*, see also under PHAKO-. Also *phako-*.

**phacocyst** \fak′əsist\ LENS CAPSULE.

**phacocystectomy** \-sistek′təmē\ [PHACOCYST + -ECTOMY] Removal of the lens capsule wholly or in part.

**phacocystitis** \-sistī′tis\ [PHACOCYST + -ITIS] Inflammation of the lens capsule. Also *phacohymenitis*.

**phacoemulsification** \fak′ō·imul′sifikā′shən\ [PHACO- + *emulsification*] A technique of cataract removal in which ultrasonic vibration of a titanium tube is employed to fragment the lens. The resulting small particles are then aspirated through the tube. ⟨"Dr. Charles D. Kelman, the ophthalmologist who invented the cataract removal procedure called phacoemulsification, plans to teach his technique, together with a new laser procedure . . ."—*New York Times* 22 Feb. 1983, C3.⟩

**phacoerysis** \fak′ō·er′əsis\ [PHACO- + Gk *erysis* a dragging, drawing] Cataract extraction with a suction-cup device.

**phacohymenitis** \-hī′mənī′tis\ [PHACO- + HYMEN + -ITIS] PHACOCYSTITIS.

**phacoid** \fak′oid\ [Gk *phakoeidēs* (from *phako(s)* lentil + *-eidēs* -like, -OID) lentiform, lentil-like] **1** Having the shape of a lens. **2** LENS.

**phacoiditis** \fak′oidī′tis\ [PHACOID + -ITIS] PHAKITIS.

**phacoidoscope** \fəkoi′dəskōp\ [PHACOID + *o* + -SCOPE] PHACOSCOPE.

**phacolysis** \fəkal′isis\ [PHACO- + LYSIS] An incision into or needling of the crystalline lens.

**phacolytic** \-lit′ik\ Pertaining to phacolysis or to liquefaction of the lens cortex.

**phacoma** \fəkō′mə\ [*phac(o)-* + -OMA] PHAKOMA.

**phacomalacia** \-məlā′shə\ Liquefaction or softening of the crystalline lens.

**phacomatosis** \-mətō′sis\ PHAKOMATOSIS.

**phacometer** \fəkäm′ətər\ [PHACO- + -METER] A device to measure the strength of an optical lens.

**phacopalingenesis** \-pal′injen′əsis\ A regrowth of lenticular substance.

**phacoscope** \fak′əskōp\ [PHACO- + -SCOPE] A device for measuring the dioptric strength of the crystalline lens. Also *phacoidoscope*.

**phacoscopy** \fəkäs′kəpē\ [PHACO- + -SCOPY] Measurement of the dioptric strength of the crystalline lens.

***Phaenicia*** \fenish′ē·ə\ A genus of blowflies (family Calliphoridae). Members of the genus are basically outdoor scavengers. The larvae develop in carrion and a wide variety of food, garbage, feces, and meat scraps. ***P. sericata*** An abundant scavenging blowfly which is attracted to necrotic tissue and suppurating wounds and can produce serious cases of myiasis, especially in injured or helpless persons. Also *Lucilia sericata*.

**phaeo-** \fē′ō-\ *Brit.* PHEO-.

**phaeochromocytoma** *Brit.* PHEOCHROMOCYTOMA.

**phage** \fāj\ [by shortening of *bacteriophage*] **1** BACTERIOPHAGE. **2** A virus that infects any kind of microorganism or protist, as, for example, a fungal virus or mycophage. Seldom used in this sense. **β-p.** A temperate phage of *Corynebacterium diphtheriae* that codes for diphtheria toxin.

**-phage** \-fāj\ [Gk *-phagos* (from *phagein* to eat) -eater] A combining form designating (1) an organism or virus that subsists on a (specified) form of nourishment or infects a (specified) form of life, as *biophage, bacteriophage;* (2) a (specified) type of phagocyte, as *macrophage*.

**phagedaena** *Brit.* PHAGEDENA.

**phagedena** \faj′ədē′nə\ [Gk *phagedaina* (from *phag(ein)* to eat) a cancerous sore, canker] A rapidly spreading ulceration. **p. gangrenosa** Phagedena proceeding to gangrene. Also *sloughing phagedena*. **geometric p.** PYODERMA GANGRENOSUM. **sloughing p.** PHAGEDENA

GANGRENOSA. **p. tropica** TROPICAL ULCER.

**phagedenic** \faj′əden′ik\ Of or relating to phagedena.

**phage-typing** \fāj′-\ The identification of bacterial strains within a species by their characteristic pattern of sensitivity to various phages.

**-phagia** \-fā′jə\ [*phag(o)-* + -IA] A combining form meaning eating or an abnormal condition associated with eating.

**phago-** \fag′ə-, fag′ō-\ [Gk *phagein* to eat, feed on] A combining form meaning eating, consuming, feeding on.

**phagocaryosis** \-kar′ē·ō′sis\ PHAGOKARYOSIS.

**phagocyte** \fag′əsīt\ [PHAGO- + -CYTE] A cell that ingests foreign particles, as microorganisms, by phagocytosis. Also *scavenger cell.* Adj. phagocytic. **alveolar p.** ALVEOLAR MACROPHAGE. **endothelial p.** MONOCYTE. **fixed p.** A phagocyte that is attached (nonmotile), as the reticulocytes of the liver, spleen, or lymph nodes. The fixed phagocytes have a phagocytic potential but are generally less phagocytically active than a free phagocyte. **free p.** A phagocyte that is unattached, thus is able to move through the circulatory system and the tissue fluid as a macrophage. Free phagocytes respond to chemotactic factors and are especially abundant in regions of infection or inflammation. They are highly phagocytic cells. **habitual p.'s** Cells, such as histiocytes and neutrophil polymorphs, that normally are capable of phagocytosis.

**phagocytic** \-sit′ik\ Of or relating to phagocytes or to their function.

**phagocytize** \fag′əsitīz′\ To ingest and usually destroy by phagocytosis. Also *phagocytose.*

**phagocytolysis** \-sītäl′isis\ Dissolution of phagocytic cells, from whatever cause, as from chemotherapy or radiation therapy, or following their entrapment in a clot. Also *phagolysis.*

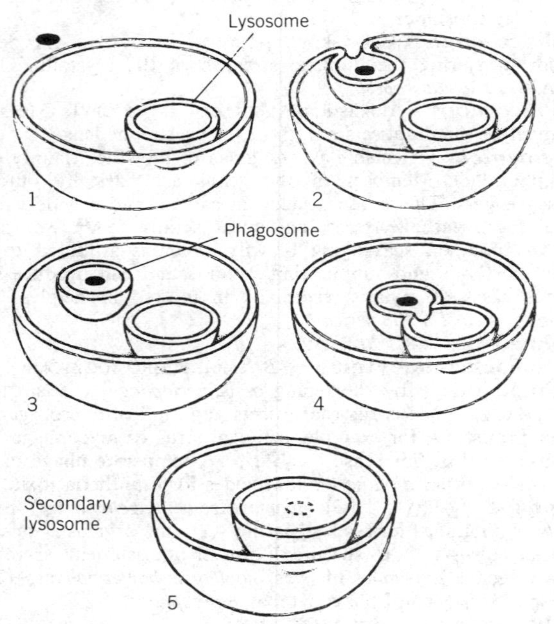


**Phagocytosis** (1) Cell and foreign particle converging; (2) particle endocytized; (3) phagosome approaching lysosome; (4) phagosome and lysosome fused; (5) particle digested in secondary lysosome.

**phagocytose** \-sī′tōs\ PHAGOCYTIZE.

**phagocytosis** \-sītō′sis\ [PHAGOCYTE + -OSIS] The process by which a cell, as a leukocyte, surrounds and engulfs a foreign particle, a bacterium or other microorganism, or another cell. The ingested particles are moved into the cytoplasm of the cell surrounded by a segment of membrane derived from the plasma membrane. The cytoplasmic vesicle, the phagosome, then combines with a lysosome, forming a secondary lysosome in which the ingested particle is digested. Also *englobement.* **spontaneous p.** Phagocytosis of a microorganism or other particle that does not require the microorganism or particle first to be coated with an opsonin. **surface p.** The ingestion, in the absence of opsonins, of bacteria or other particles trapped by phagocytes against a firm surface, such as the alveolar wall. It is believed to help limit the growth of the bacterial population during the period before the appearance of antibodies.

**phagokaryosis** \-kar′ē·ō′sis\ [PHAGO- + KARYO- + -SIS] The phagocytic action of the cell nucleus. Also *phagocaryosis.*

**phagolysis** \fəgäl′isis\ PHAGOCYTOLYSIS.

**phagolysosome** \-lī′səsōm\ A cytoplasmic vesicle produced by the fusion of a phagosome and a lysosome. The lysosomal enzymes digest most of the material within this vesicle.

**phagomania** \-mā′nē·ə\ [PHAGO- + -MANIA] BULIMIA.

**phagopyrosis** \-pīrō′sis\ [PHAGO- + PYROSIS] HEARTBURN.

**phagosome** \fag′əsōm\ [PHAGO- + Gk *sōm(a)* body] A membrane-bound cytoplasmic vesicle which contains phagocytized materials, prior to the fusion with a lysosome.

**-phagous** \-fəgəs\ [Gk *-phag(os)* (from *phagein* to eat) -eating, -eater + -OUS] A combining form meaning eating, feeding on (something specified).

**-phagy** \-fəjē\ [*phag(o)-* + -Y] A combining form meaning the eating of or subsistence on (something specified).

**phakitis** \fəkī′tis\ [*phak(o)-* + -ITIS] Inflammation of the crystalline lens. Also *phacitis, lentitis, crystallitis.*

**phako-** \fak′ō-, fak′ə-\ PHACO-.

**phakoma** \fəkō′mə\ [*phak(o)-* + -OMA] **1** A hamartomatous lesion characteristic of one of the phakomatoses; especially, a retinal phakoma. **2** A tumorlike swelling of the crystalline lens. Seldom used in this sense. For defs. 1 and 2 also *phacoma.* **retinal p.** A yellowish or gray rounded flat area of glial tissue about the size of the optic disk which may be seen in the retina in cases of phakomatoses, especially in tuberous sclerosis and in neurofibromatosis.

**phakomatosis** \fak′ōmətō′sis\ [PHAKOMA + *t* + -OSIS] (*pl.* phakomatoses) Any of a group of syndromes, including especially tuberous sclerosis and neurofibromatosis but also sometimes the Sturge-Weber syndrome and the von Hippel-Lindau syndrome in which there are either areas of glial overgrowth and proliferation or malformations of small blood vessels involving the retina and brain. Also *phacomatosis.* **Bourneville's p.** TUBEROUS SCLEROSIS.

**phalangeal** \fā′lənjē′əl, fəlan′jē·əl\ Of or relating to a phalanx.

**phalangectomy** \fal′anjek′təmē\ The surgical removal of a phalanx from either the hand or the foot.

**phalanges** \fālan′jēz\ Plural of PHALANX.

**phalangette** \fal′anjet′\ The terminal phalanx.

**phalangitis** \fal′anjī′tis\ An inflammation of the phalanx.

**phalangization** \fal′ənjīzā′shən\ The operative separation of the distal portion of fused digits without the complete division of the connecting web.

**phalanx** \fā′langks\ [L (gen. *phalangis,* from Gk *phalanx,* gen. *phalangos,* an order of battle, phalanx, round piece of wood, trunk, log, a bone of a finger or toe, spider), a pole, beam, array of soldiers in square formation] (*pl.* phalanges)

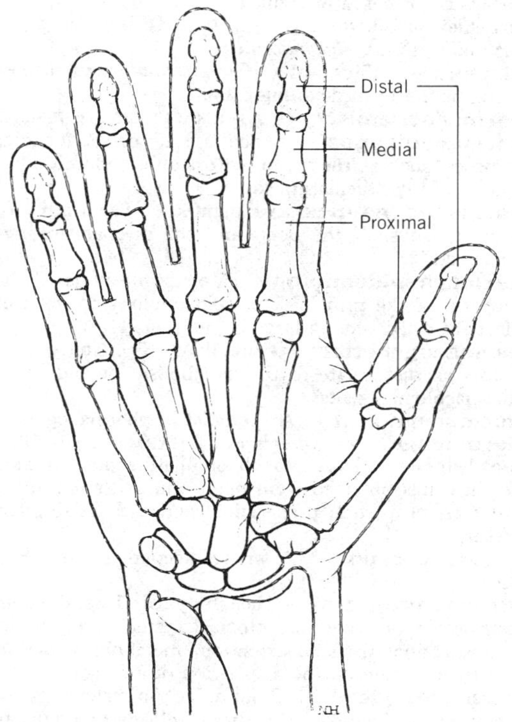


Phalanges of fingers

[NA] A long bone of the digits of the hand and foot, usually with three segments in each digit, except for the thumb and great toe. The segments are referred to as the proximal, middle, and distal segments; the thumb and great toe have only proximal and distal segments. Each bone has a base, a body or shaft, and a head. The proximal phalanx is the longest of the three. Adj. phalangeal. **Deiters phalanges** Fingerlike processes of the outer phalangeal cells of Deiters extending between the rows of the outer hair cells on the lateral side of the spiral organ of Corti. They reach up to the reticular membrane or lamina, where they end in expanded plates connected by junctional complexes to the hair cells and to the supporting cells of Hensen. Also *processus phalangeus.* **p. distalis digitorum manus** [NA] The small triangular-shaped bone at the tip of each finger, its oval base articulating with the head of the corresponding middle phalanx, except in the thumb where it articulates with the proximal phalanx. The palmar aspect of the base receives the insertion of the flexor digitorum profundus muscle, whereas the dorsal aspect receives that of the extensor digitorum muscle. The expanded head is nonarticular and flat, with a horseshoe-shaped tuberosity on its palmar aspect to which the pulp of the finger is attached by fibrous strands. Also *distal phalanx of fingers.* **p. distalis digitorum pedis** [NA] The very small, flat bone at the tip of each toe, its oval base articulating with the head of the corresponding middle phalanx except in the great toe where it articulates with the proximal phalanx. The plantar aspect of the base of the lateral four toes receives the insertion of the flexor digitorum longus muscle whereas the dorsal aspect receives that of the extensor digitorum. The corresponding aspects in the great toe receive the insertion of the flexor hallucis longus and that of the extensor hallucis, respectively. The expanded nonarticular head is flat, with a semilunar tuberosity on its plantar aspect to which the pulp of the toe is attached by fibrous strands. Also *distal phalanx of toes.* **phalanges of fingers** OSSA DIGITORUM MANUS. **p. media digitorum manus** [NA] The short middle bone of each of the medial four fingers, situated between the proximal and the distal phalanx. Its oval base has two shallow depressions for articulation with the two condyles of the head of the proximal phalanx. The dorsal surface of the base receives part of the insertion of the extensor digitorum, while the palmar aspect of the shaft receives the flexor digitorum superficialis. The head is shaped like a pulley for articulation with the base of the distal phalanx. Also *middle phalanx of fingers.* **p. media digitorum pedis** [NA] The rather short and broad middle bone of each of the lateral four toes, situated between the narrower and longer proximal phalanx and the tiny distal phalanx. The oval base has two shallow depressions separated by a fine ridge for articulation with the two condyles of the head of the proximal phalanx. The pulley-shaped head articulates with the base of the distal phalanx. The plantar aspect of the base receives the insertion of the flexor digitorum brevis while the dorsal aspect receives that of extensor digitorum. The fibrous flexor sheath is attached to the margins of the shaft. Also *middle phalanx of toes.* **middle p. of fingers** PHALANX MEDIA DIGITORUM MANUS. **middle p. of toes** PHALANX MEDIA DIGITORUM PEDIS. **p. proximalis digitorum manus** [NA] The proximal long bone of each finger, located between the corresponding metacarpal and the middle phalanx except in the thumb, where the distal articulation is with the distal phalanx. The base has a single concave oval surface for articulation with the head of the metacarpal. The palmar surface of the shaft is flat while the dorsal surface is rounded, and the fibrous flexor sheath is attached to the palmar margins. The head is pulley-shaped for articulation with the two depressions on the base of the middle phalanx. In the fifth finger and especially in the thumb, the base receives the attachment of several tendons. Also *proximal phalanx of fingers.* **p. proximalis digitorum pedis** [NA] The most posterior of the three phalanges of the lateral four toes and of the two phalanges of the great toe. It articulates proximally with the head of a metatarsal at the metatarsophalangeal joint and distally with the base of the middle phalanx of the lateral four toes and the distal phalanx of the great toe at an interphalangeal joint. It presents a concave base proximally, a trochlea-shaped head and a curved shaft that is compressed from side to side. Also *proximal phalanx of toe.* **phalanges of toes** OSSA DIGITORUM PEDIS. **tufted p.** An enlargement of the tip of the terminal phalanx, a characteristic finding in acromegaly.

**phall-** \fal-\ PHALLO-.

**phallalgia** \fəlal′jə\ [PHALL- + -ALGIA] PHALLODYNIA.

**phallanastrophe** \fal′anas′trəfē\ [PHALL- + Gk *anastrophē* a turning up or back] Upward curvature of the penis.

**phallectomy** \fəlek′təmē\ [PHALL- + -ECTOMY] PEOTOMY.

**phalli-** \fal′i-\ PHALLO-.

**phallic** \fal′ik\ [Gk *phallik(os)* pertaining to the phallus] **1** Relating to the penis. **2** In psychoanalysis, relating to

the penis during the infantile period of sexual development.
**phalliform** \falʹifôrm\ Shaped like the penis.
**phallin** \falʹin\ A hemolytic glycoside present in *Amanita phalloides.*
**phallitis** \falīʹtis\ [PHALL- + -ITIS] PENITIS.
**phallo-** \falʹō-, falʹə-\ [Gk *phallos* penis] A combining form denoting the penis. Also *phall-, phalli-.*
**phallocampsis** \-kampʹsis\ [PHALLO- + Gk *kampsis* a curving, bending] A curvature of the erect penis.
**phallocrypsis** \-kripʹsis\ [PHALLO- + Gk *krypsis* a hiding, concealment] A condition in which the penis is substantially retracted.
**phallodynia** \-dinʹē·ə\ [PHALL- + -ODYNIA] Pain affecting the penis. Also *phallalgia.*
**phalloid** \falʹoid\ Resembling a penis in appearance.
**phalloidin** \fəloiʹdin\ One of the poisons obtained from species of *Amanita,* especially from *A. phalloides.*
**phalloplasty** \falʹəplasʹtē\ [PHALLO- + -PLASTY] Any plastic operation on the penis. **reconstructive p.** The surgical reconstruction of the penis.
**phallorrhagia** \falʹôrāʹjə\ [PHALLO- + -RRHAGIA] A hemorrhage of the penis.
**phallorrhea** \falʹôrēʹə\ [PHALLO- + -RRHEA] A discharge from the penis.
**phallotomy** \falätʹəmē\ [PHALLO- + -TOMY] An incision of the penis.
**phallus** \falʹəs\ [L, from Gk *phallos* the penis] (*pl.* phalli) **1** PENIS. **2** The precursor in the embryo of the penis or clitoris before either has become sexually differentiated. It develops from the genital tubercle situated at the cranial end of the cloacal membrane.
**phanero-** \fanʹərō-\ [Gk *phaneros* visible, manifest] A combining form meaning visible, manifest.
**phanerogenic** \-jenʹik\ [PHANERO- + -GENIC] Of known origin or etiology, as a disease. Also *phanerogenetic.* Compare CRYPTOGENIC.
**phanerosis** \fanʹərōʹsis\ [PHANERO- + -SIS] **1** The processes of becoming visible. **2** The manifestation of a substance that had been inapparent because it was held in combination.
**phantasia** \fantāʹzhə\ FANTASY.
**phantasm** \fanʹtazm\ [Gk *phantasm(a)* (from *phantazein* to make visible) a phantasm, image, dream, vision, image presented to the mind by an object] An illusion or hallucination, usually recognized as such by the affected individual.
**phantogeusia** \fanʹtəjooʹsē·ə\ PSEUDOGEUSIA.
**phantom** **1** A mass of material that simulates living tissue, particularly the tissue's characteristic absorption and scattering of radiation. **2** Nonexistent but being the apparent source of sensation, especially pain that appears to issue from the site of a limb that has been amputated, as *phantom limb.* **3** GHOST. **flood p.** A phantom uniformly filled with an appropriate concentration of radioactive material. The usual purpose is to evaluate the uniformity of the field of view of the scintillation camera. **Schultze p.** An obstetric model of a female pelvis used to demonstrate the process of vaginal delivery.
**phar** **1** pharmacy. **2** pharmaceutical. **3** pharmacopeia.
**Phar. D.** doctor of pharmacy.
**Phar. M.** *Pharmaciae Magister* (L, Master of Pharmacy).
**pharm** **1** pharmacy. **2** pharmaceutical. **3** pharmacopeia.
**pharmaceutical** \fărʹməsooʹtikəl\ [Gk *pharmakeutikos* (from *pharmakeuein* to administer drugs, from *pharmakon* a drug) of or relating to drugs] **1** Pertaining to pharmaceutics. **2** Pertaining to medicinal drugs. **3** A medicinal drug. For defs. 1, 2, and 3 also *pharmaceutic.*
**pharmaceutics** \fărʹməsooʹtiks\ The field of knowledge involving the preparation, development, usage, and distribution of drugs.
**pharmacist** \fărʹməsist\ One qualified by education and training to prepare and dispense drugs by prescription. Pharmacists are licensed in conformity with the law applying to a particular jurisdiction. Also *chemist* (British usage), *apothecary* (older term), *pharmaceutist.*
**pharmaco-** \fărʹməkō-\ [Gk *pharmakon* medicine, drug] A combining form denoting drug.
**pharmacochemistry** PHARMACEUTICAL CHEMISTRY.
**pharmacodiagnosis** The use of drugs for diagnostic purposes, such as the use of edrophonium chloride in the diagnosis of myasthenia gravis.
**pharmacodynamics** \-dīnamʹiks\ The study of the effects of drugs on the body and the mechanisms by which drugs act.
**pharmacoepidemiology** \-epʹidēʹmē·älʹəjē \ The application of the principles of epidemiology to determine the effects of drugs among large populations.
**pharmacogenetics** \-jənetʹiks\ The study of genetic factors as they relate to the metabolism of and response to pharmacologic agents.
**pharmacognosist** A specialist in pharmacognosy.
**pharmacognosy** \-kägʹnəsē\ [PHARMACO- + Gk *gnōs(is)* knowledge + -Y] A branch of pharmacology that specializes in drugs obtained from plant and other natural sources, and their properties, preparation, and uses. Also *pharmacognostics.*
**pharmacography** A written account or treatise describing drugs.
**pharmacokinetics** The study of drug dynamics; the distribution of drugs in biological systems and the influence of absorption, tissue distribution, metabolism, and elimination by excretion on the disposition of a drug.
**pharmacologic** **1** Relating to pharmacology. **2** Designating the druglike properties or effects of a substance.
**pharmacologist** A specialist in pharmacology.
**pharmacology** [PHARMACO- + -LOGY] The science of drugs, including their origin, preparation, isolation, chemistry, effects, and uses. It involves or includes some aspects of pharmacognosy, pharmacokinetics, pharmacodynamics, therapeutics, and toxicology. **biochemical p.** The branch of pharmacology concentrating on drug biotransformations and the biochemical aspects of drug metabolism and drug action at a cellular or subcellular level. **marine p.** A branch of pharmacology concentrating on the identification, isolation, and development of drugs and pharmacologically active substances from aquatic plants and animals.
**pharmacometrics** The quantitative assessment of drug activity using bioassay techniques and chemical analyses to identify the pharmacologically active components and evaluate their efficacy.
**pharmacopedia** The science of the properties and preparation of drugs. Also *pharmacopedics.*
**pharmacopeia** \-pēʹə\ [Gk *pharmakopoiia* (from PHARMACO- + Gk *poiein* to make) preparation of drugs] **1** A formulary, especially an official one and usually one having legal force in all pharmacies of a given country, containing a description of drugs in current medical practice and noting their formulas, analytical composition if known, physical constants, main chemical properties useful in identification, and mode of preparation of compound preparations. Details may also be included of assay methods to regulate purity, content of active principle, preservation of quality, and, where appropriate, biologic potency. See also BRITISH PHAR-

MACOPOEIA, EUROPEAN PHARMACOPEIA, INTERNATIONAL PHARMACOPEIA, UNITED STATES PHARMACOPEIA. **2** The entire range of drugs used in medicine. For defs. 1 and 2 also *pharmacopoeia.*

**pharmacophore** A group of atoms believed to represent the critical region within a molecule that is responsible for the pharmacologic activity of the compound.

**pharmacopoeia** PHARMACOPEIA.

**pharmacoroentgenography** \-rent′genäg′rəfē\ Roentgenography of an organ or other body structure after the administration of a drug designed to change the function or appearance of the studied part in a manner to improve the examination. Also *pharmacoradiography.*

**pharmacotherapeutics** \-ther′əpyoo′tiks\ The study of the use of drugs as therapeutic agents, their administration, pharmacokinetics, and effectiveness, and their side effects and toxicity.

**pharmacotherapy** \-ther′əpē\ The treatment of disease by means of drugs.

**pharmacy** \fär′məsē\ [Gk *pharmakeia* (from *pharmakon* a drug) the use of drugs] **1** The science, art, and practice of preparing, preserving, compounding, and dispensing medicinal drugs and giving instructions for their use. **2** A place where pharmacy is practiced. **clinical p.** That branch of pharmacy concerned with the clinical application of drugs and their therapeutic value and effectiveness.

**Pharmacy and Poisons Act** Legislation enacted in 1933 in Great Britain that provided for an organization of registered pharmacists, a Poisons Board, and the establishment of a Poisons List to indicate which poisons could be sold by pharmacists only by prescription from physicians, dentists, or veterinary surgeons, and which could be bought directly by the public without prescription.

**pharyng-** \fəring-\ PHARYNGO-.

**pharyngeal** \fərin′jē·əl\ Pertaining to the pharynx.

**pharyngectomy** \far′injek′təmē\ [PHARYNG- + -ECTOMY] Excision of the pharynx for malignant disease. In practice this is never more than partial pharyngectomy.

**pharyngi-** \fərinjē-\ PHARYNGO-.

**pharyngitis** \far′ənjī′tis\ [Gk *pharynx* (gen. *pharyngos* or *pharygos*) the throat + -ITIS] Any one of the many varieties of inflammatory disease affecting the laryngopharynx, nasopharynx, or oropharynx. **acute p.** Acute inflammation of the pharynx, usually due to viral infection although bacterial superinfection commonly follows. In most cases, it is part of a more generalized upper respiratory infection such as the common cold. **acute lymphonodular p.** An acute, self-limiting infection of the fauces and oropharynx by a strain of the coxsackievirus. It is characterized by the eruption of discrete, whitish papules, chiefly on the faucial pillars and soft palate and in the oropharynx. Unlike the lesions of herpangina, these lesions do not vesiculate or ulcerate. Patients complain of sore throat, headache, and fever. **atrophic p.** Chronic pharyngitis marked by atrophy of the pharyngeal mucosa and, in particular, of the mucus glands. The posterior pharyngeal wall assumes a dry, glazed appearance. It often occurs secondary to atrophic rhinitis. **chronic p.** Chronic inflammation of the pharynx, usually secondary to chronic infection elsewhere in the respiratory tract, for instance in the paranasal sinuses. **follicular p.** HYPERTROPHIC PHARYNGITIS. **gangrenous p.** An unusually severe variety of sore throat identified as a rare entity distinct from diphtheria and perhaps a terminal complication of unrecognized blood diseases such as agranulocytosis and the leukemias. Gangrenous destruction of the faucial and pharyngeal tissues is described with spreading sometimes to the cheeks and lips. Also *necrotic angina* (obs.). **granular p.** HYPERTROPHIC PHARYNGITIS. **p. herpetica** HERPANGINA. **hypertrophic p.** Chronic pharyngitis characterized by conspicuous hypertrophy of the lymphoid nodules of the oropharynx and of the lateral bands of lymphoid tissue. The mucous glands may become involved, with their secretions diminished in quantity and viscid in consistency. Also *granular pharyngitis, follicular pharyngitis.* **p. keratosa** KERATOSIS PHARYNGIS. **p. sicca** Pharyngitis characterized by local damage to the mucus-secreting glands with corresponding drying of the pharyngeal mucosa. It often occurs as a late stage of hypertrophic pharyngitis. *Older term.* **ulceromembranous p.** Pharyngitis, usually acute pharyngitis, characterized by sore throat with pseudomembrane formation. A number of serious diseases present in this way including glandular fever, agranulocytosis, severe streptococcal infections of the throat, Vincent's angina, diphtheria, and acute leukemia. Also *ulcerated sore throat, ulceromembranous sore throat.*

**pharyngo-** \fəring′gō-\ [Gk *pharynx* (genitive *pharyngos* or *pharygos*) throat] A combining form denoting the pharynx. Also *pharyng-, pharyngi-.*

**pharyngocele** \fəring′gōsēl\ [PHARYNGO- + -CELE[1]] HYPOPHARYNGEAL DIVERTICULUM.

**pharyngoconjunctivitis** \-kənjungk′tivī′tis\ Pharyngitis and conjunctivitis occurring at the same time, as in pharyngoconjunctival fever.

**pharyngoesophagoplasty** \fəring′gō·ēsäf′əgōplas′tē\ [PHARYNGO- + ESOPHAGO- + -PLASTY] A plastic operation on the pharynx and esophagus.

**pharyngoesophagus** \fəring′gō·ēsäf′əgəs\ PARS LARYNGEA PHARYNGIS.

**pharyngolaryngectomy** \-lar′injek′təmē\ Total laryngectomy combined with partial pharyngectomy for the resection of certain malignant tumors of the laryngopharynx and cervical esophagus. Also *laryngopharyngectomy.*

**pharyngolaryngitis** \-lar′injī′tis\ LARYNGOPHARYNGITIS.

**pharyngomaxillary** \-mak′siler′ē\ Of or relating to the pharynx and the maxilla. Also *maxillopharyngeal.*

**pharyngonasal** \-nā′zəl\ NASOPHARYNGEAL.

**pharyngoparalysis** \-pəral′isis\ PHARYNGEAL PALSY.

**pharyngopathy** \far′ing·gäp′əthē\ [PHARYNGO- + -PATHY] Disease of the pharynx.

**pharyngoplasty** \fəring′gōplas′tē\ [PHARYNGO- + -PLASTY] **1** An operation utilizing a pharyngeal flap. **2** Any plastic operation on the pharynx. **Hynes p.** Pharyngoplasty utilizing a superiorly based mucomuscular flap to narrow the pharynx and the nasopharyngeal isthmus. Its purpose is to improve speech deficiencies resulting from cleft palate.

**pharyngoplegia** \-plē′jə\ [PHARYNGO- + -PLEGIA] PHARYNGEAL PALSY.

**pharyngorhinitis** \-rīnī′tis\ Inflammation of the lining of the pharynx and of the nose. It is a common occurrence in such upper respiratory infections as the common cold. Also *rhinopharyngitis.*

**pharyngoscleroma** \-sklirō′mə\ Scleroma of the pharynx, spreading there from the nose in a small proportion of cases, and producing the same nodular granulomatous lesions as characterize rhinoscleroma.

**pharyngoscope** \fəring′gəskōp\ [PHARYNGO- + -SCOPE] ESOPHAGEAL SPECULUM.

**pharyngoscopy** \far′ing·gäs′kəpē\ [PHARYNGO- + -SCOPY] Examination of the interior of the pharynx, usually by endoscopic means.

**pharyngostenosis** \-stenō′sis\ **1** Narrowing of any of the three constituent components of the pharynx from whatever cause. **2** Cicatricial stricture of the pharynx.

**pharyngostoma** \-stō′mə\ [PHARYNGO- + Gk *stoma* mouth] The opening created by pharyngostomy. Also *pharyngostome.*

**pharyngostomy** \far′ing·gäs′təmē\ [PHARYNGO- + -STOMY] The surgical fashioning of an opening into the hypopharynx from the front or lateral side of the neck.

**pharyngotomy** \far′ing·gät′əmē\ [PHARYNGO- + -TOMY] Any operation entailing incision of the pharynx. **anterior p.** External pharyngotomy performed through a transverse incision centered on the midline at the level of the hyoid bone. The oropharynx is entered in the vallecular region, the thyrohyoid membrane having been incised transversely. The procedure is a relatively simple means of access to tumors of the lower pharynx and epilarynx. Also *transhyoid pharyngotomy, infrahyoid pharyngotomy, subhyoid pharyngotomy, transverse pharyngotomy.* **external p.** Pharyngotomy performed from without, that is by way of a skin incision in the neck. **infrahyoid p.** ANTERIOR PHARYNGOTOMY. **internal p.** Pharyngotomy performed from within the pharynx, as, for example, the peroral incision of a retropharyngeal abscess. **lateral p.** External pharyngotomy using a skin incision over the lateral aspect of the larynx and entailing removal of the ipsilateral half of the hyoid bone and posterior two thirds of the thyroid ala. The procedure is indicated for removal of limited tumors of the pharynx and supraglottic larynx. Also *transthyroid pharyngotomy.* **median p.** An external pharyngotomy performed by way of a median incision through the lower lip and submental skin and entailing the division of the mandible and splitting of the tongue and floor of the mouth in the midline. The procedure is indicated for limited tumors at the back of the tongue and on the posterior pharyngeal wall. Also *translingual pharyngotomy.* **subhyoid p.** ANTERIOR PHARYNGOTOMY. **transhyoid p.** ANTERIOR PHARYNGOTOMY. **translingual p.** MEDIAN PHARYNGOTOMY. **transthyroid p.** LATERAL PHARYNGOTOMY. **transverse p.** ANTERIOR PHARYNGOTOMY.

**pharyngotyphoid** \-tī′foid\ Typhoid ulceration of the lymphoid tissue of the pharynx, liable to occur in one to two percent of cases of typhoid fever. Also *ulceration of Daguet* (obs.).

**pharynx** \far′ingks\ [Gk, the joint opening of the gullet and windpipe, the windpipe, throat, neck] [NA] The musculomembranous tubular passage of the digestive tube that extends from the base of the cranium to the esophagus at the level of the cricoid cartilage. Anteriorly its cavity communicates with the nasal, oral, and laryngeal cavities. Posteriorly it is related to the bodies of the first six cervical vertebrae. It is subdivided into pars nasalis pharyngis, pars oralis pharyngis, and pars laryngea pharyngis. **laryngeal p.** PARS LARYNGEA PHARYNGIS. **oral p.** PARS ORALIS PHARYNGIS. **primitive p.** The early embryonic pharynx from which its related pouches develop.

**phase** [Gk *phasis* (from *phainein* to bring to light, make to appear, show) the appearance of a heavenly body, a phase of the moon] **1** An identifiable part of a process or cycle often marked by a pattern of recurrence. **2** A physically or chemically distinct state, as *liquid phase.* **3** The fractional part of a period through which a wave variable has advanced. **active p.** A period of labor characterized by the relatively rapid and progressive dilatation of the cervix. It begins when 3 or 4 cm of cervical dilatation has occurred, following the latent phase, and extends to full cervical dilatation. Also *active labor.* **alpha p.** PROLIFERATIVE PHASE. **anal p.** The phase of psychosexual development during which the libido is concentrated in the area of the anus. The characteristics of the compulsive personality are said to originate during this phase. Also *anal stage.* **apophylactic p.** NEGATIVE PHASE. **aqueous p.** The water component of a mixture containing water. **beta p.** SECRETORY PHASE. **coupling p.** COUPLING. **p. of decline** The phase in a bacterial culture, late in the stationary phase, when the number of viable organisms begins to decline. **diastolic p. of contraction** The period of relaxation of the uterine musculature following the peak of a contraction. **diastolic isometric p.** The early period of diastole between closure of the semilunar and opening of the atrioventricular valve, when the pressure of the ventricular contents is diminishing but the volume not increasing. **disperse p.** The component of an emulsion which is the analogue of the solute in a solution. Thus in Freund's adjuvant, a water-in-oil emulsion, where the aqueous phase is dispersed in oil, water is the disperse phase. **effective lethal p.** That period during development when an organism is subject to the deleterious action of a lethal gene. **erythrocytic p.** The phase in the life cycle of malarial parasites in which schizogony and gametogony occur in the red blood cells. It is the clinical phase of malaria. **estrin p.** PROLIFERATIVE PHASE. **exponential p.** The phase of the bacterial growth cycle in which the logarithm of cell mass or number is proportional to time. It is also the phase of balanced growth, in which the average cell size and composition is constant. Also *logarithmic phase.* **genital p.** The final stage of psychosexual development, during which adult genitality develops. Also *genital stage.* **inductive p.** In *in-vivo* sensitization, the time between introduction of the antigen and the appearance of a detectible immune response, either antibody production or cell-mediated immunity. Also *induction period.* **lag p.** The phase in which bacteria inoculated into fresh medium have not yet begun to multiply. The duration and even the occurrence of this phase depends on the medium and the recent history of the inoculated cells. Also *lag period.* **latency p.** LATENCY. **latent p.** The time during early labor when contractions become more frequent and regular but without rapid changes in cervical dilatation or descent of the fetal presenting part. **logarithmic p.** EXPONENTIAL PHASE. **luteal p.** SECRETORY PHASE. **meiotic p.** The period during gametogenesis during which the chromosome number of a cell is halved. Reduction occurs during the first meiotic division and results from the chromosome behavior during prophase I of meiosis. Also *reduction phase.* **menstrual p.** The time when menses occur during a menstrual cycle. **motofacient p.** The stage of muscular contraction characterized by an alteration in the external length of the muscle. **negative p.** A period of depressed antibody titer of the blood following the administration of antigens. Also *apophylactic phase.* **nephrographic p.** The aspect of a renal angiography or intravenous urography at which the renal parenchyma is maximally opacified. **nonmotofacient p.** The stage of muscular contraction during which there is altered tension but no alteration in external length of the muscle. **oedipal p.** The instinctual level during which the Oedipus complex reaches its height. Also *Oedipus period.* **oral p.** In psychoanalytic psychology, the developmental period extending from birth until approximately two years, when the main energies of the infant, including the energy of both sexual and aggressive drives, are concentrated on the mouth area and on feeding. Also *oral period, oral stage.* **oral-incorporative p.** That part of the oral phase marked by possessiveness and its derivatives, i.e., voracity, greed, and envy. Also *oral-sadistic stage.* **oral-sucking p.** PREAMBIVALENT PHASE. **phallic p.** The instinctual level during which libidinal and aggressive energies are concentrated in the genital area, typically between four and six years of age. Also *phallic stage.* **positive p.** A period of increasing antibody or opsonin titer that follows the temporary fall induced by injection of antigen into a host already immunized to that antigen. **postmeiotic p.** The phase of gametogenesis after meiosis has been completed. **postmenstrual p.** The few days just following menses in the early proliferative phase of the menstrual cycle. **preambivalent p.** The early objectless period of the oral stage. Also *oral-sucking phase.* **pregenital p.** All of the instinctual levels of psychic development preceding the genital phase, including the oral, anal, and phallic phases. **premeiotic p.** The phase of gametogenesis prior to the onset of the first division of meiosis. Also *prereduction phase.* **premenstrual p.** The last few days of the secretory phase of the menstrual cycle before the menstrual phase. **preoedipal p.** All of the instinctual levels of psychic development preceding the development of the Oedipus complex. **prereduction p.** PREMEIOTIC PHASE. **progestational p.** SECRETORY PHASE. **proliferative p.** The period in the estrous or menstrual cycle between menses and ovulation when estrogen is the dominant ovarian hormone and the endometrium begins to regenerate and grow in thickness. Also *proliferative stage, estrin phase, alpha phase.* **reduction p.** MEIOTIC PHASE. **repulsion p.** REPULSION. **secretory p.** The period in the menstrual cycle between ovulation and menses. In women it is normally 14 days, during which progesterone is the dominant ovarian hormone and the endometrium becomes more glandular and vascular in preparation for implantation of a fertilized ovum. Also *luteal phase, progestational phase, beta phase, progestational stage.* **specific p.** A characteristic of bacterial surfaces whereby only flagellar antigens are present and agglutination can be produced only by the application of antibodies specific for these antigens. **stance p.** The phase of the gait cycle during which the foot is touching the ground. It consists of three parts: heel strike, mid-stance, and push-off. **stationary p.** The phase in a bacterial culture when net growth has ceased. In the transition from the exponential phase to this phase, the cells become smaller and their RNA/DNA ratio decreases. **supernormal recovery p.** A short period of increased excitability of heart muscle following conclusion of systole and represented by the U wave of the electrocardiogram. **swing p.** The phase of the gait cycle during which the foot is not in contact with the ground. It is divided into three parts: acceleration, swing-through, and deceleration. **synaptic p.** SYNAPTENE. **systolic p. of contraction** The period of progressive contraction of the uterine musculature during labor which precedes the acme of the contraction.

**phasic** \fā′zik\ Of, relating to, or occurring in phases. • In neurophysiology, *phasic* is often used in contrast to *static* and implies rapid changes.

**phasmid** \faz′mid\ [Gk *phasm(a)* an apparition, monster + -ID[1]] **1** A member of the class Secernentea (or Phasmidia). **2** One of a pair of minute caudal organs that function as chemoreceptors with openings at the terminal fine papillae behind the anus. They are characteristic of this class of nematodes. **3** An insect belonging to the orthopteran family Phasmidae; a walkingstick.

**Phasmidia** \fazmid′ē·ə\ A former name for SECERNENTEA.

**Ph.D.** Doctor of Philosophy.

**Phe** Symbol for phenylalanine.

**Phelps** [Abel Mix *Phelps,* U.S. surgeon, 1851–1902] See under OPERATION.

**Phemister** [Dallas Burton *Phemister,* U.S. orthopedic surgeon, 1882–1951] See under OPERATION.

**phemitone** MEPHOBARBITAL.

**phen-[1]** \fen-\ PHENO-[1].

**phen-[2]** \fen-\ PHENO-[2].

**phenacaine hydrochloride** $C_{18}H_{22}N_2O_2{\cdot}HCl$. *N,N′*-Bis(4-ethoxphenyl)ethanimidamide hydrochloride. A local anesthetic applied topically to the conjunctiva.

**phenacemide** $C_9H_{10}N_2O_2$. *N*-(Aminocarbonyl)benzeneacetamide. A drug used as an anticonvulsant remedy in major and focal epilepsy. It is given orally. Also *phenacetylurea.*

**phenacetin** A commonly used analgesic drug, present in many nonprescription drug preparations. Also *acetophenetidin, acetphenetidin.*

**phenaceturic acid** *N*-(2-Phenylacetyl)glycine. This is the form in which phenylacetic acid is excreted in urine, having been conjugated with glycine.

**phenacetylurea** PHENACEMIDE.

**phenaglycodol** $C_{11}H_{15}ClO_2$. 2-(4-Chlorophenyl)-3-methyl-2,3-butanediol. A drug formerly used to treat anxiety. Its effectiveness has not been clearly demonstrated.

**phenakistoscope** \fē′nəkis′təskōp\ STROBOSCOPE.

**phenanthrene** The aromatic hydrocarbon formed by fusing two benzene rings to the 1,2- and 3,4-sides of a central one. Phenanthrene derivatives are often carcinogenic. Some phenanthrenes are formed by aromatization of steroids.

**phenazocine hydrobromide** $C_{22}H_{28}BrNO$. 1,2,3,4,5,6-Hexahydro-6,11-dimethyl-3-(2-phenethyl)-2,6-methano-3-benzazocin-8-ol. A synthetic narcotic agent with actions and uses like those of morphine. It is given orally or parenterally. Chronic use can lead to addition.

**phenazopyridine hydrochloride** $C_{11}H_{12}ClN_5$. 3-(Phenylazo)-2,6-pyridinediamine monohydrochloride. A red-violet, odorless powder used as oral tablets to reduce pain and discomfort in the urinary tract. Excretion of the drug causes the urine to be orange or red.

**phenbenicillin** α-Phenoxybenzylpenicillin. A semisynthetic penicillin that is absorbed when given orally and is resistant to acid. Also *fenbencillin.*

**phenbenzamine** $C_{17}H_{22}N_2$. *N,N*-Dimethyl-*N′*-phenyl-*N′*-phenylmethyl-1,2-ethanediamine. An antihistaminic agent usually given as the hydrochloride salt.

**phendimetrazine tartrate** $C_{12}H_{17}NO{\cdot}C_4H_6O_6$. 3,4-Dimethyl-2-phenylmorpholine tartrate. A sympathomimetic drug with actions like those of amphetamine. It is used orally as an anorectic agent in the treatment of obesity.

**phene** \fēn\ A genetically determined character that, by itself or in combination with other phenes, comprises the phenotype.

**phenelzine sulfate** $C_8H_{12}N_2{\cdot}H_2SO_4$. (2-Phenylethyl)hydrazine sulfate. A white powder with a pungent odor. It is a monoamine oxidase inhibitor and antidepressant drug which is given orally.

**phenethanol** Ph—$CH_2$—$CH_2OH$. 2-Phenylethanol, a compound important as a parent to some inhibitors and products of amine oxidases, which affect catecholamine metabolism.

**phenethicillin** $C_{17}H_{20}N_2O_5S$. A semisynthetic penicillin, the methyl analogue of penicillin V. It is resistant to acid hydrolysis.

**phenethicillin potassium** The monopotassium salt of phenethicillin. It is used orally against streptococcal and pneumococcal infections of the respiratory tract, for staphylococcal infections of the skin, and against fusospiroketosis. It has about the same uses as penicillin V. Also *α-phenoxyethylpenicillin potassium.*

**phenethyl** Ph—$CH_2$—$CH_2$—. The 2-phenylethyl group, which occurs substituted in epinephrine and related neurotransmitters.
**phenethylbiguanide** PHENFORMIN.
**phenetidin** A metabolite of phenacetin.
**phenetidinurea** DULCIN.
**phenformin** \fenfôr′min\ N′-β-Phenethylformamidinyliminourea, a condensed diguanide, formerly used as an oral hypoglycemic agent, of limited use in the treatment of diabetes mellitus. Its mechanism of action is uncertain but may involve raised peripheral glucose utilization, lowered glucose output by the liver, and interference with glucose absorption by the gut. In the United States the drug is not used because of its gastrointestinal toxicity and its tendency to cause severe lactic acidosis. Also *phenethylbiguanide.*
**phenformin hydrochloride** $C_{10}H_{15}N_5{\cdot}HCl$. *N*-(2-Phenylethyl)imidodicarbonimidic diamide monohydrochloride. An oral biguanide-type hypoglycemic agent. Because of some severe toxic effects, particularly lactic acidosis, this drug is no longer used in the United States.
**phenindamine** An antihistamine drug prescribed for the symptomatic relief of allergic disease. In contrast with the majority of such drugs, which produce drowsiness, this often has a noticeable stimulant effect and thus may be contraindicated at bedtime.
**phenindamine tartrate** $C_{23}H_{25}NO_6$. 2,3,4,9-Tetrayhdro-2-methyl-9-phenyl-1*H*-indeno[2,1-*c*]pyridine hydrogen tartate. A white powder with a bitter taste. It is given orally as an antihistaminic medication. It is less active than the promazines but does not produce drowsiness. It is also used in an ointment for relief of pruritic allergic skin conditions and insect bites or stings.
**phenindione** 2-Phenyl-1,3-indandione. An uncommonly used oral anticoagulant that blocks synthesis of prothrombin. Because hepatitis and agranulocytosis have followed its use, phenindione has not attained wide popularity in the United States.
**pheniramine** A yellowish, oily liquid with an aminelike odor, insoluble in water but solube in dilute acids, alcohol, benzene, chloroform, and ether. It is a synthetic antihistamine. Also *prophenpyridamine.*
**pheniramine maleate** $C_{16}H_{20}N_2{\cdot}C_4H_4O_4$. The maleate salt of pheniramine, used as an antihistaminic agent. It has the same pharmacologic properties as the parent drug.
**Phenistix** A paper test strip used to screen for phenylketonuria. Its behavior is based on the ferric chloride reaction for phenylpyruvic acid in urine. A proprietary name.
**phenmetrazine** $C_{11}H_{15}NO$. Tetrahydro-3-methyl-2-phenyl-1,4-oxazine. A central nervous stimulant used, usually as the hydrochloride, as an anorexic agent in dieting to correct obesity.
**pheno-**[1] \fē′nō-, fē′nə-\ [Gk *phainein* to appear, make clear] A combining form meaning appearing. Also *phen-*.
**pheno-**[2] \fē′nō-, fē′nə-, fen′ə-\ [English *phene,* from French *phène* (from Gk *phainein* to appear, make clear) benzene, from its use in illuminating gas] A combining form denoting a chemical group derived from benzene. Also *phen-*.
**phenobarbital** $C_{12}H_{12}N_2O_3$. 5-Ethyl-5-phenyl-2,4,6-(1*H*,3*H*,5*H*)pyrimidine trione. A barbiturate, administered orally, that has sedative, hypnotic, and anticonvulsant activities. Also *phenobarbitone, phenylmethylbarbituric acid, phenylethylbarbituric acid.*
**phenobarbital sodium** A white, crystalline salt of phenobarbital. It is a long-acting barbiturate with sedative and hypnotic, and anticonvulsant properties. It can be given orally, subcutaneously, intravenously, or intramuscularly. Also *sodium phenobarbital, sodium phenylethylbarbiturate.*
**phenobarbitone** PHENOBARBITAL.
**phenocopy** \fē′nəkäp′ē\ **1** A phenotype that is due largely to environmental influences but that closely resembles one of mendelian character. **2** An individual manifesting such a phenotype. Also *isophan.*
**phenol** \fē′nōl\ **1** Ph—OH. A toxic, crystalline solid. With water it forms two liquid phases, one rich in phenol. The hydroxyl group on the benzene ring has mildly acidic properties (p*K* 10). Phenol was once used as a disinfectant. Also *carbolic acid* (outmoded), *hydroxybenzene, phenyl hydrate, phenyl hydroxide.* **2** Any substance containing a hydroxyl group on an aromatic ring, such as tyrosine. **camphorated p.** An ointment containing phenol, camphor, and a liquid oily base. It has been used as a local anesthetic for toothache, but phenol may cause damage to tissues if applied in a concentrated form. **liquefied p.** A solution of phenol and water containing 80% phenol, prepared by adding water to phenol. It is a convenient form of phenol for compounding lotions and other medications. Also *phenol liquefactum.*
**phenolate** PHENOXIDE.
**phenolemia** \-lē′mē·ə\ The presence of phenols in the blood.
**phenolic** \fənō′lik\ **1** Relating to, resembling, or derived from a phenol. **2** A phenolic substance produced by plants.
**phenol oxidase** Any enzyme, such as tyrosine 3-monooxygenase, that oxidizes a phenol, usually by incorporating an oxygen atom from molecular oxygen and requiring a second reductant.
**phenolphthalein** A substance used as a pH indicator, prepared from phenol and phthalic anhydride. It loses a proton with a p*K* of 9.7 to change from colorless to reddish purple.
**phenol red** See under PHENOLSULFONPHTHALEIN.
**phenolsulfonic acid** Any of the three acids, *ortho-*, *meta-* and *para-*, of formula $C_6H_4(OH)$—$SO_3H$.
***o*-phenolsulfonic acid** A syrupy liquid, soluble in water, alcohol and glycerol. Less toxic and less caustic than phenol, it is used as an antiseptic in aqueous solutions of 2–5%.
***p*-phenolsulfonic acid** An acid forming colorless deliquescent needles, soluble in water, alcohol, and glycerol. It is used to prepare salts containing a phenolic function and used as antiseptics.
**phenolsulfonphthalein** A nontoxic, water-soluble dye that is used as a pH indicator, changing from yellow to reddish purple over the range of 6.8 to 8.4. It is used in a test of renal blood flow and renal tubular secretory capacity, in which context it is usually called PSP. When used as an indicator, it is often called phenol red. Abbr. PSP
**phenomenology** \finäm′ənäl′əjē\ [*phenomen(on)* + *o* + -LOGY] The systematic investigation of events and experiences as these occur in individual consciousness, directly and immediately as phenomena, rather than by interpretation or analysis into components or by a search for origins.

# phenomenon

**phenomenon** \finäm′ənän\ [Gk *phainomenon,* neut. pres. passive part. of *phainein* to bring to light, make to appear, show] Any event or condition apprehended by the senses, as a sign or symptom. **abstinence p.** WITHDRAWAL SYMPTOMS. **adhesion p.** IMMUNE-ADHERENCE PHENOMENON. **anaphylactoid p.** PSEUDOANAPHYLAXIS. **aqueous-influx p.** Entry of aqueous humor into an episcleral vein that has been temporarily blocked, indicating normal permeability of the trabecular meshwork. Also *Ascher's glass-rod phenomenon.* **Arthus p.** ARTHUS REACTION. **Ascher's glass-rod p.** AQUEOUS-INFLUX PHENOMENON. **Aschner's p.** OCULOCARDIAC REFLEX. **Ashman's p.** The occurrence of an aberrant ventricular beat during atrial fibrillation. It follows a short pause when the previous one has been normal or long. **Aubert's p.** The illusion of the tilting of a vertical light streak to the side opposite to the direction of the head when the head is slowly tilted in a dark room. **Austin Flint p.** See under AUSTIN FLINT MURMUR. **Babinski's p.** EXTENSOR PLANTAR RESPONSE. **Bell's p.** The reflex upward and lateral rotation of the eye associated with closure of the eyelids, that occurs when the facial nerve is paralyzed on the same side. Also *Bell sign.* **blood-influx p.** The flow of blood into an aqueous vein when its intravascular pressure is elevated, indicating a relative resistance to escape of the aqueous from the anterior chamber. **borrowing-lending hemodynamic p.** HEMATOMETAKINESIS. **Bowditch p.** STAIRCASE PHENOMENON. **break-off p.** A sensation of physical separation from earth that occurs in aircraft pilots flying alone at high altitudes. **Browning's p.** THERAPIA STERILISANS DIVERGENS. **cheek p.** Upward flexion of both arms with bending of the elbows, in patients with meningitis, when pressure is applied to both cheeks just under the zygomas. **clasp-knife p.** CLASP-KNIFE RIGIDITY. **cogwheel p.** COGWHEEL SIGN. **cold agglutination p.** The agglutination or clumping of erythrocytes that occurs at temperatures less than 32°C in the presence of certain immunoglobulins, usually of IgM type, called cold agglutinins. **critical epileptic phenomena** ICTAL EPILEPTIC MANIFESTATIONS. **crossed phrenic nerve p.** After hemisection of the cord above the origin of the phrenic nerve the hemidiaphragm on the same side is paralyzed, but if the opposite phrenic nerve is then divided or blocked the paralyzed hemidiaphragm again begins to contract. **crus p.** KERNOHAN SYNDROME. **Cushing's p.** The rise in systemic arterial blood pressure which follows a sudden and usually much greater rise in intracranial pressure. **Davenport p.** ORIGINAL ANTIGENIC SIN. **declamping p.** Sudden hypotension on release of a clamp on a large artery, especially the aorta, due to massive vasodilation in the area of previous ischemia. **Dejerine-Lichtheim p.** LICHTHEIM SIGN. **diaphragm p.** Changes in thoracic contour resulting from movement of the diaphragm during respiration. Also *Litten sign, diaphragm sign, phrenic phenomenon, Litten's diaphragm phenomenon, diaphragmatic phenomenon, phrenic wave.* **diaphragmatic p.** DIAPHRAGM PHENOMENON. **doll's head p.** OCULOCEPHALIC REFLEX. **Donath p.** Hemolysis of blood that occurs when a blood specimen is chilled to 5°C and then warmed to 37°C. The phenomenon is characteristic of the type of cold hemolysins that occur in paroxysmal cold hemoglobinuria, and is the basis of the Donath-Landsteiner test for this disease. **Doppler p.** DOPPLER EFFECT. **double pain p.** The dual sensation arising from a noxious stimulus, consisting of fast, pricking pain conveyed by thinly myelinated afferent axons and a dull, slow, persistent pain conveyed via unmyelinated axons. **Erb's p.** In a patient with tetany, during electrical stimulation of a muscle the anodal opening current is more effective in obtaining a response than the anodal closing current. **Erben's p.** ERBEN'S REFLEX. **erythrocyte adherence p.** The quality of red cells of sticking to other cells or particulate matter coated with an immune complex and complement, particularly with C3. **escape p.** MARCUS GUNN PUPILLARY PHENOMENON. **face p.** CHVOSTEK SIGN. **facialis p.** CHVOSTEK SIGN. **fern p.** CERVICAL MUCUS ARBORIZATION. **flicker p.** The occurrence of a steady visual image in response to intermittent flashes of light. **Foix and Thévenard p.** A sign of mild spasticity of the legs. When the patient stands upright, his feet together or slightly apart, and his chest is pressed lightly, both on the front and back, there is initially contraction of the tibialis anterior muscles, which may be followed by dorsiflexion of the great toe and sometimes of the other toes. **Fregoli's p.** FREGOLI'S ILLUSION. **Galassi's pupillary p.** ORBICULARIS PHENOMENON. **glass-rod p.** Occlusion of an aqueous vein by pressure with a glass rod will normally result in an inflow of aqueous humor from the limbal side of the vessel. **Goldblatt p.** GOLDBLATT HYPERTENSION. **Grasset's p.** The inability of a patient suffering from hemiparesis to lift both arms or both legs simultaneously, although he can lift each arm or leg separately. Also *Grasset sign, Grasset-Gaussel phenomenon, Grasset-Bychowski sign.* **great-toe p.** EXTENSOR PLANTAR RESPONSE. **Gunn's p.** MARCUS GUNN SYNDROME. **Gunn's pupillary p.** MARCUS GUNN PUPILLARY PHENOMENON. **halisteresis p.** Osteomalacia due to withdrawal of calcium salts from bone. **Hamburger p.** CHLORIDE SHIFT. **hand p.** RAIMISTE SIGN. **Hata p.** An exacerbation of an infectious disease when a small dose of a chemotherapeutic agent is administered. **Hayflick p.** The findings that mammalian diploid cells, when cultured *in vitro* have finite life-spans and that cells derived from embryonic tissue have longer life-spans than cells derived from adult tissue. ⟨*Experimental Cell Research* 37:614, 1965.⟩ **Hertwig-Magendie p.** SKEW DEVIATION. **hip-flexion p.** Reflex flexion of the hips in paraplegics with spasticity; a form of flexor withdrawal reflex. **Hochsinger's p.** In tetany, spontaneous flexion of the fingers at the metacarpophalangeal joints, as in the Trousseau sign, when digital pressure is applied over the medial aspect of the biceps brachii. **Hoeppli p.** An eosinophilic hyaline fringe sometimes observed around schistosome eggs found in granulomas or pseudotubercles. It is thought to be a complex of host globulin and egg antigen. **Hoffmann's p.** Lowered threshold of a sensory nerve to electrical and mechanical stimulation. It is seen in some forms of tetany. **Holmes rebound p.** When a patient with cerebellar dysfunction carries out a movement against resistance, if that resistance is suddenly withdrawn the limb moves rapidly and forcibly in the direction in which the force was being applied by the patient, who finds it difficult to arrest the movement. Also *Thomas sign, Holmes phenomenon, Holmes-Stewart phenomenon, rebound phenomenon, Holmes sign.* **Houssay p.** 1 Hypoglycemia and increased sensitivity to insulin following pituitary ablation in pancreatectomized experimental animals. 2 Increased insulin sensitivity in subjects who suffer destructive lesions of the pituitary, such as infarction, tumor, or pituitary apoplexy. **Huebener-Thomsen-Friedenreich p.** Agglutination of red blood cells induced by ABO-compatible serum and caused by anti-T and anti-Tn antibodies which are present in the serum of all individuals except infants. This polyagglutination phenomenon is associated with contamination of red cell suspensions with certain neuraminidase-producing bacteria. The enzyme exposes the T-antigen, which is a public cryptoantigen. Also *Thomsen* *phenomenon, Thomsen-Friedenreich phenomenon.* **Hunt's paradoxical p.** In torsion dystonia, extension of the affected foot in response to passive flexion and flexion in response to attempted passive extension. Also *paradoxical phenomenon of dystonia.* **iceberg p.** The supposition that the known or declared prevalence of disease is but a part of the total prevalence, on analogy with the small visible portion of an iceberg above the water level. **ideomotor p.** IDEOMOTION. **immune-adherence p.** The property in an antigen-antibody reaction in which activated complement factors adhere to red cell membranes. Also *adhesion phenomenon, red cell adherence phenomenon.* **inattention p.** A sign sometimes observed in lesions of the parietal lobe: sensory stimuli applied independently to one half of the body are experienced normally, but when two comparable points on opposite sides are stimulated simultaneously the sensation upon the side of the body contralateral to the lesion is not felt or is ignored. Also *sensory inattention, extinction.* **intercritical epileptic phenomena** INTERICTAL EPILEPTIC MANIFESTATIONS. **interference p.** **1** The interference of one drug with the action of another, particularly in the case of drug-fastness of a parasite toward a full dose of one therapeutic agent, caused by subtherapeutic doses of another. **2** The interference with replication or reduction of virulence of a virus by simultaneous infection with another. **interictal epileptic phenomena** INTERICTAL EPILEPTIC MANIFESTATIONS. **inverse Marcus Gunn p.** MARIN AMAT SYNDROME. **inverted Marcus Gunn p.** MARIN AMAT SYNDROME. **irradiation p.** The overestimation of the size of an object that is caused by a difference in illumination between the object and its background. **Isakower p.** BLANK HALLUCINATION. **jaw-winking p.** MARCUS GUNN SYNDROME. **Jod-Basedow p.** IODINE-INDUCED HYPERTHYROIDISM. **Kanagawa p.** The $\beta$-hemolysis of *Vibrio parahaemolyticus* on a special blood agar. **Kleist's opposition motor p.** MAYER-REISCH PHENOMENON. **Köbner's p.** ISOMORPHIC EFFECT. **Kühne's muscular p.** Progression of a wave of contraction from the positive to the negative pole upon passage of a direct current through muscular tissue or a muscle fiber. Also *Porret's phenomenon.* **Lavrentiev's p.** The concept that each vagal axon to the GI tract innervates numerous postganglionic cells. Also *multiplication phenomenon of Lavrentiev.* **LE cell p.** The demonstration of the ability of polymorphonuclear leukocytes to ingest and display as a large homogeneous inclusion nuclear material in the presence of antinucleoprotein antibody and complement. The LE cell phenomenon is characteristically positive in patients with systemic lupus erythematosus, but is not specific for this disease. **Leede-Rumpel p.** RUMPEL-LEEDE PHENOMENON. **leg p.** SCHLESINGER SIGN. **Lichtheim's p.** LICHTHEIM SIGN. **lip p.** LIP REFLEX. **Litten's diaphragm p.** DIAPHRAGM PHENOMENON. **Lucio p.** The distinctive reactional state occurring in patients with Lucio leprosy. Also *erythema necroticans, lepra manchada, spotted leprosy.* **Lust's p.** LUST SIGN. **Lyon p.** In female eutherian mammalian embryos, at a particular stage of embryogenesis (usually at the blastocyst stage) one of their two X chromosomes is inactivated on a random basis. Consequently, during subsequent development the individual is a mosaic for heterozygous X-linked genes, and since once inactivation of either the maternally or paternally derived X chromosome takes place, all cells that develop from this small group of stem cells will have the same X chromosome inactivated. By this mechanism, dosage compensation for X-linked genes is brought about so that the same level of X-linked gene activity will be present in both male and female somatic cells. The inactive X chromosome usually replicates its DNA later in the cell cycle than the active X chromosome and the autosomes, is genetically inactive and heterochromatic, and may be seen in certain interphase cells as the sex chromatin (or Barr) body. All X chromosomes in excess of one are normally inactivated. Also *Lyon-Russell hypothesis, Lyon hypothesis, lyonization, inactive X hypothesis.* **Marcus Gunn p.** MARCUS GUNN SYNDROME. **Marcus Gunn pupillary p.** Recognition of a quantitative difference in the pupillary light reflex between the two eyes by means of alternately illuminating the pupils of the two eyes and observing the difference in pupillary constriction. Also *Gunn's pupillary phenomenon, Gunn's pupillary sign, Marcus Gunn pupillary sign, Kestenbaum sign, swinging flashlight sign, escape phenomenon.* **Marin Amat p.** MARIN AMAT SYNDROME. **Mayer-Reisch p.** Resistance to passive movement, comprising either extension or flexion of a limb according to the passive movement performed. This may be present in some degree in normal subjects. It is more marked in infants and may be exaggerated in patients with frontal lobe lesions. Also *Kleist's opposition motor phenomenon.* **Meirowsky p.** The darkening of existing melanin in the skin of living subjects within minutes of exposure to long-wave ultraviolet radiation or in skin taken post mortem when warmed to normal body temperature. **multiplication p. of Lavrentiev** LAVRENTIEV'S PHENOMENON. **neck p.** LHERMITTE SIGN. **negative glass-rod p.** Occlusion of an aqueous vein by pressure with a glass rod will normally result in an inflow of aqueous humor from the limbal side of the vessel. When this does not occur, the cause may be increased resistance to flow across the trabecular meshwork. **Negro's p.** COGWHEEL SIGN. **Neisser-Wechsberg p.** COMPLEMENT DEVIATION. **Neufeld's p.** The lysis of pneumococci by bile salts. **Orbeli p.** ORBELI EFFECT. **orbicularis p.** Contraction of the pupil followed by dilatation of the pupil after vigorous contraction of the orbicularis oculi. Also *Piltz-Westphal phenomenon, Galassi's pupillary phenomenon, Westphal-Piltz phenomenon, Westphal's phenomenon.* **Orgel p.** ERROR CATASTROPHE. **paradoxical diaphragm p.** A paralyzed diaphragm or hemidiaphragm moves upwards on inspiration and downwards on expiration, i.e. in the opposite direction to normal. **paradoxical p. of dystonia** HUNT'S PARADOXICAL PHENOMENON. **peroneal-nerve p.** LUST SIGN. **Perroncito's p.** Random and aberrant proliferation of axons in the proximal stump of a divided nerve. Also *apparatus of Perroncito, Perroncito spirals.* **Pfeiffer p.** Lysis of *Vibrio cholerae* in the peritoneal cavity of a guinea pig previously immunized against cholera. Also *Pfeiffer reaction.* **phi p.** APPARENT MOVEMENT. **phrenic p.** DIAPHRAGM PHENOMENON. **Piltz-Westphal p.** ORBICULARIS PHENOMENON. **Porret's p.** KÜHNE'S MUSCULAR PHENOMENON. **postcritical epileptic phenomena** POSTICTAL EPILEPTIC MANIFESTATIONS. **precritical epileptic phenomena** PREICTAL EPILEPTIC MANIFESTATIONS. **prezone p.** PROZONE PHENOMENON. **private cinema p.** Formed visual hallucinations of remembered people or scenes, as if in a cinema, experienced sometimes in attacks of temporal lobe epilepsy but more often in the phobic-anxiety-depersonalization syndrome. **pronation p.** **1** A form of synkinesia seen in patients with spastic flexion contracture of the arm at the elbow. Active flexion at this joint is accompanied by involuntary pronation, and voluntary elevation of the shoulder provokes abduction of the arm, with pronation and flexion of the forearm. Also *von Strümpell sign, Strümpell sign.*

2 In patients with hemiplegia, the paralyzed forearm and hand involuntarily assume a prone position when passively placed in a supine position. **prozone p.** The diminution or abrogation of an antigen-antibody reaction because the antibody is present in excess. It is seen most frequently in immunodiffusion techniques where precipitation will be absent or suboptimal in areas of antibody excess. Pronounced antibody excess may also affect agglutination by interfering with lattice formation, the second stage of agglutination, although it does not inhibit antibody attachment, the first stage of agglutination. Also *prezone phenomenon, prozone reaction.* **Purkinje p.** PURKINJE EFFECT. **Queckenstedt's p.** QUECKENSTEDT'S TEST. **quellung p.** QUELLUNG REACTION. **radial p.** The reflex wrist dorsiflexion elicited by phalangeal flexion and dependent on radial nerve innervation. **Raynaud's p.** A syndrome of unknown cause characterized by episodic "tricolor" changes of the skin of the digits: blanching, with numbness and pain; cyanosis; then redness with cutaneous burning. These changes probably represent digital vasospasm followed by capillary stasis and finally the vasodilatation of reactive hyperemia. In contrast to Raynaud's disease, Raynaud's phenomenon is frequently associated with an underlying collagen (vascular) disease, such as scleroderma. Also *Raynaud syndrome, symmetric asphyxia.* **rebound p.** See under HOLMES REBOUND PHENOMENON. **reclotting p.** THIXOTROPY. **red cell adherence p.** IMMUNE-ADHERENCE PHENOMENON. **release p.** The increased muscle tone and hyperreflexia following some supraspinal disruption or pathology involving the extrapyramidal system. **Riddoch's p.** MASS REFLEX. **R-on-T p.** The occurrence in an electrocardiogram of a ventricular premature beat on the T wave of the preceding conducted beat. It is associated with an increased risk of ventricular fibrillation. **Rumpel-Leede p.** The formation of petechiae distal to a tourniquet producing venous obstruction on the arm for a period of ten minutes. It is characteristic of hemorrhagic diastheses and certain infectious diseases such as scarlet fever. Also *Rumpel-Leede sign, bandage sign, endothelial symptom, Leede-Rumpel phenomenon.* **Sanarelli's p.** SHWARTZMAN PHENOMENON. **satellite p.** The occurence of satellite colonies; syntrophism. **Schlesinger's p.** SCHLESINGER SIGN. **Schramm's p.** A funnel-like deformity of the bladder neck and posterior urethra seen usually in the neurogenic bladder of tabes dorsalis, less often in neurogenic bladder dysfunction due to other spinal cord lesions. Also *funnel-neck prostate.* **second-set p.** The accelerated rejection by the recipient of a second allogenic graft of tissue from the same donor as a result of the primary immune response to the first graft. Also *second-set reaction.* **setting sun p.** RISING SUN SIGN. **Sherrington p.** A slow muscle contraction in response to sciatic nerve stimulation that occurs after allowing time for nerve degeneration following a section of the nerve roots. **shot-silk p.** WATERED-SILK RETINA. **Shwartzman p.** A cutaneous reaction in which an area of skin previously exposed to an intradermal endotoxin undergoes hemorrhagic necrosis if the animal receives, 18 to 36 hours later, a small intravenous dose of endotoxin. The endotoxin-induced activation of complement, platelets, and neutrophils does not involve antibodies, and can be prevented by aspirin or heparin. Also *Shwartzman reaction, Shwartzman-Sanarelli phenomenom, Sanarelli's phenomenom, Sanarelli-Shwartzman reaction.* **Solovieff's p.** A spasm of the diaphragm occurring in tetany. **Soret p.** SORET EFFECT. **staircase p.** Successive increased amplitude of cardiac muscle contraction in response to appropriately spaced electrical shocks of equal intensity. Also *treppe effect, Bowditch phenomenon, staircase.* **Strassman's p.** Continued engorgement of the umbilical veins following delivery of an infant. It is a sign of failure of the placenta to detach. **p. of successive contrast** The appearance of an image of complementary color but of the same size and shape immediately following the removal of a visual stimulus. **Sulzberger-Chase p.** The inhibition of contact hypersensitivity to an antigen by prior oral feeding of the antigen. It is thought to be mediated by the induction of antigen-specific T suppressor cells from Peyer's patches in the intestinal mucosa. **Thomsen p.** HUEBENER-THOMSEN-FRIEDENREICH PHENOMENON. **Thomsen-Friedenreich p.** HUEBENER-THOMSEN-FRIEDENREICH PHENOMENON. **tibial p.** STRÜMPELL SIGN. **tip-of-the-tongue p.** The experience of being unable to recall a certain word, name, book title, etc., although quite certain that one knows it, and firmly rejecting suggestions that do not fill this gap in memory properly even though the item is not otherwise retrievable. The fact that incorrect elements come to mind which are related in some way to the unsuccessfully sought memory is taken as evidence that material in the long-term memory store is organized. **toe p.** EXTENSOR PLANTAR RESPONSE. **tongue p.** A persistent depression in the tongue following a sharp blow, seen in myotonia. **treadmill p.** FELTON'S PARALYSIS. **Trousseau's p.** TROUSSEAU SIGN. **Tullio p.** Vertigo induced by loud high-pitched sounds. The sounds produce stimulation of the ampullary cristae of the semicircular canals of the inner ear and thus vertigo. Patients who underwent the fenestration operation were often subject to the Tullio phenomenon even though the stapes remained mobile. **Tyndall p.** TYNDALL EFFECT. **Wartenberg's p.** In patients with facial paralysis a vibratory movement that can be felt when the eyeball is lightly pressed through the closed eyelid. This movement is less on the affected than on the unaffected side. *Seldom used.* Also *Bergara-Wartenberg sign.* **Wassermann-Takaki p.** The neutralization of tetanus toxin by brain fractions containing the ganglioside that binds the toxin to the cell membrane. **Wedensky's p.** The failure of a muscle to contract in response to repetitive electrical stimuli at too rapid a rate for membrane recovery, though at slower rates larger amplitudes of contraction can occur with multiple than with single shocks. **Wenckebach's p.** WENCKEBACH BLOCK. **Westphal's p.** ORBICULARIS PHENOMENON. **Westphal-Piltz p.** ORBICULARIS PHENOMENON. **Wever-Bray p.** COCHLEAR MICROPHONICS. ⟨Wever, E.G. and Bray, C.W., *Psychological Review* 37:365, 1930.⟩ **zone p.** An observation applicable to agglutination, precipitation, or toxin neutralization reactions. It is based on the fact that optimum end points occur when an antigen and an antibody are present in optimal proportions, called the equivalence zone, whereas reduced activity occurs in the zones of antibody excess or antigen excess. Prezones (prozones) and postzones are test conditions showing reduced or absent agglutination in the zones of, respectively, antibody excess and antigen excess.

**phenothiazine** A drug of the neuroleptic class of psychotropic drugs. The phenothiazines are major tranquilizers and are commonly subdivided on the basis of chemical structure into aliphatic, piperidine, and piperazine groups. Also *dibenzothiazine.*

**phenotype** \fē′nətīp\ [PHENO-[1] + TYPE] **1** Any identifiable or observable structural or functional characteristic of an organism. It is determined by the combined influences of the genotype and the environment. **2** The total presentation of an organism, due to the collective influences of the entire genome and the environment. **Bombay p.** A very rare phenotype characterized by red cells which lack the A, B, and H antigenic determinants. Individuals with this phenotype usually develop the corresponding ABH antibodies. The Bombay red cells lack the H gene product which is responsible for the formation of the H antigen. Although the appropriate A and B transferases are present in the cells, they are unable to induce production of A and B antigens because of the lack of the precursor substance, H antigen.

**phenotypic** \-tip′ik\ **1** Of or pertaining to the phenotype. **2** Designating nongenetic, reversible responses to the environment, as opposed to genotypic changes.

**phenoxide** The anion produced by removing the hydroxyiic proton from a phenol. Also *phenolate.*

**phenoxy-** [PHEN- + OXY-] A combining form denoting the group Ph—O—.

**phenoxybenzamine hydrochloride** $C_{18}N_{22}ClNO$. *N*-(2-Chloroethyl)-*N*-(1-methyl-2-phenoxyethyl)benzylamine. An irreversible, alkylating agent used as an antihypertensive drug. The vasodilatation resulting from its use is due to its α-blocking action, preventing catecholamines from activating smooth muscle α-receptors that produce the normal degree of vasoconstriction.

**α-phenoxyethylpenicillin potassium** PHENETHICILLIN POTASSIUM.

**phenoxymethylpenicillin** PENICILLIN V.

**phenprocoumon** $C_{18}H_{16}O_3$. 4-Hydroxy-3-(1-phenylpropyl)-2*H*-1-benzopyran. An orally administered synthetic anticoagulant with longer lasting activity than dicoumarol. Its effects persist several days after treatment is discontinued.

**phensuximide** $C_{11}H_{11}NO_2$. *N*-Methyl-2 phenylsuccinimide. An analogue of ethosuximide, but not as potent as the latter. It is used in the treatment of petit mal epilepsy. The drug is given orally.

**phentermine hydrochloride** $C_{10}H_{16}ClN$. α,α-Dimethylbenzeneethanamine hydrochloride. An adrenergic amine very similar in structure and pharmacologic activity to amphetamine. It is given orally as an anorexic agent to treat obesity.

**phentolamine** 2-(*N′*-*p*-Tolyl-*N′*-*m*-hydroxyphenylaminomethyl)imidazoline. A compound with adrenergic blocking activity. It has been used in the treatment of hypertension as well as in the diagnosis of pheochromocytoma.

**phenyl** The group $C_6H_5$—, derived from benzene by removal of one hydrogen atom.

**phenylalanine** Ph—$CH_2$—$CH(NH_2)COOH$. One of the twenty amino acids that are incorporated into proteins. It is essential in the human diet.

**phenylalanine ammonia-lyase** An enzyme (EC 4.3.1.5) that catalyzes the removal of ammonia from L-phenylalanine forming a double bond in *trans*-cinnamate. The enzyme also acts on L-tyrosine.

**phenylalanine hydroxylase** PHENYLALANINE 4-MONOOXYGENASE.

**phenylalaninemia** \fen′ilal′ənin**ē′**mē·ə\ The presence of abnormally high levels of phenylalanine in the blood, as in newborn infants with phenylketonuria.

**phenylalanine 4-monooxygenase** The enzyme (EC 1.1.4.16.1) that catalyzes the conversion of phenylalanine into tyrosine, using molecular oxygen and concomitantly oxidizing a tetrahydropteridine. The disease phenylketonuria results from congenital lack of this enzyme. Also *phenylalanine hydroxylase.*

**phenylbutazone** $C_{19}H_{20}N_2O_2$. 4-Butyl-1,2-diphenyl-3,5-pyrazolidinedione. An analogue of antipyrine with analgesic, antipyretic, anti-inflammatory, and uricosuric properties. It has been used for acute arthritic conditions, bursitis, and other rheumatic conditions. Also *diphebuzol.*

**phenylene** The bivalent group $C_6H_4$=, derived from benzene by removal of two hydrogen atoms.

***p*-phenylene diamine** A compound used as a hair dye and as a dye for furs, hosiery, and blouses, and in photographic developing. It is a powerful allergen, causing dermatitis and asthma. Less commonly it causes systemic effects including subacute necrosis of the liver and a macrocytic type of anemia.

**phenylephrine hydrochloride** $C_9H_{13}NO_2{\cdot}HCl$. (*R*)-3-Hydroxy-α-[(methylamino)methyl]benzene methanol hydrochloride. An adrenergic agent with strong α-agonistic activity. It is used as a vasoconstrictor, a decongestant, and as a drug to produce mydriasis without cycloplegia in the eye. It has also been used to maintain the blood pressure during anesthesia. It is given intramuscularly, intravenously, or in eye drops.

**phenylethylbarbituric acid** PHENOBARBITAL.

**phenyl hydrate** PHENOL.

**phenylhydrazine** Ph—NH—$NH_2$. A reagent for carbonyl compounds, including sugars.

**phenylhydrazone** Ph—NH—N=CRR′. The compound formed by reaction of phenylhydrazine with a carbonyl compound.

**phenyl hydroxide** PHENOL.

**phenylketonuria** \fen′ilk**ē′**tənoo**′**rē·ə\ An autosomal recessive inborn error of phenylalanine metabolism due to a deficiency of the hepatic enzyme phenylalanine hydroxylase. Characteristic features are hyperphenylalaninemia, the urinary excretion of phenylpyruvate and hydroxyphenylacetate, microcephaly, moderate or severe mental retardation, fair skin and hair, and EEG abnormalities. It can be detected through newborn genetic screening programs and satisfactorily treated by reducing phenylalanine intake. Also *Fölling's disease* (outmoded), *phenylpyruvic oligophrenia.* Abbr. PKU **maternal p.** Physical and mental retardation with microcephaly seen in offspring of mothers with atypical phenylketonuria or those whose condition has been effectively controlled by treatment. The children of mothers with atypical phenylketonuria may or may not be phenylketonuric but many die in infancy and some may have congenital heart disease.

**phenyllactic acid** Ph—$CH_2$—CHOH—COOH. A metabolite of phenylalanine, formed reversibly from phenylpyruvate by dehydrogenases.

**phenylmercuric nitrate** $C_{12}H_{11}Hg_2NO_4$. An organic mercurial compound with antibacterial and antifungal properties. It is used as a preservative in very low concentration for solutions to be injected, eye drops, and other similar preparations.

**phenylmethylbarbituric acid** PHENOBARBITAL.

**phenylosazone** A compound formed by reaction of a sugar with phenylhydrazine. Since phenylosazones are crystalline and have defined melting points they were formerly extensively used for identifying sugars.

**phenylpropanolamine hydrochloride** $C_9H_{14}ClNO$. α-(1-Aminoethyl)benzenemethanol hydrochloride. A sympathomimetic drug that is used as a nasal decongestant and also for its bronchodilator properties.

**phenylpyruvate** Ph—$CH_2$—CO—$COO^-$. A substance formed metabolically from phenylalanine and present in blood and urine in phenylketonuria.

**phenylpyruvate tautomerase** The enzyme (EC 5.3.2.1) that increases the rate of interconversion of the keto and enol forms, Ph—$CH_2$—CO—COOH and Ph—CH=C(OH)—COOH, of phenylpyruvic acid. It occurs in animal tissues but its function is not clear.

**phenylpyruvic acid** Ph—$CH_2$—CO—COOH. A metabolite produced by transamination of phenylalanine. It is present in the urine in phenylketonuria, when hydroxylation of phenylalanine to form tyrosine in deficient. Urine is tested for it soon after birth so that treatment by restriction of phenylalanine in the diet may be started in time to avoid mental deficiency.

**phenylquinoline** $C_6H_5C_9H_6N$, a compound derived from quinoline and resembling quinine in action.

**phenyl salicylate** $C_{13}H_{10}O_3$. A white crystalline compound used in creams and ointments as a protective agent against sunburn. It has also been used in enteric coating for tablets and as an analgesic and antipyretic. Also *salol.*

**phenylthiocarbamide** $C_6H_5NHCSNH_2$. A compound used in the demonstration of mendelian variation and in genetic linkage studies in humans. The ability to taste this substance as bitter, present in about 70% of individuals, is due to the taster allele being present at the PTC locus in either the heterozygous or homozygous state. Tasting is thus a dominant trait. Inability to taste PTC requires the presence of homozygosity of the nontaster allele and is an autosomal recessive trait. Also *phenylthiourea.* Abbr. PTC

**phenylthiohydantoin** Ph—N—CS—NH—$CH_2$—CO—. Used particularly of derivatives in which one of the methylene hydrgen atoms is substituted. These derivatives are formed from the terminal residues of peptides and proteins when these are successively removed by treatment with phenylthiocyanate and then with acid.

**phenylthiourea** PHENYLTHIOCARBAMIDE.

**phenytoin** $C_{15}H_{12}N_2O_2$. 5,5-Diphenyl-2,4-imidazolidinedione. An anticonvulsant and antiepileptic agent. Practically insoluble in water, it is usually administered as the sodium salt. Also *diphenylhydantoin.*

**phenytoin sodium** The sodium salt of phenytoin. It is a commonly used form of this medication and has the same uses and properties as the parent compound. Also *sodium diphenylhydantoin, diphenylhydantoin sodium.*

**pheo-** \fē′ō-\ [Gk *phaios* twilight hue, dusky, dun] A combining form meaning brown or yellowish brown. Also *phaeo-* (British spelling).

**pheochrome** \fē′əkrōm\ Having the capacity to stain brown with chromic acid or dichromates by the formation of a precipitate containing chromium oxide; chromaffin.

**pheochromoblast** \-krō′məblast\ An embryonic cell which is the precursor of a pheochromocyte.

**pheochromocyte** \-krō′məsīt\ A cell which contains chromaffin or pheochrome material. In the adult such cells are restricted to the adrenal medulla, to small cell groups in the brainstem and to certain cells, enterochromaffin cells, in the intestinal mucosa. In the fetus they are more widely spread and can be found in sympathetic ganglia and paraganglia, which like the adrenal medulla are developed from the neural crest.

**pheochromocytoma** \-krō′məsītō′mə\ [*pheochromocyt(e)* + -OMA] A benign paraganglioma of the adrenal medulla or urinary bladder. Many secrete epinephrine and/or norepinephrine with resulting paroxysmal or continuous arterial hypertension. The tumor cells usually show a strong chromaffin reaction. Also *medullary paraganglioma, chromaffinoma, medullosuprarenoma, chromaffin-cell tumor, chromophil tumor.* **malignant p.** The malignant form of a pheochromocytoma.

**pheresis** \fərē′sis\ A widely used but incorrect term for HEMAPHERESIS. • See note at APHERESIS.

**pheromone** \fer′əmōn\ [Gk *pher(ein)* to bear, carry + *(hor)mone*] A body secretion that regulates the behavior of other individuals in a population, serving such functions as sex attractant, trail marker, or warning signal. Also *exohormone, ectohormone.*

**phial** \fī′əl\ VIAL.

**-phil** \-fil\ [Gk *-philos* -loving, from *philos* a friend] A combining form meaning one attracted to or fond of (something specified). Also *-phile.*

**-phile** \-fīl, -fil\ -PHIL.

**-philia** \-fil′ē·ə\ [Gk *philia* (from *philos* friend) love, friendship] A combining form signifying (1) a tendency or propensity; (2) excessive or morbid attraction to or fondness for.

**-philic** \-fil′ik\ [Gk *philia* love, friendship] A combining form meaning attracted to or fond of.

**Philip** [Sir Robert William *Philip,* Scottish physician, 1857–1939] Philip's glands. See under GLAND.

**Philippe** [Claudien *Philippe,* French anatomist, 1866–1903] Tract of Philippe-Gombault, triangular tract of Philippe-Gombault, Gombault-Philippe triangle. See under FASCICULUS TRIANGULARIS.

**philtrum** \fil′trəm\ [Gk *philtron* a love charm or potion, dimple of the upper lip] [NA] The vertical median groove on the external surface of the upper lip which represents the fused boundary zone between the median nasal processes of the fetus. In addition, some believe that the maxillary mesenchyme may contribute to its formation. Also *filtrum.*

**phimosiectomy** \fīmō′sē·ek′təmē\ [*phimosi(s)* + -ECTOMY] Circumcision employed as a treatment for phimosis.

**phimosis** \fimō′sis\ [Gk *phimōsis* (from *phimoun* to muzzle, gag, shut up as with a muzzle, from *phimos* a muzzle, nose band of a bridle + *-ōsis* -OSIS) a closing up, muzzling] Inability to retract the preputial skin behind the glans penis; unretractile foreskin. The tightness of the foreskin is usually of congenital origin, but may result from inflammation or edema. Also *capistration.* **labial p.** Swelling and scarring of the circumoral tissue to a degree that precludes opening the mouth sufficiently to accomplish normal oral functions. Also *oral phimosis.* **p. vaginalis** Abnormal smallness or narrowness of the vagina.

**phleb-** \fleb-\ PHLEBO-.

**phlebalgia** \flebal′jə\ [PHLEB- + -ALGIA] Pain arising from a vein or varix.

**phlebangioma** \fleb′anjē·ō′mə\ [PHLEB- + ANGIOMA] A venous aneurysm.

**phlebectasia** \fleb′ektā′zhə\ [PHLEB- + -ECTASIA] A chronic dilatation of veins. Also *phlebectasis, venectasia.*

**phlebectomy** \fləbek′təmē\ [PHLEB- + -ECTOMY] The removal of a vein. Also *venectomy.*

**phlebectopia** \fleb′ektō′pē·ə\ The location of one or more veins in an unusual anatomic site.

**phlebitic** \fləbit′ik\ Pertaining to or characterized by phlebitis.

**phlebitis** \fləbī′tis\ [PHLEB- + -ITIS] Inflammation of a vein. **adhesive p.** Phlebitis in which inflammation of the walls leads to their adherence with a tendency to obliteration of the vessel. Also *plastic phlebitis, proliferative phlebitis.* **blue p.** PHLEGMASIA CERULEA DOLENS. **p. migrans** A condition in which a number of peripheral veins are successively affected by phlebitis. Also *migrating phlebitis, phlebitis saltans.* **migrating p.** PHLEBITIS MIGRANS.

**obstructive p.** Phlebitis which leads to occlusion of a vein. Also *obliterating phlebitis.* **plastic p.** ADHESIVE PHLEBITIS. **productive p.** PHLEBOSCLEROSIS. **proliferative p.** ADHESIVE PHLEBITIS. **puerperal p.** Phlebitis, usually of the deep leg or pelvic veins, occurring during the postpartum period. **p. saltans** PHLEBITIS MIGRANS. **septic p.** SUPPURATIVE THROMBOPHLEBITIS. **sinus p.** Inflammation of an intracranial venous sinus. **suppurative p.** Phlebitis in which an infection becomes purulent. Also *suppurative venous thrombosis.*

**phlebo-** \fleb′ō-, fleb′ə-, flē′bō-\ [Gk *phleps* (genitive *phlebos*) vein] A combining form meaning vein. Also *phleb-.*

**phleboclysis** [PHLEBO- + Gk *klysis* (from *klyzein* to wash, wash away) a washing out] The intravenous injection of fluids. **drip p.** INTRAVENOUS DRIP. **slow p.** INTRAVENOUS DRIP.

**phlebodynamics** \-dīnam′iks\ The study of force and motion in the veins.

**phlebodynamometry** \-dī′nəmäm′ətrē\ A measurement of pressure gradients between venous segments, either at rest or after exercise.

**phlebofibrosis** \-fībrō′sis\ PHLEBOSCLEROSIS.

**phlebogenous** \flebäj′ənəs\ [PHLEBO- + -GENOUS] Of venous origin.

**phlebography** \flebäg′rəfē\ VENOGRAPHY.

**phlebolith** \fleb′əlith\ [PHLEBO- + -LITH] A concretion in a vein, probably due to calcification of a venous thrombus, occurring most commonly in the pelvis and visualized radiologically. Also *vein stone.*

**phlebolithiasis** \-lithī′əsis\ The presence of multiple phleboliths.

**phlebology** \flebäl′əjē\ [PHLEBO- + -LOGY] The study of the veins and the diseases affecting them.

**phlebomanometer** \-manäm′ətər\ [PHLEBO- + MANOMETER] An instrument for measuring venous blood pressure.

**phlebometritis** \-mētrī′tis\ [PHLEBO- + METRITIS] Inflammation of the uterus with thrombosis of blood vessels.

**phlebophlebostomy** \-flebäs′təmē\ A vein-to-vein anastomosis. Also *venovenostomy.*

**phleboplasty** \fleb′əplas′tē\ [PHLEBO- + -PLASTY] A plastic or reconstructive operation on a vein or veins.

**phleborheography** \-rē·äg′rəfē\ [PHLEBO- + RHEO- + -GRAPHY] A technique for diagnosing proximal venous occlusions by measuring the changes in limb volume with distal cuff inflation.

**phleborrhaphy** \flebôr′əfē\ [PHLEBO- + -RRHAPHY] Repair or reconstruction of a vein by suturing its wall.

**phlebosclerosis** \-sklirō′sis\ Fibrous thickening of a vein resulting from collagen deposition in the venous walls as a response to external trauma or venous hypertension. Also *venous sclerosis, venosclerosis, proliferative endophlebitis, productive phlebitis, venofibrosis, phlebofibrosis.* **portal p.** Fibronodular hardening of the portal vein.

**phlebostasis** \flebäs′təsis\ Stasis in a vein due either to pathological venous distension or as a result of the application of a tourniquet. When resulting from the application of tourniquets in order to reduce the central circulation, it is called bloodless phlebotomy. *Seldom used.*

**phlebostenosis** \-stenō′sis\ [PHLEBO- + STENOSIS] The narrowing or stenosis of a vein.

**phlebothrombosis** \-thrämbō′sis\ Venous thrombosis in the absence of inflammation.

**phlebotomist** \flebät′əmist\ One who draws blood from a vein, usually for testing purposes.

***Phlebotomus*** \fləbät′əməs\ [Gk *phlebotomos* vein-cutting (adj.), vein-cutter. See PHLEBOTOMY.] A genus of tiny sandflies (family Psychodidae) characterized by hairy wings held upward and outward that make a 60° angle with one another and the body. The females have bloodsucking mouthparts and feed on a variety of hosts ranging from frogs to humans. The group is of considerable medical interest as the Old World vector of species of *Leishmania* causing visceral and cutaneous leishmaniasis. Some 15 species have been incriminated. Species of *Phlebotomus* also transmit the bunyavirus of sandfly fever as well as orbiviruses of the Changuinola complex. ***P. argentipes*** A strongly anthropophilic species that transmits *Leishmania donovani,* the causative agent of kala-azar in India. ***P. chinensis*** The chief vector of kala-azar in northern and northeastern China, southern Manchuria, and central Asia. ***P. flaviscutellatus*** *LUTZOMYIA FLAVISCUTELLATA.* ***P. intermedius*** *LUTZOMYIA INTERMEDIA.* ***P. orientalis*** The sandfly vector of *Leishmania donovani* in the Sudan, cause of severe outbreaks of kala-azar in that region. Also *Phlebotomus langeroni* var. *orientalis..* ***P. papatasii*** A species that serves as the vector of *Leishmania tropica,* agent of the classical, urban, or dry type of cutaneous leishmaniasis in North Africa and the eastern Mediterranean. It is the principal vector in Iran and the Soviet Union for *L. major,* agent of the moist or rural zoonotic form of cutaneous leishmaniasis. It is also one of the vectors that can transmit the virus of sandfly fever. ***P. pessoai*** *LUTZOMYIA PESSOAI.* ***P. sergenti*** The principal transmitter of *Leishmania tropica,* the causal agent of urban or dry cutaneous leishmaniasis in the Middle East, the Soviet Union, and India and a secondary vector of *L. donovani* in northeast China, the cause of visceral leishmaniasis in that region. ***P. verrucarum*** *LUTZOMYIA VERRUCARUM.*

**phlebotomy** \flebät′əmē\ [Gk *phlebotomia* (from *phleps,* gen. *phlebo(s)* vein + *tomē* cutting, section) venesection, bloodletting] The insertion of a needle or cannula into a vein, usually for the purpose of removing blood. Also *venesection.* **bloodless p.** See under PHLEBOSTASIS.

**phlegm** \flem\ [Gk *phlegma* (from *phlegein* to burn) inflammation, heat, phlegm] **1** One of the four elemental body humors believed by the ancients to be the basis of health and disease. See under HUMORALISM. **2** Thick mucinous expectoration. *Popular.*

**phlegmasia** \flegmā′zhə\ [Gk (from *phlegma* the phlegmatic humor) inflammation, phlegmon] Severe inflammation. Also *phlegmonosis.* **p. alba dolens** Gross edema of the leg following parturition due to lymphatic obstruction associated with deep venous thrombosis. The swelling is unaccompanied by reddening. Also *cruritis, whiteleg, white leg, galactophlebitis, milk leg, thrombotic phlegmasia.* **cellulitic p.** Swelling of the leg in the postpartum period secondary to cellulitis in the soft tissues. **p. cerulea dolens** Acute and painful deep venous thrombosis associated with edema, cyanosis, purpuric areas, and petechiae, often complicated by circulatory collapse and shock. Also *blue phlebitis.* **thrombotic p.** PHLEGMASIA ALBA DOLENS.

**phlegmatic** \flegmat′ik\ Unemotional, dull, and somewhat sluggish in temperament, as if affected by an excess of phlegm, the humor in ancient physiology responsible for such characteristics.

**phlegmon** \fleg′män\ [Gk *phlegmonē* (from *phlegein* to burn, scorch, inflame) an inflammation, a festering] Suppurative inflammation of skin and subcutaneous tissues, usually caused by pyogenic microorganisms, particularly *Staphylococcus aureus.* It often progresses to ulceration, necrosis, and abscess formation. Also *phlegmona.*

**phlegmonosis** \fleg′mənō′sis\ PHLEGMASIA.

**phlegmonous** \fleg′mənəs\ Pertaining to or characterized by a phlegmon.

**phlogistic** \flōjis′tik\ PHLOGOGENIC.

**phlogo-** \flō′gō-, fläg′ō-\ [Gk *phlox,* gen. *phlogos* flame, fire] A combining form meaning inflammation, inflammatory.

**phlogocyte** \flō′gəsīt\ [PHLOGO- + -CYTE] Any white cell that participates in the inflammatory response. *Obs.*

**phlogogen** \flō′gəjən\ [PHLOGO- + -GEN] Any substance capable of producing inflammation.

**phlogogenic** \flō′gəjen′ik\ [PHLOGO- + -GENIC] Capable of causing an inflammatory response. Also *phlogistic.*

**phlorhidzin** A plant glycoside that damages the kidneys, lowering the renal threshold for glucose. Also *phlorizin, phlorrhizin, phloridzin.*

**phlorhidzinize** \flôr′ədzənīz′\ To treat an animal with phlorhidzin so that it excretes glucose, usually in order to study whether a substance to be investigated is transformed into glucose.

**phloridzin** PHLORHIDZIN.

**phlorizin** PHLORHIDZIN.

**phlorrhizin** PHLORHIDZIN.

**phloxine** \fläk′sin\ An acid red synthetic dye that is chemically related to eosin and is used to identify various intracytoplasmic structures.

**phlycten** \flik′tən\ [Gk *phlyktain(a)* blister] *Seldom used* BURN BLISTER.

**phlyctena** \flikté′nə\ [Gk *phlyktaina* blister] *Seldom used* BURN BLISTER.

**phlyctenula** \flikten′yələ\ [New L (from Gk *phlyktain(a)* blister + L *-ula,* fem. diminishing suffix)] (*pl.* phlyctenulae) A small blister or vesicle.

**phlyctenular** \flikten′yələr\ Pertaining to or characterized by phlyctenulae.

**phlyctenulosis** \flikten′yəlō′sis\ [*phlyctenul(a)* + -OSIS] Any condition characterized by the formation of small blisters or vesicles. **allergic p.** An immunologic proliferation in a sector of the cornea or conjunctiva associated with *Mycobacterium tuberculosis* infection. Also *tuberculous phlyctenulosis.*

**phobia** \fō′bē·ə\ [Gk *phob(os)* (from *phobein* to terrify) fear, terror + -IA] Pathologic fear, dread, avoidance, or abhorrence. **school p.** Pathologic fear of school related to separation fears and concern about the safety of the mother. Such a phobia may result in an inability to attend school because of pervasive anxiety and various somatic complaints. **social p.** Pathologic avoidance of certain situations for fear that they might reveal one's inadequacies or expose one to shame and humiliation. Some of the most common social phobias are fear of public speaking, of eating in public, of writing in front of others, of blushing, and of using public lavatories when other people are present. **street p.** AGORAPHOBIA.

**-phobia** \-fō′bē·ə\ [Gk *phobos* fear] A combining form meaning an excessive or morbid fear or dread of.

**phobism** \fō′bizm\ [Gk *phob(os)* fear + -ISM] *Outmoded* ANXIETY HYSTERIA.

**phocomelia** \fō′kəmē′lyə\ [New L (from Gk *phōk(ē)* a seal, sea calf + *o* + *mel(os)* limb + -IA)] A limb reduction defect in which all long bone segments are absent in one or more limbs so that the hands or feet attach directly to the trunk through their respective girdles. Compare HEMIMELIA.

**phocomelus** \fōkäm′ələs\ A fetus or postnatal individual with phocomelia.

**pholcodine tartrate** $C_{23}H_{30}N_2O_4$. 7,8-Didehydro-4,5α-epoxy-17-methyl-3-(2-morpholinoethoxy)morphinan-6α-ol. A narcotic with little analgesic or euphoriant activity. It is used primarily in cough medicines as an antitussive medication. Chronic use may lead to habituation or addiction.

**phon** \fän\ [Gk *phōnē* sound, voice] A subjective unit of loudness based on the decibel and designed to produce a scale proportional to loudness. 40 phons = 1 sone. See also SONE.

**phon-** \fōn-\ PHONO-.

**phonal** \fō′nəl\ [PHON- + -AL] **1** Designating those consonantlike and vowel-like segmental sounds articulated by the infant in the developmental stage prior to the utterance of identifiable words, after which they may be referred to as phonemes. **2** Pertaining to the voice; phonic.

**phonangiography** \fōnan′jē·ag′rəfē\ A method for quantifying the degree of arterial stenosis present by mathematical analysis of the flow turbulence recorded near the stenosis by a sensitive microphone.

**phonasthenia** \fō′nesthē′nē·ə\ MYASTHENIA LARYNGIS.

**phonation** \fōnā′shən\ [PHON- + -ATION] The utterance of vocal sounds by the coordination of respiratory and vocal fold activity, the basis of speech. Compare ARTICULATION.

**phonatory** \fō′nətôr′ē\ Pertaining to phonation.

**phoneme** \fō′nēm\ [Gk *phōnēm(a)* (from *phōnein* to produce a sound or tone) a sound made, voice, thing spoken, word] The basic segmental phonologic unit of a spoken language, identified in terms of a particular vowel or consonant. It is a category or group of sounds all of whose variants are treated as the same by the listener, and which contrast with other phoneme categories.

**phonemic** \fōnē′mik\ Relating to the analysis of speech by phoneme identification.

**phonetic** \fōnet′ik\ [Gk *phōnētik(os)* (from *phōnē* sound, voice) pertaining to sounding or speaking] Descriptive of the sounds of speech, with accurate identification of the various forms of each particular vowel or consonant, regardless of whether or not these have contrastive or categorical significance.

**phonetics** \fōnet′iks\ The study and analysis of speech sounds, including their articulatory, acoustic, and auditory features. General phonetics is not language-specific, but aims to provide an adequate framework for describing the phonological system of any particular language and, in speech pathology, deviations therefrom.

***Phoneutria*** \fōnʸoo′trē·ə\ A genus of wandering spiders. One species found in South America, *P. nigriventer* (also known as *P. fera, Ctenus ferus,* or *C. nigriventer*) is aggressive and quite poisonous. Its very painful bite may cause heart irregularities, difficulty in breathing, weakness, and temporary blindness. Some deaths of young children have been reported.

**phoniatrician** \fō′nē·ətrish′ən\ One who specializes in phoniatrics.

**phoniatrics** \fō′nē·at′riks\ [PHON- + -IATRICS] The analysis, assessment, and management of disorders of spoken language.

**phonic** \fō′nik, fän′ik\ [PHON- + -IC] Pertaining to the voice, particularly aspects of the hearing of speech sounds.

**phonics** \fō′niks, fän′iks\ [PHON- + -ICS] A systematized approach to teaching reading, in which the sound values of individual written letters are identified and put together to form words.

**phono-** \fō′nō-\ [Gk *phōnē* sound, voice] A combining form meaning sound, voice. Also *phon-.*

**phonocardiogram** \-kär′dē·əgram′\ A graphic record of heart sounds. Abbr. PCG

**phonocardiograph** \-kär′dē·əgraf′\ [PHONO- + CARDIOGRAPH] An instrument for recording heart sounds and murmurs. **logarithmic p.** A phonocardiograph that attenuates the lower vibrations so as to emphasize those of higher frequency.

**phonocardiographic** \-kär′dē·əgraf′ik\ Pertaining to phonocardiography.

**phonocardiography** \-kär′dē·äg′rəfē\ The technique and study of the graphic recording of heart sounds and murmurs. **intracardiac p.** The graphic registration of sounds and murmurs by means of a microphone situated in a cardiac cavity.

**phonocatheter** \-kath′ətər\ A catheter with a microphone at its tip for recording heart sounds and murmurs within the heart and great vessels.

**phonomyoclonus** \-mī′əklō′nəs\ The intermittent sound which may be heard when a stethoscope is applied to the skin over a muscle afflicted by myoclonic jerks.

**phonomyography** \-mī·äg′rəfē\ The acoustic recording of sounds produced during muscular activity, usually supplementing visual oscillographic display.

**phonopathy** \fōnäp′əthē\ [PHONO- + -PATHY] Any structural or functional disorder of the component parts of the speech apparatus.

**phonophores** \fō′nəfôrz\ *Outmoded* OSSICULA AUDITUS.

**phonopsia** \fōnäp′sē·ə\ [PHON- + -OPSIA] The condition of eliciting color sensations by acoustic stimulation.

**phonoreceptor** \-risep′tər\ A sound receptor.

**phonoscopy** \fōnäs′kəpē\ [PHONO- + -SCOPY] **1** The use of a stethoscope and percussion to determine the borders of the solid and hollow organs. **2** The results of such an examination.

**phor-** \fôr-\ PHORO-.

**phorbin** \fôr′bin\ The dihydro derivative of porphin with the addition of an extra ring. Chlorophylls are magnesium complexes of compounds derived from phorbin. Phorbin is a metal-free ring system composed of four pyrrole rings. Fused to one of these rings is a cyclopentane ring.

**-phore** \-fôr\ [Gk *phoros* bearing, carrying] A combining form designating a carrier or bearer of (something specified).

**phoresis** \fôrē′sis\ [Gk *phorēsis* (from *phoreein* to carry constantly, a frequentative of *pherein* to carry) a being carried] A symbiotic relationship in which one organism is transported by another. Also *phoresy, epizoic commensalism.*

**-phoresis** \-fôrē′sis, -fôr′əsis\ [See PHORESIS.] A combining form meaning the act or process of being carried or conveyed; transmission.

**phoresy** \fôr′əsē\ PHORESIS.

**phoria** \fôr′ē·ə\ [New L (from *-phoria*, combining form denoting a carrying, from *-phor(os)*, combining form denoting carrying + *-ia* -IA)] A latent misalignment of the two eyes, masked by fusion reflexes and made evident by interruption of fusion, as by covering one eye. Also *latent strabismus, suppressed strabismus.*

**-phoria** \-fôr′ē·ə\ [Gk *phor(os)* bearing, carrying + -IA] A combining form meaning (1) the state of bearing or conveying; (2) direction.

***Phormia regina*** \fôr′mē·ə rəjī′nə\ The black blowfly, a broadly feeding scavenger fly that causes a form of cutaneous myiasis or sheep strike in Canada and cooler areas of the United States. The larvae were formerly used in the treatment of septic wounds. Also *Lucilia regina.*

**phoro-** \fô′rə-, fôr′ō-\ [Gk *phoros* bearing, carrying] A combining form meaning carrying, bearing, conveying. Also *phor-.*

**phoroblast** \fôr′əblast\ FIBROBLAST.

**phorocyte** \fôr′əsīt\ FIBROBLAST.

**phorology** \fôräl′əjē\ [PHORO- + -LOGY] The study of the role of carriers in conveying disease.

**phorometer** \fôräm′ətər\ A device for measuring ocular alignment with the aid of lenses and prisms.

**phorometry** \fôräm′ətrē\ Measurement of latent ocular deviations with a phorometer.

**phoro-optometer** \-äptäm′ətər\ [PHORO- + OPTOMETER] A device to measure extraocular muscle balance and refractive error. Also *skiascope-optometer.*

**phorozoon** \-zō′än\ [PHORO- + Gk *zōon* living being, animal] The nonsexual phase or generation of an organism in which an alternation of generations or sequence of reproductive modes is involved.

**phose** \fōz\ [Gk *phōs*, contraction of *phaos* light, daylight] A sensation, especially of light or color.

**phosis** \fō′sis\ [Gk *phō(s)* (contraction of *phaos*) light, esp. daylight + -SIS] The production of subjective sensations of light or color.

**phosphagen** \fäs′fəjen\ [*phospha(te)* + -GEN] A substance capable of phosphorylating ADP and thus acting as a reserve of ATP. The main phosphagens are phosphocreatine in vertebrates and phosphoarginine in invertebrates.

**phosphataemia** *Brit.* PHOSPHATEMIA.

**phosphatase** Any enzyme that catalyzes hydrolysis of an ester of phosphoric acid to form a hydroxyl compound and free (ortho)phosphate.

**phosphate** **1** Any salt of phosphoric acid or the anions it contains, including $PO_4^{3-}$, $HPO_4^{2-}$, or $H_2PO_4^-$; orthophosphate. **2** Any ester of phosphoric acid or its salt or anions. **3** A salt, anion, or ester in which one or more phosphorus atoms are joined to several other atoms, e.g., diphosphate, $P_2O_7^{4-}$. **high-energy p.** An ester, amide, or anhydride of phosphoric acid, whose Gibbs energy of hydrolysis is strongly negative under biologic conditions, usually below −30kJ/mol. Such compounds, e.g. ATP, are good donors of the phospho group. Also *energy-rich phosphate.* **low-energy p.** An ester of phosphoric acid whose Gibbs energy of hydrolysis under biologic conditions is only moderately negative, usually not more negative than −20 kJ/mol. Such compounds are not powerful donors of the phospho group. **triple p.** A calcium, ammonium and magnesium salt of phosphoric acid sometimes found in the urinary sediment.

**phosphate acetyltransferase** An enzyme (EC 2.3.1.8) that transfers acetyl groups between coenzyme A and orthophosphate. Also *phosphotransacetylase* (outmoded).

**phosphatemia** \fäs′fətē′mē·ə\ [English *phosphate* + -EMIA] The presence of phosphates in the blood.

**phosphatidate** The salt, anion, or ester of a phosphatidic acid.

**phosphatidic acid** A derivative of glycerol phosphate in which both the remaining hydroxyl groups of the glycerol are esterfied with fatty acids. Also *phosphatide.*

**phosphatidyl** The group $R—CO—O—CH_2—CH(—O—CO—R)—CH_2—O—PO(OH)—$, derived from phosphatidic acid by removal of a hydroxyl group. Phosphatidyl derivatives of serine, choline, and 2-aminoethanol are important constituents of biologic membranes.

**phosphatidylcholine** The choline ester of a phosphatidic acid. It is one of the main constituents of many biologic membranes, especially on the outside of mammalian cell membranes. It is formed by methylation of a phosphatidylethanolamine. Also *lecithin.* Symbol: PtdCho

**phosphatidylethanolamine** The ester of a phosphatidic acid with 2-aminoethanol (trivial name ethanolamine). It can be formed biologically by synthesis from a diacylglycerol or by decarboxylation of phosphatidylserine. It occurs largely on the inside of mammalian cell membranes. Symbol: PtdEtn

**phosphatidylethanolamine methyltransferase** The enzyme (EC 2.1.1.17) responsible for the biosynthesis of phosphatidylcholines by transferring methyl groups from *S*-adenosylmethionine onto a phosphatidylethanolamine.

**phosphatidylglycerol** The glycerol ester of a phosphatidic acid, therefore containing two glycerol residues. It is an intermediate in the biosynthesis of a diphosphatidylglycerol (cardiolipin).

**phosphatidylinositide** A derivative of a phosphatidylinositol. It is formed, for example, by phosphorylation of one or more of the hydroxyl groups of the inositol residue.

**phosphatidylinositol** The inositol ester of a phosphatidic acid. It occurs in small amounts in many biologic membranes.

**phosphatidylserine** The ester of a phosphatidic acid with serine, formed by substitution on the 3-hydroxyl group of serine. A constituent of mammalian cell membranes, it occurs largely on their inside surface.

**phosphatidyltransferase** Any enzyme that catalyzes the transfer of the phosphatidyl group. Such enzymes, e.g. phosphatidylserine synthase, are important in phospholipid biosynthesis.

**phosphaturia** \fäs′fətoo′rē·ə\ Excretion of abnormal levels of phosphates in the urine. Also *phosphuria, phosphoruria.* **renal p.** Increased excretion of phosphates in urine due to their decreased reabsorption by the renal tubules. One of the main actions of parathyroid hormone is to inhibit tubular reabsorption of phosphates, thus inducing phosphaturia.

**phosphene** \fäs′fēn\ [Gk *phōs* light + *-phene,* combining form from *phainein* to appear, make clear] An entoptic visual sensation induced by mechanical or electrical stimulation rather than by light.

**phospho** \fäs′fō\ $(HO)_2P({=}O)$—. The phosphono group when joined to a heteroatom. Also *phosphoryl* (imprecise).

**3′-phosphoadenosine 5′-phosphosulfate** The donor of the group $—SO_3^-$ in most biologic sulfations, such as heparin biosynthesis. It is made by 3′-phosphorylation of adenosine 5′-phosphosulfate, i.e. adenylyl sulfate, which is formed by attack of sulfate on ADP or ATP.

**phosphocozymase** *Obs.* NICOTINAMIDE ADENINE DINUCLEOTIDE PHOSPHATE.

**phosphocreatine** $^{2-}O_3P—NH—C({=}NH_2^+)—N(CH_3)—CH_2—COO^-$. A high-energy phosphate compound which is present in vertebrate muscle tissue and which is hydrolyzed under anaerobic conditions to provide energy for muscle contraction. It is formed when the nitrogen of a guanine molecule bonds covalently with the phosphorus of a phosphate group, producing a high-energy phosphate bond. Also *creatine phosphate* (incorrect).

**phosphodiester** A compound of the type R—O—P(=O)(OH)—O—R′. **p. bond** The covalent bonding of phosphoric acid when it is doubly esterified as R—O—P(O)(OH)—O—R′, especially in a polynucleotide chain, forming an ester with the 3′-hydroxyl group of ribose in one nucleotide and an ester with the 5′-hydroxyl group of ribose in the next nucleotide.

**phosphodiesterase** Any enzyme that catalyzes the hydrolysis of a phosphodiester to an alcohol and an *O*-substituted phosphoric acid. Although the term may be used to include nucleases, it is used most often for enzymes hydrolyzing cyclic phosphates. It is inhibited by dipyridamole. **p. I** An enzyme that removes nucleotides sequentially beginning at the 3′-hydroxy terminus of oligonucleotides, by hydrolysis of phosphodiester bonds, producing 5′-nucleotides. Also *5′-exonuclease.*

**phosphodihydroxyacetone** DIHYDROXYACETONE PHOSPHATE.

**phosphoenolpyruvate** Any salt or ester of phosphoenolpyruvic acid.

**phosphoenolpyruvate carboxykinase** An enzyme responsible for the transfer of a phospho group from a nucleoside triphosphate to oxaloacetate with formation of phosphoenolpyruvate and carbon dioxide. It is involved in a pathway of sugar formation that involves the intermediate formation of oxaloacetate, but not in the corresponding catabolic pathway.

**phosphoenolpyruvate carboxylase** The enzyme (EC 4.1.1.31), found in plants and many microorganisms, that catalyzes the reaction of phosphoenolpyruvate with carbon dioxide and water to yield orthophosphate and oxaloacetate. Its action provides oxaloacetate for the functioning of the citric acid cycle and for the biosynthesis of aspartate.

**phosphoenolpyruvic acid** $CH_2{=}C(—COOH)—O—PO(OH)_2$. An intermediate in the Embden-Meyerhof glycolytic pathway. It donates a phospho group to ADP and, in anaerobic bacteria, to hexoses. Also *phosphopyruvic acid.*

**phosphofructaldolase** An enzyme which catalyzes the breakdown of fructose 1,6-diphosphate to glyceraldehyde phosphate and dihydroxyacetone phosphate. The concentration of this enzyme in serum is elevated in subjects with viral hepatitis.

**phosphofructokinase** Fructose-6-phosphate kinase. A glycolytic enzyme (EC 2.7.1.56) which catalyzes the formation of fructose 1,6-diphosphate from fructose 6-phosphate and adenosine triphosphate. The enzyme is inhibited by high levels of adenosine triphosphate and citrate. It is activated by adenosine monophosphate and adenosine diphosphate. These effects of metabolites enable the rate of glycosis to respond to the requirements of the cell. Also *phosphohexokinase* (outmoded).

**phosphofructomutase** An enzyme which catalyzes the reversible conversion of fructose 1-phosphate to its isomer fructose 6-phosphate.

**phosphogalactoisomerase** Hexose-1-phosphate uridylyltransferase. An enzyme system which catalyzes the reversible interconversion of glucose 1-phosphate and galactose 1-phosphate. It is now known to involve the combined actions of two enzymes, one of which interconverts UDPglucose and UDPgalactose. *Obs.*

**phosphogalactose uridylyltransferase** GALACTOSE-1-PHOSPHATE URIDYLYLTRANSFERASE.

**phosphoglucokinase** An enzyme (EC 2.7.1.10) that catalyzes the conversion of adenosine triphosphate and D-glucose 1-phosphate into adenosine diphosphate and D-glucose 1,6-bisphosphate.

**phosphoglucomutase** An enzyme (EC 2.7.5.1) which catalyzes the interconversion of glucose 1-phosphate and glucose 6-phosphate.

**6-phosphogluconate** The product of dehydrogenation at C-1 of glucose 6-phosphate in the metabolic pathway leading to ribose derivative for nucleic acid synthesis.

**phosphogluconate dehydrogenase** The enzyme (EC 1.1.1.43) responsible for dehydrogenation of 6-phosphogluconate at C-3, with decarboxylation, forming ribulose 5-phosphate, a reaction of the pentose phosphate pathway.

**6-phosphogluconic acid** The product of the action of glucose-6-phosphate dehydrogenase and the hydrolysis of the lactone first formed. It is an intermediate in the pentose phosphate pathway. It is further converted into a pentose phosphate by the action of 6-phosphogluconate dehydrogenase, with concomitant reduction of $NADP^+$.

**phosphoglyceracetal** PLASMALOGEN.

**3-phosphoglyceraldehyde** GLYCERALDEHYDE 3-PHOSPHATE.

**2-phosphoglycerate** An anionic form of HOCH$_2$—CH(—O—PO$_3$H$_2$)—COOH, an intermediate in the glycolytic pathway.

**3-phosphoglycerate** An anionic form of (HO)$_2$-PO—O—CH$_2$—CHOH—COOH, an intermediate in the glycolytic pathway.

**phosphoglycerate kinase** The enzyme (EC 2.7.2.3) responsible for the transfer of a phospho group from ATP to 3-phosphoglycerate to form ADP and 3-phosphoglyceroyl phosphate, (HO)$_2$PO—O—CH$_2$—CHOH—CO—O—PO-(OH)$_2$.

**phosphoglyceric acid** Either of two compounds, 2- or 3-phosphoglyceric acid, that are enzymatically interconvertible via 2,3-bisphosphoglyceric acid, and are biologically important in the Embden-Meyerhof pathway from glucose to pyruvate.

**3-phosphoglyceric acid** The 3-phosphate of glyceric acid. It is an intermediate in the glycolytic pathway, being formed when a phosphate group is transferred from 3-phosphoglyceroyl phosphate onto ADP yielding ATP. It is further metabolized by isomerization to the 2-phosphate.

**phosphoglycerides** Molecules that are formed when glycerol forms ester bonds with two molecules of phosphatidic acid, the third hydroxyl of glycerol being esterified with a phosphate group. The phosphate group is capable of forming secondary ester bonds with choline, ethanolamine, or serine. Phosphoglycerides are amphipathic molecules and are important components of membranes.

**phosphoglyceromutase** An enzyme (EC 2.7.5.3) that catalyzes the interconversion of 2-phosphoglycerate and 3-phosphoglycerate in the presence of 2,3-bisphosphoglycerate, a reaction of the glycolytic pathway.

**3-phosphoglyceroyl phosphate** *P*—O—CH$_2$—CHOH—CO—O—*P*. The acyl phosphate formed in the glycolytic pathway by the action of glyceraldehyde-phosphate dehydrogenase on glyceraldehyde 3-phosphate, inorganic phosphate and NAD$^+$. It is a powerful phosphate donor, and can react with ADP to form ATP and 3-phosphoglycerate, this reaction being catalyzed by phosphoglycerate kinase.

**phosphoguanidine** The compound (HO)$_2$P(O)—NH—C(=NH)—NH$_2$ and its zwitterionic forms. The term usually denotes its substituted derivatives phosphocreatine and phosphoarginine. Also *guanidine phosphate* (incorrect).

**phosphohexoisomerase** GLUCOSE-PHOSPHATE ISOMERASE.

**phosphohexokinase** *Outmoded* PHOSPHOFRUCTOKINASE.

**phosphoinositide** A phosphorus-containing derivative of inositol, such as a phosphatidylinositol.

**phosphoketolase** An enzyme (EC 4.1.2.9) that catalyzes the conversion of D-xylulose 5-phosphate and orthophosphate to acetyl phosphate, D-glyceraldehyde 3-phosphate, and water.

**phosphokinase** *Outmoded* PHOSPHOTRANSFERASE.

**phospholipase** Any enzyme that catalyzes hydrolysis of a phospholipid, e.g., phosphatidylcholine. Phospholipase A$_1$ catalyzes removal of the terminal acyl group and phospholipase A$_2$ that of the 2-acyl group. The name phospholipase B was once used for the combined activities of phospholipases A$_1$ and A$_2$. Phospholipase C splits between glycerol and phosphate, yielding a diacylglycerol and phosphocholine from a phosphatidylcholine, and phospholipase D splits the other side of the phospho group, yielding a phosphatidic acid and choline. Also *lecithinase* (obs.). **platelet p.** A phospholipase present in blood platelets. It is released following platelet aggregation and digests phospholipids, especially of cell membranes. Arachidonic acid is one of the products that results, and this is therefore an initial step in prostaglandin synthesis.

**phospholipid** A lipid containing phosphoric acid as a monoester or diester. Phospholipids are major components of biologic membranes.

**phospholipidemia** \fäs′fōlip′idē′mē·ə\ The presence of phospholipids in the blood.

**phosphomevalonate** Usually 5-phosphomevalonate, the intermediate in the formation of isopentenyl pyrophosphate from mevalonate. It is formed by mevalonate kinase from mevalonate and ATP, and it is then further phosphorylated to give 5-diphosphomevalonate. These steps are part of the pathway of steroid and terpene biosynthesis.

**phosphomevalonate kinase** The enzyme responsible for transfer of a phospho group from ATP onto 5-phosphomevalonate to form 5-diphosphomevalonate (mevalonic acid 5-pyrophosphate). This reaction is in the pathway of the biosynthesis of sterols and terpenes.

**phosphomolybdic acid** A complex formed between one molecule of phosphoric acid and twelve of molybdic acid. It is easily reduced to an intensely blue material, whose color is due to charge transfer effects between molybdenum atoms of different oxidation states. This feature forms the basis of sensitive tests for reducing agents (tyrosine residues of proteins in the Folin test) and for phosphate.

**phosphomonoesterase** Any enzyme that catalyzes the hydrolysis of an ester of type R—O—PO(OH)$_2$ to orthophosphate and the alcohol R—OH.

**phosphomutase** Any enzyme that catalyzes the transfer of a phospho group from one hydroxyl group to another within the same molecule.

**phosphonate** A salt or ester of phosphonic acid.

**phosphonecrosis** \fäs′fōnekrō′sis\ [*phospho(rus)* + NECROSIS] PHOSSY JAW.

**phosphonic acid** **1** The acid H—P(=O)(OH)$_2$. Also *phosphorous acid,* (older term). **2** Any of the substituted derivatives of this acid of the type R—PO$_3$H$_2$.

**phosphono** The group (HO)$_2$P(=O)—. It is usually known as *phospho* in biochemical contexts when on a heteroatom, so that use of the name *phosphono* may signify that it is on carbon.

**phosphonoacetic acid** H$_2$O$_3$P—CH$_2$—COOH. An experimental antiviral substance that inhibits the DNA replication of herpesviruses such as herpes simplex and Marek's disease viruses and cytomegalovirus, mainly by its inhibition of the viral specified, DNA-dependent DNA polymerase. This inhibition may be due to its acting as an analogue of pyrophosphate.

**phosphonolipid** A lipid containing a carbon-bound phosphono group (free or esterified), and hence a stable C-P bond. Some such lipids are artificial, but marine invertebrates contain lipids in which aminoethylphosphonic acid NH$_2$—CH$_2$—CH$_2$—PO$_3$H$_2$ residues replace the more usual aminoethyl phosphate NH$_2$—CH$_2$—CH$_2$—O—PO$_3$H$_2$ residues.

**phosphonomycin** 1,2-Epoxypropylphosphonic acid. An antibiotic analogue of phosphoenolpyruvate. It inhibits incorporation of the lactyl group of muramic acid and hence blocks peptidoglycan synthesis. Also *fosfomycin*.

**phosphonuclease** NUCLEOTIDASE.

**phosphopantetheine** A constituent of coenzyme A and of acyl carrier protein, containing the thiol group responsible for acyl group carriage in the biosynthesis and breakdown of fatty acids and in acetate metabolism.

**4′-phosphopantetheine** Pantetheine phosphorylated on O-4 of its residue of pantoic acid. This is the form in which pantetheine is bound in coenzyme A, the phosphate group being linked to the 5′-phosphate of adenosine 3′,5′-bisphosphate. It is also the form in which pantetheine occurs in some proteins, with the phosphate group linked to a serine residue.

**phosphoprotein** A protein containing phospho groups, usually as serine and threonine phosphates.

**phosphoptomaine** Any of a group of nonspecific bases that may be present in phosphorus poisoning.

**phosphopyruvic acid** PHOSPHOENOLPYRUVIC ACID.

**phosphor** \fäs′fôr\ [Gk *phōsphor(os)* (from *phōs*, contraction of *phaos* light, esp. daylight + *phoros* bearing, carrying) bearing or giving light] A material that can accept energy from incident radiation and release it shortly thereafter as radiation in the visible and ultraviolet range. The screen of a cathode-ray tube is a phosphor.

**phosphorescence** \fäs′fôres′əns\ [Gk *phōsphor(os)* (from *phōs* light + *-phoros*, suffix denoting carrying, bearing, from *pherein* to carry) bearing light + -ESCENCE] **1** Photoluminescence in which the initial state of the radiative transition is a triplet state. **2** Any photoluminescence in which the output light continues to be emitted for a substantial period (from the order of seconds to several hours) after the stimulating radiation has ceased. *Imprecise.* Compare FLUORESCENCE.

**phosphoribokinase** A transferase enzyme (EC 2.7.1.18) which catalyzes the conversion of ATP and ribose 5-phosphate to ADP and ribose 1,5-diphosphate.

**phosphoribose** RIBOSE 5-PHOSPHATE.

**phosphoribose isomerase** RIBOSEPHOSPHATE ISOMERASE.

**5-phosphoribosylamine** An intermediate in purine nucleotide biosynthesis, as the purine ring is built up on the nitrogen atom. It is formed enzymatically by nucleophilic attack of ammonia, from glutamine, on 5-phosphoribosyldiphosphate (5-phosphoribosyl pyrophosphate).

**5-phosphoribosylglycinamide synthase** The enzyme of purine nucleotide biosynthesis responsible for converting the amino group of 5-phosphoribosylamine into an —NH—CO—$CH_2$—NH group by reaction with glycine and with concomitant conversion of ATP into ADP and orthophosphate.

***N*-(5-phosphoribosyl)glycineamide** GLYCINAMIDE RIBONUCLEOTIDE.

**5-phosphoribosyl 1-pyrophosphate** 5-Phosphoribosyl diphosphate, an intermediate in nucleotide biosynthesis. It is made enzymatically by transfer of a diphospho group from ATP onto O-1 of ribose 5-phosphate. The diphosphate can be displaced by various nucleophiles according to the pathway of nucleotide synthesis being followed. Symbol: PRPP

**phosphoribosyltransferase** An enzyme which catalyzes the conversion of hypoxanthine and guanine to inosinic and guanylic acids. A deficiency of this enzyme results in the Lesch-Nyhan syndrome.

**phosphoribulokinase** An enzyme (EC 2.7.1.19) that catalyzes the conversion of D-ribulose-5-phosphate and adenosine triphosphate into ribulose 1,5-bisphosphate and adenosine diphosphate. It is a key enzyme in the Calvin cycle of photosynthetic fixation of carbon dioxide.

**phosphoribulose** RIBULOSE 5-PHOSPHATE.

**phosphoric** \fäsfôr′ik\ Concerning or containing phosphorus, particularly in its quinquevalent state.

**phosphoric acid** **1** $H_3PO_4$. It has three identical OH groups. Proton loss from one group affects the dissociation of the others, so that it has three well-separated p$K$ values of 2, 7, and 12. It is of great biologic importance. Also *orthophosphoric acid.* **2** Any acid with phosphorus atoms joined to other atoms, such as diphosphoric acid, $(HO)_2P({=}O)$-—O—$P({=}O)(OH)_2$. **diluted p.** A solution of phosphoric acid in purified water. It contains 10% weight for weight of $H_3PO_4$, and it is used as a solvent in a number of pharmaceutical preparations.

**phosphorism** \fäs′fôrizm\ PHOSPHORUS POISONING.

**phosphorolysis** \fäs′fôräl′isis\ The breakage of a bond between two parts of a molecule by reaction with phosphoric acid so that —OH is added to one part and —$PO(OH)_2$ to the other. Hence phosphorolysis of polysaccharides leads to the formation of glycosyl phosphates, as in the conversion of glycogen and orthophosphate into glucose 1-phosphate.

**phosphoruria** \fäs′fôroo′rē·ə\ PHOSPHATURIA.

**phosphorus** \fäs′fərəs\ A widely distributed nonmetallic element having atomic number 15 and atomic weight 30.974. It is never found uncombined. Besides the sole stable isotope (phosphorus 31), there are six radioactive isotopes. Four or more allotropic forms exist, the commonest being the white and red forms. Ordinarily, elemental phosphorus occurs as the white form, an exceedingly poisonous, waxy yellowish solid, transparent and colorless if pure. It ignites spontaneously in air. If this form is exposed to sunlight or heated in its own vapor to 250°C, it changes to the less dangerous red phosphorus, which slowly reverts to the white or yellow form. Valences are 3 and 5. Phosphates are widely used as fertilizer. Phosphorus is an essential component of all cell protoplasm, having a key role in biochemical synthesis and energy transfer. It is a constituent of nervous tissue and bone. Symbol: P

**phosphorus 32** A radioisotope of phosphorus emitting purely beta radiation, used in superficial radiotherapy, as for cutaneous lesions such as eczema, and for systemic therapy of leukemia and polycythemia. It is not widely used in diagnostic nuclear medicine. Physical half-life 14.45 days. Symbol: $^{32}P$

**phosphoryl** [*phosphor(us)* + -YL] **1** The tervalent group PO. **2** *Imprecise* PHOSPHO. • Although often used in this second sense, the phosphoryl group is only part of the phospho group, $PO_3H_2$.

**phosphorylase** Any enzyme that catalyzes phosphorolysis, and, more specifically (EC 2.4.1.1) the degradation of glycogen to glucose 1-phosphate. There are two forms: phosphorylase a, an active form produced by phosphorylation of a serine residue, normally in response to hormonal stimulation of the cell containing it; and phosphorylase b, an unphosphorylated form active only in the presence of effectors likely to accumulate when the cell requires ATP and therefore the breakdown of glycogen.

**phosphorylase kinase** The enzyme (EC 2.7.1.38) that catalyzes the transfer of a phospho group from ATP to the enzyme phosphorylase. This activates phosphorylase, and is a step in the hormone-mediated control of the rate of glycolysis.

**phosphorylase kinase phosphatase** An enzyme that hydrolyzes serine phosphate residues in phosphorylase kinase to release orthophosphate and convert the enzyme into an inactive form. This allows the ending of the hormone-stimulated activation by protein kinase which leads to the stimulation of glycolysis.

**phosphorylase phosphatase** The enzyme (EC 3.1.3.17) that hydrolyzes phosphorylase a to form orthophosphate and phosphorylase b. This reaction renders the glucagon-stimulated activation of glycolysis temporary.

**phosphorylation** \fäs′fôrilā′shən\ [PHOSPHORYL + -ATION] The process of substitution of a hydrogen atom by a phospho group or other substituted phosphoryl group. **oxidative p.** The production of adenosine triphosphate from inorganic phosphates and adenosine diphosphorylates by the electron transport chain, using oxygen as the terminal electron acceptor. **substrate-level p.** The process of ATP synthesis when it does not require functioning of the respiratory chain, but occurs as a direct consequence of the reactions of a metabolic pathway, rather than by the passage of reducing equivalents from metabolites to oxygen or another terminal acceptor. The formation of ATP from ADP and phosphoenolpyruvate in glycolysis, catalyzed by pyruvate kinase, is an example.

**phosphoserine** $(HO)_2PO—CH_2—CH(—NH_2)—COOH$. Serine in which the hydroxyl group has been esterified with phosphate. Phosphoserine residues occur in many phosphoproteins.

**phosphosphingoside** SPHINGOMYELIN.

**phosphothreonine** $O^3$-phosphothreonine, an amino acid whose residues are found in some phosphoproteins.

**phosphotransacetylase** *Outmoded* PHOSPHATE ACETYLTRANSFERASE.

**phosphotransferase** Any enzyme that transfers a phospho group. Also *phosphokinase*.

**phosphotriose** TRIOSE PHOSPHATE.

**phosphotungstic acid** A mineral acid which precipitates proteins and many organic bases. It is used for shadowing biologic objects for electron microscopy.

**phosphuria** \fäs′fyoo′rē·ə\ PHOSPHATURIA.

**phosvitin** \fäsvī′tin\ A protein from the yolk of hens' eggs. It is rich in phospho groups on serine residues.

**phot** \fōt\ [Gk *phōs*, gen. *phōt(os)*, light] The CGS derived unit of illuminance equal to one lumen per square centimeter; $10^4$ lux. Symbol: ph

**phot-** \fōt-\ PHOTO-.

**photic** \fō′tik\ Relating to or involving light.

**photism** \fō′tizm\ [PHOT- + -ISM] A visual sensation of color evoked by or associated with an auditory, olfactory, gustatory, or tactile stimulus.

**photo-** \fō′tō-, fō′tə-\ [Gk *phōs*, gen. *phōtos* light, daylight] A combining form meaning (1) light; (2) ultraviolet and infrared radiation; (3) photograph, photography. Also *phot-*.

**photoallergen** \-al′ərjən\ Any substance capable of producing an allergic sensitivity to light.

**photoallergy** \-al′ərjē\ [PHOTO- + ALLERGY] A reaction of the skin to light that is dependent on immunological mechanisms.

**photocathode** \-kath′ōd\ An electrode in a phototube which emits electrons by photoelectric emission when irradiated with light.

**photocauterization** \-kô′tərīzā′shən\ A procedure in which tissue is destroyed by using a light beam such as a laser.

**photoceptor** \-sep′tər\ [PHOTO- + *(re)ceptor*] A cell capable of perceiving the presence of light.

**photochemical** \-kem′ikəl\ **1** Denoting a chemical change initiated by the absorption of light or ultraviolet radiation. **2** Relating to photochemistry.

**photochemistry** \-kem′istrē\ The chemistry of substances when they are irradiated. Absorption of a light quantum by a molecule excites one of its electrons to a normally vacant orbital and changes the chemical properties of the molecule, rendering it more reactive. Photochemistry includes the study of the properties and reactions of such excited molecules.

**photochromogen** \-krō′məjən\ A mycobacterium that forms yellow or orange colonies when grown in the light.

**photochromogenic** \-krō′məjen′ik\ Forming pigment when cultured in the light. This characteristic is useful for classifying pathogenic mycobacteria.

**photocoagulation** \-kō·ag′yəlā′shən\ [PHOTO- + COAGULATION] The use of an intense beam of light from a xenon bulb or from a laser for the purpose of destruction of tissue or the formation of adhesive scars within the eye.

**photocoagulator** \-kō·ag′yəlā′tər\ A laser device that projects an intense beam of light into the interior of the eye and generates heat that coagulates vessels, as in treatment of detached retina.

**photoconductivity** \-kän′duktiv′itē\ [PHOTO- + CONDUCTIVITY] The increase in electrical conductivity caused by illumination.

**photocutaneous** \-kyootā′nē·əs\ Of or relating to cutaneous changes induced by light.

**photodensitometer** \-den′sitäm′ətər\ [PHOTO- + DENSITOMETER] An instrument for measuring the extent of darkening of processed x-ray or photographic film by determining the transmission of light through selected areas of the film, usually with the use of a photoelectric cell.

**photodermatitis** \-dur′məti′tis\ Dermatitis induced by light. **polymorphous p.** POLYMORPHOUS LIGHT ERUPTION.

**photodermatosis** \-dur′mətō′sis\ [PHOTO- + DERMATOSIS] Any abnormality of the skin induced by light.

**photodiode** \-dī′ōd\ A semiconductor that yields a current output proportional to light input.

**photodisintegration** \-disin′təgrā′shən\ The interaction of a nucleus with a quantum of radiation whose energy exceeds the separation energy of one or more of the constituents of the nucleus, resulting in the emission of charged particles or neutrons.

**photoelectric** \-ilek′trik\ Giving rise to charged particles or electricity by the absorption of light.

**photoelectron** \-ilek′trän\ An electron ejected from its orbit by collision with a photon.

**photoemission** \-imish′ən\ The ejection of electrons from a material by the action of light. The mechanism is that electrons in the atoms of the material gain energy by absorption of the light. They may then have sufficient energy to escape from the material.

**photoerythema** \-er′ithē′mə\ Erythema induced by light exposure.

**photoesthetic** \-esthet′ik\ Possessing or pertaining to the sensation elicited by photons (light).

**photofission** \-fish′ən\ [PHOTO- + FISSION] The splitting of a nucleus into two or more fragments resulting from the absorption of a high-energy photon, as might be produced in cosmic ray bombardment.

**photofluorogram** \-flôr′əgram\ The photograph obtained during photofluorography.

**photofluorography** \-flôräg′rəfē\ The recording of fluoroscopic images on small film, e.g., the recording on 100 mm film of the image produced on the output phosphor of an image intensifier tube. Also *fluorography, fluororoentgenography*.

**photofluoroscope** \-flôr′əskōp\ A type of fluoroscope adapted to allow production of photographs of the fluoroscopic images.

**photofluoroscopy** \-flôräs′kəpē\ The technique of photographing the image produced by x rays on a fluorescent screen.

**photofraction** \-frak′shən\ PEAK-TO-TOTAL RATIO.

**photogene** \fō′təjēn\ [PHOTO- + *-gene*, variant of -GEN] AFTERIMAGE.

**photogenesis** \-jen′əsis\ The production of light, as by bioluminescence. Adj. photogenic, photogenous.

**photogenic** \-jen′ik\ **1** Produced by light, as *photogenic epilepsy*. **2** Producing or emitting light such as the phosphorescence of certain bacteria.

**photography** \fōtäg′rəfē\ [PHOTO- + -GRAPHY] The process by which images are formed on a sensitized surface by the chemical action of radiant energy, especially light. **fluorescein fundus p.** Serial photography to record the passage of intravenously injected sodium fluorescein through the vessels of the ocular fundus. This discloses valuable information about the rate of circulation and the distribution and permeability of blood vessels.

**photohapten** \-hap′tən\ A substance, produced by the action of light on a photosensitive molecule (photoallergen), that combines with particular skin proteins to form a photoantigen which, in turn, initiates photodermatitis.

**photokinesis** \-kīnē′sis\ The change in movement or activity by an organism as a response to light.

**photolabile** \-lā′bīl\ Having the property of being broken down by light or by ultraviolet radiation.

**photoluminescence** \-loo′mines′əns\ Luminescence caused by exposure to light. In lower vertebrates it results from the reflection of light by iridophores in the skin. Adj. photoluminescent.

**photolysis** \fōtäl′isis\ The breakage of a chemical bond in a molecule as a consequence of absorption of a light quantum. Adj. photolytic.

**photomagnetism** \-mag′nətizm\ [PHOTO- + MAGNETISM] The process of magnetization caused by illumination.

**photometer** \fōtäm′ətər\ [PHOTO- + -METER] **1** An instrument that measures photometric quantities such as luminance, luminous intensity, luminous flux, and illumination. **2** An instrument that measures the visual threshold for light. **flame p.** An instrument for measuring quantities of an element by flame emission spectrophotometry. **flicker p.** An optical device that compares two variable visual stimuli by alternate exposure. When the alternating stimuli are adjusted so as to be perceived as being equal, the sensation of flicker will disappear. Also *flicker meter*. **Förster's p.** A device to measure the least amount of light with which the test object becomes visible.

**photometry** [PHOTO- + -METRY] The measurement of radiation based on the visual effect it produces. **internal standard flame p.** A measurement of the concentration of elements performed by using a flame photometer in which the spectral lines generated by the test specimen are compared against those produced by a standard of known concentration that undergoes the same procedure simultaneously.

**photomicrograph** \-mī′krəgraf\ An enlarged photograph of a minute object, usually taken through a microscope. Also *microphotograph, micrograph*.

**photomicroscope** \-mī′krəskōp\ An instrument that combines a microscope and a camera for taking photomicrographs.

**photomotor** \-mō′tər\ [PHOTO- + MOTOR] Describing or pertaining to a motor response to a visual stimulus. Constriction of the pupil in response to light is an example of a photomotor response.

**photomyoclonus** \-mī′əklō′nəs\ Myoclonus evoked by visual (photic) stimuli. **hereditary p.** **1** Hereditary essential myoclonus in which the myoclonic jerks are evoked or accentuated by visual stimuli. **2** Myoclonus in patients with inherited diabetes mellitus with nephropathy.

**photon** \fō′tän\ [PHOT- + *-on*, suffix denoting an elementary particle] The quantum of electromagnetic radiation, having zero charge and zero inertial mass, and having energy equal to the product of the frequency of the radiation and Planck's constant. By definition, it travels at the speed of light. **gamma p.** A quantum of electromagnetic radiation corresponding to a wavelength of about 0.1 nm or less. Gamma photons are those generated by unstable nuclei as they settle down to some lower energy state.

**photoneutron** \-n$^y$oo′trän\ [PHOTO- + NEUTRON] A neutron emitted from a nucleus as a result of the interaction of an energetic photon on the nucleus.

**photonuclear** \-n$^y$oo′klē·ər\ [PHOTO- + NUCLEAR] Pertaining to the action of a photon on a nucleus of an atom.

**photo-ophthalmia** \-äfthal′mē·ə\ [PHOTO- + OPHTHALMIA] Ocular inflammation, especially of the conjunctiva, due to intense light. Also *photophthalmia*.

**photo-oxidation** An oxidation achieved photochemically. For example, residues in proteins may be oxidized by adding dyes and illuminating the solution. The dye molecule absorbs a light quantum which expels an electron to leave an oxidized form of the dye, which reacts with the protein.

**photopathologic** \-path′əläj′ik\ Characterized by or pertaining to any abnormality resulting from excessive exposure to light.

**photopeak** A peak in the pulse-height spectrum of some radiation of interest, such as gamma or x rays.

**photoperiodism** \-pir′ē·ədizm\ A property of living organisms wherein biochemical, physiological and behavioral changes occur in response to systematic variation in light and darkness, as with the seasons or day and night. Also *photoperiodicity*.

**photophobia** \-fō′bē·ə\ [PHOTO- + -PHOBIA] An abnormal intolerance of light, usually due to inflammation of the iris and ciliary body. Adj. photophobic.

**photophosphorylation** \-fäs′fôrilā′shən\ The production of adenosine triphosphate from adenosine diphosphate and inorganic phosphate using light energy from the reactions of photosynthesis. It occurs in a cyclic or a noncyclic series of reactions involving an electron transport system. **cyclic p.** Formation of adenosine triphosphate coupled with liberation of the energy arising from molecular excitation following the absorption of light by chlorophyll, the electrons being recycled without replenishment by external donors.

**photophthalmia** \fō′täfthal′mē·ə\ PHOTO-OPHTHALMIA.

**photopia** \fōtō′pē·ə\ [PHOT- + -OPIA] PHOTOPIC VISION.

**photopic** \fōtäp′ik\ Characterized by or pertaining to light-adapted vision, as served by function of the cones.

**photopigment** \-pig′mənt\ The light-sensitive chemicals in the outer segments of the rods and cones.

**photoplethysmograph** \-plethis′məgraf\ A blood-pressure pulsation monitor that transmits light either into the finger pad where it reflects off bone, or through the aural pinna. The detected light indicates heart rate and presence of circulation.

**photoprotection** Protection from the effects of short wavelength ultraviolet light on a cell conferred by prior exposure to long wavelength ultraviolet light.

**photoproton** \-prō′tän\ A proton emitted as a result of the action of a photon on a nucleus.

**photopsia** \fōtäp′sē·ə\ [PHOT- + -OPSIA] Entoptic or neural visual sensations of light, resulting from various diseases of the vitreous body and the visual pathways; phosphenes due to stimulation of the visual system by causes other than the incidence of light upon the retina. Also *photopsy, visus lucidus*.

**photopsin** The protein component of the visual pigments of retinal cones, as distinguished from the other opsin, scotopsin, of the pigment of rods.
**photopsy** \fōtäp′sē\ PHOTOPSIA.
**photoptarmosis** \fō′tōtärmō′sis\ [PHOTO- + Gk *ptarmo(s)* a sneezing + -SIS] Sneezing evoked by bright light. *Seldom used.*
**photoptometer** \fō′täptäm′ətər\ A device for measuring the least illumination required for eyesight.
**photoreception** \-risep′shən\ The detection and response to light by an organ or organism.
**photoreceptive** \-risep′tive\ Sensitive to visible radiant energy.
**photoreceptor** \-risep′tər\ The light-sensitive rod and cone cells.
**photorespiration** \-res′pirā′shən\ [PHOTO- + RESPIRATION] The respiration that takes place in a plant cell at the same time as photosynthesis. It occurs primarily in the peroxisomes.
**photoretinopathy** \-ret′inäp′əthē\ [PHOTO- + RETINOPATHY] Thermal damage to the retina by intense light. Also *photoretinitis.*
**photoscan** \fō′təskan\ [PHOTO- + SCAN] A rectilinear recording of gamma rays emitted by a radioisotope in which a light source exposes a photographic film.
**photoscintigram** \-sin′tigram\ [PHOTO- + SCINTIGRAM] A photographic representation of scintigraphic data.
**photosensitization** \-sen′sətīzā′shən\ The process by which the skin or other tissue, as the cornea of the eye, is rendered abnormally sensitive to light. **contactant p.** Increased sensitivity of the skin to light, induced by external contact with sensitizing agents such as acridine or anthracene and their derivatives.
**photostethoscope** \-steth′əskōp\ A device for monitoring the fetal heartbeat which emits a flash of light at each beat.
**photosynthesis** \-sin′thəsis\ The process of obtaining metabolic energy by converting radiant energy, absorbed by chlorophyll, into a reduced product of low redox potential (ferredoxin) and an oxidized product. In the higher plants, algae, and cyanobacteria the oxidized product is free oxygen, derived from the oxidation of water. In more primitive bacterial photosynthesis the potential difference can oxidize only compounds of lower potential, such as hydrogen sulfide or an organic compound. The energy and reducing power provided by these reactions are used to reduce carbon dioxide to the level of carbohydrate.
**phototaxis** \-tak′sis\ [PHOTO- + Gk *taxis* an arranging, ordering] The movement of a cell in response to a light stimulus. Positive phototaxis is movement toward the light, negative phototaxis is away from the light. Adj. phototactic.
**phototherapy** \-ther′əpē\ Exposure to light for therapeutic purposes. Also *lucotherapy.*
**photothermal** \-thur′məl\ [PHOTO- + THERMAL] Pertaining to heat produced by radiant energy.
**photothermy** \fō′təthur′mē\ [PHOTO- + THERM- + -Y] The effects of heat resulting from the interaction with the energy of electromagnetic waves, such as x rays, gamma rays, radio waves, and visible light waves.
**phototopia** \-tō′pē·ə\ [PHOTO- + *t* + -OPIA] Vision with the eyes adapted to normal bright daylight.
**phototoxicity** \-täksis′itē\ [PHOTO- + TOXICITY] The property of rendering the skin abnormally sensitive to light.
**phototoxis** \-täk′sis\ [PHOTO- + TOX- + *-(s)is*] The condition resulting from damage by light.
**phototropism** \-trō′pizm\ The property exhibited by some cells or organisms of changing position or orientation in response to light.
**photoxylin** \fōtäk′silin\ CELLOIDIN.
**phren** \fren\ DIAPHRAGMA.
**phren-** \fren-\ PHRENO-.
**phrenatrophia** \fren′ətrō′fē·ə\ *Outmoded* CEREBRAL ATROPHY.
**phrenectomy** \frenek′təmē\ [PHREN- + -ECTOMY] The resection of all or part of the diaphragm.
**phreni-** \fren′i-\ PHRENO-.
**-phrenia** \-frē′nē·ə\ [Gk *phrēn* diaphragm, heart, breast, mind, reason, seat of life + *-ia* suffix denoting state or condition] A combining form denoting a condition of (1) the mind; (2) the diaphragm.
**phrenic** \fren′ik\ [PHREN- + -IC] **1** DIAPHRAGMATIC. **2** Of or relating to the mind.
**phrenicectomy** \fren′isek′təmē\ [*phrenic(o)-* + -ECTOMY] Excision or resection of the phrenic nerve.
**phrenico-** \fren′ikō-\ PHRENO-.
**phrenicocostal** \-käs′təl\ COSTOPHRENIC.
**phrenicoexeresis** \-ekser′əsis\ [PHRENICO- + EXERESIS] Avulsion of the phrenic nerve.
**phrenicotomy** \fren′ikät′əmē\ [PHRENICO- + -TOMY] Division of the phrenic nerve.
**phrenitis** \frenī′tis\ [Gk (from *phrēn* the mind) inflammation of the brain, brain fever, delirium] *Obs.* ENCEPHALITIS.
**phreno-** \fren′ə-, fren′ō-\ [Gk *phrēn* diaphragm, heart, breast, mind, reason, seat of life] A combining form denoting (1) mind; (2) the diaphragm; (3) the phrenic nerve. Also *phren-, phrenico-, phreni-.*
**phrenocolopexy** \-kō′ləpek′sē\ A surgical procedure in which the large intestine is suspended from the diaphragm to prevent ptosis and torsion of the colon.
**phrenocostal** \-käs′təl\ COSTOPHRENIC.
**phrenograph** \fren′əgraf\ [PHRENO- + -GRAPH] An instrument used for the graphic recording of diaphragmatic movement.
**phrenologist** \frenäl′əjist\ An adherent of the doctrine of phrenology.
**phrenology** \frenäl′əjē\ [PHRENO- + -LOGY] A medical doctrine of the 18th century stating that the seat of the intellect, emotions, and instincts was the brain, and that the configuration of the skull could be used to determine the particular site of these faculties.
**phrenoptosis** \fren′äptō′sis\ [PHRENO- + -PTOSIS] An abnormal downward displacement of the diaphragm.
**phrenosin** $CH_3—[CH_2]_{12}—CH{=}CH—CHOH—CH(—CH_2—O—Gal)—NH—CO—CHOH—[CH_2]_{21}—CH_3$. 1-(β-Galactosyl)-*N*-(2 hydroxytetracosyl)sphingosine. A cerebroside found in cell membranes, especially of nerve cells.
**phrenospasm** \fren′əspazm\ Spasm of the diaphragm.
**phronema** \frōnē′mə\ [Gk *phronēma* the mind, will, spirit] The association areas of the cerebral cortex and those believed to be concerned with mentation. *Outmoded.*
**phrynoderma** \frin′ədur′mə\ [Gk *phryno(s)* a toad + -DERMA] Dry skin with horny follicular papules which is a manifestation of a dietary deficiency of vitamin A or of essential fatty acids. Also *phrynoderma.*
**PHS** Public Health Service.
**phthalocyanine** A pigment structurally somewhat similar to a porphyrin, made by heating 1,2-dicyanobenzene with magnesium oxide.
**phthalylsulfacetamide** $C_{16}H_{14}N_2O_6S$. 2-[[[4[(Acetylamino)sulfonyl]phenyl]amino]carbonyl]benzoic acid. A sulfonamide that is practically not absorbed from the gastrointestinal tract. It is used to treat infections in the intestine.

**phthalylsulfathiazole** A sulfonamide conjugated at the $N^4$-position. It is inactive until hydrolyzed to sulfathiazole by intestinal tract bacteria. It has been used to reduce the bacterial population of the intestinal tract prior to bowel surgery, but the efficacy of this use of the drug remains uncertain.

**phthinoid** \thī′noid\ [Gk *phthin(ein)* to decline, waste away, decay + -OID] **1** Resembling or characteristic of tuberculosis (phthisis). **2** Having dull or impaired resonance on percussion: said of chest sounds.

**phthiriasis** \thirī′əsis\ [Gk *phtheiriasis* (from *phtheir* a louse + -IASIS) infestation with lice] **1** PTHIRIASIS. **2** Infestation with any type of human lice; pediculosis. **p. capitis** PEDICULOSIS CAPITIS. **p. corporis** PEDICULOSIS CORPORIS. **p. inguinalis** See under PTHIRIASIS. **pubic p.** See under PTHIRIASIS.

***Phthirus*** \thir′əs\ *PTHIRUS.*

**phthisic** \tiz′ik\ **1** Tuberculous; phthisical. **2** A tuberculous or phthisical individual. **3** Phthisis; tuberculosis. **4** Any of various other chronic pulmonary diseases, such as asthma. *Obs.*

**phthisiology** \tiz′ē·äl′əjē\ [*phthisi(s)* + *o* + -LOGY] The study of phthisis (tuberculosis). *Obs.*

**phthisis** \thī′sis, this′is\ [Gk *phthisis* (from *phthinein*, also *phthiein* to decline, waste away, decay) a wasting away, decay, consumption] **1** Any disease process characterized by a generalized wasting of the body or a part thereof. **2** Tuberculosis, especially pulmonary tuberculosis. An obsolete usage. Adj. phthisical. **bacillary p.** Phthisis caused by the tubercle bacillus; tuberculosis. *Obs.* **black p.** *Obs.* COAL WORKERS' PNEUMOCONIOSIS. **p. bulbi** Softening and shrinkage of an entire eye due to failure of the ciliary body to secrete an adequate amount of aqueous humor. This is a manifestation of irreparable ocular disease; atrophy of the eye. Also *ophthalmatrophia, ocular phthisis.* **colliers' p.** *Obs.* COAL WORKERS' PNEUMOCONIOSIS. **p. corneae** Opacification and atrophy of the cornea. **dorsal p.** Tuberculosis affecting the dorsal spine. **Mediterranean p.** MALTA FEVER. **p. nodosa** MILIARY TUBERCULOSIS. **nonbacillary p.** Pulmonary tuberculosis, or presumed tuberculosis, in which tubercle bacilli have not been demonstrated. **ocular p.** PHTHISIS BULBI. **p. pancreatica** Generalized wasting due to pancreatic disease.

**phyco-** \fī′kō-\ [Gk *phykos* seaweed, alga] A combining form denoting seaweed.

**phycomycete** \-mī′sēt\ [PHYCO- + *-mycete(s)*] Any fungus having nonseptate hyphae.

**phycomycetosis** \fī′kōmī′sətō′sis\ MUCORMYCOSIS.

**phycomycosis** \fī′kəmīkō′sis\ [*phycomyc(ete)* + -OSIS] MUCORMYCOSIS. **cerebral p.** Infection of the brain with the organism of rhinophycomycosis, giving rise to cerebral infarction and/or meningitis due to spreading of the infection along the ophthalmic or internal carotid arteries. The infection is usually seen in diabetic subjects. **p. entomophthorae** RHINOPHYCOMYCOSIS. **subcutaneous p.** A deep mycosis described in Africa and Asia, and caused by *Basidiobolus meristosporus*, which lives in decaying vegetation and soil. The spores enter subcutaneous tissues by direct inoculation. This is frequently a disease of children and may be associated with malnutrition and immunosuppression.

**phyla** \fī′lə\ Plural of PHYLUM.

**phylactotransfusion** \fīlak′tōtransfyoo′zhən\ IMMUNOTRANSFUSION.

**phylaxis** \filak′sis\ [Gk (from *phylax* a guard, sentinel) guarding, protection] An organism's defenses against infection, notably by phagocytosis, the formation of antibodies, and various other immunologic processes. Adj. phylactic.

**phyletic** \fīlet′ik\ [Gk *phyletik(os)* (from *phylet(ēs)* one of the same tribe + *-ikos* -IC, from *phylē* a class, tribe) pertaining to the same tribe] **1** Pertaining to an evolutionary lineage. **2** Pertaining to a phylum.

**phyllo-** \fil′ō-\ [Gk *phyllon* leaf] A combining form meaning leaf, leaves.

**phyllode** \fil′ōd\ Having a leaflike appearance: used of tumors.

**phylloid** \fil′oid\ [*phyll(o)-* + -OID] Resembling a leaf, as in shape.

**phylloquinone** \fil′əkwin′ōn\ VITAMIN $K_1$.

**phylloquinone reductase** An NAD(P)H dehydrogenase (quinone), i.e. an enzyme that catalyzes oxidation of NADH or NADPH with reduction of a quinone. *Obs.*

**phylogenesis** \fī′lōjen′əsis\ PHYLOGENY.

**phylogenetic** \fī′lōjənet′ik\ Of or pertaining to a phylogeny. Also *phylogenic.*

**phylogeny** \fīläj′ənē\ [Gk *phyl(ē)* a class, tribe + *o* + -GEN + -Y] **1** The evolutionary history of a lineage or lineages; the continuous history of evolution and speciation resulting in a taxon. Compare ONTOGENY. **2** The origin and evolution of higher taxa. For defs. 1 and 2 also *phylogenesis.*

**phylum** \fī′ləm\ [New L, from Gk *phylon* race, stock, kind] (*pl.* phyla) A major taxonomic group, ranking between kingdom and class. It is in turn divided into classes.

**physaliferous** \fis′əlif′ərəs\ [Gk *physali(s)* a bladder, bubble + -FEROUS] Having vacuoles or bubbles: used of the cells of a chordoma, which have a characteristic vacuolated cytoplasm. Also *physaliphorous.*

**physaliform** \fisal′ifôrm\ [Gk *physali(s)* a bladder, bubble + -FORM] Having the shape of a bubble or small bleb.

**physaliphorous** \fis′əlif′ərəs\ PHYSALIFEROUS.

**physeal** \fiz′ē·əl\ Of or relating to growth that takes place at the growth cartilage (cartilago epiphysialis) of a tubular bone. *Outmoded.*

**physi-** \fiz′ē-, fis′ē-\ PHYSIO-.

**physiatrician** \fiz′ē·ətrish′ən\ PHYSIATRIST.

**physiatrics** \fiz′ē·at′riks\ A term used chiefly in the U.S. and Canada for PHYSICAL MEDICINE AND REHABILITATION.

**physiatrist** \fiz′ē·at′rist\ A specialist in physical medicine and rehabilitation (physiatrics). Also *physiatrician.*

**physiatry** \fizī′ətrē\ A term used chiefly in the U.S. and Canada for PHYSICAL MEDICINE AND REHABILITATION.

**physic** \fiz′ik\ [Old French *fisique* (from L *physica, physice* natural science (in Med L, medicine), from Gk *physikē*, fem. of *physikos* natural, physical, from *physis* nature, being) medical science] **1** The art or practice of medicine. *Outmoded.* **2** A medicinal drug, especially a cathartic. **3** To treat with a medicine, especially a cathartic. • In the 16th century *physic* (or *physick*) referred to natural philosophy or natural science, which embraced the subject known as *physics* as well as that of medicine.

**physical** **1** Of or relating to the body. **2** Of or relating to physics or material things. **3** A physical examination. *Popular.*

**physician** [Middle English and Middle French *fisicien*, from Old French *fisique* medical science. See PHYSIC.] A person authorized to practice the art of healing; a licensed practitioner of medicine or osteopathy. • *Physician* is often used to make a distinction between medical practitioners and *surgeons*, but in a general sense *physician* is applied to both groups. **admitting p.** The physician responsible for the admission of a patient to a hospital or other inpatient health care facility. **attending p.** The physician legally responsible for the care given a patient in a hospital or health care program. **family p.** 1 A physician who assumes continuing responsibility for supervising the health and coordinating the care of all family members. 2 A physician who is board eligible or board certified as qualified and trained in family practice as a medical specialty. **forensic p.** See under MEDICAL EXAMINER.

**physicist** \fiz′isist\ A person who is professionally engaged in physics. **radiological p.** A person professionally engaged in physics as applied to radiology.

**Physick** [Philip Syng *Physick*, U.S. surgeon, 1768–1837] See under TONSILLOTOME.

**physicochemical** \fiz′ikōkem′ikəl\ Relating to physical chemistry.

**physicogenic** \fiz′ikōjen′ik\ Having a physical cause.

**physicotherapeutics** \fiz′ikōther′əpyoo′tiks\ *Obs.* PHYSIOTHERAPY.

**physicotherapy** \fiz′ikōther′əpē\ *Rare* PHYSIOTHERAPY.

**physics** [See under PHYSIC.] The branch of science that deals with those relationships between matter and energy that do not involve the change of the chemical nature of the matter. **nuclear p.** The science which studies the transformations undergone by the nucleus of the atom both natural and induced, the series of reactions which follow, the radioactive constants, and the application of these phenomena to the production of energy.

**physinosis** \fiz′inō′sis\ A disease of physical origin.

**physio-** \fiz′ē·ō-\ [Gk *physis* nature, natural order, creature] A combining form meaning (1) nature or natural function; (2) relating to the body, physical; (3) physiological. Also *physi-*.

**physiognomy** \fiz′ē·äg′nəmē\ [Gk *physiognōm(ia)* (from *physi(s)* nature, inborn quality + *o* + *gnōm(ōn)* a rule or guide, gnomon + *-ia* -IA) the art of judging one by the features + -Y] 1 The configuration of the face and features, regarded as significant in revealing character. 2 An assessment of character or disposition based on an analysis of the facial configuration.

**physiologic** \-läj′ik\ 1 Of or relating to physiology. 2 Within the normal range; nonpathologic. Also *physiological.*

**physiology** \fiz′ē·äl′əjē\ [Gk *physiologia* (from *physi(s)* nature, constitution, from *phyesthai* to grow + *-logia* -LOGY) the study of natural causes and phenomena] 1 The study of the functioning, especially the normal functioning, of living organisms. 2 The normal functions of living organisms. Adj. physiologic. **animal p.** Physiology as applied to animals, usually other than humans. Also *zoophysiology, zoodynamics.* **antenatal p.** The physiology of the mother and fetus from conception to the onset of labor. **applied p.** The physiology of man as it relates to interaction with the environment. **aviation p.** A branch of physiology concerned with the body's response to the special conditions which occur during flying. **cellular p.** CYTOPHYSIOLOGY. **comparative p.** The study of the similarities and differences of the physiology of different animal species. **developmental p.** The physiology of the processes of development during embryonic life. **human p.** The study of the phenomena associated with the function of human beings. Also *hominal physiology.* **pathologic p.** PHYSIOPATHOLOGY.

**physiolysis** \fiz′ē·äl′isis\ HISTOLYSIS.

**physioneurosis** \-n^y^ŭrō′sis\ ACTUAL NEUROSIS.

**physiopathology** \-pəthäl′əjē\ The study of the changes in body functions induced by disease. Also *functional pathology, pathologic physiology.* Adj. physiopathologic.

**physiotherapeutic** \-ther′əpyoo′tik\ Relating to physiotherapy.

**physiotherapeutist** \-ther′əpyoo′tist\ PHYSICAL THERAPIST.

**physiotherapist** \-ther′əpist\ PHYSICAL THERAPIST.

**physiotherapy** \-ther′əpē\ [PHYSIO- + THERAPY] The health science concerned with utilization of physical modalities such as electricity, heat, cold, sound, and light, as well as physical activity, exercise, and massage, for therapeutic purposes. Also *physical therapy, physicotherapy* (rare), *physicotherapeutics* (obs.).

**physique** \fizēk′\ [French (from L *physic(us)* physical, natural, from Gk *physikos*, from *phys(is)* nature, inborn powers + *-ikos* -IC), physiognomy, exterior of a person, man's natural constitution] The physical development, structural organization, and proportions of the body, and the appearance thereof; body constitution.

**physo-** \fī′sō-\ [Gk *physa* bellows, breath, air] A combining form signifying the presence of gas.

**physohematometra** \fī′sōhem′ətōmē′trə\ [PHYSO- + HEMATO- + Gk *mētra* uterus] An accumulation of blood and gas in the uterus.

**physohydrometra** \fī′sōhī′drəmē′trə \ [PHYSO- + HYDRO- + Gk *mētra* uterus] PNEUMOHYDROMETRA.

**physometra** \fī′sōmē′trə\ [PHYSO- + Gk *mētra* uterus] The presence of gas in the uterus. The condition is most commonly caused by gas-forming bacteria. Also *uterine tympanites.*

***Physopsis africana*** \fisäp′sis\ *BULINUS AFRICANUS.*

**physopyosalpinx** \fī′sōpī′əsal′pingks\ [PHYSO- + PYO- + SALPINX] An accumulation of pus and gas in a uterine tube.

**physostigmine** \fī′sōstig′min\ $C_{15}H_{21}N_3O_2$. An alkaloid obtained from the dry, ripe seeds of the poisonous plant *Physostigma venenosum*, Calabar bean, or ordeal bean. It inhibits the action of cholinesterase, and it is used in opthalmology as a miotic agent. It has also been used to treat glaucoma. Also *eserine.*

**physostigmine salicylate** $C_{15}H_{21}N_3O{\cdot}C_7H_6O_3$. The salicylate salt form of physostigmine. It is used as a cholinergic agent in the treatment of glaucoma to produce miosis and decrease the intraocular pressure. It may be applied topically to the conjunctiva or administered intramuscularly or intravenously to reverse the toxicity of anticholinergic drug poisoning to the central nervous system.

**physostigmine sulfate** $(C_{15}H_{21}N_3O_2)_2{\cdot}H_2SO_4$. The sulfate salt form of physostigmine. It is used in the treatment of ophthalmic conditions, such as glaucoma, as a cholinergic agent. It produces a decrease in intraocular pressure when applied topically to the conjunctiva.

**physostigminism** \fī′sōstig′minizm\ Physostigmine poisoning. Symptoms include restlessness, nausea, vomiting, weakness, epigastric pain, lacrimation, sweating, palpitation, convulsions, and collapse. Death may occur due to asphyxia through central nervous system depression and bronchial spasm.

**phyt-** \fīt-\ PHYTO-.

**phytagglutinin** \fī′təgloo′tinin\ PHYTOHEMAGGLUTININ.

**phytanic acid** 3,7,11,15-Tetramethyl-hexadecanoic acid. A fatty acid which accumulates in the peripheral nerves and other tissues of subjects with Refsum's disease.

**phytate** Any of the salts, anions, or esters of phytic acid.

**phytic acid** Inositol hexaphosphoric acid. Its anions bind calcium and magnesium ions strongly to form the complex phytin.

**phytid** \fī′tid\ [PHYT- + -ID[2]] An allergic reaction of the skin secondary to an inflammatory fungal infection, usually ringworm, that appears elsewhere on the skin surface.

**phytin** Any of the the salts of phytic acid, found in plants, including the calcium salt and the mixed calcium and magnesium salt; phytate.

**phyto-** \fī'tō-\ [Gk *phyton* a plant, tree, a thing that has grown] A combining form denoting plant. Also *phyt-*.

**phytobezoar** \-bē'zôr\ A gastric bezoar composed of vegetable matter. Also *hortobezoar*.

**phytoderma** \-dur'mə\ [PHYTO- + Gk *derma* skin] A parasitic fungal growth on or into the skin.

**phytohemagglutinin** \-hem'əgloo'tinin\ A lectin isolated from the red kidney bean (*Phaseolus vulgaris*). It is a tetrameric protein, with each subunit capable of binding *N*-acetylgalactosamine. In low concentrations it binds erythrocytes, causing agglutination. In higher concentrations it binds leukocytes and stimulates mitotic activity. Also *phytagglutinin*.

**phytoid** \fī'toid\ [PHYT- + -OID] Having plantlike characteristics: said of certain animal organisms, as the sponges and corals.

**phytol** A plant alcohol, found esterified in chlorophyll. It is (*E*)-(7*R*,11*R*)-3,7,11,15-tetramethylhexadec-2-en-1-ol, and is thus based on four isoprene units.

**phytomelin** \-mē'lin\ RUTIN.

**phytomenadione** VITAMIN $K_1$.

**phytomitogen** A lectin derived from certain plants and capable of inducing mitosis in human cells. It produces lymphocyte transformation with concomitant mitotic proliferation of the resulting blast cells, similar to that produced by antigenic stimulation.

**phytonadione** \-nədī'ōn\ VITAMIN $K_1$.

**phytonosis** \fītän'əsis\ [New L *phytonosus* (from PHYTO- + Gk *nosos* illness, disease) with the ending assimilated to the suffix -OSIS] Any disease caused by plants.

**phytotherapy** Therapeutic treatment of disease states by the use of plants.

**phytotoxic** \-täk'sik\ [PHYTO- + TOXIC] **1** Pertaining to or characteristic of a phytotoxin. **2** Toxic to plants.

**phytotoxin** \-täk'sin\ Any of various toxins, such as abrin, ricin, or robin, elaborated in the metabolic or growth processes of certain plants.

**phytotrichobezoar** \-trī'kōbē'zôr\ A gastric bezoar composed of hair mixed with vegetable matter.

**phytylmenaquinone** VITAMIN $K_1$.

**PI** **1** protamine insulin. **2** periodontal index.

**pI** Symbol for isoelectric point.

**pia** \pī'ə\ PIA MATER.

**pia-arachnitis** \-ar'aknī'tis\ [*pia (mater)* + ARACHNITIS ] LEPTOMENINGITIS.

**pia-arachnoid** \-ərak'noid\ LEPTOMENINGES.

**pia-glia** \-glī'ə\ The innermost portion of the pia mater, together with the basement membrane and glial processes on the external surface of the brain and spinal cord. Also *pia-intima*.

**pial** \pī'əl\ [*pi(a mater)* + -AL] Pertaining to the pia mater. Also *piamatral*.

**pia mater** \pī'ə mā'tər\ [Med L, lit., devoted mother, distorted translation of Arabic *al-'umm ar-raqīqa* the delicate covering (from *'umm* mother, matrix, protective covering + fem. of *raqīq* thin, delicate, tender, gentle). See also DURA MATER.] The innermost of the three investing meninges, which adheres closely to the surfaces of the brain and spinal cord. Also *pia*. Adj. pial, piamatral. **p. encephali** [NA] The pia mater covering of the brain. Also *cranial pia mater*. **p. spinalis** [NA] The pia mater covering the spinal cord. Also *spinal pia mater*.

**piamatral** \pī'əmā'trəl\ PIAL.

**pian** \pē'ən\ [French (from Tupi *pi'ã* lit., raised skin) yaws] YAWS. **p. bois** A form of cutaneous leishmaniasis seen in Guiana. Ulcerating swellings occur, usually in the legs, and there is inguinal lymphadenopathy. A minority progress to nasal involvement with deformities similar to those of mucocutaneous leishmaniasis. Also *forest yaws*.

**piarachnitis** \pī'əraknī'tis\ [*piarachn(oid)* + -ITIS] LEPTOMENINGITIS.

**piarachnoid** \pī'ərak'noid\ LEPTOMENINGES.

**piastrinemia** \pī'astrinē'mē·ə\ THROMBOCYTHEMIA.

**Pic** [Adrian *Pic*, Algerian physician, born 1863] Bard-Pic syndrome. See under SYNDROME.

**pica** \pī'kə\ [New L (from L, jay, magpie), transl. of Gk *kissa* jay, magpie, craving for strange food (from the omnivorous habits of these birds)] An appetite for and the eating of matter not fit for food, such as sand, clay, or paint. Iron deficiency anemia appears to be a cause in some young children. Also *paroxia, perverted appetite, allotriophagy, xenorexia* (older term).

**Picchini** [Luigi *Picchini*, Italian physician, flourished late 19th century] See under SYNDROME.

**Piccolomini** [A. *Piccolomini*, Italian anatomist, 1526–1605] Striae of Piccolomini. See under STRIAE MEDULLARES VENTRICULI QUARTI.

**Pick** [Arnold *Pick*, Czech physician, 1851–1924] **1** See under BUNDLE. **2** Pick bodies. See under BODY. **3** Pick syndrome, Pick's gyral atrophy, Pick's convolutional atrophy. See under PICK'S DISEASE.

**Pick** [Friedel *Pick*, Czech physician, 1867–1926] **1** Pick syndrome. See under DISEASE. **2** Pick syndrome. See under AUTOTOPOAGNOSIA.

**Pick** [Ludwig *Pick*, German physician, 1868–1935] **1** Tubular adenoma of Pick. See under TUBULAR ANDROBLASTOMA. **2** Niemann-Pick lipid. See under SPHINGOMYELIN. **3** Niemann-Pick disease. See under DISEASE. **4** Pick's cell. See under NIEMANN-PICK CELL.

**Pickering** [George White *Pickering*, English scientist, born 1904] Lewis and Pickering test. See under TEST.

**pico-** \pī'kə-, pī'kō-, pē'kō-\ [Italian *piccolo* small] A combining form denoting $10^{-12}$: used with SI units. Symbol: p

**picoampere** \-am'pir\ [PICO- + AMPERE] A unit of electric current equal to $10^{-12}$ ampere. Symbol: pA

**picocurie** \-kyoo'rē\ [PICO- + CURIE] A unit of activity of a radionuclide or of a radioactive source equal to $10^{-12}$ curie; $3.7 \times 10^{-2}$ becquerel exactly. Also *micromicrocurie* (outmoded). Symbol: pCi

**picogram** \pī'kōgram\ [PICO- + GRAM] A unit of mass or weight equal to $10^{-12}$ gram. Also *micromicrogram* (outmoded). Symbol: pg

**picoliter** \pī'kōlē'tr\ [PICO- + LITER] A unit of volume or capacity equal to $10^{-12}$ liters, $10^{-15}$ cubic meter, or $10^{-9}$ cubic centimeter. Symbol: pl

**picomole** \pī'kōmōl'\ [PICO- + MOLE[3]] An amount of substance equal to $10^{-12}$ mole. Symbol: pmol

**Picornaviridae** \pīkôr'nəvir'idē\ [PICO- + *RNA* + *vir(us)* + -IDAE] A family of small animal viruses which contain single-stranded infectious RNA enclosed in a naked, ether-resistant, icosahedral capsid which is 20–30 nm in diameter. This family includes the polioviruses, coxsackieviruses, enteroviruses, and rhinoviruses.

**picornavirus** \pikôr'nəvī'rəs\ Any virus of the family Picornaviridae.

**picramic acid** 2-Amino-4,6-dinitrophenol. A compound formed by the replacement of one $NO_2$ radical in picric acid by $NH_2$. Its toxic properties are similar to those of 2-4-dinitrophenol, which is readily absorbed through intact skin or, as vapor, through the respiratory tract. It may cause dermatitis, cataracts, granulocytopenia, polyneuropathy, increased metabolism, collapse, and death. Also *dinitroaminophenol.*

**picric acid** $C_6H_2(NO_2)_3OH$. 2,4,6-Trinitrophenol. An acid consisting of rhombohedral platelets of pale yellow color and very bitter taste. it is quite a strong acid (p$K$ 1.0) It is a dye, has antiseptic properties, and is used to preserve samples for histologic investigation. It is explosive when dry and is used in the manufacture of explosives and rocket fuels. Occupational exposure sometimes results in a condition resembling jaundice. It is also used in treatment of burns and some skin infections.

**picro-** \pik′rə-\ [Gk *pikros* sharp, pungent, bitter] A combining form meaning bitter.

**picrogeusia** \pik′rəjoo′sē·ə\ [PICRO- + Gk *geus(is)* taste + -IA] An abnormal, bitter taste in the mouth.

**picrotoxin** $C_{30}H_{24}O_{13}$. A glycoside obtained from the seed of *Anamirta cocculus* (Menispermaceae). It is employed to stimulate the respiratory center of the medulla, and is used to treat central and respiratory poisoning due to drugs such as barbiturates. It blocks presynaptic inhibition of neural impulses in the central nervous system. Also *cocculin.*

**picrotoxinism** \pik′rətäk′sinizm\ Poisoning by picrotoxin, which is used as an antidote to barbiturates. Symptoms are recurrent convulsive movements, usually clonic in nature, although a large dose may be followed by a short series of clonic movements followed by a tonic convulsion.

**PIE** pulmonary infiltration with eosinophilia (the Löffler syndrome).

**piebaldism** \pī′bôldizm\ [*pie* magpie (from L *pica* the spotted bird, magpie) + English *bald* + -ISM] A rare hereditary disorder in which many patches of skin are devoid of pigment. Also *partial albinism, piebald albinism.*

**piece / Fd p.** FD FRAGMENT. **middle p.** The region of a spermatozoon behind the head. It usually contains the centrioles, mitochondria, and the axoneme of the flagellum, surrounded by the plasma membrane. Also *middlepiece, mid-piece.* **secretory p.** A component of immunoglobulins secreted across mucosal surfaces that distinguish them from their plasma counterparts. It is a polypeptide of 58 000 molecular weight synthesized by the epithelial cells across which the immunoglobulin (usually IgA dimer but sometimes IgM polymer) is secreted and becomes bound noncovalently to the immunoglobulin during this process. Also *transport piece, transport polypeptide chain, T chain.*

**pie crusting** The placement of multiple small incisions in a skin graft in hopes of providing egress for any fluid or blood that may accumulate under the graft.

**piedra** \pē·ā′drə\ [Spanish, stone (referring to the nodules on the hair shaft)] A superficial fungal infection of the hair shaft. Also *chignon disease.* **white p.** A fungal infection of the hair shaft without invasion of the follicle. It is characterized by soft white or cream nodules on the hair surface and shafts that are fragile and swollen from internal invasion. The causative organism is *Trichosporum beigelii.* The disease occurs sporadically in both tropical and temperate areas. Also *Beigel's disease, chignon.*

**Pierini** [Luigi E. *Pierini,* Italian dermatologist, flourished 20th century] Pasini-Pierini syndrome. See under IDIOPATHIC ATROPHODERMA OF PASINI AND PIERINI.

**Pierre Marie** See under MARIE.

**piesesthesia** \pī·ē′zesthē′zhə\ The sensation of pressure. Also *piezesthesia.*

**piesimeter** \pī′ēsim′ətər\ PIEZOMETER.

**piezesthesia** \pī·ē′zesthē′zhə\ PIESESTHESIA.

**piezoelectric** \pī·ē′zō·ilek′trik\ Of or relating to piezoelectricity or the piezoelectric effect.

**piezoelectricity** \pī·ē′zō·ē′lektris′itē\ [Gk *piez(ein)* to press, squeeze + *o* + English *electricity*] Electricity generated by the mechanical stressing of certain crystalline material. See also PIEZOELECTRIC EFFECT.

**piezometer** \pī′ēzäm′ətər\ [Gk *piez(ein)* to press, squeeze + *o* + -METER] An instrument for measuring pressure sensibility. Also *piesimeter.*

**PIF** prolactin inhibiting factor (prolactin inhibiting hormone).

**pigbel** \pig′bel\ [possibly pidgin English for *pig* + *bel(ly)*] An acute form of enteritis necroticans, principally afflicting children, and marked by acute gastrointestinal symptoms, including bloody diarrhea and severe hemorrhagic jejunitis. The disease, which may often result in death, is caused by the enterotoxin *Clostridium perfringens* type *C.* which is usually ingested in contaminated meat. In Papua New Guinea, where recent research has been carried out, the infection has been traced to cooked pork left over and eaten long after its preparation for a feast. Pigbel has been reported in several tropical countries, including Uganda and Thailand. A vaccine is now available.

**pigment** \pig′mənt\ [L *pigmentum* (from *pingere* to paint, draw, stain, dye + *-mentum* -MENT) a paint, color] A colored substance with a biologic function, such as melanin. **age p.** LIPOFUSCIN. **bile p.** One of several linear tetrapyrroles derived from the catabolism of heme and found in bile. Small concentrations are also found in urine, and provide its color. Such compounds include bilirubin and biliverdin. Also *biliary pigment.* **blood p.** A colored compound in blood, usually responsible for oxygen carriage. The normal blood pigment of vertebrates is hemoglobin. **cone p.** Any of the substances present in cones of the retina that is capable of absorbing light and initiating a nerve impulse. They consist of 11-*cis*-retinal bound to various proteins. **respiratory p.** A colored substance capable of carrying oxygen to animal tissues. The human respiratory pigment is hemoglobin. **visual p.** Any of the substances present in rods and cones of the retina that are capable of absorbing light and initiating a nerve impulse. They consist of 11-*cis*-retinal bound to various proteins, which modify its absorption spectrum. Also *retinal pigment.*

**pigmentation** \pig′məntā′shən\ [PIGMENT + -ATION] Coloration by a pigment. Also *chromatosis.* **addisonian dermal p.** Darkening of the skin occurring in about 60% of patients with Addison's disease. It often starts as unduly long persistence of a suntan, with browning most pronounced over pressure points, as the elbows, on the external genitalia, and in the palmar creases. Vitiligo is occasionally seen, as are blue-black discolorations (so-called ink spots) in the buccal mucosa, especially the gums. The cause is raised concentrations of circulating adrenocorticotropin and perhaps of melanocyte-stimulating hormone and its precursors, all of which induce increased dermal deposition of melanin. **arsenic p.** A distinctive pattern of increased melanin pigmentation due to the ingestion of inorganic arsenic over a long period. **exogenous p.** Pigmentation caused by substances introduced from outside the body. **gingival p.** Deposition of coloring material within the tissues of the gingiva. **hematogenous p.** A discoloration of the skin by hemosiderin and other blood pigments. **vagabonds' p.** VAGRANTS' DISEASE.

**pigmentodermia** \pig′məntōdur′mē·ə\ [PIGMENT + *o* + -DERMIA ] Any condition in which pigmentation of the skin is evident.

**pigmentogenesis** \pig′məntōjen′əsis\ The formation of pigment.

**pigmentophore** \pigmen′təfôr\ CHROMATOPHORE.

**pigmy** \pig′mē\ See under PYGMY.
**PIH** prolactin inhibiting hormone.
**piitis** \pī·ī′tis\ [*pi(a mater)* + -ITIS] Inflammation of the pia mater.
**pil.** *pilula(e)* (L, pill(s)).
**pila** \pī′lə\ [L, a pillar, mole, pier] A pillar or structure resembling a pillar: formerly used in reference to a trabecula of spongy bone.
**pilae** \pī′lē\ Plural of PILA.
**pilaster** \pīlas′tər\ [French *pilastre* (from Italian *pilastro,* prob. from L *pil(a)* column + *-aster,* suffix denoting partial similarity) pilaster, square pillar standing against a wall] An unusually thick linea aspera femoris, usually associated with anterior bowing of the femur.
**pilation** \pīlā′shən\ [L *pil(us)* a hair, short hair + -ATION] A hairline fracture which may be found in skull bones. Also *pilatio.*
**pile**[1] [L *pila* a ball] A single hemorrhoid: usually used in the plural. **sentinel p.** Thickening of the mucous membrane at the lower end of an anal fissure. It resembles a hemorrhoid. **thrombosed p.** See under THROMBOSED HEMORRHOID.
**pile**[2] [L *pila* a pillar, mole, pier] **thermoelectric p.** THERMOPILE.
**piles** [L *pila* a ball; source of *pile* a hemorrhoid] HEMORRHOIDS.
**pileus** \pī′lē·əs\ CAUL.
**pili** \pī′lī\ Plural of PILUS.
**piliation** \pī′lē·ā′shən\ [L *pil(us)* hair + *i* + -ATION] The formation and growth of hair.
**piliform** \pi′liform\ [L *pil(us)* hair + *i* + -FORM] Resembling the hair in appearance.
**pilimiction** \pī′limik′shən\ [New L *pilimictio* (from L *pil(us)* a hair, short hair + *i* + Late L *mictio* urination)] The passage in the urine of hairs or hairlike structures, such as threads of mucus. Also *pilimictio.*
**pilin** \pī′lin\ The protein that aggregates in chains to form hollow pili.
**pill** A tablet or a spherical or ovoid solid form of medication intended to be swallowed intact. Most pills are manufactured with a coating that protects the medicament and disguises the taste. **birth control p.** ORAL CONTRACEPTIVE. **combined oral contraceptive p.** COMBINATION ORAL CONTRACEPTIVE. **enteric p.** A pill that is enteric-coated. **morning-after p.** A contraceptive preparation of estrogenic compounds in relatively high doses to be taken orally, following unprotected intercourse during the second half of the menstrual cycle. **pep p.'s** Pills containing any of various stimulants, such as amphetamine. *Popular.* **radio p.** ENDORADIOSONDE. **sequential oral p.** SEQUENTIAL ORAL CONTRACEPTIVE.
**pillar** A structure likened to an architectural column in function or shape. **anterior p. of fauces** ARCUS PALATOGLOSSUS. **anterior p. of fornix** COLUMNA FORNICIS. **p.'s of Corti** Within the organ of Corti, the two rows of epithelial cells that, with the basilar membrane, form a triangular tunnel. Together the pillars support the inner and outer hair cells and the reticular lamina of the cochlea. **p.'s of diaphragm** The crus dextrum and crus sinistrum of the pars lumbalis diaphragmatis. **p.'s of the fauces** The arcus palatoglossus and arcus palatopharyngeus. **posterior p. of fauces** ARCUS PALATOPHARYNGEUS. **posterior p. of fornix** CRUS FORNICIS.
**pillet** A small pill.
**pillow** / **Frejka p.** FREJKA PILLOW SPLINT.
**pill-rolling** PILL-ROLLING TREMOR.
**pilo-** \pī′lō-\ [L *pilus* hair] A combining form denoting hair.
**pilobezoar** \-bē′zôr\ TRICHOBEZOAR.
**pilocarpine** $C_{11}H_{16}N_2O_2$. (3*S-cis*)-3-Ethyldihydro-4-[(1-methyl-1*H*-imidazol-5-yl)methyl]-2(3*H*)-furanone. An alkaloid derived from the leaves of *Pilocarpus jaborandi* or *P. microphyllus* and having cholinergic activity.
**pilocarpine hydrochloride** The monohydrochloride salt form of pilocarpine. It is used as a miotic and to decrease intraocular pressure in ophthalmic diseases such as glaucoma. It is applied topically to the conjunctiva.
**pilocystic** \-sis′tik\ Describing a cystic cavity containing hair as in a dermoid cyst.
**pilocytic** \-sit′ik\ Having a morphologic similarity to cells that are involved in the synthesis of hairs.
**piloerection** \-irek′shən\ The erection of hairs, as in response to cold. Also *horripilation.* See also PILOMOTOR REFLEX.
**pilojection** \-jek′shən\ [PILO- + *(in)jection*] The introduction of hair into an aneurysm to promote obliteration by producing thrombosis in the aneurysm.
**pilology** \pīläl′əjē\ [PILO- + -LOGY] TRICHOLOGY.
**pilomatrixoma** \-mā′triksō′mə\ [PILO- + MATRIX + -OMA] A benign tumor of the skin, arising from the hair matrix and containing cells resembling those of basal cell carcinoma and eosinophilic ghost cells. Calcification and ossification may occur. The face and upper extremities are the usual sites. Also *pilomatricoma, calcified epithelioma, benign calcifying epithelioma, Malherbe's epithelioma, Malherbe's tumor.*
**pilomotor** \-mō′tər\ Producing or relating to movement of the hair.
**pilonidal** \-nī′dəl\ Having hair as the focus or cause, as in a pilonidal cyst.
**pilose** \pī′lōs\ [*pil(o)-* + -OSE[1]] Bearing hair; hairy.
**pilosebaceous** \-sēbā′shəs\ Pertaining to the unit comprising a hair follicle and a sebaceous gland.
**Piltz** [Jan *Piltz,* Austrian neurologist, 1871–1930] **1** Piltz sign. See under ATTENTION REFLEX OF PUPIL. **2** Westphal-Piltz phenomenon, Piltz-Westphal phenomenon. See under ORBICULARIS PHENOMENON. **3** Westphal-Piltz reflex. See under REFLEX.
**pilula** \pil′yələ\ [L, a little ball, dim. of *pila* a ball] (*pl.* pilulae) A small pill or pillet.
**pilular** \pil′yələr\ Pertaining to or resembling a pill.
**pilule** \pil′yool\ A pill of reduced size; a pillet.
**pilus** \pī′ləs\ [L, a hair, short hair] (*pl.* pili) **1** One of the threadlike appendages of the skin consisting of a slender, flexible shaft of cornified cells embedded by its root in a follicle; hair. It is present in varying numbers in different parts of the body surface but it is absent in others such as the palms of the hands, soles of the feet, glans penis, inner surfaces of clitoris, and labia minora. It also varies in length, thickness, color, shape, and waviness in different parts of the body and in different individuals. See illustration at HAIR. **2** One of the fine, threadlike or filamentous projections from the surface of some kinds of bacteria. **F p.** A special pilus, distinct from the numerous somatic pili, that is coded for by the transfer operon of a conjugative plasmid. It initiates contact with a recipient cell. Whether it serves as the route of DNA transfer, or whether this contact leads to formation of a stronger bridge in aggregated cells, is not clear. With most conjugative plasmids its formation is repressed in most cells. Also *sex pilus, conjugal pilus.* **p. incarnatus recurvus** An ingrown hair that has reentered the skin after emerging from the surface of the skin. **pili multigemini** Multiple hairs formed by separate papillae

that emerge from a single follicle. **sex p.** F PILUS. **pili torti** A structural defect in which the hairs are twisted on their own axes.

**pimel-** \pimel-\ PIMELO-.

**pimelic acid** HOOC—$[CH_2]_5$—COOH. Heptanedioic acid. It was originally derived from the oxidation of fat. Although not itself important biologically, its 2,6-diamino derivative is important as a cross-linking residue in the peptides of bacterial cell walls.

**pimelo-** \pim′əlō-\ [Gk *pimelē* soft fat] A combining form meaning fat, fatty. Also *pimel-*.

**pimeloma** \pim′əlō′mə\ [PIMEL- + -OMA] LIPOMA.

**pimelopterygium** \-terij′ē·əm\ [PIMELO- + PTERYGIUM] A fatty deposit on the conjunctiva.

**pi-meson** \pī′-mē′zän\ An elementary particle with a mass about 270 times that of an electron. It is thought to be involved in holding nuclei together. When produced by cosmic rays, pi-mesons are very short-lived. They may have either a positive or a negative charge or none. They decay into mu-mesons or very high-energy photons. Also *pion.*

**pimetine hydrochloride** $C_{16}H_{26}N_2$. *N,N*-Dimethyl-4-(phenylmethyl)-1-piperidineethanamine. A drug with antilipemic activity.

**pimozide** $C_{28}H_{29}F_2N_3O$. 1-[1-[4,4-Bis(4-flurophenyl)-butyl]-4-piperidinyl]-1,3-dihydro-2*H*-benzimidazol-2-one. A tranquilizing agent used in the management of schizophrenic disorders.

**pimple** [Middle English *pimplis, pimplis* (plurals), prob. from Old English *piplian* to break out in pimples] **1** *Popular* PAPULE. **2** *Popular* PUSTULE.

**pin** **1** A straight slender metal rod used to transfix bone. **2** In dentistry, a small metal rod used to reinforce the retention of a filling or crown. **friction-retained p.** A retention pin fixed by being forced into a cavity, in the dentine, of smaller diameter than itself. **incisal guide p.** A rod on the upper arm of an articulator that contacts an inclined table on the lower arm. It maintains the incisal guidance angle. **retention p.** A small pin fitting in a drilled-out cavity in dentin and used to help in the retention of a dental restoration. It may be first fixed in the dentin and then have plastic material built around it, or it may be part of a cast restoration. **self-threading p.** A threaded friction-retained pin. **sprue p.** A metal rod used, in investing a wax pattern, to form a channel for the flow of molten metal to the interior of the mold. Also *spruefomer.* **Steinmann p.** A smooth metal rod that is passed through bone transcutaneously in order to attach a traction system for the stabilization of long bone fractures. It is commonly inserted into the lower femur or upper tibia to permit skeletal traction for femoral shaft fractures.

**Pinard** [Adolphe *Pinard,* French obstetrician, 1844–1934] See under SIGN, MANEUVER.

**pincers** [Middle English *pinsours, pynsours,* from Middle French *pincier* to pinch] A surgical forceps with two blades that are used to grasp tissue.

**pinch** / **devil's p.'es** *Popular* PURPURA SIMPLEX. **key p.** The apposition of the pulp of the thumb to the radial border of the index finger; the grip used in turning a key. **pulp p.** Apposition of the pulp of the thumb against the pulp of any of the other fingers of the same hand.

**Pindborg** [Jens Jorgen *Pindborg,* Danish oral pathologist, born 1921] Pindborg tumor. See under CALCIFYING EPITHELIAL ODONTOGENIC TUMOR.

**pindolol** $H_{20}N_2O_2$. 1-(1*H*-Indol-4-yloxy)-3-[(1-methylethyl)amino]-2-propanol. A $\beta$-adrenergic blocking drug with properties similar to those of propranolol.

**pineal** \pin′ē·əl\ [Middle French *pineal* (from L *pine(a)* pinecone, from *pinea,* fem. of *pineus* pertaining to pinecones, + Middle French *-al* -AL) pertaining to pinecones] **1** Of, pertaining to, or having the characteristics of the pineal body. **2** CORPUS PINEALE.

**pinealectomy** \pin′ē·əlek′təmē\ [PINEAL + -ECTOMY] Surgical removal of the pineal gland.

**pinealoblastoma** \pinē′əlōblastō′mə\ PINEOBLASTOMA.

**pinealocyte** \pinē′əlōsīt′\ Any of the parenchymal cells of the pineal body. They are epithelioid cells characterized by light-staining cytoplasm, large multilobular nuclei, and prominent nucleoli. Also *pineal cell.*

**pinealocytoma** \pinē′əlōsītō′mə\ PINEOCYTOMA.

**pinealoma** \pin′ē·əlō′mə\ [PINEAL + -OMA] **1** A tumor of pineal cells. **2** A tumor arising in the pineal gland. • Germinomas are relatively common in the pineal region but should not be called pinealomas.

**pinealopathy** \pin′ē·əläp′əthē\ [PINEAL + *o* + -PATHY ] Any disorder or disease of the pineal body.

**pineo-** \pin′ē·ō-\ [L *pinea* (from *pinus* a pine) pine cone] A combining form denoting the pineal body.

**pineoblastoma** \-blastō′mə\ A rare tumor of small, poorly differentiated pineal cells which microscopically resemble medulloblastoma. Also *pinealoblastoma.*

**pineocytoma** \-sītō′mə\ [PINEO- + *-cyt(e)* + -OMA] A tumor of pineal cells. Also *pinealocytoma.*

**pinguecula** \ping·gwek′yələ\ A developmental nodule of elastic tissue situated in the interpalpebral conjunctiva on either side of the cornea. When irritated by ultraviolet light or dryness it may transform into a pterygium. Also *interpalpebral spot.* Also *pinguicula.*

**pinkeye** ACUTE CONTAGIOUS CONJUNCTIVITIS.

**pinlay** \pin′lā\ [contraction of *pin* + *(in)lay*] A metal inlay restoring the palatal surface of an upper incisor or canine and having integral retention pins. It is used as an abutment for a bridge or to restore tissue lost by attrition.

**pinna** \pin′ə\ [L (akin to *penna* a feather, quill), a feather, wing, fin] (*pl.* pinnae) **1** AURICULA. **2** A feather, wing, or fin.

**pinnal** \pin′əl\ AURICULAR.

**pinocytosis** \pī′nəsītō′sis\ [Gk *pin(ein)* to drink + CYT- + -OSIS] The process by which cells engulf fluids and solids to form vacuoles, which then move through the cell and discharge their contents from another region of the cell surface. Also *ultraphagocytosis.* **reverse p.** EXOCYTOSIS.

**Pins** [Emil *Pins,* Austrian physician, 1845–1913] Pins sign. See under EWART SIGN.

**pins-and-needles** Paresthesia which feels as if the skin were being lightly pricked with a pin or needle.

**pinselhaare** \pin′zəlhä′rə\ [German *Pinsel* a brush + *Haare,* pl. of *Haar* a hair] TRICHOSTASIS SPINULOSA.

**pint** [Old French *pinte* an old liquid measure equal to 0.93 liter in Paris] **1** In the United States, a liquid pint or a dry pint. **2** In Great Britain, a unit of capacity equal to $^1/_8$ (UK) gallon; 20 fluid ounces; 0.568 261 liter. Also *imperial pint.* Symbol: pt **dry p.** In the United States, a unit of capacity for dry measure only, equal to 0.5 (US) dry quart, $^1/_{64}$ (US) bushel; 0.550 610 liter. Symbol: dry pt **imperial p.** PINT. **liquid p.** In the United States, a unit of capacity for liquid measure only equal to 0.5 (US) quart, $^1/_8$ (US) gallon; 0.473 176 liter. Symbol: liq pt

**pinta** \pēn′tə\ [American Spanish, from *pinto* spotted, speckled, from *pintar* to paint, color] A chronic nonvenereal treponematosis caused by *Treponema carateum* and characterized by pigmentary changes, especially hypopigmentation, and hyperkeratosis in the late stages of disease. An initial lesion at the site of infection is a small, erythematous papule, usually on the legs or face. It is limited to the skin. The disease is now confined to South and Central America and Mexico. Its precise mode of transmission is unclear, but several years of close personal contact seem essential. As living standards improve, the disease becomes rare. Treatment is with intramuscular penicillin. Family contacts also should be treated. Also *azul, lota, pinto, pannus carateus* (seldom used), *painted sickness, mal del pinto, mal de los pintos, carate, spotted sickness, tina.*

**pinto** PINTA.

**pinus** \pī′nəs\ CORPUS PINEALE.

**pinworm** A nematode worm of the superfamily Oxyuroidea. The worms exist worldwide and occur as parasites in many animals and man. **human p.** A nematode worm of the species *Enterobius vermicularis.*.

**pion** \pī′än\ PI-MESON.

***Piophila casei*** \pī·äf′ilə kā′sē·ī\ A fly that deposits its eggs on cheese or other foods. The larvae, known as cheese skippers, are sometimes accidentally ingested, causing intestinal myiasis that results in vomiting, pain, and diarrhea.

**Piotrowski** [Aleksandr *Piotrowski,* German neurologist, born 1878] See under SIGN.

**pipamazine** $C_{21}H_{24}ClN_3OS$. 2-Chloro-10-[*C*-(4-carbamoylpiperidinyl)propyl]phenothiazine. A phenothiazine drug that is used as an antiemetic agent.

**pipamperone** $C_{21}H_{30}FN_3O_2$. 1-[3-(4-Fluorobenzoyl)-propyl]-4-piperidinopiperidine-4-carboxamide. A tranquilizer that has been used in the treatment of schizophrenia.

**pipazethate** $C_{21}H_{25}N_3N_3S{\cdot}HCl$. 1-Azaphenothiazine-10-carboxylic acid 2-(2-piperidinoethyoxy)ethyl ester hydrochloride. A non-narcotic phenothiazine derivative, used as an antitussive agent. It is less effective than codeine.

**pipenzolate bromide** $C_{22}H_{28}BrNO_3$. 3-Benziloyl-oxy-1-ethyl-1-methylpiperidinium bromide. A quaternary ammonium anticholinergic agent used in the treatment of gastric and duodenal ulcer and gastrointestinal spasm.

**Piper** [E. B. *Piper,* U.S. obstetrician, 1881–1935] See under FORCEPS.

**piperacetazine** $C_{24}H_{30}N_2O_2S$. A phenothiazine tranquilizer, very similar to chlorpromazine in its actions and uses.

**piperazine** $C_4H_{10}N_2$. An anthelmintic agent against pinworm (enterobiasis) and roundworm (ascariasis) infections. It is available as the hexahydrate and various salts, such as citrate, adipate, and phosphate.

**piperazine calcium edetate** A chelated compound composed of piperazine, calcium carbonate, and edetate. It has the same uses as piperazine hydrate.

**piperazine estrone sulfate** $C_4H_{10}N_2{\cdot}C_{18}H_{22}O_5S$. An odorless, white, crystalline powder slightly soluble in water. The synthetic estrogen conjugate has properties and uses like those of estradiol. It is given orally and the conjugate is hydrolyzed slowly in the body to release the estrogenic drug.

**piperazine hexahydrate** $C_4H_{10}N_2{\cdot}6H_2O$. A colorless, deliquescent crystalline compound, very soluble in water. Piperazine hexahydrate and its salts are used as an anthelmintic against roundworms (*Ascaris*) and pinworms (*Enterobius*).

**piperazine tartrate** The tartrate salt of piperazine. It has the same uses as piperazine hydrate.

**piperidolate hydrochloride** $C_{21}H_{25}NO_2HCl$. 1-Ethylpiperid-3-yl-$\alpha$,$\alpha$-diphenylacetate hydrochloride. A white, crystalline powder that is used orally as an anticholinergic drug to treat spasm of the upper gastrointestinal tract.

**piperocaine hydrochloride** $C_{16}H_{23}NO_2{\cdot}HCl$. 3-(2-Methylpiperidine)propylbenzoate hydrochloride. A local anesthetic used for regional block, and for surface anesthesia of the eye, ear, nose, and throat, using the drug in appropriate solutions.

**piperoxan hydrochloride** $C_{14}H_{19}NO_2$. 2-Piperidino-1,4-benzodioxan hydrochloride. An $\alpha$-adrenergic blocking agent like phentolamine. It was formerly used to diagnose and treat patients during the operation to remove pheochromocytomas, to prevent hypertensive episodes. Also *Fourneau 933.*

**pipette** \pīpet′\ [French (dim. of *pipe* tube, pipe), a small tube for taking samples of a fluid] A cylindrical tube, often graduated or calibrated, that is used to transport or deliver measured amounts of fluid. It is usually controlled by regulating the flow of the column of air above the fluid. Also *pipet.* **Pasteur p.** A cotton-plugged, glass tube drawn out to a fine tip, used for sterile transfer of small volumes of fluid.

**pipobroman** $C_{10}H_{16}Br_2N_2O_2$. 1,4-Di(3-bromopropionyl)-piperazine. An alkylating nitrogen mustard antineoplastic agent. It is used to treat polycythemia vera and chronic granulocytic leukemia.

**piposulfan** $C_{12}H_{22}N_2O_8S_2$. 1,4-Di($\beta$-methanesulfonyloxy-propionyl)-piperazine. A nitrogen mustard antineoplastic drug closely related chemically to pipobroman.

**$\gamma$-pipradol** AZACYCLONOL.

**pipradrol hydrochloride** $C_{18}H_{21}NOHCl$. $\alpha$,$\alpha$-Diphenyl-$\alpha$-piperid-2-ylmethanol hydrochloride. A central nervous stimulant like amphetamine. It has been used in the treatment of certain forms of depression.

**piptonychia** \pip′tənik′ē·ə\ ONYCHOMADESIS.

**piqûre** \pēkoor′, pēkYr′\ [French (from *piquer* to prick, from L *piccus,* also *picus* woodpecker), a puncture] PUNCTURE.

**piracetam** $C_6H_{10}N_2O_2$. $\alpha$-(2-oxypyrrolidin1-yl)acetamide. A drug claimed to have a selective and beneficial action on the highest integrating mechanism of the brain.

**Pirie** [George A. *Pirie,* Scottish radiologist, 1864–1929] See under BONE.

**piriform** \pir′ifôrm\ [L *pir(um)* pear + *i* + -FORM] Resembling a pear in shape. Also *pyriform.*

**piromen** A sterile, nonprotein, nonallergenic extract of *Pseudomonas aeruginosa* and *Proteus vulgaris.* The bacterial polysaccharides in the preparation are used in the treatment of some allergic, dermatologic, and ophthalmic disorders by means of the pyrogenic effects of this agent.

***Piroplasma*** \pī′rəplaz′mə\ *BABESIA.*

**piroplasmosis** \pī′rəplazmō′sis\ [*Piroplasm(a)* + -OSIS] *Obs.* BABESIOSIS.

**Pirquet** [Clemens Peter von *Pirquet,* Austrian pediatrician, 1874–1929] Pirquet's test, von Pirquet's test. See under REACTION.

**piscicide** \pis′isīd\ [L *pisci(s)* a fish + -CIDE ] Any substance poisonous to fish.

**pisiannularis** \pī′sē·an′yəlar′is\ An occasional fasciculus of the abductor digiti minimi muscle that is attached to the flexor retinaculum.

**pisiform** \pī′sifôrm\ [L *pis(um)* pea + *i* + -FORM] **1** Resembling a pea. **2** OS PISIFORME.

**pisimetacarpus** \pī′simet′əkär′pəs\ An occasional fasciculus of the abductor digiti minimi muscle that is inserted into the fifth metacarpal bone.

**Piskacek** [Ludwig *Piskacek,* Hungarian obstetrician, 1854–1933] See under UTERUS, SIGN.

**piston** A rod and attached disk fitting tightly within a cylinder designed to increase and relax pressure of the fluid it confines by its movement within the cylinder. **McGee p.** A stapedectomy piston made of stainless steel. **Shea p.** A stapedectomy piston made of Teflon. **stapedectomy p.** A piston-shaped prosthesis used in stapedectomy. It is approximately 4.5 mm in length and up to 0.8 mm in diameter. It is interposed between the long process of the incus and an opening through the stapes foot plate with the object of restoring the sound-conduction mechanism.

**pit** [Old English *pytt,* from L *puteus* a well, pit] Any depression in or indentation of a surface; fovea. **anal p.** PROCTODEUM. **arm p.** FOSSA AXILLARIS. **auditory p.** The invagination of the ectodermal acoustic placode situated on each side of the rhombencephalon. It eventually develops the rough form of the future internal ear, to which it gives rise. Also *auditory placode, otic pit, otic placode.* **chrome p.** CHROME ULCER. **costal p. of transverse process** FOVEA COSTALIS PROCESSUS TRANSVERSUS. **ear p.** A small hollow immediately anterior to the anterior incisure of the auricle. It may be the site of a congenital preauricular cyst or fistula. **gastric p.'s** FOVEOLAE GASTRICAE. **gastric p.'s of Frey** FOVEOLAE GASTRICAE. **Herbert's p.'s** In trachoma, the characteristic defects which remain on the cornea after limbal follicles have healed. **inferior articular p. of atlas** FACIES ARTICULARIS INFERIOR ATLANTIS. **inferior costal p.** FOVEA COSTALIS INFERIOR. **lens p.** A small depression on the outside of the head of an embryo in the ectoderm of the lens placode. It marks the site of formation of the lens vesicle. **nasal p.** OLFACTORY PIT. **oblong p. of arytenoid cartilage** FOVEA OBLONGA CARTILAGINIS ARYTENOIDEAE. **olfactory p.** The depression bounded by an elevated margin resulting from the invagination of each olfactory placode. Later it becomes the olfactory sac in the upper part of which the specialized olfactory epithelial cells develop. Also *nasal pit.* **optic p.** A small depression which develops in the optic plate of the front end of the neural tube and from which the optic vesicle develops. **otic p.** AUDITORY PIT. **postanal p.** FOVEOLA COCCYGEA. **primitive p.** A dimple at the front end of the embryonic primitive streak marking a distinct turning inward of cells. **pterygoid p.** FOVEA PTERYGOIDEA MANDIBULAE. **p. of the stomach** REGIO EPIGASTRICA. **superior articular p. of atlas** FACIES ARTICULARIS SUPERIOR ATLANTIS. **triangular p. of arytenoid cartilage** FOVEA TRIANGULARIS CARTILAGINIS ARYTENOIDEAE.

**pitch** [ME *picchen* pitch] The tonal attribute of a sound, which may be correlated with a location in a musical scale from low to high. It is the subjective attribute of the frequency of a sound wave, with which it bears a complex relationship. **absolute p.** The ability of an individual to identify the precise pitch of a tone or note when played on a musical instrument or sung.

**pitchblende** \pich′blend\ A black, pitchlike ore containing uranium oxides and decay products. It is the chief source of uranium and radium.

***Pithecanthropus*** \pith′əkan′thrəpəs\ [Gk *pithēk(os)* ape + *anthropos* a man, mankind] A fossil genus of the family Hominidae represented by remains first discovered at Trinil, Java, in 1891. Subsequently other examples were found near Peking, China, and in North Africa. It is included today within the genus *Homo.*

**pithing** \pith′ing\ The thrusting of a blunt, metal probe into the spinal cord below the brainstem in order to destroy the connections between the brain and the spinal cord. This functional transection of the neuraxis allows an investigator to carry out experimental procedures below the lesion without inflicting pain.

**Pitkin** [George Philo *Pitkin,* U.S. surgeon, 1885–1943] See under MENSTRUUM.

**Pitocin** A proprietary name for oxytocin.

**Pitres** [Jean-Albert *Pitres,* French physician, 1848–1927] **1** Pitres sections. See under SECTION. **2** See under SIGN.

**Pitressin** A proprietary name for vasopressin.

**pitting** The formation of a small depression, either by disease, as is seen in the nails in cases of psoriasis, or by pressure, as in edema.

**pituicyte** \pitʸoo′isīt\ A fusiform cell in the posterior lobe of the pituitary that lies parallel to the axons of the hypothalamo-hypophyseal tract.

**pituitarium** \pitʸoo′iter′ē·əm\ [New L, from *pituitary*] PITUITARY GLAND. **p. anterius** ADENOHYPOPHYSIS. **p. posterius** NEUROHYPOPHYSIS.

**pituitary** \pitʸoo′iter′ē\ [L *pituitarius* (from *pituita* mucus, phlegm, resin) pertaining to mucus or phlegm (an early conjecture about the gland)] **1** Of, pertaining to, or having characteristics of the pituitary gland. **2** The pituitary gland. **3** A hormone-containing extract of animal pituitary glands. **anterior p.** **1** Of, pertaining to, or having characteristics of the anterior pituitary gland. **2** The anterior pituitary gland. **3** A hormone-containing extract of bovine, ovine, or porcine anterior pituitary glands. **pharyngeal p.** ADENOHYPOPHYSIS. **posterior p.** **1** Of, pertaining to, or having characteristics of the posterior pituitary gland. **2** The posterior pituitary gland. **3** A hormone-containing extract of posterior pituitary glands of cattle, pigs, or sheep.

**Pituitrin** A proprietary name for posterior pituitary injection.

**pityriasis** \pit′ərī′əsis\ [Gk (from *pityron* bran, husks, chaff) a branny or scurfy skin condition] **1** A branny scaling of the skin. **2** Any skin condition marked by branny scaling. **p. alba** A chronic eczema that produces round or oval pink plaques which subside to leave a persistent fine scaling and depigmentation. Also *impetigo pityroides, pityriasis simplex, pityriasis maculata.* **p. amiantacea** A condition marked by layers of asbestoslike scale that complicate some inflammatory disorders of the scalp. It particularly affects children. Also *tinea amiantacea, abestoslike tinea.* **p. capitis** Fine superficial scaling of the hairy scalp. Also *pityriasis furfuracea, dandruff* (popular), *pityriasis vulgaris, scurf.* **p. circinata** **1** PITYRIASIS ROSEA. **2** Pityriasis rosea in which the lesions are few and large. **p. disseminata** *Obs.* PITYRIASIS ROSEA. **p. furfuracea** PITYRIASIS CAPITIS. **Gibert's p.** PITYRIASIS ROSEA. **p. lichenoides** A disease of unknown origin in which crops of papular lesions, predominantly on the trunk and limbs, undergo hemorrhagic necrosis. In a chronic form of the disease the lesions are firm, reddish-brown, lichenoid papules. Scraping detaches the surface scale and exposes a shining brown surface. This is used as a diagnostic sign. Also *Mucha-Habermann syndrome, guttate parapsoriasis, Habermann's disease, Mucha-Habermann disease.* **p. lichenoides et varioliformis acuta** PARAPSORIASIS VARIOLIFORMIS. **p. maculata** PITYRIASIS ALBA. **p. rosea** A common, self-limiting, exanthematous disease, possibly of viral origin, characterized by oval, reddish, scaly lesions that typically follow the creases of the skin. The disorder is often marked by an initial prominent lesion (the herald patch) on the trunk or upper limbs and occurs typically in spring or autumn. Also *Gibert's disease, pityriasis circinata, pityriasis disseminata, Gibert's pityriasis.* **p. rotunda** A skin disorder marked by circular patches of dry ichthyosiform scaling, occurring in certain adult populations. Its cause is unknown. **p. simplex** PITYRIASIS ALBA. **p. steatoides** SEBORRHEIC DERMATITIS. **p. versicolor** A mild superficial fungal infection that usually affects the skin of the trunk and is characterized by fine brown scaling and hyperpigmentation or hypopigmentation. It is found mainly in young adults and is especially common in warm climates. The causative organism is the yeast *Malassezia furfur* (*Pityrosporum furfur*). Also *liver spot* (popular). **p. vulgaris** PITYRIASIS CAPITIS.

**pityroid** \pit′iroid\ [Gk *pityr(on)* bran, corn husk + -OID] Branlike; flaky.

***Pityrosporum*** \pit′iräs′pərəm\ *Obs.* MALASSEZIA.

**pivampicillin hydrochloride** Ampicillin pivaloyloxymethyl ester hydrochloride. A derivative of ampicillin having the same antibiotic spectrum and uses.

**pivot** *Outmoded* DOWEL. **occlusal p.** An artificial premature contact used in the treatment of certain types of malocclusion.

**pixel** \pik′səl\ A picture element; one of the square components into which image information is divided for storage and display in digital imaging systems.

**p*K*** The negative logarithm of the dissociation constant (expressed in moles per liter) of an acid. This is also the pH at which the acid and its conjugate base are present in equal concentrations. Occasionally the subscript B is applied to a p*K* merely to mean the second of two p*K* values under discussion.

**p*K′*** The apparent value of a p*K*, especially at high concentrations of the dissociating species.

**p$K_A$** An alternative expression to p*K*, used to emphasize that the dissociation constant is that of an acid.

**PKU** phenylketonuria.

**PLA-carbon** Carbon mesh laminated on a matrix of polylactic acid, which acts as a fibrous scaffold material that stimulates regrowth of injured ligaments and tendons.

**placebo** \pləsē′bō\ [L (from *placere* to please, be pleasing) I shall please, gratify] An inactive material identical in appearance to a drug undergoing testing and given to the test subjects or patients under similar conditions. Any placebo effects are assumed to be psychological, or suggested by the process of taking a medicine. Such effects are discounted from the real actions of the drug under study.

**placement** The position of a tooth relative to the dental arch. It is used in conjunction with a directional prefix such as *bucco-* or *linguo-*. **lingual p.** LINGUOVERSION.

**placenta** \pləsen′tə\ [L, from Gk *plakoenta*, accus. of *plakoeis* (from *plax*, gen. *plakos* a flat, broad object) a flat cake] (*pl.* placentas, placentae) An extension of the fetus, representing the differentiated part of the chorion (frondosum), formed of cotyledons composed of numerous villi which, in man, are bathed by maternal blood. The human placenta is, therefore, hemochorial in type, the maternal and fetal blood being separated only by the endothelium of the fetal vessels and by the chorionic epithelium covering the villi. An organ with many physiologic functions destined to assure the development of the fetus, the placenta undergoes important modifications during pregnancy. During the first months important metabolic exchanges are carried out by virtue of the activities of the trophoblastic cells covering the villi. During later months the covering becomes thin and irregular, the fetal viscera start to function, and placental transfer is probably more by diffusion. The placenta is also an important endocrine organ, secreting steroid hormones (estrogen and progesterone) which may help to maintain the uterine mucosa during pregnancy, and also chorionic gonadotrophins which affect the maternal endocrine organs and allow continuation of pregnancy. Biological assays for excreted gonadotrophins are used in pregnancy tests. After delivery the placenta is a flat, platelike fleshy mass weighing about 600 g. The amnion is spread out over its fetal surface and the umbilical cord is usually inserted near the center. **accessory p.** SUCCENTURIATE PLACENTA. **p. accreta** A very rare, abnormal, adherent placenta in which separation from the uterine wall after delivery is impossible. Due to absence or thinning of the decidua basalis, the chorionic villi penetrate the uterine muscle. Spontaneous or manual separation of the placenta cannot be accomplished and hysterectomy is often necessary to control subsequent hemorrhage. **adherent p.** A placenta so intimately fused with the uterine wall that a plane of separation is slow in appearing and delivery of the placenta is delayed. **allantoic p.** A placenta having a relationship with the allantois, from which it obtains its vessels. It is essentially the placental type of mammals and of man. Also *chorioallantoic placenta.* **annular p.** A placenta characteristic of Carnivora, where the placental tissue is in a ringlike form arranged like a cuff or muff about the midriff of the fetus. It has occasionally occurred in human pregnancy. Also *zonary placenta, zonular placenta.* **battledore p.** A placenta which has the umbilical cord attached to its margin and not to the center. **bidiscoidal p.** A placenta subdivided into two almost equal lobes. The condition occurs normally in some monkey species and occasionally in human pregnancy. **bilobate p.** A placenta composed of two lobes which are not completely separated from each other. Also *bilobed placenta, bipartite placenta.* **central p. previa**

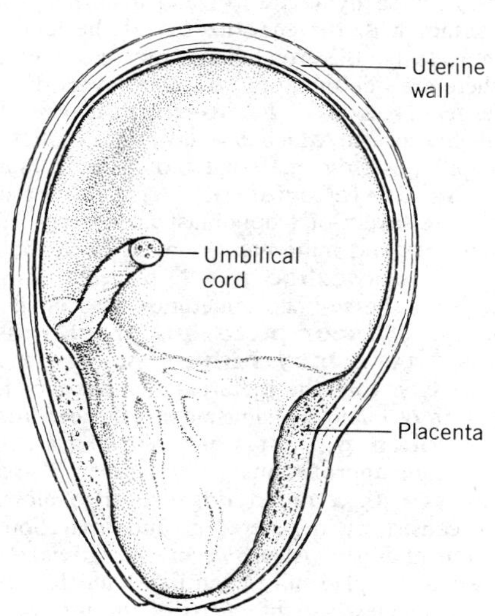


**Central placenta previa**

A placenta situated in the lower uterine segment, with the main mass directly over the internal os even when the os is fully dilated. The condition results from implantation of the blastocyst near the internal os of the uterus. Also *complete placenta previa, total placenta previa, placenta previa first degree, placenta previa centralis.* **chorioallantoic p.** ALLANTOIC PLACENTA. **circumvallate p.** A placenta in which the fetal membranes are not attached to the periphery of the disk but are inserted on the fetal aspect some distance from its edge, thus leaving a circumferential border or margin. Also *placenta circumvallata.* **cirsoid p.** A placenta with sinuous and seemingly varicose vessels on its fetal surface. Also *placenta cirsoides.* **complete p. previa** CENTRAL PLACENTA PREVIA. **deciduate p.** A placenta which fuses so intimately with the maternal (decidual) elements of the uterus that at delivery, after birth of the fetus, a substantial amount of uterine tissue is lost from the uterus with the expulsion of the placenta (as in man). Also *deciduous placenta.* **discoid p.** A placenta which is present only on a limited area of the chorion, as in man. **duplex p.** A placenta divided into two distinct lobes separated by membranous chorion, as in some primates. **fenestrated p.** A placenta in which there are areas where the placental tissue is absent or reduced to a simple membrane. Also *placenta fenestrata.* **fetal p.** That part of the placenta derived from chorionic (fetal) elements. **fundal p.** A placenta situated in the fundus of the uterus. This is the usual site of attachment. **furcate p.** A placenta which appears to be composed of lobes and in which the umbilical vessels separate some distance away from the main mass of the placenta and seem to supply distinct lobes. **hemochorial p.** A placenta in which the chorionic villi are bathed directly by circulating maternal blood. The trophoblast may be composed of one layer, as in man, or of two or three layers, as in other animals. The layers of trophoblast are interposed between the fetal capillaries and the maternal blood. **hemodichorial p.** A hemochorial placenta in which two layers of trophoblast are interposed between fetal capillaries and maternal blood, as in rabbits. **hemoendothelial p.** A placenta in which the chorionic epithelium and mesenchyme are lost and maternal blood makes direct contact with the endothelium of the fetal vessels, as in certain rodents. Electron microscopy has revealed, however, that there are one or more very thin layers of chorion covering the fetal vessels. **hemomonochorial p.** A hemochorial placenta in which one layer of trophoblast separates fetal capillaries from maternal blood, as in man and guinea pig. **hemotrichorial p.** A hemochorial placenta in which three layers of trophoblast are interposed between fetal capillaries and maternal blood, as in the rat, mouse, and hamster. **horseshoe p.** A placenta with a crescentic shape like a horseshoe, sometimes associated with a twin pregnancy. **incomplete p. previa** PARTIAL PLACENTA PREVIA. **labyrinthine p.** A placenta having a structure such that the maternal bloodstream flows through a labyrinth of channels, sinusoids, or spaces lined by trophoblast. **lobed p.** A placenta showing a subdivision into two or more approximately equal lobes. **marginal p.** A placenta with a raised ridgelike edge along its margin, usually caused by degeneration and infarction followed by deposition of fibrin. Also *placenta marginata.* **marginal p. previa** A placenta previa in which the edge of the placenta just reaches the interal os of the uterus. Also *placenta previa second degree, placenta previa marginalis.* **p. marginata** MARGINAL PLACENTA. **maternal p.** That part of the placenta derived from the decidua basalis and which is usually shed along with the fetal elements. **p. membranacea** A human placenta which is thinner than usual and spread over a greater area within the uterus than that occupied by a normal discoidal type. **monochorionic monoamniotic p.** A placenta of monozygotic twins, with a single chorion and with the twin fetuses enclosed within a single amnion. **multilobate p.** A placenta exhibiting four or more separate lobes. Also *multilobed placenta, placenta multipartita.* **nondeciduate p.** A placenta which in some mammals does not fuse intimately with the uterine mucosa and which separates easily, without loss of uterine tissue and without hemorrhage, after expulsion of the fetus. Also *nondeciduous placenta.* **partial p. previa** A placenta previa where the internal os of the uterus is only partially covered by the placenta, especially when the os is fully dilated. Also *placenta previa third degree, incomplete placenta previa.* **p. praevia** *Brit.* PLACENTA PREVIA. **p. previa** A placenta situated centrally in the inferior segment of the uterus. Also *placental presentation.* • The term is used loosely to apply to any faulty positioning of the placenta over the inferior segment of the uterus and more or less covering the internal os of the cervix. **p. previa centralis** CENTRAL PLACENTA PREVIA. **p. previa first degree** CENTRAL PLACENTA PREVIA. **p. previa second degree** MARGINAL PLACENTA PREVIA. **p. previa third degree** PARTIAL PLACENTA PREVIA. **p. reflexa** A placenta with a raised, turned-in margin as if it had been folded in on itself at the edges. **reniform p.** A placenta having the shape of a kidney. **retained p.** A placenta which remains within the cavity of the uterus after delivery of the fetus and after separation of the placenta, due to irregular or weak uterine contractions. Also *trapped placenta.* **p. spuria** An accessory portion of placental tissue in which there are no blood vessels supplied from the placenta proper. **succenturiate p.** A fragment of placental tissue, composed of one or more cotyledons, separated from the main placental mass by a membranous bridge carrying blood vessels. Also *accessory placenta, placenta succenturiata.* **total p. previa** CENTRAL PLACENTA PREVIA. **trapped p.** RETAINED PLACENTA. **trilobate p.** A placenta composed of three more or less independent lobes. Also *trilobed placenta.* **tubal-cornual p.** A placenta located in the uterine tube and extending into the horn of the uterus. **uterine p.** That part of a placenta derived from maternal tissue and which is decidual in origin. Also *pars uterina placentae.* **varicose p.** A placenta with convoluted, dilated blood vessels having a varicose appearance. **velamentous p.** A placenta in which the umbilical cord inserts into the chorion some distance from the placental margin, and from where the umbilical vessels fan out before reaching the edge of the placenta. **villous p.** A placenta formed from a chorion on which villi develop, such as the human chorion frondosum. **zonary p.** ANNULAR PLACENTA. **zonular p.** ANNULAR PLACENTA.

**placental** \pləsen′təl\ 1 Of or relating to a placenta. 2 Having a placenta.

**placentation** \plas′entā′shən\ The development of the placenta.

**placentiform** \pləsen′tifôrm\ Having the shape of a placenta.

**placentitis** \plas′entī′tis\ [*placent(a)* + -ITIS] Inflammation or infection of the placenta.

**placentogenesis** \pləsen′təjen′əsis\ [*placent(a)* + *o* + GENESIS] The origin, developmental stages, and growth of the placenta until it is fully formed.

**placentoid** \pləsen′toid\ Resembling a placenta in shape or structure or in some other feature.

**placentologist** \plas′entäl′əjist\ A person who studies the structure and function of the human or animal placenta in health and disease.

**placentology** \plas′entäl′əjē\ [*placent(a)* + *o* + -LOGY] The scientific study of the placenta, including its structure and function in health and disease. **comparative p.** The study of placentas from different animal types, including their structural and functional differences, especially in relation to histologic and ultrastructural characteristics and possible phylogenetic relationships.

**placentopathy** \plas′entäp′əthē\ [*placent(a)* + *o* + -PATHY] Any disease process involving the placenta.

**placentosis** \plas′entō′sis\ [*placent(a)* + -OSIS] Thrombosis in the intervillous spaces of the placenta.

**placentula** \pləsen′tyələ\ [L (dim. of PLACENTA), a small placenta] A tiny placenta.

**Placido** [Antonio *Placido* da Costa, Portuguese oculist, 1848–1916] See under DISK.

**placode** \plak′ōd\ [Gk *plakōdēs* (from *plax,* gen. *plakos* a broad, flat object, plate) like a plate or consisting of plates] An ectodermal thickening which gives rise to nerve ganglia, to sense organs, or to certain of their constituents. Because of certain morphologic characteristics and also of their evolution, the placodes can be considered as neuroblastic elements isolated early on from neuroblast forming the neural tube. Adj. placodal. **auditory p.** AUDITORY PIT. **dorsolateral p.'s** A series of ectodermal thickenings in the head region of the embryo lateral to the neural plate and neural crest. These placodes contribute to cranial nerve sensory ganglia and possibly also to structures such as chemoreceptors in the carotid body. **epibranchial p.** Each of the ectodermal thickenings situated in the branchial region (posterosuperior side of the branchial clefts) and participating in the constitution of several cranial ganglia: trigeminal, acousticofacial, glossopharyngeal, and vagospinal. **lens p.** An ectodermal thickening situated in front of the optic cup and partially induced by it. A depression forms in the placode and invagination results in the formation of a hollow lens vesicle, or rudiment of the lens, which is transformed into the lens proper by a lengthening of the cells on its posterior wall and their conversion into the lens fibers. Also *optic placode.* **olfactory p.** Each of two oval areas of thickened ectoderm on the ventrolateral aspects of the head above the stomatodeum. In the human embryo these are first seen on the 30th day (about 28-somite stage) and constitute the first indication of the olfactory organs. Also *nasal placode.* **optic p.** LENS PLACODE. **otic p.** AUDITORY PIT.

**plagiocephaly** \plā′jē·əsef′əlē\ [Gk *plagio(s)* slantwise, askance + CEPHAL- + -Y] Asymmetrical craniostenosis owing to premature closure of the coronal and lambdoidal sutures of the skull on one side. It results in grossly unequal curvatures of the skull on the two sides.

**plague** \plāg\ [L *plaga* (akin to Gk *plēgē* a blow, stroke, wound, from root *plēg* of *plēssein* to strike, smite) a stroke, blow, wound] **1** A severe infectious disease caused by *Yersinia pestis* and spread to humans by fleas which have bitten infected rodents (bubonic and septicemic plague) or by inhalation of virulent encapsulated organisms during close contact with another human case (primary pneumonic plague). The disease is characterized by rapid development of fever, chills, prostration, headache, vomiting, diarrhea, and, in bubonic plague, lymphadenopathy, especially in the inguinal and axillary areas. Also *pestis.* **2** Any widespread epidemic disease associated with high mortality. **3** Any large-scale infestation of a geographic area by pestiferous organisms. **ambulatory p.** A mild form of bubonic plague. Also *pestis minor, pestis ambulans.* **black p.** A severe hemorrhagic form of bubonic plague: used especially in reference to the epidemics of plague which ravaged Europe from the fourteenth through the seventeenth centuries. Also *black death* (popular). **bubonic p.** The common form of plague, in which buboes or swellings of lymph nodes appear in the inguinal, axillary, cervical, or epitrochlear areas. If untreated, the mortality is 50–60 percent. Also *pestis bubonica, malignant polyadenitis, glandular plague.* **domestic p.** URBAN PLAGUE. **glandular p.** BUBONIC PLAGUE. **hemorrhagic p.** A severe form of bubonic plague characterized by numerous hemorrhages into the skin and mucous membranes. **murine p.** *Yersinia pestis* infection of rodents which is transmitted among rodents and from rodents to man by fleas. This organism also infects rabbits and cats. **Pahvant Valley p.** TULAREMIA. **pneumonic p.** A severe, often rapidly fatal form of plague acquired by inhalation of virulent encapsulated *Yersinia pestis.* It is characterized by fever, malaise, and pneumonia. Death may occur by the second or third day of illness. Also *pulmonary plague, plague pneumonia.* **septicemic p.** An often fatal form of plague in which *Yersinia pestis* invades the blood stream, causing intense bacteremia and toxemia. In untreated cases, endotoxic shock may lead to death. Septicemic plague accounts for 5–10% of all plague cases. Also *pestis siderans, siderating plague, plague septicemia.* **sylvatic p.** *Yersinia pestis* infection among wild rodents in rural areas, the principal source of urban infection via transfer of infected fleas from dying wild rodents to *Rattus* species in settled areas, or directly to humans. **tarbagan p.** Bubonic plague endemic in eastern Siberia and Mongolia, so called because it affects a marmotlike rodent locally referred to as a tarbagan, from which the infection is transferred to man-biting fleas and thence to humans. **urban p.** Plague occurring when *Yersinia pestis* is transmitted to man by fleas from infected domestic rats. Epidemic outbreaks of disease may result. Also *domestic plague.* **white p.** *Obs.* TUBERCULOSIS.

**plana** \plā′nə\ Plural of PLANUM.

**Planck** [Max Karl Ernst Ludwig *Planck,* German physicist, 1858–1947] **1** See under THEORY, CONSTANT. **2** Planck's quantum relation. See under RELATION.

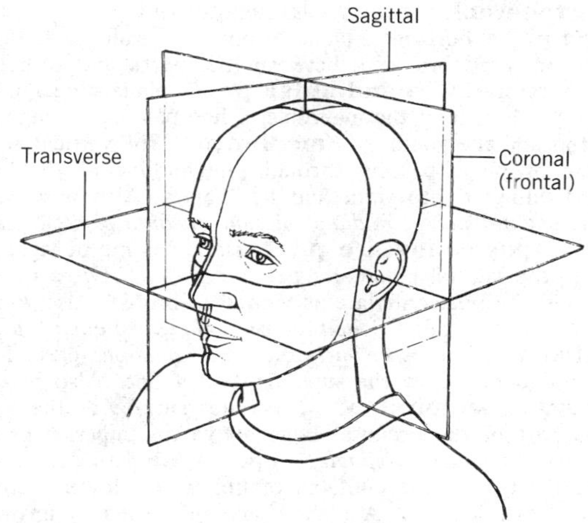


**Planes of the body**

**plane** [L *planum.* See PLANUM.] **1** A flat surface. **2** An imaginary flat surface projected along a line joining two or more points or along an axis. For defs. 1 and 2 also *planum.* **Addison's p.'s** A series of planes used clinically to divide the surface of the abdomen and thorax into topographic areas. **Aeby's p.** A plane used in craniometry that passes through the nasion and basion at right angles to the median plane. **auricular p. of sacral bone** FACIES AURICULARIS OSSIS SACRI. **auriculoinfraorbital p.** FRANKFORT HORIZONTAL PLANE. **axial p.** A plane parallel to the long axis of the body or a structure. **axial p. of tooth** Any plane passing through or parallel to the long axis of a tooth. **axial wall p.** A type of chisel used in operative dentistry. **Baer's p.** A plane that passes through the upper margins of the zygomatic arches. **Bolton p.** NASION-POSTCONDYLARE PLANE. **Bolton-nasion p.** NASION-POSTCONDYLARE PLANE. **Broadbent-Bolton p.** NASION-POSTCONDYLARE PLANE. **Broca's p.** VISUAL PLANE. **Camper's p.** CAMPER'S LINE. **coronal p.** A vertical plane, at right angles to the median plane, that divides the body into anterior and posterior portions. Also *frontal plane.* **datum p.** An arbitrary plane of reference. It is used in craniometry for making measurements. **Daubenton's p.** A plane including the midpoint of the posterior margin of the foramen magnum and the floor of the orbits. **facial p.** 1 The plane along the nasion-pogonion line, used to determine the bony profile of the face. 2 Any one of several planes passing through specific landmarks in the head, such as the Frankfort plane and the nasion-postcondylare plane. **first parallel pelvic p.** APERTURA PELVIS SUPERIOR. **Frankfort horizontal p.** A plane including the lowest parts of the orbital margins and the highest parts of the auditory meatuses. Also *auriculoinfraorbital plane.* **frontal p.** CORONAL PLANE. **p. of greatest pelvic dimension** PELVIC PLANE OF GREATEST DIMENSIONS. **Hensen's p.** H BAND. **Hodge's p.'s** A series of four parallel oblique pelvic planes that are parallel to the plane of the apertura pelvis superior. **horizontal p.** Any plane across the body at right angles to both the median and the coronal planes. Also *transverse plane.* **p. of inlet of pelvis** APERTURA PELVIS SUPERIOR. **intercristal p.** TRANSTUBERCULAR PLANE. **intertubercular p.** TRANSTUBERCULAR PLANE. **Ludwig's p.** A horizontal plane through the trunk at the level of the intervertebral disk between the fourth and fifth thoracic vertebrae. **mandibular p.** A plane tangential to the lower border of the mandible; a line passing through the menton and the gonion. **median p.** The vertical anteroposterior plane passing through the midline of the body and dividing it into right and left halves. Also *midsagittal plane, sagittal plane, midline, mesion, median sagittal plane.* **nasion-postcondylare p.** A plane passing at right angles to the sagittal plane along a line drawn between the nasion and the postcondylare as viewed in profile. Also *Broadbent-Bolton plane, Bolton-nasion plane, Bolton plane.* **nuchal p.** The outer surface of the squamous part of the occipital bone below the superior nuchal line. Also *planum nuchale.* **occipital p.** The outer surface of the squamous part of the occipital bone above the superior nuchal line. Also *planum occipitale.* **p. of occlusion** 1 A plane formed by the contacts of upper and lower teeth in centric occlusion. 2 A plane touching the maximum number of cusp tips. For defs. 1 and 2 also *occlusal plane, line of occlusion.* **orbital p.** VISUAL PLANE. **parasagittal p.** Any vertical plane parallel to the median plane. Also *paramedian plane, sagittal plane* (seldom used). **pelvic p.** Any plane passing through specified bony landmarks of the pelvis. **pelvic p. of greatest dimensions** The plane passing through the middle of the symphysis pubis anteriorly and the junction of the second and third sacral vertebrae posteriorly. It represents the level of greatest capacity of the pelvis from an obstetric point of view. It lies at a slightly higher level than the pelvic plane of least dimensions. Also *wide pelvic plane, plane of greatest pelvic dimension.* **pelvic p. of inlet** APERTURA PELVIS SUPERIOR. **pelvic p. of least dimensions** The plane that passes through the lower part of the symphysis pubis anteriorly, the tips of the ischial tuberosities laterally, and the apex of the sacrum posteriorly. It inclines slightly below the pelvic plane of greatest dimensions. Also *midplane.* **pelvic p. of outlet** The somewhat angulated plane of the apertura pelvis inferior. The anterior ischiopubic part inclines downwards and backwards to the line joining the lowest point of the ischial tuberosities, while the posterior portion of the plane inclines downwards and forwards along the sacrotuberous ligaments to the above line. **principal p.** In radiology, the plane containing the central ray of a beam of radiation. **p.'s of reference** Any planes used to specify a location, as of anatomical structures or other planes. **p. of regard** VISUAL PLANE. **sagittal p.** 1 MEDIAN PLANE. 2 *Seldom used* PARASAGITTAL PLANE. **SN p.** A line joining nasion and sella. **spinous p.** A horizontal plane at the level of a line around the trunk that passes through the anterior superior iliac spines. **sternal p.** A vertical plane along the anterior surface of the sternum. Also *planum sternale.* **subcostal p.** A horizontal plane along a line around the trunk that passes through the lowest points of the tenth costal cartilages. Posteriorly it passes through the upper part of the body of the third lumbar vertebra. **suprasternal p.** A horizontal plane at the level of the suprasternal or jugular notch. **temporal p.** A depressed area below the inferior temporal line on the side of the cranium. Also *planum temporale.* **thoracic p.** A horizontal plane at the level of the fourth intercostal spaces. **transpyloric p.** A horizontal plane along a line around the trunk at the level of a point midway between the suprasternal or jugular notch and the top of the symphysis pubis, or approximately midway between the lower end of the body of the sternum and the umbilicus. Posteriorly it passes through the lower part of the body of the first lumbar vertebra and usually it intersects the lateral line at the tip of the ninth costal cartilage. **transtubercular p.** A horizontal plane at the level of a line that passes around the trunk through the tubercles on the iliac crests. Also *intertubercular plane, intercristal plane.* **transverse p.** HORIZONTAL PLANE. **umbilical p.** A horizontal plane through the umbilicus. **vertical p.** A plane in the long axis of the body at right angles to any horizontal plane. It passes either anteroposteriorly, such as the median plane, or from side to side, such as a coronal plane. **visual p.** The two-dimensional area on the same level and direction as the lines of sight of the two eyes. Also *plane of regard, orbital plane, Broca's plane, planum orbitale.* **wide pelvic p.** PELVIC PLANE OF GREATEST DIMENSIONS.

**planigraphy** \plənig′rəfē\ [*plan(us)* + *i* + -GRAPHY] A radiographic technique to allow clear delineation of structures in a selected plane of tissue or other material by blurring image details in other planes. Also *body section roentgenography, planography, tomography, laminagraphy, laminography.*

**planing** DERMABRASION. **root p.** The removal of infected cementum and contaminated dentin from the surface of roots involved in chronic periodontitis. Also *root curettage.*

**planithorax** \plan′ithôr′aks\ A diagram of the front and back of the thorax that uses a plane projection.

**planning** / **family p.** Planning by parents or prospective parents with or without clinical counseling, as to how many children to have and when to have them; birth control.

**plano** \plā′nō\ [L *planus* flat] Without dioptric power; flat: said of a lens.

**plano-** \plā′nō-\ [L *planus* flat] A combining form meaning plane or flat, as one side of a lens.

**planocellular** \-sel′yələr\ Composed of flat cells.

**planoconcave** \-kän′kāv\ [PLANO- + CONCAVE] Flat on one surface and concave, having minus power, on the other surface: said of a lens.

**planoconvex** \-kän′veks\ [PLANO- + CONVEX] Flat on one surface and convex, having plus power, on the other surface: said of a lens.

**planocyte** \plan′əsīt\ [Gk *plano(s)* wandering + -CYTE] WANDERING CELL.

**planography** \plənäg′rəfē\ PLANIGRAPHY.

**planorbid** \planôr′bid\ **1** Of or belonging to the family Planorbidae. **2** A member of the family Planorbidae.

**Planorbidae** \planôr′bidē\ [L *plan(us)* flat + *orb(is)* a ring + -IDAE] A family of freshwater snails (suborder Basommatophora, subclass Pulmonata) containing numerous species that are intermediate hosts of trematodes parasitic in humans. The genera *Biomphalaria, Planorbis, Bulinus,* and *Helisoma* are included.

***Planorbis boissyii*** \planôr′bis boi′sē·ī\ A former name of *BIOMPHALARIA ALEXINDRINA.*

**planovalgus** \-val′gəs\ [PLANO- + VALGUS] A postural abnormality of the foot in which the longitudinal arch is flattened and the entire foot is everted.

**plantaginis semen** \plantaj′inis sē′mən\ PSYLLIUM.

**planta pedis** \plan′tə pē′dis\ [NA] The region of the undersurface of the foot. Also *sole, vola pedis* (outmoded).

**plantar** \plan′tər\ [L *plantaris* (from *planta* the sole of the foot) pertaining to the sole] Pertaining to the sole of the foot. Also *pelmatic.*

**plantaris** \plantar′is\ MUSCULUS PLANTARIS.

**plantiflexion** \plan′tiflek′shən\ PLANTAR FLEXION.

**plantigrade** \plan′tigrād\ Walking on the sole of the foot, that is, with the tarsal and metatarsal area in contact with the ground at some point in the gait cycle. It is characteristic of humans and, to some extent, other mammals such as bears.

**planum** \plā′nəm\ [L (from *planus* flat) a flat surface] PLANE. **p. nuchale** NUCHAL PLANE. **p. occipitale** OCCIPITAL PLANE. **p. orbitale** VISUAL PLANE. **p. popliteum femoris** FACIES POPLITEA FEMORIS. **p. semilunatum** An area of tall epithelium that appears semilunar in cross-section and is located between each crest and the side wall of an ampulla of a semicircular duct in the membranous labyrinth. **p. sternale** STERNAL PLANE. **p. temporale** TEMPORAL PLANE.

**planuria** \plānoo′rē·ə\ [Gk *plan(os)* wandering + -URIA] Passage of urine through an abnormal outlet.

**plaque** \plak\ [French (from Low German *placken* to patch, stick on), a thin sheet or leaf of metal] **1** Any flat lesion. **2** In microbiology, an area of clearing in a confluent cell culture, caused by viral lysis. **3** See under TERMINAISON EN PLAQUE. **argyrophile p.'s** SENILE PLAQUES. **atheromatous p.** A localized area of atheromatous tissue visible on the intimal surface of an artery. **bacterial p.** DENTAL PLAQUE. **bacteriophage p.** A clear area initiated by a phage particle in a lawn of growing sensitive indicator bacteria in soft agar on the surface of a culture plate. It is used to enumerate particles and to screen for mutants. **dental p.** A specific but highly variable material resulting from the colonization and growth of microorganisms on the surfaces of teeth and consisting of numerous microbial species and strains embedded in an extracellular matrix. Clinically, it occurs supragingivally and subgingivally and may also be found on other solid surfaces, such as restorations and oral appliances. Also *bacterial plaque, mucinous plaque, mucin plaque, gelatinoid plaque.* **fibromyelinic p.'s** Areas in the cerebral cortex of proliferation of myelinated nerve fibers and of glial fibrils, occurring in cerebral ischemia. **gelatinoid p.** DENTAL PLAQUE. **Hollenhorst p.** Glistening cholesterol crystals within the retinal arterioles, denoting embolization from the carotid intima. Also *Hollenhorst bodies.* **Lichtheim p.'s** Demyelination in the cerebral white matter in subjects with pernicious anemia. **mucin p.** DENTAL PLAQUE. **mucinous p.** DENTAL PLAQUE. **mucous p.** MUCOUS PATCH. **opaline p.** MUCOUS PATCH. **Peyer's p.'s** PEYER'S PATCHES. **senile p.'s** Focal accumulations of argyrophilic fibers replacing or lying between neuronal cell bodies in the cerebral cortex, seen as a consequence of normal aging but greatly increased in number in Alzheimer's disease. Also *argyrophile plaques.* **shagreen p.** SHAGREEN SKIN. **talc p.'s** Smooth excrescences on the pleural membrane occurring in persons exposed, usually occupationally, to talc dust.

**-plasia** \-plā′zhə\ [Gk *plas(is)* a shaping, molding + -IA] A combining form meaning a process of molding or forming.

**plasm** \plazm\ [Gk *plasma.* See PLASMA.] Either cytoplasm or any kind of protoplasm. Also *plasma.* **germ p.** The genetic material contained in the germ cells; the genes.

**-plasm** \-plazm\ [Gk *plasma* anything molded, shaped, or formed] A combining form designating one of the categories of material that form or are formed by living cells, as *cytoplasm, nucleoplasm, deuteroplasm.*

**plasma** \plaz′mə\ [Gk (from *plassein* to form, mold), a thing molded or modeled in clay or wax, an image] **1** The fluid component of circulating blood, in which formed elements are suspended. Also *blood plasma, liquor sanguinis.* **2** The fluid component of lymph. **3** PLASM. **4** A state of matter in which extreme high temperatures produce stripped nuclei and excess free electrons, as in thermonuclear reactions. **citrated p.** Plasma rendered incoagulable by the addition of citrate. **dried human p.** DRIED HUMAN PLASMA PROTEIN FRACTION. **fresh frozen p.** Plasma that is separated from red cells and frozen within six hours of a phlebotomy. It contains 100% levels of all coagulation proteins, as well as other constituents present in normal plasma. It can be stored at −20°C or colder for up to a year without loss of procoagulant activity. **hyperimmune p.** Plasma from an animal or human subject repeatedly immunized with an antigen to produce the highest antibody titer possible. Hyperimmune plasma is used to confer passive immunity to subjects who are not actively immune. **normal human p.** Sterile plasma obtained by removal and pooling of the liquid portion of anticoagulated whole blood from approximately 10 donor units. It is used as a plasma volume expander. **oxalated p.** Plasma rendered incoagulable by the addition of oxalate. **pooled p.** HUMAN PLASMA PROTEIN FRACTION. **true p.** Plasma separated from freshly drawn whole blood so that its gas content does not change during the separation.

**plasma-** \plaz′mə-\ PLASMO-.

**plasmablast** \plaz′məblast\ The precursor of the plasma cell that is the most immature, yet identifiable. It is probably a differentiated derivative of the lymphoid stem cell. Also *lymphoblastic plasma cell.*

**plasmacrit** \plaz′məkrit\ The relative volume of plasma to erythrocytes in blood, usually determined by subtracting the hematocrit from unity, or if expressed in percent, 100% minus hematocrit (%).

**plasmacyte** \plaz′məsīt\ [PLASMA + -CYTE] PLASMA CELL.

**plasmacytoid** \-sī′toid\ Resembling or having the characteristics of a plasma cell.

**plasmacytoma** \plaz′məsītō′mə\ [PLASMACYTE + -OMA] MYELOMA. **cutaneous p.** A cutaneous aggregate of plasma cells. **extramedullary p.** MYELOMA. **peripheral p.** MYELOMA. **solitary p.** MYELOMA.

**plasmacytosis** \-sītō′sis\ **1** The appearance of plasma cells in the peripheral blood. **2** An increased number or proportion of plasma cells in the bone marrow or other tissues.

**plasmagel** \plaz′məjel\ That portion of the cytoplasm which is in the gel state.

**plasmagene** \plaz′məjēn\ [PLASMA + GENE] Any genetic locus that occurs on non-nuclear DNA. This includes mitochondrial DNA, chloroplast DNA, and DNA that is taken into the cytoplasm from outside the cell but is not yet incorporated into nuclear DNA or degraded. Also *cytogene, plasmon.*

**plasmalemma** \-lem′ə\ PLASMA MEMBRANE.

**plasmalogen** A glycerophospholipid in which the glycerol moiety bears an alk-1-enyl ether group. Lipid from the central nervous system contains a high proportion of plasmalogen. Also *phosphoglyceracetal.*

**plasmanic acid** A substituted glycerol 3-phosphate in which O-1 bears a saturated alkyl group (as an ether) and O-2 is acylated.

**plasmapheresis** \-fer′əsis\ Selective hemapheresis of plasma. It may be performed to obtain plasma donation or as a therapeutic measure to remove toxins, medications, antibodies, or other harmful substances. Also *plasma depletion.*

**plasmat-** \plazmat-\ PLASMO-.

**plasmatic** \plazmat′ik\ Of or relating to plasma. Also *plasmic.*

**plasmato-** \plaz′mətō-\ PLASMO-.

**plasmatogamy** \-täg′əmē\ PLASMOGAMY.

**plasmatorrhexis** \-tôrek′sis\ PLASMORRHEXIS.

**plasmenic acid** A substituted glycerol 3-phosphate in which O-1 bears an alk-1-enyl group and O-2 is acylated.

**plasmic** \plaz′mik\ PLASMATIC.

**plasmid** \plaz′mid\ [PLASM + -ID[1]] An extrachromosomal hereditary determinant of bacteria that replicates and is transferred independently of the chromosome. Some plasmids code for a mechanism for their own transfer by conjugation, and some are readily integrated into the chromosome. Plasmids often carry genes for traits that are valuable in some circumstances but are not essential for cell growth (e.g. drug resistance, bacteriocin production, or toxin production). **conjugative p.** A plasmid, such as the F agent, that carries the genes (the *tra* locus) for making a conjugation bridge. Also *sex factor, self-transmissible plasmid, transmissible plasmid.* **F p.** F FACTOR. **R p.** R FACTOR. **self-transmissible p.** CONJUGATIVE PLASMID. **transmissible p.** CONJUGATIVE PLASMID.

**plasmin** \plaz′min\ A proteolytic enzyme (EC 3.4.21.7) formed from its precursor, plasminogen, which occurs in blood. It is responsible for the removal of fibrin clots. The two polypeptide chains formed when plasminogen is cleaved to form plasmin are joined by a disulfide bond.

**plasminogen** \plazmin′əjən\ A plasma protein of molecular 81 kDa. It is converted into plasmin by hydrolysis of an Arg-Val bond. Also *profibrinolysin, proplasmin.*

**plasmo-** \plaz′mə-\ [Gk *plasma* (genitive *plasmatos*) anything molded, shaped, or formed] A combining form denoting plasm or plasma. Also *plasma-, plasmat-, plasmato-.*

**plasmocyte** \plaz′məsīt\ [PLASMO- + -CYTE] PLASMA CELL.

**plasmocytoma** \-sītō′mə\ MYELOMA.

**plasmodia** \plazmō′dē·ə\ Plural of PLASMODIUM.

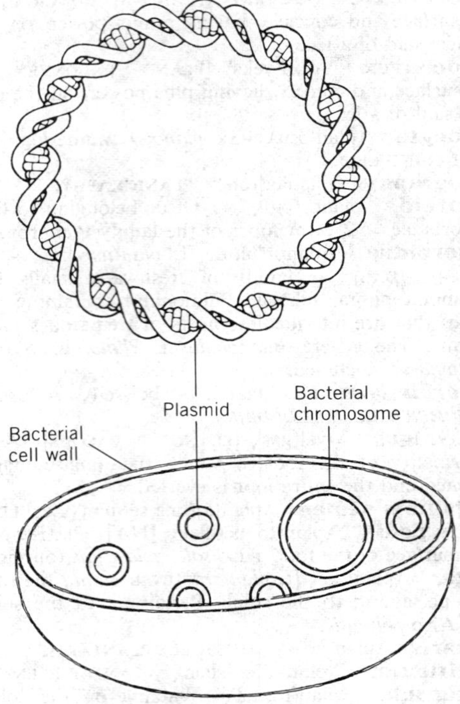


**Plasmid**

**plasmodial** \plazmō′dē·əl\ Pertaining to or caused by a member of the genus *Plasmodium.*

**plasmodiblast** \plazmō′diblast\ SYNCYTIOTROPHOBLAST.

**plasmodicidal** \plaz′mədicī′dəl\ Destructive to plasmodia; malaricidal.

**plasmodicide** \plazmō′disīd\ [*plasmodi(um)* + -CIDE] An agent that kills plasmodia.

**Plasmodiidae** \plazmō′dē·idē′\ [*plasmodi(um)* + -IDAE] A family of protozoa in the suborder Haemosporina, order Eucoccidiida, subclass Coccidia, class Sporozoea, phylum Apicomplexa. It encompasses the extremely important genus *Plasmodium,* containing the agents of human and other malarias, and the genera *Haemoproteus, Hepatocystis,* and *Leucocytozoon,* which are of considerable veterinary and biologic interest.

**plasmoditrophoblast** \-diträf′əblast\ SYNCYTIOTROPHOBLAST.

***Plasmodium*** \plazmō′dē·əm\ [New L (from *plasm(a)* + Gk *-ōd(ēs)* -like or pertaining to + L noun suffix *-ium*) something plasmalike or ameboid] A genus of sporozoan red blood cell parasites in the family Plasmodiidae, suborder Haemosporina, subclass Coccidia. It includes the four malarial parasites of man and other species found not only in primates, birds, and rodents, but also in lizards, frogs, and toads. The life cycle of the organism includes a sexual cycle followed by sporogony in the mosquito intermediate host and schizogonic cycles in the final host, first in the liver and subsequently in the red blood cells. Male and female gametocytes develop during the erythrocytic cycle, are ingested by mosquitoes with the blood meal, then rapidly emerge as female gametes (macrogametes) which are quickly fertilized by male gametes (microgametes). A zygote is formed, becomes a motile ookinete, and penetrates the gut wall of the mosquito to the outer layer. There, in the greatly enlarged structure, the oocyst, sporocysts, and, later, great numbers of sporozoites are formed. Upon release from the oocyst, the sporozoites migrate to the salivary glands, ready to be injected and infect a new host. Only *Anopheles* mosquitoes transmit the infection to humans, culicine mosquitoes serving as vectors for bird plasmodia. ***P. falciparum*** The agent of falciparum, or malignant tertian, malaria, characterized by small, often double-nucleated rings in the erythrocyte, general absence of all stages except rings and gametocytes from the peripheral blood, arc-shaped (falciform) gametocytes in the blood, the lack of host red cell enlargement and frequent presence of Maurer's clefts or dots. This organism is probably the greatest single cause of human misery, morbidity, and mortality of any infectious agent. Also *Plasmodium falciparum quotidianum, Plasmodium perniciosum, Laverania falcipara, Plasmodium aethiopicum, Plasmodium tenue.* ***P. malariae*** The agent of quartan malaria, which has a 72-hour schizogonic cycle in human erythrocytes. The parasites differ from the other agents of human malaria by the frequently formed band-shaped trophozoites, failure to enlarge the host red cell or to produce Schüffner's dots, and the rosette form of eight or nine merozoites formed by the schizont along with the black, coarse pigment. Natural infections of chimpanzees have been found in western Africa, strengthening the view that human malaria is a zoonosis. ***P. ovale*** A species found commonly in Africa, especially in western Africa, where it largely replaces *P. vivax.* The malarial fevers are tertian, as are the production and release of merozoites. The morphology and life cycle is much like that of *P. vivax,* except that stippling of host red cells appears somewhat earlier, the enlarged infected cells become distorted and often fimbriated, and only eight merozoites are produced per schizont. ***P. perniciosum*** PLASMODIUM FALCIPARUM. ***P. tenue*** PLASMODIUM FALCIPARUM. ***P. vivax*** The causative agent of vivax, or benign tertian, malaria. An erythrocyte infected with this species is characteristically enlarged and its cytoplasm stippled with Schüffner's dots. The schizont contains brown pigment granules grouped into a single mass, and forms 16 to 32 irregularly arranged merozoites.

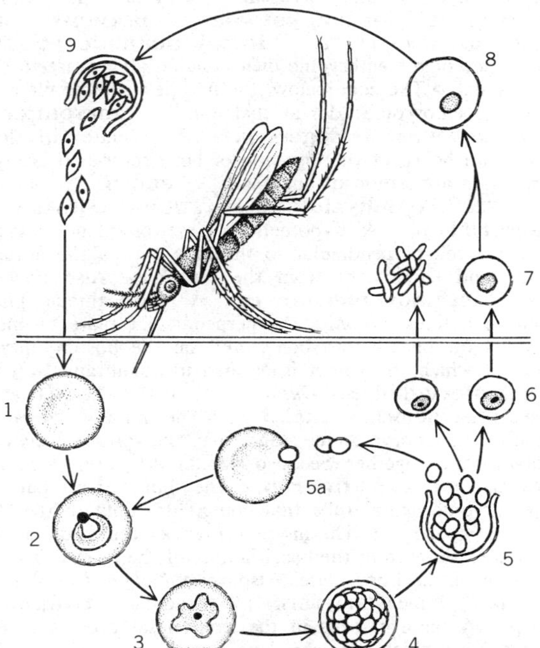


**Life cycle of *Plasmodium*** (1) Sporozoite invading red blood cell; (2) "ring" stage of development; (3) ameboid stage of development; (4) asexual division; (5) cell rupture with release of spores; (5a) reinfection of red blood cell by some spores; (6) development of other spores into sexual forms; (7) development into egg and sperm cells after mosquito sucks them in; (8) fertilized cell developing into cyst; (9) ruptured cyst releasing sporozoites.

**plasmodium** (*pl.* plasmodia) **1** A member of the genus *Plasmodium*; a malarial parasite. **2** A multinucleate protoplasmic mass.

**plasmogamy** \plazmäg′əmē\ [PLASMO- + GAM- + -Y] Fusion of the cytoplasm of two cells without nuclear fusion. It occurs in fungi and protozoa. Also *plasmatogamy.*

**plasmology** \plazmäl′əjē\ [PLASMO- + -LOGY] The scientific study of the minute structure of living protoplasm.

**plasmolysis** \plazmäl′isis\ **1** Dissolution of the protoplasm of the cell. Also *protoplasmolysis.* **2** The separation of the cytoplasm from the cell wall due to the removal of water from the protoplast by osmosis.

**plasmoma** \plazmō′mə\ MYELOMA.

**plasmon** \plaz′män\ PLASMAGENE.

**plasmonucleic acid** RIBONUCLEIC ACID.

**plasmorrhexis** \plaz′môrek′sis\ [PLASMO- + -RRHEXIS] Rupture of the plasma membrane and loss of the protoplasm resulting from an increase in internal pressure. Also *plasmatorrhexis.*

**plasmosome** \plaz′məsōm\ *Obs.* NUCLEOLUS.

**plasmotrophoblast** \-träf′əblast\ SYNCYTIOTROPHOBLAST.

**-plast** \-plast\ [Gk *plastos* molded, shaped, or formed] A combining form meaning an organized living particle or primitive cell.

**plaster** [L *(em)plastrum* (from Gk *emplastron* coated, from *emplassein* to plaster up, daub over) calcareous stone fired and reduced to powder] A semisolid substance that becomes adhesive when its temperature is raised by application to the skin. Plasters are used to hold dressings in place and to apply medicaments to the skin where they may be absorbed into the circulation. **adhesive p.** ADHESIVE TAPE. **dental p.** Superfine plaster of Paris used for making dental casts. Also *model plaster.* **impression p.** Plaster of Paris mixed with substances that reduce the setting time and expansion. It is also colored so that it is more easily separated from the cast. **model p.** DENTAL PLASTER. **mustard p.** **1** A folk remedy consisting of a poultice containing volatile oils distilled from black mustard seed, used as a counterirritant in the treatment of congestive lung disease and muscle pain. **2** Any of various locally applied rubefacients. **p. of Paris** Exsiccated calcium sulphate dihydrate that is milled to a fine powder. The addition of water produces a creamy mass which solidifies by an exothermic reaction. It is used either to make casts and molds of body surfaces or, when impregnated into bandages, to immobilize parts of the body. **sterile adhesive p.** STERILE ADHESIVE TAPE.

**plastic** [Gk *plastik(os)* (from *plassein* to form, mold, shape) suitable for molding, well formed] **1** Capable of being molded. **2** Serving to shape or reshape tissues, as in *plastic surgery.* **modeling p.** MODELING COMPOUND.

**plasticity** \plastis′itē\ The property of being plastic.

**plastid** \plasʹtid\ [Gk *plastis*, gen. *plastidos*, fem. of *plastēs* sculptor, molder] Any of a category of cytoplasmic organelles found in plant cells. They include the chloroplasts, which are involved in photosynthesis, and other related bodies, such as the chromoplasts, which are associated with food storage. Also *trophoplast*.

**plastin** \plasʹtin\ The protein forming the linin or spongioplasm of the cell.

**plastination** \plasʹtināʹshən\ A procedure for the preservation of biological specimens involving permeation of the object with a polyester resin or other plastic material, which then hardens.

**plastochromanol** A compound formed from reduced plastoquinone by a cyclization reaction of one phenolic hydroxyl group with the first isoprenoid unit of the side chain. A number may be added to the term to indicate the number of isoprenoid units in its side chain.

**plastocytemia** \plasʹtəsītēʹmē·ə\ THROMBOCYTHEMIA.

**plastocytopenia** \plasʹtəsīʹtəpēʹnē·ə\ THROMBOCYTOPENIA.

**plastocytosis** \plasʹtəsītōʹsis\ THROMBOCYTHEMIA.

**plastron** \plasʹträn\ [French (from Italian *piastrone* a large plate, augmentative of *piastra* a thin plate, plaster), a metal breastplate] The sternum together with its attached costal cartilages.

**-plasty** \-plasʹtē\ [Gk *plastos* molded, shaped, or formed] A combining form meaning a molding or shaping, especially by plastic surgery.

# plate

**plate** [French *plate* (fem. of *plat* flat, prob. from Gk *platys* flat, wide) flat] **1** A thin flat structure or layer. In anatomy it may be used to refer to a lamina or lamella. **2** A Petri dish or other vessel containing a shallow layer of solid culture medium. **3** To spread, streak, or pour (an inoculum) on an expanse of solid culture medium. **alar p.** The embryonic dorsal (i.e., sensory) portion of the neural tube above the sulcus limitans. **anal p.** The membrane that closes the posterior end of the gut during early embryonic development of vertebrates. It subsequently breaks down to form the anus or the gut aperture into the cloaca. **basal p.** A cartilaginous plate representing the primordium of the base of the skull. Chondrification takes place in three regions: chordal, hypophysial, and interorbitonasal. Also *craniofacial axis, basal cartilage, parachordal plate.* **basal p. of the cranium** The cartilaginous base plate of the embryonic skull. It is equivalent to the fused parachordal cartilages of lower types. **basal p. of Winckler** A superficial compact layer of the shed placenta composed almost entirely of decidual cells. Also *placental bed.* **base p.** BASEPLATE. **bite p.** BITEPLATE. **blood p.** *Older term* PLATELET. **bone p.** A flattened metal bar, with perforations for bone screws, that is used to immobilize a fractured or osteotomized bone. **butt p.** DISPERSIVE ELECTRODE. **cardiogenic p.** A transversely disposed bar of splanchnic mesoderm at the anterior end of the embryonic disk in front of the buccopharyngeal membrane. After the ventral folding of the ends of the embryo it comes to lie near the middle region. It will form the precursor of the heart proper and will lie below the ventral wall of the foregut. Also *cardiogenic area.* **cerebellar p.** A transversely oriented thickening formed by the union of the rhombic lips of the neural groove in the region of the developing hindbrain. It differentiates at about the twelve week stage into a median portion, the future vermis, and two lateral portions, the cerebellar hemispheres. **chordal p.** The invagination of mesodermal material axial to the node of Hensen, giving rise to a canal, a transitory stage appearing during gastrulation along the chordal axis. The momentary opening up of the inferior aspect of the canal results in the axial mesoderm seeming to become incorporated in the underlying endoderm. Also *notochordal plate.* **chorionic p.** An embryonic structure formed from several elements which together compose the fetal aspect of the placenta. From the inside to the outside of the conceptus they consist of the amnion, the extraembryonic mesenchyme (in the midst of which the chorioallantoic vessels fan out), and then the two layers of the trophoblast (cytotrophoblast or Langhans layer, and the syncytotrophoblast) which line the intervillous space. It is on this chorionic plate that villus-bearing trunks are situated. Also *chorial plate.* **cortical p.** The thick outer shell of dense bone of the alveolar part of the body of the mandible. *Outmoded.* **cough p.** A plate on which there is a microbiological culture medium used for isolation of pertussis bacteria in the diagnosis of whooping cough. The patient coughs onto the plate. **cribriform p. of ethmoid bone** LAMINA CRIBROSA OSSIS ETHMOIDALIS. **cuticular p.** The expanded free end of the phalangeal process of the supporting cells of the spiral organ of the internal ear, which takes part in the formation of the tectorial membrane. **cutis p.** DERMATOME. **decidual p.** That part of the decidua basalis which is directly in contact with the chorion frondosum. It undergoes a reaction (decidual) resulting in the appearance of decidual cells to form the compact layer of the decidua. **dental p.** *Older term* DENTURE **dermomyotome p.** DERMOMYOTOME. **dorsal p.** ROOF PLATE. **dorsal thalamic p.** The dorsal zone of the embryonic diencephalon giving rise to the epithalamus. • The zone below, the middle thalamic plate, is called the embryonic "dorsal thalamus." **dorsolateral p.** ALAR LAMINA. **Eggers p.** A bone plate with slots rather than holes for the insertion of bone screws. It is used to maintain apposition of bone ends. **end p.** See under ENDPLATE. **epiphysial p.** CARTILAGO EPIPHYSIALIS. **equatorial p.** A hypothetical plate or plane passing through a cell perpendicular to the long axis of the mitotic spindle and equidistant from the centrioles. Also *nuclear plate.* **ethmovomerine p.** A cartilaginous plate which, in a fetus, becomes the perpendicular plate, or mesethmoid, of the ethmoid bone, and on the posteroinferior aspect of which the vomer is ossified in membrane. **external pterygoid p.** *Outmoded* LAMINA LATERALIS PROCESSUS PTERYGOIDEI. **facial p.** The initially flat facial region of the embryo at the stage when the various processes involved come together. See also MAXILLARY PROCESS, FRONTONASAL PROCESS. **floor p.** The thin, ventral part of the embryonic neural tube that contributes only to the formation of ependyma. The motor centers of the medulla and spinal cord develop in the basal lamina of the neural tube on each side of the floor plate. Also *ventral plate, bodenplatte.* **foot p.** **1** BASIS STAPEDIS. **2** PEDICEL. **frontonasal p.** A plate of cells in the frontonasal process of the embryo from which the central part of the external nose develops. **growth p.** CARTILAGO EPIPHYSIALIS. **horizontal p. of palatine bone** LAMINA HORIZONTALIS OSSIS PALATINI. **inner p. of cranial bones** LAMINA INTERNA CRANII. **internal pterygoid p.** *Outmoded* LAMINA MEDIALIS PROCESSUS PTERYGOIDEI. **Kühne's terminal p.'s** The endplates on fusimotor fibers in skeletal muscle. **Lane p.'s** Narrow metal bone plates with perforations for screws that are used to hold fractured or osteotomized bones in apposition. **lateral mesoblastic p.** The unsegmented part of the intraembryonic mesoderm, which forms a sheet, or plate, lateral to the paraxial mesoderm on each side of the midline. It becomes split by the coelom to form an inner visceral layer and an outer parietal layer. **lateral pterygoid p.** LAMINA LATERALIS PROCESSUS PTERYGOIDEI. **lateral p. of pterygoid process** LAMINA LATERALIS PROCESSUS PTERYGOIDEI. **lingual p.** **1** The lingual cortical bone of the mandible. **2** A lingual connector of a partial denture, made of thin cast metal and covering all or part of the lingual surfaces of the lower anterior teeth. **location p.** A wax or acrylic baseplate containing variously shaped pieces of wire and used as an aid in locating buried teeth or roots by radiography. **meatal p.** An embryonic cellular mass which grows inward from the ectoderm of the first branchial groove toward the middle ear cavity. It eventually becomes the outer layer of the tympanic membrane. **medial p.** The intermediate cell mass of mesoderm that lies between the somites and the lateral plate mesoderm. *Outmoded.* **medial pterygoid p.** LAMINA MEDIALIS PROCESSUS PTERYGOIDEI. **medial p. of pterygoid process** LAMINA MEDIALIS PROCESSUS PTERYGOIDEI. **medullary p.** NEURAL PLATE. **metaphase p.** The plane in the equatorial region of the cell at which the chromosomes reach equilibrium during metaphase of mitosis or meiosis. **motor p.** MOTOR ENDPLATE. **nail p.** STRATUM CORNEUM UNGUIS. **nephrotome p.** A mesodermal plate laying just lateral to the somites of an embryo. It gives rise to the uriniferous tubules of the embryonic kidney systems. **neural p.** A midline, axial thickening of ectoderm on the dorsal aspect of the embryonic disk above the notochord. It is brought about by the differentiation of ectodermal cells into medulloblasts which proliferate to form stem cells for neurons and supporting cells. The neural plate is wider at the front, demonstrating from the start the predominance of the head end. It corresponds in some ways to the neurula stage which immediately follows gastrulation and plays an important part in the complex processes of the delimitation of embryonic regions in development. The plate gives rise to the neural groove, the lips of which will close over and fuse to establish the neural tube, from which the brain and spinal cord will develop. Also *medullary plate.* **notochordal p.** CHORDAL PLATE. **nuclear p.** EQUATORIAL PLATE. **optic p.** The thickening at the anterior end of the neural tube from which the optic vesicle is developed in the embryo. **orbital p. of ethmoid bone** LAMINA ORBITALIS OSSIS ETHMOIDALIS. **orbital p. of frontal bone** PARS ORBITALIS OSSIS FRONTALIS. **outer p. of cranial bones** LAMINA EXTERNA CRANII. **palatal p.** A palatal connector of a partial denture, made of cast metal and covering a part of the palate. **parachordal p.** BASAL PLATE. **parietal p.** The layer of extraembryonic mesoderm lining the trophoblast, and covering the sides of the amnion, derived from the lateral plate mesoderm, which with the associated ectoderm forms the somatopleure. In lower vertebrates, it is the outer layer of the intermediate cell mass after that structure has been divided by the coelom. **patient p.** DISPERSIVE ELECTRODE. **perpendicular p. of ethmoid bone** LAMINA PERPENDICULARIS OSSIS ETHMOIDALIS. **perpendicular p. of palatine bone** LAMINA PERPENDICULARIS OSSIS PALATINI. **pour p.** A culture in which the agar medium has been melted, cooled to about 45°C, mixed with the bacterial inoculum, and poured into a Petri dish. **prechordal p.** The region directly in front of the notochord which, unlike the rest of this structure, is not obviously separated from the underlying endoderm. Separating the notochord from the pharyngeal membrane, it represents the axis of all that which will form by delimitation of the frontal region. Furthermore, it plays an important inductive role in controlling the normal development of the forebrain, the hypophysis, the base of the skull, and the facial mass. **primitive joint p.** A thickening of mesenchyme between the cartilaginous precursors of bones at the place where a joint forms as the fetus grows. It disappears from synovial articulations but may persist in nonsynovial ones. **prochordal p.** Localized thickening of endoderm, in didermic embryos, situated in the midline cephalic to the anterior end of the head process. It is in close contact with the overlying ectoderm. At the time of gastrulation the close adhesion of the two layers prevents cephalic prolongation. The membrane so formed rotates downwards and becomes the pharyngeal (buccopharyngeal) membrane which forms the floor of the stomodeum. **quadrigeminal p.** LAMINA TECTI MESENCEPHALI. **retaining p.** RETAINER. **reticular p.** A finely corrugated nerve ending found in the ciliary body. **roof p.** The dorsal wall of the developing neural tube, which is initially thinner than other parts of the tube wall. In some parts of the nervous system, the roof plate becomes thickened but in others it becomes modified to form the tela choroidea of the third and fourth ventricles. Foramina appear on the roof of the fourth ventricle, connecting the cavity with the subarachnoid space. Also *dorsal plate.* **safety p.** DISPERSIVE ELECTRODE. **secondary spiral p.** LAMINA SPIRALIS SECUNDARIA. **segmental p.** A mesoblastic plate on each side of the notochord. The segmental plates give rise to the somites. Also *segmental zone.* **skin p.** DERMATOME. **spiral p.** LAMINA SPIRALIS OSSEA. **spread p.** A bacteriologic culture dish with an inoculum spread uniformly over the surface by a bent glass rod. **streak p.** A microbiologic culture plate containing a solid medium upon which the inoculum is distributed by streaking motions of a loop or rod. It is used to disperse organisms so that discrete colonies will develop. **Tarin's p.** VELUM MEDULLARE CAUDALE. **tarsal p.'s** The tarsus superior palpebrae and tarsus inferior palpebrae. Also *tarsal cartilages, palpebral cartilages.* **terminal p.** LAMINA TERMINALIS. **tympanic p.** The tympanic part of the temporal bone that forms the inferior, anterior, and most of the posterior parts of the bony part of the external acoustic meatus. At birth it is represented by the tympanic ring. **urethral p.** A thickening of endoderm which grows forwards from the walls of the cloaca and urogenital sinus of embryo into the phallus. The lower margin of the plate is in contact with the ectoderm lining and primary urethral groove which appears along the caudal surface of the phallus. Its raised margins are called the genital folds. **vascular foot p.** See under SUCKER FOOT. **ventral p.** FLOOR PLATE. **ventrolateral p.** BASAL LAMINA. **vertical p. of palatine bone** LAMINA PERPENDICULARIS OSSIS PALATINI. **visceral p.** SPLANCHNIC MESODERM. **wing p.** ALAR LAMINA.

**plateau** [French (from *plat* flat, prob. from Gk *platys* flat, wide), a tray, plain situated in a high place] **1** In a process, a stage during which there is no apparent growth, progression, or other change. **2** A level portion of a linear graph, which represents such a stage. **3** Any raised, flat structure. **4** In a radiation detector, an operating region within which the output count rate, for a given radiation input, is relatively independent of the applied voltage. **Geiger p.** Part of the characteristic curve (count rate against anode voltage) of a Geiger-Müller tube: the relatively level portion toward the upper end of the curve, where the count rate (from a constant radiation source) rises little as the voltage is increased. The slow rise indicates that each entering particle or photon, whatever its energy, causes a full Townsend avalanche to occur, so that all the tube's output pulses have essentially the same height. **tibial p.** Either the medial or the lateral superior articular surface of the proximal end of the tibia. *Outmoded.*

**platelet** \plat′lit\ [PLATE + *-let,* dim. suffix] A fragment of megakaryocyte cytoplasm that is normally present in large numbers in blood and which plays an important role in blood clotting. A platelet is about 1 μm in diameter, lacks a nucleus, and has a life-span in circulating blood of less than 10 days. It contains a number of activities related to hemostasis and has on its surface receptors for various plasma factors. Its properties of aggregation and adhesion permit it to initiate hemostasis when vascular endothelium is damaged and also to initiate clotting. Normal blood contains 140–400 $\times 10^9$ platelets per liter. Also *blood platelet, Bizzozero's corpuscle, Bizzozero cell, dust corpuscle, Hayem's elementary corpuscle, blood plate* (older term), *thrombocyte, soterocyte* (obs.), *Deetjen's body.* **blood p.** PLATELET. **giant p.** A larger than normal blood platelet (e.g. 7–15 μm in diameter). Giant platelets are characteristically seen in myeloproliferative disorders, such as myeloid metaplasia with myelofibrosis, or polycythemia vera. Also *megaloplastocyte.*

**plateletpheresis** \plat′litfer′əsis\ The selective removal of platelets by hemapheresis. It may be performed to obtain platelet donation or as a therapeutic measure in patients with thrombocytosis. Also *thrombocytapheresis.*

**platinectomy** \plat′inek′təmē\ [French *platin(e)* (from Spanish *platina* plate) plate, footplate of the stapes + -ECTOMY] PORTMANN INTERPOSITION OPERATION.

**plating** 1 The technique of distributing a bacterial inoculum in a solid medium, either by pouring together or by spreading or streaking on the surface of the hardened agar. 2 The fastening of fractured bones to a metal plate to keep them in alignment. **replica p.** A technique of obtaining multiple copies of a culture plate by transferring cells from all the colonies on a plate to sterile velveteen or close-packed needles and thence to multiple test plates.

**platinum** \plat′ənəm\ Element number 78, having atomic weight 195.09. A silvery white, corrosion-resistant metal, platinum occurs native and in certain ores. The metal is used in many technologic applications and in dentistry. Finely divided platinum is an important catalyst in research and industry. Symbol: Pt

**platode** \plat′ōd\ [*plat(y)-* + *-ode,* combining form from Gk *-ōdes* -OID ] PLATYHELMINTH.

**platy-** \plat′i-\ [Gk *platys* flat, broad] A combining form meaning flat, broad.

**platybasia** \-bā′zhə\ [PLATY- + *bas(e)* + -IA] A developmental defect of the skull in which the floor of the posterior fossa is elevated in the region around the foramen magnum so that the entire cranial base appears somewhat flatter than usual. Also *basilar invagination.*

**platycephaly** \-sef′əlē\ [PLATY- + CEPHAL- + -Y ] A condition in which the head is wide and flat, with a breadth-height index of less than 70. Also *platycrania.*

**platycnemia** \plat′ik·nē′mē·ə\ [PLATY- + Gk *knēm(ē)* tibia + -IA] A condition characterized by a tibia that is abnormally broad and flat. Also *platyknemia.*

**platycrania** \-krā′nē·ə\ PLATYCEPHALY.

**platycyte** A tuberculous multinucleated giant cell containing fewer nuclei than usual. . *Obs.*

**platyglossal** \-gläs′əl\ Possessing an abnormally broad, flattened tongue.

**platyhelminth** \-hel′minth\ [PLATY- + HELMINTH] A flatworm; a member of the phylum Platyhelminthes. Also *platode.*

**Platyhelminthes** \-helmin′thēz\ [PLATY- + Gk *helminthes,* pl. of *helmins* a worm] A phylum of bilaterally symmetric worms characteristically flattened and leaflike in shape. Having no true body cavity, the phylum is part of the acoelomate group and most forms are hermaphroditic. There are three classes, Turbellaria, Trematoda, and Cestoidea. The medically important species in humans and other animals are found in the subclass Cestoda of the class Cestoidea and in the subclass Digenea of the class Trematoda. The Turbellaria are free-living or endocommensals in various invertebrates.

**platyhieric** \-hī′er′ik\ Having an abnormally broad, flattened sacrum.

**platyknemia** \plat′ik·nē′mē·ə\ PLATYCNEMIA.

**platymorphia** \-môr′fē·ə\ [PLATY- + MORPH- + -IA ] A broad, flat shape or, as in the eye, a short anterior-posterior axis.

**platyonychia** \-ōnik′ē·ə\ [PLATY- + ONYCH- + -IA ] An abnormal breadth and flatness of the nails.

**platyopia** \-ō′pē·ə\ [PLATY- + *-op(e)* + -IA] A marked broadness of the face, specifically with a nasomalar index less than 107.5.

**platypellic** \-pel′ik\ Having a pelvis that is both wide and flattened, with a pelvic index of below 90.

**platypnea** \platip′nē·ə\ [PLATY- + -PNEA] Shortness of breath experienced in the standing or seated position. Also *orthostatic dyspnea.* Compare ORTHOPNEA.

**platyrrhine** \plat′ərīn\ [PLATY- + Gk *rhis,* gen. *rhinos,* the nose] **1** Having a nose broad in proportion to its length. **2** Possessing a skull that has a nasal index between 53 and 58.

**platysma** \platiz′mə\ [Gk (from *platys* broad, flat) a flat object, plate; short for *platysma myōdes* muscular plate] [NA] A broad flat muscle in the subcutaneous tissue of the neck that arises from the fascia overlying the upper parts of the pectoralis major and deltoid muscles and extends upwards to the lower face. The most anterior fibers interlace with those of the opposite side over the chin, and the adjacent fibers insert into the inferior margin of the mandible. The more posterior fibers pass forward over the lower part of the masseter muscle to insert into the skin and subcutaneous tissue of the lower part of the face and the angle of the mouth, blending with other muscles there. It is supplied by the cervical branch of facial nerve. Acting singly or together with the opposite side it depresses the angle of the mouth and lower lip and lifts and tightens the skin over the neck and the chest. It can also depress the mandible. Also *platysma muscle, tetragonus.*

**platyspondylia** \-spändil′ē·ə\ [PLATY- + SPONDYL- + -IA] An abnormal flatness of the vertebral bodies.

**platystaphyline** \-staf′ilin\ [PLATY- + STAPHYL- + -INE] Characterized by an unusually broad, flat palate.

**platytrope** \plat′itrōp\ Either of two lateral homologues, or symmetrical parts on opposite sides of the body.

**pleasure** / **function p.** The enjoyment gained from performing an act or exercising one's capacities without anxiety. **organ p.** In psychoanalytic psychology, the excitement and satisfaction that occur in extragenital erogenous zones, such as the oral and anal regions.

**plectrum** \plek′trəm\ [L (from Gk *plēktron* an instrument for striking the lyre, a cock's spur), an instrument for striking the harp] **1** *Outmoded* UVULA PALATINA. **2** *Outmoded* MALLEUS.

**pledget** \plej′ət\ [origin unknown] A small, dense pad of absorbent material used during surgical procedures to arrest bleeding or to buttress sutures.

**plegaphonia** \pleg′əfō′nē·ə\ [Gk *plēg(ē)* stroke + APHONIA] Auscultation of the chest through the use of nonlaryngeal vibrations in those instances where the subject is unable to talk. The vibrations are usually induced by gentle tapping over the upper trachea.

**plegia** \plē′jə\ [from the combining form -PLEGIA] **1** Paralysis of abrupt onset. **2** Any type of paralysis.

**-plegia** \-plē′jə\ [Gk *plēgē* a blow, stroke + -IA] A combining form denoting paralysis.

**pleio-** \plī′ō-\ PLEO-.

**pleiotropia** \plī′ətrō′pē·ə\ PLEIOTROPISM.

**pleiotropic** \plī′əträp′ik\ Pertaining to a phenotype characterized by multiple features due to a single genetic locus. Also *polyphenic*.

**pleiotropism** \plī′ətrōpizm\ The presence of multiple, seemingly unrelated, characters due to the action of a single genetic locus. Also *pleiotropy, pleiotropia, polypheny*.

**pleo-** \plē′ō-, plē′ə-\ [Gk *pleōn* (also *pleiōn*) more, larger, greater] A combining form meaning (1) multiple; (2) excessive. Also *pleio-*.

**pleochromocytoma** \-krō′mōsītō′mə\ [PLEO- + *chromocyt(e)* + -OMA] A tumor of cells with different colors.

**pleoconial** \-kō′nē·əl\ Having an increased size and number of mitochondria in the cell cytoplasm: said of a form of metabolic myopathy.

**pleocytosis** \-sītō′sis\ [PLEO- + CYT- + -OSIS ] An abnormally large number of cells in the cerebrospinal fluid.

**pleomorphic** \-môr′fik\ **1** Distinguished by having more than one form during a life cycle. **2** Having multiple spore forms: used especially of fungi. For defs. 1 and 2 also *pleomorphous*.

**pleomorphism** \-môr′fizm\ POLYMORPHISM.

**pleomorphous** \-môr′fəs\ PLEOMORPHIC.

**pleonasm** \plē′ənazm\ [Gk *pleonasm(a)* superfluity or *pleonasm(os)* superabundance, excess] An excessive size or number of parts.

**pleonosteosis** \-näs′tē·ō′sis\ Abnormally excessive bone formation. **Léri's p.** DYSCHONDROSTEOSIS.

**pleoptics** \plē·äp′tiks\ [PLEO- + *(o)ptics*] A treatment for suppression amblyopia that relatively enhances macular vision by dazzling the paramacular area with a ring of light accurately localized by a pleoptophor. Also *Bangerter's method*.

**pleoptophor** \plē·äp′təfôr\ [PLEO- + *(o)pto-* + -PHOR] A device for treating eccentric fixation by dazzling the perimacular retina, thereby relatively enhancing the visual capability of the fovea.

**plerocercoid** \plir′əsur′koid\ [Gk *plēr(ēs)* full + *o* + *kerk(os)* tail + -OID] The second or final larval stage of certain tapeworms of fish or fish-eating animals. It is characterized by an invaginated scolex at one end and a wormlike, sometimes quite elongate unencysted body in the tissues of various fish hosts, the ingestion of which transmits them to the intestine of the final host. This larval stage follows the procercoid stage in the first host, usually a crustacean.

**plesiognathus** \plē′sē·əgnath′əs\ [Gk *plēsio(s)* near + *gnathos* the jaw, esp. the lower jaw] A fistulous opening on the skin in the parotid region that is sometimes described as an accessory mouth. Such an opening is usually a branchial fistula connecting with the pharynx or nasopharynx and representing a persistent embryonic first branchial cleft.

***Plesiomonas*** \plē′sē·äm′ənəs\ A genus of vibrios consisting of a single species, *P. shigelloides*. It closely resembles *Aeromonas* but does not excrete toxins.

**plesiomorphism** \plē′sē·əmôr′fizm\ [Gk *plēsio(s)* near + MORPH- + -ISM] A resemblance in form or shape.

**plesiopia** \plē′sē·ō′pē·ə\ [Gk *plēsi(os)* near + -OPIA] MYOPIA.

**plessimeter** \plesim′ətər\ PLEXIMETER.

**plessor** \ples′ər\ PLEXOR.

**plethora** \pleth′ərə\ [Gk *plēthōrē* (from *plēthein* to be or become full; akin to *pleos* full, filled) fullness, satiety] **1** A fullness, overabundance, or excess. **2** Vascular dilatation or congestion causing a red or ruddy appearance, especially of the face. Also *panhyperemia*. Adj. plethoric.

**plethysmogram** \plethiz′məgram\ A recording obtained from a plethysmograph.

**plethysmograph** \plethis′məgraf\ [Gk *plēthysmos* (from *plēthynein*, also *plēthyein* to increase) an increase + -GRAPH] An instrument used to measure the variations in volume of a part, limb, organ, or the whole body. **body p.** An airtight box in which a subject is confined so that changes in body volume may be determined by measuring changes of gas volume or pressure within the box. It is used to measure airway resistance, functional residual capacity of the lung, and tracer gas uptake in the measurement of cardiac output. Also *aeroplethysmograph*. **finger p.** A photoplethysmograph or an impedance plethysmograph that detects blood-pressure pulsations in the finger. Also *digital plethysmograph*.

**plethysmography** \pleth′ismäg′rəfē\ A technique for recording measurements of changes in volume in an organ or part of the body by a plethysmograph. **air cuff p.** The measurement of volume flow in the deep veins by observation of the changes in pressure in an air-inflated circumferential cuff. **impedance p.** The measurement of changes in electrical impedance between electrodes placed on the skin to indicate volume changes of organs, as in diagnosing venous occlusions of the extremities by measuring the rate of venous outflow as manifested by changes in limb blood volume, following release of a proximal pneumatic cuff. Electrodes on the chest detect respiration or cardiac output. Those on the leg detect deep vein thrombosis; on the finger, the pulse; and on the scalp, vessel occlusion in the brain. **strain gauge p.** The determination of blood flow to a limb or digit by observing the changes in volume of the limb as indicated by the changes in the length of mercury-in-rubber tubes that are wrapped around the limb or digit. **tympanic p.** A test employed to differentiate between glomus jugulare tumors and intratemporal carotid aneurysms. The external auditory meatus is connected to a pressure transducer and recording system by means of a well-fitting aural speculum and a polyethylene tube. The tracings obtained in the two diseases show characteristic differences. **venous-occlusion p.** A technique for measuring the blood flow in a limb or digit by placing a cuff around the proximal part and inserting the distal part in water or air, and measuring the changes in volume when the cuff is inflated above venous pressure but below arterial diastolic pressure.

**plethysmometer** \pleth′izmäm′ətər\ [Gk *plēthysmo(s)* an increase + -METER] An apparatus for measuring the amount of swelling of a blood vessel.

**pleur-** \plUr-\ PLEURO-.

**pleura** \plUr′ə\ [Gk *pleura* a rib, in pl. *pleurai* ribs, the side or sides] [NA] A serous membrane that forms a closed invaginated sac. The visceral layer invests each lung and the parietal layer lines the thoracic cavity. **cervical p.** CUPULA PLEURAE. **p. costalis** [NA] The part of the parietal pleura that lines the internal aspect of the sternum, ribs, and transversus thoracis muscle, and the sides of the bodies of the thoracic vertebrae. It is continuous superiorly with the cervical pleura, inferiorly with the diaphragmatic pleura, and medially with the mediastinal pleura. Also *costal pleura.* **p. diaphragmatica** [NA] The thin parietal pleura that covers the part of the upper surface of the diaphragm below each lung. Along its outer periphery it is continuous with the costal pleura at the costodiaphragmatic line of reflection, and medially it is continuous with the mediastinal pleura where the diaphragm is attached to the pericardium. Also *diaphragmatic pleura.* **p. mediastinalis** [NA] The portion of the parietal pleura that lines the lateral aspect of the structures located in the interpulmonary region. Above the root of the lung on each side it forms a continuous layer between the vertebral column and the sternum, and at the root it becomes continuous with the visceral layer ensheathing the structures there. Below the root it forms the pulmonary ligament. Also *mediastinal pleura.* **p. parietalis** [NA] The serous membrane that forms the outer layer of the pleural cavity. It is subdivided according to the regions of the thoracic cavity that it lines, namely, pleura costalis, pleura diaphragmatica, and pleura mediastinalis. It extends into the root of the neck over the apex of the lung to form the cupula pleurae. Also *parietal pleura.* **pericardiac p.** The portion of the mediastinal pleura that is firmly attached to the outer surface of the pericardium. Also *pleura pericardiaca* (outmoded). **p. visceralis** [NA] The serous membrane that lines all the surfaces of the lung and the fissures between the lobes except at the root of the lung and along the attachment of the pulmonary ligament, where it is continuous with the parietal pleura. Also *visceral pleura.*

**pleura-** \plŭr′ə-\ PLEURO-.

**pleuracentesis** \plŭr′əsentē′sis\ THORACENTESIS.

**pleurae** \plŭr′ē\ Plural of PLEURA.

**pleural** \plŭr′əl\ Relating to the pleura.

**pleuralgia** \plŭral′jə\ [PLEUR- + -ALGIA] Pain originating in the pleura.

**pleurapophysis** \plŭr′əpäf′isis\ [PLEUR- + APOPHYSIS] A rib.

**pleurectomy** \plŭrek′təmē\ The surgical excision of the pleura. Also *stripping of the pleura.*

**pleurisy** \plŭr′isē\ [Old French *pleurisie,* from Late L *pleurisis,* from Gk *pleuritis* (short for *pleuritis nosos,* from *pleuritēs* costal, lateral, from *pleura* rib, side, + *nosos* illness) pleurisy] Inflammation or irritation of the pleura, which usually causes either pain during breathing or accumulation of pleural fluid. **acute p.** Inflammation of the pleura of sudden onset, indicating an acute infective, irritative, or inflammatory process. **adhesive p.** Pleurisy in which there is adherence between the visceral and parietal pleura. **basal p.** Inflammation of the pleura at the base, or caudal end, of the chest. **benign dry p.** Dry pleurisy of good prognosis. **blocked p.** ENCYSTED PLEURISY. **chronic p.** Persisting pleural inflammation or irritation. **chyliform p.** Pleurisy accompanied by milky fluid. Also *chyloid pleurisy.* **chylous p.** Pleurisy with milky effusion due to the presence of fat droplets. **diaphragmatic p.** Inflammation of the part of the pleura overlying the diaphragm. **double p.** Bilateral pleurisy; pleurisy affecting both right and left pleurae. **dry p.** Pleurisy without accumulation of effusion in the pleural cavity. Also *plastic pleurisy.* **p. with effusion** Pleurisy with accumulation of an abnormal quantity of fluid in the pleural cavity. Also *exudative pleurisy, wet pleurisy.* **encysted p.** Pleurisy with a localized, trapped collection of fluid. Also *blocked pleurisy, sacculated pleurisy.* **epidemic p.** EPIDEMIC PLEURODYNIA. **epidemic benign dry p.** EPIDEMIC PLEURODYNIA. **epidemic diaphragmatic p.** EPIDEMIC PLEURODYNIA. **exudative p.** PLEURISY WITH EFFUSION. **fibrinous p.** Pleurisy with deposition of fibrin in the pleural space. **hemorrhagic p.** Pleurisy with a bloody pleural effusion. **ichorous p.** Pleurisy with thin watery effusion. **interlobular p.** Pleurisy with fluid loculated between lobes of the lung. **mediastinal p.** Pleurisy involving the part of the pleura overlying the mediastinum. **metapneumonic p.** Pleurisy following pneumonia. **plastic p.** DRY PLEURISY. **primary p.** Pleurisy which is not recognizably the result of other disease such as pneumonia. **pulmonary p.** VISCERAL PLEURISY. **sacculated p.** ENCYSTED PLEURISY. **secondary p.** Pleurisy developing in the course of another illness. **serofibrinous p.** Pleurisy with a watery pleural effusion and with deposition of fibrin on the pleural membranes. **serous p.** Pleurisy with a watery pleural effusion. **visceral p.** Pleurisy involving the visceral pleura. Also *pulmonary pleurisy.* **wet p.** PLEURISY WITH EFFUSION.

**pleuritic** \plŭrit′ik\ Relating to or affected with pleurisy.

**pleuritis** \plŭrī′tis\ [Gk, pleurisy. See PLEURISY.] Inflammation of the pleura.

**pleuro-** \plŭr′ō-\ [Gk *pleura* rib (in plural, side or sides)] A combining form denoting (1) the pleura; (2) a side; (3) rib. Also *pleur-, pleura-.*

**pleurocentesis** \-sentē′sis\ THORACENTESIS.

**pleurodesis** \-dē′sis\ [PLEURO- + -DESIS] A surgical operation to produce adhesion of two layers of pleura, for prevention of the recurrence of pneumothorax.

**pleurodynia** \-din′ē·ə\ [PLEUR- + -ODYNIA] Pleuritic pain without pleural effusion, of unknown cause. **epidemic p.** An acute infectious disease caused by coxsackieviruses of group B (and rarely echoviruses and group A coxsackieviruses) and characterized by paroxysms of fever and sharp pleuritic pain in the chest or upper abdomen. About 25% of patients experience multiple recurrences after the initial 4–6 days of illness. Also *Bornholm disease, Daae's disease, Daae-Finsen disease, devil's grip, Dabney's grip, epidemic myalgia, epidemic myositis, epidemic pleurisy, epidemic benign dry pleurisy, epidemic diaphragmatic pleurisy, epidemic transient diaphragmatic spasm, Sylvest's disease.*

**pleurohepatitis** \-hep′ətī′tis\ Hepatitis with extension of the inflammation to that portion of the pleura near the liver.

**pleurolysis** \plŭräl′isis\ The detachment of the pleura from its adhesions by surgical means.

**pleuromelus** \-mē′ləs\ [PLEURO- + Gk *melos* a limb] An embryo, fetus, or postnatal individual with a supernumerary limb arising from the lateral aspect of the trunk.

**pleuroparietopexy** \-pərī′ətōpek′sē\ The procedure of attaching the visceral pleura to the parietal pleura in order to fix the lung to the chest wall.

**pleuropericardial** \-per′ikär′dē·əl\ Relating both to the pleura and the pericardium.

**pleuropericarditis** \-per′ikärdī′tis\ Inflammation of both the pleura and the pericardium.

**pleuroperitoneal** \-per′itənē′əl\ Relating to or connecting the pleura and the peritoneum.

**pleuroperitoneum** \-per′itənē′əm\ The pleura and the peritoneum considered as a unit.

**pleuropneumonia** \-n$^y$oomō′nē·ə\ Pneumonia associated with pleurisy.

**pleuropneumonolysis** \-n$^y$oo′mōnäl′isis\ THORACOPLASTY.

**pleuropulmonary** \-pul′mәner′ē\ Relating both to the pleurae and to the lungs.

**pleurorrhea** \plŭr′ôrē′ə\ PLEURAL EFFUSION.

**pleuroscopy** \plŭräs′kəpē\ [PLEURO- + -SCOPY] Inspection of the pleural cavity through a viewing scope inserted through the chest wall.

**pleurosoma** \-sō′mə\ [PLEURO- + SOMA] The defective development of the body wall in the thoracic and/or abdominal regions, permitting variable eventration of viscera. It is usually associated with meromelia on the same side of the body as the defect. Also *pleurosomatoschisis.*

**pleurotome** \plUr′ətōm\ A segmental subdivision of the lung supplied by the sensory nerve fibers of a single spinal nerve.

**plexectomy** \pleksek′təmē\ [*plex(us)* + -ECTOMY] The resection of a part or all of a nervous, venous, or lymphatic plexus.

**plexiform** \plek′sifôrm\ Resembling or forming a plexus.

**pleximeter** \pleksim′ətər\ [Gk *plēxi(s)* a stroke, blow + -METER] A small plate of hard material, such as ivory or hard rubber, which is placed against the body and struck in mediate percussion. Also *plessimeter, plexometer.*

**plexitis** \pleksi′tis\ [*plex(us)* + -ITIS] Inflammation of the nerves or roots which contribute to a plexus. **acute p.** GUILLAIN-BARRÉ SYNDROME.

**plexometer** \pleksäm′ətər\ PLEXIMETER.

**plexor** \plek′sər\ [New L (from Gk *plēx(is)* a stroke, blow + L *-or* -OR)] Any of various small hammers, typically with a rubber head, used in percussion of the chest or of deep tendon reflexes. Also *plessor.*

# plexus

**plexus** \plek′səs\ [L, past part. of *plectere* to braid, plait] (*pl.* plexus, plexuses) An interlacing network, as of nerves, blood vessels, or lymphatic vessels. **abdominal aortic p.** PLEXUS AORTICUS ABDOMINALIS. **annular p.** A delicate network of sensory filaments deriving from ciliary nerves and located in the substantia propria around the periphery of the cornea. **anococcygeal p.** PLEXUS COCCYGEUS. **p. anserinus** PLEXUS INTRAPAROTIDEUS. **anterior bronchial p.** PLEXUS PULMONALIS ANTERIOR. **anterior cardiac p.** PLEXUS CORONARIUS CORDIS ANTERIOR. **anterior coronary p. of heart** PLEXUS CORONARIUS CORDIS ANTERIOR. **anterior esophageal p.** PLEXUS ESOPHAGEUS ANTERIOR. **anterior pulmonary p.** PLEXUS PULMONALIS ANTERIOR. **anterolateral p. of Santorini** PLEXUS PROSTATICUS. **p. aorticus abdominalis** [NA] A network of autonomic nerves lying on the ventral and lateral surfaces of the aorta between the superior and inferior mesenteric arteries. It is formed by the right and left celiac plexuses and the lumbar splanchnic nerves. Also *abdominal aortic plexus.* **p. aorticus thoracicus** [NA] A network of autonomic and sensory nerves surrounding the thoracic aorta and continuous with the plexus aorticus abdominalis through the aortic hiatus of the diaphragm. Also *thoracic aortic plexus, plexus aorticus thoracalis.* **p. arteriae cerebri anterioris** Terminal filaments from the internal carotid and cavernous plexuses that accompany the anterior cerebral arteries and can be traced to the pia mater. Also *plexus of cerebral artery anterior.* **p. arteriae cerebri mediae** Sympathetic filaments from the internal carotid and cavernous plexuses that surround the middle cerebral arteries and extend to the pia mater. Also *plexus of cerebral artery middle, middle plexus of cerebral artery* (obs.). **p. arteriae choroideae** Sympathetic nerve fibers from the plexus arteriae cerebri mediae that accompany the choroid arteries to the choroid plexus of the inferior horns of the lateral ventricles. Also *plexus of choroid arteries.* **p. arteriae ovaricae** *Outmoded* PLEXUS OVARICUS. **Auerbach's p.** PLEXUS MYENTERICUS. **p. auricularis posterior** Sympathetic nerve filaments derived from the superior cervical ganglion and located on the posterior auricular artery. Also *posterior auricular plexus.* **p. autonomici** [NA] Plexuses composed of sympathetic and parasympathetic portions of the autonomic nervous system combined with visceral afferent fibers in the thorax, abdomen, and pelvis. These great networks are the cardiac, celiac, and pelvic plexuses. Also *autonomic plexuses, plexus sympathici.* **p. basilaris** [NA] Interconnecting veins located between the two layers of the dura mater on the clivus. It connects the cavernous sinuses as well as the two inferior petrosal sinuses and communicates with the internal vertebral venous plexuses. Also *basilar plexus.* **Batson's p.** VERTEBRAL-VENOUS SYSTEM. **p. brachialis** [NA] A network formed by the ventral primary divisions of the fifth to eighth cervical and first thoracic nerves. It gives origin to the nerves of the upper extremity. Also *brachial plexus.* **bulbar p.** A network of nerve fibers close to the embryonic bulbus cordis. **p. cardiacus** [NA] A network of autonomic nerve fibers situated at the base of the heart close to the arch of the aorta. It is composed of preganglionic parasympathetic vagal fibers, postganglionic sympathetic fibers, and scattered groups of ganglion cells. It is divided into the plexus cardiacus profundus and superficialis. Also *cardiac plexus.* **p. cardiacus profundus** The deep part of the cardiac plexus, formed by cardiac branches of both the vagus nerve and sympathetic trunk lying deep to the arch of the aorta and giving rise to the anterior and posterior coronary plexuses of the heart. Also *deep cardiac plexus, great cardiac plexus.* **p. cardiacus superficialis** The superficial part of the cardiac plexus, formed by superior cardiac branches of the left vagus nerve and left sympathetic trunk. It lies in the aortic arch near the bifurcation of the pulmonary trunk, and sends branches to the deep cardiac, anterior coronary, and left anterior pulmonary plexuses. Also *superficial cardiac plexus.* **p. caroticus communis** [NA] Sympathetic fibers that emerge from the middle cervical ganglion and descend along the common carotid artery to join the cardiac plexus. Also *common carotid plexus.* **p. caroticus externus** [NA] Postganglionic sympathetic fibers that emerge from the superior cervical ganglia as the external carotid nerves and surround the external carotid arteries and their branches. Also *external carotid plexus.* **p. caroticus internus** [NA] A network of postganglionic sympathetic fibers that arises in the superior cervical ganglia, accompanies the internal carotid arteries, and sends branches to the cranial meninges, the eyes, and glands of the head region. Also *internal carotid plexus, carotid plexus.* **p. cavernosi concharum** [NA] The rich venous plexuses in the mucous membrane overlying the nasal conchae, especially thick on the inferior concha, which resemble modified erectile tissue. Also *cavernous plexuses of conchae.* **p. cavernosus** The continuation of the plexus caroticus internus that accompanies the part of the internal carotid artery enclosed by the cavernous sinus. It supplies sympathetic fibers to the eye. Also *cavernous plexus.* **p. cavernosus clitoridis** Autonomic nerve filaments that originate in the plexus prostaticus and supply the corpora cavernosa clitoridis. Also *cavernous plexus of clitoris.* **cavernous p.** PLEXUS CAVERNOSUS. **cavernous p. of clitoris** PLEXUS CAVERNOSUS CLITORIDIS. **cavernous p.'es of**

**conchae** PLEXUS CAVERNOSI CONCHARUM. **p. celiacus** [NA] A dense network of autonomic nerve fibers, along with two large ganglionic masses called the celiac ganglion. It is composed of preganglionic parasympathetic vagal fibers and preganglionic sympathetic nerves, the greater and lesser splanchnic nerves. It is situated on the abdominal aorta surrounding the roots of the celiac and superior mesenteric arteries, and extends on to the surfaces of the diaphragmatic crura. Also *solar plexus, plexus coeliacus, epigastric plexus, celiac plexus.* **cephalic ganglionated p.** A network composed of parasympathetic nerve fibers relaying in the ciliary, sphenopalatine, otic, and submandibular ganglia along with sympathetic fibers derived from the superior cervical ganglion, constituting the autonomic innervation to the head region. *Rare.* **p. of cerebral artery anterior** PLEXUS ARTERIAE CEREBRI ANTERIORIS. **p. of cerebral artery middle** PLEXUS ARTERIAE CEREBRI MEDIAE. **p. cervicalis** [NA] A network formed by ventral primary divisions of the first to fourth cervical nerves. It communicates with the tenth, eleventh, and twelfth cranial nerves and the superior cervical ganglion, and gives rise to cutaneous sensory and deep muscular branches. **p. chorioideus** PLEXUS CHOROIDEUS. **choroid p.** PLEXUS CHOROIDEUS. **p. of choroid arteries** PLEXUS ARTERIAE CHOROIDEAE. **p. choroideus** A network of convoluted vascular villi, derived from pia mater, that protrudes from the ventricular walls into the cavities of the third, fourth, and lateral ventricles. It is the site of cerebrospinal fluid production. Also *choroid plexus, plexus chorioideus, choroid gland, tela vasculosa.* **p. choroideus ventriculi lateralis** [NA] A highly vascularized fringe, composed of pia mater and ependymal lining, that projects from the medial aspect of the body and inferior horns of the lateral ventricle and produces cerebrospinal fluid. Also *choroid plexus of lateral ventricle, lateral plexus, paraplexus, proplexus* (seldom used) . **p. choroideus ventriculi quarti** [NA] A highly vascularized fringe of pia mater and ependymal lining that produces cerebrospinal fluid and is located on the posterior roof and in the lateral recesses of the fourth ventricle. Also *choroid plexus of fourth ventricle, inferior choroid plexus.* **p. choroideus ventriculi tertii** [NA] A highly vascularized evagination of pia mater and ependyma projecting from the undersurface of the tela choroidea, where it forms the roof of the third ventricle. It produces cerebrospinal fluid. Also *choroid plexus of third ventricle, diaplex, diaplexus* (outmoded). **choroid p. of fourth ventricle** PLEXUS CHOROIDEUS VENTRICULI QUARTI. **choroid p. of lateral ventricle** PLEXUS CHOROIDEUS VENTRICULI LATERALIS. **choroid p. of third ventricle** PLEXUS CHOROIDEUS VENTRICULI TERTII. **ciliary ganglionic p.** PLEXUS GANGLIOSUS CILIARIS. **coccygeal p.** PLEXUS COCCYGEUS. **coccygeal vascular p.** GLOMUS COCCYGEUM. **p. coccygeus** [NA] A delicate network of sensory nerves formed by the coccygeal nerve and the fourth and fifth sacral nerves. It lies on the sacrotuberous ligament and gives rise to the anococcygeal nerve which supplies the skin near the coccyx. Also *anococcygeal plexus, coccygeal plexus.* **p. coeliacus** PLEXUS CELIACUS. **common carotid p.** PLEXUS CAROTICUS COMMUNIS. **corneal p.** Sensory nerve filaments derived from the ciliary branches of the ophthalmic nerve that form the annular plexus around the periphery of the cornea and then enter the substantia propria to form the stroma plexus. **p. coronarius cordis anterior** [NA] Autonomic nerves derived from the deep portion of the cardiac plexus that accompany the right coronary artery and distribute to the right atrium and ventricle. Also *anterior coronary plexus of heart, right coronary plexus of heart, anterior cardiac plexus.* **p. coronarius cordis posterior** [NA] Autonomic nerve fibers derived from the deep portion of the cardiac plexus that lie along the left coronary artery and are distributed to the left atrium and ventricle. Also *posterior coronary plexus of heart, left coronary plexus of heart.* **crural p.** PLEXUS FEMORALIS. **Cruveilhier's p.** POSTERIOR CERVICAL PLEXUS. **cystic p.** An extension of the hepatic plexus that passes along the cystic artery to supply autonomic innervation to the gall bladder. **deep cardiac p.** PLEXUS CARDIACUS PROFUNDUS. **deep cervical p.** The deep set of the cervical plexus comprising branches distributed mainly to the muscles, including a medial group to the rectus capitis anterior, rectus capitis lateralis, longus capitis, longus colli, and the diaphragm, and a lateral group to the sternocleidomastoid, trapezius, levator scapulae, and scalenus medius muscles. It also sends branches to the ansa cervicalis and various communicating branches. **deep stroma p.** The deep portion of the stroma plexus in the substantia propria of the cornea. Also *fundamental plexus.* **p. deferentialis** [NA] A network of autonomic nerve fibers that arise from the lower portion of the inferior hypogastric plexus and supply the seminal vesicles and ductus deferens in males. Also *plexus of vas deferens.* **p. dentalis inferior** [NA] A network of sensory fibers derived from the inferior alveolar or dental nerve, located near the roots of the lower teeth, and dividing into dental and gingival twigs. Also *inferior dental plexus.* **p. dentalis superior** [NA] A network of sensory fibers derived from the superior alveolar (dental) branches of the infraorbital nerve, situated at the roots of the maxillary teeth, and giving rise to dental and gingival twigs. Also *superior dental plexus, Bochdalek's pseudoganglion.* **diaphragmatic p.** PLEXUS PHRENICUS. **dorsal venous p. of foot** RETE VENOSUM DORSALE PEDIS. **dorsal venous p. of hand** RETE VENOSUM DORSALE MANUS. **p. entericus** [NA] A network of sensory and autonomic nerve fibers and scattered cell bodies located within the various layers of the intestinal wall and subdivided into submucosal, myenteric, and subserosal plexuses. **epigastric p.** PLEXUS CELIACUS. **p. esophageus** [NA] A network of parasympathetic vagal fibers partially embedded in the adventitial coat of the esophagus and communicating with the splanchnic nerves and sympathetic trunk. Also *esophageal plexus.* **p. esophageus anterior** Nerve filaments derived from the vagus nerve and the second, third, and fourth sympathetic ganglia that descend from the posterior pulmonary plexus along the front of the esophagus. Also *anterior esophageal plexus.* **p. esophageus posterior** Nerve filaments derived from the vagus nerve and the second, third, and fourth sympathetic ganglia that arise from the posterior pulmonary plexus and descend along the posterior surface of the esophagus. Also *posterior esophageal plexus.* **Exner's p.** MOLECULAR PLEXUS. **external carotid p.** PLEXUS CAROTICUS EXTERNUS. **external iliac p.** PLEXUS ILIACUS EXTERNUS. **external maxillary p.** PLEXUS FACIALIS. **p. facialis** Postganglionic sympathetic fibers surrounding the facial artery. These fibers originate in the superior cervical ganglion and are part of the external carotid plexus. Also *plexus of facial artery, plexus maxillaris externus, external maxillary plexus.* **p. femoralis** [NA] Autonomic nerve fibers accompanying the femoral artery into the lower extremity as the continuation of the abdominal aortic and the common and external iliac plexuses. Also *crural plexus.* **fundamental p.** DEEP STROMA PLEXUS. **p. gangliosus ciliaris** A rich network of myelinated and unmyelinated nerve fibers and ganglion cells in the ciliary body. It contains parasympathetic fibers from the oculomotor nerve, cervical sympathetic fibers transmitted by the ciliary nerves, and sensory fibers from the ophthalmic nerve. Also *ciliary ganglionic plexus.* **p. gastrici** [NA] The portions of the celiac plexus that communicate with branches of the vagus nerves and accompany the gastric arteries and their branches to the greater and lesser curvatures of the stomach. Also *plexus gastrici systematis autonomici, gastric plexuses, gastric coronary plexuses, superior coronary plexuses of stomach.* **p. gastricus anterior** RAMI GASTRICI ANTERIORES NERVI VAGI. **p. gastricus inferior** Sympathetic fibers from the celiac plexus that accompany the gastroepiploic arteries to the greater curvature of the stomach. They communicate with branches of the vagus nerve. Also *inferior gastric plexus, gastroepiploic plexus, left gastroepiploic plexus.* **p. gastricus posterior** RAMI GASTRICI POSTERIORES NERVI VAGI. **p. gastricus superior** Sympathetic nerve filaments that accompany the left gastric artery along the lesser curvature of the stomach and communicate with the left vagus nerve. Also *superior gastric plexus.* **gastroepiploic p.** PLEXUS GASTRICUS INFERIOR. **great cardiac p.** PLEXUS CARDIACUS PROFUNDUS. **p. haemorrhoidalis medius** PLEXUS RECTALES MEDII. **p. haemorrhoidalis superior** PLEXUS RECTALES SUPERIORES. **Heller's p.** A network of small arteries in the tela submucosa of the intestine. **hemorrhoidal p.** *Outmoded* PLEXUS VENOSUS RECTALIS. **p. hepaticus** [NA] A prolongation of the celiac plexus that ramifies on the hepatic artery and portal vein passing into the liver. Extensions innervate the pancreas and gallbladder. **Hovius p.** A small network of veins in the pectinate ligament of the iridocorneal angle which is connected to the sinus venosus sclerae. Also *Leber's plexus.* **p. hypogastricus** A network of autonomic nerve fibers situated on the front of the sacrum and divided into the plexus hypogastricus superior and plexus hypogastricus inferior. Branches supply blood vessels and viscera of the pelvis. **p. hypogastricus inferior** [NA] A network formed by sympathetic fibers, the hypogastric nerves, and parasympathetic fibers, the pelvic splanchnic nerves, along with several small ganglia lying on the anterior surface of the sacrum. The plexus supplies the viscera and vasculature of the pelvis. Also *inferior hypogastric plexus, plexus pelvinus, pelvic plexus.* **p. hypogastricus superior** [NA] A network formed by the union of fibers from the aortic plexus and the third and fourth lumbar splanchnic nerves. It lies in front of the bifurcation of the aorta and gives rise to the right and left hypogastric nerves. Also *superior hypogastric plexus, presacral nerve, nervus presacralis.* **ileocolic p.** A continuation of the superior mesenteric plexus along the ileocolic artery. It supplies autonomic nerve fibers to the ileocecal region of the large intestine. **p. iliaci** [NA] A network of autonomic nerve fibers derived from the aortic plexus and accompanying the common iliac arteries. Also *iliac plexuses.* **p. iliacus externus** Autonomic nerve fibers, derived from the aortic plexus by way of the iliac plexus, that accompany the common iliac arteries. Also *external iliac plexus.* **inferior choroid p.** PLEXUS CHOROIDEUS VENTRICULI QUARTI. **inferior dental p.** PLEXUS DENTALIS INFERIOR. **inferior gastric p.** PLEXUS GASTRICUS INFERIOR. **inferior hypogastric p.** PLEXUS HYPOGASTRICUS INFERIOR. **inferior mesenteric p.** PLEXUS MESENTERICUS INFERIOR. **inferior rectal p.** PLEXUS RECTALES INFERIORES. **inferior thyroid p.** PLEXUS THYROIDEUS INFERIOR. **inferior vesical p.** The lower part of the plexus venosus vesicalis in the female, corresponding to the prostatic plexus in the male. **infraorbital p.** Sensory fibers from the superior labial branches of the infraorbital nerve that join motor fibers from the buccal branches of the facial nerve to form a network supplying the region of the upper lip and cheek. **p. intercavernosus** A plexus of veins on the inner surface of the base of the skull that interconnects the two cavernous plexuses across the midline. Included are both anterior and posterior intercavernous channels located in front of and behind the stalk of the pituitary gland, forming a venous circle around it just above the diaphragma sellae that covers the sella turcica. Also *intercavernous plexus.* **intermediate p.** The fine nerve plexus found between that of the bulbus cordis and that of the developing atrium of the embryonic heart. It is the midsection of the periodontal ligament where the periodontal fibers appear to interweave. It may have a role in tooth eruption. **p. intermesentericus** [NA] A loose network of four to twelve nerve branches situated along the aorta between the origins of the superior and inferior mesenteric arteries and continuous above with the celiac plexus and below with the superior hypogastric plexus. Also *lumboaortic intermesenteric plexus.* **internal carotid p.** PLEXUS CAROTICUS INTERNUS. **internal carotid venous p.** PLEXUS VENOSUS CAROTICUS INTERNUS. **internal maxillary p.** PLEXUS MAXILLARIS. **interradial p.** BAILLARGER'S LINES. **intramural p.** Autonomic vasomotor and secretomotor nerve fibers found within the walls of the gastrointestinal and urogenital systems. **p. intraparotideus** [NA] The terminal branches of the facial nerve, emerging from the parotid gland to supply the muscles of facial exression. Also *pes anserinus, plexus anserinus, plexus parotideus nervi facialis, parotid plexus of facial nerve, parotid plexus, plexus parotideus.* **ischiadic p.** PLEXUS SACRALIS. **Jacobson's p.** PLEXUS TYMPANICUS. **Jacques p.** The intrinsic nerve plexus of the muscular layer of the uterus. **lateral p.** PLEXUS CHOROIDEUS VENTRICULI LATERALIS. **Leber's p.** HOVIUS PLEXUS. **left colic p.** A continuation of the inferior mesenteric plexus surrounding the left colic artery and supplying autonomic nerve fibers to the left part of the transverse colon, descending colon, and sigmoid colon. **left coronary p. of heart** PLEXUS CORONARIUS CORDIS POSTERIOR. **left gastroepiploic p.** PLEXUS GASTRICUS INFERIOR. **p. lienalis** [NA] Autonomic fibers from the left vagus nerve and celiac ganglion that follow the splenic artery to the spleen and send filaments to the pancreas. Also *splenic plexus.* **p. lingualis** Sympathetic nerve fibers that accompany the lingual artery and its branches. **p. lumbalis** [NA] A network formed by the anterior primary divisions of the first three lumbar nerves and situated on the posterior abdominal wall among fibers of the psoas major muscle. Also *lumbar plexus.* **lumboaortic intermesenteric p.** PLEXUS INTERMESENTERICUS. **p. lumbosacralis** [NA] The combination of all anterior primary divisions of the lumbar, sacral, and coccygeal nerves. **p. lymphaticus** [NA] A network of lymph capillaries situated in the tissue spaces which absorbs colloid material. The capillaries unite to form larger vessels that drain to lymph nodes. Also *lymphatic plexus.* **mammary venous p.** A venous network starting in the circulus venosus at the base of the nipple and extending through the breast towards its circumference to terminate in the axillary and internal thoracic veins. **p. maxillaris** Autonomic nerve fibers that accompany the maxillary artery and its branches. Also *maxillary plexus, internal maxillary plexus, plexus maxillaris internus.* **p. maxillaris externus** PLEXUS FACIALIS. **p. maxillaris internus** *Seldom used* PLEXUS MAXILLARIS. **maxillary p.**

PLEXUS MAXILLARIS. **Meissner's p.** PLEXUS SUBMUCOSUS. **meningeal p.** PLEXUS MENINGEUS. **p. meningeus** Vasomotor sympathetic fibers that accompany the middle meningeal artery. Also *meningeal plexus.* **p. mesentericus inferior** [NA] A cluster of autonomic fibers surrounding the inferior mesenteric artery. It is composed of sympathetic fibers from the abdominal aortic plexus and sacral parasympathetic fibers that distribute with arterial branches to the left colon, sigmoid colon, and rectum. Also *inferior mesenteric plexus.* **p. mesentericus superior** [NA] A continuation of the celiac plexus that surrounds the superior mesenteric artery. It receives fibers from the right vagus nerve and divides into secondary autonomic plexuses that accompany branches of the superior mesenteric artery. Also *superior mesenteric plexus.* **middle p. of cerebral artery** *Obs.* PLEXUS ARTERIAE CEREBRI MEDIAE. **middle colic p.** A continuation of the superior mesenteric plexus that accompanies branches of the middle colic artery to the transverse colon. **middle hemorrhoidal p.** PLEXUS RECTALES MEDII. **middle rectal p.** PLEXUS RECTALES MEDII. **molecular p.** A dense tangential fiber plexus, located superficially in the molecular or plexiform layer of the cerebral cortex (layer I) and formed by dendritic ramifications of pyramidal and fusiform cells from deeper layers, and axonal endings of Martinotti cells. Also *Exner's plexus.* **p. myentericus** [NA] A network of autonomic nerve filaments and ganglia situated between and supplying the circular and longitudinal muscle layers of the alimentary tract. Also *Auerbach's plexus.* **nasopalatine p.** A network of general sensory and autonomic nerve fibers derived from the nasopalatine and anterior palatine nerves that supplies the mucous membrane of the anterior part of the hard palate. **p. nervorum spinalium** [NA] A network of interconnecting bundles of nerve fibers including the cervical, brachial, and lumbosacral plexuses. Also *plexus of spinal nerves.* **obturator p.** PLEXUS SUBSARTORIALIS. **p. occipitalis** Postganglionic sympathetic fibers that arise in the superior cervical ganglion and accompany the occipital artery. **p. ophthalmicus** A network of sympathetic nerve fibers derived from the plexus caroticus internus and accompanying the ophthalmic artery and its branches. **p. ovaricus** [NA] A network of autonomic fibers formed by the renal and aortic plexuses superiorly and supplemented by the superior and inferior hypogastric plexuses inferiorly. It is situated along the ovarian artery and supplies the ovary and uterine tubes. Also *ovarian plexus, plexus arteriae ovaricae* (outmoded), *plexus of ovarian artery.* **p. pampiniformis** [NA] In the male, a convoluted network of veins from the testis and epididymis which ascends in front of the ductus deferens in the spermatic cord. Near the superficial inguinal ring it terminates in about four veins that enter the inguinal canal. In the female, it is a mass of veins that leave the hilum of the ovary to form the ovarian vein. Also *pampiniform plexus.* **pancreatic p.** PLEXUS PANCREATICUS. **pancreaticoduodenal p.** The portion of the pancreatic plexus that accompanies the superior pancreaticoduodenal artery. **p. pancreaticus** [NA] Autonomic nerve fibers to the pancreas that are derived from the hepatic and superior mesenteric plexuses and accompany the pancreatic branches of the hepatic and superior mesenteric arteries. Also *pancreatic plexus.* **Panizza's p.** A lymphatic plexus situated in each of the two lateral fossae of the prepuce of the penis, one on each side of the frenulum. **parotid p.** PLEXUS INTRAPAROTIDEUS. **p. parotideus** PLEXUS INTRAPAROTIDEUS. **p. parotideus nervi facialis** PLEXUS INTRAPAROTIDEUS. **parotid p. of facial nerve** PLEXUS INTRAPAROTIDEUS. **p. patellae** A network of sensory nerve fibers distributed to the skin in front of the patella, and formed by the union of the anterior and lateral femoral cutaneous nerves with the infrapatellar branch of the saphenous nerve. Also *patellar plexus.* **pelvic p.** PLEXUS HYPOGASTRICUS INFERIOR. **p. pelvinus** PLEXUS HYPOGASTRICUS INFERIOR. **p. periarterialis** [NA] Sympathetic and sensory nerve fibers accompanying and innervating an artery. Also *perivascular plexus, plexus perivascularis.* **pericorneal p.** A circumcorneal anastomosis between branches of the anterior conjunctival arteries at the sclerocorneal junction. **periesophageal p. of veins** A plexus of veins on the external surface of the esophagus. The cervical part drains into the inferior thyroid veins, the thoracic part into the azygos, hemiazygos, and accessory hemiazygos veins, while the abdominal part drains into the azygos and left gastric veins. **perivascular p.** PLEXUS PERIARTERIALIS. **p. perivascularis** PLEXUS PERIARTERIALIS. **pharyngeal p.** PLEXUS PHARYNGEUS NERVI VAGI. **pharyngeal p. of vagus nerve** PLEXUS PHARYNGEUS NERVI VAGI. **p. pharyngeus 1** [NA] A venous plexus overlying the pharyngeal constrictors that communicates with the pterygoid venous plexus and drains into the retromandibular or posterior facial vein. Also *pharyngeal venous plexus.* **2** PLEXUS PHARYNGEUS NERVI VAGI. **p. pharyngeus ascendens** Sympathetic filaments from the middle and inferior cervical ganglia accompanying the ascending pharyngeal artery and contributing to the plexus pharyngeus nervi vagi. **p. pharyngeus nervi vagi** A network formed by pharyngeal branches of the vagus nerve, pharyngeal branches of the glossopharyngeal nerve, and sympathetic fibers from the superior cervical ganglion. It lies on the middle pharyngeal constrictor and supplies autonomic, sensory, and motor innervation to the pharynx. Also *pharyngeal plexus, plexus pharyngeus, pharyngeal plexus of vagus nerve.* **p. phrenicus** Autonomic nerve fibers arising from the celiac plexus that accompany the inferior phrenic artery to the diaphragm and suprarenal glands. It communicates with the phrenic nerve and may contain a small phrenic ganglion. Also *diaphragmatic plexus.* **p. popliteus** Autonomic vasomotor nerve filaments derived from the intermesenteric (aortic) plexus and surrounding the popliteal artery. Also *popliteal plexus.* **posterior auricular p.** PLEXUS AURICULARIS POSTERIOR. **posterior bronchial p.** PLEXUS PULMONALIS POSTERIOR. **posterior cervical p.** The dorsal rami of the upper four cervical nerves that are distributed to the skin and muscles of the back of the neck. *Seldom used.* Also *Cruveilhier's plexus.* **posterior coronary p. of heart** PLEXUS CORONARIUS CORDIS POSTERIOR. **posterior esophageal p.** PLEXUS ESOPHAGEUS POSTERIOR. **posterior pulmonary p.** PLEXUS PULMONALIS POSTERIOR. **preaortic p.'es** PREVERTEBRAL PLEXUSES. **prevertebral p.'es** The large plexuses of the autonomic nervous system that are composed of sympathetic and parasympathetic nerve filaments and ganglia and are located along the aorta and its major branches in the thoracic, abdominal, and pelvic cavities. From these plexuses branches supply thoracic, abdominal, and pelvic viscera. They include the cardiac, pulmonary, celiac, mesenteric, and hypogastric plexuses. Also *preaortic plexuses.* **primary p.** The plexus of vessels that interconnects the superior and inferior hypophysial arteries and the hypophysial portal system of veins. This plexus participates in the vascular supply to the median eminence, infundibulum, and lobes of the pituitary gland. **prostatic p.** PLEXUS PROSTATICUS. **prostaticovesical p.** Plexus venosus vesicalis in the male.

**p. prostaticus** [NA] Autonomic nerve fibers derived from the inferior hypogastric plexus that supply the prostate gland, seminal vesicles, urethra, corpora cavernosa, and corpus spongiosum penis. Also *prostatic plexus, anterolateral plexus of Santorini, Santorini's plexus.* **prostatic venous p.** PLEXUS VENOSUS PROSTATICUS. **p. pterygoideus** [NA] A considerable venous network that lies within the infratemporal fossa. Its tributaries follow branches of the maxillary artery. It joins the facial vein and drains into the internal jugular vein. **pudendal p.** PLEXUS PUDENDUS. **p. pudendus** A network formed by the second, third, and fourth sacral nerves, located in the posterior pelvis on the piriformis muscle and supplying the pelvic viscera and external genitalia. Also *pudendal plexus.* **p. pulmonalis** [NA] A network of autonomic fibers formed by branches of the vagus nerve and the second to fifth thoracic sympathetic nerves. It surrounds the roots of the lung and is divided into an anterior and posterior plexus. Also *pulmonary plexus.* **p. pulmonalis anterior** A network of autonomic nerve filaments on the anterior surface of the root of the lung formed by the union of sympathetic filaments and anterior bronchial (pulmonary) branches of the vagus nerve. Also *anterior pulmonary plexus, anterior bronchial plexus.* **p. pulmonalis posterior** A network of autonomic and visceral afferent fibers to lungs and bronchi lying on the posterior surface of the root of the lung. It is formed by posterior bronchial (pulmonary) branches of the vagus nerve and sympathetic nerve fibers. Also *posterior pulmonary plexus, posterior bronchial plexus.* **pulmonary p.** PLEXUS PULMONALIS. **Quénu's hemorrhoidal p.** A lymphatic plexus in the circumanal skin which drains to the superficial inguinal lymph nodes. **Ranvier's p.** *Seldom used* SUPERFICIAL STROMA PLEXUS **p. rectales inferiores** [NA] Sympathetic and sacral parasympathetic nerve fibers derived from the pelvic plexus and accompanying the inferior rectal artery to the anal region. Also *inferior rectal plexus.* **p. rectales medii** [NA] Sympathetic and sacral parasympathetic fibers derived from the inferior hypogastric plexus and supplying the rectum. Also *middle hemorrhoidal plexus, plexus haemorrhoidalis medius, middle rectal plexus, nervi haemorrhoidales medii.* **p. rectales superiores** [NA] Sympathetic and sacral parasympathetic fibers derived from the inferior mesenteric plexus and accompanying the superior rectal artery to the distal colon and rectum. Also *superior rectal plexus, plexus haemorrhoidalis superior, superior hemorrhoidal plexus.* **rectal venous p.** PLEXUS VENOSUS RECTALIS. **Remak's p.** PLEXUS SUBMUCOSUS. **p. renalis** [NA] A rich network formed by filaments from the celiac and renal plexuses and containing small clusters of nerve cells. It follows branches of the renal artery into the kidney and supplies vasomotor innervation to blood vessels and renal glomeruli and tubules. Also *renal plexus.* **right colic p.** A continuation of the superior mesenteric plexus that accompanies branches of the right colic artery to the ascending colon. **right coronary p. of heart** PLEXUS CORONARIUS CORDIS ANTERIOR. **p. sacralis** [NA] A network formed from part of the lumbosacral trunk, from the fourth and fifth lumbar nerves and the first three sacral nerves. It lies against the posterior and lateral portions of the pelvis and gives rise to the sciatic nerve. Also *ischiadic plexus, sciatic plexus, rami ventrales nervorum sacralium.* **sacral venous p.** PLEXUS VENOSUS SACRALIS. **Santorini's p.** PLEXUS PROSTATICUS. **Sappey subareolar p.** A lymphatic plexus under the areola of the breast which drains the skin of the areola and the nipple. **sciatic p.** PLEXUS SACRALIS. **sinocarotid p.** Fine filaments of the intercarotid or sinus branch of the glossopharyngeal nerve that surround the carotid sinus and function in the regulation of blood pressure. **solar p.** PLEXUS CELIACUS. **spermatic p.** PLEXUS TESTICULARIS. **sphenoid p.** The sympathetic nerve filaments surrounding the internal carotid artery within the middle cranial fossa. *Obs.* **p. of spinal nerves** PLEXUS NERVORUM SPINALIUM. **splenic p.** PLEXUS LIENALIS. **Stensen's p.** A venous network surrounding the parotid duct. **stroma p.** Nerve filaments derived from the annular plexus that enter the substantia propria of the cornea and divide into superficial and deep networks. **sub-basal p.** SUPERFICIAL STROMA PLEXUS. **p. subclavius** [NA] Autonomic nerve filaments surrounding the subclavian artery and derived from the cervicothoracic (stellate) ganglion and the ansa subclavius. Also *subclavian plexus.* **subendocardiac p.** A plexus of nerves deep to the endocardium which is formed by branches from the coronary plexuses that traverse the myocardium. **subepithelial p.** A nerve plexus beneath the corneal epithelium that carries impulses to the ciliary branch of the ophthalmic nerve. **submolecular p.** Tangential nerve fibers in layer I of the cerebral cortex lying deep to the molecular (Exner's) plexus. **p. submucosus** [NA] The portion of the autonomic plexus entericus that lies within the submucosal layer of the intestinal wall. Also *Meissner's plexus, Remak's plexus, submucosal plexus, submucous plexus, submucous intestinal plexus.* **suboccipital venous p.** PLEXUS VENOSUS SUBOCCIPITALIS. **subpapillary p.** A network of arterial anastomoses that arise from a cutaneous plexus and extend into the papillary layer of the dermis where it gives off capillary tufts into the papillae of the dermis. **subpapillary venous p.** A superficial capillary plexus at the junction of the reticular and papillary layers of the dermis which receives blood from the rete cutaneum and drains into an intermediate network in the middle of the reticular layer. **subpericardial p.** A plexus of nerves formed by branches of the coronary plexuses on the surface of the heart. **p. subsartorialis** A plexiform network formed by sensory branches of the femoral, saphenous, and obturator nerves. It lies beneath the fascia lata, at the lower border of the abductor longus. Also *obturator plexus.* **p. subserosus** [NA] The subserosal component of the plexus entericus in the intestinal wall. Also *subserosal plexus.* **subtrapezius p.** A network of nerve fibers formed from the accessory nerve and branches of the third and fourth cervical nerves, located under the anterior border of, and innervating, the trapezius muscle. Also *subtrapezial plexus.* **superficial cardiac p.** PLEXUS CARDIACUS SUPERFICIALIS. **superficial cervical p.** The superficial set of the cervical plexus comprising those nerves which pierce the cervical fascia and innervate the skin, the ascending group being the greater auricular, lesser occipital, and transverse cutaneous nerves while the descending group consists of the supraclavicular nerves. **superficial stroma p.** The superficial portion of the stroma plexus of nerves in the substantia propria of the cornea. Also *sub-basal plexus, Ranvier's plexus* (seldom used). **superior coronary p.'es of stomach** PLEXUS GASTRICI. **superior dental p.** PLEXUS DENTALIS SUPERIOR. **superior gastric p.** PLEXUS GASTRICUS SUPERIOR. **superior hemorrhoidal p.** PLEXUS RECTALES SUPERIORES. **superior hypogastric p.** PLEXUS HYPOGASTRICUS SUPERIOR. **superior mesenteric p.** PLEXUS MESENTERICUS SUPERIOR. **superior rectal p.** PLEXUS RECTALES SUPERIORES. **superior thyroid p.** PLEXUS THYROIDEUS SUPERIOR. **supraradial p.** BEKHTEREV'S LAYER. **p. suprarenalis** [NA] Autonomic nerve fibers, principally preganglionic sympathetic fibers, that pass through the celiac ganglion and distribute to the adrenal medulla. **p. sympathici** PLEXUS AUTONOMICI. **p. temporalis superficialis** Autonomic vasomotor fibers that accompany the superficial temporal artery. **p. testicularis** [NA] Autonomic vasomotor fibers accompanying the testicular artery, formed from branches of the aortic, renal, superior, and inferior hypogastric plexuses. Branches supply the epididymus and ductus deferens. Also *spermatic plexus.* **thoracic aortic p.** PLEXUS AORTICUS THORACICUS. **p. thyreoideus impar** PLEXUS THYROIDEUS IMPAR. **p. thyreoideus inferior** PLEXUS THYROIDEUS INFERIOR. **p. thyreoideus superior** PLEXUS THYROIDEUS SUPERIOR. **p. thyroideus impar** [NA] A network of veins lying on the front of the trachea, draining the isthmus of the thyroid gland, and uniting to form the thyroid impar vein. Also *plexus thyreoideus impar, unpaired thyroid plexus, thyroid venous plexus.* **p. thyroideus inferior** Sympathetic branches from the middle cervical ganglion accompanying the inferior thyroid artery to supply the thyroid gland. Also *inferior thyroid plexus, plexus thyreoideus inferior.* **p. thyroideus superior** Sympathetic fibers from the superior cervical ganglion that accompany the superior thyroid artery to supply the thyroid gland. Also *superior thyroid plexus, plexus thyreoideus superior.* **thyroid venous p.** PLEXUS THYROIDEUS IMPAR. **tonsillar p.** A nerve plexus surrounding and supplying the palatine tonsil, formed by tonsillar branches of the glossopharyngeal nerve and the middle and posterior palatine nerves. Filaments from this plexus are distributed to the soft palate and the fauces. **Trolard's p.** PLEXUS VENOSUS CANALIS HYPOGLOSSI. **p. tympanicus** [NA] A plexus of sensory and autonomic nerve fibers that ramify on the promontory of the middle ear, formed from the tympanic branch of the glossopharyngeal nerve and the superior and inferior caroticotympanic nerves. Also *Jacobson's plexus.* **unpaired thyroid p.** PLEXUS THYROIDEUS IMPAR. **p. uretericus** [NA] Autonomic nerves derived from the renal, superior, hypogastric, and inferior hypogastric plexuses and thought to influence the motility of the ureter. **uterine p.** PLEXUS UTERINUS. **uterine venous p.** PLEXUS VENOSUS UTERINUS. **p. uterinus** The portion of the uterovaginal plexus that accompanies the uterine arteries to the uterus. Also *uterine nerves, uterine plexus.* **p. uterovaginalis** [NA] The portion of the inferior hypogastric plexus that lies in the base of the broad ligament and supplies autonomic innervation to the uterus, vagina, ovaries, urethra, and vestibule via the uterine and vaginal nerves. Also *uterovaginal plexus.* **uterovaginal venous p.** Plexus venosus uterinus and plexus venosus vaginalis considered together. **p. vaginalis** NERVI VAGINALES. **vaginal venous p.** PLEXUS VENOSUS VAGINALIS. **p. vasculosus** [NA] A network of anastomosing blood vessels, either veins or arteries. Also *vascular plexus.* **p. of vas deferens** PLEXUS DEFERENTIALIS. **p. venosus** [NA] A mass of interconnecting veins which may or may not be associated with arteries. Also *venous plexus.* **p. venosus areolaris** [NA] A network of fine veins in the areola and around the base of the nipple of the breast which drains to the lateral thoracic and axillary veins. Also *circulus venosus, venous circle of mammary gland, venous ring of Haller.* **p. venosus canalis hypoglossi** [NA] A plexus of veins within the hypoglossal canal that allows communication of venous blood between the occipital sinus on the inner aspect of the cranial cavity and the vertebral vein in the deep neck as well as the vertebral plexus of veins in the upper part of the spinal column. Also *Trolard's plexus, venous plexus of hypoglossal canal, Trolard's net* (seldom used), *rete canalis hypoglossi* (outmoded). **p. venosus caroticus internus** [NA] A venous plexus accompanying the internal carotid artery in the carotid canal of the petrous part of the temporal bone and connecting the cavernous sinus with the internal jugular vein. Also *internal carotid venous plexus.* **p. venosus foraminis ovalis** [NA] A plexus of veins that interconnects the cavernous plexus on the inner aspect of the base of the skull with the pterygoid and pharyngeal plexuses in the deep face through the foramen ovale. Also *rete foraminis ovalis, venous plexus of foramen ovale, emissary veins of foramen ovale.* **p. venosus prostaticus** [NA] A venous plexus embedded in the fascial sheath of the prostate and situated in front of the bladder and behind the arcuate pubic ligament. It receives the deep dorsal vein of the penis and tributaries from the adjacent bladder and prostate and it drains into the internal iliac and vesical veins. Also *prostatic venous plexus, Santorini's labyrinth.* **p. venosus rectalis** [NA] A venous plexus around the rectal wall which is linked anteriorly with the vesical plexus in the male and the vaginal and uterine plexuses in the female. It is divided into an internal plexus in the submucosa and an external plexus situated outside the muscular layer below the level of peritoneal reflection. The plexuses drain into the superior, middle, and inferior rectal veins and communicate with each other, thereby forming communications between the portal and systemic venous systems. Also *rectal venous plexus, hemorrhoidal plexus* (outmoded). **p. venosus sacralis** [NA] The venous plexus linking the lateral sacral veins across the front of the sacrum. Also *sacral venous plexus.* **p. venosus suboccipitalis** [NA] The venous plexus in the region of the suboccipital triangle that drains into the vertebral veins. Also *suboccipital venous plexus.* **p. venosus uterinus** [NA] The plexus of veins around each side of the uterus within the broad ligament. It communicates with the vaginal and ovarian plexuses and drains into two uterine veins on each side. Also *uterine venous plexus.* **p. venosus vaginalis** [NA] A venous plexus surrounding the vagina which communicates with the uterine, rectal and vesical venous plexuses and drains into a vaginal vein on each side to end in the internal iliac vein. Also *vaginal venous plexus.* **p. venosus vertebralis externus anterior** [NA] An extensive longitudinal venous plexus that is situated on the front of the bodies of the vertebrae. It receives tributaries from the bodies of the vertebrae and communicates with the basivertebral and intervertebral veins as well as with the posterior external vertebral venous plexus and both internal vertebral venous plexuses. The veins have no valves. **p. venosus vertebralis externus posterior** [NA] An extensive longitudinal venous plexus that is situated around the spines and the transverse and articular processes and on the back of the laminae of the vertebrae. It communicates with the intervertebral veins as well as with the anterior external and both internal vertebral venous plexuses. Its veins have no valves and they drain into the posterior intercostal, vertebral, and lumbar veins. **p. venosus vertebralis internus anterior** [NA] An extensive longitudinal venous plexus that is situated in the vertebral canal between the dura mater and the vertebrae. It comprises two longitudinal veins, or sinuses, one on each side of the posterior longitudinal ligament. They are connected by transverse anastomoses and receive basivertebral veins and anterior spinal veins. It communicates freely with the posterior internal vertebral venous plexus as well as with the anterior external vertebral venous plexus. Superiorly it communicates with the basilar plexus, occipital and sigmoid sinuses, condylar emissary veins, and the venous plexus of the hypoglossal canal. Its veins have no valves. **p. venosus vertebralis internus posterior** [NA] An extensive longitudinal venous plexus that is situated in the vertebral canal between the dura mater and the vertebrae. It comprises two longitudinal veins, or sinuses, lying on the inner surface of the laminae and ligamenta flava, one on each side of the midline. They anastomose transversely with each other and with the posterior external vertebral venous plexus by veins piercing the ligamenta flava. It receives the posterior spinal veins and also anastomoses with the anterior internal vertebral venous plexus. Superiorly it communicates with the basilar plexus, the occipital and sigmoid sinuses, condylar emissary veins, and the venous plexus of the hypoglossal canal. Its veins have no valves. **p. venosus vesicalis** [NA] A venous plexus surrounding the lower portion of the urinary bladder, as well as the base of the prostate in the male. It communicates with the vaginal plexus in the female and the prostatic plexus in the male and is drained by a number of vesical veins which unite before ending in the internal iliac vein. Also *vesical venous plexus.* **venous p.** PLEXUS VENOSUS. **venous p. of foramen ovale** PLEXUS VENOSUS FORAMINIS OVALIS. **venous p. of hypoglossal canal** PLEXUS VENOSUS CANALIS HYPOGLOSSI. **venous p. in foramen magnum** An annular network of veins around the foramen magnum and on the anterior and lateral surfaces of the lower part of the medulla oblongata, formed by communications between the anterior and posterior internal vertebral venous plexuses, the vertebral veins, basilar plexus, occipital and sigmoid sinuses, and the venous plexus of the hypoglossal canal and the condylar emissary veins. **vertebral p.** **1** PLEXUS VERTEBRALIS. **2** One of the venous plexuses surrounding or within the vertebral column. **p. vertebralis** [NA] Autonomic nerve filaments on the vertebral artery derived mainly from the cervicothoracic (stellate) ganglion. Branches from the plexus join the anterior rami of the upper five or six cervical spinal nerves. The plexus continues into the posterior cranial fossa along the basilar artery. Also *vertebral plexus.* **vertebral venous p.** Any of four plexuses: (1) plexus venosus vertebralis externus anterior; (2) plexus venosus vertebralis externus posterior; (3) plexus venosus vertebralis internus anterior; (4) plexus venosus vertebralis internus posterior. **p. vesicales** [NA] The portion of the inferior hypogastric plexus that follows the vesical arteries to the bladder. Also *vesical plexus, plexus vesicalis.* **p. vesicalis** PLEXUS VESICALES. **vesical venous p.** PLEXUS VENOSUS VESICALIS. **vitelline p.** An arrangement of blood vessels visible on the surface of the yolk sac.

# plica

**plica** \plī′kə\ [New L (from L *plicare* to fold; akin to Gk *plekein* to twine, twist, braid), a fold] (*pl.* plicae) A fold or ridge. **plicae alares** [NA] Folds of synovial membrane attached to the lower part of the medial and lateral margins of the articular surface of the patella which pass posteriorly to form the infrapatellar synovial fold. Also *alar folds.* **p. aryepiglottica** [NA] The fold of mucous membrane extending from the side of the epiglottis to the apex of the arytenoid cartilage on each side and containing fibers of the aryepiglottic and thyroepiglottic muscles and, on the posterior part of its free margin, the cuneiform and corniculate cartilages. Also *aryepiglottic fold, arytenoepiglottidean fold, arytenoepiglottic ligament.* **plicae caecales** [NA] Folds of peritoneum extending on each side of the retrocecal recess from the cecum to the posterior abdominal wall. Also *cecal folds.* **p. caecalis vascularis** [NA] A peritoneal fold which arches over the anterior cecal branch of the ileocecal artery in its course in front of the cecum to the ileocecal junction. The fold forms the anterior wall of the superior ileocecal recess. Also *vascular fold of cecum, Treves fold.* **p. chordae tympani** [NA] A fold of mucous membrane of the middle ear which invests the chorda tympani nerve on the inner surface of the tympanic membrane where it forms the upper boundary of the anterior and posterior recesses of the tympanic membrane. **p. choroidea** A fold in the roof plate, marking the beginning of the choroid plexuses of the brain. The fold is formed after the vascular pia mater comes in close contact with the ependyma in a region where the roof plate of the developing neural tube is thin, as in the third and fourth ventricles. **plicae ciliares** [NA] Small elevated ridges in the furrows between successive ciliary processes of the corona ciliaris to which some of the longer zonular fibers are attached and which extend anteriorly from the dentate processes of the ora serrata. Also *ciliary folds.* **plicae circulares** [NA] Crescentic or circular folds of mucous membrane which project into the lumen of the small intestine whether it is empty or distended. They may extend either partly or totally around the circumference of the lumen. They commence to appear in the descending part of the duodenum and are most numerous in the proximal half of the jejunum, after which they start decreasing in size and number so that they are absent in the terminal ileum. The circular fibers of the lamina muscularis mucosae extend into the folds. Also *circular folds, Kerckring's folds of small intestine, Kerckring's valves.* **p. duodenalis inferior** [NA] A nonvascular, triangular fold of peritoneum which extends from the left side of the lower part of the ascending portion of the duodenum to the posterior abdominal wall and forms the anterior boundary of the inferior duodenal recess. Also *inferior duodenal fold, duodenomesocolic fold.* **p. duodenalis superior** [NA] A crescentic fold of peritoneum which extends laterally from the left side of the upper part of the ascending portion of the duodenum to the posterior abdominal wall where it merges with the peritoneum over the front of the left kidney. At the left edge of its free margin the inferior mesenteric vein courses upwards deep to the peritoneum. It forms the anterior boundary of the superior duodenal recess. Also *superior duodenal fold, duodenojejunal fold.* **p. fimbriata** [NA] A fringed fold of mucous membrane running towards the apex of the tongue on each side of the frenulum and lateral to each deep lingual vein. Also *fimbriated fold, fimbriated crest, fimbriae of tongue.* **plicae gastricae** [NA] Numerous longitudinal folds of the mucous membrane of the stomach which are more regular along the lesser curvature forming the gastric canal but are most numerous and obvious along the greater curvature near the pyloric portion. The folds flatten out and partly disappear when the stomach is distended. Also *gastric folds, rugae of stomach.* **p. gastropancreatica** [NA] A crescentic fold of peritoneum situated over the left gastric artery as it passes from the posterior abdominal wall to the lesser curvature of the stomach. It is at the junction of the superior and inferior recesses of the omental bursa on which it encroaches. Also *gastropancreatic fold, pancreaticogastric fold.* **p. glossoepiglottica lateralis** [NA] A fold of mucous membrane extending between the lateral wall of the pharynx and the upper part of the anterior surface of the epiglottis and forming the lateral boundary of each vallecula. Also *lateral glossoepiglottic fold.* **p. glossoepiglottica mediana** [NA] The fold of mucous membrane extending in the midline between the pharyngeal part of the tongue and the upper part of the anterior surface of the epiglottis and serving as a septum between the two valleculae. Also *middle glossoepiglottic fold, median glossoepiglottic fold.* **p. hepatopancreatica** [NA] A crescentic fold of peritoneum situated over the common hepatic artery as it passes forwards from the posterior abdominal wall to the dorsal surface of the hepatoduodenal ligament. It is at the junction of the superior and inferior recesses of the omental bursa on which it encroaches. Also *hepatopancreatic fold.* **p. ileocaecalis** [NA] A peritoneal fold extending from the antimesenteric border of the terminal part of the ileum to the front of the appendix or mesoappendix and becoming adherent to the cecum. Also *ileocecal fold, Treves fold, avascular fold of Treves.* **p. incudis** [NA] A vascular fold of mucous membrane extending from the roof of the tympanic cavity to the upper margin of the body of the incus after investing the head of the malleus. Also *incudal fold.* **p. interarytenoidea** [NA] A fold of mucous membrane stretching across the incisura interarytenoidea between the corniculate cartilages and apices of the arytenoid cartilages and limiting the aditus laryngis posteriorly. Also *interarytenoid fold.* **p. interureterica** A fold of mucous membrane overlying a muscular ridge on the inner surface of the bladder, joining the two ureteral orifices and thus forming the base of the trigonum vesicae. Also *bar of bladder, interureteric bar, Mercier's bar, Mercier's barrier, interureteric ridge, interureteric crest, interureteric fold.* **plicae iridis** [NA] Numerous radiating endothelial folds on the posterior surface of the iris of the eye which push up against the pectinate ligament when the iris is fully dilated, thus sometimes interfering with drainage of the aqueous humor. Also *iridial folds.* **p. lacrimalis** [NA] A fold of mucous membrane of the nasolacrimal duct serving as a valve just above its lower opening into the inferior meatus of the nose. Also *lacrimal fold, Hasner's fold, Hasner's valve, Bianchi's valve, Huschke's valve, Rosenmüller's valve.* **p. longitudinalis duodeni** [NA] A fairly distinct longitudinal fold of mucous membrane on the medial wall of the descending portion of the duodenum about halfway down, at the lower end of which it forms a hoodlike fold above the greater duodenal papilla. Also *longitudinal fold of duodenum.* **p. mallearis anterior membranae tympani** [NA] A fold of mucous membrane of the middle ear that extends from the front extremity of the tympanic notch over the anterior process and ligament of the malleus to be attached to the lateral process of the malleus thereby helping to separate the pars flaccida of the tympanic membrane from the pars tensa below. Also *anterior mallear fold of tympanic membrane, plica mallearis anterior tunicae mucosae cavitatis tympani.* **p. mallearis posterior membranae tympani** [NA] A fold of mucous membrane of the middle ear that extends from the posterior extremity of the tympanic notch and over the lateral ligament of the malleus to be attached to the lateral process of the malleus thereby helping to separate the pars flaccida of the tympanic membrane from the pars tensa below. Also *posterior mallear fold of tympanic membrane, plica mallearis posterior tunicae mucosae cavitatis tympani.* **p. nervi laryngei** [NA] A fold in the laryngeal mucosa overlying the laryngeal nerve. **plicae palatinae transversae** [NA] Several transverse ridges of mucoperiosteum of the anterior part of the oral surface of the hard palate which extend laterally from the median palatine raphe. Also *transverse palatine folds.* **plicae palmatae** [NA] Small oblique folds of mucous membrane that extend sideways and upwards from the longitudinal ridges on the anterior and posterior walls of the canal of the cervix uteri. They are especially obvious in nulliparous females. Also *palmate folds.* **p. palpebronasalis** [NA] A vertical semilunar fold of skin that extends downwards from the anterior surface of the upper eyelid to cover the medial angle and caruncle. It occurs normally in many Mongoloid populations and may also be present in other populations as a congenital anomaly, as in the Down syndrome. Also *palpebronasal fold, epicanthic fold, epicanthus.* **p. paraduodenalis** [NA] A sickle-shaped peritoneal fold to the left of the ascending part of the duodenum containing the inferior mesenteric vein and the accompanying ascending branch of the left colic artery in its free margin. The latter overlies the wide mouth of the paraduodenal recess which faces the right side. Also *paraduodenal fold.* **p. rectouterina** [NA] A crescentic fold of peritoneum on each side of the rectouterine pouch which extends from the cervix uteri backwards around the side of the rectum to the sacrum. It encloses the uterosacral ligament on each side as well as the rectouterine muscle fibers that are continuous anteriorly with those of the uterus and posteriorly with those of the rectum. Also *rectouterine fold, Douglas fold, Douglas ligament, uterosacral fold.* **p. salpingopalatina** [NA] A small vertical fold of pharyngeal mucous membrane extending from the anterosuperior part of the tubal elevation of the auditory tube to the soft palate. Also *salpingopalatine fold, nasopharyngeal fold.* **p. salpingopharyngea** [NA] A prominent vertical fold of pharyngeal mucous membrane extending from the posteroinferior part of the tubal elevation of the auditory tube to the lateral pharyngeal wall. It encloses the salpingopharyngeus muscle. Also *salpingopharyngeal fold, tubopharyngeal ligament of Rauber.* **plicae semilunares coli** [NA] Crescentic ridges involving the full thickness of the wall of the colon and projecting into the lumen between the haustra. Also *semilunar folds of colon, sigmoid folds of colon, folds of large intestine, semilunar valves of colon, sigmoid valves of colon.* **p. semilunaris conjunctivae** [NA] A vertical crescentic fold of the conjunctiva with the free concave lateral edge facing the cornea and the convex side lateral to the lacrimal caruncle. Some authorities consider it to be a rudimentary representative of the nictitating membrane or third eyelid which is present as a specialization in some reptiles, amphibians, birds, and mammals. Also *semilunar fold of conjunctiva.* **p. spiralis** [NA] The mucous membrane of the cystic duct arranged in the form of a spiral fold so as to keep the lumen patent. It is usually most prominent in the proximal part of the duct. Also *spiral fold, Heister's valve, Amussat's valvula, spiral valve, spiral valve of cystic duct, spiral valve of Heister, Heister's fold, spiral fold of cystic duct.* **p. stapedis** [NA] A fold of mucous membrane of the middle ear that extends from the posterior wall to invest the stapes. Also *stapedial fold.* **p. sublingualis** [NA] A fold of mucous membrane covering the upper border of the sublingual gland in the floor of the mouth and extending forward to the caruncle at the base of the lingual frenulum. The minor ducts of the gland open on the surface of the fold. Also *sublingual fold.* **p. synovialis** A synovial fold projecting into a joint cavity from the synovial membrane. *Outmoded.* Also *synovial fold.* **p. synovialis infrapatellaris** The infrapatellar fold of synovium which passes into the intercondylar region of the knee joint and contains fat. Also *infrapatellar synovial fold, patellar synovial fold.* **plicae transversales recti** [NA] Three or four permanent horizontal folds of the mucous membrane of the rectum. One type comprises mucous membrane and the circular and some longitudinal muscle fibers, while the second does not have any longitudinal muscle fibers. The first type produces an indentation on the outer surface of the rectum. The largest and most constant is located just above the ampulla of the rectum, projecting from the right and anterior walls and is usually the middle fold. Also *transverse folds of rectum, horizontal folds of rectum, rectal folds, Kohlrausch folds, Houston's valves, Kohlrausch valves.* **p. triangularis** [NA] A fold of mucous membrane of variable size and shape located just posterior to the palatoglossal arch and usually adherent to the anterior part of the medial surface of the palatine tonsil. Also *triangular fold, triangular fold of His.* **plicae tubariae tubae uterinae** [NA] Numerous longitudinal folds in the mucous membrane of the uterine tube which are simple in the isthmus and higher and more complex in the ampulla. Also *tubal folds of uterine tube.* **plicae tunicae mucosae vesicae biliaris** [NA] The minute elevations of the mucous membrane of the gallbladder which provide it with a honeycomb appearance. Also *plicae tunicae mucosae vesicae felleae.* **p. umbilicalis lateralis** [NA] The raised fold of peritoneum produced on the lower part of the anterior abdominal wall by the inferior epigastric artery extending from its origin, medial to the deep inguinal ring, to the transversalis fascia at the arcuate line. It lies lateral to the medial umbilical fold on each side. Also *lateral umbilical fold, epigastric fold.* **p. umbilicalis medialis** [NA] The raised fold of peritoneum produced on the lower part of the anterior abdominal wall by the obliterated umbilical artery extending as a ligament from the superior vesical artery to the umbilicus. It lies on each side of the median umbilical fold and between the latter and each lateral umbilical fold. Also *medial umbilical fold.* **p. umbilicalis mediana** [NA] The raised fold of peritoneum produced on the lower part of the anterior abdominal wall by the median umbilical ligament containing the remains of the urachus and extending in the midline from the apex of the urinary bladder to the umbilicus. Also *median umbilical fold, middle umbilical fold, fold of the urachus.* **urorectal plicae** The folds which come together in an embryo to form the cloacal septum. They contain the mesonephric and paramesonephric ducts. **p. venae cavae sinistrae** A fold of visceral pericardium left behind at the point it was reflected over the retrogressing left anterior cardinal vein of the embryo. Also *fold of the left vena cava.* **p. vesicalis transversa** [NA] A transverse fold of peritoneum formed on the upper aspect of the urinary bladder when it is completely empty. Also *transverse vesical fold.* **p. vestibularis** [NA] One of two prominent rounded folds of mucous membrane, each enclosing the vestibular ligament on each side of the rima vestibuli and extending from the angle of the thyroid cartilage anteriorly to the anterolateral surface of the arytenoid cartilage above the vocal process posteriorly. It forms the lower margin of the vestibule of the larynx which is separated by it from the sinus of the larynx. Also *vestibular fold, false vocal fold, false vocal cord.* **plicae villosae gastricae** [NA] Minute ridges of the mucous membrane of the stomach which are situated between the gastric pits, or foveolae gastricae, and are so named because in section they resemble villi. Areas of pits and ridges present a mammillated appearance. Also *villous folds of stomach, plicae villosae ventriculi.* **p. vocalis** [NA] One of the two thin, sharp folds of mucous membrane that extends from the angle of the thyroid cartilage near the midline anteriorly to the vocal process of the arytenoid cartilage posteriorly. The stratified epithelium covering it is tightly adherent to the vocal ligament situated within the fold. It is pearly white in color because of the lack of a submucous layer and blood vessels. Also *vocal fold, vocal cord, true vocal cord, Ferrein's cord.*

**plicae** \plī′sē\ Plural of PLICA.

**plicate** \plī′kāt\ Folded, tucked, or plaited.

**plication** \plīkā′shən\ [L *plicat(us)* folded, from *plicare* to fold + -ION] **1** A folding or tucking in. **2** A fold. **caval p.** A technique for partial occlusion of the infrarenal inferior vena cava to prevent the embolization of large thrombi from the lower extremity veins to the lungs.

**plinth** \plinth, plint\ [Gk *plinth(os)* brick, tile, plinth] A narrow padded table to support a patient during massage or other physical therapy procedures. Also *plint.*

**-ploid** \-ploid\ [Gk *-plo(os)* -fold + *-eidēs* -like, -OID] A combining form indicating some multiple of a chromosome set.

**ploidy** \ploi′dē\ [-PLOID + -Y] The number of chromosome sets present in a cell or organism. A haploid cell with one chromosome set has a ploidy of 1.

**plosive** \plō′siv\ [back-formation from *explosive*] A consonant articulated by the build-up and sudden release of pressure behind a complete closure of the vocal tract. It may be voiced, as in /d/, or unvoiced as in /t/.

**plot** A chart or graphic display. **cot p.** A graph of nucleic acid reassociation kinetics in which the fraction of a sample that is reassociated is plotted on the ordinate and the cot value on the abscissa. **Kurie p.** A graphic method of showing the spectral distribution of beta energies emitted in beta decay. **Lineweaver-Burk p.** The plot that expresses the relation between the reciprocal of a rate of reaction $v$ and the reciprocal of substrate concentration $s$. If the reaction follows Michaelis-Menten kinetics, this relationship is linear and is expressed by the equation $1/v = 1/V + (K_m/V)(1/s)$, where $V$ is the limiting velocity approached as $s$ increases toward infinity, and $K_m$ is the Michaelis constant. Also *Lineweaver-Burk equation.*

**plototoxin** \plō′tətäk′sin\ A poison derived from the catfish *Plotosus lineatus,* that is reported to be composed of a hemotoxic fraction, plotolysin, and a neurotoxin, plotospasmin.

**plug** Something that stops up an orifice or opening, especially when inserted for that purpose or if removable. **cervical p.** MUCOUS PLUG. **Corner's p.** A section of greater omentum that is used to close a gastric or intestinal perforation when primary repair is not possible or desirable. Also *Corner's tampon* (older term). **epithelial p.** The aggregation of ectodermal cells which for a short time blocks the external narial opening in a fetus. **Imlach's fat p.** An occasional small mass of fat situated at the medial side of the base of the superficial inguinal ring. **kite-tailed p.** A surgical packing material composed of tightly wound yarn or cloth that can be easily removed by pulling on its attached string. Also *kite-tail tampon* (older term). **meconium p. in newborn** A plug of mucus in a neonate that blocks the passage of meconium, causing distension. Following an enema, the plug is usually passed, followed by a gush of normal meconium. In other cases the meconium is abnormally viscous due to cystic fibrosis. **mucous p.** A plug lying in the cervical canal during pregnancy which is formed from accumulated mucous secretions of the endocervical glands. Also *cervical plug.* **yolk p.** In the embryos of the lower vertebrates, especially the Batrachia, such as frogs and toads, a ventral mass of entoblastic cells, rich in vitellus, which is prominent in the posterior part of the gastrula cavity and forms a prominent bulge in this area.

**plugger** CONDENSER. **gold p.** FOIL CONDENSER. **root canal p.** A flat-ended endodontic instrument used to pack a gutta-percha cone into the root canal. Also *gutta-percha plugger.*

**plumbism** \plum′bizm\ [L *plumb(um)* lead + -ISM] LEAD POISONING.

**plumbotherapy** \plum′bōther′əpē\ The use of lead and lead salts for therapeutic purposes.

**Plummer** [Henry Stanley *Plummer,* U.S. physician, 1874–1937] **1** See under SIGN, TREATMENT, DILATOR. **2** Plummer-Vinson syndrome. See under SYNDROME. **3** Plummer's disease. See under TOXIC NODULAR GOITER.

**plumper** \plum′pər\ A thickened buccal or labial flange of a denture, used to restore the contours of the cheek or lip which have been altered by loss of the teeth and supporting tissues.

**pluri-** \plʊr′ē-\ [L *plus,* gen. *pluris* (comparative of *multus* many) more] A combining form meaning more, several.

**plurideficient** \-difish′ənt\ [PLURI- + *deficient*] POLYDEFICIENT.

**plurifocal** \-fō′kəl\ MULTIFOCAL.

**pluriglandular** \-glan′dyələr\ [PLURI- + GLANDULAR] Of, pertaining to, or involving several glands. Also *multiglandular, polyglandular.*

**plurigravida** \-grav′idə\ [PLURI- + GRAVIDA] MULTIGRAVIDA.

**plurilocular** \-läk′yələr\ MULTILOCULAR.

**plurinuclear** \-n^y^oo′klē·ər\ [PLURI- + NUCLEAR] MULTINUCLEAR.

**pluripara** \ploorip′ərə\ [PLURI- + PARA] MULTIPARA.

**pluriparity** \-par′itē\ [PLURI- + PARITY] MULTIPARITY.

**pluripartite** \-pär′tīt\ MULTIPARTITE.

**pluripolar** \-pō′lər\ MULTIPOLAR.

**pluripotent** \plʊrip′ətənt\ PLURIPOTENTIAL.

**pluripotential** \-pəten′chəl\ [PLURI- + POTENTIAL] **1** Having multiple developmental or functional capacities. **2** Capable of influencing more than one tissue or organ. For defs. 1 and 2 also *pluripotent.*

**pluripotentiality** \-pōten′shē·al′itē\ [PLURIPOTENTIAL + -ITY] **1** The ability to perform or develop in multiple ways. **2** The capability of influencing more than one tissue or organ.

**pluriresistant** \-rizis′tənt\ Resistant to several drugs of different types.

**plutonism** \ploo′tənizm\ Poisoning caused by exposure to radiations from plutonium. Symptoms are liver damage, bone changes, and graying of the hair.

**plutonium** \plootō′nē·əm\ Element number 94, a metal of the actinide series, having mass numbers ranging from 232 to 246. Plutonium 239, with a half-life of 24 360 years, is produced in quantity from uranium 238 in nuclear reactors. Plutonium 239 undergoes spontaneous fission and thus may be used as a nuclear fuel. It requires care in handling to avoid unintentional formation of a critical mass, whether in solid form or in solution. Plutonium is chemically active and toxic. Valences are 3, 4, 5, and 6. All of the isotopes are energetic alpha emitters. Plutonium tends to accumulate in the bone marrow, where it destroys blood-forming mechanisms. Symbol: Pu

**Pm** Symbol for the element, promethium.

**PMA** See under PMA INDEX.

**PMB** **1** polymorphonuclear basophil leukocyte. **2** postmenopausal bleeding.

**PMI** point of maximum impulse.

**PML** progressive multifocal leukoencephalopathy.

**PMN** polymorphonuclear neutrophil (leukocyte).

**PMR** proportionate mortality ratio.

**PMS** **1** pregnant mare serum. **2** postmenstrual stress.

**PMSG** pregnant mare serum gonadotropin.

**PMT** premenstrual tension.

**PN** **1** peripheral neuropathy (polyneuropathy). **2** peripheral nerve. **3** percussion note. **4** polyneuritis.

**PND** paroxysmal nocturnal dyspnea.

**PNdB** Symbol for the unit, perceived noise decibel, a unit of perceived noise level. The noise level numerically equal to the sound pressure level in dB of a band of random noise of width 1/3 to 1 octave centered on 1 kHz, which is judged by listeners to be equally noisy.

**-pnea** \-pnē·ə, -nē·ə, -pnē′ə, -nē′ə\ [Gk *pnoia,* from *pno(ē)* breath + *-ia* -IA] A combining form designating a (specified) kind of breathing. Also *-pnoea* (British spelling).

**pneo-** \nē′ō-\ [Gk *pnein* to breathe] A combining form meaning breath, breathing.

**pneodynamics** \nē′ōdīnam′iks\ PNEUMODYNAMICS.

**pneogram** \nē′əgram\ SPIROGRAM.

**pneometer** \nē·äm′ətər\ SPIROMETER.

**pneuma-** \n^y^oo′mə-\ PNEUMATO-.

**pneumarthrography** \n^y^oo′märthräg′rəfē\ PNEUMOARTHROGRAPHY.

**pneumarthrosis** \n^y^oo′märthrō′sis\ [Gk *pneum(a)* wind, air, breath + ARTHROSIS] Air in a joint space.

**pneumat-** \n^y^oomat′-\ PNEUMATO-.

**pneumathemia** \n^y^oo′məthē′mē·ə\ AIR EMBOLISM.

**pneumatic** \n^y^oomat′ik\ [Gk *pneumatik(os)* (from *pneuma,* gen. *pneumatos,* wind, air, breath + *-ikos* -IC) pertaining to wind, air, or breath] Relating to or functioning by means of air or gas.

**pneumatics** \n^y^oomat′iks\ [PNEUMAT- + -ICS] The science concerned with the mechanical properties of gases.

**pneumatinuria** \n^y^oo′mətinoo′rē·ə\ PNEUMATURIA.

**pneumatization** \n^y^oo′mətīzā′shən\ The development of epithelium-lined air spaces in bone, such as the ethmoidal and mastoid air cells. **mastoid p.** The process whereby the mesenchyme and bone marrow of the temporal bone at birth and particularly of the subsequently developing mastoid process, become replaced by air cells.

**pneumatized** \n^y^oo′mətīzd\ Containing air spaces.

**pneumato-** \n^y^oomat′ō-, n^y^oo′mətō-\ [Gk *pneuma* (genitive *pneumatos*) wind, air, breath] A combining form meaning (1) air or gas; (2) breathing, respiration. Also *pneuma-, pneumat-.*

**pneumatocardia** \-kär′dē·ə\ [PNEUMATO- + -CARDIA] The presence of gas in the heart, as a result of air embolism.

**pneumatocele** \n^y^oomat′əsēl\ [PNEUMATO- + -CELE[1]] **1** A thin-walled, air-containing cyst within the lung. Also *pneumocele.* **2** HERNIA OF THE LUNG. **3** AEROCELE. **p. cranii** A collection of air inside the skull, usually resulting from a fracture that creates a passage through a paranasal sinus. Also *intracranial pneumatocele, pneumatocephalus.* **extracranial p.** SUBGALEAL EMPHYSEMA. **intracranial p.** PNEUMATOCELE CRANII. **scrotal p.** The presence of air in a hernial sac in the scrotum. It may also follow pneumoperitoneum.

**pneumatocephalus** \-sef′ələs\ [PNEUMATO- + -CEPHALUS] PNEUMATOCELE CRANII.

**pneumatogram** \n^y^oomat′əgram\ SPIROGRAM.

**pneumatograph** \n^y^oomat′əgraf\ SPIROGRAPH.

**pneumatometer** \n^y^oo′mətäm′ətər\ SPIROMETER.

**pneumatometry** \n^y^oo′mətäm′ətrē\ SPIROMETRY.

**pneumatorrhachis** \n^y^oo′mətôr′əkis\ PNEUMORACHIS.

**pneumatosis** \n^y^oo′mətō′sis\ [PNEUMAT- + -OSIS] The abnormal presence of air or gas in a tissue, organ, or cavity. **p. cystoides intestinalis** A condition in which air-filled cysts occupy the intestinal wall. Also *pneumatosis cystoides intestinorum, pneumatosis intestinalis.*

**pneumatotherapy** \-ther′əpē\ PNEUMOTHERAPY.

**pneumatothorax** \-thôr′aks\ PNEUMOTHORAX.

**pneumaturia** \nʸoo′mətoo′rē·ə\ [PNEUMAT- + -URIA] The passage of urine with gas bubbles, secondary to a vesicovaginal or vesicoenteric fistula or infection with gas-forming bacteria. Also *pneumatinuria, pneumouria.*

**pneumectomy** \nʸoomek′təmē\ PNEUMONECTOMY.

**pneumencephalography** \nʸoo′mensef′əläg′rəfē\ PNEUMOENCEPHALOGRAPHY.

**pneumo-** \nʸoo′mō-\ [Gk *pneuma* air, breath and *pneumōn,* alter. of *pleumōn* the lungs] A combining form meaning (1) the lung or lungs, pulmonary; (2) air, gas; (3) breathing, respiration; (4) pneumonia. Also *pneumon-, pneumono-.*

**pneumoarctia** \-ärk′shē·ə\ PULMONARY VALVE STENOSIS.

**pneumoarthrography** \-ärthräg′rəfē\ [PNEUMO- + ARTHROGRAPHY] Roentgenography of a joint following the percutaneous injection of air or appropriate gas into the joint space. Also *pneumarthrography.*

**pneumobacterine** A vaccine prepared from killed pneumococcus cultures.

**pneumoblastoma** \-blastō′mə\ PULMONARY BLASTOMA.

**pneumobulbar** \-bul′bər\ Pertaining to the respiratory center of the medulla. Also *pneumobulbous.*

**pneumocardial** \-kär′dē·əl\ CARDIOPULMONARY.

**pneumocardiography** \-kär′dē·äg′rəfē\ The recording of the dimensional changes of the heart resulting, for example, from the pressure fluctuations in the bronchi.

**pneumocele** \nʸoo′məsēl\ [PNEUMO- + -CELE[1]] **1** PNEUMATOCELE. **2** AEROCELE. **3** HERNIA OF THE LUNG.

**pneumocentesis** \-sentē′sis\ PNEUMONOCENTESIS.

**pneumocephalon** \-sef′əlän\ PNEUMOCEPHALUS. **p. artificiale** Insufflation of air into intracranial fluid spaces, especially for treatment of subdural adhesions. *Rare.*

**pneumocephalus** \-sef′ələs\ [PNEUMO- + -CEPHALUS] The presence of air or other gas within the cranial cavity. Also *pneumocephalon, pneumocrania, pneumocranium, pneumoencephalocele, pneumoencephalos.*

**pneumocholecystitis** \-kō′ləsistī′tis\ EMPHYSEMATOUS CHOLECYSTITIS.

**pneumococcal** \-käk′əl\ Relating to or caused by pneumococci.

**pneumococcemia** \-käksē′mē·ə\ [*pneumococc(us)* + -EMIA] The presence of pneumococci (*Streptococcus pneumoniae*) in the bloodstream.

**pneumococci** \-käk′sī\ Plural of PNEUMOCOCCUS.

**pneumococcidal** \-käksī′dəl\ Lethal to pneumococci.

**pneumococcosis** \-käkō′sis\ [*pneumococc(us)* + -OSIS] Infection with pneumococci (*Streptococcus pneumoniae*)..

**pneumococcus** \-käk′əs\ [PNEUMO- + COCCUS] (*pl.* pneumococci) An organism of the species *Streptococcus pneumoniae.* • This term, which is still widely used, reflects an earlier classification of this organism.

**pneumocolon** \-kō′län\ **1** A condition characterized by air or gas in the colon. **2** Introduction of air into the colon for air-contrast barium enema studies.

**pneumoconiosis** \nʸoo′məkōnē·ō′sis\ [PNEUMO- + Gk *koni(s)* dust + -OSIS] (*pl.* pneumoconioses) A condition characterized by the deposition of mineral dust in the lungs as a result of occupational or environmental exposure. It may be relatively harmless, as in siderosis or stannosis, or severely disabling, as in coal-workers' pneumoconiosis and bauxite pneumoconiosis. Also *lithosis, lithicosis, pneumonoconiosis, pneumonokoniosis, pneumokoniosis.* **asbestos p.** ASBESTOSIS. **bauxite p.** A form of pneumoconiosis resulting from inhalation of fumes from the smelting of bauxite, an aluminum ore composed principally of $Al_2O_3$. It is characterized by the formation of emphysematous bullae which rupture, causing pneumothorax, and by diffuse fibrosis. Also *Shaver's disease, bauxite workers' disease, bauxite pulmonary fibrosis.* **coal workers' p.** An occupational disease of coal workers resulting fron deposition of coal dust in the lungs. It occurs in a simple form, noncollagenous pneumoconiosis, and in a complicated, or collagenous, form called progressive massive fibrosis. Also *black lung, coal miners' lung, colliers' lung, colliers' phthisis* (obs.), *black phthisis* (obs.), *bituminosis, anthracosis, melanedema, miners' asthma* (obsolete and incorrect). **collagenous p.** PROGRESSIVE MASSIVE FIBROSIS. **complicated p.** PROGRESSIVE MASSIVE FIBROSIS. **diatomaceous earth p.** A pneumoconiosis resulting from exposure to diatomite. It may be nondisabling (noncollagenous) when the exposure is to natural diatomite (amorphous silica), or disabling where the diatomite has been calcined and largely converted into quartz or crystalline silica. The disabling form is associated with nodular and confluent masses with collagenous fibrosis. Also *diatomite disease.* **noncollagenous p.** Pneumoconiosis in which there is no production of collagen fibers, as that resulting from exposure to coal or carbon. There is an accumulation of dust particles and macrophages containing dust around or near respiratory bronchioles, and reticulin fibers enmesh particles and cells. **rheumatoid p.** CAPLAN SYNDROME. **p. siderotica** SIDEROSIS. **talc p.** Pneumoconiosis resulting from exposure to talc and associated minerals, such as the amphibole group of asbestos minerals and quartz. Talc itself produces at most a mild peribronchial fibrosis, but other minerals contained in commercial talc can cause an ill-defined nodular fibrosis, diffuse interstitial fibrosis, or foreign-body granulomas. Also *pulmonary talcosis, talcosis.*

**pneumocrania** \-krā′nē·ə\ PNEUMOCEPHALUS.

**pneumocranium** \-krā′nē·əm\ PNEUMOCEPHALUS.

***Pneumocystis*** \-sis′tis\ A genus composed of a single species, *P. carinii,* which causes pneumocystosis, an interstitial plasma cell pneumonitis occurring in humans, especially in immunologically compromised individuals and in neonates. The taxonomic status of this microorganism is uncertain. Most investigators consider it a protozoan, possibly a sporozoan, though others view it as a fungus.

**pneumocystography** \-sistäg′rəfē\ [PNEUMO- + CYSTOGRAPHY] **1** Radiography of the urinary bladder after the injection of air or another suitable gas into it, either directly by needle or via a urethral catheter. **2** Radiography of a cyst, such as a renal cyst or breast cyst, after replacing its fluid contents by air or another gas. Also *aerocystography.*

**pneumocystosis** \-sistō′sis\ A disease resulting from infection with *Pneumocystis carinii.* The predominant clinical manifestations are those of pulmonary infection. Infants, immunocompromised patients, and debilitated persons are most often affected. Extrapulmonary infection is rare but has been reported in the spleen, liver, blood, and lymph nodes. See also *PNEUMOCYSTIS CARINII* PNEUMONIA.

**pneumocyte** \nʸoo′məsīt\ [PNEUMO- + -CYTE] A cell that lines the alveolar spaces in the lungs. Also *pneumonocyte, alveolar cell, pulmonary epithelial cell.* **granular p.** TYPE II PNEUMOCYTE. **membranous p.** TYPE I PNEUMOCYTE. **type I p.** Any of the squamous epithelial cells that cover the larger part of the alveolar surface of the lung. Also *type I cell, squama alveolaris, squamous alveolar cell, membranous pneumocyte.* **type II p.** Any of the rounded cells of the alveolar surface of the lung which produce pulmonary surfactant. Also *type II cell, granular pneumocyte, great alveolar cell, septal cell, niche cell.*

**pneumoderma** \-dur′mə\ A collection of air in the skin.
**pneumodynamics** \-dīnam′iks\ The dynamics of pulmonary ventilation. Also *pneodynamics*.
**pneumoempyema** \n^y^oo′mō·em′pī·ē′mə\ Empyema with gas in the pleural cavity; pneumopyothorax.
**pneumoencephalocele** \-ensef′əlōsēl′\ PNEUMOCEPHALUS.
**pneumoencephalography** \-ensef′əläg′rəfē\ [PNEUMO- + ENCEPHALOGRAPHY] Radiographic examination of the intracranial subarachnoid spaces and ventricles after the injection of air or oxygen into the subarachnoid space, usually via spinal lumbar puncture. Also *air encephalography, pneumencephalography*. **fractional p.** Roentgenography of the brain with sequential roentgenograms after incremental injections of air, each 5–10 ml, into the subarachnoid spaces and ventricular system of the brain.
**pneumoencephalomyelography** \-ensef′əlōmī′əläg′rəfē\ [PNEUMO- + ENCEPHALO- + MYELOGRAPHY] Roentgenography of the brain and spinal cord after replacement of some cerebrospinal fluid by air or gas via a lumbar puncture.
**pneumoencephalos** \-ensef′ələs\ PNEUMOCEPHALUS.
**pneumoenteritis** \-en′terī′tis\ Enteritis associated with pneumonia. Also *pneumonoenteritis*.
**pneumoerysipelas** \n^y^oo′mō·er′isip′ələs\ Pneumonia occurring in association with erysipelas. Also *pneumonoerysipelas*.
**pneumofasciogram** \-fas′ē·əgram′\ [PNEUMO- + *fasci(a)* + *o* + -GRAM] A roentgenogram of soft tissues after the injection of air into fascial planes.
**pneumogastrography** \-gasträg′rəfē\ [PNEUMO- + GASTRO- + -GRAPHY] Radiographic study of the stomach after insufflation of air into its lumen.
**pneumogastroscopy** \-gasträs′kəpē\ The direct visual examination of the stomach, employing air introduced via the gastroscope to distend the stomach.
**pneumography** \n^y^oomäg′rəfē\ [PNEUMO- + -GRAPHY] Radiographic examination of an organ after the injection of air or other gas into it. **retroperitoneal p.** Radiographic examination of the organs of the lumbar and pelvic regions after the injection of gas into the retroperitoneal tissues, used chiefly in the past for study of the kidneys and adrenal glands and now used only rarely.
**pneumohemia** \-hē′mē·ə\ AIR EMBOLISM.
**pneumohemopericardium** \-hē′mōper′ikär′dē·əm\ The presence of gas or air and blood in the pericardial cavity.
**pneumohemothorax** \-hē′mōthôr′aks\ The presence of air and blood in the pleural space.
**pneumohydrometra** \-hī′drəmē′trə\ [PNEUMO- + HYDROMETRA] An accumulation of gaseous and fluid material in the uterus. Also *hydrophysometra, physohydrometra*.
**pneumohydropericardium** \-hī′drəper′ikär′dē·əm\ The presence of gas or air and fluid in the pericardial cavity.
**pneumohydrothorax** \-hī′drəthôr′aks\ HYDROPNEUMOTHORAX.
**pneumokidney** \n^y^oo′məkid′nē\ [*pneumo-* + KIDNEY] The presence of gas in the renal pelvis, usually secondary to gas in the bladder as a result of an intestinal bladder fistula.
**pneumokoniosis** \-kō′nē·ō′sis\ PNEUMOCONIOSIS.
**pneumolith** \n^y^oo′məlith\ [PNEUMO- + -LITH] A calculus in the lung. Also *pulmolith*.
**pneumology** \n^y^oomäl′əjē\ [PNEUMO- + -LOGY] The science or study of the lungs and respiratory passages.
**pneumolysin** \n^y^oomäl′isin\ A hemolytic toxin produced by the pneumococcus. It is immunologically related to the oxygen-labile hemolysin of hemolytic streptococci.
**pneumolysis** \n^y^oomäl′isis\ PNEUMONOLYSIS.
**pneumomediastinography** \-mē′dē·əstinäg′rəfē\ [PNEUMO- + MEDIASTINOGRAPHY] GAS MEDIASTINOGRAPHY.
**pneumomediastinum** \-mē′dē·astī′nəm\ An accumulation of air or other gas in the mediastinum. Also *mediastinal emphysema*.
**pneumometer** \n^y^oomäm′ətər\ SPIROMETER.
**pneumomoniliasis** \-mō′nilī′əsis\ Pneumonia caused by *Candida* organisms, usually *C. albicans*; pulmonary candidiasis. Also *pneumonomoniliasis*.
**pneumomyelography** \-mī′əläg′rəfē\ Myelography with the use of air or an appropriate gas as the contrast medium.
**pneumon-** \n^y^oomən-\ PNEUMO-.
**pneumonectomy** \-nek′təmē\ [PNEUMON- + -ECTOMY] A cutting out of a portion of a lung or an entire lung. Also *pneumectomy, pulmonectomy*.
**pneumonere** \n^y^oo′mənir\ The dense mass of splanchnic mesenchyme enveloping the embryonic lung buds and later becoming the connective tissue layer of the visceral pleura. *Outmoded*.

# pneumonia

**pneumonia** \n^y^oomō′nya\ [Gk, alter. of *pleumonia* (from *pleumōn* the lungs + *-ia* -IA) lung disease] Inflammation of the lower respiratory tract, i.e., lower airways and alveolar spaces, caused by exposure of the lung to toxic material, chemicals, or any of a wide variety of microbial pathogens, including bacteria, mycobacteria, viruses, fungi, rickettsia, mycoplasmas, and parasites. **acute p.** Pneumonia of rapid onset. **p. alba** A fatal pneumonia of the newborn due to congenital syphilis. The lungs are nearly airless, appear pale or white, and undergo fatty degeneration. Also *white pneumonia, white lung*. **alcoholic p.** Pneumonia acquired in association with acute or chronic alcoholism. **amebic p.** Pneumonia occurring as a complication of lung abscesses caused by *Entamoeba histolytica*. Pulmonary involvement in amebiasis may be secondary to extension of an amebic abscess from the liver through the diaphragm and into the lung and pleural space. **anthrax p.** INHALATION ANTHRAX. **apical p.** Pneumonia involving the apex of the lung. Also *apex pneumonia*. **aspiration p.** Pneumonia resulting from inhalation of foreign material, usually food, into the lungs. Also *aspiration pneumonitis*. **atypical p.** MYCOPLASMAL PNEUMONIA. **bacterial p.** Any pneumonia resulting from bacterial infection, as for example by *Streptococcus pneumoniae, Staphylococcus aureus, Klebsiella* species, or *Haemophilus influenzae*. **bronchial p.** BRONCHOPNEUMONIA. **caseous p.** TUBERCULOUS PNEUMONIA. **catarrhal p.** BRONCHOPNEUMONIA. **cheesy p.** TUBERCULOUS PNEUMONIA. **chickenpox p.** Pneumonia due to infection of the lung with varicella virus in the course of chickenpox infection. **chronic fibrous p.** Persisting pneumonia resulting in fibrosis of the affected portion of the lung. **cold agglutinin p.** MYCOPLASMAL PNEUMONIA. **congenital aspiration p.** An inaccurate and outmoded term for RESPIRATORY DISTRESS SYNDROME OF NEWBORN. **contusion p.** Pneumonia resulting from a pulmonary contusion. *Seldom used*. Also *traumatic pneumonia*. **creeping p.** MIGRATORY PNEU-

MONIA. **croupous p.** LOBAR PNEUMONIA. **deglutition p.** Aspiration pneumonia resulting from a disorder of the swallowing mechanism. **desquamative p.** Pneumonia characterised by desquamation of alveolar lining cells into the alveolar lumens. **desquamative interstitial p.** A condition of unknown cause characterized by breathlessness and widespread abnormal opacities of the chest radiograph, in which alveolar wall cells are present in the lumen of alveoli. It is a variant of diffuse interstitial pulmonary fibrosis. **double p.** Pneumonia involving both lungs. **Eaton agent p.** MYCOPLASMAL PNEUMONIA. **embolic p.** Pneumonia resulting from embolism of infected material passing into the lungs. **fibrous p.** Pneumonia with fibrous scarring. Also *fibroid pneumonia.* **Friedländer's p.** *KLEBSIELLA* PNEUMONIA. **gangrenous p.** Pneumonia with gangrenous change in the lung. **giant cell p.** A rare, severe, interstitial pneumonia due to the measles virus and occurring in children with diseases of the reticuloendothelial system. The disease is characterized by the presence of multinucleate giant-cell inclusion bodies. Also *Hecht's pneumonia.* **hypostatic p.** Pneumonia occurring in aged or debilitated bedridden patients and characterized by passive congestion of the dependent portions of the lungs. **influenza p.** A severe, often fatal pneumonia due to influenza virus and characterized by fever, pharyngitis, myalgia, profound dyspnea, prostration, and massive pulmonary edema, hemorrhage, and consolidation. It may be complicated by a bacterial pneumonia. Persons with cardiovascular disease and other chronic disorders seem especially susceptible, as do pregnant women. Also *influenza virus pneumonia.* **inhalation p.** Pneumonia resulting from inhalation of harmful gases or of foreign particulate material into the lungs. **interstitial p.** **1** A pneumonia, often viral, predominantly involving interstitial tissues of the lung. **2** DIFFUSE INTERSTITIAL PULMONARY FIBROSIS. **interstitial plasma cell p.** *PNEUMOCYSTIS CARINII* PNEUMONIA. **Kaufman's p.** A rare acute interstitial pneumonia which affects infants and usually causes death. ***Klebsiella* p.** An acute, bacterial, lobar pneumonia caused by *Klebsiella pneumoniae* (Friedländer's bacillus), which occurs sporadically in most tropical countries. It frequently progresses to abscess formation. If untreated, mortality is very high. The disease must be differentiated from the commonly occurring pneumococcal pneumonia which responds rapidly to penicillin treatment. The antibiotics of choice are gentamicin and streptomycin, but the tetracyclines are also effective. Alcoholism is a predisposing factor. Also *Friedländer's pneumonia.* **lipoid p.** Pneumonia resulting from inhalation of oily material into the lungs. Also *lipid pneumonia, oil-aspiration pneumonia, pneumonolipidosis.* **lobar p.** Pneumonia involving predominantly one lobe of the lung or adjacent lobes, usually caused by bacterial infection. Also *croupous pneumonia.* **lobular p.** BRONCHOPNEUMONIA. **Löffler's p.** LÖFFLER SYNDROME. **Louisiana p.** A communicable form of pneumonia encountered in Louisiana and caused by a strain of *Chlamydia psittaci.* **p. malleosa** Pneumonia occurring in association with glanders. **metastatic p.** Pneumonia resulting from blood-borne spread of infection from elsewhere in the body. **migratory p.** Pneumonia in which consolidation serially involves different parts of the lung. Also *wandering pneumonia, creeping pneumonia.* **mycoplasmal p.** Epidemic or endemic pneumonia caused by *Mycoplasma pneumoniae.* A generally mild illness, it begins insidiously after a three-week incubation period. The predominant clinical features are malaise, fever, and cough. Treatment is with tetracycline or erythromycin. All age groups are affected, with school-age children and adults especially susceptible. Also *primary atypical pneumonia, atypical pneumonia, Eaton agent pneumonia, cold agglutinin pneumonia.* **obstructive p.** Pneumonia that develops beyond an obstruction to a bronchus. **oil-aspiration p.** LIPOID PNEUMONIA. **organizing p.** Pneumonia which is progressing to fibrosis. **plague p.** PNEUMONIC PLAGUE. **plasma cell p.** *PNEUMOCYSTIS CARINII* PNEUMONIA. **pneumococcal p.** Pneumonia due to infection with *Streptococcus pneumoniae,* the most common type of community-acquired pneumonia in adults. The illness begins with a sudden chill, which is followed by fever, pleuritic chest pain, and cough. Bacteremia occurs in 20–30% of cases and pleural effusion in 10–20% of cases. Penicillin is the drug of choice. A pneumococcal vaccine became available in 1977 and has been successful in preventing pneumococcal infections in certain high-risk groups, including the elderly and persons with chronic diseases such as diabetes, renal disease, congestive heart failure, or alcoholism with cirrhosis. ***Pneumocystis carinii* p.** A pneumonia occurring in infants, immunocompromised patients, and other debilitated persons and caused by *Pneumocystis carinii.* It is seen in fully half of all patients who are in the advanced stages of acquired immune deficiency syndrome. Also *pneumocystis pneumonia, interstitial plasma cell pneumonia, plasma cell pneumonia.* **primary atypical p.** MYCOPLASMAL PNEUMONIA. **purulent p.** Pneumonia associated with production of purulent sputum. **rheumatic p.** RHEUMATIC PNEUMONITIS. **secondary p.** Pneumonia developing as a complication of another disease. **staphylococcal p.** A severe pneumonia caused by *Staphylococcus aureus.* It may be complicated by lung abscess. **streptococcal p.** Pneumonia caused by *Streptococcus* species, chiefly *S. pneumoniae* and, less often, *S. pyogenes.* **suppurative p.** Pneumonia with development of abscesses. **terminal p.** Pneumonia developing just before death in an old or otherwise very sick person. **toxemic p.** Systemic infection with *Streptococcus pneumoniae* in which there is limited lung involvement. **transplantation p.** Pneumonitis affecting recipients of organ transplants. It may be the result of direct immune reaction in the lung or an opportunistic infection secondary to therapeutic immunosuppression. Also *transplant lung syndrome.* **traumatic p.** CONTUSION PNEUMONIA. **tuberculous p.** **1** A bronchial or lobar pneumonia due to *Mycobacterium tuberculosis.* Also *caseous pneumonia, cheesy pneumonia.* **2** Pneumonia occurring as the host's initial reaction to infection with the tubercle bacillus. **tularemic p.** Pneumonia caused by *Francisella tularensis.* It may be primary, from inhalation of the infectious agent, or secondary, transmitted to the lungs via the bloodstream in patients with ulceroglandular tularemia. The mortality is approximately 30 percent in untreated cases. **typhoid p.** Pneumonia complicating typhoid fever, due either to *Salmonella typhi* or *Streptococcus pneumoniae.* Also *pneumotyphoid.* **unresolved p.** Pneumonia which persists. **varicella p.** Pneumonia due to the varicella virus. Developing 2–6 days after appearance of the varicella rash, the illness may be mild or severe. It usually occurs in adults and is seldom seen in normal children with varicella. It may lead to pulmonary calcification. **viral p.** Pneumonia caused by any of a number of viruses, including adenoviruses, cytomegalovirus, influenza virus, measles virus, and varicella virus. It often occurs in the course of or consequent to a systemic viral infection. Viral pneumonia may be complicated by secondary bacterial pneumonia. **wandering p.** MIGRATORY PNEUMONIA. **white p.** PNEUMONIA ALBA. **woolsorters' p.** INHALATION ANTHRAX.

**pneumonic** \nʸoomän′ik\ [Gk *pneumonikos* (from *pneumōn* lungs) pulmonary] **1** Relating to pneumonia. **2** Relating to or affecting the lungs.
**pneumonitis** \nʸoo′mōnī′tis\ [PNEUMON- + -ITIS] Inflammation of the lung from any cause. Also *pulmonitis*. **aspiration p.** ASPIRATION PNEUMONIA. **chemical p.** An acute inflammatory condition of the lungs caused by exposure to certain chemical compounds, such as those of beryllium, cadmium, manganese, osmium, and vanadium. **eosinophilic p.** LÖFFLER SYNDROME. **interstitial p.** A pneumonia characterized by an acute inflammatory infiltrate in the interstitium of the lung. It is accompanied by interstitial edema. It is caused by numerous infectious agents as well as by chemicals, neoplasia, collagen vascular diseases, and pulmonary hypersensitivity to inhaled antigen such as seen in farmer's lung. **irradiation p. and fibrosis** Pulmonary inflammation leading to scarring with fibrosis as a sequel to irradiation. **lipid p. and fibrosis** Pulmonary consolidation with scarring from fibrosis resulting from inhalation of lipid material. **malarial p.** A pneumonitis caused by the malarial parasite *Plasmodium falciparum*. Also *pneumonopaludism*. **oil p. and fibrosis** Pulmonary consolidation with scarring from fibrosis resulting from inhalation of oil particles. ***Pneumocystis* p.** Pneumonitis resulting from *Pneumocystis carinii* infection. See also PNEUMOCYSTOSIS. **rheumatic p.** Pulmonary infiltrates and rales associated with acute rheumatic fever. Also *rheumatic pneumonia*. **uremic p.** *Imprecise* UREMIC LUNG.
**pneumono-** \nʸoo′mənō-, nʸoomō′nō-\ PNEUMO-.
**pneumonocele** \nʸoomän′əsēl\ [PNEUMONO- + -CELE[1]] HERNIA OF THE LUNG.
**pneumonocentesis** \-sentē′sis\ [PNEUMONO- + -CENTESIS] The insertion of a needle into a lung, usually for the aspiration or drainage of fluid. Also *pneumocentesis*.
**pneumonoconiosis** \-kō′nē·ō′sis\ PNEUMOCONIOSIS.
**pneumonocyte** \nʸoomän′əsīt\ [PNEUMONO- + -CYTE] PNEUMOCYTE.
**pneumonoenteritis** \-en′terī′tis\ PNEUMOENTERITIS.
**pneumonoerysipelas** \-er′isip′ələs\ PNEUMOERYSIPELAS.
**pneumonography** \nʸoo′mənäg′rəfē\ Roentgenography of the lungs. *Seldom used*.
**pneumonokoniosis** \-kō′nē·ō′sis\ PNEUMOCONIOSIS.
**pneumonolipoidosis** \-lip′oidō′sis\ LIPOID PNEUMONIA.
**pneumonolysis** \nʸoo′mənäl′isis\ [PNEUMONO- + LYSIS] The division of adhesions between the lung and the chest wall. Also *pneumolysis*.
**pneumonometer** \nʸoo′mənäm′ətər\ SPIROMETER.
**pneumonomoniliasis** \-mō′nilī′əsis\ PNEUMOMONILIASIS.
**pneumonopaludism** \-pal′yədizm\ MALARIAL PNEUMONITIS.
**pneumonopexy** \nʸoo′mənōpek′sē\ Fixation of the lung to the chest wall. Also *pneumopexy*.
**pneumonophthisis** \nʸoo′mənäfthī′sis\ PULMONARY TUBERCULOSIS.
**pneumonoresection** \-risek′shən\ The excision of part or all of a lung. Also *pneumoresection*.
**pneumonorrhaphy** \nʸoo′mənôr′əfē\ [PNEUMONO- + -RRHAPHY] Suturing of the lung.
**pneumonotomy** \nʸoo′mənät′əmē\ Surgical incision into the lung. Also *pneumotomy*.
**pneumo-orbitography** \-ôr′bitäg′rəfē\ [PNEUMO- + ORBIT + *o* + -GRAPHY] Roentgenography of the orbital contents after the injection of air or an appropriate gas into the orbital, extrabulbar area.
**pneumopericarditis** \-per′ikärdī′tis\ Pericarditis with gas or air in the pericardial cavity. **purulent p.** Purulent pericarditis with gas in the pericardial cavity.
**pneumopericardium** \-per′ikär′dē·əm\ The presence of gas in the pericardial cavity.
**pneumoperitoneal** \-per′itənē′əl\ Relating to the presence of air in the peritoneal cavity.
**pneumoperitoneum** \-per′itənē′əm\ The presence of air within the peritoneum. **transabdominal p.** The injection of air percutaneously through the abdominal wall into the peritoneal cavity, to allow roentgenographic demonstration of intraperitoneal viscera and masses as well as the undersurface of the diaphragm.
**pneumoperitonitis** \-per′itənī′tis\ Peritonitis associated with air in the cavity, as may occur with a ruptured viscus.
**pneumopexy** \nʸoo′məpek′sē\ PNEUMONOPEXY.
**pneumophagia** \-fā′jə\ AEROPHAGIA.
**pneumoplethysmography** \-pleth′izmäg′rəfē\ OCULOPNEUMOPLETHYSMOGRAPHY.
**pneumopleuroparietopexy** \-plʊr′ōpərī′ətōpek′sē\ A procedure by which the lung is sutured along with its parietal pleura to the margin of a thoracic incision.
**pneumopyelography** \-pī′əläg′rəfē\ [PNEUMO- + PYELOGRAPHY] Radiography of the kidney after the injection of air or another suitable gas into its pelvis, such as by direct needle puncture or via a ureteral catheter.
**pneumopyopericardium** \-pī′əper′ikär′dē·əm\ The presence of gas or air and pus in the pericardial cavity.
**pneumopyothorax** \-pī′əthôr′aks\ The presence of air and pus in the pleural cavity.
**pneumorachicentesis** \-rā′kēsentē′sis\ [PNEUMO- + RACHI- + CENTESIS] Myelography with air or gas as the contrast agent.
**pneumorachis** \-rā′kis\ The presence of gas within the spinal canal, either in the subarachnoid or extradural space. The gas may be injected as part of a roentgenographic examination. Also *pneumatorrhachis*.
**pneumoradiography** \-rā′dē·äg′rəfē\ [PNEUMO- + RADIOGRAPHY] PNEUMOROENTGENOGRAPHY.
**pneumoresection** \-risek′shən\ PNEUMONORESECTION.
**pneumoroentgenography** \-rent′genäg′rəfē\ [PNEUMO- + ROENTGENOGRAPHY] Roentgenography of an organ, structure, or tissue into which air or gas has been injected. Also *pneumoradiography*.
**pneumosilicosis** \-sil′ikō′sis\ The presence of silica-containing particles in the lung; silicosis.
**pneumotaxic** \-täk′sik\ Concerning the regulation of the pulmonary respiration rate.
**pneumotherapy** \-ther′əpē\ [PNEUMO- + THERAPY] **1** The use of air or oxygen, especially by insufflation, in the treatment of disease. **2** An obsolete treatment based on inhalation of air under either reduced or increased pressure. Also *pneumatotherapy*.
**pneumothermomassage** \-thur′mōməsäzh′\ The use of hot air currents to produce a massagelike effect.
**pneumothorax** \-thō′raks\ [PNEUMO- + THORAX] The presence of air in the pleural cavity. Also *pneumatothorax*. **artificial p.** Therapeutic or diagnostic introduction of air into the pleural cavity. Also *induced pneumothorax*. **clicking p.** Pneumothorax in which the patient or physician can hear a clicking sound which is synchronous with the heart beat. **closed p.** Pneumothorax in which the layers of pleura are intact. **diagnostic p.** The introduction of air into the pleural space as an aid to diagnosis. **extrapleural p.** A collapsing of the lung by installation or formation of air pockets between the parietal pleura and the chest wall. **induced p.** ARTIFICIAL PNEUMOTHORAX. **open p.** Pneumothorax in which the pleural

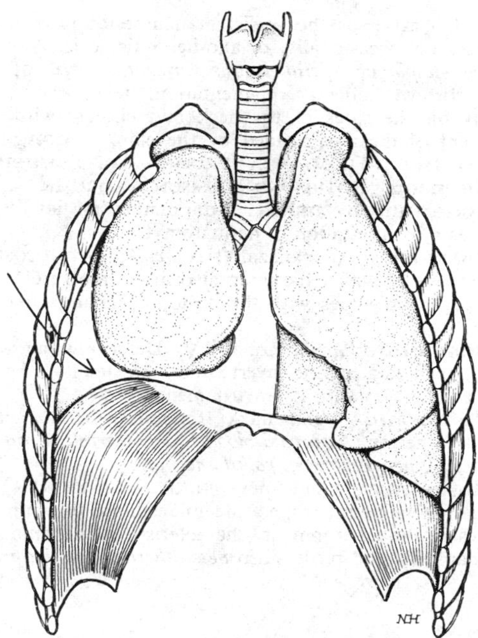

**Pneumothorax** (caused by penetrating wound of chest wall)

space is in open communication with the exterior through a hole in the chest wall. **pressure p.** TENSION PNEUMOTHORAX. **spontaneous p.** Pneumothorax developing without any known predisposing event. **sucking p.** Pneumothorax due to a wound in the chest wall which allows air to enter the pleural space during inspiration. **tension p.** Pneumothorax in which the air in the pleural space is at greater than atmospheric pressure. Also *pressure pneumothorax.* **therapeutic p.** Pneumothorax induced for therapeutic purposes. **traumatic p.** Pneumothorax resulting from trauma to the lung or chest wall. **valvular p.** Pneumothorax in which air can escape from the lung but cannot then leave the pleural space.

**pneumotomy** \n$^y$oomät′əmē\ PNEUMONOTOMY.

**pneumotropic** \-träp′ik\ Having an affinity for the lung: said principally of infective agents.

**pneumotyphoid** \-tī′foid\ TYPHOID PNEUMONIA.

**pneumouria** \n$^y$oo′mōyoo′rē·ə\ PNEUMATURIA.

**pneumoventricle** \-ven′trikəl\ [PNEUMO- + VENTRICLE] Air or other gas in the cerebral ventricles. Also *pneumoventriculi.*

**pneumoventriculography** \-ventrik′yəläg′rəfē\ [PNEUMO- + VENTRICULOGRAPHY ] Roentgenography of the brain after direct injection of air or gas into the cerebral ventricular system.

**pneumovirus** \n$^y$oo′mōvī′rəs\ [PNEUMO- + VIRUS] Any of a genus (*Pneumovirus*) of the Paramyxoviridae family which contains human and bovine respiratory syncytial viruses. They are membrane-bound and are believed to contain single-stranded RNA. Clinically they cause upper respiratory disease including bronchiolitis and pneumonia.

**PNH** paroxysmal nocturnal hemoglobinuria.

**-pnoea** \-pnē·ə, -nē·ə, -pnē′ə, -nē′ə\ *Brit.* -PNEA.

**PNPB** positive-negative pressure breathing.

**Po** Symbol for the element, polonium.

**po** *per os* (L, by mouth; orally).

**pock** [Old English *poc*] A pustule: used especially of those found in smallpox and other poxvirus disease.

**pocket** [dim. of *poke,* variant of POUCH] **1** An enclosed or definable space that functions as a receptacle or cul-de-sac and can be distinguished from the material surrounding it. **2** In dentistry, a pathologically altered gingival sulcus, lined to a variable extent with pocket epithelium. Clinically, a pocket is diagnosed when the depth from the gingival margin on gentle probing exceeds 3 mm. Also *pyorrhea pocket.* **absolute p.** PERIODONTAL POCKET. **complex p.** A serpiginous periodontal pocket with a narrow marginal opening. **compound p.** A periodontal pocket involving more than one surface of the tooth. **endocardial p.'s** Recesses in the mural endocardium, particularly in the left ventricular septum, usually associated with aortic regurgitation. Also *regurgitant pockets.* **gingival p.** A pocket that does not extend beyond the realm of the gingival tissues and may not be associated with bone loss. Also *pseudopocket, relative pocket, false pocket, supragingival pocket, supracrestal pocket.* **intrabony p.** A periodontal pocket in which the apical termination of the surrounding tissue destruction is within the alveolar process, i.e. apical to the adjacent alveolar crest. Also *infrabony pocket, intra-alveolar pocket, infracrestal pocket, subcrestal pocket.* **nuclear p.** NUCLEAR HOF. **periodontal p.** A pocket that extends beyond the realm of the gingiva, reaching into deeper and at least partially destroyed periodontal tissues. Also *absolute pocket, true pocket.* **pyorrhea p.** POCKET. **regurgitant p.'s** ENDOCARDIAL POCKETS. **relative p.** GINGIVAL POCKET. **retraction p.** A saucerlike depression in the tympanic membrane, usually in the posterosuperior quadrant, indicative of past chronic secretory otitis media. **subcrestal p.** INTRABONY POCKET. **suprabony p.** A periodontal pocket in which the apical termination of the surrounding tissue destruction is coronal to the alveolar crest. This condition is usually associated with horizontal bone loss. **supracrestal p.** GINGIVAL POCKET. **supragingival p.** GINGIVAL POCKET. **true p.** PERIODONTAL POCKET. **p.'s of Zahn** Pockets with apparent leaflets in the endocardium of the left ventricle in the presence of aortic regurgitation.

**pockmark** The scar that results from a lesion of smallpox.

**pocul.** *poculum* (L, cup).

**poculiform** \päk′yəlifôrm′\ Cup-shaped.

**poculum** \päk′yələm\ [L, a drinking cup] A cup; a cup-shaped structure. **p. diogenis** The hollow of the palm when the hand is cupped.

**pod-** \päd-, pōd-\ PODO-.

**-pod** \-päd, -pəd\ [Gk *pous,* gen. *podos* foot] A combining form meaning (1) a foot or footlike appendage; (2) having feet or legs of a (specified) kind.

**podagra** \pōdag′rə\ [Gk (from *pous,* gen. *pod(os)* foot + *agra* the chase, hunt, seizure) a foot trap, gout in the foot] Acute inflammation of the great toe, most commonly at the metatarsophalangeal joint but also at the interphalangeal joint, occurring as a characteristic manifestation of acute gout.

**podalgia** \pōdal′jə\ [POD- + -ALGIA] Pain at the metatarsophalangeal joint of the great toe.

**podalic** \pōdal′ik\ Of, pertaining to, or involving the feet, as *podalic version.*

**podarthritis** \päd′ärthrī′tis\ [POD- + ARTHRITIS] Arthritis of the first metatarsophalangeal joint of the foot.

**podencephalus** \päd′ensef′ələs\ [POD- + Gk *enkephalos* the brain] An extreme form of exencephaly in which the herniated brain is connected to the skull by only a pedicle.

**podia** \pō′dēə\ Plural of PODIUM.

**podiatrist** \pōdī′ətrist\ A practitioner of podiatry; a health professional responsible for foot care, including the diagnosis, treatment, and prevention of foot problems. The podiatrist may perform certain types of surgery and prescribe drugs and medical devices related to foot care. Also *chiropodist, podologist.*

**podiatry** \pōdī′ətrē\ [POD- + -IATRY] The medical specialization concerned with the foot, including its anatomy, mechanics, and pathology, and the diagnosis and treatment of its disorders. Also *chiropody, podology.*

**poditis** \pōdī′tis\ [POD- + -ITIS] An inflammation of the foot.

**podium** \pō′dē·əm\ [L (from Gk *podion* a small foot, dim. of *pous* foot), a balcony] A footlike expansion.

**podo-** \päd′ə-, pō′dō-\ [Gk *pous,* gen. *podos* (akin to L *pes,* gen. *pedis* foot) the foot] A combining form denoting the foot. Also *pod-.*

**podocyte** \päd′əsīt\ GLOMERULAR EPITHELIAL CELL.

**pododynamometer** \-dī′nəmäm′ətər\ An instrument for measuring the strength of the foot and leg muscles.

**pododynia** \-din′ē·ə\ [POD- + -ODYNIA] A pain in the sole of the foot and heel.

**podogram** \päd′əgram\ **1** A tracing of the margins of the foot. **2** A foot print used to measure the areas of weight-bearing as well as the foot arches.

**podography** \pädäg′rəfē\ The study of the foot by means of podograms.

**podologist** \pädäl′əjist\ PODIATRIST.

**podology** \pädäl′əjē\ PODIATRY.

**podometer** \pädäm′ətər\ PEDOMETER.

**podophyllin** \-fil′in\ PODOPHYLLUM RESIN.

**podopompholyx** \-päm′fōliks\ [PODO- + POMPHOLYX] Pompholyx that is confined to the feet.

**pogonion** \pōgō′nē·ən\ [Gk *pōgōnion* a small beard, dim. of *pōgōn* the beard] The most anterior point on the bony chin viewed from the lateral aspect. Also *mental point.*

***Pogonomyrmex*** \pōgō′nəmur′meks\ A genus of harvester ants that are economically important in agricultural areas of the United States and Mexico because of the numerous low, bare mounds they construct, which reduce vegetation for grazing animals. They have a painful bite which can be seriously poisonous when they attack animals or humans in large numbers. Some species serve as intermediate hosts of helminths. Various pathogens may also be passively carried by these ants.

**-poiesis** \-poi·ē′sis\ [Gk *poiēsis* (from *poiein* to make, form, create) a making, a forming] A combining form meaning development or production.

**poikilo-** \-poi′kəlō-\ [Gk *poikilos* many-colored, spotted, mottled, varied] A combining form meaning variegated, varied. Also *pecilo-.*

**poikilocyte** \poi′kilōsīt′\ [POIKILO- + -CYTE] An erythrocyte of irregular shape. Several types of poikilocytes are recognized, including spherocytes, elliptocytes, echinocytes, dacryocytes, schistocytes, and acanthocytes.

**poikilocytosis** \-sītō′sis\ The presence of many poikilocytes in blood. Also *poikilocythemia.*

**poikiloderma** \-dur′mə\ [POIKILO- + -DERMA] The association, in variable degree, of atrophy of the skin with macular or reticulate pigmentation and with telangiectasia. **p. atrophicans vasculare** The pattern of poikiloderma that arises as the persistent manifestation of mycosis fungoides or, occasionally, of another reticulosis. Also *parapsoriasis en plaques, perakeratosis variegata.* **p. of Civatte** Brown reticular pigmentation, telangiectasia, and atrophy on the sides of the neck and cheeks, without involvement of the area shaded by the chin. **congenital p.** ROTHMUND-THOMSON SYNDROME. **p. congenitale of Thomson** ROTHMUND-THOMSON SYNDROME.

**poikilodermatomyositis** \-dur′mətōmī′əsī′tis\ Poikiloderma as a manifestation of dermatomyositis.

**poikilosmosis** \poi′kiläzmō′sis\ [*poikil(o)-* + OSMOSIS] The process by which the internal osmotic pressure of a cell or an organism varies with the osmotic pressure of its environment.

**poikilosmotic** \poi′kiläzmät′ik\ Describing an aquatic animal, such as a marine invertebrate, that tends to be in osmotic equilibrium with its environment.

**poikilothermic** \-thur′mik\ Exhibiting or characterized by poikilothermy. Also *cold-blooded, ectothermic, exothermic, exothermal, heterothermic, poikilothermal.*

**poikilothermy** \-thur′mē\ [POIKILO- + THERM- + -Y] Fluctuation in body temperature in response to temperature changes in the environment, characteristic of all animals except mammals and birds. Also *heterothermy, ectothermy.*

# point

**point** [Old French *point* (from L *punctum,* substantive from neut. sing. past part. of *pungere* to prick, puncture, stab; a pricking, little hole, point, spot) a pricking, sting, point, dot] **1** A particular position, as in a series or scale. **2** A tapering or sharp end. **3** A fine cone used in endodontic treatment or periodontal diagnosis. **4** The working end of an instrument. It may not be pointed. **5** To move towards the surface: said of an abscess about to discharge. **6** A spot or minute orifice; punctum. **7** In anthropometry, a designated locus, usually related to the skeleton, to or from which measurements are made. **absolute near p.** NEAR POINT. **absorbent p.** A fine cone, made of rolled thin paper, used in endodontics to dry a root canal or to introduce medicaments into it. Also *paper point.* **Addison's p.** The midpoint of the epigastric region. **alveolar p.** PROSTHION. **Barker's p.** A point 32 mm behind and 32 mm above the auriculare; a site used in drainage of temporosphenoidal abscess. **p. of Béclard** The appearance of a distal, femoral, epiphyseal center of ossification during the latter part of the last trimester of pregnancy, usually two weeks before birth. The point of Béclard is a useful index of fetal maturity. **Boas p.** An area of tenderness located to the left of the twelfth thoracic vertebra in cases of gastric ulcer. **boiling p.** The temperature at which a pure substance is transformed from the liquid to the gas phase, at a given atmospheric pressure. At the boiling point, an equilibrium exists between the vapor pressure of the liquid phase and the ambient atmospheric pressure. Abbr. b.p. **Bolton p.** The highest point on the notch behind the occipital condyle as seen in lateral skull radiographs. Also *point Bo, postcondylare.* **Bolton registration p.** The midpoint of a line from the sella perpendicular to the Bolton plane. Also *registration point, R point.* **Cannon's p.** On the barium enema, a point of contraction at about the midportion of the transverse colon, indicating the point of junction between the primitive hindgut and midgut as well as the point of joining of two separate neurologic plexuses. **cardinal p.'s** 1 The two principal foci, two principal points, and two nodal points of an optical system. 2 In obstetrics, the two sacroiliac articulations and two iliopectineal eminences of the female bony pelvis. *Seldom used.* **p. of centricity** The central point on a pantographic tracing. This indicates centric position. **cold-rigor p.** The temperature at which cell activity first ceases and the cell passes into the narcotic state as the temperature is lowered. **condenser p.** NIB. **contact p.** CONTACT AREA. **p. of convergence** The given location at which the eyes fixate binocularly. **convergence near p.** The closest distance upon which the eyes can bifixate. **craniometric p.** Any one of a number of agreed points on the skull from which measurements are taken in craniometry. **critical p.** The condition of temperature and pressure at which the gas and liquid states of a pure substance have the same density and are thus indistinguishable. **crossover p.** The point in a metabolic pathway on either side of which the effects of a treatment differ. Most commonly, metabolites before such a point rise in concentration when metabolites after it fall in concentration, and vice versa. It gives an indication of a point at which the pathway is controlled, since a rise in concentration of metabolites before it and a fall of those after it suggests a slowing of the reaction at that point. **p. D** The center of the body of the symphysis of the mandible when observed in a lateral skull radiograph. **deaf p.** One of several points near the ear where a vibrating tuning fork cannot be heard. **Desjardins p.** A point on the surface of the abdomen overlying the head of the pancreas and located 5–7 cm from the umbilicus on an imaginary line between the umbilicus and the anterior fold of the right axilla. **p. of direction** An arbitrary location on the presenting part of a fetus used to relate the position of the fetus to the maternal pelvis. **p. of dispersion** VIRTUAL FOCUS. **dorsal p.** A point of tenderness between the vertebral column and the right scapular border at the level of the fourth intercostal space, found in subjects with hepatic colic. Also *Pauly's point.* **E p.** The peak of the major wave of the apex cardiogram. **p. of election** A stage in an operation at which the surgeon must choose among alternative courses before continuing. **end p.** The culminating reaction, change, or event in an analytic procedure that can be observed or measured to give the result for which the procedure was undertaken. **Erb's p.** A point 2–3 cm above the clavicle, lateral to the posterior border of the sternomastoid muscle, at which the upper cord of the brachial plexus ($C_5$–$C_6$) can be stimulated electrically. **far p.** The most remote site of accommodation, convergence, or fusion. Also *punctum remotum.* **fixation p.** The point upon which vision is directed; the object regarded by the eye. **flash p.** The temperature, constant for a given liquid, at which the vapors of a volatile liquid will ignite spontaneously. **focal p.** FOCUS. **freezing p.** The temperature at which a substance changes from the liquid to the solid state. Abbr. f.p. **fusion p.** MELTING POINT. **Galliot's p.** A point located at the intersection of a horizontal line passing 4 cm above the greater trochanter of the femur and a vertical line drawn at the junction of the medial two-thirds and the lateral third of the gluteal region. It was considered to be the ideal site for intramuscular injections. **glenoid p.** The midpoint of the glenoid cavity of the scapula. **growing p.** REPLICATION FORK. **gutta-percha p.** GUTTA-PERCHA CONE. **Hallé's p.** The intersection of the spinous plane and a vertical line drawn upward from the pubic tubercle, marking the point where the ureter crosses the pelvic brim. **Hartmann's critical p.** POINT OF SUDECK. **heat-rigor p.** The temperature at which cell death is first observed as the cell temperature is raised. Cell death is usually due to coagulation of the protoplasm. **hinge axis p.** One of the two places where the hinge axis passes through the skin. **Hirschfeld silver p.** A silver cone with a radiographically visible scale used for recording probing depth. **homologous p.** The identical anatomic point on a pair of stereoscopic roentgenograms. **image p.** In an optical system, the location that is conjugate with the object. **incisal p.** A point between the incisal edges of the lower central incisor teeth. Also *incisor point.* **isoelectric p.** The pH at which the molecules of a specified substance have no net charge, i.e. they have equal numbers of positive and negative charges. A protein has minimum solubility at its isoelectric point. This point may be determined by plotting electrophoretic mobility against pH and interpolating to find the pH at which the mobility is zero. Also *isoelectric pH.* **isoionic p.** The pH at which a molecule carrying both positive and negative charges has an equal number of each. **J p.** The point of junction between the QRS complex and the ST segment. Also *ST junction.* **lacrimal p.** PUNCTUM LACRIMALE. **Lanz p.** A point one-third of the distance from the right anterior superior iliac spine along a line between it and the left spine, denoting the surface projection of the position of the vermiform appendix. **Mackenzie's p.** An area of tenderness in the cephalad portion of the rectus abdominis muscle, associated with disease of the gallbladder. **p. of maximum impulse** The point at which the maximum thrust of the left ventricle is felt on the chest wall. Abbr. PMI **McBurney's p.** A superficial landmark on the abdominal wall located approximately one third the distance from the right anterior superior iliac spine to the umbilicus. It is said to be tender in cases of acute appendicitis. **McEwen's p.** A point just below the medial part of the supraorbital margin which is painful in acute frontal sinusitis. **median mandibular p.** A point at the anteroposterior center of the alveolar ridge of the mandible in the sagittal plane. **Méglin's p.** The site where the greater palatine nerve exits from the palatine foramen. **melting p.** The temperature at which a pure substance changes from the solid phase to the liquid phase. Also *fusion point.* **mental p.** POGONION. **metopic p.** GLABELLA. **midinguinal p.** The midpoint between the anterior superior iliac spine and the symphysis pubis. **motor p.** A point on the skin corresponding approximately to the entrance of a motor nerve into a muscle, and the site at which contraction of that muscle can be elicited at the lowest threshold of electrical stimulation. Such points are the sites of election for therapeutic application of electrical muscle stimulation. Also *Ziemssen's motor point.* **near p.** In ophthalmology, the closest site of accommodation, convergence, or fusion. Also *punctum proximum, absolute near point.* **neutral p.** The pH at which there are neither free hydrogen ions nor free hydroxyl ions, designated as pH 7. **nodal p.'s** Two points on the axis of an optical system such that an incident ray passing through one of the points will emerge through the other point, parallel to the incident ray. **object p.** In an optical system, the origin of the rays of light. **occipital p.** OPISTHOCRANION. **p. of ossification** The point at which ossification starts, appearing either in the middle of a cartilaginous matrix (endochondral ossification) or in that of a fibrous membrane (intramembranous ossification). **paper p.** ABSORBENT POINT. **Pauly's p.** DORSAL POINT. **phrenic-pressure p.** A point along the right phrenic nerve believed to display excessive sensibility to palpatory compression in disease of the gallbladder. **preauricular p.** A point on the posterior root of the zygomatic arch just anterior to the auriculare on the base line. **pressure p.** 1 A point on the skin which is exceptionally sensitive to pressure. 2 A point on the body surface overlying large superficial vessels where pressure may be applied for the control of hemorrhage from an artery. Also *pressure area.* **pressure-arresting p.** A point on the skin at which the application of pressure arrests or relieves spasm of the underlying muscles. **pressure-exciting p.** A point on the skin at which the application of pressure elicits spasm of the underlying muscle or muscles. **principal p.'s** The anterior and posterior intersection of the optic axis with the principal planes. **p. of proximal contact** CONTACT AREA. **R p.** BOLTON REGISTRATION POINT. **Ramond's p.** In gallbladder disease, a tender area between the heads of the sternocleidomastoid muscle. **reflection p.** A point at which a ray of light is reflected. **refraction p.** A point at which a ray of light is refracted. **registration p.** 1 In a lateral radiograph of the skull, the midpoint of a perpendicular line drawn from the middle of the sella turcica to the Bolton plane. 2 Any point taken as fixed for a pattern of analysis. **retromandibular tender p.** A point behind the pinna of the ear and in front of the mastoid process which is exceptionally tender in subjects with meningitis. **silver p.** An endodontic point, made of silver, for filling a root canal. **start p.** The first nucleotide of an RNA transcript. **p. of Sudeck** A section of the rectum that lies below the last sigmoid artery and above the bifurcation of the superior hemorrhoidal artery. This point was once erroneously thought to be critical in providing an adequate blood supply to the rectum following resection. Also *Sudeck's critical point, Hartmann's critical point.* **supra-auricular p.** A point on the posterior root of the zygomatic arch just above the auriculare. **supraclavicular p.** A point in the supraclavicular fossa where electrical stimulation will elicit contraction of those muscles innervated by the upper cord of the brachial plexus, including the deltoid, biceps, brachialis and brachioradialis. **sylvian p.** A point on the outer surface of the head about 30 mm behind the zygomatic process of the frontal bone and about 45 mm above the center of the zygomatic arch, marking the junction of the anterior rami with the posterior ramus of the lateral, or sylvian, fissure of the cerebrum. **thermal death p.** The temperature required to sterilize in 10 minutes a standard aqueous suspension of a given microorganism at neutral pH. **trigger p.** 1 A circumscribed area of the body where stimulation will produce a specific sensation, such as pain. Compare TRIGGER AREA. 2 A localized point of tenderness found during muscle spasm that is thought to contribute to prolongation of the spasm by a reflex mechanism. This concept has led to various therapeutic modalities directed specifically at the alleviation of trigger points, such as trigger point injection and trigger point massage. **Trousseau's p.** A tender point overlying a vertebral spinous process, sometimes noted when the corresponding spinal nerve is compressed or inflamed or when neuralgic pain is experienced along its course. *Obs.* Also *Trousseau's apophysiary point.* **vital p.** The zone of the medullary respiratory center the damage of which results in arrest of respiration and death. **Voillemier's p.** A point in the midline 6.5 cm below the line joining the anterior superior iliac spines. It is where the bladder may be punctured in edematous or obese patients. **Weber's p.** A point in the midline of the pelvic surface of the sacrum one centimeter below the promontory, stated by Weber to represent the center of gravity of the body. **p. Z** The point where a line from nasion to menton would be intersected by a perpendicular line from the anterior nasal spine. **Ziemssen's motor p.** MOTOR POINT.

**pointer** A contusion at a bony protuberance. **back p.** A device used in radiotherapy to indicate, on the exit side of the patient, the central axis of the beam.

**Poirier** [Paul-Julien *Poirier,* French surgeon and anatomist, 1853–1907] See under GLAND, LINE.

**Poiseuille** [Jean-Leonard-Marie *Poiseuille,* French physiologist, 1799–1869] 1 Poiseuille's equation. See under LAW. 2 See under SPACE.

**poison** [French (from L *potio* a drinking, drink, potion, draught of poison, from *potus,* past part. of *potare* to drink, drink heavily), a poison] A substance or mixture of substances capable of producing adverse effects in biologic systems, impairing function, or causing death. **acrid p.** A poison which produces irritation and inflammation of skin and mucous membranes. **arrow p.** A powerful poison applied to arrowheads and used primarily for hunting. Prey that is hit but not felled by the arrow itself can be followed until it succumbs to the poison. Primitive peoples in many parts of the world have used arrow poisons obtained from a variety of plant and animal sources. Some of these poisons, curare for example, have turned out to be of considerable importance in modern medicine and biomedical research. **contact p.** A substance which exerts a toxic effect by external contact. Exposure to pyrethrum insecticides and chlorophenoxy herbicides, for example, can cause dermatitis. Human poisonings have resulted from skin absorption of pentachlorophenol used as a fungicide. Many plants, notably poison ivy, and some animal venoms exert their poisonous effects through skin contact. **corrosive p.** Any substance that, in contact with living tissue, causes destruction of the tissue by chemical action. **fish p.** 1 Any of the natural toxins elaborated by fish, including venoms and ichthyosarcotoxins. 2 Any substance, usually a natural plant product, used to poison or stun fish in the water, generally for the purpose of catching them. An ambiguous term. **gonyaulax p.** Any of a group of toxins produced by the genus *Gonyaulax* and related dinoflagellates. Ingestion of shellfish which feed on these organisms may cause a variety of neurologic and neuromuscular manifestations including diplopia, dysphagia, variable pareses, and paresthesia in the limbs. Also *paralytic shellfish poison.* **hemotropic p.** Any poison having an affinity for, or producing injury to, blood or its cellular components. **irritant p.** Any substance which, on immediate, prolonged, or repeated contact with normal living tissue, induces a local inflammatory reaction. **mitotic p.** A substance that prevents or blocks mitosis. **paralytic shellfish p.** GONYAULAX POISON. **sedative p.** Any poison that depresses the functions of the central nervous system and of other vital organs.

**poisoning** 1 Exposure to a poison. 2 The condition resulting from exposure to a poison. **alcohol p.** A morbid condition resulting from excessive ingestion of alcohol. The chief adverse effects of ethyl alcohol are on the central nervous system, producing impaired vision, muscular incoordination, lengthened reaction time, dizziness, and nausea. Ingestion of methyl alcohol produces similar initial effects, but after a latent period of 6 to 36 hours, sudden headache may ensue, followed by dizziness and nausea and progressing to partial or total blindness, delirium, and coma. In nonfatal cases, the eye effects may persist for many months. See also ACUTE ALCOHOLISM, CHRONIC ALCOHOLISM. **aminopyrine p.** Poisoning from acute or chronic ingestion of aminopyrine. Persons sensitive to the drug may develop agranulocytosis or skin eruptions following the administration of even small doses. **amphetamine p.** Poisoning from the injudicious use of amphetamine, usually in diet pills. The symptoms of overdose are hyperpyrexia, hypertension, and severe central nervous system stimulation. **aniline p.** See under ANILISM. **antimony p.** Poisoning from excessive exposure to antimony. Exposure may occur in mining or in refining the ore in the production of antimony alloys or in medicinal preparations for the treatment of certain tropical diseases. Symptoms include headache, nausea, and vomiting. The most toxic compound is stibine ($SGH_3$), released as a gas when alloys are treated with acid. Poisoning with stibine (stibialism) can also result in hematuria and hemolytic anemia. **arsenic p.** Poisoning due to exposure to arsenic and causing irritation of the gastrointestinal tract with vomiting, diarrhea, colic, and collapse. Acute poisoning occurs most often in homicide or suicide cases. See also ARSENICALISM. **aspirin p.** Poisoning from accidental ingestion or overzealous therapeutic use of aspirin. Individuals differ in tolerance, some being particularly sensitive to the compound. Symptoms include nausea and vomiting, tinnitus, severe headache, rapid pulse, and increased respiration. **barbital p.** BARBITURISM. **barbiturate p.** BARBITURISM. **benzene p.** A condition that may be the result of acute or chronic exposure to benzene. Acute exposure results in central nervous system depression with headaches and dizziness. Convulsions, coma, and death may follow. Chronic exposure causes blood changes which may lead to aplastic anemia and granulocytic or lymphocytic leukemia. Benzene is a dangerous myelotoxic agent. Also *benzolism.* **beryllium p.** BERYLLIOSIS. **blood p.** SEPTICEMIA. **botulism food p.** Systemic botulism resulting from ingestion of food contaminated with preformed botulinum toxin (type A, B, or E). Most cases are associated with home-canned foods, but commercially canned or smoked foods are sometimes implicated. The illness presents as a neurologic disorder, with diplopia and difficulty in swallowing being common early manifestations. Progressive, symmetrical descending weakness or paralysis, lassitude, and dizziness develop 12–36 hours after ingestion of contaminated food. Treatment consists primarily of respiratory support and administration of trivalent ABE antitoxin of equine origin (available in the United States only from the Centers for Disease Control). Recovery is gradual, taking weeks or months. The case-fatality ratio, even with aggressive treatment, is approximately 25 percent. Also *food-borne botulism.* **bromide p.** A condition caused by prolonged or excessive therapeutic use of bromides. It may be characterized by such manifestations as confusion, tremor, headache, anorexia, memory loss, and an acneiform eruption, or by an organic mental syndrome such as hallucinosis, delirium, dementia, or delusional reaction. Also *bromidism.* **carbon monoxide p.** Poisoning occurring when carbon monoxide, acting as a chemical asphyxiant, combines with hemoglobin to form carboxyhemoglobin, which then reduces the oxygen-carrying capacity of the blood, thus causing tissue hypoxia. Typical signs and symptoms at 30–40 percent carboxyhemoglobin concentration are severe headache, vertigo, nausea, vomiting, irritability, and impaired judgment. At 40–50 percent, symptoms become more severe, including fainting on exertion. At 50–60 percent, loss of consciousness occurs, with depression of the respiratory center leading to death. Numerous deaths have been caused by carbon monoxide poisoning from a car engine running in a closed space or from the fumes in a closed car. It is the commonest form of industrial gassing accident. **carbon tetrachloride p.** Poisoning resulting from inhalation of carbon tetrachloride fumes. It produces a narcotic effect with central nervous system disturbance. At low exposures it causes liver and kidney damage. Pathologic changes include centrilobular liver necrosis and fatty degeneration. In the kidney there is proximal tubular necrosis. **cheese p.** TYROTOXICOSIS. **chemical fume p.** Poisoning produced by toxic fumes, such as may be produced from the burning of certain synthetic substances used in the stuffing of furniture and in toys, and in some modern building materials. In large fires the fumes have sometimes resulted in heavy loss of life. ⟨"Accounts of hotel infernos . . . routinely attribute deaths to smoke inhalation when they are more properly described as 'due to chemical-fume poisoning.'" —Jeanne M. Stellman, *New York Times,* 11 Dec. 1980, A34⟩ **chloral hydrate p.** A morbid condition caused by overuse of chloral hydrate as a sedative hypnotic agent. Symptoms are hypotension, dyspnea, cyanosis, irritation of the gastric mucosa, hepatic damage, and stupor or coma. Use of chloral hydrate has been largely replaced by the barbiturates. **corn cockle p.** GITHAGISM. **coyotillo p.** BUCKTHORN POLYNEUROPATHY. **cyanide p.** A morbid condition resulting from inhalation of cyanide, or ingestion of the seeds of stone fruits such as the bitter almond, *Prunus amygdalus* var. *amara,* containing a glucoside, amygdalin, which upon hydrolysis yields hydrocyanic acid. Poisoning is common among herbivorous animals that eat plants containing cyanogenic glucosides. Signs and symptoms are tachypnea, dyspnea, and respiratory paralysis which result from general inhibition of cellular respiration. Hydrocyanic acid combines with cytochrome oxidase in mitochondria. Large doses cause death within a few minutes. **fish p.** See under ICHTHYOSARCOTOXISM. **food p.** Any of a group of acute illnesses resulting from ingestion of food or water contaminated with pathogenic microorganisms, microbial toxins, or toxic chemicals of nonmicrobial origin. Common microbial agents include multiple serotypes of *Salmonella enteritidis, Staphylococcus aureus, Bacillus cereus, Clostridium perfringens, C. botulinum, Shigella* species, invasive and enterotoxigenic *E. coli, Vibrio parahemolyticus, Yersinia enterocolitica, Giardia lamblia,* rotaviruses, hepatitis A virus, and Norwalklike agents. Types of chemical food poisoning include heavy metal poisoning (copper, zinc, tin, cadmium), monosodium-L-glutamate poisoning (Chinese restaurant syndrome), fish poisoning (such as ciguatera), paralytic and neurotoxic shellfish poisoning, and a variety of mushroom poisoning syndromes. Also *sepsis intestinalis.* See also BOTULISM FOOD POISONING. **fugu p.** TETRODOTOXISM. • *Fugu* is the Japanese name for the puffer fish, various species of which are highly valued as gastronomic delicacies despite the risk of lethal poisoning from accidental contamination of the flesh during its preparation. **iron p.** Poisoning from ingestion of or chronic parenteral medication with iron salts. Acute toxic effects include vomiting and retching due to the astringent action on the gastric mucosa. A peculiar gray cyanosis has been seen in cases of ferrous sulfate poisoning, caused by the rapid rise in plasma iron and toxic effects on the central nervous system. Numerous cases of ferrous sulfate poisoning have been reported in children, attracted by the sweet coating on the tablets. Hemochromatosis is a potential hazard from long-continued parenteral medication, particularly in persons who do not have an iron deficiency. **lead p.** The toxic effects of various types of exposure to lead and its compounds. It is one of the commonest occupational diseases, arising from the inhalation of lead dust and fumes and from the absorption through intact skin of organic lead alkyl compounds added to gasoline. Symptoms include abdominal pain, constipation, and vomiting. In severe poisoning neuropathy and encephalopathy occur. Anemia occurs only in inorganic lead poisoning and only late in the disease. Psychiatric manifestations, such as disturbances in sleep and hyperexcitability, are more common in organic lead poisoning. A major hazard is to young children who ingest lead from flaking paint on woodwork or from lead paint flakes in soil and dust. Also *saturnine poisoning, plumbism, saturnism* (older term). **manganese p.** A disease resulting from exposure to manganese dust. The acute phase involves the lungs and is characterized by epithelial necrosis. The chronic phase involves the central nervous system, with marked irritability, difficulty in walking, speech disturbances, and various types of psychiatric disorders. The neurologic signs are due to damage of the basal ganglia, and resemble those of Parkinson's disease. Also *manganism.* **mercury p.** Poisoning from metallic mercury or its vapor leading to stomatitis, erethrism, and tremor. Skin contact with mercury fulminate causes dermatitis. Methyl and ethyl mercury compounds attack the nervous system, causing severe ataxia, dysarthria, and restriction of visual fields. Also *mercurialism, mercury toxicity, hydrargyria, hydrargyrism, hydrargyrosis.* **mushroom p.** Poisoning due to toxins contained in mushrooms which act following ingestion. Four types are known: poisoning causing cellular destruction, liver and kidney damage, and sometimes death; that affecting the autonomic nervous system; that affecting the central nervous system; and poisoning causing gastrointestinal irritation. Also *mycetism* (older term), *mycetismus* (older term). **mussel p.** Poisoning by the ingestion of mussels contaminated by the gonyaulax poison saxitoxin. **nutmeg p.** Poisoning from the dried, ripe seed of *Myristica fragrans.* Narcosis with hallucinations, delirium, and excitability may occur within an hour of ingestion of as little as one teaspoon of powdered nutmeg. Consumed in large quantities, it may produce drowsiness, stupor, and death. **$O_2$ p.** See under OXYGEN TOXICITY. **paraldehyde p.** 1 Poisoning from excessive chronic use of paraldehyde, resulting in symptoms similar to those of chronic alcoholism; paraldehydism. 2 Acute poisoning from an excessive dose of paraldehyde or from decomposed paraldehyde. Deaths have occurred from respiratory and circulatory failure after doses of 10 ml or more, and severe irritation of the mucous membranes and some deaths have followed oral or rectal administration of the decomposed product. Acute poisoning is rare because of the availability of other hypnotic agents with less objectionable odor and taste. **phenol p.** Poisoning which occurs by ingestion or absorption through the skin of phenol. It can cause a local irritative or corrosive reaction or more general symptoms of weakness and collapse. Following ingestion, there is intense burning of the mouth and throat and marked abdominal pain. Collapse may occur a few minutes after ingestion or skin absorption. Death is caused by respiratory failure. **phenytoin p.** A pathological condition brought on by overdosage with phenytoin. The principal effects are on the central nervous system and include ataxia, incoordination, tremors, nystagmus, diplopia, irritability, insomnia, and apathy. **phosphorus p.** Any of the toxic effects of exposure from inhalation or ingestion of phosphorus. These include anorexia, toothache, and phossy jaw. Other symptoms are anemia and fatty degeneration of the liver. **potato p.** Poisoning from the ingestion of potatoes containing excessive amounts of solanine. The principal signs are nausea, vomiting, and abdominal cramps. **puffer p.** TETRODOTOXISM. **salmon p.** A disease that affects primarily dogs and other canids but may also affect humans and other fish-eating mammals. Common along the northwest coast of North America, it is caused by ingestion of raw salmon infected with the encysted form of the fluke *Nanophyetus salmincola (Troglotrema salmincola),* which parasitizes the intestine and transmits the causal agent *Neorickettsia helminthoeca,* which produces a usually severe and commonly fatal hemorrhagic enteritis. Also *salmon disease.* **salmonellal food p.** Poisoning from food contaminated with any of various strains of *Salmonella.* Poultry and poultry products, meat and meat products, and dairy products are the foods most susceptible to contamination. The illness is characterized by nausea, vomiting, diarrhea, chills, fever, and abdominal pain. **saturnine p.** LEAD POISONING. **sausage p.** ALLANTIASIS. **scombroid p.** Poisoning from ingestion of spoiled or inadequately preserved fish of the suborder Scombroidea, which includes tuna, bonito, and mackerel. When spoilage occurs, the histidine present changes to histamine, producing an allergic type of reaction. Symptoms include abdominal pain, nausea, vomiting, intense itching, and difficulty in swallowing. **shellfish p.** Poisoning by any of the gonyaulax poisons. **silver p.** ARGYRIA. **spider p.** ARACHNIDISM. **staphylococcal food p.** Poisoning from ingestion of food containing *Staphylococcus aureus,* often found in creamed foods, pork, beef, and poultry products. Symptoms are headache, nausea, vomiting, gastrointestinal distress, and diarrhea. **tetraodon p.** TETRODOTOXISM. **thorn apple p.** Poisoning from ingestion of seeds or other parts of the thorn apple or jimson weed, *Datura stramonium,* which contains atropine and hyoscamine. The main signs of poisoning are dilated pupils, nervous excitement followed by incoordination, collapse, coma, and death. **tobacco p.** A morbid state produced by the inhalation of tobacco dust or from excessive use of tobacco or tobacco products in the form of cigarettes or snuff. The effects are progressive and include bronchitis, emphysema, and lung cancer. Also *tabagism, tobaccoism, tabacosis, tabacism.* **whelk p.** Poisoning from ingestion of, or stinging by, whelks, mollusks of the class Gastropoda. Toxic symptoms from ingestion include gastrointestinal distress, dizziness, and severe headache. Envenomation produces a sharp pain followed rapidly by cyanosis, tingling of the skin, numbness spreading over the body, paralysis, and coma. **zinc p.** Poisoning due to excessive intake of zinc. In humans, accidental oral poisoning has been reported as a result of consuming acidic food or beverages from galvanized containers. Symptoms are fever, vomiting, stomach cramps, and diarrhea. Industrial exposure to fumes results in metal-fume fever. Dermal toxicity may result from handling zinc salts, symptoms being a gray cyanosis, dermatoses, and ulceration of the nasal passages. Poisoning of other animals, as pigs, can result from their being fed foods such as milk and whey through zinc pipes, thus forming zinc lactate. Also *zincalism.*

**poisonous** 1 Having the characteristics of a poison. 2 Characterized by or containing poison.

**Poisson** [Simeon-Denis *Poisson,* French mathematician, 1781–1840] 1 Poisson-Pearson formula. See under FORMULA. 2 See under DISTRIBUTION.

**Poland** [Alfred *Poland,* English physician, 1820–1872] Poland syndrome. See under ANOMALY.

**polar** [L *pol(us)* the pole, north pole, end of an axis + *-aris* -AR ] 1 Of or relating to a pole or end of a structure. 2 Representing an extreme or the extremes in a range or continuum. 3 Of a molecule, having its electric charges separated, so that it is a dipole, and, by extension, any substance, especially a liquid, composed of such molecules. Such liquids tend to dissolve ionic or polar substances. 4 Denoting any directional effect, e.g., the effect of a mutation, which may affect the expression of genes transcribed after it.

**polarimeter** \pō′lərim′ətər\ An instrument that measures the plane of polarization of light passing through a material or the amount of polarized light transmitted.

**polarity** \pōlar′itē\ **1** The possession of either of two opposite qualities, as a positive or negative electric charge. **2** The characteristic occurrence of two poles, as the animal and vegetative poles of an ovum. **3** The ability of a terminative mutation within a gene to impair translation of distal genes of the same operon. **4** The directionality in the flow of current where the two poles of reference are the cathode and the anode. **operon p.** In some operons, a normally less frequent transcription of distal genes relative to proximal genes.

**polarization** \pō′lərīzā′shən\ **1** The establishment of a relative displacement of positive and negative charges in a body by application of an electric field. **2** A measure of such polarization, given by the dipole moment per unit volume. **3** The change in voltage of an electrochemical cell due to accumulation of gases at the surfaces of the electrodes. **4** A regularity in the direction of the electric vector, or a regular relationship between its direction and its instantaneous magnitude, in an electromagnetic wave; especially, a uniformity in the directions of the spins of a majority of a collection of atoms or subatomic particles. **5** Any process by which such changes or regularities occur. **circular p.** The polarization of light in such a way that its wave motion rotates in circles around the axis of the direction of the propagated light. **elliptical p.** The polarization of light such that its wave motion rotates in an ellipse around the axis of the direction of the propagated light. **plane p.** A polarization of light that results in a wave motion in one plane. **rotatory p.** The polarization of light resulting in a wave motion rotating in a circular or elliptical fashion around the axis of the direction of the propagated light rather than in a single plane.

**polarizer** \pō′lərī′zər\ An apparatus which brings about the polarization of light.

**polarogram** \pōlar′əgram\ The record of current flow related to applied voltage that is obtained during polarography.

**polarography** \pō′ləräg′rəfē\ A method for determining the concentration of reducible elements in a solution by measuring the electric current between electrodes immersed in the solution. An external voltage source varies the electrical potential between electrodes. Different substances react and allow current to flow at different potentials.

**poldine methylsulfate** $C_{22}H_{29}NO_7S$. 2-[[(Hydroxydiphenylacetyl)oxy]methyl]-1,1-dimethylpyreolidinium methylsulfate (salt). A synthetic quaternary anticholinergic drug used in the treatment of peptic ulcer and hypermotility of the gastrointestinal tract. It is given orally.

**pole** [L *polus.* See POLUS.] Either end of an axis of a body or of a rounded organ; the point on a curved surface farthest from the center; polus. **animal p.** The pole of the ovum where the two polar bodies are formed in succession and where segmentation begins. In medialecithal and also megalecithal ova, this pole is less rich in yolk material (vitellus). Also *apical pole, germinal pole.* **anterior p. of eyeball** POLUS ANTERIOR BULBI OCULI. **anterior p. of lens** POLUS ANTERIOR LENTIS. **apical p.** ANIMAL POLE. **caudal p. of testis** EXTREMITAS INFERIOR TESTIS. **cephalic p.** The end of the embryo which will become the head. **cranial p. of testis** EXTREMITAS SUPERIOR TESTIS. **frontal p. of cerebral hemisphere** POLUS FRONTALIS HEMISPHERII CEREBRI. **germinal p.** ANIMAL POLE. **inferior p. of kidney** EXTREMITAS INFERIOR RENIS. **inferior p. of testis** EXTREMITAS INFERIOR TESTIS. **negative p.** CATHODE. **nutritive p.** VEGETATIVE POLE. **occipital p. of cerebral hemisphere** POLUS OCCIPITALIS HEMISPHERII CEREBRI. **pelvic p.** The breech end of the fetus in its elliptic position. **placental p.** The site of the placenta in the uterus. **positive p.** ANODE. **posterior p. of eyeball** POLUS POSTERIOR BULBI OCULI. **posterior p. of lens** POLUS POSTERIOR LENTIS. **temporal p. of hemisphere of cerebrum** POLUS TEMPORALIS HEMISPHERII CEREBRI. **upper p. of kidney** EXTREMITAS SUPERIOR RENIS. **upper p. of testis** EXTREMITAS SUPERIOR TESTIS. **vegetative p.** The pole of the ovum opposite to the animal pole. In medialecithal or megalecithal ova it is the part where the yolk (vitellus) is most abundant. Also *vegetal pole, nutritive pole, vitelline pole.* **vitelline p.** VEGETATIVE POLE.

**poli** \pō′lī\ Plural of POLUS.

**policeman's tip** The typical posture of the hand in patients with the Duchenne-Erb syndrome. The hand and fingers are markedly flexed at the wrist and the forearm is inverted so that the palm faces backward and upward.

**policy[1]** [Middle French *police* (from Old Italian *polizza* certificate), certificate] A contract of insurance specifying the terms under which a party is insured. **catastrophe p.** See under CATASTROPHIC HEALTH INSURANCE. **master p.** The complete specification of a health insurance policy which covers a group of people.

**policy[2]** [L *politia* administration] A course of action or system of government. **open-door p.** The theory that minimal or no restriction of movement provides the ideal setting for treatment of mental disorders, and that rooms or wards should be locked only under special circumstances.

**poliencephalitis** \-ensef′əlī′tis\ POLIOENCEPHALITIS.

**poliencephalomyelitis** \-ensef′əlōmī′əlī′tis\ POLIOENCEPHALOMYELITIS.

**polio** \pō′lē·ō\ ACUTE ANTERIOR POLIOMYELITIS.

**polio-** \pō′lē·ō-\ [Gk *polios* gray] A combining form meaning (1) gray; (2) the gray matter of the brain and spinal cord.

**poliocidal** \-sī′dəl\ Capable of destroying polioviruses.

**polioclastic** \-klas′tik\ Having a selective affinity for and/or destroying the neurons in the gray matter of the central nervous system.

**poliodystrophia** \-distrō′fē·ə\ POLIODYSTROPHY. **p. cerebri progressiva infantalis** ALPERS SYNDROME.

**poliodystrophy** \-dis′strəfē\ [POLIO- + DYSTROPHY] Any degenerative disease of gray matter in the central nervous system. Also *poliodystrophia.* **p. cerebri** Any degenerative disease of cerebral gray matter. **Christensen-Krabbe progressive infantile cerebral p.** KRABBE'S DISEASE. **progressive cerebral p.** ALPERS SYNDROME.

**polioencephalitis** \-ensef′əlī′tis\ [POLIO- + ENCEPHALITIS] **1** Any inflammatory process involving predominantly the gray matter of the brain and brainstem. **2** Poliomyelitis predominantly involving the motor cranial nerve nuclei. For defs. 1 and 2 also *poliencephalitis.* **p. acuta hemorrhagica** WERNICKE'S DISEASE. **acute bulbar p.** BULBAR POLIOMYELITIS. **p. hemorrhagica superiore** *Incorrect* WERNICKE'S DISEASE. **p. infectiva** ENCEPHALITIS LETHARGICA. **inferior p.** BULBAR POLIOMYELITIS. **p. of Marie-Strümpell** ACUTE INFANTILE HEMIPLEGIA. **superior hemorrhagic p.** WERNICKE'S DISEASE. **Wernicke's acute hemorrhagic upper p.** WERNICKE'S DISEASE.

**polioencephalomeningomyelitis** \-ensef′əlōməning′-gōmī′əlī′tis\ [POLIO- + ENCEPHALO- + MENINGO- + MY-

ELITIS] Inflammation of the gray matter of the brain and spinal cord, associated with inflammation of the meninges. *Seldom used.*

**polioencephalomyelitis** \-ensefʹəlōmīʹəlīʹtis\ [POLIO- + ENCEPHALOMYELITIS] Inflammation of the gray matter of the brain and spinal cord. *Seldom used.* Also *poliencephalomyelitis, poliomyelencephalitis, poliomyeloencephalitis.*

**polioencephalomyelopathy** \-ensefʹəlōmīʹəläpʹəthē\ [POLIO- + ENCEPHALO- + MYELOPATHY] Any pathologic process or disorder of function which predominantly involves the neurons rather than the glia or white matter of the brain and spinal cord. **carcinomatous p.** Progressive encephalomyelopathy, predominantly involving gray matter and occurring in subjects with malignant disease which is not invading the central nervous system.

**polioencephalopathy** \-ensefʹəläpʹəthē\ [POLIO- + ENCEPHALOPATHY] Any disease affecting predominantly the gray matter of the brain. **Alpers p.** ALPERS SYNDROME.

**polioencephalotropic** \-ensefʹəlōträpʹik\ Showing a special affinity for the neurons and gray matter of the central nervous system.

**poliomyelencephalitis** \-mīʹəlensefʹəlīʹtis\ POLIOENCEPHALOMYELITIS.

**poliomyelitic** \-mīʹəlitʹik\ Of or relating to poliomyelitis.

**poliomyeliticidal** \-mīʹəlīʹtisīʹdəl\ Capable of destroying the polioviruses which cause poliomyelitis.

**poliomyelitis** \-mīʹəlīʹtis\ [POLIO- + MYELITIS] ACUTE ANTERIOR POLIOMYELITIS. • Formerly, this term was sometimes used to denote any process of inflammation of the gray matter of the spinal cord. It has also been used incorrectly to identify degenerative disorders of the anterior horn cells. Thus motor neuron disease was once called by some authorities, especially in French, *chronic anterior poliomyelitis.* Adj. poliomyelitic. **abortive p.** Acute anterior poliomyelitis in which the symptoms and signs are those of a nonspecific febrile illness without meningitis or paralytic manifestations. **acute anterior p.** An infectious disease, once occurring in epidemics, particularly in summer and autumn, due to one of three poliovirus types which attack predominantly the anterior horn cells of the spinal cord and the motor nuclei of the brainstem. It occurs in abortive, meningitic, and paralytic forms. The abortive form usually presents as a nonspecific febrile illness, the meningitic with headache, fever, and neck stiffness and with a pleocytosis (at first polymorphonuclear, later lymphocytic) in the spinal fluid. Such cases may be impossible to distinguish clinically from other lymphocytic meningitides, except by isolation of the causal virus. In the paralytic form there may be diffuse or localized muscle pain followed by asymmetrical flaccid paralysis of individual muscles or muscle groups. In severe cases there may be widespread paralysis involving respiratory and bulbar muscles. Some residual paralysis usually persists after the acute phase and may lead to contractures, deformity, and skeletal atrophy. The virus is usually transmitted by enteric spread. Once a disease predominantly of early childhood, it became more prevalent in adults as hygiene improved. Following active programs of immunization with live attenuated virus, it is now much less common. Rarely, cases are caused by coxsackieviruses. Also *Heine-Medin disease, infantile paralysis, acute spinal paralysis, infantile flaccid and atrophic spinal paralysis, Little's paralysis* (seldom used), *Medin's disease, epidemic myeloencephalitis, epidemic infantile palsy, acute infectious paralysis, acute wasting paralysis, anterior spinal paralysis, atrophic spinal paralysis, epidemic infantile paralysis, infantile spinal paralysis, poliomyelitis, polio, anterior poliomyelitis, spodiomyelitis.* **ascending p.** Acute anterior poliomyelitis in which paralysis extends progressively upwards to involve respiratory and bulbar muscles. **bulbar p.** Acute anterior poliomyelitis affecting the bulbar nuclei, usually giving rise to dysphagia and respiratory paralysis with variable involvement of other cranial nerves. Also *acute bulbar polioencephalitis, inferior polioencephalitis, cerebral poliomyelitis, encephalitic poliomyelitis.* **bulbospinal p.** Acute anterior poliomyelitis involving the brainstem and the spinal cord. Also *spinobulbar poliomyelitis.* **cerebral p.** BULBAR POLIOMYELITIS. **chronic anterior p.** See under POLIOMYELITIS. **encephalitic p.** BULBAR POLIOMYELITIS. **endemic p.** Poliomyelitis occurring repeatedly in small clusters or outbreaks within a geographic region. It once recurred each year in the spring or summer in many countries. **nonparalytic p.** Acute anterior poliomyelitis with clinical manifestations of fever, and perhaps headache and symptoms of meningitis, but without muscular paralysis. **paralytic p.** Poliomyelitis in which muscular paralysis occurs. Also *acute atrophic paralysis.* **postinoculation p.** Poliomyelitis following an injection for prophylactic inoculation against some other disease. There is evidence that in an individual incubating poliomyelitis the trauma of injection may precipitate paralysis of the limb in which the injection was given. Also, poliomyelitis caused by the vaccine strain of virus may occur as a rare complication of inoculation with live polio vaccine. Also *postvaccinal poliomyelitis.* **post-tonsillectomy p.** Poliomyelitis, usually of the bulbar type, following tonsillectomy. **postvaccinal p.** POSTINOCULATION POLIOMYELITIS. **spinal paralytic p.** The classical form of acute anterior poliomyelitis, with an onset marked by asymmetrical flaccid paralysis of one or of several extremities. **spinobulbar p.** BULBOSPINAL POLIOMYELITIS.

**poliomyeloencephalitis** \-mīʹəlō·ensefʹəlīʹtis\ POLIOENCEPHALOMYELITIS.

**poliosis** \pōʹlē·ōʹsis\ [Gk *poliōsis* (from *polios* gray) the process of becoming gray] Premature loss of pigment in hair. **p. circumscripta** An absence or deficiency of pigment in a group of contiguous hair follicles which gives rise to a strand or mesh of white hair.

**poliovirus** \-vīʹrəs\ Any of three viruses of the *Enterovirus* genus in the Picornaviridae family that can cause a spectrum of manifestations in humans ranging from subclinical infection to aseptic meningitis and poliomyelitis. They are separated immunologically into types 1, 2, and 3. Also *poliomyelitis virus.* • The term is sometimes used more loosely, including certain enteroviruses that have similar effects in other mammals. **p. muris** MURINE ENCEPHALOMYELITIS VIRUS.

**Politzer** [Adam *Politzer,* Austrian otologist, 1835–1920] See under BAG, TREATMENT.

**politzerization** \pälʹitsərīzāʹshən\ [after Adam *Politzer,* Austrian otologist, 1835–1920] A procedure resulting in inflation of the middle ear. The patient takes a little water into the mouth. A strong rubber bag is applied to one nostril through a rubber connection and the nose pinched close around it. As the patient swallows the water, a sharp squeeze to the bag forcibly raises the pressure in the nasopharynx and thus in the middle ears via the eustachian tubes. **negative p.** Politzerization using negative instead of positive pressure at the moment when the patient swallows. It is generally regarded as a dangerous procedure. Also *reverse politzerization.*

**pollakidipsia** \pälʹəkēdipʹsē·ə\ [Gk *pollaki(s)* many times + *dips(a)* thirst + -IA] An abnormal condition in which thirst occurs with excessive frequency.

**pollakiuria** \päl′əkēyoo′rē·ə\ [Gk *pollaki(s)* many times + -URIA] Abnormally frequent urination. Also *pollakisuria, sychnuria.*

**pollenosis** \päl′ənō′sis\ POLLEN ALLERGY.

**pollex** \päl′eks\ [L, the thumb, great toe] [NA] The thumb; the first digit of the hand. Also *first finger, digitus I, digitus primus.* **p. extensus** The hyperextension of the thumb. **p. flexus** Flexion deformity of the thumb. **p. pedis** HALLUX. **p. valgus** A deviation of the thumb away from the palm. **p. varus** The deviation of the thumb towards the palm.

**pollicization** \päl′isīzā′shən\ The reconstruction of a thumb by using another digit from either the hand or foot.

**pollinic** \pälin′ik\ Pertaining to pollen.

**pollinosis** \päl′inō′sis\ POLLEN ALLERGY.

**pollodic** \pälō′dik\ PANTHODIC.

**pollution** [Late L *pollutio* (from *polluere* to defile, soil, taint, from *pol-*, variant of *per-*, intensive prefix, + root *lu* as in *lutum* mud, dirt) uncleanness, defilement] **1** The act or process of making impure or unwholesome, as by mixing with a harmful substance. **2** An unwholesome condition resulting from such a process. **noise p.** Any disturbance of the environment by sound of an intensity or pitch capable of producing a harmful or stressful effect on humans subject to it, as damage to the organ of hearing or to mental or emotional stability.

**polonium** \pōlō′nē·əm\ Element number 84, having mass numbers ranging from 192 to 218. Polonium is a very rare metallic element occurring in minute traces in uranium ores. It is produced in milligram amounts in nuclear reactors by the neutron bombardment of various nuclides. For example, bombardment of bismuth 209 gives rise to bismuth 210, the parent of polonium 210, which has a half-life of 138.39 days. There are 27 known isotopes. All of them are exceedingly intense emitters of alpha particles and gamma rays, and their decay generates a great deal of heat. Polonium has a few specialized technologic applications, though it is exceedingly dangerous to handle. Also *radium F.* Symbol: Po

**polster** \pōl′stər\ A small bulge or a rounded protrusion. *Outmoded.*

**polus** \pō′ləs\ [L, from Gk *polos* (from a root meaning to turn, revolve) a pivot, pole] (*pl.* poli) Either end of an axis of a body or of a rounded organ; pole. **p. anterior bulbi oculi** [NA] The central point of the anterior curvature of the eyeball forming the anterior point of the optic axis. Also *anterior pole of eyeball.* **p. anterior lentis** [NA] The central point of the anterior convex surface of the lens of the eye forming the anterior point of the axis of the lens. Also *anterior pole of lens, stella lentis iridica* (outmoded), *stella lentis hyaloidea* (outmoded). **p. frontalis hemispherii cerebri** [NA] The frontal pole of the cerebral hemisphere; the most rostral extension of each frontal lobe. Also *frontal pole of cerebral hemisphere.* **poli lienalis inferior et superior** Extremitas anterior splenis and extremitas posterior splenis. *Outmoded.* **p. occipitalis hemispherii cerebri** [NA] The caudal projection of the occipital lobe. Also *occipital pole of cerebral hemisphere.* **p. posterior bulbi oculi** [NA] The central point of the posterior curvature of the eyeball forming the posterior point of the optic axis. Also *posterior pole of eyeball.* **p. posterior lentis** [NA] The central point of the posterior convexity of the lens of the eye forming the posterior point of the axis of the lens. Also *posterior pole of lens.* **poli renales inferior et superior** Extremitas inferior renis and extremitas superior renis. *Outmoded.* **p. temporalis hemispherii cerebri** [NA] The anterior projection of the human temporal lobe. Also *temporal pole of hemisphere of cerebrum.*

**poly** \päl′ē\ SEGMENTED NEUTROPHIL.

**poly-** \päl′i-, päl′ē-\ [Gk *polys* many, much] **1** A combining form meaning (1) much, many; (2) too much or too many, excessive. **2** Denoting a polymer.

**poly(A)** A polynucleotide of adenylate residues joined as in RNA. Messenger RNA in eukaryotes normally contains a sequence of poly(A) at its 3′-terminus.

**Polya** [Jeno *Polya*, Hungarian surgeon, 1876–1944] See under OPERATION.

**polyacrylamide gel** A gel formed by polymerization of acrylamide, $CH_2{=}CH{-}CO{-}NH_2$, and some cross-linking agent. It is much used as a medium for electrophoresis of proteins, since the gel allows electrophoretic movement but prevents disturbances due to convection.

**polyadenitis** \-ad′ənī′tis\ [POLY- + ADENITIS] Inflammation of several glands. **malignant p.** BUBONIC PLAGUE.

**polyadenomatosis** \-ad′ənō′mətō′sis\ [POLY- + *adenomat(a)*, pl. of ADENOMA + -OSIS] The presence of multiple adenomas.

**polyadenopathy** \-ad′ənäp′əthē\ Enlargement of several lymph nodes, usually in more that one region.

**polyadenylation** \-ad′ənilā′shən\ The attachment of polyadenylate, which is not synthesized through transcription, to the 3′ end of precursor mRNA in eukaryotes.

**polyagglutinability** \-əgloo′tinəbil′itē\ A condition of red cells in which there is agglutination following exposure to normal serum from adult humans with no immunizing exposure to red cell antigens. It reflects the alteration of surface molecules, either *in vivo* or *in vitro*, such that groups are exposed to and react with universally present immunoglobulins. Different forms result from various genetic or pathologic events, and they can be distinguished by differential agglutination patterns with plant lectins.

**polyamide** Polymerized acrylamide ($CH_2{=}CH{-}CO{-}NH_2$), often used as a stationary phase for thin-layer chromatography.

**polyamine** An amine containing several amino groups, especially spermine and spermidine, the amines often associated with nucleic acids.

**polyangiitis** \-an′jē·ī′tis\ [POLY- + ANGIITIS] Widespread inflammation of blood vessels.

**polyarteritis** \-är′tərī′tis\ A necrotizing arteritis involving many blood vessels, occurring as a systemic illness or as a complication of rheumatic disease such as rheumatoid arthritis, lupus erythematosus, or Wegener's granulomatosis. Clinical manifestations include skin and visceral infarcts, neuropathy, and hypertensive renal disease. Also *panarteritis, necrotizing vasculitis.* **p. nodosa** A generalized arteritis characterized by necrosis of medium-sized and small arteries and involving many organs including the heart, gastrointestinal tract, muscles, and kidneys. It is one of the connective tissue disorders. Also *periarteritis nodosa, arteritis nodosa, disseminated necrotizing periarteritis, Kussmaul's disease, Kussmaul-Maier disease, necrotizing arteritis.* • The term is used when there is no other associated rheumatic disease.

**polyarthric** \-är′thrik\ Of or involving multiple joints.

**polyarthritis** \-ärthrī′tis\ Arthritis of multiple joints. Compare MONARTHRITIS, OLIGOARTHRITIS. **benign p.** Multiple joint inflammation that resolves completely without residual joint damage. **chronic p.** Multiple joint inflammation that gives rise to permanent joint changes, as is commonly seen in rheumatoid arthritis. **chronic osteolytic p.** End-stage rheumatoid arthritis marked by bone erosion of the affected joints. **chronic villous p.** A chronic inflammation of the synovial membranes of several joints. **p. destruens** Erosive arthritis of any cause, such as rheumatoid or psoriatic arthritis. **infectious p.** An inflammation of several joints resulting from the presence of pathogenic organisms. **p. rheumatica acuta** RHEUMATIC FEVER. **rheumatoid p.** Symmetric multiple joint inflammation that is characterized by histologic changes in the synovium. **tuberculous p.** HYPERTROPHIC PULMONARY OSTEOARTHROPATHY. **vertebral p.** An inflammation of the disk spaces at several levels with no involvement of the vertebral bodies. **xanthomatous p.** An inflammation of multiple joints as a result of the presence of yellow nodules in the synovium that contain lipid-laden histiocytes.

**polyarthropathy** \-ärthräp′əthē\ Any disease process that affects many joints.

**polyarthrosis** \-ärthrō′sis\ An abnormality affecting many joints. **progressive p.** A disease process that affects many joints and results in joint destruction.

**polyarticular** \-ärtik′yələr\ MULTIARTICULAR.

**polyauxotroph** \-ôk′səträf\ A microorganism, often a mutant, with multiple requirements for specific growth factors.

**polyavitaminosis** \-āvī′təminō′sis\ [POLY- + AVITAMINOSIS] A condition resulting from a dietary deficiency of more than one vitamin.

**polyaxon** \-ak′sän\ A nerve cell that gives rise to several axons derived from the soma or from primary dendrites.

**polyaxonic** \-aksän′ik\ Possessing several axons.

**polyblast** \päl′iblast\ Any of a group of free phagocytic cells, or macrophages, associated with an inflammation of connective tissue.

**polycentric** \-sen′trik\ Having many centers.

**polycheiria** \-kī′rē·ə\ [POLY- + CHEIR- + -IA] The presence of supernumerary hands. Also *polychiria.*

**polychemotherapy** \-kē′mōther′əpē\ [POLY- + CHEMOTHERAPY] The use of several chemotherapeutic agents in a treatment schedule.

**polychiria** \-kī′rē·ə\ POLYCHEIRIA.

**polychlorinated biphenyl** Any of a series of stable compounds in which the hydrogen atoms in biphenyls are replaced by chlorine. They are serious toxic pollutants of the environment because they are stable, accumulate in animal tissues, and pass upward in food chains. In many countries their industrial use is prohibited or limited to enclosed systems. Abbr. PCB

**polychondritis** \-kändrī′tis\ [POLY- + CHONDRITIS] Inflammation of cartilage in multiple areas. **chronic atrophic p.** Degeneration of cartilage in multiple areas, such as might be found in advanced osteoarthritis or certain metabolic diseases of cartilage. Also *polychondritis chronica atrophicans.* **relapsing p.** An illness characterized by inflammatory destruction of multiple cartilage areas, especially the bridge of the nose, the pinnae, the trachea, and the aorta. The disease is of unknown cause and occurs episodically over many years. Also *Meyenburg-Altherr-Uehlinger syndrome, Meyenburg's disease.*

**polychondropathy** \-kändräp′əthē\ Abnormality of cartilage in multiple areas. Also *polychondropathia.*

**polychrest** \päl′ikrest\ [Gk *polychrēst(os)* (from *poly(s)* much, many + *chrēst(os)* useful) useful to many or for many purposes] **1** Effective in the treatments of many diseases. **2** A polychrest remedy.

**polychromasia** \-krōmā′zhə\ An increase in the proportion of erythrocytes in a blood film that exhibit a blue or blue-gray color when stained with Romanowsky-type stains. Polychromasia reflects the presence of ribonucleic acid in erythrocytes, and is an index of a young population of cells. Also *polychromatocytosis, polychromatia, polychromatosis, polychromia, polychromocytosis, polychromatophilia, polychromophilia.*

**polychromatic** \-krōmat′ik\ Having a variety of colors; multicolored. Also *polychromic.*

**polychromatocyte** \-krō′mətōsīt′\ POLYCHROMATIC CELL.

**polychromatocytosis** \-krō′mətōsītō′sis\ POLYCHROMASIA.

**polychromatophil** \-krō′mətōfil′\ **1** Having an affinity for both acidic and basic dyes. Also *polychromatophilic, polychromophil.* **2** POLYCHROMATIC CELL.

**polychromatophilia** \-krō′mətōfil′yə\ POLYCHROMASIA.

**polychromatophilic** \-krō′mətōfil′ik\ POLYCHROMATOPHIL.

**polychromatosis** \-krō′mətō′sis\ POLYCHROMASIA.

**polychromia** \-krō′mē·ə\ POLYCHROMASIA.

**polychromic** \-krō′mik\ POLYCHROMATIC.

**polychromocytosis** \-krō′məsītō′sis\ POLYCHROMASIA.

**polychromophil** \-krō′məfil\ **1** POLYCHROMATOPHIL. **2** POLYCHROMATIC CELL.

**polychromophilia** \-krō′məfil′yə\ POLYCHROMASIA.

**polycistronic** \-sisträn′ik\ POLYGENIC.

**polyclinic** \-klin′ik\ [POLY- + CLINIC] **1** A clinic offering health care in many specialties. **2** A hospital in which clinical instruction in many specialties is given.

**polyclonal** \-klō′nəl\ Related to several groups or populations of cells, usually in tissue culture, each group derived from a common ancestor by mitosis. Also *multiclonal.* Compare MONOCLONAL.

**polycoria** \-kôr′ē·ə\ [POLY- + *cor(e)-* + -IA] Multiple pupillary openings in the same iris. In true polycoria, which is a developmental condition, each pupil has its own pigment frill. Also *double pupil, multiple pupil.* **p. spuria** The presence of several holes in the iris, not all of which are encircled by a sphincter muscle. **p. vera** The presence of multiple pupils, each with its own sphincter, in the same eye.

**polycystic** \-sis′tik\ Containing or composed of multiple cysts.

**polycyte** \päl′isīt\ A segmented neutrophil with six or more nuclear lobes; a hypersegmented neutrophil.

**polycythemia** \-sīthē′mē·ə\ [POLY- + *-cyt(e)* + -HEMIA] A greater than normal number of erythrocyes, and often also of leukocytes and platelets, in blood. Also *erythroleukothrombocythemia, hematocytosis, polyglobulism, polyglobulia* (obs.). **absolute p.** A true polycythemia that is due to greater than normal number of erythrocytes in the blood and greater than normal total erythrocyte mass in blood, in contrast to spurious or "relative" polycythemia, in which the erythrocyte count and hemoglobin concentration of blood are elevated due to decrease in plasma volume. **benign p.** Polycythemia due to any cause except polycythemia vera. **chronic splenomegalic p.** POLYCYTHEMIA VERA. **compensatory p.** An increase in the number of erythrocytes in the blood as compensation for a lower than normal oxygen content of arterial and capillary blood, as in congenital heart disease, chronic pulmonary disease, residence at high altitude, and some abnormal hemoglobins. Also *erythropoietin polycythemia, anoxemic erythrocytosis.* **familial p.** The clustering of erythrocytosis in a family, often due to an inherited hemoglobinopathy. **p. hypertonica** STRESS ERYTHROCYTOSIS. **myelopathic p.** POLYCYTHEMIA VERA. **primary p.** POLYCYTHEMIA VERA. **relative p.** Apparent erythrocytosis due to decrease in plasma volume, as in stress erythrocytosis. Also *spurious polycythemia.* **p. rubra** POLYCYTHEMIA VERA. **p. rubra vera** POLYCYTHEMIA VERA. **secondary p.** Erythrocytosis resulting from nonhematopoietic disease, including appropriate response to tissue hypoxia, inappropriate erythropoietin production (as in renal disease and some neoplasia), and adenocorticosteroid or androgen excess. **splenomegalic p.** POLYCYTHEMIA VERA. **spurious p.** RELATIVE POLYCYTHEMIA. **stress p.** STRESS ERYTHROCYTOSIS. **p. vera** A chronic myeloproliferative disorder of unknown cause, manifested by an increased red cell mass despite normal oxygen saturation and often by splenomegaly, leukocytosis, thrombocytosis, and elevated leukocyte alkaline phosphatase activity. Myelofibrosis and extramedullary hematopoiesis are characteristic of longstanding disease. Also *splenomegalic polycythemia, chronic splenomegalic polycythemia, myelopathic polycythemia, primary polycythemia, polycythemia rubra, polycythemia rubra vera, Osler's disease, Vaquez disease, Vaquez-Osler disease, Osler-Vaquez disease, erythremia, chronic erythremia, hyperglobulia, hyperglobulism, polyemia polycythaemica.*

**polydactyly** \-dak′tilē\ [POLY- + DACTYL- + -Y] The presence of more than the normal number of digits or parts thereof on a hand or foot. Also *hyperdactyly, dicheiria, diplocheiria.*

**polydeficient** \-difish′ənt\ Deficient of more than one nutrient, as a marasmic child. Also *plurideficient.*

**polydentia** \-den′shə\ POLYDONTIA.

**polydipsia** \-dip′sē·ə\ [POLY- + -DIPSIA] The drinking of water in abnormally large volume. It may be psychogenic, or secondary to dehydration due to any cause, or an attempt to keep up with a sustained polyuria, as in diabetes insipidus or diabetes mellitus.

**polydontia** \-dän′shə\ [POLY- + *-(o)dontia*] The condition of having more than the normal number of teeth in the mouth. Also *polydentia, hyperdontia.*

**polydysplasia** \-displā′zhə\ [POLY- + DYSPLASIA] The abnormal development of several types of tissue within the same organ or organism.

**polydysspondylism** \-dispän′dilizm\ The malformation of several vertebrae and the sella turcica. It is associated with mental retardation and dwarfism.

**polydystrophy** \-dis′trəfē\ The presence of multiple developmental disorders in connective tissues. **pseudo-Hurler p.** MUCOLIPIDOSIS III.

**polyelectrolyte** \-ilek′trəlīt\ A substance whose molecule contains many charged groups.

**polyembryoma** \-em′brē·ō′mə\ [POLY- + EMBRYOMA] A very rare germ cell tumor of the testis or ovary composed predominantly of embryoid bodies.

**polyembryony** \-embrī′ənē, -em′brē·ənē\ [POLY- + EMBRYONY] The development of many embryos from a single fertilized egg. It is exhibited by some worms and insects and by the armadillo. Some maintain that monozygotic twins in man are a special case of polyembryony in that the division into two separate embryos is produced as the result of the first cleavage of the fertilized ovum into two separate individuals.

**polyemia** \-ē′mē·ə\ [POLY- + -EMIA] An abnormal increase in circulating blood volume. **p. hyperalbuminosa** HYPERALBUMINEMIA. **p. polycythaemica** POLYCYTHEMIA VERA.

**polyendocrine** \-en′dəkrin\ Of, pertaining to, or involving several endocrine glands.

**polyendocrinoma** \-en′dəkrinō′mə\ MULTIPLE ENDOCRINE NEOPLASIA.

**polyene** \pälē′ēn\ A substance containing several carbon-carbon double bonds in its molecular structure.

**polyene acids** Acids containing several double bonds, especially the group of fatty acids essential in the diet.

**polyesthetic** \-esthet′ik\ Pertaining to several of the senses.

**polyethylene glycol** The polymer $H—[O—CH_2—CH_2—]_nOH$. It has many uses in biology, from inducing cell fusion to being a stationary phase for gas-liquid chromatography. A number appended to the name signifies the mean relative molecular mass of the sample, and hence the degree of polymerization.

**polygalactia** \-gəlak′shə\ [POLY- + GALACT- + -IA] Excessive secretion of breast milk.

**polygalin** SENEGENIN.

**polyganglionic** \-gang′glē·än′ik\ Affecting or pertaining to several ganglia.

**polygene** \päl′ijēn\ Any of a particular group of genes that determines a phenotype in which the effects of individual genes is not discernible. Also *cumulative gene.*

**polygenic** \-jē′nik\ **1** Determined by the effect of many genes whose individual effects are not discernible: said of a phenotype. **2** Of or relating to a messenger RNA, in bacteria, that contains transcripts of the multiple structural genes present in the corresponding operon. Also *polycistronic.*

**polyglandular** \-glan′dyələr\ PLURIGLANDULAR.

**polyglobulia** \-gläbyoo′lē·ə\ [POLY- + *globul(e)* + -IA] *Obs.* POLYCYTHEMIA.

**polyglobulism** \-gläb′yəlizm\ POLYCYTHEMIA.

**polygraph** \päl′igraf\ [POLY- + -GRAPH] **1** An instrument that simultaneously records several different physiologic variables such as the blood pressure, radial pulse, and electrocardiogram. **2** An electronic instrument used to detect deception on the part of a subject by measuring physiologic responses that occur in the subject and vary with the degree of emotional arousal elicited by verbal questions. The instrument simultaneously measures and records mechanical and electrical impulses generated by changes in the subject's respiration, pulse, blood pressure, and galvanic skin reflex. Polygraph examinations are generally regarded as a reliable basis for the diagnosis of truth or deception, but they have never been accepted as evidence in courts of law in the United States. Also *lie detector* (popular), *Keeler's lie polygraph.* **Keeler's lie p.** POLYGRAPH.

**polygyria** \-jī′rē·ə\ A condition in which the gyri on the surface of the cerebral hemispheres are abnormally numerous. The individual gyri are usually small. Also *micropolygyria.*

**polyheteroxenous** \-het′əräk′sənəs\ [POLY- + HETEROXENOUS] Having many intermediate hosts.

**polyhidrosis** \-hidrō′sis\ HYPERHIDROSIS.

**polyhydramnios** \-hīdram′nē·əs\ HYDRAMNIOS.

**polyhydric** \-hī′drik\ Containing many hydroxyl groups: used of alcohols.

**polyhydruria** \-hīdroo′rē·ə\ [POLY- + HYDR- + -URIA] The condition of having excessively diluted urine.

**poly-IC** One of the synthetic RNA polymers which induce local production of interferon. It has been used experimentally, with some benefit, as a topical treatment for acute herpes infections of the cornea.

**polyinfection** Infection by several kinds of organism; mixed infection.

**polykaryocyte** \-kar′ē·əsīt\ A large, multinuclear cell.

**polyketide** \-kē′tīd\ Any of various antibiotics, such as the macrolides, whose main component is a long chain or ring of acetyl residues in which the carbonyl is not fully reduced as it is in fatty acid biosynthesis.

**polylecithal** \-les′ithəl\ MEGALECITHAL.

**polyleptic** \-lep′tik\ [POLY- + LEPT- + -IC] Characterized by numerous phases of exacerbation and remission.

**polylobular** \-läb′yələr\ MULTILOBULAR.

**polylysine** Any polymer of various numbers of lysine residues, joined by amide linkage between C-1 and N-2. It is produced by systems that synthesize protein when they are supplied with polyuridylic acid as an artificial mRNA, and it adopts a helical conformation in solution when the pH is raised to remove charges from its side chains.

**polymastia** \-mas′tē·ə\ [POLY- + MAST- + -IA] The presence of more than two mammae in a human or other primate which typically has only two. Also *polymazia, multimammae, supernumerary breasts.*

**polymastigote** \-mas′tigōt\ [alteration of *polymastigate,* from POLY- + Gk *mastix,* gen. *mastigos,* a whip + L *-atus* -ATE] A flagellate with more than two flagella, usually located at the anterior end of the organism.

**polymazia** \-mā′zhə\ POLYMASTIA.

**polymelia** \-mē′lyə\ [POLY- + MEL-[1] + -IA] The presence of accessory limbs or parts of limbs attached directly or indirectly to the same trunk.

**polymenia** \-mē′nē·ə\ POLYMENORRHEA.

**polymenorrhea** \-men′ôrē′ə\ [POLY- + MENORRHEA] Unusually frequent occurrence of menses. Also *polymenia.*

**polymer** \päl′imir′\ [POLY- + Gk *mer(os)* a part, portion, lot] A substance whose molecules are formed by the combination of several molecules of a simpler substance, often forming long chains.

**polymerase** \-mer′ās, pälim′ərās\ Any enzyme which catalyzes polymerization, as nucleotides to polynucleotides.

**polymeria** \-mir′ē·ə\ [POLY- + *mer(o)-*[1] + -IA] The presence of supernumerary parts, organs, or appendages.

**polymeric** \-mir′ik\ Occurring as a polymer.

**polymerization** \-mir′īzā′shən\ The formation of a polymer from a monomer or monomers.

**polymerize** \päl′əmərīz′\ To react or cause to react with similar molecules to form a polymer.

**polymetacarpia** \-met′əkär′pē·ə\ [POLY- + *metacarp(al bones)* + -IA] The presence of supernumerary metacarpal bones.

**polymetatarsia** \-met′ətär′sē·ə\ [POLY- *metatars(al bones)* + -IA] The presence of supernumerary metatarsal bones.

**polymicrolipomatosis** \-mī′krəlip′ōmətō′sis\ Multiple small lipomas in the subcutaneous tissue.

**polymorph** \päl′imôrf\ [short form of POLYMORPHONUCLEAR] SEGMENTED NEUTROPHIL.

**polymorphic** \-môr′fik\ Characterized by polymorphism. Also *polymorphous.*

**polymorphism** \-môr′fizm\ [POLY- + MORPH- + -ISM] **1** The characteristic of occurring in a variety of forms, often in shape or size, either as adults within a species or during development of individuals. Also *pleomorphism.* **2** The presence of any one of two or more genetically distinct phenotypes within a species, the least common of which occurs with a frequency that cannot be maintained by recurrent mutation alone (the frequency commonly and arbitrarily stated as being 0.01 or more). The term may be used in reference to nucleotide sequences, alleles, proteins, or chromosomes. **balanced p.** A condition in which an allele is present in a frequency that is both relatively high (0.01 or greater) and stable over many generations. In most instances, both features are due to selective superiority of the heterozygote over those homozygous for either allele. **chromosome p.** A condition in which is found any of two or more structural variations in a given chromosome within a species, the least common of which is not maintained by recurrent mutation. By convention, it is not associated with clinical syndromes. It is detectable cytologically as the presence or absence of satellites, variation in size of satellites, centromeric heterochromatin, bands, or in rearrangements of bands. **genetic p.** The simultaneous existence in a given breeding population of two or more alleles at a specific genetic locus at frequencies that cannot be maintained solely by mutation. The rarest occurs at a frequency greater than 0.01. **transient p.** The presence of multiple alleles, each with a frequency that cannot be maintained by mutation alone while in transition to a new equilibrium.

**polymorphocellular** \-môr′fəsel′yələr\ Pertaining to or comprised of cells of different types.

**polymorphocyte** \-môr′fəsīt\ POLYMORPHONUCLEAR LEUKOCYTE.

**polymorphonuclear** \-môr′fən^y^oo′klē·ər\ [POLY- + MORPHO- + NUCLEAR] Having a lobulated or segmented nucleus: used of segmented neutrophils as well as mature eosinophils and basophils. Also *polynuclear.* **filament p.** Having a nucleus that is segmented into distinct lobes, with the lobes being connected by fine strands or filaments of chromatin. *Seldom used.* **nonfilament p.** Having a nucleus that is lobulated, with the lobules not separated by narrow filaments of chromatin, as in a band neutrophil. *Seldom used.*

**polymorphous** \-môr′fəs\ POLYMORPHIC.

**polymyalgia** \-mī·al′jə\ [POLY- + MYALGIA] Pain in multiple muscles. **p. arteritica** POLYMYALGIA RHEUMATICA. **p. rheumatica** An acute illness of older persons, characterized by an abrupt onset of polymyalgia, sometimes with fever, anemia, and weight loss, and universally characterized by a high erythrocyte sedimentation rate. Also *rheumatic gout* (imprecise), *polymyalgia arteritica.*

**polymyoclonus** \-mī′əklō′nəs\ Repetitive myoclonic jerks, as sometimes seen in myoclonic epilepsy or hereditary myoclonus, or as a manifestation of various forms of subacute encephalitis. Also *polymyoclonia.*

**polymyopathy** \-mī·äp′əthē\ Any myopathy involving many muscles.

**polymyositis** \-mī·əsī′tis\ [POLY- + MYOSITIS] An inflammatory autoimmune disorder of muscle, related to other disorders of the collagen or connective tissue group. It can occur at any age, and may be acute, subacute, or chronic. Muscle pain and tenderness occur in some cases but others present with signs of a subacute progressive myopathy, usually involving predominantly proximal limb muscles. The serum creatine kinase activity is usually raised, the electromyogram is myopathic, and a muscle biopsy demonstrates muscle fiber necrosis, regeneration, and interstitial and/or perivascular inflammatory cell infiltration. The syndrome is often but not always associated with skin changes (dermatomyositis), and is sometimes seen with acute viral, bacterial, or parasitic infections. It may develop in middle-aged or elderly adults in association with occult malignant disease. The condition usually responds to treatment with corticosteroid drugs. Also *multiple myositis.* **acute p. with myoglobinuria** Polymyositis which is so acute and severe that it causes extensive muscle fiber destruction and hence myoglobinuria. **hemorrhagic p.** An inflammation of skeletal muscles characterized by hemorrhages into the substance of the muscle together with edema and dermatitis. **trichinous p.** TRICHINOSIS.

**polymyxin** Any of a group of five polypeptide antibiotics derived from strains of the water and soil bacterium *Bacillus polymyxa,* each one possessing specific activity against certain types of Gram-negative bacteria. **p. B** One of the polypeptide antibiotics obtained from *Bacillus polymyxa.* It is effective against Gram-negative bacteria and is used in the treatment of dermatologic, ocular, and ear infections.

**polyneural** \-nʸʊr′əl\ Affecting or pertaining to many nerves, used primarily in the context of neuropathology. *Seldom used.* Also *polyneuric.*

**polyneuralgia** \-nʸʊral′jə\ Neuralgia occurring in the distribution of many nerves.

**polyneuric** \-nʸʊr′ik\ POLYNEURAL.

**polyneuritis** \nʸʊrī′tis\ [POLY- + NEURITIS] 1 Any inflammatory process involving peripheral nerves. 2 POLYNEUROPATHY. 3 An inflammation of many nerves due to a variety of causes. Adj. polyneuritic. **acute febrile p.** GUILLAIN-BARRÉ SYNDROME. **acute idiopathic p.** GUILLAIN-BARRÉ SYNDROME. **acute infective p.** GUILLAIN-BARRÉ SYNDROME. **acute postinfectious p.** GUILLAIN-BARRÉ SYNDROME. **alcoholic p.** ALCOHOLIC NEUROPATHY. **anemic p.** Polyneuropathy in vitamin $B_{12}$ deficiency, usually occurring in association with subacute combined degeneration of the spinal cord. **ascending p.** The Guillain-Barré syndrome in which the weakness begins in the lower limbs and later ascends to involve the trunk and upper limbs. **cranial p.** Polyneuritis or polyneuropathy involving only the cranial nerves. It may represent a variant of the Guillain-Barré syndrome but may also result from granulomatous or carcinomatous meningitis and from a number of other causes. Also *polyneuritis cranialis, cranial polyneuropathy.* **diabetic p.** DIABETIC POLYNEUROPATHY. **endemic p.** BERIBERI. **p. endemica** BERIBERI. **Guillain-Barré p.** GUILLAIN-BARRÉ SYNDROME. **infectious p.** GUILLAIN-BARRÉ SYNDROME. **Jamaica ginger p.** JAMAICA JAKE PARALYSIS. **postinfectious p.** GUILLAIN-BARRÉ SYNDROME. **progressive hypertrophic p.** HEREDITARY HYPERTROPHIC INTERSTITIAL NEUROPATHY. **triorthocresyl phosphate p.** TRIORTHOCRESYL PHOSPHATE NEUROPATHY.

**polyneuromyositis** \-nʸʊr′ōmī′əsī′tis\ [POLY- + NEURO- + MYOSITIS] Polyneuritis associated with myositis. Also *neuromyositis.*

**polyneuronitis** \-nʸʊr′ōnī′tis\ [POLY- + NEURONITIS] Inflammation of multiple neurons; a form of axonal polyneuropathy in which the cell bodies are also involved.

**polyneuropathy** \-nʸʊräp′əthē\ [POLY- + NEUROPATHY] Any systemic affection of the peripheral nerves of toxic, metabolic, or unknown etiology. Some forms are predominantly demyelinating in type with relative sparing of the axons, others predominantly axonal, sometimes with "dying-back" of the axon from the periphery. Most types show varying combinations of demyelination and axonal degeneration. Nerve conduction velocity is markedly slowed in demyelinating neuropathy, but normal, at least initially, in the axonal type. Clinically, some forms are predominantly motor, others sensory, but usually there is a combination of motor and sensory symptoms and signs. Weakness and wasting of muscles with areflexia affect predominantly the distal parts of the limbs, and sensory impairment is often seen in "glove and stocking" distribution. In severe cases, proximal limb, trunk, and respiratory and bulbar muscles may be involved and sometimes other cranial nerves (cranial polyneuropathy). Causes include hypersensitivity, vitamin deficiency, many metabolic and toxic processes, inherited and degenerative disease processes, remote and presumably metabolic complications of neoplasia, and others. Also *polyneuritis, peripheral neuritis, multiple neuritis, peripheral neuropathy.* **acromegalic p.** Asymptomatic or symptomatic involvement of peripheral nerves in association with acromegaly. There may be mechanical encroachment upon nerves, as in entrapment neuropathy of the cauda equina or of the median nerve with consequent carpal tunnel syndrome. The involvement may consist of overgrowth of nerve trunks and nerve sheaths in response to growth hormone excess, producing palpable enlargement or peripheral nerves accompanied by fibrous hypertrophy of endoneurium and perineurium. **acute febrile p.** GUILLAIN-BARRÉ SYNDROME. **acute postinfectious p.** GUILLAIN-BARRÉ SYNDROME. **alcoholic p.** ALCOHOLIC NEUROPATHY. **amyloid p.** AMYLOID NEUROPATHY. **buckthorn p.** An ascending form of polyneuropathy due to eating the fruit of the buckthorn *Karwinskia humboldtiana.* The toxic principle of the fruit is an incompletely characterized quinone. Also *coyotillo poisoning.* **carcinomatous p.** Any form of polyneuropathy occurring in a subject with malignant disease. Only rarely is this due to direct carcinomatous infiltration of peripheral nerves. More often it takes the form of a sensorimotor polyneuropathy, sometimes associated with a myopathy, and represents one of the several nonmetastatic neurologic complications of malignant disease. Also *paraneoplastic polyneuropathy.* **cranial p.** CRANIAL POLYNEURITIS. **diabetic p.** Polyneuropathy occurring in patients with diabetes mellitus. There are four principal forms. In one, presumed to be of metabolic origin, sensorimotor polyneuropathy occurs in young and middle-aged diabetic subjects. In the second, occurring in elderly subjects often with mild diabetes, pain, sensory loss, and areflexia occur especially in the lower limbs. This may be secondary to ischemia of the lower limbs and may resemble tabes dorsalis, as the pupils may fail to react to light (diabetic pseudotabes). In the third variety, isolated mononeuropathies of cranial or peripheral nerves (especially the oculomotor and femoral) occur due to ischemia, as in diabetic amyotrophy due to femoral neuropathy. Fourthly, a diabetic autonomic neuropathy is sometimes seen, as in the intrinsic neural plexuses of the gut. Also *diabetic polyneuritis.* **erythredema p.** PINK DISEASE. **familial recurrent p.** An uncommon relapsing variety of demyelinating polyneuropathy, sometimes involving more than one member of a family but not demonstrating any consistent clinical picture or mode of inheritance. **isoniazid p.** A predominantly axonal variety of sensorimotor polyneuropathy due to conditioned deficiency of pyridoxine (vitamin $B_6$) in patients receiving isoniazid, usually for the treatment of tuberculosis. In the general population, some individuals acetylate the drug more slowly than others and it is the slow acetylators who are likely to develop polyneuropathy. Also *isoniazid neuropathy.* **lead p.** Polyneuropathy due to chronic lead poisoning. A symmetrical sensorimotor polyneuropathy may occur, but more often there is localized weakness with little or no sensory loss, such as wrist drop and finger drop. **paraneoplastic p.** CARCINOMATOUS NEUROPATHY. **recurrent p.** RELAPSING POLYNEUROPATHY. **relapsing p.** A form of subacute demyelinating polyneuropathy in which remissions and relapses may occur spontaneously. Relapse during pregnancy has been described. In some such cases hypertrophy of peripheral nerves ultimately develops and in many the condition appears to be steroid-responsive. Also *recurrent polyneuropathy.* **uremic p.** An axonal sensorimotor polyneuropathy which frequently develops in subjects with chronic renal failure. It may improve as a result of renal dialysis or transplantation. Also *uremic neuropathy.*

**polyneuroradiculitis** \-nʸʊr′ōrədik′yəlī′tis\ Inflammation which simultaneously involves the spinal root ganglia, spinal nerve roots, and the peripheral nerves.

**polynuclear** \-nʸoo′klē·ər\ 1 MULTINUCLEAR. 2 POLYMORPHONUCLEAR.

**polynucleolar** \-nʸooklē′ələr\ Having more than one nucleolus in the cell nucleus.

**polynucleosis** \-nʸoo′klē·ō′sis\ 1 The presence of large numbers of polymorphonuclear leukocytes in exudate, a characteristic of bacterial abscesses or empyemas. 2 Neutrophilia of the blood. *Seldom used.*

**polynucleotide** \-nʸoo′klē·ətīd′\ A polymer of nucleotide residues. RNA and DNA are polynucleotides.

**polynucleotide ligase** An enzyme which catalyzes the repair of polynucleotide chains. It unites the free 5′-phosphate and free 3′-hydroxyl ends. It is also responsible for the lengthening of polynucleotide chains by the joining of Okazaki fragments.

**polynucleotide phosphorylase** POLYRIBONUCLEOTIDE NUCLEOTIDYLTRANSFERASE.

**polynychia** \-nik′ē·ə\ POLYONYCHIA.

**polyoma** \-ō′mə\ Any neoplasm associated with a polyomavirus.

**polyomavirus** \-ō′məvī′rəs\ [POLY- + -OMA + VIRUS] An oncogenic virus (genus *Polyomavirus*) belonging to the Papovaviridae family which produces neoplasia of several types in newborn mice. It contains double-stranded circular DNA enclosed in a 72-capsomer naked icosahedral capsid, 45–55 nm in diameter. It is widespread in wild and laboratory mouse populations. Also *mouse parotid tumor virus* (outmoded).

**polyonychia** \-änik′ē·ə\ [POLY- + ONYCH + -IA] The presence of supernumerary nails on fingers or toes. Also *polynychia, polyunguia.*

**polyopia** \-ō′pē·ə\ [POLY- + -OPIA] The seeing of multiple images of a single object. Also *polyopsia, polyopy, multiple vision.*

**polyorchidism** \-ôr′kidizm\ [POLY- + *orchid(o)-* + -ISM] The condition of having supernumerary testes. Also *polyorchism.*

**polyorexia** \-ôrek′sē·ə\ BULIMIA.

**polyostotic** \-ästät′ik\ Pertaining to or involving more than one bone. Compare MONOSTOTIC.

**polyotia** \-ō′shə\ [POLY- + OT- + -IA] The presence of a supernumerary auricle on one or both sides of the head or neck.

**polyovulatory** \-äv′yələtôr′ē\ Releasing more than one ovum in a single ovarian cycle. Also *polyovular.*

**polyp** \päl′ip\ [L *polypus,* from Gk *polypous* (from *poly(s)* many + *pous* foot) many-footed; an octopus or cuttlefish, nasal polyp (likened to tentacles)] Any mass of tissue that protrudes outward from a surface, usually an epithelium. Lesions that may take the shape of a polyp include neoplasms, malformations, and inflammatory foci. Also *polypus* (obs.). **adenomatous p.** A tubular adenoma typically of the gastrointestinal tract. **antrochoanal p.** A single nasal polyp having its origin within the maxillary sinus from which, having passed into the semilunar hiatus, it is carried backward into the choana and thence into the postnasal space. It is an unusual variety. Occasionally one will prolapse into the oropharynx, appearing there from behind the soft palate. It occurs most commonly in the second decade of life. **aural p.** A polyp arising from the middle ear in the course of certain cases of chronic suppurative otitis media, often with cholesteatoma. It passes through the tympanic perforation to present in the external auditory meatus, frequently reaching such a size as to appear at the entrance to the meatus. Nowadays it is removed using microsurgical techniques. **cardiac p.** A polyp attached inside the heart by a pedicle, most commonly an atrial myxoma. **cervical p.** A growth usually emanating from the endocervical canal and composed of a core of connective tissue and an outer layer of endocervical or columnar epithelium. **choanal p.** A nasal polyp that has extended backward to occupy or pass through the corresponding choana. Many such polyps prove to be antrochoanal. **cutaneous fibrous p.** A benign polypoid cutaneous lesion with a core of fibrous connective tissue covered by epidermis. Also *skin tag, soft wart, cutaneous tag, senile fibroma.* **endometrial p.'s** Sessile growths arising from the endometrium with a core of connective tissue. They occur most commonly in the perimenopausal period. **fibrous p.** A polyp in which the covering epithelium is attenuated, occurring in the vagina, cervix, or uterus. Also *fibrinous polyp.* **fleshy p.** A sessile growth composed primarily of loose connective tissue and blood vessels, seen in the vagina, the cervix, and the uterus. **gum p.** A small pedunculated growth from the gingiva. **inflammatory p.** A polyp composed of granulation tissue such as those seen in chronic ulcerative colitis. **juvenile p.'s** Hamartomatous polyps that occur as a familial condition. They are not considered premalignant. Also *retention polyps.* **laryngeal p.** A smooth, rounded, translucent lesion arising close to the anterior laryngeal commissure of the vocal cord, usually from the subglottic aspect and bilateral in 20 percent of cases. It is a common cause of chronic hoarseness in adults, probably, in most cases, related to vocal abuse. The treatment is surgical. **lipomatous p.** A polypoid lipoma. **lymphoid p.'s** Benign colonic polyps composed of lymphoid tissue. **myomatous p.** A growth composed primarily of smooth muscle and connective tissue. **nasal p.** The typical lesion of nasal polyposis. Most patients present with several polyps, often on both sides of the nose. The polyps, usually somewhat piriform and 1–2 cm long, appear as smooth, pale, glistening, mobile structures, growing out from the middle meatus, frequently coming to occupy most or all of the nasal cavity. **osseous p.** A polyp that consists of or contains bone. **pedunculated p.** A polyp connected to the tissue of origin by a stalk. **retention p.'s** JUVENILE POLYPS. **sessile p.** A polyp with a broad base that rests flat against the tissue from which it originates. **tooth p.** The outgrowth of granulation tissue from a pulp exposure in chronic open hyperplastic pulpitis.

**polypapilloma tropicum** \-pap′ilō′mə träp′ikəm\ YAWS.

**polypectomy** \päl′ipek′təmē\ [POLYP + -ECTOMY] The excision of a polyp.

**polypeptide** \-pep′tīd\ [POLY- + PEPTIDE] 1 A substance whose molecule consists of a single chain of amino-acid residues joined by amide bonds. 2 Denoting a molecule small enough so that its different foldings are interconvertible. **gastric inhibitory p.** A polypeptide consisting of 43 amino acids and having a molecular weight of 5105, localized in the K cells of the human duodenum and jejunum and in various parts of the gut in other species. It is released by a standard meal and by oral glucose, amino acids and fat. It inhibits gastric acid secretion, pepsin secretion, motility, and gastrin release, and stimulates intestinal secretion and the release of insulin and glucagon. It is probably a true gastrointestinal hormone. Abbr. GIP **vasoactive intestinal p.** A peptide consisting of 28 amino acids and having a molecular weight of 3381. It is found in specific cells, the H cells of the gut, especially in the colon, and exerts multiple physiologic actions. These include lowered peripheral resistance and hypotension with increased splanchnic blood flow, lipolysis, and glycogenolysis, inhibition of all gastric functions, and stimulation of pancreatic and intestinal secretion of volume and electrolytes. Abbr. VIP

**polyperiostitis** \-per′ē·ästī′tis\ A periosteal inflammation of several bones.

**polyphagia** \\-fā′jə\\ BULIMIA.
**polyphalangia** \\-fəlan′jē·ə\\ [*poly-* + *phalang(es)*, pl. of PHALANX + -IA] The presence of supernumerary phalanges in a digit. Also *hyperphalangia, hyperphalangism*.
**polypharmaceutic** \\-färməsoo′tik\\ Of or relating to the simultaneous administration of multiple drugs.
**polypharmacy** \\-fär′məsē\\ **1** The administration of multiple drugs at the same time. **2** The excessive administration of drugs. Also *polypragmasy*.
**polyphenic** \\-fē′nik\\ PLEIOTROPIC.
**polypheny** \\-fē′nē\\ PLEIOTROPISM.
**polyphosphate** \\-fäs′fāt\\ Any substance of formula HO—[PO(OH)—O—]$_n$—H or its derived anions and esters.
**polyphyletic** \\-fīlet′ik\\ [POLY- + PHYLETIC] Pertaining to descent by independent evolutionary lineages or development from separate origins.
**polyphyletism** \\-fī′lətizm\\ [*polyphylet(ic)* + -ISM] The doctrine, once commonly held, that each of the types of blood cells is derived from a separate earliest precursor or stem cell.
**polyphyletist** \\-fī′lətist\\ One who adheres to the concept of polyphyletism.
**polypi** \\päl′ipī\\ Plural of POLYPUS.
**polypiferous** \\päl′ipif′ərəs\\ Bearing polyps.
**polyplastic** \\-plas′tik\\ Exhibiting several changes in form or shape.
**polypleurodiaphragmotomy** \\-plur′ōdi′əfragmät′əmē\\ A surgical procedure in which the dome of the liver or the upper left quadrant of the abdomen is exposed in a transthoracic approach that divides the diaphragm and one or more ribs.
**polyploid** \\päl′iploid\\ **1** Pertaining to or distinguished by polyploidy. **2** A cell or an organism characterized by polyploidy.
**polyploidy** \\päl′iploi′dē\\ [POLY- + -PLOID + -Y] The state of a single cell, a cell line, or all cells of an organism in which more than two complete haploid sets of paired, homologous chromosomes are present.
**polypnea** \\päl′ipnē′ə\\ TACHYPNEA.
**polypneic** \\päl′ipnē′ik\\ Pertaining to polypnea.
**polypodia** \\-pō′dē·ə\\ [POLY- + POD- + -IA] The condition of having supernumerary feet.
**polypoid** \\päl′ipoid\\ PEDUNCULATED.
**polyposis** \\päl′ipō′sis\\ [POLYP + -OSIS] The presence of multiple polyps on any part of the body. **acquired multiple p.** Multiple adenomatous polyps of the colon that occur sporadically and are not a part of any well-defined familial disorder. **adenomatous p. coli** The presence of numerous polypoid adenomas in the colon. At least 100 and often as many as 1000 tumors are present. It is a familial condition and is associated with a high risk of carcinoma in the colon or rectum. Also *polyposis coli, familial polyposis, familial polyposis coli, familial intestinal polyposis*. **p. coli** ADENOMATOUS POLYPOSIS COLI. **familial p. coli** ADENOMATOUS POLYPOSIS COLI. **familial intestinal p.** ADENOMATOUS POLYPOSIS COLI. **gastric p.** The presence of multiple polyps in the stomach. Also *polyposis gastrica, polyposis ventriculi*. **intestinal p.** The presence of multiple polyps in the small intestine. Also *polyposis intestinalis*. **nasal p.** A common and widespread disease in which the nose becomes increasingly obstructed by nasal polyps, arising usually from the mucous membrane lining of the ethmoidal air cells but sometimes from the lining of other sinuses, such as the maxillary sinus or the mucosa of the nasal cavity itself. The cause is unknown, and although allergy and infection may be relevant they are often absent. Treatment is usually surgical, but recurrence is almost inevitable and most patients undergo many operations. **p. ventriculi** GASTRIC POLYPOSIS.
**polypous** \\päl′əpəs\\ Pertaining to or characterized by polyps.
**polypragmasy** \\-prag′məsē\\ POLYPHARMACY.
**polypus** \\päl′əpəs\\ *Obs.* POLYP.
**polyradiculitis** \\-rədik′yəlī′tis\\ [POLY- + RADICULITIS] A diffuse inflammatory process involving spinal nerve roots.
**polyradiculoneuritis** \\-rədik′yəlōn$^y$urī′tis\\ [POLY- + RADICULO- + NEURITIS] Any inflammatory process involving multiple nerve roots and peripheral nerves. **acute idiopathic p.** GUILLAIN-BARRÉ SYNDROME.
**polyradiculoneuropathy** \\-rədik′yəlōn$^y$uräp′əthē\\ [POLY- + RADICULO- + NEUROPATHY] Any disorder of nerve roots and peripheral nerves. **acute postinfective p.** GUILLAIN-BARRÉ SYNDROME. **inflammatory acute p.** GUILLAIN-BARRÉ SYNDROME.
**polyribonucleotide nucleotidyltransferase** The enzyme (EC 2.7.7.8) capable of breaking down RNA by reaction with orthophosphate to liberate a nucleoside diphosphate from the 3′ end. Also *polynucleotide phosphorylase*.
**polyribosome** \\-rī′bəsōm\\ A string of ribosomes held together by a strand of mRNA. Also *ergosome*.
**polysaccharidase** Any enzyme that catalyzes hydrolysis of a polysaccharide.
**polysaccharide** \\-sak′ərīd\\ [POLY- + SACCHARIDE] A class of carbohydrates in which the molecule results from the polymerization of monosaccharide subunits. A polysaccharide usually contains 5 or more monosaccharide subunits, joined to each other by glycoside links. Glycogen and starch are examples. **p. A** A species-specific surface antigen of *Staphylococcus aureus*, identified as a ribitol teichoic acid substituted with *N*-acetylglucosamine and with D-alanine. **p. B** A teichoic acid with glucose determinants, carried on the surface of *Staphylococcus epidermidis*. **core p.** In lipopolysaccharides, a branched sequence of about seven sugar residues that connects the O polysaccharide and lipid A. A heptose is characteristic. The core polysaccharide varies among different enterobacteria. **gastric p.** The mucopolysaccharide which is contained in gastric mucus. **O-specific p.** The outermost portion of the lipopolysaccharide in the outer membrane of Gram-negative bacteria. It consists of chains of ten or more repeating units, each containing three or four different sugar residues. In salmonellae, the variety of these sugars and their specific linkages provide many hundreds of different O antigens, used in typing. **pneumococcal p.** A type-specific capsular polysaccharide (S antigen) of *Streptococcus pneumoniae*. Over 80 types are known, most with repeat units of two to four sugars or sugar derivatives.
**polyscelia** \\-sē′lē·ə\\ [POLY- + Gk *skel(os)* leg + -IA] The condition of having more than the normal complement of two legs or legs and feet.
**polysclerosis** \\-sklirō′sis\\ MULTIPLE SCLEROSIS.
**polyserositis** \\-sir′ōsī′tis\\ [POLY- + SEROSITIS] Inflammation with serous effusions of multiple serosal structures, as is seen in collagen diseases. **familial recurrent p.** Polyserositis occurring in a genetically identifiable pattern and characterized by periodic occurrences of polyserositis and fever. **periodic p.** RECURRENT POLYSEROSITIS. **recurrent p.** Polyserositis occurring at predictable intervals often associated with fever and with a recognizable familial pattern. Also *periodic polyserositis*. **tuberculous p.** Polyserositis due to infection with *Mycobacterium tuberculosa*.
**polysomaty** \\-sō′mətē\\ The state of having reduplicated

nuclear chromatin, both in the sense of an increased chromosome number, as in endopolyploidy, and in the sense of increased amount of chromatin per chromosome, as in polyteny.

**polysome** \-päl′isōm\ [POLY- + Gk *sōm(a)* body] A number of ribosomes attached to a single linear molecule of messenger RNA. Compare MONOSOME.

**polysomia** \-sō′mē·ə\ [POLY- + Gk *sōm(a)* the body + -IA] The union of conjoined twins in which two bodies are identifiable but imperfectly formed. *Imprecise.*

**polysomic** \-sō′mik\ Characterized by polysomy.

**polysomus** \-sō′məs\ An embryo, fetus, or postnatal individual with polysomia.

**polysomy** \päl′isō′mē\ The existence of more than two of a particular chromosome or homologous pair in the same nucleus, as in trisomy or tetrasomy.

**polyspermia** \-spur′mē·ə\ POLYSPERMY.

**polyspermy** \päl′ispur′mē\ [POLY- + SPERM + -Y] **1** The penetration of the ovum by several spermatozoa at the time of fertilization. Exceptional under natural circumstances, it can be produced experimentally by use of chemical agents (ether, chloroform) or by exposure of the ovum to high concentrations of spermatozoa. Usually only one male pronucleus fuses with the female pronucleus and the additional male ones are absorbed. **2** Emission of an excessive number of spermatozoa. For defs. 1 and 2 also *polyspermia.*

**pathologic p.** The penetration of an ovum at fertilization by more than one spermatozoon when normally only one gains entrance. Abnormal development or death results.

**physiologic p.** A situation which occurs normally in certain species in which more than one spermatozoon enters the ovum. Transformation of the various sperm heads often occurs to form male pronuclei, but normally only one is involved in the development of the embryo. The abnormal situation, where more than one male pronucleus is involved in subsequent development, gives rise to a polyploid individual that rarely survives beyond the early embryonic period.

**polyspike-wave** \päl′ispīk-\ In electroencephalography, a complex pattern made up of a polyspike associated with one or more slow waves. This is a variant of the irregular spike-wave complex.

**polysplenia** \-splē′nē·ə\ [POLY- + SPLEN- + -IA] The presence of two or more separate masses of splenic tissue in the abdominal cavity.

**polystichia** \-stik′ē·ə\ [POLY- + Gk *stich(os)* a line, row + -IA] The condition of having more than one row of eyelashes on a single eyelid.

**polysynaptic** \-sinap′tik\ Involving the interaction of two or more neurons.

**polysynbrachydactyly** \-sinbrak′ēdak′tilē\ [POLY- + SYN- + BRACHYDACTYLY] A condition in which there are two or more instances in the same individual of fused, shortened digits.

**polysyndactyly** \-sindak′tilē\ A condition in which there are two or more instances in the same individual of side-to-side fusion of digits.

**polysyphilide** \-sif′ilīd\ [POLY- + SYPHIL- + -IDE$^2$] A syphilitic rash characterized by a variety of lesions.

**polytendinitis** \-ten′dənī′tis\ [POLY- + TENDINITIS] Inflammation of multiple tendons or tendon sheaths.

**polytene** \päl′itēn\ Of or relating to polyteny.

**polytenization** \-tēnīzā′shən\ The process through which polyteny occurs in the cell nucleus of certain cells in a few species.

**polyteny** \-tē′nē\ [POLY- + L *taen(ia)* a band, strip + -Y] **1** The reduplication of the chromatids without separation or cell division during interphase of some cells in certain species, notably the salivary glands of *Diptera.* The resulting chromosome is often greatly enlarged, possesses a characteristic banding pattern in cytologic preparations, and contains $2^n$ times the normal DNA content, where *n* is the number of reduplications. **2** The state of a chromosome being reduplicated without chromatid separation. **3** The state of a cell having reduplicated chromosomes.

**polythelia** \-thē′lē·ə\ [POLY- + THEL- + -IA] The presence of more than one nipple on either side of the body. It is the normal state in subprimate mammalian species that regularly produce litters and it occurs abnormally in humans. Also *polythelism, hyperthelia.*

**polytocous** \-tō′kəs\ [POLY- + *toc(o)-* + -OUS] Giving birth to more than one offspring at a time.

**polytrichia** \-trik′ē·ə\ [POLY- + TRICH- + -IA] The condition of excessive hairiness, especially in comparison with persons of the same race and sex. Also *polytrichosis.*

**polytypic** \-tip′ik\ Having two or more immediately subordinate categories: said of a taxonomic category.

**poly U** POLYURIDYLIC ACID.

**polyunguia** \päl′ē·ung′gwē·ə\ [POLY- + *ungu(is)* + -IA] POLYONYCHIA.

**polyunsaturated** \-unsach′ərā′tid\ Containing many carbon-carbon double bonds: used especially of the essential fatty acids, because these contain two or more —CH=CH— groups, separated by methylene groups.

**polyuria** \päl′ēyoo′rē·ə\ [POLY- + -URIA] The formation of urine in abnormally large volume, reflected by frequency and as well as by volume of urination. Also *hyperuresis.*

**polyuridylic acid** A homopolymer of uracil-containing nucleotides. In an *in vitro* system the polyuridylic acid acts as mRNA to direct the synthesis of polyphenylalanine. Also *poly U.*

**polyvalent** \-vā′lənt\ MULTIVALENT.

**polyvinyl-** \-vī′nəl-\ [POLY- + VINYL] A combining form denoting the presence in a polymerized form of several vinyl groups in a molecule. • This is often written as an independent word, as in *polyvinyl chloride.*

**polyvinyl alcohol** A spongy plastic material that was once used for prosthetic vascular grafts. It is now used in small fragments as deliberate emboli to halt bleeding from damaged or abnormal arteries.

**polyvinylpyrrolidone** POVIDONE.

***Pomatiopsis*** \pōmat′ē·äp′sis\ A genus of widely distributed amphibious freshwater snails of the family Pomatiopsidae (formerly placed in the family Hydrobiidae). It is very similar to the genus *Oncomelania,* host of *Schistosoma japonicum,* with which it now shares familial status. It is the initial intermediate host of lung flukes (genus *Paragonimus)* in North America.

**Pomeroy** [Ralph Hayward *Pomeroy,* U.S. gynecologist, 1867–1925] See under OPERATION.

**pompholyx** \päm′fōliks\ [Gk *pompholyx* the boss of a shield] The presence of bullae on the palms and soles, usually as a result of an eczematous reaction, or, rarely, caused by sweat retention.

**Poncet** [Antonin *Poncet,* French surgeon, 1849–1913] Poncet's rheumatism. See under DISEASE.

**pond.** *pondere* (L, by weight).

**ponesiatrics** \pōnē′sē·at′riks\ [Gk *ponēs(is)* toil, exertion + -IATRICS] A technique of training dependent on perception of errors by observation of physiological parameters; biofeedback training. *Rare.*

**pons** \pänz\ [L (gen. *pontis*), a bridge] **1** Any tissue or process joining two parts of an organ or bridging a space. **2** [NA] A rounded prominence of the brainstem located between the cerebral peduncles above and the medulla oblongata below, and separated from the latter by a transverse furrow exposing the abducent, facial and vestibulocochlear nerves. Its anterior surface rests against the dorsum sellae of the sphenoid bone and the contiguous basilar part of the occipital bone. The posterior surface is ventral to and covered by the cerebellum. Also *pons cerebelli, pons varolii.* Adj. pontile, pontine. **p. cerebelli** PONS. **p. hepatis** A bridge of liver tissue that can be present over the fossa vena cava, so that the latter resembles a canal. Also *ponticulus hepatis.* **p. tarini** SUBSTANTIA PERFORATA POSTERIOR. **p. varolii** PONS.

**pontes** \pän′tēz\ Plural of PONS.

**pontibrachium** \pän′tibrā′kē·əm\ PEDUNCULUS CEREBELLARIS MEDIUS.

**pontic** \pän′tik\ [L *pons*, gen. *pontis*, bridge + -IC] The part of a bridge or partial denture which is a substitute for a missing tooth. It may be made of porcelain, acrylic resin, or gold.

**ponticulus** \päntik′yələs\ [L (dim. of *pons*, gen. *pontis*, a bridge), a little bridge] Any of various small ridgelike or bridgelike anatomic structures. **p. auriculae** An oblique ridge on the eminentia cochleae of the auricular cartilage to which the auricularis posterior muscle is attached. **p. hepatis** PONS HEPATIS. **p. nasi** *Outmoded* BRIDGE OF THE NOSE.

**pontile** \pän′til\ PONTINE.

**pontine** \pän′tīn\ [L *pons*, gen. *pont(is)* bridge + -INE] Pertaining to the pons. Also *pontile.*

**pontobulbar** \pän′təbul′bər\ Affecting or pertaining to the pons and medulla oblongata.

**pontomedullary** \pän′təmed′yəler′ē\ Pertaining to or connecting the pons and medulla oblongata.

**pontopeduncular** \pän′təpidungk′yələr\ Pertaining to the region of the pons containing fibers from the cerebral peduncle.

**Pool** [Eugene Hillhouse *Pool*, U.S. surgeon, 1874–1949] Pool-Schlesinger sign. See under SCHLESINGER SIGN.

**pool** **1** A combining of resources or skills, as for improved efficiency. **2** The total volume of liquid in an organ tissue or the whole body, especially blood. **abdominal p.** The volume of blood in the vessels of the abdomen. It increases in shock. **gene p.** The total collection of all genetic loci and alleles at those loci among members of a given population who are capable of sexual reproduction. **metabolic p.** All the substances in the body that take part in metabolism. **metabolite p.** The small molecules that can be released from bacterial cells by abrupt lysis, as by pouring into boiling water or into trichloroacetic acid solution. **recirculating lymphocyte p.** The population of lymphocytes which migrates from the blood to the lymph nodes either directly through the postcapillary venules or indirectly through the tissues and afferent lymphatics, returning to the bloodstream by way of the efferent lymphatics and the major lymphatic trunks. Lymphocyte recirculation occurs analogously through the spleen. Both T cells and B cells are found in the recirculating pool.

**poples** \päp′lēz\ [L (prob. akin to *plicare* to bend, fold) the ham of the knee, the knee] FOSSA POPLITEA.

**popliteal** \päplit′ē·əl, päp′litē′əl\ [New L *poplite(us)* (from L *poples*, gen. *poplitis*, the hollow of the leg, the knee) pertaining to the ham + -AL] Relating to the posterior surface of the knee.

**popliteus** \päp′litē′əs\ MUSCULUS POPLITEUS. **p. minor** A rare accessory slip of the popliteus muscle arising from the back of the femur medial to the plantaris muscle's attachment and inserting into the oblique popliteal ligament of the knee joint.

**POPOP** 1,4-Bis-(5-phenoxazol-2-yl)benzene. A scintillation secondary solute, used in liquid scintillation counting, that shifts the emission wavelength of the primary solute toward the central portion of the sensitivity range of the photomultiplier tube.

**population** [Late L *populatio* (from L *populus* the people) a populace, multitude] **1** The aggregate of the inhabitants of a given area. **2** The number of individuals in such an aggregate. **3** SUBPOPULATION. **4** In statistics, an aggregate of separate entities. Also *universe.* **closed p.** A population in which there is no migration. **Segi's p.** A standard population, used initially for computing age-adjusted death rates from cancer, consisting of the total age-sex distribution of the combined populations of 46 countries around the year 1950. **standard p.** The age-sex distribution of an actual population, for example, the total population of the United States at the 1960 census, or of a hypothetical population, used for the purpose of direct or indirect standardization. It is often the practice to scale the distribution to a convenient total, such as one million.

**poradenitis** \pôr′adənī′tis\ [*por(o)-* + ADENITIS] An inflammatory disease of the lymph nodes in which there is formation of multiple small abscesses. Also *poradenia.*

**poradenolymphitis** \pôrad′ənōlimfī′tis\ [*por(o)-* + ADENO- + LYMPH + -ITIS] LYMPHOGRANULOMA VENEREUM.

**porcelain** A hard, white ceramic ware, usually translucent. **aluminous p.** A dental porcelain containing a significant amount of recrystallized alumina. **high fusing p.** Dental porcelain which is fused at 2350°F to 2500°F (1288°C to 1371°C). **metal-bonding p.** A dental porcelain with a coefficient of expansion similar to that of the metal with which it can be bonded. **synthetic p.** SILICATE CEMENT.

**pore** [L *porus* (from Gk *poros* a ford, ferry, passageway, passage, pore) a passage or channel in the body] A minute hole or opening in a surface or within a structure; porus. **alveolar p.** PORE OF KOHN. **birth p.** GENITAL PORE. **external osseous acoustic p.** PORUS ACUSTICUS EXTERNUS. **genital p.** An external opening in certain tapeworms and most trematodes through which the eggs exit, often passing through a terminal metraterm before leaving the worm. Also *birth pore.* **gustatory p.** PORUS GUSTATORIUS. **interalveolar p.** PORE OF KOHN. **internal osseous acoustic p.** PORUS ACUSTICUS INTERNUS. **p. of Kohn** One of the openings in alveolar walls in the lung providing communication between adjacent alveoli. Also *alveolar pore, interalveolar pore, pulmonic alveolar vent.* **mammary p.** An opening of a lactiferous duct onto the surface of a nipple. **nuclear p.** A region of the nuclear envelope where the two membranes fuse. The perimeter (annulus) of the pore has eight granules associated with the inside face and eight granules associated with the outside face. The space in the pore is filled with material (annular material). The nuclear pore is believed to allow a selective interchange of substances between the nucleus and the cytoplasm. **slit p.** A narrow gap between adjacent foot processes that is applied to the external aspect of the glomerular capillary basement membrane. **sweat p.** PORUS SUDORIFERUS. **taste p.** PORUS GUSTATORIUS. **urinary p.** The distal opening of a collecting duct on the apex of a renal papilla. **p.'s of Vieussens** FORAMINA VENARUM MINIMARUM CORDIS.

**porencephalia** \pôr′ensəfā′lyə\ PORENCEPHALY.

**porencephalic** \pôr′ensəfal′ik\ Characterized by porencephaly. Also *porencephalous.*

**porencephalous** \pôr′ensef′ələs\ PORENCEPHALIC.

**porencephaly** \pôr′ensef′əlē\ [*por(o)-* + ENCEPHAL- + -Y] The presence of one or more cavities within one cerebral hemisphere, usually communicating with the lateral ventricle. This may be a congenital malformation (primary porencephaly), or a consequence of localized cerebral atrophy or scarring due to birth injury, infarction, or trauma (secondary porencephaly). Also *cerebral porosis, porencephalia, spelencephalia, perencephaly.* **schizocephalic p.** SCHIZENCEPHALY. **traumatic p.** The formation of a localized cyst or diverticulum associated with one or more cerebral ventricles consequent upon focal scarring and cerebral atrophy, resulting from a focal brain injury or contusion. Also *traumatic internal pseudohydrocephalus.*

**pori** \pôr′ī\ Plural of PORUS.

**porin** \pôr′in\ A protein of the outer membrane of Gram-negative bacteria that adheres closely to the underlying murein, forming trimers surrounding a pore that serves as a molecular sieve. Also *matrix protein.*

**pork** The flesh of swine prepared as food. **measly p.** Pork infected with cysticerci of the tapeworm, *Taenia solium,* a tapeworm of man.

**poro-** \pôr′ō-\ [Gk *poro(s)* a passage, pore] A combining form meaning pore, small opening, or small cavity.

**porocele** \pôr′əsēl\ [Gk *pōrokēlē* (from *pōro(s)* stone, calculus + *kēlē* hernia, swelling) a scrotal calculus] Hernia of the scrotum with resultant hardening of the testicular tissues.

**porocephaliasis** \-sef′əlī′əsis\ [*Porocephal(us)* + -IASIS] Infection with pentastome parasites of the genus *Porocephalus.* Adults occur in the lungs of reptiles, but immature forms are found in a variety of vertebrates, usually encysted in the mesenteries, liver, or other visceral organs. Also *porocephalosis.*

***Porocephalus*** \pôr′ōsef′ələs\ A genus of pentastomes (phylum Pentastomida, class Porocephalida, family Porocephalidae) parasitic in the respiratory system of reptiles with larvae usually in small mammals. The larvae of certain species, however, lack host specificity and may cause porocephaliasis in other animals including humans.

**porokeratosis** \pôr′ōker′ətō′sis\ [Gk *poros* a pore + KERATOSIS] A condition marked by an acquired circumscribed warty lesion that is characterized histologically and sometimes also clinically by a peripheral horny lamella. **disseminated superficial actinic p.** A condition marked by multiple atopic cutaneous lesions having a firm raised border and a depressed center. It is usually seen in the skin of those who have had many years of exposure to the sun. **p. excentrica** POROKERATOSIS OF MIBELLI. **p. of Mantoux** A nonfamilial dyskeratosis, seen in young adults, in which crops of nodules develop on the palms and soles and have a pigmented central punctum that is shed to leave a crater. **p. of Mibelli** A cutaneous disorder that is characterized by single or multiple atrophic lesions surrounded by a firm raised border. Histologically a dyskeratosis is present, characterized by a break in the granular layer of the epidermis and a parakeratotic plug that arises from this area. Also *porokeratosis excentrica.* **p. palmaris et plantaris disseminata** A hereditary disease characterized by multiple porokeratotic lesions of the palms and soles.

**poroma** \pôrō′mə\ [Gk *pōrōma* (from *pōr(os)* a stone or calculus) a callus] **1** An eccrine acrospiroma occurring on the foot. **2** A callus. **eccrine p.** ECCRINE ACROSPIROMA.

**poroplastic** \-plas′tik\ Porous and plastic.

**porosis** \pôrō′sis\ [*por(o)-* + -OSIS] Cavity formation within a tissue. **cerebral p.** PORENCEPHALY.

**porosity** \pôräs′itē\ The degree to which a material is porous, expressed in terms of either the number or the size of its pores.

**porotic** \pôrät′ik\ Pertaining to or characterized by porosis.

**porotomy** \pôrät′əmē\ MEATOTOMY.

**porous** \pôr′əs\ Allowing the passage of molecules dissolved in a fluid medium, thus implying the presence of pores or small openings in a structure.

**porphin** \pôr′fən\ Unsubstituted porphyrin. *Outmoded.*

**porphobilin** Any of several colored substances found in urine in certain porphyrias, especially after urine samples containing porphobilinogen have stood for some time. It is not certain that every substance so described was in fact formed from porphobilinogen.

**porphobilinogen** 2-Aminomethyl-4-(2-carboxyethyl)-3-carboxymethylpyrrole. It is the pyrrole intermediate in the biosynthesis of porphyrins. It is made from two molecules of 5-aminolevulinate with the production of two molecules of water, a reaction catalyzed by porphobilinogen synthase. It is polymerized into hydroxymethylbilane, a linear tetrapyrrole, with production of four molecules of ammonia, a reaction catalyzed by hydroxymethylbilane synthase. Small amounts normally occur in urine, but large amounts, present when some enzymes are congenitally low in activity, cause the urine to darken with formation of porphobilin.

**porphobilinogen deaminase** The enzyme (EC 4.3.1.8) that catalyzes the conversion of four molecules of porphobinogen into four molecules of ammonia and one of hydroxymethylbilane, a linear tetrapyrrole, later cyclized in the pathway of porphyrin biosynthesis.

**porphyria** \pôrfi′rē·ə, -fir′ē·ə\ [*porphyr(in)* + -IA] Any of several inborn errors of metabolism characterized by increased urinary excretion, or increased blood concentration, of porphyrins or porphyrin precursors such as porphobilinogen and δ-aminolevulinic acid. Also *porphyrinopathy* (obs.), *hematoporphyria* (obs.). • Unless otherwise qualified, acute intermittent porphyria is usually meant. **acquired p.** A disturbance of porphyrin metabolism resulting from liver damage due to alcohol or drugs. **acute p.** ACUTE INTERMITTENT PORPHYRIA. **acute intermittent p.** A hereditary disorder of autosomal dominant transmittance characterized by recurrent attacks of severe abdominal pain, vomiting, constipation, urinary retention, tachycardia, postural hypotension, and sweating; sensorimotor polyneuropathies, paraplegia, quadriplegia, and respiratory paralysis; psychotic episodes; and markedly increased urinary excretion of porphilinogen. The metabolic defect is a reduction in the enzyme, porphobilinogen deaminase. Also *acute porphyria, Swedish porphyria, Swedish genetic porphyria, pyrroloporphyria.* Abbr. AIP **congenital erythropoietic p.** A very rare hereditary disorder, of autosomal recessive transmittance, characterized by hemolytic anemia beginning in infancy, cutaneous photosensitivity with blistering and scarring, alopecia, conjunctivitis, keratitis and ectropion, and marked increase in urinary excretion of uroporphyrin. The metabolic defect may be deficiency of uroporphyrinogen cosynthetase. Also *erythropoietic porphyria, congenital photosensitive porphyria.* **congenital photosensitive p.** CONGENITAL ERYTHROPOIETIC PORPHYRIA. **p. cutanea tarda** A disorder of porphyrin metabolism that may be hereditary or acquired and is characterized by severe cutaneous photosensitivity with blistering and scarring following exposure to sunlight, cutaneous depigmentation, hirsutism, hepatic dysfunction or cirrhosis, and increased urinary excretion of uroporphyrin and coproporphyrin. Also *cutaneous porphyria, urocoproporphyria.* **p. cutanea tarda hereditaria** VARIEGATE PORPHYRIA. **p. cutanea tarda**

**symptomatica** VARIEGATE PORPHYRIA. **cutaneous p.** PORPHYRIA CUTANEA TARDA. **erythropoietic p.** CONGENITAL ERYTHROPOIETIC PORPHYRIA. **hepatic p.** A category of disorders of porphyrin metabolism, so designated on the assumption that the liver is the organ principally affected. Hepatic porphyrias include acute intermittent porphyria, variegate porphyria, hereditary coproporphyria, and porphyria cutanea tarda. Also *porphyria hepatica.* **p. hepatica** HEPATIC PORPHYRIA. **mixed p.** VARIEGATE PORPHYRIA. **ovulocyclic p.** Attacks of porphyria associated with menses. **photosensitive p.** A porphyria that has as a typical feature a marked tendency of the skin to form blisters, often followed by scarring, following exposure to sunlight that would be harmless for normal persons. Photosensitivity characteristically accompanies congenital erythropoietic porphyria and porphyria cutanea tarda. **South African p.** VARIEGATE PORPHYRIA. **South African genetic p.** VARIEGATE PORPHYRIA. **Swedish p.** ACUTE INTERMITTENT PORPHYRIA. **Swedish genetic p.** ACUTE INTERMITTENT PORPHYRIA. **p. variegata** VARIEGATE PORPHYRIA. **variegate p.** A hereditary disorder of autosomal dominant transmittance, characterized by neuropathy, intermittent attacks of abdominal pain, photosensitivity that results in blistering and scarring of skin, and increased urinary excretion of uroporphyrin and fecal excretion of protoporphyrin and coproporphyrin. The metabolic defect is unknown. Also *mixed porphyria, porphyria variegata, South African porphyria, South African genetic porphyria, porphyria cutanea tarda symptomatica, porphyria cutanea tarda hereditaria, protocoproporphyria.*

**porphyrin** \pôr′firin\ [Gk *porphyr(a)* purple + -IN] A macrocyclic ring system of four pyrrole rings joined by methine bridges. It is the parent compound of many substituted porphyrins found naturally as their chelates with metal ions, such as iron in heme and magnesium in chlorophyll. Two of the four nitrogen atoms carry hydrogen atoms, which are displaced as hydrogen ions on replacement by metal ions.

**porphyrinogen** Hexahydroporphyrin. It consists of four pyrrole rings joined in a macrocycle by methylene groups. One porphyrinogen, uroporphyrinogen, is the first tetrapyrrole macrocycle formed in the pathway of biosynthesis of natural porphyrins.

**porphyrinopathy** \pôr′firinäp′əthē\ *Obs.* PORPHYRIA.

**porphyrinuria** \pôr′firinoo′rēə\ [PORPHYRIN + -URIA] The excretion of abnormal quantities of porphyrins in urine, as may occur in the congenital porphyrias and in such acquired conditions as lead poisoning, hemolytic anemias, viral hepatitis, and alcoholism in which there is either deranged heme synthesis or impaired hepatic metabolism. Also *porphyuria.*

**porphyrism** \pôr′firizm\ The abnormal accumulation of one or more metabolic intermediates in the anabolism or catabolism of heme, usually stemming from an inborn error of metabolism. *Obs.*

**porphyruria** \pôr′firoo′rē·ə\ PORPHYRINURIA.

**porrigo** \pôri′gō\ [L, a cutaneous disease, scurf, scab, dandruff] Any disease of the scalp. *Obs.* **p. favosa** *Obs.* FAVUS. **p. lupinosa** *Obs.* FAVUS. **p. scutulata** *Obs.* FAVUS.

**porta** \pôr′tə\ [L (akin to *portare* to carry, and to Gk *porthmos* a strait, passage and *peran* to carry overseas for sale, to sell), a gate] The opening or hilum in an organ through which pass the main vessels or other structures supplying or draining the organ. **p. hepatis** [NA] A transverse fissure on the visceral surface of the liver located between the quadrate and the caudate lobes and containing the hepatic ducts, hepatic artery, and portal vein within the hepatoduodenal ligament. Also *hepatic portal, portal fissure, transverse fissure.* **p. labyrinthi** *Outmoded* FENESTRA COCHLEAE. **p. renis** *Outmoded* HILUM RENALE.

**portacaval** \pôr′təkā′vəl\ Connecting the portal vein and vena cava.

**portal** [L *portalis* (from *port(a)* a gate + *-alis* -AL) pertaining to a gate] **1** Pertaining to a porta, specifically porta hepatis. **2** Pertaining to the portal vein (vena portae hepatis) and its circulatory system. **3** Pertaining to any circulatory system of the portal vein type. See also PORTAL CIRCULATION. **4** An entrance or gateway; porta. **anterior intestinal p.** See under INTESTINAL PORTAL. **p. of entry** The characteristic site of entry (mouth, lungs, skin abrasion, genital tract, etc.) of an infecting microorganism. **hepatic p.** PORTA HEPATIS. **intestinal p.** Either of two orifices present inside the developing embryonic intestine when it becomes tubular as the result of modeling of the endoderm. The anterior intestinal portal leads into the foregut diverticulum and the posterior intestinal portal marks the opening into the hindgut. They lead away from the intermediate portion (midgut) which remains distended because of its wide connection with the yolk sac. **posterior intestinal p.** See under INTESTINAL PORTAL.

**porte-aiguille** \pôrt′āgēl′\ [French, from *porte(r)* to carry + *aiguille* (from L *acus* a needle) a needle] A device designed to hold needles for suturing during a surgical operation.

**porte-polisher** \pôrt′-\ A dental hand instrument used to hold small pieces of cane or orange wood for polishing the proximal surfaces of teeth.

**Porter** [Curt Culwell *Porter,* U.S. biochemist, born 1914] **1** Porter-Silber chromogens test. See under 17-HYDROXYCORTICOSTEROID TEST. **2** Porter-Silber chromogens. See under CHROMOGEN.

**Porter** [Thomas Cunningham *Porter,* British scientist, 1860–1933] Ferry-Porter law. See under LAW.

**Porteus** [Stanley David *Porteus,* Australian-born psychologist active in Hawaii, born 1883] Porteus maze test. See under TEST.

**portio** \pôr′shō\ [L (prob. akin to *pars* a part), a share, portion] (*pl.* portiones) A particular morphological portion of an organ or structure; a part. Also *portion.* **p. dura paris septimi** *Outmoded* NERVUS FACIALIS. **p. intermedia nervi acustici** *Outmoded* NERVUS INTERMEDIUS. **p. major nervi trigemini** *Outmoded* RADIX SENSORIA NERVI TRIGEMINI. **p. minor nervi trigemini** *Outmoded* RADIX MOTORIA NERVI TRIGEMINI. **p. mollis paris septimi** *Outmoded* NERVUS VESTIBULOCOCHLEARIS. **p. supravaginalis cervicis** [NA] The proximal part of the cervix uteri above the anterior wall of the vagina, separated from the bladder anteriorly by the parametrium, related laterally to the uterine arteries and the ureters, and covered posteriorly by peritoneum. **p. vaginalis cervicis** [NA] The portion of the cervix uteri that protrudes through the anterior wall of the vagina forming the fornices. At its lower extremity is the external os of the uterus. Also *vaginal part of cervix, intravaginal part of cervix.*

**portion** PORTIO.

**portiones** \pôrshō′nēz\ Plural of PORTIO.

**portiplexus** \pôr′tiplek′səs\ The choroid plexus extending through the interventricular foramen.

**portography** \pôrtäg′rəfē\ Radiographic study of the portal vein after the injection of a radiopaque contrast material either directly into the portal system at surgery or by means of splenoportography or by high volume contrast injection into the superior mesenteric artery. Also *portovenog-*

*raphy, portal venography.* **percutaneous transhepatic p.** The visualization of the portal system by using contrast material injected through a catheter inserted percutaneously into a portal vein radicle within the liver. **portal p.** Portography accomplished by injecting the contrast medium directly into the superior mesenteric vein or one of its branches after surgical exposure of the vein. **splenic p.** SPLENOPORTOGRAPHY. **umbilical p.** Radiographic study of the intrahepatic portal system after the injection of a radiopaque contrast agent through a catheter in the umbilical vein.

**portosystemic** \pôr′təsistem′ik\ Relating to a connection between the portal vein and systemic veins.

**portovenography** \pôr′təvēnäg′rəfē\ PORTOGRAPHY.

**porus** \pôr′əs\ [L, pore. See PORE.] (*pl.* pori) A minute natural aperture; pore. **p. acusticus externus** [NA] The rounded external opening of the bony external acoustic meatus bounded by the tympanic part of the temporal bone except superiorly where the posterior root of the zygomatic process limits it. Also *external osseous acoustic pore, orifice of external acoustic meatus.* **p. acusticus internus** [NA] A rounded opening near the center of the posterior surface of the petrous part of the temporal bone. It is the internal orifice of the internal acoustic meatus running transversely and laterally from it and giving passage to the facial and vestibulocochlear nerves, nervus intermedius, and labyrinthine vessels. Also *internal osseous acoustic pore, internal auditory foramen.* **p. crotaphiticobuccinatorius** A foramen which is occasionally formed by a bar of bone between the base and lateral surface of the lateral pterygoid lamina, on the one side, and the greater wing of the sphenoid bone just lateral to the foramen ovale, on the other side. It transmits most or all of the motor fibers of the trigeminal nerve. Also *pterygoalar foramen, Hyrtl's foramen.* **p. gustatorius** [NA] The small aperture through which a taste bud opens on the surface of the epithelium of the tongue, palate, or epiglottis. Also *gustatory pore, taste pore.* **p. opticus** 1 A depression in the center of the discus nervi optici marking the point of entrance of the central retinal artery. 2 OPTIC FORAMEN OF SCLERA. **p. sudoriferus** The external opening on the surface of the skin of a duct of a sweat gland. Also *sweat pore.*

**Posada** [Alejandro *Posada,* Argentinian parasitologist, 1870–1920] Posada-Wernicke disease. See under COCCIDIOIDOMYCOSIS.

# position

**position** [L *positio* (from *positus,* past part. of *ponere* to lay, put, place) placement, posture] 1 A bodily posture or arrangement of bodily parts, such as one maintained by or imposed upon a patient in the course of a particular diagnosis or treatment. 2 In obstetrics, the bodily posture or attitude of the fetus in relation to the pelvis of the mother. **acromion anterior p.** A shoulder presentation of the fetus prior to delivery where the scapula faces towards the anterior portion of the mother's pelvis, called *acromion left* (or *right*) *anterior position* depending on whether the fetal scapula faces the left (or right) portion of the mother's pelvis. Also *scapuloanterior position, scapula anterior position.* **acromion posterior p.** A shoulder presentation of the fetus prior to delivery where the scapula faces towards the posterior portion of the mother's pelvis, called *acromion left* (or *right*) *posterior position* depending on whether the fetal scapula faces the left (or right) portion of the mother's pelvis. Also *scapuloposterior position, scapula posterior position.* **anatomical p.** The recognized orientation of the human body for standardizing description of parts, positions, and relationships according to anatomical nomenclature, namely, the erect position with the upper limbs pendent and the eyes, palms of the hands the toes facing forward. **Bozeman's p.** A position in which the patient rests on the knees and elbows (the knee-elbow position) and is supported by straps. **bronchoscopic p.** A position with the neck extended for passage of a rigid bronchoscope. **brow anterior p.** A brow presentation in which the fetal brow points towards the mother's symphysis pubis, called *brow left anterior position,* or *left frontoanterior position* (LFA), if the fetal brow is directed slightly to the left of the midline of the symphysis pubis, and *brow right anterior position,* or *right frontoanterior position* (RFA), if slightly to the right. Also *frontal anterior position, frontoanterior position.* **brow posterior p.** A brow presentation in which the fetal brow points towards the mother's sacrum, called *brow left posterior position,* or *left frontoposterior position* (LFP), if the fetal brow is directed slightly to the left of the midline of the sacrum, and *brow right posterior position,* or *right frontoposterior position* (RFP), if slightly to the right. Also *frontal posterior position, frontoposterior position.* **brow transverse p.** A brow presentation in which the fetal brow points towards one side of the maternal pelvis. It is called *brow left transverse position,* or *left frontotransverse position* (LFT), when the fetal brow is directed toward the left portion of the mother's pelvis and the chin toward the right portion, and *brow right transverse position,* or *right frontotransverse position* (RFT), when the fetal brow is directed toward the right portion of the mother's pelvis and the chin toward the left portion. Also *frontal transverse position, frontotransverse position.* **cadaveric p.** The position of the completely paralyzed vocal cord midway between adduction and abduction. **Casselberry's p.** A prone position which allows a patient, after intubation, to drink without risking entry of the liquid into the tube. **centric p.** The position of the mandible in which the condyles are in the most posterior unstrained position and in an established vertical relationship to the maxilla. Also *centric relation, unstrained jaw relation.* **cis p.** See under CIS. **coiled p.** A position in which the patient lies on one side with knees bent and thighs drawn up close to the chest. **decerebrate p.** DECEREBRATE POSTURE. **decorticate p.** DECORTICATE POSTURE. **decubitus p.** See under DECUBITUS. **Depage's p.** A prone position in which the pelvis is raised so that the trunk and legs form an inverted V. **depressive p.** The level of psychological development during which the child is said to fear destroying and then losing the beloved and indispensable object. The depressive position is at its peak around the sixth month of life. **dorsal p.** The position of lying on one's back; a supine position. **dorsal elevated p.** The dorsal position with head and shoulders elevated. **dorsal recumbent p.** A supine posture with lower limbs flexed and rotated outward. **dorsal rigid p.** The dorsal position with the knees bent and the thighs drawn up to the chest. **dorsosacral p.** A dorsal position in which both the thighs and calves are in a flexed position. Also *lithotomy position.* **Duncan's p.** The position of the placenta with its uterine surface at the vaginal introitus at the time of placental delivery. **eccentric p.** The position of the mandible relative to the maxilla when one or both condyles are in a forward position. Also *eccentric relation.* **Edebohls p.** A dorsal position, the knees and thighs drawn up, legs flexed on thighs and thighs flexed on the belly, the hips raised and the thighs abducted. Also *Simon's position.* **electrical heart p.** The position of the heart as determined by the electrical axis in the frontal plane. Also *heart position.* **Elliot's p.** A supine position facilitating surgery on the kidney system, in which the costal margin is elevated by a posteriorly placed support. **emprosthotonos p.** See under EMPROSTHOTONOS. **English p.** LATERAL RECUMBENT POSITION. **flipper p.** [from the superficial resemblance to the normal posture of the flippers of a seal] DECEREBRATE POSTURE. **Fowler's p.** A dorsal position in which the knees and the head and shoulders are elevated, thus forming a V with the pelvis at the apex. **frontal anterior p.** BROW ANTERIOR POSITION. **frontal posterior p.** BROW POSTERIOR POSITION. **frontal transverse p.** BROW TRANSVERSE POSITION. **frontoanterior p.** BROW ANTERIOR POSITION. **frontoposterior p.** BROW POSTERIOR POSITION. **frontotransverse p.** BROW TRANSVERSE POSITION. **p. of function** The attitude adopted by the hand when gripping a small object in the palm. The metacarpophalangeal joints and interphalangeal joints are semiflexed and the wrist is dorsiflexed. **genucubital p.** KNEE-ELBOW POSITION. **genufacial p.** A position in which the patient rests on the knees and face. **genupectoral p.** KNEE-CHEST POSITION. **heart p.** ELECTRICAL HEART POSITION. **high pelvic p.** TRENDELENBURG'S POSITION. **hinge p.** The position of the condyle which permits of a purely hinge movement, the condyle being in the glenoid fossa. Also *terminal hinge position.* **horizontal p.** A dorsal position with legs extended. **intercuspal p.** The position of the mandible when the teeth are in centric occlusion. **jackknife p.** A position in which the patient is on his back, with shoulders elevated, legs flexed, and thighs perpendicular to the abdomen. It is used for urethral instrumentation. **knee-chest p.** A position in which the patient rests on the knees and chest. Also *genupectoral position.* **knee-elbow p.** A position in which the patient rests on the knees and elbows. Also *genucubital position.* **kneeling-squatting p.** A squatting position in which the body is erect with the thighs pressed against the abdomen. **lateral recumbent p.** The position of a patient lying on one side with the underarm behind the back and with both the hips and the knees flexed, with the greater degree of flexion being in the topmost leg. Also *English position, obstetrical position.* **lateroabdominal p.** A position of resting on one side, the thigh and knee drawn up. **leapfrog p.** A stooping position for rectal examination, resembling the characteristic position in the game of leapfrog. **ligamentous p.** The position of the mandible when tooth contact occurs in the retruded arc of closure. **lithotomy p.** DORSOSACRAL POSITION. **Mayo-Robson p.** ROBSON'S POSITION. **mentum anterior p.** A face presentation in which the fetal chin points towards the mother's symphysis pubis, called *mentum left anterior position,* or *left mentoanterior position* (LMA), if the fetal chin is directed slightly to the left of the midline of the symphysis pubis, and *right mentum anterior position,* or *right mentoanterior position,* (RMA), if slightly to the right. Also *mentoanterior position.* **mentum posterior p.** A face presentation in which the fetal chin points towards the mother's sacrum, called *mentum left posterior position,* or *left mentoposterior position* (LMP), if the fetal chin is directed slightly to the left of the midline of the sacrum, and *mentum right posterior position,* or *right mentoposterior position* (RMP), if slightly to the right. Also *mentoposterior position.* **mentum transverse p.** A face presentation in which the fetal chin points towards one side of the maternal pelvis, called *mentum left transverse position,* or *left mentotransverse position* (LMT), if the fetal chin is directed towards the left side, and *mentum right transverse position,* or *right mentotransverse position* (RMT), if directed towards the right. Also *mentotransverse position.* **nuchal hitch p.** The fetal position with one or both arms extended behind the head during a breech delivery. **obstetrical p.** LATERAL RECUMBENT POSITION. **occiput anterior p.** A vertex presentation of the fetus during labor with the occiput directed towards the mother's symphysis pubis and the chin towards the sacrum, called *occiput left anterior position,* or *left occipitoanterior position* (LOA), if the fetal occiput is directed slightly to the left of the midline of the symphysis pubis, and *occiput right anterior position,* or *right occipitoanterior position* (ROA), if slightly to the right. Also *occipitoanterior position.* **occiput posterior p.** A vertex presentation of the fetus during labor with the occiput directed towards the mother's sacrum and the chin towards the symphysis pubis, called *occiput left posterior position,* or *left occipitoposterior position* (LOP), if the fetal occiput is directed slightly to the left of the midline of the sacrum, and *occiput right posterior position,* or *right occipitoposterior position* (ROP), if slightly to the right. Also *occipitoposterior position, occipitosacral position.* **occiput sacral p.** OCCIPUT POSTERIOR POSITION. **occiput transverse p.** A vertex presentation of the fetus during labor with the occiput directed towards one side of the maternal pelvis. It is called *occiput left transverse position,* or *left occipitotransverse position* (LOT), when the fetal occiput is directed towards the left side, and *occiput right transverse position,* or *right occipitotransverse position* (ROT), when directed towards the right. Also *occipitotransverse position.* **occlusal p.** The position of the mandible when the teeth are in maximum contact. **opisthotonos p.** See under OPISTHOTONOS. **orthopnea p.** A position, assumed for relief of orthopnea, in which the patient sits leaning forward propped up by his arms. **orthotonos p.** See under ORTHOTONOS. **persistent occiput posterior p.** The position of the fetus in a vertex presentation in which there is no spontaneous rotation from an occiput posterior position to an occiput transverse or occiput anterior position during the course of labor. **physiologic rest p.** REST POSITION. **primary p. of gaze** The orientation of an eye in straight-ahead gaze, when the head is also oriented in a straight-ahead position. **prone p.** A position in which the patient lies face down. **protrusive p.** The position of the mandible in cases of normal occlusion when the incisors are in edge-to-edge occlusion. **rest p.** The position of the mandible relative to the maxilla when the patient is sitting or standing upright and the muscles of mastication are relaxed. It corresponds with the most posterior unstrained position of the condyles. Also *physiologic rest position.* **Robson's p.** A position that enhances exposure for surgery on the biliary system in which a sandbag is placed posteriorly below the right costal margin. **Rose p.** A dorsal position with the head hanging over the end of the table in full extension to prevent aspiration of blood, such as during oral surgery. **sacrum anterior p.** A breech presentation in which the fetal sacrum points towards the mother's symphysis pubis, called *left sacrum anterior position,* or *left sacroanterior position* (LSA), when the fetal sacrum is directed slightly to the left of the midline of the symphysis pubis, and *right sacrum anterior position,* or *right sacroanterior position* (RSA), when directed slightly to the right. Also *sacroanterior position.* **sacrum posterior p.** A breech presentation in which the fetal sacrum points towards the mother's sacrum, called *left sacrum posterior position,* or *left sacroposterior position* (LSP), when the fetal sacrum is directed slightly to the left of the midline of the maternal sacrum, and *right sacrum posterior position,* or *right sacroposterior position* (RSP), when directed slightly to the right. Also *sacroposterior position.* **sacrum transverse p.** A breech presentation in which the fetal sacrum points towards one side of the maternal pelvis. It is called *sacrum left transverse position,* or *left sacrotransverse position* (LST), when the fetal sacrum is directed towards the left side, and *sacrum right transverse position,* or *right sacrotransverse position* (RST), when directed towards the right. Also *sacrotransverse position.* **scapula anterior p.** ACROMION ANTERIOR POSITION. **scapula posterior p.** ACROMION POSTERIOR POSITION. **scapuloanterior p.** ACROMION ANTERIOR POSITION. **scapuloposterior p.** ACROMION POSTERIOR POSITION. **scorbutic p.** The position adopted by an infant with advanced scurvy and pseudoparalysis of the legs. The infant is supine, with hips externally rotated and semiflexed and with knees semiflexed. **semiprone p.** The position of lying on the left side with the right knee and thigh drawn up while the left leg is kept straight. Also *Sims position.* **Simon's p.** EDEBOHLS POSITION. **Sims p.** SEMIPRONE POSITION. **supine p.** A position in which the patient lies on the back with face up. **terminal hinge p.** HINGE POSITION. **trans p.** See under TRANS. **Trendelenburg's p.** A position in which the subject lies supine with the knees, higher than the rest of the body, hanging over the edge of a supporting surface and forming the apex of a right angle so that the body forms an inverted V with the pelvis elevated above the head. Also *high pelvic position.*

**positioner** \pəzish′ənər\ A removable appliance for effecting minor tooth movement and retention at the end of orthodontic treatment. It consists of a thin resilient cover for the whole arch. Also *tooth positioner.*

**positive** [L *positiv(us)* (from *posit(us),* past part. of *ponere* to place, set + *-ivus* -IVE) arbitrarily imposed] **1** Indicating one of two opposing values (the other being negative) considered to have significantly more of a given property or characteristic than the other value. **2** Characterized by or signifying the presence of a condition, especially one being tested, or the occurrence of a particular response. **3** A positive finding or result. **biologic false p.** A false positive serologic test result due to cross-reactive material in the serum rather than to technical error. It reflects the imperfect specificity of the test procedure, especially in serologic tests for syphilis. **false p.** A test result that is positive when the correct result would be negative.

**positronium** \päs′itrō′nē·əm\ An unstable and extremely short-lived combination of an electron and a positron.

**posologic** \päsəläj′ik\ Pertaining to dosage of a drug.

**posology** \pəsäl′əjē\ [Gk *poso(s)* how much?, how great? + -LOGY] The science of dosage. Adj. posologic.

**Possum** [*p(atient-)o(perated) s(elector) m(echanism)*] A proprietary name for a device selector switch and controller to assist the disabled that is actuated by a patient-operated switch. For example simple respiratory movements into a puff-and-sip switch enable the patient to turn on appliances, use the telephone, and type a letter.

**post** [Old English, from common West Germanic, from L *postis* a door post] **1** A supporting part underlying a podiatric orthotic device. **2** DOWEL. **implant p.** NECK OF IMPLANT SUBSTRUCTURE.

**post-** \pōst-\ [L *post* after, behind] A prefix meaning (1) situated behind, posterior; (2) subsequent to, next after.

**postabortal** \-əbôr′təl\ Following an abortion.

**postacidotic** \-as′idät′ik\ Following acidosis.

**postanesthetic** \-an′esthet′ik\ Referring to the recovery period after general or local anesthesia.

**postapoplectic** \-ap′əplek′tik\ Following apoplexy.

**postauditory** \-ô′ditôr′ē\ Continuing or occurring after cessation of the relevant auditory stimulus.

**postaxial** \-ak′sē·əl\ Behind or caudal to an axis, usually used in reference to the region of a developing embryonic limb situated caudal to its longitudinal or median axis.

**postbrachial** \-brā′kē·əl\ Denoting segmental levels caudal or inferior to the brachial plexus, especially in designating the level of spinal cord injury.

**postbulbar** \-bul′bər\ Caudal to the medulla oblongata.

**postcapillary** \-kap′iler′ē\ **1** Beyond the capillaries. **2** VENOUS CAPILLARY.

**postcardinal** \-kär′dinəl\ Pertaining to one of the pair of veins which drain the posterior parts of an embryo and which unite with the anterior cardinal veins to form the common cardinal veins entering the sinus venosus.

**postcardiotomy** \-kär′dē·ät′əmē\ Following a cardiac operation.

**postcava** \-kā′və\ VENA CAVA INFERIOR.

**postcaval** \-kā′vəl\ Relating to the inferior vena cava.

**postcecal** \-sē′kəl\ **1** Behind the cecum; retrocecal. **2** In the colon distal to the cecum.

**postcentral** \-sen′trəl\ Behind a center or central region: said of the gyrus and sulcus behind the central sulcus of the cerebral hemisphere.

**postchroming** \-krō′ming\ The treatment with potassium dichromate of material already fixed or stained with some other substance.

**postcibal** \-sī′bəl\ Following the ingestion of food.

**post cibum** [L *post* after + *cibum,* accus. of *cibus* food] After meals: used in prescription writing.

**postcisterna** \-sistur′nə\ CISTERNA CEREBELLOMEDULLARIS.

**postcoital** \-kō′itəl\ Occurring after coitus or pertaining to the period following coitus. Also *postcoitus.*

**post coitum** \pōst kō′itəm\ After sexual intercourse.

**postcoitus** \-kō′itəs\ [POST- + COITUS] POSTCOITAL.

**postconceptual** \-kənsep′shoo·əl\ Occurring after conception.

**postcondylare** \-kän′dilar′ē\ BOLTON POINT.

**postconvulsive** \-kənvul′siv\ POSTEPILEPTIC.

**postcornu** \-kôr′noo\ CORNU POSTERIUS VENTRICULI LATERALIS.

**postcranial** \-krā′nē·əl\ Behind or below the skull, usually used to denote the skeletal parts below (in humans) or behind (in quadrupeds) the head.

**postdamming** \pōst′daming\ The act of creating a posterior palatal seal.

**postdicrotic** \-dīkrät′ik\ Following the dicrotic segment of the pulse wave.

**postdiphtheritic** \-difthərit′ik\ Occurring after or as a sequel to diphtheria. Also *postdiphtheric.*

**postductal** \-duk′təl\ Beyond the insertion of the ductus arteriosus into the descending aorta: often used to describe the site of the common type of coarctation of the aorta.

**postembryonic** \-em′brē·än′ik\ Occurring after the embryonic period in development, which ends in humans at the eighth week of intrauterine life when the fetal period commences.

**postencephalitic** \-ensef′əlit′ik\ Following encephalitis.

**postepileptic** \-ep′ilep′tik\ Following an attack of epilepsy. Also *postconvulsive.*

**posteriad** \pästir′ē·ad\ Toward the posterior surface of a body, part, or organ; posteriorly.

**posterior** \pästir′ē·ər\ [L (comparative of *posterus* following, next, from *post* after, behind), later, following after] **1** Pertaining to the hind parts of a body or to the back surface of a body or part. **2** Situated behind or to the rear of other comparable structures or parts. Also *posticus* (older term). • In human anatomy, *posterior* is used with reference to the "anatomical position" and corresponds roughly to *dorsal.*

**postero-** \päs′tərō-\ [L *posterus* coming after, following, next] A combining form meaning posterior.

**posteroanterior** \-antir′ē·ər\ **1** Directed or oriented back to front. **2** Characterizing an x-ray projection in which the radiation beam enters the back of the patient and the film is close to the front of the patient. Abbr. P-A

**posteroclusion** \päs′təräkloo′zhən\ [POSTERO- + *(oc)clusion*] MANDIBULAR RETRUSION.

**posteroexternal** \-ikstur′nəl\ *Outmoded* POSTEROLATERAL.

**posterointernal** \-intur′nəl\ *Outmoded* POSTEROMEDIAL.

**posterolateral** \-lat′rəl\ Behind and to the lateral side. Also *posteroexternal* (outmoded).

**posteromedial** \-mē′dē·əl\ Behind and to the medial side. Also *posterointernal* (outmoded).

**posteromedian** \-mē′dē·ən\ Behind and in the midline of a body, organ, or part.

**posterosuperior** \-səpir′ē·ər\ Both behind and above.

**posterotemporal** \-tem′pərəl\ Pertaining to or located in the posterior part of the temporal bone or lobe of the cerebrum.

**postesophageal** \-ē′səfā′jē·əl\ Behind the esophagus; retroesophageal.

**postexposure** \-ikspō′zhər\ Following exposure; designating conditions or developments after exposure.

**postfebrile** \-feb′rəl\ Occurring after a fever. Also *metapyretic.*

**postganglionic** \-gang′glē·än′ik\ Denoting the nerve cells and unmyelinated nerve fibers arising from autonomic ganglia innervating smooth and cardiac muscle and glands.

**postglomerular** \-glōmer′yələr\ Located or taking place distal to the glomerulus.

**posthemiplegic** \-hem′iplē′jik\ Following hemiplegia.

**posthepatic** \-hepat′ik\ **1** Behind the liver. **2** Pertaining to venous outflow from the liver.

**posthepatitic** \-hep′ətit′ik\ Occurring after the resolution of hepatitis.

**postherpetic** \-hərpet′ik\ Occurring after or as a consequence of herpes zoster or a herpes simplex infection.

**posthioplasty** \päs′thē·ōplas′tē\ [Gk *posthio(n),* dim. of *posthē* penis, prepuce + -PLASTY] A plastic operation on the prepuce. Adj. posthioplastic.

**posthippocampal** \-hip′əkam′pəl\ Situated behind the hippocampus.

**posthitis** \pästhī′tis\ [Gk *posth(ē)* penis, prepuce + -ITIS] Inflammation of the prepuce.

**postholith** \päs′thəlith\ [Gk *posth(ē)* penis, foreskin + *o* + -LITH] PREPUTIAL CONCRETION.

**posthumous** \päs′chəməs\ [L *postumus* (superl. of *posterus* subsequent, next, future) last, last-born, born after the father's death, final. Later L *posthumus* posthumous derives by folk etymology from *post* after + *humus* earth] **1** Arising or occurring after death. **2** Describing a child born by cesarean section following its mother's death.

**posthypoglycemic** \-hī′pōglīsē′mik\ Occurring as a result of or following hypoglycemia.

**posthypoxic** \-hipäk′sik\ Following hypoxia.

**postictal** \-ik′təl\ Following an ictus.

**posticus** \päs′tikəs\ *Older term* POSTERIOR.

**postinfective** \-infek′tiv\ Following an infection.

**postmalarial** \-məler′e·əl\ Occurring after malaria. Also *postpaludal.*

**postmature** \-mətyoor′\ [POST- + MATURE] Having a prolonged gestation such that postmaturity is a possible outcome.

**postmaturity** \-mətyoor′itē\ [POST- + MATURITY] An obstetric syndrome characterized by a duration of gestation longer than 42 weeks, with skin and nutritional changes present in the fetus that are thought to represent sequelae of diminished placental function.

**postmaxillary** \-mak′siler′ē\ **1** Situated behind the maxilla. **2** Pertaining to the posterior part of the maxilla: applied to one of the two main centers of ossification which develop in membrane on the surface of the nasal capsule to formthe maxilla. Situated behind that of the os incisivum (premaxilla), it develops an external facial (zygomatico-orbital) process and a medial one to form the palatine process.

**postmediastinal** \-mē′dē·astī′nəl, -mē′dē·as′tənəl\ **1** Pertaining to the posterior mediastinum. **2** Behind the mediastinum.

**postmediastinum** \-mē′dē·astī′nəm\ MEDIASTINUM POSTERIUS.

**postmeiotic** \-mī·ät′ik\ Following or occurring after meiosis.

**postmenopausal** \-men′əpô′səl\ Occurring after menopause.

**postmitotic** \-mītät′ik\ Following or occurring after mitosis.

**postmortal** \-môr′təl\ [POST- + MORTAL] POSTMORTEM.

**post mortem** \pōst môr′təm\ [L *post* after + *mortem,* accus. of *mors* death] After death.

**postmortem** \-môr′təm\ [L *post mortem* after death] **1** Pertaining to or occurring in the period following death. Also *postmortal.* **2** AUTOPSY.

**postnaris** \-ner′is\ CHOANA.

**postnatal** \-nā′təl\ [POST- + NATAL[1]] Occurring after birth or pertaining to the period following birth.

**postneuritic** \-n$^y$urit′ik\ Following neuritis.

**postoperative** \-äp′ərətiv\ Occurring or done after a surgical operation.

**postovulatory** \-äv′yələtôr′ē\ Following ovulation: said of a phase of the menstrual cycle.

**postpaludal** \-pal′yədəl\ POSTMALARIAL.

**postparalytic** \-per′əlit′ik\ Following paralysis.

**post partum** \pōst pär′təm\ [L *post* after + *partum* (accusative of *partus,* substantive from past part. of *parere* to bear or bring forth young) a bringing forth, birth] After childbirth.

**postpartum** \-pär′təm\ [English adj. from the L adverbial phrase *post partum* after giving birth] Occurring after childbirth or pertaining to the period following delivery or childbirth.

**postphlebitic** \-flebit′ik\ Following phlebitis.

**postpituitary** \-pit′$^y$oo′iter′ē\ Of, pertaining to, or arising from the posterior lobe of the pituitary gland.

**postpleuritic** \-plurit′ik\ Following pleurisy.

**postpneumonic** \-n$^y$oomän′ik\ Following pneumonia.

**postpontile** \-pän′til\ Caudal to the pons.

**postprandial** \-pran′dē·əl\ Occurring after a meal, especially after dinner.

**postpyramidal** \-pīram′idəl\ Caudal to the decussation of the pyramidal tract.

**postrenal** \-rē′nəl\ **1** Behind the kidney. **2** In the urinary tract distal to the kidney.

**postrolandic** \-rōlan′dik\ Posterior to the sulcus centralis cerebri (fissure of Rolando); postcentral.

**postscarlatinal** \-skär′lətī′nəl\ Occurring after or as a consequence of scarlet fever.

**post sing. sed. liq.** *post singulas sedes liquidas* (L, after every loose stool).

**postsphenoid** \-sfē′noid\ The posterior part of the body of the embryonic sphenoid, of which the centers of ossification are distinct from those of the anterior part (presphenoid). There are eight centers of ossification in the postsphenoidal part which eventually give rise to the basisphenoid, the greater wings and the pterygoid plates.

**postsphygmic** \-sfig′mik\ Occurring after the completion of the pulse wave.

**poststenotic** \-stenät′ik\ Distal to a stenosis.

**postsylvian** \-sil′vē·ən\ Caudal to the sylvian (lateral) fissure.

**postsynaptic** \-sinap′tik\ Situated or occurring distal to a synapse.

**postsystolic** \-sistäl′ik\ Occurring after systole.

**post-tecta** \-tek′tə\ Distal to the duodenum.

**post-thrombotic** \-thrämbät′ik\ Occurring following thrombosis.

**post-traumatic** \-trômat′ik\ Occurring as a result of or following an injury.

**post-trematic** \-trēmat′ik\ Denoting any structure, such as a nerve, situated in the tissue caudal to, or behind, a gill slit.

**post-tussis** \-tus′is\ After a cough.

**postulate** \päs′tyəlāt\ [L *postulatum* (from *postulare* to claim, ask, demand, require, akin to *poscere* to ask earnestly) a demand, petition] An assumption proffered as an evident truth, especially because it is necessarily implied as a basis for an interpretation or theory. **Ehrlich's p.** SIDE CHAIN THEORY. **Koch's p.'s** KOCH'S LAW.

**posture** [Italian *postura* (from L *positura* a placing, situation, posture, from *positus*, past part. of *ponere* to lay, place, put) a posture, situation] The physical disposition of the body. **decerebrate p.** A posture assumed by a patient suffering a transverse lesion of the brainstem caudal to the superior colliculi. All four limbs are rigidly extended, the hands are usually clenched, the forearms pronated, and tonic neck reflexes are present. Also *decerebrate position, flipper position.* **decorticate p.** The position assumed by a subject with a transverse lesion of the brainstem above the superior colliculi. The arms are flexed at the elbows and the fists clenched, the legs are fully extended and rigid. Also *decorticate position.*

**postvaccinal** \-vak′sinəl\ Occurring after or as a consequence of vaccination.

**postvaccinial** \-vaksin′ē·əl\ Occurring after or as a consequence of vaccinia.

**postzone** \pōst′zōn\ [POST- + ZONE] A failure of agglutination or precipitation in circumstances of antigen excess. • The term was apparently designed to describe a phenomenon complementary to the prozone phenomenon, but the events are not comparable and the use of this term is misleading.

**postzoster** \-zäs′tər\ Occurring after or as a sequel to herpes zoster.

**potash** \pät′ash\ **sulfurated p.** Potassium polysulfides and potassium thiosulfate in a mixture that contains 12.8% sulfur in the form of sulfide. It is used as a source of sulfide in medicinal preparations, and as an external treatment of the skin for scabies, acne, and psoriasis. Also *potassa sulfurata.*

**potassa** \pōtas′ə\ **p. sulfurata** SULFURATED POTASH.

**potassemia** \pät′əsē′mē·ə\ HYPERKALEMIA.

**potassium** \pōtas′ē·əm\ Element number 19, having atomic weight 39.0983. The second lightest metal (after lithium) and the seventh element in abundance in the lithosphere, potassium is a soft, silvery metal of the alkali group. It decomposes on contact with water, forming the hydroxide. The valence is 1. There are two naturally occurring stable isotopes, the more abundant (93.1%) being potassium 39. The other is potassium 41 (6.88% natural abundance). A third naturally occurring isotope is potassium 40, with a half-life of $1.25 \times 10^9$ years. Six unstable synthetic isotopes have been identified. Potassium is an essential constituent of biologic systems. About 0.06% of the atoms in the human body are potassium atoms. The potassium ion is the principal cellular cation. Symbol: K

**potassium acid tartrate** CREAM OF TARTAR.

**potassium bitartrate** CREAM OF TARTAR.

**potassium ferricyanide** $K_3Fe(CN)_6$. Potassium hexacyanoferrate(III), a yellow-orange salt. It is commonly used as a mild oxidizing agent, as for iron(II) in heme and occasionally for thiol groups in proteins. • This substance is increasingly being called by its systematic name.

**potassium oxalate** A colorless water-soluble crystal that is used in reagents as a source of oxalic acid. It has anticoagulant properties and is a constituent of balanced-oxalate anticoagulant preparations.

**potassium penicillin G** PENICILLIN G POTASSIUM.

**potassium permanganate** A commonly used permanganate that dissolves in water to give a deep purple solution with strongly oxidizing properties. It has been used as a disinfectant.

**potassium phenoxymethyl penicillin** PENICILLIN V POTASSIUM.

**potassium sodium tartrate** $C_4H_4KNaO_6 \cdot 4H_2O$. An agent used therapeutically as a mild cathartic.

**potassium sorbate** $C_6H_7KO_2$. The potassium salt of 2,4-hexadienoic acid, used as a pharmaceutical preservative because of its ability to inhibit the growth of mold and yeast.

**potency** \pō′tənsē\ [L *potentia* (from *potens*, gen. *potentis*, pres. part. of *posse* to be able) power, ability] **1** The capacity of a drug to produce a strong physiologic effect. **2** The ability of a male to perform during sexual intercourse. **3** Inherent capacity to grow and develop, as an embryo or embryonic part. **prospective p.** All the developmental possibilities potentially available to an embryonic part. **reactive p.** The ability of an embryonic cell to respond normally to the influence of an inductor by the production of appropriate differentiated cell types. Also *competence.*

**potent** Endowed with effective power or strength.

**potential** [Late L *potentialis* (from *potentia* power, ability) powerful, capable, possible] The charge or change in charge between two points, measured in volts. In biological tissues these potentials arise primarily across cell membranes. **action p.** The propagated depolarization of nerve and muscle membrane; the potential propagated along nerve or muscle fibers. Also *action current, negative variation* (obs.). **after p.** See under AFTERPOTENTIAL. **average evoked p.** The electrical changes resulting from multiple action potentials of a nerve or group of nerve cells in response to stimulation. The effect of a single stimulus is difficult to detect in isolation because of its very low voltage, thus the stimulus is repeated hundreds of times and the changes of potential summed and averaged. Also *average evoked response.* **bioelectric p.** **1** The electromotive force existing between the inside and outside of a cell. **2** The varying electric potential which accompanies all biochemical processes, such as that recorded in an electrocardiogram or electroencephalogram. For defs. 1 and 2 also *biopotential.* **biotic p.** INTRINSIC RATE OF NATURAL INCREASE. **chemical p.** The partial molar Gibbs energy of a substance. It is analogous to a potential because, for example, the condition of equilibrium for a substance between two phases is that its partial molar Gibbs energies in the two phases should be equal. **cochlear microphonic p.** Recorded oscillatory voltage changes from the round window or scalae that reproduce the frequencies of acoustic stimulation. Also *Wever-Bray effect.* **compound action p.** The electrical signal recorded from a whole nerve when excited by a single electrical pulse, consisting of a sum of the impulses of axons, each conducting at a defined velocity. **demarcation p.** The voltage difference between the surface of a nerve or muscle and a cut or injured end, used in early studies as an approximate indication of the membrane potential. Also *injury potential.* **early vertex p.** MIDDLE LATENCY RESPONSE. **earth p.** The British term for GROUND POTENTIAL. **electrocortical p.** Any potential recorded directly from the cerebral cortex during electrocorticography. **electrotonic p.** A local, subthreshold, decremental, nonpropagated, passive spread of electrical current. **endocochlear p.** The sum of the negative and positive direct current electrical potentials in the endolymph and perilymph. **evoked p.** **1** A wave of depolarization, either propagated or stationary, induced by a stimulus acting on an excitable membrane like that of a muscle or nerve cell. **2** An electrical response recordable from the cerebral cortex upon stimulation of peripherally located receptors. Certain of these responses, such as the photic and auditory evoked potentials, are more localized and recordable over the cortical sensory receiving areas, and seem to reach the cerebral cortex over the classical afferent pathways for those modalities. Others are more diffuse and seem to be relayed through the nonspecific nuclei of the thalamus. Use of the evoked potential technique has allowed neuroscientists to map the cortical sensory receiving areas. Also *evoked response.* **evoked cortical p.'s** Electrical potentials which are recordable from the cerebral cortex or, using an averaging technique, from the overlying surface of the skull as the consequence of visual, auditory, or somatic stimuli. **excitatory postsynaptic p.** An electrical potential change characterized by a depolarization of the membrane of a postsynaptic neuron as the result of a threshold stimulus arising presynaptically. Abbr. EPSP **fasciculation p.** An electrical potential resembling a motor unit potential, which can be recorded in the electromyogram, and corresponding to spontaneous fasciculation, which can be observed clinically. **fibrillation p.'s** Spontaneous, small, spikelike potentials (20–300 μV) of irregular form and timing that appear in an individual muscle fiber within days or even hours after denervation. They are the electrical concomitant of fibrillation and may persist for months or until reinnervation. **generator p.** The graded potential which arises as the result of depolarization of a neural receptor resulting from any physical stimulus and which, when of sufficient amplitude, gives rise to an action potential. Also *receptor potential.* **giant p.** A motor unit potential observed in electromyography of higher than normal amplitude and longer than normal duration, observed when the total area occupied by a single motor unit is increased, as following reinnervation. **ground p.** The electric potential of a large body such as the earth which serves as a common return for an electrical circuit and is used as a standard reference for measurements. A term used chiefly in the U.S. Also *earth potential* (British usage). **hyperpolarizing p.** A membrane potential change toward the resting level, usually associated with inhibition. **inhibitory equilibrium p.** The membrane potential evoked in the postsynaptic neuron of an inhibitory synapse which is of insufficient intensity to cause either depolarization or hyperpolarization. **injury p.** DEMARCATION POTENTIAL. **late vertex p.** The changes in the vertex potential occurring at about 150 msec after an auditory stimulus. • The usage is ambiguous since there are other changes, of both theoretical and practical importance, which occur much later. **life p.** **1** The expectation of life for one individual according to his or her age. **2** The sum of the expectations of life of the members of a given population. **membrane p.** A voltage difference between two compartments separated by a membrane. A cell membrane generally has a membrane potential of 10–100 millivolts due to the differences in ion concentrations on the two sides of the membrane. Also *transmembrane potential.* **miniature endplate p.'s** Small (~0.5 mV) fluctuations of similar shape as endplate potentials, found only at the muscle endplate, randomly distributed in time, and believed to reflect the spontaneous quantal release of the neurotransmitter acetylcholine from the motor nerve ending. **morphogenetic p.** The appropriate developmental capacity of a region, determined as the result of fertilization of an ovum. **motor unit p.** The potential change in the electromyogram which accompanies the activation of a motor unit. **myopathic p.** An abnormal motor unit action potential, observed in myopathic conditions, having a smaller than normal amplitude and duration resulting from a dropout of motor fibers. **negative summating p.** The decrease in potential across the cochlear duct induced by acoustic stimulation. **Nernst p.** An electrical potential gradient across a membrane due to differences in ion concentration on the two sides of the membrane. The potential can be calculated with the Nernst equation. **nerve p.** In electromyographic recording using needle electrodes, a spike or wavelike potential arising from an intramuscular nerve branch. It must be distinguished from the more common potentials arising in the muscle tissue. **oxidation-reduction p.** A measure of the oxidizing and reducing strength of a system. It is the potential of an electrode that can accept electrons from the system or donate them to it, measured against a standard hydrogen electrode. Biologic values range from about −O.5 V at the most reducing to about +O.8 V at the most oxidizing. Also *redox potential, oxidoreduction potential.* **pacemaker p.** The diastolic depolarization characteristic of pacemaker cells in the heart. **polyphasic p.** An electromyographically observed muscle potential of more than four phases occurring as the summation of more than one potential source, seen most frequently following reinnervation. **polyspike p.** In electroencephalography, a complex pattern made up of several spikes, often of variable amplitude, following each other in rapid succession. **postsynaptic p.'s** The indication of synaptic transmission produced by voltage and conductance changes across the membrane of a postsynaptic neuron. **receptor p.** GENERATOR POTENTIAL. **redox p.** OXIDATION-REDUCTION POTENTIAL. **reinnervation p.'s** In electromyography, polyphasic and prolonged potentials produced by motor units that have been reinnervated. The atypical activity reflects abnormal clustering and increased numbers of muscle fibers in the reinnervated units. **reproductive p.** INTRINSIC RATE OF NATURAL INCREASE. **resting p.** The metabolically-dependent potential across a cell membrane when unexcited by an input or spontaneous activity. **ripple p.** The slight periodic variation of a nominally constant voltage potential. Also *ripple voltage.* **spike p.** The fast, initial component of the conducted action potential of neurons. **spinal evoked p.** The evoked potential recordable over the spinal column following the application of a sensory stimulus to an extremity. **streaming p.** The electrical potential created when flow occurs in a solution of charged particles. **summating p.** The direct current change in endocochlear potential arising during exposure to sound. **transmembrane p.** MEMBRANE POTENTIAL. **utricular DC p.** The direct current potential within the utricle, analogous to the endocochlear potential. **vertex p.** The changes of electrical potential resulting at the vertex as a result of an auditory or other stimulus, usually repeated many times. **visual evoked p.** The evoked potential which can be recorded from the scalp overlying the occipital cortex following one or more visual stimuli.

**potentialization** \pōten′shəlizā′shən\ The enhancement of drug effects by administering two drugs in combination so that the resulting action is greater than the sum of each component given by itself.

**potentiation** \pōten′shē·ā′shən\ [*potenti(a)* + -ATION] A phenomenon in which the effect produced when two agents act together is greater than the sum of their effects when they act separately. **paradoxical p.** POST-TETANIC POTENTIATION. **post-tetanic p.** A marked increase, often more than twofold, in the amplitude of the evoked muscle potential from a limb muscle which can be elicited by electrical stimulation of its motor nerve at tetanic rates (50 Hz or more). This is sometimes seen in myasthenia gravis but is much commoner in the myasthenic syndrome of Eaton and Lambert. Also *paradoxical potentiation.*

**potentiator** \pōten′shē·ātər\ A drug or agent that enhances the effects of another drug so that the combined effects of both are greater than the sum of the separate effects.

**potentiometer** \pōten′shē·äm′ətər\ **1** A three-terminal rheostat, or a resistor with an adjustable sliding contact that functions as an adjustable voltage divider. **2** A voltage-measuring instrument that uses a potentiometer to provide a known voltage that is balanced against an unknown voltage.

**potentize** \pō′təntīz\ **1** To cause a drug or agent to be more effective or potent. **2** In homeopathy, to increase the potency or efficacy of a drug by dilution.

**potion** [L *potio*, gen. *potionis* (from *potare* to drink), the act of drinking] A dose of a liquid medication, usually an amount in excess of a few milliliters, such as an ounce or two.

**potomania** \pō′tōmā′nē·ə\ [L *pot(us)*, past part. of *potare* to drink + *o* + -MANIA] **1** DIPSOMANIA. **2** *Obs.* DELIRIUM TREMENS.

**Pott** [Percivall *Pott*, English surgeon, 1713–1788] **1** Pott's disease. See under TUBERCULOUS SPONDYLITIS. **2** Pseudo-Pott's disease. See under DISEASE. **3** Pott's paralysis. See under PARAPLEGIA. **4** See under ABSCESS, CURVATURE, FRACTURE, DWARFISM. **5** Pott's puffy tumor. See under TUMOR.

**Potter** [Edith Louise *Potter*, U.S. pathologist, born 1901] See under FACIES.

**Potter** [Hollis Elmer *Potter*, U.S. radiologist, born 1880] Potter-Bucky diaphragm, Bucky-Potter diaphragm, Potter-Bucky grid. See under BUCKY DIAPHRAGM..

**Potter** [Irving White *Potter*, U.S. obstetrician, 1868–1956] Potter version. See under PODALIC VERSION.

**Potts** [Willis John *Potts*, U.S. pediatric surgeon, 1895–1968] **1** Potts-Smith-Gibson operation. See under POTTS OPERATION. **2** Potts clamps. See under CLAMP. **3** See under PROCEDURE.

**potus** \pō′təs\ [L (from *potare* to drink), a drinking, drink, potion] A potion.

**Pötzel** [Otto *Pötzel*, Austrian psychiatrist, 1877–1962] See under SYNDROME.

**pouch** [French *poche* (of Germanic origin) bag] A small pocketlike or saclike cavity. **abdominovesical p.** The region between the abdominal wall and the bladder. **allantochorionic p.'es** Pedunculated invaginations of the chorioallantois near the base of the pregnant uterine horn in the mare. They contain a greenish brown material, derived from the secretions and detritus of the subjacent endometrial cup, with a high content of pregnant mare serum gonadotropin. **anterior p. of Tröltsch** RECESSUS MEMBRANAE TYMPANI ANTERIOR. **branchial p.'es** PHARYNGEAL POUCHES. **Broca's p.** A rounded mass of fat and connective tissue surrounded by some elastic fibers, said to be situated in each labium majus. Also *pudendal sac.* **craniobuccal p.** CRANIOPHARYNGEAL POUCH. **craniopharyngeal p.** An ectodermal diverticulum which grows from the roof of the primitive mouth. Its distal end differentiates into the adenohypophysis, which includes pars anterior, pars intermedia, and pars tuberalis of the hypophysis, while its stalk usually loses connection with the stomodeum. Traces can occasionally be found, as a craniopharyngeal duct, which indicate the tract followed by the pouch. Also *Rathke's pouch, craniobuccal pouch, pituitary diverticulum.* **p. of Douglas** EXCAVATIO RECTOUTERINA. **gill p.** A lateral evagination of the pharynx of a vertebrate embryo. When the endoderm of the pharynx meets the overlying ectoderm and breaks down, an opening, the gill cleft, may form. **Hartmann's p.** A pouch at the junction of the gallbladder and the cystic duct. Also *ampulla of the gallbladder.* **Heidenhain p.** An experimentally constructed gastric pouch that is vagally denervated but sympathetically innervated. **hepatorenal p.** RECESSUS HEPATORENALIS. **hyomandibular p.** The first of the series of pharyngeal pouches of the vertebrate embryo, located between the mandibular and hyoid arches. **laryngeal p.** SACCULUS LARYNGIS. **Morison's p.** RECESSUS HEPATORENALIS. **paracystic p.** FOSSA PARAVESICALIS. **pararectal p.** The lateral portion of excavatio rectouterina. **paravesical p.** FOSSA PARAVESICALIS. **Pavlov p.** An experimentally constructed gastric pouch that receives both vagal and sympathetic nerve supplies. Also *miniature stomach, Pavlov stomach.* **pharyngeal p.'es** Paired sacculations of endoderm on the lateral aspects of the embryonic pharynx. Also *branchial pouches, visceral pouches.* See also BRANCHIAL FISTULA. **posterior p. of Tröltsch** RECESSUS MEMBRANAE TYMPANI POSTERIOR. **Prussak's p.** RECESSUS MEMBRANAE TYMPANI SUPERIOR. **Rathke's p.** CRANIOPHARYNGEAL POUCH. **rectouterine p.** EXCAVATIO RECTOUTERINA. **rectovaginal p.** EXCAVATIO RECTOUTERINA. **rectovesical p.** EXCAVATIO RECTOVESICALIS. **Seessel's p.** An endodermal diverticulum situated immediately behind the oral (buccopharyngeal) membrane and thus behind the ectodermal pouch of Rathke. Projecting upwards from the cephalic end of the foregut towards the brain, it may form a part of the hypophysis in some marsupials but in man it is considered to disappear entirely. **superficial perineal p.** SPATIUM PERINEI SUPERFICIALE. **uterovesical p.** EXCAVATIO VESICOUTERINA. **vesicouterine p.** EXCAVATIO VESICOUTERINA. **visceral p.'es** PHARYNGEAL POUCHES. **Willis p.** *Outmoded* OMENTUM MINUS. **Zenker's p.** HYPOPHARYNGEAL DIVERTICULUM.

**poudrage** \poodräzh′\ [French (from *poudrer* to powder,

from *poudre* dust, powder) act of powdering] The application of a powder to surfaces to promote fusion. **pleural p.** The instillation of a powder such as talc into the pleural space in order to promote fusion of the visceral and parietal pleurae.

**poultice** \pōl′tis\ [earlier *pultes,* from Med L *pultes* thick pap, from L *pultes,* pl. of *puls* a pap, from Gk *poltos* porridge] A folk remedy consisting of a soft, hot, moist application made of flour or similar vegetal substances and thought to have curative properties when applied to sores or inflamed body parts.

**pound** [Old English *pund,* from prehistoric Germanic source taken from L adverb *pondo* in weight, akin to *pondus* a weight and to *pondere* to weigh] **1** A unit of mass or weight equal to 16 ounces avoirdupois and 12 ounces troy. See under POUND AVOIRDUPOIS, POUND TROY. **2** See under IMPERIAL POUND. Symbol: lb • When *pound* is used without qualification it is usually taken to mean *pound avoirdupois.* **p. avoirdupois** A unit of mass or weight equal to 16 ounces or 7000 grains; 0.453 592 37 kilogram exactly: widely used for commercial trading in the United States and Great Britain. Symbol: lb **p. troy** A unit of mass or weight equal to 12 ounces or 5760 grains; 0.373 242 kilogram. Symbol: lb tr

**pound-force** The unit of force in the British gravitational system, equal to that force which, acting on a mass of one pound, will give to it an acceleration equal to the internationally agreed acceleration of free fall, 9.806 65 meters per second squared; 32.1740 feet per second squared approximately; 4.448 22 newtons. Symbol: lbf

**Poupart** [François *Poupart,* French anatomist and surgeon, 1661–1708] **1** See under LINE. **2** Poupart's ligament. See under LIGAMENTUM INGUINALE.

**Pourfour du Petit** [François *Pourfour du Petit,* French anatomist and surgeon, 1664–1741] Petit's canal. See under SPATIUM ZONULARE.

**povidone** 1-Ethenyl-2-pyrrolidinone homopolymer. It is used as a pharmaceutic aid because of its ability as a dispersing and suspending agent. It is also used in tablets as a binding and granulating material. Also *polyvinylpyrrolidone.*

**povidone iodine** Iodine complexed with povidone polymer, which releases iodine slowly and is effective as a topical anti-infective preparation.

**powder** [French *poudre* (from L *pulvis,* gen. *pulveris,* dust, powder) powder] A dry, finely ground, homogeneous dispersion of one or more substances for external or internal use. Some dry drugs are dispensed in single-dose, paper packets as powders. **absorbable dusting p.** A dusting powder composed primarily of cornstarch that is used inside surgical rubber gloves. **aluminum hydroxide p.** Dried aluminum hydroxide gel, a white, tasteless powder used externally as a dusting powder and internally as an antacid. Also *aluminum hydrate powder.* **blood-plasma p.** DRIED HUMAN PLASMA PROTEIN FRACTION. **compound effervescent p.'s** A mixture of sodium bicarbonate, potassium sodium tartrate, and tartaric acid, used as a cathartic. Also *Seidlitz powders.* **dusting p.** A fine, dry powder applied to the skin or mucous membranes as a medication or protective agent, containing talc, kaolin, or some similar compound. **impalpable p.** A powder composed of particles so fine that the individual fragments cannot be felt as distinct components. **Seidlitz p.'s** COMPOUND EFFERVESCENT POWDERS. **Sippy p. No. 1** A proprietary name for sodium bicarbonate and calcium carbonate powder. **Sippy p. No. 2** A proprietary name for sodium bicarbonate and magnesium oxide powder. **sodium bicarbonate and calcium carbonate p.** A powder which is a combination of precipitated calcium carbonate and sodium bicarbonate. This mixture is used for its antacid properties. It is widely used in combination with sodium bicarbonate and magnesium oxide powder in the treatment of peptic ulcers. **talcum p.** See under TALC. **tissue p.** A lyophilized preparation of homogenized tissue material often used as a nonspecific absorbent for fluorescent antibody preparations.

**power** [Old French *poeir* (from Vulgar L *potere* to be able, from L *potis* able) to be able, ability] **1** Ability to act; capability; strength. **2** The degree of magnification of a lens, expressed in diopters. **3** The rate of transfer or transformation of energy, expressed in watts. **acoustic p.** Acoustic energy transmitted per unit time. **buffering p.** The extent to which a buffer solution resists changes in pH, as measured by the inverse of the slope of a graph of pH change against concentration of added acid or alkali. **carbon dioxide-combining p.** An outdated test measuring the volume of carbon dioxide absorbed by plasma at a partial pressure of carbon dioxide of 40 millimeters of mercury. **defining p.** RESOLVING POWER. **dioptric p.** The property of an optical component or system to change the vergence of light, expressed in diopters. Converging is taken as positive (or plus) dioptric power and diverging as negative (or minus) dioptric power. For a thin lens, the dioptric power is equal to the reciprocal of the focal length in meters. Also *dioptric strength.* **resolving p.** The visual ability to discern detail. Also *defining power.* **stopping p.** **1** The ability of an absorber to attenuate or absorb incident radiation. **2** The energy lost per unit distance traveled by a charged particle in passing through matter.

**pox** [variant of *pocks,* pl. of *pock* (Old English *poc*) a pustule] **1** Any of various exanthematous diseases, especially those caused by viruses. **2** *Obs.* SYPHILIS. **chicken p.** VARICELLA. **cow p.** See under COWPOX. **Kaffir p.** ALASTRIM. **rickettsial p.** See under RICKETTSIALPOX. **wart p.** VARIOLA VERRUCOSA.

**Poxviridae** \päksvir′idē\ [POX + *vir(us)* + -IDAE] A family of very large, brick-shaped, double-stranded DNA viruses with complex morphology, including a central nucleoid surrounded by two membrane layers covered with tubules. They possess virion-associated enzymes, including a DNA-dependent RNA polymerase, nucleases, and ATPase. They are relatively resistant to chemical and physical inactivation. The family has been divided into the genera *Orthopoxvirus, Parapoxvirus, Avipoxvirus, Entomopoxvirus, Capripoxvirus,* and *Leporipoxvirus.*.

**poxvirus** \päksvī′rəs\ [POX + VIRUS] Any virus of the Poxviridae family. **p. bovis** COWPOX VIRUS. **p. muris** MOUSEPOX VIRUS. **p. myxomatis** MYXOMA VIRUS. **p. officinalis** VACCINIA VIRUS.

**$PP_i$** A symbol for free pyrophosphate (diphosphate).

***PP*** A symbol for the diphosphate group, usually used in combination. It is an abbreviation of the strictly constructed symbol *POP,* in which O is the atomic symbol, and *P* has its usual significance of $—PO_3H_2$, or —PO(OH)—, or their ionized forms.

**p.p.** **1** *punctum proximum* (L, near point of accommodation: as it pertains to vision). **2** *post prandium* (L, after meals). **3** post partum.

**ppb** parts per billion.

**PPCA** proserum prothrombin conversion accelerator (factor VII).

**PPCF** plasmin prothrombin converting factor (factor V).

**PPD** purified protein derivative (of tuberculin).

**PPD-Seibert** PURIFIED PROTEIN DERIVATIVE OF TUBERCULIN.

**ppGpp** 3′-pyrophosphoryl-guanosine-5′-diphosphate. A compound that represses the synthesis of ribosomal RNA in bacteria. It is synthesized on translating ribosomes that encounter a codon for which the aminoacyl-tRNA is not available. A 5′-triphosphate (ppGppp) is also formed.

**pphm** parts per hundred million.

**ppht** parts per hundred thousand.

**PPLO** pleuropneumonialike organism (mycoplasma).

**ppm** parts per million.

**PPO** 1 2,5-diphenyloxazole. 2 preferred provider organization.

**ppt.** precipitate.

**PQ** 1 plastoquinone. 2 permeability quotient.

**PR** 1 prosthion. 2 partial remission.

**Pr** 1 Symbol for the element, praseodymium. 2 production rate (of steroid hormones in blood or urine).

**p.r.** 1 *punctum remotum* (L, far point of accommodation: as it pertains to vision). 2 *per rectum* (L, by way of the rectum).

**PRA** plasma renin activity.

**practice** [Middle English *practik* (from Old French *practique*, from Med L *practica* from Gk *praktikē* practical science, from *praktikos* pertaining to action, effective; akin to *prassein* to accomplish, effect) practice, custom] 1 The conduct of one's professional activity. 2 Direct involvement in health care services, as distinguished from research, teaching, or administrative activities. **family p.** The practice of a family physician. This is a relatively recent field of specialization, not to be equated with general practice. Also *family medicine* (popular). **general p.** The practice of medicine by a physician, or occasionally by another health care professional such as a nurse, in which the provider does not specialize in any particular field within the profession. **group p.** A formal association of health care professionals, often physicians or dentists, providing services with the income from the practice pooled and redistributed to all members of the group according to a prearranged plan and in which all resources, such as facilities, personnel, and medical records, as well as expenses, are shared. **individual p.** SOLO PRACTICE. **prepaid group p.** An arrangement whereby a group of health care professionals, usually physicians, provides a defined set of services to individuals for a specified period of time according to a contractual agreement in return for a fixed periodic payment made in advance of the provision of services. **private p.** Medical or other health care practice in which the practitioner and the practice are independent of any external policy or managerial control. Private practitioners are usually self-employed or in an independent group practice. **solo p.** The lawful practice of a health care profession, such as medicine or dentistry, by a self-employed individual not associated in practice with other practitioners of the same profession. Also *individual practice*.

**practitioner** \praktish′ənər\ [from early English *practition*, variant of *practician* (from Med French *praticien* practitioner, from *pratique* execution of rules and principles) one qualified to practice + -ER] A provider of health care services, such as a physician, nurse, or dentist. **general p.** A health care professional such as a physician or dentist who does not specialize in any particular field of that profession, is not subject to specialty board certification, and who usually provides primary care. **indigenous p.** A health care provider such as a medicine man or shaman, who is not professionally trained or certified and who functions outside the established health care system but usually within the traditional system of an indigenous regional culture. Also *indigenous worker*. **nurse p.** See under NURSE-PRACTITIONER.

**Prader** [Andrea *Prader*, Swiss pediatrician, born 1919] Prader-Labhart-Willi syndrome. See under PRADER-WILLI SYNDROME.

**praeputium** \prēpyoo′shē·əm\ [L, the foreskin] PREPUTIUM.

**Praesapiens** \prēsā′pē·əns\ Characterizing a group of human fossils from the European Paleolithic represented by Swanscombe man and Fontéchevade man (and others according to various authors) which antedate the Neanderthalers yet are though to bear closer resemblances to modern *Homo sapiens* than to *H. neanderthalensis*.

**pragmatagnosia** \prag′matagnō′zhə\ [Gk *pragma*, gen. *pragmat(os)* a thing + AGNOSIA] A loss of ability to recognize objects that were once familiar.

**pragmatamnesia** \prag′matamnē′zhə\ [Gk *pragma*, gen. *pragmat(os)* a thing + AMNESIA] The inability to remember what objects look like.

**pramoxine** $C_{17}H_{27}NO_3$. 4-[3-(4-Butoxyphenoxy)propyl]-morpholine, a local anesthetic agent that is usually used as the hydrochloride. Its potency is approximately equal to that of benzocaine.

**prandial** \pran′dē·əl\ [L *prandi(um)* breakfast, luncheon + -AL] Pertaining to a meal, especially a dinner.

**praseodymium** \prā′zē·ōdim′ē·əm\ Element number 59, having atomic weight 140.9077. It is a soft, silvery, ductile metal belonging to the lanthanide series. Symbol: Pr

**p. rat. aetat.** *pro ratione aetatis* (L, in proportion to age).

**pratique** \prätēk′, prat′ik\ [French (from Med L *practica* practice, intercourse, dealings) permission for a ship to enter and do business at a port] An official document stating that an incoming ship or airplane has been freed of quarantine requirements.

**Prausnitz** [Carl Willy *Prausnitz*, German bacteriologist, born 1876] Prausnitz-Küstner test. See under PRAUSNITZ-KÜSTNER REACTION.

**praxis** \prak′sis\ [Gk *praxis* a doing, acting, a certain state] Acquisition of the ability to perform skilled movements. Loss of such skills in the absence of paralysis is known as *apraxia*.

**praziquantel** $C_{19}H_{24}N_2O_2$. Hexylcarbonyl-1,2,3,6,7,11b-hexahydropyrazino[2,1-α]isoquinolin-4-one, an anthelmintic effective against tapeworm and schistosomiasis.

**prazosin** \praz′əsin\ $C_{19}H_{21}N_5O_4$. An antihypertensive agent that has been found useful on occasion in peripheral arterial vasospasm because of its vasodilatory effects. Also *furazosin*.

**pre-** \prē-, prə-\ [L *prae* before, prior] A prefix meaning (1) situated before, anterior; (2) prior to, preceding.

**preagonal** \prē·ag′ənəl\ Immediately preceding death. Also *preagonic*.

**pre-AIDS** See under ACQUIRED IMMUNE DEFICIENCY SYNDROME.

**prealbumin** [PRE- + ALBUMIN] *Obs.* TRANSTHYRETIN. • The name derives from the fact that its electrophoretic mobility is greater than that of albumin, but it was abandoned since the prefix *pre-* became largely restricted to designating precursors of proteins. **thyroxine-binding p.** A protein having a molecular weight of about 50 000, present in human plasma in a concentration of 25 mg per 100 ml. It binds plasma thyroxine to a single binding site. It accounts for no more than 25% of plasma protein binding of thyroxine under normal conditions, the major role being played by thyroxine-binding globulin. Abbr. TBPA

**preamplifier** \-am′plifī′ər\ A low-noise amplifier designed to amplify low-level signals, as from electrocardiographic electrodes or a blood-pressure transducer, to a level sufficient to drive a monitor or recorder.

**preanesthesia** \prē′anesthē′zhə\ PREANESTHETIC MEDICATION.

**preanesthetic** \prē′anesthet′ik\ Referring to the period before induction of general or local anesthesia.

**preaortic** \prē′ā·ôr′tik\ Situated anterior to the aorta.

**preaxial** \-ak′sē·əl\ Anterior to or cephalad to an axis: usually used in reference to the region of a developing embryonic limb situated cephalad to its longitudinal or median axis.

**prebase** \prē′bās\ The back of the dorsal surface of the tongue, situated just above the root, or base, in the anterior wall of the oral pharynx.

**prebetalipoproteinemia** \-bā′təlip′əprō′tēnē′mē·ə\ HYPERPREBETALIPOPROTEINEMIA.

**prebladder** \-blad′ər\ A space situated in front of the neck of the urinary bladder within the prostatic sheath. *Outmoded.*

**prebrachial** \-brā′kē·əl\ Denoting the brachium of the superior colliculus.

**prebrachium** \-brā′kē·əm\ BRACHIUM COLLICULI SUPERIORIS.

**precancer** \-kan′sər\ [PRE- + CANCER] **1** A lesion which becomes a cancer. **2** A condition associated with the later development of cancer. **3** A lesion with a tendency to become malignant.

**precancerosis** \-kan′sərō′sis\ A precancerous state or condition.

**precancerous** \-kan′sərəs\ [PRE- + CANCEROUS] Describing a lesion or condition which precedes a cancer, which develops into a cancer, or which has a high risk of becoming a cancer, such as actinic keratosis, xeroderma pigmentosum, or adenomatous polyposis coli. Also *premalignant.*

**precapillary** \-kap′iler′ē\ METARTERIOLE.

**precarcinogen** \-kär′sənəjən\ [PRE- + CARCINOGEN] A natural or synthetic compound that may become carcinogenic.

**precardinal** \-kär′dinəl\ Pertaining to the paired veins draining the cranial half of the early embryo into the common cardinal vein.

**precardium** \-kär′dē·əm\ PRECORDIUM.

**precartilage** \-kär′tilij\ Embryonic cartilaginous tissue giving rise to skeletal elements, formed from young connective tissue (mesenchyme) with nuclei arranged in straight rows one against the other and with each nucleus surrounded by cytoplasm of its own.

**precava** \-kā′və\ VENA CAVA SUPERIOR.

**precementum** \-simen′təm\ CEMENTOID.

**precentral** \-sen′trəl\ In front of a center, as, specifically, the precentral gyrus in front of the central sulcus of the cerebrum.

**precession** \prisesh′ən\ The slow gyration of the rotational axis of a spinning body about another intersecting axis such that the axis of the body describes a cone. This motion is caused by the application of a torque that tends to change the direction of the rotational axis.

**prechordal** \prēkôr′dəl\ Placed anterior to the embryonic notochord. Also *prochordal.*

**precipitant** \prisip′itənt\ An agent for precipitating a substance from solution. Protein precipitants include perchloric acid and trichloroacetic acid.

**precipitate** \prisip′itāt\ [L *praecipitatus* (from *praecipitare* to cause to fall or sink, from *praeceps* falling steeply, lit., head first, from *prae-* forward + *-ceps,* from *caput* head) fallen, sunken] **1** A solid formed from a substance in solution, sometimes by chemical reaction, and sometimes by an alteration of the solution so that the solubility of the substance falls. Likewise, a liquid formed in a gaseous medium is a precipitate. **2** To form or cause to form a precipitate. **alum p.** The material harvested when antigenically active proteins are adsorbed by exposure to aluminum-containing substances. When injected into an experimental animal, the adsorbed protein is a more effective immunogen than the native protein. **keratic p.'s** Small nodular clumps of cells deposited on the back surface of the cornea as a manifestation of severe uveitis. **mutton-fat keratic p.'s** Clumps of inflammatory cells on the posterior surface of the cornea. **pigmented keratic p.'s** Melanin debris on the posterior surface of the cornea.

**precipitation** \prisip′itā′shən\ [L *praecipitatio* a headlong fall. See PRECIPITATE.] **1** The formation and descent of solid particles from substances in solution; the act or process of precipitating. **2** IMMUNOPRECIPITATION. **electrostatic p. of dust** The removal of airborne dust particles by passing the air through an ionizing field maintained at high voltage. The particles become positively charged and adhere to earthed plates, where they accumulate and are removed by periodic washing. The method is used to remove smoke from chimney effluents and from gold mines that are free of explosive gases. In air pollution technology, the same principle is used in a device that determines the concentration of particles in the atmosphere. **isoelectric p.** The process of precipitating a substance, almost always a protein, by adjusting the pH of the solution to the isoelectric point of the substance, where it is least soluble. **salt p.** SALTING-OUT.

**precipitin** \-sip′itin\ An antibody that is detected by precipitation of the agent with which it reacts. *Older term.* Also *immunoprecipitin* (older term), *precipitating antibody* (outmoded). • Names like *precipitin* (as well as *agglutinin, lysin,* and *antitoxin*) were used to describe antibodies in terms of the reactions by which they were detected before it was realized that all the reactions are properties of immunoglobulins, albeit sometimes of different classes. Some of the names have remained in common use and some have not.

**precision** \prisizh′ən\ The reproducibility of a quantifiable result, expressed as variance or standard deviation.

**preclinical** \-klin′ikəl\ **1** Pertaining to the period, as of a disease, that precedes development of clinical signs and symptoms. **2** Pertaining to the period in medical education that precedes clinical training.

**preclival** \-klī′vəl\ Rostral to the clivus of the cerebellum.

**preclotting** \-klät′ing\ The immersion of a knitted vascular prosthesis in an amount of a patient's blood in order to fill the graft interstices with clot prior to insertion in the arterial system.

**precocious** \-kō′shəs\ [L *praecox,* gen. *praecocis* (from *praecoquere* to ripen prematurely, lit., to pre-cook) early-ripening, maturing too early] **1** Developing or occurring earlier than normal, as a physical characteristic or an ability. **2** Exhibiting such early development.

**precocity** \prikäs′itē\ [See PRECOCIOUS.] Exceptionally early or premature development of mental, physical, or sexual attributes. **heterosexual p.** Premature development of the secondary sexual characters opposite to those expected on the basis of the genetic sex of the child, as in precocious virilization in a girl or precocious thelarche in a boy. Compare ISOSEXUAL PRECOCITY. **isosexual p.** Premature development of the secondary sexual characters expected on the basis of the genetic sex of the child. Compare HETEROSEXUAL PRECOCITY. **sexual p.** PRECOCIOUS PUBERTY. **skeletal p.** Accelerated bone growth with early fusion of epiphyses, and attainment of physical maturity at a younger age than normal. **true sexual p.** PRECOCIOUS PUBERTY.

**precollagenous** \-kōlaj′inəs\ Of or relating to an early and incomplete stage in the development of collagen.

**precoma** \-kō′mə\ [PRE- + COMA] A state which precedes coma.

**precommissural** \-kəmish′ərəl\ Denoting a structure rostral to the cerebral anterior commissure as precommissural fornix.

**precommissure** \-käm′ishur\ CORNU ANTERIUS VENTRICULI LATERALIS.

**preconscious** \-kän′shəs\ The mental elements that are not in consciousness at any given moment but can be called into consciousness at will. Also *coconscious* (obs.).

**precordia** \-kôr′dē·ə\ PRECORDIUM.

**precordial** \-kôr′dē·əl\ Pertaining to the precordium.

**precordium** \-kôr′dē·əm\ That part of the chest wall which is anterior to the heart. Also *precardium, precordia, antecardium, anticardium.*

**precornu** \-kôr′noo\ CORNU ANTERIUS VENTRICULI LATERALIS.

**precritical** \-krit′ikəl\ Occurring before a crisis; preceding a crisis.

**precuneal** \-kyoo′nē·əl\ Rostral to the gyrus cuneus. Also *precunial.*

**precuneate** \-kyoo′nē·āt\ Pertaining to the gyrus precuneus.

**precuneus** \-kyoo′nē·əs\ [NA] A small, wedge-shaped convolution on the medial surface of the human cerebrum bounded rostrally by the paracentral lobule and caudally by the cuneus. Also *quadrate gyrus, quadrate lobule, quader, quadrate lobe of cerebral hemisphere.*

**precunial** \-kyoo′nē·əl\ PRECUNEAL.

**precursor** \-kur′sər\ [L *praecursor* (from *prae-* PRE- + *curs(us),* past part. of *currere* to run + *-or* -OR) one that goes before] Anything that precedes, produces, or develops into a specified thing, such as a less differentiated cell or a substance occurring in an earlier stage of a metabolic pathway. Thus, an erythroblast is a precursor of an erythrocyte, and $\beta$-carotene is a precursor of vitamin A. Also *antecedent.* **mast-cell p.** A mesenchymal cell that is capable of differentiating into a mast cell.

**predentin** \-den′tin\ [PRE- + DENTIN] A layer of unmineralized dentin adjacent to the pulp of a tooth. Also *dentinoid.*

**prediabetes** \-dī′əbē′tēz\ A condition presumed to be a forerunner of diabetes mellitus, in which carbohydrate intolerance can be demonstrated only by one or another provocative test and in which all the diagnostic criteria for diabetes mellitus are not yet established. Adj. prediabetic.

**predigestion** \-dijes′chən\ [PRE- + DIGESTION] The initiation of the processes of breaking down food elements prior to ingestion.

**predispose** \-dispōz′\ To make susceptible or vulnerable.

**predisposing** \-dispō′sing\ Increasing susceptibility, especially to disease.

**predisposition** \-dis′pəzish′ən\ Special susceptibility to a disease or disorder, as from genetic constitution or environmental influences. **convulsive p.** An inherent or acquired condition predisposing the patient to suffer generalized convulsive epileptic attacks (chiefly myoclonic or tonicoclonic) which may be precipitated by brain injury or disease. Predisposition to convulsions should not necessarily be equated with predisposition to epilepsy. Certain patients, such as some schizophrenics or hysterics, have a low convulsive threshold, without ever suffering a spontaneous epileptic attack. **epileptic p.** An inherent or acquired condition predisposing the patient to epileptic attacks when subjected to brain injury or disease. If the stimulus is transient and causes merely a transient cerebral dysfunction, it may give rise to one or several fortuitous epileptic attacks, as in hyperthermic convulsions in a predisposed infant, but if the stimulus causes permanent brain damage or a focal lesion, the result may be chronic epilepsy. This explains why certain subjects are more prone to develop epilepsy than are others when subjected to the same stimulus. This inherent tendency is often inherited. Predisposition to epilepsy should not be wholly equated with predisposition to convulsions. The convulsive threshold is often, but not always, lowered in epileptic patients.

**prednisolone** 11-$\beta$-17-$\alpha$-21-Trihydroxypregna-1,4-diene-3,20-dione. A semisynthetic glucocorticoid derived from cortisol. It is administered orally for the treatment of rheumatoid arthritis, allergic conditions, neoplastic and gastrointestinal diseases, and blood dyscrasias. It is a general anti-inflammtory medication. Also *metacortandralone.*

**prednisolone acetate** A white, crystalline powder which is the 21-acetate ester of prednisolone. It has an anti-inflammatory activity similar to that of prednisolone, and is administered by intra-articular or intramuscular routes.

**prednisolone butylacetate** PREDNISOLONE TEBUTATE.

**prednisolone sodium phosphate** The sodium phosphate ester salt of prednisolone. It is a white powder or granular material with the same actions and uses as prednisolone as an anti-inflammatory medication. It may be administered intravenously or intramuscularly for rapid effect, or may be applied topically.

**prednisolone-21-stearoylglycolate** $C_{41}H_{64}O_8$. Prednisolone with glycolic acid stearate, occurring as a white, crystalline powder soluble in alcohol, acetone, and methanol. It is a glucocorticoid, with a longer duration of action than prednisolone, and it is used in creams and ointments for external local application. Also *prednisolone steaglate.*

**prednisolone succinate** The succinate ester of prednisolone. It is a creamy white powder that, when mixed with sodium carbonate, forms prednisolone sodium succinate. The latter can be administered intravenously or intramuscularly to produce a rapid onset of anti-inflammatory activity.

**prednisolone tebutate** $C_{27}H_{38}O_6$. The butylacetate ester of prednisolone, which has the same properties and uses as the parent drug. It provides a prolonged effect and is suitable for intra-articular or intralesional injection. Also *prednisolone butylacetate.*

**prednisone** $C_{21}H_{26}O_5$. 17,21-Dihydroxypregna-1,4-diene-3,11,20-trione. A synthetic steroid with glucocorticoid activity and pronounced anti-inflammatory action. It is used in the treatment of rheumatoid arthritis and related conditions, asthma, and a variety of ocular inflammatory diseases, dermatoses, and allergic disorders. Also *metacortandracin.*

**predormital** \dôr′mitəl\ Occurring before sleep; hypnagogic.

**preductal** \-duk′təl\ Immediately proximal to the orifice of the ductus arteriosus in the aorta: often used to describe the site of one type of coarctation of the aorta.

**preeclampsia** \prē′iklamp′sē·ə\ [PRE- + ECLAMPSIA] An obstetric condition occurring in the second half of pregnancy, characterized by hypertension, proteinuria, and usually edema. The condition may develop before the 20th week in association with trophoblastic disease. It is usually a disorder of primigravidas. The renal lesion is characterized by swollen, glomerular, capillary, endothelial cells, often associated with deposition of fibrin aggregates. Renal blood flow and glomerular filtration rate are reduced. In severe cases, there may be associated diffuse intravascular coagulation with infarction of the kidney, liver, or other organs. The condition is self-limiting, in that delivery of the fetus and placenta results in improvement and a return to prepregnancy status. Also *preeclamptic toxemia, eclampsism.* See also ECLAMPSIA. Adj. preeclamptic. **superimposed p.** Preeclampsia superimposed on hypertensive or renal disease which preceded the pregnancy.

**preeclamptic** \prē′iklamp′tik\ Pertaining to or exhibiting signs of preeclampsia.

**preeruptive** \prē′irup′tiv\ Pertaining to the initial period after the development of an infection before the appearance of a characteristic rash or other eruption.

**preexcitation** \prē′eksītā′shən\ [PRE- + EXCITATION] The premature electrical activation of the myocardium due to accelerated conduction. It is an intrinsic feature of the Wolff-Parkinson-White syndrome, in which an anomalous accessory pathway bypasses the atrioventricular node and the physiological delay which this node imposes. **ventricular p.** Preexcitation of part of a ventricle as a result of an accessory pathway.

**pre-exposure** \-ikspō′zhər\ Prior to exposure; designating conditions or developments before exposure.

**prefibrotic** \-fībrät′ik\ Preceding the deposition of collagen, as in an inflammatory reaction.

**preformation** \-fôrmā′shən\ [PRE- + FORMATION] A theory according to which the adult forms of an animal or vegetable are already constituted in miniature within the ovum, and likewise in the ova of successive offspring. This theory is opposed to epigenesis, which is more generally accepted.

**prefrontal** \-frän′təl\ Pertaining to or affecting the anterior part of the frontal lobe.

**preganglionic** \-gang′glē·än′ik\ Denoting the neurons, and their axons, supplying a ganglion, generally referring to the motor neurons of the spinal cord whose myelinated fibers innervate the prevertebral and paravertebral autonomic ganglia.

**pregeniculatum** \-jənik′yəlā′təm\ The small nucleus in the external medullary lamina capping the thalamic lateral geniculate nucleus. *Outmoded.*

**pregenital** \-jen′ətəl\ See under PREGENITAL PHASE.

**preglomerular** \-glōmer′yələr\ Located or occurring proximal to the glomerulus.

**pregnancy** [See under PREGNANT.] The state of a female from the time of conception until delivery of the products of conception. Also *gravidity.* **abdominal p.** An ectopic pregnancy in which the fertilized ovum implants on a surface within the peritoneal cavity and the gestation develops within that same cavity. Also *intraperitoneal pregnancy, coeliocyesis.* **ampullar p.** A tubal ectopic pregnancy located in the ampulla of the fallopian tube. **angular p.** INTERSTITIAL PREGNANCY. **bigeminal p.** TWIN PREGNANCY. **broad ligament p.** An ectopic pregnancy located between the leaves of the broad ligament. Also *intraligamentous pregnancy.* **cervical p.** An ectopic pregnancy located at the uterine cervix. **combined p.** A twin pregnancy in which one is intrauterine and the other is an ectopic pregnancy. Also *heterotopic pregnancy, compound pregnancy.* **cornual p.** 1 An ectopic pregnancy which develops in a rudimentary horn of the uterus. 2 INTERSTITIAL PREGNANCY. **ectopic p.** A pregnancy in which implantation of the blastocyst and subsequent development occur outside the uterine cavity. Also *extrauterine pregnancy, exfetation.* **exochorial p.** An intrauterine pregnancy in which the fetus develops outside the chorionic sac. Also *membranous pregnancy.* **extra-amniotic p.** An intrauterine pregnancy in which the fetus develops within the chorion but, as a result of rupture in early pregnancy, the amnion shrinks until it is located only around the insertion of the umbilical cord into the placenta. **extrauterine p.** ECTOPIC PREGNANCY. **fallopian p.** TUBAL PREGNANCY. **false p.** PSEUDOCYESIS. **gemellary p.** TWIN PREGNANCY. **heterotopic p.** COMBINED PREGNANCY. **hydatid p.** A pregnancy in which a hydatidiform mole develops. **hysterical p.** PSEUDOCYESIS. **incomplete p.** A pregnancy which is not carried to term. **interstitial p.** An ectopic pregnancy that occurs in the interstitial portion of a fallopian tube. Also *angular pregnancy, mural pregnancy, intramural pregnancy, parietal pregnancy, cornual pregnancy.* **intraligamentous p.** BROAD LIGAMENT PREGNANCY. **intramural p.** INTERSTITIAL PREGNANCY. **intraperitoneal p.** ABDOMINAL PREGNANCY. **intrauterine p.** A pregnancy that occurs within the uterine cavity. This is the normal site for a pregnancy. **isthmic p.** An ectopic pregnancy that occurs in the isthmic portion of the fallopian tube. **membranous p.** EXOCHORIAL PREGNANCY. **molar p.** A pregnancy resulting in the formation of a hydatidiform mole. **multiple p.** A pregnancy with two or more fetuses. Also *plural pregnancy.* **mural p.** INTERSTITIAL PREGNANCY. **ovarian p.** An ectopic pregnancy that is located on or within the ovary. Also *ovariocyesis.* **oviductal p.** TUBAL PREGNANCY. **parietal p.** INTERSTITIAL PREGNANCY. **plural p.** MULTIPLE PREGNANCY. **primary ovarian p.** An ectopic pregnancy which develops when an ovum is fertilized within the ovary before ovulation has occurred. **prolonged p.** A pregnancy whose duration is abnormally long for a given species. In man a prolonged pregnancy is one longer than 42 weeks calculated from the first day of the last menstrual period. **spurious p.** PSEUDOCYESIS. **tubal p.** An ectopic pregnancy that occurs within the fallopian tube. This type of ectopic pregnancy accounts for about 95% of human ectopic pregnancies. Also *fallopian pregnancy, oviductal pregnancy.* **twin p.** A pregnancy with two fetuses. Also *bigeminal pregnancy, gemellary pregnancy.*

**pregnane** The parent saturated hydrocarbon of progesterone and the adrenal cortical steroids. It is a $C_{21}$-molecule with four rings, three 6-membered and one 5-membered, with two angular methyl groups, C-18 and C-19, as well as one ethyl substituent, C-20 and C-21, on C-17 of the ring system.

**pregnanediol** Usually $5\beta$-pregnane-$3\alpha,20\alpha$-diol, which is the main breakdown product of progesterone found in urine, partly free and partly as its glucuronide. It is formed by reduction of all three double bonds of progesterone, including those of its carbonyl groups.

**pregnanetriol** Any of several different substances that have been isolated from natural sources, e.g. two 3,16,20-triols, of different stereochemistry, believed to be progesterone metabolites, and 3,17,20-triols, believed to be metabolites of adrenal steroids. Its presence in high concentrations in the urine is indicative of impaired, partially blocked cortisol biosynthesis.

**pregnant** [L *praegna(n)s,* gen. *praegna(n)tis* (from *prae-* PRE- + root of *genere* or *gignere* to produce, create) carrying young, bearing fruit] Carrying the products of conception; gravid.

**pregnene** $C_{21}H_{34}$. A polycyclic unsaturated steroid containing three 6-carbon rings and one 5-carbon ring. The $\Delta^4$- and $\Delta^5$-pregnene configuration characterizes progesterone and most of the biologically active corticosteroids and androgens.

**pregneninolone** ETHISTERONE.

**pregnenolone** 3-Hydroxypregn-5-en-20-one. The compound formed from cholesterol by scission of its side chain between C-20 and C-22, in the pathway of biosynthesis of the steroid hormones.

**prehallux** \-hal′uks\ A supernumerary digit that arises from the medial border of the foot at the true hallux or, rarely, the navicular bone.

**prehensile** \prihen′sil\ Capable of seizing or gripping.

**prehepatic** \-hepat′ik\ [PRE- + HEPATIC] **1** Relating to the condition in the embryo before the development of the liver, when it is only an undifferentiated mass of connective tissue and when other structures such as the developing placenta carry out liver function. **2** Pertaining to the portal circulation before it enters the liver.

**prehormone** \-hôr′mōn\ Any substance that is a natural precursor of an active, circulating hormone. Also *prohormone.*

**prehyoid** \-hī′oid\ In front of the hyoid bone: usually used in reference to accessory thyroid glands.

**prehypophysis** \-hīpäf′isis\ *Rare* ADENOHYPOPHYSIS.

**preictal** \-ik′təl\ Occurring before the ictus.

**preinduction** \-induk′shən\ Any process through which phenotypic alterations are produced in individuals of one generation because of environmental factors interacting with the grandparental gametes.

**preinsula** \-in′s^y^ələ\ The rostral portion of the insular cortex within the sulcus lateralis. *Rare.*

**preinvasive** \-invā′siv\ [PRE- + INVASIVE] Happening before invasion: used of a tumor which has not yet spread beyond its original site, such as carcinoma in situ.

**Preiser** [Georg Karl Felix *Preiser,* German orthopedic surgeon, 1879–1913] See under DISEASE.

**prekallikrein** \-kal′ikrē′in\ A glycoprotein of 88 000 MW that normally circulates in plasma in a 1:1 complex with high molecular weight kininogen. The complex is a cofactor in the activation of factor XII to XIIa. Factor XIIa in turn cleaves prekallikrein into two fragments, one of which is the serine protease kallikrein. Also *Fletcher factor* (original term), *proactivator, kallikreinogen.*

**prelacteal** \-lak′tē·əl\ [PRE- + LACTEAL] Prior to the onset of full lactation.

**preleptotene** \-lep′tətēn\ A stage at the beginning of meiosis, prior to the onset of chromosome thickening during the leptotene stage of meiosis.

**preleukemia** \-lookē′mē·ə\ Any of several dysmyelopoietic syndromes which often portend the appearance of acute granulocytic leukemias. They include refractory anemia, refractory anemia with ringed sideroblasts, refractory anemia with excess blasts, refractory anemia with excess blasts in transformation, and chronic myelomonocytic leukemia.

**preleukemic** \-lookē′mik\ Pertaining to, characteristic of, or resulting from preleukemia.

**prelocalization** \-lō′kəlīzā′shən\ The location of the site of future activity in the early embryo, where development or differentiation will occur when the appropriate stimulus acts.

**premalignant** \-məlig′nənt\ [PRE- + MALIGNANT] PRECANCEROUS.

**premature** \-mətyoor′\ [L *praematur(us)* (from *prae-* PRE- + *maturus* ripe, mature) ripe before the usual time] Born well before the normal 40 weeks' gestation: said of an infant. Also *preterm.* See also PREMATURE INFANT. • *Premature* is variously and ambiguously used. It may refer simply to birth significantly before the normal term, and in this sense is synonymous with *preterm.* It is also used to refer to a birth weight of less than 2500 grams regardless of the gestation period, but as commonly used refers to both duration of gestation and birth weight.

**prematurity** \-mətyoo′ritē\ [PRE- + MATURITY] PREMATURE OCCLUSAL CONTACT.

**premaxilla** \-maksil′ə\ [PRE- + MAXILLA] OS INCISIVUM.

**premaxillary** \-mak′siler′ē\ **1** Pertaining to the premaxilla. **2** Situated anterior to the maxillary bones.

**premedical** \-med′ikəl\ Preceding and designed to prepare one for the professional study of medicine. Also *premed* (popular).

**premedicant** A drug or agent used to facilitate the administration of another drug to be given later, such as the preanesthetic medication given before the anesthetic agent.

**premedication** \-med′ikā′shən\ PREANESTHETIC MEDICATION.

**premeiotic** \-mī·ät′ik\ Occurring or existing prior to the onset of meiosis.

**premelanosome** \-mel′ənōsōm′\ The incompletely melanized precursor of the melanosome. It is ovoid in shape and is destined to accumulate the melanin pigment characteristic of this cell type.

**premenarche** \-mənär′kə\ [PRE- + MENARCHE] The stage of development before the onset of menstruation. Adj. premenarchal, premenarcheal.

**premenopausal** \-men′əpô′səl\ Pertaining to or being at the stage of life before menstruation stops.

**premenstrual** \-men′stroo·əl\ Occurring before menstruation.

**premitotic** \-mītät′ik\ Occurring or existing prior to the beginning of mitosis.

**premolar** \-mō′lər\ [PRE- + MOLAR] BICUSPID.

**premonitory** \-män′itôr′ē\ [Late L *praemonitorius* (from L *praemonere* to forewarn, from *monere* to warn) giving advance warning] Occurring as a presentiment or aura, as that preceding an attack.

**premonocyte** \-män′əsīt\ PROMONOCYTE.

**premorbid** \-môr′bid\ Occurring before the appearance of pathologic signs and symptoms.

**premortal** \-môr′təl\ Occurring shortly before death.

**premyeloblast** \-mī′əlōblast′\ MYELOBLAST.

**premyelocyte** \-mī′əlōsīt′\ PROMYELOCYTE.

**prenares** \-ner′ēz\ (*sing.* prenaris) NARES.

**prenatal** \-nā′təl\ [PRE- + NATAL] Occurring or existing after conception but before birth, as *prenatal fetal development.*.

**preneoplastic** \-nē′əplas′tik\ Preceding the development of a neoplasm.

**prenyl** The isopentenyl group, $CH_2{=}C(CH_3){-}CH_2{-}CH_2{-}$, or the polymers of it, such as geranyl and farnesyl.

**preoccipital** \-äksip′itəl\ Denoting the cortex or the sulcal notch rostral to the occipital lobe of the human cerebrum.

**preoedipal** \prē·e′dipəl\ See under PREOEDIPAL PHASE.

**preoperative** \-äp′ərətiv\ Occurring or done before a surgical operation.

**preoperculum** \-ōpur′kyələm\ The frontal cerebral cortex forming the rostral part of the dorsal lip of the Sylvian (lateral) sulcus.

**preovulatory** \-äv′yələtôr′ē\ Preceding ovulation: said of a phase of the menstrual cycle.

**preparalytic** \-per′əlit′ik\ Pertaining to the initial phase of an illness which usually gives rise to paralysis, but in which there is no evidence of muscular weakness.

**preparation** **1** The process of making or becoming ready. **2** Something that has been prepared or made ready for use, as an anatomic or histologic specimen or a medicinal substance. 3 An organ or part removed from an experimental animal to reduce extraneous factors, demonstrate a physiologic or morphologic relationship, or test a function or behavior. 4 An animal so modified, especially through surgery. **allergenic protein p.'s** Extracts prepared from allergenic substances and used in the testing and hyposensitization of individuals suspected of or subject to allergy. Their strength is measured in terms of their protein-nitrogen content. **anemic decerebrate p.** An experimental technique for destroying functional activity of the brain above the mesencephalon by bilateral ligation of the internal carotid arteries. The intact vertebral-basilar artery system maintains function of the brainstem. **bulbospinal p.** OBLONGATA PREPARATION. **cavity p.** The removal of caries from a dental cavity and the shaping of the cavity to make the restoration as permanent as possible. **cerveau isolé p.** An animal with its neuraxis experimentally transected at any of various levels that leave the forebrain intact. Experimental emphasis is on the continued functioning of the forebrain, in distinction to a decerebrate preparation. **corrosion p.** An anatomical specimen prepared by injecting the parts to be saved and destroying the remaining tissue by immersion in a corrosive substance. **coverglass p.** A film of blood or other body fluid prepared by placing the material between two cover slips, which are then pulled apart. **cytologic filter p.** A specimen prepared for cytologic examination by concentrating cellular elements from their suspending fluid, using a filter with a pore size smaller than the diameter of the cells under study. **decerebrate p.** An experimental preparation in which the brainstem is surgically separated from the more rostral diencephalon and forebrain at the supracollicular or intercollicular level. **decorticate p.** A preparation with the neocortex and most of the hippocampus removed, while the basal ganglia and brainstem remain intact. **diencephalic p.** THALAMIC PREPARATION. **hanging-drop p.** A fluid specimen prepared for microscopic examination that is in the form of a drop held by surface tension on the underside of a slide or cover glass. **heart-lung p.** An animal preparation in which the output of the left ventricle is returned through an artificial system to the right atrium. The circulation in the heart and lungs is thus preserved but there is no circulation to the remainder of the body unless the preparation is used as a pump and oxygenator for the perfusion of an isolated organ. **hemispherectomized p.** A preparation in which the neocortex, neostriatum, and most of the hippocampus are removed on one side, with most of the medial rhinencephalon, diencephalon, and lower brainstem remaining intact. **high cerveau isolé p.** A preparation with section at the diencephalic-mesencephalic junction. **hypothalamic p.** A preparation in which the cerebral hemispheres and most of the thalamus and caudate nucleus have been removed, leaving the hypothalamus and brainstem intact. **intercollicular p.** A preparation in which there is section of the brainstem along a plane between the inferior and superior colliculi and through the lower mesencephalon. This is the classical decerebrate preparation with emphasis on functions below the lesion. Also *low mesencephalic preparation, Sherringtonian decerebrate preparation.* **Langendorff p.** A preparation of an isolated mammalian heart in which the aorta is cannulated and perfused, thus supplying blood flow to the coronary circulation. Also *Langendorff's method.* **low mesencephalic p.** INTERCOLLICULAR PREPARATION. **low-thoracic p.** An animal preparation in which the neuraxis (the spinal cord) has been transected at the $T_{12}$ level. **mid-pontine p.** A preparation in which there is transection of the neuraxis in front of or anterior to the trigeminal nerve. **mid-thoracic p.** An animal preparation in which the neuraxis (the spinal cord) has been transected at the $T_6$ level. **oblongata p.** A preparation in which there is transection of the neuraxis at the caudal limit of the pons. Also *bulbospinal preparation, prebulbar preparation.* **Pollack-Davis p.** An animal deprived of forebrain function due to ischemia produced by ligating the common carotid arteries and the basilar artery at the level of the upper pons. A key result is loss of the blood supply to the anterior lobe of the cerebellum. It is a form of anemic decerebrate preparation. **postcollicular p.** A preparation in which there is transection of the neuraxis behind or posterior to the inferior colliculus. **prebulbar p.** OBLONGATA PREPARATION. **premamillary p.** A preparation in which the brainstem is transected just rostral to the mamillary bodies. **proteolytic p.'s** Proteolytic enzymes from such sources as papaya and pineapple that supply papain and bromelain as well as chymotrypsin. These have been used in attempts to hasten healing in areas of trauma and tissue damage. The effectiveness of such treatment is questioned, however, and allergic sensitivities to these proteins have been reported. **Sherringtonian decerebrate p.** INTERCOLLICULAR PREPARATION. **surgical p.** The preparation of the skin of a patient or the hands of the operating team prior to surgery. A combination of mechanical washing plus an antibacterial soap or solution is usually employed. **thalamic p.** A preparation with most of the cerebral hemispheres removed, and the thalamus, basal ganglia, and brainstem remaining intact. Also *diencephalic preparation.*

**preparetic** \-pəret′ik\ Preceding paresis.

**prepartal** \-pär′təl\ Occurring at a time just prior to the onset of labor.

**prepatellar** \-pətel′ər\ Situated anterior to the patella.

**prepatency** \-pā′tənsē\ [PRE- + PATENCY] The time interval between the acquisition of a parasite and its detectability in the new host. Also *prepatent period.* Adj. prepatent.

**preperitoneal** \-per′itənē′əl\ Pertaining to the layer of the abdominal wall between the parietal peritoneum and the fascia transversalis.

**preplacental** \-pləsen′təl\ Relating to embryonic stages before the development of the placenta.

**prepollex** \-päl′eks\ A supernumerary bone of the hand that grows from the lateral border of the thumb.

**preponderance** \pripän′dərəns\ Greater force, weight, or importance. **ventricular p.** Greater hypertrophy of one cardiac ventricle relative to the other as revealed by the electrocardiogram.

**prepotential** \-pōten′shəl\ The slow depolarization which takes place in the pacemaker cells prior to the rapid depolarization of the action potential.

**preprandial** \-pran′dē·əl\ Occurring before a meal, especially before dinner.

**preprocessing** \-präs′əsing\ Signal processing prior to storage. In digital imaging systems, it includes assignment of a number to be stored which corresponds to some characteristic, usually amplitude, of a received signal.

**preprohormone** \-prōhôr′mōn\ A biosynthetic precursor of a prohormone, as preproparathyroid hormone. The preprohormone molecule is generally larger than that of the prohormone.

**preproinsulin** \-prō·in′sʸəlin\ The primal molecular form in which insulin is synthesized within the beta cell of the pancreatic islet. It is a single chain 110-amino acid polypeptide. The N-terminal 24 residues are removed after biosynthesis and after they have directed the protein to specific sites within the beta cell, proinsulin remains.

**prepubertal** \-pyoo′bərtəl\ Characteristic of prepuberty.

**prepuberty** \-pyoo′bərtē\ [PRE- + PUBERTY] The period of life before puberty.

**prepubescence** \-pyoobes′əns\ [PRE- + PUBESCENCE] The physical and emotional state of one approaching puberty; prepuberty. Adj. prepubescent.

**prepubescent** \-pyoobes′ənt\ [PRE- + PUBESÇENT] Characteristic of the physical appearance, emotional state, or hormonal development of one approaching puberty.

**prepuce** \prē′pyoos\ [L *praeputium* foreskin] PREPUTIUM. **p. of clitoris** PREPUTIUM CLITORIDIS. **p. of penis** PREPUTIUM PENIS.

**prepucotomy** \-pyookät′əmē\ PREPUTIOTOMY.

**preputial** \-pyoo′shəl\ Of or pertaining to the prepuce.

**preputiotomy** \-pyoo′shē·ät′əmē\ [*preputi(um)* + *o* + -TOMY] Surgical incision of the prepuce for treatment of phimosis. Also *prepucotomy*.

**preputium** \-pyoo′shē·əm\ [L *praeputium* foreskin] An enveloping free fold of skin. Also *prepuce*. Also *praeputium*. **p. clitoridis** [NA] The hoodlike free fold of skin covering the glans clitoridis and formed by the union anteriorly of the lateral portions of the two labia minora. Also *prepuce of clitoris*. **p. penis** [NA] The anterior end of the skin of the penis that is folded over itself at the neck of the penis and covers the glans for a varying length. At the neck the inner layer is continous with the skin adherent to the glans as far as the external urethral orfice. In the midline of the urethral surface of the penis it forms the frenulum. Also *prepuce of penis, foreskin, acrobystia, acroposthia* (outmoded).

**prepyloric** \-pīlôr′ik\ Anterior or proximal to the pylorus of the stomach.

**prerectal** \-rek′təl\ Anterior or proximal to the rectum.

**prerenal** \-rē′nəl\ [PRE- + RENAL] Located or occurring proximal to the kidneys: often used of renal failure or insufficiency due to shock, congestive heart failure, or renal artery obstruction.

**prerennin** \-ren′in\ RENNINOGEN.

**prereproductive** \-rē′prəduk′tiv\ [PRE- + REPRODUCTIVE] Preceding puberty.

**preretinal** \-ret′ənəl\ Located in the space between the retina and the vitreous humor.

**presby-** \pres′bē-\ [Gk *presbys* old man] A combining form meaning old age. Also *presbyo-*.

**presbyacusis** \-əkyoo′sis\ PRESBYCUSIS.

**presbyatrics** \-at′riks\ [PRESBY- + *-(i)atrics*] GERIATRIC MEDICINE.

**presbycusis** \-kyoo′sis\ [PRESBY- + *(a)cusis*] A slowly increasing sensorineural hearing loss, worse in the higher frequencies and associated with increasing age. Its pathogenesis is uncertain, with several etiologic factors involved. Also *presbyacusis, senile deafness* (incorrect).

**presbyo-** \pres′bē·ō-\ PRESBY-.

**presbyope** \pres′bē·ōp\ [PRESBY- + -OPE] One affected by presbyopia; one who has lost accommodative ability due to aging.

**presbyophrenia** \-frē′nē·ə\ [PRESBYO- + -PHRENIA] A form of senile dementia characterized by marked disorientation, puerile confabulations, and ceaseless motion without accomplishing anything. Also *Kahlbaum-Wernicke syndrome*.

**presbyopia** \pres′bē·ō′pē·ə\ [PRESBY- + -OPIA] A loss of accommodation of the eyes due to aging, caused by the diminished capacity of the crystalline lens to change its shape. Also *presbytia, presbytism, old sight, visus senilis*. Adj. presbyopic.

**prescapula** \-skap′yələ\ The plate of bone cephalad to the line of attachment of the spine of the scapula from the medial margin to the glenoid cavity.

**prescribe** To order for use in the treatment or prevention of a disease or injury, as a drug, diet, or regimen.

**prescription** [L *praescriptio* (from *praescribere* to set before in writing, prescribe, from *prae-* PRE- + *scribere* to write) an inscription, preamble, prescription] A written direction or order for the preparation and provision of a drug or other item used in treating or preventing a disease or injury. **shotgun p.** A poorly designed prescription with a large number of components included in the hope that, by chance, one or more of them might be effective.

**presecretory** \-sē′krətôr′ē\ Referring to those structures, as subcellular organelles or droplets, and biochemical processes which precede the actual physical secretion or extrusion of an endocrine product from the cell into the circulation.

**presegmenter** \-segmen′tər\ [PRE- + SEGMENT + -ER] A mature asexual malarial schizont in the erythrocytic stage marked by an accumulation of pigment into masses in the red cells just before segmentation occurs. Also *presegmenting body*.

**present** [French *present(er)* (from L *praesens*, gen. *praesentis*, aiding, ready, present, pres. part. of *praeesse* to be present, preside) to tender, offer] **1** To appear at the uterine cervix during labor: used especially of a fetal part. **2** To become manifest: used especially of a disease as first noticed by the patient from early symptoms.

**presentation** [French *présentation* action or manner of presenting. See PRESENT.] **1** The relationship of the long axis of the fetus to the long axis of the mother. **2** PRESENTING PART. See also POSITION. **3** Production and display of an image, as on an oscilloscope screen. **acromion p.** SHOULDER PRESENTATION. **arm p.** An abnormal presentation of the fetus in which the fetal arm appears first in the uterine cervix. **breech p.** A presentation of the fetus in which the fetal buttocks or feet appear first in the uterine cervix. Also *pelvic presentation*. **brow p.** A cephalic presentation of the fetus in which the fetal forehead appears first in the uterine cervix. **cephalic p.** A presentation of the fetus in which the fetal head is the lowest part and appears first in the uterine cervix. This is the most common presentation of a human fetus during labor. Also *head birth*. **complete breech p.** A breech presentation of the fetus in which both the buttocks and feet appear first in the uterine cervix. **compound p.** A presentation of the fetus in which there is prolapse of an extremity alongside another presenting part into the vagina or uterine cervix. **p. of the cord** The prolapse of the umbilical cord into the vagina prior to delivery of an infant. The condition is associated with a high incidence of fetal demise due to compression of the cord vessels unless recognized promptly and managed actively through the use of cesarean section. Also *funic presentation*. **double breech p.** COMPLETE BREECH PRESENTATION. **double footling p.** An incomplete breech presentation of the fetus in which both feet appear first at the uterine cervix or prolapse into the vagina. **face p.** A cephalic presentation of the fetus in which the face appears first in the uterine cervix. **footling breech p.** An incomplete breech presentation of a fetus in which one or both feet are presenting parts, called, respectively, single footling (breech) presentation and double footling (breech) presentation. Also *footling presentation*. **frank breech p.** A breech presentation of the fetus in which only the buttocks present at the uterine cervix while the lower extremities are flexed at the hips and extended at the knees. Also *single breech presentation*. **fu-**

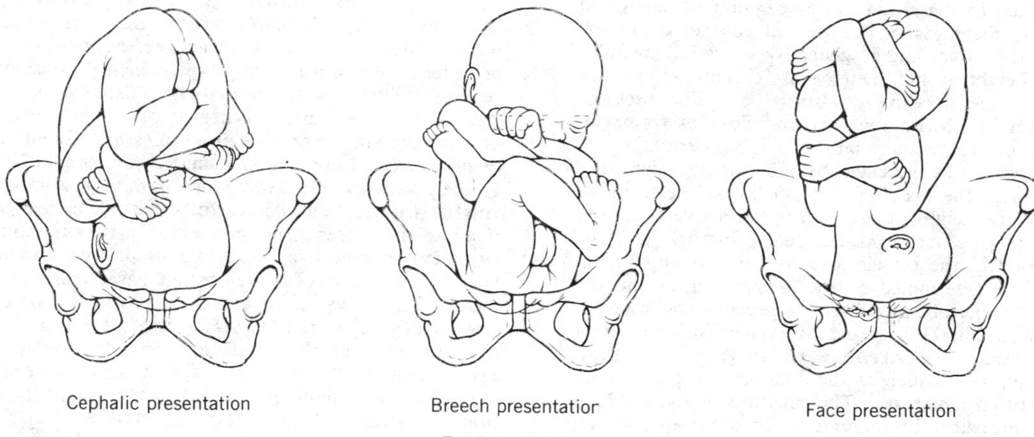

**Fetal presentations**

**nic p.** PRESENTATION OF THE CORD. **hand and head p.** A compound presentation of the fetus in which both a hand and the fetal skull appear first at the uterine cervix. **incomplete breech p.** A breech presentation of the fetus in which one or both feet or knees appear first in the uterine cervix or vagina. **longitudinal p.** A fetus whose trunk is parallel to the long axis of the mother such that either the fetal head or breech is the presenting part at the level of the uterine cervix. Also *polar presentation.* **oblique p.** SHOULDER PRESENTATION. **pelvic p.** BREECH PRESENTATION. **placental p.** PLACENTA PREVIA. **polar p.** LONGITUDINAL PRESENTATION. **shoulder p.** An abnormal presentation of a fetus in which the fetal shoulder appears first in the uterine cervix. Also *oblique presentation, acromion presentation.* **single breech p.** FRANK BREECH PRESENTATION. **single footling p.** An incomplete breech presentation of the fetus in which the foot of one lower extremity appears first at the uterine cervix or prolapses into the vagina. **torso p.** TRANSVERSE LIE. **transverse p.** TRANSVERSE LIE. **trunk p.** TRANSVERSE LIE. **vertex p.** A cephalic presentation of the fetus in which the vertex of the fetal skull is the lowest part and appears first in the uterine cervix. This is the most common cephalic presentation.

**presomite** \-sō′mīt\ [PRE- + SOMITE] Denoting the stage before the development of a somite.

**prespermatid** \-spur′mətid\ SECONDARY SPERMATOCYTE.

**presphenoid** \-sfē′noid\ **1** The part of the body of the sphenoid bone in front of the tuberculum sellae with which the lesser wings are continuous. It fuses with the postsphenoid part in the eighth month of fetal life. **2** In front the sphenoid bone.

**presphygmic** \-sfig′mik\ Preceding a pulse wave; specifically, relating to the isovolumetric phase of ventricular contraction in the cardiac cycle.

**prespondylolisthesis** \-spän′dilōlisthē′sis\ [PRE- + SPONDYLOLISTHESIS] A developmental defect of the pedicles or other parts of the last lumbar vertebra that predisposes to displacement of the vertebral body.

**press** / **French p.** A device used to disrupt bacteria and other cells by forcing a suspension under high pressure (5000–15 000 psi) through a narrow orifice controlled by a needle valve.

**pressometer** \presäm′ətər\ [*press(ure)* + *o* + -METER] MANOMETER.

**pressor** [*press(ure)* + -OR] Tending to increase blood pressure; characterized by the ability to increase arterial pressure.

**pressoreceptive** \pres′ôrisep′tiv\ Sensitive to pressure, especially blood pressure. Also *pressosensitive.*

**pressoreceptor** \pres′ôrisep′tər\ BARORECEPTOR.

**pressosensitive** \pres′ōsen′sitiv\ PRESSORECEPTIVE.

**pressosensitivity** \pres′ōsen′sətiv′itē\ The state of being sensitive to changes in pressure. **reflexogenic p.** The ability to alter or control blood pressure through visceral reflexes initiated by the action of baroreceptors that cause autonomic responses.

# pressure

**pressure** [L *pressura* (from *press(us),* past part. of *premere* to press, squeeze) a pressing, pressure] **1** A force exerted against resistance. **2** Ratio of force to area, for a force applied over an extended area. **absolute p.** Fluid pressure reckoned from perfect vacuum as datum. In many cases it is the sum of the prevailing atmospheric pressure and the pressure which a pressure-measuring instrument is indicating. **airway p.** The pressure in the airway of a lung or in a mechanical ventilator relative to the ambient pressure, in any phase of the respiratory cycle. **alveolar p.** The pressure in the terminal air unit of the lung. **ambulatory venous p.** Measurement of the pressure in a foot vein during walking or foot exercise. When values are compared with those recorded at rest, the presence and severity of proximal venous disorders can be inferred. **amniotic p.** The pressure inside the amniotic sac secondary to a uterine contraction. **arterial p.** The blood pressure in the systemic arteries. Also *arteriotony, arterial tension.* **atmospheric p.** The absolute pressure exerted by the atmosphere. It is equal to the gravity force per unit of horizontal area, exerted by the mass of the vertical column of air extending above that area, and is generally expressed in millibars or as the height, in millimeters, of a column of mercury producing the same pressure. **back p.** The pressure caused upstream by obstruction to blood flow, as from valvular stenosis or ventricular failure. **barometric p.** Atmospheric pressure as indicated by a barometer. For comparative purposes, the reading is sometimes corrected to compensate for the height of the instrument above mean sea level. **biting p.** OCCLUSAL FORCE. **blood p.** The pressure of blood in the vessels, usually used to imply arterial pressure. It is determined by the cardiac output and the resistance of the peripheral vessels, especially the arteries. Also *hematopiesis* (rare). **capillary p.** The tension of blood in capillaries. **central venous p.** Blood pressure in the major veins, such as the inferior or superior vena cava. **cerebrospinal p.** The pressure of the cerebrospinal fluid as measured by manometry or other appropriate technique. In the recumbent patient the normal pressure in the subarachnoid space as measured by lumbar puncture is 100–150 mm of fluid. Also *intrathecal pressure, intraspinal pressure.* **colloid osmotic p.** ONCOTIC PRESSURE. **continuous positive airway p.** A technique of artificial ventilation in which pressure within the lung airways is maintained above atmospheric pressure throughout the respiratory cycle. Also *constant positive airway pressure.* Abbr. CPAP **critical closing p.** That pressure within the lumen of a vessel or tube below which wall elasticity causes collapse and closure. **diastolic p.** Pressure in a vessel or chamber of the heart during diastole. **endocardial p.** Pressure exerted within the endocardium. **expiratory p.** The pressure of gas in the airway during exhalation, as in a patient receiving artificial ventilation. **filtration p.** The pressure responsible for filtration through a membrane. In relation to the capillary wall it is the resultant of the hydrostatic blood pressure less the sum of the oncotic pressure and interstitial tissue pressure. **hyperbaric p.** Pressure exceeding one atmosphere. **p. of ideas** Rapid or uncontrolled thinking leading to an inability to control or channel such thoughts properly. The subject finds himself saying things that even to him seem only tenuously related. It may appear in manic states as a flight of ideas as well as in other mental disorders. Also *thought pressure, pressured thinking.* **imbibition p.** Pressure in a gel resulting from the uptake of liquid. **inspiratory p.** Pressure applied to gas during inspiration, as in a patient receiving artificial ventilation. **inspiratory triggering p.** The negative pressure necessary, at onset of inspiration, to induce tidal volume in an individual on a mechanical ventilator. **interstitial p.** The pressure within a tissue or organ but outside of the blood vessels of the tissue or organ. **intracranial p.** The pressure within the skull. It can be estimated by measuring the pressure in the subarachnoid space. **intramyometrial p.** The pressure within the uterine myometrium secondary to uterine contractions. **intraocular p.** The result within the eye of the forcible secretion of aqueous humor by the ciliary processes and the resistance to outflow by the trabecular meshwork, usually ranging between 10 to 20 mm of mercury. Also *intraocular tension.* **intrapulmonary p.** The pressure within the air passages of the lungs. **intraspinal p.** CEREBROSPINAL PRESSURE. **intrathecal p.** CEREBROSPINAL PRESSURE. **intrathoracic p.** The pressure within the thoracic cage. **intratympanic p.** The air pressure within the middle-ear cleft, normally approximating atmospheric pressure. **intraventricular p.** The pressure within a cardiac ventricle. **jugular venous p.** Blood pressure in the jugular veins. **maximum safety p.** The upper limit of positive pressure allowable in an anesthesia-breathing system or other related apparatus, a limit which if exceeded is unacceptably hazardous to the patient. Also *maximum working pressure.* **minimum safety p.** The lower limit of positive pressure allowable in an anesthesia-breathing system or other related apparatus, a limit below which the system is unlikely to work effectively. Also *minimum working pressure.* **mutation p.** The degree to which allele frequency is derived solely by recurrent mutation. **nasal continuous positive airway p.** Continuous positive airway pressure applied by means of a well-sealed nasal mask in the treatment of excessive snoring and, in particular, of obstructive sleep apnea. Also *nasal CPAP.* **negative p.** A pressure that is lower than that of the ambient atmosphere. **negative end-expiratory p.** Subatmospheric pressure produced at the end of expiration, as during artificial ventilation. **occlusal p.** OCCLUSAL FORCE. **oncotic p.** The osmotic force across a capillary wall created by the higher concentration of protein in the plasma than in the interstitial fluid. Part of this force is attributable to a Donnan effect. Also *colloid osmotic pressure.* **osmotic p.** The pressure resulting from the passage of solvent from a solution of lower particle concentration to one of higher particle concentration across a membrane which is impermeable or semipermeable with respect to the solute. **partial p.** The tension exerted by an individual component of a gas mixture proportionate to its concentration. **perfusion p.** The pressure perfusing an organ, being the difference between arterial and venous pressures. **portal venous p.** The blood pressure within the abdominal portal venous system. Also *portal pressure.* **positive p.** A pressure higher than that of the ambient atmosphere. **positive end-expiratory p.** Greater than atmospheric pressure produced at the end of expiration during artificial ventilation. Such pressure is thought to hold partially collapsed alveoli open and to prevent further atelectasis, as in the treatment of adult respiratory distress syndrome. Abbr. PEEP **pulmonary p.** Blood pressure in the pulmonary artery. **pulmonary artery wedge p.** The pressure recorded from the tip of a catheter wedged in a small branch of the pulmonary artery. The pressure so obtained usually corresponds with the pressure in the pulmonary capillaries and the left atrium. Also *pulmonary wedge pressure.* **pulmonary capillary p.** The pressure within the pulmonary capillaries. **pulmonary wedge p.** PULMONARY ARTERY WEDGE PRESSURE. **pulse p.** The difference between peak systolic pressure and the lowest diastolic pressure. **radiation p.** The pressure exerted on a body by radiation incident on it. It is equal to the ratio of radiation force to surface area. **selection p.** The intensity of any form of selection in altering genotype frequencies in a given breeding population. **solution p.** The pressure that tends to bring into solution the molecules of a solid in a solvent. **splenic pulp p.** A technique once used for quantifying portal hypertension by direct percutaneous puncture of the spleen and manometric recording of pressures. **standard p.** STANDARD ATMOSPHERE. **subambient p.** A pressure below that of the environment. **subatmospheric p.** A pressure less than that of the atmosphere. **surface p.** The force exerted per unit length of barrier by molecules adsorbed on a surface. It shows as a diminution of surface tension, and is analogous for a surface to pressure in a volume. Detergent molecules exert a large surface pressure. Other adsorbed molecules do so when compressed. **systolic p.** The pressure in the arteries or in the chambers of the heart during systole, generally measured as the maximum pressure during systole. **thought p.** PRESSURE OF IDEAS. **tissue p.** Interstitial hydrostatic pressure that is measured by needles or catheters inserted directly into the tissue. **transairway p.** The difference between the air pressure in the lung alveoli and that in the surrounding atmosphere. **transmural p.** The pressure transmitted across the wall of an organ such as the heart or a blood vessel. **transthoracic p.** The pressure difference between intrathoracic air-containing organs and the surrounding atmosphere. **vapor p.** The pressure exerted by the gaseous phase of a substance. **venous p.** Blood pressure within the veins. Also *intravenous tension.* **ventilator p.** The positive or negative pressure, in a mechanical ventilator, by which inspiration and expiration are regulated. **water vapor p.** The partial pressure of water vapor. **wedge p.** The pressure recording obtained when a catheter occludes a small vessel. **wedged hepatic p.** The indirect measurement of portal pressure by wedging of a percutaneously-introduced catheter in a hepatic vein radicle. **zero end-expiratory p.** The situation at the end of expiration during artificial ventilation of the lungs when pressure in the airway is at atmospheric level.

**presternum** \-sturʹnəm\ *Outmoded* MANUBRIUM STERNI.

**prestriate** \-strīʹāt\ Referring to the occipital lobe cortex lying rostral to the striate cortex and including both parastriate and peristriate areas.

**presubiculum** \-soobikʹyələm\ A histologically distinctive field of cerebral allocortex forming part of the transitional region extending from the rhinal fissure to the subiculum proper.

**presumptive** \-zumpʹtiv\ Referring to an embryonic cell or tissue whose probable later identity in the fully developed organism is known on the basis of established fate mapping.

**presuppurative** \-supʹyərāʹtiv\ Occurring before suppuration, as an early stage in an inflammatory process.

**presylvian** \-silʹvē·ən\ Denoting the region rostral to the sylvian fissure or to the region surrounding its anterior branch.

**presymptom** \-simpʹtəm\ PRODROME.

**presymptomatic** \-simpʹtəmatʹik\ Existing before symptoms are manifest, or pertaining to such a period in the course of a disease.

**presynaptic** \-sinapʹtik\ Proximal to a synapse.

**presystole** \-sisʹtəlē\ [PRE- + SYSTOLE] The period immediately preceding the onset of ventricular systole.

**presystolic** \-sistälʹik\ Relating to presystole; immediately preceding the onset of ventricular systole.

**pretarsal** \-tärʹsəl\ Situated anterior to the tarsus.

**pretecta** \-tekʹtə\ The region of the duodenum just proximal to the part where it is covered by the transverse mesocolon meeting the root of the mesentery, that is, at approximately the junction of the horizontal and ascending parts. *Outmoded.*

**pretectum** \-tekʹtəm\ [PRE- + L *tectum* roof] PRETECTAL AREA.

**preterm** \-turmʹ\ [PRE- + TERM] PREMATURE.

**preterminal** \-turʹmənəl\ **1** Occurring just before death. **2** Affected by a disease that is likely to become terminal. ⟨"Among 14 'preterminal' patients treated . . . in the past 18 months, the longest survival was three weeks after [surgery]." —*Medical World News,* 23 Jan. 1978, 24⟩

**pretuberculosis** \-t^yUburʹkyəlōʹsis\ [PRE- + TUBERCULOSIS] The initial stage of tuberculosis when infection has occurred but before symptoms are apparent. *Obs.*

**pretuberculous** \-t^yUburʹkyələs\ Preceding the onset of tuberculosis.

**prevalence** \prevʹələns\ [L *praeval(entia)* (from *praevalens,* gen. *praevalentis,* pres. part. of *praevalere* to be very strong, prevail, from *prae-* PRE- + *valere* to be strong) a prevailing + *-entia* -ENCE] **1** The number of cases of disease, of sick persons, or of other eventualities such as accidents, which exist or which occur in a population at or during a given time, expressed as a rate with the total population as denominator. Also *prevalence rate.* **2** POINT PREVALENCE. **period p.** Prevalence as recorded over a given period of time, expressed as a rate with the total population at any time during the period or the estimated number at the midpoint of the period as denominator. Period prevalence is useful in relation to sickness benefits and hospital usage statistics, being related in general to longer-term illness. • The term is usually qualified by some reference to a time period, as "prevalence during July." **point p.** Prevalence as recorded at a given moment, expressed as a rate with the population at the relevant time as denominator. Point prevalence is widely used in epidemiology and health statistics. • The term is usually qualified by some reference such as "prevalence on January 1." Also *prevalence.*

**prevention** / **primary p.** Prevention of the occurrence of disease by such measures as immunization or by the provision of a wholesome water supply. **secondary p.** Prevention of the development of disease through early detection, for example by screening. **tertiary p.** Prevention of the progression of established disease or disability by appropriate treatment.

**preventive** \privenʹtiv\ Tending or intended to prevent. • Though often used as synonymous with *prophylactic,* it has been suggested that *preventive* be applied to actions and *prophylactic* to substances.

**preventriculosis** \-ventrikʹyəlōʹsis\ ACHALASIA OF THE CARDIA.

**preventriculus** \-ventrikʹyələs\ The entrance to the stomach at the cardioesophageal junction.

**prevermis** \-vurʹmis\ Rostral to the cerebellar vermis.

**prevertebral** \-vurʹtəbrəl\ In front of the vertebral column or a vertebra.

**prevertiginous** \-vərtijʹinəs\ Preceding vertigo.

**prevesical** \-vesʹikəl\ Located in front of the bladder.

**previtamin** PROVITAMIN. **p. H** CAROTENE.

**Prévost** [Jean Louise *Prévost,* Swiss physician, 1838–1927] See under SIGN.

**Preyer** [Thierry Wilhelm *Preyer,* German physiologist and physiologic chemist, 1841–1897] See under REFLEX.

**prezone** \prēʹzōn\ PROZONE.

**prezonular** \-zänʹyələr\ Located anterior to the suspensory ligament of the lens (zonule of Zinn).

**PRF** prolactin releasing factor (prolactin releasing hormone).

**PRH** prolactin releasing hormone.

**priapism** \prīʹəpizm\ [Gk *priapism(os)* (from *Priap(os)* god of fertility and procreation + *-ismos* -ISM) lewdness] A persistent, usually painful, erection of only the corpora cavernosa, unrelated to sexual stimulation. The condition may be transitory and of short duration or it may persist. Also *mentulagra.* **secondary p.** Priapism due to obstruction of the dorsal vein of the penis.

**priapitis** \prīʹəpīʹtis\ [*priap(us)* + -ITIS] Inflammation of the penis.

**priapus** \prīʹəpəs\ [L (after *Priapus,* from Gk *Priapos,* god of procreation) a phallus] PENIS.

**Price** [Ernest Arthur *Price,* English biochemist, born 1882] Carr-Price test. See under TEST.

**Price-Jones** [Cecil *Price-Jones,* English hematologist, 1863–1943] See under METHOD, CURVE.

**prickles** CROSS-BRIDGES.
**Priestley** [John Gillies *Priestley,* British physiologist, 1880–1941] Haldane-Priestley sampling. See under SAMPLING.
**prilocaine hydrochloride** $C_{13}H_{21}ClN_2O$. *N*-(2-Methylphenyl)-2-(propylamino)-propanamide hydrochloride. A local anesthetic similar in its pharmacologic effects to lidocaine. It is used by infiltration, for peripheral nerve block and for epidural anesthesia.
**primacy** \prī′məsē\ The state of being first in rank or importance. **genital p.** The subjugation of early instinctual manifestations to the apparatus of the genital phase with pregenital expressions relegated to the status of parts of ordinary physiologic function or of sexual foreplay. **phallic p.** The instinctual level at which the phallus becomes the most important organ, supplanting the earlier importance of the oral and anal phases. Phallic primacy is at its height at about the fifth year of life.
**primal** \prī′məl\ [Med L *primalis* (from L *prim(us)* first + *-alis* -AL) concerning the first period] Primary or earliest in time.
**primamycin** HAMYCIN.
**primaquine** An 8-aminoquinoline antimalarial compound used for the radical cure of vivax malaria. It is usually administered as the phosphate salt.
**primary** 1 Occurring earlier; original, as a disease, as distinguished from a secondary disease or complication. 2 First in importance; principal.
**primate** \prī′māt\ Any member of the mammalian order Primates.
**Primates** \prī′mātēz\ [Late L, pl. of *primas* one of the first, from L *primus* first] The order of the class Mammalia that includes the prosimians, the monkeys, the apes, and man, and their extinct predecessors.
**primed** \prīmd\ Made immunologically responsive by original exposure to antigen, as a lymphocyte or other cell of the immune system. Upon subsequent exposure to antigen a primed cell is capable of dividing into other primed cells, synthesizing antibody, or taking part in a cell-mediated immune reaction.
**primer** \prī′mər\ [L *prim(us)* first + -ER] A substance which prepares a material or surface for the action of another substance. **cavity p.** CAVITY LINER.
**primidone** $C_{12}H_{14}N_2O_2$. 5-Ethyldihydro-5-phenyl-4,6-(1*H*,5*H*)-pyrimidinedione. A compound closely related chemically to the barbiturates. It is metabolized to phenobarbital and phenylethylmalonamide. It is used to treat generalized seizures and focal seizures and may be used with phenytoin. It is given orally.
**primigravid** \prī′migrav′id\ [L *prim(us)* first + *i* + *gravid(us)* heavy, pregnant] Being pregnant for the first time.
**primigravida** \prī′migrav′idə\ [L *prim(us)* first + *i* + GRAVIDA] A woman who is pregnant for the first time. Also *unigravida.* **elderly p.** A primigravida who is more than 30 years of age.
**primipara** \prīmip′ərə\ [L, from *prim(um)* for the first time + *par(ere)*] A woman who has had one pregnancy carried to the stage of viability, regardless of whether the fetus was born dead or alive or whether the gestation was single or multiple. Also *unipara.* See also PARA.
**primitivation** \prim′itivā′shən\ [*primitiv(e)* + -ATION] Regression of the ego to early instinctual levels of development with consequent loss of higher and more mature ego functions, as may occur in traumatic neurosis or schizophrenia.
**primitive** [L *primitiv(us)* (from *primit(us)* first of its kind, foremost + *-ivus* -IVE) primitive] 1 Exhibiting a close relationship to an ancestral form or earlier evolutionary development; unspecialized. 2 Occurring early in development; infantile.
**primordial** \prīmôr′dē·əl\ 1 First in time; primitive. 2 Relating to a primordium.
**primordium** \prīmôr′dē·əm\ [L (from *primus* first, prime + *ordiri* to begin, commence, akin to *ordo* a series, row, order + *-ium* noun suffix), the first beginning, origin] (*pl.* primordia) The region in a fertilized ovum of which the cellular elements will give rise to an organ by a series of complex inductive processes, of multiplication and of differentiation, and sometimes of secondary regression. See also ANLAGE, BLASTEMA. **genital primordia** The part of the embryo which gives rise to the genital glands and organs of the adult. The primordium of the genital glands develops in a ridge (genital ridge) which becomes evident on the dorsal wall of the coelomic cavity. The precursors of the genital ducts are the paired mesonephric ducts and paramesonephric ducts. The primordia of the external genital organs will be completed ultimately by mesodermal contributions of perineal and caudal origin. Sexual differentiation of the entire assemblage is determined by hormonal secretion from the sex glands and by the genetic constitution of the embryo. **lens p.** The invagination of the ectodermal lens placode overlying the optic vesicle to occupy the cavity of the optic cup and from which the lens develops. Also *lens vesicle.*
**princeps** \prin′seps\ [L (from *primus* first, prime + *-ceps,* combining form from *capere* to take, seize), first, foremost; as substantive, a leader] 1 Principal; main. 2 The main stem or branch, as of a vessel.
**principle** 1 A fundamental generalization or assumption describing natural phenomena and forming the basis of other generalizations or theory. See also entries under RULE and LAW. 2 A chemical or important drug constituent, especially one that confers the main pharmaceutical properties to the drug. **active p.** The main component of a drug, which confers its specific medicinal properties. This designation is of importance in regard to drugs obtained from crude, natural sources that may contain many distinctive components. **Bragg-Gray p.** The principle basic to the use of ionization chambers for radiation dosimetry: if a solid material containing a small gas-filled cavity is uniformly irradiated with x rays or gamma rays, the energy absorbed by the material may be determined, with certain assumptions, by a measurement of the ionization produced by secondary electrons in the cavity. **conservation of energy p.** The concept that energy can be neither created nor destroyed but only converted from one form to another. **Doppler p.** DOPPLER EFFECT. **Fick p.** The principle that the cardiac output may be calculated by dividing the oxygen consumption by the arteriovenous oxygen difference. It is an application of the law of diffusion. **follicle stimulating p.** *Older term* FOLLICLE STIMULATING HORMONE. **Huygens p.** A theory of wave propagation, which states that every point on a wave front acts as a point source for the production of secondary wavelets, that the new wave front is the envelope of all the secondary wavelets, and that the amplitude at any point is the superposition of the wavelets at that point. **luteinizing p.** *Older term* LUTEINIZING HORMONE. **mass action p.** In the rat, learning is dependent more on the action of large segments of the cortex than on particular areas or subloci. **melanophore dilating p.** *Older term* MELANOCYTE STIMULATING HORMONE. **pleasure-pain p.** The belief that there is a regulatory mechanism of mental life that seeks to gain maximal pleasure or contentment for the organism or, at the very least, to avoid pain, suffering, dysphoria, and

discontent. It antedates the development of the reality principle. **reality p.** The assumption that the ego's main function is to temper the discharges of the libido in accordance with the demands of reality and subsequently in accordance with the incorporated parts of reality that have become the superego. **repetition-compulsion p.** The need to recreate and dramatize an earlier and usually painful experience. **Venturi p.** The principle that when a liquid or gas flows through a constriction in a tube, a fall in pressure occurs proportionate to rate of flow. Thus a specially designed tube (Venturi tube) can meter a supply of anesthetic gas or oxygen.

**Pringle** [John James *Pringle,* English dermatologist, 1855–1922] Bourneville-Pringle syndrome. See under TUBEROUS SCLEROSIS.

**print / voice p.** See under VOICEPRINT.

**Prinzmetal** [Myron *Prinzmetal,* U.S. internist, born 1908] See under ANGINA.

**prion** \prī′än\ [coined from *proteinaceous infection particle*] The smallest known infectious particle, a tiny viruslike entity highly resistant to inactivation, composed entirely of a hydrophobic protein and containing no DNA or RNA. Its molecular weight is 50 000 or less. Isolated in 1983 from brain tissue of sheep with scrapie, prions are postulated to be the agents of scrapie and possibly of certain slow central nervous system infections of man which resemble scrapie, especially kuru and Creutzfeldt-Jakob disease. It is not known whether prions can reproduce themselves. Compare VIROID.

***Prionurus*** \prī′ənʸoo′rəs\ [New L (from Gk *priōn* a saw + *oura* the tail, hinder parts)] A genus of scorpions with a venomous, painful sting. Well-known species of this genus include *P. citrinus* and *P. australis* of North Africa. An effective broad-spectrum antivenin has been prepared from venom of the latter species.

**prism** \priz′m\ [Gk *prisma* (from *priein* to saw) something sawn, a prism] A transparent solid whose ends are equal, parallel-plane polygons (usually triangles) and whose faces are parallelograms (usually rectangles), used to refract light beams and especially to produce spectra. Also *prisma.* Adj. prismatic. **enamel p.'s** The microscopic units of enamel, appearing as columns running from the amelodentinal junction to the surface of the enamel and related to the orientation of the crystallites. Also *enamel columns, adamantine prisms, prismata adamantina, enamel rods.* **Maddox p.** An optical testing device consisting of two prisms joined at their bases.

**prisma** \priz′mə\ [Gk, prism. See PRISM.] (*pl.* prismata) PRISM. **prismata adamantina** ENAMEL PRISMS.

**prismata** \priz′mətə\ Plural of PRISMA.

**prismatic** \prizmat′ik\ Of, pertaining to, or resembling a prism in shape or function.

**prismoid** \priz′moid\ Resembling a prism.

**privacy** The right of a patient to control the amount of information divulged about himself or herself and the right to control subsequent dissemination of that information.

**-prival** \-prī′vəl\ [L *priv(are)* to deprive + -AL] A combining form meaning pertaining to deprivation or nonfunction of a (specified) gland or organ, as *thyroprival, renoprival.*. Also *-privic, -privous.*

**-privic** \-priv′ik\ -PRIVAL.

**privilege / admitting p.'s** The right to admit patients to a health care facility. See also STAFF PRIVILEGES. **conversion p.** The right given the insured in group health care plans to change coverage to some form of individual policy, without medical examination, upon the termination of the group policy coverage. **staff p.'s** The right, granted by an inpatient health care facility to a physician or other professional, to admit patients and utilize the facilities.

**p.r.n.** *pro re nata* (L, as required; whenever necessary).

**Pro** Symbol for proline.

**pro-** \prō-, prə-\ [Gk *pro* before, in front of] **1** A prefix meaning (1) situated before, anterior; (2) prior to, preceding. **2** A chemical prefix used of proteins, meaning having a form that requires removal of part of the molecule by proteolysis before attaining its functional form, e.g., as an enzyme or hormone.

**proaccelerin** \prō′aksel′ərin\ FACTOR V.

**proactinium** PROTACTINIUM.

**proactivator** \-ak′tivā′tər\ PREKALLIKREIN.

**proal** \prō′əl\ [PRO- + -AL] Concerning forward movement.

**proangiotensin** ANGIOTENSIN I.

**proantigen** \-an′təjən\ *Outmoded* HAPTEN.

**proatlas** \-at′las\ [PRO- + *atlas,* after Atlas, the Gk god] The last of the occipital vertebrae developed in the interatlanto-occipital mesenchyme. In man, it normally disappears partly by incorporation in the occipital. It participates in the construction of the periphery of the foramen magnum, where one can often find some important remnants: basal processes or tubercles, postcondylar tubercle, posterior paramedian tubercle, postglenoid tubercle, paracondylar process, occipito-odontoid process, interoccipito-odontoid ossicle.

**probability** The chances that an event will happen or that a proposition is true, expressed as a fraction having a value between zero (impossibility) and one (certainty). **birth order p.** The probability that a woman of parity $n$ will give birth to another child in a specified time interval. It is estimated from the number of births of order $n$ in a given period, usually one year, per 1000 women of parity $n-1$ at the beginning of the period. It may be made specific for duration of marriage, maternal age, etc. **conditional p.** The probability that an eventuality will be realized given some other eventuality. For example, the probability that diagnosis A is correct given that a laboratory test B proves positive is a conditional probability. **posterior p.** The probability, resulting from the application of Bayes theorem, that a hypothesis is correct. It is the result of combining information obtained from observation or experiment with a prior probability. For example, the probability that a preliminary diagnosis will remain valid in the light of subsequent test results is a posterior probability. **prior p.** The probability as employed in the Bayes theorem to express the strength of belief in the truth of a hypothesis before additional evidence bearing on that belief has become available. Prior probabilities are usually founded on subjective opinions derived from past experience but not in the immediate context based on observation or experimental data. An example is the probability that a preliminary diagnosis made in advance of the results of confirmatory tests becoming available is correct. **reproduction p.** The ratio of the average number of offspring born to two parents, at least one of whom has a particular genotype (in humans, usually a heritable disorder), to the average number of offspring born to parents who are similar except that both lack the genotype of interest. Also *effective fertility.*

**probacteriophage** \-baktir′e·əfāj′\ PROPHAGE.

**proband** \prō′band\ [L *proband(us)* gerundive of *probare* to try, prove, test] The first patient introducing a cluster of patients with a similar illness to the medical profession, especially the individual (usually in a family) first identified as manifesting a given heritable trait. Also *propositus.* See also INDEX CASE.

**probang** \prō′bang\ [earlier *provang* of unknown origin]

An instrument for probing or applying medication to the esophagus or for the blind removal of esophageal foreign bodies, in general use prior to the introduction of endoscopic techniques at the turn of the century. It consisted of a flexible strip, originally of whale bone, carrying one of a variety of ends (sponge, bristles, etc.). Often these instruments were made with such an arrangement at one end and a coin-catcher at the other. When used for the blind removal of foreign bodies the risk of injury to the esophagus was considerable.

**probarbital** $C_9H_{14}N_2O_3$. 5-Ethyl-5-(1-methylethyl)-2,4,6-(1*H*,3*H*,5*H*)-pyrimidinetrione. A barbiturate of intermediate duration. It is used as a sedative and hypnotic, usually as the calcium or sodium salt.

**probe** [Med L *proba* (from L *probare* to make or find good, judge by a certain standard, show, prove) an examination] A slender, flexible, tapered instrument having a blunt or nodular end for exploring a wound or cavity. Also *explorer*. **blood flow p.** Any of a variety of devices used to measure the rate of volume flow through a blood vessel. **blunt p.** A long, narrow surgical instrument with a handle and a single dull blade that is used for exploration and dissection. **bullet p.** A surgical instrument formerly used for locating a bullet by insertion into the tract created by the projectile. **calibrated p.** PERIODONTAL PROBE. **drum p.** A surgical instrument that emits a tapping sound when it comes in contact with a foreign body. **electric p.** A surgical probe used to locate foreign objects in a wound. On contact with a foreign object, an electric circuit is completed and the probe emits a sound. Also *Girdner's probe, telephonic probe*. **eyed p.** A long, thin surgical instrument with a small opening at one end, designed to facilitate the placement of ligatures in a deep wound. **Girdner's p.** ELECTRIC PROBE. **heat p.** A device introduced into a tumor such as a glioma of the brain, whereby temperature is raised to about 42°C for the purpose of destroying tumor cells. **lacrimal p.** A thin wire intended for passage through the tear drainage channels to relieve blockage. Also *lacrimal sound*. **memory p.** A technique for examining retention in short-term memory. The subject is presented with a series of items, then cued by a repeat of one item from the list and asked to recall the item immediately following it in the original series. **periodontal p.** A blunt dental probe, usually calibrated in millimeters, used to measure the depth of the gingival sulcus or of periodontal pockets. Also *calibrated probe, pocket probe*. **scintillation p.** A device for the detection of electromagnetic radiation, such as gamma rays or x rays, that uses a crystal or plastic scintillator for the conversion of photons into visible light and then in turn converts the light to an electronic pulse. **telephonic p.** ELECTRIC PROBE. **ultrasound p.** An ultrasound transducer, especially one used for diagnostic purposes. **uterine p.** UTERINE SOUND. **WHO periodontal p.** A ball-shaped diagnostic probe marked with a band between 3.5 and 5.5 mm from its end. It is used by the World Health Organization for assessing the community periodontal index of treatment needs.

**probenecid** An orally effective uricosuric pharmaceutic agent, commonly used in gout for the treatment of hyperuricemia. It was formerly used to inhibit the excretion of some antibiotics, such as penicillin.

**probit** \prō′bit\ [contraction of *prob(ability) (un)it*] See under METHOD.

**problem** A conflict, abnormality, or unresolved question whose continued existence poses some degree of discomfort, uncertainty, or threat to the subject. **mind-body p.** The philosophic and psychological issue of the exact relationship existing between the entities of mind and body, and of mental and physiologic processes. Although solutions of the problem have been attempted since the time of Aristotle, all of the suggested resolutions remain theoretical today.

**proboscis** \-bäs′is, -bäs′kis\ [Gk *proboskis* (from *pro* before + *bosk(ein)* to feed, graze) an elephant's trunk] **1** A malformation of the nasal primordia of the embryo such that a tubular projection replaces the nose, as in cyclopia. **2** A tubular feeding organ with the opening at its tip, with complex biting and sucking mouthparts, as in mosquitoes and certain leeches, and retractile mouthparts, as in planarians.

**procainamide hydrochloride** $C_{13}H_{21}ClN_2O_2$. 4-Aminobenzoic acid 2-(diethylamino)ethyl ester hydrochloride. A local anesthetic agent that is rapidly metabolized by plasma cholinesterase. It is used by infiltration for local block, nerve block, and subarachnoid anesthesia.

**procaine** $C_{13}H_{20}N_2O_2$. 4-Aminobenzoic acid 2-(diethylamino)ethyl ester. A base that is slightly soluble in water and soluble in alcohol, benzene, and chloroform. It is a local anesthetic, usually administered as the hydrochloride or some other salt.

**procaine borate** $C_{13}H_{20}N_2O_2 \cdot 5BO_2$. A water-soluble salt of procaine, more active than the hydrochloride and used as a local anesthetic in ophthalmic and dental practice. Also *borocaine*.

**procaine hydrochloride** $C_{13}H_{21}ClN_2O_2$. A substance occurring as crystals that are very soluble in water and alcohol, slightly soluble in chloroform, and almost insoluble in ether. It is used as a local anesthetic. Its duration of action is relatively short because of enzymatic hydrolysis in blood and tissues. Also *ethocaine, syncaine*.

**procaine penicillin G** The procaine salt of penicillin G. It has a more prolonged action than penicillin G alone. Also *benzylpenicillin procaine*.

**procallus** \-kal′əs\ Granulation tissue that forms in the hematoma around a fracture in a bone and subsequently develops into fracture callus.

**procarbazine** $C_{12}H_{19}N_3O$. *N*-(1-Methylethyl-4-[(2-methylhydrazino)methyl]benzamide. An antineoplastic drug used mainly in the treatment of Hodgkin's disease. It is administered orally in the form of a monochloride salt.

**procarbazine hydrochloride** $C_{12}H_{19}N_3O \cdot HCl$. *N*-Isopropyl-α-(2-methylhydrazino)-*p*-toluamide. An antineoplastic agent used in the treatment of Hodgkin's disease and other lymphomas. It is usually given with other antitumor drugs, such as one of the vinca alkaloids.

**procarboxypeptidase** A zymogen of pancreatic secretion. It occurs as two forms, of sedimentation coefficients 5 and 6 svedbergs respectively. The larger has three subunits, the smaller, two. One of these subunits gives rise to carboxypeptidase A upon activation by trypsin in the intestine.

**procarcinogen** \-kär′sənəjən\ A substance which is carcinogenic after being chemically altered in the host. Most known chemical carcinogens fall into this category, such as benzo[a]pyrene or 3-methycholanthrene.

**procaryote** \-kar′ē·ōt\ PROKARYOTE.

**procaryotic** \-kar′ē·ät′ik\ PROKARYOTIC.

**procatarctic** \-kətärk′tik\ **1** Pertaining to or in the nature of procatarxis. **2** Predisposing. An outmoded usage.

**procatarxis** \-kətärk′sis\ **1** The production, by some activating cause, of a disease in one who is predisposed to it. **2** A predisposing or exciting cause. An outmoded usage.

**procedure** An activity directed at or performed on an individual with the object of improving health, treating disease or injury, or making a diagnosis. **Brock's p.** TRANSVENTRICULAR CLOSED VALVOTOMY. **Cockett p.**

The operative management of chronic venous stasis by the subcutaneous ligation of incompetent perforating veins draining into the posterior arch vein in the lower leg. **Dale p.** PALMA PROCEDURE. **Ewart's p.** A means of detecting tracheal tug by elevating the larynx with the thumb and forefinger. **exteriorization p.** A surgical procedure in which an organ, usually a hollow viscus, is brought out through the skin to permit drainage, allow observation, or bypass a distal obstruction. **Feulgen p.** FEULGEN METHOD. **Hassab p.** A nonshunt technique for treating bleeding esophageal varices that utilizes proximal gastric devascularization and a splenectomy. **Husni p.** An operative technique for bypassing a superficial femoral vein occlusion by means of the ipsilateral greater saphenous vein. Also *May procedure.* **Kazanjian's p.** RIDGE EXTENSION. **Kuhnt-Szymanowski p.** KUHNT-SZYMANOWSKI OPERATION. **Ladd's p.** A surgical procedure for treating proximal bowel obstruction secondary to malrotation of the cecum and midgut volvulus. It is accomplished by reducing the volvulus and by lysis of the peritoneal bands which obstruct the duodenal sweep. **Linton p.** A technique for relief of chronic venous stasis syndrome that involves the subfascial ligation of perforating veins in the lower leg. **May p.** HUSNI PROCEDURE. **Mikulicz p.** Reconstruction of the cervical esophagus by means of skin flaps taken from the neck. **Mustard p.** In congenital heart disease, a surgical procedure designed as a definitive repair for a complete transposition of the great arteries. The native atrial septum is excised and the atrium is partitioned with a baffle to redirect blood flow. Also *Mustard's operation.* **Palma p.** The use of the contralateral saphenous vein, which is dissected free, divided distally, tunneled subcutaneously in the suprapubic region, and anastomosed to the femoral vein, to relieve iliac vein obstruction. Also *Dale procedure, Palma-Dale procedure.* **periodic acid/Schiff p.** PERIODIC ACID-SCHIFF STAIN. **Potts p.** A surgical procedure in which complex cyanotic heart disease is palliated by creating a communication between the descending thoracic aorta and the left pulmonary artery, thereby increasing pulmonary blood flow. **pushback p.** PALATAL PUSHBACK OPERATION. **second-look p.** An operative approach involving a planned formal reoperation in 24 to 48 hours, usually following an initial operation for ischemic bowel. If tissue of marginal viability is left *in situ* at the initial operation, its fate and further management can be evaluated at the time of second-look. **Senning p.** In congenital heart disease, a surgical procedure used as a definitive treatment for a complete transposition of the great arteries, in which the atrium is refashioned with a patch or baffle and the pulmonary venous drainage is directed into the right atrium. **shelf p.** KÖNIG'S OPERATION. **stereotaxic p.** STEREOTAXY. **Sugiura p.** The extensive nonshunt devascularization of the distal esophagus and proximal stomach to treat bleeding esophageal varices. It also includes a near-total transection and reanastomosis of the distal esophagus, a splenectomy, and a pyloromyotomy. **Swenson pull-through p.** A surgical procedure used to treat congenital megacolon in the neonate. The aganglionic segment of the colon is resected and the distal margin of the normal colon is anastomosed to the anus. It is frequently done as a staged procedure with a diverting colostomy. **Tanner p.** A method of nonshunt devascularization for bleeding varices, including porto-azygous disconnection and gastric division. **Valsalva's p.** VALSALVA MANEUVER. **Womack p.** An operation to halt bleeding from esophagogastric varices in portal hypertension that includes a splenectomy and proximal gastric devascularization.

**proceedings / care and protection p.** Intervention by a court on behalf of a child whose parents or caretakers are unwilling or unable to provide adequately for the child's health, education, or general welfare.

**procelia** \-sē′lyə\ PROCOELIA.

**procelous** \-sē′ləs\ Concave on the anterior surface. Also *procoelous.*

**procentriole** \-sen′trē·ōl\ A cytoplasmic body which serves as a precursor of centrioles and basal bodies of cilia. It generally develops in proximity to an existing centriole.

**procephalic** \-səfal′ik\ Pertaining to the anterior part of the head.

**procercoid** \-sur′koid\ [PRO- + Gk *kerk(os)* tail + -OID] A larval stage of certain tapeworms which develops in aquatic crustaceans, often copepods, from the swimming first-stage coracidia eaten by the crustaceans, and which develops further into a plerocercoid, or final larval stage, after the crustacean is eaten by a fish.

**procerus** \-sir′əs\ [L (from *pro-* forward, outward + root *cer-*, akin to *crescere* to grow, + *-us*, masc. sing. suffix) long, tall] **1** Long, slender. **2** MUSCULUS PROCERUS.

# process

**process** [L *processus.* See PROCESSUS.] **1** A prominence, outgrowth of tissue, or projection; processus. **2** A sequence of events or gradual change whereby something passes, or is caused to pass, from one state to another. **accessory p. of lumbar vertebrae** PROCESSUS ACCESSORIUS VERTEBRARUM LUMBALIUM. **acromial p.** ACROMION. **alveolar p. of mandible** PARS ALVEOLARIS MANDIBULAE. **alveolar p. of maxilla** PROCESSUS ALVEOLARIS MAXILLAE. **ameloblastic p.** TOMES PROCESS. **anterior articular p. of axis** FACIES ARTICULARIS ANTERIOR AXIS. **anterior clinoid p.** PROCESSUS CLINOIDEUS ANTERIOR. **anterior p. of malleus** PROCESSUS ANTERIOR MALLEI. **articular p.** PROCESSUS ARTICULARIS. **articular p. of sacrum** PROCESSUS ARTICULARIS SUPERIOR OSSIS SACRI. **auditory p.** The dilated rough lateral lip of the osseous part of the external acoustic meatus to which the cartilaginous part is firmly attached. **basilar p.** PARS BASILARIS OSSIS OCCIPITALIS. **caudate p. of caudate lobe** PROCESSUS CAUDATUS HEPATIS. **ciliary p.'es** PROCESSUS CILIARES. **Civinini's p.** PROCESSUS PTERYGOSPINOSUS. **cochleariform p.** PROCESSUS COCHLEARIFORMIS. **condylar p.** A knuckle-shaped projection on the surface of a bone. **condylar p. of mandible** PROCESSUS CONDYLARIS MANDIBULAE. **coracoid p. of scapula** PROCESSUS CORACOIDEUS SCAPULAE. **coronoid p. of mandible** PROCESSUS CORONOIDEUS MANDIBULAE. **coronoid p. of ulna** PROCESSUS CORONOIDEUS ULNAE. **costal p.** **1** PROCESSUS COSTALIS VERTEBRAE. **2** The embryonic mesenchymal primordium of a rib, being a ventrolateral outgrowth of the caudal part of a sclerotome. **deep p. of the submandibular gland** An extension of the submandibular gland which passes forward from the deep surface of the gland around the posterior border of the mylohyoid muscle to lie between the latter and the hyoglossus muscle, running parallel to the submandibular duct as far as the back of the sublingual gland. **Deiters p.** AXON. **dendritic p.** A branching extension of the neuron soma, providing a site for synaptic contact. **ensiform p. of sternum** PROCESSUS XIPHOIDEUS. **ethmoid p.** PROCESSUS ETHMOIDALIS CONCHAE NASALIS INFERIORIS. **ethmoidal p. of inferior nasal concha** PROCESSUS ETHMOIDALIS CONCHAE NASALIS INFERIORIS. **facial p. of the parotid** The triangular anterior surface of the superficial part of the parotid gland which extends over the masseter muscle and is often continuous with the accessory parotid gland. **falciform p. of cerebellum** FALX CEREBELLI. **falciform p. of cerebrum** FALX CEREBRI. **falciform p. of sacrotuberal ligament** PROCESSUS FALCIFORMIS LIGAMENTI SACROTUBERALIS. **floccular p.** FLOCCULUS. **p. of Folius** PROCESSUS ANTERIOR MALLEI. **foot p.** PEDICEL. **frontal p. of maxilla** PROCESSUS FRONTALIS MAXILLAE. **frontal p. of zygomatic bone** PROCESSUS FRONTALIS OSSIS ZYGOMATICI. **frontonasal p.** An assembly of components on the superior wall of the buccal cavity constituted, towards the ninth week of human embryonic development, by the fusion of the two medial (internal) nasal folds. It comprises a labial component which gives rise to the upper lip, gingival component (incisive process) which bears the four upper incisors, and a palatal component represented by the primary palate. Also *prominentia frontonasalis.* **frontosphenoidal p.** PROCESSUS FRONTALIS OSSIS ZYGOMATICI. **globular p.** In the human embryo, an inferoexternal protuberance of the medial nasal fold which develops from the frontonasal process before the fifth week. Eventually it fuses with the maxillary process, when the latter has crossed the caudal end of the olfactory pit, and thus closes off the lower part of the primitive anterior naris. **Gottstein's basal p.** An outward prolongation or a basal process connecting a hair cell of the spiral organ to the basilar membrane. In the light of present knowledge, this is probably a phalangeal cell supporting the hair cell or a nerve fiber. **hamular p. of sphenoid bone** HAMULUS PTERYGOIDEUS. **head p.** A midline outgrowth of the primitive node of the early embryo which will become the notochordal plate. Also *notochordal process.* **incisive p.** MEDIAN NASAL PROCESS. **inferior articular p.** PROCESSUS ARTICULARIS INFERIOR VERTEBRAE. **infraorbital p.** The sharp anterior angle of the zygomatic bone that articulates with the maxilla and occasionally roofs over the infraorbital foramen. **infundibular p.** INFUNDIBULUM HYPOTHALAMI. **intercondylar p. of tibia** EMINENTIA INTERCONDYLARIS. **intrajugular p. of occipital bone** PROCESSUS INTRAJUGULARIS OSSIS OCCIPITALIS. **intrajugular p. of temporal bone** PROCESSUS INTRAJUGULARIS OSSIS TEMPORALIS. **jugular p.** PROCESSUS JUGULARIS OSSIS OCCIPITALIS. **jugular p. of occipital bone** PROCESSUS JUGULARIS OSSIS OCCIPITALIS. **lacrimal p.** PROCESSUS LACRIMALIS CONCHAE NASALIS INFERIORIS. **lateral p. of calcaneus** 1 TROCHLEA PERONEALIS CALCANEI. 2 PROCESSUS LATERALIS TUBERIS CALCANEI. **lateral p. of malleus** PROCESSUS LATERALIS MALLEI. **lateral nasal p.** A projecting elevation on the lateral (external) aspect of the frontonasal process separated from the median part by the nasal (olfactory) pit. As the pit deepens its lateral and medial margins become raised to form the lateral and medial nasal folds. The margins of the lateral nasal process and the maxillary process fuse to establish the side and the ala of the nose and the cheek, respectively. **lateral p. of talus** PROCESSUS LATERALIS TALI. **lateral p. of tuberosity of calcaneus** PROCESSUS LATERALIS TUBERIS CALCANEI. **lenticular p. of incus** PROCESSUS LENTICULARIS INCUDIS. **lentiform p.** PROCESSUS LENTICULARIS INCUDIS. **long p. of malleus** PROCESSUS ANTERIOR MALLEI. **lumbocostal p. of lumbar vertebra** The processus costalis which is incorporated in the transverse process of a lumbar vertebra. **malar p.** PROCESSUS ZYGOMATICUS MAXILLAE. **mamillary p. of vertebrae** PROCESSUS MAMMILLARIS VERTEBRARUM LUMBALIUM. **mandibular p.** PROMINENTIA MANDIBULARIS. **marginal p. of malar bone** TUBERCULUM MARGINALE OSSIS ZYGOMATICI. **mastoid p.** PROCESSUS MASTOIDEUS OSSIS TEMPORALIS. **maxillary p.** A triangular process in the embryo which grows caudally from the cephalic aspect of the dorsal end of the first (mandibular) branchial arch to fuse with the lateral nasal process. Part of the dorsal portion in the maxillary process becomes chondrified as a small mass behind the orbital region, and its posterior part represents the pterygoquadrate bar of lower vertebrates. This part is considered by some to be the rudiment of the incus. **maxillary p. of inferior nasal concha** PROCESSUS MAXILLARIS CONCHAE NASALIS INFERIORIS. **maxillary p. of the palatine bone** The projecting front part of facies maxillaris laminae perpendicularis ossis palatini that forms the posterior portion of the medial wall of the maxillary sinus. **medial angular p. of the frontal bone** The angulated junction of the nasal margin or notch of the frontal bone and the medial end of the supraorbital margin. **medial p. of tuberosity of calcaneus** PROCESSUS MEDIALIS TUBERIS CALCANEI. **median nasal p.** The central part of the outside of the frontonasal process on its lower aspect and partially dividing the roof of the primitive stomodeum. It forms the medial margin of the nasal (olfactory) pit where an elevation develops as the medial nasal fold (or process). This fold grows caudally and the mesenchyme of its extension into the stomodeal roof forms the globular process. Meanwhile the maxillary process extends medially beyond the lateral nasal process and crosses the caudal or lower edge of the nasal (olfactory) pit to fuse with the downgrowth of the medial nasal folds (globular process) and so form the upper lip. The deeper cranial part of the median nasal process continues backwards as the primitive nasal septum. Also *incisive process.* **median palatine p.** The small triangular premaxillary process that lies in the front part of the developing palate between the lateral palatine shelves which fuse with it as well as with each other and with the nasal septum on their cephalic aspect. The extent of its derivation from the medial nasal process is disputed. **mental p.** PROTUBERANTIA MENTALIS. **middle clinoid p.** PROCESSUS CLINOIDEUS MEDIUS. **muscular p. of arytenoid cartilage** PROCESSUS MUSCULARIS CARTILAGINIS ARYTENOIDEAE. **nasal p. of frontal bone** PARS NASALIS OSSIS FRONTALIS. **notochordal p.** HEAD PROCESS. **odontoblastic p.** A peripherally directed, slender process projecting from the cell body of each odontoblast. It comes to lie within each dentinal tubule and provides nutriment to the dentin. Also *Tomes fiber, dentinal fiber.* **odontoid p. of axis** DENS AXIS. **olecranon p. of ulna** OLECRANON. **orbital p. of palatine bone** PROCESSUS ORBITALIS OSSIS PALATINI. **palatal p.** PALATINE PROCESS. **palatine p.** A horizontal plate of tissue in the embryo which develops from the inner border of each maxillary process. The two processes grow together and make contact along the midline, passing below the primitive choanae, thus forming the posterior part of the palate, and eventually isolating the nasal fossae from the buccal cavity. Also *palatal process, palatine shelf.* **palatine p. of maxilla** PROCESSUS PALATINUS MAXILLAE. **papillary p. of liver** PROCESSUS PAPILLARIS HEPATIS. **paramastoid p. of occipital bone** PROCESSUS PARA-

MASTOIDEUS OSSIS OCCIPITALIS. **postauditory p.** A portion of the squamous part of the temporal bone that forms the lateral wall of the mastoid antrum and part of the posterior wall of the external acoustic meatus. In the adult it corresponds to the suprameatal triangle on the lateral surface of the skull. Also *postmeatal process of temporal bone.* **posterior p. of cartilage of nasal septum** PROCESSUS POSTERIOR CARTILAGINIS SEPTI NASI. **posterior clinoid p.** PROCESSUS CLINOIDEUS POSTERIOR. **posterior p. of the talus** PROCESSUS POSTERIOR TALI. **postglenoid p.** POSTGLENOID TUBERCLE. **postmeatal p. of temporal bone** POSTAUDITORY PROCESS. **primary p.** The laws of the unconscious, characterized by immediate gratification, extreme lability of cathexis, lack of negatives or conditionals, and the absence of a sense of time. The laws of the primary process result from the forces of the pleasure principle. **pterygoid p.** PROCESSUS PTERYGOIDEUS OSSIS SPHENOIDALIS. **pterygopalatine p.** A posterior prolongation of one of the palatine processes, which will give rise to the posterior portion of the bony vault of the palate. This is formed by the horizontal plate of the palatine bones, the pyramidal process of which fits into an interval between the pterygoid plates. **pterygoquadrate p.** The posterior part of the maxillary process, which is considered to give rise during development to the incus of the middle ear. **pterygospinous p.** PROCESSUS PTERYGOSPINOSUS. **pyramidal p. of palatine bone** PROCESSUS PYRAMIDALIS OSSIS PALATINI. **random p.** STOCHASTIC PROCESS. **restiform p. of Henle** *Outmoded* PEDUNCULUS CEREBELLARIS INFERIOR. **retromandibular p.** The medial portion of the parotid gland that extends into the lateral pharyngeal space between the posterior margin of the ramus of the mandible and the mastoid process. **secondary p.** The laws governing the operation of the preconscious and ego, resulting from the reality principle. **sphenoidal p.** PROCESSUS POSTERIOR CARTILAGINIS SEPTI NASI. **sphenoidal p. of palatine bone** PROCESSUS SPHENOIDALIS OSSIS PALATINI. **spinous p.** The embryonic precursor of the spinous process of the vertebrae. Until puberty the ends of the spinous processes are cartilaginous. Secondary centers then appear in them and fuse with the rest of the bone at about age 25 in man. **spinous p. of tibia** EMINENTIA INTERCONDYLARIS. **spinous p. of vertebra** PROCESSUS SPINOSUS VERTEBRAE. **Stieda's p.** PROCESSUS POSTERIOR TALI. **stochastic p.** A process whose development can be predicted only in terms of probability, rather than deterministically. Formally, a stochastic process is one in which a variate at time $t$ has a value $x_0$ and by a later time $t$ may assume any one of a set of values $(x_1, x_2, x_3,... x_n)$ with a stated probability. Also *random process.* **styloid p. of fibula** APEX CAPITIS FIBULAE. **styloid p. of radius** PROCESSUS STYLOIDEUS RADII. **styloid p. of temporal bone** PROCESSUS STYLOIDEUS OSSIS TEMPORALIS. **styloid p. of third metacarpal bone** PROCESSUS STYLOIDEUS OSSIS METACARPALIS TERTII (III). **styloid p. of ulna** PROCESSUS STYLOIDEUS ULNAE. **sucker p.** SUCKER FOOT. **superior articular p.** PROCESSUS ARTICULARIS SUPERIOR VERTEBRAE. **superior articular p. of sacrum** PROCESSUS ARTICULARIS SUPERIOR OSSIS SACRI. **supracondylar p. of humerus** PROCESSUS SUPRAEPICONDYLARIS HUMERI. **temporal p. of zygomatic bone** PROCESSUS TEMPORALIS OSSIS ZYGOMATICI. **Tomes p.** The slender projection of cytoplasm from each ameloblast of the enamel organ, which takes part in the process of enamel deposition during the formation of a tooth. Also *ameloblastic process.* **transverse p. of sacrum** CRISTA SACRALIS LATERALIS. **transverse p. of vertebra** PROCESSUS TRANSVERSUS VERTEBRAE. **trochlear p. of calcaneus** TROCHLEA PERONEALIS CALCANEI. **uncinate p. of ethmoid bone** PROCESSUS UNCINATUS OSSIS ETHMOIDALIS. **uncinate p. of pancreas** PROCESSUS UNCINATUS PANCREATIS. **vaginal p.** **1** VAGINA PROCESSUS STYLOIDEI. **2** PERITONEOVAGINAL CANAL. **vaginal p. of sphenoid bone** PROCESSUS VAGINALIS OSSIS SPHENOIDALIS. **vaginal p. of styloid** VAGINA PROCESSUS STYLOIDEI. **vaginal p. of temporal bone** VAGINA PROCESSUS STYLOIDEI. **vermiform p.** APPENDIX VERMIFORMIS. **vermiform p. of cerebellum** VERMIS CEREBELLI. **vertebral p.** Any process projecting from a vertebra, such as the transverse, spinous, superior articular, or inferior articular process. **vocal p.** PROCESSUS VOCALIS. **xiphoid p.** PROCESSUS XIPHOIDEUS. **zygomatic p. of frontal bone** PROCESSUS ZYGOMATICUS OSSIS FRONTALIS. **zygomatic p. of maxilla** PROCESSUS ZYGOMATICUS MAXILLAE. **zygomatic p. of temporal bone** PROCESSUS ZYGOMATICUS OSSIS TEMPORALIS.

**processing** The set of computer operations involving input, transformation, storage, and retrieval of coded information. **signal p.** Alteration of an electrical signal by processes such as amplification, filtering, and rectification.

**processor** **1** The central arithmetic unit of a computer that performs calculations and does not include memory or peripherals. **2** A computer program that performs the compiling, assembling and translating functions for a specific programing language such as FORTRAN.

# processus

**processus** \prōses′əs\ [L (from *processus,* past part. of *procedere* to go before, go forth, proceed, grow out, from *pro-* PRO- + *cedere* to go, happen), a going forth, advance, outgrowth, protuberance] (*pl.* processus) A prominence, outgrowth of tissue, or projection; a process. **p. accessorius vertebrarum lumbalium** [NA] A small distally directed eminence located posteroinferiorly to the base of each transverse process of the lumbar vertebrae, being especially well developed in the second to the fourth. Also *accessory process of lumbar vertebrae, accessory tubercle.* **p. alveolaris maxillae** [NA] The thick, spongy crescentic inferior border of the maxilla that contains eight sockets on each side for the roots of the upper teeth in the adult. The buccinator muscle arises from its outer surface behind the premolars. Also *alveolar process of maxilla, basal ridge.* **p. anterior mallei** [NA] A slender bony process projecting anteriorly from the neck of the malleus and connected to the petrotympanic fissure by ligamentous fibers. Also *anterior process of malleus, long process of malleus, apophysis of Rau.* **p. articularis** [NA] Either processus articularis inferior vertebrae or processus articularis superior vertebrae. Also *zygapophysis, articular process.* **p. articularis inferior vertebrae** [NA] One of a pair of projections from the vertebral arch extending downwards from the inferior aspect of the junction of the pedicles and the laminae and presenting an articular facet facing forwards and medially for articulation with the superior articular process of the vertebra below. Also *inferior articular process.* **p. articularis superior ossis sacri** [NA] One of two rounded prominences projecting posterosuperiorly from the dorsal surface of the base of the sacrum on each side of the sacral canal and bearing a concave articular facet facing posteromedially for articulation with the inferior articular process of the fifth lumbar vertebra. Lateral to each facet is a well-marked rough mamillary process. Also *superior articular process of sacrum, articular process of sacrum.* **p. articularis superior vertebrae** [NA] One of a pair of projections from the vertebral arch, extending upwards from the superior aspect of the junction of the pedicles and the laminae and presenting an articular facet facing posteriorly and usually laterally for articulation with the inferior articular process of the vertebra above. Also *superior articular process, diapophysis.* **p. calcaneus** [NA] A process that projects posteriorly from the inferior surface of the cuboid bone at its junction with the inferomedial angle of the proximal surface. It supports the anterior end of the calcaneus. **p. caudatus hepatis** [NA] A narrow strip of liver substance connecting the lower right border of the caudate lobe to the right lobe of the liver and lying behind the porta hepatis to form the superior relation of the epiploic foramen. Also *caudate process of caudate lobe.* **p. ciliares** [NA] About eighty ridges on the ringlike corona ciliaris which radiate outwards in a meridional direction from the base of the iris towards the orbicularis ciliaris of the ciliary body. In the grooves between the ridges zonular fibers of the lens extend towards the orbicularis ciliaris. Also *ciliary processes.* **p. clinoideus anterior** [NA] The prolonged medial tip of the posterior border of the lesser wing of the sphenoid bone to which the anterior end of the free border of the tentorium cerebelli is attached. Sometimes it is joined by a strip of bone to the middle clinoid process to form the caroticoclinoid foramen. Also *anterior clinoid process.* **p. clinoideus medius** [NA] A small projection at each posterolateral end of the tuberculum sellae and on each side of the hypophyseal fossa between and below the anterior and posterior clinoid processes. It may be absent. Also *middle clinoid process.* **p. clinoideus posterior** [NA] One of two projections at the superolateral angles of the dorsum sellae of the body of the sphenoid bone, to each of which the fixed edge of the tentorium cerebelli is attached. Also *posterior clinoid process.* **p. cochleariformis** [NA] The laterally curved posterior end of the bony septum between the semicanal for the tensor tympani and the bony canal of the auditory tube. It projects from the anterior wall of the tympanic cavity and provides a pulley for the tendon of the tensor tympani muscle. It is located just above the fenestra vestibuli. Also *cochleariform process.* **p. condylaris mandibulae** [NA] The anteroposteriorly flattened and superiorly rounded upward projection of the posterior margin of the ramus of the mandible comprising the head and neck of the mandible. Also *condylar process of mandible, mandibular condyle, condyle of mandible, head of mandible.* **p. coracoideus scapulae** [NA] A fingerlike process projecting forwards and laterally from the upper border of the neck of the scapula. Its root meets the upper part of the glenoid cavity at the supraglenoid tubercle and its lateral tip or apex, which can be palpated below the lateral third of the clavicle, provides origin for the coracobrachialis and the short head of the biceps brachii muscles. Also *coracoid process of scapula.* **p. coronoideus mandibulae** [NA] A flattened triangular projection at the anterosuperior angle of the ramus of the mandible, its anterior margin being continuous with the anterior margin of the ramus and its posterior margin forming the mandibular incisure. The temporalis muscle is inserted into its margins and medial surface. Also *coronoid process of mandible.* **p. coronoideus ulnae** [NA] A curved projection from the front of the proximal end of the ulna forming the distal part of the trochlear notch, its superior articular surface being continuous with the anterior surface of the olecranon. The upper part of its lateral surface bears the radial notch while the rough inferior surface has the tuberosity of the ulna. During flexion of the elbow joint the tip of the process fits into the coronoid fossa of the humerus. Also *coronoid process of ulna.* **p. costalis vertebrae** [NA] A rounded bar of bone projecting laterally from the front of the body of a cervical vertebra comprising the anterior root of the transverse process and forming the anterior boundary of the foramen transversarium. It terminates laterally in the anterior tubercle and corresponds to the vertebral end of a rib. Also *costal process.* **p. e cerebello ad medullam** PEDUNCULUS CEREBELLARIS INFERIOR. **p. e cerebello ad pontem** PEDUNCULUS CEREBELLARIS MEDIUS. **p. e cerebello ad testes** PEDUNCULUS CEREBELLARIS SUPERIOR. **p. ethmoidalis conchae nasalis inferioris** [NA] A thin bony plate projecting upwards and posteriorly from the middle of the superior border of the inferior nasal concha to articulate with the uncinate process of the ethmoid bone across the opening of the maxillary sinus. Also *ethmoidal process of inferior nasal concha, ethmoid process.* **p. falciformis ligamenti sacrotuberalis** [NA] The crescentic continuation of the sacrotuberous ligament from the ischial tuberosity along the medial surface of the ischial ramus, the curved edge of which is continuous with the fascial sheath of the internal pudendal vessels and pudendal nerve. Also *falciform process of sacrotuberal ligament, falciform ligament, falx ligamentosa* (outmoded), *ligamentous falx* (outmoded). **p. frontalis maxillae** [NA] An upward projection from the body of the maxilla anteriorly, the lateral surface being continuous with the anterior surface of the body and the medial surface forming part of the lateral wall of the nasal cavity. The superior border articulates with the nasal part of the frontal bone, the anterior border articulates with the nasal bone, and the posterior border is dimpled by the lacrimal notch and articulates with the lacrimal bone. Also *frontal process of maxilla, prefrontal bone of von Bardeleben.* **p. frontalis ossis zygomatici** [NA] The thick curved upward projection of the zygomatic bone that articulates superiorly with the frontal bone and behind with the greater wing of the sphenoid bone forming the lateral margin of the orbit. On its superolateral border is the marginal tubercle, while on its medial aspect is the orbital surface. Also *frontal process of zygomatic bone, frontosphenoidal process.* **p. intrajugularis ossis occipitalis** [NA] A small bony spike projecting forwards and laterally in the jugular notch of the occipital bone that is situated opposite a projection with the same name in the jugular notch of the temporal bone. Together they subdivide the jugular foramen into two parts, one for the sigmoid sinus and the other containing the glossopharyngeal, vagus, and accessory nerves and the inferior petrosal sinus. Also *intrajugular process of occipital bone.* **p. intrajugularis ossis temporalis** [NA] A small bony ridge in the jugular notch in the petrous part of the temporal bone that is situated opposite a spicule with the same name in the jugular notch of the occipital bone. Together they subdivide the jugular foramen into two parts, one containing the sigmoid sinus and the other the glossopharyngeal, vagus and accessory nerves and the inferior petrosal sinus. Also *intrajugular process of temporal bone.* **p. jugularis ossis occipitalis** [NA] A quadrangular plate of bone jutting out laterally from the posterior half of the occipital condyle and grooved anteriorly by the jugular notch which forms the back of the jugular foramen. Laterally it articulates with the petrous part of the temporal bone.

Also *jugular process of occipital bone, jugular process.* **p. lacrimalis conchae nasalis inferioris** [NA] A small pointed projection near the front of the superior border of the inferior nasal concha, the tip or apex of which articulates with a downward projection of the lacrimal bone while its margins meet the edges of the nasolacrimal groove on the back of the frontal process of the maxilla helping to form the wall of the nasolacrimal canal. Also *lacrimal process.* **p. lateralis mallei** [NA] A small conical lateral projection from the root of the handle of the malleus, attaching to the upper part of the tympanic membrane and forming the malleal prominence. Also *lateral process of malleus.* **p. lateralis tali** [NA] A nonarticular projection located inferiorly to the apex of the triangular lateral surface of the talus that articulates with the lateral malleolus. Also *lateral process of talus, lateral tubercle of talus.* **p. lateralis tuberis calcanei** [NA] A rounded projection on the lateral side of the plantar aspect of the calacaneal tuberosity, separated by a notch from the broader medial process and giving partial origin to the abductor digiti minimi muscle. Also *lateral process of tuberosity of calcaneus, lateral process of calcaneus.* **p. lenticularis incudis** [NA] A small nodule at the free terminal end of the long process of the incus which is covered with cartilage and articulates with the head of the stapes. Also *lenticular process of incus, lentiform process.* **p. mammillaris vertebrarum lumbalium** [NA] A small rough tubercle on the posterior border of each superior articular process of the lumbar vertebrae that provides attachment for the multifidus and medial intertransverse muscles. It is homologous with the superior tubercle of the twelfth thoracic vertebra. Also *mamillary process of vertebrae, mamillary tubercle of vertebrae, metapophysis.* **p. mastoideus ossis temporalis** [NA] A conical projection downward and forward from the petrous part of the temporal bone behind and below the external acoustic meatus. Its lateral surface provides attachment for the sternocleidomastoid, splenius capitis, and longissimus capitis muscles while its medial surface is grooved by the mastoid notch. It contains the mastoid air cells. Also *mastoid process, mastoid bone, mastoid, mastoideum* (outmoded), *mastoidea* (outmoded). **p. maxillaris conchae nasalis inferioris** [NA] A thin curved plate of bone projecting downwards and laterally from the middle of the superior border of the inferior nasal concha to articulate with the maxilla and the maxillary process of the palatine bone so as to form part of the medial wall of the maxillary sinus and attach the concha to the lateral wall of the nasal cavity. Also *maxillary process of inferior nasal concha.* **p. medialis tuberis calcanei** [NA] The distal extension of the medial part of the plantar aspect of the calcaneal tuberosity, broader than the lateral process and separated from it by a notch. It gives attachment medially to the flexor retinaculum and the abductor hallucis muscle and anteriorly to the plantar aponeurosis and the flexor digitorum brevis muscle. Also *medial process of tuberosity of calcaneus.* **p. muscularis cartilaginis arytenoideae** [NA] The rounded and prominent lateral angle of the base of the arytenoid cartilage which projects posterolaterally to give attachment to the lateral cricoarytenoid muscle anteriorly and the posterior cricoarytenoid muscle posteriorly. Also *muscular process of arytenoid cartilage.* **p. orbitalis ossis palatini** [NA] The irregular, upward projection of the front of the perpendicular plate of the palatine bone, separated from the posteriorly situated sphenoidal process by the sphenopalatine notch and presenting three articular surfaces, namely, maxillary, sphenoidal, and ethmoidal, as well as two nonarticular surfaces, namely, orbital and lateral. Also *orbital process of palatine bone.* **p. palatinus maxillae** [NA] A thick arched plate of bone projecting medially from the inferior part of the body of the maxilla and meeting the corresponding process of the opposite side in the midline to form the anterior three-fourths of the bony palate inferiorly and most of the floor of the nasal cavity superiorly. It has numerous foramina, canals, and grooves for vessels and nerves. The serrated posterior border articulates with the horizontal plate of the palatine bone to complete the bony palate. Also *palatine process of maxilla, palatine lamina of maxilla.* **p. papillaris hepatis** [NA] A short, rounded eminence at the portal or anterior end of the caudate lobe of the liver, situated to the left of the caudate process and separated from it by a notch. It lies opposite the tuber omentale of the left lobe and in fetal life it is relatively much larger and related through the lesser omentum to the pancreas. Also *papillary process of liver.* **p. paramastoideus ossis occipitalis** [NA] A bony eminence extending downward from the inferior surface of the jugular process of the occipital bone, rarely reaching the transverse process of the atlas in humans. Also *paramastoid process of occipital bone.* **p. phalangeus** DEITERS PHALANGES. **p. posterior cartilaginis septi nasi** [NA] A narrow posterior projection of the septal cartilage of the nose, especially marked in children, extending for a varying distance between the vomer and the perpendicular plate of the ethmoid bone. Also *posterior process of cartilage of nasal septum, sphenoidal process.* **p. posterior tali** [NA] The posterior projection of the posterior surface of the talus, grooved by the sulcus for the tendon of the flexor hallucis longus muscle which divides it into unequal medial and lateral tubercles for attachment of ligaments. Also *posterior process of the talus, Stieda's process.* **p. pterygoideus ossis sphenoidalis** [NA] An elongated bony mass extending perpendicularly downwards on each side from the junction of the body of the sphenoid bone and the greater wing and comprising parallel medial and lateral plates or laminae. The plates are fused in their upper parts anteriorly but they diverge posteriorly to enclose the pterygoid fossa containing the medial pterygoid and tensor veli palatini muscles. Their fused anterior surface is broad superiorly where it forms the posterior boundary of the pterygopalatine fossa. Also *pterygoid process, pterygoid apophysis, pterygoid bone.* **p. pterygospinosus** [NA] A backward projection from the posterior border of the lateral pterygoid plate to which is attached the pterygospinous ligament connecting it to the spine of the sphenoid bone. Also *pterygospinous process, Civinini's process, Civinini spine.* **p. pyramidalis ossis palatini** [NA] A triangular bony prominence projecting posteriorly, inferiorly, and laterally from the junction of the perpendicular and the horizontal plates of the palatine bone to fit into the pterygoid notch or incisure. Also *pyramidal process of palatine bone, pyramidal tuberosity of palatine bone.* **p. sphenoidalis ossis palatini** [NA] A narrow, compressed upward extension of the posterior margin of the perpendicular plate of the palatine bone, smaller than and separated from the orbital process by the sphenopalatine notch. Superiorly it articulates with the sphenoidal concha and the base of the medial pterygoid plate, helping to form the palatovaginal canal. Also *sphenoidal process of palatine bone.* **p. spinosus vertebrae** [NA] The elongated projection extending posteriorly from the junction of the laminae of the vertebral arch. It varies in direction, often extending downwards, shape and size, and provides attachment for muscles and ligaments. Also *spinous process of vertebra, spine of vertebra, vertebral spine, neural spine.* **p. styloideus ossis metacarpalis tertii (III)** [NA] The short, pointed prominence projecting proximally from the lateral side of the posterior surface of the base of the third metacarpal bone. Occasionally it has a separate ossification center and may remain separated from the base as the styloid bone. Also *styloid process of third metacarpal bone.* **p. styloideus ossis temporalis** [NA] A slender rounded projection extending downwards, medially, and forward from the junction of the petrous part of the temporal bone and the tympanic plate on the inferior surface. Its proximal part, or tympanohyal, is ensheathed by an extension of the tympanic plate, and its distal part, or stylohyal, provides attachment for the stylopharyngeus, styloglossus, and stylohyoid muscles as well as the stylohyoid and stylomandibular ligaments. It varies in length and lies deep to the parotid gland, while the jugular foramen is medial to it and the stylomastoid foramen behind it. Also *styloid process of temporal bone.* **p. styloideus radii** [NA] A blunt conical projection extending distally from the lateral surface at the lower end of the radius. It is subcutaneous and partly concealed by tendons, while the tip gives attachment to the radial collateral ligament. Also *styloid process of radius.* **p. styloideus ulnae** [NA] A short, rounded projection extending distally from the posterior margin at the lower end of the ulna and located posteromedial to the head of the ulna. To its subcutaneous tip the ulnar collateral ligament of the wrist is attached and to the lateral side of its base the apex of the triangular articular disk is attached. Also *styloid process of ulna.* **p. supraepicondylaris humeri** [NA] A curved bony spine of variable size occasionally located on the anteromedial surface of the humerus about 5 cm proximal to the medial epicondyle to which it is connected by a fibrous band. In the space deep to the band the median nerve passes alone or with the brachial artery, being the homologue of the entepicondylar foramen found in many animals. Also *supracondylar process of humerus.* **p. temporalis ossis zygomatici** [NA] The posteriorly directed projection of the zygomatic bone that has an oblique serrated border for articulation with the zygomatic process of the temporal bone, forming the zygomatic arch. Also *temporal process of zygomatic bone.* **p. transversus vertebrae** [NA] The lateral projection from the junction of the pedicle and the lamina on each side of the vertebral arch, providing attachment to muscles and ligaments and, in the thoracic region, articulating with the ribs. Also *transverse process of vertebra.* **p. uncinatus ossis ethmoidalis** [NA] An irregular curved plate of bone projecting inferiorly and posteriorly from the anteroinferior part of the labyrinth at the front of the orbital plate of the ethmoid bone. It articulates with the ethmoidal process of the inferior nasal concha, forming part of the medial wall of the maxillary sinus, while its upper free edge forms the medial boundary of the hiatus semilunaris in the middle nasal meatus. Also *uncinate process of ethmoid bone, hamulus of ethmoid bone.* **p. uncinatus pancreatis** [NA] The lower left portion of the head of the pancreas that extends upwards and to the left posterior to the superior mesenteric vessels. Also *uncinate process of pancreas, lesser pancreas, unciform pancreas, Winslow's pancreas, Willis pancreas.* **p. vaginalis ossis sphenoidalis** [NA] A thin plate of bone projecting medially from the base of the medial pterygoid plate and along the inferior surface of the body of the sphenoid bone to articulate anteriorly with the sphenoidal process of the palatine bone and medially with the wing of the vomer. On its superior surface are two longitudinal furrows helping to form the palatovaginal and vomerovaginal canals. Also *vaginal process of sphenoid bone.* **p. vaginalis peritonei** PERITONEOVAGINAL CANAL. **p. vaginalis testis** A thick cellular cord in male embryos formed by a peritoneal prolongation from the lower end of the saccus vaginalis or lateral inguinal fossa down the inguinal canal along the gubernaculum testis. As the testis descends through the inguinal canal towards the genital swellings to gain the future scrotum it draws peritoneum into the processus vaginalis. The distal part of the processus vaginalis forms the tunica vaginalis testis. The proximal part within the inguinal canal and scrotum, which is included within the spermatic cord, is usually obliterated. See also PERITONEOVAGINAL CANAL. **p. vocalis** [NA] The pointed anterior angle of the arytenoid cartilage which projects horizontally forward, providing attachment for the the vocal ligament. Also *vocal process.* **p. xiphoideus** [NA] A flat elongated downward projection at the lower end of the sternum, lying between the seventh costal cartilages and being cartilaginous in youth, partly ossified in the adult, and totally ossified and fused with the body of the sternum in old age. It is highly variable in length, shape, and curvature, and provides attachment to both thoracic and abdominal muscles. Also *xiphoid process, ensiform process of sternum, ensisternum, xiphoid cartilage, ensiform cartilage, xiphoid appendix, ensiform appendix, xiphoid bone, xiphisternum.* **p. zygomaticus maxillae** [NA] A pyramidal projection from the junction of the anterior, orbital, and infratemporal surfaces of the body of the maxilla, articulating superiorly with the zygomatic bone. Also *zygomatic process of maxilla, malar process.* **p. zygomaticus ossis frontalis** [NA] The thick and prominent lateral extremity of the supraorbital margin of the frontal bone that articulates with the zygomatic bone to form the lateral margin of the orbit. Posteriorly the temporal line extends back from it. Also *zygomatic process of frontal bone.* **p. zygomaticus ossis temporalis** [NA] A narrow elongated and curved bar of bone projecting forwards from the lower border of the temporal surface of the squamous part of the temporal bone to articulate by its narrow serrated anterior end with the temporal process of the zygomatic bone to form the zygomatic arch. The broad laterally projecting base comprises three roots, namely, anterior, middle, and posterior. Also *zygomatic process of temporal bone.*

**prochlorperazine** $C_{20}H_{24}ClN_3S$. 2-Chloro-10-[3-(4-methylpiperazin-1-yl)propyl]-phenothiazine. A clear, yellow liquid, very soluble in water. It is a phenothiazine tranquilizer and antiemetic like chlorpromazine, but more potent. It is also less active than chlorpromazine as an antihistaminic and antispasmolytic agent. It is administered rectally as suppositories, and its salts are given orally. Also *prochlorpemazine.*

**prochlorperazine edisylate** The ethanedisulfonate salt of prochlorperazine. It is given by mouth or by intramuscular or intravenous injection, and it has the same action and uses as prochlorperazine. Also *prochlorperazine ethanedisulfonate.*

**prochlorperazine maleate** The dimaleate salt of prochloroperazine. It is given orally for the same indications as prochlorperazine.

**prochondral** \-kän′drəl\ [PRO- + CHONDRAL] Existing prior to the development of cartilage, usually in an embryo.

**prochordal** \-kôr′dəl\ PRECHORDAL.

**procidentia** \-siden′shə\ [L (from *procidere* to fall down or out, from *pro-* forward or downward + *cadere* to fall) a displacement or prolapse] Prolapse, especially of the uterus. **p. uteri** PROLAPSE OF UTERUS.

**proclination** \-klinā′shən\ [PRO- + *clin(o)-* + -ATION] An abnormal labial tipping of anterior teeth.

**procoagulant** \-kō·ag′yələnt\ **1** Any precursor of an active coagulation factor, such as factor X (the precursor of factor Xa) or prothrombin (the precursor of thrombin).

2 Any substance that fosters coagulation of blood.

**procoelia** \-sē′lē·ə\ [New L, from *pro(sencephalon)* + Gk *koilia* a cavity] 1 The precursor of the lateral ventricle of the brain, formed by an outpouching of the cavity of the prosencephalon. 2 *Outmoded* VENTRICULUS LATERALIS CEREBRI. For defs. 1 and 2 also *procelia.*

**procoelous** \-sē′ləs\ PROCELOUS.

**procollagen** \-käl′əjən\ [PRO- + COLLAGEN] A soluble precursor of collagen which is synthesized in the cell and then secreted. Enzymes in the extracellular space remove a portion of both the amino and carboxyl ends of the molecule, allowing the spontaneous formation of collagen fibrils.

**proconceptive** \-kənsep′tiv\ An agent or process that facilitates conception.

**procondylism** \-kän′dilizm\ Anterior deviation of the mandibular condyles.

**proconvertin** \-kənvur′tin\ FACTOR VII.

**procreative** \-krē·ā′tiv\ Of or relating to procreation.

**proct-** \präkt-\ PROCTO-.

**proctalgia** \präktal′jə\ [PROCT- + -ALGIA] Pain in the rectum. **p. fugax** A sudden attack of pain of brief duration occurring from time to time in the lower rectum and anus, sometimes associated with transient tenesmus. It is a benign condition of unknown origin. Emotional tension appears to be one precipitating factor. It affects both sexes at any age but is commoner in women.

**proctectasia** \präk′tektā′zhə\ [PROCT- + ECTASIA] A condition in which the anal opening or the rectum is dilated.

**proctectomy** \präktek′təmē\ [PROCT- + -ECTOMY] RECTECTOMY.

**proctitis** \präktī′tis\ [PROCT- + -ITIS] Inflammation of the rectal mucosa. Also *rectitis* (seldom used). **epidemic gangrenous p.** A disease marked by ulceration of the anus and rectum, which becomes gangrenous. It is sometimes epidemic. It is associated with pyrexia, prostration, tenesmus, and the passage of bloody stools. This disease particularly afflicts children, and there is a significant mortality. It is found in India, the Pacific region, and South America. Also *Indian sickness* (an Indian usage). **ulcerative p.** Ulcerative colitis limited to the rectum.

**procto-** \präk′tə-\ [Gk *prōktos* anus] A combining form denoting (1) the anus; (2) the rectum. Also *proct-*.

**proctocele** \präk′təsēl\ [PROCTO- + -CELE[1]] RECTAL PROLAPSE.

**proctoclysis** \präktäk′lisis\ [PROCTO- + Gk *klysis* a washing off or away] Irrigation of the rectum by the infusion of fluid. Also *rectoclysis.*

**proctococcypexy** \-käk′sipek′sē\ RECTOCOCCYPEXY.

**proctocolectomy** \-kōlek′təmē\ The surgical removal of the entire colon and rectum and creation of an end ileostomy.

**proctocolitis** \-kōlī′tis\ Inflammation of the rectum and colon; coloproctitis.

**proctocolonoscopy** \-kō′lənäs′kəpē\ The direct visual examination of the rectum and colon.

**proctocolpoplasty** \-käl′pəplas′tē\ [PROCTO- + COLPOPLASTY] The surgical repair and reconstruction of a rectovaginal fistula, often performed along with a transverse colostomy to provide for fecal diversion.

**proctocystocele** \-sis′təsēl\ [PROCTO- + CYSTOCELE] Hernial protrusion of the urinary bladder into the rectum.

**proctocystoplasty** \-sis′təplas′tē\ A closure by surgical means of a rectovesical fistula.

**proctocystotome** \-sis′tətōm\ A surgical instrument used in creating a communication between the rectum and the urinary bladder.

**proctocystotomy** \-sistät′əmē\ [PROCTO- + CYSTOTOMY] RECTOCYSTOTOMY.

**proctodaeum** \-dē′əm\ *Brit.* PROCTODEUM.

**proctodeum** \-dē′əm\ [New L *proctodaeum,* from PROCT- + Gk *(h)odaion* (from *hodos* way) on the way] A depression on the surface ectoderm of an embryo opposite the anal part of the cloacal membrane, where eventually the anal orifice will develop. Also *anal pit.*

**proctodynia** \-din′ē·ə\ [PROCT- + -ODYNIA] Pain in the anus or rectum; proctalgia.

**proctologic** \-läj′ik\ Pertaining to proctology.

**proctologist** \präktäl′əjist\ A specialist in proctology.

**proctology** \präktäl′əjē\ [PROCTO- + -LOGY] The study of the diseases of the rectum and anus.

**proctoparalysis** \-pəral′isis\ [PROCTO- + PARALYSIS] Paralysis of the anal and lower rectal musculature. Also *proctoplegia.*

**proctoperineoplasty** \-per′inē′əplas′tē\ A plastic operation on the perineum, anus, and rectum. Also *proctoperineorrhaphy, rectoperineorrhaphy.*

**proctoperineorrhaphy** \-per′inē·ôr′əfē\ PROCTOPERINEOPLASTY.

**proctopexy** \präk′təpek′sē\ [PROCTO- + -PEXY] An operation to replace or maintain the rectum in its normal position by fixation to some adjacent structure. Also *rectopexy.*

**proctoplasty** \präk′təplas′tē\ [PROCTO- + -PLASTY] A plastic operation on the rectum. Also *rectoplasty.*

**proctoplegia** \-plē′jə\ PROCTOPARALYSIS.

**proctoptosis** \präk′täptō′sis\ [PROCTO- + PTOSIS] Prolapse of the anus and rectum.

**proctorrhagia** \präk′tôrā′jə\ [PROCTO- + -RRHAGIA] The passing of blood per rectum.

**proctorrhaphy** \präktôr′əfē\ RECTORRHAPHY.

**proctorrhea** \präk′tôrē′ə\ [PROCTO- + -RRHEA] Mucous drainage from the rectum.

**proctoscope** \präk′təskōp\ [PROCTO- + -SCOPE] A speculum used to permit inspection of the internal portion of the anus and the distal rectum. Also *anoscope, rectoscope.*

**proctoscopy** \präktäs′kəpē\ [PROCTO- + -SCOPY] Visual examination of the anus and distal rectum utilizing a proctoscope.

**proctosigmoid** \-sig′moid\ RECTOSIGMOID.

**proctosigmoidectomy** \-sig′moidek′təmē\ RECTOSIGMOIDECTOMY.

**proctosigmoiditis** \-sig′moidī′tis\ Inflammation of the rectum and sigmoid colon. Also *rectosigmoiditis.*

**proctosigmoidopexy** \-sig′moi′dəpek′sē\ The fixation of the rectum and sigmoid colon to a rigid, fixed structure, such as the sacrum, to prevent or repair rectal prolapse.

**proctosigmoidoscope** \-sigmoi′dəskōp\ An instrument used for direct visual examination of the rectum and sigmoid colon. The classic rigid proctosigmoidoscope is 25–30 cm long, while a flexible fiberoptic instrument is 35–60 cm long. Also *rectoromanoscope.*

**proctosigmoidoscopy** \-sig′moidäs′kəpē\ Visual inspection of the rectum and sigmoid colon utilizing a sigmoidoscope. Also *rectosigmoidoscopy, rectoromanoscopy.*

**proctostat** \präk′təstat\ [PROCTO- + -STAT] A radium-containing tube which is inserted into the rectum via the anus for treatment of carcinoma of the rectum.

**proctostenosis** \-stenō′sis\ 1 RECTAL STRICTURE. 2 ANAL STRICTURE.

**proctostomy** \präktäs′təmē\ RECTOSTOMY.

**proctotomy** \präktät′əmē\ [PROCTO- + -TOMY] A surgical incision made into the rectum. Also *rectotomy.* **external p.** A surgical incision into the rectum via a transperineal route. **internal p.** A surgical incision into the rectum via a transabdominal exposure. **linear p.** A lengthwise incision into the rectum.

**proctovalvotomy** \-valvät′əmē\ A surgical procedure in which one or more of the rectal valves are incised or rendered incompetent.
**procumbent** \-kum′bənt\ PRONE.
**procurvation** \-kərvā′shən\ A state of bending forward, as posture.
**procyclidine hydrochloride** $C_{19}H_{27}NO{\cdot}HCl$. 1-Cyclohexyl-1-phenyl-3-(pyrrolidin-1-yl)-propan-1-ol hydrochloride. An anticholinergic agent with activities like those of atropine. It is given orally in the treatment of parkinsonism to reduce rigidity and increase muscular coordination.
**procyclidine methochloride** $C_{20}H_{32}ClNO$. An anticholinergic agent with properties and activities resembling those of atropine. Also *tricyclidine methochloride*.
**prodroma** \-drō′mə\ PRODROME.
**prodromal** \-drō′məl\ Of, relating to, or of the nature of a prodrome. Also *prodromic, proemial*.
**prodromata** \-drō′mətə\ Plural of PRODROMA.
**prodrome** \prō′drōm\ [Gk *prodromos* (from *pro-* before, ahead + *dromos* a race, running) forerunner, precursor] An early symptom suggestive of the onset of an attack or disease; a premonitory event. Also *prodroma, presymptom*. **epileptic p.** Disturbance of mood or behavior or some other vague symptom such as headache which sometimes precedes by several hours or days the onset of an attack in an epileptic patient. Such a prodrome must be distinguished from an aura, which heralds the onset of an attack.
**prodromic** \-drō′mik\ PRODROMAL.
**product** 1 In mathematics, the quantity obtained by multiplying two or more other quantities. 2 A substance formed in a reaction or process. **addition p.** The product of an addition reaction. **cleavage p.** The product of a cleavage reaction. **decay p.** A nuclide that results from the radioactive decay of a parent nuclide. Often there is a series of decay products, the intermediaries being themselves radioactive and the end product stable. **fission p.'s** Nuclides produced either by nuclear fission or by the radioactive disintegration of nuclides formed in nuclear fission. **primary gene p.** The substance that is the functional product of the information encoded in a given genetic locus. It is usually polypeptide but occasionally is RNA.
**production** 1 The act or process of producing. 2 An amount produced. **ectopic hormone p.** Biosynthesis and release into the circulation of native hormones, or substances closely resembling them in chemical structure, by organs not ordinarily thought to secrete endocrine substances. Two examples are the secretion of adrenocorticotropin by an oat-cell carcinoma of the lung, and the elaboration of parathyroidlike hormone by renal cell carcinoma. Secretion of hormones from these nonglandular sites is not usually governed by customary regulatory mechanisms. The process is not strictly ectopic, since all tissues may be viewed as being totipotential, i.e., capable of secreting hormones as well as performing most other functions in the face of neoplastic derepression. **pair p.** A process whereby a high-energy photon, carrying at least 1.02 MeV, interacts with the electric field near an atomic nucleus to convert the photon's energy into matter, a positron-electron pair. The two particles share kinetic energy equal to the excess of the photon's energy over 1.02 MeV. They can therefore ionize the absorbing material. The positron quickly picks up a stray electron and undergoes annihilation, producing two 511-keV photons. See also ANNIHILATION RADIATION. Also *materialization*.
**productive** 1 Tending to produce; fruitful. 2 Producing new tissue, as an inflammation. 3 Producing mucus or sputum, as a cough.
**proelastase** The inactive precursor of elastase, as found in pancreatic secretion. It is activated by proteolysis.
**proemial** \-ē′mē·əl\ PRODROMAL.
**proencephaly** \-ensef′əlē\ [PRO- + ENCEPHAL- + -Y ] Exencephaly in which partial herniation of the brain occurs through a developmental defect in the frontal bone.
**proenzyme** \-en′zīm\ A protein that can give rise to an enzyme by covalent, usually proteolytic, modification. It is usually enzymatically inactive, but sometimes has low activity.
**proerythroblast** \prō′irith′rəblast\ PRONORMOBLAST.
**proestrus** \-es′trəs\ [PRO- + ESTRUS] The time of increased follicular activity that precedes estrus in mammals. Also *proestrum*.
**Proetz** [Arthur Walter *Proetz*, U.S. otolaryngologist, born 1888] 1 Proetz treatment. See under DISPLACEMENT. 2 See under OLFACTOMETER.
**Profeta** [Giuseppe *Profeta*, Italian physician, 1840–1911] See under LAW.
**profibrinolysin** PLASMINOGEN.
**profilactin** A complex of actin with profilin whose formation prevents the polymerization of actin into fibrils.
**profile** 1 A longitudinal or cross-sectional aggregation of medical care data, sometimes used for quality assurance or reimbursement of physicians and other providers. 2 An outline or contour, such as a lateral view of the face. **biochemical p.** The results of chemical tests (often 12, 18, or 20) that are performed on a single subject. **blood p.** COMPLETE BLOOD COUNT. **facial p.** 1 A side view of the face. 2 The outline of a sagittal section of the head. **health p.** A set of coefficients used in military or occupational medicine to provide an assessment of an individual's psychologic, physical, and physiologic attributes as an indication of fitness for military service or work. The factors usually taken into account are general condition, vision, hearing, the state of the upper and lower limbs, intelligence, and behavior. Each factor is assigned an arbitrary weight or score. **histochemical p.** The percentage composition of a muscle in terms of the histochemical types of fibers. **personality p.** 1 A graphic representation of the unique configuration of test scores or behavior ratings which describe the personality traits characteristic of an individual. 2 A verbally rendered extraction of two or three of the cardinal features discernible in the habitual behavior of an individual, used to classify or assign that person to some known subclass or personality type. *Popular.* **urethral pressure p.** A clinical test which measures the closing pressure in the urethra at intervals of a half or one centimeter from the internal to the external urethral meatus. It also measures the urethral length.
**profiler** / **beam p.** A device that plots three-dimensionally the amplitude of reflected waves from various locations in an ultrasonic beam.
**profilin** A peptide that binds actin and thereby prevents its polymerization.
**proflavin** 2,8-Diaminoacridine, usually as its hydrochloride. It is one of the acridines commonly used as a mutagen.
**profluvium** \-floo′vē·əm\ An outward flow; discharge. **p. seminis** Vaginal discharge of the semen deposited during coitus.
**profundaplasty** \-fun′dəplas′tē\ The reconstruction of the proximal profunda femoris artery, either by endarterectomy, patch angioplasty, or, rarely, by bypass graft.
**profundus** \-fun′dəs\ [L, deep, profound] Deep; in anatomy, designating a structure located at a deeper level from the surface than another. Compare SUPERFICIALIS.

**progastrin** A presumed precursor of the various forms of gastrin, in which the gastrin molecule is N-terminal. One gastrin would be formed from it by proteolysis, followed by amide formation of the C-terminal phenylalanine residue thereby produced.

**progenia** \-jē′nē·ə\ [Gk *progen(eios)* (from *pro* before + *geneion* the chin, from *genys* the underjaw) with prominent chin + -IA] MANDIBULAR PROGNATHISM.

**progenital** \-jen′ətəl\ On the exposed, outer surface of the genitals.

**progenitor** \-jen′itər\ A parent, begetter, or any ancestor.

**progeny** \präj′ənē\ [L *progeni(es)* (from *progignere* to beget) descent, child, children] Offspring; issue.

**progeria** \-jir′ē·ə\ [Gk *progēr(ōs)* (from *pro-* before, ahead + *gēras* old age) prematurely old + -IA] A syndrome of premature senility as evidenced by physical characteristics of senility, particularly in the face of a child. In some dwarfs it is associated with craniofacial malformations. Also *Hutchinson-Gilford syndrome, Hutchinson-Gilford progeria syndrome.*

**progestational** \-jestā′shənəl\ **1** Having effects similar to progesterone. The effects are primarily creation of a secretory endometrium and the maintenance of pregnancy. **2** Referring to the secretory phase of the endometrium during the menstrual cycle. **3** Delineating a class of synthetic pharmaceutical agents which have effects like those of progesterone.

**progesterone** \-jes′tərōn\ $C_{21}H_{30}O_2$. Pregn-4-ene-3,20-dione. The hormone of the corpus luteum, also secreted by the placenta, and in the adrenal cortex an essential precursor in the biosynthesis of cortisol and other corticosteroids. Its function in the menstrual cycle is to prepare the endometrium for implantation of the fertilized ovum, and in pregnancy it plays a crucial role in the maintenance of the utero-placentofetal unit and in the development of the fetus. For therapeutic purposes, synthetic and semisynthetic progestins are used in place of the native hormone. Also *progestational hormone, luteohormone* (older term), *corpus luteum hormone, luteal hormone.*

**α-progesterone** 17A-HYDROXYPROGESTERONE.

**progestin** \-jes′tin\ **1** The crude corpus luteum hormone, the isolate of which is progesterone. **2** Any natural, semisynthetic or synthetic progestational agent.

**progestogen** \-jes′təjən\ Any substance having progestational activity. Also *gestagen.*

**proglottid** \-glät′id\ [New L *proglottis,* gen. *proglottidis* (from Gk *proglōttis* tip of the tongue, from *pro-* fore + *glōttis* the tongue)] A segment of a tapeworm that is complete with reproductive organs and sometimes capable of independent movement, as in *Taenia saginata.* Also *proglottis.*

**proglottis** \-glät′is\ (*pl.* proglottides) PROGLOTTID.

**prognathism** \präg′nəthizm\ [Gk *pro-* forward + *gnath(os)* the jaw + -ISM] The characteristic of having projecting jaws, the gnathic index being above 103. Adj. prognathic, prognathous. **mandibular p.** An abnormally anterior anatomic position of the mandible. Also *anteroclusion, anterior occlusion, protrusive occlusion, mesioclusion, mesio-occlusion, underhung bite, progenia, Hapsburg jaw.*

**prognose** \prägnōs′\ PROGNOSTICATE.

**prognosis** \prägnō′sis\ [Gk *prognōsis* (from *progignōskein* to know beforehand, from *pro* before + *gignōskein* to perceive, know) a perceiving beforehand, foreknowledge] (*pl.* prognoses) An informed judgment of the course and probable outcome of a disease based on a knowledge of the facts of the particular case.

**prognostic** \prägnäs′tik\ **1** Of, for, or relating to prognosis. **2** Contributing to or useful in the process of making a prognosis. **3** A prognostic sign or symptom.

**prognosticate** \prägnäs′tikāt\ To make a prognosis. Also *prognose.*

**prognostician** \präg′nästish′ən\ **1** A practitioner considered with respect to the ability to make accurate prognoses, as *a good prognostician.* **2** An expert or specialist in prognosis.

**progonoma** \-gōnō′mə\ [Gk *progon(os)* (from *pro* before + *genesthai,* 2nd aorist inf. of *gignesthai* to be born) earlier born + -OMA] A tumor representing ancestral characteristics. **melanotic p.** MELANOTIC NEUROECTODERMAL TUMOR.

**program** **1** A sequence of coded instructions that direct the operation of a computer; software. **2** To enter such a sequence into (a computer). **burn p.** As designated by the American Burn Association, a burn care facility that offers special expertise in burn care, but without any specific area of the hospital dedicated exclusively to the care of burn victims. A term used only in the U.S. **source p.** A computer program written in assembly language ready for the assembler to convert to machine code.

**programer** **1** A person who prepares sequences of instructions for a computer. **2** A device that controls the timing and sequencing of a mechanism or process, such as the automatic chemical analyzer in the clinical laboratory.

**progranulocyte** \-gran′yəlōsīt′\ PROMYELOCYTE. **early p.** TYPE II MYELOBLAST.

**progress** To move forward or advance, as a disease process, especially so as to become more severe.

**progression** [L *progressio* (from *progressus,* past part. of *progredi* to go forth, go forward, from *pro-* PRO- + *gradi* to step, walk) an advance, progress] Forward movement or advancement, as the course of a disease, often with the implication of increased severity. **cross-legged p.** SCISSOR GAIT.

**progressive** Following a general course of increasing severity or scope of involvement: used especially of a disease.

**proguanil hydrochloride** $C_{11}H_{16}ClN_5 \cdot HCl$. 1-*p*-Chlorophenyl-5-isopropylbiguanide hydrochloride. A folic acid antagonist, antimalarial drug that is effective against the exoerythrocytic forms of some strains of *Plasmodium falciparum,* but not *P. vivax.* Resistant strains of *Plasmodia* are also common in some regions. Also *chloroguanide hydrochloride.*

**prohistiocyte** \-his′tē·əsīt′\ A large reticular cell of an irregular shape, with a chromatic nucleus and eosinophilic cytoplasm. It is the precursor of a histiocyte.

**prohormone** \-hōr′mōn\ PREHORMONE.

**proinsulin** \prō·in′sʸəlin\ The immediate precursor of insulin, a polypeptide of 86 amino-acid residues having a molecular weight of 9000, and consisting of the linked A and B chains and the C- or connecting peptide in a folded spatial arrangement. When the beta cell is stimulated to release insulin, the hormone is discharged into the bloodstream along with the metabolically inactive C-peptide and some proinsulin as well. Proinsulin is much less biologically active than insulin, but may cross-react in the insulin immunoassay. The proportion of proinsulin discharged may be increased in disease, as diabetes mellitus and islet cell adenoma, an observation of diagnostic value.

**projection** \prəjek′shən\ [L *projectio* (from *proicere* to throw forth, project, from *pro-* PRO- + L *jacere* to throw, cast, hurl) a throwing forward, projection] **1** An unconscious defense mechanism of the ego, consisting of attribution to others of the impulses, or other mental material, that the subject cannot accept in himself. **2** The radiographic image determined by the specific positioning of the patient and orientation of the x-ray beam. **3** The transmission of neural impulses to a specific area of the central nervous system. **Caldwell's p.** A roentgenographic posteroanterior projection of the skull to demonstrate the paranasal sinuses, especially the frontal sinuses. **eccentric p.** REFERRED SENSATION. **essential p.** Those thalamic nuclei dependent upon the telencephalon and determined by their retrograde neuronal atrophy following ablation of their site. **geniculostriate p.** RADIATIO OPTICA. **impersonal p.** An unconscious defense mechanism of the ego consisting of the attribution to others of neutral or nonobjectionable material from one's own mind. **left anterior oblique p.** In radiology, a projection in the oblique position with the anterior left side of the patient closest to the film or fluoroscopic screen. **left posterior oblique p.** In radiology, a projection in the oblique position with the posterior left side of the patient closest to the film or fluoroscopic screen. **neuronal p.** **1** The terminal distribution of the axon(s) of a given neuron or cell group. **2** The connection of a cortical area, subcortical nucleus, or other functional entity, especially sensory and motor areas and nuclei to another group of neurons. **pontocerebellar p.** The axons arising from the pons and terminating in the cerebellar cortex. **right anterior oblique p.** In radiology, a projection in the oblique position with the anterior right side of the patient closest to the film or fluoroscopic screen. **right posterior oblique p.** In radiology, a projection in the oblique position with the posterior right side of the patient closest to the film or fluoroscopic screen. **Towne p.** In radiology, an anteroposterior projection of the skull with the patient supine, the chin depressed, and the central ray angled caudally from the vertex of the head to the x-ray film; a projection to view the occipital bone, petrous bones, and condyles of the mandible. **Waters p.** A posteroanterior projection of the skull to demonstrate the paranasal sinuses, especially the maxillary sinuses, and the facial bones. Also *Waters view*.

**prokaryoblast** \-kar′ē·əblast′\ PRONORMOBLAST.

**prokaryote** \-kar′ē·ōt\ [PRO- + *kary(o)-* + *-ote*, from Gk *-ōtēs*, combining form denoting inhabitant] A unicellular organism with a single chromosome, lacking a nuclear membrane, and usually with a rigid peptidoglycan wall. Bacteria and cyanobacteria are prokaryotes. Also *procaryote*. Compare EUKARYOTE.

**prokaryotic** \-kar′ē·ät′ik\ Pertaining to a prokaryote. Also *procaryotic*.

**prolabium** \-lā′bē·əm\ The full thickness part of the upper lip that lies below and between the nostrils in front of the central incisor teeth.

**prolactin** \-lak′tin\ An anterior pituitary hormone that prepares the breast for and sustains lactation. It is a polypeptide having a molecular weight of about 23 000, and contains 198 amino acids. The hormone is secreted throughout the day in periodic bursts. Plasma levels rise during pregnancy and during lactation. Many physiologic stimuli, as exercise, suckling and hypoglycemia, and many pharmacologic agents, as estrogens, raise plasma levels, while L-dopa and ergot alkaloids induce falls. Raised plasma concentrations of the hormone in nonpuerperal galactorrheic states are of diagnostic use. Also *lactogenic hormone, mammogenic hormone, mammotropin, luteotropin, luteotrophin, luteotropic hormone, galactin* (outmoded), *lactation hormone* (seldom used), *mammary stimulating hormone, mammotropic hormone* (outmoded), *galactopoietic hormone* (outmoded), *lactogenic factor* (outmoded), *luteotrophic gonadotrophin* (outmoded), *letdown factor* (outmoded).

**prolapse** \prō′laps\ [New L *prolapsus*. See PROLAPSUS.] **1** The downward displacement or abnormal shift in position of a body part. Also *prolapsus*. **2** To undergo prolapse. **acute cervical disk p.** Acute prolapse, either central or lateral, of a part of the nucleus pulposus of a cervical intervertebral disk, giving rise to compression either of the spinal cord or of a spinal nerve or root. **anal p.** Downward displacement of the anal mucosa into the external environment. Also *prolapsus ani*. **p. of anterior lip of cervix** Impingement of the anterior lip of the uterine cervix between a presenting fetal part and the symphysis pubis, resulting in a large, edematous, prolapsed cervix which may obstruct the progress of labor. **p. of the cord** Expulsion of the umbilical cord through the cervix and into the vagina prior to delivery of the infant. **p. of the female urethra** Protrusion of the female urethra due to inadequate support or urethral redundancy, manifested by tenderness of the protruded mass together with frequency of urination, burning, and at times hematuria. **p. of intervertebral disk** INTERVERTEBRAL DISK PROTRUSION. **lumbar disk p.** Prolapse, either central or lateral, of a part of the nucleus pulposus of a lumbar intervertebral disk, giving rise to compression either of the cauda equina or of a single lumbar root or spinal nerve. **occult p. of cord** The presentation of the umbilical cord beside another fetal part in the uterine cervix prior to or during labor. This situation is recognized only through vaginal examination. **rectal p.** The downward displacement of the rectum through the anus. Also *proctocele, hedrocele, prolapsus recti*. **p. of uterus** Descent of the uterus into the vagina. Three degrees of severity are recognized. The first degree is marked by descent of the cervix to the introitus. In the second degree, the cervix appears outside the vagina. The third degree (frank prolapse) is the complete descent of the uterus beyond the vaginal orifice. Also *prolapsus uteri, metroptosis, hysteroptosis, descensus uteri, procidentia uteri*.

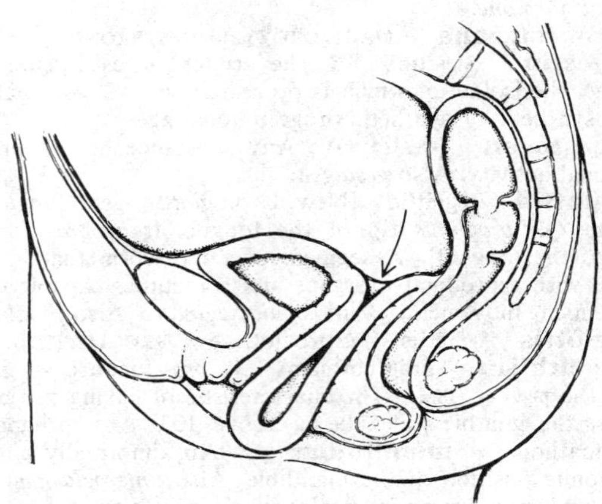

Prolapse of uterus

**prolapsus** \-lap′səs\ [New L (from L *prolapsus*, past part. of *prolabi* to glide or slide forward, fall, from *pro-* PRO- + L *labi* to glide, slide, fall), a fall, falling down] PROLAPSE. **p. ani** ANAL PROLAPSE. **p. recti** RECTAL PROLAPSE. **p. uteri** PROLAPSE OF UTERUS.

**prolatio aliformis** \-lā′shō al′ifôr′mis\ *Obs.* ALA LOBULI CENTRALIS CEREBELLI.

**Prolene** A monofilament plastic material, polypropylene, that is used for sutures. A trade name.

**proleptic** \-lep′tik\ [Gk *prolēptik(os)* (from *prolēpt(os)*, verbal of *prolambanein* to seize before, anticipate + *-ikos* -IC) pertaining to anticipation] Occurring earlier than expected or anticipated.

**prolidase** *Outmoded* PROLINE DIPEPTIDASE.

**proliferate** \-lif′ərāt\ To reproduce repeatedly; grow and increase in numbers.

**proliferation** \-lif′ərā′shən\ [French *prolifération* (from *prolifère* proliferative, from L *proles*, gen. *proli(s)* offspring + *-fère* -FER) multiplication, proliferation] The process of increasing in numbers, as by repeated cell division. **bile duct p.** A microscopic change seen in certain forms of fibrosis and cirrhosis of the liver, characterized by the regeneration and hyperplasia of bile ductules between the liver parenchyma and the fibrous septae. It is a nonspecific change, and bile never circulates through the proliferated ductules. This lesion is characteristically seen in primary biliary cirrhosis and in obstruction of large bile ducts. **mesangial p.** Proliferation of cells in the glomerular mesangial regions in response to diseases including IgA mesangial nephropathy and focal glomerulonephritis of various etiologies.

**proliferative** \-lif′ərā′tiv\ Characterized by proliferation; tending to proliferate. Also *proliferous*.

**proliferous** \-lif′ərəs\ PROLIFERATIVE.

**prolific** \-lif′ik\ [French *prolifique* (from L *proles*, gen. *proli(s)* offspring + French *-fique* -FIC) reproducing rapidly] Highly productive; producing many offspring. Also *uberous* (seldom used).

**proline** Pyrrolidine-2-carboxylic acid. It is the only one of the twenty amino acids incorporated into proteins that contains an imino, i.e. a secondary amino, group. The fact that its side chain and its amino group are part of the same five-membered ring limits the conformations it can adopt, and proline residues cause breaks in regions of $\alpha$-helix in proteins, and when abundant, as in collagen, can dictate an unusual secondary structure. Symbol: Pro, P

**proline dehydrogenase** **1** Pyrroline-5-carboxylate reductase, which can dehydrogenate proline using $NAD^+$ or $NADP^+$ and forming a double bond between N-1 and C-5, and thus forming the cyclic imine of glutamic semialdehyde, a step on the pathway of catabolism of proline to glutamate. **2** Pyrroline-2-carboxylate reductase, which similarly forms a double bond between N-1 and C-2.

**proline dipeptidase** The enzyme that catalyzes the hydrolysis of peptides containing C-terminal proline. Also *prolidase* (outmoded).

**proline-hydroxyproline-glycinuria** \pro′lin-hī′dräk′siprō′lin-glīsinoo′rē·ə\ IMINOGLYCINURIA.

**prolinemia** \prō′linē′mē·ə\ HYPERPROLINEMIA.

**prolotherapy** \prō′lōther′əpē\ A therapeutic technique that promotes proliferation of tissue, especially, a ligamentous injection procedure utilized in the nonsurgical stabilization of a joint. Also *sclerotherapy*.

**prolyl** \prō′lil\ The group derived from proline by removing a hydroxyl group from C-1. It is thus an N-terminal proline residue.

**prolymphoblast** \-lim′fəblast\ A stem cell committed to lymphoid differentiation.

**prolymphocyte** \-lim′fəsīt\ **1** Any lymphocyte displaying intermediate morphologic maturity. **2** A large lymphocyte with a prominent nucleolus, seen in prolymphocytic leukemia.

**promastigote** \-mas′tigōt\ [PRO- + MASTIGOTE] The stage of a trypanosomatid protozoan in which the flagellum arises from the kinetoplast located anterior to the nucleus and emerges from the front of the parasite. It is normally an extracellular phase found in an insect intermediate host (or in culture) as in the case of members of the genus *Leishmania*..

**promazine hydrochloride** $C_{17}H_{20}N_2S{\cdot}HCl$. *N,N*-Dimethyl-10*H*-phenothiazine-10-propanamine hydrochloride. A phenothiazine tranquilizer resembling chlorpromazine. It is used as an antipsychotic drug and an antiemetic agent. It is given orally, or by intramuscular or intravenous injection.

**promegakaryocyte** \-meg′əkar′ē·əsīt′\ A megakaryocyte precursor, with size and cytoplasmic granulation intermediate between megakaryoblast and megakaryocyte. Also *basophilic megakaryocyte, stage II megakaryocyte, lymphoid megakaryocyte*.

**promegaloblast** \-meg′əlōblast′\ The earliest recognizable erythrocyte precursor in abnormal maturation resulting from deficiencies of vitamin $B_{12}$ or folic acid, or from inherited or acquired disorders of DNA synthesis. It is characterized by larger size, deeper cytoplasmic basophilia, and less chromatin clumping when compared to its normal form, the pronormoblast. • This term has sometimes been used incorrectly as an inclusive term for all early erythrocyte precursors (both erythroblasts and megaloblasts).

**prometaphase** \-met′əfāz\ The stage of mitosis or meiosis between prophase and metaphase during which the nuclear envelope disintegrates and the centrioles reach the poles.

**promethazine hydrochloride** $C_{17}H_{21}ClN_2S$. *N,N*$\gamma$-Trimethyl-10*H*-phenothiazine-10-ethanamine hydrochloride. A phenothiazine antihistaminic agent used also as a sedative and antiemetic drug. It is used to treat nausea and vomiting with pregnancy, motion sickness or surgical procedures and it is given orally or parenterally.

**promethestrol** $C_{20}H_{26}O_2$. 4,4′-(1,2-Diethyl-1,2-ethanediyl)bis-[2-methylphenol]. A synthetic compound with properties like those of estradiol. It is effective by oral administration with actions like diethylstilbestrol. It is usually given as the dipropionate. Also *methestrol*.

**promethium** \-mē′thē·əm\ Element number 61, a rare-earth metal having 16 radioactive isotopes but no naturally occurring stable isotope. It was detected in radioactive form as a fission product of uranium, also obtained from neutron-irradiated neodymium. Half-lives range from 2.4 milliseconds to 18 years. Symbol: Pm

**prominence** \präm′ənəns\ A small projection, elevation, or protrusion; prominentia. **cephalic p.** The most prominent portion of the fetal skull that can be palpated transabdominally just above the symphysis pubis. **p. of facial canal** PROMINENTIA CANALIS FACIALIS. **laryngeal p.** PROMINENTIA LARYNGEA. **p. of lateral semicircular canal** PROMINENTIA CANALIS SEMICIRCULARIS LATERALIS. **mallear p. of tympanic membrane** PROMINENTIA MALLEARIS MEMBRANAE TYMPANI. **spiral p.** PROMINENTIA SPIRALIS. **styloid p.** PROMINENTIA STYLOIDEA. **tubal p.** TORUS TUBARIUS.

**prominentia** \präm′inen′shə\ [L (from *prominere* to project, jut out, from *pro-* forward + *-min-* root meaning bulge or jut) projection, protrusion] A small projection, elevation, or protrusion; a prominence. **p. canalis facialis** [NA] The linear bony projection on the medial wall of the tympanic cavity which is produced by the facial nerve coursing anteroposteriorly above the fenestra vestibuli and then downwards into the posterior wall above and behind the aditus to the mastoid antrum and below the prominence of the lateral semicircular canal. Also *prominence of facial canal*. **p. canalis semicircularis lateralis** [NA] The rounded eminence produced by the lateral projection of the lateral semicircular canal on the medial wall of the aditus to the antrum, above and behind the prominence of the facial canal. Also *prominence of lateral semicircular canal.* **p. foraminalis** In the chondrocranium, part of the edge of the foramen magnum, which, behind the condyle, becomes a prominence and delineates a neural demiarch. In the midline posteriorly the two prominentiae foraminales remain separated by the posterior occipital incisure. **p. frontonasalis** FRONTONASAL PROCESS. **p. laryngea** [NA] The subcutaneous angular projection in the midline of the front of the neck situated below the thyroid notch and at the upper end of the union of the laminae of the thyroid cartilage. It is more obvious in males than in females. Also *laryngeal prominence, laryngeal protuberance, protuberantia laryngea, Adam's apple* (popular), *pomum adami* (outmoded). **p. mallearis membranae tympani** [NA] A small prominence at the superior end of the stria mallearis on the external surface of the tympanic membrane produced by the lateral process of the malleus. Also *mallear prominence of tympanic membrane.* **p. mandibularis** [NA] The portion of the first branchial or visceral arch of the embryo that meets its opposite fellow to form the mandible, lower lip and gum, chin and lower cheek region. Also *mandibular process.* **p. spiralis** [NA] The surface projection of the thickened endosteum on the outer wall of the cochlear duct lying above the sulcus spiralis externus and continuing upwards as the stria vascularis. It is very vascular and contains the vas prominens. Also *spiral prominence.* **p. styloidea** [NA] A marked projection near the back of the jugular wall of the tympanic cavity corresponding to the root of the styloid process. Also *styloid prominence.*

**prominentiae** \präm′inen′shē\ Plural of PROMINENTIA.

**promonocyte** \-män′əsīt\ A maturing cell in the monocyte series, displaying size, nuclear chromatin patterns, cytoplasmic staining, and function intermediate between the monoblast and monocyte. Also *premonocyte.*

**promontorium** \präm′əntôr′ē·əm\ [L, also *promunturium* (from *prominere* to project; assimilated to *mons,* gen. *montis* mountain) a headland, spur, promontory] A projection, eminence, or prominent part. Also *promontory.* **p. cavitatis tympanicae** [NA] A rounded prominence on the medial wall of the tympanic cavity produced by the lateral projection of the basal turn of the cochlea. Its surface is grooved by the branches of the tympanic plexus of nerves. Also *promontory of tympanic cavity, tympanic promontory, promontory of the middle ear.* **p. ossis sacri** [NA] The anterior projecting edge of the upper surface of the body of the first sacral vertebra. Also *promontory of sacrum, pelvic promontory.*

**promontory** \präm′əntôr′ē\ [L *promontorium.* See PROMONTORIUM.] PROMONTORIUM. **p. of the middle ear** PROMONTORIUM CAVITATIS TYMPANICAE. **pelvic p.** PROMONTORIUM OSSIS SACRI. **p. of sacrum** PROMONTORIUM OSSIS SACRI. **tympanic p.** PROMONTORIUM CAVITATIS TYMPANICAE. **p. of tympanic cavity** PROMONTORIUM CAVITATIS TYMPANICAE.

**promoter** \prəmō′tər\ **1** A region of the genome that is the site for initiation of mRNA synthesis by binding RNA polymerase. Different promoters vary widely in their affinity for the polymerase, and they often overlap with the adjacent regulatory operator locus. **2** A substance that enhances tumor development when administered after a carcinogen. **eosinophil stimulator p.** A lymphokine that stimulates migration of eosinophils.

**promotion** Stimulation of tumor formation by a noncarcinogen (promotor) after initial exposure to a carcinogen.

**promoxolane** $C_{10}H_{10}O_3$. 2,2-Bis(1-methylethyl)-1,3-dioxolane-4-methanol. A liquid heterocyclic product used as a skeletal relaxant agent.

**promyeloblast** \-mī′əlōblast′\ A stem cell committed to myeloid differentiation.

**promyelocyte** \-mī′əlōsīt′\ A granulocyte precursor with maturation characteristics between the myeloblast and myelocyte, retaining large size and fine nuclear chromatin but displaying primary granules in the cytoplasm. Also *progranulocyte, premyelocyte.*

**pronase** \prō′nās\ A mixture of fungal proteinases, often capable of the complete degradation of a protein to amino acids. Such hydrolysis does not hydrolyze glutamine and asparagine to glutamate and aspartate, so may be used to determine them, or other acid-labile amino acids.

**pronate** \prō′nāt\ [Late L *pronat(us),* past part. of *pronare* to bend forward, from L *pronus* bending or leaning forward] **1** To rotate the forearm and hand through 180° from a position in which the palm is facing either upward or forward to one in which it is facing downward or backward, respectively. **2** To place the body in the prone position. Compare SUPINATE.

**pronation** \-nā′shən\ [*pronat(e)* + -ION] **1** Rotation of the forearm and hand so that the palm faces backward or downward. **2** Placement of the body in the prone position.

**pronatoflexor** \-nā′təflek′sər\ A muscle that is both a pronator and a flexor, such as pronator teres and brachioradialis muscles.

**pronator** \prō′nātər\ A muscle that produces pronation of a part.

**pronator-supinator** A wall-mounted handle for resisted pronation-supination exercises.

**prone** \prōn\ [L *pronus* bending forward, lying toward, prone] Lying with the face down. Also *procumbent, ventricumbent.*

**pronephron** \-nef′rän\ [PRO- + NEPHRON] One of the units of the pronephros.

**pronephros** \-nef′rəs\ [PRO- +Gk *nephros* kidney] The earliest and most cranially (anteriorly) situated kidney tissue to develop in the embryo. It is also physiologically the most primitive. Each of its segmented constituent parts (nephrotomes) in lower vertebrates contains a tubule which drains into a common, longitudinal, excretory, pronephric duct. The other end of each tubule communicates by a nephrostome with the coelom. In man it is represented by six or seven cellular cords comprising fused nephrotomes which soon involute. It is doubtful whether a longitudinal pronephric duct forms in man from pronephric elements or that it persists as the mesonephric duct, which is in fact probably derived from the first nephrotomes of the mesonephros. Also *primitive kidney, pronephric tubules.* Adj. pronephric.

**pronograde** \prō′nōgrād\ Characterized by walking or crawling in the horizontal direction of the long axis of the body: said of quadrupeds and most other animals. Compare ORTHOGRADE.

**pronormoblast** \-nôr′məblast\ [PRO- + NORMOBLAST] The earliest recognizable erythrocyte precursor, characterized by large size, finely granular chromatin, high nuclear-cytoplasmic ratio, and scant, deeply basophilic cytoplasm. Also *rubriblast, proerythroblast, macroblast of Naegeli, megaloblast of Sabin, prokaryoblast.*

**pronucleus** \-nʸoo′klē·əs\ [PRO- + NUCLEUS] (*pl.* pronuclei) **1** The precursor of the nucleus of a cell or any other type of nucleus. **2** Either the male or female pronucleus. Male and female pronuclei normally possess the haploid number of chromosomes. **female p.** The nucleus of the ovum after maturation but before fusion with the male pronucleus. **male p.** The nucleus of the spermatozoon after it has entered the ovum. Also *masculonucleus, sperm nucleus.*

**proövarium** \-ōver′ē·əm\ EPOÖPHORON.

**prop** / **dental p.** A device, made in various sizes, used to hold the mouth open by placing it between the upper and lower teeth or edentulous ridges on one side.

**propagate** \präp′əgāt\ [L *propagat(us),* past part. of *propagare* (from *propages* a slip, offspring, from *pro-* PRO- + *pangere* to set in the ground, plant) to extend, propagate] **1** To produce or cause to produce offspring. **2** To conduct, as a nerve impulse along a fiber.

**propagation** \präp′əgā′shən\ [*propagat(e)* + -ION] **1** The process of reproduction, as of a species, by which new individuals are formed and life maintained. **2** The process by which an action potential, recordable at one point on the surface of an excitable membrane, depolarizes adjacent parts of the membrane, thereby allowing the action potential to travel away from the site of the initial stimulus.

**propalinal** \-pal′inəl\ Having or pertaining to a forward and backward movement: said especially of the lower jaw, in mastication.

**propane** $CH_3—CH_2—CH_3$. The $C_3$-hydrocarbon, found in natural gas. It is easily liquefied under pressure, and is used as a fuel.

**propanol** Either of the alcohols formed by substituting propane with a hydroxyl group. Unqualified it usually refers to propan-1-ol, $CH_3—CH_2—CH_2OH$. Both are commonly used as solvents in organic chemistry. Propan-2-ol is a product of some bacterial fermentations in which acetoacetyl-CoA yields acetone, which is subsequently reduced to propan-2-ol with concomitant oxidation of NADPH. Also *propyl alcohol* (outmoded).

**propantheline bromide** $C_{23}H_{30}BrNO_3$. *N*-Methyl-*N*-(1-methylethyl)-*N*-[2-[(9*H*-xanthen-9-ylcarbonyl)oxy]ethyl]-2-propanaminium bromide. An anticholinergic drug used to treat peptic ulcer hyperacidity and hypermotility. It is given orally or parenterally.

**proparacaine hydrochloride** $C_{16}H_{27}ClN_2O_3$. 3-Amino-4-propoxybenzoic acid 2-(diethylamino)ethyl ester hydrochloride. A local anesthetic used topically in the eye.

**propargyl** The 2-propynyl group, $—CH_2—C{\equiv}C—H$. Substrate analogues containing propargyl groups can inactivate some thiol enzymes by addition of the thiol group to the triple bond.

**propene** $CH_3—CH{=}CH_2$. An unsaturated hydrocarbon whose polymers are important as plastics. Also *propylene.*

**propepsin** PEPSINOGEN.

**properdin** \-per′din\ A component of the alternative complement pathway whose function is to stabilize the alternative pathway C3 convertase with which it forms a reversible complex.

**properitoneal** \-per′itənē′əl\ Relating to an area anterior to the peritoneum.

**prophage** \prō′fāj\ [PRO- + PHAGE] A bacteriophage incorporated into the genome of a bacterial cell and replicating along with the bacterial genome. The phage genome is in the temperate phase and is not producing lysis of the infected cell. Also *probacteriophage.*

**prophase** \prō′fāz\ The first stage of nuclear division by mitosis or meiosis.

**prophenpyridamine** PHENIRAMINE.

**prophylactic** \-filak′tik\ [Gk *prophylaktikos* (from *prophylakē* advance guard, precaution, from *pro-* forward, ahead + *phylax* a guard) precautionary, prophylactic] **1** Tending or intended to prevent the occurrence of disease. • Though often used as synonymous with *preventive,* it has been suggested that *prophylactic* be applied to substances and *preventive* to actions. **2** A prophylactic agent.

**prophylaxis** \prō′fəlak′sis\ [New L, noun from Gk *prophylassein* to take precautions. See PROPHYLACTIC.] **1** The prevention of disease. **2** Specific measures taken to prevent disease in an individual or the development or spread of disease in a community. Adj. prophylactic. **chemical p.** The prevention of disease by means of chemical substances. **clinical p.** The prevention of the clinical manifestations (signs and symptoms) of disease. The disease itself may not be eradicated. Also *suppressive prophylaxis.* **dental p.** The removal, by an operator, of plaque, calculus, and stain from the teeth. Also *oral prophylaxis.* **drug p.** The prevention of disease by means of drugs. **gametocidal p.** Destruction of malarial gametocytes in the host bloodstream by means of drugs, in order to prevent transmission by inhibiting the sexual cycle in the mosquito vector. **oral p.** DENTAL PROPHYLAXIS. **serum p.** The use of specific immune serum as a means of prevention. **suppressive p.** CLINICAL PROPHYLAXIS.

**propilcillin potassium** $C_{18}H_{21}KN_2O_5S$. The potassium salt of 6(α)-phenoxybutyramido)-penicillanic acid. An antibiotic specific for Gram-negative bacteria.

**β-propiolactone** The cyclic ester of 3-hydroxypropionic acid. Its four-membered ring is highly reactive, alkylating some nucleophils with C-3 and acylating others with C-1. It is used for the inactivation of viruses and the sterilization of vaccines, grafts, and plasma. Like many alkylating agents, it is carcinogenic.

**propionate** The anion of propionic acid, or any salt or ester of this acid.

**propionibacter** \prō′pē·än′ēbak′tər\ An organism of the genus *Propionibacterium.*

***Propionibacterium*** \prō′pē·än′ēbaktir′ē·əm\ A genus of Gram-positive, nonsporulating rods included among the propionic acid bacteria. See also PROPIONIC FERMENTATION. ***P. acnes*** An anaerobic species found regularly on skin and occasionally in mixed infections. Once classified as a corynebacterium, it is now included among the propionic acid bacteria. The fermentation of lactate to propionate is evidently selected for on skin. Also *Corynebacterium acnes* (obs.).

**propionic acid** $CH_3—CH_2—COOH$. Propanoic acid. A $C_3$-carboxylic acid, of melting point −21.5°C and boiling point 140°C. It is produced by propionic acid bacteria from propionyl-CoA, the residue left after removal of a carboxyl group from methylmalonyl-CoA. It is found in some cheeses. Mammals can use it by converting it into propionyl-CoA which they convert in a pathway dependent on vitamin $B_{12}$ via methylmalonyl-CoA into succinyl-CoA.

**propionyl** $CH_3—CH_2—CO—$. The acyl group derived from propionic acid by removing a hydroxyl group from C-1.

**propionylcholine** The analogue of acetylcholine in which the acyl group is derived from propionic acid.

**propionyl-CoA** The thioester formed by acylation with propionic acid of the thiol group of coenzyme A. It is formed during catabolism of fatty acids that contain an odd number of carbon atoms, and also on activation of propionate for metabolism. It can be metabolized by carboxylation to form methylmalonyl-CoA.

**proplasmin** PLASMINOGEN.

**proplastid** \-plas′tid\ A small, colorless, cytoplasmic granule or structure which may develop into various types of plastids.

**proplexus** \-plek′səs\ *Seldom used* PLEXUS CHOROIDEUS VENTRICULI LATERALIS.

**propons** \prō′pänz\ [L *pro-* PRO- + *pons* a bridge] A

thin, myelinated axon band traversing the rostral medullary pyramid immediately behind the pons. Also *ala pontis, ponticulus.*

**proportion** / **femininity p.** The proportion of females in a population containing persons of both sexes. **masculinity p.** The proportion of males in a population containing persons of both sexes. The term is often wrongly used to mean *masculinity ratio,* the ratio of males to females in a population. **optimal p.** In immunology, that concentration of antigen and antibody that leads to a maximum association between the antigen and antibody. It is more often applied to precipitin reactions, in which the development of a visible end point totally depends upon the proportions of the reactants, than to agglutination, complement fixation, or immunofluorescence reactions in which relative proportions are less critical.

**proposita** \-päz′itə\ [L, fem. of PROPOSITUS] (*pl.* propositae) A female proband.

**propositi** \-päz′itī\ Plural of PROPOSITUS.

**propositus** \-päz′itəs\ [L (past part. of *proponere* to exhibit, set out, from *pro-* forward + *ponere* to put) exhibited, set up for consideration] (*pl.* propositi) PROBAND.

**propoxycaine hydrochloride** $C_{16}H_{27}ClN_2O_3$. 4-Amino-2-propoxybenzoic acid 2-diethylaminoethyl ester hydrochloride. A local anasthetic agent used as a local block and tissue infiltration anasthetic.

**propranolol** A substance which binds to $\beta$-receptors of epinephrine and blocks their response. It is used for treating hypertension. Chemically it is the secondary amine in which ammonia is substituted with isopropyl and 2-hydroxy-3-($\alpha$-naphthyloxy)propyl groups.

**proprietary** \prəprī′əter′ē\ **1** Privately owned or operated, as a hospital. **2** Protected by virtue of private ownership that conveys the exclusive right of manufacture and sale, as of a medicine, or of promotional use, as of a name.

**proprioception** \prō′prē·əsep′shən\ [L *propri(us)* private, proper, own + *o* + English *-ception* as in *reception*] Awareness of position, movement, or balance of the body or any of its parts. Also *proprioceptive sensation, proprioceptive sense.* Compare KINESTHESIA.

**proprioceptive** \prō′prē·əsep′tive\ Pertaining to awareness of the movement or position of body parts.

**proprioceptor** \prō′prē·əsep′tər\ [*propriocept(ion)* + -OR] A sense organ found in muscles, tendons, or joints, the excitation of which results in the sense of position or sensation of movement. It is sometimes also used to refer to sensations deriving from the vestibular apparatus.

**propriospinal** \prō′prē·əspī′nəl\ Denoting relations derived solely within the spinal cord.

**proptometer** \präptäm′ətər\ [*propto(sis)* + -METER] EXOPHTHALMOMETER.

**proptosis** \präptō′sis, prōtō′sis\ [Gk *proptōsis* (from *propiptein* to fall forward, project beyond) a falling forward] Forward displacement or prolapse, especially of the eyeball. See also EXOPHTHALMOS.

**propulsion** \-pul′shən\ ANTEROPULSION.

**propyl** \prō′pil\ **1** $CH_3—CH_2—CH_2—$. The group formed by removing a hydrogen atom from C-1 of propane. **2** ISOPROPYL.

**propyl alcohol** *Outmoded* PROPANOL.

**propylene** PROPENE.

**propylene oxide** A clearing agent that is used to facilitate the impregnation of tissues by embedding media prior to electron microscopy.

**propylhexedrine** $C_{10}H_{21}N$. *N*,$\alpha$-Dimethylcyclohexaneethanamine. An ephedrinelike adrenergic drug used as a nasal decongestant. It is administered by inhalation.

**propylthiouracil** $C_7H_{10}N_2OS$. 6-Propyl-2-thiouracil, an antithyroid drug widely used in the treatment of hyperthyroidism in Graves disease. The mechanism of action is through inhibition of iodide with consequent partial blocking of the biosynthesis of thyroid hormones, reduction of circulating thyroid hormone levels, raised secretion of pituitary thyrotropin, and consequent hyperplasia of thyroid follicle cells and goiter. Use of the drug is based on observations of the goitrogenic effects of foodstuffs, e.g., turnips and rutabagas, which contain a high concentration of thiourea derivatives.

**pro re nata** \prō rē nā′tə\ [L *pro* for + *re*, ablative of *res* thing + *nata*, fem. ablative of *natus* born to, naturally adapted to] According to circumstances; as the need arises. Abbr. p.r.n.

**prorennin** \-ren′in\ RENNINOGEN.

**prorsad** \prôr′sad\ Forward; straight ahead. *Outmoded.*

**prorubricyte** \-roo′brisīt\ BASOPHILIC NORMOBLAST.

**pros-** \präs-\ [Gk *pros* from, from the side of, near, toward, to] A prefix meaning near.

**proscillaridin** A cardiotonic glycoside found in lilies. It is a glycoside of a bufadienolide, i.e. a sterol with a six-membered lactone ring attached to C-17.

**prosect** \-sekt′\ To dissect tissues carefully for anatomical presentation.

**prosection** \-sek′shən\ An anatomical dissection carried out in an organized and detailed manner in order to demonstrate structural detail for teaching purposes.

**prosector** \-sek′tər\ A skilled person who dissects a cadaver or part for anatomical demonstration.

**prosencephalon** \präs′ensef′əlän\ [PROS- + ENCEPHALON] The wall of the forebrain vesicle which is the most rostral of three brain vesicles in the neural tube. It develops into the cerebrum. The prosencephalon can be subdivided into the telencephalon, from which the cerebral hemispheres develop, and the diencephalon, or thalamus and adjacent regions. Also *forebrain.*

**Proskauer** [Bernhard *Proskauer*, German bacteriologist, 1851–1915] **1** Voges-Proskauer reaction. See under REACTION. **2** Voges-Proskauer test. See under TEST.

**proso-** \präs′ə-, präs′ō-\ [Gk *prosō* forward, anterior] A combining form meaning forward, front.

**prosobranch** \präs′əbranch\ **1** Of or belonging to the subclass Prosobranchiata. **2** A member of the subclass Prosobranchiata, the operculate snails.

**Prosobranchiata** \präs′əbrangkē·ā′tə\ [PROSO- + L *branchi(ae)* the gills of a fish + -ATA] A subclass of gastropod mollusks, the operculate snails, in which the gills (branchiae) in the body cavity are anterior to the heart. The majority of all snails, including marine, freshwater, and land, are included in this subclass.

**prosodemic** \präs′ədem′ik\ [Gk *prosod(os)* an approach, access, interview (from *pros-* toward + *(h)odos* a way) + *-(d)emic* as in *epidemic*] Describing an infectious disease that is conveyed from one individual to another, as opposed to one transmitted from one person to several others at once through contamination of food, water, or some other vehicle.

**prosody** \präs′ədē\ [Gk *prosōdia* (from *pros* accompanying + *ōidē* a song, ode) the doctrine of accentuation, prosody] The nonsegmental features of the speaking voice, such as pitch, intonation, rhythm, and stress. It is an important component of the phonologic analysis of speech.

**prosop-** \präsəp-\ PROSOPO-.

**prosopagnosia** \präs′əpagnō′zhə\ [PROSOP- + AGNOSIA] Inability to recognize faces. Also *agnosia for faces.*

**prosopalgia** \präs′əpal′jə\ [PROSOP- + -ALGIA] TRIGEMINAL NEURALGIA.

**prosopectasia** \präs′əpektā′zhə\ [PROSOP- + ECTASIS] A disproportionate largeness of the face.

**prosopo-** \präs′əpō-\ [Gk *prosōpon* face, visage] A combining form denoting the face. Also *prosop-*.

**prosopodiplegia** \-dīplē′jə\ [PROSOPO- + DIPLEGIA] Bilateral facial paralysis.

**prosopodysmorphia** \-dismôr′fē·ə\ [PROSOPO- + DYS- + -MORPH + -IA] ROMBERG'S PROGRESSIVE FACIAL HEMIATROPHY.

**prosopopagus** \präs′əpäp′əgəs\ [PROSOPO- + -PAGUS] Unequal conjoined twins in which the parasitic member, often in the form of a tumorlike mass, is attached on the face at a site other than the jaw of the host. Also *prosopopagus parasiticus.*

**prosopoplegia** \-plē′jə\ [PROSOPO- + -PLEGIA] Paralysis affecting the face. *Seldom used.* Adj. prosopoplegic.

**prosopospasm** \präs′əpōspazm′\ [PROSOPO- + -SPASM] Spasm of the facial muscles. An imprecise and seldom used term.

**prosoposternodymia** \-stur′nədin′ē·ə\ [PROSOPO- + STERNO- + *-dym(us)* + -IA] A union of conjoined twins that results in a prosoposternopagus.

**prosoposternopagus** \-stərnäp′əgəs\ [PROSOPO- + STERNO- + -PAGUS] Equal conjoined twins joined at the face and sternum but with a single lower trunk and set of lower extremities.

**prosopothoracopagus** \-thôr′əkäp′əgəs\ [PROSOPO- + THORACO- + -PAGUS] That form of cephalothoracopagus in which union of the twins specifically involves the face and the thorax, as opposed to union of other parts of the head and the thorax.

**prostacyclin** \präs′təsī′klin\ PROSTAGLANDIN $I_2$.

**prostaglandin** \präs′təglan′din\ [*prosta(te) gland* (in the secretions of which it was first identified) + -IN] Any of several unsaturated fatty acids 20 carbons in length having an internal cyclopentane ring. They are nearly ubiquitous in tissues and body fluids, and have a high degree of structure-activity specificity and a wide range of actions, including effects on vasomotor tone, capillary permeability, nervous system function, platelet aggregation, extravascular smooth muscle, and exocrine and endocrine secretion. One of their several modes of action is regulation of cellular concentration of cyclic AMP and cyclic GMP. Prostaglandins are used experimentally to induce abortion, reduce acid secretion by the stomach, and alleviate refractory asthma. Physiologically important prostaglandins are prostaglandin $E_1$, $E_2$, $E_3$, $F_1\alpha$, $F_2\alpha$, $F_3\alpha$, and $I_2$. Abbr. PG **p. $E_1$** A prostaglandin that acts as a vasodilator and bronchodilator and an inhibitor of gastric secretion. It also inhibits platelet aggregation. **p. $E_2$** A prostaglandin that causes vasodilatation, inhibits gastric secretion, induces labor and abortion by stimulating uterine contractions, and controls renal medullary blood flow in response to vasopressin. **p. $F_2\alpha$** A prostaglandin that causes vasoconstriction and bronchoconstriction. It induces labor and abortion by stimulating uterine contractions, and also terminates pregnancy by dissolution of the corpus luteum. **p. $G_2$** The biosynthetic precursor of prostaglandins $I_2$, $F_1\alpha$, $E_2$, and $F_2\alpha$, and of platelet thromboxanes. **p. $H_2$** The biosynthetic precursor of thromboxane $A_2$. **p. $I_2$** A prostaglandin that is a potent vasodilator, an inhibitor of platelet aggregation, and an antagonist of thromboxane $A_2$. A deficiency of prostaglandin $I_2$ may be involved in atherogenesis. Also *prostacyclin, prostaglandin X, epoprostenol.* **p. $I_3$** A prostaglandin whose action inhibits platelet aggregation. **p. X** PROSTAGLANDIN $I_2$.

**Δ13-prostaglandin reductase** An enzyme that inactivates prostaglandins by reducing the double bond between carbon 13 and carbon 14.

**prostaglandin synthetase** CYCLO-OXYGENASE.

**prostanoic acid** $C_{20}H_{38}O_2$. The parent compound of the prostaglandins. Its molecule is that of icosanoic acid, with a bond between C-8 and C-12 replacing a hydrogen atom on each of them, so that a five-membered ring is formed. The side chains on this ring are *trans*-substituted.

**prostanoid** \präs′tənoid\ Any of several complex fatty acids that are 20 carbons in length, derived from arachidonic acid, and containing an internal 5- or 6-carbon ring. Prostanoids include prostanoic acid, prostaglandins, and thromboxanes.

**prostat-** \prästat-\ PROSTATO-.

**prostata** \präs′tətə\ [New L, prostate. See PROSTATE.] [NA] A conical organ composed of glandular and fibromuscular tissues that surrounds the proximal portion of the male urethra. Its flattened base is directed cranially and is contiguous with the neck of the urinary bladder while its apex is directed caudally and is related to the fascia on the superior surfaces of the sphincter urethrae and transversus perinei profundus muscles. Its anterior surface lies behind the symphysis pubis from which it is separated by the prostatic venous plexus and areolar and fatty tissue while the posterior surface is separated by its sheath and areolar tissue from the lower portion of the rectum. The inferolateral surfaces are related to the levator ani muscles. It is divided into a right and left lobe connected by the isthmus and a middle lobe comprising many compound tubuloalveolar glands the ducts of which open in the urethra traversing it. Also *prostate, prostate gland.*

**prostatalgia** \präs′tətal′jə\ [PROSTAT- + -ALGIA] Pain localized in the prostate. Also *prostatodynia.*

**prostate** \präs′tāt\ [Gk *prostatēs* (from *proistanai* to set before or in front, from *pro* before + *histanai* to make to stand) one who stands in front, a chief, leader] PROSTATA. **funnel-neck p.** SCHRAMM'S PHENOMENON.

**prostatectomy** \präs′tətek′təmē\ [PROSTAT- + -ECTOMY] Partial or total removal of the prostate. **perineal p.** Removal of the prostate through the perineum. **retropubic prevesical p.** The removal of a hypertrophied prostate by suprapubic abdominal incision without opening the bladder. **suprapubic transvesical p.** The removal of a hypertrophied prostate by suprapubic incision and opening of the bladder. **transurethral p.** Removal of a prostatic adenoma through the urethra under endoscopic control.

**prostateria** \präs′tətir′ē·ə\ PROSTATISM.

**prostatic** \prästat′ik\ 1 Pertaining to the prostate. 2 Affected by hypertrophy of the prostate.

**prostaticovesiculectomy** \prästat′ikōvesik′yəlek′təmē\ PROSTATOVESICULECTOMY.

**prostatism** \präs′tətizm\ [PROSTAT- + -ISM] A group of urinary symptoms commonly due to prostatic hypertrophy including frequency, urgency, weakening of the urine stream, and dysuria. These symptoms are not pathognomonic and may occur in other diseases such as bladder-neck obstruction. Also *prostateria.* **vesical p.** Urinary retention without prostatic disease.

**prostatitis** \präs′tətī′tis\ [PROSTAT- + -ITIS] Inflammation of the prostate gland. **bacterial p.** Acute or chronic inflammation of the prostate as a result of infection with bacteria, commonly *Escherichia coli, Klebsiella, Proteus,* or enterococci, and, less frequently, staphylococci or streptococci. *Chlamydia* may possibly be responsible for some chronic infections. The acute form is characterized by high fever, chills, perineal and back pain, and symptoms of urinary tract infection, and may progress to prostatic abscess or chronic prostatitis. The chronic form, often intractable, is characterized by focal inflammation and commonly by relapsing urinary tract infection. **fungal p.** A chronic prostatitis, frequently with abscess formation, caused by a variety of fungi, such as *Candida albicans, Coccidioides immitis,* or *Blastomyces.* Diagnosis depends on the finding of fungus in prostatic fluid.

**prostato-** \präs′tətō-\ [Gk *prostatēs* one who stands before] A combining form denoting the prostate. Also *prostat-.*

**prostatocystitis** \-sistī′tis\ [PROSTATO- + CYSTITIS] Inflammation of the prostatic urethra and the urinary bladder.

**prostatocystotomy** \-sistät′əmē\ [PROSTATO- + CYSTOTOMY] Incision of the urinary bladder and the prostate gland by a perineal approach. Also *prostocystotomy.*

**prostatodynia** \-din′ē·ə\ [PROSTAT- + -ODYNIA] PROSTATALGIA.

**prostatolith** \präs′tətōlith′\ CALCULUS OF THE PROSTATE.

**prostatolithotomy** \-lithät′əmē\ [PROSTATO- + LITHO- + -TOMY] Removal of a prostatic calculus through an incision in the prostate.

**prostatomegaly** \-meg′əlē\ [PROSTATO- + -MEGALY] Hypertrophy of the prostate gland.

**prostatomy** \prästat′əmē\ PROSTATOTOMY.

**prostatomyomectomy** \-mī′əmek′təmē\ [PROSTATO- + MYOMECTOMY] Incision of the prostate for removal of a myoma.

**prostatorrhea** \präs′tətôrē′ə\ [PROSTATO- + -RRHEA] An abnormal discharge from the prostate gland.

**prostatotomy** \präs′tətät′əmē\ [PROSTATO- + -TOMY] Incision of the prostate. Also *prostatomy.*

**prostatovesiculectomy** \-vesik′yəlek′təmē\ [PROSTATO- + VESICULECTOMY] Surgical removal of the prostate gland and the seminal vesicles. Also *prostaticovesiculectomy.*

**prostatovesiculitis** \-vesik′yəlī′tis\ [PROSTATO- + VESICULITIS] Inflammation of the prostate gland and the seminal vesicles. Also *vesiculoprostatitis.*

**prostaxia** \-stak′sē·ə\ [PROS- + Gk *tax(is)* an arranging, ordering + -IA] A stable protein distribution in the body.

**prosternation** \-stərnā′shən\ A forward flexion deformity of the trunk.

**prostheses** \prästhē′sēz\ Plural of PROSTHESIS.

**prosthesis** \prästhē′sis\ [Gk *prosthesis* (from *prostithenai* to put to, apply, add, from *pros* from, near, toward, to + *tithenai* to place, put) a putting to, adding, addition] Any artificial replacement for a body part. It may be functional or cosmetic, and attached externally or implanted surgically. Also *prothesis.* **Blom-Singer voice p.** A short, flanged, silicone tube, terminating in a simple valve, used to help restore voice after laryngectomy. The prosthesis is introduced by way of a tracheoesophageal puncture and permits the diversion of expired air into the pharynx while preventing leakage into the airway. Also *Blom-Singer valve, duckbill valve.* **caged-ball p.** BALL-TYPE VALVE. **Cronin p.** A prosthesis used in augmentation mammoplasty, consisting of a Silastic bag filled with silicone of a gel consistency. **Cutter SCDK p.** A modification of the Starr-Edwards prosthesis in which an additional cage is extended beneath the proximal chamber to increase the orifice size. **dental p.** An artificial replacement for one or more teeth or for some other oral structure. **disk valve p.** A mechanical valve for use in an intracardiac position that functions by means of a disk that floats in an enclosed cage. **endoskeletal p.** A prosthesis utilizing an interior tubular supporting structure and shaped with an exterior cosmetic cover. **exoskeletal p.** A prosthesis, such as a limb prosthesis of the more usual sort, that has a weight-bearing or supportive external structure. **feeding p.** A cleft palate prosthesis acting as an obturator to assist an infant's feeding. **knitted vascular p.** Any of the knitted textile arterial substitutes. They carry the disadvantage of requiring preclotting, but possess the advantages of good tissue ingrowth because of their large, numerous interstices and favorable suturing characteristics. **maxillofacial p.** A device worn by patients who lack a portion of the face or jaws. It is contrived to imitate as closely as possible the missing parts in texture, color, and contour. A prosthesis is chosen when a reconstructive operation is either not possible or is declined by the patient. **modular p.** A prosthesis incorporating interchangeable components, or modules, for quick assembly. **Munster p.** A prosthesis with a closely fitted socket extending above the humeral condyles for use by patients with very short below-elbow amputations. **myoelectric p.** A prosthesis whose moveable components are activated by electrical potentials generated by the patient's muscles. **ocular p.** **1** An artificial eye, made of glass or plastic. **2** *Outmoded* EYEGLASSES. **Panje voice p.** TRACHEOESOPHAGEAL FISTULA VOICE BUTTON PROSTHESIS. **pneumatic p.** A lower limb prosthesis with an inflatable socket. **Starr-Edwards p.** A form of caged-ball cardiac valve prosthesis. **Syme p.** An artificial foot with attachment to the foreleg designed for use following a Syme amputation. **tracheoesophageal fistula voice button p.** A modification of the Blom-Singer voice prosthesis. It consists of a short, biflanged silicone tube with a one-way flutter flap valve which is inserted through a previously formed tracheoesophageal fistula. Also *Panje voice button, Panje voice prosthesis.* **woven vascular p.** Any of the woven textile arterial substitutes. They are well suited for use in emergency vascular operations because they do not require preclotting, but they are technically difficult to suture and hinder tissue ingrowth for healing because of their small interstices.

**prosthetic** \prästhet′ik\ **1** Substituting for or replacing a missing part of the body; constituting an artificial component of a natural part. Also *prothetic.* **2** A prosthetic device; prosthesis. **3** Constituting the nonprotein component of a conjugated protein.

**prosthetics** \prästhet′iks\ The science and technology of the design, fabrication, and application of prostheses. **dental p.** PROSTHODONTICS.

**prosthetist** \präs′thətist\ A person engaged in the fabrication and fitting of prostheses.

**prosthion** \präs′thē·än\ [Gk *prosthion,* neut. sing. of *prosthios* (from *prosthe* (adverb) before, in front of) foremost] A craniometric point situated in the midline at the lower end of the junction between the left and right maxillary alveolar processes. Also *alveolar point, alveolare.*

**prosthodontia** \präs′thōdän′shə\ [Gk *prosth(etos)* (verbal adj. of *prostithenai* to put to, fit, add) added, fitted, applied + -ODONTIA] The study of the art of replacing lost teeth and the associated structures.

**prosthodontics** \präs′thōdän′tiks\ [*prosthodont(ia)* + -ICS] The practice of prosthodontia. Also *dental prosthetics.*

**prosthokeratoplasty** \präs′thəker′ətōplas′tē\ [*prosth(etic)* + *o* + KERATO- + -PLASTY] Transplantation of a transparent foreign substance into the opaque cornea.

**prostration** \prästrā′shən\ [Late L *prostratio* (from L *prostratus,* past part. of *prosternere* to throw down, from *pro-* PRO- + *sternere* to strew, spread) a strewing, throwing down] Utter exhaustion; a state of physical collapse. **heat p.** HEAT EXHAUSTION.

**prot-** \prōt-\ PROTO-.

**protactinium** \prōtaktin′ē·əm\ Element number 91, having atomic weight 231.036. It is a toxic, shiny metal and is produced by the loss of an alpha and beta particle from uranium 235, decaying further into actinium and finally lead. It has no stable isotope and 19 radioactive isotopes. Half-lives range from 5.7 milliseconds to 3.25 × $10^4$ years. Also *protoactinium, proactinium.* Symbol: Pa

**protamine** Any of several proteins of low molecular mass, about 5 kDa, consisting largely of arginine residues (about 30), found in association with DNA in fish sperm.

**protamine sulfate** The salt of protamine prepared by exchanging with sulfate the DNA naturally neutralizing the protamine. It is sometimes used for precipitating certain proteins.

**protan** \prō′tan\ PROTANOPE.

**protandry** \prōtan′drē\ [PROT- + ANDR- + -Y] The development of the testes earlier than the ovaries in an hermaphrodite organism. Adj. protandrous.

**protanomaly** \prō′tənäm′əlē\ [PROT- + ANOMALY] A form of partial red-green color blindness in which there is decreased appreciation of red. Also *protanomalopia, protanomalopsia.* Adj. protanomalous.

**protanope** \prō′tənōp\ [PROT- + Gk *an-* priv. + -OPE] A color-blind person who is unable to distinguish red. Also *protan.*

**protanopia** \prō′tənō′pē·ə\ [PROT- + ANOPIA] The form of red-green color blindness in which there is loss of appreciation of red. Also *protanopsia, anerythropsia.* Adj. protanopic.

**protean** \prō′tē·ən\ [L *Prote(us)* (from Gk *Prōteus*) a sea god who could take different shapes + English *-an,* suffix denoting characteristic of] Capable of assuming many different forms, as an ameba: used especially of diseases having extremely variable manifestations.

**protease** \prō′tē·ās\ PROTEINASE.

**protectin** \-tek′tin\ **1** A thin sheet of paper coated on one side with a plasterlike substance. It is often used in surgery to prevent contamination of tissues. **2** A substance in the serum which prevents hemolysis of red cells. *Outmoded.*

**protection / passive p.** PASSIVE IMMUNITY.

**protector / hearing p.** Any device which results in attenuation of the ambient sound arriving at the ear. This includes such devices as ear muffs worn over the ears and ear plugs inserted in the ear canals. The choice as to which device is used is partly determined by the frequency spectrum of the noise to which the subject is exposed. Also *ear defender.* **nipple p.** A shield used by lactating women to diminish cracking of the areolar skin.

**protein** \prō′tē·in, -tēn\ [French *protéine* (from Gk *prōteios* chief, first, primary, from *prōtos* first, earliest, foremost) protein] **1** A substance whose molecules are composed largely of amino-acid residues linked by peptide bonds and containing more than about 50 such residues. Proteins have diverse functions in living organisms, some being structural, some being enzymes, and some being hormones. **2** Composed of protein; proteinaceous. **p. A** A surface protein of many strains of *Staphylococcus aureus* that binds the F portion of many immunoglobulins and hence is useful in collecting antigen-antibody complexes. The interaction elicits various immunologic effects in animals. **autologous p.** A protein normally contained in the tissues or fluids of an individual or organism. Compare HETEROLOGOUS PROTEIN. **Bence Jones p.** A urinary protein of low molecular mass, composed of light chains of immunoglobulins, found in the urine of people with myelomas. Also *Bence Jones body, Bence Jones globulin, Bence-Jones monoclonal immunoglobulin.* **p. C** A normal plasma serine protease having a molecular weight of 45 000 which is a coagulation inhibitor. Protein C is a vitamin K-dependent factor which, when activated by thrombin, cleaves both factor VIIIa and factor Va to inactive forms. Partial deficiency of protein C has been associated with recurrent thrombophlebitis. Also *autoprothrombin IIa.* **calcium-binding p.** A protein produced in the intestinal mucosal cells on stimulation by 1,25-hydroxycholecalciferol. This protein is one of the mechanisms responsible for the transport of calcium from the luminal to the basolateral surfaces of the cell. **C4-binding p.** One of the control proteins of the complement system. C4-binding protein binds to C4b, allowing its cleavage by factor I. **α-chain p.** An abnormal protein made up of incomplete IgA heavy chains without light chains, found in alpha heavy-chain disease. **coat p.** Protein molecules packed together to form a regular array which protects the nucleic acid of a virus, and generally constituting the capsid. **conjugated p.** Any protein whose molecule contains some structure not composed of amino-acid residues, e.g. hemoglobin, which contains heme. **control p.'s** A group of proteins that are not necessary components of the complement pathways but which act as homeostatic factors in the control of complement activation. They include the C1-inhibitor, C4-binding protein, decay accelerating factor, factor I, factor H, and the complement receptor CR1. **corticosteroid-binding p.** CORTICOSTEROID-BINDING GLOBULIN. **C-reactive p.** A beta-globulin of serum that is present during the acute phase of rheumatic fever and some other inflammatory diseases. It precipitates the C substance of pneumococci as well as other phosphorylated compounds in the presence of $Ca^{2+}$. **eosinophil major basic p.** A zinc-containing protein that is the principal constituent of the large cytoplasmic granules of blood eosinophils. The major basic protein is released from eosinophil granules at sites of inflammation or allergy. It is highly cytotoxic to cells, to parasites, and to bacteria. **fibrous p.** Any protein that is a constituent of a natural fiber. Such proteins usually have long narrow molecules, and so repeat on a molecular level the structure of the fiber. **Gc p.** VITAMIN D-BINDING GLOBULIN. **globular p.** A protein whose molecules approach spherical shape in that no one dimension greatly exceeds others. **heme-thiolate p.** CYTOCHROME P-450. • The name derives from the fact that one ligand of iron is the thiolate anion of a cysteine residue. **heterologous p.** A protein of an organism of one species introduced into a member of another species. Compare AUTOLOGOUS PROTEIN. **iron-sulfur p.** A protein whose molecule contains iron ions, or iron and sulfide ions, held by ionized cysteine residues. Such proteins include rubredoxins and ferredoxins. They participate in electron-transfer reactions, as in the respiratory chain. **liquid p.** Protein in a fluid state used in liquid formulas and administered through oral and tube feedings. These liquid formulas include ones with whole protein obtained from meat, dairy products, eggs, soybean and fish protein concentrate supplemented with free amino acids and hydrolyzed casein. **M p.** **1** A type-specific protein of group A streptococci, located in fimbriae. It is antiphagocytic and contributes to virulence. More than 55 types are known. Also *M antigen.* **2** The lactose-transporting protein of the inner membrane of *Escherichia coli.* An earlier usage. **matrix p.** PORIN. **mild silver p.** A colloidal preparation of protein and 19 to 23 percent silver. It is used as a topical anti-infective agent for infections of the vaginal, rectal, ocular, urethral, otic, and nasopharyngeal regions. Casein and silver oxide are frequently used components for this preparation. **native p.** A protein in its native conformation, i.e. one that has not been denatured. **nonhistone chromosomal p.'s** Proteins other than histones which occur in association with the DNA in the cell nucleus. They are believed to play a role in the regulation of gene activity. **nonstructural p.** A viral encoded protein, expressed in infected cells, which does not become a component of the completed virus particle. Examples of nonstructural proteins are the T-antigen of the polyomaviruses and the thymidine kinase of the herpes simplex viruses. **periplasmic binding p.'s** Soluble proteins, recoverable from the periplasmic space of Gram-negative bacteria by osmotic shock or murein digestion, that specifically bind certain permeants, such as maltose. Elimination of such a protein by mutation blocks its ligand from transport into the cell, and also from chemotactic activity. **plasma p.** Any of the proteins present in the blood plasma. **retinol-binding p.** A specific protein for transporting retinol from the liver to the peripheral tissues. It has a molecular weight of 21 000, exhibits $\alpha$-mobility on electrophoresis, and contains one binding site for one molecule of retinol. It has a relatively high aromatic amino acid content. Normal levels in human plasma are 40–50 $\mu$g/ml. It forms a highly specific protein complex, with plasma prealbumin in a ratio of 1 to 2.5 respectively. The prealbumin stabilizes the binding of retinol-binding protein to retinol and decreases the losses of the protein which occurs through glomerular filtration and renal catabolism. Its constituents are determined through radioimmunoassay. Abnormalities in retinol-binding protein metabolism occur in diseases of the liver, thyroid, kidney, and pancreas, and in cystic fibrosis. Low concentrations are found in children with protein-calorie malnutrition. **p. S** A vitamin K-dependent plasma protein having a molecular weight of 69 000, which copurifies with complement component C4b. It is a coagulation inhibitor that enhances the action of protein C. **serum p.** Any protein of blood serum, i.e. any of the plasma proteins except fibrinogen and factors V and VIII. **simple p.** A protein whose molecule consists solely of amino-acid residues, without any carbohydrate, lipid, or other prosthetic group. **thyroid binding p.** Any of a group of serum proteins, which includes a globulin, an albumin, and a prealbumin, that have particular affinity for thyroid hormones and serve as carriers for them in serum. **thyroxine-binding p.** TRANSTHYRETIN. **transport p.** A protein carrier, often a permease, that transports some substance with which it forms a noncovalent complex. **p. Z** A vitamin K-dependent normal plasma protein having a molecular weight of 44 000. The function is unknown.

**proteinase** Any enzyme that catalyzes hydrolysis of a protein. Also *proteolytic enzyme, protease.*

**protein hydrolysate** A mixture obtained by submitting a protein sample to hydrolysis, which may be acid, alkaline, or enzymatic. The conditions of hydrolysis are chosen so that the hydrolysis is likely to be complete if the aim is to analyze the hydrolysate for amino acids in order to establish the composition of the protein. Alternatively, the hydrolysis may be partial if it is desired to isolate peptides as a part of establishing the sequence of the protein.

**protein kinase** 1 The enzyme (EC 2.7.1.37) that catalyzes the transfer of a phospho group from ATP onto serine residues in many proteins, including glycogen synthase and phosphorylase kinase, in response to hormonal stimulation of the cells that contain it, e.g. by epinephrine and glucagon, which activates adenylate cyclase to form cAMP. The binding of this effector to regulatory subunits of protein kinase causes their dissociation from the catalytic subunits which thereby acquire activity. It is thus a link in the process by which the hormones evoke activation of phosphorylase and inactivation of glycogen synthase. 2 Any enzyme that catalyzes this transfer onto any residue of a protein.

**protein-lysine 6-oxidase** The enzyme (EC 1.4.3.13) that catalyzes the oxidation of lysine residues, especially in collagen and elastin, to residues of allysine, by transforming their $—CH_2—NH_3^+$ groups into —CHO, a process necessary for cross-linking. Its inhibition leads to defects in connective tissue and arteries. Also *lysyl oxidase.*

**proteinosis** \prō′tēnō′sis\ [PROTEIN + -OSIS] The accumulation of greater-than-normal amounts of protein in the tissues. *Imprecise.* **lipoid p.** A rare autosomal recessive condition with onset in infancy, characterized by papules on the oropharynx, eyelids, and skin that lead to hoarseness, pruritis of the eyes, and hyperkeratosis and atrophy of affected skin. The basic defect is unknown, but cytoplasmic vacuolization and membrane-limited inclusions suggest a lysosomal storage disease. A light-sensitive form of the disease is now best regarded as erythropoietic protoporphyria. Also *Urbach-Wiethe disease, hyalinosis cutis, lipoproteinosis, lipoidproteinosis.* **pulmonary alveolar p.** A condition of unknown cause in which lipid-rich proteinaceous material accumulates in lung alveoli.

**proteinuria** \prō′tēnoo′rē·ə\ [PROTEIN + -URIA] Urinary excretion of abnormal amounts of protein. Normally up to 150 milligrams of protein may be excreted per 24 hours. Most proteins in the urine, including albumin which usually represents the major fraction, are serum proteins. However, some proteins, including Tomm-Horsfall mucoprotein, are derived from the renal tubules or the lower urinary tract. Persistent proteinuria is an important sign of renal disease, either primary or related to systemic disorders. Abnormal proteins, such as Bence-Jones protein, may be excreted in multiple myeloma. Also *albuminuria* (incorrect). **adventitious p.** Proteinuria without known renal disease. **anoxemic p.** Proteinuria associated with anoxemia, either general or local. If acute and severe, it may result in acute tubular necrosis. **asymptomatic p.** Proteinuria without any symptoms or signs of renal disease. However, absence of symptoms or signs does not rule out the possibility of underlying renal disease. Renal biopsy should be considered. **athletic p.** EXERCISE PROTEINURIA. **Bence Jones p.** The presence in urine of Bence-Jones protein, often a sign of multiple myeloma. **benign p.** Transient, exercise, orthostatic, or other varieties of proteinuria not associated with progressive renal failure. **cardiac p.** Proteinuria associated with congestive heart failure. When the heart failure is controlled, the proteinuria disappears. **effort p.** EXERCISE PROTEINURIA. **essential p.** Proteinuria of unknown origin. **exercise p.** Proteinuria following vigorous exercise, especially distance running and swimming, or contact sports. The condition is transient and of no clinical significance. Also *effort proteinuria, march proteinuria, athletic proteinuria.* **false p.** Proteinuria which is not associated with kidney disturbance. It may represent malingering. **febrile p.** Proteinuria that occurs during periods of fever and is not related to primary or systemic renal disease. **functional p.** Any proteinuria that is not associated with kidney disease. Also *physiologic proteinuria.* **gestational p.** The presence of protein in the urine during or just after a pregnancy, without evidence of hypertension, renal disease, or edema. **intermittent p.** Proteinuria which occurs at intervals. It may be functional, lordotic, or a sign of renal disease. **isolated p.** Proteinuria without any other urinary abnormality or sign of renal disease. **lordotic p.** ORTHOSTATIC PROTEINURIA. **march p.** EXERCISE PROTEIN-

URIA. **mixed p.** Proteinuria involving the excretion of two or more different proteins. *Rare.* **nonselective p.** Proteinuria characterized by the excretion of proteins with a wide range of molecular weights, usually but not exclusively associated with diffuse proliferative and membranous types of glomerulonephritis. **orthostatic p.** Proteinuria during the upright but not recumbent position. The proteinuria usually is nonselective, and occurs only during adolescence. It usually disappears by age 20 and is not associated with progressive renal disease. Also *postural proteinuria, lordotic proteinuria.* **persistent p.** The presence of protein in the urine observed on serial examination over days or weeks. It is an important sign of primary renal disease or of renal involvement in systemic disease. **physiologic p.** FUNCTIONAL PROTEINURIA. **postural p.** ORTHOSTATIC PROTEINURIA. **pyogenic p.** Proteinuria associated with pyuria. It is a sign of pyelonephritis. **selective p.** Proteinuria restricted to albumin and smaller globulins such as transferrin (molecular weight 99 000). It is usually but not exclusively seen in lipoid nephrosis. **transient p.** Proteinuria that persists only briefly, which may reflect orthostatic, exercise, or febrile proteinuria, or may be of unknown origin.

**proteinuric** \prō′tēnoo′rik\ Related to or pertaining to proteinuria.

**proteoglycan** A glycoprotein in which the protein is glycosylated with many polysaccharide chains of the glycosaminoglycan type, i.e. of alternate residues of hexosamine and uronic acid. These chains are often sulfated. Proteoglycans are found mainly in connective tissue and cartilage.

**proteolysis** \prō′tē·äl′isis\ The hydrolysis of peptide bonds in proteins. Also *peptolysis.*

**proteolytic** \prō′tē·əlit′ik\ Relating to proteolysis. Also *peptidolytic, peptolytic.*

**proteometabolism** \prō′tē·ōmətab′əlizm\ The metabolism of protein. Adj. proteometabolic.

**proteopepsis** \prō′tē·ōpep′sis\ Protein digestion.

**proteopeptic** \prō′tē·ōpep′tik\ Concerning protein digestion.

**proteopexy** \prō′tē·ōpek′sē\ [*prote(in)* + *o* + -PEXY] The incorporation or binding of protein in tissues. Also *proteopexis.*

**proteosemia** \prō′tē·ōsē′mē·ə\ The presence of partially hydrolyzed proteins in the blood.

**proteroglyphic** \prō′tərōglif′ik\ Having fixed, grooved fangs at the front of the upper jaw: used of snakes. Compare OPISTHOGLYPHIC, SOLENOGLYPHIC.

**protest / masculine p.** In adlerian psychology, any behavior or striving on the part of a man or a woman to escape or deny their feminine aspect.

***Proteus*** \prō′tē·əs\ [a sea god able to assume various shapes] A genus of enterobacteria characterized by urease production (which makes urine alkaline). They are common in soil and sewage, and are a frequent cause of urinary-tract infection. Species include *P. vulgaris* and *P. mirabilis* (which exhibit unusually high motility), *P. morganii*, and *P. rettgeri.* Certain *P. vulgaris* O antigens provide diagnostically useful serologic cross-reactions with rickettsiae.

**prothesis** \präth′əsis\ PROSTHESIS.

**prothetic** \-thet′ik\ PROSTHETIC.

**prothipendyl dihydrochloride** $C_{16}H_{19}N_3S{\cdot}2HCl$. *N,N*-Dimethyl-10*H*-pyrido[3,2-*b*]-[1,4]-benzothiazine-10-propanamine dihydrochloride. An azaphenothiazine tranquilizer with actions similar to those of chlorpromazine. It is used to treat psychotic patients and as a general tranquilizer with sedative, with antihistaminic properties.

**prothrombin** \-thräm′bin\ [PRO- + THROMB- + -IN] A plasma protein that yields thrombin upon activation by prothrombinase. Thrombin's molecular weight of 37 000 constitutes less than half of the prothrombin molecule (molecular weight 72 000). The remainder, containing 10 γ-carboxyglutamate residues, is necessary for binding with the calcium and phospholipid in prothrombinase. The normal plasma prothrombin concentration is 20 mg/dl plasma. Also *factor II.*

**prothrombinase** \-thräm′bināš\ THROMBOKINASE. **extrinsic p.** Factor Xa (thrombokinase) activity resulting from the activation of factor VII. **intrinsic p.** Factor Xa (thrombokinase) activity resulting from the activation of factor XII in the intrinsic coagulation cascade.

**prothrombinogen** \-thräm′bənəjən\ The hepatic precursor of prothrombin before its glutamate residues are converted to γ-carboxyglutamates.

**prothrombinopenia** \-thräm′binəpē′nē·ə\ HYPOPROTHROMBINEMIA.

**protides** Proteins and peptides collectively.

**protist** \prō′tist\ A single-celled organism; a member of the Protista.

**Protista** \prōtis′tə\ [Gk neut. pl. of *prōtistos* (superl. of *prōtos* first, earliest, foremost) first of all, first of the first] In one classification, a kingdom that includes the prokaryotes (bacteria) and the single-celled eukaryotic groups (algae, fungi, and protozoa).

**proto-** \prō′tə-, prō′tō-\ [Gk *prōtos* first, front, foremost] A combining form meaning (1) first, earliest; (2) primitive; (3) chief, principal. Also *prot-.*

**protoactinium** \-aktin′ē·əm\ PROTACTINIUM.

**protoblast** \prō′təblast\ [PROTO- + -BLAST] A blastomere considered as the precursor of a particular structure or organ. Adj. protoblastic.

**protochlorophyll** \-klôr′əfil\ [PROTO- + CHLOROPHYLL] A minor green pigment found in etiolated leaves that absorbs light at a wavelength of 638 μ and is thereby changed into chlorophyll.

**protochondrium** \-kän′drē·əm\ Primitive cartilagenous connective tissue that develops from precartilage and matures to become true cartilage.

**protochordate** \-kôr′dāt\ [PROTO- + CHORDATE] Any member of the groups variously classified as chordates or invertebrates.

**protocol** \prō′təkôl\ [Late or Med. L *protocol(um)* protocol, from Late Gk *prōtokollon* (from Gk *prōto(s)* first + *kollan* to glue) a first leaf glued to a manuscript describing contents, registering author, and giving other authentication] **1** The original description of the findings and conclusions of an experiment, a case history, or an autopsy. **2** A plan for the conduct of each step of a study, experiment, or treatment. **test p.** A document laying down in precise detail the tests that must be performed to determine the safety of a substance, agent, or procedure in the course of clinical, experimental, or pharmacologic study.

**protocone** \prō′təkōn\ [PROTO- + CONE] The lingual cusp of the trigon; the major, mesiolingual cusp of the mammalian upper molar tooth.

**protoconid** \-kän′id\ [*protocon(e)* + -ID[2]] The buccal cusp of the trigonid; the major, mesiolingual cusp of the mammalian lower molar tooth.

**protocoproporphyria** \-käp′rəpôrfir′ē·ə\ VARIEGATE PORPHYRIA.

**protodiastole** \-dī·as′təlē\ [PROTO- + DIASTOLE] The brief period between the end of ventricular ejection and the recording of the incisura on the aortic pressure tracing. • The term is sometimes incorrectly used to describe the end of the rapid ventricular filling phase following closure of the semilunar valves.

**protodiastolic** \-dī′əstäl′ik\ Relating to protodiastole. • The term is sometimes used incorrectly, as in *protodiastolic gallop*, to describe a gallop due to a third heart sound.

**protoduodenum** \-dʸoo′·ədē′nəm\ [PROTO- + DUODENUM] That part of the definitive duodenum developed from the foregut of the embryo. It is the proximal part extending from the pylorus to the duodenal papilla.

**protoelastin** \prō′tə·ilas′tin\ A protein having a high concentration of repeating peptide units containing glycine and proline. It is a precursor of elastin found in connective tissue.

**protofibril** \-fī′bril\ A minute fiber in the ground substance between submicroscopic fibrils of connective tissue, seen only with the electron microscope.

**protofilament** \-fil′əmənt\ AXONEME.

**protogonocyte** \-gō′nəsīt\ [PROTO- + GONOCYTE] The first sex cell formed after fertilization of an ovum and after cleavage has begun. It later divides rapidly to give rise to oogonia and spermatogonia.

**protokylol hydrochloride** $C_{18}H_{22}ClNO_5$. 4-[2-[[2-(1,3-Benzodioxol-*S*-yl)-1-methyl-ethyl]amino]-1-hydroxyethyl]-1,2-benzenediol hydrochloride. An andrenergic agent used primarily as a bronchodilator to correct bronchospasm in patients with bronchial asthma, and other conditions. It is given orally.

**Protomastigida** \-məstij′idə\ A former name for KINETOPLASTIDA.

**protometer** \prōtäm′ətər\ EXOPHTHALMOMETER.

**proton** \prō′tän\ [Gk *prōton*, neut. sing of *prōtos* first] A nuclear particle with a single positive charge numerically equal to that on an electron, $1.6 \times 10^{-19}$ coulomb, and mass of 1.008 amu, i.e. $1.67 \times 10^{-24}$ g. In solution it becomes a hydrogen ion. The proton and the neutron together form the basic building blocks for heavier nuclei.

**protonate** \prō′tənāt\ **1** To add a proton, $H^+$. **2** To add any hydrogen ion, i.e. a deuteron or a triton as well as a proton.

**proto-oncogene** \-äng′kəjēn\ Any gene in a eukaryotic cell capable of becoming an oncogene. The proto-oncogene ordinarily has a function of prime importance to normal cellular metabolism, but through mutation of its coding sequence or regulatory elements or the insertion of viral transcriptional control elements it can lose normal regulation and thus contribute to cellular transformation.

**protopathic** \-path′ik\ Denoting a hypothetical sensory system postulated (by Henry Head) to subserve "crude touch," pain, and temperature sensation. It was considered to be the first element to recover following nerve section and to be conveyed by the spinothalamic tract. Compare EPICRITIC.

**protopianoma** \-pē·ənō′mə\ [PROTO- + PIAN + -OMA] MOTHER YAW.

**protoplasm** \prō′təplazm\ [PROTO- + PLASM] The substance of the living cell, divided into the nucleoplasm and cytoplasm. Also *bioplasm*. **functional p.** The portion of the protoplasm essential for life, exclusive of the portion that serves for storage.

**protoplasmic** \-plaz′mik\ Pertaining to or composed of protoplasm. Also *protoplasmatic*.

**protoplasmolysis** \-plazmäl′isis\ PLASMOLYSIS.

**protoplast** \prō′təplast\ [PROTO- + -PLAST] **1** A bacterium from which the cell wall has been removed. The rounded protoplasmic mass is bounded by the plasma membrane and is osmotically fragile. **2** The protoplasm of a plant cell.

**protoporphyria** \-pôrfir′ē·ə\ A condition characterized by an excess of protoporphyrin. **erythropoietic p.** A hereditary disorder of autosomal dominant transmittance, characterized by cutaneous photosensitivity (with urticaria more common than blistering following sunlight exposure), scarring and depigmentation, increased erythrocyte protoporphyrin, normal urinary excretion of porphyrins, and late onset of progressive and often fatal liver disease. The metabolic defect is reduction in activity of heme synthetase, the final enzyme in the pathway of heme synthesis. Also *erythrohepatic protoporphyria, heme synthetase deficiency*.

**protoporphyrin** The prophyrin whose substituents are methyl, vinyl, methyl, vinyl, methyl, 2-carboxyethyl, 2-carboxethyl, and methyl. They are in that order in the protoporphyrin derived from hemoglobin.

**protopsis** \prōtäp′sis\ EXOPHTHALMOS.

**protospasm** \prō′təspazm\ [PROTO- + SPASM] *Outmoded* JACKSONIAN MARCH.

**protospore** \prō′təspôr\ [PROTO- + SPORE] A multinucleate spore resulting from progressive cleavage.

**protosyphilis** \-sif′əlis\ PRIMARY SYPHILIS.

**protothecosis** \-thēkō′sis\ Infection of the skin and subcutaneous tissues with species of the alga *Prototheca*. It is seen usually in a subject with an impaired immune response.

**prototroph** \prō′tətrāf\ [back-formation from *prototrophic*, from PROTO- + -TROPHIC] An organism that lacks a specific growth requirement, usually one that is the parent, or a reversion, of a given auxotroph.

**prototrophy** \prōtät′rəfē\ The state of being nonauxotrophic: usually said of the parent or a reversion of an auxotrophic mutant.

**prototropic** \-träp′ik\ Acting upon proteins: used especially of antimicrobial or antiviral agents that attack proteins.

**prototype** \prō′tətīp\ [Gk *prōtotypon* (from *prōtotypos* original, from *prōto(s)* first + *typos* form, model) an original form, archetype] **1** A type upon which the defining characteristics of a category are based. **2** An original type from which derivative types have evolved. **3** Something that serves as a model for further development or elaboration.

**protoveratrine** \-ver′ətrēn\ Either of two alkaloids isolated from *Veratrum album* and having hypotensive properties. Designated protoveratrine A and B, they are often combined for therapeutic effect. Protoveratrine B is less potent than protoveratrine A.

**protoverine** \-ver′in\ $C_{27}H_{43}NO_9$. A product from the alkaline hydrolysis of protoveratrine. It is closely related to the aglycones of the cardiac glycosides possessing hypotensive, cardiac depressant, and sedative properties.

**protovertebra** \-vur′təbrə\ [PROTO- + VERTEBRA] A precursor of a vertebra, made by the fusion of two parts, superior (or cephalic) and inferior (or caudal) of two adjacent sclerotomes.

**Protozoa** \-zō′ə\ [PROTO- + Gk *zōa*, pl. of *zōon* living being, animal] A subkingdom of the kingdom Animalia comprising the eukaryotic unicellular animals. Some protozoans aggregate but do not form true multicellular tissues, a characteristic of the other major group in the animal kingdom, the Metazoa.

**protozoa** Plural of PROTOZOON.

**protozoacide** \-zō′əsīd\ PROTOZOICIDE.

**protozoagglutinin** \-zō′əgloo′tinin\ A substance formed in the blood which can agglutinate infecting protozoa in certain protozoan infections.

**protozoan** \-zō′ən\ **1** Any member of the subkingdom Protozoa. Also *protozoon*. **2** Pertaining to or characteristic of the subkingdom Protozoa. Also *protozoal*.

**protozoiasis** \-zō·ī′əsis\ [*protozo(a)* + -IASIS] Any disease resulting from infection by protozoa. Also *protozoosis.*

**protozoicide** \-zō′isīd\ [*protozo(a)* + *i* + -CIDE] An agent that kills protozoa. Also *protozoacide.*

**protozoology** \-zō·äl′əjē\ The branch of zoology concerned with the study of protozoans. **clinical p.** The study of protozoa that cause disease in humans and domestic animals.

**protozoon** \-zō′än\ [PROTO- + Gk *zōon* living being, animal] (*pl.* protozoa) PROTOZOAN.

**protozoophage** \-zō′əfāj\ A phagocyte that ingests protozoa.

**protozoosis** \-zō·ō′sis\ PROTOZOIASIS.

**protozootherapy** \-zō′əther′əpē\ The treatment of disease caused by infection with protozoa, especially the chemotherapy of such infections.

**protract** \-trakt′\ To extend or push or draw forward (a part of the body, such as the shoulder or mandible).

**protrusio acetabuli** \-troo′zhō as′ətab′yəlī\ A deepening of the acetabulum with inward migration of the femoral head due to softening of bone. As a result the pelvic outlet is narrowed. Also *Otto pelvis, Otto's disease, sunken acetabulum, arthrokatadysis, acetabular protrusion.*

**protrusion** \-troo′zhən\ [L *protrusio* (from *protrusus,* past part. of *protrudere* to thrust forward, propel, from *pro-* PRO- + L *trudere* to push, impel) a thrusting forward] **1** A postural forward or forward and lateral movement or position of the mandible. **2** An anatomical forward position of a tooth. **acetabular p.** PROTRUSIO ACETABULI. **bimaxillary p.** Protraction of both maxilla and mandible. **intervertebral disk p.** Herniation of an intervertebral disk through the capsule, often causing impingement of a nerve root. Also *prolapse of intervertebral disk, hernia of the nucleus pulposus.* **intrapelvic p.** The distortion of the inner wall of the pelvis by the floor of the acetabulum, as is seen in the more severe forms of protrusio acetabuli. **lateral p.** Protrusive movement of the mandible with a lateral component, one condyle moving further forward than the other. Adj. lateroprotrusive.

**protrypsin** TRYPSINOGEN.

**protuberance** \-t$^y$oo′bərəns\ [Late L *protuberantia.* See PROTUBERANTIA.] A protruding or projecting part; protuberantia. **Bichat's p.** CORPUS ADIPOSUM BUCCAE. **p. of chin** PROTUBERANTIA MENTALIS. **external occipital p.** PROTUBERANTIA OCCIPITALIS EXTERNA. **frontal p.** TUBER FRONTALE. **internal occipital p.** PROTUBERANTIA OCCIPITALIS INTERNA. **laryngeal p.** PROMINENTIA LARYNGEA. **mental p.** PROTUBERANTIA MENTALIS. **natiform p.** NATES. **palatine p.** TORUS PALATINUS. **parietal p.** TUBER PARIETALE. **tubal p.** TORUS TUBARIUS.

**protuberantia** \-t$^y$oo′bəran′shə\ [Late L, a protuberance, from *protuberare* to bulge, from *pro-* PRO- + L *tuber* a swelling, hump] A protruding or projecting part; a swelling or knob; a protuberance. **p. laryngea** PROMINENTIA LARYNGEA. **p. mentalis** [NA] A raised triangular area in the midline of the anterior surface of the body of the mandible at the lower end of the symphysis menti. Its base is depressed in the center but raised on the sides by the mental tubercles. Also *mental protuberance, protuberance of chin, mental process, external mental squama* (outmoded). **p. occipitalis externa** [NA] A prominence in the midline of the external surface of the occipital bone midway between the superior angle, at lambda, and the posterior margin of foramen magnum. It gives attachment to ligamentum nuchae. Also *external occipital protuberance.* **p. occipitalis interna** [NA] An irregular prominence at the center of the cruciform eminence on the internal aspect of the squamous part of the occipital bone. Also *internal occipital protuberance.*

**Proust** [P. T. *Proust,* French physician, flourished 19th century] Proust-Lichtheim maneuver. See under MANEUVER.

***Providencia*** \präv′iden′shē·ə\ A group of enterobacteria closely related to *Proteus* but lacking rapid urea hydrolysis. They are occasionally found in urinary-tract and in burn infections.

**provider** An individual or organization that provides goods or services; in particular, a provider of health care services. **preferred p.** An affiliation of health-care providers organized to contract with employers or insurers at favorable or discounted rates, generally on a prepaid basis, to provide coverage for an enrolled population. Preferred providers are often represented by a preferred provider organization (PPO) to offer the insurance for the services they provide.

**proviral** \-vī′rəl\ Of or relating to a provirus.

**provirus** \-vī′rəs\ [PRO- + VIRUS] An early replicative intermediate of RNA tumor viruses and bacteriophages consisting of double-stranded DNA synthesized by the virion reverse transcriptase using the virion single-stranded RNA as a template. This DNA may become incorporated into the cellular DNA and serve as a permanent template for replication of viral RNA and/or a heritable gene capable of transformation of cells.

**provitamin** A substance that can give rise to a vitamin by a natural reaction. Thus, 7-dehydrocholesterol is a provitamin D, since it can form vitamin D in the skin under the action of sunlight. Also *previtamin.* **p. D** Any of the substances that form vitamin D on illumination in the skin. **p. $D_3$** 7-Dehydrocholesterol. The action of light on this substance, as by illumination of the skin, forms vitamin $D_3$ (cholecalciferol).

**provocative** \prəväk′ətiv\ Designed to elicit a diagnostic sign by deliberately provoking a pathologic reaction, as *provocative test.*

***Prowazekia*** \prō′vätsē′kē·ə\ *BODO.*

**prox-** \präks-\ PROXIMO-.

**proxemics** \präksē′miks\ [*prox(imity)* + *-emics* as in *phonemics*] The study of space and of the effect of the lack of personal space on behavior and adjustment.

**proxi-** \präk′sē-\ PROXIMO-.

**proximad** \präk′simad\ Directed proximally; towards the proximal end or part.

**proximal** \präk′siməl\ [L *proxim(us),* (superl. of *prope* near) nearest + -AL] **1** Nearest or nearer the beginning, the attached end, the center, or the midline. Compare DISTAL. **2** APPROXIMAL.

**proximalis** \präk′simā′lis\ [NA] Proximal.

**proximo-** \präk′simō-\ [L *proximus* nearest, next to] A combining form meaning proximal. Also *prox-, proxi-.*

**proxy** \präk′sē\ [Middle English *proccy,* contraction of *procuracie* procuration, from L *procuratus,* past part. of *procurare* to take care of] A variable for which data are available that is taken to represent another variable, values for which cannot be directly determined. For example, when morbidity cannot be directly measured, mortality data may have to be used as a substitute. The procedure may have obvious and serious limitations.

**prozonal** \prō′zōnəl\ Denoting a phenomenon in which a negative reaction is obtained with low dilutions of an antibody, while a positive reaction is obtained with the same antibody at higher dilutions.

**prozone** \prō′zōn\ **1** An area of antibody excess in an immunodiffusion plate where precipitation with a specific antigen is suboptimal. **2** A state of antibody excess that abrogates agglutination. For defs. 1 and 2 also *prezone, inhibition zone.*

**PRPP** 5-phosphoribosyl pyrophosphate (the donor of the 5-phosphoribosyl group in nucleotide biosynthesis).

**prurigo** \proorī′gō\ [L (akin to *prurire* to itch, be wanton or lascivious), the itch] A widespread irritable skin eruption in which the lesions have no obvious local cause. **p. agria** A severe form of prurigo. **Besnier's p.** An atopic dermatitis characterized by prurigo of the flexures and marked thickening of the skin. Also *flexural prurigo.* **dermographic p.** A condition marked by small irritable skin papules of unknown cause and wheals or excoriations that are provoked by scratching, friction, or pressure. Also *prurigo dermographica.* **p. estivalis** HUTCHINSON SUMMER PRURIGO. **flexural p.** BESNIER'S PRURIGO. **Hutchinson summer p.** A polymorphic light eruption that is characterized by excoriated papules and lichenification. The onset is prepubertal, and, although it is usually confined to exposed sites, covered areas are also often involved. Also *Hutchinson's disease, summer prurigo, summer itch, prurigo estivalis.* **p. infantilis** PAPULAR URTICARIA. **leukodermic p.** Prurigo with loss of pigment secondary to scratching. **melanotic p.** A combination of pruritis and hypermelanotic pigmentation that occurs in primary biliary cirrhosis. **p. of pregnancy** An irritable papular eruption of early pregnancy usually found on the arms, shoulders, and thighs. **p. simplex** PAPULAR URTICARIA. **summer p.** HUTCHINSON SUMMER PRURIGO. **p. vulgaris** PAPULAR URTICARIA. **winter p.** An irritable eruption characterized by intense itching, associated with chronic exposure to cold. Also *winter itch, pruritis hiemalis.*

**pruritus** \proorī′təs\ [L (from *pruritus,* past part. of *prurire* to itch), an itch, itching] **1** A condition that has as the dominant symptom a desire to scratch some part of the body to relieve irritation. **2** A sensation that elicits the desire to scratch. Also *itching.* **p. ani** Itching of the perianal skin caused by local inflammatory disorders, or without any detectable local abnormality, or more rarely by rectal abnormalities. **aquagenic p.** An itching of the skin, without visible wheal formation, that is provoked by contact of the skin with water. **autotoxic p.** Pruritus attributed to endogenous toxins, as in jaundice, uremia, and the like. **p. hiemalis** WINTER PRURIGO. **p. scroti** An itchy, irritable condition of the scrotum. **senile p.** Pruritus without discoverable cause that occurs in the elderly. **symptomatic p.** Pruritus that is a manifestation of systemic disease. **p. vulvae** Pruritus of the vulva and associated external genitalia of the female.

**Prussak** [Alexander *Prussak,* Russian otologist, 1839–1897] **1** Prussak's fibers. See under FIBER. **2** Prussak's pouch, Prussak space. See under RECESSUS MEMBRANAE TYMPANI SUPERIOR.

**psalis** \sā′lis\ *Outmoded* FORNIX CEREBRI.

**psamm-** \sam-\ PSAMMO-.

**psammism** \sam′izm\ PSAMMOTHERAPY.

**psammo-** \sam′ō-\ [Gk *psammos* sand] A combining form meaning sand, sandy. Also *psamm-.*

**psammoma** \samō′mə\ [PSAMM- + -OMA] A tumor containing psammoma bodies. . *Outmoded.* Also *acervuloma, sand tumor.*

**psammomatous** \samäm′ətəs\ **1** Containing psammoma bodies. **2** Having a sandy consistency. Also *psammous.*

***Psammophis*** [PSAMM- + Gk *ophis* a serpent, snake] A genus of venomous snakes occurring in Africa and Asia.

**psammotherapy** \sam′ōther′əpē\ [Gk *psammo(s)* sand + THERAPY] The use of heated sand, or sand baths, to alleviate painful conditions. Also *ammotherapy, psammism.*

**psammous** \sam′əs\ PSAMMOMATOUS.

**Psaume** [Jean *Psaume,* French stomatologist, flourished mid-20th century] Papillon-Léage and Psaume syndrome. See under SYNDROME.

**psauoscopy** \sô·äs′kəpē\ [Gk *psau(ein)* to touch + *o* + -SCOPY] A method of examination by touch to determine the extent of a pathologic area. In moving a fingertip lightly across the skin one detects increased skin resistance as the fingertip passes into the abnormal area.

**psellism** \sel′izm\ [Gk *psellismos* (from *psellizein* to stammer, falter in speech) stammering, inarticulateness] STUTTERING.

**pseud-** \sood-\ PSEUDO-.

**pseudacousis** \soo′dəkoo′sis\ [PSEUD- + Gk *akousis* hearing] **1** A disorder of hearing in which the subject hears his own voice altered in timbre and tonality. **2** The erroneous localization of a laterally situated source of sound. An obsolete usage.

**pseudactinomycosis** \soodak′tinōmīkō′sis\ PSEUDOACTINOMYCOSIS.

**pseudagraphia** \soo′dəgraf′ē·ə\ PSEUDOAGRAPHIA.

**pseudalbuminuria** \soo′dalbyoo′minoo′rē·ə\ [PSEUD- + ALBUMINURIA] Proteinuria which is not associated with kidney disturbance. Also *pseudoalbuminuria.*

**pseudamnesia** \soo′damnē′zhə\ [PSEUD- + AMNESIA] **1** Amnesia that is either feigned or stemming from dissociative hysteria. **2** Transitory or reversible amnesia, from any cause. An obsolete usage.

**pseudankylosis** \soo′dangkilō′sis\ FIBROUS ANKYLOSIS.

**pseudarthritis** \soo′därthrī′tis\ [PSEUD- + ARTHRITIS] Musculoskeletal pain the origin of which is not in the joint.

**pseudarthrosis** \soo′därthrō′sis\ A false joint that forms at the site of an ununited fracture. Also *pseudoarthrosis, false joint, false articulation.*

***Pseudechis*** \soodē′kis\ [PSEUD- + Gk *echis* a viper, adder] A genus of highly venomous snakes of the family Elapidae; the Australian black snake.

**pseudelminth** \soodel′minth\ PSEUDOHELMINTH.

**pseudesthesia** \soo′desthē′zhə\ [PSEUD- + *esthes(io)-* + -IA] Perception of subjective sensations, either experienced in the absence of appropriate stimuli (sensory hallucinations), or not corresponding to the provocative stimulus, or relating to an amputated limb (phantom limb). Also *pseudoesthesia.*

**pseudinoma** \soo′dinō′mə\ PHANTOM TUMOR.

**pseudo-** \soo′də-, soo′dō-\ [Gk *pseudēs* false] A combining form meaning (1) false; (2) closely resembling something else, as if in mimicry, and tending to deceive; (3) taking the place of something else; (4) abnormally present in place of something else. Also *pseud-.*

**pseudoabscess** \-ab′ses\ BENIGN INTRACRANIAL HYPERTENSION.

**pseudoacephalus** \-əsef′ələs\ [PSEUDO- + ACEPHALUS] A placentally attached parasitic twin which grossly appears to have no head but which on close examination has rudimentary cranial or facial structures.

**pseudoacromegaly** \-ak′rəmeg′əlē\ [PSEUDO- + ACROMEGALY] CHEIROMEGALY.

**pseudoactinomycosis** \-ak′tinōmīkō′sis\ A disease of the lungs simulating actinomycosis, usually due to *Nocardia.* Also *pseudactinomycosis, para-actinomycosis.*

**pseudoagglutination** \-əgloo′tinā′shən\ PSEUDOHEMAGGLUTINATION.

**pseudoaggression** \-əgresh′ən\ The denial of masochistic yearnings by creating a facade of dominance, control, or superiority.

**pseudoagrammatism** \-əgram′ətizm\ [PSEUDO- + AGRAMMATISM] SYNTACTICAL APHASIA.

**pseudographia** \-əgraf′ē·ə\ Inability to write spontaneously and legibly, although the patient is able to copy a text. Also *pseudagraphia.* • Strictly, the prefix *pseudo-* is incorrect, as this is a restricted form of agraphia.

**pseudoallele** \-əlēl′\ An allele at a genetic locus that is characterized by pseudoallelism.

**pseudoallelic** \-əlel′ik\ **1** Pertaining to two alleles or two loci that show pseudoallelism. **2** Pertaining to two alleles that appear to be located at the same locus, but are not.

**pseudoallelism** \-əle′lizm\ The state of two structurally distinct but closely linked genetic loci producing a wild-type phenotype when both are heterozygous for mutant alleles in the cis position and producing the mutant phenotype when the same mutant alleles are in the trans position.

**pseudoalveolar** \-alvē′ələr\ Simulating an alveolus in structure.

**pseudoamenorrhea** \-əmen′ôrē′ə\ [PSEUDO- + AMENORRHEA] The apparent absence of menstruation, actually resulting from blockage of menstrual flow by an imperforate hymen or by stenosis of the cervix.

**pseudoanaphylaxis** \-an′əfilak′sis\ A systemic or local reaction that resembles anaphylaxis but results from nonimmune mechanisms that lead to the release of vasoactive amines and other mediators. Also *anaphylactoid phenomenon.* Adj. pseudoanaphylactic.

**pseudoanemia** \-ənē′mē·ə\ Marked pallor without anemia.

**pseudoaneurysm** \-an′yərizm\ **1** A dilatation of a blood vessel in which the aneurysm wall is comprised of only part of the usual layers. It usually results from trauma or infection. A saccular pseudoaneurysm can occasionally form and even rupture, with life-threatening complications. **2** A dilated and tortuous blood vessel superficially resembling a true aneurysm.

**pseudoankylosis** \-ang′kilō′sis\ FIBROUS ANKYLOSIS.

**pseudoanorexia** \-an′ôrek′sē·ə\ *Seldom used* ANOREXIA NERVOSA.

**pseudoantagonist** \-antag′ənist\ A muscle that, by flexing a joint, reduces the flexion power of a second joint that is exerted by another muscle crossing the first joint.

**pseudoaphasia** \-əfā′zhə\ [PSEUDO- + APHASIA] FUNCTIONAL APHASIA.

**pseudoappendicitis** \-əpen′disī′tis\ A syndrome with abdominal pain resembling appendicitis, but without an inflamed appendix. **p. zooparasitica** A pseudoappendicitis in which parasites are harbored in the appendix.

**pseudoarthrosis** \-ärthrō′sis\ PSEUDARTHROSIS.

**pseudoastereognosis** \-əstir′ē·ägnō′sis\ [PSEUDO- + ASTEREOGNOSIS] STEREOANESTHESIA.

**pseudoathetosis** \-ath′ətō′sis\ [PSEUDO- + ATHETOSIS] Random wandering movements of the fingers and hands, when held outstretched with the eyes closed, due to loss of position and joint sense.

**pseudoatrophoderma** \-at′rəfōdur′mə\ The state of exhibiting the clinical appearance of skin atrophy but lacking the pathologic manifestations of the condition. **p. of the neck** A rare, rather poorly documented syndrome of young women that is characterized by mottled macular pigmentation, atrophy, and wrinkling of the skin of the sides of the neck.

**pseudobulbar** \-bul′bər\ Designating symptoms such as dysphagia and dysarthria, resembling those of bulbar paralysis but due to upper rather than lower motor neuron dysfunction.

**pseudocartilage** \-kär′tilij\ CHONDROID TISSUE.

**pseudocartilaginous** \-kär′tilaj′ənəs\ Composed of a substance resembling cartilage.

**pseudocast** \soo′dəkast\ FALSE CAST.

**pseudocele** \soo′dəsēl\ CAVUM SEPTI PELLUCIDI.

**pseudocephalocele** \-sef′əlōsēl′\ [PSEUDO- + CEPHALO- + -CELE[1]] Herniation of brain substance through the skull due to disease or injury or following surgery and not due to a congenital malformation.

**pseudochancre** \-shang′kər\ [PSEUDO- + CHANCRE] A chancrelike lesion. **p. redux** A chancrelike lesion at the site of a healed primary lesion of syphilis.

**pseudocholesteatoma** \-kō′lestē·ətō′mə\ A collection of caseous debris in the middle or external ear resembling the keratin accumulation of cholesteatoma.

**pseudocholinesterase** See under CHOLINESTERASE.

**pseudochromesthesia** \-krō′mesthē′zhə\ [PSEUDO- + CHROMESTHESIA] False perception of color.

**pseudochromhidrosis** \-krō′midrō′sis\ A discoloration of the axillary hair and clothing that is caused by the presence of colorific bacteria in sweat. Also *pseudochromidrosis.*

**pseudocirrhosis** \-sirō′sis\ [PSEUDO- + CIRRHOSIS] A disorder resembling cirrhosis clinically but not due to liver disease, such as constrictive pericarditis.

**pseudoclaudication** \-klô′dikā′shən\ A condition that mimics the claudication that accompanies peripheral arterial occlusive disease, with pain developing down one or both legs after exercise and easing after rest. In this condition, however, the arteries are usually normal, and the pain is a manifestation of neurologic disease, usually lumbar spinal stenosis, chronic lumbar arachnoiditis, or osteoarthritis.

**pseudocoarctation** \-kō′ärktā′shən\ A dilated and kinked vessel resembling a true coarctation in radiologic appearance but without significant obstruction. **p. of the aorta** A dilated and kinked aorta resembling coarctation of the aorta, with a slight narrowing occurring at the level of the ligamentum arteriosum.

**pseudocoel** \soo′dəsēl\ A false or partial coelom, characteristic of Nemathelminthes, in which the body cavity is partially lined with epithelium of mesodermal origin. It is also found in other members of the group of phyla formerly classified as Aschelminthes.

**pseudocoelomate** \-sē′ləmāt\ **1** Having or characterized by a pseudocoel. **2** Any member of the group of invertebrate phyla having a body cavity of the pseudocoel type.

**pseudocolloid of lips** \-käl′oid\ *Obs.* FORDYCE SPOTS.

**pseudo-corpus luteum** \-kôr′pəs loo′tē·əm\ A corpus luteum that matures but does not undergo ovulation.

**pseudocoxalgia** \-käksal′jə\ PERTHES DISEASE.

**pseudocrisis** \-krī′sis\ A sudden, temporary decrease in body temperature followed by a rise and continued fever. Also *false crisis.*

**pseudocroup** \-kroop′\ **1** LARYNGISMUS STRIDULUS. **2** LARYNGITIS STRIDULOSA.

**pseudocryptorchidism** \-kriptôr′kidizm\ [PSEUDO- + CRYPTORCHIDISM] An actively retractile testis or testes, usually in boys. The absence of true cryptorchidism can be demonstrated by observation, bringing the testis down into the scrotum by gentle pressure from above, or allowing the testis to descend spontaneously when the patient is placed in a warm bath. Also *pseudocryptorchism.*

**pseudocyesis** \-sī·ē′sis\ [PSEUDO- + CYESIS] The signs and symptoms of pregnancy in the absence of a conception. Also *pseudopregnancy, false pregnancy, spurious pregnancy, hysterical pregnancy.*

**pseudocyst** \soo′dəsist\ [PSEUDO- + CYST] **1** A false cyst; an accumulation of fluid or other material in a cystlike space that lacks a host-derived epithelial lining or outer membrane. Also *false cyst.* **2** A host cell filled with the products of rapid cell division (by endodyogeny or endopolygeny) in *Toxoplasma* or other sporozoans, resulting in an intracellular cluster of tachyzoites without the outer membrane that characterizes a true cyst.

**pseudodecidua** \-disid′yoo·ə\ [PSEUDO- + DECIDUA] A change in the endometrium resembling that seen in pregnancy.

**pseudodementia** \-dimen′shə\ [PSEUDO- + DEMENTIA] **1** Reversible cognitive dysfunction secondary to depression, which disappears when the depression clears. It is often mistaken for primary dementia in the elderly. Also *pseudosenility.* **2** A hysterical dissociation state resembling dementia. **3** Apathy due to reversible or metabolic brain disease. **4** Purposive simulation of dementia. Also *cataphrenia.*

**pseudodextrocardia** \-dek′strəkär′dē·ə\ [PSEUDO- + DEXTROCARDIA] Displacement of the heart to the right without transposition of the arteries or chambers of the heart.

**pseudodiabetes** \-dī′əbē′tēz\ LATENT DIABETES. **stress p.** Elevated blood sugar or glucosuria resulting from a sympathetic response to stress. It is characterized by hepatic glycogenolysis, gluconeogenesis, and relative insulin resistance, chiefly due to abrupt increase in the secretion of epinephrine, adrenal glucocorticoids, and possibly growth hormone.

**pseudodominance** \-däm′inəns\ The property of a heritable recessive trait to appear as if its inheritance is autosomal or X-linked dominant because of the mating of affected individuals with unaffected heterozygous carriers. Also *quasidominance.*

**pseudodysentery** \-dis′ənter′ē\ A symptom complex resembling bacillary dysentery but from a cause other than shigellosis.

**pseudoedema** \soo′dō·ēdē′mə\ Swelling of a part mimicking edema but caused by something other than the accumulation of fluid in the tissues.

**pseudoelastin** \-ilas′tin\ A protein with staining properties similar to those of elastin but which has different properties. It increases in quantity with aging and is thought to be either a degradation product or a faulty form of collagen.

**pseudoembryonic** \-em′brē·än′ik\ [PSEUDO- + EMBRYONIC] Falsely appearing to be of embryonic origin.

**pseudoendometritis** \-en′dəmētrī′tis\ A histologic appearance of inflammation of the endometrium without bacterial infection.

**pseudoephedrine** (+)-2-Methylamino-1-phenylpropan-1-ol. *d*-Pseudoephedrine, the naturally occurring isomer of ephedrine. As the hydrochloride, it is used to dilate the bronchi. Also *isoephedrine.*

***d*-pseudoephedrine hydrochloride** $C_{10}H_{16}ClNO$. α-[1-(Methylamino)ethyl]benzenemethanol hydrochloride. One of the four isomers, and one of the two natural isomers of ephedrine. It has less pressor activity and central nervous system stimulant activity than ephedrine. It is given orally as a bronchodilator and used as a nasal decongestant.

**pseudoepilepsy** \-ep′ilep′sē\ [PSEUDO- + EPILEPSY] A hysterical attack superficially resembling epilepsy.

**pseudoepiphysis** \-epif′isis\ [PSEUDO- + EPIPHYSIS] An extremity of a metacarpal which does not form part of the proper center of ossification but is characterized by a formation that may be confused with that of the diaphysis. Thus the four last metacarpals have a proximal pseudoepiphysis, while the first metacarpal has a distal pseudoepiphysis.

**pseudoerosion** \-irō′zhən\ Replacement of squamous epithelium by columnar epithelium at the cervical os, giving an appearance similar to a denuding inflammatory process.

**pseudoerysipelas** \-er′isip′ələs\ Apparent erysipelas with little or no fever or constitutional symptoms. It is often recurrent and is usually found in areas of impaired lymphatic drainage.

**pseudoesthesia** \-esthē′zhə\ PSEUDESTHESIA.

**pseudoexfoliation** \-eksfō′lē·ā′shən\ The deposition of any material on the surface of an organ or structure that makes it appear as if exfoliation has actually taken place.

**pseudoexophthalmos** \-ek′säfthal′məs\ [PSEUDO- + EXOPHTHALMOS] An apparent forward protrusion of the eye due to elongation of the globe (as in myopia) or shallowness of the orbital socket.

**pseudofolliculitis** \-fōlik′yəlī′tis\ [PSEUDO- + FOLLICULITIS] A papular eruption of the sides of the neck caused by the reentry into the skin of the tips of beard hairs that have been shaved.

**pseudofracture** \-frak′chər\ The radiographic manifestation of periosteal thickening and new bone formation that appears as an incomplete fracture related to an area of injury.

**pseudoganglion** \-gang′glē·än\ [PSEUDO- + GANGLION] An area of thickening in a nerve, resembling a ganglion. **Bochdalek's p.** PLEXUS DENTALIS SUPERIOR. **Cloquet p.** An enlargement of the palatine nerve within the anterior palatine canal. **Valentin p.** INTUMESCENTIA TYMPANICA.

**pseudogene** \soo′dəjēn\ A region of the eukaryotic genome that has molecular characteristics of a functional gene but is not transcribed and has no apparent phenotype. It lacks some of the ancillary structures necessary for transcription and translation, and may lack introns. Many may have arisen from processed mRNA by reverse transcription followed by integration into the genome. It may represent a vestigial gene sequence. **dispersed p.** Any pseudogene that occurs outside the gene cluster from which it arose. **processed p.** A pseudogene that lacks introns. It probably arises by reverse transcription of a processed mRNA and integration of the DNA transcript back in the genome.

**pseudogeusia** \-joo′sē·ə\ Dysgeusia in which recognized tastes are perceived in the absence of an appropriate stimulus or, sometimes, any stimulus. Also *pseudogeusesthesia, phantogeusia.*

**pseudoglioma** \-glī·ō′mə\ A condition in which the interior of the eye is filled with inflammatory or fibrovascular material, simulating a retinoblastoma.

**pseudoglobulin** \-gläb′yələn\ Any protein that is a globulin by the criterion that it is precipitated by half-saturation of its solution with ammonium sulfate, but is atypical of globulins in that it dissolves in water without addition of salt.

**pseudogout** \soo′dəgout\ **1** An acute arthritis occurring in older people and defined by the presence of calcium pyrophosphate dihydrate crystals within polymorphonuclear leukocytes in the joint fluid. **2** *Incorrect* CHONDROCALCINOSIS.

**pseudogynecomastia** \-gī′nəkōmas′tē·ə\ [PSEUDO- + GYNECOMASTIA] Excess of adipose tissue in the breasts of an obese male without increase in mammary glandular tissue.

***Pseudohaje*** [PSEUDO- + Arabic *ḥayya* snake] A genus of venomous snakes of the family Elapidae; the tree cobras.

**pseudohallucination** \-həloo′sinā′shən\ A hallucination that the subject recognizes as a false perception.

**pseudohelminth** \-hel′minth\ [PSEUDO- + HELMINTH] Any structure or organism resembling an intestinal worm. Also *pseudelminth.*

**pseudohemagglutination** \-hem′əgloo′tinā′shən\ The *in vitro* aggregation of adjacent erythrocytes in a fashion which resembles agglutination but differs from it in that pseudoagglutinates can be readily disaggregated. Pseudoagglutination can be caused by changes in the physicochemical properties of the milieu in which the cells are suspended as in rouleaux formation in patients with paraproteinemia. Also *pseudoagglutination.*

**pseudohematuria** \-hem′ətoo′rē·ə\ [PSEUDO- + HEMATURIA] A red coloration of urine that resembles blood but is caused by red pigments from foods such as beets or certain drugs.

**pseudohemiacardius** \-hem′ē·əkär′dē·əs\ [PSEUDO- + HEMIACARDIUS] A placental parasitic twin with no heart and usually lacking other thoracic structures. Also *pseudothorax, acephalus athorus.*

**pseudohemophilia** \-hē′məfil′yə\ [PSEUDO- + HEMOPHILIA] Any ill-defined bleeding tendency. The term originally excluded hemophilia and thrombocytopenia. *Obs.* **p. hepatica** A bleeding tendency associated with hepatic cirrhosis.

**pseudohemoptysis** \-hēmäp′tisis\ The expulsion of bloody material through the mouth from a source other than the lower respiratory tract.

**pseudoheredity** \-həred′itē\ The appearance of a phenotype among family members as a result of environmental rather than genetic factors.

**pseudohermaphrodite** \-hərmaf′rədīt\ [PSEUDO- + HERMAPHRODITE] An individual possessing gonadal tissue of one sex but whose genital ducts or external genitalia or both show one or more phenotypic characteristics of the opposite sex. **female p.** An intersexed individual with female gonads, or ovaries, but equivocal or extensively masculinized genital duct derivatives and external genitalia. The chromsomal constitution is usually of the female type. Also *androgynus, androgyne, gynandroid, female intersex.* **male p.** An individual with male gonads, or testes, but equivocal or extensively feminized genital duct derivatives and external genitalia. The chromosomal constitution is usually of the male type. Also *male intersex.*

**pseudohernia** \-hur′nē·ə\ A symptom complex resembling a strangulated hernia, but caused by inflammation of tissue within the scrotum.

**pseudohydrocephalus** \-hī′drəsef′ələs\ PSEUDOHYDROCEPHALY. **traumatic internal p.** TRAUMATIC PORENCEPHALY.

**pseudohydrocephaly** \-hī′drəsef′əlē\ The disproportionate enlargement of the cranium without concomitant enlargement of the ventricular system. Also *pseudohydrocephalus.*

**pseudohyperkalemia** \-hī′pərkəlē′mē·ə\ A spurious *in vitro* elevation of serum potassium concentration, resulting from release of potassium by platelets or blood cells after a blood sample is obtained.

**pseudohypertrichosis** \-hī′pərtrikō′sis\ [PSEUDO- + HYPERTRICHOSIS] Unusual persistence of the fine hair normally seen on an infant at birth.

**pseudohypertrophy** \-hīpur′trəfē\ An increase in the size of an organ or tissue without increase in the size of its intrinsic cells. Also *false hypertrophy.* Adj. pseudohypertrophic. **muscular p.** An appearance simulating true muscular hypertrophy but due to massive fatty infiltration, seen in certain muscles such as those of the calf in some forms of muscular dystrophy. Also *pseudomuscular hypertrophy.*

**pseudohypoaldosteronism** \-hī′pō·al′dästir′ənizm\ [PSEUDO- + HYPOALDOSTERONISM] Failure of the kidneys to respond to mineralocorticoids such as aldosterone, as in salt-losing nephropathy, giving rise to the same clinical picture as aldosterone deficiency, sodium wasting and hyperkalemia.

**pseudohyponatremia** \-hī′pōnətrē′mē·ə\ A less than normal concentration of sodium in plasma or serum as the result of increased concentration of lipids, proteins, or glucose. Hyperlipidemia may cause a volume displacement of all serum electrolytes. When there is hyperproteinemia or hyperglycemia, reduction in sodium concentration may be compensatory, to maintain normal osmolarity of plasma.

**pseudohypoparathyroidism** \-hī′pōper′əthī′roidizm\ A rare genetic disorder, inherited as an X-linked dominant trait, characterized by the biochemical abnormalities of true hypoparathyroidism, hypocalcemia, and hyperphosphatemia, but due to a failure of end-organ response to parathyroid hormone and not to deficient secretion. The clinical features are tetany, nonresponse to administered parathyroid hormone, short stature, round face, cataracts, mental retardation, short metacarpals, and ectopic calcifications.

**pseudohypothyroidism** \-hī′pōthī′roidizm\ A condition in which there is apparent failure of cellular metabolic response to thyroid hormone, not deficient secretion of the hormone. Some of the symptoms and signs of hypothyroidism are observed.

**pseudoicterus** \-ik′tərəs\ PSEUDOJAUNDICE.

**pseudoinfluenza** \-in′floo·en′zə\ Any influenzalike catarrhal illness that is distinct from the illness caused by influenza virus A or B.

**pseudointima** \-in′timə\ The inner, loosely adherent lining of a prosthetic vascular graft. It is composed of fibrin, platelets, red and white cells, and an ingrowth of fibroblasts.

**pseudoisochromatic** \-ī′sōkrōmat′ik\ [PSEUDO- + ISOCHROMATIC] Pertaining to a testing method for color blindness in which numbers or figures are formed with hues chosen so that they appear alike (isochromatic) to the color-blind individual, yet may be differentiated by the normal eye. As a result, the color-blind person cannot differentiate numbers or figures that appear obviously different to the normal person.

**pseudojaundice** \-jôn′dis\ Jaundicelike skin discoloration despite normal levels of bile pigments. It is seen with elevated serum carotene or lycopene and in chronic adrenal insufficiency. Also *pseudoicterus.*

**pseudokeratin** \-ker′ətin\ A keratin that is partially broken down by common proteolytic enzymes. Also *false keratin.*

**pseudoleukemia** \-lookē′mē·ə\ [PSEUDO- + LEUKEMIA] Any of a group of unrelated diseases having in common enlargement of the lymph nodes and/or spleen, but normal peripheral blood. *Obs.* Also *pseudoleukocythemia.*

**pseudolipoma** \-lipō′mə\ [PSEUDO- + LIPOMA] Edema of an extremity, superficially resembling a lipoma, due to a deliberate act of tying a ligature around the limb.

**pseudolithiasis** \-lithī′əsis\ A symptom complex resembling that of a calculus in an abdominal viscus.

**pseudolymphoma** \-limfō′mə\ A condition in which striking lymph node enlargement occurs, mimicking malignant lymphoma but not having the histologic or prognostic defining points of malignancy. Pseudolymphoma occurs in certain collagen diseases, such as the Sjögren syndrome and lupus erythematosus, and in some drug reactions such as that to diphenyl hydantoin.

**pseudomegacolon** \-meg′əkō′län\ A condition in which the colon is dilated to the extent that the x-ray image resembles a megacolon. The condition is sometimes due to excessive use of laxatives.

**pseudomelia** \-mē′lyə\ [PSEUDO- + MEL-[1] + -IA] PHANTOM LIMB. **p. paraesthetica** Pain and paresthesiae perceived as originating in a phantom limb.

**pseudomembrane** \-mem′brān\ A fragile, easily removable membranous structure that coats inflamed mucosal membranes. It is composed of sloughed necrotic epithelium, fibrin, bacteria, and leukocytes. It is typically seen in diphtheria and certain forms of enterocolitis. Also *false membrane, neomembrane.* Adj. pseudomembranous.

**pseudomeningitis** \-men′injī′tis\ [PSEUDO- + MENINGITIS] MENINGISM.

**pseudomenstruation** \-men′stroo·ā′shən\ [PSEUDO- + MENSTRUATION] A uterine discharge without the endometrial changes of menstruation, as that sometimes occurring in newborn babies.

**pseudomicrocephaly** \-mī′krəsef′əlē\ [PSEUDO- + MICROCEPHALY] A reduced total brain size owing to atrophy of one hemisphere, a condition not always of developmental origin.

**pseudomilium** \-mil′ē·əm\ COLLOID MILIUM.

**pseudomonad** \-mō′nad\ Any member of the genus *Pseudomonas.* • This term is sometimes used to include other nonfermenting aerobic Gram-negative rods.

**Pseudomonadaceae** \-mō′nədā′si·ē\ [*Pseudomona(s)* + -ACEAE] A family of Gram-negative, aerobic, nonfermentative, oxidase-positive rods with polar flagella.

***Pseudomonas*** \-mō′nas\ [PSEUDO- + Gk *monas* single; as substantive, a unit] The major genus of bacteria of the family Pseudomonadaceae. It comprises many species which grow on a wide variety of organic compounds and play a large role in their decomposition in nature. Most species metabolize sugars via the 2-keto-3-deoxygluconate pathway, and some accumulate poly-$\beta$-hydroxybutyrate as a reserve material. ***P. aeruginosa*** A common soil organism and a contaminant of solutions in hospitals. It is normally a minor human commensal, but is frequently dominant in opportunistic infections because of its resistance to most antibiotics. Its optimum growth occurs at a temperature of 37°C. It produces a diffusible bluish green phenazine pigment (pyocyanin) and a greenish yellow, fluorescent pteridine. Its exotoxin A inhibits protein synthesis by the same mechanism as diphtheria toxin. Also *Bacillus pyocyaneus* (obs.). ***P. cepacia*** A species widely distributed in soil and rotting plants and occasionally opportunistic in humans. Genetically it is related to *P. mallei.* ***P. fluorescens*** A species characterized by the production of a yellow fluorescent phenazine pigment. It can grow at 4°C and is hence a frequent agent of food spoilage and of contamination in hospital solutions. ***P. mallei*** A Gram-negative motile rod that causes glanders, a severe acute disease of horses and rarely of man. Also *Actinobacillus mallei* (outmoded), *Bacillus mallei* (outmoded). ***P. maltophilia*** The only oxidase-negative pseudomonad. It is an occasional opportunist. ***P. pseudomallei*** An organism, closely related to *P. mallei,* that causes melioidosis. Also *Actinobacillus pseudomallei, Malleomyces whitmori.*

**pseudomotivation** \-mō′tivā′shən\ After-the-fact rationalization for behavior, usually clearly inadequate to explain the action performed, as in the statement, "I jumped out the window to show the doctor that my room was dirty."

**pseudomotor** \-mō′tər\ Pertaining to abnormal movements.

**pseudomyasthenia** \-mī′asthē′nē·ə\ LAMBERT-EATON SYNDROME.

**pseudomycelium** \-mīsē′lē·əm\ A loosely united catenulate group of yeastlike cells formed by apical budding and resembling hyphae, especially when the cells are elongated.

**pseudomyiasis** \-mī·ī′əsis\ [PSEUDO- + MYIASIS] The presence of fly larvae in the digestive tract resulting from accidental ingestion. They may cause diarrhea or other symptoms if present in large numbers, but ordinarily they are temporary and nonpathogenic under these circumstances.

**pseudomyotonia** \-mī′ətō′nē·ə\ **1** The slow contraction and relaxation of voluntary muscle which occurs in hypothyroidism. **2** A phenomenon resembling myotonia seen in one form of myokymia. **3** In electromyography, a bizarre type of high-frequency discharges which may resemble those of myotonia but which begin and end abruptly and are seen in a number of inflammatory and metabolic disorders of muscle.

**pseudomyxoma** \-miksō′mə\ [PSEUDO- + MYXOMA] PSEUDOMYXOMA PERITONEI. **p. peritonei** The seeding of the peritoneum by mucin-secreting metastatic deposits and the filling of the peritoneal cavity by their secretion. Copious amounts of gelatinous material occupy the peritoneal cavity and may cause intestinal obstruction. This change results from metastatic spread of a mucinous cystadenocarcinoma of either ovarian or appendiceal origin. Also *pseudomyxoma.*

**pseudomyxovirus** \-mik′səvī′rəs\ Any of a group of viruses of the Paramyxoviridae family that includes the viruses of measles, canine distemper, and rinderpest.

**pseudoneoplasm** \-nē′əplazm\ A transient histological state which resembles a tumor but regresses to normal morphology.

**pseudoneuritis** \-n[y]urī′tis\ [PSEUDO- + NEURITIS] PSEUDOPAPILLEDEMA.

**pseudonucleolus** \-n[y]ooklē′ələs\ [PSEUDO- + NUCLEOLUS] KARYOSOME.

**pseudonystagmus** \-nistag′məs\ [PSEUDO- + NYSTAGMUS] Oscillatory movements of the eyes associated with fixation.

**pseudo-obstruction** \-əbstruk′shən\ A condition that clinically resembles that caused by an obstruction but is from some other cause. **idiopathic intestinal p.** A condition that appears to involve obstruction of the small bowel and colon, of unknown cause. Studies of bowel motility in these patients have indicated decreased incidence of contractions with abnormal bowel motility throughout. Also *chronic intestinal atony.*

**pseudo-ochronosis** \-ō′krənō′sis\ Dark tissue pigmentation resembling ochronosis but not due to the accumulation of homogentisic acid. Causes include chronic ingestion of Atabrine and, in the past, the application of carbolic acid dressings.

**pseudo-ovum** \-ō′vəm\ A large single nucleated cell that resembles an ovum yet is not capable of meiosis, found in granulosa-cell tumors of the ovary.

**pseudopapilledema** \-pap′ilēdē′mə\ [PSEUDO- + PAPILLEDEMA] A condition observed with the ophthalmoscope in which the optic disk appears elevated and/or hyperemic and its margins so blurred that the appearances resemble those of papilledema but the veins are not dilated. This may be seen in severe hypermetropia or it may be a developmental disorder due to the presence of hyaline bodies in the disk. Also *pseudoneuritis.*

**pseudoparalysis** \-pəral′isis\ [PSEUDO- + PARALYSIS] Impairment of movement resulting from sensory denervation of a part of the body, especially a limb, and due to loss of position and joint sense or from local pain (as in arthritis) without actual motor defect. Also *pseudoplegia, sensory paralysis* (inaccurate), *false paralysis.* **p. agitans** *Obs.* PARALYSIS AGITANS. **congenital atonic p.** MYATONIA CONGENITA. **generalized alcoholic p.** MARCHIAFAVA-BIGNAMI SYNDROME. **Parrot's p.** SYPHILITIC PSEUDOPARALYSIS. **syphilitic p.** Suppression of movement of one or more of an infant's extremities due to bony lesions of congenital syphilis. Also *Parrot's pseudoparalysis, Parrot's disease.*

**pseudoparasite** \-par′əsīt\ [PSEUDO- + PARASITE] **1** An organism, such as a commensal, that has a way of life that may be mistaken for parasitism. **2** An organism that is accidentally acquired, usually by ingestion, and may be mistaken for a parasite of the organism in which it is found. For defs. 1 and 2 also *false parasite, spurious parasite.*

**pseudoparkinsonism** \-pär′kinsənizm\ Any disorder, such as so-called atherosclerotic parkinsonism, or manganese intoxication, having clinical features resembling paralysis agitans.

**pseudopelade** \-pē′läd, -pəläd′\ [PSEUDO- + French *pelade* (from L *pilare* to remove hair) a falling off of skin, falling out of hair] A scarring, patchy alopecia that is not preceded by folliculitis. **p. of Brocq** A scalp disease of unknown origin that is characterized by the progressive development of well-defined small patches of chronic scarring alopecia. It may represent the end stage of more than one pathologic process, but there is no folliculitis at any stage that differentiates it from folliculitis decalvans.

**pseudophakia** \-fā′kē·ə\ [PSEUDO- + *phak(o)-* + -IA] A condition in which the normal substance of the lens of the eye has been replaced. **p. adiposa** Fatty degeneration of a cataract. **p. fibrosa** Connective tissue invasion of a cataract. Also *fibroid cataract.*

**pseudophlegmon** \-fleg′män\ [PSEUDO- + PHLEGMON] A condition that resembles cellulitis. **Hamilton p.** A circumscribed inflammatory swelling that does not suppurate.

**pseudophyllid** \-fil′id\ **1** Of or belonging to the order Pseudophyllidea. **2** A member of the order Pseudophyllidea. For defs. 1 and 2 also *pseudophyllidean.*

**Pseudophyllidea** \-filid′ē·ə\ An order of tapeworms having an aquatic life cycle and marked by a scolex with two opposing elongate slitlike sucking organs, or bothria. It includes the broad fish tapeworm parasitic in humans, *Diphyllobothrium latum.*

**pseudophyllidean** \-filid′ē·ən\ PSEUDOPHYLLID.

**pseudoplegia** \-plē′jə\ [PSEUDO- + *(para)plegia*] PSEUDOPARALYSIS.

**pseudopocket** \soo′dəpäkit\ [PSEUDO- + POCKET] GINGIVAL POCKET.

**pseudopod** \soo′dəpäd\ [PSEUDO- + -POD] PSEUDOPODIUM.

**pseudopodia** \-pō′dē·ə\ Plural of PSEUDOPODIUM.

**pseudopodium** \-pō′dē·əm\ [New L, from PSEUDO- + Gk *podion* a small foot] (*pl.* pseudopodia) A temporary protrusion of amebic cytoplasm used in locomotion and ingestion. Several types of pseudopodia have been described, differing in thickness and form. Also *pseudopod.* See also AXOPODIUM, FILOPODIUM, LOBOPODIUM, RHIZOPODIUM.

**pseudopolycythemia** \-päl′isīthē′mē·ə\ STRESS ERYTHROCYTOSIS.

**pseudopolymelia** \-päl′imē′lyə\ [PSEUDO- + POLYMELIA] A spontaneous, illusory somatic sensation often of movement or tingling, experienced in the fingers or toes or other peripheral parts of the body such as the ears, nose, and genitalia. **paresthetic p.** **1** Paresthesiae characterized by an impression of movement of various parts of the body. **2** An illusion that there are one or more extra limbs, as a phantom third arm or leg. *Seldom used.* Also *pseudopolymelia paraesthetica.*

**pseudopolyp** \-päl′ip\ An area of regenerating mucosa within a focus of inflammation, thus resembling a polypoid projection.

**pseudopolyposis** \-päl′ipō′sis\ A condition characterized by multiple pseudopolyps.

**pseudoporencephaly** \-pôr′ensef′əlē\ [PSEUDO- + PORENCEPHALY] Cyst formation of any cause in a cerebral hemisphere, not communicating with the lateral ventricle.

**pseudopregnancy** \-preg′nənsē\ [PSEUDO- + PREGNANCY] **1** PSEUDOCYESIS. **2** A condition of abnormal hormone secretion and endometrial histology resembling those of normal pregnancy. It may be experimentally induced by foreign bodies introduced *in utero,* stimulation of the uterine cervix, electroshock to the head, psychopharmacologic drugs, or copulation with sterile males. It is followed by prolactin secretion, persistence of the corpus luteum, and certain resemblances to human pseudocyesis. **3** The histologically observed premenstrual stage of the endometrium, resembling that seen just before implantation of a fertilized ovum.

**pseudopseudohypoparathyroidism** \soo′dəsoo′dəhī′pōpar′əthī′roidizm\ The incomplete or variant, and genetically related, form of pseudohypoparathyroidism, in which the constitutional features of the latter are present, but serum calcium and phosphate concentrations are normal.

**pseudoptosis** \soo′däptō′sis\ [PSEUDO- + PTOSIS] A lowered position of the upper eyelid due to orbicularis oculi contraction or mechanical restrictions upon movement. Also *false ptosis.*

**pseudoptyalism** \soo′dətī′əlizm\ The accumulation of saliva in the mouth or the dribbling of saliva, resulting from difficulty in swallowing rather than from excess secretion.

**pseudopuberty** \-pyoo′bərtē\ [PSEUDO- + PUBERTY] Development of secondary sexual characters at the expected time but without capacity to reproduce. It is a result of androgen or estrogen secretion in the absence of maturation of the hypothalamic-adenohypophysial-gonadal axis, hence without complete gametogenesis. An adrenocortical, ovarian, or testicular tumor secreting sex steroids may be the cause. **heterosexual p.** Pseudopuberty in which the prematurely developed secondary sexual characters are opposite to those expected on the basis of the genetic sex of the child. **isosexual p.** Pseudopuberty in which the prematurely developed secondary sexual characters are those expected on the basis of the genetic sex of the child. **precocious p.** Premature somatic growth and development of secondary sex characters in the absence of maturation of the hypothalamic-adenohypophysial-gonadal axis, without complete gametogenesis, and therefore without reproductive capacity. The condition follows untimely secretion of estrogen or androgen brought about in girls by adrenal or ovarian tumors and in boys by Leydig cell tumors. Pubescent development may be consonant with that expected on the basis of the genetic sex of the child (isosexual precocious pseudopuberty) or it may be opposite to that expected (heterosexual precocious pseudopuberty).

**pseudoreaction** \-rē·ak′shən\ A nonspecific positive reaction to a test, such as a skin test or laboratory test.

**pseudoreminiscence** \-rem′inis′əns\ PATHOLOGIC LYING.

**pseudoretinitis pigmentosa** \-ret′inī′tis\ Luetic chorioretinitis or other lesion simulating genetic retinitis pigmentosa.

**pseudorickets** \-rik′əts\ RENAL OSTEODYSTROPHY.

**pseudorosette** \-rōzet′\ A radial cluster of tumor cells, usually around a small blood vessel, seen in the histologic examination of various tumors such as ependymomas, some gliomas, and olfactory neurocytoma.

**pseudosarcoma** \-särkō′mə\ [PSEUDO- + SARCOMA] A lesion that resembles a sarcoma, especially a carcinoma with spindle-shaped cells or a lesion with a pleomorphic stroma.

**pseudoscarlatina** \-skär′lətē′nə\ An eruption that resembles the flush of scarlet fever but is not of streptococcal origin.

**pseudosclerema** \-sklirē′mə\ [*pseudo-* + SCLEREMA] *Obs.* SUBCUTANEOUS FAT NECROSIS.

**pseudoscleroderma** \-sklir′ədur′mə\ Any one of several cutaneous syndromes in which skin thickening superficially resembles scleroderma. Examples include frostbite, carcinoid syndrome, vinyl-chloride poisoning, lichen myxedematosus, and scleredema.

**pseudosclerosis** \-sklerō′sis\ [PSEUDO- + SCLEROSIS] Any of a group of degenerative disorders of the brain giving rise to progressive paralysis and rigidity and characterized pathologically by gliosis and diffuse degeneration of gray and white matter. *Outmoded.* **Jakob spastic p.** CREUTZFELDT-JAKOB DISEASE. **Neumayer's amyotrophic lateral p.** Chronic progressive myelopathy giving a clinical picture resembling that of amyotrophic lateral sclerosis, usually without sensory symptoms and signs, but resulting from chronic ischemia of the spinal cord due to atherosclerosis. *Seldom used.* Also *ischemic myelopathy.*

**pseudoscrotum** \-skrō′təm\ A thick partition that resembles a scrotum and covers the opening into the vagina in female pseudohermaphrodites.

**pseudosign** \soo′dəsīn\ **Babinski p.** Dorsiflexion of the great toe without movement of the other toes, elicited by stimulation of the outer aspect of the sole, but resulting from lower motor neuron paralysis of the plantar flexors, as in poliomyelitis, and not from an upper motor neuron lesion.

**pseudosenility** \-senil′itē\ [PSEUDO- + SENILITY] PSEUDODEMENTIA.

**pseudosmallpox** \-smôl′päks\ ALASTRIM.

**pseudostoma** \soodäs′təmə\ [PSEUDO- + Gk *stoma* mouth] A false opening between epithelial cells. It is caused artifactually by the shrinkage of tissues during section preparation.

**pseudostrabismus** \-strabiz′məs\ [PSEUDO- + STRABISMUS] The appearance of misalignment of the eyes caused by eyelid contours or corectopia.

**pseudostratified** \-strat′ifīd\ Appearing to be composed of more than one layer: said of certain columnar epithelia such as that of the respiratory tract, where the nuclei are located at different levels, giving the erroneous impression of multiple layers.

**pseudostructure** \-struk′chər\ RETICULAR SUBSTANCE.

**pseudotabes** \-tā′bēz\ [PSEUDO- + TABES] Any syndrome characterized by loss of pain sensation and of tendon reflexes in the lower limbs, with sensory ataxia, resembling tabes dorsalis but not due to neurosyphilis. Various forms of polyneuropathy can give this clinical picture, as in diabetic pseudotabes. Also *peripheral tabes.* **diabetic p.** Diabetic polyneuropathy in which the pupils fail to react to light and there is areflexia and sensory loss in the lower limbs. The clinical picture superficially resembles that of tabes dorsalis. Also *Leyden's ataxia, diabetic tabes.* **pupillotonic p.** ADIE SYNDROME.

**pseudotetanus** \-tet′ənəs\ [PSEUDO- + TETANUS] Trismus and muscular spasms resembling those of tetanus, but not due to a specific infection with *Clostridium tetani.*

**pseudothorax** \-thôr′aks\ PSEUDOHEMIACARDIUS.

**pseudotrachoma** \-trākō′mə\ Follicular conjunctivitis not due to *Chlamydia trachomatis.*

**pseudotrismus** \-triz′məs\ [PSEUDO- + TRISMUS] Difficulty in opening the mouth due to local lesions or the teeth, gums, or jaw and not resulting from spasm of the masseters.

**pseudotruncus arteriosus** \-trung′kəs\ A congenital cardiovascular defect in which there is atresia at the pulmonary valve associated with atrophy or conspicuous reduction of the proximal part of the pulmonary trunk. The pulmonary arteries are supplied from the aorta by retrograde flow through the ductus arteriosus, or else through another source of systemic supply such as major aortopulmonary collateral arteries.

**pseudotubercle** \-t$^y$oo′bərkl\ A granulomatous lesion resembling that of tuberculosis but not caused by *Mycobacterium tuberculosis.* Also *pseudotuberculoma.*

**pseudotuberculoma** \-t$^y$ubur′kyəlō′mə\ PSEUDOTUBERCLE. **silicotic p.** A pseudotuberculous lesion that is a manifestation of sarcoidosis.

**pseudotubule** \-t$^y$oo′byool\ A space, lined by hypertrophied epithelial cells of the glomerular capsule, that forms between adhesions found in the Bowman space.

**pseudotumor** \-t$^y$oo′mər\ [PSEUDO- + TUMOR] TUMOR-LIKE LESION. **p. cerebri** BENIGN INTRACRANIAL HYPERTENSION. **orbital p.** An increase of orbital volume due to a low-grade inflammatory reaction, involving especially the external ocular muscles and other orbital contents. The process is probably autoimmune and related to orbital myositis.

**pseudotympanites** \-tim′pənī′tēz\ FALSE TYMPANITES.

**pseudouridine** 5-Ribosyluracil, a nucleoside analogue found in tRNA. It is produced from uridylic acid residues by transfer of the ribosyl group from N-1 of uracil to C-5, in a reaction that occurs at specific loci.

**pseudouridylate** The anion derived from pseudouridylic acid, or salts containing this anion.

**pseudouridylic acid** A phosphoric ester, usually the 5′-phosphate, of pseudouridine.

**pseudovacuole** \-vak′yoo-ōl\ An intracytoplasmic structure resembling a vacuole, resulting from artifact or an intracellular organism.

**pseudoventricle** \-ven′trikl\ CAVUM SEPTI PELLUCIDI.

**pseudovermicule** \-vur′mikyool\ OOKINETE.

**pseudovermiculus** \-vərmik′yələs\ [PSEUDO- + L *vermiculus,* dim. of *vermis* a worm or grub] OOKINETE.

**pseudovertigo** \-vur′tigō, -vərti′gō\ [PSEUDO- + VERTIGO] Subjective feelings of faintness or dizziness, resulting from postnatal hypotension, anxiety, or a variety of metabolic disorders, but without any true sense of movement of the self or of the surroundings. These symptoms are often misconstrued as being due to vertigo.

**pseudovillus** \-vil′əs\ (*pl.* pseudovilli) A slender projection from the surface of a glomerular epithelial cell that faces the glomerular capsular space. Pseudovilli occur in cases of heavy proteinuria. Some may be true microvilli, but most are probably thin cytoplasmic bridges.

**pseudovirion** \-vir′ē·än\ [PSEUDO- + VIRION] A virus which contains cellular DNA rather than viral DNA.

**pseudovitamin $B_{12}$** A naturally occurring analogue of cobalamin in which adenine replaces dimethylbenzimidazole as one of the ligands to the cobalt atom.

**pseudovoice** \soo′dəvois\ The sound emanating from the esophagus and pharynx in the laryngectomy patient, replacing the vocal sound no longer producible.

**pseudovomiting** \-väm′iting\ Regurgitation of gastric contents without muscular effort.

**pseudoxanthoma elasticum** \-zanthō′mə ilas′tikəm\

A rare, inherited connective-tissue disorder characterized by degeneration of elastic tissue, resulting in yellowish maculopapular skin lesions and accentuation of normal skin creases. It may involve other tissues, such as the retina, heart, intestinal tract, or blood vessels, and bleeding complications are relatively common. Also *Darier's disease, Grönblad-Strandberg syndrome.*

**psilocin** \sī′ləsin\ 3-[2-(Dimethylamino)ethyl] indol-4-ol. A tryptamine compound from the fungus, *Psilocybe mexicana,* which is reported to cause hallucinogenic conditions when ingested.

**psilocybin** \sī′ləsī′bin\ A phosphorylated tryptamine compound produced by fungi of the genus *Psilocybe,* and especially from *P. mexicana.* This compound and psilocin are reputed to cause psychotropic or hallucinogenic conditions following ingestion of the mushroom fruiting bodies.

**psilosis** \sīlō′sis\ *Obs.* TROPICAL SPRUE. **p. pigmentosa** PELLAGRA.

**psittacosis** \sit′əkō′sis\ [L *psittac(us)* (from Gk *psittakos* parrot) parrot + -OSIS] An acute infectious disease caused by *Chlamydia* species and transmitted to man by psittacine birds that have not been domestically bred, such as parrots, parakeets, and cockatoos, or by other fowl such as pigeons, ducks, turkeys, and chickens. Illness may be severe, with pneumonitis, fever, pharyngitis, headache, nausea and vomiting, and hepatosplenomegaly. The mortality rate with chemotherapy is 5%. Also *parrot fever, ornithosis, parrot disease.*

**psoas** \sō′əs\ [New L (from Gk *psoa* loin; usu. in pl. *psyoai* loins, muscles of the loins] Musculus psoas major or musculus psoas minor.

**psophogenic** \sō′fəjen′ik\ [Gk *psopho(s)* an inarticulate sound + -GENIC] Triggered by intermittent loud sounds, as *psophogenic epilepsy.*

**psoralen** \sôr′ələn\ $C_{11}H_6O_3$. A coumarin occurring in many species of vascular plants. The presence of psoralen in the skin, whether it is applied locally or given systemically, enhances the pigmentary response of the skin to ultraviolet light. This property is made use of in the PUVA (psoralen, ultraviolet A) regime, which is valuable in many cases of psoriasis and some other inflammatory disorders. It is used also for vitiligo, but the response is uncertain and the long-term treatment is hazardous. Also *furocoumarin.*

**psorenteritis** \sôr′enterī′tis\ [Gk *psōra* scab, mange + ENTERITIS] An intestinal disorder seen especially in cholera, in which the villous pattern of the mucosa is lost.

**psoriasiform** \sor′ē·as′ifôrm\ Resembling psoriasis.

**psoriasis** \sôrī′əsis\ [Gk *psōriasis* (from *psōra* a cutaneous disease, the itch, scab, mange, akin to *psēn* to touch on the surface, rub, crumble + -IASIS) a skin disease] A common inflammatory skin disease of which the characteristic lesion is a well-demarcated plaque, usually dull red or dark salmon pink in color and covered with silvery scales. There are, however, many variations and atypical forms. Any part and any proportion of the skin surface may be affected. Rarely, a specific form of arthritis occurs as a complication of psoriasis. The course of the disease in unpredictable but it tends to be chronic and recurrent. The cause is unknown, but a genetic predisposition is apparent. Also *alphos* (obs.), *lepra* (obs.), *lepra alphos.* **p. annularis** PSORIASIS CIRCINATA. **arthropathic p.** PSORIATIC ARTHRITIS. **p. arthropathica** PSORIATIC ARTHRITIS. **p. buccalis** Leukoplakia of the buccal mucosa. *Obs.* **p. circinata** Psoriasis characterized by ringlike lesions with centers that are unaffected by the disease. Also *psoriasis annularis, psoriasis orbicularis, Willan's lepra.* **p. diffusa** Psoriasis affecting most or all of the body surface. **p. discoidea** Psoriasis in which the lesions are solid plaques that are rounded in outline. **erythrodermic p.** Generalized erythroderma and scaling that occurs as a manifestation of psoriasis. Also *exfoliative psoriasis.* **p. figurata** Psoriasis in which the lesions form distinct patterns. **flexural p.** Psoriasis affecting the body folds, especially the groin, natal cleft, axillae, and submammary areas. Also *inverse psoriasis.* **p. follicularis** Psoriasis in which the lesions are predominantly small and affect the skin around the orifices of sweat or pilosebaceous ducts. **p. geographica** Psoriasis in which the outline of the lesions suggests the demarcation of a coastline on a map. *Seldom used.* **guttate p.** Psoriasis in the form of small, round lesions that are widely distributed over the body. **p. gyrata** Psoriasis in which the lesions have the form of a series of arcs that have joined together, as may arise from the fusion of circinate lesions. **inverse p.** FLEXURAL PSORIASIS. **p. inveterata** Psoriasis in which the lesions are relatively resistant to treatment. They are often covered with a rough-surfaced, thick, hard, hyperkeratotic scale. **napkin p.** **1** A psoriasiform eruption affecting the diapered area in infants. It is often associated with secondary psoriasiform lesions elsewhere, and the secondary eruption alone is sometimes regarded as an adequate basis for the diagnosis, irrespective of the appearance of the diapered area. Napkin psoriasis is probably induced by external factors in a genetically predisposed infant. It is distinct from seborrheic dermatitis of the diapered area, although some cases show features of both conditions. **2** *Imprecise* DIAPER DERMATITIS. **p. orbicularis** PSORIASIS CIRCINATA. **p. ostracea** Rupioid psoriasis in which the mass of scale and crust is larger and less conical than that of typical rupioid psoriasis and has a concave inner surface. **provoked p.** Psoriasis that occurs as an isomorphic effect. **p. punctata** Psoriasis in which the lesions are small, often scaly papules. **pustular p.** Psoriasis in which the lesions contain sterile pustules that are visible to the unaided eye. It includes pustule formation within a psoriatic plaque, as is often induced by irritant medicaments, and an acute generalized pustular eruption with a systemic illness. Acral pustulosis is believed by some also to be a form of pustular psoriasis. Also *herpes pyaemicus, impetigo herpetiformis.* **rupioid p.** Psoriasis in which the lesions, found most frequently on the soles, bear conical masses composed of scale and dried exudate. The sides of the cones may be marked by concentric rings. **seborrheic p.** An eruption with clinical and histologic features of both psoriasis and seborrheic dermatitis. **ungual p.** Psoriasis of the nails. **p. universalis** Psoriasis affecting most or all of the body surface. **unstable p.** An unpredictable psoriasis in which localized pustular or ill-defined erythematous lesions appear. The condition may progress to generalized pustular psoriasis or to erythrodermic psoriasis. **volar p.** Psoriasis of the palms or soles.

**psorophthalmia** \sôr′äfthal′mē·ə\ [Gk *psōr(a)* a cutaneous disease, itch, scab, mange + OPHTHALM- + -IA] BLEPHARITIS ULCEROSA.

**psorospermosis** \sôr′ōspərmō′sis\ KERATOSIS FOLLICULARIS.

**PSRO** professional standards review organization.

**psych-** \sīk-\ PSYCHO-.

**psychanopsia** \sī′kənäp′sē·ə\ HYSTERICAL BLINDNESS.

**psychasthenia** \sī′kasthē′nē·ə\ Any of the neuroses that are not categorized as hysteria, including phobic disorders and, to a lesser extent, anxiety disorders. Also *Janet's disease.*

**psyche** [Gk *psychē* soul, spirit, mind] The mind in contradistinction to the body.

**psycheclampsia** \sīʹkiklamʹpsē·ə\ *Obs.* MANIA.

**psychedelic** \sīʹkədelʹik\ [PSYCHE + Gk *dēl(oun)* (from *dēlos* manifest) to make visible or clear + -IC] Producing an abnormal change in perception or state of consciousness: used especially of hallucinogenic agents.

**psychergograph** \sīkurʹgəgraf\ An instrument for recording responses to mental stimulation.

**psychiatric** \sīʹkē·atʹrik\ Relating to the medical specialty of psychiatry or the disorders with which it deals.

**psychiatrist** \sīkīʹətrist\ A physician with special training in the field of psychiatry. Also *psychopathist* (obs.).

**psychiatry** \sīkīʹətrē\ [PSYCH- + IATR- + -Y ] Treatment of mental and emotional disorders and behavioral dysfunctions. Also *medicopsychology, psychological medicine.* **community p.** The branch of psychiatry concerned with provision of needed psychiatric services to a specified population, with an emphasis on the environmental factors contributing to the incidence and treatment of the psychosocial disorders within that population. **comparative p.** ETHNOPSYCHIATRY. **cross-cultural p.** ETHNOPSYCHIATRY. **cultural p.** The branch of psychiatry concerned with the environmental and ecological factors within a specified group or society that contribute to the incidence, form, treatment, and prevention of biopsychosocial disorders within that society. **descriptive p.** Any system of psychiatry emphasizing the phenomenological observation and study of objective signs and symptoms of mental disorder as a way to differentiate between such disorders and devise the appropriate and special approaches required by each. Compare DYNAMIC PSYCHIATRY. **dynamic p.** Any system of psychiatry emphasizing the internal, unconscious forces or drives that give rise to the symptoms and signs of mental disorder. Such a system operates on the assumption that understanding how the disorders develop will provide the most rational approach to their treatment and prevention. Compare DESCRIPTIVE PSYCHIATRY. **existential p.** Existential analysis with emphasis on the search for the meaning of human existence. Also *phenomenological psychiatry.* **experimental p.** A branch of psychiatry focusing on the use of chemical agents and the study of biochemical interactions as a means of understanding how mental disorders develop and what treatments are best suited for the control or abolition of the symptoms they produce. **forensic p.** The branch of psychiatry concerned with the relationship between psychiatry and the law, especially the particular and often unique role of psychiatry in dealing with people whose illnesses manifest themselves in behaviors that have a direct, often adverse, effect on society. **geriatric p.** PSYCHOGERIATRICS. **industrial p.** The branch of psychiatry concerned with mental and emotional disorders occurring in the work situation, the factors of the occupational environment affecting workers' emotional and mental health, and factors promoting optimal relationships between employers and employees. Also *occupational psychiatry.* **phenomenological p.** EXISTENTIAL PSYCHIATRY. **political p.** A branch of psychiatry involving the application of psychiatric principles or data to the procedures of government and in particular to the determination of public policy affecting the mentally ill. Also *psychopolitics.* **social p.** The body of knowledge and theory upon which the methods of community psychiatry are based. It emphasizes the psychosocial nature of mental disorder and the need to include existing social structures and systems as a significant factor in effective treatment of the identified patient. **transcultural p.** That branch of psychiatry which is concerned with the effects that different cultures have on the mental health of their members and in particular the role of culture in predisposing a member to one or another kind of mental disorder.

**psychic** 1 Of or pertaining to the psyche or mind. 2 Psychologic or psychogenic rather than physical or somatic.

**psychlampsia** \sīklampʹsē·ə\ [PSYCH- + Gk *lamps(is)* a shining + -IA] *Obs.* MANIA.

**psycho-** \sīʹkə-, sīʹkō-\ [Gk *psychē* soul, spirit, mind] A combining form meaning mind, mental, psyche, psychic. Also *psych-*.

**psychoacoustics** \-əkoo͞ʹstiks\ The scientific investigation of the way in which animals, including man, hear, particularly the reception and analysis of the input signal. It is the study of the relationship between the physical characteristics of sound and its biologic processing.

**psychoactivator** A drug that produces stimulation; psychic energizer.

**psychoactive** Exerting effects on the mind or on behavior, as certain drugs.

**psychoanaleptic** \-ənəlepʹtik\ Producing a stimulating or restorative effect on mental function.

**psychoanalysis** \-ənalʹisis\ [PSYCHO- + ANALYSIS] 1 A procedure devised by Sigmund Freud for investigating mental processes. 2 A form of treatment applicable to certain kinds of mental and emotional disorder. It is based upon Freud's psychology and uses his procedure for investigating mental processes as its fundamental technique. Also *dynamic psychotherapy, psychoanalytic psychotherapy, psychoanalytic therapy.* **adlerian p.** ADLERIAN PSYCHOLOGY. **classic p.** Psychoanalysis as originally developed by Freud, with minimal if any deviation from psychoanalytic theory or psychoanalytic technique. Also *orthodox analysis.* **jungian p.** JUNGIAN PSYCHOLOGY.

**psychoanalyst** \-anʹəlist\ One who uses the methods of psychoanalysis, or one who espouses the theories of psychoanalytic psychology, or both. Usually, the psychoanalyst has had specific training in and met the curriculum, practice, and supervisory criteria of a recognized training center for psychoanalysis before he or she can assume the title of psychoanalyst.

**psychoanalytic** \-anʹəlitʹik\ Referring to or characterized by the use of psychoanalysis.

**psychoauditory** \-ôʹditôrʹē\ Relating to the conscious perception of the attributes and qualities of the sound heard.

**psychobiology** \-bī·älʹəjē\ 1 The study of psychology from a biologic point of view, emphasizing the adaptive or functional aspects of behavior that enable the organism to meet survival challenges posed by the environment. 2 An approach to the study of behavior and treatment for behavioral disorders that stresses the functional utility of psychologic processes in the adaptation of the organism to its environment. Also *Meyer system, Meyer's theory.*

**psychocatharsis** \-kəthärʹsis\ *Outmoded* CATHARSIS.

**psychodiagnosis** \-dīʹagnōʹsis\ [PSYCHO- + DIAGNOSIS] The evaluation of the personality of an individual by a systematic appraisal made of spontaneously expressed and specially elicited reactions, most often undertaken for the purpose of assessing any serious unbalance in the personality or to predict possible future reactions to severe stress or threat to the organization of the personality.

**psychodiagnostics** \-dīʹagnäsʹtiks\ [PSYCHO- + DIAGNOSTICS] A term used especially by Swiss and German writers for RORSCHACH TEST. Adj. psychodiagnostic.

**Psychodidae** \sīkädʹidē\ A family of small flies of the suborder Nematocera. It contains the genera *Phlebotomus, Lutzomyia,* and *Psychodopygus,* which include the species that are vectors of leishmaniasis.

**psychodrama** \-dram′ə\ [PSYCHO- + *drama*] A form of group psychotherapy in which personality structure and emotional conflicts are explored through dramatization. The subject acts out his problems with the help of trained auxiliary egos under the guidance of a director or therapist.

**psychodynamics** \-dīnam′iks\ The description of the development and workings of the mind, with emphasis on how the mind's hypothesized energies are distributed in the course of its adaptational maneuvers. **adaptational p.** A system of psychoanalytic psychology in which behavior disorders are viewed as disturbances of psychodynamic integration that interfere with the organism's adaptability to the social environment and its attainment of utility and pleasure.

**psychoepilepsy** \-ep′ilep′sē\ *Obs.* IDIOPATHIC EPILEPSY.

**psychogalvanic** \-galvan′ik\ Referring to changes in the electrical resistance of the skin that result from either sensory or ideational stimulation.

**psychogalvanometer** \-gal′vənäm′ətər\ Any electrical circuit designed to measure the psychogalvanic response. The readings of the degree of change in skin resistance, that is, changes in sweat gland secretion, detected by a sensitive galvanometer may be made directly and visually, or a permanent registration of the psychogalvanic response can be made by means of an ink trace or photographic recording.

**psychogender** \-jen′dər\ Psychological sexual identification; the subjectively perceived sexual identity which may or may not conform with the somatic sex of the person.

**psychogenic** \-jen′ik\ [PSYCHO- + -GENIC] Of psychological or mental origin. Also *psychogenous.* Compare SOMATOGENIC.

**psychogeriatric** \-jer′ē·at′rik\ Pertaining to mental illness in old age, commonly denoting a patient or a hospital.

**psychogeriatrician** \-jer′ē·ətrish′ən\ A psychiatrist who specializes in the treatment of emotional problems and mental disorders of the elderly.

**psychogeriatrics** \-jer′ē·at′riks\ The branch of psychiatry concerned with the changes in mental functioning associated with old age, and with mental disorders occurring in persons over the age of 65. Also *geriatric psychiatry, geropsychiatry.*

**psychohistory** The application of psychological theory, particularly psychoanalytic psychology, to history so as to understand the human forces at work in the production of past events.

**psychoinfantalism** \-infan′tilizm\ The retention of childlike mental or character traits into adulthood.

**psychokinesis** \-kīnē′sis\ The alleged induction of movement in discrete physical objects by thought processes.

**psycholeptic** \-lep′tik\ [PSYCHO- + Gk *lēptikos* (from *lambanein* to take, seize) tending to take on, accept] **1** Characterizing psychotropic agents such as minor tranquilizers, antidepressants, and hallucinogens, whose effect is primarily on mental functions rather than on psychomotor activity. **2** A psycholeptic agent.

**psycholinguistics** \-ling·gwis′tiks\ The study of the psychological aspects of language, how it is acquired, generated, and understood, and of the relationship between language and the characteristics of the individual language user, or of the language-using group.

**psychological** \-läj′ikəl\ Of or relating to psychology.

**psychologist** \sīkäl′əjist\ A person professionally trained and qualified in psychology.

**psychology** \sīkäl′əjē\ [PSYCHO- + -LOGY] The science based on the study of the behavior and mental processes of human beings, often focusing on behaviors observable among animals as a strategy for gaining an improved understanding of the processes that underlie human behavior. Contemporary psychology seeks to describe, understand, predict, and often to change the behavior of living organisms, with a particular emphasis on human behavior in its origins, development, and expression during the lifetime of the individual. Also *ergasiology, psychics* (seldom used). **abnormal p.** The branch of psychology devoted to the investigation of abnormal or unusual behaviors or mental states, with a particular interest in the insight this may offer about behaviors and mental processes falling within a more usual range. It includes the phenomena of psychopathology, mental deficiencies, and specially altered states, such as those of hypnosis, sleep deprivation, and extreme stress. Also *heteropsychology.* **adlerian p.** The theory of human personality development and behavior that emphasizes the individual as a single, coherent, and intelligible unity, whose strivings are typically related to a need to compensate for some kind of physical, psychological, or social inferiority. Also *individual psychology, adlerian psychoanalysis, Adler's theory.* **analytic p.** JUNGIAN PSYCHOLOGY. **applied p.** A utilization of the facts, methods, principles, or theories of psychology primarily for practical ends in industry, education, engineering, forensics, etc. **behavioristic p.** BEHAVIORISM. **clinical p.** That branch of psychology devoted to the study, assessment, treatment, or prevention of the disorders of behavior, maladaptive behaviors, or those problems in living that are experienced as persisting sources of psychological discomfort, pain, or anguish. Preparation for engaging in this subfield of activity includes special training in actual practice, as well as didactic instruction, and exposure to or participation in relevant programs of research. **cognitive p.** A branch of psychology that investigates cognitive processes, such as attending, perceiving, thinking, problem-solving, and remembering, which are hypothesized to play a dynamic role in human behavior by the way in which they intervene between a stimulus from the external world and a response made by the organism. **comparative p.** A branch of psychology that adopts the strategy of comparing the behavior of differing animal species as a way of discerning the principles common to behavior in general. It is also used for identifying the emergent qualities of behavior that are roughly concurrent with increasing complexity of structure. **counseling p.** A branch of applied psychology focusing on guidance for those with personal problems of a nonmedical nature, such as marital, family, social, educational, or vocational problems. **developmental p.** A branch of psychology that emphasizes those changes in behavior which can be observed to be a function of the age and growth or development of the individual, with stress on the relationship between early experience and biologic maturation. **experimental p.** The investigation of psychological phenomena, mental processes, or behavioral regularities by means of controlled experimentation. One or more independent variables is manipulated, while controlling all other related background variables as much as possible, and the effects of the manipulation on one or more dependent variables are observed. **gestalt p.** A systemic position in psychology which resists reductionism as a valid approach to an understanding of either conscious experience or behavior. Wholeness and organization are held to be features of experiential and behavioral phenomena from the start, which are not thought to be analyzable, meaningfully, by partition into more elementary units. The brain itself is held to operate in terms of integrated patterning, the cortex acting primarily as a field of force, influenced by stimuli from the environment impinging on an already ongoing field of biopsychologic activity. Also *gestaltism, gestalt* *theory.* **humanistic p.** A movement within contemporary psychology, derived from the existential and phenomenological philosophies, placing central emphasis on a holistic approach to the understanding of human behavior and mental life. The uniqueness of each individual is stressed, and free choice and spontaneity are encouraged, as is psychological growth toward maximal fulfillment of the potential of each individual. **individual p.** ADLERIAN PSYCHOLOGY. **industrial p.** A subdivision of applied psychology which attempts to find the solution to human problems arising in industrial settings. This includes worker selection or training procedures, the design of machines or conditions of work to maximize comfort and productivity, questions relating to communication with employees, morale, and rewards for work. **infant p.** The study and the interpretation of infant behavior at birth and in the first few weeks of life and the interaction of mother and baby. **Janet's p.** A forerunner of freudian psychoanalysis that recognized unconscious mental forces as significant factors in the production of dissociative states, hysteria, etc. **jungian p.** Carl Jung's system of psychology, which emphasizes that the mind is not only the result of past experience but is also a preparation for the future. A mystical and religious element in the unconscious is stressed, as well as a joining of personal experience with the collective unconscious, a distillate of fundamental ideas and trends of all mankind that may appear as archetypes which control the subject's way of perceiving reality. Also *jungian psychoanalysis, analytic psychology.* **social p.** The branch of psychology which studies the behavior of the individual as influenced by the presence of others, especially the ways in which interaction and interdependence among members of a group, or the interactions between social groups, may affect the behavior of individuals. It does not focus on the group as an entity, which is the subject matter of sociology.

**psychometrics** \-met′riks\ [PSYCHO- + Gk *metr(on)* a measure, standard + -ICS] That branch of psychology centering on the study of mental measurement, making use of psychological tests designed to reflect differences among individuals on one or more of the several dimensions of mental ability, such as intelligence, aptitudes, interests, manual abilities, special abilities, or disabilities. It includes the devising or standardization of tests and the development or application of statistical techniques particularly appropriate for the analysis of mental test data. Also *psychometry* (rare).

**psychometry** \sīkäm′ətrē\ *Rare* PSYCHOMETRICS.

**psychomotor** \-mō′tər\ [PSYCHO- + MOTOR] Denoting a combination of mental and motor events, including the production of voluntary movement and seizures giving rise to sensory auras.

**psychoneurosis** \-n$^{y}$Urō′sis\ [PSYCHO- + NEUROSIS] NEUROSIS. **compulsive-obsessive p.** OBSESSIVE-COMPULSIVE NEUROSIS. **defense p.** NEUROSIS.

**psychonomics** \-näm′iks\ The study of the relationship of the mind to the individual's internal and external environment. Also *psychonomy.*

**psychopath** \sī′kəpath\ [PSYCHO- + -PATH] A person who manifests characteristics of the antisocial personality. Also *anethopath, sociopath.* **sexual p.** **1** A person whose manifestations of an antisocial personality are predominantly in the sexual area. **2** Anyone whose sexual behavior deviates from what the culture or the observer accepts as being normal. *Incorrect.*

**psychopathia** \-path′ē·ə\ [PSYCHOPATH + -IA] PSYCHOPATHY. **p. sexualis** Sexual perversion.

**psychopathist** \sīkäp′əthist\ *Obs.* PSYCHIATRIST.

**psychopathology** \-pəthäl′əjē\ [PSYCHO- + PATHOLOGY] The study of the essential nature of mental disorder including its causes, its effects on mental structure and function, and the ways in which it manifests itself. Also *pathematology* (obs.).

**psychopathy** \sīkäp′əthē\ [PSYCHO- + -PATHY] Any mental disorder. *Imprecise.* Also *psychopathia, sociopathy.*

**psychopharmacology** \-fär′məkäl′əjē\ The study of drugs that affect mental and behavioral activity, such as psycholeptic agents.

**psychophysics** \-fiz′iks\ The branch of psychology that investigates the quantitative functional relationships between stimulus magnitudes and the sensory processes or conscious experiences they invoke.

**psychophysiology** \-fiz′ē·äl′əjē\ [PSYCHO- + PHYSIOLOGY] The study of the relationship between mental and physiologic mechanisms.

**psychopneumatology** \-n$^{y}$oo′mətäl′əjē\ *Obs.* PSYCHOSOMATIC MEDICINE.

**psychopolitics** \-päl′itiks\ POLITICAL PSYCHIATRY.

**psychoprophylaxis** \-prō′filak′sis\ A natural childbirth technique in which psychological preparation is used to condition the patient and diminish perception of pain.

**psychoses** \sīkō′sēz\ Plural of PSYCHOSIS.

**psychosexual** \-sek′shoo·əl\ [PSYCHO- + SEXUAL] Relating to the mental and emotional factors of sexuality, as distinguished from the purely physical or somatic manifestations.

**psychosexuality** \-sek′shoo·al′itē\ The mental aspects of sexual life in infantile development as well as in adulthood.

**psychosine** Any of the 1-monoglycosylsphingoids, such as glucosylsphingosine.

**psychosis** \sīkō′sis\ [PSYCH- + -OSIS] A class of mental disorders that usually includes organic mental disorders, the schizophrenias, major affect disorders, and certain paranoid states. In general, a psychosis is more severe and extensive than other forms of mental disturbance such as neurosis or character disorder. In DSM-III, psychosis indicates the presence of one or more of the following: hallucinations, delusions, grossly disorganized or catatonic behavior, and severe disturbances of thinking such as incoherence, repeated derailment or loosening of associations, poverty of thought, or markedly illogical speech. Adj. psychotic. **affective p.** A psychosis typified primarily by disturbances of mood, such as the manic-depressive psychosis. Also *affective insanity* (obs.). **alcoholic p.** Any organic mental disorder due to alcohol consumption, such as Wernicke-Korsakoff psychosis, alcoholic dementia, delirium tremens, or alcoholic hallucinosis. Also *alcoholic insanity* (outmoded). **alcoholic polyneuritic p.** WERNICKE-KORSAKOFF PSYCHOSIS. **alternating p.** MANIC-DEPRESSIVE PSYCHOSIS. **p. of association** SHARED DELUSION. **atypical p.** In DSM-III, any syndrome of psychotic symptoms that does not meet the criteria for specific mental disorder. Included are schizophreniclike or affectivelike psychotic episodes whose duration is too brief to warrant a specific diagnosis, such as monosymptomatic delusional states without other impairment in functioning. **bipolar affective p.** MANIC-DEPRESSIVE PSYCHOSIS. **bromide p.** BROMOMANIA. **buffoonery p.** A disorder characterized by hyperkinesis, facial grimacing, exaggerated gestures and postures, and clownish, foolish behavior that at times seems almost feigned. It is uncertain whether it is a catatonic excitement state or a flight into disease similar to the Ganser syndrome. Also *faxen-psychosis, buffoonery syndrome.* **chronic epileptic p.** Chronic hallucinatory paranoid psychosis occurring in epileptic patients, particularly in those with temporal lobe epilepsy. It is said to be characterized by delusions and hallucinations related especially to religious or mystic themes, and to occur more commonly in patients in whom the attacks diminish either spontaneously or as a result of therapy. The fact that psychotic symptoms may be especially common in temporal lobe epilepsy, inversely related to the severity and frequency of the attacks and seen independently of any associated brain damage, suggests that the psychotic symptoms may be epileptic in nature. On the other hand, many organic, physiological, psychological, and sociological facts may play a part in the genesis of such psychoses. **circular p.** MANIC-DEPRESSIVE PSYCHOSIS. **climacteric p.** INVOLUTIONAL MELANCHOLIA. **depressive p.** Major depression characterized by severe dejection and loss of self-esteem, difficulty in thinking, psychomotor retardation or agitation, weight loss, sleep disturbance, loss of sexual desire, brooding about death or suicide, and, in many cases, gross impairment in reality testing with hallucinations and delusions. Also *psychotic depressive reaction.* **functional p.** Any severe mental disorder for which no structural or organic basis has yet been demonstrated. At the present time, schizophrenia, manic-depressive psychosis and other major affective disorders, paranoia, and certain paranoid states are generally considered to be functional psychoses. **housewife's p.** HOUSEWIFE'S NEUROSIS. **hysterical p.** A post-traumatic stress disorder marked by hallucinations, delusions, depersonalization, and bizarre behavior. Such a disorder tends to remit spontaneously within three weeks. Culture-specific disorders such as amok, imu, lata, myriachit, and piblokto are categorized as hysterical psychoses. Also *hysteropsychosis.* **induced p.** SHARED DELUSION. **involutional p.** INVOLUTIONAL MELANCHOLIA. **Korsakoff p.** An organic disorder of the nervous system usually occurring in alcoholics and characterized by severe impairment of memory with a specific inability to record and retain new impressions and by confabulation. Also *Korsakoff syndrome, Korsakoff's disease, amnestic syndrome, amnestic-confabulatory syndrome, alcohol amnestic disorder, alcoholic dementia.* See also WERNICKE-KORSAKOFF PSYCHOSIS. **manic-depressive p.** An affective disorder consisting of acute, periodic, self-limited mood swings, with a tendency to recur. Onset is usually between the ages of 20 and 40, and characteristically there is relatively complete remission during the intervals between episodes. The episodes themselves are of manic or depressive nature, or show a mixture of both manic and depressive features at the same time. Also *alternating psychosis, bipolar affective psychosis, circular psychosis, manic-depressive disorder, periodic psychosis, erethisophrenia, manic-depressive insanity* (obs.), *cyclothymia* (imprecise), *periodic insanity* (obs.), *recurrent insanity* (obs.), *intermittent insanity* (obs.), *cyclophrenia* (obs.). **organic p.** ORGANIC BRAIN SYNDROME. **paranoiac p.** PARANOIA. **paranoid p.** PARANOIA. **periodic p.** MANIC-DEPRESSIVE PSYCHOSIS. **polyneuritic p.** WERNICKE-KORSAKOFF PSYCHOSIS. **p. polyneuritica** WERNICKE-KORSAKOFF PSYCHOSIS. **postpartum p.** Any psychosis associated with the puerperium. Also *puerperal insanity, puerperal psychosis.* **prison p.** 1 Mental disturbances precipitated by the threat of or imposition of imprisonment. 2 Any syndrome in which a conscious or partly conscious desire to escape prison leads to imitating psychosis, as in the Ganser syndrome. **puerperal p.** POSTPARTUM PSYCHOSIS. **reactive p.** Mental disorder precipitated by a clear-cut stressor or environmental factor. Such psychoses often remit spontaneously and typically are not associated with heavy genetic loading. Also *situational psychosis.* **reactive depressive p.** REACTIVE DEPRESSION. **schizoaffective p.** 1 In DSM-III, a psychotic disorder that does not fall clearly into either the affective or the schizophrenic and schizophreniform disorders. 2 In other classifications, a subtype of schizophrenia in which the predominant symptoms are those of mania or melancholia. For defs. 1 and 2 also *schizoaffective schizophrenia.* **schizophrenic p.** SCHIZOPHRENIA. **schizophreniform p.** 1 In DSM-III, a disorder that meets all the criteria for being classified as schizophrenia except that it does not last the six months required for a diagnosis of schizophrenia to be established. 2 In other classifications, such a disorder having a favorable outcome (remission) and little genetic evidence of any major relationship to schizophrenia. Also *parergasia* (obs.), *atypical schizophrenia* (imprecise). **senile p.** 1 Any psychosis appearing during the senium. 2 SENILE DEMENTIA. **situational p.** REACTIVE PSYCHOSIS. **symbiogenic p.** SYMBIOTIC PSYCHOSIS. **symbiotic p.** A pervasive developmental disorder manifested by some children at the time when they would ordinarily be able to separate from the mother. It is characterized by fantasies of omnipotence, introjection, projection, delusions, and hallucinations. Also *symbiogenic psychosis.* **tardive p.** TARDIVE DYSMENTIA. **unipolar p.** UNIPOLAR DEPRESSION. **Wernicke-Korsakoff p.** An organic disorder of the nervous system usually occurring in alcoholics, but sometimes seen in other conditions, leading to malnutrition and resulting from thiamin deficiency. It consists of Wernicke's disease (Wernicke's encephalopathy) in association with Korsakoff's psychosis. While Wernicke's disease and Korsakoff's psychosis can occur independently, it is commoner for them to occur together, and sensorimotor polyneuropathy is usually present as well. Also *Wernicke-Korsakoff syndrome, polyneuritic psychosis, alcoholic polyneuritic psychosis, psychosis polyneuritica.* **windigo p.** A culture-specific syndrome of some Canadian Indian tribes, consisting of delusions of being transformed into a windigo, a cannibalistic monster. In addition, the subject suffers from agitation, depression, and fears of inability to control sadistic impulses.

**psychosocial** Denoting the interrelationship between a person and his or her environment, in particular the psychologic and interpersonal aspects of the individual's relationship to the group.

**psychosomatic** \-sōmat′ik\ [PSYCHO- + SOMATIC] Referring to the relationship between mind and body and in particular the psychologic and emotional contributors to physical disorders such as peptic ulcer, asthma, hypertension, or migraine. Also *somatopsychic.* See also PSYCHOSOMATIC DISORDER.

**psychosurgery** \-sur′jərē\ Brain surgery for the purpose of modifying emotions or behavior, especially in the treatment of psychosis, in the absence of demonstrable organic brain disease, most commonly by means of interruption of nerve fibers connecting the frontal and limbic systems.

**psychosyndrome** \-sin′drōm\ A constellation of psychological or behavioral symptoms as they relate to the organic dysfunction of the brain. The major organic psychosyndromes are delirium, dementia, Wernicke-Korsakoff psychosis, hallucinosis, and withdrawal syndrome. **focal brain p.** Organic brain syndrome due to focal lesion of the brain. In addition to the usual symptoms of organic origin its manifestations include symptoms suggesting the location of the lesion, such as the witzelsucht resulting from frontal lobe syndromes.

**psychosynthesis** \-sin′thəsis\ The combining of individual elements of the mind into a whole, seen in jungian psychology as the constructive approach to understanding the unconscious in terms of preparing for things to come, in contrast to the reductive approach of psychoanalysis, which concerns itself almost exclusively with how the past has determined the present status of mental development.

**psychotherapeutics** \-ther′əpyoo′tiks\ PSYCHOTHERAPY.

**psychotherapist** \-ther′əpist\ One professionally trained in psychotherapy, as a psychiatrist, clinical psychologist, or counselor.

**psychotherapy** \-ther′əpē\ [PSYCHO- + THERAPY] Any form of treatment for mental disorders or emotional disturbances in which a suitably trained person establishes a professional relationship with an identified patient for the purpose of removing or modifying symptoms of the disorder, or of promoting character growth and development so as to strengthen the patient's ability to cope with the problems of living. The relationship established between patient and therapist is used to influence the patient to unlearn old, maladaptive patterns and to learn and test new approaches. Psychotherapy includes guidance, counseling, psychoanalysis, behavior therapy, conditioning, hypnotherapy, and all other forms of treatment in which the major technique employed is communication, rather than drugs or other somatic agents. Also *mental therapeutics, suggestive therapeutics, mind cure* (popular), *mental healing, psychotherapeutics, teleotherapeutics.* **brief p.** Directive psychotherapy that is typically limited to a maximum of 20 sessions and focuses on immediate crises and ways of dealing with current problems. **contractual p.** A form of brief psychotherapy in which the goals and aims of treatment, and often also the specific role that the patient and therapist will play in treatment, are explicitly agreed upon in advance. Progress is measured according to how close the treatment process has in fact achieved the goals set forth in the agreement or contract. **directive p.** A form of psychotherapy in which the therapist takes an active advisory role and suggests, persuades, or exhorts the patient to take certain approaches, adopt certain attitudes, or work toward certain goals. Also *suggestive psychotherapy, active therapy.* **dynamic p.** PSYCHOANALYSIS. **family p.** Treatment of the family as a unit rather than treatment of any single member. Focus is on relationships within the family and the influence of its style of functioning on the adjustment of individual members. Also *family therapy.* **group p.** Treatment of two or more patients at the same time by the same psychotherapist or copsychotherapists. The group is generally limited to eight to twenty patients, and the particular techniques employed are as varied as those used in individual psychotherapy. Also *group therapy, multiple therapy* (seldom used). **hypnotic p.** HYPNOTHERAPY. **psychoanalytic p.** PSYCHOANALYSIS. **suggestive p.** DIRECTIVE PSYCHOTHERAPY. **supportive p.** Any form of therapy that emphasizes development of the patient's assets by strengthening existing defenses and restoring an adaptive equilibrium, rather than trying to trace the development of those defense mechanisms and then reconstructing different methods of adaptation. **transactional p.** A form of psychotherapy used for both individuals and groups that focuses on which ego state currently dominates the patient (parent, child, or adult). Interactions are interpreted as competitive play to seek particular kinds of gratification or payoffs, and attention is directed to childhood decisions that determined such a pattern of behavior.

**psychotic** \sīkät′ik\ [PSYCH- + -OTIC[1]] **1** Characterized by symptoms of psychosis. **2** A psychotic person.

**psychotogen** \sīkät′əjən\ HALLUCINOGEN.

**psychotogenic** \sīkät′əjen′ik\ HALLUCINOGENIC.

**psychotomimetic** \sīkät′ōmimet′ik\ **1** HALLUCINOGEN. **2** HALLUCINOGENIC.

**psychotropic** \-träp′ik\ [PSYCHO- + -TROPIC[1]] Denoting any substance that affects psychic function or behavior, as *psychotropic drug.*

**psychro-** \sī′krō-\ [Gk *psychros* cold, chill] A combining form meaning cold.

**psychroesthesia** \-esthē′zhə\ [PSYCHRO- + ESTHESIA] A sense of coldness in a part of the body which nevertheless feels warm to the touch.

**psychrometer** \sīkräm′ətər\ [PSYCHRO- + -METER] HYGROMETER.

**psyllium** \sil′ē·əm\ The dried, ripe seeds of the herbs *Plantago psyllium, P. arenaria,* or *P. ovata.* The seeds contain mucilage which provides bulk and lubrication useful in treating constipation. Also *plantago seed, psyllum seed, plantaginis semen.* **p. hydrophilic mucilloid** A white or cream-colored, nearly odorless, granular powder composed of the mucilagenous portion of psyllium seeds. It is used in the treatment of chronic constipation, and is usually diluted with dextrose to improve its dispersion in liquids.

**Pt** Symbol for the element, platinum.

**pt** point.

**PTA** plasma thromboplastin antecedent (factor XI).

**PTAH** phosphotungstic acid–hematoxylin. See under STAIN.

**ptarmic** \tär′mik\ [Gk *ptarmikos* (from *ptarmos* sneezing) causing sneezing] **1** Causing sneezing; sternutatory. **2** A substance that causes sneezing; a sternutatory.

**PTC** **1** plasma thromboplastin component (factor IX). **2** phenothiocarbazine

**pter-** \ter-, tər-\ PTERO-.

**pteridine** \ter′idin\ The substance related to naphthalene by replacement of the CH groups at positions 1, 3, 5, and 8 with nitrogen atoms. It thus consists of fused pyrimidine and pyrazine rings. The term is usually used generically of substituted pteridines, which were first found in butterfly wing pigments. The biologically most important pteridines are folic acid derivatives and biopterin, and the pteridine ring is a constituent of the ring system of flavins.

**pterin** \ter′in\ 2-Amino-4-hydroxypteridine and its tautomers. Most biologically occurring pteridines are substitution products of pterin.

**pterin deaminase** The enzyme (EC 3.5.4.11) that catalyzes the hydrolysis of pterin to yield 2,4-dihydroxypteridine and ammonia.

**pterion** \tir′ē·än\ [PTER- + Gk *-ion,* diminishing suffix] (*pl.* pteria) A craniometric point situated at the midpoint of the sphenoparietal suture in the temporal fossa.

**ptero-** \ter′ō-\ [Gk *pteron* feather, in plural *ptera* feathers, wings] A combining form meaning (1) wing, winglike; (2) feather.

**pteroic acid** A component of the folic acid molecule, consisting of 2-amino-4-hydroxy-6-methylpteridine, with a *p*-aminobenzoic acid residue substituting one of the hydrogen atoms of the methyl group.

**pteroyl** A group present in folic acid, consisting of a *p*-aminobenzoyl group alkylated on its nitrogen atom by a methylene group which connects it to C-6 of pterin. In folic acid this group acylates the nitrogen of the first glutamic residue.

**pteroylglutamic acid** The simplest of the folic acids, containing a residue of pteroic acid joined in a peptide linkage to only one residue of glutamic acid.

**pterygium** \tərij′ē·əm\ [L, from Gk *pterygion* (dim. of

*pteryx* a wing) a flap, fold, pterygium] **1** A vascular tissue mass encroaching upon the superficial cornea from either side within the interpalpebral space. It arises from preexisting elastic tissue (pinguecula) in the conjunctiva in response to irritation by ultraviolet light or dryness. Also *web-eye.* **2** Any abnormal web or fold, as of skin. **p. colli** A congenital anomaly in which a web of skin, often bearing hair, extends bilaterally from the area of the mastoid process to the area of the acromial process. It is often seen in conjunction with the Turner syndrome. Also *congenital webbing of the neck.* **p. unguis** A fusion of the dorsal nail fold and the nail bed, with partial nail loss.

**pterygo-** \ter′igō-\ [Gk *pteryx* (genitive *pterygos*) a wing, anything like a wing] A combining form meaning (1) winglike, pterygoid; (2) the pterygoid process.

**pterygoid** \ter′igoid\ [Gk *pterygoeidēs* (from *pteryx,* gen. *pterygo(s)* a wing + *-eidēs* -OID) winglike] **1** Shaped like or suggestive of a wing: applied especially to the pterygoid processes of the sphenoid bone. **2** Relating directly or indirectly to the pterygoid process.

**pterygomandibular** \-mandib′yələr\ Pertaining to the pterygoid process and the mandible.

**pterygomaxillary** \-mak′siler′ē\ Pertaining to the pterygoid process and the maxilla.

**PTF** plasma thromboplastin factor.

**PTH** **1** parathyroid hormone (parathyrin). **2** parathormone (parathyrin).

**pthiriasis** \thīrī′əsis\ [See PHTHIRIASIS.] Infestation with the pubic louse, *Pthirus pubis.* Also *pthiriasis pubis, pediculosis pubis, pediculosis inguinalis.* Also *phthiriasis.* Adj. pthiriasic. **p. pubis** PTHIRIASIS.

***Pthirius*** \thī′rē·əs\ *PTHIRUS.*

***Pthirus*** \thī′rəs\ [New L, from Gk *phtheir,* gen. *phtheiros* a louse] A genus of sucking lice. Also *Pthirius, Phthirus.* • Although the etymologically correct spelling is *Phthirus,* the official name of the genus is spelled without the first *h.* ***P. pubis*** The pubic or crab louse of humans. It infests the coarse hair of the pubic region and occasionally is found on body hair of hirsute males, in axillary hair, or, rarely, in the eyebrows or eyelashes of newborn infants, who presumably acquire it from the mother at birth. Most infestations are thought to result from spread by sexual contact. Also *Pediculus pubis* (former name).

**ptomaine** \tō′mān\ [Italian *ptomaina,* from Gk *ptōma* a corpse, fallen body (from *piptein* to fall) + *-ina* -INE] Either of the naturally occurring diamines, putrescine or cadaverine, produced in decaying protein by bacterial decarboxylation of ornithine and lysine. They were once thought to be toxic, so that food poisoning due to bacterial toxins was formerly called ptomaine poisoning.

**ptomatropine** \tōmat′rəpin\ One of the ptomaines formed by the action of bacteria in the decarboxylation of amino acids.

**ptomatropism** \tōmat′rəpizm\ [*ptomatrop(ine)* + -ISM] Poisoning due to ptomatropine. The symptoms, which are similar to those of atropine poisoning, are rapid pulse, dilated pupils, and dryness of mouth. If the poisoning is severe, the subject may be restless, excited, disoriented, and even delirious.

**ptosed** \tōzd\ Marked by ptosis; drooping.

**ptosis** \tō′sis\ [Gk *ptōsis* a falling, fall] **1** The prolapse or downward displacement of an organ. **2** Abnormal downward displacement of the upper lid, as may result from paralysis of the third cranial nerve, sympathetic denervation, or injury. Also *lid drop.* Adj. ptotic. **false p.** PSEUDOPTOSIS. **traumatic p.** Drooping of an organ or part due to injury.

**-ptosis** \-tō′sis\ [Gk *ptōsis* a fall, a falling] A combining form denoting the downward movement or sinking of an organ or part.

**ptotic** \tät′ik\ Affected by or pertaining to ptosis.

**PTT** partial thromboplastin time.

**ptyal-** \tī′əl-\ PTYALO-.

**ptyalectasis** \tī′əlek′təsis\ [PTYAL- + ECTASIS] SIALECTASIS.

**ptyalism** \tī′əlizm\ [Gk *ptyalismos* (from *ptyalizein* to salivate) salivation] Excessive salivation due to any of a number of causes, such as neurologic disease, toxic causes, or lesions of the buccal cavity. Also *sialism, hypersalivation, ptyalorrhea, sialorrhea, sialosis.* **mercurial p.** Salivation due to mercury poisoning.

**ptyalo-** \tī′əlō-\ [Gk *ptyalon* saliva] A combining form denoting saliva. Also *ptyal-.*

**ptyalography** \tī′əläg′rəfē\ SIALOGRAPHY.

**ptyalolithiasis** \-lithī′əsis\ SIALOLITHIASIS.

**ptyalolithotomy** \-lithät′əmē\ SIALOLITHOTOMY.

**ptyalorrhea** \tī′əlôrē′ə\ PTYALISM.

**ptyocrinous** \tī·äk′rinəs\ Of or relating to secretion of a glandular product in the form of globules or granules rather than as a homogeneous fluid. Compare DIACRINOUS.

**Pu** Symbol for the element, plutonium.

**pubarche** \pyoobär′kē\ [L *pub(es)* puberty, pubic hair + Gk *archē* a beginning] The beginning of growth of downy pubic hair.

**puberal** \pyoo′bərəl\ PUBERTAL.

**puberphonia** \pyoo′bərfō′nē·ə\ [L *puber* arrived at adulthood + PHON- + -IA] The failure in a man to develop a normal deep voice after puberty.

**pubertal** \pyoo′bərtəl\ Pertaining to puberty or the age of puberty. Also *puberal.*

**puberty** \pyoo′bərtē\ [L *puber(tas)* (from *pubes,* also *puber* pertaining to puberty, grown up + *-tas* English *-ty*) the age or signs of maturity] The period during which secondary sexual characters develop and reproductive capacity is achieved, and during which in higher primates and humans menstruation in the female begins. In boys, the age accepted as normal for the onset of puberty is from 10 to 16, in girls from 9 to 15 years. Adj. pubertal, puberal. **delayed p.** Lack of pubertal development by the age of 15 in boys, 14 in girls. The cause may be constitutional or pathologic. Also *delayed adolescence.* **precocious p.** Development of reproductive capacity occurring in girls before the age of 8 and in boys before 10, with maturation of hormonal secretions, gametogenesis, cyclicity in females, and secondary sexual characteristics. Also *sexual precocity, true sexual precocity, true precocious puberty.*

**puberulic acid** $C_8H_6O_6$. 3,4,6-Trihydroxy-5-oxo-1,3,6-cycloheptatriene-1-carboxylic acid. An antibiotic substance produced by *Penicillium puberulum* and other *Penicillium* species.

**pubes** \pyoo′bēz\ [L, pubic hair, pubic region] **1** [NA] The hair that grows in the pubic region of the human adult; pubic hair. **2** REGIO PUBICA.

**pubescence** \pyoobes′əns\ The condition of being pubescent; being covered with short soft hairs, downy.

**pubescent** \pyoobes′ənt\ [L *pubescens,* gen. *pubescentis,* pres. part. of *pubescere* to arrive at the age of puberty] **1** Being of the age characterized by the beginning of puberty. **2** Being partly or wholly covered with epidermal down, lanugo, or fine short hairs.

**pubic** \pyoo′bik\ [*pub(es)* + -IC] Pertaining to the os pubis or the region of the pubes.

**pubis** \pyoo′bis\ [L, gen. of *pubes*: (bone) of the pubes] OS PUBIS.

**Public Health Service** A governmental agency which has responsibility for a variety of health care service obligations, including the direct provision of care in some instances, and for taking steps, within the limits imposed by statute or regulation, to safeguard, maintain, and improve the health of the population.

**pubocavernosus** \pyoo′bōkav′ərnō′səs\ COMPRESSOR VENAE DORSALIS.

**pubococcygeus** \pyoo′bōkäksij′ē·əs\ MUSCULUS PUBOCOCCYGEUS.

**puboperitonealis** \pyoo′bōper′itō′nē·ā′lis\ A variant of the transversus abdominis muscle in which some muscle bundles extend from the pubic crest to the transversus abdominis in the region of the umbilicus.

**pubotransversalis** \pyoo′bōtrans′vərsā′lis\ A variant of the transversus abdominis muscle in which muscle bundles extend from the superior pubic ramus to the transversalis fascia near the deep inguinal ring.

**pubovesicalis** \pyoo′bōves′ikā′lis\ A slender band of longitudinal muscle fibers of the external stratum of the urinary bladder that lies under the medial part of the puboprostatic ligament and merges with the retropubic connective tissue.

**pudenda** \pyooden′də\ Plural of PUDENDUM.

**pudendagra** \pyoo′dendag′rə\ [*pudend(a)* + -AGRA] Pain in the genitals, particularly female genitals.

**pudendum** \pyooden′dəm\ [neut. sing. gerundive of L *pudere* to be ashamed] (*pl.* pudenda) The external genitalia, especially those of the female; pudendum femininum. Adj. pudendal. **p. femininum** [NA] The female external genital organs including mons pubis, labium majus pudendi, labium minus pudendi, vestibulum vaginae, bulbus vestibuli, ostium vaginae, glandulae vestibulares minores, and glandula vestibularis major. Also *vulva, pudendum muliebre* (outmoded), *female pudendum, cunnus.* **p. muliebre** *Outmoded* PUDENDUM FEMININUM.

**Pudenz** [Robert H. *Pudenz,* U.S. neurosurgeon, born 1911] Pudenz-Heyer valve. See under VALVE.

**Pudlak** [P. *Pudlak,* Czech internist, flourished 20th century] Hermansky-Pudlak syndrome. See under SYNDROME.

**puericulture** \pyoo′ərikul′chər, pyoo·er′i-\ [L *puer* a child, boy + *i* + English *culture*] The art of bringing up children.

**puerperium** \pyoo′ərpir′ē·əm\ [L, (from *puer* a child, boy + *parere* to give birth) childbirth] POSTPARTUM PERIOD. Adj. puerperal.

**puff** 1 The sound of expelled air or breath, especially as heard on auscultation. 2 CHROMOSOME PUFF. **chromosome p.** An enlarged region along a polytene chromosome, the site of active transcription. Also *puff.*

**puffer** Any of the marine fishes of the family Tetraodontidae, members of which have inflatable bodies that are naked with scattered prickles. Some puffers produce the potent neurotoxin tetrodotoxin, which is present in high concentrations in the viscera and gonads at spawning. The fish has often been implicated in cases of food poisoning. Also *globefish, fugu* (Japanese). **pink p.** A patient with dyspnea due to chronic congestive pulmonary disease but with adequate oxygenation. An informal term. Compare BLUE BLOATER.

**puits de Devergie** \pʏ·ē′ də dev′ərzhē′\ In severe cases of eczema, the minute depressions on the surface of the eroded epidermis that release exudate.

***Pulex*** \pyoo′leks\ [L, a flea] A genus of fleas of the family Pulicidae. It has broad host distribution that includes humans and domestic animals, especially swine. ***P. cheopis*** *XENOPSYLLA CHEOPIS.* ***P. dugesi*** *PULEX IRRITANS.* ***P. fasciatus*** *NOSOPSYLLUS FASCIATUS.* ***P. irritans*** The common flea that is ectoparasitic on humans and many other animals, especially swine. The species is capable of transmitting the plague bacillus in experimental infections, but it is not a significant host in nature. Also *Pulex dugesi.* ***P. penetrans*** *TUNGA PENETRANS.*

**Pulfrich** [Carl *Pulfrich,* German physicist, 1858–1927] See under PENDULUM.

**pulicicide** \pyoolis′isīd\ PULICIDE.

**Pulicidae** \pyoolis′idē\ [L *pulex,* gen. *pulicis,* flea + -IDAE] A family of fleas (order Siphonaptera) including a number of significant pests of humans and domestic and wild mammals and birds, as well as vectors of plague pathogens, some suspected vectors of murine typhus in humans, and hosts for various helminth parasites.

**pulicide** \pyoo′lisīd\ [L *pulex,* gen. *pulicis,* a flea + -CIDE] Any agent that kills fleas. Also *pulicicide.*

**pulicosis** \pyoo′likō′sis\ [L *pulex,* gen. *pulicis,* a flea + -OSIS] Infestation by the human flea, *Pulex.*

**pull** 1 To strain a muscle. 2 The injury sustained when a muscle strain occurs.

**pulley** TROCHLEA MUSCULARIS.

**pulmo** \pul′mō\ [L (akin to Gk *pneumōn*) lung] (*pl.* pulmones) [NA] One of a pair of highly elastic cone-shaped organs of respiration occupying the thoracic cavity, where each is surrounded by a pleural sac and separated from the other by the heart and other contents of the mediastinum; the lung. Each lung has an apex extending into the base of the neck, and a base resting on the diaphragm, while on the mediastinal surface of each the hilus contains the blood vessels, lymphatics, and bronchi entering and leaving the lung. The left lung has two lobes, superior and inferior, separated by an oblique fissure, while the right lung has three lobes, superior, middle, and inferior, separated by oblique and horizontal fissures. They are further subdivided into bronchopulmonary segments, each of which is supplied by a segmental bronchus. In the terminal subdivisions of the segmental bronchi an exchange of gases takes place with the circulatory system. **p. dexter** [NA] The right lung. **p. sinister** [NA] The left lung.

**pulmo-** \pul′mō-\ PULMONO-.

**pulmoaortic** \pul′mō·ā·ôr′tik\ Relating to the lungs and the aorta, or to the pulmonary artery or valve and the aorta or aortic valve.

**pulmolith** \pul′məlith\ PNEUMOLITH.

**pulmometer** \pulmäm′ətər\ SPIROMETER.

**pulmometry** \pulmäm′ətrē\ SPIROMETRY.

**pulmon-** \pul′mən-\ PULMONO-.

**pulmonary** \pul′məner′ē\ [L *pulmo* (gen. *pulmonis*) lung + -ARY] Pertaining to the lungs. Also *pulmonic, pulmonal.*

**pulmonate** \pul′mənāt\ Possessing lungs or lunglike organs for breathing air.

**pulmonectomy** \-nek′təmē\ PNEUMONECTOMY.

**pulmonic** \pulmän′ik\ PULMONARY.

**pulmonitis** \-nī′tis\ PNEUMONITIS.

**pulmono-** \pul′mənō-\ [L *pulmo* (genitive *pulmonis*; akin to Gk *pneumōn,* Attic Gk *pleumōn,* from Gk *pnein* to breathe, and to L *flare* to blow, breathe) lung] A combining form meaning lung, pulmonary. Also *pulmo-, pulmon-.*

**pulmonologist** \-näl′əjist\ A physician specializing in disorders of the lungs.

**pulmonology** \-näl′əjē\ [PULMONO- + -LOGY] The science or study of the lungs.

**pulp** [L *pulpa.* See PULPA.] 1 A soft, fleshy inner part of a plant or animal such as that within a tooth, the spleen, or a fruit. Also *pulpa.* 2 Pulverized animal or vegetable matter. **coronal p.** That part of the pulp of a tooth which is contained within the crown. **dental p.** The connective tissue contained within the pulp cavity of a tooth. Also *dental nucleus, tooth pulp, pulpa dentis, endodontium.* **devitalized p.** NONVITAL PULP. **digital p.** The soft-tissue volar surface of the terminal phalanx. **enamel p.** *Outmoded* STELLATE RETICULUM. **hair p.** MEDULLA OF HAIR SHAFT. **nonvital p.** A dental pulp that has suffered complete gangrene or loss of blood supply. Also *dead pulp, devitalized pulp.* **radicular p.** That part of the pulp of a tooth which is contained within the root. **red p.** SPLENIC RED PULP. **splenic red p.** A substance that comprises the greatest part of the spleen. It consists of innumerable vascular sinusoids and a loose intervening interstitium through which blood slowly filters. Also *pulpa lienis, splenic pulp, red pulp, red substance of spleen.* **tooth p.** DENTAL PULP. **vertebral p.** NUCLEUS PULPOSUS DISCI INTERVERTEBRALIS. **vital p.** A dental pulp which is normal or, if diseased, responds to pulp tests. **white p.** Diffuse and nodular lymphatic tissue ensheathing the arteries within the interstices of the reticulum of the spleen.

**pulpa** \pul′pə\ [L, the lean part of meat, flesh of fruit, pith of stem] PULP. **p. dentis** DENTAL PULP. **p. lienis** SPLENIC RED PULP.

**pulpal** \pul′pəl\ Pertaining to the pulp, especially that of a tooth.

**pulpectomy** \pulpek′təmē\ [PULP + -ECTOMY] PULP REMOVAL. **partial p.** PULPOTOMY.

**pulpiform** \pul′pifôrm\ Having the shape of a dental pulp.

**pulpitis** \pulpī′tis\ [PULP + -ITIS] Inflammation of the dental pulp. It is the most common cause of dental pain. **acute closed p.** Acute inflammation of the dental pulp where there is not enough exposure to allow escape of the exudate. There may be localized inflammation only, giving rise to a pulp abscess, which is accompanied by chronic inflammation in the adjacent part of the pulp. More commonly, the inflammation is generalized and leads to early necrosis of the pulp. There is severe stabbing pain and hypersensitivity to heat and cold, but no sensitivity to pressure on the tooth. This is the most common type of pulpitis and is the usual cause of toothache. The pain stops when necrosis of the pulp eventually occurs. **acute open p.** Acute inflammation of a dental pulp where there is a wide enough exposure to allow escape of the exudate into the mouth. The subsequent effects are similar to those of acute closed pulpitis but the pain is not as severe. **chronic closed p.** Chronic inflammation of a closed dental pulp, as a result of infection by a relatively nonvirulent organism. The usual histologic features of chronic inflammation are seen. There is intermittent pain or no symptoms. The inflammation may be localized, with pulp abscess formation, but gradually the whole pulp is destroyed. **chronic open p.** Pulpitis which is the sequel to acute open pulpitis, if that does not end in necrosis. It takes two forms, chronic open ulcerative pulpitis and chronic open hyperplastic pulpitis. **chronic open hyperplastic p.** Chronic open pulpitis in which there is an outgrowth of granulation tissue through the exposure. This growth, called a tooth polyp, grows into the carious cavity and becomes covered with epithelium. It is painless. Also *hyperplastic pulpitis.* **hyperplastic p.** CHRONIC OPEN HYPERPLASTIC PULPITIS.

**pulpless** \pulp′lis\ Being without a pulp: said of a nonvital tooth.

**pulpotomy** \pulpät′əmē\ [PULP + *o* + -TOMY] The surgical removal of all or part of the coronal pulp of a tooth, leaving the radicular pulp. Also *partial pulpectomy, pulp amputation.*

**pulsate** \pul′sāt\ [See PULSATION.] To expand and contract rhythmically: commonly applied to blood vessels and the heart.

**pulsatile** \pul′sətil\ Characterized by pulsation.

**pulsation** \pulsā′shən\ [L *pulsatio* (from *pulsare* to strike or beat repeatedly, iterative of *pellere* to hit, push) a knocking, hammering] A rhythmic expansion and contraction, as of the pulse or the heart. **expansile p.** Pulsation of an area or a vessel which can be seen or felt to increase in size with each pulse. **suprasternal p.** A visible or palpable pulsation in the suprasternal notch.

**pulsator** \pul′sātər\ Any of various devices that produce or induce pulsatile movement, such as an apparatus to maintain artificial respiration.

**pulse** [L *pulsus* (from *pulsus,* past part. of *pellere* to beat, strike, push) a beat, stroke, beating, throbbing] **1** The rhythmical expansion of a blood vessel, especially an artery. Also *pulsus, sphygmus.* **2** A propagating disturbance (sound, light, pressure, electric current, etc.) whose duration is small compared to any characteristic response time of the system on which it impinges. **abdominal p.** The pulse of the abdominal aorta. Also *pulsus abdominalis.* **abrupt p.** A rapidly rising pulse. **allorhythmic p.** IRREGULAR PULSE. **alternating p.** PULSUS ALTERNANS. **anacrotic p.** ANADICROTIC PULSE. **anadicrotic p.** A pulse with a double upstroke, characterized by a prominent notch on the ascending limb of the pulse tracing. It is characteristic of aortic stenosis. Also *anacrotic pulse.* **arachnoid p.** THREADY PULSE. **atrial venous p.** The venous a wave, especially prominent in tricuspid stenosis. Also *atriovenous pulse.* **atriovenous p.** ATRIAL VENOUS PULSE. **biferious p.** PULSUS BISFERIENS. **bigeminal p.** A pulse characterized by beats that recur regularly in pairs. It usually consists of a premature ventricular beat following each beat of sinuatrial origin. Also *coupled pulse, digitalate pulse, pulsus bigeminus.* **bisferious p.** PULSUS BISFERIENS. **capillary p.** Rhythmical flushing and blanching of the skin, especially at the root of the nail. It occurs when there is marked vasodilatation or rapid diastolic run-off, especially in aortic regurgitation, and is best elicited by gentle pressure on the end of the nail. Also *Quincke's pulse.* **carotid p.** The pulse in the carotid artery. **catadicrotic p.** See under CATADICROTIC. **collapsing p.** A rapidly rising and falling pulse, seen particularly in aortic regurgitation but also in other conditions in which there is a rapid diastolic run-off. Also *Corrigan's pulse, waterhammer pulse.* **Corrigan's p.** COLLAPSING PULSE. **coupled p.** BIGEMINAL PULSE. **dicrotic p.** A pulse in which there is a palpable double pulsation for each heart beat as a result of accentuation of the dicrotic wave. **digitalate p.** BIGEMINAL PULSE. **entoptic p.** A visual sensation, usually a variable intensity of brightness or color, that is synchronous with the heartbeat. **epigastric p.** The pulse felt in the epigastrium due to the abdominal aorta. **febrile p.** A rapid and bounding pulse characteristic of fevers. **filiform p.** THREADY PULSE. **full p.** A pulse of large volume. Also *pulsus plenus.* **hepatic p.** Pulsation of the liver. **intermittent p.** A pulse with dropped beats. **irregular p.** A pulse in which the beats are not regularly spaced in time. Also *allorhythmic pulse, pulsus heterochronicus.* **jerky p.** A pulse with an abrupt upstroke and downstroke. **jugular p.** The pulsation in the jugular veins. **Kussmaul's p.** KUSSMAUL SIGN. **low-tension p.** A pulse which is easily obliterated by pressure. **paradoxical p.** PULSUS PARADOXUS. **parvus et tardus p.** See under PULSUS PARVUS ET TARDUS. **plateau p.**

The slow, rising and falling pulse of severe aortic stenosis, the arterial pulse tracing demonstrating a plateau. **quick p.** 1 A pulse with a fast rate. 2 A pulse with a sharp upstroke. Also *pulsus celer.* **Quincke's p.** CAPILLARY PULSE. **radial p.** The pulse felt over the radial artery. **soft p.** A pulse that is easily obliterated by pressure. Also *pulsus mollis.* **strong p.** A pulse of large volume. Also *pulsus fortis.* **thready p.** A small-volume pulse which is difficult to feel. Also *filiform pulse, pulsus filiformis, arachnoid pulse.* **trigeminal p.** A pulse with a pause after each third beat. Also *pulsus trigeminus.* See also TRIGEMINY. **unequal p.** A pulse with beats of varying time and volume. **venous p.** The pulse visible in the veins, specifically the internal jugular veins as seen in the neck. Also *pulsus venosus.* **water-hammer p.** COLLAPSING PULSE.

**pulseless** \puls′lis\ Having no pulse.

**pulsellum** \pulsel′əm\ [New L, dim. of L *pulsus* a pushing, stroke] (*pl.* pulsella) A flagellum that propels by pushing from a posterior position.

**pulsion** \pul′shən\ [Late L *pulsio* (from *pulsus,* past part. of *pellere* to impel, propel) a pushing, propulsion] A disturbance of gait comprising a tendency to fall forwards (antepulsion), to one side (lateropulsion), or backwards (retropulsion), as seen particularly in Parkinson's disease.

**pulsus** \pul′səs\ [See PULSE.] PULSE. **p. abdominalis** ABDOMINAL PULSE. **p. alternans** Pulse with alternating strong and weak beats in regular rhythm, usually found in heart failure. Also *alternating pulse, cardiac alternation.* **p. biferiens** PULSUS BISFERIENS. **p. bigeminus** BIGEMINAL PULSE. **p. bisferiens** A pulse with two systolic peaks, due to percussion and tidal waves. Commonly found in aortic regurgitation with or without aortic stenosis. May also occur in hypertrophic obstructive cardiomyopathy. Also *pulsus biferiens, bisferious pulse, biferious pulse.* **p. celer** QUICK PULSE. **p. cordis** CARDIAC IMPULSE. **p. filiformis** THREADY PULSE. **p. fortis** STRONG PULSE. **p. heterochronicus** IRREGULAR PULSE. **p. mollis** SOFT PULSE. **p. paradoxus** An arterial pulse which markedly diminishes or disappears during inspiration. This is an exaggeration of the normal inspiratory diminution in the pulse and is therefore not in fact paradoxical. It is characteristic of pericardial constriction or tamponade but is commonly seen in obstructive airways disease. Also *paradoxical pulse.* **p. parvus** A small pulse. **p. parvus et tardus** A small and prolonged pulse, typical of severe aortic stenosis. **p. plenus** FULL PULSE. **p. tardus** A pulse which is slow rising and falling. **p. trigeminus** TRIGEMINAL PULSE. **p. venosus** VENOUS PULSE.

**pulv.** *pulvis* (L, powder).

**pulverization** The rendering of a substance to a powder form.

**pulvinar** \pul′vinär\ [L (from *pulvinus* a cushion, pillow) a cushioned couch] NUCLEUS POSTERIOR THALAMI. **p. thalami** NUCLEUS POSTERIOR THALAMI.

**pulvis** [L, gen. *pulveris* (akin to *pollen* fine flour) dust, powder] Powder.

**pump** [prob. from Middle Dutch *pompe*] **1** A device that forces a gas or liquid to move in a desired direction. **2** A metabolic mechanism that moves ions or molecules. **blood p.** A device for driving blood, especially through the tubing of an extracorporeal apparatus, as is required in cardiac surgery. **breast p.** A mechanical device used to extract milk from a woman's breast. It is used when direct infant feeding is not possible, such as prematurity, or to relieve breast engorgement. **calcium p.** $Ca^{2+}$-transporting ATPase. It is found in membranes, as those of the sarcoplasmic reticulum, and pumps calcium ions into the reticulum with concomitant hydrolysis of ATP to ADP and orthophosphate. The consequence of this pumping is a rapid fall of calcium concentration in the sarcoplasm and a resultant cessation of muscular contraction. **Carrel-Lindbergh p.** A perfusion apparatus for keeping isolated organs viable. **dental p.** SALIVA EJECTOR. **infusion p.** A device for the controlled intravascular infusion of fluids. **infusion-withdrawal p.** A pump capable of both infusing and withdrawing fluids, specifically from arteries or veins. **intra-aortic balloon p.** A pump attached to a balloon which is inserted into the descending aorta to provide counterpulsation. It inflates during diastole and deflates during systole, thus increasing coronary and peripheral flow during diastole and reducing impedance to left ventricular ejection. **Lindbergh p.** A perfusion device used to preserve whole organs indefinitely. **muscle p.** The phenomenon of central return of peripheral venous blood by contraction of the muscles of the calf. The muscle pump's dysfunction with lower extremity immobilization is believed to lead to stagnation of venous blood and resulting venous thrombosis. **peristaltic p.** A pump in which usually moving rollers constrict a plastic tube resulting in a wave that pushes the contents ahead of the constriction. **rotary p.** A pump in which an eccentric cam rotates in a cylinder, forcing the fluid to move through. **saliva p.** SALIVA EJECTOR. **sodium p.** The $Na^+/K^+$-transporting ATPase. It is a protein found in cell membranes which pumps sodium ions out of cells and potassium ions in with concomitant hydrolysis of ATP to ADP and orthophosphate. **stomach p.** A suction device used to empty and lavage the stomach.

**pump-oxygenator** An apparatus consisting of an arterial pump and a blood oxygenator, used for extracorporeal circulation in cardiopulmonary bypass.

**puna** \poo′nə\ MOUNTAIN SICKNESS.

**punch** [Middle English *punchon,* from Middle French *poinçon* a rod with steel point for perforating or engraving, from L *punctum* a prick, sting] A surgical instrument used to cut out or perforate a piece of tissue. It may also be used in denting or drawing out a foreign body within the tissue. **kidney p.** See under MURPHY'S KIDNEY PUNCH. **Murphy's kidney p.** A diagnostic procedure carried out with the patient sitting with his arms folded while the examining thumb makes short jabs at the costovertebral angle. Tenderness suggests the presence of infection or inflammation of the kidney. **rubber dam p.** A punch used for making circular holes of various sizes in a rubber dam. **sphenoidal p.** A surgical instrument that punches out small pieces of bone, specially designed for removal of sphenoid bone, such as the floor of the sella turcica.

**punched-out** Resembling the sharply demarcated defect caused by a biopsy punch or trocar, frequently used to describe the radiological appearance of the osteolytic lesions of multiple myeloma.

**puncta** \pungk′tə\ Plural of PUNCTUM.

**punctate** \pungk′tāt\ **1** Having the appearance of a point or points. **2** Consisting of or characterized by minute, pointlike marks or specks, as a skin lesion.

**punctum** \pungk′təm\ [L (from *punctus,* past part. of *pungere* to prick, sting) a prick, sting, a small hole made by pricking, a point] (*pl.* puncta) A point, spot, or minute orifice. **p. convergens basalis** The nearest point to which the eyes are able to converge. Abbr. PcB **p. coxale** The highest point of the iliac crest. **p. ischiadicum** The lower part of the ischial tuberosity. *Outmoded.* **p. lacrimale** [NA] The minute orifice in the center of the lacrimal papilla which opens into the lacrimal canaliculus. It is located on the margin of each eyelid at the basal angle of the lacus lacrimalis. Also *lacrimal point.* **p. luteum** *Outmoded* MACULA RETINAE. **p. proximum** NEAR POINT. **p. remotum** FAR POINT.

**punctura** \pungkt$^y$oo′rə\ [L, a pricking, piercing, puncture. See PUNCTURE.] PUNCTURE. **p. exploratoria** EXPLORATORY PUNCTURE.

**puncture** \pungk′chər\ [L *punctura* (from *punctus,* past part. of *pungere* to prick, sting) a pricking, piercing, puncture] **1** To perforate with a sharp point. **2** A perforation made with a sharp point. Also *punctura, picqûre.* **Bernard's p.** A localized experimental lesion of the floor of the fourth ventricle that results in glycosuria. Also *diabetic puncture.* **cisternal p.** Needle puncture of the cisterna magna or suboccipital cistern through the occipitoatlantoid ligament (between the occipital bone and the atlas). It is performed in order to obtain cerebrospinal fluid for diagnosis or therapy, or in order to introduce contrast medium, when lumbar puncture is contraindicated or when it is necessary to define the upper border of a spinal lesion producing spinal block. Also *intracisternal puncture, suboccipital puncture.* **diabetic p.** BERNARD'S PUNCTURE. **epigastric p.** Pericardiocentesis in which a needle is inserted below the xiphoid cartilage and advanced toward the left shoulder and scapula. Also *Marfan's epigastric puncture.* **exploratory p.** Puncture of a site, structure, or lesion to remove the contents for diagnostic purposes. Also *punctura exploratoria.* **gland p.** The puncture of a gland or lymph node to aspirate the contents for cytologic or other analysis. **heat p.** An experimental lesion of the hypothalamus that leads to an increased body temperature. **intracisternal p.** CISTERNAL PUNCTURE. **Kronecker's p.** An experimental lesion of the medulla that decreases the heart rate. **lumbar p.** Needle puncture of the lumbar subarachnoid space, usually performed in the spaces between the spines of the third and fourth or fourth and fifth lumbar vertebrae, in order to obtain samples of cerebrospinal fluid for analysis or in order to inject material for diagnostic or therapeutic purposes. Also *spinal tap, spinal puncture, thecal puncture, rachicentesis, rachiocentesis.* Abbr. LP **Marfan's epigastric p.** EPIGASTRIC PUNCTURE. **spinal p.** LUMBAR PUNCTURE. **splenic p.** A diagnostic procedure in which a needle is inserted into the splenic parenchyma to obtain pressure measurements or to infuse radiopaque contrast material. **sternal p.** The process of entering the marrow cavity of the manubrium of the sternum with a sturdy needle, in order to obtain a sample of bone marrow. **subdural p.** The introduction of a needle into the space between the dura mater and arachnoid. The procedure may be done for injection of any diagnostic or therapeutic substance into the space or for aspiration of fluid such as cerebrospinal fluid, blood, or pus. Accidentally, the space may be entered in the performance of myelography. **suboccipital p.** CISTERNAL PUNCTURE. **suprapubic p.** A bladder puncture, for aspiration of urine or placement of a catheter, in which the needle is introduced immediately above the pubis. It is recommended in some acute cases of urinary retention. **thecal p.** LUMBAR PUNCTURE. **tibial p.** The process of entering the marrow cavity of the tibia with a sturdy needle, in order to obtain a sample of bone marrow. It is commonly used in infants and small children. **tracheoesophageal p.** In the subject after laryngectomy, the establishment of a puncture wound between the trachea, just within the stoma, and the esophagus, close to its junction with the pharynx, as the first step in the introduction of a Blom-Singer voice prosthesis. **transethmoidal p.** A method of gaining access to the inside of the skull by traversing the ethmoid bone through the nose. **ventricular p.** Needle puncture of a cerebral ventricle.

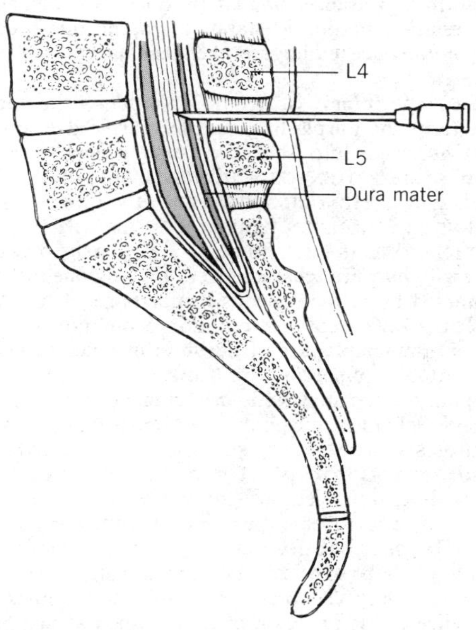


**Lumbar puncture**

**pungent** \pun′jənt\ **1** Sharp; prickly, as the spines of a plant or animal. **2** Acrid; biting; penetrating, as an odor.

**PUO** pyrexia of unknown origin.

**Puo** Symbol for a purine nucleoside, without specifying which.

**pupa** \pyoo′pə\ [L, a girl, doll] (*pl.* pupae) The stage of development that occurs between the final larval instar and the adult (or imago) of holometabolous insects. Adj. pupal.

**pupate** \pyoo′pāt\ To develop into a pupa; to pass through the pupal stage.

**pupil** [French *pupille* (from L *pupilla* a little girl, little orphan girl, the eye, dim. of *pupa* a young girl) the pupil of the eye] The central opening within the iris of the eye, through which light enters; pupilla. Adj. pupillary. **Adie's p.** ADIE SYNDROME. **Argyll Robertson p.** A miotic pupil which contracts on accommodation-convergence but not in response to light stimulation, usually due to neurologic lesions between the lateral geniculate body and the third-nerve nucleus. There is usually inequality of the two pupils, atrophy of the iris, and loss of the ciliospinal reflex. It is usually caused by syphilis. Also *Argyll Robertson pupil sign.* **artificial p.** An optical aperture created in the iris by surgical means, including the use of laser or photocoagulator beam. The need for such an opening exists if the normal pupil is displaced or occluded by a pathological condition and vision is impaired by this loss of the pupillary entry. **bounding p.** HIPPUS. **cornpickers' p.** A cycloplegic pupil due to jimson weed juice which contains stramonium. **double p.** POLYCORIA. **fixed p.** A pupil that does not react to stimuli. **Horner's p.** Miosis due to sympathetic denervation in the Horner syndrome.

**keyhole p.** A pupil on which a sector iridectomy has been performed. **multiple p.** POLYCORIA. **myotonic p.** ADIE SYNDROME. **pinhole p.** Extreme miosis, as with morphine or strong miotics. Also *pinpoint pupil.* **pseudo-Argyll Robertson p.** TONIC PUPIL. **tonic p.** The slowly reactive pupil in the Adie syndrome of hyporeflexia. Also *pseudo-Argyll Robertson pupil.*

**pupilla** \pyoopil′ə\ (*pl.* pupillae) [NA] The central orifice of the iris through which light enters the eye; the pupil. Its size is regulated by the sphincter and dilator muscles of the iris.

**pupillary** \pyoo′piler′ē\ Pertaining to the ocular pupil.

**pupillatonia** \pyoo′pilətō′nē·ə\ [*pupill(o)-* + Gk *aton(os)* slack + -IA] ADIE SYNDROME.

**pupillo-** \pyoo′pilō-, pyoopil′ō-\ [L *pupilla* (diminutive of *pupa* a young girl) a little girl, the eye] A combining form denoting the pupil.

**pupilloconstriction** \-kənstrik′shən\ [PUPILLO- + CONSTRICTION] Decrease in the diameter of the pupil of the eye.

**pupillograph** \pyoopil′əgraf\ [PUPILLO- + -GRAPH] A device that measures responses of the pupil.

**pupillography** \pyoo′pilăg′rəfē\ [PUPILLO- + -GRAPHY] The recording of pupillary responses.

**pupillometer** \pyoo′pilăm′ətər\ [PUPILLO- + -METER] An instrument for recording pupillary diameter.

**pupillometry** \pyoo′pilăm′ətrē\ [PUPILLO- + -METRY] The recording of the pupillary diameter.

**pupillomotor** \-mō′tər\ [PUPILLO- + MOTOR] Pertaining to the innervation or motility of the pupil.

**pupilloplegia** \-plē′jə\ [PUPILLO- + -PLEGIA] IRIDOPLEGIA.

**pupillostatometer** \-stətăm′ətər\ A device for measuring the interpupillary distance.

**pupillotonia** \-tō′nē·ə\ [PUPILLO- + *ton(o)-* + -IA] ADIE SYNDROME.

**Pupipara** \pyoopip′ərə\ [*pup(a)* + *i* + *-para,* combining form from L *parere* to bring forth young] A division of the suborder Cyclorrhapha, order Diptera, which includes the family Hippoboscidae, consisting of a group of related fly families in which the larva is retained in the abdomen of the female and laid as a fully developed larva ready for pupation.

**pupiparous** \pyoopip′ərəs\ [See PUPIPARA.] Pupa-bearing; designating insects that give birth to larvae ready for pupation, having passed their entire larval development within the female insect.

**pupivorous** \pyoopiv′ərəs\ [*pup(a)* + *i* + *vor(are)* to devour + -OUS] Living as a parasite in the larval and pupal stages of insects.

**Pur** Symbol for a purine, without specifying which.

**pure** [L *pur(us)* pure, unmixed, clean] **1** Containing molecules of only a single kind. **2** Containing nothing harmful for some implied purpose: used of a substance.

**purgation** \pərgā′shən\ [See PURGE.] The evacuation of the bowels by a purgative or cathartic. Also *purging.*

**purgative** \pur′gətiv\ [Late L *purgativus* purgative] **1** Causing or promoting evacuation of the bowels; cathartic. Also *lapactic.* **2** A purgative agent. **saline p.** SALINE CATHARTIC.

**purge** \purj\ [Old French *purgier* (from L *purgare* to cleanse, from *purus* clean + *agere* to do) to cleanse] **1** To administer a purgative to. **2** A purgative or cathartic, or the administration of a purgative or cathartic. *Popular.*

**purging** \pur′jing\ PURGATION.

**puriform** \pyoo′rifôrm\ Resembling pus.

**purine** \pyoo′rēn\ **1** The substance whose molecules consist of a pyrimidine ring fused by its 5,6-side to the 4,5-side of an imidazole ring. **2** Any of the substituted purines, especially adenine and guanine, which are found as constituents of nucleic acids and nucleotides.

**purinemia** \pyoo′rinē′mē·ə\ The presence of purine bases in the circulating blood. Adj. purinemic.

**purine nucleosidase** The enzyme (EC 3.2.2.1) that catalyzes the hydrolysis of an *N*-ribosylpurine to the purine and ribose.

**purine-nucleoside phosphorylase** The enzyme (EC 2.4.2.1) that catalyzes the reaction of a purine nucleoside and orthophosphate to yield the purine and ribose 1-phosphate, i.e. ribosyl phosphate.

**purity** \pyoo′ritē\ The state or quality of being pure. **radionuclidic p.** A state demanding the absence of all but one radioactive nuclide, although stable isotopes of the same element, or stable daughters, may also be present. Such purity is unusual because daughters of radioactive decay are commonly radioactive themselves and, even granted prompt chemical separation, must always be present to some degree along with the parent.

**Purkinje** [Jan Evangelista *Purkinje,* Czech physiologist, 1787–1869] **1** See under AFTERIMAGE, FIBER. **2** Purkinje's network. See under JUNCTIONAL TISSUE. **3** Purkinje layer. See under STRATUM GANGLIOSUM CEREBELLI. **4** Purkinje system. See under CONDUCTION SYSTEM OF THE HEART. **5** Purkinje phenomenon, Purkinje shift. See under EFFECT. **6** Purkinje's corpuscles. See under PURKINJE CELLS.

**Purmann** [Matthaeus Gottfried *Purmann,* German surgeon, 1648–1721] See under METHOD.

**puromycin** An antibiotic inhibitor of protein synthesis. It consists of adenosine, methylated twice on its amino group, and with its 3′-hydroxyl group replaced by an amino group acylated with 4-methoxyphenylalanine. It is thus an analogue of an aminoacyl-tRNA, and the growing peptide chain is transferred onto its free amino group and is therefore released from the ribosome. It is used in studies of protein biosynthesis.

**purple** **1** A color of the visible spectrum falling between red and blue. **2** A substance, usually a stain or dye, that is purple in appearance, or that produces a cytochemical reaction resulting in purple staining. For chemical names including *purple,* see under the chemical name. **visual p.** RHODOPSIN.

**purpura** \pur′p$^y$ərə\ [L (from Gk *porphyra* the purple fish, the dye from the purple fish, purple) purple dye, purple] A focal hemorrhage into the skin. Also *peliosis* (obs.). **p. abdominalis** HENOCH-SCHÖNLEIN PURPURA. **acute vascular p.** HENOCH-SCHÖNLEIN PURPURA. **allergic p.** HENOCH-SCHÖNLEIN PURPURA. **anaphylactoid p.** HENOCH-SCHÖNLEIN PURPURA. **p. angioneurotica** An allergic purpura characterized by angioneurotic edema accompanied by intracutaneous hemorrhage. **p. annularis telangiectodes** An eruption of unknown origin consisting of annular plaques of purpuric macules and telangiectases. Also *Majocchi's disease.* **p. arthritica** Arthropathy associated with intracutaneous hemorrhage, as in Henoch-Schönlein purpura. **athrombocytopenic p.** NONTHROMBOCYTOPENIC PURPURA. **autoimmune thrombocytopenic p.** Thrombocytopenic purpura associated with antiplatelet autoantibodies, as is seen in idiopathic thrombocytopenic purpura or lupus erythematosus. **benign hyperglobulinemic p.** PURPURA HYPERGLOBULINEMICA. **brain p.** A hyperacute hypersensitivity reaction involving the brain in anaphylactic shock or as a consequence of the injection of a drug such as arsphenamine. The condition closely resembles acute hemorrhagic leukoencephalitis but is slightly different pathologically in that there are diffuse perivascular hemorrhages throughout the brain occurring without signs of inflammation. **p. bullosa** An eruption of hemorrhagic bullae. **cachectic p.** Purpura occurring in patients with a severe decrease in skin collagen during states of cachexia. **drug p.** Purpura occurring in either thrombocytopenia or vasculitis as an adverse reaction to an ingested drug. **dysproteinemic p.** PURPURA HYPERGLOBULINEMICA. **essential p.** NONTHROMBOCYTOPENIC PURPURA. **factitious p.** Purpura deliberately induced by external agents, such as trauma, and not as a result of an illness or abnormal condition of the platelets, blood vessels, or clotting system. **hemogenic p.** Intracutaneous hemorrhage due to abnormality of the blood, such as deficiency of platelets or coagulation factors, in contrast to vascular purpura, which is due to fragility of blood vessels. **Henoch-Schönlein p.** A disease, primarily of young children, consisting of small-vessel vasculitis seen as raised red spots on the buttocks and lower legs (palpable purpura), glomerulonephritis, abdominal pain with or without intestinal infarction, sometimes diarrhea that may be bloody, fever, and arthritis. The condition is self-limited, although it tends to recur. It is thought to represent a form of allergic vasculitis. Characteristically, deposits of IgA can be found on basement membranes in biopsies of skin and renal glomeruli. Also *allergic purpura, purpura abdominalis, acute vascular purpura, anaphylactoid purpura, purpura nervosa, purpura rheumatica, Schönlein's purpura, hemorrhagic capillary toxicosis, Henoch's purpura, Henoch's disease, Schönlein's disease, Schönlein-Henoch disease, Henoch-Schönlein syndrome, Schönlein-Henoch syndrome.* **p. hyperglobulinemica** A nonthrombocytopenic purpura occurring in patients with marked hyperglobulinemia of any kind. Also *Waldenström's hyperglobinemic purpura, benign hyperglobulinemic purpura, dysproteinemic purpura.* **idiopathic thrombocytopenic p.** Thrombocytopenic purpura, usually associated with antiplatelet autoantibodies and occurring in the absence of other known causes. Also *land scurvy, essential thrombocytopenia.* **lung p.** Hemorrhage into the lung. **lung p. with nephritis** GOODPASTURE SYNDROME. **malignant p.** Extensive purpura associated with meningococcemia. See also ACUTE FULMINATING MENINGOCOCCEMIA. **mechanical p.** Purpura associated with increased intravascular pressure, as occurs in venous obstruction. **p. nervosa** HENOCH-SCHÖNLEIN PURPURA. **p. of newborn** Any of several neonatal bleeding tendencies, including thrombocytopenia and hemorrhagic disease of the newborn. **nonthrombocytopenic p.** Purpura occurring in the presence of a normal amount of platelets, and independent of specific cause. Also *athrombocytopenic purpura, essential purpura.* **orthostatic p.** Mechanical purpura occurring in the lower extremities when a patient assumes a standing position. **p. pigmentosa chronica** Recurrent intracutaneous hemorrhage associated with cutaneous hemosiderosis, causing a bronze discoloration of skin. **psychogenic p.** Intracutaneous hemorrhage ascribed to anxiety or neurosis. It was previously ascribed to autoerythrocyte sensitization. See also AUTOERYTHROCYTE SENSITIZATION SYNDROME. **p. pulicans** Petechiae resulting from the bite of insects such as fleas or other animal parasites. Also *purpura pulicosa.* **p. rheumatica** HENOCH-SCHÖNLEIN PURPURA. **Schönlein's p.** HENOCH-SCHÖNLEIN PURPURA. **p. scorbutica** A condition characterized by perifollicular hemorrhages due to vitamin C deficiency. The lesions first appear on the lower thighs and gradually spread to the buttocks, abdomen, legs, and arms. They are often followed by petechial hemorrhages developing independently of the hair follicles, especially on the feet and ankles. See also SCURVY. **secondary thrombocytopenic p.** Thrombocytopenic purpura due to a recognized cause, such as lupus erythematosus. **senile p.** Purpura induced by slight trauma in areas of chronic solar degenerative change. **p. simplex** Minor intracutaneous hemorrhage that occurs without either recognized trauma, known deficiency of clotting factors or platelets, or vascular fragility. The condition is harmless. It most commonly affects women. The lesions typically occur on the legs. Also *devil's pinches* (popular). **steroid p.** Purpura occurring in patients taking large amounts of corticosteroid hormone preparations or in patients with Cushing's disease, due to cortisol-induced atrophy of subcutaneous tissues. **symptomatic p.** Purpura that is a manifestation of a systemic disease, such as meningococcal septicemia. **thrombocytopenic p.** A bleeding disorder due to an insufficient quantity of blood platelets and usually manifested by numerous small subcutaneous hemorrhages. Also *thrombopenic purpura, thrombocytolytic purpura.* **p. thrombolytica** Intracutaneous hemorrhage due to accelerated fibrinolysis. **thrombopenic p.** THROMBOCYTOPENIC PURPURA. **thrombotic thrombocytopenic p.** A rare disorder, formerly fatal, of unknown cause, characterized by fever; neurologic abnormalities such as paralysis, dysarthria, convulsions, or coma; renal abnormalities such as proteinuria and azotemia; hemolytic anemia with negative antiglobulin test; thrombocytopenia; schistocytes in blood film; and amorphous hyaline thrombi in arterioles of affected organs, lymph nodes, or bone marrow. Not all of these features are present in all cases. Also *thrombotic thrombohemolytic purpura, febrile pleiochromic anemia, Moschcowitz disease, Moschcowitz syndrome, thrombotic microangiopathic hemolytic anemia.* **thrombotic thrombohemolytic p.** THROMBOTIC THROMBOCYTOPENIC PURPURA. **p. urticans** Intracutaneous hemorrhage that occurs at sites of urticaria. **p. variolosa** HEMORRHAGIC SMALLPOX. **vascular p.** Nonthrombocytopenic purpura due to vascular abnormalities, such as vasculitis or scurvy. **Waldenström's hyperglobulinemic p.** PURPURA HYPERGLOBULINEMICA. • This is a benign condition and should not be confused with Waldenström's macroglobulinemia.

**purpureaglycoside** One of several cardiotonic glycosides found in *Digitalis purpurea,* which yield glucose on enzymatic hydrolysis, and glucose and three molecules of digitoxose on acid hydrolysis, the latter leaving a genin, such as digitoxigenin.

**purpurin** 1,2,4-Trihydroxyanthraquinone, a colored substance found with alizarin in madder root. It can be made from alizarin by chemical hydroxylation, and has sometimes been used as a dye. It is a nuclear stain and is responsible for the red staining of new bone tissue of livestock fed with madder. Also *alizarin No. 6, alizarinopurpurin.*

**Purtscher** [Otmar *Purtscher,* German ophthalmologist, 1852–1927] See under DISEASE, RETINOPATHY.

**purulence** \pyŭrʹʸələns\ The state of being purulent. Also *purulency.*

**purulent** \pyŭrʹʸələnt\ [L *purulent(us),* from *pus,* gen. *puris,* pus] Containing, consisting of, or contributing to the formation of pus.

**pus** [L (gen. *puris;* akin to *putere* to rot, stink and to Gk *pyon* pus) foul matter, pus] An exudate composed of leukocytes, cell debris, and protein-rich fluid resulting from an acute inflammatory reaction. It is usually, but not always, caused by infectious microorganisms. **anchovy sauce p.** The characteristic exudate of amebic abscesses of the liver. Its brownish color results from a mixture of pus and old blood. **blue p.** A pus demonstrating a bluish tinge caused by the pigment pyocyanin produced by *Pseudomonas aeruginosa.* **burrowing p.** A pus that may spread a considerable distance from its origin by dissecting along preexisting anatomical planes. **cheesy p.** A semisolid, very thick pus found inside old abscesses and resulting from water absorption. **green p.** Blue pus which, not infrequently, is rather greenish blue. **laudable p.** Beneficial pus, an otherwise typical pus, so described when it first appears in an inflammatory focus indicating the onset of resolution and healing. *Seldom used.*

**pushback / palatal p.** See under PALATAL PUSHBACK OPERATION.

**pustulation** \pus′tyəlā′shən\ The formation of pustules.

**pustule** \pus′tyəl\ [L *pustula* (akin to Gk *physan* to puff, inflate) a blister, pimple; later influenced in meaning by the unrelated word *pus*] A small elevation filled with pus that is situated within or beneath the epidermis or within a pilosebaceous follicle. Also *pimple* (popular). Adj. pustular. **amniotic p.'s** AMNION NODOSUM. **compound p.** MULTILOCULAR PUSTULE. **malignant p.** See under CUTANEOUS ANTHRAX. **multilocular p.** A pustule containing more than one cavity. Also *compound pustule.* **postmortem p.** A cutaneous ulcer with pus formation, most commonly found on the hand and particularly over the knuckles of a corpse. It is caused by trauma and infection, occurring during the performance of an autopsy. **primary p.** A pustule formed with no visible preexisting lesion. **secondary p.** A pustule arising in an existing lesion. **simple p.** UNILOCULAR PUSTULE. **spongiform p. of Kogoj** A pustule formed in the upper malpighian layer by the migration of polymorphonuclear leukocytes into an edematous epidermis. It is the characteristic lesion of pustular psoriasis. **unilocular p.** A pustule containing a single cavity. Also *simple pustule.*

**pustulosis** \pus′tyəlō′sis\ [*pustul(e)* + -OSIS] Any skin disorder with lesions that are exclusively or predominantly pustular. **acral p.** A sterile pustular eruption that affects the hands and/or the feet and that usually follows a chronic relapsing course. Also *dermatitis repens, acropustulosis.* **p. palmaris et plantaris** A sterile pustular eruption affecting palms and/or soles. In the hands, the thenar and hypothenar eminences are usually affected, and in the feet, the heels and adjacent part of the insteps. The disease usually follows a chronic relapsing course. It has some features in common with psoriasis and is sometimes associated with it, but opinion is divided as to whether it should be regarded as a form of psoriasis. Also *Andrews disease.* **p. vacciniformis acuta** KAPOSI'S VARICELLIFORM ERUPTION.

**putamen** \pyootā′mən\ [L (from *putare* to cut off), a husk, shell] [NA] The large, external shell of the lentiform nucleus of the basal ganglia overlying the globus pallidus.

**Putnam** [James Jackson *Putnam,* U.S. neurologist, 1846–1918] Putnam-Dana syndrome. See under SUBACUTE COMBINED DEGENERATION OF THE SPINAL CORD.

**putrefaction** \pyoo′trəfak′shən\ The process of breakdown by bacterial action; decay. Also *mydesis* (obs.).

**putrefactive** \pyoo′trəfak′tiv\ Concerned with putrefaction.

**putrefy** \pyoo′trəfī\ [Middle French *putrefier* (from L *putrefacere,* from *putri(s)* rotten + *facere* to make) to make rotten] To be broken down by bacterial action.

**putrescentia uteri** \pyoo′tresen′shə yoo′tərī\ Gangrene of the uterus, a severe form of acute endometritis.

**putrescine** $NH_2—[CH_2]_4—NH_2$. Tetramethylenediamine, a compound produced by the decarboxylation of ornithine. This process may be bacterial, and this accounts for the presence of putrescine in putrefying material, but it is also a normal reaction of mammalian metabolism, since putrescine is a precursor of spermidine and hence of spermine.

**putrid** \pyoo′trid\ [L *putrid(us)* rotten, putrid] Undergoing putrefaction.

**Putti** [Vittorio *Putti,* Italian physician, 1880–1940] See under SYNDROME.

**putty** [Old French *potee* calcined tin, literally potful] Any of several compounds of doughlike consistency used for sealing openings. **Horsley's p.** A compound of seven parts beeswax, two parts oil, and one part carbolic acid. It is used to promote hemostasis of bleeding bony surfaces. Also *Horsley's bone wax.*

**Puussepp** [Lyudvig Martinovich *Puussepp,* Estonian neurosurgeon, 1875–1942] **1** See under OPERATION. **2** Puussepp's reflex. See under LITTLE-TOE REFLEX.

**PUVA** psoralens and longwave ultraviolet light (a form of photochemotherapy).

**PV** **1** polycythemia vera. **2** plasma volume. **3** peripheral vascular. **4** portal vein.

**PVC** **1** premature ventricular contraction. **2** polyvinylchloride.

**PVD** peripheral vascular disease.

**py-** \pī-\ PYO-.

**pyaemia** *Brit.* PYEMIA.

**pyarthrosis** \pī′ärthrō′sis\ [PY- + ARTHROSIS] Purulent joint infection, usually defined by white blood cell counts in the joint fluid of greater than 50 000 cells per cubic millimeter. Also *pyoarthrosis, arthroempyesis, arthrempyesis* (obs.), *arthropyosis, empyema articuli.*

**pycno-** \pik′nō-\ PYKNO-.

**Pyd** Symbol for a pyrimidine nucleoside, without specifying which.

**pyel-** \pī′əl-\ PYELO-.

**pyelectasis** \pī′əlek′təsis\ [PYEL- + Gk *ektasis* a stretching out] Dilatation of the renal pelvis.

**pyelitic** \pī′əlit′ik\ Pertaining to or affected by pyelitis.

**pyelitis** \pī′əlī′tis\ [PYEL- + -ITIS] An acute bacterial infection of the renal pelvis, most often due to *E. coli,* manifested by fever, flank pain, and frequent urination or dysuria when the bladder is simultaneously affected. Also *endonephritis* (outmoded). **acute p.** ACUTE PYELONEPHRITIS. **calculous p.** Pyelonephritis secondary to or associated with calculi. **chronic p.** CHRONIC PYELONEPHRITIS. **cystic p.** Chronic pyelitis characterized by the formation of multiple submucosal cysts. Also *pyelitis cystica.* **defloration p.** Infection of the female urinary tract associated with the first episode of sexual intercourse. Also *honeymoon cystitis.* **p. gravidarum** PYELONEPHRITIS OF PREGNANCY. **hematogenous p.** HEMATOGENOUS PYELONEPHRITIS. **hemorrhagic p.** Inflammation of the renal pelvis complicated by bleeding. **suppurative p.** Abscess of a renal pelvis. **urogenous p.** ASCENDING PYELONEPHRITIS.

**pyelo-** \pī′əlō-\ [Gk *pyelos* tub, vat] A combining form denoting the pelvis of the kidney. Also *pyel-.*

**pyelocaliceal** \-kal′isē′əl\ Related or pertaining to the renal pelvis and calices. Also *pyelocalyceal.*

**pyelocaliectasis** \-kal′ē·ek′təsis\ Enlargement of the renal pelvis and calices. Also *caliectasis, calicectasis, calycectasis.*

**pyelocalyceal** \-kal′isē′əl\ PYELOCALICEAL.

**pyelocystanastomosis** \-sis′tənas′təmō′sis\ PYELOCYSTOSTOMOSIS.

**pyelocystitis** \-sistī′tis\ [PYELO- + CYSTITIS] Inflammation or infection of the renal pelvis and urinary bladder.

**pyelocystostomosis** \-sistäs′təmō′sis\ [PYELO- + CYSTO- + Gk *stomōsis* (from *stoma* mouth) a surgical opening] A surgically created connection between the bladder and the renal pelvis. Also *pyelocystanastomosis*.

**pyelography** \pī′əläg′rəfē\ [PYELO- + -GRAPHY] Roentgenography of the renal pelvis after the use of a contrast agent. **air p.** Retrograde pyelography with the use of air as the contrast medium. **ascending p.** RETROGRADE PYELOGRAPHY. **excretion p.** *Outmoded* INTRAVENOUS UROGRAPHY. **intravenous p.** INTRAVENOUS UROGRAPHY. **retrograde p.** Radiologic examination of the renal pelvis and ureter after the injection of a contrast agent into the renal pelvis or ureter via a ureteral catheter. Also *ascending pyelography*.

**pyelolithotomy** \-lithät′əmē\ Extraction of calculi situated in the renal pelvis, after an incision of the pelvis. Also *pelvilithotomy, pelviolithotomy*.

**pyelonephritis** \-nefrī′tis\ [PYELO- + NEPHRITIS] Inflammation of the renal pelvis and parenchyma due to bacterial infection. Also *bacterial nephritis*. Adj. pyelonephritic. **acute p.** Acute infection of the renal pelvis and parenchyma, usually by Gram-negative bacilli such as *Escherichia coli*, species of *Proteus*, group D streptococci, and species of *Staphylococcus* and *Pseudomonas*. The onset may be abrupt, with fever, chills, flank pain, nausea, and vomiting. However, in some instances, the condition may be asymptomatic, suggested only by pyuria and bacteriuria. It may represent a new or recurrent infection, and may be secondary to calculi, obstruction, congenital anomalies, neurogenic bladder, or after urologic instrumentation. Antibiotic therapy usually is effective and recovery is the rule. Also *acute pyelitis*. **acute nonobstructive p.** Acute pyelonephritis of hematogenous or other origin unrelated to obstruction. **ascending p.** Pyelonephritis associated with retrograde infection from the bladder up a ureter. Also *urogenous pyelitis*. **asymptomatic p.** Pyelonephritis without symptoms, indicated by pyuria, bacteriuria, or characteristic radiologic signs. It may be associated with impaired renal function. **calculous p.** An infection of the renal parenchyma and pelvis superimposed upon preexisting renal calculus disease. **chronic p.** Inflammation of renal parenchyma initiated by bacterial infection and characterized by fibrosis, cellular infiltration, and secondary involvement of glomeruli and arterioles. It is difficult to distinguish from nephrosclerosis at times. The urine may exhibit only minimal proteinuria and a benign sediment. Slowly progressive renal insufficiency is common. Treatment with antibiotics may slow the progress of the condition. Also *chronic pyelitis*. **chronic bacterial p.** Chronic interstitial nephritis due to bacterial infection. **hematogenous p.** Pyelonephritis due to bacteria, usually staphylococci, carried in the bloodstream. Also *hematogenous pyelitis*. **p. of pregnancy** Acute pyelonephritis occurring during pregnancy. It is more common in patients with prior bacteriuria, and is perhaps related to dilatation of a ureter. Also *pyelitis gravidarum*. **xanthogranulomatous p.** Pyelonephritis characterized by accumulations of lipid-laden macrophages arranged in nodules in the medulla near the calices. The condition is usually associated with calculi and with infection by species of *Proteus*.

**pyelonephrosis** \-nefrō′sis\ [PYELO- + NEPHROSIS] Pyelonephritis associated with renal abscesses, usually secondary to obstruction or calculi.

**pyeloplasty** \pī′əlōplas′tē\ [PYELO- + -PLASTY] A plastic operation on the renal pelvis. Also *pelvioplasty*.

**pyelostomy** \pī′əläs′təmē\ [PYELO- + -STOMY] An operation for opening the renal pelvis for diversion of the urine, usually through a tube. Also *pelviostomy*.

**pyelotomy** \pī′əlät′əmē\ [PYELO- + -TOMY] An incision of the renal pelvis. Also *pelviotomy*.

**pyeloureteral** \-yoorē′tərəl\ Pertaining to the renal pelvis and ureter.

**pyeloureterectasis** \-yoorē′tərek′təsis\ [PYELO- + URETER + ECTASIS] Dilatation of a renal pelvis and ureter.

**pyeloureterolysis** \-yoorē′tərāl′isis\ The surgical freeing of the ureter and kidney pelvis from adjacent scar tissue.

**pyeloureteroplasty** \-yoorē′tərōplas′tē\ A plastic operation on the renal pelvis and the ureter, usually performed for relief of a stricture.

**pyelovenous** \-vē′nəs\ Pertaining to the veins of the renal pelvis.

**pyemesis** \pī·em′əsis\ [PY- + EMESIS] Vomiting in which there is purulent matter in the vomitus. Also *pyoemesis*.

**pyemia** \pī·ē′mē·ə\ [PY- + -EMIA] Septicemia caused by pyogenic bacteria and thus frequently associated with widespread abscesses. **otogenous p.** Pyemia caused by ear infection, particularly when complicated by septic thrombophlebitis of intracranial venous sinuses. **portal p.** A suppurative focus of inflammation in the portal vein.

**pyemic** \pī·ē′mik\ Pertaining to or characterized by pyemia.

***Pyemotes*** \pī′əmō′tēz\ A genus of soft-bodied mites with reduced mouthparts. It includes mites that cause dermatitis, such as the straw, or grain, itch mite *P. tritici*, which attacks stored-grain insects and can be extremely toxic to humans attacked by them. Also *Pediculoides*.

**pyencephalus** \pī′ensef′ələs\ [PY- + Gk *enkephalos* the brain] BRAIN ABSCESS.

**pyg-** \pīg-\ PYGO-.

**pygal** \pī′gəl\ Pertaining to the buttocks; natal.

**pygalgia** \pīgal′jə\ [PYG- + -ALGIA] Pain in the buttocks.

**pygo-** \pī′gō-\ [Gk *pygē* the rump, buttocks] A combining form denoting the buttocks. Also *pyg-*.

**pygoamorphus** \-əmôr′fəs\ [PYGO- + Gk *amorphos* (from *a-* priv. + *morphē* form) shapeless] An extreme degree of pygopagus parasiticus in which the parasitic member is represented by a formless mass attached to the buttocks of the host.

**pygomelus** \-mē′ləs\ [PYGO- + Gk *melos* a limb] Unequal conjoined twins in which the parasitic member is represented only by a recognizable, more or less well developed limb attached to the buttocks of the host.

**pygopagus** \pīgäp′əgəs\ [PYGO- + -PAGUS] Equal conjoined twins united solely or largely at the buttocks. They are most often oriented back to back. **p. parasiticus** Unequal conjoined twins in which the parasitic member is attached to the buttocks of the host.

**pykn-** \pikn-\ PYKNO-.

**pyknic** \pik′nik\ [PYKN- + -IC] Having a constitutional body type characterized by a short, stocky, well rounded body build and proportionately large body cavities. Also *pyknosomatic*.

**pykno-** \pik′nō-\ [Gk *pyknos* thick, compact, dense, frequent] A combining form meaning thick, compact, dense. Also *pycno-*, *pykn-*.

**pyknocyte** \pik′nəsīt\ [PYKNO- + -CYTE] A shrunken, distorted, hyperchromatic erythrocyte. Small numbers occur in normal newborns, but large numbers signify a hemolytic disorder.

**pyknocytosis** \-sītō′sis\ The presence in a blood film of many contracted erythrocytes of irregular shape and commonly exhibiting a few spicules or excrescences.

**pyknodysostosis** \-dis′ästō′sis\ An autosomal recessive

disorder of bone characterized by skull deformity, obtuse mandibular angle, short stature, partial digital agenesis, generalized osteosclerosis, and bone fragility.

**pyknolepsy** \pik′nəlep′sē\ [PYKNO- + -LEPSY] NARCOLEPSY.

**pyknomorphic** \-môr′fik\ Having a solid or compact form. Also *pyknomorphous.*

**pyknosis** \piknō′sis\ [Gk *pyknōsis* (from *pyknos* dense) condensation] A condition of shrinkage or condensation of a cell or its nucleus following cell death. Adj. pyknotic.

**pyknosomatic** \-sōmat′ik\ [PYKNO- + SOMATIC] PYKNIC.

**pyknotic** \piknät′ik\ Pertaining to or exhibiting pyknosis.

**pyla** \pī′lə\ [Gk *pylē* a gate, entrance] The opening between the third ventricle and aqueduct of Sylvius.

**pylar** \pī′lər\ Pertaining to the pyla.

**Pyle** [Edwin *Pyle,* U.S. orthopedic surgeon, born 1892] Pyle's disease, craniometaphyseal dysplasia of Pyle. See under METAPHYSEAL DYSPLASIA.

**pyle-** \pī′lə-\ [Gk *pylē* gate, entrance] A combining form denoting the portal vein.

**pylephlebitis** \-flebī′tis\ [PYLE- + PHLEBITIS] A suppurative or nonsuppurative inflammation of the portal vein, usually a result of intestinal or hepatic disease or secondary to suppurative infection of contiguous tissues. **adhesive p.** Pylephlebitis producing thrombosis.

**pylic** \pī′lik\ [*pyl(e)-* + -IC] Of or relating to the portal vein.

**PYLL** potential years of life lost.

**pylon** \pī′län\ A temporary artificial lower limb.

**pylor-** \pīlôr-\ PYLORO-.

**pyloralgia** \pī′lôral′jə\ Pain in the pyloric area.

**pylorectomy** \pī′lôrek′təmē\ [*pylor(us)* + -ECTOMY] The excision of part or all of a pylorus.

**pyloric** \pīlôr′ik\ Pertaining to the pylorus.

**pyloritis** \pī′lôrī′tis\ [*pylor(us)* + -ITIS] Inflammation of the pyloric mucosa.

**pyloro-** \pīlôr′ō-\ [Gk *pylouros* (from *pylē* gate + *ouros* keeper) gatekeeper] A combining form denoting the pylorus. Also *pylor-.*

**pylorodilator** \-dī′lātər\ A surgical tool designed to stretch the gastric pylorus.

**pylorodiosis** \-dī·ō′sis\ The correction of pyloric stricture by dilatation of the pylorus.

**pyloroduodenitis** \-doo′ədenī′tis\ Inflammation of the mucosa of the pylorus extending into the duodenum, usually due to peptic ulcer but also rarely seen in Crohn's disease.

**pylorogastrectomy** \-gastrek′təmē\ The partial resection of the stomach including the gastric pylorus. It is usually performed for distal disease in the pyloric antrum or the pyloric channel.

**pyloromyotomy** \-mī·ät′əmē\ [PYLORO- + MYOTOMY] The surgical incision of the outermost muscle fibers of the wall of the pylorus followed by blunt division of the underlying muscle fibers, allowing the constricted submucosa to resume a normal lumen, thereby relieving the pyloric obstruction. The operation is most often performed in neonates or infants for hypertrophic pyloric stenosis. Also *Fredet-Ramstedt operation, Ramstedt operation.*

**pyloroplasty** \pīlôr′əplas′tē\ [PYLORO- + -PLASTY] A gastroduodenostomy often performed to relieve a pyloric outlet obstruction. **Finney p.** A surgical procedure in which a U-shaped gastroduodenostomy is created to improve gastric emptying. Also *Finney's operation.* **Heineke-Mikulicz p.** A surgical procedure in which the pylorus is rendered incompetent by surgical division and resuture at right angles to the original linear incision. Also *Heineke-Mikulicz operation.*

**pylorospasm** \pīlôr′əspazm\ A spasm of the pyloric sphincter, causing obstruction at the pylorus. It is intermittent in nature.

**pylorostenosis** \-stenō′sis\ PYLORIC STENOSIS.

**pylorostomy** \pī′lôräs′təmē\ [PYLORO- + -STOMY] The creation of a fistula or stoma to the anterior abdominal wall by incising the stomach through the pylorus.

**pylorotomy** \pī′lôrät′əmē\ [PYLORO- + -TOMY] The incision of a pylorus, usually the gastric pylorus.

**pylorus** \pīlôr′əs\ [Gk *pylouros,* also *pylōros* (from *pylē* gate + *ouros* a keeper, guardian) gatekeeper] [NA] The terminal constricted portion of the stomach comprising the pyloric sphincter surrounding the pyloric orifice which opens into the duodenum. Its position is often marked on the surface by the prepyloric vein.

**pyo-** \pī′ō-\ [Gk *pyon* pus] A combining form denoting pus. Also *py-.*

**pyoarthrosis** \-ärthrō′sis\ PYARTHROSIS.

**pyoblennorrhea** \-blen′ôrē′ə\ [PYO- + BLENNORRHEA] A purulent discharge associated with gonorrhea. *Obs.*

**pyocalix** \-kā′liks\ Abscess of a renal calix.

**pyocele** \pī′ōsēl\ [PYO- + -CELE[1]] Distention of a body cavity with pus, as in the scrotum. **frontal sinus p.** An infected frontal sinus mucocele.

**pyocephalus** \-sef′ələs\ [PYO- + -CEPHALUS] BRAIN ABSCESS. **external p.** A purulent collection in the meningeal spaces. **internal p.** BRAIN ABSCESS.

**pyocolpocele** \-käl′pəsēl\ [PYO- + COLPO- + -CELE[1]] A pus-containing mass in the vagina.

**pyocolpos** \-käl′pəs\ [PYO- + Gk *kolpos* bosom, womb, vagina] An accumulation of purulent fluid in the vagina, usually associated with an imperforate hymen.

**pyocyanosis** \-sī′ənō′sis\ Any disease resulting from the presence of *Pseudomonas aeruginosa* (formerly *P. pyocyanea*).

**pyocyst** \pī′əsist\ A cyst filled with pus.

**pyocystis** \-sis′tis\ [PYO- + CYSTIS] The presence of pus in the bladder.

**pyocyte** \pī′ōsīt\ [PYO- + -CYTE] A polymorphonuclear leukocyte, usually a neutrophil, found in pus. Also *pus corpuscle.*

**pyoderma** \-dur′mə\ [PYO- + -DERMA] Any pyogenic skin disease. Also *pyodermia.* **chancriform p.** A sharply marginated ulcer with an indurated base, attributed to staphylococcal infection. The existence of such an entity remains in doubt. Also *pyoderma chancriforme faciei, pyoderma faciale.* **p. gangrenosum** A destructive, necrotizing, noninfective ulceration of the skin. Also *geometric phagedena.* **oral p.** A disease of the mouth characterized by widely distributed, small, elevated, pustular lesions. **primary p.** A pyogenic infection developing in previously normal skin. **secondary p.** A pyogenic infection complicating an existing skin lesion. **p. vegetans** PYODERMATITIS VEGETANS. **verrucous p.** A lymphatic verrucous reaction of the skin to chronic pyogenic infection. It is seen principally on the lower leg.

**pyodermatitis** \-dur′mətī′tis\ Dermatitis caused by pyogenic infection. Also *pyodermitis.* **p. vegetans** A chronic, vegetating hypertrophic reaction of the skin to a nonspecific bacterial infection. Also *pyoderma vegetans.*

**pyodermatosis** \-dur′mətō′sis\ [PYO- + DERMATOSIS] Any pyogenic skin disorder.

**pyodermia** \-dur′mē·ə\ PYODERMA.

**pyodermitis** \-dərmī′tis\ PYODERMATITIS.

**pyoemesis** \-em′əsis\ PYEMESIS.

**pyogenesis** \-jen′əsis\ The process by which pus is formed. Also *pyosis, pyopoiesis.*

**pyogenic** \-jen′ik\ [PYO- + -GENIC] Able to cause formation of purulent lesions in tissues: used especially of certain cocci, including staphylococci, streptococci, gonococci, and meningococci. Also *pyopoietic*.

**pyogenous** \pī·äj′ənəs\ Resulting from the presence of pus.

**pyohemothorax** \-hē′mōthôr′aks\ The presence of blood and pus in the pleural cavity.

**pyoid** \pī′oid\ [PY- + -OID] Having the appearance of pus: said of the sterile surface exudate generated by granulation tissue.

**pyometra** \-mē′trə\ [PYO- + Gk *mētra* uterus] A condition of the uterus when filled with pus. It is usually associated with an obstruction of the cervical canal from scarring or malignancy.

**pyometritis** \-mētrī′tis\ [PYO- + METRITIS] Inflammation of the wall of the uterus with purulent exudate.

**pyomyositis** \-mī′əsī′tis\ [PYO- + MYOSITIS] The presence within muscle of pus accompanied by abscess formation and sinuses. **tropical p.** A form of suppurative myositis occurring widely in the tropics, especially the humid tropics, characterized by abscess formation in one or more skeletal muscles and often septicemia with fever and jaundice. The disease is commonly associated with parasitic infections, but the causal agents are usually staphylococci that are often resistant to penicillin. If surgical drainage is performed, there is usually no residual muscle damage. Also *tropical myositis, myositis purulenta tropica*.

**pyonephritis** \-nefrī′tis\ [PYO- + NEPHRITIS] Acute pyelonephritis with abscess formation.

**pyonephrolithiasis** \ne′frəlithī′əsis\ [PYO- + NEPHRO- + LITHIASIS] Infected hydronephrosis secondary to obstruction due to a calculus.

**pyonephrosis** \-nefrō′sis\ [PYO- + NEPHROSIS] INFECTED HYDRONEPHROSIS. **calculous p.** Suppuration occurring in a kidney whose outflow tract is obstructed by a calculus. The kidney is converted into a thick-walled sac containing pus.

**pyonephrotic** \-nefrät′ik\ Related or pertaining to an infected hydronephrosis.

**pyo-ovarium** \-ōver′ē·əm\ [PYO- + OVARIUM] An ovarian abscess.

**pyopericarditis** \-per′ikärdī′tis\ Suppurative infection of the pericardium.

**pyopericardium** \-per′ikär′dē·əm\ Pus in the pericardial cavity.

**pyophthalmia** \pī′äfthal′mē·ə\ [PY- + OPHTHALMIA] An ocular infection causing a leukocytic response, usually an external infection of the conjunctiva or cornea. Also *pyophthalmitis*.

**pyophylactic** \-fīlak′tik\ **1** Protective against pus-producing organisms or against the absorption of pus. **2** A pyophylactic agent.

**pyophysometra** \-fī′sōmē′trə\ [PYO- + PHYSO- + Gk *mētra* uterus] An accumulation of gas and pus distending the uterine cavity.

**pyopneumocholecystitis** \-n^y^oo′məkō′ləsistī′tis\ Cholecystitis involving gas-producing organisms.

**pyopneumocyst** \-n^y^oo′məsist\ A collection of pus and gas within a cyst.

**pyopneumohepatitis** \-n^y^oo′məhep′ətī′tis\ Liver inflammation accompanied by pus and gas formation, usually caused by gas-producing microorganisms.

**pyopneumopericarditis** \-n^y^oo′məper′ikärdī′tis\ A pericarditis complicated by the presence of pus and gas.

**pyopneumopericardium** \-n^y^oo′məper′ikär′dē·əm\ The presence of pus and gas or air within the pericardium.

**pyopneumoperitoneum** \-n^y^oo′məper′itənē′əm\ The presence of pus and gas in the peritoneal cavity.

**pyopneumoperitonitis** \-n^y^oo′məper′itənī′tis\ A suppurative inflammation of the peritoneum accompanied by pus and gas formation, usually the result of infection by gas-producing microorganisms or of a ruptured viscus.

**pyopneumothorax** \-n^y^oo′məthôr′aks\ [PYO- + PNEUMOTHORAX] The presence of pus and air in the pleural cavity; pneumopyothorax. **subphrenic p.** The presence of air and pus under the diaphragm. *Obs.* Also *subdiaphragmatic pyopneumothorax*.

**pyopoiesis** \-poi·ē′sis\ PYOGENESIS.

**pyopoietic** \-poi·et′ik\ PYOGENIC.

**pyoptysis** \pī·äp′tisis\ [PYO- + Gk *ptysis* a spitting] The spitting of pus.

**pyorrhea** \pī′ôrē′ə\ [Gk *pyorroia* (from *pyo(n)* pus + *-rroia* -RRHEA) a discharge of pus] **1** A flow of pus. **2** *Popular* CHRONIC SUPPURATIVE PERIODONTITIS. **p. alveolaris** **1** Chronic periodontitis in which pus can be expressed from the pockets. **2** An advanced case of purulent periodontitis in which extractions are indicated. **schmutz p.** Chronic periodontitis caused by a dirty mouth. • The term derives from German *schmutz*, meaning dirt.

**pyorrhoea** *Brit.* PYORRHEA.

**pyosalpingitis** \-sal′pinjī′tis\ PURULENT SALPINGITIS.

**pyosalpingo-oophoritis** \-salping′gō-ō′əfôrī′tis\ [PYO- + SALPINGO- + OOPHORITIS] Acute exudative inflammation of the uterine tubes and ovary. Also *pyosalpingo-oothecitis*.

**pyosalpinx** \-sal′pingks\ [PYO- + SALPINX] An accumulation of pus in a uterine tube, usually resulting from pelvic inflammatory disease. Also *pus tube* (older term).

**pyosepticemia** \-sep′tisē′mē·ə\ SEPTICEMIA.

**pyosis** \pī·ō′sis\ [PY- + -OSIS] PYOGENESIS. **p. of Corlett** BULLOUS IMPETIGO. **p. of Manson** PEMPHIGUS CONTAGIOSUS.

**pyospermia** \-spur′mē·ə\ [PYO- + SPERM + -IA] The presence of pus in the seminal fluid.

**pyostatic** \-stat′ik\ An agent capable of stopping suppuration.

**pyothorax** \-thôr′aks\ The presence of pus in the pleural cavity; thoracic empyema. **subphrenic p.** An abscess immediately below the diaphragm.

**pyoumbilicus** \pī′ō·umbil′ikəs\ Suppurative infection of the umbilicus.

**pyourachus** \pī′ōyʊr′əkəs\ An accumulation of pus in the urachus.

**pyoureter** \pī′ōyʊr′ətər\ The accumulation of pus in a ureter, causing it to distend.

**pyovesiculosis** \-vesik′yəlō′sis\ [PYO- + *vesicul(a)* + -OSIS] The presence of a collection of pus in the seminal vesicles.

**Pyr** Symbol for a pyrimidine, without specifying which.

**pyr-** \pīr-\ PYRO-.

**pyrahexyl** SYNHEXYL.

**pyramid** \pir′əmid\ [Gk *pyramis*. See PYRAMIS.] **1** A polyhedron with a base and with triangular sides meeting at an apex opposite the base. **2** An anatomic structure that is roughly conical or pyramidal in shape; pyramis. **3** A system of relationships that can be represented graphically as a conical or pyramidal structure. **age-sex p.** POPULATION PYRAMID. **anterior p. of medulla oblongata** PYRAMIS MEDULLAE OBLONGATAE. **p. of cerebellum** PYRAMIS VERMIS. **p. of Ferrein** PARS RADIATA LOBULI CORTICALIS RENIS. **p. of kidney** RENAL PYRAMID. **p. of Malpighi** RENAL PYRAMID. **p. of medulla**

**oblongata** PYRAMIS MEDULLAE OBLONGATAE. **medullary p.** PYRAMIS MEDULLAE OBLONGATAE. **olfactory p.** TRIGONUM OLFACTORIUM. **population p.** A graphic representation of the age-sex structure of a population by means of horizontal bars, each corresponding to an age group, that are arranged chronologically with the youngest at the base and the oldest at the top, with the length of each bar proportional to the size of the segment of the population it represents. By convention, male age groups are to the left and female age groups to the right of the center line. Also *age-sex pyramid.* **posterior p. of medulla oblongata** FASCICULUS GRACILIS MEDULLAE OBLONGATAE. **renal p.** A conical piece of renal medulla that projects toward the renal pelvis and contains loops of Henle, vasa recta, and collecting tubules. Also *pyramid of kidney, pyramid of Malpighi.* **star p.** See under STELLATE CELLS. **p. of tympanum** EMINENTIA PYRAMIDALIS. **p. of vermis** PYRAMIS VERMIS. **p. of vestibule** PYRAMIS VESTIBULI. **Wistar's p.'s** *Outmoded* CONCHA SPHENOIDALIS.

**pyramidalis** \piram′idā′lis\ MUSCULUS PYRAMIDALIS.

**pyramides** \piram′idēz\ Plural of PYRAMIS.

**Pyramidon** A proprietary name for aminopyrine.

**pyramidotomy** \piram′idät′əmē\ PYRAMIDAL TRACTOTOMY. **spinal p.** Upper cervical division of the pyramidal tracts, sometimes employed for the relief of tremor.

**pyramis** \pir′əmis\ [Gk, gen. *pyramidos,* a pyramid] (*pl.* pyramides) A pyramid; a roughly conical or pyramidal anatomic structure. **p. cerebelli** PYRAMIS VERMIS. **p. medullae oblongatae** [NA] The wedge-shaped tracts, composed principally of corticospinal fibers, located on either side of the anterior median fissure lying on the base of the medulla oblongata. Also *medullary pyramid, anterior pyramid of medulla oblongata, pyramid of medulla oblongata.* **p. vermis** [NA] The pyramid-shaped part of the cerebellar tuber vermis and uvula. Also *pyramid of vermis, pyramis cerebelli, pyramid of cerebellum.* **p. vestibuli** [NA] The anterior portion of the vestibular crest lying just behind the spherical recess and below the elliptical recess on the medial wall of the vestibule of the internal ear. It is perforated by the macula cribrosa superior and it corresponds to the superior vestibular area at the bottom of the internal acoustic meatus. Also *pyramid of vestibule.*

**pyran** The heterocyclic compound related to benzene by replacement of two CH groups by one oxygen atom and one methylene group. It is regarded as the parent of the six-membered ring forms, the pyranose forms, of sugars.

**pyranose** The six-membered ring form of a sugar. It arises by hemiacetal formation between O-5 and C-1 of an aldose or between O-6 and C-2 of a ulose, and it is usually the predominant form of any sugar or sugar derivative in which these atoms are free to react.

**pyranoside** A glycoside in which the sugar is in the pyranose form.

**pyrantel pamoate** $C_{34}H_{30}N_2O_6S$. 1,4,5,6-Tetrahydro-1-methyl-2-[2-(2-thienyl)ethenyl]pyrimidine pamoate, an anthelmintic agent that is highly effective against ascariasis. It is also active against the hookworms *Necator americanus* and *Ancyclostoma duodenale.* It is given orally.

**pyrazinamide** $C_5H_5N_3O$. Pyrazine-2-carboxamide. A tuberculostatic agent often used in conjunction with other drugs, such as isoniazid and streptomycin. It is given orally.

**pyrazine** The heterocyclic compound related to benzene by replacement of two CH groups opposite each other in the ring by nitrogen atoms. Flavins and pteridines are biologically important compounds containing the pyrazine ring.

**pyrectic** [Gk *pyrektikos* feverish. See PYREXIA.] **1** Pertaining to or causing fever. **2** A medication that causes fever.

**pyrene** \pī′rēn\ $C_{16}H_{10}$. The tetracyclic aromatic hydrocarbon whose molecule consists of two naphthalene molecules fused so that C-2, C-1, C-8a and C-8 of one are these same atoms in the reverse order of the other. It is a yellow compound, found in coal tar.

**pyrenolysis** \pī′rənäl′isis\ [Gk *pyrēn* the stone of a fruit + *o* + LYSIS] The disruption of the nucleolus.

**pyret-** \pīret-\ PYRETO-.

**pyrethrin** Any of the esters of chrysanthemum dicarboxylic acid found in the dried flowerheads of pyrethrum (*Chrysanthemum cinerariaefolium*). These esters account for the insecticidal properties of pyrethrum.

**pyretic** \pīret′ik\ [Gk *pyretikos* (from *pyretos* fever) feverish] FEBRILE.

**pyreto-** \pī′rətō-, pīret′ō-\ [Gk *pyretos* (from *pyr* fire) burning heat, fever] A combining form meaning fever. Also *pyret-.*

**pyretolysis** \pī′rətäl′isis\ **1** The reduction of temperature in a fever. **2** The destruction of cells due to a raised temperature.

**pyretotherapy** \pī′rətōther′əpē\ [PYRETO- + THERAPY] FEVER THERAPY.

**pyrexia** \pīrek′sē·ə\ [from Gk *pyressein* (from *pyretos* burning heat, a fever, from *pyr* fire) to be feverish, sick of a fever] FEVER. **heat p.** HEATSTROKE. **Pel-Ebstein p.** PEL-EBSTEIN FEVER.

**pyrexial** \pīrek′sē·əl\ [*pyrexi(a)* + -AL] FEBRILE.

**pyrexin** \pīrek′sin\ A constituent of wound exudates capable of causing fever.

**pyridine** $C_5H_5N$. The heterocyclic compound related to benzene by replacement of one =CH— group by a nitrogen atom. It is a weak base (p*K* 5.2) and is used as a volatile buffer component in electrophoretic and chromatographic systems. It has an unpleasant smell and is harmful to breathe. Biologically important pyridines include pyridoxal and nicotinic acid.

**pyridostigmine bromide** $C_9H_{13}BrN_2O_2$. 3-Dimethylcarbamoxyloxy-1-methylpyridinium bromide, occurring as shiny, hygroscopic crystals freely soluble in water and alcohol. It is a cholinergic drug used in the treatment of myasthenia gravis. It is also used in an injectable preparation to reverse the effects of nondepolarizing muscle relaxant agents, such as curariform drugs.

**pyridoxal** Pyridine substituted with methyl, hydroxyl, formyl, and hydroxymethyl groups, in positions 2, 3, 4, and 5, respectively. It is one of the substances with vitamin $B_6$ activity. Its phosphate is a coenzyme for many enzymes that act on amino acids.

**pyridoxal kinase** The enzyme (EC 2.7.1.35) responsible for the phosphorylation of pyridoxal on its hydroxymethyl group at the expense of ATP to form pyridoxal 5′-phosphate.

**pyridoxal phosphate** Pyridoxal phosphorylated on its hydroxymethyl group. It is the prosthetic group of many enzymes that act on amino acids. It is often bound fairly tightly, but reversibly, to the apoenzyme. When the substrate binds, an imine is formed between the aldehyde group of the pyridoxal and the amino group of the substrate. Electron withdrawal by the pyridinium group through this imine bond facilitates the reaction catalyzed. Pyridoxal phosphate is also bound to phosphorylase but its physiologic role there is uncertain.

**pyridoxamine** 4-Aminomethyl-3-hydroxy-5-hydroxymethyl-2-methylpyridine. One of three equally active forms of vitamin $B_6$.

**pyridoxic acid** Either of two derivatives of pyridoxal, both of which are natural metabolites. The major one is 4-pyridoxic acid, which differs from pyridoxal by oxidation of its —CHO group to —COOH, and is produced in this way. The minor one is 5-pyridoxic acid, which differs from pyridoxine by the oxidation of C-5′ from —$CH_2OH$ to —COOH.

**pyridoxine** One of the substances with vitamin $B_6$ activity, and the first to be characterized. It differs from pyridoxal, into which mammals can convert it, by having a hydroxymethyl group where pyridoxal has a formyl group. Also *pyridoxol, adermine, rat acrodynia factor, Y factor, yeast eluate factor.*

**pyridoxine dehydrogenase** Either of two enzymes that dehydrogenate pyridoxine, the more important (EC 1.1.1.65) being the 4-dehydrogenase which forms pyridoxal with concomitant reduction of $NADP^+$, and the other (EC 1.1.99.9) being the 5-dehydrogenase which forms an isomer of pyridoxal.

**pyridoxine hydrochloride** $C_8H_{11}NO_3{\cdot}HCl$. 4-(Aminomethyl)-5-hydroxy-6-methyl-3-pyridinemethanol hydrochloride, one of the forms of vitamin $B_6$. It is used to prevent or correct a deficiency of the vitamin. Other uses are the treatment of pyridoxine responsive anemia and the prevention of peripheral neuritis resulting from administration of drugs such as isoniazid, hydralazine, and penicillamine.

**pyridoxol** PYRIDOXINE.

**pyrilamine maleate** $C_{21}H_{27}N_3O_5$. *N*-[(4-Methoxyphenyl)methyl]-*N*′,*N*′-dimethyl-*N*-2-pyridinyl-1,2-ethanediamine maleate, an antihistaminic agent that is given orally. It is less likely to cause the drowsiness usually brought on by antihistaminics. Also *mepyramine maleate.*

**pyrimethamine** $C_{12}H_{13}ClN_4$. 2,4-Diamino-5-(*p*-chlorophenyl)-6-ethylpyrimidine.A white, odorless, tasteless crystalline powder. It is a folic acid antagonist with antimalarial properties. It is used as a suppressant and to prevent malarial infections.

**pyrimidine** The heterocyclic compound related to benzene by replacing two of its =CH— groups by nitrogen atoms leaving one CH between them. The name is widely used to refer to substituted derivatives, and their tautomers, especially uracil, cytosine, and thymine, which occur in nucleic acids and nucleotides.

**pyrithione zinc** $C_{10}H_8N_2O_2S_2Zn$. Zinc 2-pyridinethiol 1-oxide. A white powder practically insoluble in water. It is a bacteriostatic and fungistatic agent used in shampoos to control seborrheic dermatitis and dandruff.

**pyro-** \pī′rō-, pī′rə-\ [Gk *pyr* fire] **1** A combining form meaning (1) fire or heat; (2) fever. **2** A prefix indicating anhydride formation between two molecules of an acid, e.g. pyrophosphoric acid, $H_4P_2O_7$, so derived from orthophosphoric acid $H_3PO_4$ by heating. It also indicates other products of dehydration induced by heat, e.g. pyroglutamic acid. Also *pyr-.*

**pyrocatechol** *Obs.* CATECHOL.

**pyrogallol** 1,2,3-Trihydroxybenzene, a phenol formed by heating gallic acid. It is very easily oxidized, and its alkaline solutions are used for removing oxygen from air.

**pyrogen** \pī′rəjən\ [PYRO- + -GEN] Any substance that induces fever. **bacterial p.** ENDOTOXIN. **endogenous p.** The mediator produced *in vivo* during inflammatory reactions that causes elevation of body temperature. It is probably the same as interleukin-1.

**pyrogenic** \-jen′ik\ [PYRO- + -GENIC] **1** Of or relating to the production of a fever. **2** Capable of producing fever.

**pyroglobulin** \-gläb′yəlin\ Any of a group of serum proteins that undergo irreversible precipitation after heating to 56°C. Elevated levels occur in many dysproteinemias, but determination rarely offers diagnostically useful information.

**pyrolysis** \pīräl′isis\ [PYRO- + LYSIS] The breaking down of a substance by heating it. Adj. pyrolytic.

**pyromania** \-mā′nē·ə\ [PYRO- + -MANIA] A compulsion to set fires. Also *incendiarism.*

**pyrometer** \pīräm′ətər\ [PYRO- + -METER] An instrument for measuring high temperatures, as those in furnaces.

**pyronine** A substance formed by oxidation of the condensation product of 3-(dimethylamino)phenol and formaldehyde. Its molecule is tricyclic, the central ring being related to benzene by the replacement of one CH group by $O^+$, and the other two fused to it are the benzene rings of the original phenol. Substitution products of the aminophenol may be used for the condensation, and give a series of substituted pyronines, which may be used as dyestuffs.

**pyroninophilia** \-nin′əfil′yə\ The ability to bind the histologic dye pyronine. It is seen particularly in the deep red staining of cells that contain abundant cytoplasmic RNA. Adj. pyroninophilic.

**pyrophos** TETRAETHYLMONOTHIONOPYROPHOSPHATE.

**pyrophosphatase** Any enzyme that hydrolyzes diphosphoric acid or its esters; usually inorganic pyrophosphatase (EC 3.6.1.1), which hydrolyzes diphosphate to form two molecules of orthophosphate.

**pyrophosphate** DIPHOSPHATE.

**pyrophosphomevalonate** Any of the anions of 5-diphosphomevalonic acid, an intermediate in the biosynthesis of steroids and terpenes from mevalonic acid.

**pyrophosphoric acid** $H_2O_3P$—O—$PO_3H_2$. Diphosphoric acid. It can be obtained by heating orthophosphoric acid. It has two low p*K* values, near 2, and values of 5.8. and 8.2. Partly neutralized solutions are often used as buffers near pH 8.

**pyrophosphorolysis** \-fäs′fôräl′isis\ A reaction in which a substrate molecule is split into two parts by reaction with diphosphate (pyrophosphate). It has the nature R—O—R′ + *P*—O— *P* → R—OH + *P*—O—P—O—R′. The reversal of the reaction of nucleic acid biosynthesis is an example. This reversal is prevented from occurring *in vivo* by the hydrolysis of diphosphate to orthophosphate.

**pyrophosphorylase** Any enzyme that catalyzes the splitting of a molecule by pyrophosphate (diphosphate) so that a diphosphate ester is among the products. Most such enzymes act physiologically in the reverse direction, with release of diphosphate, which in many cells is subsequently hydrolyzed to yield orthophosphate. An example is glucose-1-phosphate uridylyltransferase, which forms UDPglucose and diphosphate by reaction of UTP and glucose 1-phosphate, and which used to be known as UDPglucose pyrophosphorylase. However, in *Entamoeba histolytica* pyrophosphate is not readily hydrolyzed, and serves many of the functions served by ATP in higher organisms.

***Pyroplasma*** \-plaz′mə\ *BABESIA.*

**pyrosis** \pīrō′sis\ [Gk *pyrōsis* (from *pyr* fire) a burning] HEARTBURN.

***Pyrosoma*** \-sō′mə\ *BABESIA.*

**pyrotic** \pīrät′ik\ Pertaining to pyrosis (heartburn).

**pyrrobutamine** $C_{20}H_{22}ClN$. 1-[4-(4-Chlorophenyl)-3-phenyl-2-butenyl]-pyrrolidine, an antihistaminic agent that has a slow onset of action and prolonged effect of as much as 10 hours. It is given orally, usually as its diphosphate salt.

**pyrrole** A heterocyclic compound of formula $C_4H_5N$, a five-membered ring of four —CH= and one —NH— group. There are four pyrrole rings in the porphyrin ring system of heme (in hemoglobin, cytochromes) and of chlorophyll. When the porphyrin ring system is degraded to bilirubin the four pyrrole rings remain.

**pyrrolidine** A base of P*K* 11.3, the saturated derivative of pyrrole. Its molecule consists of a ring of four $—CH_2—$ groups and one —NH— group. The pyrrolidine ring is a constituent of the molecules of the amino acid proline, of various alkaloids such as nicotine, and of various synthetic medicaments.

**pyrroloporphyria** \pir′əlōpôrfir′ē·ə\ ACUTE INTERMITTENT PORPHYRIA.

**pyruvate** 1 The anion $CH_3—CO—COO^-$, or a salt containing it, derived from pyruvic acid. 2 An ester of pyruvic acid with an alcohol.

**pyruvate carboxylase** The enzyme (EC 6.4.1.1) responsible for the conversion of pyruvate and carbon dioxide into oxaloacetate with the concomitant hydrolysis of ATP. Like many other enzymes that catalyze carboxylations by carbon dioxide, it contains a biotinyl group. Some (but not all) pyruvate carboxylases are allosterically activated by acetyl-CoA. The enzyme is important in metabolism in catalyzing the net formation of oxaloacetate needed for the citric acid cycle.

**pyruvate decarboxylase** The enzyme (EC 4.1.1.1) that catalyzes the conversion of pyruvic acid into acetaldehyde and carbon dioxide. It occurs in plants and many microorganisms, but not higher animals, and is important in the pathway of ethanol production in fermentation. It contains thiamin disphosphate, and this is the group that binds the pyruvate for the catalyzed reaction.

**pyruvate dehydrogenase** Any of several enzymes that dehydrogenate pyruvic acid. The most important is pyruvate dehydrogenase (lipoamide), a component (EC 1.2.4.1) of the pyruvate dehydrogenase complex, whose overall reaction is the interaction of pyruvate, $NAD^+$ and coenzyme A to yield acetyl-CoA, NADH and carbon dioxide. The function of this component, which contains thiamin diphosphate, is to decarboxylate pyruvate with concomitant reductive acetylation of a lipoyl group on another component of the complex. **p. complex** The complex of three enzymes that together catalyze the reaction of pyruvate, coenzyme A, and $NAD^+$ to form acetyl-CoA, carbon dioxide, and NADH. It consists of a large number of subunits of each of the three proteins pyruvate dehydrogenase, lipoamide reductase, and transacetylase.

**pyruvate kinase** The enzyme (EC 2.7.1.40) that catalyzes the reaction of phosphoenolpyruvate and ADP to yield ATP and pyruvate. This is the physiologic direction of reaction, by which the enzyme is responsible for some of the ATP synthesis of glycolysis, although its name is based on the reverse reaction.

**pyruvemia** \pī′roovē′mē·ə\ Elevation of pyruvic acid levels in the blood.

**pyruvic acid** $CH_3—CO—COOH$. 2-Oxopropanoic acid. It is an important intermediate in the aerobic and anaerobic metabolism of carbohydrates of some amino acids.

**pyrvinium pamoate** $C_{52}H_{56}N_6$, $C_{23}H_{14}O_6$. A bright, orange-red to nearly black, tasteless crystalline powder, nearly insoluble in water and ether. It is used as an anthelmintic to treat enterobiasis (pinworm infection), and is active against some cases of strongyloidiasis. Also *viprynium embonate.*

**pyuria** \pīyoo′rē·ə\ [PY- + -URIA] The presence of an abnormal number of leukocytes or pus in the urine, reflecting urinary tract inflammation, such as that resulting from infection. **abacterial p.** Presence of leukocytes in the urine in the absence of documented bacterial infection. It is often associated with tuberculosis as "sterile pyuria."

**PZI** protamine zinc insulin.

**PZT** Symbol for lead zirconate titanate.

# Q

**Q** Symbol for glutamine.

**Q.** Symbol for electric quantity.

**$Q_{10}$** The symbol for the factor by which the rate of a chemical reaction increases for a rise in temperature of 10°C.

**$Q_{O_2}$** The symbol for oxygen consumption by a tissue, expressed as the number of microliters of oxygen consumed per hour, per milligram of tissue mass determined after drying.

**q.d.** *quaque die* (L, every day).

**q.h.** *quaque hora* (L, every hour).

**q.i.d.** *quater in die* (L, four times a day).

**q.l.** *quantum libet* (L, as much as desired).

**q.n.s.** *quantum non satis* (L, quantity not sufficient).

**q.p.** *quantum placeat* (L, as much as desired).

**q.q.h.** *quaque quarta hora* (L, every four hours).

**qq. hor.** *quaque hora* (L, every hour).

**QRS** See under QRS COMPLEX.

**q.s.** 1 *quantum satis* (L, sufficient quantity). 2 *quantum sufficit* (L, as much as will suffice).

**q. suff.** *quantum sufficit* (L, as much as will suffice).

**qt** Symbol for the unit, quart.

**QTc** The Q-T interval corrected for heart rate. See also BAZETT FORMULA.

**quack** \kwak\ [short for obsolete Dutch *quacksalver* (modern *kwakzalver*) (prob. from *quack(en)* to quack, chatter, prattle + *salv(en)* to anoint with salve + *-er* -ER) a charlatan] One who falsely pretends to have expertise or authority in medical practice, and who often promotes worthless treatments or remedies for financial gain; charlatan.

**quackery** \kwak′ərē\ The practice or methods of a quack.

**quacksalver** \kwak′sal′vər\ [See QUACK.] QUACK.

**quader** \kwā′dər\ [German, a squared stone, freestone, ashlar] PRECUNEUS.

**quadrant** \kwäd′rənt\ [L *quadrans*, gen. *quadrantis*, pres. part. of *quadrare* to square, from *quadrus* square, from *quatuor*, also *quattuor* four] One quarter of a circle; in anatomy, applied to one section of an area that can be divided into four equal parts by an intersecting vertical and horizontal line, for example, the surface of the anterior abdominal wall, the eardrum, or the breast. **dental q.** One of the four segments of the dentition extending from the central incisor to the most posterior molar on one side of either jaw. **q.'s of the tympanic membrane** The four areas of the tympanic membrane defined by two imaginary straight lines passing across it from side to side, one in the line of the malleus handle and the other bisecting it at right angles. The four quadrants are described clockwise as posterosuperior, posteroinferior, anteroinferior and anterosuperior.

**quadrantal** \kwädran′təl\ Pertaining to or resembling a quadrant.
**quadrantanopia** \kwädran′tənō′pē·ə\ [QUADRANT + ANOPIA] Inability to see in a 90° sector bounded by vertical and horizontal lines drawn through the fixation point. Also *quadrantanopsia.*
**quadrate** \kwäd′rət\ Four-sided or square.
**quadratus** \kwädrā′təs\ [NA] Four-sided, square, quadrate; usually used to describe four-sided muscles, for example, pronator quadratus, quadratus lumborum.
**quadri-** \kwäd′rē-\ [L prefix *quadri-* (from *quattuor* four)] A combining form meaning four.
**quadriceps** \kwäd′riseps\ [New L (from QUADRI- + *-ceps,* from *caput* head)] Having four heads: said of muscles such as quadriceps femoris. **q. femoris** MUSCULUS QUADRICEPS FEMORIS.
**quadrigemina** \-jem′inə\ **1** Plural of QUADRIGEMINUM. **2** CORPORA QUADRIGEMINA.
**quadrigeminal** \-jem′inəl\ **1** In four parts; constituting or belonging to a group of four; fourfold. **2** Pertaining to the corpora quadrigemina.
**quadrigeminum** \-jem′inəm\ (*pl.* quadrigemina) **1** Quadrigeminal; fourfold. **2** One of the corpora quadrigemina.
**quadrigeminus** \-jem′inəs\ (*pl.* quadrigemini) **1** Quadrigeminal; fourfold. **2** One of a set of four; a quadruplet.
**quadrilocular** \-läk′yələr\ Having four chambers, cavities, or cells.
**quadriparesis** \-pərē′sis\ TETRAPARESIS.
**quadriplegia** \-plē′jə\ [QUADRI- + -PLEGIA] Paralysis of the four limbs. Also *tetraplegia.* Adj. quadriplegic.
**quadriplegic** \-plē′jik\ Affected by or pertaining to quadriplegia.
**quadripolar** \-pō′lər\ [QUADRI- + POLAR] Having four poles or asters: said of a cell.
**quadrisect** \kwäd′risect\ To cut into four parts.
**quadrisection** \-sek′shən\ Division into four parts.
**quadrupl.** *quadruplicato* (L, four times as much).
**quadruplet** \kwädrup′lit, kwäd′rəplit\ [L *quadrupl(us)* fourfold + *-et* as in *doublet*] One of four fetuses or infants delivered as the product of a single gestation.
**qualimeter** \kwəlim′ətər\ [L *quali(s)* of what kind + -METER] PENETROMETER.
**quanta** \kwän′tə\ Plural of QUANTUM.
**quantitate** \kwän′titāt\ To make capable of giving quantitative results.
**quantity** A specified amount of anything. **vectorial q.** VECTOR.
**quantization** \kwän′tīzā′shən\ A process in which a continuous signal is divided into small intervals, with each interval assigned a unique code, as in an analog-to-digital converter.
**quantized** \kwän′tīzd\ Able to possess only certain values: said of a variable, such as the energy of the electrons of a molecule. A quantum of energy is therefore emitted or absorbed when this energy changes.
**quantum** \kwän′təm\ [L, neut. of *quantus* how great, how much] (*pl.* quanta) The quantity of energy that is absorbed or emitted, as electromagnetic radiation, when a molecule or submolecular particle undergoes a transformation between two states that differ in energy because of differences in electronic structure, vibrational excitation, etc.
**quantum libet** As much as desired. Abbr. q.l.
**quantum placet** As much as you please: a direction used in prescription writing.
**quantum satis** [L *quantum* as much as + *satis* enough] A sufficient quantity: used in prescription writing.
**quantum sufficit** [L *quantum* as much as + *sufficit* (third person sing. of *sufficere* to be sufficient) suffices] As much as suffices: used in prescription writing.
**quantum vis** As much as you wish. Abbr. q.v.
**quarantine** \kwôr′əntēn\ [Italian *quarantina* (from *quaranta* forty, from L *quadraginta* forty, from *quatuor* or *quattuor* four) a quarantine] **1** A restraint imposed to prevent the spread of a disease or pest. **2** A period of isolation imposed by health authorities on persons, animals, ships and aircraft, or other modes of transport, as well as on goods, cargoes, etc., coming from an area where an epidemic was in progress or where cases of a transmissible disease capable of becoming epidemic had been reported. For the quarantinable diseases the maximum periods of isolation have been laid down in the International Health Regulations. **3** To place in quarantine. **4** A place of detainment during quarantine.
**quart** [L *quart(us)* (akin to Old English *feortha*) a fourth, quarter] **1** In the United States, a unit of capacity for liquid or dry measure equal to 0.946 liter in liquid measure and 1.101 liters in dry measure. See under LIQUID QUART, DRY QUART. • When *quart* is used without qualification it is usually taken to mean *liquid quart.* **2** In Great Britain, a unit of capacity equal to 1/4 (UK) gallon; 40 fluid ounces; 1.136 522 liters. Also *imperial quart.* Symbol: qt **dry q.** In the United States, a unit of capacity for dry measure only, equal to 2 pints or 1/8 peck or 1/32 (US) bushel; 1.101 220 liters. Symbol: dry qt **imperial q.** QUART. **liquid q.** In the United States, a unit of capacity for liquid measure only, equal to 2 pints or 1/4 (US) gallon; 0.946 352 liter. Symbol: liq qt
**quartan** \kwôr′tən\ [L *quartanus* (from *quartus* fourth) pertaining to the fourth, as in *febris quartana* fourth-day fever] Characterized by recurrence every fourth day, or after 72 hours: applied especially to a type of malaria (quartan or malariae malaria) in which the febrile paroxysms recur at this rate. **double q.** Characterized by paroxysms occurring on two successive days followed by a day with no fever. Also *quartana duplex.* **triple q.** Characterized by febrile paroxysms occurring each day due to infection with three groups of quartan malarial parasites. Also *quartana triplex.*
**quartana** \kwôrtā′nə\ Quartan; quartan malaria. **q. duplex** DOUBLE QUARTAN. **q. triplex** TRIPLE QUARTAN.
**quartet** \kwôrtet′\ In cytology, the group of four gametes or gametes and other cells that result from meiosis.
**quartz** \kwôrts\ [German *Quarz,* origin unknown] A pure form of silica, often used as a material for optical apparatus such as spectrophotometer cuvettes, because it is transparent to visible and ultraviolet radiation. Also *rock crystal.*
**quasidominance** \kwā′zīdäm′inəns, kwä′sē-\ PSEUDODOMINANCE.
**quater in die** [L *quater* four times + *in* in[1] + *die,* ablative of *dies* day] Four times a day: used in prescription writing.
**quaternary** \kwät′ərner′ē, kwətur′nərē\ [L *quatern(arius)* (from *quatern(i)* four each, four at a time, from *quater* four times, + *-arius* -ARY) consisting of four each] **1** Containing four elements: said of a compound. **2** Describing an atom having 5 valence electrons (such as N, P, or As) with four bonds to organic groups and a positive charge, e.g. tetraethylammonium hydroxide, $(C_2H_5)_4N^+OH^-$, and choline, $Me_3N^+$—$CH_2$—$CH_2OH$.
**Queckenstedt** [Hans Heinrich Georg *Queckenstedt,* German physician, 1876–1918] Queckenstedt sign, Queckenstedt-Stookey test, Queckenstedt's phenomenon. See under QUECKENSTEDT'S TEST.

**quenching** [*quench*, from Middle English *quenchen*, from Old English *cwencan* to extinguish + -ING] The process of suppression; particularly, in biochemistry, suppression of fluorescence. The fluorescence of excited molecules can be quenched by the presence of molecules that can accept energy from them, thus relieving them of the need to emit this energy as light. **color q.** Inhibition of light transmission from liquid-scintillation vials due to colored chemicals whose absorption spectra overlap the emission spectra of the scintillator. **fluorescence q.** A technique for quantifying an antigen-antibody reaction by measuring the degree to which the bound antigen reduces the fluorescence emitted by a fluorescence-labeled antibody subjected to ultraviolet light. **thermal q.** The quenching that results from the absorption of beta energy by the solvent.

**Quénu** [Edouard André Victor Alfred *Quénu*, French surgeon and anatomist, 1852–1933] Quénu's hemorrhoidal plexus. See under PLEXUS.

**Quervain** See under DE QUERVAIN.

**Quetelet** [Lambert Adolph Jacques *Quetelet*, Belgian statistician and astronomer, 1796–1874] See under RULE.

**Quevenne** [Theodore *Quevenne*, French pharmacist, 1805–1855] Quevenne's iron. See under REDUCED IRON.

**Queyrat** [Louis *Queyrat*, French dermatologist, 1856–1933] See under ERYTHROPLASIA.

**Quick** [Armand James *Quick*, U.S. hematologist, born 1894] Quick's test. See under ONE-STAGE PROTHROMBIN TIME TEST.

**quick** [Old English *cwic*, *cwicu* (akin to L *vivus* alive and Gk *bios* life) alive, living] Being pregnant and able to feel fetal movements. This occurs about 16 to 20 weeks from the first day of the last menstrual period.

**quickening** [See QUICK.] The occurrence of perceived fetal movements for the first time during a pregnancy.

**quillain** SAPONIN.

**quinacrine** \kwin′əkrin\ An acridine dye that is used in cytogenetics because of its fluorescence when bound to certain regions of chromosomes.

**quinacrine hydrochloride** $C_{23}H_{30}ClN_3{\cdot}2HCl{\cdot}2H_2O$. $N^4$-(6-Chloro-2-methoxy-9-acridinyl)-*N′*,*N′*-diethyl-1,4-pentane diamine dihydrochloride dihydrate. A yellow powder used in the treatment of intestinal tapeworms and giardiasis and as an antimalarial agent. Also *mepacrine hydrochloride*.

**quinaldic acid** Quinoline-2-carboxylic acid. It is a metabolite of tryptophan, being formed by dehydroxylation of kynurenic acid. It may also be made by the oxidation of quinaldine, 2-methylquinoline. Also *quinaldinic acid*.

**quinaquina** \kwin′əkwī′nə\ *Older term* CINCHONA.

**Quincke** [Heinrich Irenaeus *Quincke*, German physician, 1842–1922] **1** Quincke's pulse, Quincke sign. See under CAPILLARY PULSE. **2** Quincke's edema. See under ANGIONEUROTIC EDEMA.

**quinhydrone** A charge-transfer complex formed by 1:1 molecular association between *p*-benzoquinone and its reduced form hydroquinone. It has a low solubility in water, and a suspension is used as a solution of standard redox potential, especially in conjunction with a platinum or gold electrode. Such an electrode was widely used for determining pH before the advent of the glass electrode.

**quinidine** A stereoisomer of quinine which has been used as an antimalarial agent. It is now used primarily in the treatment of various abnormalities of heart rhythm. Also *β-quinine, conquinine*.

**quinine** \kwī′nīn, kwinēn′\ [Spanish *quin(a)* (prob. from Quechua *kina* bark) quinine, cinchona + -INE] $C_{20}H_{24}N_2O_2$. The primary alkaloid of cinchona. In treating malaria, it is usually administered as the sulfate or dihydrochloride salt. Although it is less effective as a cure than chloroquine and some other antimalarial agents, it is useful in the treatment of malaria due to resistant strains of *Plasmodium falciparum*.

**β-quinine** QUINIDINE.

**quinine sulfate** $(C_{20}H_{24}O_2N_2)_2{\cdot}H_2SO_4$. A white, crystalline salt form of quinine, slightly soluble in water and more soluble in dilute acid solution. It is the most commonly used form of quinine.

**quininism** CINCHONISM.

**quininize** \kwin′inīz\ To treat with quinine.

**quinocide hydrochloride** $C_{15}H_{21}N_3O{\cdot}2HCl$. 8-(4-Aminopentylamino)-6-methoxyquinoline dihydrochloride. An analogue of primaquine with the same antimalarial actions and uses as primaquine phosphate.

**quinol** Any aromatic diol, such as hydroquinone, whose hydroxyl groups are so arranged that oxidation can yield a quinone.

**quinoline** A tertiary alkaloid or amine, composed of a benzene ring fused with a pyridine nucleus, yellowish to colorless and derivable from quinine, cinchonine, coal tar, bone oil and other sources. It has antiseptic and antipyretic properties, but is extremely toxic.

**quinolone** Any of a class of synthetic antimicrobial agents whose effect is due to inhibition of DNA gyrase and the resultant inhibition of DNA synthesis. Some members of this class have a broad antimicrobial spectrum and can be administered orally.

**quinone** A cyclic diketone in which the ring contains the maximum number of noncumulative double bonds, e.g. *p*-benzoquinone. The two carbonyl groups are normally conjugated with each other, sometimes through intervening carbon-carbon double bonds. Quinones are mild oxidizing agents, being reduced to aromatic diols.

**quinonoid** Having the properties of a quinone. These include color and a conjugated system of double bonds, often with parallel double bonds on opposite sides of a benzene ring, as in *p*-benzoquinone.

**quinquina** \kwinkwī′nə\ CINCHONA.

**quinsy** \kwin′zē\ [Middle English *quinaci*, from Old French *quinancie*, from Med L *quinancia*, from Gk *kynanchē* (from *kyōn*, gen. *kyn(os)* dog + *anchein* to strangle) a dog collar, severe sore throat] PERITONSILLAR ABSCESS. **lingual q.** Acute inflammation of the lingual tonsil. An incorrect and rarely used term.

**quintan** \kwin′tən\ [L *quintanus* (from *quintus* fifth) relating to the fifth or the fifth day] Recurring every fifth day: said especially of a fever or chills.

**quintuplet** \kwintup′lit, kwin′təplit\ [Late L *quintupl(ex)* fivefold + *-et* as in *doublet*] One of five fetuses or infants delivered as the product of a single gestation.

**quotid.** *quotidie* (L, daily).

**quotidian** \kwōtid′ē·ən\ [L *quotidianus* (from *quotidie* every day, from *quot* as many as + *i* + *die(s)* day) daily (adj.)] **1** Daily; recurring every day. **2** Characterized by daily recurrences, as certain kinds of fever.

**quotient** \kwō′shənt\ The result obtained by division. **Ayala's q.** A quotient derived from measuring cerebrospinal fluid pressure before and after the removal of 10 ml of fluid, once thought to be of value on assessing the volume of the fluid and the presence or absence of hydrocephalus. The pressure after removal was divided by that before removal and the result multiplied by 10. A quotient in the range of 5.5–6.5 was considered normal. Also *Ayala's index, rachidian quotient, spinal quotient, Ayala's equation*. **blood q.** MEAN CORPUSCULAR HEMOGLOBIN. **caloric q.** In metabolic processes, the ratio of the heat evolved to the oxygen consumed, expressed in calories per milligram of oxygen. **developmental q.** An estimate of the degree of psychological growth achieved by a child, based on one or more psychometric mesurements divided by the chronologic age. **D/N q.** DEXTROSE-NITROGEN RATIO. **intelligence q.** 1 An index of the level of mental development during childhood, based on the performance of a given child on an intelligence test, compared with others of the same age. It is classically expressed as a ratio of the mental and chronologic ages of that individual. 2 An index of the relative standing for a given individual on a standardized scale for measuring intelligence in the general population, in which the average score achieved is 100, with a standard deviation of approximately 16. Abbr. IQ **phonation q.** A measure of the rate of flow of air from the lungs during phonation. The quotient is based on the value of the subject's vital capacity divided by the length of time he is able to produce a vowel sound after taking a deep breath. It is used as an indicator of laryngeal dysfunction. **rachidian q.** AYALA'S QUOTIENT. **respiratory q.** RESPIRATORY EXCHANGE RATIO. **spinal q.** AYALA'S QUOTIENT.

**q.v.** *quantum vis* (L, as much as you please).

# R

**R** 1 Symbol for the unit, roentgen. 2 Symbol for gas constant. 3 rough (colony). 4 Symbol for respiratory exchange ratio. 5 Symbol for arginine. 6 Symbol for any chemical group, particularly an alkyl group.

**R.** 1 Rankine. 2 Réaumur (scale).

**−R** Symbol for Rinne's test negative (hearing test result).

**+R** Symbol for Rinne's test positive (hearing test result).

**$R_f$** The ratio of the distance moved by a spot on a chromatogram to the distance moved by the solvent front. If the front moves as fast as the moving phase generally, which it may not do because of evaporation of the moving phase, this ratio is also the fraction of the substance chromatographed that is in the moving phase at any time, and the fraction of the speed of the moving phase at which the substance travels.

**℞** *recipe* (L, take thou: written at the beginning of a prescription).

**Ra** Symbol for the element, radium.

**rabicidal** \rā′bisī′dəl\ [*rabi(es)* + *-cid(e)* + -AL] Capable of destroying rabies virus.

**rabid** \rab′id\ [L *rabid(us)* (from *rabere* to rave, rage) raving, mad, rabid] Pertaining to, affected with, or suffering from rabies.

**rabies** \rā′bēz\ [L (from *rabere* to rave, rage), madness of dogs and other animals] A usually fatal viral disease of worldwide distribution caused by a rhabdovirus and affecting wild and domestic animals, especially carnivorous mammals, and man. Human infection is almost always the result of a bite of a rabid animal. In man, an 18–60 day incubation period is followed by development of nonspecific symptoms (fever, headache, malaise, nausea, vomiting), pain or numbness at the site of exposure, and early neurological signs (anxiety, restlessness, depression). The acute neurological phase is characterized by frank nervous system involvement (hyperexcitability, agitation, delirium, confusion), hydrophobia and severe pharyngeal spasms, and paralysis. Coma usually follows, and death usually results from respiratory complications of coma. Diagnosis is confirmed by isolation of virus from saliva, cerebrospinal fluid, or urine, by demonstration of neutralizing antibody, or, at autopsy, by identification of characteristic cytoplasmic inclusion bodies (Negri bodies) in brain tissue or spinal ganglia. The disease is almost invariably fatal in man once it is clinically manifest. Rabies can be prevented with vaccination. Dogs, cats, and persons at high risk of exposure should be vaccinated at regular intervals. Prompt postexposure vaccination and passive serum therapy are recommended for persons bitten by an animal with proven or suspected rabies. Rabies vaccine prepared from human diploid fibroblast cell cultures is now used in the United States. Also *lyssa* (obs.), *hydrophobia* (popular). **dumb r.** SULLEN RABIES. **furious r.** In rabies, the clinical stage in which there is marked hyperactivity, with agitation, thrashing, running, biting, or other bizarre behavior, including hydrophobia. An animal at this stage may be vicious, lose all fear, and attack another animal or man. **paralytic r.** A stage in the clinical development of rabies, characterized by paralysis of the muscles of deglutition and, thus, drooling of saliva. Ascending paralysis, resembling that caused by transient myelitis, is a predominant or early feature. Also *paralytic hydrophobia.* **sullen r.** A stage in the clinical development of rabies characterized by a state of stupor and usually by an inability to swallow. Also *dumb rabies.*

**race** [Middle French, from Italian *razza* race, kind] A subspecies or other division or subdivision of a species. Human races are generally defined in terms of original geographic range and common hereditary traits which may be morphological, serological, hematological, immunological, or biochemical. The traditional division of mankind into several well-recognized racial types such as Caucasoid (white), Negroid (black), and Mongoloid (yellow) leaves a residue of populations that are of problematical classification, and its focus on a limited range of visible characteristics tends to oversimplify and distort the picture of human variation.

**racemase** \rā′səmās\ [*racem(ic)* + -ASE] Any enzyme that catalyzes the interconversion of enantiomers. At equilibrium it forms a racemic mixture.

**racemate** \rā′səmāt\ A mixture of a chiral compound with an equal quantity of its enantiomer. With achiral reagents, which cannot distinguish enantiomers, racemates behave like pure compounds.

**racemic** \rāsē′mik\ [L *racem(us)* a bunch of grapes + -IC; orig. used in the term *racemic acid,* the optically inactive form of tartaric acid, first found in grape juice] Having equal numbers of enantiomeric molecules: said of a mixture. A racemic mixture is optically inactive, because of the opposite effects of the two enantiomers. In chemical reactions with achiral reagents it can behave as a pure compound, because the two enantiomers react at identical rates.

**racemization** \rā′səmīzā′shən\ The process of interconverting enantiomers. This process reaches equilibrium when a racemate is formed.

**racemose** \ras′imōs\ [L *racemosus* (from *racemus* a cluster, as of grapes) having clusters] Characterized by a ramified grouping of dilated parts, suggesting a bunch of grapes.

**rachi-** \rā′ki-, rā′kē-\ [Gk *rhachis* the back, spine, backbone] A combining form denoting the spinal cord or the vertebral column. Also *rachio-*.
**rachial** \rā′kē·əl\ RACHIDIAN.
**rachicentesis** \-sentē′sis\ [RACHI- + -CENTESIS] LUMBAR PUNCTURE.
**rachidial** \rākid′ē·əl\ RACHIDIAN.
**rachidian** \rākid′e·ən\ [*rachid-*, New L stem from Gk *rachis* backbone + *-ian*, English adj. suffix] Pertaining to the vertebral column or rachis; spinal. Also *rachial, rachidial.*
**rachilysis** \rākil′isis\ [RACHI- + LYSIS] Treatment of scoliosis by combination of traction and pressure.
**rachio-** \rā′kē·ō-\ RACHI-.
**rachiocentesis** \-sentē′sis\ [RACHIO- + -CENTESIS] LUMBAR PUNCTURE.
**rachiocyphosis** \-sīfō′sis\ KYPHOSIS.
**rachiokyphosis** \-kīfō′sis\ KYPHOSIS.
**rachiopagus** \rā′kē·äp′əgəs\ [RACHIO- + -PAGUS] Equal conjoined twins joined back to back in such a way as to involve fusion of the vertebral columns. Fusion is usually limited to the cervical and/or upper thoracic regions.
**rachiotomy** \rā′kē·ät′əmē\ LAMINECTOMY.
**rachiresistance** \rā′kērizis′təns\ Failure to respond adequately to spinal anesthesia.
**rachis** \rā′kis\ [Gk, the backbone] **1** COLUMNA VERTEBRALIS. **2** An axial structure of various organisms and stages of development, such as a spinal cord, neural tube, or notochord.
**rachischisis** \rəkis′kisis, rā′kis′kisis\ [RACHI- + -SCHISIS] Any of several types and degrees of spina bifida in which the spinal meninges and spinal cord are exposed on the surface. All of these have been attributed to faulty closure of the embryonic neural tube, but this relatedness of origin has not been proved. Also *spondyloschisis, schistorachis.* **r. posterior** Spina bifida of the more usual type on the dorsal or posterior aspect, as opposed to other aspects, of the vertebral column or spinal cord. **r. totalis** A developmental cleft of the entire vertebral column and/or spinal cord. Also *holorachischisis.*
**rachitic** \rəkit′ik\ [*rachit(is)* + -IC] Of or relating to rickets. Also *rickety.*
**rachitis** \rəkī′tis\ [Gk (from *rachitēs* spinal, from *rachis* backbone) disease of the spine; adopted as a learned equivalent of RICKETS] RICKETS. **r. fetalis annularis** A prenatal inflammation resulting in enlargement of the epiphyses of the long bones. **r. fetalis micromelica** A deficient longitudinal growth of the long bones prior to birth. **r. tarda** OSTEOMALACIA.
**rachitism** \rak′itizm\ [RACHI- + *t* + -ISM] A susceptibility to rickets.
**rachitogenic** \rak′ətōjen′ik\ [*rachit(is)* + *o* + -GENIC] Giving rise to rickets.
**rachitomy** \rākit′əmē\ LAMINECTOMY.
**Racine** [Willy *Racine,* Swiss otorhinolaryngologist, 1898–1946] See under SYNDROME.
**Racouchot** [Jean *Racouchot,* French dermatologist, born 1908] Favre-Racouchot syndrome. See under NODULAR ELASTOSIS OF THE SKIN.
**rad** \rad\ [short form of *radiation*] **1** A unit of absorbed dose of ionizing radiation equal to 0.01 joule per kilogram; 0.01 gray. Also *rd.* • *Rad* may be shortened to *rd* to avoid confusion with the symbol *rad,* for radian. **2** Symbol for the unit, radian. **r. per second** A unit of absorbed dose rate of ionizing radiation, equal to $10^{-2}$ watt per kilogram; $10^{-2}$ gray per second. Symbol: rad/s, rad·$s^{-1}$
**rad.** *radix* (L, root).
**radarkymogram** \rā′därkī′məgram\ The record obtained by radarkymography.
**radarkymography** \rā′därkīmäg′rəfē\ [RADAR + KYMOGRAPHY] The recording by means of video tracking, using image intensification and closed-circuit television during fluoroscopy, to obtain a graphic tracing of heart movement.
**radiad** \rā′dē·ad\ In the direction of the radius; toward the radial side.
**radial** \rā′dē·əl\ **1** Pertaining to the radius or to the side of the upper limb in which the radius is located, that is, the lateral side. Compare ULNAR. **2** Characterized by or arranged in the form of rays or radii; symmetrically disposed around a center or axis.
**radian** \rā′dē·ən\ [*radi(us)* + *-an,* English noun suffix] The SI supplementary unit of plane angle; the plane angle between 2 radii of a circle which cut off on the circumference an arc equal in length to the radius, equivalent to 57.296 degrees. Symbol: rad
**radiant** **1** Relating to or having the character of radiation, as *radiant energy.* **2** Emitting rays of light.
**radiate** \rā′dē·āt\ **1** To extend outward in all directions from a central point. **2** To emit rays.
**radiatio** \rā′dē·ā′shē·ō\ [L (from *radiatus,* past part. of *radiare* to emit rays, radiate, from *radius* a radius, spoke of a wheel), radiation] An aggregation of nerve fibers interconnecting different portions of the brain. Also *radiation.* **r. acustica** [NA] The fiber tract extending between the medial geniculate nucleus and the transverse temporal gyrus in the human cerebrum. Also *geniculotemporal tract, acoustic radiation, auditory radiation, thalamotemporal radiation.* **r. corporis callosi** [NA] The fibers of the corpus callosum, arising from all lobes of the cerebral cortex. Also *radiation of corpus callosum.* **r. corporis striati** The fibers extending between the diencephalon and the corpus striatum. Also *striatothalamic radiation.* **r. optica** [NA] Bundles of fibers that arise from neurons in the lateral geniculate body and course through the retrolenticular part of the internal capsule to terminate principally on both gyri bounding the calcarine sulcus on the medial surface of the occipital lobe. Its fibers constitute the final relay for the conduction of visual impulses to the cerebral cortex. Also *optic radiation, radiation of Gratiolet, occipitothalamic radiation, radiatio occipitothalamica Gratioleti. visual radiation, geniculostriate tract, geniculostriate projection, geniculocalcarine tract, thalamo-occipital tract, fibers of Gratiolet, Gratiolet's radiating fibers, occipitothalamic fasciculus* (seldom used), *Wernicke's radiation.* **r. pyramidalis** The fibers projecting from the cerebral cortex to form the pyramidal (corticospinal) tract. Also *pyramidal radiation.*
**radiation** [L *radiatio.* See RADIATIO.] **1** High-speed atomic or subatomic particles, or electromagnetic quanta, photons, such as x rays, gamma rays, ultraviolet light, etc. **2** RADIATIO. **acoustic r.** RADIATIO ACUSTICA. **alpha r.** The emission of alpha particles from the nuclei of certain heavy elements, such as radium, thorium, and uranium. **auditory r.** RADIATIO ACUSTICA. **background r.** Radiation that produces a response in a detector before the source of interest is presented, or after it has been removed. Such backgrounds arise from cosmic radiation, natural radioactivity in the earth or building materials, inadequately shielded storage vaults, x-ray and teletherapy machines, spilled radioactive materials, or even patients under brachytherapy. Also *background activity.* **backscattered r.** BACKSCATTER. **beta r.** The electrons or positrons from atomic nuclei whose ratio of neutrons to protons is too large or too small for nuclear stability. **braking r.** BREMSSTRAHLUNG. **characteristic r.** The radiation emitted from an atom when an electron from

a higher energy level fills a vacancy in one of the inner electron shells. Also *characteristic ray, characteristic x ray.* **r. of corpus callosum** RADIATIO CORPORIS CALLOSI. **corpuscular r.** A beam of subatomic particles, such as electrons, protons, or neutrons. **electromagnetic r.** Radiation consisting of oscillating electric and magnetic fields traveling with a velocity of about $3 \times 10^8$ meters per second in empty space, and including radiant heat, radio waves, visible light, ultraviolet rays, x rays, and gamma rays. To explain some of its interactions, electromagnetic radiation is often considered to be a stream of uncharged particles (photons). **fractionated r.** FRACTIONATION. **gamma r.** See under GAMMA PHOTON. **geniculocalcarine r.** The axons extending between the lateral geniculate nucleus and the visual cortex of the calcarine fissure. **geniculotemporal r.** The auditory tract extending from the thalamic medial geniculate body to the auditory cortex of the superior temporal gyrus (transverse gyrus of Heschl). **r. of Gratiolet** RADIATIO OPTICA. **hard r.** X- or gamma radiation of short wavelength, high energy, and deep penetration. **heterogeneous r.** Radiation containing many wavelengths, or photons of many energy levels. **homogeneous r.** Radiation consisting of a single wavelength, or of photons of a single energy level. **infrared r.** Electromagnetic radiation of wavelength above 700 nm and so not detectable by the human eye. Much radiant heat is conveyed by such radiation. **ionizing r.** Particulate or electromagnetic radiation that displaces orbital electrons in passing through matter, producing ionized atoms or molecules. This can be done by alpha or beta particles, protons, positrons, neutrons, electrons, photons, or heavy particles. **K-r.** Characteristic radiation emitted as a result of the removal of a K-shell electron from an atom. **L-r.** Characteristic radiation emitted as a result of the removal of an L-shell electron from an atom. **nuclear r.** Any type of radiation, either electromagnetic or of particles, emitted from the atomic nucleus as the result of various nuclear processes. **occipital r.'s of corpus callosum** PARS OCCIPITALIS RADIATIONIS CORPORIS CALLOSI. **occipitothalamic r.** RADIATIO OPTICA. **optic r.** RADIATIO OPTICA. **parietal r.'s of corpus callosum** PARS PARIETALIS RADIATIONIS CORPORIS CALLOSI. **protracted r.** A technique of radiation therapy in which many individual low dose treatments are administered over a long treatment course, usually of many weeks' duration. Also *protracted treatment.* **pyramidal r.** RADIATIO PYRAMIDALIS. **striatothalamic r.** RADIATIO CORPORIS STRIATI. **supervoltage r.** X rays or gamma rays having energies greater than 1 Mev. **tegmental r.** The myelinated fibers emanating from the red nucleus. **thalamic r.** The fibers reciprocally connecting the cerebral cortex and thalamus and constituting the largest component of the internal capsule. **thalamostriate r.** A group of neural pathways coursing from the thalamus to the corpus striatum and putamen. The largest of the thalamostriate pathways originates in the nucleus centromedianus and the nucleus parafascicularis in the thalamus and traverses the internal capsule to enter the putamen. Other efferent fibers from the smaller intralaminar thalamic nuclei, such as the nucleus centralis medialis, the nucleus centralis lateralis, and the nucleus paracentralis, course to the caudate nucleus. Also *thalamostriate connections, thalamostriate fibers, thalamostriate pathways.* **thalamotemporal r.** RADIATIO ACUSTICA. **useful-beam r.** That part of the primary radiation beam which emerges from the source after collimation. **visual r.** RADIATIO OPTICA. **Wernicke's r.** RADIATIO OPTICA.

**radiationes** \rā′dē·āshē·ō′nēz\ Plural of RADIATIO.

**radical** \rad′ikəl\ [Late L *radicalis* (from L *radix*, gen. *radicis*, a root, origin, source) pertaining to a root or roots] **1** Designed to address the root cause of a disorder and by extirpating it effect a cure. Compare CONSERVATIVE. **2** A group of atoms possessing its own distinguishable identity and able to participate in a chemical reaction like a single atom, as $—CH_3$, $—C_2H_5$, $—COOH$, or $—NH_2$. • In modern chemical usage the term is increasingly restricted to the meaning of free radical. **free r.** A chemical radical which exists independently in a highly reactive, short-lived state.

**radical-ion** An entity that is a radical, in the sense of having an unpaired electron, and is also an ion, in the sense that it has electrical charge. The superoxide ion, $O_2^-$, is a biologically important example.

**radices** \rad′isēz\ Plural of RADIX.

**radicle** \rad′ikl\ RADICULA. **inferior r. of upper right pulmonary vein** *Outmoded* RAMUS LOBI MEDII VENAE PULMONALIS DEXTRAE SUPERIORIS.

**radicotomy** \rad′ikät′əmē\ [L *radix*, gen. *radicis* + *o* + -TOMY] RHIZOTOMY.

**radicul-** \rədik′yəl-\ RADICULO-.

**radicula** \rədik′yələ\ [L, dim. of *radix* a root] A structure resembling a rootlet, such as a branching venule or a fascicle of a spinal nerve root. Also *radicle.*

**radicular** \rədik′yələr\ Of the nature of or relating to a root or radicle.

**radiculectomy** \rədik′yəlek′təmē\ [RADICUL- + -ECTOMY] Excision or resection of a nerve root.

**radiculitis** \rədik′yəlī′tis\ [RADICUL- + -ITIS] Inflammation of a nerve root. Also *radicular neuritis.* **spinal r.** Inflammation of spinal nerve roots.

**radiculo-** \rədik′yəlō-\ [L *radicula* (dim. of *radix* root) a little root] A combining form meaning radicle. Also *radicul-.*

**radiculoganglionitis** \-gang′lē·ənī′tis\ [RADICULO- + GANGLIONITIS] Inflammation of spinal nerve roots and ganglia.

**radiculomedullary** \-med′ʸəler′ē\ Affecting or pertaining to nerve roots and the spinal cord.

**radiculomeningomyelitis** \-məning′gōmī′əlī′tis\ Combined inflammation of the spinal nerve roots, the meninges, and the spinal cord. Also *rhizomeningomyelitis.*

**radiculomyelopathy** \-mī′əläp′əthē\ Any disease or dysfunction of the spinal nerve roots and spinal cord.

**radiculoneuritis** \-nʸurī′tis\ [RADICULO- + NEURITIS] Inflammation of nerve roots and peripheral nerves.

**radiculoneuropathy** \-nʸuräp′əthē\ [RADICULO- + NEUROPATHY] Any disorder of nerve roots and peripheral nerves. **hypertrophic interstitial r.** HEREDITARY HYPERTROPHIC INTERSTITIAL NEUROPATHY.

**radiculopathy** \rədik′yəläp′əthē\ [RADICULO- + -PATHY] Any disease of nerve roots. **brachial r.** Any disorder of brachial nerve roots. **cervical r.** Radiculopathy caused by compression or irritation of cervical nerve roots. **spinal r.** Any disorder of spinal nerve roots.

**radii** \rā′dē·ī\ Plural of RADIUS.

**radio-** \rā′dē·ō-\ [L *radius* ray of the sun, beam of light, radius, spoke of a wheel] A combining form meaning (1) rays, radiant, radiation; (2) radius.

**radioablation** \-əblā′shən\ Ablation by means of radiation, as from a radioactive source.

**radioactive** \-ak′tiv\ Exhibiting radioactivity.

**radioactivity** \-aktiv′itē\ [RADIO- + ACTIVITY] The spontaneous rearrangement of protons and/or neutrons in an unstable atomic nucleus, in such a way that expendable energy becomes available. A proton may change into a neutron, or vice versa, or an orbital electron may be captured by the nucleus, thus altering the nuclear charge (transmutation); alpha particles, electrons, or positrons may be shot out at high speed; or the excess energy may be carried away by gamma photons or conversion electrons, leaving proton and neutron numbers unchanged (isomeric transition). There are characteristic decay processes and emitted radiations for each radionuclide. **artificial r.** INDUCED RADIOACTIVITY. **induced r.** Radioactivity resulting from the bombardment of a material with neutrons or charged particles. Such treatment induces nuclear reactions. Also *artificial radioactivity.* **natural r.** Radioactivity that occurs spontaneously in certain nuclides without human intervention.

**radioautography** \-ôtäg′rəfē\ [RADIO- + AUTO- + -GRAPHY] The technique for locating the sources of radionuclide emission in radiolabeled tissues, cells, or chromatographic fractions, by using photographic development of exposed film or emulsion.

**radiobiology** \-bī·äl′əjē\ The branch of biology concerned with the responses of living organisms and tissues to radiation, especially ionizing radiation.

**radiocarbon** \-kär′bən\ RADIOACTIVE CARBON.

**radiocarcinogenesis** \-kär′sənōjen′əsis\ [RADIO- + CARCINOGENESIS] The production of cancer by exposure to ionizing radiation. The types produced include tumors of the skin from exposure to x rays, carcinoma of the lung in miners exposed to radioactive ores, thyroid carcinoma in patients given irradiation for thymic enlargement, tumors of the reticuloendothelial system in patients given thorotrast, and different types of malignancy in survivors of nuclear bomb explosions. An increased risk of leukemia is also found in patients irradiated for ankylosing spondylitis.

**radiocardiography** \-kär′dē·äg′rəfē\ RADIONUCLIDE CARDIOGRAPHY.

**radiocarpal** \-kär′pəl\ **1** Pertaining to the radius and the carpus. Also *cubitocarpal.* **2** On the lateral side of the carpus.

**radiocarpus** \-kär′pəs\ *Outmoded* MUSCULUS FLEXOR CARPI RADIALIS.

**radiocobalt** \-kō′bôlt\ RADIOACTIVE COBALT.

**radiocolloid** \-käl′oid\ **1** A grouping of radioactive atoms in colloidal form. **2** A colloid whose particles carry a radioactive tag, such as technetium-tagged sulfur colloid.

**radiode** \rā′dē·ōd\ A sealed radium source in a thin-walled, usually metal, tube, and normally placed in another container such as a tube or a needle.

**radiodense** \-dens′\ [RADIO- + *dense*] Radiopaque at the usual diagnostic range of energies.

**radiodensity** \-den′sitē\ The degree to which something is radiolucent or radiopaque.

**radiodermatitis** \-dur′məti′tis\ RADIATION DERMATITIS.

**radiodigital** \-dij′ital\ **1** Pertaining to the radius and the fingers. **2** Pertaining to the fingers on the lateral side of the hand.

**radiodosimetry** \-dōsim′ətrē\ [RADIO- + DOSIMETRY] Measurement of radiation dose deposited by x rays or gamma radiation.

**radioelement** Any radioactive element, whether artificial or natural.

**radioepithelioma** \-ep′ithē′lē·ō′mə\ [RADIO- + EPITHELIOMA] Carcinoma secondary to exposure to elevated or repeated doses of ionizing radiation.

**radiogallium** \-gal′ē·əm\ Any of the 14 radioactive isotopes of gallium, ranging in half-life from 37 milliseconds to 68.2 months.

**radiogold** \rā′dē·ōgōld′\ RADIOACTIVE GOLD.

**radiograph** \rā′dē·əgraf′\ [RADIO- + -GRAPH] A processed film obtained during radiography. Also *roentgenograph, roentgenogram.* **bite-wing r.** A radiograph of the crowns of antagonistic teeth, taken on a bite-wing film to show approximal caries and other interdental features. Also *bite-wing film.* **cephalometric r.** A radiograph of the skull taken with a standardized technique so that mensural comparisons can be made concerning growth. **extraoral r.** An oral radiograph made with the film placed externally. **intraoral r.** An oral radiograph made with film placed in the mouth. **occlusal r.** An intraoral radiograph made with the film placed between the upper and lower teeth. Also *occlusal film.* **panoramic r.** A radiograph showing all the teeth and closely associated parts on one film as if the arches had been straightened into one plane. It is made either by having the source of x rays in the mouth and an extraoral film that is curved to fit the face, or by an orbiting panoramic apparatus. Also *panoramic x-ray film.* **periapical r.** An intraoral radiograph of the whole of a tooth and the adjacent bone. Also *periapical film.* **survey r.** SCOUT FILM. **Towne projection r.** See under TOWNE PROJECTION.

**radiography** \rā′dē·äg′rəfē\ [RADIO- + -GRAPHY] The recording on film of images produced by x rays. Also *roentgenography, röntgenography.* **body section r.** BODY SECTION ROENTGENOGRAPHY. **sectional r.** BODY SECTION ROENTGENOGRAPHY.

**radioimmunoassay** \-im′yənō·as′ā\ [RADIO- + IMMUNO- + ASSAY] Any assay procedure that employs an immune reaction, in which either the antigen or the antibody is labeled with a radionuclide to permit accurate quantification. Also *immunoradiometric assay.*

**radioimmunodiffusion** \-im′yənōdifyoo′zhən\ A method of enhancing the sensitivity of immunodiffusion by using a radiolabeled antigen or antibody, followed by autoradiographic visualization of the precipitin line.

**radioimmunoelectrophoresis** \-im′yənō·ilek′trōfôrē′sis\ A technique for separating, identifying, and roughly quantifying radiolabeled proteins by immunoelectrophoretic separation and precipitation, combined with autoradiographic visualization of the precipitin lines. Either the proteins or the antibody may be radiolabeled. The technique's usual use is the study of proteins labeled with $^{14}C$ or $^{3}H$ during cellular biosynthesis.

**radioimmunoprecipitation** \-im′yənōprisip′ətā′shn\ A precipitation technique based on the antibody-antigen reaction, in which sensitivity is enhanced by the use of a radiolabeled antigen or antibody, followed by the autoradiographic visualization of the precipitin line.

**radioindicator** \-in′dikā′tər\ [RADIO- + INDICATOR] A radioactive nuclide used as a label, which, when detected and measured with the appropriate instrument, evaluates the concentration or presence of the tracer *in vivo* or *in vitro.*

**radioiodinated** \-ī′ədinā′tid\ Labeled with any of the radioactive forms of iodine.

**radioiodine** \-ī′ədīn\ RADIOACTIVE IODINE.

**radioisotope** \-ī′sətōp\ *Incorrect* RADIONUCLIDE.

**radiolead** \rā′dē·ōled′\ RADIOACTIVE LEAD.

**radioligand** \-lig′and\ A radioactive ligand.

**radiologist** \rā′dē·äl′əjist\ A physician who has received special training to qualify as a specialist in the practice of radiology.

**radiology** \rā′dē·äl′əjē\ [RADIO- + -LOGY] The medical specialty dealing with the use of radiant energy for diagnosis and treatment. **nuclear r.** NUCLEAR MEDICINE.

**radiolucent** \-loo′sənt\ [RADIO- + LUCENT] Allowing the passage of radiant energy, such as x rays, to a varying extent depending on the nature of the object. In radiology, the differences in radiolucency are recorded on a film or displayed on a fluoroscopic screen. Also *lucent, translucent* (seldom used), *roentgenoparent.*

**radiolus** \rādē′ələs\ A sound or probe.

**radiolysis** \rā′dē·äl′isis\ [RADIO- + LYSIS] Chemical decomposition caused by radiation.

**radiomicrometer** \-mī′kräm′ətər\ An apparatus for measuring very small changes in the amount of radiant energy.

**radiomuscular** \-mus′kyələr\ Pertaining to the radius and the surrounding muscles, especially with reference to muscular branches of the radial nerve and artery. *Seldom used.*

**radiomutation** \-myootā′shən\ [RADIO- + MUTATION] A permanent change in a characteristic of a cell caused by radiation, transmissible from parent to offspring.

**radionecrosis** \-nekrō′sis\ Tissue death resulting from a large dose of ionizing radiation.

**radionephrography** \-nefräg′rəfē\ [RADIO- + NEPHROGRAPHY ] RADIORENOGRAPHY.

**radioneuritis** \-n^y^ŏŏrī′tis\ [RADIO- + NEURITIS] Inflammation of a nerve or nerves secondary to exposure to radiant energy.

**radionuclide** \-n^y^oo′klīd\ A nuclide that spontaneously exhibits radioactive decay; a radioactive nuclear species. Also *radioactive nuclide, unstable nuclide, radioactive isotope* (incorrect), *radioisotope* (incorrect). **metastable r.** A radionuclide that remains in an excited state for an appreciable time before decaying by isomeric transition. Such a radionuclide is indicated by adding m to the mass number, as in Tc 99m. **parent r.** The radionuclide, usually long-lived, that continually produces a short-lived daughter by radioactive decay.

**radiopalmar** \-pal′mər\ **1** Pertaining to the radial side of the palm. **2** Pertaining to the radius or radial artery and the palm.

**radiopaque** \-pāk′\ [*radi(o)-* + OPAQUE] Relatively impervious to x rays or other radiation, the absorbed radiation producing an image, as on a radiograph or fluoroscope. Also *roentgenopaque.*

**radiopharmaceutical** \-fär′məsoo′tikəl\ [RADIO- + PHARMACEUTICAL] A drug or other administrable agent that is tagged with a radionuclide so that its course can be traced, measured, or imaged.

**radiopharmacology** \-fär′məkäl′əjē\ The study of the development, production, use, and biologic fate of radiopharmaceuticals.

**radioplastic** \-plas′tik\ Designating a method for making a plaster cast of an organ from fluoroscopic images.

**radiopotentiation** \-pəten′chē·ā′shən\ The capacity of a drug or other agent to potentiate or enhance the desired effects of irradiation, either clinically or experimentally.

**radioreaction** \-rē·ak′shən\ [RADIO- + REACTION] A reaction to ionizing radiation, especially one involving the skin.

**radiorenography** \-rēnäg′rəfē\ [RADIO- + RENOGRAPHY] A technique for evaluation of renal function, consisting of the intravenous injection of I-131 orthoiodohippurate, an iodinated analog of *p*-aminohippurate, and the placement of an external detector over the region of each kidney and over the lumbar region for the measurement of the passage of radioactivity into and out of the kidneys. In the normal tracing, an initial sharp rise is followed by a more slowly rising second phase, and then by the disappearance of radioactivity from the kidney. The examination is useful in evaluating unilateral renal functional abnormalities. Also *emission renography, renography, radionephrography, isotope renography* (inaccurate), *isotope nephrography* (inaccurate).

**radioresistant** \-rizis′tənt\ [RADIO- + RESISTANT] Exhibiting little or no sensitivity to ionizing radiation.

**radioresponsive** \-rispän′siv\ Responding positively to radiotherapy.

**radiosensibility** \-sen′səbil′itē\ [RADIO- + SENSIBILITY] RADIOSENSITIVITY.

**radiosensitivity** \-sen′sətiv′itē\ [RADIO- + SENSITIVITY] Responsiveness of cells, tissues, or organisms to ionizing radiation, or their susceptibility to damage from it. Also *radiosensibility, radiosensitiveness.*

**radiosodium** \-sō′dē·əm\ RADIOACTIVE SODIUM.

**radiospirometry** \-spīräm′ətrē\ A method of investigating regional pulmonary function, permitting evaluation, zone by zone, of pulmonary ventilation and circulation. The examination consists of the injection of a radionuclide by catheter, directly into the superior vena cava or right atrium, or into a peripheral vein, or by the inhalation of a radioactive gas, and detection with a suitable scintillation counter of radioactivity per unit time in various pulmonary regions. The most commonly utilized radioactive gas is xenon (Xe 133).

**radiostereoassay** \-stir′ē·ō·as′ā\ A radioreceptor assay in which the tertiary protein structure and specific complementary orientation of ligand and receptor are critical for the *in vitro* interaction of the indicator and the analyte.

**radiostereoscopy** \-stir′e·äs′kəpē\ [RADIO- + STEREO- + -SCOPY] The viewing by a special apparatus of the paired roentgenograms produced by stereoroentgenography to afford a three-dimensional appearance of the object or patient area examined. Also *actinostereoscopy* (obs.).

**radiosulfur** \-sul′fər\ Any of the six radioactive isotopes of sulfur, especially sulfur 35. All decay by beta emission or annihilation radiation. Also *radioactive sulfur.*

**radiosurgery** \-sur′jərē\ Any surgical procedure in which radium or another source of high energy radiation is used.

**radiotelemetry** \-telem′ətrē\ The transmission of data by radio to a remote location. See also BIOTELEMETRY.

**radiotherapeutics** \-ther′əpyoo′tiks\ [RADIO- + THERAPEUTICS] The science of the theory and use of ionizing radiations for the treatment of disease.

**radiotherapist** \-ther′əpist\ A physician specializing in radiotherapy.

**radiotherapy** \-ther′əpē\ [RADIO- + THERAPY] The use of ionizing radiation for therapeutic purposes. Also *x-ray therapy, roentgenotherapy, roentgentherapy.* **arc r.** A type of moving radiotherapy in which the angle of movement of the beam is fixed in relation to the patient, as in a pendulum. **contact r.** Roentgen therapy with low voltage x rays and short source-skin distances, so that the x-ray tube is usually in contact with the surface of the patient. This technique is used particularly in dermatology and in the treatment of small tumors which are not very thick and easily accessible, as those in the skin, mouth, rectum, or vagina. Also *contact therapy, contact radiation therapy.* **fast neutron r.** Radiation treatment with a beam of neutrons having energies greater than 1 MeV. **interstitial r.** INTERSTITIAL RADIATION THERAPY. **intracavitary r.** Radiation therapy with the introduction of a radioactive substance or source into a natural cavity of the body. Also *intracavitary irradiation, intracavitary application brachytherapy.* **supervoltage r.** Treatment with x rays produced at energies greater than 1 MeV, or with gamma rays having photon energies greater than 1 MeV. Also *megavoltage radiotherapy, megavoltage therapy, supervoltage therapy.* **whole-body r.** Treatment by x rays or by other ionizing radiations whose source is placed at a great enough distance from the body that the totality of its surface is irradiated. Also *whole-body teleroentgentherapy.*

**radiothermy** \-thur′mē\ Radiant heating, especially as used for therapeutic purposes; diathermy. *Rare.*

**radiothyroxine** \-thīräk′sēn\ RADIOACTIVE THYROXINE.

**radiotoxemia** \-täksē′mē·ə\ [RADIO- + TOXEMIA] RADIATION SICKNESS.

**radiotracer** RADIOACTIVE TRACER.

**radium** \rā′dē·əm\ A naturally occurring radioactive element, having atomic number 88, atomic weight 226, and physical half-life 1620 years. It is a member of the radioactive series which starts with uranium 238, and thus is present wherever uranium is found. Radium has many isotopes, all radioactive. It decays into radon, a radioactive gas, followed by a series of radionuclides which together emit alpha, beta, and gamma rays. Once widely used in radiation therapy, it has been largely replaced by cesium 137 and other radionuclides. Symbol: Ra

**radium F** POLONIUM. Symbol: RaF

**radius** \rā′dē·əs\ [L, a ray, radius, spoke] (*pl.* radii) 1 [NA] The lateral bone of the forearm. It has a rounded head, a constricted neck, a shaft curved convex laterally, and an expanded distal end. It articulates proximally with the capitulum of the humerus, medially with the ulna, and distally with the scaphoid and lunate bones. Also *radial bone, spoke bone.* 2 Any straight line from the center of a circle to the periphery. **r. curvus** MADELUNG'S DEFORMITY. **r. fixus** A line drawn from the hormion to the inion of the skull. **radii lentis** [NA] Six or more faint lines or sutures representing the arrangement of lens fibers on the anterior and posterior surfaces of the lens of the eye and radiating from the poles towards the equator. Also *radii of lens, lens sutures, lens star.* **van der Waals r.** Half of the distance between the nuclei of two electrically neutral atoms when the van der Waals forces are exactly balanced by the repulsive forces. This presents a useful way of describing the physical size of the atoms.

**radix** \rā′diks\ [L, a root] (*pl.* radices) The attachment by which a structure is fixed at its base or proximal end; the root, as of a hair, nail, tooth, or nerve. **r. anterior nervorum spinalium** RADIX VENTRALIS NERVORUM SPINALIUM. **r. brevis ganglii ciliaris** RADIX OCULOMOTORIA GANGLII CILIARIS. **r. cochlearis nervi acustici** RADIX INFERIOR NERVI VESTIBULOCOCHLEARIS. **radices craniales nervi accessorii** [NA] Fibers arising from the lower end of the nucleus ambiguus, emerging as delicate rootlets from the medulla oblongata, and joining the spinal roots of the accessory nerve and filaments of the superior ganglion of the vagus nerve. Fibers are distributed, principally with the pharyngeal and recurrent laryngeal branches of the vagus nerve, to a number of muscles, among which are the musculus uvulae, levator veli palati, and the pharyngeal constrictors. Also *ramus internus nervi accessorii, internal ramus of accessory nerve, vagal accessory nerve, cranial part of accessory nerve, cranial roots of accessory nerve.* **r. dentis** [NA] ANATOMIC ROOT. **r. descendens mesencephalica nervi trigemini** TRACTUS MESENCEPHALICUS NERVI TRIGEMINI. **r. dorsalis nervorum spinalium** [NA] A dorsal nerve root of the spine containing processes of sensory neurons from its corresponding spinal ganglion. These processes project medially into the spinal cord and, laterally, they join ventral roots to form spinal nerves. Also *dorsal root of spinal nerves, posterior root of spinal nerves, sensory root of spinal nerves, dorsal root.* **r. inferior ansae cervicalis** [NA] A nerve root formed by the union of branches from the second and third cervical nerves. It lies lateral to the internal jugular vein, joins with the superior root to form the ansa cervicalis, and supplies motor innervation to the infrahyoid muscles. Also *nervus descendens cervicalis, inferior root of ansa cervicalis, descending cervical nerve, descendens cervicalis.* **r. inferior nervi vestibulocochlearis** [NA] Cochlear fibers arising from bipolar cells in the spiral ganglion and projecting peripherally to the organ of Corti and centrally to the cochlear nuclei. Also *radix cochlearis nervi acustici, cochlear root of acoustic nerve, inferior root of vestibulocochlear nerve, cochlear nerve.* **r. lateralis nervi mediani** [NA] A nerve root arising from the lateral cord of the brachial plexus and containing ventral divisions of anterior primary rami of the fifth, sixth, and seventh cervical nerves. Also *lateral root of median nerve.* **r. lateralis tractus optici** [NA] Afferent fibers that arise in the retina, undergo partial decussation in the optic chiasm, and terminate in the lateral geniculate nucleus. Also *lateral root of optic tract.* **r. linguae** [NA] The posterior surface of the tongue behind the sulcus terminalis, forming the anterior wall of the oropharynx. It is attached inferiorly to the hyoid bone and the mandible. Its covering mucous membrane is devoid of papillae and is continuous laterally with the palatine tonsils and the pharyngeal wall and posteriorly with the epiglottic folds. Also *root of tongue.* **r. longa ganglii ciliaris** RAMUS COMMUNICANS GANGLII CILIARIS CUM NERVO NASOCILIARI. **r. medialis nervi mediani** [NA] A nerve root arising from the medial cord of the brachial plexus and containing ventral divisions of anterior primary rami of the .eighth cervical and first thoracic nerves. Also *medial root of median nerve.* **r. medialis tractus optici** [NA] A nerve root situated medially in the optic tract and containing supraoptic commissural fibers. Also *medial root of optic tract.* **r. mesencephalica nervi trigemini** TRACTUS MESENCEPHALICUS NERVI TRIGEMINI. **r. mesenterii** [NA] The firm attachment of the mesentery of the jejunum and ileum to the posterior abdominal wall extending obliquely and downward from the duodenojejunal flexure on the left of the second lumbar vertebra to the ileocolic junction in the right iliac fossa. It runs anterior to the third part of the duodenum, the inferior vena cava, the right psoas major muscle, the right ureter and the right testicular or ovarian vessels. Also *root of mesentery.* **radices molles ganglii ciliaris** RAMUS SYMPATHICUS AD GANGLION CILIARE. **r. motoria nervi trigemini** [NA] A nerve bundle consisting of fibers arising in the motor nucleus of the trigeminal nerve along with some proprioceptive fibers. It exits the pons medial and anterior to the larger sensory root, and its motor fibers are distributed in the mandibular nerve. Also *portio minor nervi trigemini* (outmoded), *motor root of trigeminal nerve, nervus masticatorius.* **r. nasi** [NA] The site of continuity of the upper angle of the external nose with the forehead between the eyes. Also *root of nose.* **r. nervi facialis** A nerve root containing motor fibers and arising in the facial nucleus, exiting from the ventral surface of the pons, and supplying the muscles of facial expression (the stapedius, stylohyoid, and posterior digastric). Also *root of facial nerve.* **radices nervi spinales** Collectively the dorsal and ventral roots of single segments of the spinal cord or of multiple segments. Also *spinal nerve roots.* See also RADIX DORSALIS NERVORUM SPINALIUM, RADIX VENTRALIS NERVORUM SPINALIUM. **radices nervi trigemini** Roots of the trigeminal nerve, consisting of a large sensory and a small motor root. The sensory root contains central processes of cells in the trigeminal ganglion, and the motor root contains axons of cells in the motor nucleus of the trigeminal nerve. **r. oculomotoria ganglii ciliaris** [NA] Preganglionic parasympathetic filaments that emerge from the inferior division of the oculomotor nerve, relay in the ciliary ganglion, and innervate the ciliary and pupillary sphincter muscles. Also *radix brevis ganglii ciliaris, short root of ciliary ganglion, oculomotor root of ciliary ganglion, motor root of ciliary ganglion.* **r. penis** [NA] The two crura and the bulb by which the penis is firmly attached to the borders of the pubic arch and the perineal membrane, respectively. Also *root of penis, penile root.* **r. pili** [NA] The proximal portion of a hair that is implanted in the skin and embedded in the hair follicle, the tip forming the bulbus pili. Also *root of hair.* **r. pulmonis** [NA] The root of the lung, connecting the hilum of the lung to the heart and trachea. It comprises the primary bronchus, pulmonary and bronchial blood vessels, pulmonary nerve plexus, bronchopulmonary lymph nodes and vessels, all of which are surrounded by pleura. Also *root of lung.* **r. sensoria nervi trigemini** [NA] A sensory fiber bundle consisting of the central branches of the unipolar cells of the trigeminal ganglion that run medially below the tentorium cerebelli and enter the pons to relay in the principal sensory, spinal, and mesencephalic nuclei of the trigeminal nerve. Also *portio major nervi trigemini* (outmoded), *sensory root of trigeminal nerve.* **radices spinales nervi accessorii** [NA] Fibers that arise from motor neurons in the ventral horn of the cervical spinal cord, ascend as a trunk in the vertebral canal, enter the skull through the foramen magnum, and join the cranial roots in the foramen magnum. These fibers supply motor innervation to the sternocleidomastoid and trapezius muscles. Also *spinal roots of accessory nerve.* **r. superior ansae cervicalis** [NA] A nerve bundle containing anterior primary divisions of the first cervical nerves. It accompanies the hypoglossal nerve, joins the ansa cervicalis, and innervates the infrahyoid and geniohyoid muscles. Also *ramus descendens nervi hypoglossi, superior root of ansa cervicalis.* **r. superior nervi vestibulocochlearis** [NA] The superior, vestibular portion of cranial nerve VIII, or the nerve of equilibrium, consisting of fibers arising from cells of the vestibular ganglion. It enters the brainstem superomedial to the cochlear nerve and passes to the vestibular nuclear complex and cerebellum. Also *radix vestibularis nervi acustici, superior root of vestibulocochlear nerve, vestibular root of auditory nerve, vestibular root of acoustic nerve, vestibular branch of eighth nerve.* **radices sympathicae ganglii ciliaris** [NA] RAMUS SYMPATHICUS AD GANGLION CILIARE. **r. sympathica ganglii submaxillaris** RAMUS SYMPATHICUS AD GANGLION SUBMANDIBULARE. **r. unguis** [NA] The smaller, proximal region of a nail that is covered by the nail fold. Deep to it the germinative zone of the nail bed is thicker, proliferative and involved with growth of the nail. Also *root of nail, base of nail.* **r. ventralis nervorum spinalium** [NA] A root of spinal nerves containing axons of motor neurons and located in the ventral horns. At thoracolumbar and midsacral levels they also contain axons of preganglionic autonomic neurons found in the intermediolateral gray columns. The ventral roots join with the dorsal sensory roots to form the spinal nerves. Also *radix anterior nervorum spinalium, ventral root of spinal nerves, anterior root of spinal nerves, motor root of spinal nerves, ventral root, motor root, ventral nerve root of spinal nerves.* **r. vestibularis nervi acustici** RADIX SUPERIOR NERVI VESTIBULOCOCHLEARIS.

**radon** \rā′dän\ Element number 86, having an atomic weight of approximately 222 and a half-life of 3.83 days. Radon is the heaviest known gas, essentially inert chemically. It is the daughter of radium 226 by alpha decay. Twenty isotopes are known, all of them short-lived emitters of alpha particles giving rise to solid, unstable daughters. The natural isotopes are formed as decay products in the three series of naturally occurring radioactive elements, and radon is consequently present in minute amounts in the atmosphere. The 17 other isotopes of radon have half-lives ranging down to microseconds and mass numbers from 204 to 224. The build-up of emanations in mines and storage areas for mine tailings, ores, concentrates, and the like, is a health hazard intensified by the solid decay products which become attached to dust particles and motes in the air. Radon is packaged for therapeutic use in minute tubes, or seeds, which are implanted into certain types of tumors. Also *radium emanation.* Symbol: Rn • See note at EMANATION.

**radon 219** ACTINON.

**Radovici** [J. *Radovici,* French physician, born 1868] Radovici sign. See under PALMOMENTAL REFLEX.

**RAEB** refractory anemia with excess blasts.

**Raeder** [Johan Georg *Raeder,* Norwegian ophthalmologist, 1889–1956] Raeder syndrome. See under RAEDER'S PARATRIGEMINAL SYNDROME.

**ragocyte** \rā′gōsīt\ [*r(hematoid) a(rthritis)* + *(Ig)G* + *o* + -CYTE] A specialized cell, usually seen in cases of rheumatoid arthritis, in which polymorphonuclear leukocytes have ingested abnormal protein substances such as IgG, fibrin, and rheumatoid factor.

**Raimist** [J. M. *Raimist,* German psychiatrist, flourished 20th century] See under SIGN.

**rain / acid r.** Rain or other aqueous precipitation having a lowered pH, resulting mainly from industrial air pollution. It has had important ecological effects in countries such as Norway and Sweden where forest trees have been damaged and aquatic life in lakes and streams killed, and its effects are being widely monitored and studied elsewhere as well.

**rale** \ral\ [French *râle* (from *râler* to make a rattling sound in the throat, variant of *racler* to scrape, from Vulgar L *rasclare,* from L *radere* to scrape, shave) a rattling breath sound] An abnormal sound heard on auscultation of the chest during breathing, especially one that is caused, or seems to be caused, by air passing through fluid in the airways. Compare RHONCHUS. **atelectatic r.** A transient abnormal respiratory sound heard on auscultation, especially at the margins of the lungs, which often disappears after coughing. Also *border rale, marginal rale.* **consonating r.** A loud moist rale heard when the sound is conducted through consolidated lung. Also *metallic rale.* **crepitant r.** A fine, high-pitched rale. Also *crackling rale, vesicular rale.* **dry r.** *Outmoded* RHONCHUS. **laryngeal r.** A rale heard on auscultation of the lungs which originates in the larynx. **marginal r.** ATELECTATIC RALE. **metallic r.** CONSONATING RALE. **moist r.** A rale believed, erroneously, in the past, to be caused by air bubbling through fluid in small airways. **sibilant r.** SIBILANT RHONCHUS. **vesicular r.** CREPITANT RALE. **whistling r.** SIBILANT RHONCHUS.

**ramal** \rā′məl\ Pertaining to a ramus.

**ramex** \rā′meks\ [L, rupture] **1** A weakness in the abdominal wall or internal body cavity producing a hernia. **2** VARICOCELE.

**rami** \rā′mī\ Plural of RAMUS.

**ramicotomy** \ram′ikät′əmē\ RAMISECTOMY.

**ramification** \ram′ifikā′shən\ **1** A process or system of branching. **2** A branch, as of a nerve or vessel.

**ramiform** \ram′ifôrm\ Having the form or appearance of a branch.

**ramify** \ram′ifī\ To branch.

**ramisectomy** \ram′isek′təmē\ [*ram(us)* + *i* + L *sec(tio)* a cutting, division + -TOMY] Division of a ramus. Also *ramicotomy, ramisection.*

**ramitis** \ramī′tis\ [L *ram(us)* branch, bough + -ITIS] Inflammation of a nerve branch, or ramus.

**Ramon** [Gaston *Ramon,* French bacteriologist, 1886–1963] Anatoxin-Ramon. See under DIPHTHERIA TOXOID.

**Ramond** [Louis Jean Justin *Ramond,* French physician, 1879–1952] See under POINT.

**ramose** \rā′mōs\ **1** Branched or branching; having several branches. **2** Resembling a branch.

**rampart** \ram′pärt\ **maxillary r.** A thickening of the epithelium on the part of the maxillary process which becomes the gum of the upper jaw.

**Ramsay Hunt** See under HUNT.

**Ramstedt** [Conrad *Ramstedt,* German surgeon, 1867–1963] Ramstedt operation, Fredet-Ramstedt operation. See under PYLOROMYOTOMY.

**ramulus** \ram′yələs\ A minute branch; one of the terminal branches of a ramus.

# ramus

**ramus** \rā′məs\ [L (akin to *radix* a root) a branch, bough] (*pl.* rami) An offshoot or subdivision arising from the bifurcation of a blood vessel, lymph vessel, or nerve. Also *branch.* **r. acetabularis arteriae circumflexae femoris medialis** [NA] A branch of the medial circumflex femoral artery that runs from the upper border of adductor brevis muscle to the hip joint which it enters deep to the transverse ligament of the acetabulum to supply the fat in the fossa and the head of the femur. Also *acetabular branch of medial circumflex femoral artery, acetabular artery, artery of round ligament of hip joint.* **r. acetabularis arteriae obturatoriae** [NA] A branch of the posterior branch of the obturator artery that enters the hip joint deep to the transverse ligament of the acetabulum to supply the fat of the acetabular fossa and the head of the femur. Also *acetabular branch of obturator artery, acetabular artery.* **r. acromialis arteriae suprascapularis** [NA] A branch given off by the suprascapular artery as it crosses the superior transverse ligament of the scapula. It pierces the trapezius muscle to supply the skin over the acromion. Also *acromial branch of suprascapular artery.* **r. acromialis arteriae thoracoacromialis** [NA] A branch of the thoracoacromial artery that runs laterally over the coracoid process and deep to the deltoid muscle which it supplies and pierces to reach the acromion. Also *acromial branch of thoracoacromial artery.* **rami ad pontem arteriae basilaris** [NA] Pontine branches of the basilary artery; numerous small vessels that supply the pons. **rami alveolares superiores anteriores nervi infraorbitalis** [NA] Anterior superior alveolar branches of the infraorbital nerve, consisting of sensory and autonomic fibers to the canines, incisors, and surrounding soft tissues of the premaxilla. Also *rami dentales superiores anteriores nervi infraorbitalis, anterior superior alveolar nerves.* **rami alveolares superiores posteriores nervi maxillaris** [NA] Posterior superior branches of the alveolar nerve, consisting of general somatic afferent components supplying the upper jaw. They form part of the superior dental plexus. Also *rami dentales superiores posteriores nervi maxillaris.* **r. alveolaris superior medius nervi infraorbitalis** [NA] The middle superior alveolar branch of the infraorbital nerve, consisting of sensory and autonomic fibers to the maxillary premolars and adjacent soft tissues. Also *ramus dentalis superior medius nervi infraorbitalis, middle alveolar nerve.* **rami anastomotici ganglii otici cum nervo auriculotemporali** RAMI COMMUNICANTES GANGLII OTICI CUM NERVO AURICULOTEMPORALI. **rami anastomotici ganglii submandibularis cum nervo linguali** RAMI COMMUNICANTES GANGLII SUBMANDIBULARIS CUM NERVO LINGUALI. **rami anastomotici ganglii submaxillaris cum nervo linguali** RAMI COMMUNICANTES GANGLII SUBMANDIBULARIS CUM NERVO LINGUALI. **rami anastomotici nervi auriculotemporalis cum nervo faciali** RAMI COMMUNICANTES NERVI AURICULOTEMPORALIS CUM NERVO FACIALI. **rami anastomotici nervi lingualis cum nervo hypoglosso** RAMI COMMUNICANTES NERVI LINGUALIS CUM NERVO HYPOGLOSSO. **r. anastomoticus** RAMUS COMMUNICANS. **r. anastomoticus arteriae meningeae mediae cum arteria lacrimali** [NA] A branch given off by the middle meningeal artery in the cranial cavity where it runs anteriorly to the superior orbital fissure, through which it enters the orbit and anastomoses with the recurrent meningeal branch of the lacrimal artery. **r. anastomoticus ganglii ciliaris cum nervo nasociliari** RAMUS COMMUNICANS GANGLII CILIARIS CUM NERVO NASOCILIARI. **r. anastomoticus ganglii otici cum chorda tympani** RAMUS COMMUNICANS GANGLII OTICI CUM CHORDA TYMPANI. **r. anastomoticus ganglii otici cum nervo auriculotemporali** RAMUS COMMUNICANS GANGLII OTICI CUM NERVO AURICULOTEMPORALI. **r. anastomoticus ganglii otici cum ramo meningeo nervi mandibularis** RAMUS COMMUNICANS GANGLII OTICI CUM RAMO MENINGEO NERVI MANDIBULARIS. **r. anastomoticus nervi facialis cum nervo auriculari magno** RAMUS COMMUNICANS NERVI FACIALIS CUM NERVO AURICULARI MAGNO. **r. anastomoticus nervi facialis cum nervo auriculotemporali** RAMUS COMMUNICANS NERVI FACIALIS CUM NERVO AURICULOTEMPORALI. **r. anastomoticus nervi facialis cum nervo glossopharyngeo** RAMUS COMMUNICANS NERVI FACIALIS CUM NERVO GLOSSOPHARYNGEO. **r. anastomoticus nervi facialis cum nervo occipitali minore** RAMUS COMMUNICANS NERVI FACIALIS CUM NERVO OCCIPITALI MINORE. **r. anastomoticus nervi facialis cum nervo transverso colli** RAMUS COMMUNICANS NERVI FACIALIS CUM NERVO TRANSVERSO COLLI. **r. anastomoticus nervi facialis cum nervo vestibulocochleari** RAMUS COMMUNICANS NERVI FACIALIS CUM NERVO VESTIBULOCOCHLEARI. **r. anastomoticus nervi facialis cum plexu sympathetico** RAMUS COMMUNICANS NERVI FACIALIS CUM PLEXU SYMPATHETICO. **r. anastomoticus nervi facialis cum plexu tympanico** RAMUS COMMUNICANS NERVI FACIALIS CUM PLEXU TYMPANICO. **r. anastomoticus nervi facialis cum ramo auriculari nervi vagi** RAMUS COMMUNICANS NERVI FACIALIS CUM RAMO AURICULARI NERVI VAGI. **r. anastomoticus nervi facialis cum ramo petrosali nervi glossopharyngei** RAMUS COMMUNICANS NERVI FACIALIS CUM RAMO PETROSALI NERVI GLOSSOPHARYNGEI. **r. anastomoticus nervi glossopharyngei cum ramo auriculari nervi vagi** RAMUS COMMUNICANS NERVI GLOSSOPHARYNGEI CUM RAMO AURICULARI NERVI VAGI. **r. anastomoticus nervi lacrimalis cum nervo zygomatico** RAMUS COMMUNICANS NERVI LACRIMALIS CUM NERVO ZYGOMATICO. **r. anastomoticus nervi laryngei inferioris cum ramo**

**laryngeo interno** RAMUS COMMUNICANS NERVI LARYNGEI INFERIORIS CUM RAMO LARYNGEO INTERNO. **r. anastomoticus nervi laryngei recurrentis cum ramo laryngeo interno** RAMUS COMMUNICANS NERVI LARYNGEI INFERIORIS CUM RAMO LARYNGEO INTERNO. **r. anastomoticus nervi laryngei superioris cum nervo laryngeo inferiore** RAMUS COMMUNICANS NERVI LARYNGEI SUPERIORIS CUM NERVO LARYNGEO INFERIORE. **r. anastomoticus nervi lingualis cum chorda tympani** RAMUS COMMUNICANS NERVI LINGUALIS CUM CHORDA TYMPANI. **r. anastomoticus nervi mediani cum nervo ulnari** RAMUS COMMUNICANS NERVI MEDIANI CUM NERVO ULNARI. **r. anastomoticus nervi vagi cum nervo glossopharyngeo** RAMUS COMMUNICANS NERVI VAGI CUM NERVO GLOSSOPHARYNGEO. **r. anastomoticus peroneus nervi peronei communis** RAMUS COMMUNICANS PERONEUS NERVI PERONEI COMMUNIS. **r. anastomoticus ulnaris nervi radialis** RAMUS COMMUNICANS ULNARIS NERVI RADIALIS. **r. anterior arteriae obturatoriae** [NA] The anterior division of the obturator artery, arising outside the pelvis at the upper margin of the obturator foramen and passing anteriorly on the obturator membrane and then down along the anterior edge of the foramen supplying the adductors, obturator externus, pectineus, and gracilis muscles and anastomosing with the medial circumflex femoral artery and the posterior branch of the obturator artery. Also *anterior branch of obturator artery.* **r. anterior arteriae pancreaticoduodenalis inferioris** [NA] An arterial branch that usually arises from the inferior pancreaticoduodenal artery at the upper margin of the horizontal part of the duodenum and runs to the right in front of the head of the pancreas. It ascends in the groove between the pancreas and the duodenum to anastomose with the anterior superior pancreaticoduodenal artery and supply the duodenum and the head and uncinate process of the pancreas. Also *left inferior pancreaticoduodenal artery* (outmoded). **r. anterior arteriae recurrentis ulnaris** [NA] A branch of the ulnar artery given off just below the front of the elbow joint, running proximally between the brachialis and pronator teres muscles, supplying them and anastomosing with the inferior ulnar collateral artery anterior to the medial epicondyle. Also *anterior branch of ulnar recurrent artery, anterior ulnar recurrent artery.* **r. anterior arteriae renalis** [NA] The branch of the renal artery given off in the region of the hilum of the kidney and dividing into four segmental arteries to the superior, anterior, and inferior vascular segments of the kidney. Also *anterior branch of renal artery.* **r. anterior arteriae thyroideae superioris** [NA] The branch of the superior thyroid artery that runs distally along the anterior border of each lobe of the thyroid gland and supplies its anterior surface, anastomosing along the upper margin of the isthmus with the branch of the opposite side. Also *anterior branch of superior thyroid artery.* **r. anterior ascendens fissurae cerebri lateralis Sylvii** RAMUS ASCENDENS SULCI LATERALIS CEREBRI. **r. anterior ductus hepatici dextri** [NA] The branch of the right hepatic duct that drains the anterior segment of the right lobe of the liver. **rami anteriores arteriarum intercostalium** The anterior branches of the intercostal arteries lying in the costal grooves and passing forward to anastomose with the intercostal branches of the internal thoracic arteries. **rami anteriores nervorum cervicalium** RAMI VENTRALES NERVORUM CERVICALIUM. **rami anteriores nervorum lumbalium** RAMI VENTRALES NERVORUM LUMBALIUM. **rami anteriores nervorum sacralium** Anterior branches of sacral spinal nerves, forming the sacral plexus on the posterior wall of the pelvic cavity in front of the piriformis. **rami anteriores nervorum thoracalium** RAMI VENTRALES NERVORUM THORACICORUM. **r. anterior horizontalis fissurae cerebri lateralis Sylvii** RAMUS ANTERIOR SULCI LATERALIS CEREBRI. **r. anterior nervi auricularis magni** [NA] The anterior branch of the great auricular nerve, conveying general sensation from the skin overlying the parotid gland. Also *auriculomastoid branch of superficial branches of cervical plexus* (outmoded). **r. anterior nervi coccygei** RAMUS VENTRALIS NERVI COCCYGEI. **r. anterior nervi cutanei antebrachii medialis** [NA] The anterior branch of the medial antebrachial cutaneous nerve, conveying general sensation from the front of the medial side of the forearm. Also *ramus volaris nervi cutanei antebrachii medialis.* **r. anterior nervi laryngei inferioris** Anterior branch of the inferior laryngeal nerve, one of two terminal branches innervating intrinsic muscles on the ventral part of the larynx. **r. anterior nervi obturatorii** [NA] The anterior branch of the obturator nerve, communicating with medial cutaneous and saphenous branches of the femoral nerve to form the subsartorial plexus, which supplies the skin on the medial side of the thigh and gives rise to motor branches to adductor longus and brevis, gracilis, and pectineus. **r. anterior nervorum spinalium** RAMUS VENTRALIS NERVORUM SPINALIUM. **anterior primary rami** RAMUS VENTRALIS NERVORUM SPINALIUM. **r. anterior rami dextri venae portae hepatis** [NA] A branch of the right branch of the portal vein that supplies the anterior segment of the right lobe of the liver. Also *anterior branch of right portal branch.* **r. anterior sulci lateralis cerebri** [NA] The anterior branch of the lateral cerebral sulcus, separating the triangular and orbital portions of the inferior frontal gyrus. Also *ramus anterior horizontalis fissurae cerebri lateralis Sylvii.* **rami articulares arteriae descendentis genicularis** [NA] Branches arising from either the descending genicular artery or its muscular branches to the vastus medialis and adductor magnus and anastomosing with the medial and the lateral superior genicular arteries and anterior tibial recurrent artery for the supply of the knee joint. Also *articular branches of descending genicular artery.* **rami articulares nervi mediani** Articular branches of the median nerve, arising near the elbow joint and supplying this joint and the proximal radioulnar joint. **rami articulares nervi ulnaris** Articular branches of the ulnar nerve, consisting of several small filaments that issue from the nerve as it lies between the medial epicondyle and the olecranon. They supply the elbow joint. **r. ascendens arteriae circumflexae femoris lateralis** [NA] A branch of the lateral circumflex femoral artery arising deep to the rectus femoris muscle and passing upwards along the intertrochanteric line deep to the tensor fasciae latae muscle to anastomose with the superior gluteal, deep circumflex iliac, and medial circumflex femoral arteries, supplying the greater trochanter and the neck and head of the femur. Also *ascending branch of lateral circumflex femoral artery.* **r. ascendens arteriae circumflexae femoris medialis** [NA] A branch arising from the medial circumflex femoral artery at the proximal border of adductor brevis muscle to supply the adductors, the gracilis and obturator externus muscles, and to anastomose with the obturator artery. Also *ascending branch of medial circumflex femoral artery.* **r. ascendens arteriae circumflexae iliacae profundae** [NA] A branch arising from the deep circumflex iliac artery at the anterior superior iliac spine and ascending between the transversus abdominis and internal oblique muscles to supply them and anastomose with inferior epigastric and lumbar arteries. Also *ascending branch of deep circumflex iliac artery.* **r. ascendens sulci lateralis cerebri** [NA] The ascending branch of the lateral cerebral sulcus, separating the opercular and triangular portions of the inferior frontal gyrus. Also *ramus anterior ascendens fissurae cerebri lateralis Sylvii.* **rami atriales** Branches of the right and left coronary arteries which supply the walls of the right and left atria of the heart, respectively. **rami auriculares anteriores arteriae temporalis superficialis** [NA] Branches of the superficial temporal artery supplying the anterior part of the auricle, the lobule, and the external acoustic meatus. Also *anterior auricular branches of superficial temporal artery, anterior auricular arteries.* **r. auricularis arteriae auricularis posterioris** [NA] A branch of the posterior auricular artery that runs upwards deep to the posterior auricular muscle to supply the cranial surface and part of the lateral surface of the auricle. Also *auricular branch of posterior auricular artery.* **r. auricularis arteriae occipitalis** [NA] The auricular branch of the occipital artery, a small vessel that arises from the occipital branch of the external carotid artery and supplies the back of the pinna of the external ear, anastomosing with the posterior auricular artery. Also *auricular branch of occipital artery.* **r. auricularis nervi auricularis posterioris** [NA] The auricular branch of the posterior auricular nerve which carries motor innervation to the auricularis posterior and intrinsic muscles of the auricle. **r. auricularis nervi vagi** [NA] The auricular branch of the vagus nerve, arising from the superior vagal ganglion and joining with filaments from the inferior glossopharyngeal ganglion. It exits the temporal bone via the tympanomastoid fissure and conveys sensation from the cranial part of the auricle, the floor of the external acoustic meatus, and the outer surface of the tympanic membrane. Also *Arnold's nerve, auricular nerve of vagus.* **r. basalis medialis arteriae pulmonalis dextrae** [NA] An artery that arises from the basal part of the right pulmonary artery and supplies the medial basal, or cardiac, bronchopulmonary segment (B VII) of the inferior lobe of the right lung. **r. basalis medialis arteriae pulmonalis sinistrae** [NA] An artery that arises from the basal part of the left pulmonary artery and supplies the medial basal, or cardiac, bronchopulmonary segment (B VII) of the inferior lobe of the left lung. **rami bronchiales anteriores nervi vagi** Anterior bronchial branches of the vagus nerve, consisting of two or three nerves that join with sympathetic filaments to form the anterior pulmonary plexus on the root of the lung. They supply autonomic and visceral afferent innervation to bronchi and pulmonary vessels. **rami bronchiales aortae thoracicae** [NA] Two branches arising from the front of the thoracic aorta, the upper branch opposite the fifth thoracic vertebra and the lower one below the left bronchus. They supply the bronchial tubes, the areolar tissue of the lungs, the bronchopulmonary lymph nodes, and the esophagus. A right bronchial artery arises from either the first aortic intercostal or the upper left bronchial artery. Also *bronchial branches of thoracic aorta, bronchial arteries.* **rami bronchiales arteriae thoracicae internae** [NA] Small branches, often absent, of the internal thoracic artery supplying the bronchi and the trachea. Also *bronchial branches of internal thoracic artery, anterior bronchial arteries.* **rami bronchiales nervi vagi** [NA] Bronchial branches of the vagus nerve, supplying parasympathetic and visceral afferent innervation to the bronchi and pulmonary vessels. They join sympathetic filaments to form the anterior and posterior pulmonary plexuses on the root of the lung. **rami bronchiales segmentorum** [NA] The branches of the segmental bronchi to the bronchopulmonary segments of the lungs. Also *intrasegmental bronchial branches.* **rami buccales nervi facialis** [NA] Buccal branches of the facial nerve, divided into superficial and deep branches and supplying the muscles below the orbit and around the mouth. **rami calcanei arteriae tibialis posterioris** [NA] Branches of the posterior tibial artery that supply skin and fat around the heel and tendo calcaneus. Also *calcaneal branches of posterior tibial artery, medial calcaneal arteries.* **rami calcanei laterales nervi suralis** [NA] Lateral calcaneal branches of the sural nerve, general sensory branches to the skin of the posterior surface of the leg and the lateral surface of the foot. **rami calcanei mediales nervi tibialis** [NA] Medial calcaneal branches of the tibial nerve, general sensory branches which supply the skin of the medial and inferior surfaces of the heel. Also *medial calcaneal branches of tibial nerve.* **rami calcanei ramorum malleolarium lateralium arteriae fibularis** [NA] Branches of the lateral malleolar branches of the peroneal artery that ramify on the lateral side of the heel, anastomosing with anterior lateral malleolar arteries and, on the back of the heel, with calcaneal branches of the posterior tibial artery. Also *calcaneal branches of lateral malleolar branches of peroneal artery, calcaneal branches of peroneal artery.* **r. calcarinus arteriae occipitalis medialis** [NA] A vessel which branches from the medialoccipital artery which in turn is a branch of the posterior cerebral artery. It supplies a portion of the medial surface of the occipital lobe in the region of the calcarine sulcus. Also *calcarine artery.* **rami capsulares arteriae renalis** Extrarenal branches of the renal artery supplying the renal capsule. Also *capsular arteries, adipose arteries of kidney.* **rami cardiaci cervicales inferiores nervi vagi** [NA] Inferior cervical cardiac branches of the vagus nerve, arising at the root of the neck, and joining the superficial cardiac plexus. They contain preganglionic parasympathetic and sensory fibers. Also *rami cardiaci inferiores nervi recurrentis.* **rami cardiaci cervicales superiores nervi vagi** [NA] Superior cervical cardiac branches of the vagus nerve, arising at the upper part of the neck and communicating with the cardiac sympathetic nerves. They consist of preganglionic parasympathetic and sensory fibers that end in the deep cardiac plexus. Also *rami cardiaci superiores, supreme cardiac nerves.* **rami cardiaci inferiores nervi recurrentis** RAMI CARDIACI CERVICALES INFERIORES NERVI VAGI. **rami cardiaci inferiores nervi vagi** RAMI CARDIACI THORACICI NERVI VAGI. **rami cardiaci superiores** RAMI CARDIACI CERVICALES SUPERIORES NERVI VAGI. **rami cardiaci thoracici nervi vagi** [NA] Thoracic cardiac branches of the vagus nerve, arising from the right vagus nerve and both recurrent laryngeal nerves and ending in the deep cardiac plexus. They contain preganglionic parasympathetic and visceral afferent fibers. Also *rami cardiaci inferiores nervi vagi.* **rami caroticotympanici arteriae carotidis internae** *Outmoded* ARTERIAE CAROTICOTYMPANICAE ARTERIAE CAROTIDIS INTERNAE. **r. carpalis dorsalis arteriae radialis** [NA] A branch arising from the radial artery deep to the extensor tendons of the thumb and running medially across the back of the carpus to help form the dorsal carpal arch. Also *dorsal carpal branch of radial artery.* **r. carpalis dorsalis arteriae ulnaris** [NA] A branch arising from the ulnar artery anteriorly and proximal to the pisiform bone and running dorsally deep to the tendon of flexor carpi ulnaris muscle and then laterally deep to the extensor tendons to help form the dorsal carpal arch. Also *dorsal carpal branch of ulnar artery.* **r. carpalis palmaris arteriae radialis** [NA] A branch arising from the radial artery at the distal border of pronator quadratus muscle and passing medially across the front of the carpus and behind the flexor tendons to help form the palmar carpal arch. Also *palmar carpal branch of radial artery, anterior transverse artery of wrist.* **r. carpalis palmaris arteriae ulnaris** [NA] A branch arising from the ulnar artery at the distal border of the pronator quadratus muscle and passing laterally in front of the carpus and deep to the flexor tendons to help form the palmar carpal arch. Also *palmar carpal branch of ulnar artery, anterior transverse artery of wrist.* **rami caudati** [NA] Branches of the transverse part of the left branch of the portal vein distributed to the caudate lobe before the left branch enters the left lobe of the liver. **rami celiaci nervi vagi** [NA] Celiac branches of the vagus nerve, terminal branches of the posterior vagus that follow the left gastric artery to the celiac plexus. They contain preganglionic parasympathetic and visceral afferent fibers. Also *rami coeliaci plexus gastrici posterioris, nervi celiaci, celiac nerves, ansa of Wrisberg.* **rami centrales anterolaterales arteriae cerebri mediae** Anterolateral central branches of the middle cerebral artery. These branches consist of medial and lateral rami that arise from the sphenoid part of the middle cerebral artery. The medial rami supply the globus pallidus, caudate nucleus, and internal capsule. The lateral rami supply the putamen, internal capsule, and caudate nucleus. Also *rami lenticulostriatae arteriae cerebri mediae, lenticulostriate branches of middle cerebral artery, rami centrales arteriae cerebri mediae.* **rami centrales arteriae cerebri anterioris** [NA] Central branches of the anterior cerebral artery, a group of important vessels that arise mostly from the precommunical part of the anterior cerebral artery and include short medial and lateral central arteries as well as a long central artery or arteries. Some of these supply the optic chiasma, but most supply the anterior hypothalamus and other basal forebrain structures. **rami centrales arteriae cerebri mediae** RAMI CENTRALES ANTEROLATERALES ARTERIAE CEREBRI MEDIAE. **rami centrales arteriae cerebri posterioris** Central branches of the posterior cerebral artery. These vessels include central posteromedial and central posterolateral branches, the latter dividing into thalamic, medial posterior choroid, lateral posterior choroid and peduncular sub-rami branches. They supply the upper midbrain. **r. cervicalis nervi facialis** RAMUS COLLI NERVI FACIALIS. **rami choroidei arteriae cerebri posterioris** Choroidal branches of the posterior cerebral artery, variable in number, supplying the choroid plexuses of the third and lateral ventricles. **rami choroidei posteriores arteriae cerebri posterioris** Posterior choroidal branches of theposterior cerebral artery. These vessels include both medial and lateral posterior choroidal branches. **r. circumflexus arteriae coronariae sinistrae** [NA] A branch arising at the bifurcation of the left coronary artery and continuing along the left portion of the coronary sulcus around the left margin of the heart to the posterior interventricular groove, where it may anastomose with the right coronary artery. It supplies the left atrium and ventricle. Also *circumflex branch of left coronary artery.* **r. circumflexus fibularis arteriae tibialis posterioris** [NA] A branch arising proximally from the posterior tibial artery, and occasionally from the anterior tibial artery, and running laterally round the neck of the fibula to pierce the soleus muscle and anastomose with the lateral inferior genicular, the medial inferior genicular, and the anterior tibial recurrent arteries. Also *circumflex fibular branch of posterior tibial artery, circumflex fibular artery.* **r. clavicularis arteriae thoracoacromialis** [NA] A branch arising from the thoracoacromial artery after it has pierced the clavipectoral fascia and running superomedially between the latter and the pectoralis major muscle to supply the subclavius muscle and the sternoclavicular joint. Also *clavicular branch of thoracoacromial artery.* **r. cochlearis arteriae labyrinthi** [NA] A branch arising from the labyrinthine artery at the bottom of the internal acoustic meatus and dividing into about fourteen minute branches that pass through the canals of the modiolus and end as a network in the lamina spiralis and basilar membrane. Also *cochlear branch of labyrinthine artery.* **rami coeliaci plexus gastrici posterioris** RAMI CELIACI NERVI VAGI. **r. colicus arteriae ileocolicae** [NA] One of the terminal branches of the ileocolic artery that arises near the ileocolic junction and ascends along the medial margin of the ascending colon to supply it and anastomose with a descending branch of the right colic artery. Also *arteria ascendens* (outmoded). **r. collateralis arteriarum intercostalium posteriorum III-XI** [NA] A branch arising near the angle of a rib from each paired posterior intercostal artery in the third to eleventh intercostal spaces and running inferiorly to the superior border of the rib below along which it courses anteriorly to anastomose with an intercostal branch of either the internal thoracic or the musculophrenic artery. Also *collateral branch of posterior intercostal arteries III–XI.* **r. colli nervi facialis** [NA] The cervical branch of the facial nerve, emerging from the lower part of the parotid gland and running deep to the platysma on the front of the neck. It is motor to the platysma and joins with the transverse cervical nerve. Also *ramus cervicalis nervi facialis.* **r. communicans** Any branch that joins one nerve to another. Also *ramus anastomoticus, communicating branch.* **r. communicans arteriae fibularis** [NA] A branch arising from the peroneal artery a few inches above the lower end of the fibula and joining the communicating branch of the posterior tibial artery deep to the flexor hallucis longus muscle. Also *communicating branch of peroneal artery.* **r. communicans ganglii ciliaris cum nervo nasociliari** [NA] The communicating branch of the ciliary ganglion with the nasociliary nerve, conveying general sensation from the cornea, iris, ciliary body, and choroid through the ganglion to relay in the trigeminal sensory nuclei. Also *ramus anastomoticus ganglii ciliaris cum nervo nasociliari, sensory root of ciliary ganglion, long root of ciliary ganglion, ramus communicans nervi nasociliaris cum ganglione ciliari, radix longa ganglii ciliaris.* **r. communicans ganglii otici cum chorda tympani** [NA] An anastomotic branch connecting the otic ganglion with the chorda tympani, conveying postganglionic parasympathetic fibers to submandibular, sublingual, and lingual glands. Also *ramus anastomoticus ganglii otici cum chorda tympani.* **r. communicans ganglii otici cum nervo auriculotemporali** [NA] A communicating branch from the otic ganglion to the auriculotemporal nerve. Also *ramus anastomoticus ganglii otici cum nervo auriculotemporali.* **r. communicans ganglii otici cum ramo meningeo nervi mandibularis** [NA] A communicating branch from the otic ganglion conveying postganglionic parasympathetic fibers to the meningeal branch of the mandibular nerve. Also *ramus anastomoticus ganglii otici cum ramo meningeo nervi mandibularis.* **r. communicans nervi facialis cum nervo auriculari magno** Communicating branch of facial nerve with great auricular nerve. Also *ramus anastomoticus nervi facialis cum nervo auriculari magno.* **r. communicans nervi facialis cum nervo auriculotemporali** A branch connecting the facial nerve with the auriculotemporal nerve. Also *ramus anastomoticus nervi facialis cum nervo auriculotemporali.* **r. communicans nervi facialis cum nervo glossopharyngeo** [NA] A branch connecting the facial nerve with the glossopharyngeal nerve. Also *ramus anastomoticus nervi facialis cum nervo glossopharyngeo, ansa of Haller.* **r. communicans nervi facialis cum nervo occipitali minore** The branch connecting the facial nerve with the lesser occipital nerve. Also *ramus anastomoticus nervi facialis cum nervo occipitali minore.* **r. communicans nervi facialis cum nervo transverso colli** A branch connecting the facial nerve with the transverse cervical nerve. Also *ramus anastomoticus nervi facialis cum nervo transverso colli.* **r. communicans nervi facialis cum nervo vestibulocochleari** A branch connecting the facial nerve with the vestibulocochlear nerve. Also *ramus anastomoticus nervi facialis cum nervo vestibulocochleari.* **r. communicans nervi facialis cum plexu sympathetico** A branch connecting the facial nerve with the sympathetic plexus on the middle meningeal artery. Also *ramus anastomoticus nervi facialis cum plexu sympathetico.* **r. communicans nervi facialis cum plexu tympanico** [NA] A branch connecting the facial nerve with the tympanic plexus, a connecting filament from the facial nerve to the branch of the glossopharyngeal nerve that forms the tympanic plexus. Also *ramus anastomoticus nervi facialis cum plexu tympanico, ramus communicans with tympanic plexus.* **r. communicans nervi facialis cum ramo auriculari nervi vagi** A branch connecting the facial nerve with the auricular branch of the vagus nerve. Also *ramus anastomoticus nervi facialis cum ramo auriculari nervi vagi.* **r. communicans nervi facialis cum ramo petrosali nervi glossopharyngei** A branch connecting the facial nerve with the petrosal branch of the glossopharyngeal nerve. Also *ramus anastomoticus nervi facialis cum ramo petrosali nervi glossopharyngei.* **r. communicans nervi glossopharyngei cum ramo auriculari nervi vagi** [NA] A branch connecting the glossopharyngeal nerve with the auricular branch of the vagus nerve. Also *ramus anastomoticus nervi glossopharyngei cum ramo auriculari nervi vagi.* **r. communicans nervi lacrimalis cum nervo zygomatico** [NA] A branch connecting the lacrimal nerve with the zygomatic nerve. Also *ramus anastomoticus nervi lacrimalis cum nervo zygomatico.* **r. communicans nervi laryngei inferioris cum ramo laryngeo interno** [NA] The communicating branch of the recurrent laryngeal nerve with the internal laryngeal branch of the vagus nerve, supplying motor innervation to the arytenoideus muscle. Also *ramus communicans nervi laryngei recurrentis cum ramo laryngeo interno, ramus anastomoticus nervi laryngei inferioris cum ramo laryngeo interno, ramus anastomoticus nervi laryngei recurrentis cum ramo laryngeo interno.* **r. communicans nervi laryngei superioris cum nervo laryngeo inferiori** [NA] The communicating branch of the superior laryngeal nerve with the inferior larnygeal nerve. Also *ramus anastomoticus nervi laryngei superioris cum nervo laryngeo inferiore, Galen's nerve, Galen's anastomosis, ansa of Galen.* **r. communicans nervi lingualis cum chorda tympani** [NA] The communicating branch of the lingualnerve with the chorda tympani. Also *ramus anastomoticus nervi lingualis cum chorda tympani.* **r. communicans nervi mediani cum nervo ulnari** [NA] A branch connecting the median nerve with the ulnar nerve. Several branches from the median nerve or its anterior interosseous branch join the ulnar nerve behind the ulnar artery in the upper forearm. Also *ramus anastomoticus nervi mediani cum nervo ulnari.* **r. communicans nervi nasociliaris cum ganglione ciliari** [NA] RAMUS COMMUNICANS GANGLII CILIARIS CUM NERVO NASOCILIARI. **r. communicans nervi vagi cum nervo glossopharyngeo** [NA] A branch connecting the vagus nerve with the glossopharyngeal nerve, a connecting twig from the vagus nerve to the inferior ganglion of the glossopharyngeal nerve. Also *ramus anastomoticus nervi vagi cum nervo glossopharyngeo.* **r. communicans peroneus nervi peronei communis** [NA] A communicating branch from the common peroneal nerve that arises in the popliteal fossa, crosses the lateral head of the gastrocnemius muscle, and unites with the medial sural cutaneous nerve to form the sural nerve. Also *ramus communicans peroneus, ramus anastomoticus peroneus nervi peronei communis, peroneal communicating nerve.* **r. communicans with tympanic plexus** RAMUS COMMUNICANS NERVI FACIALIS CUM PLEXU TYMPANICO. **r. communicans ulnaris nervi radialis** [NA] The ulnar communicating branch of the radial nerve, a nerve filament that conveys sensation from the skin on adjoining sides of the middle and ring fingers. Also *ramus anastomoticus ulnaris nervi radialis.* **rami communicantes albi** The roots of the ganglia, or white communicating rami of the sympathetic chain, composed of myelinated preganglionic axons that arise from cells of the lateral gray column of the spinal cord and exit via the ventral roots in the thoracolumbar region. **rami communicantes ganglii otici cum nervo auriculotemporali** Communicating branches of otic ganglion with auriculotemporal nerve. Also *rami anastomotici ganglii otici cum nervo auriculotemporali.* **rami communicantes ganglii submandibularis cum nervo linguali** Branches connecting the submandibular ganglion with the lingual nerve. Also *rami communicantes ganglii submaxillaris cum nervo linguali, rami anastomotici ganglii submaxillaris cum nervo linguali, rami anastomotici ganglii submandibularis cum nervo linguali, motor roots of submandibular ganglion.* **rami communicantes nervi auriculotemporalis cum nervo faciali** [NA] Branches connecting the auriculotemporal nerve with the facial nerve. Also *rami anastomotici nervi auricotemporalis cum nervo faciali.* **rami communicantes nervi lingualis cum nervo hypoglosso** [NA] Branches connecting the lingual nerve with the hypoglossal nerve, forming a plexus at the anterior margin of the hypoglossus muscle. Also *rami anastomotici nervi lingualis cum nervo hypoglosso.* **rami communicantes nervorum spinalium** [NA] Branches connecting a spinal nerve withthe sympathetic chain. The white rami communicantes are myelinated preganglionic axons of the thoracolumbar outflow whose cell bodies are in the lateral gray column of the spinal cord. The gray rami communicantes are unmyelinated postganglionic axons of cell bodies in the sympathetic ganglia that accompany cutaneous branches of spinal nerves to supply arrectores pilorum muscles and sweat glands, and vasoconstrictor innervation to peripheral blood vessels. **r. coni arteriosi arteriae coronariae dextrae** [NA] A branch that arises from the right coronary artery between the pulmonary trunk and right auricle and ascends onto the front of the conus arteriosus to supply it. Also *conal branch of right coronary artery.* **r. coni arteriosi arteriae coronariae sinistrae** [NA] A branch which arises from the left coronary artery between the pulmonary trunk and the left auricle and ascends on to the conus arteriosus to supply it. It may also arise from the anterior interventricular branch. Also *conal branch of left coronary artery.* **rami corporis carotici nervi vagi** Minute branches of the vagus nerve to the carotid body that arise from the inferior ganglion, travel with pharyngeal or superior laryngeal nerves, and convey chemoreceptive sensations. **rami corticales arteriae cerebri anterioris** Cortical branches of the anterior cerebral artery. These vessels supply the medial surface of the frontal and parietal lobes of the cerebral hemispheres. **rami corticales arteriae cerebri mediae** Cortical branches of the middle cerebral artery. They supply the lateral surface of the frontal, insular, temporal, and parietal lobes of the cerebral cortex. **rami corticales arteriae cerebri posterioris** Cortical branches of the posterior cerebral artery. These vessels supply the inferomedial and inferolateral aspects of the temporal and occipital lobes as well as the medial surface of the occipital lobe. **r. costalis lateralis arteriae thoracicae internae** [NA] An inconstant branch of the internal thoracic artery that runs inferolaterally behind the ribs to supply the costal cartilages and ribs and to anastomose with corresponding posterior intercostal arteries. Also *lateral costal branch of internal thoracic artery, infracostal artery, retrocostal artery.* **r. cricothyroideus arteriae thyroideae superioris** [NA] A small branch of the superior thyroid artery that runs medially across the cricothyroid ligament to anastomose with the corresponding artery of the opposite side. Also *cricothyroid branch of superior thyroid artery, cricothyroid artery, inferior thyroid artery of Cruveilhier.* **rami cutanei anteriores nervi femoralis** [NA] Anterior cutaneous branches of the femoral nerve that convey general sensation from the front and medial aspect of the thigh and contribute branches to the subsartorial and patellar plexuses. **rami cutanei cruris mediales nervi sapheni** [NA] Medial crural cutaneous branches of the saphenous nerve, general sensory nerves that supply the skin of the medial side of the leg. **r. cutaneus anterior nervi iliohypogastrici** [NA] The anterior cutaneous branch of the iliohypogastric nerve that courses between the external and internal oblique abdominal muscles and conveys general sensation from skin on the pubis. Also *genital branch of iliohypogastric nerve* (outmoded). **r. cutaneus anterior pectoralis et abdominalis nervorum intercostalium** [NA] Anterior cutaneous branches (thoracic and abdominal) of the intercostal nerves that convey general sensation from the skin overlying the ventromedial aspect of the chest and abdomen. Also *anterior cutaneous nerve of abdomen.* **r. cutaneus lateralis** RAMUS CUTANEUS LATERALIS PECTORALIS ET ABDOMINALIS NERVORUM INTERCOSTALIUM. **r. cutaneus lateralis arteriarum intercostalium posteriorum III–XI** [NA] A branch from each paired posterior intercostal artery in the third to eleventh intercostal spaces that accompanies the lateral cutaneous branch of each corresponding thoracic spinal nerve to anastomose with other arteries and supply the skin of the thoracic and abdominal walls. Also *lateral cutaneous branch of posterior intercostal arteries III–XI, ramus cutaneus lateralis ramorum posteriorum arteriarum intercostalium, ramus cutaneus lateralis arteriarum posteriorum intercostalium.* **r. cutaneus lateralis nervi iliohypogastrici** [NA] The lateral cutaneous branch of the iliohypogastric nerve that conveys general sensation from the skin on the lateral aspect of the buttocks. Also *abdominal branch of iliohypogastric nerve* (outmoded). **r. cutaneus lateralis pectoralis et abdominalis nervorum intercostalium** [NA] Lateral cutaneous branches (thoracic and abdominal) of intercostal nerves that convey general sensation from the skin on the lateral aspect of the body wall. Also *ramus cutaneus lateralis.* **r. cutaneus lateralis ramorum dorsalium nervorum thoracicorum** [NA] The lateral cutaneous branch of the dorsal divisions of the thoracic spinal nerves, conveying sensation from the skin overlying the deep back muscles. Also *ramus cutaneus lateralis ramorum posteriorum nervorum thoracalium.* **r. cutaneus lateralis ramorum posteriorum arteriarum intercostalium** RAMUS CUTANEUS LATERALIS ARTERIARUM INTERCOSTALIUM POSTERIORUM III–XI. **r. cutaneus lateralis ramorum posteriorum nervorum thoracalium** RAMUS CUTANEUS LATERALIS RAMORUM DORSALIUM NERVORUM THORACICORUM. **r. cutaneus medialis rami dorsalis arteriarum intercostalium posteriorum III–XI** [NA] A branch of the dorsal branch of each paired posterior intercostal artery in the third to eleventh spaces that accompanies a corresponding branch of the dorsal division of an intercostal nerve to the skin over the muscles adjacent to the vertebral column. Also *medial cutaneous branch of dorsal branch of posterior intercostal arteries III–XI, ramus cutaneus medialis ramorum posteriorum arteriarum intercostalium* (outmoded). **r. cutaneus medialis ramorum dorsalium nervorum thoracicorum** [NA] Medial cutaneous branch of dorsal divisions of thoracic spinal nerves. Medial branches of upper six thoracic dorsal divisions run between semispinalis thoracis and multifidus, then pierce the rhomboids and trapezius to reach skin along vertebral spines. Medial branches of lower six thoracic dorsal divisions are distributed to multifidus and longissimus thoracis and give few filaments to skin along midline. Also *ramus cutaneus medialis ramorum posteriorum nervorum thoracalium.* **r. cutaneus medialis ramorum posteriorum arteriarum intercostalium** *Outmoded* RAMUS CUTANEUS MEDIALIS RAMI DORSALIS ARTERIARUM INTERCOSTALIUM POSTERIORUM (III–XI). **r. cutaneus medialis ramorum posteriorum nervorum thoracalium** RAMUS CUTANEUS MEDIALIS RAMORUM DORSALIUM NERVORUM THORACICORUM. **r. cutaneus nervi obturatorii** [NA] The cutaneous branch of the obturator nerve, arising as a continuation of communication between anterior cutaneous and saphenous nerves. It is distributed to the skin along the medial side of the proximal half of the leg. **r. cutaneus palmaris nervi ulnaris** RAMUS PALMARIS NERVI ULNARIS. **r. deltoideus arteriae profundae brachii** [NA] A branch arising from the profunda brachii artery and running upwards between the long and the lateral heads of the triceps to anastomose with the descending branch of posterior circumflex humeral artery. Also *deltoid branch of deep brachial artery, deltoid artery.* **r. deltoideus arteriae thoracoacromialis** [NA] A branch arising from the thoracoacromial artery and supplying the deltoid and pectoralis major muscles. Also *deltoid branch of thoracoacromial artery, deltoid artery, deltopectoral artery* (outmoded). **rami dentales superiores anteriores nervi infraorbitalis** RAMI ALVEOLARES SUPERIORES ANTERIORES NERVI INFRAORBITALIS. **rami dentales superiores posteriores nervi maxillaris** RAMI ALVEOLARES SUPERIORES POSTERIORES NERVI MAXILLARIS. **r. dentalis superior medius nervi infraorbitalis** RAMUS ALVEOLARIS SUPERIOR MEDIUS NERVI INFRAORBITALIS. **r. descendens arteriae circumflexae femoris lateralis** [NA] A large branch of the lateral circumflex femoral artery that accompanies the nerve to the vastus lateralis muscle deep to the rectus femoris muscle and along the anterior border of the vastus lateralis, supplying it and ending by anastomosing with the lateral superior genicular branch of the popliteal artery. Occasionally it arises independently from either the profunda femoris or the femoral artery. Also *descending branch of lateral circumflex femoral artery.* **r. descendens arteriae occipitalis** [NA] A large branch arising from the occipital artery as it runs in the occipital groove over the superior oblique muscle of the head. It divides into a superficial branch that runs deep to the splenius capitis muscle to supply the trapezius muscle and anastomose with the superficial cervical artery, and a deep branch that runs down between the semispinalis muscles to anastomose with the vertebral and deep cervical arteries. Also *descending branch of occipital artery, posterior cervical artery.* **r. descendens nervi hypoglossi** RADIX SUPERIOR ANSAE CERVICALIS. **r. dexter arteriae hepaticae propriae** [NA] A terminal branch of the hepatic artery proper that runs anterior to the portal vein and posterior to the hepatic duct and gives off the cystic artery to the gallbladder before dividing into two main branches that enter the right lobe of the liver. Also *right branch of proper hepatic artery.* **r. dexter venae portae hepatis** [NA] A branch of the portal vein that receives the cystic vein and enters the right lobe of the liver accompanying the right branch of the hepatic artery. Also *right branch of portal vein.* **r. digastricus nervi facialis** [NA] The digastric branch of the facial nerve, arising near the stylomastoid foramen and supplying motor filaments to the posterior belly of the digastric muscle. Also *digastric nerve.* **rami dorsales arteriae intercostalis supremae** [NA] Branches of the first and second posterior intercostal arteries derived from the highest or superior intercostal artery. Each dorsal branch follows the same course as the dorsal branch derived from posterior intercostal arteries III–XI supplying the dorsal muscles and skin over them as well as giving off a spinal branch to the vertebral canal. Also *dorsal branches of highest intercostal artery.* See also RAMUS DORSALIS ARTERIARUM INTERCOSTALIUM POSTERIORUM III–XI. **rami dorsales linguae arteriae lingualis** [NA] Small branches arising from the lingual artery and supplying the mucous membrane, the palatoglossal arch, soft palate, tonsil, and epiglottis. Also *dorsal lingual branches of lingual artery, dorsal artery of tongue.* **rami dorsales nervorum cervicalium** [NA] The dorsal rami of cervical nerves, twelve in number, that with the exception of the first divide into medial and lateral branches, and are motor to deep back muscles and sensory to the overlying skin in the neck region. Also *rami posteriores nervorum cervicalium.* **rami dorsales nervorum lumbalium** [NA] The dorsal rami of the lumbar nerves, five in number, that divide into medial and lateral branches and are motor to the multifidus and erector spinae (sacrospinalis) muscles and sensory to the skin of the posterior lumbar and gluteal regions. Also *rami posteriores nervorum lumbalium.* **rami dorsales nervorum sacralium** [NA] The dorsal rami of the sacral nerves, five in number, that divide into medial and lateral branches, supply the motor twigs to multifidus muscle, and are sensory to the skin overlying the posterior gluteal area and coccyx. Also *rami posteriores nervorum sacralium.* **rami dorsales nervorum thoracicorum** [NA] Dorsal rami of the thoracic nerves, twelve in number, that divide into medial and lateral branches and are motor to deep back muscles and sensory to the skin near the median plane. Also *rami posteriores nervorum thoracicorum.* **r. dorsalis arteriae subcostalis** [NA] A branch of the subcostal artery that runs posteriorly below the neck of the twelfth rib and lateral to the vertebral body to supply muscles of the back and the skin over them. Also *dorsal branch of subcostal artery.* **r. dorsalis arteriarum intercostalium posteriorum III–XI** [NA] A branch of each paired posterior intercostal artery of the third to eleventh spaces that runs dorsally through a gap bounded above and below by the necks of the ribs, medially by a vertebral body and laterally by a superior costotransverse ligament. After giving off a spinal branch it continues over the transverse process and supplies branches to muscles of the back and the skin over them. Also *dorsal branch of posterior intercostal arteries III–XI.* **r. dorsalis arteriarum lumbalium** [NA] A branch of each paired lumbar artery that runs dorsally between adjacent transverse processes of lumbar vertebrae to supply the muscles and skin of the back. Also *dorsal branch of lumbar arteries.* **r. dorsalis manus nervi ulnaris** RAMUS DORSALIS NERVI ULNARIS. **r. dorsalis nervi coccygei** The dorsal branch of the coccygeal nerve, conveying general sensation from the skin over the coccyx. Also *ramus posterior nervi coccygei.* **r. dorsalis nervi ulnaris** [NA] The dorsal branch of the ulnar nerve, arising about 5 cm above the wrist and reaching the dorsum of the hand by passing deep to the flexor carpi ulnaris. It divides into two or three dorsal digital branches that are sensory to the skin of the little finger and the medial side of the ring finger. Also *ramus dorsalis manus nervi ulnaris, dorsal cutaneous branch of the hand* (outmoded). **r. dorsalis nervorum spinalium** [NA] Any of the posterior primary branches of the spinal nerves, from which are derived both the motor innervation to the deep back muscles and the sensory innervation to the skin of the back. Also *ramus posterior nervorum spinalium, dorsal rami of spinal nerves.* **r. dorsalis venarum intercostalium posteriorum IV–XI** [NA] A tributary of the paired intercostal veins in the fourth to eleventh intercostal spaces. It drains the muscles and skin of the back and the vertebral venous plexuses. Also *dorsal branch of posterior intercostal veins IV–XI.* **dorsal rami of spinal nerves** RAMUS DORSALIS NERVORUM SPINALIUM. **rami duodenales arteriae pancreaticoduodenalis superioris** [NA] Branches arising from both the anterior and the posterior branches of the superior pancreaticoduodenal artery to supply the duodenum. Also *duodenal branches of superior pancreaticoduodenal artery.* **r. duralis nervi vagi** RAMUS MENINGEUS NERVI VAGI. **rami esophageales aortae thoracicae** [NA] Branches arising from the anterior aspect of the thoracic aorta and running downwards and forwards to the esophagus where they anastomose inferiorly with ascending branches of the left phrenic and left gastric arteries and superiorly with branches of the inferior thyroid arteries, supplying the whole length of the esophagus. Also *esophageal branches of thoracic aorta, esophageal arteries.* **rami esophageales arteriae gastricae sinistrae** [NA] Branches arising from the left gastric artery near the cardiac end of the stomach and running upwards through the esophageal opening of the diaphragm to anastomose with esophageal branches of the thoracic aorta, supplying the lower end of the esophagus. Also *esophageal branches of left gastric artery, inferior esophageal arteries.* **rami esophageales arteriae thyroideae inferioris** [NA] Branches of the inferior thyroid artery that descend to anastomose with esophageal branches of the thoracic aorta and supply the esophagus. Also *esophageal branches of inferior thyroid artery.* **rami esophagei nervi laryngei recurrentis** [NA] Esophageal branches of the recurrent laryngeal nerve, containing preganglionic parasympathetic and visceral afferent fibers that innervate the mucous membrane and muscular layer of the esophagus. Also *rami esophagei nervi recurrentis.* **rami esophagei nervi vagi**

[NA] Esophageal branches of the recurrent laryngeal and vagus nerves, containing preganglionic parasympathetic and visceral afferent fibers that join the esophageal plexus, from which fibers are distributed to the esophagus and the posterior surface of the pericardium. **r. externus nervi accessorii** [NA] The external branch of the accessory nerve, the portion remaining after the cranial rootlets have joined the spinal rootlets of the accessory nerve and after the internal branch of that nerve has branched from the main trunk. It descends in the neck to supply motor innervation to the sternocleidomastoid muscle, and then crosses the posterior triangle of the neck to supply the trapezius muscle. Also *spinal part of accessory nerve, external ramus of accessory nerve.* **r. externus nervi laryngei superioris** [NA] The external branch of the superior laryngeal nerve. It supplies motor innervation to the cricothyroid and inferior pharyngeal constrictor muscles. Also *external laryngeal nerve.* **r. femoralis nervi genitofemoralis** [NA] The femoral branch of the genitofemoral nerve, lying lateral to the genital branch and passing beneath the inguinal ligament to supply the skin of the upper part of the anterior thigh. Also *lumboinguinal nerve, nervus lumboinguinalis.* **rami frontales arteriae cerebri anterioris** Frontal branches of the anterior cerebral artery, supplying the corpus callosum, cingulate gyrus, paracentral lobule, and the superior and middle frontal gyri. **rami frontales arteriae cerebri mediae** Frontal branches of the middle cerebral artery, supplying the precentral and the middle and inferior frontal gyri. **r. frontalis arteriae meningeae mediae** [NA] The larger of the two terminal branches of the middle meningeal artery. It arises in a groove on the squamous part of temporal bone intracranially and then crosses the greater wing of sphenoid bone to enter another groove, or canal, in the sphenoidal angle of the parietal bone, where it divides into branches which fan out external to the dura mater, some to the vertex and others to the occipital region of the cranium. Also *frontal branch of middle meningeal artery, anterior branch of middle meningeal artery.* **r. frontalis arteriae temporalis superficialis** [NA] One of the terminal branches of the superficial temporal artery. It arises just above the zygomatic process of the temporal bone and runs in a tortuous fashion towards the frontal tuberosity supplying the skin, muscles, and pericranium of that region and anastomosing with the supraorbital and supratrochlear arteries and the corresponding artery of the opposite side. Also *frontal branch of superficial temporal artery, anterior branch of superficial temporal artery.* **r. frontalis nervi frontalis** RAMUS MEDIALIS NERVI SUPRAORBITALIS. **r. frontalis posteromedialis arteriae callosomarginalis** [NA] A branch of the callosomarginal artery which supplies the more posterior and superior cortex on the medial aspect of the frontal lobe. Also *posteromedial frontal branch.* **rami gastrici anteriores nervi vagi** [NA] Anterior gastric branches of the vagus nerve, arising from the anterior vagal trunk at the cardiac end of the stomach. They contain visceral afferent and efferent filaments that join the myenteric and submucous plexus in the fundus and body of the stomach. Also *rami gastrici nervi vagi, plexus gastricus anterior.* **rami gastrici posteriores nervi vagi** [NA] Posterior gastric branches of the vagus nerve that arise from the posterior vagal trunk, contain preganglionic parasympathetic and visceral afferent fibers and join in myenteric and submucous plexus in the posterior wall of the cardiac end, fundus and body of the stomach. Also *rami gastrici nervi vagi, plexus gastricus posterior.* **r. genitalis nervi genitofemoralis** [NA] A division (chiefly $L_2$) of the genitofemoral nerve that in the male passes through the deep inguinal ring and inguinal canal to supply the cremaster and give off filaments to the scrotum and adjacent thigh, and in the female accompanies the round ligament and ends in the skin of the mons pubis and labium majus. Also *nervus spermaticus externus, external spermatic nerve.* **rami glandulares arteriae facialis** [NA] Branches arising from the facial artery as it grooves the posterior border of the submandibular gland supplying it, adjacent lymph nodes and muscles, and the overlying skin. Also *glandular branches of facial artery.* **rami glandulares arteriae thyroideae inferioris** [NA] Two large branches, an inferior and an ascending, of the inferior thyroid artery which are distributed to the inferior and posterior portions of the thyroid gland, where they anastomose with the superior thyroid artery and the opposite inferior thyroid artery. The ascending branch gives branches to the parathyroid glands. **rami glandulares arteriae thyroideae superioris** The branches (anterior, lateral, and posterior) of the superior thyroid artery that supply the thyroid gland. **rami glandulares ganglii submandibularis** [NA] The short postganglionic parasympathetic secretory axons from the submandibular ganglion and the long sympathetic postganglionic axons innervating the submandibular salivary gland. Also *submaxillary nerves, rami submaxillares ganglii submaxillaris.* **r. glandularis anterior arteriae thyroideae superioris** [NA] The anterior branch of the superior thyroid artery which descends deep to the sternothyroid muscle along the medial margin of the superior pole of the lobe of the thyroid gland and the upper margin of the isthmus to anastomose with its fellow from the opposite side. It gives branches to the anterior surface and anastomoses with branches of the inferior thyroid artery. **r. glandularis lateralis arteriae thyroideae superioris** [NA] A small branch of the superior thyroid artery which descends along the lateral margin of the thyroid gland. When the other glandular branches are small, it may be large and then anastomoses with the inferior thyroid artery. **r. glandularis posterior arteriae thyroideae superioris** [NA] A branch of the superior thyroid artery which arises at the superior pole of the thyroid gland and descends on the posterior surface of the gland, supplying the medial, posterior, and lateral surfaces and anastomosing with the inferior thyroid artery. **rami helicini arteriae uterinae** Tortuous subsidiary branches of the uterine artery that occur in the uterine myometrium, becoming prominent during the proliferative phase of the endometrial cycle, while in the secretory phase they enlarge in length and breadth and become more coiled. Also *coiled arteries, screw arteries, spiral arteries, helicine arteries.* **rami hepatici nervi vagi** [NA] Hepatic branches of the vagus nerve, arising from the anterior and posterior vagal trunks and containing preganglionic parasympathetic and visceral afferent fibers. They course in the lesser omentum to the hepatic plexus and from there filaments are distributed to the liver, gallbladder, pancreas, stomach, and duodenum. **r. ilealis arteriae ileocolicae** [NA] A terminal branch of the ileocolic artery that arises near the ileocolic junction and runs to the left on the terminal part of the ileum, supplying it and anastomosing with the termination of the superior mesenteric artery. Also *ileal branch of ileocolic artery, terminal branch of ileocolic artery.* **r. iliacus arteriae iliolumbalis** [NA] A terminal branch of the iliolumbar artery arising behind the medial border of the psoas major muscle to supply branches to the ilium and the iliacus muscle and to the gluteal and abdominal muscles along the iliac crest. Also *iliac branch of iliolumbar artery.* **r. inferior arteriae gluteae superioris** [NA] The inferior division of the deep branch of the superior gluteal artery that curves inferolaterally between gluteus medius and gluteus minimus muscles, supplying them and anastomosing with the lateral circumflex femoral artery. Also *inferior branch of superior gluteal artery.* **rami inferiores nervi transversi colli** [NA] Inferior branches of transverse cervical nerves that are sensory, arise near the middle of the anterior border of the sternocleidomastoid muscle, pierce the platysma, and descend to the skin of the side and front of the neck as low as the sternum. Also *rami inferiores nervi cutanei colli.* **r. inferior nervi oculomotorii** [NA] The inferior branch of the oculomotor nerve, arising within the cavernous sinus and entering the orbit through the superior orbital fissure within the anulus tendineus. It divides into three motor branches to the medial rectus, inferior rectus, and inferior oblique muscles. **r. inferior ossis pubis** [NA] The short flat bar of bone that extends posteriorly and inferiorly from the lower lateral part of the body of the pubis to join the ramus of the ischium inferomedial to the obturator foramen. Also *inferior ramus of pubis.* **r. infrahyoideus arteriae thyroideae superioris** [NA] A small branch of the superior thyroid artery that runs deep to the thyrohyoid muscle along the inferior border of the hyoid bone to anastomose with the artery of the opposite side. Also *infrahyoid branch of superior thyroid artery.* **r. infrapatellaris nervi sapheni** [NA] The infrapatellar branch of the saphenous nerve, supplying sensory innervation to the skin overlying the patella. **rami inguinales arteriae femoralis** [NA] Several small branches arising from either the femoral artery or the external pudendal artery or both and supplying the inguinal lymph nodes, muscles and skin. Also *inguinal branches of femoral artery, inguinal arteries.* **rami intercostales anteriores arteriae thoracicae internae** [NA] Branches arising from the internal thoracic artery in the upper six intercostal spaces on each side. Also *anterior intercostal branches of internal thoracic artery, anterior intercostal arteries.* **rami interganglionares** [NA] Interganglionic branches connecting the ganglia of the sympathetic chains. **internal r. of accessory nerve** RADICES CRANIALES NERVI ACCESSORII. **r. internus nervi accessorii** [NA] RADICES CRANIALES NERVI ACCESSORII. **r. internus nervi laryngei superioris** [NA] The internal branch of the superior laryngeal nerve, sensory to the laryngeal mucosa as far down as the level of the vocal cords. Also *internal laryngeal nerve, internal superior laryngeal nerve.* **rami interventriculares septales arteriae coronariae dextrae** [NA] Branches of the posterior interventricular branch of the right coronary artery, which supply the posterior one-third of the interventricular septum. **rami interventriculares septales arteriae coronariae sinistrae** [NA] Branches of the anterior interventricular branch of the left coronary artery which supply the anterior two-thirds of the interventricular septum. **r. interventricularis anterior arteriae coronariae sinistrae** [NA] A branch arising at the bifurcation of the left coronary artery, descending in the anterior interventricular groove to the apex of the heart and supplying both ventricles and the anterior two-thirds of the interventricular septum. Also *anterior interventricular branch of left coronary artery, anterior interventricular artery.* **r. interventricularis posterior arteriae coronariae dextrae** [NA] A branch given off by the right coronary artery near its termination in the right portion of the coronary sulcus. It supplies branches to both ventricles and the posterior third of the interventricular septum. Also *posterior interventricular branch of right coronary artery, posterior descending coronary artery, posterior interventricular artery.* **ischial r.** RAMUS OSSIS ISCHII. **ischiopubic r.** The conjoined inferior ramus of pubis and ramus of ischium, forming one side of the pubic arch. **r. of ischium** RAMUS OSSIS ISCHII. **rami isthmi faucium nervi lingualis** [NA] Branches of the lingual nerve to the isthmus of the fauces, conveying general sensation from the oral mucosa. **rami labiales anteriores arteriae pudendae externae** [NA] Branches arising from the external pudendal arteries and piercing the fascia lata near the inferior ramus of the pubis to supply the skin of the labium majus and anastomose with the posterior labial branches of the internal pudendal artery. Also *anterior labial branches of external pudendal arteries, anterior labial arteries of vulva, anterior labial arteries.* **rami labiales inferiores nervi mentalis** [NA] Inferior labial branches of the mental nerve, conveying general sensation from the oral mucosa and skin of the lower lip. **rami labiales posteriores arteriae pudendae internae** [NA] Terminal branches of the perineal artery, which is derived from the internal pudendal artery, arising distal to the urogenital diaphragm and ramifying on the labium majus to anastomose with the anterior labial branches of the external pudendal arteries. Also *posterior labial branches of internal pudendal artery, posterior labial arteries of vulva.* **rami labiales superiores nervi infraorbitalis** [NA] Superior labial branches of the infraorbital nerve, conveying general sensation from the oral mucosa and skin of the upper lip. **r. laryngei inferior nervi vagi** NERVUS LARYNGEUS RECURRENS. **r. laryngeus recurrens nervi vagi** NERVUS LARYNGEUS RECURRENS. **rami laryngopharyngei ganglii cervicalis superioris** [NA] Laryngopharyngeal branches of the superior cervical ganglion, sympathetic branches that supply the carotid body and pass on to the sides of larynx and pharynx, where they form a plexus with the glossopharyngeal and vagus nerves. **rami laterales rami sinistri venae portae hepatis** [NA] Branches of the umbilical part of the left branch of the portal vein that accompany the lateral segmental artery of the left branch of the hepatic artery and supply the lateral segment of the left lobe and part of the caudate lobe of the liver. Also *lateral branches of left branch of portal vein.* **r. lateralis ductus hepatici sinistri** [NA] A branch of the left hepatic duct that drains the lateral segment of the left lobe of the liver. Also *lateral branch of left hepatic duct.* **r. lateralis nervi supraorbitalis** [NA] The lateral branch of the supraorbital nerve, the larger of two terminal sensory twigs, piercing the epicranial aponeurosis and supplying the skin of the scalp and the mucous membrane of the frontal sinus. **r. lateralis ramorum dorsalium nervorum cervicalium** [NA] The lateral branch of the dorsal branches of the cervical nerves, one of two terminal twigs of the dorsal branches of the eight cervical nerves. The dorsal branches are motor to deep neck muscles. Also *ramus lateralis ramorum posteriorum nervorum cervicalium.* **r. lateralis ramorum dorsalium nervorum lumbalium** [NA] The lateral branch of the dorsal branches of the lumbar nerves, consisting of terminal twigs of dorsal branches of the five lumbar nerves that supply the erector spinae muscles. Also *ramus lateralis ramorum posteriorum nervorum lumbalium.* **r. lateralis ramorum dorsalium nervorum sacralium** [NA] The lateral branch of the dorsal branches of sacral nerves, terminal branches of the dorsal rami of the upper three sacral nerves that pierce the gluteus maximus and supply the skin over the posterior gluteal area. Also *ramus lateralis ramorum posteriorum nervorum sacralium.* **rami lenticulostriatae arteriae cerebri mediae** RAMI

CENTRALES ANTEROLATERALES ARTERIAE CEREBRI MEDIAE. **rami lienales plexus celiaci** The splenic nerves from the celiac plexus. **rami linguales nervi glossopharyngei** [NA] Lingual branches of the glossopharyngeal nerve, conveying general sensation and taste from the posterior third of the tongue. **rami linguales nervi hypoglossi** [NA] Lingual branches of the hypoglossal nerve, motor to the genio-, hyo-, and styloglossus muscles and to intrinsic tongue muscles. **rami linguales nervi lingualis** [NA] Lingual branches of the lingual nerve, conveying general sensation and taste from the anterior two-thirds of the tongue and general sensation from the floor of the mouth and adjacent gingiva. **r. lingualis nervi facialis** [NA] The lingual branch of the facial nerve, often absent but sometimes arising from the stylohyoid branch, and supplying some motor twigs to the styloglossus and stylopharyngeus muscles. **r. lobi medii venae pulmonalis dextrae superioris** [NA] The vein that drains the middle lobe of the right lung and joins the three veins of the upper lobe to form the right superior pulmonary vein in the hilum of the lung. Also *middle lobe vein of right lung, inferior radicle of upper right pulmonary vein.* **r. lumbalis arteriae iliolumbalis** [NA] A terminal branch of the iliolumbar artery arising posterior to the medial border of the psoas major muscle, supplying it and quadratus lumborum muscle and anastomosing with the fourth lumbar artery. It sends a spinal branch into the vertebral canal to supply the cauda equina. Also *lumbar branch of iliolumbar artery.* **rami malleolares laterales arteriae fibularis** [NA] Terminal branches of the peroneal, or fibular, artery that pass over the posterior aspect of the tibiofibular syndesmosis and the lateral malleolus to anastomose with anterior lateral malleolar branches. Also *posterior lateral malleolar branches of peroneal artery, lateral posterior malleolar arteries.* **rami malleolares mediales arteriae tibialis posterioris** [NA] Branches arising from the posterior tibial artery and running deep to the flexor digitorum longus and tibialis posterior muscles to ramify over the medial malleolus and anastomose with the anterior medial malleolar artery in the medial malleolar rete. Also *medial malleolar branches of posterior tibial artery, medial posterior malleolar arteries, posterior medial malleolar arteries.* **rami mammarii arteriae thoracicae internae** [NA] Branches arising from the second, third, and fourth perforating branches of the internal thoracic artery, especially in the female, supplying the medial part of the breast and enlarging during lactation. Also *mammary branches of internal thoracic artery.* **rami mammarii laterales arteriae thoracicae lateralis** [NA] Branches arising from the lateral thoracic artery and running around the lateral border of the pectoralis major muscle to supply the mammary gland. In the female they are often large. Also *lateral mammary branches of lateral thoracic artery, external mammary artery, lateral mammary artery.* **rami mammarii laterales nervorum intercostalium** RAMI MAMMARII LATERALES RAMORUM CUTANEORUM LATERALIUM NERVORUM INTERCOSTALIUM. **rami mammarii laterales ramorum cutaneorum lateralium nervorum intercostalium** [NA] The mammary branches of the lateral cutaneous branches of intercostal nerves, supplying the lateral portion of the mammary glands. Also *rami mammarii laterales nervorum intercostalium.* **rami mammarii mediales ramorum cutaneorum anteriorum nervorum intercostalium** [NA] The branches of the anterior cutaneous branches of intercostal nerves supplying the medial portion of the mammary glands. Also *rami mammarii mediales nervorum intercostalium.* **r. mandibulae** [NA] A quadrilateral plate of bone continuous with and projecting upwards from the posterior end of the body of the mandible on each side. It provides attachment for the major muscles of mastication. Also *ramus of mandible.* **r. marginalis dexter cordis** [NA] A branch that arises from the right coronary artery in the coronary sulcus. It supplies branches to the anterior and posterior surfaces of the right ventricle. Also *right marginal artery of heart.* **r. marginalis mandibulae nervi facialis** [NA] The marginal mandibular branch of the facial nerve, supplying motor innervation to the risorius and depressor anguli oris muscles of the lower lip and chin and communicating with the mental nerve. **r. marginalis sinister cordis** [NA] A branch that arises from the circumflex branch of the left coronary artery in the coronary sulcus and descends along the pulmonary surface of the heart, supplying the left ventricle. Also *left marginal artery of heart.* **rami mastoidei arteriae auricularis posterioris** [NA] Branches arising in the facial canal from the stylomastoid branch of the posterior auricular artery and supplying the mastoid air cells. Also *mastoid branches of posterior auricular artery, mastoid arteries.* **r. mastoideus arteriae occipitalis** [NA] A small branch of the occipital artery that passes through the mastoid foramen into the cranial cavity to supply the mastoid air cells and anastomose with the middle meningeal artery. It may be absent or may arise from the auricular branch of the occipital artery. Also *mastoid branch of occipital artery, mastoid artery.* **rami mediales rami sinistri venae portae hepatis** [NA] Branches of the umbilical part of the left branch of the portal vein that accompany the medial segmental artery of the left branch of the hepatic artery and supply the quadrate lobe and medial segment of the left lobe of the liver. Also *median branches of left portal branch* (outmoded). **r. medialis ductus hepatici sinistri** [NA] A branch of the left hepatic duct that drains the medial segment of the left lobe of the liver. Also *medial branch of left hepatic duct.* **r. medialis nervi supraorbitalis** [NA] The medial branch of the supraorbital nerve, the smaller of two terminal twigs that pierces the frontalis muscle and supplies sensory innervation to the scalp as far as the parietal bone and the mucosa of the frontal sinus. Also *ramus frontalis nervi frontalis.* **r. medialis ramorum dorsalium nervorum cervicalium** [NA] The medial branch of dorsal rami of cervical nerves, one of two terminal twigs of dorsal rami of eight cervical nerves. It is motor to deep neck muscles and sensory to overlying skin. Also *ramus medialis ramorum posteriorum nervorum cervicalium.* **r. medialis ramorum dorsalium nervorum lumbalium** [NA] The medial branch of the dorsal rami ofthe lumbar nerves, composed of terminal motor twigs from the dorsal branches of five lumbar nerves that emerge near the articular processes of vertebrae and supply the multifidus muscle. Also *ramus medialis ramorum posteriorum nervorum lumbalium.* **r. medialis ramorum dorsalium nervorum sacralium** [NA] The more medial of the two branches into which the dorsal rami of the upper sacral nerves divide. This medial branch is small, and motor to the multifidus muscle. Also *ramus medialis ramorum posteriorum nervorum sacralium.* **r. medialis ramorum lobi medii arteriae pulmonalis dextrae** [NA] One of the two arteries to the middle lobe of the right lung which supplies the lobe's medial bronchopulmonary segment (B V). They arise from a common stem given off by the right superior pulmonary artery. **rami mediastinales arteriae thoracicae internae** [NA] Small branches of the internal thoracic artery supplying the areolar tissue, fat, lymph nodes, and thymus gland in the anterior and superior mediastina. Also *mediastinal branches of internal thoracic artery, anterior mediastinal arteries, mediastinal branches.* **rami mediastinales partis thoracicae aortae** [NA] Numerous small branches arising from the thoracic aorta and supplying pleura, nerves, and lymph nodes in the posterior mediastinum. Also *mediastinal branches of thoracic aorta, posterior mediastinal arteries, mediastinal branches, mediastinal arteries.* **r. membranae tympani nervi auriculotemporalis** [NA] The tympanic membrane branch of the auriculotemporal nerve, a sensory twig that passes between the bony and cartilaginous parts of the external acoustic meatus to supply the tympanic membrane. **r. meningeus accessorius arteriae meningeae mediae** [NA] A branch arising from either the maxillary or the middle meningeal artery and entering the cranial cavity through the foramen ovale to supply the trigeminal ganglion, dura mater, and bone. It also provides extracranial branches to neighboring muscles, sphenoid bone, and otic ganglion. Also *accessory meningeal branch of middle meningeal artery.* **r. meningeus arteriae occipitalis** [NA] One of several branches of the occipital artery that enter the cranial cavity through the jugular foramen and condylar canal to supply the dura mater and bone in the posterior cranial fossa. Also *meningeal branch of occipital artery.* **r. meningeus arteriae vertebralis** [NA] A branch arising from the vertebral artery opposite the foramen magnum and branching between the dura mater and the cranium in the cerebellar fossa to supply the falx cerebelli and the bone. Also *meningeal branch of vertebral artery.* **r. meningeus medius nervi maxillaris** [NA] The middle meningeal branch of the maxillary nerve, arising near the foramen rotundum and supplying the dura mater of the middle and anterior cranial fossae. Also *nervus meningeus medius.* **r. meningeus nervi mandibularis** [NA] The meningeal branch of the mandibular nerve, entering the middle cranial fossa via the foramen spinosum and conveying general sensation from the dura mater. Also *nervus spinosus.* **r. meningeus nervi vagi** [NA] The meningeal branch of the vagus nerve, arising from the superior ganglion and supplying the dura mater in the posterior cranial fossa. Also *ramus duralis nervi vagi, meningeal nerve.* **r. meningeus nervorum spinalium** [NA] The meningeal branch of the spinal nerves, a mixed sensory and sympathetic branch, present at all vertebral levels, that re-enters the spinal canal through the intervertebral foramen and supplies the dura mater, blood vessel walls, periosteum, ligaments, and intervertebral disks. Also *sinuvertebral nerve, nerve of Luschka, meningeal branch of spinal nerve.* **rami mentales nervi mentalis** [NA] Mental branches of the mental nerve, conveying general sensation from the skin of the chin. **r. mentalis** [NA] A branch of the inferior alveolar artery that leaves the mandibular canal through the mental foramen to supply the chin region and anastomose with the inferior labial, sublabial, and submental arteries. Also *mental artery.* **rami musculares** Collectively, small branches of a nerve or an artery that supply muscle tissue and are often unnamed. **rami musculares nervi axillaris** [NA] Muscular branches of the axillary nerve, motor to the deltoid and teres minor muscles. **rami musculares nervi femoralis** [NA] Muscular branches of the femoral nerve,motor to the quadriceps femoris. **rami musculares nervi fibularis profundi** RAMI MUSCULARES NERVI PERONEI PROFUNDI. **rami musculares nervi fibularis superficialis** RAMI MUSCULARES NERVI PERONEI SUPERFICIALIS. **rami musculares nervi iliohypogastrici** Muscular branches, considered to be general sensory, of the iliohypogastric nerve, distributed to the obliquus internus muscle. **rami musculares nervi ilioinguinalis** Muscular branches, considered to be general sensory, of the ilioinguinal nerve, distributed to the obliquus internus muscle. **rami musculares nervi ischiadici** Muscular branches of the sciatic nerve, motor and distributed to the biceps femoris, semitendinosus, and semimembranosus muscles and to the ischial head of the adductor magnus. **rami musculares nervi mediani** [NA] Muscular branches of the median nerve, arising in the proximal part of the forearm and motor to the pronator teres, flexor carpi radialis, palmaris longus, and flexor digitorum profundus muscles. **rami musculares nervi musculocutanei** [NA] Muscular branches of the musculocutaneous nerve, motor to the biceps brachii, coracobrachialis and brachialis muscles. **rami musculares nervi obturatorii** [NA] Muscular branches of the obturator nerve, motor to the obturator externus, abductor magnus, adductor longus, adductor brevis, gracilis, and sometimes the pectineus. **rami musculares nervi peronei communis** Muscular branches of the common peroneal nerve, divided into motor branches of the superficial and deep peroneal nerves. **rami musculares nervi peronei profundi** [NA] Muscular branches of the deep peroneal nerve, motor to the peroneus tertius, tibialis anterior, extensor hallucis longus, and extensor digitorum longus muscles. Also *rami musculares nervi fibularis profundi.* **rami musculares nervi peronei superficialis** [NA] Muscular branches of the superficial peroneal nerve, motor to the peroneus longus and brevis muscles. Also *rami musculares nervi fibularis superficialis.* **rami musculares nervi radialis** [NA] The muscular branches of the radial nerve, supplying motor fibers to the triceps brachii, anconeus, brachioradialis, and extensor carpi radialis longus muscles and sensory fibers to the brachialis. **rami musculares nervi tibialis** [NA] Muscular branches of the tibial nerve, motor to the posterior leg muscles, including the gastrocnemius, soleus, plantaris, popliteus, tibialis posterior, flexor digitorum longus, and flexor hallucis longus. **rami musculares nervi ulnaris** [NA] Muscular branches of the ulnar nerve, two in number, arising near the elbow and supplying motor innervation to the flexor carpi ulnaris and the medial half of the flexor digitorum profundus. **rami musculares nervorum intercostalium** Muscular branches of the intercostal nerves, supplying the intercostalis, transversus thoracis, serratus posterior superior and inferior, and the abdominal muscles. **rami musculares plexus lumbalis** Muscular branches of the lumbar plexus, distributed to the quadratus lumborum, psoas major, psoas minor, and iliacus muscles. **r. muscularis** Singular of RAMI MUSCULARES. **r. muscularis lateralis of femoral nerve** One or more of the branches of the femoral nerve that course laterally and then inferiorly in the thigh with the descending branch of the lateral femoral circumflex artery to supply the vastus lateralis portion of the quadriceps femoris muscle. **r. muscularis medialis of femoral nerve** One or more of the branches of the femoral nerve that supply the vastus medialis portion of the quadriceps femoris muscle. **r. musculi stylopharyngei nervi glossopharyngei** [NA] The stylopharyngeal muscular branch of the glossopharyngeal nerve, supplying motor innervation to the stylopharyngeus. Also *ramus stylopharyngeus nervi glossopharyngei, stylopharyngeal nerve.* **r. mylohyoideus arteriae alveolaris inferioris** [NA] A branch arising from the inferior alveolar artery proximal to the mandibular foramen. It supplies the mylohyoid muscle and anastomoses with the submental branch of the facial artery. Also *mylohyoid branch of inferior alveolar artery, mylohyoid artery.* **rami nasales anteriores nervi ethmoidalis anterioris** RAMI NASALES NERVI ETHMOIDALIS ANTERIORIS. **rami nasales externi nervi ethmoidalis anterioris** External nasal branches of the anterior ethmoidal nerve, consisting of terminal filaments that emerge at the lower border of the nasal bone and supply the skin of the ala, apex, and vestibule of the nose. **rami nasales externi nervi infraorbitalis** [NA] External nasal branches of the infraorbital nerve, supplying the skin on the side of the nose and joining with the external nasal branches of the anterior ethmoidal nerve. **rami nasales interni nervi ethmoidalis anterioris** [NA] Internal nasal branches of the anteriorethmoidal nerve, comprising two sensory branches, a medial branch to the mucosa of the anterior nasal septum and a lateral branch to the anterior part of the lateral wall of the nasal cavity. **rami nasales interni nervi infraorbitalis** [NA] Internal nasal branches of the infraorbital nerve, supplying the mucosa of the anterior mobile part of the nasal septum. **rami nasales laterales nervi ethmoidalis anterioris** [NA] Lateral nasal branches of the anterior ethmoidal nerve, mixed sensory and autonomic filaments to the anterior part of the lateral wall of the nasal cavity. **rami nasales mediales nervi ethmoidalis anterioris** [NA] Medial nasal branches of the anterior ethmoidal nerve, general sensory and autonomic filaments to the mucous membrane of the front portion of the nasal septum. **rami nasales nervi ethmoidalis anterioris** [NA] Nasal branches of the anterior ethmoidal nerve, including two internal nasal branches to the mucosa of the anterior part of the nasal cavity and an external nasal branch to the skin of the ala, apex, and vestibule of the nose. Also *rami nasales anteriores nervi ethmoidalis anterioris.* **rami nasales posteriores inferiores laterales ganglii pterygopalatini** [NA] Lateral inferior posterior nasal branches of the pterygopalatine ganglion, mixed general sensory and autonomic nerves that supply the mucosa lining the inferior nasal concha and the walls of the middle and inferior meatuses. Also *rami nasales posteriores inferiores laterales ganglii sphenopalatini.* **rami nasales posteriores superiores laterales ganglii pterygopalatini** [NA] Lateral superior posterior nasal branches of the pterygopalatine ganglion, usually six mixed general sensory and secretomotor nerves that supply the mucosa overlying the superior and middle nasal conchae and the linings of the posterior ethmoidal sinuses. Also *rami nasales posteriores superiores laterales ganglii sphenopalatini.* **rami nasales posteriores superiores mediales ganglii pterygopalatini** [NA] Two or three medial posterior superior nasal branches of the pterygopalatine ganglion. Also *posterior superior nasal branches, rami nasales posteriores superiores mediales ganglii sphenopalatini.* **r. obturatorius arteriae epigastricae inferioris** [NA] A branch of the pubic branch of the inferior epigastric artery that anastomoses with the pubic branch of the obturator artery behind the pubis and medial to the femoral ring. Also *obturator branch of inferior epigastric artery.* **rami occipitales arteriae cerebri posterioris** Occipital branches of the posterior cerebral artery, supplying the cuneus, the lingual gyrus, and the posterolateral surface of the occipital lobe. **rami occipitales arteriae occipitalis** [NA] Occipital branches of the occipital artery distributed to the posterior scalp as far forward as the vertex of the skull. **r. occipitalis arteriae auricularis posterioris** [NA] A branch arising from the posterior auricular artery in the groove between the auricular cartilage and the mastoid process. It supplies the occipital belly of the occipitofrontalis muscle and anastomoses with the occipital artery. Also *occipital branch of posterior auricular artery.* **r. occipitalis nervi auricularis posterioris** [NA] The occipital branch of the posterior auricular nerve, coursing along the superior nuchal line of the occipital bone and motor to the occipital belly of the occipitofrontalis muscle. **rami omentales arteriae gastro-omentalis dextrae** [NA] Branches of the right gastroepiploic artery that descend from the greater curvature of the stomach into the greater omentum to supply it. Also *omental branches of right gastroepiploic artery.* **rami omentales arteriae gastro-omentalis sinistrae** [NA] Branches of the left gastro-omental artery that descend from the upper part of the greater curvature of the stomach into the greater omentum to supply it. An especially large branch is given off from the terminal part of the artery. **rami orbitales arteriae cerebri anterioris** *Outmoded* ARTERIA FRONTOBASALIS MEDIALIS. **rami orbitales arteriae cerebri mediae** *Outmoded* ARTERIA FRONTOBASALIS LATERALIS. **rami orbitales ganglii pterygopalatini** [NA] Orbital branches of the pterygopalatineganglion, two or three general sensory and autonomic filaments that enter the orbit via the inferior orbital fissure and supply the periosteum and the orbitalis muscle. Also *rami orbitales ganglii sphenopalatini, orbital nerves.* **r. orbitofrontalis lateralis** ARTERIA FRONTOBASALIS LATERALIS. **r. orbitofrontalis medialis** ARTERIA FRONTOBASALIS MEDIALIS. **r. ossis ischii** [NA] A flattened bony projection from the lower extremity of the body of the ischium which extends upwards, medially, and forwards at an acute angle to join the inferior ramus of pubis on the medial side of the obturator foramen. Also *ramus of ischium ischial ramus.* **r. ovaricus arteriae uterinae** [NA] The terminal branch of the uterine artery that anastomoses with the ovarian artery near the hilum of the ovary, supplying it. Also *ovarian branch of uterine artery.* **r. palmaris nervi mediani** [NA] The palmar branch of the median nerve, arising above the flexor retinaculum, piercing the deep fascia, and supplying the skin over the thenar eminence. Also *palmar cutaneous branch of median nerve.* **r. palmaris nervi ulnaris** [NA] The palmar cutaneous branch of the ulnar nerve, arising in the forearm and following the ulnar artery into the hand. It conveys general sensation from the skin of the palm and communicates with the palmar branch of the nerve. Also *ramus cutaneus palmaris nervi ulnaris, ramus volaris manus nervi ulnaris.* **r. palmaris profundus arteriae ulnaris** [NA] A branch arising from the ulnar artery distal to the pisiform bone and passing between the hypothenar muscles to reach the proximal ends of the metacarpal bones where it anastomoses with the radial artery to form the deep palmar arch. Also *deep palmar branch of ulnar artery, deep volar metacarpal artery, deep palmar artery.* **r. palmaris superficialis arteriae radialis** [NA] A branch arising from the radial artery anterior to the distal end of the radius and running superficial to or through the thenar muscles, supplying them and anastomosing usually with the terminal part of the ulnar artery to form the superficial palmar arch. It is variable in size and termination. Also *superficial palmar branch of radial artery, superficial palmar artery, superficial volar artery.* **rami palpebrales inferiores nervi infraorbitalis** [NA] Inferior palpebral branches of the infraorbital nerve, ascending deep to the orbicularis oculi and piercing the muscle to supply the skin of the lower eyelid. **rami palpebrales nervi infratrochlearis** [NA] Palpebral branches of the infratrochlear nerve, comprising two sensory branches, a superior branch to the skin of the medial side of the upper eyelid and an inferior branch to the lower eyelid. **r. palpebralis inferior nervi infratrochlearis** The inferior branch of the rami palpebrales nervi infratrochlearis. **r. palpebralis superior nervi infratrochlearis** The superior branch of the rami palpebrales nervi infratrochlearis. **rami pancreatici arteriae gastroduodenalis** Small branches that arise from the gastroduodenal artery behind the upper part of the head of the pancreas, supplying it. Also *pancreatic branches of gastroduodenal artery of Murray.* **rami pancreatici arteriae lienalis** RAMI PANCREATICI ARTERIAE SPLENICAE. **rami pancreatici arteriae pancreaticoduodenalis superioris** [NA] Branches arising from both the anterior and the posterior superior pancreaticoduodenal arteries and supplying the front and the back of the head of the pancreas, respectively. Also *pancreatic branches of superior pancreaticoduodenal artery.* **rami pancreatici arteriae splenicae** [NA] Several branches arising from the splenic artery at varying intervals on its course along the upper margin of the pancreas and supplying the neck, body, and tail of the pancreas. Also *pancreatic branches of splenic artery, rami pancreatici arteriae lienalis.* **rami parietales arteriae cerebri anterioris** RAMI PARIETO-OCCIPITALES ARTERIAE CEREBRI ANTERIORIS. **rami parietales arteriae cerebri mediae** Parietal branches of the middle cerebral artery, consisting of anterior and posterior parietal vessels. These branches supply the lateral surface of the parietal lobe of the brain as far posteriorly as the parieto-occipital sulcus. **rami parietales arteriae hypogastricae** Parietal branches of the hypogastric artery, supplying the walls, or parietes, of the pelvis. Also *parietal branches of internal iliac artery.* **r. parietalis arteriae meningeae mediae** [NA] The parietal branch of the middle meningeal artery, arising from the middle meningeal artery in the middle cranial fossa, coursing posteriorly on the squamus part of the temporal and parietal bones, and dividing into several branches that supply the posterior part of the dura mater and cranium. **r. parietalis arteriae temporalis superficialis** [NA] The parietal branch of the superficial temporal artery. This vessel is the posterior terminal branch of the superficial temporal artery, and courses upward and backward on the side of the head to supply the scalp in the parietal region. It anastomoses across the midline with the same vessel on the opposite side, as well as with the occipital and posterior auricular arteries. Also *posterior branch of superficial temporal artery.* **rami parieto-occipitales arteriae cerebri anterioris** One or more of the terminal vessels derived from the postcommunical part of the anterior cerebral artery that supply the more posterior part of the medial surface of the parietal lobe, including the paracentral and precuneal lobules as far as the parieto-occipital sulcus. Also *parietal branches of anterior cerebral artery, rami parietales arteriae cerebri anterioris.* **r. parieto-occipitalis arteriae cerebri posterioris** [NA] One of the vessels derived from the medial cerebral artery, helping to supply the medial surface of the occipital lobe from the lingual gyrus through the cuneus to the parieto-occipital sulcus. **rami parotidei nervi auriculotemporalis** [NA] Parotid branches of the auriculotemporal nerve, containing secretomotor fibers to the parotid gland (via communication with branches of the facial nerve) and vasomotor fibers to blood vessels of the parotid gland. Also *parotid nerves.* **rami parotidei venae facialis** [NA] Small veins draining the cheek over the parotid and masseteric regions and following the parotid duct to enter the facial vein. Also *parotid branches of facial vein, anterior parotid veins.* **r. parotideus arteriae auricularis posterioris** [NA] One of several branches to the parotid gland arising from the posterior auricular artery deep to or in the substance of the gland where it is situated as it passes dorsally toward the gap between the mastoid process and the external acoustic meatus. Also *parotid branch of posterior auricular artery, parotid artery.* **r. parotideus arteriae temporalis superficialis** [NA] One of the small branches arising from the superficial temporal artery in the substance of the parotid gland, supplying it. Also *parotid branch of superficial temporal artery, parotid artery.* **rami pectorales arteriae thoracoacromialis** [NA] Branches arising from the thoracoacromial artery, running downwards between the pectoralis major and minor muscles, supplying them and the breast, especially in the female. Also *pectoral branches of thoracoacromial artery.* **r. perforans arteriae fibularis** [NA] A branch arising from the fibular, or peroneal, artery and piercing the interosseous membrane about two inches above the lateral malleolus to anastomose with the anterior lateral malleolar artery, after which it runs distally anterior to the tibiofibular syndesmosis to anastomose with the lateral tarsal artery. Also *ramus perforans arteriae peroneae, perforating branch of peroneal artery, perforating peroneal artery.* **rami perforantes arteriae thoracicae internae** [NA] Branches arising from the internal thoracic artery in the upper six intercostal spaces and piercing the internal intercostal muscle to penetrate and supply the pectoralis major muscle, through which twigs emerge close to the sternum to supply the skin. Branches to the mammary gland are given off in the second, third, and fourth spaces, especially in the female. Also *perforating branches of internal thoracic artery, perforating arteries of internal mammary artery, anterior perforating arteries.* **rami perforantes arteriarum metacarpalium palmarium** [NA] Branches in the second, third, and fourth interosseous spaces that proximally connect either the palmar metacarpal arteries or the deep palmar arch with the corresponding dorsal metacarpal arteries. Also *perforating branches of palmar metacarpal arteries, perforating arteries of hand.* **rami perforantes arteriarum metatarsalium plantarium** [NA] Branches arising distally from the four plantar metatarsal arteries proximal to their division at the webs of the toes and passing dorsally to join the corresponding dorsal metatarsal arteries. Also *perforating branches of plantar metatarsal arteries, perforating arteries of foot.* **rami pericardiaci aortae thoracicae** [NA] Small branches of the thoracic aorta that pass to the posterior surface of the pericardium to supply it and posterior mediastinal lymph nodes. Also *pericardiac branches of thoracic aorta, posterior pericardiac arteries.* **r. pericardiacus nervi phrenici** [NA] The pericardial branch of the phrenic nerve, a general sensory branch arising in the thorax and supplying the mediastinal pleura, the fibrous pericardium, and the parietal layer of serous pericardium. **rami perineales nervi cutanei femoris posterioris** [NA] Perineal branches of the posterior femoral cutaneous nerve, sensory branches to the skin of the medial side of the thigh and to skin of the scrotum (in males) or labium majus (in females). **r. petrosus arteriae meningeae mediae** [NA] The petrosal branch of the middle meningeal artery. It arises within the cranial cavity, enters the hiatus for the greater petrosal nerve, helps to supply the facial nerve and the tympanic cavity of the middle ear, and anastomoses with the stylomastoid branch of the posterior auricular artery. Also *ramus petrosus superficialis arteriae meningeae mediae.* **rami pharyngeales arteriae pharyngeae ascendentis** [NA] Branches arising from the ascending pharyngeal artery and supplying the superior and middle pharyngeal constrictor muscles, their lining mucous membrane, and the stylopharyngeus muscle. Also *pharyngeal branches of ascending pharyngeal artery.* **rami pharyngeales arteriae thyroideae inferioris** [NA] Branches of the inferior thyroid artery that supply the lower part of the pharynx and anastomose with other arteries there. Also *pharyngeal branches of inferior thyroid artery.* **rami pharyngei nervi glossopharyngei** [NA] Pharyngeal branches of the glossopharyngeal nerve, joining with sympathetic fibers and vagal branches to form the pharyngeal plexus and conveying general sensation from the mucosa of the oropharynx. **rami pharyngei nervi vagi** [NA] Pharyngeal branches of the vagus nerve, the principal motor nerves to the pharynx. **r. pharyngeus arteriae maxillaris** [NA] A small branch arising from the maxillary artery in the pterygopalatine fossa and supplying branches to the mucous membrane of the roof of the nose, upper part of the pharynx, sphenoidal sinus, and the inner end of the auditory tube. Also *pharyngeal branch of maxillary artery.* **r. pharyngeus ganglii pterygopalatini** [NA] The pharyngeal branch of the pterygopalatine ganglion, arising from the posterior part of the ganglion and entering the palatovaginal canal to supply the mucosa of the nasopharynx behind the auditory tube. Also *Bock's nerve.* **r. pharyngeus of maxillary nerve** The pharyngeal branch of the maxillary nerve. It supplies the mucous membrane of the nasopharynx posterior to the auditory tube. **rami phrenicoabdominales nervi phrenici** [NA] Phrenicoabdominal branches of the phrenic nerve, terminal branches that pass through the diaphragm, are distributed on its undersurface, and supply motor fibers to the diaphragm and sensory fibers to the peritoneum. They communicate with the phrenic and celiac plexuses. Also *phrenicoabdominal nerves.* **r. plantaris profundus arteriae dorsalis pedis** [NA] A terminal branch of the dorsalis pedis artery that passes through the heads of the first dorsal interosseous muscle into the sole of the foot. Also *deep plantar branch of dorsalis pedis artery.* **r. posterior arteriae obturatoriae** [NA] The posterior division of the obturator artery, supplying the muscles attached to the ischial tuberosity. Also *posterior branch of obturator artery.* **r. posterior arteriae pancreaticoduodenalis inferioris** [NA] A branch that usually arises from the inferior pancreaticoduodenal artery and supplies the head and uncinate process of the pancreas and the duodenum. Also *left superior pancreaticoduodenal artery* (outmoded). **r. posterior arteriae recurrentis ulnaris** [NA] A branch arising from the ulnar artery below the elbow joint and just distal to the origin of the smaller anterior ulnar recurrent artery. It supplies the two heads of flexor carpi ulnaris muscle, adjacent muscles, and the elbow joint. Also *posterior branch of ulnar recurrent artery, posterior ulnar recurrent artery.* **r. posterior arteriae renalis** [NA] The branch of the renal artery given off in the region of the hilum of the kidney and supplying the segmental artery to the posterior vascular segment of the kidney. Also *posterior branch of renal artery.* **r. posterior arteriae thyroideae superioris** [NA] A branch of the superior thyroid artery that extends from the apex of the lobe of the thyroid gland along the posterior border, supplying both lateral and medial surfaces, to anastomose with the inferior thyroid artery. Also *posterior branch of superior thyroid artery.* **r. posterior ascendens arteriae pulmonalis dextrae** [NA] A branch of the superior branch of the right pulmonary artery which supplies the upper part of the posterior bronchopulmonary segment (B II) of the right superior lobe. Also *posterior ascending branch of right pulmonary artery.* **r. posterior ductus hepatici dextri** [NA] A branch of the right hepatic duct draining the posterior segment of the right lobe of the liver. Also *posterior branch of right hepatic duct.* **rami posteriores nervorum cervicalium** RAMI DORSALES NERVORUM CERVICALIUM. **rami posteriores nervorum lumbalium** RAMI DORSALES NERVORUM LUMBALIUM. **rami posteriores nervorum sacralium** RAMI DORSALES NERVORUM SACRALIUM. **rami posteriores nervorum thoracalium** RAMI DORSALES NERVORUM THORACICORUM. **r. posterior fissurae cerebri lateralis sylvii** RAMUS POSTERIOR SULCI LATERALIS CEREBRI. **r. posterior nervi auricularis magni** [NA] The posterior branch of the great auricular nerve, constituting a general sensory nerve to the skin over the mastoid process and the back of the auricle. Also *internal auricular nerve.* **r. posterior nervi coccygei** RAMUS DORSALIS NERVI COCCYGEI. **r. posterior nervi cutanei antebrachii medialis** [NA] RAMUS ULNARIS NERVI CUTANEI ANTEBRACHIIMEDIALIS. **r. posterior nervi laryngei inferioris** The posterior branch of the inferior laryngeal nerve, one of two terminal branches that supply the intrinsic musculature of the dorsal part of the larynx. **r. posterior nervi obturatorii** [NA] The posterior branch of the obturator nerve which supplies motor innervation to the obturator externus, adductor magnus, and adductor brevis muscles. **r. posterior nervorum spinalium** RAMUS DORSALIS NERVORUM SPINALIUM. **r. posterior rami dextri venae portae hepatis** [NA] A branch of the right branch of the portal vein that runs in the liver with the posterior segmental artery of the right branch of the hepatic artery and supplies the posterior segment of the right lobe of the liver. Also *posterior branch of right branch of portal vein.* **r. posterior ramorum cutaneorum lateralium arteriarum intercostalium** The posterior branch of lateral cutaneous branches of the intercostal arteries. **r. posterior ramorum cutaneorum lateralium nervorum intercostalium** The posterior ramus of the lateral cutaneous branches of the intercostal nerves, a terminal branch that runs backward to supply the skin over the scapula and latissimus dorsi muscle. **r. posterior sulci lateralis cerebri** [NA] The posterior branch of the lateral cerebral sulcus, the continuation of the lateral cerebral sulcus posteriorly between the temporal and parietal lobes. Also *ramus posterior fissurae cerebralis lateralis sylvii.* **r. profundus arteriae cervicalis ascendentis** The deep branch of the ascending cervical artery, supplying deep musculature in the neck and often giving off spinal branches. **r. profundus arteriae circumflexae femoris medialis** [NA] A terminal branch of the medial circumflex femoral artery arising posteriorly after the latter has emerged between quadratus femoris and adductor magnus muscles and helping to supply the neck and head of femur. Also *deep branch of medial circumflex femoral artery, internal deep circumflex artery.* **r. profundus arteriae gluteae superioris** [NA] A branch arising from the superior gluteal artery outside the pelvis and running laterally on the ilium deep to gluteus medius muscle where it divides into ramus inferior arteriae gluteae superioris and ramus superior arteriae gluteae superioris. Also *deep branch of superior gluteal artery.* **r. profundus arteriae plantaris medialis** [NA] A branch of the medial plantar artery that runs distally between abductor hallucis and flexor digitorum brevis muscles, supplying them and joints and the skin on the medial side, and branching to anastomose with branches of the dorsalis pedis artery along the medial side of the foot. Also *deep branch of medial plan-*

*tar artery.* **r. profundus nervi plantaris lateralis** [NA] The deep branch of the lateral plantar nerve, supplying the second, third, and fourth lumbricales, the adductor hallucis, and interossei muscles. **r. profundus nervi radialis** [NA] NERVUS INTEROSSEUS ANTEBRACHII POSTERIOR. **r. profundus nervi ulnaris** [NA] The deep branch of the ulnar nerve. It supplies motor innervation to the hypothenar, interosseous muscles, third and fourth lumbricales, and adductor pollicis muscles. **rami prostatici arteriae vesicalis inferioris** [NA] Branches of the inferior vesical artery that anastomose with similar branches of the opposite side at the junction of the prostate and the urinary bladder and ramify tortuously in the prostatic capsule before entering the prostate. Also *prostatic branches of inferior vesical artery.* **rami pterygoidei arteriae maxillaris** [NA] Irregular branches arising from the second part of the maxillary artery and supplying the pterygoid muscles. Also *pterygoid branches of maxillary artery, pterygoid arteries.* **r. pubicus arteriae epigastricae inferioris** [NA] A branch of the inferior epigastric artery that courses from the deep inguinal ring downward behind the pubis and medial to the femoral ring to anastomose with the pubic branch of the obturator artery. In about one third of cases this anastomosis is large, lies on the lateral side of the femoral ring, and replaces the obturator artery as an "abnormal obturator artery." Also *pubic branch of inferior epigastric artery, pubic artery.* **r. pubicus arteriae obturatoriae** [NA] A branch arising from the obturator artery and passing upward behind the pubis to anastomose with the artery from the opposite side and with the pubic branch of the inferior epigastric artery medial to the femoral ring. Also *pubic branch of obturator artery, pubic artery.* **rami pulmonales systematis autonomici** [NA] Pulmonary branches of the autonomic nervous system. They supply autonomic and visceral afferent innervation, via the anterior and posterior pulmonary plexuses, to blood vessels and bronchi of the lungs. Also *rami pulmonales plexus cardiaci.* **rami renales nervi vagi** [NA] Renal branches of the vagus nerve, containing parasympathetic and sensory fibers. They arise from both vagal trunks and join the renal plexus, from which they are distributed to the kidney. Also *rami renales plexus celiaci.* **r. renalis nervi splanchnici minoris** [NA] The renal branch of the lesser splanchnic nerve, conveying preganglionic sympathetic and sensory fibers to the aorticorenal ganglion. **r. saphenus arteriae descendentis genicularis** [NA] A branch arising from the descending genicular artery and piercing the roof of the adductor canal to accompany the saphenous nerve to the medial side of the knee, where it supplies the skin on the superomedial aspect of the leg and anastomoses with the medial inferior genicular artery. Also *saphenous branch of descending genicular artery.* **rami scrotales anteriores arteriae pudendae externae** [NA] Branches arising from both the superficial and the deep external pudendal artery and supplying the skin of the scrotum and anastomosing with the posterior scrotal branches of the internal pudendal artery. Also *anterior scrotal branches of external pudendal artery, anterior scrotal branches of femoral artery, anterior scrotal arteries.* **rami scrotales posteriores arteriae pudendae internae** [NA] The small terminal branches of the perineal artery, distributed to the skin and dartos muscle of the scrotum as well as some perineal muscles. They anastomose with the anterior scrotal branches of the external pudendal artery. Also *posterior scrotal branches of internal pudendal artery, posterior scrotal arteries.* **rami septales posteriores** [NA] The terminal branches of the sphenopalatine artery, which ramify on the nasal septum and anastomose with ethmoidal arteries. Also *posterior septal branches of sphenopalatine artery, posterior septal arteries.* **r. septi nasi arteriae labialis superioris** [NA] A branch of the superior labial artery that arises near the edge of the upper lip near its center and ascends onto the lower and front part of the nasal septum to supply it and to anastomose with one of the posterior septal branches of the sphenopalatine artery. Also *septal branch of superior labial artery, anterior septal artery.* **r. sinister arteriae hepaticae propriae** [NA] A branch arising from the hepatic artery proper in the lesser omentum near the porta hepatis and proceeding in the fissure for ligamentum venosum to supply the left lobe of the liver. Also *left branch of proper hepatic artery.* **r. sinister venae portae hepatis** [NA] A branch arising from the portal vein in the right margin of the lesser omentum and supplying branches to the caudate and quadrate lobes before joining the corresponding branch of the hepatic artery to enter the left lobe of the liver. Also *left branch of portal vein.* **r. sinus carotici nervi glossopharyngei** [NA] The carotid sinus branch of the glossopharyngeal nerve, constituting a sensory nerve with pressoreceptor endings in the wall of the carotid sinus that respond to elevated arterial pressure and elicit reflex vasodilation and decreased heart rate in order to lower blood pressure. Also *sinus nerve, Hering's nerve.* **rami spinales arteriae cervicalis ascendentis** [NA] A few branches arising from the ascending cervical artery and entering the vertebral canal through the intervertebral foramina to supply the spinal cord and its membranes and the bodies of the cervical vertebrae. Also *spinal branches of ascending cervical artery.* **rami spinales arteriae intercostalis supremae** [NA] Branches arising from the dorsal branches of the first two posterior intercostal arteries and entering the vertebral canal through the intervertebral foramina to supply the spinal cord and its membranes and the vertebral bodies. Also *spinal branches of highest intercostal artery, spinal branches of superior intercostal artery.* **rami spinales arteriae vertebralis** [NA] Branches arising from the vertebral artery and entering the vertebral canal through the intervertebral foramina. Also *spinal branches of vertebral artery.* **rami spinales arteriarum sacralium lateralium** [NA] Branches arising from the superior and inferior lateral sacral arteries and supplying the spinal membranes and anastomosing with one another. Also *spinal branches of lateral sacral arteries.* **r. spinalis arteriae iliolumbalis** *Outmoded* RAMUS SPINALIS RAMI LUMBALIS ARTERIAE ILIOLUMBALIS. **r. spinalis arteriae subcostalis** [NA] A branch of the dorsal branch of the subcostal artery. It supplies the spinal cord and its membranes and the vertebrae. Also *spinal branch of subcostal artery.* **r. spinalis arteriarum lumbalium** [NA] A branch arising from the dorsal branch of each lumbar artery and entering the vertebral canal through the intervertebral foramen to supply the spinal cord and its membranes and the vertebrae. Also *spinal branch of lumbar arteries.* **r. spinalis rami dorsalis arteriarum intercostalium posteriorum III–XI** [NA] A branch of the dorsal branch of the posterior intercostal arteries (III–XI). It enters the vertebral canal through the intervertebral foramen. Also *spinal branch of dorsal branch of posterior intercostal arteries III–XI.* **r. spinalis rami lumbalis arteriae iliolumbalis** [NA] A small branch of the lumbar branch of the iliolumbar artery that enters the vertebral canal to supply the cauda equina. Also *ramus spinalis arteriae iliolumbalis* (outmoded). **r. spinalis venarum intercostalium posteriorum IV–XI** [NA] A vein accompanying the spinal branch of each dorsal branch of the posterior intercostal arteries (IV–XI) and draining the vertebral venous plexuses and bodies of the vertebrae into the dorsal branches of the posterior intercostal veins (IV–XI). Also *spinal branch of posterior intercostal veins.* **rami splenici arteriae splenicae** [NA] The terminal branches of the splenic artery that penetrate the hilum of the spleen between the two layers of the lienorenal ligament to branch throughout the spleen in the trabeculae. Also *splenic branches of splenic artery.* **r. stapedialis arteriae stylomastoideae** [NA] A branch occasionally arising from either the stylomastoid artery in the facial canal or its posterior tympanic branch and supplying the stapedius muscle and tendon. Also *stapedial branch of stylomastoid artery.* **rami sternales arteriae thoracicae internae** [NA] Branches arising from the internal thoracic artery and supplying the back of the sternum and the transversus thoracis muscle. Also *sternal branches of internal thoracic artery, posterior sternal arteries, sternal arteries.* **rami sternocleidomastoidei arteriae occipitalis** [NA] Branches of the occipital artery: an upper branch arising from it as it crosses the accessory nerve, and a lower branch, which occasionally arises from the external carotid artery. Also *sternocleidomastoid branches of occipital artery, sternocleidomastoid artery, arteria sternocleidomastoidea.* **r. sternocleidomastoideus arteriae thyroideae superioris** [NA] A branch arising from either the superior thyroid or the external carotid artery and supplying the middle of the sternocleidomastoid muscle. Also *sternocleidomastoid branch of superior thyroid artery, superior sternocleidomastoid artery, sternocleidomastoid artery.* **rami striati arteriae cerebri mediae** STRIATE ARTERIES. **r. stylohyoideus nervi facialis** [NA] The stylohyoid branch of the facial nerve, motor to the stylohyoid muscle. Also *stylohyoid nerve.* **r. stylopharyngeus nervi glossopharyngei** RAMUS MUSCULI STYLOPHARYNGEI NERVI GLOSSOPHARYNGEI. **rami submaxillares ganglii submaxillaris** RAMI GLANDULARES GANGLII SUBMANDIBULARIS. **rami subscapulares arteriae axillaris** [NA] Branches arising from the axillary artery that supply the subscapularis muscle. Also *subscapular branches of axillary artery.* **r. superficialis arteriae gluteae superioris** [NA] A branch arising from the superior gluteal artery as it leaves the greater sciatic foramen above the piriformis muscle and entering the deep surface of the gluteus maximus muscle to supply it. Also *superficial branch of superior gluteal artery.* **r. superficialis arteriae plantaris medialis** [NA] A branch arising from the medial plantar artery and dividing into twigs that run with the digital branches of the medial plantar nerve to anastomose with the medial three plantar metatarsal arteries. A twig may join the lateral plantar artery to form the superficial plantar arch. Also *superficial branch of medial plantar artery, superficial medial artery of foot.* **r. superficialis arteriae transversae cervicis** [NA] A branch arising from the transverse cervical artery of the thyrocervical trunk. It supplies the trapezius muscle, and adjacent muscles and lymph nodes. Also *superficial branch of transverse cervical artery, transverse artery of neck, superficial transverse cervical artery.* **r. superficialis nervi plantaris lateralis** [NA] The superficial branch of the lateral plantar nerve, dividing into two plantar digital nerves, sensory to the skin of the fourth and fifth toes and motor to the flexor digiti minimi brevis and the two interossei of the fourth metatarsal space. **r. superficialis nervi radialis** [NA] The superficial branch of the radial nerve, accompanying the radial artery deep to the brachioradialis muscle in the forearm. Also *superficial radial nerve.* **r. superficialis nervi ulnaris** [NA] The superficial branch of the ulnar nerve, supplying motor fibers to the palmaris brevis muscle and sensory fibers to the skin on the medial side of the hand. It divides into two palmar digital nerves. **r. superior arteriae gluteae superioris** [NA] A division of the deep branch of the superior gluteal artery lying deep to the gluteus medius muscle. Also *superior branch of superior gluteal artery.* **rami superiores nervi transversi colli** [NA] Superior branches of the transverse cervical nerves, distributed to the skin of the upper and front parts of the neck. Also *rami superiores nervi cutanei colli.* **r. superior nervi oculomotorii** [NA] The superior branch of the oculomotor nerve, ascending in the orbit lateral to the optic nerve and supplying motor innervation to the superior rectus and levator palpebrae superioris muscles. **r. superior ossis pubis** [NA] A triangular bar of bone extending posterosuperiorly and laterally above the obturator foramen from the superolateral part of the body of the pubis to the acetabulum forming about one-fifth of its articular surface. Also *superior pubic ramus.* **r. suprahyoideus arteriae lingualis** [NA] A small branch arising from the lingual artery at the greater cornu of the hyoid bone and running along its upper border superficial to the hyoglossus muscle to anastomose with its fellow from the opposite side and supply adjacent muscles. Also *suprahyoid branch of lingual artery, hyoid artery.* **r. sympathicus ad ganglion ciliare** [NA] The sympathetic branch of the ciliary ganglion. Also *radices sympatheticae ganglii ciliaris, radices molles ganglii ciliaris, sympathetic roots of ciliary ganglion.* **r. sympathicus ad ganglion submandibulare** [NA] The sympathetic branch to the submandibular ganglion. Also *radix sympathica ganglii submaxillaris.* **rami temporales arteriae cerebri mediae** Temporal branches of the middle cerebral artery, two or three in number, distributed on the lateral surface of the temporal lobe. **rami temporales arteriae cerebri posterioris** Temporal branches of the posterior cerebral artery, usually two in number, distributed to the uncus and the parahippocaudal, medial, and lateral occipitotemporal gyri. **rami temporales nervi facialis** [NA] Temporal branches of the facial nerve, motor to several facial muscles. Also *temporal facial nerve.* **rami temporales superficiales nervi auriculotemporalis** [NA] Superficial temporal branches of the auriculotemporal nerve, sensory to the skin of the temporal region. Also *subcutaneous temporal nerves.* **r. tentorii nervi ophthalmici** [NA] The tentorial branch of the ophthalmic nerve. Also *tentorial nerve, nervus tentorii, ophthalmic recurrent nerve.* **rami thalamici arteriae cerebri posterioris** THALAMOGENICULATE ARTERIES. **rami thymici arteriae thoracicae internae** [NA] Branches arising from the internal thoracic artery, and often from its mediastinal branches, that supply the remains of the thymus gland. Also *thymic branches of internal thoracic artery, thymic arteries, lateral thymic arteries.* **r. thyrohyoideus ansae cervicalis** [NA] The thyrohyoid branch of the ansa cervicalis, supplying the thyrohyoid bone muscle. Also *nerve to thyrohyoid muscle.* **rami tonsillares nervi glossopharyngei** [NA] Tonsillar branches of the glossopharyngeal nerve, sensory filaments that supply the tonsil and form a plexus with branches of the middle and posterior palatine nerves. Also *tonsillar nerves.* **r. tonsillaris arteriae facialis** [NA] A branch arising from the facial artery and ascending between the styloglossus and medial pterygoid muscles and piercing the superior pharyngeal constrictor muscle to supply the tonsil and to anastomose with other tonsillar arteries. Also *ton-*

*sillar branch of facial artery, tonsillar artery.* **rami tracheales arteriae thyroideae inferioris** [NA] Branches arising from the inferior thyroid artery to supply the trachea and anastomose inferiorly with the bronchial arteries. Also *tracheal branches of inferior thyroid artery.* **rami tracheales nervi laryngei recurrentis** [NA] Tracheal branches of the recurrent laryngeal nerve, conveying general sensation from the mucosa of the trachea. Also *rami tracheales nervi laryngei recurrentis.* **r. transversus arteriae circumflexae femoris lateralis** [NA] A branch arising from the lateral circumflex femoral artery and ending at the back of the thigh in the cruciate anastomosis. Also *transverse branch of lateral circumflex femoral artery.* **r. transversus arteriae circumflexae femoris medialis** [NA] A branch arising from the medial circumflex femoral artery as it emerges between the quadratus femoris and adductor magnus muscles at the back of the thigh, where it takes part in the cruciate anastomosis. Also *transverse branch of medial circumflex femoral artery.* **r. tubae plexus tympanici jacobsoni** RAMUS TUBARIUS PLEXUS TYMPANICI. **r. tubarius arteriae uterinae** [NA] One or more small branches arising from the termination of the uterine artery and running along the lower surface of the uterine tube, supplying it and the round ligament of uterus. Also *tubal branch of uterine artery.* **r. tubarius plexus tympanici** [NA] The tubal branch of the tympanic plexus, constituting a general sensory nerve to the mucosa of the auditory tube. Also *ramus tubae plexus tympanici jacobsoni.* **r. ulnaris nervi cutanei antebrachii medialis** [NA] The ulnar branch of the medial antebrachial cutaneous nerve. It is sensory to the skin along the posterior and medial forearm as far as the wrist. Also *ramus posterior nervi cutanei antebrachii medialis.* **rami ureterici arteriae ductus deferentis** [NA] Branches of the artery to the ductus deferens distributed to the ureter near the base of the bladder. Also *ureteral branches of artery of ductus deferens.* **rami ureterici arteriae ovaricae** [NA] Branches arising from the ovarian artery and distributed to the ureter as the latter is crossed by the artery. Also *ureteral branches of ovarian artery.* **rami ureterici arteriae renalis** [NA] Branches arising from the renal artery to supply the upper part of the ureter and the adjacent connective tissue and muscles. Also *ureteric branches of renal artery.* **rami ureterici arteriae testicularis** [NA] Branches arising from the testicular artery as it crosses the ureter mediolaterally on the posterior abdominal wall, supplying it and the adjacent retroperitoneal tissue. Also *ureteric branches of testicular artery.* **rami ventrales nervorum cervicalium** [NA] The ventral primary branches of the cervical spinal nerves, forming the cervical and part of the brachial plexuses. Also *rami anteriores nervorum cervicalium.* **rami ventrales nervorum lumbalium** [NA] The ventral primary branches of the lumbar spinal nerves, joined by gray rami communicantes of the lumbar sympathetic chain, passing through the psoas major muscle, and forming the lumbar plexus and the lumbosacral trunk. Also *rami anteriores nervorum lumbalium.* **rami ventrales nervorum sacralium** [NA] PLEXUS SACRALIS. **rami ventrales nervorum thoracicorum** [NA] The ventral branches of the twelve thoracic nerves, of which the first joins the brachial plexus, 2-12 are called intercostal nerves, and 12 is called the subcostal nerve. Also *rami anteriores nervorum thoracalium.* **r. ventralis nervi coccygei** The ventral primary ramus of the coccygeal nerve that unites with the fourth and fifth sacral nerves to form the coccygeal plexus. Also *ramus anterior nervi coccygei.* **r. ventralis nervorum spinalium** [NA] The ventral primary division of each of the spinal nerves. They supply the anterior and lateral portions of the trunk and all portions of the limbs and give rise to the cervical, brachial, lumbar, sacral, and coccygeal plexuses. Also *ramus anterior nervorum spinalium, anterior primary rami.* **rami vestibulares arteriae labyrinthi** [NA] Branches arising from the labyrinthine artery at the bottom of the internal acoustic meatus and distributed to the saccule, utricle, and semicircular ducts. Also *vestibular branches of labyrinthine artery.* **r. volaris manus nervi ulnaris** RAMUS PALMARIS NERVI ULNARIS. **r. volaris nervi cutanei antebrachii medialis** RAMUS ANTERIOR NERVI CUTANEI ANTEBRACHII MEDIALIS. **rami zygomatici nervi facialis** [NA] Zygomatic branches of the facial nerve, motor twigs to the orbicularis oculi muscle. **r. zygomaticofacialis nervi zygomatici** [NA] The cutaneous branch of the zygomatic nerve, running from the lateral orbit through the zygomatic bone. Also *zygomaticofacial nerve.* **r. zygomaticotemporalis nervi zygomatici** [NA] The zygomaticotemporal branch of the zygomatic nerve, running in the lateral wall of the orbit, exiting through the zygomaticotemporal foramen, entering the temporal fossa, and running through the temporalis muscle to the skin on the side of the forehead. Also *zygomaticotemporal nerve.*

**randomization** \ran′dəmīzā′shən\ [*random* + *-iz(e)* + -ATION] A selection of subjects or cases for study or experimentation that approximates so far as practicable one resulting by chance in order to exclude bias and minimize the influence of irrelevant factors so as to produce statistically reliable data.

**range** [French *rang* (from Middle French *rang, reng* a line, row, of Germanic origin) order of persons or things in a line] The difference between the extreme values in a statistical series. **r. of accommodation** The linear distance between the far point and the near point of accommodation. Also *range of convergence, region of accommodation, breadth of accommodation.* **r. of audibility** RANGE OF HEARING. **audiofrequency r.** The range of frequencies audible to a particular animal species, there being marked variations especially at the upper limit of hearing. In man it extends from approximately 16 Hz to 20 000 Hz, with maximal sensitivity to frequencies in the 2000 Hz region of the sound spectrum. **r. of convergence** RANGE OF ACCOMMODATION. **dynamic r.** The ratio, in decibels, of the largest to smallest amplitude, power, or intensity that a system or system component can handle. **r. of hearing** The range of frequencies of sound which an animal species is able to hear. It is characterized by a central range of sensitivity to extremely low levels of acoustic energy with the upper and lower limits requiring exponential increments of energy to remain audible. Also *range of audibility.* **interquartile r.** The distance between the upper and lower quartiles. This interval will contain one-half of the observations. **normal r.** The range of results of a test or measurement obtained in healthy persons. Also *normal values, reference range.* **particle r.** The depth to which a particle will penetrate a given substance before its kinetic energy is reduced to the value below which it can no longer produce ionization. **reference r.** NORMAL RANGE. **r. of sensibility** FECHNER'S LAW. **thermal comfort r.** A range of environmental conditions in which it is possible to work without undue thermal strain. The acceptable temperature (dry-bulb) depends on the clothing worn, the work done, and the metabolic rate of the individual. When excessive or special protective clothing is not being worn, temperatures within the range of 16–24°C are acceptable, allowing for heavy work at the low end and sedentary tasks at the warm end of the range.

**ranine** \rā′nīn\ **1** Pertaining to a ranula. **2** Pertaining to the deep lingual vein.

**ranitidine** $C_{13}H_{22}N_4O_3S$. *N*-[2-[[[5-[(Dimethylamino)-methyl]-2-furanyl]methyl]thio]ethyl]-*N′*-methyl-2-nitro-1,1-ethenediamine. A blocker of histamine $H_2$ receptors used in the treatment of duodenal and gastric ulcers and esophageal reflux. Blockage of $H_2$ receptors leads to reduction in gastric acid production. It may be administered both orally and intravenously.

**Ranke** [Karl Ernst von *Ranke*, German chemist, 1870–1926] **1** Ranke stages. See under STAGE. **2** See under THEORY.

**Ransohoff** [Joseph *Ransohoff*, U.S. surgeon, 1853–1921] See under SIGN.

**ranula** \ran′yələ\ [L (dim. of *rana* frog) a little frog] A large sublingual mucocele or cyst of the sublingual salivary gland. Also *sublingual cyst* (seldom used), *frog tongue* (seldom used), *ranine tumor* (rare). **pancreatic r.** A cyst formed by obstruction of the pancreatic duct.

**ranular** \ran′yələr\ Relating to or resembling a ranula.

**ranunculin** A glucoside from the plant *Anemone pulsatilla* that releases protoanemonin, an antibacterial substance, upon hydrolysis.

**Ranvier** [Louis Antoine *Ranvier*, French pathologist, 1835–1922] **1** Ranvier's tactile disks. See under DISK. **2** Ranvier's plexus. See under SUPERFICIAL STROMA PLEXUS. **3** Internode of Ranvier, Ranvier segment. See under INTERNODAL SEGMENT. **4** See under NODE, MEMBRANE.

**rape** [Middle English *rape(n)* to rape, from L *rapere* to seize, carry off, ravish] An unlawful, nonconsensual act of sexual intercourse carried out by force or other forms of duress. The traditional attitude that only a female can be raped has changed, and many states have enacted laws defining male rape (rape of a male by another male). Threat of violence, fraud, deceit, impairment of the victim's senses, or any other method used to overcome the physical and psychological resistance of the victim is legally interpreted as nonconsent. Unforced, nonviolent rape perpetrated by such methods may be referred to as *violation.* The legal concept of sexual intercourse, formerly referred to as carnal knowledge, is any penetration of the penis into the vulva. **statutory r.** The unlawful act of sexual intercourse with a consenting or nonconsenting female whose age is less than the age of consent as defined by statute. In most states of the United States and in most other countries, the age of consent is 16, 17, or 18 years of age. Also *rape of the second degree.*

**raphe** \rā′fē\ [Gk *rhaphē* (from *rhaptein* to sew, stitch) a seam, suture] A seam; in anatomy, the line of union of various bilateral symmetrical structures. Also *rhaphe* (outmoded). **r. of the ampulla** CRISTA AMPULLARIS. **anogenital r.** A median line of closure in the male embryo extending between the genital folds and swellings from the tip of the phallus to the anus and forming in the adult the scrotal raphe which is continued anteriorly as the raphe of the urogenital surface of the penis and posteriorly as the raphe of the perineum. **buccal r.** The ridged line of fusion between the mandibular and the maxillary processes in the buccal epithelium lateral to the angle of the mouth of the embryo. **r. corporis callosi** The stria longitudinalis lateralis corporis callosi, along with the stria longitudinalis medialis corporis callosi. **horizontal r. of the eye** The part of the horizontal meridian of the eye between the upper and lower temporal quadrants. Also *median raphe.* **lateral palpebral r.** RAPHE PALPEBRALIS LATERALIS. **median r.** HORIZONTAL RAPHE OF THE EYE. **r. medullae oblongatae** [NA] The midline union of the right and leftportions of the medulla oblongata. Also *raphe of medulla oblongata.* **r. mesencephali** The midsagittal line uniting the two halves of the midbrain. Also *raphe of midbrain.* **r. palati** [NA] A line or ridge formed by mucous membrane and the underlying periosteum in the midline of the palate, terminating anteriorly in a small papilla that overlies the bony incisive fossa and extending posteriorly in the mucous membrane of the soft palate to the tip of the uvula. Also *palatine raphe, palatine ridge, longitudinal ridge of hard palate.* **r. palpebralis lateralis** [NA] The fibrous junction of the interlacing fibers of the palpebral part of the orbicularis oculi muscle beyond the lateral angle of the eye and superficial to the lateral palpebral ligament, from which it is separated by a few lobules of the lacrimal gland. Also *lateral palpebral raphe.* **r. penis** [NA] The anterior extension of the raphe of the scrotum along the skin of the urethral surface of the penis in the median plane. **r. perinei** [NA] A midline cutaneous ridge extending anteriorly from the anus to the raphe of the scrotum. Also *raphe of perineum.* **r. pharyngis** [NA] A strong fibrous band extending downwards in the median plane from the pharyngeal tubercle on the basilar part of the occipital bone to provide attachment for the constrictor muscles of the pharynx posteriorly. Also *raphe of pharynx, pharyngeal ligament, white line of pharynx.* **r. pontis** [NA] The midline union of the two halves of the pons. Also *raphe of pons, septum pontis.* **pterygomandibular r.** RAPHE PTERYGOMANDIBULARIS. **r. pterygomandibularis** [NA] A narrow tendinous band extending from the pterygoid hamulus to the posterior end of the mylohyoid line of the mandible and giving attachment posteriorly to the superior pharyngeal constrictor muscle and anteriorly to the buccinator muscle. Also *pterygomandibular raphe, pterygomandibular ligament.* **r. scroti** [NA] A longitudinal cutaneous ridge in the median plane of the scrotum which is continuous with the raphe penis anteriorly and with the raphe perinei along the median plane of the perineum to the anus posteriorly. It represents the line of fusion of the genital folds and of the genital swellings to form the scrotum in the fetus. Also *raphe of scrotum, middle line of scrotum, Veslingius line.*

**raptus** \rap′təs\ [L (from *rapere* carry off by force, ravish, seize) a tearing off, seizure] Uncoordinated motor discharge that relieves tension, such as the motility disturbances of catatonics or the motor outbursts of patients suffering from chorea.

**rarefaction** \rer′əfak′shən\ A decrease in density. **bone r.** A decrease in density of part of a bone, especially when this causes increased radiolucence.

**RAS** reticular activating system.

**ras.** *rasurae* (L, scrapings or filings).

**rasceta** \rəsē′tə\ [Med L *raseta* lines across the wrist, from Arabic *rāḥah* the palm of the hand] The lines in the skin covering the palmar surface of the wrist.

**rash** [Old French *rasche* (from L *rasus,* past part. of *radere* to shave, scrape, scratch) a rash] An inflammatory skin eruption, usually of an extensive nature. **ammonia r.** Glazed erythema of the buttocks and other prominences in the diaper area in infants which is attributed, possibly incorrectly, to ammonia derived from urea in the urine. **antitoxin r.** SERUM RASH. **astacoid r.** LOBSTER RASH. **butterfly r.** BUTTERFLY ERUPTION. **canker r.** SCARLET FEVER. **caterpillar r.** CATERPILLAR DERMATITIS. **diaper r.** A variable inflammatory disorder on the skin of the diaper region in infants. It is caused by the chemical and physical action of urine and feces and is sometimes complicated by secondary infection. **drug r.**

DRUG ERUPTION. **enema r.** An erythematous rash of the trunk which may follow the administration of a soap enema. **heat r.** Any condition aggravated by heat, such as miliaria and intertrigo, or associated with hot weather, such as insect bites. **heliotrope r.** The purplish rash occurring about the eyes in patients with dermatomyositis. **hydatid r.** An urticarial rash produced by sensitization in response to the eruption of a hydatid cyst of the tapeworm *Echinococcus.* **lobster r.** A rash of reddish hue, suggestive of a boiled lobster, sometimes seen in serious cases of hemorrhagic smallpox. Also *astacoid rash.* **medicinal r.** DRUG ERUPTION. **mulberry r.** The blotchy eruption seen in typhus. *Older term.* **nettle r.** URTICARIA. **rose r.** ROSEOLA. **scarlet r.** Any rash resembling that of scarlet fever. **serum r.** An erythematous or urticarial rash that appears following an injection of serum. Also *antitoxin rash.* **summer r.** MILIARIA RUBRA. **vaccination r.** An allergic rash following vaccination against smallpox.

**raspatory** \ras′pətôr′ē\ [Med L *raspatorium* (from *raspare* to rasp) a rasp for scraping bone] A filelike surgical scalpel that is used to abrade tissues, especially bone. Also *scalprum, rugine.*

**RAST** radioallergosorbent test.

**Rastelli** [Gian Carlo *Rastelli,* U.S. thoracic surgeon, 1933–1970] See under OPERATION.

**raster** \ras′tər\ A comblike pattern of lines traced by the spot in a television tube to provide uniform coverage of the screen.

**rat** 1 Common name for a rodent of the genus *Rattus.*. 2 Any of the larger members of the family Muridae (rats and mice), as well as rodents in other families of the order Rodentia. **black r.** Any member of the species *Rattus rattus.* **Norwegian gray r.** The common feral rat, *Rattus norvegicus,* found worldwide. It gave origin to the common albino laboratory rat and was the first mammalian animal to be domesticated for scientific research. The color is actually brown rather than gray. Various strains have been developed by inbreeding, such as the brown Norway rat. **Sprague-Dawley r.** A strain of white laboratory rats (albino rats), developed in 1925, and used extensively for experimental purposes. The precise origin of the strain is uncertain. Most stocks of these rats are random-bred. **Wistar r.** A heterogeneous strain of white laboratory rats (albino rats), originally developed at the Wistar Institute, in Philadelphia, Pennsylvania in the United States.

# rate

**rate** [Old French, from L *rata* as in *pro rata (parte)* proportionately, from *ratus,* past part. of *reri* to reckon, suppose, judge] The amount of change in a dependent variable per unit change in the independent variable; especially, the change in a time-varying quantity per unit time. **abortion r.** The number of abortions per 1000 women of reproductive age during a given interval of time, usually one year. **absorption r.** The speed with which material of known properties will be taken up by material of other properties. **adjusted r.** A rate calculated in such a way as to allow an effect, as of mortality, to be compared in different populations after removing the influence of differences in factors, such as age structure, themselves related to the effect in question. Also *corrected rate* (incorrect). **adjusted death r.** STANDARDIZED DEATH RATE. **admission r.** The ratio, usually expressed as a percentage or per thousand, of the number of admissions to an institution providing care, during a stated period, to the population served by the institution. **age-specific birth r.** A specific birth rate related to maternal age. Conventionally, the following age ranges are used: under 15 years, the five-year age ranges from 15 years to 44 years, and over 44 years. Sometimes 17 years is used as the initial age. **age-specific death r.** The number of deaths of persons of a given age group during a stated period of time related to the average size of the group over the period in question, expressed as a rate; for example, deaths per 1000 population aged 55 to 64 years per annum. Also *age-specific mortality rate.* **age-specific fertility r.** A fertility rate specific for women in a given age group. **age-specific marital fertility r.** An age-specific fertility rate having as denominator the number of married women in the stated age range. **age-specific mortality r.** AGE-SPECIFIC DEATH RATE. **attack r.** INCIDENCE. **background counting r.** The constant baseline counting rate present at any time due either to natural radiations, as from cosmic rays, or to radioactive contamination. **basal metabolic r.** The energy expenditure of the body at complete mental and physical rest. Convention requires that the subject not attempt exercise during the hour before the test and not eat during the twelve hours preceding the test. Low values are observed in hypothyroidism, high values in thyrotoxicosis. The test is rarely used in clinical practice, but it is of historic importance. Abbr. BMR **birth r.** 1 The ratio of the number of live births occurring in a group to the number of members of the group, usually expressed as births per 1000 members. Also *natality rate.* 2 CRUDE ANNUAL LIVE BIRTH RATE. **Boeckh's r.** NET FEMALE REPRODUCTION RATE. **Boeckh-Kuczynski r.** NET FEMALE REPRODUCTION RATE. **caries r.** The incidence of new dental caries. The rate may be expressed as the number of teeth or tooth surfaces newly affected per person per annum. **carrier r.** The proportion of carriers found among apparently normal persons, usually expressed as a percentage. **case r.** MORBIDITY RATE. **case fatality r.** The number of deaths as a result of a specific disease in a well-identified group of cases, often expressed as a percentage. **cause-specific death r.** A death rate specific for a stated cause, or related group of causes, of death. **circulation r.** The velocity of blood flow. **conduction r.** The rate of transmission of a spike potential along a conducting structure such as a neuronal process, tract of axons, or muscle fiber. It is calculated from the conduction delay and the distance traveled, and is usually expressed in meters per second. **corrected r.** *Incorrect* ADJUSTED RATE. **corrected death r.** *Obs.* STANDARDIZED DEATH RATE. **corrected mortality r.** *Obs.* STANDARDIZED DEATH RATE. **corrected survival r.** A crude survival rate corrected to allow for the level of mortality from all causes. **counting r.** In radiology, the rate of occurrence of ionizing radiation events as measured by special detectors. Also *count rate.* **crude r.** GENERAL RATE. **crude annual general death r.** DEATH RATE. **crude annual live birth r.** The ratio of the number of live births occurring in a population in a year to the mean population for that year, usually expressed as live births per 1000 population. Also *birth rate.* **crude birth r.** The number of live births during a given period as related to the mean size of the total population concerned, usually expressed as live births per 1000 population. **crude death r.** The total number of deaths occurring in a population during a stated period, such number being related to the size of that population at that time, and usually expressed as deaths per 1000 population per year. Also *crude mortality rate.* • The term means the death rate from all causes unless qualified by reference to a specific cause or causes. **crude survival r.** The ratio, among persons with a given disease, of the number known to be alive at the end of a stated period to the number alive at the start of the period, usually expressed as a percentage. **death r.** 1 The ratio of the total number of deaths from all causes in a population in a year to the mean population for that year, usually expressed as deaths per 1000 population. Also *crude annual general death rate.* 2 Any rate serving as an index of the frequency of deaths in a population. Also *mortality rate, mortality.* **def r.** DEF INDEX. **discharge r.** The number of patients discharged from a hospital over a stated period in relation to the population the hospital serves. The rate is usually expressed as discharges (including deaths in the hospital) per 1000 population per year. Over a sufficiently long period, the discharge rate will approximate to the hospital's admission rate. **DMF index r.** DMF INDEX. **early neonatal death r.** The number of infant deaths occurring during the early neonatal period per 1000 live births. **effective fertility r.** A fertility rate that is specifically based on live births as numerator. **equivalent average death r.** The annual death rate of a population which would have been observed if each age group had had the same number of individuals. It is the arithmetic mean of the observed age-specific death rates up to some stated upper limit, such as 75 years. **erythrocyte sedimentation r.** The rate at which erythrocytes separate from plasma, due to their slightly greater density, when anticoagulated blood is allowed to stand in a column or tube at room temperature. The rate is measured as the number of millimeters from the meniscus of the plasma to the upper level of erythrocytes at one hour. Also *sedimentation rate, sedimentation reaction, erythrocyte sedimentation test, Fahraeus test, sedimentation time.* **evolutionary r.** The rate of change in the form and the function of descendants as compared to their ancestors. **false-negative r.** The ratio of the number of persons showing a negative result to a test applied in order to detect a given disease but who are subsequently found to have been suffering from the disease at the time of the test, to the total number of persons showing a negative result to the test. The ratio is usually expressed as a percentage. **false-positive r.** The ratio of the number of persons showing a positive result to a test applied in order to detect a given disease but who, on further investigation, are found not to be suffering from that disease, to the total number of persons giving a positive result to the test. The ratio is usually expressed as a percentage. **fatality r.** The proportion of those suffering from a given disease who die of it. The fatality rate, usually expressed as a percentage, is a measure of the gravity of a disease. Also *fatality ratio, case fatality, lethality, lethality rate.* **female reproduction r.** The number of live-born daughters that each member of a cohort of newborn females will bear on the average. **fertility r.** The number of births in a given period in relation to the number of women of reproductive age, usually expressed as births per 1000 women per year. Total fertility rates require that all births, and effective fertility rates require that live births only, be counted in the numerator. Specific fertility rates may be computed for maternal age, parity, marriage duration, etc. **fetal death r.** STILLBIRTH RATE. **five-year survival r.** See under FIVE-YEAR SURVIVAL. **frame r.** REAL-TIME RATE. **general r.** A rate based on a population considered as a whole without attention to such variables as age, sex, or economic status. Also *crude rate.* **general fertility r.** The fertility rate as computed for all women of reproductive age in a given population without attention to such variables as parity, marital status, or more limited age group. **glomerular filtration r.** The rate at which ultrafiltrate is formed from plasma passing through renal glomeruli, expressed as milliliters per minute or liters per day. For a standard adult of 1.73 $m^2$ body surface, normal is 130 ml/min or 180 l/day, representing approximately 20 percent of renal plasma flow. It is usually measured by clearance techniques, such as insulin clearance. Major determinants are renal plasma flow, permeability of glomerular basement membrane, and total surface area of available glomeruli. **gross female reproduction r.** An index of the number of live-born daughters a cohort of newborn females will bear, assuming given fertility rates and a nil mortality for the cohort from birth to the end of their reproductive period. Also *gross reproduction rate, gross reproductive rate.* **growth r.** An expression, usually in mathematical terms, to indicate increments in weight, size, or length per unit of time. Growth rates can be expressed absolutely for the whole or any part of an organism over any period of time irrespective of other factors, or relatively by comparison with increments in weight, size, or length of other organisms or their parts or in relation to specific factors. **heart r.** The frequency rate of heart beats, measured as the number of ventricular contractions per minute. **incidence r.** INCIDENCE. **infant mortality r.** The ratio of the number of deaths of infants under one year of age occurring during a given year to the number of live births registered during that year, or to the weighted mean of the number of live births registered during that year and the year preceding. In some countries the denominator would be the number of live births occurring as opposed to the number registered. The rate is customarily expressed as infant deaths per 1000 live births. **instantaneous r.** The limit to which a rate involving time approaches as the period of observation approaches zero. **instantaneous growth r.** In demography, the instantaneous rate of a population's growth. **intrinsic r. of natural increase** In demography, the constant rate of increase seen in a stable population. Also *true rate of natural increase.* **Kuczynski's r.** NET FEMALE REPRODUCTION RATE. **lethality r.** FATALITY RATE. **marital fertility r.** The total number of live births (regardless, unless otherwise stated, of the marital status or age of the mothers) per 1000 married women aged 15 to 44 years per annum. **marriage r.** NUPTIALITY RATE. **maternal mortality r.** The number of deaths due to complications of pregnancy, confinement, and the puerperium per 1000 births, live and still. Also *maternal death rate.* **mendelian r.** MENDELIAN RATIO. **morbidity r.** The ratio of the number of cases of a given disease to the total number of persons in the population, expressed either as the prevalence at a given point in time or as the incidence over a stated period. Also *case rate, sickness rate.* **mortality r.** DEATH RATE. **mutation r.** The probability that a recognizable mutation will occur in an organism per generation. **natality r.** BIRTH RATE. **r. of natural increase** The rate at which a population increases during a stated period as the result of an excess of births over deaths. **neonatal death r.** The number of infant deaths occurring during the first four weeks of life in a given year per 1000 live births in that year. Also *neonatal mortality rate.* **net female reproduction r.** An index of the number of live-born daughters that a cohort of newborn females will bear given defined rates of fertility and mortality. Also *Boeckh's rate, Kuczynski's rate, Boeckh-Kuczynski rate, replacement rate, net reproduction rate, net reproductive rate.* **nuptiality r.** The ratio of the number of marriages during a given period to the total population, expressed as a rate, usually per 1000 population per year. The rate may be made specific for age (with the number of marriageable persons of given age as denominator), for first marriages, for remarriages, etc. Also *marriage rate.* **oocyst r.** The percentage of collected wild female mosquitoes showing oocysts on the wall of the midgut. **output exposure r.** The radiation exposure rate at some calibration point under a defined set of conditions, expressed as roentgens per minute. **parasite r.** The percentage of persons in a particular age group, or area, in whom a particular kind of parasite is found. It is a measure of disease developed for epidemiological studies of malaria. Although it appears to be a simple ratio it is in fact a prevalence rate. **parity-specific birth r.** A specific birth rate calculated on the basis of parity, with only live-born infants being counted. **perinatal death r.** The number of infant deaths occurring during the first seven days of life plus the number of stillbirths occurring after 28 weeks of pregnancy in a given year per 1000 live births in that year. Also *perinatal mortality rate.* **population growth r.** The change in size of a population over a given period, usually expressed as an annual increase or decrease percent of the size at the beginning of the period. The numerical value of the average annual growth rate over a period, such as a decade, will depend on the growth curve adopted for the calculation. **postneonatal death r.** The number of infant deaths occurring during the postneonatal period per 1000 live births. **prevalence r.** PREVALENCE. **proportionate mortality r.** *Incorrect* PROPORTIONATE MORTALITY RATIO. **pulse r.** The frequency rate of the pulse, measured as the number of beats per minute that can be felt in a peripheral artery. **real-time r.** 1 The actual rate at which a physical process occurs. For example, in cineangiography, high-speed motion pictures are played back much slower than the real-time rate. 2 The number of frames per second displayed at the real-time rate. Also *frame rate.* **replacement r.** NET FEMALE REPRODUCTION RATE. **reproduction r.** See under FEMALE REPRODUCTION RATE. **respiration r.** The number of full cycles of breathing per minute. **response r.** The number of subjects replying to inquiries by interview or questionnaire out of the total number of individuals being studied, usually expressed as a percentage. The higher the response rate the more representative and reliable the results of the study. **secondary attack r.** The ratio of the number of new cases of a disease that arise within a given time (usually one incubation period) among the contacts of an initial case to the total number of contacts. **sedimentation r.** 1 ERYTHROCYTE SEDIMENTATION RATE. 2 SEDIMENTATION VELOCITY. **sex-specific death r.** A death rate specific for one sex. **sickness r.** MORBIDITY RATE. **single nephron glomerular filtration r.** The rate of glomerular filtration in a single nephron. **specific r.** A rate calculated upon a part of a population singled out as falling within some relevant category, such as a given age, sex, or economic status. **specific birth r.** The ratio of live births in a given period to mean group size in each subgroup of a population of women divided on the basis of age, parity, marital status, etc., usually expressed as births per 1000 women per year. **specific death r.** A death rate relating to a population group specified according to sex, age, or both, as opposed to a general death rate. **sporozoite r.** The percentage of collected wild female mosquitoes with sporozoites in the salivary glands. **standardized r.** A rate that, for the purpose of comparability, has been adjusted to the corresponding rate which would have prevailed in an arbitrary standard. **standardized death r.** The death rate for a population adjusted by direct or indirect standardization to render it comparable with the rates for other populations (or for the same population at different periods) similarly standardized, and thereby freed from the effects of differences in age-sex structure between the populations being compared. Also *adjusted death rate, corrected death rate* (obs.), *standardized mortality rate, corrected mortality rate* (obs.). **steroid metabolic clearance r.** The volume of blood or plasma irreversibly and totally cleared of a steroid hormone per unit time, usually expressed as liters per 24 hrs. **steroid production r.** The total quantity of a given steroid hormone made in the body per unit time, generally expressed as milligrams per day. The total includes hormone secreted by the gland of origin as well as that formed extraglandularly, as in the blood or the liver, from a variety of steroid precursors. **steroid secretory r.** The rate of secretion of a steroid hormone by its gland of origin, exclusive of the steroid formed extraglandularly, as in the blood or the liver. The rate is generally expressed as milligrams per day. **stillbirth r.** The ratio of stillbirths to all births, usually expressed as stillbirths per 1000 births, live and still. Also *fetal mortality, fetal death rate, mortinatality, natimortality.* **survival r.** The proportion, often expressed as a percentage, of persons still alive at a stated time after a given event. See also CRUDE SURVIVAL RATE, CORRECTED SURVIVAL RATE. **total fertility r.** The sum of the age-specific fertility rates over all ages of the childbearing period, approximately equal to the completed family size. It is used as a summary index for comparing fertility in different populations or at different times. **true r. of natural increase** INTRINSIC RATE OF NATURAL INCREASE.

**Rathke** [Martin Heinrich *Rathke*, German anatomist, 1793–1860] **1** Rathke's pouch. See under CRANIOPHARYNGEAL POUCH. **2** Rathke's pouch tumor, Rathke's tumor. See under CRANIOPHARYNGIOMA.

**rating / behavior r.** A notation specifying the occurrence, the nonoccurrence, or the degree of occurrence of a particular behavior pattern during a specified period of observation, such as the number of times a conversation with another person is initiated.

# ratio

**ratio** \rā′shō\ [L (from *reri* to think, consider, suppose) calculation, proportion, relation] The quotient of two numbers. **absolute terminal innervation r.** INNERVATION RATIO. **AC/A r.** The proportion between accommodative convergences and accommodations. It is of clinical importance in ocular alignment, since it determines the amount of convergence automatically resulting from the dioptric focusing of the eyes at a given distance. **A/G r.** ALBUMIN/GLOBULIN RATIO. **age dependency r.** A dependency ratio which specifies the age groups concerned, such as those under the customary age for employment or those over the usual age of retirement. **albumin/globulin r.** The ratio of serum concentrations of albumin and globulin, normally 1.5–3:1. It may be low due to either decrease in albumin concentration, reduced synthesis, accelerated loss or increased catabolism of albumin, or increase in serum globulin concentration, as may occur in chronic inflammatory disorders, in benign plasma cell hyperplasias, or in myeloma, macroglobulinemia, or related disorders. Use of the A/G ratio is now obsolete. Also *A/G ratio.* **ALT-/AST r.** The proportion between elevated levels of alanine aminotransferase (ALT) and aspartate aminotransferase (AST). In alcoholic hepatitis, AST often rises more than ALT to a ratio of 1:2 or greater, whereas toxic or viral hepatitis elevates ALT more than AST, giving a ratio of 1:1 or 2:1. **arm r.** The length of the long arm of a mitotic chromosome divided by the length of the short arm. **assimilation efficiency r.** The ratio of food energy retained to food energy consumed. **base r.** The ratio of guanine-cytosine pairs to adenine-thymine pairs in DNA, used especially to trace evolutionary relations and to classify bacteria. **base pair r.** For a given nucleic acid, the ratio between the sums of the frequencies of complementary nucleotide bases. For DNA, it is expressed symbolically by (A+T)/(G+C), where A is adenine, T is thymine, G is guanine, and C is cytosine. **beam uniformity r.** The ratio of the spatial peak intensity to the spatial average intensity. **body-weight r.** A ratio expressing the relation between the height of the body and its weight: weight in grams/height in centimeters. **cardiothoracic r.** The ratio of the maximum diameter of the heart to the internal diameter of the chest at its widest point. **cell color r.** COLOR INDEX. **channels r.** The ratio between count rates in two selected pulse-height windows in a liquid scintillation counter. It is used to cope with a quenching problem. One window is chosen for maximal count rate with an unquenched sample. The other is placed, usually, somewhat higher on the spectral hump. The ratio between them is determined with various amounts of quenching added, and the counting efficiency established for each. This permits an unknown sample to be measured, even if quenching is present. **child-woman r.** The ratio of the number of children under five years of age to the number of women of childbearing age in a population. Also *general fertility ratio.* **clinical crown–clinical root r.** The proportion of the length of the tooth exposed in the mouth to the length embedded in the tissues. **conversion r.** The ratio of the number of new fissionable atoms produced in a reactor to the number destroyed. **critical r.** In statistics, the ratio which, if exceeded, leads to the rejection of the null hypothesis on the grounds that the probability of its being true is less than a given amount. The form of the ratio depends on the statistical test being applied. **cross-products r.** ODDS RATIO. **curative r.** THERAPEUTIC INDEX. **death-to-case r.** The ratio of the number of deaths attributed to a given cause of death to the number of cases recorded in clinical records. **dependency r.** The ratio, usually expressed as a percentage, of the economically inactive to the working population. Also *economic dependency ratio.* **dextrose-nitrogen r.** The ratio of urinary dextrose to urinary nitrogen. In the carbohydrate-starved, totally pancreatectomized (i.e., insulin-deprived) animal, the average value is about 3.65, a figure approached in very severe human diabetes mellitus. It was assumed that under these experimental conditions virtually all urinary dextrose is derived from protein and that about 58% of the protein is convertible to glucose. Also *D-N ratio, glucose-nitrogen ratio, G-N ratio, D/N quotient.* **economic dependency r.** DEPENDENCY RATIO. **expiratory exchange r.** A respiratory quotient as measured by expired gas collection and equal to the volume of carbon dioxide expired divided by the volume of oxygen absorbed. **extraction r.** The difference between the arterial and venous concentrations of a substance delivered to a tissue or organ expressed as a percentage of the arterial concentration. **F r.** VARIANCE RATIO. **fatality r.** FATALITY RATE. **fetal death r.** The ratio of the number of fetal deaths to the number of live births during a stated period, usually expressed as fetal deaths per 1000 live births per year. **F:P r.** The molecular ratio of the amount of fluorochrome to protein of a fluorescein-labeled antibody. **functional terminal innervation r.** INNERVATION RATIO. **galvanic tetanus r.** The ratio between the intensity of current necessary to stimulate muscle and that necessary to tetanize the muscle. It is decreased in cases of denervation. **general fertility r.** CHILD-WOMAN RATIO. **glucose-nitrogen r.** DEXTROSE-NITROGEN RATIO. **G-N r.** DEXTROSE-NITROGEN RATIO. **grid r.** In roentgenography, the ratio of the height of the lead strips in an antiscatter grid to the distance between strips. **gyromagnetic r.** In nuclear magnetic resonance, the ratio of the angular frequency of precession to the magnetic field strength, which is a constant for each isotope. Also *nuclear magnetogyric ratio.* **holdaway r.** A cephalometric relation between the nasion, the lower incisor, and pogonium. **human blood r.** The percentage of newly fed mosquitoes in an area that on examination contain human blood. It is a measure of infection developed in the course of malarial investigations. **$^{131}$I conversion r.** A former method for estimating thyroidal secretion of hormone by measuring the appearance in serum at 48 hours after administration of protein-bound $^{131}$I. The ratio is high in thyrotoxicosis and low in hypothyroidism. Also *radioactive iodide conversion ratio.* **innervation r.** **1** The ratio of motor endplates to the total number of motoneurons innervating a given muscle, generally calculated by dividing the number of muscle fibers counted histologically by the number of efferent axons in the nerve supplying the muscle. Also *absolute terminal innervation ratio.* **2** The ratio between active motor endplates and the total capable of activation by excitation of all motoneurons innervating a given muscle. Also *functional terminal innervation ratio.* **inspiratory-expiratory phase time r.** The ratio between the time taken by inspiration and by expiration in natural breathing or, more usually, artificial ventilation. **isophane r.** The proportion in which protamine and insulin combine in preparations which contain both materials, such as NPH insulin. **K:A r.** KETOGENIC-ANTIKETOGENIC RATIO. **karyoplasmic r.** NUCLEOCYTOPLASMIC RATIO. **ketogenic-antiketogenic r.** The ratio of substances that form glucose to those that form fatty acids in the body. Also *K:A ratio.* **lecithin:sphingomyelin r.** A figure, derived from an amniotic fluid examination, that is used to evaluate the maturity of the fetal lungs. It is based on the necessity of lipid interactions for pulmonary surfactant activity. The level of sphingomyelin (S) in amniotic fluid remains fairly constant, whereas lecithin (L) increases sharply during the late phases of pulmonary maturation. When lecithin and sphingomyelin values are compared, L/S values of 2 or more indicate pulmonary maturity, and values of 1.5 or less carry a high risk of respiratory distress syndrome. Also *L/S ratio.* **male/female r.** SEX RATIO. **masculinity r.** SEX RATIO. **M/E r.** MYELOID-ERYTHROID RATIO. **mendelian r.** A ratio in one generation of phenotypes due to a given genetic locus in accordance with Mendel's laws of inheritance. Also *mendelian rate.* **middle-ear areal r.** The ratio (14:1) between the area of the tympanic membrane and that of the oval window. The ratio is of importance in explaining the function of the transformer mechanism of the middle ear.

**myeloid-erythroid r.** In a specimen of bone marrow, the ratio of cells of the granulocytic or myeloid series to cells of the erythrocytic series. The ratio normally is about 3:1. Also *M/E ratio.* **nuclear magnetogyric r.** GYROMAGNETIC RATIO. **nucleocytoplasmic r.** The ratio of nuclear volume to cytoplasmic volume in a cell. Also *karyoplasmic ratio.* **ocular micrometer r.** The ratio between a scale that is fitted into a microscope eyepiece and the corresponding distance on a microscope slide. **odds r.** The ratio of the odds in favor of an event occurring under one set of circumstances to the odds of its occurring under another. If p is the probability of occurrence in the first case and P the probability in the second, the odds ratio is $p(1-P)/P(1-p)$. An estimate of the odds ratio is provided by the ratio of the cross products in a fourfold table (*ab*/*bc*). Given statistical independence, the odds ratio is equal to one. Also *cross-products ratio, relative odds.* **ossicular lever r.** The ratio (1.3:1) between the length of the lever represented by the malleus handle and that represented by the long process of incus. It is of importance in explaining the function of the transformer mechanism of the middle ear. **parity progression r.** The proportion of women of parity $N$ who ever progress to parity $N+1$ or who do so in a given time interval. **peak-to-total r.** The number of total-absorption scintillations divided by the number of all scintillations, or, approximately, photopeak area divided by the whole spectral area. Also *photofraction, photopeak efficiency.* Symbol: P/T **P/O r.** The ratio of moles of ATP synthesized to moles of oxygen atoms reduced to water in a system in which oxidative phosphorylation is occurring. **polymorphonuclear-lymphocyte r.** The ratio of polymorphonuclear leukocytes to lymphocytes in blood. This ratio has been used as an index of serious acute radiation exposure, since neutrophils are more radiation-sensitive than are lymphocytes. **potency r.** The relative potency of two drugs expressed as the difference between the logarithms of their respective median effective doses. **primary sex r.** The ratio of males conceived to females conceived. **proportionate mortality r.** An index for comparing the age-specific mortality according to occupation of persons at ages past the normal age of retirement and devised as a means of overcoming the loss of information due to the high proportion of people in this age range described for purposes of census and death registration as unoccupied, without mention of any previous occupation. Also *proportionate mortality, proportionate mortality rate* (incorrect). Abbr. PMR **protein efficiency r.** The gain in weight shown by a young growing animal in proportion to each gram of a given protein eaten as the sole dietary protein at a standard level, such as 10 percent weight gain for 10 or more days. Zero values are found for proteins such as gelatin that are missing one essential amino acid. Egg has the highest ratio with a value of 4.4. **radioactive iodide conversion r.** $^{131}$I CONVERSION RATIO. **respiratory exchange r.** The ratio of the volume of carbon dioxide produced to that of oxygen during respiration. This value may be affected by respiratory factors as well as the nature of the food being metabolized. Also *respiratory quotient.* **risk r.** RELATIVE RISK. **saliva to plasma radioiodine r.** A test for thyroidal iodide trapping function, used in the diagnosis of congenital defects in iodide concentration. Radioiodide is given, and one hour later saliva and serum are collected. The normal ratio of $^{131}$I in an equal volume of saliva to serum is greater than 10, but is 1 or less in patients with congenital trapping defects of the thyroid gland. **sampling r.** The proportion of individual entities drawn from a population to constitute a sample. Also *sampling fraction.* **secondary sex r.** The ratio of the number of males born to the number of females born. **sex r.** The ratio of the number of males to the number of females in a population, a subgroup of a population, or an aggregate of demographic entities (births, deaths, etc.), usually expressed as the number of males per 100 females. When females predominate the ratio may be expressed as the number of females per 100 males to give a ratio greater than one. Also *male/female ratio, masculinity ratio.* **signal-to-noise r.** The ratio of the magnitude of the signal to that of the noise, useful in quantitating the degradation of signal quality by noise that is present. **standardized mortality r.** The ratio, expressed as a percentage, of the actual number of deaths in a population during a given period to the expected number as calculated by indirect standardization. Abbr. SMR **therapeutic r.** THERAPEUTIC INDEX. **variance r.** The ratio of two variances, a statistic widely used in the analysis of variance. Also *F ratio, F distribution.* Symbol: F

**ration** [L *ratio.* See RATIO.] A constant quantity of food and/or drink supplied in any given period of time, as by the day or the hour. **basal r.** A ration supplying adequate energy to meet the body's requirements but deficient in one or more vitamins.

**rationalization** \rash′ənal′īzā′shən\ A plausible explanation for behavior that conceals one's actual motives for it, often and especially from oneself as a defense mechanism.

**rattle** A series of sharp, grating sounds. **death r.** A sound of air bubbling through mucus in the throat of a severely ill person, traditionally a sign of imminent death.

**rattlesnake** Any of the snakes of the genera *Crotalus* and *Sistrurus.* The tail bears a unique rattle organ consisting of a series of loosely interlocked hollow shells which, at successive stages of growth, were each a scale covering the extreme tip of the tail. This structure produces an audible warning when vibrated.

***Rattus*** \rat′əs\ [New L, from English *rat,* Old English *ræt*] A large genus of the rodent family Muridae, containing some 570 species and subspecies of rats. These extensively varied forms include *R. rattus,* the black rat, *R. rattus alexandrinus,* the roof rat, and *R. norvegicus,* the Norwegian gray rat. Their distribution is essentially cosmopolitan as a result of commensalism with humans. They are known carriers of numerous diseases, including bubonic plague and rabies, and serious competitors for human food resources. *R. rattus* and *R. norvegicus* are commonly used for laboratory research.

**Rau** [Johann Jacob (Ravius) *Rau,* Dutch anatomist, 1668–1719] Apophysis of Rau. See under PROCESSUS ANTERIOR MALLEI.

**Rauber** [August Antinous *Rauber,* German anatomist, 1841–1917] Rauber's layer. See under PRIMITIVE ECTODERM.

**Rauscher** [Frank Joseph *Rauscher,* U.S. virologist, born 1931] Rauscher leukemia virus. See under VIRUS.

**rauwolfia serpentina** \rou·wôl′fē·ə sur′pəntē′nə, rô·wŭl′fē·ə\ The dried extracts obtained from the root, stem, and rhizome of the plant *Rauwolfia serpentina.* It contains not less than 0.15 percent of the active principle, reserpine-rescinnamine alkaloid. It has antihypertensive activity, and it has been used as a sedative and tranquilizer. In powdered form, it contains 0.15 to 0.20 percent of the active principle.

**RAV** Rous-associated virus.

**Rawson** [Arthur Joy *Rawson,* U.S. medical physicist, born 1896] Abbott-Rawson tube. See under TUBE.

**ray** [L *radius.* See RADIUS.] **1** A line of direction of radiant energy, as of light or heat. **2** One of the five mesenchymal condensations in the developing human limb bud indicating the future position of metacarpals, metatarsals and phalanges within the bud. The tissue intervening between the rays thins and breaks down, and results in the formation of the separate digits. **actinic r.** A ray at the short-wave end of the visible spectrum that produces chemical changes. Also *chemical ray.* **alpha r.'s** See under ALPHA PARTICLE. **astral r.** One of the cytoplasmic microtubules which form the spindle during mitosis or meiosis. Also *polar ray.* **beta r.'s** Radiation of high-speed electrons or positrons from a radionuclide; beta particles. **Bucky's r.'s** GRENZ RAYS. **cathode r.'s** A stream of high-energy electrons emitted from the cathode of an evacuated tube. **central r.** The straight line passing through the center of the source of radiation and the center of the beam-defining diaphragm. **characteristic r.** CHARACTERISTIC RADIATION. **chemical r.** ACTINIC RAY. **cortical r.** PARS RADIATA LOBULI CORTICALIS RENIS. **cosmic r.'s** High-energy radiation of extraterrestrial origin. Primary cosmic rays are mostly high-energy protons, which interact with the upper atmosphere to produce secondary cosmic rays, consisting of gamma rays, mesons, and many other subatomic particles. Also *ultra x rays, Millikan rays* (outmoded). **delta r.'s** Electrons with kinetic energies in the ionizing range, having been knocked out of their atomic orbits by incident charged particles with higher energies. **digital r.** The mesenchymal condensation outlining each developing digit and its associated metacarpal or metatarsal in the rounded plate at the distal end of the early embryonic limb bud. *Outmoded.* **Dorno's r.'s** The portion of ultraviolet radiation with wavelengths between 290 and 320 nm. **gamma r.'s** **1** Electromagnetic radiation emitted by an atomic nucleus because of a quantum transition between two energy levels of the nucleus. It is much more penetrating than alpha or beta radiation. **2** Electromagnetic radiation of wavelength comparable to that of nuclear radiation, from other sources (a synchroton, for example). Also *gamma radiation.* See also GAMMA PHOTON. **glass r.'s** The radiation produced in an x-ray tube when the cathode rays hit the glass wall of the tube. **grenz r.'s** Soft, poorly penetrating roentgen rays with wavelength of about 2 ångströms, sometimes used to treat lesions of the skin. Also *Bucky's rays.* **indirect r.'s** The radiation produced at the glass surface of a cathode ray tube. **infrared r.'s** Electromagnetic radiations having wavelengths longer than those of visible light but shorter than those of microwaves. **intermediate r.'s** Electromagnetic radiations of wavelengths between those of ultraviolet and x rays. Also *W rays.* **luminous r.'s** The light rays of the visible spectrum. **medullary r.** PARS RADIATA LOBULI CORTICALIS RENIS. **Millikan r.'s** *Outmoded* COSMIC RAYS. **Minin r.'s** Rays produced by incandescent light passing through dark blue glass. **paracathodic r.'s** *Obs.* X RAYS. **polar r.** ASTRAL RAY. **primary r.** A ray of an incident beam of particles or photons before it has interacted or been scattered in any way. **roentgen r.'s** X RAYS. **secondary r.'s** Radiations originating from a substance which is being irradiated by x rays. **ultraviolet r.'s** Electromagnetic radiations having wavelengths shorter than visible light but longer than x rays, i.e., with wavelengths of about 2000 to 4000 ångström units. **ultra x r.'s** COSMIC RAYS. **W r.'s** INTERMEDIATE RAYS. **x r.'s** See under X RAYS.

**Rayleigh** [Lord John W. S. *Rayleigh,* English physicist, 1842–1919] Rayleigh scattering. See under COHERENT SCATTERING.

**Raymond** [Fulgence *Raymond,* French neurologist, 1844–1910] **1** Raymond syndrome. See under INFERIOR PONTINE SYNDROME. **2** Raymond syndrome. See under SUPERIOR PONTINE SYNDROME.

**Raynaud** [Maurice *Raynaud,* French physician, 1834–1881] **1** See under DISEASE. **2** Raynaud syndrome. See under PHENOMENON.

**razor** / **Occam's r.** The principle of applying to scientific data that explanation which requires the smallest number of concepts. Also *law of parsimony.*

**Rb** Symbol for the element, rubidium.

**RBC** red blood cell (erythrocyte).

**RBE** relative biologic effectiveness.

**RBF** Renal blood flow.

**RD** **1** reaction of degeneration. **2** retinal detachment.

**Rd** Symbol for the obsolete unit, rutherford.

**rd** **1** Symbol for the obsolete unit, rutherford. **2** RAD.

**RDA** recommended daily allowance.

**Re** Symbol for the element, rhenium.

**re-** \rē-, ri-, rə-\ [L prefix *re-* back, down, again (*red-* before vowels and *h*)] A prefix meaning (1) again, once again; (2) back, backward. Also *red-*.

**reablement** \rē·ā′bəlmənt\ *Rare* REHABILITATION.

**reabsorption** \rē′əbsôrp′shən\ [RE- + ABSORPTION] RESORPTION. **facultative water r.** The reabsorption of water by renal distal tubules and collecting ducts, controlled by the antidiuretic hormone. **intestinal r.** The removal by absorption through the intestinal epithelium of a substance excreted or secreted into the gastrointestinal tract at a more proximal location. **obligatory water r.** Isosmotic reabsorption of water by proximal convoluted tubules secondary to solute reabsorption. **tubular r.** The reabsorption of water and solutes by the renal tubules. The process may be active or passive.

**reactance** \rē·ak′təns\ The part of the impedance of an alternating current circuit that is due to capacitance or inductance or both. Also *inductive resistance.*

**reactant** \rē·ak′tənt\ A substance that enters into a specified chemical reaction. **acute phase r.** A plasma protein whose concentration is increased following most forms of tissue injury. C-reactive protein is the most impressive acute phase reactant in man in that its concentration may rise a thousandfold or more. Other acute phase reactants, whose concentrations rise more modestly, include $\alpha_1$-antitrypsin, acid glycoprotein, haptoglobin, and many complement components. All acute phase reactants are synthesized in the liver, and it has been suggested that interleukin-1 may be the mediator giving rise to the increased synthesis. Also *acute phase substance.*

# reaction

**reaction** [RE- + L *actio* (from *actus,* past part. of *agere* to set in motion, drive, do, act) an action, doing] **1** Any response to a stimulus or other event. **2** A process in which a substance is changed chemically. **3** An immune response. See under RESPONSE. **acute situational r.** TRANSIENT SITUATIONAL PERSONALITY DISORDER. **adjustment r.** TRANSIENT SITUATIONAL PERSONALITY DISORDER. **alarm r.** The initial stage in the response of an animal to acute severe stress. It includes a loss of muscle tone and a fall in body temperature. Abbr. AR **allergic r.** **1** A local or general reaction elicited by a host's exposure to a substance to which he is immunologically hypersensitive. **2** A reaction to a subsequent exposure to an antigen when this is specifically altered from the reaction to the first exposure. Reactions of diminished reactivity (immunity) or of enhanced reactivity (hypersensitivity) are both allergic. • Def. 2 is the original meaning and some observers hold that it is more correct than def. 1, but the distinction it makes is infrequently observed. Def. 1 is the common usage. **anaphylactic r.** ANAPHYLAXIS. **anaplerotic r.** An enzymatic reaction that replenishes an intermediate of the tricarboxylic acid cycle that is otherwise removed because it is the precursor of a cell component. Without such replenishment the tricarboxylic acid cycle would be interrupted and could not function both to supply energy and to supply building blocks for growth. **anergastic r.** ORGANIC BRAIN SYNDROME. **annihilation r.** POSITRON ANNIHILATION EVENT. **anniversary r.** Any mental symptoms that occur on the anniversary of a significant experience and which are believed to be prompted by that experience. The relationship between the two, however, is rarely recognized by the subject. **anthrone r.** The reaction of anthrone with sugars in sulfuric acid to give a blue-green color. **antigen-antibody r.** The interaction of an immunoglobulin with its specific antigen. The biologic or serologic consequences of this interaction depend upon the location and form of the antigen, the physical state of the antibody, the site at which the interaction occurs, and the physical and biologic conditions that surround the interaction. Examples of these consequences include agglutination, precipitation, immunoglobulin coating, initiation of complement-mediated hemolysis or opsonization, neutralization of toxins, inhibition of cell-surface receptor activity, and other *in vivo* and *in vitro* events. Also *toxin-antitoxin reaction*. **antiglobulin r.** ANTIGLOBULIN TEST. **argentaffin r.** The staining of intracellular granules with silver solution without the addition of an external reducing agent. **arousal r.** A series of typical patterns or stages recorded in the electroencephalogram when a subject is in a transitional state from sleep to wakefulness. **Arthus r.** An inflammatory reaction seen following the intradermal or subcutaneous injection of an antigen to which the animal has already made antibody. The lesion is usually an ulcer marked by edema, hemorrhage, and necrosis, and is more immediate than a delayed type reaction. The reaction is secondary to the local formation of antigen-antibody complexes, activating complement and causing the accumulation of fibrin, neutrophils, and platelets, and finally plugging of the vessel with thrombi. Also *Arthus phenomenon*. See also IMMUNOLOGICAL MECHANISMS OF TISSUE DAMAGE. **Ascoli's r.** 1 ASCOLI'S TEST. 2 MIOSTAGMIN REACTION. **autoimmune complement fixation r.** The activation of complement that occurs when an autoimmune antibody reacts with an autologous antigen. It may occur *in vivo* or *in vitro*. **axon r.** Central chromatolysis in the perikaryon of a neuron following division of its axons. Also *axonal reaction, primary reaction of Nissl*. **Bachman r.** See under BACHMAN TEST. **Bekhterev's r.** Heightened sensitivity to electrical stimulation of voluntary muscles in cases of tetany. **bi-bi r.** An enzyme-catalyzed reaction in which both reactants are simultaneously bound to the enzyme at one stage, and both products at a later stage. The term thus excludes mechanisms in which one product dissociates before the second reactant binds. **biphasic r.** A response composed of opposite phases, e.g., a positive-negative electrical reaction or flexion and extension in reflexes. **biuret r.** BIURET TEST. **blocking r.** In electroencephalography, the reduction or temporary suppression of the alpha rhythm (8–13 Hz) as a result of a novel or unexpected sensory stimulus. **bombardment r.** A nuclear reaction caused by the projection of selected elementary particles or photons against a target. **Bordet and Gengou r.** COMPLEMENT FIXATION. **browning r.'s** Reactions that occur between carbohydrates and protein when food is heated, particularly when it is heated in the absence of water. They begin with glycosylation of lysine residues of the protein, and this is followed by an Amadori rearrangement, which may lead to further reactions. Brown products are eventually formed. In these reactions the lysine becomes nutritionally unavailable. **Burchard-Liebermann r.** LIEBERMANN-BURCHARD TEST. **Calmette's r.** A diagnostic test formerly used for tuberculosis in which a dilute solution of tuberculin was instilled into the conjunctival sac. The local reaction is more severe in persons affected with tuberculosis than in healthy persons or those ill from other causes. The test was inaccurate and painful, and is now obsolete. Also *Wolff-Calmette reaction, Wolff-Eisner reaction, Calmette's test, Wolff-Eisner test, ophthalmoreaction, ophthalmic reaction, conjunctival test*. **capsular r.** A reaction in which the combination of antibody with bacterial capsular antigens is manifested by swelling of the capsule. **capsule swelling r.** QUELLUNG REACTION. **capture r.** A nuclear reaction consisting of the trapping and retention of an incident particle by the target nucleus, possibly accompanied by the emission of gamma radiation. **cascade r.** A sequence of biologic interactions in which each event initiates or activates the next reaction. In many cases changes in the configuration or the composition of a molecule produce or uncover enzyme activity for which the substrate is the next reactant in the sequence. Primary examples are the activation of complement components and the initiation of the coagulation sequence. **Casoni's r.** A diagnostic test for hydatid disease in which hydatid fluid is injected intracutaneously. A positive result is seen in the immediate or delayed production of a wheal. Also *Casoni skin test, echinococcus skin test*. **chain r.** Any reaction that is capable, under appropriate conditions, of sustaining itself, in that among the products of the reaction is one or more replicas of the agent that induced it. An example is nuclear fission, which is brought about by incident neutrons and which can be made to induce further fission events, thus continuing the process, possibly at an accelerating rate. **Chopra antimony r.** A serum test formerly used for patients with kala-azar or with splenomegaly due to another cause. The patient's serum is diluted ten to one with a physiologic salt solution and a 4 percent antimony solution. Immediate appearance of a flocculant precipitate constitutes a strongly positive reaction. Also *Chopra's antimony test*. **chromaffin r.** The yellow-brown staining reaction of adrenal medullary cells that follows their treatment with chromium salts. Also *Henle's reaction*. **complement fixation r.** COMPLEMENT FIXATION. **conglutination r.** The demonstration of the existence of a complement-activating antigen-antibody reaction, either on the surface of cells or as formation of immune complexes. The reaction exploits the activity of conglutinin, a nonimmune euglobulin found in bovine serum that binds to C3b exposed by antibody-mediated activation of the complement sequence. **consensual r.** CONSENSUAL LIGHT REFLEX. **consensual light r.** CONSENSUAL LIGHT REFLEX. **Coombs and Gell r.** Any of the four types of immunological reactions described in a system devised by R. R. A. Coombs and P. G. H. Gell. See under IMMUNOLOGICAL MECHANISMS OF TISSUE DAMAGE at MECHANISM. **crisis r.** TRANSIENT SITUATIONAL PERSONALITY DISORDER. **cross r.** The interaction of an antibody with an antigen other than the one which specifically provoked its production. Because antigen-antibody reactions depend upon steric interaction of molecules with structures of complementary configuration, interaction can occur when there is partial identity or strong similarity between configurations present in different molecules. In general, the greater the similarity between the different antigens, the stronger the cross reactivity will be. **cutaneous r.** A reaction of the skin to the percutaneous absorption or intracutaneous injection of antigenic substances to which the individual is allergically sensitive. Also *dermoreaction, cutireaction, skin reaction.* **cytotoxic r.** See under IMMUNOLOGICAL MECHANISMS OF TISSUE DAMAGE. **decidual r.** The changes in the endometrium that occur as a response to increased progesterone following ovulation and which are characterized by the conversion of stromal cells to polygonal or round decidual cells. **r. of degeneration** On electrical stimulation of a muscle, loss of contraction to faradism (a stimulus of brief duration), but retention of contraction in response to galvanism (a more prolonged stimulus); a sign of denervation. Also *Erb's reaction.* **delayed r.** An immune response occurring 24 to 48 hours after contact with an antigen; a delayed hypersensitivity reaction. Also *delayed response, late reaction.* See also IMMUNOLOGICAL MECHANISMS OF TISSUE DAMAGE. **depot r.** A reddening of the skin around the site of a subcutaneous tuberculin injection. **depressive r.** *Imprecise* DEPRESSION. • Because of changes made by the International Classification of Diseases and changes in United States nomenclature, the term *depressive reaction* may refer to any affective disorder with depression as the most prominent symptom, or it may indicate reactive depression, psychoneurotic or nonpsychotic depression, or transient situational personality disorder with prominent depressive symptoms. **dermatophytid r.** -ID REACTION. **dermotuberculin r.** PIRQUET'S REACTION. **desmoplastic r.** The proliferation of dense, collagenous stroma induced by certain carcinomas, such as infiltrating ductal carcinoma of the breast, which results in a gritty, hard consistency of the tumor. **Dick r.** DICK TEST. **dopa r.** A histochemical method using dopa as a substrate for the presence of the enzyme which synthesizes melanin. **duplicative r.** A disorder of schizophrenic children who fail to develop a stable, unitary conceptualization of objects. As a result, when they see the same person in two different settings they believe that they have seen two different people. **Ebbecke's r.** DERMOGRAPHISM. **eczematoid r.** ECZEMA. **Ehrlich's benzaldehyde r.** EHRLICH'S TEST. **electric r.** Biologic response or reaction, such as muscular contraction or an evoked sensation, elicited by an electrical stimulus applied to the body. **eosinopenic r.** Depletion of peripheral blood eosinophils in response to corticosteroids. In a test formerly used to assess integrity of the adrenal cortex, injection of adrenocorticotropin was normally followed by a sharp fall in eosinophil count, whereas in the presence of Addison's disease, the eosinophil count remained unchanged. **equilibrium r.** Reflex adjustment of major parts of the body, i.e., legs, spinal column, and head, in response to lateral or anterior-posterior tilting of the supporting surface. It depends in part upon labyrinthine function. Also *tilt reaction.* **Erb's r.** REACTION OF DEGENERATION. **erythrocyte sedimentation r.** ERYTHROCYTE SEDIMENTATION. **r. of exhaustion** The raised threshold of tissue to electrical stimulation that occurs in conditions of exhaustion. **Fahraeus r.** ERYTHROCYTE SEDIMENTATION. **false negative r.** A negative or normal result in a test on materials that are, in fact, abnormal or that should give a positive result. **false positive r.** A positive or abnormal result in a test on materials that are, in fact, normal or that should give a negative result. **Felix-Weil r.** WEIL-FELIX TEST. **Fernandez r.** A delayed hypersensitivity reaction to a skin test with lepromin. **Feulgen r.** See under FEULGEN METHOD. **fight-or-flight r.** The general reaction of the sympathetic nervous system that is directed towards the preservation of the organism in the face of acute stress resulting from the perception of immediate danger or threat. These include adaptations in blood flow, metabolism, etc., to permit escape. Also *sympathetic reaction, flight reflex* (imprecise) . **first-order r.** A reaction whose rate is proportional to the concentration of one reactant. Such reactions are usually unimolecular in mechanism. **flocculation r.** See under FLOCCULATION. **Florence's r.** The formation of dark brown mahogany, rhomboid crystals when choline reacts with Florence's reagent. Since choline is a constituent of seminal fluid, this test is sometimes used to identify material as semen. **focal r.** A reaction occurring at the focus of infection or at the site of an injection. **foreign-body r.** An inflammatory immunologic reaction of tissue in the host to the introduction of foreign bodies, as that of a splinter of wood in the skin or a foreign particle lodged in the conjunctiva. **Forssman antigen-antibody r.** **1** Any immunologic reaction involving the Forssman antigen. **2** The agglutination of sheep erythrocytes, which have the Forssman antigen on their surface, by heterophil antibodies in human serum. *Imprecise.* **gemistocytic r.** A nonspecific reactive change of astrocytes that occurs in response to injury such as infarct. They are characterized by abundant, eosinophilic, homogenous cytoplasm. **Goetsch skin r.** A former test for hyperthyroidism, dependent upon the local reaction to the intradermal injection of epinephrine. Also *Goetsch's test.* **graft-versus-host r.** GRAFT-VERSUS-HOST DISEASE. **gross stress r.** POST-TRAUMATIC STRESS DISORDER. **group r.** GROUP AGGLUTINATION. **Gruber's r.** WIDAL TEST. **Gruber-Widal r.** WIDAL TEST. **GVH r.** GRAFT VERSUS HOST DISEASE. **hemagglutination-inhibition r.** Any reaction in which a positive result is the abolition of immune-mediated red cell agglutination. In a system where fluid from a viral culture agglutinates red cells, the presence of an antibody to the virus inhibits virus-mediated agglutination. In a system where antibody to a surface antigen causes agglutination, the presence of the antigen in soluble form inhibits the effect of the antibody and abolishes agglutination. **hemianopic pupillary r.** Absence of pupillary constriction in the presence of a lesion of the optic tract when a light is directed upon that half of either retina from which fibers travel through the affected tract. Also *Wernicke's reaction, Wernicke's hemianopic reaction, Wernicke symptom, Wernicke sign.* **hemoclastic r.** HEMOLYSIS. **Henle's r.** CHROMAFFIN REACTION. **Herxheimer r.** **1** Fever, intensification of skin lesions, and musculoskeletal pain occurring after the administration of penicillin to a patient with secondary syphilis. This is thought to be an allergic reaction to products of the lysed spirochete, and is considered a confirming diagnostic point. **2** The intensification of symptoms and signs of disease after the initiation of antimicrobial therapy in relapsing fever. Also *Jarisch-Herxheimer reaction, Herxheimer's fever.* **heteroclytic r.** The stronger reaction of an antibody with a cross-reacting antigen than that with the antigen used to immunize it. **heterophil antibody r.** HETEROPHIL AGGLUTINATION. **Hill r.** The evolving of oxygen when isolated chloroplasts are illuminated and an electron acceptor, e.g. a ferric salt, is reduced. This demonstration gives support to the view that light reactions of photosynthesis occur within the chloroplast. **hunting r.** A reaction of digital blood vessels to temperatures below 15°C in which there are alternating periods of vasoconstriction and vasodilatation. **hypersensitivity r.** See under IMMUNOLOGICAL MECHANISMS OF TISSUE DAMAGE. **-id r.** A diffuse skin eruption arising from a localized focus of infection. It is believed to be caused by microbial antigens to which the subject is allergically sensitive. Also *dermatophytid reaction.* **r. of identity** A qualitative demonstration that two reactants have identical immunologic specificity. Symmetrical precipitin lines form and meet precisely at a point when the materials are placed equidistant from one another and from a single, specific antibody in a double immunodiffusion plate. In a reaction of partial identity, two antigens, both of which react with the antibody but to different extents, produce asymmetrical precipitin lines which meet at a point, but one extends beyond the intersection as a spur. In a reaction of nonidentity, the precipitin lines are asymmetrical in location and intensity, and cross one another at an unpredictable intersection. **immediate r.** An immune response occurring almost immediately or within a few hours after contact with an antigen, an immediate hypersensitivity reaction. Also *immediate response.* See also IMMUNOLOGICAL MECHANISMS OF TISSUE DAMAGE. **immune r.** IMMUNE RESPONSE. **indirect-light r.** CONSENSUAL LIGHT REFLEX. **indirect pupillary r.** CONSENSUAL LIGHT REFLEX. **indophenol r.** INDOPHENOL TEST. **infusion r.** Development of fever and, occasionally, hypotension in response to the infusion of pyrogens contaminating parenteral fluids. **intracutaneous r.** The reaction resulting from the introduction into the skin, usually by injection, of a minute amount of a substance. This reaction may be of diagnostic significance, as in the tuberculin test, Schick test, and others. Also *intradermal reaction, intradermoreaction.* **involutional psychotic r.** INVOLUTIONAL MELANCHOLIA. **isomorphous provocative r.** ISOMORPHIC EFFECT. **Ito-Reenstierna r.** ITO-REENSTIERNA TEST. **Jaffé r.** JAFFÉ'S TEST. **Jarisch-Herxheimer r.** HERXHEIMER REACTION. **Jolly's r.** MYASTHENIC REACTION. **Knaus r.** The absence of response of the contracting rabbit uterus to posterior pituitary hormone after the animal has been treated with progesterone. **Kveim's r.** KVEIM-SILTZBACH TEST. **Lange's r.** COLLOIDAL GOLD TEST. **late r.** DELAYED REACTION. **lengthening r.** Upon stretch of a muscle undergoing central nervous activation, a temporary reduction in activity followed by assumption of a new level of muscle activity and stiffness appropriate to the greater length. **lepra r.** The acute, immunologically mediated, inflammatory episode that may occur in leprosy. Also *reactional leprosy.* **lepromin r.** LEPROMIN TEST. **leukemic r.** LEUKEMOID REACTION. **leukemoid r.** An elevated leukocyte count in the peripheral blood, sometimes accompanied by maturation abnormalities or alterations in other elements, suggestive of and at times indistinguishable from any of several forms of leukemia. It usually results from severe infection, intoxication, disseminated neoplasm, or brisk hemorrhage or hemolysis. Bone marrow examination usually excludes leukemia. Also *leukemic reaction.* **Lewis r.** WHEAL-FLARE REACTION. **Liebermann-Burchard r.** LIEBERMANN-BURCHARD TEST. **local r.** A reaction occurring at the point of injection or application of a drug or other substance. **local anesthetic r.** An unexpected dermal or generalized allergic response, an untoward circulatory or respiratory complication, or a seizure or coma, following the application of a topical anesthetic or the injection of a local one. **Loeb's decidual r.** The formation of a deciduoma as a reaction to a foreign body in the endometrium. It can occur only when the corpus luteum is functioning in a normal fashion. **Loewi's r.** A former, nonspecific test in which successive instillation of epinephrine into the conjunctival sac induces dilatation of the pupil in the presence of pancreatic insufficiency, hyperthyroidism, or diabetes mellitus. Also *Loewi's test.* Also *Loewi's test, Loewi symptom.* **Lohmann r.** The metabolic reaction in muscle in which the high-energy phosphate bond in ATP is transferred to creatine, forming creatine phosphate. **lymphocyte transfer r.** See under NORMAL LYMPHOCYTE TRANSFER REACTION. **macrophage disappearance r.** The diminution in number of macrophages present in peritoneal exudate of a presensitized animal following the intraperitoneal injection of a specific antigen along with a nonspecific irritant. It is a manifestation of delayed hypersensitivity, probably mediated through the migration inhibition factor. **Mantoux r.** MANTOUX TEST. **Marañón's r.** A vasomotor response observed in Graves disease when the skin over the front of the neck is stimulated. Also *Marañón sign.* **Marchi's r.** A technique of demonstrating degeneration of axons and of their myelin sheaths in the pathways of the central nervous system using osmic acid as a stain for myelin. **Mátéfy's r.** MÁTÉFY TEST. **miostagmin r.** An obsolete serologic test for syphilis, malignancies, typhoid fever, etc., based on the premise that immune complexes would lower the surface tension. Also *Ascoli's test, Ascoli's reaction.* **Mitsuda r.** LEPROMIN TEST. **mixed agglutination r.** A technique to demonstrate similar or crossreactive surface antigens on different types of cells. Indicator cells that have been coated with antibody are added to test cells. A positive result is the formation of aggregates containing both types of cells, or the adherence of the indicator cells to test cells fixed on a slide. Also *mixed cell agglutination reaction.* **mixed antiglobulin r.** A demonstration of the presence of an antibody on the surface of cells that tend to aggregate spontaneously, using as an indicator cells with antiglobulin serum attached to their surfaces. A positive reaction is indicated by the formation of mixed agglutinates that contain both antibody-coated test cells and antiglobulin-coated indicator cells. Also *mixed hemadsorption.* **mixed lymphocyte culture r.** The transformation of small lymphocytes to blast cells following the mixing of lymphocytes from two individuals in a five-day culture. The number of blast cells produced varies inversely with the histocompatibility of the two donors. Also *mixed lymphocyte reaction, mixed leukocyte reaction, mixed leukocyte culture test.* **Molisch r.** A color test for dissolved carbohydrates, performed by adding ethanolic 1-naphthol to the solution, and adding sulfuric acid so that it forms a layer under the solution. A purple color at the interface, thought to be due to the interaction of the naphthol with furfural derivatives formed by dehydration of carbohydrates indicates their presence in the sample. **Moloney r.** MOLONEY TEST. **Morelli's r.** See under MORELLI'S TEST. **myasthenic r.** A progressive reduction in the strength of a muscular contraction evoked by repetitive faradic stimulation, as seen in myasthenia gravis. Also *Jolly's reaction.* **myotonic pupillary r.** The type of pupillary reaction to light observed in the Adie syndrome. **myotonoid r.** An electrically-induced muscular contraction in which both contraction and relaxation are abnormally slow, as seen in hypothyroidism. Also *pseudomyotonic reaction.* **Nadi r.** PEROXIDASE REACTION. **Nagler's r.** Development of opalescence in human blood serum containing *Clostridium perfringens,* due to the lecithinase activity of the organism's toxin and specifically inhibited by antiserum. **near-point r.** ACCOMMODATION REFLEX. **negative supporting r.** Relaxation of antigravity extensor muscles of a limb and activation of the flexor muscles in response to passive volar flexion of the digits. It is instrumental in permitting the limb to be moved to a new position, as in ambulation. **negative therapeutic r.** Resistance, on the part of the patient, encountered in psychoanalytic treatment in which a need for punishment leads to a continued generation of symptoms and thus prevents resolution of the mental disturbances. Also *superego resistance.* **Neill-Mooser r.** SCROTAL REACTION. **Neisser's r.** A transient increase in headache in general paresis or of lightning pains in tabes dorsalis following an initial injection of an organic arsenical drug in the treatment of neurosyphilis. See also HERXHEIMER REACTION. **Neufeld r.** QUELLUNG REACTION. **neurotonic r.** A muscular contraction that lasts beyond the cessation of the stimulus. **Nile blue r.** A histochemical reaction obtained when using Nile blue sulfate to differentiate phospholipids from neutral fats. **r. of nonidentity** See under REACTION OF IDENTITY. **normal lymphocyte transfer r.** A delayed reaction to the intradermal injection of allogeneic lymphocyte into an animal. A graft-versus-host reaction, it is manifested as an erythematous lesion, its size being inversely proportional to the degree of histocompatibility between the donor and recipient. The reaction is maximal at 48 hours. **nuclear r.** Any reaction in which elementary particles, such as protons or neutrons, act on a nucleus so as to transform one nuclide into another nuclide. **obsessive-compulsive r.** OBSESSIVE-COMPULSIVE NEUROSIS. **ophthalmic r.** CALMETTE'S REACTION. **oxidase r.** 1 INDOPHENOL TEST. 2 OXIDASE TEST. **pain r.** Any of the several involuntary responses to a painful stimulus, including the withdrawal, pupillary, and pressor reflexes. **paradoxical pupillary r.** Dilatation of the pupil instead of the constriction expected in the Marcus Gunn pupillary phenomenon, a pathologic response. **Parish r.** A sometimes severe allergic reaction to the Schick test. **r. of partial identity** See under REACTION OF IDENTITY. **passive Arthus r.** A form of Arthus reaction where antigen is injected subcutaneously into an animal that has previously been injected with the homologous antibody (either locally or intravenously) rather than having made the antibody itself. **passive cutaneous anaphylaxis r.** See under PASSIVE CUTANEOUS ANAPHYLAXIS. **Pasteur's r.** PASTEUR EFFECT. **Paul-Bunnell r.** PAUL-BUNNELL TEST. **periodic acid-Schiff r.** PERIODIC ACID-SCHIFF STAIN. **peroxidase r.** The formation of insoluble colored precipitates from certain soluble dyes when incubated with hydrogen peroxide and cells, tissues, or other supporting media that contain heme proteins such as peroxidase or hemoglobin. The reaction is due to release of oxygen from hydrogen peroxide, and the consequent oxidation of the dye. The reaction is useful in distinguishing myeloblasts, which contain peroxidase, from lymphoblasts, which do not, and hence it differentiates acute granulocytic leukemia from acute lymphocytic leukemia. The peroxidase reaction is also used to detect hemoglobin in urine or feces, in the benzidine, orthotolidine and guaiac tests, and occasionally to differentiate hemoglobin variants (peroxidase positive) from carbonic anhydrase (peroxidase negative) following electrophoresis. Also *Nadi reaction.* **Petzetaki's r.** PETZETAKI'S TEST. **Pfeiffer r.** PFEIFFER PHENOMENON. **phobic r.** ANXIETY HYSTERIA. **Pinkerton-Mooser r.** SCROTAL REACTION. **Pirquet's r.** Appearance of a raised, reddened area on the skin within 24–48 hours after introduction at that site, of a small amount of old tuberculin by slight scarification. A positive test indicates sensitivity to tuberculin. Also *dermotuberculin reaction, von Pirquet's reaction, von Pirquet's cutireaction, von Pirquet's test, Pirquet's test, scarification test.* **P-K r.** PRAUSNITZ-KÜSTNER REACTION. **pneumococcus capsule swelling r.** QUELLUNG REACTION. **Porges-Pollatschek r.** An old-fashioned pregnancy test consisting of an intradermal injection of neurohypophysial solution, which produces no reaction at the injection site if the subject is pregnant. **positive supporting r.** EXTENSOR THRUST REFLEX. **Prausnitz-Küstner r.** A test used for detecting homocytotropic (IgE) antibodies functionally in man. Serum is injected into the skin of a normal (nonsensitive) subject. Two days later the appropriate antigen is injected at the same site. A wheal and flare reaction denotes a positive test. Also *Prausnitz-Küstner test, P-K reaction, P-K test.* **precipitin r.** The formation of a visible precipitate as the positive end point in a reaction between a soluble antigen and a soluble antibody. Also *precipitation test.* **primary r. of Nissl** AXON REACTION. **prozone r.** PROZONE PHENOMENON. **pseudomyotonic r.** MYOTONOID REACTION. **psychosomatic r.** PSYCHOSOMATIC DISORDER. **psychotic depressive r.** DEPRESSIVE PSYCHOSIS. **puncture r.** Swelling and erythema at the site of a subcutaneous tuberculin injection, indicative of previous exposure to tubercle bacilli. **quellung r.** An increase in refractile properties and apparent size of a microorganism that occurs when a specific antiserum reacts with the polysaccharide antigens of the bacterial capsule. This alteration of microscopic appearance is used especially to classify *Streptococcus pneumoniae.* Also *capsular swelling reaction, Neufeld reaction, pneumococcus capsule swelling reaction, quellung test, quellung phenomenon.* **rage r.** An episode of uncontrollable rage upon minimal provocation occurring as one or sometimes the sole manifestation of an attack of temporal lobe epilepsy or in the course of a neurologic illness in which there is disease or dysfunction of the anteromedial portion of a temporal lobe. **retrobulbar pupil r.** In unilateral retrobulbar neuritis, when a light is directed into the affected eye there is sluggish contraction of both pupils, but when the unaffected eye is stimulated the reaction is brisk on both sides. **reversal r.** UPGRADING REACTION. **reverse passive Arthus r.** A form of Arthus reaction where intradermal or subcutaneous injection of antibody is followed after 30 minutes to 2 hours by intravenous injection of the homologous antigen. The antigen and antibody switch locations in this reaction compared to the normal Arthus reaction. **Rubino's r.** A rarely used agglutination-sedimentation test for leprosy using sheep erythrocytes. Inactivated serum from patients at the lepromatous end of the spectrum causes the erythrocytes to agglutinate and sediment rapidly. Also *Rubino's test.* **Sanarelli-Shwartzman r.** SHWARTZMAN PHENOMENON. **sarcoid tissue r.** The formation of noncaseating granulomas, particularly as seen in a Kveim-Siltzbach test. **Schick r.** SCHICK TEST. **Schultz-Dale r.** The prompt occurrence of smooth muscle contractions when isolated strips of smooth muscle, bathed in a physiologic solution, are exposed to an antigen to which the tissue has previously been actively or passively sensitized. This *in vitro* demonstration of anaphylaxis results from release of histamine and slow-reacting substance of anaphylaxis (SRS-A) following the interaction of cell-bound IgE antibodies with the antigen. Also *Schultz-Dale technique.* **scrotal r.** Inflammation of the scrotum and tunica vaginalis in guinea pigs infected with the rickettsiae of murine or epidemic typhus. The exudate contains large mononuclear cells filled with rickettsiae. Also *Neill-Mooser reaction, Pinkerton-Mooser reaction.* **second-order r.** A reaction whose rate is proportional to the product of two concentrations, as of two reactants or of a reactant and a catalyst, or to the square of the concentration of one reactant. Many reactions between two reactants are of this type. **second-set r.** SECOND-SET PHENOMENON. **sedimentation r.** ERYTHROCYTE SEDIMENTATION RATE. **Selivanoff r.** RESORCINOL TEST. **serum r.** SEROREACTION. **shortening r.** The assumption of a new level of tonic activity and tension in a muscle following an induced quick reduction in the muscle length. It is especially evident in extensor muscles of the decerebrate preparation. **Shwartzman r.** SHWARTZMAN PHENOMENON. **skin r.** CUTANEOUS REACTION. **soluble immune complex r.** See under IMMUNOLOGICAL MECHANISMS OF TISSUE DAMAGE. **spring r.** EXTENSOR THRUST REFLEX. **startle r.** STARTLE RESPONSE. **statokinetic r.** STATOKINETIC REFLEX. Also *acceleratory reflex.* **stress r.** TRANSIENT SITUATIONAL PERSONALITY DISORDER. **supporting r.'s** The total response of limb and trunk muscles of antigravity action that makes standing possible (positive supporting reaction), or of flexor activation that permits the limbs to be moved to new positions for relaxation or locomotion (negative supporting reaction). The development of the limb rigidity for support is dependent on the stimulation of exteroceptors and proprioceptors through contact of the hands or feet with the ground. These stimuli facilitate stretch reflexes in the limb muscles. The hyperactivity of extensors in the decerebrate preparation results from a release of the positive supporting reaction, while the labile limb movements in some spinal preparations represent predominance of the negative reaction. Also *supporting reflexes.* **sympathetic r.** FIGHT-OR-FLIGHT REACTION. **thermonuclear r.** A nuclear reaction brought about by exceedingly high temperatures, for example in the sun, in which two light atomic nuclei fuse to form a heavier one, with the release of very large amounts of energy due to a shrinkage in total mass. **thread r.** FILAMENTATION. **tilt r.** EQUILIBRIUM REACTION. **toxin-antitoxin r.** ANTIGEN-ANTIBODY REACTION. **Trambusti's r.** Local reddening of the skin occurring within three days of a cutaneous injection of tuberculin that is administered by means of a needle inserted parallel to the skin surface. Also *Trambusti test, endodermoreaction.* **trigger r.** TRIGGER ACTION. **tuberculin r.** The cutaneous, and occasionally systemic, manifestations of delayed hypersensitivity that are elicited by the intradermal injection of tuberculin antigen prepared from *Mycobacterium tuberculosis.* Reddening and induration develop within 12 to 48 hours at the site of injection in an individual who has had previous immunizing exposure to the tubercle bacillus. The reaction is identical for an ongoing active case, an inactive case, a long-past case, and deliberate immunization. **tuberculin-type r.** Any cutaneous manifestation of delayed hypersensitivity elicited by the intradermal injection of a suitable antigen, such as those prepared from mumps virus, *Candida albicans,* or *Histoplasma capsulatum.* **type 1 r.** See under IMMUNOLOGICAL MECHANISMS OF TISSUE DAMAGE. **type 2 r.** See under IMMUNOLOGICAL MECHANISMS OF TISSUE DAMAGE. **type 3 r.** See under IMMUNOLOGICAL MECHANISMS OF TISSUE DAMAGE. **type 4 r.** See under IMMUNOLOGICAL MECHANISMS OF TISSUE DAMAGE. **upgrading r.** A lepra reaction associated with an increase in specific cell-mediated immunity to *Mycobacterium leprae.* Also *reversal reaction.* **vaccinoid r.** A reaction to smallpox vaccination in a person who has preexisting partial immunity to smallpox. It is characterized by abbreviated stages of illness and an overall milder course. **vital r.** In forensic medicine, any tissue or organ reaction which requires living cells and conclusively indicates that the injury initiating the reaction occurred antemortem. Enzyme histochemistry is the most reliable way to demonstrate the antemortem nature of wounds occurring very shortly before death. **Voges-Proskauer r.** A test for the products of the butanediol fermentation, particularly in *Enterobacter.* These products are oxidized by air to diacetyl, which yields a red color with $\alpha$-naphthol. See also IMVIC. **von Pirquet's r.** PIRQUET'S REACTION. **Waaler-Rose r.** ROSE-WAALER TEST. **Wassermann r.** WASSERMANN TEST. **Watson-Schwartz r.** WATSON-SCHWARTZ TEST. **Weil-Felix r.** WEIL-FELIX TEST. **Wernicke's r.** HEMIANOPIC PUPILLARY REACTION. **Wernicke's hemianopic r.** HEMIANOPIC PUPILLARY REACTION. **wheal-flare r.** A series of three sequential responses occurring in the skin following injury. Initially a circumscribed, erythematous area forms at the site of the injury as a result of capillary dilatation. This is followed by an irregular erythematous flare surrounding the site of the injury, and finally by a wheal at the site of the injury resulting from extravasation of fluid from the capillaries. Also *wheal and flare response, triple response of Lewis, Lewis reaction.* **white graft r.** HYPERACUTE REJECTION. **Widal r.** WIDAL TEST. **Wolff-Calmette r.** CALMETTE'S REACTION. **Wolff-Eisner r.** CALMETTE'S REACTION. **zero-order r.** A reaction whose rate is independent, at least over a specified concentration range, of the concentration of the reactant. **Zimmermann r.** A colorimetric reaction to 17-ketosteroids, usually in the urine. In the presence of *m*-dinitrobenzene and potassium hydroxide, 17-ketosteroids produce a color with maximum absorption at 520 m$\beta$.

**reaction-formation** An unconscious defense mechanism consisting of the development of conscious, socialized attitudes that are the opposite of existing infantile impulses that are unacceptable to the subject. Also *reversal-formation.*

**reactivate** \rē·ak′tivāt\ To make active again, as an infection.

**reactivation** \rē′aktivā′shən\ Restoration to a state of being active, especially to a state of immunologic activity, as an inactivated serum to which complement has been added.

**reactive** \rē·ak′tiv\ **1** Tending to react; responsive to a stimulus. **2** Tending to take part in a chemical reaction.

**reactivity** \rē′aktiv′itē\ **1** The tendency or ability of a substance to react, especially with a defined class of other substances. **2** The ability of an electroencephalographic tracing to be modified by a physiologic stimulus (exteroceptive or interoceptive), or by psychologic, pharmacologic, or pathologic influences. **vascular r.** The sensitivity of the systemic or pulmonary vasculature to stimuli which may increase or decrease tone. Subjects with primary hypertension or their relatives often have more than normal vascular reactivity.

**reactor** \rē·ak′tər\ [*react(ion)* + -OR] **universal r.** A person exhibiting hypersensitivity to a wide range of environmental substances, specifically associated with total allergy syndrome.

**readiness / explosion r.** Irritability and tendency to overreact with violence to minor stimuli, leading to episodic loss of control over aggressive impulses. It has most often been reported in alcoholics with suspected or demonstrated brain damage although it can be seen in other cerebral disorders as well. **reading r.** That stage during the development of the growing child, at which the maturation of the nervous system and the experiential history of the individual make it possible to profit by instruction in reading. it is considered important to begin reading instruction at just this optimal time, but this will vary for each individual. If it is undertaken too early, neural limits may be exceeded, and if started too late, an important step in cognitive development may be delayed or permanently retarded.

**reading** 1 The perception and understanding of the meaning of visual symbols, such as letters or words, by the scanning of writing or printed matter with the eyes. 2 Any of several alternative ways of interpreting symbols, such as the use of Braille or the close observation of the facial movements of a speaker (lip reading). 3 A datum indicated by an instrument that measures quantity, rate, etc. **lip r.** The interpretation of speech from information gathered not from hearing, or from hearing alone, but by attention to such visual signals as facial expression, lip movements, gestures, and contextual considerations. Although of particular importance to deaf and hearing-impaired individuals, this faculty plays a significant part in the comprehension of speech by the normally hearing. Also *speech reading*. • The term *lip reading* is unfortunate since observation of lip movements is only part of the faculty described. **speech r.** LIP READING. **wet r.** A radiologic interpretation given immediately after the film has been processed. Formerly, when films were hand-processed, the films were still wet at the time of the wet reading. Now, with machine processing, the films are dry.

**readout** 1 The process of transmitting information from a computer and displaying it. 2 The displayed information from a computer. 3 The form of presentation of computer information, such as a terminal display, printed copy, punched cards, etc. 4 The device that presents computer information, such as the terminal, printer, card punch, etc.

**readthrough** In molecular biology, transcription through a termination signal. It is usually due to the failure of RNA polymerase to recognize a termination sequence in the DNA, a consequence of mutation in a termination codon to a sense codon or presence of certain supressor tRNA molecules.

**reagent** \rē·ā′jənt\ [New L *reagens*, gen. *reagent(is)* (pres. part. of Late L *reagere* to react) reacting] Any substance capable of reacting with another, particularly if the reaction produces a change of physical properties whereby the second substance may be detected or measured. For example, dimethylglyoxime is a reagent for nickel, iron, bismuth, etc. The reagent is called selective if it indicates the presence of a small number of compounds or ions, and specific (or characteristic) if it only gives an indication with a single substance. **benzidine r.** The chromophoric reagent used in the benzidine test for heme pigments. **Bial's r.** A solution of orcinol, fuming hydrochloric acid, and ferric chloride. It turns green if pentose is present in the material, usually urine, that is added to the heated reagent. **biuret r.** An alkaline solution of copper(II) sulfate, stabilized with sodium potassium tartrate and potassium iodide, that is used in the biuret test for measuring proteins. **Cleland's r.** DITHIOTHREITOL. **diazo r.** A reagent used in Ehrlich's test for bilirubin, consisting of two solutions, A and B. Reagent A is sulfanilic acid and hydrochloric acid diluted in distilled water and reagent B is a sodium nitrite solution. They are combined in proportions of 40 to 1 immediately before use. Also *Ehrlich's diazo reagent*. **Ehrlich's aldehyde r.** A solution of 0.7 g paradimethylaminobenzaldehyde in 150 ml of concentrated hydrochloric acid, which is added to 100 ml of distilled water. It is used in Ehrlich's test for urobilinogen in the urine or feces. **Ehrlich's diazo r.** DIAZO REAGENT. **Fouchet's r.** A solution, composed of 1 g ferric chloride in a 25 g/100 ml solution of tric hloroacetic acid, that is used in testing for bilirubin in the urine. **Moro's r.** MORO'S TUBERCULIN. **Nessler's r.** An aqueous solution of potassium iodide, potassium hydroxide, and mercuric iodide that is used in measuring ammonia. Also *Nessler solution*. **Pappenheim's r.** PAPPENHEIM STAIN. **Schiff's r.** An aqueous solution of pararosaniline or basic fuchsin that is decolorized by sulfur dioxide. It is used in chemistry to detect aldehydes and in histochemistry to stain polysaccharides, nucleic acid, and proteins. **Sulkowitch's r.** A solution in distilled water of oxalic acid, ammonium oxalate, and glacial acetic acid, used in the Sulkowitch test for urinary calcium.

**reagin** \rē′əjən\ REAGINIC ANTIBODY.

**real-time** Characterized by making accessible the observation of images, events, or data as they occur or are received.

**reamer** \rē′mər\ A fine cone-shaped instrument with coarse spiral cutting edges, used for enlarging root canals by rotation.

**reamputation** \rē·amp′yətā′shən\ A surgical procedure in which an amputation is repeated at a more proximate level or a second location.

**reanimate** \rē·an′imāt\ To restore function, particularly motion.

**rearrangement** \rē′əranj′mənt\ **Amadori r.** A reaction of a glycosylamine, in which an amine, $NH_2$—R, glycosylated by a sugar, R′—CHOH—CHO, is transformed into the compound R′—CO—$CH_2$—NH—R, which itself may exist in a cyclic hemiacetal form. Such a reaction follows glucosylation of the $\beta$-chains of hemoglobin in the formation of hemoglobin $A_{Ic}$.

**reattachment** [RE- + ATTACHMENT] 1 The recementing of a dental restoration. 2 The successful replantation of a dislocated tooth. Reattachment of epithelium occurs readily, but bony ankylosis and root resorption is the usual outcome. **r. of pocket** The regaining of an organic connection between the soft tissues lining a periodontal pocket and the root of the tooth. The prognosis for surgical reattachment procedures is best when the pocket is intrabony, but most of any reattachment gained may be by epithelial rather than connective tissue.

**rebase** \rēbās′\ To make a denture base fit the underlying tissue when it has ceased to do so because of ridge resorption. A new impression is taken and plastic base material is interposed between the cast and the old denture base. Also *reline*.

**rebound** [French *rebond* (from RE- + L *bombus* a deep hollow sound) the act of rebounding] A temporary excess above control level of a behavioral, electrical, or neurophysiologic characteristic that develops following a period of suppression of the characteristic during repetitive stimulation of the preparation. Depending upon the characteristic under observation, the excess may be seen in a pattern of spontaneous acitivity or may be revealed by single presentations of the same stimulus. **REM r.** The phenomenon in which a subject deprived of REM sleep will compensate by increasing the duration of sleep and of REM sleep in the next cycle.

**rebreathing** The partial or total breathing of expired gas. Also *rehalation*.

**recall** [RE- + English *call*] The mental operation of invoking from long-term memory something previously experienced or learned. This representation may take the form of concrete imagery, or be achieved by verbal processes. **free r.** A test of memory in which retention is measured by presenting the subject with a series of items that are to be reproduced later, with the number of items remembered, rather than the specific order of their original presentation, determining the subject's score.

**recanalization** \rēkan′əlīzā′shən\ Re-establishment of

the lumen of an occluded blood vessel, usually as a result of lysis of thrombus.

**recapitulation** \rē′kəpich′əlā′shən\ Repetition of steps or stages in development. The successive appearance in vertebrate embryos of stages in development in organs such as the kidney and heart and in structures such as the branchial arches provide examples of repetition. See also RECAPITULATION THEORY.

**receptaculum** \ri′septak′yələm\ [L (from *recepta(re)* to take back, recover + *-culum* English *-cle*), a storehouse, receptacle] (*pl.* receptacula) A receptacle or container. **r. chyli** *Outmoded* CISTERNA CHYLI. **r. ganglii petrosi** FOSSULA PETROSA. **r. pecqueti** *Outmoded* CISTERNA CHYLI.

**receptoma** \rē′septō′mə\ PARAGANGLIOMA.

**receptor** \risep′tər\ [L (from *receptus,* past part. of *recipere* to receive, retain, hold back, take back, from RE- + L *capere* to take, seize, + *-or* -OR), one who receives or harbors] **1** A sensory nerve ending specialized for the reception of stimuli and capable of transmitting them in the form of nerve impulses. Also *ceptor* (outmoded). **2** A structure, usually on a membrane, with binding affinity for a particular ligand and where the ligand binding gives rise to some biologically significant effect. See illustration at RECEPTOR SITE. **3** In Ehrlich's side-chain theory, a postulated group in a cell having the property of combining with the haptophore group of a toxin. **α-r.** A site or structure on the surface of a cell at which α-adrenergic agents bind, thus producing a response. **adrenergic r.'s** A class of cellular receptors present in effector organs that receive neuronal input from postganglionic, adrenergic fibers of the sympathetic nervous system. The class is further divided into two subclasses, alpha or beta, depending on their response to agonists such as adrenaline and isoproterenol, and antagonists such as phentolamine and propranolol. **alpha-adrenergic r.** A member of a subclass of adrenergic receptors that are stimulated by adrenaline and noradrenaline and antagonized by phentolamine and phenoxybenzamine. They mediate contraction in all smooth muscles except in the nonsphincter regions of the gastrointestinal tract, where they mediate relaxation. **beta-adrenergic r.** A member of a subclass of adrenergic receptors that are characterized by their response to catecholamines and adrenergic antagonists. They are more sensitive to isoproterenol than are the alpha receptors. The beta receptors are subdivided into $beta_1$ and $beta_2$ types. The $beta_1$ is located primarily in the heart and small intestine; the $beta_2$ is found in bronchial smooth muscle, smooth muscle of the vascular system, and the uterus. **C3b r.** CR1. See under COMPLEMENT RECEPTOR. **C3d r.** CR2. See under COMPLEMENT RECEPTOR. **central r.'s** Organs or cells within the central nervous system that react to specific sensory stimuli, such as osmolality, pH, or temperature. **cholinergic r.** Membrane receptor sites in muscle and nervous tissue where the neurotransmitter acetylcholine binds to produce excitation. Specific binding with α-bungarotoxin permits its isolation and localization. **complement r.** A structure found on the surface of a variety of cells that can bind to fixed complement components and whose reactions with their ligand causes some biologically significant effect. The best defined complement receptors are those reacting with fixed C3 fragments. Three such receptors are known, designated CR1, CR2, and CR3. Receptors for fixed $C1_q$ and for fixed factor H have also been described. CR1 (immune adherence receptor or C3B receptor) is found on human erythrocytes, granulocytes, monocytes/macrophages, some B lymphocytes, and on renal podocytes. It binds fixed C3b and C4b and, more weakly, fixed iC3b, and it has a molecular mass of 190–250 kDa. CR2 (C3d receptor) is found on B lymphocytes and on many lymphoblastoid cell lines. It binds fixed iC3b, $C3d_{19}$ (the preferred ligand), and C3d, and has a molecular mass of 140 kDa. Its function is unknown. CR3 is found on granulocytes and monocytes/macrophages. It binds fixed iC3b and no other bound complement fragment. It is an important phagocytic receptor. The receptor has two chains with molecular masses of 90 and 165 kDa. **contact r.** MECHANORECEPTOR. **contiguous r.** A sense organ that requires contiguity with the stimulus, such as taste and tactile receptors. **cutaneous r.** A sense organ in the dermis or epidermis. **distance r.** A sense organ responsive (by means of sound waves, photons, olfactant molecules, etc.) to objects distant from or not immediately contiguous with the body. *Outmoded.* Also *teloreceptor, telereceptor, teleceptor, distoceptor, distance ceptor.* **equilibratory r.'s** STATIC RECEPTORS. **estrogen r.** A cellular structure possessing a specific affinity for the binding of estrogenic hormones, concentrated particularly in estrogen-sensitive tissues, as the breast and uterus. It is of clinical importance in providing an index of predictability as to whether estrogen-ablative therapy (ovariectomy) will be effective in the palliation of mammary carcinoma. **genital r.'s** CORPUSCULA GENITALIA. **gravity r.'s** STATIC RECEPTORS. **gustatory r.** A sense organ on the tongue or oropharyngeal region responsive to sapid molecules, the excitation of which gives rise to a sensation of taste. Also *taste receptor.* **immune adherence r.** CR1. See under COMPLEMENT RECEPTOR. **length r.** Any stretch receptor that is adapted primarily to gauging muscle length or, more precisely, the length of muscle fascicles in its vicinity. **muscle r.** An organized sensory organ located within the substance of a muscle, its tendon, or the epimysium. The principal receptors are muscle spindles, tendon organs and pacinian corpuscles. Also *myoreceptor* (obs.). **olfactory r.** The sensory cells of the nasal epithelium, excited by substances capable of eliciting impulses in the olfactory pathway and a sense of smell. Also *osmoreceptor* (outmoded). **pain r.** NOCICEPTOR. **Pinkus-Iggo r.** A cutaneous tactile sense organ consisting of a Merkel cell disk innervated by a myelinated axon. It responds to the magnitude of skin displacement with a proportionate slowly-adapting impulse discharge at irregular intervals. Also *touch organ.* **pressure r.** **1** Any mechanoreceptive sense organ giving rise to the sensation of pressure or touch. *Outmoded.* **2** A slowly-adapting mechanoreceptor distinguished as a Merkel cell complex or Ruffini organ. **sensory r.** A sense organ the excitation of which gives rise to conscious sensory experience. The term is also imprecisely applied to deep receptors of muscle and viscera that can be excited without resultant sensation. **static r.'s** The sense organs responsible for maintaining the organism's posture and balance, primarily the vestibular organs but strictly including muscle, tendon, and joint sense organs. Also *equilibratory receptors, gravity receptors.* **stretch r.** A sense organ, located in a muscle or tendon, whose afferent fiber discharge is determined by the magnitude of stretch. In vertebrate muscle, called a muscle spindle. **tactile r.** MECHANORECEPTOR. **taste r.** GUSTATORY RECEPTOR. **tension r.** Any stretch receptor that primarily monitors longitudinally directed stress produced within muscle or imposed on its tendon. **tissue r.** A specific pattern of molecular structure on a cell or other tissue component to which a given antibody or other defined molecule will bind. **touch r.** MECHANORECEPTOR. **visual r.** A rod or cone cell. **volume r.'s** Unidentified sense organs, inferred as responding to alterations in plasma and extracellular fluid volume, that provide the neural input underlying reflex adjustment.

**receptorology** \risep′tərä1′əjē\ [RECEPTOR + *o* + -LOGY] The study of the structure and function of receptor sites on the surface of cells, as the loci of action of drugs or hormones.

# recess

**recess** [L *recessus.* See RECESSUS.] A small hollow or space; recessus. **anterior r. of interpeduncular fossa** RECESSUS ANTERIOR FOSSAE INTERPEDUNCULARIS TARINI. **anterior r. of tympanic membrane** RECESSUS MEMBRANAE TYMPANI ANTERIOR. **Arlt's r.** An inconstant small saclike sinus occasionally found in the lower portion of the lacrimal sac. Also *Arlt sinus.* **attic r.** RECESSUS EPITYMPANICUS. **cerebellopontile r.** RECESSUS CEREBELLOPONTIS. **chiasmatic r.** RECESSUS OPTICUS. **cochlear r. of vestibule** RECESSUS COCHLEARIS VESTIBULI. **conarial r.** RECESSUS PINEALIS. **costodiaphragmatic r. of pleura** RECESSUS COSTODIAPHRAGMATICUS PLEURAE. **costomediastinal r. of pleura** RECESSUS COSTOMEDIASTINALIS PLEURAE. **duodenojejunal r.** RECESSUS DUODENALIS SUPERIOR. **elliptical r. of vestibule** RECESSUS ELLIPTICUS VESTIBULI. **epitympanic r.** RECESSUS EPITYMPANICUS. **hepatoenteric r.** A recess of the peritoneal cavity formed initially along the complete length of the right side of the dorsal mesogastrium and the stomach, and situated in a sagittal plane. Afterwards, and occurring at the time of rotation of the stomach, this third sac of the peritoneal cavity contributes to the formation of the lesser sac and its extension into the greater omentum. **hepatorenal r.** RECESSUS HEPATORENALIS. **Hyrtl's r.** RECESSUS EPITYMPANICUS. **incisive r.** A small depression on the nasal septum anterosuperior to the incisive canal and in the area of the vomeronasal organ of Jacobson when present. **inferior duodenal r.** RECESSUS DUODENALIS INFERIOR. **inferior ileocecal r.** RECESSUS ILEOCECALIS INFERIOR. **inferior omental r.** RECESSUS INFERIOR OMENTALIS. **infundibular r.** RECESSUS INFUNDIBULI. **r. of infundibulum** RECESSUS INFUNDIBULI. **interpeduncular r.** FOSSA INTERPEDUNCULARIS. **intersigmoidal r.** RECESSUS INTERSIGMOIDEUS. **labyrinthine r.** A tubular diverticulum on the medial side of the otocyst in the embryo which differentiates into the ductus and saccus endolymphaticus of the internal ear. **laryngopharyngeal r.** RECESSUS PIRIFORMIS. **lateral r. of fourth ventricle** RECESSUS LATERALIS VENTRICULI QUARTI. **lateral r. of nasopharynx** RECESSUS PHARYNGEUS. **lateral r. of rhomboid fossa** RECESSUS LATERALIS VENTRICULI QUARTI. **lienal r.** RECESSUS SPLENICUS. **mesenteric r.** PNEUMATOENTERIC RECESS. **mesocolic r.** DUODENOJEJUNAL FOSSA. **middle pharyngeal r.** BURSA PHARYNGEALIS. **nasopalatine r.** A small depression directed anteroinferiorly on the nasal septum immediately above the incisive canal. It marks the site of a canal between the nasal and oral cavities in the fetus. **neuroporic r.** A diverticulum at the anterior end of the developing brain which demarcates the region of the neuropore, which is closed by this stage. **optic r.** RECESSUS OPTICUS. **optic r. of third ventricle** RECESSUS OPTICUS. **paracolic r.'es** *Outmoded* SULCI PARACOLICI. **paraduodenal r.** RECESSUS PARADUODENALIS. **r. of pelvic mesocolon** RECESSUS INTERSIGMOIDEUS. **peritoneal r.'es** Hollows or cul-de-sacs formed by peritoneum behind or at the sides of organs or vessels in the abdominal cavity. **pharyngeal r.** RECESSUS PHARYNGEUS. **pineal r.** RECESSUS PINEALIS. **piriform r.** RECESSUS PIRIFORMIS. **pleural r.'es** RECESSUS PLEURALES. **pneumatoenteric r.** One of two peritoneal pockets appearing in the embryo on each side of the dorsal mesogastrium before the stomach rotates. The left one disappears while the right one communicates with the peritoneal cavity and extends cranially between the esophagus and the root of the right lung. With the development of the diaphragm the cranial part is detached to form the infracardiac bursa within the right pulmonary ligament, while the remaining caudal part helps to form the upper part of the omental bursa in the adult. Also *pneumoenteric recess, mesenteric recess.* **pontocerebellar r.** RECESSUS CEREBELLOPONTIS. **posterior r. of interpeduncular fossa** RECESSUS POSTERIOR FOSSAE INTERPEDUNCULARIS TARINI. **posterior r. of tympanic membrane** RECESSUS MEMBRANAE TYMPANI POSTERIOR. **Reichert's r.** RECESSUS COCHLEARIS VESTIBULI. **retrocecal r.** RECESSUS RETROCAECALIS. **retroduodenal r.** RECESSUS RETRODUODENALIS. **right subhepatic r.** RECESSUS HEPATORENALIS. **Rosenmüller's r.** RECESSUS PHARYNGEUS. **sacciform r. of distal radioulnar articulation** RECESSUS SACCIFORMIS ARTICULATIONIS RADIOULNARIS DISTALIS. **sphenoethmoidal r.** RECESSUS SPHENOETHMOIDALIS. **spherical r. of vestibule** RECESSUS SPHERICUS VESTIBULI. **splenic r.** RECESSUS SPLENICUS. **subhepatic r.'es** RECESSUS SUBHEPATICI. **subphrenic r.'es** RECESSUS SUBPHRENICI. **subpopliteal r.** RECESSUS SUBPOPLITEUS. **superior duodenal r.** RECESSUS DUODENALIS SUPERIOR. **superior ileocecal r.** RECESSUS ILEOCECALIS SUPERIOR. **superior omental r.** RECESSUS SUPERIOR OMENTALIS. **superior r. of tympanic membrane** RECESSUS MEMBRANAE TYMPANI SUPERIOR. **suprapineal r.** RECESSUS SUPRAPINEALIS. **supratonsillar r.** FOSSA SUPRATONSILLARIS. **Tarini's r.** RECESSUS ANTERIOR FOSSAE INTERPEDUNCULARIS TARINI. **r.'es of Tröltsch** Recessus membranae tympani anterior and recessus membranae tympani posterior. **tubotympanic r.** RECESSUS TUBOTYMPANICUS. **utricular r.** RECESSUS ELLIPTICUS VESTIBULI. **r. of vestibule** One of three small depressions in the bony vestibule of the inner ear: (1) recessus cochlearis vestibuli; (2) recessus ellipticus vestibuli; (3) recessus sphericus vestibuli.

**recession** \risesh′ən\ [L *recessio* (from *recedere* to recede) withdrawal. See RECESSUS.] **1** The act or an instance of receding; withdrawal. **2** A surgical repositioning (as of a tendon insertion) to a more proximal or posterior position. **3** The transplantation of an extraocular tendon to a position on the sclera behind its original insertion, performed to rotate the eye in a direction away from the operated muscle, as a correction for strabismus. Compare ADVANCEMENT. **angle r.** An anteroposterior splitting of the ciliary body due to trauma. This injury deepens the angle of the anterior chamber. **bone r.** Loss of alveolar bone from the crest associated with periodontal disease. **gingival r.** Loss of gingiva, exposing part of the root of a tooth or of several teeth. Also *gingival resorption.* **tendon r.** The surgical repositioning of a tendon insertion to a more proximal location.

**recessive** \rises′iv\ Pertaining to a phenotype, produced by a single gentic locus in diploid organisms, that is expressed only when an allele is homozygous but not when heterozygous.

**recessiveness** \rises′ivnis\ **1** The state of being recessive. **2** In genetics, a property of the phenotype such that an allele that determines the phenotype must be homozygous for expression. Compare DOMINANCE.

**recessus** \rises′əs\ [L (from *recedere* to withdraw, move back, retire, from *re-* back + *cedere* to go, depart, give way) withdrawal, a recess, indentation] (*pl.* recessus) A small hollow or fossa; recess. **r. anterior fossae interpeduncularis tarini** A diverticulum that passes under the mamillary bodies. Also *Tarini's recess, Tarin space, anterior recess of interpeduncular fossa.* **r. cerebellopontis** The angle formed at the junction of the pons and cerebellum. Also *cerebellopontile recess, pontocerebellar recess.* **r. chiasmatis** RECESSUS OPTICUS. **r. cochlearis vestibuli** [NA] A small depression on the medial wall of the bony vestibule of the internal ear, situated between the two divided limbs of the posterior end of the vestibular crest. It is pierced by foramina for the fibers of the vestibulocochlear nerve passing to the vestibular end of the cochlear duct. Also *cochlear recess of vestibule, Reichert's recess.* **r. costodiaphragmaticus pleurae** [NA] The narrow space between the costal and the diaphragmatic pleurae where they come into contact at the lower end of the thoracic cavity. Also *costodiaphragmatic recess of pleura.* **r. costomediastinalis pleurae** [NA] A narrow cleft between the costal and the mediastinal pleurae behind the sternum where the thin anterior margin of the lung does not reach the line of reflection between the pleurae. Also *costomediastinal recess of pleura.* **r. duodenalis inferior** [NA] A peritoneal fossa covered by the inferior duodenal fold. It is on the left side of the lower part of the ascending, or fourth, part of the duodenum. Its orifice faces upwards opposite that of the superior duodenal recess. Also *inferior duodenal recess, inferior duodenal fossa, fossa of Treitz.* **r. duodenalis superior** [NA] A peritoneal space under the crescentic superior duodenal, or duodenojejunal, fold and on the left side of the upper part of the ascending, or fourth, part of the duodenum. Its orifice faces downwards opposite that of the inferior duodenal recess. Also *superior duodenal recess, duodenojejunal recess, superior duodenal fossa, duodenojejunal fossa, fossa of Jonnesco.* **r. ellipticus vestibuli** [NA] A small oval depression in the roof and medial wall of the bony vestibule of the internal ear, situated above and behind the vestibular crest and lodging the utricle. Like the pyramid, it is perforated by the macula cribrosa superior, through which pass nerve fibers to the utricle and the ampullae of the lateral and superior semicircular ducts. Also *elliptical recess of vestibule, utricular recess.* **r. epitympanicus** [NA] The portion of the tympanic cavity situated above the level of the tympanic membrane and lodging the upper part of the malleus and most of the incus. Its roof is formed by the tegmen tympani and posteriorly it is continuous with the aditus to the mastoid antrum. Also *epitympanic recess, epitympanic space, Hyrtl's recess, epitympanum, tympanic attic, attic, attic recess.* **r. hepatorenalis** [NA] A deep peritoneal space extending behind the inferior surface of the right lobe of the liver and the gallbladder and in front of the right suprarenal gland and upper part of kidney, the right colic flexure, and transverse mesocolon. Superiorly it is bounded by the right triangular ligament and the inferior layer of the coronary ligament of the liver. Also *hepatorenal recess, hepatorenal pouch, right subhepatic recess, Morison's pouch.* **r. ileocecalis inferior** [NA] A peritoneal fossa behind the ileocecal fold and to the left of the cecum, bounded superiorly by the posterior surface of the ileum and its mesentery and posteriorly by the upper part of the mesoappendix. Its orifice faces to the left and inferiorly. Also *inferior ileocecal recess, inferior ileocecal fossa, Hartmann's fossa.* **r. ileocecalis superior** [NA] A narrow peritoneal space behind the vascular fold of the cecum and to the left of the ileocecal junction, bounded posteriorly by the mesentery of the ileum and inferiorly by the terminal part of the ileum. Its orifice faces to the left and downwards. It is most obvious in children and often disappears in older adults, especially obese ones. Also *superior ileocecal recess, superior ileocecal fossa, ileocolic fossa, Luschka's fossa.* **r. inferior omentalis** [NA] The lower portion of the omental bursa, lying below foramen bursae omenti majoris and behind the stomach and extending into the greater omentum. It represents the pancreaticoenteric recess in the embryo. Also *inferior omental recess, inferior fossa of omental sac, epiploic bursa.* **r. infundibuli** [NA] A downward prolongation of the floor of the third ventricle into the infundibulum. Also *infundibular recess, recess of infundibulum.* **r. intersigmoideus** [NA] A deep, funnel-shaped peritoneal space behind the upward projecting apex of the angulated attachment of the sigmoid mesocolon to the posterior abdominal wall. Its orifice faces inferiorly. The peritoneum of its posterior wall covers the left ureter crossing the bifurcation of the left common iliac artery. Also *intersigmoidal recess, intersigmoid fossa, recess of pelvic mesocolon.* **r. lateralis fossae rhomboidei** RECESSUS LATERALIS VENTRICULI QUARTI. **r. lateralis ventriculi quarti** [NA] A narrow prolongation on each side of the fourth ventricle between the inferior cerebellar and floccular peduncles. Also *lateral recess of fourth ventricle, lateral recess of rhomboid fossa, recessus lateralis fossae rhomboidei, parepicoele* (obs.). **r. membranae tympani anterior** [NA] A small pouch in the mucous membrane of the tympanic membrane situated below the plica chordae tympani and in front of the handle of the malleus. Also *anterior recess of tympanic membrane, anterior pouch of Tröltsch.* **r. membranae tympani posterior** [NA] A small pouch in the mucous membrane of the tympanic membrane situated below the plica chordae tympani and behind the handle of the malleus. Also *posterior recess of tympanic membrane, posterior pouch of Tröltsch.* **r. membranae tympani superior** [NA] A small pouch in the mucous membrane of the tympanic membrane situated between the pars flaccida and the neck of the malleus. It may be connected to the posterior recess of the tympanic membrane. Also *superior recess of tympanic membrane, Prussak's pouch, Prussak space.* **r. opticus** [NA] A small angular diverticulum of the third ventricle above the optic chiasm. Also *optic recess, chiasmatic recess, recessus chiasmatis, optic recess of third ventricle.* **r. paraduodenalis** [NA] A peritoneal fossa commonly found in the newborn but seldom in the adult. It is located to the left of the ascending part of the duodenum and behind the curved paraduodenal fold containing the inferior mesenteric vein and the ascending branch of the left colic artery in its right free margin. The orifice faces towards the right. Also *paraduodenal recess, paraduodenal fossa, Gruber-Landzert fossa, Landzert's fossa.* **r. pharyngeus** [NA] A wide slitlike pouch of variable extent in the lateral wall of the nasopharynx which is lined by mucous membrane and is situated behind the tubal elevation of the auditory tube. Also *pharyngeal recess, Rosenmüller's recess, Rosenmüller's fossa, Rosenmüller's cavity, lateral pharyngeal fossa, lateral recess of nasopharynx.* **r. phrenicomediastinalis** [NA] A recess at the junction of the diaphragmatic and the mediastinal pleurae along the line of attachment of the pericardium to the diaphragm. In this situation the phrenic nerve and its accompanying vessels form a ridge that projects into the pleural cavity. **r. pinealis** [NA] A diverticulum of the third ventricle into the stalk of the pineal body. Also *pineal recess, conarial recess, pineal ventricle.* **r. piriformis** [NA] An elongated space of the laryngopharynx situated on each side of the laryngeal orifice and bounded laterally by the thyrohyoid membrane and the lamina of the thyroid cartilage and medially by the aryepiglottic fold. Deep to the mucous membrane lining it are the branches of the internal laryngeal nerve. It is a site where foreign bodies may lodge and where abscesses may develop. Also *piriform recess, piriform fossa, piriform sinus, laryngopharyngeal recess.* **r. pleurales** [NA] Three recesses of the pleurae: recessus costodiaphragmaticus, recessus costomediastinalis, and recessus phrenicomediastinalis. Also *pleural recesses, pleural sinuses, sinus pleurae.* **r. posterior fossae interpeduncularis tarini** A diverticulum that invaginates into the pons. Also *posterior recess of interpeduncular fossa.* **r. retrocaecalis** [NA] A peritoneal fossa of variable depth lying between the cecum, and occasionally the ascending colon, anteriorly and the parietal peritoneum posteriorly and bounded on each side by the cecal folds. The orifice faces downwards and occasionally the vermiform appendix extends upwards into it for varying distances. Also *retrocecal recess, retrocecal fossa.* **r. retroduodenalis** [NA] A large peritoneal fossa occasionally found behind the horizontal, or third, and the ascending, or fourth, parts of the duodenum and anterior to the abdominal aorta. Its orifice faces to the left and downwards. Also *retroduodenal recess, retroduodenal fossa.* **r. sacciformis articulationis radioulnaris distalis** [NA] A pouch of synovial membrane projecting upward into the loose capsule of the distal radioulnar joint and lying in front of the lower portion of the interosseous membrane. Also *sacciform recess of distal radioulnar articulation.* **r. sphenoethmoidalis** [NA] A triangular fossa located above the superior concha in the lateral wall of the nasal cavity. Into its posterior part the sphenoidal sinus opens. Also *sphenoethmoidal recess.* **r. sphericus vestibuli** [NA] A small round depression on the anteroinferior part of the medial wall of the bony vestibule of the internal ear. It is situated anterior to the vestibular crest which separates it from the elliptical recess. It lodges the saccule and is perforated by the macula cribrosa media transmitting fibers of the vestibulocochlear nerve to the saccule. Also *spherical recess of vestibule.* **r. splenicus** [NA] The left portion of the omental bursa projecting towards the hilum of the spleen between the lienorenal and gastrosplenic ligaments. Also *splenic recess, lienal recess, splenic sac.* **r. subhepatici** [NA] Two peritoneal spaces below and behind the liver, the right subhepatic space being the hepatorenal recess, and the left one being the omental bursa. Also *subhepatic recesses.* **r. subphrenici** [NA] Two peritoneal spaces between the diaphragm and the liver, the right space involving the anterior, superior, and right lateral surfaces of the liver, to the right of the falciform ligament and in front of the upper layer of the coronary ligament of the liver, while the left space is to the left of the falciform ligament, in front of the triangular ligament, and above the anterior and superior surfaces of the left lobe of the liver, the anterosuperior surface of the stomach, and the diaphragmatic surface of the spleen. Also *subphrenic recesses, subphrenic spaces, suprahepatic spaces.* **r. subpopliteus** [NA] A saclike prolongation of the synovial membrane of the knee joint behind the lateral meniscus and deep to the tendon of the popliteus muscle. It may communicate distally with the superior tibiofibular joint. Also *subpopliteal recess, popliteal bursa.* **r. superior omentalis** [NA] The upper part of the omental bursa, lying above foramen bursae omenti majoris and behind the lesser omentum and the liver. Also *superior omental recess, superior fossa of omental sac.* **r. suprapinealis** [NA] A diverticulum of the epithelial roof of the third ventricle anterosuperior to the pineal recess. Also *suprapineal recess.* **r. tubotympanicus** [NA] A recess of the first pharyngeal pouch, and occasionally with a contribution from the second pouch, situated between the first and third branchial arches of the embryo which develops into the auditory tube, tympanic cavity, and mastoid antrum. The recess is at first inferolateral to the cartilaginous otic capsule but later shifts anterolaterally. Also *tubotympanic recess.*

**recidivation** \risid′ivā′shən\ [L *recidiv(us)* (from *recidere* to fall back, recur) recurring + -ATION] The recurrence of a diseased state or the relapse of a patient recovering from a disease.

**recidivist** \risid′ivist\ [L *recidiv(us)* recurring + -IST] A patient who repeatedly returns to a hospital seeking treatment for the same disease.

**reciprocation** \risip′rəkā′shən\ [L *reciprocatio* (from *reciprocare* to move back and forth, from *re(ci)-* back + *pro(c)-* forward) movement back and forth, alternation] The interaction between two parts of the framework of a removable partial denture, each acting as a counter to the effect created by the other. An example is the two opposing arms of a clasp, but reciprocation in a denture cannot be achieved unless there is an arrangement on opposite sides of the dental arch. **active r.** Reciprocation by means of another clasp arm on the same tooth. **passive r.** Reciprocation by means of a nonflexible part of a denture.

**reciprocity** \res′əpräs′itē\ [L *reciproc(us)* (from *re(ci)-* back + *pro(c)-* forth) reciprocal + -ITY] **1** A reciprocal arrangement in personal licensure whereby one jurisdiction accepts another jurisdiction's prior issuance of a license to practice medicine, and the individual is not required to demonstrate again through examination or otherwise that he or she meets minimum levels of competence required for a license. **2** An arrangement between governments whereby their nationals are entitled to certain stated medical care or other benefits on a reciprocal basis.

**Recklinghausen** [Friedrich Daniel von *Recklinghausen*, German pathologist, 1833–1910] **1** Recklinghausen's disease, von Recklinghausen's disease. See under NEUROFIBROMATOSIS. **2** Recklinghausen's disease of bone, Engel-Recklinghausen disease of bone. See under OSTEITIS FIBROSA CYSTICA. **3** Recklinghausen-Appelbaum disease. See under HEMOCHROMATOSIS.

**recognition** / **cell r.** **1** A cell's ability to recognize other similar cells. **2** The recognition of target cells by hormones and other external mediators of cell function. **immunologic r.** The process by which immunocompetent cells respond to specific antigen and undergo functional changes, including the combination of the antigen with a cell-surface receptor and activation of cellular function. **multiple codon r.** The recognition of more than one codon of messenger RNA by a single type of transfer RNA. See also WOBBLE HYPOTHESIS. **pattern r.** The detection of meaningful similarity among differently formed visual stimuli, as in identifying a given letter of the alphabet although it appears in differing typefaces or handwriting styles.

**recoil** / **passive r.** The expiratory force created during inspiration due to elastic recoil of the inflated lung.

**recombinant** \rikäm′binənt\ Designating an organism, chromosome, genetic locus, or DNA that has been produced by combining genetic material from two different sources.

**recombination** \rē'kämbinā'shən\ **1** Any process occurring during reproduction that results in an offspring with a combination of two or more genes that is distinct from the arrangement of those genes in either parent. **2** The exchange of chromosome segments between homologous chromosomes during pachytene of meiotic division I, the cytologic expression of which is crossing over. **3** CROSSING OVER. **4** In nuclear physics, the return of an ionized atom or molecule to the neutral state. **bacterial r.** **1** Any gene transfer between bacteria. **2** Molecular recombination between homologous DNA sequences in a bacterium. **intrachromosomal r.** SISTER CHROMATID EXCHANGE. **mitotic r.** SISTER CHROMATID EXCHANGE. **molecular r.** The process by which segments of DNA can be recombined *in vitro* through pairing of overlapping terminal strands, followed by covalent closure by a ligase. For multiplication of such hybrid blocks of DNA (cloning) one of the segments is the opened circle of a virus or a plasmid. The closed circle can then be replicated in a suitable host cell.

**recompression** \rē'kəmpresh'ən\ A method of treatment applied to sufferers of acute decompression sickness. Where this is suspected, the patient is taken to the nearest hyperbaric chamber.

**reconditioning** \rē'kəndish'əning\ A type of psychotherapy in which the focal point is unlearning the conditioned inhibitory reflexes that have produced faulty adaptation and replacing them, through training and practice, with adaptive excitatory reflexes.

**reconstruction** RECONSTRUCTIVE SURGERY. **Bucknall's r. of urethra** A two-stage method using matching, unmobilized strips of skin from the ventral shaft of the penis and the anterior midline of the scrotum to reconstruct the penile urethra.

**reconstructor / dynamic spatial r.** A computed-tomography scanner that simultaneously forms images of multiple slices of the body. Since it stores data on a volume, not just a slice, it can reconstruct a new slice at any angle or display a complete isolated organ. Abbr. DSR

**recontour** \rikän'toor\ To surgically impart new shape to an anatomic structure or to the body surface.

**record** [Old French (from L *recordari* to recall, bring to mind, from *cor*, gen. *cordis* the heart, mind) recollection] **1** A reviewable collection of related data. It may contain alphanumeric data, charts, radiographs, etc., as in a medical record, or it may be in a form suitable for computer storage, as a punched card. **2** To enter data into such a collection. **3** A registration of jaw relations in a plastic material. **dental identification r.** A standardized chart which records different features of the dentition of an unidentified, burned, or mutilated dead body. These features are then compared to antemortem dental records to confirm or exclude an identity. The mandible and maxilla are removed at autopsy, and detailed notations are made regarding the presence of missing, unerupted, or extracted teeth, restorations or prostheses, caries, broken teeth, malpositioned or malrotated teeth, and oddly shaped teeth. X rays are made to reveal previous root canal therapy and to delineate the pattern of bone trabeculae. In the United States, each tooth or space is individually numbered with the upper right third molar assigned number one. The count proceeds right to left with the left third molar assigned sixteen. The counting direction of the lower jaw is reversed. **face-bow r.** The registration of the hinge axis position for the purpose of reproducing it on an articulator. **interocclusal r.** A maxillomandibular record made by placing wax or setting material between bite rims or occlusal surfaces. **medical r.** A systematic record of the history of the health of a patient kept by a physician or other health practitioner. It contains clinical notes of illnesses and injuries and treatment received, the results of laboratory tests, a record of surgical procedures, notation of subjective symptoms and complaints reported by the patient, psychological sequelae to physical conditions, and other relevant medical data. **patient r.** The assemblage of documents relating to the care of a particular patient, which may, in certain countries, be subject to specific legal requirements. **protrusive r.** A maxillomandibular record in the protrusive position. **unit r.** A medical or administrative collection of information in which all items pertaining to one individual or family are held together.

**recorder** An instrument that makes a permanent record, usually graphic, of varying signals. **pulse volume r.** A recorder, using the plethysmography principle, that quantifies limb arterial pressures and blood flows. **strip-chart r.** An instrument that produces a hard-copy graphical record of one or more variables as a function of time. Moving galvanometers deflect a pen, ink-jet, heated stylus, or light beam to write the record.

**recording / depth r.** A recording of the electrical activity in the brain obtained by implanting electrodes in the deeper parts of the cerebral substance. Also *electrocorticogram* (incorrect).

**recovery** A restoration of health and strength after illness. **spontaneous r.** A phenomenon observed in classical conditioning: a conditioned response, following experimental extinction, can be observed to reappear after a period of rest. The recovery is only partial, however, and the response will be quickly extinguished again if reinforcement is not forthcoming.

**recrement** \rek'rəmənt\ [L *recrement(um)* (from *re-* again + *cre(tus)*, past part. of *cernere* to sift, separate + *-mentum* -MENT) a resifting] A secretion that is reabsorbed by the body.

**recrudescence** \rē'kroodes'əns\ [L *recrudesc(ere)* (from *re-* RE- + *crud(us)* fresh, raw) to break out afresh, be renewed + English *-ence*] The reappearance in a relatively short time of pathologic signs or symptoms that had undergone remission or disappearance.

**recrudescent** \rē'kroodes'ənt\ [See RECRUDESCENCE.] Reappearing in a relatively short time: said of pathologic signs or symptoms that have undergone remission or disappearance.

**recruitment** \rikroot'mənt\ [French *recrutement* (from *recroître* to have a new growth, from RE- + L *crescere* to come into existence, grow + *-ment* -MENT) a recruiting, a new growth] **1** In electroencephalography, any rhythmic response to repeated sensory stimulation. The most typical example is following of the alpha rhythm during photic stimulation. In those individuals in whom this phenomenon can be recorded from the frontopolar regions, it is due to ocular movements (Gastaut's oculoclonic recruitment response). **2** The addition of new individuals to a population, such as through births or immigration. The type of recruitment, such as mature female immigrants, is to be specified. **3** The incorporation of additional neurons into a stimulatory response as the result of temporal or spatial summation or through an increase in the stimulus intensity. **loudness r.** An abnormal increase of loudness over a reduced dynamic range of hearing causing the individual with a hearing loss to hear high-intensity sounds at a normal loudness level. It is a condition usually associated with cochlear pathology.

**rect.** *rectificatus* (L, rectified).

**rect-** \rekt-\ RECTO-.

**rectal** \rek'təl\ Pertaining to the rectum.

**rectectomy** \rektek′təmē\ [RECT- + -ECTOMY] The surgical removal of all or part of the rectum, often with some surrounding tissues. Also *proctectomy.*
**rectification** \rek′tifikā′shən\ In genetics, the correction of mutation by any mechanism. **full-wave r.** The transformation of alternating current to direct current by reversing the direction of flow of alternate half-cycles. **half-wave r.** The transformation of alternating electric current to direct current by elimination of alternate half-cycles. **spontaneous r.** The spontaneous conversion of a transverse lie of a fetus to a longitudinal lie prior to labor.
**rectifier** \rek′tifī′ər\ An electronic device for converting alternating current into direct current by permitting substantial current flow in one direction only.
**rectitis** \rektī′tis\ [RECT- + -ITIS] *Seldom used* PROCTITIS.
**recto-** \rek′tō-, rek′tə-\ [See RECTUM.] A combining form meaning rectum, rectal. Also *rect-.*
**rectoanal** \-ā′nəl\ ANORECTAL.
**rectocele** \rek′təsēl\ [RECTO- + -CELE[1]] Rectal prolapse into the vagina. Also *rectovaginal hernia.*
**rectoclysis** \rektäk′lisis\ PROCTOCLYSIS.
**rectococcypexy** \-käk′sipek′sē\ [RECTO- + *coccy(x)* + -PEXY] A surgical procedure in which the rectum is fixed to the anterior coccyx to treat rectal redundancy or rectal prolapse. Also *proctococcypexy.*
**rectocystotomy** \-sistät′əmē\ [RECTO- + CYSTOTOMY] An incision made into the bladder from within the rectum. Also *proctocystotomy.*
**rectolabial** \-lā′bē·əl\ Relating to or connecting the rectum and the labia.
**rectoperineorrhaphy** \-per′inē·ôr′əfē\ PROCTOPERINEOPLASTY.
**rectopexy** \rek′təpek′sē\ [RECTO- + -PEXY] PROCTOPEXY.
**rectoplasty** \rek′təplas′tē\ [RECTO- + -PLASTY] PROCTOPLASTY.
**rectoromanoscope** \rek′tərōman′əskōp\ [RECTO- + ROMANOSCOPE] PROCTOSIGMOIDOSCOPE.
**rectoromanoscopy** \rek′tərōmənäs′kəpē\ PROCTOSIGMOIDOSCOPY.
**rectorrhaphy** \rektôr′əfē\ [RECTO- + -RRHAPHY] The surgical repair and reconstruction of the rectum. It is usually performed for a rectal laceration from whatever cause. Also *proctorrhaphy.*
**rectoscope** \rek′təskōp\ [RECTO- + -SCOPE] PROCTOSCOPE.
**rectoscopy** \rektäs′kəpē\ [RECTO- + -SCOPY] Visual examination of the rectum; proctoscopy.
**rectosigmoid** \-sig′moid\ **1** Pertaining to the rectum and the sigmoid colon. **2** The rectum and sigmoid colon combined, or the region of their junction. Also *proctosigmoid.*
**rectosigmoidectomy** \-sig′moidek′təmē\ The surgical excision of the rectum and sigmoid colon along with the creation of an end colostomy. Also *proctosigmoidectomy.*
**rectosigmoiditis** \-sig′moidī′tis\ PROCTOSIGMOIDITIS.
**rectosigmoidoscopy** \-sig′moidäs′kəpē\ PROCTOSIGMOIDOSCOPY.
**rectostenosis** \-stenō′sis\ RECTAL STRICTURE.
**rectostomy** \rektäs′təmē\ [RECTO- + -STOMY] A surgical procedure in which an opening is made in the rectum to allow diversion of the fecal stream. Also *proctostomy.*
**rectotomy** \rektät′əmē\ PROCTOTOMY.
**rectovestibular** \-vestib′yələr\ Relating to or connecting the rectum and the vestibule of the vagina.
**rectovulvar** \-vul′vər\ Relating to or connecting the rectum and the vulva.
**rectum** \rek′təm\ [L, neut. sing. of *rectus* straight; short for *intestinum rectum* the straight intestine] [NA] The lower portion of the digestive tube, continuous above with the sigmoid colon at the level of the third sacral vertebra and curving downwards and forwards in the concavity of the sacrum and coccyx on to the pelvic diaphragm, which it pierces to become the anal canal in front of the tip of the coccyx.
**rectus** \rek′təs\ [L, right, straight, direct] Straight: used primarily in reference to a muscle, such as rectus femoris or rectus abdominis muscles. **r. accessorius** A rare variant of the rectus femoris muscle where a fasciculus arises from the acetabular margin and inserts into the anterior edge of the vastus lateralis muscle, being innervated by the nerve to rectus femoris.
**recumbent** \rikum′bənt\ [L *recumbens*, gen. *recumbentis*, pres. part. of *recumbere* to lie down again, recline] Lying down; reclining.
**recuperate** \rik^y^oo′pərāt\ [L *recuperat(us)*, past part. of *recuperare* (akin to *recipere* to retake, recover, from *re-* RE- + *capere* to hold, take) to regain] To recover health after illness or loss of function.
**recuperation** \rik^y^oo′pərā′shən\ The process of recuperating; convalescence.
**recuperative** \rik^y^oo′pərā′tiv\ Having to do with or tending to assist recuperation.
**recurrence** \rikur′əns\ A return or reappearance, as of a symptom.
**recurrent** \rikur′ənt\ **1** Occurring or tending to occur again. **2** Turning back on itself; running in the opposite direction, as certain nerves and vessels.
**recurvation** \rē′kərvā′shən\ A backward bending or flexure.
**recurvatum** \rē′kərvā′təm\ Bent or flexed backward.
**red** [Old English *rēad*, akin to L *ruber* red, *rufus* red, and Gk *erythros* red] **1** The color of the visible spectrum with the longest wavelength. **2** A substance, usually a stain or dye, that is red in appearance, or that produces a cytochemical reaction resulting in red staining. • For chemical names including *red,* see under the chemical name. **bordeaux r.** CERASINE. **carmine r.** CARMINE. **Congo r.** $C_{32}H_{22}N_6O_6Na_2$. An acid dye sometimes used as pH indicator, changing from blue to red at the pH range 3.0 to 5.0. It is often used as a tissue stain to demonstrate the presence of amyloid. Also *rubrum Congo.* **fast r. B** CERASINE. **neutral r.** A nontoxic dye used as a vital stain for protozoa and blood. It also has indicator properties which are utilized in bacteriological media for differentiating between different strains of bacteria. **oil r. O** $C_{22}H_{16}N_4O$. A synthetic, weakly acid, red azo dye that is widely used as a stain for neutral fat. Also *Sudan III, Sudan G.* **scarlet r.** *Ambiguous* SUDAN IV. **Sudan r.** A synthetic azo dye used for staining neutral fats, to which it gives a brilliant red color in frozen sections.
**red-** \red-, rəd-\ RE-.
**redia** \rē′dē·ə\ [after Francesco *Redi*, Italian physician and naturalist, 1626–1697] (*pl.* rediae) The larva of a trematode within its mollusk intermediate host that follows the initial sporocyst stage. It is an elongate, saclike organism with a mouth and sacciform gut. Its progeny, budded off from the inner wall of the larva, develop into daughter rediae, which leave the parent larva via a birth pore. Each daughter develops either into another redia or else directly into a cercaria, which leaves the mollusk intermediate host.
**rediae** \rē′di·ē\ Plural of REDIA.
**redifferentiation** \rē′difəren′shē·ā′shən\ The return to a fully differentiated state of a dedifferentiated tissue. This

transition allows a tissue to undertake its previous role and perform specific functions once more after a period of quiescence or nonspecific activity.

**redig. in pulv.** *redigatur in pulverem* (L, let it be reduced to a powder: used in prescription writing).

**red. in pulv.** *reductus in pulverem* (L, reduced to a powder: used in prescription writing).

**redintegration** \redin′təgrā′shən\ [L *redintegratio* (from RED- + *integratio* restoration, making whole; see INTEGRATION) renewal, revival] The evocation of a response by the application of a stimulus of much lower intensity than that which originally evoked it.

**redislocation** \rē′dislōkā′shən\ A dislocation which recurs after reduction or replacement.

**Redlich** [Emil *Redlich*, Austrian neurologist, 1866–1930] Obersteiner-Redlich line. See under OBERSTEINER-REDLICH SPACE.

**redox** \red′äks\ [*red(uction)* + *ox(idation)*] Concerned with oxidations and reductions. See also OXIDATION-REDUCTION POTENTIAL.

**reduce** 1 To combine a substance with hydrogen or to cause it to react in a way considered analogous, as by adding electrons to it. 2 To reposition so as to restore to a normal place or alignment, as a fracture; to subject to reduction.

**reductant** \riduk′tənt\ A reactant in a reaction in which it is oxidized and another substance is reduced.

**reductase** \riduk′tās\ Any enzyme that catalyzes a reaction of oxidation and reduction. The term is added to the name of the substance reduced, as in *dihydrofolate reductase.*

**reduction** [L *reductio* (from *reducere* to bring back, retract, remove, from RE- + *ducere* to tug, draw, lead) a leading back, bringing back, restoring] 1 Restoration to the normal place or position, as in the setting of a fractured bone or the surgical correction of a hernia. 2 The gain of electrons by an atom or molecule. **r. of chromosomes** The decrease in chromosome number occurring during any cell division in either or both daughter cells compared with the parental cell. It ordinarily occurs during the first meiotic division but may occur during mitosis in somatic cells. **closed r.** Realignment of bone fragments using external force without a skin incision or a need for internal manipulation. **delayed r.** Realignment of a fractured bone at a time remote from the initial injury. It may be performed days or weeks after the injury. **r. en bloc** Displacement of an unreduced hernia sac, most commonly following manipulation, resulting in disappearance of hernial swelling. Also *reduction en masse.* **hydrostatic r.** The use of fluid to reduce an intussusception. This is most commonly performed using barium given as an enema. **immediate r.** Realignment of the bone fragments close to the time of injury. **meiotic r. of chromosomes** The normal halving of the number of chromosomes in the mature gamete during the second meiotic division, from the diploid to the haploid complement. **mitotic r.** SOMATIC REDUCTION OF CHROMOSOMES. **open r.** Operative manipulation of a fracture requiring a surgical incision and direct fixation of the fragments to regain alignment. **somatic r. of chromosomes** An abnormal decrease in the number of chromosomes in one or both daughter cells during mitosis. It may occur as a spontaneous aberration or be induced experimentally. Also *mitotic reduction.* **weight r.** The loss of body weight, especially if brought about by following a particular regimen. The ideal weight reduction regimen incorporates diet, exercise, and behavior modification.

**redundancy** \ridun′dənsē\ [L *redundantia* (from *redundare* to flow back, overflow, from RED- + *unda* water, a wave, waves) an overflow, redundancy] 1 The existence of more than one system for accomplishing a task so that if all systems but one fail the remaining system ensures reliability. 2 Any condition characterized by excess or repetition beyond what is required. **gene r.** The presence of multiple copies of a gene in a genome, regardless of arrangement. Examples, in most eukaryotes, are the genes for ribosomal RNA and for histones.

**redundant** \ridun′dənt\ Exhibiting redundancy.

**reduplicated** \rid$^y$oo′plikā′tid\ Occurring twice in rapid succession rather than once, as a heart sound.

**reduplication** \rid$^y$oo′plikā′shən\ [RE- + DUPLICATION] Rapid recurrence of an event, such as a heart sound, which is then heard as two sounds rather than one.

**reduviid** \rēd$^y$oo′vē·id\ 1 Of or belonging to the family Reduviidae. 2 A member of the family Reduviidae.

**Reduviidae** \rē′d$^y$oovī′idē\ [*Reduvi(us),* name of the type genus, + -IDAE] A family of hemipterous insects (suborder Heteroptera), popularly known as kissing bugs, cone-nose bugs, or assassin bugs. Cone-nose bugs (subfamily Triatominae) are vectors of *Trypanosoma cruzi,* agent of Chagas disease. The family includes the genera *Eratyrus, Eutriatoma, Panstrongylus, Reduvius, Rhodnius,* and *Triatoma.*

***Reduvius personatus*** \rədoo′vē·əs pur′sənā′təs\ A European species, known as the masked hunter, or big bedbug, which has been introduced into the United States where it is now widespread. Its bite can cause allergic symptoms, including generalized urticaria and nausea.

**Reed** [Dorothy Mendenhall *Reed,* U.S. pathologist, 1874–1964] 1 Dorothy Reed cells, Reed-Sternberg cells. See under STERNBERG-REED CELLS. 2 Reed-Hodgkin disease. See under HODGKIN'S DISEASE.

**Reed** [Lowell Jacob *Reed,* U.S. statistician, 1886–1966] Reed and Muench method. See under METHOD.

**reef** [Middle English *riff,* from or akin to Old Norse *rif* rib] A folding or imbrication in tissue resulting from a surgical procedure.

**reefing** \rē′fing\ **stomach r.** GASTROPLICATION.

**Reenstierna** [John Libert *Reenstierna,* Swedish dermatologist, born 1882] Ito-Reenstierna reaction. See under ITO-REENSTIERNA TEST.

**reentrant** \rē·en′trənt\ Of or relating to reentry.

**reentry** \rē·en′trē\ Reactivation of a zone of cardiac muscle by a single impulse. This may occur when there is a long circuit through aberrant pathways, as in the Wolff-Parkinson-White syndrome, or when there are adjacent areas with different refractory periods, as may occur in myocardial ischemia. Reentry may lead to single or repetitive ectopic beats, or tachycardia. See also REENTRANT MECHANISM.

**reepithelialization** \rē·ep′ithē′lē·əlīzā′shən\ The stage of wound healing at which epithelial integrity is restored to the injured part by ingrowth of epithelium from the periphery of the wound or by outgrowth from surviving accessory skin structures such as hair follicles and sweat glands.

**Rees** [H. Maynard *Rees,* U.S. physician, flourished early 20th century] Rees-Ecker diluting fluid. See under REES-ECKER SOLUTION.

**reexcitation** \rē·ek′sītā′shən\ The reentry of a wave of excitation into a tissue following its recovery from a refractory state.

**reexpand** \rē′ikspand′\ To expand after having been collapsed, as a lung.

**refection** \rifek′shən\ Recovery from fatigue or hunger.

**reference** [L *refer(re)* to return, bring back again, report + -ENCE] A standard against which techniques, measurements, or other observations can be compared, or upon which inferences or calculations can be based.

**referral** \rifur′əl\ The practice of sending a patient to another health care provider, usually for specialized care, or to another organization or service agency, often for social services.

**referred** Experienced in a part of the body distant from its point of origin, as *referred pain.*

**reflect** [L *reflectere* (from *re-* back + *flectere* to bend) to bend back, turn back] **1** To bend back or turn aside, as to expose underlying structures in a surgical procedure. **2** To turn back, as light rays from a surface.

**reflection** [REFLECT + -ION] **1** A change in the direction of light rays caused by their striking a surface and returning from the surface. **2** An image perceived as it returns from a reflecting surface. **3** A turning or folding back; a fold. **4** The act or procedure of reflecting; the surgical technique of bending back or turning aside to expose underlying structures. For defs. 1–4 also *reflexion* (British spelling). **specular r.** **1** A reflection from a surface which is smooth compared to the wavelength. **2** A technique of studying surface detail by observation of the reflection of incident light from the surface.

**reflector** Any surface capable of producing a reflection. **specular r.** A reflector whose surface is smooth compared to the wavelength.

# reflex

**reflex** [L *reflexus* (from *reflectere* to bend back; see REFLECT) a turn, turning point] **1** An involuntary or stereotyped movement induced by a peripheral stimulus. **2** Any response mediated by two or more neurons, including an afferent and an efferent path. See illustration at REFLEX ARC. **3** The reflection of light from a curved smooth surface, such as the cornea, fovea centralis, or retinal arterioles. **abdominal r.** Regional contraction of the abdominal muscles in response to stroking or scratching the skin (superficial abdominal reflex) or tapping the costal margin (deep abdominal reflex). **abdominal cutaneous r.** SUPERFICIAL ABDOMINAL REFLEX. **Abrams heart r.** Contraction of the heart muscle and reduction in the cardiac outline as detected by percussion or fluoroscopy following stimulation of skin in the precordial region. Also *heart reflex.* **acceleratory r.** STATOKINETIC REFLEX. **accommodation r.** The automatic change in dioptric strength of the crystalline lens for near vision in order to maintain a clearly focused retinal image, consisting of the triad of accommodation, convergence, and pupilloconstriction. Also *near reflex, near-point reaction.* **Achilles r.** ACHILLES TENDON REFLEX. **Achilles tendon r.** Contraction of the calf muscles, especially the soleus with plantiflexion of the foot, when the Achilles tendon is struck sharply. The response is due to excitation of the muscle spindles. Also *Achilles reflex, triceps surae reflex, triceps surae jerk, ankle jerk, ankle reflex, Achilles jerk.* **acoustic r.** The reflex contraction of the intratympanic muscles on exposure to high-intensity sound, mediated at midbrain level. Also *acoustic stapedial reflex, stapedius reflex.* **acousticopalpebral r.** COCHLEOPALPEBRAL REFLEX. **acousticospinal r.** A behavioral motor response or change in sensitivity of a segmental motor reflex pathway following presentation of a sudden sound stimulus. **acoustic stapedial r.** ACOUSTIC REFLEX. **acquired r.** **1** CONDITIONED REFLEX. **2** Any reflex pattern developed as a result of experience. **acromial r.** Contraction of the biceps with flexion and supination of the forearm upon striking the acromion, or coracoid process, of the scapula, thereby phasically stretching the muscle. **adductor r. of foot** Contraction of the tibialis posterior with adduction, inversion, and plantar flexion of the foot induced by stroking the inner aspect of the sole from the base of the big toe to the heel. Also *Hirschberg's reflex, Hirschberg sign.* **adductor r. of thigh** Adduction of the initially abducted thigh upon tapping the tendon of the adductor magnus near its insertion onto the adductor tubercle. **allied r.'es** Two or more reflexes, elicited by stimuli at distinctly separate sites on or in the body, that nevertheless mutually reinforce the response by acting through the same final common pathway or on synergistic muscles. **anal r.** Contraction of the internal anal sphincter upon irritation of the overlying mucosa, as by insertion of the examining finger. Also *perianal reflex.* **ankle r.** ACHILLES TENDON REFLEX. **antagonistic r.'es** Two reflexes whose influence on a body part are of opposite effect, e.g., leading to flexion and to extension of a joint. **anticus r.** PIOTROWSKI SIGN. **antigravity r.** Any reflex that aids extensor muscles acting to support the body or its parts against the force of gravity. **aortic r.** CARDIAC DEPRESSOR REFLEX. **aponeurotic r.** SOLE-TAP REFLEX. **Aschner's r.** OCULOCARDIAC REFLEX. **attention r. of pupil** Decrease or increase in size of the pupil when the attention is drawn to a near or distant object, respectively. Also *Piltz reflex, Piltz sign.* **attitudinal r.** Any of the tonic reflexes that tend to maintain or restore the body in its normal orientation in space. The principal sensory receptors mediating these are the maculae of the utricle and saccule. Also *static attitudinal reflex, statotonic reflex.* **auditory r.** **1** Any reflex response initiated by a sudden sound, direct mechanical stimulation of the auditory apparatus, or electrical stimulation of the eighth nerve. **2** COCHLEOPALPEBRAL REFLEX. **auditory-palpebral r.** COCHLEOPALPEBRAL REFLEX. **auricular r.** Contraction of the extrinsic muscles of the ear in response to high-intensity sound. Also *postauricular response.* **auriculopressor r.** **1** Vasoconstriction and a rise in systemic blood pressure reflexly caused by a fall in blood pressure in the great veins and right auricle. Also *Pavlov's reflex.* **2** Tachycardia due to a rise in volume or pressure in the right auricle. **axon r.** A response induced at the terminal of one branch of a nerve fiber by a propagated impulse that had been initiated in another branch and then traveled antidromically to the point of bifurcation. The ramifications of the axon within the spinal cord and their synaptic connections are not necessarily involved, so the response is not a true reflex. *Imprecise.* **Babinski r.** EXTENSOR PLANTAR RESPONSE. **Bainbridge r.** BAINBRIDGE EFFECT. **Balduzzi's r.** Bilateral or contralateral elicitation of an adductor response of the foot by tapping on the dorsal surface of the ankle. **baroreceptor r.'es** The reflex arcs in which vascular tone, heart rate, force of contractility, and other vascular responses are linked to intravascular pressures. **Barkman's r.** Local contraction of the ipsilateral rectus abdominis muscle in response to stimulation of the skin below the nipple. **basal joint r.** FINGER-THUMB REFLEX. **Bekhterev's r.** **1** MENDEL-BEKHTEREV REFLEX. **2** FEMOROABDOMINAL REFLEX. **3** PARADOXICAL PUPILLARY REFLEX. **4** NASAL REFLEX. **Bekhterev-Mendel r.** MENDEL-BEKHTEREV REFLEX. **Bekhterev's deep r.** A dorsal rebound (i.e., physiological flexion) of the toes and foot together with flexor movements at the knee and hip following sudden release of the toes and foot from forceful plantiflexion. It is seen in corticospinal disease. **bending r.** Flexion of the elbow in response to passive palmar flexion of the wrist. It is exaggerated with forebrain lesions. **Benedek's r.** Plantar flexion of the foot in response to a tap over the lower, subcutaneous surface of the fibula, the ankle being slightly dorsiflexed initially to place the flexor tendons under moderate stretch. **Bezold r.** A reflex arising from response in the left ventricle of the heart and transmitted by afferent vagal nerve fibers to the medulla oblongata where vagal efferent fibers are stimulated and lead to sinus bradycardia, hypotension, and peripheral vasodilatation. Also *Bezold-Jarisch reflex, Bezold-Jarisch effect.* **biceps r.** Contraction of the biceps brachii with further flexion of the partially bent elbow when the tendon in the antecubital fossa is tapped. Also *biceps jerk.* **Bing's r.** Plantar flexion of the foot in response to striking the ankle between the two malleoli while the foot is held in the neutral position. **bladder r.** 1 The tendency of the urinary bladder to contract and empty when moderately distended, a component of the micturition reflex. In the normal individual, the bladder reflex is subject to volitional inhibition and release. Also *bladder-emptying reflex, vesical reflex.* 2 MICTURITION REFLEX. **blink r.** EYELID CLOSURE REFLEX. **body-righting r.** A righting reflex in which the initiating stimulus is pressure upon touch and other mechanoreceptors on the side of the body in contact with the supporting surface. Effects directed specifically to orientation of the head (body-on-head) and body (body-on-body) are distinguishable. Also *static adaptation reflex.* **bowing r.** BRAIN'S QUADRUPEDAL REFLEX. **brachioradialis r.** Flexion and partial supination of the initially partially pronated forearm when the styloid process or lower end of the radius is struck, thus stretching the brachioradialis muscle. In hyperreflexia, the fingers may flex also, due to deep reflex responses of the digital flexors. Also *brachioradial reflex, periosteoradial reflex, radial reflex, supinator longus reflex, styloradial reflex, supinator jerk reflex, supinator reflex, supination reflex, radioperiosteal reflex, supinator jerk.* **Brain's quadrupedal r.** In a hemiplegic patient, extension of the flexed arm upon bending over as if to assume a quadrupedal posture. Also *quadrupedal extensor reflex, bowing reflex.* **bregmocardiac r.** In an infant, slowing of the heart rate when pressure is applied over the bregmatic fontanel. **Brissaud's r.** Contraction of the tensor fasciae latae when the sole of the foot is stroked. The response may be present even in the absence of movements of the toes. **Brudzinski's r.** BRUDZINSKI SIGN. **bulbocavernosus r.** *Outmoded* BULBOSPONGIOSUS REFLEX. **bulbomimic r.** Contraction of the facial muscles when the eyeball is pressed upon. In a comatose state following a stroke the movements are seen contralateral to the lesion, while in comas of metabolic or toxic origin the response is bilateral. Also *facial reflex, Mondonesi's reflex.* **bulbospongiosus r.** 1 A stretch reflex contraction of the bulbospongiosus muscle in response to a tap to the dorsum of the penis or over the perineal surface of the penis. Also *penis reflex, penile reflex, bulbocavernosus reflex* (outmoded). 2 HUGHES REFLEX. **Capps r.** Vasomotor collapse with pallor, sweating, syncope, and irregularity of pulse and respiration, brought on by irritation of the pleura, as in thoracentesis or at the crisis stage of pneumonia. Also *pleural shock, Capps sign.* **cardiac r.** A constriction of the area of percussable cardiac dullness in response to stimulation of skin in the precardiac region. **cardiac depressor r.** Peripheral vasodilation and cardiac inhibition with consequent fall in blood pressure induced by experimental stimulation of the cardiac depressor nerve or physiological stimulation of its sensory terminals in the arch of the aorta and base of the heart. Also *aortic reflex.* **carotid body r.** CAROTID SINUS REFLEX. **carotidosympathoatrial r.** Increased contractility of the cardiac atrium resulting from sympathetic stimulation due to a fall in pressure in the carotid sinus. **carotidovagoatrial r.** Increased contractility of the cardiac atrium resulting from vagal inhibition due to a fall in pressure in the carotid sinus. **carotidoventricular r.** Increased cardiac ventricular contractility resulting from sympathetic stimulation due to a fall in pressure in the carotid sinus. **carotid sinus r.** Slowing of the heart, vasodilatation, and a fall in blood pressure due to vagal stimulation, following increased arterial blood pressure within the carotid sinus at the carotid bifurcation, or pressure upon the carotid sinus. Rarely, asystole and syncope occur. Conversely, a fall in pressure in the carotid sinus may cause an increased heart rate, vasoconstriction, and a reflex rise in blood pressure mediated by the sympathetic system. Also *carotid body reflex.* **carpophalangeal r.** Flexion of the fingers when the dorsal aspect of the wrist is tapped. It is analogous to the Mendel-Bekhterev reflex in the lower extremity. Also *milk-ejection reflex.* **celiac plexus r.** 1 In the pregnant subject, a fall in blood pressure upon assuming the supine position, thought to be due to the enlarged uterus pressing upon the celiac plexus or associated structures. 2 A sudden drop in systemic blood pressure in response to manipulation of the upper abdominal viscera and their mesenteries. It is mediated by visceral afferents and autonomic efferents coursing in the celiac plexus. **cephalopalpebral r.** Closure of the eyelids in response to percussion on the top of the head. **cerebropupillary r.** HAAB'S REFLEX. **Chaddock's r.** CHADDOCK SIGN. **chin r.** 1 An abnormal response consisting of closure of the mouth when skin over the chin is stroked. 2 JAW JERK. **chin-jerk r.** JAW JERK. **Chodzko's r.** Contractions of shoulder and proximal arm muscles in response to percussion of the manubrium sterni. **ciliary r.** Constriction of the pupil that accompanies lens accommodation as the gaze is directed from a distant to a near object. **ciliospinal r.** Dilatation of the ipsilateral pupil induced by pinching or scratching the skin over the nape of the neck. Also *pupillary-skin reflex, cutaneous pupillary reflex* (incorrect). **clasping r.** A strong, tonic flexion of the forelimbs seen in some amphibia upon cutaneous stimulation over the ventral aspect of the thorax and abdomen. It is facilitated by male sex hormones, is activated when the male grasps the female during fertilization, and is still present in a decapitated preparation. **clasp-knife r.** An extreme form of the lengthening reaction characterized by a sudden relaxation of resistance in a tonically contracting muscle under forced lengthening. It is seen chiefly in extensor muscles of decerebrate or spastic animals, and is due to excitation of tendon organs with resulting inhibition of homonymous motoneurons. **cochleopalpebral r.** Contraction of palpebral portions of the orbicularis oculi muscle in response to a sudden noise. The response is impaired by damage to the vestibulocochlear, or eighth cranial nerve. Also *cochleo-orbicular reflex, auditory-palpebral reflex, Gault's cochleopalpebral reflex, cochlear reflex, auditory reflex, acousticopalpebral reflex.* **cochleopupillary r.** A bilateral slight contraction and subsequent more prominent dilatation of the pupils in response to a sudden loud noise. Also *cochleopapillary reflex.* **cochleostapedial r.** Contraction of the stapedius muscle in response to a loud sound. By damping excursions of the footplate of the stapedius, the response protects the inner ear from excessive oscillations. Its absence results in hyperacusis. Compare TYMPANIC REFLEX. **coital r.** In some animals, e.g., cat, rabbit, ovulation in response to pituitary release of luteinizing hormone reflexly initiated by copulatory or artificial stimulation of genital parts. An intermediate step is the release of luteinizing hormone releasing hormone. **coitus r.** In a spinal animal or man, penile erection, elevation of the testes, and crinkling of the scrotum upon stimulation of the penis, especially the glans. Contraction of the flexors and adductors of the thigh may also occur. **conditioned r.** A response to a sensory stimulus that initially has no effect but comes to do so through repeated association with a second stimulus that naturally elicits that response. Also *acquired reflex*. **conjunctival r.** Forceful closure of the eyelids due to irritation of the conjunctiva. **consensual light r.** Contraction of the opposite, nonilluminated pupil, in response to a light stimulus to its fellow eye. Also *consensual reaction, indirect-light reaction, indirect pupillary reaction, consensual light reaction*. **contralateral r.** 1 A reflex response appearing on the side of the body opposite to the primary, analogous response. 2 BRUDZINSKI SIGN. **convergence r.** Contraction of the pupils upon fixing the gaze on a near object. **coordinated r.** A reflex response marked by a patterned coactivation and inhibition of appropriate muscles, sometimes acting at several joints, to yield an overall useful movement. Also *phasic reflex*. **corneal r.** A forceful closure of the eyelids when the cornea is lightly touched. It is used to gauge the depth of anesthesia. **corneomandibular r.** An abnormal contraction of the pterygoid muscles on one side with deviation of the jaw, induced by irritation of the cornea on the opposite side. Also *corneopterygoid reflex*. **coronary r.** Any alteration in the muscular tone of the coronary arteries as a result of nervous control. It may be dilatory and sympathetic mediated, constrictive due to parasympathetic activity, or result from an arrest of tonic neurovascular tone. **corticopupillary r.** HAAB'S REFLEX. **costal arch r.** Contraction of the rectus abdominis muscle in response to tapping over its attachments along the costal margin. **costal periosteal r.** A contractile response of the upper abdominal muscles with movement of the umbilicus up and outward, induced by tapping the costal cartilages, lower sternum, or costal margin. **costopectoral r.** PECTORAL REFLEX. **cough r.** 1 A sequence of actions triggered by irritation of the larynx or the tracheobronchial tree. It involves closure of the larynx, a buildup of intrathoracic and abdominal pressure, and then sudden relaxation of the larynx with release of air pressure. It serves to clear the air passages. Also *laryngeal reflex*. 2 In a urogenital examination, tightening of the anal sphincter upon coughing voluntarily. **cremasteric r.** Ipsilateral contraction of the cremaster muscle with resulting elevation of the testis, induced by scratching or stroking subinguinal or inner surfaces of the thigh. Its presence demonstrates integrity of the $L_1$ roots and spinal centers, and the response is exaggerated in spastic states. **crossed r.** A response elicited on the side of the body contralateral to that on which the stimulus was applied. **crossed adductor r.** Contraction of the ipsilateral adductor muscles with adduction and medial rotation of the thigh when the plantar surface of the foot is percussed. **crossed extensor r.** Extension of one extremity in response to elicitation of a flexor reflex in the contralateral limb. In an infant, plantiflexion (i.e., in reflex terminology, extension) of the toes on the foot contralateral to that in which toe dorsiflexion is elicited. Also *crossed extension reflex*. **crossed flexor r.** Flexion of the opposite limb, particularly a forelimb, upon elicitation of a flexor reflex in the opposite limb. It is manifested in decapitated animals and preparations in which neck and labyrinthine reflexes are excluded. **crossed r. of the pelvis** Contraction of the adductors in response to tapping the contralateral anterior superior iliac spine. Also *crossed spino-adductor reflex*. **cuboidodigital r.** TARSOPHALANGIAL REFLEX. **cutaneous r.** 1 Any reflex elicitable by stimulation of the skin, whether to local stimulation (superficial reflex) or to stimulation of the skin in general, as in cutaneous vasoconstriction on exposure to cold. 2 Contraction of the arrectores pilorum muscles with resulting goose flesh (cutis anserina) in response to cutaneous tactile stimulation. **cutaneous pupillary r.** Dilatation of the ipsilateral pupil induced by scratching or pinching the side of the neck. Also *ciliospinal reflex* (incorrect). **dartos r.** Contraction of the sympathetically innervated smooth muscle of the scrotum (tunica dartos) with wrinkling of the skin induced by application of cold to the thigh or perineum. Also *scrotal reflex, dartos muscle reflex*. **darwinian r.** The propensity of a young infant to grasp a bar and hang suspended. **dazzle r.** Closure of the eyelids in response to a bright light. It is normal in an infant. Also *Peiper's reflex*. **deep r.** A muscle contraction induced by tapping the tendon of the muscle or bones to which it attaches. Stretch transmitted to muscle spindles in the belly of the muscle excites a phasic discharge that results in a reflex stretch response. **deep abdominal r.'es** Contractions of the abdominal muscles in response to stimulation of their proprioceptors, as by tapping the costal margin or iliac crest. **deep tendon r.** Reflex contraction of a skeletal muscle evoked by a single sharp blow upon its tendon of insertion. Such reflexes are monosynaptic. The biceps, radial, triceps, knee jerk, and ankle jerk reflexes are the examples usually elicited in clinical practice. **defecation r.** A set of coordinated reactions (contraction of the rectum, relaxation of the internal and external anal sphincters, and increase of intra-abdominal pressure) stimulated by the entry of feces into the rectum. Also *rectal reflex*. **defense r.** 1 Any protective reflex, such as flexor withdrawal of a limb, or closure of the eyelids against a bright light. 2 A reflex component of a generalized alarm reaction, such as pupillary dilatation, arching of the back, cardioacceleration, protrusion of claws, etc. **deglutition r.** SWALLOWING REFLEX. **delayed r.** A reflex in which there is an unusually long interval between the presentation of the stimulus and the onset of the response. **deltoid r.** Abduction of the upper arm in response to percussion of the outer aspect of the elbow. **depressor r.** Any reflex causing the depression of a motor activity (e.g., tonic vasoconstriction). **digital r.** HOFFMAN'S REFLEX. **disynaptic r.** A reflex pathway having a single interneuron interposed between the afferent and efferent limbs, e.g., tendon organ afferent influence over homonymous motoneurons through an inhibitory interneuron. **doll's eye r.** OCULOCEPHALIC REFLEX. **dorsal r.** ERECTOR SPINAE REFLEX. **dorsocuboidal r.** TARSOPHALANGIAL REFLEX. **dorsum pedis r.** MENDEL-BEKHTEREV REFLEX. **ejaculation r.** A suddenly initiated sequence of peristaltic contractions of the vas deferens, the seminal vesicles, the prostate, the internal sphincter of the bladder, and the perineal muscles that results in ejaculation of semen. The activity is triggered when accumulative sensory inflow from mechanoreceptors of the glans penis reaches threshold. Not strictly reflex in nature, the sequence involves some of the same mechanisms as ejaculation initiated by psychic stimuli. **elbow r.** TRICEPS REFLEX. **embrace r.** MORO'S REFLEX. **enterogastric r.** Inhibition of vagally mediated gastric mobility in response to entry of irritants into the duodenum. **epigastric r.** Contraction of the upper portions of the ipsilateral rectus abdominus when skin overlying the muscle and nearby costal area is scratched. Also *supraumbilical reflex.* **Erben's r.** Slowing of the heart rate upon forcefully bending the head and neck forward, due to vagal stimulation. Also *Erben sign, Erben's phenomenon.* **erector spinae r.** Contraction of portions of the erector spinae muscle in response to tactile stimulation of the overlying skin or areas along the muscle's lateral margin. Also *dorsal reflex, lumbar reflex.* **esophagosalivary r.** Continued salivation induced by irritation of the lower esophagus, as by a tumor. Also *Roger's reflex.* **extensor r.** Any contraction in an antigravity muscle and its synergists in response to an appropriate stimulus. **extensor thrust r.** Stroking the skin behind the plantar cushion or abrupt extension of a limb elicited in the spinal animal by pressing between the cushion and the toe pads. The reflex is usually of short duration (0.2 s) and presumably contributes to the stance phase of locomotion. Also *positive supporting reaction, spring reaction.* **external auditory meatus r.** Closure of the eyelids upon thermal or tactile stimulation of the tympanic membrane or the adjacent walls of the auditory meatus. Also *Kisch reflex, Kehrer's reflex.* **external hamstring r.** Contraction of the biceps femoris in response to a tap on its tendon at the knee. **external oblique r.** OBLIQUUS REFLEX. **eyeball compression r.** OCULOCARDIAC REFLEX. **eyeball-heart r.** OCULOCARDIAC REFLEX. **eyelid closure r.** A blinking of the eyelids in response to any of a number of stimuli, including touch of the surface of the eye or eyelids, bright light, or pain. Also *sensory blinking reflex, lid reflex, reflexio palpebrarum, blink reflex, wink reflex.* ● These terms are sometimes applied more specifically to either the corneal reflex or the opticopalpebral reflex. **facial r.** BULBOMIMIC REFLEX. **faucial r.** A gag response induced by irritation of the fauces. **femoral r.** Extension at the knee and plantiflexion of the foot and toes induced by scratching the skin over the upper anterior aspect of the thigh. In reflex terminology, the movements are extensor in pattern. Also *Remak's reflex.* **femoroabdominal r.** Contraction in the ipsilateral lower abdominal wall induced by stroking the upper inner aspect of the thigh. The cremasteric reflex can be considered to be one portion of the response. Also *hypogastric reflex, Bekhterev's reflex, obliquus reflex.* **finger flexor r.** Flexion of fingers and thumb in response to flicking the nail or tapping the finger pad, occurring as a stretch reflex of the finger flexor muscles involved, as distinguished from Hoffmann's reflex, which indicates hyperexcitability of this reflex pathway. **finger-thumb r.** Opposition of the thumb with flexion of the proximal joint and extension of the distal joint when the metacarpophalangeal joint of the index or third finger is firmly flexed. Also *basal joint reflex, Mayer's reflex.* **flexion r.** A withdrawal reflex to noxious stimulation producing a flexion synergy in the upper or lower extremities. It can be used to facilitate the training of common flexion patterns. **flexion r. of leg** KNEE FLEXION REFLEX. **flexor r.** Contraction of one or a group of closely related muscles having flexor action following application of a noxious stimulus to superficial (cutaneous) or deep (e.g., joint) sensory receptors or by direct electrical stimulation of pain-mediating fibers in a nerve. **flexor withdrawal r.** Flexor withdrawal at the hip and knee in response to any stimulus applied to a lower limb in a patient with spinal cord transection or with severe bilateral lesions of the pyramidal tract in the spinal cord. **flight r.** *Imprecise* FIGHT-OR-FLIGHT REACTION. **front-tap r.** FRONT-TAP SIGN. **fundus r.** A red glow filling the pupil of an eye being viewed with an ophthalmoscope. It is not a reflex, but is the appearance produced by vascularity of the retina. **fusion r.** The mechanism whereby the two images received by the retina are merged into a single perceived image. **gag r.** Retching and gagging in response to stimulation of the mucous membrane of the fauces by a foreign body. Also *glossary reflex.* **Galant's r.** Contraction of the ipsilateral lower abdominal muscles in response to striking the anterior superior iliac spine. Also *lower abdominal periosteal reflex.* **galvanic skin r.** PSYCHOGALVANIC RESPONSE. **Gamper's bowing r.** Flexion of the head and trunk of an infant when the hip joints and knees are slowly extended from positions of flexor hypertonia, the sacrum being held steady. It is seen in anencephalic, premature, and brain-damaged infants. **gastrocolic r.** Mass evacuation of colonic contents upon entry of food into the stomach. It may be preceded by a similar movement in the small intestine. **gastroileal r.** Augmentation of peristalsis in the ileum and relaxation of the ileocolic valve following entry of food into the stomach. Also *gastroiliac reflex.* **gastropancreatic r.** An increase in pancreatic exocrine secretion induced by distension of the stomach. **gastrosalivary r.** Augmentation of salivation that occurs upon introduction of food into the stomach. **Gault's cochleopalpebral r.** COCHLEOPALPEBRAL REFLEX. **Geigel's r.** In the female, contraction of abdominal muscle fascicles located just above the inguinal ligament when the inner, upper aspect of the thigh is stroked. The response is analogous to the cremasteric reflex in the male. Also *inguinal reflex.* **genital r.** Hyperactive erection, with or without ejaculation, resulting from minor stimuli to the genitalia, e.g., as a component of the mass reflex in a spinal patient. **Gifford's r.** WESTPHAL-PILTZ REFLEX. **Gifford-Galassi r.** WESTPHAL-PILTZ REFLEX. **glabellar tap r.** GLABELLAR TAP SIGN. **glossary r.** GAG REFLEX. **gluteal r.** Contraction of the ipsilateral gluteal muscles induced by stroking the skin of a buttock. **Gordon's r.** An extensor plantar response in pyramidal tract disease produced by squeezing the calf muscles. Also *Gordon's test, paradoxical flexor reflex, Gordon sign.* **Gower-Henry r.** The postulated release of vasopressin upon depletion of atrial volume. **grasp r.** A reflex present in neonates and normally persisting for the first 6 weeks. It consists of closure of the hand on stimulation of the palm by light stroking. This primitive reflex is elicited by stroking across the palmar base of the digits, when firm grasping of the object used to apply the stimulus occurs. The reflex may return in later life as the consequence of a contralateral frontal lobe lesion. Also *grasping reflex, forced grasping, prehensory reflex, gripping reflex.* **grasping r.** GRASP REFLEX. **great toe r.** EXTENSOR PLANTAR RESPONSE. **gripping r.** GRASP REFLEX. **Guillain-Barré r.** SOLE-TAP REFLEX. **gustolacrimal r.** Lacrimation upon taking food into the mouth, as sometimes occurs during regeneration of the facial nerve. It is usually associated with the gustatory-sudorific reflex. **H r.** *Imprecise* H WAVE. **Haab's r.** Constriction of a dark-adapted pupil when attention is directed to a bright object in the periphery of the visual field, convergence and accommodation being avoided. The response is to be distinguished from a light reflex. Also *visuocortical reflex, corticopupillary reflex, cerebropupillary reflex.* **hamstring r.** Contraction of muscles on the posterior aspect of the thigh in response to a tap on the hamstring tendons at the knee. See also EXTERNAL HAMSTRING REFLEX, INTERNAL HAMSTRING

REFLEX. **heart r.** ABRAMS HEART REFLEX. **Hering-Breuer r.** A mechanism for regulation of respiration wherein vagally conducted impulses from stretch receptors of the bronchi and lungs excited during inspiration arouse inhibition of the diaphragm and other respiratory muscles, and finally arrest inspiration. Also *lung reflex.* **Hirschberg's r.** ADDUCTOR REFLEX OF FOOT. **Hoffmann's r.** Flexion of the thumb on flicking towards the palm the terminal phalanx of the middle finger. This occurs in any state of reflex hyperexcitability, but if present on one side only may indicate pyramidal tract dysfunction on that side. Also *Hoffmann sign, finger jerk, Trömner sign, Trömner's reflex, digital reflex.* **Hughes r.** Brief contraction of the bulbospongiosus muscle and downward movement of the penis when the foreskin or glans penis is pulled upward. Also *virile reflex, bulbospongiosus reflex.* **hyperactive myotactic r.** The tonic contraction of muscles in response, by mechanoreceptors, to the stimulation of sudden stretching. Also *Liddell-Sherrington reflex.* **hypogastric r.** FEMOROABDOMINAL REFLEX. **hypothenar r.** Contraction of the palmaris brevis muscle with dimpling over the hypothenar eminence in response to stimulating the skin over the pisiform bone. **ileogastric r.** Arrest of gastric motility following distension of the ileum. **inborn r.** UNCONDITIONED REFLEX. **infraspinatus r.** Contraction of the infraspinatus muscle with resulting lateral rotation and extension of the arm induced by tapping along the tendon of the muscle beneath the spine of the scapula. **inguinal r.** GEIGEL'S REFLEX. **intercoronary r.** Postulated, neurally mediated changes in the lumen of one coronary artery due to events in the other coronary artery or the muscle it supplies. **internal hamstring r.** Contraction of muscles on the posteromedial aspect of the thigh in response to a tap over the tendons at the medial border of the popliteal fossa. Participation of the semitendinosus would indicate flexor reflex sensitivity, of the semimembranosus more likely extensor (at the hip) sensitivity, though both muscles lead to flexion at the knee. **interscapular r.** SCAPULAR REFLEX. **intersegmental r.** A reflex having its afferent limb at one segmental level and its efferent outflow over another. **intestinal r.** MYENTERIC REFLEX. **intestinointestinal r.** Inhibition of activity in one portion of the intestine when another part is distended or irritated. **inverted radial r.** Flexion of the fingers in place of the normal radial reflex (brachioradialis contraction) in response to tapping the radius. It indicates an affliction affecting the motor supply to the brachioradialis, together with impairment of supraspinal control over the finger flexors. **investigatory r.** ORIENTING REFLEX. **ischemic r.** A rise in blood pressure that develops during cerebral ischemia. **jaw r.** JAW JERK. **jaw jerk r.** JAW JERK. **Juster's r.** Finger extension rather than the usual flexion when the skin of the palm is stimulated. **Kehrer's r.** EXTERNAL AUDITORY MEATUS REFLEX. **Kisch r.** EXTERNAL AUDITORY MEATUS REFLEX. **knee flexion r.** Flexion of the leg induced by tapping the tendons of the semimembranosus and semitendinosus muscles. Also *flexion reflex of leg.* **knee-jerk r.** PATELLAR REFLEX. **Kocher's r.** TESTICULAR COMPRESSION REFLEX. **labial r.** NASOLABIAL REFLEX. **labyrinthine r.** Any of several reflexes initiated by excitation of static receptors in the semicircular canals, utricle, or saccule. Also *vestibular reflex.* See also STATOKINETIC REFLEX, LABYRINTHINE RIGHTING REFLEX. **labyrinthine righting r.** Changes in tone of the neck muscles leading to righting of the head, as a result of excitation of static receptors in the labyrinth. **Laehr-Henneberg hard palate r.** Lowering of the upper lip when the hard palate is scratched, a sign of pseudobulbar paralysis. **Landau r.** A normal, two-part phenomenon wherein an infant held aloft in the prone position arches its neck and hips upward and then in response to gentle pressure downward on the head reverses the posture to flexion of the head and neck. The responses are exaggerated in hypertonic conditions and diminished in the floppy infant. **laryngeal r.** COUGH REFLEX. **latent r.** A reflex pathway and potential response inherent in a normal subject but nevertheless not evident except under some pathological condition. **let-down r.** The release of milk from the breast alveoli into the ducts as a response to suckling. This reflex is primarily mediated by oxytocin. Also *milk-ejection reflex.* **lid r.** EYELID CLOSURE REFLEX. **Liddell-Sherrington r.** HYPERACTIVE MYOTACTIC REFLEX. **light r.** In otology, the bright triangle of light reflected from the tympanic membrane at examination by the usual techniques. When the membrane is normal, the reflex is seen to lie in the anteroinferior quadrant with its apex immediately in front of the umbo, but alterations in the inclination or curvature of the membrane, irregularities caused by scars etc., and anything that diminishes the reflecting qualities of the cuticular surface may vary its appearance. Also *cone of light.* **lip r.** **1** A pouting reaction of the lips in response to a tap over the orbicularis muscle. It is a myotatic reflex evident in the embryo, in sleeping infants, and in adults with corticobulbar dysfunction. Also *snout reflex, lip phenomenon.* **2** SUCKING REFLEX. **little-toe r.** Slow abduction of the little toe in response to stroking the outer aspect of the foot, seen in upper motor neuron disorders. Also *Puussepp's reflex.* **lordosis r.** In an animal in estrus assumption of a copulatory posture (i.e., hyperextension of the back, elevation of the hindquarters, and deviation of the tail) induced by touching the back and perineal areas. **Loven's r.** Vasodilatation in an organ upon stimulation of its nerve, associated with systemic vasoconstriction and elevation in blood pressure. **lower abdominal r.** SUPRAPUBIC REFLEX. **lower abdominal periosteal r.** GALANT'S REFLEX. **lumbar r.** ERECTOR SPINAE REFLEX. **lung r.** HERING-BREUER REFLEX. **Lust's r.** LUST SIGN. **Magnus and de Kleijn neck r.** Ipsilateral extension and contralateral flexion of the limbs on the side toward which the chin is pointed when the head is rotated. Proprioceptors of the neck initiate the response, which is best seen in decerebrate preparations. **mandibular r.** JAW JERK. **Marey's r.** A neurally mediated decrease in heart rate associated with an increase in blood pressure in the aorta and carotid sinus, and the converse. **Marinesco-Radovici r.** PALMOMENTAL REFLEX. **mark-time r.** In spinal preparations with brain lesions, an alternating flexion and extension of the limbs or the hind limbs alone, resembling movements in normal locomotion. **mass r.** Flexor withdrawal of the lower limbs accompanied by evacuation of the bladder and bowels and profuse sweating below the level of the lesion which may occur on stimulation of a lower limb in a subject with spinal cord transection. Also *Riddoch's mass reflex, Riddoch's phenomenon.* **Mayer's r.** FINGER-THUMB REFLEX. **McCarthy's r.** SUPRAORBITAL REFLEX. **McCormac's r.** PATELLOADDUCTOR REFLEX. **McDowall r.** An experimentally induced decline in systemic blood pressure following arrest of vagal sensory inflow from the atria of the heart. **medioplantar r.** An abnormal response consisting of plantiflexion and fanning out of the toes in response to a tap on the instep. **mediopubic r.** Bilateral contraction of the femoral adductors in response to tapping the body of the pubic bone. **menace r.** Blinking in response to the movement of a hand or object toward the face or eyes, as in a threatened blow. **Mendel-Bekhterev r.** An abnormal reversal of the tarsophalangeal reflex response in which the toes flex rather than extend. It is seen with corticospinal tract dysfunction. Also *Bekhterev-Mendel reflex, Mendel's reflex, Bekhterev's reflex, Mendel's dorsal reflex of foot, dorsum pedis reflex.* **Mendel's dorsal r. of foot** MENDEL-BEKHTEREV REFLEX. **metacarpohypothenar r.** An abnormal response consisting of flexion of the little finger when the dorsum of the hand is struck. **metacarpothenar r.** Flexion of the thumb upon tapping the dorsum of the hand, a sign of pyramidal tract pathology. **metatarsal r.** SOLE-TAP REFLEX. **micturition r.** Any or all of the component reflexes involved in emptying the urinary bladder in response to bladder or urethral distension or urethral flow. Included are contraction of the detrusor muscle, relaxation of the urethra, and relaxation of the external sphincter. Also *urinary reflex, bladder reflex, pyelovesical reflex, renoureteral reflex.* **middle-ear r.** A reflex response mediated through the muscles of the middle ear. The muscle may be the stapedius, as in the acoustic reflex, or the tensor tympani. **milk-ejection r.** LET-DOWN REFLEX. **Mondonesi's r.** BULBOMIMIC REFLEX. **monosynaptic r.** The spikelike discharge of motoneurons to a muscle in response to a volley of impulses in those muscle spindle afferents making direct synaptic contact. The sensory axons consist mostly of the primary afferents from spindles in homonymous and synergistic muscles, together with a lesser contribution from monosynaptically connected secondary spindle afferents. The response may be monitored as an all-or-none discharge from a single motoneuron or the summated activity of the responding motoneurons as seen in the ventral root and peripheral nerve, or the H-wave in the muscle electromyograph. The tendon jerk response is largely a manifestation of the reflex. Abbr. MSR **Morley's peritoneocutaneous r.** Referral of a pain sensation to a segmentally corresponding cutaneous area when the peritoneum is locally irritated. **Moro's r.** Flexing and grasping movements of the forelimbs exhibited by a normal infant upon being subjected to a sudden short drop, jarring of the table on which it lies, or a loud noise. Also *Moro's embrace reflex, embrace reflex.* Compare STARTLE RESPONSE. **myenteric r.** An intrinsic response of the intestine consisting of contraction above and relaxation below a stimulated point. Also *intestinal reflex.* **myopic r.** In retinoscopy of a nearsighted eye, the far point image of the eye is seen to move in the opposite direction from the movement of the retinoscopic light. **myostatic r.** STRETCH REFLEX. **myotatic r.** STRETCH REFLEX. **nasal r.** Contraction of facial muscles on the side of the face on which the mucosa of the nasal passages is tickled. Also *Bekhterev's reflex.* **nasofacial r.** Sneezing induced by irritation of the nasal mucosa. Also *sneezing reflex.* **nasolabial r.** In the normal infant, retraction of the head and extension of the limbs in response to gentle, upward-sweeping stimulation of the upper lip and tip of the nose. Also *labial reflex.* **nasomental r.** Abnormal contraction of the mentalis muscle with dimpling of skin over the chin following a tap to the side of the nose. **naso-ocular r.** Dilatation of the conjunctival vessels brought on by irritation of the nasal mucosa. **nasopulmonary r.** Apnea and bronchoconstriction produced reflexly by stimulating the nasal mucosa electrically or with irritating gases such as ether. **near r.** ACCOMMODATION REFLEX. **neck r.'es** Adjustments in the posture of the limbs and trunk when the head is turned, due to excitation of receptors in the muscles and joints of the neck. Also *neck-righting reflexes.* **nociceptive r.** Any reflex, especially flexor withdrawal of a limb, elicited by a painful stimulus. Also *pain reflex.* **nose-bridge-lid r.** SUPRAORBITAL REFLEX. **nose-eye r.** SUPRAORBITAL REFLEX. **obliquus r.** 1 Contraction of the lateral abdominal muscles in response to tapping on or near their bony attachments to the lower thoracic wall. Also *external oblique reflex, upper abdominal periosteal reflex, upper deep abdominal reflex.* 2 FEMOROABDOMINAL REFLEX. **ocular counter-rolling r.** Compensatory movement of the eyes in the reverse direction from that of the head when inclined onto the shoulder. The degree of counterrotation is augmented in certain instances of vertigo and reduced if the labyrinth is inactive. Also *ocular countertorsion reflex.* **ocular fixation r.** A reflexive fixation of the eyeballs induced by various phenomena, as by movement of an object within the visual field or in response to a sound. **ocular righting r.** A tonic labyrinthine reflex consisting of rotation of the eyeballs to partially compensate for tilting of the head to the opposite side. It is obvious in the vertical pupils of a cat, but can be detected in man as well. **oculoauditory r.** Closure of both eyes induced by a loud sound. **oculocardiac r.** Slowing of the heart rate induced by pressure on the eyeball. The maneuver is sometimes used to suppress paroxysmal tachycardia. Also *Aschner's phenomenon, Aschner's reflex, eyeball-heart reflex, eyeball compression reflex.* **oculocephalic r.** Conjugate deviation of the eyes in the newborn infant in the direction opposite to that of head movement when the eyelids are held open and the head is rotated rapidly from side to side or the neck is flexed. After each such movement the eyes return to the midposition even if the altered head position is maintained. This reflex is a valuable indication of brainstem function. Also *doll's head phenomenon, doll's eye reflex, oculocephalogyric reflex, doll's eye sign, Cantelli sign.* **oculogastric r.** Nausea and dyspepsia resulting from oculomotor instability. **oculopharyngeal r.** Closure of the eyelids and swallowing in response to stimulation of the conjunctiva, as following instillation of an irritating substance in the conjunctival sac. **oculopupillary r.** Successive dilatation and contraction of the pupil in response to irritation of the cornea or conjunctiva. Also *oculosensory reflex, trigeminus reflex.* **oculovagal r.** OCULOCARDIAC REFLEX. **oculovestibular r.** VESTIBULO-OCULAR REFLEX. **olecranon r.** Flexion of the elbow when the olecranon is struck. **Oppenheim's r.** OPPENHEIM SIGN. **optical righting r.** Adjustment of the neck and limbs leading to reorientation of the head, as a response to a visual impression of the environment. **opticopalpebral r.** Contraction of the orbicularis oculi with closing of the eyelids in response to sudden presentation of an object in the visual field. Also *opticofacial winking reflex, visual orbicularis reflex.* **orbicularis oculi r.** 1 SUPRAORBITAL REFLEX. 2 WESTPHAL-PILTZ REFLEX. **orbicularis oris r.** Contraction of the levators of the upper lip in response to percussion of the upper lip or the side of the nose. **orbiculopupillary r.** WESTPHAL-PILTZ REFLEX. **orienting r.** The complex of initial, involuntary responses to a novel stimulus, including reactions of ear muscles and eyes, orientation of the head, autonomic nervous system adjustments, etc., all contributing to alert the animal and direct attention to the source. Also *investigatory reflex.* **pain r.** NOCICEPTIVE REFLEX. **palatal r.** Elevation of the soft palate or swallowing initiated by tactile stimulation of the palate. Also *palatine reflex.* **palmar r.** A flexor response of the fingers to stimulation of the palm. **palmomental r.** Contraction of the mentalis muscle on one side of the chin in response to scratching the thenar eminence on the same side. This reflex is thought to be a sign of frontal lobe disease but is often present in apparently normal old people. Also *pollicomental reflex, Radovici sign, palmchin reflex.* **palpebral r.** A turning the eyes upward during forcible closure of the eyelids for protection due to reflex association of the superior rectus and orbicularis muscles. In facial paralysis, the attempt to close the eye results in the eye turning upward (Bell phenomenon ). Also *palpebral-oculogyric reflex.* **panting r.** In dogs and other canids, rapid and shallow breathing consequent to a rise in body temperature. Evaporation, much of it from the protruding tongue, serves to dissipate heat. **paradoxical r.** A response different from and often opposite to the normal reflex pattern. **paradoxical ankle r.** Plantiflexion of the foot when the dorsum of the ankle is tapped. A stretch stimulus relayed to muscles in the vicinity would be expected to lead to dorsiflexion. **paradoxical extensor r.** EXTENSOR PLANTAR RESPONSE. **paradoxical flexor r.** GORDON'S REFLEX. **paradoxical patellar r.** 1 Adduction of the thigh when the patellar tendon is tapped. 2 Contraction of the quadriceps, i.e., upon shortening rather than extending this muscle. **paradoxical pupillary r.** Any pupillary reaction contrary to that expected to occur in the particular situation, e.g., dilatation upon exposure to light (in tabes), dilatation in response to epinephrine (when the superior sympathetic ganglion has been lesioned), and dilatation in adjustment to near vision. Also *Bekhterev's reflex.* **paradoxical triceps r.** Flexion rather than extension of the forearm when the tendon of the triceps brachii is struck. In indicates dysfunction over the triceps reflex loop through the $C_7$ and $C_8$ cord segments. **patellar r.** Contraction of the quadriceps muscle, especially the vastus intermedius head, in response to a tap on the taut patellar tendon. The reflex tests integrity of the muscle spindle stretch reflex loop over the $L_3$ and $L_4$ levels. Also *patellar tendon reflex, quadriceps reflex, knee-jerk reflex, knee jerk, quadriceps jerk.* **patelloadductor r.** Abnormal adduction of one leg when the quadriceps reflex response in the contralateral leg is elicited by tapping the patellar tendon. The response may not be a true crossed reflex, but be mediated through jarring of the pelvic origin of the adductor muscles. Also *McCormac's reflex.* **Pavlov's r.** AURICULOPRESSOR REFLEX. **pectoral r.** Adduction and medial rotation of the partially abducted arm in response to striking the humeral insertion of the pectoralis major tendon. Also *costopectoral reflex.* **Peiper's r.** DAZZLE REFLEX. **pendular r.** A knee jerk which follows a tap on the patellar tendon but in which inhibition occurs only slowly and the leg, if dependent, swings backward and forward several times like a pendulum. This reflex may be seen in a hypotonic limb, as in chorea. **penile r.** BULBOSPONGIOSUS REFLEX. **penis r.** BULBOSPONGIOSUS REFLEX. **perception r.** A behavior reaction in response to the subject's perception of a sensory stimulus or of an abruptly imposed change in his surroundings. **perianal r.** ANAL REFLEX. **pericardial r.** Vagally mediated slowing of the heart rate and systemic hypotension triggered by manipulation of the pericardium. **periosteal r.** TENDON REFLEX. **periosteoradial r.** BRACHIORADIALIS REFLEX. **peritoneointestinal r.** Inhibition of intestinal and gastric motility as a consequence of retroperitoneal hemorrhage or other irritation. **pharyngeal r.** Spastic contraction of the pharyngeal musculature upon stimulation or irritation of the oropharyngeal mucosa. Depending upon its intensity, it contributes to swallowing, gag, and vomiting reflexes. **phasic r.** COORDINATED REFLEX. **Phillipson's r.** Contraction of the quadriceps with extension of the knee following flexion of the contralateral knee forceful enough to elicit a lengthening reaction (inhibition) of its extensors. Also *thigh crossed lengthening reflex.* **pilomotor r.** Sympathetically mediated erection of the dermal papillae and hair in response to a local cold or tactile stimulus, exposure of the body to cold, or a frightening or thrilling emotion. Also *trichographism.* **Piltz r.** ATTENTION REFLEX OF PUPIL. **placing r.** PLACING RESPONSE. **plantar r.** 1 Movement of the toes upon stroking the lateral aspect of the plantar surface. Normally a plantiflexion, the response changes to dorsiflexion (positive Babinski sign) following interruption of pyramidal pathways. 2 In the experimental animal, brisk plantar flexion of the toes in response to tapping the plantar or palmar cushions. It is initiated by excitation of low-threshold cutaneous mechanoreceptors, and chiefly involves intrinsic muscles of the paw. Also *sole reflex.* **plantar flexor r.** The plantar reflex as seen in a normal individual. **platysmal r.** Constriction of the ipsilateral pupil in response to pinching the platysma muscle. **pollicomental r.** PALMOMENTAL REFLEX. **polysynaptic r.** A reflex response or pathway having interneurons, and hence several synapses, interposed between the primary afferents and the responding motoneurons. **positive supporting r.** Stiffening of extensor tone upon gentle dorsiflexion of the digits, elicited by either cutaneous or proprioceptive stimuli. It is detectable in the intact animal but exaggerated in the decerebrate preparation. **postural r.** STATIC REFLEX. **prehensory r.** GRASP REFLEX. **pressor r.** A rise in blood pressure resulting from an autonomic nervous response to excitation of nociceptors or other sensory receptors. **pressoreceptor r.** Lowering of blood pressure due to excitation of specific pressoreceptors of the carotid body and aortic arch with resulting stimulation of medullary vasodilation and cardiac inhibition centers. **Preyer's r.** In animals, an involuntary orienting movement of the pinna in response to a sound. **primitive r.** Any of a group of reflexes which are present in the young infant, disappear as the cerebral cortex matures, and may reappear as release phenomena due to degenerative cortical lesions, as in presenile or senile dementia. The grasp, sucking, snout, and rooting reflexes are examples. **pronator r.** Pronation and adduction of the hand in response to tapping the distal end of the ulna. **proprioceptive r.** Any postural or other reflex response resulting from excitation of sensory receptors in muscles, joints, or ligaments. Vestibular reflexes are sometimes included. **protective r.** Any reflex action tending to prevent harm to a body part or the body as a whole. **protective laryngeal r.** Forceful closure of the glottis in response to touch. Its disappearance is a sign of entry into the second stage of anesthesia. **psychocardiac r.** Acceleration of the heartbeat upon recalling an emotionally charged experience. **psychogalvanic r.** A change in electrical resistance across the skin associated with an emotional experience, a state of concentrated attention, etc. It is due to sympathetically mediated changes in secretory and vasomotor activity. **puboadductor r.** Contractions resulting in adduction and weak flexion of the hip when the pubis is percussed. It is enhanced by slightly abducting and medially rotating the thigh so as to stretch the adductors. **pulmonocoronary r.** Constriction of the coronary arteries caused by a traumatic event in the lung, as in pulmonary embolism. The sensory pathway is mediated by the vagus. **pupillary r.** 1 Constriction of the pupil when the eye is exposed to additional light, as in undergoing accommodation or in responding in the consensual light reflex. 2 Dilatation of the pupil as a component of the pain reaction. **pupillary-skin r.** CILIOSPINAL REFLEX. **Puussepp's r.** LITTLE-TOE REFLEX. **pyelovesical r.** MICTURITION REFLEX. **quadriceps r.** PATELLAR REFLEX. **quadrupedal extensor r.** BRAIN'S QUADRUPEDAL REFLEX. **radial r.** BRACHIORADIALIS REFLEX. **radiobicipital r.** Contraction of the biceps upon striking the radius. It may accompany the brachioradialis reflex, and should be distinguished from it. **radioperiosteal r.** BRACHIORADIALIS REFLEX. **radiopronator r.** Pronation of the forearm upon striking the radius. Compare ULNAR REFLEX. **rectal r.** DEFECATION REFLEX. **rectus abdominis r.** Contraction of the rectus abdominis in response to a pin prick or scratch of the overlying skin. The response tends to be localized to the part of the muscle beneath the stimulus. **red r.** The reddish glow seen in the pupil of a normal eye when observed with coaxial illumination, as with an ophthalmoscope. **Reimer's r.** SOLE-TAP REFLEX. **Remak's r.** FEMORAL REFLEX. **renal r.** Anuria and kidney pain in response to injury or disease of the opposite kidney and ureter or some less closely related organ. **renointestinal r.** Reflex inhibition of intestinal motility caused by irritative disease of a kidney. **renorenal r.** Pain or oliguria in a sound kidney in response to a disorder, usually acute, of the other kidney. **renoureteral r.** MICTURITION REFLEX. **retrobulbar pupillary r.** A biphasic response of the pupil consisting of constriction upon exposure to light followed by dilatation as the exposure continues, seen in retrobulbar neuritis. **retromallear r.** An abnormal light reflex sometimes observed in the posterosuperior (retromallear) quadrant of the tympanic membrane, usually indicative of a retraction pocket in this location. **Riddoch's mass r.** MASS REFLEX. **righting r.** Any of several reflexes serving to position the head, trunk, and limbs in their normal postural relationship and orientation in space, including vestibular, neck, body, and optical righting reflexes. **Roger's r.** ESOPHAGOSALIVARY REFLEX. **rooting r.** Turning of the head, pouting, and directing of the lips of an infant toward the side on which the cheek is touched. **Rossolimo's r.** Flexion of the second to fifth toes when the plantar surface of the foot is tapped so as to stretch the plantar muscles. It is a sign of hypertonia in dysfunction of the pyramidal tract. **Ruggeri's r.** Sympathetically mediated acceleration of the pulse when the eyes are focused on a very near object. **scapular r.** A contraction of muscles attaching along the medial margin of the scapula with resulting shoulder retraction, in response to a tap over the interscapular region. Also *interscapular reflex.* **scapulohumeral r.** Contraction of the subscapularis with adduction and lateral rotation of the arm when the vertebral border of the scapula is struck. Also *scapuloperiosteal reflex.* **Schäffer's r.** Dorsiflexion of the big toe (i.e., reflex flexor action) in response to pinching the Achilles tendon. It is seen in corticospinal injury. **Schunkel r.** In an animal holding one limb off the ground in partial flexion, extension of the limb when the hindquarters are pushed to that side. It is a reflex reaction to stretch of adductor muscles in the weight-supporting limb. **scratch r.** Rhythmic flexion-extension movements of a limb directed to a cutaneous locus of tickling or irritation, especially on the back or flank. It involves postural adjustments of the contralateral limb as well as reciprocal activation of muscle groups of the active limb. The response is fully developed in the spinal animal (e.g., dog). **scrotal r.** DARTOS REFLEX. **segmental r.** Any response mediated over a pathway restricted to the dorsal and ventral roots of a single spinal segment. **semimembranosus r.** See under INTERNAL HAMSTRING REFLEX. **semitendinosus r.** See under INTERNAL HAMSTRING REFLEX. **sensory blinking r.** EYELID CLOSURE REFLEX. **sexual r.** Reflex erection of the penis and seminal emission evoked by handling the organ or the genital area. The sexual reflex may occur in a patient with spastic paraplegia. **simple r.** A reflex in which the response is largely confined to a single muscle. **sinus r.** CAROTID SINUS SYNDROME. **skin r.** CUTANEOUS REFLEX. **skin pupillary r.** Dilatation of the pupil induced by pinching the skin over the ipsilateral side of the neck. **sneezing r.** NASOFACIAL REFLEX. **snout r.** LIP REFLEX. **sole r.** PLANTAR REFLEX. **sole-tap r.** In subjects with corticospinal dysfunction, plantar flexion and fanning of the toes in response to tapping on the center of the sole of the foot or on the base of the heel. It indicates hyperactive stretch reflexes of those muscles reflexly classified as extensors of the foot. Also *aponeurotic reflex, metatarsal reflex, Guillain-Barré reflex, Reimer's reflex, Weingrow's heel reflex.* **Somagyi's r.** Pupillary dilatation upon deep inspiration, and pupillary constriction upon expiration. Also *Somagyi sign.* **somatointestinal r.** Inhibition of intestinal motility resulting from irritation of the skin over the abdomen. **spinal r.** A reflex for which the sensory and motor axonal components and their central connectors are complete at spinal segmental levels. **spino-adductor r.** Activation of the thigh adductor muscles in response to tapping spinous processes of the lower lumbar vertebrae. **stapedius r.** ACOUSTIC REFLEX. **startle r.** STARTLE RESPONSE. **static r.** Any reflex contributing to the maintenance of posture and excited by a static stimulus, such as pressure on the side of the body, or position of the vestibular receptors in space. Also *postural reflex.* **static adaptation r.** BODY-RIGHTING REFLEX. **static attitudinal r.** ATTITUDINAL REFLEX. **statokinetic r.** Any of the reflexes initiated from vestibular and neck receptors that contribute to the positioning of the head, trunk, and limbs during movements such as walking. The responsible stimuli are necessarily continuously changing. Also *acceleratory reflex, statokinetic reaction.* **statotonic r.** ATTITUDINAL REFLEX. **stepping r.** STEPPING. **sternobrachial r.** Contraction of the pectoral muscles and other adductors of the arm when the sternum is tapped. **Stookey r.** Flexion of the leg in response to tapping the tendons of the semimembranosus and semitendinosus when these muscles are under moderate tension due to partial flexing of the knee. **stretch r.** Reflex contraction of a muscle induced by stretching it, as occurs in the deep tendon reflexes. Also *myotatic reflex, myostatic reflex.* **Strümpell's r.** Adduction and dorsiflexion of the foot, associated with flexion of the leg, in response to stroking the thigh and lower abdomen. It is seen in spastic paralysis. **styloradial r.** BRACHIORADIALIS REFLEX. **sucking r.** Pursing of the lips or nursing movements involving the lips, tongue, and jaw induced by tactile stimulation of the lips. It is seen in the normal infant, and in exaggeration in patients with bifrontal lobe lesions. Also *lip reflex.* **suckling r.** Secretion of milk in response to a release of pituitary prolactin triggered reflexly by mechanical stimulation of the nipple during nursing. A decrease in prolactin inhibitory hormone is probably involved. **superficial r.** A specific somatic or autonomic motor response elicitable by sensory stimulation of a localized region of the skin. See also CUTANEOUS REFLEX. **superficial abdominal r.** Contraction in a localized region of the abdominal wall musculature upon stroking the overlying skin. Also *abdominal cutaneous reflex.* **supination r.** BRACHIORADIALIS RE-

FLEX. **supinator r.** BRACHIORADIALIS REFLEX. **supinator jerk r.** BRACHIORADIALIS REFLEX. **supinator longus r.** BRACHIORADIALIS REFLEX. **supporting r.'es** SUPPORTING REACTIONS. **supraorbital r.** Contraction of the orbicularis oculi muscle with closure of the eyelids in response to a tap over the supraorbital nerve or the supraorbital ridge. Normally difficult to elicit, it may be exaggerated in lesions above the facial nucleus. Also *McCarthy's reflex, orbicularis oculi reflex, trigeminofacial reflex, nose-bridge-lid reflex, nose-eye reflex.* **suprapatellar r.** Contraction of the quadriceps induced by tapping the finger placed against the upper margin of the patella. **suprapubic r.** Deviation of the linea alba to the side on which skin in the inguinal region is stroked. It is mediated at the $T_{12}$ and $L_1$ segmental levels. Also *lower abdominal reflex.* **supraumbilical r.** EPIGASTRIC REFLEX. **swallowing r.** A sequence of movements of the upper digestive tract responsible for starting a volume of fluid or bolus of food down the alimentary canal. Involved are elevation of the base of the tongue, contraction of faucial muscles, closure of the nasopharynx, and a single peristaltic wave progressing down the pharynx and esophagus. Also *deglutition reflex.* **tactile r.** Any motor action triggered by stimulation of touch receptors in the skin or mucosa. **tarsophalangial r.** The normal response of dorsiflexion of the second to fifth toes when the area over the cuboid bone is tapped. Also *cuboidodigital reflex, dorsocuboidal reflex.* See also MENDEL-BEKHTEREV REFLEX. **tendon r.** Contraction of a muscle in response to phasic displacement of its tendon, as by a tap. Stretch-induced discharge from spindles in the muscle belly is responsible for exciting the motoneurons. Also *periosteal reflex, tendon jerk.* **tensor fasciae latae r.** Slight abduction of the thigh induced by a tap over the tensor fasciae latae muscle below its origin from the anterior superior iliac spine. **testicular compression r.** Contraction of the lower abdominal muscles in response to compression of the testicle. Also *Kocher's reflex.* **thigh crossed lengthening r.** PHILLIPSON'S REFLEX. **Throckmorton's r.** Dorsiflexion of the big toe and fanning of the others in response to a tap over the first metatarsophalangeal joint medial to the extensor hallucis tendon. A variant of the Babinski sign, the response is seen in pyramidal tract lesions. **thumb r.** Flexion of the thumb induced by a tap over the dorsal metacarpal region. **tibialis posterior r.** Inversion of the foot when the tibialis posterior tendon is tapped where it passes behind the medial malleolus. **tibioadductor r.** Adduction of the leg, and sometimes the opposite leg, upon percussing over the subcutaneous surface of the tibia. **toe r.** Contraction of the flexor muscles of the leg in response to forceful, imposed flexion of the big toe. **tonic r.** **1** Any reflex normally characterized by a relatively enduring response. **2** Any of the several neck and vestibular reflexes that form the basis of posture and attitude. **3** An abnormal response marked by exaggerated persistence of a reflex contraction after termination of the reflexogenic stimulus. **tonic plantar r.** EXTENSOR PLANTAR RESPONSE. **tonic vibration r.** A slowly mounting contraction of a muscle in response to a vibratory stimulus applied over its belly or tendon. Excitation of the primary endings of muscle spindles and reflex facilitation of the motor pool is the cause. **triceps r.** Contraction of the triceps brachii with extension of the arm when the muscle's tendon is tapped, the elbow being passively held in partial flexion. Also *elbow jerk, elbow reflex.* **triceps surae r.** ACHILLES TENDON REFLEX. **trigeminocervical r.** Contraction of homolateral neck muscles upon tapping skin over the face. **trigeminofacial r.** SUPRAORBITAL REFLEX. **trigeminus r.** OCULOPUPILLARY REFLEX. **trochanter r.** Contraction of thigh adductor muscles induced by striking the greater trochanter. **Trömner's r.** HOFFMANN'S REFLEX. **tympanic r.** Protective movement of the tympanum due to reflex contraction of middle ear muscles in response to a loud sound. Compare COCHLEOSTAPEDIAL REFLEX. **ulnar r.** Pronation and adduction of the hand in response to percussion of the styloid process of the ulna. Compare RADIOPRONATOR REFLEX. **unconditioned r.** A reflex whose mechanism and expression are intrinsic to the naive animal, and not dependent upon gradual development through association or other learning processes. Also *inborn reflex.* **unloading r.** A biphasic response in contractile and electromyographic activity of a muscle upon sudden release of its load. It consists of an initial period of silence followed by momentary rebound activity exceeding that of the control period. The mechanism probably involves a complex of phasic changes in the activity of spindles and tendon organs in the same and antagonist muscles, in Renshaw inhibition centrally, etc. **upper abdominal periosteal r.** OBLIQUUS REFLEX. **upper deep abdominal r.** OBLIQUUS REFLEX. **urinary r.** MICTURITION REFLEX. **utricular r.** Any reflex initiated by stimulation of the macula of the utricle, or of the utricle and saccule. These are principally the tonic labryinthine righting reflexes. **vagal pupillary r.** Dilatation of the pupil upon inspiration and converse narrowing upon deep expiration, mediated by receptors in the thoracic distribution of the vagus nerve. Also *vagotonic pupillary reflex.* **vagovagal r.** **1** Reflex slowing of the heart rate induced by stimulation of sensory receptors of the larynx, trachea, or lower respiratory tree, as occurs with insertion of an endotracheal tube or administration of certain gaseous anesthetic agents. **2** Reflex cardiac asystole due to distension of the esophagus. **vagus r.** Hypersensitivity to pressure along the course of the vagus nerve, seen in lung afflictions, e.g., tuberculosis. **vasomotor r.** The local response of superficial blood vessels to a cutaneous stimulus, believed to be mediated entirely via peripheral branches of visceral nerves. Also *vascular reflex.* **vasopressor r.** Any reflex pattern marked by constriction of blood vessels and elevation in blood pressure. **vasovagal r.** A visceral response mediated by the vagal nerve and triggered by irritation or stimulation of a major blood vessel. **venorespiratory r.** Increased pulmonary ventilation in response to an elevation in blood pressure in the right atrium. **vertebra prominens r.** Decrease in antigravity tone of the limbs when pressure is exerted upon the lowest cervical vertebra in a quadruped. **vesical r.** BLADDER REFLEX. **vesicointestinal r.** Inhibition of intestinal motility brought on by irritation or severe distension of the urinary bladder. **vestibular r.** LABYRINTHINE REFLEX. **vestibulo-ocular r.** An adjustment in the static position of the eyes or initiation of phasic oscillatory movements induced by stimulation of the vestibular apparatus, often indicating the nystagmus induced by unequal stimulation of the cristae in a bilateral pair of semicircular canals during acceleratory rotation of the head. Also *oculovestibular reflex.* **vestibulospinal r.** Modulation in tonic activity or reflex reactivity of motor nuclei at segmental levels in response to stimulation of one or more of the receptor areas in the vestibular apparatus. Vestibulospinal tracts play a prominent but not exclusive role in mediating the control. **virile r.** HUGHES REFLEX. **visceral r.** Any alteration of motor or sensory activity induced in a region of the body wall or distant viscus by physiological activation or irritation of a given visceral organ. **visceral**

**traction r.** 1 Laryngospasm triggered during an operation by pulling on the mesenteries, gallbladder, appendix, etc. 2 A sudden fall in blood pressure accompanying gross manipulation of abdominal viscera. **viscerocardiac r.** An alteration in heartbeat or cardiac output occasioned by sensory stimuli arising in a viscus. **visceromotor r.** Reflex spasm of somatic muscle(s) resulting from a diseased, irritated state of some viscus. Often the muscle(s) overlie the viscus. **viscerotrophic r.** Degeneration of skin, muscle, or bone attendant upon a chronic dysfunction or inflammation of some thoracic or abdominal viscus. **visual orbicularis r.** OPTICOPALPEBRAL REFLEX. **visuocortical r.** HAAB'S REFLEX. **vomiting r.** Vomiting induced by tactile or chemical stimulation of the pharynx or fauces. **von Mering r.** A decrease in tone of abdominal wall musculature after ingestion of food. **walking r.** In a subject with parkinsonism of which akinesia is a feature, initiation of the act of walking by looking down at a line on the floor or by leaning forward. Walking may then begin reflexly, and once begun it continues. **watered-silk r.** WATERED-SILK RETINA. **Weiss r.** A circular light reflection adjacent to the optic disk, commonly seen and not of definite pathologic significance. **Westphal-Piltz r.** Pupilloconstriction induced by forcible closure of the eyelids. Also *Westphal's pupillary reflex, Gifford's reflex, Gifford-Galassi reflex.* **wink r.** EYELID CLOSURE REFLEX. **withdrawal r.** A response in which a body part, as a pseudopod, tentacle, or limb, is abruptly pulled away from a source of noxious stimulation. In vertebrates the term often refers to comprehensive activation of flexor muscles in an extremity, as for example in the lower limb flexors of the hip, knee, ankle, and dorsiflexors of the toes. **wrist clonus r.** Clonus precipitated by a sudden dorsiflexion of the wrist with stretch of the flexor muscles. **wrist flexion r.** Flexion of the fingers when tendons on the volar surface of the wrist are tapped, the supinated forearm being supported to put the tendons under some initial tension. **zygomatic r.** Movement of the lower jaw to the side on which the zygoma is tapped so as to jar the masseter muscle.

**reflexion** \riflek′shən\ 1 The outmoded concept that all behavior arises out of reflex actions. *Obs.* 2 *Brit.* REFLECTION.

**reflexio palpebrarum** \riflek′shō pal′pəbrer′əm\ EYELID CLOSURE REFLEX.

**reflexogenic** \riflek′səjen′ik\ Producing, increasing, or predisposing to reflex action.

**reflexograph** \riflek′səgraf\ [REFLEX + *o* + -GRAPH] A mechanical instrument designed to record graphically the force of a reflex muscular contraction.

**reflexology** \rē′fleksäl′əjē\ 1 The analysis of motor behavior in terms of component simple and complex reflexes. 2 The study of the neurophysiologic mechanisms of reflexes in general.

**reflexometry** \rē′fleksäm′ətrē\ The technique or practice of measuring the vigor of reflex responses.

**reflexotherapy** \riflek′səther′əpē\ REFLEX THERAPY.

**reflux** \rē′fluks\ [RE- + FLUX] A retrograde or return flow; regurgitation. **abdominojugular r.** See under HEPATOJUGULAR REFLUX. **duodenogastric r.** Reflux of intestinal contents through an incompetent pyloric valve. Bile and pancreatic juices refluxed into the stomach may cause a severe gastritis. **esophageal r.** The reflux of gastric contents into the esophagus. **hepatojugular r.** Increased venous pressure in the neck veins induced by sustained compression over the liver. It is manifest by prominence and an ascending level in the neck of the jugular venous pulses. This is a normal phenomenon, and pressure in the abdomen will generally have the same result. The neck veins fill when the right atrium is temporarily overloaded because of increased venous return through the inferior vena cava. **pyelolymphatic r.** PYELOLYMPHATIC BACKFLOW. **pyelorenal r.** PYELORENAL BACKFLOW. **pyelosinus r.** PYELOSINUS BACKFLOW. **pyelotubular r.** PYELOTUBULAR BACKFLOW. **pyelovenous r.** PYELOVENOUS BACKFLOW. **vesicoureteral r.** Backflow of urine from the bladder into the ureter, unilaterally or bilaterally, during rest or especially during micturition. The condition, usually demonstrated by cystography or voiding cystourethrography, is often graded as to severity: grade I refers to reflux only into the ureter; grade II refers to reflux to the renal pelvis without dilating the pelvis; grade III refers to reflux to the pelvis with dilatation of the pelvis and calices. The condition may be secondary to obstruction of the urinary outflow tract or to any disease involving the ureteral orifices. Pyelonephritic scarring and slowly progressive renal failure are common, as in recurrent urinary tract infection. In children, vesicoureteral reflux may be idiopathic and it often disappears spontaneously. Also *ureteral reflux.*

**refract** \rifrakt′\ [L *refractus,* past part. of *refringere* to break by bending back. See REFRINGENT.] 1 To deflect by refraction, as light rays or sound waves. 2 To measure the inaccuracies of focusing of light upon the retina.

**refracta dosi** [L] In fractional or divided doses: used in prescription writing.

**refractile** \rifrak′tīl\ Having the property of refracting light.

**refraction** \rifrak′shən\ [See REFRACT.] 1 The bending of the direction of propagation of a wave as it passes from one medium to another. 2 Measurement of the optical error of the eye, as clinically performed in order to prescribe corrective lenses. **double r.** BIREFRINGENCE. **dynamic r.** A measuring of the optical correction needed by the eye when observing a near object. **ocular r.** A measuring of the optical correction needed by the eye when accommodation is relaxed. **static r.** Refraction when the eye is affected by cycloplegia; cycloplegic refraction.

**refractive** \rifrak′tiv\ Pertaining to refraction; having the capacity to refract.

**refractometer** \rē′fraktäm′ətər\ A device for measuring the refractive error of an eye.

**refractometry** \rē′fraktäm′ətrē\ The measurement of the refractive error of an eye.

**refractor** \rifrak′tər\ [REFRACT + -OR] A device containing lenses and prisms, used in determining the dioptric status of the eye.

**refractory** \rifrak′tərē\ [REFRACT + -ORY] 1 Resistant to treatment. 2 Resistant to stimulation. 3 Difficult to manage; unyielding; obstinate.

**refracture** \rifrak′chər\ 1 To fracture again. 2 A surgically created bone fracture to correct a deformity created by misalignment or improper healing of the original fracture.

**refrangible** \rifran′jibl\ Subject to refraction.

**refresh** 1 To débride. 2 To remove (tissue) to stimulate healing.

**refringent** \rifrin′jənt\ [L *refringens,* gen. *refringentis,* pres. part. of *refringere* (from *re-* back + *frangere* to break) to break by bending back] Pertaining to the ability to refract.

**refuin** ANTHRAMYCIN.

**refusion** \rifyoo′zhən\ The return of blood which has either been temporarily removed from the circulation by venesection or by obstruction through ligature of a limb.

**regard** Conscious awareness; attention.

**Regaud** [Claudius François Regaud, French radiologist, 1870–1940] **1** See under METHOD. **2** Regaud and Lacassagne technique. See under PARIS TECHNIQUE.

**Regaut** See under REGAUD.

**regeneration** \rē'jenərā'shən\ The renewal of lost or damaged tissue. It ranges from the healing of a wound, as in humans, to the replacement of an entire appendage or organ in certain other animals. The capacity is most highly developed in invertebrates and most limited in birds and mammals.

**regimen** \rej'əmən\ [L (from *regere* to steer, control) guidance, control] A course of treatment, often dealing with diet, exercise, and habits of life, prescribed with a view to maintaining or restoring health. **sanitary r.** Preventive measures or quarantine procedures formerly employed to prevent the spread of pestilential diseases.

# regio

**regio** \rē'jē·ō\ [L, gen. *regionis* (from *regere* to steer, direct, fix boundaries) a direction, line, boundary, region] (*pl.* regiones) **1** A region or portion of the body having a particular function or nervous or vascular supply. **2** An arbitrarily defined area on the surface of the body used for designating locations of structures. **regiones abdominales** [NA] The various topographical areas or subdivisions demarcated on the surface of the abdominal wall. Also *abdominal regions, abdominal zones.* **r. analis** [NA] The area of the perineum posterior to a transverse line in front of the ischial tuberosities and containing the termination of the anal canal. Also *anal region, anal triangle, rectal triangle, posterior perineum.* **r. antebrachialis anterior** [NA] The front, or anterior, surface of the forearm. Also *anterior antebrachial region, anterior forearm region, facies anterior antebrachii, regio antebrachii anterior* (outmoded). **r. antebrachialis posterior** [NA] The dorsal surface, or back, of the forearm. Also *posterior antebrachial region, posterior forearm region, facies posterior antebrachii, regio antebrachii posterior* (outmoded). **r. antebrachii anterior** *Outmoded* REGIO ANTEBRACHIALIS ANTERIOR. **r. antebrachii posterior** *Outmoded* REGIO ANTEBRACHIALIS POSTERIOR. **r. axillaris** [NA] The area of the chest and shoulder around the axilla. Also *axillary region.* **r. brachialis anterior** [NA] The front, or anterior, surface of the arm between the shoulder and the elbow joints. Also *facies anterior brachii, regio brachii anterior* (outmoded), *anterior brachial region.* **r. brachialis posterior** [NA] The dorsal surface, or back, of the arm between the shoulder and the elbow joints. Also *facies posterior brachii, regio brachii posterior* (outmoded), *posterior brachial region.* **r. brachii anterior** *Outmoded* REGIO BRACHIALIS ANTERIOR. **r. brachii posterior** *Outmoded* REGIO BRACHIALIS POSTERIOR. **r. buccalis** [NA] The area of the cheek. Also *buccal region.* **r. calcanea** [NA] The area overlying the heel bone or calcaneus; calx. Also *calcaneal region.* **regiones capitis** [NA] The various topographical areas or subdivisions of the head related to the underlying cranial bones, namely, frontal, parietal, occipital, and temporal regions. **regiones cervicales** [NA] The demarcated topographical areas or subdivisions of the neck, namely, the anterior, lateral, posterior, and sternocleidomastoid regions and their various triangles. Also *regiones colli* (outmoded). **r. cervicalis anterior** [NA] The area of the neck anterior to the sternocleidomastoid muscle and subdivided into submandibular, carotid, muscular, and submental triangles by the omohyoid and digastric muscles. Also *anterior region of neck, regio colli anterior* (outmoded), *anterior triangle of neck.* **r. cervicalis lateralis** [NA] The area of the neck bounded anteriorly by the posterior border of sternocleidomastoid muscle, posteriorly by the anterior border of the trapezius muscle, and inferiorly by the middle third of the clavicle, and including the subclavian or omoclavicular triangle. Also *regio colli lateralis* (outmoded), *posterior triangle of neck.* **r. cervicalis posterior** [NA] The area of the back of the neck lying between the anterior borders of the two trapezius muscles. Also *posterior region of neck, nuchal region, regio colli posterior* (outmoded). **regiones colli** REGIONES CERVICALES. **r. colli anterior** *Outmoded* REGIO CERVICALIS ANTERIOR. **r. colli lateralis** *Outmoded* REGIO CERVICALIS LATERALIS. **r. colli posterior** *Outmoded* REGIO CERVICALIS POSTERIOR. **regiones corporis** The anatomic regions of the body: the various topographical areas or subdivisions demarcated on the surface of the body. **r. cruralis anterior** [NA] The front, or anterior, surface of the leg between the knee and the ankle joints. Also *facies anterior cruris, regio cruris anterior* (outmoded), *anterior crural region, anterior region of leg.* **r. cruralis posterior** [NA] The dorsal surface, or back, of the leg between the knee and the ankle joints. Also *facies posterior cruris, regio cruris posterior* (outmoded), *posterior crural region, posterior region of leg.* **r. cruris anterior** *Outmoded* REGIO CRURALIS ANTERIOR. **r. cruris posterior** *Outmoded*

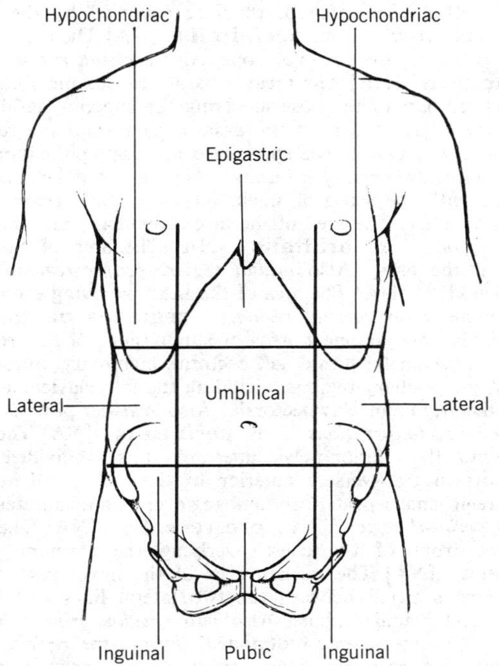


**Abdominal regions**

REGIO CRURALIS POSTERIOR. **r. cubitalis anterior** [NA] The area in front of the elbow joint. Also *regio cubiti anterior* (outmoded), *anterior cubital region.* **r. cubitalis posterior** [NA] The area posterior to the elbow joint. Also *regio cubiti posterior* (outmoded), *posterior cubital region, olecranon region, olecranal region.* **r. cubiti anterior** *Outmoded* REGIO CUBITALIS ANTERIOR. **r. cubiti posterior** *Outmoded* REGIO CUBITALIS POSTERIOR. **r. deltoidea** [NA] The area overlying the deltoid muscle and constituting the lateral aspect of the shoulder. Also *deltoid region.* **regiones dorsales** [NA] The various topographical areas or subdivisions demarcated on the posterior or dorsal surface of the trunk, namely, regio vertebralis, sacralis, scapularis, infrascapularis, and lumbalis. Also *regiones dorsi* (outmoded). **r. dorsalis pedis** DORSUM PEDIS. **regiones dorsi** *Outmoded* REGIONES DORSALES. **r. epigastrica** [NA] The upper median area of the abdomen bounded by the transpyloric plane below and the lateral line on each side. Also *epigastric region, epigastrium, epigastric zone, pit of the stomach.* **regiones faciales** [NA] The topographical areas or subdivisions of the face, namely, orbital, nasal, oral, mental, infraorbital, buccal, and zygomatic regions. Also *regiones faciei* (outmoded), *facial regions.* **r. femoralis** The thigh region, both anterior and posterior, including the femoral triangle. Also *femoral region.* **r. femoralis anterior** [NA] The front, or anterior, surface of the thigh. Also *facies anterior femoris, anterior thigh region.* **r. femoralis posterior** [NA] The dorsal surface, or back, of the thigh. Also *facies posterior femoris, posterior thigh region.* **r. frontalis** [NA] The area of the head overlying the frontal bone; the forehead. Also *frontal region.* **r. genus anterior** [NA] The area in front of the knee. Also *patellar region.* **r. genus posterior** [NA] The area behind the knee including the popliteal fossa. Also *popliteal region.* **r. glutealis** [NA] The area overlying the gluteal muscles. Also *gluteal region.* **r. hypochondriaca dextra et sinistra** [NA] The right and left upper lateral areas of the abdomen, lateral to the epigastric region, above the transpyloric plane and lateral to each lateral line. Also *hypochondriac region, hypochondrium.* **r. hypogastrica** *Outmoded* REGIO PUBICA. **r. hypothalamica anterior** [NA] The portion of the hypothalamus bounded anteriorly by the lamina terminalis and extending caudally to approximately the level of the infundibulum. It lies dorsal to the optic chiasma and contains the medial and lateral preoptic nuclei, the supraoptic and paraventricular nuclei, and the anterior hypothalamic nucleus. It is functionally predominant in parasympathetic control. Also *anterior hypothalamic region, anterior hypothalamic area.* **r. hypothalamica intermedia** [NA] The portion of the hypothalamus situated between the anterior and posterior hypothalamic regions and containing the infundibulum and tuber cinereum. Its ventral surface is bounded anteriorly by the optic chiasma and posteriorly by the mamillary bodies. Within the substance of the intermediate hypothalamic region can be found the arcuate nucleus, the tuberal nuclei, the ventromedial, dorsomedial, and dorsal hypothalamic nuclei, the intermediate part of the lateral hypothalamic area, the posterior periventricular nucleus, and the infundibular nucleus. Also *intermediate hypothalamic region, intermediate hypothalamic area.* **r. hypothalamica posterior** [NA] The portion of the hypothalamus lying caudal to the intermediate hypothalamic region and containing the medial and lateral mamillary bodies along with the posterior hypothalamic nucleus. It is a functional division concerned with control of sympathetic activation of the thoracolumbar outflow. Stimulation of this area increases metabolic rate, heart rate, respiration, and blood pressure, and results in pupillary dilatation, piloerection, and somatic activity characteristic of flight or escape. The area is also essential for control of body temperature. Also *posterior hypothalamic region, posterior hypothalamic area.* **r. infraclavicularis** *Outmoded* FOSSA INFRACLAVICULARIS. **r. inframammaria** [NA] The area on the front of the chest below each mammary gland. Also *inframammary region.* **r. infraorbitalis** [NA] The area of the face below the eye on each side of the nasal region. Also *infraorbital region.* **r. infrascapularis** [NA] The area of the back below the inferior angle of the scapula and lateral to the vertebral column. Also *infrascapular region, subscapular region.* **r. inguinalis dextra et sinistra** [NA] The right and left lower lateral areas of the abdomen on each side of the pubic region, lateral to the lateral lines and below the transtubercular plane. Also *inguinal region, iliac region, suprainguinal region.* **r. lateralis abdominis dextra et sinistra** [NA] The right and left areas of the mid-abdomen, on each side of the umbilical region and lying between the transpyloric and transtubercular planes lateral to the lateral lines. Also *lateral abdominal region, right and left lumbar region.* **r. lumbalis** [NA] The area of the back on either side of the lumbar vertebrae and between the lowest rib above and the iliac crest below; the flank. Also *lumbar region.* **r. mammaria** [NA] The area of the front of the chest related to the mammary gland. Also *mammary region.* **regiones membri inferioris** [NA] The various topographical areas or subdivisions demarcated in the lower limb, namely, regio glutealis and the regions of the thigh, knee, leg, and foot. **regiones membri superioris** [NA] The various topographical areas or subdivisions demarcated in the upper limb, namely, regio deltoidea and the regions of the arm, elbow, forearm, wrist, and hand. **r. mentalis** [NA] The area of the face overlying the chin. Also *mental region.* **r. nasalis** [NA] The area of the face occupied by the nose. Also *nasal region.* **r. occipitalis** [NA] The area of the head overlying the occipital bone. Also *occipital region.* **r. olfactoria** [NA] The area of nasal mucous membrane in the upper part of the nose involving the superior nasal concha, the adjacent part of the nasal septum, and the roof of the nose in between. The specialized mucosal epithelium contains primary sensory neurons which are bipolar and involved with the sense of smell. Also *olfactory region.* **r. oralis** [NA] The area of the face around the mouth. Also *oral region.* **r. orbitalis** [NA] The area of the face around the orbit. Also *orbital region, ocular region.* **r. parietalis** [NA] The area of the head overlying each parietal bone. Also *parietal region.* **regiones pectorales** [NA] The topographical areas or subdivisions of the front of the chest, namely, presternal, pectoral, mammary, inframammary, and axillary regions, including the infraclavicular fossa and the trigonum clavipectorale. Also *regiones pectoris* (outmoded), *pectoral regions.* **r. perinealis** [NA] The area overlying the inferior pelvic aperture. It is subdivided by a line drawn transversely anterior to the ischial tuberosities into regio analis posteriorly and regio urogenitalis anteriorly. Also *perineal region.* **r. presternalis** [NA] The area of the front of the chest overlying the sternum. **r. pubica** [NA] The median area of the lower part of the abdomen situated between the two lateral lines and below the transtubercular plane. Also *pubic region, suprapubic region, regio hypogastrica* (outmoded), *hypogastric region, hypogastrium, hypogastric zone, pubes.* **r. respiratoria** [NA] The area of mucous membrane of the nasal cavity below the olfactory region and comprising the respiratory epithelium. Also *respiratory region.* **r. sacralis** [NA] The area of the back overlying the sacrum. Also *sacral region, sacrococcygeal region.* **r. scapularis** [NA] The area of the back overlying the scapula. Also *scapular region.* **r. sternocleidomastoidea** [NA] The area of the neck overlying the sternocleidomastoid muscle and including the lesser supraclavicular fossa. Also *sternocleidomastoid region.* **r. temporalis** [NA] The area of the head overlying each temporal bone. Also *temporal region.* **r. umbilicalis** [NA] The central area of the abdomen lying between the two lateral lines, below the transpyloric plane, and above the transtubercular plane. Also *umbilical region.* **r. urogenitalis** [NA] The area of the external genital organs in the anterior part of the perineal region. Also *urogenital region, genitourinary region, anterior perineum, urogenital triangle, urogenital trigone.* **r. vertebralis** [NA] The longitudinal central area of the back overlying the vertebral column. Also *vertebral region.* **r. zygomatica** [NA] The area of the face overlying each zygomatic bone. Also *zygomatic region.*

# region

**region** [L *regio.* See REGIO.] A part or an area. See under REGIO. **abdominal r.'s** REGIONES ABDOMINALES. **r. of accommodation** RANGE OF ACCOMMODATION. **anal r.** REGIO ANALIS. **anterior antebrachial r.** REGIO ANTEBRACHIALIS ANTERIOR. **anterior brachial r.** REGIO BRACHIALIS ANTERIOR. **anterior crural r.** REGIO CRURALIS ANTERIOR. **anterior cubital r.** REGIO CUBITALIS ANTERIOR. **anterior forearm r.** REGIO ANTEBRACHIALIS ANTERIOR. **anterior hypothalamic r.** REGIO HYPOTHALAMICA ANTERIOR. **anterior r. of leg** REGIO CRURALIS ANTERIOR. **anterior r. of neck** REGIO CERVICALIS ANTERIOR. **anterior thigh r.** REGIO FEMORALIS ANTERIOR. **axillary r.** REGIO AXILLARIS. **Broca's r.** GYRUS FRONTALIS INFERIOR. **buccal r.** REGIO BUCCALIS. **C r.** CONSTANT REGION. **calcaneal r.** REGIO CALCANEA. **cervical r.** 1 See under REGIONES CERVICALES. 2 The area including and adjacent to the cervix uteri or any other cervix. **cingulate r.** The cortical zone on the medial surface of the cerebral hemisphere surrounding the corpus callosum and approximating the area of cingulate gyrus. **constant r.** That section of an immunoglobulin chain in which the amino acid sequence is identical in all molecules, except for particular allotypic marker sites. In the light chain, this region is the C-terminal portion, in the heavy chain, the C-terminal portion. Also *C region.* Compare VARIABLE REGION. Symbol: $C_H$ **core r.** The active center of a nuclear reactor, containing the fissionable material. **deltoid r.** REGIO DELTOIDEA. **dorsal lip r.** The dorsal lip of the embryonic blastopore, the mesodermal invagination of which forms a median strip in the roof of the archenteron as far as the future oral opening and later folds dorsally to form the notochord. **elbow r.** CUBITUS. **encephalic r.** ALAR LAMINA. **epencephalic r.** ALAR LAMINA. **epigastric r.** REGIO EPIGASTRICA. **extrapolar r.** Any region of the body which, in electrotherapy, is unaffected by the stimulating or ground electrodes. **facial r.'s** REGIONES FACIALES. **femoral r.** REGIO FEMORALIS. **focal r.** FOCAL ZONE. **frontal r.** REGIO FRONTALIS. **Geiger r.** A range in the anode voltage of a Geiger-Müller tube throughout which an initial ionizing event, no matter how large or small, causes avalanche ionization throughout the whole of the cathode wire. The number of electrons collected by the anode is therefore essentially independent of the incoming energy, and output pulses are closely similar. **genitourinary r.** REGIO UROGENITALIS. **gluteal r.** REGIO GLUTEALIS. **gustatory r.** The area of the oral cavity and pharynx in which taste buds are located, namely, the epithelium of the tip, sides and root of the tongue, the lower surface of the soft palate, the palatoglossal arches, the posterior wall of the oral pharynx, and the posterior aspect of the epiglottis. **hinge r.** 1 A region in the immunoglobulin molecule particularly exposed to the action of proteinases. In immunoglobulin G, it is in the heavy chains close to the attachment of the light chains. There is flexibility in this region, and the Fab regions, which bind antigens, can move relative to the Fc region, which is responsible for other functions, such as fixation of complement. 2 Any region of a protein about which relatively rigid domains can move relative to one another. **homology r.** The structural units which form the immunoglobulin molecules. Each is of approximately equal size (100 amino acid residues) and shape, containing an intrachain disulfide. Many of the same residues appear in about the same place within the unit, indicating the possibility that the primordial immunoglobulin gene coded for this polypeptide unit is of about 100 amino acids. **hypencephalic r.** BASAL LAMINA. **hypervariable r.** A short length of amino acid sequence within a variable region of immunoglobulin light and heavy chains where any of a large number of amino acids are found in different antibody molecules. These regions (of which there are three or four within a chain) contribute largely to the antibody combining site and to the idiotypic determinants. **hypochondriac r.** REGIO HYPOCHONDRIACA (DEXTRA ET SINISTRA). **hypogastric r.** REGIO PUBICA. **iliac r.** REGIO INGUINALIS (DEXTRA ET SINISTRA). **infraclavicular r.** FOSSA INFRACLAVICULARIS. **infrahyoid r.** The area of the neck directly below the hyoid bone. **inframammary r.** REGIO INFRAMAMMARIA. **infraorbital r.** REGIO INFRAORBITALIS. **infrascapular r.** REGIO INFRASCAPULARIS. **infraspinous r.** FOSSA INFRASPINATA. **inguinal r.** REGIO INGUINALIS (DEXTRA ET SINISTRA). **intermediate hypothalamic r.** REGIO HYPOTHALAMICA INTERMEDIA. **ischiorectal r.** The area between the ischium and the rectum at the pelvic outlet and containing the ischioanal fossa. **K-r.** A region of the molecule of certain polycyclic aromatic hydrocarbons, such as benz[a]anthracene, which has some character of an isolated double bond and is susceptible to epoxide formation with enzymic catalysis. This oxidation is believed to be an essential step in the carcinogenic action of such hydrocarbons. **lateral abdominal r.** REGIO LATERALIS ABDOMINIS (DEXTRA ET SINISTRA). **limbic r.** Any of several parts of the limbic lobe which consists of phylogenetically old structures on the medial and inferior aspects of the cerebrum. These parts of the brain appear to be related to homeostatic mechanisms that are important to survival of the individual and preservation of the species. Among the various functions ascribed to limbic structures are olfaction, the control of endocrine mechanisms, feeding behavior, aggressive and defensive reactions, sexual behavior, the induction of sleep, memory, fear and flight reactions, and the perception of pleasure and expression of emotions. **lumbar r.** 1 REGIO LUMBALIS. 2 REGIO LATERALIS ABDOMINIS (DEXTRA ET SINISTRA). **mammary r.** REGIO MAMMARIA. **mental r.** REGIO MENTALIS. **motor r.**

The primary motor area (Brodmann's area 4), premotor area (area 6), and supplementary motor areas in the frontal lobes of the cerebral hemispheres. Also *rolandic region*. **myotube r. of intrafusal fiber** The distal portion of the nucleated region of a nuclear bag intrafusal fiber where there is a single, central file of nuclei surrounded by myofibrillae. In appearance it resembles the myotube stage in the development of an ordinary muscle fiber. **nasal r.** REGIO NASALIS. **nuchal r.** REGIO CERVICALIS POSTERIOR. **nucleated r. of intrafusal fiber** A concentration of large, vesicular nuclei at the midlength of an intrafusal fiber in the conformation of either a cluster (nuclear bag) or chain. **occipital r.** REGIO OCCIPITALIS. **ocular r.** REGIO ORBITALIS. **olecranal r.** REGIO CUBITALIS POSTERIOR. **olecranon r.** REGIO CUBITALIS POSTERIOR. **olfactory r.** REGIO OLFACTORIA. **opticostriate r.** The caudate nucleus, lenticular nucleus, and internal capsule. **oral r.** REGIO ORALIS. **orbital r.** REGIO ORBITALIS. **parietal r.** REGIO PARIETALIS. **parotideomasseteric r.** The region of the face related to the parotid gland and masseter muscle. **patellar r.** REGIO GENUS ANTERIOR. **pectoral r.'s** REGIONES PECTORALES. **pelvic r.** PELVIS MINOR. **perineal r.** REGIO PERINEALIS. **popliteal r.** REGIO GENUS POSTERIOR. **posterior antebrachial r.** REGIO ANTEBRACHIALIS POSTERIOR. **posterior brachial r.** REGIO BRACHIALIS POSTERIOR. **posterior crural r.** REGIO CRURALIS POSTERIOR. **posterior cubital r.** REGIO CUBITALIS POSTERIOR. **posterior forearm r.** REGIO ANTEBRACHIALIS POSTERIOR. **posterior hypothalamic r.** REGIO HYPOTHALAMICA POSTERIOR. **posterior r. of leg** REGIO CRURALIS POSTERIOR. **posterior r. of neck** REGIO CERVICALIS POSTERIOR. **posterior thigh r.** REGIO FEMORALIS POSTERIOR. **precordial r.** The area of the front of the chest overlying the heart and including the upper epigastric region. **prefrontal r.** The frontal cortex in front of the precentral fissures. **pretectal r.** PRETECTAL AREA. **proportional r.** In an ionization chamber, that region of the voltage range where the gas amplification is greater than 1, and collected charge is proportional to that produced by the ionizing event. **pubic r.** REGIO PUBICA. **respiratory r.** REGIO RESPIRATORIA. **retromaxillary r.** The area behind the maxilla. **rolandic r.** MOTOR REGION. **sacral r.** REGIO SACRALIS. **sacrococcygeal r.** REGIO SACRALIS. **scapular r.** REGIO SCAPULARIS. **sensory r.** A region that includes primary and secondary somatic sensory cortex, located in the precentral and postcentral gyri and paracentral lobule of the frontal and parietal areas of the cerebral hemispheres. **sternocleidomastoid r.** REGIO STERNOCLEIDOMASTOIDEA. **submandibular r.** TRIGONUM SUBMANDIBULARE. **submental r.** TRIGONUM SUBMENTALE. **subphrenic r.** HYPOPHRENIUM. **subscapular r.** REGIO INFRASCAPULARIS. **subthalamic r.** THALAMUS VENTRALIS. **supraclavicular r.** TRIGONUM OMOCLAVICULARE. **suprainguinal r.** REGIO INGUINALIS (DEXTRA ET SINISTRA). **supraomental r.** HYPOPHRENIUM. **suprapubic r.** REGIO PUBICA. **supraspinous r.** FOSSA SUPRASPINATA. **tegmental r.** The area in the midbrain located between the cerebral aqueduct and the paired substantia nigra. **temporal r.** REGIO TEMPORALIS. **trabecular r.** A region in the developing skull where the trabecular cartilages are placed, one on each side of the pituitary gland, and where the future sphenoid bone will develop. **umbilical r.** REGIO UMBILICALIS. **urogenital r.** REGIO UROGENITALIS. **V r.** VARIABLE REGION. **$V_H$ r.** The variable region of a heavy chain polypeptide of immunoglobulins. **$V_L$ r.** The variable region of a light chain polypeptide of immunoglobulins. **variable r.** That section of an immunoglobulin in which the amino acid sequence varies among different molecules within a single class of immunoglobulins and is related to the antibody combining site. In the light chain, this region is the N-terminal half, and in the heavy chain, the N-terminal portion. Also *V region*. Compare CONSTANT REGION. **vertebral r.** REGIO VERTEBRALIS. **vestibular r.** The area of the vestibule of the nose. **volar r. of hand** *Outmoded* PALMA MANUS. **zygomatic r.** REGIO ZYGOMATICA.

**regiones** \rē′jē·ō′nēz\ Plural of REGIO.

**register / immunization r.** A documentary record of the vaccinations and immunizations which have been given to each individual in the group to which the register relates.

**registration** [Med L *registratio*, from *registratus*, past part. of *registrare* to register, list] The process of recording vital events, certifications, or other public health actions. **r. of functional form** FUNCTIONAL IMPRESSION. **medical r.** In New Zealand, the legal process by which a physician is entitled to practice medicine. **occlusal r.** A registration of tooth contacts by means of wax or articulating paper, or by mounting casts on an articulator.

**registry** \rej′istrē\ **1** The list of all registrants or enrollees in a health insurance plan. Also *panel*. **2** The list of individuals who have or have had certain diseases, as in *cancer registry*. **cancer r.** An administrative mechanism for recording relevant information about individual patients with malignant disease for the purpose of cancer control. Registries may be hospital-based or population-based, the distinction being that the coverage of the latter is more comprehensive and, because the population at risk is defined, estimates of rates of cancer incidence can be derived. Both types will allow survival rates to be determined, given adequate arrangements for follow-up at appropriate intervals of individual patients included in the registry.

**regression** \rigresh′ən\ **1** A property characterizing two variables such that a given change in one (the independent variable) is accompanied by a change in the average value of the other (the dependent variable). **2** CATABOLISM. **3** Return to an earlier level of adaptation, as from an adult to an infantile level or from genitality to orality. Also *retrogression*. **curvilinear r.** NONLINEAR REGRESSION. **multiple r.** A regression involving more than one independent variable. **nonlinear r.** A regression that involves a polynomial, trigonometric, exponential, or other nonlinear function. Also *curvilinear regression*.

**regulation** **1** The capacity of part of an early embryo to form an entire embryo. **2** The intervention of government or of another party into the health-care marketplace through the specification of rules for providers and consumers. **down r.** GENE REPRESSION. **fertility r.** BIRTH CONTROL. **ontogenetic r.** A property of various parts of the fertilized ovum of certain species of remaking, after a loss of substance, a complete normally constituted embryo. It is found in sea urchins and urodeles, and is manifested only in the first stages of division of the ovum.

**regulator** [*regulat(e)* + -OR] REGULATOR GENE.

**regulon** \reg′yəlän\ [*regul(ate)* + -ON] A group of genes that are coordinately regulated but are not contiguous on the chromosome. For example, the *ara* regulon in enteric bacteria includes six genes involved in the uptake and metabolism of arabinose, located in three operons in different regions of the genome, and possessing similar promoter and operator loci.

**regurgitant** \rigur′jitənt\ 1 Flowing or allowing to flow backward. 2 Relating to or indicative of regurgitation.

**regurgitate** \rigur′jităt\ [Med L *regurgitare* to regurgitate, from Late L *gurgitare* to engulf, from L *gurges,* gen. *gurgitis,* the gullet, a gulf, the sea] 1 To flow or allow to flow backward. 2 To bring (gastric or esophageal contents) back up into the mouth.

**regurgitation** \rigur′jitā′shən\ 1 Retrograde passage of esophageal or gastric contents into the mouth, or of the contents of any alimentary chamber into a chamber proximal to it. 2 Retrograde flow of blood through a cardiac valve. **aortic r.** The regurgitation of blood from the aorta to the left ventricle as a consequence of incomplete closure of the aortic valve cusps during diastole. Also *aortic insufficiency, aortic incompetence, Corrigan's disease.* **duodenal r.** Flow of the alkaline duodenal contents backwards into the stomach. **functional r.** Regurgitation through a valve due to a functional disorder resulting in dilatation of the vessel or chamber to which the valve is attached, rather than to an organic lesion of the valve apparatus. **mitral r.** The regurgitation of blood from the left ventricle to the left atrium as a consequence of incomplete closure of the mitral valve. **pulmonary r.** Regurgitation of blood from the pulmonary artery to the right ventricle. Also *pulmonic regurgitation.* **tricuspid r.** The reflux of blood from the right ventricle to the right atrium during systole due to incomplete closure of the tricuspid valve. **valvular r.** Backflow through a cardiac valve as a result of inadequate closure of the valve apparatus.

**rehabilitate** \rē′həbil′ităt\ [Med L *rehabilitare* rehabilitate (from RE- + L *habilitas,* gen. *habilitatis,* fitness, ability, aptitude) to rehabilitate] To restore a function or an ability to (a patient) following impairment of that function or ability.

**rehabilitation** \rē′habil′itā′shən\ 1 Restoration to a preexisting state of normal use and function following impairment of that function. Also *reablement* (rare). 2 The branch of medical practice devoted to such restoration. When in the context of physical restoration of physical function, it is identified with the specialty of physical medicine and rehabilitation. • See note at PHYSICAL MEDICINE AND REHABILITATION under MEDICINE. **alaryngeal voice r.** Any procedures used to restore the production of voice after laryngectomy. A proportion of laryngectomees will, in time, produce voice with little or no help, others will do so under instruction from speech therapists, but the remainder will remain mute unless further surgical procedures prove successful. These procedures include the introduction of a voice prosthesis or, less often, cricopharyngeal myotomy. **functional r.** The restoration of function by appropriate treatment in order to enable a person to recover, to the fullest extent possible, a capacity for employment. It would include medical and surgical treatment, physiotherapy, and occupational therapy. **mouth r.** The provision of all the treatment needed to restore the teeth, as far as possible, to normal function, especially in mouths where there has been much tooth loss and occlusal disharmony. Also *oral rehabilitation.* **occlusal r.** The restoration of occlusal function by means of equilibration, supplying of restorations and prostheses, and altering of the vertical dimension. **oral r.** MOUTH REHABILITATION.

**rehabilitee** \rē′həbil′itē′\ An individual engaged in a program of rehabilitation.

**rehalation** \rē′həlā′shən\ REBREATHING.

**rehydration** \rē′hīdrā′shən\ [RE- + HYDRATION] The restoration of water or fluid content after depletion.

**Reichert** [Frederick Leet *Reichert,* U.S. surgeon, born 1894] See under METHOD.

**Reichert** [Karl Bogislaus *Reichert,* German anatomist, 1811–1883] 1 See under CARTILAGE. 2 Reichert substance. See under SUBSTANTIA INNOMINATA. 3 Reichert's arch. See under HYOID ARCH. 4 Reichert's recess. See under RECESSUS COCHLEARIS VESTIBULI. 5 Reichert's membrane. See under LAMINA LIMITANS ANTERIOR CORNEAE.

**Reichmann** [Frieda *Reichmann,* German neurologist, flourished 20th century] Goldstein-Reichmann syndrome. See under ACQUIRED CEREBELLAR SYNDROME.

**Reichstein** [Tadeus *Reichstein,* Polish-born Swiss chemist, born 1897] Reichstein's compound Q. See under 11-DEOXYCORTICOSTERONE.

**Reid** [Robert William *Reid,* Scottish anatomist, 1851–1939] Reid's base line. See under LINE.

**Reifenstein** [Edward Conrad *Reifenstein,* Jr., U.S. endocrinologist, 1908–1975] See under SYNDROME.

**Reil** [Johann Christian *Reil,* German physician, 1759–1813] 1 Reil's ansa. See under ANSA PEDUNCULARIS. 2 Reil's triangle, trigone of Reil. See under TRIGONUM LEMNISCI. 3 Circular sulcus of Reil, Reil sulcus, sulcus circularis Reili. See under SULCUS CIRCULARIS INSULAE. 4 Island of Reil, insula of Reil. See under INSULA. 5 Band of Reil. See under TRABECULA SEPTOMARGINALIS. 6 Band of Reil. See under RIBBON OF REIL

**Reilly** [William Anthony *Reilly,* U.S. pediatrician, born 1901] Reilly bodies, Alder-Reilly bodies. See under ALDER-REILLY ANOMALY.

**reimplant** \rē·im′plant\ [RE- + IMPLANT] REPLANT.

**reimplantation** \rē′implantā′shən\ REPLANTATION.

**reinfection** \rē′infek′shən\ Repeated infection with the same pathogenic microorganism.

**reinforcement** \rē′infôrs′mənt\ 1 Anything that strengthens the occurrence of a behavior, rendering it more probable and more vigorous, exact, or frequent. 2 In classical conditioning, the experimental pairing of a conditioned stimulus with an unconditioned stimulus. 3 In operant conditioning, any event following the occurrence of an operant response that increases the likelihood of that response to reoccur. Also *positive reinforcement.* **delayed r.** 1 In classical conditioning, a conditioned response established by presenting a conditioned stimulus over an extended interval before presenting the paired unconditioned stimulus. 2 In operant conditioning, a delay imposed on the delivery of reinforcement that is contingent on the making of a particular response, until a certain period of time has elapsed after the response has been made. **differential r.** In operant conditioning, the experimental procedure of selectively reinforcing one stimulus from an array of similar stimuli. The positive reinforcement of the designated stimulus, and the nonreinforcement or punishment of all others, leads to the formation of a discriminative response. **fixed interval r.** In operant conditioning, that schedule of reinforcement in which responses are reinforced after an interval of time has elapsed that is unvarying. Also *fixed interval schedule.* **fixed ratio r.** In operant conditioning, that schedule of reinforcement in which a reward, or reinforcement, is given after a certain number of responses have been made. For example, a food pellet may be delivered to an experimental animal subject whenever ten bar presses have been completed. This would be expressed as a ratio of reinforced to nonreinforced responses of 1:10. Also *fixed ratio schedule.* **negative r.** A rewarding of the desired response in an experimental animal by the absence or termination of some form of aversive stimulus, such as an electric shock or a loud noise. **positive r.** REINFORCEMENT. • In operant conditioning, this redundant phrase is sometimes employed deliberately, to make explicit the fact that no negative reinforcement was applied. **primary r.** Presentation of a reward, such as food to a hungry animal, that strengthens a response naturally, with no need for the subject to learn the value of the reward. **r. of reflexes** Any method which is used to elicit a deep tendon reflex that at first sight appears to be absent. The subject is encouraged to relax the muscle under test by mental effort (perhaps by performing a difficult calculation) or by contracting a different group of muscles as in clenching the two hands together (Jendrassik's maneuver). Also *facilitation of reflexes.* **secondary r.** In operant conditioning, any stimulus, event, or state that gains effectiveness as a reinforcement only by association with an initial or primary reinforcement. **r. of tendon reflexes** JENDRASSIK'S MANEUVER. **variable interval r.** A paradigm used in operant conditioning, in which the time interval between response and reinforcement is not fixed, but varies randomly around a specified average interval that falls within an arbitrarily selected range. Also *variable interval schedule.* **variable ratio r.** An operant conditioning paridigm in which an experimental animal is reinforced only after it has made a number of responses, but the exact number of responses is not fixed and varies randomly between reinforcements to the next around a specified average that falls within an arbitrarily selected range. Also *variable ratio schedule.*

**reinfusion** \rē′infyoo′zhən\ A procedure in which a previously drained body fluid such as blood, bile, or gastric fluid is returned to the body.

**Reinke** [Friedrich Berthold *Reinke,* German anatomist, 1862–1919] See under EDEMA.

**reinnervation** \rē′inərvā′shən\ Restoration of the nerve supply to a viscus, organ, or muscle following denervation.

**reinoculation** \rē′inäk′yəlā′shən\ Repeated inoculation with the same type of microorganism.

**Reinsch** [Adolf *Reinsch,* German physician, 1862–1916] See under TEST.

**reinversion** \rē′invur′zhən\ [RE- + INVERSION] The restoration of an inverted uterus to its normal shape and position. The uterus may invert in the third stage of labor when there is excessive traction on the placenta.

**Reisseisen** [Franz Daniel *Reisseisen,* German anatomist, 1773–1828] Reisseisen's muscles. See under MUSCLE.

**Reissner** [Ernst *Reissner,* German anatomist, 1824–1878] **1** See under FIBER. **2** Reissner's membrane. See under PARIES VESTIBULARIS DUCTUS COCHLEARIS.

**reiterature** [L] To repeat or renew: used in prescription writing.

**Reiter** [Hans Conrad Julius *Reiter,* German physician, 1881–1969] Reiter's disease, Fiessinger-Leroy-Reiter syndrome. See under REITER SYNDROME.

**rejection** **1** An immunologic reaction against incompatible grafted tissue on the part of the host's lymphoid tissues, marked by the destruction of the graft. Also *immunologic rejection.* **2** In ultrasound imaging, elimination of small amplitude signals from a display. **acute r.** Rapid loss of an allograft or xenograft after a delay of around one week, during which the immune response gains momentum. **acute renal transplant r.** Acute rejection of a transplanted kidney, occurring most commonly during the first six postoperative months, and rarely before one week or after two years. The kidney may be swollen and tender, and pathologically is characterized by interstitial edema and hemorrhages, and vascular lesions. Clinically, the first manifestations are a decrease in creatinine clearance and lymphocyturia, followed by malaise, fever, hypertension, and oliguria. The prognosis is good, and the condition usually responds to an increase in immunosuppressive therapy. **allograft r.** The immunologic rejection of a graft by a recipient who is of the same species as the donor but genetically dissimilar. **chronic r.** Slow, protracted rejection of an allograft. **chronic renal transplant r.** A gradual decrease in renal function beginning weeks to months after transplantation, often preceded by acute rejection episodes. Usually the condition is asymptomatic. Histologic changes include interstitial fibrosis and cellular infiltration, tubular dilatation and atrophy, narrowed small blood vessels due to intimal fibrosis, and progressive hyalinization of glomeruli. Immunofluorescent techniques show deposits of IgG, IgM, complement, and fibrin in small blood vessels and glomeruli. The condition is progressive and does not respond to increased doses of steroid preparations. **first set r.** Immunologic rejection by a previously unprimed host. Compare SECOND SET REJECTION. **graft r.** Destruction by the host of an allograft or a xenograft. **hyperacute r.** An intense, early immune response to an allograft or xenograft as a result of previous sensitization to donor antigens. Also *white graft reaction.* **hyperacute renal transplant r.** Sudden rejection occurring within five to ten minutes of perfusion of a transplanted kidney with the host's blood. The kidney becomes dark and swollen. Histologically, polymorphonuclear leukocytes and platelets are sequestered in glomeruli, and fibrin thrombi form in blood vessels and glomeruli. The reaction is mediated by circulating antibodies of the host directed against endothelia in the kidneys. No treatment is known, and the affected kidney should be removed immediately. Fortunately, crossmatch of the recipient's serum and the donor's lymphocyte will reveal the likelihood of hyperacute rejection prior to transplantation. **immunologic r.** REJECTION. **second set r.** Immunologic rejection by a primed host. Compare FIRST SET REJECTION.

**rel.** relative.

**rel. ams.** relative amount of substance.

**relapse** [L *relapsus* (past part. of *relabi* to slide, glide, fall back, from RE- + L *labi* to slide, glide, fall back) having slid, glided, or fallen back] A recurrence or marked increase in severity of the symptoms of a disease, especially following a period of apparent improvement or stability. **mucocutaneous r.** A recurrence of syphilis, manifesting itself by the presence of lesions of skin and mucous membranes. **rebound r.** The recurrence of symptoms following withdrawal of treatment.

**relapsing** Characterized by relapses or recurrences, as a fever.

**relation** / **centric r.** CENTRIC POSITION. **convenience r. of teeth** ACQUIRED ECCENTRIC OCCLUSION. **cusp-fossa r.** The gnathological relationship of a stamp cusp and its fossa. **eccentric r.** ECCENTRIC POSITION. **intermaxillary r.** MAXILLOMANDIBULAR RELATION. **jaw r.** MAXILLOMANDIBULAR RELATION. **jaw-to-jaw r.** MAXILLOMANDIBULAR RELATION. **mass-energy r.** The relation giving the energy $E$ equivalent to a given mass $m$, having the form $E = mc^2$, where $c$ is the speed of light in a vacuum. **maxillomandibular r.** The relation between the mandible and the maxilla, either anatomically or functionally. Also *jaw relation, jaw-to-jaw relation, intermaxillary relation.* **object r.'s** Emotional attachment to or association with other persons or objects, the adequacy of which is a measure of adaptational level and ego strength. **occlusal jaw r.** The maxillomandibular relation in centric or acentric position when the teeth are in contact. Also *occluding relation.* **Planck's quantum r.** The relationship between the energy $E$ of a quantum of electromagnetic radiation and the frequency $\nu$ of the radiation, given by the formula $E=h\nu$, where $h$ is Planck's constant. **protrusive r.** The relationship of the jaws when the mandible is protruded. Also *protrusive jaw relation.* **range-energy r.** The relation between the distance a charged particle travels through matter before its energy is dissipated, and its initial energy. The energy loss per unit length is a complicated nonlinear function. **rest r.** REST POSITION. **unstrained jaw r.** CENTRIC POSITION. **vertical r.** The relative position of the mandible to the maxilla in the vertical direction. Also *vertical opening.*

**relationship** The connection or association between different people or situations. **blood r.** A relationship between two or more people on the basis of shared ancestry; consanguinity. **confidential r.** Any relationship in which one party places confidence and trust in a second party and relies and acts upon the advice or instructions of the second party. Such a relationship may have a legal, social, domestic, religious, or personal basis, such as the relationship existing between patient and physician, client and attorney, congregation member and cleric, husband and wife, or child and parent. **dose-effect r.** The relationship of a given dose to a quantifiable effect. The time at which the dose is measured must correspond to the time at which the effect occurs. **dose-response r.** The response of a supposedly uniform population of cells, tissues, or animals to a given dose. **linear r.** A relationship in which biologic effect is directly related to the absorbed dose of radiation.

**relative / first-degree r.** Any of the parents, siblings, and offspring of an index person. The coefficient of relationship is one half. **second-degree r.** Any of the uncles, aunts, grandparents, and grandchildren of an index person. The coefficient of relationship is one fourth. **third-degree r.** Any of the first cousins, great-aunts, great-uncles, and great-grandparents of an index person. The coefficient of relationship is one eighth.

**relax** [L *relax(are)* (from *re-* anew + *laxare* to loosen, from *laxus* slack, loose) to slacken] **1** To relieve all tension on a muscle. **2** To relieve neurally generated muscular tension, but not necessarily passive tension due to stretch. **3** To relieve from anxiety or concern.

**relaxant** \rilak′sənt\ An agent that reduces tension. **muscle r.** A drug that reduces muscle tension by affecting neurons involved in muscle innervation or the myoneural junction, such as curare or succinylcholine. **smooth muscle r.** An agent that reduces the tension of smooth muscle, such as an antispasmodic drug.

**relaxation** The state of or the action resulting in diminution of muscular tension. **isometric r.** Reduction in the level of tension of a muscle without change in its length. Also *mecystatic relaxation, isostatic relaxation.* **isovolumetric r.** Relaxation of the myocardium without change in volume of the related chamber. It occurs during the period between the closure of the semilunar valves and the opening of the atrioventricular valves. Also *isovolumic relaxation.* **mecystatic r.** ISOMETRIC RELAXATION.

**relaxin** \rilak′sin\ A polypeptide of molecular weight approximately 8000, extractable from the corpus luteum of several species but not yet proved to be present in the human female. In some animals, the substance increases in the tissues and blood during pregnancy. It has the ability to relax the symphysis pubis, inhibit uterine contractility, and soften the cervix.

**relearning** SAVINGS METHOD.

**release / contracture r.** A surgical incision made across a scar or muscle that limits function. If the scar is in the skin and a defect results, the defect is closed with a skin graft or a flap to restore function. **laryngeal r.** An operation to allow the larynx to descend in the neck so as to reduce the tension on the suture line after excision of a lengthy tracheal stricture and end-to-end anastomosis. It requires division of the superior cornu of the thyroid cartilage on either side together with the thyrohyoid muscles and thyrohyoid membrane at the upper edge of the alae of the thyroid cartilage. Also *laryngeal drop operation.*

**relief** **1** The alleviation or cessation of pain, suffering, or stress. **2** A space made between part of a denture and the underlying tissue in order to reduce pressure in that area. Also *relief space.* **gingival r.** Relief over the gingival margin, in a partial denture.

**relieve** To free wholly or partly from pain, suffering, or stress.

**reline** \rēlīn′\ REBASE.

**relucence** \riloo′səns\ [L *reluceus,* pres. part. of *relucere* to shine back] The property of partially reflected light, as occurs in any imperfectly transparent structure, such as the cornea or lens. Relucence of these structures is the basis for their visibility when illuminated by a sharply focused beam of light, as with the biomicroscope, and for the gleaming of animal eyes in a strong light at night.

**REM** rapid eye movement.

**rem** \rem\ [from *roentgen equivalent man*] A unit of radiation dose equal to the rad weighted by factors proportional to the biologic effect of each type of radiation; 1 rem = $10^{-2}$ joule per kilogram or $10^{-2}$ sievert. Symbol: rem

**Remak** [Ernst Julius *Remak,* German physician, 1849–1911] **1** Remak symptom. See under SIGN. **2** Remak's reflex. See under FEMORAL REFLEX.

**Remak** [Robert *Remak,* German anatomist and histologist, 1815–1865] **1** Remak's ganglion. See under REMAK'S GANGLION, SINOATRIAL GANGLION. **2** Remak's nuclear division. See under AMITOSIS. **3** Remak's plexus. See under PLEXUS SUBMUCOSUS. **4** Fibers of Remak. See under FIBER.

**remedy** [L *remedium* (from *re-* thoroughly + *mederi* to heal, cure, alleviate; see also MEDICAL) a means of healing, cure] Any medication that cures a disease or relieves symptoms. **specific r.** A therapeutic agent that can cure a disease rather than merely relieve symptoms.

**remineralization** \rimin′əral′īzā′shən\ The restoration of minerals to the body, as occurs in bone after doses of vitamin D are administered to a patient with osteomalacia.

**remission** \rimish′ən\ [L *remissio* (from *remittere* to send back, release, relieve, from *re-* back + *mittere* to send) remittal, release, relief, abatement] **1** A temporary but marked reduction in severity or even disappearance of the symptoms of a disease. Also *remittence.* **2** A period in the course of a disorder characterized by such remission of symptoms.

**remit** \rimit′\ To undergo remission; temporarily abate or disappear, as symptoms.

**remittence** \rimit′əns\ REMISSION.

**remittent** \rimit′ənt\ Showing recurring cycles of remission and relapse: said especially of a disease or fever.

**remnant** \rem′nənt\ Something remaining. **acroblastic r.** The darker, peripheral part of the acroblast of a spermatid, which disintegrates during spermiogenesis. **allantoic r.** The vestige of the endodermal allantoic diverticulum, present in the umbilical cord close to its attachment to the anterior abdominal wall of a human fetus. It extends through the umbilicus to connect with the urachus and the urinary bladder. **dermal r.** The combination of dead and viable dermis remaining after débridement of the blister covering a partial thickness burn.

**removal** / **pulp r.** The removal of the vital dental pulp, including the radicular pulp. Also *pulpectomy, pulp extirpation.*

**remyelination** \rē′mī·əlinā′shən\ The restoration of the myelin sheath of a nerve or nerves after demyelination.

**ren** \ren\ [L *renes* the kidneys (sing. rare and problematical in form; of unknown origin)] (*pl.* renes) [NA] One of a pair of bean-shaped organs situated on the posterior abdominal wall on either side of the vertebral column and posterior to the peritoneum; the kidney. The right one is usually slightly lower than the left and the superior extremity of each is usually more rounded, larger, and nearer the midline than the inferior extremity. It extends from the level of the upper border of the twelfth thoracic vertebra to the third lumbar vertebra. The medial margin is concave where the hilum leads into the renal sinus occupied by the renal pelvis and calices, the renal vessels and nerves, and by some fatty and areolar tissue. It is invested by a thin capsule and its substance is divided into an outer part, or cortex, and an inner part, or medulla. It produces urine from the blood and helps to maintain fluid, electrolyte, and acid-base homeostasis.

**renal** \rē′nəl\ [Late L *renalis* (from *ren(es)* the kidneys + *-alis* -AL) pertaining to the kidneys] Of or relating to the kidneys.

**renaturation** \rinā′chərā′shən\ The refolding of a protein or nucleic acid into its native state after it has been unfolded. This may sometimes be achieved by placing it in mildly denaturing conditions, e.g. dilute urea solution for proteins, enabling the less stable, wrongly folded molecules to unfold, so that the chance of reaching the native structure is increased.

**Renaut** [Joseph Louis *Renaut,* French physician, 1844–1917] **1** Renaut's layer. See under MALPIGHIAN LAYER. **2** Renaut's bodies. See under BODY.

**renculi** \ren′kyəlī\ Plural of RENCULUS.

**renculus** \ren′kyələs\ RENICULUS.

**Rendu** [Henry Jules Louis Marie *Rendu,* French physician, 1844–1902] **1** Rendu-Osler-Weber syndrome, Osler-Weber-Rendu disease. See under HEREDITARY HEMORRHAGIC TELANGIECTASIA. **2** Fiessinger-Rendu syndrome. See under STEVENS-JOHNSON SYNDROME.

**renes** \rē′nēz\ Plural of REN.

**reni-** \ren′ē-\ RENO-.

**renicapsule** \ren′ikap′sʸool\ *Outmoded* GLANDULA SUPRARENALIS.

**reniculi** \rēnik′yəlī\ Plural of RENICULUS.

**reniculus** \rēnik′yələs\ [L, dim. of *ren* kidney] (*pl.* reniculi) One of the lobuli corticales renis. . *Outmoded.* Also *renunculus, renculus.*

**reniform** \ren′iform\ [RENI- + -FORM] NEPHROID.

**renin** \rē′nin, ren′in\ The enzyme (EC 3.4.99.19) that catalyzes the hydrolytic release of angiotensin I (proangiotensin) from the N terminus of angiotensinogen. It is produced by the kidney. **r. substrate** ANGIOTENSINOGEN.

**reninoma** \ren′inō′mə\ A renin-secreting juxtaglomerular cell tumor.

**rennet** \ren′ət\ Milk coagulated by the action of chymosin (rennin) on casein.

**rennin** *Obs.* CHYMOSIN. • The name was changed because of the danger of confusion with the other proteolytic enzyme, renin.

**renninogen** \rənin′əjən\ A zymogen within the gastric glands that, upon being secreted, is converted to rennin. Also *prerennin, prorennin.*

**reno-** \rē′nō-\ [L *ren* kidney] A combining form meaning kidney, renal. Also *reni-.*

**renogenic** \-jen′ik\ [RENO- + -GENIC] NEPHROGENIC.

**renogram** \rē′nəgram\ [RENO- + -GRAM] See under RADIONUCLIDE RENOGRAM. **isotope r.** RADIONUCLIDE RENOGRAM. **radionuclide r.** A radiographic recording of kidney function obtained by external monitoring of radioactivity after the administration of an appropriate radionuclide, such as *o*-[$^{131}$I]iodohippurate. Also *isotope renogram.*

**renography** \rēnäg′rəfē\ [RENO- + -GRAPHY] RADIORENOGRAPHY. **emission r.** RADIORENOGRAPHY. **isotope r.** An inaccurate term for RADIORENOGRAPHY.

**renoprival** \-prī′vəl\ [RENO- + -PRIVAL] Related or pertaining to the absence of the kidneys, as *renoprival hypertension.*

**renotrophic** \-träf′ik\ NEPHROTROPHIC.

**renotropic** \-träp′ik\ NEPHROTROPHIC.

**renovascular** \-vas′kyələr\ Related or pertaining to the vasculature of the kidneys, as *renovascular hypertension.*

**Renshaw** [B. *Renshaw,* U.S. neurophysiologist, flourished 20th century] Renshaw inhibition. See under RECURRENT INHIBITION.

**renunculus** \rēnun′kyələs\ RENICULUS.

**Reoviridae** \rē′ōvir′idē\ [*reovir(us)* + -IDAE] The family of viruses which consist of a nonlipid, icosahedrol capsid and a multisegmented double-stranded RNA genome. It comprises three genera: *Reovirus, Orbivirus,* and *Rotavirus..*

**reovirus** \rē′ōvī′rəs\ [*r(espiratory)* + *e(nteric)* + *o(rphan)* + VIRUS] **1** Any member of the family Reoviridae. **2** A member of the genus *Reovirus* of the family Reoviridae. This genus includes three human serotypes and avian, canine, and simian reoviruses.

**rep** Symbol for the obsolete unit, roentgen equivalent physical.

**rep.** *repetatur* (L, let it be repeated).

**repair** Restoration of damaged tissue, as by surgical intervention or by natural healing. **Brown-McDowell r. of cleft lip** A modification of Mirault's operation, using a smaller full-thickness triangular flap from the lateral side of the cleft. This method was a very popular repair for many years. **Cecil-Culp r. of hypospadias** A two-stage method of reconstructing the penile urethra, first using penile skin to recreate the urethra, and then scrotal skin to replace the penile skin used in the urethral reconstruction. **excision r.** The repair of nucleic acid, usually DNA, that requires the excision of a damaged part of the chain, as of the thymine dimers produced by the absorption of ultraviolet radiation.

**reparative** \riper′ətiv\ Pertaining to or characterized by repair.

**repeat** / **long terminal r.** A nucleotide sequence directly repeated at each end of a retroviral chromosome. It contains transcriptional control elements. Abbr. LTR **tandem r.** TANDEM DUPLICATION.

**repellent** **1** Serving to repel. **2** An agent that serves to repel (pestiferous organisms). **3** Causing subsidence of swelling. An obsolete usage. **4** An agent that causes subsidence of swelling. An obsolete usage.

**repercussion** \rē′pərkush′ən\ [L *repercussio* (from *repercutere* to beat back) repulsion, deflection. See PERCUSSION.] **1** A reaction or consequence. **2** BALLOTTEMENT.

**repetatur** [L] Let it be renewed: used in prescription writing.

**replacement** / **isomorphous r.** The replacement of one atom or group in a crystal without any overall change in the crystal morphology. In simple crystals this replacement may be of one ion by another. In protein crystals, their binding of heavy atoms, when it does not change the manner in which the protein crystallizes, is included, and it may help in solving their structures by x-ray crystallography. **reciprocal r.** RETINAL RIVALRY.

**replant** [RE- + *(im)plant*] **1** To replace (an amputated part) in its original site, often requiring microvascular techniques to reattach bones, vessels, nerves, and soft tissues. **2** To replace (an avulsed tooth) in the same socket. Also *reimplant.*

**replantation** The reattachment of an amputated body part, usually requiring the microsurgical anastomosis of small blood vessels. **intentional r.** The deliberate removal of a tooth and its replantation after obturation of the root canals.

**replicase** \rep′likās\ Any enzyme that catalyzes DNA replication, such as a DNA-directed DNA polymerase.

**replicate** \rep′likāt\ [L *replicare* (from *re-* back + *plicare* to fold) to fold back, go back over] **1** To duplicate, copy, or repeat, as to produce a new strand of deoxyribonucleic acid identical to the previous strand. **2** One of the two new strands of deoxyribonucleic acid, the new strand produced being a complement of the parent strand.

**replication** \rep′likā′shən\ [See REPLICATE.] **1** The process of producing multiple copies of a molecule, each copy being identical with the original. Genetic material (DNA) is replicated by a process in which the two strands of a deoxyribonucleic acid molecule separate, and a complementary strand of each part is produced. **2** The repeating of measurements, such as chemical estimations, conducted in parallel. Replication plays an important part in the design of experiments and in the statistical analysis of experimental results. **conservative r.** A hypothetical form of replication of DNA in which the whole of the parental double helix would remain intact and a new double helix would be formed: used to contrast such a process with the actual, semiconservative one. **nonconservative r.** A model for replication of the DNA molecule in which each newly formed strand contains bases from the parental molecule interspersed with the newly added bases. This model currently receives little support while the semiconservative replication model is currently held to be correct. Also *dispersive replication.* **semiconservative r.** Replication of DNA in which the two strands of the double helix undergo a partial separation due to breakage of hydrogen bonds and a regional unwinding, thus allowing each strand to serve as a template for the synthesis of a complementary strand by specific base pairing. Each resulting daughter molecule of DNA consists of one parent strand and one new strand.

**replicon** \rep′likän\ A segment of the genome in which deoxyribonucleic acid replication is occurring.

**repolarization** \rēpō′ləriză′shən\ The recovery of polarity, as in the return of membrane potential to resting values following depolarization.

**repositioning** \rē′pəzish′əning\ **jaw r.** Changing of the position of the mandible in relation to the maxilla, usually by occlusal adjustment of natural or artificial teeth. **muscle r.** The surgical alteration of a muscle function brought about by changing the tendon origins or insertions.

**repositor** \ripäz′itər\ An instrument used to reposition organs, such as a retroflexed uterus.

**repository** \ripäz′itôrē\ A depot representing the site of a drug injection, usually intramuscularly, from which the drug is slowly released to maintain a prolonged therapeutic effect.

**representation** / **sensorimotor r.** The pattern by which different body regions are localized functionally and anatomically in the sensory receiving and motor areas of the precentral and postcentral gyri of the cerebral cortex.

**repression** \ripresh′ən\ [Late L *repressio* (from L *reprimere* to hold back, repress, from RE- + *premere* to press) a holding back, restraining] A fundamental unconscious defense consisting of the exclusion of objectionable wishes, ideas, or other material from the consciousness. **catabolite r.** The repression of the biosynthesis by glucose of a number of bacterial enzymes needed to catabolize other compounds, e.g. galactosides. This repression is mediated by a lowering of the concentration of cyclic AMP within the organism. **coordinate r.** An increase in the repressor concentration that causes a parallel reduction of more than one enzyme, either in one metabolic pathway or in several pathways. **end-product r.** The inhibition of enzymic activity in a metabolic pathway by the end product of the metabolic process. Also *enzyme repression.* **gene r.** A decrease of the activity of a gene resulting in a reduction of messenger ribonucleic acid production. The repressing agent may be a protein produced under control of a regulator gene. Also *down regulation.*

**repressor** \ripres′ər\ A molecule, usually a protein, produced under control of a regulator gene which binds to an operator gene, thus turning off transcription to the operon. **active r.** An aporepressor which combines with a corepressor to become active. It then combines with the operon, inhibiting transcription. **inactive r.** A repressor protein which has formed a complex with a metabolite and is thus unable to bind to the operator gene.

**reproduction** \rē′prəduk′shən\ [RE- + L *productio* extension, lengthening, prolongation, from *producere* to lead or bring out, from *pro-* forward + *ducere* to draw, lead, conduct] Any of the processes by which organisms produce new organisms; the production of offspring by sexual or asexual means. **asexual r.** The production of offspring by mitosis; reproduction without gametes, as in budding, fission, apomitis, and parthenogenesis. Also *asexual generation, nonsexual generation, direct generation.* **bisexual r.** SEXUAL REPRODUCTION. **cytogenic r.** Reproduction by means of spores, including either sexually or asexually formed spores. **human r.** The processes related to the creation and delivery of new human beings. **sexual r.** The union of two gametes, a sperm and an ovum, to form a zygote. Each gamete provides half of the genetic complement of the normal somatic cell of the species. Also *bisexual reproduction, syngenesis, syngamy, amphigony, sexual generation, gamogenesis.* **unisexual r.** PARTHENOGENESIS. **vegetative r.** Asexual reproduction in which the parent is a multicellular organism that divides to form two organisms.

**reproductive** \rē′prōduk′tiv\ Relating to or capable of reproduction.

**reptilase** \rep′tilās\ An enzyme that is found in the venom of *Bothrox atrops* and that clots fibrinogen by splitting off its fibrinopeptide A.

**repullulation** \ripul′yəlā′shən\ The recurrence or renewal of a morbid process.

**repulsion** \ripul′shən\ **1** The act or force of driving away. **2** In genetics, with reference to two linked, doubly heterozygous loci, the occurrence of the mutant alleles on different chromosomes. If A and B designate the wild type and a and b the mutant alleles at the two loci, then the genes are in repulsion if a and b are on different homologues (Ab/aB); that is, the genes are in trans configuration. Also *repulsion phase.* Compare COUPLING. **capillary r.** The force that tends to separate adjacent floating bodies if one can be moistened by a liquid and the other cannot.

**requirement** / **minimum daily r.** The minimum amount of each nutrient needed to prevent any sign or symptom of its nutritional deficiency disease. It varies from person to person. Abbr. MDR

**RES** reticuloendothelial system.

**rescinnamine** $C_{35}H_{42}N_2O_9$. 3,4,5-Trimethoxycinnamic acid ester of methyl reserpinate, an alkaloid from *Rauwolfia serpentina* and other *Rauwolfia* species. It has been used in the treatment of hypertension and as a tranquilizer.

**research** Scientific inquiry to discover or verify facts, test hypotheses, and elucidate theories. **clinical r.** Medical research involving patients, as in testing experimental drugs, new therapies or diagnostic techniques, or in conducting epidemiologic investigations.

**resect** \risekt′\ [L *resectus* (past part. of *resecare* to cut off, cut out, shorten, from RE- + L *secare* to cut, cut off) cut off, cut out, shortened] To excise a tissue or part of an organ.

**resectable** \risek′təbl\ Capable of being excised or resected.

**resection** \risek′shən\ [See RESECT.] Surgical removal of a part of a structure. **gastric r.** A gastrectomy in which luminal continuity is reestablished following removal of the stomach. **levator r.** A method of shortening the levator palpebri muscle in the treatment of ptosis of the upper eyelid. Utilizing either a transcutaneous or a transconjunctival approach, an appropriate length of levator tendon is excised and the remaining tendon reattached to the upper eyelid. **mandibular r.** The excision of a portion of the mandible. **maxillary r.** The excision of a portion of the maxilla. **Mikulicz r.** A nearly obsolete method of resecting tumors of the colon wherein the first stage consists of placing the tumor-bearing segment on the skin and closing the abdominal wall behind it. In the second stage the tumor is resected. **pulmonary r.** Surgical removal of all or part of a lung. **root r.** APICOECTOMY. **submucous r.** 1 The resection of any submucous structure while preserving intact the overlying mucous membrane. 2 SUBMUCOUS RESECTION OF THE NASAL SEPTUM. **submucous r. of the nasal septum** An operation for straightening the deviated nasal septum. The mucoperichondrium and mucoperiosteum of the septum is raised as a continuous sheet from either side of the enclosed cartilage and bone which is then removed to a sufficient extent to correct the deviation. Also *submucous resection.* **submucous r. of the vocal cord** An operation to improve the laryngeal airway in cases of bilateral abductor paralysis of the larynx. The mucosa is incised along the length of the cord and the subjacent fibrous and muscular components of the vocal fold removed. **transurethral r.** Prostatic resection using an instrument inserted through the urethra. **wedge r.** Surgical removal of a triangular segment of tissue.

**resectoscope** \risek′təskōp\ [RESECT + *o* + -SCOPE] An instrument used for transurethral resection of prostatic or bladder tissue.

**reserpine** \risur′pēn\ An alkaloid isolated from the root of several species of *Rauwolfia.* It decreases the concentration of 5-hydroxytryptamine in the central nervous system. It is used in the treatment of mild degrees of hypertension and as a tranquilizer for some psychoneurotic disorders.

**reserve** [L *reservare* (from RE- + L *servare* to observe, watch for, guard, preserve) to lay up, keep back, reserve] A quantity available beyond what is normally needed; a surplus of potential use in extraordinary circumstances. **alkali r.** PLASMA BICARBONATE. **alkaline r.** PLASMA BICARBONATE. **breathing r.** RESPIRATORY RESERVE. **cardiac r.** The potential of the heart to increase its function beyond its normal work load. **lifetime r.** The amount of coverage in an insurance policy, often expressed in such measures as hospital days, which are available for use over an individual's lifetime in accordance with the provisions of the policy. **respiratory r.** The difference between the ventilation of the lungs at rest and the greatest ventilation that can be attained by that subject. Also *breathing reserve.*

**reservoir** \rez′ərvwär\ [French *réservoir,* from *réserver* to reserve, from L *reservare* to lay up, keep back, reserve. See RESERVE.] 1 A space, container, or depot in which something accumulates or is kept in reserve. 2 See under RESERVOIR OF INFECTION. 3 RESERVOIR HOST. **chromatin r.** KARYOSOME. **r. of infection** Any part of the living or the inanimate environment which harbors and favors the persistence over a sufficiently long period of pathogenic organisms capable of being transmitted to humans or animals. The chief reservoir of human infection is humanity itself, but animals, plants, the soil, and inanimate objects can also act as reservoirs of infection. **Ommaya r.** A sterile plastic device consisting of a receptacle placed under the scalp and connected to a tube entering a cerebral ventricle. Therapeutic injections are made into the ventricle via the receptacle in cases of meningitis, leukemia, and some other diseases.

**reset** To restore a mechanism, device, or electronic circuit to its original state, as in restoring a counter to zero.

**resettlement** The set of medical, social, educational, and vocational measures aimed at enabling a physically or mentally handicapped person to find and retain employment. **occupational r.** A process of industrial rehabilitation whereby a person, following an incomplete recovery from an accident or disease, is placed in a new occupation better suited than the previous one to his or her present capabilities.

**residency** [*residen(t)* + *-cy,* suffix denoting position, office, rank] The training period in medicine and certain other health professions that follows formal degree programs. Residencies often last from three to seven years, are usually hospital-based, and lead to specialty board eligibility.

**resident** [L *residens,* gen. *residentis,* pres. part. of *residere* (from *re-* again + *sedere* to sit) to abide, stay] 1 Normally living in the habitat in which it is found: said of flora and fauna. 2 A health care professional who is completing a residency.

**residua** \rizij′oo·ə\ \risid′yoo·ə\ Plural of RESIDUUM.

**residue** \rez′əd$^y$oo\ [L *residuum.* See RESIDUUM.] 1 That which remains after a part has been removed. 2 In chemistry, a unit within a molecule, especially within a polymer. Thus an amino-acid residue in a peptide is that which remains of the amino-acid molecule after the condensation reaction of peptide formation, i.e., the group —NH—CHR—CO— if the residue is internal. **acceptable pesticide r.** The proportional amount of a pesticide remaining in or on food or feed that is regarded as harmless and is therefore acceptable by government regulatory agencies. **pesticide r.** The proportional amount of a pesticide that has not undergone degradation and which remains in the environment after a given period of time.

**residuum** \risid′yoo·əm\ [L (substantive from *residuum,* neut. sing. of *residuus,* past part. of *residere* to remain sitting, abide, from RE- + L *sedere* to sit, be settled, lie still), the remainder, residue] (*pl.* residua) The remainder or residue; that which remains after the removal of something else from a mixture. **gastric r.** That remaining in the stomach at a certain point in time. This most commonly refers to the gastric contents remaining during the interdigestive period, as in the morning after an overnight fast.

**resin** \rez′in\ [Middle English *recyn, resin,* from Middle

French *resine* resin, from L *resina* resin, from Gk *rētinē* (from *rhein* to run) gum, resin] **1** A sticky substance exuded by trees. **2** Any substance formed by polymerization. Thus an ion exchanger prepared from a polymer, e.g. by sulfonation of a solid polystyrene, may be called an ion-exchange resin. **activated r.** AUTOPOLYMER RESIN. **autopolymer r.** A resin that does not require heat for polymerization. Also *activated resin, cold-curing resin, self-curing resin.* **composite r.** A resin containing a high proportion of inorganic filler, used to simulate dentin and enamel. **copolymer r.** A mixture of chemically different polymers. **epoxy r.** Any of a group of substances made from epichlorohydrin and a polyhydroxy compound in the presence of hardening agents such as polyamines. Epoxy resins are resistant to heat and to chemicals and are used in coatings, adhesives, and reinforced plastics. Health problems, such as primary irritant and allergic dermatitis and asthma, arise mainly from contact with the hardeners. **ion-exchange r.** **1** An ion exchanger based on a synthetic polymer. **2** Any solid ion exchanger, such as a cellulose derivative. See also ANION EXCHANGER, CATION EXCHANGER. **jalap r.** JALAP. **phentermine r.** A complex combination of phentermine hydrochloride with an ion exchange resin in order to obtain a sustained, prolonged release of the drug. It is used orally as an anorexic medication. **podophyllum r.** The powdered mixture of resins from *Podophyllum peltatum* and *P. hexandrum.* It is a caustic for certain papillomas and it has been used as a drastic purgative and a hydragogue cathartic. Also *podophyllin.* **polyamine-methylene r.** A condensation product of phenol with polyamines to form an ion exchange resin. It has the capacity to adsorb acid and is used as an antacid treatment. It is administered orally. **polyester r.** An embedding medium for electron microscopy that is similar to the epoxy resins. **quinine carbacrylic r.** See under DIAGNEX BLUE TEST. **self-curing r.** AUTOPOLYMER RESIN. **sulfonated polystyrene r.** The ion exchanger most commonly used for chromatographic separation of amino acids. It consists of a polymer of styrene, cross-linked by inclusion of divinylbenzene, sulfonated to give it strongly acidic groups. Such resins are also used for water softening, since their sodium salts can remove calcium ions from water.

**res ipsa loquitur** [L, the thing speaks for itself] The doctrine in medical malpractice that when an injury occurs to a patient in a situation under the sole and exclusive control of the defendant and where such injury would not normally occur if the one in control had used due care, then it is presumed that the defendant is negligent.

**resistance** [L *resistens* (gen. *resistentis,* pres. part. of *resistere* to step back, stand still, stop, resist, from RE- + L *sistere* to put, place, cause to stand; akin to *stare* to stand, whence *-ance* in *resistance,* and to Gk *histanai* to set, place) stepping back, standing still, stopping, resisting] **1** The native or acquired ability of an organism to maintain its immunity to antagonistic agents in its environment. Resistance may be absolute or relative. **2** The measure of that property, expressed in ohms. Symbol: *R* **acquired radiation r.** The development of increasing tissue radioresistance, as may occur secondary to previous exposure to radiotherapy. **airway r.** The resistance to flow of air in the airways; the reciprocal of airway conductance. **basilar membrane r.** The electrical resistance of the basilar membrane of the cochlea as measured in ohm/cm$^2$, concerned with the maintenance of the observed potential difference between the scala media endolymph (+80 mV) and the scala tympani perilymph (+7 mV). **capillary r.** The resistance to unchecked blood flow that takes place in the capillaries. **cogwheel r.** COGWHEEL SIGN. **ego r.** **1** In psychiatry, the maintenance of repression resulting from fear of allowing into consciousness what has so long been denied entry. **2** In psychiatry, the maintenance of symptoms because of the epinosic gain they provide. **expiratory r.** The resistance to movement of the lung and chest wall during expiration. This involves tissue resistance and airway resistance. **hybrid r.** Resistance to infection or noxious agents in species in which there has been mixing of dissimilar genetic pools. For example, certain outbred strains of mice are relatively more resistant than inbred mice to infection. **id r.** In psychoanalytic therapy, a temporary stalemate between patient and therapist characterized by mistrust, grievance, and seemingly endless repetition of the same material on the part of the patient, no matter how many interpretations are given by the therapist and no matter how valid those interpretations might be. Id resistance is believed to be a derivative of the repetition compulsion. **inductive r.** REACTANCE. **input r.** The resistance across the cell wall of a neuron or other cell body to an intracellulary injected current pulse. **insulin r.** A subnormal or absent hypoglycemic response to administered insulin. It may be due to any of several causes, such as the presence of circulating insulin antibodies, a local allergic reaction to insulin, an acute exacerbation of chronic leukemia, or various endocrine or metabolic diseases, including the ketoacidosis of diabetes mellitus. **natural r.** NATURAL IMMUNITY. **peripheral r.** The resistance provided by the arterioles to the flow of blood through the small blood vessels. **phenotypic r.** **1** The resistance of a rare bacterial cell in a population to killing by a bactericidal agent, though its progeny are sensitive. See also PERSISTERS. **2** The reversible increase in resistance induced by subinhibitory levels of certain antibiotics (erythromycin, lincomycin), by activating a gene that methylates a base in ribosomal RNA. **pulmonary r.** The resistance to flow of air in the airways (airway resistance) plus the resistance to expansion of the lung tissues. **superego r.** NEGATIVE THERAPEUTIC REACTION. **vascular r.** The resistance to the flow of blood through blood vessels.

**resistant** \rizis′tənt\ Able to survive or flourish in spite of exposure to a substance or condition ordinarily having a noxious or destructive effect.

**resistivity** \rē′zistiv′itē\ A measure of a material's resistance to the passage of electric current, equal to the electric field intensity divided by the current density; the reciprocal of conductivity.

**resistor** \rizis′tər\ A component, usually of wire or carbon, that has electrical resistance and is placed in a circuit to limit current flow.

**resolution** \rez′əloo′shən\ [L *resolutio* (from *resolutus,* past part. of *resolvere* to unbind, loosen, open, from RE- + L *solvere* to loosen, unbind, free, from *se-* apart, aside + *luere* to liberate; akin to Gk *lyein* to loosen and to English *loose*) an unbinding, loosening dispelling] **1** The stage in a pathologic process marked by the subsidence of inflammation. **2** The ability of an optical or electronic imaging system to display separate images of two closely spaced structures. Also *definition.* **angular r.** LATERAL RESOLUTION. **axial r.** The minimal axial distance at which two targets along a beam of sound or x rays can be separately imaged. Also *range resolution, longitudinal resolution, depth resolution.* **azimuthal r.** LATERAL RESOLUTION. **depth r.** **1** The capacity of an instrument to define structures within materials as compared with surface definition. **2** AXIAL RESOLUTION. **energy r.** The process measuring the smallest relative difference between the energies of particles or photons by means of a radiation spectrometer. **lateral r.** The minimal lateral distance at which two targets along a beam of sound or x rays can be separately imaged. Also *azimuthal resolution, angular resolution, transverse resolution.* **longitudinal r.** AXIAL RESOLUTION. **range r.** AXIAL RESOLUTION. **spatial r.** 1 The minimal distance at which an optical system can distinguish two objects. 2 The maximal spatial frequency in line pairs/mm at which an optical system can distinguish a periodic pattern of parallel black and white lines. **transverse r.** LATERAL RESOLUTION.

**resolve** \rizälv'\ 1 To subside or cause to subside without suppurating: used of an inflammation. 2 To make or become normal after a pathologic process. 3 To separate or become separated into its component parts.

**resolvent** \rizäl'vənt\ An agent capable of promoting resolution of a lesion, such as an inflammatory exudate.

**resonance** \rez'ənəns\ [L *resonantia* (from *resonare* to resound, from *sonare* to sound, make a noise) echo, reverberation] 1 A condition of a mechanical or electrical system in which a small oscillating stimulus produces a large oscillation, or an impulse stimulus produces a prolonged oscillation at the natural frequency. 2 The prolonged sound that results from percussion over an air-containing viscus. 3 The phenomenon that no one formula adequately represents a molecule, but that it behaves as a hybrid of two or more formulas that differ only in the location of electrons. **amphoric r.** A sound with echoing character heard on percussion over a large lung cavity. Also *cavernous resonance.* **bell-metal r.** COIN SOUND. **cavernous r.** AMPHORIC RESONANCE. **cracked-pot r.** See under CRACKED-POT SOUND. **electron paramagnetic r.** The technique of observing the absorption of electromagnetic radiation due to a transition of an unpaired electron from its lower state to its higher state. The two states differ in energy because of the presence of an applied magnetic field. The position of the resonance, and its character, can give information about the environment of the electron. The name derives from the fact that substances with unpaired electrons, such as transition-metal ions and organic radicals, are paramagnetic. Also *electron spin resonance.* Abbr. e.p.r. **electron spin r.** ELECTRON PARAMAGNETIC RESONANCE. Abbr. e.s.r. **nasal r.** The altered quality of speech resulting from the conditions causing hypernasality or hyponasality. Also *rhinolalia, rhinism, rhinophonia, nasal speech, nasal intonation.* **nuclear magnetic r.** A phenomenon in which certain nuclei when placed in a strong magnetic field exhibit two distinct energy levels, due to the interaction of the applied magnetic field with the nuclear spin. Transitions between levels may be induced or detected by electromagnetic radiation of the proper, or resonant, frequency, thus yielding information about the nuclei present. See also MAGNETIC RESONANCE IMAGING. Abbr. NMR **proton magnetic r.** A particular case of nuclear magnetic resonance in which the nuclei of interest are those of hydrogen atoms. Abbr. p.m.r. **tympanic r.** The drumlike sound produced by percussing an air-filled cavity. **tympanitic r.** The quality of sound produced by percussion of an abdomen affected with tympanites. **vesicular r.** The resonance heard on percussion of the normal chest. **vocal r.** The sound of the voice as heard on auscultation over the chest. Abbr. VR **whispering r.** The sound of the whispering voice heard distinctly on auscultation of the chest.

**resonant** \rez'ənənt\ 1 Characterized or enhanced by resonance. 2 Prolonged or resounding: characterizing the sound produced by percussion over a hollow or air-containing viscus.

**resonator** \rez'ənā'tər\ [L *resonatus* (past part. of *resonare* to sound back, echo, ring again; see RESONANCE) sounded back, echoed + -OR] 1 A resonant electrical circuit in which oscillations are induced by a nearby circuit containing oscillations at the same frequency. 2 A hollow cavity used to intensify sounds.

**resorb** \risôrb'\ To absorb or assimilate a product of the body, such as an exudate, a cellular growth, bone, etc.

**resorbent** 1 Having the capacity to resorb. 2 A drug or agent that enhances resorption.

**resorcin** RESORCINOL. • This term is placed in front of the name of a color to name a dye of that color derived from resorcinol, e.g. *resorcin brown.*

**resorcinol** *M*-Dihydroxybenzene, a phenol. It is the only dihydroxybenzene that is nota strong reducing agent, since no quinone can be formed by its oxidation. Also *resorcin.*

**resorption** \risôrp'shən\ [L *resorpt(us),* past part. of *resorbere* to suck or draw back + -ION] The removal by absorption of a substance previously deposited, secreted, or excreted, such as dissolution of bone into body fluids or absorption by epithelia of substances which have previously been secreted or excreted. Also *reabsorption.* **apical root r.** Resorption of a root apex associated with chronic infection or excessive orthodontic movement. **bone r.** A reduction in bone mass by osteoclastic activity. It can be normal during hemostasis or abnormal during loss of bone mass. **external root r.** Resorption of a tooth root from the external, or periodontal membrane, surface. Also *surface root resorption.* **gingival r.** GINGIVAL RECESSION. **horizontal r.** A pattern of bone loss in periodontal disease in which bone is resorbed from the alveolar crest but the general level of the crest is horizontal. Any pockets developing are suprabony. **idiopathic r.** Resorption of a tooth which is not physiological and cannot be attributed to disease. **internal r.** Resorption of a tooth from the pulp. See also PINK TOOTH. **physiologic r.** Resorption associated with the remodeling of bone and with the exfoliation of deciduous teeth. **rear r.** UNDERMINING RESORPTION. **surface root r.** EXTERNAL ROOT RESORPTION. **undermining r.** Resorption of the wall of a tooth socket from the bone marrow side, and not from the side of the periodontal membrane. Also *rear resorption.* **vertical r.** A pattern of bone loss in periodontal disease in which bone resorption is irregular, parts or all of some teeth being relatively unaffected. Radiographically, vertical clefts are seen in the bone against some tooth surfaces and the periodontal pockets are often intrabony.

**respiration** [L *respiratio* (from *respiratus,* past part. of *respirare* to breathe back, draw breath, recover breath, abate, from RE- + L *spirare* to breathe, blow) a breathing, exhalation] 1 The totality of the processes of gaseous exchange between the tissues of the body and the environment in which the body exists. 2 The process of breathing. **abdominal r.** Respiration in which movement is predominantly or entirely abdominal and not thoracic. **aerobic r.** A respiratory process in which oxygen is being utilized by the tissues. **anaerobic r.** The release of energy from chemical reactions in the absence of free oxygen. **artificial r.** Respiratory movements carried out by extrinsic means such as intermittent positive pressure. *Older term.* Also *artificial ventilation.* **ataxic r.** Irregular respiration with random sequence of deep and shallow breaths observed in some subjects with lesions of the medulla oblongata. **Biot's r.** A form of breathing in which periods of apnea are interrupted by several consecutive deep breaths. It is said to be a sign of meningitis. **bronchial r.** See under BRONCHIAL BREATHING. **bronchocavernous r.** CAVERNOUS RESPIRATION. **bronchovesicular r.** A respiratory sound heard on auscultation of the lung that has characteristics of both bronchial and vesicular, or normal, breathing. **cavernous r.** An abnormally hollow or echoing respiratory sound heard on auscultation over a large air-containing lung cavity. Also *bronchocavernous respiration.* **cell r.** The release of energy from chemical reactions taking place within cells. Also *cellular respiration.* **Cheyne-Stokes r.** An extreme form of periodic breathing in which periods of shallow or absent breathing are followed by periods of hyperpnea. It is usually associated with severe lung disease, heart failure, cerebrovascular disease, or bilateral pyramidal tract damage. **cogwheel r.** Jerkiness or interruption of the inspiratory phase of breathing. Also *interrupted respiration, jerky respiration, wavy respiration.* **collateral r.** Respiratory exchange of gases in portions of the lung which are not directly ventilated through their own airways but which receive air from adjacent parts of the lung. **costal r.** THORACIC RESPIRATION. **diaphragmatic r.** See under DIAPHRAGMATIC BREATHING. **diffusion r.** Oxygenation of blood by diffusion of oxygen without respiratory movements taking place. Also *apneic oxygenation.* **direct r.** A direct gaseous exchange between living tissue and the environment without the intervention of the blood circulation. **external r.** The component of respiration that involves a gaseous exchange between the external environment and the circulating blood, across the surface of a respiratory organ as lungs or gills. **fetal r.** PLACENTAL RESPIRATION. **intermittent positive pressure r.** See under INTERMITTENT POSITIVE PRESSURE BREATHING. **internal r.** TISSUE RESPIRATION. **interrupted r.** COGWHEEL RESPIRATION. **jerky r.** COGWHEEL RESPIRATION. **Kussmaul r.** The rapid, deep, and noisy hyperpnea characteristic especially of diabetic ketoacidosis. Also *Kussmaul-Kien respiration, Kussmaul breathing, Kussmaul sign, Kussmaul symptom, air hunger.* **mouth-to-mouth r.** MOUTH-TO-MOUTH RESUSCITATION. **paradoxical r.** Respiration in which one lung becomes deflated during inspiration, usually as a result of chest trauma. **pendelluft r.** See under PENDELLUFT. **periodic r.** See under PERIODIC BREATHING. **placental r.** The process of gaseous exchange between maternal and fetal blood occurring at the placenta. Also *fetal respiration.* **spontaneous r.** Respiration occurring without physical or medicinal aid. **stertorous r.** Breathing accompanied by snoring as in deep sleep or coma. **suppressed r.** Voluntary limitation of depth of breathing, usually due to pleuritic pain. **thoracic r.** Respiration in which movement is predominantly of the thorax and not of the abdomen. Also *costal respiration.* **tidal r.** Relaxed breathing in which the tidal volume of air is breathed in each cycle. **tissue r.** 1 The process of gaseous exchange between cells and their environment. 2 The utilization of oxygen and production of carbon dioxide by a tissue. For defs. 1 and 2 also *internal respiration.* **tubular r.** An abnormal respiratory sound heard on auscultation of the lungs suggestive of the sound produced by blowing through a tube. **vesicular r.** See under VESICULAR BREATHING. **wavy r.** COGWHEEL RESPIRATION.

**respirator** \res′pərā′tər\ [L *respiratus* blown or breathed back + -OR. See RESPIRATION.] 1 A machine to deliver artificial ventilation. 2 A device which is placed over the face or head to prevent inhalation of harmful or unpleasant fumes or dusts. **demand r.** A mechanical ventilator in which onset of inspiration triggers a gas pressure or volume sufficient for a therapeutic tidal volume. **Drinker r.** TANK VENTILATOR. **Engström r.** A volume-controlled respirator used during and after the administration of anesthesia, as in open-heart surgery, to prevent hypoxia and excessive retention of carbon dioxide. It is often used to assist breathing in the immediate postoperative period. **protective r.** An appliance that covers the nose and mouth and enables the subject to breathe air through a medium that removes most of a contaminant such as dangerous dust or gas. There are five types: 1) filtering facepiece, in which the whole facepiece is made of filtering material and is disposable; 2) half-mask, in which the facepiece covers the nose and mouth and has a replaceable filter cartridge; 3) full facepiece, connected to a cannister worn on a harness; 4) powered air, a purifying respirator which draws air through a filter element, supplying purified air through a half-mask or full facepiece; and 5) powered visor, in which purified air is blown down behind a protective visor past the wearer's face. All these respirators are available with mutable filters to protect against dusts, fibers, gases, and vapors.

**respiratory** \rəspī′rətôr′ē, res′pirətôr′ē\ Of or relating to respiration.

**respirometer** \res′piräm′ətər\ SPIROMETER.

**respirometry** \res′piräm′ətrē\ SPIROMETRY.

**respondeat superior** \rispän′dē·at\ [L, let the master answer] A legal doctrine, important in cases of medical malpractice, which establishes the general rule that an employer is liable for those negligent acts of an employee which are committed in the course of employment.

**response** [L *respons(um)* (from neut. sing. of *responsus,* past part. of *respondere* to reply) a response] 1 Any organic process elicited by a stimulus, as a muscular or glandular process or a biochemical or immunochemical reaction. 2 Any mental process or behavior stimulated by a prior mental process or behavior. In psychology, mental or behavioral response is the dependent variable determined by the action of other independent variables. **allergic r.** IMMUNE RESPONSE. • See note at immune response. **anal r.** Contraction of the subcutaneous part of the external anal sphincter in response to stroking the perianal region or entry into the anal canal. It is mediated over sacral 4, 5 and coccygeal segmented levels. Also *wink response.* **anamnestic r.** 1 An antibody response of increased amplitude and more rapid onset that typically follows a second or subsequent administration of an antigen to the host. 2 An increase in antibody level to various antigens an animal has previously encountered that occurs following exposure to certain nonspecific agents, as typhoid vaccine or silica crystals. Also *recall response, booster response, memory response, secondary response, secondary immune response.* **anticipatory r.** A response, or a partial response, made in a behavioral situation before the stimulus specified as correct has been given. A runner jumping the gun would be a familiar example. **autoimmune r.** A cellular and humoral immunologic response on the part of the host to its own tissues. Although some autoimmune responses occur normally in most subjects, most autoimmune responses are regarded as pathologic and some may cause autoimmune disease. Examples include antiacetylcholine receptor antibodies in myasthenia gravis; anti-intrinsic factor antibodies in pernicious anemia; and a variety of autoantibodies to nonorgan-specific cellular components, giving rise to immune complexes in systemic lupus erythematosus. **average evoked r.** AVERAGE EVOKED POTENTIAL. **Babinski r.** EXTENSOR PLANTAR RESPONSE. **booster r.** ANAMNESTIC RESPONSE. **brainstem evoked r.** The changes in electrical potential taking place in the nuclei and neural pathways within the brainstem as a result of indirect stimulation.

**conditioned r.** A simple, learned response produced by repeatedly pairing, in a nearly simultaneous sequence, a neutral or inadequate stimulus with another stimulus that is biologically capable of arousing a response. Following repeated presentations, the neutral stimulus comes to evoke the same response or some similar variant of it. Also *conditional response.* Abbr. CR **corneal r.** See under CORNEAL TEST. **Cornell r.** The extensor plantar response evoked by scratching the dorsum of the foot medial to the extensor tendon of the great toe. **delayed r.** DELAYED REACTION. **delayed conditioned r.** In a variant of the classical conditioning procedure, the onset of the conditioned stimulus well before the unconditioned stimulus is presented, as by an interval of many seconds or a minute. The conditioned response established will at first be given at the onset of the conditioned stimulus, but with further training trials will come to be delayed until near the end of the delay interval. **disinhibition r.** In classical conditioning, a momentary increase in a conditioned response that follows the introduction of a novel and irrelevant stimulus. This effect is particularly notable when a conditioned response has undergone partial or complete extinction, and it has been interpreted as a momentary interruption of the inhibitory state of extinction. **dose r.** A measure of the degree of response following administration, by whatever route, of graded doses of a substance over a given period of time, to determine what percentage of a population exhibits an expected effect. **dynamic r.** That portion of the discharge of a stretch receptor related to acceleration and velocity of a change in length, tension, or viscoelastic status of a muscle during its stretch or release. The change in response is called positive if lengthening occurs and negative if shortening occurs. **evoked r.** EVOKED POTENTIAL. **extensor plantar r.** Dorsiflexion of the great toe on mechanical stimulation of the outer edge of the sole of the foot, usually associated with plantar flexion and fanning of the other toes. This is the inverse of the normal flexor plantar reflex. It is seen normally in infants and abnormally in others after extreme fatigue or following injury to the central nervous system, especially as a sign of a pyramidal tract lesion. Also *Babinski sign, toe phenomenon, upgoing toe, toe sign, great toe reflex, Babinski's toe sign, great-toe phenomenon, Babinski's phenomenon, Babinski's reflex, Babinski response, positive Babinski response, paradoxical extensor reflex, tonic plantar reflex, toe spread sign.* **flare r.** Local formation of a wheal due to histamine release and then by vasodilatation in the surrounding area following scratching of the skin. This is an axon reflex dependent upon the integrity of the posterior root ganglia. **frequency r.** **1** The frequency-dependent relation in both gain and phase difference between the steady-state sinusoidal input and the resultant sinusoidal output. **2** The frequency range for which the amplitude response varies less than $\pm 3$ decibels. **fright r.** A sympathetic nervous system response mediated by adrenal catecholamine release and an increased activity of the sympathetic nerves. It is characterized by sweating, pallor, tachycardia, dilated pupils, increased cardiac stroke volume, and anxiety. **ice-water r.** Contraction of the detrusor muscle, anal sphincter, and muscles of the pelvic floor upon introducing ice water into the bladder. **immediate r.** IMMEDIATE REACTION. **immune r.** The development by a host of specific cellular and/or humoral response to stimulation by an antigen. The formation of antibodies, the generation of specifically antigen-reactive lymphocytes, and the induction of specific immunological tolerance are all components of the immune response. Also *immune reaction, immunoreaction, allergic response.* ● In theory *allergic response* is the more accurate term, since reference is made not only to responses leading to reduced clinical response (immunity) but to increased clinical response (hypersensitivity) to subsequent exposure to antigen. However, in practice *allergic response* is less frequently used, especially in the United States. **lysogenic r.** The response of a bacteriophage which induces lysogeny in an infected bacterium. **lytic r.** Lysis of bacteria as a response to infection by bacteriophage, or of animal cells as a response to infection by an animal virus. **memory r.** ANAMNESTIC RESPONSE. **middle latency r.** In the electrophysiologic investigation of hearing, the evoked potentials occurring at 30–50 msec, between the end point of the brainstem-evoked response and the long latency response of the vertex potential. Also *early vertex potential.* **orienting r.** A repositioning in space of an organism as a whole in order to maximize the attention given to a source of stimulation. **placing r.** The successive flexion-extension movement of the limb of an animal that results in its paw being placed on a table top when the dorsum of the paw lightly touches the edge. It is generally thought to involve the cerebral cortex. Also *placing reflex.* **positive Babinski r.** EXTENSOR PLANTAR RESPONSE. **post-auricular r.** AURICULAR REFLEX. **primary immune r.** The immune response of the host to the initial stimulation with antigen, characterized by a longer period between exposure and antibody synthesis or cellular recognition than occurs with a secondary (anamnestic) immune response. **psychogalvanic r.** A lowering in electrical resistance of the skin triggered by pain, excitement, or other emotional states. It is due to sympathetically mediated vascular and perhaps glandular changes. Also *electrodermal response, galvanic skin response, psychogalvanic reaction, galvanic skin reflex, electric skin response.* See also PSYCHOGALVANOMETER. Abbr. PGR **quantal r.** A response that is recorded as either present or absent, such as survival or death; an all-or-none response. **rage r.** An outburst of rage which may be precipitated in an animal by electrical stimulation of a punishment center such as the perifornical region of the hypothalamus. **recall r.** ANAMNESTIC RESPONSE. **reticulocyte r.** The increase in number of reticulocytes in the blood that occurs as a result of increased rate of formation of erythrocytes, as following acute blood loss or the administration of a nutrient the lack of which is responsible for a patient's anemia. The reticulocyte response usually begins in two or three days and is maximal at seven to ten days. **Rinne r.** RINNE TEST. **secondary r.** ANAMNESTIC RESPONSE. **secondary immune r.** ANAMNESTIC RESPONSE. **second set r.** An anamnestic response, especially to a graft. **startle r.** The complex of reactions exhibited by a subject presented with a sudden alarming stimulus or situation, including muscle tensing, attitudinal movement, sympathetically mediated cardiovascular and other changes, and electroencephalographic and emotional arousal. Also *startle reaction, startle reflex, startle pattern.* Compare MORO'S REFLEX. **stretch r.** The changes in discharge of a stretch receptor induced by extension of a muscle from some given baseline length. The response may have both dynamic and static components. **thalamic r.** An increased threshold for sensory stimuli associated with a painful or abnormal response to those stimuli of above-threshold intensity, as seen in some subjects with thalamic lesions. **triple r. of Lewis** WHEAL-FLARE REACTION. **unconditioned r.** The natural or unlearned response that is evoked by a biologically adequate stimulus. An example is salivation in response to food. Compare CONDITIONED RESPONSE. Abbr. UR **vestibular placing r.** Extension of the limbs of an animal when it is suddenly dropped.

**visual evoked r.** The electrical response to patterned visual stimuli, which can be recorded, from the scalp overlying the occipital cortex. This response is of value in assessing the integrity of the visual pathway. **wheal and flare r.** WHEAL-FLARE REACTION. **wink r.** ANAL RESPONSE.

**responsibility / criminal r.** Culpability of a person, as determined by due process of law, for actions he committed that are defined as criminal. If an individual is found to have been criminally insane at the time he or she committed a crime, and therefore unable to formulate a criminal intent, the individual cannot be convicted of the crime. See also M'NAGHTEN RULE.

**rest**[1] [Medieval French *reste* (from *rester* to remain, from L *restare* to remain, stand still, from *re-* intensifying prefix + *stare* to stand) remainder] Something remaining or retained; specifically, an embryonic rest. **aberrant r.** CHORISTOMA. **adrenal r.** An embryonic rest of adrenal tissue at any site other than that of the normal gland. It is occasionally found within the kidney or gonads, or at other sites along the abdominal aorta. Also *adrenocortical rest, suprarenal rest.* **caudal medullary r.** A derivative of the enlarged caudal end of the spinal cord present in young embryos, which may persist to become involved in sacrococcygeal cysts. **embryonic r.** A small collection of embryonic cells, or a piece of embryonic tissue, which fails to develop properly and is retained within the adult. Such rests are found with some frequency at the site of embryonic origin and along the course of migration of organs that change location during embryogenesis, such as the anterior pituitary, the thyroid, the parathyroid, and the adrenal glands. It may be called epithelial rest or fetal rest depending on its nature, or when or where in development it is retained. **epithelial r.** See under EMBRYONIC REST. **fetal r.** See under EMBRYONIC REST. **r.'s of Malassez** A network of epithelial cells, remnants of the sheath of Hertwig, which are seen in histologic sections of the periodontal membrane. Also *debris of Malassez.* **mesonephric r.'s** Remnants of the fetal mesonephros which may persist in the adult. **suprarenal r.** ADRENAL REST.

**rest**[2] [Old English *ræst* (noun), *ræstan* (verb)] **1** Repose; inactivity. **2** A support or supportive structure; specifically, an extension from a partial denture, giving vertical support. **occlusal r.** A rest on an occlusal surface. Also *occlusal lug.* **precision r.** A rest fitting into a prepared rest area.

**restenosis** \rē′stenō′sis\ The recurrence of stenosis following surgical alleviation, especially of the mitral valve.

**restibrachium** \res′tibrā′kē·əm\ PEDUNCULUS CEREBELLARIS INFERIOR.

**restiform** \res′tifôrm\ [L *resti(s)* a rope, cord + -FORM] Shaped like a rope; ropelike.

**restis** \res′tis\ [L, cord, rope, halter] PEDUNCULUS CEREBELLARIS INFERIOR.

**restitutio** \res′tit^y^oo′shō\ [L (from *restitutus,* past part. of *restituere* to replace, restore, from *re-* RE- + *statuere* to set, place), a restoring] Restitution; restoration. **r. ad integrum** Recovery to complete good health.

**restitution** \res′tit^y^oo′shən\ [L *restitutio* (from *restitutus,* past part. of *restituere* to replace, restore) a restoring] The return of the fetal head to its normal position in relation to the fetal body following delivery.

**restoration** \res′tərā′shən\ [French *restauration* (from L *restauratus,* past part. of *restaurare* to rebuild, restore) a renewing, rebuilding] A repair or replacement of a tooth or teeth. **pin-ledge r.** A cast gold restoration covering the lingual surface of an incisor or canine and retained by pins recessed into small ledges.

**restorative** \ristôr′ətiv\ A medication or treatment that promotes a restoration of strength and vigor.

**restraint** \ristrānt′\ [Middle French *restrainte* (fem. of *restraint,* past part. of *restraindre* to restrain, from L *restringere* to bind back, bind tight, confine, from RE- + L *stringere* to bind, tie; Gk *strangein* to draw or bind tight) restrained, held back] Control or prevention of action, often by interfering with the physical ability of the subject to act or otherwise depriving him of freedom to act. **chemical r.** Control of a subject's action by means of a sedating or tranquilizing agent. Also *medicinal restraint.* **mechanical r.** Control of a subject's action by means of external physical agents, such as a camisole or confinement within a locked room. **medicinal r.** CHEMICAL RESTRAINT.

**restriction** [Late L *restrictio* (from *restrictus,* past part. of *restringere* to bind back, bind tight, confine; see RESTRAINT) a tightening, strictness, confining] The phenomenon in which DNA (usually phage) entering certain strains of bacteria is destroyed by double-stranded scission by an endonuclease that recognizes a short (4–8) palindromic nucleotide sequence. The host DNA is not attacked because a cognate modifying enzyme methylates a base in each strand of the palindrome. Restriction endonucleases have made possible molecular recombination of DNA.

**resuscitation** \risus′itā′shən\ [Late L *resuscitatio* (from L *resuscitatus,* past part. of *resuscitare* to revive) a reviving] Restoration or maintenance of vital signs in an organism that is in shock or predictably will go into shock. It concentrates on normalizing oxygenation, cardiac output, and blood pressure. **cardiac r.** Restoration of cardiac activity. Methods include oxygenation, correction of acidosis, use of heart stimulants, and frequently electric shock. **cardiopulmonary r.** The restoration of cardiac and respiratory function. This is most often required in the treatment of cardiac arrest and involves sternal compression and artificial ventilation. If ventricular fibrillation is responsible for the arrest, direct current countershock is usually necessary. Abbr. CPR **colloid r.** Treatment of shock with intravenous solutions of proteins, dextrans, or other relatively large molecules. In theory their advantage over crystalloid alone is their ability to remain in the vascular space by virtue of their large molecular size, but in practice this advantage is often not apparent. **crystalloid r.** Treatment of shock with intravenous solutions that have sodium chloride as their main constituent. Such solutions are inexpensive and they adequately restore fluid losses. In cases of hemorrhagic shock, they maintain circulation until blood is available. Theoretically they do not stay in the vascular space as well as colloids, but this disadvantage is not apparent in practice. **hypertonic r.** The intravenous administration of 180–300 mEq/liter hypertonic saline to burn victims. It is reported to decrease the total amount of fluid that is required to restore normal hemodynamics. **mouth-to-mouth r.** A first-aid technique for reestablishing spontaneous respiration in which the operator inflates the subject's lungs in a regular breathing rhythm by blowing directly into the subject's mouth, allowing passive expiration. The subject is supine with neck elevated and head back, and the nostrils are pinched shut during the inspiratory phase. In the case of infants and small children especially, the nose may also be covered by the operator's mouth, the subject's nostrils serving as the inspiratory air passages. Also *mouth-to-mouth breathing, mouth-to-mouth respiration, transanimation* (seldom used). **mouth-to-nose r.** A first-aid technique which is the same as mouth-to-mouth resuscitation except that the patient's nostrils, rather than the mouth, are used for insufflation. **oral r.** Administration by mouth of a saline solution. The method is used in cases of mild shock or moderate burns.

**resuscitator** \risus′itā′tər\ A person or device that can restore circulation or respiration in an individual for whom these functions have ceased, as in asphyxia, drowning, or cardiac arrest.

**retainer** \ritā′nər\ **1** The part of a bridge which is cemented to the abutment tooth. **2** The part of a partial denture which provides retention. **3** In orthodontics, an appliance for providing retention. Also *retaining appliance, retaining plate.* **continuous bar r.** An indirect retainer consisting of a cast bar on or above the cingulae of lower anterior teeth. It also acts as a minor connector. Also *continuous clasp, Kennedy bar.* **Hawley r.** HAWLEY APPLIANCE. **indirect r.** Part of a free-end partial denture acting on the opposite side of the fulcrum line to direct retainers (clasps), to prevent displacement. **intracoronal r.** INTRACORONAL ATTACHMENT. **matrix r.** A device for holding a matrix tightly around a tooth. Also *matrix holder.* **space r.** An orthodontic appliance used to retain the space between teeth, where one or more are missing, until such time as a permanent prosthesis is made, or until eruption occurs. Also *space maintainer.*

**retard** \ritärd′\ **1** Delay; retardation. **2** A delaying mechanism or device. **expiratory r.** A modification of mechanical ventilation to produce increased obstruction to expiration.

**retardate** \ritär′dāt\ [L *retardatus,* past part. of *retardare* to hinder, delay. See RETARDATION.] A mentally retarded person. **ineducable r.** A person whose degree of intellectual inadequacy is such that he cannot ordinarily be expected to be educable or even trainable. Such persons usually have severe or profound retardation, with I.Q. below 40.

**retardation** \rē′tärdā′shən\ [L *retardatio* (from *retardare* to delay, from *tardus* slow) hanging back, delay] Delayed or retarded development. **cultural-familial mental r.** Intellectual inadequacy as a result of inadequate stimulation, lack of opportunities for learning, or deprivation as a result of familial or cultural factors or both. **mental r.** Intellectual functioning that is significantly below average and is associated with impairment in social adjustment, manifested prior to maturity, usually early in life. Although not defined by intelligence measures only, mental retardation is distinguished by an IQ below 68. In about one fourth of cases, the condition is secondary to genetic chromosomal factors, infections or toxins, or other organic causes. Intellectual deficit in these cases is likely to be severe. The remaining majority of cases are without identifiable brain pathology or specific biologic causative factors. Also *mental deficiency, feeblemindedness* (older term), *hypophrenia, oligophrenia* (older term), *oligergasia* (outmoded), *aphrenia* (obs.). • The term is specifically defined in different nations and by some professional organizations, but no single definition is accepted worldwide. **psychomotor r.** **1** Delay in the attainment of motor skills, language development, and social responsiveness in infancy and childhood. A marked discordance between the degree of motor retardation and that of social response and alertness, as revealed by testing, may predict either cerebral palsy or a mainly intellectual impairment. **2** The slowness in movement or motor inertia and unresponsiveness to extrinsic or intrinsic stimuli, characteristically seen in depressive psychoses. **psychosocial r.** Mental retardation due to or exaggerated by cultural, social, and interpersonal inadequacies in the subject's environment.

**retch** \rech\ [Old English *hraecan* to clear the throat, from *hraca* a clearing of the throat] To make the involuntary, ineffective effort of vomiting.

**rete** \rē′tē\ [L, a net] (*pl.* retia) A network or meshwork of arteries or veins. **acromial r.** ACROMIAL NETWORK. **r. arteriosum** [NA] An anastomotic network formed by small arteries just prior to their becoming arterioles or capillaries. Also *arterial anastomosis, arterial network.* **r. arteriosum dermidis** [NA] A sheetlike network of arteries that derive from small arteries that pierce the superficial fascia to ramify between it and the overlying dermis or corium. Vessels from the plexus supply the subcutaneous adipose tissue, glands, and hair follicles of the skin. **r. arteriosum subpapillare** [NA] A superficial arterial plexus between the reticular and papillary layers of the dermis formed by vessels arising from the rete arteriosum dermidis and draining to another, more superficial, plexus in the middle or the reticular layer. Also *subpapillary network.* **articular r.** A network of anastomosing blood vessels around or in a joint supplying the structures of that joint. **r. articulare cubiti** [NA] A rich arterial anastomosis around the elbow joint, involving the radial collateral and middle collateral branches of profunda brachii artery anastomosing with the radial recurrent and interosseous recurrent arteries, and the superior and inferior ulnar collateral arteries anastomosing with the anterior and posterior ulnar recurrent arteries and the middle collateral branch of the profunda brachii artery. Also *articular cubital rete, anastomosis around elbow joint.* **r. articulare genus** [NA] A rich arterial anastomosis around the capsule and bones of the knee joint, formed by the descending genicular, the five genicular branches of the popliteal, the descending branch of the lateral circumflex femoral, the anterior tibial recurrent, and the circumflex fibular branch of the posterior tibial artery. Also *articular rete of knee, anastomosis around knee joint, genicular anastomosis.* **r. calcaneum** [NA] An anastomotic network of arteries around the calcaneus formed by the calcaneal and lateral malleolar branches of the peroneal artery and calcaneal branches of the posterior tibial and lateral plantar arteries. Also *calcaneal rete, calcanean network.* **r. canalis hypoglossi** *Outmoded* PLEXUS VENOSUS CANALIS HYPOGLOSSI. **r. carpale dorsale** [NA] An anastomosis on the dorsal carpal surface formed by the dorsal carpal branches of the radial and ulnar arteries and the anterior and posterior interosseous arteries. Three dorsal metacarpal arteries pass distally from this anastomosis. Also *dorsal carpal arch, posterior carpal arch, dorsal arch of wrist.* **r. foraminis ovalis** *Outmoded* PLEXUS VENOSUS FORAMINIS OVALIS. **r. malleolare laterale** An arterial network formed on and below the lateral malleolus by the anastomosis of the anterior lateral malleolar branch of the anterior tibial artery, the lateral tarsal branch of the dorsalis pedis artery, the calcaneal and perforating branches of the peroneal artery, and branches of the lateral plantar artery. Also *lateral malleolar network.* **r. malleolare mediale** An arterial anastomosis on the medial malleolus of the tibia, formed by the anterior medial malleolar branch of the anterior tibial artery, the malleolar and calcaneal branches of the posterior tibial artery, the medial tarsal branches of the dorsalis pedis artery, and branches of the medial plantar artery. Also *medial malleolar network, medial malleolar rete.* **r. mirabile** [NA] A vascular network formed in the course of an artery or a vein so that there is a single vessel on either side of the network, as in the glomerular arterioles in the kidney. **r. mirabile of kidney** See under RETE MIRABILE. **r. mucosum** GERMINATIVE LAYER OF EPIDERMIS. **r. ovarii** The rudimentary structure in the medulla of the ovary which corresponds to the tubule and duct system of the testis, and which may have imperfect connections with the mesonephric tubules. Initially, the gonadal cells in both sexes are arranged as cords, but whereas the cords become canalized in the male, they become ill-defined in the female. In some species, the rete ovarii persists into adult life as a limited system of collapsed tubules lined by epithelium situated in the hilus of the ovary. **r. patellaris** [NA] The superficial anastomosis between the skin and the fascia over the patella formed by branches of the arteries of the rete articularis genus. Also *rete of patella, anastomosis around knee joint.* **plantar venous r.** RETE VENOSUM PLANTARE. **r. testis** A network of cords which are the inward continuation of the testis cords in the male gonad. These all canalize to become the seminiferous tubules. They are linked through the rete tubules with the upper mesonephric tubules which become exceedingly convoluted to form the lobules of the head of the epididymis. **r. venosum** [NA] A network of anastomosing veins. Also *venous network.* **r. venosum dorsale manus** [NA] A superficial venous network formed on the dorsum of the hand by the three dorsal metacarpal veins and dorsal digital veins of the thumb and the index and little fingers. It is drained by the cephalic and basilic veins. Also *dorsal venous arch of the hand, dorsal venous plexus of hand.* **r. venosum dorsale pedis** [NA] An irregular superficial network of veins on the dorsum of the foot, proximal to and communicating with the dorsal venous arch and receiving tributaries from the deep veins. It is continuous with the venous network on the front of the ankle and leg. Also *dorsal venous plexus of foot.* **r. venosum plantare** [NA] A superficial network of veins in the sole of the foot, particularly dense in the fat under the heel, communicating with the distally situated plantar cutaneous arch and with the deep veins, and draining mostly into the lateral and medial marginal veins. Also *plantar venous rete.*

**retention** \riten′shən\ [L *retentio* (from *retentus,* past part. of *retinere* to hold or keep back) a holding or keeping back] **1** The stability of a denture in use. **2** The stability of a dental restoration relative to the natural tooth. **3** The holding in place of teeth which have been moved orthodontically, usually by means of an appliance. **4** The inability to empty the bladder; urinary retention. **bladder r.** URINARY RETENTION. **urinary r.** Inability to urinate, occurring despite the presence of a bladder full of urine. This condition results from urinary outflow obstruction, usually prostate hyperplasia, or neurogenic bladder dysfunction (atonic or paralytic type). Also *bladder retention, urine retention, ischuria, uroschesis.*

**retia** \rē′tē·ə\ Plural of RETE.

**retial** \rē′tē·əl\ Pertaining to or having the characteristics of a rete.

**reticul-** \rətik′yəl-\ RETICULO-.

**reticula** \retik′yələ\ Plural of RETICULUM.

**reticular** \rətik′yələr\ Pertaining to or resembling a reticulum.

**reticulate** \retik′yələt, -lāt\ In the nature of or having the appearance of a reticulum. Also *reticulated.*

**reticulated** \retik′yəlātəd\ RETICULATE.

**reticulation** \retik′yəlā′shən\ [English *reticulat(e)* (from L *reticulat(us)* resembling network, from *reticul(um),* dim. of *rete* a net + *-atus* -ATE) + -ION] In radiology, a pattern of corrugated artifacts in x-ray film emulsion due to temperature variations in the processing solutions. **dust r.** An early stage of pneumoconiosis, diagnosed by chest x ray, seen principally in coal miners.

**reticulin** \rətik′yəlin\ **1** A type of collagen found especially in the spleen and characterized by the distinctive appearance of its fibers on electron microscopy. **2** An antibiotic, a hydroxylated streptomycin.

**reticulo-** \rətik′yəlō-\ [L *reticulum* (dim. of *rete* a net) a small net] A combining form meaning reticulum, reticular. Also *reticul-.*

**reticulocyte** \retik′yəlōsīt′\ A very young erythrocyte lacking a nucleus, but containing reticular substance in its cytoplasm that stains as a fine blue network with methylene blue or similar dyes. Also *reticulated corpuscle, reticulated erythrocyte, skein cell.*

**reticulocytopenia** \-sī′təpē′nē·ə\ A fewer than normal number of reticulocytes in the blood; an absolute reticulocyte count less than $25 \times 10^9$/l. Also *reticulopenia.*

**reticulocytosis** \-sītō′sis\ A greater than normal number of reticulocytes in blood; an absolute reticulocyte count greater than $75 \times 10^9$/l. Reticulocytosis indicates an increased rate of erythrocyte formation, and may be observed in hemolytic disorders, following acute hemorrhage, or in response to treatment of anemia. Also *hyperneocytosis.*

**reticuloendotheliosis** \-en′dəthē′lē·ō′sis\ [*reticuloendotheli(um)* + -OSIS] An abnormality of the reticuloendothelial system. **leukemic r.** An uncommon leukemia characterized by pancytopenia, splenomegaly, and infiltration of bone marrow, spleen, and lymph nodes by a lymphocyte-like cell with ovoid nucleus and abundant cytoplasm that has, on special staining, numerous filamentous cytoplasmic projections. These "hairy cells" are of unknown origin, possibly of lymphocytic derivation, and characteristically display numerous cytoplasmic granules on acid phosphatase stain. The stain is not inhibited by tartrate. A small number of hairy cells may be seen in blood films. Also *hairy cell leukemia.* **systemic aleukemic r.** *Obs.* LETTERER-SIWE DISEASE.

**reticuloendothelium** \-en′dəthē′lē·əm\ RETICULOENDOTHELIAL SYSTEM.

**reticulohistiocytoma** \-his′tē·ōsītō′mə\ DERMATOFIBROMA. **r. of Crosti** A rare skin condition characterized by plaques on the skin containing fat-filled histiocytes. As both radiotherapy and steroids separately are curative, it is probably a benign condition.

**reticulohistiocytosis** \-his′tē·ōsītō′sis\ The formation of multiple reticulohistiocytomata. **multicentric r.** A rare disorder in which tumorlike nodules of histiocytes appear throughout the body, often prominently in or on tendon sheaths, joints, and elsewhere on the extremities. The etiology is unknown.

**reticuloid** \retik′yəloid\ **1** Having characteristics of or resembling reticulosis. **2** A reticuloid disorder. **actinic r.** A rare cutaneous nonmalignant disorder marked by extreme cutaneous photosensitivity. Histologic examinations reveal a lymphoid infiltrate that mimics malignant reticulosis. The disorder usually is found in males.

**reticulolymphosarcoma** \-lim′fəsärkō′mə\ A malignant lymphoma composed of cells believed to be lymphoid and histiocytic in type. Also *mixed lymphocytic-histiocytic malignant lymphoma.*

**reticulopenia** \-pē′nē·ə\ RETICULOCYTOPENIA.

**reticuloplasmocytoma** \-plaz′məsītō′mə\ [RETICULO- + PLASMO- + CYT- + -OMA] A tumor of reticulum cells and plasma cells.

**reticulosarcoma** \-särkō′mə\ [RETICULO- + SARCOMA] *Obs.* HISTIOCYTIC LYMPHOMA.

**reticulosis** \ritik′yəlō′sis\ [RETICUL- + -OSIS] (*pl.* reticuloses) Any proliferative or neoplastic disorder involving the cellular components of the reticuloendothelial system. **benign r.** CAT-SCRATCH DISEASE. **benign inoculation r.** CAT-SCRATCH DISEASE. **benign lymphocytic r.** BENIGN LYMPHOCYTOMA CUTIS. **bony r.** MALIGNANT HISTIOCYTOSIS. **familial histiocytic r.** A hereditary disease marked by anemia, granulocytopenia, and thrombocytopenia, caused in part by phagocytosis of blood cells and in part by histiocytic infiltration of bone marrow. It is inherited as an autosomal recessive trait and generally results in infant or childhood death. Also *familial hemophagocytic reticulosis.* **histiocytic medullary r.** MALIGNANT HISTIOCYTOSIS. **lipomelanic r.** A benign, nonspecific reactive change in the lymph nodes that follows chronic erythrodermic skin lesions. **primary r. of the brain** A primary lymphoma of the brain.

**reticulospinal** \-spī′nəl\ Denoting the interconnection between the reticular formation and the spinal cord.

**reticulothelium** \-thē′lē·əm\ The layer of cells that covers a reticulin framework. **agranular r.** AGRANULAR ENDOPLASMIC RETICULUM.

**reticulotomy** \retik′yəlät′əmē\ [RETICULO- + -TOMY] The production of lesions by cutting into the reticular formation of the brainstem.

**reticulum** \ritik′yələm\ [L (from *rete,* gen. *reti(s)* a net + *-culum,* instrumental and diminutive suffix) a small meshwork bag or container] (*pl.* reticula) **1** A fine mesh or network of fibers or tubules. **2** The second of the stomach chambers in a ruminant animal, having ridged interior walls resembling a honeycomb. Also *honeycomb, honeycomb stomach.* **agranular endoplasmic r.** Endoplasmic reticulum without ribosomes attached. Also *smooth endoplasmic reticulum, agranular reticulothelium.* **arachnoid r.** The precursor of the definitive subarachnoid space. The pia mater and arachnoid mater are a single vascular meninx in early development. Subsequently, particularly after cerebrospinal fluid escapes from the fourth ventricle, a space appears and two layers can be defined. The space has numerous fibrous strands, but these become less obvious as fluid accumulates. **Ebner's r.** A cellular meshwork in the seminiferous tubules. **endoplasmic r.** A network or system of folded membranes and interconnecting tubules distributed within the cytoplasm of eukaryotic cells. The membranes form enclosed or semienclosed spaces (cisternae). The endoplasmic reticulum functions in storage and transport, and as a point of attachment of ribosomes during protein synthesis. Also *Holmgren-Golgi canals.* **granular endoplasmic r.** Endoplasmic reticulum studded with ribosomes. It is found in secretory cells, such as those of the pancreas, and is particularly concerned with the synthesis of proteins for export from the cell. Also *rough endoplasmic reticulum, egastoplasm, ribosome-lamella complex.* **r. lienis** TRABECULA OF SPLEEN. **nuclear r.** The network of chromatin fibers in the nucleus of a cell. **rough endoplasmic r.** GRANULAR ENDOPLASMIC RETICULUM. **sarcoplasmic r.** The endoplasmic reticulum of a muscle fiber or cell. Also *sarcotubules.* **smooth endoplasmic r.** AGRANULAR ENDOPLASMIC RETICULUM. **splenic r.** TRABECULA OF SPLEEN. **stellate r.** A region of the enamel organ of a developing tooth which is enclosed by the inner and outer enamel epithelia and consists of a netlike arrangement of star-shaped cells. Also *enamel pulp* (outmoded). **r. trabeculare sclerae** [NA] A meshwork of fibers that extend posteriorly from the periphery of the posterior limiting lamina of the cornea onto the inner wall of the sinus venosus sclerae and to the scleral spur (forming the pars corneoscleralis) while some fine fibers pass over the inner surface of the scleral spur into the root and stroma of the iris (forming the pars uvealis). The meshwork is covered by endothelium continuous with that lining the cornea and covering the anterior surface of the iris. Between the trabecular fibers are the spaces of the iridocorneal angle. It is less developed in humans than in many other animals. Also *ligamentum pectinatum anguli iridocornealis, pectinate ligament of iridocorneal angle, Gerlach's valvula, uveal framework, Hueck's ligament, ligamentum annulare bulbi, trabecular network, trabecular meshwork.*

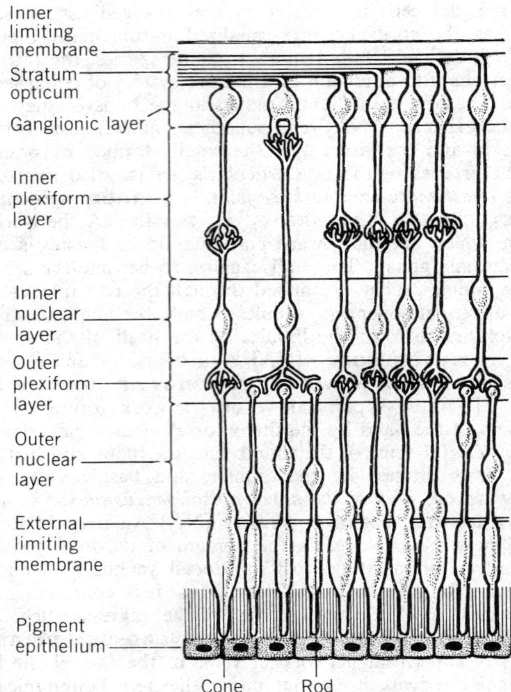


**Layers of the retina**

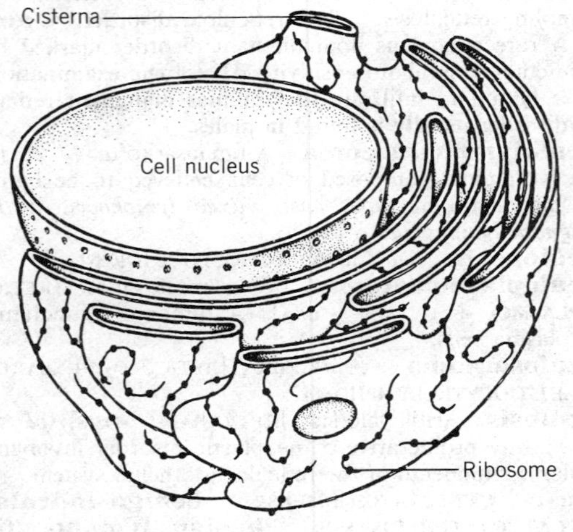


**Granular endoplasmic reticulum**

**retin-** \ret′in-\ RETINO-.

**Retin-A.** A proprietary name for tretinoin.

**retina** \ret′ənə\ [Med L (prob. from L *rete* a net), the retina] [NA] The tunica interna bulbi lying between the tunica vasculosa bulbi externally and the hyaloid membrane of the vitreous body internally. It is continuous posteriorly with the optic nerve at the discus nervi optici adjacent to the macula. It is divided into three concentric parts, namely, pars optica retinae, pars ciliaris retinae and pars iridica retinae. It is derived from the two laminae of the optic cup, the outer forming the insensitive pigment layer and the inner becoming the complex stratum nervosum (often called "retina proper") that comprises nine layers in the optic part and is specialized as a photoreceptor organ to receive visual impressions. Also *optomeninx*. Adj. retinal. **cilial r.** The portion of the retina of the eye that extends forward to cover the posterior aspect of the ciliary body. Also *ciliated epithelium*. **cilioiridial r.** The part of the optic retina that extends forward to cover the posterior aspect of the ciliary body and iris. **detached r.** See under RETINAL DETACHMENT. **iridial r.** Modified retinal tissue that covers the posterior aspect of the iris. **Kandori's fleck r.** A rare genetic condition in which the retinal pigment epithelium shows focal spots of discoloration that do not seriously handicap vision. **leopard r.** TESSELATED FUNDUS. **nasal r.** The nasal half of the retina medial to the optic disk. **shot-silk r.** WATERED-SILK RETINA. **temporal r.** The outer half of the retina lateral to the optic disk. **tigroid r.** TESSELATED FUNDUS. **watered-silk r.** The presence of diffuse glistening reflections of the surface of the retina, a normal appearance in a healthy young eye. Also *shot-silk retina, shot-silk phenomenon, watered-silk reflex*.

**retinaculum** \ret′ənak′yələm\ [L (from *retin(ere)* to hold back, check, from *tenere* to hold, + *-culum*, instrumental suffix) a tether, halter, rein] (*pl.* retinacula) **1** A fibrous strap or ligament holding another structure in place. **2** A surgical instrument used for retracting tissues. **r. capsulae articularis coxae** One of the flat bands of the deeper fibers of the capsule of the hip joint that are reflected proximally along the neck of the femur to be attached near the head. They are covered by synovial membrane. Also *Stanley's cervical ligament, retinaculum of the hip joint*. **r. caudale** [NA] A bundle of white fibrous tissue connecting the tip of the coccyx to the overlying skin, thereby forming the foveola coccygea. Also *caudal retinaculum, caudal ligament of common integument*. **retinacula cutis** [NA] Small bands of connective tissue attaching the dermis to the underlying tela subcutanea. In the mammary gland they are well developed over the upper part of the breast, forming the ligamenta suspensoria mammaria. **r. extensorum manus** [NA] A strong fibrous band comprising the distal part of the antebrachial fascia supplemented by transverse fibers and lying obliquely across the back of the wrist being attached laterally to the anterior margin of the radius, posteriorly to ridges on the radius, and medially to the pisiform and triquetral bones. It stretches across and straps down the extensor tendons and synovial sheaths of all the fingers. Also *extensor retinaculum of hand, extensor retinaculum of wrist, dorsal carpal ligament, dorsal ligament of wrist, posterior annular ligament of carpus*. **flexor r. of ankle** RETINACULUM MUSCULORUM FLEXORUM PEDIS. **flexor r. of foot** RETINACULUM MUSCULORUM FLEXORUM PEDIS. **r. flexorum manus** [NA] A strong fibrous band of the distal antebrachial fascia that spans the front of the wrist, converting the hollowed area of the carpal bones into the carpal tunnel through which run the flexor tendons of the fingers and the median nerve. It is attached medially to the hook of the hamate and the pisiform bone while laterally it splits into two layers, the superficial being attached to the tubercles of the trapezium and scaphoid bones, and the deep layer to the medial lip of the groove on the trapezium, thereby forming a tunnel for the synovial-lined tendon of the flexor carpi radialis muscle. Also *flexor retinaculum of hand, flexor retinaculum of wrist*. **r. of the hip joint** RETINACULUM CAPSULAE ARTICULARIS COXAE. **inferior extensor r. of foot** RETINACULUM MUSCULORUM EXTENSORUM PEDIS INFERIUS. **inferior peroneal r.** RETINACULUM MUSCULORUM PERONEORUM INFERIUS. **lateral patellar r.** RETINACULUM PATELLAE LATERALE. **medial patellar r.** RETINACULUM PATELLAE MEDIALE. **r. musculorum extensorum pedis inferius** [NA] A Y-shaped fibrous band overlying the front of the ankle and the dorsum of the foot. The stem is attached to the upper surface of the calcaneus and passes medially as two laminae, one superficial and one deep to the tendons of the peroneus tertius and extensor digitorum longus muscles, medial to which the laminae reunite and then diverge as the two limbs of the Y, one crossing the tendons of the extensor hallucis longus and tibialis anterior muscles superomedially to attach to the medial malleolus, while the lower limb runs inferomedially over the same tendons to blend with the plantar aponeurosis. Also *inferior extensor retinaculum of foot, anterior annular ligament of tarsus* (outmoded). **r. musculorum extensorum pedis superius** [NA] A thickened band of the distal crural fascia just above the front of the ankle joint. It is attached medially to the anterior margin of the tibia and laterally to the lower end of the anterior margin of the fibula. Deep to it pass the tendons of the muscles of the anterior compartment of the leg. Also *superior extensor retinaculum of foot, transverse ligament of leg*. **r. musculorum flexorum pedis** [NA] A broad fibrous band stretching between the medial malleolus of tibia and the medial tubercle of calcaneus, being continuous proximally with the crural fascia, especially the deep transverse layer, and distally with the plantar aponeurosis. Deep to it pass the tendons of the tibialis posterior, flexor digitorum longus, and flexor hallucis longus muscles as well as the posterior tibial vessels and tibial nerve. Also *flexor retinaculum of foot, flexor retinaculum of ankle, laciniate ligament*. **r. musculorum peroneorum inferius** [NA] A fibrous band overlying the tendons of the peroneus longus and brevis muscles and attached posteriorly to the lateral surface of the calcaneus and anteriorly to the stem of the inferior extensor retinaculum. Some fibers are attached to the peroneal trochlea of the calcaneus separating the two tendons. Also *inferior peroneal retinaculum*. **r. musculorum peroneorum superius** [NA] A fibrous band overlying the tendons of the peroneus longus and brevis muscles and extending from the lateral malleolus to the lateral surface of the calcaneus and the deep transverse fascia of the leg. Also *superior peroneal retinaculum*. **r. patellae laterale** [NA] A fibrous expansion blending with the capsule of the knee joint and extending from the distal end of the tendon of the vastus lateralis muscle to the margins of the patella, the ligamentum patellae, and condyle of the tibia, and posteriorly to the fibular collateral ligament blending with the iliotibial tract. Also *lateral patellar retinaculum*. **r. patellae mediale** [NA] A fibrous expansion blending with the capsule of the knee joint and extending from the distal end of the tendon of the vastus medialis muscle to the margins of the patella, the ligamentum patellae, and the medial condyle of the tibia, and posteriorly to the tibial collateral ligament. Also *medial pa-*

*tellar retinaculum.* **superior extensor r. of foot** RETINACULUM MUSCULORUM EXTENSORUM PEDIS SUPERIUS. **superior peroneal r.** RETINACULUM MUSCULORUM PERONEORUM SUPERIUS.

**retinal** \(1) ret′ənəl; (2) ret′inal\ **1** Of or relating to the retina. **2** The aldehyde found in visual pigments. Its molecule contains 20 carbon atoms, a 6-membered ring, and a series of conjugated double bonds that forms a chromophore. Also *retinaldehyde, retinal$_1$* (obs.), *retinene* (misleading). • The variant *retinaldehyde* is sometimes used in contexts where *retinal* might be ambiguous because of its other meaning (def. 1).

***all-trans*-retinal** The form of retinal produced from 11-*cis*-retinal when light is absorbed by rhodopsin. It dissociates from opsin and has to be isomerized before it can recombine.

**11-*cis*-retinal** Retinal with the *cis* configuration at the 11-12 double bond. In this configuration it can combine with opsin to form rhodopsin. It remains in this configuration until it absorbs light, which isomerizes it to the *trans* configuration.

**retinaldehyde** RETINAL. • See note at RETINAL.

**retinal isomerase** The enzyme (EC 5.2.1.3) that catalyzes the isomerization of the 11-12 double bond of retinal between the *cis* and *trans* forms. After excitation by light, a visual pigment releases *all-trans*-retinal from its opsin, and it can be regenerated only after this enzyme has acted to form 11-*cis*-retinal, which can recombine.

**retinal reductase** *Outmoded* ALCOHOL DEHYDROGENASE. • The name derived from the fact that the retinal-retinol interconversion was one of the aldehyde-alcohol interconversions it could catalyze.

**retinascope** \ret′inəskōp′\ RETINOSCOPE.

**retinene** A misleading term for RETINAL. • It is misleading because its ending implies that it is a hydrocarbon.

**retinitis** \ret′ənī′tis\ [*retin(a)* + -ITIS] Inflammation or degeneration of the retina. **actinic r.** Retinal macular, thermal burn caused by solar radiation. Also *actinic retinopathy.* **r. albuminurica** Renal retinitis associated with proteinuria. *Outmoded.* **apoplectic r.** Occlusion of the central retinal vein with resultant massive intraretinal hemorrhage. Also *apoplectic retinopathy.* **central angiospastic r.** CENTRAL SEROUS CHOROIDOPATHY. **r. centralis serosa** CENTRAL SEROUS CHOROIDOPATHY. **r. circinata** CIRCINATE RETINOPATHY. **circinate r.** CIRCINATE RETINOPATHY. **Coats r.** EXUDATIVE RETINITIS. **diabetic r.** DIABETIC RETINOPATHY. **exudative r.** A peripheral, vascular retinal disease consisting of focal dilatations of vessels having abnormal permeability, resulting in leakage of proteinaceous and lipoidal debris that accumulates in whitish clumps beneath the retina. It leads to progressive macular damage, retinal detachment, and may cause blindness if not treated. Also *exudative retinopathy, Coat's retinitis, Coat's disease.* **hypertensive r.** Retinitis resulting from hypertension. **Jacobson's r.** RETINITIS SYPHILITICA. **leukemic r.** LEUKEMIC RETINOPATHY. **r. pigmentosa** A progressive genetic deterioration of the ocular fundus in which melanin granules (from the broken down retinal pigment epithelium) migrate anteriorly through the retina to become deposited along the walls of the retinal vessels in a typical "bone corpuscle" pattern that is readily identified by ophthalmoscopy. Also *pigmentary retinopathy.* **r. proliferans** Massive neovascular and connective tissue growth on the inner surface of the retina, as caused by diabetes, trauma, or venous occlusion. Also *proliferating retinitis.* **punctate r.** A retinal disorder characterized by the distribution of small spots on the retina. **renal r.** Retinitis occurring in acute or advanced chronic nephritis. Retinitis in these conditions is associated with the hypertension that may be associated with nephritis, and not with the nephritis *per se.* See also HYPERTENSIVE RETINOPATHY. **splenic r.** SPLENIC RETINOPATHY. **r. stellata** Exudative debris at the macula, assuming a radiating, starlike shape because that is the contour of the Henle's fiber layer of the macula. Also *stellate retinopathy.* **suppurative r.** PURULENT RETINOPATHY. **uremic r.** Retinitis associated with advanced renal failure. In fact, the retinitis is related to the hypertension often associated with uremia and not with the uremia *per se.*.

**retino-** \ret′inō-\ [Med L *retina* (prob. from L *rete* a net) the retina] A combining form meaning retina, retinal. Also *retin-*.

**retinoblastoma** \-blastō′mə\ A malignant tumor of retinal cells which may differentiate towards photoreceptor elements. It is the commonest intraocular neoplasm of childhood. A proportion have an autosomal dominant inheritance, and these are typically bilateral. It is a highly radiosensitive and radiocurable neoplasm. Also *retinocystoma* (obs.).

**retinocerebelloangiomatosis** \-ser′əbel′ō·an′jē·ōmətō′sis\ VON HIPPEL-LINDAU SYNDROME.

**retinochoroiditis** \-kôr′oidī′tis\ [RETINO- + CHOROIDITIS] Inflammation of both retina and choroid, with the primary pathology being within the retina. **r. juxtapapillaris** Inflammation of retina and choroid adjacent to the optic disk.

**retinocystoma** \-sistō′mə\ *Obs.* RETINOBLASTOMA.

**retinodialysis** \-dī·al′isis\ [RETINO- + DIALYSIS] DIALYSIS RETINAE.

**retinoic acid** TRETINOIN.

**retinoid** \ret′inoid\ **1** Like the retina. **2** Any of a class of compounds whose molecules contain 20 carbon atoms, derived from isoprene units, and related to retinal and other compounds with vitamin-A activity.

**retinol** \ret′inôl\ A common form of vitamin A, differing from retinal only in having —$CH_2OH$ in place of the —CHO group. It is found only in foods of animal origin. It is easily converted in the body into retinal and hence incorporated into the visual pigments. Also *retinol$_1$* (obs.), *vitamin $A_1$*.

**retinol$_2$** *Obs.* VITAMIN $A_2$.

**retinopapillitis** \-pap′ilī′tis\ [RETINO- + PAPILLITIS] NEURORETINITIS.

**retinopathy** \ret′ənäp′əthē\ [RETINO- + -PATHY] A noninflammatory disease of the retina. **actinic r.** ACTINIC RETINITIS. **apoplectic r.** APOPLECTIC RETINITIS. **arteriosclerotic r.** Loss of transparency of the arteriolar walls, manifested by widening of the light reflex and arteriovenous crossing changes. Very little structural or functional change occurs in the retina because of the arteriolar wall change, inasmuch as the capillary bed continues to function. **central angiospastic r.** CENTRAL SEROUS CHOROIDOPATHY. **central serous r.** CENTRAL SEROUS CHOROIDOPATHY. **chloroquine r.** A diffuse severe pigmentary atrophy of the fundus due to selective deposition of chloroquine in melanin and its consequent toxic effect. **circinate r.** A circular subretinal deposit of whitish exudative debris surrounding a disciform degeneration. Also *circinate retinitis, retinitis circinata.* **diabetic r.** The retinal manifestation of the microangiopathy observed in the course of diabetes mellitus. The earliest lesions are retinal microaneurysms, followed later by retinal hemorrhages and exudates, and finally retinitis proliferans. It is an important cause of blindness. Also *diabetic retinitis.* **eclamptic r.** Angiospastic changes occurring in the retina of a woman with severe pre-eclampsia or eclampsia. **exudative r.** EXUDATIVE RETINITIS. **hypertensive r.** Any of various retinal abnormalities associated with hypertension, including vascular spasm, papilledema, hemorrhage, and exudation. **leukemic r.** Retinal abnormalities occurring in patients with acute leukemia, including hemorrhages and exudates, pallor of retina and choroid, and blurring of the margin of the optic disk. Also *leukemic retinitis, splenic retinitis, splenic retinopathy.* **macular r.** Retinal disease affecting the central part of the retina. **pigmentary r.** RETINITIS PIGMENTOSA. **r. of prematurity** A neovascular scarring of the retina of a prematurely born infant exposed to excessive amounts of oxygen. **proliferative r.** An overgrowth of neovascular and connective tissue upon the inner surface of the retina in association with diabetes mellitus or occlusion of the central retinal vein. **Purtscher's angiopathic r.** A severe hemorrhagic retinopathy associated with massive crushing injuries of the body. **purulent r.** A diseased condition of the retina resulting from the introduction of pyogenic organisms through an infected wound or via the blood stream. A panophthalmitis usually follows. Also *suppurative retinopathy, suppurative retinitis, septic retinopathy.* **rubella r.** A pigment granularity, especially concentrated about the macula of the retina, caused by rubella infection during the early months of gestation. **septic r.** PURULENT RETINOPATHY. **sickle cell r.** Retinal abnormalities that occur in persons with homozygous hemoglobin S disease or other severe sickling disorders. These abnormalities include microaneurysms, tortuous and dilatated retinal veins, hemorrhages and exudates, neovascularization, and retinal detachment. **splenic r.** LEUKEMIC RETINOPATHY. **stellate r.** RETINITIS STELLATA. **suppurative r.** PURULENT RETINOPATHY. **thioridazine r.** A potentially severe pigment disruption of the fundus occurring because of melanin affinity for phenothiazine derivatives and their consequent toxicity. **toxemic r. of pregnancy** Retinal edema and angiospastic changes occurring in the retina of a woman with pre-eclampsia or eclampsia.

**retinopexy** \ret′inəpek′sē\ [RETINO- + -PEXY] The surgical reattachment of a detached retina.

**retinophotoscopy** \-fōtäs′kəpē\ RETINOSCOPY.

**retinopiesis** \-pī·ē′sis\ [RETINO- + Gk *piesis* a pressing, squeezing] Replacement of a retinal detachment into its original position by internal pressure upon it.

**retinoschisis** \ret′inäs′kisis\ [RETINO- + Gk *schisis* a cleaving, parting] A splitting of the retina into two layers, with an intervening cystic space.

**retinoscope** \ret′inəskōp′\ [*retin(a)* + *o* + -SCOPE] A device for objective measurement of the refractive status of an eye by observation of the direction of movement of a beam of light reflected from the fundus of the retina. Unlike the opthalmoscope, it is not an instrument for observation of retinal structure. Also *fantascope, skiascope, striascope.* Also *retinascope.*

**retinoscopy** \ret′inäs′kəpē\ [RETINO- + -SCOPY] The objective measurement of the refractive status of an eye by observation with a retinoscope of the direction of movement of light reflected from the ocular fundus. Also *scotoscopy, skiametry, skiascopy, skiaporescopy, retinophotoscopy.*

**retinotopic** \-täp′ik\ [RETINO- + *top(o)-* + -IC] Pertaining to the topographic projection of the retina onto each of several brain regions of visual representation in the cortex, thalamus, and midbrain.

**retoperithelium** \ret′ōper′ithē′lē·əm\ [L *ret(e)* net + *o* + PERITHELIUM] A layer of cells that ensheathes a reticulin framework.

**retort** \ritôrt′\ [French *retorte* (from Med L *retorta,* fem. of *retortus,* past part. of *retorquere* to twist or bend back) a retort] A glass container, sometimes used for distillation, that consists of a rounded lower portion and an elongated neck which is angled laterally.

***Retortamonas*** \rē′tôrtam′ənəs\ [L *retorta,* fem. of *retortus,* past part. of *retorquere* to bend or twist back + Gk *monas* a unit] A genus of zoomastigophorean protozoa (family Retortamonadidae, order Retortamonadida). Members are characterized by the possession of two flagella, one anterior, and one turned posteriorly, a ventral cytosome, and a fusiform body. They occur as parasites in the intestines of many animals. Among the better known examples are *R. blattae* in cockroaches, *R. caviae* in guinea pigs, *R. ovis* in sheep, *R. cuniculi* in rabbits, and *R. intestinalis* in humans. Also *Embadomonas.*.

**retract** \ritrakt′\ To draw back; pull in, as the claws of a cat.

**retractile** \ritrak′til\ Capable of being retracted, as the claws of a cat.

**retraction** \ritrak′shən\ [L *retractio* (from *retractus,* past part. of *retrahere* to draw back, withdraw, rescue) a drawing back] **1** The act or process of retracting; a drawing back, as of the jaw (retrusion) or the gingiva. **2** Distal movement of teeth, usually achieved with an orthodontic appliance. **clot r.** The shrinking of a fibrin clot once it has formed in blood or plasma. Platelets are required for the retraction. **gingival r.** The displacement or shrinkage of the gingival margin around a tooth preparation in order to facilitate an accurate impression of this area. **head r.** Arching backward of the head and neck in infants and young children with subacute or chronic meningitis. Compare RETROCOLLIS. **lid r.** Displacement upward of the upper eyelids as seen in ophthalmic Graves disease. **mandibular r.** MANDIBULAR RETRUSION. **massive vitreous r.** The shrinking of connective tissue membranes upon the retinal surface and within the vitreous substance, developing as a sequela to retinal detachment in about five percent of cases. It is a very serious condition. **systolic r.** Indrawing of the chest wall due to systolic contraction of the heart, attributed to adherence of the pericardium to the chest wall. **uterine r.** A shortening of uterine myometrial fibers with inability to return to their normal length as long as the retraction process continues.

**retractor** \ritrak′tər\ **1** An instrument used for retracting tissues during surgical operations. **2** A device, such as a headcap and a chin cup joined by elastic, used to retract the chin during growth. **abdominal r.** A retractor that provides wider exposure to areas within the abdominal cavity. **palate r.** One of a variety of instruments for retracting and controlling the soft palate to permit examination of or certain procedures on the nasopharynx. In modern practice, such retractors have largely been replaced by two soft rubber catheters introduced through the nose and brought out through the mouth. Also *palatal elevator, posterior palate hook.* **periosteal r.** An instrument for separating and holding back the periosteum from bone. **rake r.** A small, toothed retractor used in dentistry. **rib r.** A self-retaining retractor that is used to hold the lateral aspects of a thoracotomy incision apart, thereby obtaining exposure in thoracic operations. **self-retaining r.** A retractor that maintains exposure by spring tension or by adjustment screws attached to the blades. **tonsil pillar r.** Any one of the variety of broad, blunt hooks designed to retract the anterior pillar of fauces after tonsillectomy, in order to permit inspection of the tonsil bed to

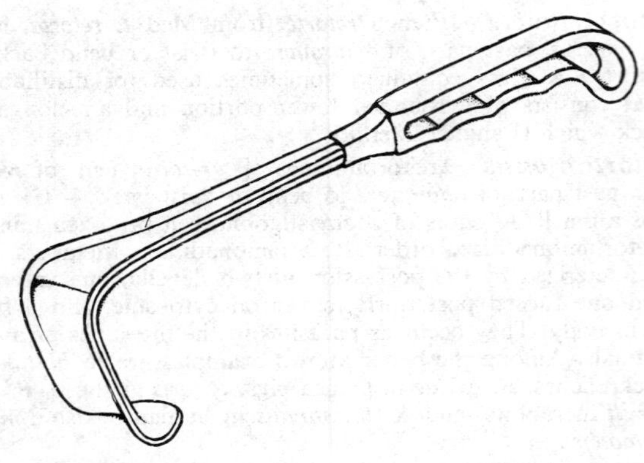

Abdominal retractor

locate bleeding points, etc. **vein r.** A small surgical device that has a smooth curved blade and is used to retract blood vessels, nerves, or other delicate structures without damaging them.

**retrad** \rē′trad\ Toward a dorsal or posterior part; posteriorly.

**retreat / vegetative r.** A psychosomatic disorder occurring in stressful situations, consisting of regression to earlier and sometimes infantile forms of visceral functioning.

**retrieval** \ritrē′vəl\ **information r.** The search for, identification of, and recovery of specific information from stored data.

**retro-** \ret′rə-, ret′rō-\ [L *retro* (adverb, from RE- + L *-tro* as in *ultro, intro*) behind, back, backward, differently, formerly] **1** A combining form meaning back, backward. **2** A combining form applied to the names of natural compounds, such as steroids or retinoids, that possess a conjugated system of double bonds. It specifies isomerization, so that the single bonds become double and the double ones single, with movement of a hydrogen atom from one end of the system to the other.

**retroaction** \-ak′shən\ Movement in a backward direction.

**retrobuccal** \-buk′əl\ **1** Pertaining to the back part of the mouth. **2** Behind the cheek.

**retrobulbar** \-bul′bər\ Behind the eyeball, in the Tenon space within the rectus muscle cone.

**retrocalcaneobursitis** \-kalkā′nē·ōbursī′tis\ ACHILLES BURSITIS.

**retrocatheterism** \-kath′ətərizm\ [RETRO- + CATHETER + -ISM] The passing of a catheter through an opening above the pubes and then through the urethra to the urinary meatus.

**retrocecal** \-sē′kəl\ Situated or occurring behind the cecum.

**retrocedent** \-sē′dənt\ Undergoing or characterized by retrocession.

**retrocession** \-sesh′ən\ [Late L *retrocessio* (from L *retrocessus*, past part. of *retrocedere* to go back) a going back] **1** A displacement backward, of an entire organ. Compare RETROFLEXION, RETROVERSION. **2** A shift in an inward direction, as of symptoms; the state of being retrocedent. **r. of uterus** Displacement of the uterus so that it occupies a position closer to the sacrum than normal.

**retroclination** \-klinā′shən\ [RETRO- + *(in)clination*] A palatal or lingual tilting of anterior teeth.

**retrocochlear** \-käk′lē·ər\ Denoting any structure situated medial or central to the cochlea of the internal ear, including the nuclei in the brainstem and the portion of the vestibulocochlear nerve between the cochlea and the brainstem: used primarily in otolaryngology.

**retrocolic** \-kō′lik\ Situated or occurring behind the colon.

**retrocollic** \-käl′ik\ Pertaining to or suffering from retrocollis.

**retrocollis** \-käl′is\ [RETRO- + *-collis* as in TORTICOLLIS] Intermittent or constant backward arching of the head and neck due to extrapyramidal disease rather than meningeal irritation or inflammation. Compare HEAD RETRACTION.

**retroconduction** \-kənduk′shən\ RETROGRADE CONDUCTION.

**retrocursive** \-kur′siv\ Stepping or running backward.

**retrodeviation** \-dē′vē·ā′shən\ [RETRO- + DEVIATION] A retroversion, retroflexion, or backward inclination.

**retrodisplacement** \-displās′mənt\ [RETRO- + DISPLACEMENT] The posterior or backward displacement of an organ, especially of the uterus.

**retroduodenal** \-d$^y$oo′ədē′nəl\ Situated or occurring behind the duodenum.

**retrodural** \-d$^y$oo′rəl\ Situated deep to the dura mater.

**retrofilling** POSTRESECTION FILLING.

**retroflexion** \-flek′shən\ [RETRO- + L *flexio* (from *flexus*, past part. of *flectere* to bend) a bending] **1** A folding or turning backward, as of an organ. Compare RETROCESSION, RETROVERSION. **2** A turning of emotion or cathexis from an object onto the self, as in the turning of rage against the object onto the self in depression. **r. of uterus** Backward deviation of the corpus uteri from its normal position.

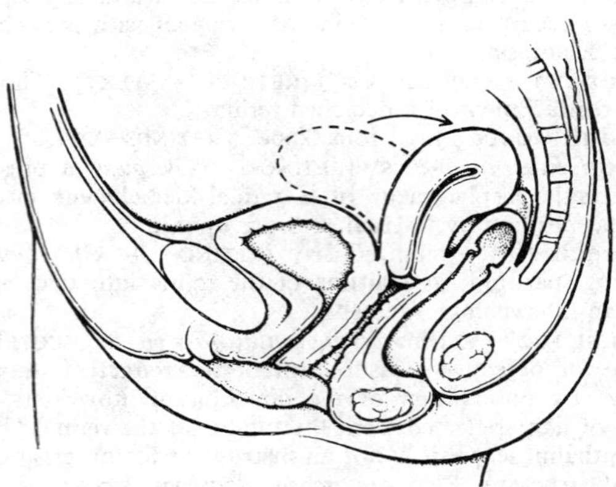

Retroflexion of uterus

**retrogasserian** \-gaser′ē·ən\ Situated or occurring caudal to the gasserian ganglion.

**retrognathism** \ret′rənath′izm\ [RETRO- + GNATH- + -ISM] A facial profile with the lower jaw, or both jaws, posterior to the normal relation to the facial frontal plane. Also *retrognathia*. See also MANDIBULAR RETRUSION. Adj. retrognathic. **Pierre Robin r.** ROBIN SEQUENCE.

**retrograde** \ret′rəgrād\ [L *retrograd(us)* (from *retro* backward + *gradi* to step) going backward] **1** Proceeding

backwards or against the normal direction of flow or current. 2 Pertaining to time preceding a given event, as *retrograde amnesia*. Compare ANTEROGRADE.
**retrography** \reträg′rəfē\ [RETRO- + -GRAPHY] MIRROR WRITING.
**retrogression** \-gresh′ən\ 1 REGRESSION. 2 CATABOLISM.
**retroillumination** \ret′rō·ilooʹminā′shən\ [RETRO- + ILLUMINATION] A technique of determining the relucence or opacity of ocular structures, as the cornea, lens, or retina, by observation of light transmitted from behind the structure. The technique is of great importance in every routine examination of the eye. Also *backlighting*.
**retroinfection** \-infek′shən\ [RETRO- + INFECTION] A maternal infection that is secondary to a primary fetal infection.
**retroinsular** \ret′rō·in′sʸələr\ Situated caudal to the insula.
**retroiridian** \ret′rō·irid′ē·ən\ Located behind the iris.
**retrojection** \-jek′shən\ [RETRO- + *(in)jection*] A flushing out of a body cavity by injection of a fluid.
**retrolenticular** \-lentik′yələr\ [RETRO- + LENTICULAR] Situated behind the crystalline lens. Also *retrolental*.
**retromastoid** \-mas′toid\ Behind the mastoid process of the temporal bone.
**retromolar** \-mō′lər\ [RETRO- + MOLAR] Situated behind the most posterior upper and lower molar tooth.
**retroperitoneal** \-per′itənē′əl\ Behind the peritoneum.
**retroperitoneum** \-per′itənē′əm\ SPATIUM RETROPERITONEALE.
**retroperitonitis** \-per′itənī′tis\ Inflammation in the retroperitoneum.
**retropharynx** \-far′ingks\ The posterior part of the pharynx.
**retroposition** [RETRO- + POSITION] A simple backward or posterior displacement of an organ or structure without other attitudinal alterations of the organ or structure.
**retropulsion** \-pul′shən\ [RETRO- + PULSION] A gait disturbance seen in some patients with parkinsonism in which the patient tends spontaneously to walk backwards, or, if he walks backwards voluntarily, he does so more and more quickly until he falls or is stopped by an obstacle. Also *opisthoporeia*. Compare ANTEROPULSION.
**retrorsine** $C_{18}H_{25}NO_6$. A poisonous alkaloid known to be mutagenic, teratogenic, and carcinogenic. It is found in species of *Senecio*. It has caused death in livestock through necrosis of the liver and damage to the kidney. The alkaloid has been identified as a toxic factor in some herbal infusions, or teas, and is the causal agent of a veno-occlusive disease of the liver in Jamaicans.
**retrosinus** \-sī′nəs\ Mastoid air cells behind the sigmoid sinus. *Outmoded*.
**retrosplenial** \-splē′nē·əl\ Situated behind the splenum of the corpus callosum.
**retrospondylolisthesis** \-spän′dilōlisthē′sis\ A bending or slipping backwards, at the posterior facet joints, of a vertebra.
**retrostalsis** \-stal′sis\ RETROGRADE PERISTALSIS.
**retrotarsal** \-tär′səl\ Behind the tarsus of the eyelid.
**retroversioflexion** \-vur′sē·ōflek′shən\ Retroversion combined with retroflexion of the uterus.
**retroversion** \-vur′zhən\ [RETRO- + VERSION] 1 A tilting backward without folding, as of an organ. Compare RETROCESSION, RETROFLEXION. 2 An abnormally posterior position of the teeth. **r. of uterus** The position in which the entire uterus is tilted backward without angulation between the corpus and cervix.
**Retroviridae** \-vir′idē\ [RETRO- + *vir(us)* + -IDAE] A family of pleomorphic, membrane-bound, single-stranded RNA viruses which possess a virion-associated, RNA-dependent DNA polymerase. The virion-associated enzyme synthesizes DNA from an RNA template, which is the reverse of the usual, DNA-to-RNA, transcription. The family contains such viruses as the murine leukosis viruses, the Rous sarcoma virus, visna virus, and the foamy viruses.
**retrovirus** \ret′rōvī′rəs\ A virus belonging to the Retroviridae family. **human lymphotrophic r.'es** Any of three viruses belonging to the oncovirus subgroup of the family Retroviridae. See under HUMAN IMMUNODEFICIENCY VIRUS.
**retrusion** \ritroo′zhən\ [L *retrus(us)*, past part. of *retrudere* to thrust back + -ION] 1 A posterior movement of the mandible. 2 A position of the mandible resulting from a retrusive excursion. **mandibular r.** An abnormally posterior anatomic position of the mandible; retrognathism. Also *posterior occlusion, posteroclusion, retrusive occlusion, mandibular retraction*.
**return** / **venous r.** The volume of blood returning to an atrium of the heart over a given period of time.
**Retzius** [Anders Adolf *Retzius*, Swedish anatomist, 1796–1860] 1 Cavity of Retzius, space of Retzius. See under SPATIUM RETROPUBICUM. 2 See under LIGAMENT, VEIN.
**Retzius** [Gustav Magnus *Retzius*, Swedish anatomist, 1842–1919] 1 Key-Retzius sheath. See under ENDONEURIUM. 2 Retzius lines. See under STRIAE OF RETZIUS.
**rev** revolution.
**revaccination** \rē′vaksinā′shən\ [RE- + VACCINATION] Repeated vaccination.
**revascularization** \rēvas′kyələrīzā′shən\ The restoration of blood flow to a part of the body.
**revehent** \rev′əhənt\ [L *revehens*, gen. *revehentis*, pres. part. of *revehere* to carry or bring back] Carrying or conveying back, as the veins draining blood from the liver to the sinus venosus of the developing heart. See also VENAE REVEHENTES.
**Reverdin** [Jacques-Louis *Reverdin*, Swiss surgeon, 1842–1929] Reverdin's operation, Reverdin's method. See under GRAFT.
**reversal** \rivur′səl\ The act or process of changing to an opposite direction or course; a complete turnabout. **epinephrine r.** REBOUND CONGESTION. **sex r.** A condition in which an organism's chromosomal sex is different from the organism's anatomic sex.
**reversal-formation** REACTION-FORMATION.
**reversible** Capable of being reversed or corrected, as the course of a disease.
**reversion** \rivur′zhən\ [L *reversio* (from *revertere* to turn back, return, from RE- + L *vertere* to turn, turn about or around) a turning back, recurrence] 1 The reappearance of a wild-type phenotype in the progeny of a cell or an organism that has a mutant phenotype. It can be caused by genotypic reversion, suppressor mutation, or phenotypic reversion. 2 ATAVISM. **genotypic r.** The reappearance of a wild-type phenotype in the progeny of a mutant cell or organism because of either a mutation at the site of the original mutation, which restores the wild-type genotype, or a mutation at another site, which counterbalances the negative effect of the original mutation. See also BACK MUTATION. **Mantoux r.** A shift from tuberculin-positive to tuberculin-negative, occasionally seen in persons immunized many years previously with BCG vaccine. It may indicate the need for reimmunization with BCG vaccine. Compare MANTOUX CONVERSION. **phenotypic r.** The reappearance of a

wild-type phenotype in the progeny of a cell of an organism that has a mutant phenotype because of nongenetic factors. The factors restore the activity of the mutated gene product or circumvent its need.

**revertant** \rivur′tənt\ An organism derived from a mutant but showing the properties of the ancestral organism before the original mutation took place.

**review** / **claims r.** The process of examining for eligibility, validity, and acceptability claims for payment submitted by enrollees, and by providers for services rendered, under the provisions of health insurance plans. **tissue r.** A review and evaluation of surgery performed in a hospital based on an assessment of the pathological diagnosis, primarily to determine the appropriateness and necessity of the procedure. It is ofter performed by a hospital committee composed of physicians.

**Revilliod** [Léon *Revilliod*, Swiss physician, 1835–1919] Revilliod sign. See under ORBICULARIS SIGN.

**revival** \rivī′vəl\ [*reviv(e)* + -AL] The restoration of life or consciousness.

**revivification** \riviv′əfikā′shən\ [RE- + VIVI- + -FICATION] **1** The restoration of life or consciousness. **2** The refreshing of a wound to promote healing; débridement.

**revolute** \rev′əloot\ Turned or curled backward.

**revolution** / **demographic r.** A process of transition seen in many populations since the eighteenth century and characterized by a marked reduction in both fertility and mortality. In several countries the fall in mortality preceded the decline in fertility, resulting in a temporary phase during which the population increased in size more rapidly than before or after the transitional period.

**revulsant** \rivul′sənt\ A substance causing an irritant reaction for purposes of counterirritant or revulsive therapy.

**revulsion** \rivul′shən\ [L *revulsio* a tearing away, from *revellere* to tear or pull away] An obsolete technique of historical interest by which blood is diverted from an afflicted area to another site by use of counterirritation.

**reward** Any stimulus, event, situation, or verbal commentary yielding a satisfaction upon successful performance of a task. A reward may be anything, from a food pellet delivered to an experimental animal on reaching the goal box of a maze to election of a human to an honor society for academic achievement. The task may be self-elected or specified by others. **token r.** A reward which does not in itself yield satisfaction but has a value which must be learned. Thus a primate may learn the value of different-colored poker chips by exchanging them for different numbers of grapes.

**rewarming** The raising of the body temperature following intentional hypothermia, such as in surface hypothermia or hypothermia induced with extracorporeal circulation.

**Reye** [Ralph Douglas Kenneth *Reye*, Australian physician, flourished 20th century] See under SYNDROME.

**Reynals** See under DURAN-REYNALS.

**Reys** [L. *Reys*, French physician, flourished 20th century] Weill-Reys-Adie syndrome, Weill-Reys syndrome. See under ADIE SYNDROME.

**RF** **1** rheumatoid factor. **2** releasing factor (releasing hormone).

**rf** radio frequency.

**RFA** right frontoanterior position (of a fetus). See under BROW ANTERIOR POSITION.

**RFP** right frontoposterior position (of a fetus). See under BROW POSTERIOR POSITION.

**RFT** right frontotransverse position (of a fetus). See under BROW TRANSVERSE POSITION.

**RH** releasing hormone.

**Rh** **1** Symbol for the element, rhodium. **2** Rhesus (factor).

**rhabd-** \rabd-\ RHABDO-.

**rhabditic** \rabdit′ik\ **1** Belonging to or characteristic of the nematode genus *Rhabditis* or closely related genera. **2** Caused by nematodes of the genus *Rhabditis* or closely related genera.

**rhabditiform** \rabdit′ifôrm\ RHABDITOID.

***Rhabditis*** \rabdī′tis\ A genus of common small nematodes (superfamily Rhabditoidea). Most species are free-living soil nematodes, but many show traits of incipient parasitism, living in cutaneous ulcers, sores, or soil-matted fur or fleece, and some are frankly parasitic during part of their life cycle or are facultative parasites. The onset of nematode parasitism is well illustrated by members of this group. Also *Rhabdonema*. ***R. strongyloides*** A species occurring in the soil which can cause dermatitis in dogs, cattle, and other animals raised in unsanitary conditions, as when the nematodes are permitted to become established in sores or mud-caked fur. Accidental or temporary parasitism of humans has also been reported.

**rhabditoid** \rab′ditoid\ **1** Similar in form to larvae of the nematode genus *Rhabditis.*. Also *rhabditiform*. **2** Characteristic of nematodes of the genus *Rhabditis* and closely related genera.

**rhabdo-** \rab′də-\ [Gk *rhabdos* a rod, stick, stripe] A combining form meaning (1) rod-shaped; (2) striped, striated. Also *rhabd-*.

**rhabdocyte** \rab′dəsīt\ *Rare* METAMYELOCYTE.

**rhabdomyoblast** \-mī′əblast\ [RHABDO- + MYOBLAST] A primitive striated muscle cell with eosinophilic cytoplasm. The cells may be rounded or straplike and may contain cross striations. They are believed to indicate differentiation in tumors toward striated muscle cells.

**rhabdomyochondroma** \-mī′əkändrō′mə\ [RHABDO- + MYO- + CHONDR- + -OMA] A benign tumor containing striated muscle cells and cartilaginous elements.

**rhabdomyolysis** \rab′dōmī·äl′əsis\ [RHABDO- + MYOLYSIS] Destruction of skeletal muscle accompanied by myoglobinemia and myoglobinuria, which may lead to acute kidney failure. This destruction may be due to many causes, such as trauma, heat stroke, seizures, hypokalemia, arterial insufficiency, compression syndromes, influenza, or toxins. **exertional r.** Rhabdomyolysis due to prolonged, intense, and unaccustomed exercise of skeletal muscle. **familial paroxysmal r.** GLYCOGEN STORAGE DISEASE V. **idiopathic r.** A syndrome of acute muscle pain and tenderness due to widespread necrosis of skeletal muscle fibers giving rise to myoglobinuria. The condition may occur in recurrent episodes, each followed by regeneration of the damaged muscle. In many cases the cause is unknown, in some the attacks follow physical exertion, and in some the cause appears to be carnitine palmityl transferase deficiency. Also *paroxysmal myoglobinuria*.

**rhabdomyoma** \-mī·ō′mə\ [RHABDO- + MYOMA] A benign tumor of striated muscle-type cells, generally consisting of polygonal, frequently vacuolated (glycogen-containing) cells having a finely granular, deeply acidophilic cytoplasm. Cells with cross-striations are fairly common. The tumor is rare, and the majority of cases have been observed in the upper neck region, the tongue, the pharyngeal wall, and the vicinity of the larynx. The heart may also be the site of origin. Also *myoma striocellulare*.

**rhabdomyosarcoma** \rab′dōmī′əsärkō′mə\ [RHABDO- + MYO- + SARCOMA] A highly malignant tumor of rhabdomyoblasts in varying stages of differentiation, with or without intracellular myofibrils, and with or without cross-striations. Cytology and growth pattern vary greatly and three types can be distinguished, embryonal, alveolar, and pleomorphic. The two former types prevail in children and adolescents. Mixed forms may occur. The embryonal and alveolar types of the tumor may arise in sites where skeletal muscle is not normally present, such as the bladder. Special staining techniques may be necessary for the demonstration of cross-striations. **embryonal r.** A subtype of rhabdomyosarcoma composed predominantly of poorly differentiated rhabdomyoblasts in a loosely structured edematous or myxomatous matrix. It may appear grossly as a grapelike structure (sarcoma botryoides). This tumor is primarily found in the bladder, vagina, orbit, and ear of children. **r. of the urinary bladder** A malignant tumor of rhabdomyoblasts of the urinary bladder. It is found mainly in children. The tumor typically appears as grapelike clusters which project into the bladder lumen, for which the term *sarcoma botryoides* has been used.

***Rhabdonema*** \-nē′mə\ *RHABDITIS.*

**rhabdosphincter** \-sfingk′tər\ A sphincter formed by striated muscle fibers. Also *striated muscular sphincter.*

**Rhabdoviridae** \-vir′idē\ [*rhabdovir(us)* + -IDAE] A family of enveloped, bullet-shaped viruses (180 × 75 nm) which contain a single-stranded RNA genome which does not serve as messenger RNA. The family contains such members as the rabies virus and vesicular stomatitis virus.

**rhabdovirus** \-vī′rəs\ [RHABDO- + VIRUS] Any member of the Rhabdoviridae family of viruses.

**rhachi-** \rā′kē-\ For words beginning *rhachi-*, see also under RACHI-.

**rhacous** \rā′kəs\ [Gk *rhakos* a strip of cloth or flesh, rag; in pl. *rhakea* wrinkles] Torn; wrinkled; cleft.

**rhaebocrania** \rē′bōkrā′nē·ə\ TORTICOLLIS.

**-rhage** \-rij\ -RRHAGE.

**rhaphe** \rā′fē\ An outmoded spelling for RAPHE.

**-rhaphy** \-rəfē\ -RRHAPHY.

**RHD** rheumatic heart disease.

**-rhea** \-rē′ə\ -RRHEA.

**rhenium** \rē′nē·əm\ Element number 75, having atomic weight 186.2. Two stable isotopes occur, widely but sparsely dispersed in minerals throughout the lithosphere. Valences are 1, 2, 3, 4, 5, 6, and 7. In elemental form, rhenium is a very dense, ductile, silvery white metal with a high melting point. Its physical properties make it valuable to technology, especially in instrumentation. Symbol: Re

**rheo-** \rē′ō-\ [Gk *rheos* a stream, current] A combining form meaning flow or current.

**rheobase** \rē′əbās\ [RHEO- + *base*] The threshold value of applied current of infinite duration that is capable of stimulating excitable tissue. Also *galvanic threshold.*

**rheoencephalography** \rē′ō·ensef′əläg′rəfē\ [RHEO- + ENCEPHALOGRAPHY] The technique of continuously recording the pulsatile changes in electrical impedance of the brain which result from vascular changes and may indicate pathology.

**rheology** \rē·äl′əjē\ [RHEO- + -LOGY] The study of the irreversible processes related to inelasticity and the flow of condensed matter.

**rheometer** \rē·äm′ətər\ [RHEO- + -METER] GALVANOMETER.

**rheometry** \rē·äm′ətrē\ [RHEO- + -METRY] Measurement of the flow of electric current or of viscous substances such as blood.

**rheonome** \rē′ənōm\ [RHEO- + Gk *nomē* (from *nemein* to distribute) a division, distribution] An instrument used to stimulate tissue with electrical current of varying strength.

**rheostosis** \rē·äs′təsis\ MELORHEOSTOSIS.

**rhesus** \rē′səs\ See under RHESUS MONKEY.

**rheum** \room\ [Gk *rheum(a)* (from *rhein* to flow) a flow] **1** A flow or discharge of mucus. **2** An upper respiratory infection.

**rheum-** \room-\ [Gk *rheuma*, gen. *rheumatos*, a flow, stream, flux (from *rhein* to flow, gush)] A combining form meaning rheumatic.

**rheuma** \roo′mə\ [Gk *rheuma* a flow, stream, flux] *Obs.* CATARRH.

**rheumatic** \roomat′ik\ [Gk *rheumatikos* (from *rheuma*, gen. *rheumatos* a flow, stream, flux) affected with a flux or discharge] **1** Pertaining to abnormalities of the musculoskeletal system. **2** Pertaining to rheumatism.

**rheumatism** \roo′mətizm\ [Gk *rheumatismos* (from *rheumatizein* to cause a flux, from *rheuma*; see RHEUM) a defluxion of rheum (to which joint pains, etc., were formerly attributed)] Any of a variety of musculoskeletal pains, including arthritis, tendonitis, bursitis, and a vast array of other complaints. *Imprecise.* **gonorrheal r.** GONOCOCCAL ARTHRITIS. **r. of the heart** RHEUMATIC HEART DISEASE. **Heberden's r.** OSTEOARTHRITIS. **inflammatory r.** RHEUMATIC FEVER. **lumbar r.** LUMBAGO. **muscular r.** NONARTICULAR RHEUMATISM. **nodose r.** Osteoarthritis with Heberden's and Bouchard's nodes. **nonarticular r.** Musculoskeletal symptoms originating in the tendons, bursae, muscles, or bones, but not involving the joints. Also *muscular rheumatism.* **palindromic r.** Episodic acute arthritis of transient duration, often occurring over several years, and sometimes being the first manifestation of a form of inflammatory arthritis. **Poncet's r.** PONCET'S DISEASE. **subacute r.** Rheumatic disease of low-grade activity and intermediate duration. **synovial r.** Rheumatic disease affecting the joints. **tuberculous r.** TUBERCULOSIS OF BONES AND JOINTS. **visceral r.** Any systemic rheumatic disease.

**rheumatismal** \roo′mətiz′məl\ RHEUMATOID.

**rheumatogenic** \roo′mətōjen′ik\ [Gk *rheuma*, gen. *rheumatos*, a flow + -GENIC] Causing or arising from rheumatic disease.

**rheumatoid** \roo′mətoid\ Pertaining to rheumatic disease, especially rheumatoid arthritis. Also *rheumatismal.*

**rheumatologic** Pertaining to the study of rheumatic disease.

**rheumatologist** A specialist in the study and treatment of rheumatic disease.

**rheumatology** \roo′mətäl′əjē\ [Gk *rheuma* (gen. *rheumatos*) a flow, stream, flux + -LOGY] The science concerned with rheumatic disease.

**-rhexis** \-rek′sis\ -RRHEXIS.

**rhigosis** \rigō′sis\ [Gk *rhigo(s)* frost, cold + -SIS] The perception of cold.

**rhin-** \rīn-\ RHINO-.

**rhinal** \rī′nəl\ NASAL.

**rhinectomy** \rīnek′təmē\ [RHIN- + -ECTOMY] Excision of the external nose, wholly or in part. • When not qualified, this is taken to mean total rhinectomy. **total r.** Radical excision of the whole external nose, usually now considered only for patients with extensive tumors of this part. Multistage plastic surgery for reconstruction has now been largely superseded by the use of custom-made prostheses attached to spectacle frames.

**rhinencephalic** \rī′nensəfal′ik\ Pertaining to the rhinencephalon.

**rhinencephalon** \rī′nensef′əlän\ [RHIN- + ENCEPHALON] Those parts of the brain concerned with olfaction, comprising the olfactory nerves, bulbs, tracts, striae, paraolfactory areas, anterior perforated substance, prepyriform cortex, amygdaloid complex, and anterior olfactory nuclei. Also *olfactory brain, olfactory area, nosebrain* (obs.), *smell-brain.*

**rhinesthesia** \rī'nesthē'zhə\ [RHIN- + ESTHESIA] The sense of smell.

**rhinism** \rī'nizm\ NASAL RESONANCE.

**rhinitis** \rīnī'tis\ [RHIN- + -ITIS] Inflammation of the lining of the nose. Symptoms common to most kinds include nasal obstruction and discharge. Sneezing and anosmia occur in a large proportion of cases. **acute r.** 1 Any rhinitis running an acute course. Also *coryza.* 2 COMMON COLD. **acute catarrhal r.** COMMON COLD. **allergic r.** Rhinitis in hypersensitized individuals caused by vasoactive amines released as the result of the antigen-antibody reaction. The disease may be seasonal, as in the case of hay fever, or perennial, as in that due to house dust. Symptoms common to both include sneezing, nasal obstruction, and watery rhinorrhea. The main lines of treatment are hyposensitization to the allergen concerned, the administration of antihistamine drugs, and the local or even general use of corticosteroids. Also *nasal allergy, atopic rhinitis.* **atopic r.** ALLERGIC RHINITIS. **atrophic r.** Chronic rhinitis characterized by progressive atrophy of the nasal mucosa and conchae, particularly of the inferior concha. The viscid secretions dry to form crusts which cause nasal obstruction and impart a foul smell to the breath. The condition, which commences at puberty especially in females, is now uncommon in both sexes. Also *ozena.* **r. caseosa** A rare variety of chronic rhinitis, usually unilateral, characterized by a granulomatous reaction in the nasal lining and the accumulation in the nose of malodorous cheesy material. The pathogenesis is uncertain. **catarrhal r.** Any variety of rhinitis in which the evidence of inflammation is confined to a simple catarrhal reaction in the absence of other more specific changes. **fibrinous r.** MEMBRANOUS RHINITIS. **gangrenous r.** CANCRUM NASI. **granulomatous r.** Rhinitis as a result of infective granulomas, such as tuberculosis or late syphilis, or of any other granulomatous disease, as Wegener's granulomatosis. **hypertrophic r.** A condition of the nasal lining in which some parts display hypertrophic changes, sometimes of a severe order. The nasal conchae are most often affected, particularly the posterior ends of the inferior conchae which may present with the nodular appearance known as mulberry hypertrophy. The pathogenesis is uncertain but chronic sinusitis, allergy, and vasomotor rhinitis have all been blamed. **infective r.** Any rhinitis caused by infection with one or more microorganisms, the commonest and most important being a variety of viruses, particularly the rhinoviruses. Bacteria, frequently found in the nose in cases of infective rhinitis such as the common cold, are usually secondary invaders colonizing the nasal mucosa already damaged by the primary viral infection. **intrinsic r.** VASOMOTOR RHINITIS. **r. medicamentosa** Rhinitis caused by local nasal medication usually applied in the form of nose drops. The symptoms are often the same as those of the disease for which the medication is employed, tempting the patient to use more, so that a vicious circle is set up. **membranous r.** Rhinitis, sometimes unilateral, characterized by the presence of a membranous exudate. In areas where diphtheria remains endemic, infection with *Corynebacterium diphtheriae* is still responsible but in rare instances. Uncommonly, infection with other organisms, including pneumococcus, staphylococcus, and streptococcus, may result in pseudomembrane formation. Also *fibrinous rhinitis, pseudomembranous rhinitis.* **perennial allergic r.** Rhinitis due to allergy and liable to occur through all seasons of the year. As the responsible allergen is present somewhere in the environment at all times, it differs, therefore, from allergens such as pollens which are present only at certain seasons. Also *nonseasonal allergic rhinitis.* **periodic r.** Rhinitis recurring at intervals. It is more likely to be the result of allergy or vasomotor instability rather than infection. **polypoid r.** Rhinitis with formation of nasal polyps. **pseudomembranous r.** MEMBRANOUS RHINITIS. **purulent r.** Rhinitis characterized by purulent nasal discharge as, for example, in the later stages of the common cold. **syphilitic r.** Rhinitis as a manifestation of nasal syphilis. • In practice the term is likely to be used in reference only to secondary syphilis as it affects the nose, this stage being accompanied as a rule by simple catarrhal rhinitis. **tuberculous r.** Rhinitis due to tuberculosis, a rare disease even where tuberculosis is still prevalent. Nodular or ulcerative forms occur, affecting the cartilaginous part of the nasal septum and, exceptionally, the lateral nasal wall. The ulcerative form is liable to produce perforation of the septum. Although primary cases have been reported, it is usually secondary to pulmonary tuberculosis. **vasomotor r.** A condition resembling rhinitis but occurring in the absence of infection, allergy, or other demonstrable cause of inflammation. It is widely regarded as due to an upset in the control of the autonomic nervous system over the blood vessels and glands of the nasal lining. Also *vasomotor rhinopathy, intrinsic rhinitis.*

**rhino-** \rī'nō-\ [Gk *rhis,* gen. *rhinos* nose] A combining form denoting the nose. Also *rhin-.*

**rhinocanthectomy** \-kanthek'təmē\ [RHINO- + CANTHECTOMY] Surgical removal of a portion of the medial canthus. Also *rhinommectomy.*

**rhinocele** \rī'nəsēl\ RHINOCOELE.

**rhinocephaly** \-sef'əlē\ [RHINO- + CEPHAL- + -Y ] A primary maldevelopment of the brain in which the rhinencephalic parts of the telencephalon are poorly developed or tend to be fused across the midline. Since some degree of rhinocephaly is always a part of the cyclopic complex, and since it is the first defect of the complex to be recognizable in the embryo, it is thought to be the underlying defect which triggers all degrees of cyclopia.

**rhinocheiloplasty** \-kī'ləplas'tē\ [RHINO- + CHEILO- + -PLASTY] A plastic operation on the nose and lips.

**rhinocoele** \rī'nəsēl\ [RHINO- + -COELE] The ventricle located in the olfactory lobe of the central nervous system. Also *rhinocele.*

**rhinodymia** \-dim'ē·ə\ [RHINO- + *-dym(us)* + -IA] Duplication of the nose in part or *in toto,* or apparent bifurcation owing to midline hypoplasia so that the nares are separated by a median depression.

**rhinoentomophthoromycosis** \-en'təmäf'thərəmīkō'sis\ [RHINO- + ENTOMOPHTHOROMYCOSIS] RHINOPHYCOMYCOSIS.

***Rhinoestrus*** \rī'nō·es'trəs\ A genus of flies (family Oestridae), larval forms of which are parasitic in the nasal passages of horses. Found in Europe, Africa, and Asia, they may cause myiasis in the human eye. These cases of human ophthalmomyiasis are usually of brief duration, with pain and inflammation and a brief conjunctivitis. Reports of extensive eye damage are probably due to other types of myiasis caused by different fly larvae.

**rhinogenous** \rīnäj'ənəs\ Originating in the nose or caused by nasal disease.

**rhinohyperplasia** \-hī'pərplā'zhə\ Hyperplasia of the nose.

**rhinolalia** \-lā'lyə\ [RHINO- + -LALIA] NASAL RESONANCE. **r. aperta** HYPERNASALITY. **r. clausa** HYPONASALITY.

**rhinolaryngology** \-lar′ing·gäl′əjē\ The branch of otorhinolaryngology concerned with the nose and larynx and with their interrelationship. Also *laryngorhinology.*

**rhinolith** \rīn′əlith\ [RHINO- + -LITH] An irregular concretion of calcium and magnesium salts formed over years around a foreign body in the nose. The foreign body is often deliberately introduced by the patient in childhood but overlooked. It may reach an overall size of several centimeters. Also *nasal calculus.*

**rhinolithiasis** \-lithī′əsis\ The disease caused by the presence of a rhinolith. The major symptoms are nasal obstruction and blood-stained nasal discharge.

**rhinologist** \rinäl′əjist\ An otorhinolaryngologist particularly experienced in rhinology.

**rhinology** \rinäl′əjē\ [RHINO- + -LOGY] The branch of otorhinolaryngology concerned particularly with the nose and paranasal regions.

**rhinomanometer** \-mənäm′ətər\ A manometer for measuring the airflow and variations in air pressure within the nose. Also *nasomanometer.*

**rhinomanometry** \-mənäm′ətrē\ The measurement of airflow and variations in air pressure within the nose. The resistance to respiration offered by the nasal soft tissues may be calculated from the results of the measurement.

**rhinommectomy** \rī′nämek′təmē\ [RHIN- + Gk *omm(a)* (from *ōmmai* perf. passive of *oran* to see, look) the eye + -ECTOMY] RHINOCANTHECTOMY.

**rhinomycosis** \-mīkō′sis\ Any one of a number of fungus diseases affecting the nose.

**rhinonecrosis** \-nekrō′sis\ Necrosis of any part of the nose.

**rhinopathy** \rīnäp′əthē\ [RHINO- + -PATHY] Any disease of the nose. **vasomotor r.** VASOMOTOR RHINITIS.

**rhinopharyngitis** \-far′injī′tis\ 1 NASOPHARYNGITIS. 2 PHARYNGORHINITIS. **r. mutilans** GANGOSA.

**rhinopharyngolith** \-faring′gəlith\ A rhinolith extending into the nasopharynx.

**rhinopharynx** \-far′ingks\ PARS NASALIS PHARYNGIS.

**rhinophonia** \-fō′nē·ə\ NASAL RESONANCE.

**rhinophycomycosis** \-fī′kōmīkō′sis\ [RHINO- + PHYCOMYCOSIS] A fungal infection of man and animals, especially horses, caused by *Entomophthora coronata* and characterized by polyp formation in the nose and paranasal sinuses. Infection may eventually disseminate to the brain via the ethmoid plate. Also *phycomycosis entomophthorae, rhinoentomophthoromycosis.*

**rhinophyma** \-fī′mə\ [RHINO- + Gk *phyma* a tumor, boil, cancer] A condition in which the external nose becomes red and swollen, with enlarged pilosebaceous orifices, as a result of hypertrophy of the sebaceous glands and connective tissue. It is usually but not invariably associated with rosacea. Also *whisky nose, strawberry nose, potato nose, copper nose.*

**rhinoplastic** \-plas′tik\ Pertaining to or achieved by rhinoplasty.

**rhinoplasty** \rī′nəplas′tē\ [RHINO- + -PLASTY] Any plastic operation on the nose. **augmentation r.** An operation in which missing or attenuated portions of the nasal skeleton are replaced or augmented by means of grafts or other implants. **Carpue's r.** INDIAN RHINOPLASTY. **English r.** A method of reconstructing the nose, utilizing flaps taken from the cheeks. **Indian r.** A method of reconstructing the nose by using a caudally based flap from the median forehead (Indian flap). Also *Indian operation, Carpue's operation, Carpue's rhinoplasty.* **Italian r.** Reconstruction of the nose by means of a distally based flap taken from the medial side of the arm (Italian flap). Also *Italian method, Italian operation, tagliacotian rhinoplasty, tagliacotian operation* (outmoded). **reconstructive r.** An operation for reconstructing the nose or a part thereof. **tagliacotian r.** ITALIAN RHINOPLASTY.

**rhinorrhea** \rī′nôrē′ə\ [RHINO- + -RRHEA] Discharge from the nose. **cerebrospinal r.** Leakage of cerebrospinal fluid through the nose due to a defect in the dura and floor of the skull, usually in the region of the cribriform plate, but sometimes of the sphenoidal sinus.

**rhinoscleroma** \-sklirō′mə\ Scleroma of the nose. Scleroma invariably originates in, and usually remains confined to, the nose.

**rhinoscope** \rin′əskōp\ [RHINO- + -SCOPE] An instrument for examining the interior of the nose, usually with an incorporated source of illumination. *Seldom used.* Also *nasoscope.*

**rhinoscopy** \rīnäs′kəpē\ [RHINO- + -SCOPY] Examination of the interior of the nose. **anterior r.** Examination of the nose by way of the anterior nares. **posterior r.** 1 Mirror examination of the posterior nares and the nasopharynx. 2 NASOPHARYNGOSCOPY.

**rhinosporidiosis** \-spôrid′ē·ō′sis\ [*Rhinosporidi(um)* + -OSIS] An exophytic granulomatous nasal mycosis caused by *Rhinosporidium seeberi* running a chronic course characterized by progressive nasal obstruction, due to friable vascular polyps, and epistaxis. Very rarely it spreads to the larynx. It is a common disease in Sri Lanka and Southern India with sporadic occurrence in Central and South America, Africa, and Italy.

***Rhinosporidium*** \-spôrid′ē·əm\ [RHINO- + New L *-sporidium*, dim. of -SPORIUM] A genus of fungi causing rhinosporidiosis and thought to belong to the class Chytridiomycetes. It is endemic in Sri Lanka and India and thought to be a fish parasite that incidentally attacks man and other mammals.

**rhinostenosis** \-stenō′sis\ NASAL STENOSIS.

**rhinotomy** \rinät′əmē\ [RHINO- + -TOMY] Any incision into the nose. **lateral r.** Rhinotomy performed to allow the surgeon better access to intranasal structures. A vertical skin incision is made alongside the nose from close to the medial palpebral canthus, skirting the ala nasi and terminating in the anterior naris. This allows the external nose on one side to be widely retracted for easier access.

**rhinotracheitis** \-trā′kē·ī′tis\ Tracheitis occurring as a complication of rhinitis.

**rhinovaccination** \-vak′sinā′shən\ Vaccination by way of the nasal mucous membrane.

**rhinovirus** \-vī′rəs\ [RHINO- + VIRUS] Any member of the *Rhinovirus* genus of the Picornaviridae family. They are small, ether-resistant, single-stranded RNA viruses. The human rhinoviruses (over 100 numbered and unnumbered serotypes) are the major known cause of the common cold. The genus also includes equine and bovine rhinoviruses.

***Rhipicephalus*** \rī′pisef′ələs\ [Gk *rhipis* a fan + *kephalē* the head] A genus of hard ticks (family Ixodidae), consisting of about 50 species, all Old World except *R. sanguineus*, the common dog tick. Both sexes have eyes and festoons, but only males have palps and ventral plates. The genus includes important vectors of disease in man and domestic animals. ***R. sanguineus*** A cosmopolitan species, the brown dog tick, parasitic on many domestic animals, particularly dogs, in the United States and elsewhere. It is probably the most widespread of all ticks, though it has rather strict temperature and humidity requirements. It is the principal vector of the agent of Rocky Mountain spotted fever in Mexico, and is also involved in transmitting *Babesia canis*, the agent of canine babesiosis. In addition, it is thought to be important in the spread of boutonneuse fever. Among the viruses spread by the brown dog tick are the Was Medarri virus, the Uukunieme group virus, and the human lymphocytic choriomeningitis virus in Ethiopia.

**rhitid-** \rit′id-\ For words beginning *rhitid-*, see under RHYTID-.

**rhitidosis** \rī′tidō′sis\ RHYTIDOSIS.

**rhiz-** \rīz-\ RHIZO-.

**rhizanesthesia** \rī′zanesthē′zhə\ SPINAL ANESTHESIA.

**rhizo-** \rī′zō-\ [Gk *rhiza* (in plural *rhizai* the roots of the eye) a root] A combining form meaning root. Also *rhiz-*.

***Rhizoglyphus*** \rīzäg′lifəs\ A genus of itch mites in the family Acaridae, responsible for occupational acarine dermatitis, such as the dermatitis of flower and onion bulb handlers caused by *R. echinopus*.

**Rhizomastigida** \-mastij′idə\ A former name for TRICHOMONADIDA.

**rhizomelia** \-mē′lyə\ [RHIZO- + MEL-[1] + -IA] **1** A relative shortening of the proximal segment of the limbs. **2** RHIZOMELIC DWARFISM.

**rhizomelic** \-mē′lik\ Of or relating to the hip joint or the shoulder joint.

**rhizomeningomyelitis** \-məning′gōmī′əlī′tis\ RADICULOMENINGOMYELITIS.

**rhizomere** \rī′zəmir\ DERMATOME.

**rhizopod** \rī′zəpäd\ [RHIZO- + -POD] **1** An ameba belonging to the superclass Rhizopoda. **2** RHIZOPODIUM.

**Rhizopoda** \rīzäp′ədə\ [New L, from *rhizopodi(um)* + *-a*, pl. suffix] A superclass of amebas (in the subphylum Sarcodina) with locomotion by lobopodia, filopodia, rhizopodia, or protoplasmic flow without forming separate pseudopodia. It consists of eight classes, the more familiar nontestate amebas being placed in the class Lobosea, subclass Gymnamoebia. Also *Rhizopodea*.

**rhizopodium** \-pō′dē·əm\ [New L, from Gk *rhiz(a)* root + Gk *podion* little foot] (*pl.* rhizopodia) A filamentous pseudopodium, with a dense inner zone and a more fluid outer layer in which granular cytoplasm can be seen to circulate. It can branch and anastomose, forming a network in which food can be trapped. This type of pseudopodium is found in the order Foraminifera. Also *rhizopod*.

**rhizotomy** \rīzät′əmē\ [RHIZO- + -TOMY] Division of a nerve root. Also *radicotomy, root section*. **anterior r.** Division of an anterior, or motor, spinal nerve root. **posterior r.** Division of a posterior, or sensory, spinal nerve root. Also *Dana's operation*. **trigeminal r.** Section of the root of the trigeminal nerve. Also *retrogasserian neurotomy, trigeminal root section*.

**rhm** Symbol for the unit, roentgen per hour at one meter.

**rhod-** \rōd-\ RHODO-.

**rhodamine** Any member of a class of dyes formed by condensation of an acid anhydride, typically phthalic anhydride or succinic anhydride, with an *m*-aminophenol. A tricyclic system is formed whose central ring contains one carbon atom from the anhydride and an oxygen atom from the phenolic groups, the other two rings being derived from two molecules of the aminophenol. These dyes give red fluorescence when excited by ultraviolet light, and they are used in immunofluorescence microscopy.

**rhodanese** THIOSULFATE SULFURTRANSFERASE.

**Rhodin** [J. A. G. *Rhodin*, Swedish-born U.S. electron microscopist, born 1922] See under FIXATIVE.

**rhodium** \rō′dē·əm\ Element number 45, having atomic weight 102.9055. Rhodium is a silvery white metal that occurs native and in ores associated with platinum. Symbol: Rh

***Rhodnius*** \räd′nē·əs\ A genus of reduviid bugs in the subfamily Triatominae, species of which are important as vectors in South America of *Trypanosoma cruzi*, the agent of Chagas disease. A well-known species is *R. prolixus*, an important vector of *T. cruzi* in Venezuela, Colombia, Central America, and Mexico.

**rhodo-** \rō′dō-\ [Gk *rhodon* the rose] A combining form meaning rose in color, red. Also *rhod-*.

**rhodogenesis** \-jen′əsis\ The formation of rhodopsin in the retina from 11-*cis*-retinal and opsin in the absence of light. Exposure to light causes rhodopsin to dissociate into opsin and *all-trans*-retinal. Also *rhodophylaxis*.

**rhodomycin** A naturally occurring antibiotic mixture derived from the species *Streptomyces purpurascens*. It contains two components, rhodomycin A, and rhodomycin B. The preparation is effective against staphylococcal infections.

**rhodophylaxis** \-fīlak′sis\ RHODOGENESIS.

**rhodopsin** \rōdäp′sin\ [RHOD- + Gk *op(sis)* sight, vision + -IN] The retinal visual pigment of the rod photoreceptors, responsible for scotopic (night) vision. Also *visual purple*. Compare IODOPSIN.

***Rhodotorula rubra*** \rō′dətôr′yələ roo′brə\ A form-species of a yeastlike fungus which is a common environmental contaminant and sometimes is a constituent of the microflora of the skin, sputum, or feces. Upon rare occasions it causes infection in immunocompromised hosts.

**rhodotorulosis** \-tôr′yəlō′sis\ [*Rhodotorul(a)* + -OSIS] A rare fungal infection caused by *Rhodotorula* species and occurring principally in debilitated persons or in those who have indwelling intravenous or urinary tract catheters. The pathogenic organisms usually enter the bloodstream via a contaminated catheter and cause nonspecific symptoms of hypotension and fever.

**rhodotoxin** \-täk′sin\ One of a group of toxic diterpenoids isolated from various species of *Rhododendron, Kalmia,* and *Leucothoe*. It is found in rhododendron flowers and in the honey.

**rhombencephalic** \räm′bensəfal′ik\ [*rhombencephal(on)* + -IC] Denoting an animal preparation in which the brainstem has been cut at the level of the upper border of the pons, i.e., below that of the classical Sherringtonian decerebration. Motor behavior differs from the latter in that there is less rigidity.

**rhombencephalitis** \räm′bensef′əlī′tis\ [*rhombencephal(on)* + -ITIS ] Encephalitis predominantly involving the brainstem.

**rhombencephalon** \räm′bensef′əlän\ [*rhomb(oid)* + ENCEPHALON] The most caudal (posterior) of the three embryonic brain vesicles which, as it becomes flexed dorsally, assumes a rhomboid shape characteristic of the definitive fourth ventricle. It comprises two parts: a cranial part or metencephalon from which is derived the pons, and a caudal part or myelencephalon which becomes the medulla oblongata. The roof of the rhombencephalon is thin and its caudal positon remains so, forming the tela choroidea of the fourth ventricle. The more cranial part of the roof is the site of development of the cerebellum. Also *hindbrain*.

**rhomboid** \räm′boid\ [Gk *rhomb(os)* a rhombus + -OID] **1** Rhombus-shaped or kite-shaped; in the shape of a parallelogram that has no right angles. **2** A structure or configuration having such a shape. **Michaelis r.** A diamond-shaped area seen over the lower end of the spine in well-developed individuals. It is outlined by joining the following points: the tip of the spine of the fifth lumbar vertebra, the cutaneous dimples over the posterior superior iliac spines, and the meeting point of the oblique medial margins of the gluteus maximus muscles. Also *rhomboid of Michaelis*.

**rhombomere** \räm′bəmir\ A neuromere in the rhombencephalon.

**rhonchal** \räng′kəl\ RHONCHIAL.

**rhonchial** \räng′kē·əl\ Relating to or characteristic of rhonchi. Also *rhonchal.*

**rhonchus** \räng′kəs\ [Late L, a snoring, from Gk *rhonchos* a snoring] (*pl.* ronchi) An abnormal sound heard on auscultation of the lungs ranging from a wheeze to a snoring sound and due to air passing through a partially obstructed or a narrowed airway. Also *dry rale* (outmoded). Compare RALE. **sibilant r.** A high-pitched wheeze heard on auscultation of the lungs. Also *sibilant rale, whistling rale.*

***Rhopalopsyllus cavicola*** \rō′pəlōsil′əs kəvik′ələ\ The cavy flea of South America, a species that transmits *Pasteurella pestis.*

**rhoptry** \räp′trē\ [Gk *rhoptr(on)* a club + -Y] One of the paired organelles found in the anterior part of sporozoites and merozoites of sporozoan protozoa. It is one of the kinds of organelle that characterize the phylum Apicomplexa. They are thought to have a glandular, proteolytic function related to the activity of the conoid or apical complex. Also *paired organelle.*

**rhotacism** \rō′təsizm\ [Gk *rhōtak(izein)* to overuse or misuse the sound of the letter ρ (rho) + -ISM] A common and usually mild form of speech defect in which there is difficulty in the pronunciation of sounds represented by *r.*

**rhythm** [Gk *rhythm(os)* (from *rheein* to flow) a measured motion, time, rhythm] **1** Movement or process conforming to a regular or periodic pattern often detectable by some corresponding indication, such as a sound or beat, temperature or electrical variation, etc. **2** Pertaining to a method of contraception making use of the alternation of periods of fertility with infertility in the menstrual cycle. See also RHYTHM METHOD. **accelerated idioventricular r.** A form of rhythm disturbance in which a relatively fast ventricular pacemaker, usually between 60 and 100 beats per minute, controls the ventricles. It is often associated with sinus bradycardia with or without atrioventricular dissociation. **agonal r.** A bizarre ventricular rhythm disturbance characteristic of the dying heart. **alpha r.** Rhythmic activity of the brain having a frequency of about 10 Hz, recorded in the parietotemporo-occipital regions, and sometimes in the rolandic region. It is seen particularly when the subject is resting physically and mentally, with the eyes closed. The rhythm may be interrupted by sensory stimuli, especially eye-opening or attention, and it reappears as soon as the eyes are closed. In the normal subject the alpha rhythm can have a frequency ranging from 8 Hz (which some authorities still consider to be abnormal) to 13 Hz or thereabouts. The upper limit of normality is less rigid than the lower. Many adjacent frequencies may be combined to form the alpha rhythm, as can be demonstrated by electronic analysis. Also *Berger's rhythm* (seldom used). **atrioventricular r.** JUNCTIONAL RHYTHM. **Berger's r.** *Seldom used* ALPHA RHYTHM. **beta r.** In electroencephalography, a rapid rhythm (14–22 Hz), usually of low voltage (5–10 $\mu$V), which can be recorded in the motor areas of the brain and sometimes in the frontal regions, especially during states of stress or anxiety or after the administration of certain drugs such as barbiturates. **bigeminal r.** See under BIGEMINY. **biologic r.** BIORHYTHM. **cardiac r.** The prevailing rhythm of the pulsations of the heart. **circadian r.** An activity cycle of approximately 24 hours that occurs as a result of the interaction of both environmental and physiologic cues. **circus r.** A cardiac rhythm which depends upon the phenomenon of reentry, whereby an electrical impulse follows itself around in a circular movement. **coronary sinus r.** A cardiac rhythm in which the pacemaker is presumed to arise adjacent to the mouth of the coronary sinus, the electrocardiographic features of which are inverted P waves in leads II and III, but with a normal or even prolonged P-R interval. **coupled r.** See under BIGEMINY. **delta r.** In electroencephalography, a slow rhythm (less than 4 Hz) made up of delta waves. **ectopic r.** A cardiac rhythm associated with a pacemaker outside the sinuatrial node. **escape r.** A form of cardiac rhythm associated with a lower pacemaker assuming dominance of the heart for one or more beats due to failure of the sinus node to do so. See also ESCAPE. **fetal r.** The rhythm of heart sounds which resembles that in the fetus in that both sounds are similar in character and intensity. Also *embryocardia.* **gallop r.** A cadence of three heart sounds which may be due either to a third or to a fourth sound, or a combination of them, in addition to the two normal sounds (first and second). It is a feature of cardiac failure, but may also be heard in healthy young people. Also *bruit de galop, Traube's murmur.* • This rhythm was named for its resemblance to that of a French dance, "le galop," and not for any similarity to the sound of a galloping horse. **gamma r.** A waveform in the electroencephalogram with a frequency of more than 22 Hz. **idionodal r.** A cardiac rhythm in which the heart is under the control of the atrioventricular node. **idioventricular r.** A cardiac rhythm disorder in which the ventricles are under the control of an independent ventricular pacemaker. **infradian r.'s** Biologic rhythms with a cycle longer than a day, usually extending for weeks or months. **junctional r.** A cardiac rhythm in which the ventricles are under the control of a pacemaker situated in the atrioventricular node or adjacent junctional tissues. Also *atrioventricular rhythm, nodal rhythm.* **nodal r.** JUNCTIONAL RHYTHM. **parasystolic r.** See under PARASYSTOLE. **quadrigeminal r.** A cardiac rhythm in which there is a pause after every fourth beat. **quadruple r.** A cadence of four heart sounds due to loud third and fourth sounds. Also *train-wheel rhythm.* **reciprocal r.** An abnormal cardiac rhythm in which the atrioventricular junctional impulse activates the ventricles twice in one cycle, producing an extra beat (echo or reciprocal beat). **reciprocating r.** A rhythm with atrial and ventricular excitation, as in AV nodal reentrant tachycardia or the circus movement tachycardias of the preexcitation syndromes. **sinus r.** The normal cardiac rhythm which is under the control of the sinuatrial node. **sinusoidal r.** In electroencephalography any rhythmic activity sufficiently regular in form to be reminiscent of a sine wave. **theta r.** A rhythm with an amplitude equal to (50 mV on average) or slightly greater than that of alpha rhythm, but which is slower than the latter (4–7 Hz) and which is usually located more anteriorly (generally in the parietotemporal region). It is normal in children but is generally pathologic in adults under standard recording and resting conditions as it usually disappears at about the age of 12 years. Theta activity is often found in adult patients with personality disorders, and may be seen posteriorly, behaving like the alpha rhythm, in some patients with cerebral metabolic disturbances. Less often it may occur focally due to a cerebral lesion. **train-wheel r.** QUADRUPLE RHYTHM. **triple r.** A cadence of three heart sounds due to the audibility of a third or fourth heart sound in addition to the normal two sounds. **ultradian r.'s** Biological rhythms with a cycle shorter than a day. **ventricular r.** A heart rhythm in which the ventricles are under the control of a ventricular pacemaker.

**rhythmic** Characterized by or of the nature of rhythm.

**rhythmicity** \riTHmis′itē\ **1** The quality of being

rhythmic. **2** The ability to generate or respond to rhythmic impulses, as of cardiac muscle.

**rhytid-** \rit′id-\ [Gk *rhytis,* gen. *rhytidos,* a wrinkle] A combining form meaning wrinkle, wrinkling.

**rhytidectomy** \rit′idek′tәmē\ [RHYTID- + -ECTOMY] The surgical removal of excess or sagging skin for the purpose of eliminating or mitigating wrinkles. Also *erugation, rhytidoplasty.*

**rhytidoplasty** \rit′idōplas′tē\ RHYTIDECTOMY.

**rhytidosis** \rit′idō′sis\ [RHYTID- + -OSIS] A wrinkling, as of the cornea. Also *rutidosis.* Also *rhitidosis.*

**RI** recession index.

**RIA** radioimmunoassay.

**rib** [Old English *rib, ribb*] One of the twenty-four curved, narrow bones that are arranged in twelve pairs on either side of the thoracic vertebrae; os costale. **abdominal r.'s** *Outmoded* COSTAE SPURIAE. **asternal r.'s** *Outmoded* COSTAE SPURIAE. **bicipital r.** **1** A bifid rib that has two heads but unites at some point in its course to continue as a single body, as is seen in hemivertebra in the thoracic region. **2** An abnormal first rib that is fused with the anterior part of the seventh cervical vertebra, in addition to having its usual articulation with the first thoracic vertebra. **bifid r.** An abnormal rib that begins as a single head but during its course the body bifurcates to continue as two or more ribs. Also *branched rib.* Compare FUSED RIB. **branched r.** **1** BIFID RIB. **2** FUSED RIB. **cervical r.** A supplementary rib attached to the transverse process of the seventh cervical vertebra above and sometimes to the first rib below. Such a rib may compress the inner cord of the brachial plexus and/or the subclavian artery. **false r.'s** COSTAE SPURIAE. **floating r.'s** COSTAE FLUITANTES. **fused r.** An abnormal rib that begins with two heads which during their courses unite to continue as a single body. Also *branched rib.* Compare BIFID RIB. **slipping r.** A rib whose anterior cartilaginous attachment is repeatedly dislocated. **spurious r.'s** COSTAE SPURIAE. **sternal r.'s** COSTAE VERAE. **sternebral r.** STERNEBRA. **true r.'s** COSTAE VERAE. **vertebral r.'s** **1** COSTAE FLUITANTES. **2** COSTAE SPURIAE. **vertebrochondral r.'s** COSTAE SPURIAE. **vertebrocostal r.'s** The eighth, ninth, and tenth ribs which have their costal cartilages connected anteriorly by capsular ligaments to the cartilage immediately above. **vertebrosternal r.'s** COSTAE VERAE. **Zahn's r.'s** LINES OF ZAHN.

**ribavirin** \rī′bәvī′rin\ 1-$\beta$-D-Ribofuranosyl-1,2,4-triazole-3-carboxamide. An experimental drug which has antiviral activity *in vivo* and *in vitro* against both RNA and DNA viruses, including influenza virus and Lassa virus.

**Ribbert** [Hugo *Ribbert,* German pathologist, 1855–1920] Ribbert's thrombosis. See under AGONAL THROMBOSIS.

**ribbon** In anatomy, a bandlike structure. **r. of Reil** The rostral medial lemniscus. Also *band of Reil.*

**Ribes** [François *Ribes,* French surgeon, 1765–1845] See under GANGLION.

**ribitol** The alcohol formed by the reduction of ribose. It is an important constituent of teichoic acids in cell walls of some bacteria. Flavins are ribitol derivatives.

**ribo-** \rī′bō-\ [See RIBOSE.] A combining form indicating (1) a relationship to ribose; (2) ribonucleic acid.

**riboflavin** \rī′bәflā′vin\ [RIBO- + FLAVIN] A water-soluble, heat-stable component of the vitamin B complex which exhibits a yellow-green fluorescence when dissolved in water and has a molecular mass of 376 daltons. Its molecule contains a benzene ring fused to a pterin, and is reducible to a colorless form. Its phosphate, often combined with AMP to form flavin adenine dinucleotide, plays a role as a coenzyme in many cellular oxidations, as the electron transport chain. Also *vitamin $B_2$, lactoflavin* (original name), *vitamin G.*

**riboflavin mononucleotide** FLAVIN MONONUCLEOTIDE.

**riboflavin phosphate** FLAVIN MONONUCLEOTIDE.

**ribofuranose** Ribose in its 5-membered-ring, hemiacetal form. This is its usual form in glycosides, e.g. in RNA.

**ribofuranosyladenine** ADENOSINE.

**ribofuranosylcytosine** CYTIDINE.

**ribofuranosylguanine** GUANOSINE.

**ribonuclease** Any enzyme that catalyzes the hydrolysis of ribonucleic acid. The site of action of the enzyme on the RNA molecule is the phosphodiester bond. Abbr. RNase **r. I** PANCREATIC RIBONUCLEASE. Abbr. RNase I **r. II** The enzyme (EC 3.1.13.1) that catalyzes hydrolysis of RNA by removal of residues from the 3′ end to yield nucleoside 5′-phosphates. Also *ribonuclease $T_2$.* Abbr. RNase II **pancreatic r.** An enzyme (EC 3.1.27.5) which catalyzes the endolytic cleavage of ribonucleic acids adjacent to uridine or cytidine, producing phosphomononucleotide and oligonucleotides and 2′,3′-cyclic phosphate intermediates. Also *ribonuclease I.* Abbr. RNase I **r. S** An enzyme that is derived by partial digestion of native pancreatic ribonuclease. Ribonuclease S in turn dissociates readily into inactive S-protein and S-peptide. **r. $T_1$** An enzyme (EC 3.1.27.3) which cleaves ribonucleic acid at the 3′,5′ linkage of a guanosine-3′-phosphate residue, producing mono- and oligonucleotides ending in guanosinephosphate with 2′,3′-cyclic intermediates. Also *guanyloribonuclease.* **r. $T_2$** RIBONUCLEASE II.

**ribonucleic acid** A long, unbranched molecule usually consisting of four types of nucleotides linked together with 3′-5′ phosphodiester bonds, synthesized in the nucleus by transcription of one strand of DNA. See also entries under RNA. Also *ribose nucleic acid, plasmonucleic acid, yeast nucleic acid.* Abbr. RNA

**ribonucleoprotein** A class of conjugated proteins containing ribonucleic acid as a prosthetic group. Also *ribose nucleoprotein.*

**ribonucleoside** A class of nucleosides in which the pentose is D-ribose.

**ribonucleoside-diphosphate reductase** The enzyme (EC 1.17.4.1) responsible for forming 2′-deoxyribonucleotides for DNA biosynthesis by reduction of ribonucleoside 5′-diphosphates. It uses the reduced forms of glutaredoxin or thioredoxin as reductants. Also *ribonucleotide reductase.*

**ribonucleotide** A class of nucleotides in which the pentose is D-ribose.

**ribonucleotide reductase** RIBONUCLEOSIDE-DIPHOSPHATE REDUCTASE.

**ribose** \rī′bōs\ [German, coined by dropping and rearranging letters from *arabinose*] An aldopentose sugar, the molecule of which occurs as a structural component of ribonucleic acid, riboflavin, and other nucleotides and nucleosides.

**ribose nucleic acid** RIBONUCLEIC ACID.

**ribose nucleoprotein** RIBONUCLEOPROTEIN.

**ribose 5-phosphate** The 5-phosphate of ribose, produced enzymatically from ribulose 5-phosphate in the pentose phosphate pathway. It is the source of ribose residues in nucleotides. It is converted into 5-phosphoribosyl pyrophosphate by reaction with ATP as the first step of building it up into nucleotides. Also *phosphoribose.*

**ribosephosphate isomerase** The enzyme (EC 5.3.1.6) responsible for the interconversion of ribose 5-phosphate and ribulose 5-phosphate. This reaction is an essential step of the pentose phosphate pathway and of the photosynthetic pathway, and it is responsible for the biosynthesis of ribose 5-phosphate for nucleotide formation. Also *phosphoribose isomerase.*

**riboside** Any glycoside formed from ribose, or an analogue in which an atom other than oxygen carries a ribosyl group. Nucleosides are therefore ribosides.

**ribosomal** \rī'bōsō'məl\ Concerned with or contained in ribosomes.

**ribosome** \rī'bəsōm\ [RIBO- + -SOME] A complex, spherical, cytoplasmic organelle about 150–250 Å in diameter with an overall composition of about three parts ribonucleic acid to two parts protein, serving as the site of protein synthesis in the cell. The ribosome can be attached to the endoplasmic reticulum or can exist as a free ribosome. Ribosomes can be dissociated into two subunits which can be separated on the basis of sedimentation. Also *Palade granule.*

**ribosuria** \rī'bəsoo'rē·ə\ Urinary excretion of D-ribose. This is one variety of pentosuria.

**ribosyl** \rī'bəsil\ The group formed from ribose by removal of a hydroxyl group from C-1 of one of its hemiacetal forms. In biology it is almost always the five-membered furanose ring form from which the hydroxyl group is removed.

**ribosylthymine** The analogue of thymidine that contains a ribosyl group in place of the 2-deoxyribosyl group; 2′-hydroxythymidine. Also *ribothymidine.*

**ribovirus** \rī'bəvī'rəs\ [RIBO- + VIRUS] RNA VIRUS.

**ribulose** A ketopentose sugar; the ketose analogue of ribose. Also *2-araboketose.*

**ribulose 1,5-bisphosphate** Ribulose phosphorylated on O-1 and O-5. This compound, made by reaction between ribulose 5-phosphate and ATP, is the substrate that reacts with carbon dioxide in photosynthesis. The product of the reaction, catalyzed by ribulose-bisphosphate carboxylase, is two molecules of 3-phosphoglycerate. Also *ribulose 1,5-diphosphate.*

**ribulose-bisphosphate carboxylase** The plant enzyme (EC 4.1.1.39) that catalyzes the reaction of ribulose 1,5-bisphosphate with carbon dioxide to form two molecules of 3-phosphoglycerate. It can accept oxygen in place of carbon dioxide to produce phosphoglycolate and phosphoglycerate. The enzyme consists of two types of subunit, one specified by nuclear DNA and the other by chloroplast DNA. It is a major protein of green leaves, and hence of animal food. Also *carboxydismutase* (original name).

**ribulose 1,5-diphosphate** RIBULOSE 1,5-BISPHOSPHATE.

**ribulose 5-phosphate** The 5-phosphate of ribulose. It is produced in the pentose phosphate pathway by dehydrogenation of 6-phosphogluconate at C-3, which is accompanied by decarboxylation. Some so produced is isomerized into ribose 5-phosphate, and some is epimerized at C-3 to give xylulose 5-phosphate, both of which are also intermediates in the pathway. Ribulose 5-phosphate is also an intermediate in the pathway of photosynthesis in plants, where it is phosphorylated by ATP at O-1 to form ribulose 1,5-bisphosphate, the compound with which carbon dioxide reacts. Also *phosphoribulose.*

**ribulosephosphate 3-epimerase** The enzyme (EC 5.1.3.1) that catalyzes the interconversion of the 5-phosphates of ribulose and xylulose by epimerization at C-3. It is essential for the function of the pentose phosphate pathway, and for the Calvin cycle of photosynthesis in plants. Also *phosphoribulose epimerase* (obs.).

**rice** [Middle English *rys,* from Old French *ris,* from Italian *riso,* from L *oryza,* from Gk *oryza,* also *oryzon,* all meaning rice. Of Oriental origin.] *Oryza sativa,* a cereal grass that is one of the chief food plants of the world and the main subsistence cereal throughout many parts of Asia. In addition to the edible seeds, the plant yields rice oil, which is expressed from the hulls by solvent extractions, and starch, which is obtained by softening and sieving the grains. When the husk is removed, brown rice remains, and when the bran (including the endosperm and germ) are also removed, white (or polished) rice remains. Brown rice contains, per 100 g, 7.5% protein, 1.8% fat, 15 mg calcium, 1.4 mg iron, 357 kcal, 0.3 mg vitamin $B_1$, 0.05 mg $B_2$, and 4.6 mg nicotinic acid. White rice contains, per 1000 g, 6.7% protein, 0.7% fat, 10 mg calcium, 1 mg iron, 360 kcal, 0.08 mg vitamin $B_1$, 0.03 mg $B_2$, and 1.6 mg nicotinic acid.

**Rich** [Arnold Rice *Rich,* U.S. pathologist, 1893–1968] Hamman-Rich disease. See under HAMMAN-RICH SYNDROME.

**Richardson** [John Clifford *Richardson,* Canadian neurologist, born 1909] Steele-Richardson-Olszewski syndrome. See under PROGRESSIVE SUPRANUCLEAR PALSY.

**Richet** [Charles Robert *Richet,* French physiologist, 1850–1935] See under FASCIA.

**Richter** [August Gottlieb *Richter,* German surgeon, 1742–1812] **1** See under SUTURE. **2** Monro-Richter line. See under LINE.

**Richter** [Ina M. *Richter,* U.S. physician, flourished 20th century] See under SYNDROME.

**ricin** \rī'sin, ris'in\ A heat-labile, antigenic phytotoxin produced by *Ricinis communis,* castor bean, or castor-oil bean, plant. It is one of the most toxic compounds known, causing death through irreversible cell damage.

**ricinism** \rī'sinizm, ris'-\ [*Ricin(us)* + -ISM] Poisoning from ingestion of seeds of the castor bean plant, *Ricinus communis.* Symptoms are hemorrhagic gastroenteritis, inflammation of the respiratory tract, and lung hemorrhages. Ingestion of even small to moderate amounts of the seeds may prove fatal.

**ricinoleic acid** 12-Hydroxyoleic acid, a fatty acid of 18 carbon atoms with a *cis* double bond between C-9 and C-10, found as the main fatty acid of the fat of the castor oil bean, *Ricinus.*

**rickets** \rik'əts\ [of unknown origin, prob. from a southwest English dialect. See also RACHITIS.] A disease, primarily of infants and children, that is brought on by a deficiency of vitamin D or its analogues in which there occurs excessive but calcium-deficient osteoid tissue formation, resulting in a softening of the bones with deformities, fractures, delayed closure of the fontanelles, and tenderness. This metabolic condition can be reversed through the administration of vitamin D, sunlight, and diet in the presence of normal parathyroid activity. Also *avitaminosis D, rachitis, Glisson's disease, English disease, infantile osteomalacia, juvenile osteomalacia.* **adult r.** OSTEOMALACIA. **celiac r.** Bony deformity and growth retardation resulting from malabsorption of vitamin D, fat, and calcium in celiac disease. Also *pancreatic rickets* (imprecise). **familial hypophosphatemic r.** Any of four forms of rickets, namely X-linked hypophosphatemia, familial hypophosphatemic osteomalacia, or either of two forms of inherited vitamin D dependent rickets. Also *renal hypophosphatemia, familial hypophosphatemia.* **familial vitamin D resistant r.** X-LINKED HYPOPHOSPHATEMIA. **fetal r.** ACHONDROPLASIA. **hemorrhagic r.** *Obs.* INFANTILE SCURVY. **hepatic r.** A condition similar to rickets which may complicate cirrhosis of the liver related to inadequate absorption of vitamin D. **late r.** OSTEOMALACIA. **pancreatic r.** *Imprecise* CELIAC RICKETS. **pseudodeficiency r.** VITAMIN D RESISTANT RICKETS. **refractory r.** VITAMIN D RESISTANT RICKETS. **renal r.** RENAL OSTEODYSTROPHY. **resistant r.** VITAMIN D RESISTANT RICKETS. **scurvy r.** INFAN-

TILE SCURVY. **tardy r.** OSTEOMALACIA. **vitamin D dependent r.** 1 Rickets due to nutritional or environmental vitamin D deficiency. 2 Rickets due to an inherited disorder of vitamin D production or action. Two forms are known and are both characterized by rickets, tetany, convulsions, and failure to thrive in infancy. In type I, plasma 1,25-$(OH)_2D_3$ levels are low due to deficiency of a renal 1-alpha-hydrolase. The condition is autosomal recessive and treatable by high doses of vitamin D or small doses of 1,25-$(OH)_2D_3$. Type II is characterized by alopecia and high levels of plasma 1,25-$(OH)_2D_3$. The defect is autosomal recessive and may be end-organ resistant. Treatment is unsatisfactory. **vitamin D resistant r.** A condition clinically resembling rickets but which does not respond to treatment with vitamin D. It is usually caused by renal phosphate loss. Also *vitamin D refractory rickets, pseudodeficiency rickets, resistant rickets, refractory rickets.*

**rickettsemia** \rik′etsē′mē·ə\ [*ricketts(ia)* + -EMIA] The presence of rickettsiae in the blood.

***Rickettsia*** \riket′sē·ə\ [after Howard Taylor *Ricketts,* U.S. pathologist, 1871–1910] A genus of microorganisms which includes the agents of typhus fever, spotted fever, tick typhus, and boutonneuse fever. ***R. akamushi*** *RICKETTSIA TSUTSUGAMUSHI.* ***R. akari*** A species that causes rickettsialpox. It is transmitted by the mite *Liponyssoides sanguineus,* an ectoparasite of the house mouse, *Mus musculus.* Transmission to man is by accidental exposure to the mite. Also *Dermacentroxenus akari.* ***R. australis*** A species that causes North Queensland tick typhus, thought to be transmitted by *Ixodes* ticks. Also *Dermacentroxenus australis.* ***R. burnetii*** *Obs. COXIELLA BURNETII.* ***R. conorii*** A species that causes boutonneuse fever in humans. It is transmitted by ticks of the genera *Rhipicephalus* and *Haemaphysalis.* Also *Dermacentroxenus conori.* ***R. diaporica*** *Obs. COXIELLA BURNETII.* ***R. mooseri*** *RICKETTSIA TYPHI.* ***R. muricola*** *RICKETTSIA TYPHI* ***R. nipponica*** *RICKETTSIA TSUTSUGAMUSHI.* ***R. orientalis*** *RICKETTSIA TSUTSUGAMUSHI.* ***R. pediculi*** *ROCHALIMAEA QUINTANA.* ***R. prowazekii*** A species that causes epidemic typhus and Brill's disease. It is transmitted by the human body louse, *Pediculus humanus humanus.* An organism indistinguishable from *R. prowazekii* has been isolated from flying squirrels in the eastern United States and occasionally causes a febrile illness. ***R. quintana*** *ROCHALIMAEA QUINTANA.* ***R. rickettsii*** The causal agent of Rocky Mountain spotted fever. It is transmitted by ticks of the genera *Dermacentor, Rhipicephalus, Amblyomma, Ixodes,* and *Haemaphysalis.* Also *Dermacentroxenus rickettsi.* ***R. sennetsui*** A species associated with a disease clinically similar (possibly identical) to infectious mononucleosis in Japan. ***R. siberica*** A species of the *Dermacentroxenus* subgenus, related to *R. conorii,* that causes Siberian tick typhus. ***R. tsutsugamushi*** The causal agent of scrub typhus or tsutsugamashi disease. It is transmitted by mites of the family Trombiculidae, genus *Leptotrombidium.* Also *Dermacentroxenus orientalis, Rickettsia akamushi, Rickettsia nipponica, Rickettsia orientalis, Theileria tsutsugamushi.* ***R. typhi*** A causal agent of murine or endemic typhus, transmitted by the common rat flea. Also *Rickettsia mooseri, Rickettsia muricola.* ***R. wolhynica*** *ROCHALIMAEA QUINTANA.*

**rickettsia** (*pl.* rickettsiae *or* rickettsias) Any of group of small (0.3–0.5 $\mu$m) coccobacillary organisms of the genera *Rickettsia* and *Coxiella.* They include several human pathogens and are mostly transmitted between mammals by arthropods. They are obligate intracellular parasites, mainly in endothelial cells, and divide by binary fission within vesicles. Adj. rickettsial.

**rickettsiae** \riket′si·ē\ Plural of RICKETTSIA.

**rickettsialpox** \riket′sē·əlpäks′\ A benign disease caused by *Rickettsia akari* and transmitted to man by the mouse mite. A characteristic eschar forms at the site of inoculation, and the infected host usually develops a vesiculopapular rash, regional lymphadenopathy, leukopenia, chills, remittent fever, sweats, headache, backache, and malaise. Weil-Felix agglutinins are absent. The disease was first reported as an outbreak in the Kew Gardens section of the borough of Queens, New York City, in 1946. Also *Kew Gardens fever, Kew Gardens spotted fever.*

**rickettsiasis** \riket′sī′əsis\ RICKETTSIOSIS.

**rickettsicidal** \riket′sisī′əl\ 1 Having the capacity to check or cure rickettsial infections. 2 A rickettsicidal drug or agent.

**rickettsiology** \riket′sē·äl′əjē\ [*rickettsi(ae)* + *o* + -LOGY] The study of rickettsiae and rickettsial diseases.

**rickettsiosis** \riket′sē·ō′sis\ [*rickettsi(a)* + -OSIS] Any infectious disease caused by rickettsiae. Also *rickettsiasis.* **north Asian tick-borne r.** Infection with the tick-borne *Rickettsia siberica* which occurs in western Siberia, the Caucasus, Mongolia, and Central Asia. The symptoms are similar to those of boutonneuse fever and Rocky Mountain spotted fever.

**rickettsiostatic** \riket′sē·ōstat′ik\ 1 Having the ability to check or control the activity of rickettsiae. 2 A rickettsiostatic drug or agent.

**rickety** \rik′ətē\ RACHITIC.

**rictal** \rik′təl\ Pertaining to a rictus or fissure.

**rictus** \rik′təs\ [L (from *rictus,* past part. of *ringi* to open the mouth wide, show the teeth), the open mouth; esp., in man, in laughter] Involuntary contraction of the musculus orbicularis oris so that the patient looks as if he were smiling. This may be seen in several organic diseases such as tetanus or encephalitis.

**RID** radioimmunodiffusion.

**Riddoch** [George *Riddoch,* English neurologist, 1888–1947] Riddoch's mass reflex, Riddoch's phenomenon. See under MASS REFLEX.

**Rideal** [Samuel *Rideal,* English chemist and bacteriologist, 1863–1929] Rideal-Walker test. See under TEST.

**ridge** [Old English *hrycg,* akin to Old Norse *hryggr* back, spine, mountain ridge] CRISTA. **alveolar r.** The ridge of bone remaining after the extraction of teeth. It is usually resorbed over a period of years. Also *edentulous ridge.* **anal r.** A ridge of tissue in the embryo situated between the urogenital membrane and the anal membrane. This is the site of the primitive perineal body. **apical ectodermal r.** In the developing embryo, a thickening of the ectoderm on the ventral side of the limb buds. This thickening directs and influences the subsequent development of the limb. **basal r.** 1 CINGULUM DENTIS. 2 PROCESSUS ALVEOLARIS MAXILLAE. **bulbar r.'s** Two endocardial elevations which become spiral ridges in the embryonic bulbus cordis and fuse together to form the bulbar septum. Also *bulbar swellings.* **carotid r.** The bony crest on which the tympanic canaliculus is situated between the rounded opening of the carotid canal anteriorly and the jugular fossa posteriorly, on the inferior surface of the petrous part of the temporal bone. **cerebral r.'s of cranial bones** JUGA CEREBRALIA OSSIUM CRANII. **deltoid r.** TUBEROSITAS DELTOIDEA HUMERI. **dermal r.'s** CRISTAE CUTIS. **digital r.'s** The distal regions of the limb buds which differentiate to form the digits. These are first seen during the second and third months of embryonic life. The digits of the hand separate first, but by the end of the third month the hindlimb digits are also clearly defined. Also *radial ridges.* **edentulous r.** ALVEOLAR RIDGE. **epipericardial r.** A bar of embryonic tissue which separates the precervical sinus from the pericardium and extends headwards medial to the lower ends of the branchial arches to reach the mandibular arch. Migration of cells along the ridge is thought to account for the course of the hypoglossal nerve. **ganglion r.** GANGLIONIC CREST. **genital r.** A thickening in the coelomic epithelium on the medial aspect of the mesonephros, constituting the primordium of the gonads and first seen in human embryos of a 4–5 mm crown-rump length. During the earliest stages of gonadal differentiation, cords of cells proliferate from the epithelium into the mesenchyme, and initially, the gonad consists of mesodermal cells of coelomic epithelial origin. Primordial germ cells (gonocytes) migrate into the region of the genital ridge from the wall of the yolk sac. The developmental changes in the genital ridges are indistinguishable in the two sexes until the end of the sixth week. Also *germ ridge, gonadal ridge.* **gluteal r. of femur** TUBEROSITAS GLUTEA OSSIS FEMORIS. **gonadal r.** GENITAL RIDGE. **interarticular r. of head of rib** CRISTA CAPITIS COSTAE. **interosseous r. of fibula** MARGO INTEROSSEUS FIBULAE. **interosseous r. of radius** MARGO INTEROSSEUS RADII. **interosseous r. of tibia** MARGO INTEROSSEUS TIBIAE. **interosseous r. of ulna** MARGO INTEROSSEUS ULNAE. **intertrochanteric r.** CRISTA INTERTROCHANTERICA. **interureteric r.** PLICA INTERURETERICA. **lateral supracondylar r.** CRISTA SUPRAEPICONDYLARIS LATERALIS. **longitudinal r. of hard palate** RAPHE PALATI. **mammary r.** A pair of external thickenings which first appear in embryos of about 7 mm crown-rump length, which extend on each side of the ventral body wall from the base of the forelimb bud to the region medial to the hindlimb bud. The intermediate portion of its cephalic one-third thickens to form the mammary primordium. Its caudal two-thirds normally disappears before the end of the embryonic period. Also *mammary line, milk line.* **marginal r.** CRISTA MARGINALIS. **medial supracondylar r.** CRISTA SUPRAEPICONDYLARIS MEDIALIS. **medullary r.** NEURAL FOLD. **mylohyoid r.** LINEA MYLOHYOIDEA MANDIBULAE. **r. of neck of rib** CRISTA COLLI COSTAE. **nephrogenic r.** A ridge of mesoderm located lateral to the somite mesoderm on each side in a vertebrate embryo. Each develops into a kidney. **neural r.** NEURAL FOLD. **oblique r.** A linear elevation running across the occlusal surface of an upper molar tooth from the mesiolingual cusp to the distobuccal cusp. **palatine r.** RAPHE PALATI. **papillary r.'s** CRISTAE CUTIS. **Passavant's r.** PASSAVANT'S BAR. **pharyngeal r.** PASSAVANT'S BAR. **pterygoid r.** CRISTA INFRATEMPORALIS. **pulmonary r.** A ridge of tissue in the embryo continuous with the septum transversum and lying close to the common cardinal vein from which the pleuropericardial membrane develops. **radial r.'s** DIGITAL RIDGES. **residual alveolar r.** An alveolar ridge which has undergone resorption. Also *residual ridge.* **rete r.'s** The downward projections of the epidermis that enclose the dermal papillae. Also *rete pegs, epithelial pegs.* **skin r.'s** CRISTAE CUTIS. **superciliary r.** ARCUS SUPERCILIARIS. **supinator r.** CRISTA MUSCULI SUPINATORIS. **supraorbital r.** ARCUS SUPERCILIARIS. **suprarenal r.** An elevation between the root of the dorsal mesentery and the mesonephros of an embryo, caused by the developing suprarenal gland. **temporal r.** LINEA TEMPORALIS OSSIS FRONTALIS. **transverse r.'s of sacrum** LINEAE TRANSVERSAE OSSIS SACRI. **transverse r.'s of vaginal wall** RUGAE VAGINALES. **urethral r.** CARINA URETHRALIS VAGINAE. **urogenital r.** A projection into the interior of the coelom of the embryo on each side of the dorsal mesentery, caused by the developing nephrogenic cord. The ridge soon extends from the developing mesonephric ridge as far as the posterior aspect of the cloaca, near which it unites with its homologue on the opposite side to form the so-called genital cord. Also *urogenital fold, urethral fold.*

**ridge lap** Part of an artificial tooth adjacent to the alveolar ridge.

**ridging** \rij′ing\ A pattern of ridges or furrows in the nails extending in the direction of the fingers, seen in association with ischemia in the aging process.

**ridit** \rid′it\ A score assigned to data arranged in ordered categories for the purpose of ridit analysis. Thus, injuries might be classified as minor, moderate, severe, and fatal. ⟨For the method of calculation of ridits, see Fliess, J. L., *Statistical Methods for Rates and Proportions,* New York, 1973.⟩

**Ridley** [Humphrey *Ridley,* English anatomist, 1653–1708] Ridley sinus. See under SINUS CIRCULARIS.

**Riedel** [Bernhard Moritz Karl Ludwig *Riedel,* German surgeon, 1846–1916] **1** Riedel's lobe. See under APPENDICULAR LOBE. **2** Riedel's disease, Riedel's thyroiditis. See under STRUMA.

**Rieder** [Hermann *Rieder,* German pathologist, 1858–1932] Rieder's paralysis. See under SYNDROME.

**Rieger** [Herwigh *Rieger,* German ophthalmologist, born 1898] Rieger's anomaly, Rieger's dysgenesis. See under RIEGER SYNDROME.

**Riehl** [Gustav Riehl, Austrian dermatologist, 1855–1943] See under MELANOSIS.

**Rietti** [Fernando *Rietti,* Italian physician, born 1890] Microelliptopoikilocytic anemia of Rietti, Greppi, and Micheli. See under ANEMIA.

**RIF** right iliac fossa.

**rifamide** $C_{43}H_{58}N_2O_{13}$. 4-*o*-[2-(Diethylamino)-2-oxoethyl]rifamycin. A semisynthetic antibiotic derived from rifamycin B, with the same actions and uses as the parent compound. It is eff ective against a wide spectrum of Gram-positive and Gram-negative bacteria and is most often used to combat respiratory and biliary tract infections.

**rifampin** $C_{43}H_{58}N_4O_{12}$. 3-[[(4-Methyl-1-piperazinyl)-imino]methyl]rifamycin, a semisynthetic antibiotic derived from rifamycin SV. It has the same general actions and uses as the parent compound. It is given orally. Also *rifampicin.*

**rifamycin** \rif′əmī′sin\ Any of a group of naturally occurring antibiotics, synthesized by a strain of *Streptomyces mediterranei,* which inhibits initiation of transcription in bacteria by binding the beta subunit of RNA polymerase. It is active against a wide variety of Gram-positive cocci, Gram-negative bacilli, and mycobacteria. The antibiotic is a mixture of five components: A, B, C, D, and E. The B component gives rise to O, S, and SV rifamycins, and rifamycin O gives rise to AG and X rifamycins. In the United States, the antibiotic mixture is used in the treatment of pulmonary tuberculosis and for asymptomatic nasopharyngeal carriers of *Neisseria meningitidis.* It is used for a broader range of organisms in other countries. Also *ansamycin.*

**Riga** [Antonio *Riga,* Italian physician, 1832–1919] Riga-Fede disease. See under FRENAL ULCER.

**right / r. to treatment** In the United States, the right of a person to receive treatment if placed in or committed to a treatment facility. The due process of law does not allow the mentally ill person who has committed no crime to be deprived of liberty by indefinite institutionalization without medical treatment.

**right-eyed** Having the right eye dominant over the left.

**rigidity** \rijid′itē\ [L *rigiditas* (from *rigidus* rigid, from *rigere* to be stiff or rigid) rigidity, stiffness] Resistance to passive movement of a limb or part of a limb resulting from increased muscular tone. **α-r.** Extensor rigidity of limbs and trunk dependent upon supraspinally initiated facilitation of segmental α-motoneurons and consequently not abolished by dorsal root section. It is characteristic of the Pollack-Davis anemic decerebrate preparation. **anatomical r.** A firmness of the cervix resulting in slow or inadequate dilatation during labor. **cadaveric r.** RIGOR MORTIS. **clasp-knife r.** An initial marked resistance to passive movement, which then suddenly gives way. This variety of increased muscle tone is characteristic of spasticity due to disease or dysfunction of the pyramidal tracts. Also *clasp-knife effect, clasp-knife spasticity, clasp-knife phenomenon.* **cogwheel r.** COGWHEEL SIGN. **decerebrate r.** Rigidity marked by extension of the head and trunk and extension hypertonia of the four limbs, with pronation of the upper limbs and adduction with internal rotation of the feet. In man it occurs as a result of severe and extensive lesions of the upper brainstem. It may be experimentally induced in animals by section of the midbrain between the superior and inferior colliculi. It is a sign of damage to the rubrospinal system and to the reticular substance (descending activating system). The hypertonia of decerebrate rigidity is associated with increased gamma motor neuron activity as opposed to that of cerebellar rigidity which is associated with increased alpha motor neuron activity. **extrapyramidal r.** Any form of increased muscular tone resulting from extrapyramidal disease or dysfunction. **γ-r.** An extensor rigidity of limbs and trunk in which fusimotor support of sensory discharge from muscle spindles is essential, so that section of the dorsal roots abolishes rigidity at that level. It is seen in the classical Sherringtonian decerebrate preparation. **hemiplegic r.** Increased muscle tone in the spastic but paralyzed limbs of a subject with hemiplegia. **hysterical r.** Increased resistance to passive movement resulting from hysteria and not from organic nervous disease. **lead-pipe r.** Constant resistance to passive movement of a limb throughout the entire range of movement, as in bending a lead pipe. This variety of increased muscle tone is observed especially in patients with parkinsonism but sometimes with other forms of extrapyramidal disease. **muscular r.** 1 MUSCLE SPASM. 2 Increased muscle tone. **nuchal r.** NECK STIFFNESS. **pallidal r.** Rigidity attributable to damage to the globus pallidus, characterized by plastic hypertonia, increased resistance to passive extension of limb muscles, and tonic persistence of tendon reflexes. This can be seen in Parkinson's disease and arteriosclerotic parkinsonism. See also PALLIDAL SYNDROME. **parkinsonian r.** Increased muscular tone in Parkinson's disease, either the lead-pipe type of rigidity or the cogwheel type, occurring in patients showing both static tremor and increased tone. **pathologic r.** Cervical stenosis or rigidity during labor as a consequence of prior injury or disease. **postmortem r.** RIGOR MORTIS. **spastic r.** SPASTICITY.

**rigor** \rig′ər\ [L (from *rigere* to be stiff) stiffness, inflexibility] 1 A shivering or shaking of the body and limbs occurring in association with fever of infectious origin; shaking chills. 2 Muscular rigidity, as *rigor mortis.* **calcium r.** Arrest of the heart in full contraction as a result of an increase of calcium in the extracellular fluid. **instantaneous r. mortis** Instantaneously developing muscular stiffening occurring at the moment of death in individuals who are engaged in strenuous physical activity immediately prior to their demise. The detection of this phenomenon is important as the body retains the position it was in at the time of death and this positioning persists until true rigor mortis develops. Also *cadaveric spasm.* **r. mortis** The postmortem stiffening of the voluntary and involuntary muscles of the body, which is usually detectable two to four hours after death and reaches completion after six to twelve hours, imparting a boardlike rigidity to the entire body. It disappears after 24 to 48 hours. The development of rigor mortis is related to the depletion of adenosine triphosphate from muscle. Antemortem conditions associated with increased oxygen utilization by tissue, such as extreme muscle activity, convulsions, and fever, deplete adenosine triphosphate and hasten its onset. Rapid cooling of the body delays its onset. Its development may be poor or incomplete in elderly, very young, or severely debilitated individuals. The shorter muscle groups develop rigor mortis more quickly than the longer muscle groups. However, muscles strongly exerted immediately prior to death develop rigor mortis first regardless of their length, a finding of potential importance in forensic medicine. Also *postmortem rigidity, cadaveric rigidity.* **r. tremens** *Outmoded* PARKINSON'S DISEASE.

**Riley** [Conrad Milton *Riley,* U.S. pediatrician, born 1913] Riley-Day syndrome. See under FAMILIAL DYSAUTONOMIA.

**Riley** [Vernon Todd *Riley,* U.S. microbiologist and virologist, born 1914] Riley virus. See under LACTIC DEHYDROGENASE VIRUS.

**rim** [Old English *rima*] An edge defining a border or margin, as the lip of a vessel or the perimeter of a circumscribed area. **r. of abrasion** ABRASION COLLAR. **occlusion r.** A wax or stent rim attached to a base and used for recording maxillomandibular relations. Also *bite rim, record rim, bite-block.*

**rima** \rī′mə\ [L (akin to *rimari* to cleave), a crack, cleft, fissure] (*pl.* rimae) [NA] A slit or cleft, often an opening between two symmetrical parts or structures. **r. glottidis** [NA] An elongated slit between the vocal folds anteriorly and the medial surfaces of the arytenoid cartilages posteriorly. It is situated at the narrowest part of the laryngeal cavity but its width and shape vary during respiration and phonation. Also *fissure of glottis, true glottis, aperture of glottis.* **r. oris** [NA] The horizontal fissure between the lips leading into the vestibule of the mouth and bounded laterally by the angles of the mouth. Also *oral fissure, buccal orifice.* **r. palpebrarum** [NA] The elliptical space between the margins of the eyelids, obvious when the eye is open. At the extremities of the gap are the angles of the eye. Also *palpebral fissure, fissure of palpebrae.* **r. pudendi** [NA] The opening or cleft between the medial surfaces of the labia majora. Also *vulvar slit, vulval cleft, pudendal cleft, pudendal fissure, urogenital fissure.* **r. vestibuli** [NA] The space between the vestibular folds situated above the rima glottidis in the laryngeal cavity. Also *false glottis, fissure of the vestibule.*

**rimae** \rī′mē\ Plural of RIMA.

**rimal** \rī′məl\ Pertaining to a rima.

**rimantadine hydrochloride** $C_{12}H_{21}N{\cdot}HCl$. α-Methyl-1-adamantanemethylamine. An antiviral agent effective in the prevention of type-A influenza viral infections.

**rimiterol hydrobromide** $C_{12}H_{17}NO_3{\cdot}HBr$. *erythro*-3,4-Dihydroxy-α-(2-piperidyl)benzyl alcohol hydrobromide, a direct-acting sympathomimetic agent that is used as a bronchodilator.

**rimose** \rī′mōs\ [L *rim(a)* a crack, cleft, fissure + -OSE[1]] Having many cracks or fissures. Also *rimous.*

**rimula** \rim′yələ\ A very small rima, usually used in reference to structures in the brain or spinal cord.

**Rindfleisch** [Georg Eduard *Rindfleisch,* German physician, 1836–1908] Rindfleisch folds. See under FOLD.

# ring

**ring** [Old English *hring*] **1** A linear structure, figure, or mark having the shape of a a circle; in anatomy, annulus. **2** An arrangement of atoms in a closed chain. For various forms of such rings, see entries under FORM. **amnion r.** The circular line of attachment of the amnion around the fetal umbilicus. **anal r.** A circular ridge surrounding the anal opening in the embryo brought about by union of the anal tubercles. **annular r.'s** In chest roentgenograms, soft-tissue rims surrounding round or oval radiolucencies, indicating pulmonary cavitation, such as in tuberculosis. Also *pleural rings.* **annular r. of Gerlach** ANNULUS FIBROCARTILAGINEUS MEMBRANAE TYMPANI. **anorectal r.** LEVATOR SLING. **Balbiani r.** A large puff of a giant chromosome which is present in larval development in the family Chironomidae of the order Diptera. The ring has a high content of ribonucleic acid and shows a rapid turnover of ribonucleic acid precursors. The ring represents a region of active transcription along a chromosome. **Bandl's r.** PATHOLOGIC RETRACTION RING. **benzene r.** See under BENZENE. **Bickel's r.** TONSILLAR RING. **Braune's r.** PATHOLOGIC RETRACTION RING. **Cabot's r.'s** Fine circular or figure-of-eight erythrocyte inclusions that stain blue with Romanowsky stains. Cabot's rings are quite rare phenomena of accelerated erythrocyte formation and occur together with polychromatophilia, basophilic stippling, and reticulocytosis. Also *Cabot's ring bodies.* **Cannon's r.** A tonic contraction ring often visible radiologically in the right half of the transverse colon, near the hepatic flexure. Also *Cannon, Boehm, and Roith sphincter* (outmoded). **casting r.** CASTING FLASK. **ciliary r.** ORBICULUS CILIARIS. **ciliary r. of iris** ANNULUS IRIDIS MAJOR. **closing r. of Winkler-Waldeyer** A thickening at the edge of the placenta as a result of the junction of fetal and maternal tissue. **common tendinous r.** ANNULUS TENDINEUS COMMUNIS. **conjunctival r.** ANNULUS CONJUNCTIVAE. **constriction r.** RETRACTION RING. **contact r.** The characteristic wound of entrance of a bullet discharged from a gun in contact with a skin surface not immediately overlying bone. **contractile r.** A ring of microfilaments encircling the cell in the cytoplasm directly beneath a division furrow. Microfilaments have contractile properties and are believed to constrict the cell during cytokinesis. **contraction r.** **1** A ringlike thickening in the wall of a hollow organ due to tonic contraction. **2** RETRACTION RING. **deep inguinal r.** ANNULUS INGUINALIS PROFUNDUS. **Döllinger's r.** SCHWALBE'S RING. **Donders r.'s** Rainbowlike halos seen around lights by glaucoma patients. **esophageal contraction r.** See under LOWER ESOPHAGEAL CONTRACTION RING. **external inguinal r.** *Outmoded* ANNULUS INGUINALIS SUPERFICIALIS. **femoral r.** ANNULUS FEMORALIS. **fibrocartilaginous r. of tympanic membrane** ANNULUS FIBROCARTILAGINEUS MEMBRANAE TYMPANI. **fibrous r.'s of heart** ANNULI FIBROSI CORDIS. **fibrous r. of intervertebral disk** ANNULUS FIBROSUS DISCI INTERVERTEBRALIS. **Fleischer keratoconus r.** A superficial corneal line of hemosiderin curving about the base of the ectatic corneal cone in keratoconus. Also *Fleischer-Strümpell ring.* **glaucomatous r.** A peripapillary halo of exposed sclera. **Graefenberg r.** A flexible oval silver wire inserted into the uterus to prevent conception. It is no longer used because of the risk of pelvic inflammation. **greater r. of iris** ANNULUS IRIDIS MAJOR. **infancy r.** An accentuated incremental line which may occur in enamel and in dentin due to a disturbance in formation of these tissues at about ten months of age. **internal inguinal r.** *Outmoded* ANNULUS INGUINALIS PROFUNDUS. **Kayser-Fleischer r.** An iridescent copper deposit in the posterior portion of the periphery of Descemet's membrane. This is virtually pathognomonic of hepatolenticular degeneration (Wilson's degeneration). **Landolt r.** See under LANDOLT RING CHART. **lesser r. of iris** ANNULUS IRIDIS MINOR. **Löwe's r.** A halo of light surrounding the central dark area perceived when observing a uniform blue field. **Lower's r.'s** ANNULI FIBROSI CORDIS. **lower esophageal contraction r.** A thin luminal narrowing at the squamocolumnar junction of the esophagus and stomach. The etiology is unknown, but such a ring is often seen in association with an axial hiatal hernia. It is often asymptomatic but may cause severe dysphagia. **lymphoid r.** TONSILLAR RING. **Maxwell's r.** The central dark disk, corresponding to the macula, perceived when observing a uniform blue field. **neonatal r.** NEONATAL LINE. **Newton's r.'s** Concentric colored rings seen on pieces of glass of different radii of curvature that are placed in contact with one another. The patterns of color that are seen on thin films or membranes, produced by the same process, are also often called Newton's rings even though they are not ring-shaped. **Ochsner's r.** An occasional thickening of the mucous membrane around the opening of the pancreatic duct where it opens into the hepatopancreatic ampulla. **pathologic retraction r.** A retraction ring which forms during a long labor. It is so exaggerated that it becomes a zone of constriction that obstructs progress in labor. Also *pathologic ring, Braun's ring, Bandl's ring, Scanzoni's second os.* **pericorneal lymphatic r.** A fine network of lymphatic vessels which is situated just deep to the pericorneal vascular capillaries and drains the bulbar conjunctiva. It communicates with a deep plexus in the fibrous layer of the conjunctiva and they drain towards the commissures to join the lymphatics of the lids. **physiologic retraction r.** A retraction ring that forms as a result of labor and which does not impede the progress of the labor. Also *physiologic ring.* **pleural r.'s** ANNULAR RINGS. **polar r.** An organelle typical of sporozoans in the subphylum Apicomplexa, part of the apical complex, consisting of an osmiophilic anterior ring formed by the inner membranous layer of the pellicle of sporozoite and merozoite stages. A single polar ring is present in most genera, two are found in *Isospora* and a few other genera, and three in *Plasmodium* merozoites. **posterior limiting r.** SCHWALBE'S RING. **retraction r.** A ringlike area of a thickening of the uterine musculature in a woman undergoing labor. It is usually located at the junction of the fundus and lower uterine segment. Also *contraction ring, constriction ring.* **Schatzki r.** A distal esophageal membrane which may cause intermittent dysphagia. It is associated with hiatal hernia. **Schwalbe's r.** The collagenous, circumferential posterior margin of the lamina limitans posterior corneae, or Descemet's membrane, from which the trabecular meshwork on the inner wall of the sinus venosus sclerae arises. Also *Döllinger's ring, Schwalbe's anterior border ring, posterior limiting ring, annu-*

*lus sclerae* (outmoded). **scleral r.** A white ring or part of a ring often seen next to the optic disk on ophthalmoscopic examination. This may be due to the margin tissue not covered by the epithelium or to the side wall of an oblique scleral canal. **signet r.** The stage of trophozoite development in the erythrocytic cycle of the malarial parasite in which the cytoplasm of the parasite stains blue around its margin and the nucleus stains red, using standard Romanowsky stains. The central vacuole remains clear (enclosing the host cell, hemoglobin being consumed), giving the parasite the appearance of a ring. Also *ring stage.* **Soemmering's r.** SOEMMERING'S RING CATARACT. **subchorial closing r.** One of the marginal structures of the human placenta devoid of chorionic vessels and marking the junction between the placenta proper and chorionic fetal membranes. **superficial inguinal r.** ANNULUS INGUINALIS SUPERFICIALIS. **terminal r.** ANNULUS. **tonsillar r.** A circular band of lymphoid tissue surrounding the pharynx and comprising the lingual tonsil anteroinferiorly, the palatine tonsils and tonsilla tubaria laterally, and the pharyngeal tonsil posterosuperiorly. Also *Bickel's ring, lymphoid ring, Waldeyer's ring.* **tracheal r.'s** CARTILAGINES TRACHEALES. **tympanic r.** ANNULUS TYMPANICUS. **umbilical r.** ANNULUS UMBILICALIS. **vascular r.** A congenital vascular anomaly consisting of an arterial ring completely encircling the trachea and esophagus, sometimes leading to pressure symptoms which impair swallowing and respiration. The ring results from persistence of the right dorsal aorta of the early embryo, together with the left dorsal aorta and both fourth branchial arch arteries. **venous r. of Haller** PLEXUS VENOSUS AREOLARIS. **r. of Vieussens** LIMBUS FOSSAE OVALIS. **Vossius lenticular r.** A ring-shaped pigment deposit, corresponding to the edge of the pupil, displaced upon the anterior surface of the lens by trauma. **Waldeyer's r.** TONSILLAR RING. **Wimberger's r.** A radiographic sign of scurvy in children, consisting of a radiopaque rim of an ossification center which has a relatively lucent center. **Zinn's r.** ANNULUS TENDINEUS COMMUNIS.

**ringbinden** \ring′bin′dən\ [German *Ring* ring + *Binden* bands] Striated muscle cells in which the outer layer of myofibrils are arranged circumferentially in a helical pattern rather than longitudinally. Such muscle cells are found occasionally in normal muscle and more commonly in myopathic conditions. Also *ring fibers.*

**ring-down / transducer r.** The process of reduction of the amplitude of oscillation during the production of an ultrasound pulse by a transducer.

**Ringer** [Sidney *Ringer,* English physiologist, 1835–1910] **1** See under INJECTION. **2** Ringer's lactate. See under LACTATED RINGER'S INJECTION. **3** Krebs-Ringer solution. See under SOLUTION. **4** Locke-Ringer solution. See under SOLUTION. **5** Ringer's mixture. See under SOLUTION.

**ring-knife** A surgical instrument consisting of a metal ring on a shaft and handle with an internal cutting edge, used in the manner of a spokeshave. The early adenoid curettes were modifications of such instruments.

**ringworm** TINEA. **animal r.** Ringworm in humans that is acquired directly or indirectly from an infected animal. Human infection with zoophilic dermatophytes are classically inflammatory in type. **anthropophilic r.** A ringworm infection caused by any species of dermatophyte that has become specialized as a human pathogen, such as *Trichophyton rubrum, Epidermophyton floccosum,* or *Microsporum audouini.* **r. of the axillae** TINEA AXILLARIS. **r. of the beard** TINEA BARBAE. **black-dot r.** Endothrix ringworm of the scalp in which the severely damaged hair shafts break off at the skin surface and create the appearance of black dots on the scalp of dark-haired subjects. **r. of the body** TINEA CORPORIS. **crusted r.** FAVUS. **ectothrix r.** A ringworm infection of hair in which the shaft is invaded by mycelia, but arthrospores are only formed on the surface. Certain dermatophyte species characteristically infect hair in this way. For example, *Microsporum canis* and *Microsporum audouinii* produce small spores in clumps, while *Trichophyton verrucosum* and *Trichophyton mentagrophytes* produce larger spores in straight chains. In ectothrix infection the hair shaft breaks a few millimeters above the scalp surface. **endothrix r.** A ringworm infection of hair in which the fungus forms both mycelia and arthrospores within the hair shaft, resulting in a marked weakening and fracture of the hair at the scalp surface. In dark-haired subjects this produces black dot ringworm. *Trichophyton tonsurans* and *Trichophyton violaceum* are two species that cause this type of hair invasion. **r. of the feet** TINEA PEDIS. **geophilic r.** Ringworm in humans caused by a dermatophyte that normally lives in soil, especially *Microsporum gypseum.* **r. of the groin** TINEA CRURIS. **hypertrophic r.** MAJOCCHI'S GRANULOMA. **r. of the nails** TINEA UNGUIUM. **r. of the scalp** TINEA CAPITIS.

**Rinne** [Heinrich Adolf *Rinne,* German otologist, 1819–1868] **1** Rinne response. See under TEST. **2** Modified Rinne test. See under TEST.

**Riolan** [Jean *Riolan,* French anatomist and botanist, 1577–1657] **1** See under MUSCLE, NOSEGAY. **2** Riolan's arch, Riolan's arcade. See under ARC. **3** Riolan's bones. See under OSSICLE.

**riomitsin** OXYTETRACYCLINE.

**ripa** \rī′pə\ [L, the bank of a river] A linear reflection or attachment of ependymal cells to the ventricular surface, corresponding to the taenia thalami along the dorsal border of the thalamus. Adj. riparian.

**riparian** \rīper′ē·ən\ Denoting a ripa or margin: used to describe ependymal attachments to cerebral ventricles.

**RISA** radioiodinated serum albumin.

**risk** [French *risque* (from Italian *rischia, risico,* or *risco* (poetic) risk, hazard, peril) danger] The probability or expected frequency of the occurrence of harmful effects as a result of the use or nonuse, incidence, or influence of a chemical, physical, or biologic agent, especially during a stated period. In toxicology, risk is the probability that a substance will produce harm under specified conditions of use. **absolute r.** In epidemiology, the difference between the incidence of, or mortality from, a disease among exposed and unexposed subgroups of a population, as distinguished from the relative risk. **assumption of r.** In negligence law, particularly as it pertains to medical malpractice, the doctrine that an individual who consents to a treatment, procedure, or omission thereof with the knowledge that injury is a reasonably foreseeable result, waives or relinquishes the future complaint that the injury was caused by the practitioner's negligence. In medical professional liability, assumption of risk is a valid defense from suit only in those cases in which medical treatment was performed with proper care. Also *volenti non fit injuria.* **attributable r.** That fraction of the total incidence of, or mortality from, a disease which can be attributed to exposure to a given factor or the possession of a given attribute. Formally, it is the difference between the incidence or mortality rates in exposed and unexposed populations. **competing r.** A risk that reduces (possibly to zero) the chances of another outcome. For example, when a disease causes a number of deaths in a population group, the separate probabilities of dying from all other causes have to be reduced accordingly. The adjustment may be important in considering cause-specific mortality when death rates are high, as in old age. **empiric r.** In clinical genetics, the probability of occurrence of a multifactorial abnormality (such as cleft palate or pyloric stenosis), given the history of the same or a closely related disorder in the family of the proband. It is determined by retrospective review of the experience of families with the same pattern of affected relatives. **insurable r.** A risk which meets the requirements for the issuance of insurance; specifically, a risk which is one of a large group of similar risks, can result in a quantifiable and defined loss, is the result of an unpredictable event (except in certain health care situations), will lead to a hardship due to the magnitude of the loss, is economically feasible to insure, and is unlikely to result in loss incurred by a large number of insured persons at once. **relative r.** In epidemiology, the ratio of the incidence of, or mortality from, a disease in a population exposed to the factor under consideration to the corresponding rate in a population not so exposed. If, as is usually the case, the disease is relatively infrequent among both exposed and unexposed persons, the relative risk may be taken to be equal to the odds ratio derived from a fourfold table, provided there has been no bias, in the selection of cases and controls, in favor of including either exposed or unexposed individuals. Also *risk ratio.*

**RIST** radioimmunosorbent test.

**risus** \rī′səs\ [L (from *ridere* to laugh) laughter] LAUGHTER. **r. sardonicus** A grimace in which the muscles of the face are fixed as if in a sardonic smile. This is seen particularly in tetanus but may also occur in some forms of poisoning, as with strychnine. Also *risus caninus, canine laugh, sardonic laugh, canine spasm, cynic spasm, spasmus caninus, trismus cynicus, trismus sardonicus.*

**Ritgen** [Ferdinand August Marie Franz von *Ritgen*, German obstetrician, 1787–1867] Ritgen's method, modified Ritgen maneuver. See under MANEUVER.

**ritodrine** $C_{17}H_{21}NO_3$. 4-Hydroxy-α-[1-[[2-(4-hydroxyphenyl)ethyl]amino]ethyl]benzenemethanol, an adrenergic agonist with specificity for beta$_2$ receptors. It is used as a uterine muscle relaxant to delay the onset of uterine contractions in premature labor.

**Ritter** [Gottfried *Ritter* von Rittershain, German physician, 1820–1883] Ritter's disease. See under PHYSIOLOGIC JAUNDICE.

**Ritter** [Johann Wilhelm *Ritter*, German physicist and physician, 1776–1810] See under FIBER.

**ritual** \rich′oo·əl\ [L *ritualis* (from *ritus* an approved usage, rite) pertaining to rites] **1** Formal behavior, such as rites or ceremonies, dictated by the culture for specific occasions. **2** In psychiatry, formalized and stereotyped behavior developed as a neurotic trait or symptom, most pronouncedly in obsessive-compulsive neurosis.

**rivalry** \rī′vəlrē\ Competition or conflict for domination or recognition. **retinal r.** The normal, spontaneous alternation of perception of the visual field between the two eyes. It is as if the occipital cortex scans portions of the visual field by alternating use of the messages from the two eyes. This is clinically recognizable by presenting to the eyes dissimilar images that cannot be fused and forcing recognition of their alternation. Also *binocular rivalry, strife rivalry, reciprocal replacement.*

**Rivers** [William Halse *Rivers*, English physician and anthropologist, 1864–1922] See under COCKTAIL.

**Rivière** [Clive *Rivière*, English physician, 1873–1929] See under SIGN.

**Rivinus** [Augustus Quirinus *Rivinus*, German anatomist and botanist, 1652–1723] **1** Rivinus incisure, notch of Rivinus, segment of Rivinus. See under INCISURA TYMPANICA. **2** Ducts of Rivinus, canals of Rivinus. See under DUCTUS SUBLINGUALES MINORES. **3** Rivinus gland. See under GLANDULA SUBLINGUALIS. **4** Rivinus membrane. See under PARS FLACCIDA MEMBRANAE TYMPANI.

**rivus** \rī′vəs\ [L, a brook, waterpipe, channel, conduit] (*pl.* rivi) A passageway for a fluid. **r. lacrimalis** [NA] The space across the conjunctival sac, usually along the groove between the edge of the lower lid and the eyeball, in which tears are conducted across the eyeball from the lacrimal ducts laterally to the lacus lacrimalis medially. Also *Ferein's canal.*

**RLF** retrolental fibroplasia.

**RLL** right lower lobe (of lung).

**RLQ** right lower quadrant (of abdomen).

**RMA** right mentoanterior position (of a fetus). See under MENTUM ANTERIOR POSITION.

**RML** right middle lobe (of lung).

**RMP** right mentoposterior position (of a fetus). See under MENTUM POSTERIOR POSITION.

**RMT** right mentotransverse position (of a fetus). See under MENTUM TRANSVERSE POSITION.

**RN** Registered Nurse.

**Rn** Symbol for the element, radon.

**RNA** ribonucleic acid. **heterogeneous nuclear R.** RNA found in the cell nucleus and consisting of long transcripts of the nuclear DNA. A large part of it consists of RNA being processed, by the excision of introns, to form messenger RNA. Also *nuclear RNA*. Abbr. hnRNA **informational R.** MESSENGER RNA. **isoacceptor transfer R.** Different transfer RNA species which are acetylated by, or accept, the same amino acid, thought to play a regulatory role in translation. **messenger R.** The RNA that carries information from the DNA to the ribosome and there determines the amino-acid sequence in peptide synthesis. It is the product of transcription of a structural gene, and in eukaryotes may differ from the initial transcript by excision of certain sequences. Also *informational RNA, template RNA*. Abbr. mRNA **nuclear R.** HETEROGENEOUS NUCLEAR RNA. Abbr. nRNA **polycistronic messenger R.** A messenger RNA that contains messages for more than one protein. **ribosomal R.** RNA of high molecular weight associated with protein to form the ribosomes. This is the most abundant type of RNA in the cell. Abbr. rRNA **soluble R.** TRANSFER RNA. Abbr. sRNA **template R.** MESSENGER RNA. **transfer R.** Any of the short-chain RNA molecules present in cells in at least 20 varieties, each capable of combining with a specific amino acid. The transfer RNA molecule recognizes the codon of messenger RNA at the ribosome and positions the amino acid in the growing polypeptide chain. Also *soluble RNA*. Abbr. tRNA

**RNAase** ribonuclease.

**RNA nucleotidyltransferase** RNA POLYMERASE.

**RNA polymerase** One of the enzymes capable of synthesizing RNA from a mixture of nucleoside triphosphates with liberation of inorganic pyrophosphate (diphosphate). One such enzyme (EC 2.7.7.6) is DNA-directed and is responsible for the formation of messenger RNA in normal animal and plant cells; another (EC 2.7.7.48) is RNA-directed and is responsible for the replication of RNA-containing viruses. Both synthesize RNA complementary in sequence to the directing nucleic acid. Also *RNA nucleotidyltransferase.*

**RNase** ribonuclease.

**RNP** ribonucleoprotein.

**ROA** right occipitoanterior position (of a fetus). See under OCCIPUT ANTERIOR POSITION.
**roach** COCKROACH.
**Robert** [Cesare-Alphonse *Robert,* French surgeon, 1801–1862] Robert's ligament. See under LIGAMENTUM MENISCOFEMORALE POSTERIUS.
**Robertshaw** [Frank Leonard *Robertshaw,* English anesthetist, flourished 20th century] See under TUBE.
**Robertson** See under ARGYLL ROBERTSON.
**Robin** [Charles Philippe *Robin,* French anatomist, 1821–1885] Virchow-Robin space. See under PERIVASCULAR SPACE.
**Robin** [Pierre *Robin,* French physician, 1867–1950] Pierre Robin anomaly, Robin anomalad, Pierre Robin syndrome, Pierre Robin retrognathism. See under ROBIN SEQUENCE.
**Robinson** [Frederick Byron *Robinson,* U.S. anatomist, 1857–1910] See under CIRCLE.
**Robinson** [Robert Alexander *Robinson,* U.S. orthopedic surgeon, born 1914] Smith-Robinson operation. See under OPERATION.
**Robison** [Robert *Robison,* English chemist, 1884–1941] Robison ester. See under GLUCOSE 6-PHOSPHATE.
**Robles** [Rudolfo *Robles,* Guatemalan dermatologist, 1878–1939] Robles disease. See under ONCHOCERCIASIS.
**roborant** \räb′ərənt\ [L *roborans,* gen. *roborantis,* pres. part. of *roborare* (from *robur* oak, hardwood) to make strong] **1** Tending to strengthen. **2** A strengthening agent.
**Robson** [Sir Arthur William Mayo-*Robson,* English surgeon, 1853–1933] See under LINE.
**robustness** In a statistical test, the degree to which the probability of drawing a wrong conclusion from the test result is not seriously affected by moderate departures from the assumptions implicit in the mathematical model on which the test is based.
**ROC** receiver operating characteristics.
***Rochalimaea*** \räsh′əlimē′ə\ A genus of organisms closely related to rickettsiae but capable of extracellular growth. ***R. quintana*** The causative agent of trench fever, transmitted by the human body louse, *Pediculus humanus humanus.* Also *Rickettsia quintana, Rickettsia pediculi, Rickettsia wolhynica.*
**Rocher** [Henri Gaston Louis *Rocher,* French surgeon, born 1876] Rocher sign. See under DRAWER TEST.
**Rochon-Duvigneaud** [André *Rochon-Duvigneaud,* French ophthalmologist, born 1863] Rochon-Duvigneaud syndrome. See under SUPERIOR ORBITAL FISSURE SYNDROME.
**Rock** [John *Rock,* U.S. gynecologist, born 1890] Hertig-Rock ova. See under OVUM.
**rod** [Old English *rodd*] **1** A straight, slender structure or shape. **2** A rod-shaped microorganism, as a bacillus. **3** Any of the photoreceptor cells of the retina serving scotopic vision. See also ROD SEGMENT. **analyzing r.** A vertical rod moving in contact with the teeth in a surveyor. **Auer r.'s** AUER BODIES. **basal r.** An internal support in the form of an organelle running along the base of the undulating membrane of certain flagellates, as in *Trichomonas.* Also *costa.* **enamel r.'s** ENAMEL PRISMS. **germinal r.** SPOROZOITE. **Harrington r.** A metal rod used in the surgical correction of scoliosis. **r.'s of Heidenhain** Rodlike cells of renal tubules. **Luque r.** A smooth metal rod used in the surgical correction of scoliosis. The rod is attached to the spine at each vertebral level by sublaminar stainless steel wires. **Maddox r.'s** Multiple, parallel, cylindrical rods of glass fused side to side and shaped into a trial lens, used to study ocular muscle balance and to measure degrees of squint. A light spot viewed through these rods by one eye interferes with binocular vision by removing the stimulus for image fusion by the two eyes. **muscle r.** MYOFIBRIL. **retinal r.'s** The visual cells that serve scotopic vision.
**rodent** [L *rodens,* gen. *rodentis,* pres. part. of *rodere* to gnaw] Any member of the mammalian order Rodentia.
**Rodentia** \rōden′shē·ə\ [RODENT + -IA] An extensive mammalian order that includes mice, rats, squirrels, woodchucks, porcupines, beavers, and other familiar animals. Their dentition is characterized by two chisel-shaped incisors and by the absence of canines. They occupy a variety of terrestrial and semiaquatic habitats worldwide. It is the largest living order, including over 6500 species.
**rodenticide** \rōden′tisīd\ [RODENT + *i* + -CIDE] Any substance or mixture of substances capable of killing rodents.
**rod-monochromat** \räd′-mänəkrō′mat\ One who is totally color blind or with no cone function.
**Roederer** [Johann George *Roederer,* German obstetrician, 1727–1763] See under ECCHYMOSIS, OBLIQUITY.
**roentgen** \rent′gən, -jən\ [after Wilhelm Konrad *Roentgen,* German physicist, 1845–1923] A unit of radiation exposure equal to $2.58 \times 10^{-4}$ coulomb per kilogram exactly. Also *röntgen.* Symbol: R, r ● Before 1975 the roentgen was the quantity of x-radiation or gamma radiation such that the associated corpuscular emission per 0.001293 gram of air produced in air ions carrying one electrostatic unit of quantity of electricity of either sign. (One cubic centimeter of dry air at 0°C and one standard atmosphere has a mass of 0.001293 gram.) **r. equivalent man** See under REM. **r. per hour at one meter** A unit of intensity of a gamma-ray source, under specified conditions of shielding, such that at a distance of one meter in air it produces an exposure rate of one roentgen per hour. Symbol: rhm **r. per second** A unit of ionization exposure rate equal to $2.58 \times 10^{-4}$ coulomb per kilogram second exactly. Symbol: R/s, $R{\cdot}s^{-1}$
**roentgenkymograph** \rent′gənkī′məgraf\ [ROENTGEN + KYMOGRAPH] The equipment used for roentgenkymography. Also *roentgenokymograph.*
**roentgenkymography** \rent′gənkīmäg′rəfē\ [ROENTGEN + KYMOGRAPHY] A radiologic technique in which the extent and speed of motions of an object or organ are recorded graphically on an x-ray film. Also *roentgenokymography.*
**roentgeno-** \rent′gənō-\ [See ROENTGEN.] A combining form denoting x rays.
**roentgenocardiogram** \-kär′dē·əgram′\ A graphic recording of cardiac pulsations derived from x rays.
**roentgenocinematography** \-sin′əmətäg′rəfē\ CINERADIOGRAPHY.
**roentgenogram** \rentgən′əgram\ [ROENTGENO + -GRAM] RADIOGRAPH.
**roentgenograph** \rent′gənōgraf′\ [ROENTGENO- + -GRAPH] RADIOGRAPH.
**roentgenography** \rent′gənäg′rəfē\ [ROENTGENO- + -GRAPHY] RADIOGRAPHY. **body section r.** A special radiologic technique to demonstrate on film the details of structures in a predetermined plane of tissue, with blurring of the details of structures in other planes. Also *planigraphy, planography, tomography, laminagraphy, laminography, body section radiography, sectional roentgenography, sectional radiography, stratigraphy.* **double contrast r.** Roentgenography of a structure, usually the surface of a cavity or lumen, with the use of two contrast media of differing radiopacities, such as barium and air. Also *double contrast visualization.* **magnification r.** A special radiographic technique in which there is increased distance between the

film and the patient, resulting in enlargement of the radiographic image of a part of the body. **mass r.** Roentgenography of large groups of people, usually for the study of a predetermined part of the body, such as the chest. **mucosal relief r.** A method for radiologic study of the mucosa, usually of the intestinal tract, by use of double contrast roentgenography, the mucosa being coated with barium and the lumen distended with air. **sectional r.** BODY SECTION ROENTGENOGRAPHY. **selective r.** Radiographic study of specific segments of the population selected on a predetermined basis, such as symptoms, occupation, age, or some other factor. **spot-film r.** Radiography of localized areas of the body during fluoroscopic study with the use of a special device adapted to the fluoroscope.

**roentgenokymograph** \-kī′məgraf\ ROENTGENKYMOGRAPH.

**roentgenokymography** \-kīmäg′rəfē\ ROENTGENKYMOGRAPHY.

**roentgenologist** \rent′gənäl′əjist\ A physician specializing in the use of roentgen rays for diagnosis.

**roentgenology** \rent′gənäl′əjē\ [ROENTGENO- + -LOGY] The medical science, a branch of radiology, dealing with the use of roentgen rays for diagnosis and therapy.

**roentgenoparent** \-par′ənt\ RADIOLUCENT.

**roentgenotherapy** \-ther′əpē\ RADIOTHERAPY.

**roentgentherapy** \rent′gənther′əpē\ [ROENTGEN + THERAPY] RADIOTHERAPY. **intraoral r.** Endoradiotherapy used within the oral cavity. **intravaginal r.** Endoradiotherapy applied in the interior of the vagina.

**roeteln** \rā′təln, ret′əln, rœ′təln\ [See RÖTELN.] RUBELLA.

**roflurane** \rōfloo′rān\ A halogenated ether containing fluorine. It is being investigated for use as a general anesthetic.

**Roger** [Georges Henri *Roger*, French physiologist, 1860–1946] Roger's reflex, Roger syndrome. See under ESOPHAGOSALIVARY REFLEX.

**Roger** [Henri Louis *Roger*, French physician, 1809–1891] **1** See under MURMUR. **2** Roger's bruit. See under BRUIT DE ROGER. **3** Maladie de Roger. See under DISEASE.

**Rohr** [Karl *Rohr*, German anatomist, born 1863] See under STRIA, LAYER.

**Rokitansky** [Karl Freiherr von *Rokitansky*, Austrian pathologist, 1804–1878] **1** Rokitansky-Aschoff sinuses of the gallbladder. See under SINUS. **2** Rokitansky-Cushing ulcer, Cushing-Rokitansky ulcer. See under CUSHING'S ULCER. **3** Rokitansky's diverticulum. See under TRACTION DIVERTICULUM OF THE ESOPHAGUS. **4** Rokitansky's disease. See under ACUTE YELLOW ATROPHY OF THE LIVER. **5** Rokitansky's pelvis. See under SPONDYLOLISTHETIC PELVIS.

**rolandic** \rōlan′dik\ [after Luigi *Rolando*, Italian anatomist, 1773–1831 + -IC] Denoting structures in the brain and spinal cord.

**Rolando** [Luigi *Rolando*, Italian anatomist, 1773–1831] **1** Column of Rolando. See under EMINENTIA TRIGEMINA. **2** Funiculus of Rolando. See under FASCICULUS. **3** Tubercle of Rolando. See under TUBERCULUM TRIGEMINALE. **4** Rolando's fibers. See under FIBRAE ARCUATAE EXTERNAE. **5** Fissure of Rolando. See under SULCUS CENTRALIS CEREBRI. **6** Rolando's gelatinous substance, substantia rolandi. See under SUBSTANTIA GELATINOSA MEDULLAE SPINALIS ROLANDI. **7** Artery of fissure of Rolando. See under ARTERIA SULCI CENTRALIS.

**role** [French *rôle* (from Med L *rotulus* a roll of parchment, roller, platen) a list, catalog] The life-style or characteristic behavior pattern developed by a person, typically determined in large part by what he perceives, as a child, as expected or demanded of him by the significant adults in his environment. **gender r.** Psychosexual differentiation, implying not only legal and social attribution of sex, but also a person's identification of self as a male or female in relation to other males and females, as expressed in mannerisms, dress, social behavior, and orientation of sexual impulses. This differentiation is the outward expression of core gender identity but may or may not be consonant with genetic, hormonal, or phenotypic sex.

**role-playing** The use, in psychotherapy or in education, of adopted roles to better understand how a given individual may see the identity and behaviors of a significant other person. The acting out by a child of the role of parent, for example, permits certain insights to be made about how that child perceives the actual parent.

**rolfing** \räl′fing\ [after Ida P. *Rolf*, U.S. biochemist and physiologist, 1896–1979 + -ING] A deep massage technique which is designed to realign the body by altering the length and tone of myofascial tissues. Also *structural integration.*

**rolitetracycline** $C_{27}H_{33}N_3O_8$. *N*-(Pyrrolidinylmethyl)tetracycline. A yellow, crystalline solid, soluble in water and alcohol. It is an antibiotic, with an antimicrobial spectrum similar to that of tetracycline hydrochloride.

**roll** [Old French *role* (from L *rotula*, dim. of *rota* a wheel, or *rotulus* a roll of parchment, roller, platen) a roll of parchment] **cotton r.** A cylinder of cotton or other cellulose fiber used to keep teeth dry during dentistry. Also *cotton-wool roll* (British usage).

**Roller** [Christian Friedrich Wilhelm *Roller*, German psychiatrist, 1802–1878] See under NUCLEUS.

**roller** A cylinder of tightly rolled material such as cotton or gauze that is used during surgical procedures. Also *roller bandage.*

**Rollier** [Auguste *Rollier*, Swiss physician, 1874–1954] See under TREATMENT, FORMULA.

**ROM** rupture of membranes.

**Romaña** [Cecilio *Romaña*, Argentinian physician active in Brazil, born 1899] See under SIGN.

**romanopexy** \rōman′əpek′sē\ [*romano-* (see ROMANOSCOPE) + -PEXY] A surgical procedure in which the sigmoid colon is secured to the abdominal wall to prevent prolapse or volvulus.

**romanoscope** \rōman′əskōp\ [*romano-* (for L *colon romanum* sigmoid colon: referring to the shape of the Roman letter S rather than the corresponding Greek Σ; see SIGMOID) + SCOPE] SIGMOIDOSCOPE.

**Romanowsky** [Dimitri Leonidovitch *Romanowsky*, Russian physician, 1861–1921] See under STAIN.

**Romberg** [Moritz Heinrich von *Romberg*, German neurologist, 1795–1873] **1** See under TEST. **2** Parry-Romberg syndrome, Romberg's disease, trophoneurosis of Romberg. See under ROMBERG'S PROGRESSIVE FACIAL HEMIATROPHY. **3** Brauch-Romberg symptom, Romberg-Howship symptom, rombergism. See under ROMBERG SIGN.

**rombergism** \räm′bərgizm\ ROMBERG SIGN.

**rongeur** \rôNzhœr′\ A cutting instrument used to resect bone, cartilage, or other hard tissues.

**ronidazole** $C_6H_8N_4O_4$. 1-Methyl-5-nitro-1*H*-imidazole-2-methanol carbamate (ester). This compound has antiprotozal activity and is used in veterinary medicine for this purpose.

**röntgen** \rent′gən\ ROENTGEN.

**röntgenography** \rent′gənäg′rəfē\ RADIOGRAPHY.

**roof** [Old English *hrōf*] Something functioning like a cover; a superior structure enclosing a space. **r. of mouth** PALATUM. **r. of orbit** PARIES SUPERIOR ORBITAE. **r. of skull** CALVARIA. **r. of tympanum** TEGMEN TYMPANI.

**room** [Old English *rūm*] A medium-sized, more or less enclosed area in a building, usually assigned to some specific use. The number of patient rooms in a health care facility is used as a measure of facility size and utilization. **birthing r.** A room in which deliveries are conducted which is less institutionally oriented and has a more homelike environment than a hospital delivery room. See also BIRTHING CENTER. **consulting r.** 1 A room where consultations are held. 2 In Great Britain, the office or examining room of a consultant, usually in a hospital. **delivery r.** A room in the maternity suite of a hospital used for vaginal deliveries. **labor r.** The area in a hospital in which women in labor are monitored prior to delivery. Also *predelivery room.* **operating r.** An enclosed area in a hospital in which operations are performed. Operating rooms differ in complexity and capabilities. **predelivery r.** LABOR ROOM.

# root

**root** [Old English *rōt*, akin to L *radix* a root, Gk *rhiza* a root] 1 The descending axis of a plant which serves to anchor the plant and to absorb and conduct water and minerals. 2 In anatomy, the attachment by which a structure is fixed at is base; radix. 3 See under ANATOMIC ROOT. **anatomic r.** That part of a tooth which is covered by cementum and devoid of enamel. In human teeth and those of many other animals, the anatomic root is demarcated from the anatomic crown by the cementoenamel junction. Also *root of tooth, radix dentis.* **anterior r. of spinal nerves** RADIX VENTRALIS NERVORUM SPINALIUM. **r. of the aorta** The commencement of the ascending aorta from the left ventricle at the base of the heart. It approximates the bulb of the aorta. **bitter r.** GENTIAN. **clinical r.** That part of a tooth which is surrounded by gingiva and periodontal membrane and is therefore not visible within the oral cavity. Also *radix clinica.* **r. of clitoris** CRUS CLITORIDIS. **cochlear r. of acoustic nerve** RADIX INFERIOR NERVI VESTIBULOCOCHLEARIS. **cranial r.'s of accessory nerve** RADICES CRANIALES NERVI ACCESSORII. **descending r. of trigeminal nerve** TRACTUS MESENCEPHALICUS NERVI TRIGEMINI. **dorsal r.** RADIX DORSALIS NERVORUM SPINALIUM. **dorsal r. of spinal nerves** RADIX DORSALIS NERVORUM SPINALIUM. **r. of facial nerve** RADIX NERVI FACIALIS. **r. of hair** RADIX PILI. **inferior r. of ansa cervicalis** RADIX INFERIOR ANSAE CERVICALIS. **inferior r. of vestibulocochlear nerve** RADIX INFERIOR NERVI VESTIBULOCOCHLEARIS. **intermediate r. of olfactory trigone** STRIA INTERMEDIA TRIGONI OLFACTORII. **internal olfactory r.** STRIA MEDIALIS TRIGONI OLFACTORII. **lateral and medial r.'s of olfactory trigone** Stria lateralis trigoni olfactorii and stria medialis trigoni olfactorii. **lateral r. of median nerve** RADIX LATERALIS NERVI MEDIANI. **lateral r. of optic tract** RADIX LATERALIS TRACTUS OPTICI. **licorice r.** GLYCYRRHIZA. **long r. of ciliary ganglion** RAMUS COMMUNICANS GANGLII CILIARIS CUM NERVO NASOCILIARI. **r. of lung** RADIX PULMONIS. **medial r. of median nerve** RADIX MEDIALIS NERVI MEDIANI. **medial r. of optic tract** RADIX MEDIALIS TRACTUS OPTICI. **mesencephalic r. of trigeminal nerve** TRACTUS MESENCEPHALICUS NERVI TRIGEMINI. **r. of mesentery** RADIX MESENTERII. **middle r. of zygomatic process** POSTGLENOID TUBERCLE. **motor r.** RADIX VENTRALIS NERVORUM SPINALIUM. **motor r. of ciliary ganglion** RADIX OCULOMOTORIA GANGLII CILIARIS. **motor r. of spinal nerves** RADIX VENTRALIS NERVORUM SPINALIUM. **motor r.'s of submandibular ganglion** RAMI COMMUNICANTES GANGLII SUBMANDIBULARIS CUM NERVO LINGUALI. **motor r. of trigeminal nerve** RADIX MOTORIA NERVI TRIGEMINI. **r. of nail** RADIX UNGUIS. **nerve r.** Bundles of nerve fibers that enter or emerge from the spinal cord and brainstem and subsequently join to form a mixed nerve. **r. of nose** RADIX NASI. **oculomotor r. of ciliary ganglion** RADIX OCULOMOTORIA GANGLII CILIARIS. **orizaba jalap r.** IPOMEA. **penile r.** RADIX PENIS. **r. of penis** RADIX PENIS. **posterior r. of spinal nerves** RADIX DORSALIS NERVORUM SPINALIUM. **posterior r. of zygomatic process** The posterior prolongation of the superior border of the zygomatic process of the temporal bone, which forms a thick ridge continuous with the suprameatal crest above the external acoustic meatus. Anteriorly it meets the anterior root at the tubercle for the attachment of the lateral ligament of the temporomandibular joint. **retained r.** The root of a tooth or part thereof which was not removed when the tooth was extracted. **sensory r. of ciliary ganglion** RAMUS COMMUNICANS GANGLII CILIARIS CUM NERVO NASOCILIARI. **sensory r. of spinal nerves** RADIX DORSALIS NERVORUM SPINALIUM. **sensory r. of trigeminal nerve** RADIX SENSORIA NERVI TRIGEMINI. **short r. of ciliary ganglion** RADIX OCULOMOTORIA GANGLII CILIARIS. **spinal r.'s of accessory nerve** RADICES SPINALES NERVI ACCESSORII. **spinal nerve r.'s** RADICES NERVI SPINALES. **spinal vestibular r.** TRACTUS VESTIBULOSPINALIS. **superior r. of ansa cervicalis** RADIX SUPERIOR ANSAE CERVICALIS. **superior r. of vestibulocochlear nerve** RADIX SUPERIOR NERVI VESTIBULOCOCHLEARIS. **sweet r.** GLYCYRRHIZA. **sympathetic r.'s of ciliary ganglion** RAMUS SYMPATHICUS AD GANGLION CILIARE. **third r. of zygomatic process** POSTGLENOID TUBERCLE. **r. of tongue** RADIX LINGUAE. **r. of tooth** ANATOMIC ROOT. **r.'s of trigeminal nerve** Radix motoria and radix sensoria nervi trigemini. **ventral r.** RADIX VENTRALIS NERVORUM SPINALIUM. **ventral nerve r. of spinal nerves** RADIX VENTRALIS NERVORUM SPINALIUM. **ventral r. of spinal nerves** RADIX VENTRALIS NERVORUM SPINALIUM. **vestibular r. of acoustic nerve** RADIX SUPERIOR NERVI VESTIBULOCOCHLEARIS. **vestibular r. of auditory nerve** RADIX SUPERIOR NERVI VESTIBULOCOCHLEARIS.

**rootlets** \root′lits\ A series of axons of cells in the ventral and lateral gray columns that unite to form a ventral root, or a series of processes of cells in the spinal ganglia that unite to form a dorsal root of a spinal nerve.

**ROP** right occipitoposterior position (of a fetus). See under OCCIPUT POSTERIOR POSITION.

**Rorschach** [Hermann *Rorschach*, Swiss psychiatrist, 1884–1922] See under TEST.

**rosacea** \rōzā′sē·ə\ [New L, fem. of *rosaceus* (from L *rosaceus* made of roses, from *ros(a)* rose + *-aceus* -ACEOUS) rose-colored] A syndrome characterized by facial erythema and a tendency to flushing, in association with inflammatory papules and pustules. It is sometimes seen along with ocular rosacea or with rhinophyma. **ocular r.** Blepharitis, conjunctivitis, or keratitis occurring as a result of rosacea.

**rosaniline** A dyestuff whose molecules contain three *p*-aminophenyl groups linked to a single carbon atom, with one of them oxidized to the quinonoid state, and with one of them carrying a methyl group *ortho* to its amino group.

**rosary / rachitic r.** The symmetrical enlargement of the costochondral junctions on the anterior chest wall of a rachitic infant. Also *rachitic beads, beading of the ribs.*

**Rose** [Edmund *Rose,* German physician, 1836–1914] **1** Rose tetanus. See under CEPHALIC TETANUS. **2** See under POSITION.

**Rose** [George Gibson *Rose,* U.S. scientist, born 1922] Waaler-Rose test, Waaler-Rose reaction. See under ROSE-WAALER TEST.

**rosella** \rōzel′ə\ RUBELLA.

**Rosenbach** [Anton Julius Friedrich *Rosenbach,* German surgeon, 1842–1923] See under ERYSIPELOID.

**Rosenbach** [Ottomar *Rosenbach,* German physician, 1851–1907] See under LAW, SIGN.

**Rosenmüller** [Johann Christian *Rosenmüller,* German anatomist, 1771–1820] **1** Rosenmüller's gland, Rosenmüller's node. See under CLOQUET'S NODE. **2** Rosenmüller's gland, Rosenmüller's node. See under PARS PALPEBRALIS GLANDULAE LACRIMALIS. **3** Rosenmüller's fossa, Rosenmüller's cavity, Rosenmüller's recess. See under RECESSUS PHARYNGEUS. **4** Rosenmüller's body, Rosenmüller's organ. See under EPOÖPHORON. **5** Rosenmüller's valve. See under PLICA LACRIMALIS.

**Rosenthal** [Curt *Rosenthal,* German psychiatrist, flourished 20th century] Melkersson-Rosenthal syndrome. See under SYNDROME.

**Rosenthal** [Friedrich Christian *Rosenthal,* German anatomist, 1780–1829] Rosenthal's vein. See under VENA BASALIS.

**Rosenthal** [Isidor *Rosenthal,* German physiologist, 1836–1915] Rosenthal's canal, spiral canal of Rosenthal. See under CANALIS SPIRALIS COCHLEAE.

**Rosenthal** [Robert L. *Rosenthal,* U.S. hematologist, born 1923] Rosenthal syndrome. See under HEMOPHILIA C.

**Rosenzweig** [Saul *Rosenzweig,* U.S. psychologist, born 1907] Rosenzweig picture frustration test. See under TEST.

**roseola** \rōzē′ələ, rō′zē·ō′lə\ [New L (from L *roseus* rosy, from *rosa* rose + *-eus* adjectival suffix), a rose-colored eruption] A pinkish red rash. Also *rose rash.* **r. infantilis** EXANTHEM SUBITUM. **r. infantum** EXANTHEM SUBITUM. **syphilitic r.** A bright pink maculoroseolar rash that is frequently the first manifestation of secondary syphilis. Also *macular syphilid, roseolar syphilid, erythematous syphilid.* **r. typhosa** The rash of typhoid fever. **r. urticata** A secondary syphilitic rash with urticarial features.

**Roser** [Wilhelm *Roser,* German surgeon, 1817–1888] Roser's line. See under NÉLATON'S LINE.

**rosette** \rōzet′\ [French, from L *ros(a)* a rose + French *-ette,* diminishing suffix] **1** A type of structure in which parts have a circular radiate arrangement, as a cluster of leaves arising from a short stem, or the fringed arrangement of merozoites in a red cell infected with *Plasmodium malariae,* holdfast of a cestode, or tumor cells arranged in a radial manner. **2** A plant disease resulting from a viral infection or a mineral deficiency. **3** One of the agglutinated borrelia cells seen in the blood when antibody appears at the end of a wave of fever in relapsing fever. **Homer Wright r.'s** Circular or spherical collections of cells which have centrally placed neurofibrils. There is no central lumen. These rosettes are seen in medulloblastomas and neuroblastomas and indicate neural differentiation. **malarial r.** A stage in the erythrocytic cycle of the malarial parasite, in which the schizont has reached maturity, divided, and arranged the progeny (merozoites) around the periphery of the cell, often in the form of a rosette. This is seen particularly in species of *Plasmodium malariae* and *P. ovale,* which usually produce only eight merozoites per schizogonic stage. Also *daisy* (informal). **Wintersteiner r.** The characteristic macroscopic arrangement of the tumor cells in retinoblastoma. The elongated cells are disposed radially around a small circular lumen which is occupied by converging neuritic processes.

**rosin** \räz′in\ The glassy, amber residue that remains after turpentine has been distilled from various species of *Pinus.* It consists mainly of abietic acid and resene, and it is used pharmaceutically to prepare cerates, plasters, and ointments. Also *colophony.*

**rosolic acid** **1** Any of a group of hydroxyphenylmethane dyestuffs, used principally as pH indicators. Although often used collectively, the term is applied specifically to monomethyl hydroxytriphenylmethane. **2** In stain technology, a mixture of rosolic acid and derivatives of pararosolic acid, used as a pH indicator which changes from yellow to red at pH 6.8 to 8.2. Also *aurin.*

**Ross** [Sir Ronald *Ross,* English protozoologist, 1857–1932] Ross cyle. See under MOSQUITO CYCLE.

**Rossbach** [Michael Josef *Rossbach,* German physician, 1842–1899] Rossbach's disease. See under HYPERCHLORHYDRIA.

**Rossolimo** [Grigoriy Ivanovich *Rossolimo,* Russian neurologist, 1860–1928] See under REFLEX, SIGN.

**Rostan** [Leon Louis *Rostan,* French physician, 1790–1866] Rostan's asthma. See under CARDIAC ASTHMA.

**rostellum** \rästel′əm\ [L, dim. of *rostrum* a beak, snout] The anterior extension of the tapeworm scolex. It may be armed with one or more rows of hooks, depending on the species.

**rostrad** \räs′trad\ **1** Toward a rostrum. **2** Toward the beak or snout end.

**rostral** \räs′trəl\ **1** Pertaining to a rostrum or any beaklike anatomical structure. **2** Resembling a rostrum. **3** Situated at or toward the snout end of an organism.

**rostralis** \rästrā′lis\ [NA] Rostral.

**rostrate** \räs′trāt\ [*rostr(um)* + -ATE] Having a beak, or beaklike process.

**rostrum** \räs′trəm\ [L, the beak or bill of a bird, snout or muzzle of a fish or animal, a hooked point] A beaklike structure or appendage. **r. corporis callosi** [NA] The narrowed anterior part of the corpus callosum that is continuous with the genu above and the lamina terminalis below. Also *rostrum of corpus callosum.* **r. sphenoidale** [NA] A triangular ridge in the midline of the inferior surface of the body of the sphenoid bone which fits into a deep cleft between the anterior parts of the alae of the vomer. Also *sphenoidal rostrum, rostrum of sphenoid, beak of sphenoid bone.* **r. of spiral lamina** *Outmoded* HAMULUS LAMINAE SPIRALIS.

**ROT** right occipitotransverse position (of a fetus). See under OCCIPUT TRANSVERSE POSITION.

**Rot** See under ROTH.

**rot** Decomposition or decay.

**rotameter** \rōtam′ətər\ [L *rota* a wheel, circuit + -METER] A tapered tube in which the position of a rotating vane indicates the rate at which liquid or gas is flowing through the tube. It is used especially to indicate flow rate of anesthetic gases.

**rotary** \rō′tərē\ Turning on its axis; rotating.

**rotate** \rō′tāt\ [See ROTATION.] **1** To turn or cause to turn on its axis. **2** To alternate.

**rotation** [L *rotatio* (from *rotatus,* past part. of *rotare* to turn around, whirl, revolve) a whirling around, turning around] Movement around an axis, especially, in obstetrics, the turning of the presenting part of a fetus around its long axis from one position to another. **clockwise r. of the heart** An electrocardiographic appearance attributed to clockwise rotation of the heart on its long axis as seen from below. Deep S waves appear in leads $V_3$ and $V_4$ and sometimes $V_5$. **counterclockwise r. of the heart** An electrocardiographic appearance in which the heart appears to have rotated in a counterclockwise direction as seen from below. **external r.** **1** The turning of the presenting part of a fetus after its delivery from one position to another. **2** LATERAL ROTATION. **internal r.** **1** The turning of the presenting part of a fetus within the birth canal prior to delivery from one position to another as an adjustment to the anatomy of the pelvic curve. **2** MEDIAL ROTATION. **lateral r.** Outward turning of a part around a longitudinal axis which is either within the same structure, such as occurs at the shoulder joint around the axis of the shaft of the humerus and at the hip joint about an axis between the femoral head and the lateral femoral condyle, or in an adjacent structure, such as occurs in the comparable movement of supination at the superior radioulnar joint where the radius swivels outward around the axis of the ulna. Also *external rotation.* **manual r.** The turning of the head of a fetus in a vertex presentation through the use of fingers or hand from one position to another. **medial r.** Inward turning of a part around a longitudinal axis which is either within the same structure, such as occurs at the shoulder joint about the axis of the shaft of the humerus and at the hip joint about an axis between the femoral head and the lateral femoral condyle, or in an adjacent structure, such as occurs in the comparable movement of pronation at the superior radioulnar joint where the radius swivels inward around the axis of the ulna. Also *internal rotation.* **molecular r.** A measure of the power of a substance in solution to rotate the plane of polarized light of specified wavelength. It is obtained from the specific rotation of the substance by multiplying by the molar mass and dividing by 100. It is sometimes quoted after multiplying by a further factor of $3/(n^2 + 2)$, where $n$ is the refractive index of the medium, to make it comparable between different solvents. **optical r.** The angle by which a specified length of solution rotates the plane of polarized light clockwise when viewed towards the light source. **renal r.** Failure of one or both kidneys to assume or maintain normal orientation with respect to the sagittal, transverse, or frontal planes of the body. Fused kidneys always involve some degrees of abnormal rotation and the fused structure may itself display further degrees of malrotation. **specific r.** A characteristic of a substance at a specified wavelength of light. It is the optical rotation of a solution of that substance divided by the path length and by the mass concentration of the substance. It is numerically the angle by which a solution of concentration 1 g/ml will rotate the plane of polarized light in a path length of 1 dm. It is positive if the rotation is clockwise when viewed towards the light source. **wheel r.** CYCLOTORSION.

**rotator** \rō′tātər\ A muscle that produces rotation of a part around a specified axis. See also LATERAL ROTATION, MEDIAL ROTATION.

**rotatory** \rō′tətôr′ē\ Relating to or characterized by rotation.

**rotavirus** \rō′təvī′rəs\ A member of the *Rotavirus* genus in the Reoviridae family. The genus is characterized by double-stranded RNA viruses which have a two-layered capsid 70–75 nm in diameter. Included in the genus are the human rotavirus, a major cause of infantile gastroenteritis worldwide, and Nebraska calf diarrhea virus, SA-11 (simian) virus, and agents of gastroenteritis in sheep and fowls. Also *duovirus* (outmoded).

**röteln** \rā′təln, ret′əln, rœ′təln\ [German (dim. pl. noun from *rot* red) lit., little red pocks] RUBELLA.

**rotenone** \rō′tənōn\ $C_{23}H_{22}O_6$. A crystalline compound that occurs in species of *Jacquinia, Derris, Lonchocarpus,* and *Tephrosia.* It is used as an insecticide and scabicide.

**rotexion** \rōtek′shən\ [*rot(ation)* + *(fl)exion*] Rotation and flexion combined.

**Roth** [Moritz *Roth,* Swiss pathologist, 1839–1914] **1** Roth spots. See under SPOT. **2** Vas aberrans of Roth. See under VAS.

**Roth** [Vladimir Karlovich *Roth,* Russian neurologist, 1848–1916] Roth's disease, Rot's disease, Roth syndrome, Bernhardt-Roth disease, Bernhardt-Roth syndrome. See under MERALGIA PARESTHETICA.

**Rothmund** [August von *Rothmund,* Jr., German physician, 1830–1906] Rothmund syndrome. See under ROTHMUND-THOMSON SYNDROME.

**Rotor** [Arturo B. *Rotor,* Philippine internist, flourished 20th century] See under SYNDROME.

**rotoscoliosis** \rō′təskō′lē·ō′sis\ STRUCTURAL SCOLIOSIS.

**rotoxamine** $C_{16}H_{19}ClN_2O$. (−)-2[(4-Chlorophenyl)(2-pyridinyl)methoxy]-*N,N*-dimethylethanamine. The active stereoisomer form of carbinoxamine. It is usually used as a tartrate salt and has activity as an antihistaminic drug.

**Rotter** [Josef *Rotter,* German surgeon, 1857–1924] Rotter's nodes. See under NODE.

**rotula** \rät′yələ\ [L, a little wheel] **1** PATELLA. **2** Any rounded bony process. **3** LOZENGE.

**rotulad** \rät′yəlad\ Toward the patella.

**rouge** \roozh\ [French (from L *rubeus* reddish), having the color of red objects] Finely powdered iron oxide used for polishing gold restorations.

**Rouget** [Charles Marie Benjamin *Rouget,* French physiologist, 1824–1904] **1** Rouget cell. See under PERICYTE. **2** Rouget's muscle. See under FIBRAE CIRCULARES MUSCULI CILIARIS. **3** Rouget's bulb. See under BULB OF OVARY.

**roughage** \ruf′ij\ Undigestible carbohydrates derived from plant foods, such as cellulose and bran. Such complex carbohydrates absorb water in the gut but are eliminated essentially unchanged. They act as laxatives and are thought to make diverticulitis unlikely. These substances absorb bile acids and their degradation products in the large bowel and so possibly protect it against carcinoma of the colon.

**Roughton** [Francis J. W. *Roughton,* British scientist, 1899–1972] Roughton-Scholander method. See under SYRINGE-CAPILLARY METHOD.

**rouleau** \roolō′\ [French, a roll] (*pl.* rouleaux) A stack of 3 to 10 or more erythrocytes resembling a stack of coins. Rouleau formation commonly indicates an increase in plasma immunoglobulin.

**rouleaux** \roolō′\ Plural of ROULEAU.

**roundworm** A worm of the phylum Nematoda; a nematode.

**Rous** [Francis Peyton *Rous,* U.S. physician, 1879–1970] **1** See under SARCOMA. **2** Rous sarcoma virus. See under VIRUS.

**Roussy** [Gustave *Roussy,* French pathologist and neurologist, 1874–1948] **1** Darier-Roussy sarcoid. See under SARCOID. **2** Dejerine-Roussy syndrome, Roussy-Dejerine syndrome. See under THALAMIC SYNDROME. **3** Lévy-Roussy syndrome. See under ROUSSY-LÉVY SYNDROME.

**routine** A subdivision of a digital computer program that performs a specific task.

**routing / contralateral r. of signals** The routing of sound across the head as an aid in reducing hearing loss. Auditory input is transferred from the side of the severely deafened ear to the less deafened or normally hearing ear by means of a hearing aid. Abbr. CROS

**Rouviere** [Henri *Rouviere,* French anatomist and embryologist, born 1875] See under NODE.

**Roux** [César *Roux,* Swiss surgeon, 1857–1926] **1** Roux's gastroenterostomy, Roux-Y gastrojejunostomy. See under ROUX EN Y GASTROENTEROSTOMY. **2** Roux-Y drainage. See under DRAINAGE. **3** Roux en Y loop. See under LOOP. **4** Roux en Y operation. See under OPERATION.

**Roux** [Pierre Paul Emile *Roux,* French bacteriologist, 1853–1933] Roux serum. See under DIPHTHERIA ANTITOXIN.

**Rovighi** [Alberto *Rovighi,* Italian physician, 1856–1919] See under SIGN.

**Rovsing** [Niels Thorkild *Rovsing,* Danish surgeon, 1862–1927] See under SIGN.

**Royle** [Norman Dawson *Royle,* Australian surgeon, died 1944] See under OPERATION.

**RPF** renal plasma flow.

**rpm** revolutions per minute.

**RPS** renal pressor substance.

**RQ** **1** recovery quotient. **2** respiratory quotient.

**-rrhachia** \-rā′kē·ə\ [Gk *rhach(is)* backbone + -IA] A combining form denoting a condition of the spinal column or spinal cord.

**-rrhage** \-rij\ [Gk *rhēgnynai* (second aorist tense *errhagēn*) to burst forth] A combining form meaning an excessive or violent flow or discharge. Also *-rhage, -rrhagia.*

**-rrhagia** \-rā′jə\ -RRHAGE.

**-rrhaphy** \-rəfē\ [Gk *rhaptein* (2nd aorist *errhaphēn*) to sew or stitch together] A combining form meaning the act of suturing. Also *-rhaphy.*

**-rrhea** \-rē′ə\ [Gk suffix *-rrhoia* (from *rhein* or *rheein* to flow) denoting a flow] A combining form meaning flow or discharge. Also *-rhea, -rrhoea* (British spelling).

**-rrhexis** \-rek′sis\ [Gk *rhēxis* (from 1st aorist *errhēxa* of *rhēgnynai* to break, burst) a breaking, bursting, cleaving] A combining form meaning a breaking, tearing apart, rupture.

**-rrhoea** \-rē′ə\ *Brit.* -RRHEA.

**rRNA** ribosomal RNA.

**R/s** Symbol for the unit, roentgen per second.

**$R \cdot s^{-1}$** Symbol for the unit, roentgen per second.

**RSA** right sacroanterior position (of a fetus). See under SACRUM ANTERIOR POSITION.

**RSP** right sacroposterior position (of a fetus). See under SACRUM POSTERIOR POSITION.

**rSr** An electrocardiographic complex characterized by a small initial r wave, a deep S wave, and a small secondary r wave.

**RST** right sacrotransverse position (of a fetus). See under SACRUM TRANSVERSE POSITION.

**RSV** **1** Rous sarcoma virus. **2** respiratory syncytial virus.

**$rT_3$** reverse triiodothyronine.

**RTA** renal tubular acidosis.

**RTF** resistance transfer factor.

**RU** rat unit.

**Ru** Symbol for the element, ruthenium.

**rub** [Middle English *rubben*] A noise generated by two serous surfaces rubbing against each other, especially as heard on auscultation. Also *friction rub, friction sound.* **pericardial r.** The noise generated by the friction between the visceral and parietal pericardium. It may have systolic, diastolic, and presystolic components or only one of these three. Also *pericardial murmur, attrition murmur, friction murmur, pericardial friction sound.* **pleural r.** A grating or rubbing sound heard during respiration on auscultation over an inflamed pleura. **pleuropericardial r.** A grating or rubbing sound heard on auscultation originating from the pleura and pericardium.

**rubber / lead r.** Rubber containing lead compounds, used as a protection against x rays, often fashioned as aprons to be worn by operators of fluoroscopic machines.

**rubefacient** \roo′bəfā′shənt\ [L *rubefaciens,* gen. *rubefacientis,* pres. part. of *rubefacere* (from *rube(r)* red + *facere* to make) to make red] **1** Causing redness of the skin. **2** An agent causing cutaneous erythema.

**rubella** \roobel′ə\ [L, fem. of *rubellus* (dim. of *ruber* red, ruddy) reddish] A mildly contagious viral disease that usually affects children 5–15 years of age. In children and adults, the illness is mild and is usually characterized by lymphadenopathy, a maculopapular rash of 3–5 days' duration, and possibly, coryza and conjunctivitis. Infection confers lifelong immunity. Congenital rubella, particularly when the fetus is infected early in gestation (first trimester), can be a disastrous disease, causing fetal death, premature delivery, and a wide range of severe congenital defects, many of which are permanent and adversely affect later development. A vaccine is available. Also *German measles, three-day measles, roeteln, röteln, rosella, rubeola notha, French measles, bastard measles.*

**rubelliform** \roobel′ifôrm\ Resembling rubella.

**rubeola** \roobē′ələ, roo′bē·ō′lə\ [New L, neut. pl. of *rubeolus,* dim. of L *rubeus* reddish, red] MEASLES. **r. notha** RUBELLA.

**rubeosis** \roo′bē·ō′sis\ [L *rube(us)* red, reddish + -OSIS] Redness, as of the skin. **r. iridis** Ischemic neovascularization of the iris, appearing as a delicate growth of tiny vessels upon the anterior surface of the iris, and also covering the trabecular meshwork. It is commonly associated with occlusion of the central retinal vein or artery, or with diabetic retinopathy. The condition may be followed by glaucoma.

**rubidium** Element number 37, having atomic weight 85.4678. It is a very reactive alkali metal with valences 1, 2, 3, and 4. The elemental metal is soft, silvery white, and melts at 38.89°C. It is the sixteenth most abundant element in the earth's crust, consisting of two isotopes of mass numbers 85 and 87 in the ratio of about 72:28. Rubidium 87 is unstable, with a half-life of $5 \times 10^{11}$ years. The beta radiation emitted by natural rubidium is energetic enough to expose x-ray film in less than 60 days. The element has some industrial applications. Symbol: Rb

**Rubin** [Isidor Clinton *Rubin,* U.S. physician, 1883–1958] See under TEST.

**rubin** \roo′bin\ ACID FUCHSIN. **basic r.** BASIC FUCHSIN.

**Rubinstein** [Jack Herbert *Rubinstein,* U.S. child psychiatrist and pediatrician, born 1925] Rubinstein-Taybi syndrome. See under RUBINSTEIN SYNDROME.

**rubivirus** \roo′bivī′rəs\ [*rub(ella)* + VIRUS] A member of the genus *Rubivirus* in the family Togaviridae. The genus includes rubella virus.

**rubor** \roo′bôr\ [L, redness] Redness of color. It is one of the cardinal signs of inflammation. **dependent r.** A purplish red coloration of the toes, feet, and sometimes the lower legs in patients with far-advanced arterial insufficiency. It is seen only when the extremities are dependent. These extremities will demonstrate elevational pallor if raised above the level of the heart.

**rubreserine** A product with a red color which arises from the decomposition of physostigmine during storage in solution. Its presence indicates this change, and a decrease in potency of the drug solution.

**rubriblast** \roo′briblast\ PRONORMOBLAST.

**rubricyte** \roo′brisīt\ POLYCHROMATOPHILIC NORMOBLAST.

**rubro-** \roo′brō-, roo′brə-\ [L *ruber*, gen. *rubr(is)* red] A combining form meaning (1) red; (2) the red nucleus (nucleus ruber).

**rubrobulbar** \-bul′bər\ RUBRORETICULAR.

**rubrocerebellar** \-ser′əbel′ər\ Denoting projections from the red nucleus that separate from the rubrospinal tract, enter the superior cerebellar peduncle, and end in the dentate nucleus of the cerebellum.

**rubrogliocladin** A dark red quinhydrone derivative of aurantiogliocladin, an antibiotic extracted from species of *Gliocladium*.

**rubro-olivary** \-äl′iver′ē\ Denoting uncrossed projections from the red nucleus to the principal inferior olivary nucleus via the central tegmental tract.

**rubroreticular** \-retik′yələr\ Denoting connections between the red nucleus and the lateral reticular nucleus of the medulla. Also *rubrobulbar*.

**rubrospinal** \-spī′nəl\ Denoting efferent fiber projections of the red nucleus that cross in the ventral tegmental decussation and descend in the lateral funiculus of the spinal cord.

**rubrothalamic** \-thəlam′ik\ Denoting efferent fibers of the red nucleus that project mainly to the ventrolateral nucleus of the thalamus.

**rubrum** \roo′brəm\ [L (neut. sing. of *ruber* red, ruddy, akin to *rubus* the blackberry, *rufus* red, tawny and *ravus* gray, russet, yellowish), red, ruddy, fiery] Red. **r. Congo** CONGO RED.

**Ruck** [Karl von *Ruck* U.S. physician, 1849–1922] Ruck's watery extract tuberculin. See under TUBERCULIN.

**ructus** \ruk′təs\ [L, a belching, eructation] An eructation; a belch; belching.

**rudiment** \roo′dəmənt\ [L *rudimentum* (from *rudis* as it is grown, raw, in its native state + *-mentum* -MENT) the first attempt or trial] The first sign of development of a part or organ as a primordium or anlage. Also *rudimentum*. **r. of corpus striatum** A thickening in the floor of each developing lateral ventricle of the telencephalon which will become the corpus striatum. **hair r.** An epidermal bud which grows down obliquely into the corium during development to give rise to a hair. Each bud consists of a core of polygonal cells and an outer columnar cell covering. **hepatic r.** A mesodermal mass in which the hepatic diverticulum develops during early embryogenesis. This thickening of splanchnic mesoderm and the adjacent mesenchyme is interposed between the hepatic diverticulum and the pericardial cavity. It originates from two mixed but distinct sources, the septum transversum anteriorly, and the tissue which migrates into the cranial part of the septum and contributes to the formation of the diaphragm. Because of the persistence of the ventral mesentery, the final relation of the liver is more towards it than to the diaphragm. **hippocampal r.** INDUSIUM GRISEUM. **lens r.** The primordium of the embryonic lens when it first appears as an ectodermal thickening in the head region of the developing embryo. **r. of vaginal process** A vestige of the vaginal process of the peritoneum, which was drawn down from the lateral inguinal fossa of the embryo through the inguinal canal into the scrotum. It may persist as a band of connective tissue in the spermatic cord. Also *rudimentum processus vaginalis*.

**rudimentary** \roo′dimen′tərē\ **1** Describing a part or organ that fails to develop fully and remains in an underdeveloped state in the adult. **2** Describing a part or organ that was well developed and functional in an ancestral form but is today nonfunctional and poorly developed.

**rudimentum** \roo′dimen′təm\ [L (from *rudi(s)* in its native state + *-mentum* -MENT), a beginning] RUDIMENT. **r. processus vaginalis** RUDIMENT OF VAGINAL PROCESS.

**Ruffini** [Angelo *Ruffini*, Italian anatomist, 1864–1929] **1** Ruffini's endings. See under RUFFINI'S CORPUSCLES. **2** Ruffini cylinders. See under CYLINDER. **3** Organ of Ruffini. See under BRUSHES OF RUFFINI.

**rufochromomycin** STREPTONIGRIN.

**ruga** \roo′gə\ [L, a crease, wrinkle] (*pl.* rugae) A fold, crease, ridge, or wrinkle, as of mucous membrane. Also *rugosity*. **rugae of scrotum** Numerous transverse and oblique ridges on the skin of the scrotum produced by contraction of the underlying dartos muscle which is directed at right angles to the ridges. **rugae of stomach** PLICAE GASTRICAE. **rugae of the urinary bladder** Folds of mucous membrane produced in the empty urinary bladder by the looseness of the submucous layer. They are absent over the trigone. **rugae vaginales** [NA] Transverse folds or ridges of mucous membrane that extend laterally from the anterior and the posterior columns of the vagina, especially on the posterior wall and near the vaginal orifice. Also *rugae of vagina, vaginal folds, transverse ridges of vaginal wall*.

**rugae** \roo′jē\ Plural of RUGA.

**Ruggeri** [Ruggero *Ruggeri*, Italian physician, died 1905] See under REFLEX, SIGN.

**rugine** \roozhēn′\ RASPATORY. **Lempert r.** A relatively small, light periosteal elevator used chiefly for endaural surgery. Also *Lempert elevator*.

**rugitus** \roo′jitəs\ [Late L (from L *rugire* to rumble), a rumbling in the bowels] A growling noise emanating from the intestines.

**rugosity** \roogäs′itē\ [Late L *rugosit(as)* (from *rugos(us)* wrinkled, from *rug(a)* a wrinkle + *-osus* -OSE) the state of being wrinkled + -Y] RUGA.

**rugous** \roo′gəs\ [*rug(a)* + -OUS] Wrinkled; marked by wrinkles.

**RUL** right upper lobe (of lung).

**rule** A principle, direction, or considered guideline, often based on an accumulation of observations. See also entries under LAW and PRINCIPLE. **American Law Institute r.** AMERICAN LAW INSTITUTE FORMULATION. **analytic r.** A direction to a patient in therapy to say everything and anything that comes to mind during the treatment session, no matter how personal or embarrassing, no matter how trivial or seemingly senseless, and no matter how unwarranted or unjustified the thought or feeling seems to be, even if those feelings and impulses involve the analyst. Also *basic rule*. **Anstie's r.** ANSTIE'S LIMIT. **Arey's r.** A method of estimating fetal length in inches according to the duration of gestation. For the first five lunar months, the fetal length in inches is equal to the sum of the lunar months since conception. For the last five lunar months, the fetal length is equal to the sum of the lunar months since conception multiplied by two. **Aston's r.** The rule that elements of odd atomic number have no more than two stable isotopes. **Bartholomew's r. of fourths** A method of determining duration of gestation according to the height of the uterine fundus above the symphysis pubis. The uterus is one-fourth the distance between symphysis pubis and umbilicus at two months after conception, one-half the distance by three months, three-fourths the distance by four months, and at the umbilicus by five months. The fundus then rises one-fourth the distance between umbilicus and xiphoid process per month until the ninth month, when it returns to the level it occupied at eight months. **basic r.** ANALYTIC RULE. **Bastedo's r.** A formula for adjusting the dosage of a drug for a child. It is determined by multiplying the adult dose by the child's age, adding 3, and dividing this sum by 30. **Clark's r.** A formula for the adjustment of a drug dosage for a child over 2 years old. It is determined by multiplying the adult dose times the weight of the child, in pounds, and dividing that product by 150. **Clark's body area r.** A formula for the adjustment of drug dosage for children. The modified dose is calculated by taking the product of the body surface area of the child times the adult dose, and dividing the product by the body surface area of the average adult (1.7 square meters). **Cowling's r.** A formula for adjusting the drug dosage for a child. It is determined by multiplying the adult dosage times the age of the child at his or her next birthday, and dividing that product by 24. **delivery date r.** NÄGELE'S RULE. **dermatomal r.** Referred visceral pain is felt in the dermatomal areas which correspond to the posterior spinal root or roots through which afferent impulses from the affected viscus enter the spinal cord. **Dilling's r.** A formula for adjusting the drug dosage for a child. It is determined by taking the product of the child's age times the adult dosage, and dividing the product by 20. **discovery r.** A requirement for malpractice litigation in some jurisdictions under which the statute of limitations does not commence to run until the wrongful act is discovered or, with reasonable diligence, should have been discovered. **Durham r.** A 1954 ruling by the United States Court of Appeals for the District of Columbia that extended the concept of not guilty by reason of insanity beyond a consideration of irresistible impulse and ability to distinguish right from wrong to all relevant psychiatric data indicating that the unlawful act was the product of mental disease or defect. The Durham rule was replaced in 1972 by the Brawner decision. Also *Durham decision.* See also AMERICAN LAW INSTITUTE FORMULATION. **Eichler's r.** A rule which states that in host-parasite complexes a larger, more varied taxonomic group tends to have a larger, more varied array of parasites than does a smaller, more uniform group of the same taxonomic rank. **Fahrenholz r.** A rule of presumed relationships in evolutionary age between host and parasite which states that the extinct ancestral forms of present-day parasites were in turn parasitic in the ancestors of present-day hosts of these parasites. **Fried's r.** A formula for adjusting the drug dosage for infants less than 2 years old. It is determined by multiplying the age of the child in months by the adult dosage and dividing the product by 150. **Fuhrman's r.** SZIDAT RULE. **Goodsall's r.** The rule in proctology that external perianal fistulas located posteriorly have their internal opening in the posterior half of the anus, while fistulas with anterior external openings usually have their primary opening in the anterior quadrant of the anus. **Haase's r.** A method of estimating fetal length in centimeters according to duration of gestation. For each lunar month since conception, during the first five months, the fetal length in centimeters is equal to the number of months since conception squared. During the last five lunar months of pregnancy, the fetal length is equal to the duration in months times five. **Hamburger's r.** A formula for adjusting drug dosage for children, determined by multiplying the child's weight in kilograms times the adult dose, and dividing that product by 70. **His r.** The duration of pregnancy in days, weeks, or months calculated from the first day of the first missed menstrual period. • The His rule is seldom used in current obstetric practice. **Jackson's r.** JACKSON'S LAW. **Knaus r.** A method of determining the estimated date of birth by calculating from the day of ovulation. The date of birth within a range of five days is one year from the date of ovulation minus three months. **McDonald's r.** A method of estimating the duration of pregnancy in lunar months by measuring the contour height of the uterine fundus above the symphysis pubis. It is applied only after the sixth lunar month, when the duration of pregnancy in lunar months is equal to the contour height above the symphysis pubis in centimeters divided by 3.5. **M'Naghten r.** A ruling stipulating that an individual accused of a crime is not criminally responsible if he "was laboring under such a defect of reason from disease of the mind as not to know the nature and quality of the act; or, if he did know it, that he did not know that what he was doing was wrong." It was promulgated in 1843 by the English House of Lords. **Nägele's r.** A method of estimating the date of birth. One counts back three months from the anniversary of the first day of the last menstrual period and adds seven days to arrive at the date. Also *delivery date rule.* **r. of nines** A formula for estimating the size of a burn as a percentage of total body surface. The body is divided into areas that represent percentage values as follows: head and neck, 9 percent; each upper extremity, 9 percent; anterior and posterior trunk, each 18 percent; each lower extremity, 18 percent; perineum, 1 percent. **r. of outlet** A method of estimating whether the maternal pelvic outlet is adequate to allow delivery of a normal-sized fetus. The sum of the internal posterior sagittal diameter and the external transverse diameter of the plane of the outlet must be at least 15 cm. **Quetelet's r.** A rule stating that, for the normal adult, the number of kilograms of body weight should equal the number of centimeters over 100 of body height. **Szidat r.** A rule of affinity between host and parasite phylogeny which postulates that specialized hosts tend to harbor specialized parasites, and primitive or generalized hosts tend to have simpler or less specialized parasites. This concept has been used to relate phylogenetic age of the host to the presumed degree of specialization of the parasite. Also *Fuhrman's rule.* **Young's r.** A formula for adjusting the drug dose for a child. It is determined by multiplying the adult dosage times the age of the child in years, and dividing that product by the sum of the child's age + 12.

**rumble** / **diastolic r.** The murmur heard at the apex in cases of mitral stenosis.

**ruminant** \roo′minənt\ [L *ruminans,* gen. *ruminantis,* pres. part. of *ruminare* to chew the cud] Any of the herbivorous animals that have four stomachs, a rumen, reticulum, omasum, and abomasum or true stomach. They have the ability to regurgitate from the rumen pellets of fibrous food, which are then rechewed. Sheep, cattle, deer, and camels are ruminants.

**rump** [Middle English *rumpe,* of Scandinavian origin] The dorsal aspect of the hindquarters of an animal; also, popularly, the buttocks of humans.

**Rumpel** [Theodor *Rumpel,* German physician, 1862–1923] Rumpel-Leede sign, Rumpel-Leede test. See under RUMPEL-LEEDE PHENOMENON.

**Rundles** [Ralph Wayne *Rundles,* U.S. internist, born 1911] Rundles-Falls syndrome. See under HEREDITARY SIDEROBLASTIC ANEMIA.

**Runeberg** [Johan Wilhelm *Runeberg,* Finnish physician, 1843–1918] Runeberg's anemia, Runeberg's disease. See under PERNICIOUS ANEMIA.

**runoff** 1 Flow into peripheral vessels. 2 Anatomically, the number and caliber of recipient vessels that are distal to an actual or proposed arterial reconstruction, as, for example, the number of tibial vessels distal to a femoral-popliteal bypass graft.

**rupia** \roo′pē·ə\ [irreg. from Gk *rhyp(os)* filth + New L *-ia* -IA] Heavily crusted sores on the skin.

**rupioid** \roo′pē·oid\ Resembling rupia.

**rupture** \rup′chər\ [L *ruptura* (from *rumpere* to break, burst; akin to English *rip*) a breaking, bursting, rupture] 1 A tear or break in any soft tissue. 2 To burst or tear. 3 *Popular* HERNIA. **extracapsular r.** A tubal ectopic pregnancy in which the wall of the fallopian tube ruptures, spilling the contents of the pregnancy into the peritoneal cavity. **r. of the gravid uterus** Disruption of the uterine musculature, most frequently at the site of a previous uterine incision, such as that of a cesarean section. The condition is associated with a high fetal mortality rate. **incidental r.** An asymptomatic, spontaneous disruption of the musculature of a gravid uterus at the site of a previous uterine scar. **intracapsular r.** A tubal ectopic pregnancy in which the amniotic sac ruptures and the embryo is expelled into the lumen of the fallopian tube. **r. of membranes** The breaking or tearing of the amniotic sac, leading to leakage of amniotic fluid through the uterine cervix and into the vagina. **premature r. of membranes** The tearing of the amniotic sac prior to the onset of labor. **prolonged r. of membranes** The tearing of the amniotic sac 24 or more hours prior to the onset of labor. **spontaneous r.** The disruption of the musculature of a gravid uterus in the absence of any trauma. The uterus may or may not have scarring from a previous incision. **spontaneous r. of membranes** Rupture of the amniotic sac without use of digital pressure or instruments. **traumatic r.** The disruption of the musculature of a gravid uterus with or without previous scarring due to the use of oxytocic agents, intrauterine manipulations, external uterine pressure, or instrumental delivery of the fetus. **r. of the tympanic membrane** Perforating injury of the tympanic membrane caused by trauma, such as that resulting from temporal bone fractures (usually longitudinal fractures), blows on the ear (particularly from the flat of the hand), blast injury (especially from exposure to bomb blast), and injury from foreign bodies introduced into the external auditory meatus. Perforations caused by otitis media are not really ruptures.

**RUQ** right upper quadrant (of abdomen).

**Russell** [Alexander *Russell*, English pediatrician, flourished 20th century] 1 Russell syndrome. See under DIENCEPHALIC SYNDROME OF INFANCY. 2 See under DWARF. 3 Silver-Russell syndrome. See under SYNDROME.

**Russell** [Frederick Fuller *Russell*, U.S. pathologist, 1870–1960] Russell's double sugar agar. See under AGAR.

**Russell** [Patrick *Russell*, English physician active in Syria, 1727–1805] 1 See under VIPER. 2 Russell's viper venom. See under VENOM.

**Russell** [R. Hamilton *Russell*, Australian surgeon, flourished early 20th century] See under TRACTION.

**Russell** [William *Russell*, Scottish physician, 1852–1940] Russell corpuscles. See under RUSSELL BODIES.

**Rust** [Johann Nepomuk *Rust*, Austrian surgeon, 1775–1840] See under SIGN.

**rust** 1 A reddish brown coat of ferric oxide or ferric hydroxide formed on iron or steel surfaces exposed to moisture. 2 To undergo oxidation into rust. 3 A parasitic fungus of the class Basidiomycetes, subclass Teliomycetidae, order Uredinales. A rust fungus seasonally produces spores of several types on leaves and/or stems of vascular plants. The clusters of spores in summer are the color of iron rust.

**rut** [Middle English *rutte*, from Old French *ruit* a noise, from Late L *rugitus* a roaring, from L *rugitus*, past part. of *rugire* to roar] A time of sexual activity in certain male animals such as deer and elephants. It is during this period that spermatogenesis and mating occur.

**ruthenium** Element number 44, having atomic weight 101.07. Ruthenium is a hard, white metal. It occurs native along with platinum and combined in various ores. It resembles osmium in that it spontaneously (under certain conditions) forms a highly toxic tetroxide, which is explosive. The metal is used as a catalyst and an alloying element. Symbol: Ru

**rutherford** \ruTH′ərfərd\ [after Sir Ernest *Rutherford*, New Zealand-born British physicist, 1871–1937] A unit of radioactivity equal to the quantity of a radioactive nuclide which undergoes $10^6$ disintegrations per second; $10^6$ disintegrations per second = 1 megabecquerel. An obsolete unit. Symbol: Rd, rd

**rutidosis** \roo′tidō′sis\ RHYTIDOSIS.

**rutin** \roo′tin\ $C_{27}H_{30}O_{16}$. A bioflavonoid found in buckwheat. Also *phytomelin, rutoside*.

**rutoside** \roo′təsīd\ RUTIN.

**Ruysch** [Frederik *Ruysch*, Dutch anatomist, 1638–1731] 1 Ruysch disease. See under CONGENITAL MEGACOLON. 2 See under TUBE. 3 Ruysch tunic, Ruysch membrane. See under LAMINA CHOROIDOCAPILLARIS. 4 Ruysch veins. See under RETZIUS VEINS. 5 Ruysch veins. See under VENAE VORTICOSAE.

**RV** residual volume.

**RVH** right ventricular hypertrophy.

**-ry** \-rē\ -ERY.

# S

**S** 1 Symbol for the unit, siemens. 2 Symbol for the unit, sone. 3 Symbol for the element, sulfur. 4 serum.

**S.** signa.

**$S_1$** first heart sound

**$S_2$** second heart sound.

**$S_f$** Svedberg flotation unit.

**s** Symbol for the unit, second (of time).

**s.** 1 *sinister* (L, left). 2 *semis* (L, half).

**$\bar{s}$** *sine* (L, without).

***S*** Symbol for the quantity, apparent power, expressed in volt-amperes.

***s*** Symbol for the quantity, length of path, expressed in meters.

**Σ** 1 The capitalized form of the eighteenth letter of the Greek alphabet, sigma. 2 Symbol for summation. 3 Symbol for syphilis.

**σ** The eighteenth letter of the Greek alphabet, sigma.

**s.a.** *secundum artem* (L, according to art).

**SAA** severe aplastic anemia.

***Sabethes*** \səbē′thēz\ A genus of New World mosquitoes related to *Aedes* that breed in treeholes, treetops, or bromeliads. *S. chloropterus* has been implicated in the sylvatic cycle of yellow fever. A species of the genus has also been implicated in the transmission of Venezuelan equine encephalomyelitis virus.

**Sabin** [Albert Bruce *Sabin*, Russian-born microbiologist active in the United States, born 1906] 1 Sabin-Feldman dye test. See under TEST. 2 Sabin vaccine. See under POLIOMYELITIS VACCINE.

**Sabin** [Florence Rena *Sabin*, U.S. anatomist, 1871–1953] Megaloblast of Sabin. See under PRONORMOBLAST.

**Sabouraud** [Raymond Jacques Adrian *Sabouraud*, French dermatologist, 1864–1938] See under AGAR.

**sabulous** \sab′yələs\ Gritty; sandy.

**sabulum** \sab′yələm\ [L, sand, gravel] ACERVULUS.

**saburra** \sabur′ə\ [L, gravel, ballast] Foul material on the lips, mouth, or teeth.

**sac** [L *saccus* (from Gk *sakkos* haircloth, sackcloth, sack, bag, from Semitic, akin to Hebrew *saq* sack, sackcloth) a sack, bag] A pouchlike structure or space; saccus or sacculus. **abdominal s.** A primitive serous sac in the embryo which will become the abdominal cavity of the fetus. **air s.** 1 Any of several thin-walled extensions of the bronchial tree in birds. These air sacs may be paired or unpaired, and they occupy most of the space between visceral organs and pneumatize the skeletal system. They serve to increase respiratory efficiency. 2 One of numerous diverticula formed by a widening of the tracheae in the respiratory system of insects. 3 The swim bladder in fishes. 4 An alveolus of the lung. **allantoic s.** ALLANTOIC VESICLE. **alveolar s.'s** SACCULI ALVEOLARES. **amniotic s.** AMNION. **aneurysmal s.** The dilated wall of an artery or ventricle due to an aneurysm. **aortic s.** A dilated vessel in human embryos formed by the fused ventral aortae. The aortic sac eventually contributes to the pulmonary trunk, the brachiocephalic trunk, and the arch of the aorta. **chorionic s.** CHORION. **conjunctival s.** SACCUS CONJUNCTIVALIS. **dental s.** A fibrocellular condensation of mesenchyme surrounding the enamel organ and dental papilla of a developing tooth. **dural s.** A continuation of the dura mater below the caudal end of the spinal cord, surrounding a wide subarachnoid space containing the cauda equina and filum terminale. **endolymphatic s.** SACCUS ENDOLYMPHATICUS. **epiploic s.** BURSA OMENTALIS. **gestation s.** CONCEPTUS. **greater s. of peritoneum** CAVITAS PERITONEALIS. **s. of Gruber** GRUBER'S CUL-DE-SAC. **heart s.** PERICARDIUM. **hernial s.** The lining of a hernia, such as the portion of peritoneum which lines an inguinal hernia. **Hilton s.** SACCULUS LARYNGIS. **lacrimal s.** SACCUS LACRIMALIS. **laryngeal s.** VENTRICULUS LARYNGIS. **lesser s. of peritoneal cavity** BURSA OMENTALIS. **Lower s.** Either bulbus venae jugularis inferior or bulbus venae jugularis superior. **lymphatic s.'s** Localized vascular islands constituting the primordia of the lymphatic channels in the embryo. **omental s.** BURSA OMENTALIS. **pericardial s.** PERICARDIUM. **peritoneal s.** A pouch of peritoneum produced normally as a recess, during development as a process or abnormally by a herniation. **pleural s.** CAVITAS PLEURALIS. **posterior lymph s.'s** Paired lymph sacs in the embryo, situated in the lumbosacral region at the junction of the iliac vein with the posterior cardinal. They drain into the cisterna chyli. **preputial s.** PREPUTIAL SPACE. **pudendal s.** BROCA'S POUCH. **retroperitoneal lymph s.** A single lymph sac in the embryo, situated at the root of the mesentery near the suprarenal glands. **serous s.** A body cavity lined by serous membrane, such as the pleural, pericardial and peritoneal cavities which comprise the intraembryonic coelom. **splenic s.** RECESSUS SPLENICUS. **synovial s.** A pouch or herniation of synovium beyond the normal confines of the joint. **tear s.** SACCUS LACRIMALIS. **tubotympanic s.** A recess, later becoming a diverticulum, which is directed laterally from the embryonic primitive pharynx, and which eventually develops into the pharyngotympanic tube and its derivatives. **vaginal s.** 1 SACCUS VAGINALIS. 2 PERITONEOVAGINAL CANAL. **vitelline s.** UMBILICAL VESICLE. **yolk s.** The extraembryonic membrane made of endoderm and splanchnic mesoderm which usually contains, in whole or in part, vitelline vessels. In reptiles and birds it surrounds the massive yolk and derives nutrition from it for the embryo. It is present in mammals, but its early history and relations vary. In many mammals endoderm spreads beneath the trophoblastic capsule and surrounds for a time a relatively large sac. In some a vascularized yolk sac placenta is formed by union with the chorion. In primates the sac is small and becomes a diminutive vesicle within the chorionic sac.

**saccade** \sakād′\ [French (from obsol. French *saquer* to pull, draw), a jerk] The rapid involuntary movement of the eyes that occurs when an image of interest falls on the retina at a distance from the fovea, as normally occurs when reading the printed page. Also *rapid eye movement, saccadic eye movement*. Adj. saccadic.

**sacchari-** \sak′əri-\ SACCHARO-.

**saccharide** \sak′ərīd\ [*sacchar(o)-* + -IDE[1]] Any substance that is either a simple sugar (aldose or ketose) or a compound of such substances in glycosidic linkage to each other. It therefore includes monosaccharides, oligosaccharides, and polysaccharides.

**saccharification** \-fikā′shən\ [SACCHARI- + -FICATION] The industrial process of transforming starch into glucose, whether with acid or with enzymes.

**saccharimeter** \sak′ərim′ətər\ [SACCHARI- + -METER] Any instrument that is used to measure sugar in a solution, usually by measuring the degree to which the solution polarizes light, by determining specific gravity, or by measuring the amount of $CO_2$ produced after fermentation. Also *saccharometer.*

**saccharin** \sak′ərin\ The cyclic imide of 2-sulfobenzoic acid. It is over 500 times as sweet as sucrose, and is used as a sweetener in foods. Also *sulfinide, sodium benzosulfimide.*

**saccharine** \sak′ərin\ Of or relating to sugar; sweet.

**saccharo-** \sak′ərō-\ [Gk *sakcharon* sugar] A combining form denoting sugar. Also *sacchari-.*

**saccharometer** \sak′əräm′ətər\ SACCHARIMETER.

**saccharum lactis** LACTOSE.

**sacciform** \sak′sifôrm\ In the shape of a pouch or sac. Also *saccular.*

**sacculated** \sak′yəlā′tid\ Possessing or characterized by saccules.

**sacculation** \sak′yəlā′shən\ **1** The process of forming a sac or saccule. **2** A saccule or a group of saccules. **cecal s.'s** HAUSTRA COLI. **colic s.'s** HAUSTRA COLI. **uterine s.** A pouch or sac in the uterine wall secondary to a thinning of the myometrium. Also *sacculated uterus.*

**saccule** \sak′yool\ [L *sacculus.* See SACCULUS.] A small sac. Also *sacculus.* **air s.'s** SACCULI ALVEOLARES. **alveolar s.'s** SACCULI ALVEOLARES. **laryngeal s.** SACCULUS LARYNGIS.

**sacculi** \sak′yəlī\ Plural of SACCULUS.

**sacculiform** \sak′yəlifôrm′\ Shaped like a saccule.

**sacculocochlear** \sak′yəlōkäk′lē·ər\ Pertaining to the sacculus and the cochlea.

**sacculotomy** \sak′yəlät′əmē\ [*saccul(e)* + *o* + -TOMY] Surgical decompression of the sacculus for the relief of the symptoms of Menière's disease. The procedure was abandoned when it was found to entail the risk of severe sensorineural deafness. Also *Fick operation.*

**sacculus** \sak′yələs\ [L, dim. of *saccus.* See SAC.] (*pl.* sacculi) **1** [NA] SACCULE. **2** [NA] A small sac of the membranous labyrinth occupying the spherical recess in the vestibule near the entrance of the scala vestibuli. Posteriorly it is continuous with the ductus endolymphaticus through which it communicates with the utricle and the saccus endolymphaticus and inferiorly it gives off the ductus reuniens which communicates with the vestibular end of the cochlear duct. In its anterior wall is the macula of the saccule. **sacculi alveolares** [NA] Saclike spaces budding outward from the terminal ends of the alveolar ducts of the lung and comprising two or more alveoli. Also *alveolar saccules, alveolar sacs, air saccules.* **s. laryngis** [NA] A fibrous pouch extending cranially from the anterior part of the laryngeal ventricle for a variable distance between the vestibular fold medially and the thyroarytenoid muscle and thyroid cartilage laterally. The mucous membrane lining it contains several mucous glands. Also *laryngeal saccule, laryngeal pouch, Hilton sac, appendage of ventricle of larynx, appendix of ventricle of larynx.*

**saccus** \sak′əs\ (*pl.* sacci) A pouchlike structure or space; a sac. **s. conjunctivalis** [NA] The potential space between the palpebral and the bulbar conjunctiva behind each eyelid, limited superiorly and inferiorly by the superior fornix and the inferior fornix of the conjunctiva, respectively. As the conjunctiva is attached to the free edges of the eyelids, the space is open anteriorly between the lids. Also *conjunctival sac.* **s. endolymphaticus** [NA] The dilated distal end of the ductus endolymphaticus, which forms a blind sac under the dura mater on the posterior surface of the petrous part of the temporal bone. Also *endolymphatic sac, Böttcher space.* **s. lacrimalis** [NA] The dilated upper extremity of the nasolacrimal duct situated in a bony fossa on the anteromedial wall of the orbit. It receives the two lacrimal canaliculi in the middle of its lateral surface and it consists of a fibroelastic wall lined by mucous membrane. Also *lacrimal sac, tear sac, dacryocyst.* **s. vaginalis** **1** [NA] A small peritoneal fossa in the lower part of the anterior abdominal wall of the embryo, from the lower end of which the processus vaginalis extends along the gubernaculum through the inguinal canal. It is present in both sexes and the site of the saccus persists postnatally as the lateral inguinal fossa. Also *vaginal sac.* **2** PERITONEOVAGINAL CANAL.

**Sachs** [Bernard Parney *Sachs,* U.S. neurologist, 1858–1944] Tay-Sachs disease. See under DISEASE.

**Sacks** [Benjamin *Sacks,* U.S. physician, 1896–1939] Libman-Sacks disease, Libman-Sacks syndrome. See under LIBMAN-SACKS ENDOCARDITIS.

**sacr-** \sākr-\ SACRO-.

**sacrad** \sā′krad\ Toward the sacrum.

**sacral** \sā′krəl\ Of or pertaining to the sacrum. Also *hieric.*

**sacralgia** \sākral′jə\ A pain in the sacral region. Also *sacrodynia.*

**sacralization** \sā′krəlīzā′shən\ ASSIMILATION SACRUM. **lumbar s.** A congenital fusion of the lowest lumbar vertebra to the sacrum.

**sacrectomy** \sākrek′təmē\ [SACR- + -ECTOMY] A surgical resection of the bony sacrum.

**sacrifice** To put to death (an experimental animal). 〈"The investigators sacrificed the animals [hamsters] and examined their brains and cervical spinal cords." —*Science News,* 22 Sept. 1979, 199.〉

**sacro-** \sā′krō-, sā′krə, sak′rō-\ [See SACRUM.] A combining form meaning sacrum, sacral. Also *sacr-.*

**sacrococcyx** \sā′krəkäk′siks\ The sacrum and the coccyx considered together.

**sacrocoxalgia** \sā′krəkäksal′jə\ A pain emanating from the sacroiliac joint.

**sacrocoxitis** \sā′krəkäksī′tis\ [SACRO- + COXITIS] Inflammation or pain deriving from the sacrum and/or coccyx.

**sacrodynia** \sā′krədin′ē·ə\ SACRALGIA.

**sacroiliac** \sā′krō·il′ē·ak, sak′rō-\ Of or pertaining to the sacrum and the ilium.

**sacroiliitis** \sā′krō·il′ē·ī′tis\ An inflammation of the sacroiliac joint, often complicating an inflammatory disease of other systems, including ankylosing spondylitis, ulcerative colitis, and Crohn's disease.

**sacrolisthesis** \sā′krəlisthē′sis\ Spondylolisthesis involving the fifth lumbar vertebra and the sacrum.

**sacrospinal** \sā′krəspī′nəl\ **1** Pertaining to the sacrum and the vertebral column. **2** Pertaining to the sacrum and the spine of the ischium.

**sacrotomy** \sākrät′əmē\ [SACRO- + -TOMY] The surgical procedure in which an incision is made into the bony sacrum.

**sacrum** \sā′krəm\ [L, neut. sing. of *sacer* sacred, short for *os sacrum,* transl. of Gk *to hieron osteon* the sacred bone; prob. so called from the importance attributed to it in the Egyptian cult of Osiris, god of resurrection] OS SACRUM. **assimilation s.** A skeletal variant in which the fifth lumbar vertebra has the characteristics of sacral vertebrae and may be completely or partially incorporated into the sacrum as the first of six segments. Also *sacralization.* **tilted s.** The forward displacement of the sacrum as a result of the separation of the sacroiliac joints.

**sactosalpinx** \sak'tōsal'pinks\ [Gk *sakto(s)* stuffed + SALPINX] HYDROSALPINX.

**saddle** DENTURE BASE. **bounded s.** A denture base with a natural tooth at each end. **free-end s.** EXTENSION BASE.

**saddlenose** A marked depression of the bridge of the nose, creating a saddlelike configuration between the nasion and the apex. It is seen with some frequency in developmental disorders of the face in which there is general hypoplasia of central facial structures, as in congenital syphilis. Also *Zaufal sign.*

**sadism** \sad'izm, sā'dizm\ [After Donatien Alphonse François, Count de *Sade*, French soldier and writer, 1740–1814] **1** A psychosexual disorder in which torture or infliction of pain or humiliation on others is a necessary condition for sexual gratification. Also *active algolagnia.* **2** Any kind of cruelty directed at others *Popular.* For defs. 1 and 2 also *tyrannism.*

**sadist** \sā'dist, sad'ist\ **1** A person with the psychosexual disorder of sadism. **2** Any cruel person. *Popular.*

**sadistic** \sədis'tik\ Characterized by sadism.

**sadomasochism** \sād'ōmas'əkizm\ **1** The coexistence of sadism and masochism in a person's sexual activity. **2** The coexistence of passive and submissive attitudes and active and aggressive attitudes in social or sexual relations with others.

**sadomasochistic** \sād'ōmas'əkis'tik\ Characterized by sadomasochism.

**Saemisch** [Edwin Theodor *Saemisch*, German ophthalmologist, 1833–1909] **1** Saemisch's ulcer. See under SERPIGINOUS CORNEAL ULCER. **2** See under SECTION.

**Saenger** [Alfred *Saenger*, German neurologist, 1860–1921] See under SIGN.

**safety** **1** Freedom from danger or risk. **2** The prevention of potentially injurious events, minimizing the chances of an injury by personal or public protection and reducing the unnecessary consequences of an injury by good first aid and medical care. Safety in the workplace involves the control of situations in which cause and effect are close in time, as in mechanically induced injury, acid burns, and gassings. The degree of public environmental safety depends largely on the design of homes and vehicles, the education of the public in utilizing safety measures, the state of repair of materials and facilities in use, and the quality of public sanitation. **3** The practical certainty that injury will not result from use of a substance or the application of a procedure under specified conditions of quantity and manner of use.

**safranine** Any of a number of dyestuffs generically known as phenylphenazonium salts, whose molecules consist of a 1,4-diazine ring with benzene rings fused 2,3 and 5,6, each carrying an amino group. Safranines can be formed by the oxidation of simple aromatic amines. One member of the group, safranine T, is prepared by oxidizing a mixture of aniline, *o*-toluidine, and *p*-phenylenediamine; it is a vivid pink.

**safranin O** An important nuclear stain that is used in histology, cytology, and botany for a variety of techniques. Its variability of color can make it unreliable, however.

**safranophilic** \saf'rənōfil'ik\ Having an affinity for safranin stains.

**sagittal** \saj'itəl\ [New L *sagittalis* (from *sagitta* an arrow) of or like an arrow] **1** Designating or pertaining to the suture between the parietal bones (sutura sagittalis). **2** Designating or pertaining to the median plane or a plane parallel to it. • It is not known exactly why this suture and the plane it lies in were named *sagittal* (of or like an arrow). Several explanations are possible, one being that an archer aims his arrow in that plane.

**sagittalis** \saj'itā'lis\ See under SAGITTAL.

**Saint** [Charles Frederick Morris *Saint*, South African roentgenologist, born 1886] See under TRIAD.

**Saint Anthony** See under ST. ANTHONY.

**sal** [L, salt] Salt: used in common names for some inorganic salts, e.g., sal soda, or sodium carbonate. **s. ammoniac** *Obs.* AMMONIUM CHLORIDE.

**s.a.l.** *secundum artis leges* (L, according to the rules of art).

**Sala** [Luigi *Sala*, Italian zoologist, 1863–1930] Sala cells. See under CELL.

**salabrasion** \sal'əbrā'zhən\ [L *sal* salt + ABRASION] A technique for the removal of tattoos whereby the anesthetized skin is briskly rubbed with moist gauze and undissolved table salt. After a waiting period, the more superficial layers of skin will slough off, carrying with them varying amounts of the tattoo pigment.

**salacetamide** ACETYLSALICYLAMIDE.

**salazosulfapyridine** SULFASALAZINE.

**salcatonin** SYNTHETIC CALCITONIN.

**salicylaldehyde** $C_6H_4(OH)CHO$. *o*-Hydroxybenzaldehyde. Salicylic aldehyde, obtained from glucosidesalicin from willow bark. It is used as an astringent and in perfumes. Also *salicylal.*

**salicylamide** *o*-Hydroxybenzamide. The amide of salicylic acid, with the same properties and uses.

**salicylate** \salis'ilāt, sal'isil'āt\ **1** An ester or salt of salicylic acid. **2** Salicylic acid and its acylated derivatives, such as aspirin.

**salicylazosulfapyridine** SULFASALAZINE.

**salicylic acid** *o*-Hydroxybenzoic acid. It occurs as a free acid in several plants and as methyl salicylate in wintergreen. It is a colorless, crystalline compound that has been used as a preservative and bactericide. In concentrated solutions it can be used to remove warts and to treat skin diseases. It is also an analgesic derivative of aspirin. Also *oxybenzoic acid.*

**salicylism** \sal'isilizm\ A series of reactions resulting from administration of salicylates, particularly in treatment of rheumatic fever and gout. Symptoms are nausea, vomiting, ringing in the ears and deafness, severe headache, and mental confusion, with quickened pulse and increased respiration. Effects disappear when the drug is discontinued.

**salicylosalicylic acid** SALYSAL.

**salicylsulfonic acid** SULFOSALICYLIC ACID.

**salicyluric acid** $CH_2{\cdot}NH_2{\cdot}CO{\cdot}O{\cdot}C_6H_4{\cdot}COOH$. An acidic metabolite of aspirin, a conjugate of salicylic acid and glycine, that is excreted in the urine.

**salient** \sā'lē·ənt\ A prominence; protuberance.

**salimeter** \səlim'ətər\ A hydrometer calibrated so that salt concentration of a solution can be read directly from the measured relative density. Also *salinometer.*

**saline** \sā'līn\ [New L *salinus* (from L *sal* salt + *-inus*, adj. suffix) of or pertaining to salt] **1** Pertaining to or containing salt. **2** A solution of salt, especially of sodium chloride. Also *saline fluid, saline solution.* **hypertonic s.** An aqueous solution of sodium chloride or other salts at a concentration of greater than 0.9%. Hypertonic salt solutions to be given intravenously should not be greater than 1.2%. **hypotonic s.** An aqueous solution of sodium chloride or other salts that is less concentrated than 0.9%. Because of the danger of hemolysis, concentrations of salt less than 0.6% are seldom used intravenously. **normal s.** A sterile, aqueous 0.9% solution of sodium chloride. It is isotonic with the blood and can be used intravenously for fluid replacement. **physiologic s.** An aqueous isotonic (0.9%) solution of sodium chloride that is used for the temporary storage of cells and cell constituents. As a sterile solution, it is used parenterally to replace fluid loss.

**salinity** \sālin′itē\ [*salin(e)* + -ITY] The concentration or content of salt in some material.

**salinometer** \sal′inäm′ətər\ SALIMETER.

**salit** An ester occurring as a brown, oily liquid that is practically insoluble in water. It has been used as a counter-irritant in the treatment of rheumatism and neuralgia from various causes. Also *bornyl salicylate.*

**saliva** \səlī′və\ [L, spittle, any viscous secretion] The mucous and serous secretion of the major and accessory salivary glands that moistens, softens and initiates digestion of food in the mouth. Certain stimuli produce copious secretions containing mostly mucus and enzymes while other stimuli produce a watery secretion. In general, it is a viscous liquid containing water, protein, inorganic salts, mucin and at least two enzymes, maltase and ptyalin. Also *sialon.* **lingual s.** Watery saliva secreted by the serous glands of the tongue. **parotid s.** Saliva secreted by the parotid glands, more watery than the saliva secreted by the submaxillary and sublingual glands. **sublingual s.** The mucinous saliva secreted by the sublingual glands. **submaxillary s.** The mucinous saliva secreted by the submaxillary glands.

**salivary** \sal′iver′ē\ Of, pertaining to, or producing saliva.

**salivate** \sal′ivāt\ To produce a secretion of saliva.

**salivolithiasis** \səlī′vōlithī′əsis\ SIALOLITHIASIS.

**Salk** [Jonas Edward *Salk*, U.S. microbiologist, born 1914] Salk vaccine. See under POLIOMYELITIS VACCINE.

***Salmonella*** \sal′mənel′ə\ [After Daniel Elmer *Salmon*, American veterinarian and pathologist, 1850–1914 + *-ella*, fem. diminishing suffix] A broad genus of motile, lactose-negative, $H_2S$-negative enterobacteria, primarily enteric pathogens causing invasive disease in vertebrates. The commonest, first-isolated serotypes were named after the animal or the disease from which they were isolated (*S. typhi; S. paratyphi* A, B, or C; *S. cholerae-suis; S. typhimurium; S. abortus ovis*), and later types were given species names for the place of origin. The 1200 such "species" are now usually designated as serotypes of *S. enteritidis*, except for *S. typhi* and *S. cholerae-suis.* Lysogenization by various phages can change the serotypes based on O (somatic) and H (flagellar) antigens. ***S. choleraesuis*** An organism that causes gastroenteritis in pigs but rarely in humans. In a classification that groups almost all Salmonellae as *S. enteritidis*, only this organism and *S. typhi* are designated as separate species. ***S. enteritidis*** A species designation now widely used to encompass most of the serotypes of *Salmonella.* Also *Bacillus enteritidis* (obs.), *Salmonella paratyphi* (outmoded). ***S. paratyphi A*** A bioserotype of *S. enteritidis* that differs from most strains in a number of biochemical characteristics. *Outmoded.* ***S. typhi*** A species of *Salmonella* that causes typhoid fever in man. It differs from other salmonellae in not forming gas. The O antigen is serotype 9,12. Also *Salmonella typhosa, Bacillus typhosus* (obs.), *Bacterium typhosum* (obs.). ***S. typhimurium*** The most common serotype of salmonella (group B, O antigens 1,4,5,12) in humans in the United States. It also causes disease naturally in mice and other animals. ***S. typhosa*** *SALMONELLA TYPHI.*

**salmonella** (*pl.* salmonellae, salmonellas) Any of the organisms of the genus *Salmonella..*

**salmonellae** \sal′mənel′ē\ Plural of SALMONELLA.

**salmonellosis** \sal′mənelō′sis\ [*Salmonell(a)* + -OSIS] Infection by bacteria of the genus *Salmonella*, either asymptomatic or symptomatic. The types of infection include gastrointestinal, bacteremic, typhoid and paratyphoid fevers, localized infection, and the convalescent or chronic carrier state.

**salol** PHENYL SALICYLATE.

**salping-** \salping-\ SALPINGO-.

**salpingectomy** \sal′pinjek′təmē\ [SALPING- + -ECTOMY] Surgical removal of a fallopian tube. Also *tubectomy.*

**salpingion** \salpin′jē·än\ A point at the apex of the inferior surface of the petrous part of the temporal bone.

**salpingitis** \sal′pinjī′tis\ [SALPING- + -ITIS] Inflammation of the fallopian tube. **chronic interstitial s.** Salpingitis marked by infiltration of plasma cells and lymphocytes. **chronic vegetating s.** Salpingitis marked by hypertrophy of the mucosa, leading to agglutination of villi, as in salpingitis isthmica nodosum. **follicular s.** PSEUDOFOLLICULAR SALPINGITIS. **gonococcal s.** Salpingitis as a result of gonococcal infection. Also *gonorrheal salpingitis.* **hemorrhagic s.** Inflammation of a fallopian tube associated with interstitial or intraluminal bleeding. **hypertrophic s.** PACHYSALPINGITIS. **s. isthmica nodosa** A lesion in which numerous, usually small, glandlike structures are dispersed through all layers of the fallopian tube, partly splitting up the thickened muscularis. The lesion is mostly localized to the isthmus of the tube and is usually bilateral. Also *adenosis, adenomyomatosis* (obs.). **mural s.** PACHYSALPINGITIS. **nodular s.** Salpingitis marked by formation of nodules in the wall and mucous lining of the uterine tube. **parenchymatous s.** PACHYSALPINGITIS. **pseudofollicular s.** Salpingitis marked by the formation of saccules resulting from mucosal agglutination. Also *follicular salpingitis.* **purulent s.** Salpingitis associated with suppuration. Also *pyogenic salpingitis, pyosalpingitis.* **tuberculous s.** An infection of the uterine tubes with *Mycobacterium tuberculosis*, resulting in a granulomatous inflammation with marked proliferation of the tubal mucosa. It has been confused with carcinoma.

**salpingo-** \salping′gō-\ [Gk *salpinx* (genitive *salpingos*) trumpet, tube] A combining form denoting (1) the fallopian tube; (2) the eustachian tube. Also *salping-.*

**salpingocele** \salping′gōsēl\ [SALPINGO- + -CELE[1]] Hernial protrusion of the fallopian tube. It can herniate into the vagina after hysterectomy, or enter into the inguinal canal.

**salpingography** \sal′ping·gäg′rəfē\ [SALPINGO- + -GRAPHY] Radiographic examination of the fallopian tubes following instillation of an opaque contrast medium via the uterine canal.

**salpingolithiasis** \-lithī′əsis\ The presence of calcium concretions in the wall of the fallopian tube.

**salpingolysis** \sal′ping·gäl′isis\ [SALPINGO- + LYSIS] A surgical procedure in which adhesions to the fallopian tubes are removed.

**salpingo-oophorectomy** \-ō′əfôrek′təmē\ The surgical removal of one or both ovaries and fallopian tubes. Also *tubo-ovariectomy, tubo-ovariotomy, oophorosalpingectomy, oothecosalpingectomy, salpingo-oothecectomy, salpingo-ovariotomy, salpingo-ovariectomy.*

**salpingo-oophoritis** \-ō′əfôrī′tis\ [SALPINGO- + OOPHOR- + -ITIS] Inflammation of a fallopian tube and ovary. Also *oophorosalpingitis, pelvic inflammatorydisease, salpingo-oothecitis, tubo-ovaritis.* **chronic s.** Chronic inflammation of the uterine tubes and ovaries. Primary infection generally occurs from the gonococcus, but may also occur from endogenous organisms when an intrauterine device is present. Also *pachysalpingo-ovaritis.*

**salpingo-oophorocele** \-ō·äf′ərōsēl′\ [SALPINGO- + OOPHORO- + -CELE] Hernia of the uterine tube and ovary, usually into the inguinal canal. Also *salpingo-oothecocele.*

**salpingo-oothecectomy** \-ō′əthēsek′təmē\ SALPINGO-OOPHORECTOMY.

**salpingo-oothecitis** \-ō′əthēsī′tis\ SALPINGO-OOPHORITIS.

**salpingo-oothecocele** \-ō′əthē′kəsēl\ SALPINGO-OOPHOROCELE.

**salpingo-ovariectomy** \-ōver′ē·ek′təmē\ SALPINGO-OOPHORECTOMY.

**salpingo-ovariotomy** \-ōver′ē·ät′əmē\ SALPINGO-OOPHORECTOMY.

**salpingopalatine** \-pal′ətīn\ **1** Pertaining to the function of the soft palate and the eustachian tube. Also *salpingostaphyline* (seldom used). **2** Related to the torus tubarius and the soft palate. For defs. 1 and 2 also *salpingopalatal.*

**salpingopexy** \salping′gəpek′sē\ [SALPINGO- + -PEXY] Attachment of the uterine tube to an adjacent structure such as the round ligament or pelvic side wall.

**salpingopharyngeal** \-fərin′jē·əl\ Pertaining to the auditory tube and the pharynx.

**salpingoplasty** \salping′gəplas′tē\ [SALPINGO- + -PLASTY] Surgical reconstruction of a fallopian tube.

**salpingorrhaphy** \sal′ping·gôr′əfē\ [SALPINGO- + -RRHAPHY] Repair and suturing of a uterine tube.

**salpingosalpingostomy** \-sal′ping·gäs′təmē\ [SALPINGO- + SALPINGO- + -STOMY] A reanastomosis of the fallopian tube.

**salpingostaphyline** \-staf′ilīn\ *Seldom used* SALPINGOPALATINE.

**salpingostomy** \sal′ping·gäs′təmē\ [SALPINGO- + -STOMY] Creation of an opening in the fallopian tube to create patency or to permit removal of contents.

**salpingothecal** \-thē′kəl\ Pertaining to the fallopian tube and the subarachnoid space.

**salpingotomy** \sal′ping·gät′əmē\ [SALPINGO- + -TOMY] An incision into a fallopian tube.

**salpinx** \sal′pinks\ [Gk *salpinx* (gen. *salpingos*) a trumpet, tube] (*pl.* salpinges) A tube.

**salsalate** SALYSAL.

**salt** [Old English *sealt,* akin to L *sal* salt and Gk *hals* (gen. *halos*) salt] Any substance composed of ions of opposite charge. Unqualified, it often refers to sodium chloride. **artificial s.** A mixture of salts prepared to mimic the composition of a natural water, such as Vichy water. **artificial Carlsbad s.** A mixture of salts of the same proportion and composition as found in natural Carlsbad water. **artificial Kissingen s.** A mixture of potassium chloride, sodium chloride, anhydrous magnesium sulfate, and sodium bicarbonate in the concentrations and proportions found in natural Kissingen water. **bile s.'s** Salts of the conjugates of bile acids with glycine and taurine. They act as emulsifying agents to aid the absorption of fat from the small intestine. **bone s.** The inorganic material that is laid down within the bone matrix as it matures. The principal mineral constituent is calcium hydroxyapatite. **Carlsbad s.** A mixture of sodium sulfate, potassium sulfate, sodium chloride, and sodium bicarbonate in the proportions found in the spring water at Carlsbad. It is a tonic water, used to treat rheumatism and having diuretic and laxative properties. **common s.** SODIUM CHLORIDE. **complex s.** A salt containing a complex ion, e.g. $Ag(CN)_2^-$, so called because it is formed from other ions, here $Ag^+$ and $CN^-$, which combine to form an ionic species. **double s.** A salt that contains more than one cation or more than one anion, e.g. $(NH_4)_2SO_4 \cdot FeSO_4 \cdot 6H_2O$. It differs from a complex salt in that all the cations and anions retain their identities and do not form complexes with each other. **effervescent s.'s** An effervescent mixture of sodium sulfate or magnesium sulfate with sodium bicarbonate and citric or tartaric acid. The mixture effervesces with the addition of water. **effervescent artificial Carlsbad s.** Artificial Carlsbad salt with the addition of sodium bicarbonate and citric and tannic acids to give an effervescent base. **effervescent artificial Kissingen s.** Artificial Kissingen salt prepared in an effervescent base. **effervescent artificial Vichy s.** A mixture of salts in the same proportion as found in natural Vichy water with the addition of sodium bicarbonate, citric acid, and tartaric acid to provide an effervescent base. **Epsom s.'s** MAGNESIUM SULFATE. **Glauber s.** A hydrated sodium sulfate, $Na_2SO_4 \cdot 10H_2O$. It crystallizes from the water of salt lakes and hot springs. **iodized s.** Salt containing 15–30 parts of iodide per million in the form of potassium iodide or sodium iodide. It also is supplemented with a small quantity of magnesium carbonate to improve its pouring qualities.

**saltation** \saltā′shən\ [L *saltatio* (from *saltatus,* past part. of *saltare* to leap, dance) a leaping, dancing] **1** Sudden, explosive, jerky, or leaping movement, as seen in chorea. **2** The method of conduction of the nerve impulse in myelinated nerves in which the impulse jumps rapidly from one node of Ranvier to the next. Also *saltatory conduction.* **3** A change in nucleotide sequence, as by mutation or unscheduled DNA replication. **4** A change in speciation during evolution.

**saltatory** \sal′tətôr′ē\ Describing or pertaining to saltation. Also *saltatorial, saltatoric, saltative.*

**Salter** [Samuel James A. *Salter,* English dentist, 1825–1897] Salter's lines. See under LINE.

**salting-in** The technique of dissolving a protein that is insoluble in pure water by adding low concentrations of inorganic salt ions. It is sometimes used to separate groups of proteins.

**salting-out** **1** A technique for precipitating proteins from solution by increasing the salt concentration. Most proteins are insoluble in water, soluble in dilute salt solutions, and insoluble at high salt concentrations. Proteins can be separated from each other by exploiting their differences in solubility at different salt concentrations. Also *salt precipitation.* **2** A technique for inducing abortion by the intra-amniotic infusion of a solution of hypertonic sodium chloride.

**salubrious** \səloo′brē·əs\ [L *salubri(s)* (from *salus* health) healthful + -OUS] Conducive to health or well-being; healthful.

**saluresis** \sal′yoorē′sis\ [L *sal* salt + Gk *ourēsis* a making water] Increased urinary excretion of salts, particularly sodium chloride.

**saluretic** \sal′yooret′ik\ **1** Any agent or condition that increases urinary excretion of salts. **2** Promoting saluresis.

**Salus** [Robert *Salus,* Austrian ophthalmologist, active in Czechoslovakia, born 1877] Koerber-Salus-Elschnig syndrome. See under AQUEDUCT OF SYLVIUS SYNDROME.

**salutary** \sal′yəter′ē\ Healthful; wholesome.

**salvarsan** [Late L *salvare* to save + L *san(itas)* health] ARSPHENAMINE.

**salvarsan copper** A combination of copper and arsphenamine, which is a yellowish-red powder. It is of historic interest since it was the first anti-infective agent proposed by Ehrlich to treat protozoan infections.

**salve** [Old English *sealf*] OINTMENT.

**salysal** $C_{14}H_{10}O_5$. 2-Hydroxybenzoic acid-2-carboxyphenyl ester. A salicylate derivative with properties and uses similar to those of aspirin. Also *salsalate, salicylosalicylic acid.*

**samarium** Element number 62, having atomic weight 150.4. It is a member of the lanthanide series of elements.

Natural samarium consists of seven isotopes, three of which are unstable with very long half-lives. Symbol: Sm

**sample** A portion of a group which is selected and observed in order to determine the statistical features of the group as a whole. **biased s.** A sample obtained by a procedure which involves systematic (as opposed to random) errors. **matched s.** A set of pairs of observations in which each member of a pair is matched with its fellow with respect to one or more variables. The object of matching is to remove the effect of confounding variables. Thus, patients and controls might be matched with respect to age, to sex, or to both. Matching may be extended so that each case has two or more matched controls. **paired s.'s** A system of testing for experimental treatment effects whereby test subjects are grouped by twos for similarity, with one being subjected to treatment and the other being used as the control. **representative s.** In statistics, a sample having, so far as certain attributes are concerned, a composition similar to that of the population from which it was drawn. **stratified s.** A sample made up of units drawn at random from each of a set of previously defined subgroups, or strata, into which the subject population has been divided. For convenience, the number of units contributed by a given stratum may (but need not) be based on the proportionate size of the stratum. **systematic s.** A sample built up by drawing members at equal intervals from a list of the aggregate to be sampled. Thus, for a one-in-ten sample one would first draw a number from 1 to 10, which might be, say, 7. The sample would then be made up of those members in the list having the ranks 7, 17, 27, etc., and comprise 10 percent of the universe.

**sample-and-hold** Designating an electronic circuit that samples a varying analog input signal at one instant of time and holds that voltage (usually on a capacitor) for conversion into a digital signal.

**sampler** A device for taking representative samples of a gas, liquid, or solid that will be used for chemical, physical, or microbiologic examination.

**sampling** The selection and observation of a sample. **chorionic villus s.** A process by which a portion of the chorion is removed and analyzed to learn about the developing fetus. It is a method for performing prenatal diagnosis in humans at an earlier stage of pregnancy (8–12 weeks gestation) than can be attempted with amniocentesis. **cluster s.** A statistical sampling procedure in which the elements making up the sample are not drawn individually but in groups, referred to as clusters. For example, cluster sampling of a human population might proceed by random selection of entire households for inclusion in the sample. **duplicate portion s.** A method of collecting food for analysis of its nutrient content. Two equal portions of a given food are collected and analyzed individually. The nutrient content is taken as the average of the two samples. **Haldane-Priestley s.** A sampling of the last part of the alveolar air expired after a sharp, deep expiration. **multistage s.** Sampling in a series of stages employing units of decreasing size, each stage but the first being the selection of a subsample from each unit drawn in the preceding stage. Thus, for example, a sampling of cities might constitute a first stage, a sampling of the wards in each selected city the second stage, a selection of streets from each selected ward the third, and so on. **quota s.** A statistical sampling procedure whereby the sample when drawn will reproduce the proportions of given characteristics designated in advance as they occur in the population being sampled. This aim is achieved by assigning to each investigator the numbers or proportions of individuals having the required characteristics which are to be included in that investigator's sample. Within the limits so set, whether of numbers or of proportions, the investigator is free to select the individuals that will make up that sample. **random s.** In statistics, selection of a sample in such a way that every entity in the population has the same determinate probability of being included in the sample. This objective may be attained by the use of a table of random numbers so that personal bias on the part of the selector is eliminated. This is the only method of selection that will enable the sampling error to be correctly estimated. Also *random selection*. **sequential s.** A method of sampling in which the individual elements of the sample (for example, patients receiving a given form of therapy) are added to the sample one at a time, or in small groups at a time, and the results emerging at each stage determine whether sampling is to continue.

**Sampson** [John Albertson *Sampson*, U.S. gynecologist, 1873–1946] Sampson cyst. See under ENDOMETRIOMA.

**Sanarelli** [Giuseppe *Sanarelli*, Italian physician, 1864–1940] Shwartzman-Sanarelli phenomenon, Sanarelli's phenomenon, Sanarelli-Shwartzman reaction. See under SHWARTZMAN PHENOMENON.

**sanatorium** \san′ətôr′ē·əm\ [Late L, neut. of *sanatorius* (from L *sanat(us)*, past part. of *sanare* to heal, cure, + *-orium* -ORY) healthful, healing] An inpatient facility for the treatment of chronic disease or for convalescence, especially one situated in a resortlike or salubrious location.

**sanatory** \san′ətôr′ē\ Tending to cure; curative.

**sancycline** 6-Demethyl-6-deoxytetracycline. An antibacterial drug of the tetracycline group of antibiotics.

**sand** [Old English *sand, sond,* akin to Gk *psammos* sand, from *psēn* to touch on the surface, rub, crumble] Soil with a particle size of 0.002–2.0 mm in diameter that is composed primarily of quartz. **brain s.** ACERVULUS. **hydatid s.** Sandlike solid material in the fluid of a hydatid cyst consisting of scoleces liberated from the ruptured brood capsules within the cyst. **intestinal s.** Small particulate matter formed in the intestine containing bacteria, bile pigment, oxides of calcium and phosphorus, and various other substances.

**sandarac** \san′dərak\ A resin obtained from *Callitris quadrivalvis.* Its principal ingredient is pimaric acid, and it is used in dentistry as a separating medium during the casting of plaster models and as a preservative varnish for casts and models. Also *gum juniper*.

**Sander** [Wilhelm *Sander*, German physician, 1838–1922] Sander's disease. See under EPIDEMIC KERATOCONJUNCTIVITIS.

**Sanders** [Clarence Elmer *Sanders*, U.S. physician, 1885–1949] See under BED.

**sandfly** A biting fly of the family Psychodidae, such as *Lutzomyia* or, especially, *Phlebotomus.* The term is sometimes applied more broadly to include flies of related families such as Heleidae and Simuliidae. Also *sand fly*.

**Sandison** [Calvin *Sandison*, U.S. surgeon, born 1899] Sandison-Clark chamber. See under RABBIT-EAR CHAMBER.

**Sandström** [Ivar Victor *Sandström*, Swedish anatomist, 1852–1889] Sandström's bodies. See under PARATHYROID GLANDS.

**sandworm** Any of the hookworms normally found in the dog or cat whose larvae cause cutaneous larva migrans in humans.

**sane** [L *san(us)* sound in body or mind] Sound of mind. A legal term.

**Sanfilippo** [Sylvester *Sanfilippo*, U.S. pediatrician, flourished 20th century] **1** See under DISEASE. **2** Sanfilippo syndrome. See under MUCOPOLYSACCHARIDOSIS III.

**Sanger Brown** [*Sanger Brown,* U.S. neuropsychiatrist, 1852–1928] See under ATAXIA.

**sangui-** \sang′gwi-\ [L *sanguis* blood] A combining form meaning blood. Also *sanguin-, sanguino-.*

**sanguicolous** \sang·gwik′ələs\ Residing in the blood.

**sanguiferous** \sang·gwif′ərəs\ Carrying or conducting blood.

**sanguification** \sang′gwifikā′shən\ *Rare* HEMATOPOIESIS.

**sanguimotor** \sang′gwimō′tər\ [SANGUI- + MOTOR] Relating to the circulation of the blood. Also *sanguimotory.*

**sanguin-** \sang·gwin-\ SANGUI-.

***Sanguinaria*** \sang′gwiner′ē·ə\ A monotypic genus of herbs of the family Papaveraceae. *Sanguinaria canadensis,* the bloodroot, Indian paint, tetterwort, red root, or puccoon root, was once used as an ingredient in compound white pine syrup. A tincture of the dried rhizome and roots has expectorant action and is used in treating respiratory disorders. It has also been applied externally to treat eczema.

**sanguine** \sang′gwin\ **1** Plethoric; ruddy. **2** Confident; anticipating success.

**sanguineous** \sang·gwin′ē·əs\ **1** Bloody. **2** Relating to blood or bloodshed. For defs. 1 and 2 also *sanguinous.*

**sanguinification** \sang·gwin′ifikā′shən\ *Rare* HEMATOPOIESIS.

**sanguino-** \sang′gwinō-\ SANGUI-.

**sanguinopoietic** \-poi·et′ik\ HEMATOPOIETIC.

**sanguinopurulent** \-pyŭr′ʸələnt\ Consisting of or resembling blood and pus.

**sanguinous** \sang′gwinəs\ SANGUINEOUS.

**sanguis** \sang′gwis\ [L, blood] BLOOD.

***Sanguisuga*** \sang′gwisʸoo′gə\ [L (from *sangui(s)* blood + *-suga* -sucker, from *sugere* to suck) a leech] HIRUDO

**sanguisuga** LEECH.

**sanguivorous** \sang·gwiv′ərəs\ HEMATOPHAGOUS.

**sanies** \sā′ni·ēz\ [L, corrupted blood] (*pl.* sanies) A serous exudate, as from a wound, that is mixed with blood and pus and is characterized by a foul smell. Adj. sanious.

**saniopurulent** \sā′nē·ōpyŭr′ʸələnt\ Sanious and purulent.

**sanioserous** \sā′nē·ōsir′əs\ Sanious and serous.

**sanious** \sā′nē·əs\ Of or characterized by sanies; composed of serum mixed with blood and pus and marked by a foul smell: said of a discharge, as from a wound.

**sanitarium** \san′itar′ē·əm\ [L *sanit(as)* health + *-arium* -ARY] An institution which promotes health. • Although the term is not precisely synonymous with sanatorium, the two are often used interchangeably now.

**sanitary** \san′itar′ē\ [French *sanitaire* (from L *sanit(as)* health + French *-aire* -ARY) sanitary] **1** Relating to the preservation or promotion of health or hygiene. **2** Free from dirt, filth, or contaminated matter that is liable to convey pathogenic microorganisms.

**sanitation** \san′itā′shən\ [English *sanit(ary)* (from French *sanitaire* sanitary, from L *sanit(as)* health + French *-aire* -ARY) + -ATION] Environmental conditions affecting, or designed to affect or promote, the protection or preservation of health. • The term is frequently used with reference to sewage or refuse disposal.

**sanitization** \san′itīzā′shən\ The process of making sanitary, as by cleaning and sterilizing.

**sanity** [L *sanitas* (from *san(us)* sound in body or mind + *-itas* -ITY) soundness] Soundness of mind. A legal term.

**Santorini** [Giovanni Domenico *Santorini,* Italian anatomist, 1681–1737] **1** Santorini's plexus. See under PLEXUS PROSTATICUS. **2** Duct of Santorini. See under DUCTUS PANCREATICUS ACCESSORIUS. **3** Santorini's concha, turbinate of Santorini. See under CONCHA NASALIS SUPREMA. **4** Santorini's cartilage. See under CARTILAGO CORNICULATA. **5** Santorini's clefts, Santorini's fissures. See under INCISURAE CARTILAGINIS MEATUS ACUSTICI. **6** Papilla of Santorini. See under PAPILLA DUODENI MAJOR. **7** Tubercle of Santorini. See under TUBERCULUM CORNICULATUM. **8** Santorini's labyrinth. See under PLEXUS VENOSUS PROSTATICUS. **9** Santorini's ligament. See under LIGAMENTUM CRICOPHARYNGEUM. **10** Santorini's muscle. See under MUSCULUS RISORIUS. **11** Santorini's muscle. See under MUSCULUS INCISURAE HELICIS. **12** See under MUSCLE. **13** Parietal emissary vein of Santorini, parietal vein of Santorini. See under VENA EMISSARIA PARIETALIS.

**sap** / **cell s.** HYALOPLASM. **nuclear s.** KARYOLYMPH.

**saphena** \səfē′nə\ [Med L *(vena) saphena* (from Arabic *ṣāfin* saphena, prob. from Gk *saph(en)ēs* clear, prominent, influenced by Arabic *ṣāf(in)* clear) the great saphenous, lit. prominent, vein] Any of three veins: (1) vena saphena magna; (2) vena saphena parva; (3) vena saphena accessoria.

**saphenectomy** \saf′ənek′təmē\ [*saphen(a)* + -ECTOMY] The removal of the saphenous vein.

**saphenous** \səfē′nəs\ Pertaining to a saphena.

**sapid** \sap′id\ [L *sapidus* (from *sapere* to have a taste) tasty] **1** Having an agreeable taste; palatable. **2** Capable of producing an effect on the organs of taste.

**sapo** \sā′pō\ [L, soap] SOAP. **s. domesticus** A soft soap prepared by saponification of animal fat with potash. Also *sapo animalis.* **s. mollis medicinalis** GREEN SOAP. **s. viridis** GREEN SOAP.

**sapo-** \sap′ō-\ SAPON-.

**sapogenin** \-jen′in\ One of several $C_{27}$-steroids, found as their glycosides (saponins) in plants. They contain two rings more than most steroids, and are acetals formed by combination of a carbonyl group at C-22 with hydroxyl groups elsewhere in the molecule.

**sapon-** \sap′ən-\ [L *sapo* (gen. *saponis*) soap] A combining form meaning soap. Also *sapo-.*

**saponifiable** \sapän′ifī′əbəl\ [*saponif(y)* + -ABLE] Containing fatty acids in ester combination: used, for example, of fats and phospholipids in contrast with sterols. The word is derived from the test applied of taking up alkali on heating, since such heating in alkali leads to hydrolysis of the ester bond and the formation of a soap.

**saponification** \sapän′ifikā′shən\ [SAPON- + *i* + -FICATION] The alkaline hydrolysis of a lipid, usually a fat, to form a soap and an alcohol, usually glycerol.

**saponify** \sapän′ifī\ [L *sapo* (gen. *saponis*) soap + English *-fy,* suffix from L *-ficare* denoting to make] To hydrolyze a lipid, usually a fat, with alkali, to yield a soap and an alcohol, usually glycerol.

**saponin** \sap′ənin\ [SAPON- + -IN] Any plant glycoside with detergent action that can be hydrolyzed to yield a carbohydrate and a steroid component that is a sapogenin. Saponins are hemolytic. Also *quillain.*

**saporosity** The quality of being sapid; savoriness.

**Sappey** [Marie Philibert Constant *Sappey,* French anatomist, 1810–1896] **1** Nucleus of Sappey. See under NUCLEUS RUBER. **2** Sappey's fibers. See under FIBER. **3** See under LIGAMENT. **4** Sappey subareolar plexus. See under PLEXUS. **5** Muscle of Sappey. See under MUSCULUS TEMPOROPARIETALIS. **6** Veins of Sappey. See under VENAE PARAUMBILICALES.

***Sappinia diploidea*** \səpin′ē·ə diploi′dē·ə\ An ameba (class Lobosea, subclass Gymnamoebia) with two closely associated nuclei with large endosomes and only a few short lobopodia. The cysts also are binucleate. It is a coprozoite, found in feces of various animals, including man.

**sapro-** \sap′rō-\ [Gk *sapros* rotten, decayed, putrid] A combining form meaning (1) rotten, putrefying; (2) decaying, decomposed; (3) saprophytic. Also *sapr-*.

**saprobe** \sap′rōb\ [SAPRO- + *-be*, suffix denoting life, irreg. from Gk *bi(os)* life, manner of life] A saprotrophic microbe or fungus. Adj. saprobic. • See note at SAPROTROPH.

**saprophagous** \səpräf′əgəs\ Subsisting on decaying organic matter; saprotrophic. Also *saprophilous*.

**saprophyte** \sap′rəfīt\ [SAPRO- + Gk *phyt(on)* a plant, tree] A saprotrophic organism, especially a fungus or microorganism. • See note at SAPROTROPH.

**saprophytic** \-fit′ik\ Of or relating to a saprophyte; saprotrophic.

**saprotroph** \sap′rəträf\ [SAPRO- + Gk *troph(ē)* nourishment] A heterotroph that decomposes nonliving organic matter to obtain nutrients, which are then absorbed through cell membranes. • The terms *saprophyte, saprobe*, and *saprozoite* denote saprotrophic plants, microbes and fungi, and animals respectively, but the boundaries are blurred in actual usage, with *saprophyte* being more widespread and traditional than the others.

**saprozoite** \-zō′īt\ [SAPRO- + Gk *zō(on)* animal, living being + -ITE] An animal, such as a protozoan, that absorbs nutrients from dead or decaying organic matter; an animal saprotroph.

**saprozoonosis** \-zō′ənō′sis\ A zoonosis whose causative agent requires both a vertebrate host and a nonanimal developmental site for its life cycle. Examples include botulism, coccidioidomycosis, ascariasis, and tungiasis.

**saralasin** A synthetic inhibitor of angiotension II. It is useful in the diagnosis of renovascular hypertension.

***Sarcina*** \sär′sinə\ [L (from *sarcire* to mend, patch), a bundle, pack, burden, luggage] A genus of Gram-positive cocci whose cells divide in three planes to form clusters like staphylococci but which are obligate anaerobes. They are not significant pathogens. *Sarcina ventriculi* has been isolated from the human stomach.

**sarcitis** \särsī′tis\ *Obs.* MYOSITIS.

**sarco-** \sär′kō-\ [Gk *sarx*, gen. *sarkos* flesh] A combining form denoting (1) flesh, soft tissue; (2) muscle tissue; (3) mesodermal or mesenchymal tissue.

**sarcoblast** \sär′kəblast\ [SARCO- + -BLAST] MYOBLAST.

**sarcocyst** \sär′kəsist\ [SARCO- + CYST] **1** One of the intramuscular tissue cysts of coccidian parasites of the genus *Sarcocystis.* Ranging in size from microscopic to 5 cm long, depending on the species, they are cylindrical with tapered ends, and contain from hundreds to many thousands of infective bradyzoites. Also *Miescher's tube* (outmoded), *Miescher's tubule* (outmoded), *sarcosporidian cyst.* **2** A member of the genus *Sarcocystis.*.

**Sarcocystidae** \-sis′tidē\ [*Sarcocyst(is)* + -IDAE] A family of coccidian protozoa in the suborder Eimeriina, order Eucoccidiida. It contains the subfamilies Sarcocystinae (genera *Sarcocystis, Arthrocystis),* Besnoitiinae (genus *Besnoitia),* and Toxoplasmatinae *(Toxoplasma, Frankelia).* Also *Toxoplasmatidae.*

***Sarcocystis*** \-sis′tis\ [New L, from SARCO- + CYST] A genus of coccidial sporozoa characterized by a schizogonic encysted stage in muscles or subcutaneous tissues of herbivores and a sexual stage in gut epithelial cells of carnivorous mammals. It is allied with the genera *Aggregata, Toxoplasma, Eimeria,* and *Isospora* in the suborder Eimeriina, subclass Coccidia, class Sporozoea, phylum Apicomplexa. The parasites form extremely long cylindrical cysts with thick walls, formerly known as Miescher's tubules, in the striated muscles of host birds, mammals, or reptiles. Cysts may be smooth, such as those found in mice, or have radial spines, such as those found in rabbits. Spores (formerly called Rainey's corpuscles) are of variable shape and thought to be sporoblasts or cytomeres that divide to produce mature forms (bradyzoites) that are motile when released. Sexual stages from intestinal cells of carnivores have recently been described with oocysts similar to those of *Isospora* and *Toxoplasma,* but usually with the sporocysts separated from their thin-walled oocysts. Also *Miescheria, Balbiania.*. ***S. hominis*** A species in which humans are the final host and cattle the intermediate host. Development of the sexual and sporogonic stages occurs in the lamina propria of the human host's intestinal mucosa. Paired sporocysts within a thin-walled oocyst are passed in the feces. The sporocysts usually separate and each encloses four infective sporozoites. When ingested by cattle, the released sporozoites penetrate the gut wall and form large spindle- to cylindrical-shaped tissue cysts with many thousands of merozoites, which are infective to humans who eat the uncooked infected beef. This organism was thought to be a species of *Isospora* until the two-host cycle was elucidated. Also *Sarcocystis bovihominis, Isospora hominis, Coccidium hominis.* ***S. lindemanni*** A species described as occurring rarely in the heart and striated muscles of humans, but thought to be acquired from sporocysts passed in the feces of dogs or other carnivores, with man the intermediate host. It is probably not a single species. ***S. suihominis*** A species in which humans are the final host and pigs the intermediate host. Except for the different intermediate host, the life cycle is similar to that of *S. hominis.*

**sarcocystosis** \-sistō′sis\ [*Sarcocyst(is)* + -OSIS] A disease caused by infection with the protozoan parasite *Sarcocystis.* It is characterized by cysts in the muscles of the intermediate host, which may be horses, cattle, sheep, pigs, birds, rodents, or humans. It is usually of low pathogenicity but *S. cruzi* in cattle can cause fever, wasting, anemia, and death. Also *sarcosporidiosis, sarcosporidiasis.*

**sarcocyte** \sär′kəsīt\ [SARCO- + -CYTE] The layer of protozoan ectoplasm between the epicyte and the myocyte. *Rare.*

**Sarcodina** \-dī′nə\ A subphylum of Protozoa, the amebas. The members are characterized by being able to produce pseudopodia, or else locomotive protoplasmic flow without discrete pseudopodia, throughout most of the life cycle. Flagella may be present during developmental stages. The body is naked or with an internal or external test or skeleton. Asexual reproduction is by fission. Sexual forms, if present, are flagellated or, rarely, ameboid gametes. All amebas are included: free-living and parasitic, and terrestrial, freshwater and marine.

**sarcogenic** \-jen′ik\ [SARCO- + -GENIC] Giving rise to muscle or to muscle fibers. Also *sarcopoietic.*

**sarcoid** \sär′koid\ [*sarc(o)-* + -OID] **1** SARCOIDOSIS. **2** Resembling sarcoma. **Boeck s.** SARCOIDOSIS. **Darier-Roussy s.** A subcutaneous nodular sarcoidosis. **multiple benign s.** SARCOIDOSIS. **Salem s.** BERYLLIUM SARCOIDOSIS. • The disease was described in employees of a manufacturer of fluorescent lamps in Salem, Massachusetts. **Schaumann s.** SARCOIDOSIS.

**sarcoidosis** \sär′koidō′sis\ [SARCOID + -OSIS] A disease of unknown cause characterized by noncaseating granulomas in many organs of the body. The most commonly involved tissues are those of the lungs, lymph nodes, and liver. Organs involved may be damaged either by the presence of granulomas or by consequent fibrosis. Also *osteitis tuberculosa cystica, osteitis tuberculosa multiplex cystoides, Besnier-*

*Boeck disease, Besnier-Boeck-Schaumann disease, Boeck's disease, Schaumann's disease, Hutchinson-Boeck disease, sarcoid, Boeck sarcoid, multiple benign sarcoid, Schaumann sarcoid, Schaumann syndrome, Danielssen-Boeck disease, Hutchinson-Boeck syndrome, Mortimer's disease, benign lymphogranulomatosis* (outmoded), *lymphogranuloma benignum* (outmoded). **beryllium s.** A disease resembling sarcoidosis and resulting from chronic beryllium poisoning. Also *Salem sarcoid.* See also BERYLLIUM POISONING. **cerebral s.** Sarcoidosis involving the brain and usually giving rise to subacute granulomatous meningitis with hydrocephalus and/or multiple cranial nerve palsies. **s. cordis** Sarcoidosis of the heart. **hypercalcemic s.** Sarcoidosis complicated by abnormal levels of calcium. **intrathoracic s.** Sarcoidosis within the chest cavity, usually in the form of pulmonary or hilar nodes. **myocardial s.** Sarcoidosis within the myocardium.

**sarcolactic acid** LACTIC ACID.

**sarcolemma** \-lem′ə\ The plasma membrane of a muscle fiber. Also *myolemma.* Adj. sarcolemmic, sarcolemmial, sarcolemmous.

**sarcolysis** \särkäl′isis\ [SARCO- + LYSIS] Destruction or disintegration of soft tissue.

**sarcolyte** \sär′kəlīt\ A cell participating in sarcolysis.

**sarcoma** \särkō′mə\ [Gk *sarkōma* (from *sarx, sarkos* flesh) a fleshy excrescence] (*pl.* sarcomas, sarcomata) A malignant tumor of connective tissue or mesenchymal cells, such as fibrous tissue, adipose tissue, muscle tissue, blood vessels, lymph vessels, synovial tissue, bone, and cartilage. The precise terminology depends on the tissue type, as fibrosarcoma, liposarcoma, rhabdomyosarcoma, hemangiosarcoma, or osteosarcoma. **alveolar soft part s.** A sarcoma with polygonal cells having granular cytoplasm and grouped into alveola-like structures surrounded by thin fibrovascular walls. **ameloblastic s.** AMELOBLASTIC FIBROSARCOMA. **s. botryoides** A form of embryonal rhabdomyosarcoma that grows as grapelike masses projecting into a cavity such as the bladder or vagina. Also *botryoid sarcoma, grapelike tumor.* **cerebral reticulum cell s.** MICROGLIOMATOSIS CEREBRI. **circumscribed cerebellar arachnoidal s.** DESMOPLASTIC MEDULLOBLASTOMA. **s. cutaneum telangiectaticum multiplex** KAPOSI SARCOMA. **deciduocellular s.** CHORIOCARCINOMA. **embryonal s.** A sarcoma composed of primitive undifferentiated cells. **endometrial stromal s.** A malignant tumor of the uterus resembling endometrial stroma. Also *stromatosis* (obs.). **Ewing s.** A highly malignant bone tumor of children with densely packed small cells without distinct cytoplasmic outlines or prominent nucleoli. The shafts and metaphyses of long bones are the common sites. Metastasis to other bones is frequent. Also *Ewing's tumor, endothelial myeloma, diffuse endothelioma.* **giant cell s.** 1 A malignant giant cell tumor. 2 A sarcoma with a prominent component of giant cells. **glandular s.** HODGKIN'S DISEASE. **granulocytic s.** A form of acute granulocytic leukemia in which nodular masses of myeloblasts are in bone marrow and other organs. When the tumors are green, the term *chloroma* is used. Also *myeloid sarcoma, myelosarcoma* (seldom used). **histiocytic s.** HISTIOCYTIC LYMPHOMA. **idiopathic multiple pigmented hemorrhagic s.** KAPOSI SARCOMA. **intracanalicular s.** CYSTOSARCOMA PHYLLODES. **Kaposi s.** A sarcoma composed of spindle-shaped cells among which are irregular vascular channels. Lesions are usually multiple in the skin and in viscera. The lower legs and feet are common sites for skin lesions where papular and plaquelike lesions occur. The tumor may be associated with malignant lymphoma. It is relatively common in parts of Africa and in those with acquired immunodeficiency syndrome (AIDS), among whom visceral lesions are relatively common. Also *idiopathic multiple pigmented hemorrhagic sarcoma, sarcoma cutaneum telangiectaticum multiplex, multiple hemorrhagic hemangioma of Kaposi, multiple idiopathic hemorrhagic sacroma, Kaposi's disease.* **Kupffer cell s.** A sarcoma of liver formerly believed to arise from Kupffer cells. It is now considered to be a hemangiosarcoma of the liver. **leukocytic s.** LEUKEMIA. **lymphangioendothelial s.** LYMPHANGIOSARCOMA. **monstrocellular s.** A malignant brain tumor with large, bizarre, multinucleated giant cells. Some consider it to be a sarcoma arising from cerebral blood vessels. Others believe it is a form of giant cell glioblastoma. **multiple idiopathic hemorrhagic s.** KAPOSI SARCOMA. **myeloid s.** GRANULOCYTIC SARCOMA. **neurogenic s.** MALIGNANT SCHWANNOMA. **osteogenic s.** OSTEOSARCOMA. **parosteal s.** PERIOSTEAL SARCOMA. **periductal s.** CYSTOSARCOMA PHYLLODES. **periosteal s.** A sarcoma arising from the periosteum. Also *parosteal sarcoma, periosteal spindle-cell sarcoma.* **s. of peripheral nerve** MALIGNANT SCHWANNOMA. **reticulum cell s.** HISTIOCYTIC LYMPHOMA. **Rous s.** A spontaneous, transmissible fibrosarcoma of the domestic chicken caused by a virus (Rous sarcoma virus). Described in 1911, this was the first neoplasm shown to be transmissible or caused by an infective agent. Also *chicken tumor I.* **spindle-cell s.** A sarcoma composed of spindle-shaped cells. **synovial s.** A sarcoma of synovium-type cells. It shows a biphasic pattern, with epithelium-like cells lining clefts and acinar spaces separated by fibrosarcomalike tissue. Most arise in young adults, usually in the vicinity of large joints. Also *malignant synovioma.* **s. of the testis** A malignant mesenchymal tumor of the testis. The most frequent form is the rhabdomyosarcoma arising in the testicular tunics. **Walker s.** A spontaneous, transplantable carcinosarcoma of rats. Also *Walker carcinosarcoma 256.*

**sarcomata** \särkō′mətə\ Plural of SARCOMA.

**sarcomatoid** \särkō′mətoid\ Resembling a sarcoma.

**sarcomatosis** \-mətō′sis\ [SARCOMA + *t* + -OSIS] **1** The presence of multiple sarcomas. Also *sarcosis.* **2** A state of widely disseminated sarcoma. **meningeal s.** Diffuse growth of sarcoma along the meninges.

**sarcomatous** \särkō′mətəs\ Describing or relating to sarcoma.

**sarcomere** \sär′kəmir\ [SARCO- + -MERE] The basic recurring structural unit of the myofibril, comprising the myofilaments and associated organelles which lie between one Z line and the next.

**sarcomesothelioma** \-mez′ōthē′lē·ō′mə \ [SARCO- + MESOTHELIOMA] A malignant mesothelioma of fibrous type.

**sarconeme** \sär′kənēm\ [SARCO- + Gk *nēm(a)* thread, yarn] MICRONEME.

***Sarcophaga*** \särkäf′əgə\ [New L, from Gk *sarkophagos* (from *sarx,* gen. *sarko(s)* flesh + *-phagos* -eating, -eater, from *phagein* to eat) flesh-eating, carnivorous] A genus of flesh flies in the family Sarcophagidae whose larvae develop in suppurating wounds, ulcers, or the nasal passages and sinuses of animals. The most important species economically is *S. haemorrhoidalis.* Others of veterinary importance are *S. carnaria, S. dux, S. fuscicauda, S. niticornis,* and *S. rubicornis.*.

**Sarcophagidae** \-faj′idē\ [*Sarcophag(a)* + -IDAE] A family of flies, order Diptera, that includes the flesh flies as well as others whose larvae develop in rotting meat. The genera *Sarcophaga* and *Wohlfahrtia* produce myiasis in humans and many domestic animals.

**sarcoplasm** \sär′kəplazm\ [SARCO- + -PLASM] The cytoplasm of a muscle cell. Also *myoplasm, myoserum*. Adj. sarcoplasmic.

**sarcoplasmic** \-plaz′mik\ Pertaining to or composed of sarcoplasm.

**sarcoplasts** \sär′kəplasts\ SATELLITE CELLS OF SKELETAL MUSCLE.

**sarcopoietic** \-poi·et′ik\ SARCOGENIC.

***Sarcopsylla penetrans*** \sär′käpsil′ə pen′ətranz\ TUNGA PENETRANS.

**sarcopsyllosis** \sär′käpsilō′sis\ [*Sarcopsyll(a)* + -OSIS] TUNGIASIS.

***Sarcoptes scabiei*** \särkäp′tēz skā′bē·ī\ The common itch mite. The female is 0.3–0.5 mm long and 0.2–0.4 wide, the male half as large. Varieties of this species are cosmopolitan in distribution and affect humans and many domestic and wild animals. Varieties are for the most part host-specific, but transitory infections can occur, particularly from animals to humans. It causes scabies in man and mange in many domestic animals. Also *Acarus scabiei*.

**sarcoptic** \särkäp′tik\ **1** Of or belonging to the genus *Sarcoptes*.. **2** Caused by mites of the genus *Sarcoptes*..

**Sarcoptidae** \särkäp′tidē\ [*Sarcopt(es)* + -IDAE] A family of mites that cause itch or mange in humans and many animals. It includes the genera *Sarcoptes, Notoedres,* and *Trixacarus*.

**sarcoptidosis** \sär′käptidō′sis\ [*Sarcoptid(ae)* + -OSIS] Infestation by mites of the family Sarcoptidae. It is characterized by dermatitis, pruritis, loss of hair, and self-mutilation by the host.

**sarcoptoid** \särkäp′toid\ Of or belonging to the superfamily of itch mites, Sarcoptoidea.

**sarcosine** $CH_3$—$NH_2^+$—$CH_2$—$COO^-$. *N*-Methylglycine, a compound originally found in starfish. It is on the pathway of degradation of choline to glycine in mammals.

**sarcosinemia** \-sinē′mē·ə\ An autosomal recessive disorder that is caused by a defect in sarcosine dehydrogenase activity. It is characterized by abnormal increases in blood and urine sarcosine and mild mental retardation.

**sarcosis** \särkō′sis\ [Gk *sarkōsis* (from *sarx*, gen. *sarkos* flesh) growth of flesh, fleshiness] **1** A state of excessive flesh formation. **2** SARCOMATOSIS.

**sarcosome** \sär′kəsōm\ [SARCO- + -SOME] A mitochondrion of a muscle fiber. Also *myomitochondrion*.

**sarcosporidiasis** \-spôr′idī′əsis\ SARCOCYSTOSIS.

**sarcosporidiosis** \-spôrid′ē·ō′sis\ SARCOCYSTOSIS.

**sarcostosis** \-stō′sis\ [*sarc(o)-* + OST- + -OSIS] Ossification of soft tissue.

**sarcotic** \särkät′ik\ **1** Causing the growth of flesh. **2** Of or relating to sarcosis.

**sarcotubules** \-t$^y$oo′byools\ SARCOPLASMIC RETICULUM.

**sarcous** \sär′kəs\ Pertaining to or consisting of muscle.

**sarin** \sär′in\ $C_4H_{10}FO_2P$. Isopropylmethylphosphonofluoridate, a nerve gas and potent cholinesterase inhibitor.

**sarmentogenin** One of the cardenolides. It contains an 11-hydroxyl group and was therefore investigated as a raw material for conversion into adrenal steroids, but no abundant source was found.

**SATA** spatial average temporal average.

**satellite** \sat′əlīt\ [L *satelles*, gen. *satellitis*, an attendant, partner] A structure closely following or associated with another, usually larger, structure. **chromosome s.** In cytologic preparations, a globoid chromatin body separated from the main body of the chromosome by a short, thin stalk. It usually occurs at the ends of the short arms of acrocentric chromosomes, but may be intercalated. In humans, the presence of a satellite on a particular acrocentric chromosome and the size of the satellite are heritable polymorphisms, having no effect on phenotype, human satellites stain positively with silver ions and contain DNA homologous with ribosomal RNA. Genes coding for ribosomal RNA are located in the stalk region. **nucleolar s.** Any of the chromosome satellites enriched in genes that encode ribosomal RNA. They stain with silver ions, their sizes are heritable polymorphic traits, and they occur at the end of the short arms of the five human acrocentric chromosomes, numbered 13, 14, 15, 21, and 22. **pericentriolar s.'s** Masses of dense material surrounding the centriole. **perineuronal s.** An oligodendroglial cell immediately adjacent to a neuronal cell body. Also *perineural satellite*. **perivascular s.** PERICYTE.

**satiation** \sā′shē·ā′shən\ [L *satiatus*, past part. of *satiare* (from *satis* enough, fully) to sate, satisfy] The complete gratification of an organismic need, sufficient to produce an insensitivity to further stimulation of the kind, and marking the point at which continued stimulation would take on a negative quality that would increase the probability of aversive and avoidant responses by the organism.

**Sattler** [Hubert *Sattler*, Austrian ophthalmologist, 1844–1928] See under VEIL, LAYER.

**saturated** \sach′ərā′tid\ **1** Brought to saturation with respect to a specified substance: said of a solution or vapor. **2** Containing no double or triple bonds and therefore unable to add further hydrogen: said of a compound.

**saturation** \sach′ərā′shən\ [Late L *saturatio* (from *saturare* to satisfy, fill, from *satur*, full, sated, akin to *satis* enough) filling, saturation] **1** The state of a solution in which no more of a specified component can dissolve, because it is in equilibrium with the pure component, or the similar state of a vapor into which no more of a specified component can vaporize. **2** The state of a substance of being unable to combine with hydrogen because it contains no double or triple bonds. **3** The state in which the population difference between the nuclear magnetic energy levels decreases to zero, as does the intensity of the absorption signal. **blood oxygen s.** The oxygen content of blood expressed as a ratio or percentage of its total oxygen-carrying capacity. **oxygen s.** See under BLOOD OXYGEN SATURATION.

**saturnism** \sat′ərnizm\ [After *Saturn(us)*, the planet, from Saturnus, Roman god of agriculture and civilization + -ISM. Lead prob. takes the name of Saturn because of the heaviness attributed to him in astrology.] *Older term* LEAD POISONING.

**satyriasis** \sat′irī′əsis\ [Gk (from *Satyr(os)* a Satyr) a satyrlike condition, esp. hypersexuality] Hypersexuality occurring in a male. Also *gynecomania, gynephilia, lagnosis, satyrism, satyromania*.

**Sauer** [Louis Wendlin *Sauer*, U.S. physician, born 1885] See under VACCINE.

**sauna** \sô′nə\ [Finnish] A specially constructed room, usually of wood, equipped with a heating device capable of raising air temperature to levels adequate to induce profuse sweating. See also SAUNA BATH.

**Saunders** [Edward Watts *Saunders*, U.S. physician, 1854–1927] See under SIGN.

**Sauvineau** [Charles *Sauvineau*, French ophthalmologist, born 1862] See under OPHTHALMOPLEGIA.

**Savage** [Henry *Savage*, English anatomist and gynecologist, 1810–1900] Savage's perineal body. See under CENTRUM TENDINEUM PERINEI.

**saw** [Old English *sagu, sage*, akin to L *secare* to cut] Any of various metal cutting instruments with teeth or serrations, used in surgical operations. **Albee s.** An electrically powered saw designed to cut wedges and slices of bone in preparation for grafting. **amputating s.** A saw used to divide bones during an amputation. **bayonet s.** A nasal saw having a small, narrow blade and an offset handle. **crown s.** TREPHINE. **Gigli s.** A flexible wire saw used for cutting bone, particularly skull. **hole s.** TREPHINE. **Stryker s.** A powered surgical saw using an electric or pneumatic source to create a reciprocating or oscillatory blade action.

**saw-tooth** SLOW SPIKE.

**saxifragant** \saksif′rəgənt\ **1** Promoting the dissolution of calculi. **2** An agent that breaks up or dissolves calculi.

**Saxtorph** [Matthias *Saxtorph,* Danish obstetrician, 1740–1800] Saxtorph's maneuver. See under PAJOT MANEUVER.

**Sayre** [Lewis Albert *Sayre,* U.S. surgeon, 1820–1900] **1** See under BANDAGE. **2** Sayre's method. See under OPERATION. **3** Sayre's jacket. See under PLASTER-OF-PARIS JACKET.

**Sb** Symbol for the element, antimony.

**SBE** subacute bacterial endocarditis.

**SC** closure of the semilunar valves.

**Sc** Symbol for the element, scandium.

**scab** [Middle English *scabbe,* of Scandinavian origin, akin to Old English *scaebb* scab, L *scabies* the mange, scab, itch, from *scabere* to scratch] A crust that forms over a surface denuded of epithelium, made up of clotted plasma and blood cells.

**scabicide** A drug or chemical agent used to combat *Sarcoptes scabiei* and effective in the treatment of scabies.

**scabies** \skā′bēz\ [L (from *scabere* to scratch), the mange, itch, scab] An infestation with the human itch or mange mite, *Sarcoptes scabiei* var. *humanus.* Skin between fingers, the knee, elbow, breasts, shoulder blades, and under the penis is most often attacked by the mites, which produce threadlike, sinuous burrows in the skin up to 1 cm long. Intense itching and rash develop in about a month caused by sensitization reactions to toxic secretions and excretions of the egg-laying females in the burrows. The lifetime of the female is about 2 months, during which time she lays eggs at 2–3 day intervals in the skin tunnels. Scabies appear in cyclic waves increasing at 15–20 year cycles, often associated with large-scale population movements. Also *seven-year itch, itch* (popular). **cat s.** Scabies in humans that is caused by cat-infesting species of notoedric mites or of *Cheyletiella.* **Norwegian s.** A modified, heavily crusted, and hyperkeratotic scabies infestation in subjects with an impaired immune response. Also *Norway itch, scabies crustosa.* **sarcoptic s.** Scabies caused by variants of the species *Sarcoptes scabiei* in the itch mite family Sarcoptidae, which infest any of a number of mammals, including man. • The same condition in nonhuman animals is more usually known as *sarcoptic mange.* Also *sarcoptic itch.*

**scala** \skā′lə\ [Late L (often in pl. *scalae* a flight of stairs, ladder; from L *scandere* to climb), a ladder, staircase] An anatomic structure resembling a winding staircase. **s. media** *Outmoded* DUCTUS COCHLEARIS. **s. tympani** [NA] A space within the cochlea of the internal ear which is filled with perilymph and is separated from the tympanic cavity by the secondary tympanic membrane and continuous with the scala vestibuli through the helicotrema at the apex of the cochlea. It is continuous with the subarachnoid space through the cochlear canaliculus. Its roof is the basilar membrane and the osseous spiral lamina, which separate it from the cochlear duct. Also *tympanic canal of cochlea.* **s. vestibuli** [NA] A space within the cochlea of the internal ear which is filled with perilymph and communicates with the anterior end of the vestibule and with the scala tympani through the helicotrema at the apex of the cochlea. Its floor is formed by the vestibular membrane and the osseous spiral lamina which separate it from the ductus cochlearis. Also *vestibular canal of cochlea.*

**scald** [Middle English *scalden* to scald, from Old French *eschalder* to scald, from Late L *excaldare* (from *ex-* intensive + *calidus* hot) to wash in hot or warm water] **1** A burn caused by hot liquid or vapor. **2** To injure tissue with a hot liquid or vapor. Water at 69°C will cause a burn in one second. Acids and alkalies at that same temperature may cause a burn in even less time.

**scale¹** **1** A thin, platelike external structure; squama. **2** A thin, flaky fragment of bone, horny epidermis, or enamel. Also *squame.* **3** Calculus on the teeth. **4** To remove calculus from (the teeth). **adhesive s.** Scale that is not easily sloughed from the surface, as in lupus erythematosus.

**scale²** [Latin *scala* ladder] **1** A set of graduations, as on an instrument, that mark units or fractions of units for measuring the magnitude of quantities. **2** In psychology, a test consisting of a graded series of questions or tasks to which quantitative score values have been assigned based on their relative difficulty as empirically determined by the average performance of a standardized group. **Apgar s.** APGAR TEST. **Berkow s.** A scale used for estimating the extent of a burn, used for the making of a diagram (Berkow diagram) of the body surface. It assumes that over twelve years of age the percentages of the body surface occupied by different regions are as follows: head and neck, 6%; trunk, 38% (comprising anterior trunk and genitals, 20%; and posterior trunk, 18%); upper extremities, 18% (comprising hands, 4.5%; and arms, 13.5%); lower extremities, 38% (comprising feet, 6.4%; legs, 12.6%; thighs and buttocks, 19%). Somewhat different values are used for children under twelve years of age. **Celsius s.** A scale of temperature on which 0 degree Celsius (0°C) is 273.15 kelvins and 100 degrees Celsius (100°C) is 373.15 kelvins. • Prior to 1948, the degree Celsius was called *degree centigrade* and the points 0 degree centigrade and 100 degrees centigrade were defined under specified conditions as the melting point of ice and the boiling point of water, respectively. **centigrade s.** *Outmoded* CELSIUS SCALE. **Charrière s.** FRENCH SCALE. **developmental s.** An itemized sequence of observations to assess the progressive changes in the structure, form, and behavior of an organism in the transition from origin to maturity. The general order of appearance of the steps or stages in growth are entirely orderly for a species, but considerable variation of patterning may be observed among individuals. A developmental scale for human postnatal development allows a comparison to be made of the maturation achieved by any given child with that of most children of the same age, by means of tabled norms of average growth. **Fahrenheit s.** A scale of temperature on which 32 degrees Fahrenheit (32°F), defined as 273.15 kelvins, represents the melting point of ice and 212 degrees Fahrenheit (212°F) represents the boiling point of water. • Though obsolescent in scientific usage, the Fahrenheit scale is still widely used in the United States in popular contexts. **French s.** A scale used for the grading by size of sounds, catheters, and similar instruments, in which each unit is equal to $^1/_3$ mm. Hence unit 30 = 1 cm. Also *Charrière scale.* **Gaffky s.** A scale based on the number of tubercle bacilli in the sputum, used to express the prognosis in tuberculosis. Also

*Gaffky table.* **Gesell developmental s.'s** Inventories for 27 age levels designed to evaluate the level of motor, linguistic, and social behavior observable during infancy and early childhood (birth–5 years). Specific items are recorded as either present or absent, and normative data tables are available to provide a basis for comparison of the degree of developmental progress observed in a given infant or preschool child. **Glasgow coma s.** A numerical scale of grades of impairment of consciousness defined according to precise clinical criteria. It involves the recording of four grades of eye opening, five of the best verbal response, and five of the best motor response. • This scale was devised in Glasgow at the Institute of Neurological Sciences **gray s.** The display of echoes of different intensity as different shades of gray, that is, different brightnesses, on an oscilloscope screen. **interval s.** A scale of measurement having a constant unit of distance between successive positions so that, for example, the interval between 0 and 1 is the same length as that between 10 and 11. The ratio of any two intervals is independent of the unit of measurement and of the zero point, both of the latter being arbitrarily fixed. For example, height, weight, age, and temperature in degrees are measured on interval scales. **Kelvin s.** The scale of temperature with intervals equal to the SI base unit of thermodynamic temperature, the kelvin. The invervals equal those of the Celsius scale, with 0 degree Celsius equal to 273.15 kelvins and 100 degrees Celsius equal to 373.15 kelvins. **Minnesota preschool s.** A series of verbal and nonverbal tests for assessing the learning ability of children aged 18 months to 6 years. **nominal s.** A scale which specifies differences among, but which does not rank, the objects to which it is applied, such as one dealing with eye or hair color rather than with size, temperature, or value. **nonlinear s.** Any scale in which the divisions corresponding to the same number of steps are not equal, such as one in which the intervals between successive positions increase logarithmically or exponentially. **ordinal s.** A scale which employs a ranking relation (for example, "greater than"), so that entities can be arranged in an ascending order, but whose successive positions are not separated by a specified constant interval. Thus, a scale on which a patient's status would be rated as cured, improved, unchanged, or deteriorated would be an ordinal scale. **pH s.** A numerical scale used to denote the hydrogen ion concentration in a solution. It is expressed as the negative logarithm of hydrogen ion concentration, with 7.00 representing neutrality. Values above 7.00 indicate alkalinity, lower figures indicate acidity. Also *Sörensen scale.* **rating s.** In psychology, a device for making systematic judgments about the degree to which certain specific traits are present, either in oneself or another person. **Sörensen s.** PH SCALE. **Stanford-Binet intelligence s.** An adaptation for American children of the French Binet-Simon scale. This English language reconstruction of the Binet-Simon scale has been revised and updated, in 1937 and 1960, to establish appropriate norms for estimating the level of general intellectual functioning of any given child, by comparing the performance attained with that of a broad sampling of American children of the same age on the same test. Also *Stanford-Binet test, Terman test.* **Vineland social maturity s.** A series of standardized developmental rating scales, varying from infancy to 30 years of age, designed to assay the social maturity of an individual in terms of the demonstrated ability for self-care, work, responsibility for behavior, and an age-appropriate ability to communicate with and relate to others in a social way. **Wechsler adult intelligence s.** An intelligence test widely used in the United States and standardized on a population of adults and older children, ages 16–64. The intelligence quotient derived from it has a mean of 100 and a standard deviation of 15. It consists of 11 subtests, six of which are verbal in nature and five of which are performance tests. Separate intelligence estimates may be based on either the verbal or performance tests, or the two may be combined into a full-scale IQ test, utilizing both verbal and nonverbal scores. Abbr. WAIS **Wechsler intelligence s. for children** An intelligence test developed for use with children between the ages of 5 and 16 years. It consists of 12 subtests including both verbal and nonverbal materials.

**scalene** \skā′lēn\ **1** Denoting a triangle with three unequal sides and angles. **2** Pertaining to one of the scalenus muscles. For defs. 1 and 2 also *scalenus.*

**scalenectomy** \skā′lənek′təmē\ The operative excising of a scalene muscle.

**scalenotomy** \skā′lənät′əmē\ The division of the scalene muscles near their insertion on the first rib. It is usually performed to relieve the compression on the neurovascular bundle that is seen in thoracic outlet syndrome.

**scalenus** \skālē′nəs\ [Late L (from Gk *skalēnos* limping, uneven; with *trigōnon* a triangle of unequal sides, akin to *skolios* crooked, bent), scalene, unequal] SCALENE. **s. anticus** *Outmoded* MUSCULUS SCALENUS ANTERIOR.

**scaler** **1** An instrument that counts the electrical pulses issuing from a detector, amplifier, or electronic window. The accumulated total is then related to the time during which the count has been run, to give an average count rate. Typically, an automatic timer is an accessory. **2** An instrument for the removal of calculus from teeth. **chisel s.** A straight-shafted scaler used interdentally with a push action. Also *watch-spring scaler.* **ultrasonic s.** An instrument for scaling teeth in which the tip is activated by ultrasonic vibrations. The instrument incorporates a water spray. **watch-spring s.** CHISEL SCALER.

**scaling** The physical removal of calculus from the teeth. **subgingival s.** The removal of calculus from within a periodontal pocket.

**scall** \skôl\ [Middle English, from Old Norse *skalli* a bald head, akin to Old English *scealu* shell] A scaly and crusted cutaneous eruption, particularly of the scalp. *Obs.* **milk s.** CRADLE CAP.

**scalloping** \skal′əping\ **vertebral s.** Multiple concavities often seen in the posterior borders of vertebral bodies in radiographs of patients with neurofibromatosis.

**scalp** [Middle English, of Scandinavian origin, akin to Old Norse *skālpr* a sheath, Dutch *schelpe* a shell, Middle French *escalope* a shell] **1** The skin and soft tissue covering of the head that bears hair in both sexes. **2** To pull or otherwise remove the scalp from.

**scalpel** \skal′pəl\ [L *scalpel(lum)* (dim. of *scalprum* a knife, chisel, from *scalpere* to cut, carve) a lancet, scalpel] A surgical cutting instrument with a small blade on a short, rigid handle. **plasma s.** A device for the simultaneous cutting and coagulation of tissue, which utilizes a jet of inert gas that has been heated and ionized by means of a direct-current arc.

**scalprum** \skal′prəm\ [L (from *scalpere* to cut, carve) a knife, chisel] RASPATORY.

**scaly** Characterized by scales. Also *squamate.*

**scan** [Middle English *scannen* (from L *scandere* to climb; to scan verse, marking its meter or rhythm with the foot as in climbing steps) to scan (verse), to examine] **1** To survey (an area or volume) by a continuous sweep of a sensing device or by a series of observations at successive points. **2** A survey of an area or volume made by scanning. **3** A display of data produced by scanning, or as if by scanning, depicting their distribution in the area or volume scanned. **B s.** An ultrasound scan in which the image is a cross-section of the object through the scanning plane. Also *B-mode scan.* **bone s.** A visualization of the topographic distribution of a radiolabeled tracer that has an affinity for bone, particularly in areas of osteolytic or obsteoblastic activity. **bone-marrow s.** A scintigram that shows the distribution of bone marrow, usually revealing the distribution of hematopoiesis. **brain s.** 1 An image of the radioactivity in the brain, obtained by moving a collimated detector back and forth across the head while an output device registers the local radioactivity. 2 Any scintigram of the head, whether made with a moving or a stationary detector. **C s.** A B scan in which the image represents a cross-section of anatomy parallel to the surface and at a depth selected by gating. Also *C-mode scan.* **CAT s.** CT SCAN. **C-mode s.** C SCAN. **compound s.** An ultrasound scan which combines at least two basic scanning motions, such as linear and sector. **CT s.** The image produced by computed tomography. Also *CAT scan.* **gamma s.** GAMMA ENCEPHALOGRAPHY. **liver s.** A scintigraphic study of the liver after injection of an appropriate radiopharmaceutical, as $^{99m}$Tc sulfur colloid, which localizes in the liver because of phagocytosis by the Kupffer cells of the reticuloendothelial system. Other tracers, such as various $^{99m}$Tc-tagged iminodiacetic acid derivatives, are excreted by the hepatic cells, and are used to visualize the biliary tract. Also *radionuclide hepatogram, emission hepatogram, isotope hepatogram* (incorrect). **mechanical compound s.** A compound scan produced by mechanical means, as by driving a transducer with a motor. **perfusion s.** A technique for diagnosing the presence of a pulmonary embolism or other pulmonary vascular problems by gamma-camera scanning of the lung fields following injection of a radionuclide into a peripheral or central vein. **radioactive s.** A scintigram, especially if made with a moving detector. **sector s.** A scan by an ultrasound system in which the sound beam is rotated through an angle. **single sweep s.** A scan completed in a single sweep of the sensing device across the area under study. **ventilation s.** A technique for diagnosing various pulmonary disorders in which the pulmonary airways are visualized by gamma camera following inhalation of a radionuclide, usually xenon.

**scandium** \skan′dē·əm\ Element number 21, having atomic weight 44.956. Scandium is widely distributed in small amounts in many minerals. The pure element is a soft, silvery white metal with specific gravity 2.989. One stable isotope, scandium 45, occurs in nature. Ten unstable isotopes are known. Symbol: Sc

**scanner** Any device that scans. **duplex s.** A device, composed of an ultrasonic echographic imager and a continuous-wave Doppler velocity flowmeter, that is used for the imaging of large and medium-sized blood vessels and the analysis of the velocity waveforms produced therein. **mechanical real-time s.** An ultrasound imaging instrument which scans the beam by mechanically driving the transducer in a repeating pattern. **multicrystal whole-body s.** A rectilinear scanner that contains several collimated detecting crystals functioning in parallel. **PET s.** An apparatus capable of performing positron emission tomography. **rectilinear s.** A device that registers the distribution of radioactive material in a living body or other target by sweeping a collimated detector back and forth across the target, each pass being stepped by a small distance at right angles to the sweep. Successive passes are combined to produce the total image, or scan. Also *scintillation scanner.* **small parts s.** An ultrasound imaging instrument designed for high-resolution imaging of anatomic areas close to the transducer. **tomographic s.** A scanner capable of presenting images of the distribution of radioactivity at a designated depth.

**scanning** Surveying an area or volume by subjecting it to the continuous sweep of a sensing device or by a series of observations at successive points. **CAT s.** COMPUTED TOMOGRAPHY. **CT s.** COMPUTED TOMOGRAPHY. **linear s.** Scanning by moving an ultrasound transducer in a straight line perpendicular to the beam. **PET s.** POSITRON EMISSION TOMOGRAPHY. **ventilation-perfusion s.** A technique for diagnosing the presence of a pulmonary embolism by administering both an inhaled and an intravenous radionuclide. Gamma-camera scanning over the lung fields may demonstrate ventilated but nonperfused segments suggestive of embolism.

**scanography** \skanäg′rəfē\ [SCAN + *o* + -GRAPHY] A special method of radiologic examination in which the x ray is directed through a slit collimator, and the x-ray tube and collimator are moved over the part to be examined so that the examination is done chiefly with the central x-ray beam, thus diminishing magnification. The technique is used primarily for measurement, as of the length of a long bone.

**scansorius** \skansôr′ē·əs\ A variable portion of the gluteus minimus muscle that is occasionally separated from the anterior margin of the muscle.

**Scanzoni** [Friedrich Wilhelm *Scanzoni,* German obstetrician, 1821–1891] 1 See under OPERATION, MANEUVER. 2 Scanzoni second os. See under PATHOLOGIC RETRACTION RING.

**scapegoating** A form of defense mechanism, which may be employed by either an individual or a group, involving the displacement of aggression onto a safe target, i.e. one unable to reply effectively. By this process a frustrated child may come to attack a relatively defenseless younger sibling, or a minority group may be blamed for economic deprivation and frustration.

**scapha** \skaf′ə\ [NA] The long, curved, narrow furrow between the helix and the anthelix of the auricle of the external ear. Also *fossa scaphoidea* (outmoded), *scaphoid fossa* (outmoded), *scapha of helix, groove of helix.*

**scapho-** \skaf′ō-\ [Gk *skaphē* anything scooped out, basin, light boat, skiff] A combining form meaning scaphoid.

**scaphocephaly** \skaf′ōsef′əlē\ [SCAPHO- + CEPHAL- + -Y] An elongated cranial case with a keel-like ridge along the midsagittal line, owing to premature ossification of the sagittal suture. Also *scaphocephalia, scaphocephalism.*

**scaphohydrocephaly** \skaf′ōhī′drəsef′əlē\ [SCAPHO- + HYDROCEPHALY] Hydrocephaly in which the skull is enlarged longitudinally due to premature closure of the sagittal suture.

**scaphoid** \skaf′oid\ [Gk *skaphoeidēs* tublike, hollowed out. See SCAPHO-.] 1 Boat-shaped. Also *navicular.* 2 OS SCAPHOIDEUM.

**scaphoiditis** \skaf′oidī′tis\ An inflammation of the scaphoid bone. **tarsal s.** KÖHLER'S DISEASE.

***Scaptocosa raptoria*** \skap′təkō′sə raptôr′ē·ə\ A species of Brazilian wolf spider that has a strong necrotizing, hemolytic venom.

**scapula** \skap′yələ\ [L (akin to *scabere* to scratch and Gk *skaptein* to dig) the shoulder blade, prob. orig. a digging tool, spade] (*pl.* scapulae) [NA] Either of two large triangular, flattened bones located on the posterior aspect of the thorax between the levels of the second to seventh ribs. It is attached to the trunk by muscles and by the clavicle through acromioclavicular and sternoclavicular joints. It presents anterior, or costal, and posterior surfaces; superior, lateral and medial margins; superior, lateral and inferior angles; and three bony processes (the coracoid, the acromion, and the spine). It articulates with the head of the humerus at its lateral angle modified to form the glenoid cavity. Also *shoulder blade, blade bone, scapular bone, omoplata* (outmoded). **alar s.** WINGED SCAPULA. **s. alata** (*pl.* scapulae alatae) WINGED SCAPULA. **Graves s.** SCAPHOID SCAPULA. **scaphoid s.** A concavity of the vertebral border of the scapula. Also *Graves scapula.* **winged s.** A scapula which stands out from the chest wall like an angel's wing, as when a patient with paralysis of one serratus anterior muscle pushes forward against a flat surface with the hand. On abduction of the arm at the shoulder the affected scapula is seen to rise up abnormally and can be seen above the calvicle when the patient is viewed from in front. Also *scapula alata, alar scapula.*

**scapular** \skap′yələr\ Of or pertaining to the scapula.

**scapulary** \skap′yəler′ē\ [SCAPULAR + -Y] A bandage or support going over the shoulders utilized to position a circumferential bandage in a manner similar to suspenders.

**scapulectomy** \skap′yəlek′təmē\ The excision of all or part of the scapula.

**scapuloclavicular** \skap′yəlōkləvik′yələr\ ACROMIOCLAVICULAR.

**scapulopexy** \skap′yəlōpek′sē\ The operative fixation of the scapula, using bone, screws, muscles, or tendons, to the chest wall or to the spinous processes of the vertebral column.

**scapus** \skā′pəs\ [L, a stalk, stem, shaft] (*pl.* scapi) A shaft or stem. **s. pili** [NA] HAIR SHAFT.

**scar** [Middle English, from Late L *eschara* (from Gk *eschara* a hearth, fireplace, scab) a scar, scab] A mark consisting of fibrous material formed in the healing process of a wound or other lesion; cicatrix. **bridle s.** A short, tight scar connecting a movable part of the body with a relatively immobile part, thus restraining or preventing movements of the former. For example, a short, tight scar from the chin to the sternum would fall into this category. **cortical s.** A scar in the cerebral or cerebellar cortex. **hesitation s.'s** See under HESITATION WOUNDS. **ice-pick s.'s** Deep, pitted scars that are usually seen on the face and are most often due to severe acne vulgaris. **mature s.** A scar in which all evidence of inflammation has subsided. It loses its induration and red color, and will no longer change in texture or appearance. **shilling s.'s** Circular, well-healed scars which appear following involution of ulcerated lesions of late secondary syphilis. **tissue-paper s.** Very thin scar tissue with the appearance of tissue paper, often forming where an ulcer has healed. It is a characteristic feature of the Ehlers-Danlos syndrome, but also occurs independently of it. **ulceration s.** 1 An immature scar that, because of thinness, is subject to shearing with even minor trauma. With the epithelial covering removed an open wound results, and if not quickly reepithelialized a chronic ulcer results. 2 The scar tissue that remains following the healing of a peptic ulcer in the stomach or duodenum. **white s. of ovary** CORPUS ALBICANS.

**scarabiasis** \skar′əbī′əsis\ [L *scarab(aeus)* a beetle + -IASIS] An intestinal infection with adult beetles. The most common form is seen in children infected by dung beetles. The condition is characterized by gastrointestinal disturbances, anorexia, and emaciation. Also *beetle disease.*

**Scardino** [Peter L. *Scardino,* U.S. urologist, born 1915] See under URETEROPELVIOPLASTY.

**scarf / Mayor s.** A triangular bandage utilized as a sling for immobilization of an upper extremity.

**Scarff** [John Edwin *Scarff,* U.S. neurosurgeon, born 1898] **1** Stookey-Scarff shunt. See under THIRD VENTRICULOCISTERNOSTOMY. **2** Stookey-Scarff operation. See under OPERATION.

**scarifier** \skar′ifī′ər\ [*scarif(y)* + *i* + -ER] An instrument with many sharp points that is used to make multiple small incisions, as for a vaccination. Also *scarificator.*

**scarify** \skar′ifī\ [Middle French *scarifier* (from Late L *scarificare* to scratch, irreg. from L *scarifare* to scratch up, from Gk *skariphos* a stylus for drawing outlines) to make incisions upon] To scratch or break a surface, such as the skin, with multiple small punctures.

**scarlatina** \skär′lətē′nə\ SCARLET FEVER. **s. haemorrhagica** A very rare, usually fatal form of scarlet fever in which hemorrhages into the skin and mucous membranes occur. **malignant s.** A usually fatal, fulminant form of scarlet fever in which the constitutional symptoms are severe and the rash appears dusky and poorly defined. **s. papulosa** Scarlet fever in which an eruption of small papules appears, especially on the legs. **s. pruriginosa** A rare form of scarlet fever in which a papular eruption occurs, causing considerable irritation. **puerperal s.** Streptococcal infection of the birth canal, with production of scarlet fever, before or shortly after childbirth. **s. pustulosa** A form of scarlet fever in which skin sepsis develops as a result of extraneous bacterial infection. **s. rheumatica** Scarlet fever associated with arthritis and other rheumatic manifestations.

**scarlatinal** \skär′lətē′nəl, skärlat′inəl\ Pertaining to, characterized by, or attributable to scarlet fever.

**scarlatinella** \skärlat′inel′ə\ [*scarlatin(a)* + -ELLA] An atypical, mild, nonfebrile form of scarlet fever.

**scarlatiniform** \skär′lətin′ifôrm\ Resembling scarlet fever: said especially of a rash. Also *scarlatinoid.*

**scarlet** **1** A brilliant red, slightly orange in hue. **2** A substance, usually a stain or dye, that is scarlet in appearance, or that produces a cytochemical reaction resulting in scarlet staining. For chemical names including *scarlet,* see under the chemical name.

**Scarpa** [Antonio *Scarpa,* Italian anatomist, orthopedist, and ophthalmologist, 1747–1832] **1** See under STAPHYLOMA, FASCIA. **2** Scarpa's ganglion. See under GANGLION VESTIBULARE. **3** Scarpa's fluid, liquor of Scarpa. See under ENDOLYMPHA. **4** Scarpa sheath. See under FASCIA CREMASTERICA. **5** Scarpa's hiatus. See under HELICOTREMA. **6** Greater fossa of Scarpa, Scarpa's triangle. See under TRIGONUM FEMORALE. **7** Scarpa's canals. See under CANALIS INCISIVUS. **8** Scarpa's nerve. See under NERVUS NASOPALATINUS. **9** Scarpa's membrane. See under MEMBRANA TYMPANI SECUNDARIA. **10** Ligament of Scarpa. See under CORNU SUPERIUS MARGINIS FALCIFORMIS.

**scarring / web s.** Scar tissue that connects parts of the body that are normally separated. Such scarring may form, for example, between two fingers. If it occurs at the neck, it can cause downward displacement of the chin onto the chest.

**SCAT** **1** sheep cell agglutination test (Paul-Bunnel test or Rose-Waaler test). **2** sickle cell anemia test.

**scat-** \skat-\ SCATO-.

**scatemia** \skətē′mē·ə\ [SCAT- + -EMIA] Poisoning from fecal matter retained within the organism, presumably related to unidentified toxins generated from within the gastrointestinal tract, perhaps by bacterial fermentation or digestion. Also *scoretemia.*

**scato-** \skat′ə-\ [Gk *skōr* (genitive *skatos*) scat, dung, feces] A combining form denoting feces. Also *scat-, skato-.*

**scatologia** \-lō′jə\ COPROLALIA.

**scatologic** \-läj′ik\ Pertaining to fecal material or scatology; coprologic. Also *skatologic.*

**scatology** \skatäl′əjē\ COPROLOGY.

**scatoma** \skatō′mə\ [SCAT- + -OMA] STERCOROMA.

**scatophilia** \-fil′yə\ COPROPHILIA.

**scatter** SCATTERING. **coherent s.** COHERENT SCATTERING. **forward s.** Scattered radiation that is restricted to an angle of 90° or less of scatter. **light s.** The irregular diffusion of light through translucent structures such as the sclera or corneal scar tissue. It is of importance in ocular biomicroscopy, since it discloses imperfections in optical structures.

**scattering** The deflection in various directions of incident radiation, particles, or photons, by a target material. The radiation may or may not impart some of its energy to the target. Scattering events are often regarded as collisions between an incident particle and an atom, its nucleus, or an electron. Also *scatter.* **coherent s.** Scattering in which the incident radiation imparts negligible energy to the target material and a definite phase relationship remains between the impinging and the scattered radiation. Also *coherent scatter, Rayleigh scattering, Thomson scattering.* **Compton s.** Scattering involving elastic collisions between incident photons and unbound or weakly bound electrons. The incident energy is shared between the scattered electron and the deflected photon. **Rayleigh s.** COHERENT SCATTERING. **Thomson s.** COHERENT SCATTERING.

**scatula** \skach′ələ\ [Med L, a rectangular paper box for holding pills or powders] A paper box designed to hold powders or pills.

**scavenger** 1 A substance that reacts with some chemical species as fast as this species is formed. A common example is a scavenger for free radicals, which can therefore inhibit radical-propagated chain reactions by removing radicals. Molecular oxygen can play such a role. 2 Designating membrane transport systems of high affinity but relatively low limiting velocity.

**Sc.D.** Doctor of Science.

**Schacher** [Polycarp Gottlieb *Schacher,* German physician, 1674–1737] Schacher's ganglion. See under GANGLION CILIARE.

**Schafer** [Erich *Schafer,* German dermatologist, born 1897] Schafer syndrome. See under PACHYONYCHIA CONGENITA.

**Schäffer** [Max *Schäffer,* German neurologist, 1852–1923] See under REFLEX.

**Schamberg** [Jay Frank *Schamberg,* U.S. dermatologist, 1870–1934] Schamberg's disease, Schamberg's dermatosis. See under PROGRESSIVE PIGMENTED PURPURIC DERMATOSIS.

**Schardinger** [Franz *Schardinger,* Austrian chemist, flourished early 20th century] Schardinger enzyme. See under XANTHINE OXIDASE.

**scharlach R** \shär′lak\ SUDAN IV.

**Schatz** [Christian Fredrich *Schatz,* German gynecologist, born 1841] See under MANEUVER.

**Schatzki** [Richard *Schatzki,* U.S. roentgenologist, born 1901] See under RING.

**Schaudinn** [Fritz Richard *Schaudinn,* German zoologist, 1871–1906] See under FIXATIVE.

**Schaumann** [Joergen *Schaumann,* Swedish dermatologist, 1879–1953] 1 Schaumann bodies. See under BODY. 2 Schaumann's disease, Schaumann syndrome, Schaumann sarcoid, Besnier-Boeck-Schaumann disease. See under SARCOIDOSIS.

**Schauta** [Friedrich *Schauta,* Austrian gynecologist, 1849–1910] 1 Schauta's operation. See under SCHAUTA-AMREICH VAGINAL OPERATION. 2 Schauta-Wertheim operation. See under WERTHEIM-SCHAUTA OPERATION.

**Schede** [Max *Schede,* German surgeon, 1844–1902] See under CLOT.

**schedule** / **fixed interval s.** FIXED INTERVAL REINFORCEMENT. **fixed ratio s.** FIXED RATIO REINFORCEMENT. **s. of reinforcement** A program of operant conditioning in which a reward is given only for a certain predetermined proportion of correct responses. The schedule may be set up on an interval or a ratio basis, and the interval may be fixed or varied. **variable interval s.** VARIABLE INTERVAL REINFORCEMENT. **variable ratio s.** VARIABLE RATIO REINFORCEMENT.

**Scheerer** [Martin *Scheerer,* German-born U.S. psychologist, 1900–1961] Weigl-Goldstein-Scheerer test. See under TEST.

**Scheie** [Harold Glendon *Scheie,* U.S. ophthalmologist, born 1909] 1 See under OPERATION. 2 Hurler-Scheie syndrome. See under MUCOPOLYSACCHARIDOSIS IH/S. 3 Hurler-Scheie compound. See under COMPOUND.

**Scheiner** [Christoph *Scheiner,* German astronomer, 1575–1650] See under EXPERIMENT.

**schema** \skē′mə\ [Gk *schēma.* See SCHEME.] (*pl.* schemata) A plan, summary, or outline, especially one in diagrammatic form. **Hamberger's s.** A model of thoracic functional anatomy based on the proposition that the external intercostal muscles are used for inspiration and the internal intercostal muscles for expiration.

**schematic** \skēmat′ik\ Of the nature of a schema; being in the form of an outline or diagram.

**schematogram** \skēmat′əgram\ A tracing of the outline of the body made by a schematograph.

**schematograph** \skēmat′əgraf\ A device for tracing an outline of the body.

**scheme** \skēm\ [Gk *schēma* (akin to Old English *sige* victory and Gk *echein* to have, hold) form, shape, manner, nature] A plan or schema.

**Scherer** [Hans Joachim *Scherer,* Austrian physician, born 1906] Van Bogaert-Scherer-Epstein syndrome. See under CEREBROTENDINOUS XANTHOMATOSIS.

**Scheuermann** [Holger Werfel *Scheuermann,* Danish orthopedist, 1877–1960] Scheuermann's disease. See under KYPHOSIS.

**Schick** [Béla *Schick,* Hungarian-born U.S. pediatrician, 1877–1967] 1 See under CONTROL, SIGN. 2 Schick reaction. See under TEST.

**Schiff** [Hugo *Schiff,* German chemist, 1834–1915] 1 See under REAGENT, TEST. 2 Schiff base. See under IMINE. 3 Periodic acid-Schiff stain. See under STAIN.

**Schilder** [Paul Ferdinand *Schilder,* German-born U.S. neurologist and psychiatrist, 1886–1940] 1 Schilder's encephalitis, Flatau-Schilder disease. See under DISEASE. 2 Schilder-Addison complex. See under ADRENOLEUKODYSTROPHY.

**Schilling** [Victor Theodore Adolf Georg *Schilling,* German hematologist, 1883–1960] 1 See under TEST, CLASSIFICATION, LEUKEMIA. 2 Schilling blood count. See under COUNT.

**Schimmelbusch** [Curt *Schimmelbusch,* German surgeon, 1860–1895] Schimmelbusch disease. See under CYSTIC MASTOPATHY.

**schindylesis** \skin′dilē′sis\ [Gk *schindylēsis* splitting, division] A fibrous joint in which the sharp edge of one bone is placed into a groove of another.

**Schiötz** [Hjalmar *Schiötz,* Norwegian physician, 1850–1927] See under TONOMETER.

**Schirmer** [Rudolph *Schirmer*, German ophthalmologist, 1831–1896] See under TEST.

**-schisis** \-skisis\ [Gk *schisis* (from *schizein* to cleave, divide) a cleaving, division] A combining form meaning a fissure or cleft.

**schistasis** \skis′təsis\ [Gk *schistē*, fem. of *schistos* split, divided + -SIS] The state of being split or cleft, particularly when the condition is of developmental origin, as in schistomelia or schistosomia.

**schistencephaly** \skis′tensef′əlē\ SCHIZENCEPHALY.

**schisto-** \skis′tə-\ [Gk *schistos* (from *schizein* to split) split, divided] A combining form meaning split, divided.

**schistocelia** \-sē′lyə\ [SCHISTO- + *-cel(e)*[2] + -IA] Any developmental fissure of the abdominal wall.

**schistocephalus** \-sef′ələs\ [SCHISTO- + -CEPHALUS] A fetus or newborn infant with a cleft or unclosed cranium.

**schistocormia** \-kôr′mē·ə\ [SCHISTO- + Gk *korm(os)* a felled tree trunk + -IA] SCHISTOSOMIA.

**schistocystis** \-sis′tis\ EXSTROPHY OF THE BLADDER.

**schistocyte** \skis′təsīt\ SCHIZOCYTE.

**schistocytosis** \-sītō′sis\ SCHIZOCYTOSIS.

**schistoglossia** \-gläs′ē·ə\ [SCHISTO- + GLOSS- + -IA] BIFID TONGUE.

**schistomelia** \-mē′lyə\ [SCHISTO- + MEL-[1] + -IA] A cleft of a limb that is of developmental origin.

**schistoprosopia** \-prōsō′pē·ə\ [SCHISTO- + PROSOP- + -IA] Any extensive or severe facial cleft, as an oblique facial cleft. Also *schizoprosopia.*

**schistorachis** \skistôr′əkis\ RACHISCHISIS.

***Schistosoma*** \shis′təsō′mə, skis′-\ [SCHISTO- + Gk *sōma* body] A genus of trematodes; the blood flukes, parasites of humans and domestic animals. As adults they are characterized by an elongate shape and sexual dimorphism. Also *Bilharzia* (former name), *Gynaecophorus* (former name), *Schistosomum* (former name). ***S. haematobium*** A species of blood fluke that is parasitic in the portal system and mesenteric veins of the bladder and rectum of humans, causing schistosomiasis haematobia. The infective fork-tailed cercariae penetrate the skin of persons coming in contact with infested water. It is especially common in the Nile delta and certain other parts of the Mediterranean region, and in the Arabian peninsula, but also occurs in all major African river systems and waterways. The egg is characterized by a terminal spine, and the intermediate hosts are snails of the subfamily Bulininae. In Egypt the chief intermediate host is *Bulinus truncatus.* Also *Distoma haematobium* (obs.). ***S. japonicum*** A highly pathogenic species infecting humans in east and southeast Asia: the cause of schistosomiasis japonica. Transmission occurs when infected human feces release eggs in water containing infective strains or subspecies of the freshwater amphibious snail, *Oncomelania hupensis.* The eggs hatch, releasing ciliated miracidia that penetrate the snail hosts, pass through several multiplying larval generations and release numerous cercariae, the stage infective to humans and other mammals by direct penetration of intact skin. The young worms enter the circulation, pass to the lungs and the liver where they develop to adult worms in about three months. The paired adults migrate to the superior mesenteric vessels and lay numerous eggs which are deposited in the large intestine and liver. ***S. mansoni*** A species found in Africa, the Middle East, South America, and the West Indies; the cause of human schistosomiasis mansoni. The eggs are characterized by a lateral spine, and the intermediate hosts are snails of the genus *Biomphalaria.*

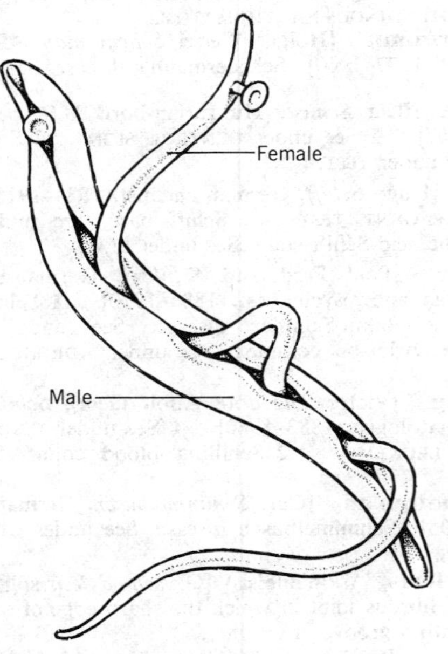

*Schistosoma mansoni* (copulating)

**schistosomacidal** \shis′təsōməsī′dəl, skis′-\ SCHISTOSOMICIDAL.

**schistosomacide** \shis′təsō′məsīd, skis′-\ SCHISTOSOMICIDE.

**schistosomal** \shis′təsō′məl, skis′-\ Relating to or caused by members of the genus *Schistosoma*.. Also *bilharzial.*

***Schistosomatium douthitti*** \shis′təsōmā′shē·əm dou′thətī, skis′-\ A species of blood fluke found in the portal veins of the vole *Microtus pennsylvanicus* and in the hare *Lepus americanus.* The species has been extensively studied in the laboratory as a model for schistosome experimental and immunological investigations that do not involve a species pathological to humans and that is easy to maintain in the laboratory.

**Schistosomatoidea** \shis′təsō′mətoi′dē·ə, skis′-\ [*Schistosomat(idae)* + *-oidea,* suffix used for higher taxa] A superfamily of trematodes of the suborder Strigeata that includes the blood flukes, namely, the families Sanguinicolidae (blood flukes of fishes), Spirorchiidae (blood flukes of turtles), and Schistosomatidae (blood flukes of mammals). All have a blood vessel habitat with elongate bodies well adapted to that site. They typically lack a muscular pharynx and an operculum, and have only sporocyst generations in the snail and a fork-tailed cercaria that penetrates the integument of its definitive host.

**schistosome** \shis′təsōm, skis′-\ A blood fluke, especially one of the genus *Schistosoma* or other genera closely related to it. Also *bilharzia worm.*

**schistosomia** \skis′təsō′mē·ə\ [SCHISTO- + Gk *sōm(a)* body + -IA] A congenital cleft of the abdominal and/or thoracic body walls associated with a reduction deformity of one or more limbs, particularly the lower limbs. Also *schistocormia.*

**schistosomiasis** \shis′təsōmī′əsis, skis′-\ [*Schistosom(a)* + -IASIS] Infection with flukes of the genus *Schistosoma,* an important and rapidly spreading helminthic infection of humans in tropical and subtropical regions of Africa, South America, the Far East, the Middle East, and the Caribbean. Current spread of the disease is caused by dams and irrigation systems which increase the expanse of fresh water harboring the intermediate hosts, freshwater snails. Infection is often asymptomatic but can be chronic and debilitating. The site of disease varies with the infecting species and is primarily due to host tissue reactions to the eggs in the form of granulation and scarring. *S. mansoni, S. japonicum, S. intercalatum,* and *S. mekongi* infection cause intestinal and liver disease, which may lead to portal hypertension. *S. haemotobium* causes urinary tract disease and has been associated with bladder cancer. Also *bilharziasis, bilharziosis, hemic distomiasis* (obs.), *snail fever, kabure itch, Sawah itch* (used in the East Indies). **Asiatic s.** SCHISTOSOMIASIS JAPONICA. **bladder s.** SCHISTOSOMIASIS HAEMATOBIA. **cerebral s.** A form of schistosomiasis due to eggs lodging in the brain, which may occur with any of the infecting species, but is most common in *Schistosoma japonicum* infections. **cutaneous s.** SCHISTOSOME DERMATITIS. **eastern s.** SCHISTOSOMIASIS JAPONICA. **s. haematobia** Infection with *Schistosoma haematobium.* Disease is a result of invasion of the urinary tract by eggs, and is characterized by cystitis and terminal hematuria. Obstructive uropathy, chronic bacteriuria, and bladder carcinoma are well-established complications. Calcification of the urinary bladder is commonly seen on abdominal radiography. Also *bladder schistosomiasis, urinary schistosomiasis, Egyptian hematuria, endemic hematuria, vesical schistosomiasis.* **hepatic s.** Schistosomiasis with accumulation of schistosome ova in the liver. The liver involvement causes fibrosis and presinusoidal portal hypertension. **intestinal s.** SCHISTOSOMIASIS MANSONI. **s. japonica** Infection with *Schistosoma japonicum,* the most severe of the infections caused by human schistosomes, confined to east and southeast Asia. Large intestine involvement is often accompanied by hepatosplenic disease and portal hypertension. There may be hypersplenism. Ascites and anemia may be complications although hepatocellular function is usually well preserved. An early acute hypersensitivity manifestation is called Katayama syndrome. Also *Asiatic schistosomiasis, urticarial fever, Japanese schistosomiasis, Oriental schistosomiasis, Kinkiang fever, Kinkian fever, schistosomiasis japonicum, Yangtze Valley fever, eastern schistosomiasis, Hankow fever.* **s. mansoni** Infection with *Schistosoma mansoni.* The disease is caused by the host tissue response to the invasion of the wall of the large intestine and liver by the eggs. There is focal granulomatous large-intestine involvement, sometimes accompanied by polyposis and protein-losing enteropathy. Heavy infections proceed to hepatosplenic disease and subsequent portal hypertension. There may also be hypersplenism. Also *intestinal schistosomiasis, Manson schistosomiasis, Manson's disease.* **oriental s.** SCHISTOSOMIASIS JAPONICA. **pulmonary s.** A type of pneumonia caused by migrating schistosome cercariae. It can also be caused by embolization of pulmonary arterioles due to eggs or adult worms. Allergic asthma or emphysema may also occur. **rectal s.** A form of schistosomiasis involving schistosome eggs in rectal blood vessels and adjoining tissues. It normally occurs in *Schistosoma mansoni* infection, but may also develop in *S. japonicum* and *S. haematobium* infections. **urinary s.** SCHISTOSOMIASIS HAEMATOBIA. **vesical s.** SCHISTOSOMIASIS HAEMATOBIA.

**schistosomicidal** \shis′təsōmisī′dəl, skis′-\ Destructive to schistosomes. Also *schistosomacidal.*

**schistosomicide** \shis′təsō′misīd, skis′-\ [*Schistosom(a)* + *i* + -CIDE] An agent that kills schistosomes. Also *schistosomacide.*

***Schistosomum*** \shis′təsō′məm, skis′-\ A former name for *SCHISTOSOMA.*

**schistosternia** \-stur′nē·ə\ [SCHISTO- + Gk *stern(on)* breast, chest + -IA] A cleft of the sternum of developmental origin. Also *sternum bifidum.*

**schistothorax** \-thôr′aks\ [SCHISTO- + THORAX] Congenital cleft of the thoracic body wall. Also *schizothorax.*

**schistotrachelus** \-trəkē′ləs\ [SCHISTO- + TRACHEL- + New L *-us,* noun suffix] A fetus or postnatal individual with a congenital cleft of the neck.

**schiz-** \skiz-\ SCHIZO-.

**schizamnion** \skizam′nē·än\ Amnion formation by the appearance of a cavity in or just above the inner cell mass, as happens in the formation of the human amnion.

**schizencephaly** \skiz′ensef′əlē\ An abnormal lobation, clefting, or other division of the brain due to defective development. Also *schistencephaly, schizocephalic porencephaly.*

**schizo-** \skiz′ə-, skiz′ō-\ [Gk *schizein* to split, divide] A combining form meaning (1) split, cleft, divided; (2) schizophrenia. Also *schiz-.*

**schizoaffective** \-əfek′tiv\ Having some schizophrenic and some affective characteristics. See also SCHIZOAFFECTIVE PSYCHOSIS, SCHIZOAFFECTIVE DISORDER.

**schizocoelic** \-sē′lik\ [SCHIZO- + *-coel(e)* + -IC] Designating an embryo in which the primitive segments are formed by the breaking into pieces of a continuous band of mesoblast. Compare ENTEROCOELIC.

**schizocortex** \-kôr′teks\ The entorhinal cortex, conceived as formed by discontinuous migration, showing a developmental split between inner and outer layers.

**schizocyte** \skiz′əsīt\ [SCHIZO- + -CYTE] An abnormally shaped erythrocyte that appears to have been the effect of shearing, tearing, or fragmentation. Schizocytes may have any of several shapes, resembling helmets (helmet cells), collar buttons, three-cornered hats, arrowheads, fish, etc. They are the result of mechanical shearing of the cells, as across a strand of fibrin, in tortuous capillaries, or in turbulent blood flow. Also *schistocyte.*

**schizocytosis** \-sītō′sis\ The presence of schizocytes in the blood. Also *schistocytosis.*

**schizogenesis** \-jen′əsis\ Reproduction or origin by fission. Also *scissiparity.*

**schizogenous** \skizäj′ənəs\ Reproducing by fission.

**schizogony** \skizäg′ənē\ [SCHIZO- + -GONY] Multiple fission in which the nucleus first divides into a number of nuclei, after which the cytoplasm is apportioned around each daughter nucleus. If the process occurs within the mother cell, it is termed endodyogeny (for two) or endopolygeny (for more than two). This type of cell division is characteristic of the asexual reproductive stage in the life cycle of *Plasmodium* and many other sporozoan protozoa. Also *agamocytogeny, agamogenesis, agamogony, merogony.*

**schizogyria** \-jī′rē·ə\ [SCHIZO- + GYR- + -IA] A dysmorphia of cerebral convolutions characterized by occasional interruptions in their continuity.

**schizoid** \skit′soid, skiz′oid\ [SCHIZ- + -OID] **1** Denoting any psychiatric disorder other than schizophrenia itself that occurs in family members of a known schizophrenic, or that occurs more frequently in families of schizophrenics than in families without a known schizophrenic member. **2** Referring to a genetically determined predisposition or vulnerability to the development of schizophrenia. **3** See under SCHIZOID PERSONALITY. **4** Employing the mechanism of splitting as a major defense.

**schizokinesis** \-kīnē′sis\ The condition of extinguishing a specific response in behavioral conditioning while the nonspecific responses persist.

**schizomycete** \-mīsēt′\ *Obs.* BACTERIUM.

**schizomycosis** \-mīkō′sis\ [SCHIZO- + MYCOSIS] Any disease caused by schizomycetes (prokaryotes); bacterial disease.

**schizont** \skiz′änt\ [SCHIZ- + Gk *ont(os)*, gen. of *ōn*, pres. part. of *einai* to be] A sporozoan trophozoite that reproduces by schizogony, producing daughter trophozoites or merozoites. Also *agamont, monont* (obs.).

**schizonticide** \skizän′tisīd\ Any antimalarial agent that destroys the parasites at the schizont stage of their life cycle, such as quinine.

**schizophasia** \skit′sōfā′zhə, skiz′ō-\ Word salad accompanied by markedly disordered thinking, seen in schizophrenics.

**schizophrenia** \skit′səfrē′nē·ə, skiz′ō-\ [SCHIZO- + -PHRENIA] Any of a group of disorders characterized by a progressive deterioration of the entire personality manifested in disorders of feeling, thinking, and conduct, and a tendency to withdraw from reality to an inner world of fantasy, preoccupation with the self, delusions, and hallucinations. The diagnostic criteria for the group vary considerably. DSM-III requires disorganization of a previous level of functioning, psychotic features such as delusions or hallucinations during the active phase, evidence of chronicity including continuous signs of the illness for at least six months, and disturbance in multiple psychological processes, such as language, thinking, perception, affect, sense of self, relationship to the external world, volition, or motor behavior. Also *schizophrenic psychosis, parergasia* (obs.), *paleophrenia* (obs.), *chronic dementia* (seldom used), *Morel-Kraepelin disease* (seldom used), *dementia praecox* (older term). **atypical s.** **1** *Imprecise* UNDIFFERENTIATED SCHIZOPHRENIA. **2** *Imprecise* SCHIZOPHRENIFORM PSYCHOSIS. **catatonic s.** A subgroup of schizophrenia characterized by stupor, negativism, rigidity or other bizarre posturing, or catatonic excitement. Also *catatonic dementia.* **childhood s.** *Outmoded* EARLY INFANTILE AUTISM. **hebephrenic s.** A subtype of schizophrenia characterized by general disorganization manifested as marked incoherence of speech, inappropriate or blunted affect, and lack of systematization of delusions. Also *hebephrenic dementia* (older term). **iatrogenic s.** TARDIVE DYSMENTIA. **latent s.** A subtype of schizophrenia in which acute psychotic symptoms and gross break with reality have not developed but the subject's overall life-style, thinking, and affect, including insecure or inadequate object relationships, suggest an underlying schizophrenia. In addition, there is often an overlay of multiple neurotic symptoms or antisocial behavior. Also *prepsychotic schizophrenia, prodromal schizophrenia, pseudoneurotic schizophrenia, pseudopsychopathic schizophrenia.* **paranoid s.** A subgroup of schizophrenia characterized by persecutory or grandiose delusions or hallucinations or delusional jealousy, with a tendency toward systematization of delusions. Also *dementia paranoides* (outmoded), *heboid paranoia* (obs.). **prepsychotic s.** LATENT SCHIZOPHRENIA. **prodromal s.** LATENT SCHIZOPHRENIA. **pseudoneurotic s.** LATENT SCHIZOPHRENIA. **pseudopsychopathic s.** LATENT SCHIZOPHRENIA. **residual s.** The condition of a subject following an acute episode of schizophrenia, when evidence of the basic disorder remains but prominent psychotic symptoms are lacking. **schizoaffective s.** SCHIZOAFFECTIVE PSYCHOSIS. **simple s.** A subgroup of schizophrenia characterized by insidious psychic impoverishment, estrangement, blunting of affect, and banality of thought without prominent psychotic symptoms such as hallucinations or delusions. Also *schizophrenia simplex, heboidophrenia* (outmoded). **undifferentiated s.** A subgroup of schizophrenia characterized by prominent delusions, hallucinations, or gross disorganization of thought or behavior, and a mixture of other symptoms so that it does not readily fit into the classical subgroups of hebephrenic, paranoid, or catatonic schizophrenia. Also *atypical schizophrenia* (imprecise).

**schizophrenic** \skit′səfren′ik, skiz′ō-\ **1** Having the characteristics of schizophrenia. **2** A schizophrenic person.

**schizophreniform** \skit′səfren′ifôrm, skiz′ō-\ Resembling schizophrenia.

**schizoprosopia** \-prōsō′pē·ə\ SCHISTOPROSOPIA.

**schizothorax** \-thôr′aks\ SCHISTOTHORAX.

**schizotonia** \-tō′nē·ə\ [SCHIZO- + *ton(o)-* + -IA] The distribution of muscle tone between flexors and extensors of one or more extremities.

**schizotropic** \-träp′ik\ [SCHIZO- + -TROPIC] Having a special affinity for schizonts.

**schizotrypanosis** \-trip′ənō′sis\ CHAGAS DISEASE.

**schizotrypanosomiasis** \-trip′ənōsōmī′əsis\ CHAGAS DISEASE.

***Schizotrypanum cruzi*** \-trip′ənəm kroo′zī\ *TRYPANOSOMA CRUZI.*

**schizozoite** \-zō′īt\ [SCHIZO- + *zo(o)-* + -ITE] MEROZOITE.

**schlafkrankheit** \shläf′krängk′hīt\ [German *Schlaf* sleep + *Krankheit* sickness] GAMBIAN TRYPANOSOMIASIS.

**schlafsucht** \shläf′zukht\ [German (from *Schlaf* sleep + *Sucht* sickness), lethargy] KLEINE-LEVIN SYNDROME.

**Schlatter** [Carl *Schlatter,* Swiss surgeon, 1864–1934] Schlatter's disease, Schlatter sprain. See under OSGOOD-SCHLATTER DISEASE.

**Schlemm** [Friedrich S. *Schlemm,* German anatomist, 1795–1858] Schlemm's canal. See under SINUS VENOSUS SCLERAE.

**schlepper** \shlep′ər\ CARRIER.

**Schlesinger** [Hermann *Schlesinger,* Austrian physician, 1868–1934] Schlesinger's phenomenon, Pool-Schlesinger sign. See under SCHLESINGER SIGN.

**Schlösser** [Carl *Schlösser,* German ophthalmologist, 1857–1925] See under TREATMENT.

**Schmidt** [Henry D. *Schmidt,* U.S. anatomist and pathologist, 1823-1888] **1** Schmidt-Lanterman segment. See under MEDULLARY SEGMENT. **2** Schmidt-Lanterman clefts, incisures of Lanterman-Schmidt. See under SCHMIDT-LANTERMAN INCISURES.

**Schmiedel** [Kasimir Christoph *Schmiedel,* German anatomist and botanist, born 1716] **1** Schmiedel's ganglion. See under INFERIOR CAROTID GANGLION. **2** Schmiedel's anastomoses. See under ANASTOMOSIS.

**Schmincke** [Alexander *Schmincke,* German pathologist, 1877–1953] See under TUMOR.

**Schmorl** [Christian Georg *Schmorl,* German pathologist, 1861–1932] **1** See under FURROW. **2** Schmorl body. See under NODULE.

**Schnabel** [Isidor *Schnabel,* Austrian ophthalmologist, 1842–1908] **1** Schnabel's caverns. See under CAVERN. **2** See under ATROPHY.

**Schneider** [Conrad Viktor *Schneider,* German anatomist, 1610–1680] Schneiderian membrane. See under TUNICA MUCOSA NASI.

**Schoemaker** [Jan *Schoemaker,* Dutch surgeon, 1871–1940] See under LINE.

***Schoengastia*** \shān·gas′tē·ə, shōn-\ A genus of chigger mites. Species of this genus cause scrub itch, a characteristic dermatitis. *S. lynni* and *S. pusilla* are typical examples.

**Scholander** [Per Fredrik *Scholander,* Swedish-born U.S. physiologist, born 1905] **1** See under APPARATUS.

2 Roughton-Scholander method. See under SYRINGE-CAPILLARY METHOD.

**Scholte** [A. J. *Scholte*, Austrian physician, flourished early 20th century] Cassidy-Scholte syndrome. See under CARCINOID SYNDROME.

**Scholz** [Willibald Oscar *Scholz*, German neurologist and psychiatrist, born 1889] Scholz disease, Scholz-Greenfield disease, Scholz metachromatic leukoencephalitis, Scholz-Bielschowsky-Henneberg diffuse cerebral sclerosis, Scholz cerebral sclerosis. See under METACHROMATIC LEUKODYSTROPHY.

**Schönlein** [Johann Lukas *Schönlein*, German physician, 1793–1864] **1** Schönlein-Henoch purpura nephritis. See under NEPHRITIS. **2** Schönlein's disease, Schönlein-Henoch disease, Schönlein's purpura, Schönlein-Henoch purpura, Schönlein-Henoch syndrome, Henoch-Schönlein syndrome. See under HENOCH-SCHÖNLEIN PURPURA.

**Schottmüller** [Hugo A. G. *Schottmüller*, German physician, 1867–1936] Schottmüller's disease. See under PARATYPHOID FEVER.

**Schramm** [Hilary *Schramm*, Polish physician, born 1857] See under PHENOMENON.

**Schreger** [Christian H. T. *Schreger*, Danish anatomist, 1768–1833] Bands of Schreger, bands of Hunter-Schreger, Schreger striae. See under SCHREGER'S LINES

**Schroeder** [Jacob Ludwig Conrad *Schroeder* van der Kolk, Dutch physiologist, 1797–1862] **1** Schroeder's fibers. See under STILLING'S FIBERS. **2** Van der Kolk's law. See under SCHROEDER VAN DER KOLK'S LAW.

**Schroetter** [Leopold von *Schroetter*, Austrian laryngologist, 1837–1908] Paget-von Schroetter syndrome. See under EFFORT THROMBOSIS.

**Schuchardt** [Karl A. *Schuchardt*, German surgeon, 1856–1901] See under INCISION.

**Schüffner** [Wilhelm August Paul *Schüffner*, German pathologist active in Indonesia, 1867–1949] Schüffner stippling. See under SCHÜFFNER'S GRANULES.

**Schüller** [Artur *Schüller*, Austrian neurologist, born 1874] Schüller's disease, Schüller-Christian disease, Hand-Schüller-Christian syndrome, Schüller syndrome, Schüller-Christian syndrome. See under HAND-SCHÜLLER-CHRISTIAN DISEASE.

**Schüller** [Karl Heinrich Anton Ludwig Max *Schüller*, German surgeon, 1843–1907] **1** Schüller's glands, Schüller's ducts. See under DUCTUS PARAURETHRALES. **2** Schüller's glands. See under GLAND.

**Schultz** [Werner *Schultz*, German internist, 1878–1947] **1** Schultz-Dale technique. See under SCHULTZ-DALE REACTION. **2** Schultz disease, Werner Schultz disease, Schultz syndrome. See under AGRANULOCYTOSIS.

**Schultze** [Bernard Sigismund *Schultze*, German obstetrician and gynecologist, 1827–1919] See under MECHANISM.

**Schultze** [Friedrich *Schultze*, German physician, 1848–1934] **1** See under ACROPARESTHESIA. **2** Schultze-Chvostek sign. See under CHVOSTEK SIGN.

**Schultze** [Max Johann Sigismund *Schultze*, German histologist and zoologist, 1825–1874] **1** Bundle of Schultze, Schultze's tract, comma tract of Schultze. See under FASCICULUS INTERFASCICULARIS. **2** See under SIGN.

**Schumm** [Otto *Schumm*, German biochemist, born 1874] **1** See under TEST. **2** Schumm's test. See under BENZIDINE TEST.

**Schütz** [Hugo *Schütz*, German neurologist and anatomist, flourished early 20th century] Schütz bundle, tract of Schütz. See under FASCICULUS LONGITUDINALIS DORSALIS.

**Schwabach** [Dagobert *Schwabach*, German otologist, 1846–1920] See under TEST.

**Schwalbe** [Albert Gustav *Schwalbe*, German anatomist and anthropologist, 1844–1917] **1** Schwalbe's fissure. See under FISSURA CHOROIDEA. **2** See under LINE, HIATUS. **3** Schwalbe's nucleus. See under NUCLEUS VESTIBULARIS MEDIALIS. **4** Schwalbe spaces. See under SPATIA INTERVAGINALIA NERVI OPTICI. **5** Schwalbe's corpuscle. See under CALICULUS GUSTATORIUS. **6** Schwalbe's anterior border ring. See under SCHWALBE'S RING.

**Schwann** [Theodor *Schwann*, German anatomist, 1810–1882] **1** Schwann's membrane, sheath of Schwann. See under NEURILEMMA. **2** Schwann hyperplasia. See under HEREDITARY HYPERTROPHIC INTERSTITIAL NEUROPATHY. **3** Schwann's white substance. See under SUBSTANTIA ALBA. **4** See under CELL. **5** Schwann cell tumor. See under NEURILEMMOMA.

**schwannoglioma** \shwän′ōglī·ō′mə\ [*schwanno(ma)* + GLIOMA] NEURILEMMOMA.

**schwannoma** \shwänō′mə\ [*Schwann (cell)* + -OMA] NEURILEMMOMA. **granular cell s.** GRANULAR CELL TUMOR. **malignant s.** A densely cellular tumor, consisting of plump, spindle-shaped or ovoid cells of Schwann cell type, generally showing little cellular pleomorphism and often accompanied by collagen fibers. Nuclear palisading, as well as an arrangement of the cells in groups, nests, cords or whorls, are features helpful in the differential diagnosis. Origin from a preexisting neurofibroma is frequent. Metastases are frequent. Also *malignant neurinoma, malignant neurofibroma, fibrosarcoma of the nerve sheath, neurofibrosarcoma, malignant neuroma, neurosarcoma, schwannosarcoma, neurogenic sarcoma, sarcoma of peripheral nerve, malignant peripheral glioma.*

**Schwartman** See under SHWARTZMAN.

**Schwartz** [Oscar *Schwartz*, U.S. pediatrician, born 1919] Schwartz-Jampel syndrome. See under CHONDRODYSTROPHIC MYOTONIA.

**Schwartz** [Samuel *Schwartz*, U.S. physician, born 1916] Watson-Schwartz reaction. See under TEST.

**Schwartz** [William Benjamin *Schwartz*, U.S. physician, born 1922] Bartter-Schwartz syndrome. See under SCHWARTZ-BARTTER SYNDROME.

**Schwartze** [Hermann Hugo Rudolf *Schwartze*, German otologist, 1837–1910] **1** Schwartze mastoidectomy, Schwartze's operation. See under SIMPLE MASTOIDECTOMY. **2** See under SIGN.

**Schwartzman** See under SHWARTZMAN.

**Schweigger-Seidel** [Franz *Schweigger-Seidel*, German physiologist, 1834–1871] See under SHEATH.

**schwelle** \shvel′ə\ [German, threshold] THRESHOLD.

**scia-** \sī′ə-\ SKIA-.

**scialyscope** \sī·al′iskōp\ [SCIA- + *ly(sis)* + -SCOPE] An optical device used to project the image of a surgical field into a darkened room adjacent to the operating room.

**sciatic** \sī·at′ik\ [Late L *sciaticus* (from Gk *ischiadikos* ischial, of the hip) pertaining to the hip or to pain in the hip] Of or relating to the hip joint or the ischium; ischial.

**sciatica** \sī·at′ikə\ A sciatic neuralgia with pain in the lumbosacral region that radiates down the back of the thigh, the lateral aspect of the leg, and into the foot. It results from involvement of the sciatic nerve roots or trunk by tumor, intervertebral disk, or inflammation. It may be accompanied by a neurologic deficit of the reflexes, muscle power, or sensation in the involved lower extremity. Also *ischiatitis* (obs.), *sciatic neuritis, sciatic neuralgia, Cotugno's disease.*

**SCID** severe combined immunodeficiency.

**science** [L *scientia* (from *sciens*, gen. *scientis*, pres. part. of *scire* to know + *-ia* -Y) knowledge, science] Knowledge of facts and phenomena subject to verification, as by experimentation, and the formulation of theory to account for them and to predict other relationships subject to verification. **food s.** 1 The study of the chemical, physical, biochemical, and biophysical properties of foods and their constituents. 2 The study of the preparation and processing of foods and the impact of these processes on their nutrient content. **forensic s.** The application of scientific principles, theory, and practice to problems encountered in law enforcement and the administration of justice. Also *criminalistics.* **life s.'s** All of those sciences dealing with life forms, including the biological sciences and branches of the physical sciences relating to the composition and environment of living organisms. **natural s.** Any of the sciences dealing with the physical universe, as physics, chemistry, or biology.

**scientist** One trained in the methods of science.

**scilla** \sil′ə\ SQUILL.

**scinti-** \sin′ti-, sin′tē-\ [L *scintilla* a spark] A combining form denoting scintillation.

**scintiangiography** \sin′tē·an′jē·äg′rəfē\ Scintigraphy of the vascular tree and its branches. It can be performed by intra-arterial injection of a radiopharmaceutical, but more commonly is performed with an intravenous injection and rapid imaging with a gamma camera over the area of interest.

**scintigram** \sin′tigram\ [SCINTI- + -GRAM] SCINTISCAN.

**scintigraph** \sin′tigraf\ SCINTISCAN.

**scintigraphy** \sintig′rəfē\ [SCINTI- + -GRAPHY] A clinical diagnostic procedure consisting of the injection, usually intravenous, of a solution containing a radioactive agent with a specific affinity for an organ or tissue of interest, followed by the determination, with the aid of a special external detector (scintiscanner or gamma camera) of the distribution of radioactivity.

**scintillant** \sin′tilənt\ SCINTILLATOR.

**scintillation** \sin′tilā′shən\ [L *scintillatio* (from *scintillatus,* past part. of *scintillare* to sparkle, emit sparks, from *scintilla* a spark) a sparkling, emitting of sparks] A tiny flash of light, especially one produced in certain substances (scintillators) when a photon or an ionizing particle deposits energy in the scintillator by ionizing one or more atoms. The resulting electron vacancies are promptly filled in again, with the emission of light quanta, usually in the visible or ultraviolet wavelengths. Typically there is one scintillation for each ionizing event. The flashes can be counted electronically, and the average count rate then measures the intensity of the incident radiation.

**scintillator** \sin′tilā′tər\ A substance that emits light under the influence of ionizing radiation, such as x radiation or gamma radiation, or of ionizing particles. As electrons cascade into the vacant shells of the ionized atoms, the liberated energy is emitted in the form of visible and/or ultraviolet light. Crystalline sodium iodide (thallium activated) is a widely used scintillator in nuclear medicine. There are also organic scintillators, such as anthracene, plastic scintillators, and the liquid scintillators for the low-energy beta emitters. Also *scintillant.*

**scintiphotograph** \sin′tifō′təgraf\ A photographic image obtained by using a scintillation camera depicting the distribution of a radioactive material. Also *scintiphoto.*

**scintiphotography** \sin′tifōtäg′rəfē\ The process of recording on photographic film the radioactivity detected by a scintillation imaging system.

**scintiscan** \sin′tiskan\ [SCINTI- + SCAN] A representation on paper or film of the distribution in a patient or in an organ of a radioactive substance, as detected by a scintillation scanner or gamma camera. Also *scintigraph, scintigram, gamma image.*

**scintiscanner** \sin′tiskan′ər\ A motor-driven scintillation probe with an automatic recording device, producing an image on paper or on x-ray film. The detector is often interfaced with a computer that processes the data to give a more informative reading.

**scion** \sī′ən\ [Middle English *ciun, sioun,* from Old French *cion* a bud, shoot] A part or tissue of one embryo experimentally grafted to a second embryo of the same or a different species. See also CHIMERA.

**sciopody** \sī·äp′ədē, skī-\ [*sci(a)-* + *o* + -POD + -Y] Abnormally large feet, particularly in children.

**scirrhoma** \skirō′mə\ SCIRRHOUS CARCINOMA.

**scirrhous** \sir′əs, skir′əs\ Hard, indurated; relating to a scirrhus.

**scirrhus** \skir′əs\ [New L, from Gk *skiros* or *skirrhos* gypsum, stucco, a hard tumor] SCIRRHOUS CARCINOMA.

**scissile** \sis′īl\ [L *scissil(is)* (from *sciss(us),* past part. of *scindere* to split, cut + *-ilis* -ILE) capable of being split] Capable of being cut or split.

**scission** \sizh′ən\ [L *scissio* (from *scissus,* past part. of *scindere* to cut, tear, divide) a cutting, tearing, dividing] The process of breaking, particularly as applied to a chemical bond between two atoms.

**scissiparity** \sis′ipar′itē\ SCHIZOGENESIS.

**scissoring** \siz′əring\ SCISSOR GAIT.

**scissors** [Old French *cisoires* cutters, from Late L *cisoria,* pl. of *cisorium* a cutting instrument, from L *caedere* to cut. English spelling was altered by L *scissor* a cutter, from *sciss(us),* past part. of *scindere* to split, cut] A cutting implement consisting of a pair of opposing blades that pivot so that their cutting edges come together to exert a shearing force on a material placed between the blades. **Liston s.** LISTON SHEARS. **stitch s.** A surgical device with two blades and handles that is used to facilitate the placement of stitches during the course of an operative procedure.

**scissors-bite** An occlusion in which the crowns of all the lower teeth are completely internal, i.e. lingual to the upper teeth.

**scissura** \sizhŏŏr′ə\ [L (from *sciss(us),* past part. of *scindere* to cut, tear, + *-ura* -URE), a tearing, rending, dividing] An incision or splitting of tissues or organs.

**scissural** \sizh′ərəl\ Pertaining to a cleft or fissure.

**scler-** \sklir-, skler-\ SCLERO-.

**sclera** \sklir′ə\ [New L (from Gk *sklēros* hard)] (*pl.* sclerae, scleras) [NA] That part of the outer fibrous coat of the eyeball which covers its posterior five-sixths and is continuous anteriorly with the cornea and posteriorly with the sheaths of the optic nerve. It comprises the lamina episcleralis, substantia propria and lamina fusca. Also *sclerotic coat, sclerotica, tunica sclerotica, white of the eye, albuginea oculi* (outmoded). Adj. scleral. **blue s.** A hereditary trait characterized by a blue color of the sclera. It is transmitted by a dominant gene.

**scleradenitis** \sklir′adənī′tis\ Sclerous inflammation of a gland.

**scleratitis** \sklir′ətī′tis\ SCLERITIS.

**sclerectoiridodialysis** \sklirek′tō·ir′idōdī·al′isis\ [SCLER- + ECTO- + IRIDO- + DIALYSIS] Removal of a portion of the sclera and separation of the underlying ciliary body from the sclera.

**sclerectome** \sklirek′tōm\ [SCLER- + Gk *ektomē* a cutting out] A surgical instrument for cutting the sclera.

**sclerectomy** \sklirek′təmē\ [SCLER- + -ECTOMY] The removal of a small portion of the anterior sclera to permit aqueous escape as a treatment for glaucoma. Also *scleroticectomy.*

**scleredema** \sklir′ədē′mə\ [SCLER- + EDEMA] An induration of the skin, especially of the face, neck, and upper trunk, that follows an infection. It is a rare disease of unknown origin. Also *scleredema adultorum, Buschke scleredema, sclerema cutis.* **s. neonatorum** SCLEREMA NEONATORUM.

**sclerema** \sklirē′mə\ [SCLER- + *(ed)ema*] A sclerotic state of a tissue. **s. adiposum** SCLEREMA NEONATORUM. **s. adultorum** 1 SCLERODERMA. 2 PROGRESSIVE SYSTEMIC SCLEROSIS. **s. cutis** SCLEREDEMA. **s. neonatorum** Sclerema occurring in severely ill infants, often premature, suffering from diarrheal or other acquired diseases. The subcutaneous tissues become hard with the overlying skin pale, smooth, and cold. Metabolic changes in fat are thought to lead to its solidification. Recovery is rare. Also *Underwood's disease, scleredema neonatorum, sclerema adiposum, sclerema of the newborn, sclerema oedematosum, scleroderma neonatorum.*

**scleriritomy** \sklir′īrit′əmē\ [SCLER- + IRITOMY] Incision through sclera and iris, as for relief of angle-closure glaucoma.

**scleritic** \sklirit′ik\ SCLEROUS.

**scleritis** \sklirī′tis\ [SCLER- + -ITIS] Inflammation of the sclera. Also *leucitis, logaditis, scleratitis, sclerotitis.* **annular s.** Inflammation of the sclera in a ring distribution around the limbus.

**sclero-** \sklir′ō-, sklir′ə-, skler′ō-\ [Gk *sklēros* dry, hard] A combining form meaning (1) hard, hardened; (2) the sclera. Also *scler-, sklero-.*

**scleroblastema** \-blastē′mə\ [SCLERO- + BLASTEMA] Tissue from which the bones of the embryo develop. Adj. scleroblastemic.

**sclerochoroiditis** \-kôr′oidī′tis\ [SCLERO- + CHOROIDITIS] Inflammation of sclera and choroid. Also *scleroticochoroiditis.*

**scleroconjunctivitis** \-kənjungk′tivī′tis\ [SCLERO- + CONJUNCTIVITIS] Inflammation of the sclera and conjunctiva.

**sclerocornea** \-kôr′nē·ə\ [SCLERO- + CORNEA] The outer coats of the eye considered as a unit.

**sclerodactyly** \-dak′tilē\ [SCLERO- + DACTYL- + -Y] Tapering and cutaneous sclerosis or atrophy occurring distal to the proximal interphalangeal joint of the fingers or toes in patients with Raynaud's phenomenon, mixed connective tissue disease, lupus erythematosus, dermatomyositis, vinylchloride poisoning, frostbite, ergotism, scleroderma, and other conditions. When sclerosis occurs on the proximal fingers of the hand, scleroderma is more likely. Also *acroteric morphea, sclerodactylia.*

**scleroderma** \sklir′ədur′mə\ [SCLERO- + DERMA] A local or generalized hardening of the skin, as in progressive systemic sclerosis. Also *disseminated trophoneurosis, primary systemic sclerosis, chorionitis* (obs.), *hidebound disease, skinbound disease, sclerosis dermatis, sclerema adultorum.* **annular s.** Scleroderma occurring as a circular patch or ring; morphea. **circumscribed s.** Scleroderma limited to one or more small areas of the skin, as in morphea. **diffuse s.** Scleroderma covering large areas of the skin, in either a contiguous or noncontiguous fashion. **generalized s.** Widespread scleroderma without systemic involvement. **linear s.** Circumscribed scleroderma in a linear distribution, either paramedian of the face and scalp, where it is often associated with facial hemiatrophy, or in a limb, where it is commonly associated with ipsilateral hypoplasia. Also *linear morphea.* **localized s.** MORPHEA. **s. neonatorum** SCLEREMA NEONATORUM. **paramedian s.** Scleroderma that develops in a band at the side of the median line of the forehead and extends into the scalp. See also LINEAR SCLERODERMA. **progressive s.** PROGRESSIVE SYSTEMIC SCLEROSIS. **pulmonary s.** Fibrosis and vascular damage to the lung as a manifestation of scleroderma. **systemic s.** PROGRESSIVE SYSTEMIC SCLEROSIS.

**sclerodermatitis** \-dur′mətī′tis\ SCLERODERMITIS.

**sclerodermatomyositis** \-dur′mətōmi′əsī′tis\ An illness containing features of both scleroderma and dermatomyositis; scleroderma with prominent inflammatory muscle features.

**sclerodermatous** \-dur′mətəs\ Pertaining to or characterized by scleroderma.

**sclerodermitis** \-dərmī′tis\ Sclerosis that follows inflammatory changes in tissues, as in some cases of stasis eczema. Also *sclerodermatitis.*

**sclerogummatous** \-gum′ətəs\ Pertaining to a sclerosing gumma.

**sclerogyria** \-jī′rē·ə\ [SCLERO- + GYR- + -IA] Sclerotic hardening of a convolution of the cerebrum.

**scleroid** \sklir′oid\ [SCLER- + -OID] Hard in texture; indurated; tough.

**scleroiritis** \sklir′ō·īrī′tis\ [SCLERO- + IRITIS] Inflammation of the sclera and iris.

**sclerokeratitis** \-ker′ətī′tis\ [SCLERO- + KERATITIS] Inflammation of both the sclera and cornea.

**sclerokeratoiritis** \-ker′ətō·īrī′tis\ [SCLERO- + KERATO- + IRITIS] Inflammation of sclera, cornea, and iris.

**sclerokeratosis** \-ker′ətō′sis\ [SCLERO- + KERATOSIS] Cornification of the scleral surface.

**scleroma** \sklirō′mə\ [SCLER- + -OMA] A progressive granulomatous disease of the upper respiratory tract, usually confined to the nose, and generally considered to be due to *Klebsiella rhinoscleromatis.* It occurs mainly in subtropical localities where the standard of domestic hygiene is poor. A stage resembling atrophic rhinitis is followed by the formation of firm nodules and, later, scarring, deformity, and stenosis. Prolonged treatment with antibiotics and steroids may help but radical surgery has also been advocated.

**scleromalacia** \-məlā′shə\ [SCLERO- + MALACIA] A thinning of the sclera, seen clinically by visibility of the uvea through the sclera, most commonly associated with chronic rheumatoid arthritis.

**scleromeninx** \-mē′ningks\ DURA MATER.

**scleromere** \sklir′əmir\ [SCLERO- + -MERE] A dense, mesenchymatous mass grouped around the notochord, and resulting from the migration of the sclerotome from the corresponding somite at the same metameric level. The scleromere, proof of the segmental origin of the vertebral axis, eventually participates in the construction of two adjacent vertebrae, and of the intervertebral disk that separates them. As a result, the definitive vertebral bodies have an intersegmental constitution.

**scleronyxis** \-nik′sis\ SCLEROTOMY.

**sclero-oophoritis** \-ō′əfôrī′tis\ [SCLERO- + OOPHORITIS] Ovarian inflammation associated with a thick ovarian capsule.

**sclerophthalmia** \sklir′äfthal′mē·ə\ [SCLER- + OPHTHALMIA] A developmental abnormality of the eye in which the opacity of the sclera has encroached upon the cornea to the extent that a much reduced area of transparency remains near the center of the cornea.

**scleroprotein** \-prō′tēn\ In an old classification of proteins, any that could not be dissolved in acid or alkali. This included collagen and keratin.

**sclerosal** \sklirō′səl\ SCLEROUS.

**sclerosant** A chemical irritant that produces inflammation and subsequent fibrosis and obliteration of the lumen when injected into a vein. It is used in the treatment of varicose veins.

**sclerose** \sklirōz′\ To undergo sclerosis; harden.
**sclerosed** \sklirōzd′\ Characterized by sclerosis; indurated.
**sclérose en plaques** \sklärōz′ äN pläk′ \ MULTIPLE SCLEROSIS.
**sclerosing** \sklirō′zing\ Tending to sclerose: used especially of disorders characterized by sclerosis.

# sclerosis

**sclerosis** \sklirō′sis\ [Gk *sklērōsis* (from *sklēros* hard) hardening, solidification] **1** A hardening of the interstitial connective tissue following damage to the parenchyma of an organ. The hardening is due to increases in the amount of interstitial fibrous connective tissue. **2** In the brain and spinal cord, any of a number of pathologic processes of varying etiology characterized in varying degree by degeneration, or demyelination, of white matter, and usually to a lesser extent of gray matter, with consequent gliosis. **acute diffuse familial infantile cerebral s.** KRABBE'S DISEASE. **Alzheimer s.** ALZHEIMER'S DISEASE. **amyotrophic lateral s.** One form of motor neuron disease in which the earliest manifestations are usually those of spastic paraparesis due to degeneration in the pyramidal tracts and signs of muscular weakness, atrophy, and fasciculation. Bulbar paralysis due to involvement of the anterior horn cells of the spinal cord or the motor nuclei of the cranial nerves usually appear later. A familial variety, often associated with a parkinsonian syndrome, has been described in the Chamorro race on the island of Guam. Also *lateral cord and associated anterior cornual syndrome, progressive lateral sclerosis, Charcot syndrome.* • Whereas it is generally agreed that three main types of clinical presentation (progressive bulbar palsy, progressive muscular atrophy, and amyotrophic lateral sclerosis) commonly occur in motor neuron disease, some authors, especially in the United States, use the term *amyotrophic lateral sclerosis* to identify the disease as a whole. **annular s.** Sclerosis occurring in a ringlike distribution around the periphery of the spinal cord. **anterolateral s.** Sclerosis of the anterior and lateral columns of the spinal cord. Also *ventrolateral sclerosis.* **arterial s.** ARTERIOSCLEROSIS. **arteriocapillary s.** ARTERIOSCLEROSIS. **arteriolar s.** ARTERIOLOSCLEROSIS. **atrophic s.** PICK'S DISEASE. **Baló's concentric s.** BALÓ'S DISEASE. **bone s.** EBURNATION. **bulbar multiple s.** Multiple sclerosis in which the brunt of the pathologic process falls upon the brainstem. **Canavan's diffuse s.** VAN BOGAERT'S FAMILIAL AXONAL SPONGY DEGENERATION. **central areolar choroidal s.** AREOLAR CHOROIDOPATHY. **cerebral centrolobar s.** SCHILDER'S DISEASE. **cerebral diffuse s.** Any of a group of degenerative disorders of the brain, many of which are genetically determined and all of which give rise to progressive sclerosis. Also *diffuse cerebral sclerosis, aplasia axialis corticalis congenita.* **cerebrospinal s.** MULTIPLE SCLEROSIS. **choroidal s.** A degenerative change of the choroid in which diffuse loss of pigment occurs, along with thickening and opacification of the vessel walls. **combined s.** SUBACUTE COMBINED DEGENERATION OF THE SPINAL CORD. **s. of corpora cavernosa** PEYRONIE'S DISEASE. **dentinal s.** SCLEROTIC DENTIN. **s. dermatis** SCLERODERMA. **diaphyseal s.** PROGRESSIVE DIAPHYSEAL DYSPLASIA. **diffuse cerebral s.** CEREBRAL DIFFUSE SCLEROSIS. **diffuse cortical s.** ALPERS SYNDROME. **diffuse infantile familial s.** Any familial form of cerebral diffuse sclerosis occurring in infancy, such as Krabbe's disease. **diffuse mesangial s.** Increase in mesangial matrix and resultant widening of the mesangial stalk (diffuse glomerulosclerosis), or of peripheral lobules (nodular glomerulosclerosis). Diffuse mesangial sclerosis is a feature of several glomerular disorders, including focal glomerulosclerosis, diabetic glomerulosclerosis, hypertensive disease, hepatic disease, and others. **diffuse systemic s.** PROGRESSIVE SYSTEMIC SCLEROSIS. **disseminated s.** MULTIPLE SCLEROSIS. **dorsolateral s.** Sclerosis, demyelination, or degeneration of the posterior and lateral columns of the spinal cord. **Erb s.** PRIMARY LATERAL SCLEROSIS. **familial centrolobar s.** PELIZAEUS-MERZBACHER DISEASE. **familial centrolobular s.** PELIZAEUS-MERZBACHER DISEASE. **focal s.** MULTIPLE SCLEROSIS. **gastric s.** LINITIS PLASTICA. **glomerular s.** GLOMERULOSCLEROSIS. **hereditary spinal s.** FRIEDREICH'S DISEASE. **insular s.** MULTIPLE SCLEROSIS. **Krabbe type diffuse s.** KRABBE'S DISEASE. **laminar cortical s.** Sclerosis involving specific layers (laminae) of the central cerebral white matter. **lateral s.** Any degenerative or demyelinating disease involving the lateral white columns of the spinal cord and especially the pyramidal tracts. Also *lateral spinal sclerosis.* **lateral spinal s.** LATERAL SCLEROSIS. **lobar s.** PICK'S DISEASE. **mantle s.** Nodular gliosis of the cerebral cortex as seen in some individuals with cerebral palsy. **Marie s.** MARIE'S HEREDITARY CEREBELLAR ATAXIA. **mesial temporal s.** Sclerosis of the medial part of one temporal lobe, involving particularly the hippocampal gyrus and the amygdala. It is important in the pathogenesis of temporal lobe epilepsy and thought to be due to birth trauma or perinatal hypoxia. **Mönckeberg s.** A degenerative arteriosclerosis involving the medium-sized peripheral arteries, especially such arteries as the brachial, radial, and leg arteries, with fibrotic and calcific changes in the medial coat with little effect on the intima or lumen of the vessel. Also *Mönckeberg's degeneration, Mönckeberg's mesarteritis, Mönckeberg's arteriosclerosis, Mönckeberg's medial sclerosis, medial arteriosclerosis, medial calcification.* **multiple s.** A demyelinating disease of the central nervous system, common in cold and temperate climates, rare in the tropics, and usually developing in young adults, though it can present at any age and in either sex. The condition gives rise to plaques of demyelination with relative sparing of axons, scattered throughout the brain and spinal cord. It is believed to be due to a process of hypersensitivity which may be precipitated by infection with one or more viruses, but a slow virus infection has also been postulated as the direct cause. Typically it gives rise to recurring episodes of neurologic dysfunction followed by remission, and though many benign cases of long duration have been reported, in many cases the course is ultimately steadily progressive. Among the common presenting symptoms are retrobulbar neuritis, loss of proprioceptive sensation in one or more limbs, spastic weakness of the legs, vertigo, cerebellar ataxia, and many more. Charcot's triad (dysarthria, nystagmus, intention tremor) is rare, occurring only in those cases presenting with a predominantly cerebellar affliction. The average duration of the illness is between 10 and 40 years. In cases demonstrating the final common path of spastic paraparesis and sensory loss, sphincter dysfunction and consequent urinary infection are common. Epilepsy is an uncommon manifestation, while dysphasia and hemiplegia are rare. Euphoria or depression is common, and some few patients show a progressive dementia. Also *multilocular sclerosis, disseminated sclerosis, multilocular neuraxitis, polysclerosis, insular sclerosis, sclérose en plaques, cerebrospinal sclerosis, focal sclerosis.* **nodular s.** ATHEROSCLEROSIS. **nuclear s.** NUCLEAR CATARACT. **Pelizaeus-Merzbacher s.** PELIZAEUS-MERZBACHER DISEASE. **Pelizaeus-Merzbacher type diffuse s.** PELIZAEUS-MERZBACHER DISEASE. **posterior s.** TABES DORSALIS. **posterior spinal s.** TABES DORSALIS. **presenile s.** PRESENILE DEMENTIA. **primary lateral s.** Degeneration of the pyramidal tracts in the lateral column of the spinal cord, giving rise to spastic paraparesis. It is of unknown cause but usually proves ultimately to be due to either multiple sclerosis or amyotrophic lateral sclerosis. Also *Erb sclerosis, primary spastic paraplegia.* **primary systemic s.** SCLERODERMA. **progressive lateral s.** AMYOTROPHIC LATERAL SCLEROSIS. **progressive systemic s.** An illness of unknown cause, characterized by cutaneous sclerosis, Raynaud's phenomenon, telangiectasia, esophageal dysmotility, and, often, muscle, cardiac, pulmonary, and renal disease. The illness is related to and classified with the collagen diseases. Also *systemic scleroderma, diffuse systemic sclerosis, systemic sclerosis, progressive scleroderma, sclerema adultorum.* **Scholz-Bielschowsky-Henneberg diffuse cerebral s.** METACHROMATIC LEUKODYSTROPHY. **Scholz cerebral s.** METACHROMATIC LEUKODYSTROPHY. **subendocardial s.** 1 ENDOCARDIAL FIBROELASTOSIS. 2 ENDOMYOCARDIAL FIBROSIS. **sudanophilic diffuse s.** Diffuse cerebral sclerosis in which there is an accumulation of sudanophilic lipid within the degenerating white matter of the brain. **systemic s.** PROGRESSIVE SYSTEMIC SCLEROSIS. **systemic duodenal s.** Duodenal dilatation occurring in progressive systemic sclerosis. **systemic s. of the kidney** Systemic sclerosis involving the kidney. Characteristic vascular lesions include severe intimal thickening of the interlobular and arcuate arteries due to increased amounts of metachromatic loose connective tissue, resulting in a characteristic "onion skin" appearance. Fibrinoid necrosis is common in the arterioles, as is interstitial fibrosis. Manifestations include slight proteinuria, renal hypertension, and rapidly progressive renal failure. **s. tuberosa** TUBEROUS SCLEROSIS. **tuberous s.** A familial disease, inherited as a dominant trait and giving rise to epilepsy, variable paresis of the limbs and, rarely, cerebellar ataxia along with mental retardation, personality disorders or psychosis, and symmetrical facial sebaceous adenomas. In infancy, it may present with infantile spasms. In the brain there are widespread areas of glial cell proliferation, sometimes including projections into the cerebral ventricles which may be seen on pneumoencephalography. In addition there may be tumors of the viscera, of developmental type, affecting the kidney, heart, stomach, pancreas, or adrenals; polycystic pulmonary degeneration; para- or juxtaventricular intracranial calcification; retinal phakomata; Koenen's tumors; mucous membrane defects; disorders of the skin, teeth, hair, and nails; and other congenital malformations. Also *Bourneville syndrome, Bourneville's disease, Sherlock's epiploitis, epiloia, Bourneville's phakomatosis, Bourneville-Crouzon disease, Bourneville-Pringle syndrome, Bourneville-Brissaud disease, Bourneville-Pelizzi syndrome, sclerosis tuberosa, neurogliosis gangliocellularis diffusa.* **unicellular s.** Fibrosis occurring between glandular cells. **vascular s.** ARTERIOSCLEROSIS. **venous s.** PHLEBOSCLEROSIS. **ventrolateral s.** ANTEROLATERAL SCLEROSIS.

**scleroskeleton** \-skel′ətən\ Bony elements of the skeleton produced by ossification of tendons, ligaments, or fasciae.

**sclerostenosis** \-stenō′sis\ Stenosis marked by induration.

**sclerosteosis** \skliräs′tē·ō′sis\ An inherited autosomal recessive syndrome characterized by osteosclerosis with hyperostosis chiefly of the calvaria, skull base, and mandible. The condition is associated with digital abnormalities and, frequently, with sensorineural deafness and facial paralysis. Also *van Buchem's disease.*

***Sclerostoma*** \skliräs′təmə\ [SCLERO- + Gk *stoma* the mouth] *STRONGYLUS.* ***S. duodenale*** *ANCYLOSTOMA DUODENALE*

**sclerostomy** \skliräs′təmē\ [SCLERO- + -STOMY] SCLEROTOMY.

**sclerotherapy** \-ther′əpē\ 1 A technique utilizing sclerosing solutions to cause obliteration of pathologic blood vessels, as in the treatment of hemorrhoids and varicose veins. 2 PROLOTHERAPY. **endoscopic s.** A nonoperative technique for controlling bleeding esophageal varices in patients with portal hypertension in which sclerosing agents are injected into or around the varices during esophagoscopy. **injection s.** A technique for obliterating veins by injecting a scarifying substance. It is used to treat hemorrhoids, varicose veins of the lower extremities, and esophageal varices.

**sclerotic** \sklirät′ik\ 1 Of, characterized by, or relating to sclerosis. 2 Pertaining to the sclera.

**sclerotica** \sklirät′ikə\ SCLERA.

**scleroticectomy** \sklirät′isek′təmē\ SCLERECTOMY.

**scleroticochoroiditis** \sklirät′ikōkôr′oidī′tis\ SCLEROCHOROIDITIS.

**scleroticotomy** \sklirät′ikät′əmē\ SCLEROTOMY.

**sclerotis** \sklirō′tis\ SCLEROTIUM.

**sclerotitis** \-tī′tis\ SCLERITIS.

**sclerotium** \sklirō′shē·əm\ [Gk *sklērot(ēs)* hardness + L *-ium*, noun suffix] (*pl.* sclerotia) A hard, resting body of fungi which is resistant to unfavorable conditions. It may remain dormant for long periods and germinate on the return of favorable conditions, as with rye ergot or the resistant fruiting structure of some myxomycetes. Also *sclerotis.*

**sclerotized** \sklir′ətīzd\ Made sclerotic; hardened and thickened.

**sclerotome** \sklir′ətōm\ [SCLERO- + -TOME] A surgical instrument used to cut the sclera.

**sclerotomy** \sklirät′əmē\ [SCLERO- + -TOMY] A surgical incision of the sclera. Also *sclerostomy, scleronyxis, scleroticotomy.*

**sclerous** \sklir′əs\ Indurated; hard in texture. Also *sclerosal, scleritic.*

**scobinate** \skäb′ināt\ Possessing an irregular, rough surface.

**scoleces** \skō′ləsēz\ Plural of SCOLEX.

**scoleciform** \skōles′ifôrm\ Resembling a scolex. Also *scolecoid.*

**scoleco-** \skō′ləkō-\ [Gk *skōlēx* (genitive *skōlēkos*) worm] A combining form meaning worm.

**scolecoid** \skō′ləkoid\ SCOLECIFORM.

**scolecology** \skō′ləkäl′əjē\ [SCOLECO- + -LOGY] HELMINTHOLOGY.

**scolex** \skō′leks\ [Gk *skōlēx* a worm] (*pl.* scoleces, scolices) The head, anterior, or holdfast end of a tapeworm by which it attaches in the intestine. It is formed within the cysticercus of *Taenia*, the cysticercoid of *Hymenolepis* tapeworms, on the sparganum of *Diphyllobothrium*, or within the cyst fluid of a hydatid (hydatid sand), among many examples. Particularly complex scoleces are found among the Tetrathyridea and Trypanorhyncha cestodes of sharks.

**scolio-** \skō′lē·ō-\ [Gk *skolios* crooked, bent, curved, winding] A combining form meaning crooked, twisted.
**scoliokyphosis** \-kīfō′sis\ A combined lateral (scoliotic) and posterior (kyphotic) curvature of the spine that is structural in nature.
**scoliolordosis** \-lôrdō′sis\ A combined lateral (scoliotic) and anterior or flattening (lordotic) curvature of the spine.
**scoliometer** \skō′lē·äm′ətər\ An instrument for measuring curvatures of the spine. Also *scoliosometer*.
**scoliosis** \skō′lē·ō′sis\ [Gk *skoliōsis* (from *skolios* crooked, twisted) obliquity, crookedness] A curvature of the spine in which there is an observable and measurable lateral deviation of part of the spine from the normally straight vertical line.

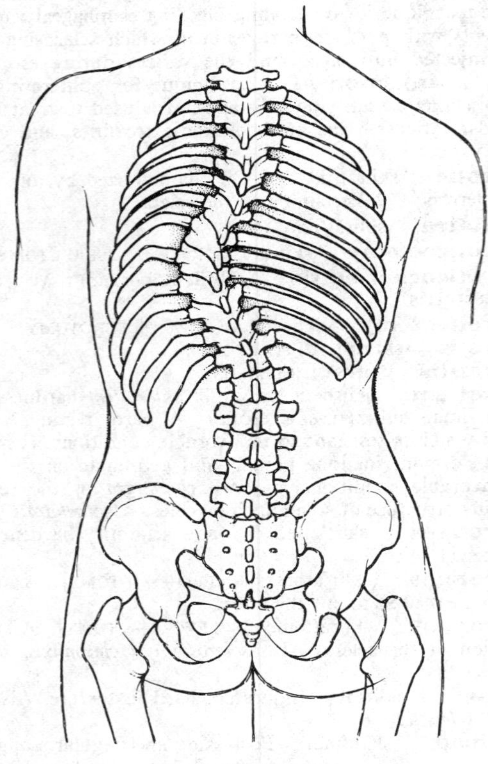
Scoliosis

There may be one curve with secondary compensatory curves above and below the primary curve. The curve may be functional, or postural, disappearing on lying down or on suspension, or it may be structural, when correction by postural change does not take place. Also *lateral curvature*. **cicatricial s.** Scoliosis resulting from the contraction of scar tissue. **congenital s.** Scoliosis that is present at birth. It can be attributed to abnormal segmentation defects, from the abnormal fusion of vertebrae, or the absence of entire vertebral bodies or parts thereof. **coxitic s.** Scoliosis, often postural, that is a consequence of pelvic tilt caused by hip joint disease. **fixed s.** Scoliosis that cannot be passively corrected because of muscle and/or bone deformity. **functional s.** See under SCOLIOSIS. **habit s.** Scoliosis thought to result from a poor sitting posture. **inflammatory s.** Scoliosis due to vertebral disease or infection. **mobile s.** Scoliosis that can be passively corrected by suspension, traction, or lateral bending of the spine. **myopathic s.** Scoliosis resulting from segmental muscle imbalance and weakness due to cerebral palsy, poliomyelitis, or muscular dystrophy. Also *muscular scoliosis, paralytic scoliosis, myogenic scoliosis*. **ophthalmic s.** A tilting of the cervical spine secondary to ophthalmic dysfunction. Also *ocular scoliosis*. **organic s.** STRUCTURAL SCOLIOSIS. **osteopathic s.** Scoliosis due to a disease or congenital abnormality of the vertebral column. **paralytic s.** MYOPATHIC SCOLIOSIS. **structural s.** A lateral deviation of the spine resulting from a disease or disorder of the spinal unit that cannot be corrected passively or by exercise. Also *organic scoliosis, rotoscoliosis*.
**scoliosometer** \-säm′ətər\ SCOLIOMETER.
**scoliotic** \skō′lē·ät′ik\ Relating to or exhibiting scoliosis.
***Scolopendra*** \skō′lōpen′drə\ A genus of centipedes (class Chilopoda) whose venom may cause severe local inflammation, pain, glandular enlargement, fever, vomiting, and vertigo. Species found in the United States include *S. heros* and *S. morsitans*.
**scoop** [Middle English *scope*, from Middle Dutch *schope* a vessel for bailing water, *schoppe* a shovel] A spoonlike surgical implement for lifting small particulate material or fluid, as from a cavity or cyst.
**-scope** \-skōp\ [Gk *skopein* to look at, contemplate, survey] A combining form meaning an instrument for viewing or observing, or providing a means for examination by any method.
**scopolagnia** \skō′pōlag′nē·ə\ VOYEURISM.
**scopolamine** $C_{17}H_{21}NO_4$. 6,7-Epoxytropine tropate. It is a viscous liquid which decays on standing. It is used therapeutically as an anticholinergic agent and as a sedative, as well as a preanesthetic medication. Its actions are similar to those of atropine. Also *hyoscine*.
**scopolamine hydrobromide** $C_{17}H_{22}BrNO_4$. An anticholinergic agent which has been used in veterinary medicine as a preanesthetic medication. It is used in the control of motion sickness and is given subcutaneously or intravenously, or applied topically to the conjunctiva.
**scopomorphinism** Addiction to both scopolamine and morphine.
**scopophilia** \skō′pōfil′yə\ VOYEURISM.
**scoptolagnia** \skäp′təlag′nē·ə\ VOYEURISM.
**scoptophilia** \skäp′təfil′yə\ VOYEURISM.
**-scopy** \-skəpē\ [Gk *skopein* to look at, contemplate, survey] A combining form meaning observation or examination, especially by means of an instrument designed for that purpose.
**scorbutic** \skôrbyoo′tik\ [*scorbut(us)* + -IC] Pertaining to, suffering from, or causing scurvy.
**scorbutigenic** \skôrbyoo′tijen′ik\ [*scorbut(us)* + *i* + -GENIC] Inducing scurvy.
**scorbutus** \skôrbyoo′təs\ [Med L. See SCURVY.] SCURVY.
**score** / **Apgar s.** A numerical index of well-being applied to a newborn infant based on the Apgar test. See under APGAR TEST. Also *recovery score*. **Donaldson s.** A measure of a disabled patient's capabilities in activities of daily living. The system includes self-care and mobility variables and grades 147 separate test items. **Kurtzke disability status s.** One of several scoring systems in use to assess in numerical terms the degree of disability in patients with multiple sclerosis at any moment in time. **LAP s.** See under LEUKOCYTE ALKALINE PHOSPHATASE STAIN. **recovery s.** APGAR SCORE. **standardized**

**s.** A transformation of the data in a frequency distribution such that the transformed variables are distributed around a mean of zero with unit variance.

**scoretemia** \skôr′ətē′mē·ə\ SCATEMIA.

***Scorpio*** \skôr′pē·ō\ A genus of scorpions of north Africa (family Scorpionidae, order Scorpionida). A particularly venomous example is *S. maurus.*

**scorpion** [L *scorpio,* also *scorpius* (Gk *skorpios* a scorpion) a scorpion, a salt-water fish] A venomous terrestrial arthropod in the class Arachnida, order Scorpionida. It is characterized by a five-segmented, flexible, tail-like postabdomen ending in the aculeus or stinger which is carried arched forward over the head. There are four pairs of legs and a large anterior pair of pedipalps with strong distal chelae or pincers. They are nocturnally active predators feeding on other arthropods and similar prey. A pair of venom glands connects via fine ducts to the tip of the stinger. Some 1100 to 1900 people, mostly young children, are said to die annually from scorpion stings in Mexico. In North Africa, deaths from scorpion stings greatly exceed those from snakebite. **devil s.** A scorpion of the genus *Vejovis.* **hairy s.** A scorpion of the genus *Hadrurus.*

**scoto-** \skō′tō-\ [Gk *skotos* darkness] A combining form meaning darkness.

**scotochromogen** \-krō′məjən\ A mycobacterium that forms pigmented colonies even in the dark.

**scotoma** \skōtō′mə\ [Gk *skotōma* (from *skotoun* to darken, blind, from *skotos* darkness) vertigo, dizziness] (*pl.* scotomata) A circumscribed area of blindness or reduced vision within the visual field. Also *aphose.* Adj. scotomatous. **annular s.** A ring-shaped defect of the visual field with intact vision in its center. Also *ring scotoma.* **arcuate s.** An arch-shaped visual-field defect corresponding to the distribution of the temporal nerve fiber layer of the retina. **Bjerrum s.** A type of arcuate scotoma characteristically associated with glaucomatous optic atrophy. Also *Bjerrum sign.* **central s.** A central visual field defect corresponding to the area of the macula. Also *central blindness.* **centrocecal s.** A field defect corresponding to the area of the macula and optic disk and the intervening space. **color s.** A defect in the visual field within which differences in spectral wavelength and the sense of color cannot be recognized. **cuneate s.** A fan- or wedge-shaped scotoma extending laterally from the blind spot and resulting from a lesion involving those fibers of the optic nerve which enter the nasal portion of the optic disk. **flittering s.** TEICHOPSIA. **hemianopic s.** A scotoma involving half of the central field of an eye, whether temporal, nasal, or altitudinal. **insular s.** Any scotoma, wherever situated in the visual field, which is surrounded by areas in which visual perception is normal. **negative s.** A visual field defect of which the individual is unaware. **paracecal s.** A visual field defect adjacent to the blind spot. **paracentral s.** A scotoma involving the visual field close to, but not actually including, the central fixation point. **pericecal s.** A visual field defect surrounding the blind spot. Also *peripapillary scotoma.* **positive s.** A visual field defect of which the individual is aware. **relative s.** A visual field defect in which more intense stimuli are visible. **ring s.** ANNULAR SCOTOMA. **scintillating s.** TEICHOPSIA. **suppression s.** A scotoma, usually permanent, and due to suppression of images from the nonfixating eye in a subject with a concomitant squint. **zonular s.** A central scotoma encircling the fixation point.

**scotomagraph** \skōtō′məgraf\ A type of perimeter used to identify and chart scotomata.

**scotomata** \skōtō′mətə\ Plural of SCOTOMA.

**scotomatous** \skōtō′mətəs\ Pertaining to or affected by a scotoma.

**scotometer** \skōtäm′ətər\ [SCOTO- + -METER] An instrument for recording and measuring the size of scotomata. **Bjerrum s.** A Bjerrum screen, when used for identifying and charting a scotoma.

**scotometry** \skōtäm′ətrē\ [SCOTO- + -METRY] The technique of identifying and measuring scotomata.

**scotomization** \-mīzā′shən\ **1** The development of scotomata in the visual field. **2** The development of figurative blind spots resulting in the suppression of certain items of information and knowledge. *Outmoded.*

**scotopia** \skōtō′pē·ə\ [*scot(o)-* + -OPIA] Vision under conditions of dark adaptation.

**scotopic** \skōtäp′ik\ [*scot(o)-* + *-op(e)* + -IC] Designating the dark-adapted state of vision, in which color perception is replaced by shades of black and white. It is served by the rod photoreceptors.

**scotopsin** The apoprotein of rhodopsin. *Seldom used.*

**scotoscopy** \skōtäs′kəpē\ [SCOTO- + -SCOPY] RETINOSCOPY.

**Scott** [Sir Henry Harold *Scott,* English physician, 1874–1956] Strachan-Scott syndrome. See under SYNDROME.

**scraper** An abrading instrument.

**scrapie** \skrā′pē\ [Scottish Border dialect; prob. so called from the sheep's scraping themselves against things to relieve the itching] An insidious, invariably fatal spongiform encephalopathy of sheep and, rarely, goats, characterized by intense pruritus and severe tremors. It is believed to be a slow infection caused by a prion, and is characterized by an incubation period of two to seven years. See also PRION.

**scraping** A specimen obtained for cytologic or microbiologic examination by abrading the affected area.

**screen** To examine systematically in order to detect from a large group those individuals displaying certain characteristics, such as evidence of a particular disease, for treatment or study. **Bjerrum s.** A large black screen which is used for mapping the central part of the field of vision and which is particularly useful in the identification and charting of scotomata. Also *campimeter screen.* **dream s.** BLANK HALLUCINATION. **fluorescent s.** Any screen impregnated with a material, such as zinc sulfide, which produces light when exposed to x rays. Also *fluoroscopic screen.* **intensifying s.** A screen containing a material such as calcium tungstate which fluoresces when exposed to x rays, and which, when placed in contact with a photographic emulsion, increases the photographic effect of the x rays. In industrial radiography and in radiography with supervoltage x rays and gamma rays, thin sheets of lead are sometimes used as intensifying screens, since electrons knocked out of the lead by the radiation increase the photographic effect. **oral s.** A thin sheet of acrylic resin, metal, or soft rubber molded to fit the dental arches and worn in the oral vestibule as an activator or to prevent mouth breathing. Also *oral shield, vestibular screen.* **tangent s.** A flat testing surface for plotting the visual field. Also *compimeter.* **vestibular s.** ORAL SCREEN.

**screening** The presumptive identification of an unrecognized disease or defect by means of tests, examinations, or other procedures which can be applied rapidly. Screening tests differentiate apparently well persons who may have a disease from those who probably have not. A screening test is not intended to be diagnostic but should be sufficiently sensitive and specific to reduce the proportion of false results, positive or negative, to acceptable levels. Persons with positive or suspicious findings must be referred to their physician for diagnosis and necessary treatment. **chest s.**

A systematic method of obtaining chest radiographs of a certain population in order to screen for lung diseases, especially tuberculosis, or cardiac abnormalities. **genetic s.** Any process used to identify individuals within a population as having a specific genotype. It may be either implicit, as in screening for disease phenotypes known to be inherited as mendelian traits, or explicit, as in screening nucleotide sequences in the genome. The process may be used in population genetic research or in medical genetic services and public health. **multiphasic s.** A form of screening in which a person is subjected to several tests on each occasion, generally for the purpose of screening large numbers of people for a wide range of health conditions or possible illnesses. Multiphasic screening is used, for example, in routine antenatal supervision and school health examinations. Also *multiple screening.* **neonatal s.** The evaluation of a newborn for the symptomatic or asymptomatic presence of various congenital conditions, especially those that can be treated if detected early to prevent or ameliorate their deleterious effects. Conditions for which large-scale screening has been advocated include galactosemia, phenylketonuria, congenital hypothyroidism, and congenital dislocation of the hip. **prenatal s.** 1 The examination of amniotic fluid, fetal cells, or maternal serum for laboratory findings suggestive or diagnostic of congenital abnormalities. 2 The examination of serum from a pregnant woman for the presence of unexpected alloantibodies that might cause a hemolytic disease of the newborn.

**screw / dentin s.** A threaded wire or pin placed in dentin for additional retention of a plastic filling. **expansion s.** A turn-screw incorporated into a removable orthodontic appliance and used to expand the arch, the screw being turned a little way at frequent intervals by the wearer.

**screwworm** The flesh-feeding larva of any of various kinds of calliphorid or sarcophagid flies. *Cochliomyia hominivorax* is responsible for most cases of screwworm myiasis in the Americas. *Chrysomyia bezziana* occupies a similar position in the Pacific and Indian Ocean regions, and the sarcophagid, *Wohlfahrtia magnifica* is found in warmer parts of the Paleoarctic region. **primary s.** A myiasis fly larva that feeds directly upon living flesh rather than necrotic tissues. This type of maggot is an obligate tissue parasite, reaching its host through minute openings as well as wounds or mucous membrane surfaces. Examples include *Cochliomyia hominivorax, Chrysomya bezziana,* and *Wohlfahrtia magnifica.* **secondary s.** A type of screwworm that invades a prior wound, feeding on infected or necrotic tissues. It is a facultative parasite. The adult is a scavenger fly that lays eggs in open sores. The larva feeds on damaged tissues or on the decaying bodies of dead animals or on organic debris. An example is *Cochliomyia macellaria,* the American secondary screwworm fly.

**Scribner** [Belding *Scribner,* U.S. nephrologist, born 1921] See under SHUNT.

**scrobiculate** \skrōbik′yəlāt\ Characterized by pits and cavities.

**scrobiculus** \skrōbik′yələs\ (*pl.* scrobiculi) A pit, cavity or small depression.

**scrofula** \skräf′yələ\ [Late L, dim. of L *scrofa* a brood sow] A syndrome characterized by primary tuberculosis of the cervical lymph nodes, with or without ulceration. *Older term.*

**scrofuloderma** \skräf′yəlōdur′mə\ [*scroful(a)* + *o* + DERMA] 1 TUBERCULOSIS CUTIS. 2 Involvement of the skin overlying tuberculous glands of the neck. Also *tuberculosis colliquativa.* **s. gummosa** TUBERCULOUS GUMMA. **papular s.** LICHEN SCROFULOSORUM. **tuberculous s.** Cutaneous tuberculosis overlying tuberculous lymphatic glands. **ulcerative s.** An ulceration of the skin overlying tuberculous lymphatic glands. **verrucous s.** Verrucous tuberculosis of the skin, particularly in relation to underlying tuberculous glands.

**scrofulous** \skräf′yələs\ Pertaining to or characterized by scrofula.

**scrotal** \skrō′təl\ Of or relating to the scrotum.

**scrotectomy** \skrōtek′təmē\ [*scrot(um)* + -ECTOMY] Surgical removal of all or part of the scrotum.

**scrotocele** \skrō′təsēl\ [*scrot(um)* + *o* + -CELE[1]] SCROTAL HERNIA.

**scrotum** \skrō′təm\ [L (variant of *scrautum* a skin quiver for arrows) the scrotum] (*pl.* scrota, scrotums) [NA] A fibromuscular sac containing the two testes and adjoining parts of the spermatic cords and suspended externally below the symphysis pubis. It consists of skin, the dartos muscle, and the three coats of the spermatic cord that are continuous with it. The skin has transverse ridges and a median raphe continuous with the septum internally, which divides it into right and left compartments. Also *bursula testium, bursa of testes, marsupium, testicular bag, oschea.* **watering-can s.** A multiple fistula of the perineal urethra draining into the scrotum, usually as a result of urethral stricture and infection.

**scruple** \skroo′pəl\ An apothecaries' unit of mass or weight equal to 20 grains, 1/24 apothecaries' ounce, or 1.295 98 gram. An obsolete unit in Great Britain. Symbol: scruple

**SCUBA** self-contained underwater breathing apparatus.

**Scultetus** [Jan *Scultetus,* German surgeon, 1595–1645] See under BANDAGE.

**scultetus** \skultē′təs\ [after Jan *Scultetus* (L form of Schultz), German surgeon, 1595–1645] SCULTETUS BANDAGE.

**scurf** \skurf\ [Middle English, from Old Norse, akin to Old English *sceorf* scurf] PITYRIASIS CAPITIS.

**scurvy** \skur′vē\ [early modern English, assimilated to the adjective *scurvy* but akin to French *scorbut* (New L *scorbutus*) and Dutch *scheurbuik* (akin to Middle Low German *schorbūk,* apparently from *schor(en)* to break + *būk* belly) scurvy, prob. orig. confused with other diseases] A deficiency disease due to a lack of vitamin C in the diet. It is characterized by soft, spongy, swollen gums, particularly in the regions of the papillae between the teeth. The swelling is accompanied by some infection and an offensive mouth odor. Patients without teeth have normal gums. Other symptoms are cutaneous bleeding beginning on the lower thighs as perifollicular hemorrhages (purpura scorbutica) and spreading to the buttocks, abdomen, legs, and arms; petechial hemorrhages arising as a result of ruptured capillary vessels; large spontaneous bruises anywhere in the body; ocular hemorrhages; drying of salivary and lachrymal glands; parotid swelling; femoral neuropathy; edema of the lower extremities; psychological disturbances; anemia; osteoporosis; and sudden death from heart failure. The bleeding is due to the breakdown of intercellular cementing substances which allows seepage of blood from the capillaries. The psychological changes are probably due to the permissive function of ascorbic acid in neurotransmitter synthesis. The bone changes and impaired wound healing are due to some effect on the growth of fibroblasts, osteoblasts, and odontoblasts as well as to the impaired collagen synthesis resulting from an inability to hydroxylate proline and lysine. Also *sea scurvy, scorbutus.* **alpine s.** PELLAGRA. **biochemical s.** A condition in which no vitamin C can be detected in the white blood corpuscles. **infantile s.** The form scurvy takes in infancy, in which the typical manifestation is hemorrhage into bones, particularly of the legs, giving rise to severe local tenderness and pain with pseudoparalysis. Dissecting hematomas occur under the periosteum, and the infant cries on movement. The condition is rapidly curable with the administration of vitamin C and preventable with supplements to cow's milk, which contains little vitamin C. It is rare except in the poorest parts of the world. Also *Barlow's disease, hemorrhagic rickets* (obs.). • At one time scurvy and rickets were confused, and the lesions of bone manifestations of scurvy in infancy were erroneously attributed to rickets. **land s.** IDIOPATHIC THROMBOCYTOPENIC PURPURA. **sea s.** SCURVY. • This was the original name, as it was frequently seen among seamen. **subclinical s.** A condition characterized by low levels of ascorbic acid in the blood and tissues. It is present in many people, especially elderly people, who often have diets containing little fresh fruit or vegetables. Some authorities believe that it is partly responsible for the anemia and other nondescript symptoms of ill health commonly found in old people. Also *subscurvy state.*

**scutate** \skyoo′tāt\ [L *scutat(us)* (from *scut(um)* a shield + *-atus* -ATE) armed with a shield] Shaped like a disk or shield.

**scute** \skʸoot\ A squama, thin lamina, or any scalelike structure. Also *scutum.* **tympanic s.** A thin bony plate forming the lateral wall of the epitympanic recess and separating it from the mastoid air cells.

**scutiform** \skʸoo′tifôrm\ In the shape of a shield.

***Scutigera*** \skyootij′ərə\ A genus of centipedes found in the eastern United States, including the eastern house centipede *S. cleopatra.*

**scutulum** \skʸoo′chələm\ [L, dim. of *scutum* a buckler, shield] (*pl.* scutula) A cup-shaped crusting around the base of infected hairs occurring in favus and caused by *Trichophyton schoenleinii.* Also *favus cup, godet.*

**scutum** \skʸoo′təm\ [L, a shield, protection] (*pl.* scuta) **1** A chitinous plate characteristic of ixodid ticks that covers the entire dorsum of the male. On females or immature ticks, it forms a shield behind the capitulum. **2** SCUTE. **s. pectoris** *Outmoded* STERNUM.

**scybala** \sib′ələ\ [Late L, pl. of *scybalum* (from Gk *skybalon* filth, refuse) dung] (*sing.* scybalum) Dry, hard masses of fecal matter in the intestine, usually associated with constipation.

**scybalum** \sib′ələm\ Singular of SCYBALA.

**scyphoid** \sī′foid\ Cup-shaped. Also *scyphiform.*

***Scytalidium hyalinum*** \sī′təlid′ē·əm hī′əlī′nəm\ A white saprophytic mold capable of causing a ringwormlike infection of the skin and nails similar to that produced by *Hendersonula toruloidea.*

**SD** **1** standard deviation. **2** streptodornase. **3** skin dose. **4** sudden death.

**SDA** **1** specific dynamic action. **2** sacrodextra anterior (a fetal position).

**SDE** specific dynamic effect (specific dynamic action).

**SE** standard error.

**Se** Symbol for the element, selenium.

**seal** [Middle English *seel,* from L *sigillum* (dim. of *signum* a mark, seal, sign) a little image, a figure embossed in a signet] Something used to close or secure firmly. **border s.** PERIPHERAL SEAL. **peripheral s.** The close contact of the margin of a denture with the underlying tissues. Also *border seal.* **velopharyngeal s.** The apposition of the soft palate to the posterior pharyngeal wall as the result of the action of the palatopharyngeal sphincter which seals off the nasopharynx from the oropharynx during swallowing, speaking, singing, etc.

**sealant** \sē′lənt\ **pit and fissure s.** A substance that blocks up the pits and fissures of a tooth without drilling, as a preventive measure against caries.

**sealer** \sē′lər\ A varnish used in filling a root canal.

**sealing** / **fissure s.** The occlusion of developmental pits and fissures in teeth by resins, cements or filling materials to prevent caries at these sites. An acid etch technique is often employed.

**seam** A line of union; raphe. **pigment s.** A finely notched pigmented layer of epithelium that edges the pupillary border of the iris. It comprises branched fibroblasts and melanocytes.

**sea onion** SQUILL.

**Seashore** [Carl Emil *Seashore,* U.S. psychologist, 1866–1949] See under TEST.

**seasickness** Motion sickness brought about in susceptible individuals by the pitching and rolling of a vessel on water. Also *nausea marina.* Also *sea sickness.*

**seatworm** The human pinworm, *Enterobius vermicularis.*

**sebaceous** \sibā′shəs\ [L *sebace(us)* (from *sebum* suet, tallow) of tallow + -OUS] Of or relating to sebum.

**sebi-** \sē′bē-\ SEBO-.

**sebiagogic** \seb′ē·əgäj′ik\ [SEBI- + *-agog(ue)* + -IC] SEBOTROPHIC.

**Sebileau** [Pierre *Sebileau,* French anatomist, 1860–1953] **1** Sebileau suspensory ligaments. See under SUSPENSORY APPARATUS OF THE PLEURA. **2** Sebileau's bands. See under BAND. **3** See under HOLLOW, MUSCLE.

**sebo-** \sē′bō-\ [L *sebum* suet, tallow, fat, grease] A combining form meaning (1) fat, fatty (2) sebum. Also *sebi-.*

**sebopoiesis** \-poi·ē′sis\ [SEBO- + -POIESIS] The production of sebum.

**seborrhea** \seb′ərē′ə\ [SEBO- + -RRHEA] The abnormally copious excretion of sebum. It usually causes the skin to appear oily and it predisposes to the development of acne vulgaris. Also *seborrhea adiposa, hypersteatosis.* **eczematoid s.** SEBORRHEIC DERMATITIS. **nasolabial s.** A redness and scaling in the nasolabial creases typical of vitamin $B_6$ deficiency. **s. sicca** SEBORRHEIC DERMATITIS. **s. squamosa neonatorum** Seborrheic dermatitis occurring in a newborn infant. *Outmoded.*

**seborrheic** \seb′ôrē′ik\ Characterized or affected by seborrhea. Also *seborrhoic, seborrheal.*

**seborrheid** \seb′ôrē′id\ Extensive seborrheic dermatitis characterized by widely scattered lesions.

**seborrhoic** \seb′ôrō′ik\ SEBORRHEIC.

**sebotrophic** \-träf′ik\ [SEBO- + TROPHIC] Stimulating sebaceous secretion. Also *sebiagogic.*

**sebum** \sē′bəm\ [L, suet, tallow, fat, grease] The secretion of the sebaceous glands. It consists mainly of triacylglycerols, wax esters and squalene, with little or no free fatty acid. During the process of excretion, anaerobic bacteria in the pilosebaceous follicles break down some of the triacylglycerol to form free fatty acids. Also *sebum cutaneum.* **s. palpebrale** LEMA. **s. preputiale** Smegma secretion beneath the prepuce.

***sec-*** [*sec(ondary)*] An obsolescent prefix used in organic chemistry to designate the class of isomer known as secondary, i.e., with a branch in the molecule.

**Secernentea** \sē′sərnen′tē·ə\ A class of nematodes characterized by the presence of minute lateral canals opening into the excretory system, and phasmids. Most of the common nematode parasites of humans and domestic animals belong to this group. Also *Secernentasida, Phasmidia* (former name).

**Seckel** [Helmut Paul George *Seckel,* German physician, born 1900] **1** Seckel dwarf. See under ATELIOTIC DWARF. **2** See under SYNDROME.

**seclusio pupillae** \sikloo′zē·ō pyoopil′ē\ A total blocking of the pupillary opening by a 360° posterior synechia (complete adherence of the pupil margin to the lens).

***seco-*** [L *sec(are)* to cut + English *o*] A prefix indicating the breaking of a bond in a chemical structure and its replacement by two hydrogen atoms. It is used in specifying the structure of vitamin D and its derivatives, in which ring B of the steroid skeleton is broken.

**secobarbital** 5-Allyl-5-(1-methylbutyl)barbituric acid. A short to intermediate-acting barbiturate used as a sedative and hypnotic.

**secobarbital sodium** SODIUM SECOBARBITAL.

**secodont** \sē′kōdänt\ SECTORIAL.

**second** [L *secund(us)* following, the second] **1** A unit of time. The SI base unit of time is defined as the duration of 9 192 631 770 periods of the radiation corresponding to the transition between the two hyperfine levels of the ground state of the caesium 133 atom. Symbol: s **2** A unit of plane angle equal to $^1/_{60}$ minute of angle. Symbol: ″ **inverse s.** RECIPROCAL SECOND. **reciprocal s.** **1** A unit of frequency (of a wave or periodic phenomenon) equal to one per second. Also *inverse second.* Symbol: $s^{-1}$ • An obsolete unit. Instead the term *hertz* is usually employed. **2** A unit of activity (of a radionuclide) equal to one per second. • This unit is now generally called *becquerel.* Symbol: $s^{-1}$

**secondaries** \sek′ənder′ēs\ Metastases. See under METASTASIS.

**secondary** \sek′ənder′ē\ **1** Dependent on and following from the occurrence of an existing disease or injury: said of another disease or complication. **2** Second in order of occurrence, as a stage of disease.

**secosteroid** \sē′kōstir′oid\ A steroid in which one ring is opened by breaking a bond within it. Vitamin D and its derivatives are important secosteroids.

**secreta** \sikrē′tə\ [Med L, substantive from L *secreta,* neut. pl. of *secretus,* past part. of *secernere* to sever, separate.] The products of secretion.

**secretagogue** \sikrē′təgäg\ **1** Stimulating a secretory action, especially of exocrine glands. **2** A drug or chemical that promotes or stimulates secretion. For defs. 1 and 2 also *succagogue, secretogogue.*

**secrete** \sikrēt′\ [L *secret(us),* past part. of *secernere* to sever, separate.] To synthesize and extrude or emit, as a gland *secreting* a hormone.

**secretin** \sikrē′tin\ A basic polypeptide secreted by the duodenal and jejunal mucosa in response to acid in the lumen of the intestine. It enters the bloodstream and stimulates the pancreas to secrete a watery juice high in ionic content but low in digestive enzymes, and it promotes, to a lesser extent, the secretion of bile and succus entericus. Also *incretin* (seldom used), *oxykrinin* (obs.). **gastric s.** *Older term* GASTRIN.

**secretion** \sikrē′shən\ [L *secretio* (from *secretus,* past part. of *secernere* to put apart, separate, sever) a separation] **1** The process by which a substance is extruded from cells or glands in the form of a fluid, solute, semisolid, or solid. **2** A material extruded from cells or glands. **external s.** A secretion as through a duct by an exocrine gland into an environment other than the blood or interstitial fluid. **gastric s.** A secretion that consists of the enzymes pepsin, rennin, and lipase as well as mucin and hydrochloric acid (0.16N or 0.5–0.6%). The acid is secreted by the parietal cells and supplies an acid medium for pepsin which is produced by the chief cells and degrades protein to proteoses. Rennin coagulates milk and lipase splits a small fraction of dietary fat. Mucin is produced by the mucous cells. **internal s.** **1** Secretion directly into the blood or an interstitial fluid. **2** HORMONE. **neurohumoral s.** A chemical transmitter substance secreted at synaptic or neuromuscular junctions. **paralytic s.** Secretion that is induced by denervation of a gland.

**secretogogue** \sikrē′təgäg\ SECRETAGOGUE.

**secretoinhibitory** \sikrē′tō·inhib′itôr′ē\ ANTISECRETORY.

**secretomotor** \sikrē′tōmō′tər\ Denoting nerves that stimulate glandular secretion.

**secretor** \sikrē′tər\ **1** An individual who secretes a water-soluble form of the ABO blood group antigens in the saliva and other body fluids. This is an autosomal dominant trait (secretor trait). Eighty percent of the population consists of secretors. **2** The genetic locus, designated *Se* and mapped to human chromosome 19, that determines secretion of the ABO antigens. Also *secretor factor.*

**sectile** \sek′til\ Capable of being cut or cut off from a larger structure.

**sectio** \sek′tē·ō, sek′shē·ō \ [L (from *sectus,* past part. of *secare* to cut) a cutting, section] SECTION. **s. cadaveris** AUTOPSY. **sectiones cerebelli** [NA] Anatomical subdivisions of the cerebellum. **sectiones hypothalami** [NA] Anatomical subdivisions of the hypothalamus. **sectiones isthmi** SECTIONES MESENCEPHALI. **s. mediana** MEDIAN LITHOTOMY. **sectiones medullae oblongatae** [NA] Structural subdivisions of the medulla oblongata. **sectiones medullae spinalis** [NA] Structural subdivisions of the spinal cord. **sectiones mesencephali** [NA] Anatomical subdivisions of the midbrain. Also *sectiones isthmi, sectiones pedunculi cerebri.* **sectiones pontis** [NA] Internal structural subdivisions of the pons. **sectiones telencephali** [NA] Anatomical subdivisions of the telencephalon. **sectiones thalamencephali** Anatomical subdivisions of the thalamencephalon.

**section** [L *sectio.* See SECTIO.] **1** The procedure of making an incision into an organ or tissue. **2** The cut flat surface of tissues or organs. **3** A subdivision of an organ or tissue; a parcel. For defs. 1, 2, and 3 also *sectio.* **abdominal s.** LAPAROTOMY. **cervical cesarean s.** A cesarean section in which the uterine incision is made either transversely or vertically through the lower uterine segment. Also *low cesarean section.* **cesarean s.** The use of an abdominal and uterine incision to deliver the fetus and placenta. Also *cesarean.* **classic cesarean s.** A cesarean section in which the uterine incision is made vertically through the fundus. Also *corporeal cesarean section.* **coronal s.** A vertical section along any coronal plane. Also *frontal section.* **corporeal cesarean s.** CLASSIC CESAREAN SECTION. **cross s.** **1** An incision into tissue or an organ that is perpendicular to the long axis. Also *transection, transsection.* **2** See under CROSS-SECTION. **extraperitoneal cesarean s.** A cesarean section in which the abdominal and uterine incisions are made without entering the peritoneal cavity. This form of cesarean section was most frequently utilized when there was a high likelihood of postoperative infection. **frontal s.** CORONAL SECTION. **frozen s.** A thin slice of tissue that is hardened by freezing and then cut with a microtome. Such sections can be used to provide rapid diagnosis during the course of surgical operations. **ground s.** A thin slice of bony tissue that is prepared by meticulously grinding a flat plate of bone down to a thin wafer. **Latzko cesarean s.** A form of extraperitoneal cesarean section in which the uterine incision is made towards one side of the uterus lateral to the bladder. **low cervical cesarean s.** A cesarean section in which the uterine incision is made either transversely or vertically through the lowest part of the lower uterine segment, the cervix. **low cesarean s.** CERVICAL CESAREAN SECTION. **paraffin s.** A thin slice of tissue that is embedded in paraffin wax and cut with a microtome. **perineal s.** EXTERNAL URETHROTOMY. **Pitres s.'s** An interrupted series of six coronal sections of the brain taken at the prefrontal (one), frontal (two), parietal (two), and occipital (one) lobes. **pituitary stalk s.** Division of the hypophysial stalk. **postmortem cesarean s.** A cesarean section performed in an effort to salvage the fetus following death of the mother. **radical caesarean s.** CESAREAN HYSTERECTOMY. **root s.** RHIZOTOMY. **Saemisch s.** A corneal incision that is supposed to halt the spread of an ulcer. **sagittal s.** A vertical section along the median, or sagittal, plane of the body. **semithin s.** A section of tissue that is embedded in resin and cut at a thickness of approximately one micron, thus making it suitable for examination by light microscopy. **serial s.** A histologic section that is immediately adjacent to the last one prepared, thus permitting an examination of the continuity of a structure. **step s.** One of a series of several histologic sections prepared at roughly even distances through a block of tissue. **transperitoneal cesarean s.** The use of a uterine incision at the uterovesical fold in performing a cesarean section. **transverse s.** A horizontal section through the body or a structure at right angles to both the median and coronal planes. **trigeminal root s.** TRIGEMINAL RHIZOTOMY. **ultrathin s.** A tissue section that is sufficiently thin, measuring 50 to 100 nm in thickness, to permit the transmission of the electron beam in an electron microscope.

**sectiones** \sek′shē·ō′nēz\ Plural of SECTIO.

**sectioning** \sek′shəning\ **surgical s.** Splitting a tooth, especially an impacted tooth, so that it can be removed in several pieces, thus preserving more surrounding bone.

**sector** \sek′tər\ **1** A part of a circular area included within an arc and two radii. **2** In bacteriology, to develop a mutant early in the growth of a colony, resulting in the formation of a sharply defined sector different in appearance (as in color or roughness) from the rest of the colony. **Sommer s.** A region in the pyramidal cell layer of the hippocampal gyrus which is especially vulnerable to hypoxia.

**sectorial** \sektôr′ē·əl\ **1** Of or relating to a sector. **2** Having sharp cutting edges: used especially of molars or premolars. The bite is enhanced by a shearing movement between counterparts in the opposing jaws. Carnivores, insectivores, and bats have dentition of this kind. Also *secodont*.

**secundigravida** \səkun′digrav′idə\ [L *secund(us)* + *i* + GRAVIDA] A woman who is pregnant for the second time.

**secundines** \sek′əndēnz\ [L *secund(us)* following, the second + *-inae*, fem. of *-inus* adjectival suffix] The placenta and fetal membranes.

**secundipara** \sek′əndip′ərə\ [L *secund(us)* following, the second + *i* + PARA] A woman who has had two pregnancies carried to the stage of viability, regardless of whether the fetus was born dead or alive or whether the gestation was single or multiple. Also *deuteripara, duipara*. See also PARA.

**SED** skin erythema dose.

**sedate** \sidāt′\ To calm by treating with a sedative drug.

**sedation** \sidā′shən\ [L *sedatio* (from *sedare* to soothe, allay; see SEDATIVE) assuagement] **1** The production of a calm and restful state, as by the administration of a drug. **2** The influence of a sedative drug, as in *to place under sedation*. **conscious s.** Sedation in which the subject is conscious but free of fear and anxiety by the action of drugs.

**sedative** [New L *sedativ(us)* (from L *sedatus*, past part. of *sedare* to settle, soothe, allay; causative verb for *sedere* to sit, be settled) settling, calming] **1** Producing calmness; relaxing. **2** A drug or agent that produces calmness, relaxes, and reduces excitement. Also *contrastimulant*. **cerebral s.** Any sedative drug whose principal effect is upon the brain. **general s.** A drug or medication that affects all organs and functions in its sedative actions. **respiratory s.** Any drug which suppresses the activity of the respiratory center and of respiratory reflexes and organs.

**sedentary** \sed′ənter′ē\ [L *sedentarius* (from *sedens*, gen. *sedentis*, pres. part. of *sedere* to sit + *-arius* -ARY) working while sitting] **1** Concerning the sitting position. **2** Of or relating to activity that is not physically strenuous.

**sedigitate** \sedij′itāt\ [L *sedigit(us)* (from *se(x)* six + *digitus* finger) six-fingered + -ATE] SEXDIGITATE.

**sediment** \sed′əmənt\ [L *sedimentum* (from *sedere* to sit, lie low + *-mentum* -MENT) a settling, sinking down] A deposit of matter on the bottom of a liquid. **urinary s.** The particulate material present in urine, separated either by gravity settling or, more often, by centrifugation. It consists of cells, casts, crystals, and sometimes microorganisms. The quantity and composition of urine sediment undergo characteristic changes in many renal and nonrenal conditions so that microscopic examination of the sediment of freshly passed urine is often a useful diagnostic procedure.

**sedimentation** \sed′iməntā′shən\ The settling of particles through a fluid in a gravitational, or other accelerational, field. This process occurs when substances are separated in centrifuges. **erythrocyte s.** The gradual settling of red cells which occurs in an undisturbed sample of anticoagulated whole blood. Also *erythrocyte sedimentation reaction, Fahraeus reaction*. See also ERYTHROCYTE SEDIMENTATION RATE. **formalin-ether s.** A technique used to detect parasites in feces. Samples are centrifuged twice, the first time diluted, then with the addition of formalin and ether. The final sediment is examined directly as a wet mount.

**sedimentometer** \sed′iməntäm′ətər\ An instrument for photographic recording of the erythrocyte sedimentation rate.

**sedoheptulose** A $C_7$-ketose, found originally in plants of the genus *Sedum*. Its phosphate is an intermediate in the pentose phosphate pathway and in the Calvin cycle of photosynthesis. The configuration at C-3, C-4, and C-5 of D-sedoheptulose is the same as that of D-fructose; that at C-6 is that of a D-sugar.

**sedoheptulose 7-phosphate** An intermediate in the pentose phosphate pathway and in photosynthesis. It can be formed by the transfer of a glycolaldehyde unit from any of several ketose phosphates onto ribose 5-phosphate, under the influence of transketolase, which carries the group transferred in combination with thiamin diphosphate. It can also be formed by transfer of a dihydroxyacetone (i.e. glycerone) unit onto erythrose 4-phosphate under the influence of transaldolase.

**seed** [Old English *sæd*] **1** To inoculate with microorganisms, as a culture. **2** Semen. **plantago s.** PSYLLIUM. **psyllium s.** PSYLLIUM. **radiogold s.** A small cylinder similar in size to a radon seed but composed of radioactive gold 198 (half-life 2.8 days), and used for interstitial radiation therapy. **radon s.** A hollow gold tube, several millimeters in length and less than a millimeter in diameter, filled with radon gas and used for interstitial radiation therapy.

**Seessel** [Albert *Seessel,* U.S. embryologist, 1850–1910] See under POUCH.

**segment** \seg′mənt\ [L *segmentum.* See SEGMENTUM.] **1** A portion of a larger part or structure, separated by naturally or artificially demarcated boundaries, such as a somite or a metamere. **2** To undergo or cause to undergo segmentation or cleavage. **3** FRAGMENT. • Used in immunology, as in *Fc segment* for *Fc fragment.* **arterial s.'s of kidney** SEGMENTA RENALIA. **body s.** METAMERE. **bronchopulmonary s.'s** SEGMENTA BRONCHOPULMONALIA. **ceratobranchial s.** One of the intermediate portions of the skeleton of a branchial arch, as in the second arch where it becomes the lesser horn of the hyoid. **connecting s.** CONNECTING TUBULE. **differential s.** **1** In cytogenetics, any of those regions of partially homologous chromosomes, such as sex chromosomes and translocation chromosomes, that never align during synapsis; hence, recombination does not occur between loci in these regions. Compare PAIRING SEGMENTS. **2** A region of a chromosome that is inherited without recombining because a homologous segment is not present in the genome (as with the X and Y chromosomes in mammals), because a structural rearrangement prevents synapsis (as in translocated chromosomes), or because of the inviability of the recombined chromosome. Such a region results in a supergene. **epibranchial s.** One of the intermediate portions of the skeleton of a branchial arch, as in the second arch where it gives rise to the stylohyoid ligament. **hepatic s.'s** SEGMENTA HEPATIS. **hypobranchial s.** The lower portion of the skeleton of a branchial arch, as is shown in the second arch where the lower segment becomes part of the body of the hyoid. **internodal s.** The interval between two nodes of Ranvier along a myelinated nerve fiber. Also *interannular segment, Ranvier segment, internode of Ranvier, internode, segmentum internodale.* **s.'s of kidney** SEGMENTA RENALIA. **s.'s of liver** SEGMENTA HEPATIS. **lower uterine s.** The thinned-out isthmic portion of the pregnant uterus which lies just above the cervix. **medullary s.** The part of the myelin sheath of a nerve fiber between two incisures of Schmidt-Lanterman. Also *Schmidt-Lanterman segment.* **mesodermal s.** SOMITE. **muscle s.** MYOTOME. **neural s.** NEUROMERE. **pairing s.'s** Those regions of partially homologous chromosomes, such as sex chromosomes and translocation chromosomes, that align during synapsis. The human X and Y chromosomes pair only at the termini of their short arms, or not at all, indicating quite restricted pairing segments. Compare DIFFERENTIAL SEGMENT. **pharyngobranchial s.** The upper portion of the skeleton of a branchial arch, such as in the second arch where it becomes the styloid process. Between the upper portion and the hyobranchial lower segment lie the intermediate portions called the epibranchial and ceratobranchial segments. **postcommunical s.** PARS POSTCOMMUNICALIS. **PR s.** The segment of the electrocardiogram that extends between the end of the P wave and the beginning of the QRS complex. **primitive s.** SOMITE. **Ranvier s.** INTERNODAL SEGMENT. **renal s.'s** SEGMENTA RENALIA. **rivinian s.** INCISURA TYMPANICA. **s. of Rivinus** INCISURA TYMPANICA. **rod s.** One of the two segments that form a rod process in the retina of the eye. The outer segment is refractile, positively birefringent, contains rhodopsin, and consists of a regular series of discoid double membrane lamellae surrounded by a cell membrane. The thicker inner segment has a fibrillar structure, stains deeply and is divisible into an outer ellipsoid of longitudinally oriented mitochondria and an inner myoid region containing particulate glycogen. The two segments are connected by a constriction containing a cilium. **RS-T s.** ST SEGMENT. **Schmidt-Lanterman s.** MEDULLARY SEGMENT. **spinal s.** A segment of the spinal cord that gives rise to the dorsal and ventral rootlets forming a single spinal nerve. **ST s.** The segment of the electrocardiogram between the end of the QRS complex and the beginning of the T wave. Also *ST-T segment, RS-T segment.* **thin s.** Any one of the narrow, thin-walled segments along the length of the ascending and descending limbs of the loop of Henle in the kidney. **upper uterine s.** The fundal portion of a pregnant uterus, consisting of hypertrophied musculature. **uterine s.** Either of the differentiated parts of the pregnant uterus, the upper or the lower uterine segment. **venous s.'s of the kidney** Portions of the kidney drained by veins accompanying the terminal branches of the renal artery. However, the intrarenal veins have no true segmental organization as they anastomose freely with each other. See also SEGMENTA RENALIA. **venous s.'s of the liver** The segments of the liver drained by the hepatic veins. However, each of the hepatic veins drains more than one of the four recognized segments (segmenta hepatis) and only the left lateral segment is drained by a single major vein, namely, the left hepatic.

**segmenta** \segmen′tə\ Plural of SEGMENTUM.

**segmental** \segmen′təl\ Pertaining to a segment. Also *segmentary.*

**segmentation** \seg′məntā′shən\ [SEGMENT + -ATION] The division of a structure, such as a cell or a fertilized ovum, into similar parts (segments). See also CLEAVAGE. **complete s.** HOLOBLASTIC CLEAVAGE. **haustral s.** The indentation of the lumen of the colon by projecting folds of the mucosa. **metameric s.** METAMERISM. **partial s.** MEROBLASTIC CLEAVAGE. **regular s.** EQUAL CLEAVAGE. **rhythmic s.** Rhythmic sequences of ringlike contractions occurring in the small intestine. **unequal s.** UNEQUAL CLEAVAGE.

**segmenter** \seg′mentər\ A mature schizont in the erythrocytic cycle of the malarial parasite just prior to cell rupture and merozoite release.

**segmentum** \segmen′təm\ [L (from *secare* to cut + *-mentum* -MENT), a piece cut off, shred] (*pl.* segmenta) A section of an organ or part that is a structurally and functionally independent unit; a segment. **segmenta bronchopulmonalia** [NA] The subdivisions of the lobes of the lung. These are independent entities, usually separated from each other by connective tissue septa, each receiving its own bronchus and its own branches from the right or left pulmonary artery. They are designated according to their anatomical position in each lobe and by Roman numerals, from S I through S X. Also *bronchopulmonary segments.* **segmenta hepatis** The subdivision of the lobes of the liver into segments according to the subdivisions of the right and left branches of the common hepatic duct, portal vein and hepatic artery to the respective lobes, each segment being served by main branches of the duct and vessels, namely, segmentum anterius and segmentum posterius of the right lobe and segmentum mediale and segmentum laterale of the left lobe. *Outmoded.* Also *hepatic segments, segments of liver.* **s. internodale** INTERNODAL SEGMENT. **segmenta renalia** [NA] The subdivisions of the substance of the kidney according to the distribution of the interlobar arteries which serve as the end-arteries of the renal artery, as their branches do not anastomose with each other. The segments include segmentum superius, segmentum anterius superius, segmentum anterius inferius, segmentum inferius and segmentum posterius. Also *renal segments, arterial segments of kidney, segments of kidney.*

**segregation** \seg′rəgā′shən\ 1 The separation, in an organism that is heterozygous at a given genetic locus, of the two alleles at meiosis and distribution to two different gametes. 2 The separation of homologous chromosomes during the first meiotic division. **nuclear s.** The process of separating multiple nuclei by division of a bacterial cell. This segregation is necessary before a recessive mutation in one nucleus can be phenotypically expressed.

**segresome** \seg′rəsōm\ A lysosome that contains partly digested organelles and metabolic waste of endogenous origin.

**Seip** [Martin Fredrik *Seip*, Norwegian pediatrician, born 1921] Seip-Lawrence syndrome, Lawrence-Seip syndrome, Berardinelli-Seip syndrome. See under SEIP SYNDROME.

**seisesthesia** \sīz′esthē′zhə\ VIBRATORY SENSIBILITY.

**seismesthesia** \sīz′mesthē′zhə\ VIBRATORY SENSIBILITY.

**Seitelberger** [Franz *Seitelberger*, Austrian neuropathologist, born 1916] Seitelberger's disease. See under INFANTILE NEUROAXONAL DYSTROPHY.

**seizure** [Middle English *seisure* (from *seisen* to seize, from Old French *saisir* to seize, from Med L *sacire* to grasp, take legal possession, akin to Germanic *satjan* to set) a seizing, seizure] 1 A sudden attack of disease. 2 An epileptic convulsion. • See note at FIT. **absence s.** PETIT MAL. **audiogenic s.** An attack of reflex auditory epilepsy. Also *audioepileptic seizure*. **cerebral s.** FOCAL EPILEPSY. **complex partial s.** An attack of minor epilepsy in which loss or impairment of consciousness is accompanied by more complex and dramatic clinical phenomena often regarded as being typical of temporal lobe epilepsy. Also *complex absence*. **cough s.** COUGH SYNCOPE. **drop s.** 1 DROP ATTACK. 2 An attack of akinetic epilepsy. **erotic s.** An attack of focal epilepsy, usually originating in the temporal lobe leading to spontaneous orgasm. **generalized s.** MAJOR MOTOR SEIZURE. **jackknife s.** INFANTILE MASSIVE SPASM. **major motor s.** An attack of major epilepsy. Also *generalized seizure*. **minor motor s.** An attack of minor epilepsy in which there are motor manifestations not amounting to a generalized convulsion. **myoclonic s.** An attack of epilepsy accompanied or characterized by myoclonus. **paralytic s.** An attack of focal epilepsy in which there is inability to speak or to move a part of the body. **photogenic s.** An attack of photic epilepsy. **psychomotor s.** Any of a variety of recurrent attacks of focal epilepsy giving rise to complex behavioral and motor manifestations. The attacks may be affective, confusional, stuporous, or hallucinatory, and may be accompanied by movements of a highly organized but semiautomatic character. Most psychomotor seizures are due to temporal lobe lesions. **reflex anoxic s.** WHITE BREATH-HOLDING. **tonic-clonic s.** An attack of major epilepsy beginning with tonic contractions of muscles followed by repeated clonic contractions of the musculature. **traumatic s.** A seizure due to an epileptogenic focus within the brain resulting from head injury. Also *traumatic convulsion*. **uncinate s.** An attack of focal epilepsy, originating in the uncal area of the temporal lobe, in which the subject experiences an abnormal sensation of smell and/or taste.

**sejunction** \sijungk′shən\ [L *sejunctio* (from *se-* apart, DIS- + *junctio* union, junction) separation, dissociation] BLOCKING OF THOUGHT.

**selection** The process through which some individuals in a population produce more offspring (positive selection) or fewer offspring (negative selection) than others in the population and thus affect the composition of the gene pool. When individuals with favorable phenotypes reproduce more abundantly than others in the population, the genotypes causing the preferred phenotype accrue while other genotypes become less frequent or are eliminated. Natural, or darwinian, selection (that occurring in nature, free of human interference) is a major determinant of the evolution of species. **artificial s.** Any process directed or applied for the purpose of altering the genotype of a breeding population of a particular species. It is usually performed to enhance or increase specific phenotypes through controlled matings of individuals that possess the desired characteristics. Also *selective breeding*. **complete s.** COMPLETE ASCERTAINMENT. **darwinian s.** See under SELECTION. **directional s.** One of the three classes of natural selection, in which occurs a systematic shift in population mean for a trait and in genotype frequencies that favor clustering of phenotypes about the new mean. It is similar to stabilizing selection, except that a new optimum mean phenotype is favored. **disruptive s.** One of the three classes of natural selection in which a breeding population is subjected to a variety of environmental forces that result in more than one optimum phenotype. The genotypes enable these heterogenous phenotypes to reach polymorphic equilibria, in which intermediate genotypes become rare. **germinal s.** 1 The process by which certain phenotypes become more prevalent because certain gametes are more likely to become involved in reproduction. For example, a gonial line containing a mutation may not proliferate as well as the nonmutant line, thus resulting in selection of the wild type trait. 2 A form of artificial selection in which only certain gametes are chosen to be used in the propagation of a species, usually domesticated animals and plants. It is a potential method of positive eugenics in humans. **incomplete s.** INCOMPLETE ASCERTAINMENT. **multiple s.** MULTIPLE ASCERTAINMENT. **natural s.** See under SELECTION. **normalizing s.** STABILIZING SELECTION. **random s.** RANDOM SAMPLING. **sexual s.** A component of selection that favors those dimorphic characteristics of the sexes that serve to attract mates and encourage breeding. **single s.** SINGLE ASCERTAINMENT. **stabilizing s.** One of the three classes of natural selection in which deviant individuals in a population are rejected, or selected against. This process preserves genotypes that produce phenotypes of proven adaptive value and high fitness, reduces phenotypic variance, and eliminates alteration due to mutation, drift, recombination, and immigration. Also *normalizing selection*. **truncate s.** TRUNCATE ASCERTAINMENT.

**selene** \silē′nē\ [Gk *selēnē* the moon] (*pl.* selenai) An object or structure suggestive of a moon or half-moon; lunula. **s. unguium** LUNULA.

**selenium** \silē′nē·əm\ A nonmetallic element having atomic number 34, atomic weight 78.96. It exists in several allotropic forms. There are six natural, stable isotopes and 14 radioactive nuclides and isomers. The element has photoelectric properties that make it technologically useful, as in xerography and in solar cells. It resembles sulfur chemically. Valences are 2, 4, and 6. Some selenium compounds are very toxic, but traces of selenium are essential for liver function. Symbol: Se

**selenium sulfide** A bright orange powder containing 52–55% selenium, used in shampoos to treat dandruff and in medicinal preparations for the treatment of seborrheic dermatitis.

**selenocysteine** The selenium analogue of cysteine. It occurs naturally in some proteins.

**selenomethionine** The analogue of methionine in which selenium replaces sulfur. It can be incorporated into proteins in cell-free systems in place of methionine.

**selenosis** \sē′lēnō′sis\ [*selen(ium)* + -OSIS] Poisoning with selenium, usually due to an excess of sodium selenite.

**self** 1 That aspect of a person which is coherent and enduring, which serves as the integrating core of the personality, and which carries out action and directs behavior. 2 The conscious perception or awareness a person has of his or her body, personality, and characteristic modes of behavior; in psychoanalytic usage, the ego. 3 Those antigens that are a normal constituent of the body of a given individual and to which immunologic responses are normally suppressed. It is based on the concept that the immune system is capable of distinguishing between self and nonself. ⟨"Flawed lymphocytes can turn up with an inability to distinguish between self and nonself, and replication of these can bring down the entire structure with the devastating diseases of autoimmunity." —Lewis Thomas, *The Youngest Science*, 1983, p. 85.⟩ Compare NONSELF. **idealized s.** The person a neurotic believes himself to be, often based on identification with an idealized image of what he feels he should be. **true s.** The total of a person's potentialities that might be developed under the most favorable conditions.

**self-absorption** \-əbsôrp′shən\ Absorption within the body of a radioactive source, so that not all of the generated radiation succeeds in escaping. In radioactivity measurements, counting procedures must take self-absorption into account, especially with beta emitters.

**self-care** Health care which the individual provides to himself or herself without outside professional assistance. Such care may be based on instructions provided by professionals.

**self-consciousness** \-kän′shəsnis\ 1 The awareness of one's own identity and existence. 2 A heightened sense of self-awareness, embarrassment, or oversensitivity to the possibly negative reactions of others to one's appearance or behavior.

**self-differentiation** \-dif′ərən′shē·ā′shən\ In embryology, continued development along a predetermined course independent of the effect of external influences which may arise from local change of environment or transfer to ectopic location.

**self-esteem** \-estēm′\ The level of appreciation of one's true worth, devoid of neurotic or unwarranted feelings of guilt or inadequacy.

**self-extinction** \-ikstingk′shən\ In psychiatry, behavior marked by living vicariously through the actions of others, subsequently the individual has no character traits that can be deemed as originating from within.

**self-fertilization** \-fur′tilīzā′shən\ Fertilization of an ovum by a spermatozoon produced by the same organism. Also *endomixis.*

**self-image** \-im′ij\ The concept each person has of his or her body and the ways it functions, including inner mental processes, memories, and associated affects.

**selfing** \sel′fing\ Self-fertilization, as between different proglottids of a tapeworm.

**self-limiting** \-lim′iting\ Tending to be limited in duration or course by its own characteristics: said especially of a disease. Also *self-limited.*

**self-recognition** \-rek′əgnish′ən\ Immunologic recognition of autoantigen.

**self-suggestion** AUTOSUGGESTION.

**self-tolerance** Immunologic tolerance to autoantigens. Also *horror autotoxicus.*

**selfwise** Developing in a previously determined manner despite relocation in an unusual or ectopic site: said of embryonic cells or tissues.

**Selivanoff** [Feodor Fedorovic *Selivanoff* (Seliwanow), Russian chemist, born 1859] Selivanoff reaction, Selivanoff's test. See under RESORCINOL TEST.

**sella** \sel′ə\ [L (from *sedere* to sit) a seat, chair, saddle] A saddle-shaped depression. **empty s.** The extension of the arachnoid and subarachnoid spaces into the sella turcica so that, on pneumoencephalogram, air appears to fill all or part of the cavity of the sella. Also *empty sella syndrome.* **s. turcica** [NA] The saddle-shaped body of the sphenoid bone located in the center of the middle cranial fossa. Adj. sellar.

**sellae** \sel′ē\ Plural of SELLA.

**sellar** \sel′ər\ Denoting the sella turcica of the sphenoid bone.

**Sellick** [Brian A. *Sellick*, English anesthetist, flourished 20th century] See under MANEUVER.

**Selter** [Paul *Selter*, German pediatrician, 1866–1941] Selter's disease. See under PINK DISEASE.

**semeiography** \sē′mī·äg′rəfē\ [Gk *semeio(n)* a mark by which something is known + -GRAPHY] A description of the symptoms of a disease. Also *semiography.*

**semeiology** \sē′mī·äl′əjē\ SYMPTOMATOLOGY.

**semeiotic** \sē′mī·ät′ik\ [Gk *semeiotik(os)* (from *semei(oun)* to mark, interpret as a sign + *-ōtikos* for *-otikos* -IC) suitable for marking; as substantive, the science of symptoms in medicine] Relating to signs or symptoms.

**Semelaigne** [Georges *Semelaigne*, French pediatrician, flourished 20th century] Kocher-Debré-Semelaigne syndrome. See under DEBRÉ-SEMELAIGNE SYNDROME.

**semen** \sē′mən\ [L (akin to *serere* to sow, beget and to Old English *sāwan* to sow), seed of vegetables, animals, man] The viscid, whitish secretions, bearing spermatozoa, of the male reproductive organs, specifically of the testes, the seminal vesicles, the prostate, and bulbourethral glands. Also *sperma, seminal fluid.*

**semenuria** \sē′mənoo′rē·ə\ SEMINURIA.

**semi-** \sem′ē-\ [L prefix (akin to Gk *hēmi-* half) half] A prefix meaning (1) partly, partially, not fully; (2) exactly half.

**semialdehyde** A designation added to the end of the name of a dicarboxylic acid in place of the word *acid* to indicate the half aldehyde, i.e. reduction of one of the two carboxy groups to an aldehyde group. Thus malonic acid is HOOC—$CH_2$—COOH, whereas malonic semialdehyde is HCO—$CH_2$—COOH.

**semiapochromat** \-ap′ōkrō′mat\ SEMIAPOCHROMATIC OBJECTIVE.

**semicanal** \-kənal′\ [SEMI- + CANAL] A tubular channel that does not form a complete circle, being half open along its length. Also *semicanalis.* **s. of auditory tube** SEMICANALIS TUBAE AUDITIVAE. **s. of tensor tympani muscle** SEMICANALIS MUSCULI TENSORIS TYMPANI.

**semicanales** \-kənā′lēz\ Plural of SEMICANALIS.

**semicanalis** \-kənā′lis\ [SEMI- + CANALIS] (*pl.* semicanales) SEMICANAL. **s. musculi tensoris tympani** [NA] The upper of two parallel canals opening into the upper part of the anterior wall of the tympanic cavity just above the fenestra vestibuli. It contains the tensor tympani muscle running from its anterior end in the angle between the petrous and squamous portions of the temporal bone. It is separated from the semicanalis tubae auditivae by the septum canalis musculotubarii. Also *semicanal of tensor tympani muscle, canal for tensor tympani muscle.* **s. tubae auditivae** [NA] The lower of two parallel canals opening into the upper part of the anterior wall of the tympanic cavity and forming the osseous part of the auditory tube. It is separated from the semicanalis musculi tensoris tympani by the septum canalis musculotubarii. Also *semicanal of auditory tube, tubal canal.*

**semicarbazide** $H_2N—NH—CO—NH_2$. A simple hydrazide related to urea. It is used as a reagent for carbonyl compounds, for which it has a high affinity and with which it forms semicarbazones.

**semicarbazone** The hydrazone formed by combination of any carbonyl compound with semicarbazide. It has the structure $H_2N—CO—NH—N{=}CRR'$, where $R—CO—R'$ is the original carbonyl compound.

**semicoma** \-kō′mə\ Loss of consciousness with retention of reflex responses to painful stimuli. Also *semisopar, semisomnus.* Adj. semicomatose. ● As many current definitions of *coma* embrace such a state, *semicoma* is now being increasingly applied to much milder degrees of impaired consciousness.

**semicomatose** \-kō′mətōs\ Pertaining to or being in a state of semicoma.

**semiconductor** \-kənduk′tər\ An electronic conductor such as silicon and germanium whose resistivity lies between that of metals and insulators. Semiconductors are used in making transistors, thermistors, and photodiodes.

**semiconscious** \-kän′shəs\ Partly conscious.

**semicrista** \-kris′tə\ (*pl.* semicristae) A small or undeveloped ridge or crest.

**semidecussation** \-dē′kusā′shən\ Partial or imcomplete crossing of nerve fibers, as in the optic chiasm of man.

**semidominance** \-däm′inəns\ INCOMPLETE DOMINANCE.

**semiflexion** \-flek′shən\ **1** A position midway between flexion and extension. **2** The act of moving to a position midway between flexion and extension.

**semih.** *semihora* (L, half an hour).

**semilunar** \-loo′nər\ Shaped like a half moon; crescent-shaped.

**semiluxation** \-luksā′shən\ SUBLUXATION.

**semimembranous** \-mem′brənəs\ Formed in part by a thin layer of connective tissue.

**semination** \sem′inā′shən\ [L *seminat(us),* past part. of *seminare* to sow, breed, + -ION] INSEMINATION.

**seminiferous** \sem′inif′ərəs\ [*semini(s),* gen. of SEMEN, + -FEROUS] Producing or conducting semen.

**seminoma** \sem′ənō′mə\ [L *semen,* gen. *seminis,* seed + -OMA] A malignant germ cell tumor of the testis composed of uniform cells having well-defined cell borders and resembling primitive germ cells. It is the most frequent malignant testis tumor and is highly radiosensitive. Also *seminal carcinoma, spermatocytoma, spermocytoma.* **ovarian s.** DYSGERMINOMA. **spermatocytic s.** An uncommon form of testicular seminoma composed of cells of varying size rather than showing the uniformity of typical seminomas.

**seminuria** \sem′inoo′rē·ə\ [SEMEN + -URIA] The excretion of semen in the urine. Also *semenuria.*

**semiography** \sē′mī·äg′rəfē\ SEMEIOGRAPHY.

**semiology** \sē′mi·äl′əjē\ SYMPTOMATOLOGY.

**semiparasite** \-par′əsīt\ An organism that is found as both a parasite and a saprophyte; a facultative parasite.

**semipenniform** \-pen′ifôrm\ UNIPENNATE.

**semipermeable** \-pur′mē·əbəl\ Having selective permeability, especially permeability to water but not to salts: said of a membrane.

**semiplegia** \-plē′jə\ HEMIPLEGIA.

**semiprivate** \-prī′vət\ [SEMI- + PRIVATE] Characterizing a hospital room with more than one, and usually with two, beds.

**semipronation** \-prōnā′shən\ Partial pronation.

**semiprone** \-prōn′\ Bent forward in a position approaching prone.

**semiquinone** A substance intermediate in oxidation state between a quinone and a quinol. It may be prepared by adding one electron to a quinone molecule, forming a radical-anion. Semiquinones may be important intermediates in biologic oxidations.

**semirecumbent** \-rikum′bənt\ Being in a position midway between sitting up and lying down.

**semis** One-half. Abbr. ss.

**semisomnus** \-säm′nəs\ SEMICOMA.

**semisopor** \-sō′pôr\ SEMICOMA.

**semispinalis** \-spīnā′lis\ MUSCULUS SEMISPINALIS.

**semistarvation** \-stärvā′shən\ The consumption of less food than is necessary to meet the nutrient requirements of a person. Also *subalimentation.*

**semisulcus** \-sul′kəs\ (*pl.* semisulci) A groove on a structure, which when joined to a similar groove on an adjacent structure forms a single sulcus.

**semisupination** \-soo′pinā′shən\ Partial supination.

**semisynthetic** Derived by synthetic steps from natural compounds: said of a substance. Making use of natural compounds in such syntheses may greatly shorten the synthetic route.

**semitendinous** \-ten′dinəs\ Partly or considerably tendinous in structure, as in *semitendinous muscle.*

**semitertian** \-tur′shən\ [SEMI- + TERTIAN] Characterizing a malarial fever in which two paroxysms occur on one day and one paroxysm occurs on the following day.

**Semon** [Sir Felix *Semon,* English laryngologist, 1849–1921] Semon-Rosenbach law. See under SEMON'S LAW.

**Senear** [Francis Eugene *Senear,* U.S. dermatologist, 1889–1958] Senear-Usher syndrome. See under SYNDROME.

**senega** \sen′əgə\ The dried root of *Polygala senega,* which contains polygalin, senegenin, and oils. It is used as an emetic and expectorant. Also *Seneca snakeroot, senega snakeroot.*

**senegenin** $C_{30}H_{45}ClO_6$. 12-(Chloromethyl)-2$\beta$,3$\beta$-dihydroxy-27-norolean-13-ene-23,28-dioic acid, the active principle, with polygalic acid, in senega root, which has properties of an emetic and expectorant. Extracts have been used with other ingredients for treatment of chronic bronchitis. Also *polygalin.*

**senescence** \sənes′əns\ [L *senescens,* pres. part. of *senescere* (from *senex* old) to grow old] The normal process of aging or growing old, as distinguished from the effects of disease in old age. Adj. senescent.

**Sengstaken** [Robert William *Sengstaken,* U.S. surgeon, born 1923] Sengstaken-Blakemore tube. See under TUBE.

**senility** \sənil′itē\ [*senil(e)* + -ITY] Old age, with the implication that involution, degeneration, or some degree of pathologic alteration has taken place in one or more functions or organ systems.

**senium** \sē′nē·əm\ [L (from *sen(ex)* old, aged + *-ium,* neut. noun suffix), old age, esp. the weakness of old age] That stage of life which constitutes the years of old age. ● The term is sometimes used to indicate feebleness or generalized debility in old age, although some authors prefer the term *senility* for such a connotation. **s. praecox** Premature senility and the presenile disorders associated with it.

**senna** \sen′ə\ [Arabic *sanā* Cassia plant] The dried leaflets of any of various species of the genus *Cassia* in the Leguminosae family, from which a cathartic drug is prepared.

**senography** \senäg′rəfē\ [Spanish or Italian *sen(o)* bosom, breast (from L *sinus* fold, bosom) + -GRAPHY] A radiographic technique, consisting of low voltage and constant potential, used for soft-tissue examinations, especially mammography.

**senopia** \senō′pē·ə\ [L *sen(ium)* weakness, decline, old age + -OPIA] SECOND SIGHT.

**sensation** [L *sensatio* (from *sensus*, past part. of *sentire* to feel, experience, perceive + *-atio* -ATION) perception] The subjective experience elicited by excitation of a sense organ or related neural pathways. **articular s.** JOINT SENSE. **chromatic s.** COLOR SENSE. **cincture s.** ZONESTHESIA. **common s.** BODY SENSE. **concomitant s.** An accompanying sensation unrelated to the primary stimulus, e.g., touch and temperature sensations are derived concomitantly from cutaneous contact. **cutaneous s.** Any of the sensory impressions arising from excitation of the skin, including touch, pressure, pain, and temperature sensations. Also *skin sensation, dermal sensation, cutaneous sensibility.* **delayed s.** A sensation that is not perceived immediately after the initial stimulus presentation but after a brief interval. **dermal s.** CUTANEOUS SENSATION. **eccentric s.** A sensation deviating from the expected reaction generally corresponding to the nature of the stimulus. **external s.** The sensory experience induced by a physical stimulus through sense organ excitation. **general s.** BODY SENSE. **generalized epileptic somatic s.** An abnormal but vague sensation at the onset of some epileptic attacks, such as a feeling of weakness, restlessness, coldness, etc., affecting the whole body but especially the limbs. It usually arises in the temporal lobe, the median frontal region, the secondary sensory area, or the supplementary sensory area. Also *generalized somatic aura.* **girdle s.** ZONESTHESIA. **gnostic s.** Sensation derived from sense organs believed to be more highly developed and differentiated or of more recent phyletic origin. *Outmoded.* Also *new sensation* (outmoded), *gnostic sensibility.* **internal s.** VISCERAL SENSE. **joint s.** JOINT SENSE. **kinesthetic s.** KINESTHESIA. **new s.** *Outmoded* GNOSTIC SENSATION. **palmesthetic s.** VIBRATORY SENSIBILITY. **primary s.** Sensation directly referrable to stimulus properties. **proprioceptive s.** PROPRIOCEPTION. **protopathic s.** The perception of painful or thermal sensations that are not well localized but are related generally to regions of the body. **radiating s.** Any sensation which spreads from the diseased or affected area to one which is unaffected by the pathologic process. **referred s.** Sensation identified as occurring at a bodily site other than that where the stimulus has been applied, especially visceral excitation referred to cutaneous sites, e.g., cardiac damage referred to arm and shoulder. Also *reflex sensation, transferred sensation, eccentric projection.* **secondary s.** A sensation distinct from that primarily or initially induced by a stimulus, e.g., paradoxical cold and visual afterimages. **skin s.** CUTANEOUS SENSATION. **subjective s.** Any internal sensory experience, including those reportedly different from what might be expected given the nature of the physical stimulus, as a sensation of heat from ice or the misnaming of hues by color-blind subjects. **tactile s.** The sensation that is perceived when tactile receptors in the skin are stimulated; the sense of touch. **transferred s.** REFERRED SENSATION. **visceral s.** VISCERAL SENSE. **s. of warmth** Sensation of a localized or general body increase in temperature derived from heat stimuli or peripheral vasodilatation.

**sense** [L *sensus* (from *sensus*, past part. of *sentire* to feel, experience, perceive) sensation, feeling, perception, sense, idea] A quality of experience; a modality of impressions, i.e., sensations, received from either within or without the organism that represent more or less direct transductions of physical phenomena, such as light or sound, and are distinguishable from experience of an affective or ideational nature. An immediate awareness, when the appropriate receptor has been stimulated, is characteristic, as is neural conduction over particular nerves and projection onto more or less specific brain regions. More senses exist than the five of traditional usage. Vision, audition, smell, taste, touch, kinesthesia, pain, temperature, sense of equilibrium, and vibratory sensibility are presently distinguished. **body s.** General somatic sensation. The sensory experience derived from excitation of sense organs in the skin, muscles, joints, tendons, and ligaments. Also *general sensation, common sensation, common sensibility, somesthesia, somatesthesia, cenesthesia* (obs.), *sixth sense* (popular). **color s.** The capacity of discriminate chromatic visual stimuli in terms of hue. Also *chromatic sensation.* **dermal s.** The sensations mediated by receptors in the skin; these include sensations of heat and cold, pain and touch. **s. of equilibrium** The sense of balance derived from sense organs of the vestibular organ. Also *equilibratory sense, vestibular sense, static sense.* **internal s.** VISCERAL SENSE. **interoceptive s.'s** VISCERAL SENSE. **joint s.** The sense of limb or joint position and movement. Also *arthresthesia, articular sensibility, joint sensibility, joint sensation, articular sensation.* **kinesthetic s.** 1 KINESTHESIA. 2 *Imprecise* MUSCLE SENSE. **labyrinthine s.** The aspects of the maintenance of body equilibrium for which the vestibular sense organs are responsible. The generally accepted view is that the labyrinth does not, under normal circumstances, give rise to sensation recognized in consciousness. It is a proprioceptor rather than an exteroceptor. **muscle s.** Awareness of muscle movement or tension, ascribed probably incorrectly to muscle spindle afferent discharge. The sensory basis for this sense remains obscure, except for muscle nociception. Also *muscular sense, kinesthetic sense* (imprecise), *muscular sensibility.* **obstacle s.** The ability of blind people to detect the presence and position of obstacles, probably based on echolocation. **pain s.** The detection of noxious stimuli resulting in subjective sensation of pain. Also *nociception.* **s. of pitch** The ability to detect alterations in the pitch of a note or tone. The normal ability to detect frequency change is more sensitive than that needed to detect the relatively large intervals of frequency change in standard musical notation. Also *tone sense.* **posture s.** The ability to detect the orientation of the body in space, dependent upon vestibular and proprioceptive sense organs. **pressure s.** The sense of weight or pressure. Also *baresthesia, baryesthesia.* **proprioceptive s.** PROPRIOCEPTION. **seventh s.** VISCERAL SENSE. **sixth s.** *Popular* BODY SENSE. **space s.** The sense of the relations and position of objects in three-dimensional space. **special s.** Any of the senses attributable to the sense organs of placodal origin, e.g., vision, hearing, and smell. **static s.** SENSE OF EQUILIBRIUM. **stereognostic s.** The tactile sense of the form and texture of objects. **tactile s.** Contact sensation derived from sensitive mechanoreceptors of the epidermis and dermis and related appendages and orifices, including that of contact, velocity, displacement, force, and lateral movement of skin. Also *touch sensibility.* **temperature s.** The cutaneous sense of warmth or cold. **time s.** 1 The ability to sense time intervals and frequencies of repetitive stimuli. 2 Rhythmic sense for acoustic stimuli, especially music. **tone s.** SENSE OF PITCH. **vestibular s.** SENSE OF EQUILIBRIUM. **visceral s.** Sensation of pain, pressure, and movement of the internal body organs, mediated by specific internal sense organs. Also *internal sensation, interoceptive senses, interoceptive sensibility, internal sense, interoception, visceral sensation, splanchnesthesia, seventh sense.*

**sensibiligen** \sen′sibil′əjən\ *Obs.* ALLERGEN.

**sensibilisinogen** \sen′sibil′isin′əjən\ *Obs.* ALLERGEN.

**sensibility** \sen′səbil′itē\ [Late L *sensibilitas* (from L *sensibil(is)* perceptible by the senses + *-itas* -ITY) sensibility] The ability to feel and perceive sensory stimuli consciously. **articular s.** JOINT SENSE. **binaural s.** Auditory directional sensation, dependent upon phase differences in sounds presented to the two ears. **bone s.** VIBRATORY SENSIBILITY. **common s.** BODY SENSE. **cutaneous s.** CUTANEOUS SENSATION. **deep s.** Bodily sensations derived from sense organs other than those in skin, especially pressure, pain, movement, and position sense. **dissociation s.** The defect in pain and temperature sensation with preservation of tactile and kinesthetic sensibilities, or the reverse, resulting from injury of the anterolateral or lemniscal systems respectively. **epicritic s.** The cutaneous sensations underlying fine discriminations, especially touch. **gnostic s.** GNOSTIC SENSATION. **interoceptive s.** VISCERAL SENSE. **joint s.** JOINT SENSE. **kinesthetic s.** KINESTHESIA. **mesoblastic s.** MYESTHESIA. **muscular s.** MUSCLE SENSE. **myotatic s.** The ability to perceive muscle stretch. **nervous s.** The capacity of nervous tissue to respond to a physical stimulus. **pallesthetic s.** VIBRATORY SENSIBILITY. **palmesthetic s.** VIBRATORY SENSIBILITY. **protopathic s.** Collectively, crude sensations of pain, temperature, and touch essential for defense against pathologic tissue changes. **somesthetic s.** Sensory experience derived from cutaneous and deep receptors, generally including mechanical, thermal, pain, position, and movement sensations. **splanchnesthetic s.** Sensation derived from visceral receptors innervated by the splanchnic nerve. **touch s.** TACTILE SENSE. **two-point s.** TWO-POINT DISCRIMINATION. **uterine s.** Responsiveness of a pregnant uterus to oxytocic drugs. **vibratory s.** The sensation derived from the high frequency repetitive mechanical displacement of mechanoreceptors. Also *pallesthesia, palmesthesia, bone sensibility, palmesthetic sensation, palmesthetic sensibility, pallesthetic sensibility, seismesthesia, seisesthesia.*

**sensibilization** \sen′sibil′īzā′shən\ The process of becoming more sensitive to subsequent stimuli, as in the increased sensitivity of the skin following a burn injury. Also *sensitization.*

**sensible** \sen′səbl\ [See SENSIBILITY.] Perceptible to sense organs and possessing the capacity to elicit sensory experience.

**sensitive** \sen′sətiv\ **1** Responsive to stimuli or to minimal stimuli. **2** Possessing acute and rapid responsiveness, often implying abnormally keen or exaggerated perception. **3** Possessing a low threshold to a given physical stimulus parameter. **4** In immunology, exhibiting hypersensitivity.

**sensitivity** \sen′sətiv′itē\ [SENSITIVE + -ITY] **1** The quality or state of being responsive to a given stimulus. **2** The quality or state of possessing a low threshold to a given physical or psychic stimulus parameter, or that of possessing acute and rapid responsiveness, often implying abnormally keen or exaggerated perception. **3** The ability of an imaging system to detect weak signals. **antibiotic s.** A measure of the effectiveness of an antibiotic. It is the lowest concentration required to suppress the growth of an organism under standard test conditions. **autoerythrocyte s.** A condition consisting of periodic inflammation of subcutaneous tissue, thought to be due to immunologic reactivity to one's own red blood cells when, as from minor trauma, blood vessels are displaced from their vascular bed. **deep s.** The state or quality of responding to or perceiving noncutaneous sense organ excitation, including visceral, muscle, tendon, and joint receptor stimulation. **delayed s.** Responsiveness to a stimulus at some time considerably later than its initial application. **diagnostic s.** The probability of a positive diagnostic test result in the presence of the disease for which the test is designed to detect. It is equal to the number of true positives divided by the sum of true positives and false negatives multipled by 100. Compare DIAGNOSTIC SPECIFICITY. **differential s.** The discrimination of increments in a continuum of intensities in a given sensory modality. **primaquine s.** An inherited deficiency in erythrocyte glucose-6-phosphate dehydrogenase, associated with an unusual susceptibility to drug-induced hemolysis. Primaquine, a number of other antimalarial drugs, a variety of sulfonamides, analgesics, and antibacterial agents all can provoke the same response in these patients. The genetic trait is X-linked, and primaquine sensitivity occurs much more frequently in male than in female subjects. **suxamethonium s.** PSEUDOCHOLINESTERASE DEFICIENCY. **thermal s.** THERMESTHESIA. **trophic s.** The quality of responding to and being maintained by a chemical substance derived from neural innervation. **vibratory s.** SEISMOGENIC EXCITABILITY.

**sensitization** \sen′sitīzā′shən\ **1** The process by which an immune response is stimulated on first being exposed to an antigen, with the consequence of preparing the body's immune system for a stronger (anamnestic) response upon reexposure to the same antigen, as in a hypersensitivity reaction. **2** A condition in which the response to later stimuli is greater than the response to the original stimulus. **3** SENSIBILIZATION. **active s.** ACTIVE IMMUNIZATION. **autoerythrocyte s.** See under AUTOERYTHROCYTE SENSITIZATION SYNDROME. **passive s.** PASSIVE IMMUNIZATION. **photodynamic s.** Damage to a bacterium or to a macromolecule by visible light, in the presence of certain dyes that can absorb that light and transfer the absorbed energy to another molecule. **Rh s.** Immunization with antigens of the Rh blood group, especially the immunization of an $Rh_0$(D)-negative mother by pregnancy with an $Rh_0$(D)-positive fetus.

**sensitizer** \sen′sətī′zər\ **1** *Obs.* ANTIBODY. **2** A substance capable of inducing an allergic sensitivity.

**sensitizin** \sen′sitī′zin\ *Obs.* ALLERGEN.

**sensomotor** \sen′sōmō′tər\ SENSORIMOTOR.

**sensoparalysis** \sen′sōpəral′isis\ [*sens(e)* + *o* + *paralysis*] **1** Loss of sensibility. **2** Pseudoparalysis of a limb or part due to loss of proprioceptive sensation.

**sensor** \sen′sər\ **1** A sense organ. **2** A device that responds to a specific physical stimulus such as heat, light, or motion and generates a corresponding electrical signal for measurement or control.

**sensorial** \sensôr′ē·əl\ Pertaining to a sensorium or sensory organ.

**sensoriglandular** \sen′sərēglan′dyələr\ Pertaining to glandular secretion elicited by sensory nerve stimulation.

**sensorimetry** \sen′sərim′ətrē\ The measurement of sensation magnitude.

**sensorimotor** \sen′sərēmō′tər\ Denoting sensory and motor functions occurring together, as in a mixed nerve or sensorimotor cortex. Also *sensomotor.*

**sensorimuscular** \sen′sərēmus′kyələr\ Denoting a reflex muscle response to a sensory stimulus.

**sensorineural** \sen′sərēn^yUr′əl\ Pertaining to a sensory nerve or a sensory mechanism.

**sensorium** \sensôr′ē·əm\ A sensory organ or organ of perception. Also *perceptorium, impressorium.* **general s.** The condition of an individual with respect to mental clarity or consciousness.

**sensory** \sen′sərē\ [L *sens(us),* past part. of *sentire* to feel, perceive, be sensible of + English *-ory,* adjectival suffix] **1** Relating to, conveying, or characteristic of sensation. **2** Of or relating to the senses. • See note at AFFERENT.

**sentence / Babcock s.** Any of a series of sentences designed to test immediate recall of verbal spoken information. The one most commonly used, which a normal individual can repeat correctly in not more than three attempts, is, "One thing a nation must have to be rich and great is a large, secure supply of wood."

**sentient** \sen′shənt\ [L *sentiens,* gen. *sentientis,* pres. part. of *sentire* to feel, perceive, be sensible of] Capable of sensation or feeling; possessing consciousness.

**separation / A/C joint s.** KNOCKED-DOWN SHOULDER. **eschar s.** The sloughing of a burn eschar from its granulating bed by bacterial autolysis. It occurs in untreated burns as a result of bacterial proliferation. **s. of placenta** The cleavage of the placenta and membranes from the wall of a pregnant uterus.

**separator** \sep′ərā′tər\ A device used to force contiguous teeth temporarily out of contact.

**Sephadex** Beads of cross-linked dextran, used experimentally for gel filtration chromatography. Various bead sizes allow for the separation of substances of different molecular weight. A proprietary name.

**sepsis** \sep′sis\ [Gk *sēpsis* putrefaction] A syndrome resulting from overwhelming invasion of the circulation by pathogenic microorganisms or the toxins they produce. **s. agranulocytica** Any infection occurring in the absence of granulocytes. **burn wound s.** Systemic sepsis originating in an infected burn wound. **gas s.** Sepsis due to *Clostridium perfringens* or other gas-forming bacteria in the blood or body tissues. **incarcerated s.** A latent infection remaining after apparent healing of a primary lesion and apt to be made active by trauma. **s. intestinalis** FOOD POISONING. **s. lenta** Infection, usually bacteremia, with α-hemolytic streptococci which results in a febrile condition. Subacute endocarditis is often present if bacteremia is protracted. **postabortal s.** An infection, usually endometritis, following an abortion. In addition to the uterine infection, the bloodstream usually contains bacteria or bacterial products. **puerperal s.** PUERPERAL FEVER.

**sept-** \sept-\ **1** SEPTI-. **2** SEPTO-.

**septa** \sep′tə\ Plural of SEPTUM.

**septal** \sep′təl\ Of or relating to a septum.

**septan** \sep′tən\ [SEPT- + *-an* as in *quartan*] Occurring every seven days: said especially of a fever.

**septate** \sep′tāt\ Partitioned or compartmented by a septum; having a septum or septa.

**septation** \septā′shən\ **1** Partitioning by a septum. **2** *Outmoded* SEPTUM.

**septemia** \septē′mē·ə\ SEPTICEMIA.

**septi-** \sep′tē-\ [L *septem* seven] A combining form meaning seven. Also *sept-*.

**septic** \sep′tik\ [Gk *sēptikos* (from *sēpsis* putrefaction + *-ikos* -IC) putrefying] Pertaining to, caused by, or characterized by sepsis.

**septic-** \sep′tik-\ SEPTICO-.

**septicaemia** *Brit.* SEPTICEMIA.

**septicemia** \sep′tisē′mē·ə\ [SEPTIC- + -EMIA] Severe generalized infection resulting from hematogenous dissemination of pathogenic microorganisms and their toxins. Also *blood poisoning, hematosepsis, ichoremia, ichorrhemia, pyosepticemia, septemia, microbemia, microbiemia.* **acute fulminating meningococcal s.** WATERHOUSE-FRIDERICHSEN SYNDROME. **Bruce's s.** UNDULANT FEVER. See under BRUCELLOSIS. **cryptogenic s.** Septicemia in which the primary focus of infection is not discovered. **metastasizing s.** SEPTICOPYEMIA. **plague s.** SEPTICEMIC PLAGUE. **puerperal s.** PUERPERAL FEVER.

**septicemic** \sep′tisē′mik\ Pertaining to or characterized by septicemia.

**septico-** \sep′tikō-\ [Gk *sēptikos* (from *sēpsis* putrefaction + suffix *-ikos* forming adjectives) putrefying] A combining form meaning sepsis or putrefaction. Also *septic-*.

**septicopyemia** \sep′tikəpī·ē′mē·ə\ [SEPTICO- + PYEMIA] Septicemia associated with metastatic pyogenic abscesses. Also *metastasizing septicemia.*

**septicopyemic** \sep′tikōpī·ē′mik\ Pertaining to or characterized by septicopyemia.

**septiform** \sep′tifôrm\ Resembling a septum.

**septile** \sep′til\ Pertaining to a septum.

**septimetritis** \sep′timētrī′tis\ [*septi(co)-* + METRITIS] Pyogenic infection of the uterus.

**septo-** \sep′tō-\ [L *saeptum* or *septum.* See SEPTUM.] A combining form meaning septum. Also *sept-*.

**septomarginal** \-mär′jinəl\ Pertaining to the margin of a septum.

**septoplasty** \sep′təplas′tē\ [SEPTO- + -PLASTY] **1** An operation for straightening a deviated nasal septum by refashioning the septal cartilage or replacing parts of it. This procedure is often combined (in septorhinoplasty) with operations to correct associated deformities of the external nose. **2** Any operation to repair a perforation of the nasal septum.

**septorhinoplasty** \-rī′nəplas′tē\ An operation combining the correction of both the deviated nasal septum (septoplasty) and a deformity of the external nose that often accompanies it. This operation is frequently preferred to submucous resection of the nasal septum.

**septostomy** \septäs′təmē\ [*sept(um)* + *o* + -STOMY] A surgical procedure in which an opening is created in an anatomical partition or septum.

**septulum** \sep′tʸələm\ (*pl.* septula) A very small septum. **septula testis** [NA] Numerous incomplete septa of fibrous tissue that extend from the mediastinum testis to be attached to the deep aspect of the tunica albuginea on the surface of the testis. They divide the substance of the testis into a large number of lobules. Also *trabecula testis* (outmoded), *septa of testis.*

## septum

**septum** \sep′təm\ [L, variant of *saeptum* (from *saepire* to fence in, enclose, from *saepes* a hedge, fence) an enclosure, partition, barrier] (*pl.* septa) A partition or a dividing wall. Also *septation* (outmoded). **anterior intermuscular s. of leg** SEPTUM INTERMUSCULARE CRURIS ANTERIUS. **aorticopulmonary s.** A partition which divides the embryonic truncus arteriosus into aortic and pulmonary channels. It is formed by the fusion of spiral cushions and then extends into the upper part of the bulbus cordis. Its proximal end fuses with the distal edge of the bulbar septum, which separates the conus arteriosus of the right ventricle from the aortic vestibule, and which will eventually fuse with the interventricular septum. The spiral form of the aorticopulmonary septum is brought about by rotation of the bulbus cordis and truncus arteriosus. Rotation in the reverse direction leads to a serious defect in which the connections of the aorta and pulmonary trunk to their respective ventricles are transposed (transposition of the great vessels). Also *spiral septum.* **s. atrioventriculare cordis** [NA] The posterior portion of the membranous part of the interventricular septum of the heart, which lies between the aortic vestibule of the left ventricle and the right atrium near the anterior horn of the limbus fossae ovalis. Also *atrioventricular septum of heart.* **Bigelow s.** CALCAR FEMORALE. **bucconasal s.** BUCCONASAL MEMBRANE. **bulbar s.** A partition which develops during embryonic life and divides the bulbus cordis in two, thus resulting in the formation of the infundibulum connecting the right ventricle to the pulmonary trunk and a vestibule whereby the left ventricle communicates with the aorta. The bulbar septum is formed from two bulbar ridges which fuse with each other, and it fuses above the spiral aorticopulmonary septum which divides the single truncus arteriosus, and below with the interventricular septum. **s. canalis musculotubarii** [NA] A thin bony lamella that separates the semicanalis musculi tensoris tympani from the semicanalis tubae auditivae. Its posterior end extends into the tympanic cavity where it hooks laterally to form the processus cochleariformis. Also *septum of musculotubal canal.* **s. cervicale intermedium** [NA] A thin pia-glial partition separating the fasciculi gracilis and cuneatus of the dorsal funiculi of the cervical spinal cord. Also *intermediate cervical septum.* **cloacal s.** The mesenchymal wedge forming between the lower adjacent walls of the allantois ventrally and hindgut dorsally which grows down in the embryo towards the cloacal membrane. It finally divides the cloaca into the ventral bladder and urogenital sinus and the dorsal rectum by the end of the seventh week in human development. Also *urorectal membrane, urorectal septum, Douglas septum.* **s. corporum cavernosorum clitoridis** [NA] An incomplete fibrous layer that separates the two corpora cavernosa in the body of the clitoris. **dorsal median s.** SEPTUM POSTICUM. **Douglas s.** CLOACAL SEPTUM. **enamel s.** ENAMEL CORD. **s. endovenosum** A vestige of the embryonic separation between veins that later unite to form the definitive trunk. *Outmoded.* Also *endovenous septum.* **s. femorale** [NA] A mass of extraperitoneal fatty tissue containing a lymph node and covered by peritoneum that fills the femoral ring but allows the passage of lymph vessels that drain the deep inguinal lymph nodes into the external iliac lymph nodes. Also *femoral septum.* **s. of frontal sinuses** SEPTUM SINUUM FRONTALIUM. **gingival s.** That part of the gingiva which lies between adjacent teeth in the same dental arch. Also *gum septum.* **s. glandis penis** [NA] A mass of fibroelastic tissue around the fossa navicularis of the urethra which forms a partition in the midline within the glans penis. Posteriorly it joins the tunica albuginea of the distal ends of the corpora cavernosa and ventrally it provides attachment to the frenulum of the prepuce. It divides the erectile tissue of the glans into two unequal parts. Also *septum of glans penis.* **gum s.** GINGIVAL SEPTUM. **iliopectineal s.** ARCUS ILIOPECTINEUS. **s. inferius** A muscular partition which develops from the floor of the bulboventricular region of the embryonic heart as early as the fourth week and becomes continuous with the atrioventricular cushion mass (septum intermedium) and with the spiral aorticopulmonary septum. It forms a large part of the definitive interventricular septum. **s. interatriale cordis** [NA] An oblique partition between the right and left atria of the heart. Also *interatrial septum of heart.* **intermediate cervical s.** SEPTUM CERVICALE INTERMEDIUM. **s. intermedium** A fibrous mass which develops in the atrioventricular canal of the fetal heart and partitions the latter into right (tricuspid) and left (mitral) channels. It arises as two separate subendocardial cushions. Subsequently it unites with the interatrial septum primum and with the muscular part of the interventricular septum (septum inferius). **intermuscular s.** A fascial sheet which separates two muscles or two groups of muscles. In the neck and limbs it is continuous externally with the deep fascia and internally it is attached to bone. It may provide extensive attachment for muscle fibers on each side of it. Also *septum intermusculare.* **s. intermusculare brachii laterale** [NA] A fibrous sheet extending from the brachial fascia to the lower part of the lateral ridge of the intertubercular sulcus, the whole length of the lateral supracondylar ridge, and the lateral epicondyle of the humerus. It provides attachment to adjacent muscles and is pierced by the radial nerve and its accompanying vessels. Also *lateral intermuscular septum of arm.* **s. intermusculare brachii mediale** [NA] A fibrous sheet extending from the brachial fascia to the lower part of the medial ridge of the intertubercular sulcus, the whole length of the medial supracondylar ridge, and the medial epicondyle of the humerus. It provides attachment to adjacent muscles and is pierced by the ulnar nerve and its accompanying vessels. Also *medial intermuscular septum of arm.* **s. intermusculare cruris anterius** [NA] A fibrous sheet extending from the crural fascia to the anterior margin of the fibula, separating the extensor muscles of the anterior compartment from the peroneal muscles of the lateral compartment of the leg. Also *anterior intermuscular septum of leg.* **s. intermusculare cruris posterius** [NA] A fibrous sheet extending between fascia cruris and the posterior margin of the fibula and separating the peroneal muscles of the lateral compartment from the soleus muscle in the posterior compartment of the leg. Also *posterior intermuscular septum of leg.* **s. intermusculare femoris laterale** [NA] A strong fibrous sheet extending from the fascia lata to the linea aspera and its prolongation upward to the gluteal tuberosity and downward to the lateral condyle of the femur, and separating the vastus lateralis muscle anteriorly from the short head of the biceps femoris muscle posteriorly. Also *lateral intermuscular septum of thigh.* **s. intermusculare femoris mediale** [NA] A fibrous sheet extending from the fascia lata to the linea aspera of the femur and separating the vastus medialis muscle from the adductor group of muscles. Also *medial intermuscular septum of thigh.* **interradicular s.** A partition of bone which separates the socket of one root of a multirooted tooth from that of an adjacent root of the same tooth. Also *septum interradiculare, septum intra-alveolarium.* **intersegmental s.** A partition made of mesenchyme lying between two adjacent somites. **s. interventriculare cordis** [NA] A partition between the right and left ventricles of the heart, composed mostly of a thick muscular part and a small membranous part near the root of the aorta. Also *interventricular septum of heart, ventricular septum.* **s. intra-alveolarium** INTERRADICULAR SEPTUM. **intraplacental septa** Incomplete partitions separating the lobes, or cotyledons, of the maternal surface of the placenta. They develop as ingrowths of the cytotrophoblastic layer which are covered by syncytium, but later the maternal tissues add reticulum fibers and associated cells, decidual cells, fibrinoid material, and blood vessels. They extend from the basal plate of the intervillous spaces towards but do not reach the chorionic plate. **Körner s.** The lateral margin of the tegmen tympani that turns down to meet the squamous part of the temporal bone in the fusion of the petrosquamosal suture. **lateral intermuscular s. of arm** SEPTUM INTERMUSCULARE BRACHII

LATERALE. **lateral intermuscular s. of thigh** SEPTUM INTERMUSCULARE FEMORIS LATERALE. **s. linguae** [NA] A median fibrous partition situated vertically in the tongue, dividing it into right and left halves and providing attachment for some of the intrinsic muscles. Inferiorly it is attached to the body of the hyoid bone. Also *lingual septum.* **s. lucidum** SEPTUM PELLUCIDUM. **medial intermuscular s. of arm** *Outmoded* SEPTUM INTERMUSCULARE BRACHII MEDIALE. **medial intermuscular s. of thigh** SEPTUM INTERMUSCULARE FEMORIS MEDIALE. **mediastinal s.** MEDIASTINUM. **membranous s. of nose** PARS MEMBRANACEA SEPTI NASI. **s. mobile nasi** *Outmoded* PARS MOBILIS SEPTI NASI. **mobile s. of nose** PARS MOBILIS SEPTI NASI. **s. musculare ventriculorum cordis** *Outmoded* PARS MUSCULARIS SEPTI INTERVENTRICULARIS CORDIS **s. of musculotubal canal** SEPTUM CANALIS MUSCULOTUBARII. **nasal s.** SEPTUM NASI. **s. nasi** [NA] A median partition dividing the nasal cavity and the external nose into right and left halves and comprising the pars membranacea, pars cartilaginea, and pars ossea. On each side its mucous membrane contains the vomeronasal organ. Occasionally it is deviated to one side or the other. Also *nasal septum.* **s. nasi osseum** [NA] The vertical bony plate forming the osseous part of the nasal septum, extending between the roof and the floor of the nasal cavity and comprising mainly the vomer posteroinferiorly and the perpendicular plate of the ethmoid bone anterosuperiorly. Also *osseous septum of nose.* **neural s.** Part of the basal telencephalon that contains the septal nuclei. Also *septum verum, true septum.* **s. orbitale** [NA] A thin, fibrous sheet lining the inner surface of the orbicularis oculi muscle and blending with the superficial lamella of the aponeurosis of levator palpebrae superioris muscle in the upper eyelid and with the anterior surface of the tarsus in the lower eyelid. It is attached to the margin of the orbit, where it becomes continuous with the periosteum. Also *orbital septum, tarsal membrane, palpebral fascia.* **osseous s. of nose** SEPTUM NASI OSSEUM. **s. pellucidum** [NA] A thin vertical partition attached above to the body of the corpus callosum and below to the rostrum of the corpus callosum and the fornix. It consists of two laminae separated by a narrow cavity. Also *septum lucidum, pellucid septum.* **s. penis** [NA] A median fibrous partition formed by the fusion of the contiguous deep fibers of the tunica albuginea that surround each of the corpora cavernosa penis independently. It is thick proximally but incomplete distally in the penis. **pericardioperitoneal s.** A thin, horizontal partition derived from part of the septum transversum which separates the embryonic liver from the pericardial cavity. **pericardiopleural s.** PLEUROPERICARDIAL MEMBRANE. **placental s.** One of the partitions which incompletely divide the human placental intervillous space into subdivisions or lobes of placental tissue called cotyledons. **pleuroperitoneal s.** A septum in the embryo which separates the pleura from the peritoneum and which contributes to the formation of the diaphragm, formed by fusion of the dorsal mesentery and the pleuroperitoneal fold. **s. pontis** RAPHE PONTIS. **posterior s.** SEPTUM POSTICUM. **posterior intermuscular s. of leg** SEPTUM INTERMUSCULARE CRURIS POSTERIUS. **posterior median cervical s.** The midline neuroglial septum between the posterior funiculi of the cervical spinal cord. **s. posticum** The thin neuroglial partition located on the midline between the posterior or dorsal funiculi. Also *dorsal median septum, posterior septum.* **s. primum** A partition which is the first (about the 32nd day of intrauterine life) of two septa participating in the division of the primitive atrium into a definitive right atrium and left atrium. It is relatively thin and grows in crescentic fashion from the cranial wall of the atrium towards the atrioventricular cushions. For a short time there is a communication between the septum primum and the cushions (ostium primum). Later the septum undergoes partial resorption of its superior part to create a second communication uniting the atria (ostium secundum), which will be overlapped later by a new partition, the septum secundum. **s. rectovaginale** [NA] A layer of areolar tissue extending between the rectum and the vagina from the central tendon of the perineum inferiorly to the base of the rectouterine pouch superiorly. It is the equivalent in the female of the rectovesical septum in the male. Also *rectovaginal septum, rectovaginal fascia.* **s. rectovesicale** [NA] A fascial layer extending from the central tendon of the perineum, where it is continuous with the prostatic sheath, to the floor of the rectovesical pouch of peritoneum and the fascia of the rectum, thereby separating the prostate and the base of the urinary bladder with the seminal vesicles and deferent ducts anteriorly from the ampulla of the rectum posteriorly. Also *rectovesical septum, rectovesical fascia, Denonvilliers aponeurosis, Denonvilliers fascia, Tyrrell's fascia, Denonvilliers ligament.* **s. scroti** [NA] A fibromuscular partition composed of the deep fibers of the dartos muscle and all the layers of the scrotal wall deep to the skin and extending upward between the two testes to divide the scrotum into two compartments. Superficially it attaches to the raphe of the scrotum. Also *septum of scrotum.* **s. secundum** A partition which develops at an early stage in embryonic life and participates with the septum primum in the division of the primitive atrium into the definitive right and left atria. It is more substantial than the septum primum and lies to the right of the latter. It grows from the cranial wall of the atrium towards the inferior vena cava and overlaps the opening (ostium secundum) created by resorption of part of the septum primum. The septum secundum directs most of the blood from the inferior vena cava through the ostium secundum into the left atrium, the aperture now being called the foramen ovale. Also *crista dividens.* **s. sinuum frontalium** [NA] A thin bony partition separating the right and left frontal sinuses of the frontal bone. It is occasionally deflected from the median plane. Also *septum of frontal sinuses.* **s. sinuum sphenoidalium** [NA] A thin bony partition dividing the sphenoidal sinus in the body of the sphenoid bone into two cavities, often unequal, each of which opens into the corresponding sphenoethmoidal recess in the nasal cavity. Also *sphenoidal septum, septum of sphenoidal sinuses.* **spiral s.** AORTICOPULMONARY SEPTUM. **s. spurium** A projection in the embryonic right atrium, above the sinuatrial opening and adjacent to the upper part of the interatrial septum secundum. It becomes inconspicuous during later development. **subarachnoidal s.** A connective tissue partition that interconnects the arachnoidea and the pia mater along the posterior median sulcus of the cervical and thoracic spinal cord. **septa of testis** SEPTULA TESTIS. **s. of testis** MEDIASTINUM TESTIS. **tracheoesophageal s.** Tissue placed between the developing trachea and esophagus. The original laryngotracheal diverticulum grows out of the ventral wall of the pharynx. From this outgrowth, the trachea extends caudally, lying ventral to and roughly parallel to the esophagus. The intervening mesodermal tissue constitutes the tracheoesophageal septum which may in rare cases break down to cause a tracheoesophageal fistula. **transverse s.** SEPTUM TRANSVERSUM. **transverse s. of ampulla** CRISTA AMPULLARIS. **s. transversum** A thin mesodermal septum placed between the pericardial cavity and the primitive yolk sac. In mammals it gives rise to most of the diaphragm. Also *transverse septum.* **true s.** NEURAL SEPTUM. **urorectal s.** CLOACAL SEPTUM. **ventricular s.** SEPTUM INTERVENTRICULARE CORDIS. **s. verum** NEURAL SEPTUM.

**septuplet** \septup′lit\ [Late L *septupl(us)* (from *septem* seven) consisting of seven + English *-et,* diminishing suffix] One of seven offspring born at the termination of a pregnancy.

**seq. luce.** *sequenti luce* (L, the following day: used in prescription writing).

**sequela** \sikwē′lə, sikwel′ə\ [L (from *sequi* to follow) a consequence] (*pl.* sequelae) A condition that follows the occurrence of a disease: used especially of diseases or other morbid conditions resulting from the preceding disease. Also *sequel.*

**sequelae** \sikwē′lē, sikwel′ē\ Plural of SEQUELA.

**sequence** [Late L *sequentia* (from *sequi* to follow) succession] **1** The order in which a number of items are arranged, or the imposition of an arrangement of items in a determined order. **2** A pattern of multiple anomalies that stem from a single known or presumed cause. The pattern is generally consistent but potentially variable. Also *anomalad* (outmoded). **amino acid s.** See under AMINO ACID. **base s.** The order of the nucleotides in a polynucleotide denoted by the purine or pyrimidine bases they contain. The base sequence of the deoxyribonucleic acid molecule contains the information needed to determine the amino acid sequence in a protein. The base sequences for nucleic acid molecules can now be readily determined. **canonical s.** CONSENSUS SEQUENCE. **coding s.** EXON. **complementary base s.** A nucleotide sequence that is determined, through base pairing rules, by a preexisting polynucleotide. **consensus s.** A derived, idealized sequence of nucleotides in which each position represents the base most often found when actual sequences of similar function within the same or different genomes are compared. Also *canonical sequence.* **deformation s.** A pattern of anomalies that results directly or indirectly from a primary mechanical force acting on normal tissue, such as oligohydramnios on the fetus. Also *deformation.* **disruption s.** A pattern of anomalies that results directly or indirectly from the breakdown of normal tissue, such as an amniotic band. Also *disruption.* **intervening s.** INTRON. **leader s.** In operons regulated by attenuation, the DNA sequence that codes for the leader peptide. **malformation s.** A pattern of anomalies that results directly or indirectly from a primary defect in development or tissue formation, such as a myelomeningocele. Also *malformation.* **nearest neighbor s.** With reference to nucleic acids, the chemical nature of the nucleotide bases adjacent to any given nucleotide. It is usually expressed as a nearest neighbor frequency. **regulatory s.** A region of DNA involved in the regulation of expression of a particular gene, including operators and promoters. **Robin s.** A congenital association of cleft palate, micrognathia, and glossoptosis of diverse cause. It is found in multiple heritable syndromes such as the Stickler syndrome and is frequently seen with cardiac defects. Also *Robin anomalad* (outmoded), *Pierre Robin anomaly, Pierre Robin retrognathism, Pierre Robin syndrome.* **termination s.** A DNA sequence that signals RNA polymerase to discontinue transcription. Also *stop codon, termination codon, termination factor.*

**sequential** \sikwen′shəl\ Characterized by a sequence.

**sequester** \sikwes′tər\ [Late L *sequestrare* to remove, set aside] To separate out or segregate; to isolate (a portion) from the whole.

**sequestra** \sikwes′trə\ Plural of SEQUESTRUM.

**sequestral** \sikwes′trəl\ Of or relating to a sequestrum.

**sequestration** \sēkwestrā′shən\ **1** The development of a sequestrum. **2** Isolation or segregation. **biochemical s.** The inability of the immune system to recognize certain determinants (hidden determinants) on a molecule. Under certain conditions, sequestration can be reversed and the determinants exposed to elicit an immune response. **bronchopulmonary s.** A congenital condition in which there is a separate mass or lobe of lung tissue with an independent bronchus outside of the lung on that side and that derives its blood supply from a systemic branch of the thoracic aorta.

**sequestrectomy** \sē′kwestrek′təmē\ [*sequestr(um)* + -ECTOMY] Removal of a fragment of dead or infected bone. Also *sequestrotomy.*

**sequestrum** \sikwes′trəm\ [L (from *sequi* to follow), the placing of a disputed thing in the hands of a third person, a deposit] (*pl.* sequestra) A fragment of necrotic tissue which has become detached from the surrounding viable tissue. This is a characteristic finding of pyogenic osteomyleitis in which a piece of bone becomes necrotic due to a combination of suppuration and ischemia. The surrounding healthy bone then proliferates, forming an ensheathing layer (involucrum).

**sequoiosis** \sē′kwoi·ō′sis\ Allergic alveolitis resulting from inhalation of sawdust from redwood trees (*Sequoia*) in which the bark is infected with *Graphium* fungi.

**SER** **1** smooth endoplasmic reticulum (agranular endoplasmic reticulum). **2** sensory-evoked response.

**Ser** Symbol for serine.

**sera** \sir′ə\ Plural of SERUM.

**serangitis** \sir′anjī′tis\ [Gk *sēranx,* gen. *sērangos,* a hollow rock + -ITIS] CAVERNITIS.

**serapheresis** \sir′əferē′sis\ The preparation of serum by coagulation of plasma obtained by plasmapheresis. Also *seropheresis.*

**serempion** \sirem′pē·än\ A fatal type of measles indigenous to the West Indies and occurring mainly in children.

**serial** \sir′ē·əl\ **1** Arranged in a series. **2** Occurring in a series at intervals.

**serialograph** \sir′ē·al′əgraf\ An x-ray apparatus used for making a series of radiographs, usually of the same patient area, such as the duodenal cap during a gastrointestinal examination.

***Sericopelma*** \ser′ikōpel′mə\ A genus of very large hairy mygalomorph spiders (family Theraphosidae). ***S. communis*** A very large, black bird spider or "tarantula" found in Panama. Its bite is venomous to humans, though the effect is local, with pain and numbness in the affected area.

**series** \sir′ēz\ [L (from *serere* to put in a row, join or bind together), a row, number, series, order] **1** A succession of events or order of things leading consecutively from one to the next. **2** A number of steps or stages in a process, as in determining a diagnosis. **3** A group of things sharing some characteristic by which they may be regarded as a set and usefully distinguished from others, as a group of chemical compounds. **electrochemical s.** The chemical elements arranged in order of their standard redox potentials. **erythrocytic s.** The erythrocytes and their precursor cells. **gastrointestinal s.** A series of radiographs made as barium advances in the gastrointestinal tract in a gastrointestinal examination. *Older term.* Also *GI series.* See under GASTROINTESTINAL EXAMINATION. **granulocytic s.** All of the blood and bone marrow leukocytes that are or will become polymorphonuclear leukocytes, including all the maturational stages of neutrophils, eosinophils, and basophils. Also *myelocytic series, myelogenous series, myeloid series* (outmoded). **leukocytic s.** All the kinds of leukocytes and their precursor cells. **lymphocytic s.** The lymphocytes and their precursor cells, i.e. lymphocytes, prolymphocytes, and lymphoblasts. Also *lymphoid series.* **myelocytic s.** GRANULOCYTIC SERIES. **myelogenous s.** GRANULOCYTIC SERIES. **myeloid s.** *Outmoded* GRANULOCYTIC SERIES. **natural radioactive s.** A radioactive series starting with a naturally occurring element such as uranium or thorium. **neptunium s.** An artificial radioactive series of heavy elements beginning with neptunium 237, half-life $2 \times 10^6$ years, and ending with stable bismuth 209. **neutrophilic s.** All the leukocytes, at various stages of maturation, that are recognizable as neutrophils, including neutrophilic myelocytes, neutrophilic metamyelocytes, neutrophilic band cells, and mature neutrophils. **radioactive s.** Any of four groups of radioactive elements such that each element in the group is formed from the preceding one by a radioactive disintegration, either alpha or beta emission. Three of the groups consist of naturally occurring nuclides headed by a very long-lived isotope and ending with an isotope of lead. The fourth consists entirely of artificially produced nuclides and ends with the only stable isotope of bismuth. **thorium s.** A natural radioactive series of heavy elements beginning with thorium 232, and ending with stable lead, lead 208.

**serine** \sir′in\ $CH_2OH—CH(NH_3^+)—COO^-$. One of the twenty amino acids that are incorporated into proteins. It is not essential, being synthesized in the body from 3-phosphoglycerate. Symbol: Ser, S

**serine dehydratase** The enzyme (EC 4.2.1.13) that catalyzes the catabolic breakdown of serine into pyruvate and ammonia. It contains pyridoxal phosphate, which assists loss of a hydrogen ion from C-2, allowing loss of a hydroxide ion from C-3. The 2-aminopropenoic acid thus formed spontaneously decomposes to pyruvate and ammonia. Also *serine deaminase* (obs.).

**serine hydroxymethyltransferase** The enzyme (EC 2.1.2.1) that catalyzes transfer of the hydroxymethyl group from serine to tetrahydrofolate, yielding glycine and 5,10-methylenetetrahydrofolate, i.e. a bound form of formaldehyde. This enzyme is responsible for the interconversion of serine and glycine.

**serine proteinase** Any enzyme of the group EC 3.4.21, which hydrolyze proteins by a reaction of the enzyme with the substrate in which a unique serine residue of the enzyme is acylated and an amine is liberated. In a subsequent step the acylenzyme is hydrolyzed, so that the hydrolysis of the peptide bond of the substrate is completed. Most such enzymes are inactivated by acylating reagents such as phenylmethylsulfonyl fluoride and diisopropylphosphorofluoridate. Examples are trypsin, chymotrypsin, and elastase.

**seriscission** \ser′isish′ən\ [L *seri(cum)* silk + SCISSION] A surgical procedure in which soft tissues are divided by tightly tying an encircling heavy silk ligature.

**sero-** \sir′ō-\ [L *serum* whey] A combining form meaning serum, serous.

**seroalbuminous** \-albyoo′minəs\ Containing serum protein.

**serocolitis** \-kəlī′tis\ Inflammation of the colonic serosa.

**seroconversion** \-kənvur′zhən\ The production in a host of specific antibodies as a result of infection or immunization. The antibodies can be detected in the host's blood serum following, but not preceding, infection or immunization.

**serocystic** \-sis′tik\ Composed of cysts that are lined by cells secreting a thin proteinaceous fluid.

**seroenteritis** \-en′terī′tis\ Inflammation of the intestinal serosa.

**seroepidemiology** \-ep′idē′mē·äl′əjē \ The use of serologic techniques, such as surveys to determine the serologic patterns of population groups, in the study of the epidemiology of diseases due to or associated with microorganisms.

**seroflocculation** \-fläk′yəlā′shən\ The formation of pronounced turbidity upon addition of an antigen to a specimen of blood serum, thus demonstrating the presence of antibody in the serum.

**serofluid** \-floo′id\ SEROUS FLUID.

**serohemorrhagic** \-hem′ôraj′ik\ SEROSANGUINEOUS.

**serolipase** \-lī′pās\ The lipase present in blood serum.

**serologic** \-läj′ik\ Of or relating to serology.

**serologist** \siräl′əjist\ A specialist in serology.

**serology** \siräl′əjē\ [SERO- + -LOGY] The study of serum, originally for the presence of antibodies but now also applied to examination of serum for the presence of circulating antigens and, by extension, to study other body fluids for antibodies or antigens. **forensic s.** The application of serologic principles, theories, and practices to problems encountered in law enforcement and the administration of justice. Forensic serology is chiefly concerned with the identification and antigen analysis of blood, semen, and saliva and their stains and residues.

**serolysin** \siräl′isin\ The lysin present in blood serum.

**seromembranous** \-mem′brənəs\ Of or relating to a tunica serosa, or serous membrane.

**seromucoid** \-myoo′koid\ The $\alpha_1$-acid glycoprotein of blood plasma. *Obs.*

**seronegative** \-neg′ətiv\ Lacking antibodies or other immunologic markers for the organism under consideration, usually due to the absence of previous exposure or infection: said of an immunocompetent individual.

**seroperitoneum** \-per′itənē′əm\ ASCITES.

**seropheresis** \-ferē′sis\ SERAPHERESIS.

**seropneumothorax** \sir′ōnʸoo′məthôr′aks\ HYDROPNEUMOTHORAX.

**seropositive** \-päz′itiv\ Possessing antibodies or other immunologic markers for the particular organism under consideration as a result of a previous or ongoing immunizing exposure to the organism, either from clinical illness, subclinical infection, or deliberate immunization.

**seroprognosis** \-prägnō′sis\ Prognosis of an infectious disease based upon observations of immunologic reactivity in serum.

**seropurulent** \-pyoor′ʸələnt\ Serous and purulent; composed of serum infiltrated with pus.

**seropus** \sir′ōpus′\ Serum and pus; a serous exudate infiltrated with pus.

**seroreaction** \-rē·ak′shən\ An *in vitro* test result indicating the presence, in serum, of immunologically active material, usually an antibody but sometimes an antigen. Also *serum reaction.*

**seroresistance** \-rizis′təns\ The failure of a seroreaction to become negative or to fall in titer after treatment.

**seroresistant** \-rizis′tənt\ Pertaining to or characterized by seroresistance.

**seroreversal** \-rivur′səl\ A reduction in serologic titer as a result of treatment.

**serosa** \sirō′sə\ [*ser(um)* + L *-osa,* fem. of *-osus* suffix denoting full of] TUNICA SEROSA.

**serosanguineous** \-sang·gwin′ē·əs\ Consisting of a mixture of whole blood and serum. Also *serohemorrhagic.*

**seroserous** \-sir′əs\ Pertaining to two or more serous membranes.

**serositis** \-sī′tis\ [*seros(a)* + -ITIS] Inflammation of a serous membrane. **adhesive s.** An inflammation of serous membranes causing mobile organs to stick together.

**serosynovitis** \-sin′əvī′tis\ Noninflammatory joint effusion.

**serothorax** \-thôr′aks\ A serous pleural effusion.

**serotonergic** \ser′ətänur′jik\ [*seroton(in)* + *erg(o)-* + -IC] Concerning, containing, producing, or activated by serotonin.

**serotonin** \-tō′nin\ 5-Hydroxytryptamine. It is formed by the decarboxylation of 5-hydroxytryptophan. It is a neurotransmitter, with action on blood vessels. It also acts as a hormone.

**serotype** \sir′ətīp\ [SERO- + TYPE] SEROVAR.

**serous** \sir′əs\ Of, pertaining to, or containing serum.

**serovaccination** \-vak′sinā′shən\ Administration of immune serum to produce immediate passive immunity, together with vaccination with bacterial vaccine to induce more prolonged, active immunity.

**serovar** \sir′əver′\ [SERO- + *var(iant)*] A subgroup within a bacterial species, defined by reaction of one or more antigens with the corresponding antiserums. Also *serotype.*

**serozyme** \sir′əzīm\ The residual prothrombin remaining in serum after coagulation. See also PROTHROMBIN CONSUMPTION TEST.

**serpent** \sur′pənt\ SNAKE.

**serpentaria** \sur′pənter′ē·ə\ The dried roots and rhizome of any of various *Aristolochia* species. It is used as a bitter tonic. Also *snakeroot.*

**serpentine** \sur′pəntēn, -tīn\ SINUOUS.

**serpiginous** \sərpij′ənəs\ [Med L *serpigo,* gen. *serpiginis* (from L *serpere* to creep), a creeping + -OUS] Extending by creeping.

***Serratia marcescens*** \serā′shē·ə märkes′əns\ A species of bacteria in the Enterobacteriaceae family, found in nature and rarely causing disease. They are Gram-negative and motile, and ferment lactose slowly or not at all. Production by the organism of a red pigment, prodigiosin, has made it useful in studying the mechanical spread of bacteria. • It is probably the cause of the red stigmata whose appearance on religious paintings was considered miraculous; hence the former name *Bacillus prodigiosus* (miraculous).

**serration** \serā′shən\ **1** The condition of being serrate or notched like a saw. **2** A notched or saw-toothed edge.

**Serres** [Antoine Etienne Renaud Augustin *Serres,* French physiologist, 1786–1868] Serres glands. See under GLAND.

**serrulate** \ser′ʸəlāt\ Having fine serrations.

**Sertoli** [Enrico *Sertoli,* Italian histologist, 1842–1910] **1** Sertoli cell tumor. See under TUBULAR ANDROBLASTOMA. **2** Sertoli-Leydig cell tumor. See under TUMOR. **3** Sertoli-cell-only syndrome. See under SYNDROME. **4** Columns of Sertoli. See under SERTOLI CELLS.

**serum** \sir′əm\ [L (akin to Gk *oros,* also *orrhos* whey, serum), serum, whey] (*pl.* sera, serums) **1** The watery liquid that separates from coagulated blood; blood serum. **2** A blood serum that has been inoculated with toxins and developed antibodies for them. **3** The clear, watery portion of any animal fluid. **alkaline blood s.** Blood serum to which sodium hydroxide has been added. Also *Lorrain Smith's blood serum.* **antianthrax s.** Serum derived from the blood of a horse or cow immunized with *Bacillus anthracis..* **antibotulinus s.** BOTULISM ANTITOXIN. **anticholera s.** A serum obtained from horses which have been injected with *Vibrio cholerae* or the toxins thereof. **anticomplementary s.** Serum that on its own gives rise to consumption of complement or interferes with manifestations of complement activation. Because it interferes with the end point, such sera cannot be subjected to any tests that employ complement fixation. **anticrotalus s.** *CROTALUS* ANTITOXIN. **antidiphtheria s.** DIPHTHERIA ANTITOXIN. **anti-gas-gangrene s.** Serum derived from horses immunized with toxins elaborated by the anaerobic organisms which cause gas gangrene. Monovalent preparations active against *Clostridium perfringens, C. septicum, C. oedematiens, C. sporogenes,* and *C. sordelli* were formerly available as was a multivalent preparation combining four monovalent serums. These preparations are of limited, if any, value in therapy. Also *gas gangrene antitoxin.* **antiglobulin s.** Serum containing antibodies directed against immunoglobulins. It is used to detect bound antibody in a wide variety of immunologic assays. It was used originally to detect blood group antibodies (particularly against the Rhesus antigens) that do not themselves agglutinate the red blood cells with which they react. Also *Coombs serum.* **antilymphocyte s.** A blood component capable of reacting specifically with lymphocytes, generally by cytotoxicity. **antimeningococcus s.** A serum obtained from animals injected with *Neisseria meningitidis.* It has been superseded in use by sulfonamides. **antiophidic s.** ANTISNAKEBITE SERUM. **antiplague s.** A serum obtained from animals injected with *Yersinia pestis.* **antiplatelet s.** A blood component capable of reacting specifically with platelets through agglutination, lysis, or cytotoxicity. **antipneumococcus s.** Serum obtained from animals, usually horses or rabbits, injected with various strains of pneumococci. **antirabies s.** A sterile solution of antiviral substances obtained from the blood or plasma of healthy animals, primarily horses, that have been immunized against rabies by vaccination. It is given in a single dose to prevent rabies in patients who were bitten by rabid animals or animals suspected of being rabid. It is preferable, however, to inject antirabies immunoglobulin for this purpose. **antireticular cytotoxic s.** A serum obtained from horses which have been inoculated with extracts of human bone marrow or spleen. When injected into human beings, it supposedly stimulates the reticuloendothelial system. Large doses, however, depress the reticuloendothelial system. Also *Bogomolets serum.* **anti-Rh s.** Serum containing antibodies directed against the Rh blood group antigens. It may occur naturally in maternal serum as a result of sensitization to Rh antigens on fetal red blood cells or as a result of immunization with Rh antigens by blood transfusion or by intentional administration of the Rh positive red blood cells. **antisnakebite s.** Antivenin used for treating bites of poisonous snakes. Also *antiophidic serum.* **antitetanus s.** TETANUS ANTITOXIN. **antitoxic s.** A serum containing antitoxin. **antitubercle s.** A serum obtained from animals injected with *Mycobacterium tuberculosis* or some preparation thereof. **antitularense s.** A serum obtained from animals injected with *Francisella tularensis* and formerly used in the treatment of tularemia. Also *Foshay serum.* **articular s.** SYNOVIA. **Behring s.** DIPHTHERIA ANTITOXIN. **blister s.** The fluid contained within a blister. Its composition is slightly different from that of pure serum. **blood s.** **1** The straw-colored fluid that separates from whole blood during coagulation. **2** Chemically or mechanically defibrinated blood plasma. **Bogomolets s.** ANTIRETICULAR CYTOTOXIC SERUM. **Calmette s.** An antivenomous serum developed in 1891. • Calmette's pioneer work in obtaining immunity in experimental animals served as the basis for serum therapy against snake bites. **convalescent s.** Serum obtained from persons convalescing from an acute infectious disease (e.g., measles, scarlet fever) and administered by injection to other persons as a means of disease prophylaxis. **Coombs s.** ANTIGLOBULIN SERUM. **Felix Vi s.** An antityphoid serum rich in antibodies to the Vi antigens of *Salmonella typhi. Outmoded.* **Felton s.** An antipneumococcal serum in concentrated form. **Flexner s.** A serum that has been used in the treatment of bacillary dysentery. **foreign s.** Serum obtained from an animal that is genetically distinct from the animal providing the other constituents of the experiment or study. **Foshay s.** ANTITULARENSE SERUM. **glycerin s.** A culture medium for tubercle bacilli, consisting of 95% blood serum and 5% glycerin. **hyperimmune s.** An antiserum having an unusually high level of specific antibodies, as from repeated exposure to the antigen stimulating such antibodies. **immune s.** ANTISERUM. **inactivated s.** Serum from which complement activity has been removed, usually by heating to 56°C for 30 minutes. **s. lactis** WHEY. **Löffler's s.** LÖFFLER'S CULTURE MEDIUM. **Lorrain Smith's blood s.** ALKALINE BLOOD SERUM. **monospecific s.** MONOVALENT ANTISERUM. **monovalent s.** MONOVALENT ANTISERUM. **multipartial s.** POLYVALENT ANTISERUM. **muscle s.** The fluid that remains following coagulation of muscle plasma for extraction of the muscle proteins myosin and actin. *Seldom used.* **normal human s.** Serum from a healthy individual. • The term is usually applied to serum used as a control to compare with that of individuals exposed to the antigens or organisms being studied. **North American antisnakebite s.** Polyvalent snakebite antivenin used for treating venenations of North American snakes, especially pit vipers such as rattlesnakes and cottonmouth moccasins. **pericardial s.** PERICARDIAL FLUID. **polyvalent s.** POLYVALENT ANTISERUM. **pooled s.** A collection of two or more sera from different donors or sources. **pregnant mare's s.** See under PREGNANT MARE SERUM GONADOTROPIN. **prophylactic s.** Serum containing antibodies reactive to specifically chosen antigens, for use in prevention of disease by passive immunity. **quality control s.** Serum used to establish the accuracy or reproducibility of a testing procedure. Analyte levels or test results are determined for the batch or lot of serum, and aliquots are used in periodic testing. Serums may be prepared to give known normal results or known abnormal values. **Roux s.** DIPHTHERIA ANTITOXIN. **truth s.** A drug, such as sodium thiopental or amobarbital, that is administered to a subject who is then interrogated in an attempt to elicit truthful answers. • The term is a misnomer, since no serum is given, and these agents do not assure that truthful answers will be given by the subjects. **Yersin s.** An antiplague serum, the first such serum developed.

**service** A unit of measure of health care; an activity conducted for a community or population with the object of improving health or providing treatment for or preventing disease or injury. **ancillary s.'s** Services in an inpatient facility or program other than room and board and professional services. They include such items as radiology, drugs, and laboratory services. **basic s.'s** The more commonly used diagnostic and therapeutic services which in health insurance coverage may be supplemented by major medical coverage for more expensive and complex care. **extended care s.'s** Services in a skilled nursing facility for a limited duration of time after a hospital stay. **homemaker s.'s** Nonmedical services which provide support at home to patients who are unable to perform certain routine tasks such as food preparation and bathing by themselves. **industrial health s.'s** Health care services that are provided for the physical well-being of industrial workers in relation to their work environment. **occupational health s.'s** Services provided for the physical, mental, and social well-being of a working population in relation to its work environment. **social s.'s** Services usually provided by social workers which aid the patient in dealing with social and related problems, such as in applying for medical reimbursement, adapting to difficult home situations and family interpersonal problems.

**servomechanism** \sur′vōmek′ənizm\ A regulatory control system that uses negative feedback to minimize the error between the desired input and the controlled output.

**sesamoid** \ses′əmoid\ Having the appearance of a sesame seed.

**sesqui-** \ses′kwē-\ [L *sesqui* (possibly from *semis* the half of anything + *quis* any, or *-que* suffix denoting *and*) half as much again] A combining form meaning multiplication by a factor of one and a half.

**sesquih.** *sesquihora* (L, an hour and a half).

**sesquihora** [SESQUI- + L *hora* hour] An hour and a half, used in prescription writing.

**sessile** \ses′il\ [L *sessilis* (from *sessus*, past part. of *sedere* to sit) fit to sit upon] Attached by a broad base, and not pedunculated.

**sesunc.** *sesuncia* (L, an ounce and a half).

**set** **1** A readiness, usually only temporary, to respond in a predetermined way; the organism is prepared and poised to make a more or less specific response on receiving an appropriate signal from the environment for that activity. See also ATTITUDE. **2** To reposition in normal place or alignment, as fractured bones. **mental s.** A readiness to respond in a particular way that is the result of instructions received or of expectation derived by the individual from prior experience. **phalangeal s.** Repositioning of the small toes by capsular incisions and manipulation. **preparatory s.** A temporary condition of readiness to respond in a given way to certain stimuli. It is usually induced by the immediately preceding experience of the subject, but it may be evoked by verbal instruction as well.

**seta** \sē′tə\ [L, a bristle] (*pl.* setae) A bristlelike hair.

**setaceous** \sētā′shəs\ [L *set(a)*, also *saet(a)* a bristle + -ACEOUS] Resembling a bristle.

**setiferous** [L *set(a)*, also *saet(a)* a bristle + *i* + -FEROUS] Covered with bristles; having setae. Also *setigerous.*

**seton** \sē′tän\ [Med L, a bristle, silk, prob. from L *seta* a bristle] A guide wire or similar object utilized to create a passage through tissues for the establishment of a sinus, creation of a fistula, or to aid in the penetration of an instrument.

**setting / discriminator s.** In a pulse-height analyzer, the highest and lowest voltages that a pulse can have and still be passed on to the counting system. Also *energy window.* **energy peak s.** **1** The setting of a narrow window in a pulse-height analyzer such that the count rate reaches maximum over a specified primary gamma peak. **2** The setting of a broad energy window to make it cover most of a primary gamma peak.

**setup** The placing of teeth, attached with wax to a denture base, so that a try-in can be carried out.

**Sever** [James Warren *Sever*, U.S. orthopedic surgeon, born 1878] See under DISEASE.

**sevoflurane** \sē′vōfloo′rān\ A halogenated ether containing fluorine, of possible use as a general anesthetic.

**sevum** \sē′vəm\ [variant of L *sebum* fat, tallow] Suet, usually prepared from omental fat, consisting of triglycerides of stearic, palmitic, and oleic acids. It is used as an ointment base.

**sex** [L *sexus* (akin to *secus* a sex, *secare* to cut) a sex] **1** The fundamental division of organisms into male and female based on genetic differences that determine the functional role of the organism in the reproductive process by which new organisms of its kind are engendered. **2** Male or female characteristics. **3** Males or females, collectively. **chromosomal s.** GENETIC SEX. **endocrinologic s.** Phenotypic sexual characteristics following from the effects of hormones secreted by the gonads of an individual, such as the development of the phallus in the male or the breasts in the female. **genetic s.** The sex of an organism based on which sex chromosomes are present in its karyotype, regardless of phenotype. In humans, the presence of two X chromosomes specifies female genetic sex and the presence of an X and a Y chromosome specifies male genetic sex. Also *chromosomal sex.* **gonadal s.** The sex of an individual as distinguished by the presence of either ovaries or testes. **morphological s.** The sex of an individual as determined by the form and structure of the external genital organs.

**sex-** \seks-\ [L prefix (from *sex* six) six] A prefix meaning six.

**sex-conditioned** \-kəndish′ənd\ SEX-INFLUENCED.

**sexdigitate** \-dij′itāt\ [L *sex* six + DIGIT + -ATE] Having an extra digit on one or more hands or feet. Also *sedigitate.*

**sexduction** \-duk′shən\ F-DUCTION.

**sex-influenced** Of or pertaining to a trait whose phenotypic expression is determined in some measure by the sex of the individual. For example, male-pattern baldness is inherited as an autosomal dominant trait but has full expression in heterozygotes only in men. Also *sex-conditioned.*

**sex-linked** Of or relating to a phenotype that is determined by a gene located on a sex chromosome.

**sex-specific** \-spəsif′ik\ **1** Pertaining exclusively to males or to females. **2** Differentiating between the sexes: said of statistical data or analysis.

**sextan** \seks′tən\ [New L *sextana* (fem. of *sextanus* relating to the sixth or the sixth day), from L *sext(us)* sixth + *-anus* English *-an*] Occurring every six days: said especially of a fever.

**sexual** \sek′shoo·əl\ [Late L *sexualis* (from L *sexu(s)* a sex + *-alis* -AL) sexual] **1** Relating to reproduction requiring the union of male and female gametes. **2** Relating to the libido or sex drive; erotic. **3** Relating to an individual's gender role.

**sexuality** \sek′shoo·al′itē\ [SEXUAL + -ITY] The quality of being sexual. **infantile s.** The childhood components of sexuality, including the oral, anal, and genital stages of development. **pregenital s.** Those aspects of sexuality manifested before establishment of genital primacy in adolescence.

**sexualization** \sek′shoo·əlīzā′shən\ The act of sexualizing or endowing with libidinal cathexis.

**Sézary** [Albert *Sézary*, French physician, 1880–1956] **1** Sézary's disease, Sézary reticulosis syndrome. See under SÉZARY SYNDROME. **2** See under CELL.

**SF** **1** spinal fluid. **2** synovial fluid (synovia).

**SGOT** serum glutamic oxaloacetic transaminase.

**SGPT** serum glutamic pyruvic transaminase.

**shadow** [Old English *sceaduwe, sceadwe*, akin to Gk *skotos* darkness] **1** In radiology, the image created on film or other recording medium by the interruption of x rays by radiopaque objects or structures. **2** UNCONSCIOUS. **3** GHOST. **acoustic s.** A region of reduced echo amplitude owing to the presence of reflectors or scatterers that lie behind a strongly reflecting or attenuating structure. Also *sound shadow.* Compare ACOUSTIC ENHANCEMENT. **bat's wing s.** An appearance on a posteroanterior or anteroposterior roentgenogram of the chest, consisting of soft-tissue densities in both lungs radiating from the hilar regions and sparing the periphery, apices, and bases, as seen classically in pulmonary edema. **sound s.** ACOUSTIC SHADOW.

**shadow-casting** A method for increasing the definition of ultramicroscopic particles under the electron microscope in which the particles are coated from one direction only using a heavy metal such as gold.

**shaft** A long, slender, rodlike anatomic structure, such as the diaphysis of a long bone or the scapus of a hair. **s. of femur** CORPUS OSSIS FEMORIS. **s. of fibula** CORPUS FIBULAE. **hair s.** The main portion of a hair, which projects above the bulb. Also *scapus pili.* **s. of humerus** CORPUS HUMERI. **s. of metacarpal bone** CORPUS METACARPALIS. **s. of metatarsal bone** CORPUS METATARSALIS. **s. of penis** CORPUS PENIS. **s. of phalanx of fingers** CORPUS PHALANGIS DIGITORUM MANUS. **s. of phalanx of toes** CORPUS PHALANGIS DIGITORUM PEDIS. **s. of radius** CORPUS RADII. **s. of rib** CORPUS COSTAE. **s. of tibia** CORPUS TIBIAE. **s. of ulna** CORPUS ULNAE.

**shakes** [Old English *sceacan* to shake] **1** A paroxysm of trembling, such as that which occurs during the chills of an intermittent fever. **2** Any of various acute or chronic conditions characterized by a tremor. A popular term. **hatter's s.** A coarse, jerky tremor resulting from mercury poisoning and affecting first the fingers, lips, tongue, and eyelids and later the arms and legs. It formerly occurred among workers in the hat industry who used mercuric nitrate as a carotting agent in making felt hats and in fur processing. Also *Danbury shakes.* **helium s.** *Popular* HIGH-PRESSURE NEUROLOGIC SYNDROME. • This term is used by divers in the mistaken belief that the helium mixture breathed to enable descent to greater depths is responsible for the condition.

**shank** [Middle English *shanke*, from Old English *scanca*] **1** The leg, tibia, or shin. **2** A structure resembling a leg.

**shaping** A procedure in operant conditioning by which a highly specific response is elicited by first reinforcing behavior that is only very generally of the kind desired and then gradually narrowing the range of behaviors reinforced to approach more and more closely the particular response required. Also *method of successive approximations.*

**Sharpey** [William *Sharpey*, Scottish anatomist, 1802–1880] Sharpey's fibers. See under BONE FIBERS.

**shave / lip s.** A vermilionectomy performed on one entire lip, usually the lower one. Also *lip peel.*

**Shaver** [Cecil Gordon *Shaver*, Canadian physician, born 1901] Shaver's disease. See under BAUXITE PNEUMOCONIOSIS.

**shear** **1** An applied force that gives rise to a tangential parallel and opposite gliding motion within the planes of a body. **2** The strain generated from applying such a force.

**shears** A large cutting implement resembling scissors. **bandage s.** Short-bladed scissors used for cutting wound dressings. They have blunt tips and a flat extension on the lower blade to slide between the dressing and the skin without risking injury to the skin. The blades join the handles at an obtuse angle. **Liston s.** Strong shears used to cut plaster casts. Also *Liston scissors.* **malleus s.** A small, strong shears, either in the form of short-bladed scissors or a miniature guillotine, used for amputating the diseased malleus head in modified radical mastoidectomy and similar operations.

# sheath

**sheath** [Old English *scēath, scæth*] A tubular structure enveloping a muscle, tendon, nerve, blood vessel, or other organ; vagina. **arachnoid s.** The delicate arachnoid mater surrounding the optic nerve. **axillary s.** A tubular extension of the prevertebral layer of deep cervical fascia that surrounds the proximal part of the axillary vessels and brachial plexus. **bulbar s.** VAGINA BULBI. **carotid s.** VAGINA CAROTICA FASCIAE CERVICALIS. **caudal s.** Microtubules arranged about the caudal pole of the nucleus in a maturing spermatid, a transient structure ensuring protection during the elongation period. Also *manchette.* **common synovial flexor s.** VAGINA SYNOVIALIS COMMUNIS MUSCULORUM FLEXORUM. **common s. of tendons of peroneal muscles** VAGINA MUSCULORUM PERONEORUM COMMUNIS. **dentinal s.** NEUMANN SHEATH. **dural s.** VAGINA EXTERNA NERVI OPTICI. **enamel rod s.** PRISM SHEATH. **endoneurial s.** ENDONEURIUM. **epithelial s.** SHEATH OF HERTWIG. **external s. of optic nerve** VAGINA EXTERNA NERVI OPTICI. **s. of eyeball** VAGINA BULBI. **fascial s. of prostate** An extension of the endopelvic fascia, enveloping the prostate and containing a venous plexus. **femoral s.** The funnel-shaped fascia surrounding the femoral vessels for about two inches below the inguinal ligament and formed by fascia transversalis anteriorly and fascia iliaca posteriorly. It contains three compartments occupied by the femoral canal medially, the femoral artery laterally, and the femoral vein in between. It is pierced anteromedially by the great saphenous vein and lymphatic vessels. **fibrous s.** A coating or covering of fibrous connective tissue around an organ or structure. **fibrous s.'s of digits of foot** VAGINAE FIBROSAE DIGITORUM PEDIS. **fibrous s.'s of digits of hand** VAGINAE FIBROSAE DIGITORUM MANUS. **fibrous s.'s of fingers** VAGINAE FIBROSAE DIGITORUM MANUS. **fibrous s. of kidney** FASCIA RENALIS. **fibrous flexor s.'s of tendons of fingers** VAGINAE FIBROSAE DIGITORUM MANUS. **fibrous s. of liver** TUNICA FIBROSA HEPATIS. **fibrous flexor s.'s of tendons of toes** VAGINAE FIBROSAE DIGITORUM PEDIS. **fibrous s. of optic nerve** VAGINA EXTERNA NERVI OPTICI. **fibrous s. of tendon** VAGINA FIBROSA TENDINIS. **fibrous tendon s.'s of muscles of fingers** VAGINAE FIBROSAE DIGITORUM MANUS. **fibrous tendon s.'s of muscles of toes** VAGINAE FIBROSAE DIGITORUM PEDIS. **fibrous s.'s of toes** VAGINAE FIBROSAE DIGITORUM PEDIS. **s. of Hertwig** An investing layer, derived from the outer enamel epithelium and the inner enamel epithelium, which surrounds the developing root of a tooth. Also *epithelial sheath, root sheath.* **Huxley s.** HUXLEY'S LAYER. **inner meningeal s. of optic nerve** VAGINA INTERNA NERVI OPTICI. **internal s. of optic nerve** VAGINA INTERNA NERVI OPTICI. **Key-Retzius s.** ENDONEURIUM. **lamellar s.** PERINEURIUM. **Mauthner s.** AXOLEMMA. **medullary s.** MYELIN SHEATH. **meningeal s.'s of optic nerve** VAGINAE NERVI OPTICI. **microfilarial s.** The membrane that surrounds certain microfilariae such as *Wuchereria, Brugia,* and *Loa.* It is thought to derive from the vitelline membrane. **myelin s.** A covering on some nerve fibers composed of compacted layers of cell membrane formed by the spiraling of the Schwann cell around the axon. Also *medullary sheath, myelin investment.* **Neumann s.** The tissue surrounding the tubular space produced by a collapse of the matrix surrounding an odontoblast process when dentin is demineralized. Also *dentinal sheath.* **neurilemmal s.** NEURILEMMA. **notochordal s.** The primitive covering of the notochord, made of fibrillar connective tissue. **nucleated s.** NEURILEMMA. **s.'s of optic nerve** VAGINAE NERVI OPTICI. **outer meningeal s. of optic nerve** VAGINA EXTERNA NERVI OPTICI. **periesophageal s.** TUNICA ADVENTITIA ESOPHAGI. **perivascular s.** The pial-glial covering around blood vessels within the brain. **pial s.** The pia mater covering the optic nerve. **plantar tendinous s. of long peroneal muscle** VAGINA TENDINIS MUSCULI PERONEI LONGI PLANTARIS. **s. of plantar tendon of long peroneal muscle** VAGINA TENDINIS MUSCULI PERONEI LONGI PLANTARIS. **prism s.** A region in enamel where there is an abrupt change in the orientation of crystallites together with a relatively high concentration of organic material. It partly or completely separates one prism from another. Also *prism cuticle, enamel rod sheath.* **rectus s.** VAGINA MUSCULI RECTI ABDOMINIS. **s. of prostate** FASCIA PROSTATAE. **s. of rectus abdominis muscle** VAGINA MUSCULI RECTI ABDOMINIS. **root s.** SHEATH OF HERTWIG. **Scarpa s.** FASCIA CREMASTERICA. **s. of Schwann** NEURILEMMA. **Schweigger-Seidel s.** An ellipsoid consisting of a mass of concentrically arranged reticular cells and macrophages forming a sheath around the penicilli in the red pulp of the spleen and narrowing the lumen of these sheathed arterioles. The sheath is well developed in some mammals and only poorly developed in humans. See also SHEATHED ARTERIES. **s. of styloid process** VAGINA PROCESSUS STYLOIDEI. **synovial s.'s** VAGINAE SYNOVIALES. **synovial s. of bicipital groove** VAGINA TENDINIS INTERTUBERCULARIS. **synovial s. of extensor carpi radialis longus and brevis muscles** VAGINA TENDINUM MUSCULORUM EXTENSORUM CARPI RADIALIUM. **synovial s. of extensor digiti minimi** VAGINA TENDINIS MUSCULI EXTENSORIS DIGITI MINIMI. **synovial s. of extensor hallucis longus** VAGINA TENDINIS MUSCULI EXTENSORIS HALLUCIS LONGI. **synovial s. of flexor carpi radialis** VAGINA SYNOVIALIS TENDINIS MUSCULI FLEXORIS CARPI RADIALIS. **synovial s. of flexor digitorum longus of foot** VAGINA TENDINUM MUSCULI FLEXORIS DIGITORUM PEDIS LONGI. **synovial s. of flexor pollicis longus** VAGINA TENDINIS MUSCULI FLEXORIS POLLICIS LONGI. **synovial s. of intertubercular groove** VAGINA TENDINIS INTERTUBERCULARIS. **synovial s. of the peronei** VAGINA MUSCULORUM PERONEORUM COMMUNIS. **synovial s. of superior oblique muscle** VAGINA SYNOVIALIS MUSCULI OBLIQUI SUPERIORIS. **synovial s. of tendon** VAGINA SYNOVIALIS TENDINIS. **synovial s. of tendon of extensor carpi ulnaris** VAGINA TENDINIS MUSCULI EXTENSORIS CARPI ULNARIS. **synovial s. of tendon of flexor hallucis longus** VAGINA SYNOVIALIS TENDINIS MUSCULI FLEXORIS HALLUCIS LONGI. **synovial s. of tendons of abductor pollicis longus and extensor pollicis brevis** VAGINA TENDINUM MUSCULORUM ABDUCTORIS LONGI ET EXTENSORIS BREVIS POLLICIS. **synovial s. for tendons of extensor digitorum and extensor indicis** VAGINA TENDINUM MUSCULORUM EXTENSORIS DIGITORUM ET EXTENSORIS INDICIS. **synovial s. of tendons of extensor digitorum longus of foot** VAGINA TENDINUM MUSCULI EXTENSORIS DIGITORUM PEDIS LONGI. **synovial s.'s of tendons**

**of foot** VAGINAE SYNOVIALES TENDINUM DIGITORUM PEDIS. **synovial s. of tibialis anterior** VAGINA TENDINIS MUSCULI TIBIALIS ANTERIORIS. **synovial s. of tibialis posterior** VAGINA SYNOVIALIS TENDINIS MUSCULI TIBIALIS POSTERIORIS. **tendinous s.'s of flexor muscles of fingers** VAGINAE FIBROSAE DIGITORUM MANUS. **tendinous s.'s of flexor muscles of toes** VAGINAE FIBROSAE DIGITORUM PEDIS. **tendon s.** A fibrous covering or sheath that is lined by synovial membrane. This outer sheath is separated from the tendon by a thin layer of synovial fluid to minimize friction and facilitate movement. **tendon s. of anterior tibial muscle** VAGINA TENDINIS MUSCULI TIBIALIS ANTERIORIS. **tendon s. of long extensor muscles of toes** VAGINA TENDINUM MUSCULI EXTENSORIS DIGITORUM PEDIS LONGI. **tendon s. of long flexor muscles of toes** VAGINA TENDINUM MUSCULI FLEXORIS DIGITORUM PEDIS LONGI. **tendon s. of posterior tibial muscle** VAGINA SYNOVIALIS TENDINIS MUSCULI TIBIALIS POSTERIORIS. **s. of thymus** A delicate fibrous capsule which surrounds each lobe of the thymus and sends septa into the parenchyma, dividing each lobe into irregular lobules. Superiorly the capsule may be continuous with the pretracheal fascia ensheathing the thyroid gland. **thyroid s.** A sheath surrounding the thyroid gland. It is derived from the pretracheal layer of the deep cervical fascia and is continuous posteriorly with the buccopharyngeal fascia. Superiorly it is attached to the arch of the cricoid cartilage while inferiorly it extends into the superior mediastinum with the inferior thyroid veins. It is separated from the capsule of the gland by loose connective tissue and blood vessels.

**Sheehan** [Harold Leeming *Sheehan,* English pathologist, flourished 20th century] See under SYNDROME.

**sheet** [Old English *scēte*] **1** A large, usually rectangular piece of linen, cotton, or other material used as bedding. **2** A flat, thin structure or layer. **β-pleated s.** One of the common secondary structures of polypeptide chains in proteins, having the chains almost fully extended. The chain has the form of an almost flat, but slightly pleated, ribbon. The C═O and N—H groups stick out to the sides and can form hydrogen bonds with parallel or antiparallel chains.

**Sheldon** [Joseph Harold *Sheldon,* English pediatrician, flourished 20th century] Freeman-Sheldon syndrome. See under WHISTLING FACE–WINDMILL VANE HAND SYNDROME.

**Sheldon** [Sir Wilfrid S. *Sheldon,* English pediatrician, born 1901] Luder-Sheldon syndrome. See under SYNDROME.

**shelf** A broad projecting structure with a flat surface. **Blumer s.** A shelflike mass felt in the rectum resulting from neoplastic or inflammatory infiltration of the pouch of Douglas. Also *rectal shelf, Strauss sign.* **buccal s.** A shelf of bone which appears on the mandible following resorption of the alveolar process. It connects the residual alveolar ridge to the lateral oblique line in the buccal sulcus. **mesocolic s.** The mesocolon transversum and omentum majus considered together. **palatine s.** PALATINE PROCESS. **rectal s.** BLUMER SHELF.

**shell** / **electron s.** A group of orbitals around an atom which form a stable structure when filled with electrons. The first electron shell can contain two electrons, the second can contain eight, and the third eighteen. They are sometimes known as the K, L, M, etc., shells.

**shellac** LAC².

**shell shock** See under SHOCK.

**Shenton** [Edward Warren Hine *Shenton,* English radiologist, 1872–1955] Shenton's arch. See under LINE.

**Shepherd** [Francis John *Shepherd,* Canadian surgeon, 1851–1929] See under FRACTURE.

**Sherren** [James *Sherren,* English surgeon, 1872–1945] See under TRIANGLE.

**Sherrington** [Charles Scott *Sherrington,* English physiologist, 1856–1952] **1** Sherrington's law. See under RECIPROCAL INNERVATION. **2** Liddell-Sherrington reflex. See under REFLEX. **3** See under PHENOMENON.

**shiatsu** \shē·ät′soo\ [Japanese *shiatsu-ryōhō* (from *shi-* finger-, digital + *atsu* pressing, pressure + *ryōhō* cure, treatment) digital pressure treatment] A system of massage, evolved in Japan, in which pressure is applied with the finger tips or a small pointed device to small, well-defined areas of the body. It is closely related to acupuncture in its theory and in some of its therapeutic applications. Also *acupressure.*

**shield** [Old English *scield*] Anything serving as a barrier to the passage or penetration of a force or substance, as for protection from injury. **amputation s.** A metal disk used to hold back the soft tissues surrounding a bone that is to be divided. **Buller s.** A transparent protective bandage placed over the eye. **circumcision s.** A device placed over the penis to aid the operation of circumcision. It may take the form of a piece of metal, slotted to receive the prepuce and so guarding the glans penis. Another form is a plastic dome which is placed beneath the prepuce, around which a ligature is then tied. **heat s.** A device that focuses radiant heat directly onto a patient, thus warming the patient without making the environment uncomfortable for those working with the patient. **nipple s.** A protective device that fits around the nipple of a pregnant or postpartum woman to prevent irritation of the nipple. **oral s.** ORAL SCREEN. **phallic s.** A device to protect the penis during circumcision. **skull s.** A metal or plastic plate worn over a cranial defect for protection, especially postoperatively.

**shielding** Enclosure of electronic circuits and wires within continuous or braided metal to minimize entry of interfering signals.

**shift** A movement or change in position. **antigenic s.** The major variation that arises in either the hemagglutinin or neuraminidase of influenza A and which usually heralds a pandemic due to lack of antibody to the new virus types. Examples of this shift are a change in the hemagglutinins $H_0$, $H_1$, $H_2$ and $H_3$, and the neuraminidases $N_1$ and $N_2$. **axis s.** The outmoded concept that the Bennett movement is due solely to a shift in the axis. **chloride s.** A movement of chloride from plasma to erythrocyte interior, or vice versa, that counterbalances the uptake or release of bicarbonate by hemoglobin, thus maintaining osmotic and ionic equilibrium. Also *Hamburger phenomenon, shift of Hamburger.* **Doppler s.** DOPPLER EFFECT. **s. down** A change in the growth medium of cells in such manner as to diminish their rate of growth. **frame s.** See under FRAME-SHIFT MUTATION. **s. of Hamburger** CHLORIDE SHIFT. **isohydric s.** The uptake or release of protons by hemoglobin without change in pH of blood. This buffering mechanism is mediated by the imidazole nitrogen of histidyl residues, and accompanies the uptake and release of bicarbonate by hemoglobin, thus facilitating carbon dioxide transport. **s. to the left** An increase in the proportion of band or nonsegmented neutrophils in the blood. Also *regenerative blood shift.* See also ARNETH CLASSIFICATION. **permanent threshold s.** The irreversible deterioration of hearing consequent upon exposure to excessive noise or ototoxic medication. **phase s.** The time difference between corresponding points in similar waveforms expressed in degrees of lag (delay) or lead (advance). **Purkinje s.** PURKINJE EFFECT. **regenerative blood s.** SHIFT TO THE LEFT. **s. to the right** An increase in the proportion of segmented neutrophils, especially of those with five or more nuclear lobes, in the blood. **temporary threshold s.** Hearing deterioration immediately following exposure to loud noise or to certain ototoxic drugs. In such cases, hearing is found to recover entirely, or to a certain degree, with the passage of time. **threshold s.** An alteration of the auditory threshold, either temporary or permanent.

**Shiga** [Kiyoshi *Shiga*, Japanese bacteriologist, 1870–1957] **1** See under TOXIN. **2** Shiga's dysentery. See under BACILLARY DYSENTERY.

***Shigella*** \shigel′ə\ [after Kiyoshi *Shiga*, Japanese bacteriologist, 1870–1957 + *ella*, L fem. diminishing suffix] A genus of Enterobacteriaceae, of the family Escherichea, that invade intestinal epithelial cells and cause bacillary dysentery. Unlike the closely related *Escherichia coli*, they lack motility and do not ferment lactose, form gas from glucose, or decarboxylate lysine. There are four species, differentiated biochemically and serologically. ***S. boydii*** Group C shigella, with 15 serotypes. The disease it causes, most prevalent in the tropics, is moderately severe. ***S. dysenteriae*** Group A shigella, with 10 serotypes, differentiated from other shigellae by lack of mannitol fermentation. It excretes an exotoxin and causes severe disease. Also *Shigella shigae* (obs.), *Bacillus dysenteriae* (obs.). ***S. flexneri*** Group B shigella, with 6 serotypes. It causes moderately severe disease. ***S. shigae*** *Obs.* *SHIGELLA DYSENTERIAE.* ***S. sonnei*** Group D shigella, differentiated from other shigellae by ornithine decarboxylation and slow lactose fermentation. It causes mild disease.

**shigella** (*pl.* shigellae) An organism of the genus *Shigella*. Also *dysentery bacillus*.

**shigellae** \shigel′ē\ Plural of SHIGELLA.

**shigellosis** \shig′əlō′sis\ [*Shigell(a)* + -OSIS] Any intestinal infection caused by bacteria of the genus *Shigella*. Clinical presentation ranges from asymptomatic disease or mild, watery diarrhea to fatal attacks of dysentery, usually caused by *S. dysenteriae I*. The infections are worldwide and highly contagious, transmitted by the fecal-oral route. Incubation period ranges from 1–6 days. Diagnosis is by stool or rectal-swab culture. Antibiotics are indicated in severe cases.

**shin** [Old English *scinu*] The anterior surface of the leg or of the tibia; shank. Also *anticnemion*. **saber s.** A prominence of the anterior border of the tibia that is caused by cortical or subperiosteal new bone formation of the anterior tibia. It is seen in osteitis deformans, syphilis, and yaws. Also *Fournier sign, saber tibia, saber-scabbard tibia, saber-shaped tibia*.

**shinbone** TIBIA.

**shingles** [Middle English *schingles*, alteration of Med L *cingulus* (from L *cingulum* a belt, girdle, from *cingere* to gird, tie about) translation of Gk *zōnē* a girdle, shingles] HERPES ZOSTER.

**shiver** **1** To exhibit an involuntary contraction of muscles either from fear, exposure to cold, or during the onset of fever. **2** A slight tremor or chill.

**shivering** The involuntary contraction of skeletal muscles that occurs either as a consequence of fear or exposure to cold, or during the onset of fever.

**shock** [French *choc* (from *choquer* to shock, akin to Dutch *schokken* to jolt) a·shock] **1** A clinical syndrome of which the major characteristics are a low blood pressure, poor peripheral perfusion, mental dulling, and oliguria. It may result from many various circumstances including trauma, fluid loss, burns, contact with electric current, and sudden diminution in cardiac function, as in myocardial infarction. **2** A jarring or jolting impact. **3** A state of profound but usually transitory disturbance or stupefaction. **acoustic s.** Dizziness, pain, and sometimes nausea caused by a sudden or continuous loud sound. **anaphylactic s.** A constellation of sudden and very severe symptoms which occur following a second injection of antigen in an individual or animal with (usually) IgE antibodies to that antigen. In humans, manifestations are acute respiratory distress and hypotension. It may be rapidly fatal if untreated. Also *anaphylactoid shock, allergic shock, anaphylactic intoxication*. **apoplectic s.** APOPLEXY. **asthmatic s.** Severe asthma with circulatory collapse. **burn s.** Hypovolemic shock resulting from a major burn. A generalized capillary permeability is created, allowing plasma to leak into the interstitial spaces and markedly decreasing the effective circulating blood volume. If fluids are not given intravenously, renal failure or death results. **cardiac s.** Shock secondary to a cardiac disorder. **cardiogenic s.** Shock arising because of impaired myocardial function, especially myocardial infarction. Also *heart shock*. **cerebral s.** Terminal hypotension following a devastating head injury in which cardiovascular centers have been destroyed. **culture s.** The impression of disorientation felt when one is removed from a familiar culture and abruptly immersed in another, especially when the pattern of customs and norms and the accepted rules governing interpersonal exchange are very different. **declamping s.** Shock that results from the sudden restoration of blood flow to a major part of the body. It occurs as a result of the redistribution of flow, reflex response, and the release of toxic metabolic products from the previously ischemic area. Also *release syndrome*. **delayed s.** A state of psychologic abnormality related to but remote in time from the original traumatic stimulus. Also *deferred shock*. **diastolic s.** The palpable impact of the heart during diastole. **electrotherapeutic s.** See under ELECTROCONVULSIVE THERAPY. **endotoxic s.** The syndrome caused by the presence of the endotoxins of Gram-negative bacteria in the bloodstream. Its features include fever with rigors, circulatory collapse, and disseminated intravascular coagulation. The pathogenetic mechanisms include intense activation of complement and the Hageman factor dependent pathways. **Forssman s.** A severe cytotoxic reaction produced by the intravenous injection of anti-Forssman antibody into guinea pigs. Guinea pigs have Forssman antigen on their endothelial cells but not on their erythrocytes, so that severe damage to blood vessels occurs, with internal bleeding and death ensuing. Although the clinical picture in the guinea pig shows some resemblance to anaphylaxis, this reaction is immunologically a Coombs and Gell type 2 (cytotoxic) and not a type 1 (anaphylactic) reaction. Also *inverse anaphylaxis* (inaccurate). **heart s.** CARDIOGENIC SHOCK. **hematogenic s.** HEMORRHAGIC SHOCK. **hemoclastic s.** A hypotensive state accompanied by severe hemolysis. The condition may result from hemolytic transfusion reactions or from hemolytic toxins, as following ingestion of fava beans by susceptible persons. **hemorrhagic s.** A state of inadequate organ and tissue perfusion resulting from severe bleeding. A healthy supine human can compensate for a loss of about 15–20% of blood volume but will go into shock with greater losses. Also *hematogenic shock, hemogenic shock*. **histamine s.** Anaphylactic shock that follows intravenous injection of large amounts of histamine. Histamine causes dilatation of arterioles and veins accompanied by a marked increase in capillary permeability and loss of plasma fluid to tissue spaces. These changes are associated with a drastic fall in blood pressure. Bronchoconstriction is also seen. **hypoglycemic s.** INSULIN SHOCK. **hypovolemic s.** A state of inadequate organ and tissue perfusion resulting from a loss of effective circulating blood volume. Besides hemorrhage, loss may occur with burns, peritonitis, sepsis, severe diarrhea, and any other cause of fluid loss. Also *oligemic shock*. **insulin s.** Peripheral circulatory failure caused by insulin overdosage, with rapid drop in blood glucose concentration, apprehension, tremor, sweating, vertigo, psychic disturbance, convulsions, collapse, and coma. The clinical condition may also accompany endogenous secretion of excessive insulin, as in islet cell adenoma of the pancreas. Also *hypoglycemic shock*. **irreversible s.** Shock that is so prolonged or so severe that vital signs cannot be adequately restored. **neural s.** Temporary loss of nervous function after an acute lesion of the central nervous system. Spinal shock is the commonest example. **neurogenic s.** Shock resulting from vasodilatation due to increased activity of the sympathetic nervous system. **obstetric s.** Shock occurring in the immediate postpartum period, usually secondary to hemorrhage. **oligemic s.** HYPOVOLEMIC SHOCK. **osmotic s.** The bursting of phages when the medium in which they are suspended is rapidly diluted. Their nucleic acid is then released into the medium. **paralytic s.** Neural shock accompanying other symptoms as a result of any lesion of the nervous system which causes paralysis. **peptone s.** PROTEIN SHOCK. **pleural s.** CAPPS REFLEX. **primary s.** Shock directly related causally and temporally to the inciting event. **protein s.** A severe, acute reaction to the intravenous administration of a protein or a protein-containing substance. It is manifested by chills and fever, bronchial constriction, cardiovascular collapse, and death. Also *peptone shock*. **secondary s.** Shock that develops gradually or at a time remote from the inciting event. **septic s.** Shock occurring in the presence of a severe infection, usually associated with the release of endotoxins by Gram-negative bacteria. **serum s.** SERUM SICKNESS. **spinal s.** **1** A condition of temporary total flaccidity or severe hypotension and areflexia of the limbs below the level of the lesion following acute spinal cord injury. This state usually passes off in a few days or weeks when spasticity, hyperreflexia, and extensor plantar responses then appear. **2** Hypotension resulting from loss of sympathetic tone following injury to the spinal cord or induction of spinal anesthesia. **surgical s.** A state of shock that occurs during or immediately after a surgical procedure. **traumatic s.** Shock accompanying injury. Although it is usually hemorrhagic, a search must be made for other factors.

**Shohl** [Alfred Theodore *Shohl*, U.S. pediatrician, born 1889] See under SOLUTION.

**Shone** [John Desmond *Shone*, English cardiologist, flourished 20th century] Shone syndrome. See under ANOMALY.

**Shope** [Richard Edwin *Shope*, U.S. physician, 1902–1966] See under PAPILLOMA, PAPILLOMAVIRUS.

**shortsighted** MYOPIC.

**shortsightedness** MYOPIA.

**short-windedness** Shortness of breath; dyspnea.

**shot** A hypodermic injection. *Popular*. **booster s.** A booster dose administered by injection. *Popular*.

**shotty** \shät′ē\ Having a hard, granular texture on palpation, suggestive of small lead pellets.

**shoulder** [Old English *sculdor*, akin to German *Schulter* shoulder] The area lateral to the junction of the neck and trunk, comprising the structures of the girdle of the upper extremity and of the region around the articulation of the humerus. **s. blade** SCAPULA. **drop s.** Downward displacement of one shoulder below the level of the normal side. **knocked-down s.** A dislocation or separation of the acromioclavicular joint that results from a physical contact injury, such as those incurred while playing football. Also *A/C joint separation*. **linguogingival s.** In dental cavity preparation in an anterior tooth, the region of the junction of the gingival and lingual walls. **loose s.** A condition seen in muscular dystrophy and other neuromuscular diseases characterized by weakness and/or hypotonia of the suspensory muscles of the shoulder, thus making it impossible, for example, for a child with this condition to be lifted by his upraised arms. **round s.'s** A forward inclination of the shoulder joints, which occurs in postural round back deformity.

**show** The discharge of blood-tinged mucus from the cervical canal of a pregnant woman just prior to labor or of a nonpregnant woman as an antecedent to menses.

**Shrapnell** [Henry Jones *Shrapnell*, English anatomist, 1761–1841] Shrapnell's membrane, flaccid membrane of Shrapnell. See under PARS FLACCIDA MEMBRANAE TYMPANI.

**shrinkage** \shring′kij\ The condition of drawing up or contracting, as in response to temperature change.

**shrinker** / **stump s.** An elastic device pulled over an amputation stump to reduce edema and shape the stump.

**shudder** **1** To tremble or shake, as from cold or in fear. **2** A brief tremor.

**shuffle** / **exon s.** The rearrangement of exons within a gene to generate a diversity of products from a locus as, for example, at the immunoglobulin loci.

**shunt** [Middle English *shunten*] **1** A sidetracking of flow, as of blood, urine, nerve impulses, or cerebrospinal fluid, by relocation or by anastomosis of structures, that occurs as a result of developmental defect, physiologic readjustment, or surgery. **2** A surgical procedure by which fluid flow is directed, as in *portocaval shunt*. **3** The new connection or conduit created by such a procedure, as in *Scribner shunt*. **4** To divert (blood or another fluid) by means of a shunt. **5** To provide with a surgical shunt.

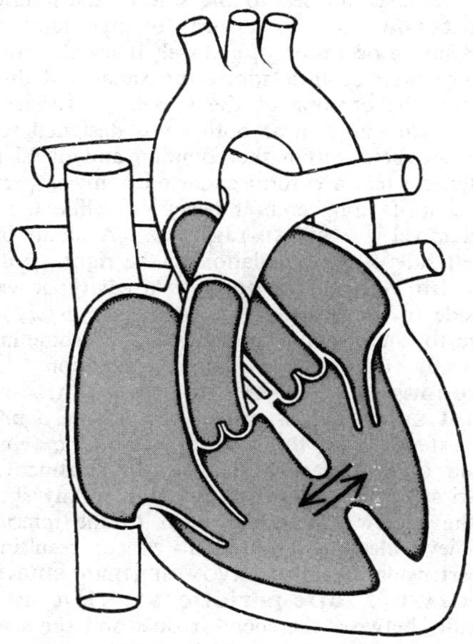

**Cardiovascular shunt** (caused by septal defect)

**6** A natural passage between two anatomical channels. **arteriovenous s.** **1** A communication between an artery and a vein, usually by means of an external or subcutaneous tube or prosthetic conduit. It is most often constructed to provide vascular access. **2** Any of the microscopic communications that occur naturally between arteries and veins in the microcirculation. Also *arteriovenous communication.* **cardiovascular s.** The shunting of blood between two parts of the circulation as a result of an abnormal communication, as in septal defects of the heart or a persistent ductus arteriosus. **cavomesenteric s.** A mesocaval shunt used in pediatric surgery in which the inferior vena cava is divided and its cephalic end anastomosed to the side of the superior mesenteric vein. **central splenorenal s.** The anastomosis of the splenic vein to the left renal vein, often after a splenectomy, for the relief of bleeding esophageal varices resulting from portal hypertension. **dialysis s.** The creation of an arteriovenous communication for dialysis, usually by external or subcutaneous prosthetic conduits. **distal splenorenal s.** The anastomosis of the splenic vein to the left renal vein, with the ligature of the more central splenic vein immediately distal to its juncture with the mesenteric veins. It is designed to relieve bleeding esophageal varices that result from portal hypertension. Also *Warren shunt.* **Drapanas s.** MESOCAVAL H GRAFT. **endolymphatic s.** **1** A fistula created between the saccus endolymphaticus and the subarachnoid space of the posterior cranial fossa for the relief of the symptoms of Menière's disease. **2** The operation to create such a fistula. **endolymphatic-mastoid s.** **1** A fistula established surgically between the saccus endolymphaticus and the excavated mastoid process as a means of decompressing the saccus for the relief of Menière's disease. A small Silastic tube is inserted to drain the saccus into the mastoid cavity which is then filled with a free or pedicled muscle graft. **2** The operation to create such a fistula. **end-to-side s.** The anastomosis of the end of one vessel to a stoma in the side of another nearby vessel. It is most commonly used in operations for portal hypertension in which the portal vein is divided, its cephalic end ligated, and its caudal end anastomosed to the side of the inferior vena cava. **internal s.** A device for maintaining distal blood flow during occlusion of a vessel. It usually consists of a plastic tube inserted into normal proximal and distal vessels following the opening of the vessel. **Javid s.** A plastic tube with knurls near both ends, designed to be inserted into and held within the common and distal internal carotid arteries while a carotid endarterectomy is performed. It maintains ipsilateral cerebral perfusion while the carotid artery is clamped. **left-to-right s.** A shunt of blood from the left side of the circulation to the right, as from the left atrium, left ventricle, or aorta to a cavity or vessel on the right side of the heart or the pumonary artery. This is usually due to a congenital anomaly, but is sometimes created surgically as in the Blalock operation. **lymphaticovenous s.** LYMPHATICOVENOUS ANASTOMOSIS. **mesoatrial s.** A bypass, usually employing a prosthetic graft, that extends from the superior mesenteric vein to the right atrium of the heart. It is used in treatment of the Budd-Chiari syndrome. **mesocaval s.** Any shunt that connects the superior mesenteric vein to the inferior vena cava to relieve bleeding esophageal varices resulting from portal hypertension. See also CAVOMESENTERIC SHUNT, MESOCAVAL H GRAFT. **otic-periotic s.** **1** A fistula created surgically between the cochlear duct and the scala tympani as a means of treating Menière's disease. A tiny platinum tube is inserted through the basilar membrane of the basal turn of the cochlea. **2** The operation to create such a fistula. **peritoneosubarachnoid s.** A connection between the subarachnoid space and the peritoneal cavity, made by insertion of a tube. Also *peritoneothecal shunt.* **peritoneothecal s.** PERITONEOSUBARACHNOID SHUNT. **peritoneovenous s.** A prosthetic device composed of plastic tubing with an interposed one-way valve. It is used to relieve ascites by transmitting the fluid from the peritoneal cavity into the central venous circulation. **portacaval s.** The anastomosis of the portal vein and the inferior vena cava. **portarenal s.** The anastomosis of the portal and renal veins, usually to treat portal hypertension. **portasystemic s.** An anastomosis of the portal vein or one of its tributaries to a systemic vein, usually the inferior vena cava or one of its tributaries. It is most often performed to treat portal hypertension. **pulmonary s.** The portion of the pulmonary blood flow which bypasses the alveoli or which perfuses unventilated alveoli and which does not therefore participate in gas exchange. **renal-splenic venous s.** SPLENORENAL SHUNT. **reversed s.** A right-to-left shunt, especially one where there has previously been a left-to-right shunt, as in a ventricular septal defect. **right-to-left s.** A shunt of blood from the right side of the heart or pulmonary artery to the left side or arterial circulation. **salpingothecal s.** A connection made between the spinal subarachnoid space and a uterine tube by insertion of a tube. **Scribner s.** A conduit of Teflon-tipped silicone rubber tubing that is inserted into an artery and a nearby vein to produce an arteriovenous fistula that can be used for vascular access in patients requiring hemodialysis. **side-to-side s.** The anastomosis of a stoma in the side of one vessel to a stoma in the side of a nearby vessel. It is most commonly used in operations for portal hypertension, where the portal vein is connected side-to-side with the inferior vena cava. **splenorenal s.** **1** The anastomosis of the splenic vein and the left renal vein to treat portal hypertension. Also *renal-splenic venous shunt.* **2** The anastomosis of the splenic artery to the left renal artery in order to bypass a proximal renal artery stenosis or occlusion. **Stookey-Scarff s.** THIRD VENTRICULOCISTERNOSTOMY. **subduroperitoneal s.** A shunt providing drainage of the cranial subdural space into the peritoneal cavity. **subduropleural s.** A shunt providing drainage of the cranial subdural space into the pleural cavity. **Thomas appliqué s.** A prosthetic arteriovenous shunt anastomosed to the femoral artery and vein. **Torkildsen s.** Introduction of a bypass between a lateral ventricle and the cisterna magna for treatment of obstruction of the aqueduct of Sylvius. Also *Torkildsen's operation, ventriculocisternal anastomosis.* **total s.** Any of the portal decompression operations that completely divert flow in the portal vein away from the liver. **ureterothecal s.** A shunt providing drainage of fluid from the spinal subarachnoid space to a ureter. The operation requires sacrifice of a kidney. **ventriculoatrial s.** Drainage of ventricular fluid directly into the right cardiac atrium. A surgical procedure is required to establish a tube between the two cavities via the jugular vein and a valve interposed either outside the skull or in the atrial tip of the tube to prevent back flow. **ventriculojugular s.** A ventriculovenous shunt for the treatment of hydrocephalus in which cerebrospinal fluid is drained into the jugular vein by means of a subcutaneous plastic tube. **ventriculoperitoneal s.** A subcutaneous tube providing drainage of ventricular fluid to the peritoneal cavity. **ventriculopleural s.** A subcutaneous tube providing drainage of ventricular fluid to the pleural cavity. **ven-**

**triculovenous s.** A treatment for hydrocephalus in which cerebrospinal fluid is drained from the cerebral ventricles into the central circulation by means of a plastic shunt. **Warren s.** DISTAL SPLENORENAL SHUNT.

**shuttle** A mechanism for carrying a substance back and forth, generally across a membrane. **glycerol phosphate s.** A mechanism for transport of electrons and protons across the inner mitochondrial membrane. The shuttle involves glycerol phosphate as a carrier and is unidirectional. It is present in tissues where $NADH^+$ is used to reduce dihydroxyacetone phosphate to glycerol phosphate which is then reoxidized within the mitochondrion by a flavoprotein. The shuttle is most studied in insect flight muscles.

**Shwartzman** [Gregory *Shwartzman,* U.S. physician, 1896–1965] Shwartzman reaction, Sanarelli-Shwartzman reaction, Shwartzman-Sanarelli phenomenon. See under SHWARTZMAN PHENOMENON. • The erroneous spellings *Schwartsman* and *Schwartman* are also sometimes used in these terms.

**Shy** [George Milton *Shy,* U.S. physician, 1919–1967] Shy-Drager syndrome. See under SYNDROME.

**SI** **1** Système International d'Unités. **2** soluble insulin.

**Si** Symbol for the element, silicon.

**Sia** [R. H. P. *Sia,* Chinese physician, flourished 20th century] Sia water test. See under TEST.

**SIADH** [From *syndrome of inappropriate antidiuretic hormone* (vasopressin) *secretion*] SCHWARTZ-BARTTER SYNDROME.

**sial-** \sī′əl-\ SIALO-.

**sialaden** \sī·al′əden\ A salivary gland.

**sialadenectomy** \sī′alad′enek′təmē\ Excision of any one of the salivary glands, usually one of the major salivary glands, particularly the parotid and submandibular glands. Also *sialoadenectomy.*

**sialadenitis** \sī′alad′enī′tis\ Inflammation of a salivary gland or glands. **chronic nonspecific s.** Chronic inflammatory swelling of a major salivary gland, often characterized by recurrent exacerbations. It is sometimes the result of infection secondary to duct obstruction, for instance by a calculus.

**sialadenography** \sī′alad′enäg′rəfē\ SIALOGRAPHY.

**sialadenotomy** \sī′alad′enät′əmē\ Incision into a salivary gland. It may be performed to drain an abscess or remove a calculus. Also *sialoadenotomy.*

**sialagogic** \sī′aləgäj′ik\ [SIAL- + *-agog(ue)* + -IC] Stimulating salivation. Also *sialogogic.*

**sialagogue** \sī·al′əgäg\ [SIAL- + -AGOGUE] An agent which stimulates the flow of saliva. Also *sialogogue.*

**sialangiography** \sī′alan′jē·äg′rəfē\ SIALOGRAPHY.

**sialectasia** \sī′alektā′zhə\ SIALECTASIS.

**sialectasis** \sī′alek′təsis\ [SIAL- + ECTASIS] Fusiform dilatation of the minor ducts of the salivary glands indicative of and consequent on chronic infection. Also *ptyalectasis, sialectasia, sialoangiectasis.*

**sialic acid** Any acylated neuraminic acid. It is a component of the carbohydrate part of many glycoproteins.

**sialidase** The enzyme (EC 3.2.1.18) that catalyzes the hydrolytic splitting off of sialic residues (residues of acetylated neuraminic acid) from glycoproteins, as from glycoprotein receptors on cells. Also *neuraminidase.*

**sialism** \sī′əlizm\ PTYALISM.

**sialo-** \sī′əlō-\ [Gk *sialon* saliva] A combining form denoting (1) saliva; (2) the salivary glands. Also *sial-.*

**sialoadenectomy** \-ad′ənek′təmē\ SIALADENECTOMY.

**sialoadenography** \-ad′ənäg′rəfē\ SIALOGRAPHY.

**sialoadenotomy** \-ad′ənät′əmē\ SIALADENOTOMY.

**sialoaerophagia** \-er′əfā′jə\ AEROPHAGIA.

**sialoaerophagy** \-eräf′əjē\ AEROPHAGIA.

**sialoangiectasis** \-an′jē·ek′təsis\ SIALECTASIS.

**sialoangiitis** \-an′jē·ī′tis\ SIALODOCHITIS.

**sialoangiography** \-an′jē·äg′rəfē\ SIALOGRAPHY.

**sialoangitis** \-anjī′tis\ SIALODOCHITIS.

**sialodochitis** \-dōkī′tis\ [SIALO- + Gk *doch(ē),* also *doch(os)* a receptacle + -ITIS] Inflammation of a salivary duct. Also *sialoangitis, sialoangiitis, sialoductitis.*

**sialodochoplasty** \-dō′kəplas′tē\ Plastic surgery of a salivary duct, as, for example, to correct cicatricial stenosis.

**sialoductitis** \-duktī′tis\ SIALODOCHITIS.

**sialogogic** \-gäj′ik\ SIALAGOGIC.

**sialogogue** \sī·al′əgäg\ SIALAGOGUE.

**sialography** \sī′əläg′rəfē\ [SIALO- + -GRAPHY] Radiography of the salivary glands after the instillation of opaque contrast medium into the ducts. Also *sialadenography, sialangiography, sialoadenography, sialoangiography, ptyalography.*

**sialolithiasis** \-lithī′əsis\ The disease characterized by the formation of salivary calculi. Symptoms depend on the site of the calculus or calculi and whether or not infections, sometimes recurrent, are concerned. In the submandibular salivary gland, the site of 90 percent of cases, large calculi are likely to obstruct the duct and result in swelling of the gland while eating. Also *ptyalolithiasis, salivolithiasis.*

**sialolithotomy** \-lithät′əmē\ Incision into a salivary duct or, uncommonly, into a salivary gland, for the removal of a calculus. The great majority of such incisions are made from within the mouth to remove a calculus from the submandibular salivary duct. Also *ptyalolithotomy.*

**sialometer** \sī′əläm′ətər\ [SIALO- + -METER] An instrument for measuring the rate of secretion of saliva from the major salivary glands. It comprises an arrangement for attachment to the opening of the salivary duct, by suction or cannulation, and a drop counter or other means of measuring the weight or volume of the secretions.

**sialometry** \sī′əläm′ətrē\ [SIALO- + -METRY] The measurement of the rate of secretion of saliva, usually from the parotid and submandibular salivary glands, done for physiologic purposes and for the investigation of salivary gland disease.

**sialon** \sī′əlän\ SALIVA.

**sialophagia** \-fā′jə\ [SIALO- + -PHAGIA] The excessive swallowing of saliva.

**sialoprotein** Any glycoprotein containing sialic acid.

**sialorrhea** \sī′əlôrē′ə\ PTYALISM.

**sialosis** \sī′əlō′sis\ PTYALISM.

**sialostenosis** \-stenō′sis\ Stenosis of the duct of a major salivary gland, usually cicatricial stenosis.

**sib** \sib\ [Middle English *sib, sibbe,* from Old English *sibb* related] **1** A brother or sister; sibling: used without regard to sex. **2** A blood relation.

**sibbens** \sib′ənz\ [variant of *sivvens*; adaptation of local Gaelic *suibhean* raspberry] A treponemal skin infection which was prevalent in Scotland during the seventeenth and eighteenth centuries, now considered to have been endemic, nonvenereal syphilis.

**sibilant** \sib′ilənt\ [L *sibilans,* gen. *sibilantis,* pres. part. of *sibilare* to hiss, whistle] Characterized by a hissing or whistling sound.

**sibling** \sib′ling\ [SIB + *-ling,* diminishing suffix] A brother or sister: used without regard to sex.

**sibship** \sib′ship\ **1** A group of two or more children having one or both parents in common. **2** The state of being a sib.

**Sibson** [Francis *Sibson,* English anatomist, 1814–1876] **1** Sibson's groove. See under FURROW. **2** Sibson's aponeurosis, Sibson's fascia. See under MEMBRANA SUPRAPLEURALIS. **3** Sibson's vestibule. See under VESTIBULE OF AORTA. **4** Sibson's muscle. See under MUSCULUS SCALENUS MINIMUS.

**Sicard** [Jean Athanase *Sicard,* French physician, 1872–1929] Sicard syndrome, Sicard's posterior condylar syndrome. See under COLLET-SICARD SYNDROME.

**siccant** \sik′ənt\ [L *siccans,* gen. *siccantis,* pres. part. of *siccare* to dry] **1** Drying. **2** An agent that causes drying. *Obs.* For defs. 1 and 2 also *siccative* (obs.).

**siccolabile** \sik′ōlā′bīl\ Altered or destroyed when subjected to drying: said of a substance.

**siccostabile** \sik′ōstā′bīl\ Remaining stable when subjected to drying; not siccolabile: said of a substance.

**siccus** \sik′əs\ [L, dry] Dry.

**sick** [Old English *seoc*] **1** Affected by or suffering from a disease. **2** Affected by nausea or the compulsion to vomit.

**sickle** To undergo sickling: used especially of erythrocytes.

**sicklemia** \siklē′mē·ə\ SICKLE CELL ANEMIA.

**sicklemic** \siklē′mik\ Pertaining to or having sickle cell anemia.

**sickler** \sik′lər\ A person whose erythrocytes can be made to sickle: usually used colloquially for a patient who suffers from sickle-cell anemia.

**sickling** \sik′ling\ The formation of sickle-shaped erythrocytes, usually occurring under conditions of low oxygen tension, low pH and high solute concentration.

**sickness** **1** The state of being sick; a diseased condition. **2** A disease; illness. **acute serum s.** See under SERUM SICKNESS. **acute sleeping s.** RHODESIAN TRYPANOSOMIASIS. **aerial s.** AIR SICKNESS. **African sleeping s.** **1** GAMBIAN TRYPANOSOMIASIS. **2** RHODESIAN TRYPANOSOMIASIS. **air s.** Motion sickness occurring among passengers and crew in air travel. Also *aerial sickness, aviation sickness.* **altitude s.** A condition resulting from anoxia due to low oxygen pressure at high altitudes (above approximately 11 000 feet). Symptoms include dyspnea, palpitations, giddiness, nausea, headache, malaise, thirst, and oliguria. The severity depends on the height, duration, and degree of acclimatization. Also *altitude disease, altitude anoxia.* **aviation s.** AIR SICKNESS. **black s.** KALA-AZAR. **Ceylon s.** BERIBERI. **chronic serum s.** See under SERUM SICKNESS. **chronic sleeping s.** GAMBIAN TRYPANOSOMIASIS. **decompression s.** A condition caused by the rapid reduction of ambient pressure which leads to the formation of gas bubbles, chiefly nitrogen, in the blood or body tissues. It occurs with rapid ascent to high altitudes in open aircraft or with rapid return from high pressures below sea level or in compressed air chambers to normal atmospheric pressure. Symptoms include pain in limbs and joints (the bends) and chest (the chokes), skin irritation, tingling and numbness of limbs, and vertigo. Later sequelae are aseptic necrosis of bone and paralysis of limbs. Also *caisson disease, decompression disease, aerobullosis, aeroemphysema, tunnel disease.* **drug-induced serum s.** An allergic reaction having the clinical characteristics of serum sickness and caused by an administered drug. **East African sleeping s.** RHODESIAN TRYPANOSOMIASIS. **falling s.** MAJOR EPILEPSY. **Gambian sleeping s.** GAMBIAN TRYPANOSOMIASIS. **green s.** CHLOROSIS. **Indian s.** An Indian term for EPIDEMIC GANGRENOUS PROCTITIS. **jumping s.** *Outmoded* CHOREOMANIA. **laughing s.** PSEUDOBULBAR PARALYSIS. **microwave s.** Adverse effects from chronic exposure to microwave radiation, including cataract and thermal damage to the eye and possibly premature senility. **mid-African sleeping s.** RHODESIAN TRYPANOSOMIASIS. **morning s.** Nausea and sometimes vomiting occurring in pregnant women, usually in the early mornings during the first trimester. Also *nausea gravidarum.* **motion s.** Sickness, characterized chiefly by nausea, vertigo, and sometimes vomiting, induced in susceptible individuals by motion. The motion is such as to produce contradictory evidence to the senses involved with equilibrium. Also *kinesis, kinesia, mechanical vertigo.* **mountain s.** Altitude sickness occurring in high mountainous regions, such as the Andes. Also *Acosta's disease, puna, mountain disease, Monge's disease.* **ozone s.** The headache, drowsiness, and eye irritation brought on by ozone poisoning. It is associated with ozone leakage into jet aircraft flying at high altitudes (greater than 12.2 Km, or 40 000 feet). **painted s.** PINTA. **radiation s.** A toxic state following exposure to or ingestion of a source of ionizing radiation. Also *radiation illness, roentgen intoxication, radiotoxemia, x-ray sickness.* • *Radiation syndrome* is more general than *radiation sickness* and is the preferred term. *Radiation sickness* is too restricted and nonspecific and fails to signify dose-dependent features. **Rhodesian sleeping s.** RHODESIAN TRYPANOSOMIASIS. **sea s.** SEASICKNESS. **secondary radiation s.** Disease due to a graft-versus-host reaction after transplantation of lymphoid cells to irradiated recipients, as that occurring in radiation chimera. Also *secondary disease.* **serum s.** **1** An illness formerly resulting from the treatment of bacterial infections in man with antibacterial antiserum raised in animals. It results from antibody formation to the xenogeneic serum proteins and the consequent formation of immune complexes. Its manifestations are those of a systemic, circulating, immune complex disease with the main target organs being the skin (urticaria and other rashes), the joints (arthralgia), and the kidneys (glomerulonephritis). Also *serum disease, serum shock, serum intoxication.* **2** An immune complex reaction to any exogenous antigen which resembles the reaction formerly found in serum sickness. **sleeping s.** **1** GAMBIAN TRYPANOSOMIASIS. **2** RHODESIAN TRYPANOSOMIASIS. **spotted s.** **1** PINTA. **2** CEREBROSPINAL MENINGITIS. **talking s.** ENCEPHALITIS LETHARGICA. **West African sleeping s.** GAMBIAN TRYPANOSOMIASIS. **x-ray s.** RADIATION SICKNESS. **Zambezi sleeping s.** RHODESIAN TRYPANOSOMIASIS.

**Sidbury** [J. B. *Sidbury,* Jr., U.S. pediatrician, born 1922] Sidbury syndrome. See under ISOVALERICACIDEMIA.

**side** **1** Either of the two halves of the body as divided by the median plane. **2** Either of the two lateral surfaces or aspects of the body between front and back. **balancing s.** In mastication, the side opposite to the working side. **working s.** In mastication, which is usually unilateral at any one time, the side of the mouth to which the mandible moves in order to act on the bolus of food.

**side-effect** A secondary effect of a drug produced along with the intended therapeutic one. The additional effect need not be adverse, but undesirable or toxic effects are usually implied. Also *side effect.*

**sideramine** \sid′əram′ēn\ A hydroxamic acid derivative formed by some bacteria. It solubilizes the $Fe^{3+}$ ion and interacts with specific membrane receptors to promote its uptake.

**sidero-** \sid′ərō-\ [Gk *sidēros* iron] A combining form denoting iron.

**sideroblast** \sid′əroblast′\ A nucleated erythrocyte precursor with stainable iron granules in the cytoplasm. **ringed s.** An erythrocyte precursor, or normoblast, that when stained by the Prussian blue method, displays numerous large blue granules, approximately 0.1 microns in diameter, in a ring around the nucleus. The granules are mitochondria stuffed with iron in an amorphous state as a result of a defect in heme synthesis. Ringed sideroblasts are found in bone marrow in many disorders, including hereditary sideroblastic anemia, idiopathic sideroblastic anemia, and erythroleukemia, or as a result of exposure to such drugs or toxins as isonicotinic acid hydrazide, cycloserine, or lead.

**siderochrome** \sid'ərōkrōm'\ SIDEROPHORE.

**siderocyte** \sid'ərōsīt'\ A mature erythrocyte with stainable iron granules in the cytoplasm.

**siderocytosis** \-sītō'sis\ The presence of siderocytes in the peripheral blood.

**sideroderma** \-dur'mə\ A bronze or brown discoloration of the skin due to deposition of iron pigments.

**siderogenous** \sid'əräj'ənəs\ **1** Producing iron. **2** Derived from iron.

**sideromycin** \-mī'sin\ Any of a group of antibiotic analogues of sideramine that interfere with its action in facilitating uptake of $Fe^{3+}$ by bacteria.

**sideropenia** \-pē'nē·ə\ IRON DEFICIENCY.

**sideropenic** \-pē'nik\ [SIDERO- + Gk *pen(ia)* poverty + -IC] Relating to or characterized by a deficiency of iron.

**siderophil** \sid'ərōfil'\ **1** A cell or tissue which absorbs or contains iron. Also *siderophile.* **2** SIDEROPHILOUS.

**siderophile** \sid'ərōfīl'\ **1** SIDEROPHIL. **2** SIDEROPHILOUS.

**siderophilous** \sid'əräf'ələs\ Having an affinity for iron: used especially of a cell or tissue. Also *siderophil, siderophile.*

**siderophore** \sid'ərōfôr'\ Any of various compounds produced by bacteria that chelate $Fe^{3+}$ and interact with specific membrane receptors to promote its uptake. They include citrate, sideramines, and enterobactins. Their competition with host transferrin may be important in pathogenesis. Also *siderochrome.*

**sideroscope** \sid'ərōskōp'\ [SIDERO- + -SCOPE] A magnetic device used for detecting the presence and location of iron embedded in the eyeball.

**siderosilicosis** \-sil'ikō'sis\ SILICOSIDEROSIS.

**siderosis** \sid'ərō'sis\ A benign form of pneumoconiosis in which small, dense opacities are seen in the chest roentgenogram. It is caused by exposure to dust or fumes of metallic iron and iron oxide. There are no symptoms or loss of lung function. It occurs among welders, hematite miners, and workers using iron oxide powder to polish silver or steel. Also *pneumoconiosis siderotica.* Adj. siderotic. **hematogenous s.** Increased iron in any organ or tissue as a result of destruction of erythrocytes rather than from increased iron absorption. **nutritional s.** NUTRITIONAL HEMOSIDEROSIS.

**side-shift** LATEROTRUSION.

**SIDS** sudden infant death syndrome.

**Siegbahn** [Karl Manne Georg *Siegbahn,* Swedish physicist, born 1886] Siegbahn unit. See under X UNIT.

**Siegert** [Ferdinand *Siegert,* German pediatrician, 1865–1946] See under SIGN.

**Siegle** [Emil *Siegle,* German otologist, 1833–1900] Siegle's pneumatic ear speculum. See under SIEGLE'S OTOSCOPE.

**Siemens** [Hermann Werner *Siemens,* German dermatologist, born 1891] **1** Christ-Siemens syndrome. See under ANHIDROTIC ECTODERMAL DYSPLASIA. **2** Hallopeau-Siemens syndrome. See under EPIDERMOLYSIS BULLOSA DYSTROPHICA (RECESSIVE).

**siemens** \sē'mənz\ [after Ernst Werner von *Siemens,* German electrical engineer, 1816–1892] Special name for the reciprocal ohm, the SI derived unit of electrical conductance; one siemens is a conductance of one ampere per volt. Symbol: S

**sieve** \siv\ A utensil equipped with a mesh for sifting substances.

**sievert** \sē'vərt\ Special name for the SI derived unit joule per kilogram when used in the field of ionizing radiation for the measurement of dose equivalence; 1 sievert = 1 joule per kilogram = 100 rems. Symbol: Sv

**SIg** surface immunoglobulin.

**Sig.** *signetur* (L, let it be labeled). It precedes the part of a prescription in which instructions are given to the patient as to the frequency and amount of the medicine to be taken.

**sighing** Characterized by slow, deep inspiration and audible expiration: said of a type of respiration. Also *suspirious.*

**sight** The act or faculty of seeing; vision. **day s.** PHOTOPIC VISION. **far s.** HYPEROPIA. **long s.** HYPEROPIA. **near s.** MYOPIA. **night s.** SCOTOPIC VISION. **old s.** PRESBYOPIA. **second s.** The onset of myopia because of development of a nuclear cataract in a person with presbyopia, with the happy consequence that the person is enabled to read without spectacles. Also *gerontopia, senopia.* **short s.** MYOPIA.

**sigma** \sig'mə\ The name of the eighteenth letter of the Greek alphabet. Symbol: $\sigma$, $\Sigma$

**sigmoid** \sig'moid\ [Gk *sigmoeidēs* (from *sigm(a),* name of the letter $\Sigma$, $\sigma$, + *-eidēs* -like, -OID) sigma-shaped. The actual shape referred to was originally that of a variant form of sigma, like a Roman C, i.e., crescentic; later it was understood as referring to the Roman S.] **1** Having the shape of the letter S, as does the sigmoid colon. **2** Relating to the sigmoid colon or flexure. **3** Denoting a graph whose slope first increases and then decreases, as, for example, the plot of the saturation of hemoglobin against oxygen concentration, where the shape is due to the fact that the first molecule of oxygen to bind facilitates the binding of others. **4** Denoting the kinetics of enzymes with similar graphs of velocity against substrate concentration or effector concentration. This behavior is common with enzymes whose rates control metabolic pathways.

**sigmoidectomy** \sig'moidek'təmē\ [SIGMOID + -ECTOMY] A surgical procedure in which all or part of the sigmoid colon is resected.

**sigmoiditis** \sig'moidī'tis\ Inflammation of the sigmoid flexure, most frequently associated with radiation injury after treatment of the cervix or body of the uterus.

**sigmoidopexy** \sigmoi'dəpek'sē\ [SIGMOID + *o* + -PEXY] A surgical procedure in which the sigmoid colon is resuspended for purposes of treatment of rectal prolapse.

**sigmoidoproctostomy** \sigmoi'dəpräktäs'təmē\ A surgical procedure in which a communication is established between the sigmoid colon and the rectum. Also *sigmoidorectostomy.*

**sigmoidorectostomy** \sigmoi'dərektäs'təmē\ SIGMOIDOPROCTOSTOMY.

**sigmoidoscope** \sigmoi'dəskōp\ [SIGMOID + *o* + -SCOPE] A speculum for examining the sigmoid colon. Also *romanoscope.*

**sigmoidoscopy** \sig'moidäs'kəpē\ [SIGMOID + *o* + -SCOPY] Endoscopic inspection of the interior of the sigmoid colon using a sigmoidoscope.

**sigmoidosigmoidostomy** \sigmoi'dōsig'moidäs'təmē\ The surgical creation of a communication between two portions of the sigmoid colon. It is usually performed to bypass an obstruction or following resection of the sigmoid colon.

**sigmoidostomy** \sig'moidäs'təmē\ [SIGMOID + *o* + -STOMY] A surgical procedure in which a communication is established between the sigmoid colon and the abdominal wall.

**sigmoidotomy** \sig′moidät′əmē\ [SIGMOID + *o* + -TOMY] A surgical incision made into the sigmoid colon.

**Sigmund** [Karl Ludwig *Sigmund*, Austrian physician, 1810–1883] Sigmund's glands. See under NODI LYMPHATICI CUBITALES.

# sign

**sign** [L *sign(um)* a mark, sign, proof, token] Any manifestation of disease which can be objectively ascertained by a physician or another observer, as by examination of the subject. Signs are often intentionally elicited for diagnostic purposes. Compare SYMPTOM. **Aaron s.** A feeling of pain or discomfort in the epigastric or precordial region while pressing over McBurney's point in appendicitis. **Abadie s.** Loss of deep pressure pain sensation in the Achilles tendon, seen in patients with tabes dorsalis. **Abrahams s.** Acute pain produced in biliary lithiasis when pressure is applied midway between the umbilicus and the ninth right costal cartilage. **accessory s.** A sign that accompanies a disorder but that is not pathognomonic. Also *assident sign.* **Achilles tendon s.** Loss of the ankle jerk in sciatica. Also *Babinski sign.* **Ahlfeld s.** A presumptive sign of pregnancy consisting of irregular but circumscribed uterine contractions after the first trimester of pregnancy. **air-cushion s.** Roentgenographic demonstration of air-containing dilated intestine in the right lower quadrant, present in some patients with chronic appendicitis. Also *Klemm sign.* **Alri s.** SLOCUM'S TEST. **anatomical snuff-box s.** Obliteration of the anatomical snuff-box, which is usually clearly visible when an attempt is made to abduct the thumb fully. This is a sign of a radial nerve lesion, due to paralysis of the abductor pollicis longus. **antecedent s.** A premonitory sign, indicating the onset of disease. **anterior tibial s.** STRÜMPELL SIGN. **anterior tibial muscle s.** STRÜMPELL SIGN. **anticus s.** STRÜMPELL SIGN. **Argyll Robertson pupil s.** ARGYLL ROBERTSON PUPIL. **Arroyo s.** ASTHENOCORIA. **assident s.** ACCESSORY SIGN. **associated abduction s.** RAIMISTE SIGN. **associated adduction s.** RAIMISTE SIGN. **auscultatory s.** A definitive sign of pregnancy consisting of identification of the fetal heartbeat. **Babinski s.** 1 EXTENSOR PLANTAR RESPONSE. 2 PRONATION SIGN. 3 Reduced contraction of the platysma during movements of the jaw and face on the affected side in subjects with hemiplegia. 4 ACHILLES TENDON SIGN. 5 In a hemiplegic subject who tries to sit up from the supine position, spontaneous flexion of the hemiplegic thigh and possibly lifting of the heel on the same side. Also *Babinski's test.* **Babinski's toe s.** EXTENSOR PLANTAR RESPONSE. **Ballance s.** Resonance to percussion over the right flank with the patient lying in the left lateral decubitus position. The effect is seen in splenic rupture. **Ballet s.** Malfunction of the extraocular muscles in the thyrotoxicosis of Graves disease. **Bamberger s.** ALLOESTHESIA. **bandage s.** RUMPEL-LEEDE PHENOMENON. **Bárány s.** Nystagmus induced by irrigating the external ear canal with either hot or cold water in the caloric test. With cold water, the direction of the nystagmus is away from the irrigated ear. With hot water, the direction is towards the irrigated ear. **Barré's pyramidal s.** Inability to hold the legs flexed at right angles while lying prone, a sign of a lesion of the pyramidal tracts. **Battle s.** An ecchymosis behind the ear, indicating a basilar skull fracture. **Beccaria s.** Painful pulsations felt in the back of the head by a woman who is pregnant. **Béclard s.** An indication of fetal maturity consisting of a center of ossification in the lower femoral epiphysis. **Beevor s.** Upward displacement of the umbilicus on lifting the head from the pillow, due to paralysis of the lower abdominal muscles, seen particularly in patients with a lesion of dorsal spinal cord. **Bell s.** BELL'S PHENOMENON. **Bergara-Wartenberg s.** WARTENBERG'S PHENOMENON. **Bespaloff s.** Reddening of the tympanic membrane and postnasal catarrh seen at the onset of measles. **Bikele s.** Resistance to passive extension of the elbow when the arm is fully abducted and externally rotated. It is seen in subjects with cervical intervertebral disk prolapse, brachial plexus lesions, or meningitis. **Bing s.** An extensor plantar response evoked in a subject with a pyramidal tract lesion by pricking the dorsum of the foot with a pin. **Bing's entotic s.** A sign, obtained by applying Bing's entotic test, whereby stapes fixation may be differentiated from fixation of the malleus and incus in cases of conductive hearing impairment. **Biot s.** See under BIOT'S RESPIRATION. **Bjerrum s.** BJERRUM SCOTOMA **Blatin s.** HYDATID THRILL. **Blumberg s.** Pain felt on sudden release of steady abdominal pressure in an area of suspected pathology, indicative of peritonitis. Repeated performance of this maneuver with comparison of the pain elicited may indicate increasing or decreasing peritonitis. **Boas s.** An area of hyperesthesia over the right lumbar region in acute cholecystitis. **Bordier-Fränkel s.** Rolling upward and outward of the eyeball on the affected side in facial paralysis. **Borsieri s.** BORSIERI'S LINE. **Boston s.** EYELID LAG. **Bouillaud s.** Chronic retraction of the chest wall due to adhesive pericarditis. **Bouveret s.** Distention of the cecum and right iliac fossa in colonic obstruction. **Boyce s.** A gurgling sound produced by pressing on the side of the neck, occurring in diverticulum of the esophagus. **Braun von Fernwald s.** An early sign of pregnancy consisting of asymmetric enlargement of the uterus with the sides separated by a longitudinal furrow. **Braunwald s.** The presence of a weak pulse rather than a stong pulse when a sinus beat follows a ventricular ectopic beat, a feature of obstructive hypertrophic cardiomyopathy. **Braxton Hicks s.** BRAXTON HICKS CONTRACTION. **Brenner s.** A metallic rub heard over the twelfth left rib posteriorly, due to air bubbles collecting between the stomach and diaphragm, occurring in cases of gastric perforation. **Broadbent s.** Systolic retraction in the lower chest posteriorly due to adhesive pericarditis. **Brockenbrough s.** Decrease in the pulse pressure accompanying a sinus beat immediately following a ventricular ectopic beat, a feature of idiopathic hypertrophic subaortic stenosis. **Brown Kelly s.** The subjective sensation of light experienced when the normal maxillary sinus is transilluminated. **Brown-Séquard s.** BROWN-SÉQUARD SYNDROME. **Brudzinski s.** 1 NUCHAL SIGN. 2 In a subject with meningitis, repetition in one leg of the movement brought about by passive flexion of the contralateral knee. Also *Brudzinski's reflex, thigh sign, contralateral sign, contralateral reflex.* **Bruns s.** Intermittent attacks of headache, vertigo, and vomiting, precipitated by abrupt movements of the head, occurring in patients with cerebral cysticercosis in the region of the fourth ventricle. **Burton s.** A blue line along the gums seen in chronic copper or lead poisoning. The first appearance is in the extreme lingual edge of the gum opposite the bicuspids and lower molars. Also *Burton's line.* See also LEAD LINE. **Calkins s.** An indication of separation of the placenta from the uterine wall, consisting of a change in uterine shape from an ovoid to a discoid configuration. **camelot s.** WATER LILY SIGN. **candlewax s.** A yellowish or brownish discoloration of the nails reminiscent of the effect of wax or oil on paper or fabric. It is regarded as virtually pathognomonic for psoriasis. Also *oil-drop sign*. **Cantelli s.** OCULOCEPHALIC REFLEX. **Capps s.** CAPPS REFLEX. **cardinal s.'s** The classical features of acute inflammation: calor (a sign of heat), rubor (redness), dolor (pain), tumor (swelling), and functio laesa (loss of function). **Carman meniscus s.** MENISCUS SIGN. **Carnett s.** Tenderness to abdominal palpation performed while the patient tenses his anterior abdominal musculature, showing that the tenderness is parietal in location because the tense abdominal muscles will keep the examiner's fingers from palpating the underlying viscera. **Case's pad s.** On gastrointestinal series, a smooth localized pressure defect on the inferior aspect of the duodenal bulb or gastric antrum, usually secondary to enlargement of the pancreas. It is accentuated in the prone position. **caviar s.** In pedal lymphangiography, a radiographic sign of lymphangiogram dye within small veins of the lower extremity. It signifies misidentification of a foot vein as a lymphatic. **Cestan s.** A sign of lower motor neuron facial paralysis: when the patient tries to close his eyes while looking forward, there is slight elevation of the upper eyelid on the affected side, attributable to the action of the levator palpebrae superioris. Also *Dupuy-Dutemps and Cestan sign*. **Chaddock s.** Extension of the big toe induced by percussion of the external submalleolar or malleolar region at the ankle, a sign of a pyramidal tract lesion. Also *Chaddock's reflex, external malleolar sign*. **Chadwick s.** Bluish discoloration of the vaginal wall and the cervix secondary to venous engorgement, a presumptive sign of pregnancy. This finding is noted in the second half of the first trimester of pregnancy. Also *Kluge sign*. **Charcot s.** Elevation of the eyebrow in patients with lower motor neuron facial paralysis, and depression of the eyebrow in patients with facial contracture. **Chaussier s.** Severe epigastric pain as a prodrome of eclampsia. **Cheyne-Stokes s.** See under CHEYNE-STOKES RESPIRATION. **chin-retraction s.** A backward or downward chin movement synchronous with inspiration. It is indicative of respiratory obstruction, deep general anesthesia, or respiratory insufficiency. **Chvostek s.** Contraction of the orbicularis oris and buccinator muscles, induced by percussion of the temporofacial branch of the facial nerve at the midpoint of a line joining the ear lobe to the corner of the mouth, and formerly considered to be a pathognomonic sign of neuromuscular hyperexcitability due to tetany. The practical value of the Chvostek sign is nowadays disputed because it is not invariably found in cases of tetany and it may be elicited in about 10% of apparently normal subjects. Nevertheless, the presence of this sign should be taken as indicative of tetany, particularly in children. Also *face phenomenon, facialis phenomenon, Chvostek-Weiss sign, Schultze-Chvostek sign, Chvostek symptom*. **Clark s.** Obliteration of hepatic dullness when there is tympanitic distention of the abdomen. **Claude s.** CLOSED FIST SIGN. **clavicular s.** Enlargement of the inner third of the clavicle. It tends to occur unilaterally and is a sign of late congenital syphilis. Also *Higouménakis sign*. **claw hand s.** Resistance and accentuated flexion of the fingers in a hemiplegic patient when one attempts to extend the fingers passively. **clenched fist s.** A characteristic gesture of a patient with angina pectoris who clenches his fist in front of the sternum to indicate the constricting quality of the discomfort. Also *Levine's clenched-fist sign*. **closed fist s.** In a patient with a lesion of the median nerve, loss of ability to oppose the thumb and to flex the terminal two phalanges of the index and middle fingers, preventing him from closing the fist completely. Also *Claude sign*. **cobra head s.** A smooth oval defect in the opacified bladder, seen during urography and representing a ureterocele. **Codman s.** In a rupture of the supraspinatus tendon at the rotator cuff, passive abduction of the shoulder is painless. Attempted active abduction, however, causes pain and hunching of the shoulder due to contraction of the deltoid muscle. **cogwheel s.** In parkinsonism, a jerky pattern of movement with intermittent resistance giving an impression of a cogwheel being moved, elicited by passive flexion or extension of a limb at a joint such as the elbow. This is thought by some to be a specific form of hypertonia, by others to be due to the superimposition of parkinsonian tremor upon a state of plastic rigidity. Also *cogwheel phenomenon, Negro's phenomenon, cogwheel rigidity, cogwheel resistance*. **coin s.** See under COIN SOUND. **Cole s.** On gastrointestinal roentgenography, deformity of the duodenal cap due to an ulcer. **Comby s.** The appearance of thin, whitish patches on the gums and buccal mucous membrane, seen in measles. **commemorative s.** A sign of a previous illness or disease, as one discovered fortuitously in a diagnostic test. **complementary opposition s.** GRASSET-GAUSSEL-HOOVER SIGN. **compressed tissue s.** The accentuation of an ultrasound echo pattern beyond an anechoic area, such as the urine-filled bladder, appearing as an increased echo density. **Conillaud s.** Prominent and reddened fungiform and filiform papillae of the tongue, seen in ascariasis. **contralateral s.** BRUDZINSKI SIGN. **Cope s.** **1** In appendicitis, tenderness elicited by compressing the femoral artery in Scarpa's triangle. **2** FEMORAL SIGN. **coughing s.** HUNTINGTON SIGN. **Courtois s.** Automatic flexion of the leg on the thigh, and of the thigh on the pelvis, induced in a hemiplegic comatose patient, on the side of the cerebral lesion, by flexion of the neck. **Courvoisier s.** A palpable, nontender gallbladder in a jaundiced patient, suggesting biliary obstruction as a result of malignancy. Obstruction by a common bile duct stone rarely causes dilatation of the gallbladder because in this case the gallbladder is usually scarred and nondistensible. **crescent s.** A sign seen during intravenous urography, most commonly in chronic hydronephrosis, in which a crescent-shaped collection of contrast medium appears in the renal parenchyma bordering a dilated calix. It represents opacified collecting ducts deviated circumferentially by the dilated calix. **Cruveilhier s.** On palpating the groin of a subject who is coughing, a perceptible tremor is felt, an indication of the existence of varices of the saphenous vein. *Seldom used*. **Cullen s.** Bluish discoloration around the umbilicus, usually indicative of acute hemorrhagic pancreatitis or a ruptured ectopic pregnancy, occasionally of intraperitoneal hemorrhage. Also *blue navel, Hellendall sign, hematomphalus*. **Cumbo s.** On a chest roentgenogram, the air crescent seen typically in a pulmonary echinococcus cyst. **curtain s.** A sign of unilateral paralysis of the superior constrictor muscle of the pharynx, caused by a lesion of the corresponding pharyngeal branch of the vagus nerve: the posterior wall of the pharynx is displaced towards the unaffected side when the patient says "Ah." The same displacement can be seen on attempting to elicit the gag reflex. **cushingoid s.'s** The signs characteristic of the Cushing syndrome or due to hypercortisolism of any cause. They include plethora; obesity of the centripetal type; buffalo hump; thin skin; easy bruising; abdominal, gluteal, and intercrural purplish striae; and sometimes hirsutism in women. **Dance s.** The absence of palpable viscera in the right lower quadrant: a sign of intussusception. **Danforth s.** Referred pain in the shoulder originating in irritation of the diaphragm caused by intra-abdominal bleeding, indicative of a ruptured ectopic pregnancy. **Darier s.** Dermographism limited to the skin lesions in urticaria pigmentosa. **Davidsohn s.** Diminished illumination of the pupil on transillumination of the maxillary sinus as an indication of fluid or tumor within the sinus. **Dejerine s.** Radicular pain is elicited in nerve root irritation when intraspinal pressure is raised by such incidents as coughing or sneezing. **de Musset s.** Rhythmical systolic nodding of the head due to vigorous arterial pulsation in aortic regurgitation. Also *Musset sign.* **Dennie s.** MORGAN'S LINE. **Diakiogiannis s.** A variant of the extensor plantar response in which light scratching of the skin over the outer aspect of the tibia and on the dorsum of the foot produces extension of the great toe. **diaphragm s.** DIAPHRAGM PHENOMENON. **doll's eye s.** OCULOCEPHALIC REFLEX. **double contour s.** The appearance on a posteroanterior or anteroposterior chest radiograph of a double contour of the right border of the heart, the extra contour representing the border of an enlarged left atrium. **doublet s.** In electromyography, motor unit action potentials occurring in pairs during minimal voluntary contraction, as may be seen in tetany. Similar paired or grouped action potentials, occurring spontaneously on recording from a relaxed muscle, may be seen in myokymia. **drawer s.** DRAWER TEST. **DTP s.** [distal tingling on pressure] TINEL SIGN. **Dubois s.** The shortened little finger of congenital syphilis. **Duchenne s.** A sign of radial nerve paralysis due to lead poisoning: a protrusion is formed by contraction of the unimpaired brachioradialis muscle when the patient flexes the forearm at the elbow against resistance. **Dupuy-Dutemps s.** LEVATOR SIGN. **Dupuy-Dutemps and Cestan s.** CESTAN SIGN. **Dupuytren s.** In cases of congenital dislocation of the hip, the femur moves freely on axial intermittent traction of the femur. **Duroziez s.** See under DUROZIEZ MURMUR. **Dutemps-Cestan s.** See under CESTAN SIGN. **echo s.** Santini's booming sound; a sound heard on percussion over a hydatid cyst suggestive of an echo from a fluid-filled chamber. **Elliot s.** 1 An induration of the edge of skin lesions in syphilis. 2 Enlargement of the blind spot by coalescent scotomata such as the small nerve fiber defects of glaucoma. **Erb s.** Hyperexcitability on galvanic electrical stimulation of muscles, as seen in tetany, with a reduction in the excitation threshold to the current caused by closing the cathode or opening the anode. *Obs.* **Erben s.** ERBEN'S REFLEX. **Escherich s.** 1 Contraction of the orbicularis oris muscle giving a pouting appearance of the lips, induced by tapping the closed lips. This may be seen in patients with latent tetany, but the snout reflex, a primitive reflex released in degenerative processes involving the frontal lobes, is similar. 2 Lightning contraction of one orbicularis oculi muscle, induced by tapping the external angle of the orbit on the same side, sometimes seen in tetany. **Ewart s.** Dullness at the left lung base in pericardial effusion, attributed to collapse of the left lower lobe because of compression. Also *Pins sign.* **external malleolar s.** CHADDOCK SIGN. **extinction s.** The extinction of the erythema of scarlet fever around the site of injection of serum from an immune subject. **eyelash s.** Movement occurring in hysterical pseudocoma when evoked by stroking the eyelashes. In deep coma due to organic brain disease no such movement occurs. **Faget s.** FAGET'S LAW. **Fajersztajn's crossed sciatic s.** In cases of sciatica, the hip joint may be flexed without pain when the knee is flexed, but pain will be elicited when the knee is held fully extended. Flexing the hip and extending the knee on the asymptomatic side causes pain on the affected side. Also *Fajersztajn's test, Fajersztajn sign.* **Federici s.** On auscultation of the abdomen, heart sounds are audible in cases of intestinal perforation with gas in the peritoneal cavity. **femoral s.** In acute appendicitis, pain elicited by passive hyperextension of the hip due to irritation of the psoas major muscle. Also *Cope sign.* **finger spread s.** Lack of prominence of the long extensor tendons of the fingers when the fingers are forcibly abducted, with the hand flat on a table. It is one sign of a radial nerve lesion. **fistula s.** Nystagmus and/or vertigo elicited by applying the fistula test in cases where a fistula exists between the middle and inner ears. **flag s.** The change in hair color which occurs in kwashiorkor. Alternating bands of red and black coloration are seen in a single hair strand. Also *signe de la bandera.* **Foerster s.** An infant, held suspended under the shoulders by the examiner's hands, rigidly flexes the hips and knees. **fontanel s.** A bulging or tenseness of the fontanel in infants with raised intracranial pressure, as in meningitis. **forearm s.** LÉRI SIGN. **formication s.** TINEL SIGN. **Fournier s.** 1 The sharp margination of a syphilitic lesion on the skin. 2 SABER SHIN. **Friedreich s.** Diastolic collapse of the jugular veins in pericardial constriction. **Froment s.** 1 Footdrop attributable to paralysis of the common peroneal nerve, which becomes more apparent when the patient's leg is briskly flexed at the knee while the patient lies on his face. Also *leg flexion sign.* 2 Flaccidity of the calf muscles and Achilles tendon when the patient puts his weight on the affected leg, seen in patients with paralysis of the medial popliteal nerve. 3 NEWSPAPER SIGN. 4 ROGER'S COUNTER SIGN. **Froment's paper s.** NEWSPAPER SIGN. **front-tap s.** Reflex contraction of the calf muscles of the extended leg induced by a brisk tap on the stretched anterior tibial muscles or the tibia, as seen in some patients with reflex hyperexcitability as a result of pyramidal tract disease. Also *front-tap reflex.* **Fuchs s.** Retraction of the upper eyelid on looking downwards, which may occur when the eye has stopped moving, or at the start of the movement. This may be seen during recovery from a third nerve palsy. **Gangolphe s.** In strangulated hernia, a serosanguineous effusion present intraperitoneally. **glabellar-tap s.** A sign elicited by tapping with a finger or blunt instrument over the glabella, on the forehead above and between the eyes. Blinking occurs in response to the first two or three taps and then ceases in the normal individual. In subjects with parkinsonism, the blinking may continue rhythmically in time with the taps. Also *glabellar tap reflex.* **Gobiet s.** Dilatation of the transverse colon in acute pancreatitis. **Golden s.** Paleness of the cervix as a finding in association with a tubal ectopic pregnancy. **Goldstein s.** Increased space between the great toe and the second toe found in subjects with the Down syndrome and cretinism. **Gonda s.** Extension of the great toe induced by flexion of the second, third, fourth, and fifth toes, seen in patients with severe pyramidal tract lesions. **Goodell s.** A softening of the cervix and vagina as observed during pregnancy. Also *Goodell's law.* **Gordon s.** 1 GORDON'S REFLEX. 2 The pendular knee jerk, a characteristic but variable sign of chorea. **Gorissenne s.** Failure of the pulse rate to increase when rising from a horizontal to a sitting position, as observed in early pregnancy. **Gottron s.** Erythematous papules occurring over the extensor surfaces of the metacarpophalangeal and proximal interphalangeal joints in patients with dermatomyositis. **Gowers s.** 1 In weakness of the pelvic girdle and proximal lower limb muscles, as seen in Duchenne muscular dystrophy and in some other neuromuscular diseases, the subject rises from the floor by "climbing up his own legs," using pressure with the hands on the extended knees and then on the thighs to assume the upright position. 2 In tabes dorsalis, before the Argyll Robertson pupil is fully developed, a light shone into the eye may elicit hippus. **Graefe s.** EYELID LAG. **Grasset s.** GRASSET'S PHENOMENON. **Grasset-Bychowski s.** GRASSET'S PHENOMENON. **Grasset-Gaussel-Hoover s.** A sign of hemiplegia: when the patient who is lying on his back is asked to try to raise the paralyzed limb, the examiner's hand placed on the healthy limb feels greater resistance than is felt in a healthy subject. *Seldom used.* Also *complementary opposition sign.* **Grey Turner s.** TURNER SIGN. **Griesinger s.** A fixed dilated pupil on the same side as a subdural hematoma. **grip s.** The grasp of the examiner's finger by a patient suffering from hemiparesis is relaxed when the patient's wrist is flexed. **Grisolle s.** A papule caused by measles becomes impalpable when the surrounding skin is stretched, whereas a papule due to smallpox can still be felt. **Grocco s.** Extension of the area of liver dullness to the left of the midspinal line, indicating enlargement of the organ. **Gubler s.** A swelling of the synovial sheaths on the back of the hand, seen in cases of chronic lead poisoning. See also GUBLER'S TUMOR. **Gunn's pupillary s.** MARCUS GUNN PUPILLARY PHENOMENON. **Günzberg s.** A resonant abdominal area, localized between the pylorus and the gallbladder, with borborygmi, observed in duodenal ulcer. **Guye s.** GUYE'S APROSEXIA. **Hahn s.** Continuous head-rolling seen in children with cerebellar disease. *Seldom used.* **Halban s.** An increase in the growth of fine hair on the mother's body as observed during pregnancy. **Hamilton s.** Long hairs on the antitragus of the pinna, a common finding in normally virilized males after the age of 30. **harlequin s.** HARLEQUIN COLOR CHANGE. **Harris s.** ATAXIC NYSTAGMUS. **Haudek s.** HAUDEK'S NICHE. **Heberden s.** HEBERDEN'S NODES. **Hefke-Turner s.** OBTURATOR SIGN. **Hegar s.** A softening of the lower uterine segment detected by bimanual examination, a sign of pregnancy. Also *Rasch sign, Loenen sign, Ladin sign.* **Hellendall s.** CULLEN SIGN. **Hertwig-Magendie s.** SKEW DEVIATION. **Hicks s.** BRAXTON HICKS CONTRACTIONS. **Higouménakis s.** CLAVICULAR SIGN. **Hochsinger s.** Closure of the hand on compression of the biceps muscle in tetany. **Hoehne s.** Absence of uterine contractions during labor or delivery despite the use of oxytocic drugs, suggestive of uterine rupture. **Hoffmann s.** 1 HOFFMANN'S REFLEX. 2 Increased excitability of sensory nerves to mechanical stimuli, seen in tetany. **Holmes s.** HOLMES REBOUND PHENOMENON. **Homans s.** Pain in the calf and behind the knee on passive dorsiflexion of the foot with the knee bent. It is suggestive but not diagnostic of deep calf vein thrombosis. **Hoover s.** A sign found in some cases of organic hemiplegia: if the patient is asked, when lying on his back, to press the affected leg down on to the bed, the opposite leg shows an involuntary lifting movement. This is absent in cases of hysterical paralysis. **Horn s.** In acute appendicitis, pain caused by traction on the right spermatic cord. **Horner s.** SPALDING SIGN. **Hoyne s.** With the patient supine, the head falls back when the shoulders are raised, described in patients with poliomyelitis. **Hueter s.** The lack of transmission of osseous vibration across a bone fracture, indicating an interposition of soft tissue. **Huntington s.** In a patient lying supine with the legs allowed to hang over the edge of the bed or couch, so that they are flexed at the knees, if coughing evokes flexion at one or both hips and knee extension, an upper motor neuron lesion is present on the side or sides upon which the sign occurs. Also *coughing sign.* **Hutchinson s.** The interstitial keratitis and redness of the cornea that are seen in congenital syphilis. **Jackson s.** In paralysis of the intercostal muscles, the upper chest is drawn in during inspiration instead of the reverse, due to the action of the diaphragm. **Jacquemier s.** Blue discoloration of the vagina secondary to vascular engorgement, suggestive of pregnancy. **Jellinek s.** Brownish pigmentation seen on the margins of the eyelids in some subjects with hyperparathyroidism. Also *Rasin sign, Jellinek symptom.* **Jolly s.** Inability to adduct the arm at the shoulder when the forearm is flexed at the elbow and the shoulder is held in abduction. This may be seen in patients with lesions of the seventh cervical segment of the spinal cord or of the seventh spinal nerve. **jugular s.** QUECKENSTEDT'S TEST. **Jürgensen s.** Light crepitation heard on auscultation in acute pulmonary tuberculosis. **Kanavel s.** With infection of the flexor tendon sheath of the little finger, there is maximal tenderness just proximal to the transverse palmar crease at the ulnar border of the palm. **Kanter s.** Failure to elicit fetal movement by pressure on the fetal head either transabdominally or transvaginally, suggestive of fetal death. **Kantor s.** STRING SIGN. **Kehr s.** Pain referred to the left shoulder after rupture of the spleen. **Kerandel s.** KERANDEL SYMPTOM. **Kergaradec s.** UTERINE SOUFFLE. **Kernig s.** A sign of meningitis or of other forms of meningeal irritation, as in subarachnoid hemorrhage: with the patient lying supine, the leg is flexed passively at the knee and the thigh at the hip. With the thigh held flexed at the hip, any attempt to extend the leg at the knee meets resistance and causes pain. **Kestenbaum s.** MARCUS GUNN PUPILLARY PHENOMENON. **Kleist s.** Flexion of all of the fingers, resulting in a clawlike posture when passive extension is attempted. This may be a variant of the grasp reflex and can be seen as the result of a contralateral frontal lobe lesion. *Seldom used.* **Klemm s.** AIR-CUSHION SIGN. **Klippel-Feil s.** Rapid passive extension of the flexed fingers evokes flexion and adduction of the thumb in the presence of a pyramidal tract lesion. **Kluge s.** CHADWICK SIGN. **Koplik s.** KOPLIK SPOTS. **Krisovski s.** Scars radiating from the lips in congenital syphilis. Also *Silex sign.* **Kussmaul s.** 1 Paradoxical inspiratory filling of the neck veins as seen in pericardial constriction. Also *Kussmaul's pulse.* 2 KUSSMAUL RESPIRATION. **Kustner s.** A cystic tumor on the median line anterior to the uterus in cases of ovarian dermoids. **Ladin s.** HEGAR SIGN. **Lasègue s.** Pain and resistance induced by attempted passive flexion of the fully extended leg and thigh at the hip. This sign is characteristic of sciatica due to intervertebral disk prolapse, but can also be seen in patients with meningitis or meningeal irritation. Also *Lasègue's test, sciatic stretch test.* **Lasègue's contralateral s.** EVOKED CONTRALATERAL PAIN. **Laugier s.** In a fracture of the distal radius, the radial and ulnar styloid processes are at the same level. **leg s.** 1 NERI SIGN. 2 SCHLESINGER SIGN. **Le Gendre s.** Increased resistance to passive elevation of the eyebrow on the unimpaired side, compared with that on the affected side, in a patient with peripheral facial paralysis. **leg flexion s.** FROMENT SIGN. **Lennhoff s.** In echinococcal liver cyst, a furrow present on deep inspiration below the lowest rib and above the liver cyst. **Léri s.** A sign of hemiplegia: passive flexion of the hand and wrist do not lead to spontaneous flexion of the elbow on the paralyzed side in a hemiplegic patient, whereas elbow flexion does occur when the same maneuver is carried out on the unaffected side, or in a normal subject. *Seldom used.* Also *forearm sign.* **Leser-Trélat s.** The rapid development of numerous pruritic seborrheic keratoses as a manifestation of a systemic malignant disease. **levator s.** In unilateral facial palsy of lower motor neuron type, a slight elevation of the upper eyelid on the paralyzed side if the subject looks downward and then closes the eyes slowly. Also *Dupuy-Dutemps sign.* **Levine's clenched-fist s.** CLENCHED FIST SIGN. **Lhermitte s.** Electric-shocklike paresthesiae radiating down the arms or, more often, down the trunk and legs on head and neck flexion. It is most often observed in multiple sclerosis, but sometimes occurring in cervical cord compression. Also *neck phenomenon.* **Lichtheim s.** The ability of a patient with pure motor aphasia to indicate the number of syllables in a word which he is unable to pronounce, thus demonstrating that he has retained some verbal comprehension. Also *Lichtheim's phenomenon, Dejerine-Lichtheim's phenomenon.* See also LICHTHEIM'S APHASIA. **ligature s.** The appearance of ecchymoses on an extremity distal to the site of application of a ligature or tourniquet. It is seen in various bleeding disorders. **Liget s.** In acute appendicitis, hyperesthesia of the skin of the anterior abdominal wall bounded by lines joining the umbilicus, pubic tubercle, and the anterior superior iliac spine, when it is lifted and pinched gently. **Litten s.** DIAPHRAGM PHENOMENON. **Lockwood s.** With appendiceal adhesions, intestinal gas which can be palpated trickling through the ileocecal valve. **Loenen s.** HEGAR SIGN. **Lombardt s.** The development of varicose veins around the spinous processes of the seventh cervical and first three thoracic vertebrae, described in early pulmonary tuberculosis. **Lorenz s.** A sign of early tuberculosis that is positive if the thoracolumbar spine is rigid. **Ludloff s.** In an avulsion fracture of the lesser trochanter, there appears swelling and bruising at the base of Scarpa's triangle. In addition, the subject is unable to raise the thigh when sitting. **Lust s.** Contraction of the tibialis anterior muscle with dorsiflexion, abduction, and eversion of the foot induced by tapping the common peroneal nerve near the neck of the fibula, seen in patients with tetany. Also *Lust's phenomenon, peroneal-nerve phenomenon, Lust's reflex.* **Macewen s.** A hyperresonant note on percussing the side of the skull, indicating internal hydrocephalus or cerebral abscess. **Magendie s.** SKEW DEVIATION. **Magendie-Hertwig s.** SKEW DEVIATION. **Magnan s.** FORMICATION. **Marañón s.** MARAÑÓN'S REACTION. **Marcus Gunn pupillary s.** MARCUS GUNN PUPILLARY PHENOMENON. **Marie s.** Tremor of the extremities or of the body, seen in Graves disease. **Marie-Foix s.** A withdrawal reflex of the leg, comprising flexion at the knee and hip, induced by transverse pressure on the instep or by forced flexion of the toes, a sign of a pyramidal tract lesion. *Seldom used.* **McBurney s.** In acute appendicitis, tenderness to palpation at a point midway between the umbilicus and the anterior superior iliac crest. **McCarthy s.** Exaggeration of McCarthy's reflex, indicating the presence of a pyramidal tract lesion. **McClintock s.** Maternal tachycardia with a rate exceeding 100 beats per minute in the immediate postpartum period, suggestive of postpartum hemorrhage. **McMurray s.** In a torn meniscus of the knee, rotatory manipulation gives rise to a painful click that can be felt at the joint margin adjacent to the injured meniscus. Also *McMurray's test.* **meniscus s.** A radiographic sign in malignant gastric ulcer: when the stomach is compressed, barium caught within the central ulceration assumes a half-moon configuration (a meniscus), separated from the main column of barium by a broad crescentic rim of tumor with irregular nodular margins, the rounded border of the barium collection in the ulcer being convex toward the lumen of the stomach. Also *Carman meniscus sign.* **Meunier s.** A progressive reduction in body weight observed for several days preceding the appearance of symptoms in measles. **Mingazzini s.** A group of three signs of organic hemiparesis: when the patient stretches out both arms horizontally in front of him with the fingers spread out, the arm on the affected side drifts downwards; the patient shows a greater degree of resistance to forcible opening of the closed eye and closed mouth on the unimpaired than on the affected side; and if both legs are flexed at the hip and knee to a right angle at each joint, the affected leg may fall away quickly. **Mirchamp s.** Pain in the parotid gland when sharp or highly flavored food or drink is taken, an early sign in mumps. *Rare.* **Möbius s.** Inability to maintain convergence of the eyes, seen in Graves disease. **Mosler s.** Sternal tenderness in acute granulocytic leukemia. **moulage s.** The clumping of barium into sausage-shaped masses upon radiographic examination of the small bowel. It is thought to be related to the presence of excess mucus stimulated by fatty acids or lactic acid and is found in idiopathic steatorrhea. **Moutard-Martin s.** EVOKED CONTRALATERAL PAIN. **Murat s.** Discomfort and vibration of the affected side of the chest during speech in patients with pulmonary tuberculosis. **Murphy s.** In acute cholecystitis, pain and inability to take a deep breath when the right subcostal region is palpated. **Musset s.** DE MUSSET SIGN. **Myerson s.** A sign of parkinsonism: tapping over the lower forehead between the eyes causes rhythmic blinking which continues in time with the taps. See also GLABELLAR-TAP SIGN. **neck s.** NUCHAL SIGN. **Negro s.** A sign of peripheral facial paralysis: when the patient looks upward without moving his head and eyeball on the affected side rises further and may deviate outwards due to overaction of the superior rectus and inferior oblique. **Neri s.** **1** In a supine subject with hemiplegia, elevation of the affected leg causes reflex flexion at the knee. Also *leg sign.* **2** Flexion of the knee on the affected side occurs in a subject with sciatica following flexion of the trunk at the hips. Also *Lasègue's maneuver.* **3** In a supine subject with hemiplegia, if the forearms are pronated and placed on a flat surface, passive flexion at the elbow joints causes supination of the affected arm only. **newspaper s.** The flexing of the terminal phalanx of the thumb against the flexed index finger, as in holding a piece of paper, observed in patients who are unable to adduct the thumb because of an ulnar nerve lesion with paresis of the adductor pollicis. Also *Froment sign, thumb sign, Froment's paper sign, signe de journal.* **niche s.** HAUDEK'S NICHE. **Nikolsky s.** The extension of a bulla through the use of pressure. It can be demonstrated by drawing a finger with firm pressure over apparently normal skin or mucous membrane. **nostril s.** Reflex enlargement of the anterior naris on the side of a diseased lung. Also *nostril reflex.* **Nothnagel s.** Paralysis of emotional movement of the facial muscles on the opposite side, seen in a patient with a thalamic tumor. **nuchal s.** A sign of meningitis: flexion of the head causes spontaneous flexion of the thighs and legs. Also *Brudzinski sign, neck sign.* **Ober s.** An indication of the integrity of the tensor fascia lata muscle. With the patient in the lateral position, the uppermost leg is tested by the examiner's supporting it in abduction and full extension. With the sudden withdrawal of the examiner's hand, the leg remains under its own support if the tensor fascia lata is functioning. Also *Ober's test.* **objective s.** PHYSICAL SIGN. **obturator s.** 1 In radiology, a widening of the soft-tissue density of the obturator muscle as seen on a roentgenogram of the pelvis or hip, usually indicative of disease of the hip joint. Also *Hefke-Turner sign.* 2 External or internal rotation of the hip with the knee flexed produces pelvic pain due to irritation of the medial obturator internus muscle caused by a pelvic abscess. **oil-drop s.** CANDLEWAX SIGN. **Oppenheim s.** A sign of a lesion of the pyramidal tract: extension of the big toe with fanning out of the other toes can be seen on applying pressure progressively more distally along the length of the tibial crest. Also *Oppenheim's reflex.* **orange-peel s.** Dimpling of the skin over a lipoma when the tumor is pinched between thumb and fingers. Also *signe de peau d'orange.* **orbicularis s.** The inability of a hemiplegic patient to close the eye on the paralyzed side without at the same time closing the other eye. Also *Revilliod sign.* **Ortolani's s.** A test for the existence of congenital dislocation of the hip. The thighs of the supine infant are flexed to a right angle with the body and brought together. They are then parted by slight outwardly-directed pressure on the knees. A distinct jerk (not a "click") that is elicited on one side or, occasionally, on both sides denotes the slipping of the femoral head over the acetabular rim and re-entry of the head into the acetabulum. **Osiander s.** Pulsation of the vagina at a rate corresponding to the maternal heartbeat as a finding in early pregnancy. **Osler s.** See under OSLER NODES. **Parkinson s.** The masklike facial appearance characteristic of parkinsonism. **Parrot s.** Bony nodes on the outer table of the neonatal skull, giving it an irregular shape, seen in congenital syphilis. Also *Parrot's node.* **Pastia s.** PASTIA'S LINES. **patent bronchus s.** The roentgenographic finding of an air-containing patent bronchus supplying a collapsed lung, pulmonary lobe, or pulmonary segment. **peroneal s.** An indication of incipient tetany. A tapping of the common peroneal nerve as it passes around the fibular neck with the knee slightly flexed causes abduction and dorsiflexion of the foot. **Petruschky s.** Tenderness or pain over the interscapular area as a result of tuberculous inflammation of the parabronchial or paratracheal lymph nodes. **Phalen s.** Paresthesiae in the distribution of the median nerve caused by sustained flexion of the wrist in patients with carpal tunnel syndrome. Also *Phalen's test.* **physical s.** A sign that can be detected and perceived directly by physical examination of the patient. Also *objective sign.* **Piltz s.** ATTENTION REFLEX OF PUPIL. **Pinard s.** An indication suggestive of a breech presentation: pressure on the uterine fundus after the sixth month of pregnancy produces pain. **Pins s.** EWART SIGN. **Piotrowski s.** Plantar flexion occurring on tapping over the muscles between the head of the fibula and the tibial tuberosity. If this flexion is exaggerated it may be a sign of a pyramidal tract lesion. *Seldom used.* Also *anticus reflex.* **Piskacek s.** Asymmetric enlargement of the uterine fundus detected during bimanual examination as a finding in early pregnancy. **Pitres s.** Lack of testicular sensation on pressure, seen in patients with tabes dorsalis. **pivot-shift s.** A sign of ligamentous injuries of the knee. While extending the knee from a flexed position and exerting torsion on the tibia, the tibia slips forward on the femoral condyles. **placental s.** Vaginal bleeding at the time of implantation of a blastocyst in the uterine cavity. **platysma s.** In patients with peripheral facial paralysis there is a stronger contraction of the platysma on the healthy than on the affected side. This is demonstrated by asking the patient, with his head flexed, to extend the head against resistance and then to open his mouth widely or to attempt to whistle. **Plummer s.** Partial or complete inability to step up onto a chair or to climb stairs owing to weakness of the quadriceps muscles, a manifestation of thyrotoxic myopathy in Graves disease. **pneumatic s.** Nystagmus and/or vertigo produced by the application of the pneumatic test. **Pool-Schlesinger s.** SCHLESINGER SIGN. **Prehn s.** A sign of epididymo-orchitis: pain is eased by supporting the scrotum. **Prévost s.** Conjugate deviation of the eyes and head towards the damaged hemisphere and the unparalyzed side, in a patient with hemiplegia. **pronation s.** If a forearm and arm affected by spastic paralysis is passively supinated, it then pronates spontaneously. Also *Babinski sign.* **pseudo-Babinski s.** A modified Babinski reflex, observed in poliomyelitis, in which only the big toe is extended because of the paralysis of all foot muscles except the dorsiflexors of the big toe. **puddle s.** A sign indicating the location of small amounts of free abdominal fluid: the patient is positioned on all fours and one flank is percussed with repeated light flicks of the finger. Auscultation is carried out beginning with the most dependent portion of the abdomen and moving towards the opposite flank. A sharp increase in the intensity of the sound picked up by the stethoscope indicates the position of the fluid. **Queckenstedt s.** QUECKENSTEDT'S TEST. **Quincke s.** See under CAPILLARY PULSE. **radialis s.** STRÜMPELL SIGN. **Radovici s.** PALMOMENTAL REFLEX. **railroad track s.** A phlebographic sign of thrombus within a vein, with contrast material appearing as a thin peripheral rim around the central nonopacified thrombus within the vein. **Raimiste s.** 1 Abrupt flexion and pronation of the hand when the hand and forearm are held vertical with the elbow resting on a table, seen in patients with flaccid organic paresis of the arm. Also *hand phenomenon.* 2 Reflex adduction or abduction in a paralyzed lower limb, induced by a corresponding but active movement of the unaffected leg, performed by the patient while lying on his back. This is seen in some patients with a spastic hemiplegia caused by a pyramidal tract lesion. Also *associated adduction sign, associated abduction sign.* **Ransohoff s.** A yellow color in the periumbilical region indicating rupture of the common bile duct. **Rasch s.** HEGAR SIGN. **Rasin s.** JELLINEK SIGN. **rebound s.** STEWART-HOLMES SIGN. **Remak s.** Slowness of pain perception, noted in patients with tabes dorsalis. Also *Remak symptom.* **reservoir s.** In cases of profuse otorrhea, the observation that the accumulation of discharge within the external auditory meatus or the concha, when mopped away or aspirated, rapidly reappears, suggesting the presence of coalescent mastoiditis. **Revilliod s.** ORBICULARIS SIGN. **rising sun s.** Downward displacement of the eyeballs in subjects with hydrocephalus so that the irises in relation to the lower lids look like the sun rising or setting over the horizon. Also *setting sun phenomenon, setting sun sign.* **Rivière s.** A change in percussion denoting a band of greater density across the back in the area of the spinous processes of the fifth, sixth, and seventh thoracic vertebrae. It is described in patients with pulmonary tuberculosis. **Roche s.** Inability to distinguish between the epididymis and testis by touch; a sign of torsion of the testis. **Rocher s.** DRAWER TEST. **Roger's counter s.** In Parkinson's disease, the accentuation of hypertonia, and sometimes of tremor, in the arm opposite to the one which is making a purposive movement, such as that used in picking up a glass from a counter. Also *Froment sign.* **Romaña s.** Unilateral palpebral edema, conjunctivitis, and regional lymphadenopathy, seen in acute Chagas disease. This occurs around the primary lesion, the chagoma, and may be accompanied by malar and temporal edema also. **Romberg s.** A sign of sensory ataxia, elicited by Romberg's test, due to loss of proprioceptive sensibility in the lower limbs: the patient, standing upright with his heels together, is unable to maintain his balance when he closes his eyes, and sways or may even fall. Patients with cerebellar or labyrinthine disturbances may be slightly more unsteady with the eyes closed, but this is not true rombergism. Also *rombergism, Brauch-Romberg symptom, Romberg-Howship symptom.* **rope s.** The appearance of the weakened or paralyzed hyoid muscles between the chin and cricoid cartilage seen in bulbar poliomyelitis, resembling a rope in the sharp angle thus formed. *Obs.* **Rosenbach s.** Loss of abdominal cutaneous reflexes in multiple sclerosis. **Rossolimo s.** Flexion and adduction of the toes in response to tapping the plantar surface of the toes, associated with injury of the corticospinal tract. **Rovighi s.** Fremitus felt on palpation and percussion over the liver in the presence of a superficial hydatid cyst. **Rovsing s.** In appendicitis, typical pain at McBurney's point elicited by pressure in the left lower quadrant over the point corresponding to McBurney's point. **Rucker s.** Retinal periphlebitis seen in patients with multiple sclerosis. **Ruggeri s.** Cardioacceleration elicited by near-focus ocular convergence. **Rumpel-Leede s.** RUMPEL-LEEDE PHENOMENON. **Rust s.** In diseases that cause bone destruction of the upper cervical vertebrae, the patient will support his head with his hands when rising from or returning to the recumbent position. **Saenger s.** In subjects with forms of neurosyphilis other than tabes dorsalis, the temporary restoration of the pupillary reaction to light after a long enough period in the dark for gradual dilatation to have occurred. **Saunders s.** Opening and clenching movements of the hand associated with wide opening of the mouth in children. Also *mouth-and-hand synkinesis.* **Schick s.** Stridor heard during exhalation in an infant with bronchial lymph node tuberculosis. **Schlesinger s.** A sign of muscular hyperexcitability in tetany: abrupt passive flexion of the leg on the thigh, while holding the knee, is followed by reflex extension of the knee with slight eversion of the foot. Also *Schlesinger's phenomenon, leg sign, Pool-Schlesinger sign, leg phenomenon.* **Schultze s.** A sign of tetany: traction upon the tongue evokes reflex contraction of its musculature. *Obs.* **Schultze-Chvostek s.** CHVOSTEK SIGN. **Schwartze s.** A sign sometimes observed in cases of otosclerosis: a pink flush is observed on otoscopic examination, corresponding to the central area of the drumhead, due to increased vascularity over the promontory showing through the normal membrane. It is seen in two percent of the cases. Also *flamingo flush.* **scimitar s.** An arteriographic sign of encroachment upon the popliteal or femoral artery lumen by adventitial cystic disease. **setting sun s.** RISING SUN SIGN. **Siegert s.** The inwardly curved, shortened fifth finger seen in subjects with the Down syndrome. **Silex s.** KRISOVSKI SIGN. **Simon s.** **1** Retraction or immobility of the umbilicus on inspiration, seen in patients with incipient meningitis. **2** Lack of the normal relationship between movements of the diaphragm and of the muscles of the thoracic cage, seen in patients with incipient meningitis. *Obs.* **Skeer s.** Episcleritis occurring around the corneal margins, sometimes seen in patients with tuberculous meningitis. *Obs.* Also *Skeer symptom.* **soft s.'s** Subtle signs of dysfunction, in particular the aggregation of borderline abnormalities found in neurologic examination of children with minimal brain dysfunction. These deviations would be of little significance if they occurred alone. **Somagyi s.** SOMAGYI'S REFLEX. **Spalding s.** The radiographic appearance of the fetal head *in utero* in which there is overlapping of the bones of the skull when the mother is not in labor. This is a sign of fetal death. Also *Horner sign.* **Spurling s.** Pain produced or increased in the neck and/or arm upon passive flexion of the head to the affected side, as if to approximate the ear to the shoulder. This is indicative of lateral prolapse of a cervical intervertebral disk. **Stellwag s.** Retraction of the upper eyelids giving the appearance of a widened palpebral fissure, together with infrequent blinking and incomplete closure of the eye, seen in Graves disease. Also *Stellwag symptom.* **Stewart-Holmes s.** A sign of dysfunction of the ipsilateral cerebellar hemisphere or cerebellar tracts: when the elbow rests on the table and the forearm is flexed at the joint against the examiner's resistance, if the forearm is suddenly released there is sudden exaggerated flexion because of hypotonia of the antagonists. Also *rebound sign.* **Stierlin s.** A radiographic sign of intestinal tuberculosis, seen with frequent emptying of the cecum on barium enema. Residual barium is seen in the terminal ileum and transverse colon, related to cecal irritation. **Stimson s.** A linear marginal inflammation of the conjunctiva of the eyelid seen in the prodromal stages of measles. **Strauss s.** **1** Increase of fat following the ingestion of fatty foods in chylous ascites. **2** BLUMER SHELF. **string s.** A persistent thin ribbonlike appearance of the small bowel or colon at barium study, indicating stenosis or continued spasm. It is seen most commonly in the terminal ileum involved with Crohn's disease. Also *Kantor sign.* **Strümpell s.** **1** The dorsiflexion of the foot that occurs spontaneously when the thigh is flexed passively at the hip. It is thought to indicate a corticospinal tract lesion. Seldom used in this sense. Also *anterior tibial muscle sign, tibial phenomenon, anticus sign, tibialis sign, anterior tibial sign.* **2** An inability to make a fist without noticeable dorsiflexion of the wrist, a sign of dubious significance. Also *radialis sign.* **3** PRONATION PHENOMENON. **subjective s.** A symptom that can be detected only by the patient. **swinging flashlight s.** MARCUS GUNN PUPILLARY PHENOMENON. **tapir snout s.** A pouting appearance of the lips seen in the myopathic facies of facioscapulohumeral muscular dystrophy. **Tarnier s.** A straightening of the angle at the junction of the uterine fundus and the lower uterine segment, suggestive of impending abortion. **Tay s.** CHERRY-RED SPOT. **thigh s.** BRUDZINSKI SIGN. **Thomas s.** HOLMES REBOUND PHENOMENON. **Thomson s.** PASTIA'S LINES. **thumb s.** NEWSPAPER SIGN. **thumb print s.** The radiographic appearance of the colon after administration of a barium enema in which the colon looks as if a thumb had compressed one or more segments. This is due to local edema or hemorrhage in the wall of the colon, as may occur with ischemic colitis. **tibialis s.** STRÜMPELL SIGN. **Tinel s.** A sign of regeneration of a peripheral nerve after injury: tapping sharply over the trunk of the nerve induces paresthesiae in its area of cutaneous innervation distal to the lesion. Also *formication sign, distal tingling on percussion, DTP sign.* **toe s.** EXTENSOR PLANTAR RESPONSE. **toe spread s.** EXTENSOR PLANTAR RESPONSE. **Traube s.** Pistol-shot sounds over large arteries in aortic regurgitation. **Trendelenburg s.** A sign of hip abnormalities that appears when the subject is standing. In the normal state, the pelvis is held horizontally when the subject is standing on one leg. If the pelvis tilts toward the opposite side, the sign is positive and is an indication of such conditions as congenital dislocation of the hip or weakness of the hip abductor muscles. Also *Trendelenburg symptom, Trendelenburg's test.* **Troisier s.** SENTINEL NODE. **Trömner s.** HOFFMAN'S REFLEX. **Trousseau s.** An early sign of tetany: when an arm is rendered ischemic by the application of a tourniquet above arterial blood pressure, the fingers flex at the metacarpophalangeal joints but are otherwise extended and the extended thumb is opposed to their tips. Also *Trousseau's phenomenon.* **Turner s.** Ecchymosis appearing in the flank region, usually on the left side, several days after the beginning of acute pancreatitis. Also *Grey Turner sign.* **Uhthoff s.** A sign of multiple sclerosis: vasodilatation resulting from exposure to heat, as in a hot bath, or resulting from exertion, may cause transient visual impairment in one or both eyes due to enlargement of central scotomata. Occasionally other manifestations of the disease are temporarily aggravated also in this manner. Also *Uhthoff symptom.* **Uriolla s.** The presence of minute black granules of blood pigment in the urine of patients with malaria. It is a sign of limited practical value. **Vedder s.'s** Calf-muscle pain in response to pressure, anesthesia over the anterior surface of the legs, loss of patellar reflexes, and inability to rise from the squatting position without the use of the hands, all often seen in beriberi. **Vermel s.** Pulsation of the temporal artery, visible during an attack of migraine. **Vipond s.** A generalized lymphadenopathy that occurs during the incubation period for various exanthematic fevers in children. **vital s.'s** The pulse, blood pressure, respiration, and temperature. **vitropression s.** An abnormal coloration of the skin made visible by compression of the skin with a glass slide to exclude blood from the area being viewed. **von Graefe s.** EYELID LAG. **von Strümpell s.** See under STRÜMPELL SIGN. **Wartenberg s.** **1** A sign of a corticospinal tract lesion: active flexion of the terminal phalanges of the fingers against resistance from the examiner's fingers. Also *Wartenberg symptom.* **2** Reduction or loss of swinging movements of one arm when walking, resulting from an ipsilateral cerebellar lesion. Seldom used in this sense. **water lily s.** A radiographic image on chest x ray characteristic of hydatid disease of the lung in which there is irregularity of the surface of the fluid level within the cyst. The irregularity represents scolices which are floating in fluid outlined by air which has entered the cyst. Also *camelot sign.* **Weber s.** WEBER SYNDROME. **Weill s.** Absent or diminished expansion of the chest below one clavicle, indicative of pneumonia affecting the lung on that side. **Weiss s.** Simultaneous contraction of the orbicularis oculi and the occipitofrontalis muscles, elicited by light tapping at the external angle of the orbit. This can be seen in tetany, and is a variant of the Chvostek sign. **Wernicke s.** HEMIANOPIC PUPILLARY REACTION. **Westermark s.** Hyperlucency of a portion of lung on x ray caused by decreased flow of blood, usually due to obstruction of a pulmonary artery by an embolus. **Wilson's pronator s.** Pronation of the forearms and hands so that the palms face outwards as a result of hypotonia, when the arms are lifted vertically above the head. This sign is characteristic of Sydenham's chorea. **Winterbottom s.** Hypertrophy of the posterior cervical lymph nodes, observed in the Gambian form of African trypanosomiasis. Occasionally, it also occurs in *Trypanosoma rhodesiense* infections (Rhodesian trypanosomiasis). **Zaufal s.** SADDLENOSE.

**signa** [L, pl. of *signum* a mark, sign] Mark, or indicate, a direction used in prescription writing. It indicates the signature of a prescription which provides directions for taking the medicine. Abbr. S.

**signal** / **Doppler velocity s.** DOPPLER EFFECT. **sensory s.** Afferent input to the central nervous system derived from peripheral sense organs.

**signal-symptom** SIGNAL SYMPTOM.

**signature** [Late L *signatura* (from L *signatus*, past part. of *signare* to write, mark, seal) a writing, sealing, signing] The part of a prescription that gives directions for the patient about taking the medicine.

**signe** \sēn′yə\ [French (from L *sign(um)* a mark, sign), sign] Sign. **s. de journal** NEWSPAPER SIGN. **s. de la bandera** FLAG SIGN. **s. de peau d'orange** ORANGE-PEEL SIGN.

**significance** \signif′ikəns\ **statistical s.** An expression in terms of probability which affords objective grounds for a decision to accept or to reject a statistical hypothesis. The decision rests on the probability that an observed difference could, according to the hypothesis, be entirely attributed to random fluctuation arising from the sampling process. If the probability is equal to or less than an amount which has been decided upon in advance, called the significance level, the difference is said to be statistically significant and the hypothesis is rejected. The risk of that decision being in error is equal to the significance level. Conventionally, risks of error of 5% or 1% are usually regarded as acceptable limits.

**sig. n. pro.** *signa nomine proprio* (L, label with the proper name, a direction used in prescription writing).

**siguatera** \sig′wəter′ə\ CIGUATERA.

**Silastic** A medical grade silicone rubber, which is biologically inert and used in implanted prostheses. A trade name.

**Silber** [Robert Howard *Silber*, U.S. biochemist, born 1915] **1** Porter-Silber chromogens test. See under 17-HYDROXYCORTICOSTEROID TEST. **2** Porter-Silber chromogens. See under CHROMOGEN.

**silence** / **electrical s.** An absence of cerebral electrical activity in an electroencephalographic recording at the usual amplification. This may reflect local or diffuse suppression of the brain waves caused by disease, but if localized can also be the result of the potentials recorded at each of a pair of electrodes being equal but opposite in phase.

**silent** Not manifested by any detectable signs or symptoms: said of a disease or disorder.

**Silex** [Paul *Silex*, German ophthalmologist, 1858–1929] Silex sign. See under KRISOVSKI SIGN.

**silica** \sil′ikə\ [New L, from L *silex*, gen. *silicis* flint] $SiO_2$. A mineral, used for scientific purposes in the preparation of optical apparatus, such as cuvettes. It is transparent down to wavelengths below 200 nm. It occurs in crystalline form as quartz, tridymite, and cristobalite, which on inhalation causes silicosis. The amorphous form of silica does not cause silicosis or lung disease. **s. gel** The precipitated and dried granular form of silicic acid. It is used as a dehydrating agent and as an absorbent.

**silicate** Any complex anion, or the salt containing it, that possesses a central silicon atom; in particular, the ion $SiO_4^{4-}$ and its derivatives.

**silicatosis** \sil′ikətō′sis\ SILICOSIS.

**siliceous** \silish′əs\ Of, relating to, or containing silica. Also *silicious.*

**silicon** \sil′ikən\ [*silic(a)* + *-on* as in *carbon*] A nonmetallic element having atomic number 14 and atomic weight 28.086. It is second only to oxygen in abundance, forming almost 26 percent by weight of the lithosphere, combined chiefly with oxygen in sand and rock. The three natural isotopes are stable. Like carbon, it has valence 4, and has to some degree a similar chain-forming propensity. Silicon is incorporated in the shells of diatoms and is found in the ash of plant tissue and the human skeleton. Trace amounts have been found essential for normal bone development and full growth in chicks. Symbol: Si

**silicon carbide** SiC. A compound in which each silicon atom is coordinated tetrahedrally with four carbon atoms, and vice versa. It thus possesses a structure like that of diamond. It is extremely hard, and is used as an abrasive. Also *carborundum*.

**silicon dioxide** The systematic name for silica. **colloidal s.** A finely dispersed form of silicon dioxide, obtained by vapor-phase hydrolysis of silicon compounds. It is used in medicinal tablets and as a suspending and thickening ingredient.

**silicone** Any polymeric substance in which the repeating unit is —O—$SiR_2$—, where R is an alkyl group. Silicones are used as plastics and lubricants. Depending on the polymer length, the number of cross-linkages, and the addition of fine silica powder, the consistency can vary from watery to rubbery. The rubbery, or elastomeric, silicones are available in the form of adhesives, sponges, solid blocks, or gels.

**siliconoma** \sil′ikənō′mə\ [*silicon(e)* + -OMA] Swelling due to a granulomatous inflammatory response to injected silicone.

**silicosiderosis** \sil′ikōsid′ərō′sis\ A modified form of silicosis caused by exposure to both quartz and iron dust, as may occur in hematite mining and iron foundry work. Lesions similar to those of the progressive massive fibrosis in coal-workers' pneumoconiosis may occur. Also *siderosilicosis*.

**silicosis** \sil′ikō′sis\ [*silic(a)* + -OSIS] Pneumoconiosis caused by exposure to silica usually in the form of quartz or flint. The lungs bear characteristic nodules with concentric (onion-skin) arrangement of collagen fibers. The nodules are 2–6 mm in diameter. They are seen as opacities in chest roentgenograms. Breathlessness occurs as the disease advances. Silicosis predisposes the victim to the development of pulmonary tuberculosis. Silicosis occurs among workers in many occupations, including quarrying and tunneling siliceous rock, stonecutting, and ceramics manufacture. Also *silicatosis*. Adj. silicotic.

**silicotuberculosis** \sil′ikōt$^y$ubur′kyəlō′sis\ Pulmonary tuberculosis occurring in association with silicosis. Also *tuberculosilicosis, infective silicosis*.

**silk** [Old English *sioloc, seolc*, from Baltic or Slavic, akin to Russian *shëlk* silk, akin to Mongolian *sirkek*, prob. originally from Chinese *sī (szu)* silk] The fine, proteinaceous filaments produced by silkworms in spinning their cocoons, or similar natural or artificial material. **floss s.** Dental floss made of natural silk fibers. **surgical s.** A permanent surgical suture material made of braided silk.

**Silvadene** A proprietary name for silver sulfadiazine.

**Silver** [Henry K. *Silver*, U.S. pediatrician, born 1918] See under SILVER-RUSSELL SYNDROME.

**silver** A metallic element having atomic number 47 and atomic weight 107.868. Pure silver is a better thermal and electric conductor than any other metal. It occurs native and in various ores. The metal is used in dental alloys. Valences are 1 and 2. Light-sensitive silver compounds are essential to photography. Most silver salts are germicidal and toxic to higher organisms. Symbol: Ag **mild s. protein** A preparation of colloidal silver containing 19–23% silver. The protein-containing colloidal suspension is dark brown or black, and it is used as a topical anti-infective medication for various epidermal regions of the body, such as the ocular, vaginal, urethral, otic, or nasal surfaces.

**silver iodide** AgI. A compound once used to treat syphilis and other diseases. It is no longer used systematically, but a colloidal solution, stabilized by the addition of gelatin, is used as an antiseptic to treat sores of the mucous membranes.

**Silverman** [Irving *Silverman*, U.S. surgeon, born 1904] **1** See under NEEDLE. **2** Vim-Silverman needle. See under NEEDLE.

**Silverman** [William Aaron *Silverman*, U.S. physician, born 1917] Caffey-Silverman syndrome. See under INFANTILE HYPEROSTOSIS.

**silver nitrate** $AgNO_3$. An anti-infective compound used in eye drops to prevent infantile purulent conjunctivitis (ophthalmia neonatorum), in other preparations as a caustic to treat skin growths, including warts, and in solutions to decrease the risk of infection in burns. Also *lapis imperialis, lapis lunaris, lapis infernalis*. **ammoniacal s. solution** An ammoniated solution of silver nitrate used in an attempt to arrest dental caries. The solution is applied to the carious surface and is reduced with oil of cloves, causing the precipitation of silver within the enamel or dentin. Also *Howe's silver nitrate*. **toughened s.** A caustic agent, prepared by fusing silver nitrate with HCl, NaCl, or potassium nitrate. Such products contain about 95% silver nitrate and are usually in the form of rods or sticks, which can be used in the removal of warts, as caustic medication. Also *lunar caustic*.

**Silverskiöld** [Nils Otto *Silverskiöld*, Swedish physician, 1888–1957] See under SYNDROME.

**silver sulfadiazine** A colloidal suspension of metallic silver and sulfadiazine used as an antibacterial agent of low toxicity in the topical treatment of burns.

***Silvius*** \sil′vē·əs\ A genus of horseflies (family Tabanidae) found in Australia.

**simethicone** A combination of dimethicones and silicon dioxide. It is a translucent, viscous fluid containing 4–7% w/w of silicon dioxide. It is a constituent of some skin creams, given orally to prevent gas in gastroscopy, and in pharmaceuticals as a releasing agent.

**Simmonds** [Morris *Simmonds*, German physician, 1855–1925] **1** See under SYNDROME. **2** Simmonds disease. See under PANHYPOPITUITARISM.

**Simon** [Charles Edmund *Simon*, U.S. physician, 1866–1927] See under SIGN.

**Simon** [Gustav *Simon*, German surgeon, 1827–1876] Simon's position. See under EDEBOHLS POSITION.

**Simon** [Theodore *Simon*, French psychologist, 1873–1961] Binet-Simon test. See under TEST.

***Simonea folliculorum*** \sī′mənē′ə fälik′yəlôr′əm\ *DEMODEX FOLLICULORUM*.

**Simons** [Arthur *Simons*, German physician, born 1877] Barraquer-Simons syndrome. See under PROGRESSIVE LIPODYSTROPHY.

**simple** **1** Not attended by complications. **2** Consisting of a single part, system, or type of cell.

**Simpson** [Sir James Y. *Simpson*, Scottish obstetrician, 1813–1870] See under FORCEPS.

**Simpson** [William Speirs *Simpson*, English civil engineer, died 1917] Simpson light. See under SIMPSON LAMP.

**Sims** [J. Marion *Sims*, U.S. gynecologist, 1813–1883] **1** Sims position. See under SEMIPRONE POSITION. **2** See under SPECULUM.

**simul** [L, at the same time] At once; at the same time, used in prescription writing.

**simulation** \sim′yəlā′shən\ **1** The act of feigning illness. **2** A close similarity or apparent mimicking of the symptoms of one disease by those of another.

**simulator** \sim′yəlā′tər\ 1 In radiotherapy, an apparatus containing a diagnostic x-ray tube, and capable of simulating the treatment beam of a radiation treatment unit. It is used for treatment planning purposes. 2 Any apparatus or instrument designed to imitate in some way the function of another. **space s.** An enclosed chamber used at ground level to simulate space conditions, such as reduced atmospheric pressure. It is used to study the effects of space travel on human beings and animals.

***Simuliidae*** \sim′yəlī′idē\ [*Simuli(um)* + -IDAE] A family of small, hump-backed, bloodsucking flies, known as blackflies or buffalo gnats, of the suborder Nematocerca in the order Diptera. Distributed from subarctic and north temperate zones to the tropics, there are over 1200 species, some of which, particularly those in the tropics, are medically important in the transmission of disease (for example, onchocerciasis in Africa, Mexico, and Central and South America). The female is characterized by bladelike, piercing mouthparts that inflict painful bites.

***Simulium*** \sīmyoo′lyəm\ [New L, from L *simulare* to simulate] A genus of blackflies (family Simuliidae) which includes species that are important pests of domestic mammals and birds. Several species are important vectors of human disease, especially onchocerciasis. ***S. damnosum*** A species of blackfly which is the most important vector of onchocerciasis in central Africa. ***S. neavei*** A significant vector of onchocerciasis in east and central Africa. Larvae and pupae develop on the shells of fast-moving crabs of the genus *Potamonautes,* hence presence of this species brings onchocerciasis into nonmountainous areas of Africa. This is in contrast to areas where there are fast-moving mountain streams in which other important onchoceriasis vector species of *Simulium* breed. ***S. ochraceum*** One of the most important blackfly vectors of onchocerciasis in Guatemala and Mexico. It is a highly anthropophilic species and an efficient vector of human infection.

**simultagnosia** \sī′multagnō′zhə\ Visual agnosia in which the patient has the ability to describe the story told by a picture and to discuss the action represented but is not capable of naming individual objects appearing in the picture.

**sin / original antigenic s.** The phenomenon observed following reinfection with a virus closely related to the original infecting virus, in which the antibody formed is still directed against the first virus. Also *Davenport phenomenon.* • The allusion to biblical original sin refers to the permanent taint induced by partaking of the fruit of the tree of knowledge.

***Sinanthropus pekinensis*** \sinan′thrəpəs pē′kinen′sis\ See under PEKING MAN.

**sincalide** $C_{49}H_{62}N_{10}O_{16}S_3$. 1-De(5-oxo-L-proline)-2-de-L-glutamide-5-L-methioninecaerulin, a choleretic agent that, when injected intravenously, causes the gallbladder to contract. It is used diagnostically to evaluate the biliary system.

**sinciput** \sin′siput\ [NA] The anterior and upper part of the head. Also *synciput.* Compare OCCIPUT.

**sinew** \sin′yoo\ [Old English *sinu, seonu*] A tendon.

**sing.** *singulorum* (L, of each, used in prescription writing).

**single-blind** [Formed on analogy with DOUBLE-BLIND] Characterized by knowledge of the experimenter but concealment from the subjects as to which subjects are exposed to the variable being tested and which are functioning as controls.

**singultation** \sing·gultā′shən\ [L *singultatus,* past part. of *singultare* to sob, hiccup] 1 Hiccuping. 2 HICCUP.

**singultus** \sing·gul′təs\ [L, a sob, hiccup] HICCUP.

**sinister** \sin′istər\ [L, left, on the left hand, sinister] Designating a structure situated on the left side of the body or the left one of two similar structures.

**sinistr-** \sin′istr-\ SINISTRO-.

**sinistrad** \sinis′trad, sin′istrad\ Toward the left side.

**sinistral** \sinis′trəl, sin′istrəl\ Pertaining to the left side. Also *sinistrous.*

**sinistrality** \sin′istral′itē\ [SINISTR- + -AL + -ITY ] The preferential or dominant use of the left member of the paired organs of the body, such as eye or hand, especially in voluntary motor acts. Also *sinistration.*

**sinistro-** \sin′istrō-\ [L *sinister* (feminine *sinistra*) left, on the left hand] A combining form meaning left, to or on the left. Also *sinistr-.*

**sinistrocardia** \-kär′dē·ə\ [SINISTRO- + -CARDIA] Displacement of the heart to the left.

**sinistrocerebral** \-ser′əbrəl\ Denoting the cerebral hemisphere on the left side.

**sinistrocular** \sin′isträk′yələr\ [SINISTR- + OCULAR] Pertaining to a dominant left eye.

**sinistrous** \sin′istrəs, sinis′trəs\ SINISTRAL.

**sinoatrial** \sī′nō·ā′trē·əl\ SINUATRIAL.

**sinoauricular** \sī′nō·ôrik′yələr\ SINUATRIAL.

**sinography** \sīnäg′rəfē\ Roentgenography of a sinus tract after instillation of a radiopaque contrast medium.

**si non val.** *si non valeat* (L, if it be not sufficient, used in prescription writing).

**sinospiral** \sī′nōspī′rəl\ Having a spiral course in relation to the sinus venosus.

**sinoventricular** \sī′nōvəntrik′yələr\ Pertaining to the sinus venosus and the ventricle of the heart. Also *sinuventricular.*

**sinuatrial** \sī′nʸoo·ā′trē·əl\ 1 Of or relating to the sinus venosus and the atrium of the heart. 2 Of or relating to the sinuatrial node (nodus sinuatrialis). For defs. 1 and 2 also *sinoatrial, sinoauricular, sinuauricular.*

**sinuose** \sin′yoo·ōs\ SINUOUS.

**sinuosity** \sin′yoo·äs′itē\ A bending, winding, or folding.

**sinuous** \sin′yoo·əs\ Having bends or folds; winding. Also *serpentine, sinuose.*

# sinus

**sinus** \sī′nəs\ [L, a curve, fold, hollow, bay, cavity] (*pl.* sinus, sinuses) 1 [NA] A cavity or hollow space filled with air, as in the cranial bones. 2 [NA] A channel or cavity containing venous blood or lymph. 3 [NA] A dilatation in a blood vessel. 4 Pertaining to or originating in the sinuatrial node of the heart, as *sinus rhythm.* Compare NODAL. **accessory s.'es of the nose** SINUS PARANASALES. **air s.** A cavity or hollow space containing air and situated within a bony structure. **alveolar s.** A sinus connecting an infected tooth root with the oral cavity, the nasal cavity, or the skin. Also *alveolar fistula, dental sinus.* **s. anales** [NA] The small recesses, deepest on the mucous membrane of the posterior wall of the anal canal, located above the anal valves between the lower ends of the vertical anal columns. Also *anal sinuses, anal crypts.* **s. aortae** [NA] Any of three dilatations in the wall of the ascending aorta, one opposite each semilunar valvule, and from two of which the coronary arteries arise. Also *aortic sinus, sinus of*

*Valsalva.* **Arlt s.** ARLT'S RECESS. **barbers' hair s.** A pilonidal sinus in the web between the fingers, which occurs in barbers as a result of implantation of a hair in the skin of that area while holding hair tightly between the fingers during cutting. Also *barbers' pilonidal sinus.* **branchial s.** A lateral depression at the base of the side of the primitive pharynx, considered to be a rudiment of the fifth branchial pouch. **s. caroticus** [NA] A dilatation in the terminal portion of the common carotid artery and in the commencement of the internal carotid artery. The tunica media is rather thin, while the tunica adventitia is relatively thick and contains a number of sensory nerve endings received from the carotid branch of the glossopharyngeal nerve. The walls are sensitive to changes in arterial blood pressure, reflexly regulating the pressure. Also *carotid sinus, bulbus caroticus.* **s. cavernosus** [NA] One of a pair of intracranial venous sinuses of the dura mater situated on the sides of the body of the sphenoid bone and extending from the superior orbital fissure anteriorly to the apex of the petrous part of the temporal bone posteriorly. In its lateral wall are the oculomotor, trochlear, ophthalmic, and maxillary nerves, while the internal carotid artery and abducent nerve lie in the center of the space, supported by interwoven trabecular filaments. Anteriorly it receives the superior ophthalmic vein, and posteriorly it is drained by the superior and inferior petrosal sinuses. Also *cavernous sinus.* **cerebral s.'es** SINUS DURAE MATRIS. **cervical s.** A small cavity formed in the embryo by the folding over of the second branchial arch over the third and fourth arches. At the time of the straightening of the head, this zone is carried backwards into the middle part of the lateral region of the neck. Normally, this sinus is obliterated rapidly by coalescence of its walls. In some cases it can be the origin of cervical cysts or of lateral fistulas of the neck. **s. circularis** Anastomosing venous channels around the hypophysial fossa formed by the right and left cavernous sinuses and the anterior and posterior intercavernous sinuses. Also *circular sinus, Ridley sinus, circulus venosus ridleyi* (outmoded). **coccygeal s.** PILONIDAL SINUS. **congenital lip s.'es** A congenital variant consisting of symmetrically placed sinuses on either side of the midline of the lower lip, penetrating the orbicularis oris muscle to depths up to 2.5 cm. Approximately 70 percent of patients with congenital lip sinuses have an associated cleft lip and/or palate. **s. coronarius** [NA] A large venous channel situated in the posterior part of the atrioventricular groove of the heart, draining most of the cardiac veins and ending in the right atrium between the right atrioventricular orifice and the opening of the inferior vena cava. Its termination is protected by a semicircular valve. Also *coronary sinus.* **s. of corpus callosum** SINUS SAGITTALIS INFERIOR. **cortical s.** A lymphatic sinus in the cortex of a lymph node. **cranial s.'es** SINUS DURAE MATRIS. **s. of Cuvier** COMMON CARDINAL VEIN. **dental s.** ALVEOLAR SINUS. **dermal s.** An epidermally lined sinus at any point along the line of closure of the embryonic neural tube, but particularly in the lumbar and sacral regions, where it may communicate by an epithelial tract either with the exterior or with the central canal of the cord or with the subarachnoidal space. It results from failure of neural tube closure. **draining s.** A pathologic opening, usually in the skin, that emits body fluids and most often is diagnostic of a deep infectious process. **s. durae matris** [NA] Venous channels that drain blood from the brain and the bones of the cranium. They are located between the two layers of dura mater, are lined with endothelium, and lack valves. Also *venous sinuses of dura mater, cranial sinuses, cerebral sinuses.* **s. epididymidis** [NA] A narrow recess of the tunica vaginalis testis situated between the lateral surface of the testis and the body of the epididymis. Also *sinus of epididymis.* **s. ethmoidales** [NA] Thin-walled air spaces in the ethmoidal labyrinth situated between the orbit and upper part of the nasal cavity on each side. They vary in size and number and are usually divided into three groups, anterior, middle, and posterior, which open into the lateral wall of the nasal cavity at variable sites, but mostly into the superior and middle meatuses. Also *ethmoidal sinuses, ethmoid antra.* **external branchial s.** A small opening or cleft on the lateral aspect of the neck from which secretions may exude. The opening is the external termination of an epithelially lined tract that represents an unobliterated vestige of the embryonic cervical sinus. **falcial s.** *Outmoded* SINUS SAGITTALIS INFERIOR. **falciform s.** *Outmoded* SINUS SAGITTALIS INFERIOR. **s. frontalis** [NA] One of two spaces on either side of the midline between the inner and outer tables of the frontal bone, situated behind the superciliary arches. Usually a bony septum separates the two sides and often each space is subdivided into smaller interconnecting compartments. It is variable in size and shape. It is lined by mucous membrane and opens inferiorly into the front of the middle meatus through either the frontonasal duct or the ethmoidal infundibulum. Also *frontal sinus.* **Guérin s.** LACUNA MAGNA. **Huguier s.** A fossa on the medial wall of the middle ear situated between fenestra vestibuli and fenestra cochleae. **inferior longitudinal s.** *Outmoded* SINUS SAGITTALIS INFERIOR. **inferior petrosal s.** SINUS PETROSUS INFERIOR. **inferior sagittal s.** SINUS SAGITTALIS INFERIOR. **s. intercavernosi** [NA] The two communicating channels, one anterior and the other posterior, between the two cavernous sinuses. They have no valves. Also *intercavernous sinuses.* **internal branchial s.** A small opening or cleft in the lateral wall of the pharynx, usually near the tonsillar fossa. It is the internal termination of a cervical sinus. **s. of jugular vein** BULBUS INFERIOR VENAE JUGULARIS. **s. of kidney** SINUS RENALIS. **s. lactiferi** [NA] Dilatations in the lactiferous ducts of the mammary gland located deep to the areola and narrowing to terminate on the surface of the papilla. They function as reservoirs of milk. Also *lactiferous sinuses.* **laryngeal s.** VENTRICULUS LARYNGIS. **s. of larynx** VENTRICULUS LARYNGIS. **lateral s.** SINUS TRANSVERSUS DURAE MATRIS. **Luschka s.** SINUS PETROSQUAMOSUS. **lymphatic s.'es** Spaces for the passage of lymph, extending through the reticular meshwork of a lymph node from the afferent lymph vessels in the cortex to the efferent lymph vessels in the medulla. The cells lining the spaces are continuous with the endothelial lining of the afferent vessels. Also *lymph channels, sinus lymphatici.* **s. of Maier** A short stemlike depression adjacent to the openings of the lacrimal canaliculi in the lacrimal sac. **marginal s.'es** Irregular dilatations at the periphery of the human placental intervillous space, once considered to form a functional component of the venous drainage of the space but now considered more likely to be localized extensions or "lakes" of blood from the subchorial space. **mastoid s.** One of the cellulae mastoideae. **s. maxillaris** [NA] One of the paired paranasal sinuses, and the largest, which is situated in the body of the maxilla and communicates with the hiatus semilunaris in the middle nasal meatus through an opening in the anterosuperior part of its medial wall. Its roof is the floor of the orbit, while its floor is the alveolar process of the maxilla. Also *maxillary sinus, sinus maxillaris highmori, antrum of Highmore, maxillary antrum, genyantrum* (outmoded). **medullary s.** An irregular channel that carries lymph through the medulla of a lymph node and toward the efferent lymphatic vessel. **s. meyeri** A shallow fossa in the floor of the external acoustic meatus near the tympanic membrane. *Outmoded.* Also *Meyer sinus.* **s. of Morgagni** 1 One of the sinus anales. 2 VENTRICULUS LARYNGIS. 3 The gap between the base of the skull and the superior constrictor muscle of the pharynx. **mucous s.'es of male urethra** LACUNAE OF MORGAGNI. **nasal s.'es** SINUS PARANASALES. **s. obliquus pericardii** [NA] A blind sac, open below and running obliquely upward and formed by the serous pericardium of the heart. It encloses the superior and inferior venae cavae and the four pulmonary veins behind the left atrium. Also *oblique sinus of pericardium.* **s. occipitalis** [NA] A venous sinus located in the attached margin of the falx cerebelli, beginning near the foramen magnum and draining into the confluence of the sinuses. Also *occipital sinus.* **omphalomesenteric s.** A tract or sinus that is an abnormal remnant of the omphalomesenteric duct, bridging the umbilicus and the distal ileum. It may be blind, or it may communicate at one or both ends of the residual duct. **Palfyn s.** A small space stated to be within the crista galli and communicating with the ethmoidal and frontal sinuses. This is not a generally recognized anatomical entity.

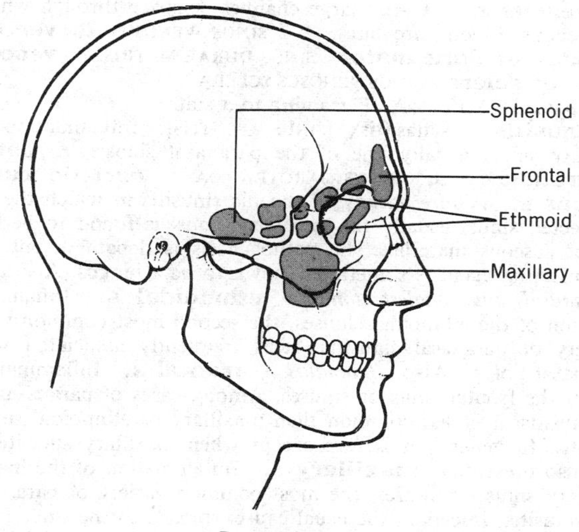


**Paranasal sinuses**

**s. paranasales** [NA] The accessory air chambers of the nasal cavity, which open into it and arise in the fetus as evaginations of the mucous membrane of the superior and middle meatuses. They include the ethmoidal, frontal, maxillary, and sphenoidal sinuses. Also *paranasal sinuses, nasal sinuses, accessory sinuses of the nose.* **parasinoidal s.** LACUNAE LATERALES. **petro-occipital s.** An occasional vein situated outside the skull along the inferior surface of the petro-occipital suture. It connects the cavernous sinus with either the ectocranial terminal part of the inferior petrosal sinus or the internal jugular vein. **s. petrosquamosus** A cavity located in a groove along the junction of the squamous and petrous parts of the temporal bone. It communicates anteriorly with the retromandibular vein through the postglenoid foramen, and opens posteriorly into the transverse sinus. Also *petrosquamous sinus, Luschka sinus.* **s. petrosus inferior** [NA] One of a pair of intracranial venous sinuses running posteriorly in a groove between the petrous part of the temporal bone and the basilar part of the occipital bone and extending from the cavernous sinus, which it drains, to the internal jugular vein, which it enters by passing through the anterior part of the jugular foramen. It receives tributaries from neighboring parts of the brain and the inner ear. Also *inferior petrosal sinus.* **s. petrosus superior** [NA] One of a pair of intracranial venous sinuses running posterolaterally in the attached margin of tentorium cerebelli and in a groove on the superior margin of the petrous part of the temporal bone and extending from the cavernous sinus, which it drains, to the transverse sinus just before the latter forms the sigmoid sinus. It receives tributaries from adjacent parts of the brain and the middle ear. Also *superior petrosal sinus.* **pilonidal s.** A hairy pit which may occur above the anal opening and overlying the lower septum on the coccyx. It is liable to inflammation. The older view was that such a sinus represented the developmental residue of the connection between skin and spinal cord at the site of closure of the posterior neuropore. More recently, it has been suggested that pilonidal sinuses are acquired lesions due to the penetration of hairs into the skin. Also *coccygeal sinus, pilonidal cyst.* **piriform s.** RECESSUS PIRIFORMIS. **s. pleurae** RECESSUS PLEURALES. **pleural s.'es** RECESSUS PLEURALES. **pleuroperitoneal s.** PLEUROPERICARDIAL HIATUS. **s. posterior cavitatis tympanicae** [NA] A small fossa on the mastoid wall of the tympanic cavity situated between the pyramidal eminence and the posterior canaliculus for the chordae tympani nerve laterally and lying below the fossa incudis. Also *posterior sinus of tympanic cavity.* **preauricular s.** A small sinus tract opening on the skin near the anterior aspect of the external ear, caused by incomplete fusion of those parts of the first and second branchial arches that form the ear. Also *fistula auris congenita, congenital preauricular fistula, preauricular fistula, earpit.* **s. prostaticus** [NA] A shallow recess on each side of the urethral crest in the prostatic part of the urethra, in the floor of which are the openings of the prostatic ducts. Also *prostatic sinus.* **s.'es of pulmonary trunk** SINUS TRUNCI PULMONALIS. **s. rectus** [NA] A venous sinus located in the junction of the falx cerebri and the tentorium cerebelli. It runs backward to join the transverse sinus on the left side. Also *straight sinus, tentorial sinus.* **renal s.** SINUS RENALIS. **s. renalis** [NA] The central cavity within the kidney. It is lined by the continuation of the renal capsule and occupied by the renal pelvis and calices, the renal vessels and nerves, and small amounts of areolar and adipose tissue. The walls are indented by the renal papillae. Also *renal sinus, sinus of kidney.* **rhomboid s.** CAVUM SEPTI PELLUCIDI. **rhomboid s. of Henle** VENTRICULUS TERMINALIS MEDULLAE SPINALIS. **Ridley s.** SINUS CIRCULARIS. **Rokitansky-Aschoff s.'es of the gallbladder** Outpouchings of the gallbladder mucosa, extending through the lamina propria and the muscular layer, that develop in association with calculus obstruction of the cystic duct. They are considered to be pathological. Also *Luschka's crypts* (incorrect). See also ADENOMYOMATOSIS OF THE GALLBLADDER. **sagittal s.** Either sinus sagittalis inferior or sinus sagittalis superior. **s. sagittalis inferior** [NA] A venous sinus located in the posterior half or two-thirds of the lower, free margin of the falx cerebri that joins the sinus rectus. Also *inferior sagittal sinus, inferior longitudinal sinus* (outmoded), *sinus of corpus callosum, falcial sinus* (outmoded), *falciform sinus* (outmoded). **s. sagittalis superior** [NA] A venous sinus located along the attached convex margin of the falx cerebri. It begins at the crista galli and extends backward to the internal occipital protuberance, where it joins the transverse sinus, usually on the right side. Also *superior sagittal sinus, superior longitudinal sinus.* **s. sigmoideus** [NA] The direct continuation of the transverse sinus, curving downward and medially on the mastoid part of the temporal bone to become the superior bulb of the internal jugular vein in the jugular foramen. Also *sigmoid sinus.* **soleal s.'es** SOLEAL SINUSOIDS. **s. sphenoidalis** [NA] One of the paired paranasal air chambers situated in the body of the sphenoid bone and separated from its fellow by a thin bony septum. It varies in size and shape, is seldom the same size as its fellow, and may extend into surrounding bones. It opens through an aperture anteriorly into the sphenoethmoidal recess of the nasal cavity. Also *sphenoidal sinus.* **s. sphenoparietalis** [NA] One of a pair of intracranial venous sinuses situated below the posterior margins of the lesser wings of the sphenoid bone, draining the surrounding dura mater and the middle meningeal vein and ending in the front part of the cavernous sinus. Also *sphenoparietal sinus.* **s. splenicus** [NA] One of the numerous and complex venous channels connecting arterial capillaries in the red pulp of the spleen with venous tributaries of the splenic veins. They are lined by flattened endothelial cells and surrounded by reticular fibers. Also *sinus of spleen.* **straight s.** SINUS RECTUS. **subarachnoidal s.'es** CISTERNAE SUBARACHNOIDEALES. **subcapsular s.** The portion of a lymphatic sinus beneath the capsule of a lymph node. It is continuous with the trabecular and the medullary sinuses. **superior longitudinal s.** SINUS SAGITTALIS SUPERIOR. **superior petrosal s.** SINUS PETROSUS SUPERIOR. **superior sagittal s.** SINUS SAGITTALIS SUPERIOR. **s. tarsi** [NA] The tunnel located between the os calcis and the talus. It contains the interosseous talocalcaneal ligament. Also *tarsal canal, tarsal sinus.* **tentorial s.** SINUS RECTUS. **terminal s.** 1 A vein which encircles the periphery of the area vasculosa of chick embryos. 2 An arterial circle at the periphery of the vascular system of the yolk sac of mammals. **tonsillar s.** FOSSA TONSILLARIS. **transverse s. of dura mater** SINUS TRANSVERSUS DURAE MATRIS. **transverse s. of pericardium** SINUS TRANSVERSUS PERICARDII. **s. transversus durae matris** [NA] A venous channel that begins at the internal occipital protuberance and is continuous on the right side with the superior sagittal sinus and on the left side with the sinus rectus. It passes laterally and forward to the petrous temporal bone, where it curves downward as the sinus sigmoideus. Also *transverse sinus of dura mater, lateral sinus.* **s. transversus pericardii** [NA] A horizontal, curved communicating passage between the right and left sides of the pericardial cavity, passing in front of the superior vena cava and left atrium and behind the aorta and pulmonary trunk. Also *transverse sinus of pericardium, Theile's canal.* **traumatic s.** A sinus resulting from injury. **s. trunci pulmonalis** [NA] Three small dilatations in the wall of the pulmonary trunk at its origin and opposite the semilunar cusps of the pulmonary valve. Also *sinuses of pulmonary trunk.* **s. tympani** [NA] A furrow in the medial wall of the tympanic cavity, situated behind the promontory and above the subiculum promontorii and corresponding to the location of the ampulla of the posterior semicircular canal in the internal ear. Also *tympanic sinus.* **s. unguis** The area immediately under the advancing nail. **urogenital s.** The ventral portion of the embryonic cloaca which becomes partitioned from the dorsal part, the primitive rectum, by the downgrowth of a mesodermal urorectal septum. In the male it contributes to the length of urethra between the prostatic utricle and the bulbourethral ducts, while in the female it forms the vestibule and the lower part of the vagina. **uterine s.** A venous channel in a pregnant uterus. **uteroplacental s.** Any of the blood channels situated between the placenta and the uterine sinuses in pregnancy. **s. of Valsalva** SINUS AORTAE. **s. venarum cavarum** [NA] The smooth posterior portion and lateral wall of the cavity of the right atrium of the heart, which extends anteriorly to the crista terminalis and contains the openings of the superior and inferior venae cavae and the coronary sinus and the foramina venarum minimarum. Its fetal origin is from the absorbed right horn of the sinus venosus. Also *sinus of venae cavae.* **s. venosus** The most caudal chamber of the primitive cardiac tube which receives the principal embryonic venous channels and opens into the primitive atrium. It comprises right and left horns. The right horn is incorporated into the back wall of the definitive right atrium while the left horn is the precursor of the coronary sinus opening into the right atrium after the partitioning of the primitive atrium. Also *venous sinus.* Abbr. SV **s. venosus sclerae** [NA] An endothelium-lined canal running circularly in the substance of the sclera close to the sclerocorneal junction. The inner wall comprises loose trabecular tissue containing the spaces of the iridocorneal angle. The sinus drains externally into the anterior ciliary veins. Also *venous sinus of sclera, Schlemm's canal, Lauth's canal.* **venous s.** 1 Any large channel or space through which venous blood circulates. 2 SINUS VENOSUS. **venous s.'es of dura mater** SINUS DURAE MATRIS. **venous s. of sclera** SINUS VENOSUS SCLERAE.

**sinusal** \sī′nəsəl\ Pertaining to a sinus.

**sinusitis** \sī′nəsī′tis\ [SINUS + -ITIS] Inflammation of any sinus, usually one of the paranasal sinuses. **barotraumatic s.** SINUS BAROTRAUMA. **chronic caseous s.** A rare variety of chronic sinusitis in which the affected sinus, usually the maxillary sinus, is found to be full of caseous material. The pathogenesis is debatable but the infecting agent is sometimes shown to be a fungus. Also *paranasal sinus cholesteatoma.* **ethmoidal s.** Inflammation of the ethmoidal sinuses, the second most common variety of paranasal sinusitis. It is frequently associated with nasal polypi. Also *ethmoiditis.* **frontal s.** Inflammation of the frontal sinus or sinuses. Among cases of paranasal sinusitis, it is less common than maxillary or ethmoidal sinusitis. In general, it is rare except when maxillary sinusitis is also present. **maxillary s.** Inflammation of the maxillary sinus or sinuses, the most common variety of paranasal sinusitis. Infection, the usual cause, spreads to the sinus from the nose except in about 10 percent of cases, in which carious teeth are to blame. Also *antritis.* **papillary s.** An uncommon variety of sinusitis characterized by metaplasia of the lining into stratified squamous or transitional epithelium with papillary hypertrophy. It may be mistaken for a transitional cell neoplasm. Virus infection has been suggested as the cause. **paranasal s.** Inflammation of one or more of the paranasal sinuses. **serous s.** *Incorrect* PARANASAL SINUS MUCOCELE. **sphenoidal s.** Inflammation of the sphenoidal sinus or sinuses. It is a relatively rare variety of paranasal sinusitis. Also *sphenoiditis.*

**sinusoid** \sī′n$^{y}$əsoid\ 1 Resembling a sinus. 2 A space or channel, lined by reticuloendothelium, for the passage of blood, as in the spleen, liver, suprarenal glands, parathyroid glands, bone marrow, and adenohypophysis. **hepatic s.** Any of the terminal branches of the portal venous system that correspond to hepatic capillaries. Obstruction around or near the hepatic sinusoid causes the portal hypertension seen in most types of cirrhosis. **myocardial s.'s** The slitlike spaces containing capillaries and situated between the myocardial fibers of the heart. *Outmoded.* **soleal s.'s** Capacious valveless veins within the soleal muscle of the calf. They are believed by some to be the site of stagnant venous blood flow which leads to calf vein thrombosis. Also *soleal sinuses.*

**sinusoidalization** \sī′nəsoi′dəlīzā′shən\ The administration of a sinusoidal current.

**sinuventricular** \sī′nʸoovəntrik′yələr\ SINOVENTRICULAR.

**siomycin** \sī′ōmī′sin\ A mixture of antibiotics closely related in structure and function to thiostrepton.

**si op. sit** *si opus sit* (L, if it be necessary: used in prescription writing).

**siphon** \sī′fən\ [L *sipho*, also *siphon* (from Gk *siphōn* a tube, siphon) a tube or pipe from which water springs out] **1** A bent tube with two extremities of unequal length, utilizing atmospheric pressure to transfer liquids from a higher to a lower level. **2** A bottle containing a liquid charged with carbonic acid. Release of a stopcock allows the liquid to be forced out by the carbonic acid gas. **carotid s.** The portion of the internal carotid artery that passes through the petrous portion of the temporal bone before becoming truly intracranial.

***Siphunculina*** \sīfun′kyəlī′nə\ A genus of biting gnats (order Diptera, family Chloropidae) that are important pests. Some species are of medical importance as mechanical vectors of conjunctivitis. ***S. funicola*** A species that is widespread in India, Sri Lanka, Java, and elsewhere in the Far East. It transmits conjunctivitis and possibly trachoma.

**Sipple** [John H. *Sipple*, U.S. physician, born 1930] See under SYNDROME.

**Sippy** [Bertram Welton *Sippy*, U.S. physician, 1866–1924] **1** Sippy method, Sippy treatment. See under DIET. **2** Sippy powder No. 1. See under POWDER. **3** Sippy powder No. 2. See under POWDER.

**sirenoform** \sī′rənōfôrm′\ Exhibiting the characteristics of sirenomelia.

**sirenomelia** \sī′rənōmē′lyə\ [*siren* (from Gk *seirēn* a Siren) a mermaid + *o* + MEL- + -IA] Any of several degrees of side-to-side fusion of the lower extremities and concomitant midline reduction of the pelvis. The thighs and calves are usually united as regards soft tissues but the long bones may display a range of union from none to total. The feet may be absent, completely fused or largely separate. Digestive and genitourinary viscera of the pelvis tend to be reduced or absent and the anus and external genitalia are often absent. Also *mermaid deformity, symmelia, symelia.*

**SIRS** soluble immune response suppressor.

**sirup** SYRUP.

**-sis** \-sis, -səs\ [Gk derivative noun suffix] A suffix usually denoting a process or condition, in nouns that are often derived from verbs ending in *-ze*, or *-se* in British spelling, (as *paralysis* from *paralyze*) or adjectives ending in *-tic* (as *peristalsis* from *peristaltic*). See also -IASIS, -OSIS.

**sisomycin** An aminoglycoside antibiotic obtained from *Micromonospora inyoensis*, with properties very similar to those of gentamicin.

**sister** A female nurse, especially the head nurse in a hospital ward. • The term is used in this sense in Great Britain, Australia, India, and South Africa, and until about 1970 was also current in New Zealand, where it is now obsolescent. Derived from reference to women in religious orders providing nursing care, the term now has no reference to religious affiliation but typically implies supervisory rank, as in *ward sister* or *theatre sister* (one in charge of a ward or surgical theatre, respectively).

**Sistrunk** [Walter Ellis *Sistrunk*, U.S. surgeon, 1880–1933] See under OPERATION.

***Sistrurus*** \sistroo′rəs\ [L *sistr(um)* a rattle used in the worship of Isis + New L *-urus*, combining form denoting tail] A genus of venomous snakes of the subfamily Crotalinae; the pigmy rattlesnakes.They occur in North America.

**site** [L *situs*. See SITUS.] A place, location, or position. **active s.** That region of the molecule of a catalyst, such as an enzyme or a membrane carrier, to which a substrate binds and at which it undergoes the reaction, i.e. is transformed into product or is translocated. Also *active center.* **allosteric s.** A region on an enzyme molecule, other than the active site, at which an effector (noncompetitive inhibitor or an activator) may bind. The binding of the effector molecule results in intramolecular conformational changes which modify the activity of the enzyme. **antibody combining s.** The site on immunoglobulin antibody that combines specifically with its corresponding antigenic determinant. It is present in the Fab portion of the molecule and appears to include the variable regions of both heavy and light chains of the molecule. Also *binding site, antibody site, paratope, combining site, antigen recognition site.* **binding s.** The specific site on a cell surface or macromolecule to which other molecules and ions bind. • In im-

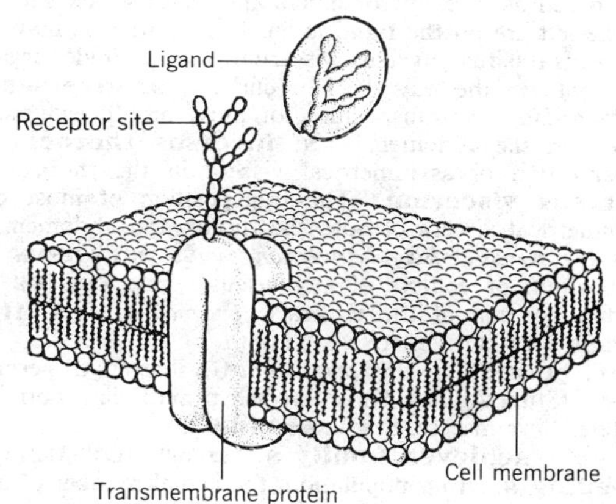

**Cell receptor site**

munology, the *binding site* of an antibody molecule which combines with antigen is called *antibody combining site* or simply *combining site.* **catalytic s.** The site on an enzyme molecule where the catalyzed reaction occurs. **combining s.** ANTIBODY COMBINING SITE. **donor s.** An area of the body from which a graft or transplant has been removed or could be removed. Also *donor area, graft donor site.* **fragile s.** See under CHROMATID GAP. **graft donor s.** DONOR SITE. **hypersensitive s.** In molecular genetics, a region of DNA in chromatin that is highly susceptible to digestion by deoxyribonuclease. It corresponds to transcriptionally active regions of the genome, especially regulatory elements of their structural genes. **immunologically privileged s.'s** See under PRIVILEGED SITES. **marker s.** See under CHROMATID GAP. **mutable s.** Any location on a chromosome or in the genome that is capable of mutation. **nucleotide replacement s.** The location of a point mutation with respect to a codon. **privileged s.'s** Those sites of the body lacking lymphatic drainage and in which antigens or tissue grafts can be placed without evoking an immune response. Examples include the central nervous system, the anterior chamber of the eye, and the cheek pouch of the hamster. **receptor s.** A cell surface component which specifically reacts with a molecule in the cell's environment, as with a hormone, or virus. The specificity is the result of complementary shapes of the receptor and the molecule being bound (the ligand). **recipient s.** The location in which a graft is placed. Also *recipient area.*

**sitiomania** \sit′ē·ōmā′nē·ə\ *Obs.* BULIMIA.

**sito-** \sī′tō-\ [Gk *sitos* or *sition* grain, bread, food] A combining form meaning food.

**sitomania** \-mā′nē·ə\ *Outmoded* BULIMIA.

**sitotaxis** \-tak′sis\ [SITO- + Gk *taxis* an arranging, ordering] The movement of a cell or organism in response to a food stimulus, whether toward the food (positive sitotaxis) or away from the food (negative sitotaxis). *Obs.* Also *sitotropism.*

**sitotherapy** \-ther′əpē\ [SITO- + THERAPY] DIET THERAPY.

**sitotropism** \sītät′rəpizm\ SITOTAXIS.

**situs** \sī′təs\ [L (substantive from *situs*, past part. of *sinere* to place, leave) site, position, arrangement] **1** Site; situation; position; location. **2** A layout or arrangement. **s. inversus** An arrangement of body parts in which they are transposed as in a mirror image and those which should be on the left are on the right, as in dextrocardia. It may affect all viscera (situs inversus viscerum), or a single organ or part, or even the way the hair curls. **s. inversus abdominalis** A transposition of most or all asymmetrical viscera in the abdomen. **s. inversus thoracis** The transposition of asymmetrical viscera in the thorax. **s. inversus viscerum** The transposition of most or all asymmetrical viscera of both the thorax and abdomen. Also *situs transversus, visceral inversion.* **s. perversus** The malposition or ectopia of any viscus. **s. solitus** The normal position of the viscera. *Outmoded.* **s. transversus** SITUS INVERSUS VISCERUM.

**si vir. perm.** *si vires permittant* (L, if strength permit).

**Siwe** [Sture August *Siwe*, Swedish pediatrician, born 1897] Letterer-Siwe disease. See under DISEASE.

**size** / **achieved family s.** COMPLETED FAMILY SIZE. **breeding s.** In a population, the actual number of organisms or individuals that engage in sexual reproduction. Symbol: N **completed family s.** **1** The number of children born alive into a family by the time family formation has been completed. Also *achieved family size.* **2** In demography, the total number of children that 1000 women will bear during their lifetime. It is approximately equal to the total fertility rate. **effective breeding s.** A breeding size that is adjusted mathematically to account for such factors as population size, age distribution, sex ratio, inbreeding, and nonrandom sampling to permit comparisons between disparate groups. Also *effective population size.* Symbol: $N_e$ **field s.** In radiology, the size of the body area which is exposed to ionizing radition being used for diagnosis or treatment. **French s.** A number in a system of measurement of catheters. For a thick-walled catheter, the French size equals three times the outer diameter in millimeters. **sample s.** In statistics, the size of sample required to detect a difference of given magnitude with a stated degree of probability in samples whose variability is known at least approximately.

**Sjögren** [Karl Gustaf Torsten *Sjögren*, Swedish physician, born 1896] **1** Marinesco-Sjögren-Garland syndrome. See under MARINESCO-SJÖGREN SYNDROME. **2** Sjögren-Larsson syndrome. See under SYNDROME.

**Sjöqvist** [Carl Olof *Sjögvist*, Swedish neurosurgeon, 1901–1954] **1** Sjöqvist tractotomy. See under TRIGEMINAL TRACTOTOMY. **2** See under OPERATION.

**skato-** \skat′ə-\ SCATO-.

**skatole** \skat′ōl\ 3-Methylindole, a compound found in the mammalian body and formed by the action of intestinal bacteria on tryptophan. It is partly responsible for the odor of feces.

**skatologic** \skatəläj′ik\ SCATOLOGIC.

**skatology** \skatäl′əjē\ COPROLOGY.

**skeletal** \skel′ətəl\ Of or relating to the skeleton.

**skeletofusimotor** \skel′ətōfyoo′simō′tər\ Denoting motoneurons that innervate both extrafusal and intrafusal muscle fibers (β-efferents).

**skeletogeny** \skel′ətäj′ənē\ [*skeleto(n)* + -GEN + -Y] The history, in all its aspects, of the formation, evolution and development of the parts and the whole of a skeleton. Adj. skeletogenous.

**skeletography** \skel′ətäg′rəfē\ A description of the skeleton and its parts.

**skeletology** \skel′ətäl′əjē\ The study of the skeleton and its parts.

**skeletomotor** \skel′ətōmō′tər\ Denoting efferent axons or motoneurons that exclusively innervate extrafusal fibers in a skeletal muscle (α-fibers).

**skeleton** [neut. sing. of Gk *skeletos* dried up, withered, from *skellein* to dry up, parch, wither] **1** The bony and some of the cartilaginous framework of the body of animals; the endoskeleton in vertebrates and the exoskeleton in invertebrates. **2** All the bones of the body considered together. **appendicular s.** The bones of the upper and the lower limbs. Also *skeleton appendiculare.* **articulated s.** A skeleton mounted on a stand, usually by wires, nylon cord, and pins, so as to resemble the normal position and articulation of the bones of the various parts and permit their movement. **axial s.** The cranium and the vertebral column with its associated ribs and sternum. **cardiac s.** A condensation of dense connective tissue forming fibrous rings, or annuli fibrosi, around the valvular orifices and providing attachments for the muscles of the heart, as well as firmness to the roots of the aorta and the pulmonary trunk. It also includes the membranous part of the interventricular septum. **gill arch s.** The branchial arch cartilages which resemble the gill skeleton of certain fishes and which include Meckel's cartilage and cartilages in the second, third, and fourth arches. **s. membri inferioris liberi** [NA] The bones of the thigh, leg, and foot. **s. membri superioris liberi** [NA] The bones of the arm, forearm, wrist, and hand. **s. of nose** The bony and cartilaginous support of the external nose, the walls of the nasal cavity, and the paranasal sinuses. **s. of partial denture** FRAMEWORK. **visceral s.** **1** Bony elements derived from the branchial arches, such as ear ossicles, part of the mandible, the hyoid bone, and possibly the laryngeal, tracheal, and bronchial cartilages. **2** Bones protecting the viscera, such as the pelvic bones, the ribs, and the sternum. For defs. 1 and 2 also *visceroskeleton.*

**skeletopia** \skel′ətō′pē·ə\ The location of an organ in relation to the skeleton. Also *skeletopy.*

**Skene** [Alexander Johnston Chalmers *Skene*, Scottish-born U.S. gynecologist, 1838–1900] **1** Skene's tubules, Skene's glands, Skene's ducts. See under DUCTUS PARAURETHRALES. **2** Skene's glands. See under GLANDULAE URETHRALES URETHRAE FEMININAE.

**skenitis** \skēnī′tis\ [*Sken(e's glands)* + -ITIS ] Inflammation of Skene's glands (the paraurethral glands).

**skewfoot** \skyoo′fůt\ Any deformity of the foot in which the forward end of the heel-toe axis is deviated more laterally than is seen in the usual range of positions.

**skewness** \skyoo′nis\ A measure of the asymmetry of a unimodal distribution. See also SKEW DISTRIBUTION.

**skia-** \skī′ə-\ [Gk *skia* shadow, shade] A combining form meaning shadow, as that seen in a roentgenogram. Also *scia-*.

**skiametry** \skī·am′ətrē\ [SKIA- + -METRY] RETINOSCOPY.

**skiaporescopy** \-pôres′kəpē\ RETINOSCOPY.

**skiascope** \skī′əskōp\ [SKIA- + -SCOPE] RETINOSCOPE.

**skiascope-optometer** PHORO-OPTOMETER.

**skiascopy** \skī·as′kəpē\ [SKIA- + -SCOPY] RETINOSCOPY.

**skimming / plasma s.** The rheological characteristic of blood flow whereby a thin layer of plasma separates erythrocytes from the intima of blood vessels.

**skin** [Old Norse *skinn* (from Germanic *skinth-* to flay, peel off, akin to L *secare* to cut) skin, hide] **1** The principal layers, comprising the epidermis and dermis, of the integumentum commune; cutis. **2** A rind, peel, covering, or outer layer. **bronzed s.** Brown skin of the peculiar shade seen in many patients with Addison's disease and in hemochromatosis. **citrine s.** Skin that has been yellowed and thickened through elastotic degeneration caused by excessive exposure to sunlight. **collodion s.** The skin of newborn infants with ichthyosis congenita. **elastic s.** Skin of unusual stretchability, as seen in the Ehlers-Danlos syndrome. **farmers' s.** SAILORS' SKIN. **freeze-dried s.** LYOPHILIZED SKIN. **glabrous s.** **1** That part of the skin without hair follicles. **2** That part of the skin without terminal hair. *Popular.* **loose s.** CUTIS LAXA. **lyophilized s.** A skin graft that has had the water content removed. Such a graft can be stored at room temperature. Although not living, when reconstituted it forms a useful temporary biologic dressing for large wounds or burns. Also *freeze-dried skin.* **nail s.** CUTICLE. **parchment s.** Dry, thin, atrophic skin. **piebald s.** A disorder of autosomal dominant inheritance in which patches of skin totally devoid of pigment are present from birth. The term has sometimes been incorrectly applied to vitiligo. **pig s.** Thickened dimpled skin, as that seen in lymphedema. **sailors' s.** Skin that shows the premature aging effects of prolonged exposure to sunshine. Also *farmers' skin.* **shagreen s.** A slightly elevated, irregularly thickened plaque that appears, usually in the lumbosacral region, in patients with tuberous sclerosis. Also *shagreen plaque, shagreen patch, shark skin.*

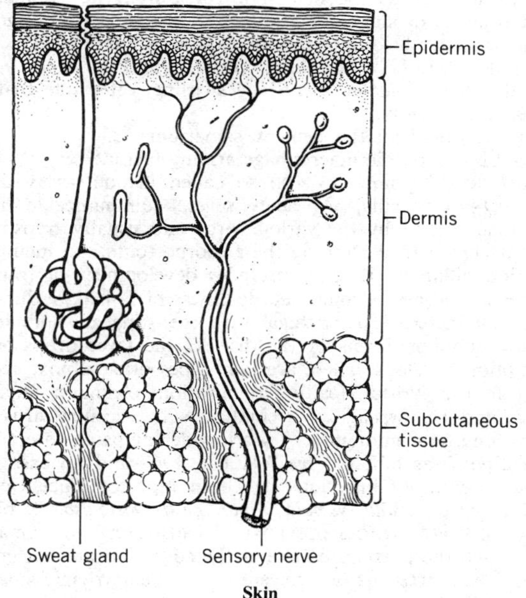

**Skin**

**Skinner** [Burrhus Frederic *Skinner,* U.S. psychologist, born 1904] See under BOX.

**skipper / cheese s.** The larva of the cheese fly, *Piophila casei,* family Piophilidae, that infests foods such as cheese, bacon, dried fish, cured meat, and other protein foods, and is an important cause of enteric myiasis from accidental ingestion. Also *cheese maggot.*

**sklero-** \sklir′ō-, sklir′ə-, skler′ō-\ SCLERO-.

**Sklowsky** [E. L. *Sklowsky,* German physician, flourished 20th century] See under SYMPTOM.

**Skoog** [Torsten Olof *Skoog,* Swedish otolaryngologist, born 1894] **1** See under OPERATION. **2** Skoog's operation. See under SKOOG'S METHOD.

**skull** [Middle English *skulle,* of Scandinavian origin] **1** CRANIUM. **2** The cranium and mandible. **3** The cranium cerebrale and the cranium viscerale. **Apert s.** The characteristic skull deformity of acrocephalosyndactyly Type I (Apert syndrome). **hot cross bun s.** See under BOSSING OF THE CRANIUM. **lacuna s.** CRANIOFENESTRIA. **maplike s.** The appearance of areas of lucency with irregular borders, resembling outlines on a map, seen typically in roentgenograms of the skull in Hand-Schüller-Christian disease. **membranous s.** The peripheral membranous (mesenchymal) layer which surrounds the developing brain of the embryo or fetus and in which appear the one or several centers of ossification proper to each bone forming the vault of the skull. **stenobregmatic s.** A skull characterized by abnormal narrowness in the bregmatic region. **West's lacuna s.** A defective development of the bones of the vault of the skull, which has a honeycomb appearance on roentgenography. It is often associated with neural tube closure defects. Also *West-Engstler skull.*

**skullcap** CALVARIA.

**slant / s. of occlusal plane** The angle between the occlusal plane and the axis-orbital plane.

**SLE** systemic lupus erythematosus.

**sleep** [Old English *slæp*] A natural, periodic behavioral state during which the body rests itself and its physiological powers are restored. It is characterized by a loss of reactivity to the environment, and during it certain physiological processes of both the body and the brain function differently than they do during alert wakefulness. Normal sleep consists of at least two quite different behavioral states: synchronized sleep, during which the electroencephalogram consists of slow waves of high amplitude, and desynchronized sleep (DS) or activated sleep characterized by rapid eye movements (REM sleep), in which the EEG pattern is characterized by waves of high frequency and low amplitude. Four stages are usually described within the human synchronized sleep cycle, followed by a period of activated sleep. Each cycle lasts between 80 and 120 minutes, and during a normal night's sleep four such cycles are experienced. **activated s.** DESYNCHRONIZED SLEEP. **active s.** DESYNCHRONIZED SLEEP. **crescendo s.** Sleep characterized by motor behavior of the limbs and body that increases in intensity during the sleep cycle. **deep restful s.** SYNCHRONIZED SLEEP. **delta-wave s.** SYNCHRONIZED SLEEP. **desynchronized s.** The stage of sleep during which the electroencephalogram shows a low voltage and fast rhythm and which is characterized by rapid eye movements (REM), irregular heart rate and respiration, periods of involuntary muscular jerks and movements, and a higher threshold for arousal. Periods of desynchronized sleep last 5–20 minutes and occur at about 90-minute intervals during a normal night's sleep. It is the stage of sleep during which dreaming frequently occurs and is believed by some to be the most refreshing form of sleep. Also *activated sleep, REM sleep, paradoxical sleep, emergent stage I, D state, rhombencephalic sleep, pontine sleep, dreaming sleep, active sleep*. Abbr. DS Compare SYNCHRONIZED SLEEP. **dreamless s.** SYNCHRONIZED SLEEP. **electric s.** Somnolence that has reportedly been induced by the application of electrical currents through the brain. It is believed by some investigators that sleep can be initiated by electrical stimulation across the temporal lobes or by applying current through the base of the brain from the frontal to the occipital poles. Whether this phenomenon is a loss of consciousness or physiological sleep has not been established. **hypnotic s.** HYPNOSIS. **NREM s.** SYNCHRONIZED SLEEP. **orthodox s.** SYNCHRONIZED SLEEP. **paradoxical s.** DESYNCHRONIZED SLEEP. **paroxysmal s.** NARCOLEPSY. **pontine s.** DESYNCHRONIZED SLEEP. **REM s.** DESYNCHRONIZED SLEEP. **rhombencephalic s.** DESYNCHRONIZED SLEEP. **rolandic s.** In birds, behavior resembling sleep following ablation of the cerebral cortex. **slow-wave s.** SYNCHRONIZED SLEEP. **synchronized s.** The stages of sleep during which the electroencephalogram shows a high voltage and slow rhythm and which is characterized by slow and regular respiration and by relatively constant heart rate and blood pressure. Synchronized sleep is usually described as consisting of four stages, in which delta waves predominate. Also *deep restful sleep, dreamless sleep, delta-wave sleep, delta state, slow-wave sleep, orthodox sleep, NREM sleep*. Compare DESYNCHRONIZED SLEEP.

**sleeplessness** INSOMNIA.

**sleepwalking** SOMNAMBULISM.

**slice** [Old French *esclisse* a splinter, thin piece of wood, of Germanic origin] An inlay cavity in which the proximal surface of the tooth has been flattened, using a fine abrasive disk.

**slide / histology s.** MICROSCOPE SLIDE. **microscope s.** A rectangular plate of glass upon which specimens are mounted prior to examination with a microscope.

**sling** 1 A looped bandage, usually made of cloth with the ends tied behind the neck, used to support the forearm. 2 Tissue or artificial material used as a suspensory support for a tissue or an organ. **Glisson s.** A leather head halter used to apply traction to the spine. The halter passes around the neck and under the chin, where it is attached to an extension apparatus over a pulley at the head of the bed. **levator s.** 1 The supportive mechanism formed by the two levator veli palatini muscles meeting in the midline of the soft palate. 2 The puborectalis portion of the levator ani muscle on each side that meets the fibers of the opposite muscle and those of the anal sphincters behind the anorectal flexure, forming a supportive loop or sling. Also *anorectal ring*.

**slit** 1 A long, narrow surgical incision. 2 To create such an aperture. **gill s.** GILL CLEFT. **pharyngeal s.** GILL CLEFT. **stenopeic s.** A narrow slit serving to exclude peripheral rays of poorly focused light, thereby serving to improve the visual acuity of an eye with refractive error. This is comparable to the pinhole camera effect. **vulvar s.** RIMA PUDENDI.

**slit lamp** See under LAMP.

**slope** 1 An inclined plane, at an angle to both the vertical and the horizontal planes; a slanting surface. 2 Agar slant. A British usage. See under SLANT CULTURE.

**slough** \sluf\ 1 Necrotic tissue. 2 To separate spontaneously, as dead tissue from its living base. **graft s.** The shedding of graft tissue following death of the transplanted tissue, whether due to poor blood supply, infection, mechanical disruption, or rejection.

**sloughing** \sluf′ing\ The spontaneous separation of necrotic tissue from its living base.

**Sluder** [Greenfield *Sluder*, U.S. physician, 1865–1925] 1 See under METHOD. 2 Sluder's neuralgia, Sluder syndrome. See under SPHENOPALATINE NEURALGIA.

**sludge** \sluj\ A thick suspension of solid matter deposited on the bed of or, occasionally, floating on the surface of, a liquid medium. **biliary s.** A suspension of solid and semisolid particles within the gallbladder.

**slug** Any of various shell-less terrestrial or aquatic gastropods, some of which serve as intermediate hosts of human parasites such as the nematode *Angiostrongylus cantonensis*. Land snails or slugs are members of the subclass Pulmonata and sea slugs belong to the subclass Opisthobranchia.

**slurry** \slur′ē\ [Middle English *slory*, from *slore* a thin mud] A suspension formed by swirling, often one that settles fairly rapidly.

**Sm** Symbol for the element, samarium.

**SMAF** specific macrophage arming factor.

**smallpox** [*small* + POX; so called in contrast with the *(great) pox* syphilis] An acute, severe, communicable disease of man caused by the variola virus and usually transmitted from person to person via the airborne route. An incubation period of about 12 days precedes development of transient viremia and a prodromal febrile illness of 2–4 days' duration. The characteristic centrifugal rash then appears and, in the more common forms of the disease, the fever drops as the eruption develops. There are four types of smallpox, according to the World Health Organization: ordinary, modified, flat, and hemorrhagic. Vaccination with vaccinia virus confers long-term immunity. A worldwide campaign to eradicate smallpox was initiated by WHO in 1967 and no case other than laboratory infections has been reported since October 1975. Also *variola, variola major, pestis variolosa*. **black s.** HEMORRHAGIC SMALLPOX. **coherent s.** Smallpox in which the pustules cohere at the edges but are not confluent. **confluent s.** Severe flat or hemorrhagic smallpox in which the vesicles appear to run together. **discrete s.** Smallpox in which the pustules are separate and distinct from one another. **flat s.** A frequently fatal form of smallpox in which fever may persist after the rash appears and in which the rash, a dusky, papular erythema of the face, arms, and trunk, fails to mature. Vesicles form in 10–12 days, but scabbing does not develop. Instead, the epidermis may peel in sheets. Death may occur in the second week of illness as a result of encephalitislike or extensive hemorrhagic manifestations or secondary bacterial infection. **hemorrhagic s.** A usually fatal, fulminant form of smallpox which may be mistaken for a hemorrhagic blood dyscrasia. The prodrome, marked by high fever and myalgia, is prolonged. Fever persists throughout the illness. The rash is a dusky erythema on the face and trunk. Petechiae, purpura, or large ecchymoses of the skin and mucosa develop and bleeding from any or all orifices may ensue. A vesicular rash may not appear. Death usually occurs 7–14 days after onset of illness. Also *black smallpox, malignant smallpox, variola hemorrhagica, purpura variolosa.* **inoculation s.** Smallpox contracted from the deliberate, direct transmission of blister fluid from a person with the disease to the skin of a healthy person. Before the development of vaccination (with vaccinia or cowpox), the procedure was widely used to prevent subsequent severe, disfiguring smallpox. **malignant s.** HEMORRHAGIC SMALLPOX. **mild s.** ALASTRIM. **modified s.** A form of smallpox occurring in previously immunized persons with residual immunity. The rash resembles that of varicella and is sparse and superficial but still distinctly centrifugal in distribution. This type of smallpox is very seldom fatal.

**smear** A specimen for microscopic study prepared by spreading the material to be examined onto a glass slide. The material, usually a drop of a body secretion or fluid, is spread very thinly over the slide surface with the help of a loop, a swab, or the edge of another glass slide. The smear may be examined fresh or may be fixed and stained prior to examination. **bronchoscopic s.** A smear of lower respiratory tract material collected at bronchoscopy to be examined for abnormal cells or microorganisms. **buccal s.** A preparation of superficial cells that are scraped from the buccal mucosa and spread onto a microscope slide. **cervical s.** Preparation of cervical secretions for diagnosis of infertility, infection, or ovulation. **cul-de-sac s.** Aspirate of fluid from the Douglas cul-de-sac for diagnosis of infection, bleeding, or neoplasm. **cytologic s.** CYTOSMEAR. **FGT cytologic s.** Any specimen from the female genital tract prepared for cytologic examination. **Papanicolaou s.** In the Papanicolaou test, a smear taken of vaginal or cervical epithelial cells that is placed on a glass slide and stained with Papanicolaou stain. Also *Pap smear.* **Tzanck s.** A diagnostic test in which scrapings taken from the base of lesions of the skin or mucous membranes are stained with Giemsa or Wright stain to reveal the multinucleated giant cells typical of infection with either the varicella-zoster virus or the herpes simplex virus. **VCE s.** The cytolgic diagnostic test for female hormone activity and for cancer of the cervix, consisting of material obtained from the vagina, ectocervix, and endocervix prepared for microscopic study.

**smegma** \smeg′mə\ [Gk *smēgma,* also *smēma* unguent, soap] The secretion of the Tyson's glands. It tends to accumulate under the prepuce as a white cheesy material. **s. embryonum** VERNIX CASEOSA.

**smegmolith** \smeg′məlith\ [*smegm(a)* + *o* + -LITH] A concretion in the smegma.

**smell** 1 The special sense perceived by receptors in the olfactory mucous membrane of the roof of the nose and a cortical center in the prepyriform cortex and amygdaloid nucleus. 2 The quality of substances that excites the sense of smell. 3 To perceive by the sense of smell.

**smell-brain** RHINENCEPHALON.

**Smellie** [William *Smellie,* Scottish obstetrician, 1697–1763] 1 See under METHOD. 2 Mauriceau-Smellie-Veit maneuver. See under MANEUVER.

**Smith** [David W. *Smith,* U.S. pediatrician, born 1921] Smith-Lemli-Opitz syndrome. See under SYNDROME.

**Smith** See under FERRIS SMITH.

**Smith** [Gardner Watkins *Smith,* U.S. surgeon, born 1931] Smith-Robinson operation. See under OPERATION.

**Smith** [Henry *Smith,* Irish-born British military surgeon active in India, 1862–1948] See under OPERATION.

**Smith** [Robert William *Smith,* Irish surgeon, 1807–1873] See under DISLOCATION.

**Smith** [Sidney *Smith,* U.S. surgeon, born 1912] Potts-Smith-Gibson operation. See under POTTS OPERATION.

**Smith** [William Henry *Smith,* U.S. bacteriologist, flourished 19th century] See under STAIN.

**Smith-Petersen** [Marius Nygaard *Smith-Petersen,* Norwegian-born U.S. orthopedic surgeon, 1886–1953] See under NAIL.

**Smithwick** [Reginald Hammerick *Smithwick,* U.S. surgeon, born 1899] Smithwick's operation. See under LUMBODORSAL SPLANCHNICECTOMY.

**smoke** [Old English *smoca*] 1 A suspension in the atmosphere of particulate matter emitted as a result of combustion. 2 An atmospheric aerosol of solid or liquid particles resulting from combustion, evaporation, or thermal decomposition. • For air quality control, many countries have formulated legal definitions of smoke. **mainstream s.** The tobacco smoke that is inhaled by the smoker. **sidestream s.** The smoke that is given off by a cigarette, pipe, or cigar between puffs and is not directly inhaled by the smoker.

**smoking / passive s.** The exposure of a nonsmoking person to tobacco smoke produced by others.

**SMR** 1 standardized mortality ratio. 2 submucous resection.

**Sn** Symbol for the element, tin.

**s.n.** *secundum naturam* (L, according to nature).

***sn-*** [*s(tereospecific) n(umbering)*] A prefix applied to glycerol and its derivatives to indicate stereospecific numbering of its carbon atoms. Thus the naturally occurring glycerol phosphate, which has 2*R* configuration, and could equally well be called L-(glycerol 3-phosphate) and D-(glycerol 1-phosphate), is designated *sn*-glycerol 3-phosphate.

**snail** [Old English *snægl*] A member of the order Gastropoda, phylum Mollusca. Many freshwater species are medically important for their role as intermediate hosts of parasitic trematodes, particularly in the tropics.

**snake** [Old English *snaca*] Any member of the reptilian suborder Serpentes. Also *serpent.* **brown s.** The venomous snake *Pseudonaja textilis* of the family Elapidae. **coral s.** Any member of the elapid genera *Micrurus* and *Micruroides..* Also *harlequin snake.* **hair s.** HORSEHAIR WORM. **harlequin s.** CORAL SNAKE. **lyre s.** Any of the black-fanged poisonous snakes of the genus *Trimorphodon* found in the southwestern United States. **tiger s.** Any member of the elapid genus *Notechis.*

**snakeroot** SERPENTARIA. **Seneca s.** SENEGA. **senega s.** SENEGA.

**snap** A quick, sharp sound. **opening s.** An abrupt sound early in diastole, associated with mitral valve opening in cases of mitral stenosis. Also *mitral click.*

**snare** \sner\ [Old Norse *snara* a snare] A surgical instrument consisting of a wire loop designed to be tightened at the end of a slender hollow shaft by means of a finger grip. It is used to remove polyps or polypoid parts by crushing and cutting through their base. **basket s.** A surgical snare having more than one loop, often used by urologists for removing calculi from the ureter during cystoscopy. **nasal s.** A snare for removing nasal polyps or, occasionally, other polypoid structures in the nose. The principal varieties are the cutting and avulsing snares. **tonsil s.** A snare used in dissection tonsillectomy to crush through the pedicle or lingual attachment. This completes the excision after the bulk of the tonsil has been previously dissected.

**Sneddon** [Ian Bruce *Sneddon,* English dermatologist, born 1915] Sneddon-Wilkinson disease. See under SUBCORNEAL PUSTULAR DERMATOSIS.

**sneeze** [Middle English *snesen,* alteration of *fnesen* (prob.

because of confusion between Middle English written *f* and *s*), from Old English *fneosan,* akin to Gk *pnein* to breathe] **1** To expel air involuntarily and explosively through the nose and mouth in response to some irritation, usually in the nose. **2** The act of sneezing.

**Snellen** [Hermann *Snellen,* Dutch ophthalmologist, 1834–1908] See under EYE, CHART, TEST.

**Snider** [Thomas H. *Snider,* U.S. physician, born 1925] Snider match test. See under MATCH TEST.

**snore** To breathe in noisily through the mouth while asleep. The coarse, rasping sound is caused by inspiration being somewhat obstructed by the relaxed walls of the oropharynx, particularly the back of the tongue. A period of apnea may precede the noisy inspiration.

**snowblindness** See under BLINDNESS.

**SNS** sympathetic nervous system.

**snuff** Any powder, especially powdered tobacco, taken by applying it to the mucous membranes of the nasal passages.

**snuffbox / anatomical s.** A triangular depression on the back of the radial side of the wrist produced by extending the fingers and thumb. The space is bounded posteriorly by the tendon of the extensor pollicis longus and anteriorly by the tendons of extensor pollicis brevis and abductor pollicis longus, which are crossed superficially by the palpable digital rami of the superficial branch of the radial nerve. The floor is formed by the scaphoid and trapezium bones, which are crossed here by the radial artery. Orthopedic surgeons exert digital pressure in this space to test for suspected fracture of the scaphoid bone. Also *tabatière anatomique* (French).

**snuffles** Noisy breathing through the partly blocked nose, particularly when this occurs in babies and the obstruction interferes with normal feeding. The term is applied especially to cases of congenital syphilis when such manifestations may be present at birth due to syphilitic rhinitis. It is also a common early manifestation of the Down syndrome.

**Snyder** [Marshall L. *Snyder,* U.S. microbiologist, born 1907] See under TEST.

**SOAP** subjective, objective, assessment, plan (headings of the problem-oriented medical record).

**soap** [Old English *sāpe* (from West Germanic *saipōn-,* which is prob. the source of L *sapo* soap) soap, hair dye] The salt of a fatty acid, usually one of about 12 to 18 carbon atoms. It is produced by the alkaline hydrolysis of fats. Also *sapo.* **green s.** A soap prepared by saponification of vegetable oils, except coconut oil and palm oil, with potassium hydroxide. Glycerin is retained in the product. Also *medicinal soft soap, potash soap, soft soap, sapo mollis medicinalis, sapo viridis.* **hexachlorophene liquid s.** A 0.225–0.26% w/w solution of hexachlorophene in a 10–13% solution of a potassium soap. Hexachlorophene is well absorbed through the skin, and there is evidence that in babies there may be brain damage from excessive exposure to this agent. Many countries limit the use of hexachlorophene in soaps, powders, and cleansing preparations. **medicinal soft s.** GREEN SOAP. **potash s.** GREEN SOAP. **soft s.** GREEN SOAP.

**soapstone** TALC.

**SOB** shortness of breath.

**sobbing** A form of breathing usually associated with weeping, in which breathing movements occur in a convulsive manner with spasmodic closure of the glottis and contractions of the diaphragm, usually producing a characteristic sound.

**socia** \sō′shē·ə\ [L, a female associate or partner] A detached, or accessory, part of an organ.

**sociacusis** \sō′shē·əkʸoo′sis\ SOCIOACUSIS.

**socio-** \sō′sē·ō-, sō′shē·ō-\ [L *socius* associated, sharing in, allied; a companion, associate] A combining form meaning (1) social, relating to society; (2) relating to sociology.

**socioacusis** \-əkʸoo′sis\ [SOCIO- + -ACUSIS] Hearing loss induced by exposure to loud noise encountered in everyday life, apart from occupational noise. Amplified music is an example of such a noise. Also *sociacusis.*

**sociodrama** \-dram′ə\ Psychodrama focusing on the entire therapy group and aiming at the active restructuring of attitudes to better fit the social mores of the society.

**sociopath** \sō′sē·əpath′\ [SOCIO- + -PATH] PSYCHOPATH.

**sociopathy** \sō′sē·äp′əthē\ [SOCIOPATH + -Y] PSYCHOPATHY.

**sociotherapy** \-ther′əpē\ Any treatment with major emphasis on the socioenvironmental and interpersonal factors that affect adjustment, such as milieu therapy or as is used in a therapeutic community.

**socket** [Anglo-French, dim. of Old French *soc* a plowshare, of Celtic origin] A hollow or concavity into which a corresponding part fits, such as a tooth socket or the component of a prosthesis into which an amputation stump fits. **adjustable s.** A prosthetic socket, fabricated with flexible material, that can be adjusted to accommodate stump volume and shape changes. **dry s.** ALVEOLITIS. **Dundee s.** A total-contact socket for a below-knee prosthesis. **eye s.** ORBITA. **infected s.** ALVEOLITIS. **partial-contact s.** A prosthetic socket that only partially contacts the amputation stump. **plug-fit s.** An old-fashioned socket for above-knee prostheses following the contour of the stump, so that the body weight is borne on the entire circumferance of the upper thigh. **septic s.** ALVEOLITIS. **suction s.** A prosthetic socket for above-knee amputations that utilizes suction as a means of suspension. **tooth s.'s** DENTAL ALVEOLI. Also *dental alveoli, alveolar cavities.* **total-contact s.** A prosthetic socket for above-knee amputees in which the stump is in complete contact with the socket, allowing for greater sensory "feedback" from the prosthetic limb.

**soda** [Italian, perhaps from Med L *sodanum* barilla, a plant] **1** Any of the alkaline materials containing sodium, namely sodium hydroxide, sodium carbonate, and sodium bicarbonate. **2** Water containing dissolved carbon dioxide, this gas sometimes being prepared by acidifying sodium carbonate. **baking s.** SODIUM BICARBONATE. **bicarbonate of s.** SODIUM BICARBONATE. **caustic s.** SODIUM HYDROXIDE. **washing s.** SODIUM CARBONATE.

**soda lime** A mixture of calcium oxide and sodium hydroxide made by adding powdered lime to molten sodium hydroxide. Since, unlike sodium hydroxide itself, it is not deliquescent, it is used for the absorption of carbon dioxide, as in breathing circuits during the administration of general anesthetics or in inhalation therapy apparatus.

**sodio-** \sō′dē·ō-\ [New L, from SODA] A combining form indicating replacement of hydrogen in a compound by sodium.

**sodium** \sō′dē·əm\ [New L, from SODA] Element number 11, having atomic weight 22.99. It is a soft, bright, very reactive metal that is lighter than water. Of the seven isotopes known, sodium 23 is the only stable one. It constitutes about 2.6% of the lithosphere, usually in the form of sodium chloride, though other minerals are known. The valence is 1. Sodium is essential in all living systems. It is the principal extracellular cation. About 0.03% of the atoms in the human body are sodium atoms. It plays a vital part in maintaining the liquid volume of blood and other fluid systems. Symbol: Na **s. channel** A pathway through cell membranes which permits passage of sodium ions. It is commonly envisaged as a protein-lined, hydrophilic pore functioning like a valve to open and close the channel. **exchangeable s.** The quantity of sodium in the body that is readily miscible with administered labeled sodium over a period of 24 hours. Normally, exchangeable sodium is approximately 42 mEq per kg body weight, or 70 percent of total body sodium. The 18 mEq of nonexchangeable sodium is located in the dense long bones. **radioactive s.** Any of the 11 radioactive isotopes of sodium, ranging in half-life from 20.1 milliseconds to 2.6 years. Also *radiosodium.*

**sodium 22** A radioactive isotope of sodium emitting positrons and high-energy photons. It has been used in biological and medical research for the study of ion transports, particularly of total body sodium metabolism. Physical half-life is 2.58 years. Symbol: $^{22}Na$

**sodium 24** A radioactive isotope of sodium, emitting electrons and high-energy photons. It was the first radionuclide used for the evaluation of extracellular water. However, since sodium enters the body cells, including bone and cartilage, it is not a reliable tracer for extracellular water and has been replaced by radiosulfate and radiobromide. Physical half-life is 15.4 hours. Symbol: $^{24}Na$

**sodium acetarsol** $C_8H_9AsNNaO_5{\cdot}5H_2O$. The pentahydrate of the sodium salt of acetarsol. It is a parenteral form of acetarsol for subcutaneous or intravenous administration.

**sodium acetate** $CH_3COONa{\cdot}3H_2O$. A colorless or white crystalline salt used as a source of sodium ions in hemodialysis. It is also used in association with other salts to correct acidosis and replace electrolyte loss. It has been given orally to alkalinize the urine and promote a mild diuresis.

**sodium acetazolamide** $C_4H_5N_4NaO_3S_2$. The sodium salt of acetazolamide, used in a sterile preparation suitable for parenteral administration. It is a carbonic anhydrase inhibitor and a diuretic agent, is used in the treatment of glaucoma, and has anticonvulsant activity in patients with epilepsy.

**sodium acid citrate** $C_6H_6NaO_7{\cdot}1{\cdot}5H_2O$. A white, odorless powder with a salty taste. It is used as an anticoagulant, usually in combination with dextrose, for preserving blood. The salt has been given orally to produce less acid urine and promote a mild diuresis.

**sodium acid phosphate** $NaH_2PO_4{\cdot}H_2O$. An odorless, colorless or white, crystalline powder. It is poorly absorbed from the gastrointestinal tract, and oral doses act as a saline cathartic. It is given rectally as an enema.

**sodium alginate** ALGIN.

**sodium *p*-aminohippurate** A derivative of hippuric acid that is given intravenously to assess the status of renal function, particularly renal plasma flow and tubular excretion capacity.

**sodium *p*-aminosalicylate** The sodium salt of aminosalicylic acid. It is used orally in the treatment of tuberculosis.

**sodium amobarbital** $C_{11}H_{17}N_2NaO_3$. The sodium salt of amobarbital, used as a hypnotic and sedative. Also *sodium isoamylethyl barbiturate.*

**sodium ampicillin** The monosodium salt of ampicillin. It can be given intramuscularly or intravenously for the same indications as ampicillin.

**sodium *n*-amylpenicillinate** AMYLPENICILLIN SODIUM.

**sodium antimonyltartrate** ANTIMONY SODIUM TARTRATE.

**sodium antimonyl-thioglycollate** $CO_2^-$—$CH_2$—S—$Sb^+$—S—$CH_2$—$COO^-Na^+$. A compound of antimony. Its main use is in therapy of granuloma inguinale.

**sodium ascorbate** $C_6H_7NaO_6$. The monosodium salt form of ascorbic acid. It is used in the parenteral administration of vitamin C.

**sodium aurothiomalate** $C_4H_3AuNa_2O_4S{\cdot}H_2O$. A soluble form of gold given by intramuscular injection in the treatment of rheumatoid arthritis and of lupus erythematosis in varieties other than the disseminated form.

**sodium aurothiosuccinate** AUROTHIOMALATE DISODIUM.

**sodium azide** $NaN_3$. A toxic salt, sometimes used to prevent bacterial growth in aqueous solutions. It is also used as a reagent in organic chemistry, since the azide ion is nucleophilic, and sodium azide is one of the few azides that is not dangerously explosive.

**sodium benzoate** $C_7H_5NaO_2$. The sodium salt of benzoic acid, used as an antifungal agent in the preservation of pharmaceuticals and food. It is also used as a test of liver function, i.e., for the liver's ability to conjugate it with glycine to form hippuric acid.

**sodium benzosulfimide** SACCHARIN.

**sodium bicarbonate** $NaHCO_3$. A white, crystalline powder used as an antacid in the stomach and to produce alkalinity of the urine. It is also used in baking, since it slowly releases carbon dioxide when heated, and thus lightens the dough. Also *baking soda, bicarbonate of soda.*

**sodium biphosphate** $NaH_2PO_4{\cdot}H_2O$. The monosodium monohydrate salt form of phosphoric acid, occurring as a colorless or white crystalline powder. It is given orally with sodium phosphate as an antihypercalcemic treatment, orally and rectally with sodium phosphate as a cathartic agent, and orally to acidify the urine.

**sodium bisulfite** $NaHSO_3$. An agent used an an antioxidant in many pharmaceutical preparations. It is a white or yellowish powder.

**sodium butabarbital** $C_{10}H_{15}N_2NaO_3$. 5-*sec*-Butyl-5-ethylbarbiturate. A barbiturate with sedative and hypnotic properties.

**sodium calcium edetate** EDETATE CALCIUM DISODIUM.

**sodium carbonate** $Na_2CO_3{\cdot}H_2O$. An alkalizing agent used in various pharmaceutical preparations. It has also been employed as a lotion or bath in the treatment of skin conditions. Also *washing soda.* **monohydrated s.** $Na_2CO_3{\cdot}H_2O$. An odorless, colorless crystalline powder that becomes anhydrous when heated to 100°C. It is used as a pharmaceutical aid, as an alkalizing agent.

**sodium caseinate** Buffered casein hydrolysate used in parenteral feeding and some formula diets.

**sodium chloride** NaCl, the usual form of dietary sodium. Excess intake of sodium chloride can result in poisoning in domestic animals, especially in swine, poultry, and cattle. Salt poisoning is closely related to water intake. Also *common salt.*

**sodium citrate** $C_6H_5Na_3O_7$. The trisodium salt of citric acid, occurring as a colorless, crystalline powder and used as an anticoagulant in the storage of blood or in blood fractionation. It is also given orally as a urinary alkalizer.

**sodium colistimethate** COLISTIN SULFOMETHATE SODIUM.

**sodium cyclamate** The sodium salt of cyclamic acid, formerly used as a non-nutritive sweetener. It was banned in the United States in 1969, but is still permitted in several other countries.

**sodium dextrothyroxine** $C_{15}H_{10}I_4NNaO_4{\cdot}XH_2O$. The sodium salt of the dextrorotatory isomeric form of thyroxine. It is employed as an anticholesterolemic agent in the treatment of euthyroid patients possessing high blood cholesterol levels. It is given orally.

**sodium diphenylhydantoin** PHENYTOIN SODIUM.

**sodium dithionate** SODIUM THIOSULFATE.

**sodium dodecyl sulfate** The sodium salt of dodecyl sulfate, and the form in which it is normally used.

**sodium fusidate** $C_{31}H_{47}NaO_6$. The sodium salt of fusidic acid, used by itself or in association with other antibiotics, such as penicillin, as an anti-infective agent. It is specific for certain strains of staphylococci that are not responsive to other antibiotics.

**sodium hydroxide** NaOH. A caustic, alkaline solid, used as an alkalinizing agent in various pharmaceutical preparations. Also *caustic soda, sodium hydrate.*

**sodium hypochlorite** ClNaO. The sodium salt of hypochlorous acid. It is used as a bleach and a disinfectant in an aqueous solution.

**sodium hyposulfite** SODIUM THIOSULFATE.

**sodium iodide** NaI. A binary halide compound occurring as a white cyrstalline powder and used as a source of iodine. **thallium-activated s.** Crystalline sodium iodide to which a fractional percentage of thallium has been added to produce a scintillation detector. Pure sodium iodide does not scintillate. The high density, 3.67 g $cm^{-3}$, and the high proton number of iodine, 53, combine to make this material effective in gamma spectrometry. Symbol: NaI(Tl)

**sodium iothalamate** A compound that can be used for glomerular filtration studies by scintillation imaging when labeled with an appropriate radionuclide.

**sodium ipodate** IPODATE SODIUM.

**sodium isoamylethyl barbiturate** SODIUM AMOBARBITAL.

**sodium levothyroxine** The sodium salt of L-3,3′,5,5′-tetraiodothyronine, the biologically more active isomer of thyroxine. It is used in thyroid replacement therapy and in the suppression of thyroid nodules.

**sodium liothyronine** The sodium salt of L-3,5,3′-triiodothyronine. The main, if limited, clinical use is in the emergency treatment of myxedema coma. It is suitable for oral or parenteral administration.

**sodium metabisulfite** $Na_2O_5S_2$. A white, crystalline powder with an odor of sulfur dioxide. It is used in an aqueous solution as an antioxidant. Also *sodium pyrosulfite.*

**sodium methicillin** METHICILLIN SODIUM.

**sodium nitrite** $NaNO_2$. A compound used as an antidote for cyanide poisoning, for the relief of pain in angina pectoris, and in the treatment of Raynaud's disease and other conditions, such as lead colic and spastic colitis.

**sodium nitroprusside** $Na_2[Fe(CN)_5NO]{\cdot}2H_2O$. An antihypertensive agent used where continuous monitoring of the blood pressure is possible. It is used to lower the blood pressure in a hypertensive crisis by intravenous infusion of the agent. Also *sodium nitroferricyanide.*

**sodium oxacillin** $C_{19}H_{18}N_3NaO_5S{\cdot}H_2O$. 5-Methyl-3-phenyl-4-isoxazolylpenicillin sodium salt monohydrate. A semisynthetic penicillin, resistant to the actions of penicillinase. It is used in the treatment of infections due to staphylococci with penicillinase and is also used to treat infections resistant to benzylpenicillin. It is given orally, intramuscularly, or intravenously.

**sodium penicillin G** PENICILLIN G SODIUM.

**sodium pentobarbital** PENTOBARBITAL SODIUM.

**sodium pertechnetate** See under PERTECHNETATE.

**sodium phenobarbital** PHENOBARBITAL SODIUM.

**sodium phenylethylbarbiturate** PHENOBARBITAL SODIUM.

**sodium phenytoin** $C_{15}H_{11}N_2NaO_2$. 5,5-Diphenyl-2,4-imidazolidinedione. An anticonvulsant and antileptic drug commonly used to treat convulsant disorders.

**sodium phosphate** $Na_2HPO_4{\cdot}7H_2O$. The heptahydrate disodium salt form of phosphoric acid. It is administered orally as a cathartic, alone or in combination with sodium biphosphate. **dibasic s.** $Na_2HPO_4$. Disodium hydrogen phosphate. A hygroscopic powder which takes up 2 to 7 mols of water in a humid atmosphere. It has some medical use as a cathartic. **dried s.** $Na_2HPO_4{\cdot}XH_2O$. A salt, nearly anhydrous after drying at 105°C for four hours, that is administered as an oral cathartic. Also *exsiccated sodium phosphate.* **effervescent s.** A mixture of citric acid, dried sodium phosphate, and sodium bicarbonate, dried and granulated, which is given as an oral cathartic. **exsiccated s.** DRIED SODIUM PHOSPHATE. **monobasic s.** $H_2NaPO_4$. Sodium dihydrogen phosphate. A white, odorless crystalline powder, usually a monohydrate salt. It has been given to acidify the urine.

**sodium polyethylene sulfonate** LYAPOLATE SODIUM.

**sodium polystyrene sulfonate** A cation exchange resin, each gram of which exchanges 110–135 mg of potassium. It is used in the treatment of hyperkalemia.

**sodium pyrosulfite** SODIUM METABISULFITE.

**sodium salicylate** The monosodium salt of salicylic acid. It is used as an antipyretic and antirheumatic drug.

**sodium secobarbital** $C_{12}H_{17}N_2NaO_3$. Sodium 5-allyl-5-(1-methylbutyl)barbiturate. A short to intermediate-acting barbiturate with hypnotic and sedative properties. Abuse may lead to addiction. Also *secobarbital sodium.*

**sodium sulfacetamide** $C_8H_9N_2O_3S{\cdot}H_2O$. The very soluble sodium salt of sulfacetamide (*N′*-acetylsulfanilamide), which easily penetrates the skin, cornea, and conjunctiva, and, via the blood, enters the cerebrospinal fluid.

**sodium sulfadiazine** $C_{10}H_9N_4NaO_2S$. 4-Amino-*N*-2-pyrimidinyl-benzenesulfonamide monosodium salt. A well-absorbed, long acting, and effective agent against many Gram-positive and Gram-negative bacteria. It is useful in prophylaxis of streptococcal infections in patients with rheumatic fever and sensitivity to penicillin.

**sodium sulfoxone** $C_{14}H_{14}N_2Na_2O_6S_3$. 4,4′-Diaminodiphenylsulfone disodiumformaldehyde sulfoxylate. A sulfone derivative with antibacterial activity. It is used in the treatment of leprosy, and is hydrolyzed in the gastrointestinal tract to dapsone.

**sodium [$^{99m}$Tc]pertechnetate** See under PERTECHNETATE.

**sodium thiamylal** A sulfur derivative of the barbiturate series. It is used in intravenous induction of general anesthesia and produces rapid onset and recovery. Also *thiamylal sodium.*

**sodium thiopental** A sulfur derivative of the barbiturate series, used in intravenous induction of general anesthesia. The anesthetic state is characterized by rapid onset and recovery. Also *thiopentone.*

**sodium thiosulfate** $Na_2O_3S_2$. An antidote, used intravenously for cyanide poisoning, in solution as a preventive for ringworm infections in public swimming pools and showers, and topically for fungal diseases of the skin. It is also used in measuring extracellular fluids of the body and as a fixer in photographic processes. Also *sodium dithionate, sodium hyposulfite.*

**sodium tolbutamide** The sodium salt of tolbutamide. It is suitable for intravenous use for diagnostic purposes.

**sodium warfarin** The sodium salt of warfarin. It has the anticoagulant actions of the parent drug and it may be given orally, intravenously, or intramuscularly.

**sodokosis** \sō'dōkō'sis\ SODOKU.

**sodoku** \sō'dōkoo\ [Japanese, from *so* rat + *doku* poison] A form of rat-bite fever caused by *Spirillum minor.* See under RAT-BITE FEVER. Also *spirillary fever, spirillum fever, spirillar fever, sodokosis, sokosho.*

**sodomy** \säd'əmē\ [after *Sodom,* also Sodoma, the principal City of the Plain in ancient Palestine, which was destroyed by fire and brimstone from heaven because of its widespread carnal wickedness; + -Y] **1** Anal intercourse between two males. **2** Anal intercourse with a partner of either sex. **3** Sexual intercourse of any variety between two males. **4** Any sexual activity labeled abnormal or deviant by the particular culture. An imprecise and outmoded term.

**Soemmering** [Samuel Thomas von *Soemmering,* German anatomist, 1755–1830] **1** See under CATARACT, LIGAMENT. **2** Soemmering's nerve. See under NERVUS PUDENDUS. **3** Soemmering spot. See under MACULA RETINAE. **4** Soemmering's muscle. See under MUSCULUS LEVATOR GLANDULAE THYROIDEAE.

**Soemmering** [Wilhelm *Soemmering,* German physician, 1793–1885] See under RING.

**softening** The process of becoming soft or softer, especially as part of a pathological process. **anemic s.** A pale area of cerebral infarction. Also *white softening.* **green s.** Softening in which the degenerating area assumes a green color because of the presence of pus. **s. of the heart** CARDIOMALACIA. **inflammatory s.** Softening due to the edema and cellular infiltrate that accompanies inflammation. **mucoid s.** MYXOMATOUS DEGENERATION. **red s.** HEMORRHAGIC INFARCT. **red s. of the brain** Encephalomalacia with red patches due to hemorrhage or congestion. **white s.** ANEMIC SOFTENING.

**software** **1** Computer programs, routines, programming languages, and related documentation, as distinguished from hardware. **2** Instructions or text associated with the use of hardware such as audiovisual equipment.

**soja bean** \sō'yə\ SOYBEAN.

**sokosho** \sōkō'shō\ [Japanese, from *so* rat + *kō* to bite + *shō* disease] SODOKU.

**sol** \säl\ [English *sol(ution)*] A colloidal solution, particularly one of fibrous molecules, capable of setting to form a gel.

**solanidine** An alkaloid whose molecule contains the steroid skeleton, with a nitrogen-containing ring system fused to ring D at C-16 and C-17. It occurs as its glycoside solanine.

**solanine** A toxic glycoside found in plants of the order Solanaceae, such as tomato and potato plants. It is solanidine glycosylated by a branched trisaccharide. Also *solanin.*

**solanism** \sō'lənizm\ [L *solan(um)* nightshade + -ISM] Poisoning from ingestion of foods from solanaceous plants that contain excessive amounts of solanine.

**solanoid** \sō'lənoid\ Having the consistency of a raw potato.

**solapsone** $C_{30}H_{28}N_2Na_4O_{14}S_5$. 1,1′-[Sulfonylbis (*p*-phenyleneimino)]bis[3-phenyl-1,3-propanedisulfonic acid] tetrasodium salt. It is a derivative of dapsone with the same actions and uses as the latter. It is less toxic than dapsone and used to treat leprosy, orally or by intramuscular injection. Also *solasulfone.*

**solar** \sō'lər\ [L *solaris* (from *sol* the sun) pertaining to the sun] Denoting the coeliac plexus of sympathetic ganglia and radiating nerve fibers. • The term derives from the resemblance of the plexus and associated radiating nerve fibers to a stylized representation of the sun.

**solasodine** \sō'ləsō'din\ $C_{27}H_{43}O_2N$. A steroidal alkaloid obtained primarily from species of the genus *Solanum.* It has been used as a starting substance for hormone synthesis.

**solasulfone** SOLAPSONE.

**solder** \säd'ər\ An alloy that can be easily melted for fusing metal parts.

**sole** [L *solea* (akin to *solum* the bottom or lowest part, ground, the sole of a foot or shoe) a leather sole strapped on the foot, sandal] PLANTA PEDIS.

**soleal** \sō'lē·əl\ Pertaining to the soleus muscle.

**soleno-** \sō'lənō-\ [Gk *sōlēn* channel, gutter, pipe] A combining form meaning channel, groove.

**Solenoglypha** \sō'lənäg'lifə\ VIPERIDAE.

**solenoglyphic** \sō'lənōglif'ik\ [SOLENO- + Gk *glyph(ein)* to carve + -IC] Having elongated, hollow poison fangs at the front of the upper jaw: used of snakes. The maxillary is short, deep, and articulated so that the fangs project forward when the mouth is open, folding back along the upper jaw when the mouth is closed. Upon striking, muscular contraction forces venom through the fangs. This efficient mechanism for delivering venom makes solenoglyphic snakes potentially more dangerous than other venomous snakes. Compare PROTEROGLYPHIC, OPISTHOGLYPHIC.

**solenonychia** \sō'lənōnik'ē·ə\ [*solen(o)-* + ONYCH- + -IA] MEDIAN CANALIFORM DYSTROPHY OF THE NAIL.

**solenopsin A** \sō'lənäp'sin\ *Trans*-2-Methyl-6-*n*-undecylpiperidine. The active principle in the venom of fire ants, genus *Solenopsis.*

***Solenopsis*** \sō'lənäp'sis\ A genus of ants known as fire ants, which can inflict painful burning stings that cause local and occasionally systemic reactions. *S. geminata* is a species native to the United States. *S. saevissima* has been introduced in the southern United States from South America and over the past two or three decades has extended its range in spite of extensive poisoning campaigns against it.

**Solente** [G. *Solente,* French physician, flourished 20th century] Touraine-Solente-Golé syndrome. See under PACHYDERMOPERIOSTOSIS.

**solid** **1** Having a definite shape and tending to retain its shape against stress. **2** A solid substance; a substance that is neither liquid nor gas.

**solipsism** \säl'ipsizm\ [L *sol(us)* alone + *ips(e)* self + -ISM] The theory that since only knowledge of the self is possible, reality for each individual consists of himself only.

**solubility** \säl'yəbil'itē\ The concentration that a substance can achieve in solution in a specified solvent when the solution is saturated.

**soluble** \säl'yəbəl\ [L *solubilis* soluble, from L *solvere* (for *se-luere,* from *se-,* prefix denoting apart + *luere* to lave, free, akin to Gk *lyein* to loosen) to loosen, untie, dissolve] Able to dissolve in a specified liquid.

**solum** \sō'ləm\ [L, the lowest part of a thing, ground, soil, sole of the foot.] The bottom; the lowest part.

**solute** \säl'yoot, sō'loot\ [L *solut(us),* past part. of *solvere* to loosen, untie, dissolve] A dissolved substance.

# solution

**solution** [L *solutio* (from *solutus,* past part. of *solvere* to loosen, untie, akin to *luere* to wash, purge, to Gk *lyein* to loosen, and to English *loosen*), a loosening] A liquid phase containing at least two substances. **alkaline sodium hypochlorite s.** A dilute (0.4 to 0.5%) solution of the oxidizing agent sodium hypochlorite buffered with sodium bicarbonate, sometimes used to irrigate and disinfect wounds. Also *Dakin solution*. **Alsever s.** A solution of citrate, dextrose, and sodium chloride that is used to suspend and preserve reagent red blood cells. **aluminum acetate s.** A solution containing a mixture of aluminum subacetate, glacial acetic acid, and water. The solution has 4.8–5.8 g of aluminum acetate in each 100 ml. It is diluted to a strength of from 1:10 to 1:30 and used topically as an astringent, antiseptic, and antipruritic agent. Also *Burow's solution*. **aluminum subacetate s.** A mixture of aluminum sulfate, acetic acid, precipitated calcium carbonate and water. The solution contains 2.3–2.6 g of aluminum oxide and 5.43–6.13 g of acetic acid in each 100 ml. It is used topically as an astringent and antiseptic, and is applied as a wet dressing for various skin diseases. **amaranth s.** A clear, intense red solution containing 0.9–1.1 g of amaranth in each 100 ml. Purified water is used as the solvent. The solution is used as a coloring agent. Also *liquor amaranthi*. **aminoacetic acid sterile s.** A sterile, aqueous solution containing 95–105% of the labeled amount of aminoacetic acid, i.e., glycine. It is used as a nutrient. **ammonium acetate s.** A clear, colorless solution containing ammonium acetate. It is used as a diaphoretic and diuretic agent. Also *spirit of Mindererus*. **antazoline phosphate ophthalmic s.** A sterile, aqueous solution containing 90–100% of the labeled amount of antazoline phosphate. It is instilled in the eye as an antihistaminic agent. **anticoagulant acid citrate dextrose s.** *Outmoded* ANTICOAGULANT CITRATE DEXTROSE SOLUTION. **anticoagulant citrate dextrose s.** A sterile solution containing 95–105% of the labeled amounts of citric acid, sodium citrate, and dextrose. The solution is used as an anticoagulant for storage of whole blood for transfusions. Also *anticoagulant acid citrate dextrose solution* (outmoded). **anticoagulant citrate phosphate dextrose s.** A sterile solution containing anhydrous citric acid, dihydrous sodium citrate, monohydrous sodium biphosphate, and monohydrous dextrose. It is used as an anticoagulant solution for the storage of whole blood. **anticoagulant heparin s.** A sterile solution containing heparin sodium 75 000 units in sufficient sodium chloride in water for injection to yield 1000 ml. It is used as an anticoagulant medication. **antipyrine and benzocaine s.** A solution containing 90–110% of the labeled amounts of antipyrine and benzocaine in glycerin. It is used in the ear as a local anesthetic. **antiseptic s.** A clear, colorless solution containing boric acid, thymol, chlorothymol, menthol, eucalytol, methyl salicylate, thyme oil, alcohol, and purified water. It is used as an antibacterial medication both externally and orally. **aqueous s.** A class of pharmaceutical preparations in which solid inorganic salts or drug hydrates are dissolved in water. These may be sterile and used for injection, or used as eye washes, gargles or for other special purposes. **atropine sulfate ophthalmic s.** A sterile aqueous solution containing 93–107% of the labeled amount of atropine sulfate. It is instilled in the eye for its anticholinergic properties. **auxiliary s.** In psychiatry, a temporary or partial solution to intrapsychic conflict such as compartmentalization or intellectualization. **benzalkonium chloride s.** A clear, colorless aqueous solution that has an aromatic odor and a slightly bitter taste. The solution contains 95–105% the labeled amounts of benzalkonium chloride, if the concentration is 1% or more, and 93–107% of the labeled amount if the concentration is less than 1%. It is used topically as an antiseptic medication. **benzethonium chloride s.** A clear, colorless, odorless solution with a slightly bitter taste. The liquid contains 95–105% of the labeled amount of benzethonium chloride. It is used topically as an antiseptic medication. **borax-carmine s.** A solution of carmine in aluminium hydroxide with aluminium chloride, which stains epithelial mucin. Also *alum-carmine stain*. **boric acid s.** A clear, colorless, odorless solution containing at least 4.25 g of boric acid in each 100 ml. It is used as an external antibacterial medication. **Bouin s.** BOUIN'S FLUID. **buffer s.** See under BUFFER. **Burnett s.** A concentrated aqueous solution of zinc chloride. **Burow s.** ALUMINUM ACETATE SOLUTION. **calcium cyclamate and calcium saccharin s.** A clear, colorless solution containing 90–110% of the labeled amounts of calcium cyclamate and calcium saccharin. It is used in some countries as a non-nutritive sweetening agent. **carbachol ophthalmic s.** A sterile, isotonic, aqueous solution containing 95–105% of the labeled amount of carbachol. It is instilled in the eye for its cholinergic properties. **cetylpyridinium chloride s.** A clear solution containing 95–105% of the labeled amount of cetylpyridinium chloride. It is used topically as an antiseptic agent. **citrated Locke s.** An aqueous solution of sodium, potassium, and calcium chlorides, together with sodium citrate, that is adjusted to pH 7.4. **coal tar s.** A solution containing 200 g of coal tar, 50 g of polysorbate 80, and sufficient alcohol to give a total volume of 1000 ml. It is diluted for use as a topical antieczema medication. **Cohn s.** A synthetic medium for growing yeasts and fungi, used principally before commercial media became available. **colloidal s.** The dispersion of finely divided particles or large molecules in a solvent such that there is not a homogeneous single phase, but the dispersed materials remain suspended indefinitely. **compound amaranth s.** A solution containing 90 ml of amaranth solution, 100 g of caramel, 250 ml of alcohol, and sufficient purified water to give a total of 1000 ml. It is used as a coloring agent. **compound cresol s.** SAPONATED CRESOL SOLUTION. **compound iodine s.** STRONG IODINE SOLUTION. **comprehensive s.** The avoidance of psychologic conflict by holding the unrealistic belief that one is the idealized self. **crystal violet s.** GENTIAN VIOLET SOLUTION. **cyanocobalamin Co 60 s.** A solution of cyanocobalamin, vitamin $B_{12}$, in which stable cobalt has been at least partly replaced by cobalt 60. It is used in tests for intestinal malabsorption, particularly in cases of pernicious anemia. **cyclopentamine hydrochloride s.** A sterile solution containing 95–105% of the labeled amount of cyclopentamine hydrochloride in an appropriate isotonic vehicle. It is administered intramuscularly, intravenously, or intranasally for its vasoconstricting properties. **cyclopentolate hydrochloride ophthalmic s.** A sterile solution which contains 95–105% of the labeled amount of cyclopentolate hydrochloride in a buffered, isotonic, aqueous medium. It is instilled in the eye for its anticholinergic properties. **Czapek-Dox s.** CZAPEK-DOX AGAR. **Dakin s.** ALKALINE SODIUM HYPOCHLORITE SOLUTION. **Darrow s.** A solution of electrolytes used in fluid therapy and for fluid replacement. It is enriched with potassium. **demecarium bromide ophthalmic s.** A sterile aqueous solution containing 92–108% of the labeled amount of demecarium bromide. It is instilled in the eye for its cholinergic properties. **dexamethasone sodium phosphate ophthalmic s.** A sterile aqueous solution containing 90–115% of the labeled amount of dexamethasone phosphate. It is instilled in the eye as a glucocorticoid anti-inflammatory medication. **diethyltoluamide s.** A solution containing 92–108% of the labeled amount of diethyltoluamide in alcohol or isopropyl alcohol. It is applied to the skin and clothing to repel insects. **diluted ammonia s.** A transparent, colorless, alkaline solution containing 9–10 g of ammonia in each 100 ml. It is used as a pharmaceutic necessity. Also *ammonia water, diluted ammonium hydroxide solution, liquor ammoniae dilutus.* **diluted ammonium hydroxide s.** DILUTED AMMONIA SOLUTION. **diluted lead subacetate s.** An aqueous solution containing lead acetate and lead monoxide. It is used as an astringent and as a local sedative. Also *liquor plumbi subacetatis dilutus.* **diluted sodium hypochlorite s.** MODIFIED DAKIN SOLUTION. **dioctyl calcium sulfosuccinate s.** A clear solution containing 95–105% of the labeled amount of dioctyl calcium sulfosuccinate. It is used as a wetting agent and as a nonlaxative stool softener. **dioctyl sodium sulfosuccinate s.** A solution containing 95–105% of the labeled amount of dioctyl sodium sulfosuccinate. It is used as a stool softener. **diphenoxylate hydrochloride and atropine sulfate s.** A solution containing 93–107% of the labeled amount of diphenoxylate hydrochloride. It also contains 80–120% of the labeled amount of atropine sulfate. It is used for its antidiarrheal action. **disclosing s.** A solution of a dye, commonly erythrosin, that stains dental plaque so that it becomes more observable. **dyclonine hydrochloride s.** A sterile aqueous solution containing 92–108% of the labeled amount of dyclonine hydrochloride. It is used topically for its anesthetic properties. ***dl*-ephedrine hydrochloride s.** RACEPHEDRINE HYDROCHLORIDE SOLUTION. **ephedrine sulfate s.** A clear, colorless solution containing ephedrine sulfate. The solution may range from neutral to acidic, and it is used for its vasoconstricting properties. **epinephrine s.** A nearly colorless solution containing 90–115 mg of epinephrine in each 100 ml. Purified water is used as the solvent, with hydrochloric acid acting as a solubilizing agent. The solution is used for its vasoconstricting properties. **epinephrine bitartrate ophthalmic s.** A solution containing epinephrine bitartrate and boric acid in purified water. It is used for its adrenergic properties to dilate the pupil and in the treatment of some types of glaucoma. **Fehling s.** A solution of copper(II) sulfate in alkaline tartrate. The tartrate ions chelate the copper ions and prevent their precipitation as copper(II) hydroxide. It is used to test for reducing agents, especially reducing sugars, which convert the copper(II) into copper(I) when the solution is heated. This conversion is detected by the appearance of a red precipitate of copper(I) oxide. **fixative s.** See under FIXATIVE. **Flemming s.** FLEMMING'S FIXING FLUID. **formaldehyde s.** An aqueous solution containing at least 37% formaldehyde, used as a disinfectant. Also *formalin, formal, liquor formaldehydi.* **Fowler s.** POTASSIUM ARSENITE SOLUTION. **gentian violet s.** A purple solution, in a mixture of alcohol and water, containing 0.95–1.05 g of gentian violet in each 100 ml. It is used topically as an antiseptic agent. Also *crystal violet solution, methylrosaniline chloride solution.* **haloperidol s.** A solution containing 90–110% of the labeled amount of haloperidol. It is used as a major tranquilizer. **Hamdi s.** A preservative solution that contains sodium sulfate, salt, glycerine, and water and that is used for museum specimens when color preservation is important. **Hanks s.** A physiologic or balanced salt solution that is used for tissue culture. **hardening s.** A solution used to stabilize a hydrocolloid impression. **Hartman s.** An intravenous solution composed of electrolytes mimicking extracellular fluid. **Hayem s.** An aqueous solution of mercury bichloride, sodium chloride, and sodium sulfate used as a diluent in enumerating blood cells. It is of historical interest because of previous widespread use. **hexylcaine hydrochloride s.** A clear, colorless, aqueous solution containing 93–107% of the labeled amount of hexylcaine hydrochloride. It is utilized topically for its anesthetic properties. **homatropine hydrobromide ophthalmic s.** A sterile, buffered, aqueous solution containing 95–105% of the labeled amount of homatropine hydrobromide. The solution is instilled in the eye for its anticholinergic properties. **hydrogen dioxide s.** HYDROGEN PEROXIDE SOLUTION. **hydrogen peroxide s.** A solution containing 2.5–3.5 g of hydrogen peroxide in each 100 ml of liquid. It is applied to the skin and mucous membranes for its anti-infective actions. Also *liquor hydrogenii peroxidi, hydrogen dioxide solution.* **hydroxyamphetamine hydrobromide ophthalmic s.** A sterile, buffered, aqueous solution containing 0.95–1.05% of hydroxyamphetamine hydrobromide. It is instilled in the eye for its adrenergic properties. **hypertonic s.** A solution having a higher osmotic pressure than the solution with which it is compared. **hypotonic s.** A solution having a lower osmotic pressure than the solution with which it is compared, ordinarily physiologic saline solution or normal plasma. **idoxuridine ophthalmic s.** A sterile, aqueous solution containing 0.09–0.11% of idoxuridine. It is instilled in the eye for its antiviral properties. **iodine s.** A reddish-brown solution containing 1.8–2.2 g of iodine and 2.1–2.6 g of sodium iodide in each 100 ml. It is used locally as an anti-infective medication. **isobaric s.** ISOBARIC SPINAL ANESTHESIA. **isofurophate ophthalmic s.** A sterile solution containing 0.09–0.11% of diisopropyl phosphorofluoridate in an appropriate vegetable oil. It is used as eye drops in the treatment of some types of glaucoma. **isotonic s.** An isosmotic solution in which cells can be immersed without changing their size and shape. **Krebs-Ringer s.** A solution in which mammalian cells and tissues may be bathed for study. The original (Ringer's) solution contained salts such as NaCl, KCl, $CaCl_2$, and $NaHCO_2$ to make a solution isotonic with extracellular fluid and close to it in ionic composition. Its composition was subsequently modified by the addition of magnesium sulfate and by buffering with phosphate. **Labarraque s.** A solution composed of equal parts of sodium hypochlorite solution and water. **liver s.** A preparation of mammalian liver containing cyanocobalamin. Also *liquid liver extract.* **Locke s.** An aqueous solution of sodium, potassium, and calcium chlorides combined with sodium bicarbonate and dextrose. **Locke-Ringer s.** A physiologic solution containing 9 g sodium chloride, 0.24 g of calcium chloride, 0.42 g of potassium chloride, 0.20 g of magnesium chloride, 0.5 g of sodium bicarbonate, 0.5 g of glucose, and sufficient water to make the final volume to 1000 ml. **Lugol s.** STRONG IODINE SOLUTION. **magnesium citrate s.** A clear, colorless to slightly yellow, effervescent solution containing magnesium carbonate 15 g, anhydrous citric acid 27.4 g, syrup 60 ml, talc 5 g, lemon oil 100 μl, potassium bicarbonate 2.5 g, and sufficient purified water to yield a total of 1000 ml. Each 100 ml contains 1.55–1.9 g of magnesium oxide. It is used as a cathartic medication. **major s.** A neurotic solution to psychologic conflict consisting of either repression and denial of traits that do not conform with the idealized self or withdrawal into resignation. **Mayer s.** MAYER'S HEMALUM. **methylrosaniline chloride s.** GENTIAN VIOLET SOLUTION. **modified Dakin s.** Sodium hypochlorite solution diluted to a strength of 0.45–0.5%. Also *diluted sodium hypochlorite solution, surgical solution of chlorinated soda.* **naphazoline hydrochloride s.** A buffered, aqueous solution containing 45–55 mg of naphazoline hydrochloride in each 100 ml. It is used for its adrenergic vasoconstricting properties. **neomycin sulfate oral s.** A solution containing an amount of neomycin sulfate equivalent to 78.75–109.375 mg of neomycin base in each 5 ml. It is used as an antibiotic medication. **Nessler s.** NESSLER'S REAGENT. **nitrofurazone s.** A clear, light yellow solution containing 190–210 mg of nitrofurazone in each 100 g. The viscous liquid is used locally as an anti-infective agent. **normobaric s.** ISOBARIC SPINAL ANESTHESIA. **Orth s.** A compound fixative containing potassium dichromate and formaldehyde. It has been recommended for the presentation of mitotic figures, bone, and colloid. Also *formol-Müller fluid, Orth stain.* **oxymetazoline hydrochloride s.** An aqueous solution containing 95–115% of the labeled amount of oxymetazoline hydrochloride. The solution is adjusted to an appropriate pH and tonicity and instilled intranasally as a vasoconstrictor. **paramethadione s.** A water-alcohol solution containing 282–318 mg of paramethadione in each ml. It is used as an anticonvulsant medication. **parathyroid s.** PARATHYROID INJECTION. **phenylephrine hydrochloride s.** A clear, colorless to slightly yellow solution containing 95–105% of the labeled amount of phenylephrine hydrochloride. It is used because of its adrenergic properties. **phenylephrine hydrochloride ophthalmic s.** A buffered, sterile, aqueous solution containing 90–115% of the labeled amount of phenylephrine hydrochloride. It is instilled in the eye for its adrenergic properties. **pilocarpine hydrochloride ophthalmic s.** A sterile, buffered, aqueous solution containing 90–110% of the labeled amount of pilocarpine hydrochloride. It is instilled in the eye for its cholinergic properties. **pilocarpine nitrate ophthalmic s.** A sterile, buffered, aqueous solution containing 90–110% of the labeled amount of pilocarpine nitrate. It is instilled in the eye for its cholinergic properties. **pituitary s.** POSTERIOR PITUITARY INJECTION. **posterior pituitary s.** POSTERIOR PITUITARY INJECTION. **potassium arsenite s.** A solution of arsenic trioxide, potassium bicarbonate, alcohol, and water, formerly used in treatment of some leukemias and dermatoses. Also *Fowler solution.* **potassium iodide s.** A clear, colorless, neutral to alkaline solution containing 97–103 g of potassium iodide in each 100 ml. It is used as an antigoitrogenic and expectorant agent. Potassium iodide has also been used in the treatment of certain mycotic infections, and it has some value in the treatment of the cutaneous-lymphatic form of sporotrichosis. **povidone-iodine s.** A transparent, reddish brown solution which consists of povidone iodine, water, and sometimes alcohol. It contains 85–120% of the labeled amount of iodine. The solution is used topically in the form of cleaning solutions, sprays, ointments, foams, and gels as an anti-infective agent. **prednisolone sodium phosphate ophthalmic s.** A sterile, buffered, aqueous solution of prednisolone sodium phosphate. It contains 90–115% of the labeled amount of prednisolone phosphate. The solution is used in the eye as an anti-inflammatory steroidal agent. **proparacaine hydrochloride ophthalmic s.** A sterile, aqueous solution containing 95–110% of the labeled amount of proparacaine hydrochloride. It is instilled into the eye as an anesthetic agent. **racemic ephedrine hydrochloride s.** RACEPHEDRINE HYDROCHLORIDE SOLUTION. **racephedrine hydrochloride s.** A clear, colorless solution consisting of racephedrine hydrochloride, chlorobutanol, and Ringer solution. It contains 0.93–1.07 g of racephedrine in each 100 ml. The solution is used for its adrenergic properties. Also *dl-ephedrine hydrochloride solution, racemic ephedrine hydrochloride solution.* **Rees-Ecker s.** An anticoagulant fluid once popular for diluting whole blood in order to count platelets. It consists of sodium citrate, formalin, and brilliant cresyl blue. Also *Rees and Ecker diluting fluid, Ecker's fluid.* **Ringer s.** A clear, colorless solution containing sodium chloride 8.6 g, potassium chloride 300 mg, calcium chloride 330 mg, and sufficient recently boiled, purified water to yield a total of 1000 ml. It is used topically as a physiologic salt solution. Also *liquor chloridorum trium isotonicus, Ringer's mixture.* **saline s.** SALINE. **saponated cresol s.** A solution composed of cresol, vegetable oil, potassium hydroxide, alcohol, and water. It contains 46–52 ml of cresol in each 100 ml. The solution is used as a disinfectant. Also *compound cresol solution.* **sclerosing s.** An irritating solution injected into a vein or a cavity to cause inflammation and scarring. **Shohl s.** A solution containing 14 g citric acid and 9.8 g sodium citrate hydrate and distilled water to make 100 ml. It is used in patients with renal tubular acidosis to correct the electrolyte abnormality. **silver nitrate ophthalmic s.** A buffered aqueous solution containing 0.95–1.05% of the labeled amount of silver nitrate. It is applied in the conjunctival sac in newborn infants for the prophylaxis of *ophthalmia neonatorum.* Silver nitrate is particularly effective against gonococci, and is superior to penicillin for this purpose. **sodium chloride s.** A sterile aqueous solution containing 0.85–0.95%, sodium chloride. It is used as an isotonic vehicle. **sodium cyclamate and sodium saccharin s.** A clear, colorless solution containing 90–110% of the labeled amounts of sodium cyclamate and sodium saccharin. It is used in some countries as a non-nutritive sweetener. Cyclamates have been banned in many countries following the report of studies in rats that linked bladder tumors with the intake of cyclamate. **sodium fluorescein ophthalmic s.** A sterile solution containing 1.86–2.10 g of sodium fluoroscein in each 100 ml. The solution also contains appropriate buffering and antimicrobial agents. It is instilled into the eye as an indicator of corneal scratches and other types of surface damage. **sodium hypochlorite s.** A clear, pale, greenish yellow solution containing 4–6% sodium hypochlorite. It is used as a disinfectant, although it is not suitable for direct application to wounds. Sodium hypochlorite has also been used as a deodorant and as a bleaching agent. **sodium phosphate s.** A clear, colorless solution containing 71–79 g of sodium phosphate for each 100 ml. The solution has a salty taste and the consistency of thick syrup. It is used as a mild, saline cathartic. **sodium sulfacetamide ophthalmic s.** A sterile solution containing 28.5–31.5% sodium sulfacetamide in water. It is instilled in the eye as an antibacterial agent. **sorbitol s.** A clear, colorless solution containing 69–71 g of total solids, consisting mainly of sorbitol, and a small amount of mannitol and other isomeric polyhydric alcohols in each 100 g. It is a syrupy liquid with a sweet taste, used as a component in many pharmaceutical preparations, creams, and toothpastes, and as an osmotic diuretic. **strong ammonia s.** A strongly alkaline, colorless, transparent solution containing 27–30% of ammonia. It is used as a solvent and a source of ammonia. Also *liquor ammoniae fortis, stronger ammonium hydroxide solution.* **stronger ammonium hydroxide s.** STRONG AMMONIA SOLUTION. **strong iodine s.** A transparent, deep brown solution containing 4.5–5.5 g of iodine and 9.5–10.5 g of potassium iodide in each 100 ml. It is used as a therapeutic source of iodine. It is also used to fix a basic dye in the Gram stain. Also *compound iodine solution, Lugol solution, liquor iodi fortis.* **Suby's G s.** A solution containing citric acid, magnesium oxide, and sodium carbonate, used to dissolve phosphate stones in the urinary tract. **surgical s. of chlorinated soda** MODIFIED DAKIN SOLUTION. **tetrahydrozoline hydrochloride s.** An aqueous solution containing 90–110% of the labeled amount of tetrahydrozoline hydrochloride. It is adjusted to an appropriate tonicity and utilized as a vasoconstrictor in 0.05 or 0.1% solution as nasal drops or spray, and in 0.05% solution in the eye. **thimerosal s.** A clear solution containing thimerosal 1 g, alcohol 525 ml, acetone 100 ml, ethylenediamine 200 mg, monoethanolamine 1 g, sodium chloride 8 g, sodium borate 1.4 g, and sufficient purified water to yield a total of 1000 ml. The solution has a characteristic odor and is applied topically as an anti-infective agent. **thioridazine hydrochloride s.** A solution containing 2.7–3.3 g of thioridazine hydrochloride in each 100 ml. It is used as a major tranquilizer. **tolnaftate s.** A solution containing 90–115% of the labeled amount of tolnaftate. It is used topically as an antifungal medication. **tribromoethanol s.** A clear, colorless solution containing 95–105 g of tribromoethanol in each 100 ml. Amylene hydrate is used as the solvent. The solution has a camphorlike odor. It is administered rectally as a general anesthetic. It has been used in convulsive disorders and to manage excited psychiatric patients. Also *bromethol, tribromoethyl alcohol solution.* **tribromoethyl alcohol s.** TRIBROMOETHANOL SOLUTION. **trimethadione s.** A solution containing 94–106% of the labeled amount of trimethadione. It is used as an anticonvulsant medication. **triple antibiotic s.** A solution made of the antibiotics bacitracin, polymyxin, and neomycin. It is used to irrigate wounds to decrease the likelihood of infection. **tropicamide ophthalmic s.** A sterile, buffered, aqueous solution containing 95–105% of the labeled amount of tropicamide. It is instilled in the eye as an anticholinergic agent. **tuaminoheptane sulfate s.** A solution containing sodium hydroxide 227 mg, phenylmercuric nitrate 20 mg, monobasic potassium phosphate 6.8 g, sodium chloride 900 mg, tuaminoheptane sulfate 10 g, and sufficient purified water to yield a total of 1000 ml. It is used intranasally to relieve congestion. **Tyrode s.** An aqueous solution of sodium, potassium, calcium, and magnesium chloride combined with sodium barcarbonate and disodium hyrodgen phosphate. **Weigert s.** WEIGERT'S IRON HEMATOXYLIN. See under HEMATOXYLIN. **xylometazoline hydrochloride s.** A solution containing 90–110% of the labeled amount of xylometazoline hydrochloride in water. It is adjusted to an appropriate pH and tonicity. It is applied intranasally as a vasoconstrictor to relieve congestion. **Zenker s.** ZENKER'S FLUID. **zinc sulfate ophthalmic s.** A sterile, isotonic, aqueous solution containing 95–105% of the labeled amount of zinc sulfate. It is instilled in the eye to treat certain types of conjunctivitis.

**solv.** *solve* (L, dissolve), a direction used in prescription writing.

**solvate** \säl′vāt\ [*solv(ent)* + -ATE] To form a complex with solute molecules: said of a solvent molecule.

**solvation** \sälvā′shən\ [*solvat(e)* + -ION] The process by which a solute molecule may bind solvent molecules.

**solvency** \säl′vənsē\ The state or characteristic of being a solvent.

**solvent** \säl′vənt\ [L *solvens* (gen. *solventis,* pres. part. of *solvere* to loosen, untie; see SOLUTION) loosening, untying] A liquid in which another substance can dissolve. **lipid s.** Any solvent capable of dissolving lipids. Such solvents are usually nonpolar liquids, often immiscible with water, such as hydrocarbons. **polar s.** A solvent in which positive and negative charges are physically or functionally separated, such that there is a high dielectric constant, high chemical activity and a tendency to form coordinate covalent bonds.

**soma** \sō′mə\ [Gk *sōma* (gen. *sōmatos*) the body] **1** All the body tissues except the germ cells. **2** The axial part of the body, excluding the limbs. **3** The body as distinct from the mind or psyche. **4** The main body of a nerve cell, from which other structures may project.

**somal** \sō′məl\ Relating to the body or soma; somatic.

**somaplasm** \sō′məplazm\ SOMATOPLASM.

**somat-** \sōmat-\ SOMATO-.

**somatagnosia** \sō′mətagnō′zhə\ [SOMAT- + AGNOSIA] Lack of awareness of one's own body.

**somatesthesia** \sō′mətesthē′zhə\ BODY SENSE.

**somatesthetic** \sō′mətesthet′ik\ SOMESTHETIC.

**somatic** \sōmat′ik\ [Gk *sōmatikos* (from *sōma* a body) bodily, corporeal] **1** Relating to or involving the skeleton or skeletal muscle, as distinct from the viscera of the body. **2** Relating to or involving the body as distinct from the mind or psyche. **3** Relating to the nongenetic components of an organism, as distinct from the germ plasm or germ cells.

**somatico-** \sōmat′ikō-\ SOMATO-.

**somatization** \sō′mətīzā′shən\ CONVERSION.

**somato-** \sō′mətō-, sōmat′ō-\ [Gk *sōma,* gen. *sōmatos* body] A combining form meaning body or somatic. Also *somat-, somatico-.*

**somatoblast** \sōmat′əblast, sō′mətō-\ A plestomere which participates in the formation of the somatic cells, as opposed to those destined to be concerned in reproduction.

**somatochrome** \sōmat′əkrōm\ Any neuron whose perikaryal and proximal dendritic cytoplasm contains prominent and stainable Nissl substance.

**somatocyte** \sōmat′əsīt\ A cell derived from a somatoblast that helps to form the tissues of the body.

**somatodymia** \-dim′ē·ə\ [SOMATO- + *-dym(us)* + -IA] A condition displayed by equal conjoined twins in which the trunks are united but the heads and sometimes the lower extremities are duplicated.

**somatoform** \sōmat′əfôrm, sō′mətō-\ **1** Manifesting in symptoms of organic disease. **2** Mimicking a disease of one or more organs or body parts.

**somatogenesis** \-jen′əsis\ **1** The development of the body tissues from somatic cells. **2** The acquisition of bodily characteristics.

**somatogenic** \-jen′ik\ [SOMATO- + -GENIC] Having its origin in the body (soma); organic. Compare PSYCHOGENIC.

**somatology** \sō′mətäl′əjē\ The study of the body, including its anatomy and physiology.

**somatomammotropin** \-mam′ətrō′pin\ [SOMATO- + MAMMOTROPIN] HUMAN PLACENTAL LACTOGEN. **human chorionic s.** HUMAN PLACENTAL LACTOGEN.

**somatomedin** \-mē′din\ Any of a few peptides found in the blood, secreted by the liver, and possibly by other organs, in response to stimulation by somatotropin, and mediating some of its actions, especially on connective tissue. These peptides stimulate cell division and the biosynthesis of protein, DNA, and RNA. Also *sulfation factor* (outmoded).

**somatomegaly** \-meg′əlē\ [SOMATO- + -MEGALY] GIGANTISM.

**somatometry** \sō′mətäm′ətrē\ [SOMATO- + -METRY] The measurement of bodily size and proportions using defined landmarks on the living human body.

**somatopagus** \sō′mətäp′əgəs\ [SOMATO- + -PAGUS] Equal conjoined twins united to greater or lesser degree in the trunk regions.

**somatopathic** \-path′ik\ Having or characterized by an organic disease rather than a psychological one.

**somatopathy** \sō′mətäp′əthē\ [SOMATO- + -PATHY] A disease of the body, as distinguished from one of psychological nature.
**somatophrenia** \-frē′nē·ə\ [SOMATO- + -PHRENIA] HYPOCHONDRIASIS.
**somatoplasm** \sō′mətōplazm′\ **1** Protoplasm of the somatic cells, as opposed to that of the germ cells. Also *somaplasm.* **2** The substance of heredity that is present in somatic cells. It is now known to be DNA. An obsolete usage.
**somatopleure** \sō′mətōplʊr′\ [SOMATO- + Gk *pleur(a)* a rib, side] The external or parietal layer of the ventral portion of the mesoderm. Primitively backing onto the ectoderm, it will be separated from it secondarily by a ventral extension of the myotomes, while largely participating in the production of the deep mesenchyme. Its internal surface will maintain the characteristics of a serous membrane, in continuation at the root of the mesentery with the splanchopleure applied to the viscera. It thus forms the parietal pericardium, the parietal peritoneum, and the vaginalis testis. Also *somatic layer, parietal wall.*
**somatopsychic** \-sī′kik\ PSYCHOSOMATIC.
**somatoschisis** \sō′mətäs′kisis\ [SOMATO- + Gk *schisis* a cleaving, division] A developmental defect characterized by a fissure of the trunk, particularly on the ventral aspect.
**somatoscopy** \sō′mətäs′kəpē\ [SOMATO- + -SCOPY] Visual examination of the body.
**somatosensory** \-sen′sərē\ Pertaining to awareness of stimuli exciting sense organs of the skin and deep tissues of the body.
**somatostatin** \-stat′in\ A hypothalamic tetradecapeptide, the hypophysiotropic hormone that inhibits the release of anterior pituitary growth hormone and acts directly on the pancreas to inhibit insulin and glucagon release. The active and synthetic forms have identical biologic activity and have been shown experimentally to induce reduction in the serum concentration of growth hormone in patients with acromegaly. Also *growth hormone inhibiting hormone, growth hormone release inhibiting hormone, growth hormone inhibitory factor.*
**somatotherapy** \-ther′əpē\ [SOMATO- + THERAPY] **1** Treatment directed at physical disorders of the body, as opposed to treatment of psychological or emotional disorders. **2** The use of physical or chemical modalities in the treatment of emotional or psychiatric disorders.
**somatotopagnosia** \-täp′agnō′zhə\ [SOMATO- + *top(o)*- + AGNOSIA] Inability to recognize or identify the parts of the body and their interrelationship.
**somatotopic** \-täp′ik\ [SOMATO- + *top(o)*- + -IC] Denoting the organized topographical pattern of representation of the body in the sensory and motor areas of the central nervous system.
**somatotroph** \sō′mətōträf′\ The most numerous cell type of the anterior pituitary, specifically synthesizing and releasing growth hormone. Formerly known as a special type of acidophilic cell, it has a typical appearance including secretory granules. Tumors comprising these cells cause acromegaly and gigantism.
**somatotrophic** \-träf′ik\ SOMATOTROPIC.
**somatotrophin** \-träf′in\ GROWTH HORMONE.
**somatotropic** \-träp′ik\ [SOMATO- + -TROPIC[1]] **1** Tending to stimulate the body or cells or tissues of the body. **2** Of or relating to somatotropin (growth hormone). Also *somatotrophic.*
**somatotropin** \-trō′pin\ GROWTH HORMONE.
**somatotype** \sō′mətōtīp′\ Body type, especially the body conformation or habitus of an individual expressed proportionately in terms of ectomorphy, mesomorphy, and endomorphy.
**somatropin** \sō′mətrō′pin\ GROWTH HORMONE.
**Sombulex** A proprietary name for hexobarbital.
**-some** \-sōm\ [Gk *sōma* body] A combining form denoting (1) an intracellular or infracellular body or structure; (2) an organism or individual with a (specified) type of body.
**somesthesia** \sō′mesthē′zhə\ BODY SENSE.
**somesthetic** \sō′mesthet′ik\ Pertaining to sensory awareness of the body. Also *somatesthetic.*
**somite** \sō′mīt\ [*som(a)* + -ITE] One of the mesodermal segments arranged in pairs, left and right, alongside the developing notochord and spinal cord of the vertebrate embryo. Transverse clefts subdivide the thickening mesoderm

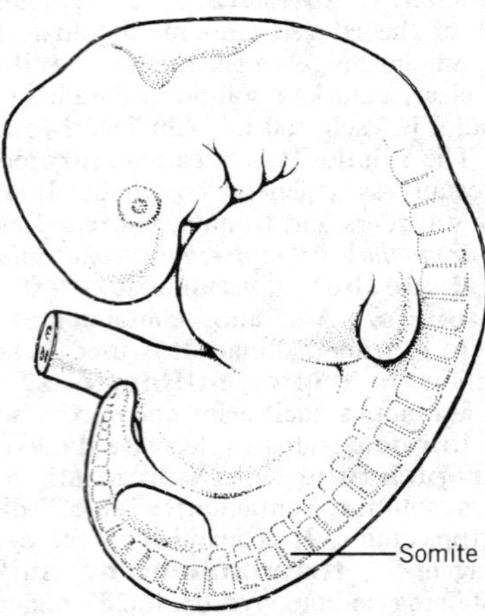


**Somites** (showing 29-day human embryo)

into blocks. Each somite provides a muscle mass supplied by a spinal nerve and also contributes to a vertebra. Each has a blood supply from the aorta and possesses a primitive kidney tubule. Somites are therefore each composed of a dermatome, myotome, and sclerotome, and they indicate the fundamental metameric construction of vertebrates. In the human embryo they are formed in groups from the central region in cranial-caudal directions. Thus, a five, ten, or fifteen somite embryo to about a forty-three somite stage, are described. Also *mesodermal segment, mesomere.* Adj. somitic. **cranial s.** One of the paired segments of paraxial mesoderm that develop at the head end of the embryo. In shark embryos three pairs of hollow somites, often called preoptic because of their position, have been demonstrated in the orbital region. They give rise to the orbital muscles. In human embryos only four pairs of occipital somites are discernible in the cranial region. The first pair soon disappears, but the other three are considered to contribute through their hypaxial divisions to the tongue musculature. **occipital s.'s** About four poorly-defined somites in the human embryonic occipital region, three of which contribute to the development of the tongue musculature.
**somitic** \sōmit′ik\ Relating to a somite.
**somnambulism** \sämnam′byəlizm\ [German *somnambulismus* (from L *somn(us)* sleep + *ambul(are)* to walk + *-ismus* -ISM) sleepwalking] A disorder consisting of partial arousal from sleep, usually during sleep stages three and four and not during REM sleep. During the arousal period the

subject may walk for relatively long distances, return to bed, fall back into sleep, and awake the next morning with no memory of having wandered. Also *délire oneirique, sleep-walking, somnambulance, oneiric delirium, noctambulation, somnambulistic trance, oneirodelirium.*

**somni-** \säm'nē-\ [L *somnus* (akin to Gk *hypnos* sleep) sleep] A combining form denoting sleep.

**somnial** \säm'nē·əl\ [Late L *somnialis* (from L *somnium* a dream, from *somnus* sleep) pertaining to dreaming] Relating to sleep or dreaming.

**somnifacient** \säm'nifā'shənt\ **1** Promoting sleep; soporific. Also *somniferous, somnific.* **2** A drug or agent that promotes sleep.

**somniferous** \sämnif'ərəs\ SOMNIFACIENT.

**somnific** \sämnif'ik\ SOMNIFACIENT.

**somnolence** \säm'nələns\ [Middle English *sompnolence,* from Middle French, ultimately from L *somnus* sleep] Unnatural sleepiness or drowsiness. Adj. somnolent.

**Somogyi** [Michael *Somogyi,* Austrian-born U.S. biochemist, 1883–1971] See under METHOD.

**sonar** \sō'när\ [*so(und) na(vigation) r(anging)*] A system that emits sound at regular intervals and by measuring the round trip acoustic delay for the return signal determines the distance of the reflecting object. It is used in medicine to detect movement of the mitral valve and to study the anatomy of the eye and brain. Bats use it for navigation.

**Sondermann** [R. *Sondermann,* German ophthalmologist, flourished 20th century] Sondermann's canals. See under CANAL.

**sone** \sōn\ [L *son(us)* a sound] A subjective unit of loudness designed to produce a scale proportional to loudness. A sound of frequency one kilohertz, 40 dB above a listener's threshold, gives a loudness of one sone; 1 sone = 40 phons. Symbol: S

**sonic** \sän'ik\ [L *son(us)* sound + -IC] Of, relating to, or affected by sound.

**sonicate** \sän'ikāt\ [SONIC + -ATE] To expose to sound or ultrasound. See also SONICATION.

**sonication** \sän'ikā'shən\ [SONIC + -ATION] The exposure of a material to high-frequency sonic or ultrasonic waves. Sonication of phospholipid suspensions, cells, or viruses is usually done for the purpose of dispersing, disrupting, or inactivating them. See also SONOCHEMISTRY.

**Sonne** [Carl *Sonne,* Danish bacteriologist, 1882–1948] See under DYSENTERY.

**sonochemistry** \sō'nəkem'istrē\ Chemical applications of sound or ultrasound, as to alter or to analyze chemical reactions.

**sonogram** \sō'nəgram\ ULTRASONOGRAM.

**sonographer** \sōnäg'rəfər\ A specialist or technician in sonography.

**sonography** \sōnäg'rəfē\ [L *son(us)* a sound, note + *o* + -GRAPHY] **1** The visual representation of the acoustic characteristics of the human voice, used in the study of voice disorders. **2** ULTRASONOGRAPHY.

**sonoinversion** \sō'nō·invur'zhən\ A variety of tympanoplasty, the principle of which is the inversion of the course of the sound waves within the ear. As the result of the reconstruction of the middle ear, sound waves impinge directly on the round window, the oval window being protected by a suprapromontorial air space. Also *sound inversion.*

**sonologist** \sōnäl'əjist\ A specialist in sonology; a specialist in the interpretation of ultrasound images.

**sonology** \sōnäl'əjē\ [L *son(us)* a sound + *o* + -LOGY] The field or study of imaging with sound or ultrasound.

**sonoscope** \sō'nəskōp\ ULTRASONOGRAPH.

**sonotomogram** \sō'nətō'məgram\ ULTRASONOGRAM.

**sonotomography** \sō'nətəmäg'rəfē\ ULTRASONOGRAPHY.

**sophisticate** To adulterate (food or medicines).

**sophistication** The intentional alteration or adulteration of food or medicines.

**sopor** \sō'pər\ [L (akin to *somnus* for *sopnus* sleep), deep sleep] A profoundly deep sleep.

**soporific** \säp'ərif'ik\ [French *soporifique* (from L *sopor* sleep + *i* + French *-fique* English *-fic,* suffix denoting making, from L *facere* to make) sleep-inducing] HYPNOTIC.

**s. op. s.** *si opus sit* (L, if it is necessary).

**sorbefacient** \sôr'bifā'shənt\ **1** Aiding or promoting absorption. **2** A sorbefacient agent.

**sorbic acid** $C_6H_8O_2$. 2,4-Hexadienoic acid. A naturally occurring compound obtained from the berries of the mountain ash *Sorbus aucuparia* as the lactone, parasorbic acid. It is used as an inhibitor of mold and yeast growth in foods.

**sorbitol** \sôr'bitôl\ The alcohol formed by reduction of the —CHO group of glucose to —$CH_2$OH. It is used as a sweetening agent. Also *glucitol.*

**sordes** \sôr'dēz\ [L, dirtiness, dirt, shabbiness] Crusts occurring in and about the mouth, particularly on the lips, teeth, and gingivae in severe chronic debilitating illness and in feverish states, as in typhoid fever. *Older term.* **s. aurium** *Obs.* CERUMEN. **s. gastricae** Foul material accumulating in the stomach consisting of a mixture of food, epithelial matter, and microorganisms.

**sore** [Old English *sār* affliction, disease, a wound, sore] **1** A circumscribed skin lesion, usually marked by some loss of tissue. **2** Tender; painful. **bed s.** See under BEDSORE. **chrome s.** CHROME ULCER. **Cochin s.** TROPICAL ULCER. **cold s.** A vesicular lesion of herpes simplex which appears on the mucosa or skin of the lip or around the nostrils, lasts 3–10 days, and may recur either at the same site or nearby. Also *fever blister, coldsore.* **Delhi s.** CUTANEOUS LEISHMANIASIS. **denture s.** A traumatic ulcer of the oral mucosa caused by a denture. **desert s.** VELDT SORE. **Gallipoli s.** VELDT SORE. **Naga s.** TROPICAL ULCER. **oriental s.** CUTANEOUS LEISHMANIASIS. **pressure s.** BEDSORE. **primary s.** TRUE CHANCRE. **soft s.** CHANCROID. **Umballa s.** VELDT SORE. **veldt s.** An ulcerative skin condition similar in appearance to a varicose ulcer, and usually occurring on exposed parts of the body, often the leg but also the face and hands. The cause is unknown, although the diphtheria bacillus can sometimes be isolated. Diphtheritic involvement of the central nervous system may also be present. The condition occurs in the tropics and subtropics where desert conditions predominate, particularly in southern Africa, regions of the Middle East, and northern Australia. Penicillin is effective in treatment. Also *desert sore, Barcoo disease, Gallipoli sore, Umballa sore, dermatitis veldtis.* **venereal s.** An ulcer acquired through sexual contact and characteristic of a sexually transmitted disease.

**Sörensen** [Sören Peer Lauritz *Sörensen,* Danish biochemist, 1868–1939] Sörensen scale. See under PH SCALE.

**Soret** [C. *Soret,* French radiologist, died 1931] See under BAND.

**Soret** [Charles *Soret,* French physicist, 1854–1904] Soret phenomenon. See under EFFECT.

**soroche** \sōrō'che\ [South American Spanish (from Quechua *surúchi* a sulfide mineral) mineral sickness, mountain sickness] A form of mountain sickness identified in the Andes. At one time it was attributed to antimony and other metallic effusions from local mining operations.

**sorption** \sôrp'shən\ [back formation from ABSORPTION and ADSORPTION] The uptake of liquid molecules by adsorption, absorption, or both.

**s.o.s.** *si opus sit* (L, if it be necessary): used in prescription writing.

**soterocyte** \sō′tərōsīt′\ *Obs.* PLATELET.

**Sotos** [Juan Fernandez *Sotos*, Spanish-born U.S. pediatrician, born 1927] See under SYNDROME.

**Sottas** [Jules *Sottas*, French neurologist, 1866–1943] Dejerine-Sottas syndrome. See under HEREDITARY HYPERTROPHIC INTERSTITIAL NEUROPATHY.

**souffle** \soo′fəl\ [French (from L *sufflare* to blow at or against, puff up, from SUB- + L *flare* to blow, sound, breathe), a blowing or puffing through the mouth] A soft, blowing murmur, especially an extracardiac murmur. **cardiac s.** A soft, blowing cardiac murmur. **fetal s.** A sharp, blowing sound, secondary to blood flow in the umbilical vessels and synchronous with the fetal heartbeat, heard by auscultation over the pregnant uterus. Also *umbilical souffle, funicular souffle, funic souffle.* **funic s.** FETAL SOUFFLE. **funicular s.** FETAL SOUFFLE. **placental s.** A sound similar to a uterine souffle but due to blood flow through placental blood vessels. **splenic s.** A soft blowing sound sometimes heard on auscultation over a diseased spleen. **umbilical s.** FETAL SOUFFLE. **uterine s.** A rushing sound, heard by auscultation of the pregnant uterus, synchronous with the maternal heartbeat and due to blood flow through the uterine vasculature. Also *Kergaradec sign.*

**Soulier** [Jean Pierre *Soulier*, French hematologist, born 1915] Bernard-Soulier syndrome. See under SYNDROME.

**sound[1]** [Old French *son*, from L *sonus* noise, sound] **1** Waves of pressure (and the concomitant density variation) in the frequency range to which the human ear is sensitive, roughly 20–20 000 Hz. **2** The sensation evoked in the listener's hearing by physical activity taking place within his auditory space, possibly at some considerable distance. This activity induces patterns of alternating pressure in the air, which radiate out in all directions from the sound source. **atrial s.** A sound generated within the heart as a consequence of atrial contraction; the fourth heart sound. It may arise in the atrium or, more commonly, by the distension of the ventricle by atrial systole. **auscultatory s.** Any sound heard by auscultation of the chest or abdomen. **bell s.** COIN SOUND. **bronchial breath s.'s** Abnormally harsh and clear breath sounds heard on auscultation over a consolidated lung. **cardiac s.** HEART SOUND. **cavernous voice s.** A hollow sound heard during phonation on auscultation of the chest over a lung cavity. **coin s.** A ringing sound heard on auscultation over a pneumothorax when a coin placed against the chest is struck with another coin. Also *bell sound, bell note, bell-metal resonance.* **cracked-pot s.** The sound, likened to that elicited from a cracked pot, evoked by percussion of the skull in a child with severe hydrocephalus, or of the chest over a lung cavity that is in communication with a bronchus. Also *bruit de pot fêlé.* **diastolic s.** An additional heart sound heard in diastole, usually the third sound. **dive-bomber s.** A note in the loudspeaker like a dive-bomber or a dog snarling, produced by electric discharges upon movement in the muscle of the exploring needle electrode during electromyography upon an apparently relaxed and resting muscle in a subject with myotonia. **eddy s.'s** Sounds superimposed on the continuous murmur of persistent ductus arteriosus. **ejection s.** EJECTION CLICK. **first s.** The heart sound that is due to closure of the mitral and tricuspid valves. It is low-pitched and likened to the sound "lub." It may be split, even in health, the first component deriving from the mitral valve and the second component, from the tricuspid. **fourth s.** The heart sound which occurs at the time of atrial systole, immediately before the first sound. It is low-pitched and seldom heard in health, but becomes pronounced if the atria contract more forcefully, or if the related ventricle is hypertrophied. **friction s.** RUB. **gallop s.** An additional heart sound, either the third or fourth sound, which gives rise to gallop rhythm. **heart s.** One of the four auscultatory sounds corresponding to events in the cardiac cycle. The first sound ($S_1$) is due to closure of the mitral and tricuspid valves, the second ($S_2$) is caused by closure of the aortic and pulmonary valves, the third ($S_3$) corresponds to the end of the phase of rapid filling, and the fourth ($S_4$) occurs at the time of atrial systole, immediately before the first sound. Also *cardiac sound, heart tone.* **hippocratic s.** The splashing sound heard in hippocratic succussion. **Korotkoff s.'s** The sounds heard as compression of an artery is released, in the auscultatory method of determining blood pressure. They are divided into five successive phases corresponding to the declining pressure: Phase 1 is characterized by clear tapping sounds which start when the pressure has fallen to the peak systolic pressure. In phase 2 swishing sounds or murmurs are heard, which are accentuated in phase 3. In phase 4 the sounds become muffled, and in phase 5 they disappear. Phase 5 corresponds most closely to true diastolic pressure in most cases. **muscle s.** A fine crackling sound that is heard over a contracting muscle. **percussion s.** The note produced by percussion. **pericardial friction s.** PERICARDIAL RUB. **pistol-shot s.** An abrupt sound heard with the stethoscope over peripheral arteries in aortic regurgitation. **post-tussis suction s.** A blowing or whistling sound heard after a cough on auscultation over some pulmonary cavities. **pulmonic second s.** The second heart sound derived from the pulmonic valve. **respiratory s.** Any auscultatory sound produced by breathing. **Santini's booming s.** An auscultatory echo sound heard on percussion over a hydatid cyst as a sonorous booming. **second s.** The heart sound that is caused by closure of the aortic and pulmonary valves. It is likened to the sound "dup." Usually single on expiration, it splits on inspiration, the aortic component preceding the pulmonary. **succussion s.'s** Splashing noises heard on auscultation when the patient's body is shaken, indicative of abnormal amounts of fluid and gas in a hollow organ, especially the stomach. They may also be heard over the lung in hydropneumothorax. Also *succussion splash, clapotement.* **third s.** A heart sound that corresponds to the end of the phase of rapid filling. It is a normal finding in the young, but in older persons it is usually associated with ventricular failure or high flow into a ventricle. It is low-pitched, and usually best heard with the bell of the stethoscope just internal to the apex beat. **vesicular breath s.'s** The auscultatory breath sounds heard over healthy lungs. **waterwheel s.** MILL WHEEL MURMUR. **white s.** WHITE NOISE. **xiphisternal crunching s.** A crunching sound heard on auscultation over the xiphisternum in a patient with mediastinal emphysema.

**sound[2]** [Middle French *sonde* line for sounding] A probe-like surgical instrument, especially one used to determine the direction and caliber of a passage such as the urethra. **Bellocq s.** A device for drawing a lint or gauze plug into the nasopharynx, once used in cases of severe epistaxis. Also *Bellocq's cannula.* **esophageal s.** A long, flexible instrument introduced into the esophagus to detect a foreign body or dilate a stricture. **lacrimal s.** LACRIMAL PROBE. **uterine s.** A calibrated probe to determine the length and position of the uterus. Also *uterometer, hysterometer, uterine probe.*

**source** [French (from *sourdre* to spring up, from L *surgere* to rise up, from SUB- + L *regere* to erect, direct) a spring of water] 1 The place or thing from which something originates. 2 The device or substance from which radiation is emitted, as from a discrete quantity of radioactive material. **point s.** A source of light or other rays, which is so small as to be considered without dimensions.

**southernwood** ABROTANUM.

**soybean** *Glycine max* of the Leguminosae family, a legume that is cultivated for food and fodder. It is high in calories and contains stigmasterol, a starting substance for hormone synthesis. It is also an excellent source of protein, with a high biological value. The fixed oil expressed from soybeans, soybean oil, consists mainly of oleic and linoleic acids. Also *soja bean, soya.*

**sp.** 1 specific. 2 spirit. 3 species.

# space

**space** [Old French *espace*, from L *spatium*. See SPATIUM.] SPATIUM. **alveolar dead s.** An effective dead space created in lung alveoli by a higher-than-normal ratio of ventilation to blood perfusion, resulting in underperfusion of some alveoli, which therefore do not contribute to gas exchange. **anatomical dead s.** The space within the respiratory passages through which air must pass before reaching gas-exchanging alveolar surfaces. Also *anatomical airway.* **antecubital s.** FOSSA CUBITALIS. **anterior perforated s.** SUBSTANTIA PERFORATA ANTERIOR. **axillary s.** FOSSA AXILLARIS. **Bogros s.** An area between the peritoneum and the fascia transversalis bounded inferiorly by the inguinal ligament in which the lower part of the external iliac artery may be reached without penetrating the peritoneum. Also *spatium retroinguinale, retroinguinal space.* **Böttcher s.** SACCUS ENDOLYMPHATICUS. **Bowman s.** The space between the glomerular capillary loops and the glomerular capsule which collects the glomerular filtrate and passes it on to the lumens of the renal tubules. Also *filtration space, capsular space.* **bregmatic s.** *Outmoded* ANTERIOR FONTANEL. **capsular s.** BOWMAN SPACE. **cartilage s.** CARTILAGE LACUNA. **chloride s.** The calculated volume of body fluid or of tissue in which a dose of labeled chloride ion is distributed as determined by the isotope dilution technique. **Colles s.** SPATIUM PERINEI SUPERFICIALE. **complemental s.** The parts of the pleural cavity which are not occupied by the lungs. **Cotunnius s.** The space within the membranous labyrinth. **cupola s.** PARS CUPULARIS RECESSUS EPITYMPANICI. **Czermak s.'s** INTERGLOBULAR SPACES. **dead s.** 1 Any unobliterated space in the body capable of being filled by exudate. 2 That region of a system through which gases or liquids flow without alteration. **deep perineal s.** SPATIUM PERINEI PROFUNDUM. **Disse s.** PERISINUSOIDAL SPACE. **distal pulp s.** A closed multilocular connective tissue space over the distal two-thirds of the palmar aspect of a distal phalanx produced by strong fibrous bands between the periosteum and the skin. Also *distal closed space, pulp space.* **s. of Donders** A space between the dorsum of the tongue and the undersurface of the palate when the mandible is in the rest position. **Douglas s.** EXCAVATIO RECTOUTERINA. **epicerebral s.** A potential space between pia mater and the surface of the brain. **epidural s.** CAVITAS EPIDURALIS. **episcleral s.** SPATIUM EPISCLERALE. **epispinal s.** A potential space between pia mater and the surface of the spinal cord. **epitympanic s.** RECESSUS EPITYMPANICUS. **extradural s.** CAVITAS EPIDURALIS. **filtration s.** BOWMAN SPACE. **follicular s.** ANTRUM FOLLICULARE. **Fontana s.'s** SPATIA ANGULI IRIDOCORNEALIS. **free-way s.** INTEROCCLUSAL DISTANCE. **globular s.'s of Czermak** INTERGLOBULAR SPACES. **haversian s.** HAVERSIAN CANAL. **Henke s.** SPATIUM RETROPHARYNGEUM. **His-Held s.** PERIVASCULAR SPACE. **His perivascular s.** PERIVASCULAR SPACE. **interarytenoid s.** PARS INTERCARTILAGINEA RIMAE GLOTTIDIS. **intercostal s.** SPATIUM INTERCOSTALE. **intercristal s.** The space contained within the inner mitochondrial membrane. **intercrural s.** The triangular interval between the crura cerebri. **interdental s.** INTERDENTAL EMBRASURE. **interglobular s.'s** Regions in dentin bounded by the curved outlines of spheres of mineralization which have not coalesced. Also *interglobular areas, Czermak spaces, globular spaces of Czermak, spatia interglobularia.* **interlamellar s.'s** The potential spaces between the layers of the cornea. **intermesoblastic s.** COELOM. **intermetacarpal s.'s** SPATIA INTEROSSEA METACARPI. **intermetatarsal s.'s** SPATIA INTEROSSEA METATARSI. **interosseous s.'s of metacarpus** SPATIA INTEROSSEA METACARPI. **interosseous s.'s of metatarsus** SPATIA INTEROSSEA METATARSI. **interpeduncular s.** FOSSA INTERPEDUNCULARIS. **interpleural s.** MEDIASTINUM. **interproximal s.** A space between the proximal surfaces of adjacent teeth in the dental arch, especially the region rootward of the contact area. **interseptal s.** A small recess lying between the septum spurium, which is formed from the valves of the sinus venosus, and the septum primum in the embryonic right atrium. **interstitial s.** Connective tissue between formed structures in organs or tissues consisting of interstitial fluid, fibroblasts, collagen and other fibrils. **intervaginal s.'s of optic nerve** SPATIA INTERVAGINALIA NERVI OPTICI. **intervillous s.** The cavernous space in the human placenta containing a mass of interconnecting and free villi, bathed in 160–180 ml of maternal blood which is delivered from the nozzlelike openings of arterioles which pierce the decidua basalis, the blood being drained by collecting veins in each subdivision or cotyledon which connects with uterine veins. The intervillous space develops from lacunae which develop in the trophoblast and as the result of erosion of the decidua. Also *intervillous lacuna.* **intra-adventitial s.** A potential space between the cells and fibers of the adventitia of a blood vessel. **intracapsular s.** PERIAXIAL SPACE. **intracristal s.** The space outside of the inner mitochondrial membrane but between the folds of this membrane. **intrapial s.** One of the small spaces between the two layers of the pia mater that communicates with the subarachnoid space. **s.'s of iridocorneal angle** SPATIA ANGULI IRIDOCORNEALIS. **Kiernan s.'s** PORTAL CANAL. **Kiesselbach s.** KIESSELBACH'S AREA. **Kretschmann s.** A small recess in the mucous membrane of the tympanic membrane, situated just below the recessus membranae tympani superior. **Kuhnt s.'s** A series of radiating recesses between the ciliary processes and the ciliary zonule which open into the posterior chamber of the eye. **Larrey s.** MORGAGNI'S FORAMEN. **Lesshaft s.** SUPERIOR LUMBAR TRIANGLE. **s. of Littre** A dilated pit in the wall of the penile urethra which may trap the end of a catheter passed toward the bladder. **lymph s.** 1 A thin-walled lymphatic channel. 2 *Imprecise* PERIAXIAL SPACE. **lymphatic s.** PERIAXIAL SPACE. **Magendie s.** CAVITAS SUBARACHNOIDEA. **marrow s.** CAVITAS MEDULLARIS OSSIUM. **mechanical dead s.** The volume of an apparatus through which a subject must breathe during respiratory testing or therapy. **Meckel's s.** CAVUM TRIGEMINALE. **medullary s.** CAVITAS MEDULLARIS OSSIUM. **meningeal s.** CAVITAS SUBARACHNOIDEA. **midpalmar s.** The space in the palm of the hand between the intermediate and medial palmar septa. It is roofed over by the central part of the palmar aponeurosis, and the floor is formed by the third, fourth, and fifth metacarpal bones, the fascia covering the interosseous muscles between these bones and part of the transverse head of the adductor pollicis muscle. Proximally is found the common flexor synovial sheath, and distally the space is continuous with the subcutaneous tissues of the webs of the medial three fingers. **Mohrenheim s.** FOSSA INFRACLAVICULARIS. **Nuel s.** A space between the outer rods of Corti and the outer hair cells of the spiral organ in the cochlear duct of the internal ear. It communicates with both the inner and the outer tunnels through intercellular gaps. **Obersteiner-Redlich s.** The zone of transition between the peripheral and central nervous systems, demarcated by a basal lamina separating Schwann cells and collagen from the central neuroglia. It is not actually a space. Also *Obersteiner-Redlich line*. **palmar s.** The space between the thenar and the hypothenar eminences and lying behind the central part of the palmar aponeurosis in the palm of the hand. It is divided by the intermediate palmar septum into the thenar space laterally and the midpalmar space medially. **parapharyngeal s.** PHARYNGOMAXILLARY SPACE. **pararenal s.** The space between the posterior layer of the renal fascia and the anterior layer of the thoracolumbar fascia in front of the quadratus lumborum muscle which is occupied by pararenal, or retroperitoneal, fat. It is closed superiorly by the attachment of the renal fascia to the diaphragm and medially by the fascia covering the large prevertebral vessels, while it is open inferiorly and laterally. **parasinoidal s.'s** The intradural lacunae lying lateral to the superior sagittal sinus and containing arachnoid villi and meningeal and diploic veins. **paraxial s.** The portion of a muscle spindle within the internal capsule. It is not a free space like the periaxial space, but is filled by the axial bundle of intrafusal muscle fibers and associated nerve endings. **Parona s.** A space between the deep flexor tendons in the forearm and the anterior surface of the pronator quadratus muscle. It is continuous distally with the midpalmar space and the common flexor synovial sheath. **pelvocrural s.** The lacuna musculorum and lacuna vasorum combined. **periaxial s.** The fluid-filled space between the lamellated external capsule of a muscle spindle and the delicate internal capsule ensheathing its axial bundle. Also *lymph space* (imprecise), *lymphatic space, intracapsular space*. **perichoroidal s.** SPATIUM PERICHOROIDEALE. **perilymphatic s.** SPATIUM PERILYMPHATICUM. **perineural s.** PERIVASCULAR SPACE. **perinodal s.** The space between the endoneurium and the neurilemma at the indentation of a node of Ranvier. **perinuclear s.** The space between the inner and outer membranes of the nuclear envelope. Also *cisterna caryothecae*. **periotic s.** SPATIUM PERILYMPHATICUM. **peripharyngeal s.** SPATIUM PERIPHARYNGEUM. **periportal s. of Mall** A space around the vessels and bile ductules in the portal canals at the periphery of a liver lobule where the lymph vessels of the liver originate. It is continuous with the space of Disse. **perisinusoidal s.** A space lying between the wall of the hepatic sinusoids and the hepatocytes bordering them and containing blood plasma. Microvilli from adjacent phagocytic cells and hepatocytes protrude into and across the space, which is continuous with the periportal space of Mall at the periphery of the lobule. Also *Disse space*. **peritoneal s.** Any of the several spaces, fossae, or recesses formed in the peritoneal cavity by the reflections between the parietal and visceral layers. **perivascular s.** The space between the two layers of the leptomeningeal sheath around the small blood vessels entering the brain substance, continuous with the subarachnoid space. It separates the vessels from the neurons, and becomes attenuated at the level of the arterioles and venules. Also *Virchow-Robin space, His perivascular space, His-Held space, perineural space, perivascular channel, perineural channel*. **perivitelline s.** The space lying between the perivitelline membrane and the zona pellucida of an ovum. Also *vitelline space, yolk space*. **personal s.** The hypothesis that each individual is surrounded by an invisible bubble of space regarded as one's own. According to this idea, a nonverbal communication, usually negative in nature, occurs when another enters that space. Infringements on one's personal space by strangers, for example, will cause most people to back away. **pharyngomaxillary s.** The space situated between the side wall of the pharynx medially, the medial pterygoid muscle laterally, and the cervical vertebrae posteriorly. Also *parapharyngeal space*. **physiologic dead s.** The portion of the respiratory tidal volume that does not participate in gaseous exchange with pulmonary blood. This encompasses alveolar dead space and anatomic dead space. Also *respiratory dead space*. **pia-arachnoid s.** CAVITAS SUBARACHNOIDEA. **placental blood s.** Any of the intervillous spaces of the placenta. **plantar s.** Any one of the four compartments in the foot that is enclosed by fascia. They confine infection or tumor and prevent spread to other parts of the foot. **pleural s.** CAVITAS PLEURALIS. **pleuroperitoneal s.** The portion of the coelom in the embryo lying between the peritoneal and the pericardial cavity. It is the precursor of the pleural cavity. **pneumatic s.** A part of a bone containing air cells or hollowed out to contain air, such as the paranasal sinuses. **Poiseuille s.** The peripheral part of the lumen of a blood vessel, adjacent to its wall, where the movement of the blood cells is reduced to a minimum. **popliteal s.** FOSSA POPLITEA. **posterior perforated s.** SUBSTANTIA PERFORATA POSTERIOR. **postnasal s.** PARS NASALIS PHARYNGIS. **postperforated s.** SUBSTANTIA PERFORATA POSTERIOR. **postpharyngeal s.** SPATIUM RETROPHARYNGEUM. **preputial s.** A cleft separating the prepuce from the glans penis and containing a fossa on each side of the frenulum. Also *preputial sac*. **prevesical s.** SPATIUM RETROPUBICUM. **prezonular s.** That portion of the posterior chamber of the eyeball anterior to the zonula ciliaris. **Prussak s.** RECESSUS MEMBRANAE TYMPANI SUPERIOR. **pterygomandibular s.** The gap between the medial surface of the ramus of the mandible and the pterygoid process of the sphenoid bone. **pulp s.** DISTAL PULP SPACE. **quadrangular s.** A gap in the posterior wall of the axilla, bounded by the teres major muscle below, the long head of triceps muscle medially, the surgical neck of the humerus laterally, and the subscapularis and teres minor muscles and capsule of the shoulder joint above. It transmits the axillary nerve and the posterior circumflex humeral vessels. **quadrilateral s. of Marie** A space situated between the cortex of the brain externally and the internal capsule medially and within the limits of the insula. Through this area course the fibers of the external capsule that connect Broca's area with the other language centers that control speech. Hence a lesion here results in aphasia. **relief s.** RELIEF. **respiratory dead s.** PHYSIOLOGIC DEAD SPACE. **retrobulbar s.** The space situated behind the bulbar sheath and containing orbital fat, muscles, nerves, and vessels. **retromylohyoid s.** The region of the sulcus on the lingual aspect of the lower jaw behind the attachment of the mylohyoid muscle. **retroperitoneal s.** SPATIUM RETROPERITONEALE. **retropharyngeal s.** SPATIUM RETROPHARYNGEUM. **retropubic s.** SPATIUM RETROPUBICUM. **s. of Retzius** SPATIUM RETROPUBICUM. **Schwalbe s.'s** SPATIA INTERVAGINALIA NERVI OPTICI. **semilunar s.** TRAUBE'S SEMILUNAR SPACE. **septal s.** The space between the contact area of adjoining teeth and the crest of the interdental septum of bone. **subarachnoid s.** CAVITAS SUBARACHNOIDEA. **subchorial s.** A region beneath the chorionic plate of the human placenta which is devoid of villi and where the intervillous space is therefore more extensive than elsewhere. **subdural s.** SPATIUM SUBDURALE. **subepicranial s.** A zone of loose cellular tissue between the epicranial aponeurosis and the underlying pericranium, permitting movement of the aponeurosis. **subphrenic s.'s** RECESSUS SUBPHRENICI. **superficial perineal s.** SPATIUM PERINEI SUPERFICIALE. **suprahepatic s.'s** RECESSUS SUBPHRENICI. **suprapubic s.** A triangular space above the pubis, bounded anteriorly by the posterior surface of the rectus abdominis muscle and posteriorly by the fascia transversalis of the posterior layer of the rectus sheath on each side of the linea alba. The transversalis fascia separates it from the upper part of the retropubic space posteriorly. **suprasternal s.** The cleft formed by the splitting of the investing layer of deep cervical fascia so that the superficial layer attaches to the anterior margin of the manubrium sterni and the deep layer to the posterior margin and the interclavicular ligament. It contains some areolar tissue, the lower parts of the anterior jugular veins, the jugular arch, and the sternal heads of the sternocleidomastoid muscle. Also *suprasternal fossa.* **Tarin s.** RECESSUS ANTERIOR FOSSAE INTERPEDUNCULARIS TARINI. **Tenon s.** SPATIUM EPISCLERALE. **thenar s.** The space in the palm of the hand lying between the lateral and the intermediate palmar septa. It is posterior to the central part of the palmar aponeurosis and anterior to the fascia over the transverse head of adductor pollicis muscle and the first dorsal interosseous muscle. Proximally it is continuous with the carpal tunnel and distally with the subcutaneous tissue of the web of the thumb. Also *thenar area.* **thiocyanate s.** An expression of extracellular fluid volume that is derived from calculations made following the intravenous injection of a measured dose of sodium thiocyanate, which diffuses uniformly into all aspects of the extracellular fluid. **third s.** The large fluid volumes required of an individual suffering from shock, sepsis, or burns. Fluid becomes sequestered in a nonfunctional extracellular/intracellular compartment, and unless it is replaced exogenously further hypovolemia results. **thyrohyal s.** The depressed area between the laryngeal prominence of the thyroid cartilage and the body of the hyoid bone above. **s. of Traube** A semilunar area on the anterior chest wall where the percussion sound is normally resonant. It is situated at the base of the left side of the thorax over the fundus of the stomach and the costodiaphragmatic recess. It is bounded below by the costal margin, above by a curved line, convex upwards, between the fifth and sixth left costal cartilages and the anterior end of the tenth rib. **Traube's semilunar s.** An area on the left side of the chest anteriorly and inferiorly over which the air in the stomach produces a vesiculotympanic sound on auscultation. Also *semilunar space.* **Tröltsch s.'s** Recessus membranae tympani anterior and recessus membranae tympani posterior. **Verga s.** CAVUM PSALTERII. **Virchow-Robin s.** PERIVASCULAR SPACE. **vitelline s.** PERIVITELLINE SPACE. **web s.** The space between the proximal ends of digits that may be partially occupied by a web, or fold of skin. **Westberg s.** The space formed between the reflection of the parietal pericardium and the commencement of the ascending aorta. **yolk s.** PERIVITELLINE SPACE. **zonular s.** SPATIUM ZONULARE.

**spacer** In molecular biology, any of the DNA sequences that are not transcribed, that are without known function, and that separate gene units.

**Spalding** [A. B. *Spalding,* U.S. gynecologist, born 1874] See under SIGN.

**spallation** \spôlā′shən\ [*spall,* from Middle English *spalle* an edged fragment chipped from a hard substance + -ATION] A type of nuclear reaction in which a target nucleus, struck by a high-energy projectile (usually a proton, but also possibly a neutron, deuteron, or alpha particle) breaks up in such a way as to form a number of relatively small fragments (mostly protons and neutrons) plus a single, relatively large remainder.

**span** The distance between two points in space or time; extent or reach. **attention s.** **1** The greatest amount of visually perceived material, most often digits or objects or pictures of objects, that can be apprehended during a single brief display. **2** The length of time for which a person can continue to concentrate on a single subject. *Popular.* **auditory s.** The number of digits, letters, or words that can be correctly repeated after one hearing, a measure of immediate memory.

**spar** A nonmetallic but lustrous, crystalline mineral.

**sparganosis** \spär′gənō′sis\ [*spargan(um)* + -OSIS] Infection with a sparganum, usually of the genus *Spirometra.* The infection is characterized by inflammation and fibrosis of subcutaneous tissues, and is derived from swallowing infected copepods in contaminated drinking water, or from eating raw or inadequately cooked frogs, or through the application of an infected frog poultice, especially to the eye. The body heat stimulates the nonencysted sparganum to migrate into the wound or the eye. **ocular s.** Infection of the eye with the sparganum larva of *Spirometra mansoni,* resulting from the application of a poultice of infected uncooked frog flesh against the eye, a practice common in parts of southeast Asia.

**sparganum** \spär′gənəm\ [Gk *sparganon* a swaddling band] (*pl.* spargana) A plerocercoid larva of a tapeworm of the order Pseudophyllidea. It is an unencysted juvenile worm with the typical pair of sucking grooves (dibothria) of the adult scolex, but without segmentation or sexual maturation. This stage develops from a procercoid larva in a copepod, the first intermediate host, and is usually found free in the flesh of a fish or other aquatic vertebrate.

**sparing** / **macular s.** In homonymous hemianopia due to a lesion of the primary visual cortex, apparent preservation of vision in half of the field subtended by the macula on the affected side. This has been shown usually to be an artifact due to impaired fixation during the charting of the fields. **sacral s.** Comparative sparing of cutaneous sensation in the area of the perineum and buttocks, as seen for a time in some patients with spinal cord lesions in whom the sensory "level" on the lower limbs and trunk is slowly ascending.

**sparsomycin** \spär′səmī′sin\ An antibiotic produced by

*Streptomyces sparsogenes* which inhibits protein synthesis in both prokaryotic and eukaryotic cells. It binds to the larger ribosomal subunit and inhibits peptide bond formation.

**spartism** \spär′tizm\ Poisoning caused by ingestion of sparteine, an alkaloid obtained from the dried tops of *Cytisus scoparius*.

# spasm

**spasm** \spaz′m\ [Gk *spasmos* (from *span* to draw, tear, rend) a convulsion, spasm] **1** An involuntary contraction of muscle. Also *spasmus*. **2** A contraction of smooth muscle in the wall of an artery, as in an intracranial vessel as a result of trauma or irritation in subarachnoid hemorrhage or due to malignant hypertension. **arterial s.** Abnormal and excessive increase in tone in an artery. **athetoid s.** ATHETOSIS. **Bell s.** FACIAL SPASM. **blacksmiths s.** MOBILE SPASM. **bowing s.** INFANTILE MASSIVE SPASM. **bronchial s.** BRONCHOSPASM. **cadaveric s.** INSTANTANEOUS RIGOR MORTIS. **canine s.** RISUS SARDONICUS. **carpopedal s.** Spasmodic contraction of the muscles of the hands and feet, occurring in patients with tetany, or hypocalcemia. It is seen most frequently in children. Also *carpopedal contraction*. **clonic s.** A clonic muscular contraction as in clonus or myoclonus. *Outmoded*. **clonic facial s.** FACIAL HEMISPASM. **cynic s.** RISUS SARDONICUS. **diffuse esophageal s.** A condition of abnormal esophageal motor function characterized by intermittent substernal pain and dysphagia, often induced by eating or drinking, or by stress. When studied roentgenographically or manometrically, high-pressure, simultaneous (nonperistaltic) contractions can be seen throughout the esophagus. Also *Barsony-Teschendorf syndrome*. **epidemic transient diaphragmatic s.** EPIDEMIC PLEURODYNIA. **esophageal s.** Involuntary contraction of smooth muscle portion of esophagus, often producing pain; esophagospasm. See also DIFFUSE ESOPHAGEAL SPASM. **facial s.** Any involuntary contraction of the facial muscles, especially facial hemispasm. Also *Bell spasm*. • The term is sometimes incorrectly applied to facial tics, which are not truly involuntary. **fatigue s.** OCCUPATIONAL CRAMP. **flexion s.** INFANTILE MASSIVE SPASM. **flexor s.** A flexor withdrawal movement of the lower limbs occurring spontaneously or on cutaneous stimulation in subjects with spastic paraplegia. **functional s.** OCCUPATIONAL CRAMP. **glottic s.** LARYNGOSPASM. **habit s.** TIC. **histrionic s.** A facial tic producing bizarre and changing facial expressions. Also *mimic spasm*. **infantile s.** INFANTILE MASSIVE SPASM. **infantile massive s.** A brief, tonic, epileptic attack of infants, characterized by sudden violent flexion of the trunk and limbs, each spasm lasting two to four seconds, sometimes occurring singly and sometimes in runs of ten or more. The spasms are not myoclonic. The symptom is generally associated with a progressive encephalopathy giving rise to mental retardation, but may be a manifestation of tuberous sclerosis or phenylketonuria. The EEG usually shows continuous, generalized, irregular, spike-wave discharge (hypsarrhythmia). The baby becomes socially unresponsive, develops gaze avoidance, and may become autistic. This may be averted and normal development resumed if treatment with adrenocorticotropic hormone or corticosteroid is started within two weeks of onset. Early recognition is essential. Also *jackknife seizure, flexion spasm, infantile spasm, jackknife spasm, salaam spasm, bowing spasm, generalized flexion epilepsy, epileptic jerk, saltatory spasm, saltatory chorea, static convulsions, Bamberger's disease, Nickkrampf, West syndrome, saltatory tic, eclampsia nutans* (obs.), *massive myoclonic jerk, salaam convulsion*. **intention s.** Any of various forms of involuntary muscular contraction precipitated by movement. For example, in tetanus the facial muscles may be involved when the patient attempts to speak (risus sardonicus), and similar facial grimacing accentuated by speaking is seen in some cases of Wilson's disease (wilsonian spasm). Myoclonic jerks of the limbs precipitated by movement occur in intention myoclonus, most often seen after anoxic brain damage. *Imprecise*. **lock s.** WRITERS' CRAMP. **massive s.** A convulsion in which most of the musculature of the body is involved. **masticatory s.** TRISMUS. **mimic s.** HISTRIONIC SPASM. **mobile s.** Posthemiplegic choreoathetosis. Also *blacksmiths spasm*. **muscle s.** An involuntary and prolonged muscular contraction. Also *myotonus, muscular rigidity, spasmus muscularis*. **myopathic s.** A spasm that occurs in conjunction with a disease of the muscle. **nictitating s.** BLEPHAROSPASM. **nodding s.** SPASMUS NUTANS. **occupation s.** OCCUPATIONAL CRAMP. **oculogyric s.** Tonic contraction of the extraocular muscles producing forced conjugate movements such as fixed upward gaze. **pantomimic s.** TIC. **pedal s.** Spasm of the foot or the great toe or both in anteflexion. It is usually seen together with carpal spasm as a manifestation of the tetany of hypocalcemia, or severe metabolic or respiratory alkalosis. **perineal s.** VAGINISMUS. **phonatory s.** Spasm of the adductor muscles of the vocal folds and sometimes of the musculature of the entire laryngeal inlet, preventing speech. **postparalytic facial s.** Facial spasm developing after a unilateral facial palsy. **professional s.** OCCUPATIONAL CRAMP. **progressive torsion s.** DYSTONIA MUSCULORUM DEFORMANS. **recruitment s.** A tetanic spasm in a limb or part induced by voluntary movement of the affected part in local tetanus. **respiratory s.** **1** Sudden difficulty in breathing. **2** Involuntary contraction of the muscles of respiration. **retrocollic s.** Spasmodic contraction of the posterior neck muscles producing intermittent retrocollis. **rotatory s.** Rotatory movements of the head caused by intermittent contraction of the splenius muscle, as seen in some patients with senile tremor. More often there is a rhythmic side-to-side or anteroposterior movement (titubating tremor). Similar movements may occur less often in severe cases of essential tremor in young adults and occasionally in cases of cerebellar degeneration. **salaam s.** INFANTILE MASSIVE SPASM. **saltatory s.** INFANTILE MASSIVE SPASM. **sewing s.** SEAMSTRESSES' CRAMP. **spinal accessory s.** SPASMODIC TORTICOLLIS. **stutter s.** The inhibition of speech which takes place in the more extreme forms of stuttering, usually in conjunction with a variety of associated motor activities related to respiration, facial grimacing, and other movements. **tailors s.** TAILORS' CRAMP. **tetanic s.** **1** A muscular spasm characteristic of tetanus. **2** *Seldom used* TONIC CONVULSION. **tonic s.** *Seldom used* TONIC CONVULSION. **tonoclonic s.** A repetitive spasmodic movement with alternating tonic and clonic features. **torsion s.** DYSTONIA MUSCULORUM DEFORMANS. **toxic s.** TOXIC CONVULSION. **vascular s.** VASOSPASM. **vasomotor s.** Spasm of the small arteries. **winking s.** BLEPHAROSPASM. **writers' s.** WRITERS' CRAMP.

**spasmo-** \spaz′mō-\ [Gk *spasmos* convulsion, spasm] A combining form meaning spasm.

**spasmodic** \spazmäd′ik\ [New L *spasmodicus* (from Gk *spasmōdēs* spasmodic, from *spasmos* spasm + L *-icus* -IC) spasmodic] **1** Characterized by muscular spasm, or relating to such spasm. **2** *Obs.* SPASTIC.

**spasmogen** \spaz′məjən\ [SPASMO- + -GEN] A substance capable of causing spasm. Adj. spasmogenic.

**spasmolygmus** \-lig′məs\ HICCUP.

**spasmolysant** \spazmäl′isənt\ **1** Helping to relax or relieve spasms; antispasmodic. **2** An agent that relieves spasms.

**spasmolysis** \spazmäl′isis\ [SPASMO- + LYSIS] Relief of spasm, of spasticity, or of a convulsive episode.

**spasmolytic** \-lit′ik\ A method, drug, or technique that induces spasmolysis.

**spasmophilia** \-fil′yə\ [SPASMO- + -PHILIA] Latent or overt tetany. *Obs.* Also *spasmodic diathesis.*

**spasmus** \spaz′məs\ [L, from Gk *spasmos.* See SPASM.] SPASM. **s. agitans** PARKINSON'S DISEASE. **s. caninus** RISUS SARDONICUS. **s. coordinatus** TIC. **s. muscularis** MUSCLE SPASM. **s. nictitans** BLEPHAROSPASM. **s. nutans** A stereotyped movement disorder consisting of repetitive head-nodding, even, in rare cases, compulsive knocking of the head against a cot or wall, observed in infants and young children, especially those who are socially deprived and confined to orphanages or other institutions. The child sits in his cot and the head and neck, or even sometimes the trunk, move rhythmically backwards and forwards. This syndrome is never epileptic and must be distinguished from infantile spasms. Also *rocking tic, nictatio spastica, bowing tic, nodding spasm, head-nodding, epilepsia nutans* (obs.).

**spastic** \spas′tik\ [Gk *spastik(os)* (from *spast(os),* verbal of *span* to draw out, tear out or away + *-ikos* -IC) pulling, stretching] **1** Describing, pertaining to, or affected by a state of hypertonia in which there is increased resistance to passive stretching of muscles, usually associated with increase of both alpha and gamma motor neuron excitability. This state is usually the result of dysfunction or disease of the upper motor neurons releasing various reflexes from their normal inhibitory influence. **2** *Obs.* SPASMODIC.

**spasticity** \spastis′itē\ **1** The state of being spastic; a spastic condition. **2** That type of hypertonia with hyperreflexia which results from a lesion of the corticospinal tract. Also *spastic rigidity.* **cerebral s.** Spasticity due to disease or dysfunction of the brain. **clasp-knife s.** CLASP-KNIFE RIGIDITY.

**spatia** \spā′shē·ə\ Plural of SPATIUM.

**spatial** \spā′shəl\ Of, relating to, or involving space.

**spatic** \spā′tik\ Pertaining to a space.

**spatium** \spā′shē·əm\ [L (prob. akin to *patere* to be or stand open, extend, *pandere* to stretch, extend, Gk *petannynai* to spread, expand, and English *fathom*), a space, distance, extent] (*pl.* spatia) [NA] A demarcated open area or cleft, either potential or actual. Also *space.* **spatia anguli iridocornealis** [NA] The spaces in the loose trabecular tissue in the inner wall of the sinus venosus sclerae through which the aqueous humor in the anterior chamber of the eye filters into the sinus and then into the bloodstream via the anterior ciliary veins. Also *spaces of iridocorneal angle, Fontana spaces, ciliary canals.* **s. episclerale** [NA] The narrow space located between the inner surface of the bulbar sheath and the outer surface of the sclera and containing delicate bands of connective tissue connecting the walls. It acts like a bursa, permitting limited movement of the eyeball within the sheath. Also *episcleral space, Tenon space.* **s. intercostale** [NA] The space intervening between adjacent ribs posterolaterally and between adjacent costal cartilages anteriorly. There are eleven in number, and each is occupied by intercostal muscles, membranes, nerves, and vessels. They are wider in front than behind. Also *intercostal space.* **spatia interglobularia** INTERGLOBULAR SPACES. **spatia interossea metacarpi** [NA] The four gaps between the five metacarpal bones, occupied mostly by the interosseous muscles and ligaments. Also *interosseous spaces of metacarpus, intermetacarpal spaces.* **spatia interossea metatarsi** [NA] The four gaps between the five metatarsal bones, occupied mostly by the interosseous muscles and ligaments. Also *interosseous spaces of metatarsus, intermetatarsal spaces.* **spatia intervaginalia nervi optici** [NA] The subdural and subarachnoid spaces surrounding the optic nerve. Also *Schwalbe spaces, intervaginal spaces of optic nerve.* **s. perichoroideale** [NA] The sum total of the tiny cleftlike mesothelium-lined spaces between the nonvascular lamellae of the suprachoroid lamina which attaches the choroid to the deep surface of the sclera. The presence of mesothelium-lined interstices is not supported by recent observations and some authorities consider the space to be that area occupied by the suprachoroid lamina. Also *perichoroidal space.* **s. perilymphaticum** [NA] The space separating the bony from the membranous labyrinths of the internal ear and containing a clear fluid (perilymph). Also *perilymphatic space, periotic space.* **s. perinei profundum** [NA] The region above the membrana perinei that extends superiorly to the dense endopelvic fascia of the floor of the pelvis. It contains the transversus perinei profundus, sphincter urethrae, compressor urethrae, and sphincter urethrovaginalis muscles. It is now considered that there is no layer of superior fascia of the urogenital diaphragm, fascia diaphragmatis urogenitalis superior, that separates the sphincter urethrae muscle from the prostate gland, and that this muscle rises on the prostate almost to the base of the bladder. Thus the commonly described flat sandwich of the urogenital diaphragm, or diaphragma urogenitale, does not actually exist. Also *deep perineal space, deep perineal pouch.* **s. perinei superficiale** [NA] The pouch or gap between the membranous layer of the superficial fascia of the perineum and the perineal membrane containing the root of the penis or clitoris and the bulbospongiosus, ischiocavernosus, and tranversus perinei superficialis muscles. Also *superficial perineal space, superficial perineal pouch, Colles space.* **s. peripharyngeum** [NA] The potential space that partially surrounds the pharyngeal part of the buccopharyngeal fascia and is continuous with the space surrounding the esophagus. It is normally filled with loose connective tissue and is subdivided into spatium retropharyngeum and spatium lateropharyngeum. Also *peripharyngeal space.* **s. retroperitoneale** [NA] The space situated between the parietal peritoneum and the muscles of the posterior abdominal and pelvic walls and occupied by the organs, nerves and vessels located there. Also *retroperitoneal space, retroperitoneum.* **s. retropharyngeum** [NA] The portion of the peripharyngeal space that lies between the lamina prevertebralis of the cervical fascia posteriorly and the buccopharyngeal fascia and pharynx anteriorly. Superiorly it extends to the base of the skull and inferiorly it is continuous with the space behind the esophagus. Laterally it is closed by the carotid sheath. It is filled with loose connective tissue, and it may be subdivided by the alar fascia. Also *retropharyngeal space, postpharyngeal space, Henke space.* **s. retropubicum** [NA] The space filled with extraperitoneal tissue and a venous plexus and located between the lateral portions of the inferior surface of the urinary bladder, covered by umbilical prevesical fascia, and the symphysis pubis, lined internally by transversalis fascia. It is bounded above by peritoneum reflected on to the anterior abdominal wall, below by the puboprostatic ligaments, and laterally by the parietal fascia covering the levator ani and obturator internus muscles. Also *retropubic space, space of Retzius, cavity of Retzius, prevesical space.* **s. subdurale** [NA] A cleft or potential space between the dura mater and arachnoid linings of the brain and spinal cord. Also *subdural space, cavum subdurale, subdural cavity.* **s. zonulare** [NA] The cleft bounded by the two layers of the ciliary zonule, or suspensory ligament of the lens, and the lens border, the one layer being attached to the front of and the other behind the equator of the lens. Also *zonular space, Petit's canal, Hannover's canal.*

**spatula** \spat′chələ\ [L, dim. of *spatha* (from Gk *spathē* any broad blade) a broad, two-edged sword without a point] An instrument with a flat, blunt, often flexible tip. It is used to mix up the ingredients of ointments and masses and for spreading plasters. **tongue s.** TONGUE DEPRESSOR.

**spatulate** \spach′ələt\ Shaped like a spatula. Also *spatular, spatuliform.*

**spatulation** \spach′əlā′shən\ [*spatul(a)* + -ATION] The preparation of a smooth, homogeneous mixture of ingredients by mixing them on a glass plate or similar flat surface and blending the components by turning and scraping them together many times.

**spatuliform** \spach′əlifôrm′\ SPATULATE.

**Spatz** [Hugo *Spatz,* German neuropathologist, 1888–1969] Hallervorden-Spatz syndrome. See under HALLERVORDEN-SPATZ DISEASE.

**spay** \spā\ [Middle English *spayen,* from Old French *espeer* to cut with a sword, from L *spatha* an unpointed broadsword] To remove the ovaries of an animal by surgery.

**SPCA** serum prothrombin conversion accelerator (factor VII).

**Spearman** [Charles Edward *Spearman,* English psychologist, 1863–1945] G factor of Spearman. See under FACTOR.

**spec.** **1** specimen. **2** special. **3** specific.

**specialist** A professional person, as a health practitioner, whose practice or research is limited to a particular branch of a field of study, usually after having acquired the appropriate special training and experience.

**specialization** \spesh′əlīzā′shən\ **1** Adaptation to more special or more limited circumstances or habitats. **2** The process of practicing as or becoming a specialist. **3** The process of becoming divided or further divided into specialties.

**specialize** To limit one's practice or research to a particular branch of a profession or field of study, usually after having acquired special training and experience in that branch or field.

**specialty** \spesh′əltē\ A field or practice in which one specializes.

**speciation** \spē′sē·ā′shən\ The evolutionary process whereby new species are developed; the separation of a population into genetically isolated segments which become recognized as new species populations.

**species** \spē′shēz, -sēz\ [L (from *specere* to see, observe) a sight, aspect, appearance, form, type, particular kind] (*pl.* species) **1** A taxonomic collection of interbreeding populations that are reproductively isolated from other such collections. A group of closely related species forms a genus. **2** A particular type of molecule, ion, etc., represented by many identical numbers. **morphological s.** A species which is recognizable as such on the basis of features like structure, color, and proportions. **polytypic s.** A species which is divided into subspecies on the basis of morphologic and color variations in different geographic regions, the subspecies often interbreeding at the common margins of adjacent ranges. **type s.** The species used in the original description of a genus. When a new genus is erected or described it receives the oldest legitimate generic name of its earliest species.

**species-specific** \-spəsif′ik\ Affecting a particular species or the cells or tissues of a particular species, as an antigen.

**specific** \spəsif′ik\ [L *speci(es)* (see SPECIES) + -FIC] **1** Of or relating to a species. **2** Caused by a particular infectious agent: said of a disease. **3** A remedy for a particular disease; a medicine intended for a particular disease or pathogen. **4** Able to discriminate between related phenomena or substances. In immunology, specific responses are able to distinguish one antigen from another.

**specificity** \spes′ifis′itē\ **1** The fact, quality, or condition of being specific, as of an antigen to its corresponding antibody. **2** The ability of a screening test to correctly identify a person who is disease-free. If $d$ is the number of persons tested who are both free of disease and negative on screening and $b$ those free of disease but positive on screening the specificity of the screening test is defined as $d/(b + d)$. **carrier s.** The phenomenon whereby antibody formation to a hapten is produced only in response to injection of the hapten coupled to an antigen (the carrier) to which the antibody-former shows a T-helper cell response. **diagnostic s.** The probability of a negative diagnostic test result in the absence of the disease for which the test is designed to detect. It is equal to the number of true negatives divided by the sum of false positives and true negatives multiplied by 100. Compare DIAGNOSTIC SENSITIVITY. **neuronal s.** The invariant functional arrangement, location, connections, and neurotransmitters of a given neuron.

**specillum** \spəsil′əm\ [L (from *specere* to see), a surgical instrument for probing wounds and ulcers] A small surgical probe or sound.

**specimen** \spes′imən\ [L (from *specere* to spy, look at, see, akin to Gk *skeptesthai* to look at or into), a proof, token, mark, pattern, example, specimen] A small sample of a tissue, substance, or material obtained with the purpose of determining its nature or making a diagnosis. **cytologic s.** A sample of individual cells that is obtained from solid tissue. It is spread over the surface of a microscope slide prior to staining and examination.

**speckle** The granular appearance seen in images using ultrasound and lasers.

**SPECT** single photon emission computed tomography.

**spectacles** EYEGLASSES. **compound s.** Eyeglass frames that will receive interchangeable or additional lenses or filters. **decentered s.** A prism effect obtained by displacing the optical center away from the pupillary center. **half-glass s.** Reading glasses for presbyopes, corresponding to the lower bifocal portion of presbyopic glasses, the upper half being absent. **stenopeic s.** Eyeglass frames containing only a narrow slit through which the patient may look. See also STENOPEIC SLIT. **wire frame s.** Protective spectacles made of wire gauze with a fine mesh to protect against foreign bodies entering the eye.

**spectinomycin** $C_{14}H_{24}N_2O_7$. Decahydro-4*a*,7,9-trihydroxy-2-methyl-6,8-bis(methylamino)-4*H*-pyrano[2,3-*b*]-[1,4]benzodioxin-4-one. An aminocyclitol antibiotic differing in structure from the aminoglycosides. It is bacteriostatic rather than bacteriocidal, and it inhibits protein synthesis. It is used to treat *Neisseria gonorrhoeae* infections where penicillin is contraindicated. Also *actinospectacin.*

**spectinomycin hydrochloride** $C_{14}H_{26}Cl_2N_2O_7$. The dihydrochloride pentahydrate salt of spectinomycin. It has the same actions and uses as the parent drug. It can be given intramuscularly and thus is useful in treating some gonorrheal infections.

**spectra** \spek′trə\ Plural of SPECTRUM.

**spectral** Concerning a spectrum.

**spectrin** \spek′trin\ A filamentous protein which is part of the erythrocyte cytoskeleton. Spectrin is composed of $\alpha$ and $\beta$ subunits and may exist either as an $\alpha\beta$ dimer of MW 250 000 or as a tetramer of MW 500 000. Together with actin and other cytoskeleton proteins it forms a network that confers shape and flexibility to the erythrocyte membrane.

**spectro-** \spek′trə-\ [L *spectrum* specter, image] A combining form meaning spectrum, spectral.

**spectrocolorimeter** \-kul′ərim′ətər\ A color-matching device using a spectral light source.

**spectrofluorometer** \-flooräm′ətər\ An analytic instrument that performs fluorescence spectrometry of high selectivity by subjecting emitted fluorescent light to analysis of the emission spectrum.

**spectrogram** \spek′trəgram\ [SPECTRO- + -GRAM] A photograph or diagram of a spectrum, such as obtained from a spectrograph. **olfactory s.** A graphic representation of a subject's ability to detect a range of odors. A number of different odors are presented using a blast olfactometer, and the minimum perceptible odor is charted for each. Also *odorogram.*

**spectrograph** \spek′trəgraf\ [SPECTRO- + -GRAPH] An instrument for displaying or recording spectra, as from electromagnetic or sound waves. **mass s.** MASS SPECTROMETER. **x-ray s.** 1 An apparatus for analysis of crystal structure by x rays. 2 The photographic recording of the results of crystal analysis by x rays.

**spectrometer** \spekträm′ətər\ [SPECTRO- + -METER] 1 A device used for measuring the wavelengths of light, often involving a prism that refracts the various wavelengths to different degrees, followed by a slit that selects only those wavelengths of interest to the experimenter. 2 A device used in the study of x radiation or gamma radiation to measure the photon energies, particularly when these need to be sorted so that photons in an energy band of interest can be picked out for special study. 3 Any instrument that similarly processes neutrons or other particulate radiations. **mass s.** An instrument that can analyze isotopes by separating nuclei differing in their charge-to-mass ratios by passing them through electrical and magnetic fields. Also *mass spectrograph.* **pulse-height s.** PULSE-HEIGHT ANALYZER. **x-ray s.** An apparatus used to analyze substances by means of x rays reflected or scattered from the substance.

**spectrometry** \spekträm′ətrē\ [SPECTRO- + -METRY] The measurement of wavelength distribution of light and other electromagnetic radiations by means of a spectrometer. **x-ray emission s.** The analysis of substances by the detection of the characteristic x rays emitted when the substances are irradiated.

**spectrophotofluorometer** \-fō′tōflooräm′ətər\ A spectrophotometer that uses the technique of fluorimetry to measure the fluorescence spectrum of a substance.

**spectrophotometer** \-fōtäm′ətər\ An instrument that measures the intensity of light transmitted by a substance in different parts of the ultraviolet, visible, or infrared spectrum. It contains a light source, a wavelength selector, a sample holder, and a photometer, and determines the amount of absorbing substance in the sample. Adj. spectrophotometric.

**spectrophotometry** \-fōtäm′ətrē\ Analysis using a spectrophotometer. **atomic absorption s.** An analytical technique in which light of a specific wavelength corresponding to the element to be analyzed is absorbed by the analyte in an amount proportional to its concentration in the sample. The resultant decrease in light intensity is then measured. In clinical chemistry the element to be analyzed is usually metallic. **flame emission s.** An analytic method in which light passing through a chemical solution that is vaporized by a flame emits radiations of various wavelengths, the length and intensity of which can be measured.

**spectropolarimeter** \pō′lərim′ətər\ An instrument for measuring in a substance the optical rotation of plane-polarized light at different wavelengths.

**spectroscope** \spek′trəskōp\ [SPECTRO- + -SCOPE] An instrument that disperses light into its spectrum, magnifies it, and displays it for observation. **direct vision s.** A small spectroscope used for spectroscopic examination of the blood *in vivo,* as from the earlobe or web of the thumb.

**spectroscopy** \spekträs′kəpē\ [SPECTRO- + -SCOPY] The identification of compounds singly or in mixtures according to their ability to absorb radiant energy at specific wavelengths. Also *microabsorption spectroscopy.* **infrared s.** The study of the absorption patterns produced when substances are exposed to electromagnetic radiation in the infrared region of the spectrum, especially of wavelength 2.5–15$\mu$m (4000–670 cm$^{-1}$). Quanta of the energy corresponding to this range excite molecular vibrations, and hence the absorption patterns provide information about the configuration of various atomic groupings within the molecule. **microabsorption s.** SPECTROSCOPY.

**spectrum** \spek′trəm\ [L (from *specere* to spy, look at, see, akin to Gk *skeptesthai* to look at or into), a specter, image, phantom, vision] (*pl.* spectra, spectrums) 1 A visual display of the distribution of intensities of radiation as a function of wavelength, or energy. 2 See under ANTIBIOTIC SPECTRUM. 3 Any continuous range of values, qualities, or orderable entities. Adj. spectral. **absorption s.** The graph obtained by plotting the absorbance of a material, usually a solution, against the wavelength of electromagnetic radiation absorbed. It is sometimes presented as a plot of transmission against wavelength. **antibiotic s.** The range of microorganisms against which a given antibiotic is effective. Also *antimicrobial spectrum.* **chromatic s.** The range of wavelengths of electromagnetic vibrations that gives rise to color sensation. Also *color spectrum.* **diffraction s.** A spectrum that is produced by passing light through a diffraction grating. Also *grating spectrum.* **electromagnetic s.** The complete range of wavelengths of electromagnetic radiations, including radio waves, infrared waves, visible light, ultraviolet rays and x rays. **excitation s.** Those wavelengths of light absorbed by photoluminescent material that excite the material to fluorescence. **fluorescence s.** The characteristic wavelengths of light emitted by material that has been excited by absorption of light. The photons emitted have lower energy and longer wavelengths than those of the light absorbed. **fortification s.** TEICHOPSIA. **grating s.** DIFFRACTION SPECTRUM. **normal s.** A diffraction spectrum in which the deviation of each color from the direction of the incident light is proportional to its wavelength. **pure s.** A range of wavelengths of electromagnetic vibrations that is not associated with color mixing. **thermal s.** That range of wavelengths of electromagnetic vibrations comprising the infrared rays. **visible s.** The range of the electromagnetic spectrum, from about 390 nm to about 770 nm, capable of stimulating the visual system.

**speculum** \spek′yələm\ [L (from *specere* to spy, look at, see + *-ulum,* dim. or instrumental suffix) a mirror] (*pl.* specula, speculums) A surgical instrument used for exploring the interior of a body passage or cavity. **anal s.** A surgical instrument used for exploring the inside of the anal canal or rectum. **Aufricht's s.** A retractor to provide exposure of the nasal dorsum during rhinoplasty. **aural s.** One of a variety of specula for examining or treating the ear by way of the external auditory meatus. **Brinkerhoff s.** A surgical rectal speculum having a sliding lateral panel to explore the rectal canal walls. **duck-billed s.** SIMS SPECULUM. **esophageal s.** A speculum with built-in proximal illumination for examining the interior of the hypopharynx and upper esophagus. It is particularly useful for the removal of foreign bodies or the taking of biopsy specimens from these regions. Also *hypopharyngoscope, pharyngoscope.* **eye s.** A surgical device for holding the eyelids apart. **Hartmann s.** **1** A bivalve nasal speculum in which the blades separate when the handles are approximated. **2** A variety of aural speculum. **s. helmontii** *Outmoded* CENTRUM TENDINEUM. **Kelly s.** A surgical speculum consisting of a metal cylinder and obdurator. It is designed to visualize the anorectal area. **Killian nasal s.** A nasal speculum with long blades separated by approximating the handles and maintained in the separated position by a screw. It is of use particularly in operations on the nose. **Martin and Davy s.** A surgical rectal speculum consisting of a conical metal tube and matching obdurator. **nasal s.** A speculum for dilating the anterior nares or the nasal cavity when examining or operating on the interior of the nose. **nasopharyngeal s.** A speculum passed through the mouth of an anesthetized patient to expose the posterior wall of the nasopharynx and the fossae of Rosenmüller. It is rarely used today. Also *Yankauer speculum.* **Pedersen s.** A vaginal speculum with narrow flattened blades. **rectal s.** Any

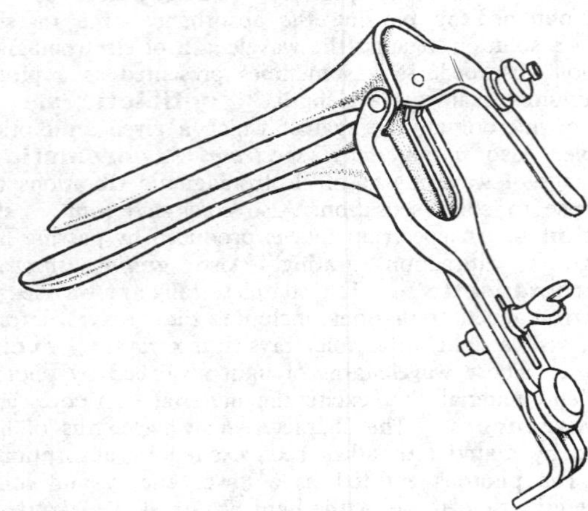

Pedersen speculum

speculum designed to explore the rectal canal walls for diagnostic and therapeutic purposes. **Siegle's pneumatic ear s.** SIEGLE'S OTOSCOPE. **Sims s.** A vaginal speculum with two blades with each resembling the bill of a duck. Also *duck-billed speculum.* **stop s.** A device used in ophthalmic surgery for separating the edges of an incision, and capable of being set to arrest the size of the opening at a predetermined distance. **Thudichum s.** A simple nasal speculum consisting of two small blades connected by a U-shaped spring. **urethral s.** An instrument for exposing the urethra. **vaginal s.** An instrument for exposing the vagina and portio of the cervix. **Yankauer s.** NASOPHARYNGEAL SPECULUM.

**Spee** [Ferdinand Graf von *Spee,* German embryologist, 1855–1937] See under CURVE.

**speech** [Old English *spæc, spræc*] Spoken discourse or language. **ataxic s.** Dysarthria in which there is incoordination of the muscles controlling articulation so that speech becomes slurred and often jerky, as in cerebellar ataxia. Also *cerebellar speech.* **clipped s.** Speech in which the words or syllables are clipped short. Also *scamping speech.* **echo s.** ECHOLALIA. **esophageal s.** The speech characteristic of the postlaryngectomy patient. Laryngeal activity is replaced by hypopharyngeal control of an air reservoir in the upper esophagus, created by swallowing air. **interjectional s.** Speech consisting largely of expletives or other disjointed but infrequent utterances, in expressive aphasia. **jumbled s.** JARGON APHASIA. **mirror s.** A speech defect in which letters or syllables of words, or the words of a phrase, are spoken in the reverse order. **nasal s.** NASAL RESONANCE. **scamping s.** CLIPPED SPEECH. **scanning s.** Ataxic speech in which there is marked slurring of the words but also with undue separation of the individual syllables. **scattered s.** Speech characterized by irrelevant and illogical utterances, neologisms, and incomprehensible condensations of multiple ideas, as seen in hebephrenic schizophrenia when there is marked loosening of associations. **slurred s.** Speech of the kind where words are pronounced indistinctly and run together, as in the dysarthria of alcoholic intoxication. **spastic s.** Dysarthria which often has a somewhat explosive character due to spasticity of the muscles which control articulation. **staccato s.** Speech in which the words and syllables are unduly separated and sometimes abbreviated so that features of both clipped and scanning speech are present. This type of speech is sometimes observed, for example, in subjects with multiple sclerosis. Also *syllabic speech.* **telegraphic s.** Abbreviated speech or writing with poverty of words and omission of prepositions and of anything other than simple nouns, verbs, and adjectives, as in composing a telegram. This may be one manifestation of motor or expressive aphasia. It is also typical of the early stages in normal language development, between two and three years of age. Also *telegrammatism.*

**spelencephalia** \spē′lənsəfā′lyə\ [L *spel(aeum)* a cave, cavern + ENCEPHAL- + -IA] PORENCEPHALY.

**spell** [early modern English (from Old English *spala* a substitute) relief, shift, turn] In morbidity statistics, a continuous period during which an individual is in a given state, as a spell of sickness, disability, or hospitalization. **breath-holding s.** See under BREATH-HOLDING.

**Spemann** [Hans *Spemann,* German biologist, 1869–1941] See under INDUCTION.

**Spence** [James *Spence,* Scottish surgeon, born 1812] Tail of Spence, axillary tail of Spence. See under AXILLARY TAIL OF BREAST.

**Spencer** [Roscoe Roy *Spencer,* U.S. physician, born 1888] Spencer-Parker vaccine. See under VACCINE.

**Spengler** [Carl *Spengler,* Swiss physician, 1860–1937] **1** Spengler's fragments. See under FRAGMENT. **2** See under TUBERCULIN.

**Spens** [Thomas *Spens,* Scottish physician, 1769–1842] Spens syndrome. See under ADAMS-STOKES SYNDROME.

**sperm** \spurm\ [Gk *sperma* seed, semen] SPERMATOZOON. **muzzled s.** Spermatozoa that are unable to adhere to the surface of the ovum.

**sperm-** \spurm-\ SPERMATO-.

**sperma** \spur′mə\ [Gk *sperma* seed, semen] SEMEN.

**spermacrasia** \spur′məkrā′zhə\ [SPERM- + Gk *akrasia* (from *a-* priv. + *kratos* force, power) weakness, impotence] An abnormally low number of spermatozoa in the semen. Also *spermatacrasia.*

**spermagglutination** \spur′magloo′tinā′shən\ [SPERM + AGGLUTINATION] Immobilization of sperm secondary to antibody production causing agglutination usually prior to ejaculation. The clumping of a number of spermatozoa usually results from the binding of a large molecule (fertilizin) to a smaller molecule (antifertilizin) on the plasma membrane of the spermatozoon.

**spermat-** \spurmat-\ SPERMATO-.

**spermatacrasia** \spur′mətəkrā′zhə\ SPERMACRASIA.

**spermateliosis** \spur′mətē′lē·ō′sis\ [Gk *sperma* seed, semen + *teleiōsis* (from *telos* end, accomplishment) development, attainment] SPERMIOGENESIS.

**spermatemphraxis** \spur′mətemfrak′sis\ [SPERMAT- + Gk *emphraxis* blockage] Blockage of the discharge of semen.

**spermatic** \spərmat′ik\ Pertaining to, transporting, or resembling sperm or semen.

**spermaticidal** \spur′mətisī′dəl\ [SPERMAT- + *i* + *-cid(e)* + -AL] Destructive or lethal to spermatozoa. Also *spermicidal, spermatocidal.*

**spermaticide** \spərmat′isīd\ [SPERMAT- + *i* + -CIDE] Any substance that destroys or is lethal to spermatozoa. Also *spermatozoicide, spermatocide, spermicide.*

**spermatid** \spur′mətid, spərmat′id\ [SPERMAT- + -ID] A male sex cell formed by division of a secondary spermatocyte in spermatogenesis, and giving rise to a spermatozoon during spermiogenesis. Also *spermatoblast, spermid, spermoblast, androcyte, nematoblast.*

**spermatism** \spur′mətizm\ [SPERMAT- + -ISM] The passage or formation of semen.

**spermatitis** \spur′mətī′tis\ [SPERMAT- + -ITIS] Inflammation of the funiculus spermaticus.

**spermato-** \spur′mətō-, spərmat′ō-\ [Gk *sperma* (genitive *spermatos*) seed, semen] A combining form meaning (1) seed; (2) spermatozoa; (3) semen. Also *sperm-, spermo-.*

**spermatocele** \spur′mətōsēl′, spərmat′ə-\ [SPERMATO- + -CELE[1]] An intrascrotal cyst containing spermatozoa, palpable as a round scrotal mass and resulting from a partial obstruction of the spermatic tubules. The etiology is unknown. Also *hydrospermatocele, spermatocyst.*

**spermatocelectomy** \-sēlek′təmē\ Excision of a spermatocele.

**spermatocidal** \-sī′dəl\ SPERMATICIDAL.

**spermatocide** \spərmat′əsīd, spur′mətō-\ SPERMATICIDE.

**spermatocyst** \spərmat′əsist, spur′mətō-\ [SPERMATO- + CYST] **1** VESICULA SEMINALIS. **2** SPERMATOCELE.

**spermatocystectomy** \-sistek′təmē\ [SPERMATOCYST + -ECTOMY] Surgical excision of the vesicula seminalis.

**spermatocystitis** \-sistī′tis\ [SPERMATOCYST + -ITIS] SEMINAL VESICULITIS.

**spermatocystotomy** \-sistät′əmē\ [SPERMATOCYST + *o* + -TOMY] Incision of a seminal vesicle, especially to allow drainage.

**spermatocyte** \spərmat′əsīt, spur′mətō-\ [SPERMATO- + -CYTE] A male sex cell situated in the wall of the seminiferous tubules of the testis and resulting from the division of a spermatogonium (type B). The production of spermatocytes is effected only from the start of puberty, and their transformation is marked by a relatively small but rapid increase in volume of the cell. **primary s.** A male sex cell resulting from division of a type B spermatogonium in the seminiferous tubules of the testis at the start of spermatogenesis. Primary spermatocytes have a diploid number of chromosomes. Also *spermiocyte.* **secondary s.** A male sex cell derived from a primary spermatocyte during spermatogenesis. During this process a primary spermatocyte, with $2n$ chromosomes, becomes two secondary spermatocytes, with $n$ chromosomes, accompanied by a large reduction in volume of the cell. The secondary spermatocytes in turn divide into two spermatids. Also *prespermatid.*

**spermatocytogenesis** \-sī′təjen′əsis\ [*spermatocyt(e)* + *o* + GENESIS] The first stage of spermatogenesis during which the spermatogonia are transformed first into spermatocytes and then into spermatids.

**spermatocytoma** \-sītō′mə\ [*spermatocyt(e)* + -OMA] SEMINOMA.

**spermatogenesis** \-jen′əsis\ [SPERMATO- + GENESIS] A series of stages in cellular differentiation which result in the formation of spermatozoa. Two stages are often recognized, spermatocytogenesis and spermiogenesis. Also *spermatogeny.*

**spermatogenic** \-jen′ik\ **1** Relating to spermatogenesis. **2** Producing spermatozoa.

**spermatogenous** \spur′mətäj′ənəs\ Able to produce spermatozoa.

**spermatogeny** \spur′mətäj′ənē\ SPERMATOGENESIS.

**spermatogonia** \-gō′nē·ə\ Plural of SPERMATOGONIUM.

**spermatogonium** \-gō′nē·əm\ [New L, from SPERMATO- + GON-[2] + *-ium,* noun suffix] A male sex cell arising by mitotic division of the primordial germ cells in the embryonic testis. Each germ cell divides into two dark type A spermatogonia. Each of these later divides into a dark type A spermatogonium and a light type A spermatogonium. The former repeats the process whereas the latter divides to produce two type B spermatogonia; it is these which then divide to produce the primary spermatocytes.

**spermatolysin** \spur′mətäl′isin\ [SPERMATO- + LYSIN] A substance capable of decomposing spermatozoa.

**spermatolysis** \spur′mətäl′isis\ [SPERMATO- + LYSIS] Dissolution of spermatozoa. Also *spermolysis.*

**spermatolytic** \-lit′ik\ Capable of causing dissolution of spermatozoa. Also *spermolytic.*

**spermatorrhea** \spur′mətôrē′ə\ [SPERMATO- + -RRHEA] Excessive and involuntary emission of semen without orgasm. Also *spermorrhea, gonacratia.* **s. dormientum** NOCTURNAL EMISSION. **false s.** Involuntary and excessive discharge of seminal fluid lacking spermatozoa.

**spermatotoxin** \-täk′sin\ A toxin destructive to spermatozoa, especially an antibody specific for spermatozoa. Also *spermotoxin, spermolysin, spermatotoxin.* Adj. spermatotoxic.

**spermatovum** \spur′mətō′vəm\ [SPERMAT- + OVUM] An ovum that has been fertilized by a spermatozoon.

**spermatoxin** \spur′mətäk′sin\ SPERMATOTOXIN.

**spermatozoa** \-zō′ə\ Plural of SPERMATOZOON.

**spermatozoicide** \-zō′isīd\ SPERMATICIDE.

**spermatozoon** \-zō′än\ [SPERMATO- + Gk *zōon* living being, animal] (*pl.* spermatozoa) A male sex cell which, after having passed through the stages in spermatogenesis of spermatogonium, primary and secondary spermatocytes, and spermatid, reaches maturity and could become capable of fertilizing an ovum. It develops from a spermatid, which is held in the wall of the seminiferous tubule where it develops a flagellum. It is then liberated into the lumen of the tubule as a spermatozoon, and undergoes a further ripening process

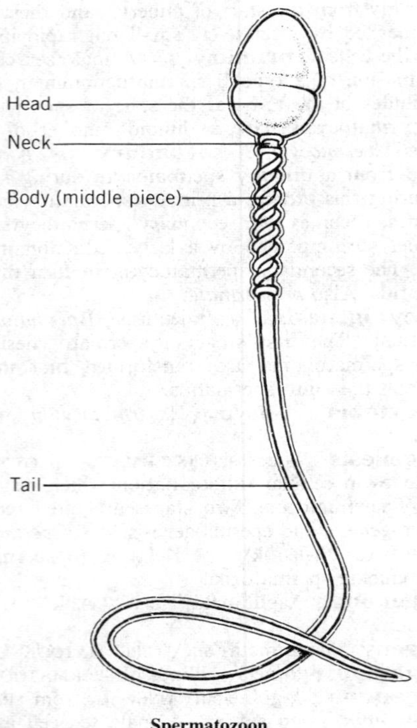

**Spermatozoon**

by its passage through the male genital tract, to be completed by capacitation in the female genital tract. In man it has an ovoid head 4 μm long, a very short neck (0.3 μm), a middle piece (4 μm), and a principal piece or a tail about 40 μm long. Also *sperm, sperm cell, zoosperm.*

**spermectomy** \spərmek′təmē\ [SPERM- + -ECTOMY] Surgical excision of a portion of the funiculus spermaticus.

**spermiation** \spur′mē·ā′shən\ [New L *spermi(um)* (prob. from Gk *spermeion* sperm, seed, from *sperma* sperm, seed) spermatozoon + -ATION] The release of spermatozoa from the Sertoli cells of the testes.

**spermicidal** \spur′misī′dəl\ SPERMATICIDAL.

**spermicide** \spur′misīd\ SPERMATICIDE.

**spermidine** $NH_2—[CH_2]_3—NH—[CH_2]_4—NH_2$. One of the polyamines, existing in neutral solution as its triply charged cation. This occurs bound to DNA, which it stabilizes. Its biosynthesis involves transfer of the 3-aminopropyl group from decarboxylated *S*-adenosylmethionine onto putrescine.

**spermiduct** \spur′midukt\ The excretory duct for spermatozoa; both ductus deferens and ductus ejaculatorius.

**spermine** $NH_2—[CH_2]_3—NH—[CH_2]_4—NH—[CH_2]_3—NH_2$. One of the polyamines, existing in neutral solution as its quadruply charged cation. This occurs bound to DNA, which it stabilizes. Its biosynthesis involves transfer of the 3-aminopropyl group from decarboxylated *S*-adenosylmethionine onto spermidine.

**spermiogenesis** \spur′mē·ōjen′əsis\ [New L *spermi(um)* (from Gk *spermeion* sperm, from *sperma* seed, germ) spermatozoon + *o* + GENESIS] The second stage of spermatogenesis during which the spermatids become transformed into spermatozoa by a complicated process of differentiation. Also *spermateliosis.*

**spermioteleosis** \spur′mē·ōtel′ē·ō′sis\ [New L *spermi(um)* + *o* + Gk *teleiōsis* completeness, development] The successive changes through which a cell derived from a spermatogonium becomes a mature spermatozoon, that is, from primary to secondary spermatocyte to spermatid. Adj. spermioteleotic.

**spermo-** \spur′mə-, spur′mō-\ SPERMATO-.

**spermocytoma** \-sītō′mə\ [SPERMO- + CYT- + -OMA] SEMINOMA.

**spermolith** \spur′məlith\ [SPERM- + *o* + -LITH] A stone located in a seminal duct.

**spermoloropexis** \-lôr′ōpek′sis\ SPERMOLOROPEXY.

**spermoloropexy** \-lôr′ōpek′sē\ [SPERM- + *o* + Gk *lōro(n)* a thong + -PEXY] Surgical attachment of the funiculus spermaticus to the pubic periosteum in correcting an undescended testicle. Also *spermoloropexis.*

**spermolysin** \spərmäl′isin\ SPERMATOTOXIN.

**spermolysis** \spərmäl′isis\ SPERMATOLYSIS.

**spermolytic** \-lit′ik\ SPERMATOLYTIC.

**spermophlebectasia** \-fleb′ektā′zhə\ [SPERMO- + PHLEB- + ECTASIA] The presence of varices in the spermatic veins.

**spermoplasm** \spur′məplazm\ [SPERMO- + -PLASM] Protoplasm contained within a spermatid, which is gradually used up or transformed during spermiogenesis.

**spermorrhea** \spur′môrē′ə\ SPERMATORRHEA.

**spermosphere** \spur′məsfir\ [SPERMO- + *sphere*] The closely arranged group of spermatids formed by division of secondary spermatocytes.

**spermotoxin** \-täk′sin\ SPERMATOTOXIN.

**spes phthisica** \spēs tiz′ikə\ [L *spes* hope + New L *phthisica* phthisic] A characteristic feeling of hopefulness noted in some tuberculosis patients about the prospect of recovery.

**sphacelation** \sfas′əlā′shən\ [Gk *sphakel(os)* gangrene + -ATION] The formation of gangrene.

**sphacelinic acid** One of the active principles isolated from ergot.

**sphacelism** \sfas′əlizm\ A gangrenous condition.

**sphaceloid** \sfas′əloid\ Resembling gangrene; gangrenous.

**sphacelus** \sfas′ələs\ [Gk *sphakelos* gangrene] A gangrenous or necrotic mass of tissue; slough. Adj. sphacelous.

**sphagiasmus** \sfā′jē·az′məs\ [Gk *sphagiasmos* (from *sphagē* slaughter, sacrifice, the throat) a slaying, sacrifice] **1** PETIT MAL. **2** Tonic or clonic contraction of neck muscles in an attack of epilepsy.

**sphenic** \sfē′nik\ SPHENOID.

**spheno-** \sfē′nō-\ [Gk *sphēn* a wedge] A combining form meaning (1) wedge, wedge-shaped; (2) sphenoid bone.

**sphenobasilar** \-bas′ilər\ Pertaining to the sphenoid bone and the basilar part of the occipital bone.

**sphenocephaly** \-sef′əlē\ [SPHENO- + CEPHAL- + -Y] A condition marked by a wedge-shaped appearance of the head or cranium. It is most often a form of oxycephaly.

**sphenoid** \sfē′noid\ [*sphen(o)-* + -OID] **1** Wedge-shaped. Also *sphenic.* **2** OS SPHENOIDALE.

**sphenoidal** \sfēnoi′dəl\ Pertaining to the sphenoid bone.

**sphenoiditis** \sfē′noidī′tis\ SPHENOIDAL SINUSITIS.

**sphenoidostomy** \sfē′noidäs′təmē\ An operation to enlarge the ostium of the sphenoidal sinus by the transnasal route. It is performed in order to provide or improve drainage in cases of sphenoidal sinusitis.

**sphenoidotomy** \sfē′noidät′əmē\ An incision made to gain access to the sphenoidal sinus by one of three routes: through the nose, between the layers of the nasal septum following submucous resection of the septum, or by way of the exenterated ethmoidal labyrinth.
**sphenoparietal** \-pərī′ətəl\ Of or pertaining to the sphenoid and the parietal bone.
**sphenosis** \sfēnō′sis\ [SPHENO- + -SIS] A wedging of the fetus into the pelvis during labor.
**sphenotic** \sfēnō′tik\ **1** Pertaining to a center of ossification in the developing sphenoid bone which gives rise to the lingula covering the carotid groove. **2** Pertaining to the strip of cartilage joining the periotic cartilage to the sphenoid.
**sphenotribe** \sfē′nōtrīb\ [SPHENO- + Gk *trib(ein)* to rub, pound, grind] An instrument used to crush the base of the fetal skull.
**sphenotripsy** \sfē′nōtrip′sē\ [SPHENO- + -TRIPSY] The crushing of the fetal skull with a sphenotribe.
**sphenoturbinal** \-tur′binəl\ Of or relating to the concha sphenoidalis.
**sphere** \sfir\ [L *sphaera,* from Gk *sphaira* a ball, sphere, globe] **1** A round three-dimensional body in the shape of a ball; globe. **2** A range or field of interest or activity. **conflict-free ego s.** That part of the ego whose energies derive from deneutralization of the sexual and aggressive drives, and which is thus available for dealing with reality in a constructive and creative rather than rigidly constricted way. **Morgagni s.'s** Aberrant globular lens fibers following extracapsular cataract extraction. **neurosecretory s.** NEUROSECRETORY GRANULE.
**spherical** \sfir′ikəl, sfer′-\ Relating to or shaped like a sphere.
**sphero-** \sfir′ō-\ [Gk *sphaira* ball, globe] A combining form meaning sphere, spherical. Also *spher-*.
**spherocylinder** \-sil′indər\ [SPHERO- + CYLINDER] TORIC LENS. Adj. spherocylindrical.
**spherocyte** \sfir′əsīt\ A spherical erythrocyte, characteristic of hereditary spherocytosis and some acquired immune hemolytic disease. Also *fragilocyte, microspherocyte.*
**spherocytic** \-sit′ik\ Pertaining to or characterized by spherocytosis.
**spherocytosis** \-sītō′sis\ [*spherocyt(e)* + -OSIS] The presence in blood of spherical, rather than the normal biconcave, erythrocytes. Spherocytosis is observed following transfusion of normal blood, following severe burns, as a feature of autoimmune hemolytic anemia, and as an inherited disorder (hereditary spherocytosis). Also *fragilocytosis, microspherocytosis.* **hereditary s.** An inherited hemolytic disorder resulting from a defect in the erythrocyte cytoskeleton that confers an abnormal spherical shape to erythrocytes. Hereditary spherocytosis exhibits autosomal dominant inheritance. Also *congenital hemolytic anemia, chronic familial icterus, congenital familial icterus, congenital hemolytic icterus, familial hemolytic icterus, congenital hemolytic jaundice, Minkowski-Chauffard syndrome.*
**spheroid** \sfir′oid\ [SPHERE + -OID] **1** Resembling a sphere, as in shape. Also *spheroidal.* **2** A spheroid body or structure.
**spheroidin** \sfiroi′din\ TETRODOTOXIN.
**spherometer** \sfiräm′ətər\ [SPHERO- + -METER] An instrument for measuring the curvature of a surface such as an optical lens.
**spherophakia** \-fā′kē·ə\ [SPHERO- + PHAK- + -IA ] Abnormal smallness and roundness of the lens, as in the Marchesani syndrome. Also *microphakia, microlentia.*
**spheroplast** \sfir′əplast\ [SPHERO- + -PLAST] A Gram-negative bacterium from which the cell wall is partially removed, allowing the organism to assume a spherical, osmotically sensitive form. The adherent outer membrane and wall fragments differentiate it from a protoplast.
**spherule** \sfer′ʸool\ A small sphere; a globule. **rod s.** The invagination at the base of retinal rods forming the synaptic region contacted by bipolar and horizontal cells.
**sphincter** \sfingk′tər\ [Gk *sphinktēr* (from *sphingein* to bind tight, bind in or together, squeeze) a tight binder, lace, band] MUSCULUS SPHINCTER. **anatomic s.** A ringlike band of muscle fibers that constricts or closes an orifice. **s. angularis** The circular muscle fibers of the stomach wall at the angular incisure which may mark the commencement of the pyloric antrum. No anatomical sphincter or sphincteric action is, in fact, present here. *Outmoded.* Also *angular sphincter.* **artificial s.** A mechanical or surgically constructed substitute for a natural sphincter. **s. of bile duct** MUSCULUS SPHINCTER DUCTUS CHOLEDOCHI. **s. of Boyden** MUSCULUS SPHINCTER DUCTUS CHOLEDOCHI. **canalicular s.** A sphincter surrounding a duct or tubular structure along its course at a site other than its orifice. *Outmoded.* **Cannon, Boehm, and Roith s.** *Outmoded* CANNON'S RING. **cardiac s.** Well-developed oblique muscle fibers near the cardiac orifice of the stomach, where they are continuous with the deep circular fibers of the esophagus. Although there is no true anatomical sphincter, they serve as a functional sphincter for some hold-up of food before entering the stomach. Also *cardioesophageal sphincter.* **choledochal s.** MUSCULUS SPHINCTER DUCTUS CHOLEDOCHI. **s. of common bile duct** MUSCULUS SPHINCTER DUCTUS CHOLEDOCHI. **cricopharyngeal s.** PARS CRICOPHARYNGEA MUSCULI CONSTRICTORIS PHARYNGIS INFERIORIS. **s. of duct of Wirsung** MUSCULUS SPHINCTER DUCTUS PANCREATICI. **duodenal s.** MUSCULUS SPHINCTER AMPULLAE HEPATOPANCREATICAE. **external s. of anus** MUSCULUS SPHINCTER ANI EXTERNUS. **s. of eye** MUSCULUS ORBICULARIS OCULI. **Giordano s.** MUSCULUS SPHINCTER DUCTUS CHOLEDOCHI. **Glisson s.** MUSCULUS SPHINCTER AMPULLAE HEPATOPANCREATICAE. **hepatic s.** Longitudinal muscle bundles in the tunica adventitia of the hepatic veins which are thickened prior to their entry into the inferior vena cava, providing the incorrect perception of a sphincter. **s. of hepatopancreatic ampulla** MUSCULUS SPHINCTER AMPULLAE HEPATOPANCREATICAE. **ileal s.** A thickening of the circular and longitudinal muscle fibers in the terminal ileum which form a part of the free margin of the ileocolic valve. **internal s. of anus** MUSCULUS SPHINCTER ANI INTERNUS. **laryngeal s.** The vital sphincter mechanism closing the laryngeal inlet to the lower airways during deglutition. It consists of three parts: the inlet or aryepiglottic sphincter, the false vocal cord sphincter, and the true vocal cord or glottic sphincter. **Lütkens s.** An occasional thickening of the muscle fibers around the neck of the gallbladder. **Nélaton s.** NÉLATON'S FOLD. **O'Beirne s.** An external constriction, more apparent in the living, at the rectosigmoid junction. There is no anatomical sphincter present. Also *O'Beirne's valve.* **Oddi s.** MUSCULUS SPHINCTER AMPULLAE HEPATOPANCREATICAE. **ostial s.** A sphincter surrounding a natural orifice. **palatopharyngeal s.** The sphincter closing off the nasopharynx from the oropharynx on swallowing and during vocalizing. It is formed by a constant band of muscle fibers running transversely in the posterolateral wall of the pharynx and extending from the anterolateral aspect of the upper surface of the palatine aponeurosis to the inner surface of the superior constrictor muscle of the pharynx with which it fuses near the upper

border. When the soft palate is elevated it produces a visible, rounded ridge, or Passavant's bar, on the pharyngeal wall. It lies at a higher level than musculus palatopharyngeus. **pancreatic s.** An occasional ring of muscle fibers surrounding the termination of the main pancreatic duct, which usually become interwoven with those of the musculus sphincter ductus choledochi. Also *sphincter pancreaticus.* **physiologic s.** A region in which constriction or closure of an orifice is achieved in the absence of an obvious ringlike band of muscle fibers. **s. pupillae** MUSCULUS SPHINCTER PUPILLAE. **pyloric s.** MUSCULUS SPHINCTER PYLORICUS. **segmental s.** A sphincter surrounding a segment of a duct or tubular structure. **smooth muscle s.** An annular arrangement of unstriped muscle around an orifice such as the anus, the entrance of the esophagus into the stomach, and the entrance of the bile and pancreatic ducts into the duodenum. **striated muscular s.** RHABDOSPHINCTER. **tubal s.** **1** Fibers of the myometrium around the intramural, uterine part of the uterine tube which do not constitute a sphincter. **2** The circular muscle fibers in the isthmus of the uterine tube which are thickened and narrow the lumen considerably and are considered to produce a sphincterlike mechanism in slowing down the progress of the zygote towards the uterine cavity. **s. urethrae** MUSCULUS SPHINCTER URETHRAE. **s. vaginae** Musculus bulbospongiosus in the female.

**sphincteral** \sfingk′tərəl\ Of or pertaining to a sphincter. Also *sphincteric.*

**sphincteralgia** \-al′jə\ [SPHINCTER + -ALGIA] Pain in the region of the anal sphincter, generally of a spastic nature.

**sphincterectomy** \-ek′təmē\ [SPHINCTER + -ECTOMY] Surgical cutting of the sphincter muscle of the iris. Also *sphincterolysis.*

**sphincteric** \sfingkter′ik\ SPHINCTERAL.

**sphincterismus** \-iz′məs\ [SPHINCTER + L *-ismus* -ISM] Spasm of the muscles of a sphincter, particularly the anal sphincter.

**sphincteritis** \-ī′tis\ [SPHINCTER + -ITIS] Inflammation of a sphincter.

**sphincterolysis** \-äl′isis\ SPHINCTERECTOMY.

**sphincteroplasty** \sfingk′tərōplas′tē\ [SPHINCTER + *o* + -PLASTY] A surgical procedure to repair a damaged or nonfunctional naturally occurring sphincter.

**sphincteroscope** \sfingk′tərōskōp′\ A surgical speculum designed to expose a sphincter, such as the anal sphincter, to examination.

**sphincteroscopy** \-äs′kəpē\ Visual inspection of a sphincter, especially the anal sphincter.

**sphincterotome** \sfingk′tərōtōm′\ A surgical instrument designed to incise a muscular sphincter, frequently the anorectal sphincter.

**sphincterotomy** \-ät′əmē\ A surgical incision into or through a muscular sphincter. **internal s.** A surgical procedure in which all or part of the internal rectal sphincter is divided.

**sphinganine** $CH_3$—$[CH_2]_{14}$—CHOH—$CH(NH_2)$—$CH_2OH$. (2*S*,3*R*)- 2-Aminooctadecane-1,3-diol, a component of natural lipids. It is produced by the reduction of the ketone 3-dehydrosphinganine, synthesized from palmitoyl-CoA and serine. It is dehydrogenated with the formation of a 4(5)-*trans* double bond to give sphingosine.

**sphingo-** \sfing′gō-\ [See SPHINGOSINE.] A combining form designating a sphingoid or a relationship to sphingosine.

**sphingoid** Any of a class of compounds including sphinganine and its homologues and stereoisomers and their hydroxy and unsaturated derivatives.

**sphingolipid** Any lipid consisting of a combined sphingoid. Sphingolipids are important components of cellular membranes.

**sphingolipidoses** \sfing′gōlip′idō′sēz\ Plural of SPHINGOLIPIDOSIS.

**sphingolipidosis** \sfing′gōlip′idō′sis\ Any of the many inborn errors that may occur in sphingolipid metabolism, as in Niemann-Pick disease. Those now known involve an abnormal tissue accumulation of catabolic intermediates that cannot be degraded further because of a specific enzyme deficiency. Also *sphingolipodystrophy.* **late onset cerebral s.** ADULT CEROID-LIPOFUSCINOSIS.

**sphingolipodystrophy** \sfing′gōli′pōdis′trəfē \ SPHINGOLIPIDOSIS.

**sphingomyelin** \sfing′gōmīəlin\ Ceramide-1-phosphocholine, i.e. an *N*-acylated sphingoid esterified on C-1 with phosphoric acid, which is also esterified with choline. It is an important constituent of mammalian cell membranes. It is stored in abnormal amounts in the affected cells in Niemann-Pick disease. Also *phosphosphingoside, Niemann-Pick lipid.*

**sphingomyelinosis** \sfing′gōmī′əlinō′sis\ NIEMANN-PICK DISEASE.

**sphingophospholipid** A sphingolipid containing esterified phosphate.

**sphingosine** \sfing′gōsēn\ [Gk *Sphinx*, gen. *Sphingos*, the Sphinx + -INE; so named because of its enigmatic nature when first isolated] $CH_3$—$[CH_2]_{12}$—CH═CH—CHOH—$CH(NH_2)$—$CH_2OH$. The compound formed from sphinganine by dehydrogenation to introduce a 4(5)-*trans* double bond. It is one of the most important sphingoids of mammalian sphingolipids.

**sphygm-** \sfigm-\ SPHYGMO-.

**sphygmic** \sfig′mik\ [SPHYGM- + -IC] Relating to the pulse.

**sphygmo-** \sfig′mō-\ [Gk *sphygmos* throbbing, pulsation] A combining form denoting pulse. Also *sphygm-*.

**sphygmochronograph** \-krō′nəgraf\ A sphygmograph that records graphically the heartbeat and the waveform of the pulse to determine the delay between them.

**sphygmochronography** \-krōnäg′rəfē\ The simultaneous graphic recording of the heartbeat and the waveform of the pulse to determine the delay between them.

**sphygmodynamometer** \-dī′nəmäm′ətər\ An instrument that measures the force of the pulse.

**sphygmogenin** \sfigmäj′ənin\ *Older term* EPINEPHRINE.

**sphygmogram** \sfig′məgram\ [SPHYGMO- + -GRAM] The recording obtained by a sphygmograph.

**sphygmograph** \sfig′məgraf\ [SPHYGMO- + -GRAPH] An instrument for recording characteristics of the pulse wave.

**sphygmography** \sfigmäg′rəfē\ [SPHYGMO- + -GRAPHY] The use of the sphygmograph. **jugular pulse s.** The recording of the pulse wave from the jugular vein.

**sphygmomanometer** \-manäm′ətər\ [SPHYGMO- + MANOMETER] An instrument for measuring the blood pressure. A bladder within a cuff encircling the arm is inflated to occlude the artery. Air is bled off until a tapping sound is heard by auscultation, which indicates systolic pressure. A muffled or disappearing sound indicates diastolic pressure. Also *hemomanometer, sphygmometer.*

**sphygmomanometry** \-manäm′ətrē\ The measurement of blood pressure by means of a sphygmomanometer.

**sphygmometer** \sfigmäm′ətər\ SPHYGMOMANOMETER.

**sphygmoscope** \sfig′məskōp\ [SPHYGMO- + -SCOPE] An

instrument such as a sphygmograph which displays the pulse wave.

**sphygmus** \sfig′məs\ [Gk *sphygmos* throbbing, pulsation] PULSE.

**spica** \spī′kə\ SPICA BANDAGE.

**spicule** \spik′yool\ [L *spiculum.* See SPICULUM.] A spine-like projection. Also *spiculum.* **cemental s.** A slender projection of cementum from the root of a tooth. Also *cemental spike.*

**spiculum** \spik′yələm\ [L (dim. of *spicum* a spike, ear of corn, tuft or head of corn-shaped plant, akin to SPINA), a point, sting, dart, arrow] (*pl.* spicula) SPICULE.

**spider** 1 An arachnid of the order Araneida, with four pairs of legs, a single cephalothorax separated from the abdomen by a constriction, a cluster of up to eight eyes, and three or four pairs of spinnerets. Venom glands are usually present. Spiders are primarily insectivorous or feed on other arthropods and small animals. While the vast majority are harmless to humans, a few kinds are capable of inflicting a dangerous or even lethal bite. These include spiders of the genera *Latrodectus, Loxosceles, Atrax, Trechona, Phoneutria, Sericopelma,* and a few others. 2 A form or structure suggestive of a spider or a spider's web, as for example a telangiectasia. **arterial s.** SPIDER TELANGIECTASIS. **banana s.** A spider of the species *Heteropoda venatoria.* **black widow s.** A spider of the species *Latrodectus mactans.* **brown recluse s.** A spider of the species *Loxosceles reclusa.* **funnel-web s.** A spider of the family Dipluridae. **lynx s.** A hunting spider of the family Oxyopidae. See also *PEUCETIA VIRIDANS.* **tree funnel-web s.** A very aggressive Australian mygalomorph spider of the species *Atrax formidabilis.* **vascular s.** SPIDER TELANGIECTASIS. **wolf s.** Any member of the Lycosidae, a large cosmopolitan family of ground-dwelling hunting spiders. The well-known European tarantula, *Lycosa tarentula,* is a large wolf spider of southern Europe.

**Spiegelberg** [Otto *Spiegelberg,* German gynecologist, 1830–1881] Spiegelberg's criteria for ovarian pregnancy. See under CRITERION.

**Spiegler** [Eduard *Spiegler,* Austrian dermatologist, 1860–1908] Spiegler's tumors. See under ECCRINE DERMAL CYLINDROMA.

**Spielmeyer** [Walter *Spielmeyer,* German neurologist and physician, 1879–1935] Spielmeyer-Vogt disease, Vogt-Spielmeyer disease. See under JUVENILE CEROID-LIPOFUSCINOSIS.

**Spigelius** [Adrian *Spigelius* (van der Spieghel), Flemish botanist and anatomist, 1578–1625] Spieghel's line, Spigelius line. See under LINEA SEMILUNARIS.

**spike** [Middle English *spik* a head of grain, from L *spica* a spike, ear of corn (akin to SPINA). L *spica* is a variant of *spicum* spike.] 1 The electrical accompaniment of a nerve impulse. 2 In electroencephalography, a brief electrical discharge (20–40 ms) which appears as a pointed wave in the electroencephalogram. It must have an amplitude at least 50 percent greater than that of the basal rhythm. Generalized spike discharges may occur in idiopathic epilepsy, while focal spike discharges suggest the presence of an epileptogenic focus beneath the recording electrodes of the channel in which it is recorded. 3 In immunoelectrophoresis, a sharply angled upward deflection on a densitometric tracing. The principal deflection of an action potential, as recorded from a nerve fiber or neuron and observed oscilloscopically, in contrast to the smaller afterdischarges or afterpotentials; spike potential. **cemental s.** CEMENTAL SPICULE. **focal s.'s** In electroencephalography, spike discharges arising in a specific area of the brain and remaining localized there. **M s.** MONOCLONAL PEAK. **multiple s.'s** In electroencephalography, a burst of several successive spikes. **physiologic occipital s.'s** Sharp waves of medium amplitude, lacking the acute sharpness and high amplitude of the spike discharges normally associated with epilepsy and occurring in the occipital regions, especially during saccadic eye movements. Also *lambda waves.* **slow s.** A wave of sharp outline in the electroencephalogram, usually lasting for more than 40 ms, with an acute rise and slower fall, in some respects resembling the tooth of a saw. Some such waves are due to an epileptic discharge arising subcortically. Also *sawtooth, sharp wave.*

**spill** An overflow or escape of a substance from its normal confines. **cellular s.** The spreading of cells, particularly cancer cells in body cavities, as a result of manipulation, as during surgery.

**Spiller** [William Gibson *Spiller,* U.S. neurologist, 1863–1940] 1 Frazier-Spiller operation. See under OPERATION. 2 Spiller syndrome. See under SUBACUTE NECROTIC MYELITIS.

**spillway** \spil′wā\ One of the spaces between antagonistic occlusal surfaces which permit food to escape during compression in mastication. **occlusal s.** A spillway that does not extend to an axial surface.

**spilus** \spī′ləs\ [Gk *spilos* stain, spot, blemish] NEVUS.

**spin** 1 An intrinsic angular momentum (independent of translatory motion) possessed by several elementary particles, as if the particle were rotating about its axis. Each variety of elementary particle has its characteristic spin quantum number, which can be only a positive integer or half-integer. 2 The total angular momentum of an atomic nucleus, compounded of the spins of the nucleons and the angular momentum of their orbital motions.

**spin-** \spīn-\ [L *spina* thorn, spine] A combining form meaning (1) spine, spinal cord, spinal; (2) shaped like a spine, spiny, pointy. Also *spini-, spino-.*

**spina** \spī′nə\ [L (akin to *spica* spike) a thorn, spine] (*pl.* spinae) 1 [NA] A pointed, sharp bony process or projection. 2 The vertebral column: used in some clinical terms. For defs. 1 and 2 also *spine.* **s. bifida** A family of developmental defects characterized by absence of the vertebral arch, usually in a number of contiguous vertebrae. The spinal meninges and cord may herniate through the defect but remain covered by skin and subcutaneous tissue, as in me-

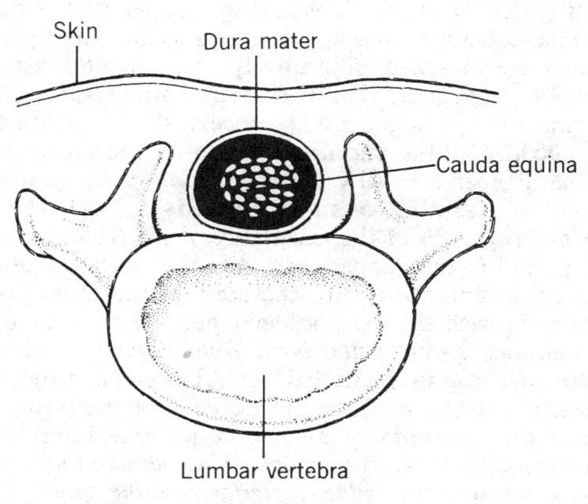

**Spina bifida occulta**

ningocele or meningomyelocele, or be exposed on the surface, as in rachischisis. Also *hydrocele spinalis, cleft spine.* **s. bifida anterior** A developmental defect of the anterior (ventral) wall of the spinal canal associated with defective development of the vertebral bodies in the thoracic and abdominal regions. **s. bifida aperta** A spina bifida that is open on the surface of the back, exposing to view nervous and meningeal tissues. **s. bifida cystica** A protruding, circumscribed mass on the back representing herniated meninges filled with cerebrospinal fluid, as in spinal meningocele, or herniated meninges containing spinal cord and cerebrospinal fluid, as in meningomyelocele. The herniated mass is usually covered by skin although the skin may be thin and transparent or may have been abraded. **s. bifida occulta** Spina bifida in which the neural arches are missing but in which the spinal cord and meninges remain *in situ* and there is no surface abnormality except the depression resulting from the absence of vertebral spines. **s. helicis** [NA] A small cartilaginous projection at the anterior extremity of the helix of the auricle just before it curves upwards. Also *spine of helix, apophysis helicis.* **s. iliaca anterior inferior** [NA] A small rounded projection at the lower end of the anterior border of the ilium situated just above the margin of the acetabulum and providing attachment for the straight head of rectus femoris muscle and the iliofemoral ligament. Also *anterior inferior iliac spine.* **s. iliaca anterior superior** [NA] The subcutaneous rounded projection at the anterior extremity of the iliac crest which provides attachment for the lateral end of the inguinal ligament and the sartorius muscle below. Also *anterior superior iliac spine.* **s. iliaca posterior inferior** [NA] The small wide projection at the lower end of the posterior border of the ilium which bends sharply forward there to form the upper margin of the greater sciatic notch. Also *posterior inferior iliac spine.* **s. iliaca posterior superior** [NA] The slight projection at the posterior extremity of the iliac crest which provides attachment for the sacrotuberous and posterior sacroiliac ligaments. Also *posterior superior iliac spine.* **s. ischiadica** [NA] A marked triangular process projecting downward and medially from the posterior margin of the body of the ischium, separating the greater sciatic notch from the lesser and having the sacrospinous ligament attached to its margins and the coccygeus and levator ani muscles attached to its pelvic surface. Also *ischial spine, spine of ischium, sciatic spine.* **s. meatus** SPINA SUPRAMEATUM. **s. mentalis** [NA] A small bony projection above the anterior ends of the mylohyoid lines and behind the lower part of the symphysis menti which is usually divided into upper and lower parts, or genial tubercles, to which the genioglossus and geniohyoid muscles are attached, respectively. Also *mental spine, genial tubercles.* **s. nasalis anterior maxillae** [NA] An anteriorly projecting pointed process at the junction of the two maxillae in the middle of the lower margin of the anterior nasal aperture. Also *anterior nasal spine, spine of maxilla.* **s. nasalis ossis frontalis** [NA] The pointed inferior projection of the nasal part of the frontal bone forming part of the upper end of the nasal septum and articulating anteriorly with the crest of the nasal bones and posteriorly with the perpendicular plate of the ethmoid bone. Also *nasal spine of frontal bone, frontal spine.* **s. nasalis posterior ossis palatini** [NA] A small projecting process at the junction of the medial ends of the posterior margins of the horizontal plates of the palatine bones providing attachment to musculus uvulae. Also *nasal spine of palatine bone, posterior nasal spine, posterior palatine spine.* **s. ossis sphenoidalis** [NA] A small downward projecting process in the posterior part of the infratemporal surface of the greater wing of the sphenoid bone, located just posterior to foramen spinosum and providing attachment for the sphenomandibular ligament at its tip and for fibers of tensor veli palatini muscle. It is grooved medially by the chorda tympani nerve. Also *spine of sphenoid bone, sphenoidal spine.* **spinae palatinae** [NA] Obliquely longitudinal ridges on the posterolateral part of the inferior surface of the palatine process of the maxilla, between which are sulci for the greater palatine vessels and nerves. Also *palatine spines.* **s. scapulae** [NA] A triangular plate of bone joined by its root to and projecting posteriorly from the upper part of the dorsal surface of the scapula. The medial end of the root meets the medial margin of the scapula, while the lateral border of the spine forms the raised spinoglenoid notch. The posterior crest of the spine is subcutaneous and is continuous laterally with the acromion. The spine provides attachment for several muscles. Also *spine of scapula.* **s. suprameatum** An occasional bony spicule at the anterior border of a shallow depression situated immediately above and behind the external acoustic meatus and lying within the suprameatal triangle. *Outmoded.* Also *spina meatus, meatal spine, suprameatal spine, spine of Henle.* **s. trochlearis** [NA] A tiny bony projection behind the medial end of the supraorbital margin and lateral to the frontolacrimal suture serving as the attachment for the fibrocartilaginous trochlea of the superior oblique muscle of the eyeball. When absent, it is replaced by a shallow depression or fovea trochlearis. Also *trochlear spine, trochlear hamulus.* **s. tympanica major** [NA] The pointed anterior end of the tympanic notch at the upper part of the tympanic sulcus located at the medial end of the external acoustic meatus. It provides partial attachment for the anterior malleolar fold. Also *greater tympanic spine, anterior tympanic spine.* **s. tympanica minor** [NA] The pointed posterior end of the tympanic notch at the upper part of the tympanic sulcus located at the medial end of the external acoustic meatus. It provides partial attachment for the posterior malleolar fold. Also *lesser tympanic spine, posterior tympanic spine.* **s. ventosa** Dactylitis that is seen in young children with endosteal bone resorption and subperiosteal new bone formation. It sometimes occurs in cases of tuberculosis.

**spinae** \spī′nē\ Plural of SPINA.

**spinal** \spī′nəl\ **1** Pertaining to the spinal cord. **2** Pertaining to the vertebral column. **3** Of or relating to a spine or spinous process. **4** Characterized by the functioning of the spinal cord independently of the brain, as from accident, disease, or, in the case of animals, experimental transection, as in *a spinal animal* or *preparation.*

**spinalgia** \spīnal′jə\ Pain related to or emanating from the spinal column.

**spinalis** \spīnā′lis\ [New L, from *spina* a spine] Spinal.

**spindle** [Old English *spinel,* from *spinnan* to spin] **1** A waveform of constant frequency in electroencephalography, which waxes and wanes in amplitude in a regular sequence. This usually occurs as the subject is falling asleep. **2** An elongated structure observed in a dividing cell. It consists of microtubules extending between the centrioles and serves in the movement of the chromosomes to the daughter nuclear regions. **aortic s.** A dilatation occurring in the arch of the aorta just beyond the ligamentum arteriosum when the isthmus aortae is well marked. Also *His spindle.* **Axenfeld-Krukenberg s.** KRUKENBERG SPINDLE. **cleavage s.** The spindle observed during nuclear division in the cells (blastomeres) of the dividing fertilized egg during cleavage. **complex muscle s.** A mammalian muscle spindle having one or more secondary endings distal to each end of the primary ending. **enamel s.** A fusiform structure which projects a short distance into the enamel from the amelodentinal junction. **His s.** AORTIC SPINDLE. **intermediate muscle s.** A mammalian muscle spindle that contains only a single secondary ending in addition to the primary ending. **Krukenberg s.** A vertical deposit of uveal pigment granules deposited upon the posterior cornea by the aqueous convection currents. Also *Axenfeld-Krukenberg spindle.* **Kühne s.** *Obs.* MUSCLE SPINDLE. **mitotic s.** The spindle composed of microtubules extending between two centrioles during mitosis. The chromosomes attach to some of the tubules and are moved toward the centriole. **monofibral s.** A spindle with a single intrafusal fiber, characteristic of some reptilian spindles. **muscle s.** A length receptor in skeletal muscles of amphibians and higher vertebrates. Lying parallel to the extrafusal fibers, it consists of a multilaminar capsule through which passes an axial bundle of one or more specialized muscle fibers (intrafusal fibers), bearing the wrappings of one or more sensory fibers. Spindles in mammals have a prominent intracapsular space, three types of intrafusal fibers, a dual motor supply, and two types of sensory endings (primary and secondary), which differ in their sensitivity to steady and dynamic changes in muscle length. Also *neuromuscular spindle, fusus intermuscularis, Kühne's fiber, Kühne spindle* (obs.). **neurotendinous s.** *Rare* TENDON ORGAN. **simple muscle s.** A mammalian muscle spindle with a primary ending but no secondary ending. **sleep s.'s** In electroencephalography, rhythmic waveforms at about 14 Hz which wax and wane in the early stages of sleep. **tandem s.** One of two or more muscle spindles arranged in series and having at least one interfusal fiber in common, or the total serial arrangement of muscle-spindle units. **tendon s.** TENDON ORGAN.

**spine** 1 SPINA. 2 COLUMNA VERTEBRALIS. **anterior inferior iliac s.** SPINA ILIACA ANTERIOR INFERIOR. **anterior nasal s.** SPINA NASALIS ANTERIOR MAXILLAE. **anterior superior iliac s.** SPINA ILIACA ANTERIOR SUPERIOR. **anterior tympanic s.** SPINA TYMPANICA MAJOR. **bamboo s.** POKER SPINE. • It is so called because of its resemblance in x ray to a bamboo shoot. **basilar s.** TUBERCULUM PHARYNGEUM. **cervical s.** The seven cervical vertebrae considered as a unit. **Civinini s.** PROCESSUS PTERYGOSPINOSUS. **cleft s.** SPINA BIFIDA. **frontal s.** SPINA NASALIS OSSIS FRONTALIS. **greater tympanic s.** SPINA TYMPANICA MAJOR. **s. of helix** SPINA HELICIS. **s. of Henle** SPINA SUPRAMEATUM. **hysterical s.** RAILWAY BRAIN. **ischial s.** SPINA ISCHIADICA. **s. of ischium** SPINA ISCHIADICA. **kissing s.'s** Spinous processes of adjacent vertebrae that come into contact with each other and may give rise to bone sclerosis and pain. Also *Baastrup's disease, Baastrup syndrome.* **lesser tympanic s.** SPINA TYMPANICA MINOR. **s. of maxilla** SPINA NASALIS ANTERIOR MAXILLAE. **meatal s.** SPINA SUPRAMEATUM. **mental s.** SPINA MENTALIS. **nasal s. of frontal bone** SPINA NASALIS OSSIS FRONTALIS. **nasal s. of palatine bone** SPINA NASALIS POSTERIOR OSSIS PALATINI. **neural s.** PROCESSUS SPINOSUS VERTEBRAE. **palatine s.'s** SPINAE PALATINAE. **peroneal s. of os calcis** TROCHLEA PERONEALIS CALCANEI. **pharyngeal s.** TUBERCULUM PHARYNGEUM. **poker s.** The anklyosed spine in anklyosing spondylitis. Also *poker back, rigid spine, bamboo spine.* **posterior inferior iliac s.** SPINA ILIACA POSTERIOR INFERIOR. **posterior nasal s.** SPINA NASALIS POSTERIOR OSSIS PALATINI. **posterior palatine s.** SPINA NASALIS POSTERIOR OSSIS PALATINI. **posterior superior iliac s.** SPINA ILIACA POSTERIOR SUPERIOR. **posterior tympanic s.** SPINA TYMPANICA MINOR. **rigid s.** POKER SPINE. **s. of scapula** SPINA SCAPULAE. **sciatic s.** SPINA ISCHIADICA. **sphenoidal s.** SPINA OSSIS SPHENOIDALIS. **s. of sphenoid bone** SPINA OSSIS SPHENOIDALIS. **s. of Spix** LINGULA MANDIBULAE. **suprameatal s.** SPINA SUPRAMEATUM. **thoracic s.** The twelve thoracic vertebrae considered as a single unit. **s. of tibia** TUBEROSITAS TIBIAE. **tibial s.** TUBEROSITAS TIBIAE. **tibial s. of MacEwen** A bony projection on the tibia which is situated at the attachment of the tibial collateral ligament of the knee in bowlegged adolescents. **trochlear s.** SPINA TROCHLEARIS. **typhoid s.** Osteomyelitis of the spinal column subsequent to typhoid fever. **s. of vertebra** PROCESSUS SPINOSUS VERTEBRAE. **vertebral s.** PROCESSUS SPINOSUS VERTEBRAE.

**Spinelli** [Pier Giuseppe *Spinelli,* Italian gynecologist, 1862–1929] See under OPERATION.

**spini-** \spī′ni-\ SPIN-.

**spiniform** Resembling or shaped like a spine.

**spinifugal** \spīnif′yəgəl\ Conducting or moving away from the spinal cord, as impulses in efferent fibers of spinal nerves.

**spinipetal** \spīnip′ətəl\ Conducting or moving toward the spinal cord, as impulses in afferent fibers of spinal nerves. Also *spinopetal.*

**spinitis** \spīnī′tis\ [SPIN- + -ITIS] **1** *Obs.* MYELITIS. **2** *Obs.* SPINAL MENINGITIS.

**spinnbarkeit** \shpin′bärkīt′\ [German *spinnbar* fit for spinning + *-keit* -NESS] The condition of reduced viscosity of the cervical mucus at the time of ovulation, such that a long thread can be produced when it is pulled away from a glass slide.

**spino-** \spī′nō-\ SPIN-.

**spinobulbar** \-bul′bər\ Denoting connections from the spinal cord to the medulla oblongata.

**spinocerebellar** \-ser′əbel′ər\ Pertaining to or affecting the nerve fiber pathways which connect the spinal cord and cerebellum.

**spinocollicular** \-kälik′yələr\ SPINOTECTAL.

**spinocostalis** \-kästā′lis\ The serratus posterior superior and serratus posterior inferior muscles considered as a single unit.

**spinogalvanization** \-gal′vənīzā′shən\ External galvanic stimulation of the spinal cord.

**spinoglenoid** \-glē′noid\ Of or pertaining to the spine of the scapula and the glenoid cavity.

**spinomuscular** \-mus′kyələr\ Pertaining to the spinal cord and its ventral roots innervating striated muscle. *Seldom used.*

**spinoneural** \-nʸŭr′əl\ Pertaining to the spinal cord and its nerve roots. *Seldom used.*

**spinopetal** \spīnäp′ətəl\ SPINIPETAL.

**spinosal** \spīnō′səl\ Of or pertaining to the foramen spinosum in the greater wing of the sphenoid bone.

**spinose** \spī′nōs\ SPINOUS.

**spinotectal** \-tek′təl\ Denoting pathways from the spinal cord to the midbrain roof. Also *spinocollicular.*

**spinotransversarius** \-trans′vərsar′ē-əs\ The splenius capitis and obliquus capitis superior muscles considered as a single unit.

**spinous** \spī′nəs\ **1** Resembling a spine; acanthoid. **2** Pertaining to a spine. **3** Possessing a spine or spines. Also *spinose.*

**spintharicon** \spinthar′ikän\ An instrument utilizing a spark chamber, used for directly viewing the distribution of low-energy radiation from radiopharmaceuticals such as iodine 125 during thyroid scans.

**spir.** *spiritus* (L, spirit).

**spir-** SPIRO-[1].

**spiracle** \spir′əkl\ [L *spiracul(um)* (from *spirare* to breathe) a breathing hole] An aperture for air breathing in arthropods, or for respiratory intake of water in sharks, skates, rays, and other cartilaginous fishes.

**spiradenoma** \spī′radənō′mə\ [*spir(o)-*[1] + ADENOMA] ECCRINE SPIRADENOMA. **cylindromatous s.** An eccrine spiradenoma that shows some histologic features of a cylindroma. **eccrine s.** A benign tumor of the coiled epithelial duct or secretory segment of the sweat gland apparatus. Also *spiroma, spiradenoma.*

**spiral** \spī′rəl\ [Med L *spiralis* (from L *spira* a coil) coiled] **1** Winding and advancing around a central axis like the thread of a screw; helical. **2** Coiled in a single plane. **3** A spiral structure or design. **Curschmann s.** A coiled mucinous body sometimes observed in the sputum of a patient with bronchial asthma. **Herxheimer s.'s** Spiral fibers in the malpighian layer of the skin. Also *Herxheimer's fibers.* **Perroncito s.'s** PERRONCITO'S PHENOMENON.

**spiramycin** \spī′rəmī′sin\ An antibiotic with aminosugars substituted on a macrolide ring. Its action resembles that of erythromycin.

**spireme** \spī′rēm\ [Gk *speirēma* wreath, coil] The nuclear chromatin during early prophase of mitosis or meiosis, when it has a threadlike appearance.

**spirillosis** \spī′rilō′sis\ [*Spirill(um)* + -OSIS] Any disease resulting from infection with microorganisms of the genus *Spirillum.* One species, *S. minor,* is pathogenic in man, causing sodoku, a type of rat-bite fever.

***Spirillum*** \spīril′əm\ A genus of spiral, Gram-negative microaerophils whose motion is effected by flagella rather than by flexion of the cell body as in spirochetes. They are related metabolically to the pseudomonads. ***S. minor*** A rigid spiral organism, with polar flagella, that is carried by apparently healthy rats and is found in ponds. It causes one form of rat-bite fever in man. The organism has not been cultivated but can be recovered after inoculation in the blood of mice. Also *Spirillum minus.*

**spirillum** [New L, dim. of L *spira* a coil] Any bacillus of the genus *Spirillum.*

**spirit** [L *spiritus.* See SPIRITUS.] An alcoholic or hydroalcoholic solution containing a volatile substance. It is usually prepared through simple solution or by the mixing of ingredients. Also *spiritus.* **aromatic ammonia s.** An alcoholic solution containing 1.7–2.1 g of ammonia and 3.5–4.5 g of ammoniumcarbonate in each 100 ml. The solution is compounded by mixing ammonia, ammonium carbonate, strong ammonia solution, lemon oil, lavender oil, myristica oil, alcohol, and purified oil. It is used as a respiratory stimulant in weakness, syncope, or threatened faint. Also *ammonia spirit, spirit of sal volatile.* **industrial methylated s.** A solution containing 95% ethyl alcohol to which sufficient impure methyl alcohol has been added to occupy $^1/_{19}$ of the total volume. The addition of methyl alcohol as a denaturant renders the solution unsafe to drink. **methylated s.** Ethanol containing a small quantity of methanol, added to make it undrinkable. Methylated spirit usually also contains a purple dye to indicate its toxicity. **s. of Mindererus** AMMONIUM ACETATE SOLUTION. **s. of nitre** NITRIC ACID. **rectified s.** Aqueous ethanol concentrated by distillation; in some countries, indicating a solution of ethanol of a specified concentration. **s. of sal volatile** AROMATIC AMMONIA SPIRIT.

**spiritus** [L (from *spirare* to breathe, blow), a breathing, breath, breeze, mind, energy, spirit] SPIRIT. • Prior to 1953 the official designation of all spirits was *spiritus.*

**spiro-**[1] \spī′rə-, spī′rō-\ [L *spira* (from Gk *speira* something coiled or twisted) a coil] A combining form meaning coil, coiled, or twisted. Also *spir-.*

**spiro-**[2] [L *spirare* to breathe, blow, exhale] A combining form meaning breathing, respiration.

***Spirochaeta*** \-kē′tə\ A genus of free-living, anaerobic or facultative organisms of the family Spirochaetaceae.

**Spirochaetaceae** \-kētā′si·ē\ A family of bacteria (order Spirochaetales) that includes the genera *Spirochaeta, Cristispira, Treponema, Leptospira,* and *Borrelia.*

**spirochetal** \-kē′təl\ Pertaining to spirochetes or to infection by spirochetes.

**spirochete** \spī′rəkēt\ [SPIRO-[1] + Gk *chaitē* long flowing hair] Any bacterium of the family Spirochaetaceae, which includes two genera of free-living nonpathogens (*Spirochaeta* and *Cristispira*) and three genera of pathogens (*Treponema,*

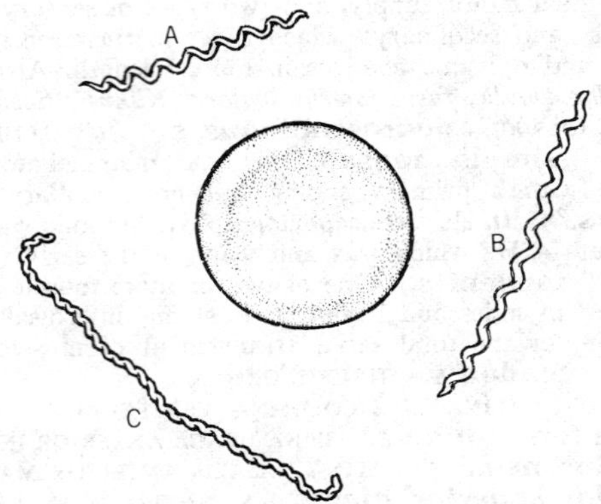


**Spirochetes** (shown for size comparison with red blood cell) (A) *Treponema;* (B) *Borrelia;* (C) *Leptospira.*

*Borrelia,* and *Leptospira*). The peptidoglycan wall, when isolated, retains the helical configuration of the cell. Motion, by flexion and by rotation like a corkscrew, is particularly adapted to highly viscous media. It is effected by axial fibrils located between the wall and a surrounding outer envelope and attached to each end of the helical protoplasmic cylinder. There are many spirochetes that have not been cultivated. Also *spirochaete.* **Dutton s.** A blood spirochete of the species *Borrelia duttoni,* a frequent cause of endemic relapsing fever in Africa.

**spirochetosis** \-kētō′sis\ Any spirochetal infection. **bronchopulmonary s.** BRONCHOSPIROCHETOSIS. **icterogenic s.** *Obs.* ICTERIC LEPTOSPIROSIS. **s. icterohemorrhagica** ICTERIC LEPTOSPIROSIS. **s. riverensis** A type of meningitis described in Brazil and thought to be the result of a chronic spirochetal infection.

**spirochetotic** \-kētät′ik\ Pertaining to or characterized by spirochetosis.

**spirogram** \spī′rəgram\ [SPIRO-[2] + -GRAM] A graphic representation of the volumes of air inhaled and exhaled during the respiratory cycle. Also *pneogram, pneumatogram.*

**spirograph** \spī′rəgraf\ A device that records spirograms. Also *pneumatograph.*

**spirography** \spīräg′rəfē\ The process or method of recording spirograms.

**spiroid** \spī′roid\ Resembling a spiral.
**spiroma** \spīrō′mə\ [*spir(o)-*[1] + -OMA] ECCRINE SPIRADENOMA.
**spirometer** \spīräm′ətər\ An apparatus used to measure the volumes of inhaled or exhaled gas. Also *respirometer, ventilometer, anapnometer* (obs.), *pneumometer, pneumonometer, pneumatometer, pneometer, pulmometer.*
***Spirometra*** \spī′rōmē′trə\ [SPIRO-[1] + Gk *mētra* the womb, uterus] A genus of tapeworms (family Diphylobothriidae, order Pseudophyllidea) parasitic in mammals, exceptionally in reptiles. The procercoid larva develops in copepods, and the plerocercoid, or sparganum, in amphibians, reptiles, or small mammals. See also SPARGANOSIS. ***S. mansoni*** A species common in wild and feral cats. The larvae of the species can cause sparganosis in humans. Widely prevalent in man in the Far East, it has been reported in other areas as well. Also *Bothriocephalus mansoni, Diphyllobothrium mansoni.*. ***S. mansonoides*** A species found in cats, especially bobcats, and in dogs. Heavy infections can cause diarrhea and anemia. Larvae may cause human sparganosis. Procercoids develop in copepods (*Cyclops*), spargana in watersnakes (*Natrix*) and experimentally in mice and other rodents, and in rabbits. Also *Bothriocephalus mansonoides, Diphyllobothrium mansonoides.*
**spirometry** \spīräm′ətrē\ The process or method of using a spirometer. Also *ventilometry, pneumatometry, pulmometry, respirometry.* **bronchoscopic s.** BRONCHOSPIROMETRY.
**spironolactone** $C_{24}H_{32}O_4S$. 7-(Acetylthio)-17-hydroxy-3-oxo-pregn-4-ene-21-carboxylic acid γ-lactone. A synthetic analogue, and an antagonist, of aldosterone. It is a diuretic agent, and it produces hyponatremia, hyperkalemia, and increased circulating angiotensin concentrations in the blood.
**spiroscope** \spī′rəskōp\ A type of spirometer which permits the subject to observe the effectiveness of breathing exercises, correlating to the amount of air moved by the lungs during breathing. It has been used to assist patients learning therapeutic breathing exercises.
**spittle** [Old English *spætl, spatl,* akin to Old English *spittan* to spit] Saliva or sputum ejected from the mouth.
**Spitz** [S. *Spitz,* U.S. pathologist, flourished 20th century] Spitz nevus. See under EPITHELIAL AND/OR SPINDLE CELL NEVUS.
**Spitzer** [Alexander *Spitzer,* Austrian anatomist, 1868–1943] See under THEORY.
**Spitzka** [Edward Charles *Spitzka,* U.S. neurologist and psychiatrist, 1852–1914] Spitzka's marginal zone. See under TRACTUS DORSOLATERALIS.
**Spix** [Johann Baptist von *Spix,* German zoologist and anatomist, 1781–1826] Spine of Spix. See under LINGULA MANDIBULAE.
**splanchn-** \splangkn-\ SPLANCHNO-.
**splanchnapophysis** \splangk′nəpäf′isis\ A bony process attached to a viscus or the alimentary canal.
**splanchnectopia** \splangk′nektō′pē·ə\ [SPLANCHN- + ECTOPIA] Abnormal location of any of the viscera, usually congenital.
**splanchnesthesia** \splangk′nesthē′zhə\ VISCERAL SENSE.
**splanchni-** \splangk′ni-\ SPLANCHNO-.
**splanchnic** \splangk′nik\ [Gk *splanchnikos* (from *splanchna* inward parts) of or for the bowels] Pertaining to the viscera; visceral.
**splanchnicectomy** \splangk′nisek′təmē\ [*splanchnic (nerve)* + -ECTOMY] Excision of splanchnic nerves. **lumbodorsal s.** Bilateral resection of the lumbodorsal sympathetic chain and splanchnic nerves, for the treatment of hypertension. Also *lumbodorsal sympathectomy, Smithwick's operation.*
**splanchnicotomy** \splangk′nikät′əmē\ [*splanchnic (nerve)* + *o* + -TOMY] Division of splanchnic nerves.
**splanchno-** \splangk′nə-\ [Gk *splanchnon* (mostly in plural *splanchna*) viscera, inward parts, especially heart, lungs, and liver] A combining form denoting the viscera. Also *splanchn-, splanchni-.*
**splanchnocele** \splangk′nəsēl\ [SPLANCHNO- + -CELE[1]] Herniation of any of the abdominal viscera.
**splanchnocoele** \splangk′nəsēl\ [SPLANCHNO- + -COELE] That part of the embryonic coelom which persists in the adult and gives rise to the definitive pericardial, pleural, and peritoneal cavities. • The term must not be confused with *splanchnocele,* which has sometimes been used for a protrusion or hernia of an abdominal viscus.
**splanchnocranium** \-krā′nē·əm\ [SPLANCHNO- + CRANIUM] That part of the embryonic cranium from which the facial skeleton is derived. It is formed as early as the fifth week in human embryonic life, by the cartilaginous axes of the two first branchial arches, to which membrane bones will next be added, partially replacing the cartilages. The first centers of ossification appear at the end of the fourth month. Morphologically the splanchnocranium corresponds with the gill arch skeleton of ancestral vertebrates, and can be distinguished from the neurocranium, which gives rise to the skull proper. Also *viscerocranium, splanchnoskeleton.*
**splanchnography** \splangk·näg′rəfē\ [SPLANCHNO- + -GRAPHY] Visceral descriptive anatomy.
**splanchnology** \splangk·näl′əjē\ [SPLANCHNO- + -LOGY] Study of the visceral organs.
**splanchnomegaly** \-meg′əlē\ [SPLANCHNO- + -MEGALY] Abnormal enlargement of any or all visceral organs; visceromegaly. Also *organomegaly, splanchomegalia.*
**splanchnomicria** \-mī′krē·ə\ [SPLANCHNO- + MICR- + -IA] Abnormally small size of viscera.
**splanchnopathy** \splangk·näp′əthē\ [SPLANCHNO- + -PATHY] Any disease process involving abdominal viscera.
**splanchnopleure** \splangk′nəplUr\ [SPLANCHNO- + Gk *pleur(a)* a rib, side] The internal or visceral layer of the ventral portion of the mesoderm. It covers the primitive intestine and its derivatives, and produces a considerable amount of "splanchnic" mesenchyme making contact with the endoderm. It is continuous at the root of the mesentery with the somatopleure, and gives rise to the visceral layer of the pericardium (including the myocardium, which is derived from it), the visceral pleura of the lungs, and the visceral peritoneum. Also *splanchnic layer, splanchnic wall, visceral wall.*
**splanchnoptosis** \splangk′näp·tō′sis, -nōtō′sis\ VISCEROPTOSIS.
**splanchnoskeleton** \-skel′ətən\ **1** Any of the bony structures forming within or connected to viscera or organs, as in the tongue, gills and penis of some animals. Also *visceroskeleton.* **2** SPLANCHNOCRANIUM.
**splanchnosomatic** \-sōmat′ik\ Both splanchnic and somatic; relating to the viscera and the body wall. Also *viscerosomatic.*
**splash** / **gastric s.** See under SUCCUSSION SOUNDS. **succussion s.** SUCCUSSION SOUNDS.
**S-plasty** A type of Z-plasty wherein the tips of the triangular flaps are rounded rather than pointed.
**splay** \splā\ [Middle English *splayen,* short for *displayen* to display, from L *displicare* to scatter] A phenomenon created by nephron heterogeneity with respect to the ratio of renal glomerular filtration rate and renal tubular absorption capacity for a solute. It may be characterized by the portion

of a curve relating the rate of tubular reabsorption of a solute and its plasma concentration that lies between the highest plasma concentration, at which the rate of tubular reabsorption equals the rate of glomerular filtration of the solute, and the lowest plasma concentration, at which the tubular transport maximum for the solute is achieved; or by the portion of a curve relating urinary excretion of a solute and its increasing plasma concentration that lies between the lowest plasma concentration at which the solute first appears in urine and the lowest plasma concentration at which the tubular transport maximum for the solute is achieved.

**splayfoot** \splā′fŭt\ TALIPES PLANUS.

**spleen** [Old French *esplen*, from L *splen*. See SPLEN.] The elongated accessory lymphatic organ of the vascular system; splen. **accessory s.** SPLEN ACCESSORIUS. **aguecake s.** CHRONIC MALARIAL SPLENOMEGALY. **diffuse waxy s.** LARDACEOUS SPLEEN. **floating s.** An abnormally mobile spleen due to lax ligaments. Also *wandering spleen, movable spleen, lien mobilis.* **Gandy-Gamna s.** SIDEROTIC SPLENOMEGALY. **lardaceous s.** One of two patterns of amyloidosis of the spleen, characterized by deposition of amyloid within the red pulp with relative sparing of the lymphoid follicles. Grossly, the cut surface is diffusely firm and waxy. Also *waxy spleen, diffuse waxy spleen.* Compare SAGO SPLEEN. **movable s.** FLOATING SPLEEN. **sago s.** One of two patterns of amyloidosis of the spleen, characterized by the presence, on gross inspection, of uniformly distributed, whitish, tapiocalike granules. Microscopically, the amyloid deposits are largely restricted to the splenic follicles, with sparing of the red pulp. Compare LARDACEOUS SPLEEN. • *Sago,* derived from the Malay word *sagu,* is a grainy starch used in food preparations especially in tropical regions where its sources, the sago palm and related trees, are abundant. **wandering s.** FLOATING SPLEEN. **waxy s.** LARDACEOUS SPLEEN.

**splen** \splen\ [L, from Gk *splēn* (akin to L *lien* spleen) the spleen] [NA] The elongated accessory lymphatic organ of the vascular system; the spleen. Variable in size but commonly the size of a large clenched fist, it is located in the upper part of the abdominal cavity opposite the posterior parts of the left ninth, tenth, and eleventh ribs from which it is separated by the diaphragm, left pleural sac, and the base of the lung. It is completely invested by peritoneum except at its hilum, and it is separated from the fundus of the stomach by the greater sac. The fibroelastic capsule sends in trabeculae which branch to form a network internally that ensheathes the splenic vessels and their branches, becoming continuous with a fine reticulum, in the interstices of which is the red and white pulp. It is involved in phagocytosis through its macrophages, stores blood and iron, produces blood cells in the fetus and certain antibodies, and is able to undergo slow, rhythmic contractions. Also *lien.* **s. accessorius** [NA] Any of the small, encapsulated masses of splenic tissue either attached to the spleen by thin bands of splenic tissue or found in the neighborhood of the spleen, often in the lienorenal ligament or the greater omentum, or located elsewhere in the abdominal cavity. Also *accessory spleen, lien accessorius, lien succenturiatus, lienunculus, lienculus, splenunculus, spleniculus, splenculus, splenulus, splenule, spleneolus.*

**splen-** \splēn-, splen-\ SPLENO-.

**splenalgia** \splēnal′jə\ [SPLEN- + -ALGIA] Pain in the spleen.

**splenauxe** \splēnôk′sē\ SPLENOMEGALY.

**splenculus** \spleng′kyələs\ [L, dim. of *splen* the spleen] SPLEN ACCESSORIUS.

**splenectomy** \splēnek′təmē\ [SPLEN- + -ECTOMY] A surgical procedure in which all or part of the spleen is resected. Also *lienectomy.* **subcapsular s.** A surgical procedure in which all or part of the spleen is removed via a subcapsular approach, thus leaving the emptied capsule.

**splenectopia** \splē′nektō′pē·ə\ [SPLEN- + ECTOPIA] Abnormal position of the spleen or of splenic tissue. Also *splenectopy.*

**splenectopy** \splēnek′təpē\ SPLENECTOPIA.

**spleneolus** \splēnē′ələs\ SPLEN ACCESSORIUS.

**splenetic** \splinet′ik\ **1** Of or relating to the spleen; splenic. **2** Suffering from disease of the spleen. An obsolete usage. **3** Irritable; bad-tempered.

**splenial** \splē′nē·əl\ Denoting the splenium of the corpus callosum or the splenius muscle.

**splenic** \splen′ik\ Of or relating to the spleen.

**spleniculus** \splenik′yələs\ SPLEN ACCESSORIUS.

**spleniform** \splen′ifôrm\ Resembling the spleen. Also *splenoid.*

**splenin** \splē′nin\ A crude and poorly characterized extract of splenic tissue which affects blood coagulation. Small amounts shorten bleeding time while large amounts increase it.

**spleniserrate** \splen′iser′āt\ Of or pertaining to the serratus and the splenius muscles.

**splenitis** \splēnī′tis\ [SPLEN- + -ITIS] Inflammation of the spleen, usually from bacterial infection. Also *lienitis.* **spodogenous s.** Enlargement and inflammation of the spleen due to uptake of foreign material.

**splenium** \splē′nē·əm\ [L, from Gk *splēnion* a pad, compress] **1** A long dressing for a wound. **2** A thickened, bandlike structure. **s. corporis callosi** [NA] The thick, rounded caudal extremity of the corpus callosum. Also *tuber corporis callosi.*

**spleno-** \splē′nō-, splen′ə-\ [Gk *splēn* spleen] A combining form denoting the spleen. Also *splen-.*

**splenoblast** \splen′əblast\ An undifferentiated cell from which the splenocyte originates.

**splenocele** \splen′əsēl\ [SPLENO- + -CELE[1]] **1** Herniation of the spleen. **2** A tumor or cyst of the spleen; splenoma.

**splenocleisis** \-klī′sis\ Induction of a new fibrous capsule around the spleen by irritating the surface.

**splenocolic** \-kō′lik\ Having to do with both the spleen and the colon, as splenocolic ligament.

**splenocyte** \splen′əsīt\ A macrophage of the white or red pulp of the spleen.

**splenodynia** \-din′ē·ə\ [SPLEN- + -ODYNIA] Splenic pain; splenalgia.

**splenogenous** \splenäj′ənəs\ [SPLENO- + -GENOUS] Originating or formed in the spleen.

**splenogranulomatosis siderotica** \-gran′yəlō′mətō′-sis sid′ərät′ikə\ SIDEROTIC SPLENOMEGALY.

**splenography** \splēnäg′rəfē\ [SPLENO- + -GRAPHY] Radiographic examination of the spleen after the injection of a radiopaque agent either into the splenic artery or splenic parenchyma. Also *lienography.*

**splenohepatomegaly** \-hep′ətōmeg′əlē\ HEPATOSPLENOMEGALY.

**splenoid** \splē′noid\ SPLENIFORM.

**splenolaparotomy** \-lap′ərät′əmē\ LAPAROSPLENOTOMY.

**splenology** \splēnäl′əjē\ The study of the spleen.

**splenolymphatic** \-limfat′ik\ Pertaining to the spleen and lymph nodes.

**splenolysin** \splēnäl′isin\ [SPLENO- + LYSIN] A material that specifically destroys splenic tissue, usually an antibody.

**splenolysis** \splēnäl′isis\ [SPLENO- + LYSIS] Dissolution or destruction of splenic tissue.

**splenoma** \splēnō′mə\ [SPLEN- + -OMA] A tumor of the spleen.
**splenomalacia** \-məlā′shə\ Abnormal softening of splenic consistency. Also *lienomalacia.*
**splenomedullary** \-med′yəler′ē\ Originating in or involving the spleen and bone marrow. Also *lienomedullary, lienomyelogenous, splenomyelogenous.*
**splenomegaly** \-meg′əlē\ [SPLENO- + -MEGALY] Enlargement of the spleen. Also *splenauxe, megalosplenia.* **chronic congestive s.** Splenomegaly due to passive congestion, as in splenic vein thrombosis or portal hypertension. Also *congestive fibrosplenomegaly.* See also BANTI SYNDROME. **chronic malarial s.** An enlarged condition of the spleen, developing after repeated attacks of acute malaria. The spleen is hard, dark in color, and fibrotic. In the presence of an aberrant immune response, massive splenomegaly may occasionally result. Also *ague-cake spleen.* See also TROPICAL SPLENOMEGALY SYNDROME. **congestive s.** See under CHRONIC CONGESTIVE SPLENOMEGALY. **Egyptian s.** Splenomegaly resulting from schistosomiasis mansoni in Egypt. There is usually hepatomegaly, with Symmers pipestem fibrosis. Ascites is often present. **febrile tropical s.** KALA-AZAR. **hemolytic s.** Splenic enlargement associated with any hemolytic disorder, formerly restricted to hereditary spherocytosis. **hypercholesterolemic s.** The rare occurrence of splenomegaly due to hypercholesterolemia. **siderotic s.** Enlargement of the spleen accompanied by marked fibrosis and focal accumulations of iron and calcium (Gamna bodies). It is seen in hemochromatosis, sickle cell disease, and congestive splenomegaly. Also *Gandy-Nanta disease, Gandy-Gamna spleen, Gandy-Gamna disease, Gamna's disease, splenogranulomatosis siderotica.* **thrombophlebitic s.** Enlargement of the spleen due to splenic vein thrombosis. Also *Opitz disease.* **tropical s.** See under TROPICAL SPLENOMEGALY SYNDROME.
**splenomyelogenous** \-mī′əläj′ənəs\ SPLENOMEDULLARY.
**splenomyelomalacia** \-mī′əlōməlā′shə\ Abnormal softness of both spleen and bone marrow. Also *lienomyelomalacia.*
**splenopancreatic** \-pan′krē·at′ik\ Pertaining to both the spleen and the pancreas; lienopancreatic.
**splenopathy** \splēnäp′əthē\ [SPLENO- + -PATHY] Any disease process of the spleen.
**splenopexy** \splē′nəpek′sē\ [SPLENO- + -PEXY] A surgical procedure in which a mobile spleen is fixed in a stationary position. Also *splenopexia, splenopexis.*
**splenoportography** \-pôrtäg′rəfē\ Radiographic examination of the portal system after the percutaneous injection of a radiopaque material into the splenic parenchyma with opacification of the splenic and portal veins. Also *splenic portography, splenic venography.*
**splenoptosis** \splē′näp·tō′sis\ [SPLENO- + -PTOSIS] Prolapse of the spleen. Also *splenoptosia.*
**splenorenopexy** \-rē′nōpek′sē\ A surgical procedure in which the spleen and left kidney are fixed to each other in a stationary position.
**splenorrhagia** \splē′nôrā′jə\ [SPLENO- + -RRHAGIA] Bleeding or hemorrhage from the spleen, as after rupture.
**splenorrhaphy** \splēnôr′əfē\ [SPLENO- + -RRHAPHY] A surgical procedure in which a damaged spleen is repaired by suturing rather than being resected.
**splenotomy** \splēnät′əmē\ [SPLENO- + -TOMY] A surgical incision into the spleen.
**splenotoxin** \-täk′sin\ Any toxin which acts upon or is produced by the spleen.
**splenule** \splen′yool\ SPLEN ACCESSORIUS.
**splenulus** \splen′yələs\ SPLEN ACCESSORIUS.
**splenunculus** \splēnung′kyələs\ SPLEN ACCESSORIUS.
**splice** **1** To join end-to-end two pieces of nucleic acid, or the ends of a linear nucleic acid, to form a circle. It may be performed either chemically or enzymatically. **2** The actual nucleotide sequences involved in the splicing process in mRNA.
**splicing** \splī′sing\ The natural process by which transcribed mRNA matures to become mRNA that will be translated. The process involves excising transcribed intron regions and rejoining the ends of each transcribed exon region. **alternative s.** The generation of two or more different mature mRNA's from the same primary transcript through variation in the sites of splicing. It is a method of producing structurally and functionally distinct proteins from the same gene and a method of developmental regulation. **gene s.** See under GENE-SPLICING. **RNA s.** The process by which a precursor mRNA has transcribed intervening sequences removed and the final mRNA generated.
**splint** [Middle Low German and Dutch *splinte* splint] **1** An apparatus for the immobilization or support of a part. **2** A device for reducing a fracture. **3** To immobilize by using a splint. **acrylic resin bite-guard s.** A removable splint which covers the occlusal surfaces and incisal edges of teeth. It separates antagonistic teeth and so temporarily relieves occlusal disharmony. **air s.** A plastic inflatable splint used to temporarily immobilize a joint or a fracture. **airplane s.** A splint that is used to hold the arm in abduction, with the forearm partly flexed. **anchor s.** A splint for fracture of the mandible or maxilla in which loops of wire are fastened onto an external bar. **Anderson s.** An external splint with intraosseous cross

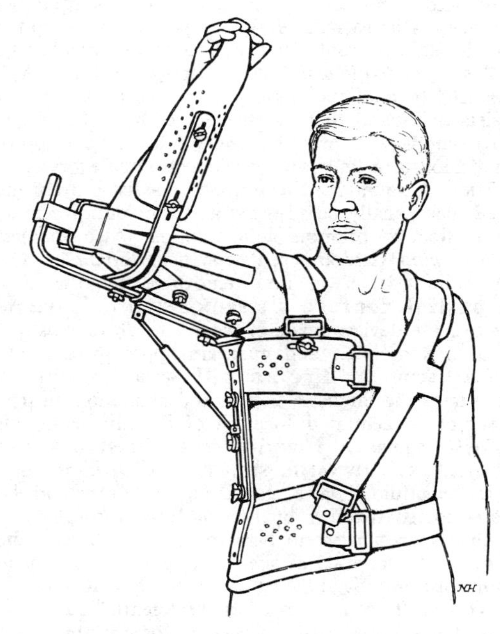

Airplane splint

pins or screws that are inserted above and below the fracture and fixed to plates on either side of the limb. **Angle s.** A splint that holds the mandible together by using the teeth. **Asch s.** A tubular splint that is used for a nasal fracture. **Balkan s.** BALKAN FRAME. **banjo traction s.** A splint made of a metal hoop shaped like a banjo body. It is used to maintain an extended position of the fingers. **bridge s.** A bridge which also acts as a splint. Also *fixed partial denture splint, splint-bridge.* **caliper s.** CALIPER. **cap s.** **1** A jaw splint of cast metal covering the crowns of the teeth in one jaw and cemented in place. **2** A provisional splint of acrylic or other resin covering the crowns of the teeth and used to stabilize fractured or avulsed teeth, or teeth loosened by periodontitis. **cast bar s.** A provisional splint consisting of facial and lingual continuous clasps made to fit the teeth at the contour line. If it is made in one piece it may be used as a removable splint, otherwise it needs to be cemented on to the teeth and/or wired interdentally. Also *continous clasp splint, Friedman splint, crib splint.* **cast cap s.** A method of fixation in fractures of the jaw by fitting to the teeth an exactly conforming negative mold. Several molds may be used, adjacent molds being connected with adjustable bars. **Chandler felt collar s.** A bulky, soft dressing that is wrapped around the neck to limit motion of the cervical spine. **coaptation s.'s** Splints that fit tight to the skin to immobilize a fracture site. **cockup s.** A splint designed to hold the wrist in extension. **continuous clasp s.** CAST BAR SPLINT. **Cramer s.** A splint made with two stout parallel wires as edges and wire crosspieces that resemble the rungs of a ladder. Also *ladder splint.* **crib s.** CAST BAR SPLINT. **Denis Brown s.** An aluminum splint that incorporates shoes to hold a corrected position in a talipes equinovarus deformity. **diodontic s.** A tapering metal rod, implanted through the root canal of a tooth to increase its stability. Also *endodontic stabilizer.* **drop foot s.** An apparatus used to hold the ankle joint in the neutral position. It consists of a band that is attached to the calf and an extension from the calf into the heel of the shoe. It prevents plantar flexion in a limb with weakened dorsiflexors. **dynamic s.** A splint used to initiate or assist movements of a joint. It can usually be adjusted and provide force in a desired direction to promote joint motion. Also *therapeutic splint, live splint* (seldom used), *functional splint.* **fixed s.** A splint which is not removable by the wearer. **fixed partial denture s.** BRIDGE SPLINT. **fracture s.** Any of the devices made of wood, metal, or plastic that are used to immobilize and maintain approximation of the ends of a fracture. **Frejka pillow s.** A soft pillow that maintains the thighs in flexion and abduction during the treatment of congenital dislocation of the hip in an infant. Also *Frejka pillow.* **Friedman s.** CAST BAR SPLINT. **functional s.** DYNAMIC SPLINT. **Gunning s.** A splint for edentulous jaws, consisting of upper and lower baseplates joined together by two or three vertical columns which have spaces between them to allow feeding. **hayrake s.** A device used as skeletal traction for the hand to maintain position, but allowing access to the hand. It is useful for skin grafting in cases of circumferential burns to the hand, or hand burns with associated forearm burns. Also *hayrake.* **Hodgen s.** A modified Thomas splint with rings to provide balanced suspension and a flexed position of the knee. Also *Hodgen's apparatus.* **interdental s.** A splint which is attached to the teeth on the facial, lingual or occlusal aspects to provide anchorage for traction, or fixation. **Kanavel's cockup s.** A cockup splint that has a finger extension. **Kirschner wire s.** An internal splint of sterile wire that is driven through bone to immobilize a fracture or small joint, as in the phalanges or metacarpals. **ladder s.** CRAMER SPLINT. **live s.** *Seldom used* DYNAMIC SPLINT. **Morris external fixation s.** A splint used to stabilize the mandible following a fracture or during reconstruction utilizing bone grafts. The splint consists of threaded pins that are placed into the angle of the mandible on each side, the pins then being attached to an external, rigid, curved acrylic bar. **nasal s.** Any of a variety of splints used to protect and stabilize the nasal bones following rhinoplasty or correction of nasal fractures. **open cap s.** A cap splint for the jaw in which the occlusal surfaces are exposed. **opponens s.** A splint that maintains the thumb in abduction. **pillow s.** A bulky fabric or inflatable splint. **plaster s.** A splint made from gauze impregnated with plaster of Paris. **plastic s.** **1** A splint made of plastic. **2** Any of a number of splints that can be molded to conform to the area to be splinted. **poroplastic s.** A splint that can be softened with water and molded to conform to the treated part. **Porzett s.** A splint used to control the movements of the arms and head of a child following an operation to correct a cleft lip. **Roger-Anderson extraoral s.** A splint used in stabilizing complex mandibular fractures and in increasing bony length wherein threaded steel pins are placed percutaneously into the fragments of bone, and the protruding ends of the pins are then joined by means of special connectors and small steel rods. Also *Roger-Anderson pin fixation appliance.* **surgical s.** An artificial device used to prevent motion during or after a surgical procedure. **Taylor s.** A metal brace that is used to immobilize the spine following trauma or disease of the spine. Also *Taylor's apparatus.* **therapeutic s.** DYNAMIC SPLINT. **Thomas knee s.** An apparatus that is used to transfer weight-bearing forces directly to the perineal and ischial regions, thus removing stresses across the knee joint. **Tobruk s.** A Thomas splint with skin traction that is encased in plaster of Paris bandaging for a fractured femur. **traction s.** A splint that allows a longitudinal pull to a fracture site.

**splinting** Immobilization by the use of splints. Also *splintage.*

**splints / shin s.** ANTERIOR TIBIAL SYNDROME.

**splitting** **1** The breaking of a bond in a molecule or the resultant breaking of the molecule. **2** In psychiatry, the dividing of psychic structure into suborganizations, sometimes seen as a defense against ambivalent feelings which would be mutually contradictory were they not relegated to separated portions of the ego. Also *splitting of the ego.* **fee s.** A process, often viewed as unethical, under which one provider will share a fee with another provider in return for having received a referral of a patient. **s. of heart sounds** The duplication of first or second heart sounds. A split first heart sound is due to asynchronous closure of mitral and tricuspid valves, a frequent normal finding. Splitting of the second heart sound is due to asynchronous aortic and pulmonary closure sounds. This is normal on inspiration but splitting usually disappears on expiration. **sagittal s. of mandible** The making of an anteroposterior cut near the angle of the mandible so that it can be lengthened or shortened by sliding the cut surfaces on one another.

**spodiomyelitis** \spō′dē·ōmī′əlī′tis\ ACUTE ANTERIOR POLIOMYELITIS.

**spodogenous** \spōdäj′ənəs\ [Gk *spodo(s)* ashes + -GENOUS] **1** Containing foreign mineral matter that yields ash upon spodography: said of tissue samples. **2** Characterized by spodogenous tissue.

**spodography** \spōdäg′rəfē\ [Gk *spodo(s)* ashes +

-GRAPHY] The incineration of a very small amount of tissue and the subsequent examination of the remaining ash to identify the mineral content of cells and tissues.

**spokeshave** \spōk′shāv\ [*spoke* + *shave*] A tool consisting of a blade set between two handles. Several surgical instruments are of this kind, particularly certain nasal instruments in which the blade is at right angles to the two shafts supporting it.

**spondyl-** \spän′dil-\ SPONDYLO-.

**spondylarthritis** \-ärthrī′tis\ [SPONDYL- + ARTHRITIS] SPONDYLARTHROSIS. **s. ankylopoietica** ANKYLOSING SPONDYLITIS.

**spondylarthrosis** \-ärthrō′sis\ Arthritis of the intervertebral joints. Also *spondylarthritis.*

**spondylitis** \spän′dəlī′tis\ [SPONDYL- + -ITIS] An inflammation of one or more vertebrae. **ankylosing s.** An illness, generally seen in young men, consisting of inflammatory arthritis leading to anklyosis of the sacroiliac joints, lumbar spine and, later, thoracic and cervical spine. This disease is often associated with the presence of the histocompatability antigen HLA B27. Also *rheumatic arthritis of spine* (outmoded), *Bekhterev's arthritis, Bekhterev syndrome, Bekhterev spondylitis, Marie-Strümpell spondylitis, rheumatoid spondylitis* (obs.), *Marie-Strümpell arthritis, Marie-Strümpell disease, rhizomelic spondylitis* (obs.), *spondylitis deformans, spondylitis rhizomelica* (obs.), *spondylitis chronica ankylopoietica, rhizomelic spondylosis.* **hypertrophic s.** A degenerative disease of the vertebrae with marked osteophyte and new bone formation. **Kümmell s.** KÜMMELL'S DISEASE. **Marie-Strümpell s.** ANKYLOSING SPONDYLITIS. **post-traumatic s.** KÜMMELL'S DISEASE. **rheumatoid s.** *Obs.* ANKYLOSING SPONDYLITIS. **rhizomelic s.** *Obs.* ANKYLOSING SPONDYLITIS. **s. rhizomelica** *Obs.* ANKYLOSING SPONDYLITIS. **traumatic s.** An injury of the spine producing an inflammation. **tuberculous s.** Infection of the spinal column by *Mycobacterium tuberculosis.* It can destroy the vertebral bodies and result in kyphosis, which may be complicated by paraplegia. Also *Pott's disease, tuberculous spinal osteomyelitis.*

**spondylo-** \spän′dilō-\ [Gk *spondylos* or *sphondylos* vertebra] A combining form meaning vertebra, vertebral. Also *spondyl-.*

**spondylodesis** \spän′diläd′əsis\ The fusion of adjacent vertebrae.

**spondylodidymia** \-didim′ē·ə\ [SPONDYLO- + *didym(us)* + -IA] The occurrence of equal conjoined twins joined at the vertebral columns.

**spondylolisthesis** \-listhē′sis\ [SPONDYL- + Gk *olisthēsis* slippage, dislocation] A forward displacement of one vertebra upon the other, usually in the lower lumbar spine, due to either a traumatic or a congenital weakness defect of the pars interarticularis. Also *spondyloptosis.*

**spondylolisthetic** \-listhet′ik\ Relating to or caused by spondylolisthesis.

**spondylolysis** \spän′diläl′isis\ [SPONDYLO- + LYSIS] 1 Ankylosis of a vertebral joint. 2 Osteoarthritic degeneration that affects the intervertebral disk space or the posterior facet joints.

**spondylomalacia** \-məlā′shə\ The softening of vertebrae. **s. traumatica** KÜMMELL'S DISEASE.

**spondylopathy** \spän′diläp′əthē\ Any disease or disorder of the vertebrae. **traumatic s.** KÜMMELL'S DISEASE.

**spondyloptosis** \spän′dilōtō′sis\ SPONDYLOLISTHESIS.

**spondyloschisis** \spän′diläs′kisis\ [SPONDYLO- + -SCHISIS] RACHISCHISIS.

**spondylosis** \spän′dəlō′sis\ [SPONDYL- + -OSIS] A noninflammatory disease of the spine, usually osteoarthritis and/or degenerative disk disease. **cervical s.** Spondylosis of the cervical spine. **s. chronica ankylopoietica** ANKYLOSING SPONDYLITIS. **degenerative s.** Osteoarthritis of the posterior facet joints of the spine, accompanied by disk degeneration and syndesmophyte formation. Also *degenerative vertebral arthropathy.* **hyperostotic s.** Spondylosis with excess bone growth or osteophyte formation. **rhizomelic s.** ANKYLOSING SPONDYLITIS.

**spondylosyndesis** \-sin′dəsis\ SPINAL FUSION.

**spondylotomy** \spän′dilät′əmē\ LAMINECTOMY.

**spondylus** \spän′diləs\ VERTEBRA.

**sponge** [L and Gk *spongia* a sponge] 1 A pad of gauze, cotton, or other absorbent material used in surgical operations to soak up blood or other fluids or as a dressing. 2 A common name of the sessile marine organism of the genus *Euspongia,* phylum Porifera. The light fibrous skeleton, when the living material is removed, readily absorbs water and is used in cleansing and as an absorbent. **absorbable gelatin s.** A sterilized preparation of gelatin, obtained by hydrolysis of collagen, that swells and absorbs up to ten times its weight of water to form an absorbable hemostatic gel. Also *spongia gelatina absorbenda.* **gauze s.** An absorbent surgical pad fashioned from sterile gauze material. **sodium s.** A theorized characteristic of damaged tissues whereby excessive amounts of sodium are absorbed relative to the quantity of fluid that is sequestered. Some believe that the volume of fluids can be limited by giving sodium in excess of isotonic for resuscitation of shock due to burns. **spermicidal s.** A contraceptive device consisting of a discoid sponge impregnated with a spermicide. The device is placed against the uterine cervix prior to sexual intercourse. Also *vaginal sponge.*

**spongeitis** \spän′jē·ī′tis\ SPONGIOSITIS.

**spongi-** \spän′jē-\ SPONGIO-.

**spongia** Sponge. **s. gelatina absorbenda** ABSORBABLE GELATIN SPONGE.

**spongiitis** \spän′jē·ī′tis\ SPONGIOSITIS.

**spongio-** \spän′jē·ō-\ [Gk *spongia* sponge] A combining form meaning sponge, spongy. Also *spongi-.*

**spongioblast** \spän′jē·ōblast′\ [SPONGIO- + -BLAST] Embryonic cell type of the mantle layer of the neural tube which gives rise to astrocytes and oligodendrocytes of the neuroglia. Also *amacrine cell, glioblast.* **s. of the retina** An embryonic neuroglial cell in the retina which gives rise to its sustentacular fibers.

**spongioblastoma** \-blastō′mə\ A tumor of spongioblasts. Also *spongiocytoma.* **s. multiforme** GLIOBLASTOMA. **polar s.** A very rare brain tumor of children, composed of unipolar or bipolar glial cells forming palisading patterns. Also *spongioblastoma polare, spongioblastoma unipolare.* **s. unipolare** A spongioblastoma with unipolar cells.

**spongiocyte** \spän′jē·ōsīt′\ [SPONGIO- + -CYTE] 1 A cell in the adrenal cortex which appears vacuolated when lipids are removed in preparation for microscopic examination. 2 A neuroglial cell. *Outmoded.*

**spongiocytoma** \-sītō′mə\ [SPONGIO- + CYT- + -OMA] SPONGIOBLASTOMA.

**spongiosa** \spän′jē·ō′sə\ SUBSTANTIA SPONGIOSA OSSIUM.

**spongiose** \spän′jē·ōs\ With many holes, like a sponge; spongy.

**spongiosis** \spän′jē·ō′sis\ Epidermal edema that separates the malpigian cells of the spongy layer.

**spongiositis** \-sī′tis\ [L *spongios(um)* (neut. of *spongiosus*) spongy + -ITIS] Inflammation affecting the corpus spongiosum penis. Also *spongeitis, spongiitis.*

**spongy** \spun′jē\ Resembling a sponge in appearance or texture.

**spoon** [Old English *spōn,* akin to Gk *sphēn* a wedge] A spoon-shaped instrument. **marrow s.** A surgical scooplike instrument designed for removing marrow from a bone marrow cavity.

**spor-** \spôr-\ SPORO-.

**sporadic** \spôrad′ik\ [Gk *sporadikos* (from *sporas,* gen. *sporados,* scattered, from *speirein* to sow) scattered, strewn] Appearing infrequently as an isolated event: said of a disease that is neither endemic nor epidemic at a given time or place.

**sporadin** \spôr′ədin\ [Gk *sporas,* gen. *sporados,* scattered + -IN] The free (nonattached) trophozoite adult stage of gregarine parasites in the invertebrate host intestine. Also *sporodin, sporont.*

**spore** [Gk *spora* (from *speirein* to sow) a sowing, begetting of children, seedtime, seed] **1** A minute propagative unit, in fungi, usually unicellular, with the potential for developing into an adult without fusion with another cell. **2** A dormant or resting stage of certain bacteria and blue-green algae, highly resistant to heat. **bacterial s.** A differentiated cell type formed by some Gram-positive bacilli and clostridia under conditions of poor nutrition. The specialized integument and composition make spores highly resistant to killing by heat and by disinfectants. **black s.** A degenerating blood parasite, such as a malarial parasite, found in the mosquito stomach.

**spori-** \spôr′i-\ SPORO-.

**sporicidal** \-sī′dəl\ Lethal to spores.

**sporicide** \spôr′isīd\ An agent or drug lethal to spores.

**-sporium** \-spôr′ē·əm\ [New L, from Gk *spor(a)* seed + L *-ium,* noun suffix] A combining form meaning (1) a layer of a spore wall; (2) a plant so characterized.

**sporo-** \spôr′ə-, spôr′ō-\ [Gk *sporos* a sowing, seed, crop] A combining form meaning seed or spore. Also *spori-, spor-.*

**sporoagglutination** \-agloo′tinā′shən\ A serologic diagnostic test used to identify *Sporothrix schenckii* by spore agglutination.

**sporoblast** \spôr′əblast\ [SPORO- + -BLAST] A developmental stage within the oocyst in sporozoan life cycles which precedes the formation of the sporocyst and which is differentiated from the sporocyst by absence of a cyst wall. This stage often occurs after passage of oocysts in the feces of the host. Also *zygotomere.*

**sporocyst** \spôr′əsist\ [SPORO- + CYST] **1** A saclike larval form of digenetic flukes that develops from a miracidium in the snail intermediate host, and contains germinal cells that develop into other sporocysts or rediae. **2** The developmental stage that follows formation of the sporoblast in the oocyst of coccidia and gregarines. Each sporocyst then produces one or more sporozoites.

**sporodin** \spôr′ədin\ SPORADIN.

**sporogony** \spôräg′ənē\ [SPORO- + -GONY] The production of sporozoites in sporozoan development. In many forms it is preceded by sexual fusion and formation of oocysts, within which the sporozoites are formed. Also *sporogeny.*

**sporont** \spôr′änt\ [*spor(e)* + *-ont,* combining form from Gk *ōn,* gen. *ontos,* pres. part. of *einai* to be] **1** The stage of sporozoan development that results in spore formation. A sporont that gives rise to a single spore is a monosporoblastic sporont. If two spores are formed, it is a pansporoblastic or disporoblastic sporont. In Myxosporidia, host tissue surrounding the sporont becomes hypertrophied, then degenerates and produces a cyst wall. In Coccidia, it is an inner mass within the oocyst that gives rise to the sporoblast, which in turn forms the sporocysts, within which the sporozoites develop. **2** SPORADIN.

**sporoplasm** \spôr′əplazm\ [SPORO- + -PLASM] The protoplasm of a spore.

**sporotheca** \-thē′kə\ The envelope or membrane within which spores are found, as seen in many different forms of fungi and among sporozoan protozoa.

**sporotrichosis** \-trikō′sis\ A worldwide disease of several animal species and man, caused by infection with the fungus *Sporothrix schenckii,* which is usually introduced into the body via puncture wounds. Cutaneous ulcers or nodules are usual and, rarely, internal organs may be affected in focal or disseminated infections.

**Sporozoa** \-zō′ə\ [SPORO- + Gk *zōa,* pl. of *zōon* living being, animal] A former class in the former phylum Protozoa that corresponds to the present class Sporozoea in the protozoan phylum Apicomplexa.

**sporozoa** Plural of SPOROZOON.

**sporozoan** \-zō′ən\ **1** Of or relating to sporozoa, or the class Sporozoea. **2** A member of the class Sporozoea.

**Sporozoea** \-zō′ē·ə\ [SPORO- + *zō(o)-* + *-ea,* suffix denoting a class] A class in the protozoan phylum Apicomplexa characterized by a complete conoid in most forms, sexual and asexual reproduction, oocysts with infective sporozoites resulting from sporogony, lack of motor organelles, movement by gliding, and body flexion or undulation of longitudinal ridges. It includes the subclasses Gregarinia, Coccidia, and Piroplasmia.

**sporozoite** \-zō′īt\ [SPORO- + *zo(o)-* + -ITE] A motile elongate reproductive body responsible for invasion of cells of the final host of many sporozoan parasites. It is the product of sporogony, usually following repeated nuclear division within an oocyst. Infection of the final host follows ingestion of infective oocysts or inoculation of sporozoites into the host, as in mosquito transmission of malarial parasites. Also *gametoblast* (obs.), *oxyopore, germinal rod, zygotoblast.*

**sporozooid** \-zō′oid\ A falciform body observed in some cancerous tumors that resembles a sporozoan spore.

**sporozoon** \-zō′än\ [SPORO- + Gk *zōon* living being, animal] (*pl.* sporozoa) An individual sporozoan organism; a member of the class Sporozoea.

**sport** [Middle English, short for *disport,* from Middle French *desport* (from *des-* DIS-[1] + *port(er)* to carry, from L *portare* to carry) a playing, diversion] An individual that varies significantly from the mean of its stock, strain, or species. If the variations are transmitted to the descendants, the sport represents a new mutation. If not transmitted to any offspring, the sport is a teratic manifestation of abnormal embryogenesis.

**sporular** \spôr′yələr\ Of or pertaining to spores.

**sporulation** \spôr′ʸəlā′shən\ The process of forming a spore within a vegetative bacterial cell. **endogenous s.** Sporulation in protozoa that occurs within the host, as seen in the mosquito phase of the plasmodial parasite causing malaria. **exogenous s.** Sporulation that results in the completion of sporulation outside the host, as seen in many coccidial oocysts. The sporulation phase precedes infection of the next host.

**sporule** \spôr′yool\ [French, from New L *sporul(a),* dim. of Gk *spora* a seed] A small spore.

**spot** **1** A small circumscribed area that differs, usually in color, from its surroundings. **2** Any small circumscribed skin lesion. *Popular.* **Bitot s.'s** Small, foamy deposits upon the conjunctiva on either side of the cornea, within the interpalpebral space, commonly containing *Bacillus xerosis.* Although they are traditionally associated with vitamin A deficiency, this clinical association is not usually present. Also *conjunctival spots, Bitot's patches.* **blind s.** The normal visual field defect corresponding to the location of the optic disk, the exit point of the optic nerve from the eyeball, which is insensitive to light stimuli. It is situated at approximately 12–15° to the nasal side of the horizontal plane. **blue s.** 1 MACULAE CAERULEAE. 2 MONGOLIAN SPOT. **Brushfield s.'s** Pale spots of the peripheral iris, occurring most frequently in the Down syndrome. **café-au-lait s.'s** Areas of coffee-colored cutaneous pigmentation. Those of smooth outline are sometimes associated with neurofibromatosis, those of irregular outline with polyostotic fibrous dysplasia. **Campbell de Morgan s.** CHERRY ANGIOMA. **Cayenne pepper s.'s** Tiny telangiectatic spots within the dermal papillae of the lesions of angioma serpiginosum and elastosis perforans serpiginosum. Also *papillary varices.* **cherry-red s.** The normal redness of the macula seen as a spot in contrast to the surrounding abnormally white retina, as in occlusion of the central retinal artery or in Tay-Sachs disease. Also *Tay sign, Tay spot.* **Christopher s.'s** MAURER'S DOTS. **cold s.** A region in a radioisotopic scan which shows decreased activity or none relative to the level of adjacent radioactivity. **conjunctival s.'s** BITOT SPOTS. **cotton wool s.'s** COTTON WOOL PATCHES. **De Morgan s.** CHERRY ANGIOMA. **eye s.** The early appearance of the developing eye in the embryo as an identifiable speck seen on the outside of the embryonic head. **flame s.'s** FLAME-SHAPED HEMORRHAGES. **focal s.** In radiology, the area of the anode of an x-ray tube on which the electrons are focused, and consequently the area which is the source of the x rays. **Forchheimer s.'s** An enanthema, consisting of small red macules which may appear on the soft palate, either preceding or accompanying the eruption of the rash in rubella. **Fordyce s.'s** Sebaceous glands in the oral mucous membrane, usually in the cheeks. They are visible as cream spots beneath the epithelium, which is slightly raised over them. Also *Fordyce granules, pseudocolloid of lips* (obs.), *Fordyce disease.* **genital s.** GENITAL AREAS. **germinal s.** The area germinativa or germinal vesicle, the round place on one side of the vitelline membrane where development of the embryo commences. **gift s.'s** LEUKONYCHIA. **ink s.'s** Blue-black discolorations in the buccal mucosa, especially the gums, of patients with addisonian dermal pigmentation. **interpalpebral s.** PINGUECULA. **Koplik s.'s** Small, irregular red spots with central gray or bluish-white specks which appear on the oral mucosa during the prodromal period of measles. Also *Koplik sign.* **lenticular s.'s** ROSE SPOTS. **liver s.** 1 *Popular* PITYRIASIS VERSICOLOR. 2 A brown patch on the face, as is seen in chloasma. *Popular.* **Maurer s.'s** MAURER'S DOTS. **Maxwell s.** The dark central area seen when looking at a uniform luminous purplish background. **milk s.'s** White or gray-white, slightly opaque spots or patches on the right ventricular epicardium occasionally seen as incidental findings at autopsy in middle-aged or older people. They are areas of fibrous thickening of the epicardium, possibly resulting from healed, circumscribed pericarditis, although their etiology is uncertain. Also *milk patches, white patches, soldiers' patches, soldiers' spots, tendinous spots.* **mongolian s.** A pigmented macular lesion commonly seen in the sacral area in infants. The pathologic abnormality is an increase in the number of dermal melanocytes. Also *mongolian macula, blue spot, sacral spot.* **Mueller s.'s** Spots occasionally observed on the iris of a person who has had smallpox. **mulberry s.** A globular phacoma on the retina which may be seen in tuberous sclerosis or in the other phacomatoses. **orange s.** A round, pinkish orange spot, a few millimeters in diameter, often observed on the tympanic membrane in cases of secretory otitis media. It is due to the presence, on the inner surface of the membrane, of a small polypoid granuloma. Several such spots may be observed in the same case. Also *Smith-McGuckin spot.* **pain s.'s** The discontinuous punctate zones from which nociceptive fibers can be excited and which give rise to fast, pricking pain sensations. **pink s.** PINK TOOTH. **plague s.'s** Ecchymoses or purpura appearing on the skin of a person with plague. **rose s.'s** Rose-colored lesions, 2–4 mm in diameter, which occur in small numbers on the upper abdomen during typhoid fever. They are usually observed during the second week of illness. Also *typhoid spots, lenticular spots.* **Roth s.'s** Round or oval retinal hemorrhages with white centers which are sometimes observed in bacterial endocarditis, collagen diseases, leukemia, dysproteinemia, and pernicious anemia. **saccular s.** MACULA SACCULI. **sacral s.** MONGOLIAN SPOT. **Smith-McGuckin s.** ORANGE SPOT. **Soemmering s.** MACULA RETINAE. **soldiers' s.'s** MILK SPOTS. **Stephen s.'s** MAURER'S DOTS. **Tardieu s.'s** 1 The multiple, often confluent petechiae and ecchymoses which are found on skin and mucous membrane areas of intense livor mortis. The spots form as a result of excessive congestion of capillaries, with subsequent rupture and extravasation of blood. They are commonly found on the face, conjunctivae, eyelids, feet, and ankles of hanging victims. 2 The subendothelial petechiae found on pleural surfaces. These form as a result of increased capillary permeability associated with venous congestion. They were formerly considered pathognomonic of asphyxial death. **Tay s.** CHERRY-RED SPOT. **temperature s.'s** Discontinuous cutaneous loci the excitation of which gives rise to thermal sensation, usually cold. **tendinous s.'s** MILK SPOTS. **touch s.** A cutaneous locus demonstrating a relatively low threshold to punctate tactile stimulation. It marks the position of a touch sensory organ. **trigger s.** The zone from which a nervous reflex can be elicited, e.g., a zone of dense trigeminal cutaneous innervation from which a paroxysm of trigeminal neuralgia can be triggered. **typhoid s.'s** ROSE SPOTS. **warm s.'s** Cutaneous loci the thermal or electrical stimulation of which gives rise to a sensory report of warmth. **Willner s.'s** Numerous small spots which develop rapidly into pustules, appearing on the internal layer of the prepuce in the early stages of smallpox. **yellow s.** MACULA RETINAE.

**spotting** Scanty vaginal bleeding occurring unexpectedly during pregnancy or between menses.

**spp.** species (as a plural form).

**sprain** [possibly Old French *espreindre* to squeeze, from L *exprimere* to squeeze or press out] An injury to joint ligaments usually resulting from a sudden wrenching or twisting motion that overstretches or tears fibers and may rupture blood vessels but leaves the structural integrity of the ligaments intact. **acromioclavicular s.** A tearing of part of the acromioclavicular ligament above the shoulder joint. **deltoid s.** An incomplete tearing of the fibers of the deltoid muscle at its insertion into the humerus. **riders' s.** A sprain of the adductor muscle group at their insertion into the femur above the knee. It is often seen in horseback riders. **Schlatter s.** OSGOOD-SCHLATTER DISEASE. **tibiofibular s.** An incomplete tearing of the ligaments after injury to either the superior or the inferior tibiofibular joint. **vertebral cervical s.** POST-TRAUMATIC CERVICAL SYNDROME.

**spray** Liquid medicine dispersed into very minute droplets, or mist, which can be inhaled or applied to surfaces such as the skin, mucous membranes, or other regions of the body.

**spread** To be disseminated or become epidemic: said of an infectious disease. **electrotonic s.** In cells or tissues with polarized cellular membranes, such as muscle and nerve, the decremental transmission of a change in potential in accord with cable properties of the structure. It does not involve the tramsmission of spikelike waves of depolarization. **gene s.** GENE FLOW. **secondary s.** **1** Spread of a localized infection to distant sites, usually by the hematogenous route. **2** The widespread dissemination of previously localized eczema. Also *autoeczematization, autosensitization dermatitis.*

**spreader** **1** An instrument used for distributing a substance over a surface. **2** An instrument used for clearing or maintaining a space within a structure or between parts. **gutta-percha s.** A fine tapering instrument used to condense gutta-percha points in a root canal. Also *root canal spreader.*

**Sprengel** [Otto Gerhard Karl *Sprengel,* German surgeon, 1852–1915] See under DEFORMITY.

**spring** [Old English, akin to *springan* to spring] An elastic wire, usually incorporating a coil, used to exert a force on a tooth or teeth in orthodontic treatment. **auxiliary s.** A simple wire arm attached to an orthodontic appliance and used to move one or two teeth. Also *finger spring.* **Weiss s.'s** Stainless steel springs used in the surgical correction of scoliosis.

**sprout** [Old English *sprūtan* to sprout] **1** New growth. **2** To send out new growth. **nodal s.** A new branch or sprout arising from a node of Ranvier of the parent axon. **syncytial s.'s** Small, multinucleated elevations on the surface of human placental chorionic villi. Two kinds are recognized. One is the precursor of a new villus, the other becomes constricted at its point of attachment and eventually breaks free into the intervillous space, and may be deported into the maternal venous system. Also *placental syncytial buds.* ⟨Hamilton and Boyd, *The Human Placenta,* 1970⟩

**sprouting** The proliferation of new branches on the telodendron of an axon, presumably induced by trophic influences arising from some change in the muscle or nervous cells in or near the area the axon supplies. It is often a response to partial denervation of the area, and the new connections are functional.

**sprue** \sproo\ [Dutch *spruw* sprue] **1** Either of two malabsorption syndromes, tropical and nontropical sprue. Also *catarrhal dysentery* (obs.). **2** In dentistry, the hole in a mold through which molten metal or other material is poured or forced, or the wax, wood, or plastic used to form the hole. **3** The part of the casting that fills a dental sprue. **celiac s.** CELIAC DISEASE. **nontropical s.** CELIAC DISEASE. **tropical s.** A disease usually acquired in a tropical country, characterized by malabsorption of dietary components and test substances, and accompanied by weight loss, sore tongue, anemia, folic acid deficiency, and, in advanced cases, edema. It usually begins with acute or subacute diarrhea. Although the cause is unknown, there is overgrowth of coliform bacteria in the small intestine, accompanied by jejunal and ileal mucosal changes which occur as the disease progresses. Treatment is with broad-spectrum antibiotics and folic acid supplements. Also *psilosis* (obs.), *cachexia aphthosa* (outmoded). See also TROPICAL STOMATITIS.

**sprue-former** SPRUE PIN.

**spt.** *spiritus* (L, spirit, used in pharmacy).

**SPTA** spatial peak temporal average.

**spud** \spud\ [Middle English *spudde*] A small surgical instrument with a broad flat blade that is used for blunt dissection or for locating and removing foreign bodies.

**Spumavirinae** \spʸooʹməvīʹrinē\ [*Spumavir(us)* + *-inae,* suffix denoting a subfamily] A subfamily of the Retroviridae. It includes membrane-bound RNA viruses with reverse transcriptase such as the syncytium-forming foamy viruses of man, cats, cattle, hamsters and the spumavirus F primate (foamy virus type 1 of monkey).

**spumavirus** \spʸooʹməvīʹrəs\ [L *spuma* foam, froth + VIRUS ] A member of the *Spumavirus* genus of the Spumavirinae subfamily of the Retroviridae. Spumavirus F is a foamy virus that infects monkeys.

**spur** [Old English *spora, spura*] **1** A part abruptly projecting from a surface, as of bone. **2** A piece of metal projecting from a dental appliance. **3** The extension of a curved precipitin line past the point at which, in a double diffusion test, it would intersect with a perfectly symmetrical line caused by an identical antigen-antibody reaction, indicating a reaction of partial identity. **calcaneal s.** A traction exostosis on the lower surface of the calcaneus at the attachment of the long plantar ligament. Also *heel spur.* **cementum s.** A spiked projection of cementum from the cervical region of a tooth. **enamel s.** A tongue-shaped projection of enamel occasionally found at the level of bifurcation in multirooted teeth. **heel s.** CALCANEAL SPUR. **occipital s.** Abnormal formation of bone on the basilar process of the occipital bone. **olecranon s.** An osteophyte or exostosis on the olecranon at the insertion of the triceps muscle.

**spurious** \spyooʹrē·əs\ Having a superficial resemblance to something real or genuine, but actually false or fake; counterfeit.

**Spurway** [John *Spurway,* English physician, flourished late 19th century] Spurway syndrome. See under LOBSTEIN SYNDROME.

**sputum** \spyooʹtəm\ [L (from *spuere* to spit, spit out, akin to Gk *ptyein* to spit, spit out, and to English *spit, spew*) spittle, spit] Material coughed up from the lungs, bronchi, or trachea. **s. aeruginosum** GREEN SPUTUM. **s. cruentum** Blood-tinged sputum. **green s.** Sputum of a green color, usually indicating that the sputum is infected. Also *sputum aeruginosum.* **mucoid s.** Colorless sputum of gelatinous consistency. Also *mucous sputum.* **nummular s.** Sputum containing lumps that take on a flattened, discoid shape on the bottom of a sputum cup. **rusty s.** Sputum with a brown discoloration from the presence of denatured blood.

**SQ** subcutaneous.

**squalene** $H{-}[CH_2{-}C(CH_3){=}CH{-}CH_2{-}]_3{-}[{-}CH_2{-}CH{=}C(CH_3){-}CH_2]_3{-}H$. A hydrocarbon found in plants and animals, where it is the biosynthetic precursor of steroids. It is formed metabolically from two molecules of farnesyl diphosphate with concomitant oxidation of NADPH.

**squalene monooxygenase** The enzyme (EC 1.14.99.7) that catalyzes the conversion of squalene into its 2,3-epoxide with uptake of dioxygen and concomitant oxidation of another substance, a step in the biosynthesis of steroids.

**squama** \skwāʹmə\ [L, a scale of a fish or a serpent] (*pl.* squamae) A scalelike or thin platelike structure. Also *squame.* **s. alveolaris** TYPE I PNEUMOCYTE. **external mental s.** *Outmoded* PROTUBERANTIA MENTALIS. **s. frontalis** [NA] The smooth convex portion of the frontal bone above the supraorbital margins forming the forehead. The internal surface is related to the frontal lobes of the cerebrum. Also *frontal squama, squama of frontal bone, perpendicular squama* (outmoded). **occipital s.** SQUAMA OCCIPITALIS. **s. occipitalis** [NA] The broad, convex superior and posterior portion of the occipital bone extending from lambda to the posterior margin of the foramen magnum, continuous with the two lateral portions of the occipital bone and presenting paired lambdoid and mastoid margins. Also *occipital squama, squame of occipital bone, squamous part of occipital bone, occipital part of occipital bone.* **perpendicular s.** *Outmoded* SQUAMA FRONTALIS. **temporal s.** PARS SQUAMOSA OSSIS TEMPORALIS. **s. of temporal bone** PARS SQUAMOSA OSSIS TEMPORALIS.

**squamae** \skwā′mē\ Plural of SQUAMA.

**squamate** \skwā′māt\ [*squam(o)-* + -ATE] SCALY.

**squamatization** \skwā′mətīzā′shən\ The process of becoming squamous cells: said of other types of cells.

**squame** \skwām\ [L *squam(a),* a scale of a fish or a serpent] **1** SCALE. **2** SQUAMA. **s. of occipital bone** SQUAMA OCCIPITALIS.

**squamo-** \skwā′mō-\ [L *squama* scale of fish or serpent] A combining form meaning scale or squama.

**squamofrontal** \-frun′təl\ Pertaining to the squama frontalis.

**squamoid** \skwā′moid\ Resembling a squama.

**squamomandibular** \-mandib′yələr\ Of or pertaining to the squama of either the frontal, the temporal, or the occipital bones and of the mandible.

**squamomastoid** \-mas′toid\ Of or pertaining to the squamous part and the mastoid process of the temporal bone.

**squamo-occipital** \-äksip′itəl\ Of or pertaining to the squama occipitalis.

**squamoparietal** \-pərī′ətəl\ Pertaining to the squamous part of the temporal bone and to the parietal bone. Also *squamosoparietal, parietosquamosal.*

**squamosa** \skwāmō′sə\ PARS SQUAMOSA OSSIS TEMPORALIS.

**squamosal** \skwāmō′səl\ **1** One of the three pieces of bone which constitute the temporal bone in the embryo (the other two being the tympanic and the petrous temporal). It develops in membrane and gives rise to the zygomatic process, the squama, and the anterior part of the mastoid process. **2** Referring to the squamous temporal bone.

**squamosoparietal** \-sōpərī′ətəl\ SQUAMOPARIETAL.

**squamotemporal** \-tem′pərəl\ Pertaining to the pars squamosa ossis temporalis.

**squamotympanic** \-timpan′ik\ Of or pertaining to the squamous and the tympanic parts of the temporal bone.

**squamous** \skwā′məs\ [*squam(o)-* + -OUS] **1** Bearing scales; scaly. **2** Of or relating to a squama.

**squamozygomatic** \-zī′gəmat′ik\ Pertaining to the squamous part and the zygomatic process of the temporal bone.

**square / Punnett s.** A matrix for determining the possible genotypes at a given locus or loci and their relative frequencies in progeny when the parental alleles are known. Each row of the matrix represents the haploid gametes of one parent, and the columns, the gametes of the other. The squares of the grid then contain the progeny genotypes. Also *checkerboard.*

**squash-bite** A maxillomandibular record made by biting into a piece of softened material.

**squill** \skwil\ [L *scilla* (from Gk *skilla* a sea onion or squill) a sea onion, sea leek, squill] The sliced and dried scale leaves of the bulb of the white variety of *Urginea maritima,* used as an expectorant. A variety from *U. indica* (red squill) has been used effectively as a rat poison. Also *scilla, sea onion, Mediterranean squill, white squill.* **red s.** See under SQUILL. **white s.** SQUILL.

**squillitic** Pertaining to or containing squill.

**squint** [Middle English *asquint* (prob. from Dutch or Low German) sidewise, obliquely] STRABISMUS. **comitant s.** CONCOMITANT STRABISMUS. **concomitant s.** CONCOMITANT STRABISMUS. **convergent s.** ESOTROPIA. **divergent s.** EXOTROPIA.

**Sr** Symbol for the element, strontium.

**sr** Symbol for the unit, steradian.

**SRBC** sheep red blood cells.

**SRF** **1** somatotropin releasing factor (growth hormone releasing hormone). **2** skin reactive factor.

**SRH** somatotropin releasing hormone (growth hormone releasing hormone).

**sRNA** soluble RNA.

**SRS-A** slow-reacting substance of anaphylaxis.

**SRT** **1** sedimentation rate test. **2** speech reception threshold.

**ss.** *semis* (L, one-half).

**Ssabanejew** [Ivan *Ssabanejew,* Russian surgeon, born 1856] Ssabanejew-Frank operation. See under FRANK'S OPERATION.

**SSS** sick sinus syndrome.

**s.s.s.** stratum super stratum (L, layer upon layer).

**s.s.v.** *sub signo veneni* (L, under a poison label).

**ST** **1** stable toxin. **2** survival time. **3** standardized test. **4** skin test.

**St** Symbol for the unit, stokes.

**stab[1]** [Middle English *stabbe,* of obscure origin] **1** To penetrate by means of a rapid thrust with a pointed object. **2** See under STAB CULTURE.

**stab[2]** [German *Stab* staff, rod] BAND NEUTROPHIL.

**stabilimeter** \stāb′ilim′ətər\ [*stabili(ty)* + -METER] An instrument designed to record and measure bodily sway of a subject who has been instructed to remain as motionless as possible while standing upright with the eyes closed or covered. Also *stabilograph.*

**stability** \stəbil′itē\ The quality or condition of being stable, or the degree to which something is stable; resistance, or the degree of resistance, to chemical or physical change or disruption. **denture s.** See under RETENTION.

**stabilizer** \stā′bilī′zər\ **1** A chemical substance that inhibits the decomposition of another. **2** A substance that favors the stability of a colloidal suspension. **endodontic s.** DIODONTIC SPLINT.

**stabilograph** \stəbil′əgraf\ STABILIMETER.

**stable** **1** Not easily changed or likely to vary; steady. **2** Designating a substance that does not easily decompose.

**stachydrine** *N,N*-Dimethylproline, a widely occurring alkaloid.

**stachyose** A crystalline tetrasaccharide found in many plants. It consists of sucrose glycosylated on O-6 of its glucose residue by a disaccharide of two α1,6-linked galactose residues.

**Stacke** [Ludwig *Stacke,* German otologist, 1859–1918] **1** See under MEATOPLASTY. **2** Stacke's operation. See under OPERATION.

**stactometer** \staktäm′ətər\ [Gk *stakto(s)* (from *stazein* to drip) oozing or dripping + -METER] A pipette with a small bore, used to measure drops of fluid.

**Staderini** [Rutilio *Staderini,* Italian neuroanatomist, flourished 19th century] Nucleus of Staderini. See under NUCLEUS INTERCALATUS.

**stadium** \stā′dē·əm\ [L, from Gk *stadion,* a unit of distance (about 600 feet), a racecourse of this length; used in New L as a transl. of STAGE (an unrelated word)] A stage, phase, or period, as of a disease. **s. acmes** The peak of activity of a disease. **s. caloris** The hot stage of a fever or a febrile illness. **s. decrementi** The stage of a disease marked by a lessening intensity of symptoms, such as fever. **s. defervescentiae** The stage of a disease marked by an abatement of fever. Also *defervescent stage.* **s. frigoris** The cold, shivering stage of a disease, especially of an intermittent fever. **s. sudoris** The sweating stage of a disease or fever.

**staff** [Old English *stæf*] **1** A wooden or metallic grooved director along which a knife may be passed. **2** A supporting rodlike structure. **3** The personnel of an organization, such as a hospital. **s. of Aesculapius** The symbol of medicine, a staff encircled by a single snake, used as an emblem by many organizations. Aesculapius is the Greek god of medicine. Compare CADUCEUS. **closed s.** The professional staff of a health care organization whose membership is not open to all practitioners in the community. **s. of Wrisberg** A somewhat cylindrical elevation often to be seen at the junction of the lateral and posterior walls of the superior vestibule of the larynx overlying the cartilage of Wrisberg (the cuneiform cartilage). As well as marking the site of the cartilage, this feature is formed in part by an unusual accumulation of mucous glands.

**Stafne** [Edward Christian *Stafne*, U.S. oral pathologist, born 1894] See under CAVITY.

**stage** [Old French *estage* (from L *stare* to stand) stage, place, position] **1** A distinct phase or period in any process, such as the life of an organism, the course of a disease, a physiologic cycle, or a procedure. The extent of spread of cancer is often described as a stage of the disease and classified as stages I–IV, corresponding to degrees of local, regional, and distant spread. **2** A platform, such as that of a microscope, on which an object can be placed for observation or manipulation. **algid s.** A condition characterized by subnormal temperature, flickering pulse, hypotension, and neurologic symptoms, as may be observed in diseases marked by massive intestinal discharges, such as cholera or falciparum malaria. **anal s.** ANAL PHASE. **bell s.** The stage of tooth development when the enamel organ attains a bell-like form. **cap s.** An early stage of tooth development when the enamel organ forms a cap on the surface of the dental papilla. **cold s.** The initial stage of a malarial paroxysm, characterized by intense chills and rigor. **crithidial s.** *Outmoded* EPIMASTIGOTE. **defervescent s.** STADIUM DEFERVESCENTIAE. **developmental s.** A time in human growth when certain kinds of behavior begin to emerge, governed by the unfolding of a genetic master plan of development for the species. Examples include Freud's successive stages of psychosexual growth, Gesell's stages of childhood development, or Piaget's stages of cognitive development. **dictyotene s.** The state of the primary oocytes in the ovary at the time of birth. This stage represents the end of the prophase of the first meiotic division, during which the oocyte still possesses the diploid number of chromosomes, a condition that persists until puberty for a few oocytes and continues for much longer for others until ovulation ceases. **emergent s. I** DESYNCHRONIZED SLEEP. **exoerythrocytic s.** Any stage in the development of malarial parasites that occurs outside of erythrocytes. In human malaria this is ordinarily a preerythrocytic stage occurring in parenchymal cells of the liver. See also CRYPTOZOITE, METACRYPTOZOITE. **expulsive s.** SECOND STAGE OF LABOR. **s. of fervescence** PYROGENETIC STAGE. **first s. of labor** The period in labor from the onset of regular uterine contractions until the cervix is fully dilated. The average duration is about 12 hours for primigravidas and about seven hours for multiparas. **genital s.** GENITAL PHASE. **Gillespie s.'s of anesthesia** A variation of Guedel stages of general anesthesia, with emphasis on progressive obtundation of reflex responses to stimuli. **Guedel s.'s of general anesthesia** The depth of narcosis according to physiologic signs and symptoms. The three traditional stages, best seen with diethyl ether, are: (1) the stage of altered consciousness and some analgesia; (2) the stage marked by loss of consciousness with uninhibited responses; and (3) the stage at which surgery is performed. This third stage is divided into four planes according to the degree of muscle relaxation needed for the operation. A fourth stage, moribundity, has been added to the traditional ones. **hot s.** The febrile stage of a malarial paroxysm. **imperfect s.** The asexual (usually conidial) stage of a fungus. **incubative s.** INCUBATION PERIOD. **s. of invasion** INCUBATION PERIOD. **s.'s of labor** The three or four distinct periods of labor that mark its progress. The first stage lasts from the onset of labor until full dilatation of the uterine cervix. The second stage proceeds from full dilatation through delivery of the infant. The third stage extends from delivery of the infant until placental delivery. An optional fourth stage covers the first hour or so following delivery of the placenta. **s. of latency** **1** A quiescent period during the course of an infectious disease, the pathogen being temporarily dormant. **2** INCUBATION PERIOD. **mechanical s.** A microscope stage that permits the microscope slide to be moved on the stage in either of two horizontal planes, thus facilitating the detailed examination of all parts of the slide. **microscope s.** A platform for holding a microscope slide while it is being examined with the microscope. **oral s.** ORAL PHASE. **oral-sadistic s.** ORAL-INCORPORATIVE PHASE. **perfect s.** The spore-forming stage following sexual fusion in fungi. **phallic s.** PHALLIC PHASE. **placental s.** THIRD STAGE OF LABOR. **preeruptive s.** The phase in the course of a disease between infection and the appearance of an eruption. **preerythrocytic s.** A stage in the development of malarial parasites which precedes their invasion of erythrocytes; exoerythrocytic stage. In human malaria this occurs in parenchymal cells of the liver. **premenstrual s.** The status of the endometrium between ovulation and menses, during which it undergoes changes initiated by the corpus luteum. **prodromal s.** The early phase of a disease which follows the incubation period and in which some clinical manifestations appear, but in which the characteristic symptoms and signs are not yet present. **prodromal s. of labor** The period immediately preceding the first stage of labor when uterine contractions have become regular but before rapid cervical dilatation has begun. **progestational s.** SECRETORY PHASE. **proliferative s.** PROLIFERATIVE PHASE. **pyretogenic s.** PYROGENETIC STAGE. **pyrogenetic s.** The stage of a disease during which fever develops and intensifies. Also *pyretogenic stage, stage of fervescence.* **Ranke s.'s** The three stages of tuberculosis: primary infection, generalized infection, and chronic infection. **rest s.** The status of the endometrium immediately following menstruation. **ring s.** SIGNET RING. **rotation s. of labor** The rotation of the fetal presenting part during labor in conformity with the dimensions of the birth canal. **second s. of labor** The period of labor from full cervical dilatation until delivery of the infant. The average duration is about 50 minutes for primigravidas and about 20 minutes for multiparas. Also *ex-*

*pulsive stage.* **Tanner s.'s** A system for correlating degrees of development of the secondary sex characteristics during puberty with chronologic age in girls and boys. In girls, breast development and pubic hair are factors; in boys, external genitalia and pubic hair. **third s. of labor** The period of labor following delivery of the infant through delivery of the placenta. The duration is usually about five minutes. Also *placental stage.* **tissue s.** A stage in the development of malarial parasites that takes place in vertebrate host tissues (other than the blood); exoerythrocytic stage. In human malaria this occurs in the parenchymal cells of the liver. **trypanosome s.** TRYPOMASTIGOTE. **vegetative s.** A stage in the life cycle of plant cells or microorganisms during which cells are dividing, usually by mitosis, into daughter cells, in contrast to the reproductive stage in which organisms form seeds or spores.

**staging** \stā′jing\ Any classification of the extent and severity of a malignant disease. **clinical s. of cancer** A system for classifying patients with cancer according to extent of disease. Widely used is the TNM system, in which the extent of cancer is defined by T (for tumor), which indicates size and local invasiveness of the primary tumor; N (for node), which indicates the extent of lymph node involvement; and M (for metastases), which gives the extent of distant metastases. In this scheme, $T_0$ means no evidence of primary tumor, $T_{IS}$ means carcinoma in situ, and $T_1$–$T_4$ indicate increasing tumor size and local invasiveness; $N_0$ means no evidence of lymph node involvement, $N_{1a}$ or $N_{2a}$ means one or two regional nodes are involved and metastases not suspected, $N_{1b}$, $N_{2b}$, etc., means one, two, etc., regional nodes are involved and metastases are suspected, and $N_X$ means the lymph nodes cannot be accessed clinically; $M_0$ means there is no evidence of distant metastases, and $M_1$, $M_2$, etc., indicate an increasing number of distant metastases. Numerous staging schemes are used for different malignancies. Many of these are similar to that for staging of carcinoma of the uterine cervix, in which Ia means cancer in situ, i.e. confined to the epithelium; Ib means invasion of the uterine cervix only; II means invasion of the uterus, adnexa, or regional lymph nodes only; and III means distant metastases. **clinical s. of lymphomas** A classification of the extent of malignant lymphoma, done without biopsy verification: Stage I is for lymphoma limited to a single lymph node or group of adjacent nodes, stage $I_E$ represents localized extranodal lymphoma; stage II is for lymphoma involving two or more contiguous lymph node areas on the same side of the diaphragm; stage III is for lymphoma involving multiple lymph node areas both above and below the diaphragm; and stage IV is for generalized lymphoma involving bone marrow or other nonlymphatic organs. In addition, B indicates that the patient has constitutional signs such as fever or weight loss, while A indicates absence of constitutional signs. Thus, stage IVB indicates advanced lymphoma with organ involvement and weight loss or fever. **pathological s. of lymphomas** A classification identical to the clinical staging of lymphomas, but with the extent of disease verified by biopsy and histologic examination, usually with laparotomy to ascertain involvement of retroperitoneal lymph nodes. **Rai s.** A scheme for classification of chronic lymphocytic leukemia according to degree of severity: stage 0 is for cases with lymphocytosis only, of blood and bone marrow; stage I is for lymphocytosis and lymphadenopathy; stage II is for lymphocytosis together with either hepatomegaly or splenomegaly or both, with or without lymphadenopathy; stage III is for lymphocytosis and anemia, irrespective of enlargement of liver, spleen, or lymph nodes; stage IV is for lymphocytosis and thrombocytopenia, irrespective of other abnormalities.

**Stahl** [Friedrich Karl *Stahl,* German physician, 1811–1873] **1** No. 1 Stahl ear. See under EAR. **2** No. 2 Stahl ear. See under EAR.

**Stähli** [Jean *Stähli,* Swiss ophthalmologist, born 1890] Stähli's line, Stähli pigment line. See under HUDSON-STÄHLI LINE.

**Stahr** [Hermann *Stahr,* German anatomist and pathologist, born 1868] See under GLAND.

**St. Aignon** [*St. Aignon,* French bishop, died 453] St. Aignon's disease. See under FAVUS.

## stain

**stain** [short for earlier *distain,* from Old French *desteindre* to discolor, from *des-* DIS-[1] + *teindre* to color, tint, from L *tingere* to dip, soak, dye (akin to Gk *tengein* to dip, soak, and to Old High German *thunkōn,* also *dunkōn,* to dip, soak, whence Pennsylvania German *dunke,* American English *dunk*)] **1** Any dye, reagent, or other chemical substance used to produce coloration in living or fixed tissues, microorganisms, or smears so that they or parts thereof are more easily visible or identifiable on microscopic examination. **2** To give color to living or fixed tissues, microorganisms, or smears in order to facilitate their microscopic examination. **3** A procedure or method utilizing the technique of staining. For terms not found under *stain,* see also under *method, procedure, reaction, technique,* and *test.* **acid s.** A dye with an anionic chromophore that, when combined with a cation such as sodium, forms a salt that may well have a basic reaction when dissolved in water. Also *acidic dye.* • Although widely used, this is a misleading term. **acid-fast s.** A staining method for demonstrating acid-fast microorganisms, that is, all *Mycobacterium* species and certain *Nocardia* species. After staining with carbolfuchsin, the microorganisms resist decolorization by strong mineral acid solutions while the decolorized portions of the specimen can be stained by a counterstain. The Ziehl-Neelsen and fluorochrome staining methods are types of acid-fast staining. **acid fuchsin s.** ACID FUCHSIN. **acid phosphatase s.** A histochemical technique used to identify enzymes that will hydrolyze organic phosphate esters at approximately pH 5.0. **alkaline phosphatase s.** A histochemical technique used to identify enzymes that will hydrolyze organic phosphate esters at approximately pH 9.0. **alum-carmine s.** BORAX-CARMINE SOLUTION. **Alzheimer s.** A mixture of methylene blue and eosin used to demonstrate Negri bodies. **amido black B s.** NAPHTHOL BLUE BLACK STAIN. **amido schwartz s.** NAPHTHOL BLUE BLACK STAIN. **aniline blue black s.** NAPHTHOL BLUE BLACK STAIN. **basic s.** A dye with a cationic chromophore that, when combined with an anionic group such as chloride, forms a salt that may well have an acidic reaction when dissolved in water. Also *basic dye.* • Although widely used, this is a misleading term. **basic fuchsin s.** BASIC FUCHSIN. **benzidine and nitroprusside peroxidase s.** A cytochemical or histochemical stain for peroxidase, in which the nitroprusside enhances and stabilizes the blue color formed in the reaction of benzidine with oxygen released from peroxides by peroxidases of cells or tissues. **Best's carmine s.** A stain in which carmine is dissolved in concentrated ammonia. The high pH achieved increases the solubility of carmine, inhibits tissue staining, and results in the deep red staining of any glycogen present. **Bielschowsky s.** A silver impregnation technique for demonstrating reticulin fibers. Also *Bielschowsky's method.* **Biondi-Heidenhain s.** A staining method for the demonstration of spirochetes, using a diluted mixture of saturated aqueous solutions of acid fuchsin or rubin, methyl green, and orange G. **Bunge-Trantenroth s.** A staining method for differentiating tubercle and smegma bacilli, using alcohol, chromic acid, hot carbolfuchsin, sulfuric acid, and alcoholic methylene blue. Tubercle bacilli stain red, while smegma bacilli are decolorized. **carbol-aniline fuchsin s.** A histologic staining technique that is used to demonstrate the presence of both parasitic protozoa and bacteria. **carbol-gentian violet s.** A histologic staining technique that has been used to demonstrate mycobacterial organisms. **certified s.** COMMISSION CERTIFIED STAIN. **chloracetate esterase s.** A histochemical technique that is used to identify cells of the myeloid series by demonstrating a lysosomal enzyme that is capable of hydrolyzing chloroacetate compounds. **Commission Certified s.** A batch of stain that has been certified as to its quality by the Biological Stain Commission, an independent nonprofit organization. Also *certified stain.* **contrast s.** COUNTERSTAIN. **Coomassie blue s.** A general protein stain commonly used to demonstrate protein bands in supportive media, such as agar or polyacrylamide gels, following electrophoresis. **counter s.** See under COUNTERSTAIN. **cytochemical s.** A stain used to localize and identify a chemical substance in a cell. The stain immobilizes and stains a chemical or enzyme at the site it occupies in the living tissue. **Davenport s.** DAVENPORT'S ALCOHOLIC SILVER NITRATE METHOD. **differential s.** A dye that, although it stains tissues nonselectively, can be extracted with a solvent at different rates from different structures to leave a selective staining pattern. **double s.** A combination of two selective stains that are used in a single technique. Usually one is concerned with distinquishing nuclei from cytoplasm. **Ehrlich's neutral s.** A stain for blood cells that is composed of methylene blue and acid fuchsin, now very rarely used. **Ehrlich's triple s.** A trichrome stain that contains orange G, acid fuchsin, and methyl green. It is used to stain blood cells. Also *Ehrlich's triacid stain.* **electron dense s.** Any staining solution that renders part of a tissue section visible by obstructing the passage of the electron beam in an electron microscope. Also *electron stain.* **fluorescent s.** A stain that, when illuminated, will emit light of a greater wavelength and therefore of a different color. This property is enhanced by the use of ultraviolet light. Such stains can be used to label a specific antibody and thus identify a specific tissue protein. **fluorochrome s.** A method of acid-fast staining using the fluorochrome dyes rhodamine and auramine. Acid-fast bacilli appear as fluorescent spots at relatively low magnification. **Fontana s.** A staining method for the demonstration of spirochetes, using ammoniacal silver nitrate solution. **Giemsa s.** A variant of the Romanowsky stain, in which azure II eosin, azure II, and glycerin are dissolved in methanol. The Giemsa stain is widely used for staining blood films and bone marrow aspirates, for staining specimens for protozoa such as *Leishmania* or trypanosomes, for *Leptospira* and *Borrelia*, rickettsiae, or viral inclusion bodies. It is also widely used for staining chromosomes to demonstrate characteristic banding patterns. **Gimenez s.** A staining method for the demonstration of rickettsiae, using carbolfuchsin and malachite green (method A) for most rickettsiae or carbolfuchsin, ferric nitrate, and fast green (method B) for *R. tsutsugamushi.* **gold chloride s.** A solution used in gold toning. **Gomori s.** GOMORI'S METHOD. **Gomori methenamine silver nitrate s.** A staining method for the demonstration of fungi, especially *Histoplasma capsulatum,* in fixed specimens, using chromic acid and methenamine silver nitrate. Fungi stain black against a green background. **Gram s.** A staining method for the classification of bacteria. Smears or tissue sections are stained with crystal violet, treated with an iodine solution, decolorized with alcohol, and then counterstained, usually with safranin. Microorganisms retaining the crystal violet stain are Gram-positive, while those which lose the primary stain by decolorization but stain with the counterstain are Gram-negative. Also *Gram's method.* **green s.** A greenish brown stain formed principally on the gingival third of the labial surfaces of maxillary incisors, usually in children. When it is removed the surface of the enamel is seen to be demineralized. **Gridley fungus s.** A staining method for the demonstration of fungi in fixed specimens, using chromic acid and, as a counterstain, either metanil yellow or Harris hematoxylin. The fungus will stain deep rose to purple and the background will be yellow. **Grübler s.** PAPPENHEIM STAIN. **Guenther s.** A staining method for demonstrating spirochetes, using an acetic acid solution, ammonia fumes, and Ehrlich's aniline gentian violet. **Gutstein s.** An aqueous solution of methyl violet and sodium bicarbonate, used to stain smears of material obtained from the skin lesions of smallpox. **Hale's iron s.** A histologic technique that uses a colloidal iron preparation to bind onto acid mucopolysaccharides. The iron can be demonstrated by the formation of Prussian blue. Also *Rinehart and Abul-Haj stain.* **heavy-metal s.** A staining solution that contains a heavy metal such as lead or uranium which will be visible in the electron microscope by virtue of its ability to obstruct the electron beam. **Heidenhain's iron hematoxylin s.** HEIDENHAIN'S IRON HEMATOXYLIN. **hemalum s.** A histologic stain which stains nuclei a deep purple. It is prepared from hematoxylin and alum. **hematoxylin and eosin s.** The most widely used staining technique in histology and histopathology. Hematoxylin stains nuclei blue-black with good intranuclear detail, and eosin binds to the cytoplasmic proteins and connective-tissue fibers, giving a range of pink, orange, or red hues depending on the nature of the substance stained. For other stains utilizing hematoxylin, see under HEMATOXYLIN. Abbr. H and E **hematoxylin-eosin-azure II s.** A histologic stain for bone marrow, composed of alum-hematoxylin and azure II-eosin. The stain facilitates identification of granulocytes and mast cells. Also *Maximow's method.* **Hiss capsule s.** An early technique, now modified, for demonstrating the presence of bacterial capsules by a combination of positive and negative staining. **histochemical s.** A stain or reaction used to localize and identify a chemical substance or an enzyme in a tissue. The stain or reaction immobilizes and stains a chemical or enzyme at the site it occupied in the living tissue. **immunofluorescent s.** An antibody or antigen to which a fluorochrome has been added. It permits location of antigen-antibody reactions in tissue sections. **immunoperoxidase s.** A general technique for specific identification of proteins in the cytoplasm of cells, based on complexing between the protein and monoclonal immunoglobulin specific for the protein. In this technique, the immunoglobulin is also complexed with a peroxidase. Then, if the peroxidase reaction is positive, it indicates the presence of the specific protein in cell cytoplasm. The procedure is used for recognition of cells characteristically seen in certain malignancies. **India ink s.** INDIA

INK METHOD. **intravital s.** A stain suitable for use within the intact living organism. Compare SUPRAVITAL STAIN. **iron s.** A stain for demonstration of iron pigment, such as hemosiderin, in tissue, based on the reaction in which iron reacts with a ferrocyanide salt to form Prussian blue. Also *Perls stain, Prussian blue stain.* **Kinyoun s.** PONDER-KINYOUN STAIN. **Kleihauer-Betke s.** A stain for hemoglobin F in erythrocytes that is based on elution of other hemoglobins such as hemoglobin A from a blood smear that has been immersed for a few minutes in a solution of citric acid and sodium citrate prior to staining with hematoxylin. Cells that contain hemoglobin F stain darkly; other cells appear as colorless ghosts. The procedure is used to determine the volume of blood that passes from fetus to mother during delivery and for identification of hereditary persistence of fetal hemoglobin. **lactophenol cotton blue s.** A staining method for demonstrating fungi in nonfixed tissue specimens, using lactophenol cotton blue dye. **Laidlaw s.** A histologic staining technique that uses a lithium silver solution for the impregnation of reticulin fibers. **Leifson's flagella s.** A stain that aggregates and mordants bacterial flagella, making them visible in the light microscope. **Leishman s.** A variant of the Romanowsky stain, containing methylene blue and eosin in absolute methanol. It is similar in applications and results to the Wright stain. **Lendrum's inclusion-body s.** A histologic staining technique in which phloxine, tartrazine, and hematoxylin are used to identify various inclusion bodies within cells. **leukocyte alkaline phosphatase s.** A stain for the presence of alkaline phosphatase in leukocyte cytoplasm, usually based on hydrolysis by alkaline phosphatase of naphthol AS BI phosphate to arylnaphtholamide which precipitates in the cytoplasm with a diazonium dye. The intensity of the reaction is scored. Normally neutrophils have a score of 40–100. When neutrophilia is due to infection or polycythemia vera, the leukocyte alkaline phosphatase (LAP) score is increased, whereas in chronic granulocytic leukemia the LAP score is usually 0 or nearly 0. **lipoid s.** A stain that binds to or dissolves in any conjugated or unconjugated lipid substance. **lithium-carmine s.** A stain for nuclei utilizing the mordant property of lithium to enhance the staining properties of carmine. **Macchiavello s.** A staining method formerly used to demonstrate rickettsiae. The method was unpredictable and was modified extensively and has been largely replaced by the Gimenez stain. Other, minor modifications of the Macchiavello stain have rendered it suitable for demonstrating *Chlamydia* species: the fixed specimen is stained with basic fuchsin, decolorized with dilute citric acid, and counterstained with aqueous methylene blue. The elementary bodies of *Chlamydia* species stain deep red. **Mallory's acid fuchsin, orange G, and aniline blue s.** MALLORY'S TRIPLE STAIN. **Mallory's phosphotungstic acid-hematoxylin s.** A technique that uses a hematoxylin solution containing phosphotungstic acid as a mordant. The solution can be naturally ripened over several months or chemically oxidized, and is used to demonstrate muscle striations, fibrin, cilia, and glial fibers. Also *PTAH stain, phosphotungstic acid-hematoxylin stain.* **Mallory's triple s.** A trichrome stain that contains acid fuchsin, orange G, and aniline blue and that is used to demonstrate connective tissue fibers and membranes. Also *Mallory's acid fuchsin, orange G, and aniline blue stain.* **Mann s.** MANN'S METHOD. **Masson's trichrome s.** A trichrome stain for detecting connective tissue fibers and membranes that contains ponceau R, acid fuchsin, and aniline blue or light green. Also *Masson stain, Masson's trichrome method.* **Mayer mucicarmine s.** A staining method for demonstrating epithelial mucins and some capsulated fungi, especially *Cryptococcus neoformans,* using carmine and aluminum hydroxide, or aluminum chloride which is diluted in water and alcohol. Mucins and fungi stain red. *Blastomyces dermatitidis* and *Histoplasma capsulatum* do not pick up this stain. **May-Grünwald s.** A neutral solution of methylene blue and eosin in methanol. It is one of the several varieties of Romanowsky stain commonly used for staining blood films. **metachromatic s.** METACHROMATIC DYE. **methyl green-pyronine s.** PAPPENHEIM STAIN. **MGP s.** PAPPENHEIM STAIN. **MSB s.** A trichrome stain containing Martius yellow, brilliant crystal scarlet, and soluble blue which is used for the demonstration of fibrin. **multiple s.** The combining of two, three, or four selective stains into a single technique in order to illustrate different tissue components simultaneously. **naphthol blue black s.** A general protein stain commonly used for demonstration of protein bands in supportive media, such as agar gel, following electrophoresis. Also *aniline blue black stain, amido black B stain, amido schwartz stain.* **negative s.** INDIA INK METHOD. **neutral s.** A combination stain derived from an acidic and a basic dye where both the cation and anion contain chromophore groups. **nonspecific esterase s.** A histochemical technique used to identify a range of lysosomal enzymes that can hydrolyze carboxylic acids. **nuclear s.** A stain that has a particular affinity for nuclear chromatin such as hematoxylin. **Orth s.** ORTH SOLUTION. **Paltauf s.** A modification of the Gram stain in which aniline oil and Gruebler's gentian violet are added to a mixture of absolute alcohol and distilled water. **Papanicolaou s.** A multiple stain containing Ehrlich's hematoxylin, orange G, phosphotungstic acid, light green, Bismarck brown, and eosin Y. It is used to identify subtle abnormalities or differentiations in the cells in vaginal and cervical smears. **Pappenheim s.** A histologic staining technique in which a solution of two basic dyes, methyl green and pyronin, are used to differentiate between DNA, which stains blue-green, and RNA, which stains red. Also *Grübler stain, Pappenheim's reagent, methyl-green pyronine stain, MGP stain.* **PAS s.** PERIODIC ACID-SCHIFF STAIN. **periodic acid-Schiff s.** A reaction that uses periodic acid to oxidize the aldehyde groups of carbohydrates in order that they will subsequently convert colorless Schiff's reagent to magenta. It is useful for demonstrating glycogen, basement membranes, and neutral mucopolysaccharides. Also *PAS stain, periodic acid-Schiff reaction, periodic acid/Schiff procedure.* **Perls s.** IRON STAIN. **peroxidase s.** Any histochemical or cytochemical stain for the demonstration of peroxidase. Benzidine and its derivatives are commonly used as chromogens in peroxidase stains. **phloxine-methylene blue s.** A double staining method particularly useful for demonstrating the presence of intracytoplasmic granules. **phosphotungstic acid-hematoxylin s.** MALLORY'S PHOSPHOTUNGSTIC ACID-HEMATOXYLIN STAIN. **plasma s.** A stain that has a particular affinity for cell cytoplasm. Also *plasmatic stain, protoplasmic stain, plasmic stain.* **Ponceau S s.** A general protein stain commonly used to demonstrate protein bands in supportive media, such as cellulose acetate, following electrophoresis. **Ponder-Kinyoun s.** A staining method for demonstrating *Corynebacterium diphtheriae,* using toluidine blue, methylene blue, and azure A dyes. Also *Kinyoun stain.* **port-wine s.** A congenital abnormality of the cutaneous vasculature that gives rise to flat red areas on the surface of the skin. Also *port-wine nevus, Unna's nevus.* **potassium hydroxide s.** A method of demonstrating fungi in unfixed specimens, using a solution of potassium hydroxide which dissolves mammalian cells or renders them translucent, whereas the polysaccharides of fungal cell walls are relatively resistant to the alkali. **progressive s.** A histologic staining method in which the reaction is allowed to proceed until the required intensity of color is achieved. **protoplasmic s.** PLASMA STAIN. **Prussian blue s.** IRON STAIN. **PTAH s.** MALLORY'S PHOSPHOTUNGSTIC ACID-HEMATOXYLIN STAIN. **regressive s.** A histologic staining method in which the reaction, once achieved, is allowed to continue and the excess dye is then removed selectively by differentiation. **Rinehart and Abul-Haj s.** HALE'S IRON STAIN. **Romanowsky s.** A combination of eosin with a saturated methanol solution of methylene blue. It is the basis for the most commonly used stains for blood, such as the Wright stain and the Giemsa stain. When blood films are treated with these Romanowsky-type stains, cytoplasm is blue to gray, nuclei are dark purple, erythrocytes are red, and cytoplasmic granules or inclusions may be purple, blue, or red. **selective s.** A stain that binds preferentially to one tissue component. This property can often be modified by altering the pH or electrolyte concentration of the stain solution. The binding may depend on Van der Waal's forces, coulombic attractions, hydrogen bonding, or covalent bonding. **Seller s.** A staining method for demonstrating Negri bodies, using alcoholic solutions of methylene blue and basic fuchsin. The Negri bodies stain bright red against a purplish pink background. It is a rapid means of diagnosing rabies. **simple s.** A dye that is used on its own to give a variable pattern of staining according to the affinity of the dye for various tissue components. **Smith s.** A staining method for demonstrating pneumococci in sputum, using aniline-oil gentian violet, a solution of iodine, a mixture of alcohol and ether, aqueous eosin, and Loeffler's methylene blue. **Stirling's modification of the Gram s.** A variation of Gram's method of staining for bacteria, using gentian violet, alcohol, aniline oil, and distilled water. **substantive s.** A permanent stain that does not require a mordant. **successive s.** A histologic staining method in which the dyes are applied sequentially rather than simultaneously. **supravital s.** A stain used for living cells detached from their source. Compare INTRAVITAL STAIN. **tartrate-resistant acid phosphatase s.** A cytochemical stain that tests the ability of tartrate to inhibit the acid phosphatase activity of cytoplasm. It is especially useful for identification of the hairy cells of leukemic reticuloendotheliosis, which contain a tartrate-resistant acid phosphatase. Other leukocytes contain tartrate-inhibitable acid phosphatase. The abnormal histiocytes of Gaucher's disease and epithelioid cells of sarcoidosis and Hodgkin's disease also contain tartrate-resistant acid phosphatase. **tetrachrome s.** A staining method in which four different stains are used. **trichrome s.** Any of several procedures for staining tissue sections in which a combination of three contrasting dyes is used to delineate nuclei, collagen, and muscle. Also *triple stain.* **triple s.** TRICHROME STAIN. **tumor s.** An area of increased density seen during angiography, due to the opacification of small abnormal vessels and occurring most commonly in neoplasms. It is best demonstrated during the capillary and venous phases of angiography. **Unna s.** Polychrome methylene blue, which is a mixture of methylene blue with the oxidation products that are created by boiling methylene blue with an alkali. **Unna-Pappenheim s.** A variation of the methyl green-pyronine stain. **van Gieson s.** A histologic stain that contains picric acid and acid fuchsin. It is used to identify mature collagen fibers, which will stain red. **Verhoeff s.** A histologic technique in which hematoxylin is used to identify elastic connective tissue fibers. **vital s.** A dye used for staining living cells, being absorbed through physiologic processes. Also *vital dye.* See also INTRAVITAL STAIN, SUPRAVITAL STAIN. **von Kossa s.** A histologic technique in which silver nitrate is used to substitute for and identify calcium salts in tissues. **Warthin-Starry silver s.** A staining method for demonstrating spirochetes in tissue, using silver nitrate. **Weigert's fibrin s.** A histologic stain containing crystal violet and basic fuchsin that is used to demonstrate amyloid in tissues. **Weigert's iron hematoxylin s.** WEIGERT'S IRON HEMATOXYLIN. See under HEMATOXYLIN. **Weigert's myelin sheath s.** A histologic technique that uses chromium salts as a mordant between hematoxylin and myelin sheaths of nerve fibers. **Weil s.** A form of iron hematoxylin in which iron alum is used as a combined oxidant and mordant for staining myelin. **Wright s.** A mixture of eosin and methylene blue in absolute methanol. It is a variant of the Romanowsky stain and is the most commonly used stain for blood films and bone marrow aspirates. It is also used for staining certain microorganisms, such as malarial parasites. **Ziehl-Neelsen s.** A method of acid-fast staining using carbolfuchsin and aqueous methylene blue. Acid-fast bacilli stain bright red, while other bacteria stain blue. Also *Ziehl-Neelsen carbolfuchsin, Ziehl-Neelsen technique.*

**staining** **1** Localized coloring of artificial teeth to simulate natural defects or of denture base to simulate vessels. **2** The use of a stain on a substance to be examined microscopically. For specific stains, see under STAIN. **negative s.** A technique for light or electron microscopy in which an object can be visualized more easily by increasing the color or electron density of the area around the object. **postvital s.** The staining of tissues in which physiologic processes have ceased. **simple s.** Histologic staining using only one dye. Contrast is achieved according to the affinity for the dye of the various tissue components. **vital s. of teeth** The staining of dentin during tooth formation by abnormal substances in the bloodstream such as tetracycline, or bile pigments in Rhesus factor incompatibility.

**staircase** STAIRCASE PHENOMENON.

**stalk** [prob. from Old Norse, akin to Norwegian dial. *stalk* and Old English *stalu* post] A slender, elongated stemlike structure connected to or supporting an anatomic organ or another structure. **allantoic s.** The stalk of the allantois, placed between the point of its outgrowth from the hindgut, later the urogenital sinus, to where it joins the allantoic vesicle. Also *allantoic duct.* **body s.** CONNECTING STALK. **cerebellar s.** The cerebellar peduncles, collectively. **connecting s.** A mesodermal stalk attaching the embryo to the wall of the chorion, formed at the time of appearance of the extraembryonic coelom as the result of mesodermal condensation, partly about the embryo and its two vesicular appendages and elsewhere on the deep surface of the trophoblastic shell. It is at first placed dorsocaudally, but with the growth, folding, and delimitation of the embryo it becomes more caudal, then ventral, and finally incorporates the shrinking vitellointestinal duct. The allantois develops within its confines, as well as the placental vessels. It becomes the umbilical cord but only the placental vessels persist within its substance to continue functioning until term. Also *embryonic stalk, body stalk.* **embryonic s.** CONNECTING STALK. **s. of the epiglottis** PETIOLUS EPIGLOTTIDIS. **hypophysial s.** INFUNDIBULUM HYPOTHALAMI. **mesangial s.** Tissue in the glomerulus located between capillary loops which forms the centers of the lobules. It contains mesangial cells and matrix, and is covered by a layer of basement membrane and epithelial cells. **neural s.** INFUNDIBULUM HYPOTHALAMI. **optic s.** A diverticulum arising from the diencephalon at the extremity of which the optic vesicle develops, opposite the lens placode. **pineal s.** PEDUNCULUS CORPORIS PINEALIS. **pituitary s.** INFUNDIBULUM HYPOTHALAMI. **s. of Rathke's pouch** The narrow, hollow inferior part of Rathke's pouch by which the pouch opens on to the wall of the stomodeum. Remnants of the stalk can persist to form the pharyngeal hypophysis or accessory hypophyses which develop along the course of the craniopharyngeal canal. **yolk s.** 1 The stalk connecting the yolk sac to the ventral aspect of the embryo. It becomes progressively incorporated in the connecting stalk at the same time at which the extraembryonic coelom disappears and when the allantois grows out from the embryo accompanied by its vessels, the future umbilical vessels. Thus the yolk stalk is eventually included within the definitive umbilical cord while the yolk sac regresses. 2 A term used chiefly in the U.S. for OMPHALOMESENTERIC CANAL.

**staltic** \stal′tik, stôl′tik\ STYPTIC.

**Stamey** [Thomas A. *Stamey,* U.S. urologist, born 1928] See under TEST.

**stammer** STUTTER.

**stammering** STUTTERING.

**stanch** \stônch, stanch\ [Old French *estancher* to stop, prob. from Vulgar L *standicare* to bring to a standstill, from L *stans,* pres. part. of *stare* to stand] To stop, cause to stop, or quell. Also *staunch.*

**standard** [Old French *estendard* (prob. from Frankish, from *stand* upright posture + *hard* firm) a standard, ensign] 1 A unit, level, or specification established as a reference for purposes of comparison or control, or for securing uniformity. 2 Serving as a model or magnitude against which similar entities, performances, or quantities may be compared. 3 A generally accepted measure of the unit of a quantity. **Aub-Dubois s.'s** DUBOIS STANDARD. **Dubois s.** The normal metabolic rate for a given age and sex expressed as calories per square meter per hour. Also *Aub-Dubois standard.* **Harris and Benedict s.** A set of equations and tables used to predict the basal metabolism of men and women. **international biological s.** An international unit for a therapeutic substance that gives the amount of activity present in an internationally agreed weight of the substance (in milligrams), prepared and stored under specified conditions. Some have special names, such as the Voegtlin unit for pituitary extract, but most are defined by the mass of the standard. **nylic s.** A standard specifying "ideal" body weight according to age, height, and sex. • The term *nylic* is derived from the *New York Life Insurance Company,* from whose records the specifications were originally developed **radioactive s.** A radioactive material of which the radioactivity at a certain point in time is known and which for that reason is used for calibration of radiation detectors or dose calibrators. **reference s.** A representative substance of known strength and purity that can be used as a basis for comparison against other similar materials, using specified tests, such as those given in the United States Pharmacopeia or the National Formulary.

**standardization** \stan′dərdīzā′shən\ 1 The act or process of introducing standards, as of measure, quality, or effectiveness, or of bringing values into conformity with a standard. 2 A statistical procedure applied to sets of data to render them directly comparable. Also *adjustment.* **biologic s.** The standardization of drugs or biologic agents by measuring their pharmacologic action on animals, in comparison with suitable reference compounds. Also *physiologic standardization.* **direct s.** A process of adjusting a rate (for example, a death rate) by applying the group-specific (for example, age-specific) rates of a study population to the group-specific distribution of a standard population. If the distribution of the standard population is scaled to some convenient figure, say one million, the procedure yields a directly standardized rate per million. **indirect s.** A process of adjusting a rate (for example, a death rate) by applying to the specific groups (for example, age groups) in the study population the set of group-specific rates of a standard population to yield an expected number. The crude rate of the study population multiplied by the ratio of the actual number of events observed to the expected number gives the indirectly standardized rate for the study population. **physiologic s.** BIOLOGIC STANDARDIZATION.

**standardize** 1 To establish standards for. 2 To evaluate according to an established reference standard.

**standby** Denoting primary equipment that is warmed up and usable in a shorter time than if turned on from a cold start.

**standing / reflex s.** In a decerebrate or spinal preparation, activation of tonic stretch reflexes in antigravity muscles sufficient to sustain standing.

**standstill** Cessation of action. **atrial s.** Cessation of atrial action, as in sinus arrest or sinuatrial block. Also *auricular standstill.* **cardiac s.** Complete cessation of cardiac action. **sinus s.** SINUS ARREST. **ventricular s.** Cessation of cardiac ventricular activity.

**Stannius** [Friedrich Hermann *Stannius,* German physician and physiologist, 1808–1883] See under LIGATURE.

**stannosis** \stanō′sis\ [L *stann(um)* tin + -OSIS] A benign form of pneumoconiosis caused by exposure to tin dust or fumes or to inorganic tin compounds in respirable form. Tin is radiopaque and gives rise to very dense opacities in the chest roentgenogram, which are scattered evenly throughout the lung tissue. The condition causes no symptoms or clinical signs.

**stannous fluoride** $F_2Sn$. Tin difluoride. It is used as an ingredient of toothpastes to help prevent dental caries.

**stanozolol** $C_{21}H_{32}N_2O$. 17-Methyl-2′*H*-androst-2-eno-[3,2-*c*]pyrazol-17-ol. An androgenic steroid used primarily as an anabolic agent.

**St. Anthony** [*St. Anthony,* Egyptian monk of the 3rd–4th century] St. Anthony's disease. See under CHOREA.

**Stanton** [Sir Thomas Ambrose *Stanton,* English physician, born 1875] Stanton's disease. See under MELIOIDOSIS.

**stapedectomy** \stā′pədek′təmē\ [Med L *stapes,* gen. *stapedis,* a stirrup + -ECTOMY] Removal of part or of the whole of the stapes. This operation may be performed for the relief of deafness in otosclerosis. In such cases sound conduction is restored using one of a number of very small prostheses, such as pistons made of biocompatible materials including teflon and stainless steel. **partial s.** 1 Stapedectomy in which only part of the stapes is removed, as in most current forms of the operation. 2 A variety of stapedectomy in which the stapes superstructure is removed and the foot plate, which is fractured, is left *in situ.* The sound conduction mechanism is restored by means of a small polythene tube inserted between the lenticular process of the incus and the fragmented foot plate.

**stapedial** \stāpē′dē·əl\ Pertaining to the stapes.

**stapediolysis** \stāpē′dē·äl′isis\ STAPES MOBILIZATION.

**stapediotenotomy** \stāpē′dē·ōtənät′əmē\ The division of the tendon of the stapedius muscle. Also *stapedial tenotomy.*

**stapediovestibular** \stāpē′dē·ōvestib′yələr\ Of or pertaining to the stapes and the vestibule of the internal ear.

**stapes** \stā′pēz\ [New L, from Med. L, a stirrup, prob. from Germanic (as in English *step*) but assimilated to L *sta(re)* to stand + *pes* foot] [NA] The innermost of the three auditory ossicles, resembling a stirrup and consisting of a head, for articulation with the lenticular process of the incus, a neck, two limbs and a base. The latter is attached to the margin of the fenestra vestibuli by the annular ligament. Also *stirrup, stirrup bone, pedistibulum* (outmoded) . Adj. stapedial.

**staphyl-** \stafəl-\ STAPHYLO-.

**staphylectomy** \staf′ilek′təmē\ UVULOTOMY.

**staphyline** \staf′ilīn\ UVULAR.

**staphylinus** \staf′əli′nəs\ [New L, from STAPHYL- + *-inus* suffix meaning pertaining to] Any of several muscles of the soft palate and uvula.

**staphylo-** \staf′əlō-\ [Gk *staphylē* bunch of grapes, uvula] A combining form meaning (1) forming grapelike clusters; (2) staphylococci; (3) the uvula. Also *staphyl-*.

**staphylocoagulase** \-kō·ag′yəlās\ COAGULASE.

**staphylococcemia** \-käksē′mē·ə\ The presence of staphylococci in the bloodstream. Also *staphylohemia*.

**staphylococci** \-käk′sī\ Plural of STAPHYLOCOCCUS.

**staphylococcolysin** \-käkäl′isin\ STAPHYLOLYSIN.

**staphylococcosis** \-käkō′sis\ [*staphylococc(us)* + -OSIS ] Infection with staphylococci.

***Staphylococcus*** \-käk′əs\ [STAPHYLO- + COCCUS] A genus of facultatively anaerobic, Gram-positive cocci that often separate incompletely at cell division, yielding three-dimensional clusters. ***S. albus*** *STAPHYLOCOCCUS EPIDERMIDIS*. ***S. aureus*** A pathogenic species that is distinguished from other staphylococci by its formation of coagulase, its failure to ferment mannitol, the yellow to orange color of its colonies (due to carotenoids), and the presence of polysaccharide A. It also forms several hemolysins. Its virulence varies over a wide range and probably involves several major factors. It is often carried in the anterior part of the nasopharynx. Also *Staphylococcus pyogenes*. ***S. epidermidis*** A species that closely resembles *S. aureus* but usually forms white colonies and instead of polysaccharide A it carries polysaccharide B. It is a normal inhabitant of the skin and causes minor abscesses, but in compromised subjects it may cause systemic disease. Also *Staphylococcus albus*. ***S. pyogenes*** *STAPHYLOCOCCUS AUREUS*. ***S. saprophyticus*** A micrococcus recently reclassified as a staphylococcus. It does not ferment glucose. It may cause urinary-tract infections.

**staphylococcus** (*pl.* staphylococci) A microorganism of the genus *Staphylococcus*.

**staphyloderma** \-dur′mə\ [STAPHYLO- + -DERMA] Any skin disorder caused by staphylococci.

**staphylohemia** \-hē′mē·ə\ STAPHYLOCOCCEMIA.

**staphylohemolysin** \-hēmäl′isin\ STAPHYLOLYSIN.

**staphyloleukocidin** \-loo′kəsī′din\ A toxin found in cultures of staphylococci that destroys leukocytes.

**staphylolysin** \staf′iläl′isin\ Any of a set of hemolysins ($\alpha$, $\beta$, $\gamma$, or $\delta$), lytic also for other cells, produced by *Staphylococcus aureus*. The $\alpha$-hemolysin is particularly implicated in virulence for humans. Also *staphylococcolysin, staphylohemolysin*.

**staphyloma** \staf′əlō′mə\ [Gk *staphylōma* (from *staphylē* a bunch of grapes) a defect in the eye inside the cornea] A localized outward bulging of the sclera or cornea, including an inner lining of uveal tissue. Adj. staphylomatous. **anterior s.** Staphyloma of the sclera near the limbus. **s. corneae racemosum** Staphyloma of the cornea, with a dark nodular appearance due to numerous iris prolapses through small corneal perforations. **posterior s.** A thinning and bulging of the sclera, located at the back of the eye. Also *staphyloma posticum*. **s. posticum** POSTERIOR STAPHYLOMA. **Scarpa s.** Staphyloma of the sclera, located at the back of the eye, due to myopic degeneration.

**staphylomatous** \staf′iläm′ətəs\ Pertaining to or affected by staphyloma.

**staphyloplasty** \staf′əlōplas′tē\ [STAPHYLO- + -PLASTY] Surgical repair of the soft palate and uvula. Also *staphylorrhaphy, veloplasty*.

**staphylorrhaphy** \staf′ilôr′əfē\ [STAPHYLO- + -RRHAPHY] STAPHYLOPLASTY.

**staphyloschisis** \staf′iläs′kisis\ [STAPHYLO- + -SCHISIS] A bifid uvula which may or may not be associated with a cleft of the soft palate.

**staphylotomy** \staf′ilät′əmē\ UVULOTOMY.

**star** [Old English *steorra*, akin to L *stella* star and Gk *astēr* star] An aster or any radiate structure. **lens s.** RADII LENTIS. **s.'s of Verheyen** VENULAE STELLATAE RENIS.

**starch** [Old English *stearc* stiff, strong] $(C_6H_{10}O_5)_n$. A water-insoluble polysaccharide stored in plants, consisting of amylose and amylopectin. Also *amylum*. **soluble s.** Starch made soluble by boiling an aqueous suspension.

**starch glycerite** A mixture of starch, benzoic acid, water, and glycerin. It is used as a vehicle for drug preparations used externally.

**Starling** [Ernest Henry *Starling*, English physiologist, 1866–1927] **1** See under LAW. **2** Frank-Starling curve. See under STARLING'S CURVE. **3** Frank-Starling mechanism. See under MECHANISM.

**Starr** [Albert *Starr*, U.S. surgeon, born 1926] Starr-Edwards prosthesis. See under PROSTHESIS.

**Starry** [Allen C. *Starry*, U.S. pathologist, born 1890] Warthin-Starry silver stain. See under STAIN.

**starter** A pure culture of a specific microorganism, usually yeasts, used to initiate fermentations.

**starvation** [*starv(e)* + -ATION] Deprivation of food for an extended period. **salt s.** The deprivation of salts which may result in renal failure and consequent retention of nitrogen in the blood as well as alkalemia. This may be followed by fatigue, muscle cramps, dyspnea, and mental apathy.

**starve** [Middle English *sterven*, from Old English *steorfan* to die, akin to German *sterben* to die] To deprive of food to such a degree as to impair body function and, if prolonged, cause death.

**stasimorphy** \stas′imôr′fē\ [*stasi(s)* + MORPH- + -Y] A teras or birth defect attributable to premature arrest of embryonic development.

**stasis** \stā′sis\ [Gk (from *histanai* to cause to stand or stop) placement, position, standstill, state] A cessation or reduction in flow or movement, as of blood or lymph. **intestinal s.** A slowing of the movement of contents through the intestine, as seen in pathologic conditions such as autonomic dysfunction of various causes. Also *enterostasis*. **papillary s.** PAPILLEDEMA. **pressure s.** Vascular stasis due to pressure on vessels. **venous s.** Stasis due to venous obstruction or compression.

**-stasis** \-stā′sis, -stəsis\ [See STASIS] A combining form meaning (1) stoppage, arrest, or inhibition, as of growth or movement; (2) equilibrium, stability, or maintenance; (3) placement, establishment.

**stat.** *statim* (L, immediately): used in prescription writing.

**stat-¹** \stat-\ STATO-.

**stat-²** \stat-\ [contraction of *(electro)stat(ic)*] A combining form meaning electrostatic: used with units in the CGS electrostatic system.

**-stat** \-stat\ [Gk *-statēs* (akin to *histanai* to cause to stop or stand) -stabilizer, -inhibitor] A combining form meaning something that stops, makes stable, or inhibits the growth or motion of (something specified).

**state** [Old French *estat* (from L *status* a standing, posture, condition, state, substantive of *status*, past part. of *stare* to stand) a state, condition] Condition; status. **absent s.** A dreamlike state with fixed stare and vacant facies, sometimes seen as a manifestation of complex partial (temporal lobe) epilepsy and more prolonged than an absence seizure. **alcoholic paranoid s.** ALCOHOLIC PARANOIA. **altered s.'s of consciousness** Modified states of awareness differing from that of normal wakefulness, yet falling within the range of nonpathologic mental experience, such as the various dream states, drug-induced states, and special states which can be brought about by meditation or hypnosis. **aneuploid s.** The state of a nucleus in which the number of chromosomes differs by one or a few from the normal number. **carrier s.** The state of a person or animal that is host to a pathogenic microorganism or parasite and, without being affected by the disease or showing clinical evidence thereof, is capable of transmitting the infection to others. **catelectrotonic s.** A state of heightened excitability in the region next to the cathode when a nerve is being stimulated by a direct current. **central excitatory s.** A state of heightened excitability of neurons in the central nervous system following the arrival of one or more subthreshold stimuli. **central inhibitory s.** A state of decreased excitability of neurons in the central nervous system. It may be due either to increased activity in inhibitory neurons or to a reduced input of those subliminal stimuli which maintain a central excitatory state. **compulsive s.** OBSESSIVE-COMPULSIVE NEUROSIS. **convulsive s.** STATUS EPILEPTICUS. **correlated s.** STEADY STATE. **D s.** DESYNCHRONIZED SLEEP. **delta s.** SYNCHRONIZED SLEEP. **dreamy s.** Prolonged depersonalization, detachment, or feelings of unreality as if the patient were living in a dream or fantasy world, resulting from prolonged epileptic discharge arising in the temporal lobe. Associated illusions or visual hallucinations are common. Also *prolonged epileptic depersonalization, dream state.* **entatic s.** The state of one region of a protein molecule in which groups are more reactive than they would be if the interacting parts of the region were free to rearrange in position, whereas they are constrained by the overall folding of the protein. **epileptic s.** STATUS EPILEPTICUS. **epileptic clouded s.** A psychotic reaction that occurs before or following an epileptic convulsion, usually manifesting some degree of confusion and attention deficit no matter what other accompanying symptoms there may be. **epileptic twilight s.** TWILIGHT EPILEPTIC STATE. **euploid s.** EUPLOIDY. **excited s.** Any state of a molecule whose energy is greater than that of the ground state. **Ganser s.** GANSER SYNDROME. **ground s.** The lowest energy level of a nucleus, atom, or molecule. **haploid s.** HAPLOIDY. **hypnagogic s.** The transition period between wakefulness and sleep characterized by a state of quiet relaxation and dreamlike mentation. **hypnopompic s.** The transition period between sleep and wakefulness characterized by a state of semiconsciousness; the period immediately preceding waking from sleep. **lacunar s.** A form of cerebral vascular disease, usually but not invariably associated with severe arterial hypertension and arteriosclerosis, in which small microinfarcts or lacunae are formed, often successively, in the brainstem, basal ganglia, or internal capsules. Associated clinical syndromes include motor or sensory hemiplegia and the dysarthria-clumsy hand syndrome. Multiple lacunae are often associated with the clinical manifestations of arteriosclerotic parkinsonism and/or pseudobulbar palsy. Also *lacunar syndrome, status lacunosus, status lacunaris.* **local excitatory s.** A state of heightened excitability in a peripheral nerve or in a localized area of the nervous system induced by one or more subthreshold stimuli. **marble s.** ÉTAT MARBRÉ. **obsessive-ruminative s.** OBSESSIVE-COMPULSIVE NEUROSIS. **persistent vegetative s.** A prolonged state of grossly impaired consciousness, following severe head injury or brain disease, in which the subject is incapable of speech and of voluntary or purposive acts but will respond reflexly to painful stimuli. **pluripotent s.** The state of the zygote or parts of the early embryo which have the potential to develop in any one of several possible ways. Also *plastic state.* **postepileptic s.** A transient state of confusion or impaired consciousness following an attack of epilepsy. **refractory s.** A changing state of an excitable tissue or cell marked by absolute unresponsiveness and then relative elevation in threshold as a sequel of a discharge. **resting s.** A phase in which an excitable cell or tissue is not subject to excitation or to the aftereffects of excitation. **singlet s.** An unstable, excited state of an atom or molecule upon absorbing light radiation, in which the electron is unchanged in spin, and so still of opposite spin to the electron with which it was paired before excitation. All of the energy can be released as light (fluorescence) and/or heat, returning the atom or molecule to the ground state. If a portion of the energy is released, the atom or molecule can remain excited in a more stable triplet state. **split-brain s.** A state of disconnection of the two cerebral hemispheres resulting from division of the corpus callosum in whole or in part and strictly involving division of the optic chiasm as well. This state has been produced for experimental purposes in animals, and partial surgical division of the corpus callosum has sometimes been used in man for the treatment of intractable epilepsy. The resulting clinical syndromes have often been called disconnection syndromes. **steady s.** Any condition that remains constant at a given point in time because of the presence of opposite forces or processes that cancel out one another's effects; dynamic equilibrium. Also *correlated state.* **subscurvy s.** SUBCLINICAL SCURVY. **triplet s.** An excited state of an atom or molecule following the absorption of light radiation. The singlet state is first produced, and upon loss of some of the absorbed energy, the electron, still remaining dislocated, reverses its spin to give the triplet state, thus increasing the stability of the excited atom or molecule. **twilight s.** A state of disordered consciousness characterized by automatism and the performance of acts of which the subject subsequently has no recollection. This may be a manifestation of temporal lobe epilepsy (twilight epileptic state) but it can also occur, though rarely, in delirium. **twilight epileptic s.** A transient mental disturbance occurring during, or towards the end of, an epileptic attack, and marked by lessening of awareness and impaired consciousness, giving the patient's surroundings a fuzzy or "opaque" appearance. This condition is intermediate between epileptic confusion, in which consciousness is more severely impaired, and dreamy states of prolonged depersonalization. Also *epileptic twilight state.* **vegetative s.** The state of phage development in which its components are actively multiplying in the host cell, but in which infective phage is not being produced.

**statement** / **antemortem s.** A statement made by

an individual immediately before his death, which is considered as legally binding as a sworn statement provided the individual acknowledges his impending death. **uncertainty s.** An expression of the inherent limitations of an analytic method, based upon observations of the method's precision, specificity, and freedom from systematic error.

**static** \stat′ik\ [Gk *statikos* (from *histanai* to cause to stand or stop) causing to stand or stop, pertaining to the resting state] **1** Characterized by lack of motion or change. **2** Pertaining to maintenance of a fixed position. **3** Relating to or caused by stasis. **4** Pertaining to the standing position. **5** Pertaining to posture or equilibrium. **6** BACTERIOSTATIC.

**-static** \-stat′ik\ [See STATIC.] A combining form meaning arresting or inhibiting (a specified process or pathogen).

**statim** [L, immediately] At once, immediately: used in prescription writing. Abbr. stat.

**station** [L *statio* (from *stat(us)*, past part. of *stare* to stand + *-io* -ION) a standing still, post, station] The position of the presenting part of the fetus in the birth canal in relation to the ischial spines. **s. of the fetus** STATION. **olfactory s. of Broca** DIAGONAL BAND.

**statistic** \stətis′tik\ **1** A number defining some characteristic of a sample or of a population, such as average, percentage, rate, or standard deviation. **2** A single observed value or datum in a set of statistics. **kappa s.** A statistic to express the measure of agreement between the ratings awarded to a set of entities, such as x-ray findings or examination marks, each of which is reported upon independently by each observer. If $K = 0$, there is no more agreement between observers than would be expected to occur by chance, while $K = 1$ indicates perfect agreement.

**statistics** \stətis′tiks\ [German *statistik* (from New L *statistic(us)* pertaining to politics, from L *stat(us)* the state + *-isticus* English *-istic*) statistics + *s*] **1** A set of quantitative data concerning the members of an aggregate. **2** The science whose object is the investigation by numerical methods, such as enumeration, census-taking, classification, or tabulation, of observations on aggregates of individuals of like kind. **3** A mathematical methodology for the analysis and interpretation of data from observations. By a characteristic inductive process these methods lead to precise statements in probability terms about the degree of uncertainty attaching to the conclusions drawn. **4** The numerical properties of an aggregate of individual entities of a similar kind. • The term was probably introduced by Achenwald, of Gottingen in Germany, in 1748. **Bose-Einstein s.** A system of statistics used in theoretical quantum physics to describe the behavior of particles of integral spin, such as photons and helium nuclei. **distribution-free s.** NONPARAMETRIC STATISTICS. **Fermi-Dirac s.** A system of statistics used in theoretical quantum physics to describe the behavior of particles of nonintegral spin, such as electrons and protons. **health s.** Statistics used for the analysis of the health status of populations and their need for and use of curative, caring, and preventive health services. **medical s.** The branch of statistics concerned with the study of quantitative information relating to the course or management of disease processes, vital events, including births and deaths, and more generally to the causes of morbidity and mortality. **nonparametric s.** Statistics for drawing inferences from samples without having to make assumptions about the form of the underlying distribution. In general the methods, many of which are based on ranking the sample observations in order of size, are less powerful than the corresponding parametric procedures. Also *distribution-free statistics.* **vital s.** Data related to births, deaths, marriage, and health and disease. Also *biostatistics* (outmoded).

**stato-** \stat′ə-, stat′ō-\ [Gk *statos* (from *histanai* to make to stand, to set, place) standing, placed, stopped] A combining form meaning (1) stasis, inhibition, or fixation; (2) balance, equilibrium. Also *stat-*.

**statoconia** \stat′əkō′nē·ə\[STATO- + Gk *konia* dust, sand] (*sing.* statoconium) [NA] Minute crystalline particles composed of calcite and protein and suspended in a gelatinous mass forming the membrana statoconiorum into which project the sterocilia and kinocilia of the hair cells of the maculae of the utricle and sacculus of the inner ear. These particles are under the influence of gravity and exert traction on the cilia of the hair cells during movements of the head and body, being involved in statotonic, statokinetic, and other reflexes. They form large stones in the ears of fishes, in which they are more commonly called otoliths or statoliths. Also *otoconia, otoconites, otolites, otosteons, ear crystals.*

**statoconium** \-kō′nē·əm\ Singular of STATOCONIA.

**statocyst** \stat′əsist\ A vesicle found in many invertebrates and functioning as a receptor organ for the perception of position of the body in space. It is analogous to the macula of the utricle and sacculus of the inner ear in humans. See also STATORECEPTOR.

**statokinetic** \-kinet′ik\ Pertaining to the maintenance of physical stability and equilibrium during movement.

**statokinetics** \-kinet′iks\ The science concerned with the reflex adjustments in bodily posture such as are made during movement in order to maintain stability and equilibrium.

**statolith** \stat′əlith\ See under STATOCONIA.

**statolon** A macromolecular, polyanionic polysaccharide containing galacturonic acid, galactose, galactosamine, glucose, arabinose, xylose, and rhamnose. It is produced by *Penicillium stoloniferum* var. ATCC 14586. It is active, prophylactically, against a wide range of viruses, and it has antitumor activity in experimental leukemia and sarcomas.

**statometer** \statäm′ətər\ [STATO- + -METER] A device for measuring the anteroposterior position of the eye within the orbit.

**statoreceptor** \-risep′tər\ A receptor concerned with static balance, or the sense of position in space, such as the maculae of the utricle and sacculus of the inner ear in humans and the statocyst in invertebrates.

**statural** \stach′ərəl\ Of or relating to stature.

**stature** \stach′ər\ The height of a person in the upright posture.

**status** \stā′təs, stat′əs\ [L (substantive from *status*, past part. of *stare* to stand), a standing, state, condition] State; condition. **s. anginosus** Recurrent attacks of angina pectoris at rest which are unresponsive to treatment; one form of unstable angina. **s. asthmaticus** A severe and persistent attack of asthma. **s. convulsivus** STATUS EPILEPTICUS. **s. cribrosus** A sievelike or honeycomb appearance of the cerebral substance resulting from dilatation of perivascular spaces or from perivascular demyelination. Also *status cribralis, état criblé.* **s. degenerativus** The presence of multiple foci of degeneration in a single individual. **s. dysgraphicus** DYSGRAPHIA. **s. dysmyelinatus** HALLERVORDEN-SPATZ DISEASE. **s. dysmyelinisatus** HALLERVORDEN-SPATZ DISEASE. **s. dysrhaphicus** A condition marked by failure of closure of midline embryonic tubular or bipartite organs (dysraphia) such as the neural tube, sternum, palate, and scrotum. Also *arrhaphia.* **s. epilepticus** A state which may sometimes develop in epileptic patients either in an exceptionally prolonged single attack or much more often as a consequence of repeated attacks occurring so frequently that the patient does not recover between them, so that there is usually prolonged unconsciousness and the EEG often shows almost continuous epileptic discharge. This complication usually occurs in patients with tonicoclonic major epilepsy (grand mal) but petit mal status may rarely occur. Severe continuing impairment of consciousness between the repeated attacks is the most important diagnostic feature. The condition is grave if not treated rapidly, as hypoxic brain damage and hyperthermia are important complications, and it is sometimes fatal. Also *epileptic state, convulsive state, continuous epilepsy, status convulsivus.* • The term is usually confined to cases of generalized epilepsy, though it can occur in patients with a focal aura or onset to the attacks which subsequently becomes generalized. **s. fibrosus** A cerebral abnormality of the newborn period affecting the basal nuclei of the brain. Loss of nerve cells with gliosis leads to shrinkage of the tissues and the crowding together of the remaining myelinated fibers, giving the impression of abnormally rich myelination. **focal s.** CONTINUOUS PARTIAL EPILEPSY. **s. lacunaris** LACUNAR STATE. **s. lacunosus** LACUNAR STATE. **s. lymphaticus** A condition of hyperplasia of lymphatic tissue, at one time thought to be a common cause of sudden death in infants. Also *status thymicolymphaticus, lymphatism.* **s. macrobioticus multiparus** ESSENTIAL TREMOR. **s. marmoratus** ÉTAT MARBRÉ. **mental s.** The level of intellectual and psychological functioning of an individual, which may be determined through examinations or tests geared to such an assessment. **myoclonic s.** Continuous or rapidly recurring myoclonic jerking in a subject with myoclonic epilepsy. **nutrition s.** The physical state of an individual, as it pertains to nutrient intake. Such information is determined through a set of four evaluations. A dietary record is kept and assessment is made as to whether or not the diet is adequate with respect to all nutrients. Anthropometry is used to discern if the patient is underweight or, in the case of a child, growth-retarded. A clinical examination will determine if a nutritional deficiency disease exists. Biochemical tests are used to discover if there are low concentrations of one or more nutrients in the blood or urine. **petit mal s.** Prolonged episodes of petit mal absence sometimes associated with continuous spike-and-wave discharge in the EEG but more often with rhythmic generalized spike-wave or multispike discharges interrupted by generalized slow activity. Clinically the principal manifestation is impairment of consciousness (vagueness, dreaminess, dullness, or detachment) or confusion, lasting for hours, in rare cases for days. This condition, due to continuous epileptic activity, must be distinguished from postepileptic confusional states, which can occur in any form of epilepsy. Also *petit mal status epilepticus, intellectual petit mal* (incorrect), *epileptic stupor* (obs.), *spike-wave stupor.* **s. praesens** The present state; the condition of a patient at the time when he or she is examined. **psychomotor s.** Continuous and prolonged or rapidly recurring attacks of temporal lobe epilepsy. **s. spongiosus** A spongy state of the cerebral substance such as may occur in many degenerative brain diseases including Canavan's disease and some cases of Creutzfeldt-Jakob disease. **s. thymicolymphaticus** STATUS LYMPHATICUS. **s. verrucosus** A pathologic state in which the cerebral cortex acquires a warty appearance. Tuberous sclerosis is one cause. **s. vertiginosus** Persistent vertigo. *Older term.*

**staunch** \stônch\ STANCH.

**stauroconidium** \stôr′ōkənid′ē·əm\ [Gk *stauro(s)* a stake, pole, in pl. palisade + CONIDIUM] (*pl.* stauroconidia) A radially lobed, stellate conidium of certain fungi of the form-class Deuteromycetes. Also *staurospore.*

**stauroplegia** \stôr′əplē′jə\ [Gk *stauro(s)* a stake, pole, cross + -PLEGIA] CROSSED HEMIPLEGIA.

**staurospore** \stôr′əspôr\ STAUROCONIDIUM.

**stay** **1** A narrow supporting structure. **2** A firm rod or strip, as of plastic, aluminum, or steel, used to reinforce a trunk orthosis. **s. of white line** *Outmoded* ADMINICULUM LINEAE ALBAE.

**St. Clair Thomson** [Sir *St. Clair Thomson,* English laryngologist, 1859–1943] See under CURETTE.

**STD** **1** standard test dose. **2** skin test dose.

**steal** [Old English *stelan* to steal] The combining of communications between two vascular beds and the occluding of direct blood flow to one of the beds, resulting in a diversion of blood flow from the second bed. **extracranial s.** The diversion of blood from one extracranial artery to another due to arterial stenosis or occlusion. **intracerebral s.** The diversion through anastomotic channels, due to arterial stenosis or occlusion, of blood normally passing into the brain territory supplied by one intracranial artery into the area normally supplied by the diseased vessel or vessels. **subclavian s.** The filling of a subclavian artery which is obstructed proximal to the origin of its vertebral artery by means of retrograde flow down its vertebral artery. The vertebral artery receives its supply from the contralateral vertebral artery via the basilar artery. This may be observed during angiography of the contralateral vertebral or subclavian artery. **vascular s.** A condition in which, due to vascular stenoses or occlusions, blood flow may be diverted preferentially to areas not usually so served, often by retrograde flow down nearby branch arteries.

**stear-** \stē·ər-\ STEARO-.

**stearate** The anion, a salt, or an ester of stearic acid.

**stearic acid** $CH_3$—$[CH_2]_{16}$—COOH. Octadecanoic acid. It is one of the major natural fatty acids.

**stearo-** \stē′ərō-\ [Gk *stear* hard fat, tallow, suet] A combining form meaning fat. Also *stear-.*

**steatadenoma** \stē′ətadənō′mə\ [*steat(o)-* + ADENOMA] SEBACEOUS ADENOMA.

**steato-** \stē′ətō-\ [Gk *stear,* gen. *steatos* hard fat, tallow, suet] A combining form meaning fat.

**steatocele** \stē′ətōsēl, stē·at′əsēl\ [STEATO- + -CELE[1]] A mass of fatty tissue in the scrotum.

**steatocystoma** \-sistō′mə\ A cyst arising from the sebaceous gland apparatus. **s. multiplex** A hereditary syndrome in which numerous small sebaceous cysts develop on the head, trunk, and limbs. Also *steatomatosis.*

**steatolysis** \stē′ətäl′isis\ LIPOLYSIS.

**steatolytic** \-lit′ik\ LIPOLYTIC.

**steatoma** \stē′ətō′mə\ [*steat(o)-* + -OMA] A tumor of the sebaceous gland apparatus.

**steatomatosis** \-mətō′sis\ STEATOCYSTOMA MULTIPLEX.

**steatomatous** \stē′ətäm′ətəs\ [STEATOMA, pl. *steatomat(a),* + -OUS] LIPOMATOUS.

**steatopygia** \-pij′ē·ə\ [STEATO- + PYG- + -IA] An exaggerated deposition of fat in the buttocks.

**steatorrhea** \stē′ətôrē′ə\ [STEATO- + -RRHEA] The presence of excess fat in the stool, measured either as an absolute amount or, preferably, related to the fat intake on a standard diet. It is generally an indication of malabsorption. **congenital pancreatic s.** *Older term* CYSTIC FIBROSIS. **familial s.** The occurrence of malabsorption symptoms in related individuals for any of a number of reasons, including celiac sprue and cystic fibrosis. **idiopathic s.** CELIAC DISEASE.

**steatosis** \stē′ətō′sis\ [*steat(o)-* + -OSIS] The accumulation of fat. **s. cordis** FATTY HEART.

**Steele** [John C. *Steele*, Canadian physician, flourished 20th century] Steele-Richardson-Olszewski syndrome. See under PROGRESSIVE SUPRANUCLEAR PALSY.

**Steell** [Graham *Steell*, English physician, 1851–1942] Steell's murmur. See under GRAHAM STEELL'S MURMUR.

**Steidele** [Raphael Johann *Steidele*, Austrian obstetrician, 1737–1823] See under COMPLEX.

**Stein** [Irving Freiler *Stein*, U.S. gynecologist, born 1887] Stein-Leventhal syndrome. See under SYNDROME.

**Steinbrinck** [W. *Steinbrinck*, German physician, flourished mid-20th century] Steinbrinck's anomaly, Chédiak-Steinbrinck-Higashi anomaly. See under CHÉDIAK-HIGASHI ANOMALY.

**Steiner** [Ludwig *Steiner*, German physician, flourished 20th century] Steiner's tumors. See under TUMOR.

**Steinmann** [Fritz *Steinmann*, Swiss surgeon, 1872–1932] See under EXTENSION, PIN.

**stella** \stel′ə\ [L (prob. from earlier *sterla*, akin to Gk *astēr* star and Old English *steorra*) a star or starlike object] (*pl.* stellae) A radiating or star-shaped structure; star. **s. lentis hyaloidea** *Outmoded* POLUS POSTERIOR LENTIS. **s. lentis iridica** *Outmoded* POLUS ANTERIOR LENTIS.

**stellate** \stel′āt\ **1** Star-shaped; radiating from a center. **2** Grouped like a cluster of stars; resembling a rosette.

**stellectomy** \stelek′təmē\ [*stell(ate ganglion)* + -ECTOMY] Excision of the stellate ganglion.

**stellula** \stel′yələ\ [Late L (dim. of L *stella* a star) a little star, asterisk] (*pl.* stellulae) A small star. **stellulae of Verheyen** *Outmoded* VENULAE STELLATAE RENIS. **stellulae verheyenii** *Outmoded* VENULAE STELLATAE RENIS.

**stellulae** \stel′yəlē\ Plural of STELLULA.

**Stellwag** [Carl von Carion *Stellwag*, Austrian ophthalmologist, 1823–1904] See under SIGN.

**stem** [Old English *stefn, stemn* stem of a plant or ship] **1** The ascending axis of a plant, either above ground or below ground level. **2** The main axis of a structure. **3** A supporting structure, as the brainstem. **brain s.** See under BRAINSTEM. **infundibular s.** The stalk by which the posterior lobe of the pituitary is attached to the hypothalamic tuber cinereum.

**Stenediol** A proprietary name for methandriol.

**Steno** See under STENSEN.

**steno-** \sten′ō-, stē′nō-\ [Gk *stenos* narrow] A combining form meaning narrow or constricted.

**stenocardia** \-kär′dē·ə\ [STENO- + -CARDIA] ANGINA PECTORIS.

**stenocephaly** \-sef′əlē\ [STENO- + CEPHAL- + -Y ] An abnormal narrowness of the head.

**stenocrotaphy** \-krät′əfē\ [STENO- + Gk *krotaph(os)* the temple of the head + -Y] An abnormal narrowness of the cranium in the temporal region.

**stenopaeic** *Brit.* STENOPEIC.

**stenopeic** \-pē′ik\ Having a narrow slit or hole to restrict light.

**stenose** \stənōz′, stənōs′\ To cause stenosis in.

**stenosed** \stənōzd′\ Narrowed or constricted.

**stenosis** \stənō′sis\ [Gk *stenōsis* (from *stenoun* to narrow, from *stenos* narrow + *-osis* -OSIS) a narrowing] A narrowing of an orifice or the lumen of a canal or tubular organ. **adult pyloric s.** **1** Pyloric narrowing due probably to hypertrophy of the pyloric musculature of unknown etiology. It is manifested by gastric dilatation, postprandial pain and vomiting, and signs of gastric outlet obstruction. **2** Gastric outlet obstruction due to narrowing of the pylorus from any cause, most typically cancer and peptic ulcer disease. **aortic s.** A narrowing of the aortic valve orifice, affecting either the cusps themselves or occurring above or below them. Abbr. AS **aortic valve s.** Narrowing of the aortic valve cusps. Also *aortic valvular stenosis.* **aqueduct s.** Narrowing, either congenitally or in infancy, of the cerebral aqueduct, resulting in hydrocephalus. Also *aqueductal stenosis.* **arterial s.** Narrowing of the lumen of an artery. **bronchial s.** BRONCHOSTENOSIS. **buttonhole mitral s.** Stenosis of the mitral valve in which the valve cusps have become adherent and contracted so as to form an orifice of buttonhole shape. **calcified aortic s.** Aortic stenosis associated with calcification of the leaflets. **caroticovertebral s.** Stenosis affecting the carotid and vertebral arteries. **carotid s.** Stenosis of the common carotid artery or its internal or external branches. **choanal s.** Narrowing of one or both posterior nares (choanae). **congenital aortic s.** Congenital narrowing of the aortic valve itself (valvular), of the adjacent outflow tract of the left ventricle (subvalvular), or of the proximal part of the ascending aorta (supravalvular). **congenital hypertrophic pyloric s.** Pyloric stenosis in infants due to hypertrophy of the muscular wall, forming a tumorlike mass that can be palpated. Symptoms appear ten days to several weeks after birth. Vomiting of feeds, characteristically projectile, leads to wasting and dehydration. Incidence in Caucasians is about 0.3 percent of all births, with males accounting for 80 percent of cases. Inheritance is multifactorial. Treatment by pyloromyotomy (Ramstedt operation) is effective. **coronary s.** Stenosis affecting the coronary arteries, usually the consequence of atherosclerosis. **coronary ostial s.** Narrowing of the orifice of the coronary arteries, most frequently due to syphilitic aortitis. **critical s.** In mammalian hemodynamic systems, that point at which a vessel stenosis has encroached enough upon the lumen to reduce flow. It is roughly equivalent to an 80 percent reduction in cross-sectional area, or a 50 percent diameter reduction. **cystic duct s.** A condition characterized by either chronic dull right upper quadrant pain or intermittent attacks of right upper quadrant pain typical of gallbladder disease, but in which the gallbladder appears entirely normal by oral cholecystography. The etiology and pathogenesis of this condition is not clear, but it is thought by some to be due to forceful contraction of the wall of the gallbladder to overcome partial anatomic or functional obstruction of the cystic duct. **fishmouth mitral s.** Severe mitral stenosis with the orifice appearing to have the shape of a fish's mouth. **hypertrophic pyloric s.** Pyloric stenosis due to hypertrophy of the pyloric musculature, either congenital or, in adults, idiopathic. See also CONGENITAL HYPERTROPHIC PYLORIC STENOSIS, ADULT PYLORIC STENOSIS. **idiopathic hypertrophic subaortic s.** A form of obstructive hypertrophic cardiomyopathy in which there is a systolic pressure difference between the apex and subaortic areas of the left ventricle. Also *hypertrophic subaortic stenosis, muscular subaortic stenosis, muscular subvalvular stenosis.* **infundibular pulmonary s.** A narrowing of the outflow tract of the right ventricle below the pulmonary valve cusps. It is often a component of tetralogy of Fallot. Also *infundibular stenosis.* **laryngeal s.** Narrowing of the airway through the larynx, such as may complicate laryngeal trauma. The treatment is surgical and presents many difficulties. Also *laryngostenosis.* • In ordinary usage the term refers specifically to cicatricial stenosis (cicatricial stricture). **lumbar canal s.** A marked narrowing of the lumbar vertebral canal usually due to hypertrophy of the bony laminae. Clinically the condition usually causes the syndrome of intermittent claudication of the cauda equina. Also *lumbar stenosis.* **mitral s.** A narrowing of the mitral valve orifice, usually a consequence of rheumatic fever. It may also be of developmental origin. Also *mitral valve stenosis.* **muscular subaortic s.** IDIOPATHIC HYPERTROPHIC SUBAORTIC STENOSIS. **muscular subvalvular s.** IDIOPATHIC HYPERTROPHIC SUBAORTIC STENOSIS. **nasal s.** Narrowing of the airway through the nose, either on one side or both. Also *rhinostenosis.* **posterior s. of the urethra** MARION'S DISEASE. **post-tracheostomy s.** A narrowing of the trachea by scar or granulation tissue following a tracheostomy. **pulmonary s.** Stenosis of the pulmonary outflow tract between the right ventricle and the distal pulmonary artery, usually localized at the pulmonary valve or within the infundibulum of the right ventricle. **pulmonary artery s.** Stenosis of one or more of the pulmonary arteries. **pulmonary valve s.** Stenosis affecting the pulmonary valve apparatus. Also *pneumoarctia.* **pyloric s.** Marked narrowing of the pylorus or of the lumen at the pyloric valve. It may be acquired, most typically from scarring in peptic ulcer disease, or congenital and hypertrophic. Also *pylorostenosis.* See also CONGENITAL HYPERTROPHIC PYLORIC STENOSIS, ADULT PYLORIC STENOSIS. **renal artery s.** A narrowing of a renal artery or its branches by atherosclerosis or fibromuscular disease. The condition may cause hypertension, or if mild may be an incidental finding. **subvalvular aortic s.** Stenosis in the outflow tract to the left ventricle below the aortic valve. It may be membranous or muscular. Also *subvalvar aortic stenosis, subaortic stenosis.* **supravalvular aortic s.** A rare form of congenital aortic stenosis in which there is a narrowing above the aortic valve. There are three main types: hourglass, hypoplastic, and intermediate. It may be associated with other abnormalities of the aorta and pulmonary arteries. See also SUPRAVALVULAR AORTIC STENOSIS SYNDROME. **tracheal s.** Narrowing of the tracheal airway from any of a variety of causes but usually referring to cicatricial stricture. The incidence rose sharply following the increased used of cuffed tracheostomy tubes for respiratory support. Also *tracheostenosis.* **tricuspid s.** Stenosis affecting the tricuspid valve apparatus. **valvular s.** Stenosis affecting one of the cardiac valves. **vertebral s.** Stenosis of one or both vertebral arteries.

**stenostomia** \-stō′mē·ə\ [STENO- + STOM- + -IA] An abnormal narrowness of the mouth.

**stenothorax** \-thôr′aks\ [STENO- + THORAX] An abnormal narrowness of the thoracic region.

**stenotic** \stənät′ik\ Having a reduced transverse dimension; characterized by stenosis.

**stenoxenous** \stenäk′sənəs\ [STENO- + *xen(o)-* + -OUS] Restricted to a narrow range of hosts: said of parasites that are limited to one or a few host species.

**Stensen** [Niels *Stensen* (Nicolaus Steno), Danish anatomist, 1638–1686] **1** Lateral nasal gland of Stensen. See under GLAND. **2** See under EXPERIMENT, PLEXUS. **3** Stensen's canal, Stensen's duct, duct of Steno. See under DUCTUS PAROTIDEUS. **4** Stensen's veins. See under VENAE VORTICOSAE.

**Stent** [Charles R. *Stent,* English dentist, died 1901] **1** Stent's mass. See under STENT DRESSING. **2** See under GRAFT.

**stent** \stent\ [after Charles R. *Stent,* English dentist, d. 1901.] **1** A molded appliance used to hold a graft in place or act as an obturator. **2** An impression of the mouth taken in impression composition.

**step** / **rate-controlling s.** RATE-LIMITING STEP. **rate-determining s.** The rate-limiting step in a sequence when this step is also the first of the sequence. **rate-limiting s.** In a series of reactions, a particular step that meets the condition that the rate of the process is approached by the rate constant of that step multiplied by a function of the concentrations of the starting materials and of the equilibrium constants of all preceding steps. Its existence implies that all preceding steps approach equilibrium, and that the flux through the pathway is controlled by the rate constant for that step. Also *rate-controlling step, rate-determining step.*

**stephanial** \stēfā′nē·əl\ Of or pertaining to the stephanion.

**stephanion** \stēfā′nē·än\ A craniometric point on the side of the cranium at the intersection of the coronal suture and the inferior temporal line.

**Stephenson** [William *Stephenson,* Scottish obstetrician, 1837–1908] See under WAVE.

**steppage** \step′ij, stepäzh′\ [French, from English *step* + French *-age* -AGE] See under STEPPAGE GAIT.

**stepping** Alternating flexion-extension movements of the pelvic limbs as seen in a spinal animal or man. It may be triggered by stimulating the plantar surface of one foot, spreading the toes, squeezing one foot, etc., and in its fullest development is sustained by the interplay of proprioceptive feedback and a central pattern generator for locomotion. Comparable tentative ambulation may be elicited in a normal infant when the sole of the foot is placed in contact with the floor and the body is advanced with each step. Also *steppage, stepping reflex, stepping movements, running movements.* **air s.** Ambulatory movements of the hindlegs of a spinal animal when it is held aloft with the legs dependent. Stretch of the inguinal skin folds is the triggering stimulus.

**steradian** \stirā′dē·ən\ [*ste(re)-* + RADIAN] The SI supplementary unit of solid angle; the solid angle which, having its vertex in the center of a sphere, cuts off an area of the surface of the sphere equal to that of a square with sides of length equal to the radius of the sphere. A complete sphere subtends a solid angle of $4\pi$ steradians at its center. Symbol: sr

**sterco-** \stur′kō-\ [L *stercus* feces, dung] A combining form denoting feces.

**stercobilin** \-bī′lin\ The linear tetrapyrrole formed from urobilin by hydrogenation of a double bond in each of the terminal pyrrole rings. It is formed by intestinal bacteria from bilirubin, and is one of the main pigments of feces.

**stercobilinogen** A colorless, reduced form of stercobilin, in which the pyrrole rings are joined by $—CH_2—$ groups. It is oxidized by air to the colored stercobilin. Also *urobilinogen.*

**stercolith** \stur′kəlith\ FECALITH.

**stercoraceous** \stur′kôrā′shəs\ Relating to or consisting of feces; fecal; stercoral.

**stercoral** \stur′kərəl\ Pertaining to feces; fecal. Also *stercorous.*

**stercorolith** \stur′kərōlith′\ *Seldom used* FECALITH.

**stercoroma** \stur′kôrō′mə\ [L *stercus,* gen. *stercor(is)* dung + -OMA] A mass of fecal material resembling a tumor in the rectum. Also *coproma, scatoma, fecaloma, fecal tumor, stercoral tumor.*

**stercorous** \stur′kərəs\ STERCORAL.

**stere-** \ster′ē-, stir′ē-\ STEREO-.

**stereo-** \ster′ē·ō-, stir′ē·ō-\ [Gk *stereos* stiff, firm, solid; of bodies and quantities, cubic] A combining form meaning (1) firm, solid; (2) three-dimensional. Also *stere-.*

**stereoagnosis** \-agnō′sis\ [STEREO- + Gk *a-* priv. + *gnōsis* knowledge] TACTILE AGNOSIA.

**stereoanesthesia** \-an′esthē′zhə\ [STEREO- + ANESTHESIA] An inability to recognize shape and size due to impairment of tactile sensation. Also *pseudostereognosis.*

**stereoblastula** \-blas′tyələ\ (*pl.* stereoblastulae) A blastula with a cavity or blastocoele that has become virtual because of the great development of certain blastomeres.
**stereocampimeter** \-kampim′ətər\ A binocular device for the measurement of visual fields.
**stereochemical** \-kem′ikəl\ Concerning stereochemistry.
**stereochemistry** \-kem′istrē\ The branch of chemistry that deals with the relative positions of atoms in space.
**stereocilia** \-sil′ē·ə\ Plural of STEREOCILIUM.
**stereocilium** \-sil′ē·əm\ (*pl.* stereocilia) A nonmotile tuft or microvillus projecting from an epithelial cell. Stereocilia are seen in the epidymis of the male reproductive tract.
**stereocognosy** \-käg′nəsē\ STEREOGNOSIS.
**stereocolpogram** \-käl′pəgram\ [STEREO- + COLPO- + -GRAM] A magnified picture of vaginal portion of the cervix displayed as a three-dimensional image.
**stereocolposcope** \-käl′pəskōp\ [STEREO- + COLPO- + -SCOPE] The instrument used to view the cervix in a three-dimensional image.
**stereoencephalotome** \-ensef′əlōtōm′\ [STEREO- + ENCEPHALOTOME] A device used to cut or destroy specific brain structures and placed in the desired area by stereotaxy.
**stereoencephalotomy** \-ensef′əlät′əmē\ [STEREO- + ENCEPHALOTOMY] The division or destruction of specific areas of the brain by means of stereotaxy.
**stereognosis** \ster′ē·ägnō′sis\ [STEREO- + Gk *gnōsis* a recognizing, knowledge] The faculty of being able to recognize by touch the shape, size, and texture of an object placed in the hand. Also *stereocognosy*. Adj. stereognostic.
**stereognostic** \ster′ē·ägnäs′tik\ Pertaining to stereognosis.
**stereogram** \ster′ē·əgram′\ [STEREO- + -GRAM] One of a pair of roentgenograms made by stereoroentgenography.
**stereoisomer** \-ī′səmər\ An isomer that differs from another molecule in the positions its constituents occupy in space, but not in how these constituents are linked to each other.
**stereoisomerism** \-īsäm′ərizm\ The phenomenon that molecules of identical constituents linked similarly can differ by the relative positions of these constituents in space.
**stereology** \ster′ē·äl′əjē\ The study of objects, which are usually microscopic in size, in three dimensions.
**stereometry** \ster′ē·äm′ətrē\ [STEREO- + -METRY] The measurement of volume or capacity.
**stereomonoscope** \-män′əskōp\ [STEREO- + MONO- + -SCOPE] An optical instrument that projects two images on the same spot on a screen, giving the impression of a third dimension.
**stereophantoscope** \-fan′təskōp\ [STEREO- + Gk *phanto(s)* (from *phainein* to bring to light) visible + -SCOPE] A binocular device in which the phenomenon of apparent motion is produced by a stroboscopic presentation.
**stereophorometer** \-fôräm′ətər\ A device for measurement and training of the vergence movements of the eyes.
**stereophoroscope** \-fôr′əskōp\ A device for evaluation of the vergence movements of the eye.
**stereopsis** \ster′ē·äp′sis\ [STERE- + -OPSIS] The ability to discern depth by means of binocular vision.
**stereoroentgenography** \-rent′genäg′rəfē\ [STEREO- + ROENTGENOGRAPHY] A technique of roentgenography producing paired, stereoscopic roentgenograms which, when viewed by a special instrument, afford three-dimensional presentation of the radiographed object or part of body. Also *stereoradiography*.
**stereoroentgenometry** \-rent′genäm′ətrē\ [STEREO- + ROENTGENOMETRY] A method of measuring the dimensions of an object or patient area by the use of stereoscopic roentgenograms.
**stereoscopic** \-skäp′ik\ [STEREO- + *-scop(e)* + -IC] Pertaining to the visual perception of three-dimensionality, as embodied in relief and solidity.
**stereoscopy** \ster′ē·äs′kəpē\ [STEREO- + -SCOPY] The viewing by a special apparatus, the stereoscope, of the paired roentgenograms produced by stereoroentgenography to afford a three-dimensional appearance of the object or patient area examined.
**stereospecific** \-spəsif′ik\ Specific for one stereoisomer rather than another: said of a reaction or interaction between molecules.
**stereospecificity** \-spes′ifis′itē\ Specificity for one stereoisomer rather than another.
**stereostroboscope** \-strō′bəskōp\ An instrument that uses interrupted light to observe successive phases of an object moving in three dimensions. Also *strobostereoscope*.
**stereotactic** \-tak′tik\ Pertaining to stereotaxy.
**stereotaxy** \-tak′sē\ [STEREO- + -TAXY] Surgery of the brain utilizing a device that guides the three-dimensional placement of an instrument in a specific or circumscribed area. Also *stereotaxis, stereotaxic surgery, stereotaxic procedure*. Adj. stereotactic, stereotaxic.
**stereotropic** \-trō′pik\ Pertaining to or exhibiting stereotropism.
**stereotropism** \-trō′pizm, ster′ē·ät′rəpizm\ [STEREO- + TROPISM] Growth or movement of the whole or part of a living organism towards or away from a solid object. There may be attraction towards such an object (positive stereotropism) or repulsion from it (negative stereotropism).
**stereotypy** \ster′ē·ətī′pē\ [STEREO- + *typ(e)* + -Y] The incessant repetition of an action, such as repeated rubbing of a part of the body.
**steric** \stir′ik\ [*ster(e)-* + -IC] Denoting an effect due to spatial configuration. For example, steric hindrance is the slowing of a reaction due to blocking by certain atoms of the approach of a reactant.
**sterilant** \ster′ilənt\ Any agent that causes failure of reproduction through interference with oogenesis or spermatogenesis, cessation of production of live gametes, or induction of fatal mutations. The term usually refers to chemical substances employed in the control of harmful insects. See also CHEMOSTERILANT.
**sterile** \ster′il\ [L *sterilis* barren, sterile] **1** Aseptic; free from living microorganisms. **2** Infertile; incapable of reproducing.
**sterility** \stəril′itē\ [L *sterilitas* (from *sterilis* barren) barrenness, sterility] **1** Inability to produce offspring. **2** The state of being free from living microorganisms; asepsis. **absolute s.** Sterility due to a condition that cannot be corrected. **aspermatogenic s.** Sterility resulting from nonproduction of viable spermatozoa. **dyspermatogenic s.** Sterility resulting from abnormal spermatogenesis. **normospermatogenic s.** Sterility in a male which is not due to a defect in production of spermatozoa. It may result, for example, from seminiferous tube blockage. **partial s.** RELATIVE STERILITY. **primary s.** Sterility in a couple who have never achieved conception. **relative s.** Inability to produce children due to an abnormality which is probably correctable, such as varicocele in the male. Also *revocable sterility, partial sterility*. **secondary s.** Sterility in a couple who have previously achieved conception.
**sterilization** \ster′əlīzā′shən\ [*steril(e)* + *-iz(e)* + -ATION] **1** Destruction or elimination of the microorganisms in a material, as by chemical agents (disinfection), phys-

ical agents (heat, ultraviolet radiation, ionizing radiation), or by filtration. 2 Destruction or elimination of an organism's reproductive capacity, such as performing a fallopian tube ligation in a woman or a vasectomy in a man. **tubal s.** A form of permanent contraception in which the fallopian tubes are surgically obstructed, as with plastic materials, or in which caustic chemicals are applied to the tubes.

**sterilize** \ster′iliz\ **1** To expose to a physical or chemical treatment that destroys the viability of all microbes present. **2** To render incapable of reproduction.

**sterilizer** \ster′əlīzər\ **s. for root canal instruments** A small sterilizer that depends on the application of high temperature for a few seconds, thus enabling instruments to be sterilized at the chairside during treatment. The sterilizer is kept at its working temperature during the treatment visit. It may contain molten metal, small glass beads, salt, or sand, into which the working end of the instrument is plunged when necessary. **steam s.** A device that uses live steam under atmospheric pressure in an enclosed space to make objects within it sterile and aseptic.

**stern-** \sturn-\ STERNO-.

**sternad** \stur′nad\ Toward the sternum.

**sternal** \stur′nəl\ Pertaining to the sternum.

**sternalis** \stərnā′lis\ MUSCULUS STERNALIS.

**Sternberg** [Carl von *Sternberg*, Austrian pathologist, 1872–1935] **1** Reed-Sternberg cells. See under STERNBERG-REED CELLS. **2** Sternberg's disease. See under HODGKIN'S DISEASE.

**Sternberg** [William H. *Sternberg*, U.S. pathologist, born 1913] Albright-McCune-Sternberg syndrome. See under ALBRIGHT'S DISEASE.

**sternebra** \stur′nəbrə\ [New L, from *stern(um)* + *-ebra* as in *vertebra*] (*pl.* sternebrae) One of the centers of ossification in the embryo that give rise by fusion to the sternum. Also *sternebral rib, sternal vertebra.*

**sternebrae** \stur′nəbrē\ Plural of STERNEBRA.

**sternen** \stur′nən\ Pertaining to the sternum itself.

**sterno-** \stur′nō-\ [Gk *sternon* breast, chest] A combining form denoting the sternum. Also *stern-*.

**sternoclavicular** \-kləvik′yələr\ Of or pertaining to the sternum and the clavicle. Also *cleidosternal, sternocleidal, sternoclavicularis.*

**sternoclavicularis** \-kləvik′yəler′is\ An occasional muscle band extending from the upper margin of manubrium sterni to the clavicle either between the pectoralis major muscle and the clavipectoral fascia or behind the sternocleidomastoid muscle. Also *supraclavicularis.*

**sternocleidal** \-klī′dəl\ STERNOCLAVICULAR.

**sternocleidomastoid** \-klī′dōmas′toid\ [STERNO- + CLEIDO- + MASTOID] Of or pertaining to the sternum, the clavicle, and the mastoid process.

**sternocoracoid** \-kôr′əkoid\ Of or pertaining to the sternum and the coracoid process of the scapula.

**sternocostal** \-käs′təl\ Of or pertaining to the sternum and the ribs.

**sternocostalis** \-kästā′lis\ MUSCULUS TRANSVERSUS THORACIS.

**sternodymus** \stərnäd′iməs\ [STERNO- + -DYMUS] STERNOPAGUS.

**sternohyoid** \-hī′oid\ Of or pertaining to the sternum and the hyoid bone.

**sternohyoideus azygos** \-hī·oi′dē·əs az′igəs\ An occasional muscle band in the midline of the neck extending from the posterior surface of manubrium sterni to the hyoid bone.

**sternoid** \stur′noid\ Resembling the sternum.

**sternomastoid** \-mas′toid\ Of or pertaining to the sternum and the mastoid process of the temporal bone.

**sterno-omphalopagus** \-äm′fəläp′əgəs\ [STERNO- + OMPHALO- + -PAGUS] Equal conjoined twins united at the sternal and umbilical regions.

**sternopagus** \stərnäp′əgəs\ [STERNO- + -PAGUS] Equal conjoined twins united at the sternal region. Also *sternodymus.*

**sternopericardial** \-per′ikär′dē·əl\ Of or pertaining to the sternum and the pericardium.

**sternoscapular** \-skap′yələr\ Of or pertaining to the sternum and the scapula.

**sternothyreoideus** \-thī′rē·oi′dē·əs\ MUSCULUS STERNOTHYROIDEUS.

**sternothyroid** \-thī′roid\ Of or pertaining to the sternum and the thyroid gland or the thyroid cartilage.

**sternotomy** \stərnät′əmē\ [STERNO- + -TOMY] A surgical incision into or through part or all of the bony sternum.

**sternotracheal** \-trā′kē·əl\ Of or pertaining to the sternum and the trachea.

**sternoxiphoid** \-zī′foid\ Of or pertaining to the sternum and the xiphoid process.

**sternoxiphopagus** \-zīfäp′əgəs\ [STERNO- + *xipho(id)* + -PAGUS] Equal conjoined twins united throughout the sternum, including the xiphoid region.

**sternum** \stur′nəm\ [New L (from Gk *sternon* the male breast, chest, breastbone, akin to *storennynai* to spread out, stretch and to L *sternere* to strew, spread)] [NA] A long, flat, bladelike bone composed of several fused segments, forming the central anterior wall of the thorax and having the costal cartilages of the true ribs articulated at its sides and the clavicles articulated at its upper end. It consists of three parts: the manubrium, corpus (or body), and xiphoid process. The anterior surface is subcutaneous, while the posterior surface is related to the adjacent contents of the thoracic cavity. Also *breast bone, xiphoid bone* (outmoded), *scutum pectoris* (outmoded). **s. bifidum** SCHISTOSTERNIA.

**sternutator** \stur′nyətā′tər\ [Back formation from *sternutatory*] An agent that can induce sneezing, such as some of the war gases.

**sternutatory** \stərnyoo′tətôr′ē\ [Late L *sternutatorius* pertaining to sneezing, from L *sternutat(us)*, past part. of *sternutare* to sneeze often + *-orius* -ORY] **1** Related to or causing sneezing. **2** A substance that causes sneezing.

**sternzellen** \stern′tsel′ən, shtern′-\ [German *Stern* star + *Zellen* cells] STELLATE CELLS.

**steroid** \stir′oid\ [*ster(ol)* + -OID] Any of a class of compounds containing a cyclopentanoperhydrophenanthrene ring system, with great variety in degree of saturation of the steroid nucleus and of keto-, hydroxyl-, and other substituents and side chains. The class includes sterols, bile acids, cardiac aglycones, plant sapogenins, carcinogenic hydrocarbons, toad poisons, and the steroid hormones. **anabolic s.** Any of a class of synthetic or semisynthetic steroid hormones that possess only limited virilizing potency but that promote the biosynthesis of tissue protein. Their use in treating various catabolic disease states and in stimulating muscle growth in competitive athletes is controversial. **s. nucleus** The system of four rings that is contained in the steroid molecule.

**steroid monooxygenase** Any enzyme that catalyzes the hydroxylation of a steroid with concomitant reduction of dioxygen and oxidation of a coreductant. Such enzymes are involved in introducing the hydroxl groups of bile acids and adrenal cortical hormones. Also *steroid hydroxylase* (obs.).

**steroidogenesis** \stiroi′dəjen′əsis\ [STEROID + *o* + GENESIS ] The biosynthesis of steroids.

**steroidogenic** \stiroi′dəjen′ik\ [STEROID + *o* + -GENIC] Relating to the biosynthesis of steroids.

**sterol** \stir′ôl\ [back-formation from CHOLESTEROL] The simplest type of steroid. It is an alcohol without other functional groups. Cholesterol is an example.

**stertor** \stur′tər\ [New L, from L *stert(ere)* to snore + *-or* as in *clamor, stridor*] The coarse, snoring sound liable to occur during inspiration, especially in the sleeping or comatose individual obliged to breath through the mouth. The noise usually occurs when the tongue falls back and obstructs the airway through the mouth immediately proximal to the fauces. Adj. stertorous.

**stertorous** \stur′tərəs\ Characterized by stertor.

**steth-** \steth-\ STETHO-.

**stethalgia** \stethal′jə\ [STETH- + -ALGIA] Pain in the chest.

**stetho-** \steth′ō-, steth′ə-\ [Gk *stēthos* breast, chest] A combining form denoting the chest. Also *steth-*.

**stethocyrtograph** \-sir′təgraf\ An instrument for measuring and recording the curvatures of the chest wall. Also *stethocyrtometer, stethokyrtograph.*

**stethogoniometer** \-gō′nē·äm′ətər\ An instrument for measuring the curvatures of the chest wall.

**stethograph** \steth′əgraf\ [STETHO- + -GRAPH] An apparatus for the continuous recording of respiratory chest movement.

**stethokyrtograph** \-kir′təgraf\ STETHOCYRTOGRAPH.

**stethoscope** \steth′əskōp\ [STETHO- + -SCOPE] An instrument used for conducting sounds originating within the patient's body to the ear of the examiner. **binaural s.** A stethoscope that is connected to both ears. Also *Cammann stethoscope.* **DeLee-Hillis obstetric s.** An instrument worn on the observer's head to auscultate the fetal heartbeat. **electronic s.** A microphone and amplifier for detecting sounds such as heart murmurs and increasing the sound applied to the ears. **Leff s.** An instrument to auscultate the fetal heartbeat.

**stethoscopic** \-skäp′ik\ Relating to or produced by a stethoscope.

**stethoscopy** \stethäs′kəpē\ [STETHO- + -SCOPY] The technique of auscultation by means of the stethoscope.

**Stevens** [Albert Mason *Stevens,* U.S. pediatrician, 1884–1945] Stevens-Johnson disease. See under STEVENS-JOHNSON SYNDROME.

**Stewart** [Douglas Hunt *Stewart,* U.S. surgeon, 1860–1933] Stewart-Morel syndrome, Morgagni-Stewart-Morel syndrome. See under HYPEROSTOSIS FRONTALIS INTERNA.

**Stewart** [Fred Waldorf *Stewart,* U.S. pathologist, born 1894] Stewart-Treves syndrome. See under SYNDROME.

**Stewart** [James Purves *Stewart,* English physician, 1869–1949] **1** Holmes-Stewart phenomenon. See under HOLMES REBOUND PHENOMENON. **2** Stewart-Holmes sign. See under SIGN.

**Stewart** [Kenneth C. *Stewart,* U.S. audiologist, born 1917] Doerfler-Stewart test. See under TEST.

**STH** somatotropic hormone.

**sthen-** \sthen-\ STHENO-.

**stheno-** \sthen′ō-, sthen′ə-\ [Gk *sthenos* strength] A combining form meaning strength. Also *sthen-*.

**sthenometry** \sthenäm′ətrē\ [STHENO- + -METRY] The measurement of muscular strength.

**stibamine glucoside** $C_{36}H_{49}N_3NaO_{22}Sb_3$. Sodium *p*-aminobenzenestibonate glucoside. It occurs as a light buff powder, and has antiprotozoal activity.

**stibenyl** Sodium 4-acetamidobenzenestibonate. The prototype pentavalent antimonial drug once used in the treatment of leishmaniasis.

**stibialism** \stib′ē·əlizm\ [L *stibi(um)* antimony + -AL + -ISM] See under ANTIMONY POISONING.

**stibiated** Treated with or containing antimony.

**stibine** $SbH_3$. Antimonious hydride. A poisonous gas formerly used as a fumigating agent.

**stibinic acids** Acids of pentavalent antimony, $H_3SbO_5$, $HSbO_3$, and $H_4Sb_2O_7$, used in organoantimony compound preparation. The last two are used as antiprotozoal agents.

**stibocaptate** \stib′ōkap′tāt\ Sodium antimony dimercaptosuccinate, a toxic trivalent antimony compound used in an intramuscular injection for the treatment of schistosomiasis. It is being replaced by less toxic drugs such as metrifonate, oxamniquine, and praziquantel.

**stibophen** $C_{12}H_4Na_5O_{16}S_4Sb{\cdot}7H_2O$. Bis[4,5-dihydroxy-1,3-benzenedisulfonato(4-)-$O^4$,$O^5$]-antimonato(5-)pentasodium heptahydrate. One of the trivalent antimony compounds employed as anthelmintics, mainly in the treatment of schistosomiasis caused by *S. mansoni, S. haematobium,* and *S. japonicum.* It occurs as a white or yellow crystalline powder, and is given either intramuscularly or intravenously. Also *neoantimosan.*

**stick / sponge s.** A rolled surgical sponge in a ring forceps.

**Sticker** [Georg *Sticker,* German physician, 1860–1960] Sticker's disease. See under ERYTHEMA INFECTIOSUM.

**Stieda** [Alfred *Stieda,* German surgeon, 1869–1945] Stieda's disease, Köhler-Pellegrini-Stieda disease. See under PELLEGRINI-STIEDA DISEASE.

**Stieda** [Ludwig *Stieda,* German anatomist, 1837–1918] Stieda's process. See under PROCESSUS POSTERIOR TALI.

**Stierlin** [Eduard *Stierlin,* German surgeon, 1878–1919] See under SIGN.

**stiffness** The quality of having a subnormal ability to move a joint, muscle, or the skin. **congenital spasmodic limb s.** LITTLE'S DISEASE. **neck s.** Rigidity of the posterior neck muscles resulting in resistance and pain when an attempt is made to passively flex the subject's head and neck. It is commonly seen as a sign of meningeal irritation in meningitis or subarachnoid hemorrhage. Also *nuchal rigidity.*

**stigma** \stig′mə\ [Gk *stigma* (from *stizein* to prick, puncture) a prick or puncture of a pointed instrument, a mark, spot] (*pl.* stigmata, stigmas) **1** A mark or spot upon the skin or other surface. **2** A visible or otherwise obvious sign that is pathognomonic or typical of a given disease. See also STIGMATA. **s. of degeneracy** Any physical, nervous, or psychic abnormality that is premonitory of or regularly associated with a degenerative state. **follicular s.** The site of ovulation as visualized on the ovarian surface. **Koplik s. of degeneration** An unusual prominence of the pisiform bone. It is seen in some instances of sporadic cretinism. **malpighian stigmata** The points of opening of the smaller or pulp veins into the trabecular veins in the spleen. *Outmoded.* **professional stigmata** Marks made on the surface of the body as a result of one's profession or occupation. They include callosities, scars, bursae, telangiectases, tattoo marks, deformities of the nails and teeth, and color changes of the skin and hair. **syphilitic stigmata** The physical signs usually associated with congenital syphilis.

**stigmata** \stigmä′tə, stig′mətə\ **1** Plural of STIGMA. **2** Marks on the hands and feet resembling the wounds of the crucified body of Christ, sometimes categorized as examples of conversion hysteria.

**stigmatism** \stig′mətizm\ [STIGMA + *t* + -ISM] A condition caused by or characteristic of stigmas.

**stigmatization** \stig′mətīzā′shən\ **1** The process of being marked by a stigma. 2 The process of developing, or of being identified as possessing indicators or pathognomonic signs that justify the labeling and consequently the treatment of a person as special or unusual. • At one point, *stigmatization* referred specifically to the development of marks resembling the stigmata of the crucified body of Christ and was assumed to be a sign of divine favor. Later, *stigmatization* referred to the production of similar marks created exogenously (by suggestion or hypnosis) or endogenously (as a form of conversion hysteria). Current usage often conveys the implication of contrived discrimination against the person or group to whom reference is made, as because of mental disorder or abnormal behavior.

**stilalgin** MEPHENESIN.

**stilbazium iodide** $C_{31}H_{36}IN_3$. 1-Ethyl-2,6-bis(*p*1-pyrrolidinylstyryl)pyridinium iodide. A compound with anthelmintic properties.

**stilbene** A cyclic hydrocarbon, of formula $C_6H_5$—CH═CH—$C_6H_5$ (*trans-*), composed of colorless, monoclinic crystals. It is soluble in ethanol and ether, and has a melting point of 124–125°C. It is the starting point for the synthesis of diethylstilbestrol, the synthetic estrogen.

**stilbestrol** \stilbes′trôl\ DIETHYLSTILBESTROL.

**stilboestrol** *Brit.* STILBESTROL.

**Stiles** [Walter Stanley *Stiles,* English physiologist, born 1901] Stiles-Crawford effect. See under EFFECT.

**stilet** \stīlet′\ STYLET.

**stilette** \stīlet′\ STYLET.

**stili** \stī′lī\ Plural of STILUS.

**Still** [Sir George Frederick *Still,* English physician, 1868–1941] 1 See under MURMUR, DISEASE. 2 Chauffard-Still syndrome, Still-Chauffard syndrome. See under CHAUFFARD SYNDROME.

**stillbirth** The death *in utero* of the products of conception after a gestation exceeding a minimum period which differs according to law from country to country but in general is of the order of six months. Also *dead birth.*

**stillborn** Designating a fetus of given gestation which is dead when it issues forth or is extracted from its mother. The period of gestation varies according to the law in different countries from 20 to 28 weeks.

**stillicidium** \stil′isid′ē·əm\ A falling or flowing of drops or tears. **s. lacrimarum** *Outmoded* EPIPHORA.

**Stilling** [Benedikt *Stilling,* German anatomist, 1810–1879] 1 See under COLUMN. 2 Stilling sacral nucleus, Stilling's nucleus. See under SACRAL NUCLEUS. 3 Canal of Stilling, central canal of Stilling. See under CANALIS HYALOIDEUS. 4 Stilling's fibers. See under FIBER. 5 Stilling's nucleus. See under NUCLEUS THORACICUS. 6 Nucleus dorsalis stillingi. See under NUCLEUS DORSALIS CLARKII.

**Stilling** [Jakob *Stilling,* German ophthalmologist, 1842–1915] 1 Nucleus amygdaliformis of J. Stilling. See under NUCLEUS SUBTHALAMICUS. 2 Stilling-Turk-Duane syndrome, Stilling syndrome. See under DUANE SYNDROME.

**stillingia** \stilin′jē·ə\ The dried root of *Stillingia sylvatica.* It has been used as a tonic, diuretic, and laxative. Also *yaw root.*

**stilus** \stī′ləs\ 1 STYLUS. 2 STYLET.

**stimulant** \stim′yələnt\ [L *stimulans* gen. *stimulantis* (from *stimulare* to goad, incite; see STIMULATE) stimulating, inciting] 1 Causing stimulation of nervous tissue or, indirectly, muscle tissue. 2 An agent that causes stimulation. Also *stimulator.* **alcoholic s.** A stimulant having ethanol as the active ingredient, such as wine or other alcoholic beverages. **central s.** A drug, technique, or method which enhances the activity of the central nervous system. Also *nervous stimulant.* **cerebral s.** Any drug, technique, or method which enhances the activity of the brain. **diffusable s.** A stimulant that acts for only a short time. **general s.** A stimulant that acts throughout the body. **local s.** A stimulant that affects only or mainly the area where it is applied. Also *topical stimulant.* **nervous s.** CENTRAL STIMULANT. **respiratory s.** A drug or other substance that increases depth or frequency of respiration. **topical s.** LOCAL STIMULANT. **uterine s.** An oxytocic drug used to stimulate uterine contractions.

**stimulate** \stim′yəlāt\ [L *stimulare* (from *stimulus* a goad) to goad, incite] To excite in a manner that, if of sufficient magnitude, can elicit activity.

**stimulation** \stim′yəlā′shən\ [L *stimulatio* (from *stimulare* to goad, incite) incitement] The process or act of exciting to produce some form of functional activity. **biocular s.** Independent photic excitation of each eye. **cerebellar s.** Electric stimulation of the cerebellum. It is sometimes used as a means of relieving spasticity. **direct s.** Excitation of a muscle by action of the stimulus on the muscle substance, rather than through its nerve. **faradic s.** The application of a stimulus consisting of an alternating current of electricity produced by an induction coil. **indirect s.** Induction of contraction in a muscle by applying a stimulus to its nerve. **intermittent photic s.** An activating technique used in electroencephalography in which flickering light from a stroboscope is used to excite the retina at different frequencies. The presence or absence of following in the alpha rhythm may be of diagnostic value and, especially in children, epileptic discharges may be elicited in the recording. **nonspecific s.** Excitation of a sense organ by a form of energy to which it is not optimally sensitive, e.g., pressure excitation of the retina to produce a sensory experience of light. Also *paraspecific stimulation.* **paradoxical s.** The apparently anomalous phenomenon that arises when stimulation of a cutaneous cold spot with a warm or hot object evokes a sensation of coldness. **paraspecific s.** NONSPECIFIC STIMULATION. **photic s.** In electroencephalography, the use of flickering stroboscopic illumination at varying frequencies in an attempt to evoke latent or subclinical epileptic discharges. **punctual s.** Excitation of a sense organ by applying a stimulus to a restricted locus in the receptive field of a given neuron. Also *punctate sensory stimulation.* **transcutaneous electrical nerve s.** A technique used for treating intractable pain in which electrodes are firmly attached to the skin over the painful area and intermittent electric stimulation is delivered via a portable stimulator controlled by the patient, who can vary the duration and intensity of the stimulation according to need. Abbr. TENS

**stimulator** \stim′yəlātər\ 1 STIMULANT. 2 Any of various devices for delivering electrical stimuli to parts of the body. **cerebellar s.** A device for the continuous administration of low voltage stimulation to the cerebellar cortex through electrodes placed surgically on the surface of the anterior and posterior lobes, and connected by subcutaneous leads with a receiver, which in turn is activated through a transmitter. Claims are made for the beneficial effect of this procedure on epilepsy and cerebral spasticity, but the results are controversial. **dorsal column s.** A device for delivering low voltage impulses to the dorsal aspect of the spinal cord, used for the alleviation of distal pain. **interdental s.** A fine, tapered stick made of wood or plastic, for rubbing between the teeth. In addition to removing dental plaque, the massaging action on the gums may increase keratinization and improve the blood supply. **long-acting thyroid s.** An immunoglobulin G autoantibody to the thyrotropin receptor. This antibody mimics the effect of thyrotropin but its effect is more prolonged. Long-acting thryoid stimulator is present in the blood of most patient with Graves disease. Abbr. LATS **nerve s.** An electrode used in the surgical exploration of nerves, whereby electrical stimulation establishes the nerve's identity by the sensory or motor response produced. It also establishes the presence or absence of conductivity of a nerve that may be damaged.

**stimuli** \stim′yəlī\ Plural of STIMULUS.

**stimulus** \stim′yələs\ [L (prob. akin to *stilus* a pointed instrument) a goad, spur] Any form of energy capable of eliciting a reaction in a sense organ or in any excitable tissue; a signal that alerts an organism or leads to responsive action. **adequate s.** The specific form of stimulus energy to which a given sense organ is optimally sensitive. Also *homologous stimulus.* **aversive s.** 1 A painful stimulus. 2 A stimulus that elicits avoidance or escape. **chemical s.** A chemical substance capable of eliciting excitation or one of several sensations such as taste, smell, and irritation. **conditioned s.** The originally neutral and ineffective stimulus which, by means of repeated pairing with an unconditioned stimulus during classical conditioning, becomes capable of eliciting the conditioned response. Also *conditioning stimulus.* Abbr. CS **conditioning s.** 1 Any stimulus that precedes a second test stimulus of the same or different nature and modifies the response which the test stimulus would have elicited if given alone. Such interrelationship need not be related to conditioned learning. 2 CONDITIONED STIMULUS. **discriminative s.** In operant conditioning, a stimulus which becomes the signal for the release of a particular response as the result of prior association, but which would not otherwise serve as an adequate stimulus to elicit that response. **heterotopic s.** A stimulus to electrical activity in the heart outside the sinuatrial node. **homologous s.** 1 ADEQUATE STIMULUS. 2 A stimulus applied to a corresponding locus on the opposite side of the body. **inadequate s.** A form of stimulus energy to which a sense organ is relatively insensitive, e.g., mechanical excitation of the retina to produce a sensation of light. **latent s.** A subliminal stimulus that is not recognized as such or is viewed as inadequate to elicit a response. **liminal s.** THRESHOLD STIMULUS. **manifest s.** An overt stimulus, recognized as having elicited a response. **maximal s.** The stimulus magnitude that produces the maximal response. **mechanical s.** Any applied-force stimulus, as the displacement of skin or stretching of muscle. **minimal s.** THRESHOLD STIMULUS. **morphogenetic s.** Any stimulus by one part of an embryo on another that results in the affected part undergoing some morphogenetic alteration. **nomotopic s.** A stimulus to the sinuatrial node. **square wave stimuli** Pulselike electrical stimuli in which the current is suddenly changed from zero to a preset intensity, held there for a predetermined duration, then suddenly returned to zero. They are useful in determining strength/duration curves. **subthreshold s.** A stimulus below the magnitude for effectiveness or detection. Also *subliminal stimulus, subminimal stimulus.* **supraliminal s.** A stimulus magnitude significantly above the threshold range. **supramaximal s.** A stimulus magnitude exceeding that producing the maximal response. **thermal s.** A cold or heat stimulus producing excitation. **threshold s.** 1 A stimulus of sufficient magnitude to be effective or detectable. 2 A sensory stimulus recognized in 50 percent of trials. Also *liminal stimulus, minimal stimulus.* **unconditioned s.** A stimulus, often used in a classical conditioning paradigm, which automatically elicits a response, usually by means of a biologically based reflex mechanism, without any need for learning or prior experience. An example is a tap on the patellar tendon. Abbr. US

**stimulus-response** A bond or linkage existing between an event and an organism's response to that event. The event or action may be any objectively defined situation, occurring within or outside the organism, which elicits an objectively definable response. Abbr. S-R

**sting** 1 A sudden, sharp pain produced by pricking or puncturing the skin, usually caused by certain species of arthropods, venomous fish, and some plants. 2 The organ or part causing the lesion.

**stippling** \stip′ling\ [Dutch *stippelen* to spot, dot + -ING] 1 The presence of multiple tiny erosions of the corneal epithelium. 2 The appearance of small granules or dots, as in a tissue or a cell. **basophilic s. of erythrocytes** The presence of numerous tiny blue dots in erythrocytes that have been stained with a Romanowsky dye such as the Wright stain. This phenomenon is due to the presence of ribosomal RNA in erythrocytes and is characteristically increased in chronic lead or arsenic poisoning, thalassemias, and hemolytic anemias. Also *punctate basophilia, polychromatophilic degeneration.* **gingival s.** The presence of small pits in the surface of the attached gingiva. The appearance is similar to that of orange peel and is related to the shape of the underlying epithelioconnective tissue junction. With inflammation and edema the stippling disappears. **malarial s.** SCHÜFFNER'S GRANULES. **Maurer s.** MAURER'S DOTS. **Schüffner s.** SCHÜFFNER'S GRANULES.

**Stirling** [William *Stirling*, English histologist and physiologist, 1851–1932] Stirling's modification of the Gram stain. See under STAIN.

**stirrup** \stur′əp\ [Old English *stigrāp*] 1 STAPES. 2 A device used to attach a brace to a shoe. It is affixed to the sole of the shoe, and two lateral projections reach to the level of the ankle joint to receive the brace. **Finochietto s.** A device for applying skeletal traction in lower extremity fractures. **swivel s.** An orthopedic device for applying traction in lower extremity fractures.

**stitch** 1 SUTURE. 2 A sharp sudden pain, especially in the flank of one one side of the abdomen. **glover s.** LOCK-STITCH SUTURE.

**stithe** \stīth\ *Outmoded* INCUS.

**stochastic** \stōkas′tik\ [Gk *stochastik(os)* (from *stochazesthai* to surmise, from *stochos* a conjecture) able to guess or aim] Susceptible to random influences and thus subject to the laws of probability; the opposite of deterministic. See also STOCHASTIC PROCESS.

**stock** The mating population from which a particular line descends. It may be a naturally occurring population of animals or plants or a population maintained by humans for selective breeding or experimentation.

**stockinet** \stäk′inet′\ An undergarment of woven cloth similar to that used for stockings, manufactured in a tubelike form of uniform diameter and used to cover an extremity or other part of the body before application of a plaster cast, splint, or other device.

**stoicheiometric** \stoi′kē·əmet′rik\ STOICHIOMETRIC.

**stoicheiometry** \stoi′kē·äm′ətrē\ STOICHIOMETRY.

**stoichiometric** \stoi′kē·əmet′rik\ 1 Relating to stoichiometry. 2 Designating a reaction in which it is shown that a whole number of molecules results from each molecule reacting, and that the equation, and absence of side reactions, are thereby established. For defs. 1 and 2 also *stoicheiometric.*

**stoichiometry** \stoi′kē·äm′ətrē\ [Gk *stoicheio(n)* a first beginning, principle, or element; in pl., primary matter or elements + -METRY] The branch of chemistry that studies the precise quantitative relations in amount of substance between the various products formed and reactants converted in any chemical reaction. A chemical reaction involves well-defined proportions of participating substances which reflect the numbers of molecules reacting and produced. Also *stoicheiometry.*

**Stokes** [Sir William *Stokes,* Irish surgeon, 1839–1900] Stokes operation, Stokes amputation. See under GRITTI-STOKES AMPUTATION.

**Stokes** [William *Stokes,* Irish physician, 1804–1878] **1** Stokes-Adams disease, Adams-Stokes disease, Stokes-Adams syndrome, Stokes syndrome, Morgagni-Adams-Stokes syndrome. See under ADAMS-STOKES SYNDROME. **2** Adams-Stokes syncope. See under SYNCOPE. **3** Cheyne-Stokes breathing, Cheyne-Stokes sign. See under CHEYNE-STOKES RESPIRATION.

**Stoll** [Norman Rudolph *Stoll,* U.S. parasitologist, born 1892] See under TEST, METHOD.

**stom-** \stōm-\ STOMATO-.

**stoma** \stō′mə\ [Gk, the mouth] (*pl.* stomas, stomata) **1** [NA] A small orifice or pore, especially on a surface. **2** An intercellular aperture in the endothelium of a capillary or a lymph channel. **3** A surgically created orifice.

**stomach** [Gk *stomachos* (from *stoma* mouth, orifice) the esophagus, entry of any hollow viscus, the stomach] **1** GASTER. **2** *Incorrect* ABDOMEN. **bilocular s.** HOURGLASS STOMACH. **cardiac s.** PARS CARDIACA GASTRIS.

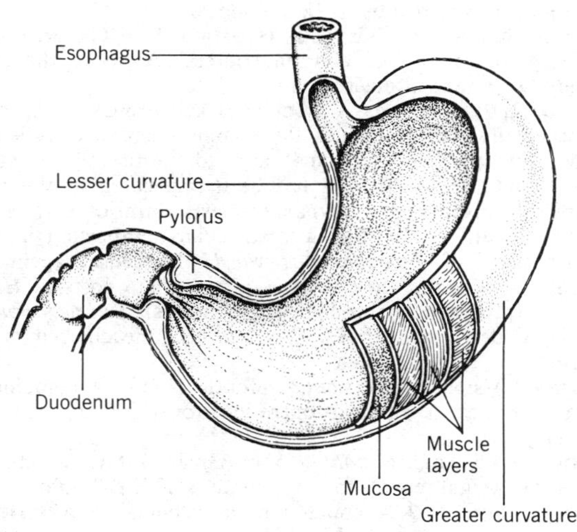


**Stomach**

**cascade s.** A bilocular appearance of the stomach on gastrointestinal series in which the radiopaque barium rapidly spills inferiorly out of the proximal portion and empties into the more dependent distal portion. Also *physiologic hourglass stomach, waterfall stomach.* **dumping s.** See under POSTGASTRECTOMY SYNDROME. **honeycomb s.** RETICULUM. **hourglass s.** A stomach with a constriction at the midportion, producing a radiographic image suggestive of an hourglass. The constriction may be either functional, and reversible, or the result of scarring, and irreversible. Also *bilocular stomach.* **miniature s.** PAVLOV POUCH. **Pavlov s.** PAVLOV POUCH. **physiologic hourglass s.** CASCADE STOMACH. **powdered s.** An antianemic agent produced by the drying, defatting, and pulverizing of the stomach wall of the hog *Sus scrofa.* It is used as a source of intrinsic factor. **primitive s.** ARCHENTERON. **sclerotic s.** LINITIS PLASTICA. **thoracic s.** A stomach that is partially or completely contained in the thorax due to a hiatal hernia. **trifid s.** A stomach divided into three pouches by the formation of two constrictions in it. **upside-down s.** Gastric volvulus resulting in an inverted position of the stomach, as in a paraesophageal hernia. **waterfall s.** CASCADE STOMACH.

**stomachache** Pain in the area of the stomach. Also *gastralgia, gastrodynia.*

**stomachic** \stōmak′ik\ A stomach tonic or stimulant.

**stomal** \stō′məl\ **1** Of or pertaining to a stoma or stomata. Also *stomatal.* **2** ORAL.

**stomat-** \stōmat-\ STOMATO-.

**stomata** \stō′mətə\ Plural of STOMA.

**stomatal** \stō′mətəl\ STOMAL.

**stomatic** \stōmat′ik\ ORAL.

**stomatitis** \stō′mətī′tis\ [STOMAT- + -ITIS] Any generalized inflammatory disease of the oral mucosa, comprising that of the tongue, palate, cheeks, gums, lips, and floor of the mouth. **acute necrotizing s.** CANCRUM ORIS. **acute ulcerative s.** Necrotizing ulcerative gingivitis which has extended beyond the gingiva to other regions of the mouth. **angular s.** ANGULAR CHEILITIS. **aphthous s.** A common variety of stomatitis characterized by the occurrence of painful, shallow apthae (recurrent aphthae) anywhere in the mouth or sometimes in the pharynx. The ulcers, usually a few millimeters in size, may occasionally be 2 to 3 cm across. They tend to recur in susceptible individuals, seeming sometimes to follow minor trauma. The cause is uncertain, there is no specific treatment but spontaneous healing takes place within a week or two. **bismuth s.** The extension of bismuth gingivitis to involve regions of the oral mucosa in contact with accumulations of plaque on the teeth. **contact s.** Stomatitis occurring in susceptible or sensitized individuals from the contact of one of a number of substances with the oral mucous membrane. The responsible agent may be in many forms including mouthwashes, toothpaste, medication, certain foodstuffs, or even the patient's dentures. **denture s.** Stomatitis confined to the oral mucous membrane in contact with dentures, i.e. the mucosa of the hard palate or alveolar processes or both. It may be associated with angular cheilitis, and in both conditions infection with *Candida albicans* occurs frequently. The affected areas are red and swollen but seldom painful. Treatment includes the prolonged use of antifungal preparations. Also *stomatitis prosthetica* (older term), *denture sore mouth.* **fusospirochetal s.** NECROTIZING ULCERATIVE GINGIVITIS. **gangrenous s.** CANCRUM ORIS. **herpetic s.** Stomatitis due to either herpes simplex or herpes zoster. The lesions, shallow painful ulcers which soon replace the initial vesicles, are clinically identical in both cases and tend to occur on the hard palate behind the teeth. The disease runs a short, acute feverish course often with bright red swelling of the gingivae and enlargement of the regional lymph nodes. Also *herpetic gingivostomatitis.* **lead s.** Inflammation of the soft tissues of the mouth due to dental plaque associated with chronic lead poisoning. Symptoms and signs include a lead line and a metallic taste in the mouth. **s. medicamentosa** Stomatitis occurring as a side-effect of ingested drugs. It may be part of a widespread reaction involving the skin and other mucosal surfaces or confined to the mouth or part of it, particularly the gingivae. Drug allergy or idiosyncrasy may be involved or it may result from local irritation as in contact stomatitis. **mercurial s.** Inflammation of the soft tissues of the mouth due to dental plaque and associated with absorption of mercury. Other symptoms are foul breath, soreness of the gums, a mercurial line along the gingival margins, and discoloration of adjacent buccal mucosa. **mycotic s.** Any one of the several varieties of stomatitis due to fungus infection. The most common cause is *Candida albicans* while the oral lesions caused by other pathogenic fungi are rare and usually associated with disseminated disease. Also *stomatomycosis.* **necrotizing ulcerative s.** CANCRUM ORIS. **s. nicotina** Keratinization and hyperkeratinization of the oral mucosa accompanied by inflammation of the minor salivary glands, caused by smoking. Also *nicotinic stomatitis.* **s. prosthetica** DENTURE STOMATITIS. **recurrent herpetic s.** Stomatitis due to the virus herpes simplex, recurring often after minor trauma to the site, as from a toothbrush. **recurrent ulcerative s.** Stomatitis, either aphthous or that caused by herpes simplex, liable to periodic recurrence in susceptible individuals. **s. scarlatina** The oral manifestations of scarlet fever, chiefly the strawberry or raspberry tongue and stippled palate and usually also the characteristic tonsillitis. *Older term.* **s. scorbutica** The oral manifestations of scurvy, chiefly apparent in the edentulous gingivae, which may become swollen, spongy and, because of the characteristic purpura, purple. In advanced cases bleeding and ulceration of the gums occur with nauseating fetor. Also *scorbutic stomatitis.* **syphilitic s.** Any of the oral manifestations of syphilis, usually the mucous patches of the secondary stage. **traumatic s.** Stomatitis consequent on trauma to the mouth. More commonly than from major trauma, this may arise from ill-fitting dentures, jagged teeth, cheek biting, thermal injury, the vigorous use of a stiff toothbrush, etc. The initial minor lesion often becomes the site of shallow ulceration. **tropical s.** The oral changes that may occur in tropical sprue, such as the development of a red and raw tongue, atrophy of the mucous membrane and papillae, and aphthous ulcerations. **ulcerative s.** Any one of the many varieties of stomatitis characterized by ulcer formation. **Vincent s.** NECROTIZING ULCERATIVE GINGIVITIS.

**stomato-** \stō′mətō-\ [Gk *stoma* (genitive *stomatos*) mouth] A combining form meaning mouth, mouthlike. Also *stomat-, stom-.*

**stomatocyte** \stō′mətōsīt′\ [STOMATO- + -CYTE] An abnormally shaped human erythrocyte in which the normal area of central pallor is replaced by a long ellipsoidal zone of pallor oriented on a diameter of the cell and resembling a fish mouth. Electron microscopy indicates that the deformity is due to concave or cup-shaped change in erythrocyte shape. Stomatocytes are often technical artifacts.

**stomatocytosis** \-sītō′sis\ The presence of numerous stomatocytes in a blood film as a result of either technical artifact, alcoholism, or inheritance, the latter being an autosomal dominant condition.

**stomatodeum** \-dē′əm\ STOMODEUM.

**stomatoglossitis** \-gläsī′tis\ Any of the varieties of stomatitis in which the tongue presents conspicuous features of the disease, as in many nutritional disorders, for example vitamin B complex and folic acid deficiencies.

**stomatologist** \stō′mətäl′əjist\ A specialist in stomatology.

**stomatology** \stō′mətäl′əjē\ [STOMATO- + -LOGY] The study of the mouth in health and disease; the branch of medicine concerned with diseases of the mouth.

**stomatomenia** \-mē′nē·ə\ [STOMATO- + Gk *mēn* month + -IA] Bleeding from the mucous membrane of the mouth during monthly menstruation.

**stomatomycosis** \-mīkō′sis\ MYCOTIC STOMATITIS.

**stomatonecrosis** \-nekrō′sis\ CANCRUM ORIS.

**stomatonoma** \-nō′mə\ *Seldom used* CANCRUM ORIS.

**stomatopathy** \stō′mətäp′əthē\ [STOMATO- + -PATHY] Any disease of the mouth.

**stomatoplastic** \-plas′tik\ Pertaining to stomatoplasty.

**stomatoplasty** \stō′mətōplas′tē\ [STOMATO- + -PLASTY] The surgical repair or reconstruction of the mouth.

**stomatorrhagia** \stō′mətôrā′jə\ [STOMATO- + -RRHAGIA] Bleeding from the mouth.

**stomatotyphus** \-tī′fəs\ The hemorrhagic macular eruption which may sometimes spread from the face to involve the inside of the mouth in severe cases of typhus fever. *Seldom used.*

**stomocephalus** \stō′mōsef′ələs\ [STOM- + *o* + -CEPHALUS] A fetus or newborn with poorly developed face and jaws and an ill-defined mouth, often with associated cyclopia.

**stomodeum** \stō′mōdē′əm\ [New L *stomodaeum,* from Gk *stom(a)* mouth + *(h)odaion* (from *hodos* way) on the way] **1** A depression in the head ectoderm destined to form the primitive mouth of an embryo. It lies in front of the anterior end of the primitive intestine, at first separated from it by the buccopharyngeal membrane. When this membrane breaks down, the mouth is formed. The stomodeal cavity of higher vertebrates is eventually subdivided into the nasal fossa and the definitive mouth. Also *stomatodeum.* **2** The anterior part of the digestive tube of ectodermal origin in certain invertebrates, especially arthropods, consisting of mouth, buccal cavity, pharynx, esophagus, crop (if present), and proventriculus. Adj. stomodeal.

**stomoschisis** \stōmäs′kisis\ [STOM- + *o* + Gk *-schisis,* a cleaving, division] An abnormal lateral extent of the oral fissure, as is seen in macrostomia.

***Stomoxys calcitrans*** \stōmäk′sis kal′sitrənz\ A species of stable fly that resembles the common housefly. It is an important pest of humans and domesticated animals throughout the world, and has been implicated in the mechanical transmission of trypanosomiasis, anthrax, and vesicular stomatitis. Stable flies are particularly important in the transmission of *Trypanosoma evansi,* the causal agent of surra in cattle, and they serve as intermediate hosts of *Habronema* (producing habronemiasis in horses), *Setaria cervi* (a filaria of deer), and *Hymenolepis carioca,* the chicken tapeworm.

**-stomy** \-stəmē\ [Gk *stom(a)* mouth + -Y] A combining form denoting a surgical operation to make an artificial opening.

**stone** [Old English *stān*] **1** In Great Britain, a unit of mass or weight equal to 14 pounds; 6.350 29 kilograms. Symbol: stone **2** A concretion or calculus. **artifical s.** DENTAL STONE. **bladder s.** VESICAL CALCULUS. **chalk s.** TOPHUS. **dental s.** A hard type of plaster of Paris. Also *artificial stone.* **diamond s.** A lathe stone with industrial diamonds embedded in the surface, or a small version for use in the mouth. **ear s.** An otolith. See under STATOCONIA. **kidney s.** RENAL CALCULUS. **lathe s.** A cylinder of abrasive material driven by a lathe. Also *lathe wheel.* **metabolic s.** CHOLESTEROL CALCULUS. **pulp s.** DENTICLE. **struvite s.** STRUVITE CALCULUS. **urate s.** URIC ACID CALCULUS. **ureteral s.** URETERAL CALCULUS. **vein s.** PHLEBOLITH. **wheel s.** A small abrasive wheel mounted on a mandrel and used for grinding teeth. **womb s.** A calcified mass in the uterus that could be derived from fetal remnant or a leiomyoma.

**Stookey** [Byron Polk *Stookey,* U.S. neurosurgeon,

1887–1966] **1** Stookey-Scarff shunt. See under THIRD VENTRICULOCISTERNOSTOMY. **2** Stookey-Scarff operation. See under OPERATION. **3** Queckenstedt-Stookey test. See under QUECKENSTEDT'S TEST.

**stool** [Old English *stōl* chair, seat] The matter discharged from the bowels; feces. **bilious s.** The brown to green stool seen in bile-salt-induced diarrhea. **lienteric s.** Stool containing undigested food particles. **spinach s.** An abnormal, dark green stool of infants, supposed to resemble cooked spinach.

**stop** / **glottal s.** A sudden brief interruption of phonatory sound effected by closure of the glottis, as in the middle of the exclamation *oh-oh!* It is a standard speech sound in many languages and may replace certain plosive consonants in dialects of others, or it may result from the speaker's inability to produce the normal sound, especially in childhood. **short s.** The fixing solution used in film processing to clear the film and stop further development.

**stopping** / **temporary s.** A thermoplastic material, mainly gutta-percha, used to seal a dressing in a tooth.

**storax** A balsam occurring as a a brown, viscous liquid, and derived from the trunk of *Liquidambar orientalis*, a tree native to western Asia, or *L. styraciflua*, native to North America. It contains the ingredients used in compound benzoin tincture, and it has the properties of an expectorant and parasiticide. Also *sweetgum*.

**storesinol** A resin derived from storax. It may be in a free form or combined with cinnamic acid. Also *storesin*.

**storiform** \stôr′ifôrm\ [L *stori(a)* rush matting + -FORM] Characterized by an irregular whorl pattern: said of fibrous histiocytomas.

**storm** A sudden, sharp increase in the severity of symptoms in the course of a disease; crisis. **thyroid s.** THYROTOXIC CRISIS. **thyrotoxic s.** THYROTOXIC CRISIS.

**STP** standard temperature and pressure.

**stp** standard temperature and pressure.

**STPD** standard temperature and pressure, dry.

**strabismus** \strəbiz′məs\ [New L, from Gk *strabismos* (from *strabos* squint-eyed, akin to *strephein* to twist, turn) a squint, cast in the eye] A constant misalignment of the eyes, particularly of the visual axes, evident without such interruption of fusion as the covering of one eye. Also *heterotropia, heterotropy, squint, cast* (popular), *periphoria*. Adj. strabismic, strabismal. **A s.** Strabismus characterized by being more convergent (or less divergent) above, and more divergent (or less convergent) below. Compare V STRABISMUS. **accommodative s.** Strabismus related to hyperopia or faults in the AC/A ratio. **binocular s.** Strabismus in which either eye may be used spontaneously. Also *alternating strabismus, bilateral strabismus*. **concomitant s.** Manifest ocular deviation of the same amount in all positions of gaze. Also *comitant strabismus, concomitant squint*. **convergent s.** ESOTROPIA. **s. deorsum vergens** Strabismus marked by a turning downward of the deviating eye, the other eye being used for fixation. Compare STRABISMUS SURSUM VERGENS. **divergent s.** EXOTROPIA. **dynamic s.** INTERMITTENT STRABISMUS. **external s.** EXOTROPIA. **incomitant s.** Manifest ocular deviation in which the angular separation of the eyes varies with the position of gaze. Also *noncomitant strabismus*. **intermittent s.** Strabismus that is inconstantly present. Also *dynamic strabismus*. **internal s.** ESOTROPIA. **kinetic s.** Sudden and transient strabismus attributed to central nervous system irritation of the innervation of the extraocular muscles. **latent s.** PHORIA. **mechanical s.** Strabismus due to structural factors, as of muscles and ligaments. Also *muscular strabismus*. **monocular s.** Strabismus in which it is always the same eye that deviates. Also *unilateral strabismus, uniocular strabismus*. **muscular s.** MECHANICAL STRABISMUS. **noncomitant s.** INCOMITANT STRABISMUS. **relative s.** Strabismus changing in amount with respect to the position of the eyes. **seesaw s.** SKEW DEVIATION. **spasmodic s.** Strabismus caused by secondary contractures of the extraocular muscles. **suppressed s.** PHORIA. **s. sursum vergens** Strabismus marked by a turning upward of the deviating eye, the other eye being used for fixation. Compare STRABISMUS DEORSUM VERGENS. **unilateral s.** MONOCULAR STRABISMUS. **uniocular s.** MONOCULAR STRABISMUS. **V s.** Strabismus characterized by being more divergent (or less convergent) above, and more convergent (or less divergent) below. Compare A STRABISMUS.

**strabotomy** \strəbät′əmē\ [Gk *strabo(s)* squint-eyed + -TOMY] The cutting of a tendon of an extraocular muscle.

**Strachan** [William Henry Williams *Strachan*, English physician, 1857–1921] Strachan syndrome, Strachan's disease. See under STRACHAN-SCOTT SYNDROME.

**strain¹** [Middle French *estraindre* (from L *stringere* to draw tight or close, tie, from Gk *strangein* to draw or bind tight and *stranx*, gen. *strangos*, a drop squeezed out) to draw tight] **1** An overstretching of a muscle or ligament, or the injury resulting from it. **2** To subject to strain, as by overexercising; damage by overtaxing, as a muscle or muscle group. **high-jumpers' s.** A strain resulting from excessive use or injury to the rotator muscle groups of the thigh. **left ventricular s.** The electrocardiographic appearance, often associated with left ventricular hypertrophic changes, in which there is ST segment depression with T wave inversion in the electrocardiographic leads over the left ventricle. **right ventricular s.** The electrocardiographic appearance associated with right ventricular hypertrophy or right ventricular overload, in which there is ST segment depression and T wave inversion over the right chest leads. **vertebral cervical s.** POST-TRAUMATIC CERVICAL SYNDROME.

**strain²** [Old English *strēon* procreation, progeny] **1** A mating population, usually derived from one organism or pair of sexual partners, that is partially or completely maintained by artificial means because of certain favorable characteristics and that is used for experimentation, horticulture, or animal husbandry. **2** In microbiology, a clone of organisms that differs in one or more inheritable characteristics from other organisms assigned to the same species. **cell s.** A line of cells which may differ in some characteristics from other lines in the same microbial species, or from the same class of differentiated cells in tissue cultures. **congenic s.** In experimental genetics, a strain of organisms that is developed by inserting, through selective breeding, a small portion of the genome of one strain (the source) into a highly inbred strain (the background). The technique is used to study the effect of the background genome on the expression of a single locus. **$F^+$ s.** A strain of *Escherichia coli* carrying the F factor and hence capable of conjugation and chromosomal transfer. Also *male strain*. **$F^-$ s.** A strain of *Escherichia coli* lacking the F factor and hence serving as recipient in conjugation with an $F^+$ strain. Also *female strain*. **heterologous s.** A microbial strain different from the one originally tested. **Hfr s.** See under HFR. **inbred s.** A strain of experimental animals produced by successive brother-sister matings. The genetic identity is a reflection of the degree of inbreeding of the members of the strains. After the 20th or more generation, the animals are so inbred that grafts can be exchanged without rejection.

**isogenic s.** A mating population that is of uniform genotype, having been constructed artificially through intensive inbreeding. **male s.** F⁺ STRAIN. **neotype s.** A specimen selected as a standard for the description and characterization of a strain when the original type strain is no longer available. **prime s.** A strain of a virus that is poorly neutralized by antibody prepared to a previously characterized strain (prototype) but induces antibody in experimentally inoculated animals which neutralizes both the prime and prototype strains equally well. **prototrophic s.'s** Strains of microorganisms having nutritional requirements similar to those of the wild-type strains of the species as found in nature. **R s.** ROUGH STRAIN. **recombinant inbred s.** A strain of experimental eukaryotic organisms that is derived by systematic inbreeding of the offspring of two preexisting highly inbred strains. Each member of a recombinant inbred strain will have received one half of its autosomal loci from each of the progenitor strains. Such strains are powerful tools in segregation and linkage analysis. **rough s.** A bacterial strain that forms rough colonies, and usually is less virulent, because it lacks a surface component, such as a capsule or a lipopolysaccharide O antigen, present on smooth strains of the same species. Also *R strain*. **smooth s.** A bacterial strain that forms smooth colonies. Also *S strain*. **T-s.** See under *UREAPLASMA*. **type s.** A strain whose characteristics are used as a basis for identifying a group of closely related organisms. **wild-type s.** **1** The strain of a particular species that predominates in any natural population. The strain may be defined by its phenotype, but it is more appropriately defined by its genotype. **2** Any strain of microorganism that is isolated from natural sources and not cultivated or selected in the laboratory: originally used to distinguish an original isolated from the less virulent strains arising from it during transfer in laboratory media or in new animal hosts. **3** A parental strain from which mutants are deliberately isolated, such as auxotrophs from prototrophs or drug-resistant organisms from drug-sensitive ones. For defs. 1, 2, and 3 also *wild type*.

**strait** [L *strictus* (past part. of *stringere* to draw tight or close) drawn tight or close, narrow] A narrow passage. **inferior pelvic s.** APERTURA PELVIS INFERIOR. **superior pelvic s.** APERTURA PELVIS SUPERIOR.

**stramonium** \strəmō′nē·əm\ The dried leaves, flowers, and fruits of *Datura stramonium*, containing a parasympatholytic principle similar in action to belladonna. Stramonium is rich in the tropane alkaloids scopolamine, hyoscyamine, and atropine, and is used as an antispasmodic, mydriatic, and antisialagogue. Also *jimson weed, apple of Peru, thorn apple, devil's apple*.

**strand** A thread, fiber, or filamentous structure. **Billroth s.** TRABECULA OF SPLEEN. **lateral enamel s.** The lateral border of the dental lamina which often appears to be separated from the rest of the lamina in a histologic section of a developing tooth. Also *buccal lamina*. **plus s.** A strand of RNA of a bacteriophage that is used as a template for transcription and for the production of a complementary (minus) strand of RNA. The plus and minus strands form double-stranded RNA, which is the replicative form. Some viruses package the plus strand and others the minus strand in the virion.

**Strandberg** [James Victor *Strandberg*, Swedish physician, born 1883] Grönblad-Strandberg syndrome. See under PSEUDOXANTHOMA ELASTICUM.

**strangulated** \strang′gyəlā′tid\ Having circumferential constriction severe enough to cause circulatory embarrassment: used especially of hernias.

**strangulation** \strang′gyəlā′shən\ The obstruction or cessation of respiration by strangling.

**strangury** \strang′gyərē\ [Gk *strangouria* (from *stranx*, gen. *strang(os)*, that which oozes or is squeezed out + *ouron* urine) retention of the urine] Difficult micturation, characterized by slow, intermittent passage of urine with associated pain and tenesmus. Also *stranguria*.

**strapping** **1** The application of strips of adhesive plaster to cover, to position, to oppose, or to compress. **2** The adhesive plaster so applied.

**Strassman** [Paul F. *Strassman*, German gynecologist, 1866–1938] See under PHENOMENON.

**strata** \strā′tə, strat′ə\ Plural of STRATUM.

**stratification** \strat′ifikā′shən\ A procedure for handling confounding variables, such as age and sex, in the statistical analysis of the results of epidemiologic studies. The total data are broken down into groups or strata corresponding to these variables and the distribution within each stratum is separately analyzed before the results are combined and interpreted.

**stratified** \strat′ifīd\ Formed or arranged in superimposed layers or strata.

**stratiform** \strat′ifôrm\ Resembling the arrangement or composition of strata.

**stratigraphy** \stratig′rəfē\ [*strat(um)* + -GRAPHY] BODY SECTION ROENTGENOGRAPHY.

# stratum

**stratum** \strā′təm, strat′əm\ [L (substantive from *stratus*, past part. of *sternere* to stretch out, strew, spread; akin to Gk *storennynai* to strew, spread) a coverlet, bed, pavement] (*pl.* strata) [NA] A layer or sheet of cells or tissue, usually one of several differentiated superimposed layers. **s. adamantinum** ENAMEL. **strata alba colliculi cranialis** The white layers of the cranial (superior) colliculus. The cranial or superior colliculus of the mesencephalon is a laminated structure, and its several layers are formed principally by nerve fibers or by neuronal cell bodies. Those that are essentially fibrous in nature constitute the strata alba colliculi cranialis, and comprise the stratum zonale, the stratum opticum, and two laminae of the stratum lemnisci, the stratum album medium and stratum album profundum. Also *strata alba colliculi superioris*. **s. album profundum corporis quadrigemini** The deep myelinated fiber layer underlying the superior colliculus. Also *lamina medullaris transversa corporis quadrigemini, deep white stratum of quadrigeminal body*. **s. basale endometrii** [NA] The thin and deepest layer of the uterine endometrium, containing the blind ends of the tubelike uterine glands. It is involved very little in the cyclic changes and is not shed at either menstruation or parturition. Also *basal layer*. **cerebral s. of retina** STRATUM NERVOSUM RETINAE. **s. cinereum** STRATUM GRISEUM COLLICULI SUPERIORIS. **s. cinereum colliculi superioris** STRATUM GRISEUM COLLICULI SUPERIORIS. **s. circulare membranae tympani** [NA] The deeper of the two fibrous layers between stratum cutaneum and stratum mucosum in the pars tensa of the tympanic membrane. Its filaments are arranged concentrically and are best developed at the periphery. It is closely applied to the outer radiate fibrous layer. Also *circular layer of tympanic membrane, circular layer of eardrum*. **s. circulare tunicae muscularis coli** [NA] The thin inner layer of circular smooth muscle fibers of the muscular coat of the colon. It is thicker in the gaps between the sacculations or haustra. Also *circular stratum of muscular tunic of colon.* **s. circulare tunicae muscularis ductus deferentis** [NA] The internal layer of circular smooth muscle fibers that forms the intermediate layer at the commencement of the deferent duct, where there is an external and and internal longitudinal layer on either side of it. **s. circulare tunicae muscularis gastricae** [NA] A uniform layer of circular smooth muscle fibers deep to the outer longitudinal fibers of the muscular coat of the stomach. It is continuous with the circular muscle fibers of the esophagus, and at the pylorus it becomes markedly thickened to form the pyloric sphincter. The circular muscle fibers of the stomach are separated from those of the duodenum by connective tissue. Also *circular layer of muscular tunic of stomach, inner muscular layer of stomach.* **s. circulare tunicae muscularis intestini tenuis** [NA] The thick inner layer of circular smooth muscle fibers of the muscular coat of the small intestine, thicker in the more cranial part than in the caudal part of the intestine. Also *circular layer of muscular tunic of small intestine.* **s. circulare tunicae muscularis recti** [NA] The thick inner layer of circular smooth muscle fibers of the muscular coat of the rectum. Also *circular layer of muscular tunic of rectum.* **s. circulare tunicae muscularis tubae uterinae** [NA] The internal layer of circular smooth muscle fibers of the muscular coat of the uterine tube. It is thickest at the isthmus narrowing the lumen of the tube. **s. circulare tunicae muscularis ureteris** [NA] The outer circular layer of smooth muscle fibers of the muscular coat of the ureter, but in the lower third of the ureter a third additional outer layer of longitudinal muscle fibers is found covering the circular layer while the inner longitudinal layer becomes indistinct. **s. circulare tunicae muscularis vesicae urinariae** [NA] The middle layer of circular smooth muscle fibers located between the external and the internal layers of longitudinal fibers in the muscular coat of the urinary bladder. The fibers are thinly and unevenly scattered but at the neck of the bladder they are arranged in a circular fashion to form the sphincter vesicae around the internal urethral orifice. **s. compactum endometrii** [NA] The relatively narrow superficial zone of the endometrium containing the necks of the uterine glands and becoming particularly obvious during the progestational or secretory phase of the menstrual cycle and pregnancy when it is separated by a grossly edematous lamina propria from the underlying spongy layer. It may be partly shed during menstruation or at parturition. Also *compact layer, compacta.* **connective tissue s. of mesentery** The layer of connective tissue between the two peritoneal layers of the mesentery. **s. corneum epidermidis** [NA] The outer keratinized layer of the epidermis, composed of many sheets of compressed opaque squames or scalelike remnants of cells the contents of which have been entirely replaced by keratin and tonofibril remains. The cells in the more superficial sheets loosen and break away. Also *horny layer of epidermis.* **s. corneum unguis** [NA] The nail proper, composed of a plate of hard, fused keratinized squames or cornified cells and analogous to stratum corneum epidermidis but more comparable in composition to stratum lucidum epidermidis. Also *horny layer of nail, nail plate.* **cortical s. zonale** STRATUM MOLECULARE. **s. cutaneum membranae tympani** [NA] The hairless outer layer of the tympanic membrane, being a modified thin layer of skin lining the external acoustic meatus and composed of stratified epithelium and a number of small blood vessels. Also *cutaneous layer of tympanic membrane, dermic layer.* **deep white s. of quadrigeminal body** STRATUM ALBUM PROFUNDUM CORPORIS QUADRIGEMINI. **s. fibrosum periostei** [NA] The outer layer of the periosteum composed of dense fibrous connective tissue and a network of blood vessels. **s. functionale endometrii** [NA] The combined compact and spongy layers of the uterine endometrium, which may be partly or wholly shed during menstruation and at parturition. These layers only become obvious during the progestational or secretory phase of the cycles. Also *functional layer of endometrium.* **s. ganglionare retinae** The ganglionic cell lamina of the retina in which the cells are multipolar and form the second neurons in the visual pathway. Their axons converge on the optic disk. Also *stratum ganglionare nervi optici, ganglionic layer of retina, ganglionic stratum of retina, ganglionic stratum of optic nerve.* **s. gangliosum cerebelli** The thin layer of large neurons (Purkinje cells) within the border of the thick granular layer of the cerebellar cortex. Also *stratum Purkinje, Purkinje layer, ganglionic layer of cerebellum.* **s. germinativum unguis** [NA] The layer of living cells on the surface of the nail bed deep to stratum corneum unguis and composed of the stratum spinosum and stratum basale. Functionally the layer deep to the root and the lunula of the nail differs from the rest of the nail bed distally in that it is thicker and actively proliferative while the distal part is not involved in nail growth, merely providing a base over which the growing nail moves. Also *germinative layer of nail.* **s. granulosum cerebelli** [NA] The thick layer of small granule cells, the principal neuronal constituents of the cerebellar cortex. Also *granular layer of cerebellum.* **s. granulosum folliculi ovarici secundarii** [NA] The layer of cells that lines the outside of the antrum folliculi and the inside of the tunica interna of the theca folliculi from which it is separated by a basement membrane in the secondary or vesicular ovarian follicle. Also *granular layer of follicle of ovary.* **strata grisea colliculi cranialis** The gray layers of the cranial (superior) colliculus. The cranial or superior colliculus of the mesencephalon is a laminated structure, and its layers are formed principally by neuronal cell bodies or by nerve fibers. Those that consist essentially of neuronal cell bodies constitute the strata grisea colliculi cranialis, comprising the stratum cinereum (or superficial gray layer), and two laminae of the stratum lemnisci, the stratum griseum medium (or intermedium) and the stratum griseum profundum. Also *strata grisea colliculi superioris.* **s. griseum centrale cerebri** SUBSTANTIA GRISEA CENTRALIS CEREBRI. **s. griseum colliculi superioris** The thick, most superficial neuronal layer of the superior colliculus, consisting of visual system neurons. Also *gray layer of superior colliculus, stratum cinereum, stratum cinereum colliculi superioris, superficial gray layer.* **s. intermedium** A thin layer of cells between the inner enamel epithelium and the stellate reticulum of a developing tooth. **s. interolivare lemnisci** The myelinated fiber tract formed by the medial condensation of arcuate fibers between the inferior olives. It arises from the cuneate and gracile nuclei, and becomes the medial lemniscus. Also *stratum lemnisci.* **s. lacunosum** The most superficial neuronal layer of the hippocampus. **s. lemnisci** STRATUM INTEROLIVARE LEMNISCI. **s. limitans externum** EXTERNAL LIMITING MEMBRANE. **s. limitans internum** INTERNAL LIMITING MEMBRANE. **s. longitudinale externum tunicae muscularis ductus deferentis** [NA] The outer layer of longitudinal smooth muscle fibers of the thick muscular coat of the deferent duct. **s. longitudinale externum tunicae muscularis ureteris** [NA] The outer layer of longitudinal smooth muscle fibers added to the outside of the circular layer of the muscular coat in the lower third of the ureter and becoming particularly prominent as the ureter passes through the wall of the bladder, where their contraction keeps the ureter's lumen open. **s. longitudinale externum tunicae muscularis vesicae urinariae** [NA] The external longitudinal smooth muscle fibers of the muscular coat of the urinary bladder which pass down over its base to blend with the capsule of the prostate or the anterior wall of the vagina. Some fibers pass anterior to the rectum as the rectovesical muscle while others enter the medial puboprostatic ligaments to form the pubovesical muscles. **s. longitudinale internum tunicae muscularis ductus deferentis** [NA] The internal layer of longitudinal smooth muscle fibers on the inner aspect of the circular fibers of the muscular tunic of the deferent duct. **s. longitudinale internum tunicae muscularis ureteris** [NA] The inner layer of longitudinal smooth muscle fibers of the muscular coat in the renal pelvis and upper two-thirds of the ureter. Proximally it extends to the junction of the minor calices and the renal papillae, while in the distal third of the ureter it becomes less distinct as a third outer layer of longitudinal fibers is added. **s. longitudinale internum tunicae muscularis vesicae urinariae** [NA] The thin internal layer of longitudinal smooth muscle fibers of the three-layer muscular coat of the urinary bladder. **s. longitudinale tunicae muscularis coli** [NA] The layer of longitudinal smooth muscle fibers that forms a continuous sheet on the outer aspect of the colon but thickens anteriorly, posteromedially, and posterolaterally to form the taeniae coli, which are absent on the sigmoid colon. On the latter the longitudinal fibers are somewhat scattered over the surface. Also *longitudinal layer of muscular tunic of colon.* **s. longitudinale tunicae muscularis gastricae** [NA] The outer layer of longitudinal smooth muscle fibers of the muscular coat of the stomach. The fibers are arranged in two series, the one continuous with longitudinal fibers of the esophagus and located most markedly along the greater and lesser curvatures, while the second extends to the right from the body of the stomach, being thickest near the pylorus and the deeper fibers participating in the pyloric sphincter. Also *longitudinal layer of muscular tunic of stomach.* **s. longitudinale tunicae muscularis intestini tenuis** [NA] The thin outer layer of longitudinal smooth muscle fibers of the muscular coat of the small intestine. Also *longitudinal layer of muscular tunic of small intestine.* **s. longitudinale tunicae muscularis recti** [NA] The outer layer of longitudinal smooth muscle fibers of the muscular coat of the rectum. It is continuous with the same layer of the sigmoid colon, but the fibers form two broad bands, one on the anterior surface and the other on the posterior surface of the rectum. At the rectal ampulla a few fasciculi of the anterior group extend anteriorly to the perineal body as the rectourethralis muscle. Also *longitudinal layer of muscular tunic of rectum.* **s. longitudinale tunicae muscularis tubae uterinae** [NA] The outer layer of longitudinal smooth muscle fibers of the muscular coat of the uterine tube. In some parts of the tube there is an additional layer of longitudinal fibers internally. **s. lucidum epidermidis** [NA] A homogeneous layer of closely packed cells containing flattened atrophied nuclei and eleidin, located superficial to the stratum granulosum epidermidis and deep to stratum corneum. Also *clear layer of skin, Oehl's layer.* **s. lucidum hippocampi** The pyramidal cell soma layer of the hippocampus. **s. moleculare** The superficial layer of the cerebral and cerebellar cortices, consisting principally of dendrites, axons, glia, and very few neurons. Also *molecular layer, marginal layer, plexiform layer, zonal lamina, layer I, cortical stratum zonale, peripheral layer.* **s. moleculare cerebelli** [NA] The most superficial layer of the cerebellar cortex, containing numerous axodendritic synapses, glia, and a few stellate neurons. It extends down to include the Purkinje cells. Also *molecular layer of cerebellum, zonal layer of cerebellum, lamina zonalis of cerebellum, molecular layer of cerebellar cortex.* • It is called the molecular layer with reference to the small, nonneuronal nuclei of glial cells and vascular elements. **s. moleculare hippocampi** A fibrous and the most superficial layer of the hippocampal cortex. **s. mucosum membranae tympani** [NA] The inner of the three layers of the tympanic membrane, being part of the mucous membrane lining the tympanic cavity and thickest at the superior part of the membrane. Also *mucous layer of tympanic membrane.* **s. nervosum retinae** A multilayered stratum of the pars optica retinae the inner surface of which is in contact with the vitreous body and bears the macula and optic disk. Also *cerebral stratum of retina, nervous layer.* **s. neuroepitheliale retinae** [NA] The layer of the stratum nervosum retinae which contains the rods and cones serving as the photosensitive receptors of light stimuli. Also *neuroepithelial layer of retina, columnar layer, layer of rods and cones, Jacob's membrane.* **s. nucleare externum** [NA] One of the ten layers (usually classified as the fourth) that are distinguished in the retina of the eye. It is situated between the external, or outer, limiting layer, or membrane, and the outer plexiform layer. It contains the tightly packed nuclei and bodies of the photoreceptor cells (rods and cones) and the narrow outer fibers of their processes. Also *outer nuclear layer.* **s. nucleare internum** [NA] One of the ten layers (usually classified as the sixth) that are distinguished in the retina of the eye. It is situated between the outer and the inner plexiform layers. It contains rows of cell bodies and nuclei, namely, from without in, those of the horizontal cells, bipolar cells, and the retinal gliocytes (Müller cells). In addition, most internally are the somata of the amacrine neurons, the neurites of which pass into the adjacent inner plexiform layer. Each of the horizontal, bipolar, and amacrine neurons comprise several types of cells which are recognized more by their patterns of connections than by their cytologic appearances. Also *inner nuclear layer.* **s. nucleare medullae oblongatae** The gray matter of the medulla oblongata constituting the sensory and motor cranial nerve nuclei. **s. opticum** **1** The innermost layer of the retina, formed by fibers of the optic nerve. **2** The optic layer of the superior colliculus, lying beneath the superficial gray layer (stratum cinereum) and containing fibers of the optic tract and nerve cells. **s. oriens** A sublayer of the cornu ammonis, containing axons and collateral branches of fibers entering and exiting the hippocampus. **s. osteogeneticum** [NA] The deep, or inner, layer of periosteum, adjacent to the bone and composed of osteoblasts and loose collagenous bundles, some of which enter bone as Sharpey's fibers in the adult. During growth and development this layer develops penetrating buds of osteogenetic tissue, containing osteocytes and osteoblasts, whereby secondary deposits of bone are laid down as osteons. Also *Ollier's layer, osteogenetic layer, cambium layer, osteoblastic layer.* **s. papillare corii** [NA] The superficial of the two layers of the dermis, comprising numerous vertically projecting and irregular papillae the apices of which fit into corresponding concavities on the deep surface of the epidermis. Also *papillary layer of corium, papillary zone.* **s. pigmenti corporis ciliaris** *Outmoded* EPITHELIUM PIGMENTOSUM PARTIS CILIARIS RETINAE. **s. pigmenti**

**iridis** *Outmoded* EPITHELIUM POSTERIUS PIGMENTOSUM PARTIS IRIDICAE RETINAE. **s. pigmentosum partis opticae retinae** [NA] A single layer of pigmented cells extending from the periphery of the optic disk to the ora serrata, where they become continuous with the ciliary epithelium. Also *pigmented layer of retina, pigmented layer of optic part of retina.* **s. plexiforme** Either stratum plexiforme externum or stratum plexiforme internum. **s. plexiforme externum** [NA] The layer of the retina in which the axons of the rod and cone cells form an intricate pattern of synapses with the dendrites and axons of the bipolar and horizontal neurons of the internal nuclear layer. Also *outer plexiform layer of the retina, external plexiform lamina.* **s. plexiforme internum** [NA] A layer of the retina between the internal nuclear layer and the lamina of ganglion cells and consisting of the branched axonal endings of the bipolar cells on the interconnecting dendrites and on the cell bodies of the ganglion cells of the innermost cellular layers of the retina, and on the processes of horizontal and amacrine cells of the ganglionic cell layer. Also *inner plexiform layer of the retina, internal plexiform lamina.* **s. Purkinje** STRATUM GANGLIOSUM CEREBELLI. **s. pyramidale** Either of the two layers of cerebral cortex containing pyramidal neurons, the external pyramidal layer (layer III) or the internal pyramidal layer (layer V). **s. pyramidalis** A sublayer of the cornu ammonis containing large and small pyramidal cells and located beneath the stratum oriens. **s. radiatum** [NA] A sublayer of the cornu ammonis located beneath the stratum pyramidalis and composed of apical dendrites of neurons in the stratum pyramidalis, along with associated axons. **s. radiatum membranae tympani** [NA] The superficial layer of fibers radiating outward from the handle of the malleus in the fibrous layer between the stratum cutaneum and the stratum mucosum membranae tympani. It is closely applied to the deeper circular fibers of the fibrous layer. Also *radiate layer of tympanic membrane.* **s. reticulare corii** [NA] The deeper of the two layers of the dermis comprising interlacing dense bands of connective tissue fibers, both collagenous and elastic, the spaces between them being filled by fat and sweat glands. It is superficial to the subcutaneous areolar tissue. Also *reticular layer of corium, proper coat of corium.* **s. spinosum epidermidis** [NA] A thin layer composed of several sheets of living polyhedral prickle cells situated superficial to stratum basale epidermidis and deep to stratum granulosum epidermidis. The prickle cells are joined to each other by spindle-shaped desmosomes attached to cytoplasmic tonofibrils. Contrary to previous concepts, these filamentous fibrils do not pass through intercellular bridges into adjacent cells. Also *spinous layer of epidermis, prickle-cell layer.* **s. spongiosum endometrii** [NA] The subepithelial or middle layer of the uterine endometrium, lying deep to the compact layer and composed of very cellular connective tissue that contains blood vessels, lymphatic spaces and the tortuous parts of the uterine glands. These layers become obvious during the progestational phase of the menstrual cycle and pregnancy. Also *spongy layer.* **s. spongiosum urethrae of the female urethra** A thin layer of spongy erectile tissue containing a venous plexus, bundles of smooth muscle fibers, and elastic fibers and situated deep to the mucous membrane of the female urethra. **s. subendotheliale endocardii** [NA] A thin layer of collagenous and some elastic fibers situated immediately deep to the endothelium of the heart. It is also present in the wall of arteries. Also *subendothelial coat.* **s. submucosum** [NA] The thin inner layer of the myometrium, firmly adherent to the overlying endometrium of the uterus and composed mostly of longitudinal muscle fibers and also some circular and oblique fibers. Also *submucous stratum.* **s. subserosum** [NA] The thin outermost layer of the myometrium, underlying the serous coat of the uterus and comprising longitudinal muscle fibers. **s. supravasculosum** [NA] The layer of the myometrium situated between the stratum vasculosum and the stratum subserosum and comprising circular and longitudinal muscle fibers. **s. vasculosum** [NA] The thick middle layer of the myometrium, the fibers of which run longitudinally, transversely and obliquely. It contains many blood vessels, mostly veins. **s. vasculosum iridis** [NA] The thick vascular layer of the stroma iridis of the eye. It lies deep to the thin, nonvascular stromal layer situated immediately beneath the mesenchymal epithelium on the anterior surface of the iris. It contains numerous spiraling, thick-walled branches of the circulus arteriosus iridis major, loose collagenous tissue, networks of nerve fibers, and scattered chromatophores. Also *vessel layer of the iris.* **s. zonale corporis quadrigemini** A layer of nerve fibers from the lateral lemniscus overlying the inferior colliculi, and nerve fibers derived from the occipital cortex overlying the superior colliculi. Also *zonal layer of quadrigeminal body.* **s. zonale thalami** A layer of myelinated axons covering the superior surface of the thalamus. Also *zonal layer of thalamus.*

**Strauss** [Hermann *Strauss,* German physician, 1868–1944] **1** See under SIGN. **2** Strauss sign. See under BLUMER SHELF.

**streak** [Old English *strica* a line, streak, akin to L *stria* a furrow, groove] A line, stripe, or furrow; stria. **angioid s.** An ophthalmoscopically visible linear break in the lamina vitrea that resembles an underlying choroidal blood vessel. It is associated with degenerative diseases of elastic tissue, such as pseudoxanthoma elasticum. Also *Knapp streak* (ambiguous), *Knapp stria* (ambiguous). **germinal s.** PRIMITIVE STREAK. **Knapp s.** ANGIOID STREAK. • The original description attributed the appearance to retinal hemorrhage, but Knapp streaks are probably the same as angioid streaks. **primitive s.** A thickened linear opacity which develops in front of the posterior edge of the embryonic germinative area in birds and mammals, the appearance of which marks the start of differentiation of the embryonic germ layers. The first manifestation of morphogenesis, it represents a transitory condensation following a furrow of the embryogenic area. It results from the migration towards this region of the cells included in the primary ectoderm, which then get inserted between this layer and the primary endoderm. Also *primitive groove, germinal streak.*

**streaking** Inoculation of bacteria on an agar plate by a loop, usually in a manner that yields isolated colonies in some region.

**stream** [Old English *strēam,* akin to Gk *rheuma* a flow] A current or continuous flow. **axial s.** The stream of rapid flow in the center of a channel such as a blood vessel. **blood s.** BLOODSTREAM. **s. of consciousness** The sequence or flow of ideas and images in the mind, which is continuous rather than made up of easily separable states. The flow of thought is conceived of as ever moving and changing, from moment to moment, yet possessed of an evident continuity as is true of a stream of flowing water. • The term, originally used by William James, is now mainly of historical interest in medicine, and is used more often in literary than medical contexts **hair s.'s** FLUMINA PILORUM.

**streaming** / **cytoplasmic s.** PROTOPLASMIC STREAMING. **protoplasmic s.** The moving or streaming of protoplasm, as the protoplasmic mass of a slime mold, the movement of cytoplasm in an ameba, or the movement of cytoplasm below the cell wall of certain algae and plant cells.

**Streiff** [Enrico Bernard *Streiff*, Italian-born Swiss ophthalmologist, born 1908] Hallermann-Streiff-François syndrome. See under HALLERMANN-STREIFF SYNDROME.

**strength** **1** The capacity to respond to force without serious structural or functional impairment. **2** Potency or degree of concentration, as of a drug or solution. **biting s.** MASTICATORY FORCE. **dioptric s.** DIOPTRIC POWER. **ego s.** The effectiveness with which the ego maintains its functions even in the face of wide variations in the drive energy with which it is supplied. **ionic s.** A measure of the electrostatic interactions between the ions of an electrolyte solution. It is equal to the sum of the valence of each ion squared divided by two. A number of biochemically important events, e.g., protein solubility, and enzymatically catalyzed reaction rates vary depending on the ionic strength of the solution.

**strephenopodia** \stref′ənōpō′dē·ə\ TALIPES VARUS.

**strephexopodia** \stref′eksəpō′dē·ə\ TALIPES VALGUS.

**strephopodia** \stref′əpō′dē·ə\ TALIPES EQUINUS.

**strephosymbolia** \stref′əsimbō′lyə\ [Gk *streph(ein)* to turn, twist + English *symbol* + -IA] **1** Visual agnosia in which objects perceived are reversed as if seen in a mirror. **2** MIRROR WRITING.

**strepitus** \strep′itəs\ [L, a noise, rustling] A noise, especially on auscultation.

**strepsitene** \strep′sitēn\ *Obs.* PACHYTENE.

**strepticemia** \strep′tisē′mē·ə\ [*strept(o)-* + -IC + -EMIA] STREPTOCOCCEMIA.

**streptidine** A substance related to inositol, from which it is synthesized in some living organisms by replacement of two of the hydroxyl groups by guanidino groups. It occurs glycosylated in the streptomycin molecule.

**strepto-** \strep′tə-\ [Gk *streptos* (from *strephein* to twist, turn) easily bent or twisted, pliant] A combining form meaning (1) twisted, coiled, or forming flexible, chainlike configurations; (2) *Streptococcus*; (3) *Streptomyces*.

***Streptobacillus moniliformis*** \-basil′əs mänil′ifôr′-mis\ A facultative, Gram-negative, nonmotile bacillus that tends to form filaments with yeastlike swellings. In crowded cultures on solid media, the bacilli tend to form defective walls. L-forms were discovered with this organism. A normal inhabitant of the mouth of rodents, it is one cause of rat-bite fever. It can also infect humans through abrasions or ingestion. Also *Haverhillia multiformis, Actinomyces muris* (obs.).

**streptocerciasis** \-sərkī′əsis, -sərsī′əsis\ Infection with the filarial nematode *Mansonella streptocerca* (previously designated *Dipetalonema streptocerca*). Distributed throughout west and central Africa, it is transmitted by the biting midge *Culicoides grahami*, and is probably a zoonosis. Skin changes resemble those of onchocerciasis, and a chronic itching dermatitis results. Treatment is with diethylcarbamazine.

**streptococcal** \-käk′əl\ Of, pertaining to, or caused by any streptococcus.

**streptococcemia** \-käksē′mē·ə\ [*streptococc(us)* + -EMIA] The presence of streptococci in the bloodstream. Also *strepticemia*.

**streptococci** \-käk′sī\ Plural of STREPTOCOCCUS.

**streptococcosis** \-käkō′sis\ [*streptococc(us)* + -OSIS] Infection with streptococci.

***Streptococcus*** \-käk′əs\ [STREPTO- + COCCUS] A genus of Gram-positive, mostly facultative, catalase-negative cocci, usually growing in pairs or chains held together by incomplete wall separation. They form D-lactic acid homofermentatively. Various species are important in milk fermentation, such as *S. lactis* or *S. cremoris*, and in many diseases. The pathogens are classified according to the type of hemolysis on blood agar ($\alpha$, $\beta$, or $\gamma$) and they are further divided into groups A to O on the basis of a carbohydrate antigen (Lancefield classification). ***S. faecalis*** A nonhemolytic, group D streptococcus, frequently found in the human intestine and oropharynx; enterococcus. It is relatively resistant to heat, high salt concentration, azide, and many antimicrobial drugs. It is an important cause of endocarditis. ***S. hemolyticus*** The $\beta$-hemolytic group of *S. pyogenes*. *Obs.* ***S. mitis*** A species of $\alpha$-hemolytic streptococci sometimes associated with bacterial endocarditis. ***S. mutans*** A nonhemolytic streptococcus that forms polysaccharides from sucrose. These are slimy and promote adhesion of dental plaque to the tooth surface. The organism also produces organic acids that are involved in the initiation of the carious process. It may also be a a cause of endocarditis. ***S. pneumoniae*** A species that is a major cause of pneumonia and of various other pyogenic infections; the pneumococcus. It is often present as a commensal in the upper respiratory tract. Its classification among the streptococci is recent. It does not belong to a Lancefield group and it tends to appear in culture as lancet-shaped diplococci rather than as chains. Growth requirements are fastidious and autolysis occurs easily, stimulated by bile or deoxycholate. Colonies on blood agar are $\alpha$-hemolytic. Virulence depends on an antiphagocytic polysaccharide capsule. Over 80 types are known. Type transformation, from R to S, was the basis for the discovery that DNA is the genetic material. Also *Diplococcus pneumoniae* (outmoded). ***S. pyogenes*** A species of group A streptococci causing a variety of human pyogenic infections and also acute glomerulonephritis and rheumatic fever. Many of the strains produce a large capsule of hyaluronic acid. Their colonies are mucoid and become matt (flat and rough) when the capsule dries out. Variants without a capsule are glossy. More than 55 immunologic types are distinguished, differing in their M protein. Also *Fehleisen streptococcus*. ***S. salivarius*** One of the commonest of the $\alpha$-hemolytic streptococci. ***S. sanguis*** A nonhemolytic streptococcus very similar to *S. mutans* and likewise adherent to teeth. ***S. viridans*** The $\alpha$-hemolytic (viridans) group of streptococci. A vague term which no longer designates a particular species.

**streptococcus** \-käk′əs\ (*pl.* streptococci) Any microorganism of the genus *Streptococcus*. **$\alpha$ s.** $\alpha$-HEMOLYTIC STREPTOCOCCUS. **anaerobic streptococci** A group of streptococci that are anaerobic, usually nonhemolytic, and smaller than the other streptococci. They are normal inhabitants of the female genital tract. Of low virulence, they produce a fetid odor in abscesses. **$\beta$ s.** $\beta$-HEMOLYTIC STREPTOCOCCUS. **Fehleisen s.** *STREPTOCOCCUS PYOGENES*. **$\gamma$ s.** Any of various streptococci that produce no hemolysis on blood agar. They are of low pathogenicity, except for those associated with bacterial endocarditis, such as *Streptococcus faecalis*. **green s.** $\alpha$-HEMOLYTIC STREPTOCOCCUS. **group A streptococci** The major group of pathogenic $\beta$-hemolytic streptococci. The characteristic group A carbohydrate is composed of rhamnose with terminal *N*-acetyl glucosamine. **hemolytic s.** $\beta$-HEMOLYTIC STREPTOCOCCUS. **$\alpha$-hemolytic s.** Any streptococcus whose colonies on blood agar are surrounded by an inner zone of partial hemolysis and a narrow outer zone of complete hemolysis. The colonies often are surrounded by a greenish zone, due to an unknown conversion of hemoglobin. This group has not been well classified. There are numerous immunologic types, mostly outside the Lancefield classification. They are regular commensals of the mouth and throat.

They are of low pathogenicity except when they attach to a damaged endocardial surface, causing subacute bacterial endocarditis. *Streptococcus salivarius* is the most common species. Also *α streptococcus, green streptococcus, viridans streptococcus.* **β-hemolytic s.** Any of the streptococci, mostly of group A, whose colonies on blood agar are surrounded by a wide, clear zone of hemolysis. Streptolysin O (oxygen-labile) and streptolysin S (oxygen-stable) are both responsible. *Streptococcus pyogenes* is the commonest β-hemolytic pathogen. Also *β streptococcus, hemolytic streptococcus.* **s. MG** A strain of nonhemolytic streptococci that cross-reacts with antibodies formed by a large percentage of patients with mycoplasmal pneumonia. **viridans s.** α-HEMOLYTIC STREPTOCOCCUS.

**streptodermatitis** \-dur′mətī′tis\ Dermatitis caused by streptococci.

**streptodornase** \-dôr′nās\ Deoxyribonuclease from streptococci, used along with streptokinase to liquefy thick, purulent exudates (enzymatic débridement).

**streptogenin** Any of a number of peptides, obtained by partial hydrolysis of various proteins, that stimulate the growth of certain microbes, including *Lactobacillus casei. Seldom used.* Also *chick growth factor S, chick growth factor.*

**streptokinase** \-kī′nās\ An enzyme released by streptococci that converts plasminogen to plasmin, which lyses blood clots. The reaction may promote spread of the organisms, and the purified enzyme has been used to dissolve clots in coronary arteries. • The name has been abandoned by some scientists because it wrongly suggests that the enzyme is a kinase.

**streptokinase-streptodornase** A mixture of enzymes from streptococci used as a proteolytic and fibrinolytic agent in removing clotted blood and purulent accumulations due to trauma or inflammation.

**streptoleukocidin** \-loo′kəsī′din\ The leukocidin elaborated by some species of streptococci. It is an exotoxin which causes degranulation and death of leukocytes.

**streptolydigin** \-lī′dəjin\ An antibiotic that inhibits bacterial RNA polymerase at the stage of chain elongation, in contrast to inhibition of initiation by the rifamycins.

**streptolysin** \streptäl′isin\ [STREPTO- + LYSIN] A hemolysin excreted by various streptococci. **s. O** An antigenically active hemolysin produced by group A streptococci. It produces hemolysis only in the reduced state, hence is inactivated in the presence of oxygen. It has some direct cardiotoxic effect experimentally but there is little evidence of its direct role in human disease. It is clinically significant in that it induces antibodies which have diagnostic importance in detecting a previous streptococcal infection. See also ANTISTREPTOLYSIN O TEST. **s. S** An oxygen-stable, nonimmunogenic hemolysin of *Streptococcus pyogenes.* It is largely cell-bound, and extractable by serum albumin.

***Streptomyces*** \-mī′sēz\ A genus of actinomycetes of the Streptomycetaceae family, comprising more than 400 species. They grow with aerial mycelia that form species-characteristic spores. They are the source of about 90% of useful antibiotics. They are major agents in the breakdown of organic matter in the soil. They occasionally cause subcutaneous mycetomas much like those due to other actinomycetes.

**streptomycete** \-mī′sēt\ Any organism of the genus *Streptomyces.*

**streptomycin** \-mī′sin\ $C_{21}H_{39}N_7O_{12}$. A naturally occurring antibiotic produced by the actinomycete *Streptomyces griseus.* It is generally used as the sulfate for tuberculosis and a number of other infectious diseases such as plague, tularemia, and brucellosis.

**streptomycin sulfate** $(C_{21}H_{39}N_7O_{12})_2 \cdot 3H_2SO_4$. The sulfate salt of streptomycin, given intramuscularly for the same indications as streptomycin.

**streptomycosis** \-mīkō′sis\ [*Streptomyc(es)* + -OSIS] An infection caused by pathogenic actinomycetes, especially of the genus *Streptomyces.*

**streptonigrin** $C_{25}H_{22}N_4O_8$. An antibiotic isolated from *Streptomyces flocculus.* It has antineoplastic activity, but causes severe, prolonged bone marrow depression. Also *rufochromomycin.*

**streptonivicin** \-nivī′sin\ NOVOBIOCIN.

**streptose** 5-Deoxy-4-*C*-formylpentofuranose. A sugar derivative which occurs in the streptomycin molecule, in which it glycosylates streptidine and is glycosylated by *N*-methyl-L-glucosamine on C-3.

**streptotrichosis** \-trikō′sis\ Infection with organisms belonging to the former genus *Streptothrix. Outmoded.* Also *streptothricosis.* See also ACTINOMYCOSIS, NOCARDIOSIS, STREPTOMYCOSIS.

**stress** [Middle English *stresse,* short for *distresse* (from L *districtus,* past part. of *distringere* to draw asunder, stretch here and there) distress] **1** A physical, chemical, or psychological factor or combination of factors that poses a threat to the homeostasis or well-being of an organism, and that produces a defensive response, as, for example, physical or emotional trauma or infection. **2** In dentistry, the force exerted in mastication by the upper teeth upon the lower. **g s.** Stress on the human body due to rapid large changes in speed and/or direction. It is experienced by the crews of aircraft or spacecraft. **occlusal s.** Pressures on the teeth produced directly or indirectly by teeth of the opposing jaw. **post-traumatic s.** See under POST-TRAUMATIC STRESS DISORDER.

**stress-breaker** In a dental prosthesis, a device allowing partial movement of the free-end saddle relative to the clasp so that the clasped tooth is not loosened by leverage.

**stress-strain** Describing the elements of viscoelasticity of a material.

**stretcher** A conveyance for carrying the sick or injured. The traditional stretcher consisted of two wooden poles acting as a frame for a canvas bed. Now they are made in many different designs and of varied materials.

**stretching / pulse s.** Increase in pulse duration due, for example, to inadequate high-frequency response.

**stria** \strī′ə\ [L, a furrow, groove] (*pl.* striae) A narrow line, thin band, or furrow; streak. Also *stripe.* **acoustic striae** STRIAE MEDULLARES VENTRICULI QUARTI. **striae albicantes gravidarum** STRIAE GRAVIDARUM. **striae arcuatae olivarum** Those internal arcuate fibers of the medulla oblongata which originate in the inferior olive, decussate, and project via the corpus restiforme to the cerebellum. **striae atrophicae** Irregularly linear atrophic streaks, common on the thighs and buttocks at puberty and on the abdominal wall in pregnancy. They can also occur when genetically susceptible skin is subjected to raised cortisol levels, whether endogenous or exogenous. At first the striae are red or purple, but they later become white. Also *striate atrophy of the skin, traction atrophy, lineae atrophicae.* **auditory striae** STRIAE MEDULLARES VENTRICULI QUARTI. **striae of Baillarger** BAILLARGER'S LINES. **brown striae** STRIAE OF RETZIUS. **striae ciliares** Radial pigmentation of the pars plana extending posteriorly from the valleys between the ciliary processes. **s. fornicis** STRIA MEDULLARIS THALAMI. **s. of Gennari** GENNARI'S BAND. **striae gravidarum** Striae atrophicae of the abdominal wall in pregnancy. Also *striae albicantes gravidarum.* **habenular s.** STRIA MEDULLARIS THALAMI. **striae of Held** STRIAE MEDULLARES

VENTRICULI QUARTI. **s. intermedia trigoni olfactorii** A small bundle of olfactory tract fibers, visible in some brains, passing from the central part of the olfactory trigone to the anterior perforated substance. Also *intermediate stria of olfactory trigone, intermediate root of olfactory trigone.* **s. kaesbekhterevi** BEKHTEREV'S LAYER. **Knapp s.** ANGIOID STREAK. • The original description attributed the appearance to retinal hemorrhage, but Knapp striae are probably the same as angioid streaks. **s. lancisii** STRIA LONGITUDINALIS MEDIALIS CORPORIS CALLOSI. **Langhans s.** A layer of canalized fibrin on the surface of the chorionic place in the intervillous space of the human placenta. A homogenous zone has been considered as fibrinoid derived from fetal cells, whereas canalized fibrin is probably derived from maternal blood protein. **s. lateralis trigoni olfactorii** The olfactory tract arising from the olfactory bulb and dividing into a trigone of three bands, the lateral of which terminates principally in the periamygdaloid and prepyriform cortex. Also *lateral olfactory tract, lateral olfactory stria.* **lateral longitudinal s. of corpus callosum** STRIA LONGITUDINALIS LATERALIS CORPORIS CALLOSI. **lateral olfactory s.** STRIA LATERALIS TRIGONI OLFACTORII. **s. longitudinalis lateralis corporis callosi** [NA] A strand of longitudinally oriented nerve fibers coursing within the indusium griseum along the dorsal surface of and near each lateral border of the corpus callosum, beneath the cingulate gyrus. Also *lateral longitudinal stria of corpus callosum, stria tecta, taenia tectae.* **s. longitudinalis medialis corporis callosi** [NA] A band of longitudinally oriented nerve fibers found on each side of the median plane coursing along the dorsal surface of the corpus callosum within the overlying thin gray layer, the indusium griseum. Also *medial longitudinal stria of corpus callosum, stria lancisii.* **s. mallearis membranae tympani** [NA] A whitish streak extending upwards from the attached tip of the handle of the malleus in the center of the tympanic membrane and produced by the attached manubrium shining through the membrane. Also *mallear stria of tympanic membrane, stria malleolaris membranae tympani* (outmoded). **s. medialis trigoni olfactorii** A bundle of olfactory tract fibers that emerges from the medial part of the olfactory trigone, extends toward the medial surface of the cerebral hemisphere, and becomes continuous with the subcallosal (or parolfactory) region. Also *internal olfactory root.* **medial longitudinal s. of corpus callosum** STRIA LONGITUDINALIS MEDIALIS CORPORIS CALLOSI. **medial olfactory s.** The medial division of the striae olfactoriae, including components to the opposite olfactory bulb and the hypothalamus. **striae medullares ventriculi quarti** [NA] Several bands of nerve fibers that transversely cross the floor of the fourth ventricle. The nerve fibers are thought to arise in the arcuate nucleus, ventromedial to the pyramid in the medulla oblongata. They partially decussate, and then course dorsally in the medulla near the midline to reach the ventricular floor, where they enter the inferior cerebellar peduncle and pass to the flocculus of the cerebellum. Also *striae medullares acusticae, striae medullares fossae rhomboideae, arcuatofloccular tract, medullary striae of fourth ventricle, striae of Held, striae of Piccolomini, medullary striae of rhomboid fossa, striae of Monakow, auditory striae, acoustic striae, taeniae acusticae.* **s. medullaris thalami** [NA] A bundle of nerve fibers arising from the amygdaloid nuclei (by way of the stria terminalis), the hippocampal formation (by way of the fornix, the olfactory tubercle, the pre-optic, systal and anterior perforated regions) as well as other forebrain structures, and terminating in the habenular nuclei, with some fibers coursing in the habenular commissure to nuclei of the opposite side. The bundle becomes visible near the anterior end of the thalamus, and courses backward along the border between the dorsal and medial thalamic surfaces beneath the taenia thalami. Also *medullary stria of thalamus, habenular stria, stria fornicis, acies thalami optici* (obs.), *stria pinealis* (obs.), *stria ventriculi tertii.* **medullary striae of fourth ventricle** STRIAE MEDULLARES VENTRICULI QUARTI. **medullary striae of rhomboid fossa** STRIAE MEDULLARES VENTRICULI QUARTI. **medullary s. of thalamus** STRIA MEDULLARIS THALAMI. **striae of Monakow** STRIAE MEDULLARES VENTRICULI QUARTI. **striae of Nitabuch** MEMBRANE OF NITABUCH. **striae olfactoriae** Three (medial, intermediate, and lateral) bundles of olfactory tract nerve fibers that diverge from the posterior end of the olfactory trigone. The medial olfactory stria is covered by a layer of gray matter, the medial olfactory gyrus, and courses toward the diagonal band of Broca; the intermediate olfactory stria (when present) passes to the anterior perforated substance; and the lateral olfactory stria courses into the limen insulae and terminates in the corticomedial part (gyrus semilunaris) of the amygdaloid complex. Also *olfactory striae.* **striae parallelae** STRIAE OF RETZIUS. **striae of Piccolomini** STRIAE MEDULLARES VENTRICULI QUARTI. **s. pinealis** *Obs.* STRIA MEDULLARIS THALAMI. **striae of Retzius** Incremental lines visible in histologic sections of enamel which are associated with a periodic bending of enamel prisms. Also *striae parallelae, brown striae, Retzius lines.* **Rohr s.** Threads of fibrin or fibrinoid related to the decidua and the syncytiotrophoblast. They may become directly exposed to the intervillous space in the placenta and they have connections with the Nitabuch stria. **Schreger striae** SCHREGER'S LINES. **s. semicircularis** STRIA TERMINALIS. **s. spinosa** A groove, frequently found on the medial aspect of the spine of the sphenoid bone, caused by the chorda tympani nerve as it emerges from the skull. Also *groove of Lucas.* **s. tecta** STRIA LONGITUDINALIS LATERALIS CORPORIS CALLOSI. **s. terminalis** [NA] A discrete bundle of finely myelinated nerve fibers interconnecting the corticomedial part of the amygdaloid complex with the septum, the preoptic and anterior hypothalamic regions, the anterior perforated substance, and other basal forebrain regions. Most of its fibers are amygdalofugal, some coursing to the opposite amygdala by way of the anterior commissure, but other fibers within the bundle course to the amygdala from lower centers. Also *stria semicircularis, fasciculus of Foville, taenia semicircularis corporis striati, Tarin's taenia.* **striae transversae corporis callosi** Transversely oriented fascicles of myelinated nerve fibers seen on the dorsal surface of the corpus callosum. **s. vascularis ductus cochlearis** [NA] The thick strip of low stratified columnar epithelium on the inner surface of the specialized periosteal area lining the outer wall of the cochlear duct and extending from the spiral prominence to the attachment of the vestibular membrane. The connective tissue deep to the epithelium contains numerous blood vessels with which penetrating processes of the epithelial cells come into contact. The strip is involved in the production of endolymph. Also *psalterial cord, stria vascularis of Huschke.* **s. ventriculi tertii** STRIA MEDULLARIS THALAMI. **Wickham striae** A characteristic pattern of white dots and lines that is seen on typical papules of lichen planus.

**striae** \strī′ē\ Plural of STRIA.

**striascope** \strī′əskōp\ RETINOSCOPE.

**striatal** \strī·ā′təl, strī′ətəl\ Pertaining to the corpus striatum.

**striate** \strī′āt\ STRIATED.

**striated** \strī′ātid\ Marked by striae, usually parallel; striped. Also *striate.*

**striation** \strī·ā′shən\ [New L *striat(us),* from L *stria* a furrow, groove + -ION] 1 The state of being striated. 2 A stria or scratch. **Baillarger s.'s** BAILLARGER'S LINES. **basal s.'s** A series of infoldings of the cell membrane at the base of certain cells, such as the renal tubular epithelial cells. **s.'s of Frommann** Successive bands and clear spaces extending distalward from a node of Ranvier or locus of injury seen in an axon stained with silver nitrate. The appearances are artifactual, and probably comparable to the rings of Liesegang. Also *Frommann's lines.* **tigroid s.** A grossly visible change of the heart muscle due to fatty change and characterized by alternating strips of yellow and reddish brown myocardium.

**striatonigral** \strī′ətōnī′grəl\ Denoting the interconnection between the corpus striatum and the substantia nigra, such as the striatonigral nerve fibers that project from both the caudate nucleus and putamen of the striatum to the substantia nigra. Also *strionigral.*

**striatopallidal** \strī′ətōpal′idəl\ Denoting the interconnection between the corpus striatum (caudate nucleus and putamen) and the globus pallidus, as in striatopallidal nerve fibers. Also *striopallidal.*

**striatum** \strī·ā′təm\ NEOSTRIATUM.

**stricture** \strik′chər\ [L *strictura* (from *strictus* drawn tight or close, narrow, past part. of *stringere* to draw tight or close) a stripping, gathering, a mass of unwrought iron] An abnormal narrowing of the interior passageway within a tubular structure, as a vessel or duct. **anal s.** Abnormal narrowing of the anus. Also *proctostenosis.* **annular s.** A bandlike constriction completely encircling a tubular structure. Also *ring stricture.* **contractile s.** RECURRENT STRICTURE. **esophagus s.** A narrowing of the esophageal lumen secondary to inflammatory, traumatic, malignant, or degenerative causes. It most often involves the gastroesophageal junction. **functional s.** Obstruction of a tubular structure due to spasm of the muscular wall. Also *spasmodic stricture, spastic stricture, false stricture, temporary stricture.* **hysterical s.** Functional stricture of the esophagus due to muscle spasm in hysterical individuals. **irritable s.** A stricture that is excessively sensitive to stimuli so as to aggravate the narrowed segment. **linear s.** A stricture from a fibrous scarring that extends down the length of a tubular structure rather than around it. **organic s.** A stricture resulting from structural change rather than from a transient event or reversible cause. **rectal s.** Narrowing in the rectum, usually due to tumor, prior surgery, or inflammation. Also *proctostenosis, rectostenosis.* **recurrent s.** A stricture appearing again or refractory to medical and surgical management, such as mechanical dilatation, operative repair, or resection. Also *contractile stricture.* **ring s.** ANNULAR STRICTURE. **spasmodic s.** FUNCTIONAL STRICTURE. **spastic s.** FUNCTIONAL STRICTURE. **string s.** Narrowing of the colon or other tubular lumen due to a concentrically growing lesion, especially a carcinoma. **temporary s.** FUNCTIONAL STRICTURE.

**stridor** \strī′dər\ [L (from *stridere* to utter a shrill or grating sound, creak, rustle) a shrill or grating sound, creaking] A harsh, high-pitched noise on breathing, especially on inspiration, indicative of a degree of obstruction of the airway, especially of the larynx or trachea. Adj. stridulous. **congenital laryngeal s.** Inspiratory stridor in the newborn, due to disease present at birth, in particular laryngomalacia. Also *congenital stridor.* **expiratory s.** Quiet phonation sometimes noticed during expiration in the lightly anesthetized subject. It is therefore not truly stridor. **inspiratory s.** Stridor synchronous with inspiration and indicative of upper airway obstruction or laryngeal spasm. Also *crowing inspiration.* **laryngeal s.** Stridor from partial laryngeal obstruction due to one of the many causes of laryngeal stenosis.

**stridulous** \strij′ələs\ Producing or associated with stridor.

**striocerebellar** \strī′ōser′əbel′ər\ Pertaining to the corpus striatum and cerebellum.

**striomotor** \strī′ōmō′tər\ 1 Pertaining to the motor functions of the corpus striatum. 2 Relating to the voluntary or striated muscular or neuromuscular system.

**strionigral** \strī′ōnī′grəl\ STRIATONIGRAL.

**striopallidal** \strī′ōpal′idəl\ STRIATOPALLIDAL.

**strip** 1 To treat by tearing away or removing one tissue from another, as in the excision of varicose veins from the leg. 2 To milk or express a fluid from (an anatomic or synthetic conduit). 3 To reduce the mesiodistal width of (teeth) in order to improve alignment. **abrasive s.** A fine linen strip coated with abrasive on one side, used in dentistry. **amalgam s.** A fine nonabrasive linen strip used for finishing newly placed amalgam restorations. **lightning s.** A fine metal strip coated on one side with abrasive and used interdentally. Also *separating strip.* **moving s.** In radiotherapy, a technique in which a rectangular beam of radiation is sequentially applied to adjacent or slightly overlapping areas of the abdomen or thorax. **plastic s.** A strip of thin transparent plastic material used to shape cement restorations in anterior teeth. **polishing s.** An abrasive strip coated with a finely powdered abrasive. **separating s.** LIGHTNING STRIP.

**stripe** STRIA. **Baillarger s.'s** BAILLARGER'S LINES. **s. of Gennari** GENNARI'S BAND. **Hensen s.** A band situated in the center of the inferior surface of the membrana tectoria of the internal ear and opposite the tunnel of Corti. **s. of Kaes-Bekhterev** BEKHTEREV'S LAYER.

**stripper** 1 An instrument for stripping. 2 VEIN STRIPPER. **external s.** A long metallic vein stripper with a ring mounted at its end that is just larger than the vein, used to remove the greater or lesser saphenous (or other) veins by bluntly dividing venous tributaries as it is passed vigorously along the vein. **internal s.** A long, olive-tipped metallic or plastic device used for stripping the greater or lesser saphenous (or other) veins. From a venotomy near the ankle it is passed proximally out the central end of the divided vein, which, after being tied tightly around the end of the stripper, is briskly extracted from the leg, everted, from below. **vein s.** An instrument used to remove a vein. It is threaded through the vein, fixed at the distal end, and then pulled back with the vein in train. Also *stripper.*

**stripping** / **s. of the membranes** The maneuver of gently pushing away the fetal membranes from their attachment to the cervix during cervicovaginal examination of a pregnant woman at or near term. This maneuver is believed by some to be occasionally a means of inducing labor. **s. of the pleura** PLEURECTOMY.

**strobila** \strō′bilə, strōbī′lə\ [Gk *strobilē* (from *strobilos* a pinecone) a piece of lint twisted like a pinecone] (*pl.* strobilae) The chain of segments (proglottids) that forms the body of a tapeworm, exclusive of the head (scolex) and the unsegmented neck.

**strobilation** \strō′bilā′shən\ The formation of a strobila or any sequence of metameric units, or of zooids, disks, or gemmules. Also *strobilization.*

**strobilocercus** \strō′bilōsur′kəs\ The larval form of certain tapeworms of the genus *Taenia*, resembling a cysticercus but everted, with a pseudosegmented neck, scolex, and a small terminal bladder. An example is the larva of *Taenia taeniaeformis*, which is known as *Cysticercus fasciolaris*.

**strobiloid** \strō′biloid\ Resembling the strobila of a tapeworm.

**stroboscope** \strō′bəskōp\ [Gk *strobo(s)* a top, a whirling + -SCOPE] An instrument that uses interrupted light to observe successive phases of a moving object. Also *phenakistoscope, zoescope*.

**strobostereoscope** \strō′bōster′ē·əskōp′\ STEREOSTROBOSCOPE.

**Strohl** [André *Strohl*, French physician, born 1887] Guillain-Barré-Strohl syndrome. See under GUILLAIN-BARRÉ SYNDROME.

**stroke** [Middle English, akin to Old English *strīcan* to strike and to L *stringere* to draw tight or close] **1** A thrusting or swinging movement of a body part or mechanical device, or one part or excursion of a cyclic movement. **2** An attack or seizure. **3** CEREBROVASCULAR ACCIDENT. **apoplectic s.** APOPLEXY. **cerebral s.** APOPLEXY. **completed s.** A neurologic deficit that follows the deprivation of cerebral blood flow. Unlike a transient ischemic attack or a reversible ischemic neurologic deficit, central neurologic function does not return to normal. **heat s.** See under HEATSTROKE. **lacunar s.** A stroke resulting from the occlusion of a small artery supplying the brain or brainstem and associated with the formation of a tiny cavity or lacuna within the brain substance. These strokes usually occur in patients with arterial hypertension, and several syndromes, including the dysarthria-clumsy hand syndrome, have been associated with lacunar infarction. **lightning s.** A syndrome caused by being struck by lightning. To varying degrees, the subject suffers severe burns, unconsciousness, cardiac arrhythmias, and frequently death. **paralytic s.** Paralysis resulting from cerebral hemorrhage or infarction. **progressive s.** Cerebral hemorrhage or infarction in which there is a slow progressive evolution of symptoms and signs due to gradual extension of the pathologic process. Also *stroke-in-evolution*. **sun s.** See under SUNSTROKE.

**stroke-in-evolution** PROGRESSIVE STROKE.

**stroma** \strō′mə\ [New L, from Gk *strōma* (from *stornynai* to spread) something spread out to lie or sit upon (akin to L *stratum*, same orig. meaning, from *sternere* to spread, and to L *structura* structure, from *struere* to arrange, construct)] (*pl.* stromata) [NA] The supporting and binding framework or matrix, usually connective tissue, of an organ. Compare PARENCHYMA. **s. of cornea** SUBSTANTIA PROPRIA CORNEAE. **erythrocyte s.** ERYTHROCYTE GHOST. **s. glandulae thyroideae** [NA] The connective tissue extending as septa from the inner capsule of the thyroid gland into the lobes dividing the substance into irregular lobules and further forming a reticular meshwork supporting the follicles. Also *stroma of thyroid gland, stroma glandulae thyreoideae* (outmoded). **s. iridis** [NA] The anterior part and bulk of the structure of the iris, comprising many blood vessels and nerves and supported by spongy connective tissue containing fluid, fibroblasts, and melanocytes, and, near the periphery of the pupil, the circular and radial smooth muscle fibers of the sphincter pupillae and dilator pupillae, respectively. Also *stroma of iris, Kölliker's layer, mesiris*. **lymphatic s.** The reticulin framework of lymphoid tissue. **s. ovarii** [NA] The interstitial connective tissue framework of the ovary, that of the cortex consisting of dense reticular fiber networks with spindle-shaped cells while that of the medulla comprises loose connective tissue, elastic fibers, nonstriated muscle cells, and many blood vessels. Also *stroma of ovary*. **s. of thyroid gland** STROMA GLANDULAE THYROIDEAE. **s. vitreum** [NA] The delicate fibrillar meshwork filled with vitreous humor and supporting the vitreous body of the eyeball. Also *vitreous stroma*.

**stromal** \strō′məl\ Of or pertaining to a stroma. Also *stromatic*.

**stromata** \strō′mətə\ Plural of STROMA.

**stromatic** \strōmat′ik\ STROMAL.

**stromatogenous** \strō′mətäj′ənəs\ Originating in the stroma of an organ.

**stromatosis** \strō′mətō′sis\ *Obs.* ENDOMETRIAL STROMAL SARCOMA.

**stromuhr** \shtrōm′oor′, strōm′-\ [German, from *Strom* stream, flow + *Uhr* clock, meter] FLOWMETER.

**Strong** [Richard Pearson *Strong*, U.S. physician and parasitologist, 1872–1948] See under VACCINE.

**Strongylata** \strän′jilā′tə\ STRONGYLIDA.

**strongyl-** \strän′jil-\ STRONGYLO-.

**strongyle** \strän′jīl\ Of or belonging to the nematode superfamily Strongyloidea, or similar to worms of this superfamily.

**Strongylida** \stränjil′idə\ [*Strongyl(us)* + *-ida*, suffix used for orders] A large order of heavy-bodied intestinal nematodes in the class Secernentea that includes many of the most pathogenic parasites of humans and domestic mammals and birds. It includes the bursate strongyle worms, including hookworms (superfamily Ancylostomatoidea), the trichostrongyles of herbivores (superfamily Trichostrongyloidea), and the metastrongyle lungworms (superfamily Metastrongylioides) among other parasitic forms. Also *Strongylata, Strongylorida*.

**strongyliform** \stränjil′ifôrm\ Similar in form to worms of the genus *Strongylus* and related genera and especially to the third-stage larval form, which is comparable to the filariform, infective third-stage larvae of hookworms.

**strongylo-** \strän′jilō-\ [Gk *strongylos* round, rounded] A combining form meaning round. Also *strongyl-*.

**Strongyloidea** \strän′jiloi′dē·ə\ A superfamily of parasitic nematodes in the order Strongylida. Now limited to the family Strongylidae with the genera *Strongylus* and *Cyathostomum* of special veterinary importance, it formerly included the hookworms, gapeworms, trichostrongyles, and lungworms, now classified in separate superfamilies.

***Strongyloides*** \strän′jiloi′dēz\ [New L, from *Strongyl(us)* + Gk *-o(e)idēs* -like] A genus consisting of about 38 species of small nematodes in the family Rhabditidae (Strongyloididae according to some workers) superfamily Rhabditoidea; the threadworms. They are parasitic in the small intestine of higher vertebrates, chiefly mammals. These nematodes are of special interest as they exhibit both a parasitic cycle that is initiated by skin penetration (as with hookworms), and an atavistic free-living soil cycle, reminiscent of their rhabditoid ancestors. ***S. stercoralis*** An intestinal threadworm of humans and other primates and of dogs, cats, and several other mammals; the cause of human strongyloidiasis. Several host-adapted strains may exist. The human strain is widely distributed but is especially common in rural tropical communities with poor sanitary facilities and in eastern Europe. It has been shown to be present in 10–20 percent of former war prisoners in southeast Asia during World War II (1939–1946), having persisted by autoinfection. Infection is from fecally contaminated soil or water in which the infective filariform larvae are found. The female embeds in the small-intestine mucosa of man and produces numerous eggs. Then follows a complex life cycle. Larvae and/or eggs are excreted in feces. Also *Anguillula stercoralis, Strongyloides intestinalis.*

**strongyloidiasis** \strän′jiloidī′əsis\ [*Strongyloid(es)* + -IASIS] Infection by nematode worms of the genus *Strongyloides,* usually with reference to *S. stercoralis,* the human threadworm. Infection in central and eastern Africa and Papua New Guinea is with *S. fulleborni.* While infection is often asymptomatic, heavy infection in humans can result in an intensely pruritic urticarial dermatitis in the invasion stage, and lung damage, host sensitization response, and pneumonitis in the pulmonary stage, and mucosal destruction, abdominal pain, and fibrotic changes in chronic cases in the intestinal stage. A malabsorption syndrome associated with jejunal mucosal abnormalities is present in a minority of infected individuals. There is often an eosinophilia during the invasive stage of the disease. Autoinfection in immunologically suppressed or compromised individuals is the most dangerous form of the disease, resulting in systemic spread of larvae, toxic effects, and, in especially heavy infections, death. Also *strongyloidosis.*

**Strongylorida** \strän′jilôr′idə\ STRONGYLIDA.

***Strongylus*** \strän′jələs\ [New L, from Gk *strongylos* round, rounded] A genus of heavy-bodied nematodes of the family Strongylidae, parasitic in horses and other equids. Many important nematode parasites of domestic animals were originally placed in this genus and have since been transferred to other genera. ***S. gigas*** *DIOCTOPHYMA RENALE.* ***S. renalis*** *DIOCTOPHYMA RENALE.*

**strontium** \strän′shē·əm\ Element number 38, having atomic weight 87.62. In nature it is usually found associated with barium, never in the free state. The four natural isotopes are stable. Symbol: Sr

**strontium 90** A radioisotope of strontium, produced by the fission of uranium 235, emitting purely beta radiation. Its daughter is yttrium 90, also a pure beta emitter. An equilibrium solution of strontium 90 and yttrium 90 is used in the treatment of ophthalmologic lesions. Because of its fixation in the osseous system, and its long biologic half-life of 7 years, strontium 90 is a particularly dangerous contaminant resulting from radioactive fallout. Physical half-life is 28 years. Symbol: $^{90}$Sr

**strophanthidin** One of the cardenolides whose glycosides occur naturally and are cardiotonic. It differs from digitoxigenin by having —CHO in place of —$CH_3$ at C-19, and in possessing a 5$\beta$-hydroxyl group.

**strophocephaly** \sträf′əsef′əlē\ [Gk *stroph(ē)* a turning, twisting + *o* + CEPHAL- + -Y] A nonspecific term for a developmentally distorted face and head, as that of a cyclops or stomocephalus.

**strophosomia** \sträf′əsō′mē·ə\ [Gk *stroph(ē)* a turning, twisting + *o* + *som(a)* + -IA] An extreme degree of thoracoceloschisis in which the thoracic and abdominal viscera are herniated through a large ventral body wall defect and the trunk tends to be twisted on its longitudinal axis.

**strophulus** \sträf′yələs\ [New L, copy error for Med L *scrophulus* (a variant and misapplication of SCROFULA) a skin eruption] A papular eruption, usually seen in children. *Outmoded.* • The term has been variously applied to miliaria and to papular urticaria. **s. albidus** MILIUM.

**structure** [L *structura* (from *struere* to arrange, construct) arrangement, construction, structure] **1** The manner of organization or arrangement of the components of an object such as an organ, a body, a molecule, etc. **2** Any constructed or formed part or whole, as an organ or other anatomical entity. **fine s.** Any of the detailed cellular and intercellular structures that can be identified with the electron microscope. Also *ultrastructure.* **primary s.** The first level of organization of a polypeptide or polynucleotide chain, that is the amino-acid sequence of the protein, and the nucleotide sequence of the nucleic acid. **quaternary s.** The fourth level of organization within a protein molecule, which represents the orientation and bonding between the different polypeptide chains that make up the molecule. **secondary s.** The second level of organization within a polypeptide or polynucleotide chain. It is the structure formed when the relationship in space of one residue to the next is constant over a length of chain. The two commonest secondary structures in proteins are the $\alpha$-helix and the $\beta$-pleated sheet. **tertiary s.** The third level of organization within a protein molecule, representing the orientation and bonding interaction between regions of secondary structure within the same polypeptide chain. The side groups of the amino acids are important in the establishment of tertiary structure. **toroid s.** The secondary molecular structure of the superhelical circular DNA molecule of the bacteriophage $\phi$X174.

**struggle / death s.** Myoclonic jerking or twitching of the limbs which often occurs just prior to death.

**struma** \stroo′mə\ [L, scrofula, goiter] GOITER. **s. baseos linguae** LINGUAL GOITER. **s. calculosa** A goiter that has become calcified. **cast iron s.** RIEDEL STRUMA. **s. colloides cystica** A colloid goiter in which large cysts have formed through the breakdown of the walls of follicles. **s. endothoracica** INTRATHORACIC GOITER. **s. fibrosa** Goiter caused by overdevelopment of the connective tissue in the gland. Also *struma hyperplastica.* **Hashimoto s.** HASHIMOTO'S DISEASE. **s. hyperplastica** STRUMA FIBROSA. **ligneous s.** RIEDEL STRUMA. **s. lingualis** LINGUAL GOITER. **s. lymphatica** *Seldom used* HASHIMOTO'S DISEASE. **s. lymphomatosa** HASHIMOTO'S DISEASE. **s. ovarii** A teratoma of the ovary in which thyroid tissue is a prominent component. Most are benign. **s. parenchymatosa** COLLOID GOITER. **retrosternal s.** SUBSTERNAL GOITER. **Riedel s.** A very rare form of chronic thyroiditis in which the symptoms and signs are more mechanical than functional, with asymmetric, stony enlargement and fibrosis of the thyroid and fibrosis of adjacent structures but no inflammatory signs. Also *Riedel's disease, cast iron struma, ligneous thyroiditis, ligneons struma, chronic fibrous thyroiditis, invasive thyroiditis, Riedel's thyroiditis, woody thyroiditis, iron-hard tumor.* **substernal s.** SUBSTERNAL GOITER. **thymus s.** Persistence of a sizable thymus gland beyond childhood, when it usually undergoes atrophy.

**strumectomy** \stroomek′təmē\ [*strum(a)* + -ECTOMY] The surgical removal of an enlarged gland or tumor, as a goitrous thyroid gland. **median s.** ISTHMECTOMY.

**strumiform** \stroo′mifôrm\ **1** Resembling a goiter. **2** Resembling scrofula. *Older term.*

**strumitis** \stroomī′tis\ [*strum(a)* + -ITIS] THYROIDITIS.

**strumous** \stroo′məs\ [*strum(a)* + -OUS] Of, relating to, resembling, or caused by goiter.

**Strümpell** [Ernst Adolph Gustav Gottfried von *Strümpell,* German neurologist, 1853–1925] **1** Strümpell's disease, Strümpell-Leichtenstern disease, Marie-Strümpell disease, Strümpell-Marie disease. See under ACUTE INFANTILE HEMIPLEGIA. **2** Fleischer-Strümpell ring. See under FLEISCHER KERATOCONUS RING. **3** See under REFLEX, SIGN. **4** Marie-Strümpell arthritis, Marie-Strümpell disease, Strümpell-Marie disease, Marie-Strümpell spondylitis. See under ANKYLOSING SPONDYLITIS. **5** Strümpell-Leichtenstern encephalitis. See under ACUTE HEMORRHAGIC LEUKOENCEPHALI-

TIS. **6** Strümpell sign. See under PRONATION PHENOMENON.

**strychnine** \strik′nin\ $C_{21}H_{22}N_2O_2$. A highly toxic alkaloid, formed biologically by reaction of tryptamine with a monoterpene.

**strychninism** \strik′ninizm\ Poisoning with strychnine. Human illness has been reported with doses as small as 15 mg. The usual fatal dose for oral ingestion is about 60 to 90 mg. Symptoms, which begin in one-half to several hours, include muscle tightness about the face and neck, tonic seizures, intense muscle cramps, then a depressed flaccid state. Further seizures may follow with death due to respiratory paralysis. Also *strychnism.*

**strychninization** \strik′ninīzā′shən\ **1** The application or administration of strychnine. **2** The state of having received strychnine.

**strychnism** \strik′nizm\ STRYCHNINISM.

**STS** **1** serologic test for syphilis (used especially for the Wasserman antibody). **2** standard test for syphilis.

**STU** skin test unit.

**Stuart** [Kenneth Lamont *Stuart,* English physician active in the West Indies, flourished 20th century] Stuart-Bras syndrome. See under SYNDROME.

**study / case-control s.** An epidemiologic study in which two or more groups are compared with respect to the frequency of a characteristic of interest. In its simplest form, one group would consist of persons displaying an abnormality, such as a stated disease or a given congenital anomaly, while the other would consist of individuals known not to be abnormal in that sense. Also *retrospective study* (incorrect). **cohort s.** An epidemiologic study in which the experience of one or more cohorts is investigated. **cross-sectional s.** **1** CROSS-SECTIONAL METHOD. **2** An epidemiological study in which the observations relate to the same point in time, as in determining whether the subjects studied have or have not, up to that point, been exposed to some noxious influence, have or have not developed a given disease, are alive or dead, etc. **descriptive s.** The simplest form of epidemiologic study, in which the distribution of the disease in the population under study, which may be, for example, a hospital series, is described solely in terms of the numbers affected by age and sex, date of onset, or some other characteristic. **dynamic studies** Intensive studies in which the time course of the tracer content (or concentration) in an organ is followed in order to monitor the function of the organ, for example the heart, lung, brain, or kidney. To extend the scope of the observations, the organ may be subjected to stress by exercise, drugs, etc. **experimental s.** **1** In biological and epidemiological studies, an investigation in which the variables can be controlled so that the resulting effect may be measured, typically in a laboratory procedure using experimental animals or tissue cultures, as in the large-scale trials of vaccines against poliomyelitis. Also *preventive trial.* **2** INTERVENTION STUDY. • See note at INTERVENTION STUDY. **gastrointestinal s.** GASTROINTESTINAL EXAMINATION. **intervention s.** In epidemiology, an investigation in which the level of the factor being studied in a population is deliberately changed in order to test a hypothesis, typically involving a human population. • *Intervention study* is used mainly of human populations, *experimental study* of animal population tissue cultures. Also *experimental study.* **longitudinal s.** LONGITUDINAL METHOD. **prospective s.** An investigation in which information about disease, injury, or vital events occurring in a group of persons is collected over a period of time so that the occurrences can be related to the characteristics of the individuals as ascertained at the initiation of the study. **retrospective s.** **1** Any inquiry or examination of events after the period of time during which the events occurred. **2** *Incorrect* CASE-CONTROL STUDY.

**stump** [Middle English *stumpe,* from the Germanic] **1** The most distal part of an extremity left after amputation. **2** The base or pedicle of a tumor, organ, or vessel that remains after partial excision. **ischial-bearing s.** An above-knee amputation stump short enough to allow body weight to be borne primarily by the ischial tuberosity and the gluteal muscles.

**stun** To render unconscious or immobile by a blow or other violent force.

**stunt** [Middle English, dull, stupid, from Old English, akin to Old Norse *stuttr* short] To retard the growth or development of.

**stupe** \st^y^oop\ [L *stupa,* also *stuppa* (from Gk *styppē* tow) the coarse part of flax, tow, oakum] A soft cloth or sponge, dampened and frequently medicated, applied as adjunctive treatment in the relief of local pain.

**stupefacient** \st^y^oo′pəfā′shənt\ [L *stupefaciens,* gen. *stupefacientis,* pres. part. of *stupefacere* (from *stupe(re)* to be amazed + *facere* to make) to stupefy, stun, astonish] An agent, drug, or physical change, producing mental obtundation or varying degrees of coma.

**stupefactive** \st^y^oo′pəfak′tiv\ Causing mental obtundation or varying degrees of coma, as a stupefacient.

**stupor** \st^y^oo′pər\ [L (from *stupere* to be insensible, to be amazed) insensibility, dullness] A state of deadened sensibilities and awareness in which there is clouding of consciousness and diminished responsivity. It is most commonly of organic origin. Also *obnubilation, psychocoma* (obs.), *apsychosis* (obs.). **benign s.** DEPRESSIVE STUPOR. **Cairns s.** AKINETIC MUTISM. **catatonic s.** A state of total withdrawal and unresponsiveness seen in catatonic schizophrenia and often accompanied by catalepsy and negativism. Also *akinetic autism* (obs.), *Kahlbaum's disease, Kahlbaum syndrome, delusion stupor* (older term) . **depressive s.** The most severe form of depression in manic-depressive psychosis. Also *benign stupor, stuporous melancholia, melancholic stupor.* **epileptic s.** **1** Postepileptic confusion so severe as to lead to stupor. **2** *Obs.* PETIT MAL STATUS. **melancholic s.** DEPRESSIVE STUPOR. **spike-wave s.** PETIT MAL STATUS. **s. vigilans** CATALEPSY.

**Sturge** [William Allen *Sturge,* English physician, 1850–1919] Sturge-Weber encephalotrigeminal angiomatosis, Sturge's disease, Sturge-Weber disease, Sturge-Weber-Dimitri disease. See under STURGE-WEBER SYNDROME.

**Sturm** [Ernst *Sturm,* U.S. physician, flourished mid-20th century] Murphy-Sturm lymphosarcoma. See under LYMPHOSARCOMA.

**Sturm** [Johann Christopher *Sturm,* German mathematician, physician, and philosopher, 1635–1703] See under CONOID.

**Sturmdorf** [A. *Sturmdorf,* U.S. gynecologist, 1861–1934] See under OPERATION.

**stutter** **1** To speak in utterances characterized by involuntary halts, breaks, and often with repetition of the initial consonant sound of a word or syllable; engage in or be afflicted with stuttering. **2** An instance of stuttering. Also *stammer.*

**stuttering** A speech disorder affecting the fluency of production, often characterized by repetitions of certain sounds, syllables, words or phrases, and by the prolongation of sounds and blocking of the articulation of words. Severer forms may be associated with facial grimacing, limb and postural gestures, involuntary grunts, or impaired control of airflow. The severity of symptoms may vary with the speaker's situation and audience. Stuttering usually begins in childhood and is commoner in males than in females. It is unusual to find evidence of neurological dysfunction in the confirmed adolescent or adult stutterer. Management varies from attempts to control respiratory activity, or in the measured production of syllables and words, to psychotherapy aimed at readjusting the self-image of the individual and his place in the community. Often several therapeutic methods are used in combination. Also *stammering, psellism, lingual titubation, battarism* (seldom used), *batturismus* (seldom used), *dysphemia* (seldom used), *dysarthria literalis* (seldom used), *dysarthria syllabaris spasmodica* (seldom used), *balbuties* (obs.). **urinary s.** Involuntarily intermittent flow during urination.

**St. Vitus** [*St. Vitus*, Christian martyr of 3rd–4th century] St. Vitus dance. See under SYDENHAM'S CHOREA.

**stye** \stī\ [Old English *stīgend*, from *stīgan* to rise] A small abscess which forms on the cutaneous or conjunctival surface of the eyelid as a result of infection, usually staphylococcal, of a sebaceous gland adjacent to an eyelash follicle. Also *hordeolum*. Also *sty*. **meibomian s.** A stye involving a meibomian gland and usually occurring on the conjunctival surface of the eyelid. **zeisian s.** A stye involving a zeisian gland and usually occurring on the surface of the skin at the edge of the eyelid.

**stylet** \stī'lət\ [French (from Italian *stiletto*, dim. of L *stilus* a sharp-pointed instrument, stylus) a sharp-pointed dagger] A slender wire or probe that is passed through a flexible catheter in order to increase its rigidity, thus facilitating the passage of the catheter. Also *stilus, style, stilet, stilette*. **endotracheal s.** A curved stylet, now rarely used, for introduction into an endotracheal tube so as to render it similarly curved and simplify its introduction between the vocal cords in peroral endotracheal anesthesia. **lacrimal s.** A slender wire probe that is used to cannulate the lacrimal duct.

**styliform** \stī'lifôrm\ STYLOID.

**stylo-** \stī'lō-\ [Gk *stylos* pillar and L *stilus* stylus. See STYLOID.] A combining form meaning styloid, especially styloid process.

**styloglossal** \-gläs'əl\ Of or pertaining to the styloid process of the temporal bone and the tongue.

**styloglossus** \-gläs'əs\ MUSCULUS STYLOGLOSSUS.

**stylohyal** \-hī'əl\ A constituent part of the hyoid chain, derived from the posterior portion of the second arch cartilage and forming in the adult the greater part of the styloid process of the temporal bone.

**stylohyoid** \-hī'oid\ **1** Of or pertaining to the styloid process of the temporal bone and to the hyoid bone. **2** MUSCULUS STYLOHYOIDEUS.

**styloid** \stī'loid\ [Gk *styloeidēs* (from L *stilus* a stylus, confused with Gk *stylos* a pillar) styluslike, slender and sharp-pointed] **1** Pillar-shaped or peg-shaped. **2** Long and pointed, as a bony process. For defs. 1 and 2 also *styliform*.

**styloiditis** \sti'loidī'tis\ Inflammation or irritation around a styloid process.

**stylomandibular** \-mandib'yələr\ Of or pertaining to the styloid process of the temporal bone and the mandible. Also *stylomaxillary*.

**stylomastoid** \-mas'toid\ Of or pertaining to the styloid and the mastoid processes of the temporal bone.

**stylomaxillary** \-mak'siler'ē\ **1** Of or pertaining to the styloid process of the temporal bone and the maxilla. **2** *Outmoded* STYLOMANDIBULAR.

**stylomyloid** \-mī'loid\ Of or pertaining to the styloid process of the temporal bone and the area around the lower molar teeth.

**stylopodium** \-pō'dē·əm\ [STYLO- + PODIUM] The first skeletal elements to be recognized in a developing amphibian limb, namely the humerus and femur. The order of appearance of the elements is usually proximal to distal, stylopodium, zeugopodium, and then autopodium, but in higher vertebrates the sequence is disturbed by the larger components differentiating earlier and more rapidly than the smaller.

**stylostaphyline** \-staf'ilīn\ Of or pertaining to the styloid process of the temporal bone and the uvula.

**stylosteophyte** \stīläs'tē·əfīt'\ A post-shaped bony outgrowth that forms an exostosis.

**stylostixis** \-stik'sis\ ACUPUNCTURE.

**stylus** \stī'ləs\ [L *stilus* stylus for incising or writing; influenced by Gk *stylos* pillar] (*pl.* styli) **1** A penlike instrument used to apply medicine topically. Very often it is impregnated with a caustic agent, such as silver nitrate. **2** A finely pointed, needlelike device used to trace a graphic recording on paper, as in an electrocardiogram. Also *pen*. For defs. 1 and 2 also *stilus*.

**stymatosis** \stī'mətō'sis\ [Gk *styma*, gen. *stymat(os)* priapism, stiffness + -OSIS] Priapism in which associated hemorrhage into the urethra produces a bloody discharge.

**stypage** \stī'pij, stēpäzh'\ [French, from Gk *styp(ē)* tow, the coarse part of flax or hemp + French *-age* -AGE] The application of a pledget soaked with a topical anesthetic to induce local anesthesia.

**stype** \stīp\ [Gk *stypē* tow, the coarse part of flax or hemp] A pledget or tampon made of absorbent material.

**stypsis** \stip'sis\ [Gk (from *styphein* to contract, be astringent) contraction, astringency] **1** The property of being astringent (styptic) or possessing astringent activity. **2** The treatment of disease states with astringent compounds.

**styptic** \stip'tik\ [Gk *styptikos* (from *styphein* to contract, be astringent) astringent] **1** Having the property of arresting bleeding, either mechanically or chemically; astringent. Also *staltic*. **2** A hemostatic medication with astringent properties. **Binelli s.** A styptic preparation composed of creosote in an aqueous solution. It is used to stop a small hemorrhage. **chemical s.** A styptic material that checks hemorrhage by means of coagulation induced by chemical action. **mechanical s.** Any hemostatic device or material that facilitates coagulation of bleeding vessels. **vascular s.** A styptic material that arrests hemorrhage by acting as a vasoconstrictor on blood vessels of relatively small size.

**styramate** $C_9H_{11}NO_3$. Carbamic acid β-hydroxyphenethyl ester. A drug employed as a centrally-acting skeletal muscle relaxant in treating skeletal-muscular disorders. It has actions similar to those of mephenesin.

**styrene** Ph—CH=$CH_2$. Ethenylbenzene. A hydrocarbon used as a raw material for making plastics. It can be polymerized to form polystyrene. Also *styrol*.

**su.** *sumat* (L, let him take).

**suA** Symbol for polarity suppressor.

**sub-** \sub-, səb-\ [L *sub* (akin to Gk *hypo* under, from under; *sub-* as prefix often assimilated before *m* and *r* as *sum-* and *sur-* and regularly before *c, f, g*, and *p* as *suc-, suf-, sug-*, and *sup-* and sometimes *sus-* before *c, p*, and *t*) under, from under, below, incompletely] A prefix meaning (1) under, beneath, below; (2) almost, slightly, somewhat, incompletely; (3) secondary, next below in rank or scope, subordinate, lesser. Also *suc-, suf-, sug-, sum- sup-, sur-, sus-*.

**subabdominal** \-abdäm'inəl\ Below the abdomen.

**subabdominoperitoneal** \-abdäm'inōper'itənē'əl\ Beneath the abdominal peritoneum. Also *subperitoneoabdominal*.

**subacetabular** \-as′ətab′yələr\ Below the acetabulum.
**subacromial** \-əkrō′mē·əl\ Below the acromion.
**subacute** \-əkyoot′\ Intermediate in character between acute and chronic; moderately severe: said especially of a disease.
**subalimentation** \-al′iməntā′shən\ SEMISTARVATION.
**subanconeus** \-angkō′nē·əs\ [SUB- + ANCONEUS] An inconstant muscle composed of a few fibers of the deep aspect of the medial head of the triceps brachii muscle, arising from the distal end of the posterior surface of the humerus and inserting into the adjacent capsule of the elbow joint. Also *articularis cubiti.*
**subapical** \-ap′ikəl, -ā′pikəl\ Below an apex, as of the lung.
**subarachnoid** \-ərak′noid\ Deep to the arachnoid membrane, as *subarachnoid space.*
**subarachnoiditis** \-ərak′noidī′tis\ [SUB- + ARACHNOIDITIS] LEPTOMENINGITIS. **acute curable juvenile s.** *Seldom used* LYMPHOCYTIC CHORIOMENINGITIS.
**subarcuate** \-är′kyoo·āt\ Slightly curved or arched.
**subatomic** \-ətäm′ik\ Pertaining to the particles which constitute the atom.
**Subbarow** [Yellapragada *Subbarow,* U.S. biochemist, born 1896] Fiske and Subbarow method. See under METHOD.
**subbasal** \-bā′səl, -bā′zəl\ Below or beneath any base or basal membrane.
**subbrachial** \-brā′kē·əl\ Pertaining to the brachium of the inferior colliculus.
**subcalcarine** \-kal′kərīn\ Deep to the calcarine sulcus, like the subcalcarine or infracalcarine gyrus.
**subcallosal** \-kalō′səl\ Deep to the corpus callosum, like the subcallosal gyrus.
**subcapsular** \-kap′s$^y$ələr\ Located just internal to the capsule of the crystalline lens.
**subcartilaginous** \-kär′tilaj′ənəs\ **1** Beneath a cartilage. **2** Not wholly cartilaginous.
**subcerebellar** \-ser′əbel′ər\ Under (ventral to) or below (inferior to) the cerebellum.
**subcerebral** \-ser′əbrəl\ Beneath the cerebrum.
**subchronic** \-krän′ik\ More nearly chronic than acute, but not fully chronic.
**subclass** \sub′klas\ [SUB- + CLASS] The taxonomic category intermediate between class and superorder.
**subclavian** \-klā′vē·ən\ Beneath the clavicle.
**subclinical** \-klin′ikəl\ Without clinical manifestations; not manifesting itself in overt illness but capable of being detected or inferred by appropriate investigation, such as serology: said of a disease or infection, such as one in its early stage. A subclinical infection may or may not be transmissible.
**subcollateral** \-kəlat′ərəl\ Deep to the collateral gyrus of the cerebral cortex.
**subconscious** \-kän′shəs\ [SUB- + CONSCIOUS] Those mental processes, or the contents of mind, that lie just outside personal awareness and of which the individual is but dimly aware. Such elements may be brought into consciousness at times, for example by the prompting of related memories. In other instances they may be shown to exert a direct influence on the behavior of an individual but not to become available to conscious awareness, for example in the phenomenon of posthypnotic suggestion.
**subcortex** \-kôr′teks\ **1** Tissue deep to the cortex, found in several organs, such as the brain. **2** Neural tissue of the cerebrum beneath, or deep to, the cerebral cortex.
**subcortical** \-kôr′tikəl\ Situated deep to the cerebral cortex.
**subcranial** \-krā′nē·əl\ Beneath the cranium.
**subcrepitant** \-krep′itənt\ Somewhat coarser or lower-pitched than a sound that would be described as crepitant: applied primarily to rales.
**subcurative** \-kyUr′ətiv\ Denoting a dose smaller than that believed to be curative.
**subcutaneous** \-kyootā′nē·əs\ [SUB- + CUTANEOUS] Being, applied, or used beneath the skin. Also *hypodermic, hypodermatic, subdermal.*
**subcuticular** \-kyootik′yələr\ SUBEPIDERMAL.
**subdermal** \-dur′məl\ SUBCUTANEOUS.
**subdiaphragmatic** \-dī′əfragmat′ik\ SUBPHRENIC.
**subduction** \-duk′shən\ [SUB- + DUCTION] A downward movement, especially of an eye; infraduction.
**subdural** \-d$^y$oo′rəl\ Deep to the dura mater; between the dura mater and the arachnoid membrane.
**subendothelial** \-en′dəthē′lē·əl\ Of or relating to a zone that is immediately external to the vascular endothelium. It may become infiltrated by material derived from the blood vascular system.
**subependymal** \-epen′diməl\ Situated deep to the ependyma.
**subependymoma** \-epen′dimō′mə\ An ependymoma containing dense glial fibers and admixed astrocytes.
**subepidermal** \-ep′idur′məl\ Beneath the epidermis. Also *subcuticular.*
**suberosis** \soo′bərō′sis\ [L *suber* cork tree, cork oak + -OSIS] A form of extrinsic allergic alveolitis caused by exposure to moldy cork dust. The causative agent is *Penicillium frequentans.*
**subfalcial** \-fal′sē·əl\ **1** Beneath the falx cerebri. **2** Beneath the falx cerebelli.
**subfamily** \sub′fam′ilē\ A category in biological taxonomy that is used, when appropriate, to subdivide a family into groups within which genera are more closely related to each other than to other genera of the family.
**subfecundity** \-fikun′ditē\ [SUB- + FECUNDITY] A condition in which the ability to reproduce or become pregnant is reduced.
**subfertility** \-fərtil′itē\ Less than normal fertility.
**sub fin. coct.** *sub finem coctionis* (L, toward the end of boiling).
**subfissure** \-fish′ər\ A cortical sulcus, or fissure, that is not visible from the surface of the cerebral cortex.
**subfoliar** \-fō′lē·ər\ Pertaining to a subfolium, especially of the cerebellum.
**subfolium** \-fō′lē·əm\ A secondary or tertiary infolding of any cerebellar folium.
**subfornical** \-fôr′nikəl\ Beneath or ventral to the fornix, like the subfornical organ.
**subfrontal** \-frun′təl\ Beneath, or deep to, the frontal gyri or frontal lobe of the brain.
**subgenus** \sub′jēnəs\ A category in biological taxonomy that is used, when appropriate, to subdivide a genus into groups within which species are more closely related to each other than to other species of the genus.
**subgerminal** \-jur′minəl\ Lying beneath the germinal, or embryonic, disk.
**subgingival** \-jin′jivəl\ Situated between the apex of a tooth and the gingival margin.
**subglenoid** \-glē′noid\ INFRAGLENOID.
**subglottic** \-glät′ik\ INFRAGLOTTIC.
**subglottis** \-glät′is\ *Outmoded* CAVITAS INFRAGLOTTICA.
**subgyrus** \-jī′rəs\ Any gyrus of the cerebral cortex lying deep to the cortical surface that is partially or completely concealed by more superficial gyri.
**subhepatic** \-hepat′ik\ Located beneath the liver.
**subhyaloid** \-hī′əloid\ Situated between the vitreous humor and the retina of the eye.

**subhyoid** \-hī′oid\ INFRAHYOID.
**subhyoidean** \-hī·oi′dē·ən\ INFRAHYOID.
**subicteric** \-ikter′ik\ [SUB- + ICTERIC] **1** Characterized by bilirubinemia too slight for jaundice to be apparent. **2** Very slightly jaundiced.
**subicular** \subik′yələr\ Pertaining to the subiculum cornu ammonis.
**subiculum** \səbik′yələm\ [L (dim. of *subex*, gen. *subicis*, support, from *subjicere* to throw, set, or place under, from SUB- + L *iacere* to throw, hurl), a support] An underlying or supporting structure. **s. cornu ammonis** The superior portion of the parahippocampal gyrus, adjacent to the hippocampal fissure and contiguous with the hippocampal fields, or cornu ammonis. Also *subiculum hippocampi*. **s. hippocampi** SUBICULUM CORNU AMMONIS. **s. promontorii cavi tympani** SUBICULUM PROMONTORII CAVITATIS TYMPANICAE. **s. promontorii cavitatis tympanicae** [NA] A smooth projection posterior to the promontory on the medial wall of the tympanic cavity and forming the lower border of the tympanic sinus. Also *subiculum promontorii cavi tympani, subiculum of promontory of tympanic cavity, support of the promontory.*
**subiliac** \-il′ē·ak\ **1** Below the ilium. **2** Of or pertaining to the subilium.
**subilium** \-il′ē·əm\ The lowest part of the ilium. *Outmoded.*
**subintern** \-in′tərn\ A medical student in the fourth and final year of medical school, which typically involves performing clinical duties in a hospital. A term used only in the U.S. ● In New Zealand, *student intern* is sometimes used with this meaning.
**subinvolution** \-in′vəloo′shən\ [SUB- + INVOLUTION] Failure of the postpartum uterus to return to its normal size before the pregnancy. **chronic s. of uterus** Failure of the uterus to return to its normal nonpregnant size after pregnancy. The uterus may remain symmetrically enlarged for prolonged periods of time and the woman may experience menorrhagia.
**subjacent** \-jā′sənt\ Underlying; situated directly beneath.
**subject** A person or animal that undergoes observation, treatment, experimentation, or dissection.
**subjective** \-jek′tiv\ [Med L *subjectivus* (from L *subjectus*, past part. of *subicere* or *subjicere* to throw or place under, + *-ivus* -IVE) brought under] Designating those psychological processes that are dependent on the experience of an individual subject and that are not directly observable by others.
**subjee** \sub′jē\ MARIHUANA.
**subkingdom** A category in biological taxonomy that is used, when appropriate, to subdivide a kingdom into groups within which phyla are more closely related among themselves than to other phyla of the kingdom.
**sublabial** \-lā′bē·əl\ Beneath the lip, usually the upper lip.
**sublatio** \-lā′shō\ [L, from *sublatus*, past part. of *tollere* to raise, carry away] SUBLATION. **s. retinae** RETINAL DETACHMENT.
**sublation** \-lā′shən\ [L *sublatio*. See SUBLATIO.] The detachment or elevation of a part from the whole. Also *sublatio.*
**sublimate** \sub′limāt\ [L *sublimatus* (past part. of *sublimare* to raise up, from *sublimis* high, lifted up, lofty) raised up] **1** The solid formed from vapor produced directly from a solid without passing through a liquid phase. **2** To undergo or cause to undergo sublimation. Also *sublime.* **corrosive s.** MERCURIC CHLORIDE.
**sublimation** \sub′limā′shən\ [*sublimat(e)* + -ION] **1** The process of forming a vapor from a solid without melting of the solid, sometimes also including the further condensation of the vapor to form a solid again. **2** The unconscious process of deflecting an instinct or drive into acceptable channels so that discharge is possible, avoiding the repression of instinctual impulse, typically occurring in association with defense mechanisms. In psychoanalytic terms, ego assists id rather than opposes it in expressing impulse.
**sublime** \səblīm′\ SUBLIMATE.
**subliminal** \-lim′inəl\ Below the limen, or absolute threshold, of a sensation or perception, used especially of situations in which the presentation of a known stimulus is not sufficient to result in conscious awareness of the stimulus yet influence of some kind on the behavior of the subject can be demonstrated. Also *subthreshold.*
**sublimis** \-lī′mis\ [L (prob. akin to *limen* threshold) high, lofty] Superficialis; superficial.
**subline** \sub′līn′\ A strain of inbred organisms that differs genetically from the parent inbred strain on account of mutation, incomplete inbreeding, or contamination from outcrossing. Also *substrain.*
**sublobe** \sub′lōb′\ Any division of a lobe.
**subluxation** \-luksā′shən\ [SUB- + LUXATION] An incomplete dislocation in which the joint surfaces remain in partial contact. Also *semiluxation, partial dislocation, incomplete dislocation.* **congenital s. of the hip** A congenital partial or recurrent dislocation of the hip. It may be detectable clinically at birth by the Ortolani sign. If untreated the hip may become truly dislocated. See also CONGENITAL DISLOCATION OF THE HIP. **Volkmann s.** A specific knee deformity due to tuberculosis, characterized by flexion contracture, external rotation, valgus deformity, and curvature of the upper tibia.
**submania** \-mā′nē·ə\ HYPOMANIA.
**submaxilla** \-maksil′ə\ *Outmoded* MANDIBULA.
**submaxillary** \-mak′siler′ē\ **1** Below the maxilla. **2** Of or pertaining to the mandible. An outmoded usage.
**submeningeal** \-mənin′jē·əl\ Deep to or beneath the meninges of the brain or spinal cord.
**submetacentric** \-met′əsen′trik\ **1** In cytogenetics, having the centromere somewhat toward one end of the chromosome, but less than in an acrocentric position. The centromeric index is between 25 and 45. **2** A chromosome with a centromere somewhat off-center. In humans, this would include chromosomes of groups B, C, and E.
**submicroscopic** \-mī′krəskäp′ik\ ULTRAMICROSCOPIC.
**submucosa** \-myookō′sə\ TELA SUBMUCOSA.
**submucosal** \-myookō′səl\ Of or pertaining to the tela submucosa.
**subnatant** \-nā′tənt\ **1** Located below or at the bottom of a structure. **2** INFRANATANT.
**subneural** \-n$^y$ʊr′əl\ Deep to or beneath a nerve or some other neural structure, like the subneural course of the popliteal vessels in the popliteal fossa.
**subnotochordal** \-nō′təkôr′dəl\ Lying beneath the notochord.
**subnucleus** \-n$^y$oo′klē·əs\ A smaller group or collection of neuron cell bodies into which a larger nucleus within the central nervous system may be divided. Also *secondary nucleus.*
**subnutrition** \-n$^y$ootrish′ən\ Nutrition that does not provide required nutrients in their optimal amounts, as occurs in obesity or vitamin deficiency states.
**suboperculum** \-ōpur′kyələm\ The region of the cere-

bral cortex lying deep to and concealed by the frontal, frontoparietal, and temporal opercula and corresponding to the insular region, or island of Reil.
**suboptic** \-äp′tik\ **1** Deep to or under the optic nerve. **2** Below or ventral to the orbit.
**suboptimal** \-äp′timəl\ Less than optimal.
**suborbital** \-ôr′bitəl\ INFRAORBITAL.
**suborder** \sub′ôrdər\ A taxonomic assemblage of closely related families within an order.
**suboxidation** \-äk′sidā′shən\ *Rare* HYPOXIA.
**subparalytic** \-par′əlit′ik\ Pertaining to or affected by incomplete paralysis.
**subpatellar** \-pətel′ər\ INFRAPATELLAR.
**subpeduncular** \-pidung′kyələr\ Beneath or under the cerebral or cerebellar pendunces.
**subperiosteal** Beneath the periosteum.
**subperitoneoabdominal** \-per′itənē′ō·abdäm′inəl\ SUBABDOMINOPERITONEAL.
**subpetrosal** \-petrō′səl\ **1** Deep to the petrous portion of the temporal bone. **2** Deep to or under one of the petrosal venous sinuses at the base of the skull.
**subphrenic** \-fren′ik\ Below the diaphragm. Also *subdiaphragmatic.*
**subphylum** \-fī′ləm\ (*pl.* subphyla) The highest taxonomic category within a phylum. It consists of classes among which a phylogenetic relationship below the level of phylum is implied.
**subpial** \-pī′əl\ Located deep to the pia mater of the brain or spinal cord.
**subpituitarism** \-pit^y oo′itərizm\ HYPOPITUITARISM.
**subplacental** \-pləsen′təl\ Lying beneath the placenta within the basal decidua.
**subpleural** \-plŏŏr′əl\ Immediately beneath the pleural membrane.
**subpontile** \-pän′tīl\ SUBPONTINE.
**subpontine** \-pän′tīn\ Deep to (ventral) or below (inferior to) the pons. Also *subpontile.*
**subpopulation** \-päp′yəlā′shən\ A defined fraction of a population. For example, females aged 15–44 years would form a subpopulation both of the population of all females, and of the population of all persons aged 15–44 years.
**subpubic** \-pyoo′bik\ Below the pubic symphysis or arch. Also *infrapubic.*
**subpulmonary** \-pul′məner′ē\ Below the lung: applied, for example, to pleural effusions that accumulate below the lower part of the lung.
**subpyramidal** \-piram′idəl\ Below or deep to any of numerous anatomical structures that are pyramidal in shape, such as the renal pyramids, the pyramid of the vermis in the cerebullum, or the pyramids in the medulla oblongata of the brainstem.
**subretinal** \-ret′inəl\ Located between the retinal rods and cones and the retinal pigment epithelium. • The term *subretinal,* though traditionally used in this sense, is misleading, since the location referred to is not underneath the retina but within it, in the original cavity of the embryonic optic vesicle.
**subrostral** \-räs′trəl\ Deep to or under the rostrum of the corpus callosum or the rostrum of the sphenoid bone.
**subscaphocephaly** \-skaf′ōsef′əlē\ A moderate degree of scaphocephaly.
**subsclerotic** \-sklirät′ik\ Partly sclerosed.
**subscription** The portion of a prescription that explains how the specified ingredients are to be compounded by the pharmacist.
**subserosa** \-sirō′sə\ TELA SUBSEROSA.
**subsigmoid** \-sig′moid\ Below the sigmoid flexure.
**subsonic** \-sän′ik\ Possessing a wave frequency less than that of audible sound.
**subspecies** \sub′spēshēz\ A category in biological taxonomy that is used, when appropriate, to subdivide a species into groups which differ from each other morphologically or in other respects but are fully capable of interbreeding. Sometimes referred to as races or varieties, subspecies are thought to represent a critical evolutionary step toward genetic isolation and speciation.
**subspinous** \-spī′nəs\ INFRASPINOUS.
**subsplenial** \-splē′nē·əl\ Deep to or under the rounded, posteriorly located splenium of the corpus callosum in the cerebrum.

# substance

**substance** [L *substantia.* See SUBSTANTIA.] Any material of a specified nature but of no particular shape or dimensions, as a tissue or a chemical; substantia. **A s.** A ANTIGEN. **acute phase s.** ACUTE PHASE REACTANT. **adamantine s. of tooth** ENAMEL. **agglutinating s.** AGGLUTININ. **anterior perforated s.** SUBSTANTIA PERFORATA ANTERIOR. **anterior-pituitarylike s.** CHORIONIC GONADOTROPIN. **antidiuretic s.** VASOPRESSIN. **anti-immune s.** ANTIANTIBODY. **B s.** B ANTIGEN. **basophil s.** Diffuse masses of material in the cytoplasm of cells which stain with basic dyes in a manner similar to the chromatin material within the nucleus. Examples include the Nissl substance of nerve cells and the endoplasmic reticulum (ergastoplasm) in pancreatic acinar cells. **black s.** SUBSTANTIA NIGRA. **blood group s.** A soluble substance that is the mucopolysaccharide component of an erythrocyte antigen of the ABO blood group. Blood group substances may be found in saliva and other sectetions, and the approximately 80% of people in whose secretions these substances occur are called secretors. **blood group specific s.'s** Polysaccharide material of animal origin with A or B isoagglutinogen or hapten specificity capable of neutralizing *in vivo* or *in vitro* the corresponding human isoagglutinins. **bony s. of tooth** CEMENTUM. **C s.** C ANTIGEN. **cement s.** A substance which surrounds the structural elements of a tissue. *Outmoded.* **central gray s. of cerebrum** SUBSTANTIA GRISEA CENTRALIS CEREBRI. **central intermediate s. of spinal cord** SUBSTANTIA INTERMEDIA CENTRALIS MEDULLAE SPINALIS. **chromidial s.** Iron-containing basophilic granules located in the cytoplasm as tigroid or chromophil bodies. **chromophil s.** A cell substance that is readily stained by cytoplasmic dyes. **compact s. of bones** SUBSTANTIA COMPACTA OSSIUM. **s. content** The amount of substance of a component divided by the mass of the system (mixture), expressed in moles per kilogram (mol/kg). Symbol: $n_c/m_s$ **cortical s. of bones** SUBSTANTIA CORTICALIS OSSIUM. **cortical s. of kidney** *Outmoded* CORTEX RENALIS. **cortical s. of lens** *Outmoded* CORTEX LENTIS. **cortical s. of lymph nodes** CORTEX NODI LYMPHATICI. **depressor s.** A substance which depresses blood pressure. **exophthalmos-producing s.** A material derived from crude extracts of anterior pituitary which induces exophthalmos in experimental animals. It is distinct from thyrotropin. Abbr. EPS **filar s.** RETICULAR SUBSTANCE. **gelatinous s. of spinal cord** SUBSTANTIA GELATINOSA MEDULLAE

SPINALIS ROLANDI. **glandular s. of prostate** PARENCHYMA PROSTATAE. **gray s.** SUBSTANTIA GRISEA. **gray reticular s. of medulla oblongata** SUBSTANTIA RETICULARIS GRISEA MEDULLAE OBLONGATAE. **gray s. of spinal cord** SUBSTANTIA GRISEA MEDULLAE SPINALIS. **ground s.** A secretion of connective tissue cells that forms the intercellular matrix in which the connective tissue cells and fibers are suspended. Also *interstitial substance.* **H s.** H ANTIGEN. **hyaline s.** An amorphous proteinaceous material that accumulates in the walls of arterioles as a result of aging, hypertension, or diabetes mellitus. **I s.** I ANTIGEN. **interfilar s.** HYALOPLASM. **interpeduncular perforated s.** SUBSTANTIA PERFORATA POSTERIOR. **interprismatic s.** The material between the enamel prisms of a tooth. Like the prisms, it is composed of hydroxyapatite crystals set in an organic matrix. **interstitial s.** GROUND SUBSTANCE. **ketogenic s.** Any substance that can be converted into ketone bodies, such as a fatty acid or certain amino acids. **lateral intermediate s. of spinal cord** SUBSTANTIA INTERMEDIA LATERALIS MEDULLAE SPINALIS. **s. of lens** SUBSTANTIA LENTIS. **medullary s.** 1 SUBSTANTIA ALBA. 2 MEDULLA. **medullary s. of bones** BONE MARROW. **medullary s. of kidney** MEDULLA RENALIS. **metachromatic s.** Fine particles in erythrocyte cytoplasm that stain with supravital dyes, including reticular substance and Heinz bodies. **muscular s. of prostate** SUBSTANTIA MUSCULARIS PROSTATAE. **Nissl s.** An aggregate of basophilic material within the cytoplasm of highly active neurons. Electron microscopy shows that this material corresponds to layers of rough endoplasmic reticulum. Also *Nissl bodies, Nissl granules.* **no-threshold s.'s** Substances that, when present in blood in any concentration, are excreted in the urine. Also *no-threshold bodies.* **periventricular gray s.** Neural tissue consisting of diffusely scattered neuronal cell bodies and unmyelinated nerve fibers found deep to the ependymal lining of the ventricular system of the brain. • The term frequently refers to tissue in the diencephalon adjacent to the third ventricle and, in the midbrain and pons, tissue surrounding the cerebral aqueduct, but it is also used for neural tissue immediately subjacent to the fourth ventricle in the medulla oblongata. **posterior perforated s.** SUBSTANTIA PERFORATA POSTERIOR. **pressor s.** A substance which increases blood pressure. **preventive s.** *Outmoded* ANTIBODY. **proper s. of choroid** SUBSTANTIA PROPRIA CHOROIDEAE. **proper s. of cornea** SUBSTANTIA PROPRIA CORNEAE. **proper s. of sclera** SUBSTANTIA PROPRIA SCLERAE. **red medullary s. of bones** RED BONE MARROW. **red s. of spleen** SPLENIC RED PULP. **Reichert s.** SUBSTANTIA INNOMINATA. **released s.** H ANTIGEN. **reticular s.** 1 A filamentous network seen in early erythrocytes that have been stained with a metachromatic stain such as methylene blue or crystal violet. The reticular substance is composed of ribosomes that are still functioning at this reticulocyte stage of erythrocytes. Also *Isaac's granules, filar substance, substantia metachromaticogranularis, pseudostructure.* 2 FORMATIO RETICULARIS. **Rolando's gelatinous s.** SUBSTANTIA GELATINOSA MEDULLAE SPINALIS ROLANDI. **rostral perforated s.** SUBSTANTIA PERFORATA ANTERIOR. **Schwann's white s.** SUBSTANTIA ALBA. **s. sensibilisatrice** ANTIBODY. **sensitizing s.** ANTIBODY. **slow reacting s. of anaphylaxis** See under LEUKOTRIENES. Abbr. SRS-A **specific capsular s.** The type-specific capsular polysaccharide of pneumococci. *Outmoded.* Also *capsular antigen, capsular polysaccharide.* **spongy s. of bones** SUBSTANTIA SPONGIOSA OSSIUM. **threshold s.'s** Substances that, when present in blood, appear in urine only when they exceed certain concentrations (thresholds). Also *threshold bodies.* **transmitter s.** NEUROTRANSMITTER. **white s.** SUBSTANTIA ALBA. **white reticular s.** SUBSTANTIA RETICULARIS ALBA. **white s. of spinal cord** SUBSTANTIA ALBA MEDULLAE SPINALIS. **yellow medullary s. of bones** YELLOW BONE MARROW.

**substantia** \-stan′shē-ə\ [L (from *substans*, gen. *substantis*, pres. part. of *substare* to stand firm, resist, from SUB- + L *stare* to stand, + -IA), substance, essence, being] The material of which anything is composed; tissue; substance. **s. alba** [NA] The white matter of the central nervous system, consisting principally of nerve fibers surrounded by myelin sheaths. Also *Schwann's white substance, white matter, white substance, medullary substance, medullary white matter.* **s. alba medullae spinalis** [NA] The longitudinal bundles of myelinated fibers coursing in the posterior, lateral, and anterior white columns of the spinal cord. Also *white substance of spinal cord.* **s. cinerea** SUBSTANTIA GRISEA. **s. compacta ossium** [NA] The dense ivory-like outer layers of a mature bone, covered externally by periosteum except at the articular ends and surrounding the spongy bone internally. It is porous, with small spaces between a considerable amount of solid matter that consists mainly of irregular cylindrical units or secondary osteons. Also *compact bone, solid bone, compact substance of bones.* **s. corticalis cerebelli** CORTEX CEREBELLI. **s. corticalis cerebri** CORTEX CEREBRI. **s. corticalis lentis** *Outmoded* CORTEX LENTIS. **s. corticalis lymphoglandulae** CORTEX NODI LYMPHATICI. **s. corticalis ossium** [NA] The superficial, external layer of compact bone, composed of circumferential lamellae and in contact with the periosteum. Also *cortical bone, cortical substance of bones.* **s. ferruginea** LOCUS CERULEUS. **s. gelatinosa** See under SUBSTANTIA GELATINOSA MEDULLAE SPINALIS ROLANDI. **s. gelatinosa centralis** [NA] A subependymal matrix of tissue that surrounds the central canal of the spinal cord, consisting principally of neuroglial cells, many of which are fibrous astrocytes. Also *substantia gliosa centralis.* **s. gelatinosa columnae posterioris** SUBSTANTIA GELATINOSA MEDULLAE SPINALIS ROLANDI. **s. gelatinosa medullae spinalis Rolandi** The gelatinous substance of the spinal cord (of Rolando). Previously defined as the most dorsal portion of the posterior gray horn of the spinal cord, it is now considered to be lamina II (of Rexed) and, by some authors, part or all of lamina III. Lamina II consists of tightly packed, small neurons, whereas lamina III contains larger, less tightly packed nerve cells. These two laminae, along with laminae I and IV, are known to be the principal receiving zones in the spinal cord for cutaneous exteroceptive primary afferent fibers. Also *gelatinous substance of spinal cord, Rolando's gelatinous substance, substantia rolandi, substantia gelatinosa columnae posterioris.* **s. glandularis prostatae** *Outmoded* PARENCHYMA PROSTATAE. **s. gliosa centralis** SUBSTANTIA GELATINOSA CENTRALIS. **s. grisea** [NA] The gray substance of the brain and spinal cord. It is composed principally of neuronal cell bodies, unmyelinated and lightly myelinated nerve fibers and collaterals, dendritic processes, neuroglial cells, and capillaries. Also *gray matter, gray substance, gray, substantia cinerea, cinerea.* **s. grisea centralis** SUBSTANTIA GRISEA CENTRALIS CEREBRI. **s. grisea centralis cerebri** [NA] The central gray substance of the cerebrum, especially the central gray matter of the mesencephalon that surrounds the cerebral aqueduct. Also *central gray substance of cerebrum, stratum griseum centrale cerebri, central gray, substantia grisea centralis, periaqueductal gray.* **s. grisea centralis medullae spinalis** SUBSTANTIA INTERMEDIA CENTRALIS MEDULLAE SPINALIS. **s. grisea medullae spinalis** [NA] Centrally placed continuous columns of gray matter throughout the length of the spinal cord that in cross section have the form of the letter H. In each lateral half of the cord the gray substance forms a dorsal and a ventral gray column, while in the thoracic segments there projects from the ventral column an additional triangular mass of gray substance known as the lateral column. Also *gray matter of spinal cord, gray substance of spinal cord, gray nucleus, substantia spongiosa medullae spinalis.* **s. innominata** A gray mass of neural tissue, located ventral to the lenticular nucleus and ansa lenticularis, that in large part consists of islands of large multipolar neurons forming the basal nucleus of Meynert. Its rostral part lies deep to the cortex of the anterior perforated substance. Also *Reichert substance.* **s. intermedia centralis medullae spinalis** [NA] The gray matter surrounding the central canal and extending laterally to become continuous with the substantia intermedia lateralis medullae spinalis. It forms lamina X of Rexed and contains the dorsal and ventral gray commissures and the substantia gelatinosa centralis. Also *substantia grisea centralis medullae spinalis, central intermediate substance of spinal cord, Kölliker's nucleus.* **s. intermedia lateralis medullae spinalis** [NA] Gray matter in the spinal cord that extends between the substantia intermedia centralis medullae spinalis medially and the gray substance of the dorsal and ventral horns laterally. It conforms primarily to the inner part of lamina VII of Rexed, and contains small tightly packed cells in its medial part and larger more loosely packed neurons in its lateral part. From its most lateral region in the thoracic segments extends the lateral horn. Also *lateral intermediate substance of spinal cord.* **s. lentis** [NA] The bulk of the structure of the lens of the eye, which is enclosed within the lens epithelium and the lens capsule and subdivided into the cortex and the nucleus of the lens. The basic structural unit consists of ribbonlike fibers arranged in laminae. Also *substance of lens, parenchyma of lens.* **s. medullaris glandulae suprarenalis** *Outmoded* MEDULLA GLANDULAE SUPRARENALIS. **s. medullaris lymphoglandulae** MEDULLA NODI LYMPHATICI. **s. medullaris renis** *Outmoded* MEDULLA RENALIS. **s. metachromaticogranularis** RETICULAR SUBSTANCE. **s. muscularis prostatae** [NA] The muscular tissue forming the major component of the stroma of the prostate, the connective tissue only forming a thin network for the nerves and vessels and connecting the glands. The muscle fibers are circular and dense around the periphery within the capsule and around the prostatic urethra. Also *muscular substance of prostate.* **s. nigra** [NA] A broad layer of gray matter containing darkly pigmented nerve cells and found bilaterally throughout the entire length of the mesencephalon. This large nuclear mass is interposed between the crus cerebri and the midbrain tegmentum of the cerebral peduncle, and consists of a dorsal compact black zone in which the neurons contain melanin and a ventral more diffuse reddish brown reticular zone in which the nerve cells are rich in iron but do not contain melanin. The substantia nigra receives many afferent fibers from the caudate nucleus and putamen, and its efferent projections course to the striatum and certain thalamic nuclei. Its neurons are believed to synthesize dopamine, which is then transported to other forebrain sites. Also *locus niger, body of Vicq d'Azyr, black substance.* **s. ossea dentis** CEMENTUM. **s. perforata** The anterior perforated space on the basal surface of the frontal lobe of the cerebrum. The perforations are sites of vascular invasion. Also *area perforata.* **s. perforata anterior** [NA] A diamond-shaped region of gray matter visible bilaterally on the ventral surface of the basal forebrain and located behind the olfactory trigone, between the optic tract and the lateral olfactory stria and in front of the gyrus semilunaris. It consists of an external plexiform layer of neurons, a pyramidal layer, and a polymorph layer of nerve cells within which are scattered groups of neurons called the islands of Calleja. Its surface is perforated by many small blood vessels that branch from the anterior and middle cerebral arteries. Also *anterior perforated space, locus perforatus anticus, anterior perforated substance, rostral perforated substance, substantia perforata rostralis.* **s. perforata posterior** [NA] A triangular region of gray substance in the floor of the interpeduncular fossa, located on the ventral surface of the most rostral part of the midbrain between the cerebral peduncles, in front of the roots of the oculomotor nerves, and behind the mamillary bodies. It is pierced by many fine branches from the posterior communicating arteries and the proximal portions of the posterior cerebral arteries. Also *posterior perforated substance, posterior perforated space, pons tarini, locus perforatus posticus, interpeduncular perforated substance.* **s. perforata rostralis** SUBSTANTIA PERFORATA ANTERIOR. **s. propria choroideae** [NA] The choroid of the eye internal to the suprachoroid lamina. It consists of three layers, the outermost being the lamina vasculosa, then the lamina choroidocapillaris, and the innermost being the complexus basalis. Also *choroid proper, proper substance of choroid.* **s. propria corneae** [NA] The transparent, fibrous, and tough layer of the cornea lying between the anterior limiting membrane of Bowman and the posterior limiting lamina of Descemet. It forms the bulk of the cornea and consists of many superimposed thin lamellae composed of modified connective tissue. Also *proper substance of cornea, stroma of cornea, mesocornea* (outmoded). **s. propria sclerae** [NA] The structural mass of the sclera of the eye, composed of dense, flattened bundles of white fibrous tissue with intermingling fine elastic fibers. Between the fibers are spaces containing connective tissue cells, some of which are pigmented. It contains scant vessels and branches of the ciliary nerves. Also *proper substance of sclera.* **s. reticularis** FORMATIO RETICULARIS. **s. reticularis alba** The longitudinally and transversely oriented fascicles of myelinated nerve fibers in the medial portion of the reticular formation of the medulla oblongata and pons, located dorsal to the pyramids and on either side of the midline raphe. Also *white reticular substance.* **s. reticularis alba gyri fornicati Arnoldi** A delicate reticular layer of mixed gray and white matter on the external (medial) surface of the hippocampal gyrus at the portion that adjoins the dentate gyrus. **s. reticularis alba medullae oblongatae** The medial part of the reticular formation on either side of the midline raphe in the medulla oblongata. It contains many fascicles of myelinated nerve fibers and is nearly devoid of neuron cell bodies. Also *white reticular formation.* **s. reticularis grisea medullae oblongatae** The more laterally located portion of the reticular formation in the medulla oblongata, found dorsal to the olive and composed primarily of gray substance. Also *gray reticular substance of medulla oblongata.* **s. rolandi** SUBSTANTIA GELATINOSA MEDULLAE SPINALIS ROLANDI. **s. spongiosa medullae spinalis** SUBSTANTIA GRISEA MEDULLAE SPINALIS. **s. spongiosa ossium** [NA] The meshwork of bony trabeculae within which are large and small intercommunicating spaces and around which is compact bone. In contrast to the latter, the solid matter is sparse while the spaces are large and numerous, presenting the appearance of a latticework. The spaces are filled with marrow and they communicate with the central marrow cavity. Also *spongy substance of bones, spongy bone, cancellous bone, trabecular bone, spongiosa.*

**substantiae** \-stan′shi·ē\ Plural of SUBSTANTIA.

**substernomastoid** \-stur′nōmas′toid\ Located beneath the sternocleidomastoid muscle.

**substituent** \substich′oo·ənt\ [L *substituens,* gen. *substituentis,* pres. part. of *substituere* to place under, substitute] Any group in a molecule that is introduced in place of another group. The hydroxyl group of ethanol, for example, may be regarded as a substituent of the ethane molecule.

**substitute** [L *substitutus* (past part. of *substituere* to put in the place of, from SUB- + L *statuere* to cause to stand, put, place, from *stare* to stand) made subject, put in the place of another] Something that can take the place of another. **blood s.** A sterile synthetic liquid suitable for intravenous infusion and which has the capacity to convey oxygen from the lungs to the tissues. **plasma s.** PLASMA VOLUME EXPANDER.

**substitution** [Late L *substitutio* (from *substitutus;* see SUBSTITUTE) a substitution] The process of replacement of one group in a molecule by another. **creeping s. of bone** The revascularization of bone and the deposition of new bone by osteoblastic activity that follows a disruption of the blood supply to the bone and necrosis of the bony trabeculae. **gene s.** The replacement of one allele with another, whether by natural or experimental means.

**substrain** \sub′strān\ SUBLINE.

**substrate** \sub′strāt\ [L *substratum.* See SUBSTRATUM.] Any reactant in an enzyme-catalyzed reaction.

**substratum** \-strā′təm\ [L (from *sub-* under + *stratum* layer) an underlying or background layer] A layer or part below another; a foundation.

**substructure** \-struk′chər\ A structure or part acting as an underlying support for another or for an organ; a foundation. **implant s.** IMPLANT INFRASTRUCTURE.

**subsulcus** \-sul′kəs\ A sulcus of the cerebral cortex hidden within the fold of a more superficial sulcus.

**subsylvian** \sil′vē·ən\ Located beneath or inferior to the lateral sulcus (sylvian fissure).

**subsynaptic** \-sinap′tik\ Denoting structures on the postsynaptic side of a synapse, such as the postsynaptic filamentous meshwork called the subsynaptic web.

**subtelocentric** \-tel′əsen′trik\ ACROCENTRIC.

**subtemporal** \-tem′pərəl\ **1** Beneath the temporal bone. **2** Below or in the lower part of the temporal lobe of the brain.

**subtertian** \-tur′shən\ Tending to be less regular and less distinct than tertian: said of a pattern of malarial fever, or a cycle of sporulation of the malarial parasite, that is characteristic of falciparum malaria.

**subthalamic** \-thalam′ik\ Denoting the subthalamus or structures and sites located ventral to or below the thalamus.

**subthalamus** \-thal′əməs\ THALAMUS VENTRALIS.

**subthreshold** \-thresh′ōld\ SUBLIMINAL.

**subthyroidism** \-thī′roidizm\ HYPOTHYROIDISM.

**subtilin** An antibiotic obtained from *Bacillus subtilis,* which is effective against Gram-positive bacteria, the tubercle bacillus, and other organisms.

**subtilisin** The proteolytic enzyme (EC 3.4.21.14) obtained from *Bacillus subtilis.* It is a serine proteinase and is used in studies of protein structure. Also *nagarse.*

**subtotal** Somewhat less than total; not quite complete.

**subtrigonal** \-trig′ənəl\ Located beneath the trigone of the urinary bladder.

**subtypical** \-tip′ikəl\ Not entirely typical.

**subungual** \-ung′gwəl\ Beneath the nail.

**subunit** Any recognizable unit in a molecule that is smaller than the whole molecule. In protein chemistry this usually refers to a single polypeptide chain, often capable of dissociating under some conditions from the others present in the molecule. **catalytic s.** The subunit responsible for catalysis in an enzyme molecule in which different types of subunit are responsible for catalytic activity and for the binding of effectors that regulate that activity. **regulatory s.** The subunit responsible for regulation of enzymatic activity in an enzyme molecule in which different types of subunit are responsible for catalytic activity and for the binding of effectors that regulate that activity.

**subvaginal** \-vaj′ənəl\ **1** Situated below the vagina. **2** Situated beneath a sheath.

**subvertebral** \-vur′təbrəl\ **1** Situated below (in quadrupeds) or anterior to the vertebral column. **2** Situated below a vertebra.

**subviral** \-vī′rəl\ Not constituting a whole virus: usually said of structural components of a virus such as a protein.

**subvitaminosis** \-vī′təminō′sis\ Any disease brought about by a vitamin deficiency, such as scurvy.

**subvolution** \-vəloo′shən\ [SUB- + *(in)volution*] The turning over or inversion of a tissue flap so as to prevent adhesion. The technique is used especially in the inversion of the mucous membrane in the correction of pterygium.

**suc-** \suk-, sək-\ SUB-.

**succagogue** \suk′əgäg\ SECRETAGOGUE.

**succedaneous** \suksədā′nē·əs\ Replacing or acting as a substitute.

**succenturiate** \suk′səntʸoo′rē·āt\ Being or functioning as a substitute; accessory.

**succession** [L *successio* (from *succedere* to undertake, succeed, come after, from SUC- + *cedere* to go, come, give way, cede) a succession, following] The act or process of following sequentially.

**succinate** Any anion, ester, or salt of succinic acid.

**succinate dehydrogenase** The enzyme (EC 1.3.99.1) that catalyzes the oxidation of succinate to fumarate in the citric acid cycle. It is a flavoprotein, contains iron, and uses ubiquinone or cytochrome b as hydrogen acceptor. Also *fumaric hydrogenase* (outmoded).

**succinylcholine chloride** $C_{21}H_{22}N_2O_2$. Succinyldicholine. A muscle-relaxant drug that blocks transmission at the myoneural junction. It is used as an adjunct agent during surgical anesthesia and during electroshock therapy.

**succinyl-CoA** Coenzyme A with its thiol group acylated by succinate. It is an intermediate in the citric acid cycle, being formed by the 2-oxoglutarate dehydrogenase complex.

**succinyl-CoA synthetase** Succinate-CoA ligase. One of the two enzymes (EC 6.2.1.4 and EC 6.2.1.5) that catalyze the formation of succinyl-CoA from succinate and coenzyme A with the concomitant hydrolysis of GTP or ATP respectively to orthophosphate and GDP or ADP. It operates in the reverse direction in the citric acid cycle.

**succinylsulfathiazole** $C_{13}H_{13}N_3O_5S_2{\cdot}H_2O$. A poorly absorbed sulfonamide antibiotic used in the treatment of infections of the gastrointestinal tract, and to prepare the intestinal tract for surgery. Its antibiotic activity is due to the slow release of sulfathiazole by hydrolysis.

**succorrhea** \suk′ôrē′ə\ [L *succ(us)* juice, sap + *o* + -RRHEA] An excessive secretory flow of fluid.

**succulence** \suk′yələns\ The appearance of being juicy: said of a part swollen with fluid.

**succus** \suk′əs\ [L (pref. *sucus*; akin to *sugere* to suck, imbibe) juice, sap, potion, ointment] A fluid secretion produced by a tissue or gland of the body. Also *juice*. **s. cerasi** Cherry juice. **s. entericus** INTESTINAL JUICE. **s. gastricus** GASTRIC JUICE. **s. pancreaticus** PANCREATIC JUICE. **s. prostaticus** The fluid secreted by the prostate gland. Also *liquor prostaticus*. **s. rubi idaei** Raspberry juice.

**succussion** \səkush′ən\ [L *succussio* (from *succutere* to shake, jolt, from *sub-* underneath + *quatere* to shake, cause to tremble) a shock, quake] The procedure of shaking the patient's body to produce the sound of splashing, which is heard if fluid and gas are both present in a hollow organ or body cavity. **hippocratic s.** Succussion in which a splashing sound is heard in the thorax, as with hydropneumothorax, or in the abdomen, as with a dilated stomach.

**suckle** \suk′əl\ [Middle English *sokelen*, prob. back-formation from *sokelynge* (from *suken* to suck, from Old English *sucan* to suck + Middle English *-lenge* English *-ling*, diminishing suffix) suckling] **1** To nourish by giving milk from the breast or udder. **2** To draw milk from the breast or udder.

**suckling** \suk′ling\ [See SUCKLE.] An animal that derives its nourishment wholly from milk from the breast or bottle; a baby or other animal that has not been weaned.

**Sucquet** [J. P. *Sucquet*, French anatomist, 1840–1870] Sucquet-Hoyer anastomosis. See under SUCQUET-HOYER CANAL.

**sucrase** Any enzyme that hydrolyzes sucrose.

**sucrose** \soo′krōs\ [French *sucr(e)* sugar + -OSE[2]] The nonreducing disaccharide whose molecules consist of an oxygen atom carrying both an $\alpha$-glucopyranosyl group and a $\beta$-fructofuranosyl group. It is the commonest sweetening agent used in foods, whose taste and texture it enhances. It is derived commercially from sugar cane and from sugar beet. Plants biosynthesize it by glucosylation of fructose 6-phosphate with UDPglucose and subsequent hydrolysis of the sucrose phosphate. It is hydrolyzed to glucose and fructose by $\beta$-fructofuranosidase during mammalian digestion. It is used in biochemical investigations in producing density gradients, as for centrifugation.

**sucrosemia** \soo′krəsē′mē·ə\ The presence of sucrose in the blood.

**sucrose polyester** A synthetic nondigestible fat substitute marketed as an aid to weight reduction. It is similar in taste to corn oil. It is used as a replacement for up to 900 calories of fat in the diet. Theoretically it could reduce daily caloric intake significantly. Long-term effects of using these compounds are unknown.

**sucrosuria** \soo′krəsoo′rē·ə\ [*sucros(e)* + -URIA] An extremely rare condition in which sucrose in food after alimentary absorption is excreted in the urine. A high concentration of sucrose in the urine may lead to polyuria due to osmosis, which may be complicated by dehydration and polydipsia. It thus resembles diabetes mellitus but otherwise is of no clinical significance.

**suction** [Late L *suctio* (from L *suctus*, past part. of *sugere* to suck, imbibe) a sucking, suction] The application of negative pressure, as for aspiration. **post-tussive s.** An abnormal sucking sound heard immediately after a cough on auscultation over a cavity that communicates with a bronchus. **wall s.** A mechanical device built into a wall, as plumbing, that allows attachment of hoses for aspiration of gas or fluids by means of exerting negative pressure or vacuum on a body cavity or drainage space.

**suctorial** \suktôr′ē·əl\ Adapted for or related to sucking.

**sudamen** \soodā′mən\ [New L, from L *sudare* to sweat] (*pl.* sudamina) A minute vesicle formed at a sweat pore, as in miliaria crystallina.

**sudamina** \soodam′inə\ **1** Plural of SUDAMEN. **2** MILIARIA CRYSTALLINA.

**Sudan** \soodan′\ Any of a group of azo dyestuffs that are soluble in hydrocarbons and insoluble in water. They are used in histologic preparations to stain fats and industrially to color oils and waxes. **S. III** OIL RED O. **S. IV** $C_{24}H_{20}N_4O$. A $\beta$-naphthol diazo dye similar to Sudan III except that its dimethyl formula gives it more intense staining properties. It is often used to stain fats in tissue sections. Also *scharlach R, scarlet red* (ambiguous), *scarlet R* (ambiguous). **S. G** OIL RED O.

**sudanophil** \soodan′əfil\ Any fat-containing material that combines with Sudan dyes.

**sudanophilia** \soodan′əfil′yə\ The property of readily combining with Sudan dyes, thus indicating the presence of fats.

**sudatory** \soo′dətôr′ē\ **1** Causing sweating. **2** A substance that causes sweating.

**Sudeck** [Paul Hermann Martin *Sudeck*, German surgeon, 1866–1938] **1** Sudeck's critical point. See under POINT OF SUDECK. **2** Sudeck-Leriche syndrome, Sudeck's disease, Sudeck's atrophy. See under POST-TRAUMATIC OSTEOPOROSIS.

**sudogram** \soo′dəgram\ [L *sudo(r)* sweat, toil + -GRAM] A graphic record of those areas of skin that exhibit sweating.

**sudomotor** \soo′dōmō′tər\ [L *sudo(r)* sweat, toil + MOTOR] **1** Stimulating sweating. **2** Of or relating to the nervous stimulation of sweating.

**sudor** \soo′dôr\ [L (akin to Gk *hidrōs* sweat), sweat, toil] SWEAT. **s. cruentus** *Obs.* HEMATIDROSIS. **s. sanguineus** *Obs.* HEMATIDROSIS.

**sudor-** \soo′dər-\ [L *sudor* sweat] A combining form meaning sweat.

**sudoral** \soo′dərəl\ [L *sudor* sweat, toil + -AL] Of or relating to sweat.

**sudorific** \soo′dərif′ik\ [L *sudor*, gen. *sudoris*, sweat, toil + -FIC] Producing sweat. Also *diaphoretic*.

**sudorometer** \soo′dəräm′ətər\ [L *sudor* sweat, toil + *o* + -METER] An instrument used for the detection of sweating.

**suet** [prob. Anglo-French, from Old French *sue, seu*, from L *sebum* lard, suet, tallow] The fat from the abdominal wall of a ruminant animal, used in ointments and as an emollient. Sheep suet is the form used most commonly used for pharmaceutic preparations. **benzoinated s.** A preparation containing 3% benzoin as a preservative. It is used as an antiseptic ointment base for topical application. Also *sevum benzoinatum*. **prepared s.** Sheep suet that has been processed and partly purified by melting the fat and straining the product.

**suf-** \suf-, səf-\ SUB-.

**suffocant** \suf′əkənt\ [L *suffocans*, gen. *suffocantis*, pres. part. of *suffocare*. See SUFFOCATE.] An agent that prevents breathing.

**suffocate** \suf′əkāt\ [L *suffocat(us)*, past part. of *suffocare* (from *suf-* under + *foces*, also *fauces* gullet, throat) to choke, stifle, suffocate] To prevent, or to be prevented from, breathing, usually by obstruction of the nose, mouth, or trachea.

**suffocation** \suf′əkā′shən\ [L *suffocatio*, from *suffocare*. See SUFFOCATE.] The prevention of breathing, usually from obstruction of the nose, mouth or trachea.

**suffusion** \səfyoo′zhən\ [L *suffusio* (from *suffundere* to spread out, pour out, from *suf-*, up from under + *fundere* to pour) a spreading out, pouring out] **1** The process of spreading fluid or light over a surface. **2** The permeation of fluid through tissue.

**sug-** \sug-, səg-\ SUB-.

**sugar** [Middle English and Middle French *sucre* (from Med L *succarum* sugar, from Old Italian *zucchero* sugar, from Arabic *sukkar* sugar, akin to Gk *sakcharon* sugar) sugar] Any monosaccharide or smaller oligosaccharide. **s. alcohol** Any compound of formula $CH_2OH$—$[CHOH]_n$—$CH_2OH$. Such compounds are made by the reduction of sugars. **blood s.** 1 The glucose present in mammalian blood. 2 The concentration of glucose in the blood, normally about 5mM. **milk s.** *Outmoded* LACTOSE. **reducing s.** A sugar that is capable of acting as a reducing agent in alkaline solution. All simple sugars are reducing sugars, and so are oligosaccharides unless the anomeric carbon atom of every residue is in glycosidic combination. Hence, sucrose is not a reducing sugar, since the anomeric carbon atoms of both its glucose and fructose residues are linked through an oxygen atom. **simple s.** Any sugar of formula H—$[CHOH]_n$—CO—$[CHOH]_m$—H, i.e. a monosaccharide or glycose, in distinction from an oligosaccharide formed by glycosylation of one such sugar by others. For natural sugars, *m* is either zero, in the aldoses, or unity in the ketoses. **starch s.** GLUCOSE.

**suggestibility** \səjes′təbil′itē, səgjes′-\ An openness to suggestion; a state of readiness to accept, without reflection, the opinions or directions of another.

**suggestion** \səjes′chən, səgjes′-\ [L *suggestio* (from *suggerere* to put under, carry, supply, add, from SUG- + L *gerere* to bear, have, do, make, rule) an adding, suggestion] The process of inducing an individual, usually by verbal means, to comply with and to accept uncritically the ideas, beliefs, or decisions of another. **posthypnotic s.** A suggestion given to an individual in the hypnotic state to carry out some act after emerging from the trance, typically after a specified interval or on the occurrence of some signal. There is usually an amnesia for the suggestion and no conscious realization of why the act was performed, with an attempt to rationalize the behavior.

**suggillation** \sug′jilā′shən\ [L *suggillatio*, also *sugillatio* (from *suggillatus, sugillatus*, past part. of *suggillare, sugillare* to beat black and blue) a bruise, a black-and-blue mark on the body] *Obs.* LIVEDO.

**Sugiura** [M. *Sugiura*, Japanese surgeon, flourished 20th century] See under PROCEDURE.

**suicide** \soo′isīd\ [L *sui* of oneself + -CIDE] 1 The intentional taking of one's own life. 2 A person who commits suicide. **immunologic s.** A technique for destroying a subpopulation of lymphocytes reacting with a particular antigen by reacting the whole cell population with highly radioactive antigen. This binds to the antigen receptors on the specifically immune lymphocytes and causes their death. The capacity to respond to that antigen can thus be specifically detected within the cell population.

**suicidology** \soo′isīdäl′əjē\ [*suicid(e)* + *o* + -LOGY] The study of suicide, including its causes and prevention.

**suigenderism** \soo′ijen′dərizm\ [L *sui*, gen. of *suus* one's own + GENDER + -ISM] The normal and usual preference, during childhood and early adolescence, for nonerotic social relationships with persons of one's own gender.

**suit / antiblackout s.** G SUIT. **anti-g s.** G SUIT. **g s.** A suit worn by pilots and air crew and designed to counteract the effects on the body of acceleration. For example, it prevents pooling of blood in the lower half of the body during positive acceleration. Also *anti-g suit, antiblackout suit.* **pressure s.** A suit designed to counter the effects of decreased atmospheric pressure at high altitudes. A partial pressure suit does not completely enclose the body but can exert a pressure on the body trunk in particular, in order to counteract the effects of an increased intrapulmonary pressure. A full, or total, pressure suit completely encloses the body and has a gas pressure above ambient pressure in order to maintain normal body function. **space s.** A pressure suit equipped with life-support apparatus and designed to protect astronauts operating in space outside their transporting vehicle.

**sulcal** \sul′kəl\ Pertaining to a sulcus.

**sulcate** \sul′kāt\ Grooved or furrowed; marked by a sulcus or sulci.

**sulcation** \sulkā′shən\ 1 Formation of ridges and furrows; fluting. 2 The state of being sulcate.

**sulci** \sul′sī\ Plural of SULCUS.

**sulciform** \sul′sifôrm\ Resembling a sulcus.

**sulculus** \sul′kyələs\ (*pl.* sulculi) A small sulcus.

# sulcus

**sulcus** \sul′kəs\ [L (akin to Gk *holkos* a furrow, trace, Gk *helkein* to drag, draw, and Old English *sulh* a plow) a furrow, rut, ditch] (*pl.* sulci) A linear groove, furrow, or shallow depression, especially of the cerebral hemispheres separating the convolutions or gyri; a shallow fissure or cleft. **alveolobuccal s.** ALVEOLOBUCCAL GROOVE. **s. ampullaris** [NA] A transverse groove on the external surface of the ampulla of each semicircular duct, lying opposite the ampullary crest and pierced by the ampullary branch of the vestibular part of the vestibulocochlear nerve. Also *ampullary sulcus.* **angular s.** INCISURA ANGULARIS GASTRICA. **ansate s.** In the carnivore brain, a short mediolaterally oriented sulcus formed by the bifurcation of the anterior end of the marginal gyrus. **anterior calcarine s.** SPLENIAL SULCUS. **anterior intermediate s. of spinal cord** SULCUS INTERMEDIUS ANTERIOR MEDULLAE SPINALIS. **anterior interventricular s.** SULCUS INTERVENTRICULARIS ANTERIOR. **anterior lateral s. of medulla oblongata** SULCUS LATERALIS ANTERIOR MEDULLAE OBLONGATAE. **anterior lateral s. of spinal cord** SULCUS LATERALIS ANTERIOR MEDULLAE SPINALIS. **anterior parolfactory s.** SULCUS PAROLFACTORIUS ANTERIOR. **s. anthelicis transversus** [NA] A transverse groove on the cranial surface of the cartilage of the auricle opposite the inferior crus of the anthelix on the outer surface and separating eminentia conchae from eminentia fossae triangularis. Also *transverse sulcus of anthelix.* **s. aorticus** An arched wide groove above and behind the hilum on the medial surface of the left lung formed by the arch and the descending part of the aorta. *Outmoded.* Also *aortic sulcus.* **s. arteriae occipitalis** [NA] A shallow linear groove lodging the occipital artery medial to the mastoid notch and posterior to the styloid process on the inferior surface of the petrous part of the temporal bone. Also *sulcus of occipital artery, groove for occipital artery.* **s. arteriae subclaviae** [NA] A shallow groove running obliquely anterolaterally across the superior surface of the first rib posterior to the scalene tubercle and occupied by the subclavian artery. Also *sulcus of subclavian artery.* **s. arteriae temporalis mediae** [NA] A nearly vertical groove for the middle temporal artery extending upwards on the temporal surface of the squama of the temporal bone and above the opening of the external acoustic meatus. Also *sulcus of middle temporal artery, groove for middle temporal* *artery.* **s. arteriae vertebralis atlantis** [NA] A relatively wide groove on the superior surface of the posterior arch of the atlas behind each lateral mass and lodging the vertebral artery and the first cervical spinal nerve. Also *sulcus of vertebral artery of atlas.* **sulci arteriosi** [NA] Grooves on the inner surface of the cranium corresponding to the meningeal arteries and their branches. Also *arterial sulci, arterial grooves.* **s. of auditory tube** SULCUS TUBAE AUDITIVAE. **s. auriculae posterior** [NA] A shallow depression separating the anthelix inferiorly from the antitragus of the ear pinna. Also *posterior sulcus of auricle, posterior auricular groove.* **s. basilaris pontis** [NA] A shallow, longitudinally oriented groove marking the median line of the ventral pons and along which usually courses the basilar artery. The elevations bounding the sulcus on each side are formed by the descending corticospinal tracts. Also *basilar sulcus of pons, basilar groove, sulcus basilaris.* **s. bicipitalis lateralis** [NA] A shallow longitudinal depression on the lateral side of the arm behind the lateral margin of the biceps brachii muscle, extending from the deltoid tuberosity to the cubital fossa. The cephalic vein ascends superficially in the groove. Also *lateral bicipital sulcus, lateral bicipital groove.* **s. bicipitalis medialis** [NA] A marked longitudinal groove located between the contiguous margins of biceps brachii and triceps muscles on the medial side of the arm and between biceps brachii and pronator teres muscles in the cubital fossa. It is occupied by the brachial vessels and the median nerve and it indicates the course of the basilic vein. Also *medial bicipital sulcus, medial bicipital groove.* **s. brevis** Any of several (two to four) short fissures that subdivide the more rostral portion of the insular region of the cerebral cortex into short gyri. Also *sulcus brevis insulae.* **bulboventricular s.** A sulcus on the surface of the embryonic heart which demarcates the primitive ventricular chamber from the bulbus cordis. It marks the site of the developing interventricular septum. **s. calcanei** [NA] A deep depression on the superior surface of the calcaneus, running obliquely mediolaterally between the posterior talar articular facet posteriorly and the middle and anterior talar articular facets anteromedially. In the articulated foot it lies below the sulcus tali, with which it forms the sinus tarsi. Also *calcaneal sulcus, interosseous groove of calcaneus.* **s. calcarinus** [NA] A deep fissure that courses rostrocaudally on the medial surface of the cerebral hemisphere in its lower posterior part. Situated below the splenium of the corpus callosum and ventral to the isthmus of the cingulate gyrus anteriorly, it forms a Y-shaped junction with the parieto-occipital sulcus and continues posteriorly to the occipital pole, separating the cuneus from the lingual gyrus. Also *calcarine sulcus, calcarine fissure, fissura calcarina, postcalcarine sulcus.* **callosal s.** SULCUS CORPORIS CALLOSI. **callosomarginal s.** SULCUS CINGULI. **s. callosus** SULCUS CORPORIS CALLOSI. **s. caroticus ossis sphenoidalis** [NA] A broad curved groove located superior to the junction of each greater wing and the body of the sphenoid bone and containing the internal carotid artery and the cavernous sinus. Also *carotid groove of sphenoid bone, cavernous groove of sphenoid bone.* **s. carpi** [NA] The broad, deep concavity formed by the palmar surfaces of the articulated carpal bones and converted by the flexor retinaculum bridging it into the carpal canal or tunnel through which pass the flexor tendons and the median nerve. Also *carpal sulcus.* **central s. of cerebrum** SULCUS CENTRALIS CEREBRI. **central s. of insula** SULCUS CENTRALIS INSULAE. **s. centralis cerebri** [NA] The central sulcus of the cerebrum, located on the lateral surface of each cerebral hemisphere slightly behind the midpoint between the frontal and occipital poles. It courses obliquely downward and forward from the superior margin of the hemisphere and reaches nearly to the lateral sulcus. It separates the precentral (motor) and postcentral (sensory) gyri, and is frequently considered the boundary between the frontal and parietal lobes. Also *sulcus centralis cerebri rolandi, fissure of Rolando, central sulcus of cerebrum, central fissure, rolandic sulcus.* **s. centralis insulae** [NA] A deep sulcus, visible on the lateral surface of the insula, separating the larger anterior and the smaller posterior insular regions. Anterior to this sulcus are found the gyri breves insulae (short gyri), and posterior to it is the gyrus longus insulae (long gyrus). Also *central sulcus of insula.* **sulci cerebri** [NA] The sulci, or fissures, that separate the gyri of the cerebral cortex. Also *sulci of cerebrum, cerebral sulci, fissures of cerebrum, cerebral fissures.* **s. cinguli** [NA] A curved fissure, visible on the medial surface of the cerebral hemisphere, that circumscribes the gyrus cinguli and follows the same arched course as the sulcus corporis callosi. Anteriorly, the sulcus cinguli commences below the rostrum of the corpus callosum. Successively passing forward, upward, and then backward, it separates the gyrus cinguli below, first from the medial aspect of the superior frontal gyrus and then from the paracentral lobule above. Finally, the sulcus cinguli terminates by coursing dorsally as the marginal sulcus, which reaches the superomedial margin of the cerebral hemisphere. Also *cingulate sulcus, sulcus of cingulum, callosomarginal sulcus, callosomarginal fissure.* **s. circularis insulae** [NA] A groove, actually more triangular in shape than circular, that separates the insula from the surrounding opercular cortices. It nearly encircles the insula, being incomplete frontally. Also *circular sulcus of insula, sulcus circularis Reili, circular sulcus of Reil, Reil sulcus, sulcus limitans insulae.* **s. collateralis** [NA] A longitudinally oriented sulcus that commences near the occipital pole of the cerebral cortex and courses rostrally on the inferior surface of the temporal lobe. It separates the parahippocampal gyrus and its medial extension, the uncus, from the medial occipitotemporal gyrus. More caudally, it is separated from the calcarine sulcus by the lingual gyrus. Also *collateral fissure, fissura collateralis.* **s. coronarius cordis** [NA] A groove on the surface of the heart indicating the separation between the atria and the ventricles, being interrupted anteriorly by the roots of the pulmonary trunk and aorta and lodging the coronary vessels of the heart. Also *coronary sulcus of heart, atrioventricular groove, auriculoventricular groove, atrioventricular furrow.* **s. corporis callosi** [NA] A fissure, visible on the medial surface of the cerebral hemisphere, that separates the corpus callosum from the cingulate gyrus. Anteriorly, the sulcus commences ventral to the rostrum of the corpus callosum and then curves around the dorsal aspect of the callosum. Posteriorly, the sulcus bends around the splenium of the corpus callosum to become continuous with the hippocampal sulcus in the temporal lobe. Also *sulcus callosus, callosal sulcus, sulcus of corpus callosum, callosal fissure.* **s. costae** [NA] A groove above and parallel to the lower border of the internal surface of a rib, extending from the neck to the junction of the middle and anterior thirds of the body of the rib, anterior to which the groove is absent. It lodges the intercostal vessels and nerves. Also *costal sulcus, costal groove, subcostal groove.* **cruciate s.** On the carnivore cerebrum, a major transverse fissure visible on lateral and medial aspects near the frontal pole. It separates the frontal and parietal cortices. Also *crucial sulcus.* **s. cruris helicis** [NA] A depression on the cranial surface of the auricle corresponding to the elevated crus helicis on the lateral surface. Also *sulcus of crus of helix.* **sulci cutis** [NA] Narrow curved grooves between the papillary ridges of the epidermis on the palmar surface of the hand and the plantar surface of the foot and toes. Also *cuticular sulci, skin furrows.* **dorsolateral s.** 1 SULCUS LATERALIS POSTERIOR MEDULLAE SPINALIS. 2 SULCUS LATERALIS POSTERIOR MEDULLAE OBLONGATAE. **s. ethmoidalis ossis nasalis** [NA] A longitudinal groove extending from above downward on the internal surface of the nasal bone and lodging the anterior ethmoidal nerve. Also *ethmoidal sulcus of nasal bone, ethmoidal groove, nasal groove, groove for nasal nerve.* **external spiral s.** SULCUS SPIRALIS EXTERNUS. **fimbriodentate s.** A fissure that separates the notched medial margin of the dentate gyrus from the fimbria of the fornix. **frontal s.** Either of the two sulci that separate the superior, middle, and inferior frontal gyri found in the frontal lobes of the cerebral cortex. See also SULCUS FRONTALIS INFERIOR, SULCUS FRONTALIS SUPERIOR. **s. frontalis inferior** [NA] A groove on the lower lateral aspect of the frontal lobe, directed forward and downward from the lower part of the precentral sulcus and separating the inferior frontal gyrus from the middle frontal gyrus. Also *inferior frontal sulcus, inferofrontal fissure, subfrontal fissure.* **s. frontalis superior** [NA] A groove on the upper lateral aspect of the frontal lobe that courses directly forward from the upper part of the precentral sulcus and separates the superior frontal gyrus from the middle frontal gyrus. Also *superior frontal sulcus.* **gingival s.** The shallow groove between a tooth and the most coronal part of the gingiva, extending from the junctional epithelium (bottom of sulcus) to the gingival margin. Also *gingival crevice.* **gingivobuccal s.** ALVEOLOBUCCAL GROOVE. **gingivolingual s.** ALVEOLINGUAL GROOVE. **s. glutealis** [NA] A transverse groove or crease separating the gluteal region from the upper end of the thigh externally and posteriorly and representing the posterior flexure line of the hip joint. Also *gluteal sulcus, gluteal fold, gluteofemoral crease.* **greater palatine s. of maxilla** SULCUS PALATINUS MAJOR MAXILLAE. **greater palatine s. of palatine bone** SULCUS PALATINUS MAJOR OSSIS PALATINI. **s. of greater petrosal nerve** SULCUS NERVI PETROSI MAJORIS. **s. habenulae** [NA] A small furrow, located on each lateral side of the habenular trigone, that separates the habenula from the pulvinar region of the thalamus. Also *sulcus of habenula.* **s. hamuli pterygoidei** [NA] A groove on the lateral aspect of the pterygoid hamulus around which the tendon of tensor veli palatini muscle moves. Also *sulcus of pterygoid hamulus, hamular groove, hamular notch.* **Harrison s.** HARRISON'S GROOVE. **hemispheric s.** The shallow, almost circular, cleft lying between the developing telencephalon and diencephalon in the embryo. **s. hippocampi** [NA] A shallow groove, the continuation of the sulcus of the corpus callosum, extending from the splenium forward almost to the tip of the temporal lobe. It forms the medial boundary of the parahippocampal gyrus and courses between the subicular extension of that gyrus and the dentate gyrus. Also *hippocampal fissure, fissura hippocampi, hippocampal sulcus, dentate fissure, fissura dentata, fissure of hippocampus.* **s. horizontalis cerebelli** FISSURA HORIZONTALIS CEREBELLI. **s. hypothalamicus** [NA] A shallow longitudinal groove on both lateral walls of the third ventricle, extending from the cerebral aqueduct to the interventricular foramen dividing the diencephalon into two parts. Also *sulcus hypothalamicus Monroi, sulcus of Monro, fissure of Monro.* **inferior frontal s.** SULCUS FRONTALIS INFERIOR. **inferior petrosal s.** SULCUS SINUS PETROSI INFERIORIS. **s. of inferior petrosal sinus** SULCUS SINUS PETROSI INFERIORIS. **inferior temporal s.** SULCUS TEMPORALIS INFERIOR. **s. infraorbitalis maxillae** [NA] A groove passing forward from the lower border of the inferior orbital fissure along the floor of the orbit, burrowing deeper anteriorly to become the infraorbital canal and transmitting the infraorbital nerve and vessels. Also *infraorbital sulcus of maxilla, infraorbital groove of maxilla.* **s. infrapalpebralis** The horizontal skin crease or depression below the lower eyelid. *Outmoded.* Also *infrapalpebral sulcus.* **interatrial s.** 1 A groove which appears on the outer aspect of the common embryonic atrium marking the site of attachment of the septa that will divide the single chamber into left and right atria. 2 INTERATRIAL GROOVE. **s. intermedius anterior medullae spinalis** A shallow, longitudinally oriented groove sometimes seen coursing along the anterior surface of the spinal cord between the anterior median fissure and the anterior lateral sulcus. It is more frequently seen in the fetal and immature spinal cord. Also *anterior intermediate sulcus of spinal cord, anterior paramedian groove of spinal cord.* **s. intermedius posterior medullae spinalis** [NA] A shallow longitudinal groove located on the posterior surface of the spinal cord in the upper thoracic and cervical regions. On each side, it courses in the white matter of the dorsal funiculus, separating the fasciculus gracilis from the fasciculus cuneatus. Also *posterior intermediate sulcus of spinal cord, posterior paramedian groove of spinal cord, paramedian sulcus.* **internal spiral s.** SULCUS SPIRALIS INTERNUS. **s. interparietalis** SULCUS INTRAPARIETALIS. **s. intertubercularis humeri** [NA] A longitudinal groove on the anterior surface of the upper part of the humerus, separating the greater from the lesser tubercle and extending downward with a medial lip along the medial margin of the humerus and a lateral lip along the anterior margin. The groove is occupied by the long head of the biceps brachii. Also *intertubercular sulcus of humerus, intertubercular groove of humerus, bicipital groove of humerus.* **s. interventricularis anterior** [NA] A shallow groove between the right and left ventricles on the sternocostal or anterior surface of the heart extending obliquely from the left margin near the left side of the origin of the pulmonary trunk to the right margin just to the right of the apex forming the incisura apicis cordis and becoming continuous with the posterior interventricular sulcus. It lodges the anterior interventricular branch of the left coronary artery and the great cardiac vein embedded in fat. Also *anterior interventricular sulcus, anterior interventricular groove.* **s. interventricularis posterior** [NA] A shallow groove separating the ventricles on the diaphragmatic or inferior surface of the heart and extending from the incisura apicis cordis, where it is continuous with the anterior interventricular sulcus, to the coronary sulcus. It usually lodges the posterior interventricular branch of the right coronary artery and the middle cardiac vein embedded in fat. Also *posterior interventricular sulcus, posterior interventricular groove.* **s. intraparietalis** [NA] A horizontally oriented sulcus that usually commences near the middle of the postcentral sulcus and courses posteroinferiorly on the upper lateral aspect of the cerebral cortex, dividing the parietal lobe into superior and inferior parietal lobules. Also *sulcus interparietalis, interparietal fissure, Pansch's fissure, Turner's sulcus.* **labiodental s.** A groove which develops on the oral part of the mandibular process and separates the future tooth-bearing part from the lip. **s. lacrimalis maxillae** [NA] A deep groove on the nasal surface of the maxilla lying just anterior to the maxillary sinus and directed posteroinferiorly into the inferior meatus of the nose. It forms the outer two-thirds of the wall of the nasolacrimal canal. Also *lacrimal sulcus of maxilla.* **s. lacrimalis ossis lacrimalis** [NA] A vertical groove anterior to the posterior lacrimal crest on the lateral or orbital surface of the lacrimal bone, its anterior margin articulating with the posterior margin of the frontal process of the maxilla to form the lacrimal sac. Also *lacrimal sulcus of lacrimal bone, groove of lacrimal bone.* **lacrimal s. of maxilla** SULCUS LACRIMALIS MAXILLAE. **lateral bicipital s.** SULCUS BICIPITALIS LATERALIS. **lateral cerebral s.** SULCUS LATERALIS CEREBRI. **s. lateralis anterior medullae oblongatae** A shallow longitudinal groove that courses along the anterolateral surface of the medulla oblongata as far as the pons. It is located lateral to the pyramids on each side, and along this sulcus the rootlets of the hypoglossal nerve emerge from the brain stem. It represents the upward continuation of the anterior lateral sulcus of the spinal cord, along which the ventral rootlets emerge from the anterior horn of the cord. Also *anterior lateral sulcus of medulla oblongata, anterolateral groove of medulla oblongata.* **s. lateralis anterior medullae spinalis** A longitudinal groove on the anterolateral surface of the spinal cord, forming the boundary between the anterior and lateral funiculi, and along which the ventral rootlets emerge from the substance of the spinal cord. Also *anterior lateral sulcus of spinal cord, anterolateral groove of spinal cord.* **s. lateralis cerebri** [NA] A deep groove found on the inferior and lateral surfaces of the cerebral cortex, commencing inferomedially near the anterior perforated substance and coursing anteriorly and then laterally to separate the orbital surface of the frontal lobe from the rostral portion of the temporal lobe. Upon reaching the inferolateral border of the cerebral cortex, it courses superiorly and posteriorly to separate the temporal lobe first from the frontal lobe and then from the parietal lobe. It is the largest of the cerebral sulci, and terminates in two short rami, the ascending and the anterior, which course into the frontal lobe; and one long posterior ramus, which is directed posterosuperiorly above the superior temporal gyrus toward the parietal lobe. Also *lateral cerebral sulcus, fissura cerebri lateralis Sylvii, sylvian fissure, fissure of Sylvius, lateral fissure of cerebrum, lateral cerebral fissure, sylvian fossa, fossa of Sylvius, sulcus Sylvii.* **s. lateralis mesencephali** A longitudinally oriented groove on the lateral aspect of the midbrain marking the boundary between the basal part of the mesencephalon (crus cerebri and substantia nigra) and the midbrain tegmentum. Also *sulcus lateralis pedunculi cerebri, lateral mesencephalic sulcus.* **s. lateralis posterior medullae oblongatae** The rostral extension of the posterior lateral sulcus of the spinal cord along the posterolateral surface of the medulla oblongata. It separates the posterior from the lateral regions of the medulla, and the rootlets of the glossopharyngeal, vagus, and accessory nerves attach to the brain stem in a line along this sulcus. Also *posterior lateral sulcus of medulla oblongata, posterolateral sulcus of medulla oblongata, dorsolateral sulcus.* **s. lateralis posterior medullae spinalis** A longitudinally oriented furrow located on the dorsolateral surface of the spinal cord and separating the posterior and lateral funiculi, or columns. Along this sulcus the dorsal roots of the spinal nerves penetrate and enter the spinal cord. Also *posterior lateral sulcus of spinal cord, posterolateral sulcus of spinal cord, posterolateral groove of spinal cord, dorsolateral sulcus.* **lateral mesencephalic s.** SULCUS LATERALIS MESENCEPHALI. **lateral occipital s.** SULCUS OCCIPITALIS LATERALIS. **s. of lesser petrosal nerve** SULCUS NERVI PETROSI MINORIS. **s. limitans** A longitudinal groove on the ependymal aspect of each lateral wall of the developing neural tube that marks the junction between the alar or dorsal laminae and the basal or ventral laminae. **s. limitans fossae rhomboideae** SULCUS LIMITANS VENTRICULI QUARTI. **s. limitans insulae** SULCUS CIRCULARIS INSULAE. **s. limitans ventriculi quarti** [NA] A prominent longitudinal groove, found bilaterally, extending along the entire length of the floor of the fourth ventricle and forming the lateral boundary of the medial eminence on both sides of the rhomboid fossa. Located lateral to the median sulcus, it is the rostral extension of the sulcus limitans. Also *sulcus limitans fossae rhomboideae.* **s. lunatus** [NA] A short vertical groove located in the cerebral cortex just in front of the occipital pole on the lateral surface of the occipital lobe. It is most commonly found in sub-human primates and only occasionally in the human cerebral cortex. When present, the lunate sulcus indicates the limits of the striate or visual cortex. Also *lunate sulcus, affenspalte, simian fissure* (obs.)*, ape fissure* (obs.). **malleolar s.** SULCUS MALLEOLARIS TIBIAE. **s. malleolaris fibulae** [NA] A broad groove with a prominent lateral edge on the posterior surface of the lateral malleolus of the fibula, which contains the tendons of peroneus longus and brevis muscles. **s. malleolaris tibiae** [NA] A marked vertical groove on the posterior surface of the medial malleolus at its junction with the posterior surface of the tibia which lodges the tendons of tibialis posterior and flexor digitorum longus muscles. Also *malleolar sulcus.* **marginal s.** A fissure that courses dorsally and nearly at a right angle from the sulcus cinguli as the latter reaches approximately the level of the splenium on the medial surface of the cerebral hemisphere. The marginal sulcus achieves the dorsal margin of the hemisphere as a continuation of the sulcus cinguli, and thereby separates the paracentral lobule from the precuneus. **s. matricis unguis** [NA] A crescentic groove produced by an infolding of skin in which the proximal part and sides of the nail are embedded. Also *sulcus of matrix of nail, nail groove.* **medial bicipital s.** SULCUS BICIPITALIS MEDIALIS. **s. medialis cruris cerebri** A longitudinally oriented sulcus found bilaterally along the medial surface of the crus cerebri in the mesencephalon and from which emerge the rootlets of the oculomotor nerve. Also *sulcus medialis mesencephali, sulcus mesencephali medialis, sulcus nervi oculomotorii, sulcus oculomotorius, medial sulcus of crus cerebri.* **median s. of fourth ventricle** SULCUS MEDIANUS VENTRICULI QUARTI. **median s. of tongue** SULCUS MEDIANUS LINGUAE. **s. medianus** FISSURA MEDIANA ANTERIOR MEDULLAE SPINALIS. **s. medianus linguae** [NA] A shallow median depression on the dorsum of the tongue extending from the tip to the foramen cecum. Also *median sulcus of tongue.* **s. medianus posterior medullae oblongatae** [NA] A shallow longitudinal midline groove along the posterior surface of the medulla oblongata continuous with the posterior median sulcus of the spinal cord. It separates the two fasciculi gracili. Also *posterior median sulcus of medulla oblongata, fissura mediana posterior medullae oblongatae, posterior median fissure of medulla oblongata.* **s. medianus posterior medullae spinalis** [NA] A shallow midline longitudinal groove that extends along the entire length of the spinal cord on its dorsal surface. Also *posterior median sulcus of spinal cord, posterior median fissure of spinal cord.* **s. medianus ventriculi quarti** [NA] A longitudinal midline sulcus in the floor of the fourth ventricle bordered on each side by an elevation called the medial eminence. Also *median sulcus of fourth ventricle.* **s. mentolabialis** [NA] A variable depression between the chin and the lower lip. Also *mentolabial sulcus, mentolabial furrow.* **s. mesenceph-**

**ali medialis** SULCUS MEDIALIS CRURIS CEREBRI. **middle frontal s.** An anteroposteriorly oriented sulcus that separates the two convolutions of the middle frontal gyrus in the frontal lobe of the brain. **middle temporal s.** SULCUS TEMPORALIS INFERIOR. **s. of middle temporal artery** SULCUS ARTERIAE TEMPORALIS MEDIAE. **s. of Monro** SULCUS HYPOTHALAMICUS. **s. mylohyoideus mandibulae** [NA] A groove on the medial surface of the mandibular ramus extending downwards and forwards from the mandibular foramen behind the lingula to a point on the mandibular body below the posterior end of the mylohyoid line and transmitting the mylohyoid nerve and vessels. Also *mylohyoid sulcus of mandible, mylohyoid groove.* **nasofrontal s.** The slight furrow between the developing nose and the frontal region in the embryo, marking the site where the root of the bridge of the nose will eventually form. **s. nasolabialis** [NA] A furrow running inferolaterally from the side of the nose to the angle of the mouth on each side, separating the lips from the cheeks. Also *nasolabial sulcus, nasolabial groove, nasolabial fold.* **s. nervi oculomotorii** SULCUS MEDIALIS CRURIS CEREBRI. **s. nervi petrosi majoris** [NA] A groove on the anterior surface of the petrous part of the temporal bone, extending anteromedially from hiatus canalis nervi petrosi majoris located anterior and medial to the arcuate eminence and running towards the foramen lacerum to transmit the greater petrosal nerve. Also *sulcus of greater petrosal nerve, groove of great superficial petrosal nerve.* **s. nervi petrosi minoris** [NA] An inconstant groove on the anterior surface of the petrous part of the temporal bone, extending anteromedially from a hiatus just lateral to the hiatus canalis nervi petrosi majoris toward either the foramen ovale or the canaliculus innominatus, and transmitting the lesser petrosal nerve. Also *sulcus of lesser petrosal nerve, groove of small superficial petrosal nerve.* **s. nervi radialis** [NA] A broad shallow groove commencing at the medial margin of the humerus below the surgical neck and running inferolaterally below the ridge of attachment of the lateral head of the triceps muscle on the posterior surface of the humerus and above the upper level of attachment of the medial head of the triceps muscle. The groove transmits the radial nerve and the profunda brachii vessels. Also *sulcus of radial nerve, radial groove, musculospiral groove, groove for radial nerve, spiral groove.* **s. nervi spinalis** [NA] A groove on the superior surface of the transverse process of the third through the sixth cervical vertebrae, often commencing on the pedicle and extending behind the vertebral artery in the foramen transversarium on to the costotransverse bar. It lodges the cervical spinal nerve corresponding in number to the vertebra. Also *sulcus of spinal nerve.* **s. nervi ulnaris** [NA] A shallow concavity on the posterior surface of the medial epicondyle of the humerus, lodging the ulnar nerve and superior ulnar collateral vessels. Also *sulcus of ulnar nerve, groove of ulnar nerve, ulnar groove.* **nymphocaruncular s.** A crescentic groove between the lateral attachment of the hymen vaginae or carunculae hymenales and the labium minus on each side of the vestibule. It contains the opening of the duct of the greater vestibular gland and occupies the lateral portion of the fossa vestibuli vaginae. **s. obturatorius ossis pubis** [NA] An oblique groove on the obturator or posteroinferior surface of the superior ramus of the pubis where it joins the body of the ilium. It transmits the obturator nerve and vessels. Also *obturator sulcus of pubis, obturator groove, obturator canal of pubic bone.* **s. of occipital artery** SULCUS ARTERIAE OCCIPITALIS. **sulci occipitales superiores** Short inconstant sulci sometimes seen on the superior occipital gyrus. Also *superior occipital sulci.* **s. occipitalis lateralis** A short anteroposteriorly oriented sulcus on the inferolateral surface of the occipital lobe that separates the superior and inferior occipital gyri. Also *lateral occipital sulcus.* **s. occipitalis transversus** [NA] A short sulcus on the lateral aspect of the cerebral cortex, perpendicular to the midline and posterior to the parieto-occipital sulcus in the occipital region. It is joined at about its middle by the intraparietal sulcus, and its superior part forms the posterior limit of the arcus parieto-occipitalis. Also *transverse occipital sulcus, transverse occipital fissure, Ecker's fissure.* **s. occipitotemporalis** [NA] A rostrocaudal sulcus separating the inferior temporal and lateral occipitotemporal gyri. Also *inferior temporal sulcus, sulcus temporalis inferior* (outmoded). **s. oculomotorius** SULCUS MEDIALIS CRURIS CEREBRI. **s. olfactorius lobi frontalis** An anteroposteriorly oriented groove, located on the inferior surface of the frontal lobe, along which courses the olfactory tract. The olfactory sulcus separates the gyrus rectus from the medial orbital gyrus. Also *olfactory sulcus of frontal lobe, olfactory sulcus.* **s. olfactorius nasi** [NA] A narrow groove that ascends from the atrium between the agger nasi and the roof of the nasal cavity to become continuous with the sphenoethmoidal recess. Also *olfactory sulcus of nose, olfactory groove.* **olfactory s.** SULCUS OLFACTORIUS LOBI FRONTALIS. **olfactory s. of frontal lobe** SULCUS OLFACTORIUS LOBI FRONTALIS. **olfactory s. of nose** SULCUS OLFACTORIUS NASI. **orbital s.** In the human brain, any of several irregular sulci on the orbital surface of the frontal lobe that commonly fall into a longitudinally oriented H-shaped pattern. They subdivide the surface into several orbital gyri. **sulci orbitales lobi frontalis** Somewhat irregular sulci on the inferior or orbital, surface of the frontal lobe that frequently form an H-shaped pattern and divide the region lateral to the gyrus rectus into medial, lateral, anterior, and posterior orbital gyri. Also *orbital sulci of frontal lobe.* **sulci palatini maxillae** [NA] Longitudinal grooves on the posteroinferior surface of the palatine process of the maxilla. The grooves, separated by the palatine spines, run near the lateral margins of the palate towards the incisive fossa and transmit the greater palatine nerves and vessels. Also *palatine sulci of maxilla, palatine grooves of maxilla.* **s. palatinus major maxillae** [NA] An oblique groove running anteroinferiorly from the middle of the posterior margin of the nasal surface of the maxilla across the rough surface behind the inferior nasal meatus to the junction of the maxilla's palatine process and the palatine bone. The groove is converted by the apposing sulcus palatinus major ossis palatini into a canal for the passage of the greater palatine nerves and vessels. Also *greater palatine sulcus of maxilla.* **s. palatinus major ossis palatini** [NA] A deep vertical groove on the posterior part of the maxillary surface of the perpendicular plate of the palatine bone, which meets the greater palatine sulcus of the maxilla to form a canal for the passage of the greater palatine nerves and vessels. Also *greater palatine sulcus of palatine bone, pterygopalatine fissure of palatine bone, palatine groove of palatine bone, palatomaxillary groove of palatine bone.* **s. palatovaginalis** [NA] An anteroposterior furrow on the inferior surface of the vaginal process of the medial pterygoid plate of the sphenoid bone. It participates in the formation of the palatovaginal canal. Also *palatovaginal groove, palatovaginal sulcus.* **sulci paracolici** [NA] Longitudinal hollows lateral to the lateral surfaces of the ascending and the descending colon and medial to the posterolateral abdominal wall and lined by the junction of the visceral and parietal peritoneum. Also *paracolic sulci,* *paracolic grooves, paracolic gutters, paracolic recesses* (outmoded). **paraglenoidal sulci** Narrow grooves for the attachment of capsular ligaments which are situated on the margin of an articular surface on certain bones. They are very distinct at the bases of the phalanges and also exist on certain carpal and tarsal bones, on the articular processes of vertebrae as well as around the symphyseal and auricular surfaces of the hip bone. **paramedial s.** An occasionally observed, interrupted, longitudinally oriented furrow that divides the superior frontal gyrus into upper and lower parts. *Seldom used.* **paramedian s.** SULCUS INTERMEDIUS POSTERIOR MEDULLAE SPINALIS. **parasplenial s.** The fissure surrounding the splenium of the corpus callosum. **s. parieto-occipitalis** [NA] A deep groove that commences about 5 cm anterior to the occipital pole near the midline on the superior surface of the cerebral cortex. Initially it courses medially to reach the superior margin of the cerebral hemisphere, and then it takes a vertical course downward on the medial surface of the cortex to join the calcarine sulcus. The parieto-occipital sulcus forms the boundary between the precuneus and cuneus, as well as the boundary between the parietal and occipital lobes. Also *parieto-occipital fissure, fissura parieto-occipitalis.* **s. parolfactorius anterior** A short, vertical groove, located on the medial surface of the cerebral hemisphere below the genu of the corpus callosum, that forms the anterior limit of a small triangular region of cortex, the parolfactory or subcallosal area. It separates the anterior parolfactory gyrus behind from the superior frontal gyrus in front. Also *anterior parolfactory sulcus.* **s. parolfactorius posterior** A shallow, curved sulcus located on the medial surface of the cerebral hemisphere that separates the anterior and posterior parolfactory gyri. At times this sulcus is described as lying between the subcallosal area (anterior parolfactory gyrus) and the paraterminal gyrus (posterior parolfactory gyrus). Also *posterior parolfactory sulcus.* **sulci of pharyngeal tonsil** **1** FOSSULAE TONSILLARES TONSILLAE PHARYNGEALIS. **2** CRYPTAE TONSILLARES TONSILLAE PHARYNGEALIS. **polar s.** One of two sulci (the superior and inferior polar sulci) found on the lateral surface of the occipital lobe near the limits of the lunate sulcus. The polar sulci course upward (superior) and downward (inferior) just rostral to the occipital pole. **pontobulbar s.** A transversely oriented sulcus, clearly visible on the ventral and lateral aspects of the brainstem, that separates the pons rostrally from the medulla oblongata caudally. Also *pontomedullary sulcus.* **pontopeduncular s.** A transversely oriented sulcus, visible on the ventral and ventrolateral aspects of the brainstem, that separates the cerebral peduncles and mesencephalon rostrally from the pons caudally. The oculomotor nerve emerges from the brain stem on the ventral aspect of the pontopeduncular sulcus. Also *pontomesencephalic sulcus.* **postcalcarine s.** SULCUS CALCARINUS. **s. postcentralis** [NA] A nearly vertical sulcus found on the lateral surface of the parietal lobe of the cerebral cortex coursing parallel but posterior to the central sulcus. It forms the posterior boundary of the postcentral gyrus, and separates that gyrus from the rest of the parietal lobe. Also *retrocentral sulcus, postcentral fissure.* **postclival s.** A groove, located on the posterior surface of the cerebellum, that courses transversely across the cerebellar vermis and separates the declive from the folium vermis. It is continuous laterally with the postlunate fissure. **posterior s. of auricle** SULCUS AURICULAE POSTERIOR. **posterior intermediate s. of spinal cord** SULCUS INTERMEDIUS POSTERIOR MEDULLAE SPINALIS. **posterior interventricular s.** SULCUS INTERVENTRICULARIS POSTERIOR. **posterior lateral s. of medulla oblongata** SULCUS LATERALIS POSTERIOR MEDULLAE OBLONGATAE. **posterior lateral s. of spinal cord** SULCUS LATERALIS POSTERIOR MEDULLAE SPINALIS. **posterior median s. of medulla oblongata** SULCUS MEDIANUS POSTERIOR MEDULLAE OBLONGATAE. **posterior median s. of spinal cord** SULCUS MEDIANUS POSTERIOR MEDULLAE SPINALIS. **posterior nasal s.** The shallow vertical furrow delimiting the lateral wall of the nasal cavity posteriorly and extending from the inferior aspect of the body of the sphenoid bone to the junction of the hard and the soft palates. **posterior parolfactory s.** SULCUS PAROLFACTORIUS POSTERIOR. **s. posterolateralis cerebelli** The fissure separating the flocculonodular lobe from the corpus cerebelli. It is the first cerebellar fissure in development. Also *posterolateral fissure.* **posterolateral s. of medulla oblongata** SULCUS LATERALIS POSTERIOR MEDULLAE OBLONGATAE. **posterolateral s. of spinal cord** SULCUS LATERALIS POSTERIOR MEDULLAE SPINALIS. **postnodular s.** A short, transversely oriented fissure, visible on the inferior surface of the cerebellum, that separates the nodulus from the uvula of the inferior vermis. **postolivary s.** A longitudinal groove on the posterolateral surface of the upper medulla oblongata, that represents the rostral continuation of the sulcus lateralis posterior medullae oblongatae. It bounds the prominent oval mass, called the oliva, posterolaterally. **s. praecentralis** SULCUS PRECENTRALIS. **preauricular s.** A short rough groove on the lower part of the pelvic surface of the ilium just below the posteroinferior margin of the auricular surface, usually better marked in the female and providing attachment for part of the ventral sacroiliac ligament. Also *preauricular groove of ilium.* **s. precentralis** [NA] A vertically oriented sulcus, located on the lateral aspect of the cerebral hemisphere, that courses parallel to the central sulcus but in front of the precentral gyrus. It separates the precentral gyrus from the remainder of the frontal lobe. Also *precentral fissure, prerolandic sulcus, vertical sulcus.* Also *sulcus praecentralis.* **s. prechiasmaticus** [NA] A narrow transverse groove on the superior surface of the body of the sphenoid bone that is bounded anteriorly by a ridge and posteriorly by the tuberculum sellae. Laterally, on each side, it is continuous with the optic canal. Also *chiasmatic groove, optic groove.* **preclival s.** A sulcus located on the posterior surface of the cerebellum that courses transversely across the cerebellar vermis and separates the culmen from the declive. It is continuous laterally with the primary fissure. **prelunate s.** An anteroposteriorly oriented sulcus on the lateral surface of the temporal lobe the posterior end of which opens into the lunate sulcus. The prelunate sulcus separates two of the lateral orbital gyri, and at times is continuous rostrally with the superior temporal sulcus. **prenodular s.** A fissure or sulcus in the embryo, separating the vermis from the flocculus on the outer aspect of the cerebellum. **prepyramidal s.** A fissure, located on the anterior surface of the cerebellum, that separates the biventral lobule from the inferior cerebellar lobule. Medially, it continues across the cerebellar vermis to separate the pyramid from the tuber vermis. **prerolandic s.** SULCUS PRECENTRALIS. **s. promontorii cavitatis tympanicae** [NA] A small vertical groove on the promontory on the medial wall of the tympanic cavity which lodges the tympanic branch of the glossopharyngeal nerve. **s. of pterygoid hamulus** SULCUS HAMULI PTERYGOIDEI. **s. pulmonalis thoracis** [NA] The broad, deep longitudinal groove on each side of the vertebral column inside the thoracic cavity that is produced by the posterior curve of the ribs and lodging the posterior part of the lung. Also *pulmonary sulcus of thorax.* **s. of radial nerve** SULCUS NERVI RADIALIS. **Reil s.** SULCUS CIRCULARIS INSULAE. **retrocentral s.** SULCUS POSTCENTRALIS. **rhinal s.** RHINAL FISSURE. **s. rhinalis** [NA] A groove that courses rostrocaudally on the inferior surface of the cerebral hemisphere in line with, and at times continuous with, the collateral sulcus. It separates the temporal pole from the uncus, and thereby forms the lateral limit of the piriform lobe of the cerebral cortex. The rhinal sulcus makes its appearance as early as the second month of prenatal development, and can be seen as a furrow between the developing olfactory lobe and the lateral surface of the pallium. Also *rhinal fissure, rhinal sulcus.* **rolandic s.** SULCUS CENTRALIS CEREBRI. **s. sclerae** A shallow circular groove on the outer surface of the eyeball, located at the junction of the sclera and the cornea and produced because the convexity of the cornea is greater than that of the remainder of the eyeball. Also *scleral sulcus, scleral furrow.* **s. of sigmoid sinus** SULCUS SINUS SIGMOIDEI. **s. of sigmoid sinus of occipital bone** SULCUS SINUS SIGMOIDEI OSSIS OCCIPITALIS. **s. of sigmoid sinus of parietal bone** SULCUS SINUS SIGMOIDEI OSSIS PARIETALIS. **s. of sigmoid sinus of temporal bone** SULCUS SINUS SIGMOIDEI OSSIS TEMPORALIS. **s. sinus petrosi inferioris** [NA] The groove which runs posteriorly between and on the petrous part of the temporal bone and the basilar part of the occipital bone and contains the inferior petrosal sinus commencing anteriorly in the posterolateral angle of the cavernous sinus and ending posteriorly in the superior bulb of the internal jugular vein. Also *sulcus of inferior petrosal sinus, inferior petrosal sulcus.* **s. sinus petrosi superioris** [NA] A linear groove for the superior petrosal sinus extending posterolaterally along the superior margin of the petrous part of the temporal bone from the apex to its junction with the sulcus for the sigmoid sinus where it arises from the transverse sinus. Also *sulcus of superior petrosal sinus.* **s. sinus sagittalis superioris** [NA] A longitudinal groove extending in the median plane along most of the internal surface of the calvaria from a point behind the foramen cecum anteriorly where it grooves the frontal crest, the parietal bones along the sagittal suture, and the squama of the occipital bone as far as the internal occipital protuberance. It lodges the superior sagittal sinus within the falx cerebri, which is attached to the lips of the groove. Also *sulcus of superior sagittal sinus, sagittal groove, groove for superior longitudinal sinus.* **s. sinus sagittalis superioris ossis frontalis** The frontal portion of sulcus sinus sagittalis superioris. Also *sulcus of superior sagittal sinus of frontal bone.* **s. sinus sagittalis superioris ossis occipitalis** The occipital portion of sulcus sinus sagittalis superioris. Also *sulcus of superior sagittal sinus of occipital bone.* **s. sinus sagittalis superioris ossis parietalis** The parietal portion of sulcus sinus sagittalis superioris. Also *sulcus of superior sagittal sinus of parietal bones.* **s. sinus sigmoidei** [NA] The S-shaped continuation of the lateral extremity of the sulcus of the transverse sinus, commencing at the base of the petrous part of the temporal bone where it meets the mastoid angle of the parietal bone and then turning downwards and medially grooving the mastoid portion of the temporal bone behind the mastoid antrum and crossing the occipitomastoid suture to turn anteriorly over the jugular process of the occipital bone to end at the jugular notch. The groove lodges the sigmoid sinus, is usually deeper on the right than on the left, and is pierced near its posterior margin by the mastoid foramen medial to the mastoid process. Also *sulcus of sigmoid sinus.* **s. sinus sigmoidei ossis occipitalis** [NA] The portion of the sulcus of the sigmoid sinus grooving the superior surface of the jugular process of the occipital bone and curving medially and anteriorly to the jugular notch. Also *sulcus of sigmoid sinus of occipital bone.* **s. sinus sigmoidei ossis parietalis** [NA] A short groove on the internal surface of the mastoid or posteroinferior angle of the parietal bone, being the point where the sulcus of the transverse sinus becomes the sulcus of the sigmoid sinus. Also *sulcus of sigmoid sinus of parietal bone.* **s. sinus sigmoidei ossis temporalis** [NA] A deep curved groove for the sigmoid sinus on the inner surface of the mastoid part of the temporal bone, pierced by the mastoid foramen and in close relation to the mastoid air cells. Also *sulcus of sigmoid sinus of temporal bone, sigmoid groove of temporal bone, sigmoid fossa of temporal bone.* **s. sinus transversi** [NA] A deep groove extending laterally from the internal occipital protuberance along the transverse ridge of the cruciform eminence, lodging the transverse sinus and ending at the junction of the mastoid angle of the parietal bone and the base of the petrous part of the temporal bone by continuing as the sulcus for the sigmoid sinus. The tentorium cerebelli is attached to the lips of the groove. Also *sulcus of transverse sinus, sigmoid fossa, lateral groove of occipital bone.* **sphenovomerian s.** A deep median groove on the superior border of the vomer, bounded on each side by the projecting ala, into which the rostrum of the sphenoid bone fits to form the sphenovomerian suture. **s. of spinal nerve** SULCUS NERVI SPINALIS. **s. spiralis externus** [NA] A concavity adjacent to the outer wall of the cochlear duct. It is situated between the spiral organ on the outer end of the basilar membrane and the overhanging rounded, highly vascular and thickened periosteal projection (the spiral prominence). Also *external spiral sulcus.* **s. spiralis internus** [NA] The concavity in the C-shaped projection formed by the thickened periosteal limbus laminae spiralis at the inner end of the cochlear duct, the upper overhang being formed by the vestibular lip to which the membrana tectoria is attached, while the lower prolonged part of the C is formed by the tympanic lip perforated by foramina for the branches of the cochlear nerve. Also *internal spiral sulcus.* **splenial s.** The anterior continuation of the calcarine sulcus of some primate brains, extending to the posterior limit (splenium) of the corpus callosum. It contains visual cortex. Also *anterior calcarine sulcus.* **s. of subclavian artery** SULCUS ARTERIAE SUBCLAVIAE. **subclavian s. of lung** SULCUS SUBCLAVIUS PULMONIS. **s. of subclavian vein** SULCUS VENAE SUBCLAVIAE. **s. subclavius pulmonis** A broad transverse groove on the anterior surface of the apex of the lung just below the tip produced by the subclavian artery arching over the intervening cervical pleura and suprapleural membrane. *Outmoded.* Also *subclavian sulcus of lung.* **s. subparietalis** [NA] A short variable sulcus found on the medial surface of the cerebral hemisphere that continues the direction of the cingulate sulcus posteriorly, thereby separating the precuneus of the parietal lobe from the cingulate gyrus. Also *suprasplenial sulcus.* **superior frontal s.** SULCUS FRONTALIS SUPERIOR. **superior longitudinal s.** FISSURA LONGITUDINALIS CEREBRI. **superior occipital sulci** SULCI OCCIPITALES SUPERIORES. **s. of superior petrosal sinus** SULCUS SINUS PETROSI SUPERIORIS. **s. of superior sagittal sinus** SULCUS SINUS SAGITTALIS SUPERIORIS. **s. of superior sagittal sinus of frontal bone** SULCUS SINUS SAGITTALIS SUPERIORIS OSSIS FRONTALIS. **s. of superior sagittal sinus of occipital bone** SULCUS SINUS SAGITTALIS SUPERIORIS OSSIS OCCIPITA-

LIS. **s. of superior sagittal sinus of parietal bones** SULCUS SINUS SAGITTALIS SUPERIORIS OSSIS PARIETALIS. **superior temporal s.** SULCUS TEMPORALIS SUPERIOR. **suprasplenial s.** SULCUS SUBPARIETALIS. **suprasylvian s.** A long sulcus on the lateral aspect of the carnivore cerebrum arching upward and forward parallel to the occipital and medial margins of the hemisphere. It separates the lateral gyrus from the suprasylvian gyrus. **s. Sylvii** SULCUS LATERALIS CEREBRI. **s. tali** [NA] The broad, deep, oblique groove on the plantar surface of the neck of the talus, located between the middle and the posterior articular facets for the calcaneus and forming the roof of the sinus tarsi when the bones are articulated. Also *sulcus of talus, fovea of talus.* **sulci temporales transversi** [NA] Vertically oriented sulci that separate the transverse temporal gyri located on the opercular surface of the superior temporal gyrus. Also *transverse temporal sulci.* **s. temporalis inferior** 1 [NA] The groove that separates the middle and inferior temporal gyri on the lateral surface of the temporal lobe. Also *inferior temporal sulcus, Clevenger's fissure, sulcus temporalis medius* (outmoded), *middle temporal sulcus* (outmoded). 2 A sulcus infrequently seen coursing below the inferior temporal gyrus. *Outmoded.* 3 *Outmoded* SULCUS OCCIPITOTEMPORALIS. **s. temporalis superior** [NA] A longitudinally oriented sulcus on the lateral aspect of the temporal lobe that courses parallel to the central sulcus and separates the superior and inferior temporal gyri. Also *superior temporal sulcus, supertemporal fissure.* **s. tendinis musculi flexoris hallucis longi calcanei** [NA] A deep groove on the inferior surface of the sustentaculum tali of the calcaneus for the tendon of flexor hallucis longus muscle coursing to the great toe. Also *sulcus of tendon of flexor hallucis longus muscle of calcaneus.* **s. tendinis musculi flexoris hallucis longi tali** [NA] A vertical groove between the medial and the lateral tubercles of the posterior process of the talus for the tendon of the flexor hallucis longus muscle. Also *sulcus of tendon of flexor hallucis longus muscle of talus, incisure of talus.* **s. tendinis musculi peronei longi calcanei** [NA] An oblique groove for the tendon of the peroneus longus muscle on the posteroinferior aspect of the peroneal trochlea on the lateral surface of the calcaneus. Also *sulcus of tendon of peroneus longus muscle on calcaneus.* **s. tendinis musculi peronei longi ossis cuboidei** [NA] A deep groove for the tendon of the peroneus longus muscle, commencing on the lateral surface and extending obliquely anteromedially across the plantar surface of the cuboid bone. Also *sulcus of tendon of peroneus longus muscle on cuboid bone.* **s. of tendon of flexor hallucis longus muscle of calcaneus** SULCUS TENDINIS MUSCULI FLEXORIS HALLUCIS LONGI CALCANEI. **s. of tendon of flexor hallucis longus muscle of talus** SULCUS TENDINIS MUSCULI FLEXORIS HALLUCIS LONGI TALI. **s. for tendon of peroneus brevis muscle** A shallow groove anterosuperior to the peroneal tubercle of the calcaneus for the tendon of the peroneus brevis muscle. The inferior peroneal retinaculum bridges over the groove, and tendon, converting it into an osseofibrous canal. **s. of tendon of peroneus longus muscle on calcaneus** SULCUS TENDINIS MUSCULI PERONEI LONGI CALCANEI. **s. of tendon of peroneus longus muscle on cuboid bone** SULCUS TENDINIS MUSCULI PERONEI LONGI OSSIS CUBOIDEI. **s. of tendon of Zinn** A narrow groove above the tubercle on the margin of the greater wing of sphenoid bone for the attachment of the annulus tendineus communis which is a site of origin of the extrinsic muscles of the eyeball. *Outmoded.* **s. terminalis atrii dextri** [NA] A shallow depression on the external surface of the lateral wall of the right atrium of the heart, connecting the right sides of the openings of the superior and inferior venae cavae and representing the embryonic boundary of the right horn of the sinus venosus, most of which becomes incorporated into the right atrium. Its position corresponds to that of the crista terminalis inside the right atrium. Also *terminal sulcus of right atrium.* **s. terminalis linguae** [NA] A V-shaped furrow on the dorsum of the tongue, its apex being at the foramen cecum and its limbs spreading anterolaterally to the sides of the tongue at the palatoglossal arches. It separates the anterior two-thirds or oral part from the posterior third or pharyngeal part of the tongue, and is bounded anteriorly by vallate papillae. Also *terminal sulcus of tongue.* **terminal s. of right atrium** SULCUS TERMINALIS ATRII DEXTRI. **terminal s. of thalamus** The rostrocaudally directed groove in the floor of the lateral ventricle that separates the lateral surface of the thalamus from the caudate nucleus, and along which courses the stria terminalis and the thalamostriate vein. *Seldom used.* **terminal s. of tongue** SULCUS TERMINALIS LINGUAE. **transverse s. of anthelix** SULCUS ANTHELICIS TRANSVERSUS. **transverse occipital s.** SULCUS OCCIPITALIS TRANSVERSUS. **s. of transverse sinus** SULCUS SINUS TRANSVERSI. **transverse temporal sulci** SULCI TEMPORALES TRANSVERSI. **s. tubae auditivae** [NA] A groove on the base of the skull lodging the cartilaginous part of the auditory tube between the petrous part of the temporal bone, the medial surface of the base of the spine of the sphenoid, and the greater wing of the sphenoid bone and extending from the angle of the junction of the squamous and petrous parts of the temporal bone to the posterior margin of the root of the medial pterygoid plate. Also *sulcus of auditory tube, groove for eustachian tube, pharyngotympanic groove.* **Turner s.** SULCUS INTRAPARIETALIS. **s. tympanicus ossis temporalis** [NA] A narrow circular groove, deficient superiorly, at the medial end of the osseous part of the external acoustic meatus for the attachment of the outer fibrocartilaginous ring of the tympanic membrane. Also *tympanic sulcus of temporal bone, tympanic groove.* **s. of ulnar nerve** SULCUS NERVI ULNARIS. **s. of umbilical vein** A groove or impression on the undersurface of the fetal liver, on which lies the left umbilical vein. Also *sulcus venae umbilicalis.* **uvulonodular s.** A groove on the inferior surface of the cerebellum that separates the uvula from the nodule portions of the cerebellar vermis and is continuous laterally with the posterolateral sulcus. **s. valleculae** A rostrocaudally oriented groove found on both sides of the cerebellar vermis, that separates the vermis from the laterally projecting cerebellar hemisphere. It is especially evident on the inferior surface of the cerebellum. Also *vermicular sulcus.* **s. venae cavae** [NA] A wide, deep groove on the posterior surface of the right lobe of the liver, devoid of peritoneum and lodging the inferior vena cava between the bare area on the right and the caudate lobe on the left. Also *sulcus of vena cava.* **s. venae cavae cranialis** A broad groove on the medial surface of the right lung, extending upwards and forwards in front of the hilum from the upper part of the cardiac impression to the anterior border of the lung. It lodges the superior vena cava and the lower end of the right brachiocephalic vein. **s. venae subclaviae** [NA] A broad, shallow, and oblique groove for the subclavian vein on the superior surface of the first rib anterior to the scalene tubercle. Also *sulcus of subclavian vein.* **s. venae umbilicalis** SULCUS OF UMBILICAL VEIN. **sulci venosi** [NA] Grooves, often branching, on the inner surface of the cranium that lodge meningeal veins. Also *venous sulci, venous grooves.* **s. ventralis medullae spinalis** FISSURA MEDIANA ANTERIOR MEDULLAE SPINALIS. **vermicular s.** SULCUS VALLECULAE. **s. of vertebral artery of atlas** SULCUS ARTERIAE VERTEBRALIS ATLANTIS. **vertical s.** SULCUS PRECENTRALIS. **s. vomerovaginalis** [NA] A fine groove medial to the palatovaginal canal and on the upper surface of the vaginal process of the medial pterygoid plate, which forms a canal with a similar apposing groove on the inferior aspect of the ala of the vomer. It is continuous anteriorly with the anterior end of the palatovaginal canal. Also *vomerovaginal sulcus.*

**sulfacetamide** $C_8H_{10}N_2O_3S$. *N*-[(4-Aminophenyl)sulfonyl]acetamide, a sulfonamide drug used for the treatment of urinary tract infections. It is given orally.

**sulfacetic acid** ASPIRIN.

**sulfacytine** $C_{12}H_{14}N_4O_3S$. 4-Amino-*N*-(1-ethyl-1,2-dihydro-2-oxo-4-pyrimidinyl)benzenesulfonamide. A relatively short-acting sulfonamide. It is given orally in the treatment of acute urinary tract infections due to organisms susceptible to this agent.

**sulfadiazine** One of the sulfonamide drugs, formed by acylation of 2-aminopyrimidine by sulfanilic acid. Also *sulfapyrimidine.*

**sulfadimethoxine** $C_{12}H_{14}N_4O_4S$. 4-Amino-*N*(2,6-dimethoxy-4-pyrimidinyl)benzenesulfonamide, and antibacterial sulfonamide that is relatively long acting after oral administration.

**sulfadimidine** SULFAMETHAZINE.

**sulfa drugs** Drugs related to sulfonamide, such as sulfadiazine and sulfathiazole. They have bacteriostatic properties against a number of microorganisms.

**sulfaethidole** $C_{10}H_{12}N_4O_2S_2$. 4-Amino-*N*-(5-ethyl-1,3,4-thiadiazol-2-yl)benzenesulfonamide, a sulfonamide antibiotic that is relatively short acting. It is used mainly for urinary tract antiseptic effects and is given orally.

**sulfamerazine** $C_{11}H_{12}N_4O_2S$. 4-Amino-*N*-(4-methyl-2-pyrimidinyl)benzenesulfonamide. A sulfonamide antibacterial agent which is usually used in combination with other sulfonamides to reduce the chance of crystalluria and renal toxicity.

**sulfamethazine** $C_{12}H_{14}N_4O_2S$. 4-Amino-*N*(4,6-dimethyl-2-pyrimidinyl)benzenesulfonamide. A sulfonamide antibiotic agent usually used in combination with others such as sulfadiazine and sulfamerazine to reduce the chances of crystalluria and renal damage. Also *sulfadimidine.*

**sulfamethoxazole** $C_{10}H_{11}N_3O_3S$. 4-Amino-*N*-(5-methyl-3-isoxazoly)benzenesulfonamide, a sulfonamide antibacterial agent used primarily for the treatment of urinary tract infections and dermatologic infections. It is given orally.

**sulfamethoxypyridazine** $C_{11}H_{12}N_4O_3S$. 4-Amino-*N*-(6-methoxy-3-pyridazinyl)benzenesulfonamide. A sulfonamide antibacterial agent used primarily in the treatment of urinary tract infections. It is given orally.

**sulfamido** SULFOAMINO.

**sulfan blue** $C_{27}H_{31}N_2NaO_6S_2$. The monosodium salt of 4-[α-(*p*-diethylaminophenyl)-α-(4-diethyliminiocyclohexa- 2, 5-dienylidene)methyl]benzene-1,3-disulfonic acid. A blue dye which has been used by intravenous injection to visualize vascular and lymphatic systems. The agent may cause allergic reactions in some individuals.

**sulfanilamide** \sul′fənil′əmīd\ The amide of sulfanilic acid. It is the simplest of the sulfonamide drugs, being ammonia acylated with sulfanilic acid. It owes its antibacterial action to competing with *p*-aminobenzoic acid in the biosynthesis of folic acid. In consequence bacteria are starved for that essential compound and cease to grow.

**sulfanilic acid** *p*-Aminobenzenesulfonic acid. It is a component of the molecules of sulfonamide drugs and is used as a reagent in protein chemistry, because the diazonium salt formed by treating it with nitrous acid gives characteristic colors with tyrosine and histidine.

**sulfanilylsulfanilamide** $C_{12}H_{13}N_3O_4S_2$. 4′-Sulfamoylsulfanilanilide. A topical antibacterial sulfonamide medication.

**sulfanuria** \sulf′ənoo′rē·ə\ [*sulf(o)-* + ANURIA] Blockage of the urinary passage due to excreted sulfonamide drugs.

**sulfapyrazine** One of the sulfonamide drugs, formed by acylation of 2-aminopyrazine with sulfanilic acid.

**sulfapyridine** $C_{11}H_{11}N_3O_2S$. 2-(*p*-Aminobenzenesulfonamido)pyridine. A sulfonamide with low water solubility and a variable rate of absorption after oral administration. It has been largely replaced by other, less toxic sulfonamides, but it is still used in the treatment of dermatitis herpetiformis.

**sulfapyrimidine** SULFADIAZINE.

**sulfasalazine** $C_{18}H_{14}N_4O_5S$. 2-Hydroxy-5-[[4-[(2-pyridinyl amino)-sulfonyl]phenyl]azo]benzoic acid. A sulfonamide used primarily in the treatment of ulcerative colitis. It is given orally. Also *salazosulfapyridine, salicylazosulfapyridine.*

**Sulfasuxidine** A proprietary name for succinylsulfathiazole

**sulfatase** Any enzyme that catalyzes hydrolysis of an ester of sulfuric acid; especially the enzyme arylsulfatase, which acts on phenyl sulfates.

**sulfate** **1** A salt or ester of sulfuric acid. **2** A salt of sulfuric acid in which both hydrogen ions are removed. **active s.** 3′-Phosphoadenosine 5′-phosphosulfate, the donor of the $—SO_3^-$ group in most biologic reactions in which esters of sulfuric acid are formed.

**sulfate adenylyltransferase** The enzyme (EC 2.7.7.4) that catalyzes transfer of the adenylyl group of ATP onto sulfate to form adenosine 5′-phosphosulfate, an intermediate in the formation of 3′-phosphoadenosine 5′-phosphosulfate, which is the usual donor of the $—SO_3^-$ group biologically. Sulfate adenylyltransferase (ADP) is a similar enzyme (EC 2.7.7.5) that catalyzes a similar reaction with ADP as the donor of the adenylyl group.

**sulfathiazole** One of the sulfonamide drugs, formed by acylation of 2-aminothiazole with sulfanilic acid.

**sulfatide** \sul′fətīd\ A sulfate ester (at the 3 position of D-galactose) of galactocerebroside, found in brain tissue and especially in myelin. Sulfatides usually contain fatty acids with 22 to 26 carbon atoms. The first sulfatide isolated was cerebron sulfuric acid. The degradation of sulfatides occurs by the removal of the sulfate group, thereby converting it back to galactocerebroside. This reaction is catalyzed by cerebroside sulfate sulfatase, and the lack of this enzyme causes an excess accumulation of sulfatides, which characterizes metachromatic leukodystrophy.

**sulfatidosis** \sul′fətidō′sis\ Any storage disease in which there is abnormal storage of sulfatides in the nervous system. Metachromatic leukodystrophy is an example.

**sulfenic acid** Any substance containing the group —S—OH. Such compounds are not usually stable, and they react rapidly with thiols to form disulfides.

**sulfhemoglobin** An abnormal form of hemoglobin that contains sulfur bound to heme, with iron in either the Fe(II) or Fe(III) state. The latter may be designated sulfmethemoglobin.

**sulfhemoglobinemia** \sulf′hēməglō′binē′mē·ə\ The presence of sulfhemoglobin in blood, usually the result of ingestion of drugs such as acetanilid, phenacetin or dapsone.

**sulfhydric acid** HYDROGEN SULFIDE.

**sulfhydryl** The group —S—H, derived from hydrogen sulfide. The sulfhydryl groups of cysteine residues are important in the functioning of some enzymes. They have p*K* values only slightly above neutrality and so exist partly in their strongly nucleophilic thiolate form. Sulfhydryl groups occur mainly in intracellular proteins, and being hydrophobic are often masked from solvent by the folding of the protein. When exposed, they are easily oxidized to form disulfide bonds, and these usually replace them in extracellular proteins. • In systematic nomenclature the name of this group as a prefix is *mercapto,* so it may also be called the *mercapto group.* Its name as a suffix is *thiol,* and this term is also used as the name of the group.
**sulfide** **1** Any compound of sulfur with a more electropositive element. **2** The ion $S^{2-}$ that many such compounds contain. **3** THIOETHER.
**sulfinic acid** A compound containing the group —S(O)—OH. It may be produced by oxidation of a sulfenic acid, and it is easily oxidized to form a sulfonic acid.
**sulfinide** SACCHARIN.
**sulfinpyrazone** $C_{23}H_{20}N_2O_3S$. 1,2-Diphenyl-4-[2-(phenylsulfinyl)ethyl]-3,5-pyrazolidinedione, an analogue of phenylbutazone, which is a powerful uricosuric agent. It has been used in the treatment of gout.
**β-sulfinylpyruvic acid** HOOC—CO—$CH_2$—$SO_2$H. A metabolite formed by transamination of 3-sulfinoalanine during the catabolism of cysteine and cystine to pyruvic acid.
**sulfisomidine** $C_{12}H_{14}N_4O_2S$. 4-Amino-*N*-(2,6-dimethyl-4-pyrimidinyl)-benzenesulfonamide, an antibacterial sulfonamide related to sulfamethazine. It is used to treat systemic and urinary tract infections and is given orally.
**sulfisoxazole** $C_{11}H_{13}N_3O_3S$. 4-Amino-*N*-(3,4-dimethyl-5-isoxazolyl)benzenesulfonamide, a sulfonamide antibacterial agent used to treat any of various infections. It is given orally.
**sulfite** The ion $SO_3^{2-}$ or a compound containing it or, more rarely, an ester of sulfurous acid. The sulfite ion is a powerful nucleophile and can add to cytosine in nucleic acids.
**sulfmethemoglobin** See under SULFHEMOGLOBIN.
**sulfo-** \sul′fə-, sul′fō-\ [L *sulf(ur)* + *o*] A combining form indicating the substitution of the group —$SO_3$H for —H in a compound. Also *sulf-, sulpho-, sulph-.*
**sulfoamino** The group formed from an amino group by substituting a sulfo group for one of its hydrogen atoms, i.e. $HO_3S$—NH—. It occurs in glycoproteins, where residues of amino sugars may be substituted by reaction with 3′-phosphoadenosine 5′-phosphosulfate to form this group. Also *sulfamido.*
**sulfobromophthalein** Disodium phenoltetrabromophthalein. A dye used medically as a test of liver excretory function.
**sulfobromophthalein sodium** $C_{20}H_8Br_4Na_2O_{10}S_2$. Disodium phenoltetrabromophthalein sulfonate. A sulfonated derivative of the product derived from the interaction of tetrabromphthalic anhydride and phenol. It is employed in a test of liver function by measuring how rapidly the dye is cleared from the blood by the liver.
**sulfomucin** \sul′fōmyoo′sin\ A molecule of acid mucopolysaccharide which contains sulfuric acid esters in the polysaccharide.
**Sulfonal** A proprietary name for sulfonmethane.
**sulfonamide** \sulfän′əmīd\ The amide of a sulfonic acid, especially any of the amides formed between ammonia or amines, usually aromatic amines, and sulfanilic acid. These are important chemotherapeutic agents. They or their breakdown products compete with *p*-aminobenzoic acid in the bacterial synthesis of folic acid, and they thus act by inhibiting the growth of bacteria.
**sulfonamidotherapy** \sul′fənam′idōther′əpē\ Therapy using sulfonamide drugs.
**sulfonate** A salt, anion, or ester of a sulfonic acid.
**sulfone** A compound containing the —$SO_2$— group joined to two organic groups. An example is methionine *S,S*-dioxide, often produced by oxidation of methionine before amino-acid analysis.
**sulfonic** \sulfän′ik\ Relating to the chemical group —$SO_3$H, especially containing it.
**sulfonic acid** Any substance containing the —$SO_3$H group, such as *p*-toluenesulfonic acid. Taurine is a biologic example.
**sulfonium** The species $H_3S^+$ and its substituted derivatives. *S*-Adenosylmethionine is a biologic example; the alkylation of the sulfur atom of methionine that occurs when it is formed makes it a good alkylating agent and thus endows it with its ability to serve as a methyl donor.
**sulfonmethane** $C_8H_{18}O_4S_2$. 2,2-bis(Ethylsulfonyl)butane. A crystalline solid, soluble in alcohol, slightly soluble in water. It is a hypnotic. Chronic use may lead to habituation or addiction. Also *acetone diethylsulfone.*
**sulfonyl-** \sul′fənil-\ A combining form denoting the chemical group —$SO_2$—.
**sulfonylurea** \-yoorē′·ə\ A compound of the class of arylsulfonylureas, used as oral hypoglycemic agents.
**sulfosalicylic acid** $C_7H_6O_6S$. The water-soluble compound that is used as a precipitant for proteins in the urine and as a reagent in measuring ferric ion. Also *salicylsulfonic acid.*
**sulfotransferase** Any of the enzymes (EC 2.8.2) that transfer the group —$SO^{3-}$ in exchange for a hydrogen atom. They usually have 3′-phosphoadenosine 5′-phosphosulfate as donor.
**sulfoxide** Any compound containing the —SO— group. Examples include dimethyl sulfoxide, $Me_2SO$, used in organic synthesis as a solvent and reagent, and methionine *S*-oxide, whose residues are formed when proteins are treated with hydrogen peroxide.
**sulfoxism** \sulfäk′sizm\ Poisoning from sulfuric acid, a substance corrosive to all body tissues. Eye contact may cause blindness, skin contact may cause severe necrosis, and ingestion may cause mucous membrane burns, hematemesis, abdominal pain, respiratory distress, shock, renal failure, and death.
**sulfur** \sul′fər\ [L *sulpur, sulphur,* or *sulfur* (of unknown origin) sulfur, brimstone] Element number 16, having atomic weight 32.06. Four stable isotopes occur naturally and six radioactive isotopes are known, with half-lives ranging from 0.19 seconds to 88 days. Under ordinary conditions, elemental sulfur is a yellow, odorless, brittle nonmetal in the form of rhombic crystals which melt at 112.8°C. It exists also in many different allotropic forms with unusual molecular configurations. It is found native in the vicinity of hot springs and volcanoes but it is chemically active and readily enters into innumerable compounds. Valences are 2, 4, and 6. Sulfur is used in a multitude of industrial processes and products. Oxides of sulfur, produced chiefly by the combustion of fuels, are dangerous air pollutants. Sulfur is an essential constituent of living organisms, entering into the composition of proteins and many other biologic compounds. Also *sulphur* (British spelling). Symbol: S **flowers of s.** SUBLIMED SULFUR. **lac s.** PRECIPITATED SULFUR. **s. lotum** WASHED SULFUR. **precipitated s.** Elemental sulfur in the form of a fine, pale yel-

low, microcrystalline or amorphous powder containing at least 99.5 percent sulfur. It has been used topically to treat scabies and in dermal medications to treat parasitic and fungal infections. Also *lac sulfuris, lac sulfur, milk of sulfur.* **radioactive s.** RADIOSULFUR. **sublimed s.** A yellow powder consisting of sulfur of 99.5% or greater purity. It is obtained by subliming elemental sulfur and condensing the vapors. It may be administered topically as a scabicide or parasiticide. Also *flowers of sulfur.* **washed s.** Sulfur obtained by sublimation and then washed with water in order to enhance its purity. Also *sulfur lotum.* **wettable s.** A compound of sulfur prepared from polysulfide of calcium. It contains a protective colloid such as casein, and is very easily suspended in water.

**sulfur 35** A radioisotope of sulfur, emitting purely beta radiation. It is used for labeling compounds such as steroid derivatives. Because sodium sulfate equilibrates rapidly within the extracellular water, and because sulfur 35 has a short biologic half-life, radiosulfate may be used for the determination of extracellular water volume. Physical half-life is 87.1 days. Symbol: $^{35}S$

**sulfur chloride** SULFUR MONOCHLORIDE.

**sulfur dioxide** $SO_2$. A colorless gas with a suffocating, unpleasant odor. It is used as an antioxidant in pharmaceutic preparations and has been used to get rid of lice, flies, and mosquitoes.

**sulfur hydride** HYDROGEN SULFIDE.

**sulfuric** \sulfyoo′rik\ Related to sulfuric acid.

**sulfuric acid** $H_2SO_4$. A strong colorless acid, occurring as an odorless syrupy liquid, extremely caustic, and miscible with water in all proportions. It is also miscible with many organic solvents and is decomposed by ethanol. $d = 1.834$. Its melting point is 10.49°C. The commercial product contains 98% $H_2SO_4$. It is very corrosive and it is an excellent dehydrating agent, even after some water has been added. It has been used for gastric hypoacidity or anacidity (as 10% solution) and to stimulate appetite (0.6 to 2.0 ml in 200 ml of water). Fuming sulfuric acid (oleum) contains up to 80% of $SO_3$.

**sulfur monochloride** $S_2Cl_2$. A nonflammable, light amber to yellowish red, fuming, oily liquid with a penetrating odor. It is used as a chlorinating agent in the manufacture of organic chemicals. The vapors cause irritation to eyes, nose, and throat, lacrimation, and respiratory distress. Also *sulfur chloride, disulfur dichloride, sulfur subchloride.*

**Sulkowitch** [Hirsh Wolf *Sulkowitch*, U.S. internist, born 1906] See under REAGENT, TEST.

**sulph-** \sulf-\ SULFO-. • For words beginning *sulph-*, see also under SULF-.

**sulpho-** \sul′fə-, sul′fō-\ SULFO-.

**sulphur** \sul′fər\ *Brit.* SULFUR.

**Sulzberger** [Marion Baldur *Sulzberger*, U.S. dermatologist, born 1895] Bloch-Sulzberger syndrome. See under INCONTINENTIA PIGMENTI.

**sum-** \sum-, səm-\ SUB-.

**summation** \sumā′shən\ [Med L *summatio* (from *summatus*, past part. of *summare* to sum up, from L *summa* a sum, amount) a summing up] The aggregate effect produced by a number of identical neural impulses or stimuli of like qualitative effect, when applied to an excitable tissue like a motor nucleus or nerve cell. The effect can be either incremental or decremental. **spatial s.** Summation resulting from spatially discrete but simultaneous subthreshold stimuli or neural impulses. **temporal s.** Summation resulting from subthreshold stimuli or neural impulses identical in kind but dispersed in time.

**summit** The highest point or elevation; apex.

**sunspot** FRECKLE.

**sunstroke** Heat stroke caused by exposure to the sun. Also *coup de soleil, heliosis, insolation, hyperpyrexial insolation* (obs.), *solar fever.*

**sup-** \sup-, səp-\ SUB-.

**super-** \soo′pər-\ [L *super* (akin to Gk *hyper* over, above) above, over, excessive] A prefix meaning (1) above, over, on top of; (2) higher in rank or position, superior; (3) excessive, excessively.

**superacid** Describing a bivalent or trivalent metal ion in connection with the electron withdrawal it effects, which is greater than that of the singly charged hydrogen ion, the latter being regarded as the more normal acid: used especially of the mechanisms of enzymes that contain such cations.

**superacute** \-əkyoot′\ Extremely acute.

**superalimentation** \-al′iməntā′shən\ Feeding beyond the dictates of appetite, employed as therapy in wasting diseases. Also *suralimentation.* See also HYPERALIMENTATION.

**superantigen** \-an′tijən\ Antigen that, following processing by macrophage, becomes able to stimulate an immune response even at very low concentration.

**supercallosal** \-kalō′səl\ SUPRACALLOSAL.

**supercerebellar** \-ser′əbel′ər\ SUPRACEREBELLAR.

**supercerebral** \-ser′əbrəl\ SUPRACEREBRAL.

**supercilia** \-sil′ē·ə\ **1** [NA] The hairs of the eyebrows. **2** Plural of SUPERCILIUM.

**superciliary** \-sil′ē·er′ē\ Pertaining to the eyebrow. Also *supraciliary* (outmoded).

**supercilium** \-sil′ē·əm\ [L (from *super* above + *cilium* eyelid), eyebrow] (*pl.* supercilia) [NA] The raised arch of skin with short, thick hairs surmounting each orbit and overlying the supraorbital margin; the eyebrow.

**supercoil** \soo′pərkoil\ A macromolecular structure in which a number of helical strands are coiled together, as $\alpha$-helical polypeptides forming a structural protein.

**supercooled** Designating a substance that has remained liquid below its freezing point. Although it will freeze if supplied with nuclei of the crystalline solid material, it may remain liquid if these are absent, or if conditions such as high viscosity retard crystal growth.

**superduction** \-duk′shən\ SUPRADUCTION.

**superdural** \-d^y^oo′rəl\ SUPRADURAL.

**superego** \-ē′gō\ The last of the three structural divisions of the psyche to develop. It is a split-off portion of the ego that contains representations of parental and social morality in the form of conscience, and the goals to which one aspires in the form of the ego ideal.

**superextension** \-iksten′shən\ HYPEREXTENSION.

**superfamily** A taxonomic group ranking above a family, comprising several families within an order.

**superfecundation** \-fikundā′shən\ The fertilization of two or more ova by spermatozoa from different acts of coitus, thus allowing the production of litter-mates or siblings with different fathers.

**superfemale** *Outmoded* METAFEMALE.

**superfetation** \-fētā′shən\ The presence in a uterus of two or more fetuses at different stages of gestation such as would result from fertilization of ova from different ovulatory cycles. Also *hypercyesis.*

**superficialis** \-fish′ē·ā′lis\ Situated on or closer than another to the surface of the body. Compare PROFUNDUS.

**superficies** \-fish′i·ēz\ [L (from *super-* upper + *facies* face) upper part, surface, facing] An outer surface.

**superfissure** \-fish′ər\ SUPERSULCUS.

**superflexion** \-flek′shən\ HYPERFLEXION.

**supergene** \soo′pərjēn\ A group of linked genes, the genotype of which tends to be inherited unchanged because recombination is suppressed. This may occur because chiasmata are prevented from occurring despite synapsis, or because the group is located on a differential segment.

**supergyre** \soo′pərjīr\ Any gyrus of the cerebral cortex that develops over another gyrus and overlaps it.

**superhelix** \-hē′liks\ The helix formed, as by DNA, when the strand arranged in this helix is itself a helix.

**superinduce** To induce over and above a preexisting condition of induction.

**superinfection** \-infek′shən\ A new infection which complicates the course of an existing infection, often resulting from invasion by microorganisms resistant to the antimicrobial agents being used to combat the original infection.

**superinvolution** \-invəloo′shən\ HYPERINVOLUTION.

**superior** [L (comparative of *superus* above, upper, from *super* above), higher, superior] Upper; higher; near or toward the top: used in human anatomy with reference to the upright posture and designating structures or parts nearer the vertex than other comparable structures farther from it.

**superlactation** \-laktā′shən\ HYPERLACTATION.

**superlethal** \-lē′thəl\ Extremely lethal.

**superligamen** \-ligā′mən\ A retention dressing or any bandage applied to a wound to keep a surgical dressing in place.

**supermaxilla** \-maksil′ə\ *Outmoded* MAXILLA.

**supermedial** \-mē′dē·əl\ SUPEROMEDIAL.

**supermicroscope** \-mī′krəskōp\ ELECTRON MICROSCOPE.

**supernatant** \-nā′tənt\ **1** Denoting a fluid remaining above particles, precipitate, or a fluid layer of greater density. **2** A supernatant fluid. Compare INFRANATANT.

**supernutrition** \-n$^y$ootrish′ən\ HYPERNUTRITION.

**superoccipital** \-äksip′itəl\ SUPRAOCCIPITAL.

**superolateral** \-ōlat′ərəl\ Above and at, or to, the side.

**superomedial** \-ōmē′dē·əl\ Above and toward or in the middle. Also *supermedial.*

**superovulation** \-äv′əlā′shən\ Ovulation occurring at a rate faster than normal.

**superoxide** The species $O_2^-$ and salts containing it. It is formed by the reduction of dioxygen, as when sodium burns in oxygen. It can be protonated to form the HO—O· radical, with a p$K$ of 4.7. It may be formed biologically by the reaction of reduced flavins with dioxygen, and is destroyed by the action of superoxide dismutase, which accelerates a slow, spontaneous reaction by which it forms peroxide and dioxygen. It is largely responsible for the lethal effect of oxygen on obligate anaerobic bacteria, which lack superoxide dismutase.

**superoxide dismutase** The widespread enzyme (EC 1.15.1.1) that catalyzes the reaction between two molecules of superoxide to form oxygen and hydrogen peroxide: $2O_2^- + 2H^+ \rightarrow O_2 + H_2O_2$. The enzyme is thought to have a protective function, since superoxide can generate hydroxyl radicals, which can damage proteins. Also *cerebrocuprein, erythrocuprein.*

**superparasite** \-par′əsīt\ An organism that lives by superparasitism; a member of a superparasitic population.

**superparasitic** \-par′əsit′ik\ Of or characterized by superparasitism.

**superparasitism** \-par′əsitizm\ **1** Parasitism in which there are normally too many parasites of the same species for the host to support, and frank disease or death is the usual outcome. **2** HYPERPARASITISM.

**superpetrosal** \-petrō′səl\ Located above or near the anterior surface of the petrous part of the temporal bone.

**superphosphate** A salt containing $HPO_4^{2-}$ or $H_2PO_4^-$ ions, used as a fertilizer. In contrast with salts of $PO_4^{3-}$ with alkaline earth metals, such salts are soluble.

**super-regeneration** \-rijen′ərā′shən\ Excessive repair of a wound or excessive growth of a part or an organ during the reparative process. See also PROUD FLESH.

**supersaturate** \-sach′ərāt\ To produce a solution, usually by evaporation of solvent, that is more concentrated than one in equilibrium with pure solute. This is possible, whether the solute is a solid, liquid, or gas, because such a solute needs nuclei on which to separate as a distinct phase.

**superscription** The sign ℞ that precedes a prescription.

**supersecretion** \-sikrē′shən\ HYPERSECRETION.

**supersensitive** \-sen′sətiv\ HYPERSENSITIVE.

**supersonic** \-sän′ik\ Having a velocity greater than that at which sound travels, which in air, at a temperature of 20°C at sea level, is 343 m/s (1235 km/h).

**superspecies** \soo′pərspē′shēz\ A taxonomic group comprising two or more closely related species usually located in adjacent habitats, often separated by a barrier, and with little or no interbreeding between members of the related species.

**supersphenoid** \-sfē′noid\ Located above the sphenoid bone.

**superstructure** \soo′pərstruk′chər\ **implant s.** The prosthesis which an oral implant supports.

**supersulcus** \-sul′kəs\ A sulcus in the cerebral cortex that forms over the surface of an underlying cerebral gyrus because it is overlapped by another cerebral gyrus during development or maturation. Also *superfissure.*

**supertemporal** \-tem′pərəl\ SUPRATEMPORAL.

**supervention** \-ven′shən\ [Late L *superventio* (from L *superventus,* past part. of *supervenire* to be added to, to come upon unexpectedly) a supervening] The development of an extraneous or unexpected sign, symptom, or condition in addition to and subsequent to another.

**supervitaminosis** \-vī′təminō′sis\ HYPERVITAMINOSIS.

**supervoltage** \-vōl′tij\ In radiology, voltages of one million volts or greater, used to produce x rays for radiation therapy.

**supinate** \soo′pināt\ [L *supinat(us),* past part. of *supinare* to bend or lay backward, turn face up, from *supinus* supine] **1** To rotate the forearm and hand so that the palm faces either upward or forward. **2** To place the body in the supine position. Compare PRONATE.

**supination** \soo′pinā′shən\ [*supinat(e)* + -ION] **1** Rotation of the forearm and hand so that the palm faces forward or upward. **2** Placing the body on its back so that the face, palms, and toes point upward. **s. of the foot** TALIPES VARUS.

**supinator** \soo′pinā′tər\ **1** A muscle of the upper limb that produces supination of the forearm and hand. **2** MUSCULUS SUPINATOR.

**supine** \soopīn′\ [L *supin(us)* (from *sub* under) backward, lying on the back] Lying on the back, with the face upward. Also *dorsicumbent.*

**supplemental** \sup′ləmen′təl\ Acting as a supplement; additional, as *supplemental vitamin.*

**supply** A store or reserve; a means by which something is made available. **extrinsic nerve s.** Innervation of a structure or organ derived from nerve fibers whose neuron cell bodies lie outside of that organ, such as the somatic motor innervation of a striated muscle. **intrinsic nerve s.** Innervation of a structure or organ derived from nerve fibers whose neuron cell bodies lie within the organ or structure itself, such as the postganglionic parasympathetic innervation of the musculature or glands of the intestine.

**support** [L *supportare* (from SUP- + L *portare* to carry) to carry, bring] **1** The act of sustaining or providing a basis for continued function. **2** A device that maintains or stabilizes something, such as an orthopedic appliance to reinforce the strength of a limb or to keep a body part in a fixed position. **3** An area under a denture that resists the forces of mastication, such as teeth, an edentulous ridge, or mucosa of the hard palate. **advanced cardiac life s.** The knowledge and technical skills required to diagnose and treat emergent life-threatening cardiac abnormalities. **advanced life s.** That set of skills that go beyond first aid in maintaining an airway, circulatory support, and the treatment of shock in an emergency situation. Abbr. ALS **advanced trauma life s.** The knowledge and technical skills required to treat shock, maintain an airway, set priorities, and diagnose and treat the severely injured patient. **basic life s.** The essentials of first aid, cardiopulmonary resuscitation, diagnosing and treating shock, and maintaining an airway in an emergency situation. Abbr. BLS **s. of the promontory** SUBICULUM PROMONTORII CAVITATIS TYMPANICAE.

**supportive** \səpôr′tiv\ **1** Providing support. **2** Adjunctive; supplementary.

**suppository** \səpäz′ətôrē\ [Med. L *suppositorium* (from Late L, neut. sing of *suppositorius* placed under, from L *supposit(us)*, past part. of *supponere* to place under + *-orium* -ORY) suppository] A solid body of various size, shape, and constitution used for the delivery of an agent or drug into the rectal, vaginal, or urethral orifices of the body. The cocoa-butter or gelatin base of the suppository is solid at room temperature, but melts and releases the medication at body temperature. **glycerin s.** A suppository made from a mixture of glycerin and sodium stearate. It is commonly used to produce evacuation of the lower bowel.

**suppressant** **1** Causing a suppressive change. **2** An agent that arrests secretion or excretion by some organ or tissue. Also *suppressor.*

**suppression** \səpresh′ən\ [L *suppressio* (from *supprimere* to hold down or back, suppress, from *sub-* down, under + *premere* to press) retention, withholding] **1** Conscious, intentional inhibition of an affect, idea, or impulse, in contrast to the unconscious mechanism of repression. **2** Cortical inhibition of the vision of one eye under conditions of binocular vision. **3** The restoration of correct translation of messenger RNA following a frameshift mutation. The restoration can result from an additional frameshift in the nucleotide chain or be due to a modification of transfer ribonucleic acid interaction. **otoacoustic s.** The reduction in the otoacoustic response to a stimulus due to the presence of a second competing or masker stimulus. **phenotypic s.** In a mutant with an auxotrophic or other growth-preventing mutation, restoration of growth by an agent, such as streptomycin, that increases the frequency of errors in translation. The resultant misreading of the mutant codon occasionally yields a functional protein.

**suppressor** **1** SUPPRESSANT. **2** An agent that is capable of reversing the effects of a mutation. **amber s.** A mutation in tRNA that supresses the effect of an amber mutation by causing the tRNA to insert its amino acid at UAG codons. **codon-specific s.** A tRNA that inserts its amino acid at a termination codon, thus reversing the effect of a nonsense mutation within a gene. Growth is restored because the suppressor tRNA only occasionally causes this altered reading of the termination codon, and because other tRNAs are present for the same amino acid. **crossover s.** A mutation, either in a specified gene or a chromosome structure, that inhibits crossing over—either generally or, more commonly, locally—during meiosis. **soluble immune response s.** A lymphokine that suppresses immune responses by plaque-forming cells.

**suppurate** \sup′yərāt\ [L *suppurat(us)*, past part. of *suppurare* (from *sup-* from under + *pus*, gen. *puris*, pus) to fester, suppurate] To produce pus.

**suppuration** \sup′yərā′shən\ The formation of pus. Adj. suppurative.

**supra-** \soo′prə-\ [L *supra* above, over, on the upper side] A prefix meaning above, on the upper side.

**supra-aortic** \-ā·ôr′tik\ **1** In the proximal aorta above the aortic valve. **2** Above the aorta, especially above the arch of the aorta.

**supracallosal** \-kalō′səl\ Located above, or over, the corpus callosum. Also *supercallosal.*

**supracerebellar** \-ser′əbel′ər\ Situated rostral to, over, or superficial to the cerebellum. Also *supercerebellar.*

**supracerebral** \-ser′əbrəl\ Located above, superficial to, or over the cerebrum. Also *supercerebral.*

**supracervical** \-sur′vikəl\ Above the cervix, as *supracervical hysterectomy.*

**suprachoroid** \-kôr′oid\ Between the choroid and sclera of the eye.

**suprachoroidea** \-kôroi′dē·ə\ LAMINA SUPRACHOROIDEA.

**supraciliary** \-sil′ē·er′ē\ *Outmoded* SUPERCILIARY.

**supraclavicularis** \-kləvik′yəler′is\ STERNOCLAVICULARIS.

**supraclinoid** \-klī′noid\ Above the clinoid processes in the middle cranial fossa.

**supraclusion** \-kloo′zhən\ [SUPRA- + *(oc)clusion*] The overeruption of a tooth or group of teeth from the line of occlusion. Also *supraocclusion.*

**supraduction** \-duk′shən\ [SUPRA- + DUCTION] The upward rotation of one eye. Also *sursumvergence, sursumduction, supravergence, superduction.*

**supradural** \-d$^{y}$oo′rəl\ Situated above, superficial to, or external to the dura mater. Also *superdural.*

**supraepitrochlear** \-ep′iträk′lē·ər\ Above the medial epicondyle of the humerus.

**suprageniculate** \-jenik′yəlāt\ **1** Denoting the suprageniculate nucleus. **2** Dorsal to the lateral geniculate nucleus.

**supragranular** \-gran′yələr\ Located in or denoting layers of the cerebral cortex superficial to the fourth, or internal granular, layer, usually with reference to the first three cerebral cortical layers, i.e., the plexiform, external granular, and external pyramidal layers.

**suprailiac** \soo′prə·il′i·ak\ Located at the upper end of or above the ilium; specifically, above the iliac crest.

**supralethal** \-lē′thəl\ In excess of a lethal amount.

**supraliminal** \-lim′inəl\ Greater than threshold awareness.

**supramamillary** \-mam′iler′ē\ The nuclei or region above the main hypothalamic mamillary nuclei.

**supramaxilla** \-maksil′ə\ *Outmoded* MAXILLA.

**supramaxillary** \-mak′siler′ē\ **1** Located above the maxilla. **2** Of or relating to the maxilla.

**supramaximal** \-mak′siməl\ Above a maximum; in electrodiagnosis, characterizing a stimulating current of high enough voltage so that further increase in current does not produce a greater amplitude of response.

**supranuclear** \-n$^{y}$oo′klē·ər\ Situated above a nucleus, as a lesion in a pathway impinging upon a given motor nucleus.

**supraoccipital** \-äksip′itəl\ Located above or superior to the occiput, occipital bone, occipital region, or occipital lobe of the cerebral cortex. Also *superoccipital.*

**supraocclusion** \-äkloo′zhən\ SUPRACLUSION.

**supraoptic** \-äpʹtik\ Denoting the hypothalamic nuclei or the zone above the optic chiasm.
**supraoptimum** \-äpʹtiməm\ [SUPRA- + OPTIMUM] A condition that exceeds the most favorable.
**suprapineal** \-pinʹē·əl\ Located above the pineal body. • This term is somewhat imprecise because it is used to denote the position of a structure either dorsal to the pineal body or rostral to it.
**suprapontine** \-pänʹtīn\ **1** Situated within the neuraxis above or rostral to the pons, as *suprapontine relay* (in the mesencephalon). **2** Located over, dorsal to, or superior to the pons, such as the anatomical position of the cerebellum.
**suprapromontorial** \-prōʹməntôrʹē·əl\ Situated in the tympanic cavity above the level of a horizontal line drawn through the apex of the promontory.
**suprarenal** \-rēʹnəl\ **1** Relating to the adrenal gland. **2** Located above the kidney.
**suprarenalectomy** \-rēʹnəlekʹtəmē\ *Seldom used* ADRENALECTOMY.
**suprarene** \-rēnʹ\ *Outmoded* GLANDULA SUPRARENALIS.
**suprarenotropic** \-rēʹnōträpʹik\ ADRENOTROPIC.
**suprascapula** \-skapʹələ\ **1** A rarely present ossicle that is situated above the superior angle of the scapula. **2** In congenital elevation of the scapula, either a bridge of bone that connects the scapula to the vertebral column or a bony projection from the superior border of the scapula that does not articulate with the vertebral column. **3** A cartilage of the dorsal part of the pectoral girdle in rays. **4** An unossified or incompletely ossified dorsal extension of the scapula in amphibians and some reptiles. Also *suprascapular cartilage*.
**suprascleral** \-sklirʹəl\ External to the sclera.
**suprasegmental** \-segmenʹtəl\ Referring to levels within the central nervous system which are above the characteristically segmental spinal cord, i.e., the brainstem and forebrain.
**suprasternal** \-sturʹnəl\ Situated above the sternum.
**suprasternale** \-stərnāʹlē\ An anthropometric point situated in the midline at the lowest point of the suprasternal notch.
**suprasylvian** \-silʹvē·ən\ **1** Denoting the region above the lateral (Sylvian) sulcus of the primate brain. **2** Denoting a cerebral gyrus found in several mammalian orders.
**supratemporal** \-temʹpərəl\ Located above, superficial to, or over the temporal lobe, temporal bone, or temporal region. Also *supertemporal*.
**supratentorial** \-tentôrʹē·əl\ Situated or occurring superior to the tentorium cerebelli.
**supraturbinal** \-turʹbinəl\ CONCHA NASALIS SUPERIOR.
**supravalvular** \-valʹvyələr\ Above a valve, especially the aortic or pulmonary valve.
**supraventricular** \-ventrikʹyələr\ At a higher level in the heart than the ventricles: commonly applied to disorders of cardiac rhythm and conduction relating to the atrioventricular node, atria, or sinuatrial node.
**supravergence** \-vurʹjəns\ [SUPRA- + VERGENCE] SUPRADUCTION.
**supraversion** \-vurʹzhən\ [SUPRA- + VERSION] **1** Upward coordinated movement of both eyes. Also *sursumversion, upgaze*. **2** Malposition of teeth in the occlusal direction, especially when this causes a deep overbite.
**supravital** \-vīʹtəl\ Denoting a staining method for living cells detached from their source. Compare INTRAVITAL.
**sur-** \sur-, sər-\ SUB-.
**sura** \sooʹrə\ [L, calf of the leg, shinbone, leg] [NA] The bulging fleshy region at the back of the leg below the knee formed by the gastrocnemius and soleus muscles and related tissues; the calf.
**sural** \sooʹrəl\ Pertaining to the calf of the leg.
**suralimentation** \surʹaliməntāʹshən\ SUPERALIMENTATION.
**suramin** An antitrypanosomal drug. Its molecule contains two residues of 1-aminonaphthalene-4,6,8-trisulfonate, which are acylated by residues of 3-amino-4-methylbenzoic acid, these in turn being acylated by residues of 3-aminobenzoic acid. These last are held together by a CO group joining their two amino groups in a urea structure. Also *Fourneau 309*.
**surdimutism** \surʹdēmyooʹtizm\ [L *surd(us)* deaf + *i* + *mut(us)* mute + -ISM] DEAF MUTISM.
**surdity** \surʹditē\ [L *surditas* (from *surdus* deaf) deafness] HEARING LOSS.

# surface

**surface** [French (from *sur* on, from L *super* over, on + *face* visage, from L *facies* the face) a surface] **1** The outward-facing aspect of the two-dimensional boundary of a structure such as a cell, a tooth, or an organ. **2** The portion of a surface that faces in a particular direction, as in *buccal surface*. **acromial articular s. of clavicle** FACIES ARTICULARIS ACROMIALIS CLAVICULAE. **alveolar s. of maxilla** ARCUS ALVEOLARIS MAXILLAE. **anterior s. of cornea** FACIES ANTERIOR CORNEAE. **anterior s. of eyelids** FACIES ANTERIOR PALPEBRARUM. **anterior s. of iris** FACIES ANTERIOR IRIDIS. **anterior s. of kidney** FACIES ANTERIOR RENIS. **anterior s. of lens** FACIES ANTERIOR LENTIS. **anterior s. of pancreas** FACIES ANTERIOR PANCREATIS. **anterior s. of sacrum** FACIES PELVICA OSSIS SACRI. **anterior s. of scapula** FACIES COSTALIS SCAPULAE. **anterior s. of stomach** PARIES ANTERIOR GASTRIS. **anterior s. of suprarenal gland** FACIES ANTERIOR GLANDULAE SUPRARENALIS. **anterior talar articular s. of calcaneus** FACIES ARTICULARIS TALARIS ANTERIOR CALCANEI. **anteromedial s. of humerus** FACIES ANTERIOR MEDIALIS HUMERI. **approximal s.** PROXIMAL SURFACE. **articular s. of acetabulum** FACIES LUNATA ACETABULI. **basal s. of denture** The surface of a denture base that faces the supporting tissues. Also *denture impression surface, denture foundation surface*. **buccal s.** The surface of a tooth facing the cheek or lip. Also *facial surface, labial surface, vestibular surface*. **carpal articular s. of radius** FACIES ARTICULARIS CARPI RADII. **colic s. of spleen** FACIES COLICA SPLENIS. **condyloid s. of tibia** FACIES ARTICULARIS SUPERIOR TIBIAE. **contact s.** PROXIMAL SURFACE. **costal s. of lung** FACIES COSTALIS PULMONIS. **costal s. of scapula** FACIES COSTALIS SCAPULAE. **cuboid articular s. of calcaneus** FACIES ARTICULARIS CUBOIDEA CALCANEI. **denture foundation s.** BASAL SURFACE OF DENTURE. **denture impression s.** BASAL SURFACE OF DENTURE. **diaphragmatic s. of heart** FACIES DIAPHRAGMATICA CORDIS. **diaphragmatic s. of liver** FACIES DIAPHRAGMATICA HEPATIS. **diaphragmatic s. of lung** FACIES DIAPHRAGMATICA PULMONIS. **diaphragmatic s. of spleen** FACIES DIAPHRAGMATICA SPLENIS. **distal s.** The surface of a tooth facing away from the center of the arch. Except in the case of the third molar, the distal surface of a tooth is normally in contact with the mesial surface of the tooth distal to it. **dorsal s. of scapula** FACIES POSTERIOR SCAPULAE. **extensor s.** The outer part of a limb joint that is undergoing extension or straightening. **facial s.** BUCCAL SURFACE. **flexor s.** The outer part of a limb joint, such as the knee or the elbow, that is undergoing flexion or bending. **gastric s. of spleen** FACIES GASTRICA SPLENIS. **inferior articular s. of tibia** FACIES ARTICULARIS INFERIOR TIBIAE. **inferior s. of liver** FACIES VISCERALIS HEPATIS. **inferior s. of pancreas** FACIES INFERIOR PANCREATIS. **infratemporal s. of maxilla** FACIES INFRATEMPORALIS MAXILLAE. **interlobar s. of lung** FACIES INTERLOBARIS PULMONIS. **isodose s.** In radiation therapy, a three-dimensional surface formed by the locus of all the points which receive the same dose. **labial s.** BUCCAL SURFACE. **lateral articular s. of sacral bone** *Outmoded* FACIES AURICULARIS OSSIS SACRI. **lingual s.** The surface of a denture or tooth facing the tongue. **medial s. of lung** FACIES MEDIASTINALIS PULMONIS. **mediastinal s. of lung** FACIES MEDIASTINALIS PULMONIS. **mesial s.** The surface of a tooth facing toward the center of the arch. Except in the case of the central incisors, the mesial surface of a tooth is normally in contact with the distal surface of the tooth mesial to it. **middle talar articular s. of calcaneus** FACIES ARTICULARIS TALARIS MEDIA CALCANEI. **morsal s.** OCCLUSAL SURFACE. **occlusal s.** The surface of a posterior tooth which faces towards antagonistic teeth. Also *morsal surface.* **orbital s. of sphenoid bone** FACIES ORBITALIS ALAE MAJORIS. **posterior s. of cornea** FACIES POSTERIOR CORNEAE. **posterior s. of eyelids** FACIES POSTERIOR PALPEBRARUM. **posterior s. of iris** FACIES POSTERIOR IRIDIS. **posterior s. of kidney** FACIES POSTERIOR RENIS. **posterior s. of lens** FACIES POSTERIOR LENTIS. **posterior s. of pancreas** FACIES POSTERIOR PANCREATIS. **posterior s. of sacrum** FACIES DORSALIS OSSIS SACRI. **posterior s. of scapula** FACIES POSTERIOR SCAPULAE. **posterior s. of stomach** PARIES POSTERIOR GASTRIS. **posterior s. of suprarenal gland** FACIES POSTERIOR GLANDULAE SUPRARENALIS. **posterior talar articular s. of calcaneus** FACIES ARTICULARIS TALARIS POSTERIOR CALCANEI. **proximal s.** The surface of a tooth which is in contact with an adjacent tooth in the same jaw when the teeth are in their normal alignment. Also *contact surface, approximal surface, proximate surface.* **pulmonary s. of heart** FACIES PULMONALIS CORDIS. **renal s. of spleen** FACIES RENALIS SPLENIS. **renal s. of suprarenal gland** FACIES RENALIS GLANDULAE SUPRARENALIS. **sacropelvic s. of ilium** FACIES SACROPELVICA OSSIS ILII. **sternocostal s. of heart** FACIES STERNOCOSTALIS CORDIS. **superior articular s. of atlas** FACIES ARTICULARIS SUPERIOR ATLANTIS. **superior articular s. of tibia** FACIES ARTICULARIS SUPERIOR TIBIAE. **superior s. of talus** FACIES SUPERIOR TROCHLEAE TALI. **symphysial s. of pubis** FACIES SYMPHYSIALIS. **temporal s. of frontal bone** FACIES TEMPORALIS OSSIS FRONTALIS. **tentorial s.** The part of the cerebral surface that overlies the crescentic lamina of dura mater covering the cerebellum, the tentorium cerebelli. It includes the inferior surfaces of the occipital lobes and the inferomedial surface of both temporal lobes. **total body s.** BODY SURFACE AREA. **vestibular s.** BUCCAL SURFACE. **visceral s. of liver** FACIES VISCERALIS HEPATIS. **visceral s. of spleen** FACIES VISCERALIS SPLENIS.

**surface-active** Having the ability to lower the surface tension of an air-water or oil-water interface. A compound with this property has a molecule composed of hydrophobic and hydrophilic parts, so that it is concentrated at the interface, because these parts have affinities for the different phases.

**surfactant** \sərfak′tənt\ Also *surface-active agent.* A phospholipid material present in the fluid lining the alveoli of the lung which helps to prevent collapse and aids reinflation of deflated alveoli. **pulmonary s.** A substance produced in the lungs and present in alveoli and small airways which reduces surface tension.

**surgeon** \sur′jən\ [Anglo-French *surgien,* contraction of Old French *serurgien* (*cirurgien*) a surgeon, from *cirurg(ie)* surgery (see SURGERY) + *-ien,* suffix meaning adherent or practitioner of] A practitioner of medicine or osteopathy or a related health care field who treats disease and illness or improves appearance or functioning principally by manual and operative intervention. Also *chirurgeon* (obs.). **assistant s.** A person who assists the operating surgeon but who is not primarily responsible for the patient's care. **attending s.** The surgeon who is primarily responsible for the care of the patient undergoing surgery. **dental s.** In the United States and Canada, a dentist who has completed a residency in surgery; in Great Britain, previous to 1956, a dentist who had received a recognized training. • Since 1956 all dentists in Britain have been permitted to use the title. The term is used by all dentists in Australia and South Africa. **district s.** See under MEDICAL EXAMINER. **oral s.** A dentist or doctor who, after further training, practices oral surgery. A term not used in South Africa. **orthopedic s.** A surgeon specializing in orthopedic practice. Also *orthopedist.*

**surgeon general** In certain health care organizations, systems of care, and countries, the chief health care administrator with principal responsibility for medical and related services.

**surgery** \sur′jərē\ [Old French *surgerie,* variant of *serurgie* or *cirurgie,* from L *chirurgia,* from Gk *cheirourgia* (from *cheir,* gen. *cheiro(s)* hand + *erg(on)* work) hand work, surgery] **1** That branch of the art, science, and practice of medicine that deals with the diagnosis and correction of bodily defects resulting from injury or disease and the relief of suffering by manual and instrumental procedures. **2** That craft performed by a surgeon. For defs. 1 and 2 also *chirurgery* (obs.). **3** A place where operative procedures may be performed. **4** A surgeon's office. **5** In Great Britain and South Africa, any medical practitioner's office or place of practice. See also OFFICE. **ambulatory s.** Surgery performed on an outpatient basis, either in a hospital or other freestanding facility. Also *day surgery, in-and-out surgery.* **anaplastic s.** ANAPLASTY. **antiseptic s.** Surgery using materials and methods that will prevent or inhibit the growth of microorganisms. **arthroscopic s.** A surgical procedure carried out within a joint by introducing the necessary surgical instruments through an arthroscope. **aseptic s.** Surgery carried out in a germ-free environment with sterile instruments. **aural s.** The use of surgical methods in the management of ear disease. Modern ear surgery has become increasingly dependent on the operating microscope. It is exceptional today for an ear operation to be performed without its aid. **bench work s.** *Ex vivo* surgery in which an organ, most often a kidney, is removed from the body and undergoes reconstruction, its viability maintained by perfusion, cryopreservation, or other such techniques. **cardiovascular s.** The operative treatment of disorders of the heart and major blood vessels. **clinical s.** Surgery oriented toward the treatment of patients rather than toward research. **closed s.** Manipulation of a part, organ, or tissue without making a skin incision. **closed heart s.** Repair of a cardiac abnormality without the use of a cardiopulmonary bypass. **conservative s.** Surgery concerned with restoration or preservation of diseased parts rather than removal or radical excision. Compare RADICAL SURGERY. **conservative dental s.** A British term for OPERATIVE DENTAL SURGERY. **cosmetic s.** COSMETIC OPERATION. **cryogenic s.** The destruction of tissue by the means of extreme cold. **day s.** AMBULATORY SURGERY. **definitive s.** Any surgical procedure performed for the treatment of a disease previously diagnosed. **dental s.** **1** The practice of dentistry. A British usage. **2** A dentist's office. A British and South African usage. **3** Oral surgery, especially when limited to treatment of the teeth and gums. A term used especially in the United States. **elective s.** Any surgery which does not need to be performed on an emergency basis and for which scheduling in advance will not affect the patient's health. **esthetic s.** COSMETIC OPERATION. **exploratory s.** A surgical procedure that allows the physician to view or handle internal organs of the body in order to determine the cause of an unexplained illness or to relate ambiguous symptoms to a specific disease. **featural s.** COSMETIC OPERATION. **foot-plate s.** STAPES SURGERY. **general s.** That branch of surgery that deals with surgical cases involving any body part, as opposed to more specialized surgery focusing on a specific organ or system. **in-and-out s.** AMBULATORY SURGERY. **laser s.** The use of laser beams in the destruction of bodily abnormalities, usually those located in or on the skin. The carbon dioxide laser has been used in the treatment of skin cancers and the eradication of tattoos, and the argon laser, by virtue of the differential absorption of energy from its green beam, in the treatment of capillary hemangiomas. Because of its tranparency, the eye is uniquely accessible to laser treatment of a large variety of conditions. **major s.** Surgery that is hazardous, involving the possibility of a disabling complication or death. **microvascular s.** Surgery involving procedures during which blood vessels with a diameter of one millimeter or less are anastomosed, done with high-power optical magnification, special sutures (having a diameter of 40 $\mu$m or less), and surgical tools. **minor s.** Surgery that is relatively simple to perform and is not hazardous. **Mohs s.** MOHS CHEMOSURGERY. **mucogingival s.** A surgical procedure involving gingiva and alveolar mucosa. It is generally designed to improve accessibility for the control of plaque around the teeth or to repair localized gingival recession. **open heart s.** Surgery involving the stopping and opening of the heart and therefore requiring extracorporeal circulation. **operative dental s.** Dentistry concerned with restoring teeth, and with replacing them with bridges. Also *conservative dental surgery* (British usage). **oral s.** A dental specialty consisting of the surgical treatment of diseases and malformations of the jaws, teeth, and mouth, such as those resulting from tooth impaction, maxillofacial injury, and tumors. • In South Africa, *maxillofacial surgery* is the preferred term in this sense. **orthopedic s.** A surgical specialty dealing with the injuries, diseases, and disorders of the musculoskeletal system. **palliative s.** Surgery undertaken to alleviate the symptoms or distress associated with an illness or injury, when curative surgery is not advisable or not possible. **peripheral vascular s.** That area of general surgery devoted to the management of pathologic conditions of the arteries, veins, and lymphatics. Its purview includes all blood vessels except those of the heart and the intracranial circulation. **plastic s.** **1** The surgical correction of congenital or acquired deformities of the head, neck, trunk and extremities, whether for functional or esthetic reasons. Also *structural surgery* (seldom used). **2** PLASTIC OPERATION. **radical s.** Surgery which involves major restructuring of portions of the patient's body, or removal of significant body parts. Compare CONSERVATIVE SURGERY. **reconstructive s.** A plastic operation designed to restore the form and/or function of a body part that has been lost through injury or disease. Also *reconstruction, reconstructive operation.* **sonic s.** The use of ultrasound to alter or destroy tissue. **stapes s.** The various surgical operations for the relief of otosclerosis in which a direct approach to the ankylosed stapes is made, in contrast with the earlier fenestration operation in which the lesion was bypassed. Also *foot-plate surgery.* **stereotaxic s.** STEREOTAXY. **structural s.** *Seldom used* PLASTIC SURGERY. **thoracic s.** Surgery performed upon the chest and its contents. **transsexual s.** Surgical procedures for changing the external reproductive organs to resemble those of the opposite sex.

**Surgicel** Oxidized regenerated cellulose, an absorbable hemostatic agent. A proprietary name.

**sursumduction** \sur′səmduk′shən\ SUPRADUCTION.

**sursumvergence** \sur′səmvur′jəns\ [L *sursum* upward, up and down + *verg(ere)* to bend, incline + -ENCE] SUPRADUCTION.

**sursumversion** \sur′səmvur′zhən\ [L *sursum* upward, up and down + VERSION] SUPRAVERSION.

**surveillance** \sərvā′ləns\ [French (from *surveiller* to oversee, from *sur* on, over, from L *super* over, on, + French *veiller* to watch, from L *vigilare* to watch, from *vigil* wakeful + *-ance* -ANCE), a keeping watch, overseeing] The maintenance of oversight or tracking of the whereabouts of a person known to have been or suspected of having been exposed to infection, with a view of preventing further spread and of treating the person being watched should the disease develop. **immunologic s.** The theory that the immune system is continuously monitoring for the presence of deviant host cells, which it identifies as foreign and destroys. Also *immunosurveillance.*

**survey** **1** To form a general, comprehensive view of or give such an account of. **2** To estimate or establish the relationships between two or more variables or attributes within a population. **3** A method whereby information about such relationships is obtained. **4** An estimate or determination. **market-basket s.** A survey made to ascertain food expenditure in relation to family income. Both the total and individual food expenditures are considered. Such a survey includes all foods and drinks purchased or acquired. Also *family-budget survey.* **total diet s.** A survey designed to find out what foods and drinks are consumed and in what quantities. Such a survey often obtains information pertaining to the reasons for consuming a particular diet, as in cases where socioeconomic status is found to have a correlation with the particular foods eaten.

**surveying** \sərvā′ing\ The process of studying, on a dental cast, the relative parallelism of teeth and associated structures in order to determine the best path of insertion for a restoration.

**surveyor** \sərvā′ər\ A device used for surveying teeth.

**survival** [English *survive* (from Middle French *survivre* to survive, from L *supervivere* to survive, from *super* on, over + *vivere* to live) + -AL] Continued life; the fact of living longer or living beyond the life-span of another. **s. of the fittest** The tendency of the fittest individuals of a population to survive, an idea attributed to Charles Darwin. The modern version of this concept is termed neodarwinism. **five-year s.** A measurement of survival from a disease,

especially cancer. It is expressed as a percentage of those under observation who were alive five years after diagnosis.
**survivorship** \sərvī′vərship\ The survival of one of two or more individuals following the death of the other or others. If the duration of survival is quite short, as in the case of a husband and wife who die in a collision, forensic scientists may be asked to determine if one spouse's death preceded the other, since provisions in wills and trusts are often contingent upon the order of death of the spouses.
**sus-** \sus-, səs-\ SUB-.
**susceptibility** \səsep′təbil′itē\ [Med L *susceptibilitas* (from Late L *susceptibil(is)* susceptible + *-itas* -ITY) susceptibility] The condition of being susceptible. **differential s.** A nonhomogeneous response in various regions of an embryo when the whole embryo is exposed to a diffusely applied teratogenic agent.
**susceptible** \səsep′tibəl\ [Late L *susceptibilis* (from L *suscept(us)*, past part. of *suscipere* to lift up, undergo + *-ibilis* English *-ible*) capable of undergoing, feeling, or admitting] Liable to infection or to the effects of substances, as toxins, or other influences; lacking the capacity to respond effectively to a pathogen.
**suspect** [L *suspect(us)*, past part. of *suspicere* to mistrust, suspect] A person whose history or symptoms indicate that he or she may, after an appropriate period of incubation, develop a disease or prove to have contracted it in a subclinical form.
**suspensiometer** \suspen′sē·äm′ətər\ [*suspensio(n)* + -METER] NEPHELOMETER.
**suspension** [Late L *suspensio* (from *suspensus*, past part. of *suspendere* to hang up, raise, from L *sus-* prefix denoting up, upward + *pendere* to hang) a suspending, hanging up] **1** A compound mixture in which finely divided, undissolved powders are dispersed throughout a suitable liquid vehicle. **2** Support, as by traction, so provided to a part of the body to free another part to respond to the pressure of its own weight, used therapeutically as in the treatment of certain spinal disorders. **Coffey s.** A uterine suspension operation in which the fundus is brought forward by suturing a loop of each round ligament to the anterior wall of the uterus, the loops coming together in the midline. **cuff s.** Suspension of a below-knee prosthesis to the limb using a fabric cuff attached to the socket and applied just above the patella. **extended insulin zinc s.** A long-acting insulin preparation, a sterile suspension of insulin with added zinc chloride. **insulin zinc s.** An intermediate-acting insulin preparation, a sterile suspension of insulin with added zinc chloride. Also *insulin lente.* **prompt insulin zinc s.** A rapidly-acting insulin preparation, a sterile suspension of insulin with added zinc chloride. **protamine zinc insulin s.** PROTAMINE ZINC INSULIN. **sterile epinephrine s.** A sterile suspension of epinephrine in vegetable oil at a concentration of about 2 mg/ml, for intramuscular injection. It is used in the treatment of asthma and other allergic states. **sterile estradiol s.** The suspension of native estrogen in concentrations of 0.2–1.0 mg/ml or various esters in concentrations of 0.5–40 mg/ml, the latter for prolonged duration of action. It is used for intramuscular injection as an estrogen. **sterile medroxyprogesterone acetate s.** The progestin suspended in an aqueous medium for parenteral injection, used in the treatment of constitutional sexual precocity in girls. **sterile progesterone s.** A sterile suspension of progesterone in water for injection. It is used chiefly as a test for adequacy of prior estrogenic stimulation of the endometrium. Post-progesterone uterine bleeding signifies sufficient endogenous estrogen secretion. **sterile propyliodone s.** A sterile suspension in water of propyliodone, the *n*-propyl ester of 3,5-diiodo-4-pyridone-*N*-acetic acid, used as a positive contrast medium for bronchography. Also *sterile propyliodone oil suspension.* **sterile testosterone s.** A sterile suspension of testosterone in aqueous medium, used as an intramuscular injection to produce androgenic effects.
**suspensory** \səspen′sərē\ Suspending, supporting, or holding up a part or structure, such as a muscle, bone, or ligament. Also *suspensorius.*
**suspirious** \səspī′rē·əs\ SIGHING.
**sustentacular** \sus′təntak′ələr\ **1** Pertaining to a sustentaculum. **2** Designating a supporting cell in an epithelial layer, such as the Sertoli cells in the seminiferous tubules.
**sustentaculum** \sus′təntak′yələm\ [L (from *sustentare* to keep upright, hold, support, from *sus-* prefix denoting up, upward + *tentare* for *tenere* to hold), a prop, stay, support] Any structure that supports or holds up another structure. **s. tali** [NA] A shelflike process projecting from the anterior part of the upper medial margin of the calcaneus and bearing on its upper surface the middle articular facet for supporting the talus. Its lower surface is grooved by the tendon of flexor hallucis longus. Also *sustentaculum of talus.*
**susurration** \sus′ərā′shən\ [*susurr(us)* + -ATION] MURMUR.
**susurrus** \səsur′əs\ [L, a murmuring, whispering, humming] MURMUR.
**Sutherland** [George Fraser *Sutherland*, U.S. neurophysiologist, born 1900] James-Lange-Sutherland theory. See under JAMES-LANGE THEORY.
**sutika** \soo′tikə\ [Bengali] A disease of pregnant women, consisting of gastrointestinal symptoms and fever, followed by megaloblastic anemia which usually develops after delivery. It is found in the Bengal region of India.
**Sutton** [Richard Lightburn *Sutton*, U.S. dermatologist, 1878–1952] **1** Sutton's nevus. See under HALO NEVUS. **2** Sutton's disease. See under PERIADENITIS MUCOSA NECROTICA RECURRENS.
**sutura** \soochoo′rə\ [L (from *suere* to sew, stitch up, akin to English *sew*) a seam, stitching, suture of skull bones] (*pl.* suturae) [NA] A type of fibrous joint in which the closely apposed ends of the skull bones are joined by a layer of fibrous tissue or sutural ligament which blends with the periosteum and tends towards progressive ossification at varying times during adult life, ending in obliteration of the joint and production of a synostosis. The joint is immobile and limited to the skull. Three varieties are described: serrated, squamous, and plane. Also *suture, suture joint, bony suture.* **s. coronalis** [NA] The extensive arched articulation between the serrated parietal margin of the frontal bone and the frontal margins of the two parietal bones. Also *coronal suture.* **suturae cranii** [NA] The immovable fibrous joints between the various contiguous bones of the skull. Also *cranial sutures, sutures of skull.* **s. dentata** A sutura serrata in which the serrations are small toothlike projections which often spread out at their free ends. They are usually located in parts of the lambdoid and sagittal sutures. Also *dentate suture, denticulate suture.* **s. ethmoidolacrimalis** [NA] A suture between the anterior margin of the orbital lamina of the ethmoid bone and the posterior margin of the lacrimal bone in the medial wall of the orbit. Also *ethmoidolacrimal suture, lacrimoethmoidal suture.* **s. ethmoidomaxillaris** [NA] The articulation between the lower margin of the orbital plate of the ethmoid bone and the superomedial margin of the orbital surface of the maxilla in the inferomedial part of the orbit. Also *ethmoidomaxillary suture.* **s. frontalis** [NA] The line of junction situated

in the median plane between the two halves of the frontal bone at birth and usually completely fused and obliterated within the first decade of life. Also *frontal suture.* See also SUTURA METOPICA. **s. frontoethmoidalis** 1 [NA] The U-shaped articulation in the middle of the floor of the anterior cranial fossa between the orbital part of the frontal bone and the cribriform plate of the ethmoid bone. 2 [NA] The articulation in the medial wall of the orbit between the medial margin of the orbital surface of the frontal bone and the superior edge of the orbital plate of the ethmoid bone, continuous anteriorly with the frontolacrimal suture. For defs. 1 and 2 also *frontoethmoidal suture.* **s. frontolacrimalis** [NA] The articulation in the medial wall of the orbit between the medial margin of the orbital surface of the frontal bone and the superior margin of the orbital surface of the lacrimal bone. Also *frontolacrimal suture.* **s. frontomaxillaris** [NA] The junction between the nasal margin of the frontal bone and the superior border of the frontal process of the maxilla. Also *frontomaxillary suture.* **s. frontonasalis** [NA] The junction on each side of the median plane between the nasal margin of the frontal bone and the superior margins of the two nasal bones just medial to the frontomaxillary sutures. Also *frontonasal suture, nasofrontal suture.* **s. frontozygomatica** [NA] The line of junction at the lateral end of the supraorbital margin between the zygomatic process of the frontal bone and the frontal process of the zygomatic bone. Also *frontozygomatic suture, zygomaticofrontal suture* (outmoded). **s. incisiva** [NA] An indistinct groove on the inferior surface of the palatine process of the maxilla, extending anterolaterally from the incisive fossa to the gap between the canine and lateral incisor teeth. The suture demarcates the junction between the premaxillary and the postmaxillary parts of the maxilla, is usually present at birth, and often becomes indistinct in the adult. Also *incisive suture, anterior palatine suture* (outmoded), *suture of Goethe* (outmoded), *premaxillary suture.* **s. infraorbitalis** [NA] An inconstant suture between the infraorbital foramen and the infraorbital canal, present only for a brief time after the canal is formed. Also *infraorbital suture.* **s. intermaxillaris** [NA] The line of junction in the median plane between the two maxillae, best seen between the alveolar processes and between the palatine processes. Some authorities limit this suture to the junction between the alveolar processes. Also *intermaxillary suture.* **s. internasalis** [NA] The articulation in the median plane between the medial margins of the two nasal bones. Also *internasal suture.* **s. lacrimoconchalis** [NA] The articulation between the descending conchal process of the medial wall of the vertical groove on the orbital surface of the lacrimal bone and the apex of the lacrimal process projecting up from the superior margin of the inferior nasal concha. Also *lacrimoconchal suture.* **s. lacrimomaxillaris** [NA] The articulation between the inferior margin of the lacrimal bone posterior to the posterior lacrimal crest and the medial margin of the orbital plate of the maxilla. Also *lacrimomaxillary suture.* **s. lambdoidea** [NA] The junction of the occipital margins of the two parietal bones and the lambdoid margin of the squamous part of the occipital bone, shaped like the Greek letter lambda. The apex is continuous with the sagittal suture. Also *lambdoid suture, lambdoidal suture, parietoccipital suture.* **s. limbosa** A sutura serrata in which there is some beveling of the interlocking surfaces. Some authorities view it as a variety of sutura squamosa in which the beveled surfaces may be serrated or ridged to facilitate interlocking. Also *limbous suture.* **s. metopica** [NA] A sutura frontalis that persists into adult life, dividing the frontal bone into two halves. Also *metopic suture.* **s. nasomaxillaris** [NA] The articulation between the lateral margin of the nasal bone and the anterior margin of the frontal process of the maxilla. Also *nasomaxillary suture.* **s. occipitomastoidea** [NA] One of the posterolateral bifurcating continuations of the lambdoid suture, commencing at the posteroinferior angle of the parietal bone and passing between the posterior margin of the petrous part of the temporal bone and the squamous part of the occipital bone. Also *occipitomastoid suture.* **s. palatina mediana** [NA] The junction in the median plane between the apposing horizontal plates of the two palatine bones forming the posterior part of the bony palate. The suture is continuous anteriorly with the intermaxillary suture. Also *median palatine suture, middle palatine suture, interpalatine suture.* **s. palatina transversa** [NA] The transverse line of junction of the posterior margins of the palatine processes of the maxillae and the anterior margins of the horizontal plates of the palatine bones in the bony palate. Also *transverse palatine suture.* **s. palatoethmoidalis** [NA] The articulation in the inferior wall of the orbit between the medial or ethmoidal surface of the orbital process of the perpendicular plate of the palatine bone and the orbital plate of the ethmoid bone. Also *palatoethmoidal suture.* **s. palatomaxillaris** [NA] The articulation in the floor of the orbit between the anterior surface of the orbital process of the palatine bone and the medial margin of the orbital surface of the maxilla. Also *palatomaxillary suture.* **s. parietomastoidea** [NA] One of the posterolateral bifurcating continuations of the lambdoid suture, commencing at the posteroinferior angle of the parietal bone and passing horizontally between the latter and the mastoid process of the temporal bone. Also *parietomastoid suture.* **s. plana** [NA] A suture in which there is simple apposition of either smooth and regular or roughened but complementary surfaces, as in the intermaxillary and the internasal sutures. Also *plane suture, flat suture, false suture.* **s. sagittalis** [NA] The articulation between the highly serrated apposing sagittal or superior margins of the parietal bones. Also *sagittal suture.* **s. serrata** [NA] A variety of suture in which the apposing edges of the participating bones have interlocking sawlike teeth, as in most of the sagittal and lambdoid sutures. Also *serrated suture, serrate suture.* **s. sphenoethmoidalis** 1 [NA] A vertical articulation between the posterior margin of the orbital plate of the ethmoid bone and the lateral margin of the body of the sphenoid bone in the most posterior part of the medial wall of the orbit. 2 [NA] The articulation between the upper end of the sphenoidal crest of the body of the sphenoid bone and the posterior margin of the perpendicular plate of the ethmoid bone. For defs. 1 and 2 also *sphenoethmoidal suture.* **s. sphenofrontalis** [NA] The union of both the anterior margin of the lesser wing and the upper edge of the orbital surface of the greater wing of the sphenoid bone with the posterior margin of the orbital plate of the frontal bone, on each side of the floor of the anterior cranial fossa. Also *sphenofrontal suture.* **s. sphenomaxillaris** [NA] An occasional articulation between the greater wing of the sphenoid bone and the orbital surface of the maxilla resulting in the inferior orbital fissure being closed laterally. Also *sphenomaxillary suture.* **s. sphenoparietalis** [NA] The articulation at pterion in the temporal fossa between the superior tip of the greater wing of the sphenoid bone and the sphenoidal angle of the parietal bone. Also *sphenoparietal suture.* **s. sphenosquamosa** [NA] The articulation in the lateral wall of the middle cranial fossa between the concave posterolateral margin of the greater wing of the sphenoid bone and the convex anterior margin of the squama of the temporal bone. Also *sphenosquamous suture, sphenosquamosal suture.* **s. sphenovomeriana** [NA] A schindylesis between the deep median groove in the superior border of the vomer and the rostrum of the sphenoid bone. Also *sphenovomerian suture.* **s. sphenozygomatica** [NA] The articulation between the anterolateral margin of the orbital surface of the greater wing of the sphenoid bone and the upper posteromedial margin of the orbital surface of the zygomatic bone. Also *sphenozygomatic suture, zygomaticosphenoid suture, zygomaticosphenoid fissure.* **s. squamosa** [NA] A variety of suture in which the apposing edges of the participating bones are overlapping and reciprocally beveled so as to fit tightly. Also *squamous suture, squamosal suture.* **s. squamosa cranii** [NA] The articulation between the externally beveled middle portion of the inferior or squamosal margin of the parietal bone and the internally beveled convex superior margin of the squamous part of the temporal bone. Also *squamous suture of cranium, squamosoparietal suture, parietotemporal suture.* **s. squamosomastoidea** [NA] An articulation present in early postnatal life between the squamous and the petrous parts of the temporal bone of which traces are occasionally found in the adult, running obliquely on the anterolateral aspect of the mastoid process. Also *squamomastoid suture.* **s. temporozygomatica** [NA] The articulation on the zygomatic arch between the zygomatic process of the temporal bone and the temporal process of the zygomatic bone. Also *temporozygomatic suture, zygomaticotemporal suture.* **s. vera** A suture in which the apposing edges of the participating bones have reciprocal projections and hollows, resulting in immovable interlocking. Some authorities recognize three varieties: sutura serrata, sutura dentata, and sutura limbosa. *Outmoded.* Also *true suture.* **s. zygomaticomaxillaris** [NA] The articulation between the posterolaterally projecting zygomatic process of the maxilla and the anteroinferior margin as well as the lower part of the posteromedial margin of the zygomatic bone. Also *zygomaticomaxillary suture.*

**suturae** \soochoo′rē\ Plural of SUTURA.

**sutural** \soo′chərəl\ Of or pertaining to a suture.

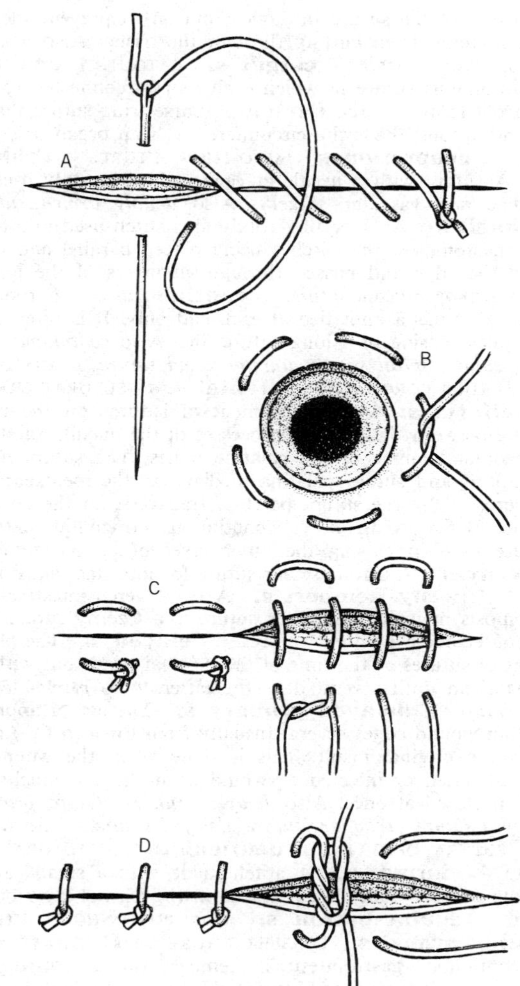


**Surgical sutures** (A) Continuous; (B) pursestring; (C) Halsted; (D) interrupted.

# suture

**suture** \soo′chər\ [L *sutura.* See SUTURA.] **1** To surgically unite or bring into apposition two surfaces or tissues by means of stitches. **2** Any of various materials used to sew the edges of a wound or tissue in approximation. **3** The product of such sewing. For defs. 1 and 3 also *stitch.* **4** SUTURA. **absorbable s.** A suture made of material that is gradually digested or hydrolyzed by the tissue and by body fluids. The material is usually catgut or tendon, sometimes coated with a substance that delays absorption. **s. of Albrecht** ENDOMESOGNATHIC SUTURE. **apposition s.** A stitch or group of stitches used to hold two tissue edges in anatomic contact without tension. Also *coaptation suture.* **approximation s.** A stitch or group of stitches used to bring two tissues together to allow healing. **atraumatic s.** A suture made with a thread that is swaged onto an eyeless needle so as to cause minimal trauma in passing through the tissue. **baseball s.** A lock-stitch suture in which the free edge of tissue (usually skin) is inverted. This is accomplished by inserting the needle through a partial thickness of skin at a point back from the free edge. When the suture is drawn firmly, the free edge will invert. **Bell s.** A lock-stitch suture whereby the needle is passed from within the wound outwardly, alternating edges of the wound in a locking fashion. **blanket s.** LOCK-STITCH SUTURE. **bolster s.** A form of retention suture that is tied over a rolled piece of gauze, a piece of rubber tubing, or a bridge. It serves to protect the skin by relieving tension on the primary suture line. **bony s.** SUTURA. **buried s.** A stitch or series of stitches used to close a wound in which the knots are buried deep within the skin edges of the wound, beneath the primary suture line. Also *implanted suture.* **button s.** A suture anchored on a button or disk so as to prevent the stitch from cutting through the flesh. **buttonhole s.** An interrupted surgical suture used to unite wound edges by passing each end of the suture through a button to prevent the suture material from cutting through the tissue. Also *double-button suture* (obs.). **catgut s.** CATGUT. **chain s.** A continuous suture in which each loop is connected to the adjacent loop. **circular s.** A pursestring suture that is wound around the entire circumference of an organ or structure. **coaptation s.** APPOSITION SUTURE. **cobbler s.** A suture with a needle at each end, commonly used in cardiac and vascular surgery. Also *doubly armed suture.* **Connell s.** An inverting continuous stitch used in intestinal anastomoses, the stitches being placed parallel and back from the edge and passed through all layers of the bowel. Also *loop-on mucosa suture.* **continuous s.** A running stitch that has a knot tied at each end only. It is often used for quick closing of a long suture line. Also *continuous running suture, spiral suture, uninterrupted suture.* **coronal s.** SUTURA CORONALIS. **cranial s.'s** SUTURAE CRANII. **cruciform s.** An arrangement of sutures on the bony palate between the palatine processes of the maxillae and the horizontal laminae of the palatine bones. The sutura intermaxillaris and sutura palatina mediana in the median plane are crossed by the sutura palatina transversa in the coronal plane. **Cushing s.** A continuous horizontal mattress suture used in closing the outer layer of an anastomosis. **Czerny s.** A seromuscular suture for intestinal anastomosis. **Czerny-Lembert s.** A two-layered intestinal anastomosis in which the inner suture is a Czerny suture and the outer one a Lembert suture. **delayed s.** The placement of sutures at the time of the original insult but without tying them until several days thereafter. Also *primo-secondary suture.* **delayed primary s.** The act of approximating wound edges several (usually from three to five) days after the original insult. This is done when the wound is contaminated or infected or would be under too much tension if closed at once. Also *delayed primary closure, primary delayed suture, secondary suture, delayed suture.* **dentate s.** SUTURA DENTATA. **denticulate s.** SUTURA SERRATA. **dermal s.** A stitch made with a small caliber needle and very fine thread placed in the dermal layer of the skin. **double-button s.** *Obs.* BUTTONHOLE SUTURE. **doubly armed s.** COBBLER SUTURE. **Dupuytren s.** A continuous gastrointestinal Lembert suture. **endognathic s.** The midline suture between one os incisivum of the maxilla and that of the other side, formed at their first appearance in fetal life. **endomesognathic s.** A suture between the endognathion (inner segment of the os incisivum) and the mesognathion (lateral segment of the os incisivum) which forms at the start of fetal life and is sometimes visible on the palatal vault in the newborn. Also *suture of Albrecht.* **end-on mattress s.** VERTICAL MATTRESS SUTURE. **epineural s.** The anastomosis of divided nerve ends by suturing the epineurium of each. **ethmoidolacrimal s.** SUTURA ETHMOIDOLACRIMALIS. **ethmoidomaxillary s.** SUTURA ETHMOIDOMAXILLARIS. **everting s.** A suture in which the inner lining of the tissues, such as endothelium or mucosa, is brought into apposition. **everting interrupted s.** An interrupted suture that turns the divided tissue outward. **false s.** SUTURA PLANA. **far-and-near s.** The closure of fascia by suturing away from and close to the edges. **figure-of-eight s.** A stitch forming the shape of the number eight, whereby a second pass of the needle crosses the first stitch at right angles. It is used as a hemostatic stitch and to approximate fascial layers. **flat s.** SUTURA PLANA. **frontal s.** SUTURA FRONTALIS. **frontoethmoidal s.** SUTURA FRONTOETHMOIDALIS. **frontolacrimal s.** SUTURA FRONTOLACRIMALIS. **frontomaxillary s.** SUTURA FRONTOMAXILLARIS. **frontonasal s.** SUTURA FRONTONASALIS. **frontozygomatic s.** SUTURA FRONTOZYGOMATICA. **Frost s.** A mattress suture placed between the upper and the lower eyelid to keep the lids closed following operations on the eye or its adnexae. **furrier s.** An inverting gastrointestinal suture made in figure-of-eight fashion, the needle being passed from within to the surface on one side of the wound and then on the other. **glovers s.** LOCK-STITCH SUTURE. **guy s.** STAY SUTURE. **Halsted s.** **1** A horizontal mattress suture that is stitched parallel to the wound on one side, with both free ends brought out on the opposite side and tied. **2** A subcuticular object placed immediately under the skin to ensure exact wound edge approximation. **hemostatic s.** A suture that approximates wound edges and also controls oozing from the edges of the wound. The danger exists, however, of its being too effective and rendering the sutured area ischemic. **horizontal mattress s.** A stitch or series of stitches used to close a wound by having the sutures pass parallel to the edge of the wound superficially, and perpendicular to the wound edges on the deeper levels. It can either be tied in an interrupted fashion or run continuously for the length of the wound. **implanted s.** BURIED SUTURE. **incisive s.** SUTURA INCISIVA. **infolding s.** INVERTING SUTURE. **infraorbital s.** SUTURA INFRAORBITALIS. **intermaxillary s.** SUTURA INTERMAXILLARIS. **internasal s.** SUTURA INTERNASALIS. **interpalatine s.** SUTURA PALATINA MEDIANA. **interrupted s.** Any stitch which is placed across two sides of skin, intestine, a vessel, or tissue, and then tied, thus approximating the edges. This technique is repeated for the length of the wound. **intradermal s.** A stitch or a series of stitches used to close a wound, placed completely within the dermal layer and running parallel to the wound. It is often used in plastic surgery. Also *subcuticular suture.* **intradermal mattress s.** A stitch or series of stitches used to close a wound by placing mattress sutures completely below the epidermis of the skin. **invaginating s.** INVERTING SUTURE. **inverting s.** A stitch or series of stitches placed so that the two edges of tissue are turned inward, thus invaginating the edge. It is usually used in an intestinal anastomosis to create a serosa-to-serosa approximation. Also *invaginating suture, infolding suture.* **lacrimoconchal s.** SUTURA LACRIMOCONCHALIS. **lacrimoethmoidal s.** SUTURA ETHMOIDOLACRIMALIS. **lacrimomaxillary s.** SUTURA LACRIMOMAXILLARIS. **lambdoid s.** SUTURA LAMBDOIDEA. **lambdoidal s.** SUTURA LAMBDOIDEA. **Lembert s.** An invaginating continuous stitch used in intestinal circular enterorrhaphy to create serosal apposition. The suture is placed through the serosa and the submucosa, but does not pierce the mucosa. It usually comprises the outer layer of a standard two-layer intestinal anastomosis, the Czerny-Lembert suture. **lens s.'s** RADII LENTIS. **limbous s.** SUTURA LIMBOSA. **lock-stitch s.** A continuous transmural stitch in which each succeeding stitch is passed beneath the loop of the last, creating a locking, blanket effect. The suture is used in intestinal surgery to preserve hemostasis. Also *glovers suture, glover stitch, blanket suture.* **loop-on mucosa s.** CONNELL SUTURE. **mattress s.** A suture that is placed back and forth through both sides of an incision. Also *quilt suture, quilted suture.* **median palatine s.** SUTURA PALATINA MEDIANA. **metopic s.** SUTURA METOPICA. **middle palatine s.** SUTURA PALATINA MEDIANA. **nasofrontal s.** SUTURA FRONTONASALIS. **nasomaxillary s.** SUTURA NASOMAXILLARIS. **nerve s.** NEURORRHAPHY. **nonabsorbable s.** A suture of a permanent nature made of materials that will withstand hydrolysis and denaturation of the body tissues. Materials possessing these qualities include stainless steel wire, nylon, silk, cotton, and various other synthetic fibers. **occipitomastoid s.** SUTURA OCCIPITOMASTOIDEA. **over-and-over s.** Any continuous stitch used to approximate tissue edges by taking equal portions of tissue on each side. The suture is used frequently because of the rapidity and ease with which it can be applied. **palatoethmoidal s.** SUTURA PALATOETHMOIDALIS. **palatomaxillary s.** SUTURA PALATOMAXILLARIS. **Paré s.** A surgical technique of uniting a wound by securing strips of cloth to the skin and then joining the strips with stitches. **parietoccipital s.** SUTURA LAMBDOIDEA. **parietomastoid s.** SUTURA PARIETOMASTOIDEA. **parietotemporal s.** SUTURA SQUAMOSA CRANII. **Parker-Kerr s.** A continuous inverting suture often used in the closure of intestinal wounds. **peg-and-socket s.** GOMPHOSIS. **petrosquamous s.** FISSURA PETROSQUAMOSA. **plane s.** SUTURA PLANA. **plastic s.** A suture made from a plastic material. **plicating s.** A stitch or series of stitches used to close a wound by folding one edge upon the other. **premaxillary s.** SUTURA INCISIVA. **presection s.** A series of surgical stitches made into tissues before incising the tissues. **primary s.** PRIMARY CLOSURE. **primary delayed s.** DELAYED PRIMARY SUTURE. **primo-secondary s.** DELAYED SUTURE. **pursestring s.** A surgical technique in which a circular stitch is placed in such a way as to draw together or invert a wound. **quilt s.** MATTRESS SUTURE. **quilted s.** MATTRESS SUTURE. **relaxation s.** A stitch or a series of stitches used to close a wound such that the stitches can later be loosened to decrease any undue tissue tension. **retention s.** One or more stitches used to close a wound by taking up large amounts of tissue in each stitch in order to relieve tension from and reinforce the primary suture line and to prevent wound disruption. Also *tension suture.* **Richter s.** An interrupted suture formerly made of silver wire and used to close an intestinal wound. **right-angle mattress s.** VERTICAL MATTRESS SUTURE. **sagittal s.** SUTURA SAGITTALIS. **secondary s.** DELAYED PRIMARY SUTURE. **seroserous s.** Any stitch or series of stitches, such as those used for Lembert sutures, that closes two serous surfaces. **serrate s.** SUTURA SERRATA. **serrated s.** SUTURA SERRATA. **s.'s of skull** SUTURAE CRANII. **sphenoethmoidal s.** SUTURA SPHENOETHMOIDALIS. **sphenofrontal s.** SUTURA SPHENOFRONTALIS. **sphenomaxillary s.** SUTURA SPHENOMAXILLARIS. **spheno-occipital s.** SYNCHONDROSIS SPHENO-OCCIPITALIS. **sphenoparietal s.** SUTURA SPHENOPARIETALIS. **sphenopetrosal s.** SYNCHONDROSIS SPHENOPETROSA. **sphenosquamosal s.** SUTURA SPHENOSQUAMOSA. **sphenosquamous s.** SUTURA SPHENOSQUAMOSA. **sphenovomerian s.** SUTURA SPHENOVOMERIANA. **sphenozygomatic s.** SUTURA SPHENOZYGOMATICA. **spiral s.** CONTINUOUS SUTURE. **squamosal s.** SUTURA SQUAMOSA. **squamosomastoid s.** SUTURA SQUAMOSOMASTOIDEA. **squamosoparietal s.** SUTURA SQUAMOSA CRANII. **squamous s.** SUTURA SQUAMOSA. **squamous s. of cranium** SUTURA SQUAMOSA CRANII. **stay s.** A large, strong suture that supports the closure of a wound. Also *guy suture.* **subcuticular s.** INTRADERMAL SUTURE. **temporozygomatic s.** SUTURA TEMPOROZYGOMATICA. **tension s.** RETENTION SUTURE. **through-and-through s.** A stitch or series of stitches placed through all layers of a closure of a wound. **transfixion s.** A hemostatic suture of a blood vessel in which the suture is first passed through the vessel, then tied around it. **transverse palatine s.** SUTURA PALATINA TRANSVERSA. **true s.** SUTURA VERA. **tympanomastoid s.** The junction between the tympanic plate and the mastoid process of the temporal bone, in line with and lateral to fissura tympanomastoidea. **uninterrupted s.** CONTINUOUS SUTURE. **vertical mattress s.** One or more stitches placed in deep and superficial layers of tissue at an angle perpendicular to the wound edge. Also *end-on mattress suture, right-angle mattress suture.* **zygomaticofrontal s.** *Outmoded* SUTURA FRONTOZYGOMATICA. **zygomaticomaxillary s.** SUTURA ZYGOMATICOMAXILLARIS. **zygomaticosphenoid s.** SUTURA SPHENOZYGOMATICA. **zygomaticotemporal s.** SUTURA TEMPOROZYGOMATICA.

**Suzanne** [Jean Georges *Suzanne,* French physician, born 1859] See under GLAND.

**SV** simian virus.

**SV40** simian virus 40.

**s.v.** *spiritus vini* (L, alcoholic spirit).

**SVC** superior vena cava.

**Svedberg** [Theodor *Svedberg,* Swedish chemist, 1884–1971] **1** Folin and Svedberg method. See under METHOD. **2** See under UNIT. **3** Svedberg coefficient. See under SEDIMENTATION COEFFICIENT.

**svedberg** \sved′bərg\ [after Theodor *Svedberg,* Swedish chemist, 1884–1971] A CGS unit of rate of sedimentation, used especially in centrifuge techniques, equal to $10^{-13}$ centimeter per second when the acceleration is one centimeter per second squared. An obsolete unit. Symbol: Sv, S

**s.v.r.** *spiritus vini rectificatus* (L, rectified, or purified, spirit of wine). The concentration of ethanol in this alcoholic preparation is 95 percent.

**s.v.t.** *spiritus vini tenuis* (L, proof spirit). In the United States, 100 proof alcohol contains 50% ethanol by volume.

**swab** \swäb\ [akin to Low German *Swabber* a mop] A mass of cotton wool, gauze, sponge, or other absorbent material at one end of a supporting stick, wire, or flexible fiber. It is used to apply or to remove fluid from surfaces, especially to collect specimens for microbiologic examination or to cleanse and medicate tissue surfaces. **NIH s.** A swab in which the collecting surface is a sticky cellophane. It is used to gather ova and other particulate material from epithelial surfaces.

**swaddler** \swäd′lər\ [Middle English *swadelen,* prob. from Old English *swethel* to swaddle; akin to Middle English *swathian* to swathe] Material in which an infant is wrapped. **silver s.** A thin sheet of metal-coated plastic material, in which an infant can be wrapped in order to minimize heat loss from radiation.

**swage** \swāj\ [Middle English, from Old French *souage* a tool for shaping metal] To adapt sheet metal to a die by pressure.

**swallow** [Middle English *swolwen,* from Old English *swelgan*] **1** To move materials from the mouth into the stomach by way of the esophagus. **2** A movement of materials from the mouth into the stomach. Also *deglutition, swallowing.* **barium s.** A radiologic examination in which the patient swallows an aqueous suspension of barium sulfate to opacify the upper gastrointestinal tract.

**swallowing** SWALLOW. **air s.** AEROPHAGIA. **infantile s.** A pattern of swallowing in which the alveolar processes (or the teeth) do not come into occlusion, the tongue is thrust forward and the circumoral musculature contracts. **tongue s.** The falling back of the tongue into the oropharynx with consequent respiratory obstruction, a risk to which the comatose patient (including particularly the anesthetized patient) is exposed when lying in the supine position.

**Swan** [Harold James C. *Swan*, U.S. cardiologist, born 1922] Swan-Ganz catheter. See under CATHETER.

**swarming** 1 The bunching together of a large number of small organisms, such as insects, commonly for breeding or the establishment of a new colony. 2 The spreading of extremely motile bacteria, such as *Proteus vulgaris*, over the surface of an agar plate, forming a thin film instead of discrete colonies.

**swearing / compulsive s.** COPROLALIA.

**sweat** [Old English *swāt*, akin to L *sudor* sweat and Gk *hidrōs* sweat] 1 The secretion produced by sweat glands. Also *perspiration*. 2 To secrete fluid from sweat glands. Also *perspire, sudor*. **bloody s.** HEMATIDROSIS. **fetid s.** BROMHIDROSIS. **night s.** Sweating which occurs during sleep or at night, as in tuberculosis.

**sweating** A state of sweat production. **insensible s.** The evaporation of body water by diffusion through the skin without discernible wetness of the skin surface. Also *transpiration, insensible perspiration*. **sensible s.** The evaporation of body water that has been actively secreted by the sweat glands and that is accompanied by discernible wetness of the skin surface. Also *sensible perspiration*.

**Swediaur** [François X. *Swediaur*, Austrian physician, 1748–1824] Swediaur's disease. See under ACHILLES BURSITIS.

**Sweet** [Robert Douglas *Sweet*, English dermatologist, flourished 20th century] Sweet syndrome. See under ACUTE FEBRILE NEUTROPHILIC DERMATOSIS.

**sweetener** A substance that provides a sweet taste. **artificial s.** A sweetening agent, such as saccharin, cyclamate, or aspartame, that is not a sugar and has no nutritional value.

**sweetgum** STORAX.

**swelling** 1 A protuberance or elevation. 2 An increase in depth and breadth, or a part so increased; enlargement or engorgement. **albuminous s.** CLOUDY SWELLING. **arytenoid s.'s** A pair of elevations which appear on the caudal margin of the developing laryngeal inlet from the pharynx. Later the arytenoid cartilages differentiate within the swellings. **blennorrhagic s.** Joint effusion due to gonococcal arthritis. **brain s.** CEREBRAL EDEMA. **bulbar s.'s** BULBAR RIDGES. **Calabar s.'s** Warm swellings, about the size of goose eggs, caused by the filarial nematode, *Loa loa*, which is very widely distributed in west Africa and to a lesser extent in other parts of tropical Africa. The swellings result from an allergic tissue reaction to the filarial toxin. Onset is acute. The swellings, which pit on pressure, last about three days. Treatment is with diethylcarbamazine. Also *Calabar edema, fugitive swellings*. **cloudy s.** A reversible form of cell injury that takes place when the cell is unable to maintain ionic and fluid homeostasis and water shifts from the extracellular space into the cell, resulting in its enlargement. This change is difficult to appreciate microscopically except for the possible capillary compression caused by the swollen cells. Also *albuminous degeneration, albuminoid degeneration, floccular degeneration, granular degeneration, parenchymatous degeneration, turbid-swelling degeneration, albuminous swelling*. **familial fibrous s. of the jaws** CHERUBISM. **fugitive s.'s** CALABAR SWELLINGS. **genital s.** In the embryo, either of two swellings, one on each side, placed below the phallus and outside the genital folds, from which they are separated by a distinct groove, and which eventually become the labia majora. Also *labioscrotal swelling*. **labioscrotal s.** GENITAL SWELLING. **lateral lingual s.'s** Oval swellings which appear on the endodermal aspect of the mandibular arch of the early embryo and fuse with the tuberculum impar to give rise to the anterior part of the tongue. **levator s.** TORUS LEVATORIUS. **premenstrual s.** Generalized edema experienced by some women in the late secretory phase of the menstrual cycle. **tubular cloudy s.** TUBULAR EDEMA. **white s.** Cool effusion of a joint, as in tuberculous arthritis. Also *tumor albus*.

**Swenson** [Orvar *Swenson*, U.S. surgeon, born 1909] See under OPERATION, PROCEDURE.

**Swift** [H. *Swift*, Austrian, flourished 20th century] Swift's disease. See under PINK DISEASE.

**swing** A suspensory sling or cradle. **mood s.'s** Oscillation from depression to elation, as seen in cyclothymic personality or, in a more extreme degree, in the alternation between manic and depressive phases of manic-depressive psychosis. **torsion s.** In otology a device for testing the vestibular reactions to accelerated rotatory movements. Two cables suspend a small chair from the ceiling while a third fixes its center point to the floor, so that only twisting movements are possible. The subject sits in the chair, which is set in motion, and the vestibular responses to the sinusoidal movements so caused are measured by electronystagmography.

**swing-bed** Pertaining to inpatient facilities or rooms which may be converted to different uses according to the type of care for which the space is most urgently needed. For example, a wing or floor of a hospital in the swing-bed system can be used for long-term care if there is a shortage of nursing homes in the community.

**switch / class s.** In immunogenetics, an alteration in a B lymphocyte that produces a change in expression of immunoglobulin class, such as from IgM to IgG. **selector s.** A switching device found on most electroencephalographs to enable recordings to be made successively from different patterns of electrodes (or montages).

**SWS** slow wave sleep (synchronized sleep).

**Swyer** [Paul Robert *Swyer*, English-born Canadian physician, born 1921] Swyer-James-Macleod syndrome, Swyer-James syndrome. See under MACLEOD SYNDROME.

**sycephalus** \sisef′ələs\ [Gk *sy(n)-* + -CEPHALUS] CEPHALOPAGUS.

**sychnuria** \sik·noo′rē·ə\ [Gk *sychn(os)* many, much, frequent + -URIA] POLLAKIURIA.

**sycosiform** \sīkō′sifôrm\ Resembling sycosis.

**sycosis** \sīkō′sis\ [Gk *sycōsis* (from *syk(on)* a fig + *-ōsis* -OSIS) a rough, figlike excrescence on the flesh, esp. the eyelids] A deep inflammation of contiguous follicles. Also *ficosis*. **s. barbae** Sycosis of the beard area. **coccogenic s.** SYCOSIS VULGARIS. **keloid s.** Chronic bacterial sycosis marked by keloid scars. Also *hypertrophic sycosis*. **lupoid s. of Brocq** Chronic bacterial sycosis associated with the formation of follicular granulomas and scars. Also *lupoid sycosis*. **s. nuchae necrotisans** Keloid acne affecting the nape of the neck. **s. vulgaris** A deep staphylococcal infection of the hair follicles. Also *sycosis staphylogenes, coccogenic sycosis*.

**Sydenham** [Thomas *Sydenham*, English physician, 1624–1689] See under CHOREA.

**syl-** \sil-\ SYN-.

**Sylvest** [Ejnar *Sylvest*, Danish physician, 1880–1931] Sylvest's disease. See under EPIDEMIC PLEURODYNIA.

**sylvian** \sil′vē·ən\ 1 Denoting or pertaining to those anatomic (primarily neuroanatomic) structures originally described by Franciscus Sylvius, Dutch anatomist, 1614–1672. 2 Pertaining to or affecting the sylvian fissure of the brain.

**sylviduct** \sil′vidukt\ *Rare* AQUEDUCTUS CEREBRI.

**Sylvius** [Franciscus *Sylvius,* Dutch physician and chemist, 1614–1672] 1 Iter of Sylvius, aqueduct of Sylvius. See under AQUEDUCTUS CEREBRI. 2 Ramus posterior fissurae cerebri lateralis sylvii. See under RAMUS POSTERIOR SULCI LATERALIS CEREBRI. 3 Sylvian aqueduct syndrome. See under AQUEDUCT OF SYLVIUS SYNDROME. 4 Fossa cerebri lateralis Sylvii, fossa of Sylvius. See under FOSSA LATERALIS CEREBRI. 5 Fossa of Sylvius, sylvian fissure, fissure of Sylvius. See under SULCUS LATERALIS CEREBRI. 6 Anterior opening of aqueduct of Sylvius. See under OPENING. 7 Valve of Sylvius. See under VALVULA VENAE CAVAE INFERIORIS.

**sym-** \sim-\ SYN-.

**symbiology** \sim'bī·äl'əjē\ [*symbio(sis)* + -LOGY] The branch of biology concerned with the study of symbiosis.

**symbiont** \sim'bē·änt\ [SYM- + -BIONT] An organism participating in a symbiotic relationship. • The term tends to be used more in reference to mutualists than to parasites, commensals, or other types of symbiont.

**symbiosis** \sim'bē·ō'sis, sim'bī-\ [Gk *symbiōsis* (from *symbi(ōnai)* to live with, from SYM- + Gk *bios* life, manner of life + *-ōsis* -OSIS) the state of living together] 1 Interdependence or mutual cooperation, as in the mother-child relationship. 2 A phase of childhood, normally extending from about the age of 3–18 months, in which the infant is not fully aware of the mother as a separate individual with her own needs, the mother functioning as an auxiliary ego. **antagonistic s.** A type of symbiosis that is beneficial to one symbiont and detrimental to another; parasitism. Also *antipathetic symbiosis.* **conjunctive s.** A symbiosis characterized by bodily union between the symbionts.

**symblepharon** \simblef'ərän\ [SYM- + BLEPHARON] Adhesion between the bulbar and palpebral conjunctiva. **anterior s.** Adhesions between the bulbar and tarsal conjunctiva that do not involve the conjunctival fornix. **posterior s.** Conjunctival adhesions located in the depths of the cul-de-sac.

**symblepharopterygium** \simblef'ərōterij'ē·əm\ [*symblepharo(n)* + PTERYGIUM] Adhesions between bulbar and palpebral conjunctiva that resemble the appearance of a pterygium.

**symbol** 1 An object that substitutes for or represents another object or concept. In psychoanalysis, symbols function as representations of unconscious content. 2 A written mark, character, or abbreviation adopted by convention to designate a chemical, a mathematical constant, a unit of measurement, etc.

**symbolism** \sim'bəlizm\ The act or process of representing one concept or thing with some other object, a common mechanism in dreams.

**symbrachydactyly** \simbrak'ēdak'tilē\ [SYM- + BRACHY- + DACTYL- + -Y] A condition in which the fingers are abnormally short and partially united, with, at minimum, webbing in the proximal segments.

**Syme** [James *Syme,* Scottish surgeon, 1799–1870] See under AMPUTATION, OPERATION, PROSTHESIS.

**symelia** \simē'lyə\ [Gk *sy(n)-* together + *mel(os)* limb + -IA] SIRENOMELIA.

**symmelia** \simē'lyə\ [See SYMELIA.] SIRENOMELIA.

**Symmers** [Douglas *Symmers,* U.S. pathologist, 1879–1952] 1 Symmers disease, Brill-Symmers disease. See under NODULAR LYMPHOSARCOMA. 2 Brown-Symmers disease. See under ACUTE INFANTILE ENCEPHALOPATHY.

**Symmers** [W. St. Clair *Symmers,* British pathologist, 1863–1937] Symmers fibrosis. See under SYMMERS PIPESTEM FIBROSIS.

**symmetrical** \simet'rəkəl\ Having symmetry.

**symmetry** \sim'itrē\ [Gk *symmetria* (from *syn-* with, together + *metr(on)* measure + *-ia* -Y) commensurability, symmetry] Similarity of structure on each side of either an axis or a plane of the body, or at opposite poles of any body; the property of divisibility into similar halves. **bilateral s.** Symmetry on two sides of a longitudinal axis of an organism. Also *bilateralism.* **inverse s.** Correspondence between one side of an organism and the opposite side of another. **radial s.** A regular arrangement of similar parts radiating from a central vertical axis.

**sympath-** \simpath-\ SYMPATHO-.

**sympathectomy** \sim'pəthek'təmē\ [*sympath(etic nerve)* + -ECTOMY] Excision of sympathetic nerves. Also *sympathetectomy, sympathicectomy.* **cervical s.** The excision of parts of the cervical sympathetic chain in order to obliterate sympathetic vascular tone to the upper extremity. It is usually performed in patients with upper extremity vasospastic disorders such as Raynaud's phenomenon or in individuals with hyperhidrosis. **lumbar s.** An excision of part of the lumbar sympathetic chain, usually its second, third, and fourth ganglia, to remove sympathetic vascular tone from the ipsilateral lower extremity and thus improve its blood supply. It is usually performed in patients with a lower extremity arterial insufficiency that is not amenable to vascular reconstruction. **lumbodorsal s.** LUMBODORSAL SPLANCHNICECTOMY. **periarterial s.** The excision of the outer tissue that surrounds an artery, thus removing sympathetic nerve fibers and producing vasodilatation distally. Also *arteriosympathectomy.*

**sympathetectomy** \simpath'ətek'təmē\ SYMPATHECTOMY.

**sympathetic** \sim'pəthet'ik\ 1 Indicating, expressing, or characterized by sympathy. 2 Pertaining to, affecting, or associated with the sympathetic nervous system. See under SYSTEMA NERVOSUM AUTONOMICUM, PARS SYMPATHICA. Also *sympathic.*

**sympathetico-** \sim'pəthet'ikō-\ SYMPATHO-.

**sympatheticomimetic** \-mimet'ik\ ADRENERGIC.

**sympatheticoparalytic** \-per'əlit'ik\ Pertaining to, producing, or affected by paralysis of a part or the entire sympathetic division of the autonomic nervous system.

**sympatheticotonia** \-tō'nē·ə\ [SYMPATHETICO- + *ton(o)-* + -IA] Overactivity of the sympathetic nervous system, producing blanching of the skin, goose flesh, generalized vasoconstriction, increased pilomotor activity, and a rise in systemic blood pressure. The oculocardiac reflex is reduced or inverted, the pupils are dilated, there is a fine rapid tremor of the hands, and insomnia often occurs. Gastrointestinal symptoms such as anorexia and constipation may also be present. This syndrome is common in thyrotoxicosis. Also *sympathicotonia, hypersympathetic dystonia, hypersympatheticotonic dystonia.*

**sympatheticotonic** \-tän'ik\ Relating to sympathicotonia. Also *sympathicotonic.*

**sympatheto-** \sim'pəthet'ō-\ SYMPATHO-.

**sympathetoblast** \sim'pəthet'əblast\ SYMPATHOBLAST.

**sympathic** \simpath'ik\ SYMPATHETIC.

**sympathicectomy** \simpath'isek'təmē\ SYMPATHECTOMY.

**sympathico-** \simpath'ikō-\ SYMPATHO-.

**sympathicoblast** \simpath'ikōblast'\ SYMPATHOBLAST.

**sympathicoblastoma** \-blastō'mə\ NEUROBLASTOMA.

**sympathicogenic** \-jen'ik\ [SYMPATHICO- + -GENIC] Denoting any manifestation of activity in the sympathetic division of the autonomic nervous system.

**sympathicolytic** \-lit'ik\ Opposing the action of sympathetic postganglionic fibers and their adrenergic transmitters, as a neural action or chemical agent; antiadrenergic. Also *sympatholytic.*

**sympathicomimetic** \-mimet′ik\ ADRENERGIC.
**sympathicotherapy** \-ther′əpē\ Treatment of certain diseases by stimulation or anesthetic blocking of the sphenopalatine ganglia, particularly applicable in psychosomatic disorders thought by some to be mediated through the sympathetic nervous system.
**sympathicotonia** \-tō′nē·ə\ [SYMPATHICO- + Gk *ton(os)* tone, tension + -IA] SYMPATHETICOTONIA.
**sympathicotonic** \-tän′ik\ SYMPATHETICOTONIC.
**sympathicotripsy** \-trip′sē\ [SYMPATHICO- + -TRIPSY] The crushing of sympathetic nerves or ganglia.
**sympathicotropic** \-träp′ik\ Denoting a neural activity or agent that principally affects the sympathetic nervous system.
**sympathicus** \simpath′ikəs\ Denoting the sympathetic nervous system.
**sympathin** \sim′pəthin\ [SYMPATH- + -IN] A neurotransmitter at sympathetic nerve synapses. The most important of these are epinephrine and norepinephrine. *Outmoded.* Also *sympathetic hormone.* • The term was coined by the American physiologist Walter B. Cannon on the incorrect presumption that the sympathetic neurotransmitter differed from norepinephrine. **s. E** *Outmoded* NOREPINEPHRINE. **s. I** The sympathetic inhibitory neurotransmitter producing vasodilatation.
**sympathizer** \sim′pəthī′zər\ The uninjured, inflamed eye in sympathetic ophthalmia.
**sympatho-** \sim′pəthō-\ [Gk *sympatheia.* See SYMPATHY.] A combining form meaning sympathetic, relating to the sympathetic division of the autonomic nervous system. Also *sympath-, sympathetico-, sympatheto-, sympathico-.*
**sympathoadrenal** \-adrē′nəl\ Denoting the relationship that exists between the sympathetic nervous system and the suprarenal (adrenal) glands. . *Seldom used.*
**sympathoblast** \sim′pəthōblast′\ [SYMPATHO- + -BLAST] The precursor of a sympathetic neuron, believed to be derived from the neural crest from where it migrates into the sympathetic ganglia. Homologous though larger cells differentiate to form chromaffin cells of organs like the adrenal medulla. Also *sympathicoblast, sympathetic neuroblast, sympathetoblast, sympathetic formative cell.*
**sympathoblastoma** \-blastō′mə\ [SYMPATHOBLAST + -OMA] NEUROBLASTOMA.
**sympathochromaffin** \-krōmaf′in\ Pertaining to or affecting the chromaffin tissue of the sympathetic nervous system.
**sympathogonia** \-gō′nē·ə\ [New L, from SYMPATHO- + Gk *gonei(es)* progenitors + L *-a,* neuter pl. suffix] SYMPATHOCHROMAFFIN CELLS.
**sympathogonioma** \-gō′nē·ō′mə\ [*sympathogoni(a)* + -OMA] NEUROBLASTOMA.
**sympathogonium** \-gō′nē·əm\ Singular of SYMPATHOGONIA.
**sympatholytic** \-lit′ik\ SYMPATHICOLYTIC.
**sympathomimetic** \-mimet′ik\ ADRENERGIC.
**sympathoparalytic** \-par′əlit′ik\ Attributable to paralysis of some component of the sympathetic nervous system.
**sympathy** [Gk *sympatheia* (from *sym-* with, together + *pathos* experience, sensation, feeling) concord, compassion, affinity] **1** A state of mutual relation or coordination existing between two body parts or structures such that a change in one is likely to produce a change in the other. **2** A phenomenon characterized by the generation of responses governed by imitation, as yawning evoked by the sight of another yawning or the spread of hysterical symptoms within a group under stress. **3** An engagement of one's emotions in sharing the feelings of another, especially feelings of suffering, fear, or loss, as a means of expressing concern and care. Adj. sympathetic, sympathic.
**symperitoneal** \sim′peritənē′əl\ Of or relating to a surgical procedure in which adhesions are induced between two parts of the peritoneal surface that are not normally attached.
**symphalangy** \simfal′ənjē\ Ankylosis of the phalanges in one or more fingers or toes as a result of end-to-end fusion of adjacent segments. It is often associated with other malformations of the hands or feet. Also *symphalangism.*
**symphyocephalus** \sim′fē·ōsef′ələs\ [Gk *symphy(ēs)* (from *syn-* together + *phyesthai* to grow) grown together + -CEPHALUS] CEPHALOPAGUS.
**symphyseal** \simfiz′ē·əl\ SYMPHYSIAL.
**symphyses** \sim′fisēz\ Plural of SYMPHYSIS.
**symphysial** \simfiz′ē·əl\ Of or relating to a symphysis. Also *symphyseal, symphysic.*
**symphysiectomy** \simfiz′ē·ek′təmē\ [*symphysi(s pubis)* + -ECTOMY] Division of the cartilage of the symphysis pubis to allow vaginal delivery of an infant. The procedure is seldom used in modern obstetrics. Also *symphysiotomy, symphysiolysis, synchondrotomy.*
**symphysis** \sim′fəsis\ [Gk *symphysis* (from *symphyesthai* to grow together, from SYM- + *phyein* to bring forth, make grow) a growing together, a natural union] **1** [NA] A cartilaginous joint in which the opposing bony surfaces are lined by thin layers of hyaline cartilage and joined by an intervening disk or pad of fibrocartilage, the thickness of which determines the degree of limited movement. The periphery of the bones are joined by fibrous ligaments that also fuse with the rim of the fibrocartilaginous pad. It is usually located at various sites in the median plane of the body. Also *fibrocartilaginous joint.* **2** An abnormal or pathologic fusion of adjacent parts. **s. ligamentosa** *Outmoded* SYNDESMOSIS. **s. menti** The midline joint between the two halves of the lower jaw. When first formed it is fibrocartilaginous, but it becomes a bony union in man from about the ninth month after birth. **s. pubica** [NA] The cartilaginous joint in the median plane between the opposing medial surfaces of the pubic bones, which are lined by hyaline cartilage and connected by the interpubic disk of fibrocartilage and by the superior and the arcuate pubic ligaments. It often contains a cavity, larger in females and rarely found before the second decade of life. Also *symphysis pubis, symphysis ossium pubis, pubic symphysis, articulation of pubis.* **sacrococcygeal s.** *Outmoded* ARTICULATIO SACROCOCCYGEA. **sacroiliac s.** *Outmoded* ARTICULATIO SACROILIACA.
**symphysitis** \sim′fisī′tis\ An inflammation of a fibrocartilaginous joint.
**symphysodactyly** \sim′fisōdak′tilē\ SYNDACTYLY.
**symphytum** \sim′fitəm\ A medicinal preparation derived from a genus of boraginaceous plants, the common comfrey, native to Europe and North America. The preparation acts as a demulcent and has astringent properties. Its pharmaceutic action has been attributed to the presence of allantoin.
**symplasm** \sim′plazm\ SYNCYTIUM.
**symplast** \sim′plast\ SYNCYTIUM.
**sympodia** \simpō′dē·ə\ [SYM- + -POD + -IA] A fusion of the feet, as in sirenomelia.
**symport** \sim′pôrt\ [SYM- + *(trans)port(er)*] A transporter in a biologic membrane that lets a molecule or ion of one substance through the membrane only in conjunction with a molecule or ion of another substance. Amino acids, for example, may be concentrated by cells that have a sym-

port for sodium ions with the amino acid, so that the sodium ion passes down an electrochemical gradient.

# symptom

**symptom** \simp′təm\ [Gk *symptōma* (from *sympiptein* to fall together, meet, happen, occur, from *sym-* with, together + *piptein* to fall) an occurrence, mishap, coincidence, attribute, symptom] Any evidence of disease or disorder which is experienced by the patient and often reported as a subjective observation, such as pain. Compare SIGN. ● If the symptom is demonstrable to an observer upon examination, it is an *objective symptom,* or, more generally, a *sign.* **accessory s.** Any symptom that accompanies a disorder but that is not pathognomonic. Also *assident symptom.* **Anton s.** Visual anosognosia; denial of blindness. Also *Anton syndrome.* **assident s.** ACCESSORY SYMPTOM. **Bekhterev s.** Paralysis or paresis of emotional as distinct from volitional facial movements. **Brauch-Romberg s.** ROMBERG SIGN. **Capgras s.** CAPGRAS SYNDROME. **cardinal s.** A symptom that is of primary significance in the identification of a disease or disorder, being the symptom, or one of those symptoms, by which the condition is known and recognized. **Castellani-Low s.** A tremor of the tongue observed in African trypanosomiasis. **characteristic s.** A symptom which is so typical of a particular disease or disorder as to guide the diagnosis when the symptom is present. Also *guiding symptom.* **Chvostek s.** CHVOSTEK SIGN. **concomitant s.** A symptom which is often though not always present and may aid the physician in making a diagnosis. **constitutional s.** A symptom which involves the whole body. Also *general symptom, systemic symptom.* **delayed s.** A symptom occurring after a considerable period has elapsed following the cause, such as trauma, that produced it. **direct s.** A symptom that can be attributed directly to a disease. Compare INDIRECT SYMPTOM. **dissociation s.** DISSOCIATED ANESTHESIA. **endothelial s.** RUMPEL-LEEDE PHENOMENON. **Epstein s.** A nervous symptom in infancy in which the upper eyelid does not move downward, making the infant appear to look frightened. **equivocal s.** A symptom that implicates no particular disease or disorder, since it may be produced by any of a number of causes. **Frenkel s.** Muscular hypotonia in tabes dorsalis. **Froin s.** Spontaneous coagulation of cerebrospinal fluid obtained by lumbar puncture, indicating a high protein content, including fibrinogen, which is never present in normal cerebrospinal fluid. **fundamental s.** Any of the pathognomonic symptoms of schizophrenia including disturbances in associations and affectivity, ambivalence, autism, and dementia. **Ganser s.** GANSER SYNDROME. **general s.** CONSTITUTIONAL SYMPTOM. **gramophone s.** The telling of an elaborate anecdote and almost as soon as one is finished, repeating it without apparent memory of having already told it, often seen in Pick's disease. **Griesinger s.** *Incorrect* GRIESINGER SIGN. **guiding s.** CHARACTERISTIC SYMPTOM. **Haenel s.** Insensitivity to pressure on the eyeballs in tabes dorsalis. Also *Haenel's variant.* **halo s.** The seeing of glare or color around lights, as occurs when the cornea is edematous, as in acute glaucoma. Also *rainbow symptom.* **indirect s.** A symptom that cannot be attributed directly to a disease but to a condition believed to be produced by it. Compare DIRECT SYMPTOM. **induced s.** A symptom intentionally induced, as for diagnostic purposes. **Jellinek s.** JELLINEK SIGN. **Jonas s.** Pyloric spasm occurring in rabies. **Kerandel s.** Severe deep pain, often delayed, and hyperesthesia, developing after a minor collision, knock, or blow to a bony protuberance, such as a shoulder. The symptom may be observed about three weeks after the onset of a trypanosomal infection of the African variety, i.e., when the parasites appear in the peripheral blood. Also *Kerandel sign.* **Kussmaul s.** KUSSMAUL RESPIRATION. **labyrinthine s.'s** Symptoms, principally vertigo, deafness, and tinnitus, characteristic of labyrinthine disease. **Lade s.** Very soft stools occurring about fourteen days before the appearance of the rash in varicella. **local s.** A symptom limited to a particular organ or part. **localizing s.** A symptom that indicates the source, focus, or location of the disease or lesion. **Loewi s.** LOEWI'S REACTION. **Magendie s.** SKEW DEVIATION. **Magnan s.** FORMICATION. **neighborhood s.** A symptom in one organ or structure caused by a lesion in a neighboring structure. **objective s.** A symptom that is demonstrable to an observer upon examination. ● See note at SYMPTOM. **passive s.** STATIC SYMPTOM. **pathognomonic s.** A symptom whose presence conclusively identifies the disease producing it. **Pel-Ebstein s.** PEL-EBSTEIN FEVER. **precursory s.** SIGNAL SYMPTOM. **premonitory s.** SIGNAL SYMPTOM. **presenting s.** The symptom that is most important in motivating the patient to seek medical advice. **prodromal epileptic s.** Any vague symptom other than the specific aura which may precede an attack of epilepsy. **rainbow s.** HALO SYMPTOM. **rational s.** SUBJECTIVE SYMPTOM. **reflex s.** A symptom occurring in a part of the body relatively remote from the site of the disorder, as a disturbance of vision caused by spasm of a cranial vessel. Also *sympathetic symptom.* **Remak s.** REMAK SIGN. **Romberg-Howship s.** 1 ROMBERG SIGN. 2 Obturator nerve neuralgia giving sharp lancinating pain down the medial aspect of the thigh in patients with strangulated obturator hernia. **signal s.** The initial symptom of an attack of focal epilepsy, sometimes becoming secondarily generalized, which may enable one to locate clinically the origin of the neuronal discharge. Thus, a tonicoclonic attack beginning with phosphenes in the left visual field can reasonably be assumed to be the result of a neuronal discharge arising in the right posterior occipital region. Also *precursory symptom, premonitory symptom.* Also *signal-symptom.* **Skeer s.** SKEER SIGN. **Sklowsky s.** A symptom suggested as an aid in the differential diagnosis of varicella and smallpox. When light pressure is exerted with the index finger on the skin near, then over, a varicellar lesion, the wall of the lesion ruptures. Under the same conditions, a smallpox lesion will not rupture. **static s.** A symptom that persists with little change in a part or organ. Also *passive symptom.* **Stellwag s.** STELLWAG SIGN. **subjective s.** A symptom evident only to the patient. Also *rational symptom.* ● See note at SYMPTOM. **sympathetic s.** REFLEX SYMPTOM. **systemic s.** CONSTITUTIONAL SYMPTOM. **Trendelenburg s.** TRENDELENBURG SIGN. **Uhthoff s.** UHTHOFF SIGN. **Wartenberg s.** WARTENBERG SIGN. **Weber s.** WEBER SYNDROME. **Wernicke s.** HEMIANOPIC PUPILLARY REACTION. **withdrawal s.'s** The substance-specific organic syndrome that follows cessation of or reduction in intake of a substance that had previously been used by the subject on a regular basis. Substances that frequently produce such a syndrome include alcohol, amphetamines, barbiturates and other sedative-hypnotics, and corticosteroids. The symptoms vary with the particular agent used, the length of use, and the amount ingested, but excitement, irritability, and psychomotor disturbances of varying intensity are common. Also *abstinence phenomenon.*

**symptomatic** \simp′təmat′ik\ **1** Being a symptom; indicative of a disease or disorder. **2** Of or relating to a symptom or symptoms, as treatment. **3** Appearing as a symptom of a disorder other than that with which the symptom is usually associated.

**symptomatology** \simp′tōmətäl′əjē\ **1** The scientific study of symptoms and their relation to disease. Also *semeiology, semiology.* **2** The complex of symptoms of a disease or of a particular case of disease.

**symptomatolytic** \simp′təmat′əlit′ik\ Bringing about the elimination of symptoms. Also *symptomolytic.*

**symptosis** \simtō′sis\ [Gk *symptōsis* (from *syn-* together + *ptōsis* a fall) a falling in, collapse] Wasting or cachexia.

**sympus** \sim′pəs\ [Gk *sympous* (from *syn-* together + *pous* foot) with the feet together] A sirenomelus displaying any degree of fusion of the feet. **s. apus** A sirenomelic individual lacking any foot structure. **s. dipus** A sirenomelic individual in which some or all elements of two feet are apparent. **s. monopus** A sirenomelic individual in which there appears to be only one foot, although on close examination this may represent the union of bilaterally symmetrical parts of two feet. Also *monopus.*

**syn** \sin\ [Gk, with, together with, jointly] A descriptor of conformation. Two groups attached to adjacent atoms are in the syn conformation when rotation about the bond between the atoms brings them as close together as possible, so that they overlap in a projection along the bond. The syn conformation of nucleosides is that in which the pyrimidine ring of a purine, or C-2 of a pyrimidine, approaches C-5 of the ribose.

**syn-** \sin-\ [Gk *syn* (as prefix assimilated before *b, p,* and *m* as *sym-*, before *l* as *syl-*, and before *s* as *sys-*) with, together with, jointly] A prefix meaning with, together, conjointly. Also *sym-, syl-, sys-.*

**synadelphus** \sin′ədel′fəs\ [SYN- + Gk *adelphos* a twin, brother] Equal conjoined twins with more or less fusion of the cephalic and thoracic regions but with four arms and four legs. Also *cephalothoracopagus.*

**synalgia** \sinal′jə\ REFERRED PAIN.

**synalgic** \sinal′jik\ Being, pertaining to, or experiencing synalgia, or referred pain.

**synanastomosis** \sin′ənas′təmō′sis\ Anastomosis among several blood vessels.

**synanche** \sinang′kē\ CYNANCHE.

**synapse** \sin′aps, sinaps′\ [New L *synapsis,* from Gk *synaptein* to join together, unite, from SYN- + Gk *haptein* to fasten to, clasp] **1** A region of structural specialization constituting a junctional site between two or more neurons or between a neuron and a muscle cell or gland cell. They permit the unidirectional transmission of nerve impulses from the presynaptic neuron to the postsynaptic neuron or effector cell. This is achieved by the liberation of specific chemical substances, called neurotransmitters, from the presynaptic element that alter the permeability characteristics of the postsynaptic membrane (chemical synapses). Transmission of impulses across certain invertebrate and lower vertebrate synapses is effected by the flow of action currents across the apposed cell membranes and apparently does not require a chemical transmitter (electrical synapses). **2** To form a synapse. **axoaxonic s.** A synapse that occurs at the site of apposition between the membranes of two axon terminals, or between an axon terminal and the initial segment of another axon. **axodendritic s.** A synapse that occurs at the site of apposition between an axon from one nerve cell (presynaptic element) and the dendrite of another nerve cell (postsynaptic element). This is the most common type of synapse found in the central nervous system and the peripheral autonomic ganglia. **axodendrosomatic s.** A synapse that occurs between the axon of one nerve cell and the dendrite and soma (cell body) of another nerve cell. **axosomatic s.** A synapse between the axon of one nerve cell and the soma (cell body) of another nerve cell. Also *pericorpuscular synapse.* **electrogenic s.** Any synapse where excitation is due to directly induced electrical depolarization, rather than through release of a chemical neurotransmitter. **false s.** A physical contact between demyelinated axons, sometimes resulting in ephaptic transmission. **neuromuscular s.** The specialized junction between a motor nerve fiber and the muscle fiber it supplies. **pericorpuscular s.** AXOSOMATIC SYNAPSE.

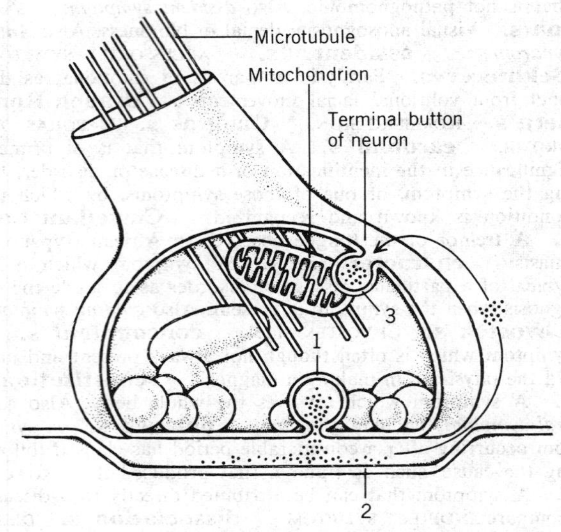


**Neuromuscular synapse** (1) Neurotransmitter released by exocytosis into intercellular space; (2) permeability of postsynaptic cell membrane altered; (3) excess neurotransmitter taken up by endocytosis.

**synapsis** \sinap′sis\ [New L. See SYNAPSE.] The pairing of homologous chromosomes during the prophase of meiosis. Also *syndesis, pairing.*

**synaptene** \sinap′tēn\ [Gk *synap(tos),* verbal of *synaptein* (from *syn-* with + *haptein* to fasten) to join together + *tain(ia)* a band, fillet] The phase of meiosis at which the homologous chromosomes align in pairs. Also *synaptic phase.*

**synaptic** \sinap′tik\ Pertaining to a synapse.

**synaptology** \sin′aptäl′əjē\ [Gk *synapto(s)* joined together + -LOGY] The field of neuroscience that deals with the study of synapses and synaptic connections in the nervous system.

**synaptosome** \sinap′təsōm\ [Gk *synapto(s)* joined together + -SOME] A synaptic terminal that has been isolated by centrifugation from homogenates of brain tissue and characteristically appears in electron microscopy as a membrane-bound structure containing synaptic vesicles.

**synarthrophysis** \sinär′thrəfī′sis\ [SYN- + ARTHRO- + PHYSIS] Ankylosis of a joint.
**synarthroses** \sin′ärthrō′sēz\ Plural of SYNARTHROSIS.
**synarthrosis** [Gk *synarthrōsis* (from *syn-* together + *arthrōsis* jointing, articulation) an immovable articulation] ARTICULATIO FIBROSA.
**syncaine** PROCAINE HYDROCHLORIDE.
**syncanthus** \sinkan′thəs\ Limitation of movement of the eye because of the adherence to the eyelids or other structures within the orbit.
**syncephalus** \sinsef′ələs\ [SYN- + -CEPHALUS] CEPHALOPAGUS. **s. asymmetros** JANICEPS ASYMMETRUS.
**syncheilia** \sinkī′lē·ə\ [SYN- + CHEIL- + -IA ] The abnormal adhesion of the lips as in microstomia or atresia of the mouth.
**synchesis** \sin′kəsis\ SYNCHYSIS.
**synchiria** \sinkī′rē·ə\ [SYN- + CHIR- + -IA] A sensory defect in which a unilateral stimulus such as a pinch or pinprick produces the sensation of an identical stimulus at the homologous point on the opposite side of the body.
**synchondrectomy** \sin′kändrek′təmē\ The excision of a synchondrosis.
**synchondroseotomy** \sin′kändrō′sē·ät′əmē\ A surgical procedure used to treat exstrophy of the bladder in which the sacroiliac joints are divided and the bladder edges are closed. Also *Trendelenburg's operation.*
**synchondroses** \sin′kändrō′sēz\ Plural of SYNCHONDROSIS.
**synchondrosis** \sin′kändrō′sis\ [SYN- + CHONDROSIS] (*pl.* synchondroses) [NA] A temporary cartilaginous joint involving the hyaline cartilage between two bones or bony parts in growth, such as the junction between diaphysis and epiphysis in the immature postcranial skeleton and also the cartilaginous junctions between the bones of the growing chondrocranium. The cartilage disappears through replacement by bone to form a synostosis at maturity. **anterior intraoccipital s.** SYNCHONDROSIS INTRAOCCIPITALIS ANTERIOR. **s. arycorniculata** See under ARYCORNICULATE JOINT. **synchondroses cranii** [NA] The unossified cartilaginous joints between the bones of the base of the skull or chondrocranium. Also *synchondroses of cranium.* **intersphenoidal s.** A cartilaginous joint between the presphenoidal and postsphenoidal parts of the body of the sphenoid bone in a fetus. Fusion occurs during the eighth month of intrauterine life but a wedge-shaped cartilage in the lower part of the synchondrosis persists until after birth. **s. intraoccipitalis anterior** [NA] The cartilaginous joint appearing between the basilar and lateral parts of the occipital bone on each side in the newborn and ossifying within a few years. Also *anterior intraoccipital synchondrosis.* **s. intraoccipitalis posterior** [NA] The cartilaginous joint appearing between the squamous and the lateral parts of the occipital bone on each side in the newborn and ossifying within a few years. Also *posterior intraoccipital synchondrosis, Budin's joint.* **s. manubriosternalis** [NA] The cartilaginous joint between the manubrium and the body of the sternum which commences as a synchondrosis and later becomes a symphysis. It may contain a cavity and is often ossified after the age of 30 years. Also *manubriosternal joint, superior sternal joint.* **s. petro-occipitalis** [NA] The cartilaginous junction between the petrous part of the temporal bone and the basilar part of the occipital bone. Also *petro-occipital synchondrosis, petro-occipital articulation.* **posterior intraoccipital s.** SYNCHONDROSIS INTRAOCCIPITALIS POSTERIOR. **sacrococcygeal s.** *Outmoded* ARTICULATIO SACROCOCCYGEA. **s. spheno-occipitalis** [NA] The cartilaginous joint between the body of the sphenoid and the basilar part of the occipital bone. Anteroposterior growth of the base of the skull occurs there until the eighteenth to twenty-fifth year, when it fuses. Also *spheno-occipital synchondrosis, spheno-occipital joint, spheno-occipital suture, basilar fibrocartilage.* **s. sphenopetrosa** [NA] The cartilaginous joint formed by the layer of fibrocartilage in the fissura sphenopetrosa. Also *sphenopetrosal synchondrosis, anterior petrosphenoid ligament, sphenopetrosal suture.* **synchondroses sternales** [NA] Synchondrosis xiphosternalis and synchondrosis manubriosternalis together. Also *sternal synchondroses, manubriogladiolar junctions.* **s. xiphosternalis** [NA] The cartilaginous joint between the xiphoid process and the body of the sternum, which is also a symphysis and often becomes synostosed after the age of about 40 years. Also *xiphisternal joint, inferior sternal joint.*
**synchondrotomy** \sin′kändrät′əmē\ SYMPHYSIECTOMY.
**synchorial** \sinkôr′ē·əl\ [SYN- + *chori(onic)* + -AL] Designating twins that are contained in a single chorionic sac. Synchorial twins are always identical, but not all identical twins are synchorial.
**synchronism** \sin′krənizm\ The synchronous occurrence of two or more events.
**synchronization** \sin′krənīzā′shən\ The act of making synchronous or the condition of being synchronous. **s. of potentials** Simultaneous firing by numerous motor units in the same muscle, as observed electromyographically. It may be related to spinal cord pathology such as anterior poliomyelitis or to stimulation of a motor nerve peripherally.
**synchronous** \sin′krənəs\ Occurring at the same time; simultaneous.
**synchrony** \sin′krənē\ [SYN- + Gk *chronos* time] The appearance of two or more separate structures at the same time, as in the development of two separate parts or organs. **bilateral s.** An electroencephalographic waveform recordable simultaneously from both cerebral hemispheres.
**synchysis** \sin′kisis\ [SYN- + Gk *chysis* a pouring, shedding] Liquefaction of the vitreous humor. Also *synchesis.* **s. scintillans** Liquefaction of the vitreous humor associated with the suspension of a myriad of multicolored, reflecting cholesterol crystals within the vitreous cavity.
**synciput** \sin′siput\ SINCIPUT.
**synclinal** \sinklī′nəl\ Leaning or bent towards a common point.
**synclitism** \sin′klitizm\ [Gk *synklinein* to lean or slope together + -ISM] The attitude of a fetus in relation to the maternal pelvis such that the fetal sagittal suture lies midway between the maternal symphysis pubis and the promontory of the sacrum. Synclitism occurs in a vertex presentation with an occiput transverse position. Also *syncliticism, synclisis.*
**syncopal** \sing′kəpəl\ Relating to or characterized by syncope. Also *syncopic.*
**syncope** \sing′kəpē\ [Gk *synkopē* (from SYN- + Gk *koptein* to cut, cut off, fell) a cutting into pieces, a fainting fit] Transient loss of consciousness due to generalized cerebral ischemia secondary to a global reduction in cerebral blood flow. Also *faint, lipsis animi.* **Adams-Stokes s.** A transient loss of consciousness of cardiac origin, usually associated with asystole. See also ADAMS-STOKES SYNDROME. **s. anginosa** Syncope associated with angina pectoris. **cardiac s.** Syncope of cardiac etiology, frequently due to a disorder of rhythm or conduction but also occurring in sudden loss of cardiac output. **carotid sinus s.** Syncope resulting from reflex bradycardia or hypotension following stimulation of the carotid sinus. **cough s.** Syncope resulting from a violent fit of coughing which, by fixing

the chest in inspiration, reduces venous return to the heart and hence cardiac output. Also *cough seizure, laryngeal syncope, tussive syncope, cough syndrome, laryngeal-vertigo syndrome, laryngeal vertigo* (incorrect). **defecation s.** Fainting during or immediately following the act of defecation. **digital s.** Spasmodic reduction of blood flow to a digit, as in Raynaud's phenomenon. **heat s.** HEAT EXHAUSTION. **laryngeal s.** COUGH SYNCOPE. **micturition s.** Reflex syncope occurring when the subject gets up at night to micturate. The subject is usually an adult male who is generally vasodilated after drinking alcohol. **orthostatic s.** POSTURAL SYNCOPE. **postural s.** Syncope on assuming the upright posture. Also *orthostatic syncope.* See also ORTHOSTATIC HYPOTENSION. **stretch s.** Syncope induced by stretching when the arms are raised and fully extended and the spine is hyperextended. **swallow s.** Syncope induced by swallowing, sometimes associated with demyelination in the trunk of the vagus nerve. **tussive s.** COUGH SYNCOPE. **vasovagal s.** The common form of faint which is associated with nausea, sweating, pallor, bradycardia, and hypotension, and is due to a sudden neurogenic loss of vascular tone. It is frequently psychogenic. Also *vasodepressor syncope, vasomotor syncope.*

**syncopic** \sinkäp′ik\ SYNCOPAL.

**syncretio** \sinkrē′shō\ [New L (irreg. from Gk *synkrētismos* a union of two parties against a third, literally, a Cretan alliance; *syncretio* prob. formed by analogy with L *concretio* concretion] *Obs.* ADHESION.

**syncytial** \sinsish′əl\ Pertaining to a syncytium.

**syncytioma** \sinsit′ē·ō′mə\ [*syncyti(um)* + -OMA] SYNCYTIAL ENDOMETRITIS. **s. malignum** CHORIOCARCINOMA.

**syncytiotoxin** \sinsit′ē-ōtäk′sin\ [*syncyti(um)* + *o* + TOXIN] A toxin having a specific effect on placental tissue.

**syncytiotrophoblast** \sinsit′ē-ōträf′əblast\ The outermost part of the trophoblast. In many species it is a more or less syncytial layer. Also *plasmoditrophoblast, plasmodiblast, plasmotrophoblast, syntrophoblast.*

**syncytium** \sinsit′ē·əm\ [New L, from SYN- + CYT- + L *-ium,* noun suffix] (*pl.* syncytia) A multinucleate mass of protoplasm which is not subdivided into individual cellular compartments. Also *symplast, symplasm, symplastic tissue.*

**syndactyly** \sindak′təlē\ [SYN- + Gk *daktyl(os)* a finger, toe + -Y] Fusion of or webbing between two or more adjacent fingers or toes. It is usually transmitted as an autosomal dominant characteristic in humans. Also *ankylodactyly, dactylosymphysis, symphysodactyly.* **complete s.** Syndactyly in which the fusion or webbing extends from the base to the tip of the affected digits. **complicated s.** Syndactyly in which bones or nails or both are involved in the fusion. **partial s.** Syndactyly in which the webbing between digits extends only part way from the base to the tips of the digits.

**syndesine** $^{-}OOC{-}CH(NH_3^{+}){-}[CH_2]_2{-}[CHOH]_2{-}CH(CHO){-}[CH_2]_2{-}CH(NH_3^{+}){-}COO^{-}$. An amino acid found in collagen, cross-linking two of its chains, formed by an aldol condensation between residues of 5-hydroxyallysine and allysine.

**syndesis** \sin′dəsis\ **1** SYNAPSIS. **2** ARTHRODESIS.

**syndesm-** \sindezm-\ SYNDESMO-.

**syndesmectomy** \sin′dezmek′təmē\ The excision of a segment of a ligament.

**syndesmitis** \sin′dezmī′tis\ An inflammation of one or more ligaments. **s. metatarsea** MARCH TUMOR.

**syndesmo-** \sin′dezmō-, sindez′mō-\ [Gk *syndesmos* (from *syndein* to bind together) ligament, bond] A combining form meaning ligament. Also *syndesm-.*

**syndesmochorial** \-kôr′ē·əl\ See under SYNDESMOCHORIAL PLACENTA.

**syndesmodiastasis** \-dī·as′təsis\ The separation of a ligament from its attachment to bone.

**syndesmologia** \-lō′jə\ *Outmoded* ARTHROLOGIA.

**syndesmology** \sin′dezmäl′əjē\ ARTHROLOGY.

**syndesmo-odontoid** \-ōdän′toid\ The posterior part of the median atlantoaxial joint, located between the anterior surface of the transverse ligament of the atlas and the posterior surface of the dens axis, the apposing surfaces being covered by fibrocartilage.

**syndesmophyte** \sindez′məfīt\ A bony protuberance from a ligamentous attachment.

**syndesmosis** \sin′dəsmō′sis\ [SYNDESM- + -OSIS] (*pl.* syndesmoses) [NA] A fibrous joint in which the apposed surfaces may be close to or some distance from each other and joined by fibrous tissue in the form of cords, ligaments, or membranes. Also *ligamentous joint, symphysis ligamentosa* (outmoded), *synneurosis* (outmoded). **s. tibiofibularis** [NA] The fibrous articulation between the triangular surface on the medial aspect of the distal end of the fibula and the fibular notch of the tibia, bound together by the anterior and the posterior tibiofibular ligaments and the interosseous membrane. Also *tibiofibular syndesmosis, tibiofibular articulation, tibiofibular joint, inferior tibiofibular joint, tibiofibular ligament.* **s. tympanostapedia** [NA] The fibrous articulation in the middle ear between the edge of the base, or footplate, of the stapes and the margin of the fenestra vestibuli which are covered by hyaline cartilage and bound together by the annular ligament of the base of the stapes. Also *tympanostapedial syndesmosis, tympanostapedial junction.*

# syndrome

**syndrome** \sin′drōm\ [Gk *syndromē* (from *syn-* together + *dromos* course, race) a concourse, concurrence, combination, combination of symptoms] The aggregate of signs, symptoms, or other manifestations considered to constitute the characteristics of a morbid entity: used especially when the cause of the condition is unknown. ● The term *syndrome* is variously used in medicine. It is sometimes argued that its scientific use should be restricted to describe only those conditions whose causes are either unknown or diverse, but this principle is widely contravened. Nevertheless, *syndrome* is more commonly applied than *disease* to any postulated morbid entity whose characteristics are not well established. However, many conditions to which *syndrome* was originally applied because of this consideration have now been systematically studied and their characteristics established, yet because the original term is still familiar to many, *syndrome* often continues in widespread use in defiance of the injunction that a distinction between *disease* and *syndrome* be made. Terms known by various designations are listed in this dictionary under the form that predominates in actual usage. For particular syndromes not found under *syndrome,* see also under DISEASE. **abdominal muscle deficiency s.** PRUNE-BELLY SYNDROME. **abruptio placentae s.** Premature separation of the placenta prior to delivery of the fetus accompanied by disseminated intravascular coagulopathy, hemorrhage, and shock. The syndrome occurs in about 30% of those instances of abruptio placentae severe enough to lead to fetal death. **abused child s.** BATTERED CHILD SYNDROME. **accelerated conduction s.**

WOLFF-PARKINSON-WHITE SYNDROME. **Achard-Thiers s.** Concurrent diabetes mellitus and hirsutism in postmenopausal women, supposed to be associated with a higher incidence of cancer of the uterus. It is not a well-defined entity. **acquired cerebellar s.** A cerebellar syndrome attributable to a lesion of the cerebellum acquired by injury, inflammation, or infarction. *Seldom used.* Also *Goldstein syndrome, Goldstein-Reichmann syndrome.* **acquired immune deficiency s.** A virus-induced immunodeficiency occurring epidemically worldwide which in the United States principally affects young, previously healthy homosexual and bisexual men and parenteral drug abusers. Also affected are persons who receive contaminated blood products (such as hemophiliacs), prostitutes and other sexual partners of infected persons, and children born to mothers infected with the virus. The condition renders patients susceptible to multiple opportunistic infections with pathogens such as *Pneumocystis carinii*, cytomegalovirus, typical and atypical mycobacteria, various fungi, *Toxoplasma gondii*, cryptosporidia, herpes group viruses, and papovavirus (progressive multifocal leukoencephalopathy); to a virulent form of Kaposi sarcoma; to a diffuse, undifferentiated non-Hodgkins lymphoma; and to central nervous system deterioration (AIDS encephalopathy). Less severe states, including a chronic lymphadenopathy syndrome, may last many months and are characterized by lymphadenopathy and, sometimes, chronic fever, diarrhea, and weight loss. Patients have profound depletion of helper T lympocytes and reduced ratios of helper to suppressor T lymphocytes. The condition has a high mortality, because even if the initial infections or malignancies are treated successfully, the underlying immunodeficiency remains and is not permanently reversible. The etiologic agent is a retrovirus, called human immunodeficiency virus (HIV), which infects and lyses T cells of the $T_4$ subset, and causes functional defects in B lymphocytes, natural killer cells, cytotoxic T cells, and central nervous system cells. The virus is present in bodily fluids (semen, blood, plasma, saliva, tears, and, probably, mother's milk) of infected persons and is transmitted by intimate exposure to genital secretions or blood and transplacentally. The virus can remain latent in the body for long periods. First recognized in the United States in 1981, the syndrome appears to have existed earlier in parts of equatorial Africa. Abbr. AIDS **acute cervical centromedullary s.** A syndrome of tetraparesis with associated sensory loss in the limbs and trunk which usually results from an acute hyperextension injury to the cervical spine, especially in the presence of preexisting spondylosis. The pathologic substrate is central softening (or hematomyelia) in the cervical cord. Rapid improvement may follow the initial severe paresis, but there is usually some permanent deficit. **acute nephritic s.** Sudden onset of hematuria, proteinuria, cylinduria, oliguria, edema, hypertension, renal insufficiency, and sometimes circulatory congestion and convulsions. It is usually due to poststreptococcal acute glomerulonephritis but also occasionally associated with lupus nephritis, rapidly progressive glomerulonephritis or malignant hypertension. **acute organic brain s.** Any reversible brain disorder such as delirium that develops rapidly and exhibits such manifestations as disturbances in consciousness, level of attention, and orientation, or distorted perceptions giving rise to hallucinations and delusions. **Adair-Dighton s.** VAN DER HOEVE-DE KLEYN SYNDROME. **Adamantiades-Behçet s.** BEHÇET SYNDROME. **Adams-Stokes s.** A syndrome characterized by episodes of syncope due to cardiac arrest. This is most commonly a complication of advanced atrioventricular block with periods of asystole, but may also be due to ventricular arrhythmias, especially ventricular fibrillation. Also *Adams-Stokes disease, Adams disease, Stokes-Adams disease, Stokes-Adams syndrome, Stokes syndrome, Morgagni-Adams-Stokes syndrome, Spens syndrome.* **adherence s.** Secondary weakness of the ocular muscle due to its adherence to the fascial sheath. **Adie s.** A benign disorder of unknown etiology, characterized by pupillary dilatation, usually unilateral but in rare cases bilateral, and often developing suddenly, particularly in young women, though males are occasionally affected. The affected pupil fails to react to light or does so very slowly and incompletely, and the accommodation-convergence reflex is also usually slow, while slight and very gradual dilatation may occur if the patient remains for some time in dark surroundings. In rare cases the pupil is not greatly dilated but shows similar abnormal reactions. The lesion responsible has been shown to be degeneration of neurons in the ciliary ganglion. In many cases the deep tendon reflexes are lost or greatly depressed, especially in the lower limbs, with abnormalities of the H reflex, but the cause of this reflex change is unknown and it is believed that some cases of constitutional areflexia without associated pupillary changes represent a variant of this syndrome. Also *pupillotonic pseudotabes, myotonic pupil, pupillotonia, pupillatonia, Holmes-Adie syndrome, Kehrer-Adie syndrome, pseudo-Argyll Robertson syndrome, Weill-Reys syndrome, Weill-Reys-Adie syndrome, Markus-Adie syndrome, Adie's pupil.* **adiposogenital s.** *Older term* FRÖHLICH SYNDROME. **adrenal virilism s.** Any of several symptom complexes associated with congenital adrenocortical hyperplasia and virilism, or with virilizing adrenocortical adenoma or carcinoma. *Imprecise.* See also ADRENAL VIRILISM. **adrenogenital s.** 1 Any virilizing syndrome, including sexual precocity in either sex, caused by excessive adrenocortical secretion of androgenic steroid hormones. 2 CONGENITAL ADRENOCORTICAL HYPERPLASIA. **Adson s.** SCALENUS ANTERIOR SYNDROME. **adult respiratory distress s.** A syndrome of pulmonary insufficiency characterized by poor oxygenation, increased functional residual capacity, decreased compliance, and a diffuse interstitial opacification pattern seen on x-ray examination of the chest. It is seen in many clinical settings besides shock. Also *shock lung, post-traumatic pulmonary insufficiency, traumatic wet lung, congestive atelectasis, Vietnam lung.* Abbr. ARDS **afferent loop s.** Pain, fullness, and tenderness caused by partial or complete acute or chronic obstruction of the proximal portion of duodenum and jejunum of a Billroth-II anastamosis between stomach and jejunum. There may also be bacterial overgrowth of the loop and subsequent malabsorption. Also *gastrojejunal loop obstruction syndrome.* **aglossia-adactylia s.** Congenital hypoplasia or agenesis of the tongue, regression of the mandible, hypoplasia of the lower alveolar ridge, with missing teeth, and partial or complete absence of digits (and sometimes other distal parts) of one or more limbs. Also *hypoglossia-hypodactyly syndrome, Hanhart syndrome.* **Ahumada-del Castillo s.** Amenorrhea and galactorrhea with reduced titers of urinary gonadotropins, not related to pregnancy or acromegaly, but with a 50% frequency of detectable pituitary tumors. **akinetic-abulic s.** A syndrome characterized by parkinsonlike tremor, bradykinesia, hypertonia, and decreased mental drive and interest. It may appear as a complication of treatment with neuroleptics. **Albright s.** 1 ALBRIGHT'S DISEASE. 2 ALBRIGHT'S HEREDITARY OSTEODYSTROPHY. **Albright-McCune-Sternberg s.** ALBRIGHT'S DISEASE. **alcoholic pseudo-Cushing s.** The clinical manifestations of Cushing syndrome associated with alcoholic hepatic disease. It is presumed to be due to failure of the disordered liver to inactivate normally secreted adrenocortical cortisol. If the hepatic disease is reversible, as in alcoholic hepatitis, the signs of hypercortisolism disappear as the hepatic disease improves. **alcohol withdrawal s.** A syndrome occurring as an abstinence reaction following cessation of alcohol intake. Withdrawal symptoms consists of craving for alcohol, coarse tremors of eyelids, hands, and tongue; nausea, weakness, autonomic hyperactivity, irritability, and sometimes delirium tremens. **Aldrich s.** WISKOTT-ALDRICH SYNDROME. **Alezzandrini s.** Retinitis, deafness, poliosis, and vitiligo, all occurring on the same side. **allergic vasculitis s.** A variable syndrome characterized histologically by a polymorphonuclear infiltrate and a fibrinoid change in small dermal blood vessels and clinically by purpura, nodules, or bullae. **Alpers s.** A familial syndrome characterized by diffuse progressive degeneration and sclerosis of the cerebral cortex, with almost total sparing of the white matter. The onset is usually in infancy or between the ages of three and five years, and the condition gives rise to microcephaly, myoclonus, seizures, and paralysis, sometimes with amaurosis and rapid progression to dementia and death. Also *Alpers disease, poliodystrophia cerebri progressiva infantalis, diffuse cortical sclerosis, progressive cerebral poliodystrophy, progressive diffuse cerebrocortical atrophy, Alpers polioencephalopathy.* **Alport s.** An autosomal dominant syndrome consisting of hereditary nephritis, often progressing to renal failure, and variable sensorineural hearing loss. It affects both sexes in successive generations. **alveolar-capillary block s.** See under ALVEOLAR-CAPILLARY BLOCK. **alveolar hypoventilation s.** CARDIOPULMONARY-OBESITY SYNDROME. **amnestic s.** KORSAKOFF PSYCHOSIS. **amnestic-confabulatory s.** KORSAKOFF PSYCHOSIS. **amniotic band s.** Bandlike formations of the placental membranes which may surround the umbilical cord or a fetal limb and which on rare occasions cause constriction severe enough to result in fetal death or amputation of the constricted limb. **amniotic fluid s.** The sudden intravascular infusion or embolism of amniotic fluid resulting in pulmonary edema, shock, and disseminated intravascular coagulopathy. The syndrome is usually diagnosed immediately postpartum following a long and vigorous labor, a traumatic or rapid delivery, or delivery of a dead or excessively large fetus. Maternal death is not uncommon. **androgen insensitivity s.** TESTICULAR FEMINIZATION. **androgenital s.** *Seldom used* CONGENITAL ADRENOCORTICAL HYPERPLASIA. **angiectid s.** The appearance of superficial intradermal clumps of venules on the posterior thigh and calf areas during the first trimester of pregnancy. The lesions are usually associated with some discomfort but disappear during or after the pregnancy. **anginal s.** ANGINA PECTORIS. **angular gyrus s.** The syndrome resulting from infarction of the angular gyrus. Sometimes if the infarct extends deeply there is a contralateral hemianopia. When the dominant hemisphere is involved, alexia, the syndrome of the isolated speech area, and apraxia may occur, but more often a lesion here results in the Gerstmann syndrome. A lesion in the nondominant hemisphere more often causes contralateral visuospatial agnosia or defects of the body image. **aniridia-Wilms tumor s.** A variable syndrome of aniridia, genitourinary abnormalities (Wilm's tumor, gonadoblastoma, renal agenesis), hemihypertrophy, and psychomotor retardation. It is associated with structural aberrations of the short arm of chromosome 11, with the common site among abnormal chromosomes from many patients being band p13. Also *WAGR syndrome, AGR triad.* **ankyloglossia superior s.** A rare condition marked by the adherence of the tip of the tongue to the hard palate or to the nasal septum through a cleft palate. The premaxilla may be hypoplastic with the upper lip and upper incisor teeth absent. Various malformations of the hands and feet may be associated. **anorectal s.** Itching and pain of the anorectal area subsequent to the administration of oral broad-spectrum antibiotics. **anterior cerebral s.** Any syndrome which is attributable to ischemia or infarction in the territory of the anterior cerebral artery. A global syndrome, caused by interruption of the anterior cerebral artery at its origin, is marked by an abrupt onset, coma, hypothalamic dysfunction, and, after recovery of consciousness, persistence of dementia (indifference, lack of initiative, loss of affective tone, and disorientation in time and space), and of contralateral hemiplegia with crural dominance, associated with sensory impairment (particularly relating to deep sensitivity), and sometimes aphasia if the dominant hemisphere is involved. Partial syndromes result from obliteration of the artery after the origin of Heubner's artery, showing less severe mental defects and no coma, and from obliteration of Heubner's artery, showing contralateral facial weakness and monoparesis involving the upper limb. **anterior chamber cleavage s.** A developmental defect of differentiation of the cornea, in which absence of the central endothelium results in a central corneal opacity. Also *Peters anomaly.* **anterior choroidal artery s.** MONAKOW SYNDROME. **anterior compartment s.** ANTERIOR TIBIAL SYNDROME. **anterior spinal artery s.** The syndrome resulting from partial or complete occlusion of the anterior spinal artery due to thrombosis or embolism. When the lesion occurs in the upper cervical region it causes the sudden onset of flaccid tetraplegia with sphincter paralysis and loss of all forms of sensation except fine touch and tactile discrimination (due to sparing of the posterior columns supplied by the posterior spinal arteries). A lesion in the dorsal region, often due to occlusion of the artery of Adamkiewicz, and commonly resulting from dissecting aneurysm of the aorta, usually results in a flaccid paraplegia with a sensory level at D10. Partial occlusion or obstruction of branches of the artery can produce very variable signs of spinal cord dysfunction, and transient ischemic episodes as well as progressive ischemic myelopathy have been described. **anterior tibial s.** A syndrome associated with overuse of the anterior tibial muscles in untrained individuals, as from running or fast walking on hard surfaces. The muscles swell and become tender in their tight fascial compartment, with severe spontaneous pain. Pain usually passes after a few weeks of rest, but there may be permanent weakness of the muscles. Rarely, muscle necrosis and myoglobinuria occur. A chronic form of the syndrome with recurrent pain on exertion, requiring surgical decompression of the compartment, has been described. Also *anterior compartment syndrome, anterior tibial compartment syndrome, shin splints.* **anterior tibial nerve s.** Atrophy of the extensor digitorum brevis and decreased sensation between the first and second toes, caused by entrapment of the anterior tibial branch of the deep peroneal nerve in the anterior tarsal tunnel of the dorsum of the foot. **anterolateral s.** Combined degeneration of the anterior horns of gray matter and of the lateral columns of the spinal cord, as seen in motor neuron disease and especially in amyotrophic lateral sclerosis. **antibody deficiency s.** The form of immunity deficiency associated with failure to produce antibody. It is characterized clinically by repeated bacterial infections, particularly with pyococci. There is no increased susceptibility to viral infections except for an increased risk of paralytic poliomyelitis, serum hepatitis, and echovirus infections of the central nervous system. Antibody deficiency syndromes may be due to primary genetic abnormalities, of which infantile sex-linked hypogammaglobulinemia (Bruton's disease) is the best known, but the acquired form of unknown etiology (common variable immunodeficiency) is much commoner. Antibody deficiency states may also be restricted to individual classes or subclasses of antibody. **Anton s.** ANTON SYMPTOM. **Anton-Babinski s.** Inability of a hemiplegic patient to realize that the affected limbs are paralyzed. This is one form of anosognosia and usually results from a lesion in the nondominant inferior parietal cortex. Sometimes it simply produces indifference of the patient to his paralysis (anosodiaphoria). The condition may be accompanied by alloesthesia or visuospatial agnosia. **anxiety s.** ANXIETY NEUROSIS. **aortic arch s.** A syndrome of arterial insufficiency chiefly affecting the head and arms, due to narrowing or occlusion of one or more of the major branches of the aortic arch. It may be due to atherosclerosis, syphilis, Takayasu's arteritis, or other cause. **aortoiliac steal s.** The pathologic diminution of visceral blood flow that results from diversion of the blood into the lower extremities following aortoiliac vascular reconstruction. **Apert s.** ACROCEPHALOSYNDACTYLY TYPE I. **Apert-Crouzon s.** ACROCEPHALOSYNDACTYLY TYPE II. **s. of approximate answers** GANSER SYNDROME. **aqueduct of Sylvius s.** A syndrome marked by a combination of the Parinaud syndrome with nystagmus on attempted vertical gaze and convergence (or retraction nystagmus or spasms of eyelid retraction), pupillary abnormalities, and unilateral or bilateral oculomotor nerve paralysis. The syndrome is due to lesions, often of vascular origin, involving the periaqueductal gray matter of the midbrain. Also *Kestenbaum syndrome, sylvian aqueduct syndrome, Koerber-Salus-Elschnig syndrome.* **argentaffinoma s.** CARCINOID SYNDROME. **Argonz-del Castillo s.** Amenorrhea and galactorrhea with subnormal levels of plasma and urinary gonadotropins. It is not associated with parturition. **arthrogryposis s.** CONGENITAL MULTIPLE ARTHROGRYPOSIS. **Ascher s.** Blepharochalasis associated with progressive enlargement of the upper lip. **Asherman s.** Partial or complete obliteration of the endometrial cavity by scar tissue, usually resulting in a reduction of menstrual flow and infertility. Also *traumatic uterine adhesions.* **asplenia s.** The congenital absence of the spleen associated with varied developmental defects of other organs and systems, particularly major cardiovascular defects and abnormal location of lungs. It may also involve defects of the central nervous system, genitourinary tract, axial skeleton, or face. Supernumerary ectopic spleens may be present. **ataxia-telangiectasia s.** ATAXIA-TELANGIECTASIA. **auriculotemporal s.** A syndrome marked by profuse sweating over one cheek, temple, and surrounding areas of the face, precipitated by eating (especially of spicy foods) or sometimes by emotion. The condition may be idiopathic, but can follow damage to the facial nerve, as after parotid surgery, and is attributable to aberrant reinnervation. It presumably results from misdirection of the autonomic fibers that normally supply the salivary glands into the pathways normally followed by facial sudomotor fibers. Also *gustatory sweating syndrome, Frey syndrome, Baillarger syndrome, Frey-Baillarger syndrome, Dupuy syndrome, gustatory hyperhidrosis.* **autoerythrocyte sensitization s.** Recurrent painful ecchymoses due to hypersensitivity to one's own erythrocytes. The condition occurs principally in women and is characterized by pruritic or erythematous ecchymoses. The lesions can be produced by intradermal or subcutaneous injection of autologous erythrocyte extract. Also *Gardner-Diamond syndrome, erythrocyte autosensitization syndrome, painful bruising syndrome.* **Avellis s.** AVELLIS PARALYSIS. **Avellis-Longhi s.** AVELLIS PARALYSIS. **Axenfeld s.** A mesodermal dysgenesis of the periphery of the anterior chamber, in which a whitish rim of tissue may be seen internal to the peripheral cornea. **Ayerza s.** AYERZA'S DISEASE. **Baastrup s.** KISSING SPINES. **Babinski s.** The combination of cardiovascular and neurologic disorders due to tertiary syphilis. Also *Babinski-Vaquez syndrome.* **Babinski-Fröhlich s.** FRÖHLICH SYNDROME. **Babinski-Nageotte s.** A syndrome resulting usually from multiple areas of infarction in the brainstem due to vertebrobasilar insufficiency and principally involving the medulla oblongata. The manifestations are variable but usually include ipsilateral paralysis of the soft palate, pharynx, larynx, and sometimes of the tongue; the Horner syndrome, cerebellar ataxia, and loss of pain sensation on the face with contralateral hemiplegia and loss of proprioceptive sensibility. **Babinski-Vaquez s.** BABINSKI SYNDROME. **Bäfverstedt s.** BENIGN LYMPHOCYTOMA CUTIS. **Baillarger s.** AURICULOTEMPORAL SYNDROME. **Balint s.** A rare syndrome characterized by loss or impairment of automatic ocular movement. The patient may begin to follow an object with his eyes, then lose it and be unable to fix upon it again. There is associated ataxia of ocular movements and often visual inattention. The condition is usually attributable to bilateral parieto-occipital lesions. Also *psychic gaze paralysis.* **Ballantyne s.** A hereditary syndrome characterized by progressive high-tone sensorineural deafness, ash-blond hair and blue eyes. It is inherited, probably, as an autosomal recessive trait. **Baló s.** BALÓ'S DISEASE. **Banti s.** Chronic splenomegaly from congestion due to portal or splenic vein hypertension, sometimes associated with anemia, thrombocytopenia, leukopenia, or gastrointestinal bleeding. Ascites and jaundice may be seen. **Bardet-Biedl s.** An autosomal recessive condition characterized by obesity, polydactyly, hypogenitalism, mental retardation, and a progressive, pigmentary retinopathy (tapetoretinal degeneration). The polydactyly and absence of spinocerebellar ataxia distinguish this entity from the Laurence-Moon syndrome. Also *Biedl syndrome.* **Bard-Pic s.** Progressive jaundice and palpable gallbladder seen in common bile duct obstruction due to cancer of the head of the pancreas. **Barlow s.** Prolapse or floppy valve syndrome of the mitral valve associated with a systolic click and late systolic murmur. **Barraquer-Simons s.** PROGRESSIVE LIPODYSTROPHY. **Barré-Guillain s.** GUILLAIN-BARRÉ SYNDROME. **Barsony-Teschendorf s.** DIFFUSE ESOPHAGEAL SPASM. **Bartter s.** A hereditary disease characterized by juxtaglomerular cell hyperplasia, hyperreninemia without hypertension, hyperaldosteronism, hypokalemic alkalosis, and sometimes by short stature and mental retardation. **Bartter-Schwartz s.** SCHWARTZ-BARTTER SYNDROME. **basal cell nevus s.** A markedly pleiotropic and variable autosomal dominant condition characterized by multiple basal cell nevi and carcinomas, palmar dyskeratosis and pits, multiple jaw cysts, rib and vertebral anomalies, and genital maldevelopment. Also *nevoid basal cell carcinoma syndrome, Gorlin-Goltz syndrome, nevoid basalioma syndrome, Gorlin syndrome, basal-cell nevus.* **Bassen-Kornzweig s.** ABETALIPOPROTEINEMIA. **Bastian s.** Flaccid paraplegia with abolition of sphincter control and tendon reflexes, attributable to a complete transverse section of the spinal cord at the level of the lumbar enlargement. *Obs.* **battered child s.** The physical condition of a baby or older child who has been the subject of maltreatment, typically recognized by multiple fractures of bones, especially ribs and shafts of long bones. Often the injuries are discovered incidental to x-raying or examination and the fractures are partially healed, indicating an earlier date of occurrence. Reporting of alleged accidents is late, and the explanation of the injuries is often inadequate or incredible. Other injuries seen are bruises of different ages, cigarette burns, scalds of an entire hand or foot, and internal injuries which may be very severe. See also CHILD ABUSE. **Baumgarten s.** *Outmoded* CRUVEILHIER-BAUMGARTEN SYNDROME. **BBB s.** A congenital malformation syndrome of telecanthus with or without hypertelorism, hypospadias, cryptorchidism, cleft lip and palate, urinary malformations, and variable mental retardation. It resembles the G syndrome, but no esophageal abnormalities are present. Inheritance is X-linked or sex-influenced autosomal dominant, and symptoms are more severe in males. Also *hypertelorism-hypospadias syndrome.* **Beau s.** ASYSTOLE. **Behçet s.** A chronic often progressive disease characterized by severe uveitis with ulceration of the mouth and genitalia, very likely due to a virus infection. Also *Behçet aphthae, Touraine's aphthosis, Behçet triple symptom complex, Behçet's disease, Adamantiades-Behçet syndrome, cutaneomucouveal syndrome, dermatostomatoophthalmic syndrome, Gilbert-Behçet syndrome, oculobuccogenital syndrome.* **Bekhterev s.** ANKYLOSING SPONDYLITIS. **Benedikt s.** Unilateral oculomotor nerve paralysis with contralateral tremor, chorea, and athetotic movements due to a lesion, usually infarction, in the region of the oculomotor nucleus and cerebral peduncle. Also *tegmental mesencephalic paralysis.* **Bennet s.** ACUTE LEUKEMIA. **Berardinelli s.** SEIP SYNDROME. **Berardinelli-Seip s.** SEIP SYNDROME. **Bernard s.** HORNER SYNDROME. **Bernard-Horner s.** HORNER SYNDROME. **Bernard-Soulier s.** A hereditary bleeding disorder of autosomal recessive transmittance, characterized by the presence of unusually large platelets that in stained blood films exhibit clumping of granules in the center of the cells (thus creating a "pseudonucleus"), prolonged bleeding time, impaired prothrombin consumption, and failure of platelets to aggregate in the presence of ristocetin, although they aggregate in the presence of collagen, epinephrine, or adenosine diphosphate. **Bernhardt-Roth s.** MERALGIA PARESTHETICA. **Bernheim s.** Right heart failure due to obstruction to flow through the right ventricle as a result of a hypertrophied septum, associated with left ventricular hypertrophy as in aortic stenosis or hypertension. **Berry-Perkins-Young s.** Male infertility due to failure of the vasa efferentia to form a normal epididymis, associated with bronchiectasis, possibly resulting from congenital polycystic disease. Also *Young syndrome.* **Bertolotti s.** Sacralization of the fifth lumbar vertebra with lumbar scoliosis and, sometimes, sciatica. **Biedl s.** BARDET-BIEDL SYNDROME. **Bielschowsky-Dollinger s.** LATE INFANTILE CEROID-LIPOFUSCINOSIS. **Biemond s.** **1** An autosomal recessive maldevelopment of multiple central nervous system structures that results in analgesia, loss of temperature sense, and loss of deep tendon reflexes. Also *Biemond syndrome type I.* **2** An autosomal recessive form of pituitary dwarfism that is associated with polydactyly, hypogenitalism, iris coloboma, and mental retardation. Also *Biemond syndrome type II.* **3** An autosomal dominant form of ataxia due to the degeneration of the posterior columns of the spinal cord. **4** The familial occurrence of brachydactyly, nystagmus, and cerebellar ataxia. **Binder s.** NASOMAXILLARY DYSOSTOSIS. **Bing-Neel s.** Macroglobulinemia with neurologic manifestations such as confusion, disorientation, dementia, coma, blurred vision, and polyneuropathy. The central nervous system manifestations are attributed to blood hyperviscosity due to marked macroglobulinemia. Coma, when present, may be called *coma paraproteinemicum.* **Biörck s.** CARCINOID SYNDROME. **Biörck-Thorson s.** CARCINOID SYNDROME. **bisected brain s.** The condition that results from surgical separation of the two cerebral hemispheres by complete transection of the corpus callosum, anterior and hippocampal commissures, and interthalamic adhesion. Such patients demonstrate that the two hemispheres are functionally independent. Perception, memory, and learned phenomena experienced by one hemisphere proceed without awareness in the other. Little or no striking change in behavior or temperament occurs, yet each hemisphere performs without regard to information stored in the other. **Björnstad s.** A genetically determined disease in which sensorineural deafness is associated with pili torti of the head including the eyebrows and eyelashes. It is probably of autosomal dominant inheritance. **Blatin s.** HYDATID THRILL. **blind loop s.** Stagnation of intestinal contents, often in a surgically created blind loop or bypassed loop of small bowel or large small-bowel diverticula, with overgrowth of bacteria and malabsorption of nutrients, especially fat and Vitamin $B_{12}$. Also *stagnant loop syndrome.* See also AFFERENT LOOP SYNDROME. **BLM s.** TARDIVE DYSKINESIA. ● The abbreviation stands for *buccal-lingual-masticatory.* **Bloch-Sulzberger s.** INCONTINENTIA PIGMENTI. **Bloom s.** A hereditary disorder characterized by stunted growth and facial erythema, and by increased mortality from leukemia in the second and third decades. **blue diaper s.** A blue color due to indoles in urine, secondary to a defect in intestinal absorption of tryptophane, permitting bacterial action to convert tryptophane to indoles. It is similar to Hartnup's disease. **blue sclera s.** LOBSTEIN SYNDROME. **blue toe s.** Toe or distal foot embolization resulting from proximal aneurysms, atherosclerotic plaques, or arterial reconstructive procedures. **body of Luys s.** HEMIBALLISMUS. **Boerhaave s.** Spontaneous rupture of the esophagus. This grave condition usually results from very forceful vomiting, often after a large meal or alcohol ingestion. **Bonnet sphenoidal foramen s.** *Seldom used* RAEDER'S PARATRIGEMINAL SYNDROME. **Bonnevie-Ullrich s.** An apparently inherited disorder marked by pterygium colli, lymphedema of the hands and feet, laxity of the skin, short stature and other congenital anomalies of the skin and bones. These features are also found in phenotypic females with XO chromosomal constitution and with the other characteristics of gonadal dysgenesis. **Bourneville s.** TUBEROUS SCLEROSIS. **Bourneville-Pelizzi s.** TUBEROUS SCLEROSIS. **Bourneville-Pringle s.** TUBEROUS SCLEROSIS. **Bouveret s.** **1** Gastric outlet obstruction secondary to a large gallstone which has eroded from the biliary tract, most often from the gallbladder, into the duodenum through a biliary fistula. **2** PAROXYSMAL TACHYCARDIA. **boxers' s.** BOXERS' ENCEPHALOPATHY. **Brachmann-de Lange s.** DE LANGE SYNDROME. **bradycardia-tachycardia s.** A form of the sick sinus syndrome characterized by bradytachycardia: the patient has at different times episodes of bradycardia (either of sinus origin or associated with sinuatrial block or sinus arrest) and atrial arrhythmias (tachycardia, flutter, or fibrillation). Also *brady-tachy syndrome* (informal). **brain s.** ORGANIC BRAIN SYNDROME. **brain death s.** A state of deep coma exceeding 24 hours in which there is no clinical or other evidence of survival of function in the cerebral hemispheres, in which spontaneous respiration and the oculocephalic and caloric brainstem reflexes are absent, and which is not a drug-induced coma, so that irreversible brain damage can be presumed even if the cardiovascular system continues to function. **Brennemann s.** Abdominal pain, fever, nausea, and vomiting occurring in children in the course of throat infections. The abdominal symptoms have been attributed to mesenteric or retroperitoneal adenitis. **Briquet s.** Hysterical dyspnea often associated with dysphonia. **Bristowe s.** A syndrome resulting from a glioma of the corpus callosum, with fits and dementia as common manifestations. *Seldom used.* **brittle bone s.** OSTEOGENESIS IMPERFECTA. **broad thumb-hallux s.** RUBINSTEIN SYNDROME. **Brock s.** MIDDLE LOBE SYNDROME. **Brown-Séquard s.** The neurologic syndrome resulting from hemisection of the spinal cord, whether resulting from trauma, tumor, or demyelination. On the side of the lesion there is paralysis of upper motor neuron type with loss of fine touch, pressure, and position sense, and tactile discrimination up to a sensory level corresponding to the spinal segment at which the lesion is present. On the opposite side there is loss of pain and temperature sense with the sensory level a few dermatomes lower. On the paralyzed side there may be a band of hyperesthesia immediately above the sensory level. Also *Brown-Séquard paralysis, Brown-Séquard disease, hemiparaplegic syndrome, Brown-Séquard sign.* **Brown sheath s.** SUPERIOR OBLIQUE TENDON SHEATH SYNDROME. **Bruns s.** A syndrome of episodic headache and vomiting, sometimes with papilledema, and of vertigo induced by change in position of the head, which may be associated with space-occupying lesions in the fourth ventricle. Similar manifestations due to intermittent hydrocephalus, but usually lacking the component of positional vertigo, occasionally occur with tumors in the lateral or third ventricles, such as colloid cyst, or in the midline of the cerebellum. **Brunsting s.** Benign mucosal pemphigoid of the head and neck area. It most often affects males of middle age. **Brushfield-Wyatt s.** *Outmoded* STURGE-WEBER SYNDROME. **bubbly-lung s.** The radiographic appearance of the lungs of infants with the Wilson-Mikity syndrome. **buccal-lingual-masticatory s.** TARDIVE DYSKINESIA. **Budd-Chiari s.** A syndrome of abdominal pain, hepatomegaly, and ascites caused by obstruction of hepatic venous flow, most commonly seen in patients with hypercoagulable states such as thrombocytosis, dysproteinemias, or estrogen therapy. Also *Chiari syndrome, Budd-Chiari disease, Budd's disease* (obs.), *Chiari's disease, endophlebitis hepatica obliterans.* **buffoonery s.** BUFFOONERY PSYCHOSIS. **Bürger-Grütz s.** FAMILIAL HYPERLIPOPROTEINEMIA TYPE I. **Burnett s.** MILK-ALKALI SYNDROME. **burning feet s.** A syndrome due to prolonged consumption of a diet deficient in protein and B group vitamins. The earliest symptom is aching, burning, or throbbing in the feet. This is replaced by paroxysmal, sharp, shooting pains that spread to the knee, are often accompanied by transient hypertension, and invariably are worse at night. Some relief may be obtained by walking or immersing the feet in cold water. Such symptoms probably arise from lesions in the dorsal root or sympathetic ganglia. Also *Gopalan syndrome.* **Buschke-Ollendorff s.** DISSEMINATED LENTICULAR DERMATOFIBROSIS. **Bywaters s.** ACUTE TUBULAR NECROSIS. **Caffey s.** INFANTILE HYPEROSTOSIS. **Caffey-Silverman s.** INFANTILE HYPEROSTOSIS. **Cairns s.** Communicating hydrocephalus following tuberculous meningitis. *Seldom used.* **calcarine artery s.** The visual field defects which arise from softening of the brain in the area supplied by the calcarine artery, comprising either a total contralateral hemianopia, or quadrantanopia affecting the upper or lower quadrant, depending on whether the softening involves both lips of the calcarine fissure (obstruction of the arterial trunk) or only one of them (obstruction of one of its branches). Bilateral softening in this distribution results in cortical blindness. **callosal s.** CORPUS CALLOSUM SYNDROME. **camptomelic s.** CAMPTOMELIC DYSPLASIA. **Canada-Cronkhite s.** CRONKHITE-CANADA SYNDROME. **Capgras s.** A condition in which the subject suffers the delusion that an impostor has replaced a person close to him, such as his wife or mother. Also *illusions of doubles, Capgras symptom.* **Caplan s.** An unusual and distinctive form of coal workers' pneumoconiosis occurring in patients who also have rheumatoid arthritis. It is characterized by multiple, large (0.5–5 cm), round, radiographic opacities. Also *rheumatoid pneumoconiosis.* **capsular thrombosis s.** Contralateral hemiplegia resulting from infarction of the anterior limb of the internal capsule, due to thrombosis of perforating branches of the middle cerebral artery. **carcinoid s.** A syndrome consisting of intermittent diarrhea, cyanotic flushing of the skin lasting for minutes or days, asthmatic attacks, heart murmurs, and hepatomegaly. It is associated with argentaffin carcinoid tumors originating in the gastrointestinal tract with hepatic metastases or, rarely, the bronchi. The syndrome is caused by excessive tumor production of serotonin and other substances, such as histamine, bradykinin, and catecholamines. Also *argentaffinoma syndrome, Biörck syndrome, Biörck-Thorson syndrome, Cassidy syndrome, Cassidy-Scholte syndrome, Hedinger syndrome, metastatic carcinoid syndrome, vasculocardiac syndrome of hyperserotoninemia.* **cardioauditory s.** JERVELL AND LANGE-NIELSEN SYNDROME. **cardiobulbar s.** Any severe cardiorespiratory defect resulting from a lesion of the medulla oblongata and including Cheyne-Stokes respiration and cardiac arrhythmia. *Seldom used.* **cardiofacial s.** A syndrome comprising partial lower facial paralysis on one side and congenital heart disease. **cardiopulmonary-obesity s.** Obesity associated with hypersomnia, muscular twitching, polycythemia, cyanosis, congestive heart failure, and arterial hypoxia and hypercapnia. Also *pickwickian syndrome, alveolar hypoventilation syndrome.* **carotid sinus s.** A syndrome caused by a hypersensitive carotid sinus. Slight pressure on one or other sinus leads to reflex bradycardia and hypotension. Also *Charcot-Weiss-Baker syndrome, sinus reflex.* **carpal tunnel s.** A syndrome of painful paresthesiae in the hands and fingers, occurring particularly in middle-aged or pregnant women and due to compression of the median nerve in the carpal tunnel. The syndrome is also seen following fracture or arthritis of the wrist, in acromegaly, myxedema, and amyloidosis. The symptoms comprise paresthesia, often with pain in the area of the index, long, and ring fingers, often particularly intense at night. In more severe cases there may be partial atrophy of the lateral half of the thenar eminence with weakness of abduction and opposition of the thumb. Also *tardy median palsy.* **Carpenter s.** See under ACROCEPHALOPOLYSYNDACTYLY. **cartilage-hair hypoplasia s.** METAPHYSEAL CHONDRODYSPLASIA, MCKUSICK TYPE. **Cassidy s.** CARCINOID SYNDROME. **Cassidy-Scholte s.** CARCINOID SYNDROME. **cat's cry s.** CRI DU CHAT SYNDROME. **cat eye s.** A congential malformation syndrome caused by trisomy or tetrasomy of part of chromosome 22 (22pter-q11). It is characterized by iris coloboma, imperforate anus, preauricular tags or fistulas, heart and urinary tract anomalies, and mild mental retardation. Also *Schmid-Fraccaro syndrome.* **Cauchois-Eppinger-Frugoni s.** Enlargement of the spleen resulting from thrombotic obstruction of the splenic vein. **cauda equina s.** A syndrome attributable to a lesion of several lumbosacral nerve roots within the spinal canal. Four main presentations can be differentiated: the sacral syndrome (S3 to S5), comprising paralysis of the gluteal muscles, abolition of the anal and bulbocavernosus reflexes, perineal anesthesia, sphincter paralysis, anesthesia of the urethral and rectal mucosae, and impotence; the medial lumbosacral syndrome (L5 to S5), which comprises in addition to the above, paralysis of the muscles of the feet and of the posterior aspect of the legs and thighs, abolition of the ankle jerk, sensory defects (L5 and S1), and considerable sphincter malfunction; the complete syndrome (L2 to S5) which comprises, in addition to the above, weakness of the quadriceps muscles, abolition of the knee jerks, sensory loss in the feet, legs, posterior aspect of the thighs, the buttocks, and the perineal region, total paralysis of the sphincters and of sexual function, and often trophic disorders; and a cauda equina hemisyndrome, which is rare and which represents a unilateral form of one of the other types. **caudal dysplasia s.** CAUDAL DYSPLASIA. **causalgia s.** See under CAUSALGIA. **cavernous sinus s.** Any syndrome resulting from damage to multiple cranial nerves (third, fourth, and sixth, and the first and second divisions of the fifth) due to a lesion, such as aneurysm or thrombosis, in the cavernous sinus. The manifestations may resemble some or all of those of the superior orbital fissure syndrome, the orbital apex syndrome, painful ophthalmoplegia, and the infraclinoid syndrome. **celiac s.** CELIAC DISEASE. **celiac band s.** Postprandial abdominal pain, severe weight loss, and position-dependent epigastric bruit that is said to arise from impingement of structures near the esophageal hiatus upon the celiac axis, with resultant intestinal ischemia. **centroposterior s.** A dissociated loss of sensation and vasomotor changes due to syringomyelic disease involving the centroposterior area of the cervical spinal cord. **cerebellomedullary malformation s.** ARNOLD-CHIARI DEFORMITY. **cerebellopontine angle s.** A syndrome of progressive unilateral deafness, nystagmus, loss of the corneal reflex and sometimes ipsilateral facial paralysis and cerebellar ataxia, due to a lesion in the cerebellopontine angle which usually proves to be an acoustic neuroma. Also *pontocerebellar angle syndrome, Cushing syndrome* (obs.). **cerebellopyramidal s.** Any syndrome in which cerebellar signs and pyramidal tract dysfunction are combined. In lesions of the medulla oblongata cerebellar signs occur on one side while those of pyramidal tract dysfunction on the other, but in lesions of the upper midbrain in the region of the cerebral and superior cerebellar peduncles, the cerebellar signs and pyramidal tract signs both occur on the side opposite to the lesion. **cerebellosympathetic s.** A syndrome caused by a lesion of the inferior cerebellar peduncle in the medulla oblongata, which also involves descending sympathetic fibers traveling from the hypothalamus to the thoracolumbar sympathetic outflow. This syndrome is characterized by the combination of a cerebellar hemisyndrome and a Horner syndrome on the same side as the lesion, and it is one of the lateral bulbar syndromes. **cerebellothalamic s.** HYPOTHALAMIC COMMISSURAL SYNDROME. **cerebrocardiac s.** KRISHABER'S DISEASE. **cerebrohepatorenal s.** A rare, severe, autosomal recessive, congenital syndrome characterized by craniofacial anomalies, generalized hypotonia, renal cortical cysts, intrahepatic biliary dysgenesis, and elevated serum long-chain fatty acids, with death in infancy. The basic defect involves peroxisomal degradation of long-chain fatty acids. Also *Zellweger syndrome.* **cervical disk s.** Brachialgia with radicular pain in the arm. It is often accompanied by numbness and muscle spasm due to compression of a cervical nerve root by protrusion of a cervical disk. Also *cervical radicular syndrome, cervical syndrome, cervical compression syndrome.* **cervical fusion s.** KLIPPEL-FEIL SYNDROME. **cervical radicular s.** CERVICAL DISK SYNDROME. **cervical rib s.** SCALENUS ANTERIOR SYNDROME. **cervical tension s.** POST-TRAUMATIC CERVICAL SYNDROME. **cervicobrachial s.** THORACIC OUTLET SYNDROME. **cervicothoracic outlet s.** THORACIC OUTLET SYNDROME. **Cestan-Chenais s.** A combination of unilateral vagal paralysis with the manifestations of the Babinski-Nageotte syndrome. It is a rare manifestation of brainstem infarction. Also *Cestan syndrome.* **Cestan-Raymond s.** SUPERIOR PONTINE SYNDROME. **chancriform s.** PRIMARY EXTRAPULMONARY COCCIDIOIDOMYCOSIS. **Charcot s.** 1 INTERMITTENT CLAUDICATION. 2 Intermittent fever, with true rigors, abdominal pain, and jaundice. It is seen in patients with acute septic cholangitis. 3 AMYOTROPHIC LATERAL SCLEROSIS. **Charcot-Marie-Tooth-Hoffmann s.** CHARCOT-MARIE-TOOTH DISEASE. **Charcot-Weiss-Baker s.** CAROTID SINUS SYNDROME. **Charlin s.** Attacks of severe pain in the head, resembling migrainous neuralgia, associated with rhinorrhea and inflammatory changes in the eye. **Chauffard s.** Juvenile rheumatoid arthritis beginning in childhood or adolescence and characterized by splenomegaly, arthritis, lymphadenopathy, arthralgia, anemia, and spiking fever. Also *Chauffard-Still syndrome, Still-Chauffard syndrome.* **Chédiak-Higashi s.** CHÉDIAK-HIGASHI ANOMALY. **Chiari s.** BUDD-CHIARI SYNDROME. **Chiari-Frommel s.** Postpartum amenorrhea, galactorrhea, and low plasma and urinary gonadotropin values which persist for at least one year after delivery without any apparent organic lesion of the pituitary or of the central nervous system. Also *Frommel-Chiari syndrome, Chiari-Frommel disease, Frommel's disease.* **Chilaiditi s.** A congenital or acquired anomaly in which part of the large bowel, or occasionally the small bowel, is trapped between the liver and the diaphragm. This is usually an asymptomatic condition discovered by radiography of the abdomen or chest, but it may give rise to abdominal pain radiating to the back or shoulders. **Chinese restaurant s.** A syndrome of sweating, flushing of the face, burning sensations in various parts of the body, abdominal or chest pains, thirst, nausea, headache, weakness, or other symptoms, which usually begin 25–35 minutes after eating food that has been lavishly seasoned with monosodium glutamate (such as the food served in some Chinese restaurants). The symptoms may last for several hours. Some people seem to be susceptible to these presumably neurotoxic effects of monosodium glutamate, and for them it takes a dose of about 25 mg to cause the symptoms. Also *Kwok's disease.* Abbr. CRS **chorea s.** PALLIDAL SYNDROME. **chorea-athetosis-agitans s.** *Obs.* HUNTINGTON'S CHOREA. **Chotzen s.** ACROCEPHALOSYNDACTYLY TYPE III. **Christian s.** HAND-SCHÜLLER-CHRISTIAN DISEASE. **Christ-Siemens s.** ANHIDROTIC ECTODERMAL DYSPLASIA. **Christ-Siemens-Touraine s.** ANHIDROTIC ECTODERMAL DYSPLASIA. **chromosome breakage s.** Any one of a small number of rare, mendelian disorders associated with an abnormal predisposition for chromosomes to break and to rearrange. Most of the disorders, such as the Bloom syndrome, Fanconi anemia, and ataxia-telangiectasia, are also associated with neoplasia, and chromosome instability may be a contributing factor to oncogenesis. **Citelli s.** The characteristic appearance of adenoid facies combined with a high-arched palate and less than average intelligence, at one time attributed to gross enlargement of the adenoids. The open mouth, due to nasal obstruction, and a degree of impaired hearing, due to middle-ear effusion, are the only features truly related to the enlarged adenoids. **Clarke-Hadfield s.** Hypoplasia of the exocrine pancreas, a rare congenital condition which causes impairment of growth in early childhood. Also *Hadfield-Clarke syndrome.* **Claude s.** INFERIOR RED NUCLEUS SYNDROME. **Claude Bernard-Horner s.** HORNER SYNDROME. **Claude and Lhermitte s.** HYPOTHALAMIC SYNDROME. **Claude-Loyez s.** INFERIOR RED NUCLEUS SYNDROME. **Claude's red nucleus s.** INFERIOR RED NUCLEUS SYNDROME. **Clérambault-Kandinsky s.** CLÉRAMBAULT-KANDINSKY COMPLEX. **click s.** The combination of a systolic click with mitral valve prolapse. It is often followed by a late systolic murmur. **closed head s.** Symptoms of injury to the brain without an associated skull fracture or penetration. **Clouston s.** HIDROTIC ECTODERMAL DYSPLASIA. **cloverleaf skull deformity s.** KLEEBLATTSCHÄDEL DEFORMITY SYNDROME. **clumsy child s.** MINIMAL BRAIN DYSFUNCTION. **Cockayne s.** An autosomal recessive phenotype of symmetric dwarfism, deafness, chorioretinitis, microcephaly, mental retardation, and features of precocious aging that are evidenced by appearance and atherosclerosis. **Cogan s.** 1 Nonsyphilitic interstitial keratitis with vertigo and tinnitus, usually resulting in profound deafness. Also *Cogan's disease, oculovestibuloauditory syndrome.* 2 OCULOMOTOR APRAXIA. **Collet-Sicard s.** Unilateral paralysis of the last four cranial nerves (ninth, tenth, eleventh, and twelfth) resulting in Vernet's paralysis combined with paralysis of the tongue muscles on the same side. Also *Collet syndrome, Sicard's posterior condylar syndrome, posterior lacterocondylar syndrome, Sicard syndrome.* **combined immunodeficiency s.** SEVERE COMBINED IMMUNODEFICIENCY. **compartment s.** The symptoms (pain, distal weakness) and signs (muscle swelling and tenderness, diminished peripheral nerve function) that result from the development of high pressures within certain fascial compartments. It is especially seen in the leg or forearm following closed fractures, electrical burns, or crush injuries. **compression s.** CRUSH SYNDROME. **concussion s.** POST-TRAUMATIC ENCEPHALOPATHY. **Condorelli s.** CONDORELLI'S ENCEPHALITIS. **congenital rubella s.** A syndrome comprising increased incidence of premature delivery and fetal death and an array of congenital defects in offspring of mothers infected with rubella virus during the first 15–20 weeks of pregnancy. The virus is transmitted transplacentally to the fetus. The incidence of single or multiple defects and the type and severity of the particular problems affecting the fetus are dependent in large part on gestational age at the time of infection. For example, 40-60% of fetuses infected during the first two months of gestation either develop multiple congenital defects or are spontaneously aborted, but only 10% of fetal infections occurring in the fourth month result in a single congenital defect. Characteristics of congenital rubella include low birth weight, deafness, cataracts or glaucoma, congenital heart disease, thrombocytopenia purpura, hepatosplenomegaly, radiolucencies in the long bones, and mental retardation with or without microcephaly. Some children appear normal at birth but develop symptoms later in childhood, including behavior and language disorders, learning disabilities, hearing loss, and diabetes mellitus. Virus persists in and is shed from infants with the congenital rubella syndrome for up to two to four years. **Conn s.** PRIMARY ALDOSTERONISM. **Conradi s.** See under CHONDRODYSPLASIA PUNCTATA. **Conradi-Hünermann s.** See under CHONDRODYSPLASIA PUNCTATA. **Conradi-Raap s.** CHONDRODYSTROPHY. **contracture s.** STIFF-MAN SYNDROME. **conus s.** A syndrome which results from a lesion of the conus medullaris. The principal clinical features are those of sphincter paralysis, saddle anesthesia, and a combination of signs of upper and lower motor neuron lesions in the lower limbs. Thus there may be substantial muscular atrophy and weakness with absent lower abdominal, cremasteric, and anal reflexes, and sometimes absence of the knee and ankle jerks, but the plantar responses are nevertheless extensor. Also *conus medullaris syndrome.* **Coote s.** SCALENUS ANTERIOR SYNDROME. **Coote-Hunauld s.** SCALENUS ANTERIOR SYNDROME. **Cornelia de Lange s.** DE LANGE SYNDROME. **coronary failure s.** UNSTABLE ANGINA. **coronary intermediate s.** UNSTABLE ANGINA. **corpora quadrigeminal s.** An ill-defined syndrome resulting from lesions in the neighborhood of the corpora quadrigemina, such as may result from tumors in the region of the pineal. The manifestations may include defects of upward conjugate gaze (Parinaud syndrome), hydrocephalus, and hemianopia if the lesion is laterally situated. **corpus callosum s.** A group of manifestations attributable to damage to the corpus callosum, usually caused by a tumor. These may include amnesia, fits, loss of ability to concentrate, sometimes a confusional state, fatigability, inattention, apathy, irritability, and sometimes left-sided motor apraxia or ataxia. A lesion of the splenium of the corpus callosum may produce pure alexia. Also *callosal syndrome.* **s. of the corpus Luysii** HEMIBALLISMUS. **s. of corpus striatum** VOGT SYNDROME. **Costen s.** TEMPOROMANDIBULAR JOINT SYNDROME. **costochondral s.** COSTOCHONDRITIS. **costoclavicular compression s.** A variant of the thoracic outlet syndrome in which compression of the subclavian artery and the cords of the brachial plexus is attributed to an abnormally narrow canal between the first rib, which may be abnormally high, and the clavicle, which may be abnormally low. Also *costoclavicular syndrome.* **cough s.** COUGH SYNCOPE. **Courvoisier-Terrier s.** Jaundice and palpable gallbladder resulting from a tumor of the ampulla of Vater. **craniocarpotarsal s.** WHISTLING FACE–WINDMILL VANE HAND SYNDROME. **Creutzfeldt-Jakob s.** CREUTZFELDT-JAKOB DISEASE. **cri du chat s.** A congenital malformation syndrome in humans caused by the deletion of the short arm of one of the chromosomes 5 ($5p^-$). The clinical manifestations include microcephaly, hypertelorism, antimongoloid slant of the palpebral fissures, epicanthal folds, strabismus, micrognathia, mental retardation, and a characteristic catlike mewing cry in infancy. Also *cri du chat, $5p^-$ syndrome, cat's cry syndrome.* **Crigler-Najjar s.** A hereditary disorder characterized by hyperbilirubinemia due to deficiency of the enzyme glucuronyl transferase in the liver. Two types are known. Type I is of autosomal recessive inheritance. Homozygotes have marked increase in unconjugated bilirubin (25 to 35 mg/dl) shortly after birth and often develop kernicterus. Type II is of autosomal dominant inheritance. Heterozygotes with type II usually exhibit mild increase in unconjugated serum bilirubin within the first decade of life, and even when jaundice occurs soon after birth, it is not severe and kernicterus is unusual. See also GILBERT SYNDROME. **crocodile tears s.** Lacrimation accompanying eating. It is usually a sequel of facial palsy, when regenerating fibers of the chorda tympani are misdirected and innervate the lacrimal gland on the affected side. **Cronkhite-Canada s.** An idiopathic, nonfamilial gastrointestinal polyposis associated with ectodermal changes such as skin pigmentation, alopecia, and onychatrophia, and with malabsorption, protein-losing enteropathy, and diarrhea. Also *Cronkhite syndrome, Canada-Cronkhite syndrome.* **Crouzon s.** CRANIOFA-

CIAL DYSOSTOSIS. **CRST s.** A subset of progressive systemic sclerosis, thought to have a more benign prognosis, consisting of calcinosis, Raynaud's phenomenon, sclerodactyly, and telangiectasia. Since laboratory tests almost universally reveal the additional presence of esophageal dysfunction, this condition is also known as the CREST syndrome. **crus s.** KERNOHAN SYNDROME. **crush s.** Acute renal failure and acute tubular necrosis secondary to a crushing injury. Also *compression syndrome.* **Cruveilhier-Baumgarten s.** Dilatation or recanalization of the paraumbilical veins resulting from portal hypertension, most often seen in hepatic cirrhosis. The auscultatory counterpart of the syndrome (Cruveilhier-Baumgarten murmur) is caused by increased flow through superficial paraumbilical veins. The caput medusae is the visual counterpart of the multiple dilated, tortuous superficial paraumbilical veins. Also *Baumgarten syndrome* (outmoded). **cryptophthalmia-syndactyly s.** A rare, autosomal recessive syndrome that is characterized by complete or partial cryptophthalmos, syndactyly, renal agenesis, craniofacial and genital abnormalities, and deafness due to ossicular maldevelopment. The palpebral fissures are absent, as are the eyelashes and eyebrows in some cases. It is usually lethal in the perinatal period. Also *Fraser syndrome.* **cubital s.** ULNAR NERVE PARALYSIS. **cubital tunnel s.** Compression of the ulnar nerve as it passes through the cubital tunnel behind the medial humeral epicondyle and between the two heads of flexor carpi ulnaris. Also *tardy ulnar palsy.* **culture-specific s.** Any of the disorders that are unique to one culture in society, such as amok and lata. **Curtis and Fitz-Hugh s.** FITZ-HUGH AND CURTIS SYNDROME. **Cushing s.** 1 A syndrome associated with hypersecretion of cortisol resulting from unilateral adrenocortical adenoma or carcinoma or to hyperfunction of both adrenal cortices. Hypersecretion of adrenocorticotropin by the anterior pituitary or by an ACTH-secreting neoplasm may also produce the syndrome. The pituitary-dependent form is called Cushing's disease. The Cushing syndrome, which is frequently fatal, is characterized by truncal obesity, muscular wasting, plethora, hirsutism, hypertension, glucose intolerance, osteopenia, weakness, impotence or amenorrhea, and severe emotional disturbance. Also *Itsenko's disease* (USSR usage), *suprarenogenic syndrome* (obs.). • Because the syndrome results from hypercortisolism, various terms conveying this sense are sometimes used to refer specifically to the syndrome. 2 *Obs.* CEREBELLOPONTINE ANGLE SYNDROME. **Cushing s. medicamentosus** IATROGENIC CUSHING SYNDROME. **cutaneomucouveal s.** BEHÇET SYNDROME. **cystic duct stump s.** Recurrent pain after cholecystectomy due to stones in the cystic duct remnant. See also POSTCHOLECYSTECTOMY SYNDROME. **Da Costa s.** NEUROCIRCULATORY ASTHENIA. **Danbolt-Closs s.** ACRODERMATITIS ENTEROPATHICA. **dancing eye–dancing feet s.** INFANTILE MYOCLONIC ENCEPHALOPATHY. **Dandy-Walker s.** Communicating hydrocephalus due to obstruction from birth of the foramina of Magendie and Luschka. All the cerebral ventricles are enlarged and the posterior fossa of the skull is small. Also *Dandy-Walker deformity.* **dead fetus s.** The retention of a dead fetus *in utero* for four weeks or longer, resulting in disseminated intravascular coagulopathy. **deafness-ear-pits s.** An autosomal dominant syndrome of which the most constant features are deafness due to middle-ear malformation and preauricular sinuses. External ear deformities, cleft palate, and severe sensorineural deafness may also occur. **Debré-de Toni-Fanconi s.** FANCONI SYNDROME. **Debré-Semelaigne s.** Myxedema in an infant or child, associated with hypertrophy of the muscles, particularly of the lower extremities, weakness, and mental retardation. Thyroid treatment is effective. Also *Kocher-Debré-Semelaigne syndrome, infantile myxedema-muscular hypertrophy syndrome.* **defibrination s.** DISSEMINATED INTRAVASCULAR COAGULATION. **Dejerine s.** 1 The syndrome of ipsilateral paralysis of the tongue or of the larynx and soft palate, with a contralateral hemiplegia, due to a lesion of the medulla oblongata. Also *Verger-Dejerine syndrome.* 2 Pain or paresthesiae, motor weakness, and sensory loss corresponding to the distribution of individual nerve roots rather than of peripheral nerves, resulting from radicular lesions. **Dejerine's anterior bulbar s.** MEDIAN MEDULLARY SYNDROME. **Dejerine's interolivary s.** MEDIAN MEDULLARY SYNDROME. **Dejerine-Klumpke s.** A syndrome resulting from birth injury to the lower or inner cord of the brachial plexus, due to traction and giving rise to paralysis of forearm and finger flexor muscles and of the small muscles of the hand. There may be an associated Horner syndrome on the same side due to damage to the stellate ganglion. Also *Klumpke's paralysis, Dejerine-Klumpke paralysis, Klumpke's palsy, Klumpke-Dejerine paralysis, Klumpke-Dejerine syndrome.* **Dejerine-Roussy s.** THALAMIC SYNDROME. **Dejerine-Sottas s.** HEREDITARY HYPERTROPHIC INTERSTITIAL NEUROPATHY. **de Lange s.** A rare form of birth defect principally characterized by low birth weight, growth retardation, hirsutism with confluent eyebrows and long eyelashes, a snub nose with anteverted nostrils and a long upper lip, microcephaly and mental retardation, small hands and feet, proximally placed thumbs, fifth finger clinodactyly, and hypertonia. The dermatoglyphs are abnormal but without a particular diagnostic feature. The chromosomes are usually normal. The etiology is uncertain. Also *Cornelia de Lange syndrome, Brachmann-de Lange syndrome.* **delayed stress s.** POST-TRAUMATIC STRESS DISORDER. **del Castillo s.** SERTOLI-CELL-ONLY SYNDROME. **dengue hemorrhagic shock s.** A disease distinguished from dengue by hemorrhagic manifestations, thrombocytopenia, hemoconcentration, circulatory failure, and shock. Death is common, especially in children. It is caused by one of the four serotypes of the dengue group B arbovirus, especially virus 2. Immunopathologic mechanisms are implicated, involving activation of complement by dengue antigen-antibody complexes. It is common in southeast Asia and may be epidemic. Rapid treatment of shock is important in management. Also *dengue shock syndrome, hemorrhagic fever syndrome.* **Denny-Brown s.** DENNY-BROWN SENSORY NEUROPATHY. **depersonalization s.** DEPERSONALIZATION. **deposed child s.** KWASHIORKOR. • The term is based on the supposition that following the birth of a new child, the last-born infant is subject to less attention, and nutritional deprivation and kwashiorkor may result. **de Quervain s.** Stenosing tenosynovitis of the long extensor muscle of the thumb and/or the short extensor muscle of the thumb. Also *Quervain syndrome, Quervain's disease, de Quervain's disease, thecostegnosis.* **dermatostomato-ophthalmic s.** BEHÇET SYNDROME. **DES s.** A congenital anomaly of the cervical transformation zone when a pregnant woman ingests diethylstilbesterol (DES). Instead of a uniform junction of squamous and columnar epithelium, the latter extends chaotically over the cervix and upper vagina. The cervix is frequently distorted and contains a hoodlike structure referred to as a coxcomb. There may also be associated uterine anomalies such as lateral strictures. In severe cases adenocarcinoma of the vagina has been identified. **De Sanctis-Cacchione s.** A syndrome of mental retardation, dwarfism, and gonadal hypoplasia associated with xeroderma pigmentosum. The phenotype can occur in patients with any of the seven currently known complementation groups of xeroderma pigmentosum. Also *xerodermic idiocy* (outmoded). **de Toni-Debré-Fanconi s.** FANCONI SYNDROME. **de Toni-Fanconi s.** FANCONI SYNDROME. **s. of deviously relevant answers** GANSER SYNDROME. **dialysis disequilibrium s.** Confusion, disorientation, headache, muscle twitching or tremors, nausea and vomiting during or following hemodialysis of a severely uremic patient. The syndrome is thought to be due to the rapid development of a large urea gradient between blood and brain tissue with resultant increases in osmotic intracellular pressure and cerebrospinal fluid pressure. Also *dysequilibrium syndrome.* **Diamond-Blackfan s.** DIAMOND-BLACKFAN ANEMIA. **diencephalic s.** Any of various disorders of endocrine and autonomic function resulting from a lesion, usually neoplastic, sited in the hypothalamus and affecting neural pathways connecting the hypothalamus and pituitary gland, other than those related to diabetes insipidus. **diencephalic s. of infancy** The development in infants, most commonly around six months, of vomiting, emaciation without loss of appetite, and pallor without anemia. Despite the emaciation, the affected infant remains paradoxically cheerful and hyperkinetic, and exhibits normal or accelerated growth. Sweating, hypoglycemia, vertical nystagmus, tremor, and disordered temperature control may occur. The usual cause is a tumor in the region of the third ventricle. Death usually occurs within a year. Also *Russell syndrome.* **DiGeorge s.** A syndrome due to absence of the thymus and parathyroid glands, associated with maldevelopment of pharyngeal pouches (branchial pouches) and hypocalcemia, and comprising impaired cell-mediated immunity but normal levels of immunoglobulins, short stature, ocular hypertelorism, and, often, deformities of the face, heart, and great vessels. Also *thymic-parathyroid aplasia, third and fourth pharyngeal pouch syndrome, third and fourth pharyngeal arch syndrome.* **Dighton-Adair s.** VAN DER HOEVE-DE KLEYN SYNDROME. **Di Guglielmo s.** ERYTHROLEUKEMIA. **Diogenes s.** The neglect of one's home or personal environment in later life, also associated with the irrational accumulation of a vast quantity of seemingly insignificant objects, such as rags or magazines. Also *senile neglect.* **disk s.** Any syndrome resulting from prolapse of an intervertebral disk. **Donath-Landsteiner s.** PAROXYSMAL COLD HEMOGLOBINURIA. **Down s.** A congenital syndrome characterized by moderate to severe mental retardation, congenital onset of growth failure, muscular hypotonicity, flat occiput, large tongue, epicanthus, slanting eyes, and simian palmar crease, with an increased incidence of intestinal stenosis, congenital heart disease (particularly endocardial cushion defects), and acute leukemia. Alzheimer's disease commonly develops in the fourth or fifth decade. It is caused by an extra chromosome 21, or at least trisomy of the distal long arm of 21, and is associated with advanced maternal age. Also *trisomy 21 syndrome, mongolism* (outmoded). **Dresbach s.** HEREDITARY ELLIPTOCYTOSIS. **Dressler s.** POST-MYOCARDIAL INFARCTION SYNDROME. **dry eye s.** The symptoms and signs associated with an inadequate tear film, as may occur in association with aging, diseases of the lachrymal glands, and certain forms of rheumatoid arthritis. **Duane s.** A developmental anomaly of simultaneous denervation of medial and lateral rectus muscles, the cocontraction of which causes retraction of the eye and an apparent paralysis of the lateral rectus muscle. Also *retraction syndrome, Stilling syndrome, Stilling-Turk-Duane syndrome, vertical retraction syndrome.*

**Dubin-Johnson s.** A familial disorder of bilirubin metabolism characterized by conjugated hyperbilirubinemia and lipofuscin pigment deposition in the liver. **Dubovitz s.** A congenital disorder characterized by short stature, peculiar facies, with hypoplasia of the supraorbital ridges, zygoma, malar eminence, and mandible; short palpebral fissures; prominent ears; thick skin with eczema; and sometimes mental retardation. **Duchenne s.** 1 PROGRESSIVE BULBAR PALSY. 2 PROGRESSIVE MUSCULAR ATROPHY. 3 Severe X-linked muscular dystrophy. See under MUSCULAR DYSTROPHY. **Duchenne-Erb s.** The syndrome attributable to birth injury of the upper cord of the brachial plexus (fifth and sixth cervical roots) causing paralysis of the deltoid, biceps, brachialis, coracobrachialis, and brachioradialis muscles, which become progressively atrophic. The other shoulder girdle muscles may become paretic. Abduction of the arm, with flexion and supination of the forearm, are lost, and so are the biceps and radial reflexes. The arm lies by the side with the forearm and hand pronated and the fingers flexed in the "policeman's tip" position. Sometimes there is initially a band of hypesthesia over the external aspect of the shoulder, arm and forearm. The finger movements are usually normal. Also *Duchenne's paralysis, Erb-Duchenne paralysis, Duchenne-Erb paralysis, Erb's paralysis, Erb's palsy, upper brachial plexus syndrome.* **dumping s.** POSTGASTRECTOMY SYNDROME. **Duplay s.** *Obs.* CALCIFIC TENDINITIS. **Dupré s.** *Obs.* MENINGISM. **Dupuy s.** AURICULOTEMPORAL SYNDROME. **dwarfism-diabetes s.** Dwarfism associated with characteristic signs and symptoms in children with diabetes mellitus and inadequate insulin treatment. The syndrome includes hepatomegaly, a pale, cool, waxy, and thick skin, and a face appearing younger than the normal for the chronologic age of the patient. **Dyke-Davidoff s.** The appearance in infants of facial asymmetry and atrophy together with paresis affecting one side of the body. It is thought to be due to a lesion on the side of the brain contralateral to the hemiparesis. **Dyke-Young s.** A form of hemolysis of unknown cause, characterized by macrocytosis of erythrocytes. **dysarthria-clumsy hand s.** A neurologic syndrome attributable to one or more small lacunar infarcts of the pons. The major clinical manifestations are dysarthria of moderate intensity, with difficulty or clumsiness in carrying out delicate or rapid alternating hand or finger movements on the side opposite to the lesion, with consequent deterioration in writing when the right hand is affected. Often there is also unilateral facial weakness, exaggeration of tendon reflexes, and an extensor plantar response on the same side as the clumsy hand, with slight difficulty in walking. The lacunae are formed from small areas of ischemic softening, generally due to severe arterial hypertension. **dysequilibrium s.** DIALYSIS DISEQUILIBRIUM SYNDROME. **dysmnesic s.** A syndrome marked by progressive general intellectual and cognitive impairment, characteristic of chronic brain syndrome or dementia. The individual suffers difficulties in adding new knowledge, perseveration, general reduction in efficiency, constructional apraxia, improvisation rather than planning, abnormal distractibility, and impairment in abstract thinking. Also *dysmnesia.* **dyssynchronous child s.** MINIMAL BRAIN DYSFUNCTION. **dystocia-dystrophia s.** Cephalopelvic disproportion in which the fetus is large and the vertex is unengaged and usually in the occiput posterior position. The syndrome is characteristically seen in the first successful and usually prolonged pregnancy of an elderly mother. **Eaton-Lambert s.** LAMBERT-EATON SYNDROME. **ectopic ACTH s.** ECTOPIC CUSHING SYNDROME. **ectopic Cushing s.** Cushing syndrome due to overproduction of ACTH by a tumor which is ectopic in the sense that it does not arise from the usual ACTH-secreting organ, the pituitary, but rather from bronchus, thymus, pancreas or other tissues. The most characteristic sign is severe hypokalemic alkalosis. Also *ectopic ACTH syndrome.* **Eddowes s.** LOBSTEIN SYNDROME. **Edwards s.** *Outmoded* TRISOMY 18 SYNDROME. **effort s.** NEUROCIRCULATORY ASTHENIA. **Ehlers-Danlos s.** Any of various heritable disorders of connective tissue, the most familiar of which is characterized by markedly hyperextensible joints, hyperextensible and fragile skin, easy bruising, and autosomal dominant inheritance. A milder form of this type is the most common of the 11 phenotypic variants of this syndrome. The most life-threatening form (the arterial, or Sack-Barabas, type) is characterized by a deficiency of type III collagen resulting in arterial fragility and death from vascular rupture or bowel perforation. Several of the autosomal recessive variants are due to deficiencies of enzymes involved in post-translational processing of type I collagen. At least one-half of those subjects with unusually extensible joints, thin skin, or poor wound-healing cannot be diagnosed as having any of the 11 variant forms currently identified, and are sometimes said to have Ehlers-Danlos syndrome, unclassified type. Also *Ehlers-Danlos disease, cutis hyperelastica.* **Eisenmenger s.** A form of cyanotic congenital heart disease in which pulmonary hypertension, due to a high pulmonary vascular resistance, complicates ventricular septal defect, atrial septal defect, or persistent ductus arteriosus. Also *Eisenmenger disease.* **Ekbom s.** RESTLESS LEGS SYNDROME. **elbow pain s.** GOLFERS' ELBOW. **elfin face s.** 1 See under SUPRAVALVULAR AORTIC STENOSIS SYNDROME. 2 See under IDIOPATHIC HYPERCALCEMIA. **Ellis-van Creveld s.** An autosomal recessive condition with variable features including short-limbed dwarfism, polydactyly, dystrophy of the fingernails, and cardiac defect, most commonly an atrial septal defect. Also *chondroectodermal dysplasia.* **emotional deprivation s.** MATERNAL DEPRIVATION SYNDROME. **empty sella s.** EMPTY SELLA. **endocrine polyglandular s.** MULTIPLE ENDOCRINE NEOPLASIA. **eosinophilic s.** HYPEREOSINOPHILIC SYNDROME. **Erb s.** MYASTHENIA GRAVIS. **Erb-Goldflam s.** MYASTHENIA GRAVIS. **Erb-Oppenheim-Goldflam s.** MYASTHENIA GRAVIS. **Erdheim s.** CYSTIC MEDIAL NECROSIS. **erythrocyte autosensitization s.** AUTOERYTHROCYTE SENSITIZATION SYNDROME. **erythroderma-atopy-bamboo hair s.** NETHERTON SYNDROME. **Estren-Dameshek s.** A variant of Fanconi's anemia in which skeletal abnormalities are not present. **$E_1$ trisomy s.** TRISOMY 13 SYNDROME. **Evans s.** Autoimmune hemolytic anemia with thrombocytopenia. **external carotid steal s.** A syndrome of transient attacks of dizziness and loss of balance caused by vertebrobasilar insufficiency. **extrapyramidal s.'s** A group of neurologic disorders resulting from lesions of the extrapyramidal nuclei and connecting pathways, giving rise to involuntary movements and other disorders of motility and tone. **Faber s.** *Obs.* ACHYLIC ANEMIA. **Fabry s.** ANGIOKERATOMA CORPORIS DIFFUSUM. **facet s.** Vertebral osteoarthritis in which the pain is thought to originate from the interarticular facets. **Fallot s.** TETRALOGY OF FALLOT. **Fanconi s.** 1 Congenital or acquired metabolic disturbances caused by a defect of proximal renal tubular function which results in urinary loss of amino acids, phosphate, sodium, potassium, bicarbonate, and in some instances glucose and protein. Acidemia, cystinosis, bone lesions, rickets, or osteomalacia result. Infantile (juvenile) and adult forms are described. Also *Debré-de Toni-Fanconi syndrome, Fanconi's disease, de Toni-Debré-Fanconi syndrome, de Toni-Fanconi syndrome, renal amino acid diabetes.* 2 FANCONI'S ANEMIA. **Favre-Racouchot s.** NODULAR ELASTOSIS OF THE SKIN. **Fazio-Londe s.** INFANTILE PROGRESSIVE BULBAR PALSY. **Fegeler s.** A syndrome characterized by the development of a capillary nevus on the face in the area controlled by the trigeminal nerve following trauma in the cervical region. The nevus is preceded by sharply defined erythema and accompanied by slight edema of the forehead and cheek. The Horner syndrome and other neurologic signs may be present. **Felty s.** A syndrome consisting of rheumatoid arthritis, splenomegaly, and leukopenia. **fetal alcohol s.** Mental retardation and/or deformity of a human fetus secondary to chronic intake of ethanol by a mother during pregnancy. ⟨"Experiments on mice . . . indicate that the extent of retardation and malformation (known in humans as fetal alcohol syndrome) is related to the alcohol levels in the pregnant mouse's blood." —*Science News,* 20 Jan. 1979, 41.⟩ **fetal aspiration s.** The entry of amniotic fluid into the bronchial tubes in excessive amounts due to premature and violent efforts to breathe by the distressed fetus in the uterus. Mucus and blood from the birth canal may also be aspirated during labor. Amniotic debris, squamae, and meconium may be found in the lungs post mortem. If the amniotic fluid is infected there is grave danger of neonatal pneumonia. Massive aspiration may be followed, after respiration has been established, by disseminated or segmental atelectasis and interstitial emphysema, surface blebs on the lung or pneumothorax. **fetal distress s.** A change in the fetal heart rate, especially a slowing, accompanied by the appearance of meconium in the amniotic fluid. These signs usually indicate fetal anoxia. **fibrosing s.** A hereditary syndrome characterized by an increased tendency to fibrosis, manifested in Peyronie's disease, Dupuytren's contracture, and the tendency to form keloid scars. **Fiessinger-Leroy-Reiter s.** REITER SYNDROME. **Fiessinger-Rendu s.** STEVENS-JOHNSON SYNDROME. **first arch s.** A poorly defined association of developmental defects in the lower face and upper neck regions. It consists mostly of hypoplasia or aplasia of structures derived from the embryonic first branchial arch, which includes the mandible, maxilla, teeth, tongue, and muscles of mastication. **Fisher s.** A type of idiopathic polyneuropathy considered to be a variant of the Guillain-Barré syndrome and characterized by marked bilateral sensory ataxia, bilateral external (and sometimes internal) ophthalmoplegia, abolition of tendon reflexes, and increased levels of protein in the cerebrospinal fluid. The syndrome may be of allergic or postinfectious etiology. The prognosis is favorable, usually with recovery within 7 to 12 weeks, and no aftereffects. Also *Miller Fisher syndrome, ophthalmoplegia-ataxia-areflexia syndrome.* **Fitz s.** See under FITZ LAW. **Fitzgerald-Gardner s.** GARDNER SYNDROME. **Fitz-Hugh and Curtis s.** Acute perihepatitis in women complicating acute salpingitis due to *Neisseria gonorrhoeae* or *Chlamydia trachomatis* infection and characterized by fever, right upper quadrant tenderness and pain, a friction rub over the liver, and elevated hepatic enzymes. Also *Curtis and Fitz-Hugh syndrome.* **fleck s.'s** A group of ocular fundus abnormalities presenting with the appearance of multiple, light-colored spots. These conditions affect the pigment epithelium of the retina. **floppy infant s.** Weakness and hypotonicity in an infant's muscles. The clinical picture may be produced by various diseases with primary lesions in brain, spinal cord, peripheral nerves, neuromuscular functions, or the muscle itself. Most commonly the lesion is in the anterior horn cells (Werdnig-Hoffman disease). Also *hypotonic infant syndrome, limp infant syndrome, infantile hypotonia.* **floppy valve s.** Mitral or aortic regurgitation resulting from myxomatous degeneration of the valve cusps. **Foix-Alajouanine s.** SUBACUTE NECROTIC MYELITIS. **Foix paramedian s.** MEDIAN MEDULLARY SYNDROME. **Forbes-Albright s.** Amenorrhea and nonpuerperal galactorrhea with low levels of gonadotropins, associated with an adenoma of the pituitary gland. **Förster s.** FÖRSTER'S DIPLEGIA. **Förster atonic-astatic s.** FÖRSTER'S DIPLEGIA. **Foster Kennedy s.** Unilateral optic atrophy, with or without anosmia, and contralateral papilledema due to a meningioma of the sphenoidal ridge region or the olfactory groove on the side of the optic atrophy. Also *Kennedy syndrome.* **four-day s.** RESPIRATORY DISTRESS SYNDROME OF NEWBORN. • The affected infant usually dies or recovers within four days. **fourth ventricle s.** A syndrome resulting from tumors in or in close relation to the fourth ventricle, giving rise to occipital headache, morning vomiting (often of projectile type), and postural vertigo, often with neck stiffness and sometimes with papilledema and signs of cranial nerve lesions. **Foville's median s.** FOVILLE'S PEDUNCULAR SYNDROME. **Foville's peduncular s.** A syndrome comprising contralateral hemiplegia and paralysis of conjugate gaze to the opposite side and attributable to damage to the central corticonuclear oculomotor tract, in the posterior region of the tegmentum pedunculi. Also *Foville superior syndrome, Foville's median syndrome.* **Foville superior s.** FOVILLE'S PEDUNCULAR SYNDROME. **fragile X s.** A syndrome, inherited as an X-linked recessive trait, that is characterized by mental retardation, macroorchidism, and mild abnormalities of connective tissue. It is associated with a fragile (marker) site on the distal long arm of the X chromosome at band Xq28, which can be detected when cells are cultured in a medium deficient in folate or thymidine. Heterozygous females are variably, but generally more mildly, affected to a much greater extent than males. Also *marker X syndrome, Martin-Bell syndrome.* **Fraser s.** CRYPTOPHTHALMIA-SYNDACTYLY SYNDROME. **Freeman-Sheldon s.** WHISTLING FACE-WINDMILL VANE HAND SYNDROME. **Frey s.** AURICULOTEMPORAL SYNDROME. **Frey-Baillarger s.** AURICULOTEMPORAL SYNDROME. **Friderichsen-Waterhouse s.** WATERHOUSE-FRIDERICHSEN SYNDROME. **Friedmann s.** BOXERS' ENCEPHALOPATHY. **Friedmann's vasomotor s.** BOXERS' ENCEPHALOPATHY. **Fröhlich s.** Obesity and hypogonadism associated with tumors of the adenohypophysis which impinge on the hypothalamus. It was formerly mistakenly attributed to hypopituitarism. Also *adiposogenital dystrophy, dystrophia adiposogenitalis, adiposis orchica, adiposogenital syndrome* (older term), *Babinski-Fröhlich syndrome, hypophysial syndrome, hypophysis syndrome, Launois-Céret syndrome, Fröhlich's adiposogenital dystrophy.* **Froin s.** The changes in the spinal fluid which result from a complete block in the spinal subarachnoid space. The CSF obtained by lumbar puncture below the block is xanthochromic, has a very high protein content, and often coagulates on standing. Also *Nonne-Froin syndrome, Lépine-Froin syndrome, loculation syndrome, spinal block syndrome.* **Frommel-Chiari s.** CHIARI-FROMMEL SYNDROME. **frontal lobe s.** The clinical manifestations which may result from a lesion of one frontal lobe. A lesion of the motor cortex may give rise to contralateral jacksonian epilepsy and hemiparesis or hemiplegia (the rolandic syndrome). One situated more anteriorly often causes amnesia, apathy, impaired attention and concentration, irritability, inappropriate jocularity, disinhibition, and, if the dominant hemisphere is involved, Broca's aphasia. Deviation of the head and eyes to the opposite side may be seen if the frontal eye field is involved, while frontal lobe ataxia, apraxia, and unilateral anosmia may occur, along with emotional and autonomic disturbances, depending upon the exact site of the lesion. **Fuchs s.** HETEROCHROMIC CYCLITIS. **G s.** A congenital malformation syndrome of hypertelorism, hypospadias, and esophageal abnormality that is inherited as either a sex-influenced autosomal dominant, with males more severely affected, or as an X-linked recessive. It may be related to the BBB syndrome. Also *hypospadias-dysphagia syndrome.* **Gaisböck s.** STRESS ERYTHROCYTOSIS. **galactorrhea-amenorrhea s.** **1** Any condition characterized by inappropriate lactation and amenorrhea, as the Forbes-Albright syndrome when a pituitary tumor is present, or the Chiari-Frommel syndrome, when such a tumor is absent. **2** OVERSUPPRESSION SYNDROME. **Ganser s.** A factitious disorder with psychologic symptoms such as inability to do anything correctly, bizarre behavior that mimics what the subject thinks is characteristic of psychosis, and variable amnesia. Also *nonsense syndrome, syndrome of approximate answers, syndrome of deviously relevant answers, Ganser state, Ganser symptom.* **Gardner s.** A dominantly inherited complex of osteomas, epidermoid cysts, adenomas of the colon, and a 95% chance of development of colonic carcinoma. Also *Fitzgerald-Gardner syndrome.* **Gardner-Diamond s.** AUTOERYTHROCYTE SENSITIZATION SYNDROME. **Gasserian s.** GASSERIAN GANGLION SYNDROME. **Gasserian ganglion s.** Pain and paresthesiae on one side of the face with loss of the corneal reflex on the affected side and hypesthesia and hypalgesia of the affected trigeminal nerve, due to a lesion of the trigeminal sensory (Gasserian) ganglion. Also *Gasserian syndrome.* **gastrojejunal loop obstruction s.** AFFERENT LOOP SYNDROME. **gay bowel s.** An assortment of bowel infections and proctocolonic problems occurring predominantly in sexually active homosexual men as a result of specific sexual practices undertaken with many casual partners. Causative agents include *Neisseria gonorrhoeae*, herpes simplex virus, shigellae, *Entamoeba histolytica*, *Chlamydia trachomatis*, papillomavirus, *Giardia lamblia*, salmonellae, and *Campylobacter* species. A patient may have a number of these infections simultaneously. **Gee-Herter-Heubner s.** INFANTILE CELIAC DISEASE. **Gélineau s.** NARCOLEPSY. **general adaptation s.** The total reactions of the body to stress. **Gerlier s.** **1** VESTIBULAR NEURONITIS. **2** PALLIDAL SYNDROME. **Gerstmann s.** A syndrome characterized by finger agnosia, left-right disorientation, and constructional apraxia, sometimes associated with dysgraphia, dyscalculia, and dyslexia. In some cases there are other associated defects such as aphasia and contralateral homonymous hemianopsia, depending upon the extent of the lesion. In most cases, the lesion responsible is in the dominant parietal lobe in the region of the angular gyrus. Also *Gerstmann-Badal syndrome.* **Gerstmann-Badal s.** GERSTMANN SYNDROME. **Gianotti-Crosti s.** INFANTILE PAPULAR ACRODERMATITIS. **Gilbert s.** A benign form of chronic or recurrent mild jaundice in which there is impaired hepatic clearance of plasma bilirubin and the serum bilirubin is not conjugated with glucuronide. The disorder is often familial and may be of autosomal dominant transmission. Several different etiologies may be responsible, and in many cases mild hemolytic anemia is present. Also *hyperbilirubinemia I, constitutional hyperbilirubinemia, constitutional jaundice, benign familial icterus, Gilbert's disease, familial cholemia, constitutional hepatic dysfunction, hereditary nonhemolytic hyperbilirubinemia.* **Gilbert-Behçet s.** BEHÇET SYNDROME. **Gilles de**

**la Tourette s.** A condition with onset usually in childhood or adolescence and marked by repetitive, violent facial tics and incoordinated, purposeless, voluntary movements. Coprolalia and echolalia occur in more than half the cases. Other frequent manifestations are palilalia, obsessive doubting, and compulsive touching. It is usually of lifelong duration but many cases have responded with some degree of relief to butyrophenones. Many authorities believe that the condition has some affinities with schizophrenia. Also *Tourette syndrome, Tourette's disorder, Tourette's disease, Gilles de la Tourette's disease, maladie des tics, convulsive tic disease.* **Gjessing s.** Episodes of catatonic excitement or stupor associated with nitrogen retention resulting from impaired metabolism of dietary protein. **glioma-polyposis s.** TURCOT SYNDROME. **s. of the globus pallidus** PALLIDAL SYNDROME. **Goldenhar s.** OCULOAURICULOVERTEBRAL DYSPLASIA. **Goldstein s.** ACQUIRED CEREBELLAR SYNDROME. **Goldstein-Reichmann s.** ACQUIRED CEREBELLAR SYNDROME. **Goltz s.** FOCAL DERMAL HYPOPLASIA. **Good s.** IMMUNODEFICIENCY WITH THYMOMA. **Goodman s.** See under ACROCEPHALOPOLYSYNDACTYLY. **Goodpasture s.** Hemorrhage into pulmonary alveoli resulting in pulmonary infiltrates and renal insufficiency associated with rapidly progressive glomerulonephritis, apparently the result of circulating antibodies against the basement membranes of the lungs and glomeruli. Clinical manifestations include hemoptysis, pulmonary infiltrates, iron deficiency anemia, and rapidly progressive renal failure. The condition affects mainly males 20–35 years of age. The prognosis has been poor, but a combination of plasmapheresis and immunotherapy has had promising results. Up to 69 percent of instances follow an influenzalike infection. Immunoglobulin and complement are deposited in a smooth linear pattern along the basement membranes, as demonstrated by immunofluorescent and electron microscopy. Antibody to glomerular basement membrane is found in the serum. Also *lung purpura with nephritis, pulmonary-renal syndrome, antiglomerular basement membrane antibody glomerulonephritis, antiglomerular basement membrane antibody nephritis.* **Gopalan s.** BURNING FEET SYNDROME. **Gordon s.** Hypertension associated with large extracellular fluid volume, low plasma renin and aldosterone levels, and hyperkalemia. Growth retardation and intermittent paralysis are clinical features. All abnormalities are reversed by prolonged sodium restriction. **Gorlin s.** BASAL CELL NEVUS SYNDROME. **Gorlin-Goltz s.** BASAL CELL NEVUS SYNDROME. **Gorlin-Psaume s.** OROFACIODIGITAL SYNDROME I. **Gottron s.** PROGRESSIVE SYMMETRICAL VERRUCOUS ERYTHROKERATODERMA. **Gougerot-Carteaud s.** CONFLUENT AND RETICULATE PAPILLOMATOSIS. **Gowers s.** VASOVAGAL ATTACK. **gracilis s.** Traumatic osteonecrosis of the pubic bone. **Gradenigo s.** A syndrome characterized by otitis media, paralysis of the abducens (sixth cranial) nerve (giving rise to strabismus and diplopia), and unilateral paroxysmal facial pain in the distribution of the trigeminal nerve. The condition is usually the result of inflammatory changes in the apex of the petrous temporal bone (petrous apicitis) consequent on mastoiditis. Also *temporal pyramid apex syndrome, Gradenigo-Lannois syndrome.* **Gradenigo-Lannois s.** GRADENIGO SYNDROME. **gray baby s.** A clinical picture resembling shock occurring particularly in preterm infants who have received chloramphenicol in high dosage. **gray platelet s.** A hereditary disorder, probably autosomal recessive in transmittance, characterized by a bleeding tendency, impaired platelet aggregation, variable thrombocytopenia, and the predominance of giant, pale gray platelets in Wright-stained blood films. The pallor of the platelets is due to absence of $\alpha$ granules. There are concomitant deficiencies of $\alpha$ granule substances (platelet factor 4, platelet-derived growth factor, and $\beta$-thromboglobulin) and also of thrombin and ADP. **gray spinal s.** The presence of abnormal changes in the gray matter of the spinal cord, giving rise to muscle atrophy and widening of the spinal canal with resulting loss of peripheral sensation and vasomotor control. **Greenfield s.** METACHROMATIC LEUKODYSTROPHY. **Greig s.** ORBITAL HYPERTELORISM. **Greither s.** A syndrome of autosomal dominant inheritance that comprises keratoderma of the palms and soles from early childhood and progressively involves the knees, ankles, and elbows. The condition reaches its greatest extent in the fifth decade and then regresses. Poikiloderma of the face and limbs is associated with it. **Grisel-Bourgeois s.** NASOPHARYNGEAL TORTICOLLIS. **Grönblad-Strandberg s.** PSEUDOXANTHOMA ELASTICUM. **Gruber s.** MECKEL SYNDROME. **Guillain-Barré s.** A syndrome of acute onset and often of rapid progression giving rise to muscular weakness beginning often in the proximal limb muscles of both the upper limbs but sometimes producing ascending weakness. Sensory symptoms are common but objective sensory loss, though sometimes severe, is more often slight or even absent. The condition is due to an autoimmune demyelinating neuropathy. The protein content of the cerebrospinal fluid is generally raised and nerve conduction velocity is slowed. The condition may be fatal due to respiratory paralysis or may require assisted respiration, but many cases are less severe. In most cases there is spontaneous improvement after weeks or months, often leading to complete recovery. No single viral or other agent has been implicated. Also *postinfective polyradiculoneuropathy, acute infectious polyneuritis, acute febrile polyneuritis, acute postinfectious polyneuritis, acute febrile polyneuropathy, acute postinfectious polyneuropathy, postinfectious polyneuritis, infectious polyneuritis, acute idiopathic polyneuritis, Guillain-Barré polyneuritis, neuromyelitis hyperalbuminotica, infective neuronitis, radiculoneuritic syndrome, acute plexitis, acute idiopathic polyradiculoneuritis, Barré-Guillain syndrome, Guillain-Barré-Strohl syndrome, Landry-Guillain-Barré syndrome, inflammatory acute polyradiculoneuropathy, acute anterior celluloneuritis.* **Gunn s.** MARCUS GUNN SYNDROME. **gustatory sweating s.** AURICULOTEMPORAL SYNDROME. **gynandrism s.** Any degree of superficial hermaphroditism. *Imprecise.* **gynecomastia-aspermatogenesis s.** *Imprecise* KLINEFELTER SYNDROME. **Haber s.** A syndrome of autosomal dominant inheritance that is characterized by an association of rosacealike eruptions and carcinoma in situ. **Hadfield-Clarke s.** CLARKE-HADFIELD SYNDROME. **Hallermann-Streiff s.** A congenital malformation syndrome that is characterized by proportionate dwarfism, psychomotor retardation, beaked nose, hypoplastic mandible, microcornea, cataracts, and hypotrichosis. The cause is probably genetic, but the condition is not clearly mendelian. Also *mandibulo-oculofacial syndrome.* **Hallervorden-Spatz s.** HALLERVORDEN-SPATZ DISEASE. **Hallgren s.** A syndrome of autosomal recessive inheritance comprising congenital deafness, retinitis pigmentosa, cerebellar ataxia, and mental retardation. **Hallopeau-Siemens s.** EPIDERMOLYSIS BULLOSA DYSTROPHICA (RECESSIVE). **Hamman s.** HAMMAN'S DISEASE. **Hamman-Rich s.** An acute form of diffuse interstitial pulmonary fibrosis. Also *Hamman-Rich disease.* **Hammond s.** *Seldom used* DOUBLE ATHETOSIS. **Hand s.** HAND-SCHÜLLER-CHRISTIAN DISEASE.

**Hand-Schüller-Christian s.** HAND-SCHÜLLER-CHRISTIAN DISEASE. **hand-shoulder s.** REFLEX DYSTROPHY OF THE UPPER EXTREMITY. **Hanhart s.** 1 PITUITARY DWARFISM III. 2 AGLOSSIA-ADACTYLIA SYNDROME. **Hanot s.** PRIMARY BILIARY CIRRHOSIS. **happy-puppet s.** A congenital disorder of unknown cause characterized by severe mental handicap, infantile spasms associated with hypsarrhythmia in the EEG, uncontrolled episodes of laughter, puppetlike ataxic and jerky movements, prognathism, and brachycephaly. **Harada s.** Uveomeningoencephalitis, choroiditis, and retinal detachment, temporary or permanent loss of hearing and visual acuity, and, sometimes, alopecia and depigmentation. Usually seen in the Far East, the syndrome may be of viral origin and may occur as a sequel to a bacterial, viral, parasitic, rickettsial, or mycotic infection. Also *Harada's disease.* **Hare s.** PANCOAST SYNDROME. **harlequin color change s.** See under HARLEQUIN COLOR CHANGE. **Hartnup s.** An autosomal recessive defect in renal and intestinal transport of certain neutral amino acids, including methionine and tryptophan. Clinical features, which are variable and episodic, include light-sensitive dermatosis, cerebellar ataxia, hyperreflexia, emotional lability, and psychosis. **Haven s.** SCALENUS ANTERIOR SYNDROME. **Hawes-Pallister-Landor s.** STRACHAN-SCOTT SYNDROME. **Head-Holmes s.** Unilateral abnormalities of sensation on the side opposite to a thalamic lesion. **heart-hand s.** HOLT-ORAM SYNDROME. **Hedinger s.** CARCINOID SYNDROME. **Heerfordt s.** Uveitis, parotitis, and facial paralysis, all frequently bilateral, and usually accompanied by low-grade fever. It is now known to be a manifestation of sarcoidosis and accompanied in the majority of cases by other evidence of this disease, either past or present, particularly pulmonary lesions and peripheral lymphadenopathy. Also *uveoparotid fever, uveoparotid syndrome, Heerfordt's disease.* **hemiconvulsive-hemiplegic s.** ACUTE INFANTILE HEMIPLEGIA. **hemiparaplegic s.** BROWN-SÉQUARD SYNDROME. **hemisphere s.** Ipsilateral ataxia, past-pointing, and a tendency to deviate to the affected side when walking, resulting from disease of one cerebellar hemisphere. Also *hemispheric syndrome.* **hemolytic uremic s.** Acute renal failure accompanied by hemolytic anemia that is characterized by fragmented erythrocytes and thrombocytopenia. It usually affects infants and young children. Other typical features include fever, hematuria, oliguria, nausea, and vomiting. The disorder may follow acute febrile diarrheal diseases of viral etiology. **hemopleuropneumonic s.** Hemoptysis, breathlessness, fever, and signs of pneumonia and pleural effusion after a penetrating wound of the chest. **hemorrhagic fever s.** DENGUE HEMORRHAGIC SHOCK SYNDROME. **Henoch-Schönlein s.** HENOCH-SCHÖNLEIN PURPURA. **hepatocerebral s.** HEPATIC ENCEPHALOPATHY. **hepatorenal s.** Renal failure secondary to severe liver failure. The renal failure is characterized by corticomedullary shunting of blood flow in the kidney. It carries a grave prognosis. Also *liver-kidney syndrome.* **Herlitz s.** EPIDERMOLYSIS BULLOSA LETALIS. **Hermansky-Pudlak s.** A rare disorder characterized by albinism, hemorrhagic diathesis, prolongation of bleeding time, and unusual phagocytic histiocytes, packed with coarse granules, in bone marrow. The cause is unknown, and the condition is not known to be hereditary. **herniated disk s.** Acute low back pain or, less commonly, cervical pain, with or without sciatica, caused by a herniated nucleus pulposus. **herpes gestationis s.** Fever, malaise, pruritis, and neuralgia in association with bullae and vesicles on the skin during the second half of pregnancy. The condition is uncommon but may recur with subsequent pregnancies. **Hertwig-Magendie s.** SKEW DEVIATION. **H.H.E. s.** ACUTE INFANTILE HEMIPLEGIA. • *H.H.E.* stands for hemiplegia, hemiconvulsions, and epilepsy. **high-pressure neurologic s.** A syndrome occurring in deep-sea divers when the maximum practicable working depth for breathing compressed air is surpassed. It is characterized by muscular tremor, disorientation, and short sleeplike periods with loss of attention. Also *helium shakes* (popular). Abbr. HPNS **Hitzig s.** A syndrome in which involuntary closure of the eye or winking may accompany other voluntary facial movements. It is due to aberrant reinnervation following a facial palsy as a result of misdirection of regenerating nerve fibers. **Hoffmann s.** Muscular hypertrophy, muscle pain and stiffness, and slowness of muscular contraction and relaxation as seen in hypothyroidism. **Hoffmann-Werdnig s.** WERDNIG-HOFFMANN DISEASE. **Holmes-Adie s.** ADIE SYNDROME. **Holt-Oram s.** A congenital disorder, transmitted as an autosomal dominant, in which the features are a hypoplastic thumb and short forearm associated with atrial or ventricular septal defects. Also *atriodigital dysplasia, heart-hand syndrome.* **Hoppe-Goldflam s.** MYASTHENIA GRAVIS. **Horner s.** Miosis, enophthalmos, ptosis, and absence of sweating on the affected side of the face due to a lesion of the ipsilateral cervical sympathetic chain or ganglia. Also *Horner-Bernard syndrome, Bernard syndrome, Bernard-Horner syndrome, Claude Bernard-Horner syndrome.* **Houssay s.** Spontaneous amelioration of diabetes mellitus in patients who incur destructive lesions of the anterior pituitary, as tumor or infarction. The experimental counterpart is the Houssay phenomenon. Also *Houssay-Biasotti syndrome.* **Houssay-Biasotti s.** HOUSSAY SYNDROME. **Hunt s.** RAMSAY HUNT SYNDROME. **Hunter s.** MUCOPOLYSACCHARIDOSIS II. **Hunt striatal s.** JUVENILE PARALYSIS AGITANS. **Hurler s.** MUCOPOLYSACCHARIDOSIS IH. **Hurler-Scheie s.** MUCOPOLYSACCHARIDOSIS IH/S. **Hutchinson s.** HUTCHINSON'S TRIAD. **Hutchinson-Boeck s.** SARCOIDOSIS. **Hutchinson-Gilford s.** PROGERIA. **hyaline membrane s.** RESPIRATORY DISTRESS SYNDROME OF NEWBORN. **hydralazine lupus s.** HYDRALAZINE LUPUS. **17-hydroxylase deficiency s.** A form of congenital adrenocortical hyperplasia, marked by adrenocortical deficiency of the enzyme steroid 17-hydroxylase, which leads to reduced estrogen and androgen secretion with resulting sexual infantilism. The compensatory hypersecretion of corticosterone and deoxycorticosterone causes hypertension and hypokalemic alkalosis. **hyperabduction s.** A neurovascular disturbance marked by blanching and paresthesia in the hand, resulting from stretching of the brachial plexus and occlusion of the subclavian artery when the arm is hyperabducted. **hyperactive child s.** A behavior disorder of children characterized by extreme overactivity, a short attention span, impulsivity, distractibility, irritability, and restlessness. The disorder is ten times more frequent in boys than in girls. The activity of such children is typically characterized by a haphazard or purposeless quality, as in uncontrollable running or climbing, and by rage when restraint is attempted. Night sleep is profound. Neurologic signs are variable and often inconclusive. The disorder is often associated with minimal brain dysfunction. Also *hyperkinetic syndrome.* Abbr. HACS **hypereosinophilic s.** Any of several states characterized by marked increase in blood eosinophils, such as pulmonary infiltrates with eosinophilia, Löffler's endocarditis, or eosinophilic fasciitis. Also *eosinophilic syndrome.* **hypergonadotropic s.** Any hypogonadal syndrome accompanied by excessive pituitary secretion of gonadotropin, with or without abnormality in chromosomal constitution. The term is usually applied to patients having a male phenotype, as in the Klinefelter syndrome. **hyperkinetic s.** HYPERACTIVE CHILD SYNDROME. **hyperkinetic heart s.** A syndrome characterized by high cardiac output of unknown cause. The features are slightly raised systolic and pulse pressures, low systemic vascular resistance and, sometimes, a systolic murmur. **hyperlucent lung s.** A syndrome in which hypoplasia or absence of pulmonary arteries leads to hyperlucent areas in the lung. **hyperophthalmopathic s.** THYROTROPIC EXOPHTHALMOS. **hypersensitive xiphoid s.** Pain elicited on compression of the xiphoid of the sternum, mimicking cardiac or gastric pain. **hypersomnia-bulimia s.** KLEINE-LEVIN SYNDROME. **hypertelorism-hypospadias s.** BBB SYNDROME. **hyperventilation s.** Breathlessness, palpitations, faintness, paresthesiae, and hyperhidrosis due to the progressive hypocapnia produced by hyperventilation that occurs as a reaction to anxiety or fear. **hyperviscosity s.** Lightheadedness, faintness, or other manifestations of central nervous system or cardiac ischemia, including dysarthria and paralysis, retinal venous congestion and hemorrhage, or cardiac failure, consequent to increased blood viscosity resulting from marked hyperglobulinemia or marked erythrocytosis. The condition is most commonly encountered when blood concentration of macroglobulin is markedly increased. **hypoglossia-hypodactyly s.** AGLOSSIA-ADACTYLIA SYNDROME. **hypo-osmolar s.** Weakness, confusion, irritability, and convulsion due to hypo-osmolarity of extracellular fluids. It may be due to administration of greater amounts of solute-free water than can be excreted by the kidneys, or secondary to inappropriate antidiuretic hormone secretion. **hypophysial s.** FRÖHLICH SYNDROME. **hypophysiodiencephalic s.** Any of a variety of syndromes due to disease or dysfunction of the pituitary gland and hypothalamus causing various combinations of endocrine disturbances, obesity, diabetes insipidus, disorders of mood and of sleep, abnormalities of growth, appetite, or temperature regulation, or a variety of autonomic disturbances. Also *tuberohypophysial syndrome, infundibulohypophysial syndrome, hypothalamohypophysial syndrome.* **hypophysis s.** FRÖHLICH SYNDROME. **hypoplastic left heart s.** A group of cardiac malformations unified by hypoplasia of the left ventricle and/or the aortic outflow tract. The outlook is determined largely by the size of the aortic outflow tract. Also *left heart hypoplasia syndrome.* • Although often considered synonymous with hypoplasia of the aortic tract complexes, this is not always the case, since rarely the left ventricle can be hypoplastic in association with a good-sized aorta. **hypospadias-dysphagia s.** G SYNDROME. **hypothalamic s.** Any of various diseases and syndromes attributable to lesions of the hypothalamus and to its efferent pathways variously characterized by sleep disorders, anorexia and cachexia, or excessive appetite, disorders of heat regulation, respiratory and cardiovascular defects, hemopoietic disturbance, major metabolic disorders, such as exophthalmic goiter, diabetes insipidus, or glycosuria, abnormalities of growth and development such as dwarfism, Simmonds disease, macrogenitosomia or adiposogenital syndrome, amenorrhea, abnormalities of sexual function, and disorders of mood, memory and intellect. Also *infundibular syndrome, tuberoinfundibular syndrome, Claude and Lhermitte syndrome.* **hypothalamic chiasmal s.** HYPOTHALAMIC COMMISSURAL SYNDROME. **hypothalamic commissural s.** A syndrome comprising contralateral hemiparesis with loss of sensation in the affected limbs, particularly affecting deep sensitivity, homonymous hemianopia which may regress, choreoathetoid movements, and unilateral cerebellar defects. The lesion responsible is between midbrain and thalamus. *Seldom used.* Also *cerebellothalamic syndrome, retrosubthalamic syndrome, hypothalamic commissural syndrome, hypothalamic decussation syndrome.* **hypothalamohypophysial s.** HYPOPHYSIODIENCEPHALIC SYNDROME. **hypotonic infant s.** FLOPPY INFANT SYNDROME. **iatrogenic Cushing s.** A syndrome resembling that of the Cushing syndrome, occurring in patients who receive large doses of corticosteroids over prolonged periods. It differs from spontaneously occurring Cushing syndrome in being associated with reduced incidences of hypertension and diabetes mellitus, and, in women, of virilism. Also *Cushing syndrome medicamentosus.* **idiopathic Fanconi s. of adults** A recessively inherited disease of middle age due to multiple transport defects in the renal tubules and characterized by proximal renal tubular acidosis, renal glycosuria, hypokalemia due to hyperkaluresis, hyperaminoaciduria, hypochloremia, hyperphosphaturic hypophosphatemia, and proteinuria of the tubular variety. Weakness and osteomalacia may develop. Cirrhosis of the liver is a rare manifestation. **idiopathic respiratory distress s.** RESPIRATORY DISTRESS SYNDROME OF NEWBORN. **iliac compression s.** The symptoms and signs of iliac vein occlusion, characterized by left foot or leg edema, resulting from extrinsic compression of the left common iliac vein by the overlying right common iliac artery. **Imerslund s.** A hereditary disorder of vitamin $B_{12}$ metabolism due to inability of the small intestine to absorb the vitamin $B_{12}$-intrinsic factor complex. Inheritance is autosomal recessive. Features include pallor, glossitis, neuropathy, mental retardation, proteinuria, megaloblastic anemia, and thrombocytopenia. Also *Imerslund-Najman-Gräsbeck syndrome.* **immobilization s.** The effect of physical immobility on an individual, including depression, constipation, osteopenia, and joint contractures. **immunodeficiency s.** Any of various disorders characterized by heightened susceptibility to infection resulting from depressed capacity to respond immunologically. **s. of inappropriate ADH secretion** SCHWARTZ-BARTTER SYNDROME. **infantile cortical hyperostosis s.** INFANTILE HYPEROSTOSIS. **infantile myxedema-muscular hypertrophy s.** DEBRÉ-SEMELAIGNE SYNDROME. **inferior pontine s.** **1** An alternating paralysis in which there is ipsilateral sixth nerve palsy (unilateral internal strabismus) and a contralateral hemiparesis, caused by a lesion that involves the sixth nerve nucleus and the pyramidal tract above its decussation. Also *inferior pontine tegmentum syndrome, Raymond syndrome.* **2** MILLARD-GUBLER SYNDROME. **inferior red nucleus s.** A syndrome attributable to a lesion of the cerebral peduncle, characterized by paralysis of the oculomotor nerve on the same side as the lesion, and by a cerebellar syndrome (asnyergia or intention tremor) on the opposite side. Also *Claude's red nucleus syndrome, Claude syndrome, Claude-Loyez syndrome, rubrospinal cerebellar peduncle syndrome.* **infraclinoid s.** Cavernous sinus syndrome resulting from an infraclinoid aneurysm of the internal carotid artery lying in the cavernous sinus and giving rise to paralysis of the third, fourth, and sixth cranial nerves and to sensory abnormalities in the distribution of the first and second divisions of trigeminus. Also *Jefferson syndrome.* **infundibular s.** HYPOTHALAMIC SYNDROME. **infundibulohypophysial s.** HYPOPHYSIODIENCEPHALIC SYNDROME. **internal capsule s.** The syndrome arising from a lesion of the internal capsule (usually vascular) characterized usually by hemiplegia which is total (affecting the whole of the opposite side of the body) and proportional, the paralysis being equally severe in each segment of the half of the body affected. The hemiplegia is initially flaccid in type, but rapidly becomes spastic. Less often there is also sensory loss in the hemiplegic limbs. The syndrome may result from hemorrhage or from occlusion of deep perforating branches of the middle cerebral artery. **internal carotid artery s.** The neurologic symptom complex attributable to obstruction or stenosis of the internal carotid artery. The consequences of total obstruction are variable, depending on the extent to which collateral circulation in the circle of Willis can compensate. Sometimes slow complete obstruction is asymptomatic, but usually it produces manifestations similar to those of the middle cerebral artery syndrome. Less frequently the opticopyramidal syndrome occurs with other variable manifestations of ischemia of the affected hemisphere, as aphasia, apraxia, or agnosia. **intestinal polyposis–cutaneous pigmentation s.** PEUTZ-JEGHERS SYNDROME. **intrauterine parabiotic s.** PLACENTAL TRANSFUSION SYNDROME. **inversed jaw-winking s.** MARIN AMAT SYNDROME. **irritable bowel s.** A disturbed state of intestinal motility for which no anatomic cause can be found. It has many manifestations including bloating, constipation, and diarrhea. Usually beginning in the first three decades of life, the disorder occurs in intermittent episodes and may be life-long, but not life-shortening. In some individuals attacks seem to be brought on by stress or emotional difficulties. Also *irritable bowel disease, irritable colon, spastic colon, mucous colitis* (outmoded), *spastic colitis* (outmoded), *mucomembranous enteritis* (outmoded), *mucous enteritis* (outmoded). **Irvine s.** Cystoid macular edema following cataract extraction. **Isaacs s.** MYOKYMIA. **Ivemark s.** Agenesis of the spleen associated with cardiovascular malformations and sometimes with situs inversus. Also *Polhemus-Schafer-Ivemark syndrome*. See also ASPLENIA SYNDROME. **Jackson s.** JACKSON'S PARALYSIS. **Jackson-Mackenzie s.** JACKSON'S PARALYSIS. **Jacod s.** PETROSPHENOID SYNDROME. **Jacod-Negri s.** PETROSPHENOID SYNDROME. **Jadassohn-Lewandowsky s.** 1 PACHYONYCHIA CONGENITA. 2 PALMOPLANTAR KERATODERMA. **Jaffe-Lichtenstein s.** See under FIBROUS DYSPLASIA. **jaw-winking s.** MARCUS GUNN SYNDROME. **Jefferson s.** INFRACLINOID SYNDROME. **jejunal s.** *Outmoded* POSTGASTRECTOMY SYNDROME. **Jervell and Lange-Nielsen s.** Congenital sensorineural deafness with ventricular fibrillation causing fainting or even sudden death. The electrocardiogram shows characteristic prolongation of the Q-T interval. Autosomal recessive inheritance is the probable cause. Also *cardioauditory syndrome, surdocardiac syndrome*. **Jeune s.** ASPHYXIATING THORACIC DYSTROPHY. **Job s.** A form of chronic granulomatous disease associated with eczema, staphylococcal abscesses and high IgE levels. Most cases have occurred in red-haired girls. **Jones-Nevin s.** CREUTZFELDT-JAKOB DISEASE. **jugular foramen s.** VERNET'S PARALYSIS. **Kahlbaum s.** CATATONIC STUPOR. **Kahlbaum-Wernicke s.** PRESBYOPHRENIA. **Kallmann s.** The hereditary concurrence of hypogonadotropic hypogonadism in males, associated with hyposmia or anosmia due to agenesis of the olfactory lobes. The endocrine disorder is caused by deficient secretion of hypothalamic gonadotropin-releasing hormone. The female counterpart, inherited as an X-linked recessive trait, is characterized by anosmia, sexual infantilism and amenorrhea with eunuchoid body proportions and normal female karyotype. It does not respond to clomiphine, but ovulation can be induced by exogenous gonadotropins. Also *olfactory genital dysplasia, hypogonadism with anosmia*. **Kanner s.** EARLY INFANTILE AUTISM. **Karroo s.** A febrile illness marked by gastrointestinal symptoms and tender cervical lymphadenopathy, seen in young adults in the Karroo region of South Africa. **Kartagener s.** A hereditary disorder, transmitted as an autosomal recessive, comprising dextrocardia, bronchiectasis, and sinusitis. Also *Kartagener's triad*. **Kasabach-Merritt s.** The association of giant cavernous hemangiomas and features of disseminated intravascular coagulation, i.e., erythrocyte fragmentation, thrombocytopenia, hypofibrinogenemia, and diminished plasma activity of prothrombin, factor V, and factor VIII. **Kast s.** MAFFUCCI SYNDROME. **Katayama s.** An acute, early manifestation of schistosomiasis japonica, marked by fever, bronchial cough, dermatitis, aches, eosinophilia, and other signs or symptoms of allergic toxemia. Also *Katayama disease*. **Kawasaki s.** A severe, exanthematous illness principally affecting children, especially from age 2 months to 9 years. It is characterized by high fever, pharyngitis, stomatitis, strawberry tongue, cervical lymphadenitis, arthralgia, diarrhea and a polymorphic exanthem in which there is induration and edema of the skin, red palms and soles and peeling of finger tips. The disease resembles toxic shock syndrome and may be fatal if the coronary arteries are involved. Complications are myocarditis, lymphocytic meningitis and icterus. Antibiotics are said to be helpful. The cause is unknown. Also *mucocutaneous lymph node syndrome, Kawasaki disease*. **Kearns-Sayre s.** Progressive paralysis of the external ocular muscles with bilateral ptosis, retinal pigmentation, and sometimes cerebellar ataxia due to a mitochondrial myopathy. Often mitochondria in the cerebellum are also abnormal. **Kehrer-Adie s.** ADIE SYNDROME. **Kennedy s.** FOSTER KENNEDY SYNDROME. **Kernohan s.** A hemiparesis, or at least an extensor response, occurring on the same side of the body as that upon which there is a space-occupying lesion of one cerebral hemisphere. The paradoxical sign of pyramidal tract dysfunction on the side of the lesion is due to the fact that the contralateral cerebral peduncle, or crus cerebri, is compressed against the free edge of the tentorium cerebelli. Also *crus phenomenon, crus syndrome, Woltman-Kernohan syndrome, Kernohan-Woltman syndrome*. **Kestenbaum s.** AQUEDUCT OF SYLVIUS SYNDROME. **kidney rejection s.** The development of vascular lesions in a transplanted kidney occurring most frequently within the first three months after transplantation. The syndrome may be acute or chronic. Features of rejection include a fall in urine volume and sodium content, an increase in fibrin degeneration products in the urine, proteinuria, pyrexia, and a rise in serum urea and creatinine. It may be associated with pulmonary complications, such as transplant lung. **Kiloh-Nevin s.** OCULAR MYOPATHY. **Kimmelstiel-Wilson s.** DIABETIC GLOMERULOSCLEROSIS. **Klauder s.** Severe erythema multiforme accompanied by extensive mucosal lesions. **kleeblattschädel deformity s.** A rare congenital malformation of the head marked by a broadening of the face and temporal region and a prominent bulge on the top of the skull in the frontoparietal region. The protrusion on top is separated from the laterally bulging face by a depression that encircles the head, thereby creating a cloverleaf shape to the head. Despite premature stenosis of the sagittal, coronal, and lambdoidal sutures, there may be marked hydrocephaly. Also seen are high arched palate, macrostomia, macroglossia, and rudimentary teeth. Also *cloverleaf skull deformity syndrome*. **Kleine-Levin s.** A syndrome marked by intermittent episodes of prolonged sleep, lasting sometimes for several days, by compulsive polyphagia, and by abnormal behavior during attacks, such as disinhibition, sexual aberrations, confusion, or hallucinations. The onset is in adolescence, more frequently affecting males, and the attacks may be precipitated by stress. The EEG is often abnormal. The prognosis is good, as the attacks generally become progressively less frequent and less severe, but full recovery may take many months. Also *periodic hypersomnia, schlafsucht, hypersomnia-bulimia syndrome, morbid hunger syndrome, periodic somnolence syndrome.* **Klinefelter s.** A syndrome that occurs in human males and is characterized by eunuchoid habitus, gynecomastia, infertility due to aspermatogenesis, small testes, and variable psychopathologic manifestations. Gonadotropin secretion can vary from normal to excessive, and testicular androgen and estrogen secretion is normal or low. The testes show fibrosis or hyalinization of the seminiferous tubules, and the Leydig cells appear normal or clumped. The syndrome is associated with a karyotype that has at least one extra X chromosome, such as XXY and XXXY, and several kinds of mosaicism, such as XXY/XY. The most common pattern is that of 47,XXY, which occurs in one of every 1000 male births. Also *XXY syndrome, gynecomastia-aspermatogenesis syndrome* (imprecise). **Klippel-Feil s.** A congenital failure of segmentation of the cervical vertebrae, causing a webbed, short neck and a low-lying hairline at the back of the neck. It is occasionally accompanied by lesions that affect the brain stem and cerebellum. Also *cervical fusion syndrome, Ostrum-Furst syndrome.* **Klippel-Trenaunay-Weber s.** An extensive capillary nevus of a limb associated with hypertrophy of the limb and phlebectasia. Also *hemangiectatic hypertrophy, angio-osteohypertrophy, congenital dysplastic angiectasia, elephantiasis congenita angiomatosa, Klippel-Trenaunay syndrome.* **Klumpke-Dejerine s.** DEJERINE-KLUMPKE SYNDROME. **Klüver-Bucy s.** An experimental syndrome induced in the rhesus monkey by ablation of the temporal limbic system, resulting in heightened oral and sexual instincts, with sexual hyperexcitability and sometimes either apathy or undue aggressiveness. An analogous syndrome has been described in man after ablation of both anterior temporal lobes or in patients with bilateral atrophy of these lobes. It can give rise to difficulty in recognizing objects by sight and touch, to a childish tendency to place even dangerous objects in the mouth, to disordered sexual behavior, emotional disturbance, and loss of the sense of fear or danger. **knee pain s.** Pain referred to the knee from hip joint disease such as tuberculosis or osteonecrosis. It is seen most often in children. **Köbberling-Dunnigan s.** FAMILIAL LIPODYSTROPHY OF LIMBS AND TRUNK. **Kocher-Debré-Semelaigne s.** DEBRÉ-SEMELAIGNE SYNDROME. **Koerber-Salus-Elschnig s.** AQUEDUCT OF SYLVIUS SYNDROME. **Korsakoff s.** KORSAKOFF PSYCHOSIS. **Kozhevnikov s.** CONTINUOUS PARTIAL EPILEPSY. **Krabbe s.** CONGENITAL GENERALIZED MUSCULAR HYPOPLASIA. **Kugelberg-Welander s.** JUVENILE FAMILIAL MUSCULAR ATROPHY. **Kulenkampff-Tarnow s.** A group of neurologic manifestations, including paroxysmal spastic torticollis, spasms of the tongue and of the pharyngeal muscles, trismus, hypersalivation, dysarthria, a fine generalized tremor, overall hyperreflexia with spasms, stiffness and athetoid movements, bradypnea, tachycardia, and anxiety with agitation. These disorders arise as a complication of treatment with chlorpromazine or other phenothiazine drugs. They may occur during the first few days of treatment, are not dose-dependent, and are usually transient. They are seen particularly in young women. In other cases similar manifestations, usually confined to the lips and tongue, develop after long-continued treatment and may persist even after drug withdrawal. Also *phenothiazine-induced dyskinesia.* **Kunkel s.** Chronic active hepatitis in young women associated with hyperproteinemia, positive antinuclear antibody, amenorrhea, and facial acne. **lacunar s.** LACUNAR STATE. **Lambert-Eaton s.** A paraneoplastic syndrome found in patients with lung cancer, but also in a few patients without evident neoplasia, characterized by muscular weakness, fatigability, and absent tendon reflexes. Also *Eaton-Lambert syndrome, myasthenic syndrome, myasthenic-myopathic syndrome, carcinomatous myasthenia, pseudomyasthenia.* **Landry s.** LANDRY'S PARALYSIS. **Landry-Guillain-Barré s.** GUILLAIN-BARRÉ SYNDROME. **Langer-Giedion s.** TRICHORHINOPHALANGEAL SYNDROME TYPE II. **Larsen s.** A heritable disorder of connective tissue, classified as an osteochondrodysplasia. Of congenital onset, it is characterized by multiple joint dislocations, marked joint laxity, short metacarpals, and abnormal facies. Both autosomal dominant and recessive forms occur. **laryngeal-vertigo s.** COUGH SYNCOPE. **lateral bulbar s.** Any of several syndromes attributable to softening of the lateral retro-olivary areas of the medulla oblongata. The symptoms vary according to the area affected. **lateral cord and associated anterior cornual s.** AMYOTROPHIC LATERAL SCLEROSIS. **lateral medullary s.** WALLENBERG SYNDROME. **lateral pontine s.** A group of neurological disorders attributable to damage to the lateral region of the pons, including transient hemiparesis, contralateral hemianalgesia, the Horner syndrome, pontine hemiplegia, isolated paralysis of the ipsilateral fifth cranial nerve (trismus, abolition of the corneal reflex) or of the eighth cranial nerve, and the Gellé syndrome. **Launois s.** PITUITARY GIGANTISM. **Launois-Cléret s.** FRÖHLICH SYNDROME. **Laurence-Moon s.** A syndrome of mental retardation, pigmentary retinopathy, hypogenitalism, and spastic paraplegia that is heritable as an autosomal recessive trait. **Läwen-Roth s.** Congenital hypothyroidism, or cretinism, with dwarfism and radiologically visible stippling of the osseous epiphyses. Also *osteochondropathia cretinoidea.* **Lawrence s.** ACQUIRED GENERALIZED LIPODYSTROPHY. **Lawrence-Seip s.** SEIP SYNDROME. **left heart hypoplasia s.** HYPOPLASTIC LEFT HEART SYNDROME. **Leitner s.** An atypical form of generalized caseous tuberculosis of the lymphohematopoietic system which affects the patient's entire constitution and is characterized by fever, disseminated soft lymphadenopathy, and hepatosplenomegaly with anemia, leukopenia, thrombocytopenia, and a greatly elevated sedimentation rate. **Lennox-Gastaut s.** Encephalopathy of unknown origin, occurring in children, usually between the ages of two and eight years, and less commonly in adolescents, and usually causing tonic epileptic attacks, atonic epileptic attacks, and atypical absences, slow diffuse spike-wave complexes in the EEG between attacks, and mental retardation and radiologic signs of cerebral atrophy. Also *Lennox syndrome, Gastaut's disease.* **LEOPARD s.** MULTIPLE LENTIGINES SYNDROME. **Lépine-Froin s.** FROIN SYNDROME. **Leriche costoclavicular outlet s.** SCALENUS ANTERIOR SYNDROME. **Leriche s.** A syndrome caused by occlusion of the terminal aorta or the iliac arteries, characterized by hip and thigh claudication, atrophy of gluteal muscles, impotence, and absent or diminished femoral artery pulses. Also *Leriche-Courty syndrome.* **Léri-Weill s.** DYSCHONDROSTEOSIS. **Lermoyez s.** A rare syndrome resembling Menière's disease. Attacks of deafness and tinnitus occur followed by vertigo. The hearing improves with the onset of the vertigo.

**Lesch-Nyhan s.** Choreoathetosis, mental retardation, and self-mutilation in early childhood due to a congenital deficiency of hypoxanthine-guanine phosphoribosyltransferase giving rise to hyperuricemia. Self-destructive behavior may include finger-biting, eye-gouging, and head-banging. The condition is due to an X-linked recessive genetic defect. Also *HGPRTase deficiency.* **Lévy-Roussy s.** ROUSSY-LÉVY SYNDROME. **Libman-Sacks s.** LIBMAN-SACKS ENDOCARDITIS. **Liddle s.** Excessive sodium reabsorption by the distal renal tubules resulting in salt retention, hypertension, and hypokalemia. It is clinically similar to the state of hyperaldosteronism, but differs in that hypoaldosteronism is characteristic. **Lightwood s.** A form of renal dysfunction in infants aged from 3 to 18 months, manifested in failure to thrive, vomiting, and dehydration. The condition was recognized in England in the 1950s but has since disappeared. A hyperchloremic acidosis was present, yet the urine did not become acid. Spontaneous recovery occurred. Ingestion of a toxic substance such as mercury may have been causative. **Lignac-Fanconi s.** CYSTINOSIS. **limp infant s.** FLOPPY INFANT SYNDROME. **liver-kidney s.** HEPATORENAL SYNDROME. **Lloyd s.** See under MULTIPLE ENDOCRINE NEOPLASIA. **Lobstein s.** Osteogenesis imperfecta when associated with blue sclera of the eyes and inherited as an autosomal dominant trait. Also *Eddowes syndrome, Eddowes disease, blue sclera syndrome, Lobstein's disease, Spurway syndrome.* **locked-in s.** A condition in which the subject is conscious and alert but tetraplegic, aphonic, and anarthric so that communication is limited to blinking or voluntary eye movements. It results from bilateral destruction of the medulla oblongata or basis pontis with sparing of the tegmentum, due to infarction or central pontine myelinolysis. **loculation s.** FROIN SYNDROME. **locus niger s.** PARALYSIS AGITANS. **Löffler s.** Evanescent pulmonary infiltrates with fever, cough, dyspnea, and eosinophilia of the peripheral blood. Also *Löffler's eosinophilia, eosinophilic pneumonitis, Löffler's pneumonia, Löffler's disease, pulmonary infiltration with eosinophilia, PIE syndrome.* See also TROPICAL PULMONARY EOSINOPHILIA. **long Q-T s.** An abnormal prolongation of the Q-T interval as recorded on the electrocardiogram. It is associated with syncope and sudden death due to cardiac dysrhythmias and may be caused by drugs, an electrolyte imbalance, or abnormalities of the central nervous system. Two hereditary forms exist. The Jervell and Lange-Nielsen syndrome is the autosomal recessive association of prolonged Q-T with congenital deafness, and the Ward-Romano syndrome is the autosomal dominant form without deafness. **Looser-Milkman s.** MILKMAN SYNDROME. **Lorain-Lévi s.** HYPOPHYSIAL DWARFISM. **Louis-Bar s.** ATAXIA-TELANGIECTASIA. **Lowe s.** OCULOCEREBRORENAL SYNDROME. **Lown-Ganong-Levine s.** SHORT PR SYNDROME. **low salt s.** SALT-DEPLETION SYNDROME. **low sodium s.** SALT-DEPLETION SYNDROME. **Lucey-Driscoll s.** A rare form of neonatal jaundice, the hyperbilirubinemia is thought to be due to a factor present in the maternal circulation which is transmitted to the infant, and which interferes with the normal conjugation of bilirubin. **Luder-Sheldon s.** A variety of the Fanconi syndrome in which defective renal tubular reabsorption of glucose and amino acids, but not of phosphate, is transmitted as an autosomal dominant. Clinically it resembles the Fanconi syndrome with osteomalacia or rickets. **Luft s.** HYPERMETABOLIC MYOPATHY. **lumbago-sciatica s.** A variable symptom complex consisting of pain in the lumbar spine region together with pain radiating down the lower limb due to prolapse of an intervertebral disk. **Lutembacher s.** The combination of atrial septal defect with mitral stenosis. Also *Lutembacher's complex, Lutembacher's disease.* **lymphadenopathy s.** Generalized lymphadenopathy sometimes noted in sexually promiscuous homosexual men and other population groups at high risk for the acquired immune deficiency syndrome (AIDS), in some instances coincidental with evidence of infection with the human immunodeficiency virus (HIV), which was originally called *lymphadenopathy-associated virus* (LAV) by researchers in France. In some but by no means all patients, the condition is one feature of the prodrome of AIDS. **lymphoproliferative s.** LYMPHOPROLIFERATIVE DISEASE. **Mackenzie s.** JACKSON'S PARALYSIS. **Macleod s.** Unilateral radiolucency of a lung or lobe in late measles pneumonitis, with diminished pulmonary vasculature, evidence of poor air exchange between inspiration and expiration, and dilatation of bronchi. Also *Swyer-James-Macleod syndrome, Swyer-James syndrome, unilateral hyperlucent lung syndrome.* **Madelung s.** MADELUNG'S DEFORMITY. **Maffucci s.** A rare, congenital malformation syndrome characterized by hemangiomata in addition to the bony deformities of Ollier's disease. The cause is unknown and inheritance is not mendelian. Also *Kast syndrome.* **malabsorption s.** A syndrome of weight loss, fatigue, diarrhea or fatty stools, and in advanced cases severe cachexia, caused by failure of intestinal absorption of nutrients. It may be the result of pancreatic exocrine failure (as in chronic pancreatitis) or intrinsic small intestinal diseases such as celiac disease, Whipple's disease, or intestinal lymphoma. **male Turner s.** NOONAN SYNDROME. **malignant hyperthermia s.** A genetically heterogeneous group of disorders which share a predisposition to rapid, often fatal, elevations of body temperature during general anesthesia, especially following administration of succinylcholine or halothane. Several of the heritable forms are associated with a chronic myopathy, skeletal anomalies suggestive of the Noonan syndrome, or both. **Mallory-Weiss s.** Hematemesis and melena due to a longitudinal mucosal tear at the gastroesophageal junction, often but not exclusively following severe retching or vomiting. **mandibulo-oculofacial s.** HALLERMANN-STREIFF SYNDROME. **Marchesani s.** WEILL-MARCHESANI SYNDROME. **Marchiafava-Bignami s.** A complication of alcoholism causing extensive demyelination confined to the central region of the corpus callosum, and giving rise to dementia or confusion, often with dysarthria, tremor, ataxia, epileptic attacks, and incontinence. The condition is usually rapidly fatal. It was first noted among wine-drinking Italian males. Vitamin $B_1$ deficiency is probably an important etiological factor, but unidentified toxic factors in the wines themselves probably play a part. Also *central degeneration of the corpus callosum, Marchiafava's disease, generalized alcoholic pseudoparalysis, callosal demyelinating encephalopathy, Marchiafava-Bignami disease.* **Marchiafava-Micheli s.** *Rare* PAROXYSMAL NOCTURNAL HEMOGLOBINURIA. **Marcus Gunn s.** Involuntary and transient unilateral ptosis associated with chewing so that with each chewing movement the subject appears to wink. Also *jaw winking, Gunn's phenomenon, Marcus Gunn phenomenon, jaw-winking phenomenon, Gunn syndrome, jaw-winking syndrome.* **Marcus Gunn inverse s.** MARIN AMAT SYNDROME. **Marden-Walker s.** A rare, autosomal recessive condition that is characterized by kyphoscoliosis, pectus carinatum, congenital joint contractures, blepharophimosis, microphthalmia, cleft palate, micrognathia, mental retardation, and myopathy. **Marfan s.** An autosomal dominant heritable disorder of connective tissue characterized by involvement of the ocular, skeletal, cardiovascular, as well as other systems. Typical features include ectopia lentis, myopia, scoliosis, arachnodactyly, tall stature with disproportionately long extremities, mitral valve prolapse, aortic root dilatation (leading to dissection and regurgitation), pneumothorax, and dural ectasia. The basic biochemical defect is unknown, but many defects of connective tissue undoubtedly produce this phenotype. **Marie s.** *Outmoded* ACROMEGALY. **Marie-Bamberger s.** HYPERTROPHIC PULMONARY OSTEOARTHROPATHY. **Marin Amat s.** Synkinesis between the orbicularis oculi (innervated by the facial nerve) and those muscles which open the mouth (innervated by the motor trigeminal nerve), leading to automatic closing of the eyes whenever the patient opens his mouth. Also *inverted Marcus Gunn phenomenon, inverse Marcus Gunn phenomenon, Marcus Gunn inverse syndrome, Marin Amat phenomenon, inversed jaw-winking syndrome.* **Marinesco-Sjögren s.** A type of inherited spinocerebellar degeneration comprising a cerebellar syndrome, with ataxia, dysarthria, and nystagmus, pyramidal signs, and sometimes signs of cranial nerve dysfunction. Most affected individuals also show early-onset cataract and oligophrenia. Also *Marinesco-Sjögren-Garland syndrome, Marinesco-Garland syndrome.* **marker X s.** FRAGILE X SYNDROME. **Markus-Adie s.** ADIE SYNDROME. **Maroteaux-Lamy s.** MUCOPOLYSACCHARIDOSIS VI. **Marshall s.** A variety of ectodermal dysplasia with congenital myopia and impaired hearing. **Martin-Bell s.** FRAGILE X SYNDROME. **Martorell s.** TAKAYASU'S ARTERITIS. **massive bowel resection s.** SHORT BOWEL SYNDROME. **maternal s.** Polyhydramnios, pruritis, and pedal edema of the mother along with impending fetal death in association with isoimmunization. The affected erythroblastotic fetus or placenta is thought to be responsible for the syndrome. **maternal deprivation s.** A syndrome of children, especially at two to five years of age, consisting of stunting of growth, infantile body proportions, pot belly, cold red hands and feet, thinning of the hair, malnutrition (easily becoming obesity with adequate feeding), an air of dejection, and catatonia. Failure of the infant to grow and thrive results from psychogenic withdrawal of the mother from the child, as from a character disorder. The picture is completely reversed under normal hospital care or care in a foster home, where the child eats voraciously and begins to thrive. If subsequently returned to the family, relapse is invariable. Also *emotional deprivation syndrome.* Abbr. MDS **maternal obesity s.** Excessive gain in weight during pregnancy or in the postpartum period, most frequently seen in association with maternal diabetes mellitus. **McCune-Albright s.** ALBRIGHT'S DISEASE. **Meckel s.** A pleiotropic, variable, autosomal recessive congenital syndrome that is lethal perinatally. Features include encephalocele, meningocele, polydactyly, polycystic kidneys and liver, microcephaly, eye anomalies, and holoprosencephaly. Also *Meckel-Gruber syndrome, Gruber syndrome.* **meconium blockage s.** Intestinal obstruction due to abnormally viscid meconium in individuals with cystic fibrosis. It may present in fetal life, in the neonatal period, or occasionally later. **meconium plug s.** A clinical picture of low intestinal obstruction in the newborn, often in a premature baby, characterized by gradual abdominal distension, anorexia, and vomiting, completely relieved after the passage of a plug of meconium of the consistency of firm putty. **medial longitudinal fasciculus s.** ATAXIC NYSTAGMUS. **median medullary s.** A syndrome resulting from a lesion of the medulla oblongata involving the nucleus of the hypoglossal nerve and the pyramidal tract, causing homolateral lingual paralysis and contralateral hemiplegia. Sometimes the medial lemniscus is also involved, resulting in contralateral reduction in tactile and proprioceptive sensitivity. Also *hemiplegia alternans hypoglossica, crossed hypoglossal paralysis, Dejerine's anterior bulbar syndrome, pyramidal and hypoglossal nerve syndrome, Dejerine's interolivary syndrome, Foix paramedian syndrome, Reynold-Revillod-Dejerine syndrome.* **megacystic s.** A condition characterized by a congenitally large bladder, usually with internally placed ureteral orifices that reflux. **megaureter-megacystis s.** Megacystic syndrome with dilatated ureters. **Meigs s.** Ascites and pleural effusion associated with a fibroma or other tumor of the ovary. **Melkersson-Rosenthal s.** Recurrent attacks of facial paralysis, facial edema, and granulomatous cheilitis, usually beginning in childhood or adolescence and often associated with migraine and ocular manifestations. The latter may include blepharochalasis, corneal opacities, and retrobulbar neuritis. Also *Melkersson syndrome.* **Melnick-Needles s.** A severe hereditary skeletal disorder characterized by flared metaphyses of long bones, S-shaped curvature of the bones of the legs, rib malformations, sclerosis of the base of the skull, and typical facies with exophthalmos, micrognathia, malalignment of teeth, and full cheeks. It is inherited as an autosomal dominant trait. Also *osteodysplasty.* **Mendelson s.** The regurgitation of gastric acid contents and aspiration during general anesthesia, resulting in bronchospasm, atelectasis, edema, and hypoxia. **Mengert shock s.** SUPINE HYPOTENSIVE SYNDROME. **Menière s.** MENIÈRE'S DISEASE. **meningeal s.** A syndrome comprising headache, frequent vomiting (often projectile), neck stiffness, and in severe cases retraction with photophobia. It is most often seen in meningitis and subarachnoid hemorrhage but can result from any process of meningeal irritation or inflammation and can be mimicked by the manifestations of a midline tumor in the posterior fossa. **meningococcic adrenal s.** WATERHOUSE-FRIDERICHSEN SYNDROME. **Menkes s.** A progressive and ultimately fatal X-linked recessive disorder of infancy, characterized by severe growth retardation, white and kinky hair, frequent epileptic seizures, and degeneration of cerebral and cerebellar gray matter. The disorder has been associated with a defect in the ability to absorb copper. Also *Menkes disease, kinky hair disease.* **metastatic carcinoid s.** CARCINOID SYNDROME. **methionine malabsorption s.** OASTHOUSE URINE DISEASE. **Michel s.** CEPHALOPATHIA SPLANCHNOCYSTICA. **middle cerebral artery s.** The neurologic syndrome attributable to obstruction of the middle cerebral (or sylvian) artery by atheroma or by an embolus, giving rise to ischemic infarction of the corresponding cerebral hemisphere. The manifestations, including various forms of aphasia and hemiplegia, and progression of the syndrome depend on the site of the obstruction and the rapidity with which it develops. Also *sylvian artery syndrome, sylvian syndrome.* **middle lobe s.** Persistent collapse of the middle lobe of the lung resulting usually from previous tuberculosis of intrathoracic lymph nodes. Also *Brock syndrome.* **midline s.** A group of manifestations attributable to tumors developing in the median sagittal plane of the posterior fossa (tumors of the cerebellar vermis and fourth ventricle). The principal features include occipital headache, often with neck stiffness, morning vomiting, postural vertigo and nystagmus, and papilledema, but in some cases the head may be held rigidly, or in an abnormal posture, and so-called tonic or cerebellar fits may occur. **Miescher s.** GRANULOMATOUS CHEILITIS. **Mikulicz s.** VON MIKULICZ SYNDROME. **Mikulicz-Radecki s.** VON MIKULICZ SYNDROME. **Mikulicz-**

Sjögren s. VON MIKULICZ SYNDROME. **milk-alkali s.** A syndrome of hypercalcemia and alkalosis attributed to the prolonged ingestion of large amounts of calcium-containing products such as milk or calcium carbonate and alkalis such as sodium bicarbonate, often taken for the relief of pain due to peptic ulcer. The condition may exist in acute, subacute, or chronic form. Features of the syndrome include lethargy, constipation, kidney stones, nephrocalcinosis, and renal insufficiency. Also *Burnett syndrome, milk-alkali disease.* **Milkman s.** Generalized osteoporosis with multiple stress fractures. The condition occurs in middle-aged women. Also *Looser-Milkman syndrome.* **Millard-Gubler s.** A syndrome resulting from a localized unilateral lesion of the anterior part of the pons, in that area where the fibers of the external oculomotor nerve cross the corticospinal (pyramidal) tract, and marked by paralysis of the third nerve and facial paralysis on the side of the lesion, associated with hemiplegia on the opposite side. Also *inferior pontine syndrome, inferior alternate paralysis, Gubler-Millard paralysis, Millard-Gubler paralysis, Gubler's hemiplegia, Gubler's paralysis.* **Miller Fisher s.** FISHER SYNDROME. **minimal brain dysfunction s.** MINIMAL BRAIN DYSFUNCTION. **minimal chronic brain s.** MINIMAL BRAIN DYSFUNCTION. **Minkowski-Chauffard s.** HEREDITARY SPHEROCYTOSIS. **minor contusion s.** POSTCONCUSSIONAL SYNDROME. **Möbius s.** 1 Congenital weakness and hypotrophy, sometimes unilateral but more often bilateral, of various muscles of the head and neck, attributable to agenesis of the motor ganglion cells of certain cranial nerves (oculomotor and external oculomotor, facial, less frequently the hypoglossal, trigeminal, and accessory nerves). The symptoms vary according to the site of the lesion and include, most often, inability to make conjugate lateral eye movements and/or bilateral facial paresis. These neurologic manifestations may be associated with various associated congenital malformations, including hypoplasia of the mandible, microphthalmia, hypoplasia or absence of lacrimal papillae, clubfoot, syndactyly, various types of generalized muscle hypoplasia, etc. It has been shown that so-called myotubular myopathy may give a similar clinical picture. Familial cases have been noted. Also *congenital facial diplegia, nuclear agenesis, congenital oculofacial paralysis, infantile nuclear paralysis* (incorrect), *oculofacial paralysis, congenital abducens-facial paralysis, congenital paralysis of horizontal gaze.* 2 OPHTHALMOPLEGIC MIGRAINE. **Moersch-Woltman s.** STIFF-MAN SYNDROME. **Mohr s.** OROFACIODIGITAL SYNDROME II. **Monakow s.** A syndrome usually including contralateral hemiparesis, hemianesthesia, and hemianopia, and resulting from occlusion of one anterior choroidal artery. Also *retrolenticular capsule syndrome, anterior choroidal artery syndrome.* **Moore s.** ABDOMINAL EPILEPSY. **morbid hunger s.** KLEINE-LEVIN SYNDROME. **Morel s.** HYPEROSTOSIS FRONTALIS INTERNA. **Morel-Wildi s.** A rare form of cerebral malformation marked by the formation of glial nodules on the surface of the frontal cortex. There are no constant clinical manifestations. Also *disseminated nodular dysgenesis of the frontal surface layer.* **Morgagni s.** HYPEROSTOSIS FRONTALIS INTERNA. **Morgagni-Adams-Stokes s.** ADAMS-STOKES SYNDROME. **Morgagni-Stewart-Morel s.** HYPEROSTOSIS FRONTALIS INTERNA. **Morquio s.** MUCOPOLYSACCHARIDOSIS IV. **Morquio-Brailsford s.** MUCOPOLYSACCHARIDOSIS IV. **Morquio-Ullrich s.** MUCOPOLYSACCHARIDOSIS IV. **Morris s.** *Seldom used* TESTICULAR FEMINIZATION **Morton s.** A congenital foreshortening of the first metatarsal ray, which gives rise to pain and deformity of the forefoot. **Morvan s.** A condition resulting in severe trophic disturbances in the fingers, and even leading to mutilation with resorption of bone suggesting that seen in leprosy. It may result from syringomyelia or from hereditary sensory neuropathy or other acrodystrophic neuropathies. Also *painless whitlow, whitlow paresoanesthesia of the upper extremities, Morvan's disease.* **Moschcowitz s.** THROMBOTIC THROMBOCYTOPENIC PURPURA. **motor radicular s.** Any clinical syndrome attributable to damage to the anterior spinal nerve roots, causing paresis or paralysis, followed by atrophy, of the muscles innervated by the damaged nerve roots. **Mount s.** A familial and hereditary condition marked by paroxysmal attacks of choreoathetosis without loss of consciousness, but with associated EEG changes in some cases resembling those of epilepsy. The presence of an atypical Kaiser-Fleischer ring suggests that there may be some connection with hepatolenticular degeneration, but no defects of copper metabolism have been found in such cases. The condition is transmitted as a dominant trait. Also *Mount-Reback syndrome, paroxysmal familial choreoathetosis.* **Mucha-Habermann s.** PITYRIASIS LICHENOIDES. **Muckle-Wells s.** A progressive heredofamilial syndrome with autosomal dominant inheritance, the principle features being recurrent urticaria, progressive sensorineural deafness, bouts of pain in the limbs, and terminal uremia. Also *heredofamilial urticaria.* **mucocutaneous lymph node s.** KAWASAKI SYNDROME. **multiple lentigines s.** An autosomal dominant syndrome whose major features include generalized lentigo, electrocardiographic changes, ocular hypertelorism, pulmonic stenosis, abnormal genitalia, retardation of growth, and deafness. Other features include hypertrophic cardiopathy and mild mental retardation in some cases. Also *cardiomyopathic lentiginosis, LEOPARD syndrome.* **Münchausen s.** A chronic factitious disorder with physical symptoms that are of such degree as to require multiple hospitalizations, even though no organic basis for the symptoms can ever be determined. The major motivation is to assume the role of patient and not, as was formerly assumed, to obtain drugs or avoid police. • Although the term is more correctly spelled Münchhausen, almost all current writers use Münchausen. **Münchmeyer s.** FIBRODYSPLASIA OSSIFICANS PROGRESSIVA. **myasthenic s.** LAMBERT-EATON SYNDROME. **myatonia congenita s.** See under MYATONIA CONGENITA. **myasthenic-myopathic s.** LAMBERT-EATON SYNDROME. **myeloproliferative s.** Any of that group of proliferative disorders of the bone marrow, having in common varying degrees of hyperplasia of erythrocyte, granulocyte, and platelet precursors, often with extramedullary hematopoiesis and splenomegaly. Included are polycythemia vera, agnogenic myeloid metaplasia, essential thrombocythemia, chronic myelocytic leukemia, acute granulocytic leukemia, erythroleukemia, and the pre leukemic syndromes. **myocardial postinfarction s.** POST-MYOCARDIAL INFARCTION SYNDROME. **myokymia-hyperhidrosis s.** Extensive, coarse, benign fasciculation of skeletal muscles associated with anxiety and excessive sweating, particularly of the extremities. **myonephropathic metabolic s.** A constellation of symptoms and signs that is seen following a crush injury or severe muscle ischemia. It is characterized by acidosis, hyperkalemia, and renal failure due to precipitated muscle pigments. **Naffziger s.** SCALENUS ANTERIOR SYNDROME. **Nager s.** NAGER'S ACROFACIAL DYSOSTOSIS. **nail-patella s.** An autosomal dominant condition characterized by nail dysplasia, hypoplastic or absent patellae, iliac horns, limited elbow motion, and nephropathy. The biochemical/developmental defect is unclear, but the genetic locus is on chromosome 9 closely linked to that controlling the ABO blood groups. Also *onycho-osteodysplasia, arthro-osteo-onychodysplasia, hereditary arthrodysplasia, Turner-Kieser syndrome.* **Nelson s.** A condition that occurs following bilateral total adrenalectomy for Cushing's disease, marked by an invasive, rapidly growing, chromophobic but granule-containing and hormone-secreting pituitary adenoma which releases very large quantities of ACTH and melanocyte-stimulating peptides into the blood, resulting in intense brown melanin pigmentation in the skin. **neocerebellar s.** A group of manifestations resulting from lesions of the cerebellar hemispheres, including hypotonia, lateropulsion towards the side of the lesion, motor incoordination, past-pointing, dysmetria, and intention tremor, predominantly involving the arms, but also evident in the legs. These disorders are proportional in intensity to the extent of the lesion or lesions and are more marked when the dentate nuclei are involved. **neonatal thymectomy s.** RUNT DISEASE. **nephrotic s.** Persistent marked proteinuria, which results in hypoalbuminemia, hypercholesterolemia, and edema. It may occur in lipoid nephrosis, focal glomerulosclerosis, membranous glomerulonephritis, lupus nephritis, diabetic glomerulosclerosis, renal amyloidosis, and other glomerular lesions. It may be associated with an increased degree of atherosclerosis due to the hypercholesterolemia and hyperlipidemia. Children with the nephrotic syndrome are more than normally susceptible to bacterial infection. Also *nephrosis.* **nerve compression s.** The successive development of pain, paresthesiae, and weakness, terminating in anesthesia and paralysis in the area supplied by a compressed nerve. **Netherton s.** A complex syndrome of autosomal recessive inheritance that is characterized by ichthyosis linearis circumflexa and trichorrhexis invaginata. Also *erythroderma-atopy-bamboo hair syndrome.* **Neumann s.** PEMPHIGUS VEGETANS. **neuroleptic malignant s.** A group of neurologic complications which may result from the administration of neuroleptic drugs, particularly phenothiazines, reserpine, and butyrophenone, marked especially by hyperpyrexia and extrapyramidal symptoms including rigidity and often involuntary movements, particularly facial dyskinesia. Recovery depends upon discontinuance of the drugs. Continued use can result in permanent impairment of brain function or death. **nevoid basal cell carcinoma s.** BASAL CELL NEVUS SYNDROME. **nevoid basalioma s.** BASAL CELL NEVUS SYNDROME. **Nezelof s.** An autosomal recessive immunodeficiency disorder marked by thymic aplasia, lymphopenia, recurrent pulmonary infections, and severe viral infections due to a lack of T cells. **night-eating s.** An eating disorder in some obese patients characterized by eating binges and insomnia at night and anorexia on waking in the morning. **nitritoid s.** NITRITOID CRISIS. **Noack s.** See under ACROCEPHALOPOLYSYNDACTYLY. **Nonne s.** SCALENUS ANTERIOR SYNDROME. **Nonne-Froin s.** FROIN SYNDROME. **Nonne-Marie s.** MARIE'S HEREDITARY CEREBELLAR ATAXIA. **nonpsychotic organic brain s.** MINIMAL BRAIN DYSFUNCTION. **nonsense s.** GANSER SYNDROME. **Noonan s.** An autosomal dominant condition characterized by moderately short stature, webbed neck, shield chest, cubitus valgus (all features of the Turner syndrome), cryptorchidism, diminished spermatogenesis, deficient Leydig cell function, and typical facies, including ptosis, low-set ears, hypertelorism, and micrognathia. Mild mental retardation and cardiac lesions, particularly pulmonic or right ventricular infundibular stenosis, occur in about half of the cases. Most subjects have a normal sex chromosome pattern, but some show XO or various mosaic constitutions. Although superficially similar to the Turner syndrome, the Noonan syndrome affects males and females equally and females are fertile. Also *pseudo-Turner syndrome, male Turner syndrome, Ullrich syndrome, Ullrich-Turner syndrome.* **Norman-Wood s.** A rare congenital type of generalized gangliosidosis which is rapidly fatal. It is marked by striking microcephaly, widespread degeneration of the cerebral white matter with lipid deposits, fatty infiltration of the liver, spleen, lymph nodes, and adrenal glands, and bilateral atrophy of the optic nerves with almost total absence of retinal vessels. **Nothnagel s.** Unilateral cerebellar ataxia and ipsilateral paralysis of the lateral rectus muscle of the eye, resulting from a lesion of the cerebellar peduncle and adjacent oculomotor nucleus on the side of the symptoms. **s. of the nucleus ambiguus and spinal fillet** AVELLIS PARALYSIS. **ocular-mucous membrane s.** Bullous erythema multiforme with extensive mucosal lesions, as in the Stevens-Johnson syndrome. **oculobuccogenital s.** BEHÇET SYNDROME. **oculocerebrorenal s.** A hereditary X-linked disorder characterized by mental retardation, hypotonia, cataracts, glaucoma, and a variety of biochemical abnormalities, including hyperaminoaciduria, proteinuria, and metabolic acidosis. Defective renal acidification of urine and hypophosphatemia with rickets are common. The condition is most common in males. Death often results from renal failure or infection. Also *Lowe's disease, Lowe syndrome, oculocerebrorenal dystrophy.* **oculocutaneous s.** VOGT-KOYANAGI SYNDROME. **oculodento-osseous s.** OCULODENTODIGITAL DYSPLASIA. **oculoglandular s.** PARINAUD'S CONJUNCTIVITIS. **oculo-otocutaneous s. of Yuge** VOGT-KOYANAGI SYNDROME. **oculopharyngeal s.** Slowly progressive ptosis and dysphagia occurring as an unusual, late-onset manifestation of muscular dystrophy. **oculovertebral s.** OCULOAURICULOVERTEBRAL DYSPLASIA. **oculovestibuloauditory s.** COGAN SYNDROME. **ODD s.** OCULODENTODIGITAL DYSPLASIA. **odor-of-sweaty-feet s.** ISOVALERICACIDEMIA. **Ogilvie s.** Dynamic ileus of the colon, especially the cecum or ascending colon, without colonic obstruction, observed in patients who are debilitated from other illnesses or surgery. Also *false colonic obstruction.* **olfactory groove s.** The syndrome which classically results from a meningioma lying in the olfactory groove beneath the frontal lobe, but which may result from other lesions in this location. Typically there is unilateral anosmia, sometimes optic atrophy if the lesion extends posteriorly to compress the optic nerve, and dementia may result from pressure upon the frontal lobe. The additional development of contralateral papilledema results in the Foster Kennedy syndrome. **OPD s.** OTOPALATODIGITAL SYNDROME. **ophthalmoplegia-ataxia-areflexia s.** FISHER SYNDROME. **Oppenheim s.** MYOTONIA CONGENITA. **opticopyramidal s.** Unilateral blindness with contralateral hemiplegia, attributable to occlusion of the internal carotid artery at a point below the origin of the ophthalmic artery. **orbital apex s.** **1** Combined paralysis of the oculomotor nerve, the ophthalmic branch of the trigeminal nerve, and the optic nerve, giving rise to ophthalmoplegia associated with blindness and corneal analgesia. The closely related superior orbital fissure syndrome of painful ophthalmoplegia gives rise to pain behind the eye, paralysis of the third, fourth, and sixth cranial nerves and similar loss of sensation in the distribution of the ophthalmic division of the fifth, but without blindness. Also *sensorimotor ophthalmoplegia* (seldom used). **2** PETROSPHENOID SYNDROME. **organic brain s.** Any psychiatric syndrome caused by or related to disturbances in brain tissue function. Abnormalities of behavior, feeling, and thinking characterize such syndromes. Also *brain disorder, organic mental disorder, organic psychosis, anergastic reaction, brain syndrome.* **orofaciodigital s.** Either of two syndromes that share congenital abnormalities of the face, mouth, and digits. Also *orodigitofacial dysostosis, dysplasia linguofacialis.* **orofaciodigital s. I** An X-linked dominant syndrome, lethal in males, that is characterized by clefts of the palate and tongue, hyperplastic frenula, broad nasal root, absence of lateral incisors, syndactyly, and variable mental retardation. Also *OFD I, Gorlin-Psaume syndrome, Papillon-Léage and Psaume syndrome.* **orofaciodigital s. II** An autosomal recessive syndrome, seen in both males and females, that is characterized by clefts of the tongue, palate, and lip; absence of the central incisors; polysyndactyly of the halluces; conductive hearing loss; and normal intelligence. Also *OFD II, Mohr syndrome.* **orogenital s.** Glossitis, corneal ulceration, and genital dermatitis, due to nutritional deficiency in Strachan syndrome. **osteomyelofibrotic s.** MYELOFIBROSIS. **Ostrum-Furst s.** KLIPPEL-FEIL SYNDROME. **otopalatodigital s.** An X-linked recessive multiple malformation syndrome defined by cleft palate, conduction deafness, characteristic facies, and widely spaced toes. Also *OPD syndrome.* **outlet s.** THORACIC OUTLET SYNDROME. **ovarian short-stature s.** *Outmoded* TURNER SYNDROME. **oversuppression s.** A condition of unknown cause marked by protracted amenorrhea and sometimes also galactorrhea, persisting long after withdrawal of a course of treatment with anovulatory agents. Also *galactorrhea-amenorrhea syndrome.* **5p⁻ s.** CRI DU CHAT SYNDROME. **Paget-von Schroetter s.** EFFORT THROMBOSIS. **painful bruising s.** AUTOERYTHROCYTE SENSITIZATION SYNDROME. **paleocerebellar s.** The clinical syndrome associated with disease of the paleocerebellum (especially the vermis and roof nuclei): the patient has difficulty in walking, tends to stagger from side to side, and also finds it difficult to stop and to turn, but there are few if any signs of ataxia or incoordination on examining the limbs individually. **paleostriatal s.** 1 PARALYSIS AGITANS. 2 PALLIDAL SYNDROME. **pallidal s.** A group of neurologic disorders attributable to damage to the globus pallidus, giving rise to slowness and reduction in the amplitude of movement, rigidity, rhythmic tremor, facial immobility, walking with short, shuffling steps, a tendency to fall, a monotonous voice, and micrographia. A typical example of a pallidal syndrome is parkinsonism. Recent work suggests that disorders of posture and tone may certainly result from pallidal lesions in animals but many of the other manifestations described are probably due to disease of the substantia nigra or of nigrostriatal pathways. Also *Gerlier syndrome, paleostriatal syndrome, syndrome of the globus pallidus, chorea syndrome.* **Pancoast s.** The Horner syndrome, muscle atrophy, and neuritic pain in the upper extremity due to involvement of the brachial plexus by tumor, especially an apical lung tumor. Also *Hare syndrome, superior sulcus tumor syndrome.* **papillary muscle s.** PAPILLARY MUSCLE DYSFUNCTION. **Papillon-Léage and Psaume s.** OROFACIODIGITAL SYNDROME I. **Papillon-Lefèvre s.** Hyperkeratosis palmaris et plantaris inherited as an autosomal recessive trait. A form of periodontosis of the deciduous and permanent dentition also occurs with this syndrome. **paralysis agitans s.** PARALYSIS AGITANS. **paramedian s.** Any syndrome resulting from brainstem infarction due to occlusion of paramedian branches of the basilar artery. **paramedian pontine s.** A syndrome attributable to a lesion of the lower part of the basis pontis, comprising contralateral hemiplegia and hemihypesthesia, sometimes with ipsilateral atrophy of the tongue. **paratrigeminal s.** RAEDER'S PARATRIGEMINAL SYNDROME. **parietal s.** Any syndrome resulting from a lesion of one parietal lobe. A lesion affecting predominantly the postcentral gyrus results in the Christiansen-Silverstein syndrome. Lesions situated more posteriorly may cause sensory inattention and, in the nondominant hemisphere, disorders of the body image including dressing apraxia and anosognosia (Anton syndrome). Lesions of the dominant parietal lobe may produce dysphasia, dyslexia, apraxia, acalculia, or the features of the Gerstmann syndrome, depending upon their exact location. **Parinaud s.** 1 Paralysis of upward conjugate ocular deviation without paralysis of convergence, due to a lesion of the superior colliculi of the midbrain. Also *Parinaud's ophthalmoplegia.* 2 PARINAUD'S CONJUNCTIVITIS. **Parkinson s.** PARKINSON'S DISEASE. **parkinsonian s.** PARKINSON'S DISEASE. **Parry-Romberg s.** ROMBERG'S PROGRESSIVE FACIAL HEMIATROPHY. **Parsonage-Turner s.** SHOULDER GIRDLE SYNDROME. **Pasini-Pierini s.** IDIOPATHIC ATROPHODERMA OF PASINI AND PIERINI. **Patau s.** TRISOMY 13 SYNDROME. **Paterson s.** PLUMMER-VINSON SYNDROME. **Paterson-Brown Kelly s.** A term preferred in Britain for PLUMMER-VINSON SYNDROME. **Paterson-Kelly s.** A term preferred in Britain for PLUMMER-VINSON SYNDROME. **Paxson s.** Reduced urinary output, the presence of urinary casts and leukocytes, sometimes shock, and a rise in the level of blood urea nitrogen. The syndrome is thought to be secondary to extravasation of blood into retroperitoneal tissue. It is seen only in association with abruptio placentae, a ruptured uterus, or a hemorrhagic twisted ovarian cyst. **peduncular s.** A group of disorders caused by lesions of the cerebral peduncles, which vary according to the region affected, including the Weber syndrome, the locus niger syndrome, the (inferior and superior) red nucleus syndrome, Foville's peduncular syndrome, the hypothalamic chiasmal syndrome, the Parinaud syndrome, or the corpora quadrigemina syndrome. **Pellizzi s.** Macrogenitosomia praecox with signs of internal hydrocephalus and absence of other neurologic symptoms, indicating a tumor of the pineal body. Also *pineal syndrome.* **pelvic congestion s.** CONGESTIVE DYSMENORRHEA. **Pendred s.** FAMILIAL GOITER WITH DEAF-MUTISM. **Penfield s.** DIENCEPHALIC AUTONOMIC EPILEPSY. **penta-X s.** PENTA-X CHROMOSOMAL ABERRATION. **Pepper s.** Large hepatic metastases from a neuroblastoma, typically of the right adrenal. **periodic s.** CYCLICAL VOMITING. **periodic somnolence s.** KLEINE-LEVIN SYNDROME. **persistent müllerian duct s.** A rare disorder of males characterized by cryptorchidism, testicular hypoplasia, normal virilization at puberty, a tendency toward malignant degeneration of the testes, and persistent müllerian duct structures presumably owing to failure of the fetal Sertoli cells to secrete müllerian regression factor. Affected subjects are of normal male genotype and phenotype. **pertussislike s.** A clinical complex resembling pertussis (whooping cough), but not caused by *Bordetella pertussis.* Adenoviruses and *B. parapertussis* have been associated with this syndrome. **petrosphenoid s.** Damage to the second, third, fourth, fifth, and sixth cranial nerves on one side, giving rise to unilateral blindness with total ophthalmoplegia and to hemifacial neuralgia with areas of hypesthesia. It is a sign of a lesion, usually a tumor involving or lying just posterior to the sphenoid bone and in relation to the petrous temporal bone. The tumor may be a meningioma, a nasopharyngeal carcinoma, or a large pituitary neoplasm. Also *petrososphenoid chiasmal syndrome, orbital apex syndrome, Jacod syndrome, Jacod-Negri syndrome.*

**Peutz-Jeghers s.** A familial syndrome of hamartomatous polyps of the small and large intestine and pigmented lesions on the skin and on the lips and buccal mucosa, complicated by intestinal bleeding or intussusception and a small increase in frequency of malignancies of the small and large intestine. It is inherited as an autosomal dominant trait. Also *intestinal polyposis–cutaneous pigmentation syndrome.* **Pfeiffer s.** ACROCEPHALOSYNDACTYLY TYPE IV. **phobic anxiety-depersonalization s.** An anxiety state in which there are specific phobias, often including agoraphobia (along with inability to leave the house alone), and episodes of panic often associated with depersonalization. **Picchini s.** An inflammation or polyserositis of the three serous membranes attached to the diaphragm, caused by a trypanosome. It also may involve the meninges, synovial sheaths, bursae, and testicular tunica vaginalis. **Pick s.** 1 PICK'S DISEASE. 2 AUTOTOPAGNOSIA. **pickwickian s.** CARDIOPULMONARY-OBESITY SYNDROME. **PIE s.** LÖFFLER SYNDROME. **Pierre Robin s.** ROBIN SEQUENCE. **pineal s.** PELLIZZI SYNDROME. **pituitary s.** ACROMEGALY. **placental dysfunction s.** Poor fetal growth and hypoxia of the fetus secondary to degenerative placental changes. Also *yellow vernix syndrome.* **placental hemangioma s.** Placental hemangiomas in association with polyhydramnios and prematurity. An increased association of stillbirth and congenital abnormalities occurs. **placental transfusion s.** Differential growth of twins *in utero* due to vascular interconnections that favor blood flow to one fetus as opposed to the other. The syndrome results in the birth of one plethoric infant and one small, anemic infant. Also *transfusion syndrome, intrauterine parabiotic syndrome.* **Plummer-Vinson s.** A syndrome characterized by difficult swallowing, postcricoid esophageal webs, and, often, spoon-shaped fingernails, occurring predominantly in middle-aged women and believed to be due to chronic iron deficiency anemia. Up to 30 percent of these cases develop postcricoid carcinoma in the course of time. Many other features associated with the syndrome, such as glossitis, angular cheilitis, and certain ocular changes, are probably nonspecific. Vitamin $B_{12}$ malabsorption and pyridoxine deficiency may be important causative factors. Also *Paterson syndrome, Paterson-Kelly syndrome* (British), *Paterson-Brown Kelly syndrome* (British), Vinson syndrome, sideropenic dysphagia, sideropenic syndrome. **plurideficiency s.** KWASHIORKOR. **pluriglandular s.** MULTIPLE ENDOCRINE NEOPLASIA. **Poland s.** POLAND'S ANOMALY. **Polhemus-Schafer-Ivemark s.** IVEMARK SYNDROME. **polycystic ovary s.** STEIN-LEVENTHAL SYNDROME. **polyglandular s.** MULTIPLE ENDOCRINE NEOPLASIA. **poly-X s.** Any of several abnormal phenotypes in human males and females caused by the presence of an excess of X chromosomes. **pontine s.** Any syndrome attributable to damage to the pons, including the Millard-Gubler syndrome, the Foville syndrome (inferior and median), and the superior pontine syndrome, and, less frequently, the lateral and paramedian pontine syndromes. The principal features consist of crossed hemiplegia (complete or partial) combined with signs of cranial nerve dysfunction (oculomotor paralysis) and often cerebellar signs. **pontocerebellar angle s.** CEREBELLOPONTINE ANGLE SYNDROME. **popliteal entrapment s.** Any of several conditions in which, because of congenitally abnormal origins of one or both heads of the gastrocnemius muscle or the popliteus muscle, the popliteal artery may become compressed or even occluded, resulting in symptoms of leg and foot ischemia. **popliteal pterygium s.** An autosomal dominant malformation syndrome of cleft palate with or without cleft lip, lower lip pits, and popliteal pterygium. Also *popliteal web syndrome.* **popliteal web s.** POPLITEAL PTERYGIUM SYNDROME. **postcardiac injury s.** POSTPERICARDIOTOMY SYNDROME. **postcardiotomy s.** POSTPERICARDIOTOMY SYNDROME. **postcholecystectomy s.** Persistence or reappearance of right-sided abdominal pain after cholecystectomy, suggesting that pain leading to cholecystectomy was not due to gallbladder disease. Other causes are retained common duct stone and stenosis of the common bile duct. **postcommissurotomy s.** POSTPERICARDIOTOMY SYNDROME. **postconcussional s.** Recurring headache, dizziness (sometimes true vertigo), irritability, anxiety, excessive fatigue, impairment of memory and concentration, and intolerance of alcohol following minor concussive head injury. There is controversy as to the extent to which this condition is organic, as in post-traumatic encephalopathy, or of emotional origin, especially when financial compensation is involved. Also *minor contusion syndrome.* **posterior cerebral artery s.** Any syndrome caused by ischemia or infarction in the territory supplied by the posterior cerebral artery. The complete syndrome, which is rare, is characterized by contralateral homonymous hemianopia, hemiparesis (sometimes with abnormal movements), hemianesthesia, and sometimes a thalamic syndrome. Where the dominant hemisphere has been damaged, there may be Wernicke's aphasia, alexia, and visual agnosia, while damage to the nondominant hemisphere sometimes gives rise to defects of the body image. Partial syndromes are caused by softening arising from damage to the branches of the posterior cerebral artery and include the thalamic syndrome, the hypothalamic decussation syndrome, and the calcarine artery syndrome. **posterior column s.** The symptoms and signs attributable to a lesion of the posterior column of the spinal cord and comprising paresthesiae, reduction or abolition of deep sensibility, sensory ataxia, and hypotonia. If the lesion is unilateral the symptoms are restricted to the same side. **posterior cord s.** Sensory ataxia with the Romberg sign resulting from any lesion or disease process involving the posterior columns of the spinal cord. **posterior cranial fossa s.** The syndrome resulting from any space-occupying lesion in the posterior fossa. Such lesions, through pressure upon the aqueduct or fourth ventricle, usually produce obstructive hydrocephalus comparatively quickly, thus giving symptoms and signs of increased intracranial pressure (headache, vomiting, and papilledema). If there is descent of the cerebellar tonsils, pain in the neck and occipital region may occur with neck stiffness. The other manifestations depend upon the exact location of the causal lesion and upon the effects which it has on adjacent structures such as the brainstem, cerebellum, or cranial nerves. **posterior inferior cerebellar artery s.** WALLENBERG SYNDROME. **posterior lacterocondylar s.** COLLET-SICARD SYNDROME. **posterolateral s.** Combined spasticity and sensory ataxia resulting from lesions of the lateral and posterior columns of the spinal cord. **postgastrectomy s.** Flushing, sweating, weakness, and abdominal distress after meals, caused by rapid emptying of large volumes of hypertonic fluids into the jejunum, in patients that have undergone gastrectomy. Also *dumping syndrome, jejunal syndrome* (outmoded). **postgonococcal urethritis s.** A recurrence of urethral exudate or pyuria, usually within 20 days after treatment of gonococcal urethritis and in the absence of reinfection. **postinfarction s.** POST-MYOCARDIAL INFARCTION SYNDROME. **postirradiation s.** The dose-dependent constellation of signs and symptoms expressed on well-defined schedules by animals or humans after whole body exposure to ionizing radiation, including hematologic, gastrointestinal, and central nervous system radiation syndromes. **postmaturity s.** The particular manifestations of the appearance of a newborn infant when pregnancy has exceeded the normal 40 weeks. The skin is dry, cracked, and may be stained yellow, and the subcutaneous fat is diminished. Such an appearance has been attributed to placental insufficiency. **post-myocardial infarction s.** A disorder occurring weeks or months after an acute myocardial infarction, characterized by fever, pleurisy, and pneumonia. It is thought to be a form of autoimmune reaction to the necrosis of infarction. Also *Dressler syndrome, myocardial postinfarction syndrome, postinfarction syndrome.* **postpartum panhypopituitary s.** SHEEHAN SYNDROME. **postpartum pituitary necrosis s.** SHEEHAN SYNDROME. **postperfusion s.** POST-TRANSFUSION MONONUCLEOSIS. **postpericardiotomy s.** A syndrome consisting of fever, chest pain, and often pleuritis or pericarditis occurring in patients after cardiac surgery or myocardial injury. Also *postcardiac injury syndrome, postcardiotomy syndrome, postvalvulotomy, postcommissurotomy syndrome.* **postphlebitic s.** Edema, dermatitis, chronic pain, and leg ulceration following deep venous thrombophlebitis. Also *post-thrombotic syndrome.* **post-transfusion s.** POST-TRANSFUSION MONONUCLEOSIS. **post-traumatic s.** POST-TRAUMATIC ENCEPHALOPATHY. **post-traumatic brain s.** Any symptoms or signs of dysfunction of the central nervous system persisting or developing after a head injury. **post-traumatic cervical s.** A symptom complex characterized by pain, muscle spasm and tenderness, headache, paresthesia, and blurred vision. It follows indirect trauma to the neck, such as a whiplash injury. Also *cervical tension syndrome, vertebral cervical strain, vertebral cervical sprain.* **postvalvulotomy s.** POSTPERICARDIOTOMY SYNDROME. **Pötzel s.** A rare neurologic syndrome caused by damage to the fifth occipital gyrus of the dominant hemisphere, particularly by obliterative endarteritis. The main clinical signs are pure alexia of abrupt onset with subsequent literal and verbal alexia, defects of color vision (inability to name colors when seen), and defects of the visual field, particularly contralateral homonymous hemianopsia or tetranopsia. **Prader-Labhart-Willi s.** PRADER-WILLI SYNDROME. **Prader-Willi s.** A syndrome of dwarfism with dysmorphic features. It is characterized by intrauterine and postnatal hypotonia, hyperphagia, mental deficiency, obesity, and hypogonadism sometimes associated with cryptorchidism. The hands and feet are small. It is associated with a high incidence of diabetes mellitus. Also *Prader-Labhart-Willi syndrome.* **preexcitation s.** WOLFF-PARKINSON-WHITE SYNDROME. **prefrontal s.** A group of disorders induced by damage to the prefrontal lobe, consisting of defects of motor coordination, apraxia, mental disorders, (euphoria, disinhibition, inappropriate jocularity, or less often depression), intellectual impairment, memory defects, and inability to concentrate. These disorders are rarely all present together. Some of the features of the prefrontal syndrome have been reproduced experimentally in chimpanzees. • This term is often wrongly used, for it seldom relates to damage which is confined exclusively to the prefrontal lobe. Defects of memory, for instance, are more often associated with temporal lobe lesions. **preinfarction s.** *Outmoded*- UNSTABLE ANGINA. **premature senility s.** See under PROGERIA. **premenstrual tension s.** Edema, headache, fatigue, nausea, and emotional instability in varying combinations occurring in the late secretary phase of the menstrual cycle. Also *premenstrual syndrome.* **prisoner of war s.** Withdrawal, apathy, and sometimes death occurring as a reaction to capture, imprisonment, and hopelessness about reunion with one's loved ones. **pronator s.** The syndrome resulting from compression of the trunk of the median nerve as it passes through the belly of the pronator teres muscle in the region of the elbow. **prune-belly s.** A syndrome consisting of absence or extreme thinning of all or one half of the musculature of the abdomen, the viscera being enclosed by thin fascia and the skin of abdomen as a result wrinkled like the surface of a prune; gross dilatation of the bladder, ureters, and renal calices; and absence or nondescent of the testes. Also *abdominal muscle deficiency syndrome, triad syndrome.* **pseudo-Argyll Robertson s.** ADIE SYNDROME. **pseudoclaudication s.** INTERMITTENT CLAUDICATION OF THE CAUDA EQUINA. **pseudo-Turner s.** NOONAN SYNDROME. **puffy hand s.** Chronic hand edema that is seen in intravenous drug abusers. It results from the destruction of veins and lymphatics in the arm and wrist by impurities in and infection resulting from injected substances. **pulmonary-renal s.** GOODPASTURE SYNDROME. **punch-drunk s.** BOXERS' ENCEPHALOPATHY. **Putnam-Dana s.** SUBACUTE COMBINED DEGENERATION OF THE SPINAL CORD. **Putti s.** An abduction contracture of the shoulder following early childhood splintage in the Duchenne-Erb syndrome. **pyramidal and hypoglossal nerve s.** MEDIAN MEDULLARY SYNDROME. **Quervain s.** DE QUERVAIN SYNDROME. **Racine s.** Swelling of the breasts and salivary glands immediately preceding menstruation. The swelling disappears after menstruation. **radial s.** RADIAL NERVE PARALYSIS. **radial aplasia-thrombocytopenia s.** A congenital disorder of unknown cause in which affected infants are born lacking the radius, usually bilaterally, and with thrombocytopenia. Many patients fail to survive infancy, but in those that do, blood composition often returns to normal. **radiation s.** A syndrome of clinically apparent signs and symptoms after whole-body or large-field exposure to ionizing radiation, usually several hundred rads or more. The most important evidence of this loosely defined syndrome is nausea, vomiting, diarrhea, fever, and increased susceptibility to infection. Lymphopenia, depressed immunoglobulin synthesis, and a maculopapular skin response, which may progress toward acute erythema, are usual. With elevated doses the syndrome may even include central nervous system effects and is rapidly fatal. See also RADIATION SICKNESS. **radicular s.** Any clinical syndrome resulting from damage to spinal motor nerve roots (motor radicular syndrome) or to sensory roots (sensory radicular syndrome). The two are often combined, producing paralysis with hypesthesia and with pain in the territory of the affected roots. **radiculoneuritic s.** GUILLAIN-BARRÉ SYNDROME. **Raeder's paratrigeminal s.** A syndrome consisting of the manifestations of the Horner syndrome but without loss of sweating on the affected side of the face. It results from division of the sympathetic fibers in the coat of the external carotid artery and may thus result from an aneurysm of or injury to the vessel in or near the cavernous sinus. Also *paratrigeminal syndrome, Raeder syndrome, Bonnet sphenoidal foramen syndrome* (seldom used). **Ramsay Hunt s.** **1** Herpes zoster auricularis with the associated infranuclear facial paralysis found to occur in 25% of these cases. In a smaller proportion, auditory symptoms (progressive sensorineural deafness and high-pitched tinnitus) and vertigo also occur. Also *Hunt syndrome.* **2** DYSSYNERGIA CEREBELLARIS MYOCLONICA. **3** JUVENILE PARALYSIS AGITANS. **Raymond s.** **1** INFERIOR PONTINE SYNDROME. **2** SUPERIOR PONTINE SYNDROME. **Ray-**

**mond-Cestan s.** SUPERIOR PONTINE SYNDROME. **Raynaud s.** RAYNAUD'S PHENOMENON. **red diaper s.** The development of red discoloration in a diaper 24 to 36 hours after soiling. The predominant intestinal organism is *Serratia marcescens.* This can be suppressed if a course of a sulfonamide drug is given. **Reifenstein s.** A hereditary condition marked by hypospadias, postpubertal atrophy of the seminiferous tubules, variable eunuchoidism and gynecomastia, low androgen excretion, and normal or elevated gonadotropins. The chromosomal constitution appears to be XY. **Reiter s.** A syndrome of unknown etiology, probably an abnormal host response to infection, characterized by nonspecific urethritis, arthritis, conjunctivitis and uveitis, the presence of the histocompatibility antigen HLA B27, and, sometimes, lesions of the skin and mucous membranes. It occurs most often in sexually active young adults and usually follows either sexually transmitted urethritis or bacterial enterocolitis. The initial episode lasts 2–6 months. Recurrence is common, and nearly half develop some degree of permanent disability. Also *Reiter's disease, Fiessinger-Leroy-Reiter syndrome.* **release s.** DECLAMPING SHOCK. **Rendu-Osler-Weber s.** HEREDITARY HEMORRHAGIC TELANGIECTASIA. **residual ovary s.** A clinical picture of continuing ovarian function after presumed surgical removal. It is usually due to an ovarian remnant from incomplete removal. **respiratory distress s. of newborn** A syndrome occurring mainly in premature infants in whom the alveoli and alveolar ducts are lined by a hyaline membrane, and in whom it is a major cause of mortality. After birth, breathing becomes labored, with indrawing of the ribs and an expiratory moan. There is progressive cyanosis. The lungs on x-ray examination appear mottled or opaque, contrasting with the air-filled bronchial passages (air bronchogram). The lungs on postmortem examination are airless. Treatment is supportive, with oxygen and, in severe cases, mechanical ventilation. Recovery after four days often takes place. Also *idiopathic respiratory distress syndrome, four-day syndrome, hyaline membrane disease, hyaline membrane syndrome, idiopathic respiratory distress of newborn, postnatal asphyxia atelectasis, congenital aspiration pneumonia* (inaccurate and outmoded). **restless legs s.** Discomfort and increasing intolerable restlessness, usually involving the legs bilaterally. The symptoms occur particularly when sitting or when lying in bed at night so that the patient is compelled to get up and to walk to relieve the discomfort. The cause is unknown. Also *Ekbom syndrome, jimmy legs, jitter legs.* **retraction s.** DUANE SYNDROME. **retrolenticular s.** THALAMIC SYNDROME. **retrolenticular capsule s.** MONAKOW SYNDROME. **retrosubthalamic s.** HYPOTHALAMIC COMMISSURAL SYNDROME. **Reye s.** An acute toxic encephalopathy of children and adolescents which follows an upper respiratory tract infection, varicella, or a gastrointestinal illness. It has been epidemiologically associated with influenza B virus, varicella-zoster virus, and, less often, influenza A virus. Annual peak incidence of the syndrome coincides with that of influenza B (winter months), and treatment of the antecedent infection with salicylates may be etiologically contributory. Reye syndrome is characterized by nausea and vomiting, central nervous system manifestations ranging from lethargy and delirium to severe obtundation, seizures, and respiratory arrest, hepatomegaly without jaundice, fatty degeneration of the liver, cerebral edema, hypoglycemia, elevated blood ammonia, and other biochemical abnormalities. Ten to 40 percent of cases are fatal. Also *encephalopathy and fatty degeneration of viscera.* **Reynold-Revillod-Dejerine s.** MEDIAN MEDULLARY SYNDROME. **Rh null s.** The homozygous state of an autosomal recessive genetic disorder that results in failure of erythrocytes to express any Rh antigens. This rare disorder is also characterized by mild hemolysis and the presence of stomatocytes in blood films. **rib-tip s.** Intercostal neuropathy resulting from abnormal mobility of the anterior ends of the lower ribs. **Richards-Rundle s.** A congenital syndrome with recessive inheritance, characterized by mental retardation, ataxia, muscle wasting, sensorineural deafness, and underdevelopment of the secondary sex characteristics. Although progressive in the early years, the disorder may become static later. **Richter s.** The transition from an indolent chronic lymphocytic leukemia to a more rapidly progressive disorder characterized by fever, increasing lymphadenopathy, hepatomegaly, and splenomegaly and the extensive infiltration of lymphatic and hematopoietic tissues with histiocytes. Richter syndrome occurs in about 3% of patients with chronic lymphocytic leukemia, is usually abrupt, and indicates a very poor prognosis. **Rieder s.** A syndrome found among soldiers, stoneworkers, and others who carry loads on their shoulders, such as haversacks or knapsacks, and due to compression of the brachial plexus in the supra- or retroclavicular region. There is sensitivity to pressure over nerve trunks in that region, and sometimes also on the outer aspect of the arm, with hypesthesia and paresthesiae, muscular weakness, and reduction of the tendon reflexes, depending upon which cord or cords of the plexus are most affected. Also *Rieder's paralysis.* **Rieger s.** A fault of mesodermal development of the anterior chamber angle in which pectinate ligaments adhere between cornea and iris. Also *Rieger's anomaly, Rieger's dysgenesis, iridocorneal mesodermal dysgenesis.* **right ovarian vein s.** Thrombosis of the right ovarian vein leading to obstruction of the right ureter. **Riley-Day s.** FAMILIAL DYSAUTONOMIA. **Rochon-Duvigneaud s.** SUPERIOR ORBITAL FISSURE SYNDROME. **Roger s.** *Seldom used* ESOPHAGOSALIVARY REFLEX. **rolandic s.** The clinical syndrome attributable to a lesion of the precentral and postcentral gyri of the rolandic operculum and paracentral lobule and marked by contralateral paralysis of the face and extremities and loss of position and joint sense, tactile discrimination and of other forms of cortical sensation with stereoanesthesia (Verger-Dejerine syndrome). In rare cases there may be impairment of the senses of crude touch, heat, and pain (Dejerine and Mouzon cortical sensory syndrome). The rolandic syndrome often includes also epileptic attacks, generally of the jacksonian type, which may be motor, sensory, or complex in nature. **Romano-Ward s.** The autosomal dominant form of the long Q-T syndrome. It is mostly commonly seen in children and is usually due to torsades de pointes. Also *Ward-Romano syndrome.* **Rosenberg-Chutorian s.** Hereditary polyneuropathy, progressive neural deafness, and bilateral progressive optic atrophy occurring in males as an autosomal sex-linked recessive syndrome. **Rosenthal s.** HEMOPHILIA C. **rotational shift s.** A condition characterized by digestive disorders, sleep anomalies, and fatigue, found to occur among those who must work on rotating shifts. **rotator cuff s.** Shoulder pain and disability elicited by attempting to hold the arm abducted from the body after there has been a tear or rupture of the tendinous cuff (rotator cuff) about the shoulder. **Roth s.** MERALGIA PARESTHETICA. **Rothmund-Thomson s.** A rare syndrome of autosomal recessive inheritance that is characterized by hyperpigmentation, telangiectasia, and atrophy. It is associated with early cataracts, saddle nose, hopogonadism, and bone defects. A mottled pigmentation develops on the cheeks and to a variable extent on the buttocks and limbs. Also *congenital* *poikiloderma, Rothmund syndrome, telangiectasia-pigmentation-cataract syndrome, poikiloderma congenitale of Thomson.* **Rotor s.** Chronic congenital conjugated hyperbilirubinemia similar to the Dubin-Johnson syndrome but without hepatic pigmentation. **Roussy-Dejerine s.** THALAMIC SYNDROME. **Roussy-Lévy s.** A type of hereditary ataxia of autosomal dominant inheritance with early onset in the young child, leading to difficulty in walking, with pes cavus, static tremor of the hands, scoliosis, progressive atrophy of distal limb muscles, and abolition or severe reduction of the tendon reflexes, with impairment of deep sensibility. Hypertrophy of peripheral nerves is rarely evident clinically but may be apparent histologically. The condition is clinically similar to Charcot-Marie-Tooth disease. Also *Roussy-Lévy disease, hereditary areflexic dysstasia, hereditary areflexia with pes cavus and amyotrophy, Lévy-Roussy syndrome.* **RSH s.** SMITH-LEMLI-OPITZ SYNDROME. **rubella s.** See under CONGENITAL RUBELLA SYNDROME. **Rubinstein s.** A congenital malformation syndrome characterized by broad terminal phalanges of the thumb and halluces, abnormal facies, developmental retardation, and cryptorchidism. The inheritance mechanism and cause are unclear. Also *broad thumb-hallux syndrome, Rubinstein-Taybi syndrome.* **rubrospinal cerebellar peduncle s.** INFERIOR RED NUCLEUS SYNDROME. **Rundles-Falls s.** HEREDITARY SIDEROBLASTIC ANEMIA. **runting s.** RUNT DISEASE. **Russell s.** DIENCEPHALIC SYNDROME OF INFANCY. **Sabinas s.** A rare, hereditary syndrome that consists of mental retardation and brittleness of the hair. It is believed by some to be a variant of trichothiodystrophy. **Saethre-Chotzen s.** ACROCEPHALOSYNDACTYLY TYPE III. **sagittal imbalance s.** VERMIS SYNDROME. **Sakati-Nyhan s.** See under ACROCEPHALOPOLYSYNDACTYLY. **salt-depletion s.** Dehydration, weakness, muscle cramps, hypovolemia, orthostatic hypotension, and shock due to loss of salt by vomiting, diarrhea, or renal salt wasting. The last may result from renal disease, adrenal insufficiency, acidosis, or osmotic diuresis as in diabetes mellitus. Salt depletion and hypovolemia lead to decreased glomerular filtration rate and azotemia. Also *low sodium syndrome, low salt syndrome, Thorn syndrome* (rare). **Sanfilippo s.** MUCOPOLYSACCHARIDOSIS III. **scalded skin s.** TOXIC EPIDERMAL NECROLYSIS. **scalenus anterior s.** A syndrome caused by compression of the subclavicular neurovascular bundle, between the scalenus anterior muscle and the first rib. There is spontaneous pain down the inner aspect of the arm, especially on pressure over the brachial plexus behind the clavicle, signs of root lesions (eighth cervical and first dorsal) and sometimes sweating and pallor of the hand with reduction of the radial pulse and edema of the forearm if the subclavian artery is compressed. In clinical practice the syndrome cannot be distinguished from that caused by a cervical rib or by a fibrous band attached to the transverse processes of the seventh cervical vertebra. In rare cases, an aneurysm of the subclavian artery may form distal to the point of compression and may be felt as a pulsatile swelling. Also *cervical rib syndrome, Naffziger syndrome, Leriche costoclavicular outlet syndrome, Coote syndrome, Coote-Hunauld syndrome, Haven syndrome, Nonne syndrome, Adson syndrome, scalenus syndrome, scalenus anticus syndrome.* **scapulocostal s.** Pain about the shoulder girdle, with variable radiation into the neck, chest, and arm, as a result of a long-standing abnormal position of the scapula on the chest wall. **Schafer s.** PACHYONYCHIA CONGENITA. **Schaumann s.** SARCOIDOSIS. **Scheie s.** MUCOPOLYSACCHARIDOSIS IS. **Schilder s.** SCHILDER'S DISEASE. **Schmid-Fraccaro s.** CAT EYE SYNDROME. **Schönlein-Henoch s.** HENOCH-SCHÖNLEIN PURPURA. **Schüller s.** HAND-SCHÜLLER-CHRISTIAN DISEASE. **Schüller-Christian s.** HAND-SCHÜLLER-CHRISTIAN DISEASE. **Schultz s.** AGRANULOCYTOSIS. **Schwachman s.** A hereditary disorder of autosomal recessive transmittance characterized by neutropenia, pancreatic insufficiency, normal sweat sodium concentration, bone marrow hypoplasia, increase in hemoglobin F concentration, and growth retardation. Anemia, thrombocytopenia, hypogammaglobulinemia, and galactosuria may also be observed in this syndrome. The disorder is distinguished from cystic fibrosis, which it resembles, by normal sweat sodium concentration and absence of pulmonary disease. Also *Schwachman-Diamond syndrome.* **Schwartz-Bartter s.** Hyponatremia, hypotonicity of plasma and other extracellular fluids, absence of dehydration, continued renal excretion of sodium, and urinary sodium concentration excessive in relation to the tonicity of the plasma. The assumed mechanism is inappropriate secretion of vasopressin. Renal and adrenocortical function are normal. The syndrome is found in association with diseases of the central nervous system and of the lung, and in certain tumors, especially oat cell carcinoma of the bronchus. Mild forms occur in Addison's disease, hypothyroidism, hepatic cirrhosis, and hypopituitarism. Also *Bartter-Schwartz syndrome, syndrome of inappropriate ADH secretion, SIADH.* **Schwartz-Jampel s.** CHONDRODYSTROPHIC MYOTONIA. **scimitar s.** A congenital disorder in which the right lower pulmonary vein drains into the inferior vena cava. It is usually associated with hypoplasia of the right lung. The abnormal vein produces a shadow on the chest x ray that suggests a scimitar. **s. of sea-blue histiocyte** A rare syndrome that is characterized by the infiltration of marrow with histiocytes containing sea-blue cytoplasmic granules. Splenomegaly and hepatic fibrosis may also occur. The storage granules can be shown to contain ceroid. The condition is often familial but is occasionally associated with chronic granulomatous, myeloproliferative, or lipid storage diseases. Also *ceroid storage disease.* **Seabright-bantam s.** Any condition marked by failure of an end organ to respond normally to a hormone, as in pseudohypoparathyroidism. • The name is derived from the *Seabright-bantam* rooster, which has tail feathers that are female in character because they do not respond to androgen. **Seckel s.** An autosomal recessive disorder characterized by intrauterine growth retardation, proportionate dwarfism, microcephaly, a prominent beaklike nose, and moderate mental retardation. Also *nanocephaly* (inexact and outmoded). **Seip s.** A syndrome characterized by virtual absence of visible adipose tissue from birth, inherited as an autosomal recessive trait. Associated features are hepatomegaly, macrogenitosomia, hypertrichosis, and acanthosis nigricans. Insulin resistance with hyperinsulinism is almost universal, and diabetes mellitus develops at puberty. Hypertriglyceridemia is common. The pneumoencephalogram may show enlarged ventricles. The basic defect is unknown, although it has been postulated to be a hypothalamic dysfunction. Also *Berardinelli syndrome, Berardinelli-Seip syndrome, total lipodystrophy and acromegaloid gigantism, congenital lipodystrophy, familial generalized lipodystrophy, generalized lipodystrophy, congenital lipoatrophic diabetes, Lawrence-Seip syndrome, Seip-Lawrence syndrome.* **Seitelberger s.** INFANTILE NEUROAXONAL DYSTROPHY. **Senear-Usher s.** PEMPHIGUS ERYTHEMATOSUS. **Sertoli-cell-only s.** A rare disorder of spermatogenesis, marked by testes of normal consistency and near-normal size, azoospermia, normal androgen production and masculinization, above-normal assay of follicle stimulating hormone with normal values for luteinizing hormone, virtual absence of germinal epithelium on testicular biopsy, and usually normal (XY) chromosome constitution. Sterility is permanent and androgen replacement therapy is not effective. Also *del Castillo syndrome, germinal cell aplasia, testicular dysgenesis syndrome.* **Sézary s.** A syndrome marked by diffuse erythroderma, lymphadenopathy, and atypical T lymphocytes (Sézary cells) with convoluted nuclei occurring in the circulating blood. The lesions represent a malignant proliferation of T lymphocytes which is believed to be caused by a retrovirus (human lymphotrophic retrovirus-1 or human T cell leukemia virus type 1, HTLV-1). Also *Sézary disease, Sézary reticulosis syndrome, cutaneous T cell lymphoma.* **Sheehan s.** A syndrome due to anterior pituitary failure and associated with postpartum pituitary necrosis following an obstetric accident such as hemorrhage or placenta previa. Lactation fails, pubic hair does not grow back, and the patient remains amenorrheic, becoming progressively lethargic, often with predominance of hypothyroid symptoms and a propensity to become severely hypoglycemic. Endocrine assays demonstrate a variable combination of low gonadal, thyroid, and adrenocortical hormones, with concomitant findings of loss of the corresponding pituitary tropic hormones, ranging from mild deficiency to panhypopituitarism. Cachexia is not typical. Also *postpartum pituitary necrosis syndrome, postpartum hemorrhagic hypopituitarism, postpartum panhypopituitary syndrome.* **Shone s.** SHONE'S ANOMALY. **short bowel s.** A syndrome of diarrhea, malabsorption, and malnutrition resulting from massive small bowel resection, usually for ischemic or inflammatory small bowel disease. The clinical syndrome depends in part on the total length of intestine resected, and in part on which functional regions are lost. Also *massive bowel resection syndrome.* **short PR s.** A form of ventricular preexcitation in which the P-R interval is less than 0.12 second while the QRS complex is usually normal. It differs from the Wolff-Parkinson-White pattern in not having a delta wave on the upstroke of a broad QRS complex, but is similarly associated with supraventricular tachycardia. Also *Lown-Ganong-Levine syndrome.* **shoulder girdle s.** A syndrome typically affecting men 20–40 years of age and characterized by intense pain of abrupt onset in the shoulder, severe for a few days but often persisting for a few weeks, followed by variable flaccid paralysis and atrophy of certain muscles of the shoulder girdle. The condition is generally unilateral, and sometimes only the deltoid or serratus anterior are involved, but weakness may be much more extensive. There may be sensory loss in the area supplied by the axillary nerve. The syndrome also occurs in women, especially in pregnancy. Recovery usually takes place within 6 months to 2 years, but occasionally paralysis is permanent. The condition resembles serum neuropathy. A viral etiology has been postulated, but it is thought more probably to be an allergic neuropathy of the brachial plexus. Also *neuralgic amyotrophy, Parsonage-Turner syndrome, Parsonage and Turner amyotrophic neuralgia, shoulder girdle neuritis, brachial neuritis, paralytic brachial neuritis.* **shoulder-hand s.** REFLEX DYSTROPHY OF THE UPPER EXTREMITY. **shoulder-neck s.** Pain and spasm in the cervical region associated with reduced range of movement in the shoulder. Also *shoulder pain syndrome.* **Shy-Drager s.** A syndrome characterized by orthostatic hypotension and by neurologic signs and symptoms attributable to widespread degenerative lesions of the central and autonomic nervous system. In its complete form the syndrome also includes double incontinence, impotence, anhidrosis, paralysis of the extrinsic ocular muscles, parkinsonian rigidity with tremor, incoordination suggesting cerebellar ataxia, and distal muscular atrophy with electromyographic evidence of neurogenic atrophy resulting from degeneration of anterior horn cells. The onset is between the fifth and sixth decades, and is often insidious, with dizzy spells, fainting, urinary disorders and loss of libido. Dementia is rare. Also *progressive multisystem degeneration, multisystem degeneration, chronic orthostatic hypotension, striatonigral degeneration.* **Sicard s.** COLLET-SICARD SYNDROME. **Sicard's posterior condylar s.** COLLET-SICARD SYNDROME. **sick sinus s.** A disorder in which there is an abnormality of sinuatrial node function leading to sinus bradycardia and sinus arrest or block; often associated with disorders of the atrioventricular node and with atrial arrhythmias, including atrial tachycardia, atrial flutter, and atrial fibrillation. **Sidbury s.** ISOVALERICACIDEMIA. **sideropenic s.** PLUMMER-VINSON SYNDROME. **Silver-Russell s.** Intrauterine growth retardation, short stature, triangular facies, short incurved little finger, single transverse palmar creases, a greater than normal frequency of genitourinary abnormalities, asymmetrical length of the limbs and delayed osseous development, incongruously associated with sexual precocity. Its etiology is unknown. The condition is closely associated with that of a Russell dwarf. **Silverskiöld s.** A variant of the mucopolysaccharidosis IV that is of autosomal dominant inheritance and is characterized by skeletal changes that affect mainly the limbs. **Simmonds s.** Severe panhypopituitarism in the absence of pituitary tumor and not a sequel of childbirth. **Sipple s.** The familial form of multiple endocrine neoplasia Type II, marked by the concurrence of medullary carcinoma of the thyroid with amyloid stroma, pheochromocytoma which is often bilateral but usually not malignant, and the occasional coexistence of parathyroid adenomas and neurofibromas. See also MULTIPLE ENDOCRINE NEOPLASIA. **Sjögren-Larsson s.** A progressive degenerative disease transmitted as a recessive autosomal trait and marked by oligophrenia, a spastic paraparesis and generalized congenital ichthyosis. In certain cases there is also macular retinal degeneration with reduced visual acuity. Also *ichthyosiform erythroderma, congenital ichthyosiform erythroderma, erythroderma ichthyosiforme congenitum.* **SLE-like s.** A condition resembling systemic lupus erythematosus, but due to a definable cause, such as virus infection or administration of a drug. **Sluder s.** SPHENOPALATINE NEURALGIA. **Sly s.** MUCOPOLYSACCHARIDOSIS VII. **small meal s.** In chronic intestinal ischemia, the symptom of severe postprandial pain that causes the subject to avoid eating. It is often accompanied by profound weight loss. **Smith-Lemli-Opitz s.** An autosomal recessive malformation syndrome characterized by small birth weight, moderate mental retardation, ptosis, anteverted nostrils, syndactyly, and male genital anomalies. Also *RSH syndrome.* **social breakdown s.** A deterioration in social abilities and interpersonal relationships occurring in psychiatric patients whose environment does not give them adequate support or otherwise fails to stimulate them toward socialization. **Sotos s.** A syndrome characterized by abnormally rapid growth of the skull and brain with early ossification resulting in dolichocephaly, macrocrania, hypertelorism, and a pointed palate. Somatic growth is also excessive, so that the birthweight may be more than 5 kg and the length more than 63 cm. Many patients have convulsions and all are mentally retarded. Pneumoencephalography shows dilatation of the cerebral ventricles, without any sign of obstruction to cerebrospinal fluid circulation. The etiology of this syndrome has not yet been elucidated. Also *cerebral gigantism.* **space adaptation s.** The symptoms, similar to motion sickness, experienced by astronauts during their first days in orbit and before adaptation to weightlessness is established. This adaptation is considered to be of the same kind as that which occurs after irreversible labyrinthine injury in otherwise healthy subjects. **Spens s.** ADAMS-STOKES SYNDROME. **spherophakia-brachymorphia s.** WEILL-MARCHESANI SYNDROME. **Spiller s.** SUBACUTE NECROTIC MYELITIS. **spinal block s.** FROIN SYNDROME. **splenic flexure s.** A syndrome of recurrent left upper quadrant abdominal pain and constipation, in patients with functional bowel disease. Also *Payr's disease.* **Spurway s.** LOBSTEIN SYNDROME. **stagnant loop s.** BLIND LOOP SYNDROME. **static cerebellar s.** The signs associated with damage to the roof nuclei, and other central cerebellar structures. The patient may sway when standing, staggers or walks on a broad base when walking and has difficulty in stopping or in turning (truncal ataxia). The signs of cerebellar ataxia in the limbs are absent. **Steele-Richardson-Olszewski s.** PROGRESSIVE SUPRANUCLEAR PALSY. **Stein-Leventhal s.** A complex of sterility, amenorrhea, obesity, and hirsutism with increased androgen secretion beginning in girls at or after puberty. The ovaries are large, pale, and polycystic, with thick, fibrous capsules. The cause is not known. Also *polycystic ovary syndrome.* **steroid withdrawal s.** A symptom complex encountered when a protracted course of corticosteroid therapy is stopped or sharply reduced. It is marked by weakness, fatigue, aching muscles, depression, and, rarely, signs resembling those of adrenal crisis precipitated by the occurrence of other illness or by surgery. The causative factors include recrudescence of the disease that had been treated with steroids, drug dependence upon steroids, and suppresion by the exogenous steroid of the hypothalamic-pituitary-adrenocortical system. **Stevens-Johnson s.** A severe form of erythema multiforme with marked constitutional symptoms. Numerous organs are involved, especially the oral and anogenital mucous membranes, conjunctiva, and more rarely the lungs. Its cause is thought to be allergic. Also *Stevens-Johnson disease, ectodermosis erosiva pluriorificialis, erythema multiforme bullosum, Fiessinger-Rendu syndrome.* **Stewart-Morel s.** HYPEROSTOSIS FRONTALIS INTERNA. **Stewart-Treves s.** A lymphangiosarcoma of a chronically swollen arm after a radical mastectomy and lymph node excision. **Stickler s.** A disorder of connective tissue that is heritable as an autosomal dominant trait and characterized by hyperextensibility of large joints, a tendency to develop degenerative arthritis, cleft palate, myopia, spontaneous retinal detachment, and radiographic evidence of mild epiphyseal dysplasia. Also *arthro-ophthalmopathy.* **stiff-man s.** Generalized progressive muscular hypertonia, which may or may not be painful, chiefly involving the trunk and the proximal muscles of the limbs, and associated with paroxysmal attacks of tetanoid spasms sometimes triggered by cold or noise. This syndrome may appear at any age and sometimes progresses to a fatal conclusion. The condition has been attributed to dysfunction of spinal cord interneurons and may respond to treatment with diazepam. Also *Moersch-Woltman syndrome, contracture syndrome.* **Still-Chauffard s.** CHAUFFARD SYNDROME. **Stilling s.** DUANE SYNDROME. **Stilling-Turk-Duane s.** DUANE SYNDROME. **stippled epiphyses s.** CHONDRODYSPLASIA PUNCTATA. **Stokes s.** ADAMS-STOKES SYNDROME. **Stokes-Adams s.** ADAMS-STOKES SYNDROME. **Strachan-Scott s.** An ill-defined form of nutritional neuropathy of undetermined etiology occurring in association with chronic liver disease or nontropical sprue, and, in rare cases, among alcoholic subjects. It causes optic atrophy and sensory ataxia with degeneration of sensory neurons and posterior root ganglia with ascending demyelination of the posterior columns of the spinal cord. *Imprecise.* Also *Strachan's disease, Hawes-Pallister-Landor syndrome, Strachan syndrome.* **straight-back s.** A disorder characterized by an abnormally straight thoracic spine, with loss of the usual anterior concavity. The associated narrow anteroposterior diameter of the thorax causes displacement of the heart to the left, possibly with some compression. **striatal s.** Any syndrome in which there is disease of or damage to the corpus striatum. **striocortical s.** CREUTZFELDT-JAKOB DISEASE. **striopallidal s.** Any syndrome in which there is disease of or damage to both the corpus striatum (lenticular and caudate nuclei) and the globus pallidus. The many causes include hepatolenticular degeneration and pseudobulbar palsy due to multiple lacunar infarcts. **Strudwick s.** SPONDYLOMETAEPIPHYSEAL DYSPLASIA. **Stuart-Bras s.** Hepatic vein occlusion seen in children in India. **Sturge-Weber s.** The association of a port-wine nevus on one side of the face, buphthalmos, glaucoma, and ipsilateral encephalomeningeal angiomatosis, the latter often causing seizures and contralateral hemiplegia. Skull radiographs show a characteristic subcortical calcification outlining the gyri of the posterior cerebral hemisphere. Its etiology is uncertain. Also *Sturge-Weber disease, Kalisher's disease, Sturge's disease, Dimitri's disease, Sturge-Weber-Dimitri disease, Weber-Dimitri disease, encephalofacial angiomatosis, oculoencephalic angiomatosis, Sturge-Weber encephalotrigeminal angiomatosis, nevoid amentia, Sturge syndrome, Sturge-Kalischer-Weber syndrome, Weber's disease, cephalotrigeminal angiomatosis, encephalotrigeminal angiomatosis, Brushfield-Wyatt syndrome* (outmoded), *Brushfield-Wyatt disease* (rare), *cephalo-oculocutaneous telangiectasia.* **subclavian steal s.** Cerebrovascular insufficiency as a result of subclavian steal, which arises when occlusive disease of the proximal part of the subclavian artery leads to diversion of blood from the brain to the distal subclavian artery during arm exercise. **subcoracoid-pectoralis minor s.** THORACIC OUTLET SYNDROME. **substantia nigra s.** An extrapyramidal neurologic syndrome, with features of parkinsonism, occurring on the side of the body opposite to a lesion of the substantia nigra. **subthalamic s.** HEMIBALLISMUS. **sudden infant death s.** The sudden and unexpected death of an infant aged up to 2 years, most commonly between 8 and 16 weeks and usually during sleep, when no significant pathologic changes can be found at autopsy and the mechanism of death is obscure. Preceding signs, if any, are trivial or their potential seriousness is not appreciated. In many cases, autopsies do, however, reveal evidence of chronic illness or a combination of abnormalities leading to death. It is unlikely that any one single agent is responsible. A very small proportion of sudden infant deaths are due to child abuse. Some of the possible final mechanisms of death include sleep apnea, nasal or lower airways obstruction, cardiac arrest, and laryngeal abnormality. Devices to detect apnea during sleep (apnea monitors) and to alert attendants or parents are sometimes used, especially when a previous infant has died from this disorder. Also *crib death, cot death* (British usage). Abbr. SIDS **Sudeck-Leriche s.** POST-TRAUMATIC OSTEOPOROSIS. **superior caval s.** SUPERIOR VENA CAVA SYNDROME. **superior cerebellar artery s.** A syndrome attributable to softening in the territory of the superior cerebellar artery, causing ipsilateral cerebellar ataxia and involuntary movements and sometimes contralateral hemianalgesia. Signs of pyramidal tract dysfunction and cranial nerve palsies are absent. **superior mesenteric artery s.** Obstruction of the third portion of the duodenum by the superior mesenteric artery where the duodenum passes through the angle formed by the aorta and that artery. The syndrome may be acute or chronic and is characterized by epigastric pain, distention, and vomiting. Also *angiomesenteric ileus.* **superior midbrain s.** WEBER SYNDROME **superior oblique tendon sheath s.** A developmental fibrosis of the sheath of the superior oblique tendon, between the trochlea and the insertion of the tendon upon the sclera, resulting in inability to move the eye up and in. Also *Brown sheath syndrome.* **superior orbital fissure s.** Paralysis of the oculomotor nerves (third, fourth, and sixth cranial nerves) and of the ophthalmic branch of the fifth cranial nerve, giving rise to total ophthalmoplegia with ptosis and mydriasis, and anesthesia of the eyeball (abolition of the corneal reflex) and of the upper eyelid, sometimes with paresis or paralysis of the nasal, frontal, and lacrimal nerves but without damage to the optic nerve. This syndrome may be attributable to inflammation, to injury, or to tumor involving the sphenoid bone or sphenoid sinus. A similar syndrome (Tolosa-Hunt syndrome) occasionally results from a granulomatous process in, or thrombosis of, the cavernous sinus or from an aneurysm of the carotid artery within the sinus. Pain behind the eye is commonly present. Also *Rochon-Duvigneaud syndrome, painful ophthalmoplegia.* See also ORBITAL APEX SYNDROME. **superior pontine s.** **1** A syndrome attributable to a unilateral lesion of the upper pons and comprising contralateral hemiplegia and hemianesthesia, sometimes ipsilateral peripheral facial paralysis, an ipsilateral cerebellar hemisyndrome, nystagmus, and conjugate deviation of the head and eyes to the side opposite the lesion, with paralysis of ocular movement towards the side of the lesion. Also *Raymond syndrome, Raymond-Cestan syndrome, Cestan-Raymond syndrome, superior pontine tegmental syndrome.* **2** WEBER SYNDROME. **superior sulcus tumor s.** PANCOAST SYNDROME. **superior vena cava s.** Venous dilatation and cyanosis of the head and neck with edema of the upper part of the body due to obstruction or compression of the superior vena cava by lesions such as neoplasm, fibrosis, and aneurysms. Also *superior caval syndrome.* **supine hypotensive s.** Dizziness and decreased blood pressure occurring when a pregnant woman lies on her back. The syndrome is due to pressure on the inferior vena cava which leads to diminution of blood flow back to the heart. Also *Mengert shock syndrome.* **suprarenogenic s.** *Obs.* CUSHING SYNDROME. **supraspinatus s.** Severe shoulder pain that is experienced in the middle third of abduction of the shoulder. It is caused by the compression of the inflamed insertion of the supraspinatus muscle against the acromion. **supravalvular aortic stenosis s.** Supravalvular aortic stenosis associated with hypercalcemia. It may be further associated with characteristic facies and known as the elfin face syndrome. See also IDIOPATHIC HYPERCALCEMIA. **surdocardiac s.** JERVELL AND LANGE-NIELSEN SYNDROME. **survivor s.** A post-traumatic stress disorder in which the subject suffers guilt feelings over surviving a particular situation while others have perished. Symptoms may include depression, insomnia, anxiety, psychosomatic complaints, and nightmares. **swallowed blood s.** The appearance of maternal blood in feces or vomitus of a neonate. Although swallowed by the baby during birth it may be attributed in error to gastrointestinal hemorrhage. Maternal and fetal blood can be differentiated by a simple test that depends on the resistance of fetal hemoglobin to alkali denaturation. Fetal hemoglobin remains in solution after exposure to pH 12.7 and adult hemoglobin is precipitated as alkaline hematin. **sweaty feet s.** ISOVALERICACIDEMIA. **Sweet s.** ACUTE FEBRILE NEUTROPHILIC DERMATOSIS. **Swyer-James s.** MACLEOD SYNDROME. **Swyer-James-Macleod s.** MACLEOD SYNDROME. **sylvian s.** MIDDLE CEREBRAL ARTERY SYNDROME. **sylvian aqueduct s.** AQUEDUCT OF SYLVIUS SYNDROME. **sylvian artery s.** MIDDLE CEREBRAL ARTERY SYNDROME. **Takayasu s.** TAKAYASU'S ARTERITIS. **tarsal tunnel s.** A syndrome characterized chiefly by pain and paresthesiae in certain toes, along the medial aspect of the foot, and in the sole, felt during the night or while walking or standing. It is attributed to irritation and compression of the branches of the posterior division of the tibial nerve as they traverse the calcaneal canal (tarsal tunnel). Superficial sensory loss is frequently encountered (particularly hypesthesia, sometimes anesthesia, and, rarely, hyperesthesia) and these usually affect only one part of the region innervated by branches of the posterior tibial nerve. Deep sensitivity may also be impaired, with loss of vibration sense in the affected toes. Reduction in the power of flexion of the toes can be detected, but this does not impede walking. Tapping and pressing on the tarsal tunnel induces pain and paresthesiae. **Taussig-Bing s.** TAUSSIG-BING MALFORMATION. **telangiectasia-pigmentation-cataract s.** ROTHMUND-THOMSON SYNDROME. **temporal pyramidal apex s.** GRADENIGO SYNDROME. **temporomandibular joint s.** A syndrome including pain in and around the temporomandibular joint and in the muscles of mastication, clicking sounds, limitation of movement and, more rarely, deafness and tinnitus. The pain is believed to be caused by spasm of the muscles, brought about by interference with the normal function of the masticatory apparatus, especially by occlusal disharmony. Treatment includes rest, bite-raising, and correction of occlusal disharmony. Also *Costen syndrome, temporomandibular syndrome.* 〈*Journal of the Michigan Dental Society* 55:673, 1956〉 **Terry s.** RETROLENTAL FIBROPLASIA. **testicular dysgenesis s.** SERTOLI-CELL-ONLY SYNDROME. **testicular feminization s.** TESTICULAR FEMINIZATION. **tetra-X s.** TETRA-X CHROMOSOMAL ABERRATION. **thalamic s.** A syndrome attributable to a thalamic lesion and marked by spontaneous, severe, burning pain, especially in the opposite side of the face and in the hand and sometimes the foot, with hyperpathia, accentuation of pain on contact, hypesthesia and hypalgesia in the affected limbs and sometimes sensory ataxia, hemiparesis, homonymous hemianopia, tremor or choreoathetosis, and excessive sweating. Also *Dejerine-Roussy syndrome, retrolenticular syndrome, Roussy-Dejerine syndrome.* **thalidomide s.** An association of developmental defects in man and simian primates that is caused by the sedative-hypnotic drug thalidomide when ingested by pregnant females during the early stages of organogenesis. The syndrome, observed to increase in occurrence in 1959–61, consisted predominantly of limb reduction defects, which usually affected one or more limbs to varying degrees ranging from minor changes of size or shape of a single bone to total absence of one or more limbs. Reduction of the lower jaw or external ears was not uncommon and abnormalities of the brain, heart, and genitourinary and gastrointestinal organs were sometimes seen. **Thibierge-Weissenbach s.** Extensive calcinosis and telangiectasia in a patient with progressive systemic sclerosis. **third and fourth pharyngeal arch s.** DIGEORGE SYNDROME. **third and fourth pharyngeal pouch s.** DIGEORGE SYNDROME **thoracic outlet s.** Any of a group of conditions in which the inner cord of the brachial plexus and/or the subclavian artery may be compressed by or angulated over a cervical rib, a fibrous band joining a prominent transverse process of the seventh cervical vertebra to the first rib, an abnormal first rib, or the edge of the scalenus anterior or scalenus medius muscle. The variable clinical manifestations may include pain and paresthesiae radiating down the medial border of the arm and forearm and the little finger, ischemia and/or embolism of the hand and arm, and atrophy of the small hand muscles, especially the thenar eminence. Pain and paresthesiae may be reproduced by digital pressure over the brachial plexus above the clavicle. Also *cervicobrachial syndrome, cervicothoracic outlet syndrome, subcoracoid-pectoralis minor syndrome, outlet syndrome.* **Thorn s.** *Rare* SALT-DEPLETION SYNDROME. **thrombopathic s.** Any bleeding tendency attributable to a qualitative platelet defect, in contrast to the quantitative defect, thrombocytopenia. **Tietze s.** COSTOCHONDRITIS. **tired housewife s.** HOUSEWIFE'S NEUROSIS. **Tolosa-Hunt s.** Unilateral recurrent retro-orbital pain, with paralysis of the extrinsic eye muscles due to involvement of the oculomotor, trochlear, and abducent nerves, sometimes with facial pain or sensory loss due to involvement of the first and second divisions of the trigeminus. The syndrome is attributable to an ill-defined granulomatous process in or near the superior orbital fissure or cavernous sinus and is often responsive to corticosteroid drugs. Also *painful ophthalmoplegia, orbital apicitis.* See also SUPERIOR ORBITAL FISSURE SYNDROME. **Tommaselli s.** TOMMASELLI'S DISEASE. **TORCH s.** The combination in the newborn infant of hepatospenomegaly, jaundice, and thromobytopenia. The syndrome may be caused by toxoplasmosis, rubella, cytomegalovirus, or herpes, from which terms it derives its name. **total allergy s.** A rare condition of hypersensitivity to a wide range of environmental substances often including synthetic materials and petrochemicals, manifested typically by severe contact hypersensitivity and hyperventilation syndrome. Psychogenic factors are believed to be an important etiologic influence. Subjects with this syndrome are sometimes called universal reactors. *Imprecise.* Also *twentieth-century syndrome.* **Touraine-Solente-Golé s.** PACHYDERMOPERIOSTOSIS. **Tourette s.** GILLES DE LA TOURETTE SYNDROME. **toxic shock s.** An acute, sometimes fatal illness characterized by rapid onset of high fever, vomiting, diarrhea, inflammation of the mucous membranes, a diffuse erythroderma, other organ system involvement, and, ultimately, severe prolonged shock and hypotension. The condition, first described in 1978, is caused by a toxin produced by *Staphylococcus aureus* and most often affects women, usually beginning during the menstrual period. **transcortical s.** A condition consisting of impairment of associative functions with aphasia, alexia, agraphia, apraxia, and agnosia as manifestations of a severe form of dementia seen in Alzheimer's disease. **transfusion s.** PLACENTAL TRANSFUSION SYNDROME. **translocation Down s.** Down syndrome that is attributed to a translocation chromosomal aberration resulting in trisomy for, at a minimum, the distal long arm of chromosome 21 (specifically, band q22). It accounts for three to five percent of Down syndrome cases, the rest being due to trisomy 21. Also *translocation mongolism* (outmoded). **transplant lung s.** TRANSPLANTATION PNEUMONIA. **traumatic vasospastic s.** VIBRATION DISEASE. **Treacher Collins s.** MANDIBULOFACIAL DYSOSTOSIS. **Treacher Collins-Franceschetti s.** MANDIBULOFACIAL DYSOSTOSIS. **triad s.** PRUNE-BELLY SYNDROME. **trichorhinophalangeal s.** A genetically heterogeneous syndrome characterized by sparse hair, bulbous nose, prominent philtrum, short stature, and cone-shaped epiphyses. At least two forms are known to exist. **trichorhinophalangeal s. type I** An autosomal dominant form of the trichorhinophalangeal syndrome. **trichorhinophalangeal s. type II** A condition distinguished from trichorhinophalangeal syndrome type I by multiple exostoses and mental retardation. Most cases are sporadic and some are associated with a deletion of part of the long arm of chromosome 8. Also *Langer-Giedion syndrome.* **triparanol s.** A syndrome represented by a constellation of disease conditions, such as alopecia, poliosis, ichthyosis, impotence, and cataracts, precipitated through the use of triparanol, a drug once used to decrease cholesterol synthesis. **triple-X s.** TRIPLE-X CHROMOSOMAL ABERRATION. **trisomy 13 s.** A severe, congenital syndrome due to the presence of an extra chromosome 13. It is characterized by microcephaly, cleft lip or palate, polydactyly, and flexion deformities of the fingers. Infants are deaf and blind and rarely survive longer than a few weeks or months. The syndrome is associated with advanced maternal age. Also *Patau syndrome, $E_1$ trisomy syndrome, trisomy $D_1$ syndrome.* **trisomy 18 s.** A severe, congenital syndrome due to the presence of an extra chromosome 18. It is characterized by growth failure, mental retardation, hypertonicity, rocker-bottom flatfoot, flexion deformities of the fingers, and renal and cardiac anomalies. Survival beyond six months is uncommon. It is associated with advanced maternal age. Also *Edwards syndrome* (outmoded), *trisomy $E_1$ syndrome* (outmoded). **trisomy 21 s.** DOWN SYNDROME. **trisomy $E_1$ s.** *Outmoded* TRISOMY 18 SYNDROME. **tropical splenomegaly s.** Splenic enlargement, often massive, that occurs in a small proportion of people in malarious areas. The liver shows sinusoidal lymphocytosis but no fibrosis, and the malarial antibody titer is high. *Plasmodium malariae* is sometimes found in the peripheral blood, and serum immunoglobulin IgM is grossly elevated. Although the immunology of the condition is not well understood, an aberrant immune response seems to be present. Also *big spleen disease.* Abbr. TSS **tuberohypophysial s.** HYPOPHYSIODIENCEPHALIC SYNDROME. **tuberoinfundibular s.** HYPOTHALAMIC SYNDROME. **Turcot s.** A familial disorder of adenomatous polyposis coli associated with malignancies of the central nervous system. Also *glioma-polyposis syndrome.* **Turner s.** A syndrome, typically found in females with complete X monosomy (45,X) that includes short stature, neck webbing, cubitus valgus, widely spaced nipples with shield chest, primary amenorrhea, sexual infantilism, and sterility. The ovaries are mere fibrous streaks. Subjects with mosaicism for X monosomy or deletions for part of an X chromosome often have less than full expression of the syndrome. Also *gonadal dysgenesis* (imprecise), *XO syndrome, ovarian short-stature syndrome* (outmoded). **Turner-Kieser s.** NAIL-PATELLA SYNDROME. **twentieth-century s.** TOTAL ALLERGY SYNDROME. **Ullrich s.** NOONAN SYNDROME. **Ullrich-Feichtiger s.** An association of developmental defects including micrognathia, polydactyly, varied genital malformations, depressed nose, microphthalmia, hypertelorism, and protruding ears. **Ullrich-Turner s.** NOONAN SYNDROME. **unilateral hyperlucent lung s.** MACLEOD SYNDROME. **Unverricht s.** PROGRESSIVE MYOCLONIC EPILEPSY. **upper brachial plexus s.** DUCHENNE-ERB SYNDROME. **Usher s.** A rare, inherited, degenerative disorder of unknown etiology causing congenital deafness and retinitis pigmentosa leading to blindness. **uveoparotid s.** HEERFORDT SYNDROME. **van Bogaert-Divry s.** A hereditary syndrome characterized by multiple cutaneous angiomata with poikiloderma and telangiectasia, and by severe abnormalities of the central nervous system giving rise to epilepsy, pyramidal and extrapyramidal motor defects, hemianopia, and dementia. The condition is transmitted as a sex-linked recessive trait. Also *diffuse corticomeningeal angiomatosis.* **van Bogaert-Scherer-Epstein s.** CEREBROTENDINOUS XANTHOMATOSIS. **Van Buchem s.** Progressive osteosclerosis and thickening of the cranium, mandible, and diaphyses of the long bones. Onset occurs after puberty, with variable development of cranial nerve compression leading to optic atrophy, deafness, and facial paralysis. Serum alkaline phosphatase levels are elevated. It is an autosomal recessive trait that is more commonly detected in males. Also *hyperostosis corticalis generalisata, endosteohyperostosis, leontiasis ossea generalisata.* **van der Hoeve s.** VAN DER HOEVE-DE KLEYN SYNDROME. **van der Hoeve-de Kleyn s.** A congenital familial disorder of bone, characterized by fragilitas ossium tarda, blue sclera, and conductive deafness which resembles but is not pathologically identical with otosclerosis. Also *van der Hoeve syndrome, Adair-Dighton syndrome, Dighton-Adair syndrome.* **vasculitis-hypersensitivity s.** Vasculitis that results from an allergic hypersensitivity to bacteria or other antigen. **vasculocardiac s. of hyperserotoninemia** CARCINOID SYNDROME. **velopalatine myoclonic s.** PALATOPHARYNGOLARYNGEAL MYOCLONUS. **Verbiest s.** INTERMITTENT CLAUDICATION OF THE CAUDA EQUINA. **Verger-Dejerine s.** DEJERINE SYNDROME. **vermis s.** Static or truncal cerebellar ataxia associated with lesions (especially tumors) situated in the vermis or other midline structures of the cerebellum. The patient staggers from side to side, and has difficulty in stopping or in turning, but there are no classical signs of cerebellar dysfunction (past-pointing, incoordination or dysmetria) in the individual limbs. The syndrome is typically seen in children with medulloblastomas. Also *sagittal imbalance syndrome.* **Verner-Morrison s.** A syndrome of watery diarrhea and hypokalemia due to a pancreatic endocrine tumor. Secretory diarrhea is thought to result from a peptide hormone secreted by the tumor. Also *pancreatic cholera.* **Vernet s.** VERNET'S PARALYSIS. **vertebrobasilar s.** The symptoms and signs resulting from recurrent and transient ischemia in the region served by the vertebral arteries and basilar trunk, including vertigo, visual defects (transient hemianopia or total blindness), dysarthria, and weakness or paresthesiae in one or more limbs. The symptoms may be precipitated in occasional cases by certain movements of the head and neck. Also *vertebrobasilar insufficiency, vertebral insufficiency, basilar insufficiency.* **vertical retraction s.** DUANE SYNDROME. **Vieusseux-Wallenberg s.** WALLENBERG SYNDROME. **Vinson s.** PLUMMER-VINSON SYNDROME. **Vogt s.** A rare type of hereditary degenerative disease developing at birth or during the first year of life, and marked by intense choreoathetoid movements of the entire body, muscular rigidity with trismus, dysphagia, and dysarthria, but with no major impairment of intelligence or of sensation. It is attributable to degeneration of the caudate nucleus and of the external segment of the lenticular nucleus. Also *syndrome of corpus striatum.* **Vogt-Koyanagi s.** Iridocyclitis, choroiditis (sometimes with retinal detachment), depigmentation of hair and skin, and associated meningitis, often with deafness and tinnitus. Also *oculocutaneous syndrome, uveocutaneous syndrome, Yuge syndrome, oculo-otocutaneous syndrome of Yuge.* **Volkmann s.** VOLKMANN'S ISCHEMIC CONTRACTURE. **von Hippel-Lindau s.** An autosomal dominant condition characterized by angiomata of the retina, hemangioblastoma of the central nervous system (usually the cerebellum), hypernephroma, pheochromocytoma, cysts and carcinoma of the pancreas, and papillary cystadenoma of the epididymis. Polycythemia may result from tumoral production of erythropoietin. Also *retinocerebelloangiomatosis.* **von Mikulicz s.** Dryness of the mouth and decreased or absent lacrimation associated with a variety of chronic diseases, such as lymphoma, leukemia, sarcoidosis and tuberculosis. Also *Mikulicz-Sjögren syndrome, Mikulicz-Radecki syndrome, Mikulicz syndrome.* **vulnerable child s.** The overly cautious parental treatment of a child who has survived severe illness. The child is treated as if she were still in danger of death. **Waardenburg s.** A congenital syndrome, inherited in an autosomal dominant manner, in which profound sensorineural deafness is associated with pigmentary upsets. Among the chief features besides deafness are abnormality of the medial palpebral canthi, disturbance of pigmentation of the irides (black children may have blue eyes), and a white forelock. **WAGR s.** ANIRIDIA-WILMS TUMOR SYNDROME. **Wallenberg s.** A common syndrome of lateral medullary infarction caused by thrombosis of one vertebral artery or of one posterior inferior cerebellar artery. Vertigo and sometimes dysphagia are common at the outset. On the affected side, there are palatolaryngopharyngeal paralysis, cerebellar ataxia, the Horner syndrome, and hypalgesia on the face. On the opposite side, there is insensitivity of the trunk and limbs to pain and temperature. Also *Vieusseux-Wallenberg syndrome, lateral medullary syndrome, posterior inferior cerebellar artery syndrome.* **Ward-Romano s.** ROMANO-WARD SYNDROME. **Wartenberg s.** CHEIRALGIA PARESTHETICA. **Waterhouse-Friderichsen s.** Septicemia and acute adrenal insufficiency resulting from bilateral adrenal hemorrhage which occurs usually in children as a complication of severe meningococcal infection or in association with anticoagulation therapy. Following the spread of the causative organism, *Neisseria meningitides,* there is generalized purpuric rash, shock, and hypertension. The disease usually occurs in epidemics in hot, dry regions, especially in West Africa. Also *meningococcic adrenal syndrome, Friderichsen-Waterhouse syndrome, acute fulminating meningococcal septicemia.* **Weber s.** A syndrome due to infarction of one cerebral peduncle resulting in a third nerve palsy on the side of the lesion and a contralateral hemiplegia. Also *superior alternate hemiplegia, Weber's paralysis, superior midbrain syndrome, Weber-Leyden syndrome, Weber symptom, superior pontine syndrome, alternating oculomotor hemiplegia, Weber sign, Weber-Dubler syndrome.* **Weber-Christian s.** RELAPSING FEBRILE NONSUPPURATIVE PANNICULITIS. **Weber-Dubler s.** WEBER SYNDROME. **Weber-Leyden s.** WEBER SYNDROME **Wegener s.** WEGENER'S GRANULOMATOSIS. **Weill-Marchesani s.** An autosomal recessive heritable disorder of connective tissue characterized by short stature, brachydactyly, joint stiffness, and congenital microspherophakia and ectopia lentis. Also *spherophakia-brachymorphia syndrome, Marchesani syndrome.* **Weill-Reys s.** ADIE SYNDROME. **Weill-Reys-Adie s.** ADIE SYNDROME. **Weingarten s.** TROPICAL PULMONARY EOSINOPHILIA. **Werdnig-Hoffmann s.** WERDNIG-HOFFMANN DISEASE. **Wermer s.** The familial form of multiple endocrine neoplasia Type I. See under MULTIPLE ENDOCRINE NEOPLASIA. **Werner s.** A hereditary disorder consisting of premature aging, shortness of stature, atrophic skin, usually severe vascular disease, testicular atrophy, and, in half the patients, mild diabetes mellitus. **Wernicke s.** WERNICKE'S DISEASE. **Wernicke-Korsakoff s.** WERNICKE-KORSAKOFF PSYCHOSIS. **West s.** INFANTILE MASSIVE SPASM. **whistling face s.** WHISTLING FACE–WINDMILL VANE HAND SYNDROME. **whistling face–windmill vane hand s.** An autosomal dominant syndrome of unknown cause characterized by an abnormal facies (sunken eyes, hypertelorism, small mouth, and long philtrum) and skeletal malformations (camptodactyly with ulnar deviation, talipes equinovarus, and scoliosis). Also *craniocarpotarsal syndrome, Freeman-Sheldon syndrome, whistling face syndrome, craniocarpotarsal dysplasia.* **Wildervanck s.** An autosomal dominant syndrome characterized by an association of profound sensorineural deafness with the Klippel-Feil malformation and certain ophthalmic disorders. Preauricular sinuses, accessory auricles, and facial and cranial asymmetry are facultative components. **Wilks s.** MYASTHENIA GRAVIS. **Willebrand s.** VON WILLEBRAND'S DISEASE. **Wilson s.** WILSON'S DISEASE. **Wilson-Mikity s.** A severe pulmonary disorder affecting premature infants in the first five weeks of life. Mortality is high. It is marked by overdistension of the alveoli and at the same time a thickening of their walls, perialveolar infiltration with monocytes, and fibrosis of interlobular septa. X rays of the lungs show a multiple cystlike pattern (bubbly-lung syndrome). The etiology is uncertain. Also *pulmonary dysmaturity.* **Wiskott-Aldrich s.** A hemorrhagic diathesis associated with recurrent infections and eczema. The small and irregularly shaped platelets have diminished numbers of organelles and they aggregate poorly *in vitro.* Cellular immunity is defective. Also *Aldrich syndrome.* **Wissler-Fanconi s.** Recurring bouts of fever, with rash, carditis, pleuritis, and pneumonia, occurring between the ages of 5 and 17 years. The cause is unknown but the illness may be a form of rheumatoid arthritis. **Wolff-Parkinson-White s.** A cardiac syndrome characterized by preexcitation due to an anomalous pathway. Characteristically, the P-R interval is abnormally short, the QRS is broadened with a delta wave on its upstroke and there are associated arrhythmias, notably atrial supraventricular tachycardia. Also *WPW syndrome, anomalous atrioventricular excitation, accelerated conduction syndrome, preexcitation syndrome.* **Woltman-Kernohan s.** KERNOHAN SYNDROME. **WPW s.** WOLFF-PARKINSON-WHITE SYNDROME. **X-linked lymphoproliferative s.** X-LINKED IMMUNODEFICIENCY WITH UNDUE SUSCEPTIBILITY TO EPSTEIN-BARR VIRUS. **XO s.** TURNER SYNDROME. **XXXX s.** TETRA-X CHROMOSOMAL ABERRATION. **XXXXY s.** A syndrome in human males with a full or mosaic 49,XXXXY karyotype, characterized by moderate mental retardation, sexual underdevelopment, and radioulnar synostosis. **XXY s.** KLINEFELTER SYNDROME. **XYY s.** *Incorrect* XYY CHROMOSOME CONSTITUTION. **yellow nail s.** A condition in which the nails become thickened, excessively curved, and yellow or green in color, with the loss of the lunula and cuticle. Growth nearly ceases and onycholysis and shedding may occur. Associated with this condition may be lymphedema, pleural effusions, and bronchiectasis. **yellow vernix s.** PLACENTAL DYSFUNCTION SYNDROME. **Young s.** BERRY-PERKINS-YOUNG SYNDROME. **Yuge s.** VOGT-KOYANAGI SYNDROME. **Zellweger s.** CEREBROHEPATORENAL SYNDROME. **Zieve s.** Hemolytic anemia and hyperlipidemia following ethanol intoxication in a patient with preexisting liver disease. **Zinser-Cole-Engman s.** DYSKERATOSIS CONGENITA. **Zollinger-Ellison s.** Severe gastric hypersecretion of hydrochloric acid and intractable peptic ulcers due to excessive secretion of gastrin by a gastrinoma.

**syndromic** \sindrō′mik\ Associated with or of the nature of a syndrome.

**syndromologist** \sin′drōmäl′əjist\ A specialist in syndromology.

**syndromology** \sin′drōmäl′əjē\ [*syndrom(e)* + *o* + -LOGY] The interdisciplinary study of the causes, mechanisms, and manifestations of syndromes, or of aggregates of signs and symptoms suspected of being associated by more than chance occurrence. Although not yet an established medical discipline, this expanding field of inquiry now represents a significant subdivision of genetics, teratology, and pediatrics.

**synechia** \sinek′ē·ə\ [Gk *synech(ein)* (from SYN- + Gk *echein* to have, hold) to hold or keep together + -IA] (*pl.* synechiae) An adhesion, especially adhesion of the iris to adjacent intraocular structures. **annular s.** Adhesion between the lens and the entire circumference of the pupil. Also *ring synechia, circular synechia.* **anterior s.** Adhesion between the iris and the cornea. **circular s.** ANNULAR SYNECHIA. **s. pericardii** ADHESIVE PERICARDITIS. **posterior s.** Adhesion between the iris and the lens. **ring s.** ANNULAR SYNECHIA. **s. vulvae** A congenital fusion of the free margins of the labia minora.

**synechiae** \sinek′i·ē\ Plural of SYNECHIA.

**synechotomy** \sin′ekät′əmē\ [Gk *synech(ein)* to hold or keep together + *o* + -TOMY] The surgical release of iris adhesions.

**synencephalocele** \sin′ensef′əlōsēl′\ [SYN- + ENCEPHALO- + -CELE[1]] Exencephaly in which brain or meningeal tissue adheres to surrounding tissues in such manner as to interfere with reduction or repair.

**synencephaly** \sin′ensef′əlē\ [SYN- + ENCEPHAL- + -Y] The condition of equal conjoined twins having two bodies and a single head.

**syneresis** \siner′əsis\ The contraction of a gel with the exudation of the fluid, as the contraction of a blood clot expelling some of the serum.

**synergism** \sin′ərjizm\ [Gk *synerg(ia)* assistance, cooperation + -ISM] The state of acting together, especially so that the combined action of all participating elements is greater than that of each element if acting separately: said of groups of muscles or chemicals. Also *synergy, synergia.*

**synergist** \sin′ərjist\ [*synerg(y)* + -IST] An agent capable of acting together with other agents to produce an effect greater than that of each agent acting separately, as the effect of a muscle or muscle group acting with other muscles or that of a drug acting with other drugs. See also SYNERGISTIC MUSCLE.

**synergy** \sin′ərjē\ [Gk *synergia* (from SYN- + Gk *erg(on)* work + -IA) assistance, cooperation] SYNERGISM.

**synesthesia** \sin′esthē′zhə\ [SYN- + ESTHESIA] A disorder of sensory perception characterized by the simultaneous perception, in addition to the normal response to a sensory stimulus, of a secondary sensation felt either in a different part of the body to that which is stimulated, or else representing a different sensory modality.

**syngamous** \sin′gəməs\ Relating to or characterized by sexual reproduction (syngamy).

**syngamy** \sin′gəmē\ [SYN- + GAM- + -Y] SEXUAL REPRODUCTION.

**syngeneic** \sin′jənē′ik\ **1** In immunology, homologous, especially when the species to which the individual belongs from which the substance is obtained is inbred, or when the substance is obtained from an identical twin: used especially of serum, tissue, cells, etc., under immunologic study. Also *syngenic.* Compare ALLOGENEIC. **2** ISOGENIC.

**syngenesiograft** \sin′jənē′sē·əgraft′\ An allograft transferred between individuals who are closely related, such as siblings, but not isogeneic.

**syngenesioplastic** \sin′jənē′sē·əplas′tik\ Pertaining to a syngenesiograft.

**syngenesis** \sinjen′əsis\ [SYN- + GENESIS] SEXUAL REPRODUCTION. Adj. syngenetic.

**syngenic** \sinjen′ik\ SYNGENEIC.

**syngnathia** \sinath′ē·ə\ Congenital union of the upper and lower jaws by fibrous bands extending between the two, a rare condition found in association with cleft palate.

**syngraft** \sin′graft\ ISOGRAFT.

**synhexyl** $C_{22}H_{32}O_2$. A synthetic analogue of tetrahydrocannabinols, the main active ingredients of cannabis. It is a viscous, odorless, resin which has had limited use as an agent to alter the mood and produce a euphoric state. It also lowers the intraocular pressure and has had limited trials in the treatment of glaucoma. Also *pyrahexyl, parahexyl.*

**synhidrosis** \sin′hidrō′sis\ [SYN- + HIDROSIS] Sweating occurring in association with another condition.

**synizesis** \sin′əzē′sis\ [Gk *synizēsis* (from *syn-* together + *(h)iz(anein)* to sit, settle) subsidence, collapse, falling together] **1** Loss of discreteness or patency; clumping; cohesion. **2** A massing of chromatin at one region in the nucleus at the onset of synapsis during meiotic division I. **s. pupillae** Occlusion of the pupil by posterior adhesions.

**synkinesis** \sin′kənē′sis\ [SYN- + Gk *kinēsis* movement, from *kinein* to move] An involuntary movement occurring in association with a voluntary movement. Also *synkinesia.* Adj. synkinetic. **brachiobrachial s.** Flexion, pronation, or supination of the forearm in a paralyzed limb, which occurs when a similar voluntary movement is made against resistance on the unaffected side; one form of coordination synkinesis. **contralateral s.** IMITATION SYNKINESIS. **coordination s.** An involuntary movement occurring in a paretic limb when a specific voluntary movement is attempted or in an unaffected limb when a similar movement is attempted in a paretic limb (imitation synkinesis). **crurocrural s.** Involuntary flexion of the leg at the knee in a paralyzed limb, which occurs when the voluntary flexion of the leg on the unaffected side is resisted; one form of coordination synkinesis. **imitation s.** An involuntary movement occurring in an unaffected limb similar to that being attempted in a paretic limb. Also *contralateral synkinesis.* **mouth-and-hand s.** SAUNDERS SIGN. **reflex s.** Any involuntary muscular contraction in a paralyzed or paretic extremity induced by an attempt to elicit a deep tendon reflex sometimes on the same side of the body but more often on the opposite side. **spasmodic s.** An involuntary movement occurring in a paralyzed limb which is evoked by and resembles a voluntary movement on the nonparalyzed side.

**synkinetic** \sin′kinet′ik\ Relating to or characterized by synkinesis.

**synnematin** CEPHALOSPORIN N.

**synneurosis** \sin′ʸurō′sis\ *Outmoded* SYNDESMOSIS.

**synonychia** \sin′ōnik′ē·ə\ [SYN- + ONYCH- + -IA ] A fusion of the nails in adjacent syndactylous fingers or toes.

**synonym** \sin′ənim\ [Gk *synōnymos* (from *syn-* with + *onoma,* also *onyma* name) of like name or meaning] **1** Any term that has the same meaning, or one of the same meanings, as another term. **2** A biological taxon, such as a species or a genus, that is judged not to be validly separable from another taxon of the same rank. In the case of synonymous species, the earliest published name ordinarily has priority and becomes the official name of the merged species.

**synonymize** \sinän′əmīz\ To equate (a biological taxon such as a genus or a species) with another taxon of the same rank; to regard (two or more taxa) as not validly separable.

**synophrys** \sinäf′ris\ [SYN- + Gk *ophrys* the eyebrow] A continuity of the eyebrows across the midline. Also *synophridia.*

**synophthalmia** \sin′äfthal′mē·ə\ [SYN- + OPHTHALM- + -IA] CYCLOPIA.

**synophthalmus** \sin′äfthal′məs\ [SYN- + Gk *ophthalmos* eye] CYCLOPS.

**synoptophore** \sinäp′təfôr\ [SYN- + OPTO- + -PHORE ] A stereoscopic device for evaluation and training of binocular functions.

**synorchidism** \sinôr′kidizm\ [SYN- + *orchid(o)-* + -ISM] The congenital fusion of the undescended testes.

**synoscheos** \sinäs′kē·əs\ [SYN- + Gk *oscheos* the scrotum] A continuity of scrotum or scrotal rudiments with the penis, as seen in some intersexes.

**synosteology** \sin′ästē·äl′əjē\ ARTHROLOGY.

**synosteosis** \sin′ästē·ō′sis\ SYNOSTOSIS.

**synosteotomy** \sin′ästē·ät′əmē\ ARTHROTOMY.

**synostosis** \sin′ästō′sis\ [SYN- + OST- + -OSIS] **1** The osseous union of two or more normally separate bones to form one. **2** The union of adjacent connected bones or parts of a bone by ossification of the connecting tissues; bony ankylosis. For defs. 1 and 2 also *synosteosis.* See also ARTHRODESIS. **cranial s.** The premature closure of the sutures of the skull by ossification. **transphalangeal s.** An interdigital fusion of phalangeal elements occurring in syndactyly. **tribasilar s.** A premature fusion of the three principal bones at the base of the skull. It often results in distortion of the definitive skull and sometimes is associated with mental retardation.

**synostotic** \sin′ästät′ik\ Pertaining to or characterized by synostosis.

**synotia** \sīnō′shə\ [SYN- + OT- + -IA] Fusion of the two ears in the midline of the lower face, one of the features of otocephaly. Also *cyclotia.*

**synovectomy** \sin′ōvek′təmē\ The excision of the synovial membrane that lines a joint or tendon sheath. Also *villusectomy.*

**synovia** \sinō′vē·ə\ [New L (coined by Paracelsus, perh. from SYN- + L *ovum* egg) orig., any of various body fluids; later restricted to joint fluid because of its resemblance to egg white] [NA] A transparent, viscous fluid, resembling egg white, secreted by synovial membrane as a lubricant and nutrient in joints, tendon sheaths, and bursae. It contains mostly mucin, albumin, cells, and salts. Also *synovial fluid, articular serum.*

**synovial** \sinō′vē·əl\ Pertaining to, secreting, or containing synovia. Also *synovialis.*

**synovialoma** \sinō′vē·əlō′mə\ SYNOVIOMA.

**synovianalysis** \sinō′vē·ənal′isis\ [*synovi(a)* + ANALYSIS] The examination of fluid extracted from a joint.

**synovin** \sin′əvin\ Synovial mucin.

**synovioblast** \sinō′vē·əblast′\ A connective-tissue cell of the synovial membrane that resembles a fibroblast.

**synoviocyte** \sinō′vē·əsīt′\ A cell found in the synovial membrane.

**synovioma** \sinō′vē·ō′mə\ [*synovi(al)* + -OMA] A tumor originating in a synovial membrane, especially when benign. Also *synovialoma.* • The malignant form is generally referred to as *synovial sarcoma.* **malignant s.** SYNOVIAL SARCOMA.

**synoviorthosis** \sinō′vē·ôrthō′sis\ The destruction of the synovial membrane by injection of a radioactive colloid. The procedure is performed in cases of arthritis that are associated with chronic synovitis.

**synoviparous** \sin′ōvip′ərəs\ Producing synovial fluid in synovial joints.

**synovitis** \sin′ōvī′tis\ [*synov(ial)* + -ITIS] An inflammation of the synovial membrane. Also *arthromeningitis.*

**bursal s.** BURSITIS. **chronic purulent s.** Chronic synovitis with pus formation due to a longstanding infection with a bacterial agent, usually *Mycobacterium tuberculosis.* **dry s.** SYNOVITIS SICCA. **filarial s.** A synovitis caused by microfilariae in or about the joints, characterized by inflammation and occasionally by fibrotic ankylosis. **s. hyperplastica** PROLIFERATIVE SYNOVITIS. **localized nodular s.** Chronic synovitis with foci of inflammation, usually lymphocytic. **pigmented villonodular s.** A disease, often affecting a knee or both knees, characterized by hemorrhagic joint fluid and a characteristic pigmented chronic inflammatory reaction. Some consider this disease to be neoplastic. Also *villonodular synovitis, villous arthritis.* **proliferative s.** Synovitis characterized by proliferation and overgrowth of synovium, such as is seen in rheumatoid arthritis. Also *synovitis hyperplastica.* **puerperal s.** Synovitis which develops as a result of sepsis occurring after childbirth. **purulent s.** The presence of pus within a joint; pyogenic arthritis. Also *suppurative synovitis, purulent arthritis.* **scarlatinal s.** Synovitis occurring as a complication of scarlet fever. **serous s.** Synovitis associated with a tense joint effusion consisting of serous fluid. **s. sicca** Synovitis characterized by relatively little joint effusion. Also *dry synovitis.* **simple s.** Synovitis marked by an effusion consisting of slightly turbid fluid. **suppurative s.** PURULENT SYNOVITIS. **tendinous s.** TENOSYNOVITIS. **transient s.** A joint effusion with synovial inflammation that completely subsides without sequelae after a period of days or weeks. Also *transitory synovitis.* **traumatic s.** Inflammation of the synovium following injury to a joint. **tuberculous s.** Synovitis resulting from direct infection with *Mycobacterium tuberculosis.* **vaginal s.** TENOSYNOVITIS. **villonodular s.** PIGMENTED VILLONODULAR SYNOVITIS.

**synovium** \sinō′vē·əm\ *Outmoded* MEMBRANA SYNOVIALIS CAPSULAE ARTICULARIS.

**synpneumonic** \sinʹʸoomän′ik\ Occurring during pneumonia.

**syntasis** \sin′təsis\ [Gk *syntasis* (from *synteinein* to stretch together, strain) a stretching together, straining] A stretching.

**syntaxis** \sintak′sis\ ARTICULATION.

**syntenic** \sinten′ik\ Of or relating to two or more genes that are present on the same chromosome regardless of whether linkage has been demonstrated between the loci.

**synteny** \sin′tənē\ [Gk *syntein(ein)* (from *syn-* SYN- + *teinein* to stretch, aim at) to increase, tend toward, aim at + -Y] The state of two or more genetic loci being present on the same chromosome, regardless of linkage.

**syntexis** \sintek′sis\ [Gk *syntēxis* a wasting away] WASTING.

**synthase** Any enzyme that catalyzes synthesis of a compound, such as citrate synthase, which catalyzes the synthesis of citrate. The term once excluded enzymes whose reactions involve breakdown of nucleoside triphosphates (i.e. synthetases), but these are now also considered synthases, e.g. glutamine synthase.

**synthermal** \sinthur′məl\ [SYN- + THERMAL] ISOTHERMIC.

**synthesis** \sin′thəsis\ [Gk *synthesis* (from root of *syntithenai* to place or put together, from SYN- + Gk *tithenai* to place, put, set) a putting together, compounding, composition] (*pl.* syntheses) The formation of a substance or molecule by chemical reaction, especially by a reaction that builds up the molecule from simpler ones. **de novo s.** Synthesis from simple starting compounds, rather than by recovery of only partly degraded material. **distributive s.** A technique of psychobiology that strives to identify the major factors whose union will provide the greatest security to the patient and the most dependable basis for coping with life. **inducible enzyme s.** The production of an enzyme whose synthesis is increased by an inducer, such as the substrate of the enzyme or an analogue thereof. **morphologic s.** HISTOGENESIS. **unscheduled DNA s.** Any synthetic activity of nuclear DNA that occurs at a time in the cell cycle when the chromosomes are not replicating; hence, occurring outside the S phase. It is usually detected by incorporation of radioactive precursors. One reason for this activity is the repair of damage, as that induced by ultraviolet or x-irradiation.

**synthesize** \sin′thəsīz\ To form (a substance or molecule) by chemical reaction, especially by a reaction that builds up the molecule from simpler ones.

**synthesizer** \sin′thəsīʹzər\ **speech s.** An electronic system that produces speech output from character input, used, for example, in reading machines for the blind.

**synthetase** Any enzyme that catalyzes synthesis of a compound with concomitant breakdown of a nucleoside triphosphate. The term is sometimes incorrectly used for synthases in general. Also *ligase.* **heme s.** FERROCHELATASE.

**synthetic** \sinthet′ik\ Produced by synthesis; especially, artificially produced by chemical synthesis rather than obtained from a natural source.

**synthetism** \sin′thətizm\ OSTEOSYNTHESIS.

**syntopy** \sin′təpē\ [SYN- + Gk *top(os)* a place + -Y] The location of an organ in relation to the surrounding organs. Also *syntopie.*

**syntrophism** \sin′trəfizm\ [SYN- + TROPH- + -ISM] CROSS-FEEDING.

**syntrophoblast** \sinträf′əblast\ SYNCYTIOTROPHOBLAST.

**syntropic** \sinträp′ik\ [SYN- + -TROPIC[1]] **1** In anatomy, turning, pointing, or arranged in the same direction: used especially of parts forming a series of segments, such as the ribs on one side or the spines of thoracic vertebrae. **2** Converging and leading in the same direction, as qualities or diseases.

**syntropy** \sin′trəpē\ The state of being syntropic. **inverse s.** Reduction (possibly to zero) of the likelihood of occurrence of one disease in a patient or group by the presence of another disease in that patient or group. For example, a person with sickle cell anemia is unlikely to contract malaria.

**synulosis** \sinʹyəlō′sis\ [SYN- + ULO-[1] + -SIS] Severe scarring. *Obs.*

**synulotic** \sinʹyəlät′ik\ [SYN- + ULO-[1] + *t* + -IC] CICATRIZANT.

***Synura*** \sinoo′rə\ A genus of flagellate protozoa (order Chrysomonadina, family Syncryptidae) often found in drinking water, sometimes imparting an unpleasant taste.

**syphil-** \sif′il-\ SYPHILO-.

**syphilemia** \sifʹilē′mē·ə\ The presence in the bloodstream of the agent of syphilis, *Treponema pallidum.*

**syphili-** \sif′əlē-\ SYPHILO-.

**syphilid** \sif′əlid\ [SYPHILIS + -ID[2]] A secondary or late-stage skin manifestation of syphilis. **acuminate papular s.** FOLLICULAR SYPHILID. **annular s.** A syphilitic rash characterized by lesions appearing as concentric rings. **ecthymatous s.** PUSTULAR SYPHILID. **erythematous s.** SYPHILITIC ROSEOLA. **follicular s.** A syphilitic infection of the hair follicles. Also *acuminate papular syphilid.* **macular s.** SYPHILITIC ROSEOLA. **papulosquamous s.** The scaling papules characteristic of secondary syphilis. **pemphigoid s.** A syphilitic blister.

**pigmentary s.** Coexistent pigmentation and depigmentation that is associated with past and present skin lesions of syphilis. **pustular s.** Rare syphilitic lesions containing or oozing pus. Also *ecthymatous syphilid.* **roseolar s.** SYPHILITIC ROSEOLA. **secondary s.** Any rash characteristic of the second stages of syphilis. **serpiginous s.** A chronic, ulcerative syphilitic lesion showing simultaneous spread and healing.

**syphilidophthalmia** \sif′ilidäfthal′mē·ə\ Ocular infection with the spirochete *Treponema pallidum*.

**syphilis** \sif′əlis\ [after *Syphilus*, chief character in poem "Syphilis sive Morbus Gallicus" by Girolamo Fracastoro (latinized as Fracastorius), published 1530. Syphilus was named from Gk *sys* a hog + *philos* loving, beloved] Infection with the spirochete *Treponema pallidum*, usually acquired during sexual contact with an infected partner or *in utero* from an infected woman. The treatment of choice for all stages is penicillin G. Also *pox* (obs.), *lues, lues venerea.* **acquired s.** Syphilis contracted during coitus. Compare CONGENITAL SYPHILIS. **cerebrospinal s.** MENINGOVASCULAR SYPHILIS. **congenital s.** An infection by *Treponema pallidum* that is spread from an expectant mother to the fetus through the placenta. At birth the disease may appear as early syphilis, and be infectious and possibly lethal. If the disease is in the late stage at birth, it is noninfectious and is characterized by stigmata or scars. Also *heredosyphilis, prenatal syphilis.* Compare ACQUIRED SYPHILIS. **s. d'emblée** Syphilis that develops with no apparent primary lesion. **early latent s.** Latent syphilis that is present within 1–4 years after the initial lesion, the specific period varying according to convention in different countries. **endemic s.** A syphilitic infection reported as having a low but consistent and regular morbidity rate. **s. hereditaria tarda** Congenital syphilis that becomes apparent some time after birth. **late s.** Any clinical, radiological, or cerebrospinal fluid manifestation of syphilis that appears five or more years after the primary stages of the disease. The skin, bones, cardiovascular system, and neurological system are most often involved. Also *tertiary syphilis, lues tarda.* **late benign s.** Late syphilis producing lesions of the skin and skeletal system only. **late latent s.** Latent syphilis that is present more than the 1–4 years after the initial lesion, the specific period varying according to convention in different countries. **latent s.** Syphilis that manifests no symptoms or signs in any system. The presence of the disease is established by repeatedly positive serological tests, clinical normality, and normal chest x ray and cerebrospinal fluid. **meningovascular s.** Tertiary syphilis giving rise to subacute granulomatous meningitis, often with associated cranial nerve palsies and endarteritis involving the vessels supplying the brain and spinal cord, often resulting in focal or generalized ischemia. Also *cerebrospinal syphilis.* **noduloulcerative s.** Syphilis marked by large, solid elevations on the skin that appear larger than half a pea and that tend to ulcerate. **nonvenereal s.** BEJEL. **parenchymatous s.** GENERAL PARESIS. **prenatal s.** CONGENITAL SYPHILIS. **primary s.** The initial stage of syphilis in which an ulceration (chancre) develops at the site of invasion by *Treponema pallidum*. The incubation period is typically 21 days, but may vary from 9 to 90 days. The disease is frequently associated with enlarged glands in the groin area and a positive blood test for antibodies. Also *protosyphilis.* **secondary s.** The stage of syphilis occurring about two months after appearance of the initial lesion and during which *Treponema pallidum* is disseminated to all organs of the body via the bloodstream, is manifested as a highly variable mucocutaneous rash and, usually, generalized lymphadenopathy. Blood tests for syphilitic antibodies are always positive. Also *mesosyphilis.* **tertiary s.** LATE SYPHILIS.

**syphilo-** \sif′əlō-\ [*syphil(is)* + *o.* See SYPHILIS.] A combining form denoting syphilis. Also *syphil-, syphili-.*

**syphilologist** \sif′iläl′əjist\ A specialist in the diagnosis, treatment, and epidemiological control of syphilis.

**syphiloma** \sif′ilō′mə\ [SYPHIL- + -OMA] A syphilitic gumma.

**syphilomatous** \sif′ilō′mətəs\ Pertaining to a syphiloma; gummatous.

**syphilonychia** \sif′ilōnik′ē·ə\ [*syphil(is)* + ONYCHIA] Papular syphilitic lesions on the nail beds of the fingers or toes. **s. exulcerans** Ulcerated syphilitic lesions around the nail beds. **s. sicca** Dried and crusted syphilitic lesions that appear under and around the nails of the fingers and toes.

**syr.** *syrupus* (L, syrup).

**syring-** \sir′ing-\ SYRINGO-.

**syringadenoma** \sir′ing·gadənō′mə\ A tumor of the ductal portion of the sweat gland apparatus. Also *syringocystoma, syringocystadenoma.* **papillary s.** SYRINGOCYSTADENOMA PAPILLIFERUM.

**syringadenosus** \sir′ing·gadənō′səs\ [SYRING- + ADEN- + L *-osus* -OSE] Relating or pertaining to the sweat glands of the skin. Also *syringadenous.*

**syringe** \sərinj′, sir′inj\ [Late L *syringa* (from Gk *syrinx*; see SYRINGO-) a fistula, a syringe] A hollow cylindrical instrument fitted with a piston or compressible bulb device such that liquids may be drawn in by creating suction and forcibly expelled as desired, and utilized for injection, withdrawal, or transfer of fluids. **aural s.** Any syringe for the ear, usually for removing cerumen, but also sometimes discharge, debris, or even foreign bodies. Many kinds have been designed, usually made of metal or rubber but some of glass, with certain of the latter intended for use by the patient. Also *ear syringe.* **chip s.** HAND AIR SYRINGE. **continuous-flow s.** A syringe adapted for refilling from an attached reservoir so that it is capable of expelling large amounts of fluid in a continuous manner. **ear s.** AURAL SYRINGE. **fountain s.** A syringe utilizing gravity as the motive force to produce injection of fluid. **hand air s.** An air syringe with a rubber bulb which is compressed in the hand. Also *chip syringe.* **hypodermic s.** A syringe designed for injections into or aspiration from the hypoderm or subcutis. **Luer s.** A glass syringe used in hypodermic and intravenous procedures that has a locking device to ensure rapid and secure fixation of the needle. Also *Luer-Lok syringe.* **probe s.** A syringe with a specially tapered point that may be used as a probe as well as for the passage of fluid, especially utilized in narrow conduits such as the lacrimal passages. **two-way s.** A syringe with an adjustable outlet valve for deviation of fluid in two directions, as may be required for aspiration from a body cavity, spinal tap, or other specific purpose. **water s.** A device used in dentistry to create a jet of water. **wound s.** A large syringe, utilized for irrigation purposes, having a rubber- or cotton-fitted piston.

**syringectomy** \sir′injek′təmē\ [SYRING- + -ECTOMY] FISTULECTOMY.

**syringo-** \siring′gō-\ [Gk *syrinx*, gen. *syringos* a pipe, whistle, airway, tube, duct, fistula] A combining form meaning tube or fistula. Also *syring-.*

**syringobulbia** \-bul′bē·ə\ [SYRINGO- + BULB- + -IA] A congenital cavitation in the medulla oblongata almost invariably the result of an upward extension of syringomyelia. It is characterized by dissociated anesthesia, with loss of pain and temperature sensation in the head and neck on one or both sides, but preservation of touch. It is associated with variable clinical evidence of involvement of the lower cranial nerves and of the ascending and descending spinal tracts.

**syringocarcinoma** \-kär′sinō′mə\ [SYRINGO- + CARCINOMA] A sweat gland carcinoma.

**syringocele** \siring′gōsēl\ [SYRINGO- + -CELE[1]] Central spinal cord cavitation in association with meningomyelocele.

**syringocystadenoma** \-sis′tadənō′mə\ SYRINGADENOMA. **s. papilliferum** A benign tumor of the apocrine sweat gland that appears clinically as a velvety red lesion, often on the scalp. It is characterized by the histologic presence of papillomatosis, cystic areas, two rows of epithelial cells, and abundant plasma cells in the stroma. Also *papillary syringadenoma.*

**syringocystoma** \-sistō′mə\ SYRINGADENOMA.

**syringoid** \siring′goid\ [SYRING- + -OID] Resembling a tube; pipelike.

**syringoma** \siring·gō′mə\ [SYRING- + -OMA] A benign tumor originating from the eccrine sweat duct and found chiefly in periorbital skin. Histologically, it is composed of groups of epithelial cells in ductlike structures. Frequently, it is formed of nests of epithelial cells with tail-like projections. Also *eruptive hidradenoma, hidradenoma eruptivum.* **chondroid s.** A benign tumor of the skin that mimics the histologic structure of a mixed tumor of the salivary glands, being composed of epithelial and mesenchymal components often resembling cartilage. Also *mixed tumor of the skin, salivary mixed cutaneous tumor, mixed tumor of salivary gland type.*

**syringomeningocele** \-məning′gōsēl\ [SYRINGO- + MENINGOCELE] A form of spina bifida consisting of a fluid-filled bulge on the back owing to a sac of meninges which has herniated through the spinal column defect but which retains a fistulous connection with the subarachnoid space. No cord or other nervous tissue is found in the sac.

**syringomyelia** \-mī·ē′lyə\ [SYRINGO- + MYEL- + -IA] A condition characterized by the formation of a central fluid-containing cavity in the substance of the spinal cord, usually occurring in the cervical region and giving rise to dissociated anesthesia (with loss of pain and temperature sensation but preservation of fine touch and tactile discrimination) often in a "half cape" over one shoulder and upper limb. It is presumed to be of developmental origin rather than a consequence of vascular insufficiency. In most cases there is atrophy and weakness of muscles in one or both hands and arms due to anterior horn cell involvement with loss of deep tendon reflexes in the affected upper limb or limbs. Often there are signs of pyramidal tract dysfunction in the legs. The commonest variety, the so-called communicating type, is often associated with the Chiari anomaly at the level of the foramen magnum. The cavity may extend up into the medulla oblongata (syringobulbia). In many cases surgical decompression at the foramen magnum is an effective treatment. Noncommunicating syringomyelia may develop at any level of the spinal cord above or below a transverse cord lesion due to trauma or in association with an intramedullary tumor. Also *hydrosyringomyelia, myelosyringocele, myelosyringosis, syringomyelus, cavitary myelitis, analgesic panaris, cavitating myelitis* (obs.). **traumatic s.** Syringomyelia resulting from injury to the spinal cord.

**syringomyelobulbia** \-mī′əlōbul′bē·ə\ Cavitation of the brain and spinal cord unrelated etiologically to interference with vascular supply; a combination of syringomyelia and syringobulbia. *Seldom used.*

**syringomyelocele** \-mī′əlōsēl′\ Central cavitation in that part of ectopic spinal cord that lies in a meningomyelocele which has herniated through a spina bifida defect and consequently bulges on the midline of the back. The cavity is continuous with the central canal of the spinal cord and is therefore a hydromyelia. *Seldom used.*

**syringomyelus** \-mī′ələs\ SYRINGOMYELIA.

**syringotomy** \sir′ing·gät′əmē\ [SYRINGO- + -TOMY] FISTULOTOMY.

**syrinx** \sir′ingks\ [Gk, a pipe, tube, airway, duct, fistula] (*pl.* syringes) A tube or pipe.

**syrosingopine** $C_{35}H_{42}N_2O_{11}$. Methyl 18-*O*-(4-ethoxycarbonyloxy-3,5-dimethoxybenzoyl)reserpate, an agent derived from reserpine by hydrolysis, followed by re-esterification. It has been used in treating hypertension.

**syrup** \sir′əp\ [Old French *sirop,* from Med L *syrupus* (from Arabic *sharāb* a beverage, fruit juice, fruit syrup, from *sharib* to drink) fruit syrup, syrup] A concentrated aqueous solution of a sugar, such as sucrose, which may contain medicinal or flavoring substances. It is most often used as a flavoring vehicle for other drugs. Also *sirup.* **acacia s.** A solution containing granular or powdered acacia 100 g, sodium benzoate 1 g, vanilla tincture 5 m, sucrose 800 g, and sufficient purified water to yield 1000 ml of fluid. It is used as a vehicle for medications. **aromatic eriodictyon s.** A solution containing eriodictyon fluidextract 32 ml, 1 in 20 potassium hydroxide solution 25 ml, compound cardamom tincture 65 ml, lemon oil 500 ml, clove oil 1 ml, alcohol 32 ml, sucrose 800 g, magnesium carbonate 5 g, and sufficient purified water to yield 1000 ml of liquid. It is used as a vehicle for medications, often to disguise the bitter taste of certain drugs. Also *aromatic yerba santa syrup, syrupus corrigens.* **bromides s.** A syrup containing ammonium, calcium, lithium, potassium, and sodium bromides. It was used for its central nervous system depressant properties in the past, but bromides have been largely replaced by less toxic, more effective agents. **cacao s.** COCOA SYRUP. **cherry s.** A solution containing cherry juice 475 ml, sucrose 800 g, alcohol 20 ml, and sufficient purified water to yield 1000 ml of liquid. It is used as a vehicle for medications. Also *syrupus cerasi.* **cocoa s.** A solution containing cocoa 180 g, sucrose 600 g, liquid glucose 180 g, sodium chloride 2 g, vanillin 200 mg, sodium benzoate 1 g, and sufficient purified water to yield 1000 ml. It is used as a flavored vehicle for medications. Also *cacao syrup.* **compound sarsaparilla s.** A solution containing sarsaparilla fluidextract, glycyrrhiza fluidextract, sassafras oil, anise oil, methyl salicylate, alcohol, and syrup. It is used as a vehicle for medications. Also *syrupus sarsaparillae compositus.* **compound white pine s.** A solution containing coarsely powdered white pine, wild cherry, aralia, poplar bud, sanguinaria, sassafras, amaranth solution, chloroform, sucrose, glycerin, alcohol, and water. It is used as a vehicle for medications and as an antitussive agent. Also *syrupus pini albae compositus.* **corn s.** LIQUID GLUCOSE. **ferrous iodide s.** A solution containing iron, iodine, hypophosphorous acid, and sucrose in purified water. It is used as a hematinic medication. **ferrous sulfate s.** A solution containing ferrous sulfate 40 g, hydrous citric acid 2.1 g, peppermint spirit 2 ml, sucrose 825 g, and sufficient purified water to yield 1000 ml of total liquid. It is used as an iron supplement. **garlic s.** SYRUPUS ALLII. **ginger s.** A solution containing strong tincture of ginger in simple syrup. Strong tincture of ginger contains 5% ginger. It is used as a carminative. **glycyrrhiza s.** A solution containing glycyrrhiza fluidextract, fennel oil, anise oil, and syrup. It is used as a flavored vehicle for medications. Also *licorice syrup.* **ipecac s.** A solution containing powdered ipecac 70 g, glycerin 100 ml, and sufficient syrup to make 1000 ml. It is used as an emetic. **lemon s.** An alcoholic solution containing an extract of fresh lemon peel, citric acid, and syrup. It is used as a flavored vehicle for medications. **licorice s.** GLYCYRRHIZA SYRUP. **s. of liquid glucose** A solution containing one part liquid glucose and two parts simple syrup. It is used in manufacturing pills. **medicated s.** A syrup to which a medicinal agent has been added. **orange s.** A solution containing sweet orange peel tincture 50 ml, anhydrous citric acid 5 g, talc 15 g, sucrose 820 g, and sufficient purified water to yield 1000 ml of liquid. It is utilized as a flavoring vehicle for medications. Also *syrupus aurantii.* **raspberry s.** A solution containing raspberry juice, sucrose, and alcohol in purified water. It is used as a flavored vehicle for medications. Also *syrupus rubi idaei.* **senna s.** A solution containing senna fluidextract 250 ml, coriander oil 5 ml, sucrose 625 g, and sufficient water to yield a total of 1000 ml. It is used as a cathartic medication. **simple s.** A syrup made up of purified water and sucrose. **s. of squills** A solution containing vinegar of squill and simple syrup. It is used in cough preparations. **Tolu balsam s.** A solution containing Tolu balsam tincture 50 ml, magnesium carbonate 10 g, sucrose 820 g, and sufficient purified water to yield a total of 1000 ml. It is used as a flavored vehicle for medications. Also *syrup of Tolu.* **white pine compound with codeine s.** A syrup containing compound white pine syrup to which codeine phosphate is added. It is used as an antitussive medication. **wild cherry s.** A solution containing a percolate of wild cherry, glycerin, sucrose, alcohol, and water. It is used as a flavored vehicle for medications.

**syrupus** \sir′əpəs\ [Med L. See SYRUP.] Syrup. **s. allii** A solution containing approximately 18 percent of the juice from *Allium sativum* (garlic). It is used in bronchitis and other pulmonary conditions for its expectorant action. Also *garlic syrup.* **s. aurantii** ORANGE SYRUP. **s. calcii lactophosphatis** A solution containing calcium lactate, phosphoric acid, and a syrup flavored with orange-flower water. It is used as a tonic. **s. cerasi** CHERRY SYRUP. **s. cocillanae compositus** A solution that contains cocillana, euphorbia liquid extracts, senega, squill, tartar emetic, codeine phosphate, menthol, and glycerin. It is used as an anticough preparation in adults. **s. corrigens** AROMATIC ERIODICTYON SYRUP. **s. papaveris** A syrup containing the liquid extract of poppy. It is used in cough preparations for its sedative properties. **s. pini albae compositus** COMPOUND WHITE PINE SYRUP. **s. pini albae compositus cum codeina** Compound white pine syrup with codeine. **s. rubi idaei** RASPBERRY SYRUP. **s. sarsaparillae compositus** COMPOUND SARSAPARILLA SYRUP.

**sys-** \sis-\ SYN-.

# system

**system** [Gk *systēma* (from *synistanai* to place or set together, combine, organize, from SYN- + Gk *histanai* to make stand, stand, set) a composite whole, what is put together] **1** A complex of anatomically related structures that perform a specific common function, such as that of digestion or blood circulation. Also *systema.* **2** A method or arrangement by which separate parts or functions are made use of so that they work together as a unit. **3** A method or plan of classification. **ABO blood group s.** A major system of red cell and tissue antigens. It comprises four antigenic types which are determined by the presence or absence of the antigens A and B, resulting in individual type A, B, AB, or O (O denoting an absent A or B antigen). Corresponding to the antigens A and B there are antibodies (isoagglutinins anti-A and anti-B, which occur in the sera of individuals whose cells lack the corresponding antigen. Thus, a person of group A has anti-B isoagglutinins, a group B person has anti-A isoagglutinin, a group O person has both anti-A and anti-B, and a group AB person has neither anti-A nor anti-B isoagglutinins. **absorbent s.** *Outmoded* SYSTEMA LYMPHATICUM. **adrenergic s.** **1** Those mechanisms in the body which have in common the use of catecholamines as chemical transmitters. **2** Pathways in the brain that utilize adrenergic substances as neurotransmitters. **alimentary s.** APPARATUS DIGESTORIUS. **anesthesia-breathing s.** A system consisting of a full-face mask, conduits, directional valves, a reservoir bag, and a carbon dioxide absorber, used, all or in part, for general anesthesia. Also *breathing system.* **arch-loop-whorl s.** The classification of fingerprints based on the arch, loop, or whorl patterns formed by the epidermal ridges on the volar surfaces of the distal phalanges. In any given population, 60–65% of individuals will have loop pattern fingerprints, 30–35% will have whorl patterns, and approximately 5% will have arch patterns. • This classification is the basis for all of the systems of 10 finger identification currently used. **ascending reticular activating s.** RETICULAR ACTIVATING SYSTEM. **association s.** Collectively, certain regions of the cerebral cortex together with the fiber systems that interconnect these regions to each other and to other cortical and certain subcortical centers, believed to be capable of integrating new incoming information with old stored information in order to effect an appropriate reaction. **autonomic nervous s.** SYSTEMA NERVOSUM AUTONOMICUM. **balanced lethal s.** In experimental genetics, a diploid strain heterozygous for two or more genes that, when any one gene is homozygous, produces a trait lethal before birth. When the heterozygous organisms are interbred, on average one half of the offspring die, or may not be recognized as having occurred at all, while one half are heterozygous. As a result, the parent appears to breed true with respect to the phenotypes determined by the genes at issue. **s. of Batson** VERTEBRAL-VENOUS SYSTEM. **biliary s.** BILIARY TRACT. **binary coded decimal s.** A numbering system that codes each decimal digit from 0 to 9 into 4-bit binary words from 0000 to 1001. **blood group s.** Inherited characters present on blood cells and in plasma which are grouped by allelic characteristics in antigen systems such as ABO, Rh, Kell, etc. See also BLOOD GROUP. **blood-vascular s.** CARDIOVASCULAR SYSTEM. **boarding-out s.** The placement of psychiatric patients in private residences rather than keeping them in hospitals. Also *villa system.* **body exhaust s.** A surgical gown and its incorporated helmet that is worn in operating rooms by hospital personnel. All air that is expired is mechanically removed from the operating environment to prevent the introduction of infection. **brain-cooling s.** Equipment for sensing brain temperature, cooling it to a predetermined temperature, and maintaining it at that temperature. **brainstem activating s.** RETICULAR ACTIVATING SYSTEM. **breathing s.** ANESTHESIA-BREATHING SYSTEM. **cardiovascular s.** The heart and blood vessels through which the blood circulates. Also *blood-vascular system.*

**case s.** A method of teaching medicine based on the careful analysis of reported clinical cases. **centimeter-gram-second s.** A system of units of mechanics in which the centimeter, gram, and second are the base units of length, mass, and time, respectively. Also *CGS system.* **central nervous s.** SYSTEMA NERVOSUM CENTRALE. **centrencephalic s.** A system of neuronal circuits integrating the functional activity of the reticular core of the medulla, pons, and mesencephalon with both cerebral hemispheres by way of diffusely projecting diencephalic-cortical pathways. **cerebellorubral s.** TRACTUS CEREBELLORUBRALIS. **cerebellorubrospinal s.** A system of pathways interconnecting the dentate, emboliform, and globose nuclei of the cerebellum, the red nucleus, and the spinal cord by way of the cerebellorubral tract and the rubrospinal tract. This system is important in modulating spinal reflexes as well as motor behavior under the control of the cerebral cortex. **cerebrospinal s.** SYSTEMA NERVOSUM CENTRALE. **CGS s.** CENTIMETER-GRAM-SECOND SYSTEM. **CGS electromagnetic s.** An aspect of the centimeter-gram-second system in which the electromagnetic unit is treated as a base unit. **chemoreceptor s.** A group of structures which sense blood levels of oxygen and carbon dioxide, for regulation of respiration. It includes the carotid body, glomus jugulare, and receptors in the aortic arch and pulmonary vessels. **chromaffin s.** Groups of chromaffin cells that, together with their associated excitatory sympathetic nerve fibers, occupy sites such as the adrenal medulla, sympathetic ganglia, and autonomic plexuses, and that secrete catecholamines. Chromaffin tissues are regarded as part of the endocrine system. **circle absorption s.** A closed-circuit, semiclosed-circuit, or semiopen anesthesia-breathing system in which inspiratory and expiratory valves direct expired air in one direction through a carbon dioxide absorber. **circulatory s.** The cardiovascular and lymphatic systems considered together. Also *vascular system.* **coherent s. of units** A system of units in which no numerical factor other than 1 is used when forming derived units by multiplication and/or division of the base units of the system. **complement s.** A group of nine plasma proteins that interact with each other, with antibodies, and with membranes to cause lysis of foreign cells or bacteria. The components of the complement system are designated C1, C2, C3, C4, C5, C6, C7, C8, and C9. Most of these components, when activated, are proteolytic enzymes. C1 is a complex of C1q, C1r and C1s. Attachment of the C1 components of complement to a membrane is initiated by attachment of immunoglobulin to the membrane. Components C2 and C4 are then deposited on the membrane, followed by deposition of C3b, a fragment of C3, and then by C5b, a fragment of C5. Components C6–C9 adhere to the membrane close to the C5b fragment, and together these components create an opening in the membrane large enough to permit cytoplasmic components to escape. In an alternate pathway, properdin activates C3 and initiates attachment of components C5–C9, bypassing the initial components of the complement system. **complete nonrebreathing s.** A nonvalvular or valvular system for producing general anesthesia in which there is a high flow of unrebreathed anesthetic gas with free escape of carbon dioxide. It is used principally in pediatric anesthesia because it is a low resistance system and the work of breathing is minimized. However, body heat and moisture are lost. Also *open system.* **conduction s. of the heart** The morphological structures that are responsible for the generation and transmission of rhythmical impulses that cause contraction of the heart muscle and the conduction of these impulses throughout the heart. These structures include the sinoatrial node, the atrioventricular node, and the atrioventricular bundle of Purkinje fibers (bundle of His). Also *systema conducens cardiacum, Purkinje system, cardionector.* **corticobulbar s.** The corticobulbar tract, considered together with its function. **corticopontine projection s.** Those fibers which originate in the frontal, temporal, parietal, and occipital cortex of the forebrain, descend through the capsula interna and crura cerebri, and terminate on cell groups of the pontine nuclei of the brainstem. **corticopontocerebellar s.** A system of nerve tracts that interconnect the cerebral cortex with the cerebellum by passing through pontine centers in the brainstem. Also *corticopontocerebellar pathways, corticopontocerebellar tracts.* **corticostrionigral s.** A system of neural connections between the cerebral cortex, the corpus striatum, and the substantia nigra. Also *corticostrionigral pathway.* **craniosacral autonomic nervous s.** SYSTEMA NERVOSUM AUTONOMICUM, PARS PARASYMPATHICA. **cutaneous s.** INTEGUMENTUM COMMUNE. **dentatorubral s.** TRACTUS CEREBELLORUBRALIS. **dermal s.** *Seldom used* INTEGUMENTUM COMMUNE. **dermoid s.** *Seldom used* INTEGUMENTUM COMMUNE. **digestive s.** APPARATUS DIGESTORIUS. **dioptric s.** A system that assists vision by refracting light through lenses, as in spectacles. **dopaminergic s.** A group of subsystems, pathways, and components in the nervous system for which dopamine is the synaptic transmitter. **dosimetric s.** A regular, organized system of designating the doses of a drug to be given. **dual-probe s.** Instrumentation composed of two scintillation detectors with appropriate electronics and recording devices for each detector, used, for example, to monitor the behavior of a radioactive tracer in two different locations in a patient. **duplex scanning s.** An ultrasound scanning system that combines real-time two-dimensional pulse echo imaging with pulse Doppler. **endocrine s.** The widely dispersed complex of glands of internal secretion. The hormones of these glands are secreted directly into the bloodstream and exert their actions on body tissues and functions generally or at remote and specific sites. The complex consisting of the hypothalamus, anterior and posterior pituitary, thyroid, adrenal cortex, and gonads operates as a true system. Other glands, acting independently of that system, are the parathyroids, the adrenal medulla, the endocrine pancreas, and the enterochromaffin cells of the gut. The endocrine roles of the thymus, the pineal, and the prostaglandins are uncertain. The general function of the endocrine glands as a group is considered to be homeostatic. Also *glandular system, hormonopoietic system* (rare). **endothelial s.** RETICULOENDOTHELIAL SYSTEM. **endovestibular s.** LABYRINTHUS VESTIBULARIS. **exteroceptive nervous s.** The system of afferent or sensory nerve fibers that carry impulses generated by stimuli from the external environment. These nerve fibers include those in the somatosensory nerves that carry impulses generated from general, or cutaneous, receptors as well as those in the special sensory nerves that respond to olfactory, visual, taste, and acoustic stimuli. **extracorticospinal s.** EXTRAPYRAMIDAL SYSTEM. **extrapyramidal s.** The basal ganglia and several related brainstem nuclei, the subthalamic nucleus, substantia nigra, red nucleus, and the reticular formation, which considered as a unit subserve aspects of motor control other than those conveyed by the pyramidal tract. A classical clinical example of disturbed function of the extrapyramidal system is parkinsonism. Also *extrapyramidal tract, extracorticospinal system, extracorticospinal tract.* **flush s.** In neurosurgery, a plastic reservoir interposed in a drainage system, used in the treatment of hydrocephalus.

The flushing of either the intraventricular and/or the distal end is accomplished by external compression of the reservoir while occluding the opposite segment of the drainage system. **fusimotor s.** A group of motoneurons (usually called $\gamma$-motoneurons) in the ventral gray matter of the spinal cord whose fibers emerge in the ventral roots and innervate the intrafusal muscle fibers of the muscle spindles. Also *gamma efferent system, gamma motor system, intrafusal motor system.* **Galton s. of classification of fingerprints** A system of classifying and recording the arch, loop, and whorl patterns of fingerprints proposed by Henry Galton in 1892, and adopted as the first system for fingerprint identification of criminals. **gamma efferent s.** FUSIMOTOR SYSTEM. **gamma motor s.** FUSIMOTOR SYSTEM. **genital s.** REPRODUCTIVE SYSTEM. **genitourinary s.** APPARATUS UROGENITALIS. **glandular s.** ENDOCRINE SYSTEM. **haversian s.** OSTEON. **hematopoietic s.** The tissues and organs in which blood cells are formed, including bone marrow, lymphglands, and spleen. **hemolytic s.** An assay system for complement fixation tests. It is made up of sheep erythrocytes coated with specific antibody usually raised in rabbits or horses and suspended in a buffered salt solution containing optimal concentrations of calcium and magnesium ions. **Henry s. of classification of fingerprints** A system of classifying fingerprints proposed by Sir Richard Henry in 1900, in which the epidermal ridge pattern on each of the ten fingers is assigned a numerical value based upon the presence of whorls, loops, and arches, and each finger is assigned a numerical value. This system, with some modifications, is currently used in most English-speaking countries. **hepatic duct s.** A system of intrahepatic and extrahepatic excretory ducts that drain bile from the various segments of the lobes of the liver where they are formed by the union of biliferous ductules and convey the bile to the common bile duct. They include the ductus hepaticus dexter, ductus hepaticus sinister, ductus hepaticus communis, ductus lobi caudati dexter, and ductus lobi caudati sinister. **hepatic portal s.** The venous network draining the spleen and gastrointestinal tract into the liver. It is part of the dual blood supply of the liver, along with the hepatic artery. **hexaxial reference s.** A system of lines resulting from the axes of the bipolar leads I, II, and III of the electrocardiogram combined with those of the unipolar limb leads. See also STANDARD LEAD. **H-2 histocompatibility s.** The major histocompatibility system in the mouse, it is composed of a number of H-2 genes which control the histocompatibility antigens on somatic cell surfaces as well as the immune responses of the animal. The antigens within a given mouse strain are controlled by arrangement of alleles of these tightly linked loci. **HL-A s.** HLA HISTOCOMPATIBILITY SYSTEM. **HLA histocompatibility s.** The major histocompatibility system in humans, containing genes which control the presence of cell surface antigens as well as the individual's ability to stimulate an immune response (Ir genes). Several major loci have been discovered, called HLA-A, B, C, and D, with many alleles at each locus. The loci are tightly linked in the major histocompatibility complex on human chromosome 6. Also *HL-A system.* **hormonopoietic s.** *Rare* ENDOCRINE SYSTEM. **hypophysioportal s.** The pituitary-portal system of veins. A group of descending veins that receive blood from the tufted capillaries in the median eminence and infundibulum of the hypothalamus, form vascular sinusoids, and carry blood into the anterior part of the pituitary gland. These vessels are frequently classified into long hypophysial veins, which drain the median eminence and the upper part of the infundibulum, and short hypophysial veins,

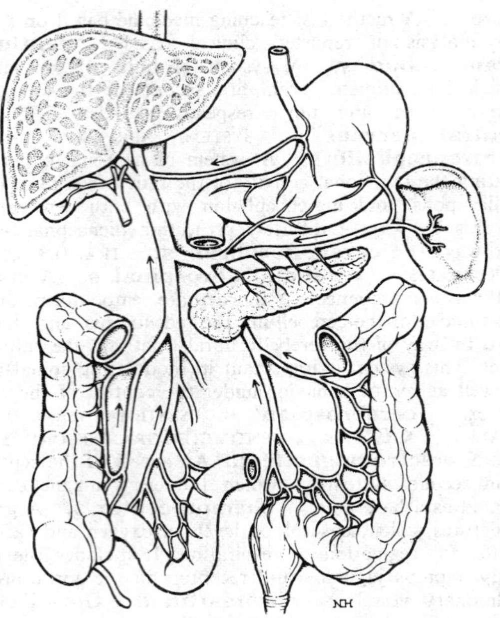

Hepatic portal system

which drain the lower infundibulum. The venous blood within the hypophysioportal system carries hormone-releasing factors from the hypothalamus to the cells of the anterior pituitary gland; hence, the system is of great functional significance. **hypothalamohypophysial s.** The anatomic and functional unit comprising several nuclei of the hypothalamus, the infundibulum, pituitary portal venous system, pituitary stalk, anterior pituitary, and the hypothalamic releasing hormones, which through long- and short-loop feedback mechanisms control the release and possibly the synthesis of the anterior pituitary hormones. **hypothalamoneurohypophysial s.** SUPRAOPTICOHYPOPHYSIAL SYSTEM. **hypoxia warning s.** Equipment that measures the partial pressure of oxygen and sets off an audible or visual alarm when it falls to a dangerous level. **immune s.** Those organs, cells, and molecules involved in the induction and manifestations of specific immune responses. **inducible s.** In the operon model of genetic regulation, a system in which an inducer substance interferes with the action of the repressor molecule, thus releasing the inhibition of transcription and permitting expression of the operon. **integumentary s.** INTEGUMENTUM COMMUNE. **International System of Units** See under SYSTÈME INTERNATIONAL D'UNITÉS. **interoceptive nervous s.** A system of sensory fibers carrying impulses generated from receptors located in the internal organs, or viscera. These visceral afferent fibers course either in somatic or in visceral nerves and, together with the visceral efferent fibers (autonomic fibers), constitute the visceral nervous system. **interofective s.** *Seldom used* VISCERAL NERVOUS SYSTEM. **interrenal s.** *Obs.* CORTEX GLANDULAE SUPRARENALIS. **intrafusal motor s.** FUSIMOTOR SYSTEM. **involuntary nervous s.** SYSTEMA NERVOSUM AUTONOMICUM. **kinesiodic s.** The great descending spinal motor pathways, along with the spinal efferent or motor elements that control the musculature. *Seldom used.* **labyrinthine s.** LABYRINTHUS VESTIBULARIS. **limbic s.** Those portions of the brain involved in controlling emotions and their autonomic effects, the activities of the autonomic nervous system generally and, through them, the viscera. Structurally, it includes a series of sub-cortical nuclei and their connections, the archeopallium, the paleopallium, and the parahippocampal and cingulate gyri of the bordering neopallium. Also *visceral brain* (outmoded). **lymphatic s.** SYSTEMA LYMPHATICUM. **macrophage s.** RETICULOENDOTHELIAL SYSTEM. **Manchester s.** In interstitial radium therapy, the method designed to facilitate the determination of the quantity of radium, expressed in milligram-hours, and the placement of various needles or tubes which must be used to provide as homogeneous a dose as possible with no point in the irradiated volume receiving less than the prescribed dose. **metameric nervous s.** Phylogenetically the oldest part of the nervous system, consisting largely of the basal ganglia and brainstem nuclei (the paleencephalon) and the gray matter of the spinal cord. **metanephric excretory s.** The collecting duct system of the metanephros, which begins to develop in the fourth week of embryonic life from the ureteric bud or diverticulum. **metanephric secretory s.** The secretory system of the embryonic kidney arising in the metanephric blastema, the caudalmost unsegmented part of the nephrogenic cord formed in the intermediate mass of mesoderm placed between the somites and the lateral plate mesoderm. **metric s.** Any decimal system of measurement based on the meter and the gram. **Meyer s.** PSYCHOBIOLOGY. **microcirculatory s.** The very small blood and lymphatic vessels that constitute the site of metabolic exchange between tissue and circulating blood. It includes pulmonary and systemic capillaries, precapillaries, arterioles, venules, and the smallest lymphatic channels. **mobile artery and vein imaging s.** A multichanneled pulsed Doppler flow detection system said to be able to provide noninvasive visualization of peripheral arteries and vascular grafts. Abbr. MAVIS **mononuclear phagocyte s.** The system of mononuclear phagocyte cells arising from promonocytes of the bone marrow and of which the macrophage is the mature cell. Some of these cells are in the tissues (fixed) while others circulate in blood and body fluids. Also *phagocytic system.* **musculoskeletal s.** All the muscles and bones in the body together with their connecting ligaments. **neokinetic s.** The great neocortical spinal motor pathways that are instrumental in the initiation of voluntary motor activity. **nervous s.** SYSTEMA NERVOSUM. **neuromuscular s.** The system of muscles throughout the body, including the cranial and spinal nerves that supply them. **nonspecific s.** RETICULAR ACTIVATING SYSTEM. **oculomotor s.** The system comprising the extraocular muscles, which are capable of moving the eyeballs, the nerves (oculomotor, trochlear, and abducens) that supply these muscles, and the central nervous system pathways mediating both involuntary and voluntary eye movements. **on-line computer s.** A computer system that acquires data directly from their source and transmits data directly to where they are used rather than converting data to other forms such as punched cards or magnetic tape. **open s.** COMPLETE NONREBREATHING SYSTEM. **pallidal s.** The large number of efferent nerve fibers that emerge from the globus pallidus and terminate in the thalamus, subthalamus, and mesencephalon. Also *pallidofugal pathways.* **palm-and-sole s. of identification** A classification of palmprints and footprints, used for the purpose of identification. **parasympathetic s.** SYSTEMA NERVOSUM AUTONOMICUM, PARS PARASYMPATHICA. **parasympathetic nervous s.** SYSTEMA NERVOSUM AUTONOMICUM, PARS PARASYMPATHICA. **peripheral nervous s.** SYSTEMA NERVOSUM PERIPHERICUM. **periventricular s.** Collectively, the elements forming the diencephalic and mesencephalic periventricular gray substance and its efferent pathways. The diencephalic periventricular system, sometimes called the dorsal longitudinal fasciculus (of Schütz), consists of vertically or obliquely arranged fibers surrounding the third ventricle that at this level interconnect preoptic and other hypothalamic regions with the dorsal thalamus. The mesencephalic periventricular system actually surrounds the cerebral aqueduct, and consists dorsally of the periaqueductal layer of the superior colliculus. Ventrolaterally, it helps form the lower end of the dorsal longitudinal fasciculus. A pathway at this level interconnects diencephalic, midbrain, and other brainstem structures. **phagocytic s.** MONONUCLEAR PHAGOCYTE SYSTEM. **pituitary portal s.** An arrangement of venous channels between the hypothalamus, the infundibulum, and the anterior lobe of the hypophysis by which certain substances produced in the hypothalamus, such as the hypothalamic releasing hormones, are transported to the cells of the anterior lobe, where their secretions, the pituitary hormones, are liberated into the bloodstream. **pneumatic s. of the temporal bone** The honeycomb of air cells occupying the mastoid process and adjacent parts of the temporal bone in four out of five adults. **portal s.** A system wherein the blood passes through two sets of capillaries or capillarylike vessels before reaching a large vessel returning the blood to the heart. **pressoreceptor s.** A group of rapidly reacting neural mechanisms that help to maintain control of arterial blood pressure. Pressoreceptors or baroreceptors located in the walls of certain large systemic arteries or in the atria of the heart respond quickly to changes in blood pressure by transmitting impulses to the brain by way of visceral afferent nerve fibers. This information then induces visceral efferent responses, by way of autonomic fibers, that alter blood pressure in the direction that would tend to re-establish homeostasis. **projection s.** Any system of neuronal pathways coursing from one region of the central nervous system to another, implying the passage of neuronal impulses in that direction, such as the thalamic projection systems to the cerebral cortex or the cerebral cortical projection systems to the brainstem and spinal cord. **Purkinje s.** CONDUCTION SYSTEM OF THE HEART. **renin-angiotensin s.** A biochemical feedback system that is an important factor in blood pressure homeostasis. Renin, a proteolytic enzyme produced and stored in the juxtaglomerular apparatus, cleaves angiotensinogen, a globulin produced by the liver, to form a decapeptide angiotensin I, which in turn is changed by converting enzyme produced mainly in the lungs, to angiotensin II. Angiotensin II, an octapeptide, is the most powerful vasoconstrictor known and also stimulates aldosterone secretion. A decrease in blood pressure stimulates renin secretion while an increase in blood pressure cuts off renin secretion. The renin-angiotensin system may be altered in several disease states, including some forms of hypertension and renal and hepatic diseases. **renin-angiotensin-aldosterone s.** A renal-plasma-adrenocortical-vasomotor system which functions to regulate blood pressure and sodium balance. The juxtaglomerular cells of the kidney secrete the enzyme renin in response to changes in blood volume and arteriolar tone. The renin enters the bloodstream and converts angiotensinogen to angiotensin, a potent vasoconstrictive substance which stimulates aldosterone secretion. The aldosterone regulates renal tubular reabsorption of sodium and secretion of potassium, thereby influencing blood volume and blood pressure. The system is overactive in conditions marked by renal ischemia, such as renovascular disorders, chronic nephritides, and malignant hypertension. It is underactive when blood volume is excessive, as in primary hyperaldosteronism when an autonomous adrenocortical adenoma hypersecretes aldosterone. **reproductive s.** The portion of the urogenital apparatus composed of the internal and external genitals of males and females and involved in reproduction of the species. Also *genital system.* **respiratory s.** APPARATUS RESPIRATORIUS. **reticular s.** FORMATIO RETICULARIS. **reticular activating s.** A physiological system located in the reticular formation of the brainstem which extends into the thalamus and projects functionally to the cerebral cortex and which is believed to be responsible for the maintenance of an activated electroencephalogram as well as behavioral wakefulness. It has been shown that the reticular formation receives collateral fibers from sensory pathways which interconnect the reticular activating system with receptors all over the body, thereby explaining how acute sensory stimulation can arouse a sleeping subject. Also *brainstem activating system, ascending reticular activating system, nonspecific system, reticular alerting system.* **reticuloendothelial s.** A scattered system of macrophage cells principally of bone marrow, spleen, and liver, but also of other organs. It includes histiocytes, monocytes, Kupffer cells, and pulmonary macrophages, among others. It is sometimes considered to include also fibroblasts, lymphocytes, and all hematopoietic cells. Also *macrophage system, endothelial system, reticuloendothelium.* **rubrospinal s.** The descending neuronal pathway which arises in the red nucleus of the midbrain, decussates, travels caudally through the brainstem and the lateral column of the spinal cord, terminating primarily upon flexor motoneurons upon which it exerts a facilitatory effect. **schlieren s.** An instrument that visualizes sound beams by using light refracted by density variations resulting from sound. **self s.** The final self that emerges from a range of possible attributes which are reduced as the child discards those that elicit rejection or fail to elicit love from the significant others in his environment. **sensory s.** Those parts of the nervous system dealing with the sensations of pain, touch, and temperature. *Outmoded.* **somatic nervous s.** That part of the nervous system concerned on the sensory side with the reception, transmission, perception, analysis, and recognition of somatic sensory information, and on the motor side with the control of movement. **somesthetic s.** The sensory component of the somatic nervous system concerned with the outer surface of the body. **stomatognathic s.** MASTICATORY APPARATUS. **supraopticohypophysial s.** A system of morphologically and functionally related structures that includes the supraoptic nucleus of the hypothalamus, the supraopticohypophysial tract, and the posterior lobe of the pituitary gland. It mediates the production, storage, and release of vasopressin, oxytocin, and the neurophysins. Also *supraopticoneurohypophysial system, hypothalamoneurohypophysial system.* **supraopticoneurohypophysial s.** SUPRAOPTICOHYPOPHYSIAL SYSTEM. **sympathetic nervous s.** SYSTEMA NERVOSUM AUTONOMICUM, PARS SYMPATHICA. **T s.** A system of branching tubular invaginations of the sarcolemma in skeletal muscle fibers that are located at the junctions between the A and I bands in higher vertebrates. They serve to carry the wave of electric depolarization of the sarcolemma into the depths of the muscle fiber when it is stimulated to contract. **thoracicolumbar autonomic nervous s.** SYSTEMA NERVOSUM AUTONOMICUM, PARS SYMPATHICA. **to-and-fro absorption s.** A closed-circuit, semiclosed-circuit or semiopen anesthesia-breathing system with no directional valves, where both inspired and expired gas pass through a carbon dioxide absorber. **triad s.** In skeletal muscle fibers, the close association of deep invaginations of the sarcolemma with pairs of sarcoplasmic reticulum channels to provide rapid conduction of the excitatory stimuli to all parts of the fibers. **urogenital s.** APPARATUS UROGENITALIS. **vagal autonomic s.** That portion of the parasympathetic component of the autonomic nervous system outflow which is mediated by the vagus nerve. Cell bodies of origin, lying in the dorsal motor nucleus of the vagus nerve in the floor of the fourth ventricle, send axons to terminal parasympathetic ganglia innervating the thoracic and abdominal viscera including the entire gastrointestinal tract as far caudally as the splenic flexure. **vascular s.** CIRCULATORY SYSTEM. **vegetative nervous s.** SYSTEMA NERVOSUM AUTONOMICUM. **vertebral-basilar s.** The formation of the basilar artery by the union of the two vertebral arteries, including their branches. **vertebral-venous s.** A network of valveless veins extending along the vertebral column from the cranial cavity to the pelvis and comprising the external and internal vertebral venous plexuses which communicate with the cranial sinuses, the azygos veins, and superior vena cava in the thorax; the ascending lumbar veins and inferior vena cava in the abdomen; and with the pelvic venous plexuses as well as with subcutaneous plexuses in the limbs. Thereby the cranial sinuses communicate with the pelvis without the blood passing through the lungs. In addition, the spread of metastases is faciliated without involving the portal, pulmonary and caval circulations. Also *system of Batson, Batson's plexus.* **vestibular s.** LABYRINTHUS VESTIBULARIS. **villa s.** BOARDING-OUT SYSTEM. **visceral nervous s.** That part of the nervous system concerned with the innervation of the internal organs of the body and the maintenance of homeostasis. It includes afferent and efferent components, the latter consisting of sympathetic and parasympathetic divisions. Also *interofective system.*

**systema** \sistē′mə\ [NA] SYSTEM. **s. conducens cardiacum** CONDUCTION SYSTEM OF THE HEART. **s. digestorium** APPARATUS DIGESTORIUS. **s. lymphaticum** [NA] That part of the circulatory system consisting of the lymph nodes and the lymphatic vessels as well as the spleen and various sites of lymphoid tissue. Also *lymphatic system, absorbent system* (outmoded). **s. nervorum centrale** SYSTEMA NERVOSUM CENTRALE. **s. nervorum periphericum** SYSTEMA NERVOSUM PERIPHERICUM. **s. nervorum sympathicum** *Obs.* SYSTEMA NERVOSUM AUTONOMICUM. **s. nervosum** [NA] The organ system including all neural structures throughout the body, allowing an organism to perceive environmental and internal stimuli, to integrate this information, and to respond reflexly or purposefully. The nervous system includes a central portion, consisting of the brain and spinal cord, and a peripheral portion composed of the cranial and spinal nerves and their associated plexuses and ganglia. Also *nervous system.* **s. nervosum autonomicum** [NA] The part of the nervous system not under voluntary control that influences the activity of all of the viscera except the brain and including the heart, lungs, and gastrointestinal and urinary organs, as well as the lacrimal, salivary, and sweat glands. It is a two-motoneuron system consisting of preganglionic and postganglionic neurons, and comprises sympathetic (pars sympathica) and parasympathetic (pars parasympathica) components. Also *autonomic nervous system, involuntary nervous system, systema nervorum sympathicum, vegetative nervous system.* **s. nervosum autonomicum, pars parasympathica** [NA] The parasympathetic division of the autonomic nervous system, the preganglionic neurons of which are found in the third, seventh, ninth, and tenth cranial nerves and the second, third, and fourth sacral nerves. The parasympathetic system tends to slow the heart, lower the blood pressure, constrict the pupils, relax the sphincters of hollow organs, promote peristalsis and is generally active during periods of calm and tranquillity. It helps promote digestion and absorption. Also *parasympathetic nervous system, craniosacral division, craniosacral autonomic nervous system, parasympathetic system, pars parasympathica systematis nervosi autonomici.* **s. nervosum autonomicum, pars sympathica** [NA] The sympathetic division of the autonomic nervous system, consisting of preganglionic fibers that arise in the lateral gray column of the thoracic and upper two or three lumbar segments of the spinal cord, relay in the ganglia of the paravertebral sympathetic trunks or in the prevertebral ganglia, and course with spinal nerves or within autonomic nerve plexuses. The sympathetic division of the autonomic nervous system tends to speed up the heart, raise the blood pressure, dilate the pupils, contract the sphincters of hollow organs, and relax the longitudinal musculature. It prepares an individual for challenging situations and is active during periods of stress and adversity. Also *thoracicolumbar autonomic nervous system, thoracolumbar outflow, sympathetic nervous system, thoracicolumbar division.* **s. nervosum centrale** [NA] The system of nerve tracts interconnecting, and comprising, the brain and spinal cord. Also *central nervous system, cerebrospinal system, systema nervorum centrale, neuraxis.* **s. nervosum periphericum** [NA] The part of the nervous system that includes the cranial and spinal peripheral nerves and their associated ganglia. Also *peripheral nervous system, systema nervorum periphericum.* **s. respiratorium** APPARATUS RESPIRATORIUS. **s. urogenitale** APPARATUS UROGENITALIS. **s. vasorum** The blood and lymph vessels of the body considered together. *Outmoded.*

**systematic** \sis′təmat′ik\ [Gk *systēmatikos* (from *systēma* a composite whole) like or forming a whole] **1** Of or relating to a system. **2** Arranged or undertaken according to a system.

**systematics** \sis′təmat′iks\ [SYSTEMATIC + pl. suffix *-s*] TAXONOMY.

**Système International d'Unités** \sēstem′ eNternasyônal′ dYnētā′\ The modern version of the metric system of units of measurement, based on the meter-kilogram-second-ampere system but expanded to include seven base units. It was adopted by the Conférence Général des Poids et Mesures, and the name was agreed upon at the 11th conference in 1960. The seven base units and the quantities they measure are: meter (*metre* in international use) for length; kilogram, for mass; second, for time; ampere, for electric current; kelvin, for thermodynamic temperature; mole, for amount of substance; and candela, for luminous intensity. Abbr. SI • In English it is commonly known as the International System of Units, but the abbreviation *SI* is used internationally, and the units are designated SI units.

**systemic** \sistem′ik\ [SYSTEM + -IC] **1** Of, relating to, or affecting the body as a whole, as *systemic infection.* **2** Designating that part of the circulation supplied by the aorta as distinct from that supplied by the pulmonary artery.

**systemoid** \sis′təmoid\ Resembling a system.

**systole** \sis′təlē\ [Gk *systolē* (from *systellein* to draw in, draw together, contract, from SYN- + Gk *stellein* to arrange, set in order) a contraction, contracting] The contraction phase of the atria or ventricles in the cardiac cycle. Also *miocardia.* Compare DIASTOLE. **atrial s.** Contraction of the atria. **end s.** The terminal part of systole. **extra s.** See under EXTRASYSTOLE. **premature s.** EXTRASYSTOLE. **ventricular s.** Contraction of the ventricles.

**systolic** \sistäl′ik\ Relating to or occurring during systole.

**systremma** \sistrem′ə\ [Gk *systremma* (from *systrephein* to twist up together) a thing twisted up together, tumor, roundness of form] A muscular cramp, usually of the calf muscles in the leg.

**syzygial** \sizij′ē·əl\ Relating to syzygy.

**syzygiology** \sizij′ē·äl′əjē\ [Gk *syzygi(a)* union, combination + *o* + -LOGY] The study of the interrelationships of the parts of a whole organism as opposed to the study of the parts in isolation.

**syzygy** \siz′ijē\ [Gk *syzygia* (from *sy(n)-* together + *zyg(on)* yoke) union, conjunction, pairing] **1** The end-to-end chain formation or lateral nonsexual pairing of certain protozoans. **2** The pairing of chromosomes in meiosis. **3** The fusion of parts or organs that retain their characteristics.

**Szondi** [Lipot *Szondi,* Swiss psychotherapist, born 1893] See under TEST.

**Szymanowski** [J. von *Szymanowski,* Russian surgeon, 1829–1868] **1** See under OPERATION. **2** Kuhnt-Szymanowski procedure. See under KUHNT-SZYMANOWSKI OPERATION.

# T

**T** **1** Symbol for tera-: used with SI units. **2** Symbol for threonine. **3** Symbol for ribosylthymine. **4** temperature.

**$T_3$** triiodothyronine.

**$T_4$** thyroxine.

**t.** **1** temporal. **2** temperature (in degrees Celsius).

**Ta** Symbol for the element, tantalum.

**tabacism** \tab′əsizm\ TOBACCO POISONING.

**tabacosis** \tab′əkō′sis\ [Spanish *tabac(o)* tobacco + -OSIS] TOBACCO POISONING.

**tabagism** \tab′əjizm\ TOBACCO POISONING.

**tabanid** \tab′ənid\ **1** Of or belonging to the family Tabanidae. **2** A fly of the family Tabanidae.

**Tabanidae** \təban′idē\ [*Taban(us)* + -IDAE] A family of strong-flying, avid-biting flies, notorious pests of horses, cattle, deer, and other animals, especially herbivores. It includes the genera *Tabanus* (horseflies) and *Chrysops* (deer flies or mangrove flies), some of which are important transmitters of a number of blood-borne parasites.

***Tabanus*** \təbā′nəs\ [L, a gadfly, horsefly] A genus of blood-sucking flies. Some species transmit important diseases of domestic animals and man, including anthrax, surra, theileriasis, and certain filarial nematodes. Important species includes *T. atratus,* the black horsefly of North America; *T. bovinus,* which attacks cattle in Asia, Africa, and South

America; *T. ditaeniatus* and *T. fasciatus,* the seroot flies of the Sudan; *T. punctifer* in the western United States and *T. sulcifrons* in the plains states; *T. quinquevittatus* and *T. nigrovittatus,* the greenhead flies; *T. lineola* and *T. similis,* the striped horseflies. All are notorious biting pest flies.

**tabatière anatomique** \tabatyer′ anatômēk′\ The French term for ANATOMICAL SNUFFBOX.

**tabefaction** \tab′əfak′shən\ [*tabe(s)* + L *factio,* gen. *factionis* (from *facere* to make, do) a making, doing] Severe wasting, either of the muscles or generally as in emaciation. Also *tabification, tabes.*

**tabella** \təbel′ə\ [L (dim. of *tabula* table), tablet] A medicated tablet.

**tabes** \tā′bēz\ [L (akin to *tabere* to melt, dissolve, disintegrate and to English *thaw*) liquefaction, disintegration, decay, wasting away] **1** TABEFACTION. **2** TABES DORSALIS. Adj. tabetic. **cerebral t.** GENERAL PARESIS. **cervical t.** Tabes dorsalis affecting predominantly the cervical portion of the spinal cord and thus affecting the upper limbs before the lower. Also *tabes superior.* **diabetic t.** DIABETIC PSEUDOTABES. **t. dorsalis** A form of neurosyphilis characterized by a syndrome including Argyll Robertson pupils with severe sensory ataxia, areflexia, insensitivity to pressure pain in the Achilles tendon, severe loss of position and joint sense in the limbs, lightning pains in the extremities, tabetic crises, and often Charcot's joint. The principal histologic changes are in the root entry zones of the posterior spinal nerve roots with consequential degeneration and atrophy of the posterior columns of the cord. Also *locomotor ataxia, posterior spinal sclerosis, posterior sclerosis, tabetic neurosyphilis, neurotabes, tabes spinalis, Duchenne's disease, tabes, myelanalosis* (outmoded), *progressive locomotor asynergy.* **t. ergotica** A toxic condition resulting from use of ergot alkaloids. Symptoms, which are usually caused by overdosage but may be due to individual susceptibility, are nausea, vomiting, weakness, tremors, confusion, convulsions, tachycardia, and mydriasis. **Friedreich's t.** FRIEDREICH'S DISEASE. **t. infantum** Tabes dorsalis in infants or children due to congenital syphilis. **t. mesenterica** Progressive wasting of the body resulting from tuberculosis of the mesenteric lymph nodes. Also *atrophia mesenterica.* **monosymptomatic t.** Tabes dorsalis manifested by a single symptom. **peripheral t.** PSEUDOTABES. **t. spasmodica** SPASTIC DIPLEGIA. **t. spinalis** TABES DORSALIS. **t. superior** CERVICAL TABES.

**tabescent** \tābes′ənt\ [L *tabescens,* gen. *tabescentis,* pres. part. of *tabescere* to waste away, decay] Becoming emaciated; wasting away.

**tabetic** \tābet′ik\ [L *tab(es)* a wasting away, decay + *-etic(us)* adjectival suffix] Pertaining to or affected by tabes dorsalis. Also *tabic, tabid.*

**tabetiform** \tābet′ifôrm\ Resembling tabes dorsalis.

**tabic** \tab′ik\ TABETIC.

**tabid** \tab′id\ TABETIC.

**tabification** \tab′ifikā′shən\ TABEFACTION.

**tablature** \tab′ləchər\ The formation of the major cranial bones by an inner and an outer table or plate of compact bone separated from each other by the diploë.

**table** [L *tabula*] **1** An arrangement of data that is designed to facilitate access to specific items in the arrangement. **2** In anatomy, a flat layer or surface, as of the outer and inner laminae of the cranial bones. Also *tabula.* **abridged life t.** A life table giving values for the basic functions for certain pivotal years only, usually spaced at five- or ten-year intervals. **Albee fracture t.** A specially designed operating table for the reduction of limb fractures and application of full-body or extensive limb plaster casts. **Bull and Fischer mortality t.'s** A statistical compilation of data used to compare mortality of burn patients by method of treatment after adjustment for age and size of burn. **complete life t.** A life table giving values for the basic functions for each year of life from birth to the last year applicable. **contingency t.** A statistical table showing the classification of an aggregate of entities according to two qualitative attributes, each attribute being divided into two or more subgroups. One attribute would be represented by the rows of the table, there being as many rows as there are subgroups of the attribute. The other attribute would be represented similarly by the columns of the table. Thus, if attribute A has *i* subgroups and attribute B has *j* subgroups, the table would have *ij* cells. Also *cross-classification table.* **Ely's t.** A table of estimated date of delivery based on counting 280 days from the first day of the last menstrual period. **fourfold t.** In statistics, a table with four cells showing how many members of a set, such as a sample of patients, possess one but not the other, both, or neither of two attributes. Conventionally, the entries in a fourfold table are designated: *a* (positive for both attributes), *b* (positive for the first and negative for the second attribute), *c* (negative for the first and positive for the second), and *d* (negative for both). **Gaffky t.** GAFFKY SCALE. **inner t.** LAMINA INTERNA CRANII. **inner t. of bones of skull** LAMINA INTERNA CRANII. **inner t. of frontal bone** *Outmoded* FACIES INTERNA OSSIS FRONTALIS. **life t.** A table indicating quantitatively the pattern of mortality associated with a particular generation. Starting with a given number of newborns it is assumed the generation will be subject at each successive age to the prevailing rates of mortality at those ages. The life table sets out how many persons will attain various ages under those conditions. A complete life table will show, for each year of age, the probability of dying before attaining the next age, the proportion surviving, and the expectation of life. **occlusal t.** The total surface of posterior teeth taking part in mastication. **outer t. of bones of skull** LAMINA EXTERNA CRANII. **tilt t.** A physical therapy treatment plinth adapted for rotation from the horizontal to the vertical position and having a footboard such that a patient may be maintained at a specific desired angle ranging from horizontal to full standing with minimal energy expenditure. It is used in the treatment of spinal cord injury and other conditions in which rapid elevation to an upright posture is detrimental, and to achieve the physiological and psychological advantages of the upright position. Also *tilting table.*

**tablespoon** A unit of capacity equal to 15 milliliters. *Popular.* Symbol: tbs, tbsp

**tablet** [French *tablette* (dim. of *table* table, from L *tabula* table) a small table] A compressed, solid, rounded disk form of oral medication, composed of one or more drugs, a disintegrating agent such as starch, suitable binding agents, and other materials that facilitate manufacture and lend desired characteristics to the product. **buccal t.** A tablet to be held between the cheek and gum to permit gradual absorption of medication through the oral mucosa. **dispensing t.** Compressed tablets of potent substances or highly concentrated drugs to be used by the dispensing pharmacist in compounding prescriptions. **enteric-coated t.** A pill with a special coating designed to prevent disintegration until it has left the stomach and entered the intestine. **hypodermic t.** A medicated tablet designed to be given by hypodermic injection after being dissolved in water. **sublingual t.** A small, flat, oval tablet to be held under the tongue to permit direct sublingual absorption of the medication. **t. triturate** A tablet containing a medication with lactose that is dissolved in sterile water just before injection.

**taboparesis** \tā'bōpərē'sis\ Simultaneous manifestations of tabes dorsalis and of general paresis occurring as a result of neurosyphilis. Also *taboparalysis.*

**tabula** \tab'yələ\ [L, table] TABLE.

**tabun** A toxic substance of formula $(CH_3)_2N$—P(=O)-(—$OC_2H_5$)—CN. It phosphorylates a reactive serine residue of acetylcholinesterase and of serine proteinases. Its effect on acetylcholinesterase is responsible for its lethal action. It has been used as an insecticide. Tabun and its derivatives are chemical warfare agents (nerve gases) prohibited by international treaty.

**tache** \täsh\ [Middle French, a stain, spot] A flat spot or mark. **t. blanche** (*pl.* taches blanches) A white spot on the liver associated with infiltration of leukocytes and bacteria in some infectious diseases. **t. motrice** MOTOR ENDPLATE. **t. noire** A black-crusted ulcer occurring at the site of the bite of an infected tick in certain tick-borne diseases such as scrub typhus or boutonneuse fever. **t.'s noires sclérotiques** The triangular, brownish, discolored area of the sclera, found when the eyelids remain open after death. The base of the triangular area coincides with the periphery of the cornea while the sides of the triangle correspond to the edges of the unclosed eyelids. This phenomenon is detectable within two to four hours following death. **t. spinale** A cutaneous blister occurring in spinal cord disease, usually as a consequence of sensory loss.

**tachistoscope** \təkis'təskōp\ [Gk *tachisto(s),* superl. of *tachys* quick + -SCOPE] A device that flashes a test pattern for only a fraction of a second, used to study visual perception. With the head held in a fixed position, the subject looks forward into a hemisphere in which light stimuli can be presented serially or simultaneously in all parts of the visual field.

**tachistoscopy** \tak'istäs'kəpē\ [Gk *tachisto(s)* (superl. of *tachys* swift) swiftest + -SCOPY] The assessment of visual perception in all parts of the visual field with a tachistoscope.

**tacho-** \tak'ō-\ [Gk *tachos* speed] A combining form meaning speed.

**tachometer** \təkäm'ətər\ [TACHO- + -METER] An instrument that measures speed or rate, such as a cardiotachometer or pneumotachometer. Also *tachymeter.*

**tachy-** \tak'ē-\ [Gk *tachys* quick, fast] A combining form meaning (1) quick, rapid; (2) abnormally rapid.

**tachyarrhythmia** \-əriTH'mē·ə\ [TACHY- + ARRHYTHMIA] A disturbance of cardiac rhythm in which the heart rate exceeds 100 beats per minute.

**tachyauxesis** \tak'i·ôksē'sis\ [TACHY- + AUXESIS] The disproportionately rapid growth of an organ or region as compared with the growth of the remainder of the body.

**tachycardia** \-kär'dē·ə\ [TACHY- + -CARDIA] A fast heart rate: applied in adults to rates exceeding 100 per minute. Also *tachyrhythmia.* **atrial t.** A disturbance of heart rhythm in which the heart beats rapidly as a result of an arrhythmia originating in the atria. **atrioventricular junctional t.** Tachycardia originating in the atrioventricular junctional tissue. Also *AV nodal tachycardia, atrioventricular tachycardia, junctional tachycardia, nodal tachycardia.* **bidirectional t.** A form of tachycardia in which the ventricular complexes alternate in their morphology, being successively negative and positive in their major direction. Most cases result from atrioventricular junctional tachycardias with aberration. **coronary sinus t.** Tachycardia originating in the coronary sinus. **double t.** The simultaneous occurrence of tachycardias from two origins, as from the atria and ventricles. **ectopic t.** A tachycardia originating from a site outside the sinuatrial node. **fetal t.** A fetal heartbeat faster than 160 beats per minute and lasting at least ten minutes. This finding is seen in association with maternal fever or in instances of hypoxia of the fetus. **junctional t.** ATRIOVENTRICULAR JUNCTIONAL TACHYCARDIA. **nodal t.** ATRIOVENTRICULAR JUNCTIONAL TACHYCARDIA. **orthostatic t.** Excessive tachycardia occurring on assuming the upright position. **paroxysmal t.** Recurrent episodes of tachycardia of sudden onset. They may arise from the atria, atrioventricular junctional tissue, or ventricles. Also *Bouveret's disease, Bouveret syndrome.* **paroxysmal atrial t.** Atrial tachycardia occurring in paroxysms. **paroxysmal nodal t.** Atrioventricular junctional tachycardia occurring in paroxysms. **paroxysmal ventricular t.** Ventricular tachycardia occurring in paroxysms. **sinus t.** A rapid heart rate due to acceleration of the sinus rate. **supranodal t.** Tachycardia arising above the level of the atrioventricular node. **supraventricular t.** Tachycardia originating above the level of the ventricles. **ventricular t.** Tachycardia originating from a focus in the ventricles.

**tachycardiac** \-kär'dē·ak\ Relating to or characterized by tachycardia. Also *tachycardic.*

**tachygenesis** \-jen'əsis\ [TACHY- + GENESIS] Acceleration of embryonic development as the result of the absence of a certain number of intermediary stages. It is seen in certain crustaceans and insects. Also *accelerated embryogenesis.* Compare BRADYGENESIS.

**tachylogia** \-lō'jə\ [TACHY- + -LOGIA] LOGOMANIA.

**tachymeter** \təkim'ətər\ TACHOMETER.

**tachyphasia** \-fā'zhə\ [TACHY- + Gk *phas(is)* (from *phanai* to speak) + -IA] LOGOMANIA.

**tachyphemia** \-fē'mē·ə\ [TACHY- + Gk *phēm(ē)* a voice, words, speech + -IA] LOGOMANIA.

**tachyphrasia** \-frā'zhə\ LOGOMANIA.

**tachyphylaxis** \-fīlak'sis\ [TACHY- + PHYLAXIS] Rapid loss of effect obtained by injection of a succession of small doses of an active substance. Using a toxin, tachyphylaxis provides protection against the injection of a much larger dose. Tachyphylaxis is also seen with some drugs and with biological mediators such as the anaphylactotoxins. Tachyphylaxis is produced by local exhaustion of receptors and/or mediators and its effect is temporary. It is not an immunologic phenomenon. Also *tachysynethia.*

**tachypnea** \tak'ipnē'ə\ [Gk *tachypnoia* (from *tachy(s)* quick, fast + *pnoē* wind, breath) quickness of respiration] Rapid breathing. Also *polypnea.*

**tachypnoea** *Brit.* TACHYPNEA.

**tachyrhythmia** \-riTH'mē·ə\ [TACHY- + RHYTHM + -IA] TACHYCARDIA.

**tachysterol** A derivative of vitamin D in which the conjugated system of double bonds, normally 5,7,10(19), is isomerized to 5(10),6,8.

**tachysynethia** \-sinē'thē·ə\ [TACHY- + Gk *synētheia* (from *syn-* with, together + *ethos* custom) habituation] TACHYPHYLAXIS.

**tachyzoite** \-zō'īt\ [TACHY- + *zo(o)-* + -ITE] A stage of development of protozoan coccidial parasites characterized by very rapid multiplication.

**tactile** \tak'til, -tīl\ [L *tactil(is)* (from *tact(us),* past part. of *tangere* to touch + *-ilis* -ILE[1]) tactile, able to be touched] Pertaining to touch or contact.

**tactor** \tak'tər\ A sensitive cutaneous mechanoreceptor or tactile sense organ.

**tactual** \tak'chəl\ [L *tactu(s)* (from *tactus,* past part. of *tangere* to touch) a touching, sense of touch or feeling + -AL] Pertaining to or resulting from touch.

***Taenia*** \tē′nē·ə\ [See TAENIA.] The most widely known genus of cyclophyllidean cestodes, including several tapeworm species of man and others in various carnivores. The larval form is a cysticercus, which encysts in tissues of herbivores, rodents, and other animals that serve as intermediate hosts. Adults are extremely large, and most species possess an armed rostellum bearing two rows of hooks. Also *Hydatigena*. ***T. armata*** *TAENIA SOLIUM*. ***T. dentata*** *TAENIA SOLIUM*. ***T. diminuta*** *HYMENOLEPIS DIMINUTA*. ***T. echinococcus*** *ECHINOCOCCUS GRANULOSUS*. ***T. elliptica*** *DIPYLIDIUM CANINUM*. ***T. hydatigena*** A species found in dogs, cats, wolves, foxes, and other carnivores. The cysticercus occurs in the liver and abdominal cavity of various ruminants, rodents, and occasionally in other animals, including man. Also *Taenia marginata*. ***T. marginata*** *TAENIA HYDATIGENA*. ***T. minima*** *HYMENOLEPIS NANA*. ***T. nana*** *HYMENOLEPIS NANA*. ***T. saginata*** The beef tapeworm; the most common large tapeworm of humans. It is found in the intestine and can measure between four and eight meters in length. The larvae (cysticerci) develop in the tissues of cattle and other ruminants, particularly in the muscles. Humans are infected by eating raw or undercooked infected beef (measly beef). Also *Taeniarhynchus saginatus*. ***T. solium*** The pork tapeworm, a parasite of the human intestine. An adult can be from one to four meters long. The larvae (cysticerci) are normally found in the muscles and other tissues of the pig, but can also occur in humans, dogs, sheep, and other animals. Infection with the adult worm results from eating undercooked infected pork. Cysticerci can become established in human tissues, causing cysticercosis, from ingestion of infective eggs or autoreinfection. Also *Taenia armata, Taenia dentata*.

**taenia** \tē′nē·ə\ [L (from Gk *tainia* a band, headband, tapeworm, ribbon, akin to *teinein* to stretch, extend), a band, tape] (*pl.* taeniae) **1** A bandlike anatomical structure. **2** A tapeworm, especially one of the genus *Taenia*. For defs 1 and 2 also *tenia*. **taeniae acusticae** STRIAE MEDULLARES VENTRICULI QUARTI. **t. choroidea** [NA] The line of attachment along which the ependyma of the lateral ventricle and the pia mater are reflected onto the choroid plexus of the lateral ventricle. This attachment line extends posterolaterally from the interventricular foramen rostrally along the dorsal surface of the thalamus to its ventrolateral border, and then along the stria terminalis to the region of the amygdala. **taeniae coli** [NA] Three thickened tapelike bands of longitudinal muscle fibers that are spread almost equidistant from each other on the surface of the large intestine from the cecum through the sigmoid colon. As they are shorter than the other coats of the large intestine, they produce the bulging sacculi or haustrations. They are not as conspicuous in the sigmoid colon. They comprise the taenia libera, taenia mesocolica, and taenia omentalis. Also *teniae coli*. **t. fimbriae** The line of attachment of the choroid plexus to the lateral border of the fimbria of the hippocampus in the inferior horn of the lateral ventricle. *Seldom used*. Also *taenia hippocampi, taenia terminalis*. **t. fornicis** [NA] The line of attachment of the choroid plexus of the lateral ventricle to the fornix. Also *taenia of fornix*. **t. of fourth ventricle** TAENIA VENTRICULI QUARTI. **t. hippocampi** TAENIA FIMBRIAE. **t. libera** One of the taeniae coli, located on the anterior surface of the cecum and the ascending, descending, and sigmoid colon, but on the inferior surface of the transverse colon. Also *free band of colon, anterior band of colon*. **t. medullaris thalami optici** TAENIA THALAMI. **medullary t. of thalamus** TAENIA THALAMI. **t. mesocolica** [NA] One of the three taeniae coli, located on the posteromedial surface of the cecum and the ascending, descending, and sigmoid colon, but on the posterior surface of the transverse colon at the attachment of the transverse mesocolon. Also *mesocolic band*. **t. omentalis** [NA] One of the three taeniae coli, located on the posterolateral surface of the cecum and the ascending, descending, and sigmoid colons but on the anterosuperior surface of the transverse colon at the attachment of the posterior layers of the greater omentum. Also *omental band*. **t. plexus choroidei ventriculi quarti** TAENIA VENTRICULI QUARTI. **t. pontis** One or two small bundles of myelinated nerve fibers that curve ventrodorsally around the rostral border of the pons to enter the cerebellum as isolated bands of fibers between the superior and middle cerebellar peduncles. These may represent displaced pontocerebellar fibers. **taeniae pylori** LIGAMENTA PYLORI. **t. semicircularis corporis striati** STRIA TERMINALIS. **t. sinus rhomboideae** TAENIA VENTRICULI QUARTI. **Tarin's t.** STRIA TERMINALIS. **t. tectae** STRIA LONGITUDINALIS LATERALIS CORPORIS CALLOSI. **t. telae** [NA] The slight thickenings seen along the lines of attachment of the tela choroidea to the ependyma of the ventricles in the brain. Also *taeniae telarum*. **t. terminalis** TAENIA FIMBRIAE. **t. thalami** [NA] A line marking the dorsomedial margin of the thalamus along which the ependyma of the third ventricle and the pia mater covering the dorsal aspect of the thalamus is reflected onto the tela choroidea of the third ventricle. Also *taenia ventriculi tertii, taenia of third ventricle, taenia medullaris thalami optici, medullary taenia of thalamus, taenia of thalamus*. **t. ventriculi quarti** [NA] A narrow white ridge extending superolaterally from the inferior angle of the fourth ventricle at the obex on each side. It serves as the line of attachment of the ependymal cells of the tela choroidea of the fourth ventricle to the ependymal cells lining the caudal part of that ventricle. Also *taenia plexus choroidei ventriculi quarti, taenia of fourth ventricle, taenia sinus rhomboideae*. **t. ventriculi tertii** TAENIA THALAMI.

**taeniacide** \tē′nē·əsīd′\ [TAENIA + -CIDE] A substance that is lethal to tapeworms. Also *tenicide*. Also *teniacide*.

**taeniae** \tē′ni·ē\ Plural of TAENIA.

**taeniafugal** \tē′nē·af′yəgəl\ [*taeniafug(e)* + -AL] Having the capability of expelling tapeworms. Also *teniafugal, tenifugal*.

**taeniafuge** \tē′nē·əfyooj′\ [TAENIA + -FUGE] An agent able to expel tapeworms. Also *tenifuge*. Also *teniafuge*.

***Taeniarhynchus*** \tē′nē·əring′kəs\ A genus of tapeworms established to include those species previously assigned to *Taenia* which have a rudimentary rostellum but no hooklets. The best-known example is *Taeniarhynchus saginatus*, still usually called *Taenia saginata*. ***T. saginatus*** *TAENIA SAGINATA*.

**taeniform** \tē′nifôrm\ [*Taeni(a)* + -FORM] Shaped like a tapeworm, especially one of the genus *Taenia* or similar forms. Also *teniform*.

**taeniid** \tē′nē·id\ [*Taeni(a)* + -ID[1]] **1** Of or belonging to the family Taeniidae. **2** A member of the family Taeniidae.

**Taeniidae** \tēnē′idē\ [*Taeni(a)* + -IDAE] A medically important family of tapeworms (order Cyclophyllidea, subclass Cestoda) parasitic in mammals. It includes the genera *Taenia, Taeniarhynchus, Multiceps, Echinococcus,* and *Cladotaenia*..

**taenioid** \tē′nē·oid\ **1** Tapewormlike; taenialike, taeniform. Also *tenioid.* **2** Belonging to, or a member of, the tapeworm superfamily Taenioidea, a taxon no longer in common use.

**taeniola** \tēnē′ələ\ [L (dim. of TAENIA), a small ribbon] A narrow, bandlike structure. Also *teniola.* **t. cinerea** A narrow grayish ridge sometimes seen in the floor of the fourth ventricle between the striae medullares ventriculi quarti and the entrance of the cochlear division of the vestibulocochlear nerve. *Rare.* **t. corporis callosi of Reil** LAMINA ROSTRALIS.

***Taeniorhynchus*** \tē′nē·ôring′kəs\ [TAENIA + *o* + Gk *rhynchos* a snout, bill, beak] *MANSONIA.*

**tag** **1** A small, sessile protuberance of the surface of an organ, usually the skin. **2** LABEL. **anal skin t.** A small appendage of skin in the perianal area related to old external hemorrhoids. **auricular t.'s** Small fleshy tubercles or appendages on the face in front of the auricle, at the site of missing limbs or parts thereof, or at the tip of the coccyx. All represent embryological remnants. **cutaneous t.** CUTANEOUS FIBROUS POLYP. **sentinel t.** A perianal skin tag found at the edge of a chronic anal fissure. **skin t.** CUTANEOUS FIBROUS POLYP.

**tagging** LABELING.

**Tagliacozzi** [Gasparo *Tagliacozzi,* Italian surgeon, 1546–1599] **1** Tagliacotian rhinoplasty. See under ITALIAN RHINOPLASTY. **2** Tagliacozzi flap. See under ITALIAN FLAP.

**tagma** \tag′mə\ [Gk *tagma* (from *tassein* to arrange) a thing ordered or arranged] (*pl.* tagmata) A molecular aggregate.

**tail** [Old English *tægel*] CAUDA. **axillary t. of breast** The prolongation of the upper outer quadrant of the breast that pierces the axillary fascia and comes to lie in the axilla at the level of the third rib adjacent to the anterior or pectoral lymph nodes. It is particularly noticeable during lactation. Also *axillary tail of Spence, tail of Spence.* **t. of epididymis** CAUDA EPIDIDYMIDIS. **t. of helix** CAUDA HELICIS. **occult t.** Rare supernumerary segments of the coccyx that can be found in the gluteal region. **t. of pancreas** CAUDA PANCREATIS. **t. of Spence** AXILLARY TAIL OF BREAST. **t. of spleen** *Outmoded* EXTREMITAS ANTERIOR SPLENIS.

**tailgut** \tāl′gut\ POSTANAL GUT.

**Taillefer** [Louis Auguste Horace Sydney Timeléon *Taillefer,* French physician, 1802–1868] See under VALVE.

**taipan** \tī′pan\ [Aboriginal Australian] Any of certain venomous snakes of the genus *Pseudechis.*

**Takahara** [Shigeo *Takahara,* Japanese otolaryngologist, flourished 20th century] Takahara's disease. See under ACATALASIA.

**Takayasu** [Michishige *Takayasu,* Japanese physician, born 1872] Takayasu's disease, Takayasu syndrome. See under TAKAYASU'S ARTERITIS.

**take** **1** The successful establishment in a graft of circulatory continuity with the recipient site. **2** To establish circulatory continuity: used especially of a graft. **3** To show signs of being effective: said of an administered vaccine. **graft t.** That portion of a graft that remains viable.

**tal.** *talis* (such a one).

**talantropia** \tal′əntrō′pē·ə\ NYSTAGMUS.

**talar** \tā′lär\ Of or relating to the talus. Also *astragalar* (outmoded).

**talbot** \tal′bət\ [after William Henry Fox *Talbot,* British physicist, mathematician, and pioneer of photography, 1800–1877] A unit of luminous energy equal to one joule of radiant energy with a luminous efficiency of one lumen per watt.

**talbutal** $C_{11}H_{16}N_2O_3$. 5-(1-Methylpropyl)-5-(2-propenyl)-2,4-6(1*H*,3*H*,5*H*)-pyrimedinetrione, an intermediate-acting barbiturate used as a sedative and hypnotic. It is given orally.

**talc** Native hydrous magnesium silicate, sometimes containing small proportions of aluminum silicate, used as a dusting powder and in cosmetic preparations. Also *soapstone, talcum.*

**talcosis** \talkō′sis\ TALC PNEUMOCONIOSIS. **pulmonary t.** TALC PNEUMOCONIOSIS.

**talcum** TALC.

**talectomy** \tālek′təmē\ The surgical removal of the talus. Also *astragalectomy.*

**tali** \tā′lī\ Plural of TALUS.

**taliped** \tal′iped\ **1** Exhibiting talipes. Also *talipedic.* **2** One afflicted with talipes.

**talipes** \tal′əpēz\ [New L (from L *tal(us)* ankle + *pes* foot); suggested by L *talipedare* to limp, walk lamely, lit., to walk on the ankles] Any congenital deformity of the foot that results in a twisted or ungainly condition. Also *clubfoot, club foot, stump foot.* • The term was originally used in reference to those deformities involving the talus, but in current usage it applies to any malformation of the foot except reduction defects. **t. adductus** TALIPES VARUS. **t. arcuatus** TALIPES CAVUS. **t. calcaneocavus** Talipes in which the characteristics of both talipes calcaneus and talipes cavus are present. **t. calcaneovalgocavus** Talipes in which the foot is deformed in such manner as to exhibit features of talipes calcaneus, talipes valgus, and talipes cavus. **t. calcaneovalgus** Talipes in which the foot exhibits the combined features of both talipes calcaneus and talipes valgus. The foot is dorsiflexed and everted. **t. calcaneovarus** Talipes in which the foot exhibits the combined features of the calcaneus and the varus deformities. **t. calcaneus** Talipes in which the foot is fixed in a dorsiflexed position so that weight is borne wholly by the heel. Also *pes calcaneus.* **t. cavovalgus** Talipes in which the foot is fixed in the combined position of cavus and valgus so that weight is borne on the medial aspect of the tarsal bones. Also *cavovalgus.* **t. cavus** Talipes in which the normal arch of the foot is exaggerated. Also *hollow foot, talipes arcuatus, talipes plantaris, equinocavus.* **t. equinocavus** Talipes in which the foot is fixed in a combined cavus and equinus position, with weight borne on the metatarsophalangeal joints. **t. equinovalgus** Talipes in which the foot is fixed in a combined equinus and valgus position, with weight borne on the metatarsophalangeal joint. Also *pes equinovalgus, equinovalgus, valgus club foot.* **t. equinovarus** Talipes in which the foot is fixed in a combined equinus and varus position, with weight borne on the fifth metatarsophalangeal joint. Also *pes equinovarus, equinovarus, equinus club foot, varus club foot.* **t. equinus** Talipes in which the foot is fixed in plantar flexion (extension), with the weight borne on the ball or metatarsophalangeal joints. Also *tip foot, strephopodia, equinus deformity.* **t. planovalgus** Talipes in which the foot is fixed in a combination of the planus and valgus positions, with weight borne along the entire medial edge of the foot, which is in eversion. Also *pes planovalgus.* **t. plantaris** TALIPES CAVUS. **t. planus** Talipes in which the natural arch of the foot is absent and weight is borne over the entire sole, which is in contact with the ground. Also *flatfoot, splayfoot, pes planus, tarsoptosis.* **spasmodic t. planus** SPASTIC FLATFOOT. **t. spasmodicus** SPASTIC FLATFOOT. **t. transversoplanus** BROAD FOOT. **t. valgus** Talipes in which the foot is fixed in an everted (abducted) position, with weight borne along the medial edge of the heel and the first metatarsophalangeal joint. Also *pes pronatus, pes valgus, pes abductus, congenital convex pes valgus, strephexopodia.* **t. varus** Talipes in which the foot is fixed in an inverted (adducted) position, with weight borne

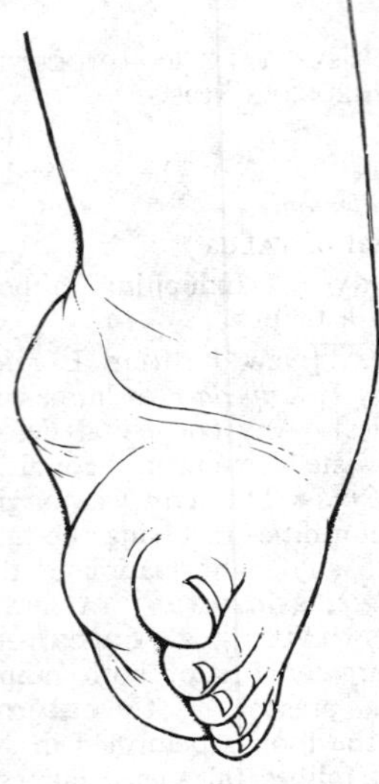

Talipes varus

along the lateral edge of the foot, except where there is a degree of equinus and/or cavus deformity as a complication. Also *crossfoot, pes adductus, strephenopodia, talipes adductus, pes varus, supination of the foot.*

**talipomanus** \tal′ipōman′əs, tal′ipäm′ənəs\ [*talip(es)* + *o* + MANUS] A congenital or acquired deformity of the hand that results in a twisted or ungainly appearance. It includes most developmental defects except reduction defects of the hand. Also *clubhand.*

**Tallerman** [Lewis A. *Tallerman,* English inventor and scientist, flourished 19th century] See under TREATMENT.

**talon** \tal′än\ [Middle French, heel, spur, from hypothetical Vulgar L *talo* heel, from L *talus* the ankle] **1** The heel. **2** A posterior extension from the trigone of an upper molar tooth. **t. noir** BLACK HEEL.

**talonid** \tal′ənid\ [TALON + -ID[2]] A posterior extension from the trigonid of a lower molar tooth.

**talus** \tā′ləs\ [L, the ankle, anklebone] [NA] The second largest bone of the tarsus which links the bones of the leg with the rest of the foot through its involvement in the talocrural joint. Superiorly it supports the tibia, medially and laterally it articulates with the malleoli, inferiorly it rests on the calcaneus, while anteriorly its head articulates with the navicular bone. Also *ankle bone, astragalus, astragaloid bone, hucklebone.*

**tambour** \tam′boor\ A drumlike instrument for recording arterial pulsations. Pressure changes within the drum bow a membrane, which moves a writing stylus or optical mirror.

**Tamm** [Igor *Tamm,* U.S. virologist, 1922–1971] Tamm-Horsfall mucoprotein. See under MUCOPROTEIN.

**tamoxifen** $C_{26}H_{29}NO$. 2-[4-(1,2-Diphenyl-1-butenyl)-phenoxy]-*N,N*-dimethylethanamine. An orally administered antiestrogen agent used in the treatment of metastatic breast cancer and for the stimulation of ovulation. In the male it has been used for the treatment of gynecomastia. It is administered as the citrate salt.

**tampan** \tam′pan\ [native South African] A tick of the species *Ornithodoros moubata.*.

**tampol** A tampon containing a medicinal substance.

**tampon** \tam′pän\ [Middle French *tampon,* also *tapon* a plug, from the Germanic] A pack or plug made of absorbent material that can be placed in a cavity to absorb blood or other fluid or to control bleeding. **Corner's t.** *Older term* CORNER'S PLUG. **Trendelenburg's t.** The inflated rubber cuff that surrounds the intratracheal part of Trendelenburg's tampon-cannula. It is designed to keep out blood from the lungs during operations on the nose and throat. Also *tracheal tampon.* **vaginal t.** A cylindrical device of cloth or paper fiber that is inserted into the vagina to absorb menstrual blood.

**tamponade** \tam′pənād′\ [French *tamponner* to stop up with a tampon] The application of external pressure to stop bleeding. Also *tamponage, tamponment.* **balloon t.** Tamponade of the esophagogastric region by a multiple-lumen tube (such as a Sengstaken-Blakemore tube) for treatment of bleeding esophageal varices. **cardiac t.** Compression of the heart due to the rapid accumulation of fluid, often blood, in the pericardial space, leading to ineffectual pumping of blood. Also *heart tamponade.* **chronic t.** Chronic compression of the heart due to fluid in the pericardial space or thickening of the pericardium. **heart t.** CARDIAC TAMPONADE.

**tamponage** \tam′pənij\ TAMPONADE.

**tamponment** \tampän′mənt\ TAMPONADE.

**tanacyte** \tan′əsīt\ A cell derived from the embryonic ependymal layer whose processes extend across the neural tube to the pia.

**tanapox** \tā′nəpäks\ An epidemic viral illness seen in the Tana River region of Kenya. There is a short febrile episode with headache, malaise, and a pocklike skin reaction. The virus is related to the yabapox virus which produces benign tumors in humans and monkeys. The disease is probably a zoonosis with a reservoir in monkeys.

**tangentiality** \tanjen′chē·al′itē\ A disturbance in association in which thought and speech digress and lose their relevance to the topic of the moment.

**tangle** A dense mass of fibrous components, as of neural filaments. **intraneural fibrillary t.** An accumulation of fibrillary material within the cytoplasm of a neuronal perikaryon. It is a consequence of aging and is also seen, in excess, in Alzheimer's disease. Also *neurofibrillary tangle, Alzheimer fibril.*

**tangoreceptor** \tang′gōrisep′tər\ A tactile sense organ.

**tank** A receptacle used especially for holding a fluid. **Hubbard t.** A specially shaped bathtub permitting a patient with abducted upper extremities to exercise while immersed in water.

**Tanner** [Ernest Ketchum *Tanner,* U.S. surgeon, born 1876] See under OPERATION.

**Tanner** [Norman Cecil *Tanner,* English surgeon, born 1906] See under PROCEDURE.

**tannic acid** A substance extracted from a Chinese tree, *Rhus,* and other plants. It is one of the simplest tannins, and consists of glucose acylated on its five hydroxyl groups by gallic acid, some of which is itself acylated on its phenolic hydroxyl groups by further residues of the same acid. It has been used as an antidote for alkaloid poisoning and was also used topically in treating burns until such treatment was found to lead often to liver failure. Also *gallotannic acid.*

**tannin** Any of a large group of compounds extracted

from plants and used to treat hides in the production of leather. Many contain gallic acid, i.e., 3,4,5-trihydroxybenzoic acid, and its derivatives, and sugars acylated by it. The phenolic hydroxyl groups are often methylated or are themselves acylated by further phenolic acids to produce chains. Complex and varied structures result.

**tanning** 1 The act of changing skin to leather by using tannic acid. 2 A former method of burn treatment using tannic acid. 3 The increase of melanin pigment in the skin induced by its exposure to sunlight.

**Tansini** [Iginio *Tansini*, Italian surgeon, 1855–1943] See under OPERATION.

**tantalum** \tan′tələm\ Element number 73, having atomic weight 180.95. Natural tantalum is very faintly radioactive, consisting principally of a single stable isotope along with traces of an unstable isotope with a half-life of over $10^{13}$ years. A gray, heavy, very hard metal, nonirritating and immune to body liquids, it is used in surgical appliances. Symbol: Ta

**tantalum 182** A radioisotope of tantalum, emitting beta and gamma radiation. It is used in therapy of superficial lesions, particularly in the eye. Physical half-life is 115.05 days. Symbol: $^{182}$Ta

**taon** \tā·än′\ A Philippine term for INFANTILE BERIBERI.

**tap¹** A surgical procedure in which fluid is drained from a space or region of the body by means of a trocar or a hollow needle. **bloody t.** The presence of blood in the cerebrospinal fluid, as that revealed by a lumbar puncture, or bloody fluid obtained by needle puncture of the brain or by erroneous introduction of a needle. **mitral t.** A tapping apex beat characteristic of mitral stenosis and associated with a loud first heart sound. **spinal t.** LUMBAR PUNCTURE. **subdural t.** Aspiration of fluid from the subdural space.

**tap²** [Middle English *tappen* to tap, from Middle French *taper* to strike with the flat of the hand, prob. of onomatopoeic origin] 1 To strike or touch lightly but often sharply. 2 A lightly given but often sharp blow or touch, commonly used in neurologic tests. **patellar t.** A maneuver that can be executed in cases of an effusion of the knee joint. The patella can be sharply tapped with the fingers against the underlying anterior surface of the distal femur. **tendon t.** A sharp, light blow delivered to the tendon of a muscle to test sensitivity of the phasic stretch reflex. The stretch releases a sensory volley from the muscle spindles which through monosynaptic connections excites the homonymous and synergistic motoneurons.

**tape** [Old English *tæppe* a narrow strip of cloth] Any long, flat strip of material, as of fabric, often used to bind or tie. **adhesive t.** A tape coated on one side with a pressure-sensitive adhesive surface, used to apply dressings or to produce immobilization. Also *adhesive plaster.* **dental t.** A fine tape of nylon or silk used for interdental cleaning in the manner of cleaning with dental floss. **sterile adhesive t.** Adhesive tape that has a protective covering strip over the adhesive surface and has been sterilized after packaging. Also *sterile adhesive plaster.*

**tapetal** \təpē′təl\ Of or pertaining to a tapetum.

**tapetum** \təpē′təm\ [L (from Gk *tapēs* a carpet, rug), an ornamental rug, tapestry] 1 A covering lamina of tissue. 2 [NA] A layer of myelinated fibers from the posterior part of the trunk and splenium of the corpus callosum that sweeps laterally and inferiorly to help form the roof and lateral wall of the posterior horn and the lateral wall of the inferior horn of the lateral ventricle. It separates the ventricle from the optic radiation. Also *tapetum ventriculi, Fielding's membrane* (obs.), *tapetum corporis callosi.* Adj. tapetal. ● In both senses, the name derives from the iridescent play of colors the structure displays. **t. corporis callosi** TAPETUM. **t. ventriculi** TAPETUM.

**tapeworm** A parasitic flatworm of the class Cestoidea. The true, or segmented, tapeworms are included in the subclass Cestoda and the unsegmented tapeworms, in the subclass of Cestodaria. **armed t.** PORK TAPEWORM.

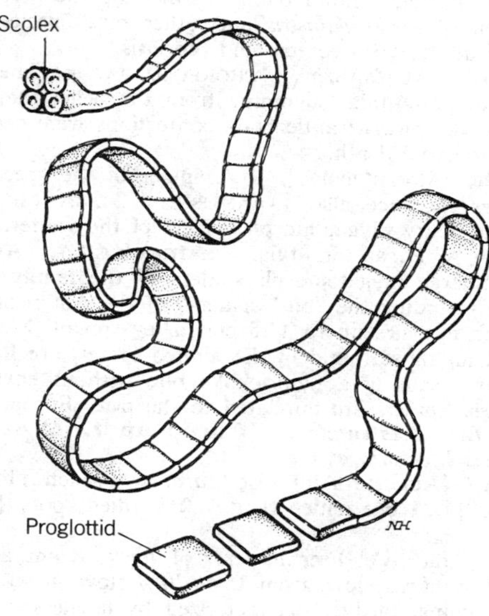


Tapeworm

**beef t.** A tapeworm of the species *Taenia saginata.* Also *hookless tapeworm, unarmed tapeworm.* **broad t.** A tapeworm of the species *Diphyllobothrium latum*; a fish tapeworm. **broad fish t.** A tapeworm of the species *Diphyllobothrium latum.* **dog t.** 1 A tapeworm of the species *Dipylidium caninum.* 2 A tapeworm of the species *Echinococcus granulosus.* **double-pored dog t.** A tapeworm of the species *Dipylidium caninum.* **dwarf t.** A tapeworm of the species *Hymenolepis nana.* **dwarf mouse t.** A tapeworm of the species *Hymenolepis nana.* **fish t.** A tapeworm of the species *Diphyllobothrium latum*; a broad tapeworm. **hookless t.** BEEF TAPEWORM. **hydatid t.** A tapeworm of the species *Echinococcus granulosus.* **Manson's larval t.** A larval tapeworm of the species *Spirometra mansonoides.* **measle t.** Any tapeworm of which the intermediate stage is a cysticercus in meat, especially *Taenia solium* or *T. saginata.* **mouse t.** A tapeworm of the species *Hymenolepis nana*; a dwarf tapeworm. **pork t.** A tapeworm of the species *Taenia solium.* Also *armed tapeworm.* **rat t.** A tapeworm of the species *Hymenolepis diminuta.* **unarmed t.** BEEF TAPEWORM.

**tapotement** \täpôtmäN′, təpät′mənt\ [French (from *tapote(r)* to tap, pat, from Middle French *taper* to slap, + French *-ment* -MENT), a tapping, patting] PERCUSSION MOVEMENTS.

**tar** [Old English *teoru*] Any dense and highly viscous organic liquid, especially coal tar. **coal t.** A black, viscid, semisolid by-product obtained by the destructive distillation of bituminous coal. It is a complex mixture of organic substances, including benzene, naphthalene, and phenols. Coal tar and its derivatives are used topically in the treatment of chronic skin diseases such as psoriasis, and in the production of food colorings. **juniper t.** A dark brown, oily liquid obtained by the destructive distillation of the wood of *Juniperus oxycedrus.* It has been used as an ointment in the treatment of psoriasis and eczema, and as an ingredient in medicated soaps and shampoos. Also *cade oil, Haarlem tar, Holland balsam, silver balsam, Haarlem oil, juniper tar oil.* **pine t.** A black liquid pitch obtained by the destructive distillation of *Pinus palustris* and other pine species. It is used topically to treat eczema and psoriasis.

**tarantism** \tar′əntizm\ CHOREOMANIA. • The term comes from tarantula, stemming from the belief that when bitten by the spider, frantic body contortions were necessary in order to avoid death.

**tarantula** \təran′chələ\ **1** A spider of the species *Lycosa tarentula.* See also TARANTISM. **2** Any of various very large, hairy mygalomorph spiders of the western hemisphere; an American tarantula. **American t.** Any of a group of large mygalomorph spiders of the family Theraphosidae including the "bird spiders" of the American tropics, which measure up to 17.5 cm in leg spread. Most species, and all those found in the United States, are harmless to humans, causing a pinpricklike bite without envenomation. These spiders are unrelated to the true (European) tarantula, *Lycosa tarentula.* **European t.** A spider of the species *Lycosa tarentula.*

**Tardieu** [Auguste Ambroise *Tardieu,* French physician, 1818–1879] **1** See under TEST. **2** Tardieu spots. See under SPOT.

**tardive** \tär′div\ [French, fem. of *tardif* (from assumed Vulgar L *tardivus* slow, from L *tard(us)* slow + *-ivus* -IVE) late in coming, tardy] Characterized by lateness or delay: said especially of a condition with late-emerging signs and symptoms.

**tare** \ter\ [Old Italian *tara* a tare, from Arabic *ṭarḥah* a thing subtracted, from *ṭaraḥa* to subtract, discard] **1** In chemistry, an empty vessel, or equivalent weight, used as a counterpoise and placed on the weight pan of a balance when determining net weight of a substance. **2** A control vessel, identical with an experimental vessel, which is subject to the same experimental conditions and is used as a basis for comparison.

**tarentism** \tar′əntizm\ CHOREOMANIA. • See note at TARANTISM.

**target** [Middle French *targette* (dim. of *targe* a shield) a small or light shield, or from Italian *targhetta* (dim. of *targa* a shield) a small shield] The object toward which an action or activity is directed, as a particular site or kind of tissue: often used attributively, as in *target organ.* **enriched t.** Target material containing a higher than normal percentage of a particular nuclide.

**targeting** \tär′gəting\ In molecular biology, the process by which a nucleotide sequence, such as a foreign gene, is inserted at a specific location in a host genome.

**tarichatoxin** \tär′ikətäk′sin\ A potent neurotoxin present in the newt *Taricha torosa.* It is chemically identical with tetrodotoxin, which is found in the puffer fish.

**Tarin** [Pierre *Tarin* (Tarinus), French anatomist and medical writer, 1725–1761] **1** Fascia of Tarin, fascia tarini. See under GYRUS DENTATUS. **2** Tarin's taenia. See under STRIA TERMINALIS. **3** Recessus posterior fossae interpeduncularis tarini. See under RECESSUS. **4** Tarinus valve, velum of Tarinus, Tarin's plate, Tarin's valve. See under VELUM MEDULLARE CAUDALE. **5** See under BAND. **6** Tarini's recess, Tarin space. See under RECESSUS ANTERIOR FOSSAE INTERPEDUNCULARIS TARINI. **7** Foramen of Tarin. See under HIATUS CANALIS NERVI PETROSI MAJORIS.

**Tarlov** [Isidore Max *Tarlov,* U.S. physician, born 1905] Tarlov cyst. See under SACRAL CYST.

**Tarnier** [Etienne Stephane *Tarnier,* French obstetrician, 1828–1897] See under SIGN.

**tars-** \tärs-\ TARSO-.

**tarsadenitis** \tär′sadenī′tis\ [TARS- + ADENITIS] Inflammation of the meibomian glands of the eyelids.

**tarsal** \tär′səl\ **1** Pertaining to any tarsus. **2** Any of the bones of the tarsus.

**tarsalgia** \tärsal′jə\ A pain in the ankle or hindfoot. Also *policeman's disease.*

**tarsalia** \tärsā′lyə\ The bones of the tarsus of the foot considered as a unit.

**tarsalis** \tärsā′lis\ **1** Tarsal. **2** Either musculus tarsalis superior or musculus tarsalis inferior.

**tarsectomy** \tärsek′təmē\ A total or partial excision of the tarsus.

**tarsen** \tär′sən\ Solely within the tarsus.

**tarsitis** \tärsī′tis\ [TARS- + -ITIS] **1** Inflammation of the tarsal plates of the eyelids. **2** Inflammatory infection of tarsal bones or joints.

**tarso-** \tär′sō-\ [New L *tarsus* (from Gk *tarsos* frame of wickerwork; broad, flat surface, as also in *tarsos podos,* the flat of the foot; the edge of the eyelid) ankle, tarsal plate of the eyelid] A combining form denoting tarsus. Also *tars-.*

**tarsocheiloplasty** \-kī′ləplas′tē\ [TARSO- + CHEILO- + -PLASTY] Any plastic operation on the margin of an eyelid.

**tarsomegaly** \-meg′əlē\ **1** A congenital malformation characterized by enlargement of a tarsal or carpal bone. **2** DYSPLASIA EPIPHYSIALIS HEMIMELICA.

**tarsometatarsal** \-met′ətär′səl\ Of or relating to the tarsus and the metatarsus.

**tarsoplasia** \-plā′zhə\ [TARSO- + -PLASIA] BLEPHAROPLASTY.

**tarsoplasty** \tär′səplas′tē\ [TARSO- + -PLASTY] BLEPHAROPLASTY.

**tarsoptosis** \tär′säptō′sis\ TALIPES PLANUS.

**tarsorrhaphy** \tärsôr′əfē\ [TARSO- + -RRHAPHY] Surgical adhesion of part of the opposing eyelid margins, performed to protect the cornea from exposure.

**tarsotomy** \tärsät′əmē\ [TARSO- + -TOMY] BLEPHAROTOMY.

**tarsus** \tär′səs\ [New L (from Gk *tarsos* a wicker frame, a broad flat surface, the foot)] **1** Either tarsus superior palpebrae or tarsus inferior palpebrae. **2** [NA] The skeleton of the posterior half of the foot, located between the distal ends of the tibia and fibula and the proximal ends of the metatarsal bones and comprising the ossa tarsi. Also *tarsus osseus* (outmoded), *bony tarsus* (outmoded). **inferior t.** TARSUS INFERIOR PALPEBRAE. **t. inferior palpebrae** [NA] A thin narrow plate of condensed fibrous tissue in which the tarsal glands are embedded in the lower eyelid. It has a free or ciliary margin and an orbital margin attached to the orbit by the orbital septum. Medially and laterally it is attached to bones of the orbit by ligaments. Also *inferior tarsus.* **t. osseus** *Outmoded* TARSUS. **superior t.** TARSUS SUPERIOR PALPEBRAE. **t. superior palpebrae** [NA] An elongated semioval plate of condensed fibrous tissue in which tarsal glands are embedded in the upper eyelid. Fibers of the levator palpebrae superioris muscle are attached to its upper and lower surfaces. It has a straight free or ciliary margin and an orbital margin attached to the orbit by the orbital septum. Medially and laterally it is attached to bones of the orbit by ligaments. Also *superior tarsus.*

**tartar** \tär′tər\ [Med L *tartarum,* from Med Gk *tartaron* tartar] **1** A substance that encrusts the inner walls of wine casks and which can be purified to yield potassium bitartrate (cream of tartar). **2** DENTAL CALCULUS.

**tartar emetic** **1** Antimony potassium tartrate. It is used in dyeing and in former times was used as an emetic and chemotherapeutic agent. **2** ANTIMONY SODIUM TARTRATE.

**tartaric acid** HOOC—CHOH—CHOH—COOH. 2,3-Dihydroxybutanedioic acid. It exists in three forms, with *RR*, *SS*, and *RS* configurations of its chiral centers at C-2 and C-3. The *RR* acid occurs naturally in many fruits. Pasteur's separation of the *RR* and *SS* acids from the racemic equimolar mixture was a pioneering step in the understanding of stereochemistry.

**tartrate** Any salt, anion, or ester of tartaric acid.

**task** / **dichotic learning t.'s** A technique of assessing auditory perception in the two cerebral hemispheres. It involves the delivery of precise auditory stimuli to each ear independently at varying time intervals.

**taste** [Old French *taster* (prob. from L *taxare*, for *taxitare*, to touch sharply, feel; equivalent to *tactare*, an intensive form of *tangere* to touch, taste) to touch, taste] The sensation evoked by sapid molecular excitation of gustatory receptors of the tongue and oropharynx, usually assigned qualities of bitter, sweet, sour, and salty. • This fourfold classification is culturally determined. Some other cultures (the Chinese, for example) have a fivefold classification of taste adding "hot," or pungent. In addition, in some east Asian languages an astringent, puckery or "styptic" taste (as of persimmons, especially the part close to the skin) is also distinguished.

**taster** **1** In studies of linkage between loci, an individual capable of tasting a specific substance when such ability is a mendelian trait. **2** An individual capable of tasting phenylthiocarbamide (PTC), due to the homozygosity or heterozygosity of the taster allele at the PTC locus. The ability to taste PTC as bitter is an autosomal dominant trait. Compare NONTASTER.

**tattoo** / **accidental t.** A tattoo caused by the deposition in the skin of pigment that was introduced by accidental trauma. Also *dirt tattoo.* **amalgam t.** Blue-black pigmentation of the alveolar mucous membrane, usually at the site of extraction of a tooth restored with silver amalgam, due to fragments of amalgam becoming included in the healing extraction wound. **dirt t.** ACCIDENTAL TATTOO.

**tattooing** [Tahitian *tatau* tattoo + -ING] **1** The injection of inks or dyes into the dermis to make designs or patterns on the skin. **2** The accidental injection of foreign matter into the dermis, causing a random design. **t. of the cornea** **1** The cosmetic darkening of a white corneal scar by infiltrating it with pigment. **2** The presence of pigmented foreign bodies in the cornea.

**taurine** $NH_3^+$—$CH_2$—$CH_2$—$SO_3^-$. Aminoethanesulfonic acid. It is formed from cysteine by oxidation of the sulfhydryl group and decarboxylation. It occurs acylated by cholic acid and related acids in the bile salts, and it seems also to be a neurotransmitter.

**taurocholate** *N*-Choloyltaurine, i.e. taurine acylated by cholic acid, forming one of the bile salts.

**taurocholemia** \tôr′ōkōlē′mē·ə\ The presence of taurocholic acid in the blood.

**taurocholic acid** The amide formed between cholic acid and taurine. It is a major constituent of bile.

**taurocyamine** $NH_2$—C(=$NH_2^+$)—NH—$CH_2$—$CH_2$—$SO_3^-$. A metabolite of taurine, containing the guanidino group in place of the amino group of taurine.

**taurodontism** \tôr′ōdän′tizm\ The property of having a tooth form in which the pulp cavity is enlarged. Compare CYNODONTISM.

**Taussig** [Helen Brooke *Taussig*, U.S. pediatrician, born 1898] **1** Taussig-Bing syndrome, Taussig-Bing disease. See under TAUSSIG-BING MALFORMATION. **2** Blalock-Taussig operation. See under BLALOCK'S OPERATION.

**tauto-** \tô′tō-\ [Gk *tauto* (from *to auto* the same) the same] A combining form meaning same.

**tautomer** \tô′təmər\ A compound that differs from its isomer, with which it readily interconverts, only in the positions of a mobile atom, frequently hydrogen, and of double bonds. A ketone containing the group —CO—$CH_2$—, for example, is a tautomer of an enol containing —C(OH)=CH—.

**tautomeral** \tôtäm′ərəl\ Denoting nerve fibers found in specific segments or parts of the spinal cord that are derived from neuronal cell bodies located in the same areas.

**tautomerase** Any enzyme that catalyzes the interconversion of tautomers.

**tautomeric** \-mir′ik\ **1** Designating substances that are tautomers of each other. **2** Designating the process of interconversion of two tautomers.

**tautomerism** \tôtäm′ərizm\ **1** The phenomenon of the existence of tautomers. **2** The process of interconversion of tautomers. **keto-enol t.** The tautomerism between the group —CO—XH— and —C(OH)=X—. In simple compounds, when X contains carbon, e.g. CH, equilibrium favors the former, keto, form, but conjugation of the C-X double bond, as in forming an aromatic ring, may displace the equilibrium.

**Tawara** [K. Sunao *Tawara*, Japanese physician, 1873–1938] His-Tawara node, node of Aschoff and Tawara, node of Tawara. See under NODUS ATRIOVENTRICULARIS.

**taxa** \tak′sə\ Plural of TAXON.

**taxis** \tak′sis\ [Gk *taxis* an ordering, arranging] Movement or growth of an animal or plant in response to a defined physical stimulus, e.g., light, surface contact, flow of a liquid. It is positive if the organism or body part approaches the stimulus and negative if it retracts.

**taxon** \tak′sän\ [back-formation from TAXONOMY] (*pl.* taxa, taxons) Any accepted taxonomic group, such as a phylum, class, order, family, genus, species, or an intermediate level (as subphylum or superclass). Additional categories such as group, division, section, or tribe are employed by specialists for more complex descriptions of related organisms.

**taxonomic** \tak′sənäm′ik\ Of or relating to taxonomy.

**taxonomy** \taksän′əmē\ [French *taxonomie* (from Gk *tax(is)* an arranging, putting in order + *onom(a)* a name + French *-ie* -Y) science of the laws of classification] **1** The analysis of variation among organisms leading to the assignment of scientific names which are intended to reflect the systematic relationships of the organisms. **2** The study of the principles and practices of biologic classification.

**-taxy** \-tak′sē, -tak′sē\ [Gk *tax(is)* (from *tassein* to arrange) arrangement + -Y] A combining form meaning arrangement, system, order.

**Tay** [Warren *Tay*, English physician, 1843–1927] **1** Tay sign, Tay spot. See under CHERRY-RED SPOT. **2** Tay's choroiditis. See under DOYNE HONEYCOMB DEGENERATION OF RETINA. **3** Tay-Sachs disease. See under DISEASE.

**Taybi** [Hooshang *Taybi*, Iranian-born U.S. radiologist, born 1919] Rubinstein-Taybi syndrome. See under SYNDROME.

**Taylor** [Charles Fayette *Taylor*, U.S. surgeon, 1827–1899] **1** Knight-Taylor brace. See under BRACE. **2** See under BRACE. **3** Taylor's apparatus. See under SPLINT.

**TB** 1 tuberculosis. 2 tubercle bacillus.
**Tb** 1 Symbol for the element, terbium. 2 tubercle bacillus.
**TBE** tuberculin bacillin emulsion (bacillary emulsion tuberculin).
**TBG** thyroxine-binding globulin.
**TBPA** thyroxine-binding prealbumin.
**TBSA** total body surface area.
**TC** 1 to contain. 2 thermal conductivity. 3 tuberculin, contagious.
**Tc** Symbol for the element, technetium.
**TCA** 1 tricarboxylic acid. 2 trichloroacetic acid.
**TD** 1 to deliver. 2 threshold of discomfort.
**tDNA** transfer DNA.
**t.d.s.** *ter die sumendum* (L, to be taken three times a day).
**Te** 1 Symbol for the element, tellurium. 2 tetanus.
**tea** [Amoy Chinese *t'e* tea] 1 The dried tip and terminal bud of the Asian shrub *Camellia sinensis.* It is made into a beverage by either steaming, yielding green tea, or fermenting, resulting in black tea. 2 Any plant that bears leaves containing terpenoid or phenolic components and, often, caffeine alkaloids. 3 An infusion prepared from the leaves of *Camellia sinensis* or another plant for use as a beverage. **beef t.** An extract made by simmering lean beef in water for two or three hours. At one time it was given to invalids to stimulate their appetite.
**Teale** [Thomas Pridgin *Teale,* English surgeon, 1801–1868] Teale's operation. See under AMPUTATION.
**team / surgical t.** A group of physicians, nurses, and paraprofessional personnel who assume the care of surgical patients before, during, and after the operative procedure.
**tear**[1] \ter\ A rip or break in a thin, flat structure. **bucket-handle t.** A longitudinal split in the meniscus of the knee. The anterior and posterior portions of the meniscus remain attached to the capsule, but the medial portion of the split becomes displaced towards the center of the joint, thus resembling a bucket handle. Also *bucket-handle injury, bucket-handle fracture.* **cemental t.** The detachment of a portion of cementum from a tooth root, seen in histologic sections.
**tear**[2] \tir\ A drop of the saline surface fluid of the eye (tears), secreted by the lacrimal glands and serving to lubricate the conjunctiva. **crocodile t.'s** See under CROCODILE TEARS SYNDROME.
**tease** To separate structural parts of (a tissue specimen) with needles for microscopic examination.
**teaspoon** A unit of capacity equal to 5 milliliters. *Popular.* Symbol: tsp
**teat** \tēt\ [Old French *tete* teat, from the Germanic root of Old English *tit* teat] PAPILLA MAMMARIA.
**technetium** \teknē'shē·əm\ Element number 43, having atomic weight 98.9062. It is a synthetic metallic element never occurring in terrestrial materials but found in the spectra of certain stars. Sixteen isotopes have been identified with mass numbers from 92 to 107. All are intensely radioactive, having half-lives up to $2.6 \times 10^6$ years. Technetium has specialized industrial applications, for which it is prepared in kilogram quantities. Also *masurium* (outmoded). Symbol: Tc
**technetium 99** The longest-lived technetium isotope, with a half-life of $2 \times 10^5$ years. It is produced by bombarding molybdenum with deuterons and neutrons, or as a fission product of uranium 235 and plutonium. It decays by beta emission of 0.292 MeV. It is useful in long-term studies where 6-hour technetium 99m would decay too rapidly. Symbol: $^{99}$Tc
**technetium 99m** An isomer of technetium 99 that decays by isomeric transition, with a half-life of 6 hours. It is particularly useful as a radiotracer in medical work because it is readily available from small laboratory generators, it forms complexes with many chemical or pharmacologic vectors, the gamma emission is in the energy range (140 KeV) favorable for scintigraphic work, the limited particulate emission restricts the radiation penalty to a patient, and its half-life makes it suitable for many clinical and research purposes. Symbol: $^{99m}$Tc
**technic** \tek'nik, teknēk'\ [French *technique.* See TECHNIQUE.] TECHNIQUE.
**technical** Of or relating to a technique or to a series of techniques.
**technician** \teknish'ən\ [TECHNIC + *-ician,* noun suffix denoting a specialist] A worker who performs procedures of an investigative, diagnostic, or clinical nature, usually under the direction of an investigator or clinician responsible for initiating and interpreting the test procedures. Also *technologist.* **audiologic t.** AUDIOMETRICIAN. **dental t.** A person who carries out the technical procedures, excluding those that must take place in the mouth, in the making of restorations and prostheses. Also *dental laboratory technician.* **physiological measurement t. in audiology** The British term for audiometrician. **radiologic t.** An individual trained and skilled in the carrying out of technical procedures pertaining to radiology. Also *radiologic technologist, x-ray technician.* **x-ray t.** RADIOLOGIC TECHNICIAN.

# technique

**technique** \teknēk'\ [French (from Gk *technikos* artistic, skilled, from *technē* art, skill) procedure followed in an art or trade] A method by which a skillful task is executed, especially a practiced method developed and refined by experience, such as those used in surgery, in the operation of diagnostic or therapeutic devices, or in laboratory testing and research. Also *technic.* **abrasion t.** DERMABRASION. **absorption-elution t.** A two-step means of separating, purifying, or identifying immunologically active material by first allowing antigen and antibody to react with one another and then dissociating the antigen-antibody complex to recover the desired constituents for subsequent manipulation. **absorption-inhibition t.** A means of identifying a soluble antigen by demonstrating that incubating the antigen with its specific antibody of known potency inhibits the antibody and causes measurable reduction in its activity level. It is often used in forensic laboratories to identify A and B antigens in stains of body fluids. **angle bisection t.** A technique for creating a radiographic image of a tooth which is equal in length to the tooth itself when the film plane is at an angle to the long axis of the tooth. Also *bisection technique.* **atrial-well t.** A techinque for transatrial repair of an atrial septal defect without use of cardiopulmonary bypass. The procedure is historically important but now obsolete. **Baermann funnel t.** A method for detecting nematode larvae, such as those of *Strongyloides stercoralis,* in feces. A fecal specimen is placed on gauze or wire mesh which just touches the surface of warmed water in a large funnel. Larvae travel through the gauze or mesh into the water and collect at the bottom of the funnel, held back by a rubber tube with a stopcock. After an hour, the bottom 10 ml of water is released, centrifuged, and the sediment studied for larvae. **bisection t.** ANGLE BISECTION TECHNIQUE. **Brock t.** TRANSVENTRICULAR CLOSED VALVOTOMY. **cerebral flow image t.** A procedure for demonstrating cerebral blood flow by scintillation camera imaging following the intravascular administration of a radiotracer. **Coffey t.** The technique of repairing exstrophy of the bladder by way of ureteral anastomosis to the sigmoid colon. The anastomosis is done between the layers of the bowel wall to prevent reflux. **competitive binding t.** An analytic technique to determine the concentration of the material to be measured by adding a labeled form of the same material and observing how the mixture of labeled and unlabeled analyte reacts with a known quantity of a binding or sorbent material. Since the measured proportion of labeled and unlabeled analyte that is bound to the indicator reflects the proportion of labeled and unlabeled material in the original mixture, the concentration of the original, unlabeled material can be calculated from the amount of labeled material that is bound. Also *displacement analysis, saturation analysis.* **Conway t.** A reduction mammoplasty in which the nipple and areola are repositioned as a full-thickness graft. **cross-fire t.** A radiotherapy technique by which various beams cross each other at the level of the lesion to be irradiated. **Cutler-Beard t.** A method of repairing a defect in an eyelid with tissues taken from the other eyelid. A full-thickness rectangular flap, not including the eyelid margin, is taken from the donor eyelid and advanced, with pedicle intact, beneath the eyelid margin into the defect of the recipient lid. After six weeks, the pedicle is divided. **dip slide t.** A useful screening technique for bacteriuria. Glass microscope slides coated with different culture media are quickly dipped in fresh urine. Excess urine is allowed to drain off, the slides are placed in capped vials at 37°C for 24 hours, and then examined for growth. **direct fluorescent antibody t.** The use of a fluorescence-labeled antibody that is specific for a particular antigen to demonstrate whether or not the unknown cells or tissue contains the antigen against which the antibody is directed. **double antibody t.** An *in vitro* radioimmunoassay procedure that utilizes an antiglobulin antibody to precipitate the primary antibody-antigen complex. **double layer fluorescent antibody t.** INDIRECT IMMUNOFLUORESCENCE. **drip infusion t.** A method of intravenous urography in which the contrast medium is administered by an infusion of a large volume of relatively dilute solution of contrast medium. **enzyme-multiplied immunoassay t.** An immunoassay technique that uses competitive binding to determine the quantity of analyte present in the test specimen. The indicator system is reagent analyte labeled with an enzyme, substrate for the enzyme, and antibody specific for the analyte. If the test specimen contains no analyte, the antibody combines with all the reagent analyte in such a way that enzyme activity is totally suppressed. Unlabeled analyte, if present, combines with antibody and displaces it from the enzyme-labeled material to a degree directly proportional to the relative quantities of labeled and unlabeled material present. **Farr t.** A means of determining the amount of antigen bound by antibody, using radiolabeled antigen and an ammonium sulfate solution that precipitates antigen-antibody complexes but not unbound antigen. Following isolation by precipitation of the antigen-antibody complexes, the level of radioactivity in the precipitated complexes can be used to quantify either the antigen or the antibody. **Fernandex t.** A method of westernizing the Oriental eyelids by removing skin and supraorbital fat from the upper eyelid, attaching the levator muscle to the overlying skin to create a supratarsal fold, and performing a Z-plasty at the medial canthus to eliminate the canthal fold. **Ferris Smith t.** MULTIPLE PARTIAL EXCISIONS. **fingerprinting t.** Any technique that identifies a substance by a number of discrete characters. It is used in protein chemistry to identify a protein by the electrophoretic or chromatographic mobilities, usually expressed by positions on a sheet of paper after separation, of the peptides formed by partial digestion of the protein. **fluorescent antibody t.** Any technique in which fluorochrome-tagged antibody is used to localize immunologically reactive material in tissue sections or on smeared cell preparations, as in direct or indirect immunofluorescence. **flush t.** A technique for measuring the systolic blood pressure in infants. The elevated arm or leg is massaged to induce blanching, an appropriate blood pressure cuff is inflated above the anticipated systolic pressure, and the arm is lowered to the horizontal position while the cuff is deflated. The pressure at which the limb becomes flushed is regarded as the systolic pressure. **Fones t.** FONES METHOD. **funicular suture t. in nerves** A microscopic nerve anastomosis performed by suture approximation of the individual nerve fascicles. **hanging drop t.** HANGING DROP. **helium dilution t.** A technique used for the determination of residual lung volume by rebreathing helium and measuring its dilution. **hemolytic plaque t.** JERNE TECHNIQUE. **Heyman's t.** A radiotherapy technique for cancer of the cervix, consisting of three series of irradiations with radium, with intervals of a week between each series. Also *Stockholm technique.* **hybridoma t.** A technique for producing monoclonal antibodies in tissue culture. Antibody-forming cells are fused with a malignant plasmacytoma and the hybrid cells subsequently cloned and grown as tumors. This technique has enormously expanded the availability of highly characterized and specific antibodies and has had a major impact on the direction and scope of immunologic research. **immunoferritin t.** A technique in which antibody is linked first to ferritin molecules and then applied to tissue sections or cell smears. Under electron microscopy, the electron dense, ferritin-labeled antibody molecules appear as dark dots. The technique is useful for high resolution determination of antigenic sites in a tissue or on a cell. **indicator-dilution t.** A method for measuring flow in a circulating system by introducing a known quantity of an indicator substance and monitoring its changing concentration over time downstream from the injection site. **indirect fluorescent antibody t.** The use of a fluorescence-labeled antiglobulin serum as the indicator to detect the attachment of an unlabeled specific antibody to a specific antigen on a cell or tissue preparation. The technique can be used if either the antigen or the antibody is the unknown. **inhibition t.** In immunology, any of those techniques which depend on the inhibition of a given reaction, as the inhibition of precipitation by haptens or the inhibition of red cell agglutination by antiviral antibody or specific antigen. **intermediate gel t.** Crossed immunoelectrophoresis in which the proteins traverse two gel strips on the second run. A reference serum can be incorporated in the intermediate strip, allowing direct comparison of qualitative and quantitative findings between reference and unknown serums. **Jerne t.** A hemolytic assay for determination of antibody-producing cells. Lymphocytes from immunized animals are mixed with erythrocytes in an agar gel and incubated, following which complement is added. A clear area of red cell lysis will form in the areas around antibody-producing cells. Also *Jerne plaque technique, hemolytic plaque technique, hemolytic plaque test.* **Kleinschmidt t.** An electron microscopical method of determining if two viral DNA molecules have homologous regions by melting and rehybridization of the DNAs to form heteroduplexes, which may show some areas of noncomplementary sequences. **Kristeller t.** KRISTELLER'S MANEUVER. **McGoon's t.** The plication of the posterior leaflet of the mitral valve in order to treat mitral insufficiency that results from a rupture of the posterior leaflet of the chordae tendinae. **Merendino's t.** A treatment of mitral insufficiency in which the valve annulus is shortened near the medial commissure by means of heavy silk sutures. **microtiter t.** A method for producing doubling dilutions with the aid of small spiral loops or solid plastic blocks calibrated to pick up small quantities of fluid and transfer them from tube to tube. The technique is used in microhemagglutination tests in which up to eight loops can be used simultaneously. Also *Takatsy technique.* **multiple pressure t.** A method for performing smallpox vaccination in which a drop of the vaccine is placed on the arm followed by the repeated application of pressure to the skin with a needle. This technique breaks the skin at the site of the needle and permits entry of the virus, and is considered preferable to scarification. **Nars-Hunter t.** The labeling of nonphenolic steroids by direct iodination of a steroid-phenol conjugate. **open-drop t.** An outmoded method of ether anesthesia in which the liquid is dripped onto a gauze-covered face mask for vaporization and inhalation. **opsonic t.** Any procedure used to measure opsonic activity, usually to evaluate the effect of antibodies or other proteins in serum applied to organisms before they are exposed to phagocytic cells. **Orr t.** ORR TREATMENT. **Ouchterlony t.** Double immunodiffusion in agar, in which antigen and antibody are placed in separate wells or troughs and are allowed to diffuse toward each other. The location and intensity of the precipitin line reflects the relative proportions of the reactants. Many different well patterns and combinations of single or multiple reactants are possible. Also *Ouchterlony test.* **parallel t.** A technique for creating a radiographic image of a tooth which is equal in length to the tooth itself by placing the film plane parallel to the long axis of the tooth. Also *right-angle technique.* **Paris t.** A method for treating carcinoma of the cervix with the use of radium tubes and vaginal cork containers retained by a colpostat. Relatively small quantities of radium are used to provide continuous irradiation for several days. Also *Regaud and Lacassagne technique.* **plaque t.** Any technique which involves the production of a hole or a plaque in a monolayer of either susceptible cells or bacteria. It may take the form of lysis by bacteriophage of areas in a confluent growth of bacteria, lysis of red cells by presensitized lymphocytes, or the lysis of virus-infected cells in a tissue-culture monolayer. **play t.** The use of games or other methods of play that are freely chosen by the child and used by the therapist as a substitute for free association in child analysis. **projective t.** A type of mental exploration making use of relatively unstructured or vague or ambiguous stimulus materials, such as ink blots or pictured scenes, which the subject is asked to describe or interpret or to use as the basis for an invented story. An analysis of the content of the response, together with certain formal characteristics of the mode of responding, makes possible an interpretation of how the individual perceives the world and directs behavior in reaction to it. **pulse echo t.** A method of imaging normally nonvisible tissues and tissue interfaces by sending pulses of ultrasound into the body and processing and displaying reflected echoes as an anatomic image. Also *pulse reflection method.* **Q t.** A method used to investigate the personality relationships between or among people by correlating the scores of different persons on an identical series of personality tests. **radioxenon t.** A technique by which regional distribution of pulmonary ventilation is measured by detecting the distribution of inhaled xenon 133 or 127. **Rebuck skin window t.** A test of the ability of a subject to mobilize white blood cells in an area that has been irritated. The test is performed by abrading the skin, covering it with a sterile glass coverslip, and, at a subsequent time, counting the number of cells that accumulate on the coverslip. Also *skin window technique.* **Regaud and Lacassagne t.** PARIS TECHNIQUE. **renal micropuncture t.** A procedure for studying the detailed activity of the kidney by inserting microcapillaries or microelectrodes into the cells, intercellular spaces, blood, or luminal spaces of the nephrons. **right-angle t.** PARALLEL TECHNIQUE. **rosette t.** Any technique in which the end point is clustering of one type of cells around cells of another type. Uses include identification of T lymphocytes by their ability to form rosettes spontaneously around unmodified sheep red blood cells; examination of antibody properties by the rosetting of cells possessing immunoglobulin receptors around antibody-coated cells; and the identification of small populations of Rh-positive human erythrocytes by their induction of rosettes of cells coated with anti-D antibody. **sandwich t.** Any immunologic procedure in which a labeled indicator is added to the specifically reacting antigen and antibody. Most often it is a solid-phase immunosorbent procedure in which the labeled reactant is immunologically similar to the immobilized reactant, thereby sandwiching the material under test between layers of known reactants. Indirect fluorescent antibody techniques are also sandwich techniques. **Schultz-Dale t.** SCHULTZ-DALE REACTION. **Seldinger t.** Percutaneous puncture of a peripheral artery or vein with a special trocar needle followed by passing a guide wire through the needle, removing the needle, leaving the wire in the vessel and passing a catheter over the wire into the vessel. Radiopaque material can then be injected through the catheter to opacify vessels. **single layer immunofluorescence t.** DIRECT IMMUNOFLUORESCENCE. **skin window t.** REBUCK SKIN WINDOW TECHNIQUE. **squash t.** A method of preparation of material for microscopic examination which involves squashing it on a microscope slide prior to staining. **Stockholm t.** HEYMAN'S TECHNIQUE. **Takatsy t.** MICROTITER TECHNIQUE. **thermal expansion t.** A casting technique using thermal expansion of of the set investment to compensate for the shrinkage of the cast metal on cooling. **thermodilution t.** A procedure for detecting flow in a circulating system by introducing a known quantity of warmer or cooler fluid and monitoring the changing temperature over time downstream from the injection site. **Warburg's t.** The study of oxygen consumption and carbon dioxide production by small portions of tissue under controlled temperature conditions. **wax expansion t.** A casting technique using thermal expansion of the wax pattern while the investment is liquid to compensate for the shrinkage of the cast metal on cooling. **Weigert-Pal t.** WEIGERT-PAL METHOD. **Ziehl-Neelsen t.** ZIEHL-NEELSEN STAIN.

**technologist** \teknäl′əjist\ [*technolog(y)* + -IST] TECHNICIAN. **medical t.** An individual trained to perform clinical laboratory determinations who has fulfilled educational requirements and passed examinations designated by appropriate regulatory agencies. **radiation therapy t.** An individual trained and skilled in the carrying out of technical procedures pertaining to radiation therapy. **radiologic t.** RADIOLOGIC TECHNICIAN.

**technology** \teknäl′əjē\ [Gk *technologia* (from *techn(ē)* art, craft + *leg(ein)* to arrange) systematic treatment] 1 The study and employment of techniques and procedures, as distinct from theoretical or conceptual studies. 2 Collectively, all the techniques employed to meet the material needs of a society.

**tectal** \tek′təl\ Pertaining to a tectum, particularly the tectum mesencephali.

**tecto-** \tek′tə-\ [L *tectum* (from *tectus,* past part. of *tegere* to cover, conceal) a roof, ceiling, room] A combining form meaning roof, rooflike.

**tectocephaly** \-sef′əlē\ SCAPHOCEPHALY.

**tectology** \tektäl′əjē\ [Gk *tekto(nia)* carpentry, construction + -LOGY] MORPHOLOGY.

**tectorial** \tektôr′ē·əl\ 1 Of or relating to a tectorium. 2 Serving as a covering or roof.

**tectorium** \tektôr′ē·əm\ A roof or covering.

**tectospinal** \-spī′nəl\ Denoting structures or physiological activity that emanates from the tectum of the mesencephalon and courses to or influences the spinal cord, such as the tectospinal tract or tectospinal effects on motor function.

**tectothalamic** \-thalam′ik\ Denoting axons extending from the optic tectum, or superior colliculus, to the thalamus.

**tectum** \tek′təm\ [L (substantive from neut. sing. of *tectus,* past part. of *tegere* to cover, akin to Gk *stegein* to cover closely), a roof, ceiling] Any rooflike or covering structure. Adj. tectal. **t. mesencephali** [NA] The portion of the mesencephalon that lies dorsal to the cerebral aqueduct, consisting principally of the two superior and two inferior colliculi, or corpora quadrigemina. Also *tectum of mesencephalon, optic tectum.* **optic t.** TECTUM MESENCEPHALI.

**TED** threshold erythema dose.

**teeth** Plural of TOOTH.

**teething** The period of eruption or cutting of the deciduous teeth.

**Teevan** [William Frederic *Teevan,* English surgeon, 1834–1887] See under LAW.

**Teflon** A synthetic polymer of tetrafluoroethylene. It is used in plastic operations and is available in the form of sheets or as solid preformed implants. A proprietary name.

**teflurane** \tef′lərān\ A halogenated ether containing fluorine. It is being studied for use as a general anesthetic.

**tegmen** \teg′mən\ [L (from *tegere* to cover, akin to Gk *stegein* to cover closely), a covering; also TEGMENTUM] Any structure that serves as a covering or roof. Also *tegumen.* **t. cruris** TEGMENTUM. **t. tympani** [NA] The thin plate of the anterior surface of the petrous part of the temporal bone that lies between the squamous part laterally and the arcuate eminence medially. It forms the roof of the tympanic cavity, of the mastoid antrum, and air cells posteriorly, and of the canal for the tensor tympani muscle anteriorly. Also *roof of tympanum.* **t. ventriculi quarti** [NA] The roof of the fourth ventricle. It is formed rostrally by the superior cerebellar peduncles and the superior medullary velum, caudally by the ependyma and tela choroidea of the fourth ventricle (which underlie the nodule of the cerebellum) and the inferior medullary velum.

**tegmental** \tegmen′təl\ 1 Pertaining to a tegmen. 2 Referring to the tegmentum in the pons, midbrain, or subthalamus.

**tegmentum** \tegmen′təm\ [L (from *teg(ere)* to cover, akin to Gk *stegein* to cover closely, + *-mentum* -MENT), a covering; also TEGUMENTUM] 1 A structure that serves as a covering. 2 [NA] The region of the mesencephalon that lies dorsal to the crus cerebri but ventral to the tectum mesencephali and cerebral aqueduct. It is continuous caudally with the tegmentum of the pons, and rostrally it merges with the caudal part of the subthalamic tegmentum. Among other nuclei and tracts, the tegmentum in the midbrain contains the large and important red nucleus. Also *tegmen cruris.* Adj. tegmental. **hypothalamic t.** SUBTHALAMIC TEGMENTUM. **t. of pons** PARS DORSALIS PONTIS. **pontile t.** PARS DORSALIS PONTIS. **t. pontis** PARS DORSALIS PONTIS. **t. rhombencephali** PARS DORSALIS PONTIS. **subthalamic t.** The portion of the tegmentum of the mesencephalon that extends rostrally into the subthalamic region of the diencephalon. Also *hypothalamic tegmentum.*

**tegumen** \teg′yəmen\ [L. See TEGMEN.] TEGMEN.

**tegument** \teg′yəmənt\ [L *tegumentum,* also *tegmentum.* See TEGMENTUM.] 1 An integument or enveloping structure. 2 Specifically, an amorphous structural component of the herpes virus located between the capsid and the envelope.

**tegumental** \teg′yəmen′təl\ [TEGUMENT + -AL] Serving as a skin or covering.

**tegumentary** \teg′yəmen′tərē\ [TEGUMENT + -ARY] Pertaining to the skin. Also *tegumentous.*

**teichoic acid** A substance found in the cell walls of Gram-positive bacteria. Its molecules have the repeating unit $—[CHOH]_n—O—PO_2^-—O—$, where $n$ may be 3 for a teichoic acid based on glycerol phosphate, or 5 for one based on ribitol phosphate. **membrane t.** LIPOTEICHOIC ACID. **streptococcal t.** Teichoic acid of group A streptococci, which consists of repeating units of glycerophosphate attached to lipids.

**teichopsia** \tīkäp′sē·ə\ [Gk *teich(os)* a wall, esp. a city wall + -OPSIA] The scintillating line of light along the boundary of a migrainous field defect; a visual shimmering. Also *fortification spectrum, flittering scotoma, scintillating scotoma, fortification figure.*

**teinodynia** \tī′nədin′ē·ə\ TENODYNIA.

**tela** \tē′lə\ [L (from *texere* to weave, plait, braid), a web, weaving, the warp] A thin, weblike membrane, layer, or tissue. **t. choroidea inferior** TELA CHOROIDEA VENTRICULI QUARTI. **t. choroidea superior** TELA CHOROIDEA VENTRICULI TERTII. **t. choroidea ventriculi laterali** A lateral extension into the lateral ventricle on each side of the tela choroidea ventriculi tertii, consisting of duplicated folds of pia mater containing blood vessels that invaginate into the ependymal lining of the lateral ventricle on each side through the choroid fissure. **t. choroidea ventriculi quarti** [NA] A duplicated fold of pia mater that helps form the roof of the part of the fourth ventricle over the medulla oblongata and provides the anchorage for the choroid plexus of the fourth ventricle. Also *tela chorioidea ventriculi quarti, tela choroidea of fourth ventricle, tela choroidea inferior.* **t. choroidea ventriculi tertii** [NA] The fused duplicated fold of pia mater that, along with a layer of ependymal cells, forms the thin roof of the third ventricle. From its inferior surface a pair of vascular processes invaginate the ependymal lining and project downward, one on each side of the midline, as the choroid plexus of the third ventricle. Also *tela chorioidea ventriculi tertii, triangular lamella, tela choroidea superior, tela choroidea of third ventricle, velum interpositum cerebri, velum interpositum, velum triangulare.* **t. elastica** *Outmoded* ELASTIC TISSUE. **t. subcutanea** [NA] A layer of irregular loose connective tissue deep to the dermis and bound to the underlying tissues by a dense fibrous layer or deep fascia. Its meshwork may contain varying amounts or no adipose cells or muscle fibers as well as the secretory parts of sweat glands. Through it pass the cutaneous nerves, blood vessels, and lymphatics. Also *hypodermis, superficial fascia, subcutaneous fascia, subcutaneous layer, fibroareolar fascia, hypoderm, subcutaneous tissue.* **t. submucosa** [NA] The layer of coarse loose connective tissue which contains some elastic fibers that is located between the tunica mucosa internally and the tunica muscularis in most of the alimentary canal. The layer is also found in parts of the respiratory and urogenital systems. Also *submucosa, submucous membrane, submucous coat, submucous layer, submucous stratum, vascular coat of viscera.* **t. submucosa bronchiorum** [NA] A layer of loose connective tissue containing mixed mucoserous and mucous glands and lying between the tunica mucosa and the rings of cartilage and dense connective tissue of the bronchi. **t. submucosa esophagi** [NA] The dense connective tissue layer which contains networks of collagenous and elastic fibers with lymphocytes that surround the glands. It lies between the tunica mucosa and the tunica muscularis of the esophagus. **t. submucosa gastrica** [NA] The layer of dense connective tissue between the tunica submucosa and tunica muscularis of the stomach. It contains fat cells, mast cells, lymphocytes, and eosinophil leukocytes as well as blood and lymph vessels and nerve and venous plexuses. Also *submucous membrane of stomach, submucous stratum of stomach, submucous layer of stomach, vascular coat of stomach.* **t. submucosa intestini tenuis** [NA] The layer of dense connective tissue containing many elastic fibers and some adipose cells that is located between the tunica mucosa and the tunica muscularis of the small intestine. In the duodenum it contains many glands. **t. submucosa pharyngis** [NA] A layer of loose connective tissue that is well developed only in the lateral wall of the nasopharynx and at the junction of the pharynx with the esophagus. Also *proper coat of pharynx.* **t. submucosa tracheae** A layer of loose connective tissue containing many blood vessels and mixed glands that lies between the tunica mucosa and the cartilages of the trachea. **t. submucosa vesicae urinariae** [NA] An irregular thin layer of loose connective tissue external to the lamina propria of the tunica mucosa of the bladder. It permits the folding of the mucous membrane in the contracted state and the flattening and decrease in number of layers during distension. **t. subserosa** The layer of connective tissue beneath the tunica serosa of some organs. Also *subserosa, subserous coat, subserous layer.* **t. subserosa gastrica** [NA] The layer of loose connective tissue that firmly joins the visceral peritoneum investing the stomach to the underlying tunica muscularis. **t. subserosa hepatis** [NA] The thin layer of loose connective tissue deep to the peritoneum that invests most of the liver and covers the thin capsule of connective tissue. **t. subserosa intestini tenuis** [NA] A fibrous layer deep to the tunica serosa of the small intestine. **t. subserosa peritonei** [NA] The layer of loose connective tissue immediately deep to the tunica serosa of the peritoneum. It is fairly extensive between the parietal peritoneum and the fascia of the abdominal walls but scant deep to the visceral peritoneum. It is directly fixed to and continuous with the fibrous tissue surrounding the viscera. Also *subperitoneal fascia, subserous layer of peritoneum.* **t. subserosa tubae uterinae** [NA] The layer of loose connective tissue containing the blood vessels and nerves of the uterine tube that lies between the tunica muscularis of the latter and the overlying peritoneum. Also *adventitious coat of uterine tube.* **t. subserosa uteri** [NA] A layer of loose connective tissue that extends along the sides of the uterus to become continuous with the subserous tissue between the two layers of the broad ligament. It separates the perimetrium from the underlying tunica muscularis. **t. subserosa vesicae biliaris** [NA] The layer of loose connective tissue immediately beneath the tunica serosa and superficial to the fibromuscular layer of the gallbladder. **t. subserosa vesicae urinariae** [NA] The layer of loose connective tissue immediately deep to the tunica serosa or peritoneum that covers the urinary bladder. **t. vasculosa** PLEXUS CHOROIDEUS.

**telae** \tē′lē\ Plural of TELA.

**telalgia** \telal′jə\ [*tel(e)-*[1] + -ALGIA] REFERRED PAIN.

**telangiectasia** \telan′jē·ektā′zhə\ [Gk *tel(os)* an end + ANGI- + ECTASIA] A vascular lesion resulting from the confluence of dilated small vessels, which may be arterial, capillary, venous, or lymphatic. Also *telangiectasis.* **cephalo-oculocutaneous t.** STURGE-WEBER SYNDROME. **familial t.** HEREDITARY HEMORRHAGIC TELANGIECTASIA. **hereditary hemorrhagic t.** A hemorrhagic disease which is inherited as an autosomal dominant disorder, although bleeding does not usually begin before the second or third decade. It is characterized by macular or nodular telangiectatic lesions occurring on the skin and mucous membranes, particularly on the tongue, lips, hands, and feet. The thin-walled blood vessels may rupture, leading to epistaxes, gastrointestinal bleeding, hemoptysis, hematuria, or cerebral hemorrhage. Polycythemia may accompany arteriovenous aneurysms that form in lungs and other viscera. Also *Rendu-Osler-Weber syndrome, Rendu-Osler-Weber disease, Osler-Weber-Rendu disease, Osler's disease, hemorrhagic familial angiomatosis, familial telangiectasia, Goldstein's disease.* **lymphatic t.** The dilatation of superficial lymphatics, as is seen in some forms of lymphangioma. Also *telangiectasia lymphatica.* **t. lymphatica** LYMPHATIC TELANGIECTASIA. **t. macularis eruptiva perstans** Urticaria pigmentosa, occurring in adults, in which telangiectasis and erythema are more evident than pigmentation. **spider t.** SPIDER TELANGIECTASIS.

**telangiectasis** \telan′jē·ek′təsis\ (*pl.* telangiectases) TELANGIECTASIA. **spider t.** A telangiectasis with small vessels radiating from a central arteriole, seen particularly in liver disease but also in pregnancy and in normal individuals. Also *spider telangiectasia, stellate telangiectsis, spider angioma, stellate angioma, vascular spider, arterial spider, stellar nevus, spider nevus, nevus arachnoideus, nevus araneus, nevus araneosus.* **stellate t.** SPIDER TELANGIECTASIS.

**telangion** \telan′jē·än\ [Gk *tel(os)* an end + *angeion* a vessel] END ARTERY.

**telar** \tē′lär\ Pertaining to or resembling a tela.

**tele-**[1] \tel′ə-\ [Gk *tēle* far away, far from] A combining form meaning far away, at a distance.

**tele-**[2] \tel′ə-\ [Gk *telos* (genitive *teleos*) an end, an end accomplished] A combining form meaning end. Also *telo-*.

**telebinocular** \-bīnäk′yələr\ An instrument that uses prisms for refraction for orthoptic training.

**telecanthus** \-kan′thəs\ [TELE-[1] + CANTHUS] An unusually great distance between the medial canthi of the eyelids. Also *canthal hypertelorism.*

**telecardiogram** \-kar′dē·əgram′\ A recording obtained by telecardiography.

**telecardiography** \-kär′dē·äg′rəfē\ The recording of the electrocardiogram from a site distant from the patient, as by radio or telephone.

**telecardiophone** \-kär′dē·əfōn′\ A device for relaying the heart sounds to auscultators at a distance from the patient.

**teleceptor** \tel′əsep′tər\ DISTANCE RECEPTOR.

**telecobalt** \tel′əkōbôlt\ See under TELECOBALT THERAPY.

**teledendrite** \-den′drīt\ TELODENDRON.

**teledendron** \-den′drän\ TELODENDRON.

**telediagnosis** \-dī'agnō'sis\ Diagnosis using electronic means such as television at a distance from the patient.
**telefluoroscopy** \-flôräs'kəpē\ [TELE-[1] + FLUOROSCOPY] The procedure of transmitting fluoroscopic images by television techniques to allow their observation at a remote site.
**telegrammatism** \-gram'ətizm\ TELEGRAPHIC SPEECH.
**teleirradiation** \-irā'dē·ā'shən\ Any form of irradiation in which the source of radiation is at a distance from the object being irradiated, as opposed to a source placed within the object.
**telemeter** \telem'ətər\ To transmit the measurement of a quantity to a distant station usually by radio where it is indicated or recorded.
**telemetry** \telem'ətrē\ The science or process of telemetering data. **cardiac t.** The transmission of the electrocardiogram to a site distant from the patient, as with cardiac monitors at a central station in an intensive care unit.
**telencephal** \telen'səfal\ TELENCEPHALON.
**telencephalic** \tel'ensəfal'ik\ Relating to the telencephalon.
**telencephalization** \tel'ensef'əlīzā'shən\ **1** The embryologic process in the later stages of vertebrate neurulation during which the telencephalon develops as a distinct part of the prosencephalon. **2** The evolutionary process by which the control of motor functions or the representation of sensory modalities becomes progressively transferred to higher centers in the brain.
**telencephalon** \tel'ensef'əlän\ [*tel(e)-*[2] + ENCEPHALON] [NA] The rostral part of the prosencephalon. It lies just behind the lamina terminalis and its cavity contributes to a small portion of the third ventricle, but this is overshadowed by the growth on each side of a telencephalic vesicle. The cavity of each vesicle forms a lateral ventricle and its wall becomes the cerebral hemisphere. Also *endbrain, telencephal.*
**teleneurite** \-n$^y$ur'īt\ **1** The terminal process of a nerve fiber. **2** The slender end of an axon.
**teleneuron** \-n$^y$ur'än\ [TELE-[2] + NEURON] The final (or end) neuron or neuronal process in a reflex arc or pathway that involves several neurons.
**teleodendron** \tel'ē·ōden'drän\ TELODENDRON.
**teleotherapeutics** \tel'ē·əther'əpyoo'tiks\ **1** PSYCHOTHERAPY. **2** HYPNOSIS.
**telepathy** \təlep'əthē\ [TELE-[1] + Gk *path(os)* experience, sensation + -Y] The alleged communication of thoughts, feelings, or mental impressions by means other than the action of the recognized channels of sense and independent of any known form of physical energy transmission. Also *thought-transference, thought-reading.*
**teleradiography** \-rā'dē·äg'rəfē\ TELEROENTGENOGRAPHY.
**teleradiotherapy** \-rā'dē·ōther'əpē\ [TELE-[1] + RADIOTHERAPY] Treatment by x rays or other ionizing rays in which the source is located at a distance from the body. Also *teleroentgentherapy.*
**teleradium** \tel'ərā'dē·əm\ [TELE-[1] + RADIUM] Radium used for radiation therapy and located at a distance from the body.
**telereceptor** \-risep'tər\ DISTANCE RECEPTOR.
**teleroentgenography** \-rent'genäg'rəfē\ [TELE-[1] + ROENTGENOGRAPHY ] Roentgenography with the distance of the x-ray tube target to the surface of the subject being at least six feet to accomplish the examination with practically parallel x rays, used to diminish magnification of the dimensions of the subject on the roentgenogram and allow more accurate direct measurements. Also *teleradiography.*
**teleroentgentherapy** \-rent'genther'əpē\ TELERADIOTHERAPY. **whole-body t.** WHOLE-BODY RADIOTHERAPY.
**telestethoscope** \-steth'əskōp\ [TELE-[1] + STETHOSCOPE] A combination of a stethoscope and an amplifier so that heart sounds may be heard by an audience.
**teletherapy** \-ther'əpē\ [TELE-[1] + THERAPY] Therapy in which the source of the therapeutic agent, such as radiation, is at a distance from the patient. ● The prefix *tele-* emphasizes that the therapeutic substance is not placed in direct contact with the patient, as in *telecobalt therapy, telecurie therapy.*
**telethermometer** \-thərmäm'ətər\ A thermometer which displays the temperature at a distance from the sensor.
**tellurism** \tel'oorizm\ [*tellur(ium)* + -ISM] A syndrome resulting from exposure to tellurium and its compounds and comprising dry mouth and skin, metallic taste, nausea, anorexia, somnolence, and vomiting. The breath of persons working with tellurium has a strong, garlicky smell.
**tellurium** \teloo'rē·əm\ Element number 52, having atomic weight 127.60. It is a brittle metal, rarely found native. The natural element comprises eight isotopes, one being unstable with a half-life of $1.2 \times 10^{13}$ years. Thirteen additional unstable isotopes have been identified. Symbol: Te
**telo-** \tel'ō-, tel'ə-\ TELE-[2].
**telobiosis** \-bī·ō'sis\ [TELO- + BIOSIS] The joining by experimental procedure of two embryos end to end.
**telocentric** \-sen'trik\ Of or relating to a chromosome with its centromere at the morphologic end.
**telocinesis** \-sīnē'sis\ TELOPHASE.
**telodendria** \-den'drē·ə\ Plural of TELODENDRION.
**telodendrion** \-den'drē·än\ TELODENDRON.
**telodendron** \-den'drän\ [TELO- + DENDRON] **1** One of many terminal arborizations into which the axon of a neuron branches; an axon ending. It is not uncommon to find many telodendria assembled into a network, but in some instances axons are seen to branch into only one or two such terminal processes. **2** The terminal branched end of a dendrite. For defs. 1 and 2 also *end-brush, telodendrion, teledendron, teledendrite, teleodendron.*
**telogen** \tel'əjən\ [TELO- + *-gen* as in *anagen*] The resting phase in the cycle of activity of the hair follicle. Compare ANAGEN, CATAGEN.
**teloglia** \teläg'lē·ə\ [TELO- + GLIA] Schwann cells that ensheath the motor terminals at a neuromuscular junction, at times projecting into the synaptic cleft.
**telognosis** \tel'ägnō'sis\ [*tel(e)-*[1] + *o* + *(dia)gnosis*] Radiographic diagnosis using a telephonic device to transmit the images.
**telokinesis** \-kīnē'sis\ TELOPHASE.
**telolecithal** \-les'ithəl\ [TELO- + Gk *lekith(os)* the yolk of an egg + -AL] Possessing moderate or much yolk. ● See note at TELOLECITHAL OVUM.
**telomere** \tel'əmir\ Either of the termini of a chromosome in a cytologic preparation from a eukaryote.
**telopeptide** [TELO- + PEPTIDE] One of the peptides from either end of a polypeptide sequence: used particularly for collagen, whose telopeptides do not possess the helical structure of most of the molecule, but are responsible for some of the stabilizing cross-links.
**telophase** \tel'əfāz\ The phase of nuclear division by mitosis or meiosis which begins as chromosomes reach the centrioles. The chromosomal constituents form a threadlike chromatin network and new nuclear envelopes are constructed around the two daughter nuclei. Also *telokinesis, telocinesis.*
**teloreceptor** \-risep'tər\ DISTANCE RECEPTOR.
**temp** temperature.

**temp. dext.** *tempori dextro* (L, to the right temple).

**temperament** [L *temperamentum* (from *temperare* to be temperate, from *tempus* time, season) disposition, middle course] The basic and enduring reactive disposition of an individual, including susceptibility to emotional stimulation, prevailing affective tone or mood, characteristic activity level, and the tendency for affiliation or sociability. Regarded as one of the raw materials from which an adult personality is shaped, temperament is thought to be largely genetically determined in the sense that it reflects such characteristics as an individual tendency toward neurophysiologic excitation or inhibition, the level of usual metabolic exchange, and a more or less permanent style of responsiveness by the endocrine system to emotion-provoking stimuli. **epileptic t.** EPILEPTIC CHARACTER.

**temperature** [L *temperatura* (from *temperare* to be temperate, from *tempus* time, season) a mixing in due proportion] **1** A measure of hotness or coldness. According to kinetic theory, the temperature of a body is proportional to the average kinetic energy of its constituent molecules. **2** An elevated body temperature; a slight fever. *Popular.* Abbr. temp. **basal body t.** The temperature of the body under conditions of complete mental and physical rest. Also *basal temperature.* **body t.** The temperature of the body, usually as observed in the axilla, rectum, or mouth in humans. **core t.** The temperature in the interior of the body. It is normally higher than the temperatures observed at superficial sites such as the axilla, rectum, or mouth. **critical t.** The highest temperature at which a particular gas can be liquefied. **normal t. and pressure** STANDARD TEMPERATURE AND PRESSURE. **optimum t.** The temperature at which an organism reaches its fastest rate of growth. It is usually close to 37°C for mammalian pathogens but lower for organisms found in the soil and on vegetation. **permissive t.** Any temperature of a culture or growth that enables an organism possessing a temperature-sensitive mutation to live or express a wild-type phenotype. **restrictive t.** Any temperature of a culture or growth that causes an organism possessing a temperature-sensitive mutation to express the mutant phenotype. **room t.** The unmodified ambient temperature in a laboratory or other indoor working space, which is usually 19 to 26°C. Incubation at room temperature implies that there is no need for exposure to refrigerator (1 to 6°C) or body (37°C) temperature. **standard t. and pressure** Any of various sets of reference conditions for the measurement of the properties of gases, for an environment, etc. The most often used is a temperature of 0°C and a pressure of one standard atmosphere (101 325 pascals). Although the standard pressure is always one standard atmosphere, standard temperatures vary, and for environments humidity is sometimes also specified. Also *normal temperature and pressure, standard conditions.* Abbr. STP, stp. • To avoid uncertainty, it is desirable to state reference conditions in full, e.g., 0°C, 1 atm; 20°C, 101.325 kPa, dry. **standard t. and pressure, dry** Standard temperature and pressure with the added requirement that the atmosphere be dry. Symbol: STPD

**temperature-sensitive** Sensitive to changes in temperature, or active only within a narrow range of temperature: commonly used to describe virus mutants which are selected for their inability to grow at 37–39°C but grow well at reduced temperatures such as 30–32°C. They are often used for genetic studies and are being evaluated for use as vaccines since they grow well in the nose but not in the lower respiratory tract and lungs because of the higher temperature.

**template** \tem′plit\ [variation of English *templet* (prob. dim. of French *temple* part of a loom) architectural support] **1** A piece of resin, plaster, or metal, having a predetermined shape, used as a guide in the setting of artificial teeth, or in the shaping of bone in alveolectomy. **2** A polymer which is able to influence the formation of another polymer, as a polynucleotide having the ability to specify the sequence of nucleotides of a replicating polynucleotide chain. **wax t.** A wax record of the occlusion of the teeth.

**temple** [from Vulgar L *tempula*, alteration of L *tempora*, pl. of *tempus* a temple of the head] In anatomy, the area of the temporal fossa above the zygomatic arch on the lateral side of the head. Also *tempus.*

**temporal** \tem′pərəl\ [Late L *temporalis* (from L *tempus*, gen. *temporis* a temple of the head) pertaining to the temples] **1** Of or relating to the temple. **2** Of or relating to the temporal bone or temporal lobe. **3** Nearer or toward the temple; lateral: applied to positions and directions in the eye or the visual field. Compare NASAL.

**temporalis** \tem′pərā′lis\ **1** Temporal. **2** MUSCULUS TEMPORALIS.

**temporo-** \tem′pərō-\ [See TEMPORAL.] A combining form meaning temple or temporal.

**temporoauricular** \-ôrik′yələr\ AURICULOTEMPORAL.

**temporofrontal** \-frun′təl\ FRONTOTEMPORAL.

**temporomandibular** \-mandib′yələr\ Of or relating to the temporal bone and the mandible.

**temporo-occipital** \-äksip′itəl\ OCCIPITOTEMPORAL.

**temporoparietal** \-pərī′ətəl\ Pertaining to the temporal and the parietal bones or regions. Also *parietotemporal.*

**temporopontile** \-pän′tīl\ Denoting connections between the temporal lobes of the cerebral hemispheres and the pons of the brainstem.

**temp. sinist.** *tempori sinistro* (L, to the left temple).

**tempus** \tem′pəs\ [L, a temple of the head] (*pl.* tempora) TEMPLE.

**tenacity** \tənas′itē\ The ability to stick fast to something else; cohesiveness. **cellular t.** The characteristic of cells which results in a continuation of cellular activities when the cellular environment is modified.

**tenaculum** \tənak′yələm\ [Late L, from L *ten(ere)* to hold + *-aculum*, suffix denoting an instrument] A hooked device for maintaining tissues in apposition.

**tendency** \ten′dənsē\ **primary reaction tendencies** Those constitutional and individual reaction tendencies that are apparent in infancy and continue through life. They appear to be governed by inheritance, and include activity level, sensitivity to stimuli, adaptability, and reaction to stress. See also TEMPERAMENT.

**tender** Painfully sensitive to pressure or touch.

**tenderness** The quality of being tender; painful sensitivity to pressure or touch. **pencil t.** Localized tenderness elicited by pressure from the tip of a pencil, a test for various conditions such as osteomyelitis or a fatigue fracture. **rebound t.** Tenderness that persists after applied pressure has been withdrawn.

**tendines** \ten′dinēz\ Plural of TENDO.

**tendinitis** \ten′dənī′tis\ [Med L *tendo*, gen. *tendin(is)* a tendon + -ITIS] Inflammation of a tendon. Also *tenonitis, tendonitis, tenontitis, tenositis.* **bicipital t.** A common form of tendinitis involving the long tendons of the long head of the biceps muscle. **calcific t.** Tendinitis associated with the deposition of hydroxyapatite. Also *periarthritis calcarea, tenontitis prolifera calcarea, periarticular calcification, Duplay syndrome* (obs.), *subdeltoid bursitis, scapulohumeral bursitis, subacromial bursitis.* **t. ossificans traumatica** Localized areas of ossification within a tendon that has been injured either by a direct blow or by avulsion from its bony insertion. Also *traumatic ossifying tendinitis.* **t. stenosans** Stenosing tenosynovitis of the flexor tendons of a finger. It results in trigger finger. Also *stenosing tendinitis.*

**tendinoplasty** \ten′dənōplas′tē\ TENOPLASTY.

**tendinosuture** \ten′dinōsoo′chər\ TENORRHAPHY.

**tendinous** \ten′dinəs\ Of, resembling, or relating to a tendon. Also *tenotic.*

**tendo** \ten′dō\ [Med L, gen. *tendonis* (later *tendinis*), from Gk *tenōn* tendon, with assimilation to L *tendere* to stretch. See also TENO-.] (*pl.* tendines) [NA] A fibrous band or cord of thick, closely packed, parallel, regularly arranged collagenous bundles that are held together by intervening loose connective tissue and are surrounded by a thick connective tissue sheath or epitendineum. It is a flexible tissue, able to resist considerable pulling force. At one end it is united to one or more muscle bellies, the collagenous bundles being continuous with the perimysium and fused by their tips with the sarcolemma so that the cone-shaped ends of the muscle fibers fit into grooves in the fibrous cord. At the other end it is attached to periosteum or perichondrium or directly to bone. Also *tendon.* **t. calcaneus** [NA] The long common tendon of insertion of both bellies of the gastrocnemius muscle and the soleus muscle. It commences below the calf at the back of the leg and attaches distally to the middle of

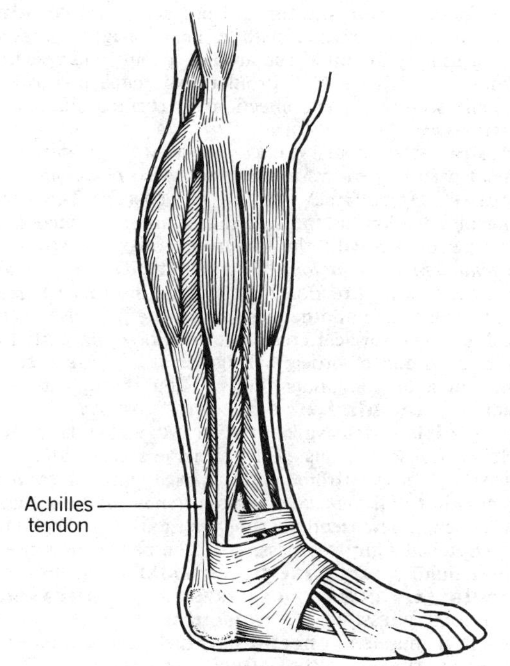


**Tendo calcaneus** (Achilles tendon)

the posterior surface of the calcaneus. Also *Achilles tendon, calcaneal tendon, cord of Hippocrates.* **t. conjunctivus** FALX INGUINALIS. **t. cricoesophageus** [NA] The stout tendon of part of the origin of the esophagus. It arises from the median vertical ridge on the posterior surface of the lamina of the cricoid cartilage and provides attachment for two bands of longitudinal muscle fibers that diverge around the sides of the esophagus to meet posteriorly in its midline. Also *cricoesophageal tendon, Gillette suspensory ligament.*

**tendo-** \ten′dō-\ [Med L *tendo* a tendon] A combining form meaning tendon.

**tendolysis** \tendäl′isis\ TENOLYSIS.

**tendon** \ten′dən\ [Med L *tendo.* See TENDO.] TENDO. **Achilles t.** TENDO CALCANEUS. **calcaneal t.** TENDO CALCANEUS. **central t. of diaphragm** CENTRUM TENDINEUM. **central t. of perineum** CENTRUM TENDINEUM PERINEI. **common t.** A tendon that receives the attachments of either more than one muscle, such as tendo calcaneus, or two or more heads of a muscle, such as that of the triceps brachii muscle. **conjoined t.** FALX INGUINALIS. **conjoint t.** FALX INGUINALIS. **t. of the conus arteriosus** A tendinous band of the fibrous base of the heart that extends forward from the anterior aspect of the aorta to the posterior surface of the conus arteriosus or infundibulum in the right ventricle. It ends by uniting with the annulus fibrosus of the pulmonary ostium. Also *tendon of infundibulum.* **coronary t.'s** The annuli fibrosi cordis of the aortic and the pulmonary trunk orifices. **cricoesophageal t.** TENDO CRICOESOPHAGEUS. **Gerlach's annular t.** ANNULUS FIBROCARTILAGINEUS MEMBRANAE TYMPANI. **hamstring t.** One of the prominent tendons on either side of the popliteal space: the tendon of insertion of the biceps femoris muscle (lateral hamstring) or of the semitendinosus and semimembranosus muscles (medial hamstrings). **t. of infundibulum** TENDON OF THE CONUS ARTERIOSUS. **intermediate t.** 1 The tendon interposed between the two bellies of either the digastric or the omohyoid muscle. 2 *Outmoded* CENTRUM TENDINEUM. **t. of origin** The attachment of a muscle to the fixed bone in a particular movement. In the limbs, this is usually the proximal attachment of a muscle. **riders' t.** A strain of the adductor tendons of the thigh that is seen in horseback riders. **snapping t.** A tendon that subluxes over a bony protuberance when active, as may occur in snapping hip. **trefoil t.** CENTRUM TENDINEUM. **t. of Zinn** ANNULUS TENDINEUS COMMUNIS.

**tendonitis** \ten′dənī′tis\ TENDINITIS.

**tendoplasty** \ten′dəplas′tē\ TENOPLASTY.

**tendosynovitis** \-sin′əvī′tis\ TENOSYNOVITIS.

**tendotome** \ten′dətōm\ TENOTOME.

**tendotomy** \tendät′əmē\ TENOTOMY.

**tendovaginal** \-vaj′ənəl\ Pertaining to a tendon and its sheath.

**tendovaginitis** \-vaj′ənī′tis\ [TENDO- + VAGINITIS] TENOSYNOVITIS. **t. granulosa** Nodular inflammation of a tendon and the tendon sheath, as seen in rheumatoid arthritis. **t. stenosans** STENOSING TENOSYNOVITIS.

***Tenebrio*** \teneb′rē-ō\ A genus of beetles the larvae of which are called meal worms. Meal worms are commonly used as food for captive insectivorous animals and birds. The common yellow meal worm, *T. molitor,* will harbor injected tubercle bacilli over successive stages. It also serves as a host for the cysticercoids of hymenolepid tapeworms such as the rat tapeworm, *Hymenolepis diminuta.*.

**tenectomy** \tenek′təmē\ [*ten(o)-* + -ECTOMY] The excision of all or part of a tendon or tendon sheath.

**tenesmus** \tenez′məs\ [L, from Gk *teinesmos* (from *teinein* to stretch, strain) a straining at defecation] A painful spasm of the anal sphincter or the sphincter vesicae accompanied by involuntary straining and a need to evacuate the rectum or bladder but with the passage of little or no fecal matter or urine.

**tenia** \tē′nē·ə\ [L *taenia.* See TAENIA.] (*pl.* teniae, tenias) TAENIA. **teniae coli** TAENIAE COLI.

**teniacide** \tē′nē·əsīd′\ TAENIACIDE.

**teniae** \tē′ni·ē\ Plural of TENIA.

**teniafugal** \tē′nē·af′yəgəl\ TAENIAFUGAL.

**teniafuge** \tē′nē·əfyooj′\ TAENIAFUGE.

**tenicide** \ten′isīd\ TAENIACIDE.

**teniform** \ten′ifôrm\ TAENIFORM.

**tenifugal** \tēnif′yəgəl\ TAENIAFUGAL.

**tenifuge** \ten′ifyooj\ TAENIAFUGE.

**tenioid** \tē′nē·oid\ TAENIOID.

**teno-** \ten′ō-\ [Gk *tenōn,* gen. *tenontos* (from *teinein* to stretch, akin to L *tendere* to stretch) tendon] A combining form meaning tendon. Also *tenon-, tenonto-.*

**tenodesis** \tenäd′əsis, ten′ədē′sis\ [TENO- + -DESIS] The surgical attachment of the end of a tendon to a bone or to another tendon.

**tenodynia** \-din′ē·ə\ [*ten(o)-* + -ODYNIA] Pain emanating from a tendon. Also *tenontodynia, teinodynia.*

**tenofibril** \-fī′bril\ TONOFIBRIL.

**tenology** \tenäl′əjē\ [TENO- + -LOGY] The study of tendons. Also *tenontology.*

**tenolysis** \tenäl′isis\ [TENO- + LYSIS] A surgical operation to cut or remove adhesions between a tendon and surrounding structures, enabling the tendon to move more freely.

**tenomyoplasty** \ten′əmī′əplas′tē\ A plastic operation on tendon and muscle. Also *myotenontoplasty, tenontomyoplasty.*

**tenomyotomy** \ten′əmī·ät′əmē\ MYOTENOTOMY.

**Tenon** [Jacques René *Tenon,* French anatomist and oculist, 1724–1816] **1** Fascia of Tenon, Tenon's capsule, Tenon's membrane. See under VAGINA BULBI. **2** Tenon space. See under SPATIUM EPISCLERALE.

**tenon-** \ten′ən-\ TENO-.

**tenonectomy** \-ek′təmē\ [TENON- + -ECTOMY] The excision of a segment of tendon and/or muscle in order to reduce its length.

**tenonitis** \ten′ənī′tis\ TENDINITIS.

**tenonometer** \ten′ənäm′ətər\ TONOMETER.

**tenonostosis** \ten′ənästō′sis\ TENOSTOSIS.

**tenontitis** \ten′əntī′tis\ TENDINITIS. **t. prolifera calcarea** CALCIFIC TENDINITIS.

**tenonto-** \tenän′tō-\ TENO-.

**tenontodynia** \ten′äntədin′ē·ə\ TENODYNIA.

**tenontolemmitis** \-lemī′tis\ TENOSYNOVITIS.

**tenontology** \ten′äntäl′əjē\ TENOLOGY.

**tenontomyoplasty** \-mī′əplas′tē\ TENOMYOPLASTY.

**tenontomyotomy** \-mī·ät′əmē\ MYOTENOTOMY.

**tenontothecitis** \-thēsī′tis\ TENOSYNOVITIS.

**tenontotomy** \ten′äntät′əmē\ TENOTOMY.

**tenopathy** \tenäp′əthē\ [TENO- + -PATHY] Any abnormality of a tendon.

**tenophyte** \ten′əfīt\ A firm bony or cartilagenous growth attached to a tendon.

**tenoplasty** \ten′əplas′tē\ [TENO- + -PLASTY] Any plastic operation on tendon. Also *tendinoplasty, tendoplasty, tenontoplasty.*

**tenoreceptor** \ten′ərisep′tər\ [TENO- + RECEPTOR] A sense organ situated in a tendon and excited by muscular contraction or stretch.

**tenorrhaphy** \tenôr′əfē\ [TENO- + -RRHAPHY] The suturing of the divided ends of a tendon. Also *tenosuture, tendinosuture.*

**tenositis** \ten′əsī′tis\ TENDINITIS.

**tenostosis** \ten′ästō′sis\ The ossification of a tendon. Also *tenonostosis.*

**tenosuspension** \ten′əsuspen′shən\ The use of a tendon, or a portion thereof, as a suspensory ligament or as a fascial sling. The tendon can be utilized as a free graft or in continuity with its related muscle.

**tenosuture** \ten′əsoo′chər\ TENORRHAPHY.

**tenosynitis** \ten′əsinī′tis\ TENOSYNOVITIS.

**tenosynovectomy** \ten′əsin′ōvek′təmē\ The excision of the synovial sheath of a tendon.

**tenosynovioma** \ten′əsinō′vē·ō′mə\ [TENO- + *synovi(al)* + -OMA] A benign tumor of synovial cells.

**tenosynovitis** \ten′ōsin′əvī′tis\ [TENO- + SYNOVITIS] An inflammation of a tendon and its sheath. Also *tenosynitis, tenontolemmitis, tenontothecitis, thecitis, tendosynovitis, tenovaginitis, tendinous synovitis, vaginal synovitis, tendovaginitis.* **adhesive t.** STENOSING TENOSYNOVITIS. **t. crepitans** An inflammation of a tendon sheath that gives rise to a crackling sound when the tendon moves. Also *crepitous tenosynovitis.* **gonococcic t.** Tenosynovitis due to gonococcal infection. Also *gonorrheal tenosynovitis.* **granulomatous t.** Granuloma formation within a tendon sheath such as occurs in tuberculosis. Also *tenosynovitis granulosa.* **ossifying t.** Bone formation within a tendon and its sheath. **stenosing t.** Tenosynovitis in which scarring of the tendon sheath prevents motion of the tendon, usually causing flexion contracture such as Dupuytren's contracture or trigger finger. Also *adhesive tenosynovitis, tendovaginitis stenosans, tenosynovitis stenosans.* **tuberculous t.** A chronic tuberculous infection that is present in the tendon sheaths and bursae. **villonodular t.** Synovial proliferation with a hemorrhagic component, occuring usually in soft tissue around a joint and resembling a tumor. **villous t.** Proliferative tenosynovitis, most commonly seen in chronic infections or rheumatoid arthritis.

**tenotic** \tenät′ik\ TENDINOUS.

**tenotome** \ten′ətōm\ [TENO- + -TOME] A surgical instrument used to perform a tenotomy. Also *tendotome.*

**tenotomy** \tenät′əmē\ [TENO- + -TOMY] The surgical cutting of a tendon, as the severing of an extraocular muscle tendon performed with the intent of correcting strabismus. Also *tendotomy, tenontotomy.* **fenestrated t.** A longitudinal incision of a tendon that is made in order to create a hole through which another tendon can be passed. **graduated t.** The surgical creation of one or more partial divisions in a tendon in order to lengthen it. **open t.** The division of a tendon under direct vision through a surgical incision. **stapedial t.** STAPEDIOTENOTOMY.

**tenovaginitis** \ten′əvaj′ənī′tis\ TENOSYNOVITIS.

**TENS** transcutaneous electrical nerve stimulation.

**tension** [L *tensio* (from *tensus,* a past part. of *tendere* to stretch; akin to Gk *teinein* to stretch, *tonos* anything that can be stretched, sinew, tendon, rope) tension] **1** The state of being stretched tight; tautness. **2** The partial pressure of a gas in a fluid. **arterial t.** ARTERIAL PRESSURE. **intraocular t.** INTRAOCULAR PRESSURE. **intravenous t.** VENOUS PRESSURE. **muscular t.** The force of stretch in a muscle. **premenstrual t.** See under PREMENSTRUAL TENSION SYNDROME. **specific t.** Tension or force developed per unit cross-sectional area of a contracting muscle. It is expressed either in newtons/$cm^2$ or g/$cm^2$. **surface t.** **1** An unbalanced cohesive force attraction of fluid molecules at the surface film that gives the film the property of a membrane. **2** A cohesive attraction which tends to minimize the surface of a fluid.

**tensor** \ten′sər, ten′sôr\ A muscle that tenses or stretches the part into which it is inserted. **t. capsularis articulationis metacarpophalangei digiti** A variant of the opponens digiti minimi muscle that is inserted into the anterior aspect of the metacarpophalangeal joint of the fifth finger. **t. ligamenti annularis** One of the rather common accessory fasciculi of origin of the supinator muscle. One, the tensor ligamenti annularis anterior, arises from the annular ligament, whereas the posterior form extends from the ulna behind the radial notch to the annular ligament.

**tent** 1 A cover or canopy enclosing the space about a patient and into which oxygen or steam, for example, can be introduced for inhalation. 2 A cylindrical wad or plug of absorbent material placed in an orifice to dilate it or in a wound to prevent premature closure while absorbing fluid discharges. **air flow t.** A large sealed enclosure within an operating room, consisting of a confined airflow system to reduce the possibility of bacterial contamination in circulating air. The surgical team works within the confined space of the air flow tent. **oxygen t.** A tent into which oxygen is fed to raise the concentration of oxygen in the air around a patient. **sponge t.** A bullet-shaped piece of compressed sponge which is inserted in the uterine cervical canal to effect dilatation. **steam t.** A tent into which steam is introduced to raise the humidity of the air around a patient.

**tentorium** \tentôr′ē·əm\ [L (from *tent(us)* a past part. of *tendere* to stretch, be in tents + *-orium* -ORY), a tent] (*pl.* tentoria) A tentlike covering, generally composed of connective tissue, serving as a roof or partition for certain structures or organs, such as the tentorium cerebelli. Adj. tentorial. **t. cerebelli** [NA] A crescentic, arched lamina of dura mater that overlies the cerebellum, forming a roof for the posterior cranial fossa and simultaneously underlying and supporting the occipital lobes of the cerebral cortex. Its U-shaped anterior margin is free and surrounds the midbrain, while its convex outer margin is attached along the superior border of the petrous part of the temporal bone and along the transverse sulci of the occipital bone. Also *tentorium of cerebellum*. **t. of hypophysis** DIAPHRAGMA SELLAE.

**tenuis** \ten′yoo·is\ [L, thin, fine, slender] Thin, slender, or delicate.

**TEPA** triethylenephosphoramide.

**ter-** \ter-, tur-, tər-\ [L *ter* thrice] A combining form meaning thrice, threefold.

**tera-** \ter′ə-\ [Gk *teras* monster] 1 TERATO-. 2 A combining form denoting $10^{12}$: used with SI units. Symbol: T

**teracurie** \ter′əkyoo′rē\ [TERA- + CURIE] A unit of activity of a radionuclide or of a radioactive source equal to $10^{12}$ curie; $3.7 \times 10^{22}$ becquerels, exactly. Symbol: TCi

**teras** \ter′as\ [Gk *teras* a monster, sign, wonder] (*pl.* terata) An embryo, fetus, postnatal individual or part thereof which is structurally malformed. Adj. teratic.

**terat-** \ter′ət-\ TERATO-.

**terata** \ter′ətə\ Plural of TERAS.

**teratism** \ter′ətizm\ [TERAT- + -ISM] The process or processes of abnormal embryogenesis by which malformed structures arise. Also *teratosis, maldevelopment, malformation*. **atresic t.** The failure of an opening, foramen, or lumen to form or to remain perforate or patent once formed, as in anorectal agenesis, imperforate hymen, or aortic atresia. **ceasmic t.** The failure of lateral halves or adjacent primordia to unite, as is seen in cleft palate or failed neural tube closure. **ectogenic t.** A teratism or malformation resulting from outside or exogenous influences. It can be caused by an environmental or nongenetic factor or factors. **ectopic t.** A teratism characterized mainly by its abnormal position, as in ectopia of the thyroid, thymus, or parathyroid glands. **ectrogenic t.** A deficiency or absence of the usual parts, as in renal agenesis, anophthalmia, or ectrodactyly. **hypergenic t.** A duplication or redundancy of parts, as in polydactyly, accessory spleens, or duodenal duplication. **symphysic t.** A teratism resulting from abnormal fusion or union of parts during development, as in fused kidneys, sirenomelia, or cyclopia. Conjoined twins could also be regarded as symphysic in nature because, regardless of the extent of union, they are presumed to have arisen, at least in part, on separate and distinct embryonic axes.

**terato-** \ter′ətō-\ [Gk *teras,* gen. *teratos* monster] A combining form meaning developmental malformation. Also *tera-, terat-*.

**teratoblastoma** \-blastō′mə\ TERATOMA.

**teratocarcinoma** \-kär′sinō′mə\ [TERATO- + CARCINOMA] 1 A malignant teratoma. Also *teratoid carcinoma*. 2 A tumor composed of teratoma and embryonal carcinoma.

**teratogen** \ter′ətəjən\ [TERATO- + -GEN] An agent or factor, such as radiation, viral infection, chemical, drug, etc., that is capable of causing the production of developmental abnormality in an embryo, fetus, or postnatal individual.

**teratogenesis** \-jen′əsis\ [TERATO- + GENESIS] The origin or mechanism of production of a developmentally abnormal embryo, fetus, postnatal individual, or part thereof. Also *teratogeny, dysmorphogenesis*. **experimental t.** The experimental production of developmental defects or malformations of an embryo, fetus, postnatal individual, or part thereof, following exposure to a teratogen.

**teratogenic** \-jen′ik\ [TERATO- + -GENIC] Tending to cause abnormal development; apt to produce malformation. Also *teratogenetic, teratogenous*.

**teratogenicity** \-jənis′itē\ The property of being teratogenic; the capacity to induce abnormal development.

**teratogeny** \ter′ətäj′ənē\ TERATOGENESIS.

**teratoid** \ter′ətoid\ [TERAT- + -OID] Resembling a teras, in the sense of a postnatally acquired defect or abnormality having similarity to a congenital one.

**teratologic** \-läj′ik\ Concerned with or in the nature of teratology.

**teratologist** \ter′ətäl′əjist\ One who practices the science of teratology.

**teratology** \ter′ətäl′əjē\ [TERATO- + -LOGY] The study of abnormal development. More particularly, it is the study of the causes, mechanisms, and manifestations of abnormal development, whether genetically, gestationally, or postnatally induced; and whether expressed as lethality, malformation, growth retardation, or functional aberration. Also *dysmorphology*.

**teratoma** \ter′ətō′mə\ [TERAT- + -OMA] A tumor that is composed of several types of tissue foreign to the site and typically representing different germ layers. The testis and ovary are the most common organs for teratomas but they may be found in a variety of locations, such as the mediastinum, or sacrococcygeal area. Their behavior generally depends on the maturity of the component tissues. Also *organoid tumor, teratoblastoma, teratoid parasite, embryoma*. Compare CHORISTOMA. **adult t.** MATURE TERATOMA. **anaplastic malignant t.** EMBRYONAL CARCINOMA. **benign t.** MATURE TERATOMA. **cystic t.** A teratoma containing grossly visible cysts. **differentiated t.** MATURE TERATOMA. **immature t.** A teratoma containing incompletely differentiated tissues, in relation to the patient's age, although mature tissues may be present. This type of teratoma is malignant. Also *malignant teratoma, intermediate malignant teratoma*. • The term *teratocarcinoma* has been used for immature teratoma as well as for a tumor containing teratoma and embryonal carcinoma. **malig-**

**nant t.** IMMATURE TERATOMA. **t. with malignant transformation** A teratoma containing a malignant component of a type typically encountered in other organs and tissues, as squamous cell carcinoma, malignant melanoma, or adenocarcinoma. This is seen both in ovary and testis. Also *dermoid cyst with malignant transformation.* **mature t.** A teratoma composed exclusively of mature differentiated tissue. It is typically benign. Also *adult teratoma, benign teratoma, differentiated teratoma.* **monodermal t.** A form of teratoma in which only one germ layer is the source of tumor tissue, such as struma ovarii, epidermoid cyst of the ovary, or carcinoid of the ovary. **t. orbitae** ORBITOPAGUS. **tridermal t.** Teratoma containing elements derived from ectoderm, mesoderm, and endoderm. Also *triphyllomatous teratoma.* **triphyllomatous t.** TRIDERMAL TERATOMA. **tropoblastic malignant t.** CHORIOCARCINOMA. **undifferentiated malignant t.** EMBRYONAL CARCINOMA.

**teratomata** \ter′ətō′mətə\ Plural of TERATOMA.

**teratomatous** \ter′ətō′mətəs\ Of the nature of or relating to a teratoma.

**teratosis** \ter′ətō′sis\ [TERAT- + -OSIS] TERATISM.

**teratospermia** \-spur′mē·ə\ [TERATO- + SPERM + -IA ] The presence of misshapen spermatozoa in the semen.

**terbium** \tur′bē·əm\ Element number 65, having atomic weight 158.925. Terbium is a silvery gray metal of the lanthanide series. It has a few technologic applications. Symbol: Tb

**tere** [L, imperative sing. of *terere* to rub] Rub, an instruction used in prescriptions.

**terebinth** \ter′əbinth\ [L *terebinthus* (Gk *terebinthos* the terebinth or turpentine tree, the resin therefrom, turpentine) the terebinth tree] A tree of the genus *Pistacia,* one of the sources of turpentine oil.

**terebinthinism** \ter′əbin′thinizm\ A morbid condition from ingestion or external application of turpentine oil, which can result in severe irritation of skin, mucous membranes, and kidneys, and in hemoglobinemia, pulmonary edema, and convulsions.

**terebrant** \ter′əbrənt\ [L, from *terebrans,* gen. *terebrantis,* pres. part. of *terebrare* to bore, pierce] Boring or piercing: said of pain. Also *terebrating.*

**terebration** \ter′əbrā′shən\ [L *terebratus,* past part. of *terebrare* to bore, pierce] *Obs.* TREPHINING.

**teres** \tē′rēz, ter′ēz\ [L, rounded, polished, smooth] Round and long: said of some muscles and ligaments.

**ter in die** Three times a day: used in prescription writing.

**term** [Old French *terme* (from L *terminus;* see TERMINUS) a boundary, limit] **1** A fixed or definite period of time. **2** The period of time in a pregnancy when the estimated date of confinement has arrived or is very near. In human pregnancies, this time arrives from 38 to 42 weeks after the first day of the last menstrual period. **3** A word or phrase used to designate a definite thing, condition, etc., as in a scientific discipline. **at t.** At or near the expiration of a term of pregnancy.

**Terman** [Lewis Madison *Terman,* U.S. psychologist, 1877–1956] Terman test. See under STANFORD-BINET INTELLIGENCE SCALE.

**terminad** \tur′minad\ **1** Toward the end. **2** Toward an extremity.

**terminaison** \ter′mināzôN′\ [French (from L *terminatio* a limit, limitation) an ending] **t.'s en grappe** GRAPE ENDINGS. **t. en ligne** An extrafusal motor endplate having a linear outline oriented along the fiber when seen in metallic stained sections. It is characteristic of amphibian and reptilian muscles. **t.'s en panier** Basketlike sensory endings that embrace the tips of muscle fibers inserted into the septa between the myotomes in selachians, fish, amphibians, and reptiles. Also *basket endings.* **t. en plaque** A motor endplate of compact, platelike form. Also *en plaque ending, en plaque terminal.* • The expression "en plaque" or simply "plaque" is often used for this term, probably because calling it a plate would cause confusion with *endplate,* which has broader application.

**terminal** [L *terminalis* marking a boundary] **1** Situated at or occurring at an end. **2** Pertaining to an extremity or end of a body or a structure. **3** Likely to lead to death; not admitting of the likelihood of recovery: said of a disease. **4** Affected by a disease likely to cause death and from which recovery is unlikely: said of a patient. **5** An ending; a distal end. **axon t.** END FOOT. **en plaque t.** TERMINAISON EN PLAQUE. **grapelike t.'s** GRAPE ENDINGS. **Wilson central t.** In electrocardiography, a terminal created by connecting resistors of equal value to the right arm, left arm, and left leg. It serves as a reference for the unipolar exploring lead when recording the precordial leads.

**terminalization** \tur′mənal′īzā′shən\ [TERMINAL + *-iz(e)* + -ATION] A progressive shift of the chiasmata along the arms of paired meiotic chromosomes from their points of origin toward the ends of the chromosomes. The process occurs between diplotene and metaphase of the first meiotic division.

**terminatio** \tur′minā′shō\ [L (from *terminare* to bound, limit, from *terminus* an end, boundary), a fixing of limits] (*pl.* terminationes) The distal end of a structure; an ending, as of a nerve or vessel. **terminationes nervorum liberae** The terminal processes of certain sensory nerve fibers that end freely in a variety of tissues and serve as neural receptors. Among many sites, they are found abundantly in the epithelium of the cornea, in the skin and mucous membranes of the respiratory tract and oral cavity, and in the connective tissue of the dermis, as well as in tissues around joints.

**termini** Plural of TERMINUS.

**terminus** \tur′minəs\ [L (from *termen* a boundary marker, limit, akin to Gk *terma* an end, limit) an end-point, limit] (*pl.* termini) **1** A term or descriptive expression. **2** An ending or terminal segment. **C t.** The portion of a polypeptide chain that is C-terminal. Also *C-terminal end.* **N t.** The portion of a polypeptide chain that is N-terminal. Also *N-terminal end.*

**ternary** \tur′nəre\ [L *ternari(us)* (from *tern(i)* three each, three + *-arius* -ARY) consisting of three] Involving the number three: used especially in chemistry of an atom with three ligands, e.g. $S^+$ as opposed to S, and N as opposed to $N^+$, and in biochemistry of a three-component complex, e.g. an enzyme with two substrate molecules bound.

**terpene** Any of the group of hydrocarbons that are oligomers of isoprene and hence have the formula $(C_5H_8)_n$. When $n = 2$ they are known as monoterpenes, when $n = 4$, diterpenes, and when $n = 3$, sesquiterpenes. Squalene, the biosynthetic precursor of sterols, is a terpene.

**terpenism** \ter′pənizm\ Poisoning from ingestion of, or skin contact with, a terpene. Some terpenes, like pinene, limonene, and phelandrene, may cause severe injury to the skin. Others, like thujone and camphor, may produce central nervous system stimulation, while others, like camomile, eucalyptus, and turpentine, exert a depressant effect and cause irritation of the kidneys and bladder.

***p*-terphenyl** 1,4-Diphenylbenzene, one of a number of fluorescent compounds used as primary solutes in a liquid-scintillation vial. It receives the excitation energy from the solvent and emits a flash of light.

**terpin** $C_{10}H_{20}O_2$. 4-Hydroxy-α,α,-trimethylcyclohexanemethanol. A product obtained by the action of nitric acid on turpentine and alcohol. The *cis*-(hydrate) form is used as an expectorant and a common ingredient in cough syrups. Also *turpentine camphor.*

**terpin hydrate** The monohydrate of terpin, *p*-menthane-1,8-diol. It is an expectorant and a common constituent of cough medicines.

**terra** \ter′ə\ EARTH. **t. alba** KAOLIN. **t. silicea purificata** Diatomaceous earth that has been boiled, washed, and calcined. It is used as an absorbent in the decolorizing and purification of some drug products, and as a dusting powder.

**terrestrial** \teres′trē·əl\ [L *terrester,* gen. *terrestri(s)* (from *terra* the earth) of or on the earth + -AL] Living or developing in or on the land.

**terrestric acid** A metabolic by-product of the fungus *Penicillium terrestre.*

**Terrier** [Louis-Felix *Terrier,* French surgeon, 1837–1908] **1** Courvoisier-Terrier syndrome. See under SYNDROME. **2** See under VALVE.

**terror** [L (from *terrere* to affright) terror, fear] Extreme fear. **day t.'s** PAVOR DIURNUS. **night t.'s** PAVOR NOCTURNUS.

**Terry** [Theodore Lasater *Terry,* U.S. ophthalmologist, 1899–1946] Terry syndrome. See under RETROLENTAL FIBROPLASIA.

***tert-*** \turt-, tərt-\ [*tert(iary)*] A prefix used in organic chemistry to designate a special class of isomer. It usually implies presence of three substituents on a single atom, for example, *tert*-butanol for $(CH_3)_3C—OH$. An outmoded usage.

**tertian** \tur′shən\ [L *(febris) tertiana,* fem. of *tertianus* relating to the third or the third day, from *tertius* third + *-anus* adjectival suffix; tertian fever] Occurring every third day, with the initial day as the first day: usually said of a malarial fever, such as the 48-hour recurrent cycle of *Plasmodium vivax.* **double t.** Characterizing an intermittent fever with two attacks, both tertian. **malignant t.** Characterizing a fever occurring in falciparum malaria in which there is usually a 48-hour periodicity, but in which the intermission may be incomplete. • The term describes the virulence of this type of malaria.

**Teschendorf** [Werner *Teschendorf,* German roentgenologist, born 1895] Barsony-Teschendorf syndrome. See under DIFFUSE ESOPHAGEAL SPASM.

**tesla** \tes′lə\ [after Nikola *Tesla,* Croatian-born American electrical engineer and inventor, 1857–1943] The special name for the SI derived unit of magnetic flux density, equal to one weber per square meter; one kilogram per second squared ampere. Symbol: T

**tessellated** \tes′əlātid\ Having a mosaiclike pattern, as does the simple squamous epithelium.

# test

**test**[1] [early modern English (from Old French, from L *testu* or *testum* an earthenware pot) a cupel, vessel for assaying precious metals, any means of assaying or testing] A procedure for determining which of two or more categories something falls into (e.g., whether a patient has a given disease or not) or for determining the position of something on a scale or continuum (specified by a grade, score, rank, or quantity). Most medical laboratory tests are designed to detect the presence of a substance or to measure its concentration by specific chemical, enzymatic, or immunologic reactions or by its effect on living organisms. **ABLB t.** ALTERNATE BINAURAL LOUDNESS BALANCE TEST. **absorption elution t.** A technique for determining the specificity and properties of antierythrocyte antibodies in serum (or bound to erythrocytes *in vivo*). Antibody is absorbed into erythrocytes of known blood group type and then eluted, often at high temperature (50°C) to recover the antibody. **acetone t.** A method to demonstrate the presence of acetone in urine. A reddish purple compound is formed when concentrated ammonia water is slowly added to urine to which a few drops of sodium nitroprusside have been added. **achievement t.** A test used to assess the degree to which training has been effective in a subject who has been trained in a particular task or area. Also *educational test.* **acidified serum t.** A test for the susceptibility of erythrocytes to lyse when exposed to serum to which a small amount of HCl has been added. The test is positive in paroxysmal nocturnal hemoglobinuria. A more specific acidified serum test ascertains whether hemolysis in acidified serum requires complement, a finding that is diagnostic of paroxysmal nocturnal hemoglobinuria. **acid-lability t.** A test that distinguishes those viruses stable at pH 3 or below (adenovirus, papovavirus, reovirus, and picornavirus) from those inactivated by low pH (myxovirus, arbovirus, herpesvirus, and poxvirus). It is sometimes used clinically to distinguish acid-labile rhinoviruses from acid-stable enteroviruses, since both are small RNA viruses resistant to ether. **acid phosphatase t.** **1** Any biochemical technique used to measure the enzymatic hydrolysis of esters of orthophosphoric acid by orthophosphoric monoester phosphohydrolase (acid phosphatase) in an acid pH medium. **2** In forensic medicine, a test used to identify seminal fluid or stains by demonstrating acid phosphatase activity. This is used in cases of alleged rape in which spermatozoa cannot be demonstrated. **ACTH stimulation t.** A measurement of the adrenal production of cortisol following intravenous or intramuscular administration of adrenal cortical tropic hormone (ACTH) which normally produces a prompt and pronounced rise in serum cortisol levels. Significant abnormalities include: primary hypoadrenalism (Addison's disease), no rise; hypoadrenalism secondary to pituitary failure, a delayed rise; hyperadrenalism (the Cushing syndrome) due to adrenal hyperplasia, an exaggerated increase in an already-high cortisol level; and hyperadrenalism due to an autonomous tumor, no effect. Also *ACTH test.* **active rosette t.** A modification of the E rosette test for identification of T lymphocytes in which the end point is the formation of high-affinity rosettes, which are formed after very brief incubation of lymphocytes with sheep erythrocytes. This figure correlates well with the level of *in vivo* cellular immunity. **acute toxicity t.** A toxicity test in which a single dose of a test substance is administered to laboratory animals, with an observation period usually of one to 14 days. **adaptation t. of Rademaker and Garcin** A test for disturbance of equilibrium in which the subject is placed on all fours, with his eyes closed, on a surface which is then tilted rapidly and successively in different directions. **Adler's t.** BENZIDINE TEST. **Adson's t.** A test for the thoracic outlet syndrome in which the patient is seated with the neck extended and the head turned to the affected side. The test is positive if the radial pulse on the affected side is diminished when the patient takes a deep breath. **afterimage t.** Evaluation of retinal correspondence by presentation of a vertical glowing filament to one eye and a horizontal filament to the other eye. Subsequent to this, eyes with normal retinal correspondence should see a positive afterimage of a light cross. Also *Hering's test.* **agglutination t.** Any of a variety of tests that are dependent on the clumping of cells, microorganisms, or particles when mixed with specific antiserum. **air conduction t.** A test of hearing using the air conduction pathway, as when a tuning fork is held near the listener's ear, or when sound stimuli are transmitted by earphone. **alkali denaturation t.** A method for measurement of the quantity of hemoglobin F in a blood specimen. A hemolysate is made alkaline by addition of NaOH (NaOH concentration of the mixture is 80 mmol/l). After two minutes, saturated solution of ammonium sulfate is added, and the mixture is filtered. The hemoglobin present in the filtrate is principally hemoglobin F, because other hemoglobins in the blood are denatured and precipitated, whereas hemoglobin F is alkali resistant. The concentration of hemoglobin in the filtrate is measured and compared with the total hemoglobin concentration in the original hemolysate to obtain the proportion of hemoglobin F as a percent of the total hemoglobin. Hemoglobin Rainier, a very rare variant, is also alkali resistant and, if present, may result in a spurious estimate of the hemoglobin F concentration. The Abt test is a semiquantitative alkali denaturation test for presence of hemoglobin F in blood-stained feces or vomit of neonates, based on the same principle. If positive for hemoglobin F, the test indicates that the blood is of fetal rather than maternal origin. **allelism t.** COMPLEMENTATION TEST. **Almén's t.** GUAIAC TEST. **alternate binaural loudness balance t.** An auditory test in which the loudness of a tone in the deafened ear is compared with or balanced against that in the normally hearing ear. The procedure is repeated for tones of increasing intensity. The test is used to establish the presence of loudness recruitment. Also *Fowler's test, ABLB test.* **alternate cover t.** Evaluation of ocular alignment by blocking the vision of first one eye, then the other, as the subject observes a fixation point. **amebocyte lysate t.** LIMULUS LYSATE TEST. **Ames t.** A method of detecting mutagens that induce reversion by using auxotrophic mutants of bacteria exhibiting several types of mutation, such as frame-shift or point mutations. The test is widely used because such mutagens are presumptive carcinogens. **amino acid t.** NINHYDRIN TEST. **Anderson and Goldberger t.** A test for typhus in which the patient's blood is injected into a guinea pig's peritoneal cavity. A typical temperature curve will result if the disease is typhus. **anesthetic t.** The initial administration of a local or general anesthetic in a small dosage to anticipate adverse effects that may occur with larger amounts. **angular deviation t.** BABINSKI-WEILL TEST. **antibiotic sensitivity t.** ANTIMICROBIAL SUSCEPTIBILITY TEST. **antibody absorption t.** A procedure to demonstrate the presence of an antigen on a cell surface by showing that the titer of the specific antibody is reduced following incubation with the cells, which absorb the antibody. **antibody screening t.** INDIRECT ANTIGLOBULIN TEST. **antiglobulin t.** Any laboratory procedure that uses an antiglobulin serum, which is antibody raised in rabbits or other hosts against globulins, often from humans. In serologic tests with red blood cells, the animal antibody is usually directed against human antibody molecules or against globulins of the complement system. Also *Coombs test, Race-Coombs test, antiglobulin reaction, antihuman serum test.* **antiglobulin consumption t.** A procedure to demonstrate that cells or other particles are coated by an antibody. **antiglobulin inhibition t.** A procedure to demonstrate the presence of globulins in a solution or, in forensic applications, in an extract made from stained material. The activity of antiglobulin serum in agglutinating antibody-coated cells will be reduced if the solution contains free globulin molecules. The species of origin of the globulin molecules is identified by using antiglobulin sera directed against globulins of different species. **antihuman serum t.** ANTIGLOBULIN TEST. **antimicrobial susceptibility t.** Any procedure to determine the effect of antimicrobial agents on the growth of microorganisms. Known concentrations of the drugs are added to microbial cultures in conditions appropriate for optimal growth, using either tube dilution cultures or drug-impregnated disks on agar cultures. Also *antibiotic sensitivity test.* **antimony trichloride t.** CARR-PRICE TEST. **antistreptolysin O t.** A test for antibodies against streptolysin O, performed by measuring the inhibitory effect of antibody-containing serum against hemolysis induced by streptolysin O. Since streptococcal exposure is widespread, only high titers of antistreptolysin O indicate recent infection or recrudescence of rheumatic fever. Cut-off levels are 250 Todd units in adults and 333 Todd units in children. Also *streptolysin O test, ASO test.* **antithrombin t.** A procedure for estimation of the inhibitory effect of a defibrinated specimen of plasma on the action of thrombin in converting fibrinogen to fibrin. **Apgar t.** A method of evaluating the well-being of a newborn infant by assigning a score of 0, 1, or 2 to each of five parameters, namely, heart rate, respiratory effort, muscle tone, reflex irritability, and color. At one minute and at five minutes, when these observations are most commonly made, the normal infant scores a total (the Apgar score) of 7 to 10. A severely asphyxiated or depressed infant scores 3 or less at either or both times of observation. Also *Apgar scale.* **Apley's t.** A test used to determine the extent of injuries to the knee. With the patient lying prone and the knee flexed to a right angle, the leg is grasped, pushed toward the knee joint, and axially rotated. Pain is elicited at the knee joint if a meniscal tear is present. Conversely, if the leg is lifted away from the knee joint along its axis, pain is elicited in lesions of the collateral ligaments. **arginine stimulation t.** A test of pituitary secretion of growth hormone. Arginine (30 g for adults, 0.5 g/kg for children) is given over one half hour and measurements of plasma growth hormone are made at 0, 30, 60, 90, and 120 minutes. An increment in growth hormone level of less than 5 ng/ml is abnormal, and of 5–10 ng/ml is considered borderline. Hyporesponsiveness characterizes primary disorder of the hypothalamus or anterior pituitary, as in idiopathic hypopituitary dwarfism. The test obviates the potential dangers of the insulin hypoglycemia test but elicits a variable response. **Ascoli's t.** **1** A precipitin test for anthrax using a tissue extract and anthrax antiserum. Also *Ascoli's reaction.* **2** MIOSTAGMIN REACTION. **ascorbate cyanide t.** A screening test for deficient glucose-6-phosphate dehydrogenase (G-6-PD) in red cells. Following incubation of red cells with sodium cyanide and sodium ascorbate, brown-colored methemoglobin is rapidly generated if there is insufficient G-6-PD to prevent oxidation by the hydrogen peroxide generated by the peroxidase activity of hemoglobin. **ASO t.** ANTISTREPTOLYSIN O TEST. **atrial pacing t.** A test in which an intracardiac electrode is positioned with its tip in the atrium in order to accelerate the heart. It is used as a stress test to induce ischemia in susceptible subjects. **auditory acuity t.** Any test to determine the auditory threshold. **augmented histamine t.** See under HISTAMINE STIMULATION TEST. **Ayer-Tobey t.** TOBEY-AYER TEST. **Babinski's t.**

BABINSKI SIGN. **Babinski-Weill t.** A patient with unilateral disease of the labyrinth, asked to take ten paces forward, then ten backward with his eyes closed and repeat this procedure five or six times, will execute star gait, that is, he will deviate to one side when moving forward and to the other side when moving backward, tracing out a star-shaped pattern. Also *angular deviation test.* **Bachman t.** A skin test for trichinosis in which a powdered extract of trichina larvae is suspended in saline and injected intradermally. An immediate wheal-and-flare reaction is definitely positive, while a delayed response (24–48 hours) may indicate either a current or past infection. **bacteriophage neutralization t.** PHAGE NEUTRALIZATION TEST. **Baermann t.** A filtration test for isolation of nematodes from soil or feces, which is especially useful for detection of *Strongyloides stercoralis* or hookworm larvae in feces. A sample is placed above a wire mesh or gauze in a warm-water-filled funnel. Rubber tubing is attached to the funnel to collect the larval nematodes as they migrate through the soil or fecal sample into the water in the funnel. The worms collect above a pinch clamp and are expelled into a dish for examination. **balance t.** A measurement and comparison of the intake and output of a substance. **Bárány's t.** A clinical test of labyrinthine function: the subject is asked to point to an object, raise his arm and then point again. This procedure is then repeated several times with the subject's eyes closed. The direction of pointing deviates progressively if vestibular function is disturbed. Also *Bárány's pointing test.* **bar-reading t.** An evaluation of binocular vision whereby a vertical barrier between the eyes and the reading matter will alternately block the vision of one eye, then the other. A person with normal binocular vision will be able to read without interruption. Also *Welland's test.* **basophil degranulation t.** A basophil test performed by incubating the serum under test, the antigen, and a preparation of basophils, either from the buffy coat of the patient or from rat peritoneal fluid. A smear of the incubated basophils is examined after supravital staining and the number of granulated cells is compared with a nonincubated control smear. A positive result is the reduction in the number of granules. **Bass-Watkins t.** A modification of the Widal test in which a drop of the patient's blood and a drop of a suspension of killed typhoid bacilli are mixed. In positive cases, agglutination occurs within two minutes. **Bender visual-motor gestalt t.** A widely used clinical test for brain damage, consisting of nine geometric designs the subject is asked to copy. Defects in reproduction are scored for their resemblance to the errors made by various classes of patients with known damage to the central nervous system. **Bennet and Cash t.** CURARE TEST. **benzidine t.** A test that exploits the peroxidase activity of heme, and is used to demonstrate the presence of blood, blood pigments, or myoglobin. In the presence of hydrogen peroxide and a saturated solution of benzidine in glacial acetic acid, heme oxidizes benzidine to a blue quinhydrone compound. Because benzidine is a carcinogen, this test is used as little as possible. Also *Adler's test, Schumm's test.* **Bernard t.** A test in which intensive antituberculosis therapy is applied to a patient with anthracosis who is suspected of having superimposed tuberculosis. Under the influence of the treatment, the radiologic signs diminish considerably if tuberculosis is associated with the anthracosis. **BG t.** COMPLEMENT FIXATION TEST. **Bial's t.** A test that demonstrates the presence of pentose in urine by the development of a green color when urine is added to freshly boiled Bial's reagent. Also *pentose test, orcinol test.* **bile acid tolerance t.** A liver function test which measures the rate at which intravenously injected bile acids are cleared from plasma. Delayed clearance is said to be a sensitive indicator of hepatocellular dysfunction. **bile esculin t.** A biochemical test used in differentiating microorganisms, especially in characterizing group D streptococci, based on the ability of organisms to grow in a medium containing bile, and to hydrolyze esculin to esculetin and glucose. **bile solubility t.** A procedure that differentiates *Streptococcus pneumoniae* from other alpha-hemolytic streptococci by demonstrating its susceptibility to lysis in the presence of bile or a bile salt reagent such as sodium deoxycholate, which activates the peptidoglycan amidase. **Binet-Simon t.** The original test of intelligence, devised in 1905 for determining the relative intellectual ability of French schoolchildren. The scale, consisting mainly of verbal tasks, was based on the level of ability shown by the average child of age three through 12. The level of competence established for any given child was expressed as the mental age, i.e., the nearest approximation to performance by a sample of children of differing chronological age. Also *Binet's test.* See also STANFORD-BINET INTELLIGENCE SCALE. **Bing t.** A tuning fork test used for the diagnosis of conductive hearing loss: the foot of a vibrating tuning fork is applied to the mastoid bone and the subject asked to say when the sound stops, at which point the external ear canal is occluded. In those with normal hearing or sensorineural hearing loss the sound becomes audible again, but not in those with conductive loss. **bithermal caloric t.** HALLPIKE'S TEST. **biuret t.** A test for peptides, or for the substance biuret, made by adding a copper-(II) salt to an alkaline solution of the specimen. Under these conditions the copper ion can displace hydrogen ions from peptide bonds and form a square planar complex, in which it is ligated by nitrogen atoms and which has a characteristic mauve color. Also *biuret reaction.* **bleeding time t.** Any of various tests that measure the time in minutes from incision of the skin until cessation of bleeding. The two basic methods are the Duke and Ivy bleeding time tests. • *Bleeding time* is often used as a shortened form for *bleeding time test.* See additional bleeding time tests listed under TIME. **blocking t.** Any agglutination inhibition procedure in which a soluble antigen combines with and inactivates an agglutinating antibody directed against cell surface antigens. **Block-Steiger t.** A tuning fork test for identifying simulated hearing loss, based on the normal ability to hear and localize a sound to the side on which it is louder. Two tuning forks of the same frequency are struck so that one is louder. One fork is held to each ear, and the subject is asked if and where he can hear the sound. **blood cholesterol t.** A test of the ability of the liver to convert cholesterol to cholic acid. **bone conduction t.** Any test of auditory function in which the bone conduction pathway is utilized. This term may refer to either the tuning fork tests such as those of Rinne and Weber, or to the bone conduction auditory threshold for pure tones. **Boyden's t.** A test to study the contrast ability and functional response of the gallbladder: gallbladder contraction is produced after administration of a fatty meal, which also serves to opacify the common bile duct. Also *post fatty meal cholecystography.* **bracelet t.** A test for rheumatoid arthritis in which lateral compression of the distal ends of the radius and ulna produces pain if the test is positive. **breath analysis t.** **1** A measurement of the amount of $^{14}CO_2$ exhaled after an oral dose of $^{14}$C-labeled aminopyrine. It is used as a test of intestinal absorptive ability and hepatic metabolism. **2** A measurement of the amount of $^{14}CO_2$ exhaled after an oral dose of $^{14}$C-D-xylose. It is used to detect bacterial overgrowth in the small intestine. **3** A measurement of exhaled hydrogen gas following an oral dose of lactose as a test of lactase deficiency. **breath-holding t.** A method of determining carbon monoxide diffusing capacity by holding the breath at total lung capacity. Also *single breath carbon monoxide diffusing capacity.* **bromphenol t.** A reagent strip test for urine protein that uses bromphenol blue as an indicator. At pH 3.0, the strip is yellow. Exposure to the $HN_2$ groups of protein causes a pH change which is manifest as a color change to blue. This test is more sensitive to albumin than to globulins. **bromsulfophthalein t.** A test of hepatic function and biliary excretion. The bromsulfophthalein (sulfobromophthalein) is injected intravenously and 45 minutes later a sample of venous blood is withdrawn at another site and photometrically analyzed for the dye. Normally less than 6% of the dose administered remains in the circulation after 45 minutes. Also *BSP test.* **BSP t.** BROMSULFOPHTHALEIN TEST. **Burchard-Liebermann t.** LIEBERMANN-BURCHARD TEST. **Caille's t.** Cessation of head nodding upon covering the eyes of a subject with spasmus nutans. **Calmette's t.** CALMETTE'S REACTION. **caloric t.** Any test of labyrinthine function in which water or air at a different temperature from blood heat is used to create a current flow in the semicircular canal system. The most commonly used test involves the sequential irrigation of each external ear canal with water above and below body temperature. See also HALLPIKE'S TEST. **CAMP t.** A procedure used to identify group B streptococci by demonstrating the presence of the CAMP factor, a material that acts to enlarge the zone of hemolysis produced by staphylococcal $\beta$-hemolysis. The streptococcus can be streaked perpendicularly to a streak of staphylococcus, or a dish procedure can be used. **capillary fragility t.** A test for hypovitaminosis C that is based on a count of cutaneous petechiae appearing after the application of a sphygmomanometer cuff to the arm at mean arterial pressure. **capillary resistance t.** GÖTHLIN'S TEST. **carbohydrate t.** SCHIFF'S TEST. **carbohydrate tolerance t.** A test that measures the body's ability to metabolize a carbohydrate by measuring the amount of substance present in blood and/or excreted in the urine after administration of a measured dose of the test sugar. **carbohydrate utilization t.** A biochemical test used in identifying bacteria or fungi. It is based on the capacity of the organism to oxidize or ferment a particular carbohydrate in the presence of an indicator for the reaction products. **carbon clearance t.** A procedure for measuring the uptake of particulate material by macrophages of the lymphoreticular system following intravenous injection of gelatin-stabilized carbon particles. Because the liver rapidly clears small numbers of particles, measuring the disappearance of low doses of carbon serves as an indication of hepatic blood flow. The disappearance of doses large enough to cause initial saturation of the liver and spleen reflects the regeneration of phagocytic capacity. **cardiolipin t.** Any of the flocculation tests for syphilis in which the substrate is cardiolipin, a lipid present in beef heart as well as other tissues. This class of serologic tests for syphilis is nonspecific and detects immunoglobulin behavior known as reagin. **carotid sinus t.** A test for angina pectoris in which one or other carotid sinus is massaged. The bradycardia induced by the massage will usually abolish angina. See also CAROTID SINUS MASSAGE. **Carr-Price t.** A standard spectrophotometric method for quantifying vitamin A. The reaction of vitamin A with antimony trichloride in chloroform produces a blue color with an absorption maximum at 620 m$\mu$. Also *antimony trichloride test.* **Casoni skin t.** CASONI'S REACTION. **catalase t.** A biochemical test that is used to differentiate bacteria such as streptococci, which do not contain catalase, from staphylococci which do have catalase. The presence of the enzyme catalase is detected by bubbles produced when hydrogen peroxide is added to the culture. **cervical posture t.** Any of the tests for nystagmus in which the head is flexed, extended, laterally inclined, or rotated. Such tests also usually employ electro-oculographic recording. **Chimani-Moos t.** A test intended to identify simulated unilateral deafness. A vibrating tuning fork is applied to the midline of the forehead or to the upper incisor teeth. The malingerer will probably claim to hear it only in the sound ear. The external meatus of this side is then firmly occluded and the malingerer is likely to insist he hears nothing, whereas a normal subject will usually state that he hears the sound in the occluded ear. **chi-square t.** See under CHI-SQUARE. **chlorpromazine stimulation t.** A diagnostic test for prolactin deficiency due to primary disease of the anterior pituitary. Chlorpromazine (25–50 mg) is given intramuscularly. In normal people, plasma prolactin rises within 15–30 minutes and reaches a plateau in 2–4 hours, with an average peak value of 25 ng/ml. Deficient response characterizes severe anterior pituitary insufficiency but is also observed in malnutrition, thyrotoxicosis, and renal failure. Hypothalamic disorders rarely if ever cause prolactin deficiency. **Chopra's antimony t.** CHOPRA ANTIMONY REACTION. **Chovstek t.** A test for the neurologic sign of spasticity of the facial musculature in which tapping the seventh nerve rostral to the ear elicits contraction of the corner of the mouth, indicating pathology. **Chrobak t.** If an eroded cervix bleeds on touch by a sound, there is a possibility that cancer is present. **chromatin t.** An examination of a cytologic preparation, usually buccal mucosal cells in humans, for one or more darkly staining regions at the nuclear periphery, known as Barr bodies, which represent inactive sex chromatin. It is used in clinical genetics for rapid determination of genetic sex and the number of X chromosomes present in somatic cells. Also *X-chromatin test.* **chronic toxicity t.** A toxicity test that is continued over a period covering a substantial portion of the lifetime of the test animal. The test substance is administered to a mouse or rat for two years, or to a dog for five to seven years. Also *long-term toxicity test, prolonged toxicity test.* **cis-trans t.** A genetic test applicable to prokaryotes for determining whether two different mutations, each with the same phenotype when present singly, are in the same or in different genes. The method involves observing the effect on phenotype when the mutant alleles are cis or trans to each other. **citrate t.** A biochemical test used to identify members of the Enterobacteriaceae family. It is based on the ability of organisms to use citrate as a carbon source, thereby forming alkaline products detectible by pH indicators. **Clark's t.** If bleeding occurs after inserting a sound into the uterine fundus, cancer should be suspected. **clomiphene t.** The measurement of pituitary gonadotropin secretion following the administration of clomiphene. The test is used in the differential diagnosis of hypogonadal states. **coagulase t.** A test for bacterial coagulase activity, expressed as gelling of plasma or fibrin-associated clumping of bacteria. **coccidioidin t.** The intradermal injection of antigens prepared from mycelial growth of *Coccidioides immitis.* A positive reaction indicates past or current coccidioidal infection. **coin t.** See under COIN SOUND. **cold agglutinin t.** A test for the presence in serum of red cell antibodies which have a temperature range of maximal activity below 37°C. Testing is usually performed at 20°C and 4°C. **cold pressor t.** The immersion of one hand in icy water, which leads to vasoconstriction and consequent transient hypertension and increased cardiac afterload. It was formerly used to test hyperreactivity in patients with suspected latent hypertension, but is now also used almost exclusively as a stress test on the heart, as for example in cardiac nuclear imaging. **coliform t.** A technique for assessing the purity of water, milk, or other dairy products by testing for the presence of the microorganism *Escherichia coli*. Its presence indicates fecal pollution and suggests a possibility of contamination by enteric pathogens of human origin. Also *coliform index*. **colloidal gold t.** A procedure to detect an abnormal globulin concentration in cerebrospinal fluid, once used to diagnose neurosyphilis and other central nervous system disorders. A colloidal gold solution, normally deep red in color, changes through lilac and blue to colorless as the gold salt precipitates. Progressively diluted cerebrospinal fluid is added to ten numbered tubes of the solution. Those tubes in which a color change occurs are recorded as a series of numbers, called the colloidal gold curve, that indicate the degree and type of abnormal protein concentration. Also *Lange's test, gold-sol test, Lange's reaction*. **complementation t.** In genetics, any process by which two mutant genes are introduced into the same cell for purposes of determining if complementation occurs. If the wild-type phenotype emerges, the mutations are nonallelic. Also *allelism test*. **complement fixation t.** A widely applicable assay for antigen-antibody interaction. The reaction is allowed to occur in the presence of a limited amount of complement, the fixation of which is assessed by the absence in the reaction mixture of hemolytic activity towards antibody-sensitized erythrocytes. Also *fixation test, B-G test*. **concentrating ability t.** URINARY CONCENTRATION TEST. **concentration t.** URINARY CONCENTRATION TEST. **concentration-dilution t.** A test or renal function in which the specific gravity of urine is measured after 18 hours of water deprivation and again several hours after a water load. Concentrating ability is related to distal tubule function and is impaired long before diluting ability. **confrontation t.** A gross method of measuring visual fields by presentation of test objects from the side, without use of a perimeter or tangent screen. **Congo red t.** A test for systemic amyloidosis. A positive result is indicated by the disappearance from the blood of more than 60 percent of an intravenously injected dose of Congo red when measured at one hour. **conjunctival t.** CALMETTE'S REACTION. **Conn's t.** CORTISONE-GLUCOSE TOLERANCE TEST. **consumption t.** Any test whose end point is the reduction of previously determined levels of an immunologic reactant following exposure to another system that contains an appropriately specific antigen or antibody. **contact t.** PATCH TEST. **contralateral straight leg raising t.** With the patient lying supine, elevation of the extended lower limb will produce pain radiating down the contralateral lower extremity in cases of sciatica. **contrast t.** The comparison of responses from two regions to an agent with simultaneous stimulation by identical quantities of the same agent. **controlled association t.** An experimental procedure devised to explore a subject's reaction to a variety of ideas by requiring a response to a verbal stimulus with another word according to some preestablished response category, such as antonyms or synonyms. **Coombs t.** ANTIGLOBULIN TEST. **corneal t.** A means of distinguishing whether an animal possesses cell-mediated or humoral immunity to an antigen by injecting the antigen into the cornea. With cell-mediated immunity, interstitial keratitis develops as a corneal reaction. The Arthus-type hypersensitivity inflammation does not occur unless the cornea has become vascularized through previous injury, because the antibodies necessary for the Arthus phenomenon cannot reach antigens injected into the avascular cornea. **Corner-Allen t.** A biologic assay for standardizing progesterone or corpus luteum preparations. The substance is injected into female rabbits whose ovaries have been removed 18 hours after mating. The stage of endometrial development is then noted. **cortisone-glucose tolerance t.** A test for the detection of latent or preclinical diabetes mellitus. The patient is fed a carbohydrate-rich diet for three days and then given 50–62.5 mg cortisone acetate by mouth $8\frac{1}{2}$ and two hours before a standard oral glucose tolerance test. In the normal subject, blood glucose value does not exceed 160 mg/100 ml at 1 hour, 140 at 2 hours. Levels above these are interpreted as indicating prediabetes. Also *Conn's test*. **cover t.** Evaluation of binocular function by occluding one eye and observing the uncovered eye. If the uncovered eye moves, it was not fixing originally. Also *screen test*. **cover-uncover t.** Evaluation of binocular function by occluding, then uncovering, one eye. If the covered eye moves away from fixation, then returns, a phoria is demonstrated. **Crafts t.** A variant of the extensor plantar response, in which a stroke with a blunt instrument applied in an upward direction over the front of the ankle evokes dorsiflexion of the great toe if pyramidal tract disease is present. **cross agglutination t.** MIXED AGGLUTINATION TEST. **crossed acoustic reflex t.** POSTAURICULAR MYOGENIC REFLEX TEST. **culture-fair t.** A psychological test specially constructed to be relatively free of biases that might result from an unequal familiarity among differing social classes or ethnic subgroups with the language used for instruction, the questions posed, or the type of task performance required. **curare t.** A test for subclinical myasthenia gravis: injection of very low doses of curare accentuates the symptoms of the disease. The test is potentially dangerous because myasthenic patients are excessively sensitive to curare and it should never be carried out unless facilities for intubation and assisted respiration are available. Modified tests involving regional perfusion after intra-arterial injection have been designed. Also *Bennet and Cash test*. **cyanide-nitroprusside t.** A qualitative test for the presence of cystine or homocystine in the urine or in renal stones. A positive result is indicated by a red-violet color after sequential exposure to sodium cyanide and nitroprusside. **cytotoxicity t.** Any test that identifies cytotoxic activity of serum or cells using the dye exclusion test as an indicator. It is usually performed to detect a complement-requiring reaction between cytotoxic antibodies and cell surface antigens. **darkroom t.** A provocative test for glaucoma, based upon the partial occlusion of a narrow angle by a dilated iris. **Davidsohn's differential t.** PAUL-BUNNELL-DAVIDSOHN TEST. **decarboxylase t.** A biochemical test used to identify bacteria, especially members of the Enterobacteriaceae and other gram negative bacilli, based on the ability of the organism to decarboxylate an amino acid such as lysine or ornithine to form alkaline amines. **dehydration t.'s** Tests for Menière's disease which depend upon reducing the degree of endolymphatic hydrops by administering agents, generally diuretics, such as glycerol and acetozolamide, capable of inhibiting fluid formation. A measurable improvement in hearing or caloric response is considered a positive result. **dehydrocholate t.** A test for circulation time between the arm and the tongue: a solution of sodium dehydrocholate is injected and the time difference between the injection and the detection of a bitter taste is noted. **delayed auditory feedback t.** A test of hearing in which the subject's speech is rerouted to his own ears by earphones after a brief time delay, causing the subject to stutter as he speaks if he can hear his delayed speech. This procedure was of considerable practical importance in the investigation of suspected nonorganic hearing loss prior to the advent of electrophysiologic tests of hearing. Also *delayed speech test.* **Denes-Naunton t.** A hearing test utilizing a comparison of the sound intensity difference threshold at 4 dB above threshold with that at 40 dB. In an individual with normal hearing the difference threshold at 40 dB is smaller than at 4 dB, whereas in a deaf patient with loudness recruitment this discrepancy is found to disappear. **dexamethazone suppression t.** A test for the integrity of the adrenal-pituitary feedback loop, in which small amounts of the potent glucocorticoid dexamethasone are given to suppress pituitary secretion of adrenocorticotropic hormone (ACTH). With normal pituitary and adrenal responsiveness, urinary steroid excretion falls within 48 hours. Continued high levels of urinary steroid indicate a failure of either pituitary or adrenal sensitivity to normal regulatory mechanisms and result in hypercortisolism. With larger doses of dexamethasone, hypercortisolism caused by adrenal hyperplasia is suppressed, but the same condition caused by autonomous tumors is unaffected. **Diagnex blue t.** A qualitative test of gastric acidity performed without intubation in which the patient swallows azuresin, or quinine carbacrylic resin, a complex of azure dye and ion exchange resin. In the presence of gastric hydrochloric acid the dye is released from the complex and ultimately appears in the urine, where the intensity of blue color can be measured. A proprietary name. Also *tubeless gastric analysis.* **Dick t.** An intracutaneous test used to determine susceptibility or immunity to scarlet fever. Erythrogenic toxin inoculation produces a reddening of the skin in 24–48 hours in susceptible individuals. Also *Dick's method, Dick reaction.* **differential t. for infectious mononucleosis** PAUL-BUNNELL-DAVIDSOHN TEST. **diffusion t.** IMMUNODIFFUSION. **dinitrophenylhydrazine t.** A screening test for the presence of maple syrup urine disease in which a white precipitate forms when an acidic solution of 2,4-dinitrophenylhydrazine is added to the urine of subjects with the disease. **direct antiglobulin t.** A procedure to demonstrate the presence of antibody or complement molecules on the surface of circulating cells, usually red blood cells, in which antiglobulin serum is added directly to a washed suspension of the cells under test. Agglutination occurs if there are globulin molecules on the cell surface with which the antiglobulin serum can react. Uncoated cells are not agglutinated. Also *direct Coombs test.* **direct Coombs t.** DIRECT ANTIGLOBULIN TEST. **direct immunofluorescence t.** IMMUNOFLUORESCENCE TEST. **distribution-free t.** NONPARAMETRIC TEST. **Dix-Hallpike t.** HALLPIKE'S TEST. **DNase t.** A biochemical test used in identifying staphylococcus species and members of the Enterobacteriaceae family, based on the presence of the enzyme deoxyribonuclease, which degrades deoxyribonucleic acid. **Doerfler-Stewart t.** A test for nonorganic hearing loss: if noise applied to the purportedly deaf ear causes a shift of threshold in the ear under test it is inferred that the ear to which the masking noise is applied is functioning. **Donath-Landsteiner t.** The diagnostic test for paroxysmal cold hemoglobinuria, in which complement-dependent antibodies are fixed to erythrocytes at low temperatures, and hemolysis occurs after warming to 37°C. Also *Donath's test.* **L-dopa response t.** A test of pituitary response to L-dopa, which normally causes increased secretion of growth hormone and decreased secretion of prolactin. Within 30–90 minutes after L-dopa administration, growth hormone levels should begin to fall, reaching half or less of baseline within 2–4 hours. This test is comparable to the insulin hypoglycemia test for diagnosing growth hormone deficiency. It is not very useful in distinguishing tumor from functional disorder as a cause of hyperprolactinemia. **Dorn-Sugarman t.** A test to determine the sex of a fetus *in utero.* A sample of the urine of the pregnant woman is administered to male rabbits and the testicular changes are observed. **double-blind t.** An experiment or test based on a double-blind study design. See under DOUBLE-BLIND. **double diffusion t.** Any immunologic procedure in which both the antigen and antibody diffuse through a gel medium such that concentrations of both reactants vary at different sites. A precipitin line will form where the antigen and antibody are in optimal proportion to each other. **Draize t.** A test designed to determine if a substance causes irritation or toxicity on contact, performed by dropping a solution of the test substance into one eye of an albino rabbit. Blistering, inflammation, or necrosis is a positive result, provided only the opposite eye, exposed only to a solvent, shows no such reaction. **draw-a-person t.** A test in which a subject's character traits or significant conflicts are inferred from the way he sketches a human figure. It is based on standards that correlate characteristics of drawings with clinical diagnostic categories. Also *Machover test.* **drawer t.** A test for rupture of the cruciate ligaments of the knee. With the knee flexed at a 90° angle, the tibia can be drawn forward on the lower femur in a rupture of the anterior cruciate ligament and backwards in a rupture of the posterior cruciate ligament. Also *drawer sign, Rocher sign.* **Dreyer's t.** An agglutination test for the differentiation of true typhoid or paratyphoid infection from other infections in persons immunized with typhoid-paratyphoid vaccine. **Duke bleeding time t.** A bleeding time test in which an incision is made in the earlobe and the time is measured until bleeding stops. Normal range is 1–5 minutes. Also *Duke's method.* **dye exclusion t.** A test for cytotoxic antibodies based on the fact that viable cells do not permit macromolecular dyes to enter the cytoplasm. When cytotoxic antibodies react with cell surface antigens, the cell loses its ability to exclude dye and becomes stained. It can be used to determine presence of cellular antigens, if the antibody specificity is known, or to detect antibodies in serum if the cell properties are known. **echinococcus skin t.** CASONI'S REACTION. **educational t.** ACHIEVEMENT TEST. **effort tolerance t.** EXERCISE TEST. **Ehrlich's t.** An assay for urobilinogen in the urine or feces, based on the red color produced by the reaction of urobilinogen with paradimethylaminobenzaldehyde. Also *Ehrlich's benzaldehyde reaction, paradimethylaminobenzaldehyde test.* **Einhorn string t.** STRING TEST. **Ellsworth-Howard t.** A test of responsiveness to injected parathyroid hormone, used to distinguish primary hypoparathyroidism from pseudohypoparathyroidism. After parathyroid hormone is injected in hypoparathyroid patients, phosphate levels in urine rise to levels 10 or more times greater than baseline. In pseudohypoparathyroidism, phosphate excretion increases very little or not at all. Also *induced phosphaturia test.* **Elsberg's t.** A method of assessing olfactory function. Samples of air containing set concentrations of volatile substances, each with a strong smell, are injected in succession into the nasal cavity during a short period in which the subject is told to suspend breathing. The minimal identifiable odor (MIO) can thus be defined. This, along with the rate of fatigue of olfactory sensibility, has been used to differentiate between intracerebral and extracerebral lesions involving the olfactory pathways.

**epithyroid iodine uptake t.** $^{131}$I UPTAKE TEST. **E rosette t.** A procedure to identify T lymphocytes by virtue of their capacity to form rosettes when incubated with unmodified sheep red blood cells. T lymphocytes have a surface receptor for sheep erythrocytes, and in a mixture of T lymphocytes and sheep red cells, the sheep cells cluster around lymphocytes to form a rosette of several sheep cells around a central lymphocyte. No antibody or immune mechanism is involved. **erythrocyte adherence t.** RED CELL ADHERENCE TEST. **erythrocyte fragility t.** OSMOTIC FRAGILITY TEST. **erythrocyte sedimentation t.** ERYTHROCYTE SEDIMENTATION RATE. **Escherich's t.** A test for tuberculin reactivity in which the tuberculin is injected subcutaneously. It is a modification of Pirquet's reaction. **estrogen stimulation t.** A test for pituitary gonadotropin reserve in amenorrheic women. Estradiol benzoate (1mg) is given intramuscularly. Some amenorrheic women show an elevation of plasma FSH/LH at 72 hours. This response predicts those patients who will respond to clomiphene. **estrogen suppression t.** A test to determine whether pituitary secretion of the gonadotropic hormone FSH/LH responds normally to levels of circulating estrogen. Administering high doses of estrogen, sometimes combined with progestin, normally causes marked reduction in urinary excretion of FSH/LH. Continuing high FSH/LH secretion in the face of high estrogen levels suggests pituitary tumor or a hypothalamic lesion. **euglobulin lysis t.** A test for increased fibrinolysin and fibrinogenolysin activity in a blood specimen, based on the fact that fibrinogen, plasmin, and plasminogen are euglobulins but the inhibitors of fibrinolysis normally present in plasma are not euglobulins. Euglobulins are precipitated by adding plasma to dilute acetic acid solution, and they are separated from other plasma components by centrifugation. The euglobulins are then redissolved and thrombin is added to induce clot formation by conversion of fibrinogen to fibrin. The time from clot formation to clot dissolution is measured. A shorter time than normal indicates increased fibrinolysin activity, as from increased plasmin activity. **exercise t.** The use of exercise to assess cardiovascular function, notably the production of ischemic ST changes on the electrocardiogram. The test is usually performed on a treadmill or bicycle ergometer. Other functions such as changes in blood pressure and pulse rate may also be evaluated. Also *exercise tolerance test, effort tolerance test.* **exercise tolerance t.** EXERCISE TEST. **F t.** A statistical test based on the ratio of two sample variances and widely used in the analysis of variance to test the homogeneity of a set of means. Also *variance ratio test.* **face-hand t.** A test for cerebral dysfunction in which the patient is asked to recognize the separateness of and to localize two stimuli presented simultaneously, one to his cheek and the other to the dorsum of one hand. **facial nerve function t.** Any of the tests used in cases of facial paralysis to assess the presence or degree of functional loss in the different branches of the affected facial nerve and the prognosis as to functional recovery. They comprise a variety of electrical tests as well as clinical assessment of movement in the muscles concerned, lacrimation and taste tests. The electrical tests include nerve excitability tests, strength-duration measurements, electroneurography, and electromyography. **Fahraeus t.** ERYTHROCYTE SEDIMENTATION RATE. **Fajersztajn's t.** FAJERSZTAJN'S CROSSED SCIATIC SIGN. **FANA t.** FLUORESCENT ANTINUCLEAR ANTIBODY TEST. **Farber's t.** The presence of swallowed vernix cells in the meconium of newborn infants who display symptoms of intestinal obstruction. The absence of such cells suggests atresia, whereas their presence rules out complete obstruction. Stenosis could exist in the latter case, however. **Fehling's t.** See under FEHLING SOLUTION. **femoral nerve stretch t.** A test to confirm the presence of nerve root compression at the third or fourth lumbar disk spaces. The test is positive if, with the subject lying in the prone position, extension of the thigh causes pain that radiates down the anterior thigh. **fern t.** A qualitative test of estrogenic activity in which dried smears of uterine cervical mucus are assessed microscopically. The degree to which a fernlike pattern emerges as the smear dries gives a rough quantitative measure of the amount of estrogen present. **ferric chloride t.** A screening test used to demonstrate a variety of substances in urine or other body fluids. Through variations in reagents and conditions, the test can be used to detect amino acids, melanin, ketone bodies, salicylates, lactic acid, and phenol derivatives. **Feulgen's t.** FEULGEN METHOD. **FIGLU t.** HISTIDINE LOADING TEST. **Finckh's t.** PROVERBS TEST. **finger-nose t.** A neurologic test to determine the ability to coordinate voluntary movements of the upper limb. The subject, with eyes closed, is asked to touch alternately the examiner's finger and the end of his nose with his index finger. **fingerprint sweat t.** A screening test for cystic fibrosis, with relatively low sensitivity and specificity. If the sweat adherent to the fingertip or palm contains excessive chloride, touching the finger or hand to the surface of an agar plate impregnated with silver salts produces a white silver chloride precipitate. **finger-to-finger t.** A clinical test of coordination and position sense of the upper limbs in which the patient is asked to approximate the tips of both index fingers in space. An intention tremor of cerebellar ataxia can be differentiated from disorders of position sense in that the latter causes a failure to carry out the test accurately with the eyes closed. **Fisher's exact t. of probability** A procedure applicable to a fourfold contingency table to test for statistical independence. The test gives the exact probability of the observed frequencies having arisen given statistical independence. The test is used when the numbers involved are small and the chi-square test is not therefore applicable. **fistula t.** The pneumatic test as applied in a case of suspected fistula in the bony labyrinth in a case of chronic otitis media. **fixation t.** COMPLEMENT FIXATION TEST. **flicking t.** A test for thrombocytopenia in which flicking of the forearm with one's finger will produce petechiae at the injury site, providing venous return has been temporarily occluded by a sphygmomanometer. **flocculation t.** See under FLOCCULATION. **fluctuation t.** A statistical analysis of the numbers of mutants in parallel bacterial cultures, which first demonstrated that mutation to resistance appear randomly and are selected, rather than induced, by phage or antibiotics. **fluorescein t.** Any of several tests using very dilute solutions of an easily identifiable fluorescein as a tracer. Such tests have been used in the body in peripheral circulatory efficiency tests and are used in environmental hygiene to trace the flow of underground water or identify possible sources of water contamination. **fluorescent antibody t.** Any test in which a fluorescence-labeled antibody is one of the reactants. In direct testing the specific antibody is labeled. In indirect testing a labeled antiglobulin antibody is used to identify and localize the attachment of an unlabeled antibody to its specific antigen. **fluorescent antinuclear antibody t.** A test that uses fluorescence-labeled antiglobulin serum to identify antinuclear antibodies in the test serum. The serum is incubated with a slide preparation of nucleated cells, and labeled antiglobulin serum is added to show the attachment of antibodies to the nuclei and the pattern of their attachment. Also *FANA test*. **fluorescent treponemal antibody t.** A test for specific antitreponemal antibodies in the serum of a patient who has had syphilis. After the serum is incubated with a slide preparation of fixed treponemal organisms, a fluorescence-labeled antiglobulin serum is added to demonstrate whether antibodies have attached to the organisms. Also *FTA test*. **fluorescent treponemal antibody t., absorbed** A more specific variant of the FTA test, in which the test serum is absorbed with nonpathogenic treponemal organisms before incubation with fixed *Treponema pallidum*. This removes antibodies reactive with other organisms and leaves antibodies specifically indicative of a syphilitic infection. Also *FTA-ABS test*. **foam t.** A qualitative test for bile pigments in urine. A positive result is indicated by the appearance of a brownish yellow foam when a test tube of the urine is shaken. **Folin and Wu t.** A test for glucose that is based on the reducing properties of the sugar. It reduces the cupric ion in an alkaline copper sulfate solution to cuprous oxide, which is dissolved with a phosphomolybdate solution and measured colorimetrically. **forced duction t.** A method of differentiating mechanical limitation of ocular movement from paralysis. Rotation of the eye by force, induced by an instrument such as a hook or forceps, is easily accomplished in conditions of paralysis. Mechanical restrictions, as from scars, resist movement. **Fowler's t.** ALTERNATE BINAURAL LOUDNESS BALANCE TEST. **fragility t.** A test of the ability of red blood cells to withstand physical stress, an indication of cell shape and membrane adequacy. Osmotic fragility is measured by exposing the cells to saline solutions of graduated tonicity. Cells that are more spherical than normal begin to hemolyze when sodium chloride concentration is 0.5 g/dl. Resistance to lysis by hypotonic saline is enhanced when erythrocytes are microcytic or hypochromic. A mechanical fragility test measures hemolysis after rapid stirring of the blood, but this test is rarely performed. **Fränkel's t.** A test for suppurative sinusitis: the patient bends forward with his head between his knees and rotated so that the side of the suspected disease is uppermost. If anterior rhinoscopy then reveals pus beneath the middle nasal concha, suppuration somewhere in the anterior group of paranasal sinuses is diagnosed. **free association t.** A word association test in which no restriction is imposed on the subject as to what the response word can be. **free urinary cortisol t.** A measurement of free (unconjugated) urinary cortisol, employed to detect Cushing syndrome of any cause. Normal values are 40–110 μg per 24 hours. Elevated values characterize the Cushing syndrome. **Friedman t.** A biologic pregnancy test in which a sample from the first passage of urine in the morning is injected into an ear vein of a mature, nonpregnant, female rabbit. If the woman is pregnant, ruptured ovarian follicles are noted in the rabbit 24 hours after injection. The test is no longer widely used now that immunologic tests are available. Also *Friedman-Lapham test*. **friend t.** A test for binocular vision in which the word FRIEND is printed in alternate red and green letters and viewed with a red filter in front of one eye, a green filter in front of the other eye. A person with binocular vision sees FRIEND. Monocular views are FIN and RED. **frog t.** MALE FROG TEST. **fructose tolerance t.** A test for any of the several enzyme deficiencies that cause the metabolic states of essential fructosuria, hereditary fructose intolerance, and hereditary fructose-1,6-diphosphatase deficiency. Fructose is administered either orally or intravenously, and the levels of blood glucose, blood fructose, urine fructose, and sometimes other serum metabolites are measured. Each of the autosomal-recessive enzyme deficiencies produces a characteristic pattern of abnormalities. **FTA t.** FLUORESCENT TREPONEMAL ANTIBODY TEST. **FTA-ABS t.** FLUORESCENT TREPONEMAL ANTIBODY TEST, ABSORBED. **fundus reflex t.** Measurement of refractive error by retinoscopy. **Gairdner's coin t.** See under COIN SOUND. **β-galactosidase t.** A color test for the enzyme β-galactosidase, using *o*-nitrophenol-β-D-galactopyranoside as a substrate. It is used in biochemical identification of many organisms, especially *Neisseria* species and the Enterobacteriaceae. Also *ONPG test*. **gallbladder function t.** CHOLECYSTOGRAPHY. **Galli Mainini t.** MALE FROG TEST. **galvanic t.** A test of vestibular function by passing a galvanic current through the ears. Using the usual binaural technique in which the positive electrode is applied on one side and the negative on the other, a response occurs in normal subjects with a current of 1–2 milliamperes. An inclination of the head toward the positive pole and nystagmus toward the negative pole are observed. **gel diffusion t.** Any test whose end point is the formation of a precipitin line following the diffusion of an antigen and/or antibody through a gel medium. **Gellé's t.** A hearing test used to assess the mobility of the ossicular chain: a vibrating tuning fork is applied to the mastoid process while the air pressure in the ear canal is varied using Siegle's otoscope. If raising the pressure diminishes the intensity of the sound heard, the ossicular chain is considered to be normally mobile; if the volume of the sound remains unchanged, the ossicular chain is considered to be fixed. **glucagon response t.** A test for responsiveness of growth hormone secretion to glucagon, which normally induces a delayed rise in growth hormone levels. Within 3 hours after injection of glucagon, growth hormone levels rise to above 5 ng/ml, sometimes to 15-20 ng/ml. In growth hormone deficiency due to hypopituitarism, the expected rise fails to occur. Also *glucagon stimulation test*. **glucose oxidase paper strip t.** A qualitative reagent strip test for urine glucose. The strip, impregnated with glucose oxidase, peroxidase, and *o*-tolidine, turns blue in the presence of glucose. Other reducing substances are not recognized. Ascorbic acid can cause a false-negative result, however. **glucose suppression t.** A test for responsiveness of growth hormone secretion to elevated glucose levels. A standard oral or intravenous glucose tolerance test is administered. Serum growth hormone values fall to levels below 5 ng/ml in normal subjects, but in patients with acromegaly, the values undergo a lesser decrease, remain unchanged, or may rise paradoxically. The paradoxical rise is not pathognomonic of acromegaly but occurs also in the neonatal period, in renal and hepatic failure, disorders of the central nervous system, malnutrition, and some carcinomas, as of the breast or lung. **glucose tolerance t.** The determination of changes in glucose concentration in timed specimens of blood and urine collected after the ingestion or injection of glucose into a subject who has fasted for 12 hours. **glycerol t.** A dehydration test in which the diuretic effect of a glycerol and water mixture, taken by mouth, is used for the diagnosis of Menière's disease. If positive, there should be an improvement of auditory threshold by 15 dB in at least one frequency between 250 to 4000 Hz, three hours after taking the mixture. There should also be a significant improvement in the speech discrimination score. **glycosylated hemoglobin t.** A measurement of the quantity of glycosylated hemoglobin in blood, usually by column chromatography. Greater than normal concentration of glycosylated hemoglobin occurs in diabetes mellitus, and the concentration of this hemoglobin fraction is proportional to the severity of hyperglycemia during the preceding several weeks. **Goetsch's t.** GOETSCH SKIN REACTION. **Gofman t.** An ultracentrifugal assay for cholesterol and related compounds. **gold-sol t.** COLLOIDAL GOLD TEST. **gonadotropin releasing hormone stimulation t.** A test for pituitary responsiveness to hypothalamic stimulation. Gonadotropin releasing hormone (GnRH) is injected and blood levels of follicle stimulating hormone (FSH) and luteinizing hormone (LH) are measured at intervals over the next several hours. Abnormal results usually indicate pituitary dysfunction, but hypothalamic lesions or the effects on the pituitary of severe hypogonadism may also cause deficient hormone secretion. **goodness of fit t.** A method of testing to determine if a set of observations conform to the predictions of a hypothetical model. **Gordon's t.** GORDON'S REFLEX. **Göthlin's t.** A test which is useful in diagnosing scurvy, based on the number of cutaneous petechiae that appear following the application of 50 mmHg cuff pressure to the arm. Also *capillary resistance test.* **Graefe's t.** A phoria measurement whereby a prism is used to separate the two images in a direction at right angles to the phoria. Alignment of these images by another prism then measures the amount of phoria present. **Graham's t.** CHOLECYSTOGRAPHY. **Gruber-Widal t.** WIDAL TEST. **guaiac t.** A test, based on the peroxidase activity of the heme group, that is used to demonstrate the presence of occult blood in the feces or gastric contents. A solution of gum guaiac and glacial acetic acid turns blue in the presence of heme and hydrogen peroxide. Also *Almén's test.* **Guthrie t.** 1 A screening test for elevated serum galactose levels, usually employed to screen newborns for galactosemia. The growth of a standardized *Escherichia coli* culture is inhibited in direct proportion to the concentration of galactose present. 2 Any of several tests for elevated levels of individual amino acids, using as the end point the inhibition of growth of *Bacillus subtilis.* **Haagensen t.** A means of detecting cancerous changes of the breasts by examining their shape as the patient leans forward. **Hallpike's t.** A quantitative type of caloric test: with the subject supine and his head slightly raised, water first at 44°C and then at 30°C is used to irrigate each ear canal for 40 seconds, and the duration of nystagmus measured. Conclusions on the presence of canal paresis and directional preponderance are drawn from the four results taken together. Also *Dix-Hallpike test, bithermal caloric test.* **Halstead-Reitan t.'s** A series of neuropsychological tests designed to measure the abilities of brain-damaged people. Neurologic diagnostic inferences are based on the pattern of performance obtained on a wide-ranging battery of tests of mental ability. Such tests have been shown to be sensitive not only to the presence or absence of cerebral lesions, but also to the location of the damage, and they may even be informative about the etiology of the cerebral nervous system disorder in individual patients. **Ham t.** A test for paroxysmal nocturnal hemoglobinuria, in which affected erythrocytes lyse after incubation in acidified serum. **Hamburger's t.** A subcutaneous tuberculin test for tuberculosis. Infiltration occurs within 24 hours in tuberculous patients. **Hammerschlag's t.** The measurement of specific gravity of blood using mixtures of benzene and chloroform. **Hamolsky's t.** *Older term* TRIIODOTHYRONINE UPTAKE TEST. **Hanfmann-Kasanin t.** A test of concept formation making use of blocks of varied shape, color, height, and width, which are sorted into categories specified by verbal instructions. A qualitative score, based on the approach to the task, solutions attempted, and discovery of solutions to the problems, is used to assess impairment or deterioration of the subject's ability to think conceptually and to verbalize his analyses. **hapten inhibition t.** A means of characterizing the structure of a complex antigenic determinant by using haptens of known composition to inhibit the interaction of the antigen with antibody known to be specific for it. **Harrison spot t.** A test to confirm the presence of bilirubin in the urine. The urine under test is adsorbed and concentrated on filter paper by precipitation with barium chloride. If after a ferric chloride-trichloroacetic acid reagent is added the paper turns green in color, the test is positive. **hatching t.** A test to detect schistosome eggs in feces or urine. These eggs will hatch only when placed in fresh water, as when feces or urine are excreted into water. The miracidia released from the egg shells are attracted to light and can thus be observed swimming at the surface of the water. **Heaf t.** An intradermal multiple-puncture test for tuberculosis in which PPD tuberculin is injected by means of six needle points. In positive cases, a number of indurated papules or a plateau appear at the injection site. Also *Sterneedle test.* **heat stability t.** A test for unstable hemoglobins, which precipitate from hemolysates within one hour of incubation at 50°C. **heel-knee t.** A neurologic test to determine the ability to coordinate voluntary movements of the lower limbs. The patient is asked to place the heel of one leg on the knee of the other and then to follow downward the anterior border of the tibia, or shin, while his eyes are closed. **heel-tap t.** A test indicative of pyramidal tract disease if a sharp tap upon the heel elicits an extensor plantar response. **Heinz body t.** The demonstration of normally invisible masses of precipitated denatured hemoglobin that are adherent to the red cell membrane by vital staining or by phase-contrast microscopic examination of unstained cells. Circulating red cells contain Heinz bodies when the patient has unstable hemoglobin or an unbalanced production of globin chains, or when there is uncorrected oxidative stress in red cells. Heinz bodies can be induced *in vitro* by oxidative stress on cells that lack adequate intrinsic reducing pathways. **hemadsorption t.** A test for infection of cells by viruses that have hemagglutinating activity and cause the presence of hemagglutinins on the surface of the infected cell. Erythrocytes added to a preparation of these cells adhere to the cell surface. **hemadsorption inhibition t.** A test for the presence of antibodies directed against hemagglutinating viruses. A positive result is abolition, by the test serum, of previously demonstrated hemadsorption to the infected cells. **hemagglutination inhibition t.** Any test whose end point is abolition of previously demonstrated agglutination. It can be used to demonstrate the presence of an antibody against hemagglutinating viral material, or to demonstrate the presence of an antigen in soluble form that reacts with and neutralizes a hemagglutinating antibody of known specificity. **hematin t.** SCHUMM'S TEST. **heme t.** SCHUMM'S TEST. **Hemoccult t.** A commercially available test for fecal occult blood, consisting of an impregnated guaiac slide and hydrogen peroxide reagent. A proprietary name. **hemolytic plaque t.** JERNE TECHNIQUE. **Hering's t.** AFTERIMAGE TEST. **Hess capillary t.** A test for capillary fragility in which a sphygmomanometer cuff is inflated to a pressure midway between the systolic and diastolic pressures for five minutes. The number of petechiae appearing in a circle 2.5 cm in diameter on the inner aspect of the arm are counted. More than 20 petechiae are regarded as abnormal. **Hirschberg's t. for strabismus** Estimation of the degree of strabismus by the location of the reflex of the fixation light upon the deviating cornea. Location of the reflex at the limbus indicates the presence of 45° of deviation. **Histalog t.** An augmented histamine test that uses the histamine analog Histalog (betazole). **histamine t.** A test of acid production by gastric parietal cells, before and after stimulation. After the subject has undergone a 12-hour fast, volume and acid content of a 1-hour specimen of gastric juice are recorded as basal acid output (BAO). Histamine or an analogue or derivative is administered and the acid content is measured in four or six 15-minute samples of gastric juice. Stimulated acid production is reported as maximal acid output (MAO) or peak acid output (PAO), values derived variously in different protocols. **histamine flare t.** A test to determine the presence of nerve damage. If the skin is scratched firmly, local blanching along the line of the scratch is soon followed by a surrounding reddening or flare, such as that following the intradermal injection of histamine. This axon reflex depends upon the integrity of sensory fibers in peripheral nerves and of posterior root ganglia and may be absent if either are diseased. **histamine stimulation t.** A test of the acid-secretory capacity of the stomach. After gastric contents are evacuated and a basal measurement of gastric acid secretion is made, a dose of histamine is given to maximally stimulate acid production, and gastric secretions are collected. True achlorhydria is indicated by absent acid production even after histamine is given. Also *gastric analysis.* • Formerly, when the standard histamine dose was lower, an *augmented histamine test* was used for additional testing in those for whom the initial test was inadequate. Now only one dosage schedule is used (for histamine phosphate), so augmentation is not necessary. **histidine loading t.** A test that demonstrates a folic acid deficiency by provoking increased excretion of formiminoglutamic acid after the administration of histidine. Excretion occurs if there is insufficient folic acid to provide coenzymes necessary for conversion of histidine to glutamic acid through the intermediary metabolite formiminoglutamic acid. Also *FIGLU test.* **histoplasmin t.** An intradermal test to demonstrate cell-mediated immunity to histoplasma organisms. Injection of a histoplasmin antigen induces induration and erythema in an individual with current or previous immunizing exposure to a histoplasma species. **Hollander t.** A test to determine whether the vagus nerves are intact, consisting of the administration of insulin to provoke hypoglycemia. As this stimulates the cephalic phase of gastric acid output, a secretion of acid indicates intact vagal nerves to the stomach. **Holmgren's t.** A test for color blindness in which the subject sorts a series of colored elements to match samples of red, green, and purple hues. **house-tree-person t.** A projective test in which inferences about the subject's character and significant conflicts are drawn from the way in which he draws a house, a tree, and a person. Also *HTP test.* **Howard t.** A renal function test designed to study urine excretion and the capacity to concentrate sodium in each kidney after bilateral ureteral catheterization. In a positive test a reduction of at least 40 percent in urine volume with either a 15 percent reduction in urine sodium or a 50 percent increase in creatinine concentrations on the same side indicates an ischemic kidney. This test is rarely used today, but is historically important. **HTP t.** HOUSE-TREE-PERSON TEST. **Huhner t.** A test for the evaluation of an infertile couple. A postcoital aspirate from the endocervix and vaginal pool is examined for motile spermatozoa. If their number is abnormal, the differential diagnosis must consider aspermia, inflammation, and a hostile cervical secretion. Also *Sim's test.* **hydrogen peroxide t.** A test for occult blood in a fluid. The existence of hemoglobin is shown by the formation of a bubbly foam when 20% hydrogen peroxide is added to the test fluid. **17-hydroxycorticosteroid t.** The measurement in the urine of steroid molecules which have hydroxyl groups at carbon 17 and 21 and a ketone group at carbon 20, reflecting degradation products of adrenal glucocorticoids. The levels are elevated in hypercortisolism of any etiology and decreased in hypoadrenalism. Also *Porter-Silber chromogens test, 17-OH-corticoids test.* **immobilization t.** Determination of antibody presence based on its ability to inhibit the motility of bacterial cells or protozoa. **immunodiffusion t.** IMMUNODIFFUSION. **immunofluorescence t.** A method of microscopically visualizing antigens by reaction with an antibody conjugated with a fluorescent chemical, usually fluorescein, so that the bound antibody can be visualized with a microscope equipped to see fluorescent labels. Also *direct immunofluorescence test.* **immunologic pregnancy t.** A pregnancy test in which the presence of chorionic gonadotropin is determined immunologically rather than by assaying its biologic activity. **indirect antiglobulin t.** A test for the presence in a serum of an antibody or complement that is capable of attaching to cell surface antigens without causing agglutination. Antiglobulin serum does not react with surface antigens but will react with immune reactants attached to the cellular antigens. The test serum is incubated with the indicator cells, which are then washed to remove unattached globulins. The addition of antiglobulin serum agglutinates the cells only if the antibody or complement from the test serum has attached to the surface. An absence of agglutination indicates that the test serum contained no antibodies reactive with the cell surface antigens. Also *indirect Coombs test, antibody screening test.* **indirect Coombs t.** INDIRECT ANTIGLOBULIN TEST. **indirect hemagglutination t.** A passive agglutination test in which the antigen is fixed to red blood cells. **indirect immunofluorescence t.** An immunofluorescence test in which a fluorescein-labeled antiglobulin antibody is used to detect antibody bound to an antigen. This technique increases the sensitivity of the assay since several antiglobulin molecules can bind to each antibody molecule, and it allows a single fluorescein-labeled reagent to be used to detect a wide variety of antigens. **indocyanine green t.** A hepatic function test that measures hepatocellular clearance of intravenously injected indocyanine green. **indole t.** A biochemical test used to identify members of the Enterobacteriaceae family and other Gram-negative bacilli, based on the ability of the organisms to produce indole from tryptophan. **indophenol t.** A cytochemical test used to identify blood cells of the granulocyte-monocyte series by demonstrating the presence of oxidizing enzymes in their cytoplasm. Also *indophenol reaction, Graff method, oxidase reaction.* **induced hypercalciuria t.** A test occasionally used for the study of parathyroid function. After intravenous administration of calcium gluconate, 60% of the dose is excreted in the urine by normal persons. **induced hypoglycemia t.** A test of insulin sensitivity in which 12 units of insulin are injected in the fasting state, and the lowest values of blood glucose are measured, usually 30 minutes after injection. Normal depression of blood glucose is about 50% compared to the fasting value, a depression of more than 60% is interpreted as insulin hypersensitivity, of less than 40% as partial insulin resistance. The test must be used with caution in suspected Addison's disease, hypopituitarism, islet cell adenoma, and other hypoglycemic states, in which the induced hypoglycemia may be prolonged and occasionally fatal. **induced phosphaturia t.** ELLSWORTH-HOWARD TEST. **inhibition t.** Any test that depends on the inhibition of an observable reaction, as the inhibition of virus-induced hemagglutination by antiviral antibody, or the inhibition of agglutination by anti-A or anti-B agglutinin in order to detect a soluble blood group. **inkblot t.** RORSCHACH TEST. **insulin-glucose tolerance t.** A test of insulin sensitivity in which the examiner assesses the glucose tolerance curve following a standard oral glucose tolerance test carried out simultaneously with insulin injection. **insulin hypoglycemia t.** A test of pituitary secretion of human growth hormone (HGH) and/or adrenocorticotropic hormone (ACTH) in response to hypoglycemia induced by insulin injection. Following the fall in blood sugar to below 40 mg/dl or to levels 50% or less of fasting levels, serum cortisol levels secreted in response to ACTH stimulation rise to double the baseline value within 40–90 minutes and HGH values rise to at least 5 ng/ml. The test is used in cases of short stature to distinguish HGH deficiency from constitutional or chromosomal abnormalities, and to evaluate overall pituitary reserve and responsiveness of the hypothalamic-pituitary axis. Because hypoglycemia may be clinically dangerous, patients should be selected carefully and kept under close surveillance. Also *insulin tolerance test.* **insulin tolerance t.** INSULIN HYPOGLYCEMIA TEST. **interfacial precipitin t.** RING TEST. **intracutaneous t.** INTRADERMAL TEST. **intracutaneous tuberculin t.** MANTOUX TEST. **intradermal t.** Any test for the presence of skin sensitivity of the delayed hypersensitivity type, elicited by injecting antigen between the layers of skin and examining 12 to 48 hours later for development of erythema and induration. Also *intracutaneous test.* **iodide-perchlorate discharge t.** A refinement of the perchlorate discharge test, enabling senstive detection of minimal impairment of thyroidal iodine binding. The conventional perchlorate discharge test is carried out, but stable iodine 127 (0.5–1.5 mg) is given along with the radioactive isotope iodine 131. **$^{131}$I-oleic acid t.** A test of mucosal absorption of fatty acids: a small amount of radioactively labeled oleic acid is ingested, and the amount of $^{131}$I that appears in the blood is a measure of the intestinal absorption of long-chain fatty acids. Absorption of fatty acids does not require pancreatic enzymes. **irrigation t.** A test for the locus of urethral infection: with the bladder full and the perineum compressed to segregate the posterior urethra, the anterior urethra is irrigated with boric acid solution. Thus any cloudiness of urine upon subsequent voiding must originate in the posterior urethra. Also *Jadassohn's test.* **Ishihara's t.** A pseudoisochromatic test using a series of plates for the detection and classification of color vision defects. **isopropanol precipitation t.** A test for the presence of unstable hemoglobins in red cells. When a freshly prepared hemolysate is incubated at 37°C with buffered isopropanol, unstable hemoglobins form a flocculent precipitate. **Ito-Reenstierna t.** An intradermal test for chancroid using a vaccine of killed *Haemophilus ducreyi.* Also *Ito-Reenstierna reaction.* **$^{131}$I uptake t.** A test of thyroid function, in which thyroidal uptake of a dose of $^{131}$I-labeled sodium iodide is measured at specified intervals after administration. Also *epithyroid iodine uptake test, RAI test, radioactive iodine test.* **Ivy bleeding time t.** A bleeding time test in which a sphygmomanometer around the upper arm is inflated to 40 mm Hg pressure, then a 5 mm deep incision is made on the flexor surface of the forearm, and the time is measured to cessation of bleeding. Normal range is 1–6 minutes. Also *Ivy's method.* **Jadassohn's t.** IRRIGATION TEST. **Jaffé's t.** A quantitative test for creatinine in diluted urine or in a protein-free filtrate of serum or plasma. Alkaline picrate in the presence of creatinine forms an intensely red color with spectrophotometric absorbance proportional to the quantity of creatinine. Also *Jaffé reaction.* **jerk t.** PIVOT SHIFT TEST. **Kato t.** A rapid method for identification and quantitation of helminth eggs, based on estimation of the number of eggs in a standard 50 mg sample of fresh feces covered with a square of plastic used to press down and spread the sample evenly. The sample is cleared in glycerine before being read. **17-ketogenic steroid t.** A test that measures the total urine levels of 17-hydroxycorticosteroids, including some that are not detected in the Porter-Silber reaction and are elevated in adrenogenital syndromes and some Cushing syndromes. The 17-hydroxyl group is converted in two steps to a 17-keto group, which can be measured by the Zimmermann reaction. The 17-ketosteroids of androgenic origin must be removed or separately measured. Also *ketogenic corticoids test, 17-ketosteroid test.* **Kjeldahl's t.** A precise but laborious method of quantifying proteins in body fluids by measuring the nitrogen content. The proteins, precipitated by acid, are oxidized by the application of hot sulfuric acid. The amount of ammonia liberated is measured by titration, and the protein concentration is calculated from the amount of nitrogen present in the ammonia, arbitrarily assigning a mean nitrogen content of 16% in the proteins under study. This method is used primarily to standarize other methods. Also *macro-Kjeldahl method, Kjeldahl's method.* **Kleihauer t.** A test for the presence of hemoglobin F in red blood cells, based on the fact that exposure to an acid solution removes adult hemoglobin from red cells on a blood smear but does not affect hemoglobin F. It is used to identify and quantify fetal red cells in the blood of pregnant or postpartum women. Also *Kleihauer-Betke test.* **knee dropping t.** A simple test for spasticity: with the patient supine, the leg is lifted by a hand beneath the knee and is then allowed to drop. In the normal state the knee flexes, the heel remains on the bed, and the leg drops quickly. If the limb is spastic, the heel rises from the bed, and the leg falls more slowly. **Knott t.** A test to detect microfilariae or other worm larvae in the blood, based on the lysis of blood cells in a 2% formalin solution, followed by centrifugation, staining with Giemsa or Wright stain, and examination of the sediment for microfilariae or larvae. **Kurzrok-Miller t.** A test of the relationship between cervical mucus and spermatozoa as part of an infertility evaluation. A drop of mucus and a drop of semen are placed side by side on a microscope slide and the ability of the spermatozoa to penetrate the mucus is determined. Also *Miller-Kurzrok test.* **Kveim t.** KVEIM-SILTZBACH TEST. **Kveim-Siltzbach t.** A diagnostic test for sarcoidosis, consisting of injection of an extract of spleen (Kveim antigen) from a patient with sarcoidosis intradermally into the subject, with subsequent determination of the presence of granuloma in a biopsy of the injected area. Also *Kveim test, Nickerson-Kveim test, Kveim's reaction.* **t. of labor** TRIAL OF LABOR. **labyrinthine t.** Any test investigating the function of the semicircular canals or utricular otolith system. **Lange's t.** COLLOIDAL GOLD TEST. **laryngeal mirror t.** A test for tuberculosis in which a laryngeal mirror is placed in the throat so that the vocal folds are visible and the patient is caused to cough. Sputum deposited on the mirror is examined for *Mycobacterium tuberculosis.* A saline wash of the mirror may be injected into a guinea pig which is sacrificed and examined after six weeks. **Lasègue's t.** LASÈGUE SIGN. **latex agglutination t.** LATEX PARTICLE AGGLUTINATION TEST. **latex fixation t.** **1** LATEX PARTICLE AGGLUTINATION TEST. **2** A test for rheumatoid factors in serum in which the antigen coated upon the latex particles is human IgG.

**latex particle agglutination t.** Any passive agglutination test in which latex particles are the inert carrier medium. Also *latex test, latex agglutination test, polystyrene latex test, latex fixation test.* **Laurell rocket t.** ROCKET IMMUNOELECTROPHORESIS. **LE cell t.** A test in which *in vitro* incubation of the blood or bone marrow causes the formation of characteristic LE cells in 75 to 80 percent of patients with systemic lupus erythematosus. Also *LE test, lupus erythematosus cell test.* **leishmanin t.** An intradermal, delayed hypersensitivity test for leishmaniasis, employing cultured promastigotes of any leishmanial species as the crude antigen source. The test is particularly sensitive to *Leishmania braziliensis, L. tropica,* and other agents of cutaneous leishmaniasis, becoming positive usually after 3–6 months in cases of active infection, and sensitive also to past infection. The test is negative in active kala-azar. *L. donovani,* the agent of visceral leishmaniasis, can usually be detected only after the disease has been cured. Also *Montenegro test, leishmanin skin test.* **lepromin t.** A test for leprosy in which intradermal injection of lepromin causes persons with cellular immunity to *Mycobacterium leprae* (including those with tuberculoid leprosy) to develop an inflammatory papule which may ulcerate. No such reaction is observed in persons with lepromatous leprosy. Also *lepromin reaction, Mitsuda test, Mitsuda reaction.* **leukocyte bactericidal t.** An *in vitro* procedure that evaluates both the phagocytic and the bactericidal capacities of circulating granulocytes by measuring the concentration of viable *Staphylococcus aureus* after exposure to a purified cell suspension under various conditions. Deficiencies may occur with congenital neutrophil disorders, with granulocytic and lymphoproliferative malignancies, with many systemic illnesses, and after exposure to certain drugs. **leukocyte migration t.** MACROPHAGE MIGRATION TEST. **Lewis and Pickering t.** A test for organic arterial occlusion by reactive hyperemia. After immersing the affected limb in warm water, the limb is elevated and a sphygmomanometer cuff applied and inflated above the systolic pressure. When the cuff is released after five minutes, the distal extremities flush in two to five seconds in a normal limb but much more slowly and patchily in the presence of organic vascular disease. **Lichtheim t.** An assessment of language retained by a patient with Broca's aphasia, with the patient asked to indicate the number of syllables there are in words he cannot speak. **Liebermann-Burchard t.** A quantitative test for cholesterol in which a green compound with a maximum absorption peak at 620 nm is generated when cholesterol is mixed with concentrated sulfuric acid and acetic anhydride. Also *Liebermann-Burchard reaction, Burchard-Liebermann reaction, Burchard-Liebermann test.* **limulus lysate t.** A sensitive *in vitro* test for the presence of lipopolysaccharide endotoxin of Gram-negative bacteria. Very small quantities of cell-wall lipopolysaccharide cause coagulation of a lysate prepared from the amebocytes of *Limulus polyphemus,* the horseshoe crab. Toxins and cell-wall products of Gram-positive bacteria do not coagulate the limulus lysate. Also *amebocyte lysate test, limulus amebocyte lysate test.* **Linzenmeier's t.** A pregnancy test in which an increase in the sedimentation rate of the woman's blood is looked for as a positive indication. **lipase t.** A diagnostic test that indicates the existence of pancreatic disease by demonstrating the presence of lipase in circulating blood. **Loewi's t.** LOEWI'S REACTION. **logrank t.** A statistical test used in the analysis of data in clinical trials of chronic diseases, especially cancer. It is based on the cumulative ratios over a sequence of time intervals of the number of patients surviving under one form of treatment compared with the number surviving under another form of treatment. **Lombard's t.** A test of hearing relying on the effect of induced noise on a subject's hearing responses. It is used in the investigation of nonorganic hearing loss. **long-term toxicity t.** CHRONIC TOXICITY TEST. **Luenbach-Koeppe t.** A pregnancy test in which the presence of anterior pituitary hormones in the woman's urine is a positive indication. **lupus erythematosus cell t.** LE CELL TEST. **Machover t.** DRAW-A-PERSON TEST. **macrophage migration t.** An *in vitro* test for the presence of cell-mediated immunity to an antigen, based upon the release of a migration inhibition factor from previously sensitized lymphocytes in the presence of the specific antigen. It is performed by observing macrophages as they move in a concentrated suspension of mononuclear cells, traveling away from the point of application in a medium containing the antigen under test. A positive result is the reduction or inhibition of normal migratory movement by macrophages. Also *leukocyte migration test, leukocyte migration inhibition test.* **male frog t.** A biologic test for pregnancy in which a male frog (genus *Rana* or *Xenopus*) or toad (genus *Bufo*) is used. Such tests are more rapid than those using female test animals. Injection of urine with adequately high levels of chorionic gonadotropin causes spermatozoa to appear within a few hours in the cloaca of the male animal used. Also *toad test, male toad test, frog test, Galli Mainini test.* **male toad t.** MALE FROG TEST. **malonate t.** A test to identify bacteria according to their ability to employ malonate as a carbon source. The end point is production of alkaline metabolites which cause the medium to change color. Aerobacter organisms utilize malonate and *Escherichia* do not. **Mancini t.** SINGLE RADIAL DIFFUSION TEST. **Mann-Whitney U t.** A statistical test of the probability that two independent sets of observations have been drawn from the same population. The test is distribution-free and may therefore be used where the t test would be inappropriate. It can also be applied to ordinal data. **manometric t.** QUECKENSTEDT'S TEST. **Mantoux t.** An intracutaneous test for tuberculosis based on a hypersensitivity reaction to increasing concentrations of tuberculin. Also *intracutaneous tuberculin test, Mantoux reaction, Mendel's test.* **Manzullo's t.** TELLURITE TEST. **Master's two-step exercise t.** An exercise test for myocardial ischemia utilizing two steps each nine inches high. It is now largely superseded by treadmill or bicycle ergometric tests. **match t.** A test for expiratory airflow obstruction in which the patient attempts to blow out a lighted match held in front of his widely open mouth. Also *Snider match test.* **Mátéfy t.** A serum test used for early diagnosis of pulmonary tuberculosis. Also *Mátéfy's reaction.* **Matzker t.** A psychoacoustic test for central auditory dysfunction. Speech material is passed through a high-frequency filter to one ear and through a low-frequency filter to the other. Failure to integrate the information and reconstitute the speech is considered evidence of a brainstem lesion. **Mazzotti t.** A test for onchocerciasis. In positive cases, a pruritic skin reaction over the subcutaneous nodules develops after oral administration of diethylcarbamazine. **McKinnon's t.** A test for smallpox. Material from the lesion of a patient is injected intradermally into an immunized rabbit and a nonimmunized rabbit. Smallpox virus produces a local lesion only in the nonimmunized animal. **McMurray's t.** MCMURRAY SIGN. **McNemar t.** A test of statistical significance applicable to a fourfold table where the individual observations are related, as where the before-after states of the same individuals are recorded, or where cases and controls have been matched as in a matched sample.

**mecholyl t.** A provocative test for pheochromocytoma. Subcutaneous injection of 25 mg mecholyl stimulates elevation of blood pressure in patients with the disease, and a fall in normal subjects. **Meltzer-Lyon t.** Instillation of $MgSO_4$ into the duodenum to retrieve gallbladder bile. Detection of cholesterol crystals in the bile aids in the diagnosis of cholesterol cholelithiasis. **Mendel's t.** MANTOUX TEST. **mercaptoethanol agglutination inhibition t.** A test to demonstrate that agglutinating antibodies are of the IgM class. The addition of the reducing agent 2-mercaptoethanol breaks the disulfide bonds necessary for the integrity of IgM pentamers, the only form of IgM that causes agglutination. If adding mercaptoethanol to an agglutinating system abolishes agglutination, it indicates that the antibodies were IgM. **metabisulfite t.** A screening test for the presence of hemoglobin S in red cells. Red cells exposed to low oxygen tensions engendered by the reducing activity of a solution of sodium metabisulfite undergo sickling if hemoglobin S is present, with or without admixture of other hemoglobins. **methylene blue t.** A test to determine the effectiveness of pasteurization of milk based on the ability of any organisms to decolorize methylene blue. **methyl red t.** One of a set of tests used to distinguish coliform bacteria from *Enterobacter* species. The mixed acid fermentation of the former, but not the butanediol fermentation of the latter, produces enough acid to lower the pH of a phosphate-buffered medium to about 4.4, which is indicated by methyl red. See also IMViC. **metoclopramide stimulation t.** A diagnostic test for prolactin deficiency. Metoclopramide, a dopamine antagonist, is given intravenously in doses of 2.5–10 mg. The normal response is a rise five to ten times the basal value of plasma prolactin. Application and usefulness of the test appear to be similar to those of the chlorpromazine stimulation test. **metyrapone t.** A test of the adequacy and integrity of the hypothalamic-pituitary-adrenocortical system in which metyrapone, which inhibits the adrenal enzyme 11-$\beta$-hydroxylase, is given according to a standard protocol. In the normal response, the adrenal cortex hypersecretes 11-deoxycortisol, the rise of which is measured in blood or urine. Failure to respond indicates a lesion either in the hypothalamus or in the anterior pituitary capacity to release ACTH in response to the test-induced deprivation of cortisol. A necessary prior assumption is that the adrenal cortex is capable of response to ACTH, which should be established by prior challenge with exogenous adrenocorticotropin. **MHA-TP t.** MICROHEMAGGLUTINATION TEST FOR *TREPONEMA PALLIDUM*. **microhemagglutination t. for *Treponema Pallidum*** A treponemal hemagglutination test that has been adapted for a microscopic technique. Also *MHA-TP test*. **Miller-Kurzrok t.** KURZROK-MILLER TEST. **Mills t.** A test for lateral epicondylitis. The test is positive if, when the wrist is flexed and the forearm fully pronated, extension at the elbow joint gives rise to pain over the external epicondyle of the humerus. **Mingazzini's t.** A procedure for revealing the presence of slight paresis of an upper or lower limb. From a sitting position the patient is asked to raise both limbs to a parallel position. The one on the paralyzed side is held lower or drifts downwards. **minimal caloric t.** A modified form of Hallpike's test in which temperature differences or the number of ear irrigations carried out is reduced. **Minnesota multiphasic personality t.** MINNESOTA MULTIPHASIC PERSONALITY INVENTORY. **Mitsuda t.** LEPROMIN TEST. **Mittelmeyer's t.** A test for vestibular disturbance in which the patient walks in place with his eyes closed. If there is a disturbance he will tend to rotate in a direction away from the dominant labyrinth. **mixed agglutination t.** A procedure that demonstrates the presence of antigenically similar material on the surface of different types of cell. A monospecific antibody will produce agglutinates that contain a mixture of cells if the antibody reacts with an antigen present on both cell types. Also *cross agglutination test*. **mixed leukocyte culture t.** MIXED LYMPHOCYTE CULTURE REACTION. **M'Naghten t.** See under M'NAGHTEN RULE. **mobility t.** A diagnostic test for assessing the movement of a tooth in relation to adjacent teeth or supporting tissues. **modified Rinne t.** A modification of the Rinne test in which the subject is asked which sounds louder, the tuning fork held near the meatus or the one placed on the mastoid bone. As the Rinne test takes longer this version of the test is frequently preferred. **Molisch t.** A test for carbohydrate, made by adding 1-naphthol to the solution under test and a layer of sulfuric acid under it. A purple ring at the interface indicates carbohydrate. It is due to reaction of a dehydration product of sugars with the naphthol. **Moloney t.** A test for delayed sensitivity to diphtheria toxoid. A minute amount of toxoid is injected intradermally. The development of a red induration within 12 to 24 hours is a positive reaction. Also *anatoxireaction, Moloney reaction, Zeller's test*. **Moloney-Underwood t.** A test for the evaluation of sensitivity to diphtheria antitoxin. It is recommended in order to identify persons in whom the antitoxin could trigger severe reactions. The test consists of an intradermal injection of 0.1 ml of diphtheria antitoxin diluted 1:1000. **monaural distorted speech t.'s** Tests of hearing in which speech may be distorted in various ways such as by filtering out certain frequencies, unduly increasing the speed of the speech signal, adding certain types of background noise, and by other means. These are of value in determining in which temporal lobe a lesion of the auditory cortex is located. **Monospot t.** A single-step test for the heterophil antibody that is characteristic of infectious mononucleosis caused by the Epstein-Barr virus. The antibody agglutinates horse red blood cells within a few minutes of contact on a slide. Absorption with guinea pig kidney, which contains Forssman antigen, removes this antibody, but absorption with beef red cells does not. A proprietary name. **Mono-Vac t.** A multiple-puncture test for tuberculosis using concentrated tuberculin. It is useful as a screening test. **Montenegro t.** LEISHMANIN TEST. **Morelli's t.** An obsolete test formerly used to distinguish transudates from exudates. When a few drops of the fluid in question were mixed in a test tube with a saturated solution of mercuric chloride, a flaky precipitate was said to result with transudates while clots indicated exudates. **Moretti's t.** A test for typhoid fever using a filtrate of the patient's urine and ammonium sulfate to which a sodium hydroxide solution is added. Production of a gold-yellow color is a positive reaction. **Moro t.** Elicitation of Moro's reflex as a test of an infant's neurologic responses. **Morton's t.** A test for metatarsalgia in which the forefoot is laterally compressed. The test is positive if the compression elicits pain. **motility t.** A test, based on microscopic observation or on the spread of growth in soft agar, used to determine if an organism has flagella and therefore is motile. This test is used in the identification of many organisms such as members of the Enterobacteriaceae family, other Gram-negative bacilli, and species of *Listeria, Bacillus,* and *Corynebacterium*. **multiple-puncture t.** A type of test for tuberculin sensitivity in which antigen is introduced into the skin by the use of several needles or tines, usually in a special instrument. See also TINE TUBERCULIN TEST, STERNEEDLE TEST,

HEAF TEST, MONO-VAC TEST. **mumps sensitivity t.** A skin test in which intradermal injection of inactivated mumps virus provokes a wheal and erythema in persons with prior immunizing contact with the virus. The test has been replaced widely by serologic tests for antibodies to mumps virus. **murexide t.** A procedure that indicates the presence of uric acid. A mixture of the specimen and nitric acid is evaporated, and the residue obtained is combined with ammonia water. A purple color develops if uric acid was present in the specimen. **Naffziger's t.** Digital pressure applied over the scalenus anterior muscle in the root of the neck reproduces the paresthesiae in the hand and fingers which are experienced spontaneously by patients with the scalenus anterior syndrome. **NBT t.** NITROBLUE TETRAZOLIUM TEST. **neuraminidase inhibition t.** A method used for identifying strains of influenza viruses that elaborate the enzyme neuraminidase. Antiserum specific for an individual strain of virus will inhibit neuraminidase activity of a viral culture of its specific strain but not of the enzyme activity of viruses of other serologic groups. **neutralization t.** Any test used to identify either specific toxins or microorganisms or the antibodies to toxins or organisms by determining the ability of an antiserum to counteract the pathogenic properties of a microorganism or its products. The Schick test for diphtheria is a neutralization test performed on the skin. **Nickerson-Kveim t.** KVEIM-SILTZBACH TEST. **nicotine t.** A test now rarely used in the diagnosis of diabetes insipidus. It involves assessing the antidiuretic effect of smoking a standard number of cigarettes after a period of prior hydration. The nicotine thus administered stimulates vasopressin (antidiuretic hormone) secretion acutely in normal people but not in patients with diabetes insipidus. **ninhydrin t.** A method to demonstrate the presence of α-amino acid nitrogen, suitable for qualitative or quantitative procedures. A purple color at the end point results when amino acids interact at an acid pH with ninhydrin. Also *amino acid test.* **nitroblue tetrazolium t.** A test of neutrophils' capacity for phagocytosis and intracellular bacterial killing. If phagocytosis and bactericidal activity are intact, adding nitroblue tetrazolium (NBT) to actively phagocytizing cells produces bluish-black clumps of reduced NBT, called formazan. It is used to diagnose neutrophil defects in chronic granulomatous disease. Also *nitroblue tetrazolium dye test, NBT test.* **nitroblue tetrazolium dye t.** NITROBLUE TETRAZOLIUM TEST. **nitrogen washout t.** A test in which the expiration of nitrogen is monitored following inspiration of 100% oxygen. The uniformity of ventilation and the volume of air in the lung can be measured. **nonparametric t.** A test of statistical significance which does not depend on the form of the underlying distribution. Also *distribution-free test.* **nonverbal intelligence t.** PERFORMANCE TEST. **Ober's t.** OBER SIGN. **obturator t.** A test for possible appendicitis in which the patient's right hip is flexed and internally rotated to elicit right lower quadrant abdominal pain. **17-OH-corticoids t.** 17-HYDROXYCORTICOSTEROID TEST. **olfactory nerve t.** A neurologic test of the sense of smell by employing a variety of chemicals at differing concentrations. **one-stage prothrombin time t.** A coagulation test in which calcium and tissue thromboplastin are added to plasma that had been anticoagulated with citrate or oxalate, and the time required for clot formation is measured. The normal range is about 12 to 16 seconds but varies with the source of tissue thromboplastin. Prolongation may be due to deficiency of prothrombin, factor VII, factor V, factor X, or fibrinogen, or to the presence of heparinlike inhibitors of coagulation. Also *prothrombin time, Quick's test.* **one-tail t.** A test of statistical significance where, *a priori,* the sample statistic under test (for example, a mean) could only be either greater than, or could only be less than, a value established by hypothesis. Also *single-tail test.* **ONPG t.** β-GALACTOSIDASE TEST. **opsonocytophagic t.** Any of a number of procedures used to study the presence in serum of opsonins, which enhance phagocytosis. It can be used to detect antibodies to specific infective agents or to detect nonspecific effects on cells mediated by broadly reactive autoantibodies or activated complement components. **Optochin t.** A test used to identify *Streptococcus pneumoniae,* whose growth, unlike that of other streptococci, is inhibited in a zone around a disk containing Optochin. Also *Optochin disk test, Optochin susceptibility test.* **oral lactose tolerance t.** A test for lactase deficiency in which 100 grams of lactose is administered orally and blood sugar levels are measured as in a glucose tolerance test. If lactase deficiency exists, the lactose will not be split to glucose and the blood sugar level will not rise more than 20 mg/dl over the fasting level. **orcinol t.** BIAL'S TEST. **orthotoluidine t.** A test that exploits the peroxidase activity of heme pigments to demonstrate the presence of blood. Heme produces a blue discoloration when orthotoluidine in 4% glacial acetic acid and hydrogen peroxide are added. **osmotic fragility t.** A measurement of the degree of hemolysis (in percent) that occurs when erythrocytes are suspended in varying concentrations of sodium chloride solution less than 0.156 mol/l or greater. The test is most commonly used to confirm hereditary spherocytosis, a condition that exhibits increased osmotic fragility of erythrocytes. Also *erythrocyte fragility test, saline fragility test.* **Ouchterlony t.** OUCHTERLONY TECHNIQUE. **ovarian hyperemia t.** An accurate biologic test for pregnancy. Serum or concentrated urine from a pregnant woman causes hyperemia of the ovaries of an immature female rat within 24 hours after intraperitoneal injection. **oxidase t.** A color test, using derivatives of *p*-phenylenediamine, for the presence of intracellular cytochrome oxidase. A positive test is found only in aerobic and facultative anaerobic bacteria, and it assists in the identification of *Neisseria* species and Pseudomonadaceae. **oxytocin sensitivity t.** A seldom-used test to determine whether a uterus is ready for induction of labor. Low doses of oxytocin are infused every minute for ten doses or until the uterus contracts. The test is positive if a strong uterine contraction occurs with a dose of 0.02 I.U. or less of oxytocin. **pancreozymin-secretin t.** SECRETIN TEST. **Pap t.** PAPANICOLAOU TEST. **Papanicolaou t.** A test for early detection of cancer of the cervix in humans that uses a Papanicolaou smear. It may also detect inclusions indicative of herpesvirus infection. Also *Pap test, smear test.* **paradimethylaminobenzaldehyde t.** EHRLICH'S TEST. **parallel swing t.** A test to demonstrate the function and status of the otolith organs of the human ear. A stretcher is suspended, parallel to the floor, on four wires and moved by compressed air. The subject lies on the stretcher and is required to identify the direction in which he is moved. The least acceleration needed to produce the sensation of motion is recorded. **parentage t.** PATERNITY TEST. **partial thromboplastin time t.** A test of the intrinsic coagulation cascade. It measures the clotting time of plasma stimulated by the addition of a plateletlike partial thromboplastin. **passive agglutination t.** A procedure used to demonstrate agglutinating antibodies against antigens that exist in soluble form. When the antigen is fixed to the surface of otherwise inert indicator particles, usually red blood cells or latex particles, the presence of a specific antigen-antibody reaction becomes apparent by agglutination of the antigen-coated indicator particles. **passive cutaneous anaphylaxis t.** See under PASSIVE CUTANEOUS ANAPHYLAXIS. **passive transfer t.** PASSIVE CUTANEOUS ANAPHYLAXIS. **patch t.** A test for hypersensitivity to various substances in which linen or gauze strips impregnated with specimens of possible allergens are applied to the skin. They are removed after 48 hours. The test site is inspected at that time and again 24 hours later. A positive skin reaction indicates hypersensitivity. The patch tests are particularly important in the investigation of allergic contact dermatitis. Also *contact test.* **paternity t.** Exclusion of paternity by comparison of genetically determined factors in the blood of a newborn and its mother to those found in the blood of one or more putative fathers. Direct exclusion of paternity occurs when a genetic marker is present in the blood of the newborn and absent in both the mother and putative father or when either one of two allelic genetic markers is absent in the child but present in the putative father. Indirect exclusion occurs when a genetic marker is homozygously present in the child, such as NN, and its allele is present in the homozygous state in the putative father, such as MM. The genetically determined factors include, in addition to the ABO, Rh and MN antigens of erythrocytes, histocompatibility antigens, erythrocyte enzymes and serum proteins. Also *parentage test.* **patting t.** A test designed to detect cerebellar ataxia. The subject is asked to pat rapidly with each hand consecutively on his knee or on the examiner's hand. Disorganization of movement or inability to maintain the speed of tapping for more than a few seconds are frequent manifestations of cerebellar disorder. **Paul's t.** A test for smallpox. Material from a lesion is rubbed into the scarified eye of a rabbit. Keratitis or epitheliosis develops within 48 hours if the material contains smallpox virus. **Paul-Bunnell t.** The classic test for the heterophil antibody characteristic of infectious mononucleosis in which a positive result is indicated by the agglutination of red blood cells of sheep. It is performed with serially diluted serum to determine the titer of the antibody. Also *Paul-Bunnell reaction, sheep cell agglutination test.* **Paul-Bunnell-Davidsohn t.** An extension of the Paul-Bunnell test in which the ability of serum to agglutinate sheep red cells is retested after absorption with beef red cells and Forssman antigen. It is used to characterize the heterophil antibody seen in infectious mononucleosis, in serum sickness, and after some upper respiratory infections. In cases of infectious mononucleosis, beef red cells markedly reduce the titer of sheep cell agglutinating antibodies, whereas Forssman antigen has no effect. In serum sickness, the Forssman antigen reduces the titer. Also *differential test for infectious mononucleosis, Davidsohn differential test.* **pendular eye-tracking t.** A test sometimes used to help differentiate brainstem and cerebellar lesions from vestibular lesions and lesions of the oculomotor pathways. The patient is required to fix his gaze on a pendulum that consumes two seconds for each excursion and has an amplitude of 15 to 20 degrees. Anomalies in the pendulum-following eye movements may be significant. Abbr. PETT **pendulousness of the legs t.** PENDULAR KNEE JERK. **pentose t.** BIAL'S TEST. **perchlorate discharge t.** A test to detect abnormalities in intrathyroidal iodide organification. Radioiodide is given as for a radioactive iodide uptake test. Counts over the thyroid are made at 15-minute intervals. Potassium perchlorate (1 g) is given by mouth. Loss of 5 percent or more of the thyroidal radioactivity within one hour after perchlorate is administered indicates an organification defect. **performance t.** A test for evaluating intelligence which minimizes the use of language. It centers instead on the manipulation of concrete objects, such as blocks, pictures, or printed mazes to be traced. Such tests examine the ability to deal with things and their relationships, rather than with relationships embodied in the meanings of linguistic and numerical symbols. Also *nonverbal intelligence test.* **Perthes t.** A test for patency of the deep veins of the leg in the presence of varicose veins. With the patient standing, a tourniquet is applied above or below the knee. If the collateral circulation is satisfactory, the varicose veins will empty when the patient walks. **Petzetaki's t.** A test for typhoid fever using the patient's urine. When combined with an alcoholic iodine solution, a golden-yellow color is produced in the upper part of the urine specimen if the test is positive. Also *Petzetaki's reaction.* **phage neutralization t.** A test for the presence of antibodies induced against a bacteriophage antigen in which the antibody becomes apparent by inhibiting the plaques of infection that develop when an unopposed bacteriophage is introduced into a culture plate of susceptible bacteria. Also *bacteriophage neutralization test.* **Phalen's t.** PHALEN SIGN. **phenolsulfonphthalein t.** An outmoded test of renal function based on the rate of excretion of phenolsulfonphthalein over four 15-minute periods following intravenous or intramuscular injection. **phentolamine t.** A nonspecific test used to diagnose pheochromocytoma, when established hypertension is present. The administration of phentolamine, an $\alpha$-adrenergic blocking agent, causes a 25–35 mm Hg drop in diastolic blood pressure if elevated catecholamines are present. **phenylalanine deaminase t.** A test to determine the ability of an organism to break down phenylalanine to phenylpyruvic acid. It is used in the biochemical identification of members of the Enterobacteriaceae family. **phosphatase t.** A test commonly used for ensuring the adequacy of the pasteurization of milk. It is based on the heat sensitivity of the enzyme phosphatase. **photostress t.** Exaggeration of a fault of retinal photochemical metabolism by exposure to a bright light. The faulty portion of retina recovers more slowly than normal. **Pirquet's t.** PIRQUET'S REACTION. **pivot shift t.** A test for anterolateral instability of the knee. The test is positive if, when the knee is extended, there is a sudden subluxation of the lateral tibial condyle upon the distal femur. Also *jerk test.* **P-K t.** PRAUSNITZ-KÜSTNER REACTION. **plantar ischemia t.** A test for vascular insufficiency of the lower leg. With the leg elevated, the plantar surface of the foot is examined for blanching after it has been alternately flexed and extended. **plasma ACTH t.** A measurement of pituitary adrenocorticotropin in plasma. Normal values range up to 80 pg/ml, and are raised in Addison's disease, pituitary-dependent Cushing syndrome, and acute physical illness. The values are very much raised in the Cushing syndrome associated with ACTH-secreting carcinomas. **plasma cortisol t.** A measurement of the plasma concentration of the principal human glucocorticoid of plasma. The range in normal subjects is 4–16 $\mu$g/100 ml at the early morning peak. Plasma cortisol, secreted in episodic bursts in response to those of pituitary corticotropin, undergoes a diurnal or circadian variation in normal subjects, with highest values observed at 6:00 A.M. and lowest values late at night. Diurnal variation is absent or abnormal in all forms of the Cushing syndrome and in patients under severe stress owing to physical or psychiatric illness. **platelet aggregation t.** Any of several procedures in which a standardized concentration of platelets is exposed to substances such as ADP, collagen, or epinephrine that cause normally reactive platelets to aggregate. The end point is increased light transmission through the previously turbid suspension of platelets. Individual platelet defects may impair aggregation to one or several aggregating agents, but not to all. **pneumatic t.** A vestibular test in which raising the pressure in the external auditory canal by pressing the tragus into the entrance of the meatus or by utilizing Siegle's otoscope may, in certain circumstances, elicit nystagmus, vertigo, or both. The test is usually employed when a fistula in the bony labyrinth is suspected in a case of chronic otitis media (fistula test). **polystyrene latex t.** LATEX PARTICLE AGGLUTINATION TEST. **porphobilinogen t.** WATSON-SCHWARTZ TEST. **Porter-Silber chromogens t.** 17-HYDROXYCORTICOSTEROID TEST. **Porteus maze t.** A performance test of intelligence consisting of a series of printed mazes of graded difficulty which the examinee is asked to trace through from beginning to end. It was originally validated against social criteria such as foresight and resourcefulness in social interaction, and social sufficiency, rather than academic success. It is held to yield a better estimate of intelligence as applied to the needs for autonomous existence than can be obtained by measures based on success in the classroom alone. **postauricular myogenic reflex t.** The electrical detection of the auricular reflex in response to sounds of known frequency and intensity. It is used in the assessment of hearing in young children, primarily as a screening procedure. Also *crossed acoustic reflex test.* Abbr. PAM **potassium cyanide t.** A test to determine the ability of an organism to reproduce in the presence of potassium cyanide. The test is used in the biochemical identification of some members of the Enterobacteriaceae family and other Gram-negative bacilli. **P and P t.** PROTHROMBIN-PROCONVERTIN TEST. **Prausnitz-Küstner t.** PRAUSNITZ-KÜSTNER REACTION. **prayer t.** A test for mobility of finger joints in which the patient is asked to press the fingers of both hands together in a position resembling that of prayer, said to have predictive value in forecasting microangiopathic complications in patients with juvenile diabetes. **precipitation t.** 1 PRECIPITIN TEST. 2 PRECIPITIN REACTION. **precipitin t.** Any test in which the end point is precipitation, such as an insoluble complex following interaction of soluble antigen and soluble antibody. Also *precipitation test.* **Prendergast's t.** A test for typhoid fever. Within 24 hours of an intradermal injection of typhoid vaccine the typhoid patient shows no reaction, whereas a patient who does not have typhoid will develop a local erythematous reaction. **projective t.** See under PROJECTIVE METHOD. **prolonged toxicity t.** CHRONIC TOXICITY TEST. **pronation-supination t.** A test of cerebellar function in which the subject is asked to pronate and supinate the forearms rapidly and successively. Incoordinate movement is a sign of dysdiadochokinesia. **prothrombin consumption t.** A measure of the residual clotting activity (prothrombin) in serum one hour after clotting has occurred under specified conditions. Also *serum prothrombin time.* **prothrombin-proconvertin t.** A modification of the prothrombin consumption test designed to increase its sensitivity to deficiencies of prothrombin and factor VII in plasma. Also *P and P test.* **proverbs t.** A test in which the subject is asked to explain what two or three common proverbs mean to him, used as a way of eliciting abnormal thinking patterns. Also *Finckh's test.* **provocative t.** Any procedure in which a suspected pathophysiologic abnormality is deliberately induced by administering an agent or by manipulating conditions know to provoke the abnormal event. For example, the water provocative test for glaucoma increases intraocular pressure by the osmotic effect of drinking a large volume of water. **psoas t.** See under FEMORAL SIGN. **psychomotor t.** A measure of the speed and/or accuracy that is characteristic of an individual in carrying out a simple sensorimotor response. In humans, such movements are usually under a degree of mental control in that they are executed under some set of instructions. For example, reaction time is most often measured as the time elapsing between the onset of a tone or a light and the instructed lift of a finger, but they are typically straightforward and direct responses, not requiring an elaborated choice or decision for action. Psychomotor activities are more complex than neuromotor reflexes or positioning responses, but are simpler than perceptuomotor actions, when a body movement is combined with a required discrimination, memory, or other cognitive process. **pulp t.** A test to determine the vitality of a dental pulp by testing its sensitivity to thermal or electrical stimuli. Also *vitality test.* **quantitative gel diffusion t.** SINGLE RADIAL DIFFUSION TEST. **Queckenstedt's t.** A test devised to reveal a blockage in the spinal canal. Bilateral compression of the jugular veins does not cause any change in the pressure of the cerebrospinal fluid when the blockage is above the level of the lumbar puncture needle. Normally, this causes an increase in pressure of about 150–250 mm of water. Also *Queckenstedt sign, Queckenstedt-Stookey test, jugular sign, manometric test, Queckenstedt's phenomenon.* **quellung t.** QUELLUNG REACTION. **Quick's t.** ONE-STAGE PROTHROMBIN TIME TEST. **Race-Coombs t.** ANTIGLOBULIN TEST. **radial diffusion t.** SINGLE RADIAL DIFFUSION TEST. **radioactive iodine t.** $^{131}$I UPTAKE TEST. **radioactive renogram t.** The measurement of glomerular filtration, tubular cell function, and/or renal blood flow by means of radiolabeled tracers. **radioallergosorbent t.** A quantitative technique to measure serum levels of an IgE antibody directed against a specific antigen. The allergen extract is coupled to a solid medium, the immunosorbent. After the IgE-containing serum is incubated with the immunosorbent, the attached antibody is identified and quantified by addition of radiolabeled rabbit antibody to human IgE. Abbr. RAST **radioimmunosorbent t.** A procedure for quantifying serum IgE levels to an accuracy of 1 ng/ml without identifying antigenic specificity. The serum under test is exposed to a solid-phase material coated with rabbit anti-IgE, and the amount of human IgE bound to the rabbit antibody is measured by the addition and counting of radiolabeled rabbit anti-IgE in soluble form. Abbr. RIST **RAI t.** $^{131}$I UPTAKE TEST. **rapid plasma reagin t.** A widely performed, nonspecific serologic test for syphilis that uses unheated plasma or serum and a modified cardiolipin reagent coupled to macroscopically visible charcoal particles. The test can be performed on pieces of cardboard in nonlaboratory settings, and it can be adapted to automated performance as the automated reagin test (ART). Also *RPR test.* **recruitment t.** A test on a hearing-impaired subject to determine if there is an abnormally rapid increase in the sensation of loudness in the affected ear. See also ALTERNATE BINAURAL LOUDNESS BALANCE TEST, LOUDNESS RECRUITMENT. **red cell adherence t.** An immune adherence procedure that depends upon the presence of receptors on primate red blood cells for the C3b component of complement. It is used to detect the presence of complement-binding antibodies against cell-surface antigens, with a positive end point being the adherence of red cells to the antibody-coated target cells. Also *erythrocyte adherence test.* **Regitine t.** A now largely obsolete test for pheochromocytoma using intravenous Regitine (phentolamine) to lower blood pressure. **Reinsch t.**

A toxicologic screening test for heavy metals in the urine and gastric system. When a clean copper strip or wire is boiled in the acidified specimen, the deposition on the copper of a discolored metallic film indicates the presence of arsenic, antimony, bismuth, mercury, selenium, or tellurium. **renin suppression t.** A diagnostic test for primary aldosteronism. The subject is maintained on a constant sodium intake over a period of days and, when sodium balance is achieved, a standardized sodium load is given. Normal subjects respond with a substantial fall in plasma renin activity, whereas patients with an autonomous primary adrenocortical tumor secreting excessive aldosterone show no such decrease. **resorcinol t.** A test for fructose in the urine. When fresh urine is boiled with hydrochloric acid and resorcinol, fructose produces a red precipitate which can be dissolved in ethyl alcohol. Also *Selivanoff reaction, Selivanoff's test, resorcinol-hydrochloric acid test.* **Rideal-Walker t.** A test for determining the phenol coefficient of a disinfectant. **ring t.** Any immunoprecipitin procedure in which antigen and antibody are layered in a tube, and a precipitin ring forms at the interface or, after diffusion, where antigen and antibody proportions are optimal. Also *interfacial test, interfacial precipitin test, ring precipitin test.* **Rinne t.** A tuning fork test of hearing in which a comparison is made of the subject's ability to hear by air conduction and by bone conduction. If the subject is able to hear the sound through air after he no longer hears it through bone, the test is positive, the reverse finding being the negative response. A positive response is found in normal subjects and those with sensorineural hearing loss, a negative response in those with conductive hearing loss. Also *Rinne response.* **Romberg's t.** A test devised to elucidate disturbances of balance. The subject stands upright with feet together and eyes are then closed. Excessive swaying or a tendency to fall forwards or backwards is indicative of severe impairment of postural sensibility in the lower limbs. The sensitivity of the test can be increased by variations such as standing on one foot only, putting one foot in front of the other, etc. Also *station test.* **Rorschach t.** A projective technique for personality assessment in which a subject is shown a series of bisymmetrical inkblots, some in black and white, others in color, and asked for each "What does this look like? What could it be?" The responses and associations offered are categorized and analyzed according to whether they contain, for example, movement, popular or very original productions, and so on, providing a description of the personality as a whole, based on the congruence between the pattern of associations produced by the subject and those obtained from individuals with known personality disturbances. Also *inkblot test, psychodiagnostics* (used especially by Swiss and German writers). **Rosenzweig picture frustration t.** A projective test consisting of line drawings depicting two persons in a patently frustrating situation, in which the verbal remarks of the offender are given, while those of the offended against are not. The subject is asked to identify with the latter figure, and to write in the reply he or she might have given in such a situation. Responses are scored in terms of the type and direction of aggression expressed. Forms considered appropriate for the age of the subject are administered. **Rose-Waaler t.** A passive hemagglutination test for rheumatoid factors in which the indicator particles are the red blood cells of sheep. The cells are coated with subagglutinating amounts of human IgG. This test is more specific but less sensitive than the latex fixation test, and it is technically much more difficult to perform. Also *sheep cell agglutination test, sensitized sheep cell test, Waaler-Rose test, Waaler-Rose reaction.* **rotation t.** A test of vestibular function in which the subject is rotated in a chair and the ensuing nystagmus measured. The procedure may be quantified by using known angular accelerations and velocities. Also *rotatory test.* **Rothera's t.** A semiquantitative test for the ketone bodies acetoacetic acid and acetone that is used on serum, plasma, or urine. Ketone bodies, in the presence of sodium nitroprusside at an alkaline pH, produce a purple color of an intensity roughly proportional to their concentration. This reaction is the basis for widely used tablet and paper strip tests for ketone bodies. **RPR t.** RAPID PLASMA REAGIN TEST. **Rubin's t.** A test used in evaluating infertility to determine whether the oviducts are patent. Carbon dioxide gas is infused transcervically. If the oviducts are patent, subdiaphragmatic accumulation of the gas produces shoulder pain at pressures of 100 mm Hg or less. **Rubino's t.** RUBINO'S REACTION. **Rumpel-Leede t.** See under RUMPEL-LEEDE PHENOMENON. **Sabin-Feldman dye t.** A serologic test for toxoplasmosis. Living toxoplasmas in the presence of a complement-like factor and specific antibody do not accept an alkaline methylene blue dye. Also *Sabin-Feldman test.* **saline fragility t.** OSMOTIC FRAGILITY TEST. **scarification t.** PIRQUET'S REACTION. **Schick t.** A test for the assessment of diphtheria immunity. Heat-inactivated toxin is injected intradermally. Unless specific antibodies are present, a red, edematous area of inflammation develops at the injection site on the fifth to seventh day. Also *Schick reaction.* **Schiff's t.** A histochemical test for the presence of polysaccharides, mucopolysaccharides, glycoproteins, or glycolipids, which are stained red-purple by Schiff's reagent. Also *carbohydrate test, Hotchkiss method.* **Schilling t.** A test of absorption of orally administered vitamin $B_{12}$, in which radiolabeled ($^{57}$Co) vitamin $B_{12}$ is administered orally after parenteral administration of nonlabeled vitamin $B_{12}$. The amount of radioactivity excreted over the ensuing 24 hours reflects absorption, provided renal function is normal and urine collection is complete. Normal excretion is 7% or more of the oral dose. If absorption is poor, the test can be repeated with the simultaneous administration of intrinsic factor, which corrects the absorptive defect in classical pernicious anemia but not in malabsorption syndromes. **Schirmer's t.** A test used to estimate the amount of lacrimal secretion. A narrow strip of filter paper is hooked over each lower eyelid and the extent to which the paper is wetted by the tears is measured. It is applied in cases of lower motor neuron paralysis to indicate the level of the lesion. A marked impairment of lacrimation on the paralyzed side suggests that the lesion involves the geniculate ganglion or the nervus intermedius. **Schumm's t.** **1** BENZIDINE TEST. **2** A quantitative test for heme in plasma, using colorimetric assay of an ether-ammonium sulfide extract. Also *heme test, hematin test.* **Schwabach's t.** A tuning fork test in which the bone conduction hearing of the subject is compared with that of the normally hearing examiner. **sciatic stretch t.** LASÈGUE SIGN. **scratch t.** A test used to study pharmacologic or immunologic reactions to test solutions in which the solution is rubbed gently into a scratch in the skin about 1 cm long. **screen t.** COVER TEST. **screening t.** **1** Any test applied to a group or population that is designed to exclude some members of the group on the basis of established criteria or to detect the existence of unrecognized disease, parasites, or other pathologic conditions in individuals. See also SCREENING. **2** A test applied to chemical compounds to determine the presence of some specific property, such as carcinogenicity. **3** A relatively imprecise test applied to an individual subject or specimen, intended to indicate the likelihood that a disease or condition is present. More expensive, difficult, or hazardous tests can then be performed to achieve a definitive diagnosis if the screening test is positive. **Seashore t.** A recorded test series for measuring an individual's relative standing on several musical capacities: pitch discrimination, rhythm, time, tonal memory, loudness discrimination, and timbre. Although originally constructed to identify musical aptitude, several of the standardized subtests have been profitably applied for evaluating deficits in auditory functioning, owing to damage occurring in either the central or peripheral mechanisms of hearing. **secretin t.** A test of pancreatic exocrine function, in which the volume and the bicarbonate level of duodenal contents are measured before and after stimulation with secretin or pancreozymin. Normal values are production of 2 to 4 ml pancreatic juice per kilogram body weight and 90 to 130 mEq/1 bicarbonate. Low levels occur in chronic pancreatitis, cystic fibrosis, extensive pancreatic carcinoma, or any other cause of exocrine damage. Also *secretin stimulation test, pancreozymin-secretin test.* **sedimentation t.** Any test in which the rate and manner in which particles (e.g., erythrocytes, barium salts) settle are used to gain information. **Selivanoff's t.** RESORCINOL TEST. **sensitized sheep cell t.** ROSE-WAALER TEST. **serologic t.** Any test performed on serum to demonstrate the presence of antibodies, especially a procedure intended to demonstrate immunizing exposure to pathogenic organisms. **sheep cell agglutination t.** **1** ROSE-WAALER TEST. **2** PAUL-BUNNELL TEST. **short increment sensitivity index t.** A test of the differential sensitivity for loudness: the subject is exposed to a pure tone of 1000 Hz the intensity of which is increased by 1 to 5 dB steps. He is asked to count the number of increments. The normal subject has a low percentage score while the score is found to be high in the presence of loudness recruitment. Also *SISI test, small increment sensitivity index test.* **short-term toxicity t.** SUBCHRONIC TOXICITY TEST. **Sia water t.** A nonspecific, minimally sensitive test for the presence of macroglobulins in serum. A drop of normal serum in a test tube of distilled water produces a faint haze, but pathologic quantities of macroglobulins produce a heavy precipitate. **sickling t.** A qualitative test for hemoglobin S, depending upon the appearance of irreversibly sickled cells after the addition of two percent sodium metabisulfite or dithionate to the blood. **Sims t.** HUHNER TEST. **single-breath oxygen t.** A nitrogen washout test used for determination of the uniformity of ventilation. **single diffusion t.** Any immunologic procedure in which the concentration of either antigen or, more usually, antibody is constant throughout the gel medium, and only a single reactant, usually the antigen, diffuses away from the point of application. The precipitin line forms at the site of optimal antigen concentration relative to the constant antibody level in the medium. **single radial diffusion t.** A procedure for detecting and quantifying a soluble antigen. The antigen is allowed to diffuse radially into a gel containing a uniformly distributed antibody. A precipitin line forms in a circle around the point at which the antigen contacts the gel, and the radius of the circle is proportional to the concentration of the antigen. Absolute figures can be derived by comparison with measurements obtained with standards of known antigen concentration. Also *quantitative gel diffusion test, radial diffusion test, Mancini test.* **single radial hemolysis t.** A test that measures antibody to influenza by measuring the radius of a ring of hemolysis that occurs around the serum-filled well as the antibody diffuses into an agar gel that contains virus-sensitized erythrocytes and complement. **single-tail t.** ONE-TAIL TEST. **SISI t.** SHORT INCREMENT SENSITIVITY INDEX TEST. **skin-puncture t.** A test employed in cases of the Behçet syndrome in which pricking of the skin with a sterile needle results in the development of a pustule within 24 hours. **slide agglutination t.** Any agglutination procedure performed on a slide or plate without centrifugation. It can be used with red cells, bacteria, or coated indicator particles and can be applied to active or passive agglutination procedures, provided a sufficiently potent agglutinating antibody is available. **slide flocculation t.** Any test performed without centrifugation on a slide or tile and whose end point is flocculation. These tests are used especially to identify antibodies to bacterial antigens. **Slocum's t.** A test for rupture of the anterior cruciate and medial collateral ligaments of the knee. The knee can be subluxed anteriorly with external rotation of the tibia, but the knee cannot be subluxed anteriorly with forced internal rotation of the tibia. Also *Alri sign.* **small increment sensitivity index t.** SHORT INCREMENT SENSITIVITY INDEX TEST. **smear t.** PAPANICOLAOU TEST. **Snellen's t.** Measurement of visual acuity with test types designed to subtend the proper visual angles. See also SNELLEN CHART. **Snider match t.** MATCH TEST. **sniff t.** A test for possible paralysis of the hemidiaphragm in which a patient is asked to sniff while diaphragmatic movement is observed fluoroscopically. **Snyder's t.** A test for caries susceptibility based on acid-producing bacteria in saliva. **spectroscopic t.** A test in which a spectroscope is used for identification of a pigment in a fluid such as blood. The spectroscope displays the refraction pattern of light. Pigments through which the light passes create distinct absorption bands. **squatting t.** A diagnostic test for beriberi in which the patient is asked to rise from a squatting position. A victim of beriberi will be unable to do so without using his hands. **Stamey t.** The differential collection of ureteral or renal urine used to detect unilateral renovascular hypertension. A positive test includes a 50 percent or more decrease in urine flow and a 20 percent or more increase in creatinine in the urine from the ischemic kidney. The test is now rarely used but it is of historical interest. **standing plasma t.** A qualitative procedure to demonstrate abnormal plasma lipid composition. After 12–16 hours of refrigeration, excessive chylomicrons rise to form a creamlike layer, and excessive very low density lipoproteins create a uniform turbidity. **Stanford-Binet t.** STANFORD-BINET INTELLIGENCE SCALE. **starch hydrolysis t.** A biochemical test used in the identification of such bacteria as *Bacillus, Corynebacterium,* and *Streptococcus* species, in which the end point is enzymatic hydrolysis of a starch solution. Also *starch test.* **station t.** ROMBERG'S TEST. **stereognostic t.** A test for peripheral nerve lesion in which different common objects are placed in the hand of the blindfolded subject. The presence of a lesion is suspected if the objects cannot be identified. **Sterneedle t.** HEAF TEST. **stiff wrist t.** A test to detect the initial stages of parkinsonism: repeated passive pronation-supination movements of the patient's wrist show that hypertonia is temporarily reduced when the patient carries out a voluntary movement, as in standing up in order to take hold of an object with the other hand. **Stoll t.** A dilution egg-counting technique used in estimation of an individual's worm burden. It is based upon the collection of a 24-hour stool specimen and the counting of ova in a standard aliquot. The technique was developed for hookworm eggs, but can be adapted to other dilution counts as well. **straight leg raising t.** A test for sciatica in which the presence is confirmed by sciatic pain radiating down the limb when the supine patient attempts to raise the straightened limb. **streptolysin O t.** ANTISTREPTOLYSIN O TEST. **stress t.** Any test of cardiovascular function in which the system is subjected to stress, such as an exercise test or an atrial pacing test. **string t.** A test to localize an area of gastrointestinal bleeding by the passage of a string per oram. Also *Einhorn string test.* **Stypven time t.** The clotting time of plasma stimulated by the addition of Stypven, a proprietary preparation of Russell viper venom. The Stypven time is prolonged in plasma lacking factor V, factor X, or platelets. **subchronic toxicity t.** A toxicity test that is continued for a period of 90 days in the rat and from 90 to 180 days in the dog, with daily administration of a test substance incorporated either in food or in drinking water, or in some cases by gavage, at specified intervals. Also *short-term toxicity test, subacute toxicity test.* **sucrose hemolysis t.** A screening test for paroxysmal nocturnal hemoglobinuria (PNH), in which the patient's erythrocytes are incubated for 60 minutes at 20°C in a mixture that contains 1 volume of normal serum, 1 volume of a 50% suspension in isotonic saline of the patient's saline-washed erythrocytes, and 18 volumes of a 97.2 g/l solution of sucrose in barbital buffer. PNH erythrocytes lyse in this medium, but normal erythrocytes do not. The test is not always positive in PNH. False negative results may occur as a result of recent prior transfusion. **sucrose tolerance t.** A test for the presence in the intestinal mucosa of the disaccharide-splitting enzyme sucrase-isomaltase, which splits sucrose into glucose and fructose. A standardized dose of sucrose is administered orally and blood glucose levels are measured at intervals thereafter as an indication that sucrose has been cleaved. Because uncleaved sucrose causes abdominal distention, cramping, and diarrhea, observation for intestinal symptoms is part of the test. **sulfosalicylic acid t.** A semiquantitative test for urinary protein that produces turbidity or precipitation of a sulfosalicylic acid solution to a degree proportional to the protein concentration. The procedure is approximately $2\frac{1}{2}$ times more sensitive to albumin than to globulin, and it does recognize Bence-Jones protein. **Sulkowitch's t.** A semiquantitative precipitation test for urinary calcium. It produces turbidity in a solution of oxalic acid, ammonium oxalate, and acetic acid to a degree proportional to the calcium concentration. A normal result is mild, or 1+, turbidity. **sweat t.** A test for cystic fibrosis in which electrolytes are measured in sweat collected after local stimulation. Chloride concentration above 50 mEq/l is abnormal in children and above 60 mEq/l is diagnostic for cystic fibrosis. Sweat chloride concentrations tend to be higher in adults. **sweating t.** The artificial induction of sweating to measure the composition or quantity of its products. The test is used to diagnose cystic fibrosis and leprosy. **Szondi t.** A projective test in which the subject's like or dislike of photographs of patients with different psychiatric conditions is used to infer his own significant conflicts or character traits. **t t.** A test of statistical significance particularly applicable to small samples, involving the ratio of a sample statistic to its standard error. **Tardieu's t.** A test formerly used to prove that extrauterine fetal respiration had occurred in a dead infant, by demonstrating the presence of air bubbles in the gastric mucosa. Now obsolete, this inaccurate method was considered evidence of extrauterine existence during the nineteenth century. **tellurite t.** A test formerly used in the diagnosis of diphtheria. Any area of the throat affected with diphtheria blackens within five to ten minutes of the application of a 2% solution of potassium tellurite. Also *Manzullo's test.* **Tensilon t.** A test for the diagnosis of myasthenia gravis in which the power of individual skeletal muscles is assessed before and after an intravenous injection of Tensilon (edrophonium hydrochloride). **Terman t.** STANFORD-BINET INTELLIGENCE SCALE. **thematic apperception t.** A technique for exploring aspects of the personality in which the subject is asked to examine a series of pictures depicting one or more human figures in an amorphous or ambiguous context and then asked to tell a story about each picture. The stories generated are later evaluated for the needs, emotions, and conflicts projected onto the story characters as a possible reflection of similar tendencies existing within the storyteller. Abbr. TAT **thermal t.** A pulp test using cold or heat. The source of cold may be a pledget of cotton soaked in ethyl chloride. The source of heat may be a piece of temporary stopping gutta percha that has been heated in a flame. **thiocyanate t.** A test of thiocyanate levels in saliva, plasma, or urine, as an index of nitroprusside toxicity. Older qualitative tests were used to detect cyanide poisoning, but current quantitative tests use ion-exchange chromatography to concentrate the ion and spectrophotometry to measure the reaction product. **Thomas t.** A maneuver to reveal a flexion contracture of the hip joint. With the patient supine on a couch, the unaffected hip is maximally flexed and the examiner's hand is placed behind the lumbar spine of the patient. When the lumbar lordosis is obliterated, flexion of the abnormal hip will indicate a positive Thomas test and the angle of flexion can be measured. **Thompson's t.** A test for urethritis in which the subject upon rising passes urine successively into two glasses. If that of the first glass is turbid but of the second clear, the anterior urethra is affected. If the urine in both glasses is turbid, the posterior urethra is affected as well. Also *two-glass test.* **Thormählen's t.** A sensitive and specific test for melanogens in urine. The successive addition of a sodium nitroferricyanide solution, a sodium hydroxide solution, and acetic acid for acidification produces a greenish blue to blue-black discoloration if melanogens are present. Shades of brown indicate the absence of melanogens. **threshold tone decay t.** TONE DECAY TEST. **thromboplastin generation t.** An elaborate test of clotting in plasma that evaluates the steps leading to the formation of prothrombinase from the steps whereby thrombin and fibrin are formed. Abbr. TGT **thyrotropin releasing hormone stimulation t.** A test of pituitary response to thyrotropin releasing hormone (TRH), which normally stimulates pituitary secretion of thyroid stimulating hormone (TSH, thyrotropin), prolactin, and human growth hormone (HGH). It is used primarily to distinguish pituitary from hypothalamic causes of thyroid disorders and sometimes to confirm diagnosis of tumors secreting growth hormone or prolactin. After injection of synthetic TRH, measurements of TSH (and HGH and prolactin if desired) are taken at intervals for 180 minutes. In hypothalamic disorders and in renal failure and anorexia nervosa, TSH rises, but more slowly than normal. With pituitary dysfunction TSH does not rise. The TSH rise is exaggerated in primary hyperthyroidism. HGH rise is exaggerated with HGH-secreting tumors. Prolactin response is highly exaggerated in functional hyperprolactinism and moderately increased with prolactin-secreting tumors. **tine t.** TINE TUBERCULIN TEST. **Tinel t.** Paresthesia in the distribution of the median nerve, elicited by tapping over the wrist or the carpal tunnel. It is suggestive of compression of or damage to the median nerve. **tine tuberculin t.** A test for tuberculin sensitivity in which a tined instrument coated with old tuberculin is used to inoculate the forearm. An area of induration 2 mm or more in diameter at the inoculation site after 48–72 hours is considered a positive reaction. Also *tine test.* **toad t.** MALE FROG TEST. **Tobey-Ayer t.** A test performed when lumbar puncture is in progress and unilateral sigmoid sinus thrombosis is suspected. Pressure on the jugular vein of the normal side will produce a quick rise of manometric pressure equivalent to the rise expected in a normal subject, but compression of the vein on the suspect side will produce little or no rise in pressure if sigmoid sinus thrombosis is present. Also *Ayer-Tobey test.* **tolbutamide tolerance t.** A provocative test for insulin-producing islet-cell tumor of the pancreas. One gram of tolbutamide is rapidly given intravenously and plasma glucose and insulin values are measured over six hours. Exaggerated increase of insulin and protracted hypoglycemia are typical of insulinoma. Whereas an exaggerated insulin response is also seen in obesity, acromegaly, and the Cushing syndrome, it is not associated with severe hypoglycemia because there is peripheral resistance to endogenous insulin. **tolerance t.** A test to estimate the capacity of the body to metabolize a nutrient, drug, or diagnostic compound and to evaluate the metabolic activity in question by the response to the test material. **tone decay t.** A test for abnormal auditory adaptation: the subject's auditory threshold may be established at 4000 Hz, the intensity is raised by 5 dB and the subject requested to press a signal indicator as long as the sound is audible. The normal subject should be able to hear this sound for 60 seconds but if the sound disappears before the alloted time the intensity is raised by 5 dB and the process repeated until the sound is heard for 60 seconds. The sum of the 5 dB increments gives the measure in dB of the degree of abnormal adaptation. Also *threshold tone decay test.* **tourniquet t.** A test using a tourniquet to evaluate a physiopathologic phenomenon, such as the Hess capillary test or the Perthes test. **toxicity t.** A test conducted on laboratory animals to determine the harmful effect of chemicals on biologic systems. **TPHA t.** TREPONEMAL HEMAGGLUTINATION TEST. **TPI t.** TREPONEMA PALLIDUM IMMOBILIZATION TEST. **traction t.** A test used to assess muscular development during the first six months of life. Traction on the arms of a supine infant enables an assessment to be made of the tone and power of the muscles of the arms and trunk, and of the degree of head lag. **Trambusti t.** TRAMBUSTI'S REACTION. **Trendelenburg's t.** 1 TRENDELENBURG SIGN. 2 A test for venous incompetence in the legs. The test is positive if, after raising the legs above the level of the heart to drain the veins and then lowering the legs quickly, the vessels rapidly become distended. **treponemal antibody t.** Any of the serologic tests for syphilis that identify antibodies specifically directed against treponemal antigens, in contrast to the nonspecific tests that identify the cardiolipin-reactive protein sometimes called reaginic antibody. **treponemal hemagglutination t.** A specific serologic test for syphilis that employs as its positive end point the agglutination of tanned sheep red blood cells coated with treponemal antigens. Also *Treponema pallidum hemagglutination test, TPHA test.* ***Treponema pallidum* immobilization t.** The first of the specific serologic tests for syphilis. It uses as its positive end point the immobilization of living, motile *Treponema pallidum* organisms following their exposure to the patient's serum and complement, which have been incubated in an atmosphere of 5% $CO_2$ and 95% nitrogen. The test is rarely performed today except in reference settings because of the difficulty in maintaining living organisms and the technical problems of reproducibility and standardization. Also *TPI test.* **$T_3$ resin uptake t.** See under TRIIODOTHYRONINE UPTAKE TEST. **trichophytin t.** An intradermal test for hypersensitivity to products of *Trichophyton* species. The test is also used as a method for establishing the capacity of a patient to exhibit delayed hypersensitivity. **triiodothyronine uptake t.** An indirect test of thyroid function that reflects the number of sites on thyroid-binding globulin (TBG) not occupied by triiodothyronine ($T_3$). Radiolabeled $T_3$ and the test serum are added to an adsorbent, which is sometimes a resin. The amount of labeled $T_3$ adsorbed rises with the level of unoccupied TBG sites. When TBG levels are normal high $T_3$ uptake indicates low circulating $T_3$, and low $T_3$ uptake indicates elevated hormone levels. Abnormal TBG levels introduce artifact. Also *$T_3$ uptake test, Hamolsky's test* (older term). **$T_3$ suppression t.** A test for subtle Graves disease in which labeled triiodothyronine is given according to a standard protocol over seven days. The thyroidal radioiodine uptake normally falls below 50 percent of the baseline value, but in cases of Graves disease it falls only slightly or remains unchanged. Also *Werner's test.* **tuberculin t.** A test for the presence of cell-mediated immunity to the tubercle bacillus, performed by intradermal injection of tuberculin, a protein filtrate of cultured tubercle bacilli. It is sometimes performed with precipitated fractions of culture filtrate called purified protein derivatives, or PPD. A positive reaction is the development of a delayed hypersensitivity reaction, manifested by induration and erythema within 12 to 72 hours. If the initial injection elicits no response, a more concentrated preparation may be injected. With especially intense reactions, the injection site may undergo necrosis. Also *tuberculin titer test.* **tuberculin patch t.** A variant of the tuberculin test in which the protein antigen is applied to the skin surface by means of an adhesive patch rather than injected into the skin. **tuberculin titer t.** TUBERCULIN TEST. **tubular reabsorption of phosphate t.** A measurement of renal tubular reabsorption of filtered phosphate, expressed as

$$\% \text{ reabsorption} = \left(1 - \frac{\text{Urine phosphate concentration} \times \text{plasma creatinine}}{\text{Urine creatinine concentration} \times \text{plasma phosphate}}\right) \times 100.$$

Values are decreased in hyperparathyroidism and increased in hypoparathyroidism. **$T_3$ uptake t.** TRIIODOTHYRONINE UPTAKE TEST. **two-glass t.** THOMPSON'S TEST. **two-stage prothrombin time t.** An assay for the amount of thrombin that is formed from prothrombin when $Ca^{2+}$ and thromboplastin from brain are added to plasma obtained from citrate-anticoagulated blood. The assay is performed by transferring samples at intervals from the citrate plasma-$Ca^{2+}$-thromboplastin mixture to tubes containing a fibrinogen solution and measuring the time required for clot formation. A standard curve is obtained by adding known amounts of thrombin to tubes containing fibrin solution and measuring time to clot formation and plotting thrombin concentration against clotting time of the fibrinogen solution. Since the time is a function of the thrombin concentration, the thrombin concentration in the plasma specimen can then be obtained from the standard curve. **two-tail t.** A test of statistical significance where, *a priori,* the sample statistic under test (for example, a mean) could be either greater than or less than a value established by hypothesis. **Tzanck t.** Microscopic examination of material from the floor of a cutaneous bulla or vesicle used in the preliminary diagnosis of herpes, varicella, and pemphigus vulgaris. A smear is prepared from material obtained from the base of an early, freshly opened bulla and stained with Giemsa stain. Herpetic conditions show characteristic intranuclear viral inclusions whereas cases of pemphigus vulgaris disclose rounded, acantholytic epidermal cells. **U t.** MANN-WHITNEY U TEST. **Unterberger's t.** A test utilizing the same procedure as Mittelmeyer's test by requiring that the patient walk in place with his eyes closed. If he rotates through more than 60 degrees in one minute, severe vestibular damage should be suspected in the ear towards which he turns. **urease t.** A quantitative test for urea in which the enzyme urease converts urea to ammonium carbonate, from which ammonia is measured colorimetrically. **Urecholine supersensitivity t.** If the increase in intravesical pressure following subcutaneous injection of 2.5 mg Urecholine exceeds that in a control subject by more than 15 cm, the bladder is neurogenic. **urinary concentration t.** Any test in which the relative density or osmolality of urine is measured after a designated period of fluid restriction, to indicate renal ability to secrete a concentrated urine. Also *concentrating ability test, concentration test.* **vaginal cornification t.** A test for estrogenic activity based on microscopic examination of vaginal secretion. The presence of cornified cells indicates estrogen stimulation. A predominance of leukocytes in the secretion indicates lack of estrogen. **Valsalva's t.** A test for tubal patency utilizing the Valsalva maneuver. The subject attempts forcibly to exhale with the mouth closed and the nose pinched. **van den Bergh's t.** The measurement of serum bilirubin, using Ehrlich's test on unmodified serum. This procedure measures only the water soluble, conjugated form of bilirubin, sometimes called direct or post-hepatic bilirubin. **vanillylmandelic acid t.** The measurement, usually by extraction and oxidation of 24-hour urinary excretion, of vanillylmandelic acid. Elevated levels are found in cases of pheochromocytoma. Also *VMA test.* **variance ratio t.** F TEST. **VDRL t.** The Venereal Disease Research Laboratory test, a nonspecific serologic test for syphilis that uses heat-inactivated serum and an antigen preparation of cardiolipin, lecithin, cholesterol, and alcohol. Flocculation as the end point, read either microscopically in the slide procedure or macroscopically in the tube technique, indicates a positive reaction. **virulence t.** A test for the toxicity or invasiveness of a pathogenic organism in which pure cultures of the organism are injected into susceptible laboratory animals. **virus neutralization t.** Any test for the presence of neutralizing antibodies specific for the virus under consideration. It is performed by adding various dilutions of serum to a test system of a constant dose of virus in a culture of susceptible cells. A positive result is indicated by the prevention of cellular infection. **visual-motor gestalt t.** See under BENDER VISUAL-MOTOR GESTALT TEST. **vitality t.** PULP TEST. **vitamin K t.** A test of the ability of hepatocytes to synthesize coagulation proteins in which the prothrombin level is measured before and 24 hours after intramuscular administration of vitamin K. A normal response would be an increase of 20% or more. **VMA t.** VANILLYLMANDELIC ACID TEST. **Voges-Proskauer t.** See under VOGES-PROSKAUER REACTION. **Vollmer's t.** A trademark for a tuberculin patch test which consists of an adhesive strip containing two pieces of filter paper with old tuberculin and one piece of filter paper with a control broth. The strip is usually applied to the forearm. **von Pirquet's t.** PIRQUET'S REACTION. **von Stein's t.** A test of static equilibrium in which the patient is required to stand on one foot with the eyes closed. Inability to remain steady suggests a labyrinthine or cerebellar lesion. **Waaler-Rose t.** ROSE-WAALER TEST. **Waldenström's t.** A screening test for porphobilinogen or urobilinogen in urine that uses Ehrlich's aldehyde reagent to produce a red color if either of the two substances are present in the urine. **Wassermann t.** A serologic test for syphilis that uses complement fixation as the end point in a reaction between the subject's serum and cardiolipin. Although the antibody recognized in this procedure is not specific for *Treponema pallidum,* the test was the first effective serologic test for syphilis. The original antigen was an extract of the tissue of a syphilitic fetus, but normal tissues were later used. Also *Wassermann reaction.* **water deprivation t.** A provocative test for activity of vasopressin (antidiuretic hormone), which causes production of increasingly concentrated urine as the body needs to conserve water, by withholding water for not more than 24 hours. Overnight water deprivation normally causes urine osmolality to reach at least 800 mOsm/kg, with decreased urine volume and preservation of normal serum osmolality. In vasopressin deficiency, urine osmolality goes no higher than 300 mOsm/kg, urine volume remains high, and serum osmolality rises because of increasing dehydration. Protocols for various periods of water deprivation and for administration of exogenous vasopressin allow discrimination among diabetes insipidus due to vasopressin deficiency, nephrogenic diabetes insipidus, and polyuria due to pathologic polydipsia. **Watson-Schwartz t.** A test for urine porphobilinogen and urobilinogen, a sign of acute intermittent porphyria, based on the formation of red coloration on combination with Ehrlich's aldehyde reagent. Porphobilinogen is insoluble in chloroform, so the pink color remains in the aqueous phase after extraction with chloroform, whereas urobilinogen enters the chloroform phase. Also *porphobilinogen test, Watson-Schwartz reaction.* **Weber's t.** A test of hearing in which the foot of a vibrating tuning fork is placed in the midline of the head at the forehead or vertex and the subject is asked where he hears the sound. The normally hearing or those with symmetrical bilateral hearing loss will hear it centrally. If it is heard better in the deafened ear the loss is conductive. If heard better on the nondeafened side the loss is sensorineural. **Weigl-Goldstein-Scheerer t.** A sorting task used to evaluate abstract thinking ability among brain-injured individuals. The subject is asked to sort the same test blocks in terms of color and shape, to shift from one basis to another, and to verbalize the basis for his action. **Weil-Felix t.** An agglutination test for previous exposure to various rickettsiae based on cross-reactivity of these antibodies with antigens of certain *Proteus* species. Also *Felix-Weil reaction, Weil-Felix reaction.* **Welland's t.** BAR-READING TEST. **Werner's t.** $T_3$ SUPPRESSION TEST. **Wheeler and Johnson t.** A qualitative test for the pyrimidine bases cytosine and uracil, which produce a green coloration when the sample is treated with bromine water. The addition of barium hydroxide will change the liquid's color to purple. **Widal t.** A diagnostic test for typhoid fever in which typhoid bacilli (*Salmonella typhi*) are agglutinated by dilutions of the patient's serum. Also *Gruber's reaction, Gruber-Widal reaction, Gruber-Widal test, Widal serum test, Widal reaction.* **Widal serum t.** WIDAL TEST. **Wilcoxon's t.** A nonparametric test for the statistical analysis of matched pairs of observations applicable when the differences between pairs can be placed in rank order. The test is also used as an alternative to the paired t test when the underlying populations cannot be assumed to be normally distributed. **wipe t.** The measurement of removable radioactive contamination from a surface, as part of radiation safety monitoring. **Wolff-Eisner t.** CALMETTE'S REACTION. **word association t.** A method applied to the investigation of thought processes, for either clinical or experimental purposes, which records the responses given to verbal stimuli of various kinds. The subject is instructed to listen to a stimulus word, and to respond with another. The response can involve either free association or controlled association. **Wright t.** A method of bacterial therapy which consists of injecting a culture of killed microorganisms belonging to the species causing the disease in order to cause specific antibodies to appear in the blood of the subject. **X-chromatin t.** CHROMATIN TEST. **xylose concentration t.** A test that distinguishes pancreatic from intestinal causes of malabsorption by observing urinary excretion of D-xylose after oral ingestion. Normal excretion, after a 25 gram dose, is 4 or more grams excreted within 5 hours. Xylose excretion is depressed with intestinal dysfunction and normal with pancreatic dysfunction. Also *D-xylose tolerance test.* **Y chromatin t.** A cytologic method for detecting the presence of human Y chromatin by staining mitotic cells with quinacrine dihydrochloride, illuminating the preparation with ultraviolet light, and observing fluorescence of the distal long arm of the Y chromosome or of this portion of Y chromatin translocated elsewhere in the genome. **Zangemeister t.** An obsolete and inaccurate test of paternity, which compared photometric light transmission of the infant's serum to that of a mixture of the infant's and putative father's serum. A decrease in light transmission through the mixture was thought to indicate parentage. **Zeller's t.** MOLONEY TEST.

**test[2]** [L *testa*. See TESTA.] **1** A shell. **2** An envelope or skeleton of certain protozoa in the subphylum Rhizopoda consisting of organic, fibrous, calcareous, silicate, strontium sulfate, or other materials, often in a highly complex form with numerous apertures through which axopodia or filopodia of cytoplasm protrude. For defs. 1 and 2 also *testa.*

**testa** \tes′tə\ [L (akin to *testu* an earthenware pot; see TEST[1]) an earthenware pot, crock, shard, shell, carapace] (*pl.* testae) TEST[2].

**testaceous** \testā′shəs\ Having a shell or test.

**testalgia** \testal′jə\ [*test(is)* + -ALGIA] ORCHIALGIA.

**testcross** In experimental genetics, a method for establishing an unknown genotype by crossing with an organism homozygous at the locus in question.

**testectomy** \testek′təmē\ [*test(is)* + -ECTOMY] ORCHIDECTOMY.

**tester** / **pulp t.** A device using small doses of electric current for testing the vitality of teeth.

**testes** \tes′tēz\ Plural of TESTIS.

**testicle** \tes′tikl\ [L *testiculus.* See TESTICULUS.] TESTIS. **retained t.** CRYPTORCHIDISM. **undescended t.** CRYPTORCHIDISM.

**testicular** \testik′yələr\ Of or pertaining to a testis, as *testicular function.*

**testiculoma ovarii** \tes′tikyəlō′mə ōver′ē·ī\ ARRHENOBLASTOMA.

**testiculus** \testik′yələs\ [L (dim. of *testis* a testicle), a testicle] (*pl.* testiculi) TESTIS.

**testimony** \tes′təmō′nē\ **expert t.** All of the sworn statements made in a legal proceeding by an expert witness, particularly the testimony given in the form of opinions or answers to hypothetical questions involving facts about which the ordinary person would be unable to form correct judgments. Also *expert evidence.*

**testing** / **histocompatibility t.** The aggregate of tests used to determine whether tissue from one individual will engraft successfully in another. Typing donor and recipient for HLA antigens is one aspect. Other important considerations include testing the recipient's serum against the donor cells for evidence of cytotoxicity, and exposing donor cells to the recipient's lymphocytes in a mixed lymphocyte culture. **nondestructive t.** Examining or analyzing materials by methods which have no deleterious effect on the material, such as by roentgenography or x-ray emission spectrometry. **reality t.** Evaluation of the outside world and objective judgment of the relationship between self and nonself. Reality testing is a fundamental ego function that makes it possible to anticipate the future and prepare for it.

**testis** \tes′tis\ [L, lit., a witness (of virility)] (*pl.* testes) **1** [NA] One of the two oval male gonads supported in the scrotum by its tissues and suspended by the spermatic cord. The convex medial and lateral surfaces, superior and inferior extremities and anterior border are covered by the visceral layer of the tunica vaginalis, whereas the posterior border is only partly invested and is attached to the epididymis and spermatic cord. Deep to the tunica vaginalis is the tunica albuginea. From its deep surface the septula spread inward to divide the substance of the gland into lobules that converge on the mediastinum posteriorly. Within the lobules are various tissues: the seminiferous tubules, whose epithelium contains cells in various stages of spermatogenesis as well as the sustentacular or supporting cells of Sertoli; and the interstitial tissue between the tubules, which contain the Leydig cells responsible for secreting testosterone, estrogens, and other androgenic steroid hormones. Also *testicle, testiculus, orchis.* **2** A male gonad of any animal organism. **abdominal t.** An undescended testis located within the abdominal cavity. **ectopic t.** A testis which has descended, usually beyond the inguinal canal, but which is not located in the scrotum. The location of an ectopic testis may be in the perineum, external to the inguinal canal, upon the abdominal wall fascia, or in the femoral region. Also *ectopia testis.* **femoral t.** A testis that is situated in the inguinal canal close to the femoral ring. **inguinal t.** A testis still situated in the inguinal canal. **inverted t.** A testis having an abnormal position in the scrotum, with the epididymis attached anteriorly. **obstructed t.** A nondescended testis whose entry into the scrotum has been blocked by a sheet of fascia. **perineal t.** A testis that is located in the region of the perineum. **t. redux** A testis that is drawn up in to the higher portion of the scrotum, as in response to exposure to cold. **retained t.** CRYPTORCHIDISM. **undescended t.** CRYPTORCHIDISM.

**testitis** \testī′tis\ [*test(is)* + -ITIS] ORCHITIS.

**test-meal** See under MEAL.

**test-object** A specimen of known properties that can be used to check the performance of a microscope.

**testopathy** \testäp′əthē\ [*test(is)* + *o* + -PATHY] ORCHIOPATHY.

**testosterone** \testäs′tərōn\ 17-β-Hydroxyandrost-4-en-3-one, the principal and most potent C-19 androgenic steroid hormone produced by the Leydig cells of the testis, and also secreted by the ovary and the adrenal cortex. Its major actions are the promotion of nitrogen retention and the induction and maintenance of the growth, development, and function of the male secondary sex characters. The secretion of the hormone is chiefly regulated by adenohypophysial luteinizing hormone. Also *orchidic hormone* (rare).

**testosterone cyclopentylpropionate** 17β-Hydroxyandrost-4-en-3-one cyclopentanepropionate, a synthetically prepared ester of testosterone used in the treatment of male hypogonadism and in the palliation of metastatic breast cancer and some forms of aplastic anemia in adults. Its action is more prolonged than that of the native steroid or of testosterone propionate, shorter than that of testosterone enanthate. Also *testosterone cypionate.*

**testosterone enanthate** $C_{26}H_{40}O_3$. A synthetically prepared ester of testosterone, used for the same indications as testosterone cypionate. It is often administered in oil so that its actions will be prolonged. Its duration of action, up to 30 days when injected intramuscularly, is the longest of the commonly used testosterone derivatives. Also *testosterone heptanoate.*

**testosterone heptanoate** TESTOSTERONE ENANTHATE.

**testosterone phenylacetate** A synthetically prepared ester of testosterone that is used for the same indications as testosterone cyclopentylpropionate.

**testosterone phenylpropionate** An ester form of testosterone with phenylpropionic acid. It has the actions of testosterone but a prolonged duration of action after injection in a suitable oil.

**testosterone propionate** $C_{22}H_{32}O_3$. A synthetically prepared ester of testosterone, having the same pharmacologic actions and indications as testosterone cypionate. Its duration of action is shorter than those of the cypionate or the enanthate.

**test type** See under TYPE.

**tetan-** \tet′ən-\ TETANO-.

**tetania** \tətā′nē·ə\ [TETAN- + -IA] TETANY. **t. gastrica** Tetany induced by alkalosis resulting from loss of hydrochloric acid as a consequence of repeated vomiting. Also *gastric tetany.* **t. neonatorum** TETANY OF THE NEWBORN. **t. parathyreopriva** PARATHYROPRIVAL TETANY.

**tetanic** \tetan′ik\ **1** Pertaining to or characterized by tetany. **2** Pertaining to or caused by tetanus.

**tetaniform** \tetan′ifôrm\ Resembling tetanus or tetany.

**tetanilla** \tet′ənil′ə\ *Seldom used* PARAMYOCLONUS MULTIPLEX.

**tetanization** \tet′ənīzā′shən\ The production of a state of continuous muscular contraction (a tetanus) in a muscle subjected to a rapid rate of recurrent electrical stimulation (50 stimuli per second).

**tetano-** \tet′ənō-\ [Gk *tetanos* stretched, strained] A combining form denoting (1) tetanus; (2) tetany. Also *tetan-*.

**tetanoid** \tet′ənoid\ [TETAN- + -OID] Resembling tetanus.

**tetanospasmin** \tet′ənōspaz′min\ The extremely potent exotoxin, elaborated by *Clostridium tetani,* which causes the neuromuscular dysfunction characteristic of tetanus. See also TETANUS TOXIN.

**tetanus** \tet′ənəs\ [Gk *tetanos* (from *teinein* to stretch) convulsive tension] **1** A severe infectious disease caused by *Clostridium tetani.* A powerful exotoxin produced by *C. tetani* causes tonic muscle spasms and hyperflexia, trismus, opisthotonos, glottal spasms, and convulsions. Tetanus may develop when the bacillus gains access to wounds which provide anaerobic conditions for growth. Also *lockjaw* (popular). **2** A sustained, tonic muscular contraction without twitching. Also *tetanic contraction.* **apyretic t.** An imprecise and outmoded term for TETANY. **artificial t.** DRUG TETANUS. **cephalic t.** A localized form of tetanus, following injury to the face or scalp, restricted to the muscles of the head and neck and usually characterized by trismus, spasm of orofacial and bulbar muscles, and often by lower motor neuron paralysis due to lesions of individual cranial nerves, such as the facial. Also *head tetanus, tetanus paradoxus, paralytic tetanus, Rose's tetanus, cephalotetanus, Janin's tetanus, Klemm's tetanus, hydrophobic tetanus, cerebral tetanus.* **chronic t.** Tetanus of long incubation and gradual development in which the spasms may continue over a prolonged period of days or weeks but in which the prognosis is normally good. Also *delayed tetanus.* **cryptogenic t.** Tetanus in which the site of entry of the organism into the body cannot be identified. Also *idiopathic tetanus, medical tetanus, rheumatic tetanus.* **delayed t.** CHRONIC TETANUS. **drug t.** Tetanic spasms produced by excessive dosage of strychnine or another drug of similar action. Also *toxic tetanus, artificial tetanus.* **head t.** CEPHALIC TETANUS. **hydrophobic t.** CEPHALIC TETANUS. **idiopathic t.** CRYPTOGENIC TETANUS. **t. infantum** TETANUS NEONATORUM. **intermittent t.** *Outmoded* TETANY **Janin's t.** CEPHALIC TETANUS. **Klemm's t.** CEPHALIC TETANUS. **localized t.** Tetanic spasm in a single area, usually in muscles near a wound. Also *local tetanus, partial tetanus, modified tetanus.* See also CEPHALIC TETANUS. **medical t.** CRYPTOGENIC TETANUS. **modified t. 1** LOCALIZED TETANUS. **2** Mild or chronic tetanus occurring in an individual who has previously been inoculated against the disease. **t. neonatorum** Tetanus in the newborn, usually a result of infection of the stump of the umbilical cord. Also *tetanus infantum.* **t. paradoxus** CEPHALIC TETANUS. **paralytic t.** CEPHALIC TETANUS. **partial t.** LOCALIZED TETANUS. **postoperative t.** Tetanus following an operation, usually a result of infection of a surgical wound. Also *surgical tetanus.* **postserum t.** Tetanus which develops subsequent to an injection of antitetanus serum. **puerperal t.** Tetanus occurring during the postpartum period. Also *uterine tetanus.* **rheumatic t.** CRYPTOGENIC TETANUS. **Rose's t.** CEPHALIC TETANUS. **splanchnic t.** Tetanus where the respiratory and pharyngeal constrictor muscles are particularly involved and dysphagia is a conspicuous symptom. **surgical t.** POSTOPERATIVE TETANUS. **toxic t.** DRUG TETANUS. **uterine t.** PUERPERAL TETANUS.

**tetany** \tet′ənē\ [TETAN- + -Y] A syndrome marked by a state of neuromuscular hyperexcitability which may cause reversible muscular contractures, particularly in the extremities. It is attributable to a lowering of the serum calcium, as in hypoparathyroidism, hypocalcemia because of impaired calcium absorption, severe renal insufficiency with calcium loss, vitamin D deficiency, etc., or in respiratory alkalosis resulting from hyperventilation or metabolic alkalosis from excessive ingestion of sodium bicarbonate, repeated vomiting with chloride loss, etc. A typical upper limb contracture results in obstetrician's hand; in the leg, it produces pedal spasm. Spasms may also affect the face (risus sardonicus, trismus) and the glottis (larynogospasm). The Chvostek and Trousseau signs are usually positive and in infants rare cases of convulsions occur. Also *tetania, apyretic tetanus* (imprecise and outmoded), *intermittent tetanus* (outmoded). **t. of alkalosis** Tetany developing in any alkalotic state. **epidemic t.** An epidemic form of tetany of acute onset, usually occurring in winter and lasting for two to three weeks. It is of unknown etiology and is now virtually unknown. **gastric t.** TETANIA GASTRICA. **hyperventilation t.** Tetany resulting from alkalosis brought about by voluntary or involuntary hyperventilation. **hypoparathyroid t.** Hypocalcemic tetany due to spontaneously occurring primary hypoparathyroidism or to ablation of, or surgical damage to, the parathyroid glands. Also *parathyroid tetany.* **infantile t.** Tetany occurring in rachitic infants. **latent t.** Tetany which can be evoked only by an appropriate maneuver, as by eliciting the Chvostek sign or the Trousseau sign. **t. of the newborn** Tetany occurring in the newborn infant, typically toward the end of the first week. It is commoner in infants fed on cow's milk, the high phosphorous content of which is considered to be an important factor. Also *neonatal tetany, tetania neonatorum.* **parathyroid t.** HYPOPARATHYROID TETANY. **parathyroprival t.** Hypocalcemic tetany due to ablation of the thyroid glands. Also *tetania parathyreopriva.* **phosphate t.** The abnormal tetanic muscular contractions induced by ingestion or injection of alkaline phosphates, resulting in a marked reduction of blood calcium levels. **postoperative t.** Hypocalcemic tetany due to ablation of, or surgical damage to, the parathyroid glands, as during thyroidectomy.

**tetarcone** \tet′ərkōn\ TETARTOCONE.

**tetartanope** \tetär′tənōp\ [Gk *tetart(os)* one quarter + *an-* priv. + -OPE] One who confuses blue and yellow colors.

**tetartanopia** \tetär′tənō′pē·ə\ [Gk *tetart(os)* one quarter + *an-* priv. + -OPIA] A faulty color vision in which blue and yellow are improperly distinguished. Also *tetartanopsia.* Adj. tetartanopic.

**tetartanopsia** \tetär′tənäp′sē·ə\ TETARTANOPIA.

**tetartocone** \tetär′təkōn\ [Gk *tetarto(s)* one quarter + *kōn(os)* cone] The distolingual cusp of an upper premolar tooth. Also *tetarcone.*

**tetartoconid** \tetär′təkō′nid\ [*tetartocon(e)* + -ID[2]] The distolingual cusp of a lower premolar tooth.

**tetra-** \tet′rə-\ [Gk prefix *tetra-* (from *tessares* or *tettares* four) denoting four] A combining form meaning four, fourfold.

**tetra-amelia** \-əmē′lyə\ [TETRA- + Gk *a-* priv. + MEL-[1] + -IA] Agenesis of all four limbs. A fleshy tab may mark the usual site of attachment of missing limbs to the trunk. Also *complete amelia.*

**tetrablastic** \-blas′tik\ Having four embryonic germ layers.

**tetrabrachius** \-brā′kē·əs\ [New L, from Gk *tetra-* four + *brachi(ōn)* arm] An individual with four arms. The condition suggests conjoined twinning in which an extreme degree of union of all external parts except the arms has obliterated other overt signs of twinning.

**tetrabromophenol blue** BROMOPHENOL BLUE.

**tetrac** 3,5,3′,5′-tetraiodothyroacetic acid, a compound formed by the oxidative deamination followed by decarboxylation of thyroxine in peripheral tissues, formerly thought to be the tissue-active form of thyroxine. It is now regarded as a metabolic product of the hormone.

**tetracaine hydrochloride** $C_{15}H_{25}ClN_2O_2$. 4-(Butylamino)benzoic acid 2-(dimethylamino)ethylester hydrochloride. A local anesthetic similar in structure to procaine, but more active than the latter. It is used for topical anesthesia of the eye and the mucous membranes of the mouth and throat, and for spinal anesthesia.

**tetrachirus** \-kī′rəs\ [New L, from Gk *tetra-* four + *cheir* hand] An individual with four hands. The condition suggests that duplication of the hands only has occurred, unless there are other indications of aberrant twinning.

**tetrachlorethane** $(CH)_2Cl_4$. A colorless liquid which smells like chloroform. It was once used as a solvent, as a parasiticide in hair washes or dyes, and as a fire extinguisher, but has been replaced because of its high toxicity. It causes a toxic hepatitis, which progresses to an acute and fatal yellow atrophy. Tetrachlorethane also causes a toxic polyneuritis, with numbness and tingling of the extremities, facial twitching, and weakness of the small muscles of the hands and feet. Also *acetylene tetrachloride.*

**tetrachloroethylene** $Cl_2C{=}CCl_2$. A colorless liquid used in the treatment of hookworm and certain trematode infections. It is also used as a dry-cleaning solvent. Excessive doses or exposure causes giddiness, vertigo, and perspiration, as well as liver damage and jaundice. Also *tetrachlorethylene, perchloroethylene, perc.*

**tetrachromic** \-krō′mik\ Pertaining to or having normal color vision in accordance with the Hering theory of four basic color receptors.

**tetracycline** 4-(Dimethylamino)-1,4,4a,5,5*a*,6,11,12*a*-octahydro-3,6,10,12,12*a*-pentahydroxy-6-methyl-1,11-dioxo-2-naphthacenecarboxamide. A broad-spectrum antibiotic obtained from a culture filtrate of several species of *Streptomyces.*

**tetracycline hydrochloride** The hydrochloride salt of tetracycline, used for the same conditions as tetracycline, but with the advantage of being very soluble in water.

**tetracycline phosphate complex** The phosphate salt of tetracycline, prepared by adding sodium metaphosphate to tetracycline or tetracycline hydrochloride. The complex is claimed to be more rapidly absorbed after oral administration than the free base or the hydrochloride.

**tetrad** \tet′rad\ TETRALOGY. **Fallot's t.** TETRALOGY OF FALLOT.

**tetradactyly** \-dak′tilē\ [TETRA- + DACTYL- + -Y ] A condition in which only four digits on one or both hands or feet are apparent.

**tetraethyl lead** $(C_2H_5)_4Pb$. An oily, colorless liquid, added to gasoline as an antiknocking agent. It is considered by some authorities to pose a health risk in the form of lead absorption from car exhaust fumes, and its use has been banned or limited in some countries. It is readily absorbed through the skin and respiratory tract and is highly toxic.

**tetraethylmonothionopyrophosphate** The sulfur analogue of tetraethylpyrophosphate. It is a potent, long-acting anticholinesterase agent that has had limited use in the treatment of glaucoma. Also *pyrophos.*

**tetraethylthiuram disulfide** DISULFIRAM.

**tetraglycine hydroperiodide** $(NH_2CH_2COOH)_4$-$HI{\cdot}1\frac{1}{4}I_2$. It is used for emergency disinfection of drinking water, yielding 8 ppm of active iodine, sufficient to destroy *Entamoeba* and *Giardia* cysts.

**tetragonum** \-gō′nəm\ A quadrangle or a quadrangular space. **t. lumbale** The quadrangular lumbar space bounded by the serratus posterior inferior muscle superiorly, internal oblique muscle of abdomen inferiorly, erector spinae muscle medially, and external oblique muscle of abdomen laterally.

**tetragonus** \-gō′nəs\ PLATYSMA.

**tetrahedron** [neut. sing. of Gk *tetraedros* four-sided, from Gk *tetra(s)* four + *hedra* a seat, base] A solid figure with four equilateral triangles as its faces, six edges, and four vertices. It is the simplest of the five regular solids. The arrangement of four atoms around C or $N^+$ is usually close to the arrangement of the vertices of a tetrahedron about its center.

**tetrahydrocannabinol** $C_{21}H_{30}O_2$. Tetrahydro -6,6,9-trimethyl-3-pentyl-6*H*-dibenzo[*b,d*]pyran-1-ol. Any of several isomers that represent the active principles of marihuana. The $\Delta^1$-3,4-*trans* isomer is the most pharmacologically active, followed by the $\Delta^6$-3,4-*trans* isomer. These chemical can produce pronounced psychological disturbances. They have been evaluated as possibly of some clinical value in the treatment of chronic glaucoma.

**tetrahydrofolate** Any of the forms of folic acid, with various numbers of glutamic residues, that have the pyrazine ring of the pteridine system hydrogenated. Such forms of folic acid comprise the coenzyme capable of accepting $C_1$ fragments by methylation, hydroxymethylation, or formylation.

**tetrahydrofolic acid** The active form of folic acid, carrying formyl, formimino, hydroxymethyl, and methyl groups in metabolism. These groups are enzymatically interconvertible when attached to tetrahydrofolic acid by one or both of its aromatic secondary amino groups.

**tetrahydrozoline hydrochloride** $C_{13}H_{16}N_2{\cdot}HCl$. 2-(1,2,3,4-Tetrahydro-1-naphthyl)-2-imidazoline monohydrochloride. A sympathomimetic agent used to reduce congestion of the nasal mucous membranes and the conjunctivae by topical application.

***Tetrahymena*** \-hī′mənə\ An abundant genus of largely freshwater free-living ciliate protozoa in the order Hymenostomatida, class Oligohymenophorea. A few species are facultative or even obligate endoparasites. ***T. pyriformis*** A species frequently used in experimental studies on protozoan nutrition, physiology, genetics, and evolution, as it is readily cultured and adaptable to various test conditions.

**tetralogy** \tetral′əjē\ [Gk *tetralogia* (from *tetra-* four + *log(os)* word, speech) a series of four dramas, a tetralogy] Any series or combination of four entities or items. Also *tetrad*. **Eisenmenger's t.** EISENMENGER'S COMPLEX. **t. of Fallot** A common form of cyanotic congenital heart malformation in which the four principal defects are infundibular pulmonary stenosis; an interventricular septal defect; a dextraposed aorta, the origin of which overides the septal defect; and right ventricular hypertrophy. Also *Fallot's tetrad, Fallot syndrome*.

**tetramastia** \-mas′tē·ə\ [TETRA- + MAST- + -IA] The presence of four breasts on one individual.

**tetramelus** \-mē′ləs\ [New L, from Gk *tetra-* four + *mel(os)* limb] Conjoined twins with four upper or lower limbs, either four arms (tetrabrachius) or four legs (tetrascelus).

**tetrameric** \-mer′ik\ Having four parts. Also *tetramerous*.

**tetramerism** \tetram′ərizm\ The condition of having four parts or groups.

**tetramerous** \tetram′ərəs\ TETRAMERIC.

**tetramethylammonium iodide** A quaternary ammonium compound with ganglionic blocking properties. It has been used in the treatment of hypertension, and has also been used as an emergency disinfectant of drinking water.

**tetramethylenediamine** The systematic name for putrescine.

**tetramethylrhodamine isothiocyanate** A fluorescent dye that can readily be conjugated to proteins. It is often used in immunofluorescence techniques. Abbr. TMRITC

**tetramitiasis** \-mītī′əsis\ CHILOMASTIGIASIS.

***Tetramitus*** \tetram′itəs\ A genus of trichomonad flagellates in the class Zoomastigophorea. ***T. mesnili*** *CHILOMASTIX MESNILI*. ***T. rostratus*** A species of trichomonads with ameboid and flagellate forms. The latter have four anterior flagella and one trailing flagellum, a large anterior cytostome, a vesicular nucleus, and a contractile vacuole. It is found in stagnant water and has been reported from human and rat feces. Also *Copromastix prowazeki*.

**tetranophthalmos** \-näfthal′məs\ [TETRA- + *n* + Gk *ophthalmos* eye] A malformed individual with four eyes, in most instances probably representing a minimal degree of twinning which is manifested mainly by duplication of the face. Also *tetraophthalmus, tetrophthalmos*.

**tetranopsia** \-näp′sē·ə\ [*tetr(a)-* + Gk *an-* priv. + -OPSIA] QUADRANTANOPIA.

**tetranucleotide** \-n$^y$oo′klē·ətīd′\ A condensation product of four nucleotides, formerly used for nucleic acids. It was once thought that nucleic acids were aggregates of tetranucleotides, only because they contain four different nucleotide residues.

***Tetranychus*** \tetran′ikəs\ [Gk *tetra-* four + *(o)nyx* (gen. *onychos*) a talon, claw, nail] A genus of spider mites or "red spiders," commonly infesting vegetation and causing considerable damage to various food crops as well as a temporary allergic dermatitis among handlers of infested material. Among species responsible for human skin reactions are *T. montensis* infesting flax, and *T. urticae, T. telarius,* and *T. molestissimus* on other crop plants.

**tetraodontoxin** \-ō′däntäk′sin\ TETRODOTOXIN.

**tetraodontoxism** \-ō′däntäk′sizm\ TETRODOTOXISM.

**tetraophthalmus** \-äfthal′məs\ TETRANOPHTHALMOS.

**tetraotus** \-ō′təs\ [New L, from Gk *tetra-* four + OT- + L *-us*, masc. noun suffix] Conjoined twins with two partially separate heads and four ears.

**tetraparesis** \-pərē′sis\ Weakness of all four limbs. Also *quadriparesis*.

**tetrapeptide** A peptide containing four amino-acid residues.

**tetraperomelia** \-per′ōmē′lyə\ [TETRA- + PEROMELIA] A severe malformation of all four limbs.

**tetraphocomelia** \-fō′kōmē′lyə\ Phocomelia on all four limbs, with both hands and both feet attached directly to the trunk.

**tetraplegia** \-plē′jə\ QUADRIPLEGIA.

**tetraploid** \tet′rəploid\ **1** Pertaining to or characterized by tetraploidy. **2** A cell, tissue, or organism that has four haploid sets of nuclear chromosomes.

**tetraploidy** \tet′rəploi′dē\ The state of having four haploid sets of chromosomes in the cell nucleus. It usually arises through duplication of the normal diploid chromosome complement.

**tetrapod** \tet′rəpäd\ [TETRA- + -POD] Any four-limbed animal, especially a vertebrate of the class Amphibia, Reptilia, Aves, or Mammalia.

**tetrapus** \tet′rəpəs\ [Gk *tetrapous* four-footed] A fetus or postnatal individual with four feet, a condition probably representing duplication of the feet alone rather than a minimal form of conjoined twinning.

**tetrascelus** \tetras′ēləs\ [Gk *tetraskelēs* four-legged, four-footed] An embryo, fetus, or postnatal individual with four legs. It usually represents duplication of the legs only rather than a minimal form of conjoined twinning.

**tetrasomic** \-sō′mik\ [TETRA- + Gk *sōm(a)* body + -IC] Having one chromosome represented four times in a cell nucleus while all other chromosomes are represented only twice.

**tetrasomy** \tet′rəsō′mē\ The condition of being tetrasomic.

**tetraspore** \tet′rəspôr\ A sexually produced (meiotic) spore of fungi of the class Basidiomycetes.

**tetraster** \tetras′tər\ [*tetr(a)-* + ASTER] An abnormal mitotic apparatus having four centrioles or four asters.

**tetrastichiasis** \-stikī′əsis\ [TETRA- + Gk *stich(os)* a row, line + -IASIS] A duplication of the eyelashes such that they appear as four rows rather than the usual two.

**tetrathionate** $^{-}O_3S—S—S—SO_3^{-}$. The anion formed on oxidation of thiosulfate by iodine in a reaction in which a disulfide bond is formed between the two thiolate groups of the thiosulfate ions.

**tetrazolium** The substance whose molecule is a five-membered ring consisting of the chain —N═NH$^+$—NH—N═ with both its ends joined to the CH group. All three hydrogen atoms are replaced, usually by aryl groups, in the tetrazolium salts commonly used. Tetrazolium salts are colorless but are easily reduced to red formazans of structure R—N═N—CR═N—NH—R, and this reaction is used to test for the action of some dehydrogenases. **blue t.** The tetrazolium in which all three aryl groups are phenyl.

**tetrodotoxin** \tet′rədōtäk′sin\ [*Tetr(a)odo(n)*, type genus of puffer fish, + TOXIN] $C_{11}H_{17}N_3O_8$. A potent neurotoxin found in the liver, skin, and ovaries of the puffer fish of the family *Tetraodontoidea*, and in the California newt, *Taricha torosa*. Also *tetraodontoxin, spheroidin*. See also TETRODOTOXISM.

**tetrodotoxism** \tet′rədōtäk′sizm\ [*tetrodotox(in)* + -ISM]

Poisoning from ingestion of improperly prepared puffer fish, family Tetraodontidae. The clinical signs include tingling of the lips and tongue, motor incoordination, numbness of the skin, salivation, muscle weakness, generalized paralysis, and death. Also *tetraodontoxism, fugu poisoning, puffer poisoning, tetraodon poisoning.*

**tetrophthalmos** \tet′räfthal′məs\ TETRANOPHTHALMOS.

**tetrose** [*tetr(a)-* + -OSE[2]] A sugar containing four carbon atoms, such as erythrose or its isomer threose.

**tetter** \tet′ər\ [Old English *teter,* akin to Late L *derbita* (whence French *dartre;* prob. from Celtic) a scaly skin eruption, and to Sanscrit *dadru* a skin eruption] Any of a number of skin diseases. An obsolete and ambiguous term. **honeycomb t.** *Popular* FAVUS.

**Teutleben** [Friedrich Ernst Karl von *Teutleben,* German physician, born 1842] Teutleben's ligament. See under LIGAMENTUM PULMONALE.

**textiform** \tek′stifôrm\ [L *text(um)* a web, weaving + *i* + -FORM] Weblike or reticular in pattern or form.

**textus** \teks′təs\ [L (from *textus,* past part. of *texere* to weave, braid, knit), woven fabric] (*pl.* textus) TISSUE. **t. adiposus fuscus** INTERSCAPULAR GLAND. **t. connectivus collagenosus** FIBROUS TISSUE. **t. connectivus elasticus** ELASTIC TISSUE. **t. connectivus fibrosus compactus** DENSE FIBROUS CONNECTIVE TISSUE. **t. connectivus fibrosus lamellaris** FIBROUS TISSUE. **t. connectivus pigmentosus** PIGMENTED CONNECTIVE TISSUE. **t. connectivus reticularis** RETICULAR TISSUE. **t. muscularis** MUSCULAR TISSUE. **t. muscularis nonstriatus** INVOLUNTARY MUSCLE. **t. muscularis striatus** MUSCULUS SKELETI. **t. muscularis striatus cardiacus** CARDIAC MUSCLE. **t. nervosus** NERVOUS TISSUE.

**TF** 1 tuberculin filtrate. 2 transfer factor. 3 tetralogy of Fallot.

**TG** thyroglobulin.

**TGC** time gain compensation (swept gain).

**TGE** transmissible gastroenteritis (of swine).

**TGF** T-cell growth factor (interleukin-2).

**T-group** ENCOUNTER GROUP.

**TGT** thromboplastin generation test.

**Th** Symbol for the element, thorium.

**thalam-** \thalam-\ THALAMO-.

**thalamectomy** \thal′əmek′təmē\ [THALAM- + -ECTOMY] THALAMOTOMY.

**thalamencephalon** \thal′amənsef′əlän\ *Obs.* DIENCEPHALON.

**thalami** \thal′əmī\ Plural of THALAMUS.

**thalamic** \thalam′ik\ Of, pertaining to, originating from, or having the characteristics of the thalamus.

**thalamo-** \thal′əmō-\ [Gk *thalamos* inner chamber, bedchamber] A combining form denoting the thalamus. Also *thalam-.*

**thalamocoele** \thalam′əsēl\ [THALAMO- + -COELE] VENTRICULUS TERTIUS CEREBRI.

**thalamocortical** \-kôr′tikəl\ Denoting nerve fibers that originate in the thalamus and are projected to the cerebral cortex, or nerve impulses that originate in or are relayed from the thalamus to the cerebral cortex.

**thalamocrural** \-kroo′rəl\ THALAMOPEDUNCULAR.

**thalamolenticular** \-lentik′yələr\ Denoting morphologic connections or physiologic interactions between the thalamus and the nucleus lentiformis of the corpus striatum.

**thalamomamillary** \-mam′iler′ē\ Denoting interconnections or physiologic interactions between the thalamus and the mamillary bodies of the posterior hypothalamus.

**thalamoparietal** \-pərī′ətəl\ Denoting neural pathways or physiologic interactions between the thalamus and the cerebral cortex of the parietal lobe.

**thalamopeduncular** \-pidungk′yələr\ Denoting anatomic relationships, nerve connections or physiologic interactions between the thalamus and the cerebral peduncles, or crura cerebri. Also *thalamocrural.*

**thalamotegmental** \-tegmen′təl\ Denoting neural pathways or physiologic interactions between the thalamus and the tegmental regions in the brainstem.

**thalamotomy** \thal′əmät′əmē\ [THALAMO- + -TOMY] The production of lesions in the thalamus, usually by stereotaxic surgery. Also *thalamectomy.*

**thalamus** \thal′əməs\ [New L, from Gk *thalamos* inner chamber, substituted for Gk *thalamē* den, lair, cave, cavity, ventricle; Galen supposed that the thalami contained "animal humors" which they supplied via the optic nerves] (*pl.* thalami) A mass of gray matter lying on either side of the third ventricle and divided by laminae into groups of anterior, medial, lateral, and posterior nuclei. Each group has a further division. Projection fibers course to the sensory cortex, and fiber tracts are received by the thalamus from the spinal cord, midbrain, optic nerves, and cerebral cortex. It provides the main input to cortex from all except olfactory sensory systems. **dorsal t.** THALAMUS DORSALIS. **t. dorsalis** [NA] The middle plate of the embryonic thalamus and the last portion to differentiate, forming the major nuclei projecting upon specific fields of cerebral cortex. Also *dorsal thalamus.* **optic t.** The dorsal diencephalic mass which receives afferent projections from all sensory systems. It was formerly thought to receive only optic fibers. **t. ventralis** [NA] The part of the diencephalon situated between the thalamus dorsalis and the tegmentum of the mesencephalon and forming a zone of transition between the two structures. It lies somewhat ventral to the thalamus, medial to the internal capsule, and lateral to and behind the thalamus. It contains, among other structures, the subthalamic nucleus, the zona incerta, and fields H, $H_1$, and $H_2$ of Forel. Fiber bundles passing through it include the lenticular, thalamic, and subthalamic fasciculi as well as the ansa lenticularis. The thalamus ventralis (especially the subthalamic nucleus) has nerve fiber connections with the globus pallidus. Also *ventral thalamus, subthalamus, subthalamic region.*

**thalassaemia** *Brit.* THALASSEMIA.

**thalassanemia** \thəlas′ənē′mē·ə\ THALASSEMIA.

**thalassemia** \thal′əsē′mē·ə\ [Gk *thalass(a)* the sea + -EMIA] Any of several hereditary conditions in which there is a reduction in rate of formation of one or more of the globin chains of hemoglobin. Also *thalassanemia, congenital microcytic anemia, familial microcytic anemia.* ● In this term Gk *thalassa,* sea, refers to the Mediterranean (which to the Greeks was simply "the sea"), from the high prevalence of β-thalassemia trait among peoples of the Mediterranean basin. **α-t.** A hereditary disorder due to reduced formation of α-globin chains in erythrocyte precursor cells of the bone marrow. The cause is deletion or partial inactivation of one or more of the four β-globin gene loci normally present in each cell. Severity of the disorder depends on the number of α loci deleted (or partially inactivated). In α-thalassemia-2 trait, one α gene locus is deleted, and there is little or no hematologic effect. In α-thalassemia-1 trait or in homozygous α-thalassemia-2, two α globin gene loci are deleted, and the effect is mild microcytosis, usually without anemia. In a more severe form of α-thalassemia, three of the four α-globin gene loci are deleted, α-globin synthesis is markedly diminished, and surplus β-globin and γ-globin chains form the tetramers hemoglobin H (resulting in hemoglobin H disease) and hemoglobin Bart's respectively. In the most severe form of α-thalassemia (Bart's hemoglobin hydrops fetalis) all four α-globin gene loci are deleted due to homozygosity for α-thalassemia-1. No α-globin chains are formed, all hemoglobin is γ-globin chain tetramer (hemoglobin Bart's), and the fetus with this disorder dies *in utero* from severe anemia and congestive heart failure. The α-thalassemias that are the effect of partially inactivated α-globin genes are those associated with hemoglobin Constant Spring or with dysfunctional α-thalassemia genes. The nature of the latter is not yet known. **β-t.** A hereditary blood disorder in which there is a reduction in the quantity of hemoglobin in erythrocytes due to diminished formation of the β-globin chains of hemoglobin. β-thalassemia is subdivided into $\beta^0$-thalassemia, $\beta^+$-thalassemia, and $\beta^{++}$-thalassemia, in which the mutant gene directs the formation of no β-globin, a small amount of β-globin, or a moderate amount of β-globin, respectively. Also *Mediterranean disease.* **βδ-t.** A hereditary blood disorder in which there is a reduction in the quantity of hemoglobin in erythrocyte due to diminished formation of both β-globin and δ-globin chains of hemoglobin. The cause is a deletion of the entire δ-β gene complex, so that the affected chromosome cannot direct the formation of either β- or δ-globin chains. **δ-t.** A hereditary blood condition due to diminished formation of the δ-globin chains of hemoglobin. It is a very rare condition, most cases having been reported from Japan. It is without any clinical or hematologic manifestations. **hemoglobin C-β-t.** A disorder that results from concurrence of hemoglobin C trait and β-thalassemia trait, in a person who has inherited a gene for hemoglobin C from one parent and a gene for β-thalassemia trait from the other parent. The condition typically causes pallor, splenomegaly, anemia and erythrocytic microcytosis with abundant target erythrocytes. Also *hemoglobin C-thalassemia disease.* **hemoglobin E-α-t.** A minor disorder that results from concurrence of hemoglobin E trait and α-thalassemia trait, a combination that is common in persons from southeast Asia. The condition results in mild erythrocytic microcytosis without anemia. **hemoglobin E-β-t.** A disorder that results from concurrence of hemoglobin E trait and β-thalassemia trait, in a person who has inherited a gene for hemoglobin E from one parent and a gene for β-thalassemia trait from the other parent. The disorder is characterized by pallor, growth retardation, splenomegaly, severe anemia, and erythrocytic hypochromia and microcytosis. **hemoglobin Lepore-β-t.** A thalassemic disorder that results from concurrence of hemoglobin Lepore trait and β-thalassemia trait, due to inheritance of a gene for hemoglobin Lepore trait from one parent and a gene for β-thalassemia trait from the other parent. **hemoglobin S-α-t.** A minor condition due to inheritance of a gene for hemoglobin S from one parent, and a gene for α-thalassemia from the other parent. The combination is common in black people. It is associated with mild erythrocytic microcytosis. **hemoglobin S-β-t.** A disorder that results from concurrence of hemoglobin S trait and β-thalassemia trait, in a person who has inherited a gene for hemoglobin S trait from one parent and a gene for β-thalassemia trait from the other parent. The condition often causes a severe sickle cell disorder with pain crises, jaundice, pallor, anemia, and microcytosis. Also *microdrepanocytosis, sickle-cell thalassemia, microdrepanocytic disease.* **heterozygous β-t.** The condition that results from inheritance of a gene for β-thalassemia from one parent and the corresponding normal gene from the other parent (β-thalassemia trait). The clinical and hematologic expression is a mild thalassemia with microcytosis of erythrocytes, but little or no anemia, i.e., thalassemia minor. **homozygous β-t.** See under THALASSEMIA MAJOR. **t. intermedia** A form of thalassemia in which the anemia is of mild to moderate degree, less severe than in thalassemia major, but more marked than in thalassemia minor. **t. major** Very severe anemia beginning in late infancy, with severe growth retardation and bone abnormalities, usually resulting in death before puberty. It is usually the result of inheritance of genes for β-thalassemia from both parents, i.e. homozygous β-thalassemia. Also *Cooley's anemia, Mediterranean anemia, familial erythroblastic anemia, erythroblastic anemia of childhood.* **t. minor** A mild thalassemia, usually due to inheritance of a thalassemia gene from only one parent (thalassemia trait). Thalassemia minor may also be the result of inheritance of a gene for β-thalassemia from one parent and of a gene for either α-thalassemia or δβ-thalassemia from the other. Also *microelliptopoikilocytic anemia of Rietti, Greppi, and Michele.* **sickle-cell t.** HEMOGLOBIN S-β-THALASSEMIA.

**thalidomide** \thalid′əmīd\ $C_{13}H_{10}N_2O_4$. A sedative-hypnotic drug which in 1961 was discovered to be a highly potent human teratogen when ingested by pregnant women between the 20th and 36th days after conception, and which was subsequently withdrawn from the market. The prevalent malformations were phocomelia and other reduction defects of the fetal limbs, although facial and internal malformations sometimes occurred. See also THALIDOMIDE SYNDROME.

**thallium** \thal′ē·əm\ A soft, heavy metallic element having atomic number 81 and atomic weight 204.37. Two stable isotopes occur naturally and numerous radioactive isotopes have been prepared, the most stable of which has a half-life of 3.8 years. Valences are 1 and 3. The element and its compounds are very toxic and are suspected of being carcinogenic. Symbol: Tl

**thallium 201** One of the radioactive isotopes of thallium, having a half-life of 73 hours and providing several gamma and x-ray photons ranging from 30 to 167 keV. Symbol: $^{201}$Tl

**THAM** A proprietary name for trihydroxymethylaminomethane (tromethamine).

**thanato-** \than′ətō-\ [Gk *thanatos* death, corpse] A combining form meaning death.

**thanatoid** \than′ətoid\ [*thanat(o)-* + -OID] Deathlike.

**thanatology** \than′ətäl′əjē\ [THANATO- + -LOGY] 1 The study of death and its effect on individuals and families. 2 In forensic medicine, the study of the circumstances under which death occurred, especially as they relate to the production of postmortem phenomena.

**thanatophobia** \than′ətōfō′bē·ə\ [THANATO- + -PHOBIA] Pathologic fear of death or dying.

**thanatopsy** \than′ətäp′sē\ AUTOPSY.

**Thanatos** \than′ətəs\ DEATH INSTINCT.

**Thane** [Sir George Dancer *Thane,* English anatomist, 1850–1930] See under METHOD.

**Thaysen** [Thornwald Einar Hess *Thaysen,* Danish physician, 1886–1936] 1 Gee-Thaysen disease. See under ADULT CELIAC DISEASE. 2 Thaysen's disease. See under CELIAC DISEASE.

**Thd** Symbol for ribothymidine (ribosylthymine).

**thea** \thē′ə\ [New L, a former genus that included the tea plant] TEA.

**theaism** \thē′ə·izm\ [THEA + -ISM] A condition produced by the caffeine in tea that is consumed in excessive amounts. Symptoms are insomnia, nervousness, headache, nausea, and vomiting. Sensitive persons may experience tachycardia, increased respiration, premature systoles, and muscular tremors.

**thebaic** \thēbā′ik\ Of or relating to opium.
**thebaine** $C_{19}H_{21}O_3N$. An alkaloid that constitutes 0.15–2% of opium and is known to cause spasms like those caused by strychnine. Also *paramorphine, dimethylmorphine.*
**Thebesius** [Adam Christian *Thebesius,* German physician, 1686–1732] **1** Thebesian valve. See under VALVULA SINUS CORONARII. **2** Veins of Thebesius. See under VENAE CARDIACAE MINIMAE.
**theca** \thē′kə\ [L (from Gk *thēkē* a case, box, akin to *tithenai* to place, put, set) a case, envelope, sheath] A protective covering, sheath, or capsule. **t. cerebri** *Obs.* DURA MATER ENCEPHALI. **t. cordis** *Outmoded* PERICARDIUM. **t. externa** [NA] The fibrous outer layer of the theca folliculi, which consists of compressed ovarian cortical stroma. Also *theca of follicle of von Baer, tunica externa thecae folliculi, external coat of capsule of graafian follicle, fibrous capsule of graafian follicle.* **t. of follicle of von Baer** THECA EXTERNA. **t. folliculi** The sheath of connective tissue that surrounds a mature ovarian follicle and consists of two layers, the theca interna and the theca externa. Also *theca of follicle.* **t. interna** The vascular and cellular inner layer of the theca folliculi. It is separated from the membrana granulosa by a basement membrane, and as the follicle fully develops, the cells produce estrogenic hormones. Also *internal coat of capsule of graafian follicle, tunica interna thecae folliculi.* **t. tendinis** VAGINA SYNOVIALIS TENDINIS. **t. vertebralis** *Obs.* DURA MATER SPINALIS.
**thecae** \thē′sē\ Plural of THECA.
**thecal** \thē′kəl\ Pertaining to a theca.
**thecitis** \thēsī′tis\ TENOSYNOVITIS.
**thecoma** \thēkō′mə\ [*thec(a)* + -OMA] A benign tumor of ovarian stromal cells many of which contain abundant, lipid-rich cytoplasm, resembling theca cells. The tumor is typically estrogenic. Also *theca cell tumor.*
**thecomatosis** \thēkō′mətō′sis\ [*thecoma* + *t* + -OSIS] Growth of spindle cells and connective tissue of the ovarian stroma, primarily seen after menopause. Also *ovarian stromal hyperplasia.*
**thecostegnosis** \thē′kōstegnō′sis\ [L *thec(a)* a sheath + *o* + Gk *stegnōsis* a making close] DE QUERVAIN SYNDROME.
**theelol** \thē′lôl\ *Older term* ESTROGEN.
**Theile** [Friedrich Wilhelm *Theile,* German anatomist, 1801–1879] **1** Theile's glands. See under LUSCHKA'S CRYPTS. **2** Theile's canal. See under SINUS TRANSVERSUS PERICARDII.
***Theileria*** \thīler′ē·ə\ [After Sir Arnold *Theiler,* Swiss-born South African veterinary biologist, 1867–1936 + -IA] A genus of parasitic protozoa of the family Theileriidae (order Piroplasmida) that contains some of the most important agents of disease of domestic animals. Transmitted by ticks, the organisms reproduce sexually in cells, especially lymphocytes, and then enter red blood cells from which they are picked up by host ticks. ***T. tsutsugamushi*** *RICKETTSIA TSUTSUGAMUSHI.*
**thel-** \thēl-\ [Gk *thēlē* nipple] A combining form meaning nipple. Also *thelo-.*
**thelarche** \thelär′kē\ [THEL- + Gk *archē* a beginning] Development of the breasts in girls. **precocious t.** Breast development in a girl before the usual age of puberty. Also *premature thelarche.*
***Thelazia*** \thelā′zē·ə\ The eye worms of mammals; a genus of nematodes in the family Thelaziidae. They superficially resemble filarial worms and are parasitic in the lacrimal ducts and on the surface of the eyes of various mammals, rarely including man. Infection occurs when larvae emerge from the mouthparts of muscoid flies, the intermediate hosts, when the fly feeds near the eyes of a final host.
**thele** \thē′lē\ PAPILLA MAMMARIA.
**theleplasty** \thē′ləplas′tē\ [Gk *thēlē* a nipple + -PLASTY] Any plastic operation on the mammary nipple. Also *mamilliplasty, mammilliplasty.* Also *thelyplasty.*
**thelerethism** \thēler′əthizm\ [THEL- + ERETHISM] An erection of the nipple, brought about by mechanical stimulation.
**thelitis** \thēlī′tis\ [THEL- + -ITIS] MAMILLITIS.
**thelo-** \thē′lō-\ THEL-.
**thelorrhagia** \thē′lôrā′jə\ [THELO- + -RRHAGIA] A hemorrhaging from the nipple.
**thely-** \thē′lē-\ [Gk *thēlys* (adjective) female] A combining form meaning female.
**thelyplasty** \thel′əplas′tē\ THELEPLASTY.
**thenad** \thē′nad\ In the direction of the thenar eminence or the palm of the hand.
**thenal** \thē′nəl\ Of or relating to the palm of the hand or the thenar eminence.
**thenar** \thē′när\ [Gk *thenar* the palm of the hand, sole of the foot] **1** [NA] The bulging mass of muscles and related tissues at the base of the thumb on the lateral aspect of the palm of the hand. Also *ball of thumb, thenar eminence, thenar area.* **2** Of or relating to the palm of the hand.
***Theobaldia*** \thē′ōbal′dē·ə\ A former name for *CULISETA.*
**theobromine** $C_7H_8N_4O_2$. 3,7-Dimethylxanthine. A white, crystalline powder, a purine derivative that occurs in the theobroma (cacao, or cocoa) bean (1.5–3%), cola nuts, and tea. It has mild diuretic properties, stimulates the myocardium, and dilates the coronary vessels. It is used to treat artiosclerosis and some peripheral vascular diseases, and it is generally administered in the form of one of its more soluble salts.
**theobromine magnesium oleate** Magnesium 3,7-dimethylxanthine oleate. The magnesium double salt of theo bromine and oleic acid. It has been administered orally to treat patients with cardiovascular disease. Diuresis and dilatation of the coronary vessels are expected from this medication.
**theophylline** $C_7H_8N_4O_2 \cdot H_2O$. 1,3-Dimethylxanthine. A white, crystalline, monohydrated methylated purine that occurs in tea leaves and is prepared synthetically. It is used as a smooth muscle relaxant and diuretic agent as well as a myocardial stimulant. Its actions as a diuretic and central nervous stimulant are intermediate between theobromine and caffeine.
**theophylline aminoisobutanol** AMBUPHYLLINE.
**theophylline calcium salicylate** A double salt or mixture of calcium theophylline and calcium salicylate (1:1), containing about two molecules of water. It is a white, almost tasteless powder that is given orally to produce a diuretic effect, stimulate the heart, and relax smooth muscles.
**theophylline cholinate** OXTRIPHYLLINE.
**theophylline ethanolamine** A soluble formulation of theophylline with ethanolamine, containing 75% theophylline by weight.
**theophylline ethylenediamine** $C_{16}H_{24}N_{10}O_4$. A white or slightly yellowish, soluble salt form of theophylline and ethylenediamine. It is used to relax bronchial smooth muscle, to stimulate respiration, and as a diuretic, and is used orally or by injection to treat asthmatic attacks. It contains 85% theophylline by weight. Also *aminophylline.*
**theophylline methylglucamine** An equimolecular combination of theophylline and *N*-methylglucamine that has been used as a smooth muscle relaxant. Also *glucophylline.*
**theophylline monoethanolamine** An equimolecular

compound of theophylline and ethanolamine which contains 75% theophylline by weight. It is a soluble formulation of theophylline.

**theophylline sodium** The sodium salt of theophylline. It is used in soluble preparations of theophylline in combination with glycine or sodium acetate.

**theophylline sodium acetate** A water-soluble preparation of theophylline sodium and sodium acetate. It contains 55% theophylline by weight.

**theophylline sodium glycinate** A soluble preparation of theophylline composed of a mixture of theophylline sodium and glycine. It contains 49% theophylline, by weight.

**theorem** \thē′ərəm\ [Gk *theōrēma* (from *theōrein* to look at, contemplate, from *theōros* a spectator, observer, from *thea* a looking at, view, spectacle) a spectacle, a principle deduced] A proposition that can be demonstrated to be true. **Bayes t.** A mathematical statement of relationships between test sensitivity and specificity and the predictive value of a positive test result:

$$p^+ = \frac{pSe}{pSe + (1-Sp)(1-p)},$$

where $p^+$ is the predictive value of a positive test, or the conditional probability of the presence of disease, given a positive test result; *Se* is the sensitivity of the test, or the probability of a positive test in the presence of disease; *Sp* is the specificity of the test, or the probability of a negative test in the absence of disease; and *p* is the prevalence rate, or prior probability, of disease in the population tested.

# theory

**theory** [Gk *theōria* (from *theōrein* to look at, contemplate) a looking at, observing, contemplation] A set of arguments or propositions formulated to account for observed phenomena or to provide a coherent basis for the interpretation of observed phenomena. **Adler's t.** ADLERIAN PSYCHOLOGY. **adsorption t. of narcosis** The theory that an anesthetic or narcotic acts at the surface of a cell membrane, thus altering the permeability of the membrane and also possibly intracellular metabolism. **aerodynamic t. of phonation** MYOELASTIC THEORY. **apposition t.** The concept that tissues expand by the surface deposition of new tissue. It is applicable particularly to growth in bone. **avalanche t.** The theory that nerve impulses traveling in approximate synchrony are reinforced by ephaptic interaction. **balance t. of sex** A theory of sex determination based on the ratio of sex chromosomes to autosomal sets. The most prevalent statement of the theory holds that female differentiation depends on a 1:1 ratio of X chromosomes to autosomal haploid sets, and male differentiation depends on a 1:2 ratio. **behavior t.** The theory that neurotic behavior consists of learned patterns of reaction that are unadaptive and should therefore be amenable to unlearning through extinction or inhibition. **Bohr's t.** The theory that the electrons in an atom can exist only in states of certain discrete energies, and that an electron remaining in any one of those states does not emit electromagnetic radiation even though, in the classical view, it is being accelerated. The transition of an electron from one state (orbit) to another is accompanied by emission of electromagnetic radiation of frequency equal to the difference in energy of the two states divided by Planck's constant. **Buergi's t.** BUERGI'S HYPOTHESIS. **Burn and Rand t.** Stimulation of preganglionic sympathetic fibers results in the release of acetylcholine which then stimulates the postganglionic fibers to release epinephrine or norepinephrine at their terminals. **Cannon's t.** The theory that the body's response in emergencies, as to situations providing fear or pain, includes the promotion of adrenal medullary secretion through the action of the sympathetic nervous system. Also *emergency theory*. **Cannon-Bard t. of emotions** A theory regarding the origin of emotion: diencephalically integrated patterns of response are evoked directly through reflex pathways at the thalamic level or indirectly by conditioned responses at the cortical level. Discharges sent upward from the activated hypothalamus to the cortex add the sensory quality of feeling to the automatic responses and the combination is the emotion. Also *Cannon hypothalamic theory of emotion*. **t. of central analysis** RUTHERFORD'S THEORY. **chemicoparasitic t.** The generally accepted theory that caries is caused by the production of acids or proteolytic enzymes by bacteria on the surface of the teeth. **chromosome t. of inheritance** The notion that chromosomes are the mediators of heredity by being the cytologic location of genes. Also *chromosome theory of heredity*. See also WEISMANN'S THEORY, MENDEL'S LAWS. ● Several hypotheses laid the foundation for this theory: Walter Sutton and Theodor Boveri in the first years of the 20th century, proposed independently the chromosomal basis of Mendel's laws, Weismann theorized a reduction chromosome division in gametogenesis, and E.B. Wilson recognized the central role of chromosomes in development. **clonal selection t. of immunity** A theory developed to explain how an animal can make antibodies to an apparently almost unlimited variety of antigens, many of which do not occur naturally. It proposes that the population of different potential antibody molecules is generated by genetic mechanisms independent of the presence of antigen and acting to produce a population of lymphocytes carrying on their surface the particular antibody combining sites of the antibodies they are capable of making. Antigen then acts to select the particular lymphocytes with whose antibodies it can react and causes them to proliferate and differentiate into antibody-producing cells. This is essentially a darwinian theory of antibody diversity and replaced earlier instructive (or lamarckian) theories. **clonic t. of phonation** NEUROCHRONAXIC THEORY. **Cohnheim's t.** **1** Emigration of leukocytes from a blood vessel to a lesion is an essential characteristic of inflammation. Also *emigration theory*. **2** Tumors arise from embryonic rests. Also *embryonal theory, fetal rest-cell theory*. **t. of concrescence** The theory that the multicuspidate teeth of mammals have evolved by fusion of several unicuspidate teeth of lower vertebrates. **contractile ring t.** The theory that cytokinesis is associated with a dense ring of microfilaments arranged circumferentially around the cell beneath the division furrow. The microfilaments slide past each other, constricting the cell like a purse string. **convergence-projection t.** An attempt to explain visceral pain referred to a cutaneous site by the convergence of visceral and skin afferent nerves on the same neuron in the dorsal horn of the spinal cord. **Dalcq-Pasteels t.** The suggestion that soon after fertilization of the vertebrate egg a definite topographic and dynamic relation is established between the arrangement of the yolk (yolk gradient) and the substances in the dorsoventral field. It was claimed that a fairly consistent representation of vertebrate morphogenesis is possible on the basis of the ideas of gradient, field, and threshold of developmentally active substances. **t. of demographic transition** An account, based on the experience of presently industrialized countries, of the demographic changes to be expected in the course of economic development from an agrarian, low-income economy characterized by high birth and death rates, through a stage when death rates, but not birth rates, fall, to a stage when both fertility and mortality rates become stabilized at a relatively low level. **drive-reduction t.** The hypothesis that motivated behavior can best be understood as an activity of the organism leading away from some aversive state of increased tension, or toward a state of reduced or eliminated tension, by the achievement of a diminished drive through the attainment of the goal. **dualistic t. of hematopoiesis** The concept that, of the blood cells, lymphocytes, granulocytes, and erythrocytes each have separate ancestral lines of precursors, without a common totipotential "stem cell," and that monocytes are derived from granulocyte precursors. **duplicity t. of vision** The view that there are separate sensory receptors in the eye for the brightness and the color of light. Regarded now as firmly established, the retinal cones are held to be primarily sensitive to the wave length or color of light and are active in daylight vision, while the rod cells are chiefly reactive to the intensity of light, and provide achromatic vision during twilight or under the low-intensity conditions of night vision. **Ehrlich side-chain t.** SIDE CHAIN THEORY. **electron-hole t.** The theory that when an electron in the valence band of a semiconductor is sufficiently excited, it enters a conduction band, where it contributes to the conduction of current. The vacancy left in the valence band is referred to as a hole, implying the absence of an electron. This hole can move under the influence of an electric field, by being filled by acquiring an electron from a neighboring atom. **embryonal t.** COHNHEIM'S THEORY. **emergency t.** CANNON'S THEORY. **emigration t.** COHNHEIM'S THEORY. **encrustation t.** The theory that the early phase of atherogenesis is the occurrence of small mural thrombi composed of such blood elements as platelets, fibrin, and leucocytes collecting in areas of arterial intimal injury and that fatty deposition is a secondary phenomenon. **extravascular t. of erythrocyte formation** A concept, widely accepted, that the formation of erythrocyte precursors occurs entirely in the interstitial zones of the bone marrow rather than within the small blood vessels. **fetal rest-cell t.** COHNHEIM'S THEORY. **frequency t.** RUTHERFORD'S THEORY. **gametoid t.** The theory that cancers arise from cells with sexual characteristics and grow as parasites in the host. **gate t.** A proposal that pain is determined by the interaction of three elements in the spinal cord: the substantia gelatinosa, dorsal column fibers, and the first central (T) cells in the dorsal horn. By this theory it is suggested that the "gate" for impulses transmitting pain may be closed by decreasing the small fiber input through an inhibitory mechanism of negative feedback by enhancing the large fiber input, whereas the "gate" is opened by small fiber input that remains uninhibited because of a lack of input from large fibers. In this manner it is proposed that non-toxic touch stimuli conducted along large fibers from adjacent regions of skin are able to inhibit pain. Also *Melzack and Wall gate control theory.* **t. of gene-culture evolution** A two-part unproven hypothesis of sociobiology that genes encode rules that determine the probability that one form of behavior or trait will be altered to another, and that this probability depends on the number of individuals in a population already expressing one trait or the other. The theory was put forth to explain the impact of genetics, environment, and their interrelationships on the shaping of cultural behavior. Also *Lumsden-Wilson theory.* **germ t.** The proposition that all infectious and contagious diseases are caused by microorganisms. **germ layer t.** The theory that there develops in an embryo three germ layers which give rise to all the organs of the adult, each organ and tissue being derived from ectoderm, mesoderm, or endoderm, or from a combination. • The theory was established by K.E. von Baer in 1828. **gestalt t.** GESTALT PSYCHOLOGY. **Golgi's t.** The theory that axons of Golgi cells and collateral dendrites of Deiters cells interconnect or synapse and that such connections are important in the interneuronal transmission of information. **group factor t.** The theory that human intelligence consists of several components or special abilities, measurably distinct from one another, which in their aggregate make up the intelligence. **Helmholtz t. of color vision** The concept that color vision is achieved by the function of three types of receptors for color (red, green, and violet) and that other colors are perceived as a combined function of these three primary colors. Also *Young-Helmholtz theory.* **Helmholtz t. of hearing** The theory of hearing which held that analysis of sound into component tones is effected in the cochlea by the transversely disposed fibers of the basilar membrane. It was assumed that these fibers were a series of tuned resonators. Also *resonance theory of hearing, static theory of hearing, place theory of hearing.* Compare RUTHERFORD'S THEORY. • The theory is not tenable since the basilar membrane fibers do not show the transverse or longitudinal variations of tension necessary to support it. It is not strictly a theory of hearing but of cochlear or end-organ function. **Hering t.** The concept that vision employs three visual substances and opponent receptors: black-white, red-green, and blue-yellow. Also *opponent-colors theory.* **humoral t.** HUMORALISM. **hydrate microcrystal t. of anesthesia** A theory used to explain narcosis. It is based on the putative reaction of anesthetic molecules to form hydrates or clothrates. The molecule, encased in a cage of water, yields a microcrystal that affects cell membrane permeability or electrical excitability. **t. of inheritance of acquired characteristics** LAMARCK'S THEORY. **inside-outside t.** The theory that blastomeres within the compact mouse morula "recognize" their position in some undefined way as being either superficial or deep and respond by differentiating as trophectoderm or inner cell mass cells respectively. See also POLARIZATION HYPOTHESIS. **instructive theories of antibody production** Those theories proposing that the specificity of cells for antigen results initially from having come in contact with antigen when no specificity existed. The antigen is believed to instruct the cell to produce antibodies against it. No molecular mechanism for such instruction that is compatible with modern molecular biology has been proposed. Compare SELECTIVE THEORIES OF ANTIBODY PRODUCTION. **intravascular t. of erythrocyte formation** A concept, not generally accepted at present, that the formation of erythrocyte precursors occurs within the small blood vessels or sinusoids of the bone marrow, from differentiation of endothelial cells into erythroblasts. See also EXTRAVASCULAR THEORY OF ERYTHROCYTE FORMATION. **Jackson's t.** The theory that the faculties most recently acquired in the process of evolution are the first to be lost as a consequence of a cerebral cortical lesion. An example is the early impairment of fine finger movement resulting from a lesion of the "hand" area of the contralateral motor cortex. **James-Lange t.** The view that emotions are really our experience of bodily changes in circulation, the viscera, and the musculature, that occur reflexively following presentation of an adequate stimulus, and that there is no particular cortical excitation involved. Also *James-Lange-Sutherland theory.* **Ladd-Franklin t.** The theory that complex photosensitive molecules in the dendrites of retinal ganglion cells release specific substances responsible for red, green, and blue color vision. **Lamarck's t.** An erroneous theory that explained evolution through inheritance of environmentally induced adaptive characteristics. Also *theory of inheritance of acquired characteristics, lamarckism.* **lateral chain t.** SIDE CHAIN THEORY. **lipoid t. of narcosis** An explanation of narcosis based on the relative solubility of general anesthetics in oil, such as oleyl alcohol or olive oil. The oil-water partition coefficient correlates with anesthetic potency. Also *Meyer-Overton theory.* **local circuit t.** The neurophysiologic theory that, as sodium ions flow across the cell membrane of a neuron, current flows from the unstimulated, positively charged area of the membrane to the stimulated negative or depolarized area, which then acts as a sink. This charge progresses along the membrane and is accompanied by a reversal of charge across the membrane as the effect of the initial stimulus moves on. **lock and key t.** A theory which states that the enzyme molecule must fit the substrate molecule as a key fits a lock before catalysis can take place. **Lumsden-Wilson t.** THEORY OF GENE-CULTURE EVOLUTION. **malthusian t.** MALTHUSIANISM. **mass action t.** The theory that large areas of the brain act in concert during the perception of sensory information, the integration of this information, and the performance of motor activity. **Melzack and Wall gate control t.** GATE THEORY. **membrane ionic t.** The concept that electrical potentials across biological membranes are the consequence of differences in the distribution of charged ions on the two sides of the membrane and of the specific permeability and transport properties of the membrane with respect to these ions. **mendelian t.** A theory of inheritance based on the principles first discovered by Gregor Mendel in 1865 and modified and expanded by knowledge of cell and molecular biology. It is found to be the usual method of inheritance in most diploid organisms. The principles of mendelian inheritance are: hereditary characters are determined by the action of genes; genes are located on specific loci on chromosomes; genes are transmitted from parent to offspring; in diploids, genes occur as a pair of alleles; each gamete receives but one allele of a given genetic locus; fertilization is a random event in that gametes carrying particular alleles are not generally favored; and provided two genetic loci are not linked, they are transmitted independently to gametes. Also *mendelism.* **metabolic t. of atherosclerosis** The theory that atherosclerosis is essentially a disturbance of lipid metabolism. **Metchnikoff's t.** A theory postulating that the purpose of inflammation was to bring phagocytes to the injured area in order to engulf and remove bacteria and other harmful elements. Proposed in 1884 by Elie Metchnikoff, the theory has proven to be generally correct, and covers the cellular factors of the inflammatory process, including margination and emigration of leukocytes, chemotaxis, and phagocytosis. **Meyer's t.** PSYCHOBIOLOGY. **Meyer-Overton t.** LIPOID THEORY OF NARCOSIS. **miasma t.** The theory once widely held that epidemics of infectious disease were caused by noxious emanations from putrescent matter in the ground which arose under certain conditions, as of temperature and humidity. **migration t.** The belief that sympathetic ophthalmia results from a factor that extends from one eye to the other via anatomic connections. **monophyletic t. of hematopoiesis** The concept that all of the types of blood cells are derived from a common ancestral "stem cell" or totipotential cell, assumed to be a tissue lymphocyte. Also *unitary theory of hematopoiesis, unitarian theory of hematopoiesis.* **t. of Morawitz** A theory of coagulation that postulated (1) conversion of prothrombin to thrombin by the action of thromboplastin, and (2) conversion of fibrinogen to fibrin, and thus the formation of a clot, by the action of thrombin on fibrinogen. This theory is the basis for subsequent concepts of coagulation. **myoelastic t.** A theory of the mechanism of phonation, now widely accepted, that vocal cord vibrations are produced by the subglottic air pressure forcing apart the vocal cords held together by the tonic contraction of laryngeal muscles. Compare NEUROCHRONAXIC THEORY. **myogenic t.** A theory contending that the contraction of cardiac muscle fibers originates from properties endogenous to the heart muscle cells themselves rather than resulting from exogenous factors such as nerve impulses coming to the heart along autonomic nerves. **neounitarian t. of hematopoiesis** The concept that the granulocytic series of blood cells ordinarily has its own precursor cell, the myeloblast, but that in abnormal conditions a lymphocyte can differentiate into cells of the granulocytic series. Also *neounitary theory of hematopoiesis.* **network t. of immunity** The theory that proposes that it is the reaction between immunoglobulin idiotypes and antibodies to them that controls the immune response. **neurochronaxic t.** A theory of the mechanism of phonation, now disproved, postulating that vocal cord vibrations are produced by rhythmic contractions and relaxations of the thyroarytenoid muscles resulting from synchronized impulses in the motor nerves concerned. Also *neuromuscular theory of phonation, clonic theory of phonation.* Compare MYOELASTIC THEORY. **neurogenic t.** The theory that cardiac rhythmicity is determined by neural control rather than by an inherent myogenic pattern. **neuromuscular t. of phonation** NEUROCHRONAXIC THEORY. **neuron t.** The theory that the nervous system consists of many neurons which are contiguous but not interconnected in a continuous manner. **nucleocytoplasmic relation t.** PLASMA RELATION THEORY. **operon t.** The theory that a segment of the DNA molecule (operator) acts as a binding site for regulatory molecules, and the operator regulates the transcription of adjacent structured genes. **opponent-colors t.** HERING THEORY. **Papez t. of emotion** A refinement of the Cannon-Bard theory of emotions proposing that the functional circle formed by the interconnections of hippocampus, fornix, mamillary bodies, anterior thalamic nuclei, and gyrus cinguli elaborates the functions of central emotion and give the sensory quality that constitutes emotional experience. **perceptual defense t.** The view that selectivity in perception is possible, and that a screening-out or selective blocking of unpleasant stimuli provides a mechanism for reducing or eliminating anxiety-provoking material that might otherwise enter awareness. **permeability t. of narcosis** The theory that anesthetic or narcotic agents decrease cell membrane permeability and thereby induce narcosis. **place t. of hearing** HELMHOLTZ THEORY OF HEARING. **Planck's t.** The fundamental law of the quantum theory: electromagnetic radiation is emitted and absorbed only in indivisible units called quanta, the energy $E$ of a single quantum associated with radiation of frequency $\nu$ being given by the formula $E = h\nu$, where $h$ is Planck's constant. **plasma relation t.** The theory that the ratio of nuclear volume to cytoplasmic volume is generally constant for a given cell type. Also *nucleocytoplasmic relation theory.* **polarization-membrane t.** A theory stating that the plasma membrane of a living cell has an electrical polarity, the inside being negative with respect to the outside, due to the unequal ion distribution across the differentially permeable membrane. **polychromatic t.** A theory that there are specific visual receptors for each of seven color stimuli, namely for crimson, orange, yellow, green, blue-green, blue, and blue-violet. **polyphyletic t. of hematopoiesis** The concept that each of the types of blood cells has its own distinct precursor cell, and that there is no common ancestral totipotential "stem cell." **population t.** Any theory dealing with the interrelationships between population dynamics on the one hand, and, on the other, biologic, economic, environmental, social, and other factors, taken singly or in combination. Examples are the Malthus population theory and the theory of demographic transition. **proteomorphic t.** The theory that the mechanism of immunity against bacterial infection is located primarily in the hematopoietic system and secondarily in all somatic cells and that the liver excretes all waste products generated by the immunizing process. **Ranke's t.** The proposition that the development of tuberculosis occurs in three stages: primary infection, generalized infection, and finally, chronic infection. **recapitulation t.** The theory propounded by Haeckel in 1866 which stated that events in the life history, or ontogeny, of an individual are an abbreviated repetition of the past evolutionary stages, or phylogeny, of that particular organism. Its fallacy lay in the fact that an embryonic descendant need not resemble the ancestral adult and an adult descendant may resemble an ancestral embryo. Also *biogenetic law, Haeckel's law, Müller-Haeckel law.* **t. of reentry** The theory that premature ectopic beats arise because of reentry of the same impulse which initiated the preceding beat. **resonance t. of hearing** HELMHOLTZ THEORY OF HEARING. **t. of rotation** Accommodation of the fetus to the bony framework of the birth canal during labor leads to internal rotation of the fetus. **Rutherford's t.** The classical theory of hearing which claims that the analysis of the signals generated in the cochlea in response to sound stimulation is carried out in the central nervous system and not in the cochlea itself. Also *theory of central analysis, telephone theory, frequency theory.* Compare HELMHOLTZ THEORY OF HEARING. **t. of saltatory conduction** The concept that a nerve impulse "jumps" between adjacent nodes of Ranvier in myelinated axons, resulting in a discontinuous electrical conduction. **selective theories of antibody production** Theories proposing that the specificity of cells for antigen inheres in the cells before contact with antigen, and that antigen acts to trigger the production of antibodies, as in the side chain theory and in the clonal selection theory. Compare INSTRUCTIVE THEORIES OF ANTIBODY PRODUCTION. **shunt muscle t.** A theory that certain muscles (shunt muscles) act primarily during rapid movement and along the long axis of the moving bone to provide centripetal force. These muscles insert far from the fulcrum and originate close to the fulcrum. Other muscles (spurt muscles), which insert close to the fulcrum and originate far from the fulcrum, produce acceleration along the curve of motion. The theory is controversial. **side chain t.** The theory, proposed by Paul Ehrlich in 1900, that cells carried receptor groups with haptophore side chains on their surfaces. Upon contact with antigen, these side chains combined with it and the receptors were thrown off the cell and replaced by new ones. The receptors released into the circulation were antibody molecules. Also *Ehrlich side-chain theory, Ehrlich's theory, lateral chain theory, Ehrlich's postulate.* **signal detection t.** A way of conceptualizing the separate contributions of sensory input and the rule governing decision, which together determine the judgment of a subject as to whether a signal has or has not been presented. The theory assumes that thresholds are not absolute, and it proposes that the ability of a subject to detect a weak signal against a noisy background will be a combined function of input stimulus intensity and the decision rule or criterion adopted, the latter being based on the relative value of gain or loss that will result from errors made in detection, whether these errors consist of missing signals or falsely perceiving nonexistent signals. **single hit t.** An explanation for the dose-response relationship of hemolysis by complement, in which the sigmoid dose-response curve for whole complement is attributed to the complexity of the complement sequence and the propensity of some of the intermediate stages to decay rather than proceed to lysis. **sliding filament t.** **1** The concept that muscular contraction involves actin and myosin filaments moving past one another. **2** A concept that the movement of a cilium or flagellum involves the movement of the microtubules of one doublet in relation to the microtubules of an adjacent doublet, the microtubules each retaining a constant length. The microtubules of adjacent doublets are connected by dynein arms which respond to the hydrolysis of ATP by bending. **somatic mutation t. of cancer** The theory that cancer is the result of a mutation in somatic cells. **sound pattern t.** The theory that analysis of sound frequency is determined by the patterns of firing in the auditory nerve fibers: since individual nerve fibers cannot convey impulses at rates greater than 300 Hz and the upper limit of audible frequencies is in excess of 10 kHz, it is considered that groups of nerve fibers respond on the volley principle and the pattern of neural excitation is dependent on the frequency and intensity of each component of the sound. **Spitzer's t.** An explanation of the partitioning of the truncoconal segment of the mammalian embryonic heart based on phylogenic considerations. Specifically, congenital heart defects involving varying degrees of transposition of the great vessels, aorta, and pulmonary trunk, were presumed to recapitulate the positions of these vessels in submammalian animals. **static t. of hearing** HELMHOLTZ THEORY OF HEARING. **structural t.** STRUCTURAL HYPOTHESIS. **surface tension t. of narcosis** The theory that an anesthetic lowers the aqueous surface tension of a cell membrane, thus enhancing its permeability, and subsequently altering intracellular metabolism. **target t.** A theory explaining biologic effects in terms of the greater sensitivity of certain sites. In the cell, special target sites may be relatively sensitive. It is often necessary to register "hits" in such targets once, twice, or more times by ionizations in order to obtain the biologic effect. Also *hit theory.* **telephone t.** RUTHERFORD'S THEORY. **template t.** An instructive theory of antibody production that proposes that antigen acts like a template with respect to antibody formation, determining the shape of the combining site of the antibody. The theory is not now regarded as tenable. **thermodynamic t. of narcosis** When equilibrium is reached in the partition of anesthetic among the lipid and aqueous phases, the same thermodynamic potential, or free molal energy, exists in all phases. **thermostat t.** A theory that a fall in body temperature activates a feeding center in the brain and a reverse effect is brought about when a rise activates a satiety center. **tonic t. of phonation** MYOELASTIC THEORY. **trialistic t. of hematopoiesis** The concept that, of the blood cells, lymphocytes, granulocytes, and erythrocytes each have separate ancestral lines of precursors, without a common totipotential "stem cell," and that monocytes are derived from tissue histiocytes. **two-sympathin t.**

The idea that two different types of substances (sympathin E and sympathin I) are released into the bloodstream following stimulation of adrenergic nerves. **unitarian t. of antibodies** UNITARIAN HYPOTHESIS. **unitarian t. of hematopoiesis** MONOPHYLETIC THEORY OF HEMATOPOIESIS. **Warburg's t.** Cancer is the result of altered cellular respiratory mechanisms with selective proliferation of cells having increased glycolytic metabolism. **wave t.** The theory that light and similar types of radiation are transmitted through space in the form of waves. **Weismann's t.** 1 The theory, enunciated in 1892, that heritable variations arise in the germ plasm. It contradicted the lamarckian theory of the inheritance of acquired characteristics and formed the foundation for the chromosome theory of inheritance. Also *weismannism.* 2 The theory, enunciated in 1887, that germ cells of organisms that reproduce sexually must undergo a reduction in chromosome number. **Young-Helmholtz t.** HELMHOLTZ THEORY OF COLOR VISION. **Yukawa t.** The theory that the force between nucleons is the result of the exchange of mesons by the nucleons.

**thèque** \tek′\ [French (from L *theca* a case, sheath), a small box or chest] An aggregate of four or more melanin-containing nevus cells in contact with the basal layer of the epidermis.

**therapeusis** \ther′əpyoo′sis\ THERAPEUTICS.

**therapeutic** \ther′əpyoo′tik\ [Gk *therapeutikos* (verbal of *therapeuein* to wait on, attend, serve, from *theraps* an attendant, servant) inclinded to serve, able to cure] 1 Of or relating to the remedial treatment of disease. 2 Tending to restore health or improve impaired function; effective as a therapy.

**therapeutics** \ther′əpyoo′tiks\ The branch of medicine that is concerned with the remedial treatment of disease. Also *therapeusis.* **alimentary t.** DIET THERAPY. **cellular t.** ORGANOTHERAPY. **empiric t.** EMPIRIC TREATMENT. **massive sterilizing t.** A general principle of treatment that attempts to find a drug capable of destroying all of the parasites in the tissues without harming the tissues of the host. Also *therapia sterilisans magna.* **mediate t.** Treatment of an infant by giving medication to a nursing mother so that the infant imbibes the medication with her milk. The method is of historical interest only. **mental t.** PSYCHOTHERAPY. **rational t.** RATIONAL TREATMENT. **specific t.** The employment of drugs with highly selective, specific actions in the treatment of disease. **suggestive t.** PSYCHOTHERAPY.

**therapeutist** \ther′əpyoo′tist\ THERAPIST.

**Theraphosidae** \ther′əfäs′idē\ A family of very large, hairy mygalomorph spiders found in warm temperate and tropical areas, but not in Europe. Most are harmless, though *Sericopelma communis* of Panama is poisonous. In America these spiders are commonly called tarantulas, though this is a misnomer. See also AMERICAN TARANTULA.

**therapia** \ther′əpē′ə\ [New L. See THERAPY.] THERAPY. **t. sterilisans covergens** The rapid reduction in the number of parasites present following the administration of a chemotherapeutic agent. **t. sterilisans divergens** An increase in the number of parasites during a course of chemotherapy, before they finally disappear. Also *Browning's phenomenon.* **t. sterilisans fractionata** The administration of small, repeated doses of a microparasiticide. A suggested regimen by some authorities in the past in cases where the microorganisms do not become resistent to the chemotherapeutic agent. **t. sterilisans magna** MASSIVE STERILIZING THERAPEUTICS.

**therapist** \ther′əpist\ [*therap(y)* + -IST] A person skilled in some form of therapy. Also *therapeutist.* **corrective t.** An allied health professional trained in physical education and restorative exercises. **occupational t.** A practitioner of occupational therapy. **physical t.** A practitioner of physiotherapy. Also *physiotherapist, physiotherapeutist.* **radiation t.** A physician specialized by training and experience in the use of ionizing radiation for treatment of disease. **speech t.** An individual formally trained in linguistics and the speech sciences, child development and other aspects of psychology, neurology, and relevant aspects of surgery, leading to a professional diploma or university degree, and registered as being competent to practice speech therapy.

# therapy

**therapy** \ther′əpē\ [New L *therapia*, from Gk *therapeia* (from *therapeuein* to attend, serve, take care of, treat, from *theraps* an attendant, servant) service, care, treatment] Systematic treatment of disease or measures to improve health, especially as undertaken according to a particular method or modality. Also *therapia.* • The word is often used with a combining form indicating modality or object of treatment, as in *chemotherapy, radiotherapy, physiotherapy, psychotherapy.* **active t.** DIRECTIVE PSYCHOTHERAPY. **alimentary t.** DIET THERAPY. **alkali t.** ALKALITHERAPY. **analytic t.** The therapeutic application of jungian psychology. **anticoagulant t.** Treatment with anticoagulants of patients who have thromboembolic problems or are at risk to develop them, e.g. postoperatively. Heparin acts directly, while the oral anticoagulants depress coagulation indirectly by restricting hepatic synthesis of several active clotting factors. **anticonvulsant t.** Any treatment to control attacks of epilepsy. **antigametocyte t.** Antimalarial therapy directed toward destruction of the plasmoidal gametes in the blood of the patient. Small doses of pamaquine do this, as do certain other antimalarial drugs. **antiplatelet t.** Pharmacologic therapy that uses various agents to suppress platelet adhesion or aggregation, in some circumstances thus improving the patency of vascular grafts or diminishing the likelihood of vascular complications. **art t.** The use of the arts such as dance, music, painting, and sculpture, either singly or in combination, as an adjunct to treatment of mental illnesses. It offers opportunities for sublimation, catharsis, distancing from the group or participation in group projects, visible accomplishment, and enhancement of self-esteem. **behavior t.** Therapy for disorders or problems associated with behavior based on the techniques of experimental psychology. It is based on the assumption that maladaptive behaviors are the result of faulty learning and can be corrected by re-educational techniques such as aversion therapy, biofeedback, shaping, systematic desensitization, and token economy. Also *learning-theory therapy, conditioning therapy.* **Bernheim's t.** *Older term* HYPNOTHERAPY. **bilateral electroconvulsive t.** The classical form of electroconvulsive therapy, in which the current is applied to both sides of the head. **blunderbuss t.** An antiquated type of drug therapy in which many drugs are given at the same time to achieve the same objective. **brief stimulus t.** A modified form of electroconvulsive therapy in which the current is applied for a shorter period of time than in the classical method. Abbr. BST **buffer t.** The use of buffer solutions as therapeutic measures to bring a hydrogen ion concentration into the normal range. **carbon dioxide t.** A method of therapy, rarely used since the 1950s, believed to be of limited usefulness in the treatment of some anxiety conditions. The patient inhales a mixture of 30% carbon dioxide and 70% oxygen, which produces unconsciousness. **Chaoul t.** Radiation therapy using x rays of lower energy, with the source-to-tissue distance being small. **client-centered t.** NONDIRECTIVE COUNSELING. **cognitive t.** An active, structured, directive psychotherapeutic approach that aims to alter the ways the patient thinks about himself, the future, and the world, reported to be of particular value in the treatment of depression. It is based on the assumption that one's behavior is determined by how one perceives and structures the world. **collapse t.** A treatment, now obsolete, for cavitary pulmonary tuberculosis in which collapse of the affected lung is brought about. **combined t.** The use of multiple therapeutic agents. Multiple antimicrobial agents with different modes of action prevent the emergence of resistant mutants. Agents acting on successive steps in a pathway, such as a sulfonamide and trimethoprim, may be used to achieve synergism. Multiple agents with similar actions may be used to decrease toxicity. **conditioning t.** BEHAVIOR THERAPY. **contact t.** CONTACT RADIOTHERAPY. **contact radiation t.** CONTACT RADIOTHERAPY. **couples t.** A type of family therapy that focuses on the marital dyad in the belief that psychopathology within the social matrix of marriage perpetuates and engenders individual psychopathology. Also *marriage therapy.* **deleading t.** The use of chelating agents to rid the body of heavy metals such as lead by mobilizing them from tissue stores and facilitating their excretion. **diathermic t.** DIATHERMY. **diet t.** Treatment of an illness or condition by means of diet. Also *sitotherapy, bromatherapy, bromatotherapy, alimentary therapy, dietotherapy, dietetic treatment, alimentary therapeutics, trophotherapy.* **duplex t.** Simultaneous use of diathermy and galvanic stimulation. Also *pulsed diathermy.* **electroconvulsive t.** The application of a small amount of electrical current for a fraction of a second to the head through two electrodes placed either bilaterally in the temporal areas (bilateral electroconvulsive therapy) or unilaterally (unilateral electroconvulsive therapy). It is of particular value in affective disorders and some forms of schizophrenia. Also *electric convulsion therapy, electroshock therapy, electric shock treatment, electroconvulsive treatment, shock therapy* (imprecise), *shock treatment.* **electromagnetic field t.** The therapeutic use of high Gauss magnetic fields, primarily in the noninvasive treatment of nonunion following bone fracture. **electron beam t.** Radiotherapy by electrons with the source located at a distance from the body. **electroshock t.** ELECTROCONVULSIVE THERAPY. **electrotherapeutic sleep t.** See under ELECTROSLEEP. **endocrine t.** Any treatment with hormonal substances. **endocrine ablative t.** 1 Treatment of a disease of an endocrine gland by removal of that gland, as of Graves disease by thyroidectomy. 2 Treatment of a disease by removal of one or more glands, as of carcinoma of the breast with metastases by ovariectomy. **family t.** FAMILY PSYCHOTHERAPY. **fango t.** The therapeutic use of fango; mud baths as originally given with mud from the thermal spring of Battaglio, Italy. **fever t.** The treatment by artificially induced fever as, for example, by induced malaria, by typhoid vaccine, or by elevated environmental temperature. Also *fever treatment, pyretotherapy.* **gametocyte t.** A means of preventing the spread of malaria (*Plasmodium* species) in which antibodies developed in the human host destroy the *Plasmodium* gametocytes and so prevent the development of infection in mosquitoes. **gamma-ray t.** Radiation therapy using gamma rays from radioactive substances, such as radium or cobalt 60. **gene t.** The introduction into an organism of one or more specific genes into the somatic cells, germ line cells, or both, in order to correct a specific defect. The transferred DNA must integrate into the genome of the recipient so as to be transferred to both parents of mitosis of somatic cells. **gestalt t.** A form of psychotherapy emphasizing wholeness in reactions and achieving optimal balance in meaningfulness between focal and background experience. **group t.** GROUP PSYCHOTHERAPY. **heat t.** The use of heat for therapeutic purposes, principally for the relief of pain and relaxation of muscle spasm. Ways in which the heat is produced and applied include conductive heating, convective heating, conversive heating, radiant heating, reflex heating, superficial heating, and deep heating. **humidification t.** The treatment of inflammatory disease of the respiratory tract by ensuring maximum humidification of the inspired air, as by special tents with ultrasonic atomizers. **hyperbaric oxygen t.** Therapeutic use of air containing oxygen at greater than normal atmospheric pressure. It may be applied to an entire room such as an operating theater to increase oxygen carrying capacity of the blood, or be applied locally to an extremity or area of tissue breakdown, as in the treatment of decubitus ulcers. A special airtight chamber (hyperbaric chamber) is sometimes used in the treatment of carbon monoxide poisoning and gas gangrene. Hyperbaric oxygen therapy has also been used as an adjunct to radiotherapy in the treatment of certain cancers. Also *hybaroxia.* **hypoglycemic t.** The treatment of mental disorder, now rarely used, utilizing intramuscular injections of insulin to produce low blood sugar and, in consequence, sleepiness, semistupor, or coma depending upon the degree of hypoglycemia produced. Also *subcoma insulin therapy, ambulatory insulin treatment.* See also INSULIN COMA THERAPY. **immunosuppressive t.** Therapy designed to suppress the immune response, as in the treatment of autoimmune disease or in conjunction with organ transplantation. Chemotherapy, antilymphocyte serum, and x-ray treatment are utilized either singly or in combination. **insulin coma t.** A form of hypoglycemic therapy, used mainly for schizophrenic disorders, consisting of the inducement of a series of comas, each lasting between five and sixty minutes. Sometimes convulsions occur spontaneously during the period of coma, and sometimes electroconvulsive therapy is administered to the patient during one of more of the insulin comas. Also *insulin shock therapy, shock therapy* (imprecise), *hypoglycemic shock treatment.* **interstitial radiation t.** A method of radiation therapy consisting of the placement directly into the tissues of needles, seeds, or other types of implants containing radioactive material. Also *interstitial radiotherapy.* **interstitial radium t.** Radium therapy with the use of radioactive needles implanted in the neoplastic tissues. **intraosseous t.** The transfusion or infusion of fluid or cells into the medullary cavity of a bone, usually the tibia or sternum. **intrathecal t.** Any treatment which involves the injection of agents into the spinal theca. **intravenous t.** The administration of liquid therapeutic agents directly into a vein. **larval t.** MAGGOT THERAPY. **learning-theory t.** BEHAVIOR THERAPY. **light t.** Therapeutic use of light rays within the visible spectrum. The original concept, now obsolete, attributed various therapeutic properties to light of different colors. In modern contexts the concept may be applicable, for example, to the stimulation of photoneuroendocrine effects. **maggot t.**

An archaic method of wound débridement that used maggots or the larvae of certain flesh flies, such as the green-bottle fly (*Phaenicia sericata*), based on the assumption that they would eat only dead tissue. Maggots do feed largely on necrotic tissue and stimulate healing by their secretion of allantoin. Also *larval therapy, surgical maggot therapy.* **malarial t.** MALARIOTHERAPY. **malarization t.** MALARIOTHERAPY. **manipulative t.** Application of accurately determined, specifically directed manual forces to the body to improve mobility of restricted joints, to relieve pain, and purportedly, to improve function elsewhere in the body and enhance the sense of well-being. **marriage t.** COUPLES THERAPY. **megavoltage t.** SUPERVOLTAGE RADIOTHERAPY. **metatrophic t.** The use of a dietary program in conjunction with the administration of a drug or therapeutic agent to enhance its effectiveness. **multiple t.** *Seldom used* GROUP PSYCHOTHERAPY. **nondirective t.** NONDIRECTIVE COUNSELING. **nonspecific t.** Treatment of infections by the injection of nonspecific substances such as proteins, serum, or vaccines in an effort to stimulate general cell activity and host defenses against infection, or to produce fever. Also *paraspecific therapy.* **occupational t.** Therapy directed toward the restoration or maintenance of the ability to accomplish daily tasks of a specific occupational nature. It is a modern allied health science based on neurodevelopmental, biomechanical, and rehabilitative concepts. **organic t.** ORGANOTHERAPY. **oxygen t.** Therapy consisting in administration of additional oxygen by inhalation. **paraspecific t.** NONSPECIFIC THERAPY. **parenteral t.** The administration of a medication by some route other than the alimentary canal, usually by injection into a vein, muscle, or the skin. **physical t.** PHYSIOTHERAPY. **play t.** The use of toys and games in the psychiatric treatment of children as a substitute for the verbal productions that provide the majority of material in the treatment of adults. **protective t.** Treatment effected by relieving an organ or body part of its normal function to facilitate natural healing. Also *sparing therapy.* **psychoanalytic t.** PSYCHOANALYSIS. **pulp canal t.** ROOT CANAL TREATMENT. **radionuclide t.** The treatment of disease by means of oral, intravenous, or interstitial application of radioactive materials. **rational t.** Cognitive behavior therapy that utilizes an action-oriented and problem-solving approach while emphasizing the subject's responsibility for creating his own problems in living. **reflex t.** Treatment utilizing a physiological reflex to achieve a specific therapeutic effect, such as vasodilatation, relaxation of muscle spasm, or other effect. Also *reflexotherapy.* See also SYMPATHICOTHERAPY. **relaxation t.** A psychotherapeutic approach aimed at reducing negative emotions that are too easily aroused, such as fear, anger, or anxiety, by inducing a state of deep muscle relaxation. **replacement t.** Treatment involving the administration of natural body products or synthetic analogues to correct a deficiency, such as the hormonal treatment of a glandular deficiency, in which small, physiologic doses of the deficient hormone or hormones are given to replace the secretion lost through disease or ablation of the gland. Also *substitution therapy.* **rhythmic sensory bombardment t.** The intermittent, rhythmic application of sonic, photic, or tactile stimuli over a one-hour period as treatment for affective disorders and some types of psychoneurosis. **root canal t.** ROOT CANAL TREATMENT. **rotation t.** A method of radiotherapy in which the external source of radiation is rotated around the patient. The tumor or tissue-volume being treated is located at the center of rotation. Also *rotational radiation therapy.* **sclerosing t.** The introduction of a sclerosing solution into a vein to induce a chemical thrombosis. **shock t.** 1 *Imprecise* ELECTROCONVULSIVE THERAPY. 2 *Imprecise* INSULIN COMA THERAPY. **short-wave t.** See under SHORT-WAVE DIATHERMY. **sleep t.** CONTINUOUS SLEEP TREATMENT. **sleep-electroshock t.** The treatment of mental illness involving the induction of sleep with sedative or hypnotic drugs before the administration of electroconvulsive therapy. This method is sometimes used in patients who are unwilling to submit to electroconvulsive therapy. **social t.** Therapy structured to provide the mental patient with an integrated, stable, coherent milieu so that the optimal combination of treatments can be administered and so that every interpersonal and treatment experience of the patient will be synergistically applied toward realistic and specific therapeutic goals. **solar t.** HELIOTHERAPY. **somatic cell gene t.** See under GENE THERAPY. **sparing t.** PROTECTIVE THERAPY. **speech t.** The clinical assessment and management of a wide variety of conditions related to impairment of voice, speech, and language. The conditions included are developmental disorders of language acquisition and childhood dyspraxias and other neuromotor disorders, adult dysphonias, speech disorders as occur in the postlaryngectomy state, and aphasias following head injury and cerebrovascular accidents. **subcoma insulin t.** HYPOGLYCEMIC THERAPY. **substitution t.** REPLACEMENT THERAPY. **supervoltage t.** SUPERVOLTAGE RADIOTHERAPY. **supplementary x-ray t.** The supplemental use of x-ray treatment to organs or parts of the body which have already been treated by radium or other radioactive agents. **supportive t.** 1 Any treatment regimen or technique that supports or facilitates another treatment or the patient's own defenses. 2 A psychotherapeutic technique based on encouragement and reinforcement of the patient's ego defenses. **surgical maggot t.** MAGGOT THERAPY. **telecobalt t.** Treatment with gamma rays obtained from a source containing a capsule of radioactive cobalt and located at a distance from the body. **total-push t.** The simultaneous use of several types of psychiatric treatment, used particularly with schizophrenics. It includes physiotherapy, irradiation, exercise and games, diets, behavior modification, socialization, and other methods that are indicated for amelioration of the patient's symptoms. Also *total-push treatment.* **ultrasonic t.** The use of ultrasound for treatment in physical medicine and rehabilitation. **unilateral electroconvulsive t.** Electroconvulsive therapy in which current is applied only to one side of the head in an effort to minimize side effects and to restrict current mainly to the nondominant side of the brain. **x-ray t.** RADIOTHERAPY. **x-ray sieve t.** The therapeutic administration of x rays with the area of treatment covered by a radiation-absorbing shield containing pores of uniform sizes.

**Theridiidae** \ther′idē′idē\ A large family of spiders, the comb-footed spiders, characterized by comblike bristles on the hind tarsi and an irregular web in which the spider hangs in an inverted position. It includes the notorious venomous black widow spider, *Latrodectus mactans.*

**therm-** \thurm-, thərm-\ THERMO-.

**thermacogenesis** \thur′məkōjen′əsis\ [THERM- + *(pharm)aco-* + GENESIS] Drug activity that elevates the temperature of the body.

**thermal** \thur′məl\ [THERM- + -AL] **1** Relating to heat or temperature. **2** Characterized by heat or warmth or having heat-conserving qualities.

**thermalgesia** \thur′maljē′zē·ə\ THERMOALGESIA.

**thermalgia** \thərmal′jə\ [THERM- + -ALGIA] CAUSALGIA.

**thermanalgesia** \thur′manaljē′zē·ə\ THERMOANESTHESIA.
**thermanesthesia** \thur′manesthē′zhə\ THERMOANESTHESIA.
**thermesthesia** \thur′mesthē′zhə\ Temperature sensation; the ability to respond to heat and cold. Also *thermoesthesia, thermal sensitivity.*
**thermesthesiometer** \thur′mesthē′zē·äm′ətər\ An instrument for measuring the sensitivity of the skin to heat. Also *thermoesthesiometer.*
**thermhyperesthesia** \thərmhīp′əresthē′zhə\ [THERM- + HYPERESTHESIA] Excessive sensitivity to heat or cold. Also *thermohyperesthesia.*
**thermhypesthesia** \thurm′hīpesthē′zhə\ Diminished sensitivity to hot or cold stimuli. Also *thermohypesthesia, thermohypoesthesia.*
**thermic** \thur′mik\ Relating to heat or temperature; thermal.
**thermion** \thur′mē·än\ [THERM- + English *ion*] An electron or other charged particle liberated from a heated surface.
**thermionics** \thur′mē·än′iks\ [THERMION + -ICS] The study of the emission of charged particles from heated surfaces.
**thermistor** \thur′mistər\ A resistive temperature sensor with a large negative temperature coefficient.
**thermo-** \thur′mō-\ [Gk *thermē* heat] A combining form meaning heat. Also *therm-.*
**thermoalgesia** \-aljē′zē·ə\ [THERMO- + ALGESIA] Pain caused by heat. Also *thermalgesia.* Adj. thermoalgesic.
**thermoanaesthesia** *Brit.* THERMOANESTHESIA.
**thermoanalgesia** \-an′aljē′zē·ə\ THERMOANESTHESIA.
**thermoanesthesia** \-an′esthē′zhə\ Loss of the normal sense of temperature, or loss of ability to differentiate between hot and cold. Also *thermoanalgesia, thermanalgesia, thermanesthesia.* Adj. thermoanesthetic.
**thermoasymmetry** \-āsim′ətrē\ A difference in temperature noted between corresponding parts of the body on the two sides as seen in unilateral lesions of sympathetic pathways.
**thermocauterectomy** \-kô′tərek′təmē\ The excision of tissue or an organ using a heated wire or cautery.
**thermocautery** \-kô′tərē\ **1** A surgical cauterization device utilizing a hot wire or pointed tool. **2** Any form of cautery using heat.
**thermochroic** \-krō′ik\ **1** Pertaining to the differential properties of heat radiation with respect to refraction, reflection, and absorption, depending on wavelength. **2** Having the property of differentially transmitting, absorbing, or changing radiant heat depending on wavelength.
**thermochroism** \-krō′izm\ **1** The differential properties of heat radiation with respect to refraction, reflection, and absorption, depending on wavelength. **2** The property of certain substances which differentially transmit, absorb, or change radiant heat depending on wavelength. For defs. 1 and 2 also *thermochrosis.*
**thermocoagulation** \-kō·ag′yəlā′shən\ Destruction and removal of tissue by coagulation utilizing high-frequency electric current.
**thermocouple** \thur′məkup′əl\ A temperature sensor formed from the junction of two dissimilar conductors and which produces an electromotive force that varies with temperature. Also *thermojunction.*
**thermodilution** \-dīloo′shən\ [THERMO- + DILUTION] A technique for measuring blood flow by the introduction of relatively cold fluid of known quantity into the circulation. By measuring the fall in temperature by a thermistor the volume in which the cold fluid has been diluted can be calculated.
**thermoduric** \-d^yoo′rik\ Able to tolerate high temperatures.
**thermodynamics** \-dīnam′iks\ [THERMO- + DYNAMICS] The branch of physics dealing with the macroscopic properties of matter, and with macroscopic transfers of energy, in situations where temperature is a significant variable.
**thermoelectricity** \-ē′lektris′itē\ Heat-generated electricity.
**thermoesthesia** \-esthē′zhə\ THERMESTHESIA.
**thermoesthesiometer** \-esthē′zē·äm′ətər\ THERMESTHESIOMETER.
**thermogenesis** \-jen′əsis\ The production of heat, especially heat production by the body. Adj. thermogenic. **dietary induced t.** A rise in body temperature occurring during digestion. It is related to the specific dynamic action of food. **nonshivering t.** A heat-producing mechanism which liberates chemical energy due to processes not involved in muscle contraction. It is controlled by the hypothalamus thermoregulatory centers and effector pathways involving the sympathetic nervous system. At target cells catecholamines have a calorigenic action. **shivering t.** Body heat production through the muscular activity of shivering. Both shivering and nonshivering thermogenesis can collectively contribute to body heat production.
**thermography** \thərmäg′rəfē\ [THERMO- + -GRAPHY] The examination or recording of an image of the variations in surface temperatures of an object by detecting the infrared radiation emitted by the object.
**thermohyperalgesia** \-hī′pəraljē′zē·ə\ Pain induced by hot or cold stimuli at thresholds lower than normal.
**thermohyperesthesia** \-hī′pəresthē′zhə\ THERMHYPERESTHESIA.
**thermohypesthesia** \-hī′pesthē′zhə\ THERMHYPESTHESIA.
**thermohypoesthesia** \-hī′pō·esthē′zhə\ THERMHYPESTHESIA.
**thermointegrator** \-in′təgrā′tər\ An apparatus for measuring the environmental warmth experienced by a living organism, which is typically in a chamber with controlled radiation, convection, and conduction.
**thermojunction** \-jungk′shən\ THERMOCOUPLE.
**thermolabile** \-lā′bīl\ Readily altered by heat.
**thermology** \thərmäl′əjē\ [THERMO- + -LOGY] The study of heat and heat-associated phenomena. Also *thermotics.*
**thermoluminescence** \-loo′mines′əns\ The phenomenon in which radiant energy absorbed by certain materials, such as lithium fluoride, is later released in the form of light when these materials are heated.
**thermolysis** \thərmäl′isis\ The breakdown of a substance induced by heating it. Adj. thermolytic.
**thermomassage** \-məsäzh′\ Massage given in conjunction with deep or superficial application of heat.
**thermometer** \thərmäm′ətər\ [THERMO- + -METER] An instrument for measuring temperature. **air t.** A gas thermometer in which air is used to measure changes in temperature. **alcohol t.** A liquid-in-glass thermometer in which alcohol is used to measure changes in temperature. Also *spirit thermometer.* **Beckmann t.** A thermometer with a fine bore that is used to measure small temperature differences. **bimetal t.** A thermometer which measures changes in temperature by alterations in the curled shape of two metals having different coefficients of expansion that are bonded together. **Celsius t.** A thermometer calibrated by the Celsius scale. See under SCALE. Also *centigrade ther-*

*mometer.* **clinical t.** A mercury thermometer designed to measure the maximum temperature at the recording site of the body. This temperature will continue to be recorded until the thermometer is shaken to reset it. It is commonly used to measure the temperature in the mouth, axilla, or rectum. Also *fever thermometer.* **depth t.** A thermometer designed to measure the temperature at sites within the tissues of the body. **differential t.** A thermometer for measuring small temperature differences. Also *thermoscope, metastatic thermometer.* **Fahrenheit t.** A thermometer calibrated by the Fahrenheit scale. See under SCALE. **fever t.** CLINICAL THERMOMETER. **gas t.** A thermometer measuring changes in temperature by the expansion or contraction of some common gas, as air, helium, or oxygen. **globe t.** A thermometer used for measuring radiant temperature and consisting of a hollow, black, nonreflecting copper sphere of about 15 cm diameter with the thermometer bulb at the center. **half-minute t.** A clinical thermometer designed to equilibrate with a water bath temperature within thirty seconds. **Kelvin t.** A thermometer calibrated by the Kelvin scale. See under SCALE. **liquid-in-glass t.** A thermometer measuring changes in temperature by the expansion or contraction of a liquid, as alcohol or mercury, within a narrow, calibrated tube. **maximum t.** A thermometer designed to record the highest temperature to which it has been exposed. **mercury t.** A liquid-in-glass thermometer in which mercury is used to measure changes in temperature. **metastatic t.** DIFFERENTIAL THERMOMETER. **minimum t.** A thermometer designed to record the lowest temperature to which it has been exposed. **spirit t.** ALCOHOL THERMOMETER. **surface t.** A thermometer designed to measure the temperature of the skin or other body surface.

**thermometry** \thərmäm′ətrē\ [THERMO- + -METRY] The measurement of temperature, most often by using a thermometer or thermocouple.

**thermopenetration** \-pen′ətrā′shən\ **1** The conversive heating of tissues at depth, as by short wave, microwave, or ultrasound. **2** The measured amount of heat produced at a given depth of tissue.

**thermophile** \thur′məfīl\ [THERMO- + -PHILE] An organism that grows at high temperatures. Some organisms found in natural hot springs can grow at 90°C.

**thermophore** \thur′məfôr\ [THERMO- + -PHORE] A substance or device capable of retaining heat that may be utilized in a therapeutic heat pack.

**thermopile** \thur′məpīl\ A temperature sensor formed from several thermocouples connected in series and more sensitive than a single thermocouple. Also *thermoelectric pile.*

**thermoplacentography** \-plas′əntäg′rəfē\ Use of thermography to determine the site of placental attachment. This site is indicated by a temperature rise caused by the large blood flow.

**thermoplegia** \-plē′jə\ [THERMO- + -PLEGIA] HEATSTROKE.

**thermopolypnea** \-päl′ipnē′ə\ An increased rate of pulmonary respiration due to pyrexia. Adj. thermopolypneic.

**thermoradiotherapy** \-rā′dē·ōther′əpē\ A method of treatment which combines the use of ionizing radiation and heat. It is based on the hypothesis that heat increases the radiosensitivity of tissues.

**thermoreceptor** \-risep′tər\ Any nerve ending or other sensory receptor which is specifically sensitive to heat or cold.

**thermoscope** \thur′məskōp\ [THERMO- + -SCOPE] DIFFERENTIAL THERMOMETER.

**thermostromuhr** \-shtrōm′oor′, -strō′moor′ \ [THERMO- + STROMUHR] An instrument for measuring blood flow in a vessel, consisting of a heating element between two thermocouples applied to the outside of the vessel.

**thermosystaltism** \-sis′təltizm\ A muscular contraction that takes place in response to heat.

**thermotics** \thərmät′iks\ THERMOLOGY.

**thermotoxin** \-täk′sin\ A poisonous material produced by living tissue as a response to heat exposure.

**thermotropic** \-träp′ik\ Exhibiting thermotropism. Also *caloritropic.*

**thermotropism** \thərmät′rəpizm\ [THERMO- + TROPISM] A condition in which cells or multicellular organisms move in response to a temperature gradient, either toward a region of warmer temperature (positive thermotropism) or toward a colder region (negative thermotropism).

**theromorph** \thir′əmôrf\ [Gk *thēr* a wild animal + *o* + -MORPH] A fetus or postnatal individual or a part thereof which bears a fancied or real resemblance to the form of a lower animal. Such a similarity has been seen between the head of the anencephalic infant and that of a monkey.

**thesaurismosis** \thē′sôrismō′sis\ [Gk *thēsaurism(a)* (akin to *tithenai* to place, put) a store, treasure + -OSIS] *Outmoded* STORAGE DISEASE. **amyloid t.** AMYLOIDOSIS. **calcium t.** CALCINOSIS.

**thesaurosis** \thē′sôrō′sis\ *Outmoded* STORAGE DISEASE.

**theta** \thāt′ə\ The name of the eighth letter of the Greek alphabet. Symbol: $\theta$

**thevetin** \thev′ətin\ A cardiac glycoside obtained from *Thevetia* species. It is similar in action to digitalis. Upon hydrolysis, it yields glucose, thevetose, and digitoxigenin. The yellow oleander contains this compound in quantities capable of causing severe poisoning and even death in man and animals.

**THF** tetrahydrofolate.

**thi-** \thī-\ THIO-.

**thiabendazole** $C_{10}H_7N_3S$. 2-(4-Thiazolyl)-1*H*-benzimidazole. A broad-spectrum anthelmintic effective against threadworms, roundworms, creeping eruption, and hookworm infections. It is the best available treatment for strongyloidiasis. It is also used for worm infestations in veterinary medicine.

**thiacetazone** $C_{10}H_{12}N_4OS$. *N*-[4- [[(Aminothiomethyl)-hydrazono]methylene]phenyl]acetamide. An antitubercular drug which is often used in combination with isoniazid. Thiacetazone decreases the degree of isoniazid resistance developing from chronic use. It is given orally.

**thiambutosine** $C_{19}H_{25}N_3OS$. 1-(4-Butoxyphenyl)-3-(4-dimethylaminophenyl)thiourea. An antileprotic drug that is given orally but is poorly (about 10%) absorbed from the gastrointestinal tract. The value of the drug is limited by the resistance that usually develops to the agent within one or two years of treatment.

**thiamin** \thī′əmin\ One of the B vitamins, making up part of the coenzyme thiamin pyrophosphate. Its molecule consist of a thiazolium ring carrying methyl and 2-hydroxyethyl substituents on C-4 and C-5 and alkylated on nitrogen by a $CH_2$ group which is also the 5-substituent on 4-amino-2-methylpyrimidine. Deficiency of this vitamin prevents the breakdown of carbohydrates, which eventually leads to beriberi. Also *vitamin $B_1$, aneurin, antineuritic factor, antiberiberi factor, antineuritic vitamin, thiamine.*

**thiamine** THIAMIN.

**thiamin pyrophosphate** The ester formed between diphosphoric acid and the hydroxyl group of thiamin. It is a component of the decarboxylase of the dehydrogenase complexes that act on pyruvate and other 2-oxoacids, and also of transketolase. It easily loses $H^+$ from C-2 of its thiazole ring to form a species capable of adding to the carbonyl group of 2-oxoacids, whose decarboxylation it catalyzes by the electron withdrawal it exerts. Also *cocarboxylase* (outmoded).

**thiamin pyrophosphatase** NUCLEOSIDEDIPHOSPHATASE.

**thiamylal sodium** SODIUM THIAMYLAL.

***Thiara*** \thī-er′ə\ [New L] A genus of snails of the family Thiaridae. The habitat is fresh water and brackish water, and the distribution is worldwide. Several species are the intermediate hosts of trematode parasites including *Paragonimus, Metagonimus, Haplorchis,* and *Prohemistomum*. Some species are ovoviviparous and bear dorsal brood pouches while many females are parthenogenetic, enabling a single individual to initiate a new colony. Also *Melanoides*.

**thiazides** A class of drugs of the basic benzene disulfonamide composition, having diuretic properties. They inhibit the renal reabsorption of sodium, and increase the tubular excretion of chloride ion, thus increasing the excretion of water. Also *benzothiadiazides*.

**thiazole** Any substance with a five-membered ring containing one sulfur atom, one nitrogen atom, and three CH groups. The term is usually restricted to 1,3-thiazole, which has sulfur and nitrogen atoms at positions 1 and 3 respectively.

**thiazolium** The cation formed by combination of $H^+$ with the nitrogen of thiazole, and hence any substance in which this added hydrogen is substituted, e.g. by an alkyl group.

**Thibierge** [Georges *Thibierge*, French physician, 1856–1926] Thibierge-Weissenbach syndrome. See under SYNDROME.

**thickness / half-value t.** HALF-VALUE LAYER.

**Thiemann** [H. *Thiemann*, Dutch surgeon, flourished early 20th century] See under DISEASE.

**thiemia** \thī-ē′mē-ə\ The presence of abnormal compounds of sulfur in the blood. *Seldom used.*

**thienamycin** $C_{11}H_{16}N_2O_4S$. 3-[(2-Aminoethyl)thio]-6-(1-hydroxyethyl)-7-oxo-1-azabicyclo-[3.2.0]-hept-2-ene-2-carboxylic acid. An antibiotic agent obtained from *Streptomyces cattleya*.

**Thiers** [Joseph *Thiers*, French physician, born 1885] Achard-Thiers syndrome. See under SYNDROME.

**Thiersch** [Karl *Thiersch*, German surgeon and embryologist, 1822–1895] **1** Thiersch operation. See under OLLIER-THIERSCH GRAFT. **2** See under KNIFE, OPERATION, CANALICULUS.

**thigh** [Old English *thēoh*] The part of the lower limb between the hip and the knee; femur. **cricket t.** Partial or complete rupture of the rectus femoris muscle or the patellar tendon.

**thigh-lift** A cosmetic operation on the thighs, usually done through circumferential incisions at the level of the groin and gluteal folds, to excise redundant skin and excess fat. The purpose is to eliminate apparent bulges and sags from the surface of the thighs, producing a better contour.

**thigmesthesia** \thig′mesthē′zhə\ [*thigm(o)-* + ESTHESIA] Touch perception.

**thigmo-** \thig′mō-\ [Gk *thigma* a touching, contact] A combining form meaning touch, contact.

**thigmotaxis** \thig′mətak′sis\ [THIGMO- + TAXIS] Organismic movement towards or away from a mechanical displacement.

**thigmotropic** \thig′mətrāp′ik\ Pertaining to thigmotropism.

**thigmotropism** \thigmät′rəpizm\ [THIGMO- + TROPISM] The orientation of an organism in response to a mechanical displacement.

**thimble** \thim′bəl\ [Old English *thȳmel*, from *thūma* thumb] COPING.

**thimerosal** $C_9H_9HgNaO_2S$. Ethyl(2-mercaptobenzoato-S)mercury sodium salt. An organomercury compound with anti-infective properties that is used locally on the skin for minor injuries and abrasions.

**thinking** The mental process of maintaining a coherent train of ideas or a series of symbolic representations of events, objects, or relationships that are available from memory, and of mentally operating on or reorganizing their configuration in a way that leads to a conclusion or to the solving of a problem. See also COGNITION. **autistic t.** Thinking that focuses on the self to the exclusion of appropriate involvement with external reality. Also *dereistic thinking*. **concrete t.** Thought processes strongly influenced by the specific instance or individual fact or event, rather than by how that instance may relate to others of the kind or to more general categories of experience. Thinking of this kind is characteristic of lowered levels of brain function, as in dementia or certain forms of brain damage. Also *concretism, concretization*. **dereistic t.** AUTISTIC THINKING. **preoperational t.** That stage in cognitive growth, between two and seven years approximately, during which the developing child begins to think in symbolic terms about aspects of the world not physically present. While the operations typical of logical thought have yet to emerge, a first step in that direction is evident in the processes of perception and intuition. **pressured t.** PRESSURE OF IDEAS.

**thio-** \thī′ə-\ [Gk *thei(on)* brimstone, sulfur] **1** A combining form used in organic chemistry, always prefixed with another combining form, to indicate substitution by a substituted sulfur atom, e.g. methylthio- for $CH_3$—S—. **2** A combining form used in organic chemistry to indicate replacement of an oxygen atom by a sulfur atom, e.g. thiourea, $NH_2$—CS—$NH_2$, thioester, R—CS—O—R′ (or, more commonly, R—CO—S—R′). Also *thi-, thion-*.

**thioarsenite** $C_{11}H_{12}AsNO_5S_2$. [[[4-(Aminocarbonyl)-phenyl]arsinidene]bis(thio)]biacetic acid. A mercaptoarsino-derivative that has been used in the treatment of intestinal amebiasis.

**thiobarbituric acid** $C_4H_4N_2O_2S$. The product resulting from the condensation of malonic acid and thiourea. It is the prototype member of the thiobarbiturate series.

**thiochrome** [THIO- + CHROME] A yellow pigment with blue fluorescence formed by oxidation of thiamin. Its formation may be used to assay the content of thiamin in a sample.

**thioctic acid** LIPOIC ACID.

**thioester** An ester containing one sulfur atom in place of an oxygen atom. Thioesters are of two types, R—CS—O—R′ and R—CO—S—R′. The latter is of great biologic importance, being an acylating agent and also capable of losing $H^+$ from the R group in some enzymatic reactions, e.g. from acetyl-CoA in the reaction of citrate synthase.

**thioether** Any compound in which a sulfur atom carries two alkyl groups. Biologically the most important is methionine. Also *sulfide*.

**thioglucose** Glucose with one of its oxygen atoms replaced by sulfur. The commonest is 5-thioglucose, in which the ring oxygen is replaced. This is used as a glucose analogue in biochemical studies; it inhibits glucose transport.

**thioglycolate** An anion, salt, or ester of thioglycolic acid.

**thioglycolic acid** HS—$CH_2$—COOH. A liquid with a

smell resembling that of hydrogen sulfide. It is miscible with water, ethanol, and organic solvents. On storage it self-esterifies. The thioesters formed are acylating agents in neutral aqueous solution. For this reason it is no longer much used as a reducing agent in protein chemistry. It has been used as a depilatory, and to soften hair by its action on reducing SS bonds of proteins. Some of its salts are also used as medicaments (bismuth and sodium, antimony and sodium, etc.).

**thioguanine** Normally 6-thioguanine, guanine in which the oxygen atom is replaced by sulfur. It is used in biochemical studies as a guanine analogue, but its base-pairing properties are unlike those of guanine. It is also used as an antineoplastic drug in the treatment of acute granulocytic anemia. Also *2-amino-6-mercaptopurine.*

**thiol** \thī′ôl\ Any compound containing the —S—H group, or that group itself. The group easily loses $H^+$ to form the powerfully nucleophilic thiolate anion. Also *mercaptan* (obs.). See also SULFHYDRYL.

**thiolase** Any enzyme that catalyzes the reaction between a compound R—R′ and a thiol R″—SH to form R—S—R″ and R′—H, especially acetyl-CoA acetyltransferase, which catalyzes the reaction of acetoacetyl-CoA with coenzyme A to form two molecules of acetyl-CoA. *Obs.*

**thiolate** The ion derived from a thiol by loss of a hydrogen ion, or a salt containing such an ion. It has the structure $R—S^-$, and is a strong nucleophile. Cysteine residues in enzymes often function after conversion into the thiolate form. Also *mercaptide* (obs.).

**thiol ester** One of the two types of thioester, the one with the grouping —CO—S—. It is the one of considerable biologic importance, as in acetyl-CoA and in the acyl enzyme of glyceraldehyde-3-phosphate dehydrogenase. Such compounds are powerful acylating agents. Formation of a thiol ester also facilitates loss of H-2 as $H^+$ from an acid, as in the condensation of acetyl-CoA with oxaloacetate to form citrate.

**thiomersalate** An organic compound of mercury, consisting of benzoate with the substituent $C_2H_5$—Hg—S— on C-2. It is used as a bacteriocide and fungicide.

**thion-** \thī′ən-\ THIO-.

**thioneine** ERGOTHIONEINE.

**thiopanic acid** $CH_2OH{\cdot}C(CH_3)_2{\cdot}CHOH{\cdot}CO{\cdot}NH{\cdot}CH_2{\cdot}CH_2SO_2OH$. A compound that acts as an inhibitor of bacterial growth in competition with pantothenic acid. Also *pantoyl taurine.*

**thiopentone** SODIUM THIOPENTAL.

**thiopropazate dihydrochloride** $C_{23}H_{28}ClN_3O_2S{\cdot}2HCl$. 4-[3-(2-Chlorophenothiazin-10-yl)-propyl]-1-piperazine-ethanol acetate dihydrochloride. A phenothiazine tranquilizer and antipsychotic drug. It is given orally.

**thioredoxin** A heat-stable protein of 108 residues, containing one disulfide bridge and occurring in organisms from bacteria to mammals. Like glutaredoxin its reduced form is capable of donating reducing equivalents in the reduction of ribonucleotides to form 2′-deoxyribonucleotides, which are required for DNA biosynthesis. Its oxidized form can be reconverted into its reduced form, which contains two sulfhydryl groups, by thioredoxin reductase, using NADPH as reductant. It is also able to reduce various disulfides to thiols.

**thioredoxin reductase** The enzyme (EC 1.6.4.5) that catalyzes the reduction of the disulfide bond of thioredoxin with concomitant oxidation of NADPH. The enzyme, like its substrate, contains a single, reducible disulfide. It is a flavoprotein.

**thioridazine** $C_{21}H_{26}N_2S_2$. 10-[2-(1-Methyl-2-piperidyl)-ethyl]-2-(methylthio)phenothiazine. A tranquilizer and antipsychotic agent with actions and uses like those of chlorpromazine. It is given orally.

**thioridazine hydrochloride** $C_{21}H_{26}N_2S_2{\cdot}HCl$. 10-[2-(1-Methyl-2-piperidyl)ethyl]-2-(methylthio)phenothiazine hydrochloride. The hydrochloride salt of thioridazine, with the same actions and uses as a tranquilizer as the parent drug. It is given orally.

**thiosemicarbazone** METHISAZONE.

**thiostrepton** \-strep′tän\ A sulfur-containing antibiotic that inhibits protein synthesis in prokaryotes by blocking the attachment of EFTu and of EFG to the ribosome.

**thiosulfate** The ion $^-S—SO_3^-$ or a salt containing it, or, rarely, a compound $R—S—SO_3$. The salt is used for titrating iodine, which oxidizes it to tetrathionate, often to determine the quantity of iodine used or produced in a reaction.

**thiosulfate sulfurtransferase** A liver enzyme (EC 2.8.1.1) that catalyzes the reaction: $S^-—SO_3^- + CN^- \rightarrow S^-—CN + SO_3^{2-}$. Its function is unknown, but may be the removal of cyanide. Also *rhodanese.*

**thiourea** \-yoorē′ə\ $NH_2—CS—NH_2$. A substance similar in properties to urea, but more easily alkylated on sulfur to form compounds of structure $NH_2—C(=NH_2^+)—S—R$, and also differing in that it can be oxidized to a dimer containing a disulfide bond.

**thioxanthene** Any of a group of tricyclic compounds having the dibenzothiopyran nucleus. They resemble phenothiazines, with a carbon atom rather than a nitrogen atom in the central ring. Chlorprothixene and thiothixene are included as psychotropic drugs of this class.

**Thiry** [Ludwig *Thiry,* Austrian physiologist, 1817–1897] Thiry fistula, Thiry-Vella fistula. See under FISTULA.

**thixotropism** \thiksät′rəpizm\ THIXOTROPY.

**thixotropy** \thiksät′rəpē\ The property, found in certain gels, of liquefying upon agitation and resuming the gel state upon standing. Also *thixotropism, reclotting phenomenon.*

**Thoma** [Richard *Thoma,* German histologist, 1847–1923] 1 Thoma-Zeiss counting cell. See under THOMA-ZEISS COUNTING CHAMBER. 2 Thoma's liquid. See under FLUID. 3 See under AMPULLA.

**Thomas** [André *Thomas,* French physician, born 1867] 1 Dejerine-Thomas atrophy. See under OLIVOPONTOCEREBELLAR DEGENERATION. 2 Thomas sign. See under HOLMES REBOUND PHENOMENON.

**Thomas** [Hugh Owen *Thomas,* English surgeon, 1834–1891] 1 See under HEEL. 2 Thomas knee splint. See under SPLINT.

**Thomas** [Theodore Gaillard *Thomas,* U.S. physician, 1831–1903] See under PESSARY.

**Thomas Morton** See under MORTON.

**Thompson** [Sir Henry *Thompson,* English surgeon, 1820–1904] See under TEST.

**Thomsen** [Asmus Julius Thomas *Thomsen,* Danish physician, 1815–1896] Thomsen's disease. See under MYOTONIA CONGENITA.

**Thomsen** [Oluf *Thomsen,* Danish physician, 1878–1940] Thomsen antibody. See under T ANTIBODY.

**Thomson** [Frederick Holland *Thomson,* English physician, 1867–1938] Thomson sign. See under PASTIA'S LINES.

**Thomson** [Sir Joseph John *Thomson,* English physicist, 1856–1940] Thomson scattering. See under COHERENT SCATTERING.

**Thomson** [Matthew Sidney *Thomson,* English dermatologist, 1894–1969] Poikiloderma congenitale of Thomson. See under ROTHMUND-THOMSON SYNDROME.

**thonzylamine hydrochloride** $C_{16}H_{23}ClN_4O$. *N*-[(4-Methoxyphenyl)methyl]-N′,N′-dimethyl-*N*-2-pyrimidinyl-1,2-

ethanediamine monohydrochloride. One of the older, ethylenediamine-type, antihistaminic agents, prescribed as a syrup or oral tablet.

**thorac-** \thôras-, thôrak-\ THORACO-.

**thoracectomy** \thôr′əsek′təmē\ [THORAC- + -ECTOMY] A resection of a segment of rib.

**thoracentesis** \thôr′əsentē′sis\ [THORAC- + -*(c)entesis*] The drainage of fluid from the pleural space, usually by needle puncture and aspiration. Also *thoracocentesis, paracentesis of the chest, pleuracentesis, pleurocentesis, paracentesis thoracis.*

**thoraces** \thôr′əsēz\ Plural of THORAX.

**thoracic** \thôras′ik\ Of or relating to the thorax. Also *thoracal.*

**thoracico-** \thôras′ikō-\ THORACO-.

**thoracicolumbar** \-lum′bär\ THORACOLUMBAR.

**thoraco-** \thôr′əkō-\ [Gk *thōrax* (genitive *thōrakos*) chest] A combining form denoting the chest or thorax. Also *thorac-, thoracico-.*

**thoracoceloschisis** \-sēläs′kisis\ [THORACO- + CELO-[2] + Gk *schisis* a cleaving, division] Failure of closure of the embryonic body wall, leaving the thoracic and abdominal cavities or major parts thereof exposed ventrally.

**thoracocentesis** \-sentē′sis\ THORACENTESIS.

**thoracocyrtosis** \-sirtō′sis\ [THORACO- + Gk *kyrt(os)* curved + -OSIS] An abnormal curvature of the chest. *Imprecise.*

**thoracodorsal** \-dôr′səl\ Pertaining to the posterior region of the external surface of the chest.

**thoracodynia** \-din′ē·ə\ [THORAC- + -ODYNIA] Any pain in the chest.

**thoracogastropagus** \-gasträp′əgəs\ [THORACO- + GASTRO- + -PAGUS] Equal conjoined twins linked in the thoracic and abdominal regions. Also *gastrothoracopagus.*

**thoracolaparotomy** \-lap′ərät′əmē\ [THORACO- + LAPAROTOMY] A surgical incision into the thoracic and abdominal cavities.

**thoracolumbar** \-lum′bär\ Pertaining to the thoracic and the lumbar portions of the vertebral column or the spinal cord: used specifically to denote the ganglia and fibers of the sympathetic part of the autonomic nervous system. Also *thoracicolumbar.*

**thoracolysis** \thôr′əkäl′isis\ [THORACO- + LYSIS] An incision of pleural adhesions.

**thoracomelus** \thôr′əkäm′ələs\ [THORACO- + Gk *melos* a limb] A fetus or postnatal individual with an extra arm or leg attached to the thorax. The extra limb, if an arm, may be the result of duplication of one of the usual arms, or it may be the only external indication of an extreme degree of union of conjoined twins. **t. parasiticus** Unequal conjoined twins in which the parasitic member is represented by a limb, probably only a leg, attached to the thorax.

**thoracomyodynia** \-mī′ədin′ē·ə\ [THORACO- + MY- + -ODYNIA] Pain originating in the muscles of the chest wall.

**thoracoomphalopagus** \thôr′əkō·am′fəläp′əgəs\ Equal conjoined twins exhibiting extensive union in the thoracic and abdominal regions but with definite duplication in the cephalic and caudal regions. It is a rare teratism.

**thoracopagus** \thôr′əkäp′əgəs\ [THORACO- + -PAGUS] Equal conjoined twins united in the thoracic region, usually at the sternum. **t. parasiticus** Unequal conjoined twins of which the parasitic member is attached to the thorax, usually at the sternum, of the host. **tribrachial t.** A thoracopagus united along the lateral aspect of the thoraces with a single arm attached at some point along the line of fusion. The unattached aspects of the respective thoraces are associated with two normal shoulder girdles and arms. Also *tribrachius.*

**thoracoparacephalus** \-par′əsef′ələs\ [THORACO- + PARA- + -CEPHALUS] A form of thoracopagus parasiticus in which the parasitic member is represented by a rudimentary head attached to the thorax of the host.

**thoracoplasty** \thôr′əkōplas′tē\ [THORACO- + -PLASTY] The removal of a segment of rib, thereby causing the chest wall to collapse inward upon a diseased lung. Also *pleuropneumonolysis.* **costoversion t.** The surgical use of removed ribs by placing them in a reversed position to provide a strut. Occasionally a rib is placed vertically to form a concaved bony framework to reduce peridoxic movement of the chest wall during healing. **lateral t.** The removal of a varying number of lower ribs to obliterate an empyema space. It is designed to avoid collapsing the apical portion of the chest wall.

**thoracoschisis** \thôr′əkäs′kisis\ [THORACO- + -SCHISIS] The failure of closure of the thoracic cavity by completion of the embryonic body wall in the region of the sternum. It is usually accompanied by ectopia cordis.

**thoracoscope** \thôrak′əskōp\ [THORACO- + -SCOPE] An instrument that is passed through the chest wall for visual inspection of the pleural spaces.

**thoracoscopy** \thôr′əkäs′kəpē\ Examination of the pleural space by means of a thoracoscope.

**thoracostomy** \thôr′əkäs′təmē\ [THORACO- + -STOMY] The surgical establishment of an opening in the chest wall for the purposes of draining the chest cavity.

**Thoraeus** [Robert *Thoraeus,* Swedish physicist, flourished 20th century] See under FILTER.

**thorax** \thôr′aks, thō′raks\ [Gk *thōrax* a breastplate, the chest] (*pl.* thoraces) The upper part of the trunk between the neck and the abdomen, which contains the heart and great vessels and the lungs, trachea, and bronchi; the chest. Its skeleton comprises the twelve thoracic vertebrae posteriorly, twelve pairs of ribs and their costal cartilages, and the sternum. It communicates with the neck through the inlet of thorax. Its outlet is closed by the diaphragm which separates it from the abdominal cavity. The pectoral girdles are attached to it at the sternoclavicular joints and by several muscles. It functions primarily during respiration. **barrel-shaped t.** BARREL CHEST.

**Thorazine** A proprietary name for chlorpromazine hydrochloride.

**Thorel** [Charles *Thorel,* German pathologist, 1868–1935] See under BUNDLE.

**thorium** \thôr′ē·əm\ Element number 90, having atomic weight 232.038. A metal in the actinide series, thorium has 12 isotopes of atomic masses 223 to 234, all of them unstable. The naturally occurring thorium 232 emits alpha particles and has a half-life of $1.41 \times 10^{10}$ years. One of its decay products is the radioactive thoron. It eventually decays to a stable isotope of lead. Symbol: Th

**thorium dioxide** $ThO_2$. A chemical substance formerly used as a positive contrast agent in roentgenography; thorotrast. This material is no longer used because of the radioactivity of thorium.

**Thormählen** [Johann *Thormählen,* German physician, flourished early 20th century] See under TEST.

**Thorn** [George Widmer *Thorn,* U.S. physician, born 1906] Thorn syndrome. See under SALT-DEPLETION SYNDROME.

**Thorn** [Wilhelm *Thorn,* German gynecologist, born 1857] See under MANEUVER.

**Thornton** [Lawson *Thornton,* U.S. surgeon, born 1884] See under NAIL.

**Thornwaldt** See under TORNWALDT.

**thoron** An alpha-emitting isotope of radon formed in the

radioactive disintegration series that begins with thorium 232 and having a half-life of 55.6 seconds. Its mass number is 220. • See note at EMANATION.

**thorotrast** A preparation containing the dioxide of thorium 232, formerly used as a contrast medium in radiography, but no longer used because of its radioactivity.

**Thorson** [Ake *Thorson*, Swedish physician, flourished 20th century] Biörck-Thorson syndrome. See under CARCINOID SYNDROME.

**thought** / **audible t.** A thought that the patient hears as being spoken inside his head, an auditory hallucination.

**Thr** Symbol for threonine.

**threadworm** A nematode worm of the genus *Strongyloides.* • The term is sometimes applied loosely to any of various other small parasitic roundworms, such as *Enterobius vermicularis.*

**threonine** \thrē′ənēn\ $CH_3$—CHOH—$CH(NH_3^+)$—$COO^-$. One of the twenty amino acids that are incorporated into proteins. It is essential in the mammalian diet. Threonine residues in enzymes may be phosphorylated in processes that control enzyme activity, and those in glycoproteins may be glycosylated. Symbol: Thr, T

**threonine dehydratase** The enzyme that catalyzes the conversion of threonine into 2-oxobutyrate and ammonia. It is a pyridoxal enzyme and first forms enzyme-bound 2-aminocrotonic acid, which spontaneously decomposes to form oxobutyrate and ammonia. In bacteria different forms exist: one, whose function is degradative, is activated by lack of glucose; another, whose function is a step in isoleucine biosynthesis, is inhibited by the presence of isoleucine.

**threose** A four-carbon aldose sugar, the D sugar having the (2*S*,3*R*)-configuration. It is thus the 2-epimer of the biologically more important sugar erythrose.

**threpsis** \threp′sis\ [Gk *threpsis* (from *trephein* to nourish) nourishment] NUTRITION.

**threshold** [Old English *threscwald*] The minimum amount of stimulus energy required to elicit a particular sensation or response in an experimental subject under otherwise optimal conditions of measurement. Also *absolute threshold, stimulus threshold, sensitivity threshold, schwelle.* **achromatic t.** 1 The minimal photic energy for detection of light. 2 The level of photic reduction of a chromatic stimulus below which hue discrimination is lost. Also *colorless visual threshold.* **alpha t.** The energy an alpha particle must have to escape the binding forces within the nucleus in alpha decay. If the binding energy released by combination of two neutrons and two protons within the nucleus is less than 28.3 MeV (the binding energy of an alpha particle), the nucleus is susceptible to alpha decay. This condition is generally true for nuclei with atomic number equal to or greater than 60, where the binding energy per nucleon is 6 MeV or less. **audiometric t.** The threshold of hearing for an individual as determined by pure tone audiometry. **auditory t.** The level of hearing at which sounds are just audible. It is possible to define this in precise, quantitative terms relevant to two basic parameters of auditory sensation, so that the frequency by intensity matrix of the pure tone audiogram is accepted as the primary measure of threshold for clinical purposes. Other thresholds refer to discrimination of small differences of one parameter as its value is changed, and to speech discrimination. **chromatic t.** The level of photic energy required for hue discrimination of colored light stimuli. **colorless visual t.** ACHROMATIC THRESHOLD. **convulsant t.** A measurement of the likelihood of any subject to suffer epileptic convulsions in response to an appropriate stimulus, expressed by the amount, per unit body weight, of a convulsant drug, such as leptazol or bemegride, which is just sufficient to induce the first clinical signs of convulsions (myoclonus), or EEG evidence of epilepsy. Other techniques using photic stimulation or a combination of photic stimulation with analeptic drugs have been used. The finding of a low convulsant threshold does not confirm the diagnosis of epilepsy, as many but not all epileptics have a low threshold and some individuals with a low threshold never develop epilepsy. Also *myoclonic threshold.* **difference t.** The least difference, usually in a quantitative aspect, that can be detected between two stimuli compared either simultaneously or successively. It is a measure of relative rather than absolute threshold, defining the barely perceptible change needed to permit a difference to be perceived between two stimuli as often as it is not. Also *just-noticeable difference, difference limen, differential threshold.* **differential t.** DIFFERENCE THRESHOLD. **differential light t.** The least discriminable increment in photic intensity. **t. of discomfort** LOUDNESS DISCOMFORT LEVEL. Abbr. TD **differential sensory t.** The smallest discernible increment in sensory stimulus magnitude. **displacement t.** The least amount of misalignment of lines that can be discerned; the limit of accuracy in perceiving the alignment of lines. Also *Vernier acuity.* **double-point t.** The least distance at which two points applied to the skin can be distinguished as separate. Also *threshold for two-point discrimination.* **epileptic t.** A measurement of the predisposition to attacks in a known epileptic patient, expressed as the amount, per unit body weight, of a convulsant or analeptic drug (leptazol, bemegride, etc.) which is just sufficient to bring on the clinical and electroencephalographic manifestations of an attack. The epileptic threshold is related to, but not identical with, the convulsant threshold. For instance, in a patient with temporal lobe epilepsy, a nonconvulsive epileptic manifestation may be induced before the convulsant threshold is reached. **erythema t.** An outmoded, qualitative indication of radiotherapy dose, being the amount of radiation necessary to produce erythema at the treatment site. **excretion t.** The level of a substance (such as glucose) in the plasma at which the substance is no longer completely extracted from the luminal fluid by the tubule cells, and at which it first appears in the urine. **flicker fusion t.** The slowest alternation of stroboscopic light that is not visible as an inconstant light. **galvanic t.** RHEOBASE. **Geiger t.** The anode voltage, applied to a Geiger-Müller tube, at which the region of limited proportionality passes into the Geiger plateau. Below this voltage, avalanche ionization is restricted to the region of the primary ionization. Above the threshold, the avalanche spreads throughout the length of the cathode in response to each ionizing event, and the output pulses are all nearly the same size. **light t.** The quantity of photic energy required for sensory detection of light. **myoclonic t.** CONVULSANT THRESHOLD. **neuron t.** The minimal stimulus required to excite a neuronal membrane and cause the discharge of a nerve impulse. **t. of nose** LIMEN NASI. **olfactory t.** The minimum molecular concentration of an odorant necessary to excite the sense of smell. There are two recognized measurements: the minimum perceptible odor and the minimum recognizable odor. Also *odor threshold.* **pain t.** The quantitative level of already existing sensation at which a change in quality to that of a noxious sensation first becomes evident, as in the transition from heat sensation to one of painful burning. **renal t.** The concentration of a substance in plasma at which it begins to appear in the urine. Also *renal* *excretory threshold.* **renal t. for glucose** The plasma level of glucose at which it first appears in the urine when the tubule cells no longer can extract all the filtered glucose. The normal threshold for glucose is approximately 180 mg/dl. The threshold may be increased when the glomerular filtration rate is decreased, or decreased in renal glycosuria. **sensitivity t.** THRESHOLD. **speech reception t.** The level of intensity measured in dB HL at which 50 percent of a standardized word list is recognized by the listener. There is variation in detailed procedure relating to numerical scoring and word and sentence list construction. Abbr. SRT **stimulus t.** THRESHOLD. **stretch t.** The minimal stretch of a muscle beyond the relaxed length required to induce its reflex contraction, or an increase in discharge from one of the stretch receptors in the muscle, its tendon, or a nearby joint. **swallowing t.** The minimal stimulus of the buccal cavity necessary to elicit reflex swallowing. **t. for two-point discrimination** DOUBLE-POINT THRESHOLD. **t. of visual sensation** The least intensity of light required for vision under given conditions of adaptation of the eye.

**thrill** A palpable fine vibration, as that associated with a loud cardiovascular murmur. **aneurysmal t.** A thrill felt over an aneurysm. **aortic t.** A thrill felt in the aortic area in the second right intercostal space. **arterial t.** A thrill felt over an artery. **arteriovenous t.** A thrill felt over an arteriovenous communication. **diastolic t.** A thrill felt in diastole, usually in the mitral area in the presence of mitral stenosis. **hydatid t.** A vibration or sensation of trembling felt on palpation of the body surface directly over a hydatid cyst. Also *Blatin sign.* **presystolic t.** A thrill felt in the presystolic period in association with the presystolic murmur of mitral stenosis. **systolic t.** A thrill felt during systole. It can be due to mitral regurgitation, aortic stenosis, pulmonary stenosis, or ventricular septal defect.

**thrix** \thriks\ [Gk, gen. *trichos,* hair] Hair; a hair. **t. annulata** RINGED HAIR.

**throat** [Old English *throte,* also *throtu*] **1** The front part of the neck. **2** FAUCES. **3** PARS NASALIS PHARYNGIS. **septic sore t.** STREPTOCOCCAL SORE THROAT. **sore t.** **1** The characteristic pain in the throat, usually on swallowing or made worse by swallowing, common to many kinds of inflammatory or malignant disease of the fauces and pharynx. **2** Nonspecific acute or chronic pharyngitis. **streptococcal sore t.** Sore throat due to a streptococcal (usually group A) infection and sometimes occurring in epidemics. The infection may be spread by droplets, either by the airborne route or by direct contact, and, less commonly, by infected food or milk. Also *septic sore throat.* **trench t.** VINCENT'S ANGINA. **ulcerated sore t.** ULCEROMEMBRANOUS PHARYNGITIS. **ulceromembranous sore t.** ULCEROMEMBRANOUS PHARYNGITIS.

**Throckmorton** [Thomas Bentley *Throckmorton,* U.S. neurologist, 1885–1961] See under REFLEX.

**throe** \thrō\ [Middle English *throwe,* prob. from Old English *thrawu* pain, akin to Gk *trauma* wound] A paroxysm or pang, especially, in the plural, the pangs of childbirth.

**thromb-** \thrämb-\ THROMBO-.

**thrombasthenia** \thräm′basthē′nē·ə\ GLANZMANN'S DISEASE. **Glanzmann's t.** GLANZMANN'S DISEASE.

**thrombectomy** \thrämbek′təmē\ [THROMB- + -ECTOMY] The removal of a thrombus from the lumen of an artery or a vein.

**thrombembolia** \thräm′bembō′lyə\ THROMBOEMBOLISM.

**thrombin** \thräm′bin\ [THROMB- + -IN] A serine protease (EC 3.4.21.5) of blood plasma, which converts fibrinogen into fibrin by splitting off N-terminal peptides from two of the three chains of the fibrinogen molecule, thus causing formation of the blood clot. Also *paraglobulin* (obs.), *fibrin ferment* (obs.). **topical t.** A preparation of thrombin for local application as a hemostatic.

**thrombo-** \thräm′bō-, thräm′bə-\ [Gk *thrombos* clot of blood] A combining form meaning blood clot or thrombus. Also *thromb-.*

**thromboangiitis** \-an′jē·ī′tis\ [THROMBO- + ANGIITIS] An inflammatory disorder of a blood vessel associated with thrombosis. **t. obliterans** A disorder of the blood vessels of the extremities associated with inflammation of medium-sized arteries and veins, resulting in vasular occlusion, peripheral gangrene, and amputation. Also *Buerger's disease.*

**thromboarteritis** \-är′tərī′tis\ Inflammation of an artery resulting from or associated with thrombosis.

**thromboclasis** \thrämbäk′ləsis\ THROMBOLYSIS.

**thromboclastic** \-klas′tik\ THROMBOLYTIC.

**thrombocytapheresis** \-sī′təfer′əsis\ PLATELETPHERESIS.

**thrombocytasthenia** \-sī′tasthē′nē·ə\ GLANZMANN'S DISEASE.

**thrombocyte** \thräm′bəsīt\ [THROMBO- + -CYTE] PLATELET.

**thrombocythemia** \-sīthē′mē·ə\ [*thrombocyt(e)* + -HEMIA] A greater than normal number of platelets per unit volume of blood; a platelet count of greater than $450 \times 10^9$/l of blood. Also *piastrinemia, plastocytemia, plastocytosis, thrombocytosis.* **essential t.** Chronic increase in platelets of venous blood, usually exceeding $1000 \times 10^9$/l, of unknown cause. The disorder may be accompanied by hemorrhagic or thrombotic phenomena. Also *Frank's essential thrombocythemia, hemorrhagic thrombocythemia, primary thrombocythemia, megakaryocytic leukemia.* **hemorrhagic t.** ESSENTIAL THROMBOCYTHEMIA. **idiopathic t.** An increase in platelet count of venous blood to greater than $450 \times 10^9$/l of unknown cause. **primary t.** ESSENTIAL THROMBOCYTHEMIA.

**thrombocytocrit** \-sī′təkrit\ **1** A device for measuring the ratio of the volume of platelets to the total volume of a blood specimen. **2** The relative volume of platelets in blood.

**thrombocytolysis** \-sītäl′isis\ Dissolution of platelets.

**thrombocytopathic** \-sī′təpath′ik\ Exhibiting thrombocytopathy.

**thrombocytopathy** \-sītäp′əthē\ Any qualitative platelet defect. **constitutional t.** Any nonacquired qualitative defect in the platelet, as in pseudohemophilia, vascular hemophilia, Glanzmann's disease (thrombasthenia), and von Willebrand's disease. *Ambiguous.*

**thrombocytopenia** \-sītəpē′nē·ə\ [*thrombocyt(e)* + *o* + -PENIA] A fewer than normal number of platelets per unit volume of blood, i.e., fewer than $130 \times 10^9$ platelets per liter. Also *thrombopenia, thrombopeny, plastocytopenia.* **essential t.** IDIOPATHIC THROMBOCYTOPENIC PURPURA. **malignant t.** Serious bleeding resulting from the thrombocytopenia of aplastic anemia. Also *aleukia hemorrhagica.* **secondary t.** A deficiency of circulating platelets secondary to such conditions as systemic lupus erythematosus, lymphoproliferative diseases, Gaucher's disease, or other splenomegalic states. It may also result from massive blood transfusions or from ingestion of drugs such as quinidine, thiazides, or drugs that cause bone marrow suppression.

**thrombocytopoiesis** \-sī′təpoi·ē′sis\ [*thrombocyt(e)* + *o* + -POIESIS] The generation of platelets by megakaryocytes in the bone marrow. Presumably the stimulus is thrombopoietin. Also *thrombopoiesis.*

**thrombocytopoietic** \-sī′təpoi·et′ik\ Relating to or characterized by thrombocytopoiesis. Also *thrombopoietic.*

**thrombocytosis** \-sītō′sis\ THROMBOCYTHEMIA.

**thromboelastograph** \thräm′bō·ilas′təgraf\ [THROMBO- + ELASTO- + -GRAPH] An instrument that, by recording changes in the shear elasticity of blood or plasma as it undergoes clot formation or fibrinolysis, allows the evaluation of the rate of formation and tensile strength of evolving fibrin.

**thromboembolectomy** \thräm′bō·em′bəlek′təmē\ [THROMBO- + *embol(us)* + -ECTOMY] The removal of an embolic thrombus from a vascular lumen or heart chamber for purposes of improving blood flow, usually by surgical means.

**thromboembolism** \-em′bəlizm\ [THROMBO- + EMBOLISM] Occlusion of a vessel by a thrombus originating from another site. Also *thromboembolia, thrombembolia.*

**thromboendarterectomy** \-end′ärtərek′təmē\ [THROMBO- + ENDARTERECTOMY] Excision of the lining of an artery together with an occluding thrombus. **coronary t.** The removal of an atherosclerotic stenosis or occlusion of a coronary artery by stripping the diseased intima and media from the underlying adventitia.

**thrombogenesis** \-jen′əsis\ [THROMBO- + GENESIS] Clot formation; production of thrombi.

**thrombogenic** \-jen′ik\ [THROMBO- + -GENIC] Tending to cause thrombosis; thrombus-forming.

**thromboid** \thräm′boid\ Resembling an intravascular clot or thrombus.

**thrombokinase** \-kī′nās\ The serine proteinase (EC 3.4.21.6) that converts prothrombin into thrombin. It is the activated form of factor X, designated factor Xa. It hydrolyzes bonds on the C-terminal side of arginine residues, with a preference for those to glycine and isoleucine residues. Also *autoprothrombin C, prothrombinase.*

**thrombokinesis** \-kīnē′sis\ The process of blood clot formation.

**thrombolysis** \thrämbäl′isis\ The dissolution of intravascular clots or thrombi. Also *thromboclasis.*

**thrombolytic** \-lit′ik\ Relating to or causing thrombolysis. Also *thromboclastic.*

**thrombopenia** \-pē′nē·ə\ THROMBOCYTOPENIA.

**thrombopeny** \thräm′bōpē′nē\ THROMBOCYTOPENIA.

**thrombophilia** \-fil′yə\ The predilection for a patient to develop thrombi and emboli.

**thrombophlebitis** \-flebī′tis\ [THROMBO- + PHLEBITIS] Inflammation of a vein associated with thrombosis. **intracranial t.** Thrombophlebitis of an intracranial vein or venous sinus. **t. migrans** The occurrence of thrombophlebitis in several sites simultaneously or sequentially. **septic t.** SUPPURATIVE THROMBOPHLEBITIS. **spinal t.** Thrombophlebitis of veins and venous plexuses within the spinal canal. **suppurative t.** A purulent infection of the superficial or deep veins, most often seen in burn patients, drug abusers, or patients with indwelling venous catheters. It is associated with signs of sepsis and is frequently fatal. When the condition is diagnosed, radical excision and drainage of the affected vein are mandatory. Also *septic thrombophlebitis, septic phlebitis.*

**thromboplastic** \-plas′tik\ Relating to thromboplastin.

**thromboplastin** \-plas′tin\ [THROMBO- + Gk *plast(os)* formed, shaped + -IN] **1** In the classic theory of coagulation of Morawitz, the substance that causes conversion of prothrombin to thrombin in the presence of calcium; i.e., thrombokinase (factor Xa). Also *factor III* (rare). **2** A phospholipid extract of brain or other tissue that converts prothrombin to thrombin. **3** Phospholipids of platelets and other cells that together with other clotting factors activate factor X and convert prothrombin to thrombin.

**thromboplastinopenia** \-plas′tinōpē′nē·ə\ *Obs.* HEMOPHILIA.

**thrombopoiesis** \-poi·ē′sis\ THROMBOCYTOPOIESIS.

**thrombopoietic** \-poi·et′ik\ THROMBOCYTOPOIETIC.

**thrombose** \thräm′bōs\ To form a blood clot, especially *in vivo.*

**thrombosed** \thräm′bōst\ Affected by thrombosis.

**thrombosis** \thrämbō′sis\ [Gk *thrombōsis* (from *thrombos* a clot) clotting, coagulation] The formation of a thrombus within a blood vessel. **agonal t.** Thrombosis occurring at the time of death. Also *Ribbert's thrombosis.* **atrophic t.** MARASMIC THROMBOSIS. **ball-valve t.** A spherical clot so located (usually in the left atrium) that it may occlude an orifice intermittently. **calcarine t.** Thrombosis of vessels supplying or situated in the neighborhood of the calcarine fissure of the brain. **cardiac t.** INTRACARDIAC THROMBOSIS. **cerebellar t.** Thrombosis of any of the arteries supplying the cerebellum. **cerebral t.** Thrombosis of an artery supplying the brain, a common cause of cerebrovascular accident. **coronary t.** Clot formation in a coronary artery, which commonly leads to myocardial infarction. **deep venous t.** The formation of a thrombus in the main conduit veins of the extremities or trunk. **effort t.** The formation of a thrombus within the axillary vein, usually associated with repetitive and strenuous muscle activity of the upper extremity or with thoracic outlet syndrome. Also *Paget-von Schroetter syndrome.* **iliofemoral t.** The formation of a thrombus in the deep vessels of the thigh and pelvis: used especially to describe an

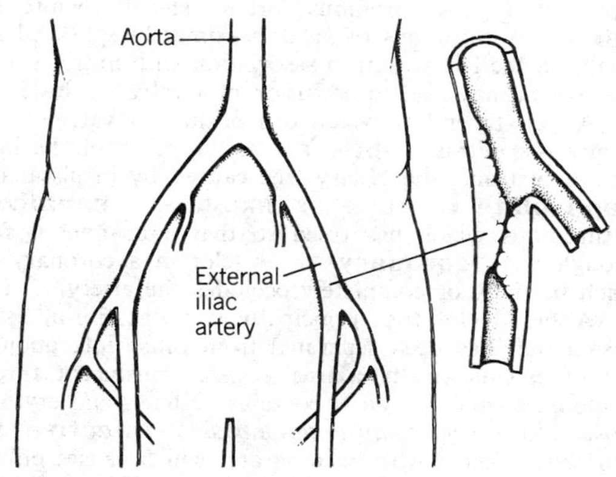


**Iliofemoral thrombosis**

occlusion by thrombus of the iliac and femoral veins of the thigh and pelvis. **infective t.** A thrombus occurring in association with infection. **intracardiac t.** Thrombosis within a cardiac chamber. Also *cardiac thrombosis.* **intraventricular t.** Thrombosis occurring within a cardiac ventricle. **jumping t.** MIGRATING THROMBOSIS. **marasmic t.** Thrombosis occurring as a result of wasting or general debility. Also *marantic thrombosis, atrophic thrombosis.* **mesenteric t.** Thrombosis occurring in a mesenteric artery. **migrating t.** Thrombosis which occurs successively in different arteries or veins. Also *jumping thrombosis.* **mural t.** Thrombosis arising from the wall of a vessel or of a cardiac chamber, especially the left ventricle, in myocardial infarction. **placental t.** Formation of a thrombus within the tissue of the placenta or within the uterine veins at the site of placental attchment. **platelet t.** The *in vivo* formation of clots that are dominated by clumped platelets usually associated with fibrin. These tend to occur in rapidly flowing arterial blood. Also *plate thrombosis.* **puerperal t.** Thrombophlebitis occurring during the postpartum period. **Ribbert's t.** AGONAL THROMBOSIS. **suppurative venous t.** SUPPURATIVE PHLEBITIS.

**thrombosthenin** \-sthē′nin\ A protein found in platelets that resembles actinomycin. It may be responsible for clot retraction.

**thrombotest** \thräm′bōtest\ A modified prothrombin time test that measures factor IX as well as the other vitamin-K-dependent clotting factors.

**thrombotic** \thrämbät′ik\ Pertaining to or characterized by thrombosis.

**thromboxane** \thräm′bäksān\ Any of a group of lipids with structures related to the prostaglandins except that the active forms have an endoperoxide ring instead of the five-carbon ring characteristic of prostaglandins. The thromboxanes are unstable, short-lived molecules.

**thrombus** \thräm′bəs\ [New L, from Gk *thrombos* a curd, lump, clot] (*pl.* thrombi) A semisolid aggregate of blood cells enmeshed in fibrin and clumps of platelets, which results from the rapid conversion of fibrinogen to fibrin, especially within a blood vessel. Also *blood clot, crassamentum* (rare). **agglutinative t.** HYALINE THROMBUS. **agonal t.** A thrombus formed in the heart or great vessels at the time of death. **annular t.** A thrombus that forms a ringlike obstruction in a vessel but, having an opening in its center, does not occlude the vessel entirely. **antemortem t.** A thrombus formed shortly before death. **ball t.** A thrombus of an approximately spherical shape, usually in the left atrium in association with mitral valve disease, which may lead to occlusion of a valve. **ball-valve t.** A ball thrombus which can occlude a valvular orifice, usually the mitral. **bile t.** A thrombus of the intrahepatic or extrahepatic biliary tree caused by inspissated bile. **blood plate t.** PLATELET THROMBUS. **canalized t.** A thrombus which has lysed so that a channel is formed through it. **coronary t.** A clot in a coronary artery which partially or completely occludes the artery. **fibrin t.** A blood clot that principally contains fibrin, as when plasma that has been separated from cells clots upon addition of calcium. **hyaline t.** A translucent thrombus occluding a small vessel. It contains platelets and erythrocyte ghosts. Also *agglutinative thrombus.* **infective t.** A thrombus infected with bacteria and which causes inflammation of the vein and adjacent tissues. **laminated t.** An organized thrombus in which there are layers that have been laid one upon another over a course of time. Also *mixed thrombus, stratified thrombus.* **lateral t.** A thrombus attached to one side of a vessel wall, not occluding the vessel. **marasmic t.** A thrombus occurring in a wasting disease. Also *marantic thrombus.* See also MARASMIC THROMBOSIS. **milk t.** Blockage by curdled milk of a lactiferous duct of the mammary gland. **mixed t.** LAMINATED THROMBUS. **mural t.** A thrombus attached to the endocardium, often as a result of myocardial infarction or in cardiomyopathy. **occlusive t.** A thrombus that occludes a vessel. Also *obstructive thrombus.* **organized t.** A thrombus that has been invaded by fibroblasts, with the formation of scar tissue. **pale t.** WHITE THROMBUS. **parasitic t.** The blocking of a blood vessel by a parasitic mass, as by malarial parasites and pigment in infected red cells in the cerebral capillaries, causing cerebral malaria. **platelet t.** A thrombus composed primarily of blood platelets. Also *plate thrombus, blood plate thrombus.* **red t.** A thrombus composed mainly of red blood corpuscles. **saddle t.** A thrombus which overlies the bifurcation of a blood vessel, as in saddle embolism of the aorta. **septic t.** A thrombus which has become secondarily infected. **stratified t.** LAMINATED THROMBUS. **traumatic t.** A thrombus arising as a consequence of injury. **valvular t.** A thrombus which is capable of acting as a valve. **white t.** An *in vivo* clot that consists of fibrin and layers of platelets and leukocytes, with few red cells. Also *white clot, pale thrombus.*

**throwback** \thrō′bak\ **1** The reversion to a specific trait or general characteristics present in distant ancestors. **2** An individual with one or more characteristics not present in recent ancestors, but suggestive of those of remote ancestors. See also ATAVISM.

**thrush** \thrush\ [of Scandinavian origin, akin to Danish and Norwegian *trøske* thrush] An infection of the oral and pharyngeal mucous membranes with *Candida* species. Also *oral candidiasis, oral moniliasis.*

**thrust** / **extensor t.** In a spinal preparation, a sudden and brief extension of a limb in response to mild mechanical pressure on the ipsilateral plantar foot pad. **tongue t.** The habitual placing of the tongue between the upper and lower teeth when swallowing. It is normal for the teeth to meet in maximum contact during swallowing.

**thujone** $C_{10}H_{16}O$. A terpene ketone, forming a major constituent of many essential oils. The molecule consists of cyclohexanone carrying methyl and isopropyl substituents on C-2 and C-5, and with a bond joining C-3 to C-5. Also *absinthol.*

**thulium** Element number 69, having atomic weight 168.9342. It is a soft, silvery gray metal, the least abundant of the lanthanide series. In common with other rare-earth elements, it has compounds that are somewhat toxic. Symbol: Tm

**thumb** [Old English *thūma*, akin to L *tumere* to swell] The first digit of the hand; pollex. **tennis t.** Tendinitis in the flexor pollicis longus. **trigger t.** A condition in which the thumb is arrested in a flexed position near the beginning of attempted extension and then suddenly released. It results from interference with the movement of the tendon within its sheath.

**thumb-sucking** The act or habit of sucking the thumb, commonplace and normal among infants and often continued for several years. If it persists or recurs in later childhood it is considered a neurotic trait or regressive manifestation. If unduly persistent, the habit can lead to malocclusion of the first and sometimes the permanent dentition.

**Thy** Symbol for thymine.

**thylakentrin** \thī′ləken′trin\ *Older term* FOLLICLE STIMULATING HORMONE.

**thym-**[1] \thīm-\ THYMO-[1].

**thym-**[2] \thīm-\ THYMO-[2].

**thymectomy** \thīmek′təmē\ [*thym(o)*-[1] + -ECTOMY] The surgical removal of all or part of the thymus gland. Also *thymusectomy.*

**thymi-** \thī′mē-\ THYMO-[1].

**-thymia** \-thim′ē·ə\ [Gk *thymos* life, breath, soul, the heart as the seat of the passions] A combining form denoting a condition associated with the mind or emotions.

**thymic** \thī′mik\ Of, relating to, or resembling the thymus.

**thymidine** \thī′midēn\ The 2′-deoxynucleoside formed

by glycosylation of thymine with 2-deoxyribose. Its 5′-phosphate is a constituent of DNA. Symbol: dThd, dT **tritiated t.** Thymidine that has incorporated tritium. It is used as a radioactive marker for metabolic reactions involving thymidine, especially in the generation of DNA.

**thymidine diphosphoric acid** Thymidine 5′-diphosphate, an intermediate in the formation of dTTP, which is the precursor of thymidylate residues in DNA. Symbol: dTDP

**thymidine kinase** The enzyme (EC 2.7.1.21) that catalyzes the formation of thymidine 5′-phosphate and ADP from thymidine and ATP. It is not on the main pathway of thymidylate synthesis, since thymidine 5′-phosphate is made by methylation of 2′-deoxyuridine 5′-phosphate, as well as by glycosylation of thimine with the 5-phospho-2-deoxyribosyl group.

**thymidine triphosphoric acid** Thymidine 5′-triphosphate, the donor of thymidylyl groups in the biosynthesis of DNA. Symbol: dTTP

**thymidylate** A salt, anion, or ester of thymidine esterified with phosphoric acid. Unless otherwise specified, thymidine 5′-phosphate is meant. It can be phosphorylated twice to form dTTP, the donor of thymidylyl groups for DNA biosynthesis.

**thymidylic acid** Thymidine 5′-phosphate. It consists of a 2-deoxyribosyl group phosphorylated on O-5 attached by C-1 to the N-1 of thymine. Its residues occur in DNA.

**thymin** \thī′min\ THYMOPOIETIN.

**thymine** \thī′mēn\ The compound 2,4-hydroxy-5-methylpyrimidine, existing largely in the form of the tautomer 1,2,3,4-tetrahydro-5-methyl-2,4-dioxopyrimidine. It is the base characteristic of DNA, RNA containing uracil instead (i.e. the corresponding compound lacks a methyl group). Its nucleoside is called ribosylthymine, and its 2′-deoxynucleoside is called thymidine. Also *5-methyluracil.* Symbol: Thy **t. dimer** A compound formed between two thymine molecules by mutual addition across their 5(6) double bonds. This process can occur in DNA, blocking replication, under the influence of ultraviolet radiation, and a repair process exists for the excision of such dimers. Also *UV-induced dimer.*

**thymitis** \thīmī′tis\ [THYM-[1] + -ITIS] Inflammation of the thymus. **autoimmune t.** Proliferation and sensitization of T lymphocytes along with histologic changes in the thymus gland, as seen in myasthenia gravis.

**thymo-[1]** \thī′mə-, thī′mō-\ [Gk *thymos* thymus] A combining form denoting the thymus. Also *thym-, thymi-.*

**thymo-[2]** \thī′mə-, thī′mō-\ [Gk *thymos* life, breath, soul, the heart as the seat of the passions] A combining form meaning soul, spirit, or emotions. Also *thym-.*

**thymocyte** \thī′məsīt\ [THYMO-[1] + -CYTE] A cell of lymphoid type found in the thymus. Thymocytes originate in the bone marrow and migrate into the thymus. After considerable cell division, cell differentiation, and cell death, a proportion of thymocytes leave the thymus to form the peripheral T lymphocyte population.

**thymol** \thī′môl\ $C_{10}H_{14}O$. A phenol obtained from *Thymus vulgaris, Monarda punctata,* and *Trachyspermum ammi,* and also made synthetically. It is used in the preparation of trichloroethylene. It has antifungal, antibacterial, and anthelmintic properties. Also *thyme camphor.*

**thymol blue** $C_{27}H_{30}O_5S$. A dyestuff used primarily as a pH indicator, turning from red to yellow at a pH 1.2 to 2.8, and from yellow to blue at a pH 8.0 to 9.6. Also *thymolsulfonphthalein.*

**thymolize** To treat with, or apply, thymol.

**thymolphthalein** A substance used as a pH indicator. It has a p*K* of about 10 and is colorless in its protonated form and blue in its deprotonated form.

**thymolsulfonphthalein** THYMOL BLUE.

**thymolysis** \thīmäl′isis\ [THYMO-[1] + LYSIS] The destruction or involution of the thymus gland, either as a normal event in mammalian maturation or as induced by glucocorticoids.

**thymoma** \thīmō′mə\ [THYM-[1] + -OMA] A tumor of thymic epithelial cells.

**thymonucleic acid** *Older term* DEOXYRIBONUCLEIC ACID. • This term was used because the thymus is rich in DNA.

**thymopoietin** \-poi·ē′tin\ A thymic polypeptide hormone of molecular weight 5562 which induces differentiation of lymphoid cells to thymocytes and blocks neuruomuscular transmission, but is probably not significant in the pathogenesis of myasthenia gravis. Also *thymin nucleosin.*

**thymoprivous** \-prī′vəs\ Deprived of the thymus; subject to the condition resulting from removal or atrophy of the thymus. Also *thymoprivic.*

**thymosin** \thī′məsin\ A protein isolated from cell-free extracts of the thymus gland, having the capacity to stimulate the development of immunologically competent lymphocytes.

**thymus** \thī′məs\ [L, from Gk *thymos* the thymus, sweetbread] [NA] The primary organ of the lymphoid system and defense mechanism of the body, comprising two unequal lobes of variable shape and size joined together by areolar tissue and situated in the anterior and superior mediastinum. Each lobe develops separately from the third pharyngeal pouch of its side, becomes pyramidal in shape, and extends up into the neck, sometimes to the thyroid gland, and down to the fourth costal cartilage. It continues to grow until puberty when it commences to involute, its parenchyma undergoing slow atrophy and replacement by fat. Each lobe is surrounded by a thin fibrous capsule from which septa penetrate the parenchyma, forming incomplete lobules. Each lobule has a peripheral cortex which is densely packed with small lymphocytes. The central paler part, or medulla, has fewer lymphocytes and is continuous with the medulla of adjacent lobules. The epithelial cells, especially in the medulla, are clumped and layered around a central hyalinizing mass, forming Hassall's corpuscles. Throughout the lobule the cellular processes are linked by desmosomes forming a reticular network in which the interstitial spaces are occupied by cells of the lymphocyte series. Also *thymus gland.* **accessory t.** Ectopic nodules of thymic tissue sometimes found along the route of migration of the embryonic thymus from its points of origin, from the third and fourth pharyngeal pouches, caudalward to the superior mediastinum.

**thymusectomy** \thī′məsek′təmē\ THYMECTOMY.

**thyreo-** \thī′rē·ō-\ THYRO-.

**thyreoitis** \thī′rē·ō·ī′tis\ *Seldom used* THYROIDITIS.

**thyro-** \thī′rō-, thī′rə-\ [See THYROID.] A combining form meaning thyroid. Also *thyreo-.*

**thyroactive** \-ak′tiv\ Stimulating thyroid gland secretion.

**thyroarytenoid** \-ar′ətē′noid\ Of or relating to the thyroid and arytenoid cartilages.

**thyrocalcitonin** \-kal′sitō′nin\ CALCITONIN.

**thyrocarditis** \-kärdī′tis\ A disorder of the heart arising as a result of thyrotoxicosis.

**thyrochondrotomy** \-kändrät′əmē\ LARYNGOFISSURE.

**thyrocricotomy** \-krīkät′əmē\ CRICOTHYROTOMY.

**thyroepiglottic** \-ep′iglät′tik\ Pertaining to the thyroid cartilage and the epiglottis.

**thyrofissure** \-fish′ər\ LARYNGOFISSURE.

**thyrogenic** \-jen′ik\ [THYRO- + -GENIC] **1** THYROGENOUS. **2** Thyroid-producing.

**thyrogenous** \thīräj′ənəs\ [THYRO- + -GENOUS] Originating in the thyroid. Also *thyrogenic.*

**thyroglobulin** \-gläb′yəlin\ The protein of the thyroid gland whose tyrosine residues may be converted into thyroxine. It is a dimer having a molecular mass of about 660 kDa. Its function is storage of thyroxine and triiodothyronine, which it releases on proteolysis. Also *iodothyroglobulin* (seldom used).

**thyroglossal** \-gläs′əl\ Of or relating to the thyroid gland and the tongue. Also *thyrolingual.*

**thyrohyal** \-hī′əl\ Pertaining to the constituent part of the hyoid apparatus derived from the third branchial arch, which in the adult forms the greater horn of the hyoid.

**thyrohyoid** \-hī′oid\ Of or relating to the thyroid cartilage and the hyoid bone. Also *hyothyroid.*

**thyroid** \thī′roid\ [earlier *thyreoid,* from Gk *thyreoeidēs* (from *thyreos* an oblong, doorlike shield with a notch for the neck, from *thyra* door) shieldlike] **1** Having the shape of a shield; scutiform, as in *thyroid cartilage.* **2** Pertaining to or near the thyroid cartilage, as in *thyroid gland.* **3** The thyroid gland. **4** Of or pertaining to the thyroid gland. **5** A medicinal extract of beef or hog thyroid which has been defatted, cleaned of connective tissue, dried, and powdered for use as replacement therapy in hypothyroidism; dessicated thyroid. **aberrant t.** Thyroid tissue that develops in an ectopic site. It is most often seen along the course of migration of the embryonic thyroglossal duct from the base of the tongue to its usual location on either side of the larynx, but is sometimes seen in the mediastinum in association with the thymic vestiges as an intrathoracic thyroid. **intrathoracic t.** A part or all of the thyroid gland that is situated in the superior mediastinum. It is presumed to have descended from its usual location when the embryonic thymus migrated from the pharyngeal region into the chest. **lingual t.** Ectopic thyroid tissue in the base of the tongue, either at or near the site of origin of the thyroid evagination from the floor of the embryonic pharynx.

**thyroidea** \thīroi′dē·ə\ THYROID GLAND. **t. ima** ARTERIA THYROIDEA IMA.

**thyroidectomy** \thī′roidek′təmē\ [THYROID + -ECTOMY] An excision of the thyroid gland. **medical t.** Nonsurgical destruction of the thyroid gland, or great reduction of its functional mass, by the administration of drugs or radioactive chemicals.

**thyroidism** \thī′roidizm\ HYPERTHYROIDISM.

**thyroiditis** \thī′roidī′tis\ [THYROID + -ITIS] Any inflammation of the thyroid gland. Also *thyreoitis* (seldom used), *strumitis.* **acute t.** Thyroiditis caused by pyogenic bacteria, such as streptococci or staphylococci and characterized by fever, dysphagia, and, sometimes, abscess formation. Also *pyogenic thyroiditis.* **acute nonsuppurative t.** SUBACUTE THYROIDITIS. **acute suppurative t.** An extremely rare condition marked by bacterial infection of the thyroid and resulting either in septicemia or extension of localized infection in the neck. **autoimmune t.** HASHIMOTO'S DISEASE. **chronic t.** HASHIMOTO'S DISEASE. **chronic atrophic t.** Infiltration and replacement of the thyroid by connective tissue due to unknown cause. This is probably the commonest etiology of myxedema in the adult. **chronic fibrous t.** RIEDEL STRUMA. **chronic lymphadenoid t.** HASHIMOTO'S DISEASE. **chronic lymphocytic t.** HASHIMOTO'S DISEASE. **de Quervain's t.** SUBACUTE THYROIDITIS. **experimental allergic t.** Thyroiditis experimentally induced in laboratory animals following injection of thyroglobulin or thyroid extract in complete Freund's adjuvant. Histopathologically, it resembles Hashimoto's disease. **focal lymphocytic t.** Focal infiltration of the thyroid gland by plasma cells and lymphocytes, a lesion perhaps related to or an early stage of Hashimoto's disease. **giant-cell t.** SUBACUTE THYROIDITIS. **granulomatous t.** SUBACUTE THYROIDITIS. **Hashimoto's t.** HASHIMOTO'S DISEASE. **invasive t.** RIEDEL STRUMA. **ligneous t.** RIEDEL STRUMA. **lymphocytic t.** HASHIMOTO'S DISEASE. **lymphoid t.** HASHIMOTO'S DISEASE. **painless t.** SILENT THYROIDITIS. **parasitic t.** Chagas disease involving the thyroid gland. **postpartum t.** Inflammation of the thyroid developing several months after childbirth and manifested either as hyperthyroidism or hypothyroidism. While the clinical course is similar to that of subacute thyroiditis, the histology is similar to that of Hashimoto's disease. **pseudotuberculous t.** SUBACUTE THYROIDITIS. **pyogenic t.** ACUTE THYROIDITIS. **Riedel's t.** RIEDEL STRUMA. **silent t.** Painless inflammation of the thyroid which follows a clinical course similar to that of subacute thyroiditis but which histologically resembles Hashimoto's disease. Also *painless thyroiditis.* **subacute t.** Inflammation of the thyroid gland presumed to be due to viral infection, as with mumps virus, adenovirus, coxsackievirus, echovirus, or influenza virus. It is characterized by gradual or sudden onset of pain, tenderness and enlargement of the thyroid, fever, and occasionally by signs of mild thyrotoxicosis, subsiding within months and usually leaving no residual deficit in thyroid function. It is not considered an autoimmune disease, and is marked by typical histopathology consisting of patchy follicular lesions, and lesions in which a central core of colloid is surrounded by multinucleated giant cells, progressing to form granulomas. Also *acute nonsuppurative thyroiditis, de Quervain's thyroiditis, giant-cell thyroiditis, granulomatous thyroiditis, pseudotuberculous thyroiditis.* **subacute diffuse t.** A form of subacute thyroiditis in which the inflammation is less patchy and more generalized than in the typical case. **woody t.** RIEDEL STRUMA.

**thyroidotherapy** THYROTHERAPY.

**thyroidotomy** \thī′roidät′əmē\ THYROTOMY.

**thyrolaryngeal** \-lerin′jē·əl\ Of or relating to the thyroid gland and the larynx.

**thyrolingual** \-ling′gwəl\ THYROGLOSSAL.

**thyrolytic** \-lit′ik\ [THYRO- + LYTIC] Destructive to the thyroid.

**thyromegaly** \-meg′əlē\ [THYRO- + -MEGALY] **1** GOITER. **2** Enlargement of the thyroid gland.

**thyronine** \thī′rənēn\ The amino acid related to tyrosine by substitution of a *p*-hydroxyphenyl group on its phenolic hydroxyl group. It is not biologically important itself but is the parent compound of thyroxine. It is formed in an iodinated state by reactions between iodinated tyrosine residues of thyroglobulin.

**thyroparathyroidectomy** \-par′əthī′roidek′təmē\ The *en bloc* removal of the thyroid and parathyroid glands.

**thyropenia** \-pē′nē·ə\ [THYRO- + Gk *penia* poverty, need] Subnormal secretion of thyroid hormone.

**thyropharyngeal** \-fərin′jē·əl\ Pertaining to the thyroid cartilage and the pharynx.

**thyroprival** \-prī′vəl\ [THYRO- + -PRIVAL] Of, resulting from, or marked by lack of thyroid function.

**thyroprivia** \-priv′ē·ə\ [*thyropriv(al)* + -IA] **1** Absence of thyroid hormones, or the condition resulting from it. **2** The state resulting from the removal of the thyroid gland. **3** HYPOTHYROIDISM.

**thyrotherapy** The treatment of certain disease states by

employing thyroid gland preparations of various domestic animals. Also *thyroidotherapy*.

**thyrotome** \thī′rətōm\ [THYRO- + -TOME] An instrument used for incising the thyroid cartilage.

**thyrotomy** \thīrät′əmē\ [THYRO- + -TOMY] An incision of the thyroid gland. Also *thyroidotomy*.

**thyrotoxic** \-täk′sik\ [THYRO- + TOXIC] Of or marked by thyrotoxicosis.

**thyrotoxicosis** \-täk′sikō′sis\ The condition resulting from hyperthyroidism due to any cause. **t. factitia** Hyperthyroidism induced by ingestion, sometimes surreptitious, of exogenous thyroid hormone or hormones. It is characterized by the peripheral symptoms and signs of overactive thyroid gland function, but without true exophthalmos or pretibial myxedema.

**thyrotrope** \thī′rətrōp\ **1** A thyrotropic substance. **2** A person with any disorder of the thyroid gland, especially with abnormal secretion of thyroid hormone.

**thyrotroph** \thī′rətrāf\ THYROTROPIC CELL.

**thyrotrophic** \-träf′ik\ THYROTROPIC.

**thyrotrophin** \-träf′in\ THYROTROPIC HORMONE.

**thyrotropic** \-träp′ik\ [THYRO- + -TROPIC[1]] Tending to act on or stimulate the thyroid gland. Also *thyrotrophic*.

**thyrotropin** \-trō′pin\ THYROTROPIC HORMONE. **human chorionic t.** The thyrotropic substance or substances that can be isolated from the human placenta. It consists of human chorionic gonadotropin which bears some chemical resemblance to human thyroid stimulating hormone and so may possess thyrotropic activity, or of a separate placental thyrotropin, or both. Abbr. hCT

**thyroxine** \thīräk′sēn\ 3,5,3′,5′-Tetraiodothyronine, one of the two principal hormones secreted by the thyroid gland, the other being triiodothyronine. The chief action of thyroxine is to stimulate the rate of oxygen consumption and of metabolism by all cells and tissues. Its secretion is excessive in hyperthyroidism, deficient in hypothyroidism, and defective in certain forms of congenital goiter. It is used in the replacement therapy for hypothyroidism. Also *thyroxin*. Symbol: $T_4$ Adj. thyroxinic. **radioactive t.** Thyroxine in which one or more of the four iodine atoms are radioactive, most commonly $^{131}I$ or $^{125}I$. It is used in the study of thyroid hormone biosynthesis, secretion, secretion rate, plasma binding, rate of turnover, peripheral metabolism, and disposition of thyroxine. Also *radiothyroxine*.

**Ti** Symbol for the element, titanium.

**TIA** transient ischemic attack.

**TIBC** total iron-binding capacity.

**tibia** \tib′ē·ə\ [L, a flute, reed-pipe, shinbone] [NA] The long bone on the anteromedial side of the leg, articulating proximally with the femur, distally with the talus, and laterally with the fibula and transmitting the weight of the trunk to the foot. Also *shin bone, shank bone, shinbone, canna major* (outmoded). **saber t.** SABER SHIN. **saber-scabbard t.** SABER SHIN. **saber-shaped t.** SABER SHIN. **t. valga** GENU VALGUM. **t. vara** GENU VARUM.

**tibiad** \tib′ē·ad\ Toward the tibia.

**tibial** \tib′ē·əl\ Of or pertaining to the tibia.

**tibiale posticum** OS TIBIALE POSTERIUS.

**tibialis** \tib′ē·ā′lis\ [L, tibial] Tibial.

**tic** \tik\ [French, possibly from Low German *tukken* to twitch] An abnormal movement which is intermittent, abrupt and aimless, caused by contraction of one or several muscles. The muscles of the face are commonly involved. The movements are often multiple and initially may be voluntary, giving relief of tension, but eventually may become so habitual as to be virtually involuntary though sometimes they can be temporarily suppressed by an effort of will. Although tics are frequently psychogenic, they also occur often in the encephalitides and can occur in any type of brain pathology that involves the motor pathways, and in particular in extrapyramidal disease. Also *habit spasm, habit tic, mimetic convulsion, mimic convulsion, habit chorea, spasmus coordinatus, pantomimic spasm*. **blinking t.** A tic involving the orbicularis oculi, causing irregular, repetitive blinking. **bowing t.** SPASMUS NUTANS. **compulsive t.** GILLES DE LA TOURETTE SYNDROME. **convulsive t.** FACIAL TIC. **diaphragmat. t.** A recurrent involuntary contraction of the diaphragm. Also *diaphragmatic chorea*. **t. douloureux** TRIGEMINAL NEURALGIA. **facial t.** Any tic involving facial muscles. Also *convulsive tic*. See also FACIAL SPASM. **habit t.** TIC. • Some writers use *habit tic* specifically to indicate tics of psychogenic origin, although strictly speaking the term is tautologic since all tics are habitual. **mimic t.** A facial tic which resembles a voluntary movement, such as voluntary winking. **motor t.** Any tic in which muscular contraction is the sole manifestation, accompanied by no evident emotional tension or anxiety. Facial, diaphragmatic, laryngeal, and other movements as well as blepharospasm are included. **rocking t.** SPASMUS NUTANS. **saltatory t.** INFANTILE MASSIVE SPASM. **wide-eyed t.** A tic marked by intermittent excessive opening of one or both eyes, giving the patient an expression of surprise. **winking t.** A form of tic marked by irregular repetitive winking of one eye. Other facial muscles are often involved.

**ticarcillin disodium** $C_{15}H_{14}N_2NA_2O_6S_2$. The disodium salt of 6-(α-carboxy-α-thien-3-ylacetamido)penicillanic acid, a penicillin similar to carbenicillin except that it is more effective against *Psuedomonas aeruginosa*. It is used as an antibacterial and may be administered intramuscularly or intravenously.

**tick** A bloodsucking ectoparasite belonging to the superfamily Ixodoidea, order Acarina, class Arachnida. The superfamily of ticks comprises the hard ticks (family Ixodidae) and the soft ticks (Argasidae). **African relapsing fever t.** Any of the ticks originally classified in the species *Ornithodoros moubata*. **castor bean t.** A tick of the species *Ixodes ricinus*. **deer t.** A tick of the species *Ixodes dammini*. **dog t.** Any of the ticks usually found on dogs, which include members of the species *Haemaphysalis leachi, Ixodes canisuga, Dermacentor variabilis*, and *Rhipicephalus sanguineus*. **hard t.** Any

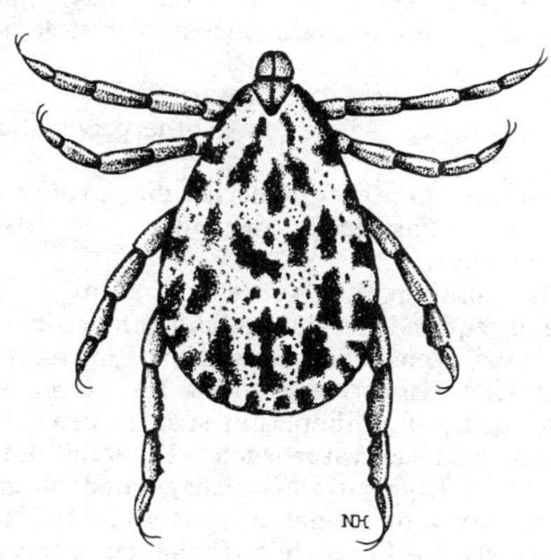

**Wood tick** (*Dermacentor*)

tick of the family Ixodidae. Also *hard-bodied tick.* **lone star t.** A tick of the species *Amblyomma americanum.* It is common in the southeastern United States, Mexico, and Central and South America. This is a three-host tick, all stages of which attach to domestic and wild animals and man. It transmits several diseases and can cause tick paralysis in both man and dogs. **Pacific coast dog t.** A tick of the species *Dermacentor occidentalis.* **pajaroello t.** A tick of the species *Ornithodoros coriaceus.* **Rocky Mountain t.** A tick of the species *Dermacentor andersoni.* **seed t.** A tick during the six-legged larval stage, which is the stage prior to its emergence as a nymph with eight legs. Heteroxenous seed ticks usually parasitize rodents or other small mammals whereas the nymphs and adults usually feed on larger animals such as herbivores. **soft t.** Any tick of the family Argasidae. Also *soft-bodied tick.* **spotted-fever t.** A tick of the species *Dermacentor andersoni.* **tampan t.** A tick of the species *Ornithodoros moubata.* **wood t.** Any of several species of hard ticks of the genus *Dermacentor,* especially *D. variabilis, D. andersoni,* or *D. occidentalis.*

**tickle** 1 To feel or cause to feel a prickling sensation, usually considered disagreeable, as by touching or scratching a sensitive area of skin, often provoking the nervous responses of laughter and immediate withdrawal from the stimulus. 2 The sensation of being tickled.

**ticpolonga** \tik′pōläng′ə\ [Sinhalese *tikpolaṅgā* (from *tik* a spot + *polaṅgā* a viper) Russell's viper] RUSSELL'S VIPER.

**t.i.d.** *ter in die* (L, three times a day).

**tide** / **alkaline t.** A transient increase in blood and urine pH associated with gastric acid secretion. **fat t.** Transient elevation of fat concentration in blood and lymph following meals. **red t.** A luminescent mass of marine protozoa of the order Dinoflagellata that may coat the surface of a body of water.

**Tiedemann** [Friedrich *Tiedemann,* German anatomist and physiologist, 1781–1861] Tiedemann's gland. See under GLANDULA VESTIBULARIS MAJOR.

**Tietze** [Alexander *Tietze,* German surgeon, 1864–1927] Tietze's disease, Tietze syndrome. See under COSTOCHONDRITIS.

**tiglic acid** $CH_3—CH=C(CH_3)—COOH$. 2-Methylcrotonic acid. Its methyl groups are *trans* to each other. It occurs esterified in plant oils. The coenzyme A thioester is an intermediate in the catabolism of isoleucine.

**tigroid** \tī′groid\ Striped like the coat of a tiger. In some disease states, the retina takes on this appearance. Also, the Nissl substance of neuronal cell bodies may appear tigroid when stained by appropriate stains in histologic preparations.

**tigrolysis** \tīgräl′isis\ CHROMATOLYSIS.

**tilt** / **pelvic t.** Movement of the pelvis about its sagittal axis.

**timbre** \teN′br, tam′bər\ The peculiar quality of a sound that gives it a character of its own. **t. métallique** BRUIT DE TAMBOUR.

**time** The duration of a process or event. **action t.** The duration required for a stimulus to the retina in order to induce a visual sensation of maximal intensity. **activated partial thromboplastin t.** A coagulation test in which a partial thromboplastin such as cephalin, calcium, and a factor XII activator such as kaolin are added to plasma obtained from citrate-anticoagulated plasma and the time required for clot formation is measured. Normal range is approximately 30–40 seconds. Prolongation occurs if there is deficiency of factor VIII, IX, XI, XII, V, or X or of prothrombin or fibrinogen, or if inhibitors are present. Abbr. APTT **adaptation t.** The time required for any receptor, stimulated at a constant intensity, no longer to show a change in the pattern of its response. **arm-lung t.** The time that it takes an indicator injected intravenously into the arm to reach the lungs. **association t.** The time elapsing between presentation of a stimulus and the production of some complex associated response established by instruction, such as the production of synonyms, antonyms, or the first word to come to mind in a word association test. **biologic t.** A period of time measured with reference to changes observed in a biological system. **bleeding t.** The time in minutes from when skin is incised until bleeding ceases. See also DUKE BLEEDING TIME TEST, IVY BLEEDING TIME TEST. **blocking t.** In electroencephalography, the time lag between the application of a stimulus and the recorded disappearance of the brain rhythm that is blocked. **circulation t.** The time that it takes for the blood or an injected indicator to flow from one point in the circulation (usually venous) to another (usually arterial). **clot retraction t.** The time required for a clot to separate from serum after it has formed in a test tube. Normally clot retraction is complete in one hour at room temperature. **clotting t.** The time from withdrawal of blood or plasma from a vein until such a firm clot has formed in a test tube that the tube can be inverted without loss of the clot. Also *coagulation time.* **conduction t.** The time, usually measured in milliseconds in which a propagated electrical impulse travels between points along a linear excitable structure such as a nerve or a planar surface such as the cortex. **counter resolving t.** That time required for a counting instrument to record one pulse and to recover electronically to a state able to accept the next pulse. **dead t.** In a radiation detector, a brief interval during which it is temporarily refractory to a new excitation. Also *insensitive time, resolving time.* **decimal reduction t.** The time required for a given concentration of disinfectant to reduce the viable number of a test organism tenfold. **deep tendon reflex relaxation t.** The time required to relax after induction of the Achilles tendon reflex. This time is markedly delayed in severe hypothyroidism with myxedema. The test is often helpful in gauging the adequacy of replacement therapy in the long-term treatment of hypothyroidism. **delay t.** The time required for a signal to pass through a system or medium, as an electric wave through a filter or an acoustic wave through water. **doubling t.** The average time required for doubling the number of cells present in a population, such as an *in vitro* culture, a zygote, or a tumor. It is usually longer than the average generation time of individual cells of the population, because not all cells divide during each doubling of the population due to nutritional constraints on some segments of the population, cell senescence, or cell death. Also *mean generation time.* Abbr. $t_D$ **euglobulin clot lysis t.** A test for *in vivo* activation of fibrinolysis. When dilute acidified plasma is chilled, there is precipitation of fibrinogen, plasminogen, plasmin, and plasminogen activator, without antiplasmins. Following a thrombin-induced conversion of fibrinogen to fibrin, the time required for spontaneous clot lysis reflects the rate of fibrinolytic activation. A deficiency of fibrinogen causes spuriously short lysis time. **expiratory pause t.** The interval between the end of expiration and the start of the next inspiration during artificial ventilation of the lungs. **filter bleeding t.** A bleeding time test in which blood is allowed to flow through a woven dacron filter until the flow of blood ceases. The time that elapses until cessation of blood flow is measured. Normal range is 1–6 minutes. The filter bleeding time reflects platelet function independently of vascular factors that may influence other bleeding time tests. **generation t.** 1 The average time required for a cell to complete one cell cycle. 2 The average length of time of the reproductive cycle of an organism; the time between generations. 3 The time required for doubling the number of cells present in a culture. The mean generation time is equivalent to the doubling time. **inertia t.** REFRACTORY PERIOD. **insensitive t.** DEAD TIME. **inspiratory pause t.** The interval between the end of inspiration and the start of the next expiration during artificial ventilation of the lungs. **lead t.** The time interval in the natural history of a chronic disease between presymptomatic recognition, as by screening tests, and clinical diagnosis. **longitudinal relaxation t.** $T_1$ RELAXATION TIME. **mean t.** MEAN EFFECTIVE LIFE. **mean generation t.** DOUBLING TIME. Abbr. MGT. **perception t.** The interval between stimulus presentation and sensory recognition of the nature of the stimulus. Also *recognition time*. **plasma clot t.** RECALCIFICATION TIME. **prothrombin t.** ONE-STAGE PROTHROMBIN TIME TEST. **pulmonary circulation t.** The time required for blood to circulate through the lungs. **reaction t.** The time interval between stimulus application and response. **real t.** See under REAL-TIME. **recalcification t.** A rarely performed clotting time test in which plasma is first separated from oxalate-anticoagulated blood and then warmed to 37°C. Then calcium is added and the time is measured until a clot forms. The test does not localize the site of coagulation disorder and is insensitive to all but the most severe deficiencies. It can be used to indicate platelet dysfunction if values for platelet-rich and platelet-poor plasma are compared. Also *plasma clot time*. **recognition t.** PERCEPTION TIME. **relaxation t.** The reciprocal of the rate constant for any process that can be described as a relaxation, such as an approach to equilibrium after the equilibrium has been disturbed. **resolving t.** DEAD TIME. **response t.** The time between the administration of a stimulus and the onset of a response to it. **retention t.** The length of time a chemical is retained in the body regardless of route of administration. Factors affecting it include rate of absorption, distribution, metabolism, and excretion. **retinocortical t.** The interval between photic excitation of retinal photoreceptors and discharge of neurons in the area striata of the cerebral cortex. **rise t.** The time for an electric pulse to rise from 10 percent to 90 percent of its peak value. **sedimentation t.** ERYTHROCYTE SEDIMENTATION RATE. **serum prothrombin t.** PROTHROMBIN CONSUMPTION TEST. **spin-lattice relaxation t.** $T_1$ RELAXATION TIME. **spin-spin relaxation t.** $T_2$ RELAXATION TIME. **stimulus-response t.** The time between the induction of a stimulus and the observed response. **survival t.** 1 The length of time that a material or cell remains present and active in the body. The material may have originated in the body, such as a hormone or a blood cell, or it may be introduced from the outside for therapeutic or experimental purposes. 2 The duration of life following a specific event, such as onset of illness, therapeutic intervention, or an experimental procedure. **synaptic transmission t.** The interval between impulse arrival at an axonal terminal and generation of a postsynaptic impulse. • Although the time can vary considerably for a given synapse, the term is conventionally used for the minimum duration of synaptic transmission. **template bleeding t.** A modification of the Ivy bleeding time test, in which a device (template) is used to make an incision of precise length and depth in the skin of the forearm. Normal range is 1–6 minutes. **thermal death t.** The time required, at a given temperature, to sterilize a suspension of an organism. It depends on the number of organisms and is a less useful measurement than the rate of killing. **thrombin t.** The length of time required for a clot to form when thrombin is added to plasma, thus bypassing all the earlier steps in coagulation and testing only the conversion of fibrinogen to fibrin. It is prolonged when there is deficiency or abnormality of fibrinogen or when fibrin degradation products or heparinlike coagulation inhibitors are present. **transit t.** The time taken for a substance, especially a tracer substance, to travel between two points, as along the bowel or from a renal artery to a vein. **transverse relaxation t.** $T_2$ RELAXATION TIME. **treadmill walking t.** The semiquantative measurement of lower extremity ischemia performed by recording the time a patient can walk at a standard treadmill rate and grade before being forced to halt due to claudication. **$T_1$ relaxation t.** In nuclear magnetic resonance, the characteristic time associated with the return to its initial value of the component of the magnetization vector along the measuring field, after a disturbance. Also *spin-lattice relaxation time, longitudinal relaxation time.* **$T_2$ relaxation t.** In nuclear magnetic resonance, the characteristic time associated with the return to its initial value of the component of the magnetization perpendicular to the measuring field, after a disturbance. Also *spin-spin relaxation time, transverse relaxation time.* **ventricular activation t.** The time from the onset of the Q wave to the peak of the R wave in the QRS complex of the electrocardiogram.

**timer** / **electronic t.** A timer in which the duration is determined by an electronic circuit. A digital timer counts clock pulses in a register. An analog timer measures the voltage increase of a capacitor charged through a high resistance. **photoelectric t.** An automatic time switch for correctly exposing x rays, which pass through the film and cause a screen to fluoresce. A photocell integrates the light and terminates the exposure when correct.

**time-sharing** 1 Apparently simultaneous use of a computer by many users whose programs are alternated. 2 Alternate use of a single beam by two displays in a dual-trace cathode-ray tube.

**tin** A metallic element of atomic number 50, atomic weight 118.69. Natural tin has nine stable isotopes and at least two allotropic forms. Below 13.2°C the ordinary lustrous white metal changes slowly to gray tin, a less dense and weaker substance. Valences are 2 and 4. Tin has several important industrial uses. It resists the action of pure water, sea water, and weak acid, and is extensively used as a thin protective coat on the so-called tin cans used in commercial food canning. Rats have been shown experimentally to need traces of tin but its function is not known. Symbol: Sn Adj. stannic, stannous.

**tina** \tē′nə\ PINTA.

**tinct.** *tinctura* (L, tincture).

**tinctorial** \tingktôr′ē·əl\ 1 Of or relating to staining properties. 2 Pertaining to the act of staining.

**tinctura** \tingktʸʊr′ə\ [L (from *tingere* to dip, immerse, dye; see also STAIN) a dying, tinting] Tincture. **t. balsamica** COMPOUND BENZOIN TINCTURE. **t. stomachica** COMPOUND CARDAMOM TINCTURE.

**tincturation** \tingk′chərā′shən\ The preparation of a tincture from a crude source of a drug.

**tincture** \tingk′chər\ [L *tinctura*. See TINCTURA.] An alcoholic or water-alcoholic solution of ingredients of animal, vegetable, or chemical origin. Tinctures are usually prepared by percolation or a similar extractive process. **aromatic rhubarb t.** An alcoholic solution of powdered rhubarb, cinnamon, clove, and myristica in glycerin and water. It is used as a cathartic. **belladonna t.** An alcoholic solution of belladonna leaf prepared so that 27–33 mg of belladonna alkaloids are contained in 100 ml of solution. It is used for its anticholinergic properties. **camphorated opium t.** PAREGORIC. **capsicum t.** A solution of powdered capsicum prepared with equal parts of alcohol and water. It is used for its irritant and carminative properties. **compound benzoin t.** An alcoholic solution containing benzoin 100 g, aloe 20 g, storax 80 g, and Tolu balsam 40 g in 1000 ml. It is used topically to protect the skin. Also *friar's balsam, tinctura balsamica, Turlington's balsam, Wade's balsam.* **compound cardamom t.** A solution in which 1000 ml contains cardamom seed 20 g, cinnamon 25 g, and caraway 12 g dissolved in glycerin and dilute alcohol. It is used as a flavoring agent. Also *tinctura stomachica.* **deodorized opium t.** OPIUM TINCTURE. **digitalis t.** A solution of finely powdered digitalis in a menstruum of alcohol and water. It is used as a cardiotonic medication. **ferric citrochloride t.** A hydroalcoholic solution containing ferric chloride and sodium citrate. It is used as a hematinic agent. **t. of fresh drugs** A tincture prepared according to the general method, by macerating 500 g of the crushed, fresh drug source in 1000 ml of alcohol, letting the mixture stand for 14 days, and filtering the alcoholic extract through paper. **glycerinated t.** A tincture prepared by the addition of glycerin to diluted alcohol. The glycerin is added in order to improve the extraction of the active agent or preserve the finished preparation. **green soap t.** An alcoholic solution that contains green soap and lavender oil. It is used as a skin detergent. Also *medicinal soft soap liniment, linimentum saponis mollis.* **t. of guaiacum** An alcoholic solution of gum guaiac that is used to demonstrate the presence of heme pigments. **iodine t.** A solution of iodine and sodium iodide in dilute alcohol, prepared so that 1.8–2.2 g of iodine and 2.1–2.6 g of sodium iodide are contained in 100 ml of solution. It is used as a topical anti-infective medication. **lemon peel t.** A hydroalcoholic extract of fresh lemon peel. It is used as a flavoring agent. **mother t.** A concentrated tincture used to make standard dilutions. It usually contains 10% of the substance involved. **nitromersol t.** A solution in which 1000 ml contains nitromersol 5 g, sodium hydroxide 1 g, and acetone 100 ml dissolved in alcohol and purified water. It is applied topically for its local anti-infective properties. **opium t.** A hydroalcoholic solution containing 0.95–1.05 of morphine in 100 ml. The tincture is prepared by percolation of granulated opium followed by concentration of the product. It is used as an antiperistaltic agent. Also *laudanum, deodorized opium tincture.* **strong iodine t.** A solution of iodine and potassium iodide in alcohol prepared so that 6.8–7.5 g of iodine and 4.7–5.5 g of potassium iodide are contained in 100 ml of solution. It is used as an irritant, and as an antibacterial and antifungal agent. **sweet orange peel t.** An alcoholic solution of the outer rind of the nonartificially colored fresh ripe fruit of *Citrus sinensis.* It is used as a flavoring agent. **thimerosal t.** A solution in which 1000 ml contains thimerosal 1 g, alcohol 525 ml, acetone 100 ml, ethylenediamine 0.2 g, and monoethanolamine 1 g dissolved in water. It is applied topically for its local anti-infective properties. **Tolu balsam t.** An alcoholic solution of Tolu balsam. It is used as a flavoring agent and as an ingredient of Tolu balsam syrup. **vanilla t.** A solution of vanilla and sucrose dissolved in equal parts of alcohol and water. It is used as a flavoring agent and as an ingredient of acacia syrup.

**tinea** \tin′ē·ə\ [New L (from L, a maggot, grub, moth worm) ringworm, once popularly attributed to a wormlike parasite] A fungal infection of the skin, hair, or nails in humans that is caused by a fungus of one of the dermatophytes: *Microsporum (Nannizzia), Trichophyton (Arthroderma),* or *Epidermophyton.* The fungal invasion is confined to the keratinized tissues, but the clinical appearance is produced by a variable degree of inflammation in the living epidermis and dermis. Central clearing leads to classic ringlike lesions, but this occurs in only a minority of cases. Also *ringworm, dermophytosis, dermomycosis, mycotic dermatitis, cutaneous mycosis.* **t. amiantacea** PITYRIASIS AMIANTACEA. **asbestoslike t.** PITYRIASIS AMIANTACEA. **t. axillaris** Tinea affecting the axillary skin. Also *ringworm of the axillae.* **t. barbae** Tinea of the beard and mustache areas that affects the skin, hair follicles, and hair shafts. It is commonly inflammatory and is usually caused by *Trichophyton verrucosum* or *Trichophyton mentagrophytes.* Also *ringworm of the beard.* **t. capitis** Tinea affecting the skin, follicles, and hairs of the scalp. It is more common in children and is characterized by broken hairs, patchy alopecia, and variable inflammation. It is caused by any of several species, including *Microsporum canis, Microsporum audouini,* and *Trichophyton schoenleinii.* Also *tinea tondens, ringworm of the scalp.* **t. circinata** **1** Tinea showing central clearing. Also *nummular erythema.* **2** Tinea corporis in which the infection is confined to the trunk rather than the limbs. **t. corporis** Tinea affecting the skin of the trunk and limbs but specifically excluding the groin, palms, and soles. Also *ringworm of the body.* **t. cruris** Tinea affecting the groin, usually seen in the adult male and commonly caused by *Trichophyton rubrum* or *Epidermophyton floccosum.* Also *eczema marginatum, gym itch, jock itch* (popular), *ringworm of the groin, tinea inguinalis.* **t. faciei** Tinea of facial skin excluding that of the beard and mustache areas in adult males. **t. favosa** FAVUS. **t. glabrosa** A scalelike tinea that affects those portions of the skin without coarse terminal hairs. *Older term.* **t. inguinalis** TINEA CRURIS. **t. interdigitalis** **1** Tinea pedis affecting the clefts between the toes. **2** Tinea due to *Trichophyton mentagrophytes* var. *interdigitale.* Also *dermatophytosis interdigitale.* **t. kerion** KERION. **t. manus** Tinea of the hands, usually caused by *Trichophyton rubrum.* Also *tinea manuum.* • The term is usually restricted to palmar infections, whereas tinea of the dorsal surfaces is commonly referred to as tinea circinata or tinea corporis. **t. pedis** Tinea of the foot, in particular the lateral clefts between the toes and the soles. This is the commonest site for dermatophyte infection in developed countries. It is usually caused by *Trichophyton rubrum, Trichophyton mentagrophytes* var. *interdigitale,* or *Epidermophyton floccosum.* Also *ringworm of the feet, athlete's foot* (popular). **t. profunda** **1** A rare, deep, mycetomalike infection with a ringworm species that involves subcutaneous tissues. **2** MAJOCCHI'S GRANULOMA. **t. tondens** TINEA CAPITIS. **t. unguium** Tinea of the nail plate of the toe or, less commonly, the finger. It is usually caused by *Trichophyton rubrum* or *Trichophyton mentagrophytes* var. *interdigitale.* Also *ringworm of the nails.* **t. vera** *Obs.* FAVUS

**Tinel** [Jules *Tinel,* French neurologist, 1879–1952] See under TEST, SIGN.

**tingible** \tin′jibəl\ [*ting(e)* + *-ible* (-ABLE)] Having a glistening appearance: applied particularly to the cytoplasmic inclusions within germinal center macrophages.

**tingle** To experience a prickling sensation.

**tingling** A prickling sensation, usually repetitive. It may be felt in a limb as a result of ischemia or of pressure or a blow upon a peripheral nerve. A similar sensation may travel up and down the back as a consequence of acute fear or of a pleasurable or exhilarating experience. **distal t. on percussion** TINEL SIGN.

**tiniadazole** $C_8H_{13}N_3O_4S$. 1-[2-(Ethylsulfonyl)ethyl]-2-methyl-5-nitroimidazole. A nitroimidazole compound closely related to metronidazole. It is used as an antiprotozoal agent.

**tinnitus** \tiniʹtəs\ [L (from *tinnire* to tinkle, jingle) a tinkling, jingling, ringing] Any form of adventitious noise arising within the ears or head and audible to the subject. The nature of the noise may be whistling, ringing, clicking, or pulsating, and in some instances may be audible to others. **t. cerebri** Tinnitus in which the sound seems to be inside the head rather than in the ears. **clicking t.** A clicking sound arising in the ear, usually repetitive and sometimes demonstrable by amplifying and recording techniques. It may arise from contractions of the intratympanic muscles. **objective t.** Tinnitus which can be heard by another person, either directly or with the aid of an auscultation tube or electronic amplification. The tinnitus is usually muscular or vascular in origin. **subjective t.** Tinnitis which is audible only to the subject. • As this is the case in all but rare instances of tinnitus, the term is used only by way of contrast with objective tinnitus.

**tip** A pointed or markedly narrowed extremity of a part of the body. **t. of nose** APEX NASI. **pinched nasal t.** PINCHED TIP DEFORMITY. **root t.** APEX RADICIS DENTIS. **t. of sacral bone** APEX OSSIS SACRI. **t. of tongue** APEX LINGUAE. **Woolner's t.** TUBERCULUM AURICULAE.

**Tiselius** [Arne Wilhelm Kaurin *Tiselius*, Swedish chemist, 1902–1971] **1** Tiselius electrophoresis cell. See under CELL. **2** See under APPARATUS.

# tissue

**tissue** [French *tissu* (from *tisser* to weave, from Old French *tistre* to weave, from L *texere* to weave) fabric, tissue] An aggregation of cells and intercellular matter that subserves a united function. Also *textus*. **accidental t.** Tissue situated in a part where it is abnormal. It may be either normal in another part of the body (analogous) or not normal in any part (heterologous). **adenoid t.** A mass of lymphoid tissue that is situated in the nasopharynx. **adipose t.** A connective tissue that is largely composed of fat cells. Also *fatty tissue*. **analogous t.** Normal tissue situated in an abnormal location, as distinguished from heterologous tissue, which is foreign to the organism as a whole. **aponeurotic t.** Regularly arranged bundles of collagen fibers and their associated fibroblasts that together form the substance of flattened tendinous sheets or aponeuroses. **areolar connective t.** A loose, irregular connective tissue that by its extensibility and elasticity allows considerable movement to occur between adjacent structures. Also *areolar tissue*. **basement t.** BASEMENT MEMBRANE. **bony t.** A skeletal or supporting connective tissue that combines hardness and resilience. The matrix is progressively mineralized and remains vascularized, providing nutrition to the included osteocytes. A characteristic feature of bony tissue is its layered or lamellar structure which is readily seen with polarized light microscopy. Also *osseous tissue*. **brown adipose t.** INTERSCAPULAR GLAND. **cancellous t.** Spongy bone that is present in the medullary cavity of all bones. In long bones it is more abundant toward the ends rather than in the central region. **cartilaginous t.** A skeletal or supporting connective tissue that combines strength with elasticity. The formative cells or chondrocytes are located within the cartilaginous matrix which becomes progressively replaced by bony tissue during development. Some cartilaginous structures persist into the adult stage in the form of articular surfaces and supporting elements, such as the nasal and bronchial cartilages. **cavernous t.** Tissue that is composed of numerous large vascular channels. **cellular t.** A tissue that contains a high proportion of cells and a low proportion of intercellular matter. **chondroid t.** A type of primitive cartilage found in an embryo. It consists of large round cells which lay down a feltwork of fine collagenous or elastic fibers. Also *vesicular supporting tissue, pseudocartilage*. **chordal t.** Cells or tissue belonging to or derived from the embryonic notochord. **chromaffin t.** Tissue consisting principally of chromaffin cells. **cicatricial t.** SCAR TISSUE. **compact t.** Dense bony tissue that forms the outer layers of all bones and constitutes the cortex. **connective t.** A composite mass of intercellular matrix, connective tissue fibers, and cells that provides the structural and supporting tissue of the body. **critical t.** The tissue showing adverse effects at the lowest dose, with no reference to the severity of the effects. **dartoid t.** A smooth muscle tissue of the type present in the dartos muscle of the scrotum. **dense fibrous connective t.** Fibrous tissue in which the collagen bundles are compacted to form a particularly strong structure, as in tendons and aponeuroses. Also *textus connectivus fibrosus compactus*. **elastic t.** A connective tissue with a high proportion of elastic fibers, which allow greater elasticity than collagen fibers. It is found particularly in the walls of large blood vessels and in the ligamenta flava of the neck. Also *fibroelastic tissue, yellow elastic tissue, textus connectivus elasticus, tela elastica* (outmoded). **embryonal connective t.** MESENCHYME. **endothelial t.** VASCULAR ENDOTHELIUM. **episcleral t.** A layer of loose connective tissue between the sclera and the overlying conjunctival membrane. **epithelial t.** A sheet of cells attached on their deep aspect to a basement membrane and covering either an external or an internal surface of the body. **epivaginal connective t.** Connective tissue surrounding an invagination, such as the sheath of the optic nerve. **erectile t.** Tissue composed of a series of cavernous spaces that, when distended with blood, increase the size and rigidity of a structure. **erectile t. of penis** A large spongelike system of irregular vascular spaces interposed between the afferent arteries and the efferent veins in the corpora cavernosa penis. In erection these fairly empty spaces are filled with blood under high pressure causing enlargement and rigidity of the penis. **extracellular t.** Connective tissue fibers and ground substance that hold the extracellular body fluid. **extraperitoneal t.** A connective tissue layer that surrounds the mesothelial lining of the peritoneum. **fatty t.** ADIPOSE TISSUE. **fibroareolar t.** An irregularly arranged connective tissue with a high proportion of collagen and elastic fibers, as is seen in the dermis. **fibrocellular t.** A connective tissue formed largely from fibers and cells with a minimum of intercellular matrix. **fibroelastic t.** ELASTIC TISSUE. **fibrohyaline t.** A fibrous connective tissue that contains hyalin material or substance. **fibrous t.** Connective tissue with a high proportion of collagen fibers and little intercellular matrix. Also *white fibrous tissue, textus connectivus collagenosus, textus connectivus fibrosus lamellaris*. **glan-**

**dular t.** A localized mass of epithelial cells that are modified to perform a secretory function. **granulation t.** Tissue formed in a wound as a result of inflammation and composed of ground substance, inflammatory cells, and capillaries. Also *proud flesh.* **gut-associated lymphoid t.** Lymphoid tissue within the subepithelial connective tissue that lines the alimentary canal. Particular aggregations are identifiable as the pharyngeal tonsils and Peyer's patches in the small bowel. **hematopoietic t.** Any tissue in which blood cells are formed. In normal adults this is the bone marrow. In the fetus the liver and spleen are involved. **heterologous t.** **1** Tissue that is foreign to the tissue with which it is being matched. **2** Tissue that is not normal in any part of the organism, as distinguished from analogous tissue, which is not foreign to the organism but is abnormally situated. **heterotopic t.** Normal tissue elements that are located in an abnormal anatomic site. **homologous t.** Tissue that is the same as that with which it is being matched. **indifferent t.** Embryonic tissue which has not begun to differentiate. **inflammatory t.** A tissue in which some features of the process of inflammation can be identified. **interstitial t.** The connective tissue that lies between and around the main functional cells of an organ. Also *interstitium.* **junctional t.** That part of the conducting system of the heart that connects the atria with the ventricles. It includes the atrioventricular node and bundle. Also *Purkinje's network.* **keratinized t.** Epithelium that has been partly converted into horny scales. **Kuhnt's intermediary t.** A layer of neuroglial tissue (probably astrocytes) interposed between the retina and the bundles of optic nerve fibers at the edge of the optic disk and oriented somewhat parallel to the optic nerve axons. **laminated t.** A tissue that is constructed in a series of layers or strata. **lymphoid t.** Tissue that is composed predominantly of lymphocytes but that often includes other cells such as plasma cells and macrophages. The cells are distributed within a loose reticular connective tissue framework, as seen in the lymph nodes, the white pulp of the spleen, and gut-associated lymphoid tissue. **mesenchymal t.** MESENCHYME. **metanephrogenic t.** Mesenchymal tissue corresponding to the aggregated nephrotomes of the sacral region and which gives rise to uriniferous tubules of the metanephros, i.e., to the definitive kidney. **mucoid t.** Connective tissue in the embryo, containing stellate fibroblasts, a jellylike substance which is metachromatic and reacts somewhat like mucin, and varying amounts of collagenous fibers. Mucoid tissue found in the umbilical cord is often called Wharton's jelly. **mucous t.** Connective tissue that has a high mucopolysaccharide content and a low fiber content. It is seen in the early embryo. **multilocular adipose t.** INTERSCAPULAR GLAND. **muscular t.** A tissue composed of cells that are highly specialized for contraction along with some intervening connective tissue. Also *textus muscularis, myoideum.* **nephrogenic t.** Part of the intermediate mesoderm of the embryo from which the embryonic and adult kidneys develop. **nervous t.** Tissue composed of neurons and their processes and neuroglial cells (including Schwann cells) and their processes, which together form the parenchyma of the neural organs that comprise the nervous system. Nervous tissue is highly specialized for the conduction and transmission of neural impulses and the production of neurally active humoral substances. Also *neural tissue, nerve tissue, textus nervosus.* **osseous t.** BONY TISSUE. **osteogenic t.** Fibrous connective tissue that contains osteoblasts with the capacity to form bony tissue. **osteoid t.** Bone matrix prior to impregation with bone salts, normally found in a thin layer on the surface of bony trabeculae. In certain bone diseases it occurs in considerably increased amounts. **parenchymatous t.** PARENCHYMA. **periapical t.** The periodontal membrane and the bone which surround the apex of the root of a tooth. **periodontal t.** The fibrovascular tissue of the periodontal membrane. **periosteal t.** A fibrous connective tissue layer that is well vascularized and covers the surface of bones apart from their articular surfaces. The cells in the deeper layers have the capacity to lay down new bone on the surface of the existing structure, either for growth, remodeling of bone, or repair of fractures. **pigmented connective t.** Connective tissue with a high elastic fiber content, as in the ligamentum flavum which appears yellow. Also *textus connectivus pigmentosus.* **pseudoerectile t.** Tissue composed of a series of cavernous vascular spaces that is similar to erectile tissue but that lacks the functional changes. **reticular t.** A connective tissue composed of reticulin fibers and reticular cells that are arranged to form an open network to faciliate movement of cells and fluids. Also *reticulated tissue, textus connectivus reticularis.* **retroperitoneal t.** Tissue on the posterior abdominal wall that is covered by a layer of peritoneum. **scar t.** An irregularly arranged mass of fibrous tissue that is formed directly from granulation tissue by the activity of fibroblasts. Also *cicatricial tissue.* **scleral t.** Dense fibrous tissue that forms the outer hard coat of the eyeball. **sclerous t.'s** Cartilage, tendon, ligament, and bone. **skeletal t.** **1** Any bone or cartilage. **2** Any connective tissue that contributes to the structural architecture of an organ. **splenic t.** The cells and connective tissues that together form the red and the white pulp areas of the spleen. **subcutaneous t.** TELA SUBCUTANEA. **subcutaneous fatty t.** PANICULUS ADIPOSUS. **sustentacular t.** A supportive tissue composed of cells and/or fibers that assist in the functioning of the principal parenchymatous cells in an organ; specifically, such supportive tissue of the retina, consisting of retinal gliocytes (Müller cells), which are elaborate neuroglial elements containing long processes that stretch radially throughout almost the entire thickness of the retina. From these vertically oriented fibers other glial processes stretch horizontally to form a neuroglial meshwork within which are located the retinal neural cells. **symplastic t.** SYNCYTIUM. **target t.** **1** Those cells subjected to humoral or cell-mediated immune reactions, either *in vitro* or *in vivo.* **2** Those particular glands, tissues, or cell masses which respond to a given hormone. **tendinous t.** Regularly arranged bundles of collagen fibers and their included fibroblasts that together provide the flexible, yet nonextensible, tissue of muscle tendons. **tuberculosis granulation t.** Tissue produced in the healing process of tuberculous infection. It contains fibroblasts and tubercles which contain concentric masses of epithelial cells, lymphocytes, and occasional Langhans giant cells. **vesicular supporting t.** CHONDROID TISSUE. **white fibrous t.** FIBROUS TISSUE. **yellow elastic t.** ELASTIC TISSUE.

**tissue-active** Physiologically active at the subcellular level: said especially of the molecular form of a hormone, as dihydrotestosterone with respect to testosterone.

**tissue-borne** Supported entirely by the oral mucosa and underlying tissues: said of partial dentures.

**tissular** \tish′ələr\ Relating to a tissue or tissues.

**titanium** \tītā′nē·əm\ Element number 22, having atomic weight 47.90. Never found free, it is present in many ores and in most igneous rock. It occurs in meteorites and moon rocks and it has been identified in the solar spectrum. It is the ninth most abundant element in the lithosphere. Elemental titanium is a very strong, lustrous white metal, less than half as heavy as steel (specific gravity, 4.54). The five natural isotopes are stable. Four radioactive isotopes are known. Valences are 2, 3, and 4. Titanium is present in plants and the human body, but it has no known biologic function. Symbol: Ti

**titanium dioxide** $TiO_2$. A white, amorphous, odorless powder. Like zinc oxide, it is used in skin medications for the treatment of pruritus and dermatologic conditions in dusting powders, creams, and pastes.

**titer** \tī′tər\ [French *titre* (from Old French *title* title, from L *titulus* title of rank) title, rank, percentage of gold or silver in an alloy] **1** The quantity of reagent, as found by titration, necessary to react with a fixed amount of another reagent. **2** The reciprocal of the highest dilution that produces a reaction. For example, if a 1:256 dilution reacts and 1:512 dilution does not, the titer is 256.

**TITh** triiodothyronine.

**titillation** \tit′əlā′shən\ [L *titillatio* a tickling, titillation] The sensation caused by tickling.

**titrant** \tī′trənt\ The material, whether solute or solution, with which another is titrated.

**titrate** \tī′trāt\ [*titr(e)* (see TITER) + -ATE] To add one solution to a sample until just enough has been added to react completely with a substance in that sample. This is normally done in order to measure the concentration of that substance in the sample, or occasionally to measure the concentration of the reactant in the solution added. It requires some method for determining which reactant is in excess, so that the addition can be controlled, and so that it can be known when the end-point has been achieved.

**titration** \tītrā′shən\ The process of titrating, or a particular act of titrating.

**titre** \tī′tər\ *Brit.* TITER.

**titubant** \tich′əbənt\ Demonstrating titubation.

**titubation** \tich′əbā′shən\ [L *titubatio* (from *titubatus*, past part. of *titubare* to stagger, totter, stammer) a staggering, wavering] **1** A syncopated gait. **2** A rhythmic tremor of the head and neck whether anteroposterior or lateral in direction, as seen in some patients with senile tremor or cerebellar degeneration. **lingual t.** STUTTERING.

***Tityus*** \tit′ē·əs\ A genus of scorpions some species of which are extremely venomous. The sting of *T. serrulatus* of Brazil has caused many human fatalities, especially among young children, in whom mortality may run as high as 15–20 percent.

**TKD** tokodynamometer (tocodynamometer).

**TKG** tokodynagraph (tocodynagraph).

**TL** **1** temporal lobe. **2** tubal ligation. **3** total lipids.

**Tl** Symbol for the element, thallium.

**TLC** **1** total lung capacity. **2** thin-layer chromatography.

**TLE** thin-layer electrophoresis.

**Tm** **1** Symbol for the element, thulium. **2** Symbol for transport maximum.

**TMIF** tumor cell migration inhibition factor.

**TMV** tobacco mosaic virus.

**Tn** Symbol for normal intraocular tension (intraocular pressure).

**TOA** tubo-ovarian abscess.

**tobacco** [Spanish *tabaco*, prob. from Taino] The dried, prepared leaves of *Nicotiana tabacum*, which contains the alkaloid nicotine.

**tobaccoism** \təbak′ō·izm\ TOBACCO POISONING.

**Tobey** [George Loring *Tobey*, U.S. otolaryngologist, 1881–1947] Ayer-Tobey test. See under TOBEY-AYER TEST.

**tobramycin** An aminoglycoside antibiotic obtained from *Streptomyces tenebrarius*, with properties much like those of gentamicin. It is particularly effective against *Pseudomonas* infections.

**toco-** \tō′kə-, tō′kō-\ [Gk *tokos* childbirth] A combining form meaning childbirth. Also *toko-*.

**tocoalgography** \tō′kō·algäg′rəfē\ TOCOGRAPHY.

**tocodynamometer** \tō′kōdī′nəmäm′ətər\ An instrument for recording the amplitude versus time of the expulsive force of uterine muscular contractions during labor. Also *tocometer, tokodynamometer.* Abbr. TKD

**tocography** \tōkäg′rəfē\ [TOCO- + -GRAPHY] The recording and interpreting of the expulsive force of uterine muscular contractions during labor. Also *tocoalgography.*

**tocol** A trivial designation for the substance 2-methyl-2-(4,8,12-trimethyltridecyl)chroman-6-ol, the parent of several natural tocopherols.

**tocometer** \tōkäm′ətər\ TOCODYNAMOMETER.

**tocopherol** \tōkäf′ərôl\ Any mono-, di-, or trimethyltocol. Several such compounds, e.g. α-tocopherol, i.e. 5,7,8-trimethyltocol, have vitamin E activity. Tocopherols function as antioxidants, but their biologic function is not well understood. They are plant products, and essential in mammalian food.

**tocopherolquinone** A quinone found in chloroplasts and derived from tocopherol by oxidative opening of its oxygen-containing ring.

**Tod** [David *Tod*, British surgeon, 1794–1856] Tod's muscle. See under MUSCULUS OBLIQUUS AURICULAE.

**Todd** [Robert Bentley *Todd*, English physician and anatomist, 1809–1860] Todd's palsy, Todd's paralysis. See under POSTEPILEPTIC PARALYSIS.

**toddler** A child in the early stages of learning to walk, usually in the second year. *Popular.*

**toe** [Old English *tā*, akin to L *digitus* finger, toe] Any one of the five digits of the foot; digitus pedis. **claw t.** A great toe that has a rounded nail resembling a claw. The condition predominates among those who wear narrow shoes with high heels. Associated calluses may be present. **great t.** HALLUX. **hammer t.** A fixed flexion deformity of the proximal interphalangeal joint of the toe with compensatory hyperextension of the metatarsophalangeal and distal interphalangeal joints. The second toe is most commonly affected. Also *mallet toe.* **little t.** DIGITUS MINIMUS. **mallet t.** HAMMER TOE. **Morton's t.** MORTON'S NEUROMA. **stiff t.** HALLUX RIGIDUS. **upgoing t.** EXTENSOR PLANTAR RESPONSE.

**toenail** The unguis that covers the dorsal aspect of the distal phalanx of the toe.

**Togaviridae** \tō′gəvī′ridē\ [L *toga* gown, toga + *vir(us)* + -IDAE] A family of enveloped RNA viruses, 40–90 nm in diameter, which were formerly known as group A and group B arboviruses because many of them were arthropod-borne. There are four genera: *Alphavirus* (formerly group A), *Flavivirus* (formerly group B), *Pestivirus,* and *Rubivirus.* Members of this family include the viruses of eastern and western equine encephalitis, yellow fever, dengue, and rubella.

**togavirus** \tō′gəvī′rəs\ Any member of the family Togaviridae.

**toilet** [French *toilette* (from *toil(e)* a fabric of flax, hemp, or cotton, from L *tela* the web of a loom, + *-ette*, fem. diminishing suffix) the act of cleansing oneself] The cleansing of a wound or part of the body.

**toko-** \tō′kə-, tō′kō-\ TOCO-.

**tolazamide** A sulfonylurea used as an oral hypoglycemic agent in the treatment of diabetes mellitus. Its duration of action is intermediate.

**tolazoline hydrochloride** $C_{10}H_{13}ClN_2$. 4,5-Dihydro-2-(phenylmethyl)-1*H*-imidazole hydrochloride. A vasodilator agent with direct relaxant activity on smooth muscle. It is used in conditions in which vasospasm is present and in peripheral vascular diseases. It is given orally or parenterally. Also *benzazoline hydrochloride*.

**tolbutamide** 1-Butyl-3-(*p*-tolylsufonyl)urea, one of the most widely used of the sulfonylurea derivatives, an oral hypoglycemic agent employed in the treatment of obese, middle-age-onset diabetes mellitus, and acting by stimulating the secretion of insulin by the pancreatic beta cell. Its duration of action is short. The use of this and related drugs is now limited to diabetic patients unwilling or unable to take insulin, because the sulfonylureas have been associated with an increased incidence of cardiovascular deaths.

**Toldt** [Karl *Toldt*, Austrian anatomist, 1840–1920] See under MEMBRANE.

**tolerance** [L *tolerantia* (from *tolerare* to endure, tolerate, akin to *tollere* to bear, raise) endurance, fortitude] **1** The capacity to undergo exposure to drugs or poisons in unusual quantity or for an appreciable time without showing the expected response or toxic effects. **2** A tendency toward a reduced level of response to the repeated activation of a stimulus. **acoustic t.** LOUDNESS DISCOMFORT LEVEL. **acquired t.** **1** Tolerance to a drug induced by prolonged use. **2** Immunologic tolerance induced by suitable exposure to nonself antigens. **adaptation t.** The interaction between host and a given parasite over evolutionary time which results in a selective diminution of the host's defenses to that parasite, usually associated with reduced virulence and a mutually compatible host-parasite balance. **adoptive t.** Immunologic tolerance induced in a subject by the transfer of lymphoid cells from a syngeneic donor who has been made tolerant to a specific antigen. **crossed t.** The development of tolerance to a compound as a consequence of tolerance from exposure to another compound. **drug t.** Tolerance to drugs that develops upon repeated administration. It is usually evident as a progressively smaller pharmacological response to each subsequent dose of the drug. **g-t.** The force of inertia that the body can tolerate without coming to harm. **high-dose t.** The induction of immunologic tolerance following the administration of either a large single dose of antigen, such as that of pneumococcal polysaccharide, or repeated doses of protein antigens, usually without the presence of adjuvants. Also *high-zone tolerance*. Compare LOW-DOSE TOLERANCE. **high-zone t.** HIGH-DOSE TOLERANCE. **immune t.** IMMUNOLOGIC TOLERANCE. **immunologic t.** Immunologic nonreactivity to specific antigens in an otherwise immunocompetent subject. The tolerance may have been caused by fetal or neonatal contact with the antigens or by administration of doses of antigen in later life. Immunity to other antigens is not affected. Also *immunotolerance, immune tolerance*. **low-dose t.** The induction of immunologic tolerance following the administration of repeated low doses of antigen below the level that would normally be immunogenic. Also *low-zone tolerance*. Compare HIGH-DOSE TOLERANCE. **low-zone t.** LOW-DOSE TOLERANCE. **species t.** The resistance or insensitivity of a particular species to the expected effects of a drug or chemical agent. **split t.** Any of several peculiarities of immunologic activity. They include an immune response to certain epitopes of an immunogenic complex but apparent tolerance to others, and the induction of either humoral immune response to an antigen in conjunction with tolerance at the level of cell-mediated immunity, or occasionally vice versa. *Imprecise*.

**tolerant** Capable of tolerance.

**tolerogen** \tōler′əjən\ Antigen used to cause specific immunologic tolerance to subsequent exposure to the same antigen.

**tolerogenic** \täl′ərōjen′ik\ Capable of inducing immunologic tolerance.

**tolidine** A dimethylbenzidine, in which each methyl group is on a different ring and *ortho* to its amino group. Like many other benzidines it is carcinogenic. It was once used as a reagent to test for oxidizing agents, which give a blue color with it.

**tolmetin sodium** $C_{15}H_{14}NNaO_3 \cdot 2H_2O$. Sodium (1-methyl-5-*p*-toluoylpyrrol-2-yl)acetate dihydrate. An anti-inflammatory drug used in the treatment of rheumatoid arthritis. It is given orally.

**tolnaftate** $C_{19}H_{17}NOS$. *O*-2-Naphthyl *m,N*-dimethylthiocarbanilate, the first chemical compound found to be an effective topical fungicide. It is usually used in a 1 percent concentration in a cream, gel, powder, or spray solution and is highly effective against tinea infections.

**Tolosa** [Eduardo *Tolosa*, Spanish cardiologist, flourished 20th century] Tolosa-Hunt syndrome. See under SYNDROME.

**toluene** \täl′yoo-ēn\ $CH_3—C_6H_5$. Methylbenzene. A substance obtained from coal tar. It is used as a solvent, especially because it is less toxic and carcinogenic than benzene, being slowly degraded by the body to benzoic acid. Like many organic solvents, however, it can cause liver damage, as by inhalation of its vapor.

**toluidine blue** A dye used in histology.

**tomatine** $C_{50}H_{83}NO_{21}$. Any of a group of compounds isolated from tomato leaves and occurring in glycosidic linkage with glucose, xylose, and galactose. It has antifungal properties and has also been used like digitonin to precipitate certain steroids. Also *lycopersicin*.

**-tome** \-tōm\ [Gk *-tomon* -cutter, cutting instrument, and *tomos* a slice, piece, from *temnein* to cut] A combining form meaning (1) instrument for cutting; (2) a section or segment.

**tomentum** \tōmen′təm\ [L, feathers, straw, and other materials for stuffing cushions or beds] The network of small and delicate nutrient vessels of the pia mater that penetrate the cerebral cortex, usually at right angles, and supply the neural substance. *Rare*. Also *tomentum cerebri*. **t. cerebri** TOMENTUM.

**Tomes** [Sir John *Tomes*, English dentist and anatomist, 1815–1895] **1** Tomes fiber. See under ODONTOBLASTIC PROCESS. **2** Granular layer of Tomes. See under LAYER.

**Tommaselli** [Salvatore *Tommaselli*, Italian physician, 1834–1906] Tommaselli syndrome. See under DISEASE.

**tomo-** \tō′mə-\ [Gk *tomos* (from *temnein* to cut) a slice, section] A combining form meaning section.

**tomogram** \-gram\ [TOMO- + -GRAM] A roentgenogram obtained by body section roentgenography.

**tomograph** \-graf\ [TOMO- + -GRAPH] Radiologic equipment for doing body section roentgenography.

**tomography** \təmäg′rəfē\ [TOMO- + -GRAPHY] BODY SECTION ROENTGENOGRAPHY. **computed t.** A radiologic examination in which a thin, collimated x-ray beam rotates about the patient with registration of photon exit doses on detectors, the exit doses then undergoing manipulation by computer to produce an image of the slice of tissue examined. Also *computerized axial tomography* (outmoded), *computerized transaxial tomography* (outmoded), *computer-assisted tomography, CT scanning, CAT scanning*. **focal plane t.** Tomography in which structures at a certain depth are sharply focused while those at other depths are blurred. **positron emission t.** The construction of tomographic images showing the location within a patient of radionuclides that decay by positron emission, and thus emit two gamma rays which can be detected by external detectors. Unlike computed tomography, positron emission tomography gives not only recordings of tissue density but in addition information about the metabolism of the tissue being scanned. Also *positron emission transaxial tomography, PET scanning.* **single photon emission computed t.** The construction of tomographic images showing the location within a patient of radionuclides of the type which decay by emitting single gamma photons. Also *single photon tomography.* Abbr. SPECT

**tomolevel** \tō′mōlev′əl\ [TOMO- + *level*] The level of the body, usually stated in centimeters from the top of the x-ray table, for a body section roentgenogram.

**-tomy** \-təmē\ [Gk *tom(ē)* a cut, incision + -Y] A combining form meaning the act of cutting, especially in a surgical operation.

**tone** [Gk *tonos* (from *teinein* to stretch, draw tight) a cord, sinew, stretch, tension, tone] **1** A healthy state of tissue marked by slight tension and associated with the capacity to function and respond normally. **2** A vocal or musical sound. **arterial t.** The state of tension in an arterial wall. **heart t.** HEART SOUND. **muscle t.** TONUS. **myogenic t.** The component of muscle tone, or resistance to passive stretch, that is thought to be independent of the nerve supply of the muscle and persists after denervation. In fact, denervated muscle is flaccid. It possesses physical elasticity but no tone. Also *myogenic tonus.* Compare NEUROGENIC TONE. **nervous t.** The level of ongoing, background nervous activity. *Imprecise.* **neurogenic t.** A state of tonus which has its origins in the nervous system, as that mediated through reflex action involving the muscle spindles. Also *neurogenic tonus.* Compare MYOGENIC TONE. **peripheral vasomotor t.** The background tension in the blood vessels, especially the arteries, that determines their degree of constriction or relaxation i.e., blood pressure.

**tongs** A hinged, two-armed surgical instrument used for grasping or holding. **Crutchfield t.** A skull tongs that consists of two hinged arms with protected points that pierce the upper sides of the skull. It is attached to a weight for traction. **skull t.** An instrument applied to the vertex of the skull to provide traction in the reduction and stabilization of a cervical vertebral fracture or dislocation. A popular form of the instrument is the Crutchfield tongs or an adaptation of it.

**tongue** [Old English *tunge*, akin to L *lingua* tongue] A muscular organ that is covered with mucous membrane on its upper and lower surfaces, is situated in the floor of the mouth and the anterior wall of the pharynx, and is involved in mastication, swallowing, taste, and speech; lingua. **adherent t.** A tongue which is abnormally attached by folds of mucous membrane to the floor of the mouth and to the alveolar processes. **antibiotic t.** Black hairy tongue as a complication of the oral use of antibiotics. **bald t.** A smooth, red, shiny state of the tongue with atrophy of the papillae, as seen in a variety of nutritional disturbances. **beefy t.** The inflamed tongue as seen in cases of pernicious anemia, in which patches over the dorsum and margins or sometimes the whole tongue assume a red coloration. Shallow ulcers may be present and glossodynia or glossopyrosis are common. Also *raw-beef tongue.* **bifid t.** A tongue the tip of which is notched or which is deeply grooved in its midsagittal surface. It is usually of developmental origin. Also *diglossia, schistoglossia, cleft tongue.* **black hairy t.** A condition in which a black or dark brown patch occurs on the dorsum of the tongue, usually on the middle one third. Because of hypertrophy of the filiform papillae the patch appears to consist of a mat of fine hairs. Pigment-producing fungi and other organisms have been isolated but are unlikely to be the cause. Excessive smoking has been blamed as one of the possible causes. Many cases are associated with the oral use of antibiotics. Also *lingua villosa nigra, lingua nigra, melanotrichia linguae.* **cleft t.** BIFID TONGUE. **coated t.** A tongue displaying an increase of coating either in extent or degree, particularly when the anterior two thirds are involved, or when the coating is associated with papillary hypertrophy or is discolored. Also *furred tongue.* **crescent t.** A crescent-shaped appearance of the tongue, due to paralysis of the hypoglossal nerve with wasting of the muscles on the concave side. **fissured t.** A condition of the tongue characterized by longitudinal and transverse furrows or grooves tending to divide the papillae into patterned groups, made more apparent by folding the tongue downwards about its long axis. Familial and congenital incidence have been reported, although the incidence increases with increasing age. It occurs particularly in the Melkersson-Rosenthal syndrome and, sometimes, in the Down syndrome. **frog t.** *Seldom used* RANULA. **furred t.** COATED TONGUE. **geographic t.** A disease in which multiple patches of superficial desquamation occur on the dorsum of the tongue, giving it a maplike appearance. The affected areas tend to heal, only to be replaced by others in different localities, as if migrating. Within the patches there is an absence of the filiform papillae. The etiology is unknown. Also *benign migratory glossitis, exfoliative glossitis, glossitis migrans.* **glazed t.** The smooth, shiny tongue as it may appear in the course of a number of varieties of chronic superficial glossitis associated with certain deficiency diseases. Also *glassy tongue.* **hobnail t.** The appearance of the tongue in some cases of atrophic or interstitial glossitis, usually due to tertiary syphilis, with contrasting patches of atrophy of the papillae, epithelial hyperplasia, and superimposed leukoplakia. **raspberry t.** A vivid red, uncoated tongue with raised papillae, seen a few days after the rash appears in scarlet fever. **raw-beef t.** BEEFY TONGUE. **smooth t.** A tongue which has lost its filiform papillae by atrophy. The condition is caused by anemia, vitamin B deficiency, candidiasis, or lichen planus. **sprue t.** The tongue in tropical sprue when folic acid deficiency may produce extreme examples of atrophy of the papillae and bald tongue. Aphthous ulceration may occur. **strawberry t.** A coated tongue with swollen, protruding papillae, seen in scarlet fever during the first 24 hours of the rash. **trombone t.** Involuntary repetitive protrusion and retraction of the tongue, seen in some patients with general paresis. The movement is often tremulous during the phase of protrusion. Also *trombone tremor of tongue, Magnan's trombone movement.*

**tongue-tie** Shortness or absence of the frenum of the tongue, usually of developmental origin. If it remains uncorrected into late infancy it is likely to interfere with speech. Also *ankyloglossia.*

**tonic** \tän′ik\ [Gk *tonikos* (from *tonos*; see TONE) tensile, contractile, tonic] **1** Of or characterized by tension. **2** Characterized by a state of continuous or prolonged muscular contraction. **3** Restorative and invigorating; healthful. **4** An agent or drug given to improve the normal tone of a tissue, organ, or organism. **bitter t.** A liquid preparation for improving the appetite and digestion that contains bitter ingredients, such as quinine, quassia, or gentian.

**tonicity** \tōnis′itē\ The property or state of having tone or being tonic. It is exemplified in tissues by muscle tone or in fluids by the characteristic that determines whether or not it will lead to passive movement of the fluid across a membrane.

**tonicize** \tän′isīz\ To make more tonic.

**tonicoclonic** \tän′ikōklän′ik\ Denoting muscular contractions which are intermittently both tonic and clonic. Also *tonoclonic.*

**tono-** \tō′nō-, tō′nə-\ [Gk *tonos* tension, stretching, tightening] A combining form meaning (1) tone, tension; (2) pressure.

**tonoclonic** \tän′ōklän′ik\ TONICOCLONIC.

**tonofibril** \tän′ōfī′bril\ A thin filament observed in the cytoplasm of an epithelial cell which is believed to bind adjacent cells together and to have a supportive function. Also *tenofibril, epitheliofibril.*

**tonofilament** \tän′ōfil′əmənt\ One of the cytoplasmic filaments, of 100 Å diameter, which are associated with the plasmalemma at the desmosome (macula adherens).

**tonogram** \tō′nəgram\ [TONO- + -GRAM] A recording of the rate of outflow of aqueous.

**tonography** \tōnäg′rəfē\ [TONO- + -GRAPHY] Measurement of the rate of outflow of the aqueous humor, as determined by the rate of softening of the eye when external pressure is applied.

**tonometer** \tōnäm′ətər\ [TONO- + -METER] **1** A device for measuring tension or pressure, as intraocular pressure. Also *tenonometer.* **2** A chamber in which blood is equilibrated at various gas tensions. **air-puff t.** A tonometer that consists of an air jet that flattens the corneal surface. The pressure is determined by instantaneous computer analysis of the amount of corneal flattening. **applanation t.** A tonometer that consists of a flat surface which apposes to and flattens the cornea by an amount that correlates with the intraocular pressure. **electronic t.** A tonometer that consists of a plunger which indents the cornea. The amount of indentation is electrically measured and recorded upon a graph. **impression t.** A tonometer utilizing a plunger that indents the cornea. **MacKay-Marg electronic t.** An applanation tonometer in which the intraocular pressure is measured by a force transducer in the center of an annular ring. **pneumatic t.** A tonometer consisting of an air pressure chamber that propels a plunger against the cornea. The intraocular pressure correlates with the amount of air pressure required for indentation. **Schiötz t.** A tonometer measuring intraocular pressure by the degree of indentation of the cornea resulting from application of a standard weight.

**tonometry** \tōnäm′ətrē\ [TONO- + -METRY] **1** The measurement of tension or pressure, especially intraocular pressure, by means of a tonometer. **2** The equilibration of blood at various gas tensions in a tonometer. **applanation t.** The most accurate clinical method of measurement of intraocular pressure, consisting of measurement of the force required to flatten a predetermined area of the cornea, usually 3.06 $mm^2$. **digital t.** A crude estimation of intraocular pressure obtained by the alternate indentation of the eye by two fingers. **impression t.** A technique of intraocular pressure measurement whereby a plunger indents the cornea.

**tonoplast** \tän′əplast\ [TONO- + -PLAST] *Obs.* VACUOLE.

**tonoscope** \tän′əskōp\ [TONO- + -SCOPE] An instrument that records ultrasonically a change in density of the brain. It is used especially on the exposed surface of the brain to locate the position of an underlying abnormality, such as a tumor.

**tonsil** [L *tonsillae* (akin to *toles* neck swelling or goiter) the tonsils] **1** An aggregation of lymphoid tissue, usually in the mucous membrane of the upper part of the digestive tract, that is well demarcated and that has the surface epithelium invaginating the tissue, as in the palatine tonsil. **2** Any of various anatomic structures that resemble the palatine tonsil. For defs. 1 and 2 also *tonsilla, amygdala.* Adj. tonsillar. **buried t.** A not uncommon conformation of the palatine tonsil, usually bilateral, in which it is scarcely visible when inspected in the usual way, almost the whole of the lymphoid mass lying out of sight between the anterior and posterior faucial pillars. **t. of cerebellum** TONSILLA CEREBELLI. **eustachian t.** TONSILLA TUBARIA. **faucial t.** TONSILLA PALATINA. **Gerlach's t.** TONSILLA TUBARIA. **lingual t.** TONSILLA LINGUALIS. **Luschka's t.** TONSILLA PHARYNGEALIS. **nasopharyngeal t.** TONSILLA PHARYNGEALIS. **palatine t.** TONSILLA PALATINA. **pharyngeal t.** TONSILLA PHARYNGEALIS. **third t.** TONSILLA PHARYNGEALIS. **t. of torus tubarius** TONSILLA TUBARIA. **tubal t.** TONSILLA TUBARIA.

**tonsilla** \tänsil′ə\ [New L, sing. of L *tonsillae* tonsils. See TONSIL.] (*pl.* tonsillae) TONSIL. **t. cerebelli** [NA] A small, circumscribed portion of the cerebellar hemisphere located on each side lateral to the uvula of the cerebellar vermis. It is found on the posterior surface of the cerebellum between the biventral lobule and the flocculus, and is bounded by the retrotonsillar and posterolateral fissures. Also *tonsilla of cerebellum, tonsil of cerebellum, amygdala of cerebellum* (seldom used). **t. of cerebellum** TONSILLA CEREBELLI. **t. lingualis** [NA] A collection of nodules of lymphoid tissue situated in the tela submucosa of the pharyngeal part of the tongue that produce small irregular elevations of the mucous membrane. Also *lingual tonsil, amygdala accessoria* (outmoded), *accessory amygdala* (outmoded). **t. palatina** [NA] A mass of lymphoid tissue, variable in size, that is situated in the tonsillar fossa in each lateral wall of the oropharynx. Its projecting medial surface is free and covered by a mucous membrane which is pitted by tonsillar crypts, while its lateral surface is covered by a capsule that separates it from the superior constrictor muscle of the pharynx. Also *palatine tonsil, faucial tonsil.* **t. pharyngea** TONSILLA PHARYNGEALIS. **t. pharyngealis** [NA] Diffuse lymphoid tissue producing projecting folds of mucous membrane that radiate forward and sideways from the pharyngeal bursa at the junction of the roof and posterior wall of the nasopharynx. It is prominent in young children but slowly atrophies towards the end of the first decade of life. It is often absent in adults. Also *pharyngeal tonsil, third tonsil, Luschka's tonsil, nasopharyngeal tonsil, tonsilla pharyngea, adenoid.* **t. tubaria** [NA] The lateral extension of the pharyngeal tonsil behind and around the pharyngeal orifice of the auditory tube on the lateral wall of the nasopharynx. Also *tubal tonsil, tonsil of torus tubarius, eustachian tonsil, noduli lymphatici aggregati tubae auditivae, Gerlach's tonsil, tubal lymphatic nodules.*

**tonsillar** \tän′silər\ Of or relating to a tonsil, especially the palatine tonsil. Also *amygdaline.*

**tonsillectomy** \tän′silek′təmē\ [L *tonsill(ae)* the tonsils + -ECTOMY] The operation of removing the palatine tonsils. The common indication is to prevent further attacks in cases of recurrent tonsillitis, most of the many other indications being controversial. **dissection t.** Tonsillectomy by deliberate dissection followed by the careful establishment of hemostasis, now almost universally preferred to guillotine tonsillectomy. **guillotine t.** Tonsillectomy using one of a number of especially designed guillotines, largely replaced by the dissection tonsillectomy.

**tonsillith** \tän′silith\ TONSILLOLITH.

**tonsillitis** \tän′səlī′tis\ [*tonsill(a)* + -ITIS] Inflammation of the tonsils, usually the palatine tonsils. **acute parenchymatous t.** Acute tonsillitis when the whole tonsil is uniformly inflamed and swollen but when exudate or pseudomembrane is absent. Also *parenchymatous tonsillitis, phlegmonous tonsillitis* (older term). **caseous t.** A condition of the palatine tonsils in which creamy-white debris accumulates in the crypts, particularly in the intratonsillar cleft, causing discomfort and often tainting the breath. It is generally regarded as a variety of chronic tonsillitis to be treated by tonsillectomy. **chronic t.** Low-grade tonsillitis persisting between attacks of acute tonsillitis. It is an ill-defined disease except in the uncommon conditions where walled-off abscesses persist within the lymphoid follicles. The treatment is tonsillectomy. **diphtheritic t.** Tonsillitis due to infection with *Corynebacterium diphtheriae*, the tonsils being covered with the characteristic diphtheritic pseudomembrane. **follicular t.** Acute tonsillitis characterized by the appearance of exudate or pseudomembrane around the opening of the tonsillar crypts. Also *lacunar tonsillitis.* **lacunar t.** FOLLICULAR TONSILLITIS. **lingual t.** Inflammation of the lingual tonsils, a rare and sometimes unilateral acute infection. **mycotic t.** TONSILLOMYCOSIS. **parenchymatous t.** ACUTE PARENCHYMATOUS TONSILLITIS. **phlegmonous t.** *Older term* ACUTE PARENCHYMATOUS TONSILLITIS. **streptococcal t.** Tonsillitis due to infection with streptococci, usually group A β-hemolytic streptococci, the most common organism identified in throat swabs from acutely infected tonsils. In the majority of cases, the streptococci are secondary invaders, the primary infection being due to a virus, usually an adenovirus. Scarlet fever is a variety of this disease. Rheumatic fever and acute glomerulonephritis are important among the systemic complications. **superficial t.** Acute tonsillitis occurring as a feature of an attack of acute pharyngitis in which the mucous membrane covering the tonsils is inflamed along with the mucous membrane elsewhere in the pharynx although specific features such as exudate or pseudomembrane are absent. **suppurative t.** Tonsillitis in which the pus-forming organisms, usually secondary invaders, lead to abscess formation within the substance of the tonsil or, rarely, purulent discharge from the tonsillar crypts. **ulceromembranous t.** Acute tonsillitis in which a confluent pseudomembrane covers the surface of the inflamed tonsil or tonsils. See also ULCEROMEMBRANOUS PHARYNGITIS.

**tonsilloadenoidectomy** \tänsil′ō·ad′ənoidek′təmē\ ADENOTONSILLECTOMY.

**tonsillolith** \tänsil′əlith\ [L *tonsill(ae)* the tonsils + *o* + -LITH] A concretion of calcium and magnesium salts deposited in and around the caseous material sometimes accumulating in tonsillar crypts but in particular in the intratonsillar cleft. It may slowly grow and eventually reach the size of the top joint of the thumb. Also *tonsillith, tonsillar calculus.*

**tonsillomycosis** \tänsil′əmīkō′sis\ Infection of the tonsils with any species of fungus. A rare occurrence. Also *mycotic tonsillitis.*

**tonsillotome** \tänsil′ətōm\ *Obs.* TONSIL GUILLOTINE. **Physick t.** A modification of the uvulotome used to remove the tonsils. It is the precursor of the tonsil guillotines.

**tonsillotomy** \tän′silät′əmē\ [L *tonsill(ae)* the tonsils + *o* + -TOMY] The amputation of the prominent part of the palatine tonsil. ● Until well into the twentieth century, the operation for removing the palatine tonsils, that is tonsillectomy, was generally called tonsillotomy.

**tonus** \tō′nəs\ [L (from Gk *tonos*; see TONE), tension, strain, tone] The normal, slightly contracted state of muscle tissue, serving to resist passive stretching and maintain readiness to respond, and in the skeletal muscles serving to maintain posture. Also *muscle tone.* **acerebral t.** A state of moderately exaggerated postural tone of muscles that is seen after loss of the cerebral hemispheres. **myogenic t.** MYOGENIC TONE. **neurogenic t.** NEUROGENIC TONE.

**Tooth** [Howard Henry *Tooth,* English physician, 1856–1925] Marie-Tooth disease, Tooth disease, Tooth's atrophy. See under CHARCOT-MARIE-TOOTH DISEASE.

# tooth

**tooth** [Old English *tōth*; akin to L *dens* (gen. *dentis*) tooth and Gk *odous* (gen. *odontos*) tooth] (*pl.* teeth) In most vertebrates, a mineralized or horny structure projecting from the jaws and used for seizing and masticating food and sometimes as a weapon of defense or attack. It is typically composed of thick, hard dentin surrounding a pulp cavity and covered by enamel on the crown and cement on the

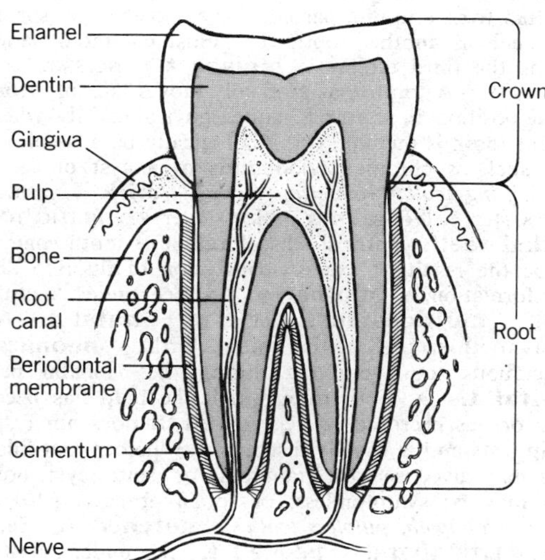


Tooth and surrounding structures

root. In invertebrates, analagous structures may occur at various places on the upper part of the digestive tract. Type and number vary greatly from one species to another. Also *dens.* **abutment t.** A tooth supporting a bridge or adjacent to a partial denture. **accessional teeth** The permanent molar teeth. They are accessional in that they have no deciduous predecessors. **accessory t.** SUPERNUMERARY TOOTH. **anchor t.** A tooth used for anchorage of an orthodontic appliance. **auditory teeth of Huschke** DENTES ACUSTICI. **t. of axis** *Outmoded* DENS AXIS. **baby t.** DECIDUOUS TOOTH. **buccal teeth** CHEEK TEETH. **canine t.** CANINE. **cheek teeth** Molar and premolar teeth. Also *buccal teeth.* **conical t.** An incompletely developed tooth, sometimes associated with partial anodontia or ectodermal dysplasia. Also *peg-shaped tooth.* **Corti's teeth** DEN-

TES ACUSTICI. **Corti's auditory teeth** DENTES ACUSTICI. **cuspid t.** CANINE. • This term is used especially of the human dentition. **cutting t.** INCISOR. **dead t.** NONVITAL TOOTH. **deciduous t.** A tooth of the first dentition which is shed and replaced by a permanent tooth. Also *dens deciduus, baby tooth, milk tooth, primary tooth, temporary tooth.* **devital t.** NONVITAL TOOTH. **diatoric t.** A porcelain artificial tooth that is retained by means of an undercut central area. Also *pinless tooth.* **drifting t.** MIGRATING TOOTH. **t. of epistropheus** *Outmoded* DENS AXIS. **eye t.** An upper canine tooth. **Fournier t.** See under SYPHILITIC TOOTH. **green teeth** Deciduous teeth having a greenish color due to neonatal hemolytic jaundice, or permanent teeth discolored green due to chronic or repeated ingestion of tetracycline or related compounds during infancy or early childhood. **hair teeth** *Outmoded* DENTES ACUSTICI. **hereditary brown t.** A tooth affected by amelogenesis imperfecta. **hereditary brown opalescent t.** A tooth affected by dentinogenesis imperfecta. In addition to the characteristic appearance, the tooth has an obliterated pulp chamber and may have a short root. **hutchinsonian t.** See under SYPHILITIC TOOTH. **Hutchinson's t.** See under SYPHILITIC TOOTH. **impacted t.** A tooth prevented from erupting partially or completely by some obstacle such as another tooth. The most commonly affected tooth is the third molar. **incisor t.** INCISOR. **migrating t.** A tooth that gradually moves laterally from its normal position in the arch, either physiologically when an adjacent tooth is missing, or pathologically because of a condition such as chronic periodontitis or a cyst of the jaw. Also *drifting tooth, wandering tooth.* **milk t.** DECIDUOUS TOOTH. **Moon's t.** See under SYPHILITIC TOOTH. **mottled teeth** Intrinsic discoloration of tooth enamel. It may be the result of excessive ingestion of fluoride during tooth formation. **mulberry t.** See under SYPHILITIC TOOTH. **multicuspid t.** MOLAR[2]. **natal t.** A deciduous tooth erupted at the time of birth. **neonatal t.** A deciduous tooth erupting during the neonatal period. **nonvital t.** A tooth from which the pulp has been removed or has necrosed or degenerated. It does not respond to pulp tests and is usually discolored. Whether root-filled or not, it may give rise to a granuloma or dental cyst, both of which may be symptomless, or to an abscess. Also *dead tooth, devital tooth, pulpless tooth.* **notched t.** See under SYPHILITIC TOOTH. **pegged t.** See under SYPHILITIC TOOTH. **peg-shaped t.** CONICAL TOOTH. **pegtop t.** See under SYPHILITIC TOOTH. **permanent t.** A tooth which is not replaced by a successor. Also *succedaneous tooth, successional tooth.* **pink t.** A tooth in which internal resorption has removed sufficient dentin to allow pink soft tissue to show through the translucent enamel. Also *pink spot.* **pinless t.** DIATORIC TOOTH. **primary t.** DECIDUOUS TOOTH. **pulpless t.** NONVITAL TOOTH. **rotated t.** A tooth that has erupted with an orientation representing a rotation about its long axis. **screwdriver t.** See under SYPHILITIC TOOTH. **shell t.** A tooth having an abnormally large pulp chamber and thin dentin. **submerged t.** An ankylosed deciduous tooth that has become surrounded by the growth of alveolar tissues. **succedaneous t.** PERMANENT TOOTH. **successional t.** PERMANENT TOOTH. **supernumerary t.** An additional tooth commonly found in the incisor region, where it may prevent the eruption of the normal tooth. It usually has a conical crown, but it may have the structure and shape of the adjacent normal tooth, in which case it is known as a supplemental tooth. Also *accessory tooth.* **supplemental t.** See under SUPERNUMERARY TOOTH. **syphilitic t.** A tooth malformed because of congenital syphilis, which causes an enamel hypoplasia in those permanent teeth formed at birth or for some time afterwards. The teeth most often affected are first incisors and first molars. Such an incisor is barrel-shaped, and the incisal edge has a deep crescentic notch. It is also called *notched tooth, pegged tooth, pegtop tooth, screwdriver tooth, Hutchinson's incisor, Hutchinson's tooth,* or *hutchinsonian tooth.* An affected molar is similarly contracted, having a dome-shaped crown and instead of the normal arrangement of cusps a rough, pitted surface or irregular nodules. This molar is also called *mulberry molar, dome-shaped molar, Moon's tooth, Moon's molar, mulberry tooth,* or *Fournier tooth.* **temporary t.** DECIDUOUS TOOTH. **tube t.** An artificial tooth which can be cemented onto a cylindrical pin on a denture base. **Turner's t.** A permanent tooth having enamel hypoplasia caused by infection from its deciduous predecessor or by injury if the latter is accidentally driven into the developing tooth germ. **vital t.** A tooth with a vital pulp. **wandering t.** MIGRATING TOOTH. **wisdom t.** THIRD MOLAR.

**toothache** Pain in or around a tooth, most commonly caused by pulpitis. Also *odontalgia.*

**tooth-borne** Supported entirely by the natural teeth: said of a partial denture.

**toothbrushing** The cleaning of the teeth with a specially designed brush and, in most western countries, dentifrice. There are various methods, such as Bass, Bell, Charters, Fones, Hirschfeld, horizontal scrub, or Stillman. In all methods the gums are necessarily brushed at the same time.

**toothed** DENTATE.

**toothpick** A fine, flat tapering instrument used to remove fibrous food particles from between the teeth. It may be made of metal, wood, plastic, or other stiff flexible material. **balsa wood t.** A type of interdental stimulator.

**top / spinning t.** A device used to check the accuracy of an x-ray exposure switch. A top, consisting of a radiopaque disk with a small hole near the rim, is spun above a film during the x-ray exposure. The number of resulting dots on the processed film indicates the number of x-ray pulses during the exposure.

**topagnosia** \täp′agnō′zhə\ [*top(o)-* + AGNOSIA] **1** TOPOANESTHESIA. **2** Inability to identify or recognize places; loss of topographic sense.

**topagnosis** \täp′agnō′sis\ [*top(o)-* + Gk *a-* priv. + *gnōsis* knowledge] TOPOANESTHESIA.

**topalgia** \täpal′jə\ [*top(o)-* + -ALGIA] Localized pain. Also *topoalgia.*

**topectomy** \täpek′təmē\ [*top(o)-* + -ECTOMY] Resection of a specific area of the cerebral cortex, usually frontal or prefrontal, as a form of psychosurgery. Also *corticectomy.*

**topesthesia** \täp′esthē′zhə\ [*top(o)-* + -ESTHESIA] The ability to localize accurately tactile stimuli applied to the surface of the body. Also *topoesthesia.*

**tophaceous** \tōfā′shəs\ Pertaining to or having tophi.

**tophi** \tō′fī\ Plural of TOPHUS.

**topholipoma** \tō′fōlipō′mə\ [*toph(us)* + *o* + LIPOMA] A lipoma with chalky deposits.

**tophus** \tō′fəs\ [L (also *tofus*), tufa, a porous, friable stone] (*pl.* tophi) An accumulation of monosodium urate deposits in soft tissues, such as the ear or tendons, or about joints, as occurs in chronic gout. Also *tophic concretion, chalk stone, tuberculum arthriticum, gouty pearl.* **auricular tophi** Small deposits of sodium urate crystals beneath the perichondrium of the pinna occurring sometimes in cases of gout. Also *tophi of the pinna.* **tophi of the pinna** AURICULAR TOPHI.

**topical** \täp′ikəl\ [Gk *topik(os)* (from *top(os)* a place, spot + *-ikos* -IC) local, pertaining to a place + -AL] Restricted to a circumscribed area, especially of skin or mucous membrane, as an application of a medication, antiseptic, or anesthetic agent.

**topo-** \täp′ō-, täp′ə-\ [Gk *topos* a place] A combining form meaning (1) place, region; (2) local, localized.

**topoalgia** \-al′jē·ə\ TOPALGIA.

**topoanesthesia** \-an′esthē′zhə\ [TOPO- + ANESTHESIA] Inability to localize accurately any tactile sensation. Also *topagnosia, topagnosis.*

**topoesthesia** \-esthē′zhə\ TOPESTHESIA.

**topographic** \-graf′ik\ Pertaining to a particular anatomical part or region or to its description.

**topography** \təpäg′rəfē\ [TOPO- + -GRAPHY] The study or description of a particular anatomical part or region, especially in relation to surrounding parts or regions.

**topoisomerase** An enzyme that converts one topological isomer of a macromolecule, usually DNA, into another.

**topology** \təpäl′əjē\ [TOPO- + -LOGY] The spatial configuration of the fetal presenting part and the birth canal. *Older term.*

**toponym** \täp′ənim\ In anatomy, the designation of a region, as distinct from the name of an organ or a structure.

**toponymy** \təpän′imē\ In anatomy, the nomenclature of regions of the body as distinct from that of organs and structures. *Outmoded.*

**topophylaxis** \-filak′sis\ Use of a tourniquet to limit an injected medication to a single limb.

**topothermesthesiometer** \-thur′mesthē′zē·äm′ətər\ An instrument that measures the variation of temperature sensitivity in local sites of the skin.

**torcular** \tôr′kyələr\ [L (from *torculum* an oil or wine press) a room for an oil or wine press] A cellarlike cavity. **t. herophili** CONFLUENS SINUUM.

**tori** \tôr′ī\ Plural of TORUS.

**toric** \tôr′ik\ **1** Of or relating to a torus. **2** Resembling a torus.

**Torkildsen** [Arne *Torkildsen,* Norwegian neurosurgeon, born 1899] Torkildsen's operation. See under SHUNT.

**Tornwaldt** [Gustav Ludwig *Tornwaldt,* German physician, 1843–1910] **1** Tornwaldt's disease. See under BURSITIS. **2** Bursa of Tornwaldt, Tornwaldt cyst. See under BURSA PHARYNGEALIS.

**torose** \tôr′ōs\ Bulging or knobby. Also *torous.*

**torous** \tôr′əs\ TOROSE.

**torpent** \tôr′pənt\ An agent that decreases irritation.

**torpidity** \tôrpid′itē\ TORPOR.

**torpitude** \tôr′pityood\ TORPOR.

**torpor** \tôr′pər\ [L (from *torpere* to be numb, inactive), numbness, torpor] **1** A state of stupor developing as a result of damage to, or dysfunction of, the central nervous system. **2** A state of dormancy or sluggishness occurring in response to environmental stress. For defs. 1 and 2 also *torpidity, torpitude.* See also HIBERNATION, ESTIVATION. **summer t.** ESTIVATION. **winter t.** HIBERNATION.

**torque** \tôrk\ A force that produces or tends to produce rotation, such as may be exerted by an orthodontic appliance.

**torr** \tôr\ [after Evangelista *Torricelli,* Italian physician, 1608-1647] A unit of pressure, used especially in vacuum technology, equal to $^{1}/_{760}$ standard atmosphere; 133.322 pascals. The torr is equal to the conventional millimeter of mercury to within one part in $10^7$. Symbol: Torr

**torrefaction** \tôr′əfak′shən\ [See TORREFY.] The process of drying by exposure to heat; roasting.

**torrefy** \tôr′əfī\ [irreg. from L *torrefacere* (from *torre(re)* to parch, dry, roast + *facere* to make) to dry or roast by fire] To dry or roast by direct exposure to fire or other source of heat; to parch.

**torsade de pointes** \tôrsäd′ də pweNt′\ [French, from *torsade* a twist, turn + *de* of + *pointes* points, peaks] A form of ventricular tachycardia in which there are phasic changes in the morphology of the QRS complexes, as if there were a twisting of the points around the axis. It is particularly associated with prolongation of the QT interval, as in the Romano-Ward syndrome and the Jervell and Lange-Nielsen syndrome.

**torsion** \tôr′shən\ [Late L *torsio,* variant of *tortio* (from *torquere* to wrench, twist, torture) twisting, torture] A twisting or rotation about a long axis. **lateral t.** EXCYCLODEVIATION. **negative t.** EXCYCLODEVIATION. **positive t.** INCYCLODEVIATION.

**torsionometer** \tôr′shənäm′ətər\ An instrument used to measure the rotation of the spinal column.

**torsiversion** \tôr′sivur′zhən\ [*torsi(on)* + VERSION] The rotation of a tooth about its long axis.

**torso** \tôr′sō\ [Italian (from L *thyrsus* from Gk *thyrsos* stalk, stem) stump, stalk, trunk] The main part of the body to which the head and limbs are attached. Also *trunk, truncus.*

**torticollis** \tôr′təkäl′is\ [L *tortus* (past part. of *torquere* to wrench, twist, writhe) wrenched, twisted + *collum,* also *collus* neck] Any condition in which the head and neck are turned and twisted to the side either permanently, intermittently, or spasmodically. Spasmodic torticollis is the commonest variety. Also *wryneck, collum valgum, collum distortum, cephaloxia, wry neck, loxia, rhaebocrania, caput distortum, trachelocyllosis.* **acute t.** Torticollis caused by a muscle spasm secondary to nerve root entrapment in the cervical spine. **congenital t.** A unilateral fibrosis of a sternocleidomastoid muscle. It appears at birth as a swelling on the side of the neck and later may subside or result in shortening of the muscle. Also *infantile torticollis.* **fixed t.** Torticollis that is not reversible. **infantile t.** CONGENITAL TORTICOLLIS. **intermittent t.** SPASMODIC TORTICOLLIS. **labyrinthine t.** Torticollis associated with unilateral labyrinthitis, the head being twisted, as a rule, toward the affected ear or sometimes, in nonsuppurative labyrinthitis, toward the sound side. Nystagmus is also present, directed usually toward the normal ear. **myogenic t.** Torticollis that is secondary to muscle spasm. It may be either a muscle spasm caused by the primary condition of the muscle or a spasm that is secondary to nerve root entrapment in the cervical spine. Also *stiff neck* (popular). **nasopharyngeal t.** Torticollis, caused by dislocation of the atlantoaxial joint, complicating retropharyngeal abscess or even, rarely, tonsillectomy. The basic pathology in these cases is rupture of the transverse ligament of the atlas. Also *Grisel's disease, Grisel-Bourgeois syndrome.* **neurogenic t.** SPASMODIC TORTICOLLIS. **ocular t.** A tilting of the head upon the neck to compensate for the cyclodiplopia of a superior oblique paralysis. **paralytic t.** SPASMODIC TORTICOLLIS. **reflex t.** Torticollis caused by a muscle spasm, usually of the sternomastoid muscle, that is associated with an inflammatory process such as suppuration of the adjacent lymph nodes. **rheumatoid t.** Torticollis due to rheumatoid arthritis. **spasmodic t.** A condition marked by rotation and tilting of the head caused by intermittent tonic, clonic, or tonicoclonic contraction of the cervical muscles, particularly the trapezius and sternomastoid muscles. This is a fractional variety of torsion spasm. It is an extrapyramidal syndrome but its pathology is poorly defined.

In occasional rare cases it is thought to be a hysterical phenomenon. Also *spastic torticollis, intermittent torticollis, paralytic torticollis, neurogenic torticollis, accessory cramp* (outmoded), *spinal accessory spasm*. **spastic t.** SPASMODIC TORTICOLLIS. **symptomatic t.** Torticollis causing pain.

**tortipelvis** \tôr′tipel′vis\ DYSTONIA MUSCULORUM DEFORMANS.

**tortua** \tôr′choo·ə\ [New L, irreg. from L *tortus,* past part. of *torquere* to wrench, twist, writhe] Agony; intense pain. **t. facies** TRIGEMINAL NEURALGIA.

**tortuous** \tôr′choo·əs\ Following an irregular, winding course marked by many turns and twists.

**toruloid** \tôr′ʸəloid\ NODULAR.

**toruloma** \tôr′ʸəlō′mə\ [*torul(us)* + -OMA] *Obs.* CRYPTOCOCCOMA.

***Torulopsis glabrata*** \tôr′ʸəläp′sis glabrā′tə\ A form-species of yeastlike fungus normally resident in the human mouth, nose, gastrointestinal tract, and vagina. It has been implicated as a low-virulence opportunistic pathogen in hospitalized patients with other serious diseases.

**torulopsosis** \tôr′ʸəläpsō′sis\ A rare fungal infection caused by *Torulopsis glabrata,* a constituent of the normal oropharyngeal, gastrointestinal, genital, and dermal flora. Infection usually occurs in persons with serious underlying diseases, or in immunocompromised patients.

**torulosis** \tôr′ʸəlō′sis\ CRYPTOCOCCOSIS.

**torulus** \tôr′ʸələs\ [L (dim. of TORUS) a small protuberance] (*pl.* toruli) A small bulge or elevation. **toruli tactiles** [NA] TACTILE ELEVATIONS.

**torus** \tôr′əs\ [L, a strand, rope, raised ridge, bulge] (*pl.* tori) **1** In anatomy, a rounded or linear bulging projection or protuberance. **2** A surface or solid figure resembling a doughnut generated by the revolution of a circle about an axis lying in its plane but not intersecting it. **buccal t.** A ridge rarely observed on the inside of the cheek, marking the line of union of the maxillary and mandibular processesof the embryo. **t. levatorius** [NA] A rounded elevation of the mucous membrane that is located in the lower margin of the pharyngeal orifice of the auditory tube in the lateral wall of the nasopharynx. It is produced by the underlying levator veli palatini muscle. Also *levator cushion, levator swelling*. **t. mandibularis** A bony mass, of variable extent, situated on the medial surface of the body of the mandible just below the lower premolars. Occasionally it is very marked and prominent. **palatine t.** TORUS PALATINUS. **t. palatinus** A bony mass, of variable extent, situated in the midline of the oral surface of the bony palate. Occasionally it is very marked and protuberant. Also *palatine torus, palatine protuberance*. **supraorbital t.** The bony ridge beneath the eyebrows. **t. tubarius** [NA] The base of the cartilaginous part of the auditory tube, which forms an elevation of the mucous membrane behind the orifice of the tube on the lateral wall of the nasopharynx. Also *tubal prominence, tubal protuberance, tubal elevation.*

**Toti** [Addeo *Toti,* Italian ophthalmologist and laryngologist, born 1861] See under OPERATION.

**totipotence** \tō′tipō′təns, tō′tip′ətəns\ TOTIPOTENCY.

**totipotency** \tō′tipō′tənsē, to′tip′ətənsē\ [L *toti(us),* gen. of *totus* entire + POTENCY] The ability of a cell to differentiate into any type of cell of the organism. The fertilized ovum is a totipotent cell capable of giving rise to every cell type in an adult body. Also *totipotence, totipotentiality*. Adj. totipotent, totipotential.

**totipotentiality** \tō′tipōten′shē·al′itē\ TOTIPOTENCY.

**touch** [French *toucher* (from Vulgar L *toccare* to knock, ring a bell) to touch] **1** The tactile sense. **2** Exploration of an object using the tactile sense. **double t.** Simultaneous pelvic and rectal digital examination. **rectal t.** Digital examination of the rectum. **vaginal t.** Manual pelvic examination by way of the vagina. **vesical t.** Digital exploration of the bladder.

**Touraine** [Albert *Touraine,* French dermatologist, born 1883] **1** Touraine-Solente-Golé syndrome. See under PACHYDERMOPERIOSTOSIS. **2** Touraine's aphthosis. See under BEHÇET SYNDROME.

**tourniquet** \tur′nəkit, toor′-\ [French, turnstile, tourniquet] Any device that can be constricted around a part with sufficient circumferential pressure to occlude the flow of blood to or from the part. **Esmarch's t.** A flat elastic bandage used to constrict circulation in a limb. **forceps t.** A surgical instrument that is used during the disarticulation of the hip, consisting of a clamp that has one pointed blade and one flat blade. The pointed blade is passed beneath the femoral artery and the flat blade lies superficially. Closure of the forceps controls femoral artery bleeding. Also *Lynn Thomas tourniquet*. **garrote t.** SPANISH WINDLASS. **Lynn Thomas t.** FORCEPS TOURNIQUET. **pneumatic t.** A broad band with an inflatable bladder that compresses a part with air pressure. **scalp t.** A tourniquet placed around the head near the edge of the hairy scalp. It has been used to reduce the epilating effect of cancer chemotherapy. **Spanish t.** SPANISH WINDLASS. **torcular t.** SPANISH WINDLASS. **windlass t.** SPANISH WINDLASS.

**Tourtual** [Caspar Theobald *Tourtual,* German anatomist, 1802–1865] Tourtual's canal. See under CANALIS PALATINUS MAJOR.

**Touton** [Karl *Touton,* German dermatologist, 1858–1934] Touton giant cell. See under CELL.

**Towne** [Edward Bancroft *Towne,* U.S. physician, 1883–1957] Towne projection radiograph. See under PROJECTION.

**Townsend** [John Sealy Edward *Townsend,* Irish physicist, 1868–1957] Townsend avalanche, Townsend ionization. See under AVALANCHE IONIZATION.

**tox-** \täks-\ TOXICO-.

**toxaemia** \täksē′mē·ə\ *Brit.* TOXEMIA.

**toxanemia** \täk′sənē′mē·ə\ TOXINEMIA.

**toxaphene** \täk′səfēn\ $C_{10}H_{10}Cl_8$. A polychlorinated hydrocarbon used as a contact agricultural insecticide. Contact with human skin may cause mild irritation. It may also be absorbed through the skin causing central nervous system stimulation with tremors, convulsions, and possibly death. It has been reported to cause liver injury in experimental animals.

***Toxascaris leonina*** \täksas′kəris lē·ənī′nə\ A species of nematode found in the intestines of domestic dogs and cats and in wild felids and canids throughout the world. The parasite differs in slight morphological details from members of the genus *Toxocara* and also in terms of the developmental cycle, which in *T. leonina* occurs completely in the gut, the larvae not migrating through the lungs of the host. Infrequently found in man, it has caused visceral larva migrans in children.

**toxemia** \täksē′mē·ə\ [TOX- + -EMIA] The presence of toxic substances in the bloodstream produced by the body or by the invasion of microorganisms. Also *toxicemia*. See also TOXEMIA OF PREGNANCY. **eclamptic t.** Hypertension, proteinuria, and edema of a pregnant woman in association with the occurrence of seizures. Also *eclamptogenic toxemia*. **hydatid t.** Toxemia caused by hydatid fluid escaping from a hydatid cyst into the peritoneal cavity. Urticaria often accompanies this condition. **preeclamptic t.** PRE-

ECLAMPSIA. **t. of pregnancy** A hypertensive disorder of women occurring during pregnancy or in the postpartum, characterized by proteinuria and edema. *Imprecise.*

**toxemic** \täksē′mik\ Pertaining to or characterized by toxemia.

**toxenzyme** \täksen′zīm\ A toxic enzyme.

**toxi-** \täk′si-\ TOXICO-.

**toxic** \täk′sik\ [Late L *toxicus* (from L *toxicum* poison, from Gk *toxikon pharmakon* arrow poison, from *toxikos* pertaining to archery, from *toxon* a bow, arch) poisonous] **1** Having the characteristics of a toxin or poison; poisonous. **2** Caused by or associated with the action of a toxin or poison. **3** Affected by or contaminated with a toxin or poison.

**toxicant** \täk′sikənt\ **1** Having a toxic or poisonous effect. **2** A toxic agent; a cause of intoxication; a poison.

**toxication** \-kā′shən\ INTOXICATION.

**toxicemia** \-sē′mē·ə\ TOXEMIA.

**toxicide** [täk′sisīd] An agent that is able to counteract the effect of a toxic substance; an antidote.

**toxicity** \täksis′itē\ **1** The quality of being toxic or the degree to which something is toxic; the capacity of substances to produce adverse effects in biologic systems. **2** A toxic condition. **antibiotic t.** Adverse reactions that may occur following the use of antibiotics. Most such reactions are allergic in nature and may be severe enough to lead to anaphylaxis and death. **bismuth t.** BISMUTH NEPHROPATHY. **cadmium t.** CADMIUM NEPHROPATHY. **digitalis t.** The toxic effect of overdosage of digitalis in the treatment of patients with cardiac disease. Symptoms include cardiac irregularities, anorexia, nausea, vomiting, and visual disturbances. Also *digitoxicity.* **iron dextran t.** Systemic reactions to iron dextran, including headache, fever, back pain, arthralgias, and in rare cases, peripheral vascular collapse. Anaphylactic reactions and death have also been reported in rare instances. Intravenous injections were formerly reported to cause severe toxic reactions and this method of administration was avoided. However, experiments indicate that only minor reactions are experienced in a few cases when the rate and volume have been carefully adjusted. **mercury t.** MERCURY POISONING. **osmotic diuretic t.** Adverse reactions from the administration of osmotic electrolytes or osmotic nonelectrolytes. In the doses employed for potassium, the increase in blood level is usually minimal if renal function is normal. In cases of renal failure, the blood level may rise sufficiently to cause serious changes in cardiac conduction. For osmotic nonelectrolytes, urea, glucose, and dextrose are generally regarded as nontoxic, but in patients with renal failure, mannitol may produce vascular overfilling with hyperosmolality and hyponatremia while sucrose may produce renal tubular necrosis. **oxygen t.** A condition resulting from breathing high partial pressures of oxygen and characterized by abnormalities in vision and hearing, difficulty in breathing, muscular twitching, anxiety, confusion, and, in severe cases, convulsions. The cause is unknown, but one possible etiologic factor is interference in enzyme activity. **phenacetin t.** The effects of large doses of phenacetin: most frequently cyanosis, a bluish-grey discoloration which is caused by formation of methemoglobin. Only the finger tips and nails may be involved or the entire body surface, including mucous membranes, may be affected. Renal injury, called phenacetin nephritis, was seen occasionally during the early years of drug use, attributed to overdosage. Other causes of the methemoglobinemia are *p*-chloroacetanilid, a contaminant of phenacetin, and hypersensitivity of the patient. **salicylate t.** Effects of overdosage with salicylates: initially, respiratory stimulation, irritability, nausea, vomiting, fever, dizziness, tinnitus, and hallucinations. Delirium, coma, and death may follow in two hours to several days. In spite of their low level of toxicity, the various forms of salicylates are responsible for many poisonings due to overdosage or accidental ingestion. **sulfonamide t.** Toxicity resulting from systemic sensitivity reactions to sulfonamides. Toxic effects are rarely seen in persons receiving sulfonamides for the first time, but with succeeding administration, reactions may occur manifested by nausea and vomiting, headache, dizziness, ataxia, irritability, and restlessness, followed by fever, anemia, dermatitis and leukopenia. Renal damage may occur caused by precipitation of crystals in the collecting tubules of the kidney which obstructs the flow of urine and may injure the tubular epithelium. Also *sulfa kidney.*

**toxico-** \täk′sikō-\ [Gk *toxiko(n pharmakon)* arrow poison. See TOXIC.] A combining form meaning poison or toxin. Also *tox-, toxi-, toxo-.*

**toxicodendrol** \täk′sikōden′drôl\ A poisonous, nonvolatile, oily phenolic resin found in the sticky sap of *Toxicodendron* species. It contains the active principle urushiol. It is not transmissible and apparently does not enter the bloodstream. Minute quantities are capable of causing dermatitis and may be carried to sensitive individuals through smoke, dust, contaminated articles, and the hair of animals.

**toxicoderma** \täk′sikōdur′mə\ [TOXICO- + -DERMA] A skin disease caused by a poison. *Outmoded.*

**toxicogenic** \täk′sikōjen′ik\ [TOXICO- + -GENIC] **1** Poison-producing. **2** TOXIGENIC.

**toxicoid** \täk′sikoid\ [TOXIC + -OID] Transiently toxic: said of a normally innocuous substance or the reaction to it. For example, the intake of large amounts of water after excessive sodium loss through sweating can produce a toxicoid reaction of cramps and convulsions.

**toxicokinetics** \täk′sikōkinet′iks\ The science that deals with the absorption, distribution, metabolism, and excretion of harmful substances, especially with reference to analysis of the concentration of such substances over a specified time.

**toxicologic** \täk′sikəläj′ik\ Pertaining to toxicology.

**toxicologist** \täk′sikäl′əjist\ A person trained in toxicology.

**toxicology** \-käl′əjē\ [TOXICO- + -LOGY] The study of the adverse effects of substances on biologic systems, and of their detection and treatment. **forensic t.** The application of the scientific principles and practice of toxicology to problems of law and the administration of justice. It is primarily concerned with identification and quantitation of toxic substances found in the tissues or body fluids of individuals whose death is believed to be caused by or related to exposure, ingestion, or injection of such substances. **predictive t.** Toxicological study aimed at providing a data base that can be used to assess the risk or hazard associated with a situation in which the toxic agent, the subject, and the exposure conditions are defined. **prospective t.** A study designed to test the validity of assumptions about the effects of a toxic agent and the validity of the biologic method of monitoring. **retrospective t.** The study of persons previously exposed to a toxic agent to evaluate the level of exposure at which the risk of health impairment is negligible.

**toxicopathic** \täk′sikōpath′ik\ Pertaining to any pathologic condition caused by a toxin or a poison. Also *toxipathic.*

**toxicopathy** \täk′sikäp′əthē\ [TOXICO- + -PATHY] A pathologic condition induced by a poison or a toxin. Also *toxipathy.*

**toxicosis** \-kō′sis\ [*toxic(o)-* + -OSIS] Any pathologic condition due to or associated with a poison. Also *nosotoxicosis, toxonosis, toxosis.* **aspergillus t.** Any mycotoxicosis caused by ingestion of food contaminated with members of the genus *Aspergillus,* especially aflatoxicosis produced by *A. flavus,* a common contaminant of cereal grains and nuts. Also *aspergillotoxicosis.* **endogenic t.** ENDOINTOXICATION. **exogenic t.** Poisoning caused by ingestion of a toxic substance or substances, particularly those present in food such as aflatoxin in peanuts. **gestational t.** Any toxemic complication occurring during pregnancy. **hemorrhagic capillary t.** HENOCH-SCHÖNLEIN PURPURA. **$T_3$-t.** Hyperthyroidism associated with greatly elevated plasma levels of triiodothyronine and only slightly raised, normal, or low values of plasma thyroxine. It is found most commonly in patients with toxic nodular goiter and persons who have had thyroid surgery. In some patients successfully treated for Graves disease with antithyroid drugs, the appearance of $T_3$-toxicosis may herald the recrudescence of typical thyrotoxicosis. Also *$T_3$-thyrotoxicosis.*

**toxiferine** \täksif′ərin\ Any of a group of potent curare alkaloids derived principally from the tropical tree *Strychnos toxifera.* The bark has been shown to contain twelve crystalline quaternary alkaloids, toxiferines I–XII. Toxiferines I and II have been found in calabash curare.

**toxiferous** \täksif′ərəs\ [TOXI- + -FEROUS] Poison-bearing; poison-producing.

**toxigenic** \-jen′ik\ [TOXI- + -GENIC] Toxin-producing: used most commonly in reference to virulent strains of exotoxin-producing microorganisms. Also *toxigenous, toxinogenic, toxicogenic.*

**toxigenicity** \-jənis′itē\ The property of being toxigenic or the degree to which something is toxigenic. Also *toxinogeny, toxinogenicity.*

**toxigenous** \täksij′ənəs\ TOXIGENIC.

**toxignomic** \täk′signō′mik\ [TOXI- + Gk *gnōm(ē)* a means of knowing, a mark + -IC] Characteristic of a toxin or poison.

**toximetry** \täksim′ətrē\ [TOXI- + -METRY] The branch of toxicology dealing with the quantitative measurement of toxicity.

**toxin** \täk′sin\ [TOX- + -IN] A substance formed by an organism (animal, plant, or microbial) that is poisonous to certain other organisms. Also *toxinum.* **animal t.** Any toxin elaborated in the metabolic and growth processes of an animal; a zootoxin. **bacterial t.** Any toxin produced by bacteria. Unless otherwise specified, the term refers to a soluble exotoxin rather than to an endotoxin. **botulinum t.** The protein exotoxin released by *Clostridium botulinum.* Seven immunologically distinct types have been recognized, of which only A, B, and E are significant causes of human botulism in the United States. Formation of some types depends on a prophage. These are the most powerful toxins known. Based on rat studies, the estimated lethal dose for the average adult human is approximately 0.01 μg. The toxins are not destroyed, and type E is activated, by gastrointestinal proteases. Crystalline type A toxin has a molecular weight of 900 000, and a neurotoxin of molecular weight 150 000 can be separated from it. The neurotoxin is absorbed from the intestine and binds to neuromuscular and peripheral autonomic presynaptic terminals, where it blocks the release of acetylcholine-containing vesicles. Gangliosides bind the toxin. Also *botulinus toxin, botulin* (seldom used). **cholera t.** An exotoxin produced by *Vibrio cholerae,* which binds to a ganglioside of intestinal epithelial cells and activates cell-membrane adenyl cyclase. The resulting excessive secretion of chloride and bicarbonate, accompanied by water, leads to severe diarrhea and dehydration. Also *choleragen.* **dermonecrotic t.** An exotoxin produced by *Staphylococcus aureus.* Intradermal injection causes extensive necrosis of the skin. Also *necrotizing toxin.* **Dick test t.** ERYTHROGENIC TOXIN. **dinoflagellate t.** Any toxin derived from marine dinoflagellates, such as saxitoxin from *Gonyaulax* species, which is responsible for much shellfish poisoning. **diphtheria t.** A protein of inolecular weight 60 000, coded for by phage $\beta$, that is secreted by *Corynebacterium diphtheriae.* It is a general cytotoxin, responsible for the cardiotoxic and neurotoxic symptoms and the mucosal damage of diphtheria. The toxin initially formed is not enzymatically active, but if it is nicked proteolytically and reduced it can be separated into an enzymatically active fragment A of molecular weight 21 150 and a binding fragment B of molecular weight 39 000. Fragment B is necessary for entry of A into the host cell, where it blocks protein synthesis by transferring ADP-ribose from NAD to elongation factor EF2. Also *diphtherotoxin.* **epidermolytic t.** EXFOLIATIN. **erythrogenic t.** An exotoxin produced by certain lysogenic strains of *Streptococcus pyogenes.* It is responsible for the characteristic rash of scarlet fever. Three immunologically distinct types (A, B, and C) are known. Intradermal injection produces inflammation, and the toxin is used in the Dick test to determine susceptibility to scarlet fever. Also *Dick test toxin, scarlatinal toxin, scarlet fever erythrogenic toxin, streptococcus erythrogenic toxin.* **fusarial t.** Any toxic substance produced by molds of the genus *Fusarium,* usually produced on food grains and introduced by ingestion. **gonococcal t.** An endotoxin present in gonococci. **labile t.** A large heat-labile enterotoxin, very similar to cholera toxin, produced by enterotoxic strains of *Escherichia coli.* A binding portion helps entry of an active portion, which activates adenylcyclase in the membrane of mucosal cells. The resulting cyclic AMP causes exudation of fluid. Compare STABLE TOXIN. Abbr. LT **meningococcal t.** An endotoxin present in meningococci. **necrotizing t.** DERMONECROTIC TOXIN. **perfringens alpha t.** A $Ca^{2+}$-dependent lecithinase (phospholipase) produced by *Clostridium perfringens.* Its presence can be recognized by the development of opacity surrounding the colony of the organism on egg-yolk agar. **perfringens theta t.** An oxygen-labile hemolysin produced by *Clostridium perfringens.* **plant t.** Any of various toxins elaborated in the metabolic and growth processes of certain plants; a phytotoxin. **rickettsial t.** A toxin in the cell wall of rickettsiae that causes endothelial damage. **scarlatinal t.** ERYTHROGENIC TOXIN. **scarlet fever erythrogenic t.** ERYTHROGENIC TOXIN. **Shiga t.** A potent exotoxin produced by *Shigella dysenteriae* type 1. It causes dysentery and is reported to be neurotoxic for laboratory animals. **stable t.** A small (MW 5000) enterotoxin produced by various bacteria. It activates guanylcyclase to produce cyclic GMP. Compare LABILE TOXIN. Abbr. ST **staphylococcal t.** A mixture of extracellular toxins formed by staphylococci, including hemotoxins, enterotoxins, leukocidins, staphylokinase, staphylocoagulase, and dermonecrotic toxins. **streptococcal t.** A mixture of extracellular toxins produced by *Streptococcus pyogenes.* These include hemolysins, streptokinase, hyaluronidase, and leukocidin. **streptococcus erythrogenic t.** ERYTHROGENIC TOXIN. **tetanus t.** A single antigenic type of toxin, released by *Clostridium tetani.* The molecular weight is 160 000. Activity is increased by proteolytic nicking. Sulfhydryl reagents then separate an $\alpha$ chain (molecular weight 55 000) and a $\beta$ chain. The latter binds to gangliosides and presumably promotes entry of the $\alpha$ chain, which blocks release of the inhibitory transmitter, glycine, at spinal motor neurons.

**toxin-antitoxin** \täk′sin-an′tētäk′sin\ A mixture of a bacterial toxin or toxoid and an equivalent or nearly neutralizing amount of its specific antitoxin. Such mixtures were formerly used for immunization.

**toxinemia** \-nē′mē·ə\ The presence in blood of a toxic substance. Also *toxanemia*.

**toxinogenic** \täk′sinōjen′ik\ TOXIGENIC.

**toxinogenicity** \täk′sinōjənis′itē\ TOXIGENICITY.

**toxinogeny** \täk′sinäj′ənē\ TOXIGENICITY.

**toxinosis** \täk′sinō′sis\ [TOXIN + -OSIS] A toxic reaction from exposure to a noxious agent of animal or plant origin.

**toxinum** \täksī′nəm\ TOXIN.

**toxipathic** \-path′ik\ TOXICOPATHIC.

**toxipathy** \täksip′əthē\ TOXICOPATHY.

**toxisterol** \täksis′tərôl\ A substance resulting from excessive irradiation of ergosterol. Although isomeric with calciferol, it has only minor antirachitic action and is extremely toxic.

**toxo-** \täk′sə-, täk′sō-\ TOXICO-.

***Toxocara*** \täk′səkar′ə\ [Gk *toxo(n)* a bow, arc + *kara* head, top, summit] A genus of ascarid nematodes that are common intestinal roundworms of carnivores, though one species, *T. vitulorum,* occurs in cattle. Members of the genus that occur in domestic pets have been implicated in visceral larva migrans of children. Also *Belascaris*.

**toxocariasis** \-kərī′əsis\ [*Toxocar(a)* + -IASIS] An infection with parasitic nematodes of the genus *Toxocara.* See also VISCERAL LARVA MIGRANS.

**toxogen** \täk′səjən\ [TOXO- + -GEN] A poison-producing agent; a toxigenic organism.

**toxoid** \täk′soid\ [TOX- + -OID] A bacterial exotoxin modified by chemical treatment (as with formaldehyde) so that it has lost its toxicity but retains the ability to elicit synthesis of, and to combine with, antitoxin. Also *anatoxin.* **adsorbed t.** A toxoid adsorbed onto alum precipitates. The alum acts as an adjuvant, and these preparations give rise to enhanced antibody responses when used to immunize humans or animals. **bacterial t.** A bacterial toxin which has lost its toxicity while retaining immunogenicity. It may occur naturally or be produced through the use of agents such as formalin. **diphtheria t.** A sterile solution obtained from formaldehyde-treated cultures of *Corynebacterium diphtheriae.* It is preserved with a nonphenolic chemical, and used as an immunizing material against diphtheria. Also *diphtheria vaccine, anatoxin-Ramon.* **diphtheria and tetanus t.'s** A sterile solution comprising both fluid diphtheria and tetanus toxoids, the proportion of each calculated to provide an active immunizing dose of both toxoids when given in the labeled amount. **formol t.** A toxin treated with formaldehyde so as to lose its toxic properties while retaining its antigenicity. **tetanus t.** A sterile liquid preparation of the growth products of *Clostridium tetani* treated with formaldehyde, serving as an active immunizing agent. Also *tetanus vaccine.*

**toxolecithin** \-les′ithin\ A lecithin combined with a toxin, as in certain snake venoms. Also *toxolecithid.*

**toxoneme** \täk′sənēm\ [Gk *toxo(n)* a bow + *nēm(a)* thread, yarn] MICRONEME.

**toxonosis** \-nō′sis\ TOXICOSIS.

**toxophore** \täk′səfôr\ [TOXO- + -PHORE] According to the side chain theory, the chemical group within a molecule of a substance, especially a toxin, by which the substance exerts its specific activity on the organism. Adj. toxophorous.

***Toxoplasma*** \-plaz′mə\ [Gk *toxo(n)* a bow, arc + PLASMA] A genus of intestinal coccidia of cats and other felids with an extremely wide range of warm-blooded intermediate hosts, including man, in which asexual multiplication is found, ending with tissue cysts. The sexual phase of the parasite, passing from schizogony to gametogony, occurs only in intestinal cells of cats, leading to production of oocysts in which infective sporozoites develop. The complex life cycle involves congenital as well as fecal transmission, and carnivorism as well, in which tissue cysts develop, particularly in rodents and herbivores. Multiplication in the nonfelid host involves production of tachyzoites, the arc-shaped, rapidly multiplying forms which develop in pseudocysts, and bradyzoites which form slowly within a true cyst membrane. Only a single valid species, *Toxoplasma gondii,* has so far been recognized in the genus. See also TOXOPLASMOSIS.

**toxoplasmatic** \-plazmat′ik\ TOXOPLASMIC.

**Toxoplasmatidae** \-plazmat′idē\ SARCOCYSTIDAE.

**toxoplasmic** \-plaz′mik\ Pertaining to or suggestive of *Toxoplasma.* Also *toxoplasmatic.*

**toxoplasmin** \-plaz′min\ An antigen prepared from embryonated eggs or peritoneal fluids of mice infected with *Toxoplasma gondii* and used to test for hypersensitivity to *Toxoplasma.*

**toxoplasmosis** \-plazmō′sis\ [*Toxoplasm(a)* + -OSIS] A worldwide disease of humans and animals caused by the sporozoan protozoan parasite, *Toxoplasma gondii.* Human disease acquired postnatally or in adulthood (acquired toxoplasmosis) is usually mild and benign, whereas *T. gondii* infection contracted transplacentally (congenital toxoplasmosis) can cause a variety of central nervous system problems and bilateral retinochoroiditis. **acquired t.** *Toxoplasma gondii* infection acquired postnatally or in adulthood through ingestion of tissue cysts in raw or undercooked meat or oocysts from infected cat feces. Infection is usually benign, with asymptomatic lymphadenopathy the most common manifestation. Central nervous system involvement and retinochoroiditis occur only rarely. However, in immunocompromised hosts, new or reactivated infection may produce severe illness commonly manifested as necrotizing encephalitis, myocarditis, and/or pneumonitis. More than half of all immunodeficient patients with toxoplasmosis have central nervous system involvement. **congenital t.** *Toxoplasma gondii* infection transmitted transplacentally to a fetus, occurring in about one-third of cases of acute acquired toxoplasmosis in pregnant women. Infection of the fetus is most common in the third trimester, but the effects on the fetus are most severe when infection occurs in the first trimester. Most infected neonates appear normal and are asymptomatic at birth, but localization of infection in the central nervous system months or years later produces effects ranging from mild diminution of vision or slight learning dysfunction to the full tetrad of signs: retinochoroiditis, hydrocephaly or microcephaly, convulsions, and intracerebral calcifications. Bilateral retinochoroiditis is the most common sequel of congenital toxoplasmosis.

***Toxorhynchites*** \täk′sôringkī′tēz\ A genus of tropical mosquitoes in the subfamily Toxorhynchitinae. The species *T. rutilus,* the larvae of which feed on other mosquito larvae, has been used with limited success as a biological control agent. Also *Megarhinus.*

**toxosis** \täksō′sis\ TOXICOSIS.

**Toynbee** [Joseph *Toynbee,* English otologist, 1815–1866] **1** Toynbee's otoscope. See under AUSCULTATION TUBE. **2** See under EXPERIMENT, MANEUVER. **3** Toynbee's corpuscles. See under CORNEAL CORPUSCLES. **4** Toynbee's law. See under GULL-TOYNBEE LAW. **5** Toynbee's ligament. See under LIGAMENTUM MALLEI ANTERIUS.

**TP** **1** tuberculin precipitation (Calmette's tuberculin). **2** threshold potential.

**TPC** thromboplastic plasma component (factor VIII).
**T-piece** AYRE'S TUBE.
**TPN** Symbol for triphosphopyridine nucleotide (now written as NADP in view of the change of this name).
**TPNH** Symbol for the reduced form of TPN (now normally symbolized NADPH).
**TQ** tocopherolquinone.
**TR** 1 tuberculin residue (new tuberculin). 2 tricuspid regurgitation.
**tr.** *tinctura* (L, tincture).
**trabecula** \trəbek′yələ\ [L (dim. of *trabs*, gen. *trabis*, a tree, beam), a little beam of wood] (*pl.* trabeculae) **1** A small beam or rib. **2** A beamlike supporting strand of tissue within a structure, such as one of the fibrous strands extending into an organ from its capsule, one of the lamellae of cancellous bone usually interconnected to form a meshwork of stress- and strain-resistant struts within bone, or any other strand of tissue forming a supporting framework. **trabeculae carneae cordis** [NA] Rounded and irregular muscular ridges projecting from most of the inner surface of the walls of the ventricles of the heart. They are more numerous in the left ventricle and are usually of three types: slight ridges, ridges fixed at both ends and free in the middle, or ridges attached by their bases to the walls while their apices project freely into the cavity and are continuous with the chordae tendineae. Also *fleshy trabeculae of heart.* **trabeculae corporis spongiosi penis** [NA] Fibroelastic partitions that extend inward from the tunica albuginea of the corpus spongiosum penis and form a network within which small cavernous spaces are situated. The partitions also contain smooth muscle fibers. Also *trabeculae of corpus spongiosum of penis.* **trabeculae corporum cavernosorum penis** [NA] Partitions composed of collagenous, elastic, and smooth muscle fibers that extend inward into the corpora cavernosa penis from the tunica albuginea and septum penis and form a dense interlacing network within which the cavernous spaces are situated. The partitions contain arteries and nerves. Also *trabeculae of corpora cavernosa of penis.* **trabeculae cranii** Two paired and lateral primordial cartilages representing the anterior portion of the cartilaginous matrix which will form the base of the skull. Situated in front of the hypophyseal cartilages (future body of the sphenoid), the trabeculae cranii will give rise to the cribriform plate of the ethmoid interposed between the cranial cavity and the nasal fossae in the anterior fossa of the base of the skull. **fleshy trabeculae of heart** TRABECULAE CARNEAE CORDIS. **t. septomarginalis** [NA] A thick band of myocardium that often extends from the interventricular septum to the base of the anterior papillary muscle in the right ventricle and contains the right crus of the atrioventricular bundle. It may also assist in preventing overdistension of the right ventricle. Also *septomarginal trabecula, moderator band, band of Reil, Leonardo's band.* **t. of spleen** A fibrous extension of the splenic capsule into the substance of the spleen. Arterial and venous channels may be found ensheathed within trabeculae. Also *reticulum lienis, splenic reticulum, Billroth strand.* **t. testis** *Outmoded* SEPTULA TESTIS.
**trabeculae** \trəbek′yəlē\ Plural of TRABECULA.
**trabecular** \trəbek′yələr\ **1** Possessing one or more trabeculae. Also *trabeculate.* **2** Of or relating to a trabecula.
**trabecularism** \trəbek′yələrizm\ The state of having trabeculae in an organ or a structure.
**trabeculate** \trəbek′yəlāt\ TRABECULAR.
**trabeculation** \trəbek′yəlā′shən\ The process of developing trabeculae in a structure or an organ. **t. of the bladder dome** In radiology, the irregularity of the outline of the opacified lumen of the urinary bladder, due most commonly to hypertrophy of the bladder wall secondary to outlet obstruction.
**trabes** \trā′bēz\ Plural of TRABS.
**trabs** \trabz\ [L, a tree trunk, beam] (*pl.* trabes) A beamlike strand of tissue that supports a structure or an organ.
**trace** [Old French, from L *tractus* a track, trail. See TRACT.] **1** A minute but detectable quantity. **2** A vestige or imprint of the past. **contact t.'s** In the commission of a criminal act, the trace evidence produced when physical material, such as blood, hairs, and fibers, is either transferred from one individual to another or from an individual to the environment as a result of physical contact. **memory t.** The hypothesized permanent change in neural tissue that is the result of experience, i.e., of a more temporary excitation to activity. The trace remaining in brain tissue, presumed to be some form of physiologic alteration, forms the basis of memory. Also *engram.*
**tracer** [*trac(e)* + -ER] **1** LABEL. **2** A device for recording movements of the mandible. **arrow point t.** STYLUS TRACER. **Gothic arch t.** STYLUS TRACER. **needle-point t.** STYLUS TRACER. **radioactive t.** A radioactive isotope used to label a compound so that its course in a chemical reaction or metabolic pathway can be traced. It is normally mixed in trace (i.e. quantitatively negligible) amounts with the unlabeled material. Also *radioactive indicator, radiotracer, radioactive label.* **stylus t.** A device for recording movements of the mandible in one plane on a plate attached to the maxilla or to the mandible. Also *needle-point tracer, arrow point tracer, Gothic arch tracer, seagull tracer.*
**trache-** \trā′kē-\ TRACHEO-.
**trachea** \trā′kē·ə\ [Med L, from Gk *(artēria) tracheia* rough (artery), from *trachys* rough. (The word *artēria* referred indiscriminately to air- and blood-conveying channels.)] [NA] The cartilaginous and membranous air passage that extends in the median plane from the larynx at the level of the sixth cervical vertebra to its termination as the right and left principal bronchi at the level of the fifth thoracic vertebra. It is composed of 16 to 20 rings of hyaline cartilage which are incomplete posteriorly where the free ends are connected by fibrous and elastic tissue and smooth muscle. The rings are linked to each other by fibrous tissue and the tube is lined internally by a mucous membrane. Also *windpipe, weasand* (obs.). Adj. tracheal. **cervical t.** PARS CERVICALIS TRACHEAE. **scabbard t.** The trachea flattened from side to side by compression from without.
**tracheitis** \trā′kē·ī′tis\ [TRACHE- + -ITIS] Inflammation of the trachea. **t. sicca** Tracheitis without sputum production.
**trachel-** \trā′kəl, trak′əl-\ TRACHELO-.
**trachelectomy** \trā′kəlek′təmē\ [TRACHEL- + -ECTOMY] The surgical excision of the uterine cervix. Also *cervicectomy.*
**trachelismus** \trā′kəliz′məs\ [TRACHEL- + Gk *ismos* -ISM] Spasmodic contraction of the neck muscles occurring in some epileptic attacks and transiently impeding circulation and respiration. *Seldom used.* Also *trachelism.*
**trachelitis** \trā′kəlī′tis\ [TRACHEL- + -ITIS] CERVICITIS.
**trachelo-** \trā′kəlō-\ [Gk *trachēlos* throat, neck] A combining form meaning neck, cervical. Also *trachel-.*
**trachelocele** \trā′kəlōsēl′\ TRACHEOCELE.
**trachelocyllosis** \trā′kəlōsilō′sis\ TORTICOLLIS.
**trachelodynia** \trā′kəlōdin′ē·ə\ CERVICALGIA.
**trachelopexy** \trā′kəlōpek′sē\ [TRACHELO- + -PEXY] A surgical procedure in which the uterine cervix is fixed in place by securing it to adjacent structures.

**tracheloplasty** \trā′kəlōplas′tē\ [TRACHELO- + -PLASTY] Any plastic operation on the uterine cervix. Also *hysterotracheloplasty.*

**trachelorrhaphy** \trā′kəlôr′əfē\ [TRACHELO- + -RRHAPHY] A surgical procedure in which a lacerated uterine cervix is repaired with sutures.

**trachelos** \trak′ələs\ COLLUM.

**tracheloschisis** \trā′kəläs′kisis\ [TRACHELO- + -SCHISIS] A congenital fissure on the neck. It is most often a cervical (branchial) fistula or sinus.

**trachelosyringorrhaphy** \trā′kəlōsir′ing·gôr′əfē\ [TRACHELO- + SYRINGO- + -RRHAPHY] The surgical repair of a cervical or vaginal fistula by suturing the uterine cervix in a fixed position in order to obtain increased stability and support.

**trachelotomy** \trā′kəlät′əmē\ [TRACHELO- + -TOMY] A surgical incision made into the uterine cervix.

**tracheo-** \trā′kē·ō-\ [Gk *tracheia* windpipe. See TRACHEA.] A combining form denoting the trachea. Also *trache-, -trachi-.*

**tracheoaerocele** \trāk′ē·ō·er′əsēl\ *Rare* DIVERTICULA OF TRACHEA.

**tracheobronchial** \-bräng′kē·əl\ BRONCHOTRACHEAL.

**tracheobronchitis** \-brängkī′tis\ Inflammation of the bronchi and trachea.

**tracheobronchomegaly** \-bräng′kōmeg′əlē\ A condition of unknown cause in which the trachea and major bronchi are abnormally wide.

**tracheobronchoscopy** \-brängkäs′kəpē\ The instrumental inspection of the interior of the tracheobronchial tree.

**tracheocele** \trā′kē·ōsēl′\ [TRACHEO- + -CELE[1]] The herniation of a portion of the mucous membrane of the trachea through a defect in its wall. Also *trachelocele.*

**tracheography** \trā′kē·äg′rəfē\ [TRACHEO- + -GRAPHY] Roentgenography of the trachea after its mucosa has been coated with a radiopaque contrast medium.

**tracheolaryngotomy** \-lar′ing·gät′əmē\ CRICOTRACHEOTOMY.

**tracheomalacia** \-məlā′shə\ Softening of the tracheal cartilages, a problem sometimes in neonates, when it may accompany laryngomalacia.

**tracheopathia** \-path′ē·ə\ TRACHEOPATHY. **t. osteoplastica** A condition of unknown cause in which hard, bonelike growths or deposits project into the lumen of the trachea.

**tracheopathy** \trā′kē·äp′əthē\ [TRACHEO- + -PATHY] Any disease of the trachea. Also *tracheopathia.*

**tracheoplasty** \trā′kē·əplas′tē\ [TRACHEO- + -PLASTY] Any plastic operation on the trachea.

**tracheorrhaphy** \trā′kē·ôr′əfē\ [TRACHEO- + -RRHAPHY] The repair of a lacerated trachea, usually by suture.

**tracheoschisis** \trā′kē·äs′kisis\ [TRACHEO- + -SCHISIS] Any fissure of the trachea.

**tracheoscope** \trā′kē·əskōp\ [TRACHEO- + -SCOPE] An instrument for directly inspecting, investigating, and providing access for the performance of certain minor operative procedures within the trachea.

**tracheoscopy** \trā′kē·äs′kəpē\ [TRACHEO- + -SCOPY] The instrumental inspection of the interior of the trachea. **percervical t.** Tracheoscopy by way of a tracheostome. **peroral t.** Tracheoscopy by the oral passageway.

**tracheostenosis** \-stenō′sis\ TRACHEAL STENOSIS.

**tracheostome** \trā′kē·əstōm′\ [TRACHEO- + Gk *stoma* mouth] A surgical opening in the midline of the neck anteriorly communicating with the lumen of the cervical trachea, indicated in a variety of circumstances: in obstruction to the airway above the level of the intended opening, in which case the procedure allows the obstruction to be bypassed; respiratory insufficiency, alleviated by providing a route for mechanical ventilatory support; inability to clear secretions from the lower airways, by providing a route for the mechanical aspiration of secretions; inhalation of pharyngeal contents, prevented by allowing the pharynx to be blocked off from the lower airways; and provision of an alternate airway after laryngectomy. The tracheostome is maintained for as long as necessary with a tracheostomy tube. Also *tracheostoma.* **end t.** A variety of tracheostome necessary after laryngectomy where the trachea, transected below the diseased larynx, is sutured to the skin of the lower neck.

**tracheostomy** \trā′kē·äs′təmē\ [TRACHEO- + -STOMY] **1** The operation to establish a tracheostome by means of an incision in the cervical trachea (tracheotomy). **2** The situation existing after such an operation.

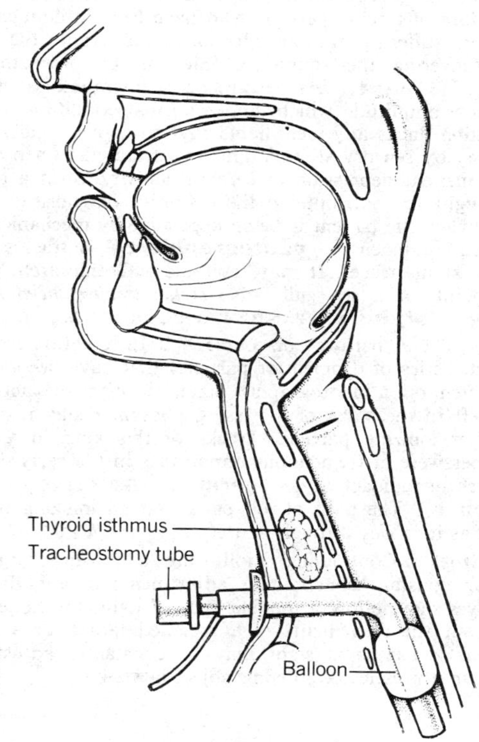


**Tracheostomy**

**tracheotomy** \trā′kē·ät′əmē\ [TRACHEO- + -TOMY] The incising of the cervical trachea through a skin incision, either vertical or transverse, in the midline of the front of the neck. • Until around the middle of the twentieth century, this was the term customarily used for what is now called tracheostomy. **inferior t.** Tracheotomy where the trachea is incised below the level of the isthmus of the thyroid gland. • Prior to the early years of the twentieth century, the thyroid isthmus was regarded by surgeons as a barrier to the upper trachea, so that if the trachea had to be opened, the opening had to be either above or below it. **superior t.** Tracheotomy where the trachea is incised above the level of the isthmus of the thyroid gland. • See note at INFERIOR TRACHEOTOMY.

**trachi-** \trā′kē-\ TRACHEO-.

**trachoma** \trəkō′mə\ [Gk *trachōma*, from *trachys* rough] Infection of the conjunctiva and cornea caused by *Chlamydia trachomatis* and occurring in nearly all developing countries, where it is endemic or hyperendemic. It is the most common ophthalmic disease in the world. Follicles and linear scarring of the conjunctivae, an active keratitis, and corneal pannus are the main signs. Antibiotic therapy is usually effective, although surgery may be necessary in advanced cases. Also *Egyptian ophthalmia, Egyptian conjunctivitis, trachomatous conjunctivitis, granular conjunctivitis.* Adj. trachomatous.

**tracing** A graphic recording made by a pen on paper, a scribe on a plate, or a beam on a cathode ray tube. **cephalometric t.** A tracing of selected parts of a cephalometric radiograph for the purpose of clarity and in order to determine certain planes and angles. **contact t.** The procedure of tracing persons who have been in contact with a patient suffering from an infectious disease, with the object of discovering the source of infection or preventing its spread. **flat t.** An electroencephalographic tracing of very low amplitude which, under normal conditions of amplification, lacks any identifiable rhythm and is totally uninfluenced by sensory stimuli. This is attributed to a transient or permanent depression of cerebral activity. Such a tracing is thought to contribute to the definitive diagnosis of brain death when the patient is being kept alive by mechanical respiration equipment. **pantographic t.** A tracing made with a stylus tracer. It may resemble a Gothic arch, an arrow point, or a sea gull. Also *stylus tracing, needle point tracing.* **stylus t.** PANTOGRAPHIC TRACING.

**track** 1 A pathway or course. 2 In radiation research, a linear series of droplets or particles that have become visible, often on a photographic plate, through the action of ions left in the wake of a passing photon, neutron, proton, or other ionizing particle. Tracks of this kind in a cloud chamber were of tremendous importance in the early days of research in radioactivity. **germ t.** GERM LINE. **ionization t.** The path of ion pairs that an ionizing particle leaves as it moves through matter.

**tracking** Continuously following a moving target by making constant concomitant adjustments of a body part. The eyes may follow a moving spot of light, the finger may trace out the movements of a specified target, or a device such as a telescopic sight may be constantly adjusted to maintain a preselected moving object in view.

# tract

**tract** [L *tractus* (substantive from *tractus*, past part. of *trahere* to draw away, drag, prolong) a drawing, dragging, tract, track, trail] 1 TRACTUS. 2 A continuous pathway through a group of organs, generally constituting a body system, along which may course fluids, solids, or air, such as the genitourinary, gastrointestinal, and respiratory tracts. **afferent t.** 1 A collection of nerve fibers that carry nerve impulses from more peripheral regions to more centrally located sites in the spinal cord or brain, such as the ascending afferent tracts in the spinal cord. Compare EFFERENT TRACT. 2 AFFERENT PATHWAY. **alimentary t.** CANALIS ALIMENTARIUS. **anterior cerebrospinal t.** TRACTUS CORTICOSPINALIS VENTRALIS. **anterior corticospinal t.** TRACTUS CORTICOSPINALIS VENTRALIS. **anterior pyramidal t.** TRACTUS CORTICOSPINALIS VENTRALIS. **anterior spinocerebellar t.** TRACTUS SPINOCEREBELLARIS VENTRALIS. **anterior spinothalamic t.** TRACTUS SPINOTHALAMICUS VENTRALIS. **arcuatofloccular t.** STRIAE MEDULLARES VENTRICULI QUARTI. **ascending t.** 1 A bundle of fibers that courses from lower to higher centers in the central nervous system. 2 The long afferent pathways in the spinal cord that convey impulses to the brainstem, cerebellum, and thalamus. 3 Fiber bundles totally within the brain that course from brainstem or diencephalic sites to the basal ganglia or cerebral cortex in the telencephalon. **ascending and descending association t.'s of cord** Collectively, fascicles of ascending and descending nerve fibers that constitute the intersegmental fiber systems in the spinal cord. Fibers in these tracts commence and terminate within the spinal cord in contrast to the long ascending and descending tracts that interconnect the spinal cord with supraspinal structures in the brain. Some examples of ascending and descending association tracts of the spinal cord include the fasciculi proprii ventrales, laterales, and dorsales, the fasciculus sulcomarginalis, the fasciculus septomarginalis, and the fasciculus interfascicularis. **ascending t.'s of spinal cord** The long ascending fiber tracts in the spinal cord that transmit afferent impulses to suprasegmental regions. These include the anterior and lateral spinothalamic tracts, the anterior and posterior spinocerebellar tracts, the fasciculi gracilis and cuneatus, and the spinotectal, spinoreticular and spino-olivary tracts. Other ascending fibers that do not reach suprasegmental levels may also be considered as helping to constitute the ascending tracts of the spinal cord, and these include all the ascending fibers in the intersegmental association tracts as well as those in the dorsolateral tract (of Lissauer). **association t.** A bundle of nerve fibers that interconnects different regions of the cerebral cortex within the same cerebral hemisphere. Association tracts are distinguished from commissural tracts, which interconnect the cerebral cortices of the two hemispheres, and projection tracts, which either arise in the cerebral cortex and terminate in subcortical centers or arise in subcortical sites and terminate in the cerebral cortex. **Bekhterev's t.** TRACTUS TEGMENTALIS CENTRALIS. **biliary t.** The channel along which bile passes from the biliary canaliculi in the liver to the termination of the common bile duct in the duodenum. It includes the gallbladder and the cystic duct. Also *biliary system, biliary apparatus.* **Bruce's t.** FASCICULUS SEPTOMARGINALIS. **t. of Bruce and Muir** FASCICULUS SEPTOMARGINALIS. **bulbospinal t.** See under TRACTUS OLIVOSPINALIS. **Burdach's t.** FASCICULUS CUNEATUS BURDACHI. **t. of Calza** A bundle of longitudinal muscle fibers in the stratum submucosum of the myometrium that encircles the anterior surface, fundus, and posterior surface of the uterus. **census t.** An area of a city treated as a statistical unit for census purposes. **central t. of acoustic nerve** CENTRAL TRACT OF COCHLEAR NERVE. **central t. of auditory nerve** CENTRAL TRACT OF COCHLEAR NERVE. **central t. of cochlear nerve** The ascending pathway in the central nervous system by which auditory impulses transmitted by fibers in the cochlear division of the vestibulocochlear nerve to the cochlear nuclei in the brainstem reach the cerebral cortex. From the cochlear nuclei most of the fibers cross the midline in the trapezoid body to ascend to the inferior colliculus in the contralateral lateral lemniscus. Some fibers, however, ascend in the ipsilateral lateral lemniscus. From the midbrain, fibers forming the ascending auditory pathway course through the inferior brachium to the medial geniculate body, through which they are relayed in the sublenticular part of the internal capsule to the auditory receiving areas in the cerebral cortex (areas 41, 42, and 22). Also *central tract of auditory nerve, central tract of acoustic nerve.* **central t. of cranial nerves** LEMNISCUS TRIGEMINALIS. **central tegmental t.** TRACTUS TEGMENTALIS CENTRALIS. **central t. of thymus** TRACTUS CENTRALIS THYMI. **central t. of trigeminal nerve** LEMNISCUS TRIGEMINALIS. **cerebellobulbar t.** FASTIGIOBULBAR TRACT. **cerebelloreticular t.** FASTIGIOBULBAR TRACT. **cerebellorubral t.** TRACTUS CEREBELLORUBRALIS. **cerebellospinal t.** A group of nerve fibers that arises in the nucleus fastigii and emerges from the cerebellum by way of the uncinate fasciculus and that is believed by some investigators to pass through the medulla oblongata to enter the ventral funiculus of the spinal cord without synapsing in the lower brainstem. The existence of this tract has been questioned. **cerebellotegmental t. of bulb** FASTIGIOBULBAR TRACT. **cerebellothalamic t.** TRACTUS CEREBELLOTHALAMICUS. **cerebellovestibular t.** A group of nerve fibers that originates in the cerebellum and terminates in the vestibular nuclei of the lower pons and upper medulla oblongata. The cerebellovestibular tract consists of fibers from the flocculus, nodule, and fastigial nucleus that course through the juxtarestiform body to terminate in the ipsilateral vestibular nuclei; fibers from the fastigial nucleus that terminate in the opposite vestibular nuclei; and fibers from Purkinje cells in the anterior and posterior regions of the vermis that do not synapse in the deep cerebellar nuclei but course directly to the lateral and inferior vestibular nuclei on the same side. **colliculorubral t.** TECTORUBRAL TRACT. **Collier's t.** That portion of the medial longitudinal fasciculus that descends through the tegmentum. *Seldom used.* **comma t.** FASCICULUS INTERFASCICULARIS. **comma t. of Schultze** FASCICULUS INTERFASCICULARIS. **commissurospinal t.** A group of fibers that arises from neurons in the nucleus of the posterior commissure (nucleus of Darkschewitsch), crosses the midline in the posterior commissure to enter the contralateral medial longitudinal fasciculus, and descends through the brainstem to the spinal cord. Some of its fibers are also thought to join the ipsilateral medial longitudinal fasciculus. **cornucommissural t.** An intersegmental tract located in the anterior part of the posterior funiculus just dorsal to the gray commissure along the lumbar and sacral spinal segments. The fibers have their cell bodies in the posterior horn of the spinal gray matter, and ascend or descend for one or more segments before terminating in the gray substance of the posterior horn. **corticobulbar t.** TRACTUS CORTICONUCLEARIS. **corticocerebellar t.** TRACTUS CORTICOPONTINUS. **corticocollicular t.** CORTICOTECTAL TRACT. **corticogeniculate t.** A descending efferent pathway that courses from the visual region in the occipital lobe of the cerebral cortex to the lateral geniculate body. The corticofugal fibers of this tract are believed to exert a modifying influence on visual afferent information arriving at the lateral geniculate body from the retina. **corticohypothalamic t.'s** TRACTUS CORTICOHYPOTHALAMICI. **corticonigral t.** Nerve fibers believed to arise in several parts of the cerebral cortex, including the pre- and postcentral gyri, the temporal lobe, the insula, and the preoccipital region, and terminate in or around the substantia nigra of the mesencephalon. The existence of these fibers, however, has been questioned by some researchers. **corticonuclear t.** TRACTUS CORTICONUCLEARIS. **corticopallidal t.** A diffuse group of fibers believed by some researchers to originate from many areas of the cerebral cortex and terminate directly upon cells in the globus pallidus. It is still uncertain whether such direct corticofugal projections to the globus pallidus exist. **corticopontile t.** TRACTUS CORTICOPONTINUS. **corticopontine t.** TRACTUS CORTICOPONTINUS. **corticopontocerebellar t.'s** CORTICOPONTOCEREBELLAR SYSTEM. **corticorubral t.** A group of nerve fibers that projects directly from the precentral and supplementary motor region of the cerebral cortex to the red nucleus in the mesencephalon. The corticorubral tract is uncrossed, and there is a somatotopic arrangement of the projection from specific sites in the motor cortex to specific parts of the red nucleus. **corticospinal t.** TRACTUS CORTICOSPINALIS. **corticospinal t. anterior** TRACTUS CORTICOSPINALIS VENTRALIS. **corticotectal t.** A collection of nerve fibers derived from the frontal, temporal, parietal and, especially, occipital lobe that descend to project into the superficial and intermediate gray layers of the superior colliculus. The corticotectal fibers from the visual cortex in the occipital lobe appear to terminate in the more rostral part of the superior colliculus, which does not receive many retinal fibers. Also *corticocollicular tract.* **corticothalamic t.** Collectively, direct projections from many regions of the cerebral cortex to the various nuclei in the thalamus. Frequently, more specific corticothalamic projections are described with respect to the cortical site from which the fibers originate and the thalamic nucleus to which they project, such as the corticothalamic connections between the prefrontal cortex in the frontal lobe and the nucleus dorsalis medialis in the medial group of thalamic nuclei. **crossed marginal t.** TRACTUS DORSOLATERALIS. **crossed pyramidal t.** TRACTUS CORTICOSPINALIS LATERALIS. **dead t.** An area of dentin with tubules devoid of odontoblast processes. **Deiters t.** TRACTUS VESTIBULOSPINALIS. **dentatothalamic t.** TRACTUS CEREBELLOTHALAMICUS. **descending t.** **1** A bundle of nerve fibers forming a pathway that courses from higher to lower centers in the central nervous system, especially the long pathways coursing from the cerebral cortex to the brainstem or spinal levels, such as the tractus corticonuclearis or the tractus corticospinalis. **2** Any tract of fibers whose cell bodies lie higher in the neuraxis than the sites of termination of the projection fibers, such as the tractus vestibulospinalis. **descending t.'s of spinal cord** Collectively, long descending fiber tracts in the spinal cord that transmit impulses from suprasegmental regions to the spinal cord. These include the anterior and lateral corticospinal tracts, the vestibulospinal, tectospinal, rubrospinal, and reticulospinal tracts, the olivospinal and solitariospinal tracts, as well as descending autonomic fibers. Other descending fibers in the spinal cord do not arise at supraspinal levels but constitute the descending elements in the insegmental association tracts, as well as the descending fibers in the dorsolateral tract (of Lissauer). **descending vestibular t.** TRACTUS VESTIBULOSPINALIS. **digestive t.** CANALIS ALIMENTARIUS. **direct cerebellar t. of Flechsig** TRACTUS SPINOCEREBELLARIS DORSALIS. **direct pyramidal t.** TRACTUS CORTICOSPINALIS VENTRALIS. **direct spinocerebellar t.** TRACTUS SPINOCEREBELLARIS DORSALIS. **direct vestibulocerebellar t.** VESTIBULOCEREBELLAR TRACT. **dopaminergic t.** A bundle of fibers in the brain or spinal cord whose terminals release dopamine as a neurotransmitter, e.g., the nigrostriatal tract. **dorsal spinocerebellar t.** TRAC-

TUS SPINOCEREBELLARIS DORSALIS. **dorsolateral t.** TRACTUS DORSOLATERALIS. **efferent t.** 1 A group of nerve fibers forming a central tract or pathway that carries nerve impulses from higher or more centrally located sites in the brain or spinal cord to lower or more peripherally located regions in the neuraxis. Compare AFFERENT TRACT. 2 EFFERENT PATHWAY. **extracorticospinal t.** EXTRAPYRAMIDAL SYSTEM. **extrapyramidal t.** EXTRAPYRAMIDAL SYSTEM. **fastigiobulbar t.** A tract of nerve fibers that have their neuronal cell bodies in the nucleus fastigii of the cerebellum and emerge from the cerebellum by way of the uncinate fasciculus and juxtarestiform body before joining the inferior cerebellar peduncle. Some fibers cross to the opposite side, while others remain uncrossed and terminate in the dorsomedial part of the lower pontine and medullary reticular formation. Also *cerebellobulbar tract, cerebelloreticular tract, fastigioreticular tract, cerebellotegmental tract of bulb.* **fastigiovestibular t.** The portion of the cerebellovestibular tract that commences in the fastigial nucleus and terminates in the vestibular nuclei. **Flechsig's t.** TRACTUS SPINOCEREBELLARIS DORSALIS. **foraminous spiral t.** TRACTUS SPIRALIS FORAMINOSUS. **fronto-occipital t.** The fasciculus occipitofrontalis superior and fasciculus occipitofrontalis inferior. **frontopontile t.** TRACTUS FRONTOPONTINUS. **frontopontine t.** TRACTUS FRONTOPONTINUS. **gastrointestinal t.** The part of the apparatus digestorius that consists of the stomach and the intestines. **generative t.** The organa genitalia femina interna and the organa genitalia femina externa considered together. **geniculocalcarine t.** RADIATIO OPTICA. **geniculostriate t.** RADIATIO OPTICA. **geniculotemporal t.** RADIATIO ACUSTICA. **genital t.** The internal and external reproductive organs of both males and females. **genitourinary t.** APPARATUS UROGENITALIS. **t. of Goll** FASCICULUS GRACILIS MEDULLAE SPINALIS. **Gowers t.** TRACTUS SPINOCEREBELLARIS VENTRALIS. **habenular t.'s** Collectively, efferent fiber pathways from the habenular nuclei to other diencephalic and brainstem centers. The largest of these is the habenulointerpeduncular tract, which courses to the interpeduncular nucleus of the midbrain. Other connections include the habenulothalamic tract to the nucleus medialis dorsalis of the thalamus and the habenulotectal and habenulotegmental fibers to the mesencephalon. **habenulodiencephalic t. of Edinger** Fibers passing from the habenular nucleus to the dorsomedial nucleus of the dorsal thalamus. **habenulointerpeduncular t.** FASCICULUS RETROFLEXUS. **habenulopeduncular t.** *Incorrect* FASCICULUS RETROFLEXUS. **Helweg's t.** TRACTUS OLIVOSPINALIS. **Hoche's t.** FASCICULUS SEPTOMARGINALIS. **hypothalamohypophysial t.** TRACTUS HYPOTHALAMOHYPOPHYSIALIS. **iliopubic t.** DEEP CRURAL ARCH. **iliotibial t.** TRACTUS ILIOTIBIALIS. **intermediolateral t.** COLUMNA INTERMEDIOLATERALIS. **internuncial t.** Any tract connecting two nuclei in the central nervous system. **interstitiospinal t.** A group of nerve fibers that arises from neurons in the interstitial nucleus (of Cajal) in the midbrain and descends in the ipsilateral medial longitudinal fasciculus. Most of the fibers are believed to terminate among internucial neurons in the medial part of the ventral horn, especially the cervical segments. **intestinal t.** INTESTINAL CANAL. **lateral cerebrospinal t.** TRACTUS CORTICOSPINALIS LATERALIS. **lateral corticospinal t.** TRACTUS CORTICOSPINALIS LATERALIS. **lateral intersegmental t.** FASCICULI PROPRII. **lateral t. of isthmus** The part of the lateral lemniscus that occupies the trigonum lemnisci (triangle of Reil). **lateral olfactory t.** STRIA LATERALIS TRIGONI OLFACTORII. **lateral pyramidal t.** TRACTUS CORTICOSPINALIS LATERALIS. **lateral spinothalamic t.** TRACTUS SPINOTHALAMICUS LATERALIS. **lenticulothalamic t.** A collection of nerve fibers that arises in the lenticular nucleus (i.e., the globus pallidus and putamen) and courses to the thalamus. Most of these fibers originate in the globus pallidus and course to the nucleus ventralis anterior, the nucleus intermedius, and the nucleus centromedianus of the thalamus and hence are called pallidothalamic fibers. **Lissauer's t.** TRACTUS DORSOLATERALIS. **Löwenthal's t.** TRACTUS TECTOSPINALIS. **lower respiratory t.** The respiratory tract below the level of the larynx. **Maissiat's t.** TRACTUS ILIOTIBIALIS. **mamillointerpeduncular t.** A small bundle of nerve fibers that courses along the ventral surface of the brain and interconnects the mamillary body with the ipsilateral interpeduncular nucleus. Also *mamillopeduncular tract.* **mamillotegmental t.** A bundle of fibers that emerges from the medial nucleus of the mamillary body in the posterior hypothalamus. It initially ascends in conjunction with the mamillothalamic tract and then curves caudally away from it, entering the midbrain ventral to the medial longitudinal fasciculus and terminating in the tegmental nuclei. **mamillothalamic t.** FASCICULUS MAMILLOTHALAMICUS. **Marchi's t.** TRACTUS TECTOSPINALIS. **mesencephalic t. of trigeminal nerve** TRACTUS MESENCEPHALICUS NERVI TRIGEMINI. **Meynert's t.** FASCICULUS RETROFLEXUS. **Monakow's t.** TRACTUS RUBROSPINALIS. **motor t.** 1 A descending bundle of nerve fibers arising in the brain and terminating on motoneurons or interneurons in the cranial nerve nuclei or in the gray matter in the ventral horn of the spinal cord. It conveys impulses influencing the activity of efferent motor fibers in the cranial nerves or in the ventral roots of the spinal cord. 2 Either the tractus corticonuclearis or the tractus corticospinalis. **nigrorubral t.** A neural pathway within the mesencephalon believed by some investigators to interconnect the substantia nigra and the red nucleus. This tract has been described as consisting of both crossed and uncrossed fibers, but not much detailed information is available about it. **nigrostriatal t.** COMB BUNDLE. **occipitopontile t.** TRACTUS OCCIPITOPONTINUS. **occipitopontine t.** TRACTUS OCCIPITOPONTINUS. **olfactohabenular t.** SEPTOHABENULAR TRACT. **olfactohypothalamic t.** Descending fibers originating in the medial olfactory region (into which fibers from the medial olfactory stria terminate) that project to the preoptic region and to much of the hypothalamus by way of the medial forebrain bundle. By this route it is believed that olfactory impulses influence hypothalamic functions, especially feeding behavior. **olfactory t.** TRACTUS OLFACTORIUS. **olivocerebellar t.** TRACTUS OLIVOCEREBELLARIS. **olivospinal t.** TRACTUS OLIVOSPINALIS. **optic t.** TRACTUS OPTICUS. **pallidoreticular t.** Descending fibers from the globus pallidus to the reticular formation of the mesencephalon. **pallidosubthalamic t.** A group of fibers that arises principally in the lateral segment of the globus pallidus, passes along the subthalamic fasciculus through the internal capsule, and terminates on cells in the subthalamic nucleus. **pallidotegmental t.** A group of pallidofugal fibers that arises from the medial segment of the globus pallidus, courses dorsomedial to the subthalamic nucleus, descends adjacent to the red nucleus, and terminates in the dorsolateral tegmental region of the lower mesencephalon. **pallidothalamic t.** A group of pallidofugal fibers that terminates in the thalamus. Pallidothalamic fibers arise in the medial segment of the globus pallidus, form a well-defined bundle (the ansa lenticularis), enter the prerubral area (field H of Forel), where they bend laterally to join the thalamic fasciculus (field $H_1$ of Forel). They are distributed to the nucleus ventralis anterior and to a lesser extent the nucleus ventralis lateralis and the nucleus centromedianus. Also *striothalamic tract.* **paraventriculohypophysial t.** TRACTUS PARAVENTRICULOHYPOPHYSIALIS. **parietopontine t.** TRACTUS PARIETOPONTINUS. **periependymal t.** FASCICULUS LONGITUDINALIS DORSALIS. **periventricular t.** FASCICULUS LONGITUDINALIS DORSALIS. **t. of Philippe-Gombault** FASCICULUS TRIANGULARIS. **pontocerebellar t.** PEDUNCULUS CEREBELLARIS MEDIUS. **portal t.** A fibrous sheath situated at the periphery of a hepatic lobule that encloses a branch of the portal vein, a branch of the hepatic artery, and an interlobular bile duct. **posterior spinocerebellar t.** TRACTUS SPINOCEREBELLARIS DORSALIS. **predorsal t.** TRACTUS TECTOSPINALIS. **prepyramidal t.** TRACTUS RUBROSPINALIS. **projection t.** PROJECTION FIBERS. **pyramidal t.** TRACTUS PYRAMIDALIS. **pyramidal t. anterior** TRACTUS CORTICOSPINALIS VENTRALIS. **pyramidoanterior t.** TRACTUS CORTICOSPINALIS VENTRALIS. **pyramidolateral t.** TRACTUS CORTICOSPINALIS LATERALIS. **respiratory t.** APPARATUS RESPIRATORIUS. **reticulobulbar t.** Diffuse fibers (not a specific bundle) from the reticular formation in the core of the brainstem that project to the motor nuclei of the cranial nerves. **reticulo-olivary t.** A group of scattered fibers with cell bodies in the bulbar and pontine reticular formation that project to the inferior olivary nucleus. These fibers probably join descending rubro-olivary fibers coursing in the central tegmental tract from the red nucleus and also destined to terminate in the inferior olive. **reticuloreticular t.** Nerve fibers derived from neurons of the reticular formation at certain levels of the brainstem that project to portions of the reticular formation at other levels. These reticuloreticular fibers do not gather into discrete tracts, but are more diffusely organized within the neuropil in the core of the brainstem. Also *reticuloreticular fibers.* **reticulospinal t.** TRACTUS RETICULOSPINALIS. **rubrobulbar t.** RUBRORETICULAR TRACT. **rubro-olivary t.** A bundle of descending uncrossed fibers that arises in the parvocellular part of the red nucleus, enters the central tegmental tract, and projects to the dorsal part of the principal inferior olivary nucleus. **rubroreticular t.** A group of nerve fibers that arise from cells in the red nucleus, decussate along with fibers of the rubrospinal tract, and terminate in the nuclei of the reticular formation. Some rubroreticular fibers reach various bulbar cranial nerve nuclei. Also *rubrobulbar tract.* **rubroreticulospinal t.** An interconnected rubroreticular and reticulospinal pathway by which neurons that arise in the parvocellular prerubral part of the red nucleus course to the spinal cord by way of synaptic connections in the reticular formation. **rubrospinal t.** TRACTUS RUBROSPINALIS. **rubrothalamic t.** An ascending group of fibers thought by some researchers to arise in the caudal part of the red nucleus and terminate in the nucleus ventralis lateralis of the thalamus. Evidence that these fibers are few in number or even nonexistent has also been published. **t. of Schütz** FASCICULUS LONGITUDINALIS DORSALIS. **Schultze's t.** FASCICULUS INTERFASCICULARIS. **semilunar t.** FASCICULUS INTERFASCICULARIS. **seminal t.** The vesicula seminalis and ductus excretorius vesiculae seminalis. **sensory t.** An afferent neural bundle of the central nervous system that conveys impulse activity essential to sensory experience. **septohabenular t.** A group of fibers interconnecting the medial olfactory region (which receives input from the medial olfactory stria) with the habenular nuclei by way of the stria medullaris thalami. Also *olfactohabenular tract.* **septomarginal t.** FASCICULUS SEPTOMARGINALIS. **solitariospinal t.** A poorly localized descending bundle of fibers taking origin from reticular neurons in the vicinity of the nucleus solitarius and innervating spinal centers concerned with innervation of respiratory muscles. **solitary t. of medulla oblongata** TRACTUS SOLITARIUS. **spinal t. of trigeminal nerve** TRACTUS SPINALIS NERVI TRIGEMINI. **spinal vestibular t.** TRACTUS VESTIBULOSPINALIS. **spinocerebellar t. anterior** TRACTUS SPINOCEREBELLARIS VENTRALIS. **spinocervical t.** A group of nerve fibers having their cell bodies in the thoracic nucleus (Clarke's nucleus) that ascends in the lateral funiculus from lumbosacral levels of the spinal cord to terminate in the lateral cervical nucleus located in the upper cervical segments. Fibers from the lateral cervical nucleus are believed to ascend to the contralateral nucleus ventralis posterolateralis of the thalamus, making the spino-cervical-thalamic pathway an adjunct to the spinothalamic tract mediating tactile and pressure modalities. **spino-olivary t.** A group of ascending fibers originating in the spinal cord and coursing in both the ventral funiculus (ventral spino-olivary tract) and the dorsal funiculus (dorsal spino-olivary tract) to terminate in the contralateral dorsal and medial accessory olivary nuclei. This tract appears to be related to the ascending spinocerebellar pathways because it projects to the bed nuclei of the olivocerebellar tract and because it can be activated by incoming afferent fibers from the skin and Golgi tendon organs. **spinospinal t.'s** FASCICULI PROPRII. **spinotectal t.** TRACTUS SPINOTECTALIS. **spinothalamic t.** Collectively, the anterior and lateral spinothalamic tracts; ascending bundles arising in the dorsal horn of the spinal cord conveying impulse activity derived from nociceptors, thermoreceptors, and sensitive mechanoreceptors. It is predominantly crossed at the spinal level and terminates in several zones of the contralateral thalamus. Also *lemniscus spinalis, spinal lemniscus.* **Spitzka's t.** TRACTUS DORSOLATERALIS. **Spitzka-Lissauer t.** TRACTUS DORSOLATERALIS. **Spitzka's marginal t.** TRACTUS DORSOLATERALIS. **strionigral t.** Nerve fibers that have been described as coursing from the putamen and caudate nucleus of the corpus striatum directly to the substantia nigra without synapsing in the globus pallidus as do most striatofugal fibers. Other reports have also denied the existence of direct strionigral fibers. Also *striatonigral tract.* **striorubral t.** Fibers of the lenticular fasciculus that arise from the medial pallidal segment and course to the prerubral field (field H of Forel). Also *prerubral fasciculus.* **striothalamic t.** PALLIDOTHALAMIC TRACT. **sulcomarginal t.** FASCICULUS SULCOMARGINALIS. **supraopticohypophysial t.** TRACTUS SUPRAOPTICOHYPOPHYSIALIS. **tectobulbar t.** TRACTUS TECTOBULBARIS. **tectocerebellar t.** Fibers thought by some investigators to arise in both the superior and inferior colliculi of the midbrain and enter the cerebellum by way of the superior medullary velum in association with the superior cerebellar peduncle. They are believed to terminate diffusely in the vermal and paravermal regions of the cerebellar cortex (including the declive, lobulus simplex, folium, tuber and pyramis) and to transmit information to the cerebellum relating to incoming visual and auditory stimuli. Other investigators have questioned the existence of direct tectocerebellar fibers, believing instead that they undergo synaptic connections in the pontine nuclei, thereby constituting a tecto-pontine-cerebellar pathway. **tectoru-**

**bral t.** A tract formed by fibers that emerge from the deep white layer of the superior colliculus, course around the periventricular gray substance of the midbrain, and enter the magnocellular portion of the red nucleus of the same side. Other fibers from the superior colliculus cross to the opposite side in the dorsal tegmental decussation to reach the contralateral red nucleus. Also *colliculorubral tract, tectotegmental tract.* **tectospinal t.** TRACTUS TECTOSPINALIS. **tectotegmental t.** TECTORUBRAL TRACT. **tegmental t.** TRACTUS TEGMENTALIS CENTRALIS. **tegmento-olivary t.** Fibers that arise in the central gray matter of the midbrain and terminate in the inferior olivary nucleus. Some of the tegmento-olivary fibers are thought to descend in the tractus tegmentalis centralis. **tegmentospinal t.** Fibers arising from cell bodies in the mesencephalic reticular formation lateral and caudal to the red nucleus that partially decussate and then descend in association with the rubrospinal tract in the lateral funiculus of the spinal cord. **temporopontile t.** TRACTUS TEMPOROPONTINUS. **temporopontine t.** TRACTUS TEMPOROPONTINUS. **thalamocortical t.** Collectively, the many fiber projections originating from cell bodies in the thalamic nuclei that course through the internal capsule to terminate in the cerebral cortex. **thalamohypothalamic t.'s** Nerve fibers that arise from the dorsomedial nucleus of the thalamus and pass to many hypothalamic nuclei by way of the periventricular system of fibers. **thalamo-occipital t.** RADIATIO OPTICA. **thalamo-olivary t.** A few fibers that descend in the substance of the tractus tegmentalis centralis to end in the olivary nucleus. **tracheobronchial t.** TRACHEOBRONCHIAL TREE. **transverse peduncular t.** A bundle of fibers, more prominent in subhuman mammals, than in man, that arises from a nuclear mass located medial to the substantia nigra in the ventral tegmental area of Tsai and courses dorsally to terminate in the oculomotor nucleus. • The tract is so named because the nucleus from which its fibers arise receives optic fibers that cross in the optic chiasma and then separate from the optic tract and recross in the fibrous portion of the cerebral peduncle before terminating. **triangular t.** TRACTUS OLIVOSPINALIS. **triangular t. of Philippe-Gombault** FASCICULUS TRIANGULARIS. **trigeminothalamic t.** LEMNISCUS TRIGEMINALIS. **tuberohypophysial t.** TRACTUS TUBEROHYPOPHYSIALIS. **tuberoinfundibular t.** TRACTUS TUBEROHYPOPHYSIALIS. **Türck's t.** TRACTUS TEMPOROPONTINUS. **uncrossed pyramidal t.** TRACTUS CORTICOSPINALIS VENTRALIS. **upper respiratory t.** The upper or proximal part of the respiratory tract comprising the nasal passages and pharynx and excluding the laryngeal, tracheobronchial, and pulmonary airways. • The term is sometimes used imprecisely to include the fauces. **upper urinary t.** The part of the urinary tract that comprises the renal pelvis and the abdominal portion of the ureter. **urinary t.** The continuous canal for the excretion of urine which extends from the renal pelvis to the external urethral orifice through the ureters, bladder, and urethra. **urogenital t.** APPARATUS UROGENITALIS. **uveal t.** TUNICA VASCULOSA BULBI. **ventral corticospinal t.** TRACTUS CORTICOSPINALIS VENTRALIS. **ventral pyramidal t.** TRACTUS CORTICOSPINALIS VENTRALIS. **ventral spinocerebellar t.** TRACTUS SPINOCEREBELLARIS VENTRALIS. **ventral spinothalamic t.** TRACTUS SPINOTHALAMICUS VENTRALIS. **vestibulocerebellar t.** A fascicle of nerve fibers consisting principally of primary afferent fibers from the vestibular part of the vestibulocochlear nerve, but also containing some fibers with cell bodies in the medial and inferior vestibular nuclei. Most of these fibers terminate in the flocculus, nodule, uvula, and lingula but some also terminate in the fastigial nuclei. They course to the cerebellum by way of the inferior cerebellar peduncle. Also *direct vestibulocerebellar tract.* **vestibulo-ocular t.** A group of fibers within the medial longitudinal fasciculus that arises from the vestibular nuclei and terminates in the nuclei of the abducens, trochlear, and oculomotor nerves. The fibers coming from the superior vestibular nucleus ascend to terminate in the ipsilateral visuomotor nuclei, while those that arise in the other vestibular nuclei partially cross to the opposite side. The chief function of this tract is to coordinate movements of the eye in response to the stimulation of vestibular receptors in the internal ear. **vestibulospinal t.** TRACTUS VESTIBULOSPINALIS. **t. of Vicq d'Azyr** FASCICULUS MAMILLOTHALAMICUS. **vocal t.** The air passage through the nose, mouth, pharynx, and larynx. *Outmoded.* **Waldeyer's t.** TRACTUS DORSOLATERALIS.

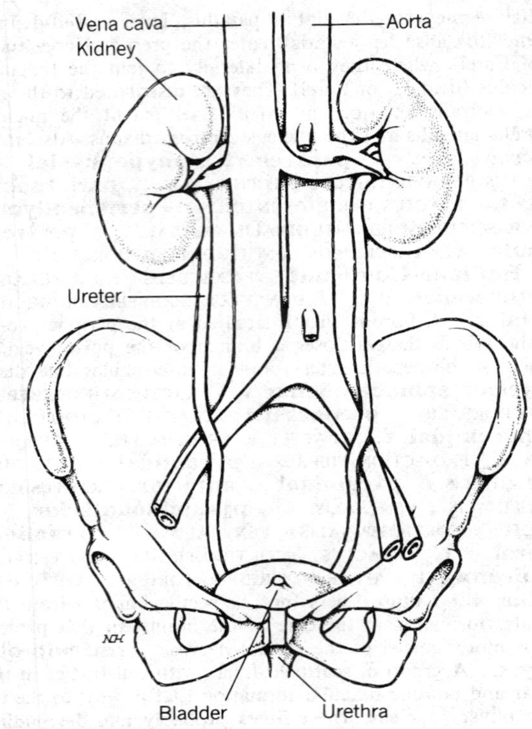


**Urinary tract**

**traction** \trak′shən\ [L *tractio* (from *tractus,* past part. of *trahere* to draw away, drag, prolong) a drawing, dragging] **1** The process of drawing or pulling, or the force exerted in such a process. **2** The tension produced by drawing or pulling, as on a body part or organ. **axis t.** Traction along the axis of the maternal pelvis during a forceps delivery of a fetus. **Bryant's t.** The application of a vertical force on the extended lower extremities of an infant with a fracture of the femur. **Buck's t.** BUCK'S EXTENSION. **elastic finger t.** A rarely used method of stabilizing finger bone fractures. **external t.** Traction applied to fracture of the jaw by a device which passes outside the oral cavity. **halo t.** Traction applied to the spine in cases of fracture or dislocation of the vertebrae, by a device consisting of two metal hoops, one of which (the halo) is pinned to the cranium while the other rests against the iliac crests. The two hoops are connected by turnbuckle rods. Also *halo-pelvic traction.* **intermaxillary t.** 1 The application of force between lower and upper arches to produce the movement of teeth in both arches. 2 Traction applied to a fractured jaw using the opposite jaw as a base. Also *maxillomandibular traction.* **intramaxillary t.** The application of a force between groups of teeth within the one arch. **intraoral elastic t.** Maxillomandibular fixation, using rubber bands between the arch bars for securing stability of fractured areas for the orthodontic movement of teeth. **isometric t.** Traction in which the body segment is immobilized, such as traction applied to the foot with the knee contained in a rigid orthosis. **isotonic t.** Traction in which the force applied is fixed and the limb or body segment free to move. **maxillomandibular t.** INTERMAXILLARY TRACTION. **Russell t.** A splint that applies horizontal forces to stabilize and reduce fractures around the knee joint or femur. **skeletal t.** A traction method in which a pin in inserted percutaneously into a bone so that strong traction can be applied to the limb. Also *nail extension, skeletal extension.* **vertebral t.** A distraction of the vertebral column that is applied manually or with an apparatus. It is used to stabilize the spine in inflammatory disorders, after injury, or for correction of a spinal deformity. **vitreous t.** Pull exerted upon the retina by adhesions between the vitreous humor and the retina. **weight t.** Traction applied to the skeleton via a system of weights and pulleys. **windlass t.** Traction applied to a limb via tapes and cord which are fixed to a Thomas splint. A bar is passed through the cord and rotated to apply increased traction to the limb.

**tractology** \traktäl′əjē\ [TRACT + *o* + -LOGY] The study of connections within the central nervous system. It includes determination of the source, trajectory, and termination of fiber bundles, their relation to other prominent neural structures, and their probable functional roles in the overall behavior of the organism.

**tractor** An instrument utilized to apply traction.

**tractotomy** \traktät′əmē\ [TRACT + *o* + -TOMY] Incision or division of a nerve tract. **descending root t.** TRIGEMINAL TRACTOTOMY. **intramedullary t.** TRIGEMINAL TRACTOTOMY. **mesencephalic t.** Division of a tract in the mesencephalon, usually the spinothalamic tract. **pyramidal t.** Division of the pyramidal tract, usually in the upper cervical region. Also *pyramidotomy.* **Sjöqvist t.** TRIGEMINAL TRACTOTOMY. **spinothalamic t.** Division of the spinothalamic tract, usually performed in the spinal cord for relief of pain distal to the level of the division; chordotomy. **trigeminal t.** Section of the descending root of the trigeminal nerve. Also *Sjöqvist tractotomy, descending root tractotomy, intramedullary tractotomy.*

**tractus** \trak′təs\ [L, tract. See TRACT.] (*pl.* tractus) [NA] A pathway coursing in the spinal cord and/or brain that consists of bundles of nerve fibers that collectively form an anatomical or functional unit. Also *tract.* See also FASCICULUS. • Tracts in the central nervous system are often named with respect to the sites of origin and termination of their constituent nerve fibers (such as the spinocerebellar tract), but others reflect the function they subserve (such as the olfactory tract) or some other specific characteristic. **t. centralis thymi** A fibrous connective tissue septum, centrally located in the thymus, along which course blood vessels and nerves and from which collagenous and reticular fibers radiate between the epithelial cells. Also *central tract of thymus.* **t. cerebellorubralis** A group of nerve fibers that have their neuronal cell bodies in the dentate, globose, and emboliform nuclei of the cerebellum and that leave the cerebellum by means of the superior cerebellar peduncle, cross to the opposite side in the caudal midbrain, and terminate in the contralateral red nucleus located in the mesencephalic tegmentum. Also *cerebellorubral tract, dentatorubral system, cerebellorubral pathway, cerebellorubral system.* **t. cerebellothalamicus** A group of nerve fibers that have their neuronal cell bodies in the dentate nucleus of the cerebellum and emerge from the cerebellum by way of the superior cerebellar peduncle. The fibers then cross to the opposite side in the midbrain and ascend to terminate in the contralateral nucleus ventralis lateralis and the nucleus ventralis anterior of the thalamus. These thalamic nuclei project to the primary motor cortex, and in this way the tractus cerebellothalamicus is capable of influencing motor activity. Also *dentatothalamic tract, cerebellothalamic tract.* **t. corticobulbaris** Descending axons derived mainly from motor cortex and contiguous with the corticospinal tract, but terminating in brainstem motor nuclei controlling head and neck muscles. It includes corticobulbar, or corticonuclear, fibers. **t. corticohypothalamici** A group of nerve fibers believed bysome investigators to originate in the posterior orbital cortex and to terminate directly in the hypothalamus. Also *corticohypothalamic tracts.* • The term, however, is not usually used for projections from the phylogenetically old periamygdaloid cortical region to the hypothalamus (medial forebrain bundle), or from the hippocampal formation to the hypothalamus (fornix), both of which are known to exist. **t. corticonuclearis** [NA] A group of fibers that forms a part of the great motor pathway from the cerebral cortex and that descends in the internal capsule to terminate in the motor nuclei of the cranial nerves in the brainstem. This tract is frequently but erroneously considered a part of the pyramidal tract, but its fibers terminate in the midbrain, pons, and medulla oblongata before arriving at the pyramidal decussation. Also *corticobulbar tract, corticonuclear tract.* **t. corticopontinus** A collection of frontopontine, temporopontine, parietopontine, and occipitopontine fibers that originate in the various lobes of the cerebral cortex, descend in the internal capsule, and terminate in the pontine nuclei on the same side. The pontine nuclei then give origin to pontocerebellar fibers that cross to the opposite side and project to the opposite cerebellar hemisphere through the middle cerebellar peduncle. It is by means of the tractus corticopontinus and the pontocerebellar path that the cerebral cortex is capable of influencing cerebellar function. Also *corticopontile tract, corticocerebellar tract, corticopontine tract, palliopontine fiber.* **t. corticospinalis** An efferent motor pathway that originates in the large pyramidal cells and other, smaller, neurons in the motor cortex and other cortical areas, descends in the rostral half of the posterior limb of the internal capsule, the intermediate three-fifths of the cerebral peduncle, and the ventral part of the pons to the pyramid in the medulla oblongata, where a large number of its fibers cross to the opposite side and continue to descend as the tractus corticospinalis lateralis in the lateral funiculus of the spinal cord. The remaining fibers descend uncrossed in the ventral funiculus of the spinal cord as the tractus corticospinalis ventralis, and then cross to the opposite side in small numbers segmentally, to terminate with fibers of the tractus corticospinalis ventralis in the gray matter of the ventral horn. The tractus corticospinalis descends without interruption from the cerebral cortex to the spinal cord, and is a most important pathway for the initiation and cortical control of voluntary movements effected through spinal motoneurons to striated musculature. Also *corticospinal tract.* See also TRACTUS PYRAMIDALIS. **t. corticospinalis anterior** TRACTUS CORTICOSPINALIS VENTRALIS. **t. corticospinalis lateralis** [NA] A descending motor pathway that courses in the lateral funiculus of the spinal cord medial to the posterior spinocerebellar tract and extends almost the entire length of the spinal cord. The fibers of the tractus corticospinalis lateralis are derived from neurons in the opposite cerebral cortex and terminate on nerve cells in the anterior gray matter of the spinal cord, and the tract is formed by those fibers of the tractus corticospinalis which cross at the pyramidal decussation in the medulla oblongata. The tractus corticospinalis lateralis represents nearly two thirds of the fibers in the entire tractus corticospinalis. Also *tractus pyramidalis lateralis, lateral corticospinal tract, crossed pyramidal tract, lateral pyramidal tract, pyramidolateral tract, lateral cerebrospinal tract, fasciculus cerebrospinalis lateralis, fasciculus pyramidalis lateralis, crossed pyramidal fasciculus, lateral cerebrospinal fasciculus, lateral pyramidal fasciculus.* **t. corticospinalis ventralis** [NA] A descending motor pathway that coursesin the anterior funiculus of the spinal cord immediately adjacent to the ventral median fissure. The fibers that constitute the tractus corticospinalis ventralis represent about one-third of the fibers in the tractus corticospinalis, specifically those that do not cross in the pyramidal decussation but do cross the spinal cord segmentally to terminate in the opposite anterior gray matter of the cervical and upper thoracic spinal segments. This tract is difficult to trace below the midthoracic region of the spinal cord, and is best represented in the subhuman primate and human central nervous system. Also *ventral pyramidal tract, anterior pyramidal tract, pyramidoanterior tract, tractus corticospinalis anterior, anterior cerebrospinal tract, anterior corticospinal tract, uncrossed pyramidal tract, ventral corticospinal tract, fasciculus of Türck, Türck's column, Türck's bundle, tractus pyramidalis anterior, fasciculus pyramidalis anterior, direct pyramidal fasciculus, fasciculus cerebrospinalis anterior, anterior pyramidal fasciculus, uncrossed pyramidal fasciculus, direct pyramidal tract, corticospinal tract anterior, pyramidal tract anterior.* See also TRACTUS CORTICOSPINALIS. **t. dorsolateralis** [NA] A small fascicle of myelinated and unmyelinated nerve fibers located between the dorsal and lateral funiculi of the spinal cord and occupying the region between the tip of the posterior gray matter and the cord surface. It is composed partially of primary afferent nerve fibers the cell bodies of which lie in the dorsal root ganglia. These incoming fibers bifurcate into ascending and descending branches that course for one or two segments and then enter the posterior gray matter and synapse with second-order neurons. They carry impulses of pain and thermal and light tactile sense. The tractus dorsolateralis also contains a large number of propriospinal fibers which are intraspinal with respect to both their origin and their termination. Also *dorsolateral tract, dorsolateral fasciculus, fasciculus dorsolateralis, crossed marginal tract, marginal bundle, Lissauer's tract, Spitzka-Lissauer tract, Spitzka's tract, Spitzka's marginal tract, Waldeyer's tract, Lissauer's marginal zone, Spitzka's marginal zone.* **t. frontopontinus** The portion of the tractus corticopontinus that arises in the gyri of the frontal lobe. Also *frontopontile tract, frontopontine tract, frontopontine fibers, Arnold's bundle.* **t. habenulointerpeduncularis** FASCICULUS RETROFLEXUS. **t. hypothalamohypophysialis** [NA] Collectively, several bundles of nerve fibers originating in various hypothalamic nuclei and terminating at different levels throughout the median eminence, infundibular lobe, and the posterior lobe of the hypophysis. It comprises the supraopticohypophysial, paraventriculohypophysial, and tuberohypophysial tracts. Also *hypothalamohypophysial tract.* **t. iliopubicus** *Outmoded* DEEP CRURAL ARCH. **t. iliotibialis** [NA] The strong thickened band of the fascia lata on the lateral side of the thigh that is split superiorly to receive the insertions of the tensor fasciae latae muscle anteriorly and most of the gluteus maximus muscle posteriorly. Superiorly the superficial layer is attached to the outer lip of the iliac crest, whereas the deep layer extends deep to the tensor fasciae latae and blends with the capsule of the hip joint. Inferiorly the fused layers attach to the lateral condyle of the tibia and join an aponeurosis of the vastus lateralis muscle. Also *iliotibial tract, tractus iliotibialis maissiati* (outmoded), *Maissiat's band, iliotibial band, Maissiat's tract, iliotibial ligament of Maissiat, ligament of Maissiat.* **t. mamillothalamicus** FASCICULUS MAMILLOTHALAMICUS. **t. mesencephalicus nervi trigemini** [NA] A longitudinally oriented bundle of nerve fibers that courses from the rostral pons to the superior colliculus adjacent to the mesencephalic nucleus of the trigeminal nerve in the brainstem. It is composed of the peripheral and central processes of primary sensory trigeminal neurons whose cell bodies lie in the mesencephalic nucleus and that transmit proprioceptive afferent impulses from receptors in striated musculature supplied by the motor division of the trigeminal nerve. Also *radix mesencephalica nervi trigemini, mesencephalic root of trigeminal nerve, radix descendens mesencephalica nervi trigemini, descending root of trigeminal nerve, mesencephalic tract of trigeminal nerve.* **t. occipitopontinus** The part of the tractus corticopontinus that arises in the gyri of the occipital lobes and terminates in the pons. Also *occipitopontile tract, occipitopontine tract.* **t. olfactorius** [NA] A narrow, elongated band of myelinated nerve fibers that projects caudally from the olfactory bulb and contains mainly centrally directed nerve fibers from the mitral and tufted cells in the olfactory bulb. The fibers in this tract convey impulses of the special sense of smell, but the tract also contains some centrifugal fibers coursing back to the olfactory bulb. Posteriorly, the olfactory tract divides into the medial, intermediate, and lateral olfactory striae. Also *olfactory tract, olfactory bundle, precommissural bundle.* **t. olivocerebellaris** [NA] A group of nerve fibers that have their neuronal cell bodies in the inferior olivary nucleus and that for the most part cross the median plane to enter the contralateral inferior cerebellar peduncle, forming the largest component of that peduncle. Olivocerebellar fibers are distributed to all parts of the cerebellar cortex and end as climbing fibers capable of exciting Purkinje cells. Also *olivocerebellar tract, fibrae cerebello-olivares, olivocerebellar fibers.* **t. olivospinalis** [NA] A small triangular bundle of descendingnerve fibers located in the upper cervical segments of the spinal cord near the surface of the lateral funiculus opposite the ventral gray column and immediately lateral to the emerging ventral rootlets. The exact origin and termination of these fibers are unknown, though at one time they were thought to derive from cells in the inferior olivary nucleus and end in the gray matter of the ventral horn. Since the evidence for this is inconclusive, some authors refer to this pathway as the bulbospinal tract, thereby being less specific with respect to the location of the neuronal cell bodies. It is known, however, that this bundle of fibers does contain ascending spino-olivary fibers that terminate in the medial and dorsal olivary nuclei of the medulla oblongata. Also *olivospinal tract, tractus triangularis, triangular tract, Helweg's tract, bulbospinal tract, bundle of Helweg* (seldom used). **t.**

**opticus** [NA] A substantial bundle of myelinated fibers that arises from the posterolateral aspect of the optic chiasma and courses backward and laterally to end in the lateral geniculate body of the metathalamus and the superior colliculus of the midbrain. Each human optic tract contains both uncrossed nerve fibers originating from ganglion neurons in the temporal retinal field of the ipsilateral eye, and crossed nerve fibers originating from the nasal retinal field of the contralateral eye. Also *optic tract, optic lemniscus* (obs.). **t. paraventriculohypophysialis** [NA] A group of nerve fibers arising from neurons in the paraventricular nucleus located in the wall of the third ventricle in the anterior hypothalamus. The fibers in this tract course through the infundibular stalk to terminate in the posterior lobe of the hypophysis, and they transport neurosecretory material that is important in the liberation of both oxytocin and vasopressin, especially oxytocin. Also *paraventriculohypophysial tract.* **t. parietopontinus** The portion of the tractus corticopontinus that arises from the parietal lobe and terminates in the pontine nuclei. Also *parietopontine tract.* **t. pyramidalis** Collectively, the descending corticospinal tract (as the motor pathway to spinal motoneurons) along with the descending corticonuclear tract (as the motor pathway to the cranial nerve nuclei). *Imprecise.* Also *pyramidal tract.* See also TRACTUS CORTICOSPINALIS, FIBRAE PYRAMIDALES MEDULLAE OBLONGATAE. ● Although many of the descending corticospinal fibers do pass through the pyramids in the medulla oblongata (for which the tract has been named), many of the descending corticonuclear fibers terminate in the cranial nerve nuclei above the level of the pyramidal decussation. Hence, use of this term is less accurate than referring to the specific pathways within the so-called pyramidal tract. **t. pyramidalis anterior** TRACTUS CORTICOSPINALIS VENTRALIS. **t. pyramidalis lateralis** TRACTUS CORTICOSPINALIS LATERALIS. **t. reticulospinalis** [NA] Collectively, the medial and lateral reticulospinal tracts. The medial reticulospinal tract arises from neurons in the pontine reticular formation and descends in a diffuse manner in the ipsilateral anterior funiculus of the spinal cord. The lateral reticulospinal tract arises from neurons in the reticular formation of the medulla oblongata, and many of these fibers cross to the opposite side and descend in the contralateral lateral funiculus, medial to the lateral corticospinal tract. Both of these tracts terminate on interneurons of the intermediate gray matter of the ventral horn. Electrical stimulation of the pontine (medial) reticulospinal fibers frequently results in a facilitation of spinal reflexes, whereas stimulation of bulbar (lateral) reticulospinal fibers inhibits spinal reflexes. Also *reticulospinal tract.* **t. rubrospinalis** [NA] A relatively compact bundle of nerve fibers located in the lateral funiculus of the spinal cord ventromedial to the lateral corticospinal tract. These fibers arise from neuronal cell bodies in the red nucleus of the midbrain and subthalamus, decussate to the opposite side and, descending through all spinal levels, terminate in the gray matter of the ventral horn. The tractus rubrospinalis is believed to help modulate the activity of spinal motoneurons. Also *Monakow's tract, prepyramidal tract, rubrospinal tract, Monakow's fibers, fasciculus aberrans of Monakow, von Monakow's fibers, Monakow's fasciculus, Monakow's bundle, extrapyramidal motor fasciculus* (an outmoded and imprecise term). **t. solitarius** [NA] A longitudinally oriented fasciculus ofdescending primary afferent nerve fibers located in the dorsolateral aspect of the lower pons and medulla oblongata. Its fibers, derived from the facial, glossopharyngeal, and vagus nerves, then leave the tractus solitarius to enter the adjacent nucleus of the tractus solitarius, conveying to it special sensory taste impulses from the tongue and palate (facial glossopharyngeal, and vagus), and general visceral afferent impulses from the pharynx, esophagus, and possibly even gastrointestinal organs in the abdomen (vagus). Also *respiratory column* (obs.), *solitary tract of medulla oblongata, funiculus solitarius, solitary fasciculus, solitary bundle, fasciculus rotundus* (seldom used), *respiratory bundle* (obs.). **t. spinalis nervi trigemini** [NA] A longitudinally oriented bundle of nerve fibers that extends from the site of entrance of the sensory root of the trigeminal nerve in the pons to the upper cervical segments of the spinal cord. The nerve fibers in this tract are descending central processes of primary sensory neurons of the trigeminal nerve that have their cell bodies in the trigeminal ganglion. These fibers terminate in the adjacent spinal nucleus of the trigeminal nerve and transmit impulses of pain, temperature, and touch from the peripheral fields of the ophthalmic, maxillary, and mandibular divisions of the trigeminal nerve. Also *spinal tract of trigeminal nerve.* **t. spinocerebellaris anterior** TRACTUS SPINOCEREBELLARIS VENTRALIS. **t. spinocerebellaris dorsalis** [NA] A flattened bundle of nerve fibers situated superficial to the tractus corticospinalis lateralis at the periphery of the posterior part of the lateral funiculus of the spinal cord. It is an ascending tract arising from second–order neurons located in the ipsilateral nucleus thoracicus (Clarke's nucleus) that extends in the lateral gray column of the spinal cord from the seventh cervical to the third lumbar segment. The fibers ascend to the medulla oblongata where they enter the inferior cerebellar peduncle and course to the cerebellum, where they terminate in the pyramis vermis and paramedian lobule. They convey proprioceptive impulses that arise in muscle spindles and tendon organs, and exteroceptive impulses from touch and pressure receptors. Also *tractus spinocerebellaris posterior, posterior spinocerebellar tract, direct spinocerebellar tract, Felchsig's tract, direct cerebellar tract of Flechsig, dorsal spinocerebellar tract, fasciculus cerebellospinalis* (imprecise), *cerebellospinal fasciculus* (imprecise). **t. spinocerebellaris ventralis** [NA] A group of ascending second-order afferent nerve fibers in the ventral aspect of the lateral funiculus of the spinal cord that in cross-section is seen as a crescent-shaped fasciculus at the periphery of the lateral white column, superficial to the lateral spinothalamic tract. The fibers are derived from neurons in the ipsilateral, but most predominantly the contralateral, posterior gray column. They ascend to the upper pons and course along the dorsal surface of the superior cerebellar peduncle to reach the anterior lobe of the cerebellum. The tract conveys proprioceptive impulses concerning movement and posture. Also *anterior spinocerebellar tract, tractus spinocerebellaris anterior, Gowers tract, fasciculus of Gowers, fasciculus anterolateralis superficialis Gowersi, ventral spinocerebellar tract, spinocerebellar tract anterior, column of Gowers, fasciculus ventrolateralis superficialis.* **t. spinotectalis** [NA] A bundle of nerve fibers that arises from neurons in the spinal gray matter, crosses to the contralateral side of the spinal cord, and ascends in the lateral funiculus medial to the ventral spinocerebellar tract. Spinotectal fibers terminate in the superior colliculus located in the tectum of the midbrain, and they participate in spinovisual reactions and reflexes, allowing the body and head to orient appropriately to visual impulses. Also *spinotectal tract.* **t. spinothalamicus anterior** TRACTUS SPINOTHALAMICUS VENTRALIS. **t. spinothalamicus lateralis** [NA] A bundle of nerve fibers located in the lateral funiculus of the spinal cord, medial and slightly ventral to the ventral spinocerebellar tract. The cell bodies of its fibers are located in the contralateral gray column, and the fibers cross the midline in the anterior white commissure before forming the lateral spinothalamic tract. The tract ascends in the brainstem dorsolateral to the olivary nuclei, giving off collateral branches to the reticular formation. It terminates in the nucleus ventralis posterolateralis of the thalamus and conveys impulses of pain and thermal sensibility. Also *lateral spinothalamic tract.* **t. spinothalamicus ventralis** [NA] A bundle of nerve fibers that courses in the most peripheral part of the white matter in the ventral funiculus at a site anterior to the ventral gray column. The cell bodies of these fibers are located in the contralateral gray column, and the fibers cross the midline in the anterior white commissure before assuming their position in the ventral funiculus. The tract, however, also contains some uncrossed fibers. In the ventral funiculus the tract ascends to the thalamus by joining the medial lemniscus in the upper pons, and terminates in the nucleus ventralis posterolateralis of the thalamus, transmitting impulses of light touch. Also *anterior spinothalamic tract, tractus spinothalamicus anterior, ventral spinothalamic tract.* **t. spiralis foraminosus** A spirally rounded area below the transverse crest at the lateral end or fundus of the internal acoustic meatus, perforated by several small orifices through which nerve fibers course from the first $1^1/_2$ turns of the cochlea. Also *foraminous spiral tract.* **t. subarcuatus** A group of small cells stated to be under the arch of the anterior semicircular canal of the internal ear. *Outmoded.* **t. supraopticohypophysialis** [NA] A group of nerve fibers that arises from clusters of neurons positioned over the lateral part of the optic chiasma (the supraoptic nucleus). The fibers course through the infundibular stalk to reach the posterior lobe of the hypophysis, and carry neurosecretory material that is important for the liberation of vasopressin and oxytocin, especially vasopressin. Also *supraopticohypophysial tract.* **t. tectobulbaris** [NA] Descending fibers that arise from neurons in the superior colliculus, cross in the tegmental decussation, and descend through the pons to the medulla oblongata near the tectospinal tract. Fibers of the tractus tectobulbaris terminate in or near the pontine nuclei and certain motor nuclei of the cranial nerves. They participate in reflex movements in response to visual stimulation. Also *tectobulbar tract.* **t. tectospinalis** [NA] A bundle of nerve fibers that arises in the deeper layers of the superior colliculus, crosses the midline in the dorsal tegmental decussation, and descends in the anterior part of the ventral funiculus of the spinal cord near the ventral median fissure. Most of the fibers terminate in the gray matter of the anterior horn in the upper four cervical segments, but some descend to lower cervical spinal levels. Also *Löwenthal's tract, Marchi's tract, predorsal tract, tectospinal tract, predorsal bundle* (obs.). **t. tegmentalis centralis** [NA] A composite bundle of nerve fibers, including the main long ascending tract of the brainstem reticular formation, extending between the medulla oblongata and the thalamus and extending through the pons, midbrain, and subthalamus. It contains descending fibers from nerve cells in the periaqueductal gray substance of the midbrain that project to the inferior olivary complex, and ascending fibers from the reticular formation in the brainstem that project to the thalamus. It occupies a large part of the bulbar tegmentum, but in the midbrain is displaced dorsally so that its fibers are located adjacent to the central gray substance. In the diencephalon it projects through the subthalamus to the intralaminar thalamic nuclei. Also *Bekhterev's tract, central tegmental fasciculus, central tegmental tract, central tegmental bundle, tegmental tract.* **t. temporopontinus** The portion of the tractus corticopontinus that arises in the temporal lobe of the cerebral cortex and terminates in the pontine nuclei. Also *temporopontile tract, Türck's tract, temporopontine tract, Türck's bundle.* **t. triangularis** TRACTUS OLIVOSPINALIS. **t. tuberohypophysialis** A group of nerve fibers that originates from neurons in the infundibular (arcuate) and other adjacent nuclei in the tuberal region of the hypothalamus and terminates in the infundibular stalk of the hypophysis. These neurons are thought to be the sites of production of releasing factors and release-inhibiting factors for hormones produced by the anterior lobe of the hypophysis. Also *tuberoinfundibular tract, tuberohypophysial tract.* **t. vestibulospinalis** [NA] A bundle of descending nerve fibers that originates from neurons in the lateral vestibular nucleus (Deiter's nucleus) and terminates on neurons in the gray matter of the ventral horn in the spinal cord. It courses the entire length of the spinal cord and is located near the surface of the anterior funiculus. Its fibers terminate in every spinal segment, but the cervical and lumbar segments receive the greatest number of vestibulospinal fibers. It is an uncrossed tract, and it conveys to the cord impulses converging on the lateral vestibular nucleus from the vestibular apparatus in the internal ear and from the cerebellum. Also *Deiter's tract, descending vestibular tract, vestibulospinal tract, spinal vestibular root, spinal vestibular tract.*

**tragacanth** \trag′əkanth\ GUM TRAGACANTH. **Indian t.** STERCULIA GUM.

**tragal** \trā′gəl\ Of or relating to the tragus.

**tragi** \trā′jī\ Plural of TRAGUS.

**tragopodia** \trag′əpō′dē·ə\ GENU VALGUM.

**tragus** \trā′gəs\ [L, from Gk *tragos* he-goat; from the hairy nature of the skin of this part of the ear] (*pl.* tragi) [NA] A small posteriorly projecting tag of the auricular cartilage situated below the crus helicis and in front of the concha where it partly covers the opening of the external acoustic meatus. Also *antilobium* (outmoded).

**train** / **t. of four** An assessment of the action of competitive neuromuscular blockers during general anesthesia, where four supramaximal electrical shocks to the ulnar nerve, 0.5 seconds apart, permit comparison of the fourth twitch response in the thumb to the first twitch response. **t. of pulses** A set number of individual stimulus pulses, as 10 or 1000. In testing for fatigue, the repetitive stimulus is usually set for and not left to fire indefinitely. In the conventional test of fatigue, a train of pulses at 30 or 100 Hz and $^1/_3$ sec duration is followed by a rest period of $^2/_3$ sec.

**training** The inculcation of specific responses by means of special procedures devised for guiding behavior. Such responses range from those developed in animal subjects for experimental purposes to the acquisition and sharpening of specific human skills. **assertiveness t.** The combining of behavior therapy and directive psychotherapy in training a subject in the expression of appropriate feelings, both positive and negative. **auditory t.** The teaching of listening and of auditory and speech perceptual skills, usually to those hearing-impaired children or adults who require hearing aids. **habit t.** The teaching of a child, or a regressed patient, the appropriate patterns of personal hygiene and social behavior. **sensitivity t.** An educational-experiential small group technique in which the members meet regularly, usually with a designated leader, to learn about themselves, about interpersonal relationships, about group process, and about larger social systems. The aim is not therapeutic. Sensitivity training focuses instead on increasing relatedness and opening communication channels between each member and the other people within that member's social system. **toilet t.** Training of the child to achieve urinary and fecal continence. It is usually carried out when the child is between one and three years of age.

**trait** [French (from L *tractus*, past part. of *trahere*; see TRACT) a feature, trait] **1** Any distinguishing characteristic, especially a genetically determined one. **2** The state of being heterozygous for an allele that determines a recessive disorder, such as sickle cell trait. **dominant t.** A phenotype expressed in an individual heterozygous for the allele that determines the trait. In strict mendelian terms, the phenotype is the same whether the allele is present in a heterozygous or homozygous state. Also *dominant character*. Compare RECESSIVE TRAIT. **Hageman t.** FACTOR XII DEFICIENCY. **recessive t.** A phenotype expressed in an individual who is homozygous for the allele that determines a trait. Also *recessive character*. Compare DOMINANT TRAIT. **secretor t.** See under SECRETOR. **sickle cell t.** The inherited heterozygous state for hemoglobin S. **single gene t.** MONOGENIC CHARACTER. **thalassemia t.** Inheritance of a gene for any of the thalassemias from one parent only. See also THALASSEMIA MINOR.

**Trambusti** [Arnaldo *Trambusti*, Italian pathologist, born 1863] Trambusti test. See under REACTION.

**trance** [French *transe* (from L *transire* to go or pass over or beyond, be transformed, take no note of, from TRANS- + L *ire* to go) a trance] A sleeplike state, such as stupor or coma, with markedly diminished responsivity to environmental stimulation. **alcoholic t.** A cataleptic condition brought on by overconsumption of alcohol. Doses sufficient to produce coma will impair the circulation because of central nervous system depression and asphyxia. Vital functions are reduced to the lowest level, and the patient ordinarily can only be roused with great difficulty. **hypnotic t.** HYPNOTIC LETHARGY. **induced t.** HYPNOTIC LETHARGY. **somnambulistic t.** SOMNAMBULISM.

**tranquilizer** \trang′kwilī′zər\ [*tranquil* + *iz(e)* + -ER] A calming agent that, unlike a sedative, produces its quieting action without primary interference with consciousness and thinking. **major t.** A tranquilizing drug, such as one of the phenothiazines, that is used in the treatment of psychotic symptoms. **minor t.** A tranquilizing drug used to treat anxiety symptoms and symptoms of psychoneurosis.

**tranquillizer** *Brit.* TRANQUILIZER.

**trans** \trans\ [L, across, through] **1** Having the configuration of being on opposite sides, in chemistry usually referring to two groups on opposite sides of a double bond or of a ring. The groups concerned are often the main chain of the compound. **2** In genetics, having both wild-type alleles of two linked, doubly heterozygous loci on different homologous chromosomes. See also REPULSION. Compare CIS.

**trans-** \trans-, tranz-\ [L *trans* across, through] **1** A prefix meaning through, across, beyond. **2** A stereochemical prefix indicating that two groups of a molecule are in the trans configuration. When used in this sense it is written *trans-*.

**transacetylase** ACETYLTRANSFERASE.

**transacylase** ACYLTRANSFERASE.

**transaldolase** The enzyme (EC 2.2.1.2) that catalyzes the transfer of the glycerone (i.e. dihydroxyacetone) unit from a ketose phosphate to an aldose phosphate. In the pentose phosphate pathway it catalyzes the interconversion of sedoheptulose 7-phosphate and glyceraldehyde 3-phosphate with fructose 6-phosphate and erythrose 4-phosphate. It carries the unit transferred as an imine with the side chain of one of its lysine residues. Protonation of this imine assists in the carbon-carbon bond breakage involved in the reaction.

**transamidation** \-am′idā′shən\ **1** Either of two reactions: R—CO—NH—R′ + R″—COOH → R—COOH + R″—CO—NH—R′, or R—CO—NH—R′ + $NH_2$—R″→ R—Co—NH—R″ + $NH_2$—R′. The latter is important in the cross-linking of fibrin in clot stabilization, in which an amide bond is formed by reaction of a lysine residue in one chain and a glutamine residue in another, with release of ammonia. **2** *Incorrect* TRANSAMINATION.

**transamidinase** AMIDINOTRANSFERASE.

**transaminase** AMINOTRANSFERASE.

**transamination** \-am′inā′shən\ The process of transfer of amino groups. Biologically the most common is the concomitant transfer of an amino group and a hydrogen atom in exchange for the oxygen atom of a carbonyl group. This process is important in the metabolism of amino acids. Also *transamidation* (incorrect).

**transanimation** \-an′imā′shən\ **1** Resuscitation, especially of a newborn that has failed to breathe spontaneously. **2** *Seldom used* MOUTH-TO-MOUTH RESUSCITATION.

**transantral** \-an′trəl\ Going across or through the maxillary sinus: used especially of a surgical approach, as in *transantral ethmoidectomy*.

**transaortic** \-ā·ôr′tik\ Across the aorta: descriptive of an operative procedure that involves an aortotomy to approach intra-aortic lesions.

**transatrial** \-ā′trē·əl\ Across the atrium: used especially in reference to open cardiac surgical procedures that are performed across the left or right atrium.

**transaxonal** \-ak′sənəl\ Through or across axons.

**transcalent** \-kā′lənt\ [TRANS- + L *calens*, gen. *calentis*, pres. part. of *calere* to be warm or hot] Permeable to heat.

**transcarbamoylase** CARBAMOYLTRANSFERASE.

**transcavitary** \-kav′iter′ē\ Moving across a cavity: said of metastasis in the peritoneal or other cavities.

**transcervical** \-sur′vikəl\ Of or relating to any diagnostic or therapeutic procedure performed through the cervical opening of the uterus.

**transcobalamin** \-kōbal′əmin\ The vitamin $B_{12}$-binding proteins of blood plasma. They are glycoproteins of relative molecular mass 60 000.

**transcondylar** \-kän′dilər\ Passing through the condyles of a bone: said especially of a surgical procedure. Also *transcondyloid*.

**transcortical** \-kôr′tikəl\ **1** Passing through the cortex of the cerebrum or cerebellum: used especially of an incision or excision. **2** Pertaining to the connections between areas of the cerebral cortex.

**transcortin** \-kôr′tin\ CORTICOSTEROID-BINDING GLOBULIN.

**transcriptase** \transkrip′tās\ Any enzyme catalyzing transcription, i.e. synthesis of RNA as a copy of a DNA template, or vice versa. It thus includes both DNA-directed RNA polymerase and RNA-directed DNA polymerase. **reverse t.** An enzyme found in viruses of the Retroviridae family. It catalyzes the formation of DNA using an RNA template, and is thus an RNA-dependent DNA polymerase. The name refers to the fact that the enzyme transcribes nucleic acids in the reverse order from the usual DNA-to-RNA transcription. It is used in genetic engineering to produce DNA suitable for introduction into a genome from an isolated species of mRNA.

**transcription** \transkrip′shən\ The process by which a strand of RNA is synthesized with its sequence specified by a complementary strand of DNA, which acts as a template. **complementary t.** A process of transcription involving both strands of the DNA molecule, in which a gene is read in one direction, then later the same segment is read in the opposite direction. This process is known to occur in the lambda phage. **reverse t.** The formation of DNA as a complementary copy of an RNA template. The formation of RNA as a copy of DNA is the common process of transcription. Reverse transcription occurs naturally in the replication of RNA-containing viruses, and the enzyme involved is much used in genetic engineering, to make DNA that can be incorporated into the genome of an organism from isolated mRNA. **symmetric t.** A process of transcription in which both strands of the DNA are used simultaneously as templates.

**transcutaneous** \-kyootā′nē·əs\ PERCUTANEOUS.

**transdermic** \-dur′mik\ PERCUTANEOUS.

**transdetermination** \-ditur′mənā′shən\ An ontogenic process in which primordial or progenitor cells for one tissue develop into another because of the activation or introduction of genes that would normally not have a developmental role at that time.

**transducer** \transd^y oo′sər\ [L *transduc(ere)* (from TRANS- + *ducere* to lead) to lead over, carry over + -ER] A device that converts energy from one form to another. Examples are strain gauge, inductive, capacitive, piezoelectric, and chemical sensors, and thermocouples, thermistors, photocells, microphones, and loudspeakers. **acoustic t.** A device which converts electrical energy to acoustic energy and vice versa. **bone conduction t.** An audiologic instrument which converts electrical activity to mechanical vibrations of the same frequency. When placed on the skull, usually in the mastoid region, acoustic energy is conveyed to the cochlea, stimulating the sense of hearing. The range and intensity of the sound frequencies used is rather less than can be achieved through air conduction audiometry. **electrochemical t.** A transducer in which a change in concentration of a chemical at the input yields a related current or voltage at the output. Examples are transducers to measure pH, partial oxygen pressure, partial carbon dioxide pressure, and metal ions. **electromechanical t.** A transducer that converts electricity to motion, as a loudspeaker, or motion to electricity, as a piezoelectric transducer. **piezoelectric t.** A transducer in which an input force deforms a crystal or ceramic material to produce a proportional electrical charge at the output. **pressure t.** An instrument that senses pressure and converts it to a proportional output voltage. For measuring intravascular blood pressure, a catheter conducts the pressure to a diaphragm, which stretches a strain gauge, forming a Wheatstone bridge. **quarter-wave t.** An ultrasound transducer which has a matching layer in front of the transducer element which is one-quarter wavelength in thickness. This matching layer reduces the reflection of ultrasound at the transducer/skin interface. **rotating t.** An ultrasound transducer assembly which utilizes a group of two to four transducer elements mounted on a rotating wheel. **ultrasound t.** A device which converts electrical energy to ultrasonic energy and vice versa.

**transductant** \-duk′tənt\ A bacterium that has been modified by transduction.

**transduction** \transduk′shən\ [L *transduct(us)*, past part. of *transucere* to lead or bring across + -ION] **1** The transfer of genetic material from a bacteriophage to a bacterium or from one bacterium to another, using a bacteriophage as a vector. **2** The transformation of physical energy by a sense organ, resulting in sense-cell membrane depolarization and axonal impulse generation. **abortive t.** The introduction of a character into a bacterium by a phage, as in transduction, but without incorporation of the phage DNA into the bacterial genome, with the result that only one of the two daughter cells inherits the character. **vestibular t.** The process whereby mechanical distortion of the vestibular end organs in the ampullae and utricle of the inner ear is converted into action potentials in the vestibular nerve.

**transduodenal** \-d^y oo′ədē′nəl\ Through the duodenum.

**transect** \transekt′\ To cut in making a cross section.

**transection** \transek′shən\ CROSS SECTION.

**transethmoidal** \-ethmoi′dəl\ Going across or through the ethmoidal labyrinth: used especially of a surgical approach.

**transfaunation** \-fônā′shən\ The passing or transfer of animal symbionts from one host to another.

**transfection** \-fek′shən\ [TRANS- + *(in)fection*] The process of infecting cells with an RNA tumor virus by the addition of DNA extracted from a cell transformed by that virus. Hypothetically, the provirus DNA is integrated into the DNA of the transformed cell and is able to replicate in the transfected cell.

**transfer** A movement or passage from one place to another. **adoptive t.** An immunologic technique in which specific reactivity to an antigen is conferred upon an animal by the injection of lymphocytes from an immune donor, usually from the same inbred strain. **egg t.** The transfer, using artificial means, of the fertilized ovum of one female to the uterus of another. **embryo t.** The transfer of an embryo from the uterus of one animal to that of another for the purpose of obtaining more offspring with known desirable characteristics provided through the ova of the real parent. **group t.** A chemical reaction in which a group is transferred from one molecule to another, or from one part of a molecule to another. **linear energy t.** For a charged particle, the average energy locally imparted to the medium in traversing a unit distance. Abbr. LET **nuclear t.** In experimental genetics and embryology, the *in vitro* manipulation of an intact nucleus from one cell and transplantation into another cell. It is often the introduction of a nucleus from a differentiated, somatic cell into an unfertilized oocyte, resulting in a zygote. **passive t.** The conferring of immunity to a nonimmune host by the injection of antibody or lymphocytes from an immune or sensitized donor. **phosphate-group t.** The process of transfer of the phospho group, —$PO_3H_2$ and its ionized forms, as from an alkyl phosphate to an alcohol, forming a new alcohol and a new alkyl phosphate. ATP is a donor in many biologic phosphate transfers. **placental t.** The passage of gases or fluids via the placenta from the maternal to the fetal circulation. **temporalis t.** An operation in which the temporal muscle (musculus temporalis) or a part of it is used to replace the functioning of paralyzed facial muscles.

**transferase** \trans′fərās\ Any of the class of enzymes capable of catalyzing the transfer of an atom or group from one molecule to another.

**transference** \transfur′əns\ In psychotherapy, the projection of libidinal or aggressive feelings, thoughts, and wishes onto the analyst, not because of the analyst's actual attitudes or appearance, but because of the patient's unconscious need to relive past experiences and to endow the analyst with the same magical powers and omniscience which he attributed to his parents in childhood. **institutional t.** The development of emotional dependence upon a facility such as the hospital or clinic to which one goes for treatment.

**transferrin** \-fer′in\ A plasma protein that reversibly binds iron and transports it to cells. It is a beta-globulin of approximate MW 80 000. Each molecule of transferrin may bind 0, 1, or 2 atoms of Fe(III) together with bicarbonate. The protein portion of transferrin is called apotransferrin.

**transfix** \-fiks′\ To pierce completely.

**transfixion** \-fik′shən\ **1** A surgical procedure in which tissue is incised from within, moving in an outward direction. **2** The surgical placement of a transfixion suture.

**transformation** 1 The change of a cell from the normal state to the malignant state. 2 In microbiology or cell biology, the entry and incorporation of naked DNA. 3 In statistics, the substitution for purposes of data analysis of a related value for an observed value, for example, square root of $X$ or log $X$ for $X$. **antigenic t.** A modification in the antigenic properties of a cell, due to the addition, modification, or deletion of antigenically active components from the cell surface. **bacterial t.** A hereditary change in a bacterium resulting from the uptake of DNA from another source. The phenomenon was discovered as a transformation of pneumococcal type, with heat-killed organisms as the donor, and was subsequently traced to DNA transfer. **blast t.** LYMPHOCYTE TRANSFORMATION. **Bliss t.** BLISS METHOD. **globular-fibrous t.** The alteration of actin from its globular to its filamentous form by association of the subunits into long chains. Also *G-F transformation.* **lymphocyte t.** The functional and morphologic changes that T or B lymphocytes undergo when activated by contact with a suitable antigen or mitogen. Transformation of lymphocytes in culture is assessed by measuring incorporation of radiolabeled thymidine, an indicator of DNA synthesis. Morphologic changes, seen *in vivo* as well as *in vitro*, include increase in overall cell size and increase in nuclear size with decrease of chromatin density. Also *lymphoblast transformation, blast transformation.* **membranous t.** The development of irregular projections of material resembling glomerular basement membrane into the external surface of the membrane. They may be separated by subepithelial or intramembranous deposits.

**transformer** A device, usually consisting of two insulated coils wound on an iron core, used to transfer electrical energy from one circuit to another, usually with a change in voltage. **filament t.** A step-down transformer used to supply current to heat the filament of an electronic tube or an x-ray tube. **resonance t.** A type of high voltage transformer used in some x-ray generators, in which the secondary winding is designed to resonate at the supply frequency. Thus, the core can be made smaller than that required for a conventional transformer. Also *resonant transformer.* **step-down t.** A transformer in which the secondary or outgoing voltage is less than the primary or incoming voltage. **step-up t.** A transformer in which the secondary or outgoing voltage is greater than the primary or incoming voltage.

**transformiminase** FORMIMINOTRANSFERASE.

**transfuse** \-fyooz′\ 1 To administer a transfusion of (blood or other fluid). 2 To administer a transfusion to (a recipient).

**transfusion** [L *transfusio* (from *transfundere* to pour from one vessel into another, from TRANS- + L *fundere* to shed, pour) a pouring over, transfusion] The transfer of blood or blood products from one individual to another. **arterial t.** A transfusion of blood or other fluid directly into an artery of the recipient. Also *intra-arterial transfusion.* **bone marrow t.** The transfusion of donor hemopoietic cells directly into the medullary cavity of a recipient. **direct t.** Transfer of blood from a donor directly to another individual by means of interconnecting cannula and tubing, with or without an intermediate receptacle and the use of anticoagulants. Also *immediate transfusion.* **drip t.** Slow transfusion of blood, appropriately prepared and conversed, by means of a container and intravenous apparatus. **exchange t.** The replacement of a patient's blood by donor blood, performed by repeated removal of the recipient's blood and transfusion of donor blood until most or all of the patient's blood has been replaced. The procedure has been most widely used in the treatment of newborns with Rh-incompatibility isoimmune hemolytic anemia (erythroblastosis fetalis). Also *exsanguination transfusion, replacement transfusion, substitution transfusion.* **fetomaternal t.** Passage of fetal blood via the placenta into the maternal circulation. The process usually occurs at the time of placental delivery. **granulocyte t.** LEUKOTHERAPY. **immediate t.** DIRECT TRANSFUSION. **indirect t.** Transfusion of blood that has been collected from a donor, treated appropriately, and stored in a container for subsequent use. Also *mediate transfusion.* **intra-arterial t.** ARTERIAL TRANSFUSION. **leukocyte t.** The intravenous infusion of leukocytes, especially granulocytes. **mediate t.** INDIRECT TRANSFUSIÓN. **placental t.** Passage of the blood contained in the placenta via the umbilical vasculature to an infant just after delivery. **replacement t.** EXCHANGE TRANSFUSION. **sternal t.** Transfusion of blood directly into the sternal bone marrow. **substitution t.** EXCHANGE TRANSFUSION.

**transfusional** \-fyoo′zhənəl\ Relating to or caused by transfusion.

**transgenic** \-jen′ik\ Of or pertaining to two different genomes, especially with respect to a DNA sequence from one genome introduced into another.

**transhemophilin** \-hē′məfil′in\ FACTOR VIIIR:AG.

**transhiatal** \-hī·ā′təl\ Through or across an opening or gap that has been either naturally acquired or surgically created.

**transhydrogenase** The enzyme that transfers hydrogen between NADH and $NADP^+$.

**transient** \tran′shənt, tran′zē·ənt\ 1 Passing quickly: said of an episode or attack of a disease. 2 Nonresident; not deeply entrenched: said of certain parasites or bacterial flora. 3 A heart sound of brief duration, such as a snap or click.

**transilient** \transil′ē·ənt\ Passing across: used especially of association fibers traversing nonadjacent convolutions of the cerebral cortex. *Seldom used.*

**transistor** \tranzis′tər\ A semiconducting device having three or more terminals and usually made of silicon. It is used for electronic amplifying and switching circuits. **field-effect t.** A voltage-controlled transistor having an extremely high input resistance.

**transition** \tranzish′ən\ Passage from one stage or condition to another. **cervicothoracic t.** The junctional zone of a throughgoing structure as it traverses the anatomical boundary between the cervical and thoracic regions of the body, such as the cervicothoracic transition of the spinal cord, which is characterized by a narrowing in the diameter of the cord in the thoracic region, compared to that in the lower cervical region. **forbidden t.** A transition between two states of a quantum-mechanical system in which the change in the spin and quantum number is forbidden by certain selection rules. Such transitions occur because the selection rules apply only to simple situations, e.g., absence of surrounding molecules, but they may occur with a frequency reduced in comparison with transitions not so forbidden. **isomeric t.** A process by which an atomic nucleus in an excited state falls toward, or into, its ground state, with no change in the mass number or the atomic number. The excess energy is released by gamma emission or internal conversion. The gamma radiation often produced by radioactive decay occurs because a daughter nucleus, initially in an excited state, proceeds toward ground state by isomeric transition. Also *isomeric level decay.*

**transitional** \tranzish′ənəl\ Passing from one stage or condition to another.

**transitozoonosis** \tran′sitōzō′ənō′sis\ A zoonosis passed to animals or humans during migratory movements, as in the brief exposure of cattle to trypanosomiasis during transit through tsetse fly belts in Africa.

**transketolase** The enzyme (EC 2.2.1.1) that catalyzes the transfer of a unit of glycolaldehyde, CHO—$CH_2OH$, from a ketose phosphate donor to an aldose phosphate acceptor. Metabolically, sedoheptulose 7-phosphate, fructose 6-phosphate, and xylulose 5-phosphate serve as donors, and ribose 5-phosphate, erythrose 4-phosphate, and glyceraldehyde 3-phosphate as acceptors. The enzyme is important in the pentose phosphate pathway and in the Calvin cycle of photosynthesis. The enzyme contains thiamin diphosphate, which carries the unit transferred as a 1,2-dihydroxyethyl group.

**translateral** \-lat′ərəl\ [TRANS- + LATERAL] In radiology, describing the view obtained by a horizontal radiation beam with the patient prone or supine.

**translation** [L *translatio* (from *translatus,* past part. of *transferre* to carry or bring over or across) a transferring] **1** The process of forming a specific protein having its amino acid sequence determined by the codons of messenger RNA. The ribosome and transfer RNA are necessary for translation. **2** Orthodontic movement of a tooth without change in inclination. **nick t.** In genetics, a process for inserting radio-labeled nucleotides into DNA using the enzyme DNA polymerase I.

**translocase** \-lō′kās\ A protein that forms a complex with GTP and the ribosome. It assists in the movement of a molecule of tRNA from its entrance (A-site) to the site where it donates its amino acid to the growing polypeptide chain (P-site). Also *transfer factor II.*

**translocation** \trans′lōkā′shən\ [TRANS- + L *loc(are)* to place, dispose (from *locus* a place) + -ATION] **1** Any chromosome rearrangement involving a shift of one or more cytologically distinct segments within the chromosome complement. It can be intra- or interchromosomal, balanced or unbalanced, reciprocal or nonreciprocal. **2** The rearrangement of a nucleotide sequence from its usual location to another in the genome. **3** In cell biology, the incorporation of a protein into, or transport across, a particular membrane. **balanced t.** Any translocation in which either no apparent loss of chromatin, or loss only of short arms of acrocentric chromosomes, occurs. Such aberrations theoretically have no effect on phenotype, but result in partial aneuploidy in a proportion of gametes. **group t.** A transport system by which entry of sugars into a prokaryotic cell is accompanied by phosphorylation of the sugar, the phosphate donor being phosphoenolpyruvate. **insertional t.** The rearrangement of one chromosome segment to a new location anywhere between the telomeres of a chromosome that is usually nonhomologous. **nonreciprocal t.** A chromosome rearrangement involving one chromosome only. **reciprocal t.** A chromosome rearrangement involving the interchange of distinct chromosome segments. **robertsonian t.** A chromosome rearrangement in which the centromeres of two acrocentric chromosomes fuse, resulting in a larger metacentric or submetacentric chromosome and usually the loss of the short arms of the acrocentrics. **unbalanced t.** Any translocation involving loss of chromatin, excepting loss of the short arms of acrocentric chromosomes. Such a translocation usually has a deleterious effect on the phenotype.

**translucent** \-loo′sənt\ *Seldom used* RADIOLUCENT.

**transluminal** \-loo′minəl\ Through or by way of the lumen, especially that of a blood vessel.

**transmeatal** \-mē·ā′təl\ Going across or through the meatus, for example the external auditory meatus. Also *permeatal.*

**transmethylase** METHYLTRANSFERASE.

**transmethylation** \-meth′ilā′shən\ The process of transfer of methyl groups. Biologically the donor is usually *S*-adenosylmethionine. Being a sulfonium salt, its methyl group is subject to nucleophilic attack, because it is on a good leaving group, and so is easily transferred.

**transmigration** \trans′mīgrā′shən\ [Late L *transmigratio* (from L *transmigratus,* past part. of *transmigrare* to move to another dwelling place, from TRANS- + L *migrare* to quit, move) a moving to another dwelling place] A movement to an opposite position, as across the body. **external t.** Transference of an ovum from the ovary on one side of the body to the uterine tube or horn of the opposite side, usually across the peritoneal cavity, but not via the uterus. **internal t.** Transference of an ovum from one uterine horn to that of the other side by passage through the common uterine chamber. It occurs in many mammalian species but with varying frequency. Also *ovular transmigration.*

**transmissibility** \-mis′ibil′itē\ The capability of being transmitted, as from one host to another or from one site to another: used especially with reference to diseases and infections.

**transmissible** \-mis′ibəl\ Capable of being transmitted, as from one host or site to another host or site: said especially of diseases and infections.

**transmission** [L *transmissio* (from *transmittere* to send over, from TRANS- + L *mittere* to send) a passing over, passage] **1** INHERITANCE. **2** In genetics, any passage of genetic information, either through inheritance or between organisms or cells through transformation, transfection, or transduction. **3** The physiologic process by which a nerve impulse passes across the synapse. **4** The passage of the agents of disease from one organism to another. **arthropod t.** The transmission of a parasite from one host to another by means of an insect or other arthropod vector. **cochlear t.** The process whereby acoustic energy is transmitted from the stapes footplate to the hair cells of the organ of Corti. **cyclical t.** Transmission of a parasite after a cycle of development within the host has been completed. **direct t.** **1** Transmission of an infectious agent directly from one host to another, as by direct contact. **2** Transmission of an agent from one host to another immediately following its acquisition by the first host, without an interval during which the organism undergoes a cycle of development in the first host, as in the mechanical transmission of African trypanosomes by bloodsucking horseflies in which no cyclical development can occur. **duplex t.** Simultaneous transmission of nerve impulses in opposite directions along a nerve fiber. **ephaptic t.** The passage of information from one axon to another via an ephapse or false synapse, as by direct physical contact between demyelinated axons. **hereditary arthropod t.** Transmission of the agents of an infection from one generation of the arthropod vector to another, as, for example, the rickettsiae of Rocky Mountain spotted fever in ticks. **horizontal t.** Transmission of disease or infection by direct contact with an infected individual, or by contact with infected excreta. **humoral t.** Transmission of a nervous impulse across a synapse through the release from the nerve ending of a chemical transmitter followed by its combination with a receptor. Also *neurohumoral transmission.* **insect t.** See under ARTHROPOD TRANSMISSION. **neurohumoral t.** HUMORAL TRANSMISSION. **placental t.** Passage of substances, disease, toxins, antigens, antibodies, drugs and their derivatives, products, or breakdown molecules, across the placenta from mother to fetus or vice versa. **synaptic t.** Propagation of an electrical impulse or chemical substance from one neural element to another or to muscle across the junctional specialization constituting a synapse. **vertical t.** The direct passage of any phenotype or disease from a parent to an offspring, regardless of method, such as genetic inheritance, transplacental migration, or perinatal infection.

**transmittance** \-mit′əns\ The ratio of the transmitted to the incident radiation.

**transmitter** A substance whose diffusion excites a cell such as a neuron.

**transmural** \-myoo′rəl\ [TRANS- + L *mur(us)* a wall + -AL] Extending through the full thickness of a wall or across a wall.

**transmutation** \-myootā′shən\ The process of transforming one nuclide into another, typically involving a change of the proton number, nuclear charge, and often of the neutron number as well. This usually takes place through natural radioactive decay, but nuclear reactions also produce such changes through collisions between the nuclei and high-speed particles. Also *conversion*.

**transonic** \transän′ik\ [*tran(s)-* + SONIC] **1** Traveling at a speed approximately equal to that of sound. **2** Pertaining to conditions encountered in the passage from subsonic to supersonic speed.

**transorbital** \-ôr′bitəl\ Indicating extent across the orbital space.

**transovarial** \-ōver′ē·əl\ By way of the ovary: said chiefly of infections that may be transmitted from a female host to eggs in her ovary and thus to her offspring, as in the case of certain viral and rickettsial infections in mites and ticks. Also *transovarian*.

**transpalatal** \-pal′ətəl\ Going through the palate: used especially of a surgical approach.

**transparietal** \-pərī′ətəl\ Passing through or across the wall of a cavity.

**transpeptidation** \-pep′tidā′shən\ A reaction in which an aminoacyl group is transferred from one amino group to another and in which both donor and product are peptides. The process is involved in the biosynthesis of some peptides, but not in that of proteins.

**transphosphorylation** The process of transfer of a phospho group.

**transpiration** \tran′spərā′shən\ INSENSIBLE SWEATING. **pulmonary t.** The passage of water through the epithelium of the lungs and formation of water vapor in the respiratory airways.

**transpire** \transpī′r\ [*tran(s)-* + L *spir(are)* to breathe, blow] To experience insensible sweating.

**transplacental** \-pləsen′təl\ Across or through the placenta.

**transplant** [TRANS- + PLANT] **1** To transfer, as tissue, from one site to another; graft. **2** That which is transplanted, as tissue or an organ. **cadaver kidney t.** A kidney transplanted from a donor who has suffered brain death. Cadaver kidney transplants are not as successful as transplants from living donors who are related to the recipient and whose blood and tissue types are matched. Nevertheless, in many major centers, the five-year kidney survival rates with cadaver kidneys are great enough to offer a reasonable alternative to chronic dialysis in the treatment of end-stage renal disease.

**transplantar** \-plan′tər\ Extending across the sole of the foot.

**transplantation** **1** The grafting of tissue from one person to another (homograft) or from one site to another on the same person (autograft). **2** The placing of an extracted tooth or tooth germ into a different socket. It may be autogenous if in the same individual or homogenous if to another human. **corneal t.** KERATOPLASTY. **heart t.** The insertion of a healthy heart into a recipient with an inadequately functioning heart. It is usually placed orthotopically, but occasionally it is positioned heterotopically as a cardiac assist mechanism. **heterotopic t.** HETEROTOPIC GRAFT. **homotopic t.** ORTHOTOPIC GRAFT. **orthotopic t.** ORTHOTOPIC GRAFT. **pancreatic t.** An experimental technique for the maintenance therapy of patients with diabetes mellitus, consisting of one of several techniques for implanting heterologous cells isolated from the islets of Langerhans into the body. Present methods do not yet permit its use in the management of human disease. **pancreaticoduodenal t.** Implantation of a homograft, comprising pancreas and duodenum, for the treatment of unstable juvenile diabetes mellitus. The procedure is technically practical, but its usefulness is limited by graft rejection. **renal t.** Transplantation of a kidney from a living donor or a cadaver to a recipient with end-stage renal disease. A kidney transplant from an identical twin is usually very successful. Kidney transplants from other living related donors, especially siblings who are good matches as to blood and tissue types, are reasonably successful but require immunosuppressive therapy after transplantation. Cadaver renal transplants are the least successful, but still are acceptable as an alternative to chronic dialysis for the maintenance of life in end-stage renal disease. **tendon t.** An operation whereby a tendon is altered in its action, either by changing the point of insertion or rerouting its line of pull. Such a procedure is carried out in neuromuscular diseases when a sound musculotendinous unit replaces a weaker one.

**transpleural** \-plʊr′əl\ Across the pleura.

**transport** Movement from one location to another, as of molecules across a membrane or of substances carried in the blood. **active t.** The movement of a particle across a cellular membrane by a process which required energy and involves transport against concentration or electrical gradients. Compare PASSIVE TRANSPORT. **active renal tubular t.** The excretion or resorption of solute by renal tubular cells by a process which requires energy and involves transport against concentration or electrical gradients. **bulk t.** Movement across the cell membrane of particles that are too large to pass through channels or pores in the

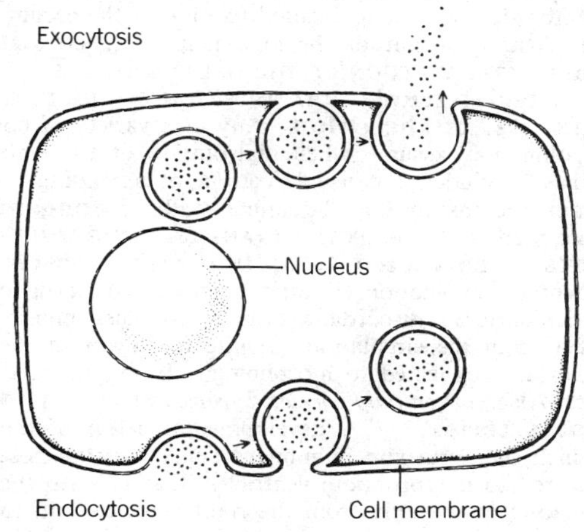


**Bulk transport**

membrane. The movement may be either into the cell (endocytosis) or out of the cell (exocytosis). **competitive t.** A transport system in which one or more substances are transferred across a cellular membrane by the same carrier molecule. The substances are said to compete for a site on the carrier because when one molecule is being transferred the others are not able to interact with the common carrier. **competitive renal tubular t.** The excretion of resorption of two or more solutes by the same transport system in renal tubular cells. **membrane t.** The process of transport of a substance across a membrane. Biologically many such processes occur at specific sites, and may be driven against a concentration gradient by coupling with the transport of another substance down its concentration gradient in the same direction or the one opposite to that of the substance transported. Alternatively, the transport may be coupled with ATP or phosphoenolpyruvate hydrolysis. **ovum t.** The passage of an ovum after ovulation into and through the oviduct until fertilization or disintegration occurs. **passive t.** The transport of a particle across a cellular membrane by a process which involves downhill movement along a pressure, concentration, or electrical gradient. Compare ACTIVE TRANSPORT. **tubal t.** The passage of spermatozoa and ova through the oviduct.

**transposase** \trans′pōsās′\ A class of enzymes that catalyzes the transposition of oligonucleotides from one site in the genome to another.

**transpose** \-pōz′\ 1 To subject to transposition. 2 To position teeth out of normal sequence in the dental arch.

**transposition** \trans′pəzish′ən\ [TRANS- + POSITION] 1 The condition of reversing or being reversed in place or order. 2 The development of an asymmetrical organ or part in the contralateral position. 3 The surgical alteration of the position of a bodily structure, such as a nerve. 4 In genetics, the movement of genetic information, in the form of oligonucleotides, between sites in the genome. **t. of affect** In psychiatry, the displacement of the affective accompaniment of an idea onto another seemingly unrelated idea, frequently seen in obsessive-compulsive and depressive disorders. **t. of the aorta** A developmental defect of the heart in which the origin of the aorta is at the right ventricle instead of its normal position at the left ventricle. • See note at TRANSPOSITION OF THE GREAT ARTERIES. **t. of the appendix** Any of several aberrant positions in which the vermiform appendix may be found when malrotation of the embryonic gut has prevented fixation of the cecum in the lower right quadrant of the abdomen. **t. of arterial stems** TRANSPOSITION OF THE GREAT ARTERIES. **t. of the arterial trunk** TRANSPOSITION OF THE GREAT ARTERIES. **t. of the colon** Any of a variety of positions the colon may assume when malrotation of the embryonic gut has precluded the usual fixation of ascending and descending colons to the abdominal wall. **congenitally corrected t.** CORRECTED TRANSPOSITION OF THE GREAT VESSELS. **corrected t. of the great vessels** The segmental combination of atrioventricular discordance and ventriculoarterial discordance which produces physiological correction of the circulations despite the fact that the great arteries are connected to morphologically inappropriate ventricles. Also *congenitally corrected transposition.* **t. of the great arteries** 1 A developmental defect of the heart in which the aorta and pulmonary trunk are transposed and connected to inappropriate ventricles, that is, with the aorta originating abnormally from the right ventricle and the pulmonary trunk from the left. Also *transposition of arterial stems, transposition of the arterial trunk, transposition of the great vessels* (imprecise). 2 Any anomaly in which the aorta is anterior to the crista supraventricularis or its remnant. • The term is ambiguous because both senses are in use. Def. 2, the older meaning, was in fact clinically associated with the condition described in def. 1, but in 1971 it was shown that the aorta could be posterior to the crista, whereupon def. 1 became the more common meaning, though it is not accepted by all. To avoid ambiguity, it is probably better to refer to the condition described in def. 1 as *ventriculoarterial discordance.* **t. of the great vessels** *Imprecise* TRANSPOSITION OF THE GREAT ARTERIES. **t. of the intestine** Situs inversus of the gastrointestinal tract. **t. of the pulmonary veins** The termination of one or more pulmonary veins at any site other than the left atrium. The most frequent sites of abnormal termination are the right atrium and the inferior vena cava. **t. of the stomach** Situs inversus of the stomach.

**transposon** \-pō′zän\ A transposable element of bacterial DNA that contains a readily detectable gene, often for drug resistance.

**transsacral** \-sā′krəl\ Across or through the sacrum: said of an approach to the structures on the inner surface of the sacrum from the posterior aspect.

**transscleral** \-sklir′əl, skler′əl\ Traversing the sclera of the eye.

**transsection** \-sek′shən\ CROSS SECTION.

**transsexual** \-sek′shoo·əl\ [TRANS- + SEXUAL] 1 Relating to or characterized by transsexualism. 2 A transsexual person.

**transsexualism** \-sek′shoo·əlizm\ [TRANS- + SEXUAL + -ISM] A condition in which one's anatomic sex is the opposite of one's gender role and sexual identity, typically with the accompanying feeling that one is in the wrong body and that the only solution is to have a sex reassignment operation (transsexual surgery).

**transsphenoidal** \-sfinoi′dəl\ Going by way of the sphenoidal sinus: usually said of the surgical approach to the hypophysial fossa.

**transsynaptic** \-sinap′tik\ Occurring across a synapse.

**transtadial** \transtā′dē·əl\ [*tran(s)-* + *stadi(um)* + -AL] From one stage to another; pertaining to transmission through more than one stage.

**transtemporal** \-tem′pərəl\ 1 Passing through the temple: used especially of a procedure requiring a temporal craniotomy. 2 Traversing the temporal lobe: used especially of a surgical procedure.

**transtentorial** \-tentôr′ē·əl\ Traversing the tentorium cerebelli: used especially of a surgical procedure.

**transthalamic** \-thalam′ik\ Passing through or crossing the thalamus.

**transthoracic** \-thôras′ik\ 1 Across the thoracic wall. 2 Through the thoracic cavity.

**transthyretin** The protein in blood serum that binds both thyroxine and retinol-binding protein. Also *prealbumin* (obs.), *thyroxine-binding protein.*

**transtracheal** \-trā′kē·əl\ Across the tracheal wall.

**transtrusion** \-troo′zhən\ [TRANS- + TRUSION] The lateral movement of the mandibular condyle during mastication.

**transtympanic** \-timpan′ik\ Going across or through the tympanic cavity: used especially of a surgical approach, for instance to the stapes.

**transudate** \trans′yədāt\ [*tran(s)-* + L *sud(are)* to sweat + -ATE] A liquid which has passed through a membrane or has been extruded by a tissue. In contrast to an exudate, a transudate has high fluidity, low protein content, and few or no cells or solid matter other than soluble salts. Examples of transudates are pleural fluid in patients with heart failure and ascitic fluid in patients with liver cirrhosis. **pleural t.** Fluid which has accumulated in the pleura by transudation through the pleural membrane.

**transuranic** \-yooran′ik\ Referring to any of the elements of atomic number greater than 92, the atomic number of uranium. They are all radioactive, with relatively short half-lives and thus do not exist naturally, but may be obtained from nuclear fission or by bombardment of other heavy elements. Also *transuranian.*

**transureteroureterostomy** \-yoorē′tərōyoorē′tə-räs′təmē\ Surgical connection of one ureter to the other to divert the passage of urine around an obstruction.

**transurethral** \-yoorē′thrəl\ Performed by way of the urethra: said of a surgical procedure.

**transvaginal** \-vaj′ənəl\ Performed through the vagina.

**transvaterian** \-vəter′ē·ən\ Across the ampulla of Vater.

**transvector** \-vek′tər\ An animal capable of transmitting a poison or other toxic substance originating from a source outside its own body. Bivalve mollusks, for example, are transvectors of the dinoflagellates and certain algae, as in the red tide, that are toxic to fish and other aquatic life and harmful to man.

**transvenous** \-vē′nəs\ Conveyed through the venous circulation or inserted by way of a vein or veins; pervenous.

**transversalis** \-vərsā′lis\ Transverse.

**transverse** Passing across the longitudinal axis of a body, an organ, or a structure; crosswise.

**transversectomy** \-vərsek′təmē\ [*transvers(e process)* + -ECTOMY] Excision of the vertebral transverse process.

**transversion** \-vur′zhən\ [*transvers(e)* + -ION] **1** The eruption of a tooth in an abnormal position. **2** In genetics, a mutation that substitutes a purine for a pyrimidine, or vice versa.

**transversocostal** \-vur′səkäs′təl\ COSTOTRANSVERSE.

**transvesical** \-ves′ikəl\ Passing through the bladder: used especially of an operation performed through a suprapubic cystostomy in order to gain access to a distal ureteral stone, neoplasm, or congenital anomaly of the urinary tract.

**transvestism** \-ves′tizm\ [TRANS- + L *vest(ire)* (from *vestis* a garment, clothes) to clothe, dress + -ISM] A condition characterized by dressing in the clothes of the opposite sex, particularly for sexual gratification. Also *transvestitism, cross-dressing, cross dressing.*

**transvestite** \-ves′tīt\ A person who practices transvestism.

**transvestitism** \-ves′titizm\ TRANSVESTISM.

**Trantas** [Alexios *Trantas,* Greek ophthalmologist, 1867–1960] Trantas dots. See under DOT.

**tranylcypromine sulfate** $C_{18}H_{24}N_2O_4S$. *trans*-(+)-2-Phenylcyclopropanamine sulfate. A monoamine oxidase inhibitor used as an antidepressant agent. It is given orally.

**trapeziform** \trəpē′zifôrm\ TRAPEZOID.

**trapezium** \trəpē′zē·əm\ [New L (from Gk *trapezion* a small table, irregular four-sided figure; dim. of *trapeza* table)] OS TRAPEZIUM.

**trapezoid** \trap′əzoid\ **1** A quadrilateral of which only two sides are parallel. **2** Resembling a quadrilateral with only two parallel sides. Also *trapeziform.* **3** OS TRAPEZOIDEUM. **4** CORPUS TRAPEZOIDEUM.

**Traube** [Ludwig *Traube,* German physician and pathologist, 1818–1876] **1** See under SIGN, SPACE. **2** Traube's murmur. See under GALLOP RHYTHM.

**traum-** \trôm-, troum-\ TRAUMATO-.

**trauma** \trou′mə, trô′mə\ [Gk (akin to *titrōskein* to wound, hurt) a wound, hurt] **1** An injury to the body, especially one resulting from an external force. **2** A psychological shock, especially one having a lasting effect on the personality. **acoustic t.** The damage caused to the cochlear structures by high-intensity acoustic stimulation and having demonstrable effects on hearing, sometimes temporary in the initial stages, but resulting in permanent threshold shift on continued exposure to noise. Also *auditory trauma.* **occlusal t.** Injury to the periodontium caused by occlusal forces transmitted through a tooth. Also *periodontal trauma, occlusal traumatism, periodontal traumatism.* **perinatal t.** Physical injury to the fetus occurring at or about the time of birth: used especially of cerebral birth trauma. **periodontal t.** OCCLUSAL TRAUMA. **primary occlusal t.** Injury to the periodontium from excessive occlusal stress to a tooth or teeth with normal supporting structures. **psychic t.** Trauma of a psychologic nature rather than a physical one, or stress resulting from fantasied or other nonphysical threats. **secondary occlusal t.** Periodontal injury from occlusal stresses on a tooth or teeth already affected by plaque-associated periodontal disease. It may cause an acceleration of the destruction process.

**traumat-** \trômat-, troumat-\ TRAUMATO-.

**traumata** \trô′mətə, trou′mətə\ Plural of TRAUMA.

**traumatic** \trô′matik\ [Gk *traumatikos* (from *trauma* a wound) relating to wounds] Of or resulting from trauma; relating to or causing physical injury or psychological shock.

**traumatism** \trou′mətizm, trô′-\ [TRAUMAT- + -ISM] The physical or psychologic state resulting from trauma. Also *traumatosis* (seldom used). **occlusal t.** OCCLUSAL TRAUMA. **periodontal t.** OCCLUSAL TRAUMA.

**traumatize** \trô′mətīz\ [Gk *traumatizein* (from *trauma* injury) to injure] To cause trauma or traumatism in.

**traumato-** \trô′mətō-, trou′mətō-\ [Gk *trauma,* gen. *traumatos* a wound, injury] A combining form meaning trauma, injury. Also *traum-, traumat-.*

**traumatogenic** \trô′mətōjen′ik\ [TRAUMATO- + -GENIC] **1** Capable of causing an injury. **2** Caused by a wound or injury.

**traumatologist** \trô′mətäl′əjist\ A person specializing in traumatology.

**traumatology** \trô′mətäl′əjē\ [TRAUMATO- + -LOGY] The study of the medical and social aspects of trauma.

**traumatosis** \trô′mətō′sis\ [TRAUMAT- + -OSIS] *Seldom used* TRAUMATISM.

**Trautmann** [Moritz Ferdinand *Trautmann,* German surgeon, 1832–1902] See under TRIANGLE.

**Travase** An enzymatic preparation that attacks dead tissue while sparing living tissue. It is used in the débridement of burns. A proprietary name.

**tray** A flat utensil with raised edges, used for conveying or holding for ready access various articles. **impression t.** A device, more or less conforming to the shape of the dental arch, used to support the plastic material when making an impression.

**TRBF** total renal blood flow.

**Treacher Collins** [Edward *Treacher Collins,* English ophthalmologist, 1862–1919] Treacher Collins-Franceschetti syndrome, Treacher Collins syndrome. See under MANDIBULOFACIAL DYSOSTOSIS.

**treat** [Old French *traitier* (from L *tractare* to drag, handle, treat, from *trahere* to draw away, drag, prolong) to treat, handle] **1** To provide with medical or surgical care. **2** To apply remedies to, as a disease.

# treatment

**treatment** [TREAT + -MENT] An action or program of action directed to the care of a patient for the restoration of health or the improvement or stabilization of function. Such measures, usually prescribed by a medical practitioner, are designed most often to counteract disease or stimulate healing. **ambulatory insulin t.** HYPOGLYCEMIC THERAPY. **Ascoli t.** A treatment formerly used for malaria, in which successive injections of epinephrine caused contractions of the spleen, thereby forcing malarial parasites into the body circulation. **Bier's t.** Passive hyperemia induced by the use of a loose tourniquet; an obsolete treatment for joint and extremity inflammation. Also *Bier's passive hyperemia*. **Brandt t.** Bimanual palpation and massage of the adnexa for the purpose of expressing pus from a pyosalpinx. **Brown-Séquard t.** ORGANOTHERAPY. **Calot's t.** The correction of tuberculous kyphosis by inserting pads under a plaster jacket through an opening in the jacket. **Castellani's t.** A treatment for elephantiasis involving bed rest, tight bandaging, and daily fibrinolysin injections. **Chervin's t.** A technique for the treatment of stuttering, based on the speaking of various sound sequences by the subject. Also *Chervin's method*. **closed t. of burns** The treatment of burns with the use of topical antimicrobial agents applied to the burn under surgical dressings. **closed-plaster t.** The application of a circumferential plaster immobilization dressing to an extremity following nonsurgical reduction of a musculoskeletal injury. **cold t. of burns** The initial treatment of thermal burns by contact with cold or cool water in an attempt to limit the amount of tissue destruction. Although useful immediately following the burn, if such treatment is delayed by more than a few minutes its effectiveness is questionable. **conservative t.** Treatment designed to restore relatively satisfactory health or function while avoiding radical therapeutic or surgical measures. Compare RADICAL TREATMENT. **continuous sleep t.** The use of sleep in treating agitated, excited, or malignantly anxious patients. Barbiturates or other drugs are used to induce sleep for 20 hours a day for two or three weeks. Also *prolonged narcosis, prolonged sleep treatment, sleep therapy*. **Cox's t.** Treatment of cholera by the intravenous infusion of large quantities of isotonic saline. **cross-fire t.** CROSS-FIRE. **dietetic t.** DIET THERAPY. **drip t.** INTRAVENOUS FEEDING. **electric shock t.** ELECTROCONVULSIVE THERAPY. **electroconvulsive t.** ELECTROCONVULSIVE THERAPY. **empiric t.** Treatment by remedies determined on the basis of experience. Also *empiric therapeutics*. **expectant t.** Symptomatic treatment in expectation of the patient's eventual unassisted recovery from the underlying condition. **fever t.** FEVER THERAPY. **fractionated t.** FRACTIONATION. **Frenkel's t.** FRENKEL'S EXERCISES. **Girard's t.** The treatment of seasickness with atropine and strychnine. **Goeckerman t.** The treatment of psoriasis with topical tar and ultraviolet light. **Hartel's t.** A treatment for trigeminal neuralgia consisting of injection of alcohol into the gasserian ganglion, using a technique in which the needle is inserted through the foramen ovale from the inside of the mouth. **hyperbaric oxygen t.** See under HYPERBARIC OXYGEN THERAPY. **hypoglycemic shock t.** INSULIN COMA THERAPY. **isoserum t.** Treatment using serum obtained from a person who has had the disease that now afflicts the patient. **Keating-Hart's t.** Treatment of superficial cancer by fulguration. **Kenny's t.** See under KENNY'S METHOD. **Lambotte's t.** The correction and stabilization of a limb fracture by an external fixation apparatus with intraosseous pins. **Leriche's t.** The periarticular injection of a local anesthetic in the treatment of joint sprains. **light t.** See under PHOTOTHERAPY. **maintenance t.** Treatment designed to maintain a patient in a stable condition, especially in cases of chronic disease when no cure is available. **Matas t.** The treatment of various forms of neuralgia by the injection of absolute alcohol into the affected ganglion, particularly injection of the gasserian ganglion in trigeminal neuralgia. **medical t.** Treatment of a disease or condition by a health care professional utilizing means other than surgery. **Murphy's t.** Treatment of peritonitis by maintaining the patient in a sitting position so that pus collects in the pelvis. **Nordach t.** Treatment of pulmonary tuberculosis involving rest, fresh air, and a nourishing diet. **open t. of burns** Treatment of burns with or without a topical antimicrobial agent, but always without a surgical dressing. **organ t.** ORGANOTHERAPY. **Orr t.** The treatment of compound infected wounds and fractures of the limbs, in which the fractured ends are aligned and coated with petrolatum gauze. The limb is then immobilized in a plaster cast. Also *Orr technique, Orr method*. **palliative t.** Treatment directed at improving a patient's tolerance of symptoms, as by reducing pain, rather than seeking to combat the disease producing such symptoms. **Pasteur t.** The original method of vaccination with extracts of dried, inactivated, infected rabbit spinal cord, used after a bite from a rabid animal. See also ANTIRABIES VACCINE OF PASTEUR. **Paul's t.** Therapeutic use of lymph percutaneously for rheumatic disorders. **Plummer's t.** The use of iodine in the treatment of thyrotoxicosis. **Politzer's t.** The use of politzerization in treatment, as of patients with difficulty in ventilating the middle ears. **preventive t.** PROPHYLACTIC TREATMENT. **Proetz t.** PROETZ DISPLACEMENT. **prolonged sleep t.** CONTINUOUS SLEEP TREATMENT. **prophylactic t.** Treatment intended to prevent the development of disease, such as the use of chemotherapy as chemoprophylaxis for close contacts of infectious disease. Also *preventive treatment*. **protracted t.** PROTRACTED RADIATION. **radical t.** Treatment designed to address the root cause of a disorder and by extirpating it effect a cure. It may or may not be innovative or experimental. It is designed to accomplish a more lasting benefit or is performed under more critical circumstances than conservative treatment, but is usually attended by greater risk. Compare CONSERVATIVE TREATMENT. **rational t.** Treatment by remedies determined on the basis of knowledge of their effects on the condition treated. Also *rational therapeutics*. **Rollier t.** A method of treating surgical tuberculosis by systematic exposure of the affected part or area to direct sunlight. **root canal t.** The removal of dental pulp, preparation of root canals, and root canal filling. Also *root canal therapy, pulp canal therapy*. **salicyl t.** The use of salicylates in the treatment of arthritis. **Schlösser's t.** Treatment of trigeminal neuralgia by the injection of alcohol into the divisions of the nerve where they emerge from the skull. **shock t.** ELECTROCONVULSIVE THERAPY. **Sippy t.** See under SIPPY DIET. **slush t.** The dermatologic application of carbon dioxide snow that has been made into a slush by adding acetone or ether. **solar t.** HELIOTHERAPY. **specific t.** Treatment directed against a specific disease or against a specific cause of a disease. **symptomatic t.** Treatment directed at counteracting symptoms rather than the disease producing them, as in cases where the disease is self-limiting. **Tallerman t.** The application of hot, dry air to symptomatic body areas, particularly bones, joints, and extremities. **thyroid t.** Any treatment involving the administration of thyroid hormone, thyroxine, or triiodothyronine. *Popular.* **total-push t.** TOTAL-PUSH THERAPY.

***Trechona*** \trēkō′nə\ A genus of funnel-web spiders in the family Dipluridae, which includes several species venomous to humans. The effective toxins are probably similar to those in snake venoms.

**tree** 1 A perennial woody plant, generally with a single stem, or trunk, at its base. 2 An anatomical structure having the form of a trunk dividing into branches and thus suggestive of the appearance of a tree, as *bronchial tree* or *vascular tree.* **arterial t.** The entire arterial system, from aorta to capillaries. **bronchial t.** ARBOR BRONCHIALIS. **laryngotracheobronchial t.** The larynx, trachea, bronchi, and their branches. **tracheobronchial t.** The part of the respiratory tract that includes the trachea, the bronchi, and the smaller divisions of the bronchi. Also *tracheobronchial tract.* **vascular t.** The vascular system considered in its entirety, from the largest vessels to capillaries. **venous t.** The entire venous system, from capillaries to venae cavae.

**Treitz** [Wenzel *Treitz,* German anatomist, 1819–1872] 1 Fossa of Treitz. See under RECESSUS DUODENALIS INFERIOR. 2 Ligament of Treitz, muscle of Treitz. See under MUSCULUS SUSPENSORIUS DUODENI. 3 See under FASCIA. 4 Vascular arch of Treitz. See under TREITZ ARCH.

**Trélat** [Ulysse *Trélat,* Jr., French surgeon, 1828–1890] Leser-Trélat sign. See under SIGN.

**trema** \trē′mə\ [Gk *trēma* a thing pierced through, hole, eye of a needle] 1 In lower vertebrates, a gill cleft which allows water to flow from the pharynx to the outside of the throat region. 2 A pharyngeal pouch in higher vertebrates including man. This meaning is now reflected in terms such as *pretrematic* and *post-trematic.*

**Trematoda** \trem′ətō′də\ [New L (from Gk *trēma,* pl. *trēmata,* + *-ōdēs* -ODE)] A class of the phylum Platyhelminthes which includes the orders Monogenea and Digenea, the latter including the parasitic flukes of man and domestic animals.

**trematode** \trem′ətōd\ [See TREMATODA. A member of the class Trematoda. Also *trematoid.*

**trematodiasis** \trem′ətōdī′əsis\ [*trematod(e)* + -IASIS] A disease caused by a trematode infection.

**trematoid** \trem′ətoid\ 1 Trematodelike. 2 TREMATODE.

**trematol** \trem′ətôl\ TREMETOL.

**tremens** \trē′məns\ [L, pres. part. of *tremere* to tremble] Associated with or characterized by trembling, shaking movements, or tremor.

**tremetol** \trem′ətôl\ $C_{13}H_{14}O_2$. A toxin found in *Eupatorium rugosum,* white snakeroot, and *Haplopappus heterophyllus.* rayless goldenrod. It causes trembles in cattle and sheep and milk sickness in humans. Also *tremetone, trematol.*

**tremogram** \trem′əgram\ A recording or tracing of tremors obtained by means of a tremograph. Also *tremorgram.*

**tremograph** \trem′əgraf\ An instrument for recording tremor electronically, either by ink-writing on moving paper or on a cathode ray screen. Also *tremorgraph.*

**tremolabile** \trem′ōlā′bīl\ 1 Liable to be affected adversely if shaken, as a solution. 2 Unusually sensitive to tremor.

**tremometer** \tremäm′ətər\ An instrument used to measure the amplitude of hand tremors.

**tremor** \trem′ər\ [L (from *tremere* to tremble, quake) a trembling, quaking] A rhythmic, repetitive involuntary movement, often, of constant amplitude and frequency, generally involving one or more limbs, sometimes the head, neck, lips, tongue, or other parts of the body. Tremor may be transient or constant, restricted or generalized, rapid or slow. Also *atelokinesia* (seldom used). **action t.** Tremor which occurs during the course of a movement. It may be either of the kinetic or attitudinal type. Also *persistent tremor, motor tremor, effort tremor.* **alternating t.** The rhythmic resting tremor, due to intermittent contraction of agonist and antagonist muscles, having a frequency of about 4 Hz, which occurs in the hands and arms but sometimes in other parts of the body in diseases involving the corpus striatum and the substantia nigra such as parkinsonism. **arsenic t.** A tremor resulting from chronic exposure to arsenic. **asynergic family t.** ESSENTIAL TREMOR. **attitudinal t.** A tremor which occurs when a motor contraction or attitude is maintained voluntarily, as when the hands and arms are held outstretched, and which vanishes at rest. It may be due to anxiety, thyrotoxicosis, drugs, or toxins, but can also occur in some extrapyramidal disorders including some cases of parkinsonism and in essential tremor. **benign familial t.** ESSENTIAL TREMOR. **bread-crumbing t.** PILL-ROLLING TREMOR. **convulsive t.** PARAMYOCLONUS MULTIPLEX. **t. cordis** PALPITATION. **effort t.** ACTION TREMOR. **essential t.** A benign familial extrapyramidal disorder, often of dominant inheritance, in which there is action tremor involving the limbs which increases in severity with age and is also accentuated by emotion. Some patients also show static tremor of the head and neck. Ethyl alcohol often relieves the tremor. Also *benign familial tremor, asynergic family tremor, familial tremor, heredofamilial tremor, status macrobioticus multiparus.* **familial t.** ESSENTIAL TREMOR. **fine t.** Any tremor in which the oscillatory movements are fine, of small amplitude, and often rapid. One such is the accentuated physiologic tremor occurring in anxiety. **flapping t.** ASTERIXIS. **heredofamilial t.** ESSENTIAL TREMOR. **intention t.** A form of action tremor which increases in amplitude as the action nears completion, as when a pointing finger approaches its target. This tremor is diagnostic of a lesion of cerebellar tracts or connections and is most often seen in multiple sclerosis. **kinetic t.** Tremor occurring during active movement. **lenticulostriate t.** PILL-ROLLING TREMOR. **t. mercurialis** Tremor due to chronic exposure to mercury or its compounds. **motor t.** ACTION TREMOR. **muscular t.** FASCICULATION. **nonintention t.** Any tremor that does not increase in severity toward the end of a movement. It may be either a static or an action tremor. **parkinsonian t.** The static tremor of Parkinson's disease, with slow (4 to 6 per second), regular oscillations, which usually cease during voluntary movement of the affected part though occasionally the tremor is also of action type. It is exacerbated by fatigue, emotion, and cold, and it can also affect the lips, lower jaw, and tongue. **passive t.** STATIC TREMOR. **persistent t.** ACTION TREMOR. **physiologic t.** A very fine, rapid tremor with a frequency of about 10–12 per second found in normal individuals. It may be just visible when the hands are outstretched, but even when not evident to the naked eye it can usually be recorded electrically. The tremors of anxiety and fatigue and essential tremor may represent an accentuation of physiologic tremor. **pill-rolling t.** Any static tremor of the hands as that seen typically in paralysis agitans in which the subject appears to be rolling a small object between the thumb and the tips of the fingers. Also *coin-counting, pill-rolling, bread-crumbing tremor, lenticulostriate tremor.* **postural t.** A tremor occurring when a limb or other part of the body is held in a specific position, as when the hand is outstretched. **t. potatorum** DELIRIUM TREMENS. **progressive cerebellar t.** DYSSYNERGIA CEREBELLARIS MYOCLONICA. **resting t.** STATIC TREMOR. **saturnine t.** A tremor resulting from chronic lead poisoning. Also *tremor saturninus.* **senile t.** Rhythmic involuntary movements, usually of the hands, occurring in a minority of the aged. It may be a physiologic tremor made more pronounced by aging. **static t.** Tremor which occurs when the affected part is at rest and which disappears during motor activity. The tremor usually occurs at a rate of four to six per second. Also *resting tremor, passive tremor.* **striocerebellar t.** A combination of static, action, and sometimes intention tremor seen in some patients with a form of hereditary ataxia such as olivopontocerebellar degeneration. **t. tendinum** An involuntary twitching of the hands and feet, as may occur in anxiety. **titubating t.** A nodding or lateral to-and-fro tremor of the head. It is sometimes seen in association with senile tremor, sometimes with cerebellar degeneration. **trombone t. of tongue** TROMBONE TONGUE.

**tremorgram** \trem′ərgram\ TREMOGRAM.

**tremorgraph** \trem′ərgraf\ TREMOGRAPH.

**tremorine** \trem′ərēn\ 1,4-Dipyrrolidino-2-butyne, a central cholinomimetic drug that is used to produce in experimental animals a model resembling parkinsonism, characterized by a profound tremor of the head and limbs, used for the study of drugs to control such signs.

**tremostable** \trem′ōstā′bəl\ Likely to remain stable in spite of being shaken, as a solution.

**tremulous** \trem′yələs\ [L *tremulus* (from *tremere* to quake, quiver) quaking, quivering] In a quivering state; trembling.

**Trendelenburg** [Freidrich *Trendelenburg,* German surgeon, 1844–1924] **1** See under TAMPON, OPERATION, POSITION. **2** Trendelenburg's operation. See under SYNCHONDROSEOTOMY. **3** Trendelenburg gait. See under GLUTEAL GAIT.

**trepan** \tripan′\ TREPHINE.

**trepanation** \treplsənā′shən\ TREPHINATION.

**trepanning** \tripan′ing\ TREPHINING.

**trephination** \tref′ənā′shən\ [*trephin(e)* + -ATION] An operation utilizing a trephine on the skull or cornea. Also *trepanation.*

**trephine** \trifīn′, -fēn′\ [earlier *trafine,* for *trefine,* from L *tres* three + *fines,* pl. of *finis* end; invented and named in early 17th century because it had three ends; it superseded the ancient trepan (from Gk *trypanon* auger, gimlet)] **1** A tubular, serrated saw with fluted sides for boring a circular hole in bone, usually the skull. The saw either flares slightly or has an adjustable stop appliance to prevent it from plunging. The bone button can be subsequently replaced. Also *hole saw, crown saw.* **2** A small, refined instrument used to make a hole in the cornea. **3** To operate on the skull or cornea with a trephine. For defs. 1, 2, and 3 also *trepan.*

**trephining** \trifī′ning\ The act or process of operating with a trephine, as on the skull or cornea. Also *trepanning, terebration* (obs.), *foration.* **sclerocorneal t.** Removal of a disk of tissue from the limbus, as in the performance of a filtering operation for glaucoma.

**trephocyte** \tref′əsīt\ [Gk *treph(ein)* to nourish + *o* + -CYTE] TROPHOCYTE.

**trepidant** \trep′idənt\ [L *trepidans,* gen. *trepidantis,* pres. part. of *trepidare* to fear, be agitated] Characterized by tremor; trembling.

**trepidatio** \trep′idā′shō\ TREPIDATION. **t. cordis** PALPITATION.

**trepidation** \trep′idā′shən\ [L *trepidatio* (from *trepidatus,* past part. of *trepidare* to hurry with alarm or in confusion) confused hurry, alarm] Agitation, tremor, palpitation. Also *trepidatio.*

***Treponema*** \trep′ənē′mə\ [Gk *trep(ein)* to turn + *o* + *nēma* thread, yarn, tissue] A genus of extremely thin spirochetes, best seen by dark-field microscopy. Various species cause a variety of human and animal infections, including syphilis. Several species are commensals in the human gingival crevice and the gastrointestinal tract, or in the genital region. These include *T. macrodentium, T. refringens, T. denticola, T. orale, T. scoliodontum,* and *T. vincentii.* ***T. carateum*** The species that causes pinta. The organism appears to be a variant of *T. pallidum.* ***T. cuniculi*** A treponeme that causes benign venereal spirochetosis in rabbits. Its presence may complicate experimental studies with human treponemes. Also *Treponema paraluis-cuniculi.* ***T. pallidum*** The treponeme that causes syphilis. It has from 4 to 14 spirals and pointed ends. It can be propagated in laboratory animals but not *in vitro.* Suspensions in suitable media can remain motile for days. Infection induces reaginic antibodies and also specific antitreponemal antibodies. The latter can be detected by immunofluorescent tests or by the TPI test. Also *Trypanosoma luis.* ***T. paraluis-cuniculi*** TREPONEMA CUNICULI. ***T. pertenue*** The species that causes yaws. The organism appears to be a variant of *T. pallidum,* altered in pathogenicity but not immunologically.

**treponemal** \trep′ənē′məl\ Of or relating to the anaerobic bacteria *Treponema.*

**treponematosis** \trep′ənē′mətō′sis\ [*TREPONEMA* + *t* + -OSIS] Infection caused by any microorganism of the genus *Treponema.* **tropical t.** Any of the tropical diseases caused by spirochetes of the genus *Treponema*; yaws, bejel, or pinta.

**treponeme** \trep′ənēm\ An organism of the genus *Treponema.*

**treponemiasis** \trep′ənēmī′əsis\ [*Treponem(a)* + -IASIS] Any infection caused by microorganisms of the genus *Treponema*; treponematosis.

**treponemicidal** \trep′ənē′misī′dəl\ Capable of destroying spirochetes of the genus *Treponema.*

**trestolone acetate** 17β-hydroxy-7α-methylestr-4-en-3-one acetate, an anticancer, androgenic, synthetic, steroid hormone.

**tretamine** TRIETHYLENEMELAMINE.

**tretinoin** $C_{20}H_{28}O_2$. 3,7-Dimethyl-9-(2,6,6-trimethyl-1-cyclohexen-1-yl)-2,4,6,8-nonatetraenoic acid. A keratolytic agent used topically in the treatment of acne. It decreases the cohesion of the horny cell layer in the epidermis, which results in peeling of the skin, and may cause erythema and dryness of the skin. Also *retinoic acid, vitamin A acid.*

**Treves** [Norman *Treves,* U.S. surgeon, 1894–1964] **1** Stewart-Treves syndrome. See under SYNDROME. **2** Avascular fold of Treves, Treves fold. See under PLICA ILEOCAECALIS. **3** Treves fold. See under PLICA CAECALIS VASCULARIS.

**Trevor** [David *Trevor,* British orthopedic surgeon, born 1906] Trevor's disease. See under DYSPLASIA EPIPHYSIALIS HEMIMELICA.

**TRF** T-cell replacing factor.

**TRH** thyrotropin releasing hormone.

**tri-** \trī-, tri-\ [L and Gk prefix *tri-* (from L *tres* three and

Gk *treis* three) denoting three] A prefix meaning three, threefold.

**triac** \trī′ak\ 3,5,3′-triiodothyroacetic acid, a compound formed by the oxidative deamination followed by decarboxylation of triiodothyronine in peripheral tissues. Formerly thought to be the tissue-active form of triiodothyronine, it is now regarded as a metabolic product of the hormone.

**triacanthine** $N^6$-(3-methylbut-2-enyl)adenine, or $N^6$-($\Delta^2$-isopentenyl)adenine. A modification of adenine found as a plant hormone and in tRNA. It is one of the cytokinens.

**triacetin** \trī·as′ətin\ Glyceryl triacetate. A compound that has been used as a superficial fungal inhibitor.

**triacetyloleandomycin** TROLEANDOMYCIN.

**triad** \trī′ad\ [Gk *trias* (gen. *triados*, from *tria*, neut. pl. of *treis* three) the number three, a triad] A close or regular association of three things, as the co-occurrence of three symptoms. **AGR t.** ANIRIDIA-WILMS TUMOR SYNDROME. **anal t.** The three traits of obstinancy, parsimony, and pedantic orderliness, frequently seen in the anal character. **Charcot's t.** A combination of dysarthria, nystagmus, and intention tremor, described as characteristic of multiple sclerosis but only rarely seen in that disease when cerebellar pathways are predominantly involved. Marburg's triad is more often noted. **Gougerot's t.** Vasculitis manifested as nodules, purpura, and bullae. **hepatic t.** The portal vein, hepatic artery, and bile duct which share a common pattern of arrangement throughout the liver, their grouped tributaries occupying the portal canals at the periphery of the liver lobules. Also *portal triad.* **Hutchinson's t.** The occurrence in a subject with congenital syphilis of interstitial keratitis, nerve deafness, and Hutchinson teeth. Also *Hutchinson syndrome.* **Kartagener's t.** KARTAGENER SYNDROME. **Marburg's t.** Spasticity of the limbs, abolition of the cutaneous abdominal reflexes, and pallor of the temporal halves of the optic disks, typically seen in the advanced stages of multiple sclerosis. **meningitic t.** Headache, vomiting, and neck stiffness, the three principal signs of meningitis. **Oppenheim's t.** Hypoacusis, loss of the corneal reflex, and damage to the sixth nerve, occurring on the same side as a tumor in the cerebellopontine angle. **portal t.** HEPATIC TRIAD. **Saint's t.** The concurrence of hiatal hernia, diverticulosis of the colon, and cholelithiasis. **Whipple's t.** The three cardinal signs of insulin-secreting islet-cell adenomas of the pancreas. They are spontaneously occurring hypoglycemia with blood glucose values below 50 mg/100 ml; the characteristic symptoms of severe, acute hypoglycemia temporally correlated with measurable low blood sugar levels; and relief of those symptoms by the administration of glucose.

**triaditis** \trī′ədī′tis\ [TRIAD + -ITIS] Inflammation in a triad or triads; specifically, portal triaditis. **portal t.** Infiltration of the portal triads (hepatic triads) with chronic inflammatory cells, as seen in chronic hepatitis.

**triage** \trē·äzh′\ [French (from *trier* to choose, sort + *-age* -AGE), process of trying, choosing, sorting] The organized sorting of casualties into predetermined categories. In a battlefield situation, the categories usually are: beyond help in the present situation, in need of immediate attention, and capable of surviving with no additional ill effects until treatment can be provided.

**trial** / **blind t.** A clinical trial in which the results obtained in one or more treatment groups are to be compared with a control or placebo group, and which is so designed that the individuals being observed are unaware, so long as the trial is in progress, of the group to which they have been allocated, the object being to ensure that the results are free from subjective bias. **cross-over t.** A clinical trial based on a cross-over study design. See under CROSS-OVER. **double-blind t.** A clinical trial based on a double-blind study design. See under DOUBLE-BLIND. **t. of labor** Nonintervention in either the initiation or continuation of labor as long as satisfactory progress is observed and no complications occur. Also *test of labor.* **preventive t.** EXPERIMENTAL STUDY. **randomized controlled t.** A form of prospective study in which subjects are allotted in a random manner to one or more treatment groups and a control group.

**trialism** \trī′əlizm\ The theory that neutrophils, monocytes, and lymphocytes arise from distinctive primitive cells.

**triamcinolone** $C_{21}H_{27}FO_6$. 9-Fluoro-11$\beta$,16$\alpha$, 17,21-tetrahydroxypregna-1,4-diene-3,20-dione. A very potent synthetic glucocorticoid. It is used in the treatment of conditions that respond to glucocorticoids, as anti-inflammatory agents. It is given orally.

**triamcinolone acetonide** The hexacetonide ester of triamcinolone. It is used as an anti-inflammatory drug by various routes of administration.

**triamcinolone diacetate** The diacetate ester of triamcinolone. It is given orally, intramuscularly, intra-articularly, or by injection in the soft tissues as an anti-inflammatory agent.

**triamcinolone hexacetonide** $C_{30}H_{41}FO_7$9-Fluoro-11$\beta$,16$\alpha$,-17,21-tetrahydroxypregna-1,4-diene-3,20-dione cyclic 16,17-acetal with acetone. An ester form of triamcinolone with the same properties and uses as the parent drug. It can be injected into, or near the lesions, or intra-articularly in arthritis.

**triamelia** \trī′əmē′lyə\ [TRI- + AMELIA] The total agenesis of three limbs.

**triamterene** $C_{12}H_{11}N_7$. 6-Phenyl-2,4,7-triamino-6-phenylpteridine. A diuretic which acts by increasing sodium and chloride secretion but does not affect potassium secretion. It is given orally.

# triangle

**triangle** [L *triangulum* (from *triangulus* three-cornered, from *tri-* three + *angulus* an angle) a triangle] **1** A geometrical figure that has three sides meeting at three angles. **2** In anatomy, any area or space that is demarcated so as to resemble a geometrical figure with three sides. Also *trigonum, trigone.* **anal t.** REGIO ANALIS. **anterior t. of neck** REGIO CERVICALIS ANTERIOR. **aortic t.** A radiologically translucent triangle bounded anteriorly by the left subclavian artery, inferiorly by the arch of the aorta, and posteriorly by the spine. **auditory t.** AREA VESTIBULARIS. **t. of auscultation** A triangular area on the back of the chest bounded by the medial margin of the scapula, the trapezius muscle, and the latissimus dorsi muscle. • Once regarded as an area of special relevance to auscultation, it is now merely a convenient means of referring to a clinical anatomic area. **Béclard's t.** A triangle bounded by the posterior belly of the digastric muscle, the posterior margin of the hyoglossus muscle, and the greater cornu of the hyoid bone. **Bolton t.** The triangle formed by connecting the nasion, the postcondylare, and the midpoint of the sella turcica. **t. of Budde** A triangular space bounded by the common hepatic duct and right hepatic duct on the left, the cystic duct on the right, and the right end of the porta hepatis above. It is usually traversed by the cystic artery. **Burow's t.'s** Triangles of skin on either side of the base of a sliding flap which are excised to facilitate movement of the flap. **Calot's t.** An area bounded by the liver, the cystic duct, and the hepatic duct in which the cystic artery, the right hepatic artery, and, occasionally, accessory hepatic ducts are located. **cardiohepatic t.** The triangular area in the right fifth intercostal space that demarcates the space between the upper margin of the liver and the heart. **carotid t.** TRIGONUM CAROTICUM. **cephalic t.** A triangle that is formed by connecting the pogonion, the glabella, and the most distal point on the occiput in the median plane. **cervical t.'s** The regio cervicalis anterior, regio cervicalis lateralis, and their subdivisions. **Codman's t.** A roentgenographic sign of a bone tumor that consists of a triangular cuff of periosteal bone at the margin of the tumor and that results from the elevation of the periosteum by the tumor. Also *lipping* (seldom used), *reactive triangle*. **crural t.** The area bounded by the inner aspect of the thighs and the symphysis pubis and comprising the inguinal, genital, and lower abdominal regions. **digastric t.** TRIGONUM SUBMANDIBULARE. **Einthoven's t.** A hypothetical equilateral triangle with the heart at its center and its apices situated in the two arms and the left leg, as formed from the three standard leads of the electrocardiogram. **Elaut's t.** A triangular area between the promontory of the sacrum below and the common iliac artery on each side. **t. of elbow** FOSSA CUBITALIS. **t. of election** TRIGONUM CAROTICUM. **extravesical t.** PAWLIK'S TRIANGLE. **Farabeuf's t.** A triangle in the neck that is formed by the internal jugular vein, the hypoglossal nerve, and the facial vein. **femoral t.** TRIGONUM FEMORALE. **fetal t.** A three-sided space formed by the fetal trunk, flexed thigh, and arm. **frontal t.** A triangle formed by connecting the two extremities of the maximum frontal diameter to each other and to the glabella. **Gombault-Philippe t.** FASCICULUS TRIANGULARIS. **Henke's t.** TRIGONUM INGUINALE. **Hesselbach's t.** TRIGONUM INGUINALE. **hypoglossal t.** TRIGONUM NERVI HYPOGLOSSI. **hypoglossohyoid t.** A triangular area bounded by the posterior margin of the mylohyoid muscle, the hypoglossal nerve and the posterior belly of the digastric muscle and situated within the submandibular triangle. **iliofemoral t.** An area bounded by a line from the anterior superior iliac spine to the top of the greater trochanter, a horizontal line from the anterior superior spine, and a vertical line from the top of the greater trochanter. **inferior carotid t.** TRIGONUM MUSCULARE. **inferior occipital t.** A triangle formed by connecting the lowest points on the mastoid processes to each other and to the inion. **infraclavicular t.** FOSSA INFRACLAVICULARIS. **inguinal t.** TRIGONUM INGUINALE. **Jackson's safety t.** An area demarcated between the anterior margins of the sternocleidomastoid muscles, with the apex being where the muscles meet in the suprasternal notch and the base being where they meet a horizontal line at the level of the lower margin of the thyroid cartilage. **Kanavel's t.** The surface marking in the palm delineating the extent of the fibrous flexor sheath. **Labbé's t.** A triangular area bounded inferiorly by a horizontal line through the lower margin of the left ninth costal cartilage, the line of the false ribs laterally, and the line of the liver to the right. It is the area in which the stomach is related to the anterior abdominal wall. **Langenbeck's t.** An area that lies behind the head of the femur between the piriformis and gluteus medius muscles. **Lesser's t.** A triangle bounded by the anterior and posterior bellies of the digastric muscle and the hypoglossal nerve. **Lieutaud's t.** TRIGONUM VESICAE. **lumbar t.** TRIGONUM LUMBALE. **lumbocostoabdominal t.** An irregular space between the external oblique muscle of the abdomen, the serratus posterior inferior muscle, the erector spinae muscle, and the internal oblique muscle of the abdomen. **Malgaigne's t.** TRIGONUM CAROTICUM. **Minor's t.** A triangular space behind the anus that is produced by the attachment of the superficial division of the sphincter ani externus to the coccyx. **muscular t.** TRIGONUM MUSCULARE. **t. of necessity** TRIGONUM MUSCULARE. **nodal t.** A triangle of enlarged lymph nodes which may be felt, usually by digital pressure, on the inner aspect of the knee in patients with infectious mononucleosis. **occipital t.** The upper subdivision of the regio cervicalis lateralis that is bounded by the sternocleidomastoid muscle anteriorly, the trapezius muscle posteriorly, and the inferior belly of the omohyoid muscle below. The accessory nerve crosses it in an anteroposterior direction near the apex. **omoclavicular t.** TRIGONUM OMOCLAVICULARE. **palatal t.** A triangle formed by connecting the extremes of the greatest breadth of the palate to each other and to the prosthion. **Pawlik's t.** A triangular area on the anterior wall of the vagina that is related to the base of the urinary bladder superficial to the trigonum vesicae. Also *Pawlik's trigone, vaginal triangle, extravesical triangle*. **Petit's t.** TRIGONUM LUMBALE. **Petit's lumbar t.** TRIGONUM LUMBALE. **popliteal t. of femur** FACIES POPLITEA FEMORIS. **posterior t. of neck** REGIO CERVICALIS LATERALIS. **pubourethral t.** A triangle in the perineum that is bounded by the ischiocavernosus muscle laterally, the bulbocavernosus muscle medially, and the transversus perinei superficialis muscle posteriorly. **reactive t.** CODMAN'S TRIANGLE. **rectal t.** REGIO ANALIS. **Reil's t.** TRIGONUM LEMNISCI. **retromandibular t.** A variable triangular hollow situated on the alveolar part of the mandible behind the last molar tooth. **Scarpa's t.** TRIGONUM FEMORALE. **Sherren's t.** An area on the right side of the anterior abdominal wall that is marked by lines joining the pubic tubercle, the umbilicus, and the highest point on the iliac crest. **sternocostal t.** MORGAGNI'S FORAMEN. **subclavian t.** TRIGONUM OMOCLAVICULARE. **submandibular t.** TRIGONUM SUBMANDIBULARE. **submental t.** TRIGONUM SUBMENTALE. **suboccipital t.** A triangle, deep to the semispinalis capitis muscle immediately below the occiput, that is bounded superomedially by the rectus capitis posterior major muscle, superolaterally by the obliquus capitis superior, and inferolaterally by the obliquus capitis inferior. The vertebral artery passes transversely across its floor on the posterior arch of the atlas and the posterior atlanto-occipital membrane. **superior lumbar t.** An occasional intermuscular space under cover of the latissimus dorsi muscle and located above and medial to the inferior lumbar triangle of Petit and between the twelfth rib or serratus posterior inferior muscle above, the lateral margin of erector spinae or the quadratus lumborum muscle medially, and the superior border of the internal abdominal oblique muscle inferolaterally. The floor is usually the conjoined three layers of the lumbodorsal fascia. Also *surgical lumbar triangle, Lesshaft space*. **suprameatal t.** A triangular bounded anteriorly by the posterosuperior margin of the external opening of the external acoustic meatus, superiorly by the supramastoid crest, and posteriorly by a vertical tangent to the curve of the posterior margin of the external opening of the external acoustic meatus. This area forms the lateral wall of the mastoid antrum in the petrous part of the temporal bone. **surgical lumbar t.** SUPERIOR LUMBAR TRIANGLE. **tracheal t.** TRIGONUM MUSCULARE. **Trautmann's t.** A triangular space in the temporal bone bounded anteriorly by a line tangential to the posterior semicircular canal, superiorly by the superior petrosal sinus (or the inferior temporal line on the cranial exterior), and posteriorly by the anterior margin of the transverse sinus. **Tweed t.** A cephalometric figure based on the Frankfort plane, the mandibular plane, and a projection of the axis of the lower incisors. **umbilicomammillary t.** A triangular area limited by three lines that connect the two nipples of the mammae and the umbilicus. **urogenital t.** REGIO UROGENITALIS. **vaginal t.** PAWLIK'S TRIANGLE. **vesical t.** TRIGONUM VESICAE. **von Weber's t.** A triangle formed by connecting the plantar aspects of the heads of the first and fifth metatarsal bones to each other and to the midpoint of the plantar aspect of the heel. **Ward's t.** A radiographically lucent area, located in the boss of the femoral neck and bounded by trabeculae, that is relatively weak and vulnerable to fracture. **Wernicke's t.** The wedge of myelinated axons formed in the pulvinar region of the thalamus, penetrating the internal capsule, and extending into the optic radiation. Also *campus of Wernicke.*

**triangular** \trī·ang′gyələr\ Of or shaped like a triangle. Also *trigonal.*

**triangularis** \trī·ang′gyəler′is\ **1** Triangular. **2** MUSCULUS DEPRESSOR ANGULI ORIS.

**triantebrachia** \trī′antēbrā′kē·ə\ [TRI- + *antebrach(ium)* + -IA] The duplication of one forearm so that, with the normal one, there are three forearms.

***Triatoma*** \trī·at′əmə\ A genus of cone-nose bugs in the family Reduviidae. A number of species, including *T. dimidiata, T.* (or *Panstronglylus) infestans,* and *T. maculata,* are important vectors of *Trypanosoma cruzi,* the agent of Chagas disease. ***T. megista*** PANSTRONGYLUS MEGISTUS. ***T. sanguisuga*** A species popularly known as the Mexican bedbug, found in the southern United States. Its painful bite causes irritation, swelling, and occasionally nausea.

**Triatominae** \trī′atām′inē\ A subfamily in the family Reduviidae; the cone-nose bugs. These bloodsucking insects are frequently serious pests of humans and domestic animals, but are most noteworthy as vectors of Chagas disease to man and other vertebrates. Of special importance for transmission to humans are species of *Triatoma, Panstrongylus,* and *Rhodnius.*

**triatrial** \trī·ā′trē·əl\ Having three atria, as the heart in cor triatrium.

**triazologuanine** AZAGUANINE.

**tribe** A taxonomic group ranking below a family and above a genus.

***Tribolium*** \tribō′lē·əm\ [Gk *tribol(os)* a prickly plant, burr + L *-ium,* neut. noun suffix] A genus of small grain beetles, or flour beetles (order Coleoptera), that destroy vast quantities of flour and cereal products. The species *T. confusum* and *T. castaneum,* reddish brown beetles about 3.5 millimeters in length, are abundant in temperate zones and serve as intermediate hosts of several members of the tapeworm genus *Hymenolepis,* including the common dwarf tapeworm of humans, *H. nana.*

**tribology** \tribäl′əjē\ [Gk *trib(ein)* to rub + *o* + -LOGY] The science and technology of surfaces that are in contact and move in relation to each other, especially those of the skeleton.

**Tribondeau** [Louis *Tribondeau,* French physician, 1872–1918] Bergonie-Tribondeau law. See under LAW.

**tribrachia** \trī·brā′kē·ə\ The possession of characteristics seen in a tribrachial thoracopagus.

**tribrachius** \trī·brā′kē·əs\ [TRI- + L *brachi(um)* the arm + New L *-us,* masc. noun suffix] TRIBRACHIAL THORACOPAGUS.

**TRIC** trachoma inclusion conjunctivitis.

**tricarboxylic acid** Any substance containing three carboxyl groups, especially, in biological contexts, citric, isocitric, or aconitic acids, because of their importance in carbohydrate catabolism.

**triceps** \trī′seps\ Characterized by three heads, as of a muscle. Also *tricipital.* **t. surae** MUSCULUS TRICEPS SURAE.

**trich-** \trik-\ TRICHO-.

**tricheiria** \trīkī′rē·ə\ [TRI- + *cheir-* + -IA] The condition of having three hands, as when one is duplicated and the other is normal.

**trichesthesia** \trik′esthē′zhə\ [TRICH- + ESTHESIA] Sensibility to cutaneous hair displacement. Also *trichoesthesia.*

**trichi-** \trik′i-\ TRICHO-.

**trichiasis** \trikī′əsis\ [TRICH- + -IASIS] A posterior misdirection of the eyelashes so that they abrade the cornea.

**trichilemmoma** \trik′ilemō′mə\ TRICHOLEMMOMA.

***Trichina*** \trikī′nə\ A former name for *TRICHINELLA.*

**trichina** [New L, from Gk *trichinos* of hair, from *thrix* a hair] (*pl.* trichinae) A nematode worm of the species *Trichinella spiralis.*

**trichinae** \trikī′nē\ Plural of TRICHINA.

***Trichinella*** \trik′inel′ə\ A genus of adenophorean nematodes in the family Trichinellidae which contains the single species *Trichinella spiralis,* the etiologic agent of trichinosis in many mammals including humans. Also *Trichina* (former name). ***T. spiralis*** The trichina worm or pork worm, a small parasitic worm, (males 1 to 1.5 mm, females 2 to 4 mm) which is the causal agent of trichinosis. It is widely distributed throughout the world, but is more common in temperate zones of the northern hemisphere. It is transmitted from host to host by ingestion of infected meat. The cysts are digested free and the young larvae excyst, molt, and mature in about a week. The adult females release larvae into the submucosa. These larvae wander through the body, eventually encyst within muscle fibers, and await another predator to continue the cycle.

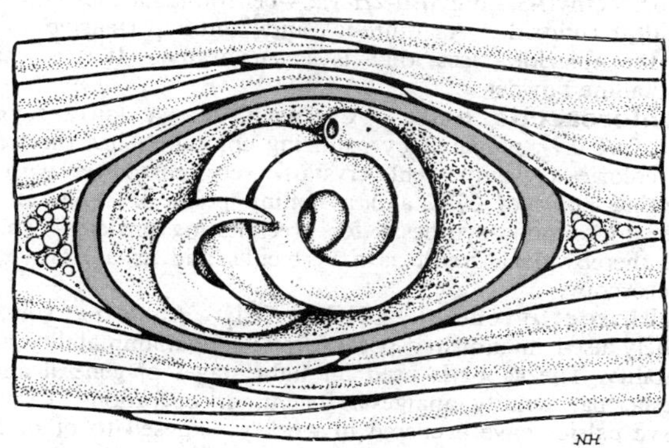

*Trichinella spiralis* (showing larva encysted in human muscle)

**trichinelliasis** \trik′inəlī′əsis\ TRICHINOSIS.

**Trichinelloidea** \trik′inəloi′dē·ə\ A superfamily of nematodes in the subclass Adenophorea which includes species that are parasitic in humans including *Trichinella spira-*

*lis, Trichuris trichiura,* and *Capillaria hepatica.* Also *Trichuroidea.*

**trichinellosis** \trik′inəlō′sis\ TRICHINOSIS.

**trichiniasis** \trik′inī′əsis\ TRICHINOSIS.

**trichiniferous** \trik′inif′ərəs\ Containing trichinae; trichinosed.

**trichinization** \trik′inīzā′shən\ The process of becoming infected with trichinae.

**trichinoscope** \trik′inəskōp′\ A magnifying glass used to inspect meat suspected of being infected with encysted trichinae. Pork is not inspected for this parasite by the United States Department of Agriculture.

**trichinosed** \trik′inōzd\ Infected with trichinae (*Trichinella* larvae).

**trichinosis** \trik′inō′sis\ [*Trichin(a)* + -OSIS] The disease induced by larvae of the trichina worm, *Trichinella spiralis,* usually acquired through ingestion of raw or insufficiently cooked meat, especially pork, infected with the worm. It is divided into three phases corresponding to periods in the life cycle of the worm. The intestinal phase occupies the time of growth and maturation of the larvae from the initial infection, and is marked by intestinal disturbance, nausea, pain, and diarrhea. The blood-migratory and muscle-penetration phase, during the migration of larvae from the next generation of worms, is characterized by fever, sweating, malaise, high eosinophilia, intense muscle pain, and rheumatic aches, usually preceded by puffiness around the eyes. Death from toxemia, respiratory distress, or other effect may occur during this phase, usually in the fourth or fifth week. The third phase is the period of worm encystment in the muscles, starting six weeks after infection, with pain, facial and sometimes generalized edema, and gradual subsidence of symptoms into a chronic course during which immunity usually develops. These severe manifestations are characteristic of cases resulting from heavy infestations. Most infections are benign to mild, depending upon host resistance as well as the quantity of infecting parasites. Also *trichinelliasis, trichinellosis, trichiniasis, trichinous polymyositis.*

**trichinotic** \trik′inät′ik\ **1** Of or referring to trichinosis. **2** Infected with trichinae; trichinosed: said of meat.

**trichinous** \trik′inəs\ Infected with or caused by trichinae.

**trichlormethiazide** $C_8H_8Cl_3N_3O_4S_2$. 6-Chloro-3-(dichloromethyl)-3,4-dihydro-2*H*-1,2,4-benzothiadiazine-7-sulfonamide-1,1-dioxide. A diuretic and antihypertensive drug of the thiazide class that is given orally. It is a white crystalline powder.

**trichloroacetic acid** $Cl_3C—COOH$. A fairly strong acid (p*K* 0.7), prepared by oxidizing chloral. It has the form of colorless, deliquescent crystals, very corrosive, with a melting point of 57°C and a boiling point of 196°C. It is used for organic synthesis, for precipitating proteins (which are thereby denatured), as a herbicide, and as a fixative in microscopy.

**trichloroethylene** $CHCL{=}CCl_2$. A toxic solvent widely used in industry because of its nonflammability and stability. The vapor is used for light stages of general anesthesia, particularly analgesia for minor operations. Cranial nerve palsies have occurred in workers exposed to or in patients administered trichloroethylene anesthesia. Contact with the skin may cause burns. Fatal liver damage has been recorded. Mild exposure produces euphoria, which may lead to addiction.

**trichloromethane** The systematic name of chloroform.

**trichloromethylchloroformate** DIPHOSGENE.

**trichlorophenol** $C_6H_3Cl_3O$. 2,4,5-trichlorophenol. An antiseptic and disinfectant more potent than phenol, but also much more toxic. It has been used as a surgical disinfectant, but the trichlorophenols have generally been replaced by less toxic agents.

**2,4,5-trichlorophenoxyacetic acid** A compound widely used as an herbicide to control woody weeds and brambles and also used in warfare to destroy food crops and defoliate enemy cover. Its main health risk comes from contamination with dioxin. 2,4,5-Trichlorophenoxyacetic acid itself is both teratogenic and fetotoxic to animals. Where dioxin content is minimal (below one part per million) there is no evidence of toxic effects on man from its use as an herbicide. See also AGENT ORANGE. Abbr. 2,4,5-T

**trichlorotrivinylarsine** $(CHCl{:}CH)_3As$. One of a group of highly toxic sternutating agents used in chemical warfare.

**tricho-** \trik′ə-, trik′ō-\ [Gk *thrix* (genitive *trichos*) hair] A combining form meaning hair, hairlike, or hairy. Also *trich-, trichi-.*

**trichobezoar** \-bē′zôr\ [TRICHO- + BEZOAR] A bezoar composed primarily of hair and usually found in the stomach. Also *pilobezoar, hairball, hair ball, hair cast, tumeur pileuse.*

***Trichobilharzia*** \-bilhär′zē·ə\ A genus of schistosomatid blood flukes, some species of which are parasitic in ducks and other aquatic birds and have been implicated in schistosome dermatitis (swimmer's itch). Some common species from freshwater snails in North American lakes associated with swimmer's itch include *T. elvae, T. ocellata, T. physellae, T. stagnicolae,* and *T. szidati.*

**trichocephaliasis** \-sef′əlī′əsis\ TRICHURIASIS.

**trichocephalosis** \-sef′əlō′sis\ TRICHURIASIS.

***Trichocephalus*** \-sef′ələs\ [TRICHO- + -CEPHALUS] An invalid name for *TRICHURIS.* • This term, however, is descriptively more accurate than the valid term.

**trichoclasis** \trikäk′ləsis\ [TRICHO- + Gk *klasis* a breaking into pieces] The fracture of the hair as a result of brittleness. Also *trichoclasia.*

**trichodarteriitis** \-därter′ē·ī′tis\ *Obs.* ARTERIOLITIS.

***Trichoderma*** \-dur′mə\ A form-genus of fungi often found as soil inhabitants and laboratory contaminants. It has occasionally been implicated in alimentary toxic aleukia.

**trichoepithelioma** \-ep′ithē′lē·ō′mə\ [TRICHO- + EPITHELIOMA] A benign skin tumor of the hair follicle simulating abortive pilar structures and containing horn cysts. It may be solitary or multiple, the latter being inherited. The face is the most common site. Also *epithelioma adenoides cysticum, Brooke's tumor.*

**trichoesthesia** \-esthē′zhə\ TRICHESTHESIA.

**trichoesthesiometer** \-esthē′zē·äm′ətər\ An apparatus for measuring sensitivity to mechanical displacement of hairs.

**trichofolliculoma** \-fəlik′yəlō′mə\ [TRICHO- + *follicul(us)* + -OMA] An organized, benign tumor, derived from a hair follicle, in which abortive hair roots appear to enter into a large central sinus. It is typically a tumor of the head and neck.

**trichographism** \trikäg′rəfizm\ PILOMOTOR REFLEX.

**trichohyalin** \-hī′əlin\ The hyalin of the hair.

**trichoid** \trik′oid\ [TRICH- + -OID] Resembling hair.

**tricholemmoma** \-lemō′mə\ [TRICHO- + *lemm(a)* + -OMA] A benign tumor derived from the lower part of the outer sheath of the hair root. The head is the most frequent site. Histologically, there are cells with clear cytoplasm rich in glycogen and arranged as solid masses. Also *trichilemmoma.*

**trichology** \trikäl′əjē\ [TRICHO- + -LOGY] The study of the hair. Also *pilology.*

**trichomalacia** \-məlā′shə\ A defect of the hair shaft

that is characterized by soft, fragile, swollen hairs. It may result from physical injury to the follicles.

**trichomegaly** \-meg′əlē\ [TRICHO- + -MEGALY] **1** The presence of hair of an abnormally large shaft diameter in relation to the site and the age of the patient. **2** The presence of abnormally long eyelashes from birth.

**trichomonacidal** \-mō′nəsī′dəl\ Having a destructive effect upon *Trichomonas* organisms. Also *trichomonadicidal.*

**trichomonacide** \-mō′nəsīd\ [*Trichomona(s)* + -CIDE] An agent used to destroy *Trichomonas* organisms.

**trichomonad** \trikäm′ənad\ A member of the genus *Trichomonas.*

**trichomonadicidal** \-mōnad′isī′dəl\ TRICHOMONACIDAL.

**Trichomonadida** \-mōnad′idə\ An order of flagellate protozoa in the class Zoomastigophorea, subphylum Mastigophora. Typical members have four to six flagella, one of which is recurrent and free or partially attached. An undulating membrane, when present, is associated with the adherent part of the recurrent flagellum. A pelta and a noncontractile oxostyle are usually present. *Trichomonas* is a typical genus. Some forms have both pseudopodia and flagella at different stages, as in *Histomonas* and *Dientamoeba.* Nearly all species are parasitic. Also *Rhizomastigida* (former name).

**trichomonal** \trikäm′ənəl\ Relating to or caused by a member of the genus *Trichomonas.*

***Trichomonas*** \trikäm′ənas\ [TRICHO- + Gk *monas* solitary, single; as substantive, a unit] A genus of parasitic, pyriform flagellates (order Trichomonadida) having four anterior flagella and one posterior flagellum along an undulating membrane. Species of medical and veterinary importance cause trichomoniasis in humans, other primates, and birds. Specificity is more related to characteristics of microhabitat than to host species. Some authorities divide this genus into the genera *Pentatrichomonas, Tritrichomonas,* and *Tetratrichomonas.* ***T. buccalis*** *TRICHOMONAS TENAX.* ***T. elongata*** *TRICHOMONAS TENAX.* ***T. hominis*** *PENTATRICHOMONAS HOMINIS.* ***T. intestinalis*** *PENTATRICHOMONAS HOMINIS.* ***T. tenax*** A species found in the mouths of humans, particularly around the tartar of teeth. It is believed to be nonpathogenic, but it is often found in diseased mouths and is associated with pyogenic organisms in the gums around the base of the teeth. Also *Tetratrichomonas buccalis, Trichomonas buccalis, Trichomonas elongata.* ***T. vaginalis*** A species commonly affecting the vagina, urethra, and possibly, the prostate. Infection is usually sexually acquired and manifests as vaginitis and, occasionally, urethritis. Infection in men is usually asymptomatic, as are some vaginal infections. Differences in pathogenicity exist among strains of the species.

**trichomoniasis** \-mənī′əsis\ [*trichomon(as)* + -IASIS] **1** Any disease caused by trichomonads. Also *trichomonosis.* **2** A disease caused by infection with *Trichomonas vaginalis*; urogenital trichomoniasis. **urogenital t.** A common infection of the genitourinary tract caused by *Trichomonas vaginalis,* a flagellated protozoon.

**trichomonicide** \-mō′nisīd\ TRICHOMONACIDE.

**trichomonosis** \-mōnō′sis\ TRICHOMONIASIS.

**trichomyces** \-mī′sēz\ [TRICHO- + -MYCES] A ringworm condition caused by fungi of the form-genus *Trichophyton,* which cause infections of hair. *Obs.*

**trichomycosis** \-mīkō′sis\ [TRICHO- + MYCOSIS] The presence of a corynebacterial infection of the axillary and pubic hair. • The term was formerly applied to any fungal infection of the hair. **t. axillaris** Lepothrix of the axillary hairs. Also *axillary trichomycosis, trichonocardiosis, trichonocardiosis axillaris, epidermophytosis axillaris.* **t. chromatica** LEPOTHRIX. **t. nodosa** LEPOTHRIX. **pubic t.** Lepothrix of the pubic hair. **t. pustulosa** A pustular ringworm infection of the scalp or beard.

**trichon** \trik′än\ TRICHOPHYTIN.

**trichonocardiosis** \trik′ənōkär′dē·ō′sis\ TRICHOMYCOSIS AXILLARIS. **t. axillaris** TRICHOMYCOSIS AXILLARIS.

**trichophytid** \-fī′tid\ A dermatophytid provoked by a *Trichophyton* organism. Also *trichophytide.*

**trichophytin** \trikäf′itin\ An extract of a *Trichophyton* species of fungus used as an allergen for intradermal testing. Cross reactions occur with *Microsporum* and *Epidermophyton* infections. A positive *Trichophyton* test, immediate or delayed, is found in inflammatory ringworm and particularly in dermatophytid reactions. The test is otherwise of little clinical value except in the investigation of defective immunity. Also *trichon.*

**trichophytobezoar** \-fī′təbē′zôr\ A bezoar made up primarily of animal hair and vegetable fibers.

***Trichophyton*** \trikäf′ətän\ [TRICHO- + Gk *phyton* a plant, tree, from *phyein* to bring forth, produce] A genus of keratinophilic, ascigerous, soil-dwelling fungi, some species of which are pathogenic dermatophytes. These are "ringworm" fungi, which attack the skin, nails, and hair. Some twenty species of *Trichophyton* are recognized, nine of which have been isolated from humans, three from animals. All species classified in the perfect (sexual) state are placed in the genus *Arthroderma..* Also *Megalosporon* (obs.). ***T. acuminatum*** *TRICHOPHYTON TONSURANS.* ***T. arloingi*** *TRICHOPHYTON MENTAGROPHTES.* ***T. asteroides*** *TRICHOPHYTON MENTAGROPHTES.* ***T. ceratophagus*** *TRICHOPHYTON SCHOENLEINII.* ***T. ectothrix*** A species of *Trichophyton,* a ringworm fungus that grows into the hair follicle, surrounds the hair shaft, and penetrates it. Spores are usually found outside of the hair cuticle. ***T. endothrix*** A species of *Trichophyton,* a ringworm fungus that grows from the epidermis into the hair follicle, penetrates the hair shaft, and grows downward within the hair shaft. ***T. epilans*** *TRICHOPHYTON TONSURANS.* ***T. flavum*** *TRICHOPHYTON TONSURANS.* ***T. gypseum*** *TRICHOPHYTON MENTAGROPHYTES.* ***T. interdigitale*** *TRICHOPHYTON MENTAGROPHYTES.* ***T. mentagrophytes*** The chief cause of inflammatory ringworm of feet, hands, and glabrous skin, especially intertriginous areas. It also causes chronic forms of tinea pedis and tinea cruris. It is widespread among animals, such as cattle, horses, dogs, cats and guinea pigs, and is frequently spread to humans. In the perfect (sexual) state it is classified as *Arthroderma benhamiae.* Also *Trichophyton asteroides, Trichophyton arloingi, Trichophyton gypseum, Trichophyton interdigitale, Trichophyton niveum, Trichophyton quinckeanum.* ***T. niveum*** *TRICHOPHYTON MENTAGROPHYTES.* ***T. purpureum*** *TRICHOPHYTON RUBRUM.* ***T. quinckeanum*** *TRICHOPHYTON MENTAGROPHYTES.* ***T. rubrum*** The most common cause of chronic dermatophytosis of the nails, glabrous skin areas, hands, and feet. It often can result in generalized involvement and may attack bearded areas. It is also responsible for Majocchi's granuloma, chiefly deep in hair follicles of the legs. Also *Trichophyton purpureum, Epidermophyton purpureum, Epidermophyton rubrum.* ***T. sabouraudi*** *TRICHOPHYTON TONSURANS.* ***T. schoenleinii*** A species that produces an endothrix infection of the hair and is the common cause of favus. Also *Trichophyton ceratophagus.* ***T. tonsurans*** A species of dermatophytic fungus common in Latin America and spread widely in the United States, initiating epidemic tinea capitis. It will also attack glabrous skin and, on rare occasions, infect the nails. The lesions are persistent but noninflammatory and, in contrast to ringworm caused by *Microsporum*, scalp infections are common in adults as well as children. Also *Trichophyton acuminatum, Trichophyton epilans, Trichophyton sabouraudi, Trichophyton sulfureum, Trichophyton flavum*.

**trichophytosis** \-fitō′sis\ [*Trichophyt(on)* + -OSIS] Any of the diseases caused by a member of the form-genus *Trichophyton*. **t. cruris** Tinea cruris due to a *Trichophyton* species, for example, *T. rubrum*. **t. of the glabrous skin** Tinea glabrosa due to a species of *Trichophyton*.

**Trichoptera** \trikäp′tərə\ [TRICHO- + Gk *ptera* wings] An order of insects with two pairs of mothlike wings that shed hairs, producing allergic symptoms in sensitive persons; caddis flies.

**trichoptilosis** \trik′ōtilō′sis, trikäp′ti-\ [TRICHO- + Gk *ptilōsis* (from *ptilon* soft feathers) plumage] The longitudinal splitting of the distal end of the hair shaft.

**trichorrhexis** \trik′ôrek′sis\ [TRICHO- + -RRHEXIS] An increased tendency of the hair to break. **t. invaginata** A structural defect of the hair shaft in which the shaft develops nodes that are formed by the telescoping of the shaft within itself. It is characteristic of the Netherton syndrome. Also *bamboo hair*.

**trichoschisis** \trikäs′kisis\ [TRICHO- + -SCHISIS] The presence of clean transverse fractures of the hair shafts.

**trichosiderin** \-sid′ərin\ A pigment occurring in human red hair.

**trichosis** \trikō′sis\ [TRICH- + -OSIS] Any abnormal state of the hair. **t. hirsuties** HIRSUTISM.

***Trichosoma*** \-sō′mə\ [TRICHO- + SOMA] *CAPILLARIA*.

**trichostasis spinulosa** \trikäs′təsis spin′yəlō′sə\ The retention, within a follicle, of hairs produced in successive cycles. The retained hairs are surmounted by a horny plug. Also *pinselhaare*.

**trichostrongyle** \-strän′jīl\ Of or related to the genus *Trichostrongylus*.

***Trichostrongylus*** \-strän′jələs\ [TRICHO- + Gk *strongylos* round, rounded] A genus of small roundworms (family Trichostrongylidae, suborder Strongylina), found in the intestine or the stomach of many herbivorous mammals and gallinaceous birds and sometimes called hairworms, black scour worms, or bankrupt worms. In large numbers, they are especially damaging to young animals, which develop persistent diarrhea, wasting, and anorexia. Worms of some species are known to infect man.

**trichothiodystrophy** \-thī′ōdis′trəfē\ [TRICHO- + THIO- + DYSTROPHY] An abnormality of the hair shaft in which the fine, brittle hairs show alternating light and dark zones when viewed under a polarizing microscope. The sulfur content of the hair is greatly reduced. The defect has been associated with several syndromes, including the Sabinas syndrome, and mental retardation has frequently been a related feature.

**trichotomy** \trīkät′əmē\ Division into three parts.

**trichromat** \trīkrō′mat\ One with normal (trichromatic) color vision.

**trichromatic** \trī′krōmat′ik\ **1** Involving three primary colors. Also *trichromic*. **2** Characterized by trichromatism.

**trichromatism** \trīkrō′mətizm\ [TRI- + CHROMAT- + -ISM] The normal ability of the eye to perceive three primary colors. Also *trichromatopsia*.

**trichromic** \trīkrō′mik\ TRICHROMATIC.

**trichterbrust** \trish′tərbrUst, triSH′-\ [German *Trichter* funnel, tunnel + *Brust* breast] PECTUS EXCAVATUM.

**trichuriasis** \trik′yərī′əsis\ [*Trichur(is)* + -IASIS] Infection with worms of the genus *Trichuris*, in particular *T. trichiura*. Human infections are usually asymptomatic and without peripheral eosinophilia, but occasionally, in heavy infections, severe diarrhea, bleeding, or rectal prolapse may occur, especially in young children. Also *trichocephalosis, trichocephaliasis*.

***Trichuris*** \trikyoo′ris\ [TRICH- + Gk *oura* the tail, hinder parts] A genus of intestinal nematodes in the family Trichuridae and superfamily Trichinelloidea; the whipworms. A number of species parasitize the large intestine and rectum of various mammals, such as *T. felis* in the cecum and colon of cats, *T. discolor* in cattle, *T. globulosa* in cattle, sheep, goats, and other herbivores, *T. leporis* in rabbits, *T. muris* in rats, *T. suis* in pigs, *T. vulpis* in dogs, *T. ovis* in sheep and cattle, and the medically important *T. trichiura* in humans. Also *Trichocephalus* (invalid). ***T. trichiura*** A species which is the causative agent of human trichuriasis, an infection of the cecum or large intestine. It is a worldwide human parasite, abundant in tropical regions and especially common in rural areas of poor sanitation.

**Trichuroidea** \trik′yəroi′dē·ə\ TRICHINELLOIDEA.

**tricipital** \trīsip′itəl\ **1** Pertaining to a triceps muscle. **2** TRICEPS.

**triclobisonium chloride** $C_{36}H_{74}Cl_2N_2$. Hexamethylenebis(dimethyl[1-methyl-3-(2,2,6-trimethylcyclohexyl)propyl]-ammonium)dichloride, a bacteriostatic compound used in the treatment of superficial skin infections and vaginal infections.

**triclosan** $C_{12}H_7Cl_3O_2$. 5-Chloro-2-(2,4-dichlorophenoxy)-phenol. A white, crystalline powder, practically insoluble in water. It is used as a bacteriostatic agent against Gram-positive and many Gram-negative organisms. It is contained in soaps, scrubs, and deodorants in concentrations of 0.1 to 0.2%.

**tricornute** \trīkôr′nʸoot\ Containing or consisting of three horns, or cornua, such as the lateral ventricle of the brain.

**tricresol** \trīkrē′sôl\ A mixture of *o*-, *m*-, and *p*-cresol, used for disinfection.

**tricresyl phosphate** $(CH_3C_6H_4)_3PO_4$. A colorless or pale liquid that exists in three isomeric forms, *ortho, meta*, and *para*. The *ortho* form is highly toxic and is contained in the commercial product. It is used as a plasticizer to make plastics more pliable, as a grinding medium for pigments, and in the recovery of phenol residues from gas-plant effluents. This *ortho* form (triorthocresyl phosphate) inhibits the action of the enzyme acetylcholinesterase, and it particularly inhibits pseudocholinesterase in the peripheral nerves and spinal cord. Persons poisoned by triorthocresyl phosphate experience mild gastrointestinal symptoms which are later followed by peripheral neuritis and upper motor neuron lesions with spasticity. Abbr. TCP

**tricrotic** \trīkrät′ik\ [Gk *trikrot(os)* (from *tri*-, prefix denoting three + *krot(ein)* to strike, beat) having a triple beat + -IC] Characterized by having three waves, with two on the downstroke: said of a pulse. Compare DICROTIC, MONOCROTIC.

**tricuspid** \trīkus′pid\ Having three cusps.

**tricyclamol chloride** PROCYCLIDINE METHOCHLORIDE.

**tridermic** \trīdur′mik\ [TRI- + DERM- + -IC] Describing an animal possessing three germ layers: ectoderm, mesoderm, and endoderm. The tridermic animals constitute the great majority of Metozoa, with the exception of sponges and coelenterates.

**tridigitate** \trīdij′ətāt\ [TRI- + DIGITATE] Having only three digits on a hand or foot.

**tridihexethyl chloride** $C_{21}H_{36}ClNO$. γ-Cyclohexyl-*N,N,N*-triethyl-γ-hydroxy-benzene propanaminium chloride. An anticholinergic agent with peripheral effects like those of atropine. It is used in the treatment of peptic ulcer and gastrointestinal hypermotility.

**tridymus** \trid′iməs\ [TRI- + -DYMUS] One of three triplets.

**triester** \trī′estər\ A derivative of an acid in which three of its acidic groups are esterified. An important method of nucleotide synthesis depends on making triesters of phosphoric acid.

**triethanolamine** $N(—CH_2—CH_2OH)_3$. A base used as a buffer because its p*K* of 7.8 is close to the pH of many biologic media. The three hydroxyl groups lower th p*K* to a value below that typical of tertiary amines.

**triethylenemelamine** A nitrogen mustard antineoplastic agent of limited use in the treatment of chronic leukemias but not used for acute leukemias. Also *tretamine.*

**triethylenephosphoramide** A nitrogen mustard compound from which triethylenethiophosphoramide is derived. Abbr. TEPA

**triethylenethiophosphoramide** A nitrogen mustard antineoplastic agent used against adenocarcinoma of the breast and ovary and malignant lymphomas. It produces a marked reduction of the bone marrow.

**trifid** \trī′fid\ Divided or cleft into three parts.

**trifluoperazine hydrochloride** $C_{21}H_{24}F_3N_3S \cdot 2HCl$. 10-[3-(4-Methylpiperazin-1-yl)propyl]-2-trifluoro-methylphenothiazine dihydrochloride. A phenothiazine tranquilizer with actions and uses very similar to those of chlorpromazine hydrochloride. It is given orally or parenterally as a tranquilizer for its rapid onset and prolonged effects. It is also an effective antiemetic drug.

**5-trifluoromethyldeoxyuridine** TRIFLURIDINE.

**trifluperidol hydrochloride** $C_{22}H_{24}ClF_4NO_2$. 4′-Fluoro-4-[4-hydroxy-4-(α,α,α-trifluoro-*m*-tolyl)piperidino]-butyrophenone hydrochloride. A phenothiazine tranquilizer which is given orally. It has also been used to treat highly active, manic subjects.

**triflupromazine** $C_{18}H_{19}F_3N_2S$. *N,N*-Dimethyl-2-(trifluoromethyl)-10*H*-phenothiazine-10-propanamine. A phenothiazine psychotropic drug used as a tranquilizer and antiemetic. It is usually administered as the hydrochloride salt.

**trifluridine** $C_{10}H_{11}F_3N_2O_5$. α,α,α-Trifluorothymidine. A pyrimidine nucleoside antimetabolite originally introduced as an anticancer drug but found to be effective against viruses. It is used to treat herpes simplex, types 1 and 2. It is applied topically for primary and recurrent herpes simplex keratitis and keratoconjunctivitis. Also *5-trifluoromethyldeoxyuridine.*

**trifocal** \trīfō′kəl\ [TRI- + FOCAL] Having three segments with different focal distances, for near, intermediate, and distant vision: said of spectacle lenses.

**trifurcate** \trīfur′kāt\ [TRI- + L *furc(a)* a fork + -ATE] Having three branches.

**trifurcation** \trī′fərkā′shən\ [*trifurcat(e)* + -ION] **1** A branching into three parts. **2** The region of division into separate roots of a three-rooted molar tooth.

**trigastric** \trīgas′trik\ Characterized by three bellies, as of a muscle.

**trigastricus** \trīgas′trikəs\ A variation of musculus digastricus in which the anterior belly is either doubled or has an extra slip.

**trigeminal** \trījem′inəl\ **1** Having three roots or origins. **2** Denoting the fifth cranial nerve or nervus trigeminus.

**trigeminus** \trījem′inəs\ [L, threefold, triple] Denoting the fifth cranial nerve, or nervus trigeminus.

**trigeminy** \trījem′inē\ [L *trigemin(us),* also *tergeminus* triple + -Y] A disorder of cardiac rhythm in which heart beats or pulses occur in threes. It may be due to a sinus beat with two premature beats following it, or to two sinus beats followed by one premature beat. After a pause, the rhythm repeats itself.

**triglyceride** A triacylglycerol; a fat.

**trigon** \trī′gōn\ TRIGONE.

**trigona** \trīgō′nə\ Plural of TRIGONUM.

**trigonal** \trī′gōnəl\ **1** Of or relating to a trigone. **2** TRIANGULAR.

**trigone** \trī′gōn\ [French (from Gk *trigōnon* a triangle, from *tri-* prefix denoting three + *gōnia* a corner, angle), presenting three angles] **1** TRIANGLE. **2** The three main cusps, namely, protocone, paracone, and metacone, viewed as a unit in the upper molars of mammals. Also *trigon.* **t. of bladder** TRIGONUM VESICAE. **carotid t.** TRIGONUM CAROTICUM. **cerebral t.** FORNIX CEREBRI. **collateral t.** TRIGONUM COLLATERALE. **collateral t. of fourth ventricle** TRIGONUM NERVI VAGI. **femoral t.** TRIGONUM FEMORALE. **t. of the fillet** TRIGONUM LEMNISCI. **t. of the habenula** TRIGONUM HABENULAE. **habenular t.** TRIGONUM HABENULAE. **Henke's t.** TRIGONUM INGUINALE. **t. of hypoglossal nerve** TRIGONUM NERVI HYPOGLOSSI. **iliopectineal t.** FOSSA ILIOPECTINEA. **inguinal t.** TRIGONUM INGUINALE. **interpeduncular t.** FOSSA INTERPEDUNCULARIS. **t. of lateral ventricle** TRIGONUM COLLATERALE. **left fibrous t. of heart** TRIGONUM FIBROSUM SINISTRUM. **Lieutaud's t.** TRIGONUM VESICAE. **lumbar t.** TRIGONUM LUMBALE. **olfactory t.** TRIGONUM OLFACTORIUM. **omoclavicular t.** TRIGONUM OMOCLAVICULARE. **Pawlik's t.** PAWLIK'S TRIANGLE. **t. of Reil** TRIGONUM LEMNISCI. **right fibrous t. of heart** TRIGONUM FIBROSUM DEXTRUM. **submandibular t.** TRIGONUM SUBMANDIBULARE. **urogenital t.** REGIO UROGENITALIS. **t. of vagus nerve** TRIGONUM NERVI VAGI. **vesical t.** TRIGONUM VESICAE.

**trigonectomy** \trī′gōnek′təmē\ [*trigon(um vesicae)* + -ECTOMY] Surgical removal of the trigonum vesicae, the base of the urinary bladder.

**trigonelline** *N*-Methylpyridinium-3-carboxylate. A substance derived by methylation of nicotinic acid. It is found in urine and is one end-product of the catabolism of nicotinamide coenzymes.

**trigonid** \trīgän′id\ [*trigon(e)* + -ID[2]] The three main cusps, viewed as a unit, in the lower molars of mammals.

**trigonitis** \trig′ənī′tis\ [*trigon(um vesicae)* + -ITIS] Inflammation localized at the bladder trigone (trigonum vesicae), producing an edematous and sometimes bulbous appearance of the mucosa of the trigone. **senile t.** The squamous transformation of areas of transitional epithelium on the female trigone associated with atrophy of this squamous epithelium presumably due to lack of estrogen.

**trigonocephaly** \trig′ənōsef′əlē\ [Gk *trigōno(s)* triangular + CEPHAL- + -Y] A developmentally abnormal head in which the skull acquires a more or less triangular configuration owing to premature synostosis of cranial bones. The cerebral hemispheres tend to be compressed.

**trigonum** \trīgō′nəm\ [L (from Gk *trigōnon* a triangle; see TRIGONE), a triangle] [NA] TRIANGLE. **t. acustici** AREA VESTIBULARIS. **t. caroticum** [NA] A subdivision of the anterior triangle of the neck, which is bounded anteroinferiorly by the superior belly of the omohyoid muscle, posteriorly by the sternocleidomastoid muscle, and superiorly by the posterior belly of the digastric muscle and the stylohyoid muscle. It contains the upper part of the common carotid artery and its terminal branches. Also *carotid triangle,* *carotid trigone, triangle of election, Malgaigne's triangle.* **t. cerebrale** FORNIX CEREBRI. **t. collaterale** [NA] A flattened triangular area that forms the floor of the lateral ventricle between the posterior and inferior horns. Also *trigone of lateral ventricle, trigonum ventriculi lateralis, collateral trigone.* **t. collaterale ventriculi quarti** TRIGONUM NERVI VAGI. **t. femorale** [NA] An area of the groin that is bounded by the medial edge of the sartorius muscle laterally, the medial edge of the adductor longus muscle medially, and the inguinal ligament superiorly. Also *femoral triangle, Scarpa's triangle, femoral trigone, greater fossa of Scarpa.* **t. fibrosum dextrum** [NA] A large mass of fibrous tissue situated at the base of the heart between the aortic arterial ring anteriorly and the atrioventricular rings posteriorly. It is part of the fibrous skeleton of the heart. Also *right fibrous trigone of heart.* **t. fibrosum sinistrum** [NA] A small mass of fibrous tissue situated at the base of the heart between the left posterior side of the aortic arterial ring and the front of the left atrioventricular ring. It is part of the fibrous skeleton of the heart. Also *left fibrous trigone of heart.* **t. habenulae** [NA] A small pyramidal region, the base of which forms a depressed triangular area situated on the lateral aspect of the posterior part of the third ventricle. It contains the medial and lateral habenular nuclei, and receives fibers from the stria medullaris thalami. Also *trigonum habenularis, trigone of the habenula, habenular trigone.* **t. hypoglossale** TRIGONUM NERVI HYPOGLOSSI. **t. hypoglossi** TRIGONUM NERVI HYPOGLOSSI. **t. inguinale** [NA] The triangular area on the internal surface of the lower part of the anterior abdominal wall. It is bounded by the inguinal ligament inferiorly, the lateral margin of the rectus abdominis muscle medially, and the inferior epigastric vessels laterally. It is the site of direct inguinal hernia. Also *inguinal trigone, inguinal triangle, Hesselbach's triangle, Henke's trigone, Henke's triangle.* **t. interpedunculare** FOSSA INTERPEDUNCULARIS. **t. lemnisci** [NA] A triangular area on the dorsal surface of the lower mesencephalon bounded inferiorly by a line along the site of attachment of the superior cerebellar peduncle with the mesencephalon, superiorly by the inferior colliculus and the brachium of the inferior colliculus, and laterally by the lateral mesencephalic sulcus. Within the triangle, the fibers of the lateral lemniscus approach the surface of the mesencephalic tectum. Also *trigone of the fillet, trigone of Reil, Reil's triangle.* **t. lumbale** [NA] A triangular area, variable in size, between the free posterior margin of the external oblique muscle of the abdomen, the lower lateral margin of the latissimus dorsi muscle, and the iliac crest. In this area the internal oblique muscle forms the floor and is subcutaneous. Also *lumbar triangle, lumbar trigone, Petit's triangle, Petit's lumbar triangle.* **t. musculare** [NA] One of the subdivisions of the anterior triangle of the neck. It is bounded by the midline anteriorly, the anterior margin of the sternocleidomastoid muscle posteroinferiorly, and the superior belly of the omohyoid muscle posterosuperiorly. Also *inferior carotid triangle, muscular triangle, triangle of necessity, tracheal triangle.* **t. nervi hypoglossi** [NA] A triangular area in the caudal part of the floor of the fourth ventricle, located just lateral to the median sulcus on the surface of the median eminence. Deep to the medial part of the triangle is located the rostal part of the hypoglossal nucleus, while deep to its lateral part is found the nucleus intercalatus. Also *trigonum hypoglossi, trigonum hypoglossale, hypoglossal triangle, trigone of hypoglossal nerve, eminentia hypoglossi, hypoglossal eminence, tuberculum hypoglossi, internal white wing.* **t. nervi vagi** [NA] A dark or ashen-colored area in the floor of the fourth ventricle that overlies the dorsal motor nucleus of the vagus nerve and is located caudal to the inferior fovea and just lateral to the hypoglossal trigone. Also *trigonum vagi, trigonum collaterale ventriculi quarti, collateral trigone of fourth ventricle, ala cinerea, eminentia vagi* (imprecise), *trigone of vagus nerve, vagal eminence, vagus area, eminentia cinerea cuneiformis, ashlike wing.* **t. olfactorium** [NA] A triangular area formed by the diverging bundles of the olfactory tract and located at the most caudal part of that tract immediately rostral to the anterior perforated substance. From the olfactory trigone course the olfactory tract fibers that form the medial, intermediate, and lateral olfactory striae. Also *olfactory pyramid, olfactory, trigone, caruncula mammillaris* (outmoded). **t. omoclaviculare** [NA] One of the two subdivisions of the regio cervicalis lateralis, which is bounded inferiorly by the middle third of the clavicle, superiorly by the inferior belly of the omohyoid muscle, and anteriorly by the posterior margin of the sternocleidomastoid muscle. Its floor is formed by the first rib, an origin of the serratus anterior muscle, and the insertion of the scalenus medius muscle, and it is crossed by the third part of the subclavian artery partly surrounded by the brachial plexus. Also *omoclavicular triangle, omoclavicular trigone, subclavian triangle, greater supraclavicular fossa, supraclavicular region.* **t. sternocostale** MORGAGNI'S FORAMEN. **t. submandibulare** [NA] The subdivision of the regio cervicalis anterior that is bounded by the base of the mandible superiorly and the anterior and posterior bellies of the digastric muscle inferiorly. Its floor is formed by the hyoglossus and mylohyoid muscles. Included in its contents are the submandibular salivary gland and the facial vein and artery. Also *submandibular trigone, submandibular triangle, digastric triangle, submandibular region.* **t. submentale** [NA] One of the triangles of the anterior cervical region which is situated in the midline and bounded on each side by the anterior belly of the digastric muscle, the base being the body of the hyoid bone. Its apex is at the mandible and its floor is formed by the mylohyoid muscle. It contains the submental lymph nodes and small veins. Also *submental triangle, submental region.* **t. vagi** TRIGONUM NERVI VAGI. **t. ventriculi lateralis** TRIGONUM COLLATERALE. **t. vesicae** [NA] A smooth triangular area on the interior of the base of the urinary bladder where the mucous membrane is firmly attached to the underlying muscle layer. Its apex, or anteroinferior angle, is the internal urethral orifice. Its posterolateral angles receive the orifices of the ureters, between which stretches the interureteric fold forming the superior border, or base. Also *trigone of bladder, Lieutaud's trigone, Lieutaud's triangle, vesical triangle, vesical trigone, Lieutaud's body.*

**trihexyphenidyl hydrochloride** $C_{20}H_{32}ClNO$. α-Cyclohexyl-α-phenyl-1-piperidinepropanol hydrochloride. An anticholinergic drug like atropine but weaker in its activity. It is used in the treatment of parkinsonism and extrapyramidal syndrome induced by drugs like reserpine or the phenothiazines. It is given orally. Also *benzhexol hydrochloride.*

**trihydroxyestrin** ESTRIOL.

**triiodomethane** IODOFORM.

**triiodothyronine** L-3,5,3′-Triiodothyronine, one of the two principal hormones secreted by the thyroid gland, the other being thyroxine. It is secreted in excess in the hyperthyroidism of Graves disease, but disproportionately or uniquely increased in $T_3$-toxicosis. It is believed by some to be the tissue-active form of thyroid hormone, thyroxine serving as a peripheral precursor through deiodination. It is used pharmaceutically in the $T_3$ suppression test for thyroid function, and in the treatment of myxedema coma. Symbol: $T_3$ **reverse t.** 3,3′,5′-triiodothyronine, an iodinated thyronine found in human and animal serum, at a concentration averaging 40 ng/100 ml in normal persons. The hormone, having a short half-life and almost no calorigenic activity, is secreted to a small extent by the thyroid, but most of it arises from the peripheral deiodination of thyroxine. Serum concentration is low in hypothyroidism, raised in hyperthyroidism. Symbol: $rT_3$

**triketohydrindene hydrate** *Obs.* NINHYDRIN.

**trilaminar** \trīlam′inər\ Comprising three layers.

**trilobate** \trīlō′bāt\ Possessing three lobes. Also *trilobed.*

**trilocular** \trīläk′yələr\ Having three compartments, chambers, or cells.

**trilogy** \tril′əjē\ Any series or combination of three entities or items. **t. of Fallot** The combination of cardiac developmental defects, consisting of atrial septal defect, pulmonary stenosis, and right ventricular hypertrophy, in distinction from the tetralogy of Fallot which additionally includes dextroposition of the aorta.

**trimagnesium phosphate** TRIBASIC MAGNESIUM PHOSPHATE.

***Trimastigamoeba*** \trīmas′tigəmē′bə\ A genus of amebas (order Schizopyrenida, subclass Gymnamoebia, class Lobosea) commonly found in stagnant water, and characterized by having an ameboid stage and a flagellate stage in the life cycle. The species *T. philippinensis* has been found in human sewage. The organism moves quickly by eruptive anterior waves of pseudopodia. It feeds on bacteria, produces oval cysts (about 13×10 μm), and has four anterior flagella in its flagellate stage.

**trimastigote** \trīmas′tigōt\ [TRI- + MASTIGOTE] **1** Having three flagella. **2** A protozoan organism with three flagella.

**trimeprazine tartrate** A phenothiazine drug with antipruritic properties. It has antihistaminic activity but it causes drowsiness, and this side effect limits its usefulness.

**trimer** \trī′mər\ A molecular structure composed of three subunits.

***Trimeresurus*** \trim′ərəsoo′rəs\ A genus of venomous snakes of the family Viperidae, subfamily Crotalinae; the habus, or tree vipers. They have prehensile tail. They are found in southeastern Asia.

**trimeric** \trimer′ik\ Composed of three subunits.

**trimester** \trīmes′tər\ A period of three months. **first t.** The first three months of a human pregnancy. **second t.** The middle three months of a human pregnancy. **third t.** The last three months of a human pregnancy.

**trimethadione** 3,5,5-Trimethyloxazolidine-2,4-dione. An anticonvulsant drug that is used only for the treatment of petit mal seizures. It is generally reserved for patients refractory to other drugs. Also *troxidone.*

**trimethaphan camsylate** $C_{32}H_{40}N_2O_5S_2$. Decahydro-2-oxo-1,3-bis(phenylmethyl)thieno[1′,2′:1,2]thieno[3,4]imidazzol-5-ium salt with (+)-7,7-dimethyl-2-oxobicyclo-[2.2.1]heptane-1-methanesulfonic acid (1:1). A short-acting ganglionic blocking agent which must be given by continuous intravenous infusion to keep the blood pressure reduced. It is used for the initial period of control to reduce blood pressure quickly.

**trimethobenzamide hydrochloride** $C_{21}H_{29}ClN_2O_5$. *N*-[(2-Dimethylaminolthoxy)benzyl]- 3,4,5-trimethoxybenzamide hydrochloride. An antiemetic agent useful in radiation sickness but not against motion sickness. It is given usually by intramuscular injection because of unpredictable absorption when given orally.

**trimethoprim** 2,4-Diamino-5-(3,4,5-trimethoxybenzyl)-pyrimidine. An effective antibacterial and antimalarial agent. It is a potent inhibitor of bacterial and protozoal dihydrofolate reductase, with much less action against the corresponding mammalian tissue enzyme.

**trimethoprim and sulfamethoxazole** A combination of five parts sulfamethoxazole and one part trimethoprim. These agents are more effective together as an antibacterial medication, particularly for urinary tract infections. The combination is also used to treat otitis media.

**trimethylene** CYCLOPROPANE.

**trimipramine maleate** $C_{20}H_{26}N_2,C_4H_4O_4$. A tricyclic antidepressant drug with actions very similar to those of imipramine, except for greater antihistaminic and sedative effects.

**trimorphic** \trīmôr′fik\ TRIMORPHOUS.

**trimorphism** \trīmôr′fizm\ [TRI- + MORPH- + -ISM] Existence in three (postembryonic) forms in the course of a life cycle, as exemplified by holometabolous insects, which appear successively as larvae, pupae, and adults.

**trimorphous** \trīmôr′fəs\ [TRI- + MORPH- + -OUS] Existing in three forms; characterized by trimorphism. Also *trimorphic.*

**trineural** \trīnʸUr′əl\ Referring to three nerves. *Seldom used.*

**trineuric** \trīnʸUr′ik\ Referring to three nerve cells or three nerves. *Rare.*

**trinitrin** NITROGLYCERIN.

**trinitroglycerin** NITROGLYCERIN.

**trinitroglycerol** NITROGLYCERIN.

**trinitrol** ERYTHRITYL TETRANITRATE.

**trinitrotoluene** 2,4,6-Trinitrotoluene. A pale yellow, crystalline solid that is an easily detonated explosive. Also *trotyl.* Abbr. TNT

**trinomial** \trīnō′mē·əl\ [TRI- + L *nomen* (gen. *nominis*) a name + -AL] A taxonomic designation comprising three names, the third being a subspecific epithet.

**trinucleotide** \trīnʸoo′klē·ətīd′\ **1** TRIPLET. **2** Any three nucleotides or deoxynucleotides covalently linked in a linear array.

**triocephalus** \trī′əsef′ələs\ [TRI- + *o* + -CEPHALUS] A fetus or newborn infant with a severely malformed head having no mouth, nose, or eyes. The head is small and rounded and contains very little brain.

**triophthalmos** \trī′äfthal′məs\ [TRI- + Gk *ophthalmos* eye] Equal conjoined twins with a single body but with two heads united side by side so that they share a single eye in the region of fusion but have two normal-appearing eyes on the free sides of the respective faces.

**triorchid** \trī·ôr′kid\ [TRI- + *orchid(os),* erroneous form for gen. of Gk *orchis,* gen. *orchios,* testicle] An individual with three testes.

**triose** \trī′ōs\ [TRI- + -OSE[2]] A sugar containing three carbon atoms in its molecule. Two such sugars exist, glyceraldehyde and glycerone (dihydroxyacetone).

**triose kinase** An enzyme (EC 2.7.1.28) which catalyzes the phosphorylation of glyceraldehyde to glyceraldehyde 3-phosphate with concomitant conversion of adenosine triphosphate to adenosine diphosphate.

**triose phosphate** Either of the two triose phosphates in the glycolytic pathway, glyceraldehyde 3-phosphate or glycerone phosphate (dihydroxyacetone phosphate). Also *phosphotriose.*

**triose-phosphate isomerase** The enzyme (EC 5.3.1.1) that catalyzes the interconversion of glyceraldehyde 3-phosphate and glycerone phosphate. A carboxyl group in the enzyme removes a hydrogen ion from either substrate to form an intermediate enediol. The enzyme works very rapidly, approaching the rate limited by diffusional encounters with its substrates. The reaction is a step in the glycolytic pathway.

**triotus** \trī-ō′təs\ [TRI- + OT- + New L *-us*, masc. sing. noun suffix] A diprosopus with a single body but with two incompletely formed heads united side by side so that a single ear structure is present in the area of union and two normal-appearing ears are visible on the free aspects.

**trioxsalen** $C_{14}H_{12}O_3$. 4,5′, 8-Trimethylpsoralen. It is used orally as a pigmentation agent in the treatment of vitiligo.

**tripalmitin** The fat, i.e. triacylglycerol, whose molecules consist of glycerol acylated on each of its hydroxyl groups by palmitic acid.

**tripara** \trip′ərə\ [TRI- + PARA] A woman who has had three pregnancies carried to the stage of viability, regardless of whether the fetus was born dead or alive or whether the gestation was single or multiple. See also PARA.

**tripartite** \trīpär′tīt\ Being in three parts.

**tripelennamine** $C_{16}H_{21}N_3$. *N,N*-Dimethyl-*N′*-(phenylmethyl)-*N′*-2-pyridinyl-1,2-ethanediamine. An effective antihistaminic agent less potent than promethazine. It is short acting and causes less drowsiness and sedation. It is generally given orally as the hydrochloride or citrate, and has been used parenterally as the hydrochloride.

**tripelennamine citrate** $C_{16}H_{21}N_3{\cdot}C_6H_8O_7$. The citrate salt form of tripelennamine. It is a white, crystalline powder, and is given orally as an antihistamine agent in the treatment of allergic disorders.

**tripelennamine hydrochloride** $C_{16}H_{21}N_3{\cdot}HCl$. The monohydrochloride form of tripelennamine. It acts as a histamine antagonist and is used in the treatment of allergic responses to many substances. It is given orally, topically, or parenterally.

**triphalangia** \trī′fəlan′jē·ə\ [TRI- + *phalang(es)*, pl. of PHALANX + -IA] Having three phalanges per digit, a condition which is abnormal in the thumb and great toe of humans.

**tripharmacon** A pharmaceutic preparation containing three drugs. Also *tripharmacum*.

**triphenylchlorethylene** $C_{20}H_{15}Cl$. 1,1,2-Triphenyl-2-chlorostilbene, a synthetic estrogen resembling diethystilbestrol.

**triphenylethylene** $C_{20}H_{16}$. $\alpha$-Phenyl-stilbene, a synthetic estrogen, not related to natural C-18 estrogens, but somewhat similar to diethylstilbestrol.

**triphosphoric acid** $H_5P_3O_{10}$. An acid resulting from the condensation of three molecules of orthophosphoric acid with elimination of two molecules of water. Its monoesters with nucleosides are biologically important.

**triplegia** \trīplē′jə\ [TRI- + -PLEGIA] Hemiplegia combined with paralysis of one limb on the opposite side of the body.

**triplet** 1 Any association of three members. 2 One of three fetuses or infants delivered as the product of a single gestation. 3 Designating the electronic state of a molecule when it has two electrons of parallel spin. The spin angular momentum couples vectorially with the orbital angular momentum in three possible ways. Atoms with paired electrons may be excited by electromagnetic radiation, usually ultraviolet or visible, by promotion of one electron from the pair in one orbital to an orbital of higher energy. After this event the spins remain parallel and the atom is in a short-lived singlet state. If it passes over from this excited singlet state into a triplet state its lifetime is prolonged, and it may then exhibit phosphorescence or photochemical reaction. 4 The group of three residues in DNA or mRNA that specify a single amino-acid residue in a protein. Also *trinucleotide*.

**triplex** \trip′leks, trī′pleks\ Having three.

**triploblastic** \trip′ləblas′tik\ [Gk *triplo(os)* triple + BLAST- + -IC] 1 Referring to the three embryonic layers: ectoderm, mesoderm, and endoderm. 2 Describing an animal having various parts derived from these three layers.

**triploid** \trip′loid\ [TRI- + -PLOID] Having three sets of chromosomes.

**triploidy** \trip′loidē\ [TRI- + -PLOID + -Y] The condition in an organism of having three sets of chromosomes in its cells.

**triplopia** \triplō′pē·ə\ [Gk *tripl(oos)* triple + -OPIA] The seeing of three images of a single object. Also *triple vision, visus triplex*.

**tripod** \trī′päd\ [Gk *tripous* (gen. *tripodos*, from TRI- + *pous*, gen. *podos*, a foot) a tripod] 1 Having three legs. 2 An object or animal with three legs.

**tripodia** \trīpō′dē·ə\ [TRIPOD + -IA] A condition seen in equal conjoined twins when there is side-to-side union of the trunks so that they share one lower extremity while each trunk has a normal-appearing lower limb on its free side.

**triprolidine hydrochloride** $C_{19}H_{22}N_2{\cdot}HClH_2O$. (*E*)-2[1-(4-Methylphenyl)-3-(1-pyrrolidinyl)-1-propenyl]-pyridine monohydrochloride monohydrate. An antihistaminic agent used in the treatment of certain allergic responses. It is given orally.

**triprosopus** \trī′prōsō′pəs\ [New L, from TRI- + Gk *prosōpon* face] A fetus or newborn infant with a single body but a malformed head on which there are three recognizable facial areas.

**tripsis** \trip′sis\ [Gk (from *tribein* to rub) rubbing, friction, wear and tear] 1 TRITURATION. 2 Rubbing; massage.

**-tripsy** \-trip′sē\ [*trips(is)* + -Y] A combining form meaning the act of crushing, especially in a surgical operation.

**tripus** \trī′pəs\ [New L, from Gk *tripous* three-footed, three-legged] Conjoined twin fetuses or newborn individuals with tripodia.

**triquetral** \trīkwē′trəl\ 1 TRIQUETROUS. 2 Pertaining to the os triquetrum.

**triquetrous** \trīkwē′trəs\ [L *triquetrus* (from *tri-* three- + a stem meaning pointed) three-cornered, three-pointed] Three-cornered; triangular. Also *triquetral*.

**triquetrum** \trīkwē′trəm\ [neuter sing. of *triquetrus*. See TRIQUETROUS.] OS TRIQUETRUM.

**triradius** \trīrā′dē·əs\ A dermatoglyphic point from which dermal ridges diverge in three directions at approximately 120° to each other.

**TRIS** Tris(hydroxymethyl)aminomethane; a buffer used to correct metabolic acidosis.

**trismic** \triz′mik\ Relating to or having the characteristics of trismus.

**trismoid** \triz′moid\ [*trism(us)* + -OID] *Obs.* TRISMUS NEONATORUM. • This term was once used for neonatal trismus erroneously thought to be due to cerebral birth injury.

**trismus** \tris′məs, triz′-\ [Gk *trismos* (from *trizein* to squeak, grate) a squeaking, grating] Spasm or contracture of the masticatory muscles, making it difficult to open the mouth, most commonly in peritonsillar abscess. This is an important early manifestation of tetanus, but there are many other causes as well, including dental disease, as pericoronitis, and hysteria. Also *masticatory spasm, lockjaw, locked jaw*. Adj. trismic. **t. cynicus** RISUS SARDONICUS. **t. dolorificus** TRIGEMINAL NEURALGIA. **t. neonatorum** Trismus in neonates due to neonatal tetanus. Also *trismus nascentium, trismoid* (obs.). **t. sardonicus** RISUS SARDONICUS.

**trisomic** \trīsō′mik\ Marked by trisomy.

**trisomy** \trī′sōmē\ A state of aneuploidy in a diploid cell or organism in which one chromosome is present in three copies. It is usually a result of nondisjunction.

**trisplanchnic** \trīsplangk′nik\ Of or relating to the cavities and organs of the skull, thorax, and abdomen. *Outmoded.*

**trisporic acids** A group of terpenoid $C_{18}$ carboxylic acids produced by the fungus *Blakeslea trispora.* It stimulates carotene synthesis in this species, and stimulates reproductive activity in *Mucor mucedo.*.

**tristichia** \trīstik′ē·ə\ [TRI- + Gk *stich(os)* a row, line + -IA] The state of possessing three rows of eyelashes on a lid.

**tristimania** \tris′timā′nē·ə\ [L *tristi(s)* sad + -MANIA] MELANCHOLIA.

**trisulcate** \trīsul′kāt\ Having three sulci.

**trisulfapyrimidines** Tablets containing sulfadiazine, sulfadimidine, and sulfamerazine in equal amounts, given as a mixture to decrease the chances of precipitation in the urinary tract.

**tritanomaly** \trī′tənäm′əlē\ Color blindness in which the sensory mechanisms for blue and yellow are defective. It occurs both as an autosomal dominant and as a less severe X-linked trait.

**tritanope** \trī′tənōp\ [Gk *trit(os)* third + *an-* priv. + -OPE] A person unable to discern blue colors.

**tritanopia** \trī′tənō′pē·ə\ [Gk *trit(os)* third + *an-* priv. + -OPIA] Inability to discern blue colors. Also *tritanopsia.* Adj. tritanopic.

**tritanopsia** \trī′tənäp′sē·ə\ TRITANOPIA.

**triticeum** \trītis′ē·əm\ CARTILAGO TRITICEA.

**tritium** \trit′ē·əm\ The radioactive isotope of hydrogen, having atomic mass 3. Its half-life is 12.3 years. Also *radioactive hydrogen, hydrogen 3.* Symbol: $^3H$

**tritocone** \trī′təkōn\ [Gk *trito(s)* third + *kōn(os)* cone] The distobuccal cusp of a maxillary premolar tooth.

**tritoconid** \trī′təkō′nid\ [*tritocon(e)* + -ID[2]] The distobuccal cusp of a mandibular premolar tooth.

**triton** \trī′tän\ The nucleus of a tritium atom, sometimes given the symbol t.

**tritubercular** \trī′tʸūbur′kyələr\ Having three tubercules or cusps.

**triturable** \trit′yərəbl\ Capable of being triturated.

**triturate** \trit′yərāt\ **1** To rub and grind to obtain a powder. **2** A substance that has been triturated. **tablet t.** A tablet made from a medicated powder that has been rubbed with lactose and triturated.

**trituration** \trit′yərā′shən\ [Late L *trituratio* (from *tritura* a threshing, treading, from *terere* to rub, grind, thresh) a rubbing, threshing, treading] The conversion of a solid to a powder by rubbing and grinding, usually with a mortar and pestle. Also *tripsis.*

**triturator** \trit′yərā′tər\ A mechanical device for triturating dental alloy and mercury, usually an oscillating capsule containing a steel ball.

**trizonal** \trīzō′nəl\ Arranged in three zones or layers.

**tRNA** transfer RNA.

**trocar** \trō′kär\ [French *trocart,* from *trois quarts* three quarters] A hollow, cylindrical instrument with a sharp tip that is designed to pierce the wall of a body cavity, organ, or hollow structure, usually to drain or infuse liquid. **Durham's t.** A trocar used as an introducer for Durham's tube, necessarily made on the same lobster-tail principle. **Lichtwitz t.** A straight trocar, fitted to a handle, for introducing a cannula into the maxillary sinus to permit irrigation of the sinus. **piloting t.** The introducer of a tracheostomy tube. **rectal t.** A curved trocar designed to drain the urinary bladder through the rectum.

**troch.** trochiscus (lozenge).

**trochanter** \trōkan′tər\ [Gk *trochantēr* (prob. akin to *trochos* wheel and *trechein* to run) a trochanter] Either of the two bony prominences at the upper end of the femur lateral to and below its neck. **greater t.** TROCHANTER MAJOR. **lesser t.** TROCHANTER MINOR. **t. major** [NA] A large quadrangular process that overhangs the junction of the shaft and neck of the femur. Its anterior and lateral surfaces provide attachment for the gluteus minimus and medius muscles, respectively, whereas the superior and medial aspects provide attachment for the short lateral rotators of the hip joint, namely, the piriform, the obturator internus, and the two gemelli and obturator externus muscles. Also *greater trochanter.* **t. minor** [NA] A medially directed conical projection at the posteromedial aspect of the junction of the neck with the shaft of the femur. It provides insertion for the iliopsoas muscle, the iliacus portion of which extends down the shaft below. Also *lesser trochanter.* **t. tertius** [NA] An occasional unusually prominent gluteal tuberosity, especially the portion opposite the lesser trochanter. It is usually found as a large prominence in many quadrupedal mammals. Also *third trochanter.*

**trochanteric** \trō′kanter′ik\ Of or relating to a trochanter. Also *trochanterian.*

**trochanteritis** \trōkan′tərī′tis\ An inflammation around the greater trochanter. It often involves the trochanteric bursa.

**trochanterplasty** \trōkan′tərplas′tē\ A surgical refashioning of the greater trochanter to form a new femoral neck.

**troche** \trō′kē, trōsh\ LOZENGE.

**trochin** \trō′kin\ *Outmoded* TUBERCULUM MINUS HUMERI.

**trochinian** \trōkin′ē·ən\ Pertaining to the tuberculum minus humeri.

**trochiscation** \trō′kiskā′shən\ The production of troches from fine powders obtained by elutration.

**trochiscus** \trōkis′kəs\ LOZENGE. Abbr. troch.

**trochlea** \träk′lē·ə\ [L (from Gk *trochileia,* from *trochos* a wheel) a pulley, pulley block] An anatomic part or structure that resembles a pulley, either in form, as that of the humerus or talus, or in function, as that of the superior oblique muscle of the eye. **t. humeri** [NA] The pulley-like grooved surface of the condyle at the distal end of the humerus that articulates with the trochlear notch of the ulna. Also *trochlea of humerus.* **t. muscularis** [NA] An anchored loop of connective tissue, either fibrous or fibrocartilaginous, through which a tendon passes to change its direction. Also *muscular trochlea, pulley.* **t. musculi obliqui superioris bulbi** [NA] The fibrocartilaginous loop attached to the trochlear fovea or spine on the orbital part of the frontal bone, through which the tendon of the superior oblique muscle passes. Also *trochlea of superior oblique muscle.* **t. peronealis calcanei** [NA] An eminence or ridge of variable size found near the anterior part of the lateral surface of the calcaneus. Located about one inch below the lateral malleolus, it is grooved posteroinferiorly by the peroneus longus tendon and anterosuperiorly by the peroneus brevis tendon. Also *peroneal trochlea of calcaneus, peroneal tubercle of calcaneus, trochlear process of calcaneus, peroneal spine of os calcis, lateral process of calcaneus.* **t. of superior oblique muscle** TROCHLEA MUSCULI OBLIQUI SUPERIORIS BULBI. **t. tali** [NA] The superior articular surface of the body of the talus for articulation with the tibia in the ankle joint. On each side its malleolar surfaces articulate with the medial and lateral malleolus of the tibia and fibula, respectively. Also *trochlea of talus.*

**trochlear** \träk′lē·ər\ **1** Of or relating to a trochlea. **2** Resembling a pulley.

**trochleariform** \träk′lē·ar′ifôrm\ In the shape of a pulley.

**trochlearis** \träk′lē·ar′is\ Trochlear.

**trochocephalia** \trō′kōsəfā′lyə\ TROCHOCEPHALY.

**trochocephaly** \trō′kəsef′əlē\ [Gk *trocho(s)* anything round or circular + CEPHAL- + -Y] A more than usually rounded contour of the head resulting from premature synostosis of the frontal and parietal bones.

**trochoid** \trō′koid\ Permitting rotation, as a wheel, pivot, or pulley.

**trochoides** \trōkoi′dēz\ ARTICULATIO TROCHOIDEA.

**Troisier** [Charles Emile *Troisier,* French physician, 1844–1919] Troisier's node, Troisier sign, lymph node of Troisier. See under SENTINEL NODE.

**troland** \trō′lənd\ [after Leonard Thompson *Troland,* 1889–1932, U.S. physicist] The unit of illumination upon the retina resulting from entry of one candela square meter through one square millimeter of pupil. Also *luxon.*

**Trolard** [Paulin *Trolard,* French anatomist, 1842–1910] **1** Trolard's net, Trolard's plexus. See under PLEXUS VENOSUS CANALIS HYPOGLOSSI. **2** Trolard's vein, anterior anastomotic vein of Trolard. See under VENA ANASTOMOTICA SUPERIOR.

**troleandomycin** The triacetyl ester of oleandomycin. It has antibiotic activity against *Streptococcus pyogenes* and *Diplococcus pneumoniae.* Because of the high incidence of hypersensitivity reactions associated with its use, it is reserved for patients sensitive to the more commonly used antibiotics. Also *triacetyloleandomycin.*

**trolnitrate phosphate** $C_6H_{18}N_4O_{17}P_2$. 2,2′,2″-Nitrilotrisethanol trinitrate(ester) phosphate (1:2) (salt). An organic nitrate given orally to decrease the number and severity of anginal attacks.

***Trombicula*** \trämbik′yələ\ A genus of mites of the family Trombiculidae, the larvae of which are commonly known as chiggers or red bugs. Larval forms are serious pests and transmit various rickettsial and possibly viral diseases to man and other animals. A number of medically important species originally included in this genus are now often referred to by subgeneric or separate generic names. See also *LEPTOTROMBIDIUM.* ***T. akamushi*** See under *LEPTOTROMBIDIUM.* ***T. alfreddugesi*** A species common in North America, especially in grassy brush areas of the southeastern United States. The larvae (chiggers) attack humans and a wide range of domestic and wild mammals, birds, reptiles, and some amphibians. In humans they cause an itching dermatitis, particularly in sensitized individuals. The species is included in the subgenus *Eutrombicula,* which is regarded by some as a separate genus. Also *Eutrombicula alfreddugesi, Trombicula irritans.* ***T. autumnalis*** The harvest mite, found in Europe in autumn. Its larvae cause skin lesions in humans and other animals. ***T. deliensis*** See under *LEPTOTROMBIDIUM.* ***T. fletcheri*** See under *LEPTOTROMBIDIUM.* ***T. irritans*** *TROMBICULA ALFREDDUGESI.* ***T. pallida*** See under *LEPTOTROMBIDIUM.* ***T. scutellaris*** See under *LEPTOTROMBIDIUM.*

**trombiculiasis** \trämbik′yəlī′əsis\ [*Trombicul(a)* + -IASIS] Infestation by mite larvae of the genus *Trombicula* or *Leptotrombidium..* Also *trombiculosis, trombidiiasis* (outmoded), *trombidiosis* (outmoded).

**trombiculid** \trämbik′yəlid\ **1** Of or belonging to the family Trombiculidae. **2** A mite of the family Trombiculidae.

**Trombiculidae** \träm′bikyoo′lidē\ [*Trombicul(a)* + -IDAE] A family of mites, commonly called chiggers during the larval stages when they feed on vertebrates. The larval stage is normally seen, while the free-living, bright red, velvety, figure-8-shaped adults of many species have not been correlated with their parasitic larval stages. Some 300 species have been described. The medically important genus *Trombicula* has been divided into several subgenera, including *Eutrombicula* and *Neotrombicula* in North America. Other important genera include *Euschoengastia, Schoengastia, Apolonia,* and *Acomatacarus* which cause chigger dermatitis in many parts of the world, and *Leptotrombidium,* which includes the important vectors of scrub typhus.

**trombiculosis** \trämbik′yəlō′sis\ TROMBICULIASIS.

**trombidiiasis** \trämbid′ē·ī′əsis\ *Outmoded* TROMBICULIASIS.

**trombidiosis** \trämbid′ē·ō′sis\ *Outmoded* TROMBICULIASIS.

***Trombidium*** \trämbid′ē·əm\ A genus of mites in the family Trombidiidae, with larvae parasitic on insects. It formerly included mites that were later classified in the genus *Trombicula,* family Trombiculidae.

**Trömner** [Ernest L. O. *Trömner,* German neurologist, born 1868] Trömner sign, Trömner's reflex. See under HOFFMAN'S REFLEX.

**tromophonia** \träm′əfō′nē·ə\ [Gk *tromo(s)* (from *tremein* to tremble) a trembling + PHON- + -IA] A tremulous or quavering and usually weak speaking voice.

**tropaeolin** \trōpē′əlin\ Any of a group of yellow and orange monoazo dyes, including methyl orange and acid orange, that are used as pH indicators. They are also occasionally used in stains. Also *tropeolin.* **t. D** METHYL ORANGE. **t. G** METANIL YELLOW.

**-trope** \-trōp\ [Gk *tropos* a turn, direction, way] A combining form meaning (1) a turn or movement in a specified direction; (2) something used to turn, as a surgical instrument.

**tropeine** \trō′pē·in\ Any of the esters of tropine, such as atropine, homatropine, and other mydriatic alkaloids.

**tropeinism** \trōpē′inizm\ Poisoning by a tropeine. Symptoms and signs include dysphagia, tachycardia, dryness of the mouth, mydriasis, hallucinations, convulsions, and death.

**tropeolin** \trōpē′əlin\ TROPAEOLIN.

**troph-** \träf-, trōf-\ TROPHO-.

**trophectoderm** \-ek′tədurm\ TROPHOBLAST.

**trophic** \träf′ik\ [Gk *trophikos* (from *trophē* nourishment) nourishing] **1** Having to do with nutrition. **2** Pertaining to that which stimulates growth and development or stimulates an increased activity. **3** Pertaining to nutritional changes in skin and other tissues which may follow impairment of nerve supply.

**-trophic** \-träf′ik, -trō′fik\ [Gk *trophikos* (from *trophē* nourishment) nourishing] A combining form meaning nutrition, nourishment. Also *-tropic.*

**tropho-** \träf′ə-, trō′fə-\ [Gk *trophē* (from *trephein* to nourish, feed) nourishment] A combining form meaning food or nutrition.

**trophoblast** \träf′əblast, trō′fə-\ [TROPHO- + -BLAST] In mammals, a layer of tissue formed by cells forming the outer covering of the blastocyst. After implantation of the blastocyst this layer is no longer cellular. At the 5th–6th day of human pregnancy, the blastocyst attaches to the luteinized endometrium and differentiates on its surface a syncytium which helps to penetrate the epithelium and then break through into the maternal mucous membrane (implantation). As early as implantation (about the 8th–9th day), the trophoblast starts to establish fetal-maternal exchange of gases and nutriments. When the blastocyst has completely penetrated into the maternal mucosa, the trophoblast consists of an external syncytial layer around the blastocyst, the syncytiotrophoblast, and an internal cellular layer, the cytotrophoblast (or layer of Langhans). A third layer of mesenchyme is rapidly added beneath, and all three form the chorion. Also *trophectoderm, trophoderm, chorionic ectoderm.* Adj. trophoblastic.

**trophoblastoma** \-blastō′mə\ [TROPHOBLAST + -OMA] CHORIOCARCINOMA.

**trophocyte** \träf′əsīt, trō′fə-\ A cell that nourishes other cells. Also *trephocyte.*

**trophoderm** \träf′ədurm, trō′fə-\ TROPHOBLAST.

**tropholecithus** \-les′ithəs\ [TROPHO- + Gk *lekithos* yolk] The nutritive yolk substance of a megalecithal ovum which exhibits partial or meroblastic cleavage. Adj. tropholecithal.

**trophoneurosis** \-n$^{y}$ŭrō′sis\ [TROPHO- + NEUROSIS] A trophic disorder occurring in a patient without organic neurologic disease, and attributed to emotional disorder. Some such manifestations are factitious, as in swelling of a hand caused by a ligature around the wrist. *Obs.* Adj. trophoneurotic. **disseminated t.** SCLERODERMA. **facial t.** ROMBERG'S PROGRESSIVE FACIAL HEMIATROPHY. **lingual t.** Hemiatrophy of the tongue. **t. of Romberg** ROMBERG'S PROGRESSIVE FACIAL HEMIATROPHY.

**trophoneurotic** \-n$^{y}$ŭrät′ik\ Pertaining to or affected by trophoneurosis.

**trophonucleus** \-n$^{y}$oo′klē·əs\ [TROPHO- + NUCLEUS] The macronucleus of ciliate protozoa.

**trophoplast** \träf′əplast\ [TROPHO- + -PLAST] PLASTID.

**trophospongia** \-spän′jē·ə\ Plural of TROPHOSPONGIUM.

**trophospongium** \-spän′jē·əm\ (*pl.* trophospongia) A network of canals found within certain cells, as the epithelial cells of the intestine. The canal system may be related to the Golgi apparatus.

**trophotaxis** \-tak′sis\ [TROPHO- + TAXIS] The movement of cells in response to nutritive materials. Also *trophotropism.*

**trophotherapy** \-ther′əpē\ [TROPHO- + THERAPY] DIET THERAPY.

**trophotropic** \-träp′ik\ Relating to that portion of the subcortical, diencephalic system that integrates parasympathetic with somatomotor activities and promotes protective, recuperative, and nurturant behavior patterns.

**trophotropism** \trōfät′rəpizm\ [TROPHO- + TROPISM] TROPHOTAXIS.

**trophozoite** \-zō′īt\ [TROPHO- + *zo(o)-* + -ITE] The active, growing stage of a protozoan organism, such as an ameba, in which it is motile and ingests food, as contrasted with the encysted stage. In certain sporozoans, such as the malarial parasites, it is the asexual or vegetative stage, between the ring form and the mature schizont.

**tropia** \trō′pē·ə\ [Gk *trop(ē)* a turning round, turn + -IA] A manifest misalignment of the eyes, present without interruption of fusion, as by covering one eye; strabismus. • *Tropia* is used in many combinations, as in *esotropia* and *exotropia.*

**-tropic**[1] \-trō′pik, -träp′ik\ [Gk *tropikos* (from *tropos* a turning, from *trepein* to turn) turning] A combining form meaning (1) turning or changing in response to a (specified) stimulus; (2) having an affinity for or stimulating a (specified) organ, tissue, or substance.

**-tropic**[2] \-träp′ik, -trō′pik\ -TROPHIC.

**tropical** \träp′ikəl\ Pertaining to that area of the earth between the Tropic of Cancer and the Tropic of Capricorn.

**tropicamide** \trōpik′əmīd\ $C_{17}H_{20}N_2O_2$. A fast-acting anticholinergic and cycloplegic. It is widely known by the proprietary name Mydriacyl.

***Tropicorbis*** \trō′pikôr′bis\ See under *BIOMPHALARIA.*

**tropine** An alkaloid found combined in plants. Its ester with tropic acid is atropine. It consists of a cycloheptanol molecule with a bridge of $—N(CH_3)—$ joining C-3 and C-6.

**tropism** \trō′pizm\ [Gk *trop(ē)* (from *trepein* to turn) a turn, turning around or *tropos* (from *trepein* to turn) a turn, direction, way + -ISM ] An automatic, unlearned orienting movement made by an organism with respect to a source of physical stimulation. Positive tropism refers to movement toward the source of stimulation, negative tropism away from it.

**tropocollagen** \trō′pōkäl′əjən\ One of the subunits of a collagen molecule. Each tropocollagen molecule is composed of three polypeptide strands twisted to form a three-stranded helix having dimensions of about 280 by 1.5 nanometers and a mass of 300 000 daltons.

**tropoelastin** \trō′pō·ilas′tin\ A monomeric unit of the protein of elastin, a connective tissue. It is first synthesized as proelastin, having high concentrations of repeating units containing glycine and proline. Proelastin, after secretion from the cell, is acted upon by enzymes and converted to tropoelastin.

**tropometer** \trōpäm′ətər\ A device to measure the amount by which an eye is rotated within the orbit.

**tropomyosin** A muscle protein whose molecule lies in the helical groove of actin filaments and prevents several actin molecules from interacting with myosin while the muscle is at rest. When the muscle is activated by a rise in the concentration of calcium ions, these are bound by the associated protein troponin, and its conformational change causes the tropomyosin to unmask the actin molecules.

**troponin** A muscle protein associated with actin filaments. It binds calcium ions when the concentration of these rises, and causes an associated molecule of tropomyosin to unmask several actin molecules, so that they can interact with myosin and initiate muscular contraction.

**trotyl** TRINITROTOLUENE.

**trough** \trôf, träf\ [Old English *trog*] A longitudinal depression or gutter. **gingival t.** GINGIVAL SULCUS. **Langmuir t.** An instrument used to study the behavior of lipid films and to determine the minimal surface area occupied by a monomolecular lipid film. **synaptic t.** A shallow depression on the surface of a striated muscle fiber within which is located the nerve terminal or axonal ending that forms the motor endplate. Also *synaptic gutter, primary synaptic cleft.* **vestibular t.** The gutter formed by the oral mucosa as it passes from the lip or cheek onto the alveolar process of the jaw. Also *vestibular sulcus.*

**Trousseau** [Armand *Trousseau,* French physician, 1801–1867] **1** Trousseau's apophysiary point. See under TROUSSEAU'S POINT. **2** See under TWITCHING. **3** Trousseau's phenomenon. See under SIGN. **4** Lallemand-Trousseau bodies, Trousseau-Lallemand bodies. See under BENCE JONES CYLINDERS.

**troxidone** TRIMETHADIONE.

**troy** \troi\ [after *Troyes,* France, where troy weight was first used] See under TROY WEIGHT.

**Trp** Symbol for tryptophan. • It replaces the earlier symbol Try, which was easily misprinted as Tyr, the symbol for tyrosine.

**truncal** \trung′kəl\ **1** Pertaining to the trunk of the body. **2** The trunk, or primary stem, of a vessel or nerve.

**trunci** \trung′kī\ Plural of TRUNCUS.

**truncoconal** \trung′kəkō′nəl\ Referring to both the

truncus arteriosus and the conus arteriosus.

**truncus** \trungʹkəs\ [L (from the adj. *truncus* trimmed, pruned) the trunk of a tree, of a human body] (*pl.* trunci) **1** [NA] The main stem of a blood or lymph vessel or a nerve from which branches arise. Also *trunk.* **2** TORSO. **t. arteriosus** The cranial portion of the primitive embryonic cardiac tube, which gives rise to the first pair of ventral aortic arches. After the formation of the midline cardiac tube (20th–22nd day in man) the truncus arteriosus undergoes the complex backward folding which affects the heart itself within its pericardial mantle, and it will become progressively more in front of and below the ventricle. At the same time it will participate in the longitudinal partitioning of the bulboventricular portion through the development within it of a helical (spiral) septum which will fuse below with the interventricular septum and the right and left endocardial bulbar ridges. This internal partitioning separates the aorta from the pulmonary trunk so that the primitive truncus arteriosus corresponds approximately to the ascending part of the definitive aortic arch beneath the pulmonary bifurcation. Persistence of the primitive truncus arteriosus accounts for the anomaly described as persistent or common truncus arteriosus. • This term has been used by some authors for the bulbus arteriosus (bulbus cordis) itself, but it is more acceptable to use it for the short prolongation of the primitive cardiac tube beyond the bulbus cordis. **t. arteriosus communis** A large vessel resulting from the failure of the ventral aorta, the common arterial trunk of the embryonic heart, to be subdivided into the ascending aorta and the pulmonary trunk of the definitive heart. The respective pulmonary arteries as well as the usual branches of the arch of the aorta arise from the persisting single arterial trunk which takes origin astride a ventricular septal defect. Also *persistent truncus arteriosus.* **t. brachiocephalicus** [NA] A large artery arising from the convexity of the arch of the aorta behind the middle of the manubrium sterni and extending upwards and posteriorly to the right in front of the trachea. It terminates in the right subclavian and common carotid arteries. Also *brachiocephalic artery, brachiocephalic trunk, innominate artery, anonymous artery.* **t. bronchomediastinalis dexter** [NA] A large lymphatic vessel that drains the tracheobronchial, sternal, and anterior mediastinal lymph nodes on the right side as well as the left inferior tracheobronchial lymph nodes. It empties either into the right lymphatic duct or independently into the junction of the right internal jugular and subclavian veins. Also *right bronchomediastinal trunk.* **t. bronchomediastinalis sinister** [NA] A large lymphatic vessel that drains the tracheobronchial, sternal, and anterior mediastinal lymph nodes on the left side, except for the inferior tracheobronchial lymph nodes. It empties either into the thoracic duct or independently into the junction of the left internal jugular and subclavian veins. Also *left bronchomediastinal trunk.* **t. coeliacus** [NA] A large arterial trunk arising from the front of the abdominal aorta just below the aortic orifice in the diaphragm and passing anteriorly above the pancreas to divide into the left gastric, hepatic, and splenic arteries. Also *celiac trunk, celiac artery, celiac axis.* **t. corporis callosi** [NA] The principal portion of the corpus callosum, arching posteriorly from the genu of the corpus callosum to the splenium. In the median plane it forms the floor of the longitudinal cerebral fissure, and overlying the truncus is a thin gray layer called the indusium griseum. Also *trunk of corpus callosum.* **t. costocervicalis** [NA] An artery that arises from the back of the subclavian artery on each side and arches posteriorly over the cervical pleura to the neck of the first rib. There it divides into the superior intercostal and deep cervical arteries. Also *costocervical trunk, costocervical artery, costocervical arterial axis.* **t. fasciculi atrioventricularis** [NA] The slender stem of the atrioventricular bundle that extends upwards from the atrioventricular node into the trigonum fibrosum dextrum and under the attachment of the septal cusp of the tricuspid valve as far as the interventricular septum. There it passes below the membranous part to reach the upper border of the muscular part and divide into right and left crura. Also *trunk of atrioventricular bundle, trunk of bundle of His.* **t. inferior plexus brachialis** [NA] The lowermost of the three trunks of the brachial plexus. It is formed by the junction of the ventral primary rami of the eighth cervical and first thoracic spinal nerves, and terminates by splitting into an anterior and a posterior division. The anterior division courses beneath the clavicle to become the medial cord of the brachial plexus, while the posterior division joins with the posterior divisions of the superior and middle trunks to form the posterior cord. Also *inferior trunk of brachial plexus.* **trunci intestinales** [NA] Large lymph vessels that convey lymph from the stomach, intestines, pancreas, spleen, and lower part of the liver to the cisterna chyli, thoracic duct, or lumbar lymphatic trunks. Also *intestinal lymphatic trunks.* **t. jugularis dexter/sinister** [NA] A large lymphatic vessel on either side of the neck that is formed by efferent vessels of the superior and inferior deep cervical nodes, joining into a single short channel which usually opens into the thoracic duct on the left side and into either the junction of the internal jugular and subclavian veins or the right lymphatic duct on the right side. **t. linguofacialis** [NA] The arterial trunk from which the facial artery fairly frequently arises in common with the lingual artery instead of independently from the external carotid artery. Also *linguofacial trunk.* **t. lumbaris dexter/sinister** [NA] Large lymphatic vessels, one on the right side of the inferior vena cava and the other on the left side of the abdominal aorta, that receive lymph from the lateral aortic lymph nodes on the corresponding sides and terminate in the cisterna chyli. Also *lumbar lymphatic trunks.* **t. lumbosacralis** [NA] A nerve trunk formed by a portion of the ventral primary ramus of the fourth lumbar nerve and the entire ventral primary ramus of the fifth lumbar nerve. The lumbosacral trunk forms along the medial margin of the psoas major muscle and descends into the pelvis to join the first sacral nerve, thereby contributing to the formation of the sacral plexus. Also *lumbosacral trunk, lumbosacral cord.* **trunci lymphatici** [NA] Large collecting lymph vessels that are formed by the union of smaller vessels and terminate in either the thoracic duct, the right lymphatic duct, or the junction of the internal jugular and subclavian veins. They include the truncus lumbaris dexter/sinister, trunci intestinales, truncus bronchomediastinalis dexter/sinister, truncus subclavius dexter/sinister, and truncus jugularis dexter/sinister. Also *lymphatic trunks.* **t. medius plexus brachialis** [NA] The middle of the three trunks of the brachial plexus. It is formed by the ventral primary ramus of the seventh cervical nerve, and terminates by splitting into an anterior and a posterior division. The anterior division of the middle trunk joins with the anterior division of the superior trunk to form the lateral cord of the brachial plexus, while the posterior division of the middle trunk joins the posterior divisions of the superior and inferior trunks to form the posterior cord. Also *middle trunk of brachial plexus.* **persistent t. arteriosus** TRUNCUS ARTERIOSUS COMMUNIS. **trunci plexus brachialis** [NA] Three nerve trunks (superior, middle, and inferior) located in the posterior triangle of the neck and formed by the ventral primary rami of the fifth, sixth, seventh, and eighth cervical nerves and the first thoracic nerve. Emerging between the scalenus anterior and scalenus medius muscles, each of the three trunks divides into an anterior and a posterior division. These six divisions then become rearranged below the clavicle in the axilla to form the medial, lateral, and posterior cords of the brachial plexus. Also *trunks of brachial plexus.* See also TRUNCUS SUPERIOR PLEXUS BRACHIALIS, TRUNCUS MEDIUS PLEXUS BRACHIALIS, TRUNCUS INFERIOR PLEXUS BRACHIALIS. **t. pulmonalis** [NA] A major artery that arises from the conus arteriosus of the right ventricle of the heart and passes upwards and backwards in front of the ascending aorta to its left side. There, below the arch of the aorta, it divides into right and left pulmonary arteries. It carries deoxygenated blood to the lungs. Also *pulmonary trunk, pulmonary artery.* **t. subclavius dexter/sinister** A lymphatic vessel at the base of the neck on each side, receiving the lymph of the upper limb from the apical lymph nodes on the corresponding side and terminating in the right lymphatic duct on the right side and the thoracic duct on the left side. The vessels on both sides may terminate in the corresponding subclavian vein, however. **t. superior plexus brachialis** [NA] The uppermost of the three trunks of the brachial plexus. It is formed by the junction of the ventral primary rami of the fifth and sixth cervical nerves, and terminates by splitting into an anterior division that helps form the lateral cord of the brachial plexus and a posterior division that assists in the formation of the posterior cord. Before dividing, however, it gives rise to the suprascapular nerve and the delicate nerve to the subclavius muscle. Also *superior trunk of brachial plexus.* **t. sympathicus** [NA] Either of the two ganglionated nerve trunks located immediately lateral to the vertebral column, one on each side. They extend from the highest levels in the neck near the base of the skull to the coccyx, and in the thoracic and upper lumbar levels receive preganglionic sympathetic nerve fibers by way of white rami communicantes from all the thoracic and the upper two or three lumbar spinal nerves. Postganglionic sympathetic fibers leave the sympathetic trunks to join the spinal nerves by way of gray rami communicantes at all segmental levels. Also arising from each sympathetic trunk are the greater, lesser and least splanchnic nerves, which course through the diaphragm into the abdomen. Also *sympathetic chain, sympathetic ganglionated trunk, sympathetic nerve, sympathetic trunk, ganglionated cord* (seldom used). **t. thyrocervicalis** [NA] A short, thick artery that arises from the anterosuperior aspect of the subclavian artery near the medial margin of the scalenus anterior muscle and usually divides into the inferior thyroid, transverse cervical, and suprascapular arteries. Also *thyrocervical trunk.* **t. transversus** COMMON CARDINAL VEIN. **t. vagalis anterior** [NA] A nerve bundle formed from the anterior esophageal plexus on the anterior aspect of the lower esophagus near the esophageal hiatus of the diaphragm. It consists principally of fibers from the left vagus nerve, though it contains some right vagal fibers as well. Gastric branches from this trunk are distributed to the anterosuperior surface of the stomach. Also *vagal trunk anterior, anterior vagal nerve, anterior gastric trunk, anterior gastric nerve.* **t. vagalis posterior** [NA] A nerve bundle formed from the posterior part of the esophageal plexus on the posterior aspect of the esophagus near the esophageal hiatus. It consists principally of fibers from the right vagus nerve, but also contains a few left vagal fibers. Upon entering the abdominal cavity, gastric branches from this trunk are distributed to the posteroinferior surface of the stomach. Also *vagal trunk posterior, posterior vagal nerve, posterior gastric nerve, posterior gastric trunk.*

**trunk** [L *truncus.* See TRUNCUS.] **1** TRUNCUS. **2** TORSO. **anterior gastric t.** TRUNCUS VAGALIS ANTERIOR. **t. of atrioventricular bundle** TRUNCUS FASCICULI ATRIOVENTRICULARIS. **basilar t.** *Outmoded* ARTERIA BASILARIS. **t.'s of brachial plexus** TRUNCI PLEXUS BRACHIALIS. **brachiocephalic t.** TRUNCUS BRACHIOCEPHALICUS. **t. of bundle of His** TRUNCUS FASCICULI ATRIOVENTRICULARIS. **celiac t.** TRUNCUS COELIACUS. **t. of corpus callosum** TRUNCUS CORPORIS CALLOSI. **costocervical t.** TRUNCUS COSTOCERVICALIS. **inferior t. of brachial plexus** TRUNCUS INFERIOR PLEXUS BRACHIALIS. **intestinal lymphatic t.'s** TRUNCI INTESTINALES. **left bronchomediastinal t.** TRUNCUS BRONCHOMEDIASTINALIS SINISTER. **linguofacial t.** TRUNCUS LINGUOFACIALIS. **lumbar lymphatic t.'s** TRUNCUS LUMBARIS DEXTER/-SINISTER. **lumbosacral t.** TRUNCUS LUMBOSACRALIS. **lymphatic t.'s** TRUNCI LYMPHATICI. **middle t. of brachial plexus** TRUNCUS MEDIUS PLEXUS BRACHIALIS. **nerve t.** A collection of myelinated and unmyelinated peripheral nerve fibers bound into a bundle by connective tissue called the epineurium. Smaller fascicles of fibers within a nerve trunk are surrounded by other layers of connective tissue called the perineurium, while strands of collagenous fibers pass from the perineurium between individual nerve fibers as the endoneurium. **posterior gastric t.** TRUNCUS VAGALIS POSTERIOR. **pulmonary t.** TRUNCUS PULMONALIS. **right bronchomediastinal t.** TRUNCUS BRONCHOMEDIASTINALIS DEXTER. **superior t. of brachial plexus** TRUNCUS SUPERIOR PLEXUS BRACHIALIS. **sympathetic t.** TRUNCUS SYMPATHICUS. **sympathetic ganglionated t.** TRUNCUS SYMPATHICUS. **thyrocervical t.** TRUNCUS THYROCERVICALIS. **vagal t. anterior** TRUNCUS VAGALIS ANTERIOR. **vagal t. posterior** TRUNCUS VAGALIS POSTERIOR.

**trusion** \troo′zhən\ [L *trus(us),* past part. of *trudere* to thrust, push + -ION] The malposition of a tooth or group of teeth.

**truss** \trus\ [French *trousser* to refold, truss, tie up to prevent dragging] A device worn to hold in place or support a hernia, especially an inguinal hernia. **yarn t.** A truss to control inguinal hernia in an infant, formed by winding yarn around the lower trunk and the thigh.

**try-in** The trial placement in the mouth of a restoration, crown, or bridge before cementation, or of a denture framework or setup before proceeding to the finishing stage.

**trypan blue** A synthetic acid dye used chiefly in vital staining techniques to assess the viability of cells, especially of the reticuloendothelial system. If the cell is dead, the dye penetrates the membrane of the cells and turns it blue. It has also been used as a trypanocide.

**trypanicide** \trīpan′isīd\ TRYPANOSOMICIDE.

**trypanid** \trī′pənid\ [*trypan(osome)* + -ID[2]] A trypanosomal dermal eruption.

**trypanocidal** \trī′pənōsī′dəl\ TRYPANOSOMICIDAL.

**trypanocide** \trīpan′əsīd\ TRYPANOSOMICIDE.

**trypanolysis** \trī′pənäl′isis\ [*trypano(some)* + LYSIS] The dissolution or destruction of trypanosomes.

**trypanolytic** \trī′pənōlit′ik\ Destructive of trypanosomes; pertaining to trypanolysis.

***Trypanosoma*** \trip′ənəsō′mə, trīpan′ō-\ [Gk *trypano(n)* gimlet, auger + *sōma* body] A genus of flagellates in the family Trypanosomatidae. It includes several hundred species which are parasitic in blood and lymph of all classes of vertebrates and a number of invertebrate hosts. Some species, such as *T. cruzi,* may invade cells. Many are pleomorphic, the species are morphologically similar, and no sexual stages are known; therefore, species determination is often difficult. ***T. ariari*** TRYPANOSOMA RANGELI. ***T. brucei*** An important African species of trypanosome that naturally infects certain antelopes, in which disease rarely results. It is highly pathogenic in a number of domestic animals and in other wild animals including Thompson's gazelle, dikdik, duiker, jackal, serval, monkey, and others. It is considered noninfective for humans, although the human trypanosomes are thought to be so closely related to it that they are often regarded as subspecies: *T. brucei rhodesiense* and *T. brucei gambiense* (the wild animal form being *T. brucei brucei*). Vast areas of Africa have been denied access to cattle and other domestic animals because of the presence of tsetse flies able to transmit *T. brucei.* Also *Trypanosoma pecaudi.* ***T. cruzi*** A trypanosome in the subgenus *Schizotrypanum* (raised to generic level by some); the causative agent of Chagas disease of man and animals. It infects a large number of mammals, many of which serve as reservoir hosts, especially opossums (*Didelphis*), armadillos (*Dasypus*), woodrats (*Neotoma*), dogs, cats, and in some areas the black rat, (*Rattus rattus*). It is widely distributed in South and Central America, and is found in woodrats, racoons, opossums, and skunks in Texas, Arizona, New Mexico, and southern California, and recently in Maryland and in several southeastern States. Some 14 mammal species have been found infected in the United States, where human cases occur as a result of the feeding and defecation habits of the triatomine cone-nose bug vectors. Infection of animals is probably by ingestion of the bug, and of humans by contact of infected bug feces with ocular, buccal, or other mucosal surfaces. Also *Schizotrypanum cruzi.* ***T. escomili*** TRYPANOSOMA RANGELI. ***T. gambiense*** A species that causes Gambian trypanosomiasis or West African sleeping sickness. It is transmitted by several species of tsetse flies, but the principal vector is *Glossina palpalis.* It is endemic in tropical regions of western and central Africa, the behavior and habits of the vectors determining disease distribution. Reservoirs of infection other than man are unknown or controversial. This trypanosome is considered by some workers to be a subspecies of *T. brucei.* Also *Trypanosoma castellani, Trypanosoma hominis, Trypanosoma nigeriense, Trypanosoma ugandense.* ***T. guatemalensis*** TRYPANOSOMA RANGELI. ***T. hominis*** TRYPANOSOMA GAMBIENSE. ***T. luis*** TREPONEMA PALLIDUM. ***T. nigeriense*** TRYPANOSOMA GAMBIENSE. ***T. pecaudi*** TRYPANOSOMA BRUCEI. ***T. rangeli*** A species found in many mammals, including man, in Central and South America. It is transmitted by triatomine bugs (*Rhodnius prolixus, Triatoma dimidiata,* and probably others). It is not known to be pathogenic in the final host, but may cause disease in the bug. It is medically important in that it may be confused with *T. cruzi,* the agent of Chagas disease, with which it may be associated. Also *Trypanosoma ariari, Trypanosoma guatemalensis, Trypanosoma escomili.* ***T. rhodesiense*** A species which causes Rhodesian trypanosomiasis, an acute form of African sleeping sickness found in Zimbabwe (Rhodesia), northeastern Zambia, and Tanzania. The principal vector is *Glossina morsitans,* and the habits of the fly define the geographic distribution of the disease. A small antelope, the bushbuck, is known to be a reservoir host. The species appears to be a derivative of the antelope-infecting *T. brucei* and is considered by some to be a subspecies of it. ***T. ugandense*** TRYPANOSOMA GAMBIENSE.

**trypanosomacide** \trīpan′ōsō′məsīd\ TRYPANOSOMICIDE.

**trypanosomal** \trīpan′ōsō′məl\ **1** Relating to or caused by trypanosomes. **2** Resembling the typical adult form of trypanosomes: said of a developmental stage of some hemoflagellates. See also TRYPOMASTIGOTE.

**trypanosomatic** \trīpan′ōsōmat′ik\ Relating to or caused by trypanosomes.

**trypanosomatid** \trīpan′ōsō′mətid\ [*Trypanosomat(idae)* + -ID[1]] **1** Of or belonging to the flagellate family Trypanosomatidae. **2** A member of the family Trypanosomatidae. For defs 1 and 2 also *trypanosomid.*

**Trypanosomatidae** \trīpan′ōsōmat′idē\ [*Trypanosoma* + *t* + -IDAE] A family of blood and tissue, intra- and extracellular flagellates in the order Kinetoplastida, class Zoomastigophorea. It includes parasites of all classes of vertebrates, of insects and leeches as well as other invertebrates, and of certain plants. The whole family probably originated as insect or leech gut parasites, as many still are, but many have acquired new hosts from the bloodsucking habits of their invertebrate hosts, thus acquiring a heteroxenous life cycle. In their development they pass through one or more of a number of stages structurally similar to forms of other genera, such as trypomastigote, opisthomastigote, choanomastigote, epimastigote, promastigote, and amastigote. Nine genera are known in the family, two of which, *Trypanosoma* and *Leishmania,* are of great medical and veterinary importance.

**trypanosomatosis** \trīpan′ōsō′mətō′sis\ TRYPANOSOMIASIS.

**trypanosomatotropic** \trīpan′ōsō′mətōträp′ik\ Having an attraction to or affinity for flagellates of the family Trypanosomatidae.

**trypanosome** \trīpan′əsōm\ [See *TRYPANOSOMA.*] **1** A flagellate protozoan of the genus *Trypanosoma* or similar genus in the family Trypanosomatidae. **2** *Outmoded* TRYPOMASTIGOTE.

**trypanosomiasis** \trip′ənōsōmī′əsis\ [*trypanosom(a)* + -IASIS] Any of a group of diseases caused by protozoa of the genus *Trypanosoma,* and characterized by irregular and chronic fevers, skin eruptions, edema, adenitis, lethargy, and, if untreated, death. In Africa the trypanosomes develop in and are spread to man by tsetse flies (*Glossina*) and mechanically by other biting flies. Triatomine (cone nose) bugs of the hemipteran family Reduviidae are responsible for transmission of *Trypanosoma cruzi,* the agent of the South American form, known as Chagas disease. Also *trypanosomatosis, trypanosomosis, trypanosome fever.* **acute t.** RHODESIAN TRYPANOSOMIASIS. **African t.** **1** GAMBIAN TRYPANOSOMIASIS. **2** RHODESIAN TRYPANOSOMIASIS. **American t.** CHAGAS DISEASE. **Brazilian t.** CHAGAS DISEASE. **chronic t.** GAMBIAN TRYPANOSOMIASIS. **Congo t.** GAMBIAN TRYPANOSOMIASIS. **Cruz t.** CHAGAS DISEASE. **t. cruzi** CHAGAS DISEASE. **East African t.** RHODESIAN TRYPANOSOMIASIS. **Gambian t.** A chronic disease caused by *Trypanosoma gambiense* and found in western and central Africa. It is spread by the bite of tsetse flies, such as *Glossina palpalis,* and is associated with riverside vegetation. The disease is characterized by chronic irregular fever and a firm, tender, red nodule at the site of the bite. The main lesions occur in the cervical lymph nodes (Winterbottom sign), the submaxillary region, mesentery, and the central nervous system. Compared to Rhodesian trypanosomiasis, the Gambian form is less acute, with the fulminating fatal central nervous system infection developing in one to two years rather than $2^1/_2$ months. Treatment is with suramin or, when there is central nervous system involvement, melarsoprol. Also *Congo trypanosomiasis, Gambian sleeping sickness, West African sleeping sickness, lethargus, African lethargy, nelavane, sleeping sickness, African sleeping sickness, African trypanosomiasis, morbus dormitivus, schlafkrankheit,*

*West African trypanosomiasis, chronic trypanosomiasis, chronic sleeping sickness.* **Rhodesian t.** An acute disease caused by *Trypanosoma rhodesiense* and found in east and southeast Africa. It is spread by the bite of savannah tsetse flies, such as *Glossina morsitans* and *G. swynnertoni.* Although the clinical picture resembles Gambian trypanosomiasis, the Rhodesian (Zimbabwean) form tends to be more severe, to pursue a more rapid course, and to involve the central nervous system more quickly. Involvement of the lymph glands is usual. The disease is a zoonosis, the reservoir hosts being antelope, especially the bushbuck. Death usually occurs within one year of infection, often before the "sleeping sickness" stage develops. Treatment is with pentamidine or suramin, and melarsoprol for the neurological late phase. Also *kaodzera, East African sleeping sickness, mid-African sleeping sickness, Rhodesian sleeping sickness, Zambezi sleeping sickness, lethargus, African lethargy, nelavane, sleeping sickness, African sleeping sickness, African tryanosomiasis, morbus dormitivus, East African trypanosomiasis, acute trypanosomiasis, acute sleeping sickness.* **South American t.** CHAGAS DISEASE. **West African t.** GAMBIAN TRYPANOSOMIASIS.

**trypanosomic** \trīpan′ōsō′mik\ Pertaining to trypanosome infection.

**trypanosomicidal** \trīpan′ōsō′misī′dəl\ Destructive to trypanosomes. Also *trypanocidal.*

**trypanosomicide** \trīpan′ōsō′misīd\ An agent or substance that kills trypanosomes. Also *trypanicide, trypanocide.* Also *trypanosomacide.*

**trypanosomid** \trīpan′ōsō′mid\ TRYPANOSOMATID.

**trypanosomosis** \trīpan′ōsōmō′sis\ TRYPANOSOMIASIS.

**trypan red** A synthetic acid dye that is used chiefly as a vital stain.

**tryparsamide** \trīpär′səmīd\ A pentavalent arsenical drug used for the treatment of trypanosomiasis and neurosyphilis. It is most effective against the early stages of trypanosomiasis before invasion of the nervous system. It is a sodium hydrogen *p*-carbamylmethylaminophenyl arsonate hemihydrate. Also *tryponarsyl, trypotan.*

**trypochetes** \trī′pōkēts\ DÖHLE BODIES.

**trypomastigote** \trī′pōmas′tigōt\ The stage of development in certain hemoflagellates in which the flagellum arises from a posteriorly placed basal granule and kinetoplast and forms an undulating membrane which runs along the length of the body. It is the infective stage for African trypanosomiasis and South American trypanosomiasis, and resembles the typical adult form of *Trypanosoma.* Also *trypanosome stage* (outmoded), *trypanosomal form* (outmoded), *trypanosome* (outmoded).

**tryponarsyl** \trī′pōnär′sil\ TRYPARSAMIDE.

**trypotan** \trī′pōtan\ TRYPARSAMIDE.

**trypsin** \trip′sin\ [Gk *trips(is)* (misspelled as *trypsis*) rubbing, friction + -IN; supposedly so called because it was first obtained by rubbing the pancreas with glycerol] A pancreatic proteinase (EC 3.4.21.4) that hydrolyzes polypeptides on the C-terminal side of arginine and lysine residues. It is formed from trypsinogen by removal of the N-terminal peptide Val—$[Asp—]_4$—Lys, under the influence of either enteropeptidase secreted by the duodenal lining or trypsin already produced. Trypsin contains just over 220 amino-acid residues and possesses six disulfide bonds. It is often used in studies of protein sequence for partial hydrolysis of polypeptides. **t. inhibitor** A polypeptide with high affinity for trypsin, inhibiting its activity. One such, of molecular mass 6 kDa and of dissociation constant from trypsin of $10^{-13}$ M, occurs in pancreatic secretion. Its function appears to be to prevent premature autocatalytic activation of trypsinogen. Another is found in plants such as soya beans.

**trypsinize** \trip′sinīz\ To treat with trypsin and therefore to hydrolyze polypeptides in the material so treated. This process breaks down connective tissue fibers and thereby separates the enclosed cells.

**trypsinogen** The secreted precursor of trypsin, from which it differs by possessing an N-terminal hexapeptide. It is almost inactive in comparsion with trypsin. Also *protrypsin.*

**tryptamine** The amine formed by decarboxylation of tryptophan. Its 5-hydroxy derivative is serotonin, but it does not appear to be a precursor of this. It is a precursor of many plant and fungal metabolites, including lysergic acid.

**tryptic** \trip′tik\ Of or relating to trypsin: used of hydrolysis catalyzed by trypsin or of material treated with trypsin, as *tryptic* digest of a protein.

**tryptone** \trip′tōn\ A commercial tryptic digest of meat, used in bacterial culture media.

**tryptophan** \trip′təfan\ One of the twenty amino acids that are incorporated into proteins. It is essential in mammalian food. It consists of indole, substituted at C-3 by the group $—CH_2—CH(NH_3{}^+)—COO^-$. It has characteristic ultraviolet absorption. Its content in proteins cannot be measured in routine amino-acid analysis, because it is usually destroyed during acid hydrolysis, being easily oxidized in strongly acid solutions. It is a precursor of serotonin in animals and of many alkaloids in plants. Also *tryptophane.* Symbol: Trp, W

**tryptophanase** The enzyme (EC 4.1.99.1) that catalyzes the breakdown of tryptophan to form indole, pyruvate, and ammonia. It contains pyridoxal phosphate, and initially catalyzes a 2,3-elimination from its substrate, yielding indole and 2-aminopropenoic acid, which is subsequently hydrolyzed to form pyruvate and ammonia.

**tryptophan 2,3-dioxygenase** The enzyme (EC 1.13.11.11) that catalyzes the oxidation of tryptophan by dioxygen with incorporation of both oxygen atoms and formation of *N*-formylkynurenine. It is the first enzyme of the normal route of tryptophan catabolism. Also *tryptophan pyrrolase* (outmoded).

**tryptophane** \trip′təfān\ TRYPTOPHAN.

**tryptophanuria** \trip′təfanyoo′rē·ə\ A hereditary disorder characterized by excess urinary excretion of tryptophan and hypopigmentation of the optic fundus.

**tryptophyl** The acyl group formed by removing OH from the carboxyl group of tryptophan.

**TS** **1** test solution. **2** tricuspid stenosis.

**tsetse** \tset′sē\ [Tswana *tsêtsê* ] TSETSE FLY.

**TSH** thyroid stimulating hormone (thyrotropic hormone).

**TSH-RF** thyroid stimulating hormone-releasing factor.

**tsp** Symbol for the unit, teaspoon.

**TSTA** tumor-specific transplantation antigen.

**tsutsugamushi** \tsʊt′səgäm′ʊshē \ [Japanese *tsutsuga* sickness + *mushi* an insect] **1** Any of the trombiculid mites that are vectors of scrub typhus. **2** An abbreviated name for tsutsugamushi disease; scrub typhus.

**TTP** **1** thymidine triphosphate. • This is also abbreviated dTTP in order to emphasize that thymidine is a 2′-deoxynucleoside. **2** thrombotic thrombocytopenic purpura.

**tuaminoheptane sulfate** $(C_7H_{17}N)_2 \cdot H_2SO_4$. 2-Hepatanamine. A topical nasal decongestant used in the form of drops.

**tub** **1** A tank. **2** To perform the daily washing and débridement of (a patient with major burns). *Popular.*

**tuba** \tʸoo′bə\ [L (akin to *tubus* a pipe or tube) a tuba, trumpet] Any elongated cylindrical structure, canal, or organ that has a hollow core. Also *tube.* **t. auditiva**

[NA] An osseocartilaginous tube through which air passes between the nasopharynx and the middle ear so as to equalize the pressure on the outer and inner surfaces of the tympanic membrane. The part leading from the middle ear is osseous, whereas that part adjacent to and ending in the lateral wall of the nasopharynx consists of fibrocartilage. Both parts are lined by mucous membrane. Also *eustachian tube, auditory tube, pharyngotympanic tube, eustachian canal.* **t. uterina** [NA] Either of a pair of slender muscular tubes that are situated in the upper margins of the broad ligament on either side of the uterus. The medial end passes through the uterine wall to open into the superior angle of the uterine cavity whereas the lateral end opens by its abdominal ostium into the peritoneal cavity close to the medial surface of the ovary. Its subdivisions include the infundibulum, ampulla, isthmus, and pars uterina. Its function is to transport ova from the ovaries to the uterine cavity. When fertilization of the ovum occurs, it usually takes place in the ampulla of the tuba uterina. Also *uterine tube, fallopian tube, oviduct, ovarian duct, hysterosalpinx.*

**tubae** \t^yoo′bē\ Plural of TUBA.

**tubal** \t^yoo′bəl\ Of, relating to, or occurring in a tube or tubes, as the fallopian tubes or the eustachian tubes.

**tubba** \tʊb′ə\ [West Indies, of African origin] FOOT YAWS.

**tubboe** \tʊb′ō\ [West Indies, of African origin] FOOT YAWS.

**Tubbs** [Oswald S. *Tubbs,* English surgeon, born 1908] See under DILATOR.

# tube

**tube** [L *tubus* (akin to *tuba* a tuba, trumpet) a pipe, tube] **1** TUBA. **2** A hollow, elongated, cylindrical, often flexible structure used for delivering, transferring, or draining fluids. **3** Any of various sealed glass or metal electronic devices, usually having a vacuum or rarified gas inside, designed for detection, amplification, conversion, etc., of electrons or electromagnetic radiation. **Abbott-Miller t.** MILLER-ABBOTT TUBE. **Abbott-Rawson t.** A double-lumen nasogastric tube used for gastric decompression or irrigation. **Aberdeen t.** A plastic tracheostomy tube designed for use in infants. **air t.** RESPIRATORY AIRWAY. **Alder Hey t.** A silver tracheostomy tube designed especially for use in children. The distinguishing features include a funnel-shaped projection on the inner tube, which is fitted with a speaking valve, and a window at the elbow of both inner and outer tubes. **auditory t.** TUBA AUDITIVA. **auscultation t.** A length of rubber or plastic tubing suitably tipped at either end through which the otologist may listen to sounds originating in the middle ear of the patient during swallowing or when air is passed into the eustachian tube via the eustachian catheter and so draw conclusions about the degree of patency of the eustachian tube. Also *Toynbee's otoscope, otophone* (obs.). **Ayre's t.** In pediatric anesthesia, a T-shaped piece connected to the endotracheal tube. Gases are insufflated via the vertical limb, and exhalation occurs at the other end of the crosspiece. Also *T-piece.* **Bowman's t.'s** CORNEAL TUBES. **breathing t.** RESPIRATORY AIRWAY. **bronchial t.** **1** An anatomic bronchus. **2** An airway inserted into a bronchus via the trachea. **buccal t.** END TUBE. **Cantor t.** A long, nonrefillable, mercury-weighted intestinal tube used to relieve mechanical obstructions of the small intestine. **capillary t.** A narrow-bore tube into which fluid will flow by capillarity. **cardiac t.** The primitive embryonic heart, formed by the fusion in the midline at the 8 somite stage of two symmetrical endocardial tubes clothed in a mantle of splanchnopleure (myoepicardial mantle). The fused tubes are suspended in a cephalic prolongation of the intraembryonic coelom, the future pericardial cavity. Only its posterior attachment, the dorsal mesocardium, will persist up to the 16 somite stage and will play a most important role in the flexion and then the bending of the heart tube on itself. **Carlens t.** A double-lumen endotracheal tube, insertion of which permits one-lung ventilation with collapse of the other during thoracic surgery under general anesthesia. **cathode ray t.** A display tube such as a television tube in which an electron beam can be deflected to any point on a fluorescent screen to display a picture, graph, or characters. Abbr. CRT **Celestin's t.** A plastic tube which is placed in the esophagus either surgically or endoscopically and which serves as a prosthesis to maintain patency in inoperable esophageal cancer. **cerebromedullary t.** NEURAL TUBE. **Chaoul t.** An x-ray tube used for superficial x-ray therapy, designed so that the anode can be placed close to the skin. **chest t.** A tube, usually hooked to underwater seal drainage, placed through the chest wall into the pleural cavity to drain air or fluid from the chest cavity. **Coolidge x-ray t.** A hot cathode x-ray tube, in which electrons are produced by thermionic emission from a heated filament. Also *Coolidge tube.* **corneal t.'s** Tubelike cleavages formed artifactually by the splitting of the stromal layers of the cornea, as from injection. Also *Bowman's tubes.* **Crookes t.** An early type of vacuum tube, used at the time of the discovery of x rays. **cuffed t.** A tracheal or tracheostomy tube modified by the application of an inflatable balloon applied in the manner of a cuff around the terminal part of it. When inflated the balloon acts to isolate the lower air passages from the upper air and food passage, permitting the application of positive pressure respiration and/or preventing the aspiration of secretions, gastrointestinal contents, or blood from any site above the level of the cuff. **Diamond's t.** A double-lumen tube that may be used in the nasogastric or nasojejunal positions for decompression or to sample the luminal contents for diagnostic purposes. **discharge t.** Any partially evacuated tube, usually made of glass, which contains metal electrodes, a cathode, and an anode, and which permits the passage of electricity through the tube when a moderately high voltage difference is applied to the electrodes. **drainage t.** A tube that facilitates the drainage of fluids from a body cavity. **drawing t.** A device attached to the side of a microscope that permits an image to be displayed on a sheet of paper so that it may be copied by drawing. **Durham's t.** The silver tracheotomy (tracheostomy) tube in wide use from 1869 until recent times. The short intratracheal part, being at right angles to the horizontal part, necessitated the design of a flexible inner tube and introducer, incorporating the distinguishing lobster-tail feature that consisted of several rigid sections linked in such a way as to render the whole flexible. Durham proposed the use of two cannulae of this sort, the temporary right-angled tube, in which the distance between the shield and the vertical part could be varied to take into account the thickness of the soft tissues, and the permanent tube without this arrangement. The tube known nowadays is the so-called temporary tube. Also *lobster-tail tube.* **electron multiplier t.** A vacuum tube containing about 10 dynodes (plates) that uses a cascade process and secondary emission to amplify small electron currents to large pulses. **embryonic fallopian t.** The anlage of the mature fallopian tube, formed from the upper segment of the paramesonephric duct. **empyema t.** A tube, usually of rubber or plastic, that is used to provide drainage of pus in thoracic empyema. **end t.** Terminal attachment on a banded molar tooth. Also *buccal tube.* **endobronchial t.** An artificial airway inserted in the bronchus via the nose or mouth. **endocardial t.'s** Cords of cells formed by the coalescence of angioblastic masses originating in the splanchnopleure of the cephalic end of the embryo and of the yolk sac. The cords rapidly gain a lumen, and early on will exhibit contractions, having already come together and fused, thus delimiting a single, midline, ventral cardiac tube. **endotracheal t.** An artificial airway placed in the trachea and inserted via the mouth or nose. Also *endotracheal airway.* **esophageal t.** A flexible tube introduced into the stomach through the esophagus for purposes of decompression or nasal feeding. **eustachian t.** TUBA AUDITIVA. **fallopian t.** TUBA UTERINA. **feeding t.** Any tube used to feed a patient unable, unwilling, or advised not to feed himself normally, the commonest being the nasogastric tube. **Fuller t.** A silver tracheotomy (tracheostomy) tube. The outer tube is split lengthways so as to permit the two parts to be squeezed together for ease of introduction, the subsequent insertion of the inner tube restoring and maintaining the full size of the lumen. **Geiger-Müller t.** The detecting device at the front end of a Geiger-Müller counter. It is an ionization chamber containing electrodes with several hundred volts between them, and a gas at low pressure (~1/100 atm). Shape and design vary widely, but typically the tube is a metal or silvered-glass cylinder with a fine wire along the axis for the positive electrode. Given an appropriate voltage, when an entering particle or photon causes an ionizing event, the intense electrostatic field around the wire produces avalanche ionization, and the resulting electrical pulse is passed on to the scaling circuits. Geiger-Müller tubes are simple, rugged, and electrically undemanding. They make good alpha and beta particle detectors, but they have poor stopping power for gamma photons, for which reason bismuth may be incorporated into the outer wall to encourage ion formation. Also *Geiger tube.* **grenz-ray t.** An x-ray tube designed to operate in the range of 10 to 20 kilovolts, to produce grenz rays for radiation therapy. **Harris t.** A mercury-weighted single-lumen tube, similar to but shorter than the Miller-Abbott tube, used for intestinal diagnostic studies. **hot cathode x-ray t.** Any x-ray tube in which the cathode consists of a spiral filament of tungsten which is heated to incandescence for the production of electrons by thermionic emission. **image intensifier t.** In radiology, a vacuum tube containing an input fluorescent screen which converts an x-ray pattern into a pattern of light photons. A photocathode converts the light pattern into an electron pattern, which is then accelerated and focused on an output fluorescent screen which converts the electron pattern into a light image of much higher luminance. **intestinal t.** The embryonic intestine after the intestinal groove has formed. **Jackson t.** A silver tracheotomy (tracheostomy) tube made in the form of a somewhat long arc of a circle. Its novel feature is the freedom from projections and the lack of bulk of the tube beyond the shield. **KCH t.** NEGUS TUBE. • This was designed at King's College Hospital, London. **Killian's t.'s** A series of improved bronchoscopes or esophagoscopes with proximal lighting, designed in 1896, that served as the prototypes of the instruments that remained standard for many years. **Kobelt's t.'s** Remnants of the mesonephric tubules in the epoophoron and the paroophoron of the female and in the paradidymis of the male. **laryngostomy t.** LARYNGOTOMY TUBE. **laryngotomy t.** A modified metal tracheostomy tube used for maintaining an airway after cricothyrotomy. The principal characteristic is that the tube is oval in cross-section, being flattened in the vertical plane. Also *laryngostomy tube.* **Levin t.** A single-lumen plastic tube inserted through the nose into the stomach and generally used for aspiration of gastric contents or for lavage. **Linton t.** A device that produces tamponade compression of esophageal varices by means of a balloon inflated within the stomach and drawn up against the gastroesophageal junction. **lobster-tail t.** DURHAM'S TUBE. **malpighian t.'s** MALPIGHIAN TUBULES. **medullary t.** NEURAL TUBE. **Miescher's t.** *Outmoded* SARCOCYST. **Miller-Abbott t.** A long double-lumen tube capped by an inflatable mercury-filled balloon, mostly used for intestinal decompression. Also *Abbott-Miller tube.* **Montgomery T t.** A T-shaped silicone tube used in the management of stenosis of the cervical trachea. The cross-limb of the T lies within the trachea and supports it, and the vertical limb serves as a tracheostomy tube. **nasogastric t.** A narrow tube passed through the nose into the stomach by way of the pharynx and esophagus, usually as a temporary measure after operations on the mouth, pharynx, larynx, esophagus, or abdominal viscera while healing is taking place. It is used to permit artificial feeding and sometimes aspiration of stomach contents. It was originally made of rubber, but now is commonly made of a plastic polymer. **nasopharyngeal t.** A soft rubber artificial airway inserted through the nose into the pharynx. **nasotracheal t.** A plastic or rubber airway inserted through the nose into the trachea. **Negus t.** A silver tracheostomy tube, in the form of an arc of a circle. The outer end is slightly funnelled so that a speaking valve may be incorporated in the inner tube without narrowing the lumen. Also *KCH tube.* **nephrostomy t.** A tube placed through the kidney parenchyma into the renal pelvis for external drainage of urine. **neural t.** A tube formed during neurulation by the fusion of the edges of the neural grooves and representing one of the embryonic stages in the development of the central nervous system. Fusion starts at the level of the fourth somite and extends cranially and caudally, but closure of the two ends of tube occurs later. As a result the neural tube communicates transitorily with the amniotic cavity through the anterior and posterior neuropores. The cephalic end of the tube will become the brain and soon exhibits its three expansions to form the primary cerebral vesicles. The remainder of the tube forms the spinal cord, and here the tube is oval in outline with the lumen a narrow vertical slit. There is a roof plate and a floor plate which contribute little but the lateral wall thickens into a ventral basal lamina and a dorsal alar lamina separated by a longitudinal sulcus limitans. The anterior and lateral columns of gray matter develop in the basal lamina, and the posterior column appears somewhat later in the alar lamina. Also *medullary tube, neuroderm, cerebromedullary tube.* **observation t.** An optical extension fitted at right angles to one eyepiece of an operating microscope or, less commonly, to a headlight. It is used to enable an observer to study the details of microsurgery or the part under examination. **orotracheal t.** A plastic or rubber airway inserted through the mouth into the trachea. **ovarian t.'s** PFLÜGER'S CORDS. **Parker t.** An obtuse-angled silver tracheotomy (tracheostomy) tube designed to take into account the fact that the trachea slants backward as it descends from the neck into the thorax.

**pharyngotympanic t.** TUBA AUDITIVA. **photomultiplier t.** An electron multiplier tube containing a photocathode which converts photons to electrons. It is used, for example, to detect the minute quantity of light from a scintillation crystal and amplify it to a large enough pulse to drive a counting circuit. Abbr. PMT **pus t.** *Older term* PYOSALPINX. **Robertshaw t.** A double-lumen endotracheal tube similar to Carlen's tube. **roentgen t.** X-RAY TUBE. **rotating anode t.** An x-ray tube in which the anode consists of a disk, usually a molybdenum alloy faced with tungsten, which rotates at speeds from 3000 to 10 000 revolutions per minute during the time that x rays are being produced. **Ruysch t.** A tiny tubular sac, about 5 mm long, identified by a minute orifice situated anteriorly in both sides of the nasal septum near a recess just above the incisive canal. It is a vestige of the fetal vomeronasal organ of Jacobson and is lined by columnar cells and many glands. In many animals it is well developed and involved with the sense of smell, but in humans it is rudimentary. **sediment t.** A tube that has one end much narrowed. It is used to collect and quantify urine sediment. Also *sedimentation tube.* **sedimentation t.** **1** A cylindrical tube used in determining the erythrocyte sedimentation rate. **2** SEDIMENT TUBE. **Sengstaken-Blakemore t.** A nasogastric double balloon tipped rubber tube passed from the nose or mouth into the stomach and used to tamponade bleeding gastroesophageal varices. **Shiner's t.** A long, flexible tube that is inserted through the nose into the small intestine under radiographic control in order to obtain small samples of jejunal mucosa. **speaking t.** A tracheostomy tube fitted with a speaking valve. **stomach t.** Any of various kinds of tubes inserted through the mouth or nose into the stomach, generally for feeding, aspiration, or lavage. **T t.** A drainage tube in the shape of a T. It is frequently used to decompress the common bile duct postoperatively. **test t.** A narrow cylindrical glass or plastic container that is open at one end. It is used to collect, store, and analyze liquids, and to hold microbiologic cultures. **thoracostomy t.** A tube that is inserted into the pleural cavity to drain fluid or air from the thoracic cavity. **Thunberg t.** A tube, used in the study of tissue oxidation, that contains the reaction mixture, which must be subjected to a partial vacuum. **tracheal t.** An orotracheal or nasotracheal tube; an endotracheal tube. **tracheostomy t.** A metal, plastic, or rubber airway inserted through the neck into the trachea during tracheostomy. Also *tracheotomy tube.* **tracheotomy t.** TRACHEOSTOMY TUBE. **Tucker t.'s** Two flexible-tipped tubes, one straight and one curved, designed to be connected by means of a rubber tube to a 20 ml syringe for injecting iodized oil into the lower air passages in bronchography. **tympanostomy t.** VENTILATION TUBE. **uterine t.** TUBA UTERINA. **vacuum t.** Any glass tube from which the air has been evacuated to a high degree of vacuum, as an electron tube. **ventilation t.** A small plastic tube, designed in various forms, for insertion through an incision in the tympanic membrane, used to provide ventilation of the middle ear after aspiration of the secretions in cases of secretory otitis media. Also *ventilating tube, tympanostomy tube, drain-tube* (incorrect), *grommet* (popular). **Venturi t.** See under VENTURI PRINCIPLE. **Voltolini's t.** A small gold tube used to maintain the patency of surgical perforations of the tympanic membrane. Such tubes were abandoned because it was found that they became extruded. They may be regarded as the precursor of modern ventilation tubes. **Wintrobe t.** See under WINTROBE METHOD. **x-ray t.** A type of discharge tube, so constructed as to produce x rays. When high velocity electrons strike the metal anode, the kinetic energy is converted mostly into heat with a small portion converted to x rays. Also *roentgen tube.*

**tubectomy** \t^yoobek′təmē\ [*tub(e)* + -ECTOMY] SALPINGECTOMY.

**tuber** \t^yoo′bər\ [L (akin to *tumere* to be puffed or blown up, swollen), a bump, swelling, protuberance] A rounded eminence; tubercle. **t. anterius hypothalami** TUBER CINEREUM. **t. calcanei** [NA] The posterior and inferior projection of the calcaneus to form the heel. Also *tuberosity of calcaneus, calcaneal tubercle.* **t. cinereum** [NA] A rounded mound of gray matter visible on the inferior surface of the hypothalamus, located rostral to the mamillary bodies and caudal to the optic chiasma. It helps form the floor of the third ventricle, and contains the tuberomamillary and lateral tuberal nuclei of the hypothalamus. Anteroinferiorly, the tuber cinereum is continuous with the infundibular stalk that interconnects the posterior lobe of the hypophysis with the hypothalamus. Also *tuber anterius hypothalami, tuberculum cinereum, gray tubercle, postchiasmatic eminence* (obs.). **t. corporis callosi** SPLENIUM CORPORIS CALLOSI. **t. dorsale** TUBER VERMIS. **t. frontale** [NA] A rounded elevation on the external surface of the frontal bone on each side of the median plane and a short distance above the supraorbital margin. It is variable between individuals and is more obvious in females and young individuals. It marks the site where ossification began in the bone. Also *frontal tuber, frontal eminence, frontal boss, frontal protuberance, frontal tuberosity.* **iliopubic t.** EMINENTIA ILIOPUBICA. **t. ischiadicum** [NA] A rough, large, curved projection at the lower part of the dorsal surface and lower extremity of the body of the ischium. Its lower part gives attachment to the adductor magnus muscle and supports the trunk in the sitting position, whereas its upper part provides attachment for the hamstring or posterior femoral muscles. It turns forward anteriorly to merge with the ramus of the ischium. Also *tuberosity of ischium, ischial tuberosity.* **t. maxillae** [NA] The rough, rounded projection at the posteroinferior angle of the infratemporal surface of the maxilla. It usually increases in prominence after eruption of the upper third molar tooth behind which it bulges. It articulates with the pyramidal process of the palatine bone and provides attachment for some fibers of the medial pterygoid muscle. Also *maxillary tuber, maxillary tuberosity, tuberosity of maxilla.* **t. omentale hepatis** [NA] A rounded prominence on the visceral surface of the left lobe of the liver just dorsal to, cranial to, and occupying the concavity of the lesser curvature of the stomach. There it is in contact with the lesser omentum, through which it is related to the tuber omentale pancreatis. Also *omental tuber of liver, omental tuberosity of liver.* **t. omentale pancreatis** [NA] A rounded bulge on the superior border at the junction of the head and body of the pancreas, lying above the lesser curvature of the stomach and in contact with the lesser omentum. Through the lesser omentum it is related to the tuber omentale hepatis. Also *omental tuber of pancreas, omental tuberosity of pancreas, tuber omentale of pancreas.* **omental t. of liver** TUBER OMENTALE HEPATIS. **omental t. of pancreas** TUBER OMENTALE PANCREATIS. **t. parietale** [NA] A slight elevation, occasionally conical, near the center of the external surface of the parietal bone and usually above the superior temporal line. It is more obvious in young individuals and in certain populations and indicates the site where ossification of the bone commenced. Also *parietal tuber, parietal eminence, parietal tuberosity, parietal protuberance.* **t. valvulae cerebelli** TUBER VERMIS. **t. vermis** [NA] The portion of the cerebellar vermis located at the most caudal part of the inferior surface of the cerebellum, between the folium vermis and the folium pyramis. Coextensive laterally with the tuber vermis on each side are the caudal (inferior) semilunar lobules. Also *tuber valvulae cerebelli, tuber dorsale.*

**tubera** \t^y oo′bərə\ Plural of TUBER.

# tubercle

**tubercle** \t^y oo′bərkl\ [L *tuberculum.* See TUBERCULUM.] **1** A small nodule or eminence, as on a bone, tooth, or other anatomic structure. Also *tuberculum.* **2** A small, rounded, nodular lesion. **3** In particular, the characteristic lesion of tuberculosis: a grayish translucent mass of small spherical cells. **accessory t.** PROCESSUS ACCESSORIUS VERTEBRARUM LUMBALIUM. **acoustic t.** *Outmoded* AREA VESTIBULARIS. **adductor t. of femur** TUBERCULUM ADDUCTORIUM FEMORIS. **amygdaloid t. of Schwalbe** *Outmoded* AREA VESTIBULARIS. **anal t.** One of the protuberances which form around the edge of the cloacal membrane, causing the latter to lie at the bottom of a depression called the proctodeum. Also *anal hillock.* **anatomical t.** TUBERCULOSIS CUTIS VERRUCOSA. **anterior t. of atlas** TUBERCULUM ANTERIUS ATLANTIS. **anterior t. of calcaneus** TUBERCULUM CALCANEI. **anterior t. of cervical vertebrae** TUBERCULUM ANTERIUS VERTEBRARUM CERVICALIUM. **anterior obturator t.** TUBERCULUM OBTURATORIUM ANTERIUS. **t. of anterior scalene muscle** TUBERCULUM MUSCULI SCALENI ANTERIORIS. **anterior t. of thalamus** TUBERCULUM ANTERIUS THALAMI. **articular t. of temporal bone** TUBERCULUM ARTICULARE OSSIS TEMPORALIS. **auricular t.** TUBERCULUM AURICULAE. **Babès t.'s** Nodules that consist of accumulations of microglia and other neuroglial cells, observed in regions of the central nervous system where neurons have undergone chromatolysis and degeneration as the result of encephalitis due to rabies or some other cause. In rabies encephalitis Babès tubercles are said to be most frequently found in the substantia nigra. Also *Babès nodules, Babès nodes, rabic nodules, rabic tubercles.* **calcaneal t.** TUBER CALCANEI. **Carabelli t.** CARABELLI CUSP. **carotid t.** TUBERCULUM ANTERIUS VERTEBRAE CERVICALIS VI. **carotid t. of sixth cervical vertebra** TUBERCULUM ANTERIUS VERTEBRAE CERVICALIS VI. **caseous t.** A tubercle which has undergone caseation necrosis. Also *yellow tubercle.* Compare GRAY TUBERCLE. **cervical t.'s** The two small protuberances at the base of the femoral neck. The superior of the two is situated at the upper end of the intertrochanteric line, whereas the inferior one is at its lower end. The superior tubercle is sometimes called the femoral tubercle, tubercle of femur, or trochanteric tubercle. **Chassaignac's t.** TUBERCULUM ANTERIUS VERTEBRAE CERVICALIS VI. **condyloid t.** A small projection at the lateral extremity of the condyle of the mandible. The lateral ligament of the temporomandibular joint is attached to it. **conoid t.** TUBERCULUM CONOIDEUM. **corniculate t.** TUBERCULUM CORNICULATUM. **costal t.** TUBERCULUM COSTAE. **cuneate t.** TUBERCULUM CUNEATUM. **cuneiform t.** TUBERCULUM CUNEIFORME. **t. of Czermak** TUBERCULUM EPIGLOTTICUM. **darwinian t.** TUBERCULUM AURICULAE. **deltoid t.** **1** TUBEROSITAS DELTOIDEA HUMERI. **2** A small rough area for the attachment of the deltoid muscle on the anterior border of the lateral third of the clavicle. **dissection t.** TUBERCULOSIS CUTIS VERRUCOSA. **dorsal t. of radius** TUBERCULUM DORSALE RADII. **ear t.** TUBERCULUM AURICULAE. **epiglottic t.** TUBERCULUM EPIGLOTTICUM. **Farre's t.'s** Tumor nodules on the hepatic surface which are detectable on physical examination. **t. of femur** See under CERVICAL TUBERCLES. **fibrous t.** A tubercle which has undergone fibrosis. **genial t.'s** See under SPINA MENTALIS. **genital t.** A conical protuberance situated above the orifice of the urogenital sinus, made of a mass of mesoderm covered by ectoderm. It gives rise to the clitoris in the female and elongates in the male to form the penis. **Ghon t.** The primary lesion of pulmonary tuberculosis consisting of localized parenchymal infiltrate or nodule associated with enlargement of the regional hilar or mediastinal lymph nodes. The nodule and regional lymph nodes are often calcified. Also *Ghon focus, Ghon's primary lesion.* **gracile t.** TUBERCULUM NUCLEI GRACILIS. **gray t.** **1** The typical gray, translucent tubercle of tuberculosis. Compare CASEOUS TUBERCLE. **2** TUBER CINEREUM. **greater t. of humerus** TUBERCULUM MAJUS HUMERI. **hepatic t.** A mass of endodermal cells situated on the ventral aspect of the embryonic intestine at the lower end of its anterior third. It gives rise to the hepatic and biliary pathways. **His t.** TUBERCULUM AURICULAE. **t. of the iliac crest** TUBERCULUM ILIACUM. **iliopectineal t.** EMINENTIA ILIOPUBICA. **iliopubic t.** EMINENTIA ILIOPUBICA. **inferior genial t.** See under SPINA MENTALIS. **inferior thyroid t.** TUBERCULUM THYROIDEUM INFERIUS. **infraglenoid t.** TUBERCULUM INFRAGLENOIDALE. **intervenous t.** TUBERCULUM INTERVENOSUM. **jugular t.** TUBERCULUM JUGULARE OSSIS OCCIPITALIS. **jugular t. of occipital bone** TUBERCULUM JUGULARE OSSIS OCCIPITALIS. **labial t.** TUBERCULUM LABII SUPERIORIS. **lacrimal t.** *Outmoded* PAPILLA LACRIMALIS. **lateral intercondylar t.** TUBERCULUM INTERCONDYLARE LATERALE. **lateral orbital t.** EMINENTIA ORBITALIS. **lateral palpebral t.** EMINENTIA ORBITALIS. **lateral t. of posterior process of talus** TUBERCULUM LATERALE PROCESSUS POSTERIORIS TALI. **lateral t. of talus** **1** TUBERCULUM LATERALE PROCESSUS POSTERIORIS TALI. **2** PROCESSUS LATERALIS TALI. **lesser t. of humerus** TUBERCULUM MINUS HUMERI. **Lisfranc's t.** TUBERCULUM MUSCULI SCALENI ANTERIORIS. **Lister's t.** TUBERCULUM DORSALE RADII. **Lower's t.** TUBERCULUM INTERVENOSUM. **Luschka's t.** CARINA URETHRALIS VAGINAE. **lymphoid t.** A tuberculous lesion containing lymphoid cells. **mamillary t. of hypothalamus** CORPUS MAMILLARE. **mamillary t. of vertebrae** PROCESSUS MAMMILLARIS VERTEBRARUM LUMBALIUM. **marginal t. of zygomatic bone** TUBERCULUM MARGINALE OSSIS ZYGOMATICI. **medial intercondylar t.** TUBERCULUM INTERCONDYLARE MEDIALE. **medial t. of posterior process of talus** TUBERCULUM MEDIALE PROCESSUS POSTERIORIS TALI. **mental t. of mandible** TUBERCULUM MENTALE MANDIBULAE. **miliary t.** One of the tubercles which form in many organs in hematogenous tuberculosis. The name is derived from the fact that in untreated cases at autopsy the lesions are frequently the size of millet seeds (approximately 2 mm in diameter). **Montgomery's t.** Any of the enlarged sebaceous glands which appear during pregnancy on the areolae of the breast. Also *Morgagni's tubercle.* **Morgagni's t.** **1** MONTGOMERY'S TUBERCLE. **2** BULBUS OLFACTORIUS. **3** CARTILAGO CUNEIFORMIS. **müllerian t.** A tubercle situated on the posterior wall of the urogenital sinus of the embryo, at the point of entrance of the mesonephric and paramesonephric ducts. **necrogenic t.** TUBERCULOSIS CUTIS VERRUCOSA. **t. of nucleus cuneatus** TUBERCULUM CUNEATUM. **t. of nucleus gracilis** TUBERCULUM NUCLEI GRACILIS. **olfactory t.** 1 *Outmoded* BULBUS OLFACTORIUS. 2 A small oval elevation situated behind the olfactory pyramid. It is prominent in rodents and insectivores but rarely seen in humans. **orbital t.** EMINENTIA ORBITALIS. **palpebral t.** EMINENTIA ORBITALIS. **paramolar t.** An accessory tubercle or cusp on the buccal aspect of the crown of an upper molar tooth. **peroneal t. of calcaneus** TROCHLEA PERONEALIS CALCANEI. **pharyngeal t.** TUBERCULUM PHARYNGEUM. **t. of philtrum** TUBERCULUM LABII SUPERIORIS. **posterior t. of atlas** TUBERCULUM POSTERIUS ATLANTIS. **posterior t. of cervical vertebrae** TUBERCULUM POSTERIUS VERTEBRARUM CERVICALIUM. **posterior obturator t.** TUBERCULUM OBTURATORIUM POSTERIUS. **posterior t. of thalamus** NUCLEUS POSTERIOR THALAMI. **postglenoid t.** 1 A conical downward projection that is situated on the inferior surface of the posterior root of the zygomatic process of the temporal bone. It separates the lateral part of the articular surface of the mandibular fossa from the anterior margin of the tympanic part of the temporal bone. Also *postglenoid process, third root of zygomatic process, middle root of zygomatic process.* 2 A rarely occurring upward projection situated on the posterior arch of the atlas behind the superior articular facet. **postmortem t.** TUBERCULOSIS CUTIS VERRUCOSA. **preglenoid t.** TUBERCULUM ARTICULARE OSSIS TEMPORALIS. **prosector's t.** TUBERCULOSIS CUTIS VERRUCOSA. **pterygoid t.** TUBEROSITAS PTERYGOIDEA MANDIBULAE. **pubic t. of pubic bone** TUBERCULUM PUBICUM OSSIS PUBIS. **rabic t.'s** BABÈS TUBERCLES. **t. of rib** TUBERCULUM COSTAE. **t. of Rolando** TUBERCULUM TRIGEMINALE. **t. of root of zygoma** A distinct projection situated at the junction of the posterior and anterior roots of the zygomatic process of the temporal bone. It is anterolateral to the articular tubercle and provides attachment for the lateral ligament of the temporomandibular joint. **t. of Santorini** TUBERCULUM CORNICULATUM. **scalene t.** TUBERCULUM MUSCULI SCALENI ANTERIORIS. **t. of scaphoid bone** TUBERCULUM OSSIS SCAPHOIDEI. **sebaceous t.** MILIUM. **t. of sella turcica** TUBERCULUM SELLAE TURCICAE. **t. for serratus anterior muscle** TUBEROSITAS MUSCULI SERRATI ANTERIORIS. **spinous t.** One of the rudimentary spinous processes on the crista sacralis mediana of the sacrum. **superior genial t.** See under SPINA MENTALIS. **superior thyroid t.** TUBERCULUM THYROIDEUM SUPERIUS. **supraglenoid t.** TUBERCULUM SUPRAGLENOIDALE. **supratragic t.** TUBERCULUM SUPRATRAGICUM. **t. of tibia** 1 TUBEROSITAS TIBIAE. 2 *Outmoded* EMINENTIA INTERCONDYLARIS. **t. of trapezium** TUBERCULUM OSSIS TRAPEZII. **trochanteric t.** See under CERVICAL TUBERCLES. **t. of upper lip** TUBERCULUM LABII SUPERIORIS. **t.'s of vertebra** The superior, inferior, and lateral tubercles in the region of a transverse process of the twelfth thoracic vertebra. They correspond to the mamillary, accessory, and transverse processes, respectively, of a lumbar vertebra. **Whitnall's t.** EMINENTIA ORBITALIS. **Wrisberg's t.** TUBERCULUM CUNEIFORME. **yellow t.** CASEOUS TUBERCLE. **t. of zygoma** TUBERCULUM ARTICULARE OSSIS TEMPORALIS. **zygomatic t.** TUBERCULUM ARTICULARE OSSIS TEMPORALIS.

**tubercul-** \tʸʊburʹkyəl-\ TUBERCULO-.

**tubercula** \tʸʊburʹkyələ\ Plural of TUBERCULUM.

**tubercular** \tʸʊburʹkyələr\ 1 Pertaining to a tubercle. 2 Characterized by tubercles. 3 *Incorrect* TUBERCULOUS.

**tuberculase** \tʸʊburʹkyəlās\ A vaccine prepared from tubercle bacilli and formerly used in tuberculosis prophylaxis.

**tuberculate** \tʸʊburʹkyələt\ Characterized by or having tubercles. Also *tuberculated, tuberculose.*

**tuberculid** \tʸʊburʹkyəlid\ [TUBERCUL- + -ID²] A widespread eruption attributed to the hematogenous dissemination of tubercle bacilli from a focus of infection in an individual already sensitized to tuberculosis. Also *tuberculoderm, tuberculide, tuberculoderma.* **papular t.** A tuberculid consisting predominantly of small papules that do not undergo necrosis. **papular necrotic t.** PAPULONECROTIC TUBERCULID. **papulonecrotic t.** A tuberculid characterized by the development, mainly on the extremities, of papules that undergo necrosis and leave scars. Also *papular necrotic tuberculid, tuberculosis papulonecrotica.* **rosacealike t.** Rosacea in which small firm granulomatous papules are present. • The condition was for many years incorrectly classified on histological grounds as a tuberculid.

**tuberculide** \tʸʊburʹkyəlīd\ TUBERCULID.

**tuberculin** \tʸʊburʹkyəlin\ [TUBERCUL- + -IN] A sterile liquid containing an extract prepared from broth cultures of *Mycobacterium tuberculosis* or other mycobacteria. It was first developed by Koch for use in the treatment of tuberculosis. Many modifications of it are used today, primarily in skin tests for tuberculin hypersensitivity and as an aid in the diagnosis of past or present tuberculosis. Also *tuberculinum.* **alkaline t.** Tuberculin prepared by extracting a broth culture of mycobacteria with an alkaline solution. It is very similar to the original tuberculin prepared by Koch. **autogenous t.** AUTOTUBERCULIN. **Behring's t.** TUBERCULASE. **Béraneck's t.** Tuberculin containing both a basiotoxin of a tubercle extract and an acidotoxin of the filtrate. **Buchner's t.** Tuberculin prepared by triturating dried tubercle bacilli with sand and expressing the material under hydraulic pressure. **Calmette's t.** Purified old tuberculin formerly used in conjunctival testing, as in Calmette's reaction. Also *tuberculin precipitation, purified tuberculin.* **Dixon's t.** A tuberculin prepared from mycobacteria treated with ether and extracted in a salt solution. **endotin t.** New tuberculin treated with xylol, ether, chloroform, and alcohol to remove inert substances. **Klemperer's t.** Tuberculin prepared from cultures of *Mycobacterium bovis.* **Koch's t.** OLD TUBERCULIN. **Landmann's t.** Tuberculin prepared from especially virulent cultures of tubercle bacilli, water, physiological salt solution, and glycerin, and which is heated gradually. **Maragliano's t.** A tuberculin containing the water-soluble extracts of tubercle bacilli. **Maréchal's t.** Old tuberculin mixed with guaiacol. **Moro's t.** An ointment consisting of equal parts of old tuberculin and lanolin, used as a tuberculin test. Also *Moro's reagent.* **old t.** A sterile solution of the concentrated soluble products of the growth of tubercle bacilli. The material is adjusted to a standard potency with glycerin and saline and used as a skin test for tuberculosis. Also *tuberculinum pristinum, original tuberculin, paratoloid, paratoloidin, Koch's tuberculin, Koch's lymph.* **original t.** OLD TUBERCULIN. **perlsucht t.** SPENGLER'S TUBERCULIN. **perlsucht t. original** SPENGLER'S TUBERCULIN. **perlsucht t. rest** PERLSUCHT BACILLEN EMULSION. **PPD t.** PURIFIED PROTEIN DERIVATIVE OF TUBERCULIN. **t. precipitation** CALMETTE'S TUBERCULIN. Abbr. TP **purified t.** CALMETTE'S TUBERCULIN. **purified protein derivative**

**of t.** A concentrate prepared from a culture of tubercle bacilli and purified by ultrafiltration and precipitation of the protein material using trichloroacetic acid. Also *PPD-Seibert, Seibert's tuberculin, PPD tuberculin.* Abbr. PPD **Ruck's watery extract t.** A concentrated tuberculin prepared by a series of filtrations and precipitations and finally diluted into a 1% aqueous solution. **Seibert's t.** PURIFIED PROTEIN DERIVATIVE OF TUBERCULIN. **Spengler's t.** Tuberculin prepared from *Mycobacterium bovis.* Also *perlsucht tuberculin, perlsucht tuberculin original.* **Vaudremer's t.** Tuberculin prepared with ground *Aspergillus fumigatus* mycelia in order to decrease its toxicity.

**tuberculination** \t$^y$ōōbur'kyəlinā'shən\ TUBERCULINIZATION.

**tuberculinization** \t$^y$ōōbur'kyəlinīzā'shən\ The use of tuberculin in tuberculosis therapy or in skin tests. Also *tuberculination.*

**tuberculinum** \t$^y$ōōbur'kyəlī'nəm\ TUBERCULIN. **t. pristinum** OLD TUBERCULIN.

**tuberculization** \t$^y$ōōbur'kyəlīzā'shən\ 1 The formation of tubercles in body tissues. 2 The process whereby a population is subjected to infection with tuberculosis over a period of years so that a degree of immunity to the disease is acquired.

**tuberculo-** \t$^y$ōōbur'kyəlō-\ [L *tuberculum* tubercle] A combining form meaning (1) tubercle; (2) tuberculosis, tuberculous; (3) the tubercle bacillus, *Mycobacterium tuberculosis.* Also *tubercul-.*

**tuberculoalbumin** \-albyoo'min\ A tuberculaselike protein extracted from tubercle bacilli.

**tuberculocele** \t$^y$ōōbur'kyəlōsēl'\ [TUBERCULO- + -CELE[1]] Testicular tuberculosis.

**tuberculocidal** \t$^y$ōōbur'kyəlōsī'dəl\ Capable of destroying *Mycobacterium tuberculosis.*

**tuberculocide** \t$^y$ōōbur'kyəlōsīd'\ Any agent lethal to *Mycobacterium tuberculosis.*

**tuberculoderm** \t$^y$ōōbur'kyəlōdurm'\ [TUBERCULO- + -DERM] TUBERCULID.

**tuberculoderma** \-dur'mə\ TUBERCULID.

**tuberculoid** \t$^y$ōōbur'kyəloid\ 1 Histologically similar to tuberculosis: used principally to designate a type of leprosy. 2 Relating to or having tuberculoid leprosy.

**tuberculoidin** \t$^y$ōōbur'kyəloi'din\ Tuberculin modified by treatment with alcohol so that it is free of bacilli.

**tuberculoma** \t$^y$ōōbur'kyəlō'mə\ [TUBERCUL- + -OMA] A mass of caseous tuberculous tissue resembling a tumor, usually found in the lungs or brain. **t. en plaque** A flat plaque of tuberculous tissue found over the surface of the brain, usually overlying the frontoparietal cortex. It sometimes appears in tuberculous meningoencephalitis. **tuberculoprotein** The protein of the tubercle bacillus, used in serologic tests. *Outmoded.*

**tuberculose** \t$^y$ōōbur'kyəlōs\ TUBERCULATE.

**tuberculosilicosis** \-sil'ikō'sis\ SILICOTUBERCULOSIS.

# tuberculosis

**tuberculosis** \t$^y$ōōbur'kyəlō'sis\ [TUBERCUL- + -OSIS] An infectious disease of man and animals which is caused by any of several *Mycobacterium* species. The organisms almost always gain access to the body through inhalation or ingestion. In man, the disease is usually due to *M. tuberculosis.* Characteristically, tubercles form in the tissues where they may grow and caseate or regress and heal. The most common primary site of infection is the lung, but any other organ or tissue may be involved, including the lymphatic system. Symptoms vary with the organ or system involved. The disease may run an acute course but is usually a chronic process. Also *white plague* (obs.). Abbr. TB **active t.** 1 Tuberculosis in which bacteriologic tests are positive. 2 Tuberculosis in which there is progression of disease associated with replication of tubercle bacilli. **acute miliary t.** An acute form of tuberculosis in which there is hematogenous dissemination of infection. Miliary tubercles form in various body organs. **adrenal t.** *Older term* ADDISON'S DISEASE. **aerogenic t.** Tuberculosis caused by inhalation of air-borne tubercle bacilli. Also *air-borne tuberculosis.* **anthracotic t.** Pulmonary tuberculosis infection occurring in persons, usually coal workers, with anthracosis of the lungs (pneumoconiosis). **attenuated t.** A mild type of chronic tuberculosis. **t. of bones** Infection of bone by *Mycobacterium tuberculosis.* Also *skeletal tuberculosis.* **t. of bones and joints** Infection of either the bones or joints by *Mycobacterium tuberculosis.* Also *tuberculous rheumatism.* **bovine t.** Tuberculosis in cattle usually affecting the lungs, caused by *Mycobacterium bovis.* It is transmissible to other animals and to man. Formerly, an important source of human infection was unpasteurized milk from infected cows. **bronchogenic t.** Pulmonary tuberculosis in which spread occurs by a bronchial route to other previously uninvolved lung tissue. **bronchopneumonic t.** A severe form of tuberculosis in which there is pneumonic consolidation. **caseous t.** Tuberculosis in which the tubercles have undergone caseation necrosis. **cerebral t.** 1 TUBERCULOUS MENINGITIS. 2 A condition characterized by intracerebral tuberculomas. **childhood t.** 1 Pulmonary tuberculosis occurring in infants and children. The primary focus of infection may be in any part of the lung parenchyma. Lymph node involvement usually occurs and lymphohematogenous spread of disease is quite common. Cavitation rarely occurs. Pulmonary and lymph node lesions frequently heal spontaneously. 2 *Outmoded* PRIMARY TUBERCULOSIS. **chronic fibroid t.** Long-standing tuberculosis in which fibrosis has occurred, usually in the lung. **chronic ulcerative t.** Pulmonary tuberculosis with ulceration of the bronchioles and alveoli which usually results in cavity formation. Ulceration may occur also in the larger bronchi or in the trachea and larynx. **t. colliquativa** SCROFULODERMA. **cutaneous t.** TUBERCULOSIS CUTIS. **t. cutis** Any tuberculous infection of the skin, including such conditions as lupus vulgaris, tuberculosis cutis verrucosa, tuberculosis cutis orificialis, scrofuloderma, and papulonecrotic tuberculid. Also *cutaneous tuberculosis, scrofuloderma.* **t. cutis orificialis** A form of tuberculosis cutis in which ulcerative tuberculous lesions develop around the body orifices. The condition is sometimes seen in persons with systemic tuberculosis. Also *tuberculosis orificialis, tuberculosis ulcerosa.* **t. cutis verrucosa** A warty granulomatous nodule occurring in an individual who has been exposed to tuberculosis. It results from infection of the skin with *Mycobacterium tuberculosis,* either from the subject's own sputum or from contact with infected dead tissue. Also *verruca necrogenica, tuberculosis verrucosa, tuberculosis verrucosa cutis, warty tuberculosis, anatomical tubercle, anatomical wart, postmortem tubercle, prosector's tubercle, necrogenic wart, pathologist's wart, postmortem wart, prosector's wart, tuberculous wart, dissection tubercle, necrogenic tubercle.* **cystic t. of bones** Tuberculosis of bones causing radiologically or pathologically visible cavitation. **disseminated t.** Tuberculosis that has spread hematogenously to various parts of the body, especially in the form of miliary tuberculosis. **endogenous t.** Tuberculosis which results from spread of infection or reactivation of infection in another area of the patient's body. The initial focus is often a primary tuberculous lesion. **endothelial t.** Tuberculosis which affects the lymphatic canals, lymph nodes, or serous membranes (for example, pleura, peritoneum, pericardium, cerebral meninges). **extrapulmonary t.** Tuberculosis in any part of the body other than the lung. **exudative t.** A simple form of pulmonary tuberculosis in which alveolar spaces and small bronchi fill with a cellular exudate containing many mononuclear cells. See also TUBERCULOUS PNEUMONIA. **fibrocaseous t.** Chronic tuberculosis in which lung tissues have become fibrous and the diseased areas have undergone caseation necrosis. **fibrosing t.** Chronic tuberculosis in which there is pronounced fibrosis but little, if any, caseation. Also *fibroid tuberculosis.* **t. fungosa cutis** Localized fungating tuberculosis affecting the skin and sometimes seen in conjunction with tuberculous infection of an underlying bone or lymph node. **genital t.** Tuberculous infection of the reproductive organs, usually the uterine tubes and endometrium. **genitourinary t.** Tuberculosis of the genitourinary system, usually the result of septic or miliary tuberculosis. **glandular t.** TUBERCULOSIS OF LYMPH NODES. **hematogenous t.** Tuberculosis in which the infective tubercle bacilli are transported by the bloodstream from the primary site of infection to other organs and tissues. **hilus t.** Tuberculosis of the lymph nodes at the hilus of the lung. **ileocecal t.** Tuberculosis of the ileum and cecum. **t. of intestines** Tuberculous infection of the intestinal tract, resulting in superficial ulcerating or hypertrophic lesions. The hypertrophic lesion can eventuate in mass or stricture formation. **laryngeal t.** TUBERCULOUS LARYNGITIS. **latent t.** Tuberculosis in which the bacteriologic findings are negative and in which no radiologic changes occur for an extended period of time. Also *quiescent tuberculosis.* **t. lichenoides** LICHEN SCROFULOSORUM. **t. luposa** LUPUS VULGARIS. **t. of lymph nodes** Tuberculous infection of the lymph nodes, especially the cervical, bronchial, and mesenteric nodes. Also *lymphoid tuberculosis, glandular tuberculosis, lymphogenous tuberculosis* (imprecise). See also SCROFULA. **lymphogenous t.** 1 Tuberculosis which spreads via the lymphatic system. 2 *Imprecise* TUBERCULOSIS OF LYMPH NODES. **lymphoid t.** TUBERCULOSIS OF LYMPH NODES. **meningeal t.** Tuberculosis involving the meninges of the subarachnoid space. **t. miliaris cutis** An uncommon form of tuberculosis cutis resulting from hematogenous spread of tubercle bacilli and deposition of bacilli in the skin so that a papular or pustular rash develops. **miliary t.** Tuberculosis of various body organs and tissues resulting from hematogenous dissemination of tubercle bacilli. The characteristic lesions are minute tubercles which develop in the affected organs and tissues. Also *phthisis nodosa.* **minimal t.** Tuberculous infiltration of the lungs in which the shadows of the infiltrate on x ray do not occupy more than the area of two intercostal spaces (the apex of the upper lobe of the lung being equal to one intercostal space). **moderately advanced t.** Tuberculosis with disseminated lesions of slight to moderate density throughout the volume of one lung or its equivalent in both lungs, or dense confluent lesions over one third of the volume of one lung. In both instances, cavitation is less than 4 cm in diameter. **open t.** Any form of tuberculosis in which the organisms are discharged from the body, as in an exudate, particularly sputum. **t. orificialis** TUBERCULOSIS CUTIS ORIFICIALIS. **t. papulonecrotica** PAPULONECROTIC TUBERCULID. **postprimary t.** REINFECTION TUBERCULOSIS. **primary t.** An initial tuberculous infection of the lungs. A pulmonary parenchymal lesion, often caseous, is associated with spread of infection to regional lymph nodes (for example, a small focus of tuberculous pneumonia with extension to hilar lymph nodes). Healing occurs with fibrosis and possibly calcification of affected tissues. If complete healing does not take place, the disease may progress to an acute or chronic infection. Hematogenous dissemination of infection may then occur with miliary disease the result. Also *childhood tuberculosis* (outmoded). **productive t.** Tuberculosis in which there is development of a new type of tissue, namely, granulomatous tissue consisting of epithelioid cells in concentric masses, lymphocytes, or Langhans giant cells at the foci of infection. **pulmonary t.** Infection of the lungs with *Mycobacterium tuberculosis.* The resulting disease may range from a small, harmless scar to widespread lung damage and destruction. Also *pneumonophthisis.* **quiescent t.** LATENT TUBERCULOSIS. **reinfection t.** A second infection with tuberculosis, usually pulmonary, occurring after healing of a previous primary infection. Also *postprimary tuberculosis.* **renal t.** Infection of one or both kidneys by *Mycobacterium tuberculosis.* Pyuria without bacteriuria is common. At first symptoms may be absent but, as the disease spreads in the urinary tract, ulcerations may lead to contraction of the bladder with concomitant frequency and hematuria. The kidneys also may be involved in miliary tuberculosis with scattered small foci of inflammation. Chemotherapy of renal tuberculosis usually is effective. **skeletal t.** TUBERCULOSIS OF BONES. **t. of spine** Tuberculosis of a vertebral body or disk. Also *spinal caries.* **surgical t.** Any form of tuberculosis (for example, tuberculosis of the bones, joints, or organs) that is amenable to surgical treatment, removal, or control. **t. ulcerosa** TUBERCULOSIS CUTIS ORIFICIALIS. **t. verrucosa** TUBERCULOSIS CUTIS VERRUCOSA. **t. verrucosa cutis** TUBERCULOSIS CUTIS VERRUCOSA. **warty t.** TUBERCULOSIS CUTIS VERRUCOSA.

**tuberculostatic** \tʸʊburʹkyəlōstatʹik\ [TUBERCULO- + -STAT + -IC] Inhibiting the growth of *Mycobacterium tuberculosis.*

**tuberculotic** \tʸʊburʹkyəlätʹik\ Pertaining to, having, or characterized by tuberculosis; tuberculous.

**tuberculotoxin** \tʸʊburʹkyəlōtäkʹsin\ Any toxin derived from *Mycobacterium tuberculosis.*

**tuberculous** \tʸʊburʹkyələs\ Pertaining to, affected with, or characterized by tuberculosis; caused by *Mycobacterium tuberculosis.* Also *tubercular* (incorrect).

**tuberculum** \tʸʊburʹkyələm\ [L (dim. of *tuber* a bump, protuberance) a small bump, swelling, protuberance] TUBERCLE. **t. acusticum** AREA VESTIBULARIS. **t. adductorium femoris** [NA] A small palpable projection at the summit of the medial surface of the medial condyle of the femur. There it meets the medial supracondylar line and is situated just above the medial epicondyle, providing attachment for the tendon of the adductor magnus muscle. Also *adductor tubercle of femur.* **t. anterius atlantis** [NA] A small median projection on the ventral surface of the anterior arch of the atlas to which the anterior longitudinal ligament and longus colli muscle are attached. Also *anterior tubercle of atlas.* **t. anterius thalami** [NA] A prominent elevation that projects slightly above the dorsal thalamic surface at the most rostral end of the thalamus and lies close to the midline on each side, helping to form the boundary of the interventricular foramen. The tuberculum anterius thalami is formed by the anterior thalamic nuclear group. Also *anterior tubercle of thalamus.* **t. anterius vertebrae cervicalis VI** [NA] The large anterior tubercle on each side of the sixth cervical vertebra against which the common carotid artery lying anterior to it may be compressed. Also *carotid tubercle, carotid tubercle of sixth cervical vertebra, Chassaignac's tubercle.* **t. anterius vertebrarum cervicalium** [NA] A small rounded projection at the free end of the anterior bar or costal process of the transverse process of the cervical vertebrae. It is situated anterolateral to the foramen transversarium and provides attachment for tendinous slips of the scalenus anterior, longus colli, and longus capitis muscles. Also *anterior tubercle of cervical vertebrae.* **t. arthriticum** TOPHUS. **t. articulare ossis temporalis** [NA] A horizontal bulge, covered with cartilage, on the posterior part of the inferior surface of the zygomatic process of the temporal bone, forming the anterior boundary of the mandibular fossa. It is in contact with the articular disk of the temporomandibular joint. Also *articular tubercle of temporal bone, preglenoid tubercle, tubercle of zygoma, zygomatic tubercle, articular eminence of temporal bone.* **t. auriculae** [NA] A small projection or pointed prominence on the incurved free margin of the ear where the upper and posterior parts of the helix meet. It is particularly prominent at about the sixth month of fetal life. Also *Woolner's tip, His tubercle, ear tubercle, darwinian tubercle, auricular tubercle, vestigial nodule.* **t. calcanei** [NA] A small rounded projection, often double, on the inferior surface of the calcaneus at the anterior extremity of the rough area for the attachment of the ligamentum plantare longum. Also *anterior tubercle of the calcaneus.* **t. cinereum** 1 TUBERCULUM TRIGEMINALE. 2 TUBER CINEREUM. **t. conoideum** [NA] A prominent projection near the posterior margin of the inferior surface of the clavicle near its lateral end. It provides attachment for the conoid part of the coracoclavicular ligament. Also *conoid tubercle.* **t. corniculatum** [NA] A prominent rounded eminence on the posterior part of the free margin of the aryepiglottic fold on each side which is produced by the underlying cuneiform cartilage. Also *corniculate tubercle, tubercle of Santorini.* **t. costae** [NA] A prominent projection on the outer surface of the posterior end of a rib at the junction of its neck and body. It is divided into a superolateral nonarticular part for the attachment of the lateral costotransverse ligament and an inferomedial, oval articular surface for articulation with the costal fovea on the transverse process of a corresponding vertebra. Also *tubercle of rib, costal tubercle.* **t. cuneatum** [NA] An elongated oval enlargement located lateral to the posterointermediate sulcus and the tuberculum gracile on each side of the posterior aspect of the medulla oblongata. The tuberculum cuneatum is formed by the nucleus cuneatus, into which project for synapse the nerve fibers of the fasciculus cuneatus. Also *tuberculum nuclei cuneati, tubercle of nucleus cuneatus, cuneate tubercle.* **t. cuneiforme** [NA] A small inconstant eminence that is situated just anterior to the corniculate tubercle on the free margin of the aryepiglottic fold on each side. It is produced by the underlying cuneiform cartilage. Also *cuneiform tubercle, Wrisberg's tubercle.* **t. dorsale radii** [NA] A prominent ridge in the center of the posterior surface of the distal end of the radius to which the extensor retinaculum is attached. Medial to it is the deep oblique groove for the tendon of extensor pollicis longus muscle, while lateral to it is a shallow groove for the tendon of extensor carpi radialis brevis muscle. Also *dorsal tubercle of radius, Lister's tubercle.* **t. epiglotticum** [NA] An elongated rounded eminence at the distal end of the posterior surface of the epiglottis. Also *epiglottic tubercle, cushion of epiglottis, tubercle of Czermak.* **t. gracile** [NA] TUBERCULUM NUCLEI GRACILIS. **t. hypoglossi** TRIGONUM NERVI HYPOGLOSSI. **t. iliacum** [NA] A palpable prominence on the outer lip of the iliac crest, two to three inches posterosuperior to the anterior superior iliac spine. Through it the transtubercular plane passes. Also *tubercle of the iliac crest.* **t. impar** A median, approximately triangular swelling, placed between paired lateral swellings of the first branchial arch in the embryo. It is a primordium of the body of the tongue just in front of the thyroid diverticulum. **t. infraglenoidale** [NA] A rough triangular area at the upper end of the lateral margin of the scapula where it meets the glenoid cavity. There it provides attachment for the long head of triceps muscle. Also *infraglenoid tubercle, infraglenoid tuberosity.* **t. intercondylare laterale** [NA] The upward projection of the lateral side of the intercondylar eminence on the superior surface of the upper end of the tibia. Also *lateral intercondylar tubercle.* **t. intercondylare mediale** [NA] The upward projection of the medial side of the intercondylar eminence on the superior surface of the upper end of the tibia. Also *medial intercondylar tubercle.* **t. intervenosum** [NA] A small eminence on the posterior wall of the right atrium of the heart, situated immediately below the opening of the superior vena cava. It is indistinct in human adults but is quite prominent in many other mammals. Also *intervenous tubercle, Lower's tubercle.* **t. jugulare ossis occipitalis** [NA] An oval projection situated on the superior surface of the condylar part of the occipital bone and above the anterolateral margin of the foramen magnum on each side. It overlies the hypoglossal canal and on its upper surface is a groove for the termination of the sigmoid sinus. Also *jugular tubercle of occipital bone, jugular tubercle, jugular eminence.* **t. labii superioris** [NA] A small prominence at the lower extent of the philtrum of the upper lip where the skin meets the mucous membrane. Also *tubercle of upper lip, labial tubercle, tubercle of philtrum.* **t. laterale processus posterioris tali** [NA] The outer and larger of the two projections bounding the groove for the tendon of the flexor hallucis longus muscle on the posterior process of the talus. Also *lateral tubercle of posterior process of talus, lateral tubercle of talus.* **t. majus humeri** [NA] The large rounded projection at the lateral side of the upper end of the humerus. It is separated from the lesser tubercle by the intertubercular sulcus on its medial side. The upper and posterior parts are separated from the head by the anatomical neck and provide attachment to the supraspinatus, infraspinatus, and teres minor muscles from front to back. Also *greater tubercle of humerus, greater tuberosity of humerus.* **t. marginale ossis zygomatici** [NA] A small, rounded, subcutaneous projection situated on the temporal, or posterosuperior, border of the zygomatic bone just below the frontozygomatic suture. Also *marginal tubercle of zygomatic bone, marginal process of malar bone, Soemmering's bone* (outmoded). **t. mediale processus posterioris tali** [NA] The inner and smaller of the two projections bounding the groove for the tendon of the flexor hallucis longus muscle on the posterior process of the talus. It provides attachment to fibers of the deltoid ligament superiorly and to the medial talocalcanean ligament inferiorly. Also *medial tubercle of the posterior process of the talus.* **t. mentale mandibulae** [NA] A raised area on each side of the depressed base of the mental protuberance at the lower end of the anterior aspect of the symphysis menti. Also *mental tubercle of mandible.* **t. minus humeri** [NA] The anterior prominence at the upper end of the humerus just distal to the anatomical neck. It is separated laterally from the greater tubercle by the intertubercular sulcus, and it is flattened for the insertion of the subscapularis muscle. Also *lesser tubercle of humerus, lesser tuberosity of humerus.* **t. musculi scaleni anterioris** [NA] A small, rough projection on the inner border of the first rib, continuous with a ridge on the superior surface separating the subclavian vein, anteriorly, from the artery, posteriorly, and providing attachment to the scalenus anterior muscle. Also *tubercle of anterior scalene muscle, Lisfranc's tubercle, scalene tubercle.* **t. nuclei cuneati** TUBERCULUM CUNEATUM. **t. nuclei gracilis** One of two elongated, ovoid enlargements located symmetrically, one on each side of the dorsal median sulcus on the posterior aspect of the medulla oblongata. It is formed by the nucleus gracilis, into which project for synapse the fibers of the fasciculus gracilis. Also *tuberculum gracile, tubercle of nucleus gracilis, gracile tubercle, eminentia gracilis, clava.* **t. obturatorium anterius** [NA] A small projection on the anteroinferior margin of the obturator foramen at the anterior end of the inferior margin of the superior pubic ramus. There the free margin of the obturator membrane is attached anteriorly. Also *anterior obturator tubercle.* **t. obturatorium posterius** [NA] A small projection on the posterosuperior margin of the obturator foramen where it meets the anterior margin of the acetabular notch, to which the free margin of the obturator membrane is attached posteriorly. Also *posterior obturator tubercle.* **t. olfactorium** The elevation on the base of the frontal lobe of most mammals, the cortex of which constitutes a major termination of the intermediate olfactory stria and for a three-layered primary olfactory cortex. **t. ossis scaphoidei** [NA] A laterally directed, rounded projection on the distal part of the palmar surface of the scaphoid bone. It provides attachment to the flexor retinaculum and part of the abductor pollicis brevis muscle. Also *tubercle of scaphoid bone, tuberosity of scaphoid bone.* **t. ossis trapezii** [NA] A prominent ridge on the palmar surface of the trapezium bone. Medial to it is a deep groove for the tendon of flexor carpi radialis muscle. It provides attachment to the flexor retinaculum and to parts of the three thenar muscles. Also *tubercle of trapezium, tuberosity of trapezium.* **t. pharyngeum** [NA] A small midline protuberance situated on the inferior surface of the basilar part of the occipital bone in front of the foramen magnum, to which the highest fibers of the superior constrictor of the pharynx and the pharyngeal raphe are attached. Also *pharyngeal tubercle, basilar crest of occipital bone, pharyngeal crest of occipital bone, basilar spine, pharyngeal spine.* **t. posterius atlantis** [NA] A median projection on the outer surface of the posterior arch of the atlas that represents a rudimentary spinous process. It provides attachment to the ligamentum nuchae and the two recti capitis posteriores minores muscles on either side. Also *posterior tubercle of atlas.* **t. posterius thalami** NUCLEUS POSTERIOR THALAMI. **t. posterius vertebrarum cervicalium** [NA] The rounded free extremity of the posterior root of the transverse process of the cervical vertebrae. It extends posterolaterally to the foramen transversarium and provides attachment for the splenius, levator scapulae, longissimus cervicis, iliocostalis cervicis, scalenus medius, and scalenus posterior muscles. Also *posterior tubercle of cervical vertebrae.* **t. pubicum ossis pubis** [NA] The rounded prominence at the lateral extremity of the pubic crest providing attachment for the medial end of the inguinal ligament and the cremaster muscle and forming the lateral boundary of the floor of the superficial inguinal ring. Also *pubic tubercle of pubic bone.* **t. sellae turcicae** [NA] A transverse bony elevation situated behind the sulcus prechiasmaticus and at the anterior boundary of the sella turcica. It marks the junction of the presphenoid and postsphenoid bones. Also *tubercle of sella turcica.* **t. supraglenoidale** [NA] A rough elevation above the glenoid cavity at its junction with the root of the coracoid process. At that point the long head of the biceps brachii muscle arises within the fibrous capsule of the shoulder joint. Also *supraglenoid tubercle, supraglenoid tuberosity.* **t. supratragicum** [NA] A small elevation occasionally located below the anterior incisure and above the tragus of the auricle of the external ear. Also *supratragic tubercle.* **t. thyroideum inferius** [NA] A small eminence situated on the inferior margin of the external surface of the thyroid cartilage at the lower end of the oblique line. Also *inferior thyroid tubercle.* **t. thyroideum superius** [NA] A small eminence situated at the upper end of the oblique line just in front of the root of the superior cornu of the thyroid cartilage. Also *superior thyroid tubercle.* **t. trigeminale** [NA] An elevation on the dorsolateral aspectof the caudal medulla oblongata between the fasciculus cuneatus and the roots of the medullary part of the accessory nerve. Slightly larger above, it tapers in width inferiorly, and is formed by the spinal tract of the trigeminal nerve. Also *tubercle of Rolando, tuberculum cinereum.*

**tuberositas** \t$^y$oo′bəräs′itas\ [Late L (from L *tuberosus* tuberous, from *tuber* a bump, swelling, protuberance + *-itas* -ITY), fullness of bumps, tuberosity] An elevation or a projection on a bone, usually having an uneven surface for the attachment of muscles or ligaments. Also *tuberosity.* **t. deltoidea humeri** [NA] A V-shaped, rough elevation at the middle of the anterolateral surface of the humerus for the insertion of the deltoid muscle. Also *deltoid tuberosity of humerus, deltoid eminence, deltoid crest, deltoid tubercle, deltoid ridge.* **t. glutea ossis femoris** [NA] A thick vertical ridge on the posterior surface of the upper third of the shaft of the femur, extending from the root of the greater trochanter to the upper end of the lateral lip of linea aspera, with which it is continuous. It provides attachment for the lower half of the gluteus maximus muscle and the pubic part of the adductor magnus muscle. Also *gluteal tuberosity of femur, gluteal crest, gluteal ridge of femur.* **t. iliaca** [NA] The large rough portion of the sacropelvic surface just below the posterior part of the iliac crest and superior to the auricular surface, comprising two depressions. They are separated by a ridge for the interosseous and dorsal sacroiliac ligaments that connect it to the sacrum. Also *iliac tuberosity.* **t. masseterica** [NA] The lateral surface of the angle and adjacent ramus of the mandible that has several oblique ridges for the attachment of the tendinous septa in the masseter muscle. Also *masseteric tuberosity.* **t. musculi serrati anterioris** [NA] A rough, well-marked elevation at the middle of the external surface of the body of the second rib for the attachment of part of the first digitation and all of the second of the serratus anterior muscle. Also *tuberosity for serratus anterior muscle, tuberosity for anterior serratus muscle, tubercle for serratus anterior muscle.* **t. ossis cuboidei** [NA] A small rounded projection on the lateral surface of the cuboid bone at the junction with its plantar surface. It is the lateral termination of the ridge posterior to the groove for the tendon of the peroneus longus muscle on the plantar surface. It has a smooth facet for the sesamoid bone or cartilage in the tendon. Also *tuberosity of cuboid bone.* **t. ossis metatarsalis primi (I)** [NA] An oval elevation on the plantar aspect of the projecting lateral angle of the base of the first metatarsal bone for the insertion of the peroneus longus muscle and some fibers of the tibialis anterior muscle. Also *tuberosity of first metatarsal* *bone.* **t. ossis metatarsalis quinti (V)** [NA] A large projection extending proximally from the lateral aspect of the base of the fifth metatarsal bone for the attachment of the peroneus brevis muscle on its dorsal surface and the plantar aponeurosis to its tip. Also *tuberosity of fifth metatarsal bone.* **t. ossis navicularis** [NA] A rounded prominence projecting plantarward from the medial surface of the navicular bone. The tibialis posterior muscle is mainly attached to it. Also *tuberosity of navicular bone.* **t. phalangis distalis manus** [NA] An elevated U-shaped roughness on the palmar aspect of the distal phalanx of each finger. Connective tissue fibers are attached to it, anchoring the soft tissues of the tip of the finger. Also *distal tuberosity of fingers.* **t. phalangis distalis pedis** [NA] A rough prominence on the plantar aspect of the distal phalanx of each toe to which connective tissue fibers are attached, anchoring the soft tissues of the tip of the toe. Also *distal tuberosity of toes.* **t. pterygoidea mandibulae** [NA] The rugged medial surface of the angle and adjacent ramus of the mandible for the insertion of the tendinous fasciculi of the medial pterygoid muscle. Also *pterygoid tuberosity of mandible, pterygoid tubercle.* **t. radii** [NA] A conical projection on the anteromedial aspect of the proximal end of the radius just distal to the neck. It has a rough posterior part for the insertion of the biceps brachii muscle and a smooth anterior part related to a bursa deep to the tendon of the muscle. Also *radial tuberosity, tuberosity of radius, bicipital tuberosity, bicipital eminence.* **t. sacralis** [NA] The rough and pitted area posterior to the auricular surface on the lateral part of the sacrum to which the interosseous and dorsal sacroiliac ligaments are attached. Also *sacral tuberosity.* **t. tibiae** [NA] A triangular projection at the upper end of the anterior margin of the shaft of the tibia, at the apex of the junction of the two tibial condyles. It presents a smooth upper portion for the attachment of the ligamentum patellae and a rough lower portion related to the subcutaneous infrapatellar bursa. Also *tuberosity of tibia, tubercle of tibia, tibial tuberosity, spine of tibia, tibial spine.* **t. ulnae** [NA] The lower part of the anterior surface of the raised coronoid process at the upper end of the ulna just proximal to its junction with the shaft. The brachialis muscle and the oblique cord are attached to it. Also *tuberosity of ulna.*

**tuberositates** \tʸoo′bəräs′itā′tēz\ Plural of TUBEROSITAS.

**tuberosity** \tʸoo′bəräs′itē\ [L *tuberositas.* See TUBEROSITAS.] TUBEROSITAS. **t. for anterior serratus muscle** TUBEROSITAS MUSCULI SERRATI ANTERIORIS. **bicipital t.** TUBEROSITAS RADII. **t. of calcaneus** TUBER CALCANEI. **t. of cuboid bone** TUBEROSITAS OSSIS CUBOIDEI. **deltoid t. of humerus** TUBEROSITAS DELTOIDEA HUMERI. **distal t. of fingers** TUBEROSITAS PHALANGIS DISTALIS MANUS. **distal t. of toes** TUBEROSITAS PHALANGIS DISTALIS PEDIS. **t. of first metatarsal bone** TUBEROSITAS OSSIS METATARSALIS PRIMI (I). **frontal t.** TUBER FRONTALE. **gluteal t. of femur** TUBEROSITAS GLUTEA OSSIS FEMORIS. **greater t. of humerus** TUBERCULUM MAJUS HUMERI. **iliac t.** TUBEROSITAS ILIACA. **infraglenoid t.** TUBERCULUM INFRAGLENOIDALE. **ischial t.** TUBER ISCHIADICUM. **t. of ischium** TUBER ISCHIADICUM. **lesser t. of humerus** TUBERCULUM MINUS HUMERI. **masseteric t.** TUBEROSITAS MASSETERICA. **t. of maxilla** TUBER MAXILLAE. **maxillary t.** TUBER MAXILLAE. **t. of navicular bone** TUBEROSITAS OSSIS NAVICULARIS. **omental t. of liver** TUBER OMENTALE HEPATIS. **omental t. of pancreas** TUBER OMENTALE PANCREATIS. **parietal t.** TUBER PARIETALE. **pterygoid t. of mandible** TUBEROSITAS PTERYGOIDEA MANDIBULAE. **pyramidal t. of palatine bone** PROCESSUS PYRAMIDALIS OSSIS PALATINI. **radial t.** TUBEROSITAS RADII. **t. of radius** TUBEROSITAS RADII. **sacral t.** TUBEROSITAS SACRALIS. **t. of scaphoid bone** TUBERCULUM OSSIS SCAPHOIDEI. **t. for serratus anterior muscle** TUBEROSITAS MUSCULI SERRATI ANTERIORIS. **supraglenoid t.** TUBERCULUM SUPRAGLENOIDALE. **t. of tibia** TUBEROSITAS TIBIAE. **tibial t.** TUBEROSITAS TIBIAE. **t. of trapezium** TUBERCULUM OSSIS TRAPEZII. **t. of ulna** TUBEROSITAS ULNAE. **ungual t.** Either the tuberositas phalangis distalis manus or tuberositas phalangis distalis pedis. Also *unguicular tuberosity.*

**tubo-** \tʸoo′bə-, tʸoo′bō-\ [L *tuba* or *tubus* tube] A combining form meaning tube.

**tuboabdominal** \-abdäm′inəl\ Pertaining to the uterine tube and the abdomen.

**tubocurarine** \-kyoorär′ēn\ [TUBO- + *curar(e)* + -INE; so called as the active principle of tube curare, the type of curare packed in bamboo tubes.] A racemic alkaloid isolated from the bark and stems of *Chondodendron tomentosum.* The compound tubocurarine chloride has been used to induce muscle relaxation in surgical procedures, in convulsive shock therapy, and in the treatment of tetanus and spastic disorders.

**tubocurarine chloride** $C_{37}H_{42}Cl_2N_2O_6$. 7′,12′-Dihydroxy-6,6′-dimethoxy-2,2′,-2′-trimethyltubocuraranium chloride. The *d*-form is a skeletal muscle relaxant that is administered intravenously. It is a nondepolarizing, competitive blocking agent and produces a flaccid paralysis of all the skeletal muscles.

**tubogastrostomy** \-gasträs′təmē\ The surgical creation, using the anterior gastric wall, of a communication between the gastric lumen and the skin.

**tuboligamentous** \-lig′əmen′təs\ Pertaining to the oviduct and broad ligament.

**tubo-ovarian** \-ōver′ē·ən\ Pertaining to the oviduct and ovary.

**tubo-ovariectomy** \-ōver′ē·ek′təmē\ SALPINGO-OOPHORECTOMY.

**tubo-ovariotomy** \-ōver′e·ät′əmē\ SALPINGO-OOPHORECTOMY.

**tubo-ovaritis** \-ō′vərī′tis\ [TUBO- + OVARITIS] SALPINGO-OOPHORITIS.

**tuboplasty** \tyoo′bəplas′tē\ [TUBO- + -PLASTY] Repair or restructuring of a damaged oviduct, usually carried out to preserve or improve the chances for future conceptions.

**tubotympanal** \-tim′pənəl\ Of or relating to the auditory tube and the tympanic cavity. Also *tubotympanic.*

**tubular** \tʸoo′byələr\ **1** Of or relating to a tubule. **2** In the shape of a tube.

**tubule** \tʸoo′byool\ [L *tubulus.* See TUBULUS.] TUBULUS. **Albarrán's t.'s** SUBCERVICAL GLANDS OF ALBARRÁN. **Bellini's t.** One of the wide tubules formed by the union of some straight collecting tubules which, in turn, open on the apex of a renal papilla. **biliferous t.** One of the ductuli biliferi. **caroticotympanic t.'s** CANALICULI CAROTICOTYMPANICI. **collecting t.'s** The tubulus renalis arcuatus and tubulus colligens rectus. **collecting t.'s of the mesonephros** EPIGENITAL DUCTS. **connecting t.** A short curved tubule that joins the distal convoluted tubule of the nephron with the commencement of the collecting tubule. Also *connecting segment, tubulus renalis arcuatus.* **convoluted t.'s** **1** The tubulus contortus proximalis and tubulus contortus distalis of the kidney considered together. Also *convoluted renal tubules.* **2** TUBULI SEMINIFERI CONTORTI. **convoluted seminif-**

**erous t.'s** TUBULI SEMINIFERI CONTORTI. **dentinal t.'s** Small tubes within the dentin of a tooth. Also *dental tubules, dentinal canals, canaliculi dentales.* **discharging t.** DUCTUS EXCRETORIUS. **distal convoluted t.** TUBULUS CONTORTUS DISTALIS. **distal straight t.** TUBULUS RECTUS DISTALIS. **t.'s of the epoöphoron** VERTICAL TUBULES. **Ferrein's t.'s** The branched collecting tubules, as well as the ascending and descending limbs of the loops of Henle, in the medullary rays in the pars radiata of the renal cortex. **galactophorous t.'s** DUCTUS LACTIFERI. **Henle's t.'s** The tubulus rectus proximalis, tubulus rectus distalis, and tubulus attenuatus. **Kobelt's t.'s** The outermost tubules of the epoöphoron. Also *outer tubules of the parovarium.* **lactiferous t.'s** DUCTUS LACTIFERI. **malpighian t.'s** Excretory structures of insects and arachnids which empty waste products into the gut from the body cavity. They vary in number and length but are generally long, slender blind tubes lying in the hemocoel and bathed in the blood of the insect or arachnid. Also *malpighian tubes.* **mesonephric t.'s** Tubules developing in the mesonephros. In most vertebrates the mesonephric tubules form temporary, functional urinary tubules which overlap the initial activity of the permanent kidney. The tubules drain into the mesonephric duct. **metanephric t.'s** Tubules which develop in the metanephrogenic cap, a condensation of mesoderm formed on the cranial end of the ureteric diverticulum. The metanephric tubules give rise to the renal corpuscles, the secreting and convoluted tubules of the permanent kidney. **Miescher's t.** *Outmoded* SARCOCYST. **outer t.'s of the parovarium** KOBELT'S TUBULES. **paraurethral t.'s** DUCTUS PARAURETHRALES. **t.'s of parovarium** VERTICAL TUBULES. **pronephric t.'s** PRONEPHROS. **proximal convoluted t.** TUBULUS CONTORTUS PROXIMALIS. **proximal straight t.** TUBULUS RECTUS PROXIMALIS. **renal t.** TUBULUS RENALIS. **segmental t.'s** Pronephric or mesonephric tubules when they exhibit a segmental arrangement. **seminiferous t.'s** The tubuli seminiferi contorti and tubuli seminiferi recti. **Skene's t.'s** DUCTUS PARAURETHRALES. **spiral t.'s** The tubulus contortus proximalis and tubulus contortus distalis. **straight t.'s** 1 The tubulus rectus proximalis, tubulus rectus distalis, and tubulus colligens rectus in the kidney. Also *straight renal tubules.* 2 Tubuli seminiferi recti in the testis. **straight collecting t.** TUBULUS COLLIGENS RECTUS. **straight renal t.'s** 1 STRAIGHT TUBULES. 2 The ascending and descending limbs of the loop of Henle. **straight seminiferous t.'s** TUBULI SEMINIFERI RECTI. **T t.** A planar and radially oriented interconnecting system of membranous tubules crossing the myofibrillar zone at two levels in each sarcomere, the level varying depending on the phylum. The tubules connect with the sarcolemma peripherally and have contacts with terminal cisterns of the endoplasmic reticulum. They carry inward the action potential that triggers Ca release and initiates the contraction mechanism. **uriniferous t.** One of a large number of structural units of the kidney held together by connective tissue containing blood vessels, nerves and lymphatics. Each unit comprises a nephron and a collecting tubule. **vertical t.'s** Those small canals, usually blind, found near the ovary in the broad ligament of the uterus ascending straight upwards towards the horizontally placed duct of the epoophoron. They are remnants of mesonephric tubules. Also *tubules of the epoöphoron, tubules of parovarium.*

**tubuli** \tʸoo′byəlī\ Plural of TUBULUS.

**tubuliform** \tʸoo′byəlifôrm′\ Having the shape of a tubule.

**tubulin** \tʸoo′byəlin\ The protein constituent of cytoplasmic microtubules, including those of the mitotic spindle. It consists of two similar 60-kDa proteins, which aggregate to form easily dissociated tubules. GTP is required for tubule assembly. Colchicine binds tightly to tubulin and thereby breaks up the tubules. This inhibits mitosis.

**tubuloacinar** \tʸoo′byəlō·as′inär\ ACINOTUBULAR.

**tubuloacinous** \tʸoo′byəlō·as′inəs\ ACINOTUBULAR.

**tubulocyst** \tʸoo′byəlōsist′\ TUBULAR CYST.

**tubulorrhexis** \tʸoo′byəlôrek′sis\ [*tubul(e)* + *o* + -RRHEXIS] Necrosis and fragmentation of the renal tubular basement membrane. It may be caused by toxins, acute tubular necrosis, or ischemia due to vascular occlusion. **ischemic t.** Necrosis and fragmentation of the renal tubular basement membrane due to ischemia, a pathologic feature of acute tubular necrosis, and renal infarct.

**tubulovillous** \tʸoo′byəlōvil′əs\ Both tubular and villous, as in *tubulovillous adenoma of the colon.*

**tubulous** \tʸoo′byələs\ Having tubules.

**tubulus** \tʸoo′byələs\ [L, dim. of TUBUS] (*pl.* tubuli) A small tube. Also *tubule.* **t. attenuatus** The lower parts of the limbs and the U-turn of a nephron, which are thinner than the rest of the loop. **t. colligens rectus** [NA] The straight portion at the commencement of the tubulus renalis colligens which is continuous proximally with the distal convoluted tubule. It is lined by lightly acidophilic cuboidal cells and is situated in the renal cortex. Also *straight collecting tubule, Bellini's duct.* **t. contortus distalis** [NA] The second or distal convolution of the renal tubule. It is continuous proximally with the tubulus rectus distalis at the macula densa and distally leads into the arcuate or straight portion of the tubulus renalis colligens. It is lined by cuboidal epithelium. Also *distal convoluted tubule.* **t. contortus proximalis** [NA] The first or proximal convolution of the renal tubule. It is situated in the renal cortex and is connected proximally to the glomerular capsule of the nephron by a short constriction and distally becomes continuous with the tubulus rectus proximalis. In it reabsorption of the glomerular filtrate commences and a secretion is added. The lumen is lined by simple cuboidal epithelium on the surface of which are tightly packed microvilli. Also *proximal convoluted tubule.* **tubuli epoophori** The short transverse ductules, ten to fifteen in number, lying in the mesosalpinx between the ovary and the uterine tube and connecting with the longitudinal duct of the epoophoron. They are remnants in the female of the tubules of the mesonephros. **t. rectus** Any of four structures: (1) tubulus rectus proximalis; (2) tubulus rectus distalis; (3) tubulus colligens rectus; (4) any of the tubuli seminiferi recti. **t. rectus distalis** [NA] The distal straight thick portion of the loop of Henle. It connects the thin ascending part of the tubulus attenuatus to the distal convoluted tubule. Also *distal straight tubule.* **t. rectus proximalis** [NA] The terminal, straight portion of the proximal convoluted tubule which becomes the proximal part of the loop of Henle and enters the outer part of the medulla to form the descending part of the tubulus attenuatus. It is lined by simple cuboidal epithelium. Also *proximal straight tubule.* **t. renalis** [NA] One of more than a million minute epithelial-lined tubes commencing at the glomerular capsule as the nephron and ending at the renal pyramid as the collecting tubule. Its various parts are specialized for resorption and excretion of the glomerular filtrate. Also *renal tubule.* **t. renalis arcuatus** [NA] CONNECTING TUBULE. **t. renalis colligens** The collecting tubule that is the continuation of each tubulus contortus distalis beyond the renal nephron. It commences as an arcuate or straight tubule in the medullary rays of the cortex and unites, in short intervals, at acute angles with similar tubules to form a wider tube, the papillary duct that opens on the apex of each papilla. Its lumen is lined by cuboidal cells. Also *collecting duct.* **tubuli seminiferi contorti** [NA] Three or four threadlike tortuous canals supported by loose connective tissue in each lobule of the testis, commencing as either free blind ends or anastomosing loops and terminating at the apex of the lobule as straight tubules. Each has a basement membrane on which rests a modified stratified cuboidal epithelium. The epithelium contains spermatogenic cells and the sustentacular cells of Sertoli. Also *convoluted seminiferous tubules, convoluted tubules.* **tubuli seminiferi recti** [NA] Twenty to thirty large straight excretory ducts formed by the union of the terminal parts of the convoluted seminiferous tubules at the apices of the lobules of the testis. They pass upward and backward into the fibrous tissue of the mediastinum testis to form an interlacing tubular network, the rete testis. The epithelium comprises tall columnar Sertoli cells containing fat droplets. Also *straight seminiferous tubules, vasa recta.*

**tubus** \tʸoo′bəs\ [L (akin to *tuba* a tuba, trumpet) a pipe, tube] (*pl.* tubi) A tube. **t. digestorius** *Outmoded* CANALIS ALIMENTARIUS. **t. vertebralis** CANALIS VERTEBRALIS.

**Tucker** [Ervin Alden *Tucker,* U.S. obstetrician, 1862–1902] Tucker-McLean forceps. See under FORCEPS.

**tucking** The surgical shortening of an extraocular muscle tendon by folding it upon itself, with the intent of rotating the eye toward the operated muscle for the correction of strabismus.

**Tuffier** [Marin Theodore *Tuffier,* French surgeon, 1857–1929] See under LIGAMENT.

**tuft** A small clump, cluster, or bunch; a coil. **enamel t.'s** Leaflike remnants of enamel matrix which project a short distance into enamel from the amelodentinal junction. **hair t.** A group of hairs arising in a single follicle. Also *barbula.* **synovial t.'s** SYNOVIAL VILLI.

**tufting** A radiographic appearance of diffuse bone resorption about the tip of the terminal phalanges of the hands. It is seen in generalized disorders of bone resorption such as hyperparathyroidism.

**tug** / **tracheal t.** A downward jerking of the trachea, produced by aneurysm of the aorta, best felt with the neck extended, the mouth closed, and the cricoid cartilage drawn upwards by the thumb and forefinger.

**tugging** / **tracheal t.** See under TRACHEAL TUG.

**tularaemia** *Brit.* TULAREMIA.

**tularemia** \tʸoo′lərē′mē·ə\ [after *Tulare* County, California, where *Francisella tularensis* was first isolated + -EMIA] An infectious disease of wild rodents and rabbits caused by *Francisella tularensis* and transmitted to man and other animals either by direct contact (including bites) or by arthropod vectors such as ticks and tabanids. The various forms of the disease including ulceroglandular, pneumonic, typhoidal, and oculoglandular, result from different routes of the infecting strain. All forms of tularemia are marked by fever, chills, headache, and myalgia. Also *rabbit fever, deer-fly fever, deer-fly disease, Pahvant Valley fever, Pahvant Valley plague, Francis disease, Ohara's disease, yatobyo* (Japanese). **oculoglandular t.** Tularemia resulting from inoculation of the conjunctival sac or ocular contact with aerosols infected with *Francisella tularensis.* There is severe, painful conjunctivitis, photophobia, a mucopurulent discharge, local granulomatous lesions (often affecting the cornea), and preauricular lymphadenopathy in addition to the general symptoms of tularemia. **pneumonic t.** A form of tularemia caused by aerogenic infection with *Francisella tularensis.* Alveolar inflammation and patchy infiltrates occur where bacteria lodge in the lungs. See also TULAREMIC PNEUMONIA. **typhoidal t.** Tularemia in which there is no local lesion or specific organ involvement. The course of illness is severe with high fever and toxemia. **ulceroglandular t.** Tularemia resulting from direct contact, with bacteria entering the skin, as by a bite, and producing a lesion at the inoculation site. This lesion ulcerates and regional lymph nodes enlarge and become inflamed. This is the most common form of tularemia.

**tularine** \tʸoo′lərin\ An antigen employed in the Foshay test for tularemia.

**tulle gras** \tʏl′ grä′, tool′ grä′\ [French *tulle* (after *Tulle,* town in south-central France) a very light, transparent fabric of cotton or silk, with round or polygonal stitching + *gras* fatty] A dressing, used mostly in Great Britain, of fine mesh gauze impregnated with Peruvian balsam, soft paraffin, and vegetable oil. It is used to protect raw surfaces. Also *tullegras gauze.*

**Tullio** [Pietro *Tullio,* Italian physician, flourished 20th century] See under PHENOMENON.

**Tulp** [Nicholas *Tulp* (Nikolaas Tulpius), Dutch anatomist, 1593–1674] Valve of Tulpius. See under VALVA ILEOCECALIS.

**tumefacient** \tʸoo′məfā′shənt\ Tending to produce swelling.

**tumefaction** \tʸoo′məfak′shən\ [Middle French (from L *tumefactus,* past part. of *tumefacere* to make to swell, inflate), an inflating] **1** The process of becoming tumescent or swollen, as from an accumulation of fluids. **2** TUMESCENCE.

**tumefy** \tʸoo′məfī\ To swell or cause to swell. Also *intumesce.*

**tumescence** \tʸoomes′əns\ [L *tumescens,* pres. part. of *tumescere* (inceptive of *tumere* to be blown up, puffed up, or tumid) to begin to swell] The state of being swollen, as from an accumulation of internal fluids. Also *tumentia, turgescence, tumefaction.*

**tumescent** \tʸoomes′ənt\ [L *tumescens,* gen. *tumescentis,* pres. part. of *tumescere* to begin to swell] Subject to swelling.

**tumeur** \tʏmœr′\ [French, a tumor] The French word for TUMOR. **t. pileuse** TRICHOBEZOAR.

**tumid** \tʸoo′mid\ Enlarged or engorged; swollen.

# tumor

**tumor** [L (from *tumere* to be puffed or blown up, to be tumid, swollen), a swelling, tumor] **1** An expanding lesion due to a progressive, apparently uncontrolled proliferation of cells; a neoplasm. Benign tumors remain localized whereas malignant tumors invade neighboring tissues and spread by lymph or blood streams to create secondary (metastatic) growths in other tissues and organs. Also *tumeur* (French). **2** A swelling of any nature; tumefaction. **Abrikosov's t.** GRANULAR CELL TUMOR. **Ackerman's t.** KERATOACANTHOMA. **acoustic nerve t.** A neurilemmoma of the acoustic nerve. **acute splenic t.** A tender abdominal mass resulting from acute inflammation of the spleen, usually in the setting of bacteremia. **adenoid t.** ADENOMA. **adenomatoid t.** A benign tumor characterized by irregular glandlike structures or spaces lined or associated with vacuolated mesotheliumlike cells. The tumor is typically found in the region of the epididymis, spermatic cord, and fallopian tube. Some consider it a benign form of mesothelioma, others suggest a mesonephric origin. Also *angiomatoid tumor.* **adenomatoid odontogenic t.** A jaw tumor in which odontogenic epithelium is arranged as ductlike structures. It may be partly or largely cystic. The anterior maxilla is the most common site. It usually occurs in children and young adults. Also *adenoameloblastoma, ameloblastic adenomatoid tumor.* **adipose t.** LIPOMA. **adrenal rest t.** A lipoid cell tumor of the ovary believed to arise from adrenal rests. Also *adrenocorticoid adenoma of the ovary, adrenocortical tumor of the ovary.* **t. albus** WHITE SWELLING. **alpha cell t.** GLUCAGONOMA. **alveolar t.** BRONCHIOLOALVEOLAR CARCINOMA. **ameloblastic adenomatoid t.** ADENOMATOID ODONTOGENIC TUMOR. **aneurysmal giant cell t.** ANEURYSMAL BONE CYST. **angiomatoid t.** ADENOMATOID TUMOR. **angle t.** PONTINE ANGLE TUMOR. **aortic body t.** A chemodectoma of the aortic body. **argentaffin carcinoid t.** A carcinoid tumor with cells giving a positive argentaffin reaction. **ascites t.** A malignant neoplasm the cells of which grow abundantly in suspension in the ascitic fluid. • The term is largely reserved for experimental tumors. **benign t.** A neoplasm which remains localized. Also *innocent tumor.* **benign mixed t.** PLEOMORPHIC ADENOMA. **benign Triton t.** NEUROMUSCULAR HAMARTOMA. **Brenner t.** A tumor of the ovary, typically benign, composed of nests of epithelial cells of transitional urothelial type, embedded in ovarian stroma. Also *oophoroma folliculare.* **Brodie's t.** CYSTOSARCOMA PHYLLODES. **Brooke's t.** TRICHOEPITHELIOMA. **brown t.** A tumorlike lesion of bone in hyperparathyroidism resembling the giant cell tumor of bone. Numerous osteoclasts are present. **brown fat t.** HIBERNOMA. **Burkitt's t.** BURKITT'S LYMPHOMA. **t. of Buschke-Loewenstein** A large condyloma acuminatum of the anogenital region. It may be locally agressive. Also *giant condyloma.* **calcifying epithelial odontogenic t.** A tumor resembling an ameloblastoma but with calcified islands. Also *Pindborg tumor.* **carcinoid t.** See under CARCINOID. **carotid body t.** A chemodectoma of the carotid body. **cerebellopontine angle t.** PONTINE ANGLE TUMOR. **chemoreceptor t.** PARAGANGLIOMA. **chromaffin-cell t.** PHEOCHROMOCYTOMA. **chromophil t.** PHEOCHROMOCYTOMA. **clear cell t.** RENAL CELL CARCINOMA. **Cock's t.** A trichilemmal cyst of the scalp marked by secondary infection and ulceration and simulating a squamous carcinoma. **Codman's t.** CHONDROBLASTOMA. **collision t.** The joining of two distinct tumors particularly of different histologic types. **colloid t.** 1 MYXOMA. 2 MUCINOUS CARCINOMA. **colloid ovarian t.** MUCINOUS CYSTADENOMA OF THE OVARY. **connective tissue t.** A tumor of connective tissue. Also *soft tissue tumor, connective tumor.* **craniopharyngeal duct t.** CRANIOPHARYNGIOMA. **cystic t.** A tumor containing prominent spaces filled with fluid. **dentinoid t.** DENTINOMA. **dermoid t.** A tumor containing multiple cutaneous components, such as hair follicles or sebaceous glands. The most usual type is a dermoid cyst. **desmoid t.** A tumorlike fibroblastic lesion which may grow in a locally aggressive manner. **dumbbell t.** HOURGLASS TUMOR. **dysontogenetic t.** 1 EMBRYONAL TUMOR. 2 A tumor caused by abnormal embryologic development. **Ehrlich t.** A transplantable undifferentiated carcinoma of mice. It grows in solid and ascites forms. It originally arose as a spontaneous mammary carcinoma. **eighth-nerve t.** A neurilemmoma of the eighth cranial nerve. **embryonal t.** A tumor of embryonic-appearing tissue, as a nephroblastoma. Also *dysontogenetic tumor, embryoplastic tumor.* **embryonal mixed t.** HEPATOBLASTOMA. **embryoplastic t.** EMBRYONAL TUMOR. **endodermal sinus t.** YOLK SAC TUMOR. **eosinophilic t. of the pituitary** ACIDOPHIL ADENOMA. **epithelial t.** A tumor of epithelial cells. **Ewing's t.** EWING SARCOMA. **extramedullary hematopoietic t.** ERYTHROBLASTOMA. **false t.** TUMORLIKE LESION. **fatty t.** LIPOMA. **fibroplastic t.** 1 FIBROMA. 2 FIBROSARCOMA. **fibrous t.** FIBROMA. **fungating t.** A tumor with the gross appearance of a large fungus or mushroom. There is usually a central necrotic area on the surface. **Furth pituitary t.** An induced, transplantable, hormone-secreting anterior pituitary tumor of mice. The commonest such tumor, mammotropic in effect, is widely used experimentally. **ganglion nodosum t.** A paraganglioma of the ganglion nodosum (vagus). **germinal t.** A tumor of germ cells, as a seminoma. **G-cell t.** GASTRINOMA. **giant cell t. of bone** An aggressive, osteolytic tumor usually involving the ends of the long bones and characterized by richly vascularized tissue consisting of rather plump, spindle-shaped or ovoid cells and by the presence of numerous giant cells of osteoclast type, which are uniformly distributed throughout the affected tissue. Relatively little collagen is present. It occurs in men and women with equal frequency and typically in those of 20–40 years of age, rarely in younger subjects. The giant cells of giant cell tumors are so similar to normal osteoclasts that they may be assumed to be the neoplastic counterparts of these cells. Giant cell tumors show a high rate of recurrence after curettage. All are potentially malignant, but it is not currently possible to predict, based on an examination of the histologic structure, whether the future course of a tumor will prove to be benign or malignant. Also *osteoclastoma.* **giant cell t. of tendon sheath** A benign lesion of tendons or synovia containing multinucleated giant cells, histiocytes, fibroblasts and lipid-laden cells. Common sites are fingers and knees. It is unclear whether it is a true neoplasm. **glomus t.** A benign tumor of the neuromyoarterial glomus. It is commonly found at the distal portion of the extremities but also occurs in the stomach. Also *angiomyoneuroma, angioneuroma* (outmoded), *glomangioma, angioneuromyoma* (outmoded). **glomus jugulare t.** A chemodectoma of the glomus jugulare. Two main varieties occur: tumors of the jugular bulb, which, when advanced enlarge the jugular foramen and may produce paralysis of one or more of the last four cranial nerves, and intratympanic tumors, giving rise to impaired hearing and tinnitus, the typical vascular polyp being visible through an intact tympanic membrane. Treatment includes surgery or radiotherapy or both. **granular cell t.** A benign tumor, probably neurogenic, made up of large, round or polygonal, finely granular, acidophilic cells with small dense nuclei. Superficially located tumors are often accompanied by pseudoepitheliomatous hyperplasia of the overlying squamous epithelium. It was previously considered to be of myoblastic origin. The tumor may occur at a variety of sites, such as the tongue, breast, or vulva. A rare malignant form has been described. Also *granular cell neurofibroma, granular cell schwannoma, Abrikossov's tumor, myoblastoma, myoblastomyoma, granular cell myoblastoma, myoblastic myoma, myoschwannoma.* **granulation t.** 1 GRANULOMA. 2 PYOGENIC GRANULOMA. **granulosa t.** GRANULOSA CELL TUMOR. **granulosa cell t.** An ovarian tumor composed of elements resembling granulosa cells. Follicular, trabecular, insular, and diffuse patterns may be present. Call-Exner bodies are typical features of the follicular variety. Theca cells are often present. Granulosa cell tumors are usually estrogenic, but may be inactive or in rare cases androgenic. Their degree of malignancy is low. Also *granulosa cell carcinoma, granulosa tumor, folliculoma, granulosa-theca cell tumor.* **granulosa-theca cell t.** GRANULOSA CELL TUMOR. **Grawitz t.** RENAL CELL CARCINOMA. **Gubler's t.** A tumorous lesion marked by a swelling (Gubler sign) of the synovial sheaths of the wrist or the back of the hand, associated with muscle paralysis and chronic lead poisoning. **gummy t.** GUMMA. **heterologous t.** A tumor containing tissues foreign to the site. Also *heterotypic tumor.* **hilar cell t.** A benign ovarian tumor with cells resembling the testicular Leydig cell tumor. **homologous t.** A tumor composed of tissue like that of its site of origin. **Hortega cell t.** A primary lymphoma of the central nervous system. **hourglass t.** A tumor whose shape resembles an hourglass or dumbbell, two masses being connected by a narrow portion. It is typically seen where a neurofibroma has grown through an intervertebral foramen with part in the spinal canal and part in the thorax. Also *dumbbell tumor, dumbbell ganglioneuroma, hourglass ganglioneuroma, dumbbell neurofibroma.* **Hürthle cell t.** A tumor of the thyroid composed of cells with abundant amounts of eosinophilic cytoplasm. It can be benign or malignant. **infiltrating t.** A tumor that invades adjacent tissues. **innocent t.** BENIGN TUMOR. **interstitial cell t.** LEYDIG CELL TUMOR. **iron-hard t.** RIEDEL STRUMA. **islet cell t.** A tumor of the islet cells of the pancreas. If benign it is an islet cell adenoma, if malignant an islet cell carcinoma. Also *nesidioblastoma.* **ivorylike t.** COMPACT OSTEOMA. **juxtaglomerular cell t.** A rare, renin-secreting tumor of the juxtaglomerular apparatus of the kidney, containing granular PAS-positive cytoplasm. Also *juxtaglomerular tumor, renal hemangiopericytoma.* **Koenen's t.** PERIUNGUAL FIBROMA. **Krompecher's t.** BASAL CELL CARCINOMA. **Krukenberg t.** A metastatic signet ring cell carcinoma in the ovary, typically originating from a primary in the stomach. **lacteal t.** GALACTOCELE. **Leydig cell t.** A testicular tumor of leydig cells. Also *interstitial cell tumor.* **t. lienis** Mild splenic enlargement detectable on physical examination. **lipoid cell t. of ovary** A rare tumor composed of lipid-containing cells resembling Leydig, lutein, or adrenal cortical cells. It is usually benign. Also *luteoma.* **Malherbe's t.** PILOMATRIXOMA. **malignant t.** CANCER. **malignant mixed t.** 1 A malignant tumor having a mixture of tissue components. 2 Carcinoma in a pleomorphic adenoma. **malignant mixed mesodermal t.** MESODERMAL MIXED TUMOR. **malignant triton t.** A tumor of peripheral nerves that is composed of Schwann cell elements and rhabdomyosarcoma. It typically occurs in patients with von Recklinghausen's disease (neurofibromatosis). • *Triton* refers to a genus of salamanders (*Triturus*) on which experiments have been conducted regarding the relation of nerves to muscle differentiation. **march t.** A swelling and inflammation of the transverse metatarsal ligaments following unaccustomed exercise, such as long marches. Also *syndesmitis metatarsea.* **melanotic neuroectodermal t.** A rare benign tumor composed of epithelial lined tubules or spaces separated by prominent amounts of fibrous stroma. Melanin is within the epithelial cells. It most frequently occurs in the maxilla of infants and is probably of neural crest derivation. It may be locally aggressive. Also *melanotic progonoma, retinal anlage tumor, melanotic ameloblastoma, pigmented epulis.* **Merkel cell t.** MERKEL CELL CARCINOMA. **mesodermal t.** A tumor derived from mesodermal tissues. **mesodermal mixed t.** A malignant tumor, typically of the uterus, with an admixture of carcinoma and sarcoma, the latter containing heterologous elements, such as osteosarcoma. Also *malignant mixed mesodermal tumor.* **metastatic t.** A malignant tumor growing at a secondary site derived from cells which spread from the original neoplasm. The cells are usually transported by the lymph or blood streams. Also *secondary tumor, metastasis.* **mixed t.** A tumor having multiple tissue components, usually epithelial and mesenchymal. **mixed t. of salivary glands** PLEOMORPHIC ADENOMA. **mixed t. of salivary gland type** CHONDROID SYRINGOMA. **mixed t. of the skin** CHONDROID SYRINGOMA. **mucoepidermoid t.** A tumor composed of an intimate admixture of squamous cells, mucus-secreting cells, and cells of intermediate type. It is typically found in the salivary glands. The tumor is usually malignant, and may then be called a mucoepidermoid carcinoma. **mucous t.** MYXOMA. **müllerian mixed t.** A category comprising mesodermal mixed tumor and carcinosarcoma of the uterus. **muscular t.** MYOMA. **Nélaton's t.** A teratoma of the abdominal wall. **neuroepithelial t.** NEUROEPITHELIOMA. **nonencapsulated sclerosing t.** A small papillary carcinoma of the thyroid with prominent fibrosis. **odontogenic t.** A tumor arising from odontogenic tissues, such as the dental lamina, tooth germ, and dental sac. **organoid t.** 1 A tumor with cells arranged in an organlike manner. 2 TERATOMA. **oxyphil cell t.** A tumor composed of cells with abundant eosinophilic cytoplasm. **pacinian t.** A benign skin or soft-tissue tumor, probably of neuroectodermal origin, containing structures resembling the pacinian corpuscles. **Pancoast's t.** A cancer of the apex of the lung or thoracic inlet which invades the brachial plexus causing the Pancoast syndrome. Also *pulmonary sulcus tumor, superior sulcus tumor, thoracic inlet tumor.* **papillary t.** A tumor with fingerlike projections. **paraffin t.** PARAFFINOMA. **parvilocular pseudomucinous t.** MUCINOUS CYSTADENOMA. **pearl t.** CHOLESTEATOMA. **phantom t.** An opacity seen on chest roentgenogram suggestive of a tumor but which subsequently disappears, usually having been caused by an infection or localized pleural effusion. Also *pseudinoma.* **phyllodes t.** CYSTOSARCOMA PHYLLODES. **Pindborg t.** CALCIFYING EPITHELIAL ODONTOGENIC TUMOR. **pineal t.** 1 A tumor of the pineal gland. 2 A tumor of intrinsic pineal cells, not of the associated glial cells in the pineal. **polypoid t.** A tumor growing in the shape of a polyp. **pontine angle t.** Any unilateral neoplasm that occupies the angle between the pons and the cerebellum. The commonest tumor is the neurilemmoma of the acoustic nerve. Others are meningioma, fifth nerve tumor, etc. Also *angle tumor, cerebellopontine angle tumor.* **Pott's puffy t.** The localized area of pitting edema overlying the diseased bone in cases of osteomyelitis of the skull, characteristically appearing in the frontal region in cases of osteomyelitis of the frontal bone secondary to frontal sinusitis. **pregnancy t.** A granulomatous epulis occurring during pregnancy as a local exacerbation of existing chronic gingivitis. **premalignant fibroepithelial t.** PREMALIGNANT FIBROEPITHELIOMA. **pseudointraligamentous t.** An ovarian tumor which appears to rest between the leaves of the broad ligament, but is merely covered by a peritoneal fold. **pulmonary sulcus t.** PANCOAST'S TUMOR. **ranine t.** *Rare* RANULA. **Rathke's t.**

CRANIOPHARYNGIOMA. **Rathke's pouch t.** CRANIOPHARYNGIOMA. **retinal anlage t.** MELANOTIC NEUROECTODERMAL TUMOR. **Ringertz t.** An inverted papilloma arising on the lateral wall of the nose and liable to spread extensively within the maxillary and ethmoid sinuses. It recurs obstinately after removal even when procedures have been radical. A small proportion undergo malignant transformation. Also *inverted nasal papilloma.* **salivary mixed cutaneous t.** CHONDROID SYRINGOMA. **sand t.** PSAMMOMA. **Schmincke t.** A lymphoepithelial carcinoma of the nasopharynx. **Schwann cell t.** NEURILEMMOMA. **secondary t.** METASTATIC TUMOR. **Sertoli cell t.** TUBULAR ANDROBLASTOMA. **Sertoli-Leydig cell t.** An ovarian tumor composed of both Sertoli cells and Leydig cells. It may be androgenic or estrogenic. **Spiegler's t.'s** ECCRINE DERMAL CYLINDROMA. **Steiner's t.'s** Gummata of tertiary syphilis found in the periarticular tissue. **superior sulcus t.** PANCOAST'S TUMOR. **teratoid t.** A teratoma or a similar growth. **thoracic inlet t.** PANCOAST'S TUMOR. **tridermic t.** A teratoma with tissues from all three germ cell layers. **true t.** NEOPLASM. **turban t.** An eccrine dermal cylindroma occurring extensively in the scalp in the shape of a turban. **varicose t.** A swelling due to venous distension. **villous t.** A tumor with many fine fingerlike projections. **Warthin's t.** ADENOLYMPHOMA. **white t.** TUBERCULOUS ARTHRITIS. **Wilms t.** NEPHROBLASTOMA. **xanthomatous giant cell t. of the tendon sheath** A giant cell tumor of the tendon sheath with a prominent number of lipid-containing cells. **yolk sac t.** A highly malignant germ cell tumor of the testis and ovary containing structures resembling those seen in the yolk sac and other embryonic tissues. Microscopically, reticular, tubular, papillary, and solid structures are seen. A loose vacuolar network is typical. It usually occurs in children. Also *endodermal sinus tumor, orchioblastoma, infantile type embryonal carcinoma, testicular adenocarcinoma of infancy.* **Yoshida t.** An induced, transplantable, undifferentiated tumor of rats which grows in ascites and solid forms. Also *Yoshida ascites tumor, Yoshida sarcoma.* **Zollinger-Ellison t.** A gastrinoma causing the Zollinger-Ellison syndrome.

**tumoricidal** \t$^y$oo′mərisī′dəl\ [TUMOR + *i* + *-cid(e)* + -AL] Causing death to tumor cells.

**tumorigenesis** \t$^y$oo′mərijen′əsis\ [TUMOR + *i* + GENESIS ] Tumor formation.

**tumorigenic** \t$^y$oo′mərijen′ik\ Causing tumor formation.

**tumorlet** \t$^y$oo′mərlit\ [TUMOR + *-let,* diminishing suffix] A microscopic tumorlike collection of cells in the lung. Such collections are often multiple and occur near scars. They may be hyperplastic bronchioloalveolar cells or minute carcinoids.

**tumorous** \t$^y$oo′mərəs\ Like a tumor.

**tumour** \t$^y$oo′mər\ *Brit.* TUMOR.

**tumultus** \t$^y$oomul′təs\ [L, a confusion, uproar, tumult] **t. cordis** PALPITATION.

***Tunga penetrans*** \tung′gə pen′ətranz\ A species of flea found in subtropical and tropical Africa and America; the chigoe. The female penetrates the human skin, often under the toenail where she becomes greatly distended with eggs, causing a painful ulcer and inflammation. This species also attacks other hosts, especially swine (feet, snout, scrotum, teats), sometimes affecting feeding and growth or causing death of piglets by disrupting milk flow. Also *Pulex penetrans, Sarcopsylla penetrans.*

**tungiasis** \tung·gī′əsis\ [*Tung(a)* + -IASIS] Infestation with the chigoe flea, *Tunga penetrans.* Also *sarcopsyllosis.*

**tungsten** Element number 74, having atomic weight 183.85. A gray metal with about the same density as gold, tungsten has the highest melting point (3410°C) of any metal. There are five naturally occurring stable isotopes and 12 unstable isotopes. Tungsten has many technologic uses. Also *wolfram.* Symbol: W

**tunic** \t$^y$oo′nik\ [L *tunica.* See TUNICA.] TUNICA. **Bichat's t.** TUNICA INTERNA VASORUM. **fibrous t.** TUNICA FIBROSA. **fibrous t. of eyeball** TUNICA FIBROSA BULBI. **fibrous t. of liver** TUNICA FIBROSA HEPATIS. **mucous t.** TUNICA MUCOSA. **muscular t.** TUNICA MUSCULARIS. **pharyngeal t.** FASCIA PHARYNGOBASILARIS. **pharyngobasilar t.** FASCIA PHARYNGOBASILARIS. **proper t.** TUNICA PROPRIA. **Ruysch t.** LAMINA CHOROIDOCAPILLARIS. **serous t.** TUNICA SEROSA. **t.'s of spermatic cord and testis** TUNICAE FUNICULI SPERMATICI ET TESTIS.

# tunica

**tunica** \t$^y$oo′nikə\ [L (from presumed earlier *ctunica,* from Semitic, whence also Gk *chitōn* tunic; akin to Hebrew *kətonet* or *kuttōneth* tunic, cloak) a tunic, a covering membrane] An investing membrane, coat or layer of tissue that covers or lines an organ, part, or space. Also *tunic.* **t. adventitia** The outermost layer of an organ or tubular structure, comprising relatively dense connective tissue. It is often derived from and blends with the connective tissue of surrounding structures. Also *tunica externa, adventitial coat, external coat of viscera, tunica fibrosa, capsula.* **t. adventitia ductus deferentis** [NA] The outermost fibrous coat that surrounds the muscular coat of the ductus deferens and blends with adjoining connective tissue. **t. adventitia esophagi** [NA] The layer of loose connective tissue that is external to the tunica muscularis of the esophagus and that blends with surrounding structures. Also *external coat of esophagus, periesophageal sheath.* **t. adventitia ureteris** [NA] A layer of fibroelastic connective tissue that surrounds the tunica muscularis of the ureter and blends with the capsule of the kidney at the pelvis and with the connective tissue of the posterior abdominal wall behind the ureter throughout its length. It contains nerve plexuses, small ganglia, and some nerve cells. Also *external coat of ureter.* **t. adventitia vasorum** TUNICA EXTERNA VASORUM. **t. adventitia vesiculae seminalis** [NA] The layer of connective tissue containing many elastic fibers that surrounds the tunica muscularis of the seminal vesicle. **t. albuginea** [NA] A dense, often opaque, white connective tissue membrane that covers certain organs or parts. Also *albugineous coat, white coat.* **t. albuginea corporis spongiosi** [NA] A dense fibrous sheath that surrounds the corpus spongiosum penis. It is thinner than that of the corpora cavernosa and has extensive elastic networks as well as some smooth muscle fibers in its inner layer. **t. albuginea corporum cavernosorum** [NA] The thick fibrous sheath that surrounds each corpus cavernosum penis, fusing to form the fibrous septum between them. The collagenous fibers are arranged in two layers, the outer longitudinal and the inner circular, with each containing elastic networks. Posteriorly the inner layer contains small veins draining the cavernous spaces. Also *fibrous coat of corpus cavernosum of penis, fibrous capsule of corpora cavernosa of penis.* **t. albuginea ovarii** [NA] A collagenous condensation of the connective tissue of the cortex immediately beneath the germinal epithelium of the ovary. It increases in density with aging. Also *fibrous coat of ovary, albuginea ovarii* (outmoded). **t. albuginea testis** [NA] A thick layer of dense fibroelastic connective tissue that contains scattered smooth muscle cells and forms the middle layer of the covering of the testis, lying beneath the tunica vaginalis and superficial to tunica vasculosa. Also *albuginea testis, perididymis, fibrous coat of testis, fibrous capsule of testis.* **t. conjunctiva** [NA] The thin mucous membrane lining the insides of the eyelids and the front surface of the eyeball. It comprises the tunica conjunctiva palpebrarum, tunica conjunctiva bulbi, the fornices, conjunctival sac and glands, and the lacrimal caruncle. Also *conjunctiva.* **t. conjunctiva bulbi** [NA] The portion of the tunica conjunctiva that lines the anterior surface of the cornea and sclera. Over the latter it is loosely attached, but over the cornea it is continuous with the corneal epithelium. Also *bulbar conjunctiva, ocular conjunctiva.* **t. conjunctiva palpebrarum** [NA] The portion of the tunica conjunctiva lining the inner surfaces of the eyelids where it is adherent to the tarsi. It is highly vascular and contains lymphoid tissue in its deeper part, especially near the fornices. At the free margins of the eyelids it is continuous with the skin and the lining membranes of the lacrimal canaliculi and the tarsal glands. Also *palpebral conjunctiva.* **t. dartos** [NA] The layer of subcutaneous areolar tissue of the scrotum that contains the fibers of the dartos muscle. Also *dartos fascia of scrotum, dartos coat.* **t. elastica** TUNICA MEDIA VASORUM. **t. externa** TUNICA ADVENTITIA. **t. externa thecae folliculi** THECA EXTERNA. **t. externa vasorum** [NA] The outermost connective tissue coat of a blood vessel, most of the elements of which are organized longitudinally. It is separated from the tunica media by the external elastic membrane and it blends with connective tissue surrounding the vessel. Its thickness and composition vary according to the type and size of the vessel. Also *tunica adventitia vasorum, external coat of vessels.* **t. fibrosa** 1 [NA] A fibrous membrane surrounding an organ or part. Also *fibrous tunic, fibrous coat.* 2 TUNICA ADVENTITIA. **t. fibrosa bulbi** [NA] The outer fibrous coat of the eyeball, comprising the sclera and the cornea. Also *fibrous tunic of eyeball, corneosclera, fibrous coat of eye.* **t. fibrosa hepatis** [NA] A fibrous connective tissue capsule surrounding the liver, covered by the mesothelium of the peritoneum except at the bare area, and extending into the porta hepatis as septa to divide the liver into lobes and lobules and form the perivascular sheaths in the portal canals. Also *fibrous tunic of liver, Glisson's capsule, fibrous sheath of liver, fibrous capsule of liver.* **t. fibrosa splenis** [NA] The capsule of the spleen that is composed of dense collagenous connective tissue, some elastic fibers, and a few smooth muscle fibers. It is thickest at the hilum, where it surrounds the blood vessels. It sends trabeculae into the spleen from its inner surface and the hilum. The outer surface is covered by a layer of mesothelium of the surrounding peritoneum. Also *fibrous capsule of spleen.* **tunicae funiculi spermatici** [NA] The connective tissue coats that envelop the spermatic cord, namely, external spermatic fascia, cremasteric fascia, and internal spermatic fascia, and extends into the scrotum. **tunicae funiculi spermatici et testis** The fascial coverings of the spermatic cord, namely, the external and internal spermatic fasciae and the cremasteric fascia, that extend from the superficial inguinal ring into the scrotum, where they also cover the testis. There the internal spermatic fascia adheres to the parietal layer of the tunica vaginalis testis, the visceral layer of which covers the tunica albuginea. Also *tunics of spermatic cord and testis.* **t. interna bulbi** [NA] The innermost, sensory coat of the eyeball comprising the retina, considered apart from the tunica fibrosa bulbi and tunica vasculosa bulbi. **t. interna thecae folliculi** THECA INTERNA. **t. interna vasorum** [NA] The innermost coat of the walls of blood vessels, comprising an inner layer of endothelial cells, a subendothelial layer of fine fibroelastic connective tissue which is usually organized longitudinally, and a variable outer layer of elastic fibers (the internal elastic membrane) which separates the coat from the tunica media. In small and medium-sized arteries the layers are clearly defined, whereas in larger arteries some smooth muscle fibers are present and the internal elastic membrane is indistinct, as the elastic fibers are located in the subendothelial layer. In small and medium-sized veins the coat is thin and the subendothelial layer is poorly defined. In large veins the coat is slightly thicker. Also *intima, Bichat's tunic.* **t. media vasorum** [NA] The middle and thickest coat of the wall of blood vessels comprising mostly circularly arranged smooth muscle fibers and some elastic and collagenous fibers. Its character determines the type of artery. The large arteries have a small amount of elastic fibers whereas the smaller arteries and arterioles have mostly smooth muscle cells. In medium-sized veins there is a thick layer of connective tissue and elastic fiber networks and a few smooth muscle fibers, being best developed in the lower limb. In large veins the coat is poorly developed and smooth muscle fibers are scant or absent. Also *tunica elastica.* **t. mucosa** The inner surface of tubular structures and hollow organs, comprising a superficial epithelial membrane which is lubricated by mucus and rests upon a basal lamina which is supported by a layer of connective tissue, the lamina propria. In the digestive tract the outer limit is formed by a thin muscular layer, the muscularis mucosae. The surface area may be increased by folds of surface projections, or villi, and there may be invaginations called intestinal glands or crypts. Also *mucous coat, mucous tunic, mucous membrane, mucosa.* **t. mucosa bronchiorum** [NA] The mucous membrane that lines the bronchi, continuous with and similar to that of the trachea and having some reticular, collagenous, and elastic fibers in the lamina propria. It shows distinctive longitudinal folds due to contraction of the smooth muscle. **t. mucosa cavitatis tympani** [NA] The mucous membrane that lines the tympanic cavity and the structures within it. It has mostly squamous or low cuboidal epithelium, except at the opening of the auditory tube where it is columnar and ciliated. Also *mucous coat of tympanic cavity.* **t. mucosa coli** The mucous membrane of the colon which has a smooth surface, lacking plicae and villi, and is lined by simple columnar epithelium. The intestinal glands are deeper and more tightly packed than in the small intestine. **t. mucosa ductus deferentis** [NA] The mucous membrane of the ductus deferens in which there is an obvious elastic network and the lamina propria forms longitudinal folds. The pseudostratified columnar epithelium bears stereocilia. **t. mucosa esophagi** [NA] The mucous membrane of the esophagus in which the stratified squamous nonkeratinizing epithelium is continuous with that of the pharynx. The lamina propria comprises loose connective tissue with fine elastic networks and scattered lymphocytes. **t. mucosa gastrica** [NA] The mucous membrane of the stomach, presenting a honeycomb appearance that is produced by folding of the mucin-secreting, tall, columnar epithelium into slitlike gastric pits. At the bottom of the pits are the openings of the gastric glands which vary in nature and function in different parts of the stomach. The gastric glands occupy the entire thickness of the mucosa and are separated from each other by a discontinuous lamina propria. Also *tunica mucosa ventriculi.* **t. mucosa intestini crassi** The mucous membrane of the large intestine in which the simple columnar epithelium has a thin striated border, villi are absent, and there are no folds. The intestinal crypts are longer and have more goblet cells than in the small intestine. **t. mucosa intestini tenuis** [NA] The mucous membrane of the small intestine in which the surface area is greatly increased by the formation of circular folds, or plicae circulares, as well as villi, at the bases of which the intestinal crypts or glands open. In addition, the columnar cells covering villi have a brush border comprising many microvilli. The lamina propria has an argyrophil framework forming the core of the villi and filling the gaps between the crypts. **t. mucosa laryngis** [NA] The mucous membrane of the larynx in which the epithelium varies in different parts. In the upper part and the vocal folds it is stratified squamous and nonkeratinizing, whereas lower in the larynx there is pseudostratified ciliated columnar epithelium with goblet cells. The lamina propria is thick and has many elastic fibers and tubuloacinar glands. **t. mucosa linguae** [NA] The mucous membrane on the surface of the tongue which differs on its various aspects. On the dorsum, the anterior two thirds is roughened by numerous small protrusions or papillae of three varieties, many of which contain taste buds. The one third posterior to the sulcus terminalis is nodular due to the lingual tonsils between which the surface epithelium has clefts or crypts. The under surface of the tongue is smooth and possesses a submucosa while elsewhere the thick lamina propria is fused with the interstitial connective tissue of the intrinsic muscles. **t. mucosa nasi** The mucous membrane lining the nasal cavity, which has a stratified squamous epithelium and some hairs in the anterior part of the vestibule, and a pseudostratified cilated columnar epithelium with many goblet cells in the rest of the respiratory region. In the olfactory region (tunica mucosa olfactoria) the nonciliated epithelium is thick and comprises olfactory receptor, supporting, and basal cells. In the respiratory region (tunica mucosa respiratoria) the lamina propria contains mucous and serous glands, and its deepest layer blends with the periosteum or perichondrium of the nasal walls. In the olfactory region it contains olfactory glands. The mucous membrane is continuous with that of the paranasal sinuses, the nasopharynx, and the nasolacrimal duct, and is thickest and highly vascular over the nasal conchae and septum. Also *schneiderian membrane.* **t. mucosa olfactoria** The part of the tunica mucosa nasi occurring in the olfactory region. Also *olfactory mucous membrane, olfactory membrane.* **t. mucosa oris** [NA] The mucous membrane of the oral cavity, the epithelium of which is of the stratified squamous nonkeratinizing type. The lamina propria has high papillae and contains small mucous glands and numerous nerve endings. **t. mucosa pharyngis** [NA] The mucous membrane that lines the pharynx and is continuous with that of the nasal cavity, mouth, larynx, and auditory tubes. In the nasopharynx the epithelium is columnar and ciliated while in the oral and laryngeal parts it is stratified squamous epithelium. There are many mucous glands in the nasopharynx, and the muscularis mucosae is replaced by a dense elastic network. **t. mucosa recti** [NA] The mucous membrane of the rectum which is thrown into a series of longitudinal folds, or rectal columns, at the lower end and at the commencement of the anal canal. Here the muscularis mucosae becomes broken up and disappears so that the lamina propria, which contains a plexus of large veins, is continuous with the submucosa. In addition, the mucous membrane forms two or more semilunar-shaped transverse or horizontal folds in the lower part of the rectum. **t. mucosa respiratoria** See under TUNICA MUCOSA NASI. **t. mucosa tracheae** [NA] The mucous membrane that lines the trachea in which the epithelium is cilated pseudostratified columnar with goblet cells, resting on a distinct basement membrane supported by a lamina propria with many elastic fibers, small glands, and lymphocytes. **t. mucosa tubae auditivae** [NA] The mucous membrane lining the auditory tube in which the epithelium is of ciliated low columnar type in the bony part and taller, ciliated pseudostratified with goblet cells near the pharynx. The lamina propria contains seromucous glands near the pharynx. **t. mucosa tubae uterinae** [NA] The mucous membrane of the uterine tube, lined by columnar ciliated epithelium and raised into numerous large plicae or folds that become higher and more complex in the ampulla. The epithelium also contains secretory and intercalary cells. At the margins of the infundibulum and fimbriae, the epithelium becomes continuous with the peritoneal epithelium. **t. mucosa ureteris** [NA] The mucous membrane lining the ureter. It is similar to that of the renal calices and pelvis and the bladder, the epithelium consisting of transitional epithelium resting upon a thin basal lamina and supported by the lamina propria with dense fibroconnective tissue and many elastic fibers. The membrane forms longitudinal folds that disappear when the ureter is distended. **t. mucosa urethrae femininae** [NA] The mucous membrane lining the female urethra, arranged in longitudinal folds and lined with stratified squamous epithelium and patches of pseudostratified columnar cells. The epithelium forms many invaginations in which glandular outpocketings with clear mucous cells are found. The lamina propria consists of loose connective tissue, many elastic networks, and cavernlike venous plexuses. **t. mucosa uteri** [NA] The mucous membrane lining the uterus. It is usually firmly bound to the underlying myometrium and composed of simple columnar epithelium containing uterine glands that extend into its total depth and are separated by connective tissue or the stroma. The structure and thickness of the mucosa vary with changes in the menstrual cycle. Also *endometrium.* **t. mucosa vaginae** [NA] The mucous membrane lining the vagina, having a thick stratified squamous epithelium, usually nonkeratinizing, and lacking glands. The dense connective tissue of the lamina propria contains a network of elastic fibers, lymphocytes, and occasional lymph nodules. **t. mucosa ventriculi** TUNICA MUCOSA GASTRICA. **t. mucosa vesicae biliaris** [NA] The mucous membrane of the gallbladder. It is thrown into numerous folds, especially in the empty state, and has a surface epithelium of tall columnar cells with oval nuclei at their bases. Simple tubuloalveolar glands are located in the lamina propria near the neck of the gallbladder. **t. mucosa vesicae urinariae** [NA] The mucous membrane of the urinary bladder, which is very similar to that of the ureter. The thick lamina propria has a deep layer of loose connective tissue permitting the mucous membrane to form numerous deep folds when the bladder is in an empty, contracted state. **t. mucosa vesiculae seminalis** [NA] The mucous membrane of the seminal vesicle, which is thrown into numerous complicated folds that project into the lumen and have secondary and tertiary foldings which may fuse with each other to produce cavities. The epithelium is highly variable and is often pseudostratified, but it may be simple columnar. Many cells contain secretion granules. The lamina propria is a loose connective tissue containing many blood vessels. **t. muscularis** Any of the middle coats, or tunics, of smooth muscle in the wall of tubular structures and hollow organs, as in the digestive, respiratory, and urogenital tracts. Usually it consists of an inner layer of circularly arranged muscle fibers and an outer layer of longitudinally directed smooth muscle fibers, which are located external to the tela submucosa and deep to the tunica serosa. Also *muscular coat, muscular tunic.* **t. muscularis bronchiorum** [NA] The muscular coat of the bronchi. The coat in the extrapulmonary bronchi is similar to that of the trachea where the smooth muscle fibers fill the gap between the ends of the cartilaginous rings posteriorly, whereas in the intrapulmonary bronchi the submucosa is supported by an outer layer of smooth muscle fibers arranged in incomplete spirals intermingled with elastic fibers. **t. muscularis coli** [NA] The muscular coat of the colon in which the outer longitudinal smooth muscle fibers are concentrated in three compact bands, or taeniae coli. **t. muscularis ductus deferentis** [NA] The muscular coat that forms most of the wall of the ductus deferens. It consists of inner and outer longitudinal layers and a thick intermediate layer of circular muscle fibers. **t. muscularis esophagi** [NA] The muscular coat of the esophagus, consisting of two layers that are composed of striated muscle with variable orientation in its upper part. In the middle part, the portion consisting of smooth muscle increases relative to the portion of striated bundles until the coat consists entirely of smooth muscle in the lower part of the esophagus, where the inner layer is circular and the outer is longitudinal. **t. muscularis gastrica** [NA] The muscular coat of the stomach comprising three layers of smooth muscle. The outer longitudinal layer is continuous with that of the esophagus and is most obvious along the greater and lesser curvatures. The thick middle layer of circular fibers is continuous with those of the esophagus, and they thicken at the pylorus to form the pyloric sphincter. The innermost layer is obliquely oriented and formed by incomplete loops that run from the cardiac orifice to the fundus and body of the stomach. **t. muscularis intestini tenuis** [NA] The muscular coat of the small intestine, comprising an inner circular and an outer longitudinal layer of smooth muscle with the sympathetic myenteric nerve plexus between them. Also *myenteron.* **t. muscularis pharyngis** [NA] The muscular coat of the pharynx which consists of an inner longitudinal and an outer circular or oblique layer of striated muscle. **t. muscularis recti** [NA] The muscular coat of the rectum, similar to tunica muscularis coli except that the outer longitudinal layer again becomes a continuous layer along the outside. **t. muscularis tracheae** [NA] The muscular coat of the trachea, which consists of a layer of interlacing transverse bundles of smooth muscle attached to the ends of the cartilage rings posteriorly and to the elastic fiber bundles. **t. muscularis tubae uterinae** [NA] The muscular coat of the uterine tube, which abuts directly on the mucous membrane. It consists of a broad inner circular and a narrow outer longitudinal layer in which the muscle bundles are scattered and embedded in loose connective tissue with elastic networks. Also *myosalpinx, muscular layer of fallopian tube.* **t. muscularis ureteris** [NA] The muscular coat of the ureter, consisting of an inner longitudinal and an outer circular layer. An additional outer longitudinal layer is added to the outer layer in the lower third of the ureter and when passing through the wall of the bladder. The layers are not clearly separated, the area of separation containing connective tissue and elastic fibers that are continuous with the lamina propria. Circular muscle fibers may be absent in the lower third of the ureter. **t. muscularis urethrae femininae** [NA] The muscular coat of the female urethra, consisting of inner longitudinal and outer circular smooth muscle fibers and strengthened by a striated muscle sphincter at its external orifice. **t. muscularis uteri** [NA] The muscular coat of the uterus, which is arranged in bundles separated by connective tissue and forms three ill-defined layers: an inner longitudinal, a thick middle layer of circular and oblique fibers with many blood vessels, and an outer thin layer of longitudinal muscle fibers under the serous coat. Also *myometrium.* **t. muscularis vaginae** [NA] The muscular coat of the vagina, comprising a thin inner layer of circular smooth muscle fibers and a thick outer layer of interlacing longitudinal fibers continuous with the uterine myometrium. In addition, at the introitus there is a sphincter of striated muscle. **t. muscularis vesicae biliaris** [NA] The muscular coat of the gallbladder, consisting of a layer of irregular smooth muscle fibers oriented in various directions. Between the layers are elastic, collagenous, and reticular fibers, as well as blood vessels and lymphatics. It is related directly to the mucous membrane. **t. muscularis vesicae urinariae** [NA] The strong and fairly thick muscular coat of the urinary bladder. It comprises three barely distinguishable layers, the outer and inner longitudinal layers separated by a marked circular layer that is thickened to form sphincters around the internal urethral orifice and to a lesser extent around the ureteric orifices. **t. muscularis vesiculae seminalis** [NA] The muscular coat of the seminal vesicle. It is thinner than that of the ductus deferens and comprises inner circular and outer longitudinal layers. **t. propria** The special covering of a particular part, as distinguished from a general investing membrane. *Outmoded.* Also *proper tunic, proper coat.* **t. sclerotica** SCLERA. **t. serosa** The membrane that lines the walls of the pleural, pericardial, and peritoneal cavities and is reflected onto the outer surface of the viscera contained in them. It consists of a relatively dense areolar connective tissue lined by a layer of mesothelial cells on the free surface, which is covered by a thin proteinaceous fluid. Also *serous membrane, serous coat, serous tunic, serosa, membrana serosa.* **t. serosa coli** The serous coat of the colon, which has taglike protuberances, or appendices epiploicae, consisting of adipose tissue on the free border of the colon. **t. serosa gastrica** [NA] The serous coat of the stomach, formed by a thin layer of loose connective tissue that contains nerves and vessels and is covered by a mesothelial layer which is continuous with the greater and lesser omenta. Also *tunica serosa ventriculi.* **t. serosa hepatis** [NA] The serous coat of the liver, formed by the peritoneum that surrounds the capsule over most of the liver except the small bare area on the posterior surface of the right lobe. **t. serosa intestini tenuis** [NA] The serous coat of the small intestine, which consists of a layer of mesothelial cells on loose connective tissue. **t. serosa peritonei** [NA] The serous coat of the peritoneum. **t. serosa splenis** [NA] The serous coat of the spleen. Also *serous capsule of spleen.* **t. serosa tubae uterinae** [NA] The serous coat of the uterine tube. **t. serosa uteri** [NA] The serous coat of the uterus. Also *perimetrium.* **t. serosa ventriculi** TUNICA SEROSA GASTRICA. **t. serosa vesicae biliaris** [NA] The serous coat of the gallbladder, consisting of peritoneum covering the area not attached to the liver and containing blood vessels and lymphatics. It is continuous with the tunica serosa hepatis. **t. serosa vesicae urinariae** [NA] The serous coat of the urinary bladder, consisting of fibroelastic tissue covered by peritoneum only on the superior surface of the bladder. **t. vaginalis testis** [NA] A closed serous sac that represents the distal part of the embryonic processus vaginalis, which is usually closed off at the deep inguinal ring at birth.

The visceral layer covers the tunica albuginea on the lateral and medial surfaces and anterior border of the testis, whereas at the posterior border it is reflected forward to form the parietal layer. The inner surface is lined with a layer of mesothelial cells. Also *serous membrane of epididymis, vaginal coat of testis.* **t. vasculosa** Any coat or layer well supplied with blood vessels. **t. vasculosa bulbi** [NA] The middle, vascular coat of the eyeball that comprises the choroid, ciliary body, and iris. Also *uvea, uveal tract, uveal coat.* **t. vasculosa lentis** A vascular mesenchymal condensation that encapsulates the lens of the developing eye by the second month of intrauterine life, the ventral part of which is the pupillary membrane. By the sixth month all the vessels supplying the capsule have atrophied so that the vascular capsule soon disappears. **t. vasculosa testis** A layer of a plexus of blood vessels on the internal aspect of the tunica albuginea of the testis that is supported by a delicate areolar connective tissue. It covers the septa and is reflected over all the lobules. Also *vascular layer of testis.*

**tunnel** In anatomy, an elongated canal or enclosed passageway usually open at both ends. **aortico-left ventricular t.** A congenital anomaly characterized by a tunnel between the ascending aorta and the left ventricle. **carpal t.** CANALIS CARPI. **cervical t.'s** The ducts of the branching cervical glands that open into the hollows between the plicae palmatae of the cervical canal of the uterus. *Outmoded.* **t. of Corti** CUNICULUS INTERNUS. **cubital t.** The gap between the two heads of the flexor carpi ulnaris muscle through which the ulnar nerve passes to the forearm. *Outmoded.* **flexor t.** CANALIS CARPI. **inner t. of Corti** CUNICULUS INTERNUS. **tarsal t.** A fibro-osseous tunnel formed by the flexor retinaculum and tarsal bones through which pass the posterior tibial vessels, tibial nerve, long flexor and tibialis posterior tendons, and their synovial sheaths.

**TUR** transurethral resection (of the prostrate).

**turbinal** \tur′bənəl\ TURBINATE. **sphenoidal t.'s** CONCHA SPHENOIDALIS.

**turbinate** \tur′bināt\ [L *turbinatus* (from *turbo,* gen. *turbinis* gyration, spinning, a spinning-top) top-shaped] **1** Shaped like a top, scroll, or spiral. Also *turbinal, turbinated.* **2** CONCHA NASALIS. **t.'s of the ethmoid** The concha nasalis superior and concha nasalis media, as well as the concha nasalis suprema, when present. **inferior t.** CONCHA NASALIS INFERIOR. **middle nasal t.** CONCHA NASALIS MEDIA. **nasal t.** CONCHA NASALIS. **t. of Santorini** CONCHA NASALIS SUPREMA. **sphenoid t.** CONCHA SPHENOIDALIS. **superior nasal t.** CONCHA NASALIS SUPERIOR. **t. of Zuckerkandl** A rarely occurring small ethmoidal concha situated above the concha nasalis suprema.

**turbinated** \tur′binā′tid\ TURBINATE.

**turbinectomy** \tur′binek′təmē\ [*turbin(ate)* + -ECTOMY] Excision of one of the nasal conchae, an operation seldom indicated except sometimes with regard to the middle concha.

**turbinotome** \tur′binətōm′\ CONCHOTOME.

**turbinotomy** \tur′binät′əmē\ [*turbin(ate)* + *o* + -TOMY] Resection of part of a concha. Also *conchotomy.*

**Türck** [Ludwig *Türck,* Austrian neurologist and laryngologist, 1810–1868] **1** Türck's bundle, Türck's tract. See under TRACTUS TEMPOROPONTINUS. **2** Türck's column. See under TRACTUS CORTICOSPINALIS VENTRALIS.

**Turcot** [Jacques *Turcot,* Canadian surgeon, born 1914] See under SYNDROME.

**turgescence** \tərjes′əns\ TUMESCENCE.

**turgid** \tur′jid\ Swollen; distended; tumid.

**turgidization** \tur′jidīzā′shən\ The establishment of turgor in a cell or tissue, as by the injection or uptake of a fluid.

**turgor** \tur′gər\ [Late L (from L *turgere* to swell) turgidity, swelling] The condition of being swollen or extended to fullness.

**turista** \toorēs′tə\ [Spanish, a tourist, touring] See under TRAVELERS' DIARRHEA.

**Turk** [Siegmund *Turk,* Swiss ophthalmologist, flourished 20th century] Stilling-Turk-Duane syndrome. See under DUANE SYNDROME.

**Türk** [Wilhelm *Türk,* Austrian hematologist, 1871–1916] Türk's irritation leukocyte. See under TÜRK CELL.

**Turner** [Daniel *Turner,* English dermatologist, 1667–1740] Turner's cerate. See under CALAMINE OINTMENT.

**Turner** [George Grey *Turner,* English surgeon, 1877–1951] Grey Turner sign. See under TURNER SIGN.

**Turner** [Henry Hubert *Turner,* U.S. endocrinologist, 1892–1970] **1** See under SYNDROME. **2** Ullrich-Turner syndrome, male Turner syndrome, pseudo-Turner syndrome. See under NOONAN SYNDROME.

**Turner** [John A. Alden *Turner,* U.S. physician, flourished early 20th century] **1** Parsonage-Turner syndrome, Parsonage and Turner amyotrophic neuralgia. See under SHOULDER GIRDLE SYNDROME. **2** Turner-Kieser syndrome. See under NAIL-PATELLA SYNDROME.

**Turner** [Joseph G. *Turner,* English dentist, died 1955] See under TOOTH.

**Turner** [V. C. *Turner,* U.S. surgeon, flourished 20th century] Hefke-Turner sign. See under OBTURATOR SIGN.

**Turner** [Sir William *Turner,* English anatomist, 1832–1916] Turner sulcus. See under SULCUS INTRAPARIETALIS.

**turning** *Older term* VERSION.

**turnsol** \turn′säl\ LITMUS.

**TURP** transurethral resection of the prostrate.

**tus.** *tussis* (L, cough).

**tussal** \tus′əl\ TUSSIVE.

**tussicular** \tusik′yələr\ TUSSIVE.

**tussis** \tus′is\ [L, a cough] COUGH. **t. convulsiva** PERTUSSIS. **t. stomachalis** STOMACH COUGH.

**tussive** \tus′iv\ [*tuss(is)* + -IVE] Relating to or caused by coughing. Also *tussal, tussicular.*

**tutamen** \tootā′mən\ [L (from *tutari* to guard, akin to *tueri* to look at, watch over), a defense, protection] (*pl.* tutamina) A protective covering. **tutamina cerebri** The protective coverings of the cerebrum, including the scalp, the bones forming the cranium, and the meninges immediately surrounding the brain. **tutamina oculi** The protective appendages of the eye, namely the eyelids, eyebrows, conjunctiva, and lacrimal apparatus. *Outmoded.*

**tutamina** \tootam′inə\ Plural of TUTAMEN.

**Tweed** [Charles H. *Tweed,* U.S. orthodontist, 1895–1970] See under TRIANGLE.

**Tween 80** A preparation of sorbitan polyoxyalkalene. It is widely used for its detergent and emulsifying properties. A trade name.

**Tween-ether** A mixture of a non-ionic detergent (Tween 80) and the lipid solvent, ether, which is useful in a number of laboratory procedures.

**tweezers** [earlier *tweez(e)* (from French *(é)tui* a small case + pl. *-s*) an instrument case, set of instruments + *-ers* as in *pincers*] A forcepslike surgical instrument used for grasping and holding under spring tension.

**twig** In anatomy, a fine terminal branch of a nerve or a blood vessel.

**twin** [Old English *getwinn*] One of two fetuses or infants or parts thereof delivered as the product of a single gestation. **acardiac t.** ACARDIUS. **binovular t.'s** DIZYGOTIC TWINS. **conjoined t.'s** Two individuals or parts of two individuals united to varying degrees and with varying extents of residual duality. The twins are always monozygotic and are presumed to have arisen as a result of the appearance of two embryonic axes on the same embryonic disk, with consequent fusion of adjacent or approximating parts. When the twins are approximately equal and union involves symmetrical fusion of discrete regions or parts, the preferred nomenclature is to use the name of the region(s) where union occurs with the suffix *-pagus*, as in thoracopagus or cephalopagus. If union is complete at one end and residual duplication is apparent at the other, the term *duplicitas*, followed by *anterior* or *posterior* to designate the duplicated end, is used. If the conjoined twins are unequal in size, the condition is named for the region on the larger to which the smaller is attached, followed by the term *parasiticus*, as in cephalopagus parasiticus. **dichorial t.'s** DIZYGOTIC TWINS. **dissimilar t.'s** DIZYGOTIC TWINS. **dizygotic t.'s** Twins developed from two fertilized ova, usually liberated from the ovaries simultaneously, which develop in separate or partially fused chorionic sacs. Three out of four of all human twins are dizygotic. Also *binovular twins, dichorial twins, dissimilar twins, false twins, fraternal twins, unlike twins, two-egg twins.* **false t.'s** DIZYGOTIC TWINS. **fraternal t.'s** DIZYGOTIC TWINS. **identical t.'s** MONOZYGOTIC TWINS. **impacted t.'s** CRYPTODIDYMUS. **incomplete conjoined t.'s** Equal conjoined twins each of which is incompletely formed, usually in the same way or to the same degree. **monoamniotic t.'s** Monozygotic twins contained within a single amnion. It is likely that they divided soon after differentiation of the embryonic disk and of the amniotic cavity. About four percent of all monozygotic twins are monochorionic monoamniotic twins. Of this proportion about five percent are conjoined twins due to failure of complete division. **monochorionic t.'s** Monozygotic twins enclosed in a single chorion. Also *monochorial twins.* **monozygotic t.'s** Twins derived from the division of a single fertilized ovum and which usually have a common chorionic sac and a common placenta. There are separate umbilical cords and usually each twin has its own amnion. About one in four of all human twins is monozygotic. The exact arrangement of chorion and amnion of each twin depends on when division of the early embryo occurs. If, for example, separation occurs at the two-cell stage of cleavage of the fertilized ovum, then the monozygotic twins will probably have a chorion each and be indistinguishable from dizygotic or dichorionic twins. Also *identical twins, monovular twins, similar twins, true twins, uniovular twins, one-egg twins.* **parabiotic t.'s** Two animals joined surgically in order to study the effect of humoral agents that are transmitted in the common circulation. **parasitic t.** The smaller or less developed member of a pair of conjoined unequal twins. **placental parasitic t.** OMPHALOSITE. **Siamese t.'s** Conjoined twins of which the members are of equal size. *Popular.* • The original highly publicized twins of this type from Siam were of the xiphopagus type. **similar t.'s** MONOZYGOTIC TWINS. **true t.'s** MONOZYGOTIC TWINS. **two-egg t.'s** DIZYGOTIC TWINS. **uniovular t.'s** MONOZYGOTIC TWINS. **unlike t.'s** DIZYGOTIC TWINS.

**twinge** \twinj\ A brief, sharp painful sensation.

**twinning** Duplication of parts or of the whole organism, which may not be entire in that conjoined parts or conjoined twins may result. Twinning can be natural and spontaneous but with the dizygotic type under hereditary control through the mother, and also experimentally induced in animals. It can result from the release at ovulation of more than one ovum either from one, or more likely from two ovarian follicles when dizygotic (fraternal or unlike) twins result, or as the result at an early stage of development of the division of the cleaving ovum or very young embryo into two so that monozygotic (identical or like) twins are obtained. The arrangement of the chorion and amnion at birth can give an indication of the type of twinning. **experimental t.** The experimental production, usually from a single zygote, of complete embryonic duplication. The embryonic stage at the time of experimental intervention generally determines the relationship between the embryo and its surrounding membranes. Thus, a pair of monozygotic twins may either be located within a single amniotic cavity or are located in two quite separate amniotic cavities. In the latter, the twinning event probably occurs at a slightly earlier stage than in the former class. **spontaneous t.** See under TWINNING.

**twitch** A brief skeletal muscular contraction. **skin t.** Superficial skeletal muscle fasciculation visible on the skin surface.

**twitching** The act or occurrence of brief skeletal muscle contraction. **fascicular t.** Repetitive contraction of bundles of skeletal muscle fibers. **fibrillar t.** Spontaneous, rhythmic contractions of a single skeletal muscle fiber which can be induced by denervation. **Trousseau's t.** Fasciculation of the muscles of facial expression.

**tylectomy** \tīlek′təmē\ [Gk *tyl(os)* callus + -ECTOMY] The surgical excision of any localized swelling or tumor.

**tylosis** \tīlō′sis\ [Gk *tylōsis* (from *tylos* a callus) a becoming or making callous or hard] The formation of diffuse keratoderma. **t. ciliaris** MARGINAL BLEPHARITIS.

**tympan-** \tim′pən-\ TYMPANO-.

**tympanal** \tim′pənəl\ TYMPANIC.

**tympanectomy** \tim′pənek′təmē\ [TYMPAN- + -ECTOMY] The excision of the tympanic membrane, the malleus, the incus, and the intratympanic portion of the tensor tympani muscle or the diseased remnants of these, as carried out as part of the radical mastoidectomy procedure.

**tympani-** \tim′pənē-\ TYMPANO-.

**tympania** \timpan′ē·ə\ TYMPANITES.

**tympanic** \timpan′ik\ **1** Pertaining to the tympanum. **2** Resonant. Also *tympanal.*

**tympanichord** \timpan′ikôrd\ CHORDA TYMPANI.

**tympanion** \timpan′ē·än\ [Gk (dim. of *tympanon* a kettledrum) a drum, roller] A point at the upper or lower end of the vertical diameter of the annulus tympanicus. *Outmoded.* **lower t.** The lowest point on the vertical diameter of the annulus tympanicus. **upper t.** The highest point on the vertical diameter of the annulus tympanicus.

**tympanites** \tim′pənī′tēs\ [Gk *tympanitēs* (from *tympanon* a kettledrum) a dropsy in which the belly is stretched tight, like a drum] Gross distension of the abdominal wall caused by the accumulation of gas in the peritoneal cavity or a part of the gastrointestinal tract. Tympany is elicited by percussion of the distended part. Also *tympania, tympanism, tympanosis, meteorism.* **false t.** Abdominal distension not due to intestinal or peritoneal gas. Also *pseudotympanites.* **uterine t.** PHYSOMETRA.

**tympanitic** \tim′pənit′ik\ **1** Affected with, pertaining to, or characteristic of tympanites. **2** Emitting a drumlike sound on percussion.

**tympano-** \tim′pənō-\ [Gk *tympanon* drum, kettledrum] A combining form denoting (1) the tympanum; (2) the tympanic membrane; (3) tympanites. Also *tympan-, tympani-.*

**tympanogram** \tim′pənōgram′\ [TYMPANO- + -GRAM]

The printout of an impedance bridge showing the stiffness or the compliance of the middle-ear structures as it varies with changes in pressure within the external ear canal.

**tympanolabyrinthopexy** \-lab'ərin'thəpek'sē\ A precursor of certain varieties of the fenestration operation for the relief of deafness.

**tympanomalleal** \-mal'ē·əl\ **1** Of or relating to the tympanic part of the temporal bone and the malleus. **2** Of or relating to the tympanic membrane and the malleus.

**tympanomastoid** \-mas'toid\ **1** Of or relating to both the tympanic and mastoid compartments of the middle-ear cleft. **2** Related to both the tympanic and mastoid parts of the temporal bone, as in the tympanomastoid suture.

**tympanomastoiditis** \-mas'toidī'tis\ Inflammation of both tympanic and mastoid compartments of the middle-ear cleft.

**tympanometry** \tim'pənäm'ətrē\ [TYMPANO- + -METRY] The measurement of air pressure in the middle-ear cleft, and of the stiffness of the ossicular chain and tympanic membrane, now readily and accurately achieved using the impedance bridge.

**tympanoplasty** \tim'pənōplas'tē\ [TYMPANO- + -PLASTY] **1** The reconstruction, by one of a variety of surgical means, of the sound-conducting mechanism of the middle ear when this has been damaged by disease or by the radical surgery necessary to excise it. **2** The excision of disease of the middle-ear cleft and the cleft's subsequent reconstruction. Used in this sense particularly in the U.S. **combined approach t.** Tympanoplasty of whatever kind performed as the final operative stage after combined approach mastoidectomy. **intact canal-wall t.** Tympanoplasty, usually combined approach tympanoplasty, in which the emphasis is on the intact preservation of the external auditory meatus, particularly of the thinned-out bone of the outer attic and posterior walls. **type 2 t.** Tympanoplasty in which sound transmission is made possible through a deformed, reconstructed, or prosthetic ossicular chain. **type 3 t.** Tympanoplasty in which the tympanic membrane, or reconstructed tympanic membrane, is brought into direct contact with a normal stapes. Hearing is maintained as a result of the columella effect. **type 4 t.** Tympanoplasty in which the mobile stapes footplate is exposed directly to the sound waves. The round window is afforded protection by the creation of a small compartment that corresponds to the lower half of the tympanic cavity and is responsible for the baffle effect. **type 5 t.** A fenestration operation modified to deal with the problem created by an ankylosed stapes encountered in the course of tympanoplasty.

**tympanosclerosis** \-sklerō'sis\ A disease of the middle ear in which plaques of collagen form in the tympanic membrane, in the lining epithelium of the middle ear, or in both. They may become calcified. It is the end result of past otitis media and is part of the healing process. When it results in fixation of the middle-ear ossicles considerable deafness is likely to follow. Also *tympanic hyalinization, tympanic hyalinosis, otitis media sclerotica* (older term).

**tympanosis** \tim'pənō'sis\ TYMPANITES.

**tympanosympathectomy** \-sim'pəthek'təmē\ Surgical excision of the tympanic plexus on the surface of the tympanic promontory, formerly performed as treatment for tinnitus. *Imprecise.* See also TYMPANIC NEURECTOMY.

**tympanotomy** \tim'pənät'əmē\ [TYMPANO- + -TOMY] MYRINGOTOMY. **posterior t.** An operation for obtaining access to the tympanic cavity by the transmastoid route. **transmeatal t.** The operation for obtaining access to the tympanic cavity by the transmeatal route, entailing the raising of a posterior tympanomeatal flap. This is the approach employed for stapedectomy.

**tympanous** \tim'pənəs\ Affected with tympanites; tympanitic.

**tympanum** \tim'pənəm\ [L (from Gk *tympanon* kettledrum), a drum, timbrel, tambourine] **1** The tympanic cavity and the tympanic membrane combined. **2** The middle ear as a whole. An outmoded usage.

**tympany** \tim'pənē\ [TYMPAN- + -Y] A low-pitched, drumlike sound produced by percussion over an air-filled region, especially in the stomach and intestine or in the peritoneal and pleural cavities. **bell t.** A ringing and resonant note sometimes heard on percussion over a pneumothorax.

**Tyndall** [John *Tyndall,* Irish physicist, 1820–1893] **1** See under LIGHT. **2** Tyndall phenomenon. See under EFFECT.

**type** [L *typus.* See TYPUS.] **1** A category or class based on shared characteristics. **2** A specimen or example of a category or class which is taken as a standard for determining membership in that category or class. See also TYPE SPECIES. **basic personality t.** The group of personality characteristics shared by most members of a particular social unit. **blood t.** See under BLOOD TYPE. **cycloid t.** CYCLOTHYMIC PERSONALITY. **Lévi-Lorain t.** HYPOPHYSIAL DWARFISM. **Lorain t.** HYPOPHYSIAL DWARFISM. **personality t.** CHARACTER. **schizoid t.** SCHIZOID PERSONALITY. **test t.** Type of various sizes used in tests designed to measure visual acuity. Also *optotype.* **wild t.** WILD-TYPE STRAIN.

**type-specific** Uniquely characteristic of a particular strain of microorganism. Type-specific substances, such as certain antigens, are often used for classification into serovars.

**typh-** \tīf-\ TYPHO-.

**typhemia** \tīfē'mē·ə\ [TYPH- + -EMIA] The presence of *Salmonella typhi* in the blood.

**typhinia** \tīfi'nē·ə\ RELAPSING FEVER.

**typhl-¹** \tifl-\ TYPHLO-¹.

**typhl-²** \tifl-\ TYPHLO-².

**typhlectasis** \tiflek'təsis\ [TYPHL-¹ + ECTASIS] Distention or dilatation of the cecum.

**typhlectomy** \tiflek'təmē\ [TYPHL-¹ + -ECTOMY] CECECTOMY.

**typhlo-¹** \tif'lō-\ [Gk *typhlon* cecum] A combining form denoting the cecum. Also *typhl-*.

**typhlo-²** \tif'lō-\ [Gk *typhlos* blind] A combining form meaning blind, blindness. Also *typhl-*.

**typhloappendicitis** \-əpen'disī'tis\ Inflammation of the cecum and appendix.

**typhlodicliditis** \-dik'lidī'tis\ [TYPHLO- + Gk *diklid(es)* folding doors + -ITIS] Inflammation of the ileocecal valve.

**typhlolexia** \-lek'sē·ə\ [TYPHLO-² + Gk *lex(is)* word + -IA] WORD BLINDNESS.

**typhlology** \tifläl'əjē\ The scientific study of blindness.

**typhlomegaly** \-meg'əlē\ [TYPHLO-¹ + -MEGALY] The presence of an enlarged cecum. *Seldom used.*

**typhlon** \tif'län\ *Obs.* CAECUM.

**typhlopexy** \tif'ləpek'sē\ [TYPHLO-¹ + -PEXY] A surgical procedure in which the cecum is fixed to the anterior abdominal wall to prevent volvulus. Also *typhlopexia.*

**typhlostomy** \tifläs'təmē\ The surgical creation of an opening in the cecum, which may communicate with the skin, for purposes of drainage or decompression.

**typhloureterostomy** \tif'lōyoorē'təräs'təmē\ The creation of an anastomosis between the ureters or a ureter and the cecum.

**typho-** \tī′fō-\ [New L *typhus*. See TYPHUS.] A combining form meaning (1) typhus; (2) typhoid. Also *typh-*.

**typhobacterin** \tī′fōbak′tərin\ TYPHOID VACCINE.

**typhoid** \tī′foid\ [*typh(us)* + -OID] **1** Similar to typhus; typhuslike. An obsolete usage. **2** TYPHOID FEVER. **3** Pertaining to typhoid fever; typhoidal. **ambulatory t.** A mild form of typhoid fever. Also *walking typhoid, latent typhoid*. **bilious t.** *Outmoded* ICTERIC LEPTOSPIROSIS. **latent t.** AMBULATORY TYPHOID. **provocation t.** The systemic symptoms occurring as a reaction to the endotoxin of the killed *Salmonella typhi* contained in the typhoid vaccine. **walking t.** AMBULATORY TYPHOID.

**typhoidal** \tīfoi′dəl\ Pertaining to or resembling typhoid fever.

**typhomania** \tī′fōmā′nē·ə\ [TYPHO- + -MANIA] The confused state seen in some patients with typhoid fever.

**typhopneumonia** \tī′fōnʸoomō′nē·ə\ Typhoid fever in which there is pulmonary involvement, usually pneumonia.

**typhous** \tī′fəs\ Related to or resembling typhus.

**typhus** \tī′fəs\ [New L, from Gk *typhos* (akin to *typhein* to smoke, smoulder) delusion, delirium, a fever with delirium or stupor, any of various fevers] Any of a group of acute infectious, arthropod-borne diseases of man and animals caused by species of *Rickettsia*, characterized in man by high fever, severe headache, malaise, and a generalized macular or maculopapular rash which erupts during the latter half of the first week of illness. Specific types of typhus are differentiated on the basis of serologic tests. Different rickettsiae are involved, as are a variety of arthropod vectors. Also *typhus fever*. ● When not further specified, the word *typhus* usually refers to epidemic louse-borne typhus or to flea-borne typhus. **African tick t.** BOUTONNEUSE FEVER. **amarillic t.** *Outmoded* YELLOW FEVER. **Australian tick t.** NORTH QUEENSLAND TICK TYPHUS. **benign t.** **1** Any mild type of typhus. **2** BRILL'S DISEASE. **chigger-borne t.** SCRUB TYPHUS. **classic t.** EPIDEMIC LOUSE-BORNE TYPHUS. **collapsing t.** A typhoid feverlike illness observed in Korea. **endemic t.** FLEA-BORNE TYPHUS. **epidemic t.** EPIDEMIC LOUSE-BORNE TYPHUS. **epidemic louse-borne t.** An acute form of typhus caused by *Rickettsia prowazekii* and transmitted to man by the louse *Pediculus humanus humanus*. An 8–12 day incubation period is followed by an abrupt onset of severe headache, high fever, chills, and myalgia. A macular or maculopapular rash appears on about the fifth day. In the second week, the disease increases in severity and may be fatal if untreated. Also *epidemic typhus, louse-borne typhus, louse typhus, classic typhus, European typhus, ship fever, exanthematous typhus, petechial typhus*. **European t.** EPIDEMIC LOUSE-BORNE TYPHUS. **exanthematous t.** EPIDEMIC LOUSE-BORNE TYPHUS. **flea-borne t.** An acute form of typhus caused by *Rickettsia mooseri* and transmitted to humans from rats by the rat flea, *Xenopsylla cheopis*. The disease is not communicable from one human being to another. The characteristic symptoms are similar to but milder than those of epidemic louse-borne typhus, and the duration of illness is shorter, the rash less extensive, and the case fatality rate lower. Also *murine typhus, endemic typhus, rat typhus, flea typhus, urban typhus, shop typhus*. **Indian tick t.** A rickettsial disease observed in India and thought to be the same as boutonneuse fever. North and northwest India and Pakistan are the areas involved. It is a mild, sporadic form of typhus. **Kenya t.** A rickettsial disease observed in Kenya in urban as well as rural settings, and closely resembling boutonneuse fever, although an eschar (tache noir) does not occur. It is transmitted by *Rhipicephalus sanguineus, R. simus, Haemaphysalis haebreum*, and larvae of *Amblyomma leachi* all of which are found on dogs. Small rodents probably form the reservoir of infections. Also *Kenya fever*. **louse-borne t.** EPIDEMIC LOUSE-BORNE TYPHUS. **mite-borne t.** SCRUB TYPHUS. **t. mitior** Any mild case of typhus. **murine t.** FLEA-BORNE TYPHUS. **north Asian tick t.** SIBERIAN TICK TYPHUS. **north Queensland tick t.** A relatively mild rickettsiosis caused by *Rickettsia australis* and thought to be transmitted to man by ixodid ticks that normally have rodents and small marsupials as hosts. It is characterized by headache, fever, rash, adenopathy, conjunctivitis, and an eschar at the site of the tick bite. Also *north Queensland tick fever, Queensland tick fever, Queensland tick typhus, Australian tick fever, Australian tick typhus*. **petechial t.** EPIDEMIC LOUSE-BORNE TYPHUS. **Queensland tick t.** NORTH QUEENSLAND TICK TYPHUS. **rat t.** FLEA-BORNE TYPHUS. **recrudescent t.** BRILL'S DISEASE. **rural t.** SCRUB TYPHUS. **São Paulo t.** ROCKY MOUNTAIN SPOTTED FEVER. **scrub t.** An acute typhuslike rickettsiosis of rural Asia caused by *Rickettsia tsutsugamushi* and transmitted to man by the bite of larval trombiculid mites (chiggers). After a 9–12 day incubation period, a papular lesion usually appears at the site of the infecting chigger bite. The lesion then enlarges, undergoes necrosis, and crusts, forming the characteristic tache noir. Regional lymphadenopathy and prodromal symptoms of headache, malaise, and anorexia may occur. The onset of illness is acute with fever, chills, headache, ocular pain, conjunctivitis, malaise, cough, and commonly interstitial pneumonitis. A macular rash appears on the trunk and limbs toward the end of the first week. In the second week, fever persists and signs of multiple system involvement appear. The mortality in untreated cases is 0–30% in different foci. Antibiotic therapy is almost always curative. Also *tsutsugamushi disease, shimamushi disease, kedani disease, kedani fever, mite fever, tsutsugamushi fever, Queensland coastal fever, river fever of Japan, Japanese flood fever, mite-borne typhus, mite typhus, chigger-borne typhus, rural typhus, yochubio*. **shop t.** FLEA-BORNE TYPHUS. **Siberian tick t.** A relatively mild spotted fever caused by *Rickettsia sibirica* and transmitted to man by *Dermacentor* or *Haemaphysalis* ticks. It is characterized by headache, fever, conjunctivitis, a maculopapular rash, and an ulcerative lesion at the site of the infecting tick bite. Also *north Asian tick typhus*. **sporadic t.** BRILL'S DISEASE. **tick t.** Any tick-borne rickettsiosis; spotted fever. **urban t.** FLEA-BORNE TYPHUS.

**typical** Characteristic or representative of a type.

**typing** The classification of microorganisms, tissues, or blood cells on the basis of their antigenic characteristics. In transplantation immunology, it is used to determine the degree of organ compatibility between a donor and recipient. In microbiology, it is used to distinguish various strains within the species. See also entries under CLASSIFICATION. **blood t.** The classification of blood on the basis of membrane antigens on the surface of red cells by use of antigen-specific sera. **colicin t.** Classification of enterobacteria on the basis of their sensitivity to killing by various colicins. **phage t.** The characterization of bacterial strains by their susceptibility to different bacteriophages. It is used for typing staphylococcal or typhoid strains for epidemiologic purposes. **tissue t.** The identification of histocompatibility antigens, usually performed by testing for HLA antigens on lymphocytes. Antibodies, usually used in cytotoxicity techniques, are used to identify antigens in the A, B, C, and DR series. Mixed lymphocyte culture tests are used for D antigens.

**typodont** \tī′pōdänt\ [*typ(e)* + -ODONT] Simulated or

natural teeth set in an artificial arch. It is used as a teaching aid.

**typology** \tīpäl′əjē\ **1** A system of classification by type. **2** The study of types, as of microorganisms.

**typus** \tī′pəs\ [L (from Gk *typos* an impress, print, mark, image), a type, figure, impression, stamp] **t. inversus** A temperature curve sometimes seen in grave cases of tuberculosis, salmonella infections, and other illnesses. The morning reading is higher than that of the evening.

**Tyr** Symbol for tyrosine.

**tyraminase** *Outmoded* MONOAMINE OXIDASE.

**tyramine** The product of decarboxylation of tyrosine. It is closely related to epinephrine, although not a precursor. It occurs in cheese, and it can have harmful effects on patients who are being treated with inhibitors of the flavin-containing amine oxidase.

**tyramine oxidase** MONOAMINE OXIDASE.

**tyrannism** \tir′ənizm\ SADISM.

**tyro-** \tī′rō-, tī′rə-\ [Gk *tyros* cheese] A combining form meaning cheese.

**tyrocidine** A constituent with gramicidin in tyrothricin, an antibiotic produced from *Bacillus brevis.*

**Tyrode** [Maurice Vejux *Tyrode,* U.S. pharmacologist, 1878–1930] See under SOLUTION.

**Tyrode-B** BAVISTER'S MEDIUM.

***Tyroglyphus*** \tīräg′lifəs, tī′rōglif′əs\ *TYROPHAGUS.* ***T. farinae*** *ACARUS SIRO.* ***T. siro*** *ACARUS SIRO.*

**tyroid** \tī′roid\ [*tyr(o)-* + -OID] Cheesy, as in texture.

***Tyrophagus*** \tīräf′əgəs\ [New L, from TYRO- + Gk *-phagos* -eating, -eater] A genus of astigmatid or soft mites in the family Acaridae; meal or grain mites. They have sucker-like or clawlike appendages and are slow moving and only weakly sclerotized. Many contribute to occupational acarine dermatitis, such as *T. putrescentiae* (formerly called *Tyroglyphus longior* var. *castellani*), which affects dock workers handling cheese as well as grocers and other food, grain, and copra handlers. Also *Tyroglyphus.* ***T. siro*** *ACARUS SIRO.*

**tyrosinase** MONOPHENOL MONOOXYGENASE.

**tyrosine** \tī′rəsēn\ The amino acid 4-hydroxphenylalanine. It can be formed in mammals from phenylalanine, but the pair are essential. They are both among the twenty amino acids incorporated into proteins. Tyrosine residues in enzymes can function as acid catalysts. The phenolic hydroxyl group has a p*K* of about 10. Symbol: Tyr, Y

**tyrosinemia** \-sinē′mē·ə\ Increased levels of tyrosine in blood due to defective tyrosine aminotransferase, associated with neuropsychiatric dysfunction and mental retardation. The condition is inherited as an autosomal recessive.

**tyrosinosis** \-sinō′sis\ An autosomal recessive disorder that takes one of two forms. The subacute form is characterized by neonatal failure to thrive and death from liver failure in infancy. The chronic form is marked by liver and renal tubular dysfunction and vitamin D-resistant rickets. In either case, hypertyrosinemia, hypermethioninemia, and excessive urinary excretion of multiple amino acids occur. The basic defect is unknown. Also *tyrosyluria.*

**tyrosinuria** \-sinoo′rē·ə\ [*tyrosin(e)* + -URIA] Urinary excretion of tyrosine.

**tyrosyluria** \-siloo′rē·ə\ **1** Increased urinary excretion of ketonic metabolites of tyrosine, such as *p*-hydroxyphenylpyruvic acid, in hypertyrosinemia, tyrosinosis, scurvy, pernicious anemia, and other disorders. **2** TYROSINOSIS.

**tyrothricin** \-thrī′sin\ An antibiotic isolated from *Bacillus brevis* and consisting mainly of gramicidin and tyrocidine. It is active against Gram-positive bacteria and is used along or in combination with other antibacterial agents for the local treatment of skin and mouth infections. It is too toxic to be used systemically.

**tyrotoxicon** \-täk′sikän\ $C_6H_5N(:N)OH$. Benzenediazonium hydroxide, a toxic compound found in contaminated cheese and other milk products.

**tyrotoxicosis** \-täk′sikō′sis\ Illness resulting from ingestion of tyrotoxicon. Symptoms are nausea, vomiting, dizziness, severe epigastral pain, dilated pupils, numbness of the limbs, prostration, and possible death. Also *cheese poisoning.*

**tyrotoxism** \-täk′sizm\ [TYRO- + TOX- + -ISM] Poisoning due to ingestion of contaminated cheese. See also TYROTOXICOSIS.

**Tyrrell** [Frederick *Tyrrell,* English surgeon, 1797–1843] **1** See under HOOK. **2** Tyrrell's fascia. See under SEPTUM RECTOVESICALE.

**Tyson** [Edward *Tyson,* English anatomist, 1649–1708] Glands of Tyson, crypts of Tyson. See under GLANDULAE PREPUTIALES.

**tysonitis** \tī′səni′tis\ [glands of *Tyson* + -ITIS] An inflammation of one or both parafrenal glands.

**tyvelose** \tī′vəlōs\ 3,6-Dideoxy-D-mannose. A sugar in O antigen determinant 9, characteristic of group D salmonellae. It was first isolated from cultures of *Salmonella typhi.*

**Tzanck** [Arnault *Tzanck,* Russian dermatologist, 1886–1954] See under CELL, SMEAR, TEST.

**tzetze** \tset′sē\ [See TSETSE.] TSETSE FLY.

# U

**U** **1** Symbol for the element, uranium. **2** Symbol for uridine. **3** Symbol for uracil.

**U.** unit.

**uarthritis** \yoo′ärthrī′tis\ [irreg. from *u(ratic) arthritis*] GOUT.

**uberous** \yoo′bərəs\ *Seldom used* PROLIFIC.

**uberty** \yoo′bərtē\ *Seldom used* FERTILITY.

**ubichromanol** The compound containing a dihydrochromene ring formed by reaction of one hydroxyl group of ubiquinol with the first double bond of the side chain. The number after it, as in ubichromanol-9, expresses the number of isoprene units in the side chain.

**ubichromenol** The compound formed by dehydrogenation of an ubichromanol with formation of a chromene ring. Such compounds are found in mammalian tissues.

**ubiquinol** The reduced form of ubiquinone.

**ubiquinone** A substituted *p*-benzoquinone, with two adjacent methoxy substituents on one side of the ring, and a methyl and polyisoprene substituent on the other. The number of isoprene units is added after the name, e.g ubiquinone-10 is the typical mammalian ubiquinone, and bacterial ubiquinone containing six isoprene units is thus ubiquinone-6. Ubiquinone functions as a hydrogen carrier in the respiratory chain. Also *coenzyme Q.* Symbol: Q

**ubiquitin** A peptide of about 75 residues, found in animals, plants, and bacteria, with little change of structure between one organism and another. ATP is used to link it covalently to proteins, so that it acylates them on lysine with its C-terminus. Such linkage stimulates their intracellular proteolysis.

**UDP** Symbol for uridine diphosphate.

**UDPG** Symbol for uridine diphosphate glucose (UDP-glucose).

**UDPgalactose** UDP carrying an α-D-galactopyranosyl group on its distal phosphate. It is interconvertible with UDPglucose by the action of an epimerase, and this provides a pathway for galactose production and utilization.

**UDPG-glycogen transglucosidase** *Outmoded* GLYCOGEN SYNTHASE.

**UDPglucose** UDP carrying an α-D-glucopyranosyl group on its distal phosphate. It is made from UTP and glucose 1-phosphate with elimination of diphosphate (pyrophosphate), and is a donor of glucosyl groups in many reactions of polysaccharide biosynthesis. It can also be epimerized to form UDPgalactose.

**UDPglucose dehydrogenase** The enzyme (EC 1.1.1.22) that oxidizes UDPglucose with the reduction of two molecules of $NAD^+$ to form UDPglucuronate required for the biosynthesis of compounds of glucuronic acid.

**UDPglucose 4-epimerase** The enzyme (EC 5.1.3.2) that catalyzes the interconversion of UDPglucose and UDP-galactose. It is involved in forming the galactosyl group for lactose synthesis. It requires $NAD^+$, and this is unusual for an enzyme not involved in an oxidative reaction. The $NAD^+$ is thought to accept H-4 as a hydride ion giving a carbonyl group at C-4 of the center epimerized, so that reversal of this reaction with hydride addition on the other side of the ring completes the epimerization.

**UDPglucuronate** UDP glycosylated on its distal phosphate by glucuronic acid. This compound is produced by dehydrogenation of UDPglucose, and is the donor of glucuronosyl residues in forming glucuronides and polysaccharides.

**UDPglucuronate epimerase** Either of two known enzymes: one (EC 5.1.3.6) interconverts UDPglucuronate and UDPgalacturonate by epimerization at C-4, and the other interconverts UDP-D-glucuronate and UDP-L-iduronate by epimerization at C-5.

**UFA** unesterified fatty acids. (Used especially of fatty acids in the blood).

**Uhl** [Henry Stephen Magraw *Uhl*, U.S. internist, born 1921] See under ANOMALY.

**Uhthoff** [Wilhelm *Uhthoff*, German ophthalmologist, 1853–1927] Uhthoff symptom. See under UHTHOFF SIGN.

**ul-[1]** \yool-\ ULO-[1].

**ul-[2]** \yool-\ ULO-[2].

**ula** \yoo′lə\ [New L, from Gk *oula* gums, gingivae] *Outmoded* GINGIVA.

# ulcer

**ulcer** \ul′sər\ [Old French *ulcere*, from L *ulcus*, gen. *ulceris* (akin to Gk *(h)elkos* a wound, festering wound, ulcer) a sore, ulcer] A depressed, well-defined area of excavation into the deeper layers of an organ, usually resulting from inflammation or ischemia. Also *ulcus, ulceration.* **acute stress u.** A shallow ulcer, usually of multiple occurrence, seen in the body or fundus of the stomach of critically ill patients. Also *stress ulcer.* **Aden u.** TROPICAL ULCER. **Allingham's u.** ANAL FISSURE. **amebic u.** An ulcer produced by infection with *Entamoeba histolytica*, especially a skin lesion of amebiasis cutis. In intestinal amebiasis, flask-shaped ulcers of the mucosa and submucosa of the large intestine commonly result from amebic abscesses. **amputating u.** A circumferential ulcer around a digit or limb that destroys the soft tissues down to the underlying bone. **anastomotic u.** A peptic ulcer occurring after gastroenterostomy or gastric resection in which the Billroth anastomosis (Billroth's operation) is used. The ulcer is typically on the jejunal side of the anastomosis. Also *stomal ulcer, stoma ulcer, marginal ulcer.* **Annam u.** CUTANEOUS LEISHMANIASIS. **aphthous u.'s** APHTHAE. **arterial u.** ISCHEMIC ULCERATION. **arteriosclerotic u.** An ulcer caused by arterial insufficiency resulting from arteriosclerosis. **atheromatous u.** Erosion of the intimal surface of an atheromatous plaque, often giving rise to thrombus formation. **Bahia u.** MUCOCUTANEOUS LEISHMANIASIS. **Barrett's u.** An ulcer occurring in columnar epithelium in the esophagus which has replaced the normally squamous epithelium, usually as the result of severe peptic esophagitis. **Bazin's u.** An ulcerated lesion of nodular tuberculosis, which usually affects the calf in young women. **Bouveret-Duguet u.** An ulcer appearing most often on the anterior part of the soft palate, more rarely on the uvula, at the outset of typhoid fever, coincident with the appearance of rose spots. Often bilateral, these ulcers heal without scarring. Also *Bouveret's ulcer.* **Buruli u.** A necrotizing ulcer caused by an acid-fast bacillus, *Mycobacterium ulcerans*, and affecting the skin and subcutaneous tissues, usually of the extremities. It is seen in Africa, Papua New Guinea, Australia, and Mexico. The organism grows saprophytically on the grass *Echinocloa pyramidalis*, and infection is probably via superficial skin abrasions. The lesion begins as a small, subcutaneous nodule and is followed by spreading noncaseous necrosis of subcutaneous tissue. The base of the ulcer contains large numbers of *M. ulcerans.* Calmette-Guérin bacillus (BCG) seems to give some protection. Treatment, although largely surgical, is facilitated with clofazimine and rifampicin. Also *mycobacterial ulcer.* • The term is named after the area of Uganda where the condition was intensively studied. **chiclero u.** A form of cutaneous leishmaniasis caused by *Leishmania mexicana* in which the ear is the principal site of ulceration. It is common among chicle workers in Mexico and Central America. Also *chicle ulcer.* **chrome u.** A deep ulcer of the skin caused by exposure to chromium compounds during plating and in the manufacture and use of chromium salts. Such ulcers follow from neglected skin abrasions. Also *chrome pit, chrome sore.* **cold u.** An ulcer that appears on the extremities as a result of ischemia. **contact u. of the larynx** LARYNGEAL CONTACT PACHYDERMIA. **creeping u.** SERPIGINOUS ULCER. **Cruveilhier's u.** *Seldom used* GASTRIC ULCER. **Curling's u.** A peptic ulcer of the stomach or duodenum originally described in association with extensive burns of the body surface. However, pathophysiology of all stress ulcers is similar. *Outmoded.* **Cushing's u.** A peptic ulcer developing acutely as the result of severe damage to the central nervous system due to head injury or brain disease. Also *Cushing-Rokitansky ulcer, Rokitansky-Cushing ulcer.* **decubital u.** BEDSORE. **decubitus u.** BEDSORE. **diphtheritic u.** Any ulcer resulting from infection with *Corynebacterium diphtheriae.* The ulcer may be on the skin or at any site of diphtherial infection. **duodenal u.** An ulcer of the duodenum due to peptic digestion. **elusive u.** HUNNER'S ULCER.

**endemic u.** Any ulcer commonly seen in a specific geographic region, such as the ulcer of cutaneous leishmaniasis. **exuberant u.** An organizing ulcer with its base covered by an excess of granulation tissue that may interfere with healing. Also *fungous ulcer.* **factitial u.** Any chronic wound that is kept from healing by patient automanipulation. **Fenwick-Hunner u.** HUNNER'S ULCER. **fissured u.** A linear ulcer, either along a surface or perpendicular to a mucous membrane, as seen in Crohn's disease. **fistulous u.** The defect caused by the opening of a fistula on a surface such as the skin or a mucous membrane. **flask u.** The typical flask-shaped colonic ulcer found associated with amebic and other forms of colitis. Also *sea anemone ulcer.* **frenal u.** Ulceration of the frenum of the tongue with granulation tissue formation, caused by repeated injury to it by the lower incisor teeth when the tongue is protuded in coughing. It is a common occurrence in whooping cough. Also *Riga-Fede disease, Fede's disease.* **fungous u.** EXUBERANT ULCER. **gastric u.** Ulceration of the mucosa of the stomach due to peptic digestion. Also *ulcus ventriculi, Cruvelhier's ulcer* (seldom used). **gastroduodenal u.** An ulcer of the stomach or duodenum; peptic ulcer. **girdle u.** An ulcer found in tuberculosis of the intestines which encircles the intestinal wall. **gouty u.** An ulcer occurring over a tophus. **gravitational u.** VARICOSE ULCER. **groin u.** LYMPHOGRANULOMA VENEREUM. **gummatous u.** An ulceration of a gumma. **herpetic u.** An ulcer of the oral mucosa or of the skin, usually around the mouth or external nares, due to herpes simplex or, less often, herpes zoster. **Hunner's u.** A painful ulcer in the bladder that is resistant to relief or control. Also *elusive ulcer, Fenwick-Hunner ulcer, ulcus simplex vesicae.* **hyperkeratotic u.** A chronic benign ulcer with hyperkeratotic margins. **hypertensive u.** An ulcer, often on the calf, attributable to infarction in the presence of severe hypertension. **hypostatic u.** An ankle ulcer attributable to an impairment of venous return from the lower leg. Also *ulcus hypostaticum.* **indolent u.** A chronic ulcer that fails to heal. **jejunal u.** A rarely occurring ulcer of the jejunum usually associated with oral potassium supplements or severe gastric hypersecretion, or secondary to gastroenterostomy. **kissing u.'s** Ulcers in direct apposition. **kurunegala u.** TROPICAL ULCER. **Lipschütz u.** LIPSCHÜTZ DISEASE. **lupoid u.** An ulcer resembling that of lupus vulgaris. **Malabar u.** TROPICAL ULCER. **marginal u.** ANASTOMOTIC ULCER. **Marjolin's u.** BURN SCAR CARCINOMA. **Meleney's u.** A progressive, infectious gangreneous ulcer caused by infection of a wound by a microaerophilic streptococcus. **mercurial u.** A deep ulcer caused by mercury compound such as mercury fulminate lodging in cracks or abrasions of the skin. **Mooren's u.** A chronic progressive necrotic erosion of the corneal surface usually occurring in elderly persons. **mycobacterial u.** BURULI ULCER. **mycotic u.** An ulcer caused by fungal growth. **neurogenic u.** NEUROTROPHIC ULCER. **neurotrophic u.** A trophic ulcer caused by loss of sensation, as in various forms of sensory neuropathy or syringomyelia. Also *neurogenic ulcer.* **Parrot's u.** The ulcer which accompanies untreated cases of thrush. **penetrating u.** An ulcer that, having involved the full thickness of the wall of an organ such as the stomach, continues to extend into an adjacent, usually solid, organ such as the pancreas. Also *ulcus penetrans.* **peptic u.** An ulcer of the upper gastrointestinal tract thought to result from gastric acid hypersecretion. **perforating u.** An ulcer that penetrates the full thickness of the wall of a hollow viscus, creating an open communication between the lumen and a serosal cavity. In the case of the stomach, for example, such an ulcer results in the discharge of gastric secretions into the peritoneal cavity and the development of peritonitis. **perforating u. of the foot** A deep, painless trophic ulcer of the sole of the foot that may penetrate to the bone. It is usually associated with sensory nerve deficits as in diabetic polyneuropathy, tabes dorsalis, leprosy, or hereditary sensory neuropathy. Also *plantar ulcer, mal perforant.* **phagedenic u.** A rapidly spreading destructive ulcer. Also *ulcus ambulans, sloughing ulcer.* **plantar u.** PERFORATING ULCER OF THE FOOT. **plantar neurotrophic u.** A chronic ulcer of the sole that develops as a result of impaired sensory innervation. **post-thrombotic u.** VARICOSE ULCER. **pudendal u.** A characteristic ulcer of granuloma inguinale. **radiation u.** An ulcer resulting, at least in part, from exposure to ionizing radiation. **rodent u.** BASAL CELL CARCINOMA. **Rokitansky-Cushing u.** CUSHING'S ULCER. **Saemisch u.** SERPIGINOUS CORNEAL ULCER. **scorbutic u.** An ulcer attributable to scurvy. Also *ulcus scorbuticum.* **sea anemone u.** FLASK ULCER. **serpiginous u.** Coexisting ulceration and healing, a characteristic manifestation of late syphilis. Also *creeping ulcer.* **serpiginous corneal u.** A very severe progressive necrosis of the cornea usually due to a virulent pneumococcal infection. Also *Saemisch ulcer, ulcus serpens corneae.* **sloughing u.** PHAGEDENIC ULCER. **stasis u.** VARICOSE ULCER. **stercoraceous u.** STERCORAL ULCER. **stercoral u.** A colonic ulcer formed by pressure from impacted feces, occasionally resulting in fistula formation. Also *stercoraceous ulcer.* **stomal u.** ANASTOMOTIC ULCER. **stress u.** ACUTE STRESS ULCER. **symptomatic u.** 1 An ulcer that produces symptoms referable to it, such as pain. 2 An ulcer that is a manifestation of a systemic disease. **syphilitic u.** HARD CHANCRE. **tanner's u.** CHROME ULCER. **transparent u. of the cornea** A noninflammatory loss of the corneal stroma, as due to collagenase activity. **trophic u.** An ulcer resulting from functional ischemia, as in a paralyzed limb. **trophoneurotic u.** An ulcer caused by interruption or degeneration of the nerves supplying a tissue or part, such as cutaneous ulcers in leprosy. **tropical u.** 1 A chronic sloughing ulcer on the leg, which occurs in the humid tropics and may be epidemic. It can destroy muscles, tendons, nerves, vessels, and even periosteum. The cause is unknown, although fusiform bacilli and the spirochete *Treponema vincentii* are often found associated with it. Also *phagedena tropica, Naga sore, Aden ulcer, Malabar ulcer, tropical phagedenic ulcer, Yemen ulcer, Zambesi ulcer, ulcus grave, ulcus tropicum, Cochin sore, kurunegala ulcer.* 2 CUTANEOUS LEISHMANIASIS. ● Many of the regional names for tropical ulcer can also apply to cutaneous leishmaniasis and vice versa. **tropical phagedenic u.** TROPICAL ULCER. **undermining u.** An ulcer, usually chronic, with overhanging borders, e.g., the ulcer of the colon associated with amebic colitis. **varicose u.** A chronic indolent ulcer of the leg associated with varicose veins, stasis, and high venous pressure, occurring as a result of chronic venous insufficiency. Also *gravitational ulcer, stasis ulcer, post-thrombotic ulcer, venous ulcer, venous stasis ulcer.* **venereal u.** CHANCROID. **venous u.** VARICOSE ULCER. **venous stasis u.** VARICOSE ULCER. **warty u.** BURN SCAR CARCINOMA. **Yemen u.** TROPICAL ULCER. **Zambesi u.** TROPICAL ULCER.

**ulcera** \ul′sərə\ Plural of ULCUS.

**ulceration** \ul′sərā′shən\ [L *ulceratio* (from *ulcerare* to cause to ulcerate) a breaking out into sores or ulcers, an ulcer] **1** ULCER. **2** The process by which an ulcer forms. Also *exulceration* (seldom used), *helcosis*. **ischemic u.** An open, nonhealing skin lesion, characteristically extremely painful, that results from chronic arterial insufficiency and is usually found in the distal foot. It has morbid prognostic implications for the limb in question. Also *arterial ulcer.* **tracheal u.** Ulceration of the tracheal lining. It is a common complication from the pressure of the cuff of cuffed endotracheal tubes. At one time tuberculous tracheobronchitis with multiple tracheal ulcers would sometimes occur.

**ulcerative** \ul′sərətiv, ul′sərā′tiv\ Characterized by ulceration.

**ulcerogangrenous** \ul′sərōgang′rənəs\ Of or relating to ulceration accompanied by gangrene.

**ulcerogenic** \ul′sərōjen′ik\ [ULCER + *o* + -GENIC] Causing ulceration. Also *ulcerogenous.*

**ulceroglandular** \ul′sərōglan′dyələr\ Characterized by local ulceration at a site of infection and by regional or generalized lymphadenopathy: said of the most common form of tularemia.

**ulceromembranous** \ul′sərōmem′brənəs\ Ulceration accompanied by exudation that forms a membrane.

**ulcus** \ul′kəs\ [L, ulcer. See ULCER.] ULCER. **u. ambulans** PHAGEDENIC ULCER. **u. cancrosum** *Obs.* BASAL CELL CARCIMONA. **u. exedens** *Obs.* BASAL CELL CARCINOMA. **u. grave** TROPICAL ULCER. **u. hypostaticum** HYPOSTATIC ULCER. **u. interdigitale** An ulceration of the skin between the toes. **u. penetrans** PENETRATING ULCER. **u. rodens** *Obs.* BASAL CELL CARCINOMA. **u. scorbuticum** SCORBUTIC ULCER. **u. serpens corneae** SERPIGINOUS CORNEAL ULCER. **u. simplex vesicae** HUNNER'S ULCER. **u. tropicum** TROPICAL ULCER. **u. tuberculosum** Any tuberculous ulcer, especially an ulcerative lesion of tuberculosis cutis. **u. venereum** CHANCROID. **u. ventriculi** GASTRIC ULCER. **u. vulvae acutum** LIPSCHÜTZ DISEASE.

**ule-**[1] \yoo′lə-\ ULO-[1].

**ule-**[2] \yoo′lə-\ ULO-[2].

**-ule** \-ʸool, -ʸəl\ [L *-ulus,* masc. dim. suffix; *-ula,* fem. dim. suffix; *-ulum,* neut. dim. suffix] A suffix meaning little of its kind, small.

**ulegyria** \yoo′ləjī′rē-ə\ [Gk *oulē* a scar + GYR- + -IA] Atrophic sclerosis of cerebral gyri. It may be congenital or postnatally acquired.

**ulerythema** \yoo′lərithē′mə\ [UL-[1] + ERYTHEMA] Erythema followed by follicular scarring. **u. ophryogenes** Keratosis pilaris rubra atrophicans of the face that primarily affects the eyebrow area. Also *honeycomb nevus.*

**uletic** \yoolet′ik\ [UL-[2] + *-etic,* adjectival suffix] *Obs.* CICATRICIAL.

**ulexine** CYTISINE.

**Ullmann** [Emerich *Ullmann,* Hungarian surgeon, 1861–1937] See under LINE.

**Ullrich** [Otto *Ullrich,* German pediatrician, 1894–1957] **1** Morquio-Ullrich syndrome. See under MUCOPOLYSACCHARIDOSIS IV. **2** Ullrich-Feichtiger syndrome. See under SYNDROME. **3** Ullrich-Turner syndrome, Ullrich syndrome. See under NOONAN SYNDROME.

**ulna** \ul′nə\ [L (akin to Gk *ōlenē* forearm) forearm] (*pl.* ulnae) [NA] The long triangular-shaped bone on the medial side of the forearm parallel to the radius with which it articulates laterally. Its proximal hook-shaped end articulates with the trochlea of the humerus, and its distal end is separated from the carpus by the articular disk of the inferior radioulnar joint. Also *cubitus.*

**ulnad** \ul′nad\ Toward the ulna.

**ulnar** \ul′nər\ Pertaining to the ulna or to the side of the upper limb in which the ulna is located, that is, the medial side. Compare RADIAL.

**ulnocarpal** \ul′nōkär′pəl\ **1** Pertaining to the ulna and the carpus. **2** Denoting the ulnar side of the wrist.

**ulo-**[1] \yoo′lō-\ [Gk *oulē* a scar] A combining form meaning scar. Also *ul-* , *ule-* .

**ulo-**[2] \yoo′lō-\ [Gk *oulon* (mostly in plural *oula*) the gums] A combining form denoting the gums. Also *ul-* , *ule-* .

**uloglossitis** \yoo′ləgläsī′tis\ [ULO-[2] + GLOSSITIS] Inflammation of the gingivae and the tongue. *Seldom used.*

**ulose** See under KETOSE. • This is also used as the ending of the name of a specified ketose, as in *xylulose.*

**ulosis** \yoolō′sis\ [Gk *oulōsis* (from *oulē* a scar) formation of scar tissue] CICATRIZATION.

**ult. praes.** *ultimum praescriptus* (L, last prescribed).

**ultra-** \ul′trə-\ [L *ultra* (for *ultera*) beyond] A prefix meaning beyond, especially beyond the normal, usual, or expected limits.

**ultracentrifugation** \-sentrif′yəgā′shən\ The use of an ultracentrifuge to separate materials for preparative or analytic purposes.

**ultracentrifuge** \-sen′trifyooj\ A centrifuge capable of generating centrifugal force at or beyond 100 000 times gravity. It is used to separate and analyze macromolecules according to their differences in molecular density.

**ultrafilter** \ul′trəfil′tər\ A filter with microscopic pores of any of various sizes, usually smaller than 400 nm. Such filters were used originally to distinguish viruses from bacteria and fungi, since only viruses could pass through the ultrafilter.

**ultrafiltrate** \-fil′trāt\ Fluid passed through a semipermeable membrane that retains colloidal material and allows passage of crystalloid solutions.

**ultrafiltration** \-filtrā′shən\ The process of filtration of a solution through a membrane whose pores are so small that they are impermeant to large molecules such as proteins. **sequential u. -hemodialysis** See under HEMODIALYSIS.

**ultraligation** \-līgā′shən\ The ligature control of a blood vessel beyond a major branch or branches.

**ultramicropipet** \-mī′krəpīpet′\ A pipet capable of measuring and delivering liquid in very small quantities, from 0.001 to 0.010 ml.

**ultramicroscope** \-mī′krəskōp\ ELECTRON MICROSCOPE.

**ultramicroscopic** \-mī′krəskäp′ik\ Of such minute size as to be visible only with an electron microscope. Also *ultravisible, submicroscopic, amicroscopic.*

**ultramicroscopy** \-mīkräs′kəpē\ ELECTRON MICROSCOPY.

**ultramicrotome** \-mī′krətōm\ A device for cutting sections that are suitable for examination in an electron microscope.

**ultraphagocytosis** \-fag′əsītō′sis\ PINOCYTOSIS.

**ultraprophylaxis** \-prō′fəlak′sis\ [ULTRA- + PROPHYLAXIS] The prevention of the birth of diseased or abnormal children by regulations prohibiting marriages of persons regarded as being physically or mentally unfit.

**ultrasonic** \-sän′ik\ [ULTRA- + SONIC] Characterized by a frequency of vibration above the audible range, especially in the range of 1 to 10 MHz; of or relating to ultrasound.

**ultrasonics** \-sän′iks\ [ULTRA- + L *son(us)* a sound, tone + -ICS] **1** The science and technology of ultrasound. **2** Ultrasonic characteristics or phenomena. **3** Instruments for removing dental calculus in which the working tip vibrates at an ultrasonic frequency.

**ultrasonogram** \-sän′əgram\ The image produced by an ultrasound imaging instrument. Also *sonogram, sonotomogram, ultrasonotomogram, echogram.*
**ultrasonograph** \-sän′əgraph\ An ultrasonic imaging instrument. Also *sonoscope, ultrasonoscope, echoscope.*
**ultrasonographic** \-sän′əgraf′ik\ Of or relating to ultrasound imaging or to an ultrasonograph.
**ultrasonography** \-sənäg′rəfē\ Imaging with ultrasound. Also *sonography, ultrasonotomography, sonotomography, echography.*
**ultrasonoscope** \-sän′əskōp\ ULTRASONOGRAPH.
**ultrasonotomogram** \-sän′ətō′məgram\ ULTRASONOGRAM.
**ultrasonotomography** \-sō′nətōmäg′rəfē\ ULTRASONOGRAPHY.
**ultrasound** \ul′trəsound\ [ULTRA- + *sound*] Vibration propagated in an elastic medium at frequencies above the range of audible sound, especially in the range of 1 to 10 MHz. **Doppler u.** The use of ultrasound to determine the velocity of moving objects, such as red blood cells, using the Doppler effect.
**ultrastructure** \ul′trəstruk′chər\ FINE STRUCTURE.
**ultraviolet** \-vī′əlet\ [ULTRA- + *violet*] Designating invisible electromagnetic radiation having a wavelength shorter than that of the violet end of the visible spectrum and longer than that of x rays, from 180 to 390 nm.
**ultravirus** \-vī′rəs\ FILTERABLE VIRUS.
**ultravisible** \-viz′ibəl\ ULTRAMICROSCOPIC.
**umbauzonen** \um′boutsō′nən\ [German *Umbau* alteration, remodeling + *Zonen* zones] LOOSER'S TRANSFORMATION ZONES.
**umbellatine** BERBERINE.
**umbilical** \umbil′ikəl\ Pertaining to the umbilicus.
**umbilicate** \umbil′ikāt\ Shaped like or resembling the umbilicus; pitted; dimpled.
**umbilication** \um′bilikā′shən\ [*umbilic(us)* + -ATION] A central depression or pit.
**umbilicus** \umbil′əkəs, umbəlī′kəs\ [L (dim. of *umbo* a boss, protuberance (akin to Gk *omphalos* the navel, a boss) the navel] [NA] The scar on the ventral abdominal wall marking the site of attachment of the umbilical cord in placental mammals. It forms a few days after the severance of the cord at or after birth. Also *omphalos, omphalus, belly button* (popular), *bellybutton* (popular). **amniotic u.** An opening present in the early embryos of many Amniota (reptiles, birds, and mammals) as long as the closure of the amniotic folds remains incomplete. **decidual u.** The scar on the endometrial surface marking the implantation site of the blastocyst after it has penetrated the uterine lining and has become embedded.
**umbo** \um′bō\ [L, a boss, protuberance, as on a shield] (*pl.* umbones) [NA] In anatomy, a rounded protuberance on a surface, like the boss of a shield. **u. membranae tympani** [NA] The center and point of maximal convexity of the inner surface of the tympanic membrane, where the tip of the handle of the malleus is attached. It corresponds to the center and point of maximal concavity of the outer surface of the membrane.
**umbonate** \um′bōnāt\ Possessing an umbo or having the rounded, protuberant shape of an umbo.
**umbra** \um′brə\ [L, a shadow] That part of the shadow of an object illuminated by an extended source into which no light from the source propagates.
**umbrella / Mobin-Uddin u.** A caval interruption device that is inserted transvenously, usually via the internal jugular vein, into the infrarenal inferior vena cava. It serves as a block to large thrombi embolizing to the central circulation.
**UMP** uridine monophosphate (uridine phosphate). Usually uridine 5′-phosphate is meant.
**un-** \un-, ən-\ [Old English, akin to L *in-* not, Gk *a-* and *an-* privative] A prefix meaning not.
**uncal** \ung′kəl\ Pertaining to the uncus.
**unciform** \un′sifôrm\ **1** UNCINATE. **2** OS HAMATUM.
**uncinal** \un′sinəl\ UNCINATE.
**uncinate** \un′sināt\ **1** Hooked; hook-shaped. Also *uncinal, unciform.* **2** Pertaining to an uncus.
**uncompensated** \unkäm′pənsā′tid\ **1** Denoting the persistence of loss in a specific function following damage to a body part or organ that normally contributes to that function, e.g., the indefinite persistence of a lurching gait in a patient who has lost use of the hip abductors, for which there are no adequate substitute muscles. **2** In experimental neurophysiology, denoting the persistence of deficient or abnormal behavior subsequent to destruction of a central nervous system structure or sensory organ, indicating failure of other nervous structures to compensate for the lost function.
**unconditioned** \un′kəndish′ənd\ **1** Not involving learning or conditioning. **2** Characterized by an absence of learning or conditioning.
**unconscious** \unkän′shəs\ [UN- + CONSCIOUS] **1** Characterized by loss of awareness and inability to perceive or apprehend stimuli, as in coma. Also *insensible.* **2** The division of the mind that contains all psychic material not within the immediate field of awareness such as the id and much of the superego and ego. Also *shadow.* **collective u.** In jungian psychology, the part of the unconscious that contains the inherited distillate of the experience of one's forbears and race, as contrasted with that which is personal or individual.
**unconsciousness** [UNCONSCIOUS + -NESS] A state of loss of awareness with inability to perceive or apprehend stimuli; coma.
**uncotomy** \ungkät′əmē\ [*unc(us)* + *o* + -TOMY ] Ablation of the uncal portion of the temporal lobe of the brain. It is usually performed as psychosurgery.
**uncoupling** The process of separating two normally concomitant reactions. It is most often applied to the oxidation of metabolites when this is normally accompanied by ATP synthesis. Uncoupling allows the oxidation to proceed, since without such uncoupling it would be inhibited once all the ADP present was converted into ATP. Uncoupling is often achieved by making the mitochondrial membrane permeable to hydrogen ions, since oxidations build up a gradient in hydrogen ions, which can normally be dissipated only by ATP synthesis.
**uncovertebral** \ung′kōvur′təbrəl\ Pertaining to the uncinate process of a vertebra. *Outmoded.*
**uncrossed** Perceived to be on the same side as the eye that receives the image: used especially of diplopia.
**unction** \ungk′shən\ [L *unctio* (from *unctus,* past part. of *ungere* to anoint) an anointing] **1** OINTMENT. **2** The process of applying an oil, salve, or ointment.
**unctuous** \ungk′choo·əs\ Oily; greasy.
**uncture** \ungk′chər\ OINTMENT.
**uncus** \ung′kəs\ [L, hook] **1** [NA] The hook-shaped rostral end of the parahippocampal gyrus, located on the inferomedial aspect of the temporal lobe and overlying the amygdaloid nuclei. It is a phylogenetically old part of the pallium and, along with the rostral part of the parahippocampal gyrus and the lateral olfactory stria, constitutes what is frequently referred to as the piriform lobe. Also *uncus gyri fornicati, uncus gyri hippocampi, uncus gyri parahippocampi, gyrus uncinatus, uncinate gyrus.* **2** Any hook-shaped struc-

ture. Adj. uncal. **u. gyri parahippocampi** UNCUS.

**undecylenic acid** $C_{11}H_{20}O_2$. Undec-10-enoic acid. A colorless liquid that is practically insoluble in water. It has antifungal activity and is used topically to treat dermatophytic infections.

**underachiever** \-achē′vər\ A person, particularly a student, whose level of performance is significantly lower than expected when judged on the basis of prior record, measured intelligence, or other known characteristics. Such a person is understood to have the capacity to improve performance.

**undercut** The hollow caused by the reduction in width of a structure, such as a tooth, toward its base.

**underhorn** CORNU INFERIUS VENTRICULI LATERALIS.

**undernutrition** \-n[y]ootrish′ən\ Inadequate nutrition due to a failure to ingest, absorb, or assimilate all the essential nutrients in adequate quantities.

**understain** To expose tissues to a dye for the time needed to react with only the fast-staining components. This permits sequential staining with a counterstain.

**undertoe** A condition whereby the great toe is situated beneath the other toes.

**underweight** A condition characterized by a loss of body tissue, especially body fat. An underweight person is one who weighs at least 10 percent less than the average body weight for people of the same nationality, age, sex, height, and body frame size.

**Underwood** [Michael *Underwood,* English pediatrician, 1736–1820] Underwood's disease. See under SCLEREMA NEONATORUM.

**undifferentiation** \un′difəren′shē·ā′shən\ A state marked by lack of differentiation. Adj. undifferentiated.

**undine** \un′dīn\ [Mod L *undina* (from L *und(a)* wave, water + *-ina* -INE) a water nymph] A small flask with a spout, used for application of eyedrops.

**undinism** \un′dinizm\ [German *Undin(e)* (from New L *Undina* a water nymph, from L *und(a)* a wave + *-ina* -INE) a water nymph + -ISM] UROLAGNIA.

**undoing** An unconscious, ego defense mechanism in which an action, thought, or feeling opposite to the one which must be denied is performed. Expiation, ceremonial rituals, and counting compulsions are often based on undoing.

**undulant** \un′dyələnt\ Rising and falling like waves, as the intensity of a fever.

**unfit to plead** The term used in Britain and New Zealand for INSANE ON ARRAIGNMENT. • In British law, an individual is adjudged *unfit to plead* if he is found to be insane at the time of trial, regardless of his mental condition at the time of the crime. Competency to stand trial is decided by a jury after hearing medical evidence.

**ung.** *unguentum* (L, ointment).

**ungual** \ung′gwəl\ Of or relating to the nails. Also *unguinal.*

**unguent** \ung′gwent\ OINTMENT.

**unguentum** \ung·gwen′təm\ [L (from *ungere,* also *unguere* to anoint, daub) an ointment, unguent] OINTMENT. **u. acidi benzoici compositum** BENZOIC AND SALICYLIC ACID OINTMENT. **u. acidi borici** BORIC ACID OINTMENT. **u. acidi carbolici** PHENOL OINTMENT. **u. acidi undecylenici compositum** COMPOUND UNDECYLENIC ACID OINTMENT. **u. adipis lanae hydrosi** OINTMENT OF HYDROUS WOOL FAT. **u. album** WHITE OINTMENT. **u. aquae rosae** ROSE WATER OINTMENT. **u. aquae rosae petrolatum** PETROLATUM ROSE WATER OINTMENT. **u. calaminae** CALAMINE OINTMENT. **u. calaminae compositum** COMPOUND OINTMENT OF CALAMINE. **u. capsici compositum** COMPOUND OINTMENT OF CAPSICUM. **u. chrysarobini** CHRYSAROBIN OINTMENT. **u. emulsificans** EMULSIFYING OINTMENT. **u. epinephrinae bitartratis ophthalmicum** EPINEPHRINE BITARTRATE OPHTHALMIC OINTMENT. **u. flavum** YELLOW OINTMENT. **u. glycolis polyethyleni** POLYETHYLENE GLYCOL OINTMENT. **u. hydrargyri ammoniati** AMMONIATED MERCURY OINTMENT. **u. hydrargyri oxidi flavi** YELLOW MERCURIC OXIDE OPHTHALMIC OINTMENT. **u. hydrocortisoni** HYDROCORTISONE OINTMENT. **u. hydrocortisoni acetatis** HYDROCORTISONE ACETATE OINTMENT. **u. hydrophilicum** HYDROPHILIC OINTMENT. **u. iodi** IODINE OINTMENT. **u. kaolini** OINTMENT OF KAOLIN. **u. lanolini** LANOLIN OINTMENT. **u. nitrofurazoni** NITROFURAZONE OINTMENT. **u. oleoresinae capsici compositum** COMPOUND OINTMENT OF CAPSICUM. **u. paraffini** PARAFFIN OINTMENT. **u. penicillini** PENICILLIN OINTMENT. **u. phenolis** PHENOL OINTMENT. **u. physostigminae** PHYSOSTIGMINE OINTMENT. **u. picis carbonis** COAL TAR OINTMENT. **u. picis liquidae** OINTMENT OF TAR. **u. picis pini** PINE TAR OINTMENT. **u. resorcini** OINTMENT OF RESORCINOL. **u. resorcini compositum** COMPOUND RESORCINOL OINTMENT. **u. resorcinolis** OINTMENT OF RESORCINOL. **u. resorcinolis compositum** COMPOUND RESORCINOL OINTMENT. **u. sedativum** COMPOUND OINTMENT OF CALAMINE. **u. simplex** SIMPLE OINTMENT. **u. sulfacetamidi sodici** SODIUM SULFACETAMIDE OPHTHALMIC OINTMENT. **u. sulfuris** SULFUR OINTMENT. **u. undecylenati** ZINC UNDECENOATE OINTMENT. **u. zinci oxidi** ZINC OXIDE OINTMENT. **u. zinci oxidi cum benzoino** OINTMENT OF ZINC OXIDE WITH BENZOIN.

**unguiculus** \ung·gwik′yələs\ [L, dim. of *unguis.* See UNGUIS.] A small nail.

**unguinal** \ung′gwinəl\ UNGUAL.

**unguis** \ung′gwis\ [L (akin to Gk *onyx,* gen. *onychos,* a talon, claw, nail), a nail of a human finger or toe, a claw of a toed animal, a bird's talon] [NA] A horny keratin structure that covers the dorsal aspect of the terminal phalanx of each digit; nail. **u. avis** CALCAR AVIS. **u. incarnatus** INGROWING NAIL. **u. ventriculi lateralis cerebri** CALCAR AVIS.

**uni-** \yoo′nē-\ [L *unus* one] A prefix meaning one, single, unitary.

**uniarticular** \-ärtik′yələr\ MONOARTICULAR.

**uniarticulate** \-ärtik′yəlit\ MONOARTICULAR.

**uniaural** \-ôr′əl\ MONOTIC.

**uniaxial** \-ak′sē·əl\ In embryology, denoting development which takes place about or along a single axis.

**unicellular** \-sel′yələr\ **1** Consisting of a single cell. **2** Characterizing a level of life-form organization in which the individual organism consists of a single cell, as bacteria or protozoa. Also *monocellular, monoplastic.*

**uniceps** \yoo′niseps\ Possessing only one belly: said of a muscle.

**uniflagellate** \-flaj′əlāt\ [L *un(us)* one + *i* + FLAGELLATE] Having only one flagellum; monotrichous.

**Uniform Anatomical Gift Act** A model statute in the United States, approved in 1968, which enables any person who is 18 or more years of age and of sound mind to donate all or part of his or her body after death for any medical purpose. • A number of other countries have enacted similar legislation, in some cases prior to the U.S. legislation, as the Human Tissue Act (1961) of the United Kingdom and an act with the same title (1964) of New Zealand, where there is no age specification but the consent of the next of kin is required. South Africa and Japan (in

May 1983) have enacted similar statutes.

**unigeminal** \-jem′inəl\ [UNI- + GEMINAL] Pertaining to one member of a twin pair.

**unigerminal** \-jur′minəl\ [UNI- + GERMINAL] Developing from a single ovum or germ.

**unigravida** \-grav′idə\ [UNI- + GRAVIDA] PRIMIGRAVIDA.

**unilaminar** \-lam′inər\ Having only one layer.

**unilateral** \-lat′ərəl\ On or affecting one side only.

**unilocular** \-läk′yələr\ Having only one cavity or compartment.

**uninuclear** \-nyoo′klē·ər\ [UNI- + NUCLEAR] MONONUCLEAR.

**uninucleate** \-n^y^oo′klē·āt\ [UNI- + NUCLEATE] MONONUCLEAR.

**uniocular** \-äk′yələr\ [UNI- + OCULAR] Pertaining to the use of one eye only.

**union** [Med L *unio,* gen. *unionis* (from *unire* to unite) unity, union] A joining together to be one or to be whole. **faulty u.** NONUNION. **immediate u.** HEALING BY FIRST INTENTION. **primary u.** HEALING BY FIRST INTENTION. **syngamic nuclear u.** The fusion of the male and female pronuclei when the ovum is fertilized; the union of gametes in sexual reproduction with simultaneous determination of the sex of the zygote.

**uniovular** \-äv′yələr\ [UNI- + OVULAR] Originating from one ovum, as monozygotic twins.

**unipara** \yoonip′ərə\ [UNI- + PARA] PRIMIPARA.

**unipennate** \-pen′āt\ [UNI- + PENNATE] Having a featherlike appearance on one side: said of a muscle whose belly resembles one half of a feather. Compare BIPENNATE. Also *semipenniform.*

**unipolar** \-pō′lər\ **1** Having a single aster or pole: said of a cell. **2** Having a single process, as a neuron with one axon. **3** In electroencephalography, recording between a scalp electrode and a distant site which may be at ground potential.

**unipotency** \-pō′tənsē\ [UNI- + POTENCY] The ability of an embryonal cell or group of cells to develop into only one specific cell type, organ, or part because its fate has been determined. Adj. unipotent, unipotential.

**unirritable** \-ir′ətəbəl\ INEXCITABLE.

# unit

**unit** [from *unity,* from L *unitas* oneness, unity, from *un(us)* one + *-itas* -ITY] **1** One person or thing. **2** A value or measure used as a standard for reckoning quantity. **3** A quantity, as of a drug, required to produce a given effect. **4** A group of health professionals working collaboratively as a separate administrative division for a specific purpose, as *coronary care unit.* **absolute u.** A unit of measurement forming part of a coherent system of units. **Allen-Doisy u.** MOUSE UNIT. **alpha u.'s** Glycogen particles in a rosette arrangement, forming nonmembrane, limited, cytoplasmic organelles composed of enzymes and polysaccharides. **androgen u.** The international unit of androgenic activity of potency, equal to 0.1 mg of crystalline androsterone, assayed by the capon comb growth test. Also *international androgen unit.* **Ångström u.** See under ÅNGSTRÖM. **antivenene u.** An expression of the potency of the antivenomous serum which is required to protect against a fatal dose of venom. **atomic mass u.** A unit of mass, used in conjunction with SI units especially in atomic and nuclear physics, equal to 1/12 of the mass of an atom of the nuclide $^{12}C$; 1.660 57$\times 10^{-27}$ kilogram, approximately. Also *unified atomic mass unit, atomic weight unit.* Abbr. amu Symbol: u **base u.** One of the arbitrarily chosen units of a system of measurement, regarded as dimensionally independent, on which the system of units is based. See also SI BASE UNIT. Compare DERIVED UNIT. **British thermal u.** A unit of heat equal to 1.055 06 kilojoules, approximately. Originally, the British thermal unit was the quantity of heat needed to raise the temperature of one pound of water through one degree Fahrenheit at or near 39.1 degrees Fahrenheit. Abbr. Btu, BTU, B.Th.U. **burn u.** A facility or area, especially one within a hospital, specializing in the care of burn victims. ● See note at BURN CENTER. *Burn unit* is widely recognized in the English-speaking world but is most commonly used in the U.S. and India, although it is also used in Japan and appears to be gaining currency elsewhere, as in South Africa. **central processing u.** The section of a computer that contains the arithmetic and logic unit, the control unit, registers, and input/output circuits. **$CH_{50}$ u.** The reciprocal of the dilution of complement-containing serum used to achieve hemolysis of 50 percent of red cells maximally coated with a complement-fixing antibody. Also *minimal hemolytic unit, hemolytic unit.* **clinical u.** A unit of estrogenic activity which is equal to approximately one sixth of an international unit. **cobalt 60 beam therapy u.** Equipment for administering radiation therapy, with the radiation beam coming from a source of cobalt 60 external to the patient. **coherent u.** A derived unit in a system of measurement formed by the multiplication and/or division of base units without the introduction of a numerical factor other than 1. **coincidence u.** An apparatus to record only two or more radiations which are detected simultaneously. **u. of convergence** A quantitative measurement of the angular degrees by which the two eyes turn toward each other. **coronary care u.** The specialized unit within a hospital that provides intensive care for patients with severe heart disease including those suspected of having sustained an acute myocardial infarction and those requiring postoperative care. **corpus luteum hormone u.** PROGESTERONE UNIT. **crossover u.** CENTIMORGAN. **dental u. 1** A tooth and its supporting structures. **2** A piece of equipment embodying the various items needed to practice dentistry, such as engine, light water spray, suction device, and bracket table. **derived u.** A unit derived by the multiplication and/or division of a base unit of a system of measurement. In some systems, certain derived units also require the introduction of a numerical factor. Some derived units are given special names, which may then be used in the formation of further derived units. See also SI DERIVED UNIT. Compare BASE UNIT. **digitalis u.** A standardized unit of digitalis potency, expressed either comparatively, against a national or international standard preparation, or quantitatively, by biological activity in an animal such as a cat. **u. of energy** See under JOULE. **estrone u.** The international unit of estrogenic potency, equal to 0.1 μg of a standard preparation of estrone. Also *international estrone unit.* **flotation u.** SVEDBERG UNIT. **u. of force** See under NEWTON. **geriatric assessment u.** A ward or part of a hospital where old people are admitted for medical diagnosis together with functional and social assessment. A British usage. **u. of heat** See under JOULE. **hemolytic u.** $CH_{50}$ UNIT. **hemorrhagin u.** An expression of the amount of snake venom required to produce hemorrhage in chick embryos. **insulin u.** INTER-

NATIONAL INSULIN UNIT. **intensive care u.** The unit within a hospital that cares for very seriously ill patients using sophisticated technology and specially trained personnel. **u. of intermedin** A semiquantitative, bioassay unit for the activity of melanocyte stimulating hormone, dependent upon the capacity of the hormone to stimulate the expansion of melanophores in the skin of a hypophysectomized frog. One unit is equal to one μg of alkali-treated USP Posterior-pituitary Reference Standard. **international u.** 1 A quantity of biological material, as of vitamins, hormones, etc., which produces a specific internationally accepted biological effect. 2 A unit defined by an international organization. Abbr. IU **international androgen u.** ANDROGEN UNIT. **international estrone u.** ESTRONE UNIT. **international u. of gonadotrophic activity** The international unit of gonadotropic potency, equal to 0.1 mg of the standard human pregnancy urine preparation preserved at and allocated by the National Institute for Medical Research, London. It is approximately the quantity required to induce vaginal cornification in the immature rat. **international u. of immunological activity** An internationally accepted amount of antiserum or antigen. It is accepted by the World Health Organization as a standard measure of potency in a number of antitoxins, vaccines, immunoglobulins, and test antigens such as tuberculin or diptheria toxoid. **international insulin u.** An international unit equal to 1/22 of a milligram of pure crystalline insulin. Also *insulin unit.* **international u. of luteinizing activity** PROGESTERONE UNIT. **international u. of male hormone** A formerly used standard equal to the androgenic, biologic activity exerted by 0.1 mg of crystalline androsterone. **international u. of penicillin** The penicillin activity of 0.6 μg of a standard sample of the sodium salt of penicillin G. Pure penicillin G contains 1667 units per milligram. Also *unit of penicillin.* **international u. of progestational activity** PROGESTERONE UNIT. **international progesterone u.** PROGESTERONE UNIT. **international prolactin u.** PROLACTIN UNIT. **international u. of vitamin A** An amount equivalent to 0.6 μg of pure β-carotene. Also *vitamin A unit.* **international u. of vitamin D** An amount equivalent to 0.025 μg of pure cholecalciferol (vitamin $D_3$). Also *vitamin D unit.* **lung u.** TERMINAL AIRWAY UNIT. **Mache u.** A unit of radioactivity equal to that quantity of radon derived from 1 liter of specified water which gives rise to a saturation current of $10^{-3}$ electrostatic unit; equivalent to $3.6 \times 10^{-10}$ curie per liter approximately, 13 becquerel per liter approximately. **map u.** CENTIMORGAN. **minimal hemolytic u.** $CH_{50}$ UNIT. **morgan u.** MORGAN. **motor u.** A motoneuron together with the muscle fibers supplied by its axonal process, i.e., together with its muscle unit. Motor units are categorized in several systems of classification according to their histochemical and contractile characteristics, nervous control, and susceptibility to pathologic conditions. Two commonly used classifications differentiated by type of muscle fiber and their related contractile characteristics are identified by the following types: fast-glycolytic, fast-oxidative-glycolytic, and slow-oxidative; fast-fatiguable, fast-fatigue resistant, and slow motor units (resistant to fatigue). **mouse u.** The smallest amount of an estrogenic substance that will produce a specific change in the vaginal epithelium of an ovarectomized mouse. This unit is used in connection with bioassay methods for estrogens and gonadotropins. Also *Allen-Doisy unit.* **muscle u.** The group of muscle fibers innervated by a single efferent axon. Compare MOTOR UNIT. **nerve u.** 1 NEURON. 2 The electrical impulse activity associated with a single axon or neuron soma. **Oxford u.** The original unit of penicillin, equivalent to 0.6 μg of penicillin G, determined by bioassay with a standard test organism. *Outmoded.* **u. of oxytocin** The oxytocic activity of 0.5 mg of a reference standard of USP posterior pituitary. 500 international units of oxytocic activity corresponds to 1 mg of synthetic oxytocin (International units are equivalent to USP units). **parathyroid u.** A unit eqivalent to 1/100 of the quantity of hormone needed to raise by 1 mg/100 ml the serum calcium concentration of normal dogs 16 to 18 hrs following injection. **u. of penicillin** INTERNATIONAL UNIT OF PENICILLIN. **peripheral resistance u.** A unit of resistance, derived by dividing the pressure drop across the peripheral arterial bed, measured in mmHg, by the blood flow through that bed in milliliters per second. **pilosebaceous u.** The hair follicle and the associated sebaceous gland. **progesterone u.** The international unit of progestational potency, equal to 1 mg of a standard preparation of pure, crystalline progesterone. Also *international unit of progestational activity, international progesterone unit, international unit of luteinizing activity, corpus luteum hormone unit, progestin unit.* **prolactin u.** The international unit of lactogenic potency, equal to 0.1 mg of the standard preparation of adenohypophysial prolactin. Also *international prolactin unit.* **psychiatric u.** A section of a hospital or clinic designed and reserved for psychiatric patients. Psychiatric units in general hospitals have grown markedly in number since the 1960s and are generally preferred to a scatter bed system in which psychiatric patients are mixed with all other types of patients in general medical units. Also *psychiatric ward* (older term). **rat u.** The smallest amount or highest dilution of an estrogenic substance that will produce cornification and desquamation of the vaginal epithelium of an ovarectomized rat. This unit is used in connection with bioassay methods for estrogens and gonadotropins. **sensation u.** The minimal discriminable increment in stimulus intensity, especially in audiometry. **SI base u.** One of the seven base units of the Système International d'Unités. They are the meter, kilogram, second, ampere, kelvin, mole, and candela. Compare SI DERIVED UNIT. **SI derived u.** In the Système International d'Unités, a derived unit formed without the introduction of a numerical factor other than unity, such as the unit of area, square meter. The SI derived units thus form a coherent system. Some SI derived units have been given special names, such as newton, joule, and watt, which may be used to form other derived units. Compare SI BASE UNIT. **Siegbahn u.** X UNIT. **SI supplementary u.** Either of the units, radian and steradian, which may be used as either a base unit or a derived unit within the Système International d'Unités. **skin test u.** The amount of a given substance which, when administered by intradermal injection, produces a positive response in a susceptible individual but no response in an immune subject. Specifically, skin test unit has been applied to the amount of scarlet-fever toxin which, on intradermal injection, elicits a positive (Dick) reaction in a person susceptible to scarlet fever and no reaction in a person immune to the disease. **slow motor u.** A motor unit resistant to fatigue. **supplementary u.** See under SI SUPPLEMENTARY UNIT. **Svedberg u.** The unit of time of $10^{-13}$ seconds, used in citing sedimentation coefficients. A particle with a sedimentation coefficient of one Svedberg unit will therefore sediment at a velocity of $10^{-13}$ $cm{\cdot}s^{-1}$ in an accelerational field of 1 $cm{\cdot}s^{-2}$. Values of about a million times this field are normally used for determining sedimentation coefficients. Also *flotation unit.* Symbol: S **terminal airway u.**

The portion of a lung distal to a terminal bronchiole. Also *lung unit*. **u. of thyrotrophic activity** The thyroid growth-stimulating activity of a given adenohypophysial extract. One unit is equivalent to that amount of extract, which, administered daily for 5 days, stimulates the thyroid of an immature, 200 gram guinea pig to attain a weight of 600 mg. **Todd u.** The unit in which the results of testing for antistreptolysin O (ASO) are expressed. It denotes the reciprocal of the highest dilution of test serum at which there continues to be neutralization of a standard preparation of the streptococcal enzyme streptolysin O. **tuberculin u.** That amount of purified protein derivative (usually 0.00002 mg of PPD) in 0.1 ml of tuberculin solution which corresponds to a 1:10 000 solution of old tuberculin. Abbr. TU **unified atomic mass u.** ATOMIC MASS UNIT. **USP u.** A unit of potency or biological activity used in the United States Pharmacopeia for antibiotics, hormones, toxins, vaccines, and other pharmaceutic preparations. The USP units have been established by international agreement in association with the Food and Drug Administration or the National Institutes of Health. **u. of vasopressin** A unit equivalent to the pressor activity of 0.5 mg of the USP posterior-pituitary reference standard. One mg of synthetic vasopressin is biologically equivalent to 600 international units. **vitamin A u.** INTERNATIONAL UNIT OF VITAMIN A. **vitamin D u.** INTERNATIONAL UNIT OF VITAMIN D. **Voegtlin u.** A unit equal to the degree of contraction induced in the isolated guinea pig uterus by 0.5 mg of the reference or standard preparation of posterior pituitary powder. **u. of work** See under JOULE. **X u.** A unit of length, used for the measurement of x-ray wavelengths, equal to $10^{-13}$ meter, approximately; 0.1 picometer, approximately. Also *Siegbahn unit*. Symbol: X, XU

**unitary** \yoo′niter′ē\ **1** Characterized or based on unity or one. **2** Of or relating to a unit or units.

**United States Adopted Names** The names for nonproprietary drugs selected by the United States Adopted Names Council, which is jointly sponsored by the American Medical Association, the American Pharmaceutical Association, and the U.S. Pharmacopeial Convention, Inc. This system of designation of drug names has been in operation since 1961. Abbr. USAN

**United States Pharmacopeia** An authoritative compendium on drugs, their preparation, and tests of their purity and identity. It was first published in 1820 by the United States Pharmacopeial Convention, Inc., and has been revised regularly every ten years, and more frequently in recent years. Abbr. USP

**univalent** \yoo′nēvā′lənt, yooniv′ələnt\ **1** Having a single valence. Also *monovalent*. **2** Containing only one strain or type of microorganism or virus.

**universe** POPULATION.

**univitelline** \-vitel′in\ [UNI- + VITELLINE] Relating or referring to a single ovum, or to what arises from a single ovum, as *univitelline twins*..

**unmedullated** \unmed′yəlā′tid\ UNMYELINATED.

**unmyelinated** \unmī′əlinā′tid\ Not surrounded by a myelin sheath, as *unmyelinated fine nerve fibers*. Also *unmedullated, nonmyelinated, nonmedullated*.

**Unna** [Paul Gerson *Unna*, German dermatologist, 1850–1929] **1** Unna's disease. See under SEBORRHEIC DERMATITIS. **2** Unna's nevus. See under PORT-WINE STAIN. **3** See under STAIN. **4** Unna-Pappenheim stain. See under STAIN. **5** Unna's boot. See under UNNA'S PASTE BOOT.

**unofficial** Designating medications that are not listed in a pharmacopeia or a similar compendium of drugs compiled by an authoritative group.

**unorganized** In embryology, lacking organ structure; displaying failure of organogenesis.

**unprimed** \unprīmd′\ Not immunologically primed; having no exposure to antigen.

**unsaturated** \unsach′ərā′tid\ **1** Able to dissolve further quantities of solute. **2** Possessing double or triple valence bonds which have two or three pairs of shared electrons and the potential to bind additional atoms or groups: used especially of carbon-carbon bonds.

**Unverricht** [Heinrich *Unverricht*, German physician, 1853–1912] Unverricht's myoclonia, Unverricht's disease, Unverricht syndrome. See under PROGRESSIVE MYOCLONIC EPILEPSY.

**upgaze** SUPRAVERSION.

**upstream** **1** In a chromosome, the nucleotide sequences 5′ to the first exon of a gene. Many of the regulatory elements, such as the CAAT box and promoter regions, are upstream. Compare DOWNSTREAM. **2** Any nucleotide sequence that is removed toward the origin of gene expression from a reference sequence; for example, the initiation codon is upstream from the coding sequences.

**uptake** The absorption and assimilation of a substance by an organ or tissue, as of cholesterol by the adrenal cortex or of iodine by the thyroid. **absolute iodine u.** A method for estimating absolute rate of iodine accumulation in the whole body, to ascertain whether abnormal values for thyroidal $^{131}$I uptake are due to reciprocal changes in the extracellular fluid content of stable iodine. Abbr. AIU **iodine-131 u.** A means of evaluating thyroid gland activity used for diagnosing hyperthyroidism, but not hypothyroidism, and Graves disease. A tracer dose of iodine 131, or preferably iodine 123, is orally administered. The percentage taken up by the thyroid gland between two and six hours and again at 24 hours is measured using a gamma counter. The normal 24-hour uptake is about 10–30%. Hyperthyroidism is evidenced by a value of over 30%. As a test for Graves disease, the suppression test, thyroid uptake is measured at 24 hours after a dose before and after an eight-day course of triiodothyronine (75–100 μg/day). Patients with Graves disease show no decline in uptake whereas healthy individuals show a decrease of up to one half of the original value as a result of suppression of thyrotropic hormone secretion by the administered triiodothyronine.

**ur-** \yoor-\ URO-.

**Ura** Symbol for uracil.

**urachal** \yʊr′əkəl\ Pertaining to the urachus.

**urachovesical** \yʊr′əkōves′ikəl\ [*urach(us)* + *o* + VESICAL] Belonging to both the urachus and the urinary bladder.

**urachus** \yʊr′əkəs\ [Gk *ourachos* (from *ouron* urine + *echein* to hold) the urinary canal of a fetus] The distal part of the allantois, directed towards the umbilicus, at first continuous with its proximal part which forms the bladder but later becoming obliterated. In human embryos, the lumen of the urachus is obliterated early in development and is soon a simple cord of cells. Later, it becomes a fibrous cord extending from the apex of the bladder to the umbilicus (the median umbilical ligament). Rarely the lumen of the urachus can persist until after birth, when urine may drain from the umbilicus (urachal fistula). If only a localized part of the lumen persists, a urachal cyst may develop. **patent u.** A persistence throughout the urachus of the embryonic allantoic lumen such that the resulting fistulous connection between the urinary bladder and umbilicus causes leakage of urine at the umbilicus.

**uracil** \yoo′rəsil\ A pyrimidine derivative. It is a tautomer of 2,4-dihydroxypyrimidine, namely 1,2,3,4-tetrahydro-2,4-dioxopyrimidine. It is one of the four bases that occur as nucleotide residues in RNA. Its derivative formed by ribosylation at N-1 is uridine. Symbol: Ura

**uraemia** *Brit.* URAEMIA.

**uragogue** \yUr′əgäg\ *Obs.* DIURETIC.

**urali** \ooräʹlē\ CURARE.

**uranisco-** \yooʹrənisʹkō-\ URANO-.

**uraniscoplasty** \yooʹrənis′kəplasʹtē\ PALATOPLASTY.

**uraniscorrhaphy** \yooʹrəniskôr′əfē\ PALATOPLASTY.

**uraniscus** \yooʹrənis′kəs\ PALATUM.

**uranium** \yoorā′nē·əm\ Element number 92, having atomic weight 238.029. Fourteen isotopes are known, all of them unstable. The most common of the three naturally occurring isotopes is uranium 238, having 99.28% natural abundance. It is found in various minerals in equilibrium with a variety of disintegration products and along with small amounts of uranium 234 and uranium 235. In elemental form, uranium is a heavy, silvery white metal. Valences are 2, 3, 4, 5, and 6. The metal and its compounds are chemically toxic and radiologically hazardous. See also RADIOACTIVE SERIES. Symbol: U **u. II** A uranium isotope having atomic weight 234, with a half-life of $2.7 \times 10^5$ years. It is produced by the beta-decay of uranium $X_2$ and of uranium Z, and it in turn decays by alpha emission. **u. $X_1$** A radioactive isotope of thorium, produced by alpha-decay of uranium. It has mass number 234 and a half-life of 24.5 days. It decays by beta emission to uranium $X_2$. Symbol: $^{234}Th$ **u. $X_2$** A radioactive isotope of protactinium, having mass number 234 and a half-life of 1.17 minutes. It is a product of uranium $X_1$ by beta-decay, and it in turn decays by beta emission to uranium II and by isomeric transition to uranium Z. Also *brevium.* Symbol: $^{234m}Pa$ **u. Y** A radioactive isotope of thorium, having mass number 231 and a half-life of 25.5 hours. It is formed by alpha-decay of uranium 235 and decays by beta emission. Symbol: $^{231}Th$ **u. Z** A radioactive isotope of protactinium, having mass number 234 and a half-life of 6.7 hours. It is produced by isomeric transition of uranium $X_1$ and decays by beta emission and isomeric transition. Symbol: $^{234}Pa$

**uranium 235** An isotope of uranium comprising approximately 0.7% of naturally occurring uranium. It has a half-life of $7.1 \times 10^8$ years and decays by alpha emission and spontaneous fission. It sustains a fission chain reaction in a thermal neutron field. Symbol: $^{235}U$

**urano-** \yooʹrənō-\ [Gk *ouranos* (diminutive *ouraniskos* palate) sky, roof of the mouth] A combining form denoting the palate. Also *uranisco-.*

**uranoplastic** \-plas′tik\ Having to do with the plastic surgery of the palate.

**uranoplasty** \yoor′ənōplasʹtē\ PALATOPLASTY.

**uranorrhaphy** \yooʹrənôr′əfē\ PALATOPLASTY.

**uranoschisis** \yooʹrənäs′kisis\ [URANO- + -SCHISIS] CLEFT PALATE.

**uranostaphyloplasty** \-staf′ilōplasʹtē\ **1** The surgical repair of both the cleft hard and soft palates. Also *uranostaphylorrhaphy.* **2** PALATOPLASTY.

**uranostaphyloschisis** \-stafʹiläs′kisis\ [URANO- + STAPHYLO- + -SCHISIS] A cleft of both the hard and soft palates. Also *uranoveloschisis.*

**uranosteoplasty** \yooʹrənäs′tē·əplasʹtē\ [*uran(o)-* + OSTEO- + -PLASTY] The surgical repair of the cleft hard palate.

**uranoveloschisis** \-vəläs′kisis\ URANOSTAPHYLOSCHISIS.

**uranyl** \yoo′rənil\ The group $UO_2$, which occurs in many compounds of uranium(VI). Some of these have giant molecules, whereas others contain the ion $UO_2^{2+}$, which has a high affinity for nucleic acids and may be used to precipitate them.

**urarthritis** \yooʹrärthrī′tis\ [*ur(ic acid)* + ARTHRITIS] GOUT.

**urate** \yoo′rāt\ The salt of uric acid.

**uratemia** \yooʹrətē′mē·ə\ HYPERURICEMIA.

**urateribonucleotide phosphorylase** An enzyme (EC 2.4.2.16) that catalyzes the conversion of urate D-ribonucleotide and orthophosphate to urate and D-ribose 1-phosphate.

**uratic** \yoorat′ik\ Pertaining to uric acid or urate.

**uratosis** \yooʹrətō′sis\ [*urat(e)* + -OSIS] The condition of deposition of urate in the form of tophi.

**uraturia** \yooʹrətyooʹrē·ə\ URICOSURIA.

**Urbach** [Erich *Urbach,* U.S. dermatologist, 1893–1946] Urbach-Oppenheim disease. See under NECROBIOSIS LIPOIDICA.

**Urd** Symbol for uridine.

**ur-defense** \oor′difensʹ\ [German *ur-,* prefix denoting primitive + English *defense*] A belief considered essential to an individual's psychic integrity, such as belief in personal survival, faith in some abstract omnipotent being, or a conviction of man's ultimate kindness to man.

**ure-** \yooʹrə-\ [Gk *ouron* urine] A combining form denoting urea or urine. Also *urea-, ureo-.*

**-ure** \-ʸər\ [L *-ura,* noun suffix denoting act, process, state of being, function] A suffix meaning (1) act or process; (2) condition; (3) rank or office.

**urea** \yooʹrē·ə\ [French *urée* (from Gk *ouron* urine) substance found in the urine] $NH_2$—CO—$NH_2$. The double amide of carbonic acid. It is the main compound in which mammals, as well as some members of the fishes, amphibia, and reptiles, excrete in the urine the nitrogen of the proteins of their food. Strong solutions of urea (8 M) are used to denature proteins, hold them in solution, and expose the groups they contain to reagents. Urea was second only to oxalic acid as an organic compound to be synthesized from an inorganic one, by heating ammonium cyanate. It is made in animals that excrete it in the urea cycle by the hydrolysis of arginine to form it and ornithine. By reacting sequentially with carbamoyl phosphate and aspartate, ornithine re-forms arginine. The process occurs in the liver, and the urea is then excreted by the kidneys, normally accounting for approximately half of the urinary solids. Thus, when renal function is decreased urea accumulates in the blood. Blood urea and the urea clearance are good indicators of renal function. It may be manufactured by heating ammonium carbamate, derived from carbon dioxide and ammonia, under pressure. Also *carbamide* (obs.). Adj. ureal. **plasma u.** The quantity of urea present in blood plasma, used as a measure of kidney function. **sterile u.** A preparation of urea suitable for parenteral administration. It is used as an osmotic diuretic agent to reduce intracranial pressure in preparation for neurosurgery.

**urea-** \yooʹrē·ə-\ URE-.

***Ureaplasma*** \yooʹrē·əplaz′mə\ A genus of mycoplasmas that liberate ammonia from urea. They were formerly known as T-strains because they form tiny colonies. The species of human occurrence, *Ureaplasma urealyticum,* is frequently found in the genital tract and may cause nongonococcal urethritis.

**urease** The enzyme (EC 3.5.1.5) that hydrolyzes urea to carbon dioxide and ammonia. The plant enzyme, particularly abundant in jack beans, is often used for determination of urea concentration. It is highly specific and was the first enzyme to be crystallized. Urease also occurs in invertebrates.

There also exists an ATP-hydrolyzing urease (EC 3.5.1.45) in yeasts and algae.

**urea stibamine** A compound of urea with stibamine used in the treatment of leishmaniasis.

**urecchysis** \yoorek′isis\ [UR- + Gk *ekchysis* (from *ekchein* to pour out) a pouring out] Infiltration of skin or other tissues by urine, the result of trauma to the bladder or a ureter, or to rupture of these organs by disease.

**uremia** \yoorē′mē·ə\ [UR- + -EMIA] A symptom complex due to renal insufficiency and characterized by azotemia, acidosis, hyperphosphatemia and hypocalcemia, hyperkalemia, nausea and vomiting, pruritus and uremic frost, anemia, mental impairment and neuropathies, osteodystrophy, hypertension, pericarditis, pulmonary edema, and a host of other abnormalities. Some features of uremia are due to abnormalities of electrolytes, while others may be related to retention of phenolic and guanidinelike compounds. **prerenal u.** Uremia associated with disorders proximal to the kidneys which impair their function, such as shock, congestive heart failure, or renal artery stenosis. Also *extrarenal uremia.*

**uremic** \yoorē′mik\ Of, relating to, or afflicted by uremia.

**ureo-** \yoo′rē·ō-\ URE-.

**ureolysis** \yoo′rē·äl′isis\ [UREO- + LYSIS] Decomposition of urea by bacteria, enzymes or chemical action into carbon dioxide and ammonia.

**ureolytic** \yoo′rē·əlit′ik\ Relating to or causing ureolysis.

**ureotelic** \yoo′rē·ətel′ik\ Excreting urea as the principal end product of nitrogen metabolism. Mammals are ureotelic.

**-uresis** \-yoorē′sis\ [Gk *ourēsis* (from *ourein* to urinate) urination] A combining form meaning excreted in the urine or denoting the excretion of urine.

**ureter** \yʊr′ətər\ [Gk *ourētēr* (from *ourein* to urinate) the ureter] [NA] A thick, rounded muscular tube that carries the urine from the renal pelvis of the kidney to the base of the bladder on each side and is subdivided into an abdominal part and a pelvic part. It is constricted at its origin from the renal pelvis, at the point where it crosses the pelvic brim and as it passes through the wall of the urinary bladder. It consists of fibrous, muscular, and mucous coats. Also *renal duct* (outmoded), *nephric duct* (outmoded). Adj. ureteral, ureteric. **aberrant u.** A ureter that sends urine into an area other than the bladder. **circumcaval u.** RETROCAVAL URETER. **double u.** A congenital anomaly consisting in the presence of two ureters on one or both sides. The ureters may lead by separate courses to the bladder or may join, draining through a single orifice. **ectopic u.** An anomalous opening of the ureter into the bladder. It is usually associated with a double ureter which may include double ureteric openings, one at or near the usual termination, the other in the urethra or bladder neck. **retrocaval u.** A ureter which passes dorsal to and then around the infrarenal vena cava on its course to the bladder. This aberrant course is due to the persistence in the embryo of a subcardinal instead of the usual supracardinal vein that is to be incorporated into the infrarenal part of the vena cava. Also *postcaval ureter, circumcaval ureter.* **retroiliac u.** A ureter that passes dorsal to a common iliac vein on its course to the bladder. This abnormal course is due to persistence of the subcardinal instead of supracardinal embryonic veins in the formation of the inferior vena cava and its major tributaries.

**ureter-** \yoorē′tər-\ URETERO-.

**ureteral** \yoorē′tərəl\ Pertaining to the ureter, as *ureteral peristalsis* or *ureteral catheter.* Also *ureteric.*

**ureteralgia** \yoo′rētəral′jə\ [URETER- + -ALGIA] Pain affecting or originating in a ureter.

**ureterectasis** \yoorē′tərek′təsis\ [URETER + ECTASIS] Dilatation of the ureter, whether congenital or acquired, as hydroureter in infants and children, and ureteral dilatation secondary to urinary tract stones or tumors in adults. Also *ureterectasia.*

**ureterectomy** \yoorē′tərek′təmē\ [URETER + -ECTOMY] Partial or total resection of the ureter, as for the excision of ureteral tumors or the correction of ureteral stricture or hydroureter. Ureterectomy is often performed in conjunction with nephrectomy (nephroureterectomy) for treatment of urothelial tumors involving the renal pelvis or caliceal system.

**ureteric** \yoo′rēter′ik\ URETERAL.

**ureteritis** \yoo′rētərī′tis\ [URETER- + -ITIS] An acute or chronic inflammation of the ureter associated with or secondary to pyelonephritis or cystitis. **u. cystica** The appearance of small cysts in the ureter in association with a long-standing inflammatory process.

**uretero-** \yoorē′tərō-\ [Gk *ourētēr* urinary canal] A combining form denoting the ureter. Also *ureter-.*

**ureterocele** \yoorē′tərōsēl\ [URETERO- + -CELE[1]] Cystic dilatation of the terminal intravesical segment of the ureter secondary to congenital stenosis of the ureteral orifice.

**ureterocelectomy** \-sēlek′təmē\ [*ureterocel(e)* + -ECTOMY] Surgical removal of a ureterocele.

**ureterocolostomy** \-kəläs′təmē\ [URETERO- + COLO- + -STOMY] Transplantation of the end of the ureter from the bladder to the colon.

**ureterocutaneostomy** \-kyootā′nē·äs′təmē\ CUTANEOUS URETEROSTOMY.

**ureterocystanastomosis** [URETERO- + CYST- + ANASTOMOSIS] URETERONEOCYSTOSTOMY.

**ureterocystoneostomy** \-sis′tənē·äs′təmē\ URETERONEOCYSTOSTOMY.

**ureterocystostomy** \-sistäs′təmē\ URETERONEOCYSTOSTOMY.

**ureteroenterostomy** \-en′təräs′təmē\ [URETERO- + ENTERO- + -STOMY] A surgical connection between the ureter and intestine. Also *ureteroenteroanastomosis.*

**ureterography** \yoorē′tərāg′rəfē\ Roentgenography of the ureter after opacification of its lumen, accomplished by retrograde or antegrade instillation of a contrast medium or during urography.

**ureteroheminephrectomy** \-hem′ēnefrek′təmē\ [URETERO- + HEMI- + NEPHRECTOMY] Surgical removal of a part of the kidney and its ureter where there is duplication of a ureter or the entire upper urinary tract.

**ureteroileostomy** \yoorē′tərō·il′ē·äs′təmē\ [URETERO- + ILEO- + -STOMY] Surgical connection of the ureters to a loop of the ileum.

**ureterolith** \yoorē′tərōlith′\ [URETERO- + -LITH] A calculus in a ureter.

**ureterolithotomy** \-lithät′əmē\ [URETERO- + LITHOTOMY] Incision of, and removal of a calculus from, a ureter.

**ureterolysis** \yoorē′təräl′sis\ [URETERO- + LYSIS] Surgical freeing of an adhering ureter.

**ureteromeatotomy** \-mē′atät′əmē\ [URETERO- + MEATOTOMY ] Surgical widening of the ureteral orifice into the bladder.

**ureteroneocystostomy** \-nē′əsistäs′təmē\ [URETERO- + NEO- + CYSTOSTOMY] Surgical relocation of the site at which the ureter opens into the bladder. Also *ureterocystanastomosis, ureterocystoneostomy, ureterocystostomy, ureterovesicostomy.*

**ureteroneopyelostomy** \-nē′ōpī′əläs′təmē\ [URETERO- + NEO- + PYELOSTOMY] Reconnection of a ureter to the renal pelvis at a newly created opening, as after division of the ureter to remove a portion containing a stricture. Also *ureteropelvioneostomy, pelvioneostomy.*

**ureteronephrectomy** \-nefrek′təmē\ [URETERO- + NEPHRECTOMY] Excision of a kidney and its ureter.

**ureteropathy** \yoorē′tərāp′əthē\ [URETERO- + -PATHY] Any diseased condition of the ureter.

**ureteropelvioneostomy** \-pel′vē·ōnē·äs′təmē\ URETERONEOPYELOSTOMY.

**ureteropelvioplasty** \-pel′vē·əplas′tē\ [URETERO- + PELVIOPLASTY] The plastic repair of the connection of the ureter with the renal pelvis. **Culp u.** Ureteropelvioplasty in which a spiral flap of renal pelvic tissue is joined with the ureter. **Foley Y-type u.** FOLEY Y-PLASTY. **Scardino u.** Ureteropelvioplasty in which a vertical flap of renal pelvic tissue is joined with the ureter.

**ureteroplasty** \yoorē′tərōplas′tē\ [URETERO- + -PLASTY] Plastic surgery on a ureter, as for treatment of stricture.

**ureteroproctostomy** \-präktäs′təmē\ [URETERO- + PROCTO- + -STOMY] Surgical connection of a ureter to the rectum. Also *ureterorectostomy.*

**ureteropyelitis** \-pī′əlī′tis\ [URETERO- + PYELITIS] Inflammation of a ureter and renal pelvis. Also *ureteropyelonephritis.*

**ureteropyeloplasty** \-pī′əlōplas′tē\ [URETERO- + PYELOPLASTY] Any plastic surgery performed on the upper ureter and the renal pelvis.

**ureterorectostomy** \-rektäs′təmē\ [URETERO- + RECTO- + -STOMY] URETEROPROCTOSTOMY.

**ureterorrhagia** \yoorē′tərôrā′jə\ [URETERO- + -RRHAGIA] Hemorrhage from a ureter.

**ureterorrhaphy** \yoorē′tərôr′əfē\ [URETERO- + -RRHAPHY] Suture of a sectioned or incised ureter.

**ureterosigmoidostomy** \-sig′moidäs′təmē\ [URETERO- + SIGMOID + -STOMY] Surgical transplantation of the outlet of the ureter from the bladder to the sigmoid colon.

**ureterostenosis** \-stenō′sis\ [URETERO- + STENOSIS] Stricture of a ureter. Also *ureterostegnosis.*

**ureterostoma** \yoorē′təräs′təmə\ A fistula of the ureter.

**ureterostomy** \yoorē′təräs′təmē\ [URETERO- + -STOMY] Surgical creation of an external opening for a ureter. Also *ureterostomosis.* **cutaneous u.** The procedure of directing the ureter to the skin usually from an incision in the iliac region. Also *ureterocutaneostomy.*

**ureterotomy** \yoorē′tərät′əmē\ [URETERO- + -TOMY] A surgical procedure involving an incision into the ureter. The incision is usually made through the ureteral wall, in the longitudinal axis of the ureter, in order to gain access to the ureteral lumen usually for purposes of removing a ureteral stone or placement of a ureteral catheter.

**ureterotrigonoenterostomy** \-trīgō′nō·en′təräs′təmē\ [URETERO- + *trigon(e)* + ENTERO- + -STOMY] Insertion of the ureter and part of the trigone of the bladder into the intestine.

**ureterotrigonosigmoidostomy** \-trīgō′nōsig′moidäs′təmē\ The insertion of the ureter and a portion of the trigone of the bladder into the sigmoid flexure.

**ureteroureteral** \yoorē′tərōyoorē′tərəl\ Pertaining to an artificial anastomosis between two segments of a ureter.

**ureteroureterostomy** \yoorē′tərōyoorē′təräs′təmē\ [URETERO- + URETERO- + -STOMY] Surgical connection of the two ureters or of parts of the same ureter. Also *van Hook's operation.*

**ureterovesical** \-ves′ikəl\ Pertaining to a ureter and the bladder, as *ureterovesical junction.* Also *vesicoureteral.*

**ureterovesicoplasty** \-ves′ikōplas′tē\ [URETERO- + VESICO- + -PLASTY] Plastic operation at the site of junction of the ureter and the urinary bladder to correct reflux.

**ureterovesicostomy** \-ves′ikäs′təmē\ [URETERO- + VESICO- + -STOMY] URETERONEOCYSTOSTOMY.

**urethane** $C_3H_7NO_2$. Ethyl carbamate, an anticancer chemical. Also *urethan.*

**urethr-** \yoorē′thr-\ URETHRO-.

**urethra** \yoorē′thrə\ [Gk *ourēthra* (from *ourein* to urinate) the urethra] A slitlike tube conveying urine from the internal urethral orifice at the apex of the trigone of the urinary bladder to the external urethral orifice. Adj. urethral. **anterior u.** PARS SPONGIOSA URETHRAE MASCULINAE. **cavernous u.** PARS SPONGIOSA URETHRAE MASCULINAE. **double u.** A congenital malformation consisting of a double urethra with separate openings. The condition is prone to urinary infection. **u. feminina** [NA] A tube about 4 cm in length extending from the internal urethral orifice at the neck of the bladder in the female and passing behind the symphysis pubis embedded in the anterior wall of the vagina to open in the vestibule behind the glans clitoridis. Also *female urethra, urethra muliebris* (outmoded). **imperforate u.** The failure of the urethral orifice to be patent at birth. It is probably the result of an excessive persistence of embryonic urethral plate tissue. **u. masculina** [NA] A slitlike canal about 20 cm long extending from the internal urethral orifice at the neck of the bladder in the male through the prostate, perineal membrane, and corpus spongiosum penis to end at the external urethral orifice at the tip of the glans penis. In its course it makes a double curve and is subdivided into pars prostatica, pars membranacea and pars spongiosa. It serves to transport both the urine and the seminal secretions. Also *male urethra, urethra virilis.* **membranous u.** PARS MEMBRANACEA URETHRAE MASCULINAE. **u. muliebris** *Outmoded* URETHRA FEMININA. **penile u.** PARS SPONGIOSA URETHRAE MASCULINAE. **posterior u.** Pars membranacea urethrae masculinae and pars prostatica urethrae masculinae. **primary u.** The vesicourethral part of the cloaca in the embryo, from which is derived the whole urethra in the female and the prostatic urethra proximal to the opening of the prostatic utricle in the male. **prostatic u.** PARS PROSTATICA URETHRAE MASCULINAE. **spongy u.** PARS SPONGIOSA URETHRAE MASCULINAE. **u. virilis** URETHRA MASCULINA.

**urethral** \yoorē′thrəl\ Pertaining to the urethra.

**urethralgia** \yoo′rēthral′jə\ [URETHR- + -ALGIA] Pain in the urethra. Also *urethrodynia.*

**urethrascope** \yoorē′thrəskōp\ URETHROSCOPE.

**urethratresia** \yoorē′thrətrē′zhə\ [URETHR- + ATRESIA] Obstruction or congenital imperforation of the urethra.

**urethrectomy** \yoo′rēthrek′təmē\ [URETHR- + -ECTOMY] Total or partial resection of the urethra, usually in conjunction with a radical cystectomy for treatment of bladder carcinoma.

**urethritis** \yoo′rəthrī′tis\ [URETHR- + -ITIS] Inflammation of the urethra. **atrophic u.** The development of immature and imperfect squamous epithelial cells in the female urethra due to estrogen deprivation occurring postmenopausally. Also *senile urethritis.* **u. cystica** Urethritis accompanied by the formation of cysts on the urethral membrane. **gonococcal u.** Urethritis due to *Neisseria gonorrhaeae*; gonorrhea in a male. Also *gonorrheal urethritis, urethritis venerea, specific urethritis.* **nonspecific u.** Urethritis that cannot be determined to have been caused by a specific microorganism, as by a gonococcal organism. Such cases are probably of viral origin, and occur in both acute and chronic forms. Also *simple urethritis.* **polypoid u.** Chronic inflammation of the mucosa of the urethra with inflammatory polyps extending into the lumen. **senile u.** ATROPHIC URETHRITIS. **simple u.** NONSPECIFIC URETHRITIS. **specific u.** GONOCOCCAL URETHRITIS. **u. venerea** GONOCOCCAL URETHRITIS.

**urethro-** \yoorē′thrō-, yoorē′thrə-\ [Gk *ourēthra* urethra] A combining form meaning urethra. Also *urethr-*.

**urethrocele** \yoorē′thrəsēl\ [URETHRO- + -CELE[1]] Descent of the female urethra from its normal subpubic attachment, frequently leading to stress urinary incontinence.

**urethrocystitis** \-sistī′tis\ CYSTOURETHRITIS.

**urethrocystocele** \-sis′təsēl\ [URETHRO- + CYSTOCELE] Herniation of the urethra and the bladder into the vaginal canal.

**urethrocystography** \-sistäg′rəfē\ [URETHRO- + CYSTOGRAPHY] Radiographic visualization of the uretha and bladder employing a contrast medium.

**urethrocystometry** \-sistäm′ətrē\ [URETHRO- + CYSTO- + -METRY] Simultaneous measurement of the pressures in the bladder and urethra.

**urethrocystopexy** \-sis′təpek′sē\ [URETHRO- + CYSTO- + -PEXY] Operative fixation of the junction of the urethra and bladder for treatment of stress incontinence.

**urethrodynia** \-din′ē·ə\ URETHRALGIA.

**urethrography** \yoo′rēthräg′rəfē\ [URETHRO- + -GRAPHY] Roentgenography of the urethra after its opacification by injecting a contrast medium at the urethral orifice or by having the patient void after the bladder urine has been opacified.

**urethrometer** \yoo′rēthräm′ətər\ [URETHRO- + -METER] A device used to measure the caliber of the urethra.

**urethrometry** \yoo′rēthräm′ətrē\ [URETHRO- + -METRY] **1** Measurement of the caliber of the urethra, as to locate and determine the extent of urethral stricture. **2** Measurement of urethral resistance to the backward flow of a fluid.

**urethropexy** \yoorē′thrəpek′sē\ [URETHRO- + -PEXY] Operative fixation of the female urethra for relief of stress incontinence.

**urethroplasty** \yoorē′thrəplas′tē\ [URETHRO- + -PLASTY] Plastic repair of the urethra.

**urethrorrhagia** \yoorē′thrôrā′jə\ [URETHRO- + -RRHAGIA] Bleeding from the urethra. Also *urethral apoplexy*.

**urethrorrhaphy** \yoo′rēthrôr′əfē\ [URETHRO- + -RRHAPHY] Surgical closure of a urethral wound or fistula.

**urethrorrhea** \yoorē′thrôrē′ə\ [URETHRO- + -RRHEA] An abnormal discharge from the urethra.

**urethroscope** \yoorē′thrəskōp\ [URETHRO- + -SCOPE] An instrument for visualizing the interior of the urethra. Also *urethrascope*.

**urethroscopy** \yoo′rēthräs′kəpē\ [URETHRO- + -SCOPY] Visual examination of the urethra with the urethroscope.

**urethroscrotal** \-skrō′tal\ Pertaining to the urethra and the scrotum, as *urethroscrotal fistula*.

**urethrospasm** \yoorē′thrəspazm\ Muscular spasm of the urethra.

**urethrostenosis** \-stenō′sis\ [URETHRO- + STENOSIS] **1** A narrowing of the urethral meatus. **2** Stricture of the urethra.

**urethrostomy** \yoo′rēthräs′təmē\ [URETHRO- + -STOMY] The surgical formation of either a permanent fistula opening into the urethra, for treatment of stricture, or a temporary opening into the urethra for introduction of instruments.

**urethrotome** \yoorē′thrətōm\ [URETHRO- + -TOME] An instrument used for incising urethral strictures. **dilating u.** A urethrotome combined with a urethral dilator.

**urethrotomy** \yoo′rəthrät′əmē\ [URETHRO- + -TOMY] An incision of the urethra, done either from inside with the help of a urethrotome (internal urethrotomy), or from the outside through the skin (external urethrotomy). **external u.** An incision into the urethra through the perineum. Also *perineal urethrotomy, perineal section*.

**urethrotrigonitis** \-trig′ənī′tis\ [URETHRO- + TRIGONITIS] Inflammation of the urethra and bladder trigone.

**urgency** \ur′jənsē\ A strong desire to urinate immediately.

**urhidrosis** \yoor′hidrō′sis\ URIDROSIS.

**URI** upper respiratory infection.

**-uria** \-[y]oo′rē·ə\ [Gk *our(on)* urine + -IA] A combining form signifying the presence in the urine of a (specified) substance, often associated with an abnormal or diseased condition.

**uric-** \yoo′rik-\ URICO-.

**-uric** [Gk *our(on)* urine + -IC] A suffix denoting the presence of acids in the urine, often implying amide formation with glycine.

**uric acid** A tautomer of 2,6,8-trihydroxypurine, namely 1,2,3,6,7,8-hexahydro-2,6,8-trioxopurine. It is the compound in which most nitrogen from nucleic acid is excreted in the urine of man, although most other mammals oxidize it to allantoin. It is the main route of nitrogen excretion of birds, and of some reptiles. It is a weak acid of p*K* 5.4, and the free acid has low solubility in water. Uric acid can crystallize in the tissues when purine catabolism is deranged in gout.

**uricacidemia** \yoo′rikas′idē′mē·ə\ HYPERURICEMIA.

**uricemia** \yoo′risē′mē·ə\ HYPERURICEMIA.

**urico-** \yoo′rikō-\ [*uric (acid)* + *o*] A combining form denoting uric acid. Also *uric-*.

**uricopoiesis** \yoo′rikōpō·ē′sis\ [URICO- + -POIESIS] The formation of uric acid.

**uricosuria** \yoo′rikōsoo′rē·ə\ [URICO- + *s* + -URIA] Urinary excretion of uric acid or urates. Also *uraturia*.

**uricosuric** \yoo′rikōsoo′rik\ **1** Stimulating the urinary excretion of uric acid or urates. **2** Any condition or agent that promotes the urinary excretion of uric acid or urates, as the drug probenecid.

**uricotelic** \yoo′rikōtel′ik\ Excreting uric acid as the principal end product of nitrogen metabolism. Birds are uricotelic.

**uridine** \yoo′ridēn\ $N^1$-$\beta$-D-Ribofuranosyluracil, the nucleoside of uracil. It is a component of RNA and of many other nucleotides. Symbol: Urd, U

**uridine diphosphate** Usually uridine 5′-diphosphate. Its glycosylated derivatives are donors of glycosyl groups in polysaccharide biosynthesis, so it is produced in such glycosylations. It can be recycled after conversion into uridine triphosphate. Abbr. UDP

**uridine diphosphate acetylgalactosamine** Uridine diphosphate carrying an *N*-acetylgalactosaminyl group on its distal phosphate. This is the donor of such groups in polysaccharide biosynthesis. It is formed by epimerization of UDP-*N*-acetylglucosamine.

**uridine diphosphate acetylglucosamine** Uridine diphosphate carrying an *N*-acetylglucosaminyl group on its distal phosphate. This is the donor of such groups in polysaccharide biosynthesis. It is made from UTP and *N*-acetylglucosamine 1-phosphate, with simultaneous formation of free diphosphate (pyrophosphate).

**uridine diphosphate galactose** See under UDPGALACTOSE.

**uridine diphosphate glucose** See under UDPGLUCOSE.

**uridine diphosphogalactose** See under UDPGALACTOSE.

**uridine diphosphoglucose** See under UDPGLUCOSE.

**uridine diphosphoglucose dehydrogenase** See under UDPGLUCOSE DEHYDROGENASE.
**uridine diphosphoglucuronate** See under UDP-GLUCURONATE.
**uridine monophosphate** See under URIDINE 5′-PHOSPHATE. Abbr. UMP
**uridine 5′-phosphate** A compound comprising a ribosyl group phosphorylated on O-5, attached by C-1 to the N-1 of uracil. Certain nucleases form it, together with other nucleoside 5′-phosphates, by hydrolysis of RNA. It is the first pyrimidine nucleotide to be biosynthesized from carbamoyl phosphate and aspartate, being formed by decarboxylation of orotidine 5′-phosphate. Also *uridylic acid.* • Unless otherwise specified, uridine monophosphate (UMP) is taken to mean uridine 5′-phosphate.
**uridine triphosphate** Uridine 5′-triphosphate. It is important as the source of uridylic acid residues in RNA, and also for the biosynthesis of many UDPsugars, which are the donors of the glycosyl groups for polysaccharide biosynthesis.
**uridrosis** \yooʹridrōʹsis\ [*ur(ea)* + *(h)idrosis*] The excretion of urea in the sweat, a process that is notably increased in cases of uremia. Also *urinidrosis.* Also *urhidrosis.* **u. crystallina** Uridrosis that is characterized by crystals of urea (uremic frost) being deposited on the skin surface.
**uridylic acid** URIDINE 5′-PHOSPHATE.
**uridylyltransferase** Any enzyme that transfers the uridylyl group, i.e. uridylic acid from whose phosphate group OH has been removed. The donor is usually UTP, and the transfer is onto a phosphate group of a sugar phosphate, so that a UDPsugar is formed, together with diphosphate (pyrophosphate). An example is glucose-1-phosphate uridylyltransferase, which is responsible for the biosynthesis of UDPglucose.
**urin-** \yooʹrin-\ URINO-.
**urinal** \yurʹənəl\ A receptacle or fixture designed to receive urine. **condom u.** A portable urinal made from a condom with an attached rubber tube. It is worn on the penis by incontinent males to lead the urine into a bag which is generally worn on the leg. Also *Texas catheter.*
**urinalysis** \yooʹrinalʹsis\ [*urin(e) (an)alysis*] A laboratory examination of urine, usually a screening routine for unselected urine specimens. Variables evaluated are color, concentration as indicated by specific gravity or osmolality, pH, and the presence of a variety of chemical constituents, especially sugar, protein, and blood. A microscopic examination of formed elements is often included.
**urinary** \yooʹrinerʹē\ Of, relating to, or for the passage of urine.
**urinate** [*urin(e)* + -ATE] To pass urine. Also *micturate.*
**urination** \yooʹrināʹshən\ [Med L *urinat(us)* (past part. of *urinare* to urinate, from L *urina* urine) urinated + -ION] The act of passing urine. Also *micturition, miction.*
**urine** [Old French, from L *urina* (remotely akin to Gk *ouron* urine) urine] The excretory product of the kidneys, originating as the ultrafiltrate of plasma passing through glomerular capillaries. Its volume and solute composition result from the absorptive and secretory activities of renal tubular epithelium which, in health, combine to maintain physiologic levels of blood volume, pH, and electrolyte composition, and to eliminate metabolic waste products. The principal normal constituents, besides water, include urea, sodium chloride, and the salts of sulfuric, phosphoric, and uric acids. Abnormalities of urine composition may reflect systemic abnormalities of metabolism or plasma constituents, or the presence of disease in any part of the kidney. **black u.** Urine of very dark color. It is caused by a variety of agents and conditions, such as melanin in patients with melanosarcoma, large amounts of bile in patients with obstructive jaundice or very severe parenchymal liver disease, homogentistic acid in alkaptonuria, hemoglobin or myoglobin in acid urine, and several drugs such as phenothiazine derivatives, metronidiazol, and others. **chylous u.** CHYLURIA. **cloudy u.** A freshly voided urine with a cloudy appearance due to pus, crystals, bacteria, blood, or to free fat globules, as in the nephrotic syndrome. Also *milky urine.* **milky u.** CLOUDY URINE. **residual u.** Urine that remains in the bladder following urination, as determined by bladder catheterization, or radiographic or radioisotopic techniques. Residual urine is thought to reflect the balance between bladder outlet resistance and the propulsive activity of the bladder.
**urine-mucoid** \-myooʹkoid\ A mucinlike material in the urine. It may represent contamination from the vagina. *Outmoded.* Also *uromucoid.*
**urinidrosis** \yooʹrinidrōʹsis\ URIDROSIS.
**uriniferous** \yooʹrinifʹərəs\ [URIN- + *i* + -FEROUS] Carrying urine: said of the renal tubules.
**urino-** \yooʹrinō-\ [L *urina* urine] A combining form denoting urine. Also *urin-.*
**urinogenous** \yooʹrinäjʹənəs\ UROGENOUS.
**urinoma** \yooʹrinōʹmə\ [URIN- + -OMA] The collection of urine within the external renal capsule, usually associated with hydronephrosis. Also *external hydronephrosis, perirenal hydronephrosis, subcapsular hydronephrosis, uronchus.*
**urinometer** \yooʹrinämʹətər\ [URINO- + -METER] A device for measuring the specific gravity of urine. A widely used model consists of a calibrated weighted float which, when placed in a container of the urine to be tested, sinks to a depth determined by the specific gravity of the specimen. Also *urometer, urogravimeter.*
**urinometry** \yooʹrinämʹətrē\ [URINO- + -METRY] The measurement of relative density of urine specimens.
**uro-** \yooʹrō-\ [Gk *ouron* urine] A combining form meaning (1) urine; (2) the urinary tract. Also *ur-, urono-.*
**urobilin** A linear tetrapyrrole on the pathway of porphyrin degradation. One step of its formation is carried out by intestinal bacteria, but some is reabsorbed into the blood and it is partly responsible for the color of urine.
**urobilinogen** STERCOBILINOGEN.
**urocanate hydratase** The enzyme (EC 4.2.1.49) that catalyzes the reaction of urocanate with water to form 3-(imidazolone)propionic acid, a step in the normal catabolism of histidine. Also *urocanase* (outmoded).
**urocanic acid** 3-(Imidazol-4-yl)propenoic acid. It is formed metabolically from histidine by loss of ammonia.
**urocele** \yooʹrəsēl\ [URO- + -CELE[1]] An enlarged scrotum from extravasation of urine. Also *uroscheocele.*
**urochezia** \-kēʹzē·ə\ [URO- + Gk *chez(ein)* to defecate + -IA] The passage of urine through the anus.
**urochrome** [URO- + Gk *chrōm(a)* color] The pigment of urine, largely a combined form of urobilin.
**uroclepsia** \-klepʹsē·ə\ [URO- + Gk *kleps(ō)*, fut. of *kleptein* to steal, do a thing secretly + -IA] The involuntary, unconscious passage of urine.
**urocoproporphyria** \yooʹrəkōprōʹpôrfirʹē·ə\ PORPHYRIA CUTANEA TARDA.
**urocystitis** \-sistīʹtis\ [UROCYST- + -ITIS] Inflammation of the urinary bladder.
**urodeum** \-dēʹəm\ The ventral division of the cloaca into which the urogenital ducts open. *Outmoded.*
**urodialysis** \-dī·alʹisis\ [URO- + DIALYSIS] Suppression of urine secretion. It may be complete or partial.

**urodynia** \-din′ē·ə\ [UR- + -ODYNIA] Pain resulting from urination.
**urodysfunction** \-disfungk′shən\ [URO- + DYSFUNCTION] Impairment or abnormality in urinary function.
**uroflowmeter** \-flō′mētər\ [URO- + FLOWMETER] An instrument used for the recording of urine flow. Also *uroflometer.*
**urogastrone** A substance found in the urine of pregnant women and capable of inhibiting the development of peptic ulcers. It is apparently a peptide.
**urogenital** \-jen′itəl\ Pertaining to the urinary and genital structures. Also *genitourinary.*
**urogenous** \yooräj′ənəs\ **1** Produced in or from the urine. **2** Capable of forming urine. For defs. 1 and 2 also *urinogenous.*
**urogram** \yoor′əgram\ [URO- + -GRAM] A roentgenogram obtained during urography.
**urography** \yooräg′rəfē\ [URO- + -GRAPHY] Roentgenography of the urinary tract after the opacification of the urine being excreted, accomplished usually by the intravenous administration of an iodine-containing contrast medium or, infrequently, by subcutaneous injection of the contrast medium. **ascending u.** *Outmoded* RETROGRADE PYELOGRAPHY. **descending u.** *Seldom used* INTRAVENOUS UROGRAPHY. **excretory u.** INTRAVENOUS UROGRAPHY. **intravenous u.** Roentgenography of the urinary tract after the intravenous administration of an iodine-containing contrast medium that is excreted in the urine. Also *excretion urography, descending urography* (seldom used), *excretory urography, excretion pyelography* (outmoded), *intravenous pyelography.* Abbr. IVU
**urogravimeter** \-gravim′ətər\ URINOMETER.
**urokinase** \-kī′nās\ A plasminogen activator enzyme excreted in urine.
**urolagnia** \-lag′nē·ə\ [URO- + Gk *lagneia* lust, desire] A paraphilia in which sexual gratification is dependent upon urinary function. It may include drinking one's own or another's urine, watching others urinate, or having the sexual partner urinate on one's body. Also *undinism, urophilia.*
**urolith** \yoo′rəlith\ URINARY CALCULUS.
**urolithiasis** \-lithī′əsis\ [URO- + LITHIASIS] The presence or formation of calculi in the urinary tract, or the diseased state associated with it.
**urolithic** \-lith′ik\ Pertaining to urinary calculi or urolithiasis.
**urolithotomy** \-lithät′əmē\ [URO- + LITHOTOMY] Removal of a calculus from the urinary tract through an incision.
**urologist** \yooräl′əjist\ A specialist in the practice of urology.
**urology** \yooräl′əjē\ [URO- + -LOGY] The branch of medicine treating the urinary tract diseases, from the medical and chiefly the surgical viewpoints and, by extension, the diseases of the male genitourinary system.
**urolytic** \-lit′ik\ Able to dissolve or decompose urinary calculi.
**urometer** \yooräm′ətər\ URINOMETER.
**uromucoid** \-myoo′koid\ URINE-MUCOID.
**uroncus** \yooräng′kəs\ URINOMA.
**uronic acid** An acid derived from a sugar by oxidation from $—CH_2OH$ to —COOH of the highest-numbered carbon atom. Polymers of such acids are present in the cell walls of plants.
**urono-** \yoo′rənō-\ URO-.
**uropathy** \yooräp′əthē\ [URO- + -PATHY] Any pathologic state of, or abnormal change in, the urinary tract. **obstructive u.** Uropathy due to obstruction of the urinary tract, usually mechanical in nature. It is characterized by dilatation of the collecting system proximal to the obstruction. Atrophy of the renal parenchyma develops if the obstruction is prolonged. Decreased urine flow, increased urinary frequency, and chronic renal failure are clinical features of obstructive uropathy. Relief in obstruction usually results in a profound but transient diuresis, and may improve renal function.
**urophan** \yoo′rəfan\ [URO- + Gk *phan(os)* visible, manifest] An ingested substance that remains unaltered after passing through the digestive system and into the urinary tract.
**urophilia** \-fil′ē·ə\ [URO- + -PHILIA] UROLAGNIA.
**uropod** \yoo′rəpäd\ [Gk *our(a)* tail + *o* + -POD] A cytoplasmic projection from a cell surface as from a lymphocyte, possibly due to locomotion or active movement of membrane components.
**uropoiesis** \-poi·ē′sis\ [URO- + -POIESIS] The formation of urine.
**uropoietic** \-poi·et′ik\ Pertaining to or entering into the formation of urine.
**uroporphyrin** A porphyrin with a carboxymethyl and a 2-carboxyethyl substituent on each pyrrole ring. A uroporphyrin is a precursor of protoporphyrin and therefore of heme in biosynthesis. A different uroporphyrin, formed without reversal of the fourth pyrrole ring on cyclization, is found in the urine in one type of congenital porphyria.
**uroporphyrinogen III** The first cyclic product in porphyrin biosynthesis. It is the porphyrinogen with the substituents carboxymethyl (Cm) and 2-carboxyethyl (Cet) in the order Cm, Cet, Cm, Cet, Cm, Cet, Cet, Cm. The cyclization is brought about by uroporphyrinogen-III synthase acting on hydroxymethylbilane, and involves reversal of the fourth pyrrole ring.
**uropsammus** \yoo′rəsam′əs\ [URO- + Gk *psammos* sand] Gravel or sediment in the urine.
**uropterin** Any urinary pterin. Xanthopterin is the main natural one.
**uroscheocele** \yooräs′kē·əsēl′\ UROCELE.
**uroschesis** \yooräs′kəsis\ [URO- + Gk *schesis* a checking, holding] *Rare* URINARY RETENTION.
**urothelium** \-thē′lē·əm\ Epithelium lining the urinary tract.
**urotoxicity** \-täksis′itē\ [URO- + TOXICITY] Toxicity related to urinary substances.
**urotoxin** \-täk′sin\ [URO- + TOXIN] Any toxic substance in the urine.
**uroureter** \yoo′rōyʊr′ətər\ [URO- + URETER] Swelling of a ureter due to retained urine.
**urticant** \ur′tikənt\ [Med L *urticans,* gen. *urticantis* (from *urticare* to sting, cause itching or burning, from L *urtica* a stinging nettle) causing stinging or itching] **1** A substance that causes wheals to form. **2** Of or relating to wheal formation.
**urticaria** \ur′təkar′ē·ə\ [New L (from L *urtica* a stinging nettle) nettle rash] An eruption of transient, edematous, circumscribed, and often itchy swellings of the skin. Also *hives, nettle rash, erythema urticans* (seldom used). Adj. urticarial, urticarious. **acute u.** **1** Urticaria of short duration, with the distinction from chronic urticaria often being drawn arbitrarily at two months. **2** Urticaria occurring within minutes of exposure to an antigen, such as penicillin or a bee sting. **aquagenic u.** Urticaria provoked by contact of the skin with water. **bullous u.** Urticaria in which the edema formation is so intense as to form bullae. **cholinergic u.** A characteristic urticaria, especially of adolescents and young adults, marked by uniform tiny wheals provoked by exertion, heat, or anything that causes sweating. It

lasts 10 to 30 minutes. Also *cholinergic dermatosis.* **cold u.** Urticaria provoked by exposure to cold. **factitious u.** DERMOGRAPHISM. **u. febrilis** Urticaria associated with fever. **giant u.** Urticaria with giant weals. Also *angioedema.* **hemorrhagic u.** Urticaria in which the wheals contain areas of hemorrhage. Also *urticaria petechialis.* **heredofamilial u.** MUCKLE-WELLS SYNDROME. **u. maritima** Urticaria induced by sea bathing and due to various causes. **papular u.** A skin eruption of wheals followed one to two days later by more persistent papules. It is usually attributed to insect bites. Also *prurigo simplex, prurigo vulgaris, prurigo infantilis.* **u. perstans** A skin eruption in which the wheal-like lesions persist for several days or weeks. **u. petechialis** HEMORRHAGIC URTICARIA. **u. photogenica** SOLAR URTICARIA. **physical u.** Any urticaria provoked by a physical agent such as cold, heat, or pressure. **u. pigmentosa** A cutaneous eruption, caused by the proliferation of mast cells, that consists of persistent macules or raised lesions which form wheals after rubbing or stroking resulting in hyperpigmentation of affected areas. **pressure u.** Urticaria that is provoked by prolonged and heavy pressure and that becomes evident hours after the pressure is relieved. **solar u.** Urticaria provoked by exposure to sunlight. Also *urticaria photogenica.*

**urticariogenic** \ur′tiker′ē·əjen′ik\ [*urticari(a)* + *o* + -GENIC] Causing urticaria or its wheals.

**urushiol** $C_{15}H_{27}{\cdot}C_6H_3(OH)_2$. 3-Pentadecadienyl catechol, the irritant principle of poison ivy and other species of the *Toxicodendron* genus.

**USAN** United States Adopted Name.

**Usher** [Barney David *Usher,* Canadian dermatologist, born 1899] Senear-Usher syndrome. See under SYNDROME.

**Usher** [Charles Howard *Usher,* English physician, 1865–1942] See under SYNDROME.

**USP** United States Pharmacopeia.

**ustilaginism** \us′tilaj′inizm\ A condition resulting from ingestion of maize infected with the smut *Ustilago maydis.* Symptoms of poisoning, which resemble those from ergot, include hyperemia, itching, profuse sweating, and a bluish coloration of the extremities with edema and a feeling of coldness.

**ustion** \us′chən\ [L *ust(us),* past part. of *urere* to burn, parch + -ION] The burning of tissue with a surgical cautery.

**ustulation** \us′tyəlā′shən\ [Med L *ustulatio* (from L *ustulare* to burn partially, char) a charring] The drying of a drug by heat so that it can be pulverized.

**uta** \oo′tə\ [Spanish, from Quechua] A mild form of cutaneous leishmaniasis found at high elevations (900–3000 meters) in the Andes of Peru, Argentina and Bolivia. It is characterized by a single lesion on the skin. The agent is *Leishmania peruviana,* and the vectors are sandflies of the genus *Lutzomyia,* and possibly *L. verrucarum* or *L. peruensis.* Dogs can act as reservoir hosts.

**ut dict.** *ut dictum* (L, as said, i.e., as directed, used in prescription writing).

**utend.** *utendus* (L, to be used, a direction used in pharmacy).

**uter-** \yoo′tər-\ UTERO-.

**utercystostomy** \yoo′tərsistäs′təmē\ [UTER- + CYSTO- + -STOMY] A communication between the uterus and bladder, a fistula. Also *uterocystostomy.*

**uteri** \yoo′tərī\ Plural of UTERUS.

**utero-** \yoo′tərō-\ [L *uterus* the womb] A combining form denoting the uterus. Also *uter-.*

**uterocystostomy** \-sistäs′təmē\ UTERCYSTOSTOMY.

**uterofixation** \-fiksā′shən\ [UTERO- + FIXATION] An operative fixation of an abnormally positioned uterus.

**uterogestation** \-jestā′shən\ [UTERO- + GESTATION] A pregnancy which lasts for the normal period of time.

**uterolith** \yoo′tərōlith′\ [UTERO- + -LITH] UTERINE CALCULUS.

**uterometer** \yoo′tərām′ətər\ [UTERO- + -METER] UTERINE SOUND.

**uteropexy** \yoo′tərōpek′sē\ [UTERO- + -PEXY] HYSTEROPEXY.

**uteroplacental** \-pləsen′təl\ Pertaining to both the uterus and the placenta.

**uteroplasty** \yoo′tərōplas′tē\ [UTERO- + -PLASTY] An operation performed on the uterus to correct a congenital anomaly, as by changing its position or shape. Also *hysteroplasty, metroplasty.*

**uterosacral** \-sā′krəl\ Pertaining to the uterus and sacrum.

**uterosalpingography** \-sal′ping·gäg′rəfē\ HYSTEROSALPINGOGRAPHY.

**uteroscope** \yoo′tərōskōp\ [UTERO- + -SCOPE] HYSTEROSCOPE.

**uterothermometry** \-thərmäm′ətrē\ [UTERO- + THERMOMETRY] The measurement of the temperature of the uterus, usually for an estimation of blood flow. Also *hysterothermometry.*

**uterotomy** \yoo′tərät′əmē\ [UTERO- + -TOMY] HYSTEROTOMY.

**uterotonic** \-tän′ik\ An agent which stimulates uterine contractions, such as ergot derivatives, oxytocics, and prostaglandins.

**uterotropic** \-träp′ik\ Having an affinity for the uterus.

**uterotubography** \-t^y^oobäg′rəfē\ [UTERO- + TUBO- + -GRAPHY] HYSTEROSALPINGOGRAPHY.

**uterovesical** \-ves′ikəl\ Pertaining to the uterus and urinary bladder.

**uterus** \yoo′tərəs\ [L (prob. remotely akin to Gk *hystera* womb) the womb, belly] [NA] A piriform, hollow muscular organ situated in the lesser pelvis between the urinary bladder anteriorly and the rectum posteriorly in the female. The fundus lies above the cornu where the uterine tubes enter it on each side, while below that level is the corpus which is demarcated from the cervix inferiorly by the isthmus. The cervical canal connects its cavity with the vagina. Its position varies with the degree of distension of the bladder and the rectum, and it is connected to these organs and to the lateral wall of the pelvis by peritoneal folds and ligaments, especially the broad ligament attaching its lateral margin on each side to the lateral pelvic wall. It serves as a site for the implantation of the fertilized ovum, and permits development of the embryo and fetus. Also *womb, hystera, metra* (outmoded). **u. acollis** A uterus lacking a cervix or with the vaginal portion much reduced in size. **arcuate u.** SADDLE-SHAPED UTERUS. **u. bicameratus vetularum** Distention of the cervical canal and endometrial cavity secondary to cervical stenosis as a result of adhesion formation. **u. bicornis** A uterus which is, to varying degrees, bifurcated at its cephalic end owing to incomplete union of the caudal segments of the two embryonic paramesonephric ducts. There is distinct external indication of subdivision of the organs into lateral horns, in contrast to uterus septus in which the internal division is not marked externally. Also *bifid uterus, bicornuate uterus, uterus bifidus.* **u. bicornis bicollis** A uterus bicornis which has two distinct cervices indicating a minimal union of the most caudal parts of the embryonic paramesonephric ducts. **u. bicornis unicollis** A uterus bicornis with only one cervix apparent in

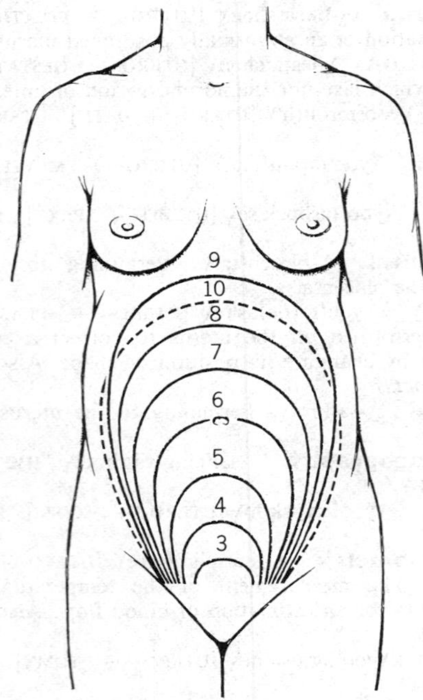


Changes in uterus during pregnancy

the vagina, indicating that the embryonic paramesonephric ducts probably united properly in all but the more cephalic region of usual fusion. **bicornuate u.** UTERUS BICORNIS. **bifid u.** UTERUS BICORNIS. **u. biforis** A uterus in which the cervix is divided by a septum. Also *double-mouthed uterus.* **u. bilocularis** UTERUS SEPTUS. **bipartite u.** UTERUS SEPTUS. **capped u.** A condition of the uterus marked by tonic contractions of the musculature of the fundus. **cochleate u.** An adult uterus in which the body is small and acutely flexed and the cervix is conical. **u. cordiformis** Uterus subseptus which has a heart-shaped external appearance because of a notch at the cephalic end of the fundus. **Couvelaire u.** A pregnant uterus having an extravasation of blood into the musculature in association with an abruptio placentae. Disseminated intravascular coagulopathy is a common associated feature. Hysterectomy may be required as treatment. Also *uteroplacental apoplexy.* **u. didelphys** A double uterus associated with double cervix and double vagina, indicating that the embryonic paramesonephric ducts underwent little or no fusion of their caudal segments during organogenesis. Also *dihysteria.* **double-mouthed u.** UTERUS BIFORIS. **u. duplex** Any uterus with a degree of duplication of the lumen, from uterus didelphys to uterus subseptus. **embryonic u.** The earliest anlage of the uterus, formed in man by fusion of the paramesonephric ducts. **fetal u.** A uterus in which the cervical canal is longer than the endometrial cavity. **fibroid u.** A leiomyoma of the uterus. **gravid u.** A pregnant uterus. **u. incudiformis** A uterus bicornis in which the cephalic margin of the fundus presents a broad, flat appearance suggestive of an anvil. Also *uterus planifundalis.* **infantile u.** A uterus of an adult which is small and underdeveloped. Also *pubescent uterus.* **u. masculinus** PROSTATIC UTRICLE. **ovoid u.** A pregnant uterus shaped like an egg. **u. parvicollis** A uterus of normal size except for an abnormally small cervix. **Piskacek u.** An asymmetric enlargement of the uterus secondary to implantation of a blastocyst in one corner. **u. planifundalis** UTERUS INCUDIFORMIS. **pubescent u.** INFANTILE UTERUS. **sacculated u.** UTERINE SACCULATION. **saddle-shaped u.** A malformation of a uterus secondary to depression of the fundus. Also *arcuate uterus.* **scarred u.** A uterus which has had a surgical procedure performed on it, such as a cesarean section, hysterotomy, or myomectomy. Compare UNSCARRED UTERUS. **u. septus** A uterus completely partitioned into two lumina by a midsagittal septum. Also *uterus bilocularis, bipartite uterus.* **u. simplex** A uterus comprising a single cavity. This is the normal type of human uterus. **u. subseptus** An incomplete uterus septus in which the septum is deficient in its caudal extent and does not reach the cervix. **u. unicornis** A one-horned uterus in which a unilateral fallopian tube connects directly with a tubular but somewhat truncated uterus. This condition is presumed to result from the development of only one paramesonephric duct in the embryo, or failure of more than one paramesonephric duct to grow caudalward into the pelvic region. **unscarred u.** A uterus which has not had a surgical procedure performed on it. Compare SCARRED UTERUS.

**UTP** uridine triphosphate.

**UTPgalactose-1-phosphate uridylyltransferase** See under GALACTOSE-1-PHOSPHATE URIDYLYLTRANSFERASE.

**UTPglucose-1-phosphate uridylyltransferase** See under GLUCOSE-1-PHOSPHATE URIDYLYLTRANSFERASE.

**utricle** \yoo′trikəl\ [L *utriculus.* See UTRICULUS.] **1** UTRICULUS. **2** Any small sac. **prostatic u.** A diverticulum up to 6 mm long extending backwards within the prostate behind its median lobe from a slitlike opening on the colliculus seminalis in the prostatic urethra. Its walls consist of stratified epithelium, muscle, and fibrous tissue, and contain openings of many small glands. It is formed from the paramesonephric ducts, but epithelium is probably derived also from the urogenital sinus by a proliferation called the sinu-utricular cord. It is analagous to the uterus and upper vagina in the female. Also *utriculus prostaticus, uterus masculinus, utriculus masculinus.* **urethral u.** PROSTATIC UTRICLE.

**utricular** \yootrik′yələr\ Pertaining to or resembling a utricle.

**utriculi** \yootrik′yəli\ Plural of UTRICULUS.

**utriculitis** \yootik′yəlī′tis\ [*utricul(us)* + -ITIS] Inflammation of the prostatic utricle.

**utriculus** \yootrik′yələs\ [L (dim. of *uter,* gen. *utris,* a skin for wine, oil, water), a small bag] [NA] A small, irregular sac of the membranous labyrinth, occupying the elliptical recess and the area below it in the posterosuperior part of the vestibule. The ampullae of the semicircular ducts open into it, while the ductus utriculosaccularis extends from its anteromedial end to the ductus endolymphaticus. Also *utricle, utriculus vestibuli, alveus communis* (outmoded). **u. masculinus** PROSTATIC UTRICLE. **u. prostaticus** [NA] PROSTATIC UTRICLE. **u. vestibuli** UTRICULUS.

**UV** ultraviolet.

**uva ursi** \yoo′və ur′sē\ The dried leaves of *Arctostaphylos uva-ursi* of the Ericaceae family. It contains a poisonous phenolic glycoside, arbutin, and it has been mixed with tobacco for smoking as well as prepared as a tonic and infusion. It has antiseptic, diuretic, and astringent properties. Also *bearberry*.

**uvea** \yoo′vē·ə\ [Med L, fem. of *uveus* (from L *uva* grapes) pertaining to grapes, short for *tunica uvea* grapy coat, for its resemblance to the skin of a grape] TUNICA VASCULOSA BULBI.

**uveal** \yoo′vē·əl\ Pertaining to the uvea.

**uveitis** \yoo′vē·ī′tis\ [*uve(a)* + -ITIS] Inflammation of all or any part of the uveal tract. Also *iridochoroiditis, iridocyclochoroiditis, choroidocyclitis, chorioidoiritis.* Adj. uveitic. **anterior u.** IRIDOCYCLITIS. **granulomatous u.** A nodular, chronic inflammation of the choroid, ciliary body, or iris. It is usually caused by the presence of microorganisms. **heterochromic u.** Mild chronic inflammation of the ciliary body and iris, associated with a developmental deficiency of melanin in the affected eye. **lens-induced u.** Inflammation of the anterior segment of the eye resulting from sensitivity to proteins of the crystalline lens. Also *phacoanaphylactic uveitis.* **nongranulomatous u.** Inflammation of the iris and ciliary body without focal nodular deposits. It is usually attributed to immunologic or viral etiology. **phacoanaphylactic u.** LENS-INDUCED UVEITIS. **posterior u.** CHOROIDITIS. **sympathetic u.** SYMPATHETIC OPHTHALMIA. **tuberculous u.** Inflammation of the interior of the eye due to infection with *Mycobacterium tuberculosis.*

**uveolabyrinthitis** \yoo′vē·ōlab′ərinthī′tis\ A simultaneous inflammation of the uveal tract and the vestibular apparatus.

**uveomeningoencephalitis** \yoo′vē·ōməning′gō·ensefəlī′tis\ Uveitis associated with meningoencephalitis. Also *uveoneuraxitis.*

**uveoneuraxitis** \yoo′vē·ōn$^{y}$Ur′aksī′tis\ [ *uve(a)* + NEURAXITIS] UVEOMENINGOENCEPHALITIS.

**uveoparotid** \yoo′vē·ōpərät′id\ Pertaining to both the uveal tract and the parotid salivary gland.

**uveoparotitis** \yoo′vē·ōpar′ətī′tis\ HEERFORDT SYNDROME.

**uviofast** \yoo′vē·ōfast′\ [*u(ltra)vio(let)* + *fast*] UVIORESISTANT.

**uviol** \yoo′vē·ôl\ [*u(ltra)viol(et)*] Glass that is highly transparent to ultraviolet radiation.

**uvioresistant** \yoo′vē·ōrizis′tənt\ [*u(ltra)vio(let)* + *resistant*] Unaffected by ultraviolet light. Also *uviofast.*

**uviosensitive** \yoo′vē·ōsen′sətiv\ [*u(ltra)vio(let)* + *sensitive*] Sensitive to ultraviolet light.

**uvul-** \yoo′vyəl-\ UVULO-.

**uvula** \yoo′vyələ\ [Med L (dim. of L *uva* a grape, bunch of grapes), a little grape or bunch of grapes, the uvula] **1** A pendulous, fleshy mass. **2** UVULA PALATINA. **bifid u.** A midline cleft of the uvula that may extend into the soft palate. Also *cleft uvula.* **u. of bladder** UVULA VESICAE. **u. cerebelli** UVULA VERMIS. **u. of cerebellum** UVULA VERMIS. **cleft u.** BIFID UVULA. **Lieutaud's u.** UVULA VESICAE. **u. palatina** [NA] A median conical mass hanging from the lower border of the soft palate and projecting into the opening between the oral and the pharyngeal cavities. It consists of a fold of mucous membrane containing the two narrow, parallel musculus uvulae, one on each side of the midline, and connective tissue. It varies in length and size. Also *palatine uvula, uvula, pendulous palate* (outmoded), *plectrum* (outmoded), *staphyle* (obs.), *cion* (outmoded). **u. vermis** [NA] The portion of the vermis of the cerebellum located between the pyramis vermis and the nodulus. It lies in the midline between the two cerebellar tonsils on the inferior surface of the cerebellum, immediately behind the dorsolateral (posterolateral) fissure. Also *uvula cerebelli, uvula of cerebellum.* **u. vesicae** [NA] A median longitudinal elevation of the mucous membrane behind the internal urethral orifice in the neck of the urinary bladder. It is especially obvious in males past middle age and is produced by the median lobe of the prostate. Also *Lieutaud's uvula, uvula of bladder, Lieutaud's luette.*

**uvular** \yoo′vyələr\ Pertaining to the uvula. Also *staphyline.*

**uvulectomy** \yoo′vyəlek′təmē\ UVULOTOMY.

**uvulo-** \yoo′vyəlō-\ [L *uvula* (diminutive of *uva* grape) uvula] A combining form denoting uvula, especially the uvula palatina. Also *uvul-.*

**uvulonodular** \yoo′vyəlōnäd′yələr\ Denoting the uvula and nodulus regions of the cerebellar vermis, as *uvulonodular sulcus.*

**uvulotomy** \yoo′vyəlät′əmē\ [UVULO- + -TOMY] Amputation of the uvula, nowadays infrequently indicated. Also *uvulectomy, staphylotomy, staphylectomy.*

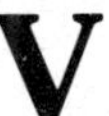

**V** **1** Symbol for the element, vanadium. **2** Symbol for the unit, volt. **3** Symbol for valine.

**V$_h$** The variable region of the immunoglobulin heavy chain.

**VA** visual acuity.

**vaccina** \vaksī′nə\ VACCINIA.

**vaccinable** \vak′sinəbl\ Susceptible to successful vaccination.

**vaccinal** \vak′sinəl\ **1** Pertaining to vaccine or vaccination. **2** Capable of conferring immunity or protection when administered by means of inoculation.

**vaccinate** \vak′sināt\ To give vaccine by injection in order to produce active immunity to disease.

**vaccination** \vak′sinā′shən\ The administration of vaccine by injection or orally in order to produce active immunity to disease. **autogenous v.** A vaccination that utilizes a vaccine prepared from organisms obtained from the patient himself. **booster v.** The administration of additional doses of vaccine, usually smaller than the initial dose, at specified intervals after the primary vaccination to maintain the individual's immunity to a disease. **jennerian v.** Vaccination with virus from cowpox lesions to immunize persons against smallpox.

# vaccine

**vaccine** \vak′sēn, -sin, vaksēn′\ [L *vaccinus* (from *vacca* a cow) of or derived from cows] An antigenic preparation used to produce active immunity to a disease. Vaccines may be living, attenuated strains of viruses or bacteria which give rise to clinically inapparent or trivial infections. Vaccines may also be killed or inactivated organisms or purified products derived from them. Formalin-inactivated toxins (toxoids) are used as vaccines against diphtheria and tetanus. Synthetic or genetically engineered antigens are currently being developed for use as vaccines. Also *vaccinum*. • The original vaccine was a preparation of cowpox (vaccinia) virus used to give immunity to smallpox. The English word *vaccine* was originally an adjective, meaning (like its Latin model) of or derived from cows. The substance used for inoculation was known as *vaccine matter, vaccine lymph*, or *vaccine virus* (1799). **adjuvant v.** A vaccine to which some form of immunopotentiator has been added, as a suspension on which antigens are adsorbed, a water-in-oil emulsion, or an emulsion containing killed mycobacteria (Freund's complete adjuvant) to increase antigenicity. **adsorbed diphtheria and tetanus toxoids and pertussis v.** A sterile suspension of the precipitate derived from treating a blend of diphtheria toxoid and tetanus toxoid with alum, aluminum hydroxide, or aluminum phosphate and mixing it with pertussis vaccine, a killed suspension of *Bordetella pertussis*. The three components are present in proportions sufficient to confer immunity to each of the diseases. The mixture is used especially for prophylaxis of diphtheria, tetanus, and pertussis in infants and young children. **adsorbed pertussis v.** A sterile bacterial fraction or suspension of *Bordetella pertussis* which has been precipitated or adsorbed by aluminum hydroxide or aluminum phosphate. It is given intramuscularly as an active immunizing agent against pertussis. **anthrax v.** A vaccine prepared from nonencapsulated spores of *Bacillus anthracis* and used to immunize persons at high risk of exposure to anthrax, as veterinarians and some industrial workers, and animals at risk of developing anthrax. **antirabic v.** RABIES VACCINE. **antirabies v. of Pasteur** A vaccine prepared from a living attenuated rabies virus. According to the original method advocated by Pasteur, treatment of rabies consisted of daily subcutaneous injections of a suspension of rabbit spinal cord in physiologic serum over a course of 15–18 days, using progressively younger and therefore more virulent spinal cord. Preparations of desiccated spinal cords have been generally abandoned in favor of phenolized rabies vaccines such as Fermi's and Semple's vaccines, although variants of Pasteur's type of rabies vaccination are still used in some countries. Also *Pasteur vaccine*. **antityphoid v.** TYPHOID VACCINE. **attenuated v.** A live bacterial or viral vaccine, carrying mutations that eliminate its pathogenicity but not its ability to elicit a protective immune response. **attenuated live measles virus v.** A sterile preparation of an attenuated line of measles virus grown in a chick embryo cell culture. It causes a mild, noncommunicable infection in most individuals after a single dose, which produces an immunity to measles that lasts at least 10 years. **autogenous v.** Bacteria (usually staphylococci) cultured from a patient, killed, and injected in the hope of eliciting strain-specific immunity. **BCG v.** A preparation containing a dried, living culture of the Calmette-Guérin strain of *Mycobacterium tuberculosis* var. *bovis* (bacille Calmette-Guérin). It is used for immunization against tuberculosis and is usually administered intracutaneously. Also *Calmette's vaccine, tuberculosis vaccine*. **Calmette's v.** BCG VACCINE. **Castañeda's v.** Typhus vaccine prepared according to Castañeda's rat-lung method. **Castellani's v.** TYPHOID AND PARATYPHOID VACCINE. **cholera v.** A sterile suspension of specific strains of killed *Vibrio cholerae* used to produce immunity to cholera. **cowpox v.** Smallpox vaccine obtained from cultures grown on the skin of cows. See also SMALLPOX VACCINE. **Cox v.** TYPHUS VACCINE. **Danysz v.** A preparation combining cultures of the normal human bowel flora. The vaccine was thought by some to exert an antianaphylactic effect in certain allergic states. It is now obsolete. **diphtheria v.** DIPHTHERIA TOXOID. **diphtheria and tetanus v.** An active immunizing agent against diphtheria and tetanus which consists of a mixture of diphtheria toxoid and tetanus toxoid. **diphtheria and tetanus toxoids and pertussis v.** An active immunizing agent against diphtheria, tetanus, and pertussis which consists of a mixture of diphtheria toxoid and tetanus toxoid (prepared using formaldehyde as the toxoiding agent) and a sterile suspension of killed *Bordetella pertussis*. Also *DPT vaccine, triple vaccine*. **DPT v.** DIPHTHERIA AND TETANUS TOXOIDS AND PERTUSSIS VACCINE. **duck embryo v.** A rabies vaccine prepared from rabies virus grown in duck embryonic tissue, inactivated with beta-propiolactone, and administered in a series of 14 daily intramuscular injections to persons exposed to rabies. This vaccine was widely used for 20 years but has been discontinued in the United States in favor of the more efficacious human diploid cell vaccine. Abbr. DEV **Durand's v.** A typhoid-paratyphoid vaccine containing a microbial suspension with an admixture of 1:1000 diethyldithiocarbamate to potassium. **Durand and Giroud v.** A vaccine against epidemic louse-borne typhus prepared from a culture of *Rickettsia prowazekii* grown on the lungs of white mice or rabbits and treated with formol. Vaccination consists of three subcutaneous injections of 1 ml each eight days apart, a booster injection being necessary one year after primary vaccination. The duration of immunity obtained is less than one year. **epidemic typhus v.** TYPHUS VACCINE. **Felix v.** A typhoid-paratyphoid vaccine containing bacteria inactivated by alcohol. **Fermi's v.** A mixed attenuated-inactivated rabies vaccine containing a suspension of 5% sheep cerebral material inoculated with fixed rabies virus in an aqueous medium that contains at the outset 1% phenol, (reduced to 0.5% in the finished vaccine). Though habitually classed among inactivated vaccines, it includes, along with the phenol-inactivated virus, titrated quantities of live virus. **Flury v.** An antirabies vaccine of chick embryo origin, of which there are two types: low egg passage (LEP) vaccine used in the vaccination of dogs, and high egg passage (HEP) vaccine used in the vaccination of other animals. **Haffkine's v.** 1 A cholera vaccine prepared from a killed culture of *Vibrio cholerae*. It is administered in two injections 7–10 days apart. The first inoculation is weaker than the second. 2 A bubonic plague vaccine prepared from a killed culture of *Yersinia pestis*. **heterologous v.** A vaccine based on one organism and used to protect another (for example, vaccinia virus and smallpox). *Older term*. **human diploid cell v.** A rabies vaccine prepared from rabies virus grown in human diploid cell culture and inactivated. It is highly immunogenic and causes few reactions. This vaccine is now the only rabies vaccine licensed for use in man in the United States. **humanized v.** A smallpox vaccine prepared from material obtained from vaccinia vesicles in humans. **Idanov and Fadeewa v.** A vaccine against measles prepared from attenuated virus grown in chick embryos. It is administered intradermally or subcutaneously. **influenza v.** A killed or inactivated sterile suspension of influenza virus grown in embryonated chicken eggs. Specific antigenic types of influenza viruses A and B are used according to the type of influenza expected to be prevalent at a given time. The vaccine may be given intramuscularly or subcutaneously to enhance resistance to influenza virus infection. Attenuated living strains of influenza virus have also been used as vaccines. Also *influenza virus vaccine.* **jennerian v.** SMALLPOX VACCINE. **Kelev's v.** A rabies vaccine prepared from a live virus (Kelev strain) and analogous to the Flury HEP vaccine. **Kolle's v.** 1 A vaccine against plague prepared from sterile suspensions of *Yersinia pestis.* 2 A cholera vaccine prepared from killed cholera vibrios. **Lépine's v.** A poliomyelitis vaccine analogous to the Salk vaccine and containing virus inactivated first by formol, then by $\beta$-propiolactone. It is administered subcutaneously in three injections, the second injection 6 weeks after the first and the third 2 to 3 months after the second. Vaccination is completed with booster injection given 1 year later. **live v.** Any vaccine containing live microorganisms or viruses whose virulence has been attenuated. **live measles, mumps, and rubella virus v.** A trivalent vaccine that contains an aqueous suspension of live, attenuated strains of measles virus, mumps virus, and rubella virus grown in chick embryo or duck embryo cells. The preparation is supplied as a lyophilized powder to be reconstituted immediately before use by adding a sterile diluent. It is used to obtain active immunization in children against all three viral diseases at the same time. Also *MMR vaccine.* **live mumps v.** A suspension of the Jeryl Lynn strain of mumps virus grown in chick embryo tissue culture. It is given subcutaneously to children older than 15 months and to adults. It brings about active immunity from a single injection and continuing protection against mumps for at least 10 years. **live oral poliovirus v.** POLIOMYELITIS VACCINE. **Lustig-Galeotti v.** A plague vaccine consisting of *Yersinia pestis* and caustic soda neutralized by acetic acid. **measles v.** A live, attenuated measles virus vaccine obtained from cultures of the virus grown in chick embryos or on canine renal tissue. It is administered subcutaneously and confers active immunity against measles. **MMR v.** LIVE MEASLES, MUMPS, AND RUBELLA VIRUS VACCINE. **monovalent v.** A vaccine made from a single dominant antigen of a given pathogen. Also *univalent vaccine.* **multivalent v.** A vaccine which contains antigens derived from several strains within a single species of pathogenic organisms. Also *polyvalent vaccine.* **mumps v.** A live, attenuated mumps virus vaccine obtained from cultures of the virus. It is administered subcutaneously and confers active immunity against mumps. **paratyphoid v.** A vaccine prepared from killed cultures of one or more of the bacilli causing paratyphoid fever, *Salmonella paratyphi A, S. schottmuelleri,* and *S. hirschfeldii.* It is given prophylactically to confer immunity against paratyphoid fever. **Pasteur v.** ANTIRABIES VACCINE OF PASTEUR. **pertussis v.** A sterile suspension or fraction of killed *Bordetella pertussis* administered to confer active immunity to pertussis. It may be combined with diphtheria and tetanus toxoids in a single trivalent injection. Also *whooping cough vaccine.* **poliomyelitis v.** 1 A sterile suspension of three types of inactivated polioviruses. The viruses are grown separately in monkey renal tissue cultures, and are then inactivated and combined. The vaccine is administered subcutaneously and confers active immunity against poliomyelitis. Also *Salk vaccine.* 2 A suspension of one or a combination of three types of live, attenuated polioviruses propagated separately in monkey kidney tissue culture. The vaccine is administered orally and is an active immunizing agent against poliomyelitis. This vaccine appears to be more efficacious than the killed vaccine in preventing the spread of epidemic poliomyelitis. Also *Sabin vaccine, live oral poliovirus vaccine.* **polyvalent v.** MULTIVALENT VACCINE. ***Pseudomonas* v.** A vaccine made from the antigens of several strains of *Pseudomonas aeruginosa* and used prophylactically to immunize patients actively against future infection with *Pseudomonas* organisms. Its effectiveness in improving the chances for survival from massive burns is controversial. **rabies v.** A sterile suspension of killed, fixed rabies virus obtained from duck embryo tissue previously infected with fixed rabies virus. The virus is inactivated by $\beta$-propiolactone. Rabies vaccine is also available prepared in human diploid cell tissue culture for those allergic to duck embryo vaccine or who do not develop adequate antibody titer to the latter. Also *antirabic vaccine.* **Rocky Mountain spotted fever v.** A sterile suspension of killed *Rickettsia rickettsii* which is prepared by growing the organism on chick embryos. The vaccine is administered subcutaneously as an active immunizing agent against Rocky Mountain spotted fever. However it has been shown to be of dubious value, conferring only limited protection against even small doses of infective rickettsiae. It is seldom used. **Sabin v.** POLIOMYELITIS VACCINE. **Salk v.** POLIOMYELITIS VACCINE. **Sauer's v.** A pertussis vaccine derived from freshly isolated strains of *Bordetella pertussis.* **smallpox v.** A suspension of living vaccinia virus obtained from cultures of a virus grown on the skin of vaccinated calves or sheep or on embryonated chick membranes. Available as a liquid or a freeze-dried preparation, the vaccine provides long-term active immunity against smallpox. In effective immunization, active viral infection is initiated in the skin by gently puncturing the skin with the side of a needle through a suspension of live virus. Also *jennerian vaccine, vaccinum vacciniae, vaccinum variolae, variolovaccine.* • This vaccine is no longer used, since smallpox has been eradicated throughout the world. **Spencer-Parker v.** Rocky Mountain spotted fever vaccine prepared from ticks infected with *Rickettsia rickettsii.* **staphylococcus v.** A vaccine prepared from cultures of one or more strains of *Staphylococcus.* It has been used in the treatment of some staphylococcal infections, especially recurrent furunculosis. **streptococcus v.** A vaccine prepared from cultures of *Streptococcus* species. **Strong's v.** A cholera vaccine prepared from nucleoproteins of *Vibrio cholerae.* **TAB v.** TYPHOID AND PARATYPHOID VACCINE. **tetanus v.** TETANUS TOXOID. **triple v.** DIPHTHERIA AND TETANUS TOXOIDS AND PERTUSSIS VACCINE. **trivalent v.** A vaccine with three strains or types of immunizing agent. For example, trivalent polio vaccine consists of polio immunotypes 1, 2, and 3. **tuberculosis v.** BCG VACCINE. **tularemia v.** A vaccine against tularemia prepared from cultures of *Francisella tularensis* inactivated by phenol, or after extraction by acetone, or from bacterial strains of little virulence. The protection conferred by the vaccine is not absolute. **typhoid v.** A sterile suspension of heat- or chemical-killed *Salmonella typhi* in a diluent containing not less than one billion typhoid bacilli per milliliter. An active immunizing agent against typhoid fever, it is administered subcutaneously to persons at high risk for the disease (for example, persons in or traveling to endemic areas, health care personnel caring for typhoid fever patients). The degree of immunity conferred is not great. Oral vaccines of killed or attenuated typhoid bacilli have also been used. Also *antityphoid vaccine, typhobacterin.* **typhoid and paratyphoid v.** A vaccine prepared from sterile suspensions of killed *Salmonella typhi, S. paratyphi A,* and *S. schottmuelleri* (formerly *S. paratyphi B.*) and administered subcutaneously as an active immunizing agent to persons at high risk for typhoid and paratyphoid fevers.

Also *typhoparatyphoid vaccine, TAB vaccine, vaccinum typhosum et paratyphosum, Castellani's vaccine.* **typhoid-paratyphoid A and B, and cholera v.** A mixture of sterile suspensions of killed *Salmonella typhi, S. paratyphi A, S. schottmuelleri* (formerly *S. paratyphi B*), and *Vibrio cholerae.* It is administered subcutaneously in an effort to confer immunity to typhoid and paratyphoid fevers and cholera in persons at high risk for these diseases. **typho-paratyphoid v.** TYPHOID AND PARATYPHOID VACCINE. **typhus v.** A sterile suspension of killed *Rickettsia prowazekii,* usually grown in embryonated chicken eggs. An active immunizing agent against epidemic louse-borne typhus, it is administered subcutaneously. Also *Cox vaccine, epidemic typhus vaccine.* **univalent v.** MONOVALENT VACCINE. **varicella v.** Live attenuated varicella virus of the Oka strain, developed in Japan as a vaccine against varicella (chickenpox) and demonstrated to be effective in conferring protection as late as three days after exposure to infection and in children with malignancies. The vaccine has been shown to be 100% efficacious in preventing varicella in healthy children before exposure. **Weigl v.** A type of typhus vaccine prepared by infecting lice rectally with rickettsiae and emulsifying the louse intestines in a solution of phenol and sodium chloride. **whooping cough v.** PERTUSSIS VACCINE. **yellow fever v.** A vaccine prepared from live, attenuated yellow fever virus grown in chick embryos and then freeze-dried. The reconstituted solution is administered subcutaneously to produce long-lasting immunity to yellow fever. **Zinsser-Castañeda v.** A typhus vaccine used in southern Mexico and derived from a combination of *Rickettsia prowazekii* and *R. mooseri* (murine rickettsiae).

**vaccinia** \vaksin′ē·ə\ [L *vaccin(us)* (from *vacca* a cow) pertaining to cows + -IA] An acute infection caused by the vaccinia virus and characterized by a localized pustular eruption. The infection stimulates antibody production which confers immunity to smallpox. A live vaccinia virus preparation is used as an active immunizing agent against smallpox. When a viral infection of this nature occurs in cattle it is called cowpox. Also *vaccina.* **chronic progressive v.** VACCINIA NECROSUM. **v. gangrenosa** VACCINIA NECROSUM. **generalized v.** A systemic infection which may occur about ten days after smallpox vaccination. The vaccinia virus appears in the bloodstream and a widespread vesicular rash erupts but leaves no scars. Also *vaccinid, vacciniola.* **v. necrosum** A severe complication of smallpox vaccination characterized by progressive necrosis at the vaccination site and at metastatic sites due to unchecked viral growth. It usually occurs in immunologically deficient subjects. Also *vaccinia gangrenosa, progressive vaccinia, chronic progressive vaccinia.* **progressive v.** VACCINIA NECROSUM.

**vaccinial** \vaksin′ē·əl\ Pertaining to or of the nature of vaccinia.

**vaccinid** \vak′sinid\ GENERALIZED VACCINIA.

**vacciniform** \vaksin′ifôrm\ [*vaccini(a)* + -FORM] Vaccinialike: said especially of a rash.

**vacciniola** \vak′sinē′ələ\ GENERALIZED VACCINIA.

**vaccinoid** \vak′sinoid\ Resembling vaccinia.

**vaccinum** \vaksī′nəm\ VACCINE. **v. typhosum et paratyphosum** TYPHOID AND PARATYPHOID VACCINE. **v. vacciniae** SMALLPOX VACCINE. **v. variolae** SMALLPOX VACCINE.

**vacuolation** \vak′yoo·əlā′shən\ The formation of development of vacuoles. Also *vacuolization.*

**vacuole** \vak′yoo·ōl\ [French (from L *vacu(us)* empty + *-ole* -OLE) a small empty space, vacuole] **1** A minute clear region in the cytoplasm of a cell. **2** A membrane-limited chamber in the cytoplasm of a cell in which fluid, storage products, or waste products may be secreted. Also *tonoplast* (obs.). Adj. vacuolar. **autophagic v.** A type of secondary lysosome which is formed as a primary lysosome engulfs a portion of the cytoplasm of a cell and in which the cytoplasmic material is digested. This process is common in cells during tissue regression and programmed cell death. **contractile v.** An osmoregulatory and possibly excretory organelle in free-living freshwater protozoa that are hypertonic to their environment. The action of the contractile vacuole is to take in the excess water and pump it out of the organism via fine ducts to the outside. Among parasitic protozoa, the ciliate *Balantidium,* parasitic suctorians, and trypanosome flagellates retain their contractile vacuoles. **digestive v.** SECONDARY LYSOSOME. **food v.** A bubblelike cytoplasmic structure seen in many protozoans, in which food inclusions are digested. **plasmocrine v.** A small crystaloid-containing vacuole in a secretory cell. **rhagiocrine v.** A small colloid-containing vacuole in a secretory cell. **secretory v.** A small, membrane-bound cytoplasmic vacuole originating in the Golgi apparatus. It fuses with the inside of the cell membrane and then opens to the exterior by the process of exocytosis. Also *secretory granule.* **water v.** A membrane-bound droplet of water located in the cell cytoplasm.

**vacuolization** \vak′yoo·əlīzā′shən\ VACUOLATION.

**Vacutainer** A vacuum-evacuated, stoppered test tube that is used with a specially adapted needle to collect blood during a phlebotomy. A trade name.

**vacuum** \vak′yoo·əm\ [L (substantive from *vacuum,* neut. of *vacuus* void, empty), an empty place] A space devoid or nearly devoid of gas or any matter.

**vacuumizing** \vak′yoo·əmī′zing\ The mixing of plaster of Paris or the firing of porcelain in a partial vacuum in order to reduce porosity.

**vadum** \vā′dəm\ [L, a shallow, shoal, ford] A gyrus, buried beneath the surface of the cerebral cortex, that forms an elevation on the floor of a cerebral sulcus, thereby altering the depth of that sulcus. An example of such an elevation may be observed in the floor of the central sulcus which, when opened, is seen to be of varying depths because of a group of small buried gyri that interlock with each other.

**vagal** \vā′gəl\ Denoting the vagus nerve.

**vagectomy** \vājek′təmē\ VAGOTOMY.

**vagi** \vā′gī, -jī\ Plural of VAGUS.

**vagin-** \vaj′in-\ VAGINO-.

**vagina** \vəjī′nə\ [L, a sheath, scabbard, the husk of grain] (*pl.* vaginae) **1** A sheath or any structure resembling a sheath. **2** [NA] The lowest part of the female genital tract, being a very dilatable fibromuscular tube lined with stratified epithelium and extending from the cervix uteri to the vestibule, where it opens posteroinferiorly to the external urethral orifice. It serves as the organ of copulation, directed posterosuperiorly to meet the uterus at an angle of more than ninety degrees. **bipartite v.** VAGINA SEPTA. **v. bulbi** [NA] The thin fibrous sheath that surrounds the eyeball from the optic nerve to the sclerocorneal junction, forming a socket for the eyeball, from which it is separated by the episcleral space. Posteriorly it separates the eyeball from the orbital fat. The sheath fuses with the sclera, both posterior to the sclerocorneal junction and where the optic nerve, posterior ciliary arteries, and ciliary nerves pierce it. It sends tubular sheaths over the extraocular muscles as they pass through it to their insertions. It is thickened inferiorly to form the suspensory ligament of the eye. Also *sheath of* *eyeball, bulbar fascia, Tenon's capsule, bulbar sheath, fascia of Tenon, Tenon's membrane.* **v. carotica fasciae cervicalis** [NA] An extension of the deep cervical fascia surrounding the internal and common carotid arteries, the internal jugular vein, the vagus nerve, and components of ansa cervicalis. Also *carotid sheath.* **v. cellulosa** *Seldom used* PERINEURIUM. **v. cordis** *Outmoded* PERICARDIUM. **embryonic v.** The more caudal portion of the fused paramesonephric ducts where it reaches the urogenital sinus in the early embryo. This primitive vagina gains a lumen, the uterovaginal canal, and by a complicated process involving bilateral sinovaginal bulbs eventually acquires a new lining which is probably almost entirely endodermal. **v. externa nervi optici** [NA] The dense collagenous and elastic outermost sheath surrounding the optic nerve, continuous with the dura mater around the brain. It is about 0.3–0.5 mm in thickness and blends anteriorly with the sclera. Blood vessels from the ophthalmic artery penetrate this external sheath to reach the internal vascular sheath and supply the optic nerve and retina. Also *external sheath of optic nerve, dural sheath, outer meningeal sheath of optic nerve, fibrous sheath of optic nerve.* **vaginae fibrosae digitorum manus** [NA] Transverse and oblique fibrous bands arching anterior to the superficial and deep flexor tendons and synovial sheaths of the fingers to be attached to the margins of the phalanges and to the palmar ligaments of the interphalangeal joints so as to form osseofibrous canals. Also *fibrous sheaths of fingers, fibrous sheaths of digits of hand, fibrous flexor sheaths of tendons of fingers, tendinous sheaths of flexor muscles of fingers, fibrous tendon sheaths of muscles of fingers.* **vaginae fibrosae digitorum pedis** [NA] Transverse and oblique fibrous bands arching below the tendons and synovial sheaths of the long and short flexors of the toes to be attached to the margins of the phalanges so as to form osseofibrous canals. Also *fibrous sheaths of toes, fibrous sheaths of digits of foot, fibrous flexor sheaths of tendons of toes, tendinous sheaths of flexor muscles of toes, fibrous tendon sheaths of muscles of toes.* **v. fibrosa tendinis** [NA] A strong arched band of fibrous tissue attached to bone to form an osseofibrous canal for a tendon and its synovial sheath. Also *fibrous sheath of tendon.* **v. interna nervi optici** [NA] Internal sheath of the optic nerve. The closely investing pia-arachnoid internal vascular covering of the optic nerve from which septa pass into the nerve. Additionally, the vagina interna nervi optici also invests the central retinal artery as far as the optic disc, and the central retinal vein from the optic disc to its point of exit from the optic nerve. Also *inner meningeal sheath of optic nerve, internal sheath of optic nerve.* **v. musculi recti abdominis** [NA] A fibrous sheath formed by the aponeuroses of the muscles of the anterolateral abdominal wall where the aponeurosis of the internal oblique muscle splits into two at the lateral margin of the rectus abdominis muscle, the anterior sheet fusing with the aponeurosis of the external oblique to form the anterior lamina, and the posterior sheet fusing with the aponeurosis of transversus abdominis to form the posterior lamina, the two laminae surrounding each rectus abdominis muscle and fusing in the midline to form linea alba. Also *rectus sheath, sheath of rectus abdominis muscle.* **v. musculorum peroneorum communis** [NA] A single synovial sheath surrounding both the peroneus longus and brevis tendons from about two inches above the lateral malleolus, passing deep to the superior extensor retinaculum and then separating around each tendon above the trochlea peronealis on the calcaneus. Also *common sheath of tendons of peroneal muscles, synovial sheath of the peronei, common peroneal bursa.* **vaginae nervi optici** The external and internal meningeal sheaths of the optic nerve, which are continuations around that nerve of the dural and pial meningeal coverings of the brain. Between these two sheaths is found an extension of the fine arachnoidea, deep to which is located the intervaginal space (spatia intervaginalia), which is continuous with the subarachnoid space. Also *meningeal sheaths of optic nerve, sheaths of optic nerve.* See also VAGINA INTERNA NERVI OPTICI, VAGINA EXTERNA NERVI OPTICI. **v. processus styloidei** [NA] The lateral part of the lower border of the tympanic part of the temporal bone which splits to enclose the root of the styloid process. Also *sheath of styloid process, vaginal process of styloid, vaginal process of temporal bone, vaginal process.* **v. septa** A partial or complete partitioning of the vagina into two lumina by a sagittally oriented septum. Also *bipartite vagina.* **vaginae synoviales** [NA] Thin, double-layered sheaths or synovial sacs usually surrounding tendons, where they lie on bony surfaces or in osseofibrous tunnels and containing synovial fluid to facilitate movement of tendons. Also *synovial sheaths.* **vaginae synoviales digitorum manus** [NA] The synovial sheaths surrounding the tendons of the fingers to their insertions. **vaginae synoviales digitorum pedis** [NA] The synovial sheaths that surround the tendons of the toes to their insertions. **vaginae synoviales tendinum digitorum manus** [NA] The synovial sheaths enveloping the tendons of the long flexors of the fingers to their points of insertion. Those of the middle three fingers commence opposite the respective heads of the metacarpal bones. **vaginae synoviales tendinum digitorum pedis** [NA] The synovial sheaths surrounding the tendons of the long and short flexors of the toes and extending from the heads of the metatarsal bones to the insertions of the tendons. Also *synovial sheaths of tendons of foot.* **v. synovialis communis musculorum flexorum** [NA] The common synovial sheath for the superficial and deep flexor tendons of the medial four fingers as they pass through the carpal tunnel, commencing about one inch proximal to flexor retinaculum and terminating about the middle of the palm except in the case of the sheath for the little finger which extends along it to the terminal phalanx. Also *common synovial flexor sheath, ulnar bursa.* **v. synovialis musculi obliqui superioris** [NA] A delicate synovial sheath surrounding the tendon of the superior oblique muscle of the orbit as it passes through the trochlea. Also *synovial trochlear bursa, synovial sheath of superior oblique muscle.* **v. synovialis tendinis** [NA] A thin, double-layered sheath, or synovial sac, enveloping a tendon, usually where it crosses a bony surface or lies in an osseofibrous tunnel, and containing synovial fluid to facilitate movement of the tendon. Also *synovial sheath of tendon, theca tendinis.* **v. synovialis tendinis musculi flexoris carpi radialis** [NA] The synovial sheath surrounding the tendon of the flexor carpi radialis muscle as it passes through the flexor retinaculum and in the groove on the trapezium bone. Also *bursa musculi flexoris carpi radialis, bursa of flexor carpi radialis muscle, synovial sheath of flexor carpi radialis.* **v. synovialis tendinis musculi flexoris hallucis longi** [NA] The synovial sheath surrounding the tendon of the flexor hallucis longus muscle and extending from the posterior aspect of the medial malleolus deep to the flexor retinaculum to the sole of the foot, where it ends as it is crossed by the tendon of flexor digitorum longus and then forms again from the middle of the first metatarsal bone to its insertion. Also *synovial sheath of tendon of flexor hallucis longus.* **v. synovialis tendinis musculi tibialis posterioris** [NA] The synovial sheath surrounding the tendon of the tibialis posterior muscle and extending from just above the medial malleolus to the insertion of the tendon. Also *tendon sheath of posterior tibial muscle, synovial sheath of tibialis posterior.* **v. tendinis intertubercularis** [NA] A sheath, derived from the synovial membrane of the shoulder joint, that surrounds the long head of the biceps muscle as it emerges from the capsule deep to the transverse humeral ligament and passes down in the intertubercular sulcus deep to a fibrous expansion of the tendon of the pectoralis major muscle. Also *synovial sheath of intertubercular groove, synovial sheath of bicipital groove, intertubercular bursa, bursa of biceps brachii muscle.* **v. tendinis musculi extensoris carpi ulnaris** [NA] The synovial sheath surrounding the tendon of the extensor carpi ulnaris muscle, commencing proximal to and passing deep to the extensor retinaculum to end at the insertion of the tendon. Also *synovial sheath of tendon of extensor carpi ulnaris.* **v. tendinis musculi extensoris digiti minimi** [NA] The synovial sheath surrounding the tendon of the extensor digiti minimi muscle, commencing proximal to and passing deep to the extensor retinaculum to end about midway along the fifth metacarpal bone. Also *synovial sheath of extensor digiti minimi.* **v. tendinis musculi extensoris hallucis longi** [NA] The synovial sheath surrounding the tendon of the extensor hallucis longus muscle, extending from above the inferior extensor retinaculum to the dorsum of the foot near the tarsometatarsal joint. Also *synovial sheath of extensor hallucis longus.* **v. tendinis musculi extensoris pollicis longi** [NA] The synovial sheath surrounding the tendon of the extensor pollicis longus, extending from just proximal to the extensor retinaculum to about the middle of the dorsum of the first metacarpal bone. **v. tendinis musculi flexoris pollicis longi** [NA] The synovial sheath surrounding the tendon of the flexor pollicis longus muscle passing deep to the flexor retinaculum from about one inch proximal to it to end at the insertion of the tendon. Occasionally the sheath communicates with the common sheath of the digital flexors deep to the retinaculum. Also *synovial sheath of flexor pollicis longus, radial bursa.* **v. tendinis musculi peronei longi plantaris** [NA] A synovial sheath of the tendon of the peroneus longus muscle that commences in the peroneal groove of the cuboid bone and ends near the medial margin of the long plantar ligament. Also *plantar tendinous sheath of long peroneal muscle, sheath of plantar tendon of long peroneal muscle.* **v. tendinis musculi tibialis anterioris** [NA] The synovial sheath surrounding the tendon of the tibialis anterior muscle and extending from above the superior extensor retinaculum to the level of the talonavicular joint. Also *tendon sheath of anterior tibial muscle, synovial sheath of tibialis anterior.* **v. tendinum musculi extensoris digitorum pedis longi** [NA] The synovial sheath surrounding the tendons of the extensor digitorum longus and peroneus tertius muscles and extending from above the inferior extensor retinaculum to the level of the cuneiform bones. Also *synovial sheath of tendons of extensor digitorum longus of foot, tendon sheath of long extensor muscles of toes.* **v. tendinum musculi flexoris digitorum pedis longi** [NA] The synovial sheath surrounding the tendon of the flexor digitorum longus muscle and extending from the posterior aspect of the medial malleolus to the point where it crosses the flexor hallucis longus muscle below the navicular bone. Also *tendon sheath of long flexor muscles of toes, synovial sheath of flexor digitorum longus of foot.* **v. tendinum musculorum abductoris longi et extensoris brevis pollicis** [NA] The synovial sheath surrounding each of the tendons of the abductor pollicis longus and extensor pollicis brevis muscles, often communicating with each other as they pass through the same compartment of the extensor retinaculum and end at the base of the first metacarpal bone. Also *synovial sheath of tendons of abductor pollicis longus and extensor pollicis brevis.* **v. tendinum musculorum extensoris digitorum et extensoris indicis** [NA] The synovial sheath surrounding the tendons of the extensor digitorum and extensor indicis muscles as they pass through a single tunnel of the extensor retinaculum to end near the middle of the dorsum of the hand. Also *synovial sheath for tendons of extensor digitorum and extensor indicis.* **v. tendinum musculorum extensorum carpi radialium** [NA] The synovial sheath surrounding each of the tendons of the extensor carpi radialis longus and brevis muscles as they pass deep to the extensor retinaculum where they usually communicate or fuse with the sheath of the extensor pollicis longus as it crosses superficial to them. Also *synovial sheath of extensor carpi radialis longus and brevis muscles.*

**vaginae** \vajī′nē\ Plural of VAGINA.

**vaginal** \vaj′ənəl\ **1** Pertaining to the vagina or any sheath. **2** Having the characteristics of a sheath.

**vaginalectomy** \vaj′inəlek′təmē\ VAGINECTOMY.

**vaginalitis** \vaj′inəlī′tis\ [*(tunica) vaginal(is testis)* + -ITIS] Inflammation of the tunica vaginalis testis.

**vaginapexy** \vaj′inəpek′sē\ [VAGINA + -PEXY] COLPOPEXY.

**vaginectomy** \vaj′inek′təmē\ [VAGIN- + -ECTOMY] **1** COLPECTOMY. **2** Surgical removal of all or part of the tunica vaginalis testis. Also *vaginalectomy.*

**vaginismus** \vaj′əniz′məs\ [VAGIN- + L *-ismus* -ISM] Painful spasm of the vagina, typically during coitus. Also *colpismus, perineal spasm, colpospasm, vulvismus.* **perineal v.** Vaginismus due to spasm of the perineal muscles. Also *superficial vaginismus, vulvar vaginismus.* **posterior v.** Vaginismus due to spasm of the levator ani. **superficial v.** PERINEAL VAGINISMUS. **vulvar v.** PERINEAL VAGINISMUS.

**vaginitis** \vaj′ənī′tis\ [VAGIN- + -ITIS] **1** Inflammation of the vagina; colpitis. **2** Inflammation of a sheath or an investing membrane. **v. adhaesiva** ADHESIVE VAGINITIS. **adhesive v.** Inflammation that results in obliteration of the vaginal mucosa, with scarring and attachment of opposing surfaces. Also *vaginitis adhaesiva.* **atrophic v.** Inflammation that appears when there is deficient estrogen effect on the vaginal mucosa. Also *postmenstrual vaginitis, senile vaginitis.* **v. cystica** Vaginitis with gaseous blebs under the mucosa. **desquamative inflammatory v.** A rare type of inflammation occurring in menstruating women in which the appearance is similar to an atrophic vaginitis. **diphtheritic v.** Inflammation of the vagina caused by *Corynebacterium diphtheriae.*. **emphysematous v.** Vaginal inflammation associated with gaseous blebs under the mucous membrane. Also *emphysematous colpitis.* **exfoliative v.** Vaginal inflammation associated with increased shedding of cells. **gonococcal v.** Vaginitis resulting from infection with gonococci (*Neisseria gonorrhoeae*), occurring usually in premenstrual girls. **granular v.** Vaginal inflammation in which the rugae are swollen and infiltrated with plasma cells and lymphocytes. Also *colpitis granulosa.* **mucous v.** Vaginal inflammation associated with mucous secretion from the cervix. **postmenstrual v.** ATROPHIC VAGINITIS. **pneumocystic v.** A vaginitis associated with multiple gas-filled cysts in the wall of the vagina. It may be caused by aerobic or anaerobic bacteria. Also *elytropneumatosis.* **senile v.** ATROPHIC VAGINITIS. **v. testis** PERIDIDYMITIS. **tri-**

**chomonas v.** Vaginitis caused by the parasite *Trichomonas vaginalis,* which may result in a frothy, purulent, yellow to greenish mucoidal exudate, pruritis, and a foul odor. The *Trichomonas* infection is common and widespread among males, usually as an asymptomatic urethritis, as well as among females, in whom it is also usually asymptomatic, especially at normal vaginal pH levels, but it may produce the acute form of vaginitis in heavy infections or where there is an altered vaginal flora and reduced acidity.

**vagino-** \vaj′inō-\ [L *vagina* sheath] A combining form denoting vagina. Also *vagin-*.

**vaginocele** \vaj′inōsēl′\ [VAGINO- + -CELE[1]] COLPOCELE.

**vaginodynia** \-din′ē·ə\ COLPODYNIA.

**vaginofixation** \-fiksā′shən\ **1** COLPOPEXY. **2** COLPOPLASTY.

**vaginography** \vaj′inäg′rəfē\ Roentgenography of the vagina after instillation of a radiopaque contrast medium into the vagina.

**vaginolabial** \-lā′bē·əl\ Pertaining to the vagina and labia.

**vaginometer** \vaj′inäm′ətər\ [VAGINO- + -METER] An instrument for measuring vaginal dimensions.

**vaginopathy** \vaj′inäp′əthē\ [VAGINO- + -PATHY] An abnormality of the vagina.

**vaginoperineal** \-per′inē′əl\ Relating to the vagina and perineum.

**vaginoperineorrhaphy** \-per′inē·ôr′əfē\ COLPOPERINEORRHAPHY.

**vaginopexy** \vaj′inōpek′sē\ COLPOPEXY.

**vaginoplasty** \vaj′inōplas′tē\ COLPOPLASTY.

**vaginoscope** \vaj′inōskōp′\ [VAGINO- + -SCOPE] An instrument used to inspect the vagina, usually in children. Usage would include searching for foreign bodies or sources of bleeding.

**vaginoscopy** \vaj′inäs′kəpē\ [VAGINO- + -SCOPY] Viewing of the vagina with a magnifying lens or after special staining; colposcopy.

**vaginotomy** \vaj′inät′əmē\ [VAGINO- + -TOMY] COLPOTOMY.

**vaginovulvar** \-vul′vər\ VULVOVAGINAL.

***Vaginulus plebeius*** \vəjin′yələs plē′bē·əs\ A gastropod slug found in Costa Rica which serves as the intermediate host of *Morerastrongylus costaricensis,* cause of human abdominal angiostrongylosis. The nematode is normally found in various wild rodents but can infect man when infected slugs are accidentally ingested.

**vagitus** \vəjī′təs\ [L (from *vagire* to wail, howl, bleat) a wail, howl] The cry of a newborn infant. *Older term.*

**vago-** \vā′gō-\ [L *vagus* wandering] A combining form denoting the vagus nerve.

**vagoaccessorius** \-ak′sesôr′ē·əs\ Denoting the vagus nerve, along with the medullary root of the accessory nerve.

**vagoglossopharyngeal** \-gläs′ōfərin′jē·əl\ Denoting, collectively, the vagus and glossopharyngeal nerves, their roots, their motor nuclei of origin, or their sensory nuclei in the brainstem.

**vagolysis** \vāgäl′isis\ [VAGO- + LYSIS] Surgical destruction of the vagus nerve. Adj. vagolytic.

**vagomimetic** \-mimet′ik\ Having or pertaining to a parasympathetic effect.

**vagosympathetic** \-sim′pəthet′ik\ Denoting the combined parasympathetic and sympathetic systems.

**vagotomy** \vāgät′əmē\ [VAGO- + -TOMY] Division of the vagus nerve. Also *vagectomy.* **medical v.** Blocking of the action of the vagus nerves with anticholinergic drugs.

**vagotonia** \-tō′nē·ə\ [VAGO- + *ton(o)-* + -IA] Hyperexcitability of the parasympathetic nervous system giving rise to vasomotor instability, hyperhidrosis, and a tendency to constipation and to muscle cramps. Also *parasympathicotonia, vagotony, parasympathotonia.* Adj. vagotonic. • This is an imprecise concept.

**vagotonic** \-tän′ik\ Pertaining to vagotonia.

**vagotonin** \-tō′nin\ A pancreatic hormonal extract with the properties of increasing vagal tone, inducing bradycardia, and promoting glycogen storage in the liver. *Older term.*

**vagotony** \vāgät′ənē\ VAGOTONIA.

**vagotropic** \-träp′ik\ Having an influence on the motor nucleus of the vagus nerve.

**vagotropism** \vāgät′rəpizm\ [VAGO- + TROPISM] Chemical affinity for neurons whose axons are conveyed in the vagus nerve.

**vagovagal** \-vā′gəl\ Denoting a reflex whose afferent and efferent arcs are conveyed by the vagus nerve.

**vagrant** \vā′grənt\ Moving or shifting unpredictably.

**vagus** \vā′gəs\ [L, wandering] Denoting the tenth cranial nerve, or nervus vagus.

**vagusstoff** \vä′gəs·shtôf′\ [German, from *Vagus* vagus nerve + *Stoff* material, substance] *Obs.* ACETYLCHOLINE.

**Val** Symbol for valine.

**val** **1** value. **2** equivalent.

**valence** \vā′ləns\ [L *valentia* (from *valens,* gen. *valentis,* pres. part. of *valere* to be strong) strength, power] The number of binding sites on a molecule that can react with ligands. Thus, the valence of an antibody is the number of antigen-binding sites it possesses, and the valence of an antigen is the number of determinants (whether identical or different) that can bind antibody. Also *valency.*

**valency** \vā′lənsē\ VALENCE.

**Valentin** [Gabriel Gustav *Valentin,* German physiologist, 1810–1883] **1** Valentin pseudoganglion. See under INTUMESCENTIA TYMPANICA. **2** Valentin's ganglion. See under GANGLION. **3** Valentin's corpuscles. See under CORPUSCLE.

**valeric acid** $CH_3$—$[CH_2]_3$—COOH. Pentanoic acid. Although it is the parent acid of natural compounds it is not itself of much natural importance.

**valethamate bromide** $C_{19}H_{32}BrNO_2$. Diethylmethyl(2-$\beta$-methyl-$\alpha$-phenylvaleryloxyethyl)-ammonium bromide. A white, crystalline powder, very soluble in water and alcohol. It is a quaternary ammonium anticholinergic agent with peripheral effects like those of atropine. It has been used for the treatment of peptic ulcers and spasm of the gastrointestinal, genitourinary, and biliary tracts.

**valetudinarian** \val′it$^y$oo′dəner′ē·ən\ [L *valetudinari(us)* (from *valetudo,* gen. *valetudinis,* state of health, from *valere* to be strong) sickly, an invalid + English *-an*] A person who is chronically weak or sickly, especially an invalid preoccupied with health problems.

**valetudinarianism** \val′it$^y$oo′dəner′ē·ənizm\ [VALETUDINARIAN + -ISM] The chronically weak or invalid condition of a valetudinarian, or the preoccupation with health problems associated with it.

**valgus** \val′gəs\ [L, bow-legged] Bending or twisting outward or away from the midline: said of a deformed part.

**validation** \val′idā′shən\ The act of making valid. **consensual v.** Comparison of one's evaluations with those of others to make certain that one's interpretations are based in reality and not idiosyncratic elaborations of one's own pathology.

**validity** \vəlid′itē\ [*valid* + -ITY] The extent to which a conclusion is justified by the facts on which it is based or a measurement is considered to be an accurate indication of whatever it is intended to measure. **face v.** An early estimate formed about whether a given test will serve as a useful measure of some variable. It is usually based on an apparent similarity between the test behaviors and the variable to be predicted, for example, a test of fingertip dexterity may be used to select those who will be proficient small-part assembly workers. A true measure of validity can only be obtained by correlating test performance scores with actual job performance, but in selecting those tests which might prove to be empirically predictive, surface or face resemblances are often used as a general guide.

**valine** \val′ēn\ $(CH_3)_2CH—CH(NH_3^+)—COO^-$. 2-Amino-3-methylbutyric acid, one of the twenty amino acids that are incorporated into proteins. It is essential in the mammalian diet and is metabolized by transamination and oxidation of the oxoacid so formed to 2-methylpropionyl-CoA, which is further metabolized to propionic acid. Symbol: Val, V

**valinemia** \val′inē′mē·ə\ Increased valine in the blood, due to a genetic deficiency of valine aminotransferase. Clinical manifestations include mental retardation, neuropsychiatric dysfunction, and protein intolerance. The mode of inheritance is not known.

**valinomycin** \val′inōmī′sin\ A depsipeptide antibiotic, consisting of the sequence of L-valine, 2-hydroxy-3-methylbutanoic acid, D-valine, and lactic acid, occurring twice to make an eight-residue cyclic molecule. It is an ionophore for potassium ions. It has been used in the study of the pumping of hydrogen ions in the electron transport chain, since by allowing potassium transport it discharges the electric field across mitochondrial membranes, and therefore allows hydrogen-ion pumping to continue until a measurable pH gradient is established.

**Valium** A proprietary name for diazepam.

**vallate** \val′āt\ [L *vallatus* (past part. of *vallare* to surround with a barrier, from *vallum* a palisade, barrier) palisaded, walled] Surrounded by a rimmed depression; cupped.

**vallecula** \vəlek′yələ\ [Late L (dim. of L *valles* or *vallis* a hollow, valley), a little valley] **1** A small depression, groove, or hollow on the surface of an organ or one of its parts. Also *valley*. **2** VALLECULA EPIGLOTTICA. **v. cerebelli** [NA] A deep, longitudinally oriented hollow on the inferior cerebellar surface between the two cerebellar hemispheres. Within the vallecula cerebelli is located the rostral part of the medulla oblongata. Also *valley of cerebellum, longitudinal fissure of cerebellum*. **v. cerebri lateralis** FOSSA LATERALIS CEREBRI. **v. epiglottica** [NA] The depression on each side of the median glossoepiglottic fold between the pharyngeal part of the tongue anteriorly and the anterior surface of the epiglottis posteriorly. Also *vallecula, glossoepiglottic fossa, vallecula linguae* (outmoded). **v. fossa sylvii** FOSSA LATERALIS CEREBRI. **v. linguae** *Outmoded* VALLECULA EPIGLOTTICA. **v. ovata** *Outmoded* FOSSA VESICAE BILIARIS. **v. for petrosal ganglion** FOSSULA PETROSA. **v. sylvii** FOSSA LATERALIS CEREBRI.

**vallecular** \vəlek′yələr\ Pertaining to a vallecula.

**valley** VALLECULA. **v. of cerebellum** VALLECULA CEREBELLI.

**vallum** \val′əm\ [L, a palisade, fortification] **1** In anatomy, a raised area; a wall. **2** The eyebrow. **v. unguis** [NA] The external wall of skin raised over the groove in which the root and sides of the nail are embedded. Also *wall of nail*.

**valproate sodium** $C_8H_{15}NaO_2$. A compound that has antiepileptic activity. It is more effective particularly against simple and complex (petit mal) absence seizures, and with bilateral massive epileptic myoclonus attacks, particularly in children.

**Valsalva** [Antonio Maria *Valsalva*, Italian anatomist and physician, 1666–1723] **1** See under TEST. **2** Aneurysm of the sinus of Valsalva. See under AORTIC SINUSAL ANEURYSM. **3** Valsalva's antrum. See under ANTRUM MASTOIDEUM. **4** Valsalva's experiment, Valsalva's procedure. See under MANEUVER. **5** Ligaments of Valsalva. See under LIGAMENTA AURICULARIA. **6** Valsalva's muscle. See under MUSCULUS TRAGICUS. **7** Sinus of Valsalva. See under SINUS AORTAE.

**value** [Middle English, from Old French, fem. of *valu*, past part. of *valoir* to be worth, from L *valere* to be strong] The magnitude of a quantity. **adaptive v.** DARWINIAN FITNESS. **biological v.** A measure of the nutritional value of a protein to animals. It is based on the content in that protein of those amino acids, such as lysine, that are essential to animals. It is expressed as the quantity of protein nitrogen retained from a given amount of dietary protein that has been digested and absorbed. It is estimated by measuring nitrogen intake ($N_I$), urinary nitrogen ($N_u$), and fecal nitrogen ($N_F$). Then biological value equals

$$\frac{N_I - N_F - N_u}{N_I - N_F}.$$

**cot v.** An expression of the sequence complexity of a nucleic acid, based on reassociation kinetic analysis, using a logarithmic scale. Low values ($10^{-4}$ to $10^{-1}$) indicate repetitive or simple-sequence nucleic acids, and high values ($10^1$ and greater) indicate nonrepetitive sequences. **cryocrit v.** The relative volume of precipitated cryoglobulin, as a percentage of the volume of the serum specimen after centrifugation of serum previously refrigerated at 4°C. **fuel v.** The potential thermal energy of food. **iodine v.** IODINE NUMBER. **lethal equivalent v.** LETHAL EQUIVALENT. **liminal v.** THRESHOLD VALUE. **normal v.'s** NORMAL RANGE. **normothetic v.** The value of a variable, such as pulse rate or blood pressure, for an individual as compared with the accepted norm for the population. **P v.** PREDICTIVE VALUE. **predictive v.** An expression of the likelihood that a given test result correlates with the presence or absence of disease. A positive predictive value considers all subjects with an abnormal, or positive, test result. It is the ratio of patients who have the disease to the entire population of individuals with a positive test result, expressed as

$$\frac{\text{True positives}}{\text{True positives} + \text{false positives}} \times 100.$$

Negative predictive value is the ratio of nondiseased patients with negative test results to the entire population of individuals with a negative result, expressed as

$$\frac{\text{True negatives}}{\text{True negatives} + \text{false negatives}} \times 100.$$

Also *P value*. **reference v.** The value for a test result that is used in assessing the significance of results found in the test subjects. It is usually expressed as upper and lower reference values, which delimit the reference range. **relative v.** A value expressed as a ratio of some other reference value. The ratio may be a proportion or a percentage. **survival v.** REPRODUCTIVE FITNESS. **threshold v.** The minimal intensity for excitation or sensory detection. Also *liminal value*.

**valva** \val′və\ [L (akin to *volvere* to roll, turn around), a leaf in a folding door] (*pl.* valvae) [NA] An anatomic valve; a membranous fold or other structure that permits or regulates the flow of the contents in a canal, tube, or hollow organ in one direction but prevents reflux of the contents in the other direction. It may be capable of closing off the opening. Compare VALVULA. **v. aortae** [NA] A valve comprising three semilunar cusps, or valvules, guarding the orifice of the aorta from the left ventricle of the heart. Designated right, left, and posterior cusps, their convex margins are attached to the wall of the orifice and each consists of a fold of endocardium with some fibrous tissue between the two layers. The nodules on the free margins are thicker and the lunules more obvious than in the cusps of the pulmonary valve. Also *aortic valve, valve of aorta.* **v. atrioventricularis dextra** [NA] The valve occupying the right atrioventricular orifice of the heart and usually comprising three triangular cusps, named anterior, posterior, and septal, attached by their bases to the fibrous ring surrounding the orifice. Their apices project into the right ventricle. Their atrial surfaces are smooth, while the ventricular surfaces are rough and provide attachment for the chordae tendineae. Also *right atrioventricular valve, tricuspid valve.* **v. atrioventricularis sinistra** [NA] The valve occupying the left atrioventricular orifice of the heart, usually comprising two unequal triangular cusps, named anterior (the larger cusp) and posterior, attached by their bases to the fibrous ring surrounding the orifice. Their atrial surfaces are smooth, while chordae tendineae are attached to the ventricular surfaces. Also *left atrioventricular valve, mitral valve, bicuspid valve.* **v. ileocecalis** [NA] A valve composed of two segments protecting the opening of the terminal ileum where it meets the large intestine at the junction of the cecum and the colon. The upper and lower segments, or lips, project into the lumen and consist of double folds of mucous membrane containing mostly circular and some longitudinal muscle fibers of the intestine. Extending laterally from the junctions of the lips are horizontal membranous ridges, or frenula. The valve serves as a sphincter and prevents reflux of cecal contents into the ileum. Also *ileocecal valve, ileocolic valve, valve of colon, Bauhin's valve, valve of Macalister, valve of Tulpius, valve of Varolius.* **v. sinus venosi** Either of the thin venous valves guarding the opening of the early sinus venosus into the right atrium. The left valve retrogresses and is incorporated in the interatrial septum. The right valve forms the crista terminalis, the valve of the coronary sinus, and much of the valve of the inferior vena cava. Also *valve of sinus venosus.* **v. trunci pulmonalis** [NA] The valve occupying the orifice of the pulmonary trunk at its junction with the right ventricle of the heart and comprising three semilunar cusps, or valvules, named anterior, right, and left, attached by their bases to the wall of the pulmonary trunk orifice. Their free margins project upwards into the lumen of the pulmonary trunk, preventing backflow of blood into the ventricle. Also *pulmonary trunk valve, pulmonary valve.*

**valval** \val′vəl\ Pertaining to a valve or valves; valvular. Also *valvar.*

# valve

**valve** [L *valva.* See VALVA.] **1** A mechanism that regulates direction or volume of flow, as in a tube or between chambers. **2** An anatomic structure that functions as a valve. See under VALVA, VALVULA. **anal v.'s** VALVULAE ANALES. **anterior urethral v.'s** URETHRAL VALVES. **v. of aorta** VALVA AORTAE. **aortic v.** VALVA AORTAE. **Ball's v.'s** VALVULAE ANALES. **ball-type v.** A prosthetic heart valve in which a free-floating caged ball provides forward flow during systole and prevents reflux during diastole. Also *caged-ball prosthesis.* **Bauhin's v.** VALVA ILEOCECALIS. **Béraud's v.** A projecting fold of mucous membrane occasionally located at the junction of the lacrimal sac and the nasolacrimal duct. Also *Krause's valve, valvule of Béraud.* **Bianchi's v.** PLICA LACRIMALIS. **bicuspid v.** **1** VALVA ATRIOVENTRICULARIS SINISTRA. **2** Any two-cusped valve, normal or abnormal. **bicuspid aortic v.** An aortic valve with two as opposed to the normal three cusps. It is a congenital abnormality affecting about 1 percent of individuals and which often proceeds to calcification and aortic stenosis in later life. **bicuspid pulmonary v.** A pulmonary valve which has only two cusps rather than the normal three. **Blom-Singer v.** BLOM-SINGER VOICE PROSTHESIS. **Bochdalek's v.** An annular mucous fold situated in the punctum lacrimale at the entrance of each lacrimal canaliculus, just proximal to Foltz valve. Also *valvule of Bochdalek.* **cardiac v.'s** Valves that regulate the flow of blood through and out of the heart, namely, the left and right atrioventricular, the aortic, and the pulmonary valves. **caval v.** VALVULA VENAE CAVAE INFERIORIS. **v. of colon** VALVA ILEOCECALIS. **congenital ureteric v.'s** Anomalous small, transverse folds of mucosa in the lower portion of the ureter especially at the ureterovesical junction. **congenital urethral v.** A rare loose fold of mucous membrane in the prostatic part of the male urethra. It may lead to obstruction. **coronary v.** VALVULA SINUS CORONARII. **v. of coronary sinus** VALVULA SINUS CORONARII. **diode v.** A thermionic valve containing a cathode and an anode, without an electronic grid system. **directional v.** A valve, in a mechanical ventilator, breathing circuit, or other related apparatus, which serves to guide the flow of gas in one direction. Also *unidirectional valve.* **duckbill v.** BLOM-SINGER VOICE PROSTHESIS. **escape v.** PRESSURE-LIMITING VALVE. **eustachian v.** VALVULA VENAE CAVAE INFERIORIS. **expiratory v.** A valve on the expiratory limb of a breathing circuit, which controls the removal of gas. **flow-control v.** An adjustable valve for the regulation of gas flow in a mechanical ventilator or breathing circuit. **Foltz v.** A fold of mucous membrane in the constricted portion situated just beyond the commencement of the vertical segment of each lacrimal canaliculus. It is located just beyond Bochdalek's valve. Also *valvule of Foltz.* **v. of foramen ovale** VALVULA FORAMINIS OVALIS. **Gerlach's v.** A projecting fold of mucous membrane of the cecum occasionally located at the opening of the vermiform appendix. Also *valve of vermiform appendix.* **Guérin's v.** VALVULA FOSSAE NAVICULARIS. **Hasner's v.** PLICA LACRIMALIS. **heart v.'s** CARDIAC VALVES. **Heister's v.** PLICA SPIRALIS. **Hoboken's v.'s** Projections into the lumen of the umbilical arteries produced by thickening of the tunica media at their bends or kinks in the umbilical cord. Also *valvulae hobokenii.* **hot cathode v.** THERMIONIC VALVE. **Houston's v.** The middle fold of the plicae transversales recti. **Huschke's v.** PLICA LACRIMALIS. **ileocecal v.** VALVA ILEOCECALIS. **ileocolic v.** VALVA ILEOCECALIS. **v. of inferior vena cava** VALVULA VENAE CAVAE INFERIORIS. **inspiratory v.** A valve on the inspiratory limb of a breathing circuit, which controls the entry of gas. **Kerckring's v.'s** PLICAE CIRCULARES. **Kohlrausch v.'s** PLICAE TRANSVERSALES RECTI. **Krause's v.** BÉRAUD'S VALVE. **left auriculoventricular v.** *Outmoded* VALVA ATRIOVENTRICULARIS SINISTRA. **LeVeen v.** A peritoneovenous shunt that is equipped with a one-way valve which, when inserted with one end in the peritoneal cavity and the other end in the venous circulation near the heart, can conduct ascites back into the circulation. **lymphatic v.** VALVULA LYMPHATICA. **v. of Macalister** VALVA ILEOCECALIS. **Mercier's v.** An occasional fold of mucous membrane which partly obstructs the orifice of the ureter in the bladder. **mitral v.** VALVA ATRIOVENTRICULARIS SINISTRA. **monocuspid aortic v.** A rare congenital abnormality of the aortic valve in which only one cusp is present and which leads to aortic stenosis if the patient survives infancy. **Morgagni's v.'s** VALVULAE ANALES. **v. of navicular fossa** VALVULA FOSSAE NAVICULARIS. **nonrebreathing v.** A valve on a breathing circuit that prevents the rebreathing of gas by allowing it to escape. **O'Beirne's v.** O'BEIRNE SPHINCTER. **oxygen flush v.** A valve used for rapidly admitting large gas flows into a mechanical ventilator, or breathing circuit, or other related apparatus. **parachute mitral v.** A congenitally deformed mitral valve that has all chordae descending to a single papillary muscle. **pop-off v.** PRESSURE-LIMITING VALVE. **posterior urethral v.'s** AMUSSAT'S VALVULA. **pressure-limiting v.** A vent utilizing controlled resistance to prevent pressure buildup in a breathing circuit, mechanical ventilator, or other related apparatus. Also *escape valve, pop-off valve, relief valve.* **Pudenz-Heyer v.** Slits placed in the distal end of a plastic tubular system for draining ventricular fluid into the heart, abdominal cavity, or pleural space, for the treatment of hydrocephalus. The slits are designed to open under pressure exerted by ventricular fluid and to close to prevent reflux. **pulmonary v.** VALVA TRUNCI PULMONALIS. **pulmonary trunk v.** VALVA TRUNCI PULMONALIS. **pyloric v.** A prominent circular fold of mucous membrane stated to be present at the pyloric orifice of the stomach when it is empty. *Outmoded.* **quadricuspid aortic v.** A congenital abnormality in which there are four cusps in the aortic valve. A quadricuspid valve is regularly seen in truncus arteriosus communis. **quadricuspid pulmonary v.** A congenital abnormality in which there are four rather than three cusps to the pulmonary valve. **relief v.** PRESSURE-LIMITING VALVE. **right atrioventricular v.** VALVA ATRIOVENTRICULARIS DEXTRA. **Rosenmüller's v.** PLICA LACRIMALIS. **semilunar v.** 1 VALVULA SEMILUNARIS. 2 A valve composed of semilunar cusps, or valvules, such as the aortic and pulmonary valves. An outmoded usage. **semilunar v.'s of colon** PLICAE SEMILUNARES COLI. **semilunar v.'s of rectum** VALVULAE ANALES. **sigmoid v.'s of colon** PLICAE SEMILUNARES COLI. **v. of sinus venosus** VALVA SINUS VENOSI. **speaking v.** A valve fitted to the outer end of the inner tube of a tracheostomy tube to enable the wearer to speak. The valve opens to permit inspiration by way of the tube, but closes at expiration so as to direct air through the glottis. **spiral v.** PLICA SPIRALIS. **spiral v. of cystic duct** PLICA SPIRALIS. **spiral v. of Heister** PLICA SPIRALIS. **Spitz-Holter v.** A plastic one-way valve interposed in a tubular system used to drain ventricular fluid into the heart, abdominal cavity, or pleural space for the treatment of hydrocephalus. The valve is designed to open at a specific pressure to discharge fluid. It closes to prevent reflux. **v. of Sylvius** VALVULA VENAE CAVAE INFERIORIS. **Taillefer's v.** A fold of mucous membrane near the middle of the nasolacrimal duct. **Tarin's v.** VELUM MEDULLARE CAUDALE. **Tarinus v.** VELUM MEDULLARE CAUDALE. **Terrier's v.** The highest oblique ridge of mucous membrane in the neck of the gallbladder. **thebesian v.** VALVULA SINUS CORONARII. **thermionic v.** An electronic tube containing a heated cathode for the emission of electrons and designed to rectify oscillating currents. Also *hot cathode valve.* **tracheostoma v.** A prosthesis for occluding the tracheostoma after laryngectomy when a Blom-Singer voice prosthesis or tracheoesophageal fistula voice button prosthesis has been introduced. While enabling the subject to breathe in through the stoma, it causes the expired air to be diverted through the voice prosthesis into the pharynx where voice is produced, usually at the pharyngoesophageal junction. **tricuspid v.** 1 VALVA ATRIOVENTRICULARIS DEXTRA. 2 Any three-cusped valve. **triode v.** A thermionic valve containing a cathode, an anode, and an electronic grid system to regulate the flow of electrons. **v. of Tulpius** VALVA ILEOCECALIS. **unidirectional v.** DIRECTIONAL VALVE. **urethral v.'s** Folds in the mucous membrane lining the urethra. Also *anterior urethral valves.* **v. of Varolius** VALVA ILEOCECALIS. **v. of veins** VALVULA VENOSA. **v. of vermiform appendix** GERLACH'S VALVE. **v. of Vieussens** 1 VELUM MEDULLARE CRANIALE. 2 A valvelike structure found at the site where the great cardiac vein enlarges to become the coronary sinus. **Willis v.** VELUM MEDULLARE CRANIALE.

**valvectomy** \valvek′təmē\ [*valv(e)* + -ECTOMY] The excision of a leaflet of a heart valve, a procedure undertaken to relieve severe pulmonary stenosis. Also *valvulectomy.*

**valvoplasty** \val′vəplas′tē\ [*valv(e)* + *o* + -PLASTY] Any reconstructive operation performed on a valve of the heart or a vein, usually to repair valvular incompetence. Also *valvuloplasty.*

**valvotome** \val′vətōm\ [*valv(a)* + *o* + -TOME ] An instrument designed to incise the commissures between heart valves.

**valvotomy** \valvät′əmē\ [*valv(a)* + *o* + -TOMY] The incision of the commissures between the heart valves. Also *cardiovalvulotomy, valvulotomy.* **closed pulmonary v.** TRANSVENTRICULAR CLOSED VALVOTOMY. **mitral v.** MITRAL COMMISSUROTOMY. **pulmonary v.** A valvotomy to relieve obstruction of the pulmonary artery due to stenosis. The pulmonary artery is incised or enlarged either by a closed technique (transventricular closed valvotomy) or under direct vision with the use of the cardiopulmonary bypass method. **rectal v.** The incision into one or more of the rectal valves. **transventricular closed v.** A valvotomy performed to correct congenital stenosis of the pulmonary artery valve by inserting a cutting instrument into the pulmonary artery through the pulmonary valve by means of an incision in the outflow tract of the right ventricle. The instrument is withdrawn from the pulmonary artery into the right ventricle to achieve valvotomy, thus obviating the need for cardiopulmonary bypass. Also *Brock's operation, Brock's procedure, Brock technique, transventricular pulmonary valvotomy, Brock's infundibulectomy, closed pulmonary valvotomy.* **transventricular pulmonary v.** TRANSVENTRICULAR CLOSED VALVOTOMY.

**valvula** \val′vyələ\ [New L (dim. of *valva* a leaf in a folding door), a little valve] (*pl.* valvulae) [NA] A small valve, as in a vein or lymphatic vessel, or, especially, a segment or cusp of a valve in the heart, as of the aortic, mitral, or pulmonary trunk valves. Also *valvule.* Compare VALVA. **Amussat's v.** 1 An anomalous fold of mucous membrane on either side of the seminal colliculus in the urethra. Also *posterior urethral valves.* 2 PLICA SPIRALIS. **valvulae anales** [NA] Small transverse crescentic folds of mucous membrane linking the lower ends of adjoining anal columns. Above each fold is an anal sinus. Also *anal valves, Ball's valves, Morgagni's valves, semilunar valves of rectum.* **v. foraminis ovalis** [NA] The septum primum of the

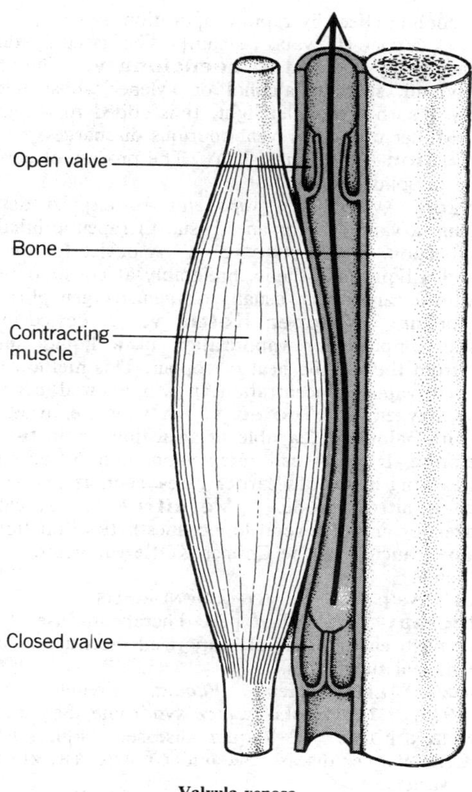

Valvula venosa

fetal heart, which forms a flaplike valve on the left atrial side of the foramen ovale situated in septum secundum. After birth, when septum primum fuses with limbus fossae ovalis to help close the foramen, the crescentic margin of the septum primum may be located adherent to the left side of the interatrial septum, persisting into adult life. Also *valve of foramen ovale.* **v. fossae navicularis** [NA] A fold of mucous membrane occasionally situated in the roof of the navicular fossa of the male urethra and separating the fossa from the lacuna magna when the latter is present. Also *valve of navicular fossa, Guérin's valve, Guérin's fold, valvule of Guérin.* **Gerlach's v.** RETICULUM TRABECULARE SCLERAE. **valvulae hobokenii** HOBOKEN'S VALVES. **v. lymphatica** [NA] One of the small valves with two or three semilunar cusps located throughout the course of lymphatic vessels at their constrictions. The valves are arranged so as to prevent backflow of lymph, and consist of a duplication of the endothelium with a fine fibrous-tissue core. Also *lymphatic valve.* **v. prostatica** MEDIAN BAR. **v. semilunaris** One of the segments or cusps of the valva aortae or the valva trunci pulmonalis, each consisting of a duplication of the endocardium with some fibrous tissue between the two layers, usually attached at the base with the apex being free and strengthened by a nodule. Also *semilunar cusp, semilunar valve.* **v. semilunaris anterior valvae trunci pulmonalis** [NA] The anterior semilunar cusp of the valve of the pulmonary trunk (valva trunci pulmonalis). **v. semilunaris dextra valvae aortae** [NA] The right semilunar cusp of the aortic valve (valva aortae). **v. semilunaris dextra valvae trunci pulmonalis** [NA] The right semilunar cusp of the valve of the pulmonary trunk (valva trunci pulmonalis). **v. semilunaris posterior valvae aortae** [NA] The posterior semilunar cusp of the aortic valve (valva aortae). **v. semilunaris sinistra valvae aortae** [NA] The left semilunar cusp of the aortic valve (valva aortae). **v. semilunaris sinistra valvae trunci pulmonalis** [NA] The left semilunar cusp of the valve of the pulmonary trunk (valva trunci pulmonalis). **v. sinus coronarii** [NA] A thin semilunar fold of endocardium over the lower part of the opening of the coronary sinus in the right atrium of the heart, protecting the sinus from reflux of blood during contraction of the atrium. Also *valve of coronary sinus, coronary valve, thebesian valve.* **v. venae cavae inferioris** [NA] A duplication of the endocardium of the right atrium with a few muscle fibers between its layers forming a semilunar valve anterior to the orifice of the inferior vena cava. Its convex base is attached to the anterior edge of the orifice while its free concave edge is attached by two horns, the left to the anterior edge of the limbus fossae ovalis while the right blends with the atrial wall. Somewhat rudimentary in the adult, it is large during fetal life, directing blood from the inferior vena cava to the left atrium through the foramen ovale. Also *valve of inferior vena cava, caval valve, valve of Sylvius, eustachian valve.* **v. venosa** [NA] A semilunar valve, either unicuspid, bicuspid, or tricuspid, composed of a double layer of endothelium-lined tunica intima with a core of connective and elastic tissue, and located in small and medium-sized veins, especially in the lower limbs. It is usually absent in very small and very large veins. On the cardiac side of the attachment of each cusp, the wall of the vein is distended to form a sinus. The valve serves to reduce reflux of blood along the column of the vein. Also *valve of veins.*

**valvulae** \val′vyəlē\ Plural of VALVULA.

**valvular** \val′vyələr\ Pertaining to or functioning as a valve.

**valvulate** \val′vyəlāt\ Having a valvule or valvules.

**valvule** \val′vyool\ VALVULA. **v. of Béraud** BÉRAUD'S VALVE. **v. of Bochdalek** BOCHDALEK'S VALVE. **v. of Foltz** FOLTZ VALVE. **v. of Guérin** VALVULA FOSSAE NAVICULARIS.

**valvulectomy** \val′vyəlek′təmē\ VALVECTOMY.

**valvulitis** \val′vyəlī′tis\ [*valvul(a)* + -ITIS] Inflammation of a valve, particularly a cardiac valve. **rheumatic v.** Rheumatic inflammation of a cardiac valve. **uricemic v.** Deposition of tophus on heart valves in patients with chronic tophaceous gout.

**valvuloplasty** \val′vyəlōplas′tē\ VALVOPLASTY.

**valvulotome** \val′vyəlōtōm′\ [*valvul(a)* + *o* + -TOME] A surgical instrument used for incising a cardiac valve. Also *cardiovalvulotome.*

**valvulotomy** \val′vyəlät′əmē\ VALVOTOMY.

**vanadate** Any anion with a central vanadium atom, or a salt containing it, especially a compound of vanadium(V), i.e. in the +5 oxidation state. At physiologic pH such ions resemble phosphate, and powerfully inhibit many enzymes, e.g. the $Na^+/K^+$-transporting ATPase of mammalian cell membranes, to which it binds with a dissociation constant of under 1 nM. Vanadate is reduced *in vivo* to ions containing vanadium(IV).

**vanadium** Element number 23, having atomic weight 50.9415. In nature it consists largely of stable vanadium 51 with a small admixture (0.24%) of the slightly radioactive vanadium 50 (half-life, 6 × $10^{15}$ years). Seven other unstable isotopes are known. Pure vanadium is a soft, ductile, bright white metal. Valences are 2, 3, 4, and 5. The metal and its compounds are toxic. Trace amounts are essential to lower plants, some marine animals, and rats. Symbol: Va

**vanadiumism** \vənā′dē·əmizm\ Poisoning from chronic exposure to vanadium or its compounds. Symptoms are respiratory tract irritation, inflammation of the conjunctiva and lungs, and blood dyscrasia.

**van Bogaert** [Ludo *van Bogaert*, Belgian neurologist, flourished 20th century] **1** Van Bogaert's encephalitis, van Bogaert sclerosing leukoencephalitis. See under SUBACUTE SCLEROSING PANENCEPHALITIS. **2** Van Bogaert-Bertrand disease. See under CANAVAN'S DISEASE. **3** Van Bogaert-Nyssen-Peiffer disease. See under METACHROMATIC LEUKODYSTROPHY. **4** Canavan-van Bogaert-Bertrand disease. See under VAN BOGAERT'S FAMILIAL AXONAL SPONGY DEGENERATION. **5** Van Bogaert-Divry syndrome. See under SYNDROME. **6** Van Bogaert-Scherer-Epstein syndrome. See under CEREBROTENDINOUS XANTHOMATOSIS.

**van Buchem** [Francis Steven Peter *van Buchem*, Dutch internist, born 1897] **1** Van Buchem's disease. See under SCLEROSTEOSIS. **2** See under SYNDROME.

**vancomycin** A glycopeptide antibiotic obtained from *Streptomyces orientalis* which is bactericidal against several Gram-positive bacteria. It is reserved for serious infections that cannot be treated with less toxic antimicrobial drugs, such as the penicillins and cephalosporins.

**van Creveld** [Simon *van Creveld*, Dutch pediatrician, born 1894] Ellis-van Creveld syndrome. See under SYNDROME.

**Van de Graaff** [Robert Jemison *Van de Graaff*, U.S. physicist, 1901–1967] **1** Van de Graaff machine. See under GENERATOR. **2** See under ACCELERATOR.

**van den Bergh** [Albert Abraham Hujmans *van den Bergh*, Dutch physician, 1869–1943] See under TEST.

**van der Hoeve** [Jan *van der Hoeve*, Dutch physician, 1878–1952] Van der Hoeve syndrome. See under VAN DER HOEVE-DE KLEYN SYNDROME.

**van der Kolk** See under SCHROEDER.

**van der Waals** [Johannes Diderik *van der Waals*, Dutch chemist, 1837–1923] See under RADIUS.

**van Gehuchten** [A. *van Gehuchten*, Belgian neurologist, 1861–1915] Cells of van Gehuchten. See under GOLGI TYPE II NEURONS.

**van Gieson** [Ira Thompson *van Gieson*, U.S. histologist and bacteriologist, 1865–1913] See under STAIN.

**van Helmont** [Jean Baptiste *van Helmont*, Flemish physician and chemist, 1577–1644] Speculum helmontii, van Helmont's mirror. See under CENTRUM TENDINEUM.

**van Hook** [Weller *van Hook*, U.S. surgeon, 1862–1933] Van Hook's operation. See under URETEROURETEROSTOMY.

**Van Hoorne** [Jan *Van Hoorne*, Dutch anatomist, 1621–1670] Van Hoorne's canal. See under DUCTUS THORACICUS.

**vanillylmandelic acid** 3-methoxy-4-hydroxymandelic acid, the major urinary metabolite of the catecholamines epinephrine and norepinephrine. Abbr. VMA

**Van Slyke** [Donald Dexter *Van Slyke*, U.S. physician and chemist, 1883–1971] Van Slyke and Neill method. See under METHOD.

**van't Hoff** [Jacobus Hendricus *van't Hoff*, Dutch chemist, 1852–1911] See under EQUATION.

**vapocauterization** \vā′pōkô′tərīzā′shən\ Cauterization by use of a hot vapor.

**vapo-coolant** \vā′pō-koo′lənt\ A highly volatile liquid, such as ether, ethyl chloride, or ethyl fluoride, used to produce a cooling effect by rapid evaporation.

**vapor** \vā′pər\ [L, vapor, steam] The gaseous state of a substance easily liquefied. **quenching v.** The vapor of a compound, such as alcohol or xylene, whose molecules strongly absorb ultraviolet light. It is added to the gas in a Geiger-Müller tube to prevent spurious discharges.

**vaporization** \vā′pərīzā′shən\ The process of converting a liquid or solid into vapor.

**vaporizer** \vā′pərīzər\ [*vaporiz(e)* + -ER] A device for producing a vapor, as for anesthesia, therapeutic inhalations, or disinfection. **anesthetic v.** A device for the evaporation of a liquid anesthetic, preferably at constant temperature, into a carrier gas, usually oxygen, oxygen plus nitrous oxide, or air. **Copper Kettle v.** A device in which the heat supplied for vaporization of a liquid anesthetic comes from the specific heat of copper. This method yields a calibrated vapor concentration in a measured carrier gas, such as oxygen. **Fluotec v.** A vaporizer used specifically with halothane, capable of adjusting to fluctuations in temperature. It yields calibrated vapor concentrations capable of existing in various carrier gases, such as oxygen or oxygen plus nitrous oxide. **Vernitrol v.** A calibrated vaporizer for any of several liquid anesthetics, functioning on the same principle as the Copper Kettle vaporizer. A proprietary name.

**vapors** \vā′pərs\ *Obs.* HYPOCHONDRIASIS.

**vapotherapy** \vā′pōther′əpē\ Therapeutic use of an aerosol or mist, either of simple vaporized moisture or containing medicinal substances.

**Vaquez** [Louis Henri *Vaquez*, French physician, 1860–1936] **1** Babinski-Vaquez syndrome. See under BABINSKI SYNDROME. **2** Vaquez disease, Vaquez-Osler disease, Osler-Vaquez disease. See under POLYCYTHEMIA VERA.

**var.** variety.

**variability** \ver′ē·əbil′itē\ The capacity to vary or to be a variable.

**variable** \ver′ē·əbəl\ **1** In mathematics, a quantity that can assume any value within a specified set of values, including, in some cases, infinity. **2** Changeable; subject to variation. **acoustic v.** One of the variables that are functions of space and time in a sonic wave: pressure, density, temperature, and particle motion. **confounding v.** An independent variable which is known to be or suspected of being related to the dependent variable but which is not of immediate interest and whose influence must be removed or allowed for in order to examine the relationship between the dependent variable and the independent variable or variables that are the subject of study. For example, in studying the relationship between smoking (independent variable) and lung cancer (dependent variable) it might be necessary to eliminate the influence of urban vs. rural residence (confounding variable). **dependent v.** A variable whose value is determined at least partly by one or more independent variables or predicted by a regression equation. **dummy v.** An arbitary variable intended to represent some qualitative characteristic and often taking the values 1 or 0 to denote the presence or absence of the attribute. **explanatory v.** An independent variable which is interpreted as causing or explaining the variation in another variable. For example, if $P$ is a patient's pulse rate and $T$ the patient's temperature, in the expression $P = a + bT$, $T$ could be regarded as an explanatory variable. **independent v.** A variable which establishes the value of another variable when a defined relationship exists between them. By convention the first former variable is designated as the independent and the latter as the dependent variable. Thus, in the simplest case, $y = a + bx$, $x$ is the independent variable and *y* is the dependent variable. By extension two or more independent variables may be involved in the relationship, each contributing to the determination of the value of the one dependent variable. Also *predictor variable.* **intervening v.** A variable located in a causal sequence between the independent and dependent variables and thus statistically associated with both. Thus, in the sequence intensity between air pollution and the incidence of chronic bronchitis, abnormalities in the respiratory epithelium could be an intervening variable. **predictor v.** INDEPENDENT VARIABLE. **random v.** A variable which may take any one of a set of possible values each having its relative frequency or distinctive probability. Each random variable has thus a related frequency function or probability function which defines the frequency or probability of occurrence of each possible value of the variable. Also *variate.*

**variance** \ver′ē·əns\ The average squared deviation of a set of values from their mean. The average is determined by dividing the sum of squared deviations by one less than the number of observations. Symbol: $\sigma^2$ **environmental v.** In population genetics, the fraction of the total phenotypic variance ascribable to differences in the environments that affect individuals in a given population. Compare GENETIC VARIANCE. Symbol: $V_e$ **genetic v.** In population genetics, the fraction of the total phenotypic variance ascribable to differences in the genotypes of individuals in a given population. It is comprised of four components: additive variances, dominance variances, variances due to assortative mating, and variances due to epistasis. Compare ENVIRONMENTAL VARIANCE. Symbol: $V_g$.

**variant** \ver′ē·ənt\ **1** Something that differs from another or others in some aspect but displays the essential characteristics of the type to which it belongs. **2** In genetics, any organism that differs in phenotype or genotype from the wild type of the species. **alpha v.** A rhythmic wave form which is of slower frequency than the normal alpha rhythm but which behaves in all other respects like an alpha rhythm. **Haenel's v.** HAENEL SYMPTOM. **L-phase v.'s** L-FORMS **petit mal v.** See under ATYPICAL ABSENCE.

**variate** \ver′ē·it\ RANDOM VARIABLE. **binary v.** A variable in which only two values can exist, such as on/off, present/absent, or zero/one. **continuous v.** A quantity that may assume any of a theoretically infinite number of values within a defined interval. **discrete v.** A quantity that may assume any of a limited number of values within a defined interval.

**variation** [L *variatio* (from *variare* to diversify, vary) diversification, divergence, fluctuation] **1** The act of varying or the extent to which something is varied; measurable change or modification. **2** Any discernible difference among individuals or groups of individuals other than deviations ascribable to age or sex. The differences may reside in phenotype or genotype or both, and may result from genetic or environmental factors or their interaction. **continuous v.** Differences in a phenotype among individuals that are so numerous and of such small degree that neither one nor several phenotypes predominate. Distinguishing whether two individuals are alike or dissimilar with respect to the phenotype is difficult. **discontinuous v.** Differences in phenotype among individuals that fall into two or more discrete classes or distributions. **genetic v.** GENOTYPIC VARIATION. **genotypic v.** Any difference in genotype among individuals, which are usually of the same or related species, or groups of individuals. The three main causes of genotypic variation within a species are mutation, selection, and drift. Also *genetic variation.* **impressed v.** The differences among individuals or groups of individuals that are caused largely by environmental factors. **inborn v.** The individual variation which is due to differences in the information contained in the genetic material. **meristic v.** In a group of organisms of the same species or family, a variation in a phenotype that has quantifiable features, such as numbers of body parts. **negative v.** *Obs.* ACTION POTENTIAL. **phase v.** A phenomenon, studied mostly in salmonellae, in which a strain can shift rapidly between two H (flagellar) antigen types. The mechanism is a reversible inversion of a region of DNA, which regulates the production of one or the other H antigen. Also *smooth-rough variation, S-R variation.* **phenotypic v.** **1** Any difference in phenotype among individuals or groups of individuals regardless of cause. **2** Differences among individuals of a species in a given trait, particularly one determined by alleles at a single gene locus. **quasicontinuous v.** The apparent continuous variation in a trait in a sample that, for many possible reasons, is actually discontinuous. **saltatory v.** Any sudden change in phenotype in an offspring compared to its parents. Also *halmatogenesis.* **sampling v.** The variation between the estimates provided by two or more samples of the value of some parameter, such as a mean or a proportion, of the population from which they have been drawn. **smooth-rough v.** PHASE VARIATION. **S-R v.** PHASE VARIATION.

**varicated** \var′ikā′tid\ Affected by varices.

**varication** \var′ikā′shən\ The presence or formation of varices.

**variceal** \vəris′ē·əl\ Related to or caused by a varix or varices.

**varicectomy** \var′isek′təmē\ [*varic(o)-* + -ECTOMY] The excision of a venous varix.

**varicella** \var′isel′ə\ [New L (irreg. dim. of *variola* smallpox), chickenpox] A contagious viral disease caused by the varicella-zoster virus, a herpesvirus, and characterized by lesions beginning as macules and developing into vesicles. The incubation period is 17 to 21 days. The disease is relatively benign in children but may be serious in infants and adults. Also *chickenpox, chicken pox.* **v. bullosa** A rare form of varicella characterized by severe itching, the formation of large cutaneous vesicles (bullae), and the development of general constitutional symptoms. **v. gangrenosa** A rare form of varicella seen in children with underlying disease, as leukemia, and characterized by skin eruptions which lead to gangrenous ulceration. **v. inoculata** Abortive varicella produced in a susceptible individual by artificial inoculation with varicella virus from a lesion in another host. This procedure is unreliable and somewhat dangerous as a means of varicella prophylaxis. Also *vaccination varicella.* **pustular v.** A rare form of varicella in which some of the vesicles become pustular and purulent as a result of secondary infection, usually with staphylococci or streptococci. Also *varicella pustulosa.* **v. pustulosa** PUSTULAR VARICELLA. **vaccination v.** VARICELLA INOCULATA.

**varicellation** [*varicell(a)* + -ATION] Prophylactic immunization against varicella (chickenpox) with the varicella-zoster virus. Also *varicellization.*

**varicelliform** \var′isel′ifôrm\ Resembling varicella: said chiefly of cutaneous eruptions.

**varicelloid** \var′isel′oid\ [*varicell(a)* + -OID] Resembling varicella.

**varices** \var′isēz\ Plural of VARIX.

**varico-** \var′ikō-, ver′ikō-\ [L *varix* (genitive *varicis*) varicose vein] A combining form meaning varix, varicosity.

**varicocele** \var′ikōsēl′\ [VARICO- + -CELE[1]] Dilated veins occurring in the spermatic cord, sometimes producing a dull, aching pain in the scrotum and often associated with oligospermia. Also *varicole, cirsocele, pampinocele, ramex.*

**varicocelectomy** \var′ikōsēlek′təmē\ [*varicocel(e)* + -ECTOMY] The operative relief of varicocele by partial excision of the dilatated veins.

**varicoid** \var′ikoid\ Resembling a varix; cirsoid.

**varicole** \var′ikōl\ VARICOCELE.

**varicophlebitis** \var′ikōflebī′tis\ [VARICO- + PHLEBITIS] Inflammation of varicose veins.

**varicose** \var′ikōs\ [L *varicosus* (from *varix,* gen. *varicis* varicose vein) having varicose veins] Pertaining to or characterized by varices.

**varicosis** \var′ikō′sis\ [VARICO- + -SIS] A condition characterized by the presence of varices.

**varicosity** \var′ikäs′itē\ **1** The quality or condition of being varicose. **2** A varix or group of varices.

**varicotomy** \var′ikät′əmē\ [VARICO- + -TOMY] Incision of a varix or a varicose vein.

**varicula** \vərik′yələ\ A varix in the conjunctiva.

**variety** [French *variét(é)* (from L *varietas* variety, from *varius* varius) diversity] A recognized taxonomic category within a subspecies; a subdivision of a species often based on differences in phenotype.

**variola** \vərī′ələ\ [Med L (prob. dim. of L *varius* spotted, of divers colors, prob. akin to *varus* a blotch, pimple), smallpox] SMALLPOX. **v. benigna** VARIOLOID. **v. crystallina** *Obs.* VARICELLA. **v. hemorrhagica** HEMORRHAGIC SMALLPOX. **v. hemorrhagica pustulosa** A form of hemorrhagic smallpox in which the hemorrhages appear within the pustules as well as between them. **v. major** SMALLPOX. **v. miliaris** A form of smallpox in which the individual skin lesions are very small. **v. minor** ALASTRIM. **v. mitigata** ALASTRIM. **v. pemphigosa** A form of smallpox in which the vesicles resemble the bullae characteristic of pemphigus. **v. siliquosa** Smallpox in which the contents of the vesicles are absorbed and the empty walls of the pustular lesions remain. **v. sine eruptione** Smallpox which is aborted by existing immunity so that the patient experiences only the febrile prodromal illness. This form of the disease is probably noncontagious and develops only in vaccinated persons intensely exposed to smallpox. Also *variola sine variolis, varioloid.* **v. sine variolis** VARIOLA SINE ERUPTIONE. **v. verrucosa** A form of smallpox in which the skin lesions do not progress beyond the papular stage. Also *wart pox.*

**variolar** \vərī′ələr\ [*variol(a)* + AR] Concerning or characterized by smallpox. Also *variolous.*

**variolate** \var′e·əlāt′\ [*variol(a)* + -ATE] To inoculate with the smallpox virus.

**variolation** \var′ē·əlā′shən\ [*variol(a)* + -ATION] Inoculation with variola virus. Formerly used for protection against natural smallpox, it was a dangerous practice and was supplanted by vaccination. Also *variolization.*

**varioliform** \var′ē·ō′lifôrm\ [*variol(a)* + *i* + -FORM] Smallpoxlike: used especially in reference to an exanthem.

**variolization** \var′ē·ō′līzā′shən\ VARIOLATION.

**varioloid** \var′ē·əloid′\ **1** Resembling smallpox. **2** A mild, abortive form of smallpox occurring in persons who have been vaccinated or have had the disease previously. Also *variola benigna.* **3** VARIOLA SINE ERUPTIONE.

**variolous** \vərī′ələs\ VARIOLAR.

**variolovaccine** \vərī′əlōvak′sēn\ SMALLPOX VACCINE.

**varix** \var′iks\ [L, a varicose vein, esp. in the leg] (*pl.* varices) A mass composed of enlarged and tortuous blood or lymphatic vessels. **anastomotic v.** A varix associated with communicating vessels. **aneurysmal v.** A form of arteriovenous aneurysm in which there are dilated and tortuous vessels. Also *aneurysmoid varix.* **arterial v.** A varix affecting an artery. **chyle v.** A varix of chyliferous lymphatic vessels near the pelvis of the ureter, as may occur in filariasis. Rupture of varices results in chyluria. **cirsoid v.** CIRSOID ANEURYSM. **esophageal varices** Dilated, tortuous, submucosal esophageal veins resulting from portal hypertension. **gelatinous v.** Nodularity of the umbilical cord due to small accumulations of gelatinous material. **lymph v.** A swelling of a lymph node due to dilated lymphatics. Also *varix lymphaticus.* **papillary varices** CAYENNE PEPPER SPOTS.

**varnish / cavity v.** CAVITY LINER.

**varolian** \vərō′lē·ən\ **1** Associated with Constanzo Varolius, anatomist from Bologna and later Rome, 1543–1575, after whom certain anatomic structures have been named. **2** Denoting the pons.

**Varolius** [Constantius *Varolius,* Italian anatomist and surgeon, 1543–1575] **1** Pons varolii. See under PONS. **2** Valve of Varolius. See under VALVA ILEOCECALIS.

**varus** \ver′əs\ [L, bent, twisted] Bending or twisting inward or toward the midline: said of a deformed part.

**vas** \vas\ [L, a vessel, container] (*pl.* vasa) A vessel; especially, a channel conducting bodily fluids such as blood, lymph, or semen. **v. aberrans** **1** *Outmoded* DUCTULUS ABERRANS SUPERIOR. **2** Any vessel having an abnormal course. **v. aberrans of Roth** An occasional diverticulum of the rete testis or of the ductuli efferentes testis. **vasa aberrantia hepatis** Atrophied remains of bile ducts found in the fibrous appendix of the liver, the edges of the left lobe and near the groove for the inferior vena cava. **v. afferens arteriae interlobularis** ARTERIOLA GLOMERULARIS AFFERENS. **v. afferens glomeruli** ARTERIOLA GLOMERULARIS AFFERENS. **vasa afferentia** Afferent vessels; vessels carrying blood to a part or lymph to a node, for example, arteriolae glomerulares afferentes, or vasa afferentia nodi lymphatici. **vasa afferentia nodi lymphatici** Vessels that convey lymph to a lymph node, entering it at various points on its periphery and losing all their coats except the endothelial layer to form a plexus in the capsule before entering the subcapsular lymph sinus. Also *afferent vessels of lymph node.* **v. anastomoticum** [NA] A vessel that connects one vessel to another, as between arteries, veins, or lymph vessels. Also *anastomotic vessel.* **vasa auris internae** [NA] The labyrinthine arteries and veins of the internal ear. **vasa brevia** ARTERIAE GASTRICAE BREVES. **v. capillare** [NA] Any side branch of the terminal arterioles beyond the precapillary sphincters that communicates with other similar branches to form a network, the nature of which varies in different tissues, and from which venules derive. See illustration at CAPILLARY BED. Also *capillary.* **v. collaterale** [NA] A branch running parallel to its parent artery of origin. Also *collateral vessel.* **vasa corona** VASOCORONA. **v. deferens** *Outmoded* DUCTUS DEFERENS. **v. efferens arteriae interlobularis** ARTERIOLA GLOMERULARIS EFFERENS. **v. efferens glomeruli** ARTERIOLA GLOMERULARIS EFFERENS. **vasa efferentia** Efferent vessels or ducts; for example, vessels conducting blood away from a part, as from the renal glomerulus to the capillary plexus around the tubules, or vessels carrying lymph away from a lymph node (vasa efferentia nodi lymphatici), or the ductules from the rete testis to the duct of the epididymis (ductuli efferentes testis). **vasa efferentia nodi lymphatici** Vessels commencing in the lymph sinuses of the medulla of a lymph node and conducting lymph away from the node through its hilum. Also *efferent vessels of lymph* *node.* **Ferrein's vasa aberrantia** Aberrant bile canaliculi that are not connected with hepatic lobules. **vasa lymphatica** [NA] Delicate valved channels commencing in networks of lymph capillaries found in most tissues and running either superficially or deeply to and between varying numbers of lymph nodes along their course, until they reach either the thoracic duct or right lymphatic duct, which discharge the lymph into the left and right brachiocephalic veins respectively. The vessels anastomose freely and the larger ones are supplied by vasa vasorum and nerve networks. Also *lymphatic vessels, lymph vessels, lymphatics, lymphatic ducts.* **vasa lymphatica profunda** [NA] Lymphatic vessels draining the deeper tissues of regions of the body and coursing along the deeply placed vessels to regional lymph nodes. Also *deep lymphatic vessels.* **vasa lymphatica superficialia** [NA] Lymphatic vessels draining the superficial capillary plexuses of the body, especially of the skin, and coursing in the subcutaneous tissues, often alongside superficial veins, near the deep fascia to reach regional lymph nodes. Vessels are also located in the subserous areolar tissues of organs, such as the liver, testis, and ovary, and of the walls of the abdomen. They anastomose freely but seldom communicate with the vasa lymphatica profunda. Also *superficial lymphatic vessels.* **v. lymphaticum** [NA] Any of the vasa lymphatica. Also *lymphangion, lymphoduct.* **vasa previa** Presentation of the umbilical vessels within the fetal membranes at the cervical os in advance of the fetal presenting part. The condition results from velamentous insertion of the umbilicus and is associated with high fetal mortality. **v. prominens ductus cochlearis** [NA] A relatively large blood vessel in the base of the spiral prominence on the lateral wall of the cochlear duct. **vasa recta** 1 ARTERIOLAE RECTAE RENIS. 2 TUBULI SEMINIFERI RECTI. **vasa sanguinea retinae** [NA] The blood vessels of the retina, including the circulus vasculosus nervi optici and all the arterioles and venules of the central artery and vein of the retina, respectively. **v. spirale** [NA] One or two large veins in the layer of vascular connective tissue of the zona arcuata of the lamina basilaris. **vasa vasorum** [NA] Minute nutrient blood vessels of the outer and middle coats of the larger arteries and veins.

**vas-** \vas-\ VASO-.

**vasa** \vā′zə\ Plural of VAS.

**vasal** \vā′zəl\ Pertaining to vasa or vessels; vascular.

**vascul-** \vas′kyəl-\ VASCULO-.

**vascular** \vas′kyələr\ [VASCUL- + -AR] Relating to or containing vessels, especially blood vessels. Also *angeial.*

**vascularity** \vas′kyəlar′itē\ The extent to which a tissue or organ contains blood vessels.

**vascularization** \vas′kyələr′izā′shən\ The formation of vascular elements or blood vessels in a tissue, an organ, or a part of a body during normal development, during repair or growth, or as a result of surgical procedures. In its full sense, vascularization implies the development of capillaries to supply oxygen and nutriment and remove waste, and thus results in proper functional activity.

**vasculature** \vas′kyələchər\ A system of vessels, or the arrangement of vessels, serving an organ or part of the body, or the body as a whole. Also *angioarchitecture.*

**vasculitis** \vas′kyəlī′tis\ [VASCUL- + -ITIS] Inflammation of blood vessels; angiitis. **allergic cutaneous v.** An immune-complex induced inflammation in the small blood vessels of the skin that occurs as a reaction to microbial or other antigens and is characterized by crops of papules, purpuric lesions, vesicles, and focal necroses. **necrotizing v.** POLYARTERITIS. **nodular v.** A subacute recurrent or chronic eruption of inflammatory nodules, principally on the lower legs. Nodular vasculitis comprises a number of distinct but overlapping clinicopathological entities. **retinal v.** Inflammation of the vessels of the retina of the eye.

**vasculo-** \vas′kyəlō-\ [L *vasculum* (diminutive of *vas* vessel) small vessel] A combining form meaning vessel, especially a blood vessel.

**vasculocardiac** \vas′kyəlōkär′dē·ak\ Pertaining to the heart and blood vessels.

**vasculogenesis** \vas′kyəlōjen′əsis\ [VASCULO- + GENESIS] The formation of the blood vessels and thus of the vascular system in its entirety.

**vasculolymphatic** \vas′kyəlōlimfat′ik\ Pertaining to blood vessels and lymphatic vessels.

**vasculum** \vas′kyələm\ (*pl.* vascula) A small vessel. **v. aberrans** *Outmoded* DUCTULUS ABERRANS SUPERIOR.

**vasectomy** \vasek′təmē\ [*vas (deferens)* + -ECTOMY] Bilateral ligation or interruption of the vas deferens. It is employed as a method of surgical contraception. Also *vasoligation, vasoligature, deferentectomy, gonangiectomy.* **crossover v.** A vasectomy involving the connection of one ductus deferens to the other.

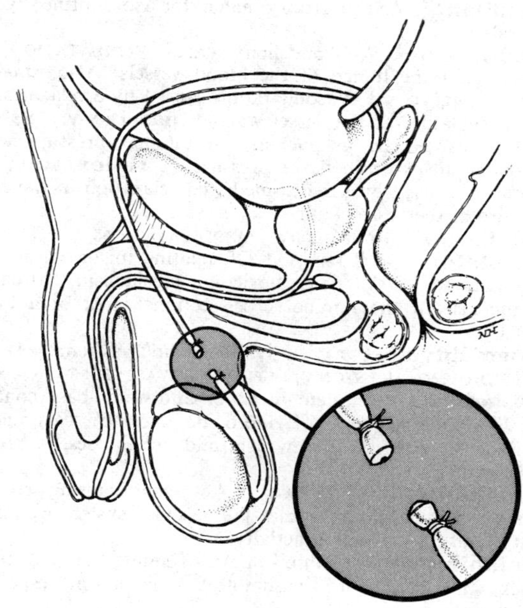

Vasectomy

**vasifaction** \vas′ifak′shən\ [VAS- + *i* + L *factio* a making, doing] The formation of blood vessels or the capacity to form them. Also *vasiformation.* Adj. vasifactive, vasoformative.

**vasiform** \vas′ifôrm\ Shaped like a vessel; tubular in form.

**vasiformation** \va′sifôrmā′shən\ VASIFACTION.

**vasitis** \vasī′tis\ [VAS- + -ITIS] An infective process of the vas deferens usually spreading from adjacent organs and caused by a variety of infective agents including *Neisseria gonorrhoeae.* **v. nodosa** A beading and nodularity of the vas deferens just above the epididymis, probably a result of previously unrecognized vasitis of unknown origin.

**vaso-** \vas′ō-\ [L *vas* vessel, receptacle] A combining form meaning vessel, especially a blood vessel. Also *vas-*.

**vasoactive** \-ak′tiv\ Exerting an effect on the vasculature.

**vasoconstriction** \-kənstrik′shən\ [VASO- + CONSTRICTION] A narrowing of the lumen of the blood vessels. **active v.** Vasoconstriction caused by contraction of the musculature of the vessel wall. **passive v.** Vasoconstriction caused by an increase in extrinsic tissue pressure or a reduction in luminal pressure.

**vasoconstrictive** \-kənstrik′tiv\ VASOCONSTRICTOR.

**vasoconstrictor** \-kənstrik′tər\ **1** Of or relating to vasoconstriction. **2** An agent that effects vasoconstriction. For defs. 1 and 2 also *vasoconstrictive*.

**vasocorona** \-kôrō′nə\ One of several annular arterial anastomoses around the spinal cord from which branches penetrate the cord in a radial fashion. *Outmoded.* Also *vasa corona*.

**vasodepression** \-dipresh′ən\ A loss of tone in blood vessels with consequent hypotension.

**vasodepressor** \-dipres′ər\ **1** Tending to lower vascular tone. **2** An agent that lowers vascular tone and blood pressure.

**Vasodilan** A proprietary name for isoxsuprine hydrochloride.

**vasodilatation** \-dil′ətā′shən\ [VASO- + DILATATION] A widening of the lumen of the blood vessels. Also *vasodilation*. **active v.** Vasodilatation caused by a relaxation of the musculature of the vessel wall. **passive v.** Vasodilatation caused by an increase in luminal pressure when compared to extrinsic tissue pressure. **reflex v.** Vasodilatation caused by a reflex-mediated relaxation in the musculature of the vessel wall.

**vasodilation** \-dīlā′shən\ VASODILATATION.

**vasodilator** \-dī′lātər\ **1** Of, relating to, or causing vasodilatation. **2** An agent, device, or mechanism that causes an increase in the luminal cross-sectional area of a blood vessel.

**vasoepididymostomy** \vas′ō·ep′idid′imäs′təmē\ [VASO- + EPIDIDYMO- + -STOMY] EPIDIDYMOVASOSTOMY.

**Vasogen** An ointment in an oil-and-water base containing 20% dimethicone, 7.5% zinc oxide, and 1.5% calamine. It is used for bedsores, diaper rash, and dermatoses. A proprietary name.

**vasoinhibitor** \-inhib′itər\ An agent causing reduced activity of musculature within the vascular system by inhibition of vasomotor neural activity.

**vasoinhibitory** \-inhib′itôr′ē\ Tending to reduce or block the action of vasomotor innervation, especially vasopressor activity.

**vasolabile** \-lā′bīl\ Of or relating to an instability of the vascular system.

**vasoligation** \-līgā′shən\ [VASO- + LIGATION] VASECTOMY.

**vasoligature** \-lig′əchər\ [VASO- + LIGATURE] VASECTOMY.

**vasomotion** \-mō′shən\ An alteration of the contractility of vessel walls in the vascular system.

**vasomotor** \-mō′tər\ Influencing the contractility of the muscular walls of the blood vessels.

**vasoneuropathy** \-n$^y$ŭräp′əthē\ AUTONOMIC NEUROPATHY.

**vaso-orchidostomy** \-ôr′kidäs′təmē\ [VASO- + ORCHIDOSTOMY] An operation forming a connection between the ductus deferens and the testis.

**vasoparalysis** \-pəral′isis\ VASOMOTOR PARALYSIS.

**vasoparesis** \-pərē′sis\ [VASO- + PARESIS] Paresis of effector organs controlled by vasomotor nerves.

**vasopressin** \-pres′in\ An octapeptide secreted by the supraoptic nuclei of the hypothalamus and stored in, and released from, the posterior lobe of the pituitary gland. Through the action of the hormone upon water reabsorption by the distal renal tubule, hydration is precisely maintained. The peptide has vasopressor and weak oxytocic effects, and stimulates intestinal contraction. The main physiologic regulator of its secretion is the osmotic pressure of the circulating plasma, but many nociceptive stimuli and pharmacologic agents stimulate its release. Endogenous deficiency of vasopressin characterizes diabetes insipidus of central origin, and it is used pharmaceutically in the treatment of diabetes insipidus. The human hormone has the sequence Cys-Tyr-Phe-Gln-Asn-Cys-Pro-Arg-Gly-$NH_2$, and has a disulfide bond between residues 1 and 6. Also *antidiuretic hormone, antidiuretic substance, β-hypophamine* (seldom used).

**vasopressinase** \-pres′inās\ OXYTOCINASE.

**vasopressin 8-lysine** LYPRESSIN.

**vasopressin tannate** A preparation of the pressor principle from the posterior lobe of the pituitary gland, containing the water-insoluble tannic acid salts. It is injected intramuscularly.

**vasopressor** \-pres′ər\ [VASO- + Late L *pressor* (from *press(us)*, past part. of *premere* to press + *-or* -OR) one who presses] **1** Producing an increase in blood pressure. **2** An agent capable of producing an increase in blood pressure.

**vasopuncture** \-pungk′chər\ Puncture of a vas deferens.

**vasoreflex** \-rē′fleks\ A reflex that involves the vascular system.

**vasorelaxation** \-rē′laksā′shən\ A decrease in blood pressure brought about by the diminution of tension in the vessel walls.

**vasoresection** \-risek′shən\ Partial excision of the ductus deferens.

**vasorrhaphy** \vasôr′əfē\ [VASO- + -RRHAPHY] A suturing of the ductus deferens.

**vasosection** \-sek′shən\ [VASO- + SECTION] The division of a vessel, especially the ductus deferens.

**vasosensory** \-sen′sərē\ Pertaining to sensory innervation of the vascular system.

**vasospasm** \vaz′ōspazm\ An excessive contraction in the muscular vessel walls of the vascular system. Also *angiospasm, vascular spasm*.

**vasospasmolytic** \-spaz′məlit′ik\ Capable of reversing a vasospasm.

**vasospastic** \-spas′tik\ Of or relating to the initiation of vasospasm. Also *angiospastic*.

**vasostimulant** \-stim′yələnt\ **1** Causing contraction of the muscle in the walls of the vessels of the vascular system. **2** An agent capable of causing such contraction.

**vasostomy** \vasäs′təmē\ [VASO- + -STOMY] The surgical creation of an opening into a ductus deferens.

**vasotomy** \vasät′əmē\ [VASO- + -TOMY] An incision of the ductus deferens. Also *Belfield's operation*.

**vasotonia** \-tō′nē·ə\ [VASO- + *ton(o)-* + -IA] The tension in the walls of the vessels of the vascular system.

**vasotonic** \-tän′ik\ **1** Of or relating to vasotonia. **2** Tending to increase vascular tension. **3** An agent that increases vascular tension. For defs. 1–3 also *angiotonic*.

**vasotribe** \vas′ōtrīb\ ANGIOTRIBE.

**vasotropic** \-träp′ik\ [VASO- + -TROPIC[1]] Producing or capable of producing an effect on blood vessels.

**vasovagal** \-vā′gəl\ Pertaining to or affecting the blood vessels and vagus nerve.

**vasovasotomy** \-vasät′əmē\ [VASO- + VASOTOMY] Anastomosis of the severed ends of the vas deferens for reversal of a vasectomy.
**vasovesiculectomy** \-vesik′yəlek′təmē\ [VASO- + VESICUL- + -ECTOMY] Excision of the ductus deferens and the seminal vesicle.
**vasovesiculitis** \-vesik′yəlī′tis\ [VASO- + VESICUL- + -ITIS] Inflammation of the ductus deferens and seminal vesicle.
**vastus** \vas′təs\ Large; broad: used in the designation of certain muscles.
**Vater** [Abraham *Vater,* German anatomist and botanist, 1684–1751] **1** Carcinoma of the ampulla of Vater. See under CARCINOMA. **2** Ampulla of Vater. See under AMPULLA HEPATOPANCREATICA. **3** Vater's corpuscles, Vater-Pacini corpuscles. See under PACINIAN CORPUSCLES. **4** See under FOLD. **5** Papilla of Vater. See under PAPILLA DUODENI MAJOR.
**vault** [French *voûte* (from L *volutus,* past part. of *volvere* to roll, turn or from *volvitatus,* past part. of *volvitare* to turn, leap) a vault] An arched roof. **cranial v.** The portion of the skull that includes the frontal, occipital, parietal, and temporal bones. **v. of pharynx** FORNIX PHARYNGIS.
**VCE** vagina, ectocervix, and endocervix (smear).
**VCG** vectorcardiogram.
**VD** venereal disease.
**VDH** valvular disease of the heart.
**VDRL** Venereal Disease Research Laboratory. See also VDRL TEST.
**vection** \vek′shən\ [L *vectio* (from *vectus,* past part. of *vehere* to carry, convey) a carrying, conveying] The active conveyance of an agent of disease from an infected host to a noninfected host by the action of a vector, usually a blood-sucking insect, mite, or tick.
**vector** \vek′tər\ [L (from *vect(us),* past part. of *vehere* to convey, bear + *-or* -OR), one who carries or bears] **1** An animal capable, without itself suffering from a disease, of conveying an infection that produces the disease from one host to another. The infecting organism may multiply within the vector or be transmitted vertically from the vector to its offspring, but an agent that passively transports infection is not a vector. **2** A quantity having direction as well as magnitude. Also *vectorial quantity.* **3** In electrocardiography, the magnitude, direction, and sense of the total electrical forces either instantaneously (instantaneous vector) or presented as a mean over a defined period, e.g., those generated during depolarization of the ventricles. **biological v.** A vector, commonly an arthropod, in which development or multiplication of the infecting organism takes place prior to its transmission to another host, as in the production of sporozoites in the life cycle of the malarial parasites in the mosquito vector. **cardiac v.** The sum of all the electrical forces during the inscription of one event in the cardiac cycle, such as ventricular depolarization (the QRS complex). **instantaneous v.** The sum of all the electrical events in the heart at one instant in time, represented by an arrow of appropriate direction, magnitude, and sense. **manifest v.** The projection of a two-dimensional or three-dimensional cardiac vector in a single plane. **mechanical v.** A disease vector in which no development of the agent takes place. This can be seen in the transfer of *Trypanosoma equinum* flagellates by the mouthparts of tabanid flies, rather than by injection of the progeny of cyclic development by the normal tsetse fly vector. **spatial v.** A vector which moves in three dimensions as in the vectorcardiogram, for which vector loops are formed in frontal, sagittal, and horizontal planes.
**vectorcardiogram** \vek′tərkär′dē·əgram′\ The registration of the moment-to-moment electromotive forces of the heart, derived from two simultaneously recorded scalar electrocardiograms. It is usually displayed as a loop on an oscilloscope. Also *vector cardiogram.* Abbr. VCG
**vectorcardiograph** \vek′tərkär′dē·əgraf\ An instrument for recording vectorcardiograms.
**vectorcardiography** \vek′tərkär′dē·äg′rəfē\ The recording of the direction, magnitude, and sense of the instantaneous vectors of the heart throughout one complete cardiac cycle. It is usually obtained in three planes. Also *cardiovectrography, vector cardiography.* **spatial v.** Representation of the cardiac vector by projection on each of the three mutually orthogonal planes, usually displayed as loops.
**vectorial** \vektôr′ē·əl\ Relating to a vector.
**Vedder** [Edward Bright *Vedder,* U.S. surgeon, 1878–1952] Vedder signs. See under SIGN.
**vegan** \vēg′an, vej′an\ [Contraction of *veg(etari)an*] One who will not consume food of animal origin.
**vegetal** \vej′ətəl\ VEGETATIVE.
**vegetarian** \vej′əter′ē·ən\ [*veget(able)* + L *-ari(us)* -ARY + English *-an,* noun suffix] One who consumes a diet composed entirely of foods of vegetable origin. Vegans strictly adhere to this regimen but other vegetarians also consume eggs (ovovegetarians), or dairy products (lactovegetarians), or both (ovolactovegetarians).
**vegetation** [Med L *vegetatio* (from L *vegetatus,* past part. of *vegetare* to grow, from *vegere* to quicken, arouse) a growing, flourishing] A vigorously growing fungoid excrescence. **adenoid v.** ADENOIDS. **bacterial v.'s** Clumps of fibrin, platelets, and bacteria, found most often on heart valves and due to infection by bacteria of platelets which have adhered to the valve. They are the characteristic lesions of bacterial endocarditis. **verrucous v.'s** Wartlike clumps of fibrin and platelets on the endocardium, especially of the heart valves, due to immunologic disease.
**vegetative** \vej′ətətiv, vej′ətā′tiv\ [Med L *vegetativ(us)* (from *vegetat(us),* past part. of *vegetare* to grow + L *-ivus* -IVE) vegetative] **1** Engaged in or relating to processes of nutrition or growth, as distinct from reproduction. Also *vegetal.* **2** Existing like a vegetable, without will or consciousness. **3** Pertaining to involuntary bodily functions or to the autonomic nervous system.
**vehicle** Any substance having little or no therapeutic action itself but used to convey or to give bulk to a medicine.
**veil** [L *velum.* See VELUM.] **1** CAUL. **2** Any anatomic structure that resembles a veil; velum. **Fick's v.** Glare or colored halos seen as a result of corneal edema from contact lens wear. **Sattler's v.** A corneal haze resulting from the anoxia induced by prolonged wearing of a contact lens. **vitreous v.'s** Very fine, filmlike sheets of tissue that have split off from the most anterior portions of the retina in juvenile retinoschisis and are faintly visible, having been displaced forward from their normal position.
***Veillonella*** \vā′yənel′ə\ A genus of Gram-negative anaerobic cocci with complex growth requirements, found in the mouth and the gastrointestinal tract of humans and other mammals. They resemble *Propionibacterium* species in producing propionic acid.

# vein

**vein** [Old French *veine,* from L *vena* a blood vessel, vein] VENA. **accessory cephalic v.** VENA CEPHALICA AC-

CESSORIA. **accessory hemiazygos v.** VENA HEMIAZYGOS ACCESSORIA. **accessory portal v.'s** Anastomotic veins between the tributaries of the portal vein and those of the caval systems. They provide important collateral channels for return of portal blood to the heart in conditions such as liver diseases that obstruct the hepatic capillaries. The paraumbilical veins, for example, may function as accessory portal veins. **accessory saphenous v.** VENA SAPHENA ACCESSORIA. **accessory suprarenal v.'s** Small veins that drain the capillary network of the cortex of the suprarenal glands. The superior veins follow the superior suprarenal arteries and end in the inferior phrenic veins, while the inferior veins of the right gland drain into the inferior vena cava and those of the left gland drain into the left renal vein. Some join veins of the pararenal fat and end in the suprarenal veins. **accessory vertebral v.** VENA VERTEBRALIS ACCESSORIA. **accompanying v.** VENA COMITANS. **accompanying v. of hypoglossal nerve** VENA COMITANS NERVI HYPOGLOSSI. **adipose v.** CAPSULAR VEIN. **afferent v.'s** Veins carrying blood to an organ. See under ARTERIAL VEIN. **allantoic v.** A vein in the embryo which drains blood from the allantois towards the general venous circulation. Towards the thirtieth day of human intrauterine life this vein gains connection with the placenta and conveys back to the fetus the oxygen and nutritive substances supplied from the maternal circulation by means of the placenta. It is then known as the umbilical vein. **angular v.** VENA ANGULARIS. **anomalous pulmonary v.'s** A congenital malformation, often associated with an atrial septal defect, in which pulmonary veins drain into some site other than the left atrium, such as the right atrium, coronary sinus great veins, or an anomalous chamber. **anterior anastomotic v. of Trolard** VENA ANASTOMOTICA SUPERIOR. **anterior auricular v.'s** VENAE AURICULARES ANTERIORES. **anterior cardiac v.'s** VENAE CARDIACAE ANTERIORES. **anterior cerebral v.'s** VENA CEREBRI ANTERIOR. **anterior ciliary v.'s** VENAE CILIARES ANTERIORES. **anterior circumflex humeral v.'s** Veins that accompany the anterior circumflex humeral artery and terminate in either the axillary vein or the brachial veins. **v. of anterior condylar foramen** An emissary vein at the base of the skull which connects the venous plexus of the hypoglossal canal with the inferior petrosal sinus or directly with the internal jugular vein. It may replace the venous plexus of the hypoglossal canal. **anterior v. of corpus callosum** A vein that follows the curvature of the corpus callosum along the medial surface of the frontal pole of the cerebral hemisphere. Rostral to the anterior wall of the third ventricle it becomes the anterior cerebral vein. Also *anterior limbic vein*. **anterior facial v.** VENA FACIALIS. **anterior intercostal v.'s** VENAE INTERCOSTALES ANTERIORES. **anterior jugular v.** VENA JUGULARIS ANTERIOR. **anterior labial v.'s** VENAE LABIALES ANTERIORES. **anterior limbic v.** ANTERIOR VEIN OF CORPUS CALLOSUM. **anterior median longitudinal v. of spinal cord** One of the venae spinales anteriores which is situated in front of the anterior median fissure of the spinal cord. It receives the anterior sulcal veins which accompany the branches of the anterior spinal artery in the cord, and communicates with the other longitudinal veins and the radicular veins. **anterior median v. of medulla** A venous channel, coursing along the ventral median fissure of the medulla oblongata that is an extension of the anterior median vein of the spinal cord leading into the brainstem. **anterior median v. of spinal cord** Either the anterior median longitudinal vein of spinal cord, or one of the anterior sulcal veins which drains the anteromedial portions of the spinal cord and ends in the anterior median longitudinal vein. **anterior parietal diploic v.** VENA DIPLOICA TEMPORALIS ANTERIOR. **anterior parotid v.'s** RAMI PAROTIDEI VENAE FACIALIS. **v.'s of anterior perforated space** A group of veins on the inferomedial surface of the frontal lobe near the anterior perforated space that drain posteriorly into the basilar venous plexus. These include the posterior orbital vein, the small veins on the orbital surface of the frontal lobe, the vein of the olfactory bulb, and the anterior vein of the corpus callosum. **anterior radicular v.'s of spinal cord** About six to twelve veins that drain the plexus between the anterior spinal veins and empty into the internal vertebral venous plexuses and the intervertebral veins. Some smaller veins, also located along some ventral nerve roots of the spinal cord, also drain the medial portion of the anterior gray column and the white substance adjacent to the anterior median fissure. **anterior scrotal v.'s** VENAE SCROTALES ANTERIORES. **anterior spinal v.'s** VENAE SPINALES ANTERIORES. **anterior spiral v.** A tributary of the labyrinthine veins that drains the apical and middle turns of the cochlea. It receives a vestibular vein anteriorly and ends in the vena aqueductus cochleae by uniting with the posterior spiral vein. **anterior temporal diploic v.** VENA DIPLOICA TEMPORALIS ANTERIOR. **anterior tibial v.'s** VENAE TIBIALES ANTERIORES. **anterior vertebral v.** VENA VERTEBRALIS ANTERIOR. **anterolateral v.'s of spinal cord** Two of the venae spinales anteriores which run longitudinally on the anterior surface of the spinal cord on either side of the emerging ventral roots, helping to drain the spinal cord and ending in the internal vertebral venous plexuses. **appendicular v.** VENA APPENDICULARIS. **v. of aqueduct of vestibule** VENA AQUEDUCTUS VESTIBULI. **arciform v.'s** VENAE ARCUATAE RENIS. **arcuate v.'s of kidney** VENAE ARCUATAE RENIS. **arterial v.** **1** A vessel arising from the heart but containing deoxygenated (venous) blood, such as truncus pulmonalis. **2** A vessel supplying blood to an organ, thereby resembling an artery but containing venous blood, such as the portal vein. **ascending lumbar v.** VENA LUMBALIS ASCENDENS. **avalvular v.'s** Veins that lack valves, usually very small or very large veins. Valves are absent in dural venous sinuses, diploic, brachiocephalic, portal, ophthalmic, urethral, pulmonary, bronchial, renal, suprarenal, uterine, umbilical and placental veins, the superior vena cava, veins of the vertebral plexuses, and others. **axillary v.** VENA AXILLARIS. **azygos v.** VENA AZYGOS. **basal v.** VENA BASALIS. **basilic v.** VENA BASILICA. **basivertebral v.'s** VENAE BASIVERTEBRALES. **brachial v.'s** VENAE BRACHIALES. **brachiocephalic v.'s** VENAE BRACHIOCEPHALICAE DEXTRA ET SINISTRA. **Breschet's v.'s** VENAE DIPLOICAE. **bronchial v.'s** VENAE BRONCHIALES. **Browning's v.** VENA ANASTOMOTICA INFERIOR. **buccal v.'s** The veins that accompany the buccal artery and are tributaries of either the pterygoid plexus, the retromandibular vein, or the facial vein. **v. of bulb of penis** VENA BULBI PENIS. **v. of bulb of vestibule** VENA BULBI VESTIBULI. **Burow's v.** **1** An occasional branch of the inferior epigastric vein that is joined by a branch from the urinary bladder to proceed to the portal vein. **2** Either of the two renal veins. **v. of calcar avis of Morand** A tributary of the internal cerebral vein that drains the calcar avis on the medial wall of the posterior cornu of the lateral ventricle of the cerebral hemisphere. **v. of canaliculus of cochlea** VENA AQUEDUCTUS COCHLEAE. **capillary v.** VENULA. **capsular v.** One of the small veins draining the adipose capsule of the kidney and communicating with the venulae stellatae before terminating in the renal vein. Also *adipose vein.* **cardiac v.'s** VENAE CORDIS. **cardinal v.'s** Either of two pairs of longitudinally-oriented veins (anterior and posterior) which are responsible for draining the intra-embryonic tissues into the heart. On each side the anterior and posterior cardinal veins unite to form a common cardinal vein (duct of Cuvier) which drains into the corresponding horn of the sinus venosus. Many sections of the cardinal vein system atrophy and disappear, particularly on the left side of the body. Nevertheless parts of the anterior cardinals are retained as the brachiocephalic veins and the superior vena cava, while the posterior cardinals contribute to the caudal end of the inferior cava and to parts of the definitive azygos venous system. **cavernous v.'s of penis** VENAE CAVERNOSAE PENIS. **central v.** A vein lying in the center of an organ or part of an organ. **central v.'s of hepatic lobules** VENAE CENTRALES HEPATIS. **central v.'s of liver** VENAE CENTRALES HEPATIS. **central v. of retina** VENA CENTRALIS RETINAE. **central v. of suprarenal gland** VENA CENTRALIS GLANDULAE SUPRARENALIS. **cephalic v.** VENA CEPHALICA. **cerebral v.'s** VENAE CEREBRI. **choroid v.** VENA CHOROIDEA. **ciliary v.'s** VENAE CILIARES. **v. of cochlear aqueduct** VENA AQUEDUCTUS COCHLEAE. **v. of cochlear canal** VENA AQUEDUCTUS COCHLEAE. **collecting v.** One of the tributaries of the hepatic veins formed by the union of several sublobular, or intercalated, veins of the liver. **common cardinal v.** Either of two symmetric venous channels formed on each side of the embryo by the union of the anterior and posterior cardinal veins. Each opens into the corresponding horn of the sinus venosus. On the right side it contributes to the superior vena cava, while on the left side it becomes reduced in size to form the oblique atrial vein of Marshall. Also *duct of Cuvier, ductus cuvieri, canal of Cuvier, sinus of Cuvier, truncus transversus.* **common femoral v.** The femoral vein proximal to the junction with the profunda femoris vein: a term used by some surgeons. Compare SUPERFICIAL FEMORAL VEIN. **common iliac v.** VENA ILIACA COMMUNIS. **companion v.** VENA COMITANS. **condylar emissary v.** VENA EMISSARIA CONDYLARIS. **v. of condyloid canal** VENA EMISSARIA CONDYLARIS. **condyloid emissary v.** VENA EMISSARIA CONDYLARIS. **conjunctival v.'s** VENAE CONJUNCTIVALES. **costoaxillary v.'s** Veins draining the circulus venosus of the breast that anastomose with intercostal veins and provide collateral communications between the lateral thoracic branches of the axillary veins, the superior vena cava, and the azygos system. **cutaneous v.** VENA CUTANEA. **cystic v.** VENA CYSTICA. **deep cervical v.** VENA CERVICALIS PROFUNDA. **deep circumflex iliac v.** VENA CIRCUMFLEXA ILIACA PROFUNDA. **deep v.'s of clitoris** VENAE PROFUNDAE CLITORIDIS. **deep dorsal v. of clitoris** VENA DORSALIS PROFUNDA CLITORIDIS. **deep dorsal v. of penis** VENA DORSALIS PROFUNDA PENIS. **deep facial v.** VENA PROFUNDA FACIEI. **deep femoral v.** VENA PROFUNDA FEMORIS. **deep lingual v.** VENA PROFUNDA LINGUAE. **deep middle cerebral v.** VENA MEDIA PROFUNDA CEREBRI. **deep v.'s of penis** VENAE PROFUNDAE PENIS. **deep temporal v.'s** VENAE TEMPORALES PROFUNDAE. **deep v. of thigh** VENA PROFUNDA FEMORIS. **deep v. of tongue** VENA PROFUNDA LINGUAE. **v.'s of dental pulp** Veins which accompany the rami dentales of the inferior alveolar, anterior superior alveolar, and posterior superior alveolar arteries and drain the pulp cavity of a tooth through the apical foramen. **v. of dentate nucleus** A vein accompanying the artery that supplies the dentate nucleus in the interior of the cerebellum. The artery is a branch of the posterior inferior cerebellar artery, and the vein, one of the inferior cerebellar veins, drains into the occipital or inferior petrosal sinus. **v.'s of diploë** VENAE DIPLOICAE. **diploic v.'s** VENAE DIPLOICAE. **dorsal digital v.'s of foot** VENAE DIGITALES DORSALES PEDIS. **dorsal lingual v.'s** VENAE DORSALES LINGUAE. **dorsal metacarpal v.'s** VENAE METACARPALES DORSALES. **dorsal metatarsal v.'s** VENAE METATARSALES DORSALES PEDIS. **dorsal scapular v.** VENA SCAPULARIS DORSALIS. **dorsal v.'s of tongue** VENAE DORSALES LINGUAE. **emissary v.** VENA EMISSARIA. **emissary v.'s of foramen ovale** PLEXUS VENOSUS FORAMINIS OVALIS. **episcleral v.'s** VENAE EPISCLERALES. **esophageal v.'s** VENAE ESOPHAGEALES. **ethmoidal v.'s** VENAE ETHMOIDALES. **external dorsal v.** A vein in the embryonic dorsal venous arcade of the lower limb which gives rise to the short (external) saphenous vein. **external iliac v.** VENA ILIACA EXTERNA. **external jugular v.** VENA JUGULARIS EXTERNA. **external mammary v.'s** Veins from the deep part of the mammary gland that drain directly into the lateral thoracic veins. **external nasal v.'s** VENAE NASALES EXTERNAE. **external pudendal v.'s** VENAE PUDENDAE EXTERNAE. **facial v.** VENA FACIALIS. **femoral v.** VENA FEMORALIS. **fetal umbilical v.** A single umbilical cord vessel which carries oxygenated blood from the placenta to the fetus. **fibular v.'s** VENAE FIBULARES. **v. of flocculus** An intracranial vein that drains the flocculus of the flocculonodular lobe of the cerebellum and flows into the inferior petrosal sinus. **v.'s of foramen cecum** Veins which occasionally pass through the foramen cecum ossis frontalis and connect the superior sagittal sinus with the veins in the nasal cavity. However, the foramen is patent in very few adults. **frontal v.'s** VENAE SUPRATROCHLEARES. **frontal diploic v.** VENA DIPLOICA FRONTALIS. **frontal v.'s of superior cerebral v.'s** VENAE FRONTALES VENARUM SUPERIORUM CEREBRI. **Galen's v.'s** **1** Vena magna cerebri and venae internae cerebri. **2** VENAE CARDIACAE ANTERIORES. **genicular v.'s** VENAE GENICULARES. **great cardiac v.** VENA CARDIACA MAGNA. **great cerebral v.** VENA MAGNA CEREBRI. **great v. of Galen** VENA MAGNA CEREBRI. **great saphenous v.** VENA SAPHENA MAGNA. **hemiazygos v.** VENA HEMIAZYGOS. **hepatic v.'s** VENAE HEPATICAE. **highest intercostal v.** VENA INTERCOSTALIS SUPREMA. **hypophyseoportal v.'s** A series of long and short portal veins draining the plexuses in the median eminence and infundibulum of the hypothalamus and communicating with plexuses in the anterior lobe of the hypophysis. **ileac v.'s** VENAE ILEALES. **ileal v.'s** VENAE ILEALES. **ileocolic v.** VENA ILEOCOLICA. **iliolumbar v.** VENA ILIOLUMBALIS. **inferior anastomotic v.** VENA ANASTOMOTICA INFERIOR. **inferior cerebellar v.'s** VENAE INFERIORES HEMISPHERII CEREBELLI. **inferior cerebral v.'s** VENAE INFERIORES CEREBRI. **inferior epigastric v.** VENA EPIGASTRICA INFERIOR. **inferior gluteal v.'s** VENAE GLUTEAE INFERIORES. **inferior hemorrhoidal v.'s** VENAE RECTALES INFERIORES. **inferior labial v.'s** VENAE LABIALES INFERIORES. **inferior laryngeal v.** VENA LARYNGEA INFERIOR. **inferior mesenteric v.** VENA MESENTERICA INFERIOR. **infe-**

**rior ophthalmic v.** VENA OPHTHALMICA INFERIOR. **inferior palpebral v.'s** VENAE PALPEBRALES INFERIORES. **inferior phrenic v.'s** VENAE PHRENICAE INFERIORES. **inferior rectal v.'s** VENAE RECTALES INFERIORES. **inferior striate v.** VENA STRIATA. **inferior thalamostriate v.** VENA STRIATA. **inferior thyroid v.** VENA THYROIDEA INFERIOR. **infrasegmental v.** PARS INTERSEGMENTALIS. **innominate v.'s** VENAE BRACHIOCEPHALICAE DEXTRA ET SINISTRA. **intercalated v.** VENA SUBLOBULARIS. **intercapital v.'s** VENAE INTERCAPITULARES. **intercapitular v.'s of foot** See under VENAE INTERCAPITULARES. **intercapitular v.'s of hand** See under VENAE INTERCAPITULARES. **interlobar v.'s of kidney** VENAE INTERLOBARES RENIS. **interlobular v.'s of kidney** VENAE INTERLOBULARES RENIS. **interlobular v.'s of liver** VENAE INTERLOBULARES HEPATIS. **internal cerebral v.'s** VENAE INTERNAE CEREBRI. **internal dorsal v.** A vein of the embryonic dorsal venous arcade of the lower limb which gives rise to the great (internal) saphenous vein. **internal iliac v.** VENA ILIACA INTERNA. **internal jugular v.** VENA JUGULARIS INTERNA. **internal pudendal v.** VENA PUDENDA INTERNA. **internal thoracic v.'s** VENAE THORACICAE INTERNAE. **intersegmental v.** PARS INTERSEGMENTALIS. **intervertebral v.** VENA INTERVERTEBRALIS. **intrasegmental v.** PARS INTRASEGMENTALIS. **jejunal v.'s** VENAE JEJUNALES. **jugular v.** Any of three veins: (1) vena jugularis anterior; (2) vena jugularis externa; (3) vena jugularis interna. **v.'s of kidney** VENAE RENIS. **Kohlrausch v.'s** Superficial veins of the penis passing from the under surface around the sides to the superficial dorsal vein. **Krukenberg's v.'s** VENAE CENTRALES HEPATIS. **Kuhnt's postcentral v.** A branch of the central vein of the retina that leaves it by piercing the optic nerve and runs posteriorly through the optic canal to terminate separately in the cavernous sinus or superior ophthalmic vein. **Labbé's v.** VENA ANASTOMOTICA INFERIOR. **v.'s of labyrinth** VENAE LABYRINTHI. **labyrinthine v.'s** VENAE LABYRINTHI. **lacrimal v.** VENA LACRIMALIS. **Latarjet's v.** VENA PREPYLORICA. **lateral circumflex femoral v.'s** VENAE CIRCUMFLEXAE LATERALES FEMORIS. **lateral marginal v. of foot** VENA MARGINALIS LATERALIS PEDIS. **lateral palpebral v.'s** Veins which drain the lateral half of the eyelids, communicate with the supratrochlear and infraorbital veins and the superior and inferior palpebral veins, and form the middle temporal vein at the lateral angle of each eye. **lateral plantar v.'s** Veins which arise from the deep plantar venous arch, run posteriorly with the lateral plantar artery, communicate with the small saphenous vein, and join the medial plantar veins behind the medial malleolus to form the posterior tibial veins. **lateral sacral v.'s** VENAE SACRALES LATERALES. **lateral sympathetic v.'s** A plexus of veins which develops on each side of the posterior body wall of the embryo lateral to the sympathetic trunk and dorsomedial to the posterior cardinal vein. It soon becomes one longitudinal trunk, having a cranial connection with the posterior cardinal vein, and a caudal connection, especially on the right side, with the corresponding subcardinal vein. Both trunks soon regress, but the more caudal portion on the right contributes to the formation of an infrarenal portion of the inferior vena cava. Also *veins of thoracolumbar line, paraureteric veins, supracardinal veins.* **lateral thoracic v.** VENA THORACICA LATERALIS. **left azygos v.** VENA HEMIAZYGOS. **left colic v.** VENA COLICA SINISTRA. **left coronary v.** VENA CARDIACA MAGNA. **left gastric v.** VENA GASTRICA SINISTRA. **left gastroepiploic v.** VENA GASTRO-OMENTALIS SINISTRA. **left hepatic v.'s** VENAE HEPATICAE SINISTRAE. **left inferior pulmonary v.** VENA PULMONALIS SINISTRA INFERIOR. **left marginal v. of heart** A vein of considerable size that accompanies the left marginal artery along the posterior aspect of the left surface of the heart and ascends to join the great cardiac vein. **left ovarian v.** VENA OVARICA SINISTRA. **left superior intercostal v.** VENA INTERCOSTALIS SUPERIOR SINISTRA. **left superior pulmonary v.** VENA PULMONALIS SINISTRA SUPERIOR. **left suprarenal v.** VENA SUPRARENALIS SINISTRA. **left testicular v.** VENA TESTICULARIS SINISTRA. **left umbilical v.** UMBILICAL VEIN. **levoatriocardinal v.** Any systemic vein, other than the left superior vena cava or coronary sinus, that enters the left atrium. It usually represents the right superior vena cava or one of its major tributaries. **lingual v.** VENA LINGUALIS. **long saphenous v.** VENA SAPHENA MAGNA. **lumbar v.'s** VENAE LUMBALES. **v. of Marshall** VENA OBLIQUA ATRII SINISTRI. **Marshall's oblique v.** VENA OBLIQUA ATRII SINISTRI. **mastoid emissary v.** VENA EMISSARIA MASTOIDEA. **maxillary v.'s** VENAE MAXILLARES. **Mayo's v.** VENA PREPYLORICA. **medial circumflex femoral v.'s** VENAE CIRCUMFLEXAE MEDIALES FEMORIS. **medial marginal v. of foot** VENA MARGINALIS MEDIALIS PEDIS. **medial plantar v.'s** Veins which arise from the deep plantar venous arch, run posteriorly with the medial plantar artery, communicate with the great saphenous vein, and join the lateral plantar veins behind the medial malleolus to form the posterior tibial veins. **medial sympathetic v.'s** Veins, lying one on each side, medial to the sympathetic ganglionic chain on the posterior thoracic and abdominal wall of an embryo. They contribute to the azygos and hemiazygos veins of the adult. Also *azygos line veins.* **median antebrachial v.** VENA INTERMEDIA ANTEBRACHII. **median basilic v.** VENA INTERMEDIA BASILICA. **median cephalic v.** VENA INTERMEDIA CEPHALICA. **median cubital v.** VENA INTERMEDIA CUBITI. **median v. of elbow** VENA INTERMEDIA CUBITI. **median v. of forearm** VENA INTERMEDIA ANTEBRACHII. **median hepatic v.'s** VENAE HEPATICAE INTERMEDIAE. **median sacral v.** VENA SACRALIS MEDIANA. **mediastinal v.'s** VENAE MEDIASTINALES. **meningeal v.'s** VENAE MENINGEAE. **middle cardiac v.** VENA CARDIACA MEDIA. **middle colic v.** VENA COLICA MEDIA. **middle hemorrhoidal v.'s** VENAE RECTALES MEDIAE. **middle hepatic v.'s** VENAE HEPATICAE INTERMEDIAE. **middle lobe v. of right lung** RAMUS LOBI MEDII VENAE PULMONALIS DEXTRAE SUPERIORIS. **middle meningeal v.'s** VENAE MENINGEAE MEDIAE. **middle rectal v.'s** VENAE RECTALES MEDIAE. **middle sacral v.** VENA SACRALIS MEDIANA. **middle temporal v.** VENA TEMPORALIS MEDIA. **middle thyroid v.'s** VENAE THYROIDEAE MEDIAE. **musculophrenic v.'s** VENAE MUSCULOPHRENICAE. **nasofrontal v.** VENA NASOFRONTALIS. **oblique v. of left atrium** VENA OBLIQUA ATRII SINISTRI. **obturator v.'s** VENAE OBTURATORIAE. **occipital v.** VENA OCCIPITALIS. **occipital diploic v.** VENA DIPLOICA OCCIPITALIS. **occipital emissary v.** VENA EMISSARIA OCCIPITALIS. **occipital emissary v. of Sperino** VENA EMISSARIA OCCIPITALIS. **v. of olfactory bulb** A vein that drains the olfactory bulb. It belongs to a group of veins in the anterior perforated substance that flow posteriorly into the basilar venous plexus. See also VEINS OF ANTERIOR PERFORATED SPACE. **om-**

**phalomesenteric v.'s** VITELLINE VEINS. **v.'s of optic chiasma** Small venous channels that drain the optic chiasma and flow into the cavernous sinus and basilar venous plexus. **palatine v.** VENA PALATINA. **palmar digital v.'s** VENAE DIGITALES PALMARES. **palmar metacarpal v.'s** VENAE METACARPALES PALMARES. **palpebral v.'s** VENAE PALPEBRALES. **pancreatic v.'s** VENAE PANCREATICAE. **pancreaticoduodenal v.'s** VENAE PANCREATICODUODENALES. **paraumbilical v.'s** VENAE PARAUMBILICALES. **paraureteric v.'s** LATERAL SYMPATHETIC VEINS. **parietal emissary v.** VENA EMISSARIA PARIETALIS. **parietal emissary v. of Santorini** VENA EMISSARIA PARIETALIS. **parietal v. of Santorini** VENA EMISSARIA PARIETALIS. **parotid v.'s** VENAE PAROTIDEAE. **parumbilical v.'s** VENAE PARAUMBILICALES. **perforating v.'s** VENAE PERFORANTES. **pericardiac v.'s** VENAE PERICARDIACAE. **pericardiacophrenic v.'s** VENAE PERICARDIACOPHRENICAE. **pericardial v.'s** VENAE PERICARDIACAE. **pericorneal v.'s** VENAE EPISCLERALES. **peroneal v.'s** VENAE FIBULARES. **pharyngeal v.'s** VENAE PHARYNGEALES. **plantar digital v.'s** VENAE DIGITALES PLANTARES. **plantar metatarsal v.'s** VENAE METATARSALES PLANTARES. **popliteal v.** VENA POPLITEA. **portal v.** VENA PORTAE HEPATIS. **postcardinal v.'s** Paired veins which appear at about the fourteenth somite stage of a human embryo in the dorsolateral part of the urogenital fold and are concerned with the drainage of the mesonephros and the trunk. Cranially, they join the anterior cardinal vein on each side to form the common cardinal vein (duct of Cuvier). Other longitudinal veins, or venous lines, soon appear, such as the subcardinals and the medial and lateral sympathetic veins to form very complicated patterns from which eventually the inferior vena cava and the renal, gonadal, and azygos veins will develop. **posterior auricular v.** VENA AURICULARIS POSTERIOR. **posterior circumflex humeral v.'s** The venae comitantes of the posterior circumflex humeral artery which terminate in the axillary vein. **posterior facial v.** VENA RETROMANDIBULARIS. **posterior intercostal v.'s** VENAE INTERCOSTALES POSTERIORES. **posterior jugular v. of Walther** A deep vein of the neck which arises in the plexus between the occipital, vertebral, and deep cervical veins and descends deep to the muscles of the neck medial to the deep cervical vein, and passes between the transverse process of the seventh cervical vertebra and the neck of the first rib to end in the brachiocephalic trunk below the vertebral vein. **posterior labial v.'s** VENAE LABIALES POSTERIORES. **posterior v. of left ventricle** VENA POSTERIOR VENTRICULI SINISTRI CORDIS. **posterior median longitudinal v. of spinal cord** One of the venae spinales posteriores which is situated behind the posterior median septum of the spinal cord. **posterior median v. of medulla** A vein that courses along the dorsal median sulcus of the medulla oblongata. It communicates laterally with variable radicular veins that follow the last four cranial nerves, and inferiorly with veins that drain the dorsal surface of the spinal cord. **posterior median v. of spinal cord** Either the posterior median longitudinal vein of spinal cord, or one of the posterior septal veins which drains the posteromedial portions of the spinal cord and ends in the posterior median longitudinal vein. **posterior parietal diploic v.** VENA DIPLOICA TEMPORALIS POSTERIOR. **posterior radicular v.'s of spinal cord** Six to twelve veins which drain the posterior funiculus and the posterior gray column of the spinal cord and the plexus on the posterior surface of the cord. They empty into the internal vertebral venous plexuses and the intervertebral veins. **posterior scrotal v.'s** VENAE SCROTALES POSTERIORES. **posterior spinal v.'s** VENAE SPINALES POSTERIORES. **posterior temporal diploic v.** VENA DIPLOICA TEMPORALIS POSTERIOR. **posterior tibial v.'s** VENAE TIBIALES POSTERIORES. **posterolateral v.'s of spinal cord** Two of the venae spinales posteriores which run longitudinally in the pia mater on the posterior surface of the spinal cord behind the dorsal nerve roots, one on each side, helping to drain the spinal cord and ending in the internal vertebral venous plexuses. **precardinal v.** VENA PRECARDINALIS. **prepyloric v.** VENA PREPYLORICA. **primary head v.** One of the veins that drain the capillary plexus of the head in the embryo and pass caudally from the medial side of the trigeminal ganglion to become continuous with the precardinal veins. Also *vena capitis primaria.* **pterygoid v.'s** Veins that drain the medial and lateral pterygoid muscles and terminate in the pterygoid plexus. **v. of pterygoid canal** VENA CANALIS PTERYGOIDEI. **pulmonary v.'s** VENAE PULMONALES. **pulp v.** VENA PULPAE RUBRAE. **radial v.'s** VENAE RADIALES. **ranine v.** 1 VENA PROFUNDA LINGUAE. 2 Vena comitans nervi hypoglossi with its tributary vena sublingualis. **renal v.'s** VENAE RENALES. **retromandibular v.** VENA RETROMANDIBULARIS. **retroperitoneal v.'s** Veins of the posterior abdominal wall and the abdominal surface of the diaphragm that drain mainly into the inferior vena cava or its tributaries, and may establish collateral circulations between the portal and systemic venous systems. **Retzius v.'s** Veins connecting the intestinal veins or those of the retroperitoneal organs, such as the pancreas and the bare area of the liver, or retroperitoneal tributaries of the portal vein with the inferior vena cava and its retroperitoneal tributaries. Also *Ruysch veins.* **revehent v.'s** **right colic v.** VENA COLICA DEXTRA. **right gastric v.** VENA GASTRICA DEXTRA. **right gastroepiploic v.** VENA GASTROOMENTALIS DEXTRA. **right hepatic v.'s** VENAE HEPATICAE DEXTRAE. **right inferior pulmonary v.** VENA PULMONALIS DEXTRA INFERIOR. **right marginal v. of heart** A vein running to the right along the lower margin of the heart and ending either in the small cardiac vein in the coronary sulcus or directly in the right atrium. **right ovarian v.** VENA OVARICA DEXTRA. **right superior intercostal v.** VENA INTERCOSTALIS SUPERIOR DEXTRA. **right superior pulmonary v.** VENA PULMONALIS DEXTRA SUPERIOR. **right suprarenal v.** VENA SUPRARENALIS DEXTRA. **right testicular v.** VENA TESTICULARIS DEXTRA. **Rosenthal's v.** VENA BASALIS. **Ruysch v.'s** 1 RETZIUS VEINS. 2 VENAE VORTICOSAE. **v.'s of Sappey** VENAE PARAUMBILICALES. **v. of septum pellucidum** VENA SEPTI PELLUCIDI. **short gastric v.'s** VENAE GASTRICAE BREVES. **short saphenous v.** VENA SAPHENA PARVA. **sigmoid v.'s** VENAE SIGMOIDEAE. **small cardiac v.** VENA CARDIACA PARVA. **smallest cardiac v.'s** VENAE CARDIACAE MINIMAE. **small v. of heart** VENA CARDIACA PARVA. **small saphenous v.** VENA SAPHENA PARVA. **sphenopalatine v.** The vein that accompanies the sphenopalatine artery, draining the greater part of the nasal cavity and ending in the pterygoid plexus. **spinal v.'s** See under VENAE SPINALES ANTERIORES, VENAE SPINALES POSTERIORES. **spiral v. of modiolus** VENA SPIRALIS MODIOLI. **splenic v.** VENA SPLENICA. **stellate v.'s of kidney** VENULAE STELLATAE RENIS. **Stensen's v.'s** VENAE VORTICOSAE. **sternocleidomastoid v.** VENA STERNOCLEIDOMASTOIDEA. **striate**

**v.** VENA STRIATA. **stylomastoid v.** VENA STYLOMASTOIDEA. **subcardinal v.'s** A pair of longitudinal veins that form in the ventromedial part of the mesonephric ridges of the embryo and become connected to the postcardinal veins. The preaortic anastomosis connects the pair of veins to each other and later forms the left renal vein. **subclavian v.** VENA SUBCLAVIA. **subcostal v.** VENA SUBCOSTALIS. **subcutaneous v.'s of abdomen** VENAE SUBCUTANEAE ABDOMINIS. **sublingual v.** VENA SUBLINGUALIS. **sublobular v.** VENA SUBLOBULARIS. **submental v.** VENA SUBMENTALIS. **superficial circumflex iliac v.** VENA CIRCUMFLEXA ILIACA SUPERFICIALIS. **superficial dorsal v.'s of clitoris** VENAE DORSALES SUPERFICIALES CLITORIDIS. **superficial dorsal v.'s of penis** VENAE DORSALES SUPERFICIALES PENIS. **superficial epigastric v.** VENA EPIGASTRICA SUPERFICIALIS. **superficial femoral v.** The femoral vein distal to the junction with the profunda femoris vein: a term used by some surgeons. Compare COMMON FEMORAL VEIN. **superficial middle cerebral v.'s** VENAE MEDIAE SUPERFICIALES CEREBRI. **superficial temporal v.'s** VENAE TEMPORALES SUPERFICIALES. **superior anastomotic v.** VENA ANASTOMOTICA SUPERIOR. **superior cerebellar v.'s** VENAE SUPERIORES HEMISPHERII CEREBELLI. **superior cerebral v.'s** VENAE CEREBRI SUPERIORES. **superior epigastric v.'s** VENAE EPIGASTRICAE SUPERIORES. **superior gluteal v.'s** VENAE GLUTEAE SUPERIORES. **superior hemorrhoidal v.** VENA RECTALIS SUPERIOR. **superior intercostal v. of Braune** A variant of the right superior intercostal vein which ascends to end in the right brachiocephalic vein. **superior labial v.** VENA LABIALIS SUPERIOR. **superior laryngeal v.** VENA LARYNGEA SUPERIOR. **superior mesenteric v.** VENA MESENTERICA SUPERIOR. **superior ophthalmic v.** VENA OPHTHALMICA SUPERIOR. **superior palpebral v.'s** VENAE PALPEBRALES SUPERIORES. **superior phrenic v.'s** VENAE PHRENICAE SUPERIORES. **superior rectal v.** VENA RECTALIS SUPERIOR. **superior thalamostriate v.** VENA THALAMOSTRIATA. **superior thyroid v.** VENA THYROIDEA SUPERIOR. **supracardinal v.'s** Paired symmetrical veins, appearing during the second month of embryonic life and assuring the venous return from the dorsal walls of the embryo. They drain into the proximal part of the posterior cardinal veins which become progressively obliterated, and in effect the supracardinals replace them. The anterior portion of the left supracardinal vein will become the hemiazygos vein and the rest usually disappears without trace. The right will become the azygos vein and through its caudal part it contributes to the infrarenal segment of the inferior vena cava. **supraorbital v.** VENA SUPRAORBITALIS. **suprascapular v.** VENA SUPRASCAPULARIS. **supratrochlear v.'s** VENAE SUPRATROCHLEARES. **sylvian v.** VENAE MEDIAE SUPERFICIALES CEREBRI. **v. of sylvian fossa** VENAE MEDIAE SUPERFICIALES CEREBRI. **systemic v.** One of the veins draining areas supplied by the aorta and its branches and conveying the blood to the right atrium of the heart. **temporomandibular articular v.'s** VENAE ARTICULARES TEMPOROMANDIBULARES. **terminal v.** VENA THALAMOSTRIATA. **thalamostriate v.** VENA THALAMOSTRIATA. **thebesian v.'s** VENAE CARDIACAE MINIMAE. **v.'s of Thebesius** VENAE CARDIACAE MINIMAE. **thoracoacromial v.** VENA THORACOACROMIALIS. **thoracoepigastric v.'s** VENAE THORACOEPIGASTRICAE. **thymic v.'s** VENAE THYMICAE. **v.'s of thymus** VENAE THYMICAE. **tonsillar v.'s** Veins which leave the lower part of the deeper aspect of the palatine tonsil to join the pharyngeal, lingual, facial, and external palatine veins. **trabecular v.** VENA TRABECULARIS. **tracheal v.'s** VENAE TRACHEALES. **transverse cervical v.'s** VENAE TRANSVERSAE CERVICIS. **transverse v. of face** VENA TRANSVERSA FACIEI. **transverse facial v.** VENA TRANSVERSA FACIEI. **transverse v.'s of neck** VENAE TRANSVERSAE CERVICIS. **Trolard's v.** VENA ANASTOMOTICA SUPERIOR. **tympanic v.'s** VENAE TYMPANICAE. **ulnar v.'s** VENAE ULNARES. **umbilical v.** The vein which in the fetus returns blood from the placenta to the left branch of the portal vein. Some of the blood flows through the liver and the rest flows through the ductus venosus into the inferior vena cava. It is the left vein of a pair of primitive umbilical veins, its counterpart having disappeared early in the second month of development. Very shortly after birth it constricts and fibroses. Its intracorporeal section remains as the round ligament (ligamentum teres of the liver) found in the lower edge of the falciform ligament. Also *vena umbilicalis, vena umbilicalis sinistra, left umbilical vein.* **uterine v.'s** VENAE UTERINAE. **v.'s of uterus** VENAE UTERINAE. **varicose v.** A dilated, tortuous vein, most often found beneath the skin of the legs. **vertebral v.** VENA VERTEBRALIS. **vesalian v.** An occasional small emissary vein draining the cavernous sinus and passing through an inconstant foramen in the greater wing of the sphenoid bone anteromedial to foramen ovale to join the pterygoid plexus. **vesical v.'s** VENAE VESICALES. **vestibular v.'s** VENAE VESTIBULARES. **vidian v.** VENA CANALIS PTERYGOIDEI. **v.'s of Vieussens** VENAE CARDIACAE ANTERIORES. **vitelline v.'s** A pair of embryonic veins which drains the yolk sac and communicates with the sinus venosus. In later development it traverses the umbilical cord and within the embryo it receives blood from the gastrointestinal tract. Its peripheral portions involute but its derivatives include the hepatic portal vein and the cardiac end of the inferior vena cava. Also *omphalomesenteric veins.* **vorticose v.'s** VENAE VORTICOSAE.

**veinlet** \vān′lit\ VENULA.

**Veit** [Gustav *Veit,* German gynecologist, born 1824] Mauriceau-Smellie-Veit maneuver. See under MANEUVER.

***Vejovis*** \vejō′vis\ A genus of the family Vejovidae found in North America; the devil scorpions. The following species are among the more important members: *V. spinigerus,* the stripe-tailed devil scorpion; *V. carolinianus,* the southern devil scorpion; and *V. flavus,* the slender devil scorpion. None of these species are believed to be lethal to humans but they are capable of stinging severely.

**vela** \vē′lə\ Plural of VELUM.

**velamen** \vəlā′mən\ (*pl.* velamina) Any membranous covering; tegument; velum.

**velamenta** \vel′əmen′tə\ Plural of VELAMENTUM.

**velamentous** \vel′əmen′təs\ [*velament(um)* + -OUS] **1** Like a veil. **2** Describing a placenta in which the umbilical cord is attached at one edge.

**velamentum** \vel′əmen′təm\ [L (from *vela(re)* to clothe, cover + *-mentum* -MENT), a covering, veil] Any fibrous or membranous covering of a viscus or any of its parts. An envelope of tissue that surrounds an organ, such as the meninges of the brain and spinal cord; a velum or capsule.

**velar** \vē′lär\ Pertaining to a velum, particularly that of the palate.

**veliform** \vel′ifôrm\ Like a velum in form; membranous.

**Vella** [Luigi *Vella,* Italian physiologist, 1825–1886] **1** See under FISTULA. **2** Thiry-Vella fistula. See under FISTULA.

**vellus** \vel′əs\ [L (akin to *vellere* to pluck, *villus* shaggy hair, and English *wool*) fleece] The short, fine, downy hair that before birth or in early infancy replaces the lanugo in all hair-bearing areas except the scalp. It is itself replaced by terminal hair in many body regions from the approach of puberty onwards.

**velocimetry** \vel′äsim′ətrē\ The measurement of velocity. **laser Doppler v.** A technique of beaming laser light at moving objects and measuring their velocities by measuring the Doppler frequency shift of the reflected light. By measuring red blood cell velocities it can transcutaneously measure microvascular perfusion. Abbr. LDV

**velocity** \vəläs′itē\ [L *velocitas* (from *velox*, gen. *velocis*, fleet, agile, akin to *volare* to fly + *-itas* -ITY) velocity] Measure of the rate of motion of a body expressed as the rate of change of its position in a particular direction with time. **conduction v.** The speed with which a wave of depolarization or a biochemical substance passes along a muscle fiber or axon or an assemblage of such units, such as a muscle, a nerve, the cortex of the brain, or deep central nervous structures. **limiting v.** The velocity of an enzyme-catalyzed reaction that is approached as substrate concentration is raised indefinitely. This quantity has sometimes been called the maximum velocity, but it is not a true maximum. Symbol: $V$, $V_{max}$ **maximum v.** See under LIMITING VELOCITY. **nerve conduction v.** The rate of conduction of an impulse along the fibers of a peripheral nerve, usually measured in meters per second. **propagation v.** Propagation speed with direction specified. **sedimentation v.** The rate at which a particle moves through a medium of fixed or graded density when subjected to centrifugal and gravitational force. It is used to describe behavior of macromolecules subjected to analytical ultracentrifugation, and expressed in Svedberg units. Also *sedimentation rate.* **sensory conduction v.** The rate of conduction of an impulse along the sensory fibers of a peripheral nerve, usually expressed in meters per second.

**veloplasty** \vē′lōplas′tē\ STAPHYLOPLASTY.

**velour** \vəloor′\ [French *velours* (from Old French *velos* hairy, shaggy, from L *villosus* hairy, shaggy, from *vill(us)* shaggy hair + *-osus* -OSE) velvet, velour] A technical modification of the knitted vascular graft in which yarn loops are at right angles to the knit, either into or away from the graft lumen, thereby improving handling and graft-healing characteristics.

**Velpeau** [Alfred Louis Armand Marie *Velpeau*, French surgeon, 1795–1867] **1** Velpeau's deformity. See under SILVER FORK DEFORMITY. **2** See under BANDAGE. **3** Velpeau's canal. See under CANALIS INGUINALIS.

**velum** \vē′ləm\ [L a veil, cover, sail] (*pl.* vela) A veil-like structure; a veil. **anterior medullary v.** VELUM MEDULLARE CRANIALE. **artificial v.** ARTIFICIAL PALATE. **caudal medullary v.** VELUM MEDULLARE CAUDALE. **cranial medullary v.** VELUM MEDULLARE CRANIALE. **inferior medullary v.** VELUM MEDULLARE CAUDALE. **v. interpositum** **1** TELA CHOROIDEA VENTRICULI TERTII. **2** VELUM MEDULLARE CRANIALE. **v. interpositum cerebri** TELA CHOROIDEA VENTRICULI TERTII. **v. interpositum rhombencephali** VELUM MEDULLARE CRANIALE. **v. medullare anterius** VELUM MEDULLARE CRANIALE. **v. medullare caudale** [NA] Caudal (inferior or posterior) medullary velum. A thin crescentic sheet of white matter and neuroglial tissue that helps form the roof of the lower part of the fourth ventricle. Rostrally it extends from the white matter of the cerebellum, and caudally it reaches the taenia of the fourth ventricle. Its inner surface is covered by ependymal cells, while its external surface is covered by pia mater. Also *velum medullare inferius, inferior medullary velum, velum medullare posterius, posterior medullary velum, velum of Tarinus, Tarinus valve, Tarin's valve, Tarin's plate, velum semilunare, caudal medullary velum.* **v. medullare craniale** [NA] Cranial (superior or anterior) medullary velum. A thin lamina of white matter that extends between the two superior cerebellar peduncles and helps to form the rostral part of the roof of the fourth ventricle. It is continuous dorsally with the central white core of the vermis, and the folia of the lingula lie just over its dorsal surface. Also *velum medullare superius, superior medullary velum, velum medullare anterius, anterior medullary velum, velum interpositum rhombencephali, Willis valve, valve of Vieussens, cranial medullary velum, velum interpositum.* **v. medullare inferius** VELUM MEDULLARE CAUDALE. **v. medullare posterius** VELUM MEDULLARE CAUDALE. **v. medullare superius** VELUM MEDULLARE CRANIALE. **nursing v.** A variety of artificial velum, enabling the infant with cleft palate to feed. **v. palatinum** PALATUM MOLLE. **pharyngeal v.** A remnant of the buccopharyngeal membrane as it regresses. **posterior medullary v.** VELUM MEDULLARE CAUDALE. **v. semilunare** VELUM MEDULLARE CAUDALE. **superior medullary v.** VELUM MEDULLARE CRANIALE. **v. of Tarinus** VELUM MEDULLARE CAUDALE. **v. transversum** A groove which marks the boundary between that part of the third ventricle derived from the diencephalon and that derived from the telencephalon. It runs dorsal to the region of the interventricular foramina of Monro, separating the epithalamic region from the telencephalon. It delineates the position where the tela choroidea of the third ventricle (velum interpositum) subsequently differentiates. **v. triangulare** TELA CHOROIDEA VENTRICULI TERTII.

# vena

**vena** \vē′nə\ [L, a blood vessel, vein] (*pl.* venae) [NA] A vessel conducting blood, usually deoxygenated, from peripheral capillary plexuses to the heart. The exceptions are those of the pulmonary circulation, which conduct oxygenated blood from the lungs to the left atrium, and those of the portal circulation, which carry blood from the abdominal portion of the alimentary canal, the spleen, and the pancreas to the liver. The wall of the vessel, comprising three coats, namely, tunica interna, tunica media, and tunica externa, is thinner than that of an artery, and the larger vessels contain valves. Also *vein.* **venae advehentes** A series of afferent veins, formed in the embryo from liver sinusoids, which receive blood from the umbilical or vitelline venous systems and pass it on through venae revehentes and then into the common hepatic vein. **v. anastomotica inferior** [NA] A vein that extends from the superficial middle cerebral vein over the temporal lobe of the brain to the transverse sinus. Also *inferior anastomotic vein, Labbé's vein, Browning's vein.* **v. anastomotica superior** [NA] A vein extending from the superficial middle cerebral vein to the superior sagittal sinus, thereby connecting the latter with the cavernous sinus. Also *superior anastomotic vein, Trolard's vein, anterior anastomotic vein of Trolard.* **v. angularis** [NA] The portion of the facial vein formed at the medial angle of the eye by the supratrochlear and supraorbital veins, and extending down the side of the root of the nose to the entrance of the superior labial vein. Also *angular vein.* **anomalous venae cavae** An anomalous connection involving the superior or inferior vena cava or both. Usually it is a case of one caval vein's being connected to the other, or an abnormal connection directly to the right atrium, such as a persistent left superior caval vein draining via the coronary sinus. Rarely, the connection may be to the morphologically left atrium. **venae anteriores cerebri** [NA] Small veins accompanying the anterior cerebral artery in the longitudinal cerebral fissure and ending in the basal vein. Also *anterior cerebral veins.* **v. appendicularis** [NA] The vein accompanying the appendicular artery of the vermiform appendix and joining tributaries from the terminal ileum and the cecum to form the ileocolic vein. Also *appendicular vein.* **v. aqueductus cochleae** [NA] A small vein that drains the sacculus, part of the utriculus, and the cochlea and leaves the basal turn of the cochlea to pass through the cochlear canaliculus with the perilymphatic duct. It ends in either the superior bulb of the internal jugular vein or the adjacent inferior petrosal sinus. Also *vein of cochlear canal, vein of cochlear aqueduct, vein of canaliculus of cochlea.* **v. aqueductus vestibuli** [NA] A vein draining the semicircular canals of the internal ear through the bony aqueduct of the vestibule into the labyrinthine veins. Also *vein of aqueduct of vestibule.* **venae arcuatae renis** [NA] Veins accompanying the arcuate arteries, forming an anastomotic arch between the cortex and medulla of the kidney, receiving the interlobular veins from the cortex and draining into the interlobar veins which ultimately form the renal vein. Also *arcuate veins of kidney, arciform veins, venous arches of kidney.* **venae articulares temporomandibulares** [NA] Veins draining the plexus surrounding the temporomandibular joint and ending in either the retromandibular or the maxillary veins. Also *temporomandibular articular veins.* **venae auriculares anteriores** [NA] Veins draining the auricle of the external ear into the retromandibular vein. Also *anterior auricular veins.* **v. auricularis posterior** [NA] A vein commencing in a plexus in the scalp behind the ear and communicating with the superficial temporal vein anteriorly and the occipital vein posteriorly before descending across the insertion of the sternocleidomastoid muscle to join the posterior division of the retromandibular vein and form the external jugular vein. Also *posterior auricular vein.* **v. axillaris** [NA] The major deep vein draining the upper limb, formed at the lower border of the teres major muscle by the confluence of the brachial and basilic veins, and accompanying the axillary artery through the axilla to end at the outer border of the first rib by continuing as the subclavian vein. Also *axillary vein.* **v. azygos** [NA] A vein arising in front of the twelfth thoracic vertebra from either the confluence of the right ascending lumbar and subcostal veins or the back of the inferior vena cava, and ascending through the aortic opening or right crus of the diaphragm along the right side of the vertebrae to the fourth thoracic vertebra, where it arches forward over the root of the right lung to end in the superior vena cava. Also *azygos vein.* **v. basalis** [NA] A vein formed at the anterior perforated substance by the union of the anterior cerebral, deep middle cerebral, and striate veins and running posteriorly around the cerebral peduncle to end in the great cerebral vein. Also *basal vein, Rosenthal's vein, vena basalis rosenthali* (outmoded). **v. basalis rosenthali** *Outmoded* VENA BASALIS. **v. basilica** [NA] A vein arising from the medial side of the dorsal venous network of the hand, passing superficially along the medial side of the forearm, and receiving the median cubital vein in the cubital fossa, before piercing the deep fascia medially in the distal half of the arm to join the brachial veins and form the axillary vein at the lower border of teres major muscle. Also *basilic vein.* **venae basivertebrales** [NA] Veins in the bodies of the vertebrae draining the cancellous tissue and passing radially to pierce the front and sides of the bodies to join the anterior external vertebral plexuses as well as the posterior surface of the bodies to join the transverse branches connecting the anterior internal vertebral plexuses. They also communicate with the intervertebral veins. Also *basivertebral veins.* **venae brachiales** [NA] Two veins accompanying the brachial artery, frequently anastomosing with each other by cross branches and terminating at the lower border of the teres major muscle by joining the basilic vein to form the axillary vein. Also *brachial veins.* **venae brachiocephalicae dextra et sinistra** [NA] Valveless veins receiving blood from the head, neck, and upper limbs and formed on each side by the union of the subclavian and internal jugular veins in the root of the neck. They end behind the right first costal cartilage by uniting with each other to form the superior vena cava. Each receives numerous tributaries as well as the right lymphatic duct on the right side and the lymphatic duct on the left at their origins. Also *brachiocephalic veins, innominate veins.* **venae bronchiales** [NA] Veins lying anterior and posterior to the bronchial arteries but only

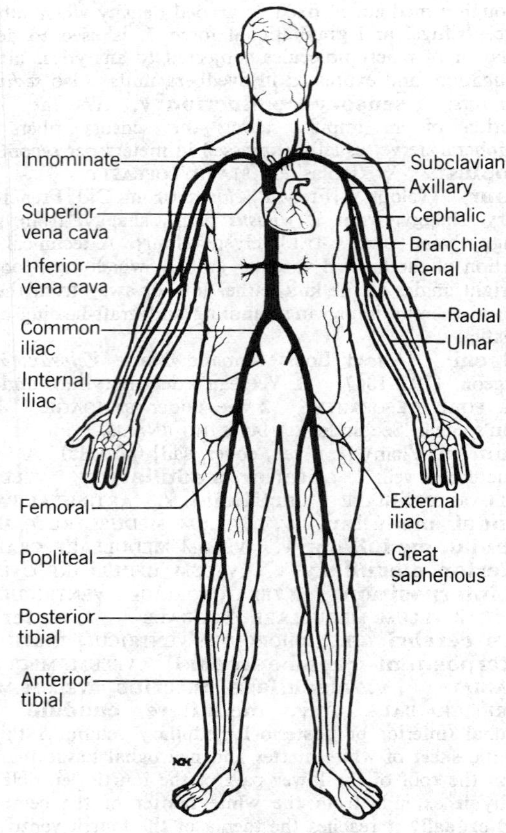

**Major veins of the body**

draining the larger subdivisions of the bronchi and structures at the roots of the lungs. On the right side they usually end in the azygos vein just before it joins the superior vena cava, while on the left they drain into either the accessory hemiazygos or the left superior intercostal veins. Also *bronchial veins.* **v. bulbi penis** [NA] A vein draining the bulb of the penis and ending in the internal pudendal vein. Also *vein of bulb of penis.* **v. bulbi vestibuli** [NA] A vein draining the bulb of the vestibule of the vagina and ending in the internal pudendal vein. Also *vein of bulb of vestibule.* **v. canalis pterygoidei** [NA] A vein that accompanies the artery of the pterygoid canal through the canal to end in the pterygoid plexus. Also *vein of pterygoid canal, vidian vein.* **v. capitis primaria** PRIMARY HEAD VEIN. **venae cardiacae anteriores** [NA] A number of small veins that drain the front of the right ventricle and usually open separately into the right atrium. Also *anterior cardiac veins, Galen's veins, veins of Vieussens.* **venae cardiacae minimae** [NA] Numerous minute veins within the walls of the heart that open mostly into the atrial cavities. Some open into the ventricles. They are devoid of valves. Also *smallest cardiac veins, thebesian veins, veins of Thebesius.* **v. cardiaca magna** [NA] A vein commencing at the apex of the heart and ascending in the anterior interventricular sulcus to the coronary sulcus, which it follows to the back of the heart to end in the beginning of the coronary sinus. Also *great cardiac vein, left coronary vein.* **v. cardiaca media** [NA] A vein commencing at the apex of the heart and ascending posteriorly in the posterior interventricular sulcus to end in the coronary sinus near its termination. It drains the ventricular walls. Also *middle cardiac vein.* **v. cardiaca parva** [NA] A vein draining the back of the right atrium and ventricle and running in the coronary sulcus posteriorly to end in the coronary sinus near its termination. Also *small cardiac vein, small vein of heart.* **v. cava inferior** [NA] A major vein draining all of the body below the level of the respiratory diaphragm. It begins in front and to the right of the body of the fifth lumbar vertebra at the confluence of the common iliac veins, ascends on the right of the abdominal aorta, grooving the posterior surface of the liver and piercing the tendinous part of the diaphragm and the fibrous pericardium, to end in the posteroinferior part of the right atrium. Also *inferior vena cava, postcava.* **v. cava superior** [NA] The major vein draining all of the upper half of the body and formed by the union of the two brachiocephalic veins behind the first right sternochondral joint. It receives the azygos vein and descends vertically to the level of the third right costal cartilage, where it enters the upper part of the right atrium of the heart after piercing the fibrous pericardium. Also *superior vena cava, precava.* **venae cavernosae penis** [NA] Several veins draining the corpus cavernosum penis that end directly in the deep dorsal vein of the penis. Also *cavernous veins of penis.* **venae centrales hepatis** [NA] Veins in the center of the polyhedral hepatic lobules joined by sinusoids that drain the interlobular branches of the portal vein and hepatic artery in the portal canals. Also *central veins of liver, central veins of hepatic lobules, Krukenberg's veins.* **v. centralis glandulae suprarenalis** [NA] A vein in the medulla of the suprarenal gland receiving venules that drain the cortex and medulla and emerging from the hilum as the suprarenal vein. Also *central vein of suprarenal gland.* **v. centralis retinae** [NA] The vein draining the superior and inferior nasal and temporal veins of the retina and accompanying the central artery of the retina in the optic nerve behind the lamina cribrosa before leaving it to run in the subarachnoid space and terminate in either the superior ophthalmic vein or the cavernous sinus. Also *central vein of retina.* **v. cephalica** [NA] A vein arising from the lateral side of the dorsal venous network of the hand and ascending subcutaneously along the anterolateral aspect of the forearm and in front of the elbow in the lateral bicipital groove to the groove between the deltoid and pectoralis major muscles, after which it pierces the clavipectoral fascia to end in the axillary vein below the level of the clavicle. Also *cephalic vein.* • The name of the vein is first recorded as Arabic *qīfāl* (in Avicenna), which was evidently an adaptation of Gk *kephalikos* cephalic. It seems to have been so called from the practice of bloodletting in which it was the vein of choice for treating maladies of the head. See also note at BASILIC. **v. cephalica accessoria** [NA] A vein that arises either from the medial side of the dorsal venous network of the hand or from a small subsidiary plexus on the back of the forearm and runs anterolaterally to join the cephalic vein below the level of the elbow. Also *accessory cephalic vein.* **venae cerebelli inferiores** *Outmoded* VENAE INFERIORES HEMISPHERII CEREBELLI. **venae cerebelli superiores** *Outmoded* VENAE SUPERIORES HEMISPHERII CEREBELLI. **venae cerebri** [NA] The numerous superficial and deep veins draining the surfaces and inner regions of the cerebral hemispheres, respectively. Also *cerebral veins.* **v. cerebri anterior** One of the venae anteriores cerebri. *Outmoded.* **venae cerebri inferiores** See under VENAE INFERIORES CEREBRI. **venae cerebri internae** See under VENAE INTERNAE CEREBRI. **v. cerebri magna** VENA MAGNA CEREBRI. **v. cerebri magna galeni** *Outmoded* VENA MAGNA CEREBRI. **v. cerebri media** *Outmoded* VENAE MEDIAE SUPERFICIALES CEREBRI. **v. cerebri media profunda** See under VENA MEDIA PROFUNDA CEREBRI. **venae cerebri superiores** See under VENAE SUPERIORES CEREBRI. **v. cervicalis profunda** [NA] A vein commencing in the suboccipital triangle in a plexus formed by the occipital vein and veins of the deep muscles of the neck. It accompanies the deep cervical artery between the semispinalis cervicis and semispinalis capitis muscles and then passes between the neck of the first rib and the transverse process of the seventh cervical vertebra to end in the vertebral vein. Also *deep cervical vein.* **v. chorioidea** *Outmoded* VENA CHOROIDEA. **v. choroidea** [NA] A vein commencing at the junction of the body and inferior horn of the lateral ventricle of the brain and running upward on the lateral side of the choroid plexus along the edge of the tela choroidea to the interventricular foramen, where it joins the thalamostriate vein to form the internal cerebral vein. Also *choroid vein, vena chorioidea* (outmoded). **venae ciliares** [NA] The veins of the eyeball that accompany the branches of the anterior and posterior ciliary arteries and drain the ciliary body into the superior ophthalmic vein. Also *ciliary veins.* **venae ciliares anteriores** [NA] The veins following the course and accompanying the branches of the anterior ciliary arteries, with which they emerge from the sclera near the sclerocorneal junction and join the muscular veins of the four recti muscles, to form a circumcorneal ring of episcleral veins. Also *anterior ciliary veins.* **venae circumflexae laterales femoris** [NA] Veins accompanying the lateral circumflex femoral artery and usually terminating in the femoral vein. Also *lateral circumflex femoral veins.* **venae circumflexae mediales femoris** [NA] Veins accompanying the medial circumflex femoral artery and usually terminating in the femoral vein. Also *medial circumflex femoral veins.* **v. circumflexa iliaca profunda** [NA] A vein formed by the union of the venae comitantes of the deep circumflex iliac artery and ending in the external iliac vein near the inguinal ligament. Also *deep circumflex iliac vein.* **v. circumflexa iliaca superficialis** [NA] A vein accompanying the superficial circumflex iliac artery and helping to drain the lower anterior abdominal wall and superolateral part of the thigh, before ending in the great saphenous vein just before the latter pierces the saphenous opening. Also *superficial circumflex iliac vein.* **v. colica dextra** [NA] The vein accompanying the right colic artery, draining the upper half of the ascending colon and right colic flexure and ending in the superior mesenteric vein. Also *right colic vein.* **v. colica media** [NA] The vein accompanying the middle colic artery, draining the transverse colon, and ending in the superior mesenteric vein. Also *middle colic vein.* **v. colica sinistra** [NA] A vein accompanying the left colic artery, draining the descending colon, left colic flexure, and the adjacent part of the transverse colon, and ending in the inferior mesenteric vein. Also *left colic vein.* **v. comitans** [NA] A vein that accompanies an artery or other structure. Also *accompanying vein, companion vein.* **v. comitans nervi hypoglossi** [NA] A vein, usually larger than the lingual vein, commencing below the tip of the tongue and accompanying the hypoglossal nerve superficial to the hyoglossus muscle to end in the lingual, facial, or internal jugular vein. It may receive the sublingual vein. Also *accompanying vein of hypoglossal nerve.* **venae comitantes** Veins accompanying an artery. **venae conjunctivales** [NA] Veins that drain the conjunctiva and terminate in the superior ophthalmic vein. Also *conjuctival veins.* **venae cordis** [NA] The veins accompanying the coronary arteries and draining the walls and tissues of the heart, mostly into the coronary sinus. Also *cardiac veins.* **v. cutanea** [NA] One of the veins draining the subpapillary or superficial plexus and connecting with two other plexuses in the skin before ending in a subcutaneous or superficial vein. Also *cutaneous vein.* **v. cystica** [NA] One or two veins arising on the neck of the gallbladder and entering the substance of the liver after communicating with veins draining the hepatic ducts and upper part of the bile ducts. Also *cystic vein.* **venae digitales dorsales pedis** [NA] Veins along the dorsal margins of each toe that unite in pairs at the clefts of the toes to form the dorsal metatarsal veins. Also *dorsal digital veins of foot.* **venae digitales palmares** [NA] Interconnecting veins along the margins and palmar aspects of the fingers that communicate between the heads of the metacarpal bones by intercapitular veins with the dorsal digital veins and then drain into the superficial palmar venous arch. Also *palmar digital veins.* **venae digitales plantares** [NA] Veins draining the plantar aspects of the toes and uniting at the clefts to form the plantar metatarsal veins. Also *plantar digital veins.* **venae diploicae** [NA] Veins located in bony canals in the cancellous tissue, or diploë, between the laminae of the cranial bones. They have thin walls composed of endothelium supported by some elastic tissue, and have no valves. They communicate with each other, the meningeal veins, the intramural venous sinuses, and pericranial veins, and terminate in four main channels, namely, frontal, anterior temporal, posterior temporal, and occipital diploic veins. Also *diploic veins, veins of diploë, Breschet's veins.* **v. diploica frontalis** [NA] A vein draining a series of veins in the anterior part of the frontal bone and emerging from the bone at the supraorbital notch, where it joins the supraorbital vein. Also *frontal diploic vein.* **v. diploica occipitalis** [NA] A large vein ramifying in the occipital bone and opening into the occipital vein or into the transverse sinus near the confluence of sinuses or into the occipital emissary vein. Also *occipital diploic vein.* **v. diploica temporalis anterior** [NA] A vein having several tributaries in the posterior part of the frontal bone and the anterior part of the parietal bone and piercing the greater wing of the sphenoid bone to end partly in the sphenoparietal sinus and partly in the anterior deep temporal vein. Also *anterior temporal diploic vein, anterior parietal diploic vein.* **v. diploica temporalis posterior** [NA] A vein ramifying in the parietal bone and running down to the mastoid angle of the bone where it either pierces the inner table or passes through the mastoid foramen into the transverse sinus. Also *posterior temporal diploic vein, posterior parietal diploic vein.* **venae dorsales linguae** [NA] Veins draining the dorsum and sides of the tongue and joining the lingual vein between the hyoglossus and genioglossus muscles. Also *dorsal lingual veins, dorsal veins of tongue.* **venae dorsales superficiales clitoridis** [NA] Superficial veins draining the prepuce and superficial tissues of the clitoris and passing posteriorly in the midline to end in the external pudendal vein. Also *superficial dorsal veins of clitoris.* **venae dorsales superficiales penis** [NA] Subcutaneous veins draining the prepuce and skin of the penis and passing posteriorly in the midline to end in the external pudendal vein. Also *superficial dorsal veins of penis.* **v. dorsalis profunda clitoridis** [NA] A vein draining the glans and corpora cavernosa of the clitoris and ending in the vesical plexus after communicating with the internal pudendal veins. Also *deep dorsal vein of clitoris.* **v. dorsalis profunda penis** [NA] A vein that drains the glans penis and corpora cavernosa penis, passes between the arcuate pubic ligament and the perineal membrane, and divides into two branches that end in the prostatic plexus after communicating with the internal pudendal veins. Also *deep dorsal vein of penis.* **v. emissaria** [NA] One of the veins connecting the dural venous sinuses with veins outside the cranium by passing through foramina in the cranium. Also *emissary vein, emissarium, emissary.* **v. emissaria condylaris** [NA] A vein passing through the posterior condylar canal and connecting the sigmoid or occipital sinus with the deep cervical or vertebral vein. Also *condylar emissary vein, vein of condyloid canal, condyloid emissary vein.* **v. emissaria mastoidea** [NA] A small vein passing through the mastoid foramen and connecting the sigmoid sinus with the occipital or posterior auricular vein. Also *mastoid emissary vein.* **v. emissaria occipitalis** [NA] An inconstant vein passing through the occipital protuberance and connecting the confluence of sinuses with the occipital vein. It may receive the occipital diploic vein. Also *occipital emissary vein, occipital emissary vein of Sperino.* **v. emissaria parietalis** [NA] A vein passing through the parietal foramen and connecting the superior sagittal sinus with the veins of the scalp. Also *parietal emissary vein, parietal vein of Santorini, parietal emissary vein of Santorini.* **venae epigastricae superiores** [NA] Paired veins accompanying the superior epigastric artery that receive tributaries from the rectus abdominis muscle in the rectus sheath and from the subcutaneous abdominal veins. They communicate with the venae communicantes of the inferior epigastric artery and unite with the musculophrenic veins to form the internal thoracic vein. Also *superior epigastric veins.* **v. epigastrica inferior** [NA] The vein formed by the union of the venae comitantes of the inferior epigastric artery which communicate with the superior epigastric veins in the rectus sheath, as well as with paraumbilical and intercostal veins. It terminates in the external iliac vein just proximal to the inguinal ligament. Also *inferior epigastric vein.* **v. epigastrica superficialis** [NA] The vein draining the lower part of the anterior abdominal wall and crossing the inguinal ligament to end in the great saphenous vein before it enters the saphenous opening. Also *superficial epigastric vein.* **venae episclerales** [NA] Veins forming a circumcorneal ring deep to the conjunctiva. They receive palpebral, conjunctival, and muscular veins and drain into the anterior ciliary veins or the superior ophthalmic vein. Also *episcleral veins, pericorneal veins.* **venae esophageales** [NA] Several veins draining the esophagus, those of the cervical part ending in the inferior thyroid and vertebral veins, those of the thoracic part ending in the azygos, hemiazygos, and accessory hemiazygos veins, while those of the abdominal part end in both the azygos and left gastric veins. Also *esophageal veins.* Also *venae oesophageales.* **venae ethmoidales** [NA] Veins accompanying the anterior and posterior ethmoidal arteries. They drain the ethmoidal sinuses and enter the orbit through the anterior and posterior ethmoidal foramina, respectively, to end in the superior ophthalmic vein. Also *ethmoidal veins.* **v. facialis** [NA] A vein formed at the medial angle of the eye by the union of the supraorbital and supratrochlear veins and then running obliquely down the side of the nose. It is joined by the anterior division of the retromandibular vein and ends in the internal jugular vein opposite the greater cornu of the hyoid bone. Also *facial vein, anterior facial vein.* **v. faciei profunda** See under VENA PROFUNDA FACIEI. **v. femoralis** [NA] The vein accompanying the femoral artery, commencing at the opening in the adductor magnus muscle as the continuation of the popliteal vein and ending behind the inguinal ligament by continuing as the external iliac vein. In the femoral triangle it receives many muscular tributaries, the medial and lateral circumflex femoral and the profunda femoris veins as well as the great saphenous vein, which joins it by piercing the cribriform fascia of the saphenous opening. It contains a number of valves. Also *femoral vein.* **venae fibulares** [NA] Veins accompanying the fibular, or peroneal, artery and communicating with the venous plexus in the soleus muscle and with superficial veins before ending in the posterior tibial vein. Also *fibular veins, peroneal veins.* **venae frontales venarum superiorum cerebri** [NA] The superficial tributaries of the superior cerebral veins draining the inferior (orbital) and anteromedial surfaces of each cerebral hemisphere, and joining those from the lateral surface to end obliquely in the superior sagittal sinus. Also *frontal veins of superior cerebral veins.* **v. gastrica dextra** [NA] A small vein running from left to right along the pyloric part of the lesser curvature of the stomach in the lesser omentum and receiving tributaries from the stomach and the proximal part of the superior part of the duodenum as well as the prepyloric vein before ending in the portal vein. Also *right gastric vein.* **venae gastricae breves** [NA] Several small veins draining the fundus and the left portion of the stomach and passing through the gastrosplenic ligament to end in the splenic vein or one of its tributaries. Also *short gastric veins.* **v. gastrica sinistra** [NA] The vein accompanying the left gastric artery, ascending in the lesser omentum along the lesser curvature toward the cardia of the stomach and ending in the portal vein. Also *left gastric vein.* **v. gastro-omentalis dextra** [NA] The vein accompanying the right gastro-omental (gastroepiploic) artery in the greater omentum along the greater curvature of the stomach, draining both surfaces of the stomach and the greater omentum, and ending in the superior mesenteric vein below the neck of the pancreas. Also *right gastroepiploic vein.* **v. gastro-omentalis sinistra** [NA] The vein accompanying the left gastro-omental (gastroepiploic) artery in the greater omentum along the greater curvature and draining both surfaces of the stomach and the greater omentum before ending in the splenic vein at its commencement. Also *left gastroepiploic vein.* **venae geniculares** [NA] The veins accompanying the genicular branches of the popliteal artery, draining the knee joint and ending in the popliteal vein. Also *genicular veins.* **venae gluteae inferiores** [NA] The venae comitantes of the inferior gluteal artery, anastomosing with the medial circumflex femoral and first perforating veins in the upper part of the back of the thigh, and passing through the greater sciatic foramen below the piriformis muscle to form a single trunk that ends in the internal iliac vein. Also *inferior gluteal veins.* **venae gluteae superiores** [NA] The venae comitantes of the superior gluteal artery that pass through the greater sciatic foramen above the piriformis muscle to join the internal iliac vein either independently or as a single trunk. They drain the area of the gluteal region supplied by the artery and its branches. Also *superior gluteal veins.* **v. hemiazygos** [NA] A longitudinal vein that arises from the junction of the left subcostal and left ascending lumbar veins, or from the posterior side of the left renal vein, or from a plexus of veins anterior to the upper lumbar vertebrae and communications from the inferior vena cava and renal vein, or from a combination of any of these. It ascends along the left border of the bodies of the lower thoracic vertebrae, receiving the lower three left posterior intercostal veins until it reaches the eighth thoracic vertebra, where it turns to the right across the vertebral body behind the aorta, esophagus, and thoracic duct to end in the azygos vein independently or in conjunction with the accessory hemiazygos vein. Also *hemiazygos vein, left azygos vein.* **v. hemiazygos accessoria** [NA] A longitudinal vein descending along the left border of the bodies of the fifth through seventh thoracic vertebrae, turning then to the right and joining the azygos vein either independently or in conjunction with the hemiazygos vein. Along its course it receives the fourth through eighth left posterior intercostal veins and occasionally the left bronchial veins. Also *accessory hemiazygos vein.* **venae hemispherii cerebelli inferiores** See under VENAE INFERIORES HEMISPHERII CEREBELLI. **venae hemispherii cerebelli superiores** See under VENAE SUPERIORES HEMISPHERII CEREBELLI. **venae hepaticae** [NA] Three veins, right, left, and anterior, draining the liver, arising from the union of the sublobular veins and converging on the posterior surface of the liver, from which they emerge to enter directly into the inferior vena cava. Also *hepatic veins.* **venae hepaticae dextrae** [NA] Veins draining the posterior segment and upper part of the anterior segment of the right lobe of the liver, and opening into the right side of the inferior vena cava either as a single trunk or two veins. Also *right hepatic veins.* **venae hepaticae intermediae** [NA] Veins draining the medial segment of the left lobe and the lower part of the anterior segment of the right lobe of the liver, forming a single stem that either enters the left side of the inferior vena cava independently or joins the stem of the left hepatic veins to form a common trunk entering the vena cava. Also *middle hepatic veins, median hepatic veins.* **venae hepaticae sinistrae** [NA] Veins draining the lateral portion of the left lobe of the liver and forming a stem that either enters the left side of the inferior vena cava independently or joins the stem of the middle hepatic veins to form a common trunk entering the vena cava. Also *left hepatic veins.* **venae ileales** [NA] Veins draining the ileum and ending in the superior mesenteric vein. Also *ileal veins, ileac veins.* **v. ileocolica** [NA] A vein accompanying the ileocolic artery and draining the cecum, vermiform appendix, terminal ileum, and the lower portion of the ascending colon, and ending in the superior mesenteric vein. Also *ileocolic vein.* **v. iliaca communis** [NA] A large vein formed in front of each sacroiliac articulation by the union of the external and internal iliac veins and extending medially and upwards to the right side of the fifth lumbar vertebra, where it joins its fellow of the opposite side to form the inferior vena cava. The right vein is shorter and less obliquely inclined than the left, and each receives the iliolumbar vein and occasionally the lateral sacral veins, while the median sacral vein joins the left common iliac vein. Also *common iliac vein.* **v. iliaca externa** [NA] The continuation of the femoral vein behind the inguinal liagment, accompanying the external iliac artery upward along the brim of the minor pelvis to the front of the sacroiliac articulation, where it joins the internal iliac vein to form the common iliac vein. Also *external iliac vein.* **v. iliaca interna** [NA] A vein formed at the upper margin of the greater sciatic foramen by the union of the tributaries corresponding to most of the branches of the internal iliac artery and ascending to the front of the sacroiliac articulation, where it joins the external iliac vein to form the common iliac vein. Also *internal iliac vein.* **v. iliolumbalis** [NA] The vein accompanying the iliolumbar artery but ending in the common iliac vein after it receives the fifth lumbar vein and tributaries from the psoas muscle and the iliac fossa. Also *iliolumbar vein.* **inferior v. cava** VENA CAVA INFERIOR. **venae inferiores cerebri** [NA] Small veins draining the under surfaces of the cerebral hemispheres. Those on the orbital surface of the frontal lobe join the superior cerebral vein and end in the superior sagittal sinus, while those on the temporal lobe terminate in the cavernous, superior petrosal, and transverse sinuses after anastomosing with the middle cerebral and basal veins. Also *inferior cerebral veins.* **venae inferiores hemispherii cerebelli** [NA] Veins passing posteriorly and laterally on the inferior surface of the cerebellum to end either in the straight sinus or one of the sigmoid sinuses as well as in the inferior and occipital sinuses. Also *inferior cerebellar veins, venae cerebelli inferiores* (outmoded). **venae intercapitulares** [NA] The intercapitular veins of the hand (venae intercapitulares manus), which connect the palmar digital veins to the dorsal digital veins by passing back between the metacarpal heads, and the intercapitular veins of the foot (venae intercapitulares pedis), which connect the plantar digital veins with the dorsal digital veins by passing between the metatarsal heads. Also *intercapital veins.* **venae intercapitulares manus** See under VENAE INTERCAPITULARES. **venae intercapitulares pedis** See under VENAE INTERCAPITULARES. **venae intercostales anteriores** [NA] Tributaries of the internal thoracic and musculophrenic veins that drain the anterior portions of the intercostal spaces. Also *anterior intercostal veins.* **venae intercostales posteriores** [NA] Veins accompanying the posterior intercostal arteries and draining most of the upper eleven intercostal spaces on each side. Near the vertebral column each receives a dorsal branch draining the skin and muscles of the back and the vertebral venous plexuses. Also *posterior intercostal veins.* **v. intercostalis superior dextra** [NA] A vein formed anterior to the heads of the ribs by the union of the second, third, and sometimes the fourth posterior intercostal veins and then descending to join the terminal part of the azygos vein. Also *right superior intercostal vein.* **v. intercostalis superior sinistra** [NA] The vein formed by the union of the second, third, and sometimes the fourth posterior intercostal veins. It ascends obliquely on the left of or across the aortic arch and ends in the left brachiocephalic vein. Also *left superior intercostal vein.* **v. intercostalis suprema** [NA] The vein that drains the first intercostal space on each side, ascends in front of the neck of the first rib, and runs forward over the pleura to end in the corresponding brachiocephalic or vertebral vein. Also *highest intercostal vein.* **venae interlobares renis** [NA] Veins draining the arcuate veins of the kidney, passing between the renal pyramids, and anastomosing with each other before converging on the hilum to form the renal vein. Also *interlobar veins of kidney.* **venae interlobulares hepatis** [NA] Terminal branches of the portal vein in the portal canals. They accompany the interlobular arteries, form sinusoids at the periphery of the lobules, and drain into the central vein. Also *interlobular veins of liver.* **venae interlobulares renis** [NA] Veins draining both the stellate venules beneath the fibrous capsule of the kidney and the venous ends of the peritubular capillary plexus and passing towards the corticomedullary junction, where they end in the arcuate veins. Just before their terminations they receive some of the terminations of the ascending vasa recta. Also *interlobular veins of kidney.* **v. intermedia antebrachii** [NA] A vein that occasionally arises from the superficial palmar venous plexus and ascends in the midline of the forearm anteriorly, receiving tributaries along its course and ending either in the median cubital or basilic vein. Also *median antebrachial vein, median vein of forearm.* **v. intermedia basilica** [NA] The medial terminal branch of a low dividing median antebrachial vein which courses proximally and medially to end in the basilic vein. Also *median basilic vein.* **v. intermedia cephalica** [NA] The lateral terminal branch of a low dividing median antebrachial vein which courses proximally and laterally to end in the cephalic vein. Also *median cephalic vein.* **v. intermedia cubiti** [NA] A branch given off by the cephalic vein distal to the elbow, passing upward obliquely across the cubital fossa, where it communicates with the deep veins of the forearm, and ending in the basilic vein proximal to the elbow. Also *median cubital vein, median vein of elbow.* **venae internae cerebri** [NA] Two veins, right and left, formed near the interventricular foramen by the union of the thalamostriate and choroid veins and continuing posteriorly between the layers of the tela choroidea of the third ventricle, to unite and form the great cerebral vein below the splenium of the corpus callosum. Together with the great cerebral vein, they are known as Galen's veins. Also *internal cerebral veins.* **v. intervertebralis** [NA] One of numerous veins that accompany the spinal nerves through the intervertebral foramina, draining the internal and external vertebral plexuses and ending in the vertebral, posterior intercostal, lumbar, and lateral sacral veins. Also *intervertebral vein.* **venae jejunales** [NA] Veins draining the jejunum and ending in the superior mesenteric vein. Also *jejunal veins.* **venae jejunales et ileales** Venae jejunales and venae ileales considered together. **v. jugularis anterior** [NA] One of a pair of veins (right and left) that begins below the chin by the confluence of several veins from the lower lip and chin region and descends in the paramedian line of the neck in the superficial fascia. Above the level of the clavicle it turns laterally deep to the sternocleidomastoid muscle to end in either the external jugular or the subclavian vein. Just above the sternum there is a communication between the right and left veins forming the jugular venous arch. Also *anterior jugular vein.* **v. jugularis externa** [NA] A superficial vein formed in the parotid gland behind the angle of the mandible by the union of the posterior division of the retromandibular vein and the posterior auricular vein, and coursing downward superficial to the sternocleidomastoid muscle into the subclavian triangle, where it pierces the deep fascia above the middle of the clavicle to end in the subclavian vein. Also *external jugular vein.* **v. jugularis interna** [NA] A deep vein commencing in the posterior part of the jugular foramen as a continuation of the sigmoid sinus and passing down the neck in the carotid sheath to the back of the sternoclavicular articulation where it joins the subclavian vein to form the brachiocephalic vein. Through its tributaries it drains the brain and parts of the face and the neck. Also *internal jugular vein.* **venae labiales anteriores** [NA] Veins draining the anterior portion of the labium majus and ending in the external pudendal veins. Also *anterior labial veins.* **venae labiales inferiores** [NA] Veins draining the lower lip and passing laterally to end in the facial vein. They communicate with the mental vein. Also *inferior labial veins.* **venae labiales posteriores** [NA] Veins draining the posterior part of the labium majus and ending in the internal pudendal vein. Also *posterior labial veins.* **v. labialis superior** [NA] A vein draining the upper lip, communicating with the infraorbital vein and running laterally to end in the facial vein. Also *superior labial vein.* **venae labyrinthi** [NA] Veins draining the semicircular canals, vestibule, and cochlea, uniting at the base of the modiolus to form one or more veins that leave through the internal acoustic meatus to end in the inferior petrosal, superior petrosal, or transverse sinus. Also *veins of labyrinth, labyrinthine veins.* **v. lacrimalis** [NA] The vein that accompanies the lacrimal artery and its branches in the orbit and drains the lacrimal gland into the superior ophthalmic vein. Also *lacrimal vein.* **v. laryngea inferior** [NA] A vein draining the lower part of the larynx and ending in the plexus thyroideus impar or in the inferior thyroid veins. Also *inferior laryngeal vein.* **v. laryngea superior** [NA] A vein draining the upper part of the larynx, accompanying the superior laryngeal artery and ending in the superior thyroid vein. Also *superior laryngeal vein.* **v. lienalis** VENA SPLENICA. **v. lingualis** [NA] The terminal trunk formed by the veins accompanying the lingual artery deep to the hyoglossus muscle. Anterior to the muscle it is called the deep lingual vein, which is joined by the sublingual vein. Posterior to the muscle it receives the dorsal lingual veins and near its termination in the internal jugular vein, opposite the greater cornu of the hyoid bone, it is joined by the vena comitans nervi hypoglossi. Also *lingual vein.* **venae lumbales** [NA] Four veins on each side accompanying the lumbar arteries. They drain the muscles and skin of the lumbar region and the walls of the abdomen as well as the vertebral venous plexuses. In front of the transverse processes of the vertebrae they are connected vertically to one another by the ascending lumbar vein. The first and second lumbar veins end in either the ascending lumbar vein or the inferior vena cava, the azygos vein, or the hemiazygos vein. The third and fourth veins end in the inferior vena cava. Also *lumbar veins.* **v. lumbalis ascendens** [NA] A paired longitudinal vein located behind the psoas major muscle and in front of the junction between the transverse processes and bodies of the lumbar vertebrae, and connecting the common iliac, iliolumbar, and lumbar veins. Superiorly it joins the subcostal vein to continue as the azygos vein on the right and the hemiazygos vein on the left. Also *ascending lumbar vein.* **v. magna cerebri** [NA] The large vein formed by the union of the two internal cerebral veins below the splenium of the corpus callosum, around which it turns upward to end in the straight sinus after receiving the right and left basal veins and the superior cerebellar veins. Also *great cerebral vein, vena cerebri magna, great vein of Galen, vena cerebri magna galeni* (outmoded).

**v. marginalis lateralis pedis** [NA] A superficial vein which is formed by the union of the superficial veins of the lateral side of the sole of the foot and runs along the lateral side of the dorsum of the foot, communicating with the dorsal venous arch and the dorsal venous network, to end behind the lateral malleolus as the small saphenous vein. Also *lateral marginal vein of foot.* **v. marginalis medialis pedis** [NA] A superficial vein which is formed by the union of the superficial veins of the medial side of the sole of the foot and runs along the medial side of the dorsum of the foot, communicating with the dorsal venous arch and the dorsal venous network, and ending in front of the medial malleolus as the great saphenous vein. Also *medial marginal vein of foot.* **venae maxillares** [NA] Veins derived from the pterygoid venous plexus and forming a trunk accompanying the first part of the maxillary artery between the neck of the mandible and the sphenomandibular ligament, and joining the superficial temporal vein in the parotid gland to form the retromandibular vein. Also *maxillary veins.* **v. media profunda cerebri** [NA] A vein receiving tributaries from the insula and the opercular gyri and lying on the floor of the lateral cerebral sulcus over the surface of the insula, before it joins the basal vein at the anterior perforated substance. Also *deep middle cerebral vein.* **venae mediastinales** [NA] Small veins accompanying the mediastinal branches of the internal thoracic artery, draining areolar tissue and lymph nodes in the anterior mediastinum and ending in the left brachiocephalic vein. Also *mediastinal veins.* **venae mediae superficiales cerebri** [NA] Veins commencing on the lateral surface of the cerebral hemisphere and running over the posterior ramus of the lateral sulcus to the inferior surface of the hemisphere, where they end in the cavernous or sphenoparietal sinus. Also *superficial middle cerebral vein, vena cerebri media* (outmoded), *sylvian vein, vein of sylvian fossa.* **venae meningeae** [NA] Veins that accompany the meningeal arteries, drain the dura mater, and communicate with the lacunae of the superior sagittal sinus, other dural sinuses, and the diploic veins. Also *meningeal veins.* **venae meningeae mediae** [NA] Veins that accompany the middle meningeal artery and its branches and communicate with the venous lacunae of the superior sagittal sinus, diploic veins, and the superficial middle cerebral veins. After leaving the skull they end in the pterygoid venous plexus. Also *middle meningeal veins.* **v. mesenterica inferior** [NA] A vein that accompanies the inferior mesenteric artery and its branches, drains the rectum, sigmoid colon, and descending colon to end behind the pancreas, usually by joining the splenic vein. Also *inferior mesenteric vein.* **v. mesenterica superior** [NA] The vein that accompanies the superior mesenteric artery from the right iliac fossa along the root of the mesentery, anterior to the third part of the duodenum and behind the neck of the pancreas, where it joins the splenic vein to form the portal vein. It drains the small intestine, cecum, vermiform appendix, ascending colon, and transverse colon. Also *superior mesenteric vein.* **venae metacarpales dorsales** [NA] Three longitudinal veins formed by dorsal digital veins of adjacent fingers joining at the webs and extending to the middle of the dorsum of the hand, to end in the dorsal venous network. Near their terminations they receive perforating branches from the palmar metacarpal veins. Also *dorsal metacarpal veins.* **venae metacarpales palmares** [NA] Venae comitantes of the palmar metacarpal arteries. They end in the deep palmar venous arch and send perforating branches between the metacarpal bones to the dorsal metacarpal veins. Also *palmar metacarpal veins.* **venae metatarsales dorsales pedis** [NA] Veins formed by dorsal digital veins of adjoining toes uniting at the clefts and running proximally along the dorsal metatarsal arteries, to end over the bases of the metatarsal bones in the dorsal venous arch. Also *dorsal metatarsal veins.* **venae metatarsales plantares** [NA] Veins formed in the sole of the foot by the plantar digital veins of adjacent toes uniting at the clefts and extending posteriorly in the spaces between the metatarsal bones, where they communicate by perforating branches with the dorsal metatarsal veins, and then join to form the deep plantar venous arch. Also *plantar metatarsal veins.* **venae musculophrenicae** [NA] Veins that accompany the musculophrenic artery, receive the seventh through ninth anterior intercostal veins and veins from the diaphragm and the adjacent anterior abdominal wall, and then join the superior epigastric veins to form the internal thoracic veins. Also *musculophrenic veins.* **venae nasales externae** [NA] Several veins on the external aspect of the nose communicating across the midline, the upper veins draining to the angular vein or the ophthalmic veins while those from the ala drain into the facial vein. Also *external nasal veins.* **v. nasofrontalis** [NA] A vein formed by connections between the supratrochlear, external nasal, and angular veins, entering the orbit lateral to the trochlea of the superior oblique muscle and usually ending in the superior ophthalmic vein. Also *nasofrontal vein.* **v. obliqua atrii sinistri** [NA] A small vein descending obliquely on the posterior aspect of the left atrium and joining the coronary sinus at its left end. Superiorly it is continuous with the ligament of the left vena cava. Also *oblique vein of left atrium, vein of Marshall, Marshall's oblique vein.* **venae obturatoriae** [NA] Veins formed by tributaries draining the obturator muscles, the hip joint, and the adductor muscles. They enter the pelvis through the obturator canal with the obturator artery and end in the internal iliac vein. Also *obturator veins.* **v. occipitalis** [NA] A vein commencing in a venous plexus in the posterior part of the scalp and piercing the cranial attachment of the trapezius muscle, to end in the suboccipital triangle by joining the vertebral and deep cervical veins. Also *occipital vein.* **venae oesophageales** VENAE ESOPHAGEALES. **v. ophthalmica inferior** [NA] A vein formed near the front of the orbit by veins draining the inferior oblique and inferior rectus muscles, the lacrimal sac, and the lower eyelid and running posteriorly along the orbital floor to end either in the superior ophthalmic vein or the cavernous sinus. It communicates through the inferior orbital fissure with the pterygoid plexus. Also *inferior ophthalmic vein.* **v. ophthalmica superior** [NA] A vein formed at the medial end of the upper eyelid by tributaries communicating with the supraorbital, supratrochlear and angular veins. It runs posterolaterally with the ophthalmic artery to the medial end of the superior orbital fissure, where it is often joined by the inferior ophthalmic vein, and then continues through the fissure to end in the cavernous sinus. Also *superior ophthalmic vein.* **v. ovarica dextra** [NA] A vein arising from the pampiniform plexus in the broad ligament near the right ovary and uterine tube, communicating with the uterine plexus and accompanying the right ovarian artery to end in the inferior vena cava. Also *right ovarian vein.* **v. ovarica sinistra** [NA] A vein arising from the pampiniform plexus in the broad ligament near the left ovary and uterine tube, communicating with the uterine plexus and accompanying the left ovarian artery to end in the left renal vein. Also *left ovarian vein.* **v. palatina** [NA] A vein arising in the soft palate, leaving near the upper pole of the palatine tonsil, and running obliquely downwards and forwards in the bed of the tonsil to pierce the superior pharyngeal constrictor muscle near its lower border and terminate in the facial vein or any of several veins in the immediate vicinity. Also *palatine vein.* **venae palpebrales** [NA] Veins draining the eyelids. They may either join the conjunctival veins to form the episcleral veins or drain directly into the superior ophthalmic vein. Also *palpebral veins.* **venae palpebrales inferiores** [NA] Veins arising in the lower eyelid, communicating with the infraorbital vein and running medially and downward to end in the angular vein. Also *inferior palpebral veins.* **venae palpebrales superiores** [NA] Veins arising in the upper eyelid and opening into the angular vein. They communicate with the middle temporal veins. Also *superior palpebral veins.* **venae pancreaticae** [NA] Small veins draining the pancreas and ending in the splenic, portal, and superior mesenteric veins. Also *pancreatic veins.* **venae pancreaticoduodenales** [NA] Veins accompanying the superior and inferior pancreaticoduodenal arteries anterior and posterior to the head of the pancreas. The veins form anastomosing arcades in the groove between the duodenum and the head of the pancreas, draining both. The anterior superior pancreaticoduodenal vein joins the right gastro-omental vein to end in the superior mesenteric vein, and the posterior superior pancreaticoduodenal vein ends in the portal vein, while the anterior inferior and posterior inferior pancreaticoduodenal veins end either singly or as a common trunk in either the first jejunal vein or the superior mesenteric vein. Also *pancreaticoduodenal veins.* **venae paraumbilicales** [NA] Veins draining the skin around the umbilicus, anastomosing with veins in the anterior abdominal wall and along the median umbilical ligament and extending along the ligamentum teres of the liver to end in the left branch of the portal vein. Also *paraumbilical veins, parumbilical veins, veins of Sappey.* **venae parotideae** [NA] Veins draining the parotid gland and ending in the retromandibular vein. Also *parotid veins.* **venae perforantes** **1** [NA] Paired veins accompanying the perforating branches of the profunda femoris artery, draining the muscles of the thigh into the profunda femoris vein and setting up communications between the popliteal vein and the inferior gluteal vein. **2** Veins passing between the metacarpal bones and connecting the palmar metacarpal with the dorsal metacarpal veins, and between the metatarsal bones connecting the plantar metatarsal and the dorsal metatarsal veins. For defs. 1 and 2 also *perforating veins.* **venae pericardiacae** [NA] Veins draining the pericardium, passing anterior to the arch of the aorta and ending in the left brachiocephalic vein and superior vena cava. Also *pericardiac veins, pericardial veins.* **venae pericardiacophrenicae** [NA] Veins draining the upper surface of the diaphragm, accompanying the pericardiacophrenic artery and phrenic nerve and ending in either the internal thoracic or the corresponding brachiocephalic veins. Also *pericardiacophrenic veins.* **persistent left v. cava superior** A systemic vein, usually small with few tributaries, that terminates in the coronary sinus after coursing along the posterior-lateral wall of the left atrium. It is a vestige of the left common cardinal vein. **venae pharyngeales** [NA] Veins forming a plexus between the prevertebral fascia and the pharyngeal constrictor muscles, communicating with the pterygoid plexus superiorly and draining into the internal jugular vein below. Also *pharyngeal veins.* **venae phrenicae inferiores** [NA] Veins draining the inferior surface of the diaphragm and accompanying corresponding arteries, that of the right side ending in the inferior vena cava while the left one has two branches, the anterior one ending in the inferior vena cava and the posterior one in the left renal or suprarenal vein. Also *inferior phrenic veins.*

**venae phrenicae superiores** [NA] Small veins on the posterosuperior surface of the diaphragm that communicate with the pericardiacophrenic veins and drain into the azygos or hemiazygos vein. Also *superior phrenic veins.* **v. poplitea** [NA] The vein superficial to the popliteal artery, with which it shares a fascial sheath, formed at the lower border of the popliteus muscle by the union of the anterior and posterior tibial veins and ending at the opening in the adductor magnus muscle where it continues as the femoral vein. Also *popliteal vein.* **v. portae hepatis** [NA] The thick vein formed by the union of the superior mesenteric and the splenic veins behind the neck of the pancreas and ascending from there into the right border of the lesser omentum, to come to lie behind the hepatic artery and the bile duct and anterior to the epiploic foramen until it reaches the porta hepatis, where it ends in right and left branches ramifying in the liver. Its other tributaries are the left and right gastric veins, prepyloric vein, paraumbilical veins, and cystic vein. Also *portal vein.* **v. posterior ventriculi sinistri cordis** [NA] A vein on the diaphragmatic surface of the left ventricle, arising near the apex and running on the left of the middle cardiac vein, usually to end in the coronary sinus though it may join the great cardiac vein. Also *posterior vein of left ventricle.* **v. precardinalis** [NA] Either of the paired veins draining the cranial half of the embryo into the common cardinal veins which open into the corresponding horns of the sinus venosus. Also *precardinal vein.* **v. prepylorica** [NA] A small vein draining the anterior surface of the pylorus, lying in a groove opposite the pyloric sphincter and ending in the right gastric vein. Also *prepyloric vein, Latarjet's vein, Mayo's vein.* **venae profundae clitoridis** [NA] Veins draining most of the glans and corpora cavernosa of the clitoris and ending mainly in the deep dorsal vein of the clitoris. Also *deep veins of clitoris.* **venae profundae penis** [NA] Veins draining the cavernous spaces of the corpora cavernosa and corpus spongiosum penis, most of which emerge from these structures and pass obliquely over their lateral surfaces to end in the deep dorsal vein of the penis. Also *deep veins of penis.* **v. profunda faciei** [NA] A communicating vein that connects the pterygoid plexus to the facial vein deep to the zygomaticus major muscle. Also *deep facial vein.* **v. profunda femoris** [NA] The vein accompanying the profunda femoris artery and receiving corresponding muscular and perforating tributaries through which anastomoses are set up between the inferior gluteal and popliteal veins. It often receives the medial and lateral circumflex femoral veins just before it joins the femoral vein. Also *deep femoral vein, deep vein of thigh.* **v. profunda linguae** [NA] A vein commencing as several branches near the tip of the tongue and accompanying the deep lingual artery to the anterior border of the hyoglossus muscle, where it continues as the lingual vein with the artery deep to the muscle. At the anterior border it may receive the sublingual vein. Also *deep lingual vein, deep vein of tongue, ranine vein.* **venae pudendae externae** [NA] Veins formed by the anterior scrotal or labial veins, joined by the superficial dorsal veins of the penis or clitoris and ending in the great saphenous vein just before it pierces the saphenous opening. Also *external pudendal veins.* **v. pudenda interna** [NA] A vein formed by the union of the deep veins of the penis or clitoris, then accompanying the internal pudendal artery to end in the internal iliac vein. Its tributaries are the posterior scrotal or labial veins, veins of the bulb of the penis or of the vestibule, and the inferior rectal veins. Also *internal pudendal vein.* **venae pulmonales** [NA] Four veins, two from each lung and devoid of valves, that carry oxygenated blood from the lungs to the left atrium of the heart. Originating in capillary plexuses in the walls of the lung alveoli, small vessels coalesce to form larger branches, such as intrasegmental and infrasegmental veins, until a single trunk is formed for each lobe, three from the right lung and two from the left. The vein from the middle lobe of the right lung usually joins that from the upper lobe so that only two veins, superior and inferior, run to the heart. Also *pulmonary veins, venous arteries.* **v. pulmonalis dextra inferior** [NA] A vein formed in the hilum of the right lung by the union of the apical (superior) branch and the common basal veins. It drains the bronchopulmonary segments of the lower lobe of the right lung and ends in the left atrium of the heart. Also *right inferior pulmonary vein.* **v. pulmonalis dextra superior** [NA] A vein formed in the hilum of the right lung by the union of four segmental veins and ending in the left atrium of the heart. The apical, anterior, and posterior segmental veins drain the upper lobe, and another drains the middle lobe, the latter having two main tributaries, a medial and a lateral vein. Also *right superior pulmonary vein.* **v. pulmonalis sinistra inferior** [NA] A vein formed in the hilum of the left lung by the union of the apical (superior) branch and the common basal veins draining the bronchopulmonary segments of the lower lobe of the left lung. It ends in the left atrium of the heart. Also *left inferior pulmonary vein.* **v. pulmonalis sinistra superior** [NA] A vein formed in the hilum of the left lung by the union of the apicoposterior, anterior, and lingular branches draining the bronchopulmonary segments of the upper lobe of the left lung. It ends in the left atrium of the heart. Also *left superior pulmonary vein.* **v. pulpae rubrae** [NA] One of the numerous veins draining the venous sinuses of the red pulp of the spleen and composed of thin walls containing elastic fibers and lined by endothelium. Also *pulp vein, vena pulparis.* **venae radiales** [NA] Veins arising from the lateral side of the superficial and deep palmar venous arches, receiving deep veins from the dorsum of the hand and accompanying the radial artery in the forearm to the front of the elbow, where they join the ulnar veins to form the brachial veins. Also *radial veins.* **venae rectae of kidney** VENULAE RECTAE RENIS. **venae rectales inferiores** [NA] Veins commencing in the lower external part of the rectal venous plexus, draining the lower part of the anal canal, and ending in the internal pudendal vein. They help to establish a communication between the systemic and portal systems of veins. Also *inferior rectal veins, inferior hemorrhoidal veins.* **venae rectales mediae** [NA] Veins commencing in the middle of the internal part of the rectal venous plexus, draining the muscular walls of the region of the rectal ampulla, and ending in the internal iliac vein after crossing the pelvic surface of the levator ani muscle. They receive tributaries from the bladder, prostate, and seminal vesicle. They help to establish a communication between the systemic and portal systems of veins. Also *middle rectal veins, middle hemorrhoidal veins.* **v. rectalis superior** [NA] A vein that drains the upper portions of both the internal and the external parts of the rectal venous plexus, commencing as about six veins extending up in the rectal submucosa and piercing the muscular wall of the rectum to form a single vessel that continues as the inferior mesenteric vein. It helps to establish a communication between the systemic and portal systems of veins. Also *superior rectal vein, superior hemorrhoidal vein.* **venae renales** [NA] Veins formed anterior to the renal arteries in the hilum of each kidney and joining the inferior vena cava at right angles. The left vein is longer than the right, receives the left suprarenal vein, the left testicular or ovarian vein, and several small tributaries. It crosses in front of the abdominal aorta and lies behind the pancreas. The right vein is behind the second part of the duodenum. Also *renal veins.* **venae renis** [NA] Intrarenal veins that form free anastomoses and arcades within the kidney. They include the stellate veins or venules and the intralobular, interlobular, straight, arcuate, and interlobar veins. Also *veins of kidney.* **v. retromandibularis** [NA] A vein formed in the parotid gland by the union of the superficial temporal and maxillary veins which then courses down in the gland deep to the facial nerve, to end behind the angle of the mandible in two branches, an anterior one that joins the facial vein and a posterior one that unites with the posterior auricular vein to form the external jugular vein. Also *retromandibular vein, posterior facial vein.* **venae revehentes** Venous channels formed from liver sinusoids in the embryo. They receive blood passing to the liver from venae advehentes and carry it to the common hepatic vein. Also *revehent veins.* **venae sacrales laterales** [NA] Veins that accompany the lateral sacral arteries, form the sacral venous plexus with branches of the median sacral vein anterior to the sacrum, and receive sacral intervertebral veins before ending in the internal iliac or superior gluteal veins. Also *lateral sacral veins.* **v. sacralis mediana** [NA] A single vein formed by the union of the venae comitantes of the median sacral artery in front of the sacrum, and ending in either the left common iliac vein or the junction of the two common iliac veins. Also *median sacral vein, middle sacral vein, vena sacralis media* (outmoded). **v. saphena accessoria** [NA] A vein commonly formed by tributaries draining the medial and posterior aspects of the thigh and communicating with the small saphenous vein before ending in the great saphenous vein in the upper part of the thigh. Also *accessory saphenous vein.* **v. saphena magna** [NA] The longest vein in the body. It commences on the medial side of the dorsal venous arch of the foot, receives branches from the plantar surface, and ascends anterior to the medial malleolus, along the medial margin of the tibia, posteromedial to the knee, and along the medial side of the thigh, to end by piercing the saphenous opening and entering the femoral vein. It contains numerous valves, communicates at several places with deep veins, and receives many tributaries draining most of the superficial area of the lower limb, the lower part of the anterior abdominal wall, and the external genitalia. Also *great saphenous vein, long saphenous vein.* **v. saphena parva** [NA] A vein arising from the lateral side of the dorsal venous arch of the foot and receiving tributaries from the lateral plantar surface before ascending behind the lateral malleolus to the popliteal fossa, where it pierces the deep fascia to end in the popliteal vein. It receives tributaries from the back of the heel and leg and communicates with the accessory saphenous vein, in which it may terminate, and the great saphenous vein. It contains several valves. Also *small saphenous vein, short saphenous vein.* **v. scapularis dorsalis** [NA] A vein accompanying the dorsal scapular artery, draining the scapular region, and passing through the brachial plexus to end in the subclavian vein. Also *dorsal scapular vein.* **venae scrotales anteriores** [NA] Veins draining the anterior part of the scrotum, anastomosing with the posterior scrotal veins, and ending in the external pudendal veins. Also *anterior scrotal veins.* **venae scrotales posteriores** [NA] Veins draining the posterior part of the scrotum, anastomosing with the anterior scrotal veins, and ending in the internal pudendal vein. Also *posterior scrotal veins.* **v. septi pellucidi** Either of the anterior and posterior veins that drain the septum pellucidum and open into the vena thalamostriata. Also *vein of septum pellucidum.* **venae sigmoideae** [NA] Veins draining the sigmoid colon and ending in the inferior mesenteric vein. Also *sigmoid veins.* **venae spinales anteriores** [NA] Veins that drain the anterior part of the spinal cord and pia mater. They comprise three longitudinal veins, one accompanying the anterior spinal artery in the anterior median fissure and two situated on the anterolateral aspects of the cord, one behind each ventral nerve root. They drain the anterior substance of the cord as well as the gray matter and end in the anterior internal vertebral venous plexus and the intervertebral veins, as well as communicating with the posterior spinal and radicular veins. Also *anterior spinal veins.* **venae spinales posteriores** [NA] Veins that drain the posterior part of the spinal cord and pia mater. They comprise three longitudinal veins, one behind the posterior median septum of the cord and two situated on the posterolateral aspects, one behind each dorsal nerve root. They drain the posterior substance of the cord and end in the posterior internal vertebral venous plexus and the intervertebral veins, and they communicate with the anterior spinal and radicular veins. Also *posterior spinal veins.* **v. spiralis modioli** [NA] A small vein coursing in the spiral modiolus of the cochlea and ending in either the labyrinthine veins or the vein of the cochlear canaliculus. Also *spiral vein of modiolus.* **v. splenica** [NA] A large vein formed at the hilum of the spleen by trabecular veins draining the spleen. It passes to the right through the lienorenal ligament, in front of the left kidney to the back of the pancreas, where it lies below the splenic artery and receives many branches draining the pancreas. It ends behind the neck of the pancreas, joining the superior mesenteric vein to form the portal vein. Also *vena lienalis, splenic vein.* **v. sternocleidomastoidea** [NA] A vein accompanying the sternocleidomastoid artery, draining the sternocleidomastoid muscle, and ending in the internal jugular vein. Also *sternocleidomastoid vein.* **v. striata** One of a group of veins that drain the corpus striatum and basal forebrain and course through the anterior perforated substance to join the basal vein on the inferior surface of the cerebrum. Also *inferior striate vein, inferior thalamostriate vein, striate vein.* **v. stylomastoidea** [NA] A vein accompanying the stylomastoid artery, draining the tympanic antrum and mastoid air cells, and passing through the stylomastoid foramen to end in the posterior auricular or the retromandibular vein. Also *stylomastoid vein.* **v. subclavia** [NA] The continuation of the axillary vein at the outer border of the first rib, the upper surface of which it crosses obliquely in front of the subclavian artery and the scalenus anterior muscle, to join the internal jugular vein and form the brachiocephalic vein. Its usual tributaries are the external jugular, dorsal scapular, and anterior jugular veins. At its termination it receives the thoracic duct on the left side and the right lymphatic duct on the right. Also *subclavian vein.* **v. subcostalis** [NA] A vein accompanying the subcostal artery and joining the ascending lumbar vein to help form the azygos vein on the right side and the hemiazygos vein on the left. Also *subcostal vein.* **venae subcutaneae abdominis** [NA] The superficial veins of the anterior abdominal wall. They form numerous plexuses that drain into the great saphenous veins and the deeper veins of the abdomen. Also *subcutaneous veins of abdomen.* **v. sublingualis** [NA] A vein accompanying the sublingual artery that may, at the anterior border of the hyoglossus muscle, either join the deep lingual vein and continue deep to the muscle as the lingual veins, or join the vena comitans nervi hypoglossi, which continues superficial to the muscle. Also *sublingual vein.* **v. sublobularis** [NA]

One of several veins formed by the union of central veins that drain the liver lobules and ending by joining one or more similar veins to form a collecting vein, a tributary of the hepatic veins. Also *sublobular vein, intercalated vein.* **v. submentalis** [NA] A vein accompanying the submental artery on the mylohyoid muscle, communicating with the anterior jugular vein in the submental triangle, and running posteriorly to end in the facial vein. Also *submental vein.* **superior v. cava** VENA CAVA SUPERIOR. **venae superiores cerebri** [NA] Numerous veins on the superolateral and medial surfaces of the cerebral hemispheres running upward to the superomedial margin of each hemisphere. Those from the medial surface join those from the outer convex surface before they enter the superior sagittal sinus. Also *superior cerebral veins.* **venae superiores hemispherii cerebelli** [NA] Veins on the superior surface of the cerebellum, some of which run laterally to end in the superior petrosal and transverse sinuses while others run forward and medially over the superior vermis to join either the straight sinus or the great cerebral vein. Also *superior cerebellar veins, venae cerebelli superiores* (outmoded). **v. supraorbitalis** [NA] A vein commencing on the forehead, where it communicates with the superficial and middle temporal veins, and running medially to the medial angle of the eye, where it pierces the orbicularis oculi muscle to join the supratrochlear vein and form the angular vein. It sends a branch into the orbital cavity to communicate with the superior ophthalmic vein and receives the frontal diploic vein and a tributary from the frontal sinus. Also *supraorbital vein.* **v. suprarenalis dextra** [NA] A vein arising in the medulla of the right suprarenal gland and emerging from the hilum to enter the adjacent inferior vena cava. Also *right suprarenal vein.* **v. suprarenalis sinistra** [NA] A vein arising in the medulla of the left suprarenal gland, emerging from the hilum to run inferomedially behind the pancreas and end in the left renal vein. Also *left suprarenal vein.* **v. suprascapularis** [NA] A vein, often double, accompanying the suprascapular artery and nerve, draining the dorsal scapular region, and ending in the external jugular vein. Also *suprascapular vein.* **venae supratrochleares** [NA] Veins commencing in a plexus on the forehead, communicating with the superficial temporal veins, and forming a single trunk that runs inferiorly near the median plane to the medial angle of the eye, where it joins the supraorbital vein to form the angular vein. Also *supratrochlear veins, frontal veins.* **venae temporales profundae** [NA] Veins accompanying the deep temporal branches of the maxillary artery, draining the deep part of the temporal muscle, and ending in the pterygoid venous plexus. Also *deep temporal veins.* **venae temporales superficiales** [NA] Anterior and posterior veins draining an extensive network in the scalp and uniting into a single trunk above the zygomatic arch. This trunk is joined by the middle temporal vein before crossing the posterior root of the arch with the superficial temporal artery to enter the parotid gland, where it joins the maxillary vein to form the retromandibular vein. It receives numerous tributaries. Also *superficial temporal veins.* **v. temporalis media** [NA] A vein lying deep to the temporal fascia, draining the temporal muscle, and communicating with the deep temporal veins. It receives the lateral palpebral veins and pierces the fascia just above the zygomatic arch to join the superficial temporal vein. Also *middle temporal vein.* **v. terminalis** VENA THALAMOSTRIATA. **v. testicularis dextra** [NA] A single vein ending in the inferior vena cava and formed at the deep inguinal ring by the coalescence of the venae comitantes of the right testicular artery, which in turn are formed by the union of several veins in the spermatic cord that drain the pampiniform plexus anterior to the ductus deferens. Also *right testicular vein.* **v. testicularis sinistra** [NA] A single vein ending at right angles in the left renal vein and formed at the deep inguinal ring by the coalescence of the venae comitantes of the left testicular artery, which in turn are formed by the union of several veins in the spermatic cord that drain the pampiniform plexus anterior to the ductus deferens. Also *left testicular vein.* **v. thalamostriata** A vein that courses in a groove between the thalamus and the caudate nucleus and drains both of these structures. Behind the anterior column of the fornix, the thalamostriate vein joins with the choroid vein to form the internal cerebral vein. Also *vena terminalis, superior thalamostriate vein, thalamostriate vein, terminal vein.* **venae thoracicae internae** [NA] Paired veins formed by the union of the musculophrenic and superior epigastric veins between the sixth costal cartilage and the transversus thoracis muscle, and ascending with the internal thoracic artery to the third costal cartilage, where they join to form a single trunk that ends in the corresponding brachiocephalic vein. The tributaries correspond to the branches of the artery. Also *internal thoracic veins.* **v. thoracica lateralis** [NA] A vein accompanying the lateral thoracic artery, draining the anterolateral thoracic wall, and communicating with the superficial epigastric veins through the thoracoepigastric veins. It receives the costoaxillary veins before it ends in the axillary vein. Also *lateral thoracic vein.* **v. thoracoacromialis** [NA] A vein accompanying the thoracoacromial artery and ending in either the axillary, subclavian, or cephalic vein. Also *thoracoacromial vein.* **venae thoracoepigastricae** [NA] Veins that connect either the superficial epigastric vein or the femoral vein with the lateral thoracic vein. They may occasionally form a single trunk. They establish a communication between the areas of drainage of the superior vena cava and the inferior vena cava. Also *thoracoepigastric veins.* **venae thymicae** [NA] Small veins draining the thymus gland and ending in the left brachiocephalic, internal thoracic, and inferior thyroid veins. Also *thymic veins, veins of thymus.* **v. thyreoidea ima** See under VENA THYROIDEA INFERIOR. **venae thyroideae mediae** [NA] Veins draining the lower part of the lobes of the thyroid gland and the adjacent larynx and trachea and crossing the corresponding common carotid artery to end in the internal jugular vein on both sides. Also *middle thyroid veins.* **v. thyroidea inferior** [NA] A vein draining each side of the lower part of the thyroid plexus on the surface of the thyroid gland and descending to end in the corresponding brachiocephalic vein. Often the veins of the two sides join in the midline to form a single trunk (formerly called vena thyreoidea ima) that ends in either the left brachiocephalic vein or the superior vena cava. Also *inferior thyroid vein.* **v. thyroidea superior** [NA] A vein formed at the upper pole of the thyroid gland by superficial and deep tributaries draining the gland and the thyroid plexus. It accompanies the superior thyroid artery and ends in the internal jugular or the facial vein. Also *superior thyroid vein.* **venae tibiales anteriores** [NA] Veins that commence as the venae comitantes of the dorsalis pedis artery and then accompany the anterior tibial artery through the anterior compartment of the leg and join the posterior tibial veins at the lower border of the popliteus muscle to form the popliteal vein. Also *anterior tibial veins.* **venae tibiales posteriores** [NA] Veins commencing in the plantar venous arch, accompanying the posterior tibial artery through the posterior compartment of the leg and receiving tributaries corresponding to branches of the artery, the largest being the fibular veins and veins from the soleus muscle. They communicate with superficial veins along their course and end by joining the anterior tibial veins at the lower border of the popliteus muscle to form the popliteal vein. Also *posterior tibial veins.* **v. trabecularis** [NA] One of the numerous veins formed by coalescence of pulp veins in the spleen and composed only of endothelium supported by the connective tissue of the trabeculae. At the hilum of the spleen they unite to form the splenic vein. Also *trabecular vein.* **venae tracheales** [NA] Numerous small branches draining the trachea, anastomosing with laryngeal and bronchial veins, and ending in either the left brachiocephalic vein or the inferior thyroid vein. Also *tracheal veins.* **venae transversae cervicis** [NA] Veins accompanying the transverse cervical artery, leaving the deep aspect of the trapezius muscle anteriorly to cross the posterior triangle of the neck and end either in the external jugular or in the subclavian vein. Also *transverse cervical veins, transverse veins of neck.* **v. transversa faciei** [NA] A vein accompanying the transverse facial artery below the zygomatic arch, draining the malar region, and communicating with the infraorbital, buccal, facial, and parotid veins before terminating in either the retromandibular or the superficial temporal vein. Also *transverse facial vein, transverse vein of face.* **venae tympanicae** [NA] Veins draining the tympanic cavity that emerge through the petrotympanic fissure to end either in the retromandibular vein or in the plexus formed by the venae articulares temporomandibulares. Also *tympanic veins.* **venae ulnares** [NA] Veins draining the medial side of the superficial and deep venous arches of the hand and accompanying the ulnar artery in the forearm to the cubital fossa, where they receive the veins of the common interosseous artery and join the radial veins to form the brachial veins. They communicate with the median cubital vein. Also *ulnar veins.* **v. umbilicalis** UMBILICAL VEIN. **v. umbilicalis sinistra** UMBILICAL VEIN. **venae uterinae** [NA] A pair of veins on each side draining the lower part of the uterine plexus located above the lateral fornix of the vagina within the broad ligament, and accompanying the uterine artery laterally to end in the corresponding internal iliac vein. Also *uterine veins, veins of uterus.* **v. vertebralis** [NA] A vein arising from the suboccipital venous plexus and tributaries from the internal vertebral plexus above the posterior arch of the atlas and entering the foramen in the transverse process of the atlas, to descend as a plexus around the vertebral artery through successive foramina in the transverse processes of the cervical vertebrae until it emerges as a single vessel from the sixth vertebra to end in the brachiocephalic vein. Also *vertebral vein.* **v. vertebralis accessoria** [NA] An inconstant small vein arising from the venous plexus around the vertebral artery in its course through the foramina transversaria and emerging from the foramen transversarium of the seventh cervical vertebra to run forward over the cervical pleura and end in the brachiocephalic vein. Also *accessory vertebral vein.* **v. vertebralis anterior** [NA] A small vein commencing in a venous plexus adjacent to the upper cervical transverse processes and accompanying the ascending cervical artery to end in the terminal part of the vertebral vein. Also *anterior vertebral vein, anterior vertebral vein of Lauth.* **venae vesicales** [NA] Several veins draining each side of the vesical plexus and ending in the corresponding internal iliac vein. Also *vesical veins.* **venae vestibulares** [NA] Small veins draining the vestibule of the internal ear and ending in the labyrinthine veins and occasionally also in the vein of the aqueduct of the vestibule. Also *vestibular veins.* **venae vorticosae** [NA] The four or five large veins of the vascular coat of the choroid that are formed by the veins accompanying the short and long posterior ciliary arteries. They converge in whorls on two superior and two inferior veins, and pierce the sclera at equidistant points about midway between the lamina cribrosa and the sclerocorneal junction. The upper two drain into the superior ophthalmic vein while the lower two end in the inferior ophthalmic vein. Also *vorticose veins, Stensen's veins, Ruysch veins.*

**venacavography** \vē′nəkəväg′rəfē\ [*vena cav(a)* + *o* + -GRAPHY] Serial roentgenography of the opacified inferior or superior vena cava.

**venae** \vē′nē\ Plural of VENA.

***Vena medinensis*** \med′inen′sis\ *DRACUNCULUS MEDINENSIS.*

**venation** \vēnā′shən\ The distribution and arrangement of the veins of a part.

**vene-**[1] \vē′nə-\ VENO-.

**vene-**[2] \ven′ə-\ [L *venenum* venom, poison] A combining form denoting venom or poison.

**venectasia** \vē′nektā′zhə\ [*ven(e)-*[1] + ECTASIA] PHLEBECTASIA.

**venectomy** \vēnek′təmē\ [*ven(e)-*[1] + -ECTOMY] PHLEBECTOMY.

**veneer** \vənir′\ [German *furnier* (from French *fournir* to supply, furnish) veneer, inlay] A thin layer of porcelain or acrylic resin, simulating dentin and used to cover all or part of a crown or pontic.

**venenation** \ven′ənā′shən\ [L *venenat(us),* past part. of *venenare* to infect with poison + -ION] Poisoning; envenomation.

**venene** \ven′ēn\ [L *venen(um)* venom, poison] A mixture of snake venoms used to produce antivenin.

**veneniferous** \ven′ənif′ərəs\ [L *venen(um)* venom, poison + *i* + -FEROUS] Producing, bearing, or transmitting poison, as venomous snakes or certain fungi. Also *venenific.*

**venenose** \ven′ənōs\ [L *venen(um)* poison, venom + -OSE[1]] VENOMOUS.

**venenous** \ven′ənəs\ [L *venen(um)* poison, venom + -OUS] VENOMOUS.

**venepuncture** \ven′ēpungk′chər\ VENIPUNCTURE.

**venereal** \vənir′ē·əl\ [L *venere(us)* (from *venus,* gen. *veneris* sexual love; personified as *Venus,* the love goddess) sexual, erotic + -AL] Associated with, disseminated by, or caused by sexual contact or intercourse. Also *genitoinfectious.*

**venereologist** \vənir′ē·äl′əjist\ A medical practitioner who specializes in the care of those with venereal and other sexually transmissible disease and in the epidemiological control of those infections.

**venereology** \vənir′ē·äl′əjē\ The medical study of venereal and other sexually acquired diseases.

**venesection** \ven′əsek′shən\ [VENE-[1] + SECTION] PHLEBOTOMY.

**venesuture** \ven′əsoo′chər\ [VENE-[1] + SUTURE] A suture of a defect in a vein. Also *venisuture.*

**veni-** \vē′nē-\ VENO-.

**venipuncture** \ven′ipungk′chər\ Puncture of a vein for aspiration of blood. Also *venepuncture.*

**venisuture** \ven′isoo′chər\ VENESUTURE.

**veno-** \vē′nō-, vē′nə-\ [L *vena* vein] A combining form meaning vein. Also *veni-, vene-.*

**venoatrial** \-ā′trē·əl\ Pertaining to a vena cava and the right atrium.

**venofibrosis** \-fībrō′sis\ PHLEBOSCLEROSIS.

**venography** \vēnäg′rəfē\ [VENO- + -GRAPHY] Roentgenography of veins after their opacification by the injection of a contrast medium. Also *phlebography.* **ascending v.**

The display of lower extremity major vein anatomy by serial radiographs of contrast material administered into a foot vein and allowed to pass centrally. **descending v.** The demonstration of the status of valves in the femoral vein by injecting a contrast dye into the vein. With placement of the patient in a semi-upright position, the passage of the dye toward the foot within the vein suggests valvular incompetence. **extradural v.** A radiologic technique of demonstrating the spinal extradural venous plexus with injected contrast medium. **impedance v.** A diagnostic test for acute venous thrombosis that is performed by recording and comparing the rate of change of calf volume expansion with inflation and deflation of a thigh cuff. **portal v.** PORTOGRAPHY. **radionuclide v.** A technique for visualizing veins, usually of the lower extremities, by using gamma-camera scanning following injection of a radioisotope. **splenic v.** SPLENOPORTOGRAPHY. **uterine v.** Radiographic visualization of the ovarian veins, periuterine veins, and veins in the broad ligament after the injection of a radiopaque contrast material into the uterine wall. **vertebral v.** The radiographic study of the epidural venous plexus by injecting a radiopaque contrast medium into a spinous process or into the ascending lumbar veins. **wedged hepatic v.** A technique of indirect measurement of portal venous pressure in which a percutaneously inserted catheter is wedged in a hepatic vein radicle. Retrograde contrast injection through the wedged catheter may also opacify the portal vein and demonstrate hepatic parenchymal architecture.

**venom** \ven′əm\ [Old French *venim* (from L *venenum* poison, potion; orig. philter, love charm, akin to *Venus*, the love goddess) a poison, venom] A poisonous substance secreted by an animal, typically from specific glands and by a specific mechanism such as stinging or biting, serving primarily to capture prey or to defend against enemies. **bee v.** The venom injected by the sting of a bee, which can cause severe anaphylactic reactions accompanied by cerebral edema and vascular congestion. Also *apisin*. **cobra v.** The venom of cobras; a complex neurotoxin made up of 61 amino acids in a single chain cross-linked by four disulfide bonds. It is rapidly absorbed from the subcutaneous tissue and causes respiratory paralysis if left untreated. **kokoi v.** The venom of a Colombian frog, *Phyllobates bicolor*, used as an arrow poison and possessing neurotoxic properties. **moccasin v.** A venom secreted by certain snakes of the family Viperidae, subfamily Crotalinae, characterized by its hemolytic activity, as the members of the genus *Agkistrodon*, including the water moccasin (cottonmouth) and copperhead of the eastern United States and the cantil or Mexican moccasin of Central America. **rattlesnake v.** Any of the venoms of the approximately 25 species of rattlesnakes, which vary widely in toxicity so that identification of the species is of major importance for effective treatment of a bite. **Russell's viper v.** A venom, from *Daboia* (Russell's viper), that accelerates the clotting of plasma containing adequate coagulation factors V and X and platelet factor 3 by converting factor X to Xa. **snake v.** The venom of any poisonous snake, a complex mixture of proteins and enzymes injected into prey through channels in the fangs in order to kill the prey or as an aid in swallowing or digesting. The venom is generally produced by modified oral glands situated in the space between the eye and the angle of the mouth. Snake venom can act on several human organ systems, but its principal effects are either hemolytic or neurotoxic. **toad v.** The poisonous secretion from the skin glands of many species of toads. Among the more toxic species are the Colorado River toad, *Bufo alvarius*, and the marine toad, *Bufo marinus*. The venom has a cardioactive digitalislike action. **viper v.** The venom of snakes of the family Viperidae, which causes injury to body tissues, both at the site of the bite and in surrounding areas, changes in red blood cells, defects in coagulation, injury to the blood vessels, and, to a lesser extent, damage to the heart, kidneys, and lungs.

**venomization** \ven′əmīzā′shən\ Treatment with snake venom.

**venomotor** \-mō′tər\ Influencing or capable of influencing the contractility of the muscle in the walls of veins.

**venomous** \ven′əməs\ [VENOM + -OUS] Producing venom. Also *venenose, venenous*.

**veno-occlusive** \-äkloo′siv\ Characterized by or relating to the occlusion of veins.

**venoperitoneostomy** \-per′itō′nē·äs′təmē\ The anastomosis of a vein, usually the greater saphenous vein, to the peritoneal cavity in order to drain ascitic accumulations.

**venopressor** \-pres′ər\ Producing or capable of producing an increase of pressure within the venous system.

**venosclerosis** \-sklirō′sis\ PHLEBOSCLEROSIS.

**venose** \vē′nōs\ [L *venosus* (from *ven(a)* vein + *-osus* -OSE[1]) full of veins] Having veins, especially prominent ones.

**venosinal** \-sī′nəl\ Pertaining to the sinus venarum of the right atrium of the heart.

**venosity** \vēnäs′itē\ **1** The quality or state of being venose; a relatively great number or fullness of veins (in a part). **2** The quality or state of being venous, or the degree to which something is venous (as blood with relatively low oxygen content).

**venotomy** \vēnät′əmē\ [VENO- + -TOMY] An incision into a vein.

**venous** \vē′nəs\ Pertaining to a vein or veins.

**venovenostomy** \-vēnäs′təmē\ PHLEBOPHLEBOSTOMY.

**vent** An opening leading to the outside, such as the anus and the cloaca. **pulmonic alveolar v.** PORE OF KOHN.

**venter** \ven′tər\ [L, the belly, womb] **1** The bulging, central part of an anatomic structure; belly. **2** The belly of a muscle; venter musculi. **3** ABDOMEN. **4** The anterior aspect of the abdomen. **5** The cavity of the uterus; womb. **6** Any cavity containing viscera. An obsolete usage. **v. anterior musculi digastrici** [NA] The anterior belly of the digastric muscle, arising from the digastric fossa adjacent to the midline on the lower border of the mandible and extending backwards to join the posterior belly at the intermediate tendon, which is usually attached to the body and greater cornu of the hyoid bone by a fibrous expansion. It is supplied by the mylohyoid branch of the inferior alveolar nerve. **v. frontalis musculi occipitofrontalis** [NA] The quadrilateral, thin front part of the occipitofrontalis muscle, extending from the galea aponeurotica in front of the coronal suture to the skin of the eyebrow and of the root of the nose. It is supplied by the temporal branches of the facial nerve. Also *frontal belly of occipitofrontal muscle, frontalis muscle, frontal muscle*. **v. inferior musculi omohyoidei** [NA] A narrow fleshy muscle belly arising from the superior margin of the scapula near the scapular notch and extending forwards across the lower part of the neck to end in the intermediate tendon of the omohyoid muscle, which is held to the clavicle and first rib by an ensheathing band of deep cervical fascia. It is innervated by the ansa cervicalis. Also *inferior belly of omohyoid muscle*. **v. musculi** [NA] The belly of a muscle; the bulging, fleshy, and contractile body of a muscle, usually located between the tendinous origin and insertion. Also *muscle belly*, *myogaster.* **v. occipitalis musculi occipitofrontalis** [NA] The quadrilateral, thin posterior part of the occipitofrontalis muscle arising from the lateral two-thirds of the supreme nuchal line of the occipital bone and from the mastoid process of the temporal bone, and inserting into the galea aponeurotica. It is supplied by the posterior auricular branch of the facial nerve. Also *occipital belly of occipitofrontal muscle, occipital muscle.* **v. posterior musculi digastrici** [NA] The posterior belly of the digastric muscle, arising from the mastoid notch of the temporal bone and extending anteroinferiorly to join the anterior belly at the intermediate tendon, which is usually attached to the body and greater cornu of the hyoid bone. It is innervated by the facial nerve. **v. superior musculi omohyoidei** [NA] A long, narrow fleshy muscle belly that extends upwards at an angle from the intermediate tendon of the omohyoid muscle to its insertion on the inferior margin of the body of the hyoid bone. It is innervated by the ansa cervicalis. Also *superior belly of omohyoid muscle.*

**ventilate** [See VENTILATION.] **1** To provide access to the free circulation of air. **2** To provide with a means of exchanging gases between the blood and the environment via the lungs, as in *ventilating a patient.*

**ventilation** [L *ventilatio* (from *ventilatus,* past part. of *ventilare* to ventilate, fan, from *ventulus* a little wind, dim. of *ventus* the wind) a fanning, winnowing] **1** The process of providing a supply of fresh air to an environment. **2** The process of gaseous exchange between the blood and the environment via the lungs. **alveolar v.** The volume of inspired air reaching the alveoli of the lungs per minute. **artificial v.** ARTIFICIAL RESPIRATION. **assisted v.** Mechanical ventilation in which a delivered gas volume is triggered by inspiration and normalizes tidal volume. **assisted-controlled v.** Mechanical ventilation used in assisting breathing when deficient, or completely assuming control of breathing in the presence of apnea. **constant positive pressure v.** A method of artificial ventilation of the lungs in which the pressure of air in the airways remains positive throughout the respiratory cycle. **controlled v.** Mechanical ventilation that takes the place of natural inspiration and expiration in management of pulmonary insufficiency. **dead space v.** The portion of minute volume used to ventilate mechanical, anatomic, and alveolar dead space: wasted ventilation. **intermittent demand v.** A method of artificial ventilation of the lungs in which the lungs are inflated mechanically only when there is insufficient spontaneous ventilation. **intermittent mandatory v.** A method of artificial ventilation of the lungs in which periods of spontaneous breathing are followed by periods of artificial ventilation. **intermittent positive pressure v.** A method of artificial ventilation in which the lungs are inflated by producing positive pressure of the inhaled gases and are deflated by removing this pressure. **maximum voluntary v.** MAXIMUM BREATHING CAPACITY. Abbr. MVV **middle-ear v.** The maintenance of atmospheric pressure within the middle-ear cleft by way of the eustachian tube, a prerequisite for normal hearing. During swallowing or yawning the eustachian tube, otherwise closed, opens briefly to permit correction of the negative pressure that tends constantly to build up within the enclosed middle-ear compartments. **minute v.** The volume of air expired per minute. **negative pressure v.** A method of artificial ventilation in which a negative or subatmospheric pressure is produced to assist expiration. **total v.** The total volume of air breathed in a stated time. **walking v.** An assessment of respiratory ventilatory function during exercise by measurement of the quantity of gas expired during the last 3 minutes of a 4-minute walk on a horizontal surface at a speed of 2 miles per hour.

**ventilator** [L (from *ventilare* to ventilate, fan; see VENTILATION), a fanner, winnower] Any device that provides ventilation. **mechanical v.** A mechanical circulator of air or gas. **pressure-cycled v.** A type of mechanical ventilator in which gas flow into the lungs is terminated when a preset airway pressure is attained. Also *pressure ventilator.* **tank v.** An apparatus for artificial ventilation of a patient who has weak or paralyzed respiratory muscles, comprising a rigid tank which encloses the body from the neck down. Changes of pressure of air within the tank bring about inspiration and expiration. Also *Drinker respirator, iron lung* (popular) . **time-cycled v.** A type of mechanical ventilator in which the time for each respiratory cycle is preset. **volume-cycled v.** A type of mechanical ventilator which is set to deliver a certain volume of air into the lungs. Also *volume ventilator.*

**ventilometer** \ven′tiläm′ətər\ SPIROMETER.

**ventilometry** \ven′tiläm′ətrē\ SPIROMETRY.

**ventplant** \vent′plant\ [*vent* + *(im)plant*] ORAL IMPLANT.

**ventrad** \ven′trad\ Toward the ventral aspect or any venter. Also *ventralward.*

**ventral** \ven′trəl\ [L *ventralis* (from *venter,* gen. *ventris,* the belly) pertaining to the belly] **1** Pertaining to the belly or abdominal surface of the body. **2** Relatively near the belly side of the body as compared with other structures or parts of the same kind nearer the back; in human anatomy, commonly equivalent to *anterior.* Compare DORSAL.

**ventralis** \ventrā′lis\ Ventral.

**ventralward** \ven′trəlwərd\ VENTRAD.

**ventri-** \ven′trē-\ VENTRO-.

**ventricle** \ven′trikl\ [L *ventriculus.* See VENTRICULUS.] VENTRICULUS. **aortic v. of heart** *Outmoded* VENTRICULUS SINISTER CORDIS. **auxiliary v.** A prosthetic pumping device that is designed to augment left ventricular function. Also *booster heart.* **v.'s of the brain** A system of intercommunicating cavities in the brain that are lined with ependyma and are filled with cerebrospinal fluid. The ventricular system communicates with the subarachnoid spaces. Each cerebral hemisphere contains a lateral ventricle; the diencephalon contains the third ventricle; and the fourth ventricle lies beneath the inferior surface of the cerebellum and overlies the caudal pons and rostral medulla oblongata. The two lateral ventricles communicate with each other and with the third ventricle by means of the interventricular foramina, and the third ventricle communicates with the fourth ventricle through the cerebral aqueduct. The caudal part of the fourth ventricle is continuous with the central canal of the spinal cord. In certain regions the ventricles contain invaginations of pia mater reflected over cords of ependyma, forming the choroid plexuses that are the source of cerebrospinal fluid. **cerebral v.** VENTRICULUS LATERALIS CEREBRI. **v. of cord** CANALIS CENTRALIS MEDULLAE SPINALIS. **double-inlet v.** A congenital anomaly in which both atria of the heart connect to only one ventricle. Almost always there is a second rudimentary ventricle present which is not connected to the atria. The ventricle which is connected may be right, left, or intermediate in its morphology. Also *single ventricle* (imprecise). **double-outlet right v.** A congenital anomaly in which more than half of both great arteries are connected to the right ventricle. This includes cases in which there are overriding arterial valves, but more usually both great arteries are exclusively connected to the right ventricle, and the

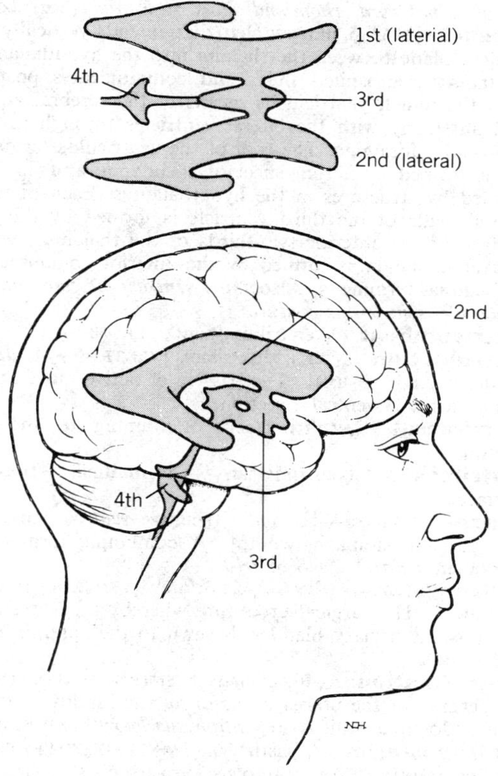


Ventricles of the brain

only exit for the left ventricle is a coexisting ventricular septal defect which may very rarely close. **fifth v.** CAVUM SEPTI PELLUCIDI. **first v. of cerebrum** VENTRICULUS LATERALIS CEREBRI. **fourth v. of cerebrum** VENTRICULUS QUARTUS CEREBRI. **Galen's v.** VENTRICULUS LARYNGIS. **v. of heart** VENTRICULUS CORDIS. **v. of larynx** VENTRICULUS LARYNGIS. **lateral v. of cerebrum** VENTRICULUS LATERALIS CEREBRI. **left v. of heart** VENTRICULUS SINISTER CORDIS. **Morgagni's v.** VENTRICULUS LARYNGIS. **optic v.** The cavity of the embryonic optic vesicle. **pineal v.** RECESSUS PINEALIS. **primitive v.** A chamber in the primitive cardiac tube extending from the atrioventricular canal to the bulboventricular sulcus. It becomes the major part of the definitive left ventricle. **right v. of heart** VENTRICULUS DEXTER CORDIS. **second v. of cerebrum** VENTRICULUS LATERALIS CEREBRI. **single v.** *Imprecise* DOUBLE-INLET VENTRICLE. **sixth v.** CAVUM PSALTERII. **terminal v. of spinal cord** VENTRICULUS TERMINALIS MEDULLAE SPINALIS. **third v. of cerebrum** VENTRICULUS TERTIUS CEREBRI. **Verga's v.** CAVUM PSALTERII.

**ventricornu** \ven′trēkôr′noo\ CORNU ANTERIUS MEDULLAE SPINALIS.

**ventricular** \ventrik′yələr\ Pertaining to a ventricle.

**ventriculi** \ventrik′yəlī\ Plural of VENTRICULUS.

**ventriculitis** \ventrik′yəlī′tis\ [*ventricul(o)-* + -ITIS] Inflammation of the cerebral ventricles.

**ventriculo-** \ventrik′yəlō-\ [L *ventriculus* (diminutive of *venter* belly) stomach, ventricle] A combining form meaning ventricle.

**ventriculoatriostomy** \-ā′trē·äs′təmē\ [VENTRICULO- + ATRIO- + -STOMY] The surgical establishment of a cerebrospinal fluid shunt from a cerebral ventricle to the right cardiac atrium via the internal jugular vein, for the relief of hydrocephalus.

**ventriculocisternostomy** \-sis′tərnäs′təmē\ [VENTRICULO- + CISTERN + *o* + -STOMY] Surgical establishment of a shunt between a ventricle and a subarachnoid cistern. **third v.** Surgical establishment of a shunt between the third ventricle and the interpeduncular cistern. Also *Stookey-Scarff shunt.*

**ventriculography** \ventrik′yəläg′rəfē\ [VENTRICULO- + -GRAPHY] Roentgenography showing the ventricles of the brain or the heart with the use of contrast medium, usually air in the brain and a radiopaque medium in the heart. **isotope v.** **1** A technique of studying the circulation of cerebrospinal fluid through the cerebral ventricles and subarachnoid space by tracing the distribution of radioactivity after injecting a labeled substance such as radioiodinated serum albumin (RISA) into the lumbar theca. **2** A technique for study of the ventricles of the heart by recording the distribution of radioactivity after injecting an appropriate radionuclide into the bloodstream.

**ventriculometry** \ventrik′yəläm′ətrē\ [VENTRICULO- + -METRY] Measurement of the volume of ventricular fluid or of the pressure within the ventricles.

**ventriculomyotomy** \-mī·ät′əmē\ The incision of a muscular hypertrophy in the aortic or pulmonary outflow tracts in order to relieve outflow obstruction.

**ventriculonector** \-nek′tər\ FASCICULUS ATRIOVENTRICULARIS.

**ventriculophasic** \-fā′zik\ Modified by ventricular contraction: applied especially to the slight alterations in atrial rhythm which may follow ventricular contraction in cases of complete atrioventricular heart block.

**ventriculoplasty** \ventrik′ylōplas′tē\ [VENTRICULO- + -PLASTY] Surgical reshaping of the ventricle of the heart.

**ventriculopuncture** \-pungk′chər\ [VENTRICULO- + PUNCTURE] Insertion of a needle or trochar into a cerebral ventricle.

**ventriculoscope** \ventrik′yəlōskōp′\ [VENTRICULO- + -SCOPE] A type of endoscope for viewing the ventricular cavities of the brain. Coagulation and biopsy of tissue in the wall of the ventricle is also made possible.

**ventriculoscopy** \ventrik′yəläs′kəpē\ Examination of the cavity of a ventricle with a ventriculoscope.

**ventriculostomy** \ventrik′yəläs′təmē\ [VENTRICULO- + -STOMY] Establishment of an opening or shunt between a cerebral ventricle and another cavity or to the exterior. **third v.** Establishment of an opening between the third ventricle and one of the surrounding subarachnoid spaces or cisterns.

**ventriculosubarachnoid** \-sub′ərak′noid\ Denoting the ventricular system of the brain along with the subarachnoid space surrounding the brain and spinal cord, within which is found the cerebrospinal fluid. The ventricular system communicates with the subarachnoid space.

**ventriculotomy** \ventrik′yəlät′əmē\ [VENTRICULO- + -TOMY] The incision of a ventricle.

**ventriculovenostomy** \-vēnäs′təmē\ [VENTRICULO- + VENO- + -STOMY] Establishment of an opening or shunt between a cerebral ventricle and a vein, such as a jugular vein.

**ventriculus** \ventrik′yələs\ [L (dim. of *venter* the belly, womb, a fetus, swelling, ventricle; see VENTER), the belly, a ventricle, the stomach] **1** A small cavity or chamber in an organ, usually filled with fluid, such as the ventricle in the brain or the right and left ventricles (lower chambers) of the heart. Also *ventricle*. **2** GASTER. **3** The midgut in the digestive tract of insects. **v. cerebri** VENTRICULUS LATERALIS CEREBRI. **v. cordis** [NA] One of the two lower chambers of the heart, namely, ventriculus dexter cordis and ventriculus sinister cordis. Also *ventricle of heart*. **v. dexter cordis** [NA] The chamber of the heart that forms most of the sternocostal surface and about half of the diaphragmatic surface of the heart. Its thick muscular walls are thinner than those of the left ventricle, from which it is separated by the interventricular septum. The rough interior is ridged by trabeculae carneae. It receives deoxygenated blood from the right atrium through the tricuspid orifice and sends the blood into the pulmonary trunk through the pulmonary orifice. Also *right ventricle of heart*. **v. laryngis** [NA] A small pouch of mucous membrane extending laterally between the vestibular and the vocal folds and upwards deep to the vestibular fold as far as the angle of the thyroid cartilage. Also *ventricle of larynx, sinus of larynx, laryngeal sinus, laryngeal sac, Galen's ventricle, Morgagni's ventricle, sinus of Morgagni*. **v. lateralis cerebri** [NA] An irregularly shaped cavity located in the inferomedial part of each of the two cerebral hemispheres, filled with cerebrospinal fluid secreted by the choroid plexuses of the lateral ventricle. Each lateral ventricle consists of a central part and frontal (anterior), temporal (inferior), and occipital (posterior) horns that extend into their respective lobes of the forebrain. The lateral ventricles develop from the embryonic central cavity of the prosencephalon, but in the adult the right and left ventricles are almost completely separated by the septum pellucidum. They do, however, communicate with each other and with the third ventricle through the interventricular foramen and, similar to the other ventricles in the brain, are lined with ependyma. Also *procoelia* (outmoded), *paracoele, paracele, cerebral ventricle, ventriculus cerebri, first ventricle of cerebrum, second ventricle of cerebrum, lateral ventricle of cerebrum*. **v. medius** VENTRICULUS TERTIUS CEREBRI. **v. quartus cerebri** [NA] A broad but shallow rhomboid-shaped space, lined with ependyma and filled with cerebrospinal fluid, situated in the hindbrain ventral to the cerebellum and dorsal to the pons and rostral medulla. The floor of the fourth ventricle, called the rhomboid fossa, is diamond-shaped, and of its four angles two are placed laterally and correspond to the lateral recesses. At its caudal angle it communicates directly with the central canal traversing the spinal cord, and at its rostral angle with the cerebral aqueduct of the midbrain. It also communicates with the subarachnoid space by way of a median (foramen of Magendie) and two lateral (foramina of Luschka) openings. Also *fourth ventricle of cerebrum*. **v. quintus** CAVUM SEPTI PELLUCIDI. **v. sinister cordis** [NA] The chamber of the heart with the thickest walls, forming the apex, the left margin, a small part of the sternocostal surface, and about half of the diaphragmatic surface of the heart. It receives oxygenated blood from the left atrium through the mitral orifice and discharges the blood into the aorta through the aortic orifice. The trabeculae carneae ridging the internal wall are more numerous than in the right ventricle, from which it is separated by the interventricular septum. Also *left ventricle of heart, aortic ventricle of heart* (outmoded). **v. terminalis medullae spinalis** [NA] A dilated saclike enlargement of the central canal in the caudal part of the conus medullaris of the spinal cord. Also *terminal ventricle of spinal cord, rhomboid sinus of Henle*. **v. tertius cerebri** [NA] A narrow cleft that extends vertically in the median plane between the thalami into the hypothalamus. It contains cerebrospinal fluid, and communicates posteriorly with the fourth ventricle by means of the cerebral aqueduct and anteriorly with the lateral ventricles through the interventricular foramina. The roof of the ventriculus tertius cerebri is formed by a thin sheet of ependyma, and its floor is formed by structures in the hypothalamus. Each of the two lateral walls of the third ventricle is formed by the medial surface of the anterior two-thirds of the thalamus, while its rostral boundary is formed by the anterior commissure and the lamina terminalis. Also *third ventricle of cerebrum, thalamocoele, ventriculus medius*.

**ventricumbent** \ven′trikum′bənt\ PRONE.

**ventriduction** \ven′triduk′shən\ [VENTRI- + L *duct(are)* to draw, lead + -ION] The passive or active movement of a body part in a ventral direction.

**ventrimesal** \ven′trimē′səl\ Pertaining to the ventrimeson.

**ventrimeson** \ventrim′əsän\ The midline of the ventral surface.

**ventro-** \ven′trə-\ [L *venter* (genitive *ventris*) belly, ventricle, paunch, stomach, womb] A combining form meaning abdomen, ventral. Also *ventri-*.

**ventrocystorrhaphy** \-sistôr′əfē\ [VENTRO- + CYSTORRHAPHY] The surgical procedure whereby a cystic structure, such as the urinary bladder, is sewn to the anterior abdominal wall.

**ventrofixation** \-fiksā′shən\ [VENTRO- + FIXATION] A suspension of the uterus by suturing the fundus to the anterior abdominal wall. Also *ventrohysteropexy, ventrosuspension*.

**ventroposterior** \-pästir′ē·ər\ ANTEROPOSTERIOR.

**ventroptosis** \ven′träptō′sis, ven′trōtō′sis\ GASTROPTOSIS.

**ventrosuspension** \-suspen′shən\ VENTROFIXATION.

**ventrotomy** \venträt′əmē\ [VENTRO- + -TOMY] VENTRAL CELIOTOMY.

**Venturi** [Giovanni Battista *Venturi*, Italian physicist, 1746–1822] **1** See under EFFECT. **2** Venturi tube. See under PRINCIPLE.

**venula** \ven′yələ\ [L (dim. of *vena* a vein), a small vein] (*pl.* venulae) [NA] One of the minute vessels that collect blood from capillaries or sinusoids and join to form veins. Also *venule, capillary vein, veinlet*. **v. macularis inferior** [NA] A venule that accompanies the branches of the inferior macular arteriole and drains the lower part of the macula retinae into the central vein of the retina. Also *inferior macular venule*. **v. macularis superior** [NA] A venule that accompanies the branches of the superior macular arteriole and drains the upper part of the macula retinae into the central vein of the retina. Also *superior macular venule*. **v. medialis retinae** [NA] A venule that drains the part of the retina situated between the optic disk and the macula and terminates in the central vein of the retina. Also *medial venule of retina*. **v. nasalis retinae inferior** [NA] The venule that accompanies the corresponding arteriole and drains the lower quadrant of the retina medial to the optic disk into the central vein of the retina. Also *inferior nasal venule of retina*. **v. nasalis retinae superior** [NA] The venule that accompanies the corresponding arteriole and drains the upper quadrant of the retina medial to the optic disk into the central vein of the retina. Also *superior nasal venule of retina*. **v. postcapillaris** VENOUS CAPILLARY. **venulae rectae renis** [NA] Minute straight vessels in the renal medulla that drain capillary plexuses around the ascending and descending limbs of Henle's loop and the collecting ducts, and end in either the arcuate or the interlobular veins. Also *straight venules of kidney, venae rectae of kidney.* **v. retinae medialis** See under VENULA MEDIALIS RETINAE. **venulae stellatae renis** [NA] Minute veins draining the most superficial parts of the renal cortex and joining to form the interlobular veins. Also *stellate venules of kidney, stellate veins of kidney, stars of Verheyen, stellulae of Verheyen* (outmoded), *stellulae verheyenii* (outmoded). **v. temporalis retinae inferior** [NA] The venule that accompanies the corresponding arteriole and drains the lower quadrant of the retina lateral to the optic disk into the central vein of the retina. Also *inferior temporal venule of retina.* **v. temporalis retinae superior** [NA] The venule that accompanies the corresponding arteriole and drains the upper quadrant of the retina lateral to the optic disk into the central vein of the retina. Also *superior temporal venule of retina.*

**venulae** \ven′yəlē\ Plural of VENULA.

**venular** \ven′yələr\ Pertaining to or involving venules. Also *venulous.*

**venule** \ven′yool\ [L *venula.* See VENULA.] VENULA. **inferior macular v.** VENULA MACULARIS INFERIOR. **inferior nasal v. of retina** VENULA NASALIS RETINAE INFERIOR. **inferior temporal v. of retina** VENULA TEMPORALIS RETINAE INFERIOR. **medial v. of retina** VENULA MEDIALIS RETINAE. **postcapillary v.'s** Small vessels through which blood flows after leaving the capillaries and before reaching the veins. It is the site of most of the leukocyte migration into inflammatory areas and is also the area of recirculation of lymphocytes from blood to lymph. **stellate v.'s of kidney** VENULAE STELLATAE RENIS. **straight v.'s of kidney** VENULAE RECTAE RENIS. **superior macular v.** VENULA MACULARIS SUPERIOR. **superior nasal v. of retina** VENULA NASALIS RETINAE SUPERIOR. **superior temporal v. of retina** VENULA TEMPORALIS RETINAE SUPERIOR.

**venulous** \ven′yələs\ VENULAR.

**verapamil** $C_{27}H_{38}N_2O_4$. 5-[(3,4-Dimethoxyphenehtyl)-methylamino]-2-(3,4-dimethoxyphenyl)-2-isoptopylvaleronitrile. An antiarrhythmic drug that interferes with calcium transport across the myocardial cell membrane. It slows impulse transmission via the A-V node and depresses spontaneous rhythmicity of the sinus node. It is used to treat superventricular tachyarrhythmias and is given orally and intravenously.

**Verbiest** [Henk *Verbiest,* Dutch neurosurgeon, born 1909] Verbiest syndrome. See under INTERMITTENT CLAUDICATION OF THE CAUDA EQUINA.

**verbigeration** \vərbij′ərā′shən\ [L *verbigeratus,* past part. of *verbigerare* (from *verb(um)* word + *i* + *-ger,* suffix from *gerere* to carry or wear) to exchange words] Stereotypy of words, phrases, or sentences, which sometimes become the only response possible for a patient to give, no matter what the stimulus. Also *catalogia.*

**verbomania** \vur′bōmā′nē·ə\ [L *verb(um)* a word + *o* + -MANIA] LOGOMANIA.

**verdoperoxidase** \vur′dōperäk′sidās\ MYELOPEROXIDASE.

**Verga** [Andrea *Verga,* Italian neurologist, 1811–1895] **1** See under GROOVE. **2** Verga's ventricle, Verga space. See under CAVUM PSALTERII.

**verge** \vurj\ Margin or edge; circumference or boundary. **anal v.** The demarcation zone between the anal canal and perianal skin.

**vergence** \vur′jəns\ [L *vergens,* pres. p. of *vergere* to turn a thing in any direction] **1** A binocular movement in which the eyes rotate in opposite directions. For example, in convergence the right eye moves to the left and the left eye moves to the right, both eyes approaching the midline. Compare DUCTION. **2** The converging or diverging direction of focused rays of light. Also *vergency.*

**Verheyen** [Philippe *Verheyen,* Flemish anatomist, 1648–1710] Stars of Verheyen, stellulae of Verheyen, stellulae verheyenii. See under VENULAE STELLATAE RENIS.

**Verhoeff** [Frederick Herman *Verhoeff,* U.S. ophthalmologist, 1874–1968] See under OPERATION, STAIN.

**verm-** \vurm-, vərm-\ VERMI-.

**vermal** \vur′məl\ VERMIAN.

**vermetoid** \vur′mətoid\ [L *verme(s),* pl. of *vermis* worm, grub + *t* + -OID] Wormlike.

**vermi-** \vur′mē-\ [L *vermis* a worm, grub] A combining form meaning worm.

**vermian** \vur′mē·ən\ **1** Pertaining to a worm or worms. **2** Denoting the vermis of the cerebellum. Also *vermal.*

**vermicidal** \vur′misī′dəl\ [*vermicid(e)* + -AL] Destructive to worms.

**vermicide** \vur′misīd\ [VERMI- + -CIDE] An agent destructive to worms, particularly the intestinal animal parasites; a helminthicide or anthelmintic.

**vermicular** \vərmik′yələr\ [*vermicul(e)* + -AR] **1** Resembling a worm in shape, appearance, or movement. Also *vermiculate, vermiculose, vermiculous.* **2** Pertaining to a wormlike anatomic structure such as the vermis of the cerebellum or the vermiform appendix.

**vermiculate** \vərmik′yələt\ VERMICULAR.

**vermicule** \vur′mikyool\ [L *vermiculus.* See VERMICULUS.] A small worm or wormlike structure. Also *vermiculus.* **traveling v.** OOKINETE.

**vermiculose** \vərmik′yəlōs\ VERMICULAR.

**vermiculous** \vərmik′yələs\ [*vermicul(e)* + -OUS] **1** VERMICULAR. **2** Infected with worms or wormy.

**vermiculus** \vərmik′yələs\ [L, dim. of *vermis* a worm, grub] (*pl.* vermiculi) VERMICULE.

**vermiform** \vur′mifôrm\ [VERMI- + -FORM] Resembling a worm in shape; vermicular.

**vermifugal** \vərmif′yəgəl\ [VERMI- + *-fug(e)* + -AL] Expelling worms; anthelmintic.

**vermifuge** \vur′mifyooj\ [VERMI- + -FUGE] An agent used to expel parasitic worms; an anthelmintic.

**vermilionectomy** \vərmil′yənek′təmē\ [*vermilion (border)* + -ECTOMY] The surgical excision of any portion of the vermilion border of the lip. Following vermilionectomy, the lip is usually resurfaced with a sliding flap contrived from the mucosa of the lip. See also LIP SHAVE.

**vermin** [Middle English, from Middle French *vermine* (from L *vermis* a worm) undesirable insects] Any animals that are regarded as pests, such as rats, lice, and bedbugs, or animals that compete with man for food, game, or territory.

**verminal** \vur′minəl\ VERMINOUS.

**vermination** \vur′minā′shən\ [VERMIN + -ATION] **1** Worm-breeding; larva production. **2** Infestation with vermin.

**verminosis** \vur′minō′sis\ [VERMIN + -OSIS] **1** Infection or infestation with worms or larvae. **2** Infestation with vermin. **3** A disease caused by the presence of worms or vermin.

**verminotic** \vur′minät′ik\ Of or relating to verminosis.

**verminous** \vur′minəs\ [VERMIN + -OUS] **1** Relating to or caused by worms or vermin. Also *verminal.* **2** Infected with worms or infested with vermin. **3** Tending to be a breeding place for vermin; filthy.

**vermis** \vur′mis\ [L (akin to *vertere* to turn, and to English *worm, writhe,* and *wriggle*) worm, grub] **1** A worm. **2** A wormlike anatomic structure, especially the vermis cerebelli. **v. cerebelli** [NA] The narrow median portion of the cerebellum that interconnects the two cerebellar hemispheres. The superior surface of the cerebellar vermis is divided by short fissures into the lingula, central lobule, culmen, declive, and folium vermis, and the inferior surface is divided into the tuber vermis, pyramis vermis, uvula vermis, and nodulus. Also *middle lobe of cerebellum, vermiform process of cerebellum, worm of cerebellum, vermiform lobe.* Adj. vermal, vermian. **inferior v.** The inferior portion of the vermis cerebelli, including, from posterior to anterior, the tuber vermis, pyramis vermis, uvula vermis, and nodulus. **superior v.** The superior portion of the vermis cerebelli, including, from anterior to posterior, the lingula, central lobule, culmen, declive, and folium vermis.

**vermix** \vur′miks\ APPENDIX VERMIFORMIS.

**vermography** \vərmäg′rəfē\ [VERM- + *o* + -GRAPHY] Roentgenography of the appendix, especially when its lumen contains a contrast medium, such as air or barium.

**vernal** [L *vernalis* (from *vern(us)* of spring, from *ver* spring, + *-alis* -AL) vernal] Of or relating to the spring season.

**Verner** [John Victor *Verner,* U.S. physician, born 1927] Verner-Morrison syndrome. See under SYNDROME.

**Vernet** [Maurice Albin *Vernet,* French physician, born 1887] Vernet syndrome. See under PARALYSIS.

**Verneuil** [Aristide Auguste Stanislas *Verneuil,* French surgeon, 1823–1895] **1** See under DISEASE. **2** Kümmell-Verneuil disease. See under KÜMMELL'S DISEASE.

**Vernier** [Pierre *Vernier,* French mathematician, 1580–1637] Vernier acuity. See under DISPLACEMENT THRESHOLD.

**vernix** \vur′niks\ [Med L, variant of *veronix* resin, varnish] **v. caseosa** Butterlike or cheesy material on the skin surface of the near-term fetus and neonate. It consists of desquamated epidermis and sebum and is washed off at the baby's first bath. Also *smegma embryonum.*

**Verocay** [José *Verocay,* Czech pathologist, 1876–1927] Verocay bodies. See under BODY.

***Veronicella leydigi*** \ver′ōnisel′ə lī′digī\ A species of slug that serves as an intermediate host of *Angiostrongylus cantonensis* in Hawaii, Tahiti, and elsewhere in the Pacific.

**verruca** \vəroo′kə\ [L, an excrescence, wart] WART. **v. acuminata** CONDYLOMA ACUMINATUM. **v. digitata** DIGITATE WART. **v. filiformis** FILIFORM WART. **v. molluSciformis** CONDYLOMA. **v. necrogenica** TUBERCULOSIS CUTIS VERRUCOSA. **v. peruviana** VERRUGA PERUANA. **v. plana** PLANE WART. **v. plantaris** PLANTAR WART. **v. seborrheica** SEBORRHEIC KERATOSIS. **v. vulgaris** COMMON WART.

**verrucae** \vəroo′sē, vəroo′kē\ Plural of VERRUCA.

**verruciform** \vəroo′sifôrm\ [*verruc(a)* + *i* + -FORM] Resembling a wart. Also *verrucoid.*

**verrucoid** \ver′ookoid\ VERRUCIFORM.

**verrucosis** \ver′ookō′sis\ [*verruc(a)* + -OSIS] The presence of large numbers of warts. **lymphostatic v.** An infectious condition of the skin of the feet as a complication of chronic lymphedema from any cause.

**verrucosity** \ver′ookäs′itē\ [*verruc(a)* + *-os(e)*[1] + -ITY] A warty protuberance.

**verrucous** \vəroo′kəs\ [*verruc(a)* + -OUS] Like or pertaining to warts; warty. Also *verrucose.*

**verruga** \vəroo′gə\ [Spanish, a wart] VERRUGA PERUANA. **v. peruana** The cutaneous lesion of the eruptive form of bartonellosis. Cherry-red hemangiomalike nodules appear on the face and limbs. Also *verruca peruviana, Peruvian wart, verruga.*

**versene** ETHYLENEDIAMINETETRAACETIC ACID.

**version** [Med L *versio* (from L *vers(us),* past part. of *vertere* to turn, turn round + *-io* -ION) a turning] **1** A binocular movement in which the eyes rotate in the same direction. For example, in *dextroversion* both eyes rotate to the right. Also *turning* (older term). **2** An obstetric maneuver utilized to change the presentation of a fetus. **abdominal v.** EXTERNAL VERSION. **bimanual v.** A combination of external and internal version to change the presentation of a fetus. Also *combined version.* **bipolar v.** Version effected by placing the hands on both the breech and vertex ends of the fetus. The operator may utilize external maneuvers alone or a combination of external and internal version. **Braxton Hicks v.** An obsolete method of bimanual manipulation to bring the fetal head into the pelvis in cases of placenta previa. **cephalic v.** Version that alters the position of a fetus from a breech to a vertex presentation. **combined v.** BIMANUAL VERSION. **external v.** Version of a fetus by maneuvers effected through pressure exerted on the maternal abdominal wall and uterus. Also *abdominal version.* Compare INTERNAL VERSION. **Hicks v.** BRAXTON HICKS VERSION. **internal v.** Transvaginal conversion of a fetus from one presentation to another by manipulation of the fetal parts through a dilated cervix. Compare EXTERNAL VERSION. **pelvic v.** Version that alters the position of a fetus from a transverse lie to a breech presentation by exerting pressure on the fetal buttocks. **podalic v.** Internal version of a fetus from a vertex to a breech presentation by pushing the head upward followed by pulling down the lower extremities into the dilated cervix. Also *Potter version.* **Potter v.** PODALIC VERSION. **spontaneous v.** The nonoperative, unassisted conversion of a fetus from one presentation to another. **Wigand's v.** WIGAND'S EXTERNAL VERSION. **Wigand's external v.** A seldom-used external version technique for converting a transverse lie to a vertex presentation. Also *Wigand's version.*

**vertebr-** \vur′təbr-\ VERTEBRO-.

**vertebra** \vur′təbrə\ [L (from *vertere* to turn, pivot) a joint, esp. of the back, a vertebra] (*pl.* vertebrae) One of a series of bony units or segments joined together by fibrocartilaginous disks to form the vertebral or spinal column. Each unit comprises a body anteriorly and a dorsal vertebral arch composed of paired pedicles and laminae and enclosing the vertebral foramen which encloses the spinal cord and its surrounding membranes. Attached to the arch are four articular processes, two transverse processes, and one spinous process. The units articulate with the ribs in the thoracic region. The bones are grouped regionally, there being seven cervical, twelve thoracic, five lumbar, five sacral, and four coccygeal vertebrae. Also *spondylus.* Adj. vertebral. **anticlinal v.** One of the lower thoracic vertebrae, usually the eleventh in humans, in which the spinous process points straight dorsally, indicating the change of direction of the spines, those above the level being inclined caudally and those below the level being directed cranially and dorsally. **butterfly v.** A sagittally cleft vertebra which appears as a butterfly-like configuration on radiographs. Also *cleft vertebra.* **cervical vertebrae** VERTEBRAE CERVICALES. **vertebrae cervicales** [NA] The upper seven vertebrae, of which the first two are named atlas and axis, constituting the cervical part of the vertebral column, which is normally curved convex forwards. The most distinctive feature is the foramen in each transverse process. Also *cervical vertebrae.* **cleft v.** BUTTERFLY VERTEBRA. **vertebrae coccygeae I–IV** [NA] The rudimentary vertebrae that fuse in the adult to form the coccyx. Also *coccygeal vertebrae, caudate vertebrae, caudal vertebrae.* **coccygeal vertebrae** VERTEBRAE

COCCYGEAE I–IV. **cranial v.** One of the metameric elements represented by modified vertebrae that is postulated to be incorporated in the bones of the skull, especially the base of the skull. **false vertebrae** Segments of the vertebral column that normally become fused into composite bones, namely, the sacral and coccygeal vertebrae, which form the sacrum and the coccyx, respectively. **vertebrae lumbales** [NA] The five large vertebrae, devoid of costal facets, that constitute the lumbar region of the vertebral column, forming the central skeletal pillar of the posterior abdominal wall, which is normally curved convex forwards.

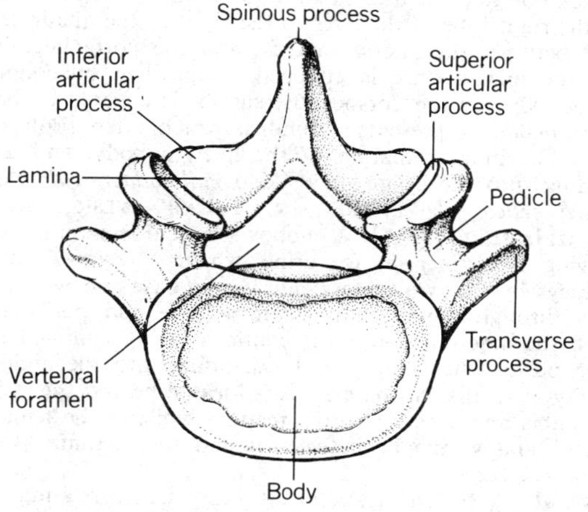


**Fifth lumbar vertebra** (top view)

Also *lumbar vertebrae.* **lumbar vertebrae** VERTEBRAE LUMBALES. **movable vertebrae** TRUE VERTEBRAE. **v. plana** The collapse and flattening of a vertebral body. It can be seen in diseases that cause bone destruction, such as eosinophilic granuloma. Also *Calvé's disease.* **primitive v.** A mass of dense mesenchymatous tissue surrounding the spinal cord formed by the fusion of two sclerotomes (right and left), and which ultimately becomes the vertebral body. **v. prominens** [NA] The seventh cervical vertebra, so named because its long spinous process makes it visible and/or palpable at the lower end of the nuchal midline. Often, however, the spinous process of the first thoracic vertebra, and occasionally that of the sixth cervical vertebra, is more prominent. Also *prominent vertebra.* **sacral vertebrae** VERTEBRAE SACRALES I–V. **vertebrae sacrales I–V** [NA] Five vertebrae situated in the posterosuperior part of the pelvis that fuse to form the os sacrum in the adult. Also *sacral vertebrae.* **sternal v.** STERNEBRA. **thoracic vertebrae** VERTEBRAE THORACICAE. **vertebrae thoracicae** [NA] The twelve vertebrae forming the thoracic region of the vertebral column, which is normally curved convex posteriorly. Their bodies and most of the transverse processes are distinguished by costal facets for articulation with the heads and tubercles of the ribs, respectively. Also *thoracic vertebrae.* **true vertebrae** The individual vertebrae in the cervical, thoracic, and lumbar regions that normally do not fuse with each other during life. Also *movable vertebrae.*

**vertebrae** \vur′təbrē\ Plural of VERTEBRA.

**vertebral** \vur′təbrəl\ [New L *vertebral(is)* concerning the vertebra] Pertaining to a vertebra or the vertebrae.

**vertebrarium** \vur′təbrer′ē·əm\ COLUMNA VERTEBRALIS.

**vertebrarterial** \vur′təbrärtir′ē·əl\ Pertaining to the vertebral artery or to a vertebra and an artery. Also *vertebroarterial.*

**Vertebrata** \vur′təbrā′tə\ [VERTEBR- + -ATA] A subphylum of the phylum Chordata, comprising fishes, amphibians, reptiles, birds, and mammals. A segmented vertebral column encloses the spinal cord and supports the body. The brain is enclosed in a skeletal cranium.

**vertebrate** \vur′təbrət\ [VERTEBR- + -ATE] **1** Any member of the subphylum Vertebrata. **2** Characterized by the presence of a vertebral column.

**vertebrectomy** \vur′təbrek′təmē\ Surgical removal of a vertebra.

**vertebro-** \vur′təbrō-\ [L *vertebra* (from *vertere* to turn) any turning joint in the body, a joint in the backbone, spinal vertebra] A combining form meaning vertebra, vertebral. Also *vertebr-.*

**vertebroarterial** \-ärtir′ē·əl\ VERTEBRARTERIAL.

**vertebrobasilar** \-bas′ilər\ **1** Pertaining to the vertebral and basilar arteries. **2** Pertaining to the vertebrae and the base of the skull.

**vertebrochondral** \-kän′drəl\ Pertaining to a vertebra and a costal cartilage.

**vertebrocostal** \-käs′təl\ Pertaining to a vertebra and a rib.

**vertebrodidymus** \-did′iməs\ [VERTEBRO- + -DIDYMUS] Conjoined twins united through the vertebral columns.

**vertebrosacral** \-sā′krəl\ Pertaining to the vertebrae and the sacrum; sacrovertebral.

**vertex** \vur′teks\ [L, also *vortex* (from *vertere* or *vortere* to revolve, turn) a whirling, whorl, hair vortex at top of head, top of head, top of anything] (*pl.* vertices) **1** An apex, especially a highest point in the vertical axis of a body or structure. **2** An osteometric point situated at the highest point in the vault of the skull in the midline with the skull orientated in the Frankfurt horizontal plane. Also *vertex cranii, vertex cranii ossei, vertex of bony cranium, mesocranium.* **v. corneae** [NA] The thin center or apex of the cornea of the eye. Also *vertex of cornea.* **v. cranii** VERTEX. **v. cranii ossei** VERTEX.

**verticalis** \vur′tikā′lis\ **1** [NA] Referring to any plane passing longitudinally through the body in the anatomical position; vertical. **2** Pertaining to the vertex.

**verticomental** \vur′tikōmen′təl\ Pertaining to the vertex and the chin: used in reference to a diameter measured in craniometry.

**vertiginous** \vərtij′inəs\ **1** Characterized by or attacked by vertigo. **2** Producing or associated with vertigo.

**vertigo** \vur′təgō, vurtī′gō\ [L (gen. *vertiginis,* from *vertere* to turn), a whirling or turning around, giddiness, dizziness] A hallucination of movement, especially of rotation, either of the subject himself or of his surroundings. It occurs in normal subjects following certain stimuli, but is particularly important as a symptom of any of various diseases affecting the vestibular apparatus. These include diseases of the ear such as Menière's disease, but also intracranial disease such as acoustic neuroma. When severe, vertigo is frequently accompanied by nausea, vomiting, or even collapse. Nystagmus is an important physical sign. Adj. vertiginous. **v. ab stomacho laeso** GASTRIC VERTIGO. **alternobaric v.** Vertigo due to sudden decrease of atmospheric pressure as when an airplane dives or when a deep sea diver comes too quickly to the surface. See also LABYRINTHINE BENDS. **apoplectic v.** Vertigo of sudden onset, particularly as a symptom of brainstem ischemia or infarction or of intracerebellar hemorrhage. *Seldom used.* **auditory v.** AURAL VERTIGO. **aural v.** Vertigo due to ear disease. Also *auditory vertigo, oticodinia* (obs.). **benign paroxysmal v. of childhood** Paroxysms of vertigo with vomiting but normal hearing in children from one to five years, in the absence of disease of the central nervous system. It is a self-limiting disorder. **benign paroxysmal positional v.** BENIGN POSITIONAL VERTIGO. **benign positional v.** Positional vertigo in cases where lesions of the central nervous system are not considered a cause. It may follow head injury, when disease of the utricle has been thought responsible. It occurs also in cases of vestibular neuronitis. Also *benign paroxysmal positional vertigo.* **central v.** Vertigo due to disease of the central nervous system. **disorientation v.** A false impression of the position of the body in space and in relation to the surroundings, as seen in some parietal lobe lesions. *Imprecise.* **epidemic v.** The epidemic form of vestibular neuronitis. **essential v.** Vertigo of undetermined cause. **gastric v.** Vertigo associated with gastric disease. *Imprecise.* Also *stomachal vertigo, vertigo ab stomacho laeso.* **height v.** A sensation of falling or faintness on looking down from a high place and sometimes also on looking up toward a height. • As this is not true vertigo this is a misleading term. **horizontal v.** Vertigo, usually positional vertigo, occurring when lying flat. **labyrinthine v.** Vertigo due to inner-ear disease as in Menière's disease. **laryngeal v.** *Incorrect* COUGH SYNCOPE. **lateral v.** A dizzy sensation experienced, usually by the occupant of a car or train, when watching the rapid passing of a series of posts, trees, etc. Also *riders' vertigo* (ambiguous). **mechanical v.** MOTION SICKNESS. **nocturnal v.** A sense of falling experienced when falling asleep. This may be due to drugs or alcohol but can occur without such factors and is of no definite pathologic significance. **objective v.** **1** Vertigo as characterized by the sensation that stationary objects are in motion. **2** Vertigo that may be appreciated by another person, not only by the patient himself, usually when there is nystagmus, unsteadiness of gait, or falling. **ocular v.** Vertigo attributed to a functional defect of the eyes. **organic v.** Vertigo due to an organic disorder of the labyrinth or central nervous system, or occurring in a healthy individual as the result of physiologic stimuli. **paralytic v.** VESTIBULAR NEURONITIS. **positional v.** Vertigo occurring when the head is moved into or maintained in a critical position, characteristically on lying down or sitting up. Also *postural vertigo.* **post-traumatic v.** Postural vertigo following concussive head injury. This is a common, self-limiting disorder. **postural v.** POSITIONAL VERTIGO. **residual v.** Mild vertigo, often evoked by change in position of the head, persisting after an acute attack of epidemic vertigo or retrobulbar neuronitis. **riders' v.** *Ambiguous* LATERAL VERTIGO. • Lateral vertigo may precipitate motion sickness **stomachal v.** GASTRIC VERTIGO. **subjective v.** Vertigo characterized by the subject's feeling that he is moving, usually rotating, rather than that external objects are in motion around him. **toxic v.** Vertigo due to the toxic effect of drugs or to metabolic disorders. **vertical v.** Vertigo characterized by a subjective sensation of movement in a vertical plane, as if rising in the air or falling into a hole. This type of vertigo may be labyrinthine in origin, but is also be noted in patients with various diseases of the nervous system, and similar sensations (pseudovertigo) may be of emotional origin. **vestibular v.** Vertigo due to disease within the vestibular labyrinth and its central connections. The vertigo of Menière's disease is an example.

**verumontanitis** \ver′oomän′tənī′tis\ [*verumontan(um)* + -ITIS] Inflammation of the colliculus seminalis (verumontanum) caused by *Neisseria gonorrhoeae* or other organisms and producing symptoms similar to prostatitis.

**verumontanum** \ver′oomәntā′nәm\ COLLICULUS SEMINALIS.

**Vesalius** [Andreas *Vesalius,* Flemish anatomist, 1514–1564] **1** Ligament of Vesalius. See under LIGAMENTUM INGUINALE. **2** Vesalian vein. See under VEIN.

**vesic-** \vesik-\ VESICO-.

**vesica** \vәsī′kә\ [L, a bladder, esp. urinary] (*pl.* vesicae) A distensible membranous sac or hollow muscular organ serving as a receptacle or reservoir for fluids; a bladder. **v. biliaris** [NA] A piriform sac that concentrates and stores bile and is situated in a fossa on the visceral surface of the right lobe of the liver to the right of the quadrate lobe and between the inferior margin and the porta hepatis. Its ventrocranial surface is attached to the liver by connective tissue, whereas the dorsocaudal surface is covered by hepatic peritoneum. It presents a fundus, which often projects beyond the inferior margin of the liver, a body, and a neck leading into the cystic duct. Also *gallbladder, gall bladder, vesica fellea, cholecystis.* **v. fellea** VESICA BILIARIS. **v. urinaria** [NA] A hollow musculomembranous sac serving as a reservoir for urine, which it receives from the kidneys by the two ureters entering its base and which it expels through the urethra. Its form, size and position vary with the amount of urine it contains, being confined to the true pelvis when empty and expanding into the abdominal cavity as it fills. In the male it is located behind the symphysis pubis and anterior to the rectum, while in the female the uterus and vagina lie between it and the rectum. Also *urinary bladder.*

**vesical** \ves′ikәl\ [*vesic(a)* + -AL] Of or relating to the urinary bladder.

**vesicant** \ves′ikәnt\ [*vesic(ate)* + *-ant,* agentive suffix] **1** Capable of inducing a serous discharge or blister. **2** A blistering agent. For defs. 1 and 2 also *vesicatory, epispastic.*

**vesicate** \ves′ikāt\ [L *vesic(a)* the bladder, a blister + -ATE] To blister or cause blistering.

**vesication** \ves′ikā′shәn\ The formation of blisters; blistering.

**vesicatory** \ves′ikәtôr′ē\ VESICANT.

**vesicle** \ves′ikl\ [L *vesicula* (dim. of *vesica* a bladder, blister) a small swelling or bubblelike formation] **1** A small sac, cyst, pouch, or follicle. **2** A fluid-filled space either within or beneath the epidermis and smaller than 1 cm in diameter; a small blister. Compare BLEB, BULLA. **3** An intracellular organelle, as, for example, a synaptic vesicle. **acoustic v.** OTOCYST. **acrosomal v.** A membrane-bound vesicle in the cytoplasm of a spermatid. It forms when proacrosomal vesicles of Golgi origin coalesce to form the acrosomal vesicle as a cap on the nucleus at the future anterior end of the cell. **air v.'s** ALVEOLI PULMONIS. **allantoic v.** A small diverticulum issuing from the posterior part of the yolk sac and which develops within the body stalk. Also *allantoic sac.* **amnioembryonic v.** AMNION. **anhidrotic v.** A characteristic lesion of miliaria. **archoplasmic v.** A small vesicle originating from the centrosome of a spermatid and which contributes to the formation of the tail of the spermatozoon. **auditory v.** OTOCYST. **Baer's v.** VESICULAR OVARIAN FOLLICLE. **blastodermic v.** BLASTOCYST. **cephalic v.'s** CEREBRAL VESICLES. **cerebral v.'s** Paired diverticula which grow out of the cranial, or telencephalic, part of the forebrain vesicle. The cavity of each cerebral vesicle forms a lateral ventricle, and its wall forms the corresponding cerebral hemisphere. Also *cephalic vesicles, telencephalic vesicles.*

**v.'s of the cerebral hemispheres** CEREBRAL VESICLES. **cervical v.** An enclosed cervical cyst or vesicle that forms, usually temporarily, at the site of the original precervical or cervical sinus. This formation may result from faulty fusion of the second arch operculum with the neck. **chorionic v.** 1 CHORION. 2 Any of the small, villus-lined pouches of the allantochorion present on the fetal aspect of an annular or other placental type. Also *vesicula serosa.* **coated v.** Any of the small invaginations of the plasma membrane that are lined with an electron dense layer and associated with the uptake of large protein molecules into the cell. It is visible only by electron microscopy. **compound v.** MULTILOCULAR VESICLE. **endocytic v.'s** Small vesicles formed from invaginations of the cytoplasmic membrane by the process of phagocytosis or pinocytosis. **lens v.** A vesicle formed from the invagination of the optic placode, precursor of the future lens. **lung v.'s** ALVEOLI PULMONIS. **Malpighi's v.'s** ALVEOLI PULMONIS. **medullary coccygeal v.** A dilated caudal expansion of the embryonic spinal cord in early embryos. **micropinocytotic v.** A small invagination of the plasma membrane that is associated with the transport of fluids into the cell. It is visible only with the aid of an electron microscope. Also *caveola.* **midbrain v.** MESENCEPHALON. **multilocular v.** A vesicle having multiple compartments, as commonly seen in eczema. Also *compound vesicle.* **Naboth's v.'s** NABOTHIAN CYSTS. **ocular v.** OPTIC VESICLE. **olfactory v.** A blind sac formed by invagination of the olfactory placode. It first forms a pit communicating externally and also with the primitive mouth. However, when the maxillary process fuses with the medial and lateral nasal processes, the olfactory pit becomes converted into a blind sac. Also *primitive nasal sac.* **optic v.** One of a pair of laterally placed, symmetrical evaginations from the prosencephalon, appearing on the 18th day of human embryonic life, even before the closure of the neural tube. It passes through a primary stage where it has the form of a spherical vesicle, then through a secondary stage where its external surface, facing the ectoderm, becomes depressed to form the optic cup. Also *ocular vesicle.* **otic v.** OTOCYST. **primitive brain v.** See under MESENCEPHALON. **pulmonary v.'s** ALVEOLI PULMONIS. **secondary cerebral v.'s** Five vesicles of the embryonic brain which are recognizable in the fifth week of gestation. The prosencephalon (forebrain) is divided into two parts, an anterior telencephalon and a posterior diencephalon. The mesencephalon (midbrain) remains unchanged while the rhombencephalon (hindbrain) is divided into an anterior metencephalon and a posterior myelencephalon. **seminal v.** VESICULA SEMINALIS. **sense v.** The saccular primordium of a sense organ, such as the optic or auditory vesicle. **synaptic v.'s** Small membrane-bound organelles, unique to nerve cells, that aggregate within the presynaptic element near the surface of the synapse. Synaptic vesicles range in diameter from 200 to 650 Å, and are believed to contain the neurotransmitter substance utilized for the transmission of the nerve impulse across the synaptic junction. With the arrival of the nerve impulse at the presynaptic terminal, the membranous walls of the vesicles appear to fuse with the presynaptic membrane, thereby allowing the substance within the vesicle to discharge into the synaptic cleft. Postsynaptic-membrane receptor molecules then combine with molecules of the transmitter to alter the ionic properties of the postsynaptic membrane, effecting the initiation of the postsynaptic potential. **telencephalic v.'s** CEREBRAL VESICLES. **umbilical v.** An extraembryonic structure, remnant of the yolk sac, attached to the umbilical cord and lined by endoderm. It retains continuity with the epithelium of the developing midgut through the vitellointestinal duct. In fishes, it results simply from the constricting off of the ventral part of the digestive tube and is full of yolk. In the amniotes, and particularly in mammals, it is formed rather differently as the result of the formation of a body stalk, and it becomes a site for hematopoiesis. Also *vitelline sac.* **Unna's v.** The teardrop vesicle filled with clear fluid which is characteristic of varicella and herpes zoster. *Obs.*

**vesico-** \ves′ikō-\ [L *vesica* bladder] A combining form meaning (1) bladder or vesica (2) vesicle. Also *vesic-*.

**vesicoabdominal** \-abdäm′ənəl\ Pertaining to the urinary bladder and either the abdominal wall or an abdominal organ.

**vesicobullous** \-bul′əs\ Marked by the presence of blisters of varying size.

**vesicocavernous** \-kav′ərnəs\ VESICULOCAVERNOUS.

**vesicocervical** \-sur′vikəl\ Pertaining to the urinary bladder and the cervix of the uterus.

**vesicoclysis** \ves′ikäk′lisis\ [VESICO- + Gk *klysis* (from *klyzein* to wash) a washing] The washing out of the urinary bladder through injections.

**vesicofixation** \-fiksā′shən\ [VESICO- + FIXATION] 1 Attachment of the uterus to the urinary bladder. 2 CYSTOPEXY.

**vesicoperineal** \-per′inē′əl\ Pertaining to the urinary bladder and the perineum, as *vesicoperineal fistula.*

**vesicopustule** \-pus′tyool\ [VESICO- + PUSTULE] A vesicle that forms a pustule.

**vesicorectostomy** \-rektäs′təmē\ [VESICO- + RECTOSTOMY] CYSTOPROCTOSTOMY.

**vesicorenal** \-rē′nəl\ Pertaining to the urinary bladder and the kidney.

**vesicosigmoid** \-sig′moid\ Pertaining to the urinary bladder and the sigmoid colon.

**vesicosigmoidostomy** \-sig′moidäs′təmē\ [VESICO- + SIGMOIDOSTOMY] Surgical creation of a connection between the urinary bladder and the sigmoid colon.

**vesicostomy** \ves′ikäs′təmē\ [VESICO- + -STOMY] CYSTOSTOMY.

**vesicotomy** \ves′ikät′əmē\ [VESICO- + -TOMY] CYSTOTOMY.

**vesicoureteral** \ves′ikōyoorē′tərəl\ URETEROVESICAL.

**vesicovaginal** \-vaj′ənəl\ Pertaining to the urinary bladder and the vagina.

**vesicul-** \vesik′yəl-\ VESICULO-.

**vesicula** \vəsik′yələ\ [L, dim. of *vesica* a bladder. See VESICLE.] (*pl.* vesiculae) A small bladder or sac; a vesicle. **vesiculae nabothi** NABOTHIAN CYSTS. **v. seminalis** [NA] One of two sacculated, tubular structures in which a single tubule is tightly folded in long loops within a capsule. It is an elongated, blunt-ended oval structure situated between the posterior surface of the bladder and the rectum and separated from its fellow by a ductus deferens which joins its excretory duct to form the ejaculatory duct on each side of the median plane in a groove at the base of the prostate. The lumen of the tube has several sacculations at irregular intervals. It produces a slightly alkaline secretion which contains vesiculase and fructose and forms part of the seminal fluid. Also *seminal vesicle, spermatocyst, gonecyst* (obs.). **v. serosa** CHORIONIC VESICLE.

**vesiculae** \vesik′yəlē\ Plural of VESICULA.

**vesicular** \vesik′yələr\ 1 Pertaining to or composed of a vesicle or vesicles. 2 Designating a soft auscultatory breath sound presumably originating in the pulmonary vesicles (alveoli pulmonis) and generally characteristic of the normal lung.

**vesiculate** \vesik′yələt\ Characterized by vesicles. Also *vesiculated.*
**vesiculation** \vesik′yəlā′shən\ [VESICUL- + -ATION] The formation of vesicles.
**vesiculectomy** \vesik′yəlek′təmē\ [VESICUL- + -ECTOMY] Excision or resection of a vesicle, especially a seminal vesicle.
**vesiculitis** \vesik′yəlī′tis\ [VESICUL- + -ITIS] **1** Inflammation of a vesicle. **2** SEMINAL VESICULITIS. **seminal v.** An inflammatory process of the seminal vesicles, usually accompanying similar processes in the prostate. Also *vesiculitis, spermatocystitis.*
**vesiculo-** \vesik′yəlō-\ [L *vesicula* (diminutive of *vesica* bladder) little bladder, vesicle] A combining form meaning vesicle. Also *vesicul-.*
**vesiculobronchial** \-brängʹkē·əl\ **1** BRONCHOVESICULAR. **2** Having both vesicular (that is, normal) and bronchial characteristics: said of auscultatory breath sounds.
**vesiculocavernous** \-kav′ərnəs\ Characterized by both vesicular and cavernous resonance: said of auscultatory breath sounds. Also *vesicocavernous.*
**vesiculography** \vesik′yəläg′rəfē\ [VESICULO- + -GRAPHY] Roentgenography of the seminal vesicle and vas deferens after their opacification by injecting a contrast medium into the ejaculatory duct or into the surgically exposed vas deferens.
**vesiculoprostatitis** \-präs′təti′tis\ PROSTATOVESICULITIS.
**vesiculotomy** \vesik′yəlät′əmē\ [VESICULO- + -TOMY] Incision of a vesicle. **seminal v.** Surgical incision of the seminal vesicles.
**Veslingius** [Johannes *Veslingius,* German anatomist and botanist, 1598–1649] Veslingius line. See under RAPHE SCROTI.
**vessel** [Old French *vaissel* (from L *vascellum* a small vase, urn, dim. of *vas* a vessel, container, utensil) a vase, vessel] A closed channel for carrying fluid; vas. **afferent v. of glomerulus** ARTERIOLA GLOMERULARIS AFFERENS. **afferent v.'s of lymph node** VASA AFFERENTIA NODI LYMPHATICI. **anastomotic v.** VAS ANASTOMOTICUM. **arterioluminal v.'s** Small unnamed branches which arise from branches of the coronary arteries in the epicardial fat of the heart and penetrate the myocardium where they form a meshwork of capillaries and sinusoids about the muscle fibers. The meshwork may drain into either the venae cardiacae minimae, or the larger cardiac veins, or directly into the ventricles through minute openings between the trabeculae. **arteriosinusoidal v.'s** Arterioluminal vessels that end in sinusoids, rather than capillaries, in the myocardium. **bile v.** Any one of the various vessels in the liver that carry bile. **blood v.** Any vessel carrying blood, namely, an artery, arteriole, capillary, venule or vein. **collateral v.** VAS COLLATERALE. **deep lymphatic v.'s** VASA LYMPHATICA PROFUNDA. **efferent v. of glomerulus** ARTERIOLA GLOMERULARIS EFFERENS. **efferent v.'s of lymph node** VASA EFFERENTIA NODI LYMPHATICI. **great v.'s** The large blood vessels entering or leaving the heart, including the aorta, pulmonary veins and trunk, superior vena cava, and inferior vena cava. **hemorrhoidal v.'s** **1** Any of the rectal veins, including venae rectales inferiores, venae rectales mediae, and vena rectalis superior. **2** Rectal veins that have become varicose. **lacteal v.'s** Central lacteals that drain the intestinal villi and conduct the chyle to the submucosal lymphatic plexus, from which the lacteals carry it to the thoracic duct. **lymphatic v.'s** VASA LYMPHATICA. **nutrient v.** ARTERIA NUTRICIA. **superficial lymphatic v.'s** VASA LYMPHATICA SUPERFICIALIA. **Warburg v.** WARBURG'S APPARATUS.
**vestibula** \vestib′yələ\ Plural of VESTIBULUM.
**vestibular** \vestib′yələr\ Pertaining to a vestibule.
**vestibule** \ves′təbyool\ [L *vestibulum* an entry court, vestibule] See under VESTIBULUM. **v. of aorta** The anterior and superior part of the left ventricle immediately below the aortic orifice, the walls of which consist mostly of fibrous tissue. Also *aortic vestibule, Sibson's vestibule, Gibson's vestibule.* **buccal v.** That part of the vestibule of the oral cavity which lies between the cheeks and the alveolar processes and teeth of the jaws. **v. of ear** VESTIBULUM. **Gibson's v.** VESTIBULE OF AORTA. **labial v.** That part of the vestibule of the oral cavity which lies between the lips and the alveolar processes and teeth of the jaws. **v. of larynx** VESTIBULUM LARYNGIS. **v. of mouth** VESTIBULUM ORIS. **nasal v.** VESTIBULUM NASI. **v. of nose** VESTIBULUM NASI. **v. of omental bursa** VESTIBULUM BURSAE OMENTALIS. **v. of oral cavity** VESTIBULUM ORIS. **Sibson's v.** VESTIBULE OF AORTA. **v. of vagina** VESTIBULUM VAGINAE. **v. of vulva** VESTIBULUM VAGINAE.
**vestibulectomy** \vestib′yəlek′təmē\ [*vestibul(e)* + -ECTOMY] LABYRINTHECTOMY.
**vestibulocerebellar** \vestib′yəlōser′əbel′ər\ Denoting the afferent vestibular fibers or impulses that course to the cerebellum from the vestibular nuclei in the brainstem, or referring more generally to the role of the cerebellum in the functioning of the vestibular system.
**vestibulocerebellum** \vestib′yəlōser′əbel′əm\ The portions of the cerebellum, i.e., the flocculus, nodulus, and uvula, involved in vestibular functions.
**vestibulocochlear** \vestib′yəlōkäk′lē·ər\ Pertaining to the vestibule and the cochlea of the internal ear.
**vestibulospinal** \vestib′yəlōspī′nəl\ Denoting the descending nerve fibers or impulses that course from the vestibular nerve or vestibular nuclei to the spinal cord, such as the vestibulospinal tract.
**vestibulotomy** \vestib′yəlät′əmē\ [*vestibul(e)* + *o* + -TOMY] Any surgical operation requiring opening the vestibule of the inner ear, as in stapedectomy.
**vestibulourethral** \vestib′yəlōyoorē′thrəl\ Pertaining to the vestibule of the vagina and the urethra.
**vestibulum** \vestib′yələm\ [L, an entrance court, porch, vestibule] (*pl.* vestibula.) **1** A small cavity or space at the entrance of a canal or leading into another cavity; a vestibule. **2** [NA] Specifically, the ovoid central portion of the bony labyrinth of the internal ear, situated behind the cochlea, in front of the semicircular canals, and medial to the tympanic cavity, with which it communicates through the fenestra vestibuli. It lodges the utriculus and the sacculus. Also *vestibule of ear, vestibulum auris.* **v. auris** VESTIBULUM. **v. bursae omentalis** [NA] The narrow portion of the omental bursa located immediately to the left of the epiploic foramen, above the first part of the duodenum and below the caudate process of the liver. It is separated from the omental bursa proper by the two gastropancreatic folds. Also *vestibule of omental bursa.* **v. laryngis** [NA] The cone-shaped part of the larynx situated between the inlet of the larynx and the level of the vestibular folds and formed anteriorly by the epiglottis, laterally by the aryepiglottic folds, and posteriorly by mucous membrane connecting the arytenoid cartilages. Also *vestibule of larynx.* **v. nasi** [NA] A small dilated recess situated immediately above and inside the external opening of the nostril and lined with skin containing vibrissae. It is bounded laterally by the ala and the major alar cartilage, medially by the medial crus of this cartilage, and superiorly by the limen nasi.

Also *vestibule of nose, nasal vestibule.* **v. oris** [NA] The part of the oral cavity that is bounded externally by the cheeks and lips and internally by the alveolar processes and teeth of the jaws. Also *vestibule of oral cavity, vestibule of mouth, external oral cavity, buccal cavity.* **v. vaginae** [NA] The cleft between the labia minora, behind the glans clitoridis, where the vaginal and external urethral orifices are situated. On its surface are the openings of the ducts of the greater and lesser vestibular glands. Also *vestibule of vagina, vestibule of vulva, vulvar canal.*

**vestige** \ves′tij\ [L *vestigium* a footprint, imprint, track, trace] An imperfectly developed or degenerate structural part in an embryo or adult organism which exhibits no obvious function. It may have had functional significance in ancestral or developing forms and could therefore be of evolutionary or phylogenetic importance. Also *vestigium.* Adj. vestigial. **caudal medullary v.** A derivative of the variably distended termination of the spinal cord in the embryo (medullary coccygeal vesicle). It may persist as a vestigial structure beneath the skin over the tip of the coccyx. **coccygeal v.** A remnant of the neural tube of the embryo situated near the tip of the coccyx. **wolffian v.'s** Derivatives of the embryonic mesonephros and its excretory duct which persist in the adult, including appendix of epididymis, efferent ductules, lobules of epididymis, paradidymis, and aberrant ductules in the male and appendices vesiculosae, epoophoron and paroophoron in the female from the mesonephros. In the male, the duct of epididymis, ductus deferens, and ejaculatory duct derive from the mesonephric duct while in the female there is the duct of epoophoron.

**vestigia** \vestij′ē·ə\ Plural of VESTIGIUM.

**vestigial** \vestij′ē·əl\ Relating to or constituting a vestige.

**vestigium** \vestij′ē·əm\ VESTIGE.

**veterinarian** \vet′ərener′ē·ən, vet′rəner′ē·ən\ A person who has graduated from an officially recognized school of veterinary medicine and who is qualified to treat animals, using medical and surgical methods. Also *veterinary surgeon (British).*

**veterinary** \vet′ərener′ē, vet′rəner′ē\ [L *veterinarius* (from *veterina* draft animals, beasts of burden, prob. from *vetus,* gen. *veteris* old) tending or treating domestic animals] Pertaining to any aspect of the study or treatment of disease in animals.

**VF** 1 vocal fremitus. 2 ventricular fibrillation. 3 visual field.

**vf** visual field.

**via** \vī′ə, vē′ä\ [L, a way, road, passage] (*pl.* viae) 1 A passage or way. 2 By way of. **viae naturales** The natural passages of the body, such as the birth canal and digestive tract. **primae viae** *Outmoded* CANALIS ALIMENTARIUS.

**viable** \vī′əbəl\ [French, from *vi(e)* (from L *vita* life) life + French *-able* -ABLE] Capable of survival: used especially of a fetus whose development permits independent life outside the uterus.

**viae** \vī′ē, vē′ē\ Plural of VIA.

**vial** [Middle English *viole, fiole,* from L *phial(a)* (from Gk *phialē* a flat, shallow bowl) a broad, shallow dish] A small bottle. Also *phial.*

**vibesate** \vī′bəsāt\ An aerosolized polyvinyl plastic adherant that serves as an occlusive topical dressing for operative wounds.

**vibex** \vī′bēks\ [L *vibex,* also *vibix* a weal] A linear subcutaneous hemorrhage.

**vibices** \vibī′sēz\ Plural of VIBEX.

**vibration** [L *vibratio* (from *vibrare* to oscillate, wave, shake, agitate) a shaking, oscillation] 1 OSCILLATION. 2 A rapid shaking or trembling. **chest wall v.** Induced vibration of the chest in physical therapy as an aid to expectoration.

**vibrator** A device for the application of mechanical vibration for therapeutic purposes. **bone conduction v.** An electromechanical transducer applied to the skin over the mastoid process of the temporal bone for transmitting sound vibrations to the internal ear via the bones of the skull, as used in bone conduction hearing aids. Also *bone vibrator.*

***Vibrio*** \vib′rē·ō\ [New L, from L *vibrare* to move quickly, agitate, shake] A genus of curved, motile, facultative, Gram-negative bacilli. Unlike Enterobacteriaceae, they are oxidase positive and have polar flagellation. Saprophytes are abundant in the environment. The main pathogen is *V. cholerae.* ***V. cholerae*** The source of a major severe epidemic diarrhea, cholera. The organism resembles Enterobacteriaceae biochemically but can grow into media too alkaline (pH 9) for most bacteria. It excretes a neuraminidase and a potent enterotoxin. The latter causes excessive fluid secretion by activating cell membrane adenyl cyclase. Also *Vibrio comma* (obs.). ***V. comma*** *Obs.* *VIBRIO CHOLERAE.* • This name was used because of the organism's shape. ***V. leonardii*** A species of bacteria that cause disease in insects. They are used in biologic control of the wax moth and the European corn borer. ***V. parahaemolyticus*** A halophilic vibrio, found in marine water and shellfish, that is a frequent cause of food poisoning, especially in Japan. It can also infect tissues through breaks in the skin. Most strains isolated from stools are $\beta$-hemolytic.

**vibrio** \vib′rē·ō\ (*pl.* vibrios, vibriones) Any microorganism of the family Vibrionaceae. **cholera v.** Any organism of the species *Vibrio cholerae.* **El Tor v.** Any of several strains of *Vibrio cholerae* that excrete a hemolysin. **noncholera v.'s** Organisms that closely resemble *Vibrio cholerae* morphologically and biochemically but differ serologically. They are found in waters and shellfish and occasionally cause diarrhea in man.

**vibriocidal** \vib′rē·ōsī′dəl\ Capable of destroying vibrios.

**vibriolysis** \vib′rē·ōlī′sis, -äl′əsis\ Lysis or destruction of vibrios.

**vibriones** \vib′rē·ō′nēz\ Plural of VIBRIO.

**vibrissae** \vībris′ē\ [New L (from *vibrissare,* variant of *vibrare* to shake, wave, trill) tactile hairs, feelers] (*sing.* vibrissa) 1 [NA] The coarse hairs in the skin lining the vestibule of the nose. 2 Large tactile hairs or bristles on the muzzle of animals, such as a cat's "whiskers," or analogous structures of certain invertebrates such as flies.

**vibromassage** \vī′brōməsäzh′\ Massage by means of a mechanical vibrating device.

***vic-*** [contraction of *vic(inal)*] A prefix used in forming chemical names to show that the two substituents named after it are attached to neighboring atoms.

**vicarious** \vīker′ē·əs\ [L *vicarius* (from *vic(e)* in place of) alternate, substitute] 1 Serving as a psychological substitute: used especially of a partial satisfaction gained by identifying in fantasy with the activities of another person. 2 Functioning at a bodily site other than the usual one, as *vicarious menstruation,* or as in the assumption of behavioral control by intact brain regions when the structures normally controlling that activity have been damaged.

**vicinal** \vī′sinəl\ [L *vicinal(is)* (from *vicin(us)* near, neighboring + *-alis* -AL) pertaining to the neighborhood] Attached to adjacent atoms within a molecule: said of two groups. Thus the two hydroxyl groups in the structure

—CHOH—CHOH— are vicinal, and such a structure is oxidized by periodate.

**vicine** \vī′sin\ $C_{10}H_{16}N_4O_7$. A crystalline glycoside isolated from seeds of vetches (genus *Vicia*) which yields glucose and a pyrimidine on hydrolysis.

**Vicq d'Azyr** [Felix *Vicq d'Azyr*, French anatomist, 1748–1794] **1** Bundle of Vicq d'Azyr, fasciculus of Vicq d'Azyr, tract of Vicq d'Azyr. See under FASCICULUS MAMILLOTHALAMICUS. **2** Body of Vicq d'Azyr. See under SUBSTANTIA NIGRA. **3** See under BAND.

**Vidal** [Jean Baptiste Emile *Vidal*, French dermatologist, 1825–1893] Vidal's disease. See under LICHEN SIMPLEX.

**vidarabine** $C_{10}H_{13}N_5O_4{\cdot}H_2O$. 9-β-D-Arabinofuranosyl-9*H*-purine-6-amine monohydrate. An antiviral agent that is a purine analogue which inhibits DNA synthesis. It is used topically in the treatment of herpes keratitis and parenterally for treatment of herpes simplex encephalitis. Also *adenine arabinoside, ara-A.*

**videognosis** \vid′ē·ägnō′sis\ [*video-*, combining form from L *videre* to see + *(dia)gnosis*] A diagnosis based on the study of roentgenographic images transmitted by television techniques.

**Vieth** [Gerhard Ulrich Anton *Vieth*, German mathematician, 1763–1836] Vieth-Müller horopter. See under HOROPTER.

**Vieussens** [Raymond de *Vieussens*, French anatomist, 1641–1715] **1** Ansa of Vieussens, loop of Vieussens, Vieussens annulus. See under ANSA SUBCLAVIA. **2** Valve of Vieussens. See under VELUM MEDULLARE CRANIALE. **3** See under VALVE, ORIFICE. **4** Opening of Vieussens. See under ANTERIOR OPENING OF AQUEDUCT OF SYLVIUS. **5** Pores of Vieussens. See under FORAMINA VENARUM MINIMARUM CORDIS. **6** Isthmus of Vieussens, limbus of Vieussens, Vieussens annulus, ring of Vieussens. See under LIMBUS FOSSAE OVALIS. **7** Veins of Vieussens. See under VENAE CARDIACAE ANTERIORES.

**view / apical lordotic v.** A roentgenographic view of the chest to project anterior structures relatively superiorly and posterior structures inferiorly, used especially to project the lung apices clear of the scapulas and ribs, and also for better demonstration of abnormalities of the middle lobe on the right side and the lingula on the left side. **coned-down v.** A technique of roentgenography in which the area radiographed is limited by the use of a metal tube collimator at the x-ray tube, to provide a roentgenogram with improved detail. **Waters v.** WATERS PROJECTION.

**vigilambulism** \vij′ilam′byəlizm\ [L *vigil* awake + *ambul(are)* to walk + -ISM] Ambulatory automatism in a patient who appears to be asleep but who cannot be aroused, possibly due to nocturnal temporal lobe epilepsy. Also *vigil ambulatory automatism.*

**vigor** [L, life, activity] Energy, strength, or drive, as that expressive of robust health or active growth.

**villi** \vil′ī\ Plural of VILLUS.

**villonodular** \vil′ōnäd′yələr\ Marked by villi and nodule formation, as in forms of proliferative synovitis.

**villose** \vil′ōs\ Covered with villi.

**villositis** \vil′ōsī′tis\ [L *villos(us)* hairy, shaggy + -ITIS] Inflammation of the placental villi.

**villosity** \viläs′itē\ **1** The state or property of being villose. **2** A villus or a group of villi.

**villous** \vil′əs\ **1** Pertaining to or characterized by villi. **2** Covered with villi; villose.

**villus** \vil′əs\ [L (akin to *vellus* wool, fleece; see VELLUS) shaggy hair] (*pl.* villi) A small fingerlike or leaflike process projecting from a surface, usually of a membrane, with a free tip at the opposite end. **amniotic v.** An irregular, flat, opaque area on the amnion of the placenta, usually noted near the insertion of the umbilical cord. **anchoring villi** Chorionic villi which project deep into the uterine mucosa (decidua basalis). They were once considered to anchor the placenta. **arachnoid villi** GRANULATIONES ARACHNOIDEALES. **villi of choroid plexus** The folds of the choroid plexuses that are formed by the invagination of pia mater into the ventricles. *Imprecise.* **chorionic villi** Cylindrical evaginations branching from the chorion, making direct contact with the maternal blood, and by means of their connective tissue-vascular layers carrying out a physiologic exchange between mother and fetus. They represent the differentiated, functional part of the placenta, and by way of their epithelial (trophoblast) covering, they perform various metabolic and endocrine functions. In human pregnancy they produce and metabolize both steroid hormones and chorionic gonadotrophin. **floating v.** A villus with its tip floating free in the intervillous space of the human placenta. **free v.** An unattached chorionic villus which floats freely in the intervillous space. **villi intestinales** [NA] Fingerlike or leaflike vascular processes projecting from the mucous membrane of the small intestine, being numerous and large in the duodenum and jejunum but fewer and smaller in the ileum. They increase the surface area of the mucosa and have a core of lamina propria covered by epithelium, but the muscularis mucosae and submucosa do not project into them. The central core of each process contains a blind-ending lymph capillary or central lacteal containing absorbed fat after a meal, and a vascular capillary network draining into a vein at the base of the villus. Also *intestinal villi, villi of small intestine.* **labial villi** PARS VILLOSA. **lingual villi** PAPILLAE FILIFORMES. **villi pleurales** Scattered microvilli situated on the free surface of the pleura, especially in the costomediastinal recess. Also *pleural villi.* **primary v.** The first stage in the development of a placental villus by an outgrowth of syncytiotrophoblast towards the decidua basalis. **secondary v.** A primary placental villus which has gained a core of cytotrophoblast and even some mesoderm, but which is not yet vascularized. **villi of small intestine** VILLI INTESTINALES. **synovial villi** Villi projecting from the synovium into the joint cavity. Also *synovial tufts, synovial glands, mucilaginous glands.* **tertiary v.** A secondary placental villus which has undergone vascularization during the fourth week of human pregnancy and is taking part in the extraembryonic circulation. **zonary villi** Villi restricted to the zonary or annular part of the chorion as seen in the Carnivora.

**villusectomy** \vil′əsek′təmē\ SYNOVECTOMY.

**vinbarbital sodium** $C_{11}H_{15}N_2NaO_3$. 5-Ethyl-5-(1-methyl-1-butenyl)-2,4,6-(1*H*,3*H*,5*H*)-pyrimidinetrione sodium salt. An intermediate acting barbiturate used as a mild hypnotic and for preoperative and preanesthetic sedation. It can be given orally, rectally, or intravenously.

**vinblastine** \vinblas′tēn\ A vinca alkaloid which binds with unpolymerized tubulin, preventing the formation of cytoplasmic microtubules. Also *vincaleukoblastine.*

**vinblastine sulfate** $C_{45}H_{58}N_4O_9{\cdot}H_2SO_4$. An antineoplastic agent used in the treatment of Hodgkin's disease and other lymphomas, usually in association with other drugs. It is given intravenously.

**vincaleukoblastine** \ving′kəloo′kəblas′tēn\ VINBLASTINE.

**Vincent** [Henri *Vincent*, French physician, 1862–1950] **1** Vincent stomatitis, Vincent's disease. See under NECROTIZING ULCERATIVE GINGIVITIS. **2** See under MIXTURE.

**3** Vincent's disease. See under ANGINA. **4** Vincent's bacillus. See under *FUSOBACTERIUM FUSIFORMIS.*

**vincristine** \vinkris′tēn\ $C_{46}H_{56}N_4O_{10}$). An alkaloid obtained from *Vinca rosea,* Madagascar periwinkle, that possesses antineoplastic properties.

**vincristine sulfate** $C_{46}H_{56}N_4O_{10}\cdot H_2SO_4$. The sulfate salt of vincristine given intravenously as an antineoplastic agent for the treatment of leukemia.

**vincula** \ving′kyələ\ Plural of VINCULUM.

**vinculum** \ving′kyələm\ [L (from *vincire* to bind, fetter), a band, bond, chain, fetter] (*pl.* vincula) A slender connecting tendinous band or fold. **v. breve** [NA] The short variety of vincula tendinum, of which there are two bands in each finger, triangular in shape and attached to the posterior surfaces of the flexor tendons near their insertions. One attaches the tendon of flexor digitorum superficialis to the front of the proximal interphalangeal joint and adjacent proximal phalanx, while the second attaches the tendon of flexor digitorum profundus to the front of the distal interphalangeal joint and adjacent middle phalanx. **vincula lingulae cerebelli** Vincula of the cerebellar lingula. A small lateral projection of the lingula of the cerebellar vermis lying on the superior (anterior) medullary velum. Also *frenulum lingulae cerebelli.* **v. longum** [NA] The long variety of vincula tendinum; two long, threadlike bands connecting each side of the superficial flexor tendon to the synovial sheath at the lateral borders of the proximal end of the proximal phalanx, while one band attaches the tendon of the flexor digitorum profundus to the posterior part of the synovial sheath at the distal end of the proximal phalanx, often blending with the vinculum breve there. **vincula tendinum** Small bands of synovial membrane attached to flexor tendons of the digits, namely, vincula tendinum digitorum manus and vincula tendinum digitorum pedis. See also VINCULUM LONGUM, VINCULUM BREVE. **vincula tendinum digitorum manus** [NA] Small threadlike bands of synovial membrane connecting the tendons of the flexor digitorum superficialis and flexor digitorum profundus muscles to the posterior walls of their synovial sheaths opposite the interphalangeal joints and phalanges of the fingers and conveying blood vessels to the tendons. They are cordlike representatives of mesotendons. There are two varieties, namely, vinculum breve and vinculum longum. Also *vincula of tendons of fingers, vaginal ligaments of fingers.* **vincula tendinum digitorum pedis** [NA] Small threadlike bands of synovial membrane connecting the tendons of the flexor digitorum longus and flexor digitorum brevis muscles to the dorsal walls of their synovial sheaths opposite the interphalangeal joints and phalanges of the toes, and conveying blood vessels to the tendons. They are cordlike representatives of mesotendons and are similar to those found in the fingers. Also *vincula of tendons of toes.*

**Vineberg** [Arthur *Vineberg,* Canadian heart surgeon, born 1903] See under OPERATION.

**vinegar** [French *vinaigre* (from *vin* wine, from L *vinum* wine + French *aigre* sharp, from L *acer* sharp) vinegar] A solution of dilute impure acetic acid resulting from fermentation of wine or cider.

**Vinson** [Porter Paisley *Vinson,* U.S. surgeon, 1890–1959] Vinson syndrome. See under PLUMMER-VINSON SYNDROME.

**vinyl** \vī′nəl\ [L *vin(um)* wine + -YL] $CH_2{=}CH{-}$. Ethenyl, the group formed by removing a hydrogen atom from ethylene. Vinyl groups occur in heme, for example.

**vinyl ether** $CH_2{=}CH{-}O{-}CH{=}CH_2$. A liquid anesthetic utilized in its vapor state. It is no longer used. Also *divinyl ether.*

**viocid** \vī′ōsid\ GENTIAN VIOLET.

**violaceous** \vī′əlā′shəs\ Violet or purplish in color, as a skin discoloration.

**violation** [L *violatio* (from *violare* to injure, violate, akin to *vis* force) violation, sexual violation] See under RAPE. • In forensic medicine, *violation* usually connotes unforced, nonviolent rape of the type perpetrated by fraud, deception, threat, or impairment of the victim's senses.

**violescent** \vī′əles′ənt\ Of a color suggesting violet.

**violet** **1** A bluish purple color. **2** A substance, usually a stain or dye, that is violet in appearance, or that produces a cytochemical reaction resulting in violet staining. For chemical names including *violet,* see under the chemical name. **crystal v.** A synthetic basic dye that is a component of methyl violet. It can be used as a nuclear, amyloid, or bacterial stain. Also *violet G, hexamethyl violet.* **v. G** CRYSTAL VIOLET. **gentian v.** An ill-defined mixture of crystal violet and methyl violet. It is no longer recognized as a certified stain by the Biological Stain Commission. Also *viocid, gentiavern.* **neutral v.** A synthetic, weakly basic dye that is similar to neutral red but, due to its greater molecular weight, appears violet instead of red. **Paris v.** METHYL VIOLET. **visual v.** IODOPSIN.

**viomycin** \vī′əmī′sin\ $C_{25}H_{43}N_{13}O_{10}$. A polypeptide antibiotic produced by *Streptomyces* species including *S. puniceus* and *S. floridae* and used for cases of tuberculosis that are resistant to the drugs of choice.

**viosterol** \vī′äs′tərôl\ ERGOCALCIFEROL.

**VIP** vasoactive intestinal polypeptide.

**viper** \vī′pər\ [L *vipera* (prob. for *vivipara* or *vivipera* live-bearing; see VIVIPAROUS) an adder, viper] Any venomous snake of the family Viperidae. • The probable origin of the name is supported by the ancient Romans' accurate observation of (ovo)viviparous reproduction in these snakes. **Gaboon v.** A large-fanged, heavy-bodied venomous snake of the species *Bitis gabonica,* found in West Africa. **pit v.** Any snake of the subfamily Crotalinae. It has characteristic heat-sensitive depressions above the nostrils. **Russell's v.** A highly venomous snake of the species *Vipera russellii,* found in central and southern Asia. Also *ticpolonga.*

**Viperidae** \vīper′idē\ [L *viper(a)* a viper + -IDAE] A large and varied family of venomous snakes, divided into two subfamilies: Viperinae, the true vipers, and Crotalinae, the pit vipers. They are characterized by elongated hollow fangs attached to the front of the upper jaw. Also *Solenoglypha.*

**Viperinae** \vīper′inē\ A subfamily of the family Viperidae; the true vipers. They are characteristically short and thick-bodied and lack heat-sensitive pits. They occur only in the Old World.

**viprynium embonate** PYRVINIUM PAMOATE.

**viraemia** \vīrē′mē·ə\ *Brit.* VIREMIA.

**viral** \vī′rəl\ Of or pertaining to viruses or caused by a virus.

**Virchow** [Rudolf Ludwig Karl *Virchow,* German pathologist, 1821–1902] **1** Virchow's disease. See under LEONTIASIS OSSIUM. **2** Virchow's corpuscles, Virchow cells. See under CORNEAL CORPUSCLES. **3** Virchow's granulations. See under GRANULATION. **4** See under LAW, LINE. **5** Virchow-Hassall body. See under HASSALL'S CORPUSCLE. **6** Virchowian leprosy. See under LEPROMATOUS LEPROSY. **7** Virchow's gland, Virchow's node. See under SENTINEL NODE. **8** Virchow cells. See under LEPRA CELLS. **9** Virchow-Robin space. See under PERIVASCULAR SPACE.

**viremia** \vīrē′mē·ə\ [*vir(us)* + -EMIA] The presence of a virus or viruses in the bloodstream. Also *virusemia.*

**virgin** [L *virgo* (gen. *virginis*) a maiden] A person who has never had sexual intercourse.

**viricidal** \vī′risī′dəl\ VIRUCIDAL.

**viricide** \vī′risīd\ VIRUCIDE.

**virile** \vir′əl\ [L *virilis* (from *vir* a man) pertaining to a man, male] **1** Of or relating to the male sex. **2** Displaying masculine characteristics.

**virilia** \viril′ē·ə\ ORGANA GENITALIA MASCULINA.

**virilism** \vir′əlizm\ [*viril(e)* + -ISM] **1** The presence of male secondary sex characters in the female, as from congenital adrenocortical hyperplasia or from ovarian tumors. The condition may be marked by hirsutism, recession of the frontal hair line, masculine body habitus, deepening of the voice, sebaceous gland stimulation with acne, and enlargement of the clitoris. **2** MASCULINITY. **adrenal v.** Virilism caused by excessive or untimely secretion of adrenocortical androgenic steroid hormones associated with hyperplasia, adenoma, or carcinoma of the adrenal cortex in adults or children. Girls become masculinized in varying degrees, whereas boys evince development of male secondary sex characters, but without enlargement of the testes.

**virility** \vəril′itē\ The possession of features that are characteristic of the male sex.

**virilization** \vir′ilīzā′shən\ [*viril(e)* + *-iz(e)* + -ATION] The induction or development of male secondary sex characters, especially in the female as a result of the presence of androgenic hormones. Also *masculinization.*

**virilize** \vir′ilīz\ [*viril(e)* + -IZE] To induce the development in the female of male secondary sex characters. Also *masculinize.*

**virilizing** \vir′ilī′zing\ Inducing virilism, as an ovarian androgen-secreting tumor.

**virion** \vir′ē·än, vī′rē·än\ [*vir(us)* + *i* + -ON] A structurally complete virus. Also *viral particle.*

**virocyte** \vī′rəsīt\ ATYPICAL LYMPHOCYTE.

**virogene** \vī′rəjēn\ The complete genome of a tumor virus.

**viroid** \vī′roid\ [*vir(us)* + -OID] An infectious agent consisting solely of nucleic acid without any capsid structure or virus particles. The prototype viroid, or pathogenic RNA, is potato spindle tuber viroid. Its molecular weight is about 130 000. Viroids usually reside in the nucleus of an infected cell, where they function as abnormal regulatory molecules, although they do not code for specific proteins. Viroid replication apparently involves reliance on the host cell's enzyme system. A helper virus is not required. About a dozen different viroids have been identified since 1971, each of which causes a particular disease of a higher plant. Compare PRION.

**virologist** \vīräl′əjist, vir-\ An expert in the field of virology.

**virology** \vīräl′əjē, vir-\ [*vir(us)* + *o* + -LOGY ] The branch of microbiology which deals with viruses and the diseases that they cause.

**viropexis** \vī′rəpek′sis\ [*vir(us)* + *o* + Gk *pēxis* a fixing, a making fast] Attachment of virus to the membrane of an animal cell and penetration by phagocytosis.

**virostatic** \vī′rəstat′ik\ VIRUSTATIC.

**virucidal** \vī′rəsī′dəl\ Capable of destroying a virus. Also *viricidal.*

**virucide** \vī′rəsīd\ [*viru(s)* + -CIDE] A material that inactivates a virus on direct contact. Also *viricide.*

**virulence** \vir′yələns\ The pathogenicity or disease-producing capacity of any infectious agent.

**virulent** \vir′yələnt\ Characterized by a relatively high degree of virulence.

**viruria** \vīroo′rē·ə\ [*vir(us)* + -URIA] The presence of virus in the urine, as cytomegalovirus or mumps virus, usually but not necessarily associated with active viral infection.

# virus

**virus** [L (akin to Sanskrit *visha* poison and Gk *ios* poison, esp. of serpents), a slimy or poisonous liquid, poison, venom] **1** Any of a number of small, obligatory intracellular parasites with a single type of nucleic acid, either DNA or RNA, and no cell wall. The nucleic acid is enclosed in a structure called a capsid, which is composed of repeating protein subunits called capsomeres, with or without a lipid envelope. The complete infectious virus particle, called a virion, lacks ribosomes or any means of generating adenosine triphosphate and consequently must rely on the metabolism of the cell it infects. Viruses are morphologically heterogeneous, occurring as spherical, filamentous, polyhedral, or pleomorphic particles. They are classified by the host infected (animal, plant, or protist), the type of nucleic acid, the symmetry of the capsid, and the presence or absence of an envelope.

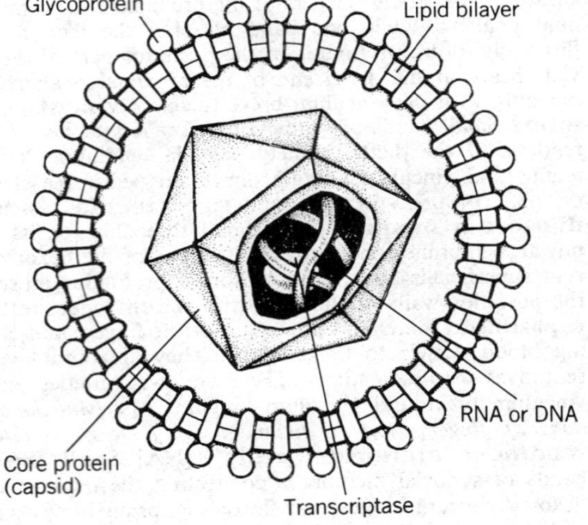


**Virus** (schematic)

**2** Any contagium or infective agent, especially one that is not identifiable as a bacterium or other full-fledged organism. An outmoded usage. See also FILTERABLE VIRUS. **acute laryngotracheobronchitis v.** Parainfluenza virus, type 2. **adeno-associated v.** Any of a group of four defective parvoviruses which replicate in the nucleus of cells that are also infected with certain adenoviruses which are serologically and chemically unrelated. Abbr. AAV **Amapari v.** A virus from Brazil in the Tacaribe group of arenaviruses. **animal v.** Any virus that infects animals. **Apeú v.** A virus of the C group of the Bunyaviridae family which is transmitted by culicine mosquitos in Brazil. Vertebrate hosts include monkeys and rodents. Infection in humans is associated with malaise, headache, generalized pain, and CNS pleocytosis. **Apoi v.** A flavivirus which was isolated from trapped rodents at the foothills of Mt. Apoi, Hokkaido, Japan. Human disease is characterized by fever, headache, stiff neck, prostration, myalgias, arthralgias, encephalitis, and paralysis. **arbor v.** ARBOVIRUS. **Argentinian hemorrhagic fever v.** JUNÍN VIRUS. **arthropod-borne v.** A virus transmitted by an arthropod vector, such as a mosquito or a tick. See also ARBOVIRUS. **attenuated v.** A virus which has lost its virulence and ability to cause disease. Attenuation is often accomplished by passing a virus through different host tissues. Other techniques, including cold adaptation, generation of temperature-sensitive mutants, and multiple passage through a single host tissue, also result in attenuation. **Australian X disease v.** MURRAY VALLEY ENCEPHALITIS VIRUS. **avian sarcoma v.** ROUS SARCOMA VIRUS. **B v.** See under HERPES B VIRUS. **bacterial v.** A virus that infects bacteria; a bacteriophage. **Bakau v.** A virus of the Bakau group of the Bunyaviridae family isolated from mosquitoes in Malaya and in Pakistan. Although serologic evidence of infection is observed, no known human disease is reported though mice die when experimentally inoculated with the virus. **Bangui v.** An unclassified virus which infects humans in central Africa and produces a syndrome characterized by fever, malaise, headache, arthralgia, and rash. **Banzi v.** A flavivirus which is transmitted by *Culex* and *Mansonia* mosquitoes in southeastern and southern Africa, Zimbabwe, Mozambique, and Kenya. Human disease is characterized by malaise, headache, and other local and generalized pain. **Batai v.** A virus in the Bunyamwera group of the Bunyaviridae family, which is transmitted by anopheles mosquitoes in Czechoslovakia, Austria, and Yugoslavia. Human infection is characterized by fever, malaise, headache, and local and generalized pain. **bat salivary gland v.** Any of various flaviviruses recovered from the salivary glands of bats. Laboratory-acquired human infections with at least one such virus have produced fever, headache, myalgia, and, in some cases, central nervous system involvement. **Bhanja v.** A virus of the Bunyaviridae family first isolated from the ticks removed from a paralyzed goat in Bhanjanagar, India. The reported human disease is a febrile illness. The geographic distribution includes India, Nigeria, Cameroon, Senegal, Italy, and Yugoslavia. The virus has been isolated from humans, cattle, sheep, and ground rodents. **Bimiti v.** A bunyavirus belonging to the Guama group, isolated in Trinidad. **BK v.** A polyomavirus which was isolated from the urine of a patient after renal transplantation. Despite widespread serological evidence of BK infection, no human disease has been identified. **Bolivian hemorrhagic fever v.** MACHUPO VIRUS. **Brunhilde v.** The prototype strain of poliovirus type 1. **Bunyamwera v.** An RNA virus belonging to the *Bunyavirus* genus of the Bunyaviridae family. It is the prototype for the Bunyamwera group viruses. It is transmitted by culicine mosquitoes and is distributed in southeastern and western Africa. It produces a febrile systemic disease with a rash in humans. **Bussuquara v.** A flavivirus (group B arbovirus of the family Togaviridae) that is transmitted by culicine mosquitoes. Monkeys and rodents are the suspected reservoirs. It is distributed in Brazil, Colombia, and Panama. **Bwamba v.** A bunyavirus transmitted by *Anopheles gambiae* in parts of central Africa. It is the cause of Bwamba fever. **Cache Valley v.** A bunyavirus belonging to the Bunyamwera group, recovered from mosquitoes in Trinidad. It has not been associated with human disease. • The term is named after *Cache Valley*, Utah. **California encephalitis v.** A virus in the California group of the Bunyaviridae family and *Bunyavirus* genus originally isolated in California from *Aedes* mosquitoes. It causes fever, meningitis, and encephalitis in humans. The virus normally causes zoonoses in ground squirrels, and humans are infected only if bitten by an infected mosquito vector. **California myxoma v.** A leporipoxvirus, closely related serologically to Shope fibroma virus, that produces fibromas in its natural host in California, the bush rabbit, *Sylvilagus bachmani.* The natural vector is *Anopheles freeborni.* **Calovo v.** A bunyavirus of the Bunyamwera group. It is transmitted by *Anopheles maculipennis* mosquitoes and is distributed in Czechoslovakia, Austria, and Yugoslavia. It produces fever, malaise, headache, and localized and generalized pain in humans. **Candiru v.** A virus belonging to the phlebotomus fever group of the Bunyaviridae, found in Brazil. It produces fever, malaise, headache, and localized and generalized pain in humans. **canine distemper v.** A paramyxovirus that causes canine distemper. Also *distemper virus.* **Caraparu v.** A bunyavirus that is prevalent in Brazil, Suriname, French Guiana, Trinidad, and Panama. It is transmitted by culicine mosquitoes, and monkeys and rodents serve as reservoirs. In humans it produces fever, headache, malaise, and localized and generalized pain. **Catu v.** A bunyavirus belonging to the Guama group and found in Brazil, French Guiana, and Trinidad. It is transmitted by culicine and anopheline mosquitoes, with monkeys, rodents, and marsupials serving as reservoirs. In humans it produces fever, malaise, headache, and localized and generalized pain. **CCA v.** RESPIRATORY SYNCYTIAL VIRUS. • The initials stand for *chimpanzee coryza agent.* **CELO v.** CELOVIRUS. **central European tick-borne encephalitis v.** A flavivirus that is a causal agent of an encephalitis in central Europe which is clinically similar to Russian spring-summer encephalitis. The tick *Ixodes ricinus* is considered the chief vector but other ixodid ticks are also involved. A wide variety of mammals and several birds have demonstrated antibodies to this virus. Human infection appears to be associated with infected milk. The virus develops rapidly in mammary glands and is active for several days at low temperatures in raw milk and uncooked milk products. **Chagres v.** A virus found in Panama belonging to the phlebotomus fever group of the Bunyaviridae family, transmitted by culicine mosquitoes and *Lutzomyia* sandflies. In humans it produces fever, malaise, headache, and localized and generalized pain. • The term is named after the Chagres River, Panama. **Chandipura v.** A rhabdovirus belonging to the vesicular stomatitis group of the *Vesiculovirus* genus. It is transmitted by sandflies (*Phlebotomus* species). Domestic animals, marsupials, and small rodents serve as reservoirs. It is prevalent in India and Nigeria. Human infection produces fever, malaise, headache, and localized and generalized pain. **Changuinola v.** A reovirus in the *Orbivirus* genus which causes a zoonosis among arboreal mammals in Panama. Infection in humans is associated with fever, headache, malaise, arthralgia, and rash. **chicken embryo lethal orphan v.** See under CELOVIRUS. **chikungunya v.** An alphavirus (group A arbovirus) that is transmitted by culicine mosquitoes. Wild birds, bats, and domestic animals serve as reservoirs. It is distributed in the southeastern, central, and western parts of Africa, and in India, Thailand, and Malaysia. In humans it produces fever, headache, malaise, arthralgia, and rash. **Coe v.** A coxsackievirus that causes acute upper respiratory illness in humans. It has caused epidemic disease in military populations. **Colorado tick fever v.** The orbivirus that causes Colorado tick fever. Also *CTF virus.* **common cold v.'es** Viruses which infect the human respiratory tract and result in the common cold. They include rhinoviruses, coronaviruses, adenoviruses, parainfluenza viruses, influenza viruses, and other viruses of diverse families and genera. **Congo v.** A virus prevalent in Nigeria, Zaire, and Uganda that belongs to the Crimean-Congo hemorrhagic fever group of the Bunyaviridae. It is transmitted by tick members of the genus *Hyalomma* and the species *Amblyomma variegatum* and *Boophilus decoloratus*. Cattle serve as a reservoir. **contagious pustular dermatitis v.** ORF VIRUS. **cowpox v.** A poxvirus that infects cattle, causing cowpox. It is presumably what was originally used for antismallpox vaccination and in this role became transformed, as a result of repeated human-to-human vaccination, into vaccinia virus. Also *poxvirus bovis*. **Coxsackie v.** COXSACKIEVIRUS. **Crimean-Congo hemorrhagic fever v.** Any virus of the Crimean-Congo hemorrhagic fever group in the Bunyaviridae family. These viruses cause zoonoses among cattle and small mammals in the Soviet Union, Bulgaria, Pakistan, Nigeria, Zaire, and Uganda, and are transmitted by ticks of the genera *Hyalomma, Amblyomma,* and *Boophilus*. See also CRIMEAN HEMORRHAGIC FEVER VIRUS, CONGO VIRUS. **Crimean hemorrhagic fever v.** A virus of the Crimean-Congo hemorrhagic fever group in the Bunyaviridae family, prevalent in the Soviet Union, Bulgaria, and Pakistan. It is transmitted by *Hyalomma* sp. and *Boophilus microplus* ticks, with small mammals and cattle serving as reservoirs. In humans it produces Crimean hemorrhagic fever. **CTF v.** COLORADO TICK FEVER VIRUS. **C-type v.** See under ONCOVIRUS. **defective v.** A virus which is incomplete in that it does not contain all of the nucleic acid and protein components which are necessary for viral replication. Often defective virions consist of empty capsids or capsid with amounts of nucleic acid insufficient for replication. **dengue v.** A flavivirus transmitted by *Aedes* mosquitoes, especially *A. aegypti,* and the cause of dengue. There are four serological types. Also *dengue hemorrhagic fever virus*. **distemper v.** CANINE DISTEMPER VIRUS. **DNA v.'es** Viruses in which the genome consists of deoxyribonucleic acid. Animal DNA viruses belong to the families Parvoviridae, Papovaviridae, Adenoviridae, Herpetoviridae, and Poxviridae. **Dugbe v.** A virus in the Nairobi sheep disease group of the Bunyaviridae family which causes zoonoses in cattle in Nigeria and the Central African Republic. It is transmitted by ticks of the *Amblyomma* genus. Infection in humans is characterized by fever, malaise, headache, and local and generalized pain. **Duvenhaga v.** A rhabdovirus related to human rabies virus which was isolated from the brain of a man bitten by a rat in South Africa. **eastern equine encephalitis v.** An alphavirus that causes eastern equine encephalomyelitis in horses and humans, primarily in eastern North America. It is transmitted by mosquitoes, chiefly by *Culiseta* and *Aëdes* species. The principal reservoir hosts are probably birds. Also *EEE virus*. **EB v.** EPSTEIN-BARR VIRUS. **Ebola v.** A pleomorphic, membrane-bound RNA virus from Sudan and Zaire. It is thought to form a new family of viruses with Marburg virus. Infection in humans occurs by person-to-person spread, probably via contact with blood, and results in fever, malaise, headache, myalgia, a maculopapular rash, hemorrhages, disseminated intravascular coagulation, and high mortality. **ECBO v.** ECBOVIRUS. **ECHO v.** ECHOVIRUS. **ECMO v.** ECMOVIRUS. **ECSO v.** ECSOVIRUS. **ectromelia v.** MOUSEPOX VIRUS. **EEE v.** EASTERN EQUINE ENCEPHALITIS VIRUS. **EMC v.** See under CARDIOVIRUS. **encephalomyocarditis v.** See under CARDIOVIRUS. **enteric v.** Any virus which infects the gastrointestinal tract. **enteric cytopathogenic bovine orphan v.** See under ECBOVIRUS. **enteric cytopathogenic human orphan v.** See under ECHOVIRUS. **enteric cytopathogenic monkey orphan v.** See under ECMOVIRUS. **enteric cytopathogenic swine orphan v.** See under ECSOVIRUS. **epidemic pleurodynia v.** A virus that causes epidemic pleurodynia: usually a group B coxsackievirus. **Epstein-Barr v.** A herpesvirus which is the major cause of infectious mononucleosis and a common subclinical illness in children and young adults which is characterized only by seroconversion to the virus, and which is associated with Burkitt's lymphoma, nasopharyngeal carcinoma, some B-cell lymphomas in immunosuppressed or immunodeficient persons, and a usually fatal progressive combined variable immunodeficiency. It was formerly thought to be transmitted as an X-linked recessive trait but has been reported in both males and females. Also *EB virus*. **equine encephalitis v.** Any virus that causes encephalitis in horses and usually also in humans. The principal viruses of this category are eastern equine encephalitis virus, western equine encephalitis virus, and Venezuelan equine encephalitis virus. **equine influenza v.** Either of two viruses that cause equine influenza. They are serologically distinct from the types that ordinarily infect humans, though the equine types also occasionally cause human illness. **Everglades v.** An alphavirus isolated from culex mosquitoes in Everglades National Park, Florida. Human illness, reported in southern Florida, is associated with fever, headache, prostration, and central nervous system involvement. **feline leukemia v.** A C-type RNA retrovirus that is a common cause of T-cell hematopoietic malignancies or immunodeficiency in cats. The virus affects principally helper T-lymphocytes. **fibroma v.** A virus of the myxoma subgroup of the poxviruses which causes benign subcutaneous tumors in rabbits, squirrels, and hares. **filamentous bacterial v.** Any of a family of bacteriophages (Inoviridae) having a filamentous morphology and single-stranded DNA. **filterable v.** A contagium or infective agent small enough to pass through an ultrafilter; a virus. *Older term*. Also *ultravirus*. ● As the study of filterable viruses intensified, they were more and more often referred to simply as *viruses*. The shortened term has generally replaced the full form, which has furthermore become outmoded since filterability is not an essential defining characteristic of viruses as they are now understood. **fixed v.** Modified rabies virus of high virulence used to infect rabbits for preparation of the original Pasteur's rabies vaccine. **foamy v.** Any of the syncytium-forming viruses in the Spumavirinae subfamily of the Retroviridae family. They have been isolated from monkeys, cats, cattle, hamsters, and humans in the latent form associated with no known disease. They are pleomorphic, membrane-bound RNA viruses which contain reverse transcriptase. **Friend leukemia v.** A murine leukosis virus belonging to the oncovirus C genus and the mammalian subgenus of the Retroviridae family. It produces leukemia in mice. **Ganjam v.** A virus of the Nairobi sheep disease group of the Bunyaviridae family isolated from ticks on healthy goats in the Ganjam district in India. It has been associated with human febrile illnesses in Africa. **gerbilpox v.** A poxvirus, isolated from the livers of apparently health gerbils captured in Dahomey, Africa. It is very closely related to the vaccinia-variola group. **German measles v.** RUBELLA VIRUS. **Germistan v.** A bunyavirus of the Bunyamwera group which causes zoonoses among rodents in South Africa, Zimbabwe (Rhodesia), Mozambique, Angola, and Uganda. It is transmitted by culex mosquitoes. Disease in humans is characterized by malaise, headache, and local and generalized pain. **Guama v.** A virus in the Guama group of bunyaviruses which causes a zoonosis transmitted by culicine mosquitoes among monkeys, rodents, and marsupials in Brazil, French Guiana, and Trinidad. Human disease is characterized by fever, malaise, headache, and local and generalized pain. **Guaroa v.** A virus in the Bunyamwera group of bunyaviruses which is transmitted by anopheles mosquitoes in Panama, Colombia, and Brazil. Human disease is characterized by fever, malaise, headache, and local and generalized pain. **Hantaan v.** A prototype of a new genus of Arenaviridae; the agent of epidemic hemorrhagic fever. Also *Korean hemorrhagic fever virus.* **Hazara v.** A virus in the Bunyaviridae family that is classified with the Crimean-Congo hemorrhagic fever group, originally isolated at Lahore, Pakistan, from ticks. **helper v.** Any of several viruses which complements defective viruses and allows them to reproduce. **hemadsorbing enteric v.** A parvovirus, isolated from the gastrointestinal tract of normal calves, which causes hemadsorption and agglutination of both human and guinea pig erythrocytes to infected tissue culture cells. No disease has been associated with this virus. **hemadsorption v.** See under PARAINFLUENZA VIRUS. **hemagglutinating v. of Japan** SENDAI VIRUS. **hemorrhagic fever v.** An epidemic form of dengue virus, a mosquito-associated flavivirus in the family Togaviridae, four serotypes of which are known. A number of large but focal outbreaks have occurred in southeast Asia, especially in Thailand, with mortality rates of up to 7 percent among hospitalized patients. **hepadna v.** Any of a family of DNA viruses which contains the hepatitis B virus of man and three other closely related viruses which cause hepatitis and/or hepatic carcinoma in animals: the woodchuck hepadna virus, the ground squirrel hepadna virus, and the Pekin duck (or duck) hepadna virus. • *Hepadna* is a contraction of *hepa(titis)* and *DNA*. **hepatitis A v.** An unclassified single-stranded RNA virus (27 nm in diameter) which is the major cause of infectious hepatitis. Maximal amounts of virus are shed in the stools of afflicted subjects just prior to the development of symptoms. Transmission occurs by the fecal-oral route via contaminated food, water, or fomites. **hepatitis B v.** A virus of a new unnamed family which is composed of a membrane-bound particle (42 nm in diameter), called a Dane particle, containing double-stranded circular DNA and a DNA polymerase. Mild detergent treatment disrupts the particle and yields a 28-nm core particle. It is one of the major causes of post-transfusion hepatitis. Human disease is characterized by acute and chronic hepatitis and an asymptomatic carrier state. Transmission is predominantly via parenteral routes or contact with infected blood. Also *serum hepatitis virus* (outmoded). Abbr. HBV **hepatitis C v.** The proposed name for one of the viruses which cause non-A, non-B viral hepatitis based on the evidence of an antigen-antibody system by immunodiffusion. **herpes v.** Any of a family of large (150 nm diameter), ether-sensitive, enveloped viruses which contain double-stranded linear DNA. It includes herpes simplex virus, varicella-zoster virus, Epstein-Barr virus, and human cytomegalovirus. **herpes B v.** A herpes virus that infects macaque monkeys usually without adverse effect but that can cause severe central nervous system disease, including encephalitis, in humans. It is sometimes given the genus-species designation *Herpesvirus simiae*. Also *herpesvirus B, herpesvirus simian B.* **herpes simplex v.** A large, enveloped DNA virus, *Herpesvirus hominis*; the cause of herpes simplex infections, including fever blisters, cold sores, and genital herpes. It contains a DNA core of 30 nm diameter, and the capsid contains 162 pentameric and hexameric double-stranded subunits arranged in 5-3-2 symmetry, and is 100 nm in diameter. The enveloped virion has a diameter of 120–150 nm. There are two types of herpes simplex virus, type 1 predominantly infecting the oral region and type 2, the genital region. Infection may be asymptomatic, and between recurrent manifestations of disease the virus remains latent in neurons of sensory root ganglia. **human immunodeficiency v.** A virus belonging to the oncovirus subgroup of the family Retroviridae, identified in 1984 as the probable etiologic agent of acquired immune deficiency syndrome (AIDS). Related to and sharing features with human T cell leukemia/lymphoma viruses 1 and 2 (HTLV-1 and HTLV-2, also called human lymphotrophic retroviruses), HIV is an enveloped virus 80–110 nm in diameter with a characteristic bar-shaped tubular core containing a dimeric, 10-kilobase RNA genome and reverse transcriptase. HIV is highly lymphotropic, infecting the $T_4$ subset of T cells, and strongly cytopathic, causing premature death of the infected $T_4$ cells. The virus or its precursor may have originated in Africa. HIV has spread rapidly throughout the world since the late 1970s. The virus is transmitted from person to person via intimate contact and blood transfusions, and is present in the bodily fluids (semen, blood cells, blood plasma, saliva, and possibly mother's milk) of infected persons. The exact mechanism of transmission by intimate contact is not known. It is not known what determines which individuals are susceptible to infection and expression of disease. Also *human T cell leukemia/lymphoma virus-3, lymphadenopathy-associated virus* (French usage). Abbr. HIV. **human papilloma v.** See under PAPILLOMAVIRUS. **human T cell leukemia/lymphoma v. -1** A virus belonging to the oncovirus subgroup of the family Retroviridae, closely associated with human T cell malignancies. It is an enveloped virus 80–110 nm in diameter which contains a 9-kilobase RNA genome, reverse transcriptase, and no oncogene. The virus apparently requires intimate person-to-person contact for transmission and is highly lymphotrophic, infecting primarily T lymphocytes of the $T_4$ subset and also, in some persons, transforming B cells. Endemic in some regions of Africa, the Caribbean basin countries, southern Japan, and the southeastern United States, the virus causes T cell leukemias and lymphomas which can be rapidly fatal and which are often manifested by lesions of the skin and bones. Abbr. HTLV-1 **human T cell leukemia/lymphoma v. -2** A virus belonging to the oncovirus subgroup of the family Retroviridae, possibly associated with leukemic reticuloendotheliosis. Like other lymphotropic retroviruses (particularly HTLV-1 and HIV), it is an enveloped virus 80–110 nm in diameter which contains an RNA genome, reverse transcriptase, and no oncogene. Little is known about this virus other than its basic structural features. Abbr. HTLV-2 **human T cell leukemia/-lymphoma v. -3** HUMAN IMMUNODEFICIENCY VIRUS. Abbr. HTLV-3 **human wart v.** HUMAN PAPILLOMAVIRUS. **Ilesha v.** A virus in the Bunyamwera group of the Bunyaviridae family. It is transmitted by anopheles mosquitoes in Ghana, Nigeria, Central African Republic, and Uganda. Human disease is characterized by fever, malaise, headache, and local and generalized pain. **Ilheus v.** A virus in the *Flavivirus* genus of the Togaviridae family. It causes zoonoses among wild birds and monkeys in Guatemala, Honduras, Panama, Colombia, Venezuela, Trinidad, Guyana, Suriname, and Brazil. It is transmitted by mosquitoes. Human disease is characterized by fever and central nervous system involvement, including severe sequelae from meningoencephalitis. **inclusion v.** Any virus which produces cytoplasmic or intranuclear inclusions. **influenza v.** Any virus belonging to the *In-*

*fluenzavirus* genus of the Orthomyxoviridae family. Viruses of this group are enveloped RNA viruses with a segmented genome and with hemagglutinin and neuraminidase glycoproteins on their surface. They include human, bovine, equine, and avian viruses, and are classified by complement fixation into types A, B, and C. Influenza A virus is further separated into many subtypes by the antigenic characteristics of its surface hemagglutinin and neuraminidase glycoproteins. The classic winter epidemics of influenza are caused by influenza viruses A and B, while type C is an infrequent contributor to common cold illnesses. **Ingwavuma v.** A bunyavirus belonging to the Simbu group. It has been associated with human disease. **Inkoo v.** A virus in the California group of the Bunyaviridae family. It causes zoonoses among large mammals, fox, and hare in Finland and is transmitted by *Aedes* mosquitoes. Human disease is characterized by malaise, headache, and pain. **insect v.** Any virus that principally infects insects. Such viruses are of increasing importance in the search for specific and environmentally safe pathogens to be used for biological control of insect pests. **Itaqui v.** A virus belonging to the *Bunyavirus* genus of the Bunyaviridae family. It is the cause of a febrile systemic illness in Brazil and is transmitted by culex mosquitoes. Monkeys and rodents are suspected as the reservoir. **Japanese encephalitis v.** A virus in the *Flavivirus* genus of the Togaviridae family. It is transmitted by culex mosquitoes in Japan, Korea, China, southeastern Asia, and India. It causes a zoonosis among pigs and herons. Human disease is characterized by fever and central nervous system involvement including severe meningoencephalitis. Also *Japanese B encephalitis virus, Russian autumn encephalitis virus.* **JC v.** One of the SV40-like human viruses of the Papovaviridae family. It has been isolated from patients with progressive multifocal leukoencephalopathy. The virus was first isolated in fetal glial cells obtained from a patient identified by the initials JC. **JH v.** A common cold virus now classified as rhinovirus type 1A. • The name is derived from *Johns Hopkins* University, Baltimore, Maryland, where it was first identified. **Junín v.** A virus of the Arenaviridae family which is carried in a chronic persistent infection by rodent species in Argentina. The human disease, Argentinian hemorrhagic fever, is contracted from infected rodent urine. Also *Argentinian hemorrhagic fever virus.* **Jurona v.** A virus belonging to the *Bunyavirus* genus of the Bunyaviridae family but unassigned as to group. **K v.** A polyomavirus of rats and mice. **Karimabad v.** A virus of the phlebotomus fever group of the Bunyaviridae family. **Kemerova v.** A virus in the *Orbivirus* genus of the Reoviridae family. It causes zoonoses among small mammals and wild birds in western Siberia and Egypt and is transmitted by *Ixodes* ticks. Human disease is characterized by fever, malaise, headache, and local and generalized pain. **Ketapang v.** A virus belonging to the Bakau group of bunyaviruses. **Keystone v.** A virus belonging to the California group of bunyaviruses. **Kilham rat v.** A rat parvovirus which induces a hemorrhagic encephalopathy in young rats. Also *latent rat virus.* **Kirk v.** A member of the Parvoviridae family and *Parvovirus* genus. It is defective and dependent on an adenovirus as a helper virus. **Korean hemorrhagic fever v.** HANTAAN VIRUS. **Kotonkan v.** A virus belonging to the Rhabdoviridae family. It is antigenically related to rabies virus and has been isolated from mosquitoes, but it is not known to cause human disease. It infects cattle, rodents, and horses in Nigeria. **Kumba v.** SEMLIKI FOREST VIRUS. **Kyasanur Forest v.** A tick-borne flavivirus that causes Kyasanur Forest disease. **LaCrosse v.** A member of the Bunyaviridae family, *Bunyavirus* genus, and the California group. It produces fever associated with central nervous system involvement, ranging from meningoencephalitis to encephalitis with sequelae. It is transmitted by *Aedes, Culex,* and *Culiseta* mosquitoes. Small mammals serve as a reservoir. It is distributed geographically in the western and north central United States as well as Texas and the southeastern states. **lactic dehydrogenase v.** A virus of mice which is ether-sensitive and contains RNA. It is believed to be a togavirus. Infection in mice results in the elevation of serum lactic dehydrogenase (lactate dehydrogenase). Also *Riley virus.* **Lagos bat v.** A virus of the Rhabdoviridae family isolated from the brains of Nigerian fruit bats on the island of Lagos. **Lansing v.** The prototype strain of poliovirus type 2. • The term is named after *Lansing,* Michigan. **Lassa v.** An arenavirus that is the agent of Lassa fever. It is carried in western Africa by rats, especially those of the species *Mastomys natalensis.* • The term is named after *Lassa,* Nigeria. **latent v.** A virus which can be recovered from a host by culturing, cocultivation, or reactivation, but which does not appear to be causing any overt pathologic disease. Mechanisms responsible for latency include inapparent persistent infections and lysogeny. Also *masked virus.* **latent rat v.** KILHAM RAT VIRUS. **LCM v.** LYMPHOCYTIC CHORIOMENINGITIS VIRUS. **Lenny v.** A poxvirus isolated from a patient with a vesicular eruption. It differs serologically from other poxviruses. **Leon v.** The prototype strain of poliovirus type 3. **leukemia v.** Any of various type C oncoviruses which cause leukemia in certain animals, such as avian leukemia virus, murine leukemia virus, and hamster leukemia virus. **leukemia-sarcoma v.** Any of various type C oncoviruses that cause leukemia and/or sarcomas in certain animals, such as murine leukemia-sarcoma viruses, feline leukemia-sarcoma viruses, primate leukemia-sarcoma viruses, and bovine leukemia-sarcoma viruses. **Lokern v.** A bunyavirus, serologically related to bunyamwera virus, that has been isolated from mosquitoes. It can produce headache, fever, and myalgia. **louping ill v.** A tick-borne flavivirus, found in Great Britain and Ireland and, the cause of ovine encephalomyelitis, or louping ill of sheep. Cattle, horses, and pigs are less commonly affected. Humans are rarely infected. In seriously affected sheep, a jumping vertigo or loup develops, and mortality can be high. The tick *Ixodes recinus* is a vector, and transmission to man is also apparently possible by close contact with sheep and sheep carcasses. **Lucké's v.** A virus of the Herpetoviridae family which almost certainly causes renal adenocarcinoma in the leopard frog (*Rana pipiens*). Virus is produced only during the winter and is excreted at higher titer in urine. During the summer months infected frogs carry the virus inapparently. **Lumbo v.** A mosquito-borne bunyavirus widely distributed throughout Africa. **lymphadenopathy-associated v.** The name originally given in France for HUMAN IMMUNODEFICIENCY VIRUS. Abbr. LAV **lymphocytic choriomeningitis v.** An arenavirus that is endemic in mice and infects humans and other mammals rarely; the causative agent of lymphocytic choriomeningitis. Also *LCM virus.* **lysogenic v.** A virus which produces lysogeny. **lytic v.** A virus that causes host cell death by lysis as a consequence of its replication. Examples include poliovirus and reovirus. **M-25 v.** A subtype of parainfluenza virus, type 4. **Machupo v.** An arenavirus of the Tacaribe sero-complex found in Bolivia, which causes hemorrhagic fever in humans. Wild rodents are the common host and humans are only occasionally infected. Also *Bolivian hemorrhagic fever virus.* **Madrid v.** A mosquito-borne bunyavirus found in Panama which infects humans and rodents and has been associated with human febrile illness. **maedi v.** A lentivirus which is the cause of ovine chronic progressive pneumonia, or maedi. It is closely related to visna virus. **mammary cancer v. of mice** MOUSE MAMMARY TUMOR VIRUS. **mammary tumor v.** MOUSE MAMMARY TUMOR VIRUS. **Mappatta v.** A virus of the Mappatta group of *Bunyaother* viruses in the Bunyaviridae family. **Marburg v.** An enveloped RNA virus with cylindrical virions 65–90 nm in diameter and 130–2600 nm in length. With the morphologically similar Ebola virus, it is believed to be distinct from all other known viruses. It infects African green monkeys (*Cercopithecus aethiops*) and provokes an often fatal hemorrhagic fever in humans. See also MARBURG VIRUS DISEASE. • The term is named after *Marburg* University, Federal Republic of Germany. **Marcy v.** An agent found in stools in cases of epidemic diarrhea which caused gastroenteritis when fed to human volunteers. Transmission studies done in the late 1940s suggested a viral agent but none was isolated *in vitro*. **Marituba v.** A virus belonging to the Bunyaviridae family and *Bunyavirus* genus, and transmitted by culex mosquitoes. Monkeys and rodents serve as reservoirs. It produces fever, malaise, and localized and generalized pain in humans in Brazil. **marmoset v.** A virus of the family Herpetoviridae which has been repeatedly isolated from the throats and autopsy materials of marmosets. **masked v.** LATENT VIRUS. **Mayaro v.** A mosquito-borne alphavirus found in Central and South America which causes fever in humans. **measles v.** A virus of the family Paramyxoviridae, genus *Morbillivirus*, which causes the common childhood disease measles and, rarely, pneumonia, encephalomyelitis, and subacute sclerosing panencephalitis. **Mengo v.** A picornavirus of mice belonging to the *Cardiovirus* genus. Carditis and encephalitis have been reported from rare cases of human infection. Also *mengovirus*. **milkers' nodule v.** PARAVACCINIA VIRUS. **MM v.** A strain of encephalomyocarditis virus. **Modoc v.** A flavivirus without a known arthropod vector found in rodents in the western United States. **Mokola v.** A rhabdovirus which has been isolated from shrews and rarely from humans. It is serologically related to rabies virus. **molluscum contagiosum v.** A large poxvirus which infects humans exclusively, causing molluscum contagiosum. Transmission is by direct contact and by fomites. **monkeypox v.** An orthopoxvirus which infects several genera of monkeys, apes, and sometimes humans, causing a smallpoxlike disease. Human infection is rare and person-to-person spread seldom occurs. **mouse hepatitis v.** A member of the Coronaviridae family that occurs as a latent infection in a varying percentage of mice. The virus causes hepatitis in newborn mice but produces only negligible hepatic damage in older mice. However, synergism between the blood parasite *Eperythrozoon coccoides*, by itself harmless, and the virus results in fatal hepatitis in older mice. Also *murine hepatitis virus*. **mouse mammary tumor v.** A group B oncovirus commonly latent in mice which causes cancers in genetically susceptible strains under appropriate hormonal conditions. The virus is abundantly present in the lactating mamma. Also *mouse mammary tumor agent, Bittner milk factor, milk factor, mouse mammary tumor factor, mammary tumor virus, murine mammary tumor virus, mammary cancer virus of mice*. Abbr. MMTV **mouse parotid tumor v.** *Outmoded* POLYOMAVIRUS. **mousepox v.** A poxvirus of the *Orthopoxvirus* genus. It causes infectious ectromelia in mice. Also *ectromelia virus, poxvirus muris*. **mouse thymic v.** A virus of the family Herpetoviridae which is probably enzootic in some stocks of laboratory mice and in wild mice. It produces nonfatal infections in newborn mice, with massive thymic necrosis. Only newborn mice are affected. **Mucambo v.** A mosquito-borne alphavirus found in Central and South America in humans, rodents, and birds. **mumps v.** A paramyxovirus that in humans causes parotitis and meningoencephalitis, orchitis, pancreatitis, and other complications. Transmission is via salivary secretions, and the incubation period is 6–21 days. The virus can be propagated in several cell culture systems, growth being indicated by hemadsorption and the formation of syncytia and eosinophilic cytoplasmic inclusions. **murine encephalomyelitis v.** The enterovirus that causes Theiler's mouse encephalomyelitis. Also *poliovirus muris*. **murine hepatitis v.** MOUSE HEPATITIS VIRUS. **murine leukemia v.** Any of a number of type C oncoviruses that produce leukemia and sometimes lymphosarcoma in mice. **murine mammary tumor v.** MOUSE MAMMARY TUMOR VIRUS. **murine sarcoma v.** A type C oncovirus that produces sarcomas in mice. **Murray Valley encephalitis v.** A mosquito-borne flavivirus found in Papua New Guinea and southeastern Australia; the cause of Murray Valley encephalitis. It has been isolated from two species of *Culex* and *Aedes*. Also *Australian X disease virus*. **Murutucu v.** A mosquito-borne bunyavirus found in Brazil which infects monkeys, rodents, and humans, causing febrile illness. **myxoma v.** A leporipoxvirus occurring naturally among wild rabbits (*Sylvilagus*) in Brazil and Uruguay and later introduced into wild and domestic rabbits (*Oryctolagus*) in Australia, Chile, and Europe, where it is widespread. In *Sylvilagus* it produces only local swelling, whereas in *Oryctolagus* it produces full-fledged myxomatosis, a disease which on first contact is more than 90 percent fatal but in time becomes less severe, perhaps due to virus attenuation or to the development of genetic resistance in the host population. Also *myxomatosis virus, rabbit myxoma virus, poxvirus myxomatis*. **myxomatosis v.** MYXOMA VIRUS. **Nebraska calf diarrhea v.** A virus belonging to the Reoviridae family and the *Rotavirus* genus. It is closely related morphologically and antigenically to human rotavirus. It produces diarrhea in cattle. **Negishi v.** A tick-borne flavivirus found in Japan which causes human encephalitis. **Nepuyo v.** A mosquito-borne bunyavirus found in Central and South America which infects rodents and bats. Serological evidence of human infection has been demonstrated. **neurotropic v.** Any virus showing an affinity for nerve cells. Also *neurovirus*. **newborn pneumonitis v.** Parainfluenza virus type 1. See under PARAINFLUENZA VIRUS. **Norwalk v.** NORWALK AGENT. **Nyando v.** A bunyavirus which has not been assigned to a group. It is transmitted by anopheles mosquitoes, and is prevalent in eastern and central Africa. It causes fever, malaise, headache, and local and generalized pain in humans. **O v.** A virus belonging to the Reoviridae family and the *Rotavirus* genus. It is related to the human rotavirus and produces diarrhea in sheep. **Omsk hemorrhagic fever v.** A tick-borne flavivirus found in southwestern Siberia; the cause of Omsk hemorrhagic fever. **oncogenic v.** Any virus capable of producing tumors, such as oncoviruses or papovaviruses. Also *tumor virus*. **O'nyong-nyong v.** A mosquito-borne alphavirus found in Africa which causes O'nyong-nyong fever. **orf v.** The parapoxvirus which causes orf. It primarily infects sheep and goats, producing lesions that progress from papules to vesicles to pustules to crusts. Human infection occurs in individuals whose occupations bring them in close contact with sheep and goats. Usually a single lesion on the hands or arms is found but occasionally generalized infection occurs. Also *contagious pustular dermatitis virus.* **Oriboca v.** A mosquito-borne bunyavirus found in Brazil, Trinidad, and Guiana which infects humans, marsupials, and rodents. Human infection has been associated with febrile illness. **Oropouche v.** A mosquito-borne bunyavirus, found in Brazil and Trinidad, which has been associated with febrile illness in humans. **orphan v.** Any virus which, when first identified, was not specifically associated with disease. **Ossa v.** A mosquito-borne bunyavirus found in Panama which infects humans and rodents. Human infection has been associated with febrile illness. **pantropic v.** A virus that replicates in tissues derived from all three embryonic layers. **papilloma v.** See under PAPILLOMAVIRUS. **pappataci fever v.** PHLEBOTOMUS FEVER VIRUS. **parainfluenza v.** Any of four types of enveloped, single-stranded RNA viruses of the genus *Paramyxovirus,* family Paramyxoviridae, that are responsible for a spectrum of illnesses, particularly in infants and young children, ranging from mild upper respiratory infections to croup, or tracheobronchitis, and pneumonia. Type 1 (originally known as hemadsorption virus type 2) is the most likely to produce laryngotracheobronchitis (croup), and type 3 (originally known as hemadsorption virus type 1), to cause bronchiolitis and pneumonia. All types cause common colds in adults. **paravaccinia v.** A parapoxvirus that causes paravaccinia, or pseudocowpox, producing cherry-red papules, which resemble those of cowpox, on the udders of cows. Like cowpox, the virus may spread to humans, causing lesions on the hands known as milkers' nodules. Also *milkers' nodule virus, pseudocowpox virus.* **pharyngoconjunctival fever v.** Any of various adenoviruses causing pharyngoconjunctival fever. *Outmoded.* **phlebotomus fever v.** A virus transmitted by sandflies (*Phlebotomus papatasi, P. sergenti,* and others) with two recognized serotypes, Naples and Sicilian. It is tentatively classified in the family Bunyaviridae and is carried only by sandflies to humans, as it undergoes transovarial transmission in the vector. The disease is nonfatal but debilitating and has appeared in mass outbreaks in Italy and north Africa. The virus is distributed from the Mediterranean and central Asia to India and southern China. Also *sandfly fever virus, pappataci fever virus.* **Piry v.** A mosquito-borne bunyavirus found in east Africa and associated with acute febrile illness in humans. **plant v.** Any of the viruses that infect plants. **pneumonia v. of mice** A pneumovirus which causes bronchopneumonia in mice. It is found in many mouse colonies in the United States. Also *PVM virus.* **poliomyelitis v.** POLIOVIRUS. **polyoma v.** See under POLYOMAVIRUS. **Powassan v.** A tick-borne flavivirus found in Canada, New York state, and New Jersey which rarely causes encephalitis in humans. • The term is named after *Powassan,* Ontario, Canada. **pox v.** See under POXVIRUS. **pseudocowpox v.** PARAVACCINIA VIRUS. **pseudorabies v.** A herpes virus, sometimes designated *Herpesvirus suis,* that naturally infects pigs, cattle, sheep, dogs, cats, and mink. It is the causative agent of pseudorabies. Infection in pigs is often asymptomatic but central nervous system involvement may occur. In other animals it is almost invariably fatal. **Punta Toro v.** A bunyavirus of the phlebotomus fever group that occurs in Panama. It is transmitted by *Lutzomyia* sandflies and produces febrile illness in humans. **PVM v.** PNEUMONIA VIRUS OF MICE. **rabbit myxoma v.** MYXOMA VIRUS. **rabbitpox v.** An orthopoxvirus closely related to if not identical with vaccinia virus and causing epidemics among laboratory rabbits, often with high fatality. Infection among wild rabbits has not been reported. **rabies v.** A rhabdovirus of the *Lyssavirus* genus; the cause of rabies. Virus is present in the saliva of infected animals and is generally transmitted via a bite. The incubation period, which usually ranges from 15 days to five months, may be as long as one year. Evidence suggests that the virus first replicates locally and then travels through the axoplasm of peripheral nerves to the central nervous system. **Rauscher leukemia v.** A strain of murine leukemia virus. **respiratory syncytial v.** A pneumovirus (family Paramyxoviridae) about 100 nm in size. It causes a respiratory infection that is mild in adults but often severe in infants, with bronchiolitis or bronchopneumonia. Also *RS virus, chimpanzee coryza agent, CCA virus.* • The word *syncytial* in the name of this virus refers to the characteristic cytopathologic effect it has in cell cultures, which is the formation of multinucleated giant cell or syncytia. **Restan v.** A mosquito-borne bunyavirus found in Trinidad and Surinam which has been associated with human febrile illness. **Rift Valley fever v.** See under RIFT VALLEY FEVER. **Riley v.** LACTIC DEHYDROGENASE VIRUS. **rinderpest v.** A virus of the Paramyxoviridae family that is closely related to measles and canine distemper viruses. It is the cause of rinderpest in cattle in parts of Africa and Asia. **RNA v.** Any virus in which the genome consists of ribonucleic acid. The families of animal viruses which are classified as RNA viruses include the Picornaviridae, Caliciviridae, Reoviridae, Orthomyxoviridae, Paramyxoviridae, Coronaviridae, Retroviridae, Togaviridae, Bunyaviridae, Arenaviridae, and Rhabdoviridae. Also *ribovirus.* **Ross River v.** A mosquito-borne alphavirus which infects birds and has been associated with epidemic human polyarthritis, a seasonal illness occurring in the area of the Ross river in southern Australia. **Rous-associated v.** A helper virus isolated from stocks of defective Rous sarcoma virus. **Rous sarcoma v.** A type C oncovirus which induces tumors when injected into chickens and transforms chicken fibroblast tissue cultures. Also *avian sarcoma virus.* Abbr. RSV **RS v.** RESPIRATORY SYNCYTIAL VIRUS. **rubella v.** A virus belonging to the Togaviridae family and *Rubivirus* genus and the causing of rubella. Transmission is via the respiratory route and the incubation period is from 14 to 17 days. Infection confers lifelong immunity. The virus can be propagated in various cell culture systems and it agglutinates red blood cells from a wide variety of species. Also *German measles virus.* **Russian autumn encephalitis v.** JAPANESE ENCEPHALITIS VIRUS. **Russian spring-summer encephalitis v.** Any of a complex of tick-borne flaviviruses found in central Europe and the USSR. It occurs in two different subtypes causing two forms of disease in humans, a western, or central European, subtype and an eastern, or taiga forest, subtype. The virus is transmitted by the tick *Ixodes persulcatus* in the *USSR* and possibly by *Haemaphysalis concinna* and *H. japonica douglasi* in northern China and the Khabarovsk region of the eastern USSR. Other tick vectors have also been incriminated. **salivary gland v.** *Outmoded* CYTOMEGALOVIRUS. **sandfly fever v.** PHLEBOTOMUS FEVER VIRUS. **scrapie v.** The causative agent of scrapie, which affects sheep and rarely goats. It is an unusually stable agent, withstanding boiling for three hours and exposure to 20% formalin for 18 hours. It may be a viroid or a prion rather than a true virus. **Semliki Forest v.** An alphavirus, found in Africa, for which the natural host and vectors remain unknown. Also *Kumba virus.* **Sendai v.** A paramyxovirus recovered from a group of newborn infants during an outbreak of pneumonia in Sendai, a city in northern Honshu, Japan. It has subsequently been shown to be identical with a virus that produces latent infection and pneumonia in laboratory mice, and it is closely related, or identical, to parainfluenza virus type 1. Also *hemagglutinating virus of Japan.* **serum hepatitis v.** *Outmoded* HEPATITIS B VIRUS. **Shope papilloma v.** SHOPE PAPILLOMAVIRUS. **simian v.** Any of the viruses isolated from monkeys and serially numbered, though they belong to many different families. Abbr. SV **simian v. 40** An oncogenic polyomavirus originally discovered in apparently normal cultures of monkey kidney cells. It is frequently used as a model for studies in molecular biology. Also *simian vacuolating virus, SV-40 virus, vacuolating virus.* Abbr. SV40 **Sindbis v.** A mosquito-borne alphavirus found in many countries in Africa, Asia, and eastern Europe, and in Australia. It is the type species of the *Alphavirus* genus. **slow v.** Any virus that produces an infection with an unusually long incubation period (months to years) before disease manifestations occur. Examples include the causative agents of progressive multifocal leukoencephalopathy, subacute sclerosing panencephalitis, Creutzfeldt-Jakob disease, kuru, scrapie, and mink encephalopathy. Also *slow infection virus.* **smallpox v.** VARIOLA VIRUS. **Spondweni v.** A mosquito-borne flavivirus, found in South Africa and Nigeria, which infects humans, sheep, and cattle. **St. Louis encephalitis v.** A mosquito-borne flavivirus found in the western United States, Canada, and Central and South America, which in humans causes a brief febrile illness and can occasionally cause encephalitis. The natural chain of infection is from wild birds to mosquitoes and back to birds. Man is an occasional dead-end host. **street v.** Virulent rabies virus isolated from domestic or wild animals that acquired the infection naturally, as distinguished from strains of the virus developed in the laboratory. **SV-40 v.** SIMIAN VIRUS 40. **Tacaribe v.** An arenavirus found in Trinidad, where bats and cricetid rodents are the usual hosts. Occasional human infection has resulted in a hemorrhagic fever. **Tahyňa v.** A mosquito-borne bunyavirus, belonging to the California group, found in Europe and Africa. It causes a febrile illness in humans. **Tataguine v.** A virus belonging to the Bunyaviridae family and the *Bunyaother* genus, but unassigned with regard to group. It produces fever, malaise, headache, and localized and generalized pain. It is transmitted by anopheline and culicine mosquitoes and is found in Senegal, Nigeria, Central African Republic, and Cameroon. **temperate v.** See under TEMPERATE BACTERIOPHAGE. **Tensaw v.** A mosquito-borne bunyavirus found in the United States which infects humans, dogs, and rabbits. Human infection has been associated with encephalitis. **Thogoto v.** A tick-borne virus belonging to the Bunyaviridae family and the *Bunyaother* genus, but unassigned as to group. It is transmitted by *Boophilus decoloratus, Rhipicephalus* species, and *Amblyomma* species. Cattle, camels, and other domestic animals serve as the reservoir. It is distributed in Egypt, Kenya, and Nigeria. It produces fever and meningoencephalitis in humans. **tick-borne encephalitis v.** Any of the tick-borne flaviviruses that produce encephalitis in humans. They include Russian spring-summer encephalitis viruses, central European encephalitis viruses, louping ill virus, and Powassan virus. **trivittatus v.** A mosquito-borne bunyavirus found in the United States. It infects cotton rats and other rodents. Serologic evidence of infection has also been demonstrated in humans, horses, and rabbits. **tumor v.** ONCOGENIC VIRUS. **type C v.** See under ONCOVIRUS. **Uganda S v.** A mosquito-borne flavivirus found in Africa and southeast Asia. It appears to infect humans but has not been associated with disease. **vaccinia v.** A poxvirus thought to be originally derived from cowpox virus and used for vaccination against smallpox. Also *virus vaccinicum, poxvirus officinalis.* **v. vaccinicum** VACCINIA VIRUS. **vacuolating v.** SIMIAN VIRUS 40. **varicella-zoster v.** A herpes virus that causes varicella (chickenpox) and herpes zoster (shingles) in humans. **variola v.** An orthopoxvirus which is the causative agent of smallpox, or variola. Also *smallpox virus.* **Venezuelan equine encephalitis v.** A mosquito-borne alphavirus in the family Togaviridae, the agent of Venezuelan equine encephalomyelitis (VEE), causing disease in humans and equines from Peru to Texas and a wider distribution of antibody. Epidemic disease in both horses and man have occurred with high mortality, especially in horses, mules, and donkeys. Also *VEE virus.* **visna v.** A lentivirus, first reported from Iceland, which is the cause of visna, an invariably fatal demyelinating encephalomyelitis of sheep and goats. It is closely related to maedi virus. **wart v.** HUMAN PAPILLOMAVIRUS. **western equine encephalitis v.** An alphavirus responsible for encephalitis of moderate severity, occurring in the eastern as well as the western United States, Canada, Mexico, Argentina, Brazil, and British Guiana. In the western United States, the principal vector is *Culex tarsalis.* Also *WEE virus.* **West Nile v.** A mosquito-borne flavivirus found in Africa, Europe, the Mediterranean area, the USSR, India, southeast Asia, and Borneo. Birds are probably the normal hosts but the virus does infect man. Although human infection is usually silent, it has also been associated with outbreaks of a short febrile illness. **whitepox v.** An orthopoxvirus that is closely related to variola virus. It has been recovered from primates but not from humans. **wyeomyia v.** A bunyavirus of the Bunyamwera group found in Panama, Colombia, Trinidad, French Guiana, and Brazil. It was discovered in *Wyeomyia* mosquitoes and subsequently has been found in other species of *Wyeomyia* as well as *Aedes, Anopheles,* and *Psorophora* mosquitoes. The virus produces fever, headache, malaise, and localized and generalized pain in humans. **yabalike disease v.** A DNA virus belonging to the Poxviridae family. It produces epidermal lesions in *Macaca mulatta* and occasionally in humans. **yabapox v.** A poxvirus that produces yabapox in rhesus monkeys. It has not been assigned to a genus. **yellow fever v.** A mosquito-borne flavivirus that is the causative agent of yellow fever. The virions have a lipoprotein envelope and are variously reported as between 29 and 38 nm in diameter. Yellow fever virus antigens cross-react serologically with other flaviviruses. **Zika v.** A mosquito-borne flavivirus found in Africa and Malaysia. It is the causative agent of Zika fever.

**virusemia** \vī′rəsē′mē·ə\ VIREMIA.

**virustatic** \vī′rəstat′ik\ [*viru(s)* + -STATIC] **1** Capable of inhibiting the replication of viruses. **2** A virustatic agent. For defs. 1 and 2 also *virostatic.*

**viscera** \vis′ərə\ Plural of VISCUS.

**viscerad** \vis′ərad\ Toward the viscera.

**visceral** \vis′ərəl\ [Late L *visceral(is)* pertaining to the *viscera*] **1** Of or pertaining to the viscera. **2** Situated near or nearer the viscera, or far or farther from the body wall. Compare PARIETAL.

**visceralgia** \vis′əral′jə\ [*viscer(o)-* + -ALGIA] Any deep pain, usually of neurologic origin, in the viscera.

**viscerimotor** \vis′ərimō′tər\ VISCEROMOTOR.

**viscero-** \vis′ərō-\ [L *viscus,* gen. *visceris* any internal body part] A combining form meaning viscus, viscera, visceral.

**viscerocranium** \-krā′nē·əm\ SPLANCHNOCRANIUM.

**viscerogenic** \-jen′ik\ Originating within the viscera.

**visceroinhibitory** \-inhib′itôr′ē\ Acting to reduce the function of internal organs of the body.

**visceromegaly** \-meg′əlē\ [VISCERO- + -MEGALY] Abnormal enlargement of the visceral organs, especially, the general enlargement of all abdominal organs which may accompany acromegaly.

**visceromotor** \-mō′tər\ Relating to or controlling the movements of internal organs of the body. Also *viscerimotor.*

**visceroptosis** \vis′əräptō′sis\ [VISCERO- + PTOSIS] Prolapse or caudal displacement of viscera, especially abdominal viscera. Also *splanchnoptosis.*

**viscerosensory** \-sen′sərē\ Of or relating to the sensory innervation of internal organs of the body.

**visceroskeleton** \-skel′ətən\ **1** SPLANCHNOSKELETON. **2** VISCERAL SKELETON.

**viscerosomatic** \-sōmat′ik\ SPLANCHNOSOMATIC.

**viscerotomy** \vis′ərät′əmē\ Incision of an organ during autopsy.

**viscerotrophic** \-träf′ik\ [VISCERO- + -TROPHIC] **1** Making use of internal organs of the body for growth: used especially of viruses. **2** Capable of stimulating the growth of internal organs of the body.

**viscerotropic** \-träp′ik\ [VISCERO- + -TROPIC[1]] Attracted to the internal organs of the body.

**viscid** \vis′id\ Gluelike in consistency and tending to adhere; sticky.

**viscidity** \visid′itē\ The condition or quality of being viscid.

**viscoelasticity** \vis′kō·ē′lastis′itē\ [*visco(sity)* + ELASTICITY] The stiffness, compliance, and stress-strain response characteristics of a material. Adj. viscoelastic.

**viscosimeter** \vis′kōsim′ətər\ [*viscosi(ty)* + -METER] An instrument used for measuring the viscosity of a fluid, usually whole blood or blood serum or plasma. **monolayer v.** A device for determining the viscosity properties of material in a monolayer configuration.

**viscosimetry** \vis′kōsim′ətrē\ [*viscosi(ty)* + -METRY] Measurement of the viscosity of a fluid, as of whole blood or of blood plasma. Factors determining viscosity include, among other things, the protein composition of the fluid, the number and nature of suspended particles (such as blood cells), and interactions among the particles and between the particles and soluble proteins. Viscosity is usually measured clinically by comparing the flow rate of the test fluid against that of distilled water or saline through a calibrated tube system at standard temperature and pressure.

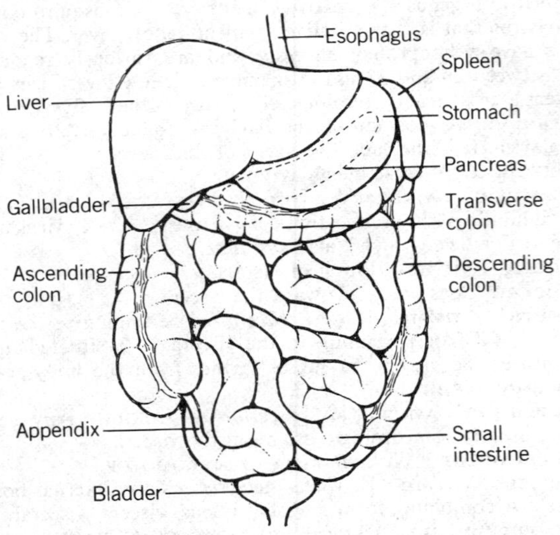


**Abdominal viscera**

**viscosity** \viskäs′itē\ [Med L *viscositas* (from Late L *viscosus* sticky) stickiness. See VISCOUS.] The resistance that a fluid offers to flow or to alteration of shape. It is a result of the molecular cohesion of materials dissolved or suspended in the fluid.

**viscous** \vis′kəs\ [Late L *viscosus* (from L *viscus* or *viscum* mistletoe, birdlime made from mistletoe berries) full of birdlime, sticky] Having high viscosity.

**viscus** \vis′kəs\ [L, any of the soft inner parts of the body] (*pl.* viscera) Any organ within a major cavity of the body, such as the abdominal or the thoracic cavity, and innervated by the autonomic nervous system. **cervical viscera** The parts of the digestive and respiratory tracts situated in the neck.

**vision** [L *visio* (from *videre* to see) sight, seeing, conception] **1** The act or power of seeing; sight. **2** Visual acuity. Abbr. V Adj. visual. **binocular v.** The simultaneous use of both eyes, resulting in cortical fusion of the images with depth perception. **central v.** The portion of the visual field near the object at which the eye is directed. **chromatic v.** COLOR VISION. **color v.** The ability to perceive the hues normally stimulated by the various parts of the visible spectrum. Also *chromatic vision.* **day v.** PHOTOPIC VISION. **double v.** DIPLOPIA. **epileptic panoramic v.** A symptom of an epileptic attack, caused by a neuronal discharge from the temporal lobe, during which events from the patient's past life are seen vividly in a panoramic fashion. This is usually an accelerated ecmnesic visual hallucination (the private cinema phenomenon). **foveal v.** Normal alignment of the center of the retina upon the point of fixation. **gun-barrel v.** TUNNEL VISION. **half v.** HEMIANOPIA. **haploscopic v.** Perception of two separate images, presented separately to the two eyes by a stereoscopic device. **multiple v.** POLYOPIA. **night v.** SCOTOPIC VISION. **peripheral v.** The area of the visual field seen by the extramacular portions of the retina. **photopic v.** The function of the eye during light adaptation; vision under light-adapted conditions. One can recognize the transition from photopic vision to scotopic (night) vision by the disappearance of color perception, which is replaced by appreciation only of shades of black and white. Also *day vision, photopia, day sight, visus diurnus.* **rod v.** SCOTOPIC VISION. **scotopic v.** The function of the eye during dark adaptation; vision under dark-adapted conditions. One can recognize the transition from photopic (day) vision to scotopic vision by the disappearance of color perception, which is replaced by appreciation only of shades of black and white. Also *night vision, rod vision, night sight, visus nocturnus.* **shaft v.** TUNNEL VISION. **triple v.** TRIPLOPIA. **tubular v.** TUNNEL VISION. **tunnel v.** A functional or hysterical disorder in which the field of vision is severely constricted to a small diameter, which is the same at all distances from the eye. Also *gun-barrel vision, shaft vision, tubular vision.* **yellow v.** XANTHOPSIA.

**visit** An encounter between a health care provider and a patient which involves either the provider's going to the patient's residence (a home visit) or the patient's going to the provider's place of practice (an office visit): a measure of health care utilization. **office v.** A visit, or encounter, between a patient and a health care provider that occurs in the provider's place of practice. A term used chiefly in the U.S., Canada, and New Zealand. • The term is not used in Australia or Japan. In the United Kingdom, the corresponding term for the general practitioner is *surgery visit*. The term does not apply to visits to consultants, who are seen in *consulting rooms*. **trial v.** The testing of a patient's ability to cope with new surroundings by allowing him to go home or to a halfway house or other facility for a weekend or other limited period of time. The visit is made with the understanding that he will return to the hospital and any problems encountered will be worked out before permanently leaving the hospital.

**visual** Pertaining to vision; pertaining to the sense of sight.

**visualization** \vizh′oo·əlīzā′shən\ 1 Any means of rendering visible some phenomenon or some region of the body; especially, the production of radiographic images with the aid of contrast media. 2 The mental perception of a visual image. **double contrast v.** DOUBLE CONTRAST ROENTGENOGRAPHY.

**visus** \vī′səs\ [L (substantive from *visus,* past part. of *videre* to see, perceive) a seeing, sight, vision] Vision. **v. brevior** MYOPIA. **v. debilitas** ASTHENOPIA. **v. decoloratus** COMPLETE COLOR BLINDNESS. **v. defiguratus** METAMORPHOPSIA. **v. dimidiatus** HEMIANOPIA. **v. diminutus** MICROPSIA. **v. diurnus** PHOTOPIC VISION. **v. duplicatus** DIPLOPIA. **v. lucidus** PHOTOPSIA. **v. nocturnus** SCOTOPIC VISION. **v. senilis** PRESBYOPIA. **v. triplex** TRIPLOPIA.

**visuscope** \viz′əskōp\ [L *visu(s),* past part. of *videre* to see + -SCOPE] An ophthalmoscope that projects a fixation target at which the patient looks. This permits determination of the part of the retina used for fixation, a fact of significance in the management of suppression amblyopia.

**vitaglass** \vī′təglas\ [L *vita* life + English *glass* ] VITA GLASS.

**vital** [L *vitalis* (from *vit(a)* life + *-alis* -AL) pertaining to life, vital] 1 Of, relating to, or characteristic of life, as *a vital process.* 2 Essential to life.

**vitality** \vītal′itē\ [L *vitalitas* (from *vitalis* pertaining to life, vital) vitality] The condition or degree in which vital processes are intact and vigorous. **pulp v.** The state of health of the dental pulp. It can range from the normal through the various stages of pulpitis, or degeneration, to necrosis.

**vitamin** [L *vit(a)* life + English *amin(e)*] Any organic substance required by animals in their diets in fairly small amounts. Physiologically, they act as precursors of cofactors in metabolic processes. Essential amino acids are not usually classed as vitamins, because animals need larger quantities of them and because they are themselves components of proteins. • The term was coined in 1912 by Casimir Funk as *vitamine.* The terminal *-e* was dropped when it was discovered that many vitamins are not amines. **v. A** A fat-soluble vitamin required for the transportation of monosaccharides in the biosynthesis of glycoproteins necessary in the maintenance of mucosal epithelium in the mouth and the respiratory and urinary tracts. It is also essential for the production of rhodopsin needed for vision in dim light. A deficiency of vitamin A results in night blindness, xerophthalmia, keratomalacia, blindness, nasopharyngeal and genitourinary-tract infections, and the stunting of growth. It consists of retinal, retinol, and some other derivatives interconvertible in the body and capable of supplying retinal for formation of visual pigments, etc. Also *antixerophthalmic vitamin, antixerophthalmia factor.* See also RETINOL, CAROTENE. **v. A acid** TRETINOIN. **v. A esters** R—$CH_2$—O—CO—R′, where R′—COOH is the esterifying fatty acid and R—$CH_2$OH is retinol. It is the storage form of vitamin A in the tissues. It is hydrolyzed by a liver enzyme, and the free retinol travels via the bloodstream to the tissue where there is a metabolic need. **v. $A_1$** RETINOL. **v. $A_2$** $C_{20}H_{28}O$. 3,4-Didehydroretinol, a form of vitamin A with half the biologic activity of retinol. It is found naturally in the retina and liver of freshwater fish as well as in invertebrates and amphibians. Also *retinol₂* (obs.). **antihemorrhagic v.** *Obs.* VITAMIN K. **antineuritic v.** THIAMIN. **antipellagra v.** NIACIN. **antirachitic v.** VITAMIN D. **antiscorbutic v.** VITAMIN C. **antisterility v.** VITAMIN E. **antixerophthalmic v.** VITAMIN A. **v. B** The vitamin B complex or any of the vitamins in the vitamin B complex. **v. B complex** The B vitamins, collectively: thiamine, riboflavin, niacin, pyridoxine, biotin, pantothenic acid, folic acid, inositol, and $B_{12}$, i.e., the main water-soluble vitamins. Although unrelated chemically, these vitamins often occur together naturally in the same foodstuffs, such as cereal germ, liver, and yeast. **v. $B_1$** THIAMIN. **v. $B_2$** RIBOFLAVIN. **v. $B_2$ complex** The water-soluble vitamins other than thiamine: riboflavin, nicotinic acid, pantothenic acid, pyridoxine, biotin, folic acid, and $B_{12}$ as well as choline, inositol, and *p*-aminobenzoic acid. All of these substances were once considered necessary for optimal health. Choline, inositol, and *p*-aminobenzoic acid are no longer considered essential dietary components by most authorities. *Outmoded.* **v. $B_2$ phosphate** FLAVIN MONONUCLEOTIDE. **v. $B_6$** Any of the water-soluble derivatives of 2-methyl pyridine, namely pyridoxine, pyridoxal, and pyridoxamine, all of which have the same potency. The vitamin is a cofactor in transamination, metabolism of tryptophan and degradation of glycogen to glucose-1-phosphate. A deficiency of vitamin $B_6$ leads to dermatitis and depression in adults and epileptiform seizures in babies. Good sources are nuts, meat, whole grains, and yeast. Also *antiacrodynia factor, antidermatitis factor of rats, eluate factor.* **v. $B_{12}$** Cyanocobalamin, i.e., cobalamin with cyanide as a ligand to cobalt(III). Vitamin $B_{12}$ is often used to describe any substance that can give cobalamin to the body, thus providing the methyl carrier for methionine biosynthesis and the coenzyme for the interconversion of methylmalonyl-CoA and succinyl-CoA that is important in the catabolism of fatty acids whose molecules contain an odd number of carbon atoms. Sources of vitamin $B_{12}$ include meat, liver, and kidney. It can be produced in culture from *Streptomyces griseus.* It is not found in vegetable products except in root nodules of legumes and some seaweeds. Vitamin $B_{12}$ requires an intrinsic factor for absorption. Deficiency leads to pernicious anemia and abnormal neurologic function. The recommended daily allowance is 3 $\mu$g. Also *extrinsic factor, animal protein factor, cow manure factor, LLD factor, antianemia factor, zoopherin.* **v. $B_{17}$** LAETRILE. • It is not a vitamin. **v. $B_t$** CARNITINE. **v. C** A cofactor of some hydroxylating enzymes. Its absence from the diet in man causes capillary fragility and, ultimately, scurvy. Also *antiscorbutic factor, reducing factor, antiscorbutic vitamin.* • The term is almost synonymous with ascorbic acid, since even small modifications of ascorbic acid render the substance inactive as a vitamin. **v. D** A mixture of hormones with antirachitic properties, especially ergocalciferol (vitamin $D_2$) and cholecalciferol (vitamin $D_3$). Food sources include egg yolk, fatty fish, and enriched milk. Also *antirachitic factor, antirachitic vitamin.* **v. $D_2$** ERGO-

CALCIFEROL. **v. $D_3$** CHOLECALCIFEROL. **v. $D_4$** Activated 22,23-dihydroergosterol, a weaker antirachitic agent than vitamins $D_2$ and $D_3$. Also *22,23-dihydroercalciol, (24S)-methylcalciol.* **v. E** Any of a group of fat-soluble compounds that act as antioxidants and are necessary for normal reproduction, muscle development, and resistance to red blood cell hemolysis in many species. The vitamin's function in humans is ill defined, and deficiency states are rare. Chemically, substances with vitamin E activity are tocopherols. The richest sources are vegetable oils. It is administered therapeutically for intermittent claudication. Also *antisterility factor, antisterility vitamin.* **v. F** Any of several essential dietary components, usually essential fatty acids, but also thiamin. *Obs.* **fat-soluble v.'s** Those vitamins that partition into fat rather than water. They were originally called vitamin A, to distinguish them from water-soluble vitamin B, but they now include vitamins A, D, E, and K. **v. G** RIBOFLAVIN. **v. H** BIOTIN. **v. K** Any of a group of fat-soluble vitamins ($K_1$, $K_2$, and $K_3$) essential for the hepatic synthesis of prothrombin and other blood-clotting factors. Deficiency leads to prolonged blood-clotting time and hemorrhage. Vitamin K is used therapeutically in obstructive jaundice, hemorrhagic states related to intestinal disease, and disease of the liver and parenterally in hypothrombinemia of the newborn either directly or via the mother during labor. Sources include spinach, cabbage, kale, cauliflower, tomatoes, soybean oil, alfalfa, egg yolk, and putrefied fish meal. As vitamin K is produced by bacteria in the intestine, dietary deficiency is not encountered except in newborns with sterile intestines and in malabsorption states. Also *antihemorrhagic factor* (obs.), *antihemorrhagic vitamin* (obs.). See also MENADIONE. **v. $K_1$** $C_{31}H_{46}O_2$. 2-Methyl-3-phytyl-1,4-napthoquinone. A fat-soluble prothrombinogenic agent first isolated from lucerne but found in other green plants. Also *phytylmenaquinone, phytomenadione, phytonadione, phylloquinone.* **v. $K_2$** MENAQUINONE. **v. $K_3$** MENADIONE. **v. P** BIOFLAVONOID. **permeability v.** BIOFLAVONOID. **therapeutic v.'s** 1 Vitamins used to correct a dietary deficiency of adequate intake to meet average requirements or to meet special nutritional needs of rapid growth, pregnancy, or lactation. 2 Very large amounts of specific vitamins administered to compensate for impaired metabolic conversion systems in the body that transform vitamins to essential cofactors of enzymes. For example, some patients with congenital methylmalonic aciduria show a dramatic response to massive doses of vitamin $B_{12}$. **water-soluble v.'s** The vitamins that are soluble in water. These are all the vitamins except vitamins A, D, E, and K, the fat-soluble ones. The water-soluble vitamins are utilized or excreted without appreciable storage in the tissues and must be consumed more regularly than the fat-soluble vitamins.

**vitellin** \vītel′in\ [*vitell(us)* + -IN] A phospholipoprotein of egg yolk.

**vitelline** \vītel′in, -ēn\ Relating to the vitellus of an ovum.

**vitellomesenteric** \vītel′ōmes′enter′ik\ Pertaining to both the yolk sac and the mesentery. Also *omphalomesenteric.*

**vitellus** \vītel′əs\ [L, the yolk of an egg] The yolk of an egg. It is the nutritive region of the protoplasm of the ovum and contains glycosides, proteins, phospholipids, and neutral fats in the granules or the vacuoles of the deutoplasm. The quantity and distribution of the vitellus in an egg are very variable according to species and have a marked influence on the early stages of embryonic development. The human ovum is virtually lacking any vitelline material. **v. ovi** Egg yolk: used in pharmaceutical preparations to emulsify fats and certain other organic compounds.

**vitiation** \vish′ē·ā′shən\ The impairment or debasement of a process.

**vitiligines** \vitilij′inēz\ [L, pl. of *vitiligo*] Areas of leukoderma, as is seen in vitiligo.

**vitiligo** \vit′əlē′gō, -lī′gō\ [L (prob. from *vitium* a blemish) tetter] A disorder of pigmentation in which the melanocytes inhibit melanogenesis and eventually disappear, resulting in a patchy loss of pigmentation. Also *acquired leukopathia, acquired albinism.* Adj. vitiliginous. **v. capitis** ALOPECIA AREATA. **Cazenave's v.** ALOPECIA AREATA. **v. iridis** A mottled and irregular patchy loss of melanin from the iris of the eye.

**vitiligoidea** \vit′iligoi′dē·ə\ [New L, from *vitilig(o)* + -OID] *Outmoded* XANTHOMA. **v. tuberosum** *Outmoded* XANTHOMA.

**vitium** \vish′ē·əm\ [L, defect, flaw, fault] A defect. **v. conformationis** A defect by which shape is conspicuously altered from the usual.

**vitodynamics** \vī′tōdīnam′iks\ BIODYNAMICS.

**vit. ov. sol.** *vitello ovi solutus* (L, dissolved in egg yolk).

**vitrectomy** \vitrek′təmē\ [*vitr(eous humor)* + -ECTOMY] Surgical removal of a portion of the vitreous humor.

**vitreoretinal** \vit′rē·ōret′ənəl\ Pertaining to the vitreous humor (or the vitreous body) and the retina.

**vitreoretinopathy** \vit′rē·ōret′ināp′əthē\ A disorder of the vitreous humor and the retina of the eye, the most severe consequences of which are usually traction phenomena leading to detachment of the retina.

**vitreous** \vit′rē·əs\ [L *vitreus* (from *vitrum* glass) of or like glass] 1 Glasslike; hyaline. 2 CORPUS VITREUM. 3 HUMOR VITREUS. **anterior v.** Material resembling jelly located in an embryo between the surface ectoderm and the lens vesicle. It contributes to the development of the cornea. **detached v.** Separation of the posterior vitreous face from the retina, a common occurrence with aging. **persistent hyperplastic primary v.** A developmental anomaly in which a portion of the embryonic vitreous remains of small size and becomes transformed into dense scar tissue. This results in severe traction deformity of the internal eye structures behind the lens or of the retina. **primary v.** Primitive vitreous humor formed between the lens and the retina as a loose reticulum derived from ectoderm. Later this is invaded by hyaloid blood vessels and mesenchyme to form the secondary vitreous. Also *primary vitreous body.* **secondary v.** Loose gelatinous tissues formed from the union of the ectodermal reticulum comprising the primary vitreous and hyaloid vessels with accompanying mesenchymal cells which enter the optic cup through the choroidal fissure. **tertiary v.** A union of embryonic zonular fibers, elements of the primary vitreous, with the basement membrane of the unpigmented epithelium of the developing ciliary body. These tissues become attached to the lens capsules and give rise eventually to the zonule of Zinn or zona ciliaris.

**vitreum** \vit′rē·əm\ CORPUS VITREUM.

**vitrina** \vitrī′nə\ [New L (from L *vitr(um)* glass, woad + *-ina* -INE; see VITREOUS)] A translucent material resembling glass. **v. auditoria** *Outmoded* ENDOLYMPHA. **v. auris** *Outmoded* ENDOLYMPHA.

**vitriol** [Med L *vitriolum* (from Late L *vitreolum*, from L *vitreus* glassy, shiny) a sulfate] *Obs.* SULFURIC ACID. **green v.** FERROUS SULFATE.

**vitropressure** \vit′rəpresh′ər\ DIASCOPY.

**vivi-** \viv′ē-\ [L *vivus* alive] A combining form meaning alive.

**viviparous** \vīvip′ərəs\ [L *viviparus* (from *viv(us)* live + *parere* to give birth) bearing live young] Having embryonic development which occurs entirely within the female reproductive tract. Nourishment of the embryo is derived directly from the mother, and the young are released at birth. Also *zoogonous*. Compare OVOVIVIPAROUS, OVIPAROUS.

**vivisection** \viv′əsek′shən\ [VIVI- + SECTION] An act of experimental surgery, performed on a live anesthetized animal. Also *biotomy* (older term).

**VLDL** very-low-density lipoprotein.

**VMA** vanillylmandelic acid.

**vocal** Pertaining to the voice or the organs of speech.

**vocalization** \vō′kəlīzā′shən\ **epileptic v.** VOCAL EPILEPSY. **iterative v.** See under VOCAL EPILEPSY.

**Voegtlin** [Carl *Voegtlin*, Swiss-born U.S. physiologist, born 1879] See under UNIT.

**Voges** [Daniel Wilhelm Otto *Voges*, German physician, born 1867] Voges-Proskauer test, Voges-Proskauer reaction. See under REACTION.

**Vogt** [Alfred *Vogt*, Swiss ophthalmologist, 1879–1943] **1** Vogt's disease. See under DOUBLE ATHETOSIS. **2** Limbal girdle of Vogt. See under GIRDLE. **3** Vogt-Koyanagi syndrome. See under SYNDROME.

**Vogt** [Oskar *Vogt*, German neurologist, 1870–1959] **1** See under SYNDROME. **2** Vogt-Spielmeyer disease. See under JUVENILE CEROID-LIPOFUSCINOSIS.

**voice** [Old French *vois* (from L *vox*, gen. *vocis*, voice, akin to *vocare* to call) a voice] **1** The characteristic, relatively low frequency sound which arises from the periodic excitation of the expiratory air flow by the alternating movements of adduction and abduction of the vocal folds. The fundamental frequency of the voice may be varied at will to produce differing patterns of intonation. **2** The component of laryngeal excitation which takes place during the articulation of voiced speech sounds, resulting in a linguistically meaningful contrast such as between the unvoiced "t" and the voiced "d." **bronchial v.** BRONCHOPHONY. **eunuchoid v.** An anomalous high-pitched or falsetto voice characteristic of some adolescent and adult male speakers. **myxedema v.** The hoarse somewhat muted voice occurring in a proportion of adults with well-established myxedema.

**voiceprint** A spectrogram that plots the frequencies of speech versus time. It permits discrimination between the different phonetic components of speech and aids in identification of the speaker, although it does not, despite the intentional analogy with "fingerprint," have the uniqueness and facility of identification of a fingerprint.

**void** To empty or evacuate; to eliminate as waste.

**Voillemier** [Léon Clémont *Voillemier*, French urologist, 1809–1878] See under POINT.

**vol** volume.

**vola** \vō′lə\ [L, the hollow of the hand or foot, palm, sole] A concave or hollow surface; palm; sole. **v. manus** *Outmoded* PALMA MANUS. **v. pedis** *Outmoded* PLANTA PEDIS.

**volar** \vō′lər\ Pertaining to the palm of the hand or sole of the foot; palmar or plantar.

**volaris** \vōler′is\ PALMARIS.

**volatile** \väl′ətəl\ [L *volatil(is)* (from *volat(us)*, past part. of *volare* to fly + *-ilis* -ILE) flying, swift, fleeting] Characterized by rapid evaporation.

**volatilize** \väl′ətəlīz′\ To evaporate, or turn into vapor from the liquid or solid state.

**volenti non fit injuria** [L, he who consents cannot receive an injury] ASSUMPTION OF RISK. See under RISK.

**volition** \vōlish′ən\ [French (from Med L *volitio* volition, from L *vol-*, stem of *velle* to wish, be willing, + *-itio* -ITION), the act by which the will makes a determination] The act or process of consciously selecting a course of action directed toward some end or goal, and of initiating and sustaining whatever behavior may be required to achieve it. Adj. volitional.

**Volkmann** [Alfred Wilhelm *Volkmann*, German physiologist, 1800–1877] Volkmann's canals. See under CANAL.

**Volkmann** [Richard von *Volkmann*, German surgeon, 1830–1889] **1** See under SUBLUXATION. **2** Volkmann's ischemic paralysis, Volkmann's paralysis, Volkmann syndrome. See under VOLKMANN'S ISCHEMIC CONTRACTURE.

**volley** [Middle French *volee* (from L *volata*, fem. of *volatus*, past part. of *volare* to fly) the act of flying, a volley] Synchronized electrical activity of several axons excited simultaneously. **antidromic v.** Nerve impulse conduction induced by electrical excitation to travel in a direction opposite to that of physiological activity.

**Vollmer** [Herman *Vollmer*, U.S. pediatrician, 1896–1959] See under TEST.

**volsella** \välsel′ə\ [L (from *vols(us)*, also *vulsus*, past part. of *vellere* to pluck, pull, + *-ella*, diminishing suffix), a pair of tweezers, pincers] VOLSELLA FORCEPS.

**volt** [after Alessandro *Volta*, Italian physicist, 1745–1827] The special name for the SI derived units of electrical potential, potential difference, and electromotive force, equal to the difference of electrical potential between two points on a conductor carrying a constant current of one ampere, when the power dissipated between these points is equal to one watt; 1 volt = 1 watt/1 ampere. Symbol: V

**voltage** [VOLT + -AGE] The electromotive force, potential, or potential difference, measured in volts, which causes current to flow in an electric circuit. **effective v.** **1** For an alternating voltage, the root-mean square voltage. **2** For a sinusoidally varying voltage, $\frac{1}{\sqrt{2}}$ times the peak voltage. **inverse v.** The half-cycle of alternating current in which there is no or minimal current flow through the electrical component or equipment. **peak v.** The maximal electric potential of a pulsating supply or of an alternating supply during the half-cycle in which flow of current occurs. **pulsating v.** An electrical potential which is unidirectional but varies in magnitude at a periodic frequency. **ripple v.** RIPPLE POTENTIAL.

**voltaic** \vältā′ik\ Pertaining to electricity produced by chemical action.

**voltammeter** \vōltäm′ətər\ A device to measure both volts and amperes.

**voltmeter** \vōlt′mētər\ An instrument for measuring electrical voltage. **electrostatic v.** A voltmeter which works by measuring the force exerted between stationary electric charges. **sphere gap v.** An instrument designed to measure high voltages by determining the distance between two metal spheres at which a spark will jump.

**volume** [L *volumen* (gen. *voluminis*, from *volvere* to wind round, roll, to make by rolling, akin to Gk *eilyein* to wrap around) a thing rolled up, volume, fold] A measure of the quantity of space occupied by something. **alveolar v.** The volume of air in the alveoli of the lungs. **alveolar dead-space v.** The volume of air ventilating unperfused alveoli and which cannot therefore participate in gas exchange. **v. content** The volume of a component of a system divided by the mass of the system, expressed in cubic meters per kilogram. Symbol: $V_C/m_S$ **v. of distribution** The volume of body fluid in which a marker or solute is uniformly distributed. It is determined by dividing the original amount of material by its concentration in an appropriate specimen after equilibrium is reached. The physical and physiologic properties of the solute determine which fluid compartments it will enter and how long it will remain. **end-diastolic v.** The volume of blood in a ventricle at the end of diastole. **end-systolic v.** The volume of blood in a ventricle at the end of systole. **expiratory reserve v.** The volume in excess of the tidal volume which can be expired from the lungs by a maximum expiratory effort. Also *supplemental air* (obs.). Abbr. ERV **forced expiratory v.** FORCED VITAL CAPACITY. **forced expired v.** FORCED VITAL CAPACITY. Abbr. FEV • *FEV* is commonly used with a numerical subscript. For example, $FEV_1$ refers to the maximal amount of air that can be expired in one second, $FEV_2$ in two seconds, etc. The most common timed periods are one and three seconds. **gram-molecular v.** The volume occupied by one mole of substance in the gaseous state at a temperature of 0°C and a pressure of one standard atmosphere. For an ideal gas, the gram-molecular volume is 22.242 liters. **inspiratory reserve v.** The volume of a gas in excess of the tidal volume that can be drawn into the lungs by a maximum inspiratory effort. Abbr. IRV **inspiratory triggering v.** In a mechanical ventilator, a predetermined volume of gas which triggers the cycle to expiration. **maximal expiratory v.** The maximum volume of air that can be exhaled. **mean corpuscular v.** The average erythrocyte volume, in cubic microns, calculated by dividing the hematocrit (times ten) by the erythrocyte count. Abbr. MCV **minute v.** The volume of gas expelled from the lungs in one minute. This is the product of tidal volume and respiratory rate. **normal v.** STANDARD VOLUME. **packed-cell v.** HEMATOCRIT. Abbr. PCV **partial v.** The volume occupied by one type of molecule or particle in a solution. It is the reciprocal of the density of the molecule or particle. **v. percent** The number of milliliters of a substance in 100 milliliters of the medium: usually applied to gas contained in blood Symbol: vol % **residual v.** The volume remaining in the lungs and respiratory passages after a maximum expiration. Abbr. RV **standard v.** The volume of one mole of gas at a temperature of 0°C and a pressure of one standard atmosphere. Also *normal volume.* **stroke v.** The quantity of blood ejected from a ventricle during systole. Abbr. SV **target v.** That volume of tissues whose irradiation is considered useful in the course of radiotherapy and which comprises the tumor and the adjacent tissues prone to being invaded by it. **tidal v.** The volume of gas expired in one breath in normal respiration.

**volumetric** \väl′yəmet′rik\ [*volum(e)* + *(m)etric*] Concerning or using the measurement of volume.

**voluntary** Subject to the will; of a human action, consciously executed or inhibited.

**voluntomotory** \vō′ləntōmō′təry\ Relating to voluntary movement.

**volute** \vō′lyoot\ [L *volut(a)*, fem. of *volutus*, past part. of *volvere* to turn or wind around, roll] **1** Rolled up. **2** A spiral turn, whorl, or twist.

**volutin** \vōlyoo′tin\ See under VOLUTIN GRANULES.

**volvulate** \väl′vyəlāt\ To form a volvulus.

**volvulosis** \väl′vyəlō′sis\ ONCHOCERCIASIS.

**volvulus** \väl′vyələs\ [New L (from L *volvere* to wind round, roll, to make by rolling; see VOLUME)] A twisting or rotation of a tubular viscus, usually a part of the alimentary tract, resulting in kinking which can cause obstruction or necrosis of the affected segment. **v. of the colon** Volvulus affecting the colon, usually the cecum or sigmoid colon. **gastric v.** Volvulus of the stomach, which can occur in an organoaxial and mesenteroaxial form. The organoaxial form is associated with paraesophageal hernia. Also *volvulus of the stomach.*

**vomer** \vō′mer\ [L, plowshare] [NA] A thin, flat trapezoid-shaped bone that forms the posteroinferior part of the nasal septum. The superior margin fits against the rostrum of the sphenoid, the posterior margin separates the choanae, and the inferior margin articulates with the nasal crest. The upper half of the anterior margin articulates with the perpendicular plate of the ethmoid bone while the lower half joins the cartilage of the nasal septum. Adj. vomerine.

**vomit** [L *vomitus* (from *vomere* to vomit, akin to Gk *emein* to vomit) vomiting, emesis] **1** To eject the stomach contents through the mouth in a sudden, forceful fashion, usually associated with nausea. **2** The ejected stomach contents. **Barcoo v.** A disease seen in southern Australia and characterized by nausea, vomiting, and excessive hunger. **bilious v.** Vomit containing bile, often associated with intestinal obstruction or occurring after gastric surgery. **black v.** COFFEE-GROUND VOMIT. **coffee-ground v.** Vomit containing blood denatured by gastric acid, resulting in black particles which resemble coffee grounds. Also *black vomit, melenemesis.*

**vomiting** The retrograde forcible expulsion of gastric contents through the mouth. Also *emesis, emesia, vomition.* **cerebral v.** PROJECTILE VOMITING. **cyclical v.** Recurrent or periodic vomiting, often associated with acidosis. It is a common disorder in children, possibly related to migraine. Also *periodic vomiting, periodic syndrome.* **dry v.** Vigorous attempts at vomiting without expulsion of gastric contents. **explosive v.** PROJECTILE VOMITING. **fecal v.** The act of vomiting malodorous, putrified material resembling feces, often associated with intestinal obstruction. Also *stercoraceous vomiting, fecal emesis, copremesis.* **morning v.** Vomiting experienced by pregnant women, usually during the first trimester and often most severely in the morning hours. The condition is felt to be secondary to rapidly increasing estrogen levels. Also *vomiting of pregnancy, vomitus gravidarum.* **periodic v.** CYCLICAL VOMITING. **pernicious v.** Excessive vomiting during pregnancy, such that the mother becomes severely dehydrated. **v. of pregnancy** MORNING VOMITING. **projectile v.** Vomiting which occurs suddenly, without antecedent nausea or retching, in meningitis and in various intracranial diseases accompanied by increased intracranial pressure. It may occur either spontaneously or when the patient changes his position. Also *cerebral vomiting, explosive vomiting.* **stercoraceous v.** FECAL VOMITING.

**vomition** \vämish′ən\ VOMITING.

**vomitive** \väm′itiv\ **1** Relating to or inducing vomiting; emetic. **2** An emetic or vomitory. An old-fashioned usage.

**vomitory** \väm′itôr′ē\ *Older term* EMETIC.

**vomiturition** \väm′ichərish′ən\ Repeated bouts of dry vomiting. *Older term.*

**vomitus** \väm′itəs\ **1** Vomit; vomited material. **2** Emesis; vomiting. **v. cruentus** Vomit containing blood; hematemesis. *Older term.* **v. gravidarum** MORNING VOMITING. **v. matutinus** Morning vomiting, as in early pregnancy, alcoholic gastritis, or certain other conditions.

**von Baer** See under BAER.

**von Economo** See under ECONOMO.

**von Gierke** [Edgar Otto Konrad *von Gierke*, German pathologist, 1877–1945] Von Gierke's disease. See under GLYCOGEN STORAGE DISEASE I.

**von Hippel** [Eugen *von Hippel*, German ophthalmologist, 1867–1939] Von Hippel-Lindau syndrome. See under SYNDROME.

**von Kossa** [Julius *von Kossa*, Hungarian pharmacologist, born 1865] See under STAIN.

**von Kupffer** See under KUPFFER.

**von Langenbeck** [Bernhard Rudolf Konrad *von Langenbeck*, German surgeon, 1810–1887] See under OPERATION, FLAP.

**von Leber** See under LEBER.

**von Mikulicz** See under MIKULICZ.

**von Monakow** See under MONAKOW.

**von Pirquet** [Clemens Freiherr *von Pirquet*, Austrian pediatrician, 1874–1929] Von Pirquet's cutireaction, von Pirquet's reaction. See under REACTION.

**von Recklinghausen** See under RECKLINGHAUSEN.

**Von Sallmann** [Ludwig *Von Sallmann*, Austrian-born U.S. ophthalmologist, 1892–1975] Witkop-Von Sallmann disease. See under DISEASE.

**von Tröltsch** [Anton Friedrich *von Tröltsch*, German otologist, 1829–1890] 1 Tröltsch spaces. See under SPACE. 2 Recesses of Tröltsch. See under RECESS. 3 Anterior pouch of Tröltsch. See under RECESSUS MEMBRANAE TYMPANI ANTERIOR. 4 Posterior pouch of Tröltsch. See under RECESSUS MEMBRANAE TYMPANI POSTERIOR.

**von Willebrand** [Erik Adolph *von Willebrand*, Finnish physician, 1870–1949] 1 Willebrand syndrome. See under VON WILLEBRAND'S DISEASE. 2 Willebrand factor. See under FACTOR VIIIR:AG.

**Voorhees** [James D. *Voorhees*, U.S. obstetrician, 1869–1929] See under BAG.

**vortex** \vôr′teks\ [L (gen. *vorticis*). See VERTEX.] (*pl.* vortices) A structure with a whorled or spiral arrangement or design. **v. coccygeus** The spiral arrangement of hairs occasionally found over the tip of the coccyx. *Outmoded.* Also *coccygeal vortex, coccygeal whorl.* **Fleischer's v.** A rare congenital anomaly affecting the lamina limitans anterior corneae such that colored lines appear to spiral outwards from its center, producing corneal opacity. **v. of heart** The area at the apex of the heart where the spirally arranged bundles of cardiac muscle fibers form a whirlpool pattern. **v. lentis** The starlike pattern on the surface of the crystalline lens of the eye produced by the radii lentis. **vortices pilorum** [NA] Spiral patterns of hair growth, as on the scalp.

**vortices** \vôr′tisēz\ Plural of VORTEX.

**vorticose** \vôr′tikōs\ Having a whorled pattern.

**v. o. s.** *vitello ovi solutus* (L, dissolved in egg yolk).

**Vossius** [Adolf *Vossius*, German ophthalmologist, 1855–1925] See under RING.

**voussure** \voosʏr′\ [French (from L *volutus*, past part. of *volvere* to turn, curve) vault, arch] Undue prominence of the precordium due to enlargement of the heart in infancy, as a consequence of congenital heart disease.

**vox** \väks\ [L, voice] The voice. **v. cholerica** The peculiar suppressed voice sometimes noted in persons with cholera.

**voyeurism** \voi′yərizm\ [French *voyeur* a watcher, onlooker, + -ISM] A paraphilia in which sexual gratification is dependent upon watching one or more people who are nude, undressing, or engaging in sexual intercourse. The watching or later recall of the scene gives the subject his gratification as he makes no attempt to establish further contact with those he observes. Also *scopophilia, scopolagnia, scoptolagnia, scoptophilia.*

**VPC** volume of packed cells (packed-cell volume).

**VPF** vascular permeability factor.

**V-plasty** \vē′-plas′tē\ A method of obtaining additional diameter in the lumen of a hollow body structure. A linear incision is made in the axial direction of the wall of the structure, and the resulting defect is filled in with a V-shaped flap.

**VPRC** volume of packed red cells.

**VR** vocal resonance.

**Vrolik** [Willem *Vrolik*, Dutch physician, 1801–1863] Vrolik's disease. See under OSTEOGENESIS IMPERFECTA CONGENITA.

**VS** 1 volumetric solution. 2 ventricular septum.

**v.s.** 1 *vide supra* (L, see above). 2 vibration second.

**VSD** ventricular septal defect.

**VT** 1 ventricular tachycardia. 2 vacuum tuberculin.

**vulgaris** \vulger′is\ [L *vulgaris* common, usual] Common; not rare.

**vulgarobufotoxin** \vul′gərōbʸoo′fōtäksin\ BUFOTOXIN.

**vulnerability** \vul′nərəbil′itē\ The state of being susceptible to pathogenic agents or to injury.

**Vulpian** [Edme-Felix-Alfred *Vulpian*, French physician, 1826–1887] 1 See under LAW, EFFECT. 2 Vulpian's conjugate deviation. See under ADVERSIVE ATTACK.

**vulsella** \vulsel′ə\ [See VOLSELLA.] VOLSELLA FORCEPS.

**vulv-** \vulv-\ VULVO-.

**vulva** \vul′və\ [L (also *volva*) the womb, vulva] PUDENDUM FEMININUM. Adj. vulvar.

**vulvectomy** \vulvek′təmē\ [*vulv(a)* + -ECTOMY] Surgical removal of the vulva.

**vulvismus** \vulviz′məs\ VAGINISMUS.

**vulvitis** \vulvī′tis\ [VULV- + -ITIS] Any inflammation of the vulva. Also *edeitis.* **adhesive v.** Inflammation of the vulva which results in synechiae. **diabetic v.** Vulvovaginitis associated with copious glycosuria in diabetes mellitus. The causative agent is most commonly *Candida albicans.* **eczematiform v.** Inflammation of the vulva associated with the formation of vesicular pustules. **intertriginous v.** Superficial dermatitis of the vulva caused by moisture and rubbing of opposing surfaces, as from obesity. **plasma cell v.** A rare inflammatory lesion of the vulva, presenting clinically as a reddish brown plaque and histologically as a plasma-cell infiltrate; a form of Zoon's erythroplasia. **ulcerative v.** Inflammation of the vulva accompanied by ulceration, as in herpes or moniliasis.

**vulvo-** \vul′vō-\ [L *vulva* womb or vulva] A combining form denoting the vulva. Also *vulv-*.

**vulvopathy** \vulväp′əthē\ [VULVO- + -PATHY] Any abnormality of the vulva.

**vulvovaginal** \vul′vōvaj′ənəl\ Pertaining to the vulva and the vagina. Also *vaginovulvar.*

**vulvovaginitis** \vul′vōvajənī′tis\ [VULVO- + VAGIN- + -ITIS] Inflammation of the vagina and vulva. **mycotic v.** Candidiasis affecting the vulva and vagina, or the vulvovaginal glands.

**v/v** volume/volume: used following a designation of concentration, as of percentage.

**vv** veins.

**VW** vessel wall.

# W

**W** 1 Symbol for the unit, watt. 2 Symbol for the element, tungsten.

**w** Symbol for the unit, watt An incorrect symbol.

**w̄** with

**Waaler** [Erik *Waaler,* Norwegian biologist, flourished 20th century] Waaler-Rose test, Waaler-Rose reaction. See under ROSE-WAALER TEST.

**Waardenburg** [Petrus Johannes *Waardenburg,* Dutch ophthalmologist, born 1886] See under SYNDROME.

**wadding** \wäd′ing\ A surgical dressing made of cotton or other absorbent material that is used to protect and cover a wound.

**Wade** [Dewitt Clinton *Wade,* U.S. physician, 1838–1904] Wade's balsam. See under COMPOUND BENZOIN TINCTURE.

**wafer** A drug preparation in which the drug is sandwiched between thin disks of flour paste, dried, and sealed. This method of formulating drugs so that they could be swallowed without tasting the ingredients has been largely replaced by capsules and coated pills.

**Wagner** [Ernst Leberecht *Wagner,* German pathologist, 1829–1888] 1 Wagner's disease. See under COLLOID MILIUM. 2 See under LINE.

**waist** [Old English *wæst* growth, akin to *weaxen* to grow] The part of the body between the twelfth ribs and the iliac crests.

**Waldenström** [Jan Goesta *Waldenström,* Swedish physician, born 1906] 1 See under TEST, MACROGLOBULINEMIA. 2 Waldenström's hyperglobulinemic purpura. See under PURPURA HYPERGLOBULINEMICA.

**Waldenström** [Johann Henning *Waldenström,* Swedish physician, born 1877] Waldenström's disease. See under PERTHES DISEASE.

**Waldeyer** [Heinrich Wilhelm Gottfried *Waldeyer,* German anatomist, 1836–1921] 1 Waldeyer's layer. See under GERMINAL EPITHELIUM. 2 See under FOSSA. 3 Waldeyer's fossa. See under MESENTERICOPARIETAL FOSSA. 4 Waldeyer's glands. See under GLAND. 5 Waldeyer's ring. See under TONSILLAR RING. 6 Zona vasculosa of Waldeyer. See under MEDULLA OVARII. 7 Waldeyer's layer. See under EPITHELIUM SUPERFICIALE OVARII.

**Walker** [Arthur Earl *Walker,* U.S. neurologist, born 1907] Dandy-Walker deformity. See under DANDY-WALKER SYNDROME.

**Walker** [George *Walker,* U.S. surgeon, born 1869] Walker carcinosarcoma 256. See under SARCOMA.

**Walker** [J. T. Ainslie *Walker,* English chemist, 1868–1930]. Rideal-Walker test. See under TEST.

**walking** / **chromosome w.** In molecular genetics, a procedure for isolating and determining the nucleotide sequence of extended regions of a chromosome by means of the sequential isolation and cloning of overlapping oligonucleotides. **heel w.** Walking on the heels to avoid pressure on hypersensitive soles, as seen in some patients with peripheral neuropathy. **reflex w.** Ambulatory movements seen in a spinal animal when it is held so that its feet contact a moving treadmill.

**wall** The boundary of a cavity, hollow organ, or cell; paries. **basal w.** *Outmoded* MUREIN. **capillary w. of glomerulus** The fenestrated layer of epithelial cells and their interdigitating pedicels resting on a basement membrane of the glomerular capsule which separates it from the endothelium of the capillaries of the renal glomerulus. **cavity w.** A part of the surface of a prepared dental cavity. **cell w.** The nonliving, rigid or semirigid covering outside the cell membrane of prokaryotic cells and plant cells. It is secreted by the cell. **gingival cavity w.** The cavity wall nearest to the gingiva. Also *gingival wall.* **inferior w. of tympanic cavity** PARIES JUGULARIS CAVITATIS TYMPANICAE. **jugular w. of tympanic cavity** PARIES JUGULARIS CAVITATIS TYMPANICAE. **labyrinthine w. of middle ear** PARIES LABYRINTHICUS CAVITATIS TYMPANICAE. **medial w. of middle ear** PARIES LABYRINTHICUS CAVITATIS TYMPANICAE. **w. of nail** VALLUM UNGUIS. **parietal w.** SOMATOPLEURE. **splanchnic w.** SPLANCHNOPLEURE. **superior w. of orbit** PARIES SUPERIOR ORBITAE. **tegmental w. of middle ear** PARIES TEGMENTALIS CAVITATIS TYMPANICAE. **tympanic w. of cochlear duct** PARIES TYMPANICUS DUCTUS COCHLEARIS. **vestibular w. of cochlear duct** PARIES VESTIBULARIS DUCTUS COCHLEARIS. **visceral w.** SPLANCHNOPLEURE.

**Wallenberg** [Adolf *Wallenberg,* German physician, 1862–1949] See under SYNDROME.

**Waller** [Augustus Volney *Waller,* English physiologist, 1816–1870] 1 See under LAW. 2 Wallerian degeneration. See under DEGENERATION.

**walleye** \wôl′ī′\ EXOTROPIA.

**Wallgren** [Arvid Johann *Wallgren,* Swedish physician, born 1898] Wallgren's aseptic meningitis. See under LYMPHOCYTIC CHORIOMENINGITIS.

**Walsham** [William Johnson *Walsham,* English surgeon, 1847–1903] See under FORCEPS.

**Walthard** [Max *Walthard,* Swiss gynecologist, 1867–1933] 1 Walthard's inclusions. See under WALTHARD'S CELL NESTS. 2 Walthard's islets. See under ISLET.

**Walther** [Augustine Friedrich *Walther,* German anatomist and botanist, 1688–1746] 1 Canals of Walther, Walther's ducts. See under DUCTUS SUBLINGUALES MINORES. 2 Walther's ganglion. See under GANGLION IMPAR.

**wandering** Movement, as of a cell, from one location to another. **w. of a tooth** The migration of a tooth.

**wanderlust** \wän′dərlust, vän′dərlŭst\ [German *wander(n)* to wander, travel + *Lust* joy] Pathologic desire, sometimes compulsive in nature, to wander and roam away from home. Also *vagabond neurosis.*

**Wangensteen** [Owen H. *Wangensteen,* U.S. surgeon, born 1898] See under DRAINAGE.

**Warburg** [Otto Heinrich *Warburg,* German biochemist and physiologist, 1883–1970] 1 See under TECHNIQUE, THEORY. 2 Warburg vessel. See under APPARATUS.

**Ward** [Frederick O. *Ward,* British osteologist, 1818–1877] See under TRIANGLE.

**ward** [Old English *weard* a watch, guard, surveillance] A large room or defined area occupied by many patients or beds in a hospital or other health care facility. **isolation w.** A hospital ward especially for persons having or suspected of having a communicable disease. **psychopathic w.** *Older term* PSYCHIATRIC UNIT.

**Wardill** [William Edward Mandall *Wardill,* English surgeon, born 1894] See under METHOD.

**warfare** / **biological w.** The use in warfare of biological agents, such as pathogenic microorganisms, toxins, or disease vectors. **chemical w.** The use in warfare of chemical agents other than explosives, such as war gases, incendiary mixtures, and defoliants.

**warfarin sodium** $C_{19}H_{15}NaO_4$. 3-(α-Acetonybenzyl)-4-hydroxycoumarin. A crystalline powder, soluble in water and alcohol, very slightly soluble in ether. It is used as a rodenticide and clinically as an anticoagulant.

**warm-blooded** HOMEOTHERMIC.

**Warren** [W. Dean *Warren*, U.S. surgeon, born 1924] Warren shunt. See under DISTAL SPLENORENAL SHUNT.

**wart** \wôrt\ [Old English *wearte*, akin to L *verruca* wart, excrescence] A benign keratotic tumor most often induced by a papovavirus. Also *verruca*. **acuminate w.** CONDYLOMA ACUMINATUM. **anatomical w.** TUBERCULOSIS CUTIS VERRUCOSA. **common w.** A benign tumor of the skin caused by an infection with the human papovavirus. It is a common tumor of childhood and young adult life. Also *verruca vulgaris*. **digitate w.** The digitate form of the common wart, seen most often on the scalp. Also *verruca digitata*. **filiform w.** A threadlike form of the common wart. It most often arises on the face. Also *verruca filiformis*. **fugitive w.** A wart of brief duration. **genital w.** CONDYLOMA ACUMINATUM. **Hassall-Henle w.'s** HASSALL-HENLE BODIES. **juvenile plane w.** PLANE WART. **mosaic w.** A group of contiguous plantar warts. **mother w.** The one wart in a group of warts that was once believed to be the progenitor of the other warts in the group. It was formerly held that the mother wart had to be eradicated in order to effect a complete eradication of the group. **mucocutaneous w.** A common wart found at a mucocutaneous junction. **necrogenic w.** TUBERCULOSIS CUTIS VERRUCOSA. **pathologist's w.** TUBERCULOSIS CUTIS VERRUCOSA. **periungual w.** A common wart at the nail fold. **Peruvian w.** VERRUGA PERUANA. **pitch w.'s** Hyperkeratotic lesions which occur on skin exposed to pitch and tar. They at first resemble keratoacanthoma, clinically and histologically, and resolve spontaneously. Later they may develop into squamous carcinoma. **plane w.** A flat form of the common wart which is seen most often on the face and the backs of the hands in children. Also *juvenile plane wart, verruca plana*. **plantar w.** A common wart on the plantar surface of the foot or the toes. Also *verruca plantaris*. **postmortem w.** TUBERCULOSIS CUTIS VERRUCOSA. **prosector's w.** TUBERCULOSIS CUTIS VERRUCOSA. **seed w.** A small wart secondary to or derived from a larger wart. **soft w.** CUTANEOUS FIBROUS POLYP. **soot w.** A lesion on the scrotum occurring in the early stage of chimney-sweeps' cancer. **telangiectatic w.** ANGIOKERATOMA. **tuberculous w.** TUBERCULOSIS CUTIS VERRUCOSA.

**Wartenberg** [Robert *Wartenberg*, German neurologist, 1887–1956] **1** Wartenberg's paresthetic neuralgia, Wartenberg's disease, Wartenberg syndrome. See under CHEIRALGIA PARESTHETICA. **2** See under PHENOMENON. **3** Wartenberg symptom. See under SIGN.

**Warthin** [Aldred Scott *Warthin*, U.S. pathologist, 1866–1931] **1** Warthin's tumor. See under ADENOLYMPHOMA. **2** Warthin-Starry silver stain. See under STAIN. **3** Warthin-Finkeldey cell. See under CELL.

**warty** \wôr'tē\ [WART + -Y] **1** Hard and rough. **2** Resembling a wart; verrucous.

**wash / jet w.** See under IRRIGATION CANNULA.

**washing** The removal of unwanted soluble material from a precipitate or suspension of cells. Fluid is added to the material, which is centrifuged. The supernatant is removed, and the cells are resuspended in fresh medium. Repeated suspension and centrifugation are often needed for complete removal of highly concentrated or tenacious material.

**Wasmann** [Adolphus *Wasmann*, German anatomist, flourished 19th century] Wasmann's gland. See under GLANDULA GASTRICA PROPRIA.

**washout / nitrogen w.** See under TEST.

**Wasmann** [Adolphus *Wasmann*, German anatomist, flourished 19th century] Wasmann's gland. See under GLANDULA GASTRICA PROPRIA.

**wasserhelle** \väs'ərhel'ə\ [German *Wasser* water + *hell* bright, clear] A cell of the parathyroid gland which has a clear swollen appearance. Such cells are abundant in adenoma of the parathyroid.

**Wassermann** [August Paul von *Wassermann*, German bacteriologist, 1866–1925] **1** See under ANTIBODY. **2** Wassermann reaction. See under TEST.

**Wassermann-fast** \was'ərmən-fast'\ Exhibiting a positive Wassermann reaction over a prolonged period in spite of treatment for syphilis.

**Wassilieff** [Nikolai Porfiryevich *Wassilieff*, Russian physician, born 1861] Wassilieff's disease. See under ICTERIC LEPTOSPIROSIS.

**wastage / birth w.** REPRODUCTIVE WASTAGE. **pregnancy w.** The spontaneous termination of pregnancy through abortion or fetal death. **reproductive w.** The combined stillbirth and infant mortality rates. Also *birth loss, birth wastage*.

**wasting** Loss of body tissues. This may be generalized, as in emaciation or cachexia, or localized, as in loss of muscle mass due to poliomyelitis. Also *macies*.

**water** [Old English *wæter* (akin to L *unda* water, the waves, Gk *hydōr* water) water] $H_2O$. A colorless liquid occurring as a constituent in all organisms and in the biological sciences widely used as a solvent. It boils at 100°C (212°F) and freezes at 0°C (32°F). **w. of adhesion** Water which is held to a solid surface by hydrogen bonds, not forming an essential part of the constitution of the molecules of the surface. **ammonia w.** DILUTED AMMONIA SOLUTION. **aniline w.** A solvent containing aniline oil in distilled water that is used to increase the solubility of certain stains. **bacteriostatic w. for injection** Sterile water for injection that contains one or more suitable bacteriostatic agents. **body w.** The water component of the body. In mammalian species including humans this is by weight approximately 73 percent of lean body mass. **cinnamon w.** A clear, saturated solution of cinnamon oil in purified water. It is used as a flavoring agent in pharmaceutic preparations. Also *aqua cinnamomi*. **concentrated anise w.** A solution prepared by mixing 2 ml of anise oil, 70 ml of 90% ethanol, and sufficient water to make a final volume of 100 ml. It is shaken with sterilized talc and filtered. It is used as a carminative and flavoring agent in cough medicines. **concentrated camphor w.** A preparation combining 4 g camphor, 60 ml of 90% ethanol, and sufficient water to make a total volume of 100 ml. It has been used as an antipruritic and mild analgesic skin medication. Also *aqua camphorae concentrata*. **concentrated caraway w.** A mixture containing 2 ml of caraway oil, 60 ml of 90% ethanol, and sufficient water to make a total volume of 100 ml. It is shaken with 5 g of sterilized talc and filtered. **deionized w.** Water chemically very pure, but not sterile, obtained by passing tap water through a column of ion exchangers. **distilled w.** Water purified by distillation. Its main impurities, therefore, are the components of dissolved air, including carbon dioxide, which renders it slightly acid. **false w.'s** A slow leakage of amniotic fluid during labor and before rupture of the fetal membranes produces a gush of fluid. **hard w.** Water containing an appreciable concentration of calcium or magnesium salts. **heavy w.** DEUTERIUM OXIDE. **w. of hydration** Water that is loosely bound to a substance, usually in definite molecular proportions, and which can be removed without changing the chemical properties of the substance. **w. for injection** Water for parenteral use that is prepared by distillation and that meets specified standards. It contains no added substances. **mineral w.** Natural spring water that has been imbibed with carbon dioxide gas. Such water contains small amounts of various minerals and is sometimes slightly alkaline. **peppermint w.** A clear, saturated solution of peppermint oil in purified water, used as a vehicle in pharmaceutic preparations. Also *aqua menthae piperitae*. **peptone w.** A solution of peptone in water which is used in the indole test for *Escherichia coli* and also as an enrichment culture medium for the isolation of *Vibrio cholerae*. **purified w.** Mineral-free water obtained by distillation or deionization and meeting the standards specified for pharmaceutical or other purposes. **rose w.** A solution of stronger rose water diluted with an equal volume of purified water. Also *aqua rosae*. **soft w.** Water that contains only a small concentration of mineral salts, particularly those of calcium and magnesium. Soft water lathers easily. **spearmint w.** A dilute aqueous solution containing spearmint oil in dilute alcohol. It is used as a carminative and flavoring agent. Also *aqua menthae viridis*. **sterile w. for injection** Water that has been sterilized and suitably packaged for injection.

**water-bite** TRENCH FOOT.

**water-borne** Spread by water, especially by contaminated water; said of communicable diseases such as typhoid fever.

**water-brash** See under BRASH.

**Waterhouse** [Rupert *Waterhouse*, British physician, 1873–1958] Waterhouse-Friderichsen syndrome. See under SYNDROME.

**Waters** [Charles Alexander *Waters*, U.S. radiologist, 1888–1961] Waters view, Waters projection. See under PROJECTION.

**waters** *Older term* AMNIOTIC FLUID.

**watershed / abdominal w.'s** The slopes in the abdominal cavity formed by the lumbar vertebrae and the brim of the pelvis, which determine the directions in which free liquid effusions gravitate when the body is supine.

**Watkins** [John Armstrong *Watkins*, U.S. physician, born 1888] Bass-Watkins test. See under TEST.

**Watkins** [Thomas James *Watkins*, U.S. gynecologist, 1863–1925] See under OPERATION.

**Watson** [Cecil James *Watson*, U.S. physician, born 1901] Watson-Schwartz reaction. See under TEST.

**Watson** [James Dewey *Watson*, U.S. molecular biologist, born 1928] **1** Watson-Crick model. See under MODEL. **2** Watson-Crick helix. See under DOUBLE HELIX.

**watt** [after James *Watt*, Scottish engineer, 1736–1819] A special name for the SI derived unit of power, radiant flux, or sound energy flux; the power which in one second gives rise to energy of one joule; 1 watt = 1 joule/second = 1 volt-ampere. Symbol: W **w. per kilogram** A unit of absorbed dose rate of an ionizing radiation, equal to one gray per second; $10^2$ rad per second. Also *joule per kilogram-second*. Symbol: W/kg, $W{\cdot}kg^{-1}$ **w. per square meter** The SI derived unit of radiant flux density, radiant exitance, irradiance, and sound intensity. Symbol: $W/m^2$, $W{\cdot}m^{-2}$ **w. per steradian** The SI derived unit of radiant intensity. For a source in a given direction, it is the radiant power leaving the source, or an element of the source, in an element of solid angle containing the given direction, divided by that element of solid angle. Symbol: W/sr, $W{\cdot}sr^{-1}$

**wattage** \wät′ij\ [WATT + -AGE] The active power output or consumption of an electric circuit in watts.

# wave

**wave** [Old English *wafian* to wave] The disturbance of particles in a medium that results in a ridge-and-trough oscillation. **a w.** The positive pressure wave in the atria or in the jugular venous pulse caused by atrial systole. **activation w.** WAVE OF EXCITATION. **alpha w.** In electroencephalography, a single wave of the alpha rhythm (8–15 Hz). **anacrotic w.** See under ANADICROTIC. **anadicrotic w.** See under ANADICROTIC. **arterial w.** The wave in the jugular venous pulse due to the transmitted impulse from the carotid arteries. **beta w.** In electroencephalography, a single wave of the beta rhythm (14–22 Hz). **brain w.'s** The waves recorded in the electroencephalogram. Also *electroencephalographic waves*. **c w.** The positive pressure wave in the atria due to reflexion of the atrioventricular valves at the commencement of ventricular systole. **cannon w.** A large venous a wave in the jugular venous pulse which occurs when the right atrium contracts against the closed tricuspid valve. It is characteristically intermittent in complete heart block but occurs with each cycle in junctional rhythm. **catacrotic w.** See under CATACROTIC. **catadicrotic w.** See under CATADICROTIC. **complex w.'s** POLYRHYTHMIC WAVES. **continuous w.** A wave emitted continuously, such as one produced by the continuous excitation of an ultrasound transducer, contrasted with a pulsed wave. Abbr. CW **contraction w.** The spreading of a contraction in a muscle from the point of stimulation, or a graphic record of such a contraction. **cove-plane T w.** Inverted T wave following a bowed ST segment elevation in acute myocardial infarction. **delta w.** **1** One of the slow brain waves, with a frequency equal to or less than 3 Hz, which may occur sporadically or may be grouped together in a delta rhythm. The waves may be monomorphic (monorhythmic waves) or polymorphic (polyrhythmic waves) if a rhythm of different frequency is superimposed. While a delta rhythm may dom inate the electroencephalogram in young infants, delta waves are always abnormal in older children or adults, occurring diffusely in disorders of cerebral metabolism or focally as a consequence of many different cerebral lesions, such as tumor or hematoma. Also *delta discharge*. **2** The initial slurred component of the R wave in the Wolff-Parkinson-White syndrome due to premature depolarization of a part of one ventricle. **dicrotic w.** The second wave in a dicrotic pulse. See under DICROTIC. **electroencephalographic w.'s** BRAIN WAVES. **electromagnetic w.'s** Waves whose propagation involves simultaneous periodic variations of the electric and magnetic field intensities, in directions perpendicular to each other and to the direction of propagation. They include radio waves, light, x rays, and gamma rays. **w. of excitation** The spreading wave of activity from the point of stimulation in an excitable tissue. Also *activation wave, stimulus wave*. **F w.** A regular "saw-tooth" wave seen in the electrocardiogram in atrial flutter. Also *flutter wave*. **ff w.'s** The low-amplitude, irregular undulations of the baseline seen in atrial fibrillation on the electrocardiogram. Also *f waves, fibrillary waves, fibrillation waves.* **fibrillary w.'s** FF WAVES. **fibrillation w.'s** FF WAVES. **flat-top w.'s** In electroencephalography, waves with a flat-topped or plateau appearance once thought to be typical of psychomotor epilepsy. Subsequently it was shown that the significant finding was not plateau or flat-topped waves going upwards, but spikes or sharp waves going downwards, and hence these waves are no longer thought to be of significance. **fluid w.** Conduction of hydromechanical force by free peritoneal fluid, used in the detection of ascites during the physical examination. **flutter w.** F WAVE. **gamma w.** In the neurogram recorded from a spinal root or peripheral nerve, the relatively small elevation formed by summation of potentials in myelinated fibers smaller in diameter and slower in conduction velocity than $\alpha$ and $\beta$ fibers. **glottal w.** The wavelike motion of the glottic soft tissues occurring during phonation. **H w.** The electromyographic wave of spikelike form representing the monosynaptic reflex response to excitation of spindle primary afferent axons by single-shock stimulation of the muscle nerve. It measures central sensitivity of the monosynaptic reflex pathway of the spindle 1a axons, exclusive of direct involvement of the peripheral sensory receptor. Also *H reflex* (imprecise). **in phase w.'s** In electroencephalography, waveforms occurring in the same direction simultaneously in a number of channels. **kappa w.'s** In electroencephalography, intermittent, slow, frontal discharges, once thought to be associated with intellectual activity such as mental arithmetic. It has since been shown that these waves are artifactual. **lambda w.'s** PHYSIOLOGIC OCCIPITAL SPIKES. **light w.'s** Electromagnetic waves capable of stimulating the retina. **longitudinal w.** A wave in which the direction of motion of particles of the medium is parallel to the direction of wave propagation. **microelectric w.** MICROWAVE. **monomorphic w.'s** MONORHYTHMIC WAVES. **monorhythmic w.'s** Brain waves which give a simple sinusoidal tracing in the EEG. A well-developed alpha rhythm may give this appearance, as may generalized delta activity. Also *monomorphic waves.* **P w.** The component of the electrocardiogram which is due to atrial activation. It is the first reflection of the electrical cardiac cycle. **papillary w.** PERCUSSION WAVE. **percussion w.** The ascending portion of the pulse wave tracing. Also *papillary wave.* **peristaltic w.** A wave of peristalsis; one of a series of contractions of a muscular tubular organ such as the alimentary tract. **phrenic w.** DIAPHRAGM PHENOMENON. **P mitrale w.** A bifid P wave on the electrocardiogram seen particularly in mitral stenosis, but also in other conditions with left atrial hypertrophy or hypertension. **polymorphic w.'s** POLYRHYTHMIC WAVES. **polyrhythmic w.'s** Complex brain waves appearing in the EEG, often with several components of different frequency. These waves may occur successively in regular or irregular patterns. Also *complex wave, polymorphic wave.* **postextrasystolic T w.** The T wave of the sinus beat following an extrasystolic beat. **P pulmonale w.** A sharply peaked P wave on the electrocardiogram characteristic of right atrial hypertension or hypertrophy. It is usually a consequence of pulmonary hypertension, but it may also be due to tricuspid stenosis. **pulse w.** The wave due to venous or arterial pulsation perceived by touch or by a graphic recording. **Q w.** The initial negative component of the QRS complex. It is usually due to septal depolarization and becomes broad and deep over an area of myocardial infarction. **QS w.** A single negative wave representing the QRS complex of the electrocardiogram, no positive R deflection being present. It may be a normal finding in certain leads, such as a VR or $V_1$, but often signifies myocardial infarction in other leads. **R w.** The positive deflection of the QRS complex of the electrocardiogram. **random w.'s** Irregular brain waves of no fixed frequency. They appear in the electroencephalogram in early sleep. **recoil w.** The second of the two waves in a dicrotic pulse. **S w.** The negative deflection which follows an R wave of the QRS complex. **sharp w.** SLOW SPIKE. **shear w.** A wave in an elastic medium in which the displacement of an element of the medium is at right angles to the direction of wave propagation. **sine w.** A waveform of periodic oscillations in which the amplitude of each point is proportional to the sine of the time and which results, for example, from an alternating current generator. **slow occipital w.'s** SLOW POSTERIOR WAVES. **slow posterior w.'s** Slow waves of delta frequency interrupting the alpha rhythm, and occurring in the posterior temporal and occipital regions, either unilaterally or bilaterally, but more especially on the right side, in some patients with behavior disorders. They are uncommon in adults but not infrequent in children and adolescents. Also *slow occipital waves.* **standing w.'s** A constant repetitive wave appearance of arteries seen occasionally during angiography. **Stephenson's w.** A surge of congestion of the vasculature of the female pelvis during the menstrual cycle. There is a gradual increase of congestion premenstrually, a stationary peak is reached during menses, and then there is a gradual decrease. **stimulus w.** WAVE OF EXCITATION. **T w.** The deflection of the electrocardiogram which is due to ventricular repolarization. It follows the QRS complex, from which it is separated by the ST segment. **theta w.** A single wave of the theta rhythm, usually used to denote an electroencephalographic wave with the frequency of 4–7 Hz. **tidal w.** The second and lesser of the two waves which comprise the main systolic arterial pulse wave. Its precise cause is uncertain. **transverse w.** A wave in which the varying quantity is a vector and is perpendicular to the direction of propagation. **traveling w.** The pattern of deformation of the basilar membrane in response to a sound stimulus. The wavelike deformation starts at the basal end of the cochlea and travels along the basilar membrane in response to high-intensity sound levels. **U w.** The deflection on the electrocardiogram following the T wave. Its genesis is uncertain. **v w.** The wave which occurs in the atria during ventricular systole. It is usually due to the filling of the atria while the atrioventricular valves are closed but in mitral or tricuspid regurgitation is augmented by the blood which regurgitates from the relevant ventricle. **$V_1$ w.** A wave representing the summation of F and H wave components of the electromyographic response to peripheral nerve stimulation as recorded from hand and other distally located muscles. **$V_2$ w.** A late wave (e.g., at 50 ms in hand muscles) in the electromyographic response to stimulation of a muscle nerve. It represents a long-loop reflex, perhaps involving the cerebral cortex. **x w.** The negative pressure wave in the atria caused by atrial relaxation. **y w.** The negative pressure wave in the atria caused by emptying of the atria following the opening of the atrioventricular valves and prior to atrial systole.

**waveform** The graphical representation of a wave obtained by plotting the magnitude of a physical variable such as voltage, pressure, or flow usually versus time. Also *waveshape.*

**wavelength** In a periodic wave, the distance between two points at the same phase in consecutive cycles. **effective w.** The wavelength of monochromatic x rays which would have the same absorption or attenuation in a specified absorber as the heterogeneous beam being considered. Also *equivalent wavelength*. **equivalent w.** EFFECTIVE WAVELENGTH. **minimum w.** The shortest wavelength in a spectrum of x rays. Also *quantum limit*.

**wavemeter** \wāv′mētər\ A device to measure the wavelength of electromagnetic radiation.

**waveshape** WAVEFORM.

**wax** [Old English *weax*] Any high-melting, hydrophobic substance; especially, in biology, any of the esters formed between long-chain fatty acids and fatty alcohols and found in plants, especially on their leaves, or formed by animals. **baseplate w.** A high-fusing wax mixture used for baseplates and occlusion rims. **bone w.** An antiseptic wax mixture used in bone surgery. **casting w.** A wax mixture used in patterns for casting in dentistry. Also *inlay wax*. **w. D** See under MYCOBACTERIAL WAX D. **emulsifying w.** A mixture of cetostearyl alcohol and sodium laural sulfate, or similar sulfated higher alcohol, used as a water-soluble base in ointments and creams for external application. **Horsley's bone w.** HORSLEY'S PUTTY. **inlay w.** CASTING WAX. **mycobacterial w. D** A glycolipid, containing peptide residues, from the basal wall of mycobacteria. It enhances the immunogenicity of other antigens. **sticky w.** An adherent yellow wax used in dentistry for the temporary fixation of components. **white w.** Bleached and purified beeswax (yellow wax), used as a component of ointments. Also *bleached beeswax*. **yellow w.** The wax obtained from the honeycomb of the bee, *Apis mellifera*. After purification and bleaching, it is used as a base and an emulsifying agent in ointments. Also *unbleached beeswax, beeswax*.

**waxing** The making of a wax pattern or denture base. Also *waxing-up*.

**waxing-up** WAXING.

**WBC** 1 white blood cell (leukocyte). 2 white blood-cell count.

**WDLL** well-differentiated lymphocytic (malignant) lymphoma (lymphocytic lymphosarcoma).

**weal** \wēl\ WHEAL.

**wean** [Middle English *wenen*, from Old English *wenian* to accustom] To change the total dependence of (the young of any mammal) from mother's milk or milk from another source to different forms of nourishment, usually including solid foods.

**wear** / **interproximal w.** The wear of proximal surfaces of teeth by the relative physiological movement of one tooth against another, especially when the diet is abrasive, producing flat opposing surfaces at the contact areas. The space formed by the loss of enamel is taken up by mesial drift. **occlusal w.** The wear of the occlusal surfaces of teeth by attrition, producing a gradual reduction in cusp and ridge height.

**weasand** \wē′zənd\ [Old English *wāsend* windpipe] 1 *Obs.* TRACHEA. 2 The throat, in general.

**web** [Old English, woven cloth, fabric] 1 The fibrillary component of cell cytoplasm. 2 Any tissue or membrane, especially when bridging a space between structures, as between the digits of an animal. **w. of duodenum** A congenital anomalous layer either of dense or of filmy tissue within the lumen of the duodenum which produces a partial or total obstruction. **esophageal w.** A congenital weblike stricture usually occurring in the lower esophagus and causing dysphagia. **subsynaptic w.** A network of fine channels penetrating into a postsynaptic cell. **terminal w.** The fibrillar cytoplasm beneath the microvilli of the absorbing cells of the intestinal mucosa.

**webbing** The appearance or formation of a web or web-like structure. **congenital w. of the neck** PTERYGIUM COLLI. **skin w.** A scar contracture joining two adjacent structures that are normally not connected. This commonly occurs between proximal fingers, the neck and chest, and the upper arm and chest wall.

**Weber** [Ernst Heinrich *Weber*, German anatomist, 1795–1878] 1 See under LAW, TEST. 2 Weber-Fechner law. See under LAW.

**Weber**

**Weber** [Sir Hermann David *Weber*, English physician, 1823–1918] Weber's paralysis. See under SYNDROME.

**Weber** [Moritz Ignaz *Weber*, German anatomist, 1795–1875] 1 Weber's glands. See under GLAND. 2 Weber zone. See under ZONA ORBICULARIS ARTICULATIONIS COXAE.

**Weber** [Wilhelm Eduard *Weber*, German physicist and physiologist, 1804–1891] 1 See under POINT. 2 Von Weber's triangle. See under TRIANGLE.

**weber** \vā′bər, web′ər\ [after Wilhelm Eduard *Weber*, German physicist and physiologist, 1804–1891] Special name for the SI derived unit of magnetic flux; the magnetic flux which, linking a circuit of one turn, produces in it an electromotive force of one volt if reduced to zero at a uniform rate in one second; 1 weber = 1 volt × 1 second. Symbol: Wb

**web-eye** PTERYGIUM.

**web-fingered** Characterized by a mild form of syndactyly of the hand in which the affected digits are connected only by a fold of skin.

**webfoot** A mild form of syndactyly of the feet in which affected digits are connected by a fold of skin.

**webspace** See under SPACE.

**Wechsberg** [Friedrich *Wechsberg*, German physician, 1873–1929] Neisser-Wechsberg phenomenon. See under COMPLEMENT DEVIATION.

**Wechsler** [David *Wechsler*, Rumanian-born psychologist active in the United States, born 1896] 1 Wechsler Adult Intelligence scale. See under SCALE. 2 Wechsler Intelligence Scale for Children. See under SCALE.

**Wedensky** [Nikolay Yevgenyevich *Wedensky*, Russian physiologist, 1852–1922] See under FACILITATION, INHIBITION, PHENOMENON.

**wedge** [Old English *wecg*] A solid material having the shape of an acute V, for insertion in a gap to hold structures apart or secure them in place. **dental w.** 1 A wooden wedge used to force open the mouth of an unconscious person. 2 A small wooden or plastic wedge used interdentally to hold a matrix band tightly against a tooth at the gingival margin.

**weed** A useless plant with low value or esteem whose growth is detrimental to desirable plants. **jimson w.** STRAMONIUM.

**Weeks** [John *Weeks*, U.S. ophthalmologist, 1853–1949] 1 Koch-Weeks bacillus. See under *HAEMOPHILUS AEGYPTIUS*. 2 Koch-Weeks conjunctivitis. See under ACUTE CONTAGIOUS CONJUNCTIVITIS.

**weep** To exude a serous fluid, particularly from a surface such as the skin or a mucous membrane, as a manifestation of inflammation or edema.

**weeping** Characterized by exudation of serum from a tissue.

**Wegener** [F. *Wegener*, German pathologist, flourished 20th century] Wegener's granuloma, Wegener syndrome. See under WEGENER'S GRANULOMATOSIS.

**Wegner** [Friedrich Rudolf Georg *Wegner*, German pathologist, 1843–1917] See under DISEASE.

**Weigert** [Carl *Weigert*, German histopathologist,

1845–1904] **1** Weigert's myelin sheath stain. See under STAIN. **2** Weigert-Pal technique. See under WEIGERT-PAL METHOD. **3** Weigert's fibrin stain. See under STAIN. **4** Weigert solution, Weigert's iron hematoxylin stain. See under WEIGERT'S IRON HEMATOXYLIN.

**weight** [Old English *wiht,* from *wegan* to carry, bear, weigh in scales, akin to L *vehere* to convey] **1** In scientific usage, the force exerted on an object by gravity, expressed in newtons. The weight of a body thus varies slightly from place to place on the earth's surface, and markedly between the earth's surface and other places, such as the surface of the moon. **2** In common usage, the apparent mass of a body when measured in air by comparison to standard masses of prescribed composition, the effects of the buoyancy of the air being ignored. **3** A piece of material, usually metal, of known mass, used as a comparison object in weighing. **4** In statistics, a procedure to assign differential importance to certain observations at the expense of others, or a numerical factor employed in applying such a procedure. **apothecaries' w.** A measurement system of weights formerly used in pharmacy. Its units are the grain (0.0648 gram), the scruple (equal to 20 grains), the dram (equal to 3 scruples), the ounce (equal to 8 drams or 240 grains), and the pound (equal to 12 ounces). **atomic w.** An imprecise but customary term for ATOMIC MASS. Abbr. at wt **avoirdupois w.** The most commonly used system of weights, based on the pound of 7000 grains or 16 ounces (0.453 kilogram). **birth w.** See under BIRTHWEIGHT. **combining w.** EQUIVALENT WEIGHT. **equivalent w.** The mass of a substance that reacts with or combines with one mole of $O^{1}/_{2}$ (8 grams) or one mole of H (1.008 grams). Also *combining weight, gram equivalent.* **fine w.** A British term for TROY WEIGHT. **gram-atomic w.** GRAM-ATOM. **gram molecular w.** *Obs.* MOLE[3]. **imperial w.** In Great Britain, weight as defined by Act of Parliament. In 1824 imperial weight was based on the troy pound, but since 1855 the avoirdupois pound has been the imperial standard. **molecular w.** See under RELATIVE MOLECULAR MASS. Abbr. mol wt **troy w.** A system of weights, used especially for weighing precious metals and gemstones, based in the United States on the pound troy of 5760 grains and in Great Britain on the ounce troy of 480 grains. Also *fine weight* (British usage).

**Weigl** [Egon *Weigl,* Romanian-born German psychologist, flourished mid-20th century] Weigl-Goldstein-Scheerer test. See under TEST.

**Weigl** [R. *Weigl,* Polish virologist, flourished 20th century] See under VACCINE.

**Weil** [Arthur *Weil,* German-born U.S. neuropathologist, born 1887] See under STAIN.

**Weil** [Edmund *Weil,* Austrian bacteriologist, 1879–1922] Weil-Felix reaction, Felix-Weil reaction. See under WEIL-FELIX TEST.

**Weil** [H. Adolf *Weil,* German physician, 1848–1916] Weil's disease, Larrey-Weil disease. See under ICTERIC LEPTOSPIROSIS.

**Weil** [Ludwig A. *Weil,* German dentist, 1849–1895] Weil's basal layer. See under SUBODONTOBLASTIC LAYER.

**Weill** [Edmond *Weill,* French pediatrician, 1858–1924] See under SIGN.

**Weill** [Georges *Weill,* French ophthalmologist, 1866–1952] **1** Weill-Reys syndrome, Weill-Reys-Adie syndrome. See under ADIE SYNDROME. **2** Weill-Marchesani syndrome. See under SYNDROME.

**Weinberg** [Wilhelm *Weinberg,* German physician, 1862–1937] **1** Hardy-Weinberg law. See under LAW. **2** Hardy-Weinberg equilibrium. See under EQUILIBRIUM.

**Weingarten** [R. J. *Weingarten,* German physician, flourished mid-20th century] Weingarten syndrome. See under TROPICAL PULMONARY EOSINOPHILIA.

**Weir** [Robert Fulton *Weir,* U.S. surgeon, 1835–1927] Weir's operation. See under APPENDICOSTOMY.

**Weir Mitchell** [Silas *Weir Mitchell,* U.S. neurologist, poet, and novelist, 1829–1914] Weir Mitchell's disease, Mitchell's disease. See under ERYTHROMELALGIA.

**Weismann** [August Friedrich Leopold *Weismann,* German biologist, 1834–1914] Weismannism. See under WEISMANN'S THEORY.

**weismannism** \wīs′mənizm\ WEISMANN'S THEORY.

**Weiss** [Leopold *Weiss,* German oculist, 1849–1901] See under REFLEX.

**Weiss** [Nathan *Weiss,* Austrian physician, 1851–1883] Chvostek-Weiss sign. See under CHVOSTEK SIGN.

**Weiss** [Soma *Weiss,* Hungarian-born U.S. physician, 1898–1942] **1** Mallory-Weiss syndrome. See under SYNDROME. **2** Charcot-Weiss-Baker syndrome. See under CAROTID SINUS SYNDROME.

**Weissenbach** [Raymond Joseph Emil *Weissenbach,* French physician, 1885–1963] Thibierge-Weissenbach syndrome. See under SYNDROME.

**Weitbrecht** [Josias W. *Weitbrecht,* German-born anatomist active in Russia, 1702–1747] **1** Weitbrecht's cartilage. See under DISCUS ARTICULARIS ARTICULATIONIS ACROMIOCLAVICULARIS. **2** Weitbrecht's cord, Weitbrecht's ligament. See under CHORDA OBLIQUA. **3** See under FORAMEN.

**Welander** [Lisa *Welander,* Swedish neurologist, born 1909] Kugelberg-Welander disease, Kugelberg-Welander syndrome. See under JUVENILE FAMILIAL MUSCULAR ATROPHY.

**Welch** [William Henry *Welch,* U.S. pathologist, 1850–1934] Welch's bacillus. See under *CLOSTRIDIUM PERFRINGENS.*

**Welcker** [Hermann *Welcker,* German anatomist, 1822–1899] **1** Welcker's angle. See under ANGULUS SPHENOIDALIS OSSIS PARIETALIS. **2** See under METHOD.

**well**[1] [Old English *wel,* akin to German *wohl* well (adverb)] Healthy; sound; not or no longer ill.

**well**[2] [Middle English *welle,* from Old English *welle, wella,* akin to *weallan* to boil and to German *Welle* a wave] **1** A shallow, sharply circumscribed depression in a flat, horizontal surface. It is usually the site at which a reactive liquid, such as serum or a suspension of antigen or antibody, is introduced into a gel for immunologic testing. **2** A concavity in a glass or porcelain plate.

**wellness** The quality or condition of being well, especially of being robustly healthy and fit. ⟨"the 'wellness' being sought is 'not simply the absence of symptoms but positive well-being, the kind of robustness that comprehends respect for the body and appreciation of its worth' " —*Medical World News,* 29 Mar. 1982, 33.⟩

**Wells** [Michael Vernon *Wells,* English physician, flourished 20th century] Muckle-Wells syndrome. See under SYNDROME.

**wen** [Old English *wenn*] **1** SEBACEOUS CYST. **2** EPIDERMAL CYST.

**Wenckebach** [Karel Frederik *Wenckebach,* Dutch internist, 1864–1940] **1** Wenckebach's phenomenon. See under BLOCK. **2** See under PERIOD.

**Wepfer** [Johann Jakob *Wepfer,* Swiss physician, 1620–1695] Wepfer's glands. See under GLANDULAE DUODENALES.

**Werdnig** [Guido *Werdnig,* Austrian neurologist, 1844–1919] Werdnig-Hoffmann paralysis, Werdnig-Hoffmann atrophy, Hoffmann-Werdnig syndrome, Werdnig-Hoffmann syndrome. See under WERDNIG-HOFFMANN DISEASE.

**Wermer** [Paul *Wermer,* U.S. physician, died 1975] See under SYNDROME.

**Werner** [C. W. Otto *Werner,* German physician, born 1879] See under SYNDROME.

**Werner** [F. F. *Werner,* German chemist, flourished early 20th century] Werner's test. See under $T_3$ SUPPRESSION TEST.

**Werner** [Heinrich *Werner,* German physician, 1874–1946] His-Werner disease, Werner-His disease. See under TRENCH FEVER.

**Wernicke** [Karl *Wernicke,* German neuropsychiatrist, 1848–1905] **1** Wernicke's reaction, Wernicke's hemianopic reaction, Wernicke symptom. See under HEMIANOPIC PUPILLARY REACTION. **2** Campus of Wernicke. See under TRIANGLE. **3** See under APHASIA, SIGN, FIELD. **4** Para-Wernicke encephalopathy. See under SUBACUTE NECROTIZING ENCEPHALOPATHY. **5** Wernicke's encephalopathy, Wernicke syndrome. See under WERNICKE'S DISEASE. **6** Kahlbaum-Wernicke syndrome. See under PRESBYOPHRENIA. **7** Wernicke-Korsakoff syndrome. See under WERNICKE-KORSAKOFF PSYCHOSIS. **8** Wernicke's radiation. See under RADIATIO OPTICA.

**Wernicke** [Robert *Wernicke,* Argentinian pathologist, 1854–1922] Posada-Wernicke disease. See under COCCIDIOIDOMYCOSIS.

**Wertheim** [Ernst *Wertheim,* German gynecologist, 1864–1920] **1** Wertheim-Schauta operation. See under OPERATION. **2** See under OPERATION.

**West** [Charles *West,* English physician, 1816–1898] **1** West syndrome. See under INFANTILE MASSIVE SPASM. **2** See under SKULL.

**Westberg** [Friedrich *Westberg,* German physician, born 1868] See under SPACE.

**Westergren** [Alf *Westergren,* Swedish physician, born 1891] See under METHOD.

**Westphal** [Alexander Karl Otto *Westphal,* German neurologist, 1863–1941] **1** Westphal's phenomenon, Westphal-Piltz phenomenon, Piltz-Westphal phenomenon. See under ORBICULARIS PHENOMENON. **2** Westphal's pupillary reflex. See under WESTPHAL-PILTZ REFLEX.

**Westphal** [Karl Friedrich Otto *Westphal,* German neurologist, 1833–1890] **1** See under MANEUVER. **2** Edinger-Westphal nucleus, Westphal's nucleus. See under NUCLEUS OCULOMOTORIUS ACCESSORIUS.

**wet-nurse** To breast-feed (a child other than one's own); work as a wet nurse.

**Wetzel** [Norman Carl *Wetzel,* U.S. pediatrician, born 1877] See under GRID.

**Wever** [Ernest Glen *Wever,* U.S. psychologist, born 1902] **1** Wever-Bray effect. See under COCHLEAR MICROPHONIC POTENTIAL. **2** Wever-Bray phenomenon. See under COCHLEAR MICROPHONICS.

**Wharton** [Thomas *Wharton,* English anatomist, 1614–1673] **1** See under JELLY. **2** Submaxillary duct of Wharton, Wharton's duct. See under DUCTUS SUBMANDIBULARIS.

**wheal** \ʰwēl\ [alteration of *wale,* from Old English *walu* weal] A transient, edematous, circumscribed, and often pruritic swelling of the skin. Also *weal.*

**wheel / Burlew w.** An abrasive rubber wheel used for polishing teeth and restorations. A proprietary name. **lathe w.** LATHE STONE.

**Wheeler** [Henry Lord *Wheeler,* U.S. chemist, 1867–1914] Wheeler and Johnson test. See under TEST.

**wheeze** [Middle English *whesen,* from Old Norse *hvaesa* to hiss] **1** To emit a high-pitched, more or less musical nonvocal sound during breathing, usually audible without auscultation and subjectively. It is usually produced by bronchial, tracheal, or laryngeal constriction or obstruction. **2** The sound produced in wheezing. **asthmatoid w.** A wheeze occurring during breathing and resembling that present in asthma.

**whey** \ʰwā\ [Old English *hwæg*] The fluid in milk that separates from the clot of casein and fat in making curds, or that separates from the milk after coagulation with rennet or from lactic acid upon souring. It contains most of the lactose in the original milk as well as the water-soluble vitamins and minerals, but is 92% water. Once a fashionable therapy for a variety of disorders, it can be used in the preparation of humanized milk, or for special diets. Also *serum lactis.*

**whiplash** See under WHIPLASH INJURY.

**Whipple** [Allen Oldfather *Whipple,* U.S. surgeon, 1881–1963] See under OPERATION, TRIAD.

**Whipple** [George Hoyt *Whipple,* U.S. physiologist, born 1878] See under DISEASE.

**whipworm** A nematode worm of the genus *Trichuris.*

**whirlbone** PATELLA.

**whisper** [Old English *hwisprian*] The speech sound produced when the vocal folds are prevented from vibrating. The myoelastic anterior portions of the folds are held together in adduction and air passes through the glottis in the posterior, arytenoid region.

**whistle / Galton's w.** A means of testing high-tone hearing, highly regarded in the early years of the twentieth century. It consisted of a cylindrical tube fitted with a moveable piston. Air was blown in to produce the whistle and the piston was moved to vary the pitch.

**White** [Paul Dudley *White,* U.S. cardiologist, 1886–1973] Wolff-Parkinson-White syndrome. See under SYNDROME.

**White** [Priscilla *White,* U.S. internist and diabetologist, born 1900] See under CLASSIFICATION.

**white** [Old English *hwīt*] A color produced by the reflection of all the rays of the spectrum. **w. of the eye** SCLERA.

**white-cap** FAVUS.

**Whitehead** [Walter *Whitehead,* English surgeon, 1840–1913] See under OPERATION.

**whitehead** MILIUM.

**whiteleg** PHLEGMASIA ALBA DOLENS.

**whitepox** \ʰwīt′päks\ ALASTRIM.

**Whitfield** [Arthur *Whitfield,* English dermatologist, 1868–1947] Whitfield's ointment. See under BENZOIC AND SALICYLIC ACID OINTMENT.

**whitlow** \ʰwit′lō\ [Middle English *whitflawe, whitflowe,* possibly from *whit* white + *flawe* flaw] PARONYCHIA. **herpetic w.** An acute infection of the paronychial tissues by the virus of herpes simplex. **melanotic w.** SUBUNGUAL MELANOMA. **painless w.** MORVAN SYNDROME. **perionychial w.** PARONYCHIA. **thecal w.** THECAL FELON.

**Whitmore** [Alfred *Whitmore,* English surgeon, 1876–1946] Whitmore's fever. See under MELIOIDOSIS.

**Whitnall** [Samuel Ernest *Whitnall,* English anatomist, 1876–1952] Whitnall's tubercle. See under EMINENTIA ORBITALIS.

**Whitney** [Donald Ransom *Whitney,* U.S. statistician, born 1915] Mann-Whitney U test. See under TEST.

**WHO** World Health Organization.

**whoop** [Middle English *whopen, houpen* to shout, from Old French *houper* to cry out, of imitative origin] A crowing sound during sudden inspiration which follows a paroxysm of coughing in pertussis.

**whooping cough** PERTUSSIS.

**whorl** \ʰwurl\ [Middle English *whorle*] A spiral arrangement, pattern, or twist, as of the dermal ridges in a fingerprint. **coccygeal w.** VORTEX COCCYGEUS. **lens w.** The bow of lens nuclei seen extending from the equator into the cortex in cross section of the crystalline lens.

**Whytt** [Robert *Whytt,* Scottish physician, 1714–1766] See under DISEASE.

**wick** / **iris w.** A faulty closure of a surgical or traumatic wound of the eye due to interposition of prolapsed iris tissue between the edges of the wound.

**Wickham** [Louis Frederic *Wickham*, French dermatologist, 1861–1913] Wickham striae. See under STRIA.

**Widal** [Georges Fernand Isidore *Widal*, French physician, 1862–1929] Gruber-Widal reaction, Widal reaction, Gruber-Widal test, Widal serum test. See under WIDAL TEST.

**Widmark** [Erik Johan *Widmark*, Swedish ophthalmologist, 1850–1909] See under CONJUNCTIVITIS.

**width** 1 Linear extent, usually measured at right angles to the length and the shorter of the two dimensions; lateral extent. 2 The magnitude of a range, as of radiofrequencies. **pulse w.** PULSE DURATION.

**Wien** [Wilhelm *Wien*, German physicist, 1864–1928] See under LAW.

**Wiethe** [Camillo *Wiethe*, Austrian otologist, 1888–1949] Urbach-Wiethe disease. See under LIPOID PROTEINOSIS.

**Wigand** [Justus Heinrich *Wigand*, German obstetrician, 1769–1817] See under MANEUVER, VERSION.

**Wilcoxon** [Frank *Wilcoxon*, Irish-born U.S. chemist and statistician, born 1892] See under TEST.

**wild** [Old English *wilde*] Originating in a natural environment; not domestic or bred or produced in captivity or in a laboratory: commonly said of infective organisms or viruses which have been isolated from a host with a naturally acquired infection, as opposed to a laboratory-adapted or mutated strain.

**Wilde** [Sir William Robert Wills *Wilde*, Irish surgeon, 1815–1876] See under INCISION.

**Wildermuth** [Hermann A. *Wildermuth*, German psychiatrist and neurologist, 1852–1907] See under EAR.

**Wildervanck** [L. S. *Wildervanck*, Dutch physician, flourished 20th century] See under SYNDROME.

**Wildi** [Erwin *Wildi*, Swiss pathologist, flourished 20th century] Morel-Wildi syndrome. See under SYNDROME.

**wild-type** Of or relating to a genetic locus or an allele that specifies a phenotype that predominates in natural populations or that is designated as normal.

**Wilkinson** [Darrell Sheldon *Wilkinson*, English dermatologist, flourished 20th century] Sneddon-Wilkinson disease. See under SUBCORNEAL PUSTULAR DERMATOSIS.

**Wilks** [Sir Samuel Baronet *Wilks*, English physician, 1824–1911] Wilks symptom complex, Wilks syndrome. See under MYASTHENIA GRAVIS.

**will** The conscious processes involved in deciding upon a course of action. See also VOLITION. **living w.** A written document specifying that in the event of the maker of the will suffering an injury or disease from which no recovery can reasonably be expected, he or she will be allowed to die and not kept alive by artificial means or extraordinary measures. In the majority of states in the United States, living wills are not considered legal documents. A term used only in the U.S. and Canada.

**Willan** [Robert *Willan*, English dermatologist, 1757–1812] Willan's lepra. See under PSORIASIS CIRCINATA.

**Willett** [John Abernathy *Willett*, English obstetrician, 1872–1932] Willett's clamp. See under FORCEPS.

**Willi** [Heinrich *Willi*, Swiss pediatrician, flourished mid-20th century] Prader-Labhart-Willi syndrome. See under PRADER-WILLI SYNDROME.

**Willis** [Thomas *Willis*, English anatomist and physician, 1621–1675] 1 Willis gland. See under CORPUS ALBICANS. 2 See under PARACUSIS. 3 Cords of Willis. See under CORD. 4 Willis valve. See under VELUM MEDULLARE CRANIALE. 5 Antrum of Willis. See under ANTRUM PYLORICUM. 6 Ophthalmic nerve of Willis. See under NERVUS OPHTHALMICUS. 7 Willis pancreas. See under PROCESSUS UNCINATUS PANCREATIS. 8 Willis pouch. See under OMENTUM MINUS. 9 Nerve of Willis. See under NERVUS ACCESSORIUS.

**Wills** [Lucy *Wills*, English scientist, flourished early 20th century] Wills anemia. See under FOLIC ACID DEFICIENCY ANEMIA.

**Wilms** [Max *Wilms*, German surgeon, 1867–1918] 1 Wilms tumor. See under NEPHROBLASTOMA. 2 Aniridia-Wilms tumor syndrome. See under SYNDROME.

**Wilson** [Clifford *Wilson*, English physician, born 1906] 1 Kimmelstiel-Wilson syndrome. See under DIABETIC GLOMERULOSCLEROSIS. 2 Kimmelstiel-Wilson lesion. See under LESION.

**Wilson** [Frank Norman *Wilson*, U.S. cardiologist, 1890–1952] See under BLOCK.

**Wilson** [Louis Blanchard *Wilson*, U.S. physician, 1866–1943] See under METHOD.

**Wilson** [Miriam Geisendorfer *Wilson*, U.S. pediatrician, born 1922] Wilson-Mikity syndrome. See under SYNDROME.

**Wilson** [Samuel Alexander Kinnier *Wilson*, U.S. neurologist, 1877–1937] 1 Wilson's pronator sign. See under SIGN. 2 Wilson's degeneration, Kinnier Wilson disease, Wilson syndrome. See under DISEASE.

**Wilson** [Sir William James Erasmus *Wilson*, English dermatologist, 1809–1884] 1 Wilson's lichen. See under LICHEN PLANUS. 2 Wilson's disease. See under SYNDROME.

**wind** / **electric w.** CONVECTIVE DISCHARGE.

**windkessel** \wind′kesəl\ [German (from *Wind* wind + *Kessel* kettle, caldron), wind chamber] A mechanism, such as a compressed air chamber in a steam engine or pump, which serves to convert a strongly pulsatile flow into a relatively smooth flow. This concept has been applied to the function of the aorta and other arteries whereby they convert the phasic flow entering from the left ventricle to a more continuous flow in the peripheral vessels.

**windlass** \wind′ləs\ **Spanish w.** A band of fabric or a handkerchief tied with a knot around the part to be constricted and then tightened by twisting with a stick. Also *Spanish tourniquet, windlass tourniquet, torcular tourniquet, garrote tourniquet, garrot.*

**window** [Middle English *windowe*, from Old Norse *vindr* wind, air + *auga* the eye] 1 The transparent opening in an x-ray tube, usually made of beryllium, which transmits a beam of x rays with little filtration. 2 An opening between two chambers or spaces, as that in a wall that separates them; fenestra. **acoustic w.** An area of good sound transmission, such as the liver or the fluid-filled bladder, over which the ultrasound transducer must be positioned in order to image deeper structures effectively. **aortic w.** In radiography of the chest in left anterior oblique position, a clear space situated between the spinal column in back, the concavity of the aortic arch on top, the aorta and the pulmonary artery in front. **aorticopulmonary w.** A congenital malformation of the heart in which a communication exists between the aorta and the pulmonary artery at the level at which the two great vessels are juxtaposed just above the semilunar valves. It results from failure of the embryonic ventral aorta to form separate aortic and pulmonary trunks. Blood flows in systole and in diastole from the aorta to the pulmonary artery, giving rise to increased pulmonary blood flow and pulmonary hypertension as a later sequel. These are effects similar to those of persistent ductus arteriosus. Also *aorticopulmonary septal defect, aortopulmonary fenestration, aortic septal defect, aortopulmonary defect.* **beryllium w.** That portion of the glass envelope of an x-ray tube that has been replaced by beryllium to allow the exit of soft x rays (i.e., less than 20 keV) for use in diagnostic radiology such as mammography, or in radiation therapy to the skin. **cochlear w.** FENESTRA COCHLEAE. **energy w.** DISCRIMINATOR SETTING. **oval w.** FENESTRA VESTIBULI. **Rebuck skin w.** See under REBUCK SKIN WINDOW TECHNIQUE. **round w.** FENESTRA COCHLEAE. **skin w.** See under REBUCK SKIN WINDOW TECHNIQUE. **vestibular w.** FENESTRA VESTIBULI.

**windowing** The cutting of a defect in a solid surface, such as a plaster of Paris cast or the cortex of bone.

**windpipe** TRACHEA.

**wing** [Middle English *winge, wenge,* from Old Norse *vængr* wing] **1** One of the vertebrate forelimbs adapted for flying, as in bats and birds. **2** Any appendage adapted for flying, as in insects. **3** Any flattened, laterally projecting process. **ashlike w.** TRIGONUM NERVI VAGI. **external white w.** AREA VESTIBULARIS. **greater w. of sphenoid bone** ALA MAJOR OSSIS SPHENOIDALIS. **w. of ilium** ALA OSSIS ILII. **w.'s of Ingrassia** WINGS OF SPHENOID BONE. **internal white w.** TRIGONUM NERVI HYPOGLOSSI. **lesser w. of sphenoid bone** ALA MINOR OSSIS SPHENOIDALIS. **major w. of sphenoid bone** ALA MAJOR OSSIS SPHENOIDALIS. **minor w. of sphenoid bone** ALA MINOR OSSIS SPHENOIDALIS. **w.'s of nose** ALAE NASI. **orbital w. of sphenoid bone** ALA MINOR OSSIS SPHENOIDALIS. **small w. of sphenoid bone** ALA MINOR OSSIS SPHENOIDALIS. **w.'s of sphenoid bone** Ala major ossis sphenoidalis and ala minor ossis sphenoidalis. Also *wings of Ingrassia.* **temporal w. of sphenoid bone** ALA MAJOR OSSIS SPHENOIDALIS. **w. of vomer** ALA VOMERIS.

**wink** [Old English *wincian* to shut the eyes] Voluntary momentary closure of one eyelid.

**Winkelman** [Nathaniel William *Winkelman,* U.S. neurologist, 1891–1956] Winkelman's disease. See under JUVENILE PARALYSIS AGITANS.

**winking** Repetitive, brief closing of the eyelids. **jaw w.** MARCUS GUNN SYNDROME.

**Winkler** [Max *Winkler,* Swiss physician, 1875–1952] Winkler's disease. See under CHRONIC NODULAR CHONDRODERMATITIS OF THE HELIX.

**Winslow** [Jakob Benigus *Winslow,* Danish-born French anatomist, 1669–1760] **1** Winslow's ligament. See under LIGAMENTUM POPLITEUM OBLIQUUM. **2** Winslow's pancreas. See under PROCESSUS UNCINATUS PANCREATIS.

**Winterbottom** [Thomas Masterman *Winterbottom,* English physician, 1765–1859] See under SIGN.

**Wintersteiner** [Hugo *Wintersteiner,* Austrian ophthalmologist, 1865–1918] See under ROSETTE.

**Wintrobe** [Maxwell Myer *Wintrobe,* Canadian-born U.S. physician, born 1901] **1** See under METHOD, HEMATOCRIT. **2** Wintrobe and Landsberg method. See under METHOD.

**wire** [Old English *wīr,* akin to L *viere* to bind with twigs, weave, and L *vitis* vine] **1** A slender, flexible length of metal, used in surgery and dentistry. **2** To secure with or subject to the action of wires, as to immobilize fractures or promote the formation of clots in an aneurysm. **alignment w.** A flexible wire arch used to move teeth in orthodontics. **alveolar w.** A wire ligature passing through the alveolar bone of fragments of a fractured jaw, to achieve immobilization. **diagnostic w.** A fine wire used in endodontics, with or without radiographs, to measure the length of a root canal. Also *measuring wire.* **Kirschner w.** A heavy wire used to join fractured bone fragments. **ligature w.** A thin, soft wire used in fixed orthodontic appliances. **measuring w.** DIAGNOSTIC WIRE. **separating w.** Wire formed into a loop around the contact area for the purpose of separating the teeth.

**wiring** The use of wire in maintaining position of a part. **aortic aneurysm w.** A method of controlling the growth of an aneurysm in which a large length of wire is inserted in the vessel, thus causing thrombosis of the aneurysm. **circumferential w.** The splinting of a fractured jaw by fixing an intraoral splint to edentulous fragments by encircling sections of bone with wires which pass into the oral cavity and around the splint. **continuous loop w.** Wiring to provide multiple eyelets with one length of wire. Also *multiple loop wiring.* **eyelet w.** A technique for splinting a fractured jaw by attaching looped wires to pairs of adjacent teeth in upper and lower jaws, forming small loops (eyelets) for the application of ligatures between the jaws. Also *Ivy loop wiring.* **interdental w.** Fixation of the maxilla by the wiring together of the teeth. **Ivy loop w.** EYELET WIRING. **multiple loop w.** CONTINUOUS LOOP WIRING. **single loop w.** Attachment of a ligature wire to a single tooth.

**Wirsung** [Johann Georg *Wirsung,* German-born anatomist active in Italy, 1600–1643] **1** Duct of Wirsung, canal of Wirsung. See under DUCTUS PANCREATICUS. **2** Sphincter of duct of Wirsung. See under MUSCULUS SPHINCTER DUCTUS PANCREATICI.

**WISC** Wechsler intelligence scale for children.

**Wiskott** [Alfred *Wiskott,* German pediatrician, born 1898] Wiskott-Aldrich syndrome. See under SYNDROME.

**Wissler** [Hans *Wissler,* Swiss pediatrician, born 1906] Wissler-Fanconi syndrome. See under SYNDROME.

**Wistar** [Caspar *Wistar,* U.S. biologist and anatomist, 1761–1818] See under RAT.

**witch hazel** HAMAMELIS.

**withdrawal** \wiTHdrô′əl\ **1** The act of retracting, retreating, or relinquishing. **2** Voluntary removal of the penis from the vagina in coitus interruptus. **3** Abstinence from a substance such as alcohol or drugs upon which the subject has become dependent. See also WITHDRAWAL SYMPTOMS. **4** In psychiatry, retreat from social relationships into solitude, sometimes to the extent of total dissolution of all bonds with others and reinvestment of those object cathexes onto the self in the form of severe hypochondriacal and autistic self-preoccupation. **thought w.** BLOCKING OF THOUGHT.

**Witkop** [Carl Jacob *Witkop,* U.S. oral pathologist, born 1920] Witkop-Von Sallman disease. See under DISEASE.

**witness** / **expert w.** A witness who, by virtue of education, training, experience, or demonstrated skill, qualifies as an authority on a particular subject and who is therefore allowed to answer hypothetical questions and to render opinions on that subject as it is considered in a court of law. Expert witnesses testify most commonly on those scientific, professional, or technical matters about which an ordinary individual of average intelligence and without special training is unable to make a correct judgment. See also MEDICAL EXPERT.

**Witts** [Leslie John *Witts,* English physician, born 1898] Witts anemia. See under IRON DEFICIENCY ANEMIA.

**Witzel** [Friedrich Oskar *Witzel,* German physician, 1856–1925] See under OPERATION.

**witzelsucht** \vit′səlzUkht, -zookt\ [German *witzel(n)* to affect wit + *Sucht* sickness] Excessive and abnormal joviality, with a marked tendency to joke and to make puns, seen particularly in patients with frontal lobe syndromes. Also *moria.*

**WMA** World Medical Association.

**$\overline{\text{wo}}$** without.

***Wohlfahrtia*** \vōlfär′tē·ə\ [irreg. after Peter *Wolfart,* German medical writer, 1675–1726 + -IA] A genus of flesh flies or screwworms of the family Sarcophagidae. The larvae of some species, dropped directly by the female fly, enter small openings in the skin and cause myiasis in wounds or sores of humans and other animals.

**Wolfe** [John Reissberg *Wolfe,* Scottish ophthalmologist, 1824–1904] Krause-Wolfe graft, Wolfe's graft, Wolfe-Krause graft. See under FULL-THICKNESS GRAFT.

**Wolff** [Julius *Wolff,* German anatomist, 1836–1902] See under LAW.

**Wolff** [Kaspar Friedrich *Wolff,* German-born embryologist, physician, and botanist active in Russia, 1733–1794] **1** Wolffian body. See under MESONEPHROS. **2** Wolffian duct. See under MESONEPHRIC DUCT. **3** Wolffian vestiges See under VESTIGE.

**Wolff** [Louis *Wolff,* U.S. cardiologist, 1898–1972] Wolff-Parkinson-White syndrome. See under SYNDROME.

**Wolff-Eisner** [Alfred *Wolff-Eisner,* German serologist, 1877–1948] Wolff-Eisner reaction, Wolff-Eisner test. See under CALMETTE'S REACTION.

**wolffian** \wʊl′fē·ən\ Associated with the work of Kaspar Friedrich Wolff.

**Wolfring** [Emilij F. von *Wolfring,* Polish ophthalmologist, 1832–1906] Glands of Wolfring. See under GLANDULAE LACRIMALES ACCESSORIAE.

**wolfsbane** \wʊlfs′bān\ ACONITE.

**Woltman** [Henry William *Woltman,* U.S. neurologist, 1889–1964] Moersch-Woltman syndrome. See under STIFF-MAN SYNDROME.

**woman** A female adult human being. **reference w.** A hypothetical woman whose anatomy, physiology, biochemistry, clinical chemistry, and hematologic values are within normal limits, and with whom all other women may be compared. Also *standard woman.* **standard w.** REFERENCE WOMAN.

**womb** \woom\ [Old English *wamb* (from common Germanic) the belly, womb] UTERUS.

**Wood** [Norman *Wood,* English physician, flourished 20th century] Norman-Wood syndrome. See under SYNDROME.

**Wood** [Robert Williams *Wood,* U.S. physicist, 1868–1955] See under GLASS, FILTER, LAMP, LIGHT.

**wood** [Old English *wudu* a tree, wood] The hard region of a stem or root between the bark and the pith. **Panama w.** The dried inner bark of *Quillaja saponaria* and other *Quillaja* species, containing alcohol-soluble saponin glycosides. It is used externally as a liquid extract or tincture for its emulsifying properties, particularly in tar preparations and some volatile oils. Also *quillaia bark, soap bark.*

**wool** **1** Sheep hair or the yarn or fabric manufactured from it. **2** Any substance having the texture or appearance of wool. **cotton w.** ABSORBENT COTTON.

**Woolner** [Thomas *Woolner,* English sculptor, 1825–1892] Woolner's tip. See under TUBERCULUM AURICULAE.

**word salad** A potpourri of jumbled, unrelated, irrelevant neologisms and phrases that are incomprehensible to the listener. It is a manifestation of a severe association disturbance.

**work** / **social w.** Social service work which, utilizing special techniques, aims to promote an improved relationship between individuals and their social environment by making use of the capabilities of the individual and the resources of the community.

**worker** / **ancillary w.** In South Africa, a paramedical worker. **indigenous w.** INDIGENOUS PRACTITIONER. **social w.** A professionally trained person who provides social services in a health care agency or other setting, including independent practice.

**working through** A psychoanalytic process during which id resistance is overcome by allowing the patient an opportunity to amalgamate new insights with other areas of his personality, to alter the balance among his defenses, to form new identifications, and to reconstruct his ego ideal.

**work-up** Any or all of the procedures used to assemble data and present a collective picture of a patient's condition in order to reach a diagnosis, often a specific diagnosis to determine a particular course of treatment. The taking of a medical history and the administration of a physical examination and laboratory tests are standard features, but often other specialized examinations are conducted as well. ⟨"preoperative work-ups to establish a diagnosis of vascular insufficiency. Before being considered for surgery, each patient is first given a detailed vascular, psychological, and neurological examination" —*Medical World News,* 3 Apr. 1978, 73.⟩

**World Health Organization** An intergovernmental organization forming part of the United Nations system and having as its aim "the attainment by all peoples of the highest possible level of health" (Article 1 of the Constitution). It is concerned in particular with major problems the solutions of which call for the cooperation of many countries, such as campaigns against transmissible diseases, cancer, and cardiovascular disease. It lays down international standards for biologic preparations and norms for substances such as insecticides, maintains an up-to-date international pharmacopeia and international health regulations, collects and disseminates epidemiologic information, and encourages the exchange of scientific knowledge. Regional programs aim to promote mental health, maternal and child care, dental health, public health administration, and education for the health professions and of the public in health matters. The World Health Organization has an extensive research program and is also involved in the coordination of research conducted at a national level, convening each year many scientific meetings and publishing periodicals and reports in several languages. It has an important role in standardization of terminology in the health field. Abbr. WHO

**Worm** [Ole *Worm,* Danish physician, 1588–1654] Wormian bones. See under OSSA SUTURALIA.

**worm** [Old English *wyrm* (akin to L *vermis* worm, grub) serpent, worm] **1** An invertebrate animal which is elongate and soft-bodied in the adult form, such as an annelid, nematode, cestode, or trematode. **2** An insect larva such as a caterpillar, grub, or maggot. *Popular.* **African eye w.** A nematode worm of the species *Loa loa..* **bilharzia w.** SCHISTOSOME. **blinding w.** A nematode worm of the species *Onchocerca volvulus..* **caddis w.** The larva of a caddis fly. Also *case worm, caseworm.* **case w.** **1** CADDIS WORM. **2** The encysted larva of an *Echinococcus* tapeworm. Also *caseworm.* **w. of cerebellum** VERMIS CEREBELLI. **dragon w.** GUINEA WORM. **eye w.** Any of various nematode worms that are parasitic in the eyes of mammals and birds, including the African eye worm *Loa loa,* and species of *Thelazia* and *Oxyspirura..* **fluke w.** FLUKE. **guinea w.** A nematode worm of the species *Dracunculus medinensis..* Also *dragon worm, Medina worm.* **horsehair w.** A worm of the genus *Gordius* or a related genus of the phylum Gordiacea (Nematomorpha). Also *hairworm, hair snake.* **kidney w.** A nematode worm of the species *Dioctophyma renale..* **meal w.** A larva of the meal moth *Asopia farinalis,* or of *Tenebrio molitor* or other grain beetle. Many of these insects are intermediate hosts of the spirurid nematode *Gongylonema* and of several tapeworms of the genus *Hymenolepis..* **Medina**

w. GUINEA WORM. **pork w.** A nematode worm of the species *Trichinella spiralis;* a trichina. **screw w.** See under SCREWWORM. **seat w.** The human pinworm, *Enterobius vermicularis.*. **tongue w.** A member of the class (or phylum) Pentastomida; a pentastome. **trichina w.** A nematode worm of the species *Trichinella spiralis.*.

**wormwood** ABSINTHIUM.

**wound** [Old English *wund,* from common Germanic] **1** An injury caused by physical means and involving a discontinuity of normal anatomy. **2** To inflict with a wound. **aseptic w.** **1** A wound created under sterile conditions. **2** A wound from which no bacteria can be grown. **avulsion w.** A wound, usually resulting from blunt force, in which the full thickness of skin and all or part of the underlying soft tissues are removed. If the tissues remain connected at one edge it is considered a flap. **blowing w.** A wound in the thorax that permits entry and exit of air. **contused w.** A wound with an element of blunt trauma, so that the edges of the wound may be devitalized. **crease w. of head** A wound created by an object that glances off the skull and injures the scalp but does not cause a skull fracture. **defense w.'s** Nonlethal wounds of the upper extremities sustained when a victim raises his arms or hands in an effort to protect his chest or face by warding off an assailant's weapon. Such wounds are usually cuts or slashes of the palms or forearms, incurred when a victim is attacked with a knife or, less commonly, a blunt instrument or gun. **entrance w.** The wound produced when a projectile, discharged from a firearm, penetrates the body. Entrance wounds vary in appearance, depending on the type of firearm and ammunition, the angle and range of fire, the presence or absence of intervening substances such as clothing, and the body site penetrated. Also *in-shoot wound.* **exit w.** The wound produced when a projectile, discharged from a firearm, completely passes through and exits from a portion of the body. It is usually more irregular and often larger than an entrance wound, due to tumbling and deformation of the projectile as well as lack of support provided by the skin through which the projectile exits. Also *out-shoot wound.* **hesitation w.'s** Superficial, nonlethal cuts or sawing wounds usually found on the anterior neck or flexor muscles of the wrists of suicide victims. These wounds represent repeated trial attempts on the part of the individual during the commission of the suicide. • If the suicide attempt fails, the scars that form are called *hesitation scars* or *hesitation marks.* **incised w.** A wound created by a sharp object that produces margins that are smooth and intact. **in-shoot w.** ENTRANCE WOUND. **lacerated w.** A jagged wound created at least in part by a tearing action, so that the edges of the wound may be damaged. **nonpenetrating w.** A wound, caused by a blow, in which the skin remains intact despite injury to the tissues beneath. **open w.** A wound that penetrates the skin and directly communicates with the tissues beneath. **out-shoot w.** EXIT WOUND. **penetrating w.** An open wound, generally one whose depth is greater than its surface extent. **perforating w.** A penetrating wound that has passed through the wall of a body cavity or a viscus. **puncture w.** A penetrating wound made by a very slender object. **septic w.** A wound that is infected with microorganisms. **seton w.** A perforating injury, commonly produced by stabbing, in which the exit wound is on the same aspect of the injured part as the entrance wound. **stab w.** In forensic medicine, an incised wound whose depth of penetration is greater than its surface length. Compare CUT. **sucking w.** A perforating wound of the chest that permits ingress of air with each respiration. Unless it is promptly covered, the affected lung will collapse and respiratory embarrassment will result. **tangential w.** A wound at a tangent to the main axis of the injured part. Also *crease.* **tetanus-prone w.** Any wound that is capable of permitting growth of anaerobic organisms, especially *Clostridium tetani.* Such wounds include puncture wounds, some stab wounds, any wound with devitalized tissue, wounds contaminated with dirt or feces, and burns.

**W-plasty** \dub′əlyooplas′tē\ A method of reorienting or revising scars by excising a series of small triangular segments from each side of the scar after which the small triangular flaps which remain are interdigitated across the wound. Also *running W-plasty.*

**WR** Wasserman reaction.

**wreath** \rēth\ A twisted band or ring of leaves or flowers or a structure resembling it. **hippocratic w.** The configuration of the scalp hair that remains into the final state of common baldness.

**Wright** [James Homer *Wright,* U.S. pathologist, 1871–1928] **1** See under STAIN. **2** Homer Wright rosettes. See under ROSETTE.

**wrinkle** A crease in the skin.

**Wrisberg** [Heinrich August *Wrisberg,* German anatomist, 1739–1808] **1** Wrisberg's ganglion. See under GANGLIA CARDIACA. **2** Ansa of Wrisberg. See under RAMI CELIACI NERVI VAGI. **3** Wrisberg's cartilage. See under CARTILAGO CUNEIFORMIS. **4** Wrisberg's ligament, posterior meniscofemoral ligament of Wrisberg. See under LIGAMENTUM MENISCOFEMORALE POSTERIUS. **5** See under STAFF. **6** Wrisberg's tubercle. See under TUBERCULUM CUNEIFORME. **7** Intermediate nerve of Wrisberg, nervus intermedius of Wrisberg, nerve of Wrisberg. See under NERVUS INTERMEDIUS. **8** Nerve of Wrisberg. See under NERVUS CUTANEUS BRACHII MEDIALIS.

**wrist** CARPUS. **tennis w.** Tenosynovitis of the wrist tendons, which is seen in tennis players.

**wristdrop** Paralysis and weakness of the extensor muscles of the wrist.

**writing** / **mirror w.** The reversal of letters or of whole words in writing, as if the written script were viewed through a mirror. This is often seen in wholly or partially left-handed children as they begin to learn to write. Also *specular writing, strephosymbolia, retrography.* **specular w.** MIRROR WRITING.

**wryneck** \rī′nek\ TORTICOLLIS.

**wt** weight.

**Wu** [H. *Wu,* Chinese biochemist, flourished late 19th and early 20th centuries.] Folin and Wu test. See under TEST.

***Wuchereria*** \voo′kərir′ē·ə\ [after Otto *Wucherer,* German physician in Brazil, 1820–1874 + -IA] A genus of filarial nematodes in the family Onchocercidae, superfamily Filarioidea, which includes the medically important human filarial worm, *W. bancrofti.* ***W. bancrofti*** The causative agent of Bancroft's filariasis. The worm is widely distributed in Asia and the western Pacific, extending to eastern Europe, the Near East, northern Africa, and Central and South America. Human cases number in the millions. Vectors are mosquitoes of the genera *Culex, Aedes, Anopheles, Mansonia,* and *Psorophora.* Little host specificity is present. Also *Filaria bancrofti, Filaria nocturna, Filaria sanguinis hominis.* ***W. malayi*** *BRUGIA MALAYI.*

**wuchereriasis** \vooker′ərī′əsis\ Infection with nematodes of the genus *Wuchereria.*

**Wunderlich** [Carl Reinhold August *Wunderlich,* German physician, 1815–1877] See under CURVE.

**w/v** weight/volume: used after a concentration to specify

that the concentration is in terms of weight per unit volume.
**w/w** weight/weight: used after a concentration to specify that the concentration is in terms of weight per unit of weight.
**Wyatt** [Walter *Wyatt*, Australian pediatrician, flourished 20th century] Brushfield-Wyatt syndrome, Brushfield-Wyatt disease. See under STURGE-WEBER SYNDROME.
***Wyeomyia*** \wīˈōmīˈyə\ A genus of culicine mosquitoes that breed in treetops and often lay their eggs in bromeliad plant axils in the upper canopy of tropical South American rain forests. These mosquitoes transmit the yellow fever virus to arboreal animals which are the source of jungle yellow fever.

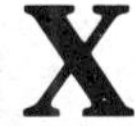

**X** **1** Symbol for unknown amino acid. **2** Symbol for the unit, Kienböck unit.
$^{A}_{Z}X$ Generalized symbol for an element, where X is the chemical symbol, A the mass number and Z the atomic number.
*X* Symbol for the quantity, reactance, expressed in ohms.
**Xaa** Symbol for unknown amino acid.
**xanth-** \zanth-\ XANTHO-.
**xanthaemia** \zanthēˈmē·ə\ *Brit.* XANTHEMIA.
**xanthelasma** \zanthilazˈmə\ [XANTH- + Gk *elasma* a metal plate] A slightly raised, yellowish plaque in the skin of the eyelids, composed of lipoidal material, often symmetrical on the two sides. Also *xanthoma palpebrarum*. **generalized x.** XANTHOMA.
**xanthelasmatosis** \zanˈthilazˈmətōˈsis\ XANTHOMA.
**xanthemia** \zanthēˈmē·ə\ HYPERCAROTENEMIA.
**xanthine** \zanˈthēn\ The tautomer of 2,4-dihydroxypurine. It is produced by oxidation of hypoxanthine and by hydrolysis of guanine in the catabolism of purines, in which it is oxidized to form uric acid. Symbol: Xan.
**xanthine dehydrogenase** The enzyme (EC 1.2.1.37) that oxidizes xanthine to uric acid with concomitant reduction of $NAD^+$. Some forms of this enzyme contain molybdenum.
**xanthinoxidase** An enzyme that produces uric acid from its interaction with xanthine and hypoxanthine.
**xanthinuria** \zanˈthinooˈrē·ə\ A rare, autosomal recessive disorder that is characterized by urinary excretion of large amounts of xanthine, the formation of xanthine calculi, and low serum uric acid as a result of a deficiency of xanthine oxidase. Also *xanthine oxidase deficiency, xanthiuria, xanthuria*.
**xanthinuric** \zanˈthinooˈrik\ **1** Pertaining to xanthinuria. **2** Of or relating to complications resulting from either an accumulation or hyperexcretion of xanthines.
**xanthism** \zanˈthizm\ [XANTH- + -ISM] Albinism in Negroid individuals. It is characterized by hair that is red or yellowish red, skin that is copper-colored, and iris pigmentation that tends to be dilute. Also *rufous albinism*.
**xanthiuria** \zanˈthēyooˈrē·ə\ XANTHINURIA.
**xantho-** \zanˈthō-\ [Gk *xanthos* yellow] A combining form meaning yellow. Also *xanth-*.
**xanthochromia** \-krōˈmē·ə\ [XANTHO- + CHROM- + -IA] A yellow coloring of the cerebrospinal fluid. Also *xanthopathy*.
**xanthochromic** \-krōˈmik\ Yellow in color.
**xanthocyanopsia** \-sīˈənäpˈsē·ə\ [XANTHO- + CYAN- + -OPSIA] Color vision anomaly in which only yellow and blue colors are visible.
**xanthocyte** \zanˈthəsīt\ [XANTHO- + -CYTE] A cell producing or containing a yellow pigment.
**xanthofibroma** \-fībrōˈmə\ FIBROUS HISTIOCYTOMA. **x. thecocellulare** *Obs.* DERMATOFIBROMA.
**xanthogranuloma** \-granˈyəlōˈmə\ [XANTHO- + GRANULOMA] A benign tumor or tumorlike lesion with histiocytes, lipid-laden cells, fibrous tissue, and often giant cells. **juvenile x.** JUVENILE XANTHOMA.
**xanthoma** \zanthōˈmə\ [XANTH- + -OMA] (*pl.* xanthomas, xanthomata) A yellow or orange papule, nodule, or plaque in the skin that is caused by a localized collection of lipid-containing cells in the dermis, most frequently found in patients with various disorders of lipid metabolism. Also *xanthelasmatosis, cholesterosis cutis* (seldom used), *generalized xanthelasma, vitiligoidea* (outmoded), *vitiligoidea tuberosum* (outmoded). **craniohypophyseal x.** A deposit of cholesterol crystals in the bones around the pituitary gland of subjects with Hand-Schüller-Christian disease and other histiocytosis conditions. **diabetic x.** XANTHOMA DIABETICORUM. **x. diabeticorum** Eruptive xanthomas on the skin of the elbows, buttocks, and dorsal surfaces of the thighs when chylomicronemia occurs in the course of uncontrolled diabetes mellitus. It is characteristic of chylomicronemia and not specific for diabetes. The lesions are small, reddish yellow papules on an erythematous base and appear in clusters. Also *diabetic xanthoma, xanthosis diabeticorum* (seldom used), *xanthosis diabetica* (seldom used). **x. disseminatum** A skin condition marked by widely distributed small xanthomata that favor the leg flexures. It is not associated with hyperlipemia. Also *xanthoma multiplex*. **eruptive x.** A condition in which cutaneous xanthomata appear suddenly as very small yellow papules. It is often a presenting feature of hyperlipidemia. Also *xanthoma eruptivum*. **generalized plane x.** A rare cutaneous xanthoma characterized by extensive plaques of infiltration and sometimes associated with lymphoreticu lar disease. **juvenile x.** A benign xanthoma that involves the skin, mucous membranes, and eyes in young children. It has no association with any abnormality of lipid metabolism, and it resolves itself within one or two years. Also *juvenile xanthogranuloma, juvenile histiocytoma*. **x. multiplex** XANTHOMA DISSEMINATUM. **x. palpebrarum** XANTHELASMA. **plane x.** A clinical pattern of cutaneous xanthomata that is characterized by macules or plaques of infiltrate. Also *planar xanthoma, xanthoma planum*. **synovial x.** A yellow, cholesterol-filled plaque found in the synovial membrane. **x. tuberosum** *Outmoded* FAMILIAL HYPERLIPOPPROTEINEMIA TYPE III. **x. tuberosum multiplex** *Outmoded* FAMILIAL HYPERLIPOPROTEINEMIA TYPE III.
**xanthomatosis** \-mətōˈsis\ [XANTHOMA + *t* + -OSIS] A condition occurring in various forms of hyperlipidemia in which lipids accumulate in nodules (xanthomata) in tendons, subcutaneous fat, skin, and elsewhere. Many forms of xanthomatosis are hereditary disorders of lipid metabolism.

**biliary hypercholesterolemic x.** Widespread xanthomatosis developing in biliary cirrhosis or chronic biliary tract obstruction associated with marked elevation of serum cholesterol. **cerebrotendinous x.** A rare familial disorder, due to the deposition of cholestanol (dihydrocholesterol) in the central nervous system, and characterized by xanthomata in the skin, in tendons, and in the lungs, bilateral cataracts, slowly progressive cerebellar ataxia and dementia, appearances of premature senility, and changes in the hair and nails. Some patients die in early adult life but in others the condition runs a very slow and indolent course following an onset in childhood. Also *van Bogaert-Scherer-Epstein syndrome.* **chronic idiopathic x.** HAND-SCHÜLLER-CHRISTIAN DISEASE. **x. generalisata ossium** HAND-SCHÜLLER-CHRISTIAN DISEASE. **x. iridis** Xanthomatosis affecting the iris of the eye. **normocholesteremic x.** HAND-SCHÜLLER-CHRISTIAN DISEASE.

**xanthomatous** \zanthäm′ətəs\ Relating to or characterized by xanthomas.

**xanthopathy** \zanthäp′əthē\ XANTHOCHROMIA.

**xanthophane** \zan′thəfān\ A yellow photoreceptor pigment.

**xanthophyll** \zan′thəfil\ $C_{40}H_{56}O_2$. Dihydroxy-α-carotene. A yellow pigment widely distributed in nature, as in green foliage, avian egg yolk, and human plasma.

**xanthopia** \zanthō′pē·ə\ XANTHOPSIA.

**xanthopsia** \zanthäp′sē·ə\ [XANTH- + -OPSIA] Faulty color vision with an exaggerated perception of yellow hues. Also *xanthopia, yellow vision.*

**xanthopsin** \zanthäp′sin\ VISUAL YELLOW.

**xanthorrhea** \zan′thôrē′ə\ [XANTHO- + -RRHEA] A yellow, serous discharge from the vagina; yellow menses.

**xanthorubin** \-roo′bin\ XANTORUBIN.

**xanthosarcoma** \-särkō′mə\ [XANTHO- + SARCOMA] MALIGNANT FIBROUS HISTIOCYTOMA.

**xanthosine** 9-*N*-β-D-Ribofuranosylxanthine, the nucleoside of xanthine. Symbol: Xao

**xanthosis** \zanthō′sis\ [XANTH- + -OSIS] A yellow discoloration, as of the skin. **x. diabetica** *Seldom used* XANTHOMA DIABETICORUM. **x. diabeticorum** *Seldom used* XANTHOMA DIABETICORUM.

**xanthotoxin** METHOXSALEN.

**xanthurenic acid** A metabolite of L-tryptophan found in urine that is present in increased quantities with a vitamin $B_6$ deficiency. It consists of 4,8-dihydroxyquinoline-2-carboxylic acid.

**xanthuria** \zanthoo′rē·ə\ XANTHINURIA.

**xantorubin** \zan′təroo′bin\ A yellow pigment which accumulates in serum after removal of the liver, largely unconjugated bilirubin. Also *xanthorubin.*

**Xao** A symbol for xanthosine.

**Xe** Symbol for the element, xenon.

**xeno-** \zē′nə-, zē′nō-, zen′ō-\ [Gk *xenos,* host, guest, stranger] A combining form meaning (1) foreign, extraneous, different, alien; (2) parasite or host.

**xenobiotic** \-bī·ät′tik\ [XENO- + BIOTIC] Not occurring in nature: used especially of certain synthetic organic compounds that are recalcitrant to biodegradation.

**xenodiagnosis** \-dī′agnō′sis\ A method of diagnosis based on feeding a laboratory-bred, infection-free potential host or vector on blood or other tissue suspected of harboring a parasite, and examining the vector or host later for presence of that parasite.

**xenogeneic** \-jənē′ik\ HETEROLOGOUS.

**xenogenic** \-jen′ik\ HETEROLOGOUS.

**xenogenous** \zenäj′ənəs\ [XENO- + -GENOUS] Originating from without the organism or caused by a substance foreign to the organism.

**xenograft** \zen′əgraft\ [XENO- + GRAFT] A tissue graft that is transferred from an organism of one species to an organism of a different species. Also *heterogenous graft, heterologous graft* (older term), *heteroplastic graft* (older term), *xenogeneic graft, heterograft, heterotransplant, heteroplastid.*

**xenology** \zenäl′əjē\ [XENO- + -LOGY] The study of host-parasite relationships.

**xenon** Element number 54, having atomic weight 131.30. Xenon is a colorless, odorless gas comprising about one part in 20 million of the atmosphere. There are nine stable isotopes and numerous short-lived radioactive isotopes. Xenon is one of the so-called inert gases, but a few highly unstable compounds have been reported. Symbol: Xe

**xenoparasite** \-par′əsīt\ [XENO- + PARASITE] A parasite which, because of weakened host resistance, becomes established in a host in which it does not ordinarily thrive, or becomes pathogenic in a host in which it is ordinarily a harmless ecosite.

**xenoplasty** \zen′əplas′tē\ [XENO- + -PLASTY] HETEROTRANSPLANTATION.

***Xenopsylla*** \-sil′ə\ [XENO- + Gk *psylla* a flea] A genus of fleas in the family Pulicidae, many species of which are important in disease transmission throughout the world. ***X. cheopis*** The oriental rat flea, a widely distributed species, particularly in the tropics where it is important in transmission of plague and murine typhus. It is closely associated with the black or roof rat, *Rattus rattus,* but also bites man readily. Transmission of plague bacilli is thought to be related to blockage of the proventriculus by a mass of bacilli, causing the host flea to probe more desperately, thus presumably facilitating passage of bacilli into the human host. Also *Pulex cheopis.*

**xenorexia** \zen′ôrek′sē·ə\ [XENO- + Gk *orex(is)* a longing for + -IA] *Older term* PICA.

**xenotope** \zen′ətōp\ An antigenic determinant present in a species foreign to the responding animal.

**xenotropic** \-träp′ik\ Of or pertaining to a virus whose genome may be integrated into the genome of the cells of a particular species, but which normally infects and is propagated in the cells of another species. Compare ECOTROPIC.

**xero-** \zir′ō-\ [Gk *xēros* dry] A combining form meaning dry.

**xerocheilia** \-kī′lē·ə\ [XERO- + CHEIL- + -IA] A dryness of the lips.

**xeroderma** \-dur′mə\ [XERO- + DERMA] Dryness of the skin. **x. of Kaposi** XERODERMA PIGMENTOSUM. **x. pigmentosum** A group of rare inherited autosomal recessive disorders in which the skin is readily damaged by ultraviolet light. This condition produces atrophy, pigmentary changes, and tumors, and predisposes to cancer of the skin. Also *angioma pigmentosum atrophicum, xeroderma of Kaposi.*

**xerography** \ziräg′rəfē\ XERORADIOGRAPHY.

**xeromenia** \-mē′nē·ə\ A condition in which the flow of menstrual blood is absent although the other symptoms of menstruation occur.

**xerophagia** \-fā′jə\ [XERO- + -PHAGIA] Consumption of dry food. Also *xerophagy.*

**xerophthalmia** \zir′äfthal′mē·ə\ [*xer(o)-* + OPHTHALMIA] Abnormal and severe dryness of the surface of the cornea and conjunctiva, as may occur in pemphigus, vitamin A deficiency, or certain autoimmune syndromes. Also *xerophthalmus, keratoconjunctivitis sicca.*

**xerophthalmus** \zir′äfthal′məs\ XEROPHTHALMIA.

**xeroradiography** \-rā′dē·äg′rəfē\ [XERO- + RADIOGRAPHY] A method of roentgenography using, instead of film, a metal plate coated with a semiconductor, such as selenium.

The image is obtained by dusting the plate with a dark powder, the particles of the powder being fixed in place by the electrical charges resulting from exposure of the plate to x rays. Also *xerography*.

**xerosis** \zirō′sis\ [*xer(o)-* + -OSIS] A dryness, as of the skin, eyes, or mucous membranes. **x. cutis** A dryness of the skin.

**xerostomia** \-stō′mē·ə\ [XERO- + STOM- + -IA] The dry state of the mouth consequent on the many conditions characterized by diminished salivary secretion, such as the von Mikulicz syndrome. Also *dry mouth*.

**xerotic** \zirät′ik\ **1** Of or relating to xerosis. **2** Dry.

**xerotocia** \-tō′sē·ə, -tō′shə\ [XERO- + *toc(o)-* + -IA] DRY LABOR.

**xiph-** \zif-, zīf-\ XIPHO-.

**xiphi-** \zif′ē-, zī′fē-\ XIPHO-.

**xiphisternum** \zif′istur′nəm\ PROCESSUS XIPHOIDEUS.

**xipho-** \zif′ō-, zī′fō-\ [Gk *xiphos* sword] A combining form meaning (1) xiphoid; (2) the xiphoid process. Also *xiphi-*, *xiph-*.

**xiphodidymus** \-did′iməs\ [XIPHO- + -DIDYMUS] XIPHOPAGUS.

**xiphodymus** \zifäd′iməs\ [XIPHO- + *-(di)dymus*] XIPHOPAGUS.

**xiphodynia** \-din′ē·ə\ XIPHOIDITIS.

**xiphoid** \zif′oid\ [Gk *xiphoeidēs* (from *xiphos* sword) sword-shaped] **1** Sword-shaped; ensiform. **2** See under PROCESSUS XIPHOIDEUS.

**xiphoidalgia** \zif′oidal′jə\ XIPHOIDITIS.

**xiphoiditis** \zif′oidī′tis\ [*xiphoid (process)* + -ITIS ] Inflammation or tenderness of the xiphoid process. Also *xiphodynia, xiphoidalgia*.

**xiphopagotomy** \zifäp′əgät′əmē\ [*xiphopag(us)* + -TOMY] The surgical separation of conjoined twins united at the xiphoid.

**xiphopagus** \zifäp′əgəs\ [XIPHO- + -PAGUS] Equal conjoined twins united at the breast bone, particularly at the xiphoid process. Also *xiphodidymus, xiphodymus*.

**X-linked** Of or pertaining to a genetic locus, or a phenotype produced by a genetic locus, on the X-chromosome of any organism.

**XO** **1** The symbolic designation in any organism, cell line, or cell for the presence of but one sex chromosome, the X. **2** In humans, a designation for the sex chromosome karyotype in the Turner syndrome. The preferred designation is 45,X.

**x-radiation** See under X RAYS.

**x rays** [*X* (as unknown factor) + RAY] The electromagnetic radiation produced by a gas tube or by a hot cathode tube, resulting from the bombardment of the anode by high velocity electrons from the cathode. Also *roentgen rays, x-radiation, paracathodic rays* (obs.). **characteristic x ray** CHARACTERISTIC RADIATION. **hard x ray** An x ray of high energy, i.e., short wavelength and great penetrating ability. **soft x ray** An x ray of low energy, i.e., long wavelength and low penetrating ability. **supersoft x.** X rays of very low energy, i.e., of very long wavelengths and very low penetrating power.

**XU** Symbol for the unit, X unit.

**xyl-** \zīl-\ XYLO-.

**xylan** Any polysaccharide composed of xylose residues. Xylans are usually 1,4-linked and occur with cellulose in wood and, particularly, in cereal straws and brans.

**xylitol** \zī′litôl\ A sugar alcohol used as an alternative sweetener to sucrose. It is used in chewing gums, as it inhibits the growth of bacteria causing tooth decay. Though equivalent in caloric content to sugar, it is as sweet as fructose, hence less xylitol than sugar need be used for an equivalent sweetening effect. It is ideally used as an additive to low-calorie food products.

**xylo-** \zī′lō-, zī′lə-\ [Gk *xylon* wood] A combining form meaning wood, woody. Also *xyl-*.

**Xylocaine** A proprietary name for lidocaine.

**xyloketose** *Obs.* XYLULOSE.

**xylometazoline hydrochloride** $C_{16}H_{24}N_2 \cdot HCl$. A white, odorless crystalline powder with sympathomimetic properties and marked α-adrenergic activity. It is used in dilute solution in nasal drops and sprays for temporary relief of nasal congestion.

**xylose** \zī′lōs\ An aldose containing five carbon atoms. It is the 3-epimer of ribose. It occurs in plant xylans from wood, and was once known as wood sugar.

**xylosuria** \zī′ləsoo′rē·ə\ [*xylos(e)* + -URIA] Urinary excretion of xylose, occurring especially after ingestion of certain fruits such as cherries, plums and grapes. It may occur in essential pentosuria.

**xylulose** A ulose containing five carbon atoms. Its chiral centers have the same configuration as those in xylose. Its 5-phosphate is an important metabolite. Also *xyloketose* (obs.).

**xylulose 5-phosphate** An intermediate in photosynthesis in plants and in the pentose phosphate pathway. It can donate a two-carbon fragment to an aldose under the action of transketolase to become glyceraldehyde 3-phosphate. It is interconvertible with ribulose 5-phosphate by enzymatic epimerization at C-3.

**L-xylulosuria** \zī′lyəlōsoo′rē·ə\ PENTOSURIA.

**xyphoid** \zī′foid\ See under XIPHOID.

**xyrospasm** \zī′rəspazm\ [Gk *xyro(n)* a razor + *spasm(os)* a convulsion, spasm] An occupational spasm or neurosis seen in barbers and involving the muscles of the forearm and wrist.

**xysma** \zis′mə\ [Gk *xysma* (from *xyein* to scratch, scrape) shavings, shreds] Shredded, sloughed intestinal mucosal tissue in the stool.

**xyster** \zis′tər\ [Gk *xystēr* (from *xyein* to scratch, scrape) a rasp, file] A surgical instrument, similar to a file, that is used to abrade bone and other firm tissues.

**X-zone** FETAL CORTEX.

# Y

**Y** 1 Symbol for the element, yttrium. 2 Symbol for tyrosine.

**-y** \-ē\ [French *-ie,* from L *-ia* and Gk *-ia, -eia,* derivative noun suffixes] A noun suffix meaning (1) a condition or quality; (2) a process or operation; (3) a field of practice or study.

**yabapox** \yab′əpäks\ A poxviral disease occurring in rhesus monkeys. Its predominant manifestations are subcutaneous tumors. Also *Yaba tumor.*

**Yates** [Frank *Yates,* English statistician, born 1902] See under CORRECTION.

**yatobyo** \yät′ōbyō′\ [Japanese (from *ya* field, rural + *to* rabbit + *byō* sickness) rabbit fever] A Japanese term for TULAREMIA.

**yaw** \yô\ [back-formation from YAWS] A skin lesion occurring in yaws. **mother y.** The initial or primary lesion of yaws. Also *buba madre, mamanpian, protopianoma.* **ringworm y.** An acircinate skin lesion of yaws simulating ringworm.

**yawn** [Middle English *yanen, yonien* from Old English *geonian,* to yawn, akin to L *hiatus* a gaping] 1 A deep, involuntary inspiration normally through an open mouth and sometimes accompanied by stretching of the arms and shoulders (pandiculation). It is usually associated with drowsiness or boredom. 2 To execute a yawn. Also *oscitate.*

**yawning** The act of producing a yawn. Also *oscitation, hiation.*

**yaws** \yôz\ [of Carib origin, akin to *yáya* (Carib of the Lesser Antilles) yaws] A nonvenereal spirochetal infection caused by *Treponema pertenue,* usually occurring in tropical regions among primitive, rural-based populations and more commonly seen in children than in adults. The primary stage is characterized by appearance of a granulomatous lesion or papule (the frambesioma or mother yaw) at the site of infection, usually on the lower leg or foot. The lesion enlarges and crusts, then heals spontaneously. In the second stage, there is a generalized eruption of granulomatous, papular, macular, or squamous lesions and, in some cases, osteitis and periositis. The late stage is characterized by appearance of cutaneous plaques, nodules, and ulcers, hyperkeratoses of the hands and feet, and gummatous lesions affecting bones. Yaws is readily cured with penicillin. Also *frambesia, framboesia, pian, bouba (Brazilian), buba (South American Spanish), parangi (Sri Lankan), Charlouis disease* (outmoded), *Breda's disease* (outmoded), *frambesia tropica, polypapilloma tropicum.* **crab y.** FOOT YAWS. **foot y.** Tertiary yaws involving the soles of the feet and sometimes the palms of the hands, and marked by hyperkeratosis, fissuring, ulcerations, and severe pain. A crablike gait may ensue. Also *dumas, tubba, tubboe, crab yaws.* **forest y.** PIAN BOIS.

**Yb** Symbol for the element, ytterbium.

**year** / **potential y.'s of life lost** See under LIFE.

**yeast** [Middle English *yest,* Old English *gist,* akin to Gk *zeein* to boil, seethe] Any of various unicellular nucleated fungi, typically saprophytic, capable of fermenting a range of carbohydrates, and generally reproducing asexually by budding. The yeasts do not constitute a taxon. Also *faex.* **dried y.** A dried tablet or powder form of *Saccharomyces cerevisiae* which is rich in protein and B vitamins and is administered in the treatment of vitamin B deficiency. Also *cerevisiae fermentum siccatum.* **false y.** Any of the yeastlike fungal forms belonging to the form-order Cryptococcales of the form-class Deuteromycetes. This fungus reproduces only by asexual budding or pseudohyphal asporogenous growth. Also *imperfect yeast.* **perfect y.** TRUE YEAST. **sporogenous y.** TRUE YEAST. **true y.** Any of the budding yeasts belonging to the class Ascomycetes. In addition to budding, these fungi reproduce sexually by producing ascospores. Included in this group are the brewers' yeasts. Also *perfect yeast, sporogenous yeast.*

**yellow** [Old English *geolu,* akin to Gk *chlōros* pale green, greenish yellow] 1 A color of the visible spectrum falling between green and orange. 2 A substance, usually a stain or dye, that is yellow in appearance, or that produces a cytochemical reaction resulting in yellow staining. For chemical names including *yellow,* see under the chemical name. **brilliant y.** An acid azo dye occasionally used in tissue stains but largely useful as an indicator, changing from yellow to orange at pH 7.4 to 8.6. **butter y.** A yellow dye once added to foodstuffs but since shown to be carcinogenic. Its molecule is diazobenzene with a dimethylamino group as a *p*-substituent in one ring. **canary y.** AURAMINE O. **Manchester y.** MARTIUS YELLOW. **Martius y.** A synthetic acid dye used as a counterstain in the MSB stain for fibrin. Also *Manchester yellow.* **rhubarb y.** CHRYSOPHANIC ACID. **visual y.** The photopigment with greatest sensitivity in the yellow portion of the spectrum. Also *xanthopsin.*

**yellow jack** *Popular* YELLOW FEVER.

**Yersin** [Alexandre John Emile *Yersin,* Swiss bacteriologist active in France, 1863–1943] See under SERUM.

***Yersinia*** \yursin′ē·ə\ [after A.J.E. *Yersin,* discoverer of the plague bacillus] A recently named genus consisting of several former members of *Pasteurella* that were reclassified into the family of Enterobacteriaceae. They are Gram-negative facultative rods with simple growth requirements. ***Y. enterocolitica*** A species widely distributed in wild and domestic animals. In humans it acts much like other enterotoxic Enterobacteriaceae, causing chiefly an acute gastroenteritis. At least 34 different O antigens have been recognized. Its temperature optimum is low. Motility and several biochemical reactions are evident at 25°C but not at 37°C. ***Y. pestis*** A species of nonmotile, short, Gram-negative rods; the plague bacillus. It tends to stain in a bipolar fashion with methylene blue. It grows well on ordinary media, with a temperature optimum of 28°C. Virulent organisms have a capsule. The VW antigens also promote resistance to phagocytosis. The organism produces a murine toxin, lethal to rats and mice. The organism is primarily a pathogen of rats, and it is transmitted by fleas from rats to humans and among humans. Also *Pasteurella pestis* (former name). ***Y. pseudotuberculosis*** A species closely resembling *Y. enterocolitica.* In humans it generally causes acute mesenteric lymphadenitis or terminal ileitis rather than gastroenteritis. Also *Pasteurella pseudotuberculosis* (former name).

**yersiniosis** \yərsin′ē·ō′sis\ Any disease caused by bacteria of the genus *Yersinia.*

**-yl** [French *-yle* from Gk *hylē* wood, material] An ending in organic chemistry which converts the name of a substance into the name of a group. If it replaces the ending *-ane* of a hydrocarbon it forms an alkyl group by removing H. If it replaces the ending *-ic acid* in the name of an acid, as in *hexanoic acid*, it forms the corresponding acyl group by removing —OH.

**-ylene** \-ilēn, -əlin\ [-YL + Gk *-ēnē*, fem. patronymic suffix] A chemical suffix. It occurs in the words *methylene*, for the group $—CH_2—$, *ethylene*, a common name for ethene, $CH_2{=}CH_2$, and *propylene*, the group $—CH(CH_3)—CH_2—$. In systematic names it replaces the ending *-ane* of a saturated hydrocarbon, or the final letter of the ending *-ene* of an unsaturated one, to indicate formation of a bivalent group by removing two hydrogen atoms from different positions in the molecule.

**yochubio** \yōchoobyō′\ [Japanese *yōchūbyō* (from *yōchū* larva + *byō* disease) scrub typhus.] SCRUB TYPHUS.

**yogurt** \yō′gərt\ [Turkish *yoğurt*] A food made from curdled milk fermented by a specific strain of lactobacillus. Yogurt is sometimes advocated as a means of improving intestinal flora.

**yoke** \yōk\ [Old English *geoc*, akin to L *jugum* yoke and Gk *zygon*, also *zygos* yoke] JUGUM. **alveolar y.'s** JUGA ALVEOLARIA. **cerebral y.'s of bone of cranium** The variable raised markings on the internal surface of the cranium formed between the impressions for the cerebral gyri. *Outmoded.* **sphenoidal y.** JUGUM SPHENOIDALE.

**yolk** \yōk\ [Middle English *yolke*, from Old English *geolca*, akin to *geolu* yellow] The nutrient material in an ovum; vitellus.

**Yoshida** [Tomizo *Yoshida*, Japanese pathologist, born 1903] See under TUMOR.

**Young** [Frank George *Young*, English biochemist, born 1908] Young syndrome. See under BERRY-PERKINS-YOUNG SYNDROME.

**Young** [Freida *Young*, English physician, flourished 20th century] Dyke-Young syndrome. See under SYNDROME.

**Young** [Thomas *Young*, English physician 1773–1829] **1** See under RULE. **2** Young-Helmholtz theory. See under HELMHOLTZ THEORY OF COLOR VISION.

**Y-plasty** \wī′plastē\ **Foley Y.** A plastic operation for obstruction of the ureteropelvic junction, in which a Y incision is closed as a V, giving additional width to the narrowed area. Also *Schweizer-Foley Y-plasty, Foley Y-type ureteropelvioplasty.* **Schweizer-Foley Y.** FOLEY Y-PLASTY.

**ys** yellow spot (macula lutea retinae).

**ytterbium** An element in the lanthanide series, having atomic number 70 and atomic weight 173.04. Symbol: Yb

**yttrium** A metallic element having atomic number 39 and atomic weight 88.9059. Yttrium 89, the only stable isotope, is found in most rare-earth minerals. Twenty unstable isotopes and isomers are known. Yttrium 90, with a half-life of 64 hours, exists in equilibrium with its parent, strontium 90, in the fallout from nuclear explosions. Symbol: Y

**Yule** [George Udny *Yule*, English statistician, 1871–1951] Greenwood-Yule method. See under METHOD.

# Z

**Z** **1** Symbol for atomic number. **2** Symbol for proton number. **3** Symbol for glutamine or glutamic acid without specifying which.

**(Z)-** [German *zusammen* together] A stereochemical prefix describing the placing of substituents about a double bond. For a detailed description of its use, see under (*E*)-.

**z** Symbol for catalytic amount.

**Zahn** [Friedrich Wilhelm *Zahn*, German pathologist, 1845–1904] **1** Pockets of Zahn. See under POCKET. **2** Lines of Zahn. See under LINE.

**Zahorsky** [John *Zahorsky*, Hungarian-born U.S. pediatrician, 1871–1963] Zahorsky's disease. See under EXANTHEM SUBITUM.

**Zander** [Jonas Gustav Wilhelm *Zander*, Swedish physician, 1835–1920] See under APPARATUS.

**Zangemeister** [Wilhelm *Zangemeister*, German gynecologist, 1871–1930] See under TEST.

**Zappert** [Julius *Zappert*, Czech-born physician active in Austria, 1867–1942] Zappert's chamber. See under HEMOCYTOMETER.

**Zaufal** [Emanual *Zaufal*, Czech rhinologist, 1837–1910] Zaufal sign. See under SADDLENOSE.

**zeatin** \zē′ətin\ A naturally occurring cytokinin found in immature corn kernels, peas, and spinach. It enhances DNA synthesis and has the highest growth-promoting activity of any of the natural cytokinins.

**Zeeman** [Pieter *Zeeman*, Dutch physicist, 1865–1943] See under EFFECT.

**zein** \zē′in\ A seed protein from corn, *Zea mays*. It is of poor nutritional value because of its low lysine content.

**Zeis** [after Eduard *Zeis*, German ophthalmologist, 1807–1868] **1** Zeisian stye. See under STYE. **2** Glands of Zeis. See under GLANDULAE SEBACEAE PALPEBRARUM.

**zeism** \zē′izm\ [New L *ze(a)* (from Gk *zeia* a coarse wheat) maize + -ISM] Any disorder arising from the consumption of a diet largely consisting of maize, such as pellagra. Also *zeismus.*

**Zeiss** [Carl *Zeiss*, German optician, 1816–1888] Abbe-Zeiss counting cell, Abbe-Zeiss counting chamber, Thoma-Zeiss counting cell. See under THOMA-ZEISS COUNTING CHAMBER.

**Zeller** [Albert *Zeller*, German surgeon, flourished late 19th century] Zeller's test. See under MOLONEY TEST.

**Zellweger** [Hans Ulrich *Zellweger*, Swiss-born U.S. pediatrician, born 1909] Zellweger syndrome. See under CEREBROHEPATORENAL SYNDROME.

**Zenker** [Friedrich Albert von *Zenker*, German pathologist and anatomist, 1825–1898] **1** Zenker's leiomyoma. See under LEIOMYOSARCOMA. **2** Zenker's diverticulum, Zenker's pouch. See under PHARYNGOESOPHAGEAL DIVERTICULUM. **3** Zenker's fixative, Zenker solution. See under FLUID. **4** Zenker-formol fixative. See under HELLY'S FLUID. **5** Zenker's degeneration. See under HYALINE NECROSIS. **6** Zenker's paralysis. See under COMMON PERONEAL NERVE PARALYSIS.

**zenkerize** \zeng′kərīz\ To fix a tissue for histologic study using Zenker's fixative.

**zeolite** Any of a group of aluminosilicate minerals. They may be used as cation exchangers, especially for softening water. Synthetic zeolites are also available for this purpose.

**zero** [French *zéro* (from Italian *zero*, contraction of *zefiro*, from Arabic *ṣifr* cipher, zero, empty) zero] **1** The numeral or symbol 0, indicating the absence of quantity. **2** The point on a graduated scale from which reckoning begins. **absolute z.** The temperature 0 kelvin, −273.15°C, −459.67°F; the temperature at which molecular motion ceases and a body has no heat energy. **audiometric z.** The 0 dB level on a pure tone audiometer. It is calibrated in dB HL as defined by the International Organization for Standardization (ISO) and refers to a statistical mean for the hearing of otologically normal young people. It is possible to have hearing better than 0 dB HL, so that it is necessary to include −10 dB HL on the attenuator.

**zeugmatography** \zoog′mətäg′rəfē\ [Gk *zeugma*, gen. *zeugmatos* a band, bond + -GRAPHY] A magnetic resonance imaging technique that uses static, radio-frequency, and gradient magnetic fields to produce a three-dimensional image of the distribution of elements such as hydrogen and phosphorus in the body.

**Z-flap** See under FLAP.

**zidovudine** $C_{10}H_{13}N_5O_4$. 3′-Azido-2′-deoxythymidine. An antiviral agent that inhibits retroviral reverse transcriptase. It is used in the treatment of human immunodeficiency virus (HIV) infection, where it has been shown to prolong life but is not curative. It is generally administered orally but also can be given intravenously. Its major toxic effect is bone marrow suppression. Also *azidothymidine.*

**Ziegler** [Samuel Lewis *Ziegler,* U.S. ophthalmologist, 1861–1925] See under OPERATION.

**Ziehen** [Georg Theodor *Ziehen,* German psychiatrist, 1862–1950] Ziehen-Oppenheim disease. See under DYSTONIA MUSCULORUM DEFORMANS.

**Ziehl** [Franz *Ziehl,* German bacteriologist, 1857–1926] Ziehl-Neelsen carbolfuchsin, Ziehl-Neelsen technique. See under ZIEHL-NEELSEN STAIN.

**Ziemssen** [Hugo Wilhelm von *Ziemssen,* German physician, 1829–1902] Ziemssen's motor point. See under MOTOR POINT.

**Zieve** [Leslie *Zieve,* U.S. physician, born 1915] See under SYNDROME.

**Zimmermann** [Wilhelm *Zimmermann,* German chemist and physician, born 1910] See under REACTION.

**zinc** Element number 30, having atomic weight 65.38. It occurs in various ores, never in the free state. Ordinary zinc is a bluish white lustrous metal consisting of five stable isotopes. Ten unstable isomers and isotopes are known. The valence is 2. The metal and its compounds have many technological uses. Compounds are used in cosmetics and pharamaceuticals. $Zn^{2+}$ ions are constituents of many enzymes, such as carbonic anhydrase and carboxypeptidase, in which they supply electron attraction, and are required in the zinc-insulin complex that is stored in pancreatic cells. Symbol: Zn **white z.** ZINC OXIDE.

**zinc 65** A radioisotope of zinc which disintegrates by electron capture, emitting a characteristic x ray of 8 keV, a beta particle, and a gamma ray. It is employed in the study of mineral metabolism and leukocyte life cycle. Physical half-life is 245 days. Symbol: $^{65}Zn$

**zinc acetate** $(CH_3CO_2)_2Zn{\cdot}2H_2O$. A zinc salt that has been used in dilute solutions as eye lotions and in eye drops in the treatment of conjunctivitis. It has also been used orally as an emetic.

**zincalism** \zing′kəlizm\ Zinc poisoning. See under POISONING.

**zinc bacitracin** A zinc salt of bacitracin, which has greater stability than does bacitracin alone. It is used in preparations for topical application.

**zinc caprylate** $C_{16}H_{30}O_4Zn$. A topical fungicide with properties very much like those of zinc propionate.

**zinc chloride** $ZnCl_2$. A white, deliquescent powder with caustic and astringent properties. It is used topically in lotions to treat chronic skin conditions.

**zinc oxide** ZnO. A white powder without taste or odor. It is used topically for skin disorders. It has mild astringent properties and it is applied in dusting powders, lotions, pastes, creams and ointments. Also *white zinc.*

**zinc permanganate** $Mn_2O_8Zn$. A medication very similar to potassium permanganate. It is used as an antiseptic and astringent solution.

**zinc peroxide** $ZnO_2$. A yellowish white powder used topically in the treatment of ulcerative skin conditions. **medicinal z.** A mixture of zinc peroxide, zinc oxide, and zinc hydroxide containing not less than 60% $ZnO_2$. It is used like hydrogen peroxide as a disinfectant and deodorizing medication, in a suspension or a cream.

**zinc stearate** The zinc salt of a mixture of stearic and palmitic acids. It is water insoluble and used as a protective medication for the skin in the treatment of chronic diseases such as eczema and acne.

**zinc sulfate** $ZnSO_4{\cdot}7H_2O$. A colorless, crystalline powder used in skin lotions because of its astringent properties.

**zincundecate** A medication composed of a mixture of undecenoic acid and zinc undecenoate. It is used to treat tinea pedis.

**zinc undecylenate** The zinc salt of undecylenic acid. It is used topically in an ointment as an antifungal treatment, and for some skin diseases such as psoriasis.

**Zinn** [Johann Gottfried *Zinn,* German anatomist and naturalist, 1727–1759] **1** Tendon of Zinn, aponeurosis of Zinn. See under ANNULUS TENDINEUS COMMUNIS. **2** See under MEMBRANE. **3** Zonule of Zinn, zone of Zinn, zonula ciliaris zinnii. See under ZONULA CILIARIS. **4** Sulcus of tendon of Zinn. See under SULCUS.

**Zinser** [Ferdinand *Zinser,* German dermatologist, 1865–1952] Zinser-Cole-Engman syndrome. See under DYSKERATOSIS CONGENITA.

**Zinsser** [Hans *Zinsser,* U.S. bacteriologist, 1878–1940] Brill-Zinsser disease. See under BRILL'S DISEASE.

**zirconium** A metallic element having atomic number 40 and atomic weight 91.22. In nature it consists of five isotopes, of which zirconium 96 is weakly radioactive, with a half-life of $3.6 \times 10^{17}$ years. Compounds of zirconium are not detectably toxic. The metal is extremely resistant to corrosion and has some use in surgical instruments. Symbol: Zr

**$z_C/m_S$** Symbol for the quantity, catalytic content, i.e., the catalytic activity divided by mass, often applied to the content of an enzyme in a tissue.

**Zn** Symbol for the element, zinc.

**zoacanthosis** \zō′akanthō′sis\ [*zo(o)-* + ACANTH- + -OSIS] A dermatosis caused by the implantation of animal hair bristles or other animal tissue into the dermis.

**zoescope** \zō′əskōp\ STROBOSCOPE.

**zoite** \zō′īt\ [*zo(o)-* + -ITE] MEROZOITE.

**Zollinger** [Robert Milton *Zollinger,* U.S. surgeon, born 1903] **1** Zollinger-Ellison tumor. See under TUMOR. **2** Zollinger-Ellison syndrome. See under SYNDROME.

**zona** \zō′nə\ [L (from Gk *zōnē* a girdle, belt, zone, herpes zoster] (*pl.* zonae) **1** An encircling region or area, usually with specific boundaries; a zone. **2** An area or part, usually delimited, with distinctive characteristics or structure; a zone, band, or layer. **3** HERPES ZOSTER. **z. arcuata** [NA] The inner, thin part of the basilar membrane extending between the limbus laminae spiralis and the bases of the outer rods of the spiral organ and forming the floor of the inner tunnel of Corti. Also *arcuate zone.* **z. cartilaginea** LIMBUS LAMINAE SPIRALIS OSSEAE. **z. dermatica** A rim of thickened skin encircling the protruded nervous tissue in spina bifida. **z. epithelioserosa** An interval of membranous tissue lying between the zona dermatica and the protruded nervous tissue in spina bifida. **z. fasciculata** FASCICULAR ZONE. **z. glomerulosa** GLOMERULAR ZONE. **z. ignea** *Older term* HERPES ZOSTER. **z. incerta** [NA] A thin strip of gray substance that also contains fine fiber bundles, located dorsal and medial to the subthalamic nucleus and separated from the ventral limit of the thalamus by the thalamic fasciculus. It receives corticofugal fibers from the precentral region of the cerebral cortex and probably also from the globus pallidus, but the functional significance of this region is still to be determined. **z. ophthalmica** HERPES OPHTHALMICUS. **z. orbicularis articulationis coxae** [NA] A ring round the neck of the femur formed by the deeper, circular fibers of the fibrous capsule of the hip joint, blending with the pubofemoral and ischiofemoral ligaments but having no direct attachment to bone. Also *orbicular zone of hip joint, annular ligament of femur, ring ligament of hip joint, zonular band, Weber zone.* **z. pectinata** [NA] The thick outer part of the basilar membrane extending from the bases of the outer rods of the spiral organ to the crista basilaris on the outer wall of the cochlear duct. Also *pectinate zone.* **z. pellucida** A relatively thick, striated, PAS-positive envelope which is formed about the primary oocyte when it is inside an ovarian follicle and which separates it from the surrounding follicular cells. The zona thickens as the follicle matures and is present after the ovum has been expelled from the follicle at ovulation. It plays a part in fertilization, when it is penetrated usually by only one spermatozoon, but how and if it excludes other spermatozoa is not fully understood. It persists while the ovum undergoes its cleavage divisions and disappears when the morula becomes a blastocyst at the time it has entered the uterine cavity. Also *zona radiata.* **z. radiata** ZONA PELLUCIDA. **z. reticularis** RETICULAR ZONE. **z. rolandica** CORTICAL MOTOR AREA. **z. serpiginosa** HERPES ZOSTER. **z. spongiosa** APEX CORNUS POSTERIORIS MEDULLAE SPINALIS. **z. vasculosa** MEDULLA OVARII. **z. vasculosa of Waldeyer** MEDULLA OVARII.

**zonae** \zō′nē\ Plural of ZONA.

**zonate** \zō′nāt\ Marked by zones.

**Zondek** [Bernhardt *Zondek*, German-born Israeli obstetrician and gynecologist, 1891–1966] Aschheim-Zondek hormone. See under LUTEINIZING HORMONE.

# zone

**zone** [L *zona*. See ZONA.] **1** An area or part, usually delimited, with distinctive characteristics or structure. **2** A girdling or encircling area or layer; a band. **abdominal z.'s** REGIONES ABDOMINALES. **z. of adhesion** Any of several hundred regions in a Gram-negative cell where the inner and the outer membrane are continuous across a hole in the murein. They are best visualized when stretched by osmotic contraction of the protoplast (plasmolysis). They appear to be sites of entry of some phages, and to play a role in the translocation of components into the outer membrane during growth. Also *Bayer patch, intermembrane junction.* **algogenic z.** DOLOROGENIC ZONE. **analgesic z.** A cutaneous area not responsive to pain sensation. **androgenic z.** FETAL CORTEX. **z. of antemortem wound** Either of the two zones of tissue reaction to injury as demonstrated by enzyme histochemistry. The central or superficial zone, located immediately adjacent to the wound edge, is an area of imminent necrosis and shows decreased enzyme activity. Increased enzyme activity occurs in the adjacent surrounding peripheral zone, and the temporal sequence of appearances of differing enzyme activities in this zone may be used as a rough guideline for timing antemortem wounds. **z. of antibody excess** See under ZONE PHENOMENON. **z. of antigen excess** See under ZONE PHENOMENON. **arcuate z.** ZONA ARCUATA. **Barnes z.** The lowermost portion of a pregnant uterus. Placental attachment at this site is likely to result in some form of placenta previa. **chondrogenic z.** The inner layer of perichondrium where proliferation of cells leads to appositional growth. **ciliary z.** *Outmoded* ANNULUS IRIDIS MAJOR. **z. of coagulation** That part of a burn where dermal vessels are destroyed or clotted. **cornuradicular z.** ROOT-CORD JUNCTION. **Cozzolino z.** FISSULA ANTE FENESTRAM. **dead z.** The depth zone closest to the ultrasound transducer, in which imaging cannot be performed. **dendritic z.** A volume of neural tissue within which lies the receptive surfaces of the dendrites of a nerve cell; the dendritic field of a neuron. **dolorogenic z.** Any trigger point which, when touched or stimulated in any way, arouses pain, such as skin areas on the face and head in trigeminal neuralgia. Also *algogenic zone.* **dorsal z. of His** ALAR LAMINA. **ectopic z.** An area on the prosencephalon of the early embryonic brain that surrounds most of the optic vesicle and from which much of the telencephalon and diencephalon arise. Also *ectopic zone of Schulte.* **ectopic z. of Schulte** ECTOPIC ZONE. **ependymal z.** EPENDYMAL LAYER. **epigastric z.** REGIO EPIGASTRICA. **equivalence z.** In precipitation reactions, that zone in which both antigen and antibody are completely combined and no uncombined antigen or antibody is present. See also ZONE PHENOMENON. **ergotropic z.** The region of the caudal hypothalamus that activates the sympathetic system to increase vasodilatation in skeletal muscle and enhance adrenergic responses in other effectors, resulting in increased blood pressure, heart rate, and cardiac output. **erogenous z.** Any part of the body which is reactive to sexual stimulation. Also *erotogenic zone.* **erotogenic z.** EROGENOUS ZONE. **extravisual z.** The area outside the portion of the visual field seen through a spectacle lens. **far z.** FAR FIELD. **fascicular z.** The wide middle zone of the adrenal cortex, consisting of large lipid-rich cells arranged radially in parallel cords. The mitochondria tend to be spherical. It is thought to be the principal adrenocortical site of glucocorticoid synthesis in some species. Also *zona fasciculata.* **fetal z.** FETAL CORTEX. **focal z.** The region of minimum diameter and area in a beam of radiation. **Fraunhofer z.** FAR FIELD. **Fresnel z.** NEAR FIELD. **gingival z.** *Outmoded* ATTACHED GINGIVA. **glomerular z.** The narrow outer subcapsular layer of the adrenal cortex, consisting of small cells arranged in indefinite clusters. The mitochondria tend to be elongated. It is thought to be the principal site of aldosterone secretion in some species. Also *zona glomerulosa.* **H z.** The zone in striated muscle where the myosin filaments do not have overlapping actin filaments. In the middle of this zone is the M line, where the myosin molecules reverse direction. **z. of hyperemia** The cutaneous area surrounding a deeper burn where dilated dermal vessels carry a greater than normal amount of blood. Such vascular dilatation is characteristic of first degree burns. **hypnogenic z.** Any region of the body that when subjected to pressure will induce a hypnotic state or sleep in susceptible subjects. *Older term.* **hypogastric z.** REGIO PUBICA. **inhibition z.** PROZONE. **interpalpebral z.** The parts of the cornea and sclera visible between the open eyelids. **Lissauer's marginal z.** TRACTUS DORSOLATERALIS. **Looser's transformation z.'s** Radiolucent lines visualized on roentgenograms of bones, believed to represent fatigue fractures taking place in some bone diseases, such as osteomalacia. *Imprecise.* Also *umbau zones, umbauzonen.* **mantle z.** MANTLE LAYER. **Marchant's detachable z.** An area on the endocranial surface of the sphenoid and occipital bones where the dura mater can be easily stripped away. **marginal z.** MARGINAL LAYER. **maturation z.** Any zone where cells acquire their fully differentiated form. **median root z.** FASCICULUS TRIANGULARIS. **medullary z.** MEDULLA RENALIS. **motor z.** Any area of the cerebral cortex whose stimulation regularly produces contraction of one or more muscles resulting in some type of movement. The movement may be limited to one muscle or may include an ensemble of muscles in the trunk and/or extremities. **multiplication z.** A region where cell division is actively taking place. **near z.** NEAR FIELD. **nephrogenic z.** The subcapsular region in the developing kidney where the metanephric blastemal cap differentiates into the renal corpuscles. **neutral z.** The place between the tongue and the cheeks where the opposing muscular forces are equal. It is assumed that natural or artificial teeth will be stable if placed in this zone. **notogenetic z.** The part of the vertebrate embryo which is sustained by the notochord. **nuclear z.** The central, harder portion of the substantia lentis which has a high refractive index and, on slit-lamp examination, is subdivided into adult, outer embryonic, and inner embryonic nuclear zones. **orbicular z. of hip joint** ZONA ORBICULARIS ARTICULATIONIS COXAE. **organizer z.** ORGANIZER. **papillary z.** STRATUM PAPILLARE CORII. **pectinate z.** ZONA PECTINATA. **perifollicular z.** An ill-defined zone of lymphocytes and dendritic reticulum cells at the periphery of a lymphoid follicle. **placental z.** The site on the surface of the gravid uterus covered by the insertion of the placenta. **z. of plateaux and furrows** Pars plana and pars plicata of the peripheral eye. **pupillary z.** The portion of the iris central to the collarette. **z. of rarefaction** A localized area of radiolucency in an x ray of bone, typically seen in juvenile scurvy. The zone of rarefaction is usually sited at the upper end of the tibial metaphysis on its medial aspect. It represents localized destruction of bone. **reticular z.** The moderately wide innermost layer of the adrenal cortex, contiguous with the adrenal medulla, and consisting of interconnected networks of cells that contain less lipid than those of the fascicular zone. The mitochondria are elongated with both tubular and flattened cristae. Also *zona reticularis.* **z. of round nuclei** In the olfactory epithelium, a deep layer of rounded nuclei that is formed by the receptor cells. **sclerotic z.** A circumcorneal vascular zone formed deep to the conjunctiva by conjunctival branches of the anterior ciliary arteries, which then pierce the sclera near the sclerocorneal junction to end in the circulus arteriosus iridis major. **segmental z.** SEGMENTAL PLATE. **Spitzka's marginal z.** TRACTUS DORSOLATERALIS. **z. of stasis** The cutaneous area in a burn where damaged vessels result in sluggish blood flow. **transition z.** 1 The point at which the previously cylindrical ultrasonic beam begins to widen into a cone. 2 See under TRANSITIONAL ZONE. **transitional z.** 1 The region of the equator of the lens of the eye where new lens fibers are continually produced by transformation of the cells of the anterior epithelium. The fibers are at first nucleated, but the nuclei disappear as the fibers develop and grow. 2 PECTEN ANALIS. **trigger z.** TRIGGER AREA. **trophotropic z. of Hess** A region in the anterior hypothalamus and preoptic area the electrical stimulation of which has induced lethargy, adynamia, and sleep behavior in animals. Additional physiologic responses were parasympathetic in nature and were subsequently interpreted as being pleasurable to animals. **umbau z.'s** LOOSER'S TRANSFORMATION ZONES. **ventral z. of His** BASAL LAMINA. **vermilion z.** VERMILION BORDER. **vermilion transitional z.** VERMILION BORDER. **Weber z.** ZONA ORBICULARIS ARTICULATIONIS COXAE. **Wernicke z.** WERNICKE CENTER. **X z.** FETAL CORTEX. **z. of Zinn** ZONULA CILIARIS.

**zonesthesia** \zōn′esthē′zhə\ [Gk *zōn(ē)* a girdle, belt + -ESTHESIA] The perception that a portion of the body, usually the trunk, is being constricted or strangled, as if by a girdle. Also *girdle sensation, cincture sensation.*

**zonifugal** \zōnif′yəgəl\ Moving away from a region or zone, as may occur when a perceived sensation becomes distributed to parts other than the central zone.

**zonipetal** \zōnip′ətəl\ Passing from the periphery inward toward a region, as a perceived sensation that appears to move into a central zone from some more distant site.

**zonula** \zōn′yələ, zän′yələ\ [L (dim. of ZONA), a little girdle] A small, usually circular, zone. Also *zonule.* **z. adherens** An adhering zone, as a belt, between adjacent cells, with filamentous material between the plasma membranes and with tonofilaments in the cytoplasm. Also *intermediate junction.* **z. ciliaris** [NA] The thick structure formed by the vitreous membrane and the radial fibers anterior to the ora serrata of the retina which then splits into two layers, a thin layer lining the hyaloid fossa of the vitreous body and a second layer comprising a series of fibers which pass over the ciliary body and attach to the capsule of the lens in front and behind the equator, thereby forming the suspensory ligament of the lens. The term is often used in reference to the second layer only. Also *ciliary zonule, zonule of Zinn, zone of Zinn, zonula ciliaris zinnii* (outmoded), *lens zonule, suspensory ligament of lens, apparatus suspensorius lentis* (outmoded). **z. occludens** A tight junction in which the region of membrane contact occurs as a band around the surface of the cell. It is usually found in the epithelial tissue of vertebrates.

**zonulae** \zōn′yəlē\ Plural of ZONULA.

**zonule** \zōn′yool\ [L *zonula.* See ZONULA.] ZONULA. **ciliary z.** ZONULA CILIARIS. **lens z.** ZONULA CILIARIS. **z. of Zinn** ZONULA CILIARIS.

**zonulitis** \zōn′yəlī′tis\ [L *zonul(a ciliaris)* + -ITIS] Inflammation of the suspensory ligaments of the crystalline lens.

**zonulolysis** \zōn′yəläl′isis\ ZONULYSIS.

**zonulotomy** \zōn′yəlät′əmē\ [*zonul(e)* + *o* + -TOMY] A cutting of the suspensory ligament of the crystalline lens.

**zonulysis** \zōn′yəlī′sis\ [*zonu(le)* + LYSIS] Dissolution of the suspensory ligament of the lens, as by the enzyme $\alpha$ chymotrypsin, used in the technique of intracapsular cataract extraction. Also *zonulolysis.*

**zoo-** \zō′ə-\ [Gk *zōon* living being, animal] A combining form meaning animal (1) animal; (2) living, alive.

**zooanthroponosis** \zō′ə·an′thrəpōnō′sis\ [ZOO- + ANTHROPONOSIS] A disease of humans transmissible to animals. Compare ANTHROPOZOONOSIS.

**zoobiology** \zō′əbī·äl′əjē\ [ZOO- + BIOLOGY] The biology of animals.

**zoodermic** \zō′ədur′mik\ Pertaining to the skin of an

animal other than man: used to refer to skin grafts made of animal skin.

**zoodynamics** \zō′ədīnam′iks\ [ZOO- + DYNAMICS] ANIMAL PHYSIOLOGY. Adj. zoodynamic.

**zoogenous** \zō·äj′ənəs\ Originating in or produced by animals. Also *zoogenic*.

**zoogonous** \zō·äg′ənəs\ [ZOO- + GON-[2] + -OUS ] VIVIPAROUS.

**zoograft** \zō′əgraft\ [ZOO- + GRAFT] ANIMAL GRAFT.

**zoology** \zō·äl′əjē\ [ZOO- + -LOGY] The branch of science that deals with the study of animals.

**Zoomastigophorea** \zō′əmas′tigōfôr′ē·ə\ [New L, from ZOO- + Gk *mastix*, gen. *mastigo(s)* a whip + -PHORE] A class of protozoan flagellates that includes many disease-causing parasites of man and animals such as the trypanosomes, leishmaniae, trichomonads and others.

**Zoon** [Johannes Jacobus *Zoon*, Dutch dermatologist, born 1902] See under ERYTHROPLASIA.

**zoonoses** \zō′ənō′sēz\ Plural of ZOONOSIS.

**zoonosis** \zō′ənō′sis\ [New L *zoonosus* (from ZOO- + Gk *nosos* disease, illness) with ending assimilated to the suffix -OSIS] (*pl.* zoonoses) A disease of animals that is capable of afflicting man. Adj. zoonotic.

**zoonotic** \zō′ənät′ik\ Of, relating to, or characteristic of a zoonosis.

**zooparasite** \zō′əpar′əsīt\ An organism that is parasitic in animals.

**zooparasitic** \zō′əpar′əsit′ik\ Parasitic in animals.

**zoophagic** \zō′əfāj′ik\ [*zoophag(ous)* + -IC] CARNIVOROUS.

**zoophagous** \zō·äf′əgəs\ [Gk *zōophagos* (from *zōo(n)* animal + *phag(ein)* to eat) living on animal food] CARNIVOROUS.

**zoopherin** \zō′əfer′in\ VITAMIN $B_{12}$.

**zoophile** \zō′əfīl\ A parasite or bloodsucking insect that prefers animals to human hosts.

**zoophilia** \zō′əfil′yə\ [ZOO- + -PHILIA] BESTIALITY.

**zoophilic** \zō′əfil′ik\ [ZOO- + -PHILIC] **1** Preferring animals to humans as hosts: said of certain bloodsucking insects. Compare ANTHROPOPHILIC. **2** Characterized by or relating to bestiality.

**zoophysiology** \zō′əfiz′ē·äl′əjē\ [ZOO- + PHYSIOLOGY] ANIMAL PHYSIOLOGY.

**zoosperm** \zō′əspurm\ [ZOO- + SPERM] SPERMATOZOON.

**zoospermia** \zō′əspur′mē·ə\ [ZOO- + SPERM + -IA] The presence of active spermatozoa in ejaculated semen. Compare NECROSPERMIA.

**zootic** \zō·ät′ik\ [ZOO- + *t* + -IC] Pertaining to animals other than humans.

**zootoxin** \zō′ətäk′sin\ An animal toxin; any toxin elaborated in the metabolic and growth processes of an animal.

**zootrophotoxism** \zō′əträf′ōtäk′sizm\ [ZOO- + TROPHO- + TOX- + -ISM] Poisoning by contaminated food of animal origin.

**zoster** \zäs′tər\ [Gk *zōstēr* a belt, girdle] HERPES ZOSTER. **z. auricularis** HERPES ZOSTER AURICULARIS. **z. facialis** Herpes zoster that affects one or more divisions of the trigeminal nerve. **z. femoralis** Herpes zoster involving the cutaneous distribution of the femoral nerve. **z. ophthalmicus** HERPES OPHTHALMICUS. **z. oticus** HERPES ZOSTER AURICULARIS. **symptomatic z. ophthalmicus** Herpes ophthalmicus associated with a neoplastic or other pathologic process involving the ophthalmic division of the trigeminal nerve.

**zosteriform** \zäster′ifôrm\ Resembling herpes zoster in distribution.

**zosteroid** \zäs′təroid\ Resembling herpes zoster in appearance.

**Z-plasty** \zē′plastē\ A method of reorienting or revising scars and/or releasing scar contractures by using a Z-flap. Also *Z-plastic relaxing operation*.

**Zr** Symbol for the element, zirconium.

**Zsigmondy** [Ruchard Adolf *Zsigmondy*, German chemist, 1865–1929] Brownian-Zsigmondy movement. See under BROWNIAN MOVEMENT.

**zuckerguss** \tsʊk′ərgʊs′\ [German, icing] A firm, white thickening of the serosal surface of certain organs, most typically the spleen and liver. It is often a nonspecific and incidental finding at autopsy that probably results from organization of peritoneal exudates.

**Zuckerkandl** [Emil *Zuckerkandl*, Austrian anatomist and physiologist, 1849–1910] **1** See under GLAND. **2** Organs of Zuckerkandl. See under ORGAN. **3** Zuckerkandl's body. See under PARAGANGLION. **4** Zuckerkandl's convolution. See under GYRUS SUBCALLOSUS.

**Zwaardemaker** [Hendrik *Zwaardemaker*, Dutch physiologist, 1857–1930] See under OLFACTOMETER.

**zwitterion** \tsvit′ərī′ən\ [German, from *Zwitter* (akin to *zwei* two) hybrid + ION] An ion with both positive and negative regions of charge.

**zyg-** \zīg-\ ZYGO-.

**zygapophysis** \zī′gəpäf′isis\ [ZYG- + APOPHYSIS] **1** The embryonic precursor of the articular process of a vertebra. **2** PROCESSUS ARTICULARIS.

**zygo-** \zī′gō-, zī′gə-\ [Gk *zygon* yoke, crossbar] A combining form meaning joining, pairing. Also *zyg-*.

**zygoma** \zīgō′mə\ [Gk *zygōma* (from *zygon* a yoke) a bolt, bar, zygomatic arch] **1** ARCUS ZYGOMATICUS. **2** OS ZYGOMATICUM.

**zygomatic** \zī′gəmat′ik\ Pertaining to the zygoma.

**zygomaticoauricular** \zī′gəmat′ikō·ôrik′yələr\ Pertaining to the zygomatic bone and the auricle of the ear.

**zygomaticofrontal** \zī′gəmat′ikōfrun′təl\ Related to the zygomatic and frontal bones, as in *zygomaticofrontal suture*.

**zygomycosis** \zī′gəmīkō′sis\ [*Zygo(mycetes)* a class of mold fungi + MYCOSIS] MUCORMYCOSIS. ● This term, although less often used, is probably more correct, since *Mucor* is only one genus of zygomycetous fungi causing this condition.

**zygonema** \zī′gənē′mə\ The thin thread of chromatin during the zygotene stage of meiosis.

**zygopodium** \zī′gəpō′dē·əm\ [New L, from ZYGO- + Gk *podion* a little foot] In embryology that part of a developing limb comprising the radius and ulna or the tibia and fibula.

**zygosity** \zīgäs′itē\ The nature of a zygote: often used in combination, as in indicating whether the genetic determinants of a specific character are identical (homozygosity) or different (heterozygosity), or, in the case of a twin pregnancy, whether development occurs from a single zygote (monozygosity) or two zygotes (dizygosity).

**zygote** \zī′gōt\ [Gk *zygōtos* (from *zygoun* to yoke a pair, akin to L *jungere* to join, unite) yoked] A diploid single cell formed in eukaryotes after fertilization by the union of the haploid male and female gametes. In effect a zygote exists from the time of pairing off of chromosomes from the male and female pronuclei after fertilization until the first cleavage division. A holozygote usually contains two complete genomes. Also *fertilized ovum*. **duplex z.** A fertilized ovum which has two identical genes for a given dominant character.

**zygotene** \zī′gōtēn\ The second stage, after leptotene, in a typical first meiotic division, when the homologous chromosomes begin to pair in a specific point-to-point fashion and become twisted about one another (synapsis). It is usually initiated at specific loci, or zygomeres, on each chromosome.

**zygotic** \zīgät′ik\ Relating to or concerning a zygote.

**zym-** \zīm-\ ZYMO-.

**zymase** \zī′mās\ A cell-free yeast extract containing the enzymes necessary for fermentation. *Obs.*

**zymo-** \zī′mō-, zī′mə-\ [Gk *zymē* leaven, ferment] A combining form denoting (1) fermentation; (2) enzyme. Also *zym-*.

**zymogen** \zī′məjən\ The inactive or nearly inactive form of an enzyme that can be converted into active enzyme by proteolysis, especially any of the precursors of the digestive enzymes that are secreted into the gut.

**zymogenesis** \zī′məjen′əsis\ The conversion of an enzyme from its precursor state.

**zymogram** \zī′məgram\ A graphic record of the electrophoretic pattern obtained on separating isoenzymes.

**zymohydrolysis** \-hīdräl′isis\ FERMENTATION.

**zymolysis** \zīmäl′isis\ FERMENTATION.

**zymosis** \zīmō′sis\ [Gk *zymōsis* (from *zymoun* to cause to ferment, from *zymē* a leaven, ferment) fermentation, leavening, swelling] **1** FERMENTATION. **2** A kind of fermentation in the host's body, or an analogous process, that was once thought to account for the pathogenesis of most infectious diseases. *Obs.*

**zymosterol** A yeast sterol containing double bonds at positions 8 and 24 like lanosterol, but saturated at position 5.

**zymotic** \zīmät′ik\ Pertaining to or caused by zymosis, as *zymotic diseases. Outmoded.*

# TABLE OF NORMAL RANGES

All stated normal ranges are dependent on the analytical method used and may vary considerably between laboratories depending on the method used and other variables. Normal ranges are generally based on mean normal value ± 2 S.D.

| SOURCE | ANALYTE OR TEST | NORMAL RANGE: TRADITIONAL UNITS | NORMAL RANGE: SI UNITS | COMMENTS |
|---|---|---|---|---|
| Serum | Acetone | Negative | Negative | |
| Urine | | Negative | Negative | |
| Plasma | Adrenocorticotropin (ACTH) | ≤60 pg/mL | ≤60 mg/L | |
| Serum | Alanine transaminase (ALT) | 8–20 × $10^{-3}$ U/mL (30°C)<br>5–35 U/mL (37°C) | 8–20 U/L (30°C)<br>5–35 U/mL (37°C) | |
| Serum | Albumin | 3.5–5.5 g/dL | 35–55 g/L | |
| Urine | Qualitative<br>Quantitative | Negative<br>10–150 mg/24 hr | Negative<br>0.010–0.150 g/24 h | |
| Serum | Aldolase | 0–11 × $10^{-3}$ U/mL | 0–11 U/L | |
| Serum | Aldosterone<br>Adult, recumbent<br>Male, standing<br>Female, standing | <br>3–10 ng/dL<br>6–22 ng/dL<br>5–30 ng/dL | <br>0.08–0.3 nmol/L<br>0.17–0.61 nmol/L<br>0.14–0.8 nmol/L | For adult on unrestricted sodium diet, no diuretics, after standing 3 hours |
| Urine | | 2–16 μg/24 hr | 6–44 nmol/24 h | On unrestricted sodium diet, no diuretics |
| Urine | δ-Aminolevulinic acid | 1.3–7.0 mg/24 hr | 10–53 μmol/24 h | |
| Serum | α-Amino nitrogen | 3.0–5.5 mg/dL | 2.1–3.9 mmol/L | |
| Plasma | Ammonia nitrogen | 15–49 μg/dL | 11–35 μmol/L | |
| Urine | | 20–70 mEq/24 hr | 20–70 mmol/24 h | |
| Serum | Amylase | 25–125 × $10^{-3}$ U/dL | 25–125 U/L | |
| Urine | | 1–17 U/hr | 1–17 U/h | |
| Urine | Amylase/creatinine clearance ratio | 1–4% | 0.01–0.04 (clearance fraction) | |
| Serum | $\alpha_1$-Antitrypsin | 150–350 mg/dL | 1.5–3.5 g/L | |
| Urine | Arsenic | <50 μg/24 hr | <0.66 μmol/24 h | |
| Blood | Ascorbic acid | 0.4–1.5 mg/dL | 23–85 mol/L | |
| Urine | | 2–10 mg/dL | 0.11–0.57 mmol/L | On adequate diet |
| Serum | Aspartate transaminase (AST) | 8–20 × $10^{-3}$ U/mL (30°C)<br>7–40 U/mL (37°C) | 8–20 U/L (30°C)<br>7–40 U/mL (37°C) | |
| Blood | Base excess | 0 ± 2 mEq/L | 0 ± 2 mmol/L | |
| Serum | Bicarbonate | 23–29 mEq/L | 23–29 mmol/L | |
| Serum | Bile acids | 0.3–3.0 mg/L | 0.6–60.0 μmol/L | |
| Serum | Bilirubin<br>Direct<br>Indirect<br>Total | <br><0.4 mg/dL<br><0.8 mg/dL<br>0.2–1.2 mg/dL | <br><6.8 μmol/L<br><13.7 μmol/L<br>3.4–20.5 μmol/L | |
| Urine | Bilirubin, qualitative | Negative | Negative | |
| Serum | Calcium | 4.5–5.5 mEq/L<br>9.0–11.0 mg/dL | 2.25–2.75 mmol/L<br>2.25–2.75 mmol/L | Slightly higher in children; varies with protein concentration |
| Urine | Low calcium diet<br>Normal diet | 50–150 mg/24 hr<br>100–250 mg/24 hr | 1.25–3.8 mmol/24 h<br>2.5–6.3 mmol/24 h | |
| Serum | Calcium, ionized | 2.1–2.6 mEq/L<br>4.25–5.25 mg/dL | 1.05–1.30 mmol/L<br>1.05–1.30 mmol/L | |
| Blood, serum, or plasma | Carbon dioxide concentration<br>Adults<br>Children | <br>24–30 mEq/L<br>20–28 mEq/L | <br>24–30 mmol/L<br>20–28 mmol/L | |
| Blood | Carbon dioxide partial pressure ($P_{CO_2}$) | 33–44 mmHg | 4.4–5.9 kPa | |
| Blood | Carboxyhemoglobin | Up to 5% of total | 0.05 of total | |
| Serum | β-Carotene | 40–200 μg/dL | 0.74–3.72 μmol/L | |
| Urine | Catecholamines<br>Epinephrine | <br><15 μg/24 hr | <br><82 nmol/24 h | |

(Continued)

TABLE OF NORMAL RANGES *(Continued)*

| SOURCE | ANALYTE OR TEST | NORMAL RANGE: TRADITIONAL UNITS | NORMAL RANGE: SI UNITS | COMMENTS |
|---|---|---|---|---|
| | Norepinephrine | <100 μg/24 hr | <590 nmol/24 h | |
| | Total free catecholamines | 4–126 μg/24 hr | 24–745 nmol/24 h | |
| | Total metanephrines | 0.1–1.6 mg/24 hr | 0.5–8.1 μmol/24 h | |
| Serum | Ceruloplasmin | 23–44 mg/dL | 1.5–2.9 μmol/L | |
| Serum | Chloride | 96–106 mEq/L | 96–106 mmol/L | |
| Urine | | 110–250 mEq/24 hr | 110–250 mmol/24 h | Varies with intake |
| Serum | Cholesterol | | | |
| | Total | 150–250 mg/dL | 3.9–6.5 mmol/L | |
| | Esters | 68–76% of total cholesterol | 0.68–0.76 of total cholesterol | |
| Serum | Cholinesterase | 8–18 U/mL | 8–18 U/mL | Units vary widely with method |
| Urine | Chorionic gonadotropin | 0 | 0 | |
| Urine | Chorionic gonadotropin, in pregnancy | 13,000 IU/24 hr | 13,000 IU/24 h | 6th week, mean |
| | | 30,000 IU/24 hr | 30,000 IU/24 h | 8th week, mean |
| | | 105,000 IU/24 hr | 105,000 IU/24 h | 12–14th week, mean |
| | | 46,000 IU/24 hr | 46,000 IU/24 h | 16th week, mean |
| | | 5,000–20,000 IU/24 hr | 5,000–20,000 IU/24 h | After week 16 |
| Blood | Citric acid | 1.2–3.0 mg/dL | 60–160 μmol/L | |
| Serum | Copper | | | |
| | Male | 70–140 μg/dL | 11–22 μmol/L | |
| | Female | 85–155 μg/dL | 13–24 μmol/L | |
| Urine | | 0–30 μg/24 hr | 0–0.48 μmol/24 h | |
| Plasma | Cortisol | | | |
| | 8 A.M. | 4–19 μg/dL | 110–520 nmol/L | |
| | 6 P.M. | 2–15 μg/dL | 50–410 nmol/L | |
| | Midnight | <5 μg/dL | <140 nmol/L | |
| Urine | Cortisol, free | 10–100 μg/24 hr | 27.6–276 μmol/24 h | |
| Serum | Creatine | 0.2–0.8 mg/dL | 15–61 μmol/L | |
| Urine | Males | 0–40 mg/24 hr | 0–305 μmol/24 h | |
| | Females | 0–100 mg/24 hr | 0–763 μmol/24 h | Higher in children and during pregnancy |
| Serum | Creatine kinase (CK, CPK) | | | |
| | Males | $12–80 \times 10^{-3}$ U/mL (30°C) | 12–80 U/L (30°C) | |
| | | $55–170 \times 10^{-3}$ U/mL (37°C) | 55–170 U/L (37°C) | |
| | Females | $10–55 \times 10^{-3}$ U/mL (30°C) | 10–55 U/L (30°C) | |
| | | $30–135 \times 10^{-3}$ U/mL (37°C) | 30–155 U/L (37°C) | |
| Serum | Creatine kinase isoenzymes | | | |
| | CK-MM | Present | Present | |
| | CK-MB, CK-BB | Absent | Absent | |
| Serum | Creatinine | 0.6–1.2 mg/dL | 53–106 μmol/L | |
| Urine | Males | 15–25 mg/kg body weight/24 hr | 133–221 mol · $kg^{-1}$ body weight/24 h | |
| | Females | 12–20 mg/kg body weight/24 hr | 106–177 mol · $kg^{-1}$ body weight/24 h | |
| Urine | Creatinine clearance | | | |
| | Males | (100–140 mL/min)/1.73 sq meter surface area | (100–140 mL/min)/1.73 $m^2$ surface area | |
| | Females | (90–130 mL/min)/1.73 sq meter surface area | (90–130 mL/min)/1.73 $m^2$ surface area | |
| Serum | Cryoglobins | 0 | 0 | |
| | Cyanocobalamin (*See* Vitamin $B_{12}$) | | | |
| Urine | Cystine, qualitative | Negative | Negative | |
| Urine | Dehydroepiandrosterone | Less than 15% of total 17-ketosteroids | Less than 0.15 of total 17-ketosteroids | |
| | Males | 0.2–2.0 mg/24 hr | 0.7–6.9 μmol/24 h | |
| | Females | 0.2–1.8 mg/24 hr | 0.7–6.2 μmol/24 h | |
| Blood | Erythrocyte count | | | |
| | Adults | | | |
| | Males | $4.6–6.2 \times 10^6$/cu mm | $4.6–6.2 \times 10^{12}$/L | |
| | Females | $4.2–5.4 \times 10^6$/cu mm | $4.2–5.4 \times 10^{12}$/L | |

TABLE OF NORMAL RANGES *(Continued)*

| SOURCE | ANALYTE OR TEST | NORMAL RANGE TRADITIONAL UNITS | NORMAL RANGE SI UNITS | COMMENTS |
|---|---|---|---|---|
| | Children | | | |
| | Birth | $3.9–5.5 \times 10^6$/cu mm | $3.9–5.5 \times 10^{12}$/L | |
| | 1–7 days | $3.9–6.0 \times 10^6$/cu mm | $3.9–6.0 \times 10^{12}$/L | |
| | 8–14 days | $3.6–6.0 \times 10^6$/cu mm | $3.6–6.0 \times 10^{12}$/L | |
| | 15–30 days | $3.0–5.5 \times 10^6$/cu mm | $3.0–5.5 \times 10^{12}$/L | |
| | 1–3 months | $2.7–5.5 \times 10^6$/cu mm | $2.7–5.5 \times 10^{12}$/L | |
| | 3–6 months | $3.1–4.5 \times 10^6$/cu mm | $3.1–4.5 \times 10^{12}$/L | |
| | 0.5–2 years | $3.7–6.0 \times 10^6$/cu mm | $3.7–6.0 \times 10^{12}$/L | |
| | 3–6 years | $4.1–5.3 \times 10^6$/cu mm | $4.1–5.3 \times 10^{12}$/L | |
| | 6–11 years | | | |
| | Males | $4.2–5.1 \times 10^6$/cu mm | $4.2–5.1 \times 10^{12}$/L | |
| | Females | $4.1–5.3 \times 10^6$/cu mm | $4.1–5.3 \times 10^{12}$/L | |
| | 12–16 years | | | |
| | Males | $4.4–5.5 \times 10^6$/cu mm | $4.4–5.5 \times 10^{12}$/L | |
| | Females | $4.1–5.2 \times 10^6$/cu mm | $4.1–5.2 \times 10^{12}$/L | |
| Blood | Erythrocyte indices | | | |
| | Mean corpuscular hemoglobin (MCH) | | | |
| | Adults | 27–31 pg | 0.42–0.48 nmol | |
| | Birth | 31–37 pg | 0.48–0.57 nmol | |
| | 1–30 days | 28–40 pg | 0.43–0.62 nmol | |
| | 1–3 months | 26–35 pg | 0.40–0.54 nmol | |
| | 3–6 months | 25–35 pg | 0.39–0.54 nmol | |
| | 0.5–2 years | 23–31 pg | 0.36–0.48 nmol | |
| | 2–6 years | 25–30 pg | 0.39–0.47 nmol | |
| | 6–11 years | | | |
| | Males | 25–30 pg | 0.39–0.47 nmol | |
| | Females | 26–30 pg | 0.40–0.47 nmol | |
| | 12–16 years | 27–31 pg | 0.42–0.48 nmol | |
| | Mean corpuscular volume (MCV) | | | |
| | Adults | 82–100 fL | 82–100 fL | |
| | Birth | 98–120 fL | 98–120 fL | |
| | 1–7 days | 88–120 fL | 88–120 fL | |
| | 8–14 days | 86–120 fL | 86–120 fL | |
| | 15–30 days | 85–110 fL | 85–110 fL | |
| | 1–3 months | 77–110 fL | 77–110 fL | |
| | 3–6 months | 74–108 fL | 74–108 fL | |
| | 0.5–2 years | 70–90 fL | 70–90 fL | |
| | 2–6 years | 74–89 fL | 74–89 fL | |
| | 6–11 years | | | |
| | Males | 76–91 fL | 76–91 fL | |
| | Females | 78–90 fL | 78–90 fL | |
| | 12–16 years | | | |
| | Males | 81–92 fL | 81–92 fL | |
| | Females | 80–92 fL | 80–92 fL | |
| Urine | Estrogens, Total | | | |
| | Males | 5–25 μg/24 hr | 5–25 μg/24 h | |
| | Females | | | |
| | Proliferative phase | 5–25 μg/24 hr | 5–25 μg/24 h | |
| | Luteal phase | 22–80 μg/24 hr | 22–80 μg/24 h | |
| | Pregnancy | <45,000 μg/24 hr | <45,000 μg/24 h | |
| | Postmenopausal | <10 μg/24 hr | <10 μg/24 h | |
| Serum | Fatty acids | 190–420 mg/dL | 7–15 mmol/L | |
| | nonesterified | 8–125 mg/dL | 0.30–0.90 mmol/L | |
| Serum | Ferritin | 20–200 ng/mL | 20–200 μg/L | |
| Plasma | Fibrinogen | 200–400 mg/dL | 5.9–11.7 μmol/L | |
| Serum | Folate | 1.8–9.0 ng/mL | 4.1–20.4 nmol/L | |
| Erythrocytes | | 150–450 ng/mL | 340–1020 nmol/L | |
| Plasma | Follicle-stimulating hormone (FSH) | | | |
| | Males | $4–25 \times 10^{-3}$ U/mL (I.U.) | 4–25 U/L | |
| | Females | $4–30 \times 10^{-3}$ U/mL (I.U.) | 4–30 U/L | |
| | Postmenopausal | $40–250 \times 10^{-3}$ U/mL (I.U.) | 4–250 U/L | |
| Serum | Gastrin | 0–200 pg/mL | 0–200 ng/L | |
| Serum | $\alpha_1$-Globulin | 0.2–0.4 g/dL | 2–4 g/L | |
| Serum | $\alpha_2$-Globulin | 0.5–0.9 g/dL | 5–9 g/L | |
| Serum | $\beta$-Globulin | 0.6–1.1 g/dL | 6–11 g/L | |

*(Continued)*

## TABLE OF NORMAL RANGES *(Continued)*

| SOURCE | ANALYTE OR TEST | NORMAL RANGE TRADITIONAL UNITS | NORMAL RANGE SI UNITS | COMMENTS |
|---|---|---|---|---|
| Serum | γ-Globulin | 0.7–1.7 g/dL | 7–17 g/L | |
| Urine | Glucose | | | |
| | As reducing substances | 0.5–1.5 g/24 hr | 0.5–1.5 g/24 h | |
| | As glucose | <0.5 g/24 hr | <2.8 mmol/24 h | |
| Blood | Glucose (fasting) | 60–100 mg/dL | 3.33–5.55 mmol/L | |
| Plasma or serum | | 70–115 mg/dL | 3.89–6.38 mmol/L | |
| | Glutamic oxaloacetic transaminase (*See* Aspartate transaminase) | | | |
| Serum | γ-Glutamyl transpeptidase | | | |
| | Males | $6–32 \times 10^{-3}$ U/mL (30°C) | 6–32 U/L (30°C) | |
| | Females | $4–18 \times 10^{-3}$ U/mL (30°C) | 4–18 U/L (30°C) | |
| Serum | Growth hormone | 0–10 ng/mL | 0–10 μg/L | |
| Serum | Haptoglobin (as hemoglobin binding capacity) | 100–200 mg/dL | 16–31 μmol/L | |
| Blood | Hematocrit | | | |
| | Adults | | | |
| | Males | 40–54 mL/dL | 0.40–0.54 | |
| | Females | 37–47 mL/dL | 0.37–0.47 | |
| | Children | | | |
| | Birth–7 days | 42–60 mL/dL | 0.42–0.60 | |
| | 8–14 days | 39–60 mL/dL | 0.39–0.60 | |
| | 15–30 days | 31–55 mL/dL | 0.31–0.55 | |
| | 1–6 months | 28–42 mL/dL | 0.28–0.42 | |
| | 0.5–6 years | 33–40 mL/dL | 0.33–0.40 | |
| | 6–11 years | | | |
| | Males | 36–42 mL/dL | 0.36–0.42 | |
| | Females | 36–43 mL/dL | 0.36–0.43 | |
| | 12–16 years | | | |
| | Males | 37–47 mL/dL | 0.37–0.47 | |
| | Females | 36–43 mL/dL | 0.36–0.43 | |
| Plasma | Hemoglobin | <5.0 mg/dL | <0.8 μmol/L | |
| Urine | | Negative | Negative | |
| Blood | Hemoglobin $A_{1c}$ | 3–5% of total | 0.03–0.05 of total | |
| Blood | Hemoglobin $A_2$ | 1.5–3.0% of total | 0.015–0.03 of total | |
| Blood | Hemoglobin concentration (venous blood) | | | |
| | Adults | | | |
| | Males, White and Asian | 14.0–18.0 g/dL | 140–180 g/L | |
| | Males, Black | 13.0–18.0 g/dL | 130–180 g/L | |
| | Females | 12.0–16.0 g/dL | 120–160 g/L | |
| | Children | | | |
| | Birth–7 days | 13.5–22.0 g/dL | 135–220 g/L | |
| | 8–14 days | 12.5–21.0 g/dL | 125–210 g/L | |
| | 15–30 days | 10.0–20.0 g/dL | 100–200 g/L | |
| | 1–3 months | 9.0–14.0 g/dL | 90–140 g/L | |
| | 3–6 months | 9.5–14.0 g/dL | 95–140 g/L | |
| | 0.5–2 years | 10.5–13.5 g/dL | 105–135 g/L | |
| | 2–6 years | 11.0–14.5 g/dL | 110–145 g/L | |
| | 6–16 years | 12.0–15.0 g/dL | 120–150 g/L | |
| Blood | Hemoglobin, fetal | <1% of total | <0.01 of total | |
| Urine | Homogentisic acid, qualitative | Negative | Negative | |
| Serum | Hydroxybutyric dehydrogenase (HBD) | $0–180 \times 10^{-3}$ U/mL (30°C) | 0–180 U/L (30°C) | |
| Plasma | 17-Hydroxycorticosteroids | 8–18 μg/dL | 0.22–0.50 μmol/L | |
| Urine | Males | 3–9 mg/24 hr | 8.3–25 μmol/24 h | |
| | Females | 2–8 mg/24 hr | 5.5–22 μmol/24 h | |
| Urine | 5-Hydroxyindoleacetic acid | | | |
| | Qualitative | Negative | Negative | |
| | Quantitative | <9 mg/24 hr | <47 μmol/24 h | |
| Serum | Immunoglobulin | | | |
| | IgG | 550–1900 mg/dL | 5.5–19.0 g/L | |
| | IgA | 60–333 mg/dL | 0.60–3.3 g/L | |
| | IgM | 45–145 mg/dL | 0.45–1.5 g/L | |
| | IgD | 0.5–3.0 mg/dL | 5–30 mg/L | |
| | IgE | <500 ng/mL | <500 g/L | Varies markedly with age in children |
| Plasma | Insulin (fasting) | $5–25 \times 10^{-6}$ U/mL | $5–25 \times 10^{-3}$ U/L | |

TABLE OF NORMAL RANGES *(Continued)*

| SOURCE | ANALYTE OR TEST | NORMAL RANGE TRADITIONAL UNITS | NORMAL RANGE SI UNITS | COMMENTS |
|---|---|---|---|---|
| Serum | Iodine, protein bound | 3.5–8.0 μg/dL | 0.28–0.63 μmol/L | |
| Serum | Iron | 75–175 μg/dL | 13–31 μmol/L | |
| Serum | Iron binding capcity | | | |
| | Total | 250–410 μg/dL | 45–73 μmol/L | |
| | Saturation | 20–55% | 0.20–0.55 | |
| Urine | 17-Ketosteroids, adults | | | |
| | Males | 6–20 mg/24 hr | 21–69 μmol/24 h | |
| | Females | 4–13 mg/24 hr | 14–45 μmol/24 h | Decreases with age |
| Blood | Lactate | | | |
| | Venous | 4.5–19.8 mg/dL | 0.5–1.2 mmol/L | |
| | Arterial | 4.5–14.4 mg/dL | 0.5–1.6 mmol/L | |
| Serum | Lactate dehydrogenase (LD, LDH) | $0–300 \times 10^{-3}$ U/mL (I.U.) (30°C) | 0–300 U/L (30°C) | Wroblewski modified |
| | | $45–90 \times 10^{-3}$ U/mL (I.U.) (30°C) | 45–90 U/L (30°C) | |
| | | $100–190 \times 10^{-3}$ U/mL (37°C) | 100–190 U/L (37°C) | |
| Serum | Lactate dehydrogenase isoenzymes | | | |
| | $LDH_1$ | 22–37% of total | 0.22–0.37 of total | |
| | $LDH_2$ | 30–46% of total | 0.30–0.46 of total | |
| | $LDH_3$ | 14–29% of total | 0.14–0.29 of total | |
| | $LDH_4$ | 5–11% of total | 0.05–0.11 of total | |
| | $LDH_5$ | 2–11% of total | 0.02–0.11 of total | |
| Serum | Leucine aminopeptidase | $14–40 \times 10^{-3}$ U/mL (30°C) | 14–40 U/L (30°C) | |
| Blood | Leukocyte count | | | |
| | Adults | | | |
| | Whites and Asians | 4500–11,000/cu mm | $4.5–11.0 \times 10^9$/L | |
| | Blacks | 3500–11,000/cu mm | $3.5–11.0 \times 10^9$/L | |
| | Children | | | |
| | Birth | 9000–30,000/cu mm | $9.0–30.0 \times 10^9$/L | |
| | 1–7 days | 9400–34,000/cu mm | $9.4–34.0 \times 10^9$/L | |
| | 8–14 days | 5000–21,000/cu mm | $5.0–21.0 \times 10^9$/L | |
| | 15–30 days | 5000–20,000/cu mm | $5.0–20.0 \times 10^9$/L | |
| | 1–3 months | 5000–15,000/cu mm | $5.0–15.0 \times 10^9$/L | |
| | 3–6 months | 5000–12,000/cu mm | $5.0–12.0 \times 10^9$/L | |
| | 0.5–2 years | 6000–11,000/cu mm | $6.0–11.0 \times 10^9$/L | |
| | 2–6 years | 5000–11,000/cu mm | $5.0–11.0 \times 10^9$/L | |
| Serum | Lipase | 0–1.5 U | 0–1.5 U | Varies widely with method |
| Serum | Lipids, total | 450–850 mg/dL | 4.5–8.5 g/L | |
| Serum | Lipoprotein cholesterol | | | |
| | Low-density (LDL) | 60–180 mg/dL | 600–1800 mg/L | |
| | High-density (HDL) | 30–80 mg/dL | 300–800 mg/L | |
| Serum | Luteinizing hormone (LH) | | | |
| | Males | $6–18 \times 10^{-3}$ U/mL (I.U.) | 6–18 U/L | |
| | Females | | | |
| | Premenopausal | $5–22 \times 10^{-3}$ U/mL (I.U.) | 5–22 U/L | |
| | Midcycle | 3 times baseline | 3 times baseline | |
| | Postmenopausal | Greater than $30 \times 10^{-3}$ U/mL (I.U.) | Greater than 30 U/L | |
| Serum | $\alpha_1$-Macroglobulin | 145–410 mg/dL | 1.5–4.1 g/L | |
| Serum | Magnesium | 1.5–2.5 mEq/L | 0.75–1.25 mmol/L | |
| | | 1.8–3.0 mg/dL | 0.75–1.25 mmol/L | |
| Urine | | 6.0–9.0 mEq/24 hr | 3.0–4.5 mmol/24 h | |
| Blood | Methemoglioblobin | <130 mg/dL | 4.7–20 μmol/L | |
| Urine | Myoglobin, qualitative | Negative | Negative | |
| Serum | 5′-Nucleotidase | $3.5–12.7 \times 10^{-3}$ U/mL (37°C) | 3.5–12.5 U/L (37°C) | |
| Serum | Nitrogen, nonprotein | 15–35 mg/dL | 10.7–25.0 mmol/L | |
| Serum | Osmolality | 285–295 mOsm/kg serum water | 285–295 mmol/kg serum water | |
| Urine | Osmolality, random | 50–1400 mOsm/kg water | 50–1400 mOsm/kg water | Varies with fluid intake |
| Urine | Osmolality ratio, urine/serum | 1.0–3.0 | 1.0–3.0 | <3.0 following 12 h fluid restriction |

*(Continued)*

TABLE OF NORMAL RANGES *(Continued)*

| SOURCE | ANALYTE OR TEST | NORMAL RANGE TRADITIONAL UNITS | NORMAL RANGE SI UNITS | COMMENTS |
|---|---|---|---|---|
| Erythrocytes | Osmotic fragility | Begins in 0.45–0.39 g/dL NaCl<br>Complete in 0.33–0.30 g/dL NaCl | Begins in 77–67 mmol/L NaCl<br>Complete in 56–51 mmol/L NaCl | |
| Blood | Oxygen capacity | 16–24 vol. % | 7.14–10.7 mmol/L | Varies with hemoglobin concentration |
| Blood | Oxygen content | | | |
| | Arterial | 15–23 vol. % | 6.69–10.3 mmol/L | |
| | Venous | 10–16 vol. % | 4.46–7.14 mmol/L | |
| Blood | Oxygen saturation | | | |
| | Arterial | 94–100% | 0.94–1.00 | |
| | Venous | 60–85% | 0.60–0.85 | |
| Blood | Oxygen partial pressure ($P_{O_2}$), arterial | 75–105 mmHg | 10.0–14.0 kPa | |
| Blood | $P_{50}$ | 25–27 mmHg | 3.33–3.60 kPa | |
| Urine | pH | Average 6; range 4.5–8.0, depending on diet | Average 6; range 4.5–8.0, depending on diet | |
| Blood | pH, arterial | 7.35–7.45 | 7.35–7.45 | |
| Serum | Phenylalanine | <3 mg/dL | <0.18 mmol/L | |
| Urine | Phenylpyruvic acid, qualitative | Negative | Negative | |
| Blood | Phosphatase, acid (leukocyte) | Total score 14–100 | Total score 14–100 | |
| Serum | Phosphatase | | | |
| | Acid | $0.11–0.60 \times 10^{-3}$ U/mL (37°C) | 0.11–0.60 U/L | |
| | Alkaline | $20–90 \times 10^{-3}$ U/mL (30°C) | 20–90 U/L (30°C) | Values are higher in children |
| Serum | Phosphate, inorganic | | | |
| | Adults | 3.0–4.5 mg/dL | 1.0–1.5 mmol/L | |
| | Children | 4.0–7.0 mg/dL | 1.3–2.3 mmol/L | |
| Serum | Phospholipids | 6–12 mg/dL | 1.9–3.9 mmol/L | As lipid phosphorus |
| Urine | Phosphorus | 0.9–1.3 g/24 hr | 29–42 mmol/24 h | |
| Blood | Platelet count | | | |
| | Adult | 150,000–350,000/cu mm | $150–350 \times 10^9$/L | |
| | Birth–2 years | 200,000–400,000/cu mm | $200–400 \times 10^9$/L | |
| | 3–6 years | 240,000–570,000/cu mm | $240–570 \times 10^9$/L | |
| | 6–16 years | 200,000–500,000/cu mm | $200–500 \times 10^9$/L | |
| Urine | Porphobilinogen | | | |
| | Qualitative | Negative | Negative | |
| | Quantitative | 0–0.2 mg/dL<br><2.0 mg/24 hr | 0–9 μmol/L<br><9 μmol/24 h | |
| Urine | Porphyrins | | | |
| | Coproporphyrin | 50–200 μg/24 hr | 75–300 nmol/24 h | |
| | Uroporphyrin | 10–40 μg/24 hr | 12–48 nmol/24 h | |
| Serum | Potassium | 3.5–5.0 mEq/L | 3.5–5.0 mmol/L | |
| Urine | | 25–100 mEq/24 hr | 25–100 mmol/24 h | Dependent on diet |
| Urine | Pregnanediol | | | |
| | Males | 0.1–1.0 mg/24 hr | 0.3–3.1 μmol/24 h | |
| | Females | | | |
| | Proliferative phase | 0.5–1.5 mg/24 hr | 1.6–4.7 μmol/24 h | |
| | Luteal phase | 2.0–7.0 mg/24 hr | 6.2–22 μmol/24 h | |
| | Postmenopausal | 0.2–1.0 mg/24 hr | 0.6–3.1 μmol/24 h | |
| | Pregnancy | <50 mg/24 hr | <156 μmol/24 h | |
| Urine | Pregnanetriol | <2.2 mg/24 hr in adults | <6.5 μmol/24 h in adults | |
| Plasma | Progesterone | | | |
| | Follicular phase | <2 ng/mL | <6 nmol/L | |
| | Luteal phase | 2–20 ng/mL | 6–64 nmol/L | |
| Serum | Prolactin | | | |
| | Males | 1–20 ng/mL | 1–20 μg/L | |
| | Females | 1–25 ng/mL | 1–25 μg/L | |
| Serum | Protein, total | 6.0–8.0 g/100 dL | 60–80 g/L | |
| Urine | Protein | | | |
| | Qualitative | Negative | Negative | |

TABLE OF NORMAL RANGES *(Continued)*

| SOURCE | ANALYTE OR TEST | NORMAL RANGE: TRADITIONAL UNITS | NORMAL RANGE: SI UNITS | COMMENTS |
|---|---|---|---|---|
| | Quantitative | 40–150 mg/24 hr | 40–150 mg/24 h (no conversion factor because of mixed proteins) | Varies with activity level |
| Erythrocyte | Protoporphyrin | 27–61 μg/dL packed RBC | 0.48–1.09 μmol/L packed RBC | |
| Blood | Reticulocyte count | 25,000–75,000/fL<br>0.5–1.5% of erythrocytes | 25–75 × $10^9$/L | |
| | Riboflavin (*See* Vitamin $B_2$) | | | |
| Serum | Sodium | 136–145 mEq/L | 136–145 mmol/L | |
| Urine | | 50–220 mEq/24 hr | 50–220 mmol/24 h | Varies with intake |
| Urine | Specific gravity | 1.003–1.030 | 1.003–1.030 | |
| Serum | Sulfates, inorganic | 0.8–1.2 mg/dL | 83–125 μmol/L | |
| Plasma | Testosterone | | | |
| | Males | 275–875 ng/dL | 9.5–30 nmol/L | |
| | Females | 23–75 ng/dL | 0.8–2.6 nmol/L | |
| | Pregnant | 38–190 ng/dL | 1.3–6.6 nmol/L | |
| Serum | Thyroid-stimulating hormone (TSH) | 0–7 × $10^{-6}$ U/mL | 0–7 × $10^{-3}$ U/L | |
| Serum | Thyroxine ($T_4$) | 4.4–9.9 μg/dL | 57–128 nmol/L | |
| Serum | Thyroxine, free | 1.0–2.1 ng/dL | 13–27 pmol/L | |
| Serum | Thyroxin binding globulin (TBG) (as thyroxine) | 10–26 μg/dL | 129–335 nmol/L | |
| Serum | Thyroxine iodine | 2.9–6.4 μg/dL | 229–504 nmol/L | |
| Urine | Titratable acidity | 20–40 mEq/24 hr | 20–40 mmol/24 h | |
| Serum | Triglycerides | 40–150 mg/dL | 0.4–1.5 g/L<br>0.45–1.71 mmol/L | |
| Serum | Tri-iodothyronine ($T_3$) | 150–250 ng/dL | 2.3–3.9 nmol/L | |
| Serum | Urate | | | |
| | Males | 2.5–8.0 mg/dL | 0.15–0.48 mmol/L | |
| | Females | 1.5–7.0 mg/dL | 0.09–0.42 mmol/L | |
| Blood | Urea | 21–43 mg/dL | 3.5–7.2 mmol/L | |
| Plasma or serum | | 24–49 mg/dL | 4.0–8.2 mmol/L | |
| Blood | Urea nitrogen | 10–20 mg/dL | 7.1–14.3 mmol/L | |
| Plasma or serum | | 11–23 mg/dL | 7.9–16.4 mmol/L | |
| Urine | | 10–20 g/24 hr | 0.36–0.71 mol/24 h | |
| Urine | Uric acid | 250–750 mg/24 hr | 1.48–4.43 mmol/24 h | On average diet |
| Urine | Urobilinogen | Up to 1.0 Ehrlich U/2 hr<br>0–4.0 mg/24 hr | Up to 1.0 Ehrlich U/2 h<br>0–6.8 μmol/24 h | 1–3 P.M. |
| Urine | Vanillylmandelic acid (VMA) (4-hydroxy-3-methoxymandelic acid) | 1–8 mg/24 hr | 5–40 μmol/24 h | |
| Serum | Viscosity | 1.4–1.8 times water | 1.4–1.8 times water | |
| Serum | Vitamin A | 20–80 μg/dL | 0.70–2.8 μmol/L | |
| Urine | Vitamin $B_1$ | 60–500 μg/24 hr | 0.18–1.48 μmol/24 h | |
| Serum | Vitamin $B_2$ | 2.6–3.7 μg/dL | 70–100 nmol/L | |
| Serum | Vitamin $B_{12}$ | 180–900 pg/mL | 133–664 pmol/L | |
| Urine | Volume | 700–1700 mL/24 hr | 0.7–1.7 L/24 h | |

Data from the following sources were used in compiling this table:


*JAMA*, Editorial, May 2, 1986, 255:17; 2331–2339.

Conn, R. B., "Laboratory Reference Values of Clinical Importance," appendix to B. F. Miller and C.B. Keane, *Encyclopedia and Dictionary of Medicine, Nursing, and Allied Health*, 4th ed. W. B. Saunders, Philadelphia, 1987.

Mayo Clinic, Department of Laboratory Medicine, Rochester, Minnesota.

Veterans Administration Medical Center, Department of Laboratory Medicine, Durham, North Carolina.

*Fundamentals of Clinical Chemistry*, edited by N. W. Tietz, 3rd ed. W. B. Saunders, Philadelphia, 1987.

*Clinical Diagnosis and Management by Laboratory Methods*, edited by J. B. Henry, 17th ed. W. B. Saunders, Philadelphia, 1984.

# TABLE OF RADIOPHARMACEUTICALS AND THEIR DIAGNOSTIC APPLICATIONS

| ORGAN SYSTEM | RADIOPHARMACEUTICAL | BIOLOGICAL BEHAVIOR | CLINICAL APPLICATION |
|---|---|---|---|
| *Cardiovascular system* | | | |
| Myocardial imaging | Thallium-201 | $K^+$ analogue-extracted in proportion to myocardial blood flow | 'Cold spot' imaging for detection of coronary artery disease<br>Diagnosis of right ventricular hypertrophy |
| | $^{99m}$Tc-pyrophosphate | Reacts with mitochondrial calcium crystals in acutely infarcted myocardial cells | 'Hot spot' imaging for detection and sizing of acute myocardial infarctions |
| Ventriculography | $^{99m}$Tc labeled red blood cells | Compartmental localization of red cells in cardiac chambers | Quantification of right and left ventricular function at rest and with exercise<br>Detection of regional cardiac wall motion abnormalities, aneurysms<br>Shunt detection and quantification<br>Quantification of valvular regurgitation<br>Measure of absolute ventricular volume |
| *Central nervous system* | | | |
| Cerebral anatomy | $^{99m}$Tc-pertechnetate ($TcO_4$)<br>$^{99m}$Tc-glucoheptinate<br>$^{99m}$Tc-diethylenetria-minepentaacetic acid (DTPA) | Localization at sites of breakdown of blood-brain barrier | Detection of neoplasms, infection (abscess or encephalitis), subdural hematoma |
| Cerebral blood flow | (same as above) | Intravascular compartmental localization | Visualize cerebral blood flow, diagnose 'brain death', vascular malformations |
| | $^{133}$Xe Gas | Washout of gas proportional to cerebral blood flow | Quantification of regional cerebral blood flow |
| Cerebrospinal fluid | $^{111}$In-DTPA<br>$^{169}$Yb-DTPA | Follows cerebrospinal fluid flow | CSF shunt patency<br>Localize CSF leaks<br>Differentiate normal pressure hydrocephalus from atrophy |
| Cerebral metabolism | $^{18}$F-deoxyglucose | Analogue for glucose metabolism | Regional glucose metabolism (requires positron emission tomography) |
| *Gastrointestinal system* | | | |
| Liver-spleen imaging | $^{99m}$Tc-sulfur colloid | Phagocytosis by reticuloendothelial cells | Organ sizing<br>Detect space-occupying disease (>2 cm)<br>Trauma |
| Spleen only imaging | Heat damaged $^{99m}$Tc labeled red blood cells | Splenic trapping of damaged red cells | Detect ectopic splenic tissue<br>Evaluate functional asplenia |
| Hepatobiliary imaging | $^{99m}$Tc iminodiacetic acid derivatives | Active transport—follows biliary conjugation and excretion pathway | Assess patency of cystic and common bile ducts<br>Differentiate congenital biliary atresia from neonatal hepatitis<br>Define biliary anatomy |
| Functional bowel studies | $^{99m}$Tc sulfur colloid<br>$^{111}$In-DTPA<br>$^{99m}$Tc-DISIDA | Compartmental localization | Esophageal transit and reflux<br>Gastric emptying<br>Bile reflux |
| Gastrointestinal bleeding | | | |
| acute | $^{99m}$Tc-sulfur colloid<br>$^{99m}$Tc-labeled red blood cells | Compartmental localization | Localization of acute GI bleeding site |
| chronic | $^{51}$Cr-labeled red blood cells | Compartmental localization | Sensitive test to quantify GI blood loss |
| Gastrointestinal protein loss | $^{51}$Cr-albumen | Compartmental localization | Sensitive test to quantify protein loss |
| Peritoneovenous shunts | $^{99m}$Tc-sulfur colloid | Compartmental localization | Determine shunt patency |
| Gastric mucosa | $^{99m}$Tc-pertechnetate | Active transport | Detection of Meckel's diverticulum and Barrett's esophagus |

(*continued*)

## TABLE—CONTINUED

| ORGAN SYSTEM | RADIOPHARMACEUTICAL | BIOLOGICAL BEHAVIOR | CLINICAL APPLICATION |
|---|---|---|---|
| Salivary glands | $^{99m}$Tc-pertechnetate | Active transport | Differentiate benign (Warthins's) from malignant tumors<br>Evaluate salivary flow and patency of ducts |
| *Genitourinary system* | | | |
| Renal function | $^{99m}$Tc-DTPA | Cleared by glomerular filtration (GFR) | Measure GFR |
| | $^{131}$I-orthoiodohippurate (OIH) | 90% cleared by GFR and tubular secretion on first pass | Measure effective renal plasma flow (ERPF) |
| | $^{99m}$Tc-dimercaptosuccinic acid (DMSA) | 50% accumulated and retained in renal cortex | Quantification of relative functional renal mass |
| Renal morphology | $^{99m}$Tc-DMSA | 50% accumulated and retained in renal cortex | Differentiate benign renal masses (column of Bertin) from cysts, tumor or infarcted tissue |
| | $^{99m}$Tc-glucoheptinate | Cleared by glomular filtration as well as retained in renal cortex | Differentiate benign renal masses (column of Bertin) from cysts, tumor or infarcted tissue |
| Renal perfusion | $^{99m}$Tc-DTPA<br>$^{99m}$Tc-glucoheptinate | Early intravascular compartmental localization | Visualize relative renal perfusion with radionuclide angiogram<br>Diagnose early rejection of renal transplants |
| Renal collecting system and ureters | $^{99m}$Tc-DTPA + Frusemide (Furosamide) | Frusemide used to rapidly increase urine flow | Diuretic 'wash out' test—used to assess mechanical obstruction |
| Bladder | $^{99m}$Tc-DTPA or glucoheptinate | Compartmental localization | Quantify bladder residuum, direct and indirect cystography to detect reflux |
| Scrotum | $^{99m}$Tc-pertechnetate | Early: intravascular compartmental localization<br>Late: localizes in extracellular fluid space | Radionuclide angiogram differentiates acute testicular torsion from epididymitis<br>Diagnose 'missed' torsion, varicocele |
| *Lacrimal system* | $^{99m}$Tc-pertechnetate | Passive transport | Assess lacrimal drainage and duct drainage |
| *Lymphatics* | $^{99m}$Tc-antimony sulfide | Passive transport in lymph flow to lymph nodes then phagocytized by RE cells in nodes | Identify lymph nodes with occult metastases for therapy<br>Direction of lymph drainage |
| *Pulmonary system* | | | |
| Ventilation | $^{133}$Xeon gas<br>$^{81m}$Kr krypton gas<br>$^{99m}$Tc aerosols (DTPA) | Distributed to lungs in proportion to regional ventilation | Demonstrate regional ventilatory abnormalities<br>Improves specificity of V-P imaging |
| Perfusion | $^{99m}$Tc macroaggregates or microspheres | Pulmonary capillary blockade | Detect pulmonary emboli<br>Detect right to left shunts<br>Preoperative quantification of relative lung function |
| Parenchymal | $^{67}$Ga-citrate | Localizes in T lymphocytes and proteinaceous fluid | Measures active alveolitis in interstitial lung disease<br>Staging of bronchogenic carcinoma |
| *Skeletal system* | $^{99m}$Tc-pertechnetate | Localizes at sites of increased extracellular fluid (ECF) | Detection of inflammatory joint disease |
| | $^{99m}$Tc polyphosphate compounds | Fixed to hydroxyapatite crystal surface of bone | Increased sensitivity over radiographs for detection of benign and malignant bone lesions |
| *Thyroid* | $^{131}$Iodine<br>$^{123}$Iodine | Active transport and organification | Evaluate size and morphology of gland<br>Determine functional status of thyroid and nodules<br>Evaluate mediastinal masses |
| | $^{99m}$Tc-pertechnetate | Active transport<br>No organification | Detect thyroid metastases, treat thyroid cancers<br>Diagnose subacute or silent thyroiditis |
| | $^{201}$Thallium | Active transport | Identify nonfunctioning thyroid cancers |
| *Tumor and inflammatory processes* | $^{67}$Gallium citrate | Nonspecific protein binding | Localize source of sepsis or fever of unknown aetiology |
| | | Some localization in granulocytes | Staging and localization of lymphomas and lung carcinomas |

(From Grainger and Allison, *Diagnostic Radiology*, Churchill Livingstone, 1986, with permission.)